PDR®

68

EDITION

2014

PHYSICIANS' DESK REFERENCE®

Executive Chairman: Edward Fotsch, MD
President: Richard C. Altus
Chief Medical Officer: Salvatore Volpe, MD, FAAP, FACP, CHCQM

Executive Vice President and Chief Financial Officer: Gary Lubin
Chief Technology Officer: David Cheng
Senior Vice President, Operations: Dawn Carfora
Senior Vice President, Sales: Jeffrey Davis
Senior Vice President, Corporate Development & General Counsel: Andrew Gelman
Senior Vice President, Marketing & Business Line Management: Barbara Senich, BSN, MBA, MPH

Associate Vice President, PDR Communications: Marjorie Jaxel
Associate Vice President, Sales: Dennis McCormack
Director, Client Services and Sales Operations: Karen Fass
Directors, Strategic Accounts: Mike Baczynski, Nick Clark, Robert Davison, Melinda Doyle, Dan Stokes

Vice President, Clinical & Regulatory Solutions: Mukesh Mehta, DPh, MBA, RPh
Director, Clinical Services: Sylvia Nashed, PharmD
Manager, Clinical Databases and Services: Christine Sunwoo, PharmD

Associate Manager, Clinical Content Development: Anila Patel, PharmD
Senior Drug Information Specialist: Pauline Lee, PharmD
Drug Information Specialists: Vanessa DeAlmeida, PharmD; Demyana Farag, PharmD; Kristine Mecca, PharmD; Autri Sajedeen, PharmD
Managing Clinical Editor: Julia Tonelli, MD
Medical Editor: Christa Mary Kronick, MA

Director, Marketing: Kim Marich
Manager, Corporate Communications: Thomas W. Eck
Manager, Art Department: Livio Udina

Senior Director, Content Operations & Manufacturing: Jeffrey D. Schaefer
Associate Director, Manufacturing & Distribution: Thomas Westburgh
Senior Production Manager, PDR: Steven Maher
Senior Manager, Content Operations: Noel Deloughery
Senior Content Operations Specialist: Allison O'Hare
Content Operations Specialist: Kiranjit Kaur
Senior Production Coordinator: Yasmin Hernández
Production Coordinator: Eric Udina
Associate Manager, Fulfillment: Gary Lew
Web Operations and Customer Service Manager: Lee Reynolds

ISBN: 978-1-56363-825-1

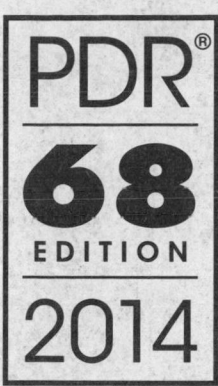

FOREWORD TO THE 68th EDITION

About PDR Network, LLC

As the nation's leading aggregator and distributor of drug labeling information, product safety alerts, and REMS programs, PDR Network® is committed to ensuring that prescribers have access to the right information at the point of prescribing. This information is distributed across channels through the PDR® suite of digital and print services, which includes the *Physicians' Desk Reference*® (*PDR*®), the most highly trusted drug information reference available in the U.S., now available in multiple book formats; PDR interactive drug services for Electronic Health Record (EHR) systems; PDR.net®, the Internet home of *PDR*; *mobile*PDR®; and PDR Drug Alerts, the only specialty-specific service that provides electronic delivery of FDA-approved Drug Alerts to physicians and other healthcare professionals.

By improving communication of important medication information and FDA-approved Drug Alerts, PDR Network's unique services enhance patient safety and may help to reduce medical liability.

For more information or to sign up for electronic PDR Drug Alerts, visit PDR.net.

About the *Physicians' Desk Reference* (*PDR*)

PDR is published by PDR Network, LLC (PDR Network) in cooperation with participating manufacturers, and contains U.S. Food and Drug Administration (FDA)-approved product labeling. In accordance with current FDA policies, *PDR* also includes prescribing information provided by manufacturers for products marketed without FDA approval, as well as information on some dietary supplements and other products.

For ease of use, *PDR* includes color-coded indices (designated with white, pink, or blue pages at the front of the book), and a Generic/Brand Cross-Reference Table in Section 2. This table can help you quickly locate the brand names associated with specific active ingredients as well as their product indications. In addition, manufacturer-supplied information on dietary supplements is listed separately in Section 6.

Each full-length product information entry in *PDR* provides you with an exact, formatted copy of the product's FDA-approved or other manufacturer-supplied labeling. Under the Federal Food, Drug and Cosmetic (FD&C) Act, a drug approved for marketing may be labeled, promoted, and advertised by the manufacturer for only those uses for which the drug's safety and effectiveness have been established. The Code of Federal Regulations [Title 21 Section 201.100(d)(1)] pertaining to labeling for prescription products requires that for *PDR* content "indications, effects, dosages, routes, methods, and frequency and duration of administration, and any relevant warnings, hazards, contraindications, side effects, and precautions" must be "*same in language and emphasis*" as the approved labeling for the products. The FDA regards the words *same in language and emphasis* as requiring VERBATIM use of the approved labeling when providing such information. Furthermore, information that is emphasized in the FDA-approved labeling by the use of type set in a box, or in capitals, boldface, or italics, must be given the same emphasis in *PDR*.

The FDA has also recognized that the FD&C Act does not, however, limit the manner in which a physician may use an approved drug. Once a product has been approved for marketing, a physician may choose to prescribe it for uses, treatment regimens, or patient populations that are not included in the approved labeling. The FDA also observes that accepted medical practice includes drug use that is not reflected in approved drug labeling. In addition, the dietary supplements listed in Section 6 are marketed under the Dietary Supplement Health and Education Act of 1994 (DSHEA). Products marketed under the DSHEA do not receive formal evaluation or approval from the FDA. The following disclaimer applies to all product information listed in Section 6, as mandated by the federal government: *These statements have not been evaluated by the Food and Drug Administration. This product is not intended to diagnose, treat, cure, or prevent any disease.*

The function of PDR Network is the compilation, organization, and distribution of this information. All product information appearing in *PDR* is made possible through the courtesy of the manufacturers whose products appear in it. The information concerning each product has been provided by such manufacturers and in each instance fully approved by such manufacturers prior to publication by PDR Network. In organizing and presenting the material in *PDR*, PDR Network does not warrant or guarantee any of the products described, or perform any independent analysis in connection with any of the product information contained herein. PDR Network does not assume, and expressly disclaims, any obligation to obtain and include any information other than that provided to it by the manufacturers. It should be understood that by making this material available, PDR Network is not advocating the use of any product described herein, nor is PDR Network responsible for the use of a product, or the use and/or misuse of a product due to typographical error. Additional information on any product may be obtained from the manufacturer.

Updates to *PDR*

The book edition of *PDR* contains the latest information available when the edition closes for new material. As new drugs are released and new research data, clinical findings, and safety information emerge throughout the year, it is the responsibility of the manufacturer to provide that information to the medical community and revise that information accordingly in PDR's database. These revisions are distributed in *PDR Updates*, on PDR.net, *mobile*PDR, and within Electronic Health Record (EHR) Systems and other healthcare IT systems where integrated. To be certain that you have the most current data, always consult the *PDR Updates*, PDR.net, *mobile*PDR, and the eDrug Updates or the applicable *PDR* modules in your EHR before prescribing or administering any product described in the following pages.

Electronic PDR Resources

PDR.net

PDR.net, a web portal designed specifically for healthcare professionals, provides trusted, professional drug information, including full FDA-approved labeling as well as concise point-of-care drug information. **PDR.net** provides prescribers with online access to the authoritative drug information they need to support their treatment decisions.

***mobile*PDR**

***mobile*PDR** provides the only source for FDA-approved full product labeling and concise point-of-care drug information from the PDR database directly on a mobile device. Prescribing information on more than 2,400 drugs, full-color product images, and weekly updates provide up-to-date drug information. ***mobile*PDR** is free for U.S.-based MDs, DOs, NPs, and PAs in full-time patient practice and can be downloaded from PDR.net. ***mobile*PDR** is available for all major mobile platforms.

PDR Drug Alerts

FDA-approved Drug Alerts are delivered electronically to physicians and other prescribers who register to receive them at PDR.net, through participating medical societies, or by returning the verification form distributed with complimentary copies of *PDR*. By ensuring that this service is used exclusively for the rapid delivery of **PDR Drug Alerts**—not advertising or marketing—PDR Network fulfills FDA guidance for electronic delivery of alerts, improves patient safety, and may help to reduce liability.

Electronic Health Records

PDR Network's services for EHRs offer prescribers a comprehensive suite of free, interactive EHR tools—including drug labeling information, boxed warnings, drug safety alerts, and patient education and financial support programs that deliver critical drug information to help you provide optimal patient care.

Supported by medical societies and medical insurance and malpractice carriers, PDR Network's services for EHRs are convenient and readily accessible for you within your workflow at no cost to you or your patients. To request PDR Network's services in your EHR, please contact your EHR vendor. PDR Network services for EHRs include:

PDR® BRIEF

PDR BRIEF offers an intuitive dashboard of full labeling information and provider resources surfacing within your EHR system to support your treatment decisions within your workflow. **PDR BRIEF** is activated when a medication is selected to ensure you have the most current full prescribing information, label updates, boxed warnings, patient education, financial support, and adherence resources available.

PDR®+ for Patients

PDR+ for Patients drug education guides are designed to help patients understand the drugs prescribed by their physician. Available in your EHR workflow, the guides are easy to hand out during an office visit or automatically send to the Patient Portal. By addressing potential concerns early on and sharing **PDR+ for Patients**, physicians can help their patients start and stay on therapy.

PDR Search™

PDR Search delivers an unparalleled interactive and searchable drug database of drug labeling and safety and product support information. **PDR Search** supplies full drug prescribing information and prescribing summaries with access to FDA and PDR Drug Alerts, as well as patient education, financial support, and adherence resources, directly through your EHR application.

Patient Financial Support

PDR® Pharmacy Discount Card

This free program provides patients with access to medications at discounted prices, helping them save up to 75% on their prescriptions at more than 60,000 pharmacies nationwide. PDR Network distributes this program via healthcare provider offices, allowing them to share the program with their patients directly. The program is offered at no cost to participating providers or their patients who benefit from it. If you are not already enrolled, call 800-232-7379 or visit PDR.net/PharmacyDiscountCard.

Other Products from PDR

PDR® Pharmacopoeia Pocket Dosing Guide

The ***PDR Pharmacopoeia Pocket Dosing Guide*** provides quick dosage confirmation in a convenient and portable print format. Only slightly larger than an index card and just half an inch thick, it fits easily into any pocket and provides you with FDA-approved dosing recommendations for more than 1,500 drugs. Unlike many other condensed drug references, the information in the ***PDR Pharmacopoeia Pocket Dosing Guide*** is drawn exclusively from the FDA-approved drug labeling as published in *PDR* or supplied by the manufacturer.

PDR® for Nonprescription Drugs, 35th Edition (NPD)

NPD is the true over-the-counter (OTC) companion to *PDR*. It is the premier source for information on the most commonly used OTC medications. These include analgesics, cough and cold preparations, fever reducers, and more. The 2014 ***NPD*** offers physicians, residents, and medical students invaluable, easily accessible content. ***NPD*** is an excellent source for OTC drugs and contains manufacturer names, product names, indications and usage, drug warnings, and comparison tables for quick, at-a-glance dosing and ingredient information.

For more information on these or any other members of the growing family of PDR Network products, please call toll-free 800-232-7379; fax 201-722-2680; or visit PDRNetwork.com. To order a PDR Network publication, visit PDRbooks.com and simply use code: L9001BK01.

CONTENTS

SECTION 1

MANUFACTURERS' INDEX

Listed in this index are all manufacturers participating in the *Physicians' Desk Reference®*. It is through their courtesy that the *PDR®* is brought to the medical profession.

Each company's entry may include the address, phone, and fax number of its headquarters and regional offices, as well as contacts for inquiries, orders, and medical emergency information. Products with entries in the Product Information section are listed with their page numbers. Other products available from the manufacturer are listed following the described products.

If an entry in the index lists multiple page numbers, the first one shown refers to photographs of the product; the last one to its prescribing information.

- **Bold page numbers** indicate full prescribing information.
- *Italic page numbers* signify partial information.
- The ◆ symbol marks drugs shown in the Product Identification Guide.

BAYER HEALTHCARE LLC 305, 636
100 Bayer Boulevard
Whippany, NJ 07981

Direct Inquiries to:
(888) 84-BAYER
(888) 842-2937
www.bayerhealthcare.com

For Medical Information contact:
Vice President, Medical Communications
(888) 84-Bayer (888) 842-2937

Products Described:
◆Desonate Gel........................ 305, 636
◆Finacea Gel......................... 305, 638
◆Nexavar Tablets..................... 305, 640
◆Stivarga Tablets.................... 305, 646
◆Xofigo Injection.................... 305, 652

BOEHRINGER INGELHEIM PHARMACEUTICALS, INC. 305, 655
A subsidiary of Boehringer Ingelheim USA Corporation
900 Ridgebury Road
P.O. Box 368
Ridgefield, CT 06877-0368

Direct Inquiries to:
(800) 243-0127
TTY (800) 246-6196

For medical information or to report an adverse drug experience contact:
(800) 542-6257 (option 4)
TTY (800) 459-9906
us.boehringer-ingelheim.com

Products Described:
◆Jentadueto Tablets.................. 305, 655
◆Tradjenta Tablets................... 305, 664

BRISTOL-MYERS SQUIBB COMPANY 305, 672
P.O. Box 4500
Princeton, NJ 08543-4500
(609) 897-2000

For Medical Information Contact: Generally:
Bristol-Myers Squibb Medical Information Department
P.O. Box 4500
Princeton, NJ 08543-4500
(800) 321-1335

To report SUSPECTED ADVERSE REACTIONS, Contact Bristol-Myers Squibb Co. at
(800) 721-5072 between 8:00 AM-8:00 PM EST

Sales and Ordering:
Orders may be placed by:
1. Calling your purchase orders in toll-free between 9:00 AM-5:00 PM EST:
(800) 631-5244

2. E-mail your purchase orders to:
customerserviceoperations@bms.com

3. Faxing your purchase orders to:
(800) 277-0988

Product information on these pages reflects product labeling on September 30, 2013. Current information on products of Bristol-Myers Squibb may be obtained at www.bms.com or www.pdr.net.

Products Described:
◆Atripla Tablets..................... 305, 672
Baraclude Oral Solution.............. 685
◆Baraclude Tablets................... 305, 685
◆Bydureon for Injectable Suspension.. 305, 692
◆Byetta Injection.................... 305, 701
Coumadin for Injection............... 712
◆Coumadin Tablets.................... 305, 712
◆Eliquis Tablets..................... 305, 718
◆Erbitux Injection................... 305, 723
◆Ixempra Kit for Injection.......... 305, 729
◆Kombiglyze XR Extended-Release Tablets..... 306, 736
◆Nulojix Injection................... 306, 746
◆Onglyza Tablets..................... 306, 754
◆Orencia for Injection............... 306, 763
◆Reyataz Capsules.................... 306, 772
◆Sprycel Tablets..................... 306, 789
◆Sustiva Capsules.................... 306, 795
◆Sustiva Tablets..................... 306, 795
Symlin Injection..................... 808
◆SymlinPen........................... 306, 808
◆Yervoy Injection.................... 306, 816

BRISTOL-MYERS SQUIBB & GILEAD SCIENCES, LLC 306, 820
333 Lakeside Drive
Foster City, CA 94404

For Medical Information:
1-888-547-4267
medicalinformation@bms-gilead.com
To Report Adverse Events:
1-800-445-3235, press option 3
For Business Operations:
1-800-445-3235, press option 8

Products Described:
◆Atripla Tablets..................... 306, 820

J. R. CARLSON LABORATORIES, INC. 306, 2566
60 W. University Drive
Arlington Heights, IL 60004-1985

Direct Inquiries to:
Customer Service
(888) 234-5656
FAX: (847) 255-1605
www.carlsonlabs.com
For Medical Information Contact: In Emergencies:
Customer Service
(888) 234-5656
FAX: (847) 255-1605

Products Described:
Norwegian Cod Liver Oil.............. 2566
Super Daily D_3 Liquid............. 2566
◆Super Omega-3 Gems Soft Gels........ 306, 2566

CPH INTERNATIONAL CORP. 2567
P.O. Box 11439
Oakland, CA 94611
U.S.A.

Direct Inquiries to:
CPHINTL@SBCGLOBAL.NET
Fax: (510) 352-6009

Products Described:
Corovasin/Cardibose/Veratrol-CV/Restrogin Tablets.......... 2567
Cyto-Sod/Chelanil/Carnisod/Probix Tablets.................. 2567
Macutein Mega-30 mg/Optigold/Catasod-Ocuxtra/Glaucofit/Neo-GPX/Eristinol Tablets....... 2567
Neurofit-Mega/Neutropin/Waxaner/Nervox-Hexa/Tiowax Tablets/Capsules............ 2567
Tofipan/Tofipan-Z/Felamon/Menomon Tablets/Capsules....... 2567

EISAI INC. 2549
100 Tice Boulevard
Woodcliff Lake, NJ 07677

Direct Inquiries to:
(888) 274-2378

Products Described:
Aciphex Delayed-Release Tablets...... 2549
Aciphex Sprinkle Delayed-Release Capsules........ 2549

FERRING PHARMACEUTICALS INC. 306, 834
4 Gatehall Drive
Parsippany, NJ 07054

Direct Inquiries to:
Ferring Pharmaceuticals Inc.
4 Gatehall Drive, Third Floor
Parsippany, NJ 07054
(888) FERRING (337-7464)

For Medical Information Contact:
Ferring Pharmaceuticals Inc.
4 Gatehall Drive, Third Floor
Parsippany, NJ 07054
(888) FERRING (337-7464)

Products Described:
◆Prepopik for Oral Solution.......... 306, 834

FLEET LABORATORIES 838
Division of C.B. Fleet Company, Incorporated
Lynchburg, VA 24502

Direct Inquiries to:
Sherrie McNamara, RN, MSN, MBA
Director, Global Medical Affairs and Pharmacovigilance
(888) 999-9711

Products Described:
Boudreaux's Butt Paste All Natural Formula Ointment......... 838
Boudreaux's Butt Paste Maximum Strength Formula Ointment........ 838
Boudreaux's Butt Paste Original Formula Ointment.............. 838
Fleet Babylax Liquid Glycerin Suppositories.................. 838
Fleet Bisacodyl Laxatives............ 839
Fleet Enema Extra.................... 839
Fleet Enema for Children............. 839
Fleet Enema.......................... 839
Fleet Glycerin Suppositories......... 838
Fleet Liquid Glycerin Suppositories.......................... 838
Fleet Mineral Oil Enema.............. 841
Fleet Pedia-Lax Chewable Tablets..... 841
Fleet Pedia-Lax Enema................ 839
Fleet Pedia-Lax Glycerin Suppositories.......................... 838
Fleet Pedia-Lax Liquid Glycerin Suppositories.......................... 838
Fleet Pedia-Lax Liquid Stool Softener............................ 841
Phazyme Ultra Strength Antigas Softgels............................ 842

FOREST PHARMACEUTICALS, INC. 306, 842
(Subsidiary of FOREST LABORATORIES, INC.)
13600 Shoreline Drive
St. Louis, MO 63045

Direct Inquiries to:
Medical Information and Communication
13600 Shoreline Drive
St. Louis, MO 63045
(800) 678-1605

Products Described:
◆Linzess Capsules.................... 306, 842
Namenda XR Extended Release Capsules.................. 846
◆Teflaro for Injection............... 306, 849
◆Tudorza Pressair for Oral Inhalation........................ 306, 855

GILEAD SCIENCES, INC. 306, 859
333 Lakeside Drive
Foster City, CA 94404

For Product Information:
(800) 445-3235, press option 2
medicalinformation@gilead.com
To Report Adverse Events:
(800) 445-3235, press option 3
For Business Operations:
(800) 445-3235, press option 8

Products Described:
◆Atripla Tablets (See Bristol-Myers Squibb & Gilead Sciences, LLC)....... *306, 859*
◆Cayston for Inhalation Solution........................ 306, 859
◆Complera Tablets.................... 306, 863
◆Letairis Tablets..................... 306, 873
◆Ranexa Extended-Release Tablets........................ 306, 878
◆Stribild Tablets.................... 306, 881
◆Truvada Tablets..................... 306, 892
◆Viread Oral Powder.................. 307, 902
◆Viread Tablets...................... 307, 902

GLAXOSMITHKLINE 913
Five Moore Drive
Research Triangle Park
North Carolina 27709
(919) 483-2100

Direct Inquiries to:
GSK Response Center
(888) 825-5249
www.gsk.com

Products Described:
Advair Diskus 100/50 Inhalation Powder............................ 913
Advair Diskus 250/50 Inhalation Powder............................ 913
Advair Diskus 500/50 Inhalation Powder............................ 913
Advair HFA 45/21 Inhalation Aerosol............................ 925
Advair HFA 115/21 Inhalation Aerosol............................ 925
Advair HFA 230/21 Inhalation Aerosol............................ 925
Amerge Tablets....................... 936
Argatroban Injection................. 940
Arixtra Injection.................... 946
Arranon Injection.................... 954
Arzerra Injection.................... 958
Avandamet Tablets.................... 961
Avandaryl Tablets.................... 971
Avandia Tablets...................... 981
Avodart Soft Gelatin Capsules........ 991
Beconase AQ Nasal Spray.............. 996
Benlysta for Injection............... 999
Bexxar Injection..................... 1002
Boostrix Injection Vaccine........... 1007
Breo Ellipta Inhalation Powder....... 1013
Ceftin for Oral Suspension........... 1021
Ceftin Tablets....................... 1021
Cervarix Injection Vaccine........... 1025
Coreg Tablets........................ 1031
Coreg CR Extended-Release Capsules........................... 1038
Dyazide Capsules..................... 1046
Engerix-B Injection Vaccine.......... 1048
Epivir-HBV Oral Solution............. 1051
Epivir-HBV Tablets................... 1051
Flolan for Injection................. 1055
Flonase Nasal Spray.................. 1059
Flovent Diskus 50 mcg................ 1063
Flovent Diskus 100 mcg............... 1063
Flovent Diskus 250 mcg............... 1063
Flovent HFA 44 mcg Inhalation Aerosol............................ 1070
Flovent HFA 110 mcg Inhalation Aerosol............................ 1070
Flovent HFA 220 mcg Inhalation Aerosol............................ 1070
Fluarix Injection Vaccine............ 1078
Fluarix Quadrivalent Injection Suspension.......................... 1082
Flulaval Injection Vaccine........... 1087
Flulaval Quadrivalent Injection Vaccine............................ 1092
Havrix Injection Vaccine............. 1097
Hycamtin Capsules.................... 1100
Hycamtin for Injection............... 1103
Imitrex Injection.................... 1108
Imitrex Nasal Spray.................. 1113
Imitrex Tablets...................... 1119
Infanrix Injection Vaccine........... 1124
Jalyn Capsules....................... 1127
Kinrix Injection Vaccine............. 1134
Lamictal Chewable Dispersible Tablets............................ 1137
Lamictal ODT Orally Disintegrating Tablets.............. 1137
Lamictal Tablets..................... 1137
Lamictal XR Extended-Release Tablets............................ 1150
Lovaza Capsules...................... 1161
Malarone Tablets..................... 1163
Malarone Pediatric Tablets........... 1163
Mekinist Tablets..................... 1171
Menhibrix Injection Vaccine.......... 1168
Mepron Suspension.................... 1176
Pediarix Injection Vaccine........... 1180
Potiga Tablets....................... 1184
Promacta Tablets..................... 1190
Raxibacumab Injection................ 1196
Relenza Inhalation Powder............ 1200
Requip Tablets....................... 1205
Requip XL Extended-Release Tablets............................ 1212
Rotarix Oral Suspension.............. 1219
Rythmol Tablets...................... 1223
Rythmol SR Extended Release Capsules........................... 1228
Serevent Diskus Inhalation Powder............................ 1233
Tafinlar Capsules.................... 1242
Timentin for Injection............... 1246
Timentin for Injection Pharmacy Bulk Package....................... 1246
Timentin Injection Galaxy Containers......................... 1246
Treximet Tablets..................... 1251
Twinrix Injection Vaccine............ 1257
Tykerb Tablets....................... 1260
Valtrex Caplets...................... 1265
Ventolin HFA Inhalation Aerosol...... 1271
Veramyst Nasal Spray................. 1277
Votrient Tablets..................... 1283
Wellbutrin Tablets................... 1290
Wellbutrin SR Sustained-Release Tablets............................ 1297
Zantac 150 Tablets................... 1304
Zantac 300 Tablets................... 1304
Zantac Syrup......................... 1304
Zofran Injection..................... 1307

◆Elocon Lotion 0.1% ... 1460
Elocon Ointment 0.1% ... 1462
◆Emend Capsules ... 307, 1463
Emend for Injection ... 1471
Follistim AQ Cartridge ... 1479
Follistim AQ Injection ... 1488
◆Foradil Aerolizer ... 308, 1494
Fosamax Oral Solution ... 1502
◆Fosamax Tablets ... 308, 1502
◆Fosamax Plus D Tablets ... 308, 1510
Ganirelix Acetate Injection ... 1517
Gardasil Vaccine ... 1519
◆Implanon Implant ... 308, 1531
◆Integrilin Injection ... 308, 1538
◆Intron A for Injection ... 308, 1543
Invanz for Injection ... 1559
◆Isentress Chewable Tablets ... 308, 1566
◆Isentress Tablets ... 308, 1566
◆Janumet Tablets ... 308, 1575
◆Janumet XR
Extended-Release Tablets ... 308, 1584
◆Januvia Tablets ... 308, 1595
◆Juvisync Tablets ... 308, 1603
◆Liptruzet Tablets ... 308, 1618
Lotrisone Cream ... 1627
◆Maxalt Tablets ... 308, 1633
◆Maxalt-MLT Orally
Disintegrating Tablets ... 308, 1633
◆Mevacor Tablets ... 308, 1638
M-M-R II Vaccine ... 1629
◆Nasonex Nasal Spray ... 308, 1644
Nexplanon Implant ... 1650
◆Nitro-Dur Transdermal
Infusion System ... 308, 1657
◆Noroxin Tablets ... 308, 1660
Noxafil Oral Suspension ... 1665
◆NuvaRing Vaginal Ring ... 308, 1674
PedvaxHIB Vaccine ... 1680
◆PegIntron Powder for
Injection ... 308, 1684
Pneumovax 23 Vaccine ... 1699
Pregnyl for Injection, USP ... 1702
Primaxin I.V. ... 1703
◆Prinivil Tablets ... 308, 1709
◆Propecia Tablets ... 308, 1713
ProQuad Vaccine ... 1718
◆Proscar Tablets ... 308, 1727
Proventil HFA Inhalation
Aerosol ... 1733
◆Rebetol Capsules ... 308, 1736
◆Rebetol Oral Solution ... 308, 1736
Recombivax HB Vaccine ... 1748
◆Remeron Tablets ... 309, 1752
◆RemeronSolTab Tablets ... 309, 1758
RotaTeq Vaccine ... 1763
◆Saphris Tablets ... 309, 1768
Sinemet Tablets ... 1776
Sinemet CR Sustained-
Release Tablets ... 1778
◆Singulair Chewable Tablets ... 309, 1781
Singulair Oral Granules ... 1781
◆Singulair Tablets ... 309, 1781
◆Stromectol Tablets ... 309, 1788
Sylatron Injection ... 1790
◆Temodar Capsules ... 309, 1796
Temodar for Injection ... 1796
◆Tice BCG Vaccine ... 309, 1805
Trusopt Sterile Ophthalmic
Solution ... 1807
Vaqta Vaccine ... 1809
Varivax Vaccine ... 1815
◆Victrelis Capsules ... 309, 1819
◆Vytorin 10/10 Tablets ... 309, 1831
◆Vytorin 10/20 Tablets ... 309, 1831
◆Vytorin 10/40 Tablets ... 309, 1831
◆Vytorin 10/80 Tablets ... 309, 1831
◆Zemuron Injection ... 309, 1842
◆Zetia Tablets ... 309, 1848
◆Zioptan Ophthalmic
Solution ... 309, 1854
◆Zocor Tablets ... 309, 1857
◆Zolinza Capsules ... 309, 1864
Zostavax Vaccine ... 1867

MERCK SHARP & DOHME CORP.
(See MERCK)

MISSION PHARMACAL COMPANY **1872**
10999 IH 10 West, Suite 1000
San Antonio, TX 78230-1355

Direct All Inquiries to:
P.O. Box 786099
San Antonio, TX 78278-6099
Toll Free: (800) 292-7364
Customer Service (M-W 7A-5:30P C.T., Th 7:30A-5P C.T.)
(210) 696-8400
FAX: (210) 696-6010
www.missionpharmacal.com

Products Described:
Avar Cleanser ... 1873
Avar LS Cleanser ... 1873
Avar-e Emollient Cream ... 1872
Avar-e LS Emollient Cream ... 1872
Binosto Effervescent Tablets ... 1874
CitraNatal Assure Capsules ... 1880
CitraNatal Assure Tablets ... 1880
CitraNatal B-Calm Tablets ... 1880
CitraNatal 90 DHA Capsules ... 1880
CitraNatal 90 DHA Tablets ... 1880
CitraNatal Harmony Gel Caps ... 1881
Eletone Cream ... 1881
Ferralet 90 Tablets ... 1881
Lithostat Tablets ... 1882
Ovace Plus Shampoo ... 1883
Ovace Plus Wash Cleansing Gel ... 1884
Thiola Tablets ... 1884
Tindamax Tablets ... 1886
Uribel Capsules ... 1889
Urocit-K Tablets ... 1890

Other Products Available:
Avar-e Green Emollient Cream
Calcet Creamy Bites Chewable Pieces
Calcet Petites Tablets
CitraNatal DHA Capsules
CitraNatal DHA Tablets
CitraNatal Rx Tablets
Compete Tablets
Dr. Smith's Diaper Ointment
Dr. Smith's Rash-N-All Ointment
Fosfree Tablets
Lycelle Head Lice Removal Kit
NataFort Prenatal Tablets
Oncovite Tablets
Ovace Plus Creme
Ovace Wash
Prednisolone Solution 25 mg/5 mL
Texacort Topical Solution
Thera-Gesic Plus Creme
Thera-Gesic Creme

MSD INTERNATIONAL GMBH
(See MERCK)

MSD OSS B.V.
(See MERCK)

NEOPHARM, CO. LTD. **309, 1892**
#928, Tamnip-dong,
Yuseong-gu, Daejon,
South Korea (Zip: 305-510)

Products Described:
◆Atopalm Moisturizing
Cream ... 309, 1892
◆Psoriapalm Non-Greasy
Psoriasis Lotion ... 309, 1893

NOVARTIS PHARMACEUTICALS CORPORATION **309, 1893**
One Health Plaza
East Hanover, NJ 07936
(for branded products)

For Information Contact (branded products):
Customer Interaction Center
(888) NOW-NOVA (888-669-6682)
www.pharma.us.novartis.com

Products Described:
◆Afinitor Tablets ... 309, 1893
Afinitor Disperz Tablets ... 1893
◆Amturnide Tablets ... 309, 1905
◆Arcapta Neohaler ... 309, 1913
◆Coartem Tablets ... 309, 1919
◆Diovan Tablets ... 309, 1925
◆Diovan HCT Tablets ... 309, 1931
◆Exelon Patch ... 310, 1937
◆Exforge Tablets ... 310, 1944
◆Exforge HCT Tablets ... 310, 1951
◆Exjade Tablets ... 310, 1958
Extavia Kit ... 1964
◆Fanapt Tablets ... 310, 1971
◆Femara Tablets ... 310, 1977
◆Focalin XR Capsules ... 310, 1984
◆Gilenya Capsules ... 310, 1989
◆Gleevec Tablets ... 310, 1995
◆Hecoria Capsules ... 310, 2007
◆Ilaris Injection ... 310, 2019
◆Myfortic Tablets ... 310, 2024
◆Neoral Oral Solution ... 310, 2032
◆Neoral Soft Gelatin
Capsules ... 310, 2032
◆Reclast Injection ... 310, 2041
Sandimmune Oral Solution ... 2049
Sandimmune Injection ... 2049
Sandimmune Soft Gelatin
Capsules ... 2049
◆Sandostatin Injection ... 310, 2054
◆Sandostatin LAR Depot ... 311, 2056
◆Simulect for Injection ... 310, 2061
◆Tasigna Capsules ... 311, 2064
◆Tekamlo Tablets ... 311, 2071
◆Tekturna Tablets ... 311, 2078
◆Tekturna HCT Tablets ... 311, 2083
◆Tobi ... 311, 2090
◆Tobi Podhaler ... 311, 2093
◆Xolair ... 311, 2098
◆Zometa Injection Concentrate
for Intravenous Infusion ... 311, 2103
◆Zortress Tablets ... 311, 2109

Other Products Available:
Comtan Tablets
Exelon Capsules
Exelon Oral Solution
Stalevo Tablets
Tegretol XR Tablets
Trileptal Oral Suspension
Trileptal Tablets

NOVO NORDISK INC. **311, 2120**
800 Scudders Mill Road
Plainsboro, NJ 08536

Direct Inquiries to:
Novo Nordisk Inc.
(800) 727-6500
8:30 AM - 6:00 PM EST M-F

In Emergencies after hours & weekends:
(609) 987-5800

Products Described:
Levemir FlexPen ... 2120
Levemir Injection ... 2120
NovoLog FlexPen ... 2129
NovoLog Injection ... 2129
NovoLog Mix 70/30
FlexPen ... 2137
NovoLog Mix 70/30
Injection ... 2137
◆Victoza Injection ... 311, 2145

NSE PRODUCTS, INC. (PHARMANEX) **2569**
75 West Center Street
Provo, UT 84601

For Information and Product Support:
1-(800) 487-1000
Website: www.nuskin.com

Products Described:
ageLOC R^2 Day Capsules ... 2569
ageLOC R^2 Night Capsules ... 2569
CordyMax Cs-4 Capsules ... 2569
LifePak Capsules ... 2569
MarineOmega Softgel Capsules ... 2570
ReishiMax GLp Capsules ... 2570
Tēgreen 97 Capsules ... 2570

ONYX PHARMACEUTICALS, INC. **311, 2156**
249 E. Grand Avenue
South San Francisco, CA 94080

Direct Inquiries to:
Phone: 877-ONYX-121 (669-9121)
Fax: 877-ONX-PHRM (669-7476)
Email: medinfo@onyx.com

Products Described:
◆Kyprolis for Injection ... 311, 2156

OTSUKA AMERICA PHARMACEUTICAL, INC. **311, 2161**
2440 Research Boulevard
Rockville, MD 20850

Direct Medical Inquiries to:
Medical Affairs
Otsuka America Pharmaceutical, Inc.
(800) 441-6763
Fax: (301) 212-8634

To Request Routine or Emergency Medical Information, or to Report an Adverse Experience:
(800) 438-9927

Products Described:
Abilify Injection ... 2161
Abilify Oral Solution ... 2161
Abilify Tablets ... 2161
Abilify Discmelt Orally
Disintegrating Tablets ... 2161
Abilify Maintena
Extended-Release Injectable
Suspension ... 2176
◆Samsca Tablets ... 311, 2184

PBM PHARMACEUTICALS, INC. **311, 2189**
200 Garrett Street, Suite O
Charlottesville, VA 22902

Direct Inquiries to:
Donnatal Tablets Customer Service
(800) 485-9828
Customer Service
(800) 858-4006 = Donnatal
Fax: (866) 234-6455

Products Described:
◆Donnatal Tablets ... 311, 2189

PERQUE INTEGRATIVE HEALTH **2570**
44621 Guilford Drive, Suite 150
Ashburn, VA 20147

Direct Inquiries to:
(800) 525-7372

Products Described:
Perque Life Guard Tabsules ... 2570
Perque Potent C Guard Powder ... 2571
Perque Repair Guard Tabsules ... 2571

PFIZER INC. **2190**
235 East 42nd Street
New York, NY 10017-5755

For updates to the product information listed below, please check the Pfizer Web site http://www.pfizerpro.com or call (800) 438-1985.

For Medical Information, Contact:
(800) 438-1985
24 hours a day, 7 days a week

Distribution:
1855 Shelby Oaks Drive North
Memphis, TN 38134
(901) 387-5200

Customer Service:
(800) 533-4535

Pfizer Companies Include:
Agouron Pharmaceuticals
King Pharmaceuticals, Inc.
Parke-Davis
Pharmacia & Upjohn
G.D. Searle & Co.
Wyeth Pharmaceuticals (see WYETH PHARMACEUTICALS)

Products Described:
Viagra Tablets ... 2190
Xeljanz Tablets ... 2195

Other Products Available:
Accupril Tablets
Accuretic Tablets
Aldactazide Tablets
Alsuma Injection
Altace Capsules
Aromasin Tablets
Arthrotec Tablets
Atgam Sterile Solution
Avinza Capsules
Azulfidine Tablets, EN-Tabs
Bicillin L-A Injection
Bosulif Tablets
Caduet Tablets
Calan Tablets, SR Caplets
Camptosar for Injection
Cardura Tablets, XL Tablets
Caverject
Celebrex Capsules
Celontin Capsules
Chantix Tablets
Cleocin HCl Capsules
Cleocin Pediatric for Oral Solution, USP
Cleocin Phosphate Sterile Solution
Cleocin T Topical Gel, Lotion, Solution
Cleocin Vaginal Cream, Ovules
Colestid Tablets, Oral Suspension
Colestid/Flavored Colestid for Oral Suspension
Cortef Tablets
Daypro Caplets
Depo-Estradiol Injectable Solution
Depo-Medrol Injectable Suspension
Depo-Provera
depo-subQ provera Injectable Suspension
Depo-Testosterone Injection
Detrol Tablets
Detrol LA Capsules
Didrex Tablets
Diflucan
Dilantin
Elelyso Injection
Ellence Injection
Embeda Extended Release Capsules
Emcyt Capsules
Eraxis for Injection
Estring Vaginal Ring
Feldene Capsules
Flagyl
Flector Patch
Gelfilm Sterile Film
Gelfoam Sterile Powder, Sponge
Genotropin Lyophilized Powder
Geodon
Glucotrol Tablets, XL Tablets
Glynase PresTab Tablets
Glyset Tablets
Halcion Tablets
Hemabate Sterile Solution (Sales restricted to hospitals only)
Idamycin
Inlyta Tablets
Inspra Tablets
Levoxyl Tablets
Lincocin Sterile Solution

Lipitor Tablets
Lomotil Tablets
Lopid Tablets
Lyrica Capsules, Oral Solution
Medrol Tablets and Dosepak
Mycobutin Capsules
Nardil Tablets
Neurontin Capsules, Tablets, Oral Solution
Nitrostat Tablets
Norpace
Norvasc Tablets
Oxecta Tablets
Pfizerpen for Injection
Prepidil Gel
Procardia Capsules, XL Tablets
Prostin E2 Vaginal Suppository
Prostin VR Pediatric Sterile Solution
Provera Tablets
Relpax Tablets
Revatio Injection, Tablets
R-Gene 10 for Intravenous Use
Skelaxin Tablets
Solu-Cortef Injection
Solu-Medrol Injection
Somavert for Injection
Sutent Capsules
Tikosyn Capsules
Toviaz Extended-Release Tablets
Unasyn
VFEND
Vibramycin
Xalatan Sterile Ophthalmic Solution
Xalkori Capsules
Xanax Tablets, XR Tablets
Zithromax
Zmax for Oral Suspension
Zoloft
Zyvox

PIVOTAL THERAPEUTICS INC. **311, 2202**
81 Zenway Blvd
Unit #10
Woodbridge, Ontario L4H 0S5
Canada
Telephone: 1-905-856-9797

Direct Inquiries to:
Pivotal Therapeutics (US), Inc.
3651 FAU Blvd., Suite 400
Boca Raton, FL 33431
United States
Telephone: 1-888-358-2080
Telephone: 1-561-288-5231
Email: info@pivotaltherapeutics.us
Website: www.pivotaltherapeutics.us

Products Described:
◆Vascazen.................... **311, 2202**

PRESTIUM PHARMA, INC. **311, 2203**
411 South State Street, Suite E-100
Newtown, PA 18940

Direct Inquiries to:
(267) 685-0340

Products Described:
◆Denavir Cream.............. **311, 2203**
◆Vusion Ointment............. **311, 2204**

PURDUE PHARMA L.P. **311, 2206**
One Stamford Forum
Stamford, CT 06901-3431

For Medical Inquiries:
(888) 726-7535

Adverse Drug Experiences:
(888) 726-7535

Customer Service:
(800) 877 5666
FAX: (800) 877-3210

Products Described:
◆Butrans Transdermal System.................... **311, 2206**
◆Dilaudid Injection............ **312, 2217**
◆Dilaudid Oral Liquid.......... **311, 2215**
◆Dilaudid Tablets............. **311, 2215**
◆Dilaudid-HP Injection......... **312, 2217**
◆Dilaudid-HP Lyophilized Powder 250 mg............ **312, 2217**
◆Intermezzo Sublingual Tablet...................... **312, 2222**
◆OxyContin Tablets............ **312, 2227**

RANBAXY LABORATORIES INC. **312, 2234**
9431 Florida Mining Boulevard East
Jacksonville, Florida 32257

Direct Inquiries to:
(609) 720-9200

Products Described:
◆Absorica Capsules........... **312, 2234**
Halog Cream...................... **2240**
Halog Ointment................... **2241**
Kenalog Spray.................... **2242**

RECORDATI RARE DISEASES, INC. **312, 2243**
100 Corporate Drive
Lebanon, NJ 08833

Direct Inquiries to:
(908) 236-0888

Products Described:
◆Chemet Capsules............. **312, 2243**
◆Panhematin for Injection...... **312, 2244**

REGENERON PHARMACEUTICALS, INC. **312, 2245**
777 Old Saw Mill River Road
Tarrytown, NY 10591

For Medical Information Contact:
(877) REGN-777 (877-734-6777)

Products Described:
◆Arcalyst Injection for Subcutaneous Use.......... **312, 2245**
◆Eylea Injection............... **312, 2251**

RLC LABS, INC. **312, 2255**
Cave Creek, AZ 85331

For Product Information:
(877) 797-7997
sales@rlclabs.com

For Customer Service & Ordering Information:
(877) 797-7997
FAX: (623) 879-8683
customerservice@rlclabs.com
www.rlclabs.com

Products Described:
◆Nature-Throid Tablets......... **312, 2255**
◆WP Thyroid Tablets.......... **312, 2257**

SALIX PHARMACEUTICALS, INC. **312, 2259**
8510 Colonnade Center Drive
Raleigh, NC 27615

Direct Inquiries to:
(866) 669-7597 Phone
(919) 862-1817 Fax
www.salix.com

For adverse events, product quality complaints and patient information requests:
Product Information Center
(800) 508-0024 Phone
(510) 595-8183 Fax
E-mail: salix@medcomsol.com

Products Described:
◆Apriso Extended-Release Capsules................... **312, 2259**
◆Fulyzaq Delayed-Release Tablets.................... **312, 2261**
◆MoviPrep Oral Solution....... **312, 2263**
◆Relistor Subcutaneous Injection.................. **313, 2266**
Solesta Syringes.................. **2274**
◆Xifaxan Tablets.............. **313, 2279**

Other Products Available:
Anusol-HC Cream 2.5%
Anusol-HC Suppository 25 mg
Azasan Tablets
Deflux
Diuril Oral Suspension
Giazo Tablets
Metozolv Orally Disintegrating Tablets
OsmoPrep Tablets
Pepcid Oral Suspension
Proctocort Cream 1%
Proctocort Suppository 30 mg

SCHERING CORP.
(See MERCK)

SMITH & NEPHEW, INC. **313, 2283**
3909 Hulen Street
Fort Worth, TX 76107

Direct Inquiries to:
(800) 441-8227

Products Described:
◆Collagenase Santyl Ointment.................. **313, 2283**
◆Regranex Gel................ **313, 2283**

STIEFEL LABORATORIES, INC. **313, 2286**
Research Triangle Park, NC 27709

Direct Inquiries to:
Professional Services Department
888 STIEFEL (888-784-3335)

Products Described:
Altabax Ointment................. **2286**
Bactroban Cream.................. **2289**
Bactroban Nasal.................. **2290**
Bactroban Ointment............... **2291**
Duac Gel......................... **2292**
Fabior Foam...................... **2293**
◆Soriatane Capsules............ **313, 2296**
Sorilux Foam, 0.005%............. **2304**
Veltin Gel....................... **2306**

Other Products Available:
Oilatum Cleansing Bar (Unscented)
PanOxyl Bar 10
SARNA Original Anti-Itch Lotion
SARNA Sensitive Anti-Itch Lotion
Zeasorb Powder
Zeasorb-AF Powder (Athlete's Foot)
Zeasorb-AF Powder (Jock Itch)

SUNOVION PHARMACEUTICALS INC. **313, 2309**
84 Waterford Drive
Marlborough, MA 01752
(508) 481-6700

For Medical Information Inquiries:
Medical Information
(800) 739-0565
minfo@sunovion.com
www.SunovionMedical.com
For Adverse Event Reporting:
(877) 737-7226
For Customer Service:
(888) 394-7377
CAC@sunovion.com

Products Described:
◆Brovana Inhalation Solution... **313, 2309**
◆Latuda Tablets.............. **313, 2315**

SUPERNUS PHARMACEUTICALS **313, 2327**
1550 E Gude Drive
Rockville, MD 20850

Direct Inquiries to:
(866) 398-0833

Products Described:
◆Oxtellar XR Tablets.......... **313, 2327**
◆Trokendi XR Capsules........ **313, 2334**

SYNERGY WORLDWIDE **313, 2571**
1955 West Grove Parkway, Suite 100
Pleasant Grove, Utah 84062

Direct Inquiries to:
(801) 769-7800

Products Described:
◆ProArgi-9+ Dietary Supplement................ **313, 2571**

TAKEDA PHARMACEUTICALS U.S.A., INC. **313, 2347**
One Takeda Parkway
Deerfield, IL 60015

Direct Inquiries to:
Sales and Ordering:
Customer Service
(877) TAKEDA7
(877) 825-3327

For Medical Information Contact:
General:
(877) TAKEDA7
(877) 825-3327
To Report Adverse Drug Experiences:
(877) TAKEDA7
(877) 825-3327

Products Described:
◆Amitiza Capsules............ **313, 2347**
Brintellix Tablets................ **2351**
◆Colcrys Tablets.............. **313, 2359**
◆Dexilant Delayed Release Capsules.................. **313, 2365**
◆Edarbi Tablets............... **313, 2370**
◆Edarbyclor Tablets........... **313, 2374**
◆Kazano Tablets.............. **313, 2379**
◆Nesina Tablets............... **313, 2387**
◆Oseni Tablets............... **313, 2395**
◆Uloric Tablets............... **313, 2406**

TEVA **314, 2411**
11100 Nall Avenue
Overland Park, KS 66221

For Company Inquiries Contact:
(800) 221-4026

For Medical Information Contact:
(888) 4-TEVA-RX
(888-483-8279)

Products Described:
◆Azilect Tablets.............. **314, 2411**
◆Copaxone Injection.......... **314, 2417**

TEVA RESPIRATORY, LLC. **314, 2421**
425 Privet Road
Horsham, PA 19044

For All Inquiries Call:
1-888-482-9522

Products Described:
◆ProAir HFA Inhalation Aerosol................... **314, 2421**
Qvar Inhalation Aerosol........... **2426**

TEVA SELECT BRANDS **314, 2430**
A Division of TEVA PHARMACEUTICALS USA
650 Cathill Road
Sellersville, PA 18960

Direct Inquiries to:
41 Moores Road
Frazer, PA 19355
(800) 292-4283

Products Described:
◆Adipex-P Capsules........... **314, 2430**
◆Adipex-P Tablets............. **314, 2430**
Proglycem Capsules............... **2432**
◆Proglycem Suspension........ **314, 2432**

TOPICAL BIOMEDICS, INC. **314, 2437**
6565 Spring Brook Avenue, Ste 11
Rhinebeck, NY 12572-0494

Direct Inquiries to:
Professional Services at Topricin
(845) 871-4900 ex 1115
Fax: (845) 876-0818
info@topicalbiomedics.com for free samples and prescription pads

Products Described:
◆Topricin Foot Therapy Cream..................... **314, 2437**
◆Topricin Junior.............. **314, 2437**
◆Topricin Pain Relief and Healing Cream............. **314, 2437**

TRIVITA, INC. **314, 2571**
16100 N Greenway Hayden Lp.
Suite #950
Scottsdale, AZ 85260

Direct Inquiries to:
(800) 991-7116
Fax: (480) 778-2992

Products Described:
◆Nopalea Superfruit........... **314, 2571**

UNICITY INTERNATIONAL, INC. **314, 2572**
The Make Life Better Company
1201 North 800 East
Orem, UT 84097

Direct Inquiries to:
(801) 226-2600
www.unicity.com
science.unicity@unicity.com
Products of Unicity International, Inc. are distributed through independent distributors.

Products Described:
Bio-C Tablets.................... **2572**
◆Bios Life Cardio Advanced Fiber and Nutrient Drink.... **314, 2572**

SECTION 2

BRAND AND GENERIC NAME INDEX

This index includes all entries in the Product Information section. Products are listed alphabetically by both brand and generic name. Generic names are underlined; brand names are not. Under each generic name, you will find a list of the brands that contain it. This enables you to find a product by either of its names. For example, the brand Amerge appears once in the A's, and again under its generic name, naratriptan hydrochloride.

Each time a brand name appears, it is followed by the manufacturer's name and the page number to consult for further information. If multiple page numbers appear, the first one refers to photographs of the product; the last one to its prescribing information. Under a generic heading, all fully described brands are listed first, followed by those with only partial information.

- **Bold page numbers** indicate full prescribing information.
- *Italic page numbers* signify partial information.
- The ◆ symbol marks drugs shown in the Product Identification Guide.

A

BRAND AND GENERIC NAME INDEX

BRAND AND GENERIC NAME INDEX

BRAND AND GENERIC NAME INDEX

U

V

BRAND AND GENERIC NAME INDEX

GENERIC/BRAND CROSS-REFERENCE TABLE

This table includes a list of more than 200 of the top prescribed products used in the retail setting, identified by generic name. For ease of use, products are listed alphabetically with reference to the corresponding brand name(s) available on the market. Additionally, the table contains indications for each product; if indications differ either by the way the drug is supplied (ie, injection, cream, etc.) or by specific brand, it is noted.

Products with full prescribing information listed in *PDR®* are in **boldface** in the Brand(s) column. Please go to **PDR.net®** to view prescribing information on a particular product.

GENERIC	BRAND(S)	INDICATION(S)
Acetaminophen/Codeine Phosphate	Tylenol with Codeine	pain
Acyclovir	Zovirax Cream, Zovirax Ointment, Zovirax Oral	Cream/Ointment: herpes, infections (viral/topical) Oral: chickenpox; herpes, infections (viral/systemic), shingles
Albuterol Tabs	Proventil	asthma, bronchospasm
Albuterol Sulfate/Ipratropium	Combivent, Combivent Respimat, Duoneb	bronchospasm, COPD
Alendronate Sodium	**Fosamax**	osteoporosis, Paget's disease
Allopurinol	Zyloprim	chemotherapy adjunct, gout, hyperuricemia, hyperuricosuria, renal calculi
Alprazolam	Niravam, Xanax, Xanax XR	Niravam, Xanax: anxiety, panic disorder Xanax XR: panic disorder
Amiodarone	Cordarone	arrhythmia
Amitriptyline	Amitriptyline HCl (generic)	depression
Amlodipine Besylate	Norvasc	angina; coronary artery disease; hypertension; revascularization, reduce risk
Amlodipine Besylate/ Benazepril HCl	Lotrel	hypertension
Amoxicillin	Amoxil, Moxatag	Amoxil: gonorrhea; *Helicobacter pylori* eradication; infections (bacterial/skin, bacterial/respiratory tract, otic, urinary tract); otitis media; ulcer, gastrointestinal Moxatag: pharyngitis, tonsillitis
Amoxicillin/Potassium Clavulanate	Augmentin, Augmentin ES-600, Augmentin XR	Augmentin: infections (bacterial/respiratory tract, bacterial/skin, otic, urinary tract), otitis media, sinusitis Augmentin ES-600: infections (otic) Augmentin XR: infections (bacterial/respiratory tract); pneumonia, bacterial; sinusitis
Amphetamine/ Dextroamphetamine	Adderall, Adderall XR	Adderall, Adderall XR: ADHD Adderall: narcolepsy
Anastrozole	Arimidex	breast cancer
Atenolol	Tenormin	angina; hypertension; myocardial infarction, postmanagement
Atenolol/Chlorthalidone	Tenoretic	hypertension
Atorvastatin Calcium	Lipitor	cardiovascular risk reduction, hypercholesterolemia, hyperlipidemia, hypertriglyceridemia

Azithromycin	**Azasite**, Zithromax, Zmax	Azasite: conjunctivitis, infections (bacterial/ophthalmic) Zithromax: cervicitis; COPD; infections (bacterial/respiratory tract, bacterial/skin, gynecological, otic, urinary tract); *Mycobacterium avium* complex; otitis media; pharyngitis; pneumonia, bacterial; sinusitis; tonsillitis; urethritis Zmax: infections (bacterial/respiratory tract); pneumonia, bacterial; sinusitis
Baclofen	Baclofen (generic), Gablofen, Lioresal Intrathecal	Baclofen: multiple sclerosis, muscle spasm Gablofen, Lioresal Intrathecal: musculoskeletal conditions
Benazepril	Lotensin	hypertension
Benzonatate	Tessalon, Zonatuss	cough
Benztropine	Cogentin	extrapyramidal disorder, Parkinson's disease
Bisoprolol/HCTZ	Ziac	hypertension
Brompheniramine/ Dextromethorphan/ Pseudoephedrine	Bromfed DM	allergy, congestion, cough
Bupropion	Budeprion XL, Wellbutrin XL	depression, major depressive disorder
Bupropion SR	**Wellbutrin SR**, **Zyban**	Wellbutrin SR: depression, major depressive disorder Zyban: smoking cessation
Buspirone HCl	Buspirone HCl (generic)	anxiety
Butalbital/Acetaminophen/ Caffeine	Esgic, Esgic-Plus, Fioricet, Zebutal	migraine/tension headache
Carbamazepine	Carbatrol, Epitol, Equetro, Tegretol, Tegretol-XR	Carbatrol, Epitol, Tegretol, Tegretol-XR: pain, seizures, trigeminal neuralgia Equetro: bipolar disorder, mania
Carbidopa/Levodopa	Parcopa, **Sinemet**, **Sinemet CR**	Parkinson's disease
Carisoprodol	Soma	musculoskeletal conditions, pain
Carvedilol	**Coreg**, **Coreg CR**	congestive heart failure; hypertension; myocardial infarction, postmanagement
Cefdinir	Cefdinir	bronchitis, infections (bacterial/respiratory tract, bacterial/skin, otic), otitis media, pharyngitis, pneumonia, sinusitis, tonsillitis
Cefuroxime Axetil	**Ceftin**	bronchitis, gonorrhea, impetigo, infections (bacterial/respiratory tract, bacterial/skin, otic, urinary tract), Lyme disease, otitis media, pharyngitis, sinusitis, tonsillitis
Cephalexin	Keflex	infections (bacterial/bone, bacterial/respiratory tract, bacterial/skin, otic, urinary tract), otitis media, prostatitis
Chlorhexidine Gluconate	Peridex, PerioGard	gingivitis
Chlorthalidone	Thalitone	congestive heart failure, edema, hypertension

Ciprofloxacin HCl	Cetraxal, Ciloxan, Cipro Oral, Cipro XR	Cetraxal: infections (otic), otitis externa Ciloxan: conjunctivitis; infections (bacterial/ophthalmic); ulcer, corneal Cipro Oral: anthrax, bronchitis, diarrhea, gonorrhea, infections (bacterial/bone, bacterial/respiratory tract, bacterial/skin, bacterial/systemic, gynecological, intra-abdominal, urinary tract), prostatitis, sinusitis, typhoid fever Cipro XR: infections (urinary tract)
Citalopram HBr	Celexa	depression
Clarithromycin	**Biaxin**, **Biaxin XL**	Biaxin: bronchitis, *Helicobacter pylori* eradication, infections (bacterial/skin, bacterial/respiratory tract, otic); *Mycobacterium avium* complex; otitis media; pharyngitis; pneumonia, bacterial; sinusitis; tonsillitis; ulcer, gastrointestinal Biaxin XL: bronchitis; infections (bacterial/respiratory tract); pneumonia, bacterial; sinusitis
Clindamycin HCl Systemic	Cleocin	infections (bacterial/respiratory tract, bacterial/skin, bacterial/systemic, gynecological, intra-abdominal), septicemia
Clindamycin Palmitate HCl Systemic	Cleocin Oral Solution	infections (bacterial/respiratory tract, bacterial/skin, bacterial/systemic, gynecological, intra-abdominal), septicemia
Clindamycin topical	Cleocin T	acne vulgaris
Clobetasol	Clobetasol Propionate (generic), Clobevate, Clobex, Cormax, Olux, Olux-E, Temovate, Temovate-E, Temovate Scalp	corticosteroid responsive dermatoses
Clonazepam	Clonazepam ODT, Klonopin	panic disorder, seizures
Clonidine	Catapres, Catapres-TTS, Duraclon Injection	Catapres, Catapres-TTS: hypertension Duraclon Injection: cancer pain; pain, neuropathic
Clopidogrel	Plavix	angina, coronary syndrome, myocardial infarction, stroke
Clotrimazole/Betamethasone	**Lotrisone**	athlete's foot, infections (fungal/topical)
Cyclobenzaprine	Amrix, Cyclobenzaprine (generic)	muscle spasm, musculoskeletal conditions, pain
Diazepam	Diastat, Diazepam Injection (generic), Valium	Diastat: seizures Diazepam Injection: alcohol withdrawal management, anxiety, muscle spasm, seizures, surgical adjunct/aid Valium: alcohol withdrawal management, anxiety, muscle spasm, seizures
Diclofenac Sodium	Diclofenac DR	ankylosing spondylitis, osteoarthritis, rheumatoid arthritis
Dicyclomine HCl	Bentyl	irritable bowel syndrome
Digoxin	Lanoxin	arrhythmia, heart failure
Diltiazem HCl ER	Cardizem CD, **Cardizem LA**, Cartia XT, Dilacor XR, Diltia XT, Taztia XT, Tiazac	angina, hypertension
Diphenoxylate/Atropine	Lomotil	diarrhea
Divalproex Sodium	Depakote, **Depakote ER**	bipolar disorder, mania, migraine/tension headache, seizures
Donepezil	Aricept	Alzheimer's disease

Please go to **PDR.net** to view Prescribing Information for these and other products.

Doxazosin	Cardura, Cardura XL	Cardura: benign prostatic hypertrophy, hypertension Cardura XL: benign prostatic hypertrophy
Doxepin	Doxepin	anxiety, depression
Doxycycline	Vibramycin, Vibra-Tabs	acne, actinomycosis, anthrax, bartonellosis, brucellosis, chancroid, cholera, conjunctivitis, gonorrhea, infections (bacterial/ophthalmic, bacterial/respiratory tract, bacterial/skin, gynecological, intra-abdominal, urinary tract), listeriosis, malaria, plague, psittacosis, Rocky Mountain spotted fever, syphilis, trachoma, tularemia, typhus, urethritis, yaws
Enalapril	Vasotec	heart failure, hypertension
Ergocalciferol	Drisdol	hypoparathyroidism, hypophosphatemia, rickets
Escitalopram Oxalate	Lexapro	anxiety, depression, major depressive disorder
Estradiol Oral	Estrace, Estradiol Tablets	cancer, breast; cancer, prostate; hypoestrogenism; menopause; osteoporosis; vaginitis, atrophic
Ethinyl Estradiol/Drospirenone	Gianvi, Loryna, Yaz	acne, contraception, PMDD
Ethinyl Estradiol/Norgestimate	Ortho-Cyclen, Ortho Tri-Cyclen, Sprintec, Tri-Previfem, Tri-Sprintec, Trinessa	Ortho-Cyclen, Sprintec: contraception Ortho Tri-Cyclen, Tri-Previfem, Tri-Sprintec, Trinessa: acne, contraception
Ethinyl Estradiol/Norgestimate/ Ferrous Fumarate	Gildess Fe, Junel Fe, Loestrin Fe, Microgestin Fe	contraception
Etodolac	Etodolac	osteoarthritis, rheumatoid arthritis, pain
Famotidine	Pepcid, **Pepcid AC**, **Pepcid Complete**, Pepcid Oral Suspension	Pepcid, Pepcid Oral Suspension: erosive esophagitis; GERD; hypersecretory conditions; ulcer, gastrointestinal; Zollinger-Ellison syndrome Pepcid AC, Pepcid Complete: heartburn
Fenofibrate	Antara, Fenoglide, Lipofen, Lofibra, **Tricor**, Triglide	hypercholesterolemia, hyperlipidemia, hypertriglyceridemia
Fentanyl Transdermal	**Duragesic**	pain
Finasteride	**Propecia**, **Proscar**	Propecia: alopecia Proscar: benign prostatic hypertrophy
Fluconazole	Diflucan	candidemia; candidiasis, esophageal; candidiasis, oropharyngeal; candidiasis, vaginal; infections (fungal/ systemic, fungal/vaginal, gynecological, urinary tract); meningitis; peritonitis; pneumonia, fungal
Fluocinonide	Fluocinonide, Fluocinonide-E, Vanos	dermatitis; inflammation, topical; pruritus, topical; psoriasis
Fluoxetine	Prozac, Prozac Weekly, Sarafem	Prozac: bipolar disorder, bulimia, depression, major depressive disorder, obsessive-compulsive disorder, panic disorder Prozac Weekly: depression, major depressive disorder Sarafem: premenstrual dysphoric disorder
Fluticasone Propionate	**Flonase**	allergy, rhinitis
Folic Acid	Folic Acid	anemia; anemia, megaloblastic
Furosemide Oral	Lasix	congestive heart failure, edema, hypertension

Gabapentin	Gralise, Horizant, Neurontin	Gralise, Neurontin: pain, neuropathic; postherpetic neuralgia Horizant: pain, neuropathic; postherpetic neuralgia, restless legs syndrome Neurontin: seizures
Gemfibrozil	Lopid	coronary artery disease, hypercholesterolemia, hyperlipidemia, hypertriglyceridemia
Glimepiride	Amaryl	diabetes
Glipizide	Glucotrol	diabetes
Glipizide ER	Glucotrol XL	diabetes
Glyburide	DiaBeta, Glynase PresTab, Micronase	diabetes
Glyburide/Metformin HCl	Glucovance	diabetes
Guanfacine	Tenex	hypertension
Hydralazine	Hydralazine HCl (generic)	hypertension
Hydrochlorothiazide	Microzide	hypertension
Hydrocodone/Acetaminophen	Anexsia, Lorcet, Lortab, Maxidone, Norco, **Vicodin**, **Vicodin ES**, **Vicodin HP**, Zydone	pain
Hydrocodone Polistirex/ Chlorpheniramine polistirex	Tussionex	allergy, cough
Hydrocortisone Acetate Topical Rx	Alacort, Anucort-HC, Anusol-HC Suppository, Cortifoam, Hemorrhoidal HC	Alacort: dermatitis; inflammation, topical; pruritus, topical Anucort HC, Anusol-HC Suppository, Hemorrhoidal HC: colitis, ulcerative; hemorrhoids; inflammation, topical; proctitis; pruritus, topical Cortifoam: proctitis
Hydromorphone HCl	**Dilaudid**, **Dilaudid-HP**, Exalgo	pain
Hydroxychloroquine	Plaquenil	lupus erythematosus, malaria, rheumatoid arthritis
Hydroxyzine	Hydroxyzine HCl (generic)	allergy; anxiety; nausea; pruritus, topical; sedation, preoperative; vomiting
Hydroxyzine Pamoate	Hydroxyzine Pamoate (generic), Vistaril	allergy; anxiety; pruritus, topical; sedation; sedation, preoperative
Ibuprofen	Advil Migraine, Caldolor, Motrin, **Motrin (Children's, Infants'**, Junior), **Motrin IB**, Neoprofen, Nuprin	Advil Migraine: migraine/tension headache Caldolor: fever, pain Motrin (Children's, Infants', Junior): fever, influenza, pain Motrin, Motrin IB: arthritis, dysmenorrhea, fever, pain Neoprofen: ductus arteriosus Nuprin: arthritis, fever, pain
Indomethacin	Indomethacin (generic), Indocin	ankylosing spondylitis, arthritis, bursitis, gout, pain, tendinitis
Ipratropium	Atrovent HFA, Atrovent Nasal	Atrovent HFA: bronchitis, bronchospasm, COPD, emphysema Atrovent Nasal: allergy, rhinitis
Irbesartan	Avapro	diabetic nephropathy, hypertension
Isosorbide Mononitrate	Imdur, Ismo, Monoket	angina

Ketoconazole	Extina, Ketoconazole Topical, Nizoral A-D, Nizoral Shampoo, Xolegel	Extina, Xolegel: dermatitis, seborrheic Ketoconazole Topical: athlete's foot; dermatitis, seborrheic; infections (fungal/topical); tinea versicolor Nizoral A-D: dandruff Nizoral Shampoo: infections (fungal/topical)
Labetalol HCl	Labetalol HCl (generic), Trandate	hypertension
Lamotrigine	**Lamictal**, **Lamictal CD**, **Lamictal ODT**, **Lamictal XR**	Lamictal, Lamictal CD, Lamictal ODT: bipolar disorder, seizures Lamictal XR: seizures
Lansoprazole	Prevacid, Prevacid Solutab	erosive esophagitis; GERD; heartburn; *Helicobacter pylori* eradication; hypersecretory conditions; ulcer, gastrointestinal; Zollinger-Ellison syndrome
Latanoprost	Xalatan	glaucoma/IOP
Levetiracetam	Keppra, Keppra XR	seizures
Levocetirizine Dihydrochloride	Xyzal	allergy, rhinitis, urticaria
Levofloxacin	Levaquin	anthrax, bacteremia, bronchitis, infections (bacterial/respiratory tract, bacterial/skin, bacterial/systemic, urinary tract), plague, pneumonia, prostatitis, sinusitis
Levothyroxine	Levothroid, Levoxyl, **Synthroid**, Unithroid	Levothroid: cancer, thyroid; diagnostic aid; goiter; hypothyroidism; surgical adjunct/aid; thyrotoxicosis; TSH suppression Levoxyl, Synthroid, Unithroid: cancer, thyroid; goiter; hypothyroidism; surgical adjunct/aid; TSH suppression
Lisinopril	**Prinivil**, Zestril	heart failure, hypertension
Lisinopril/HCTZ	Prinzide, Zestoretic	hypertension
Lithium Carbonate	Eskalith, Lithium Carbonate (generic), Lithobid	bipolar disorder, mania
Lorazepam	Ativan, Ativan Injection	Ativan: anxiety, depression Ativan Injection: anesthesia, adjunct; seizures
Losartan Potassium	Cozaar	hypertension; nephropathy, diabetic; stroke, reduce risk
Losartan Potassium/HCTZ	Hyzaar	hypertension; stroke, reduce risk
Lovastatin	Altoprev, **Mevacor**	Altoprev: angina, reduce risk; coronary artery disease; hypercholesterolemia; hyperlipidemia; hypertriglyceridemia; myocardial infarction, reduce risk; revascularization, reduce risk Mevacor: angina, reduce risk; coronary artery disease; hypercholesterolemia; hyperlipidemia; myocardial infarction, reduce risk; revascularization, reduce risk
Meclizine HCl	Antivert, Dramamine Less Drowsy, Zentrip	Antivert: motion sickness, nausea, vertigo, vomiting Dramamine Less Drowsy, Zentrip: motion sickness, nausea, vomiting
Medroxyprogesterone Acetate	Provera	amenorrhea; endometrial hyperplasia; uterine bleeding, abnormal
Meloxicam	Mobic	osteoarthritis, rheumatoid arthritis
Metformin	Glucophage, Riomet	diabetes
Metformin HCl ER	Fortamet, Glucophage XR, Glumetza	diabetes

Please go to **PDR.net** to view Prescribing Information for these and other products.

Methadone HCl Non-In	Dolophine, Methadone (generic), Methadose	detoxification, methadone maintenance, pain
Methocarbamol	Robaxin, Robaxin Injection, Robaxin-750	musculoskeletal conditions, pain
Methotrexate	Methotrexate (generic)	cancer, bone; cancer, breast; cancer, head and neck; cancer, lung; leukemia; lymphoma; psoriasis; rheumatoid arthritis
Methylphenidate	Methylin	ADHD, narcolepsy
Methylphenidate Sustained-Release	Ritalin SR	ADHD, narcolepsy
Methylprednisolone Tabs	Medrol, Medrol Dosepak	corticosteroid responsive disorders
Metoclopramide	Metoclopramide (generic), Metozolv ODT, Reglan, Reglan Injection	Metoclopramide, Reglan, Reglan Injection: chemotherapy adjunct, diagnostic aid, gastroparesis, GERD, nausea, vomiting Metozolv ODT: gastroparesis, GERD
Metoprolol Succinate ER	Toprol-XL	angina, heart failure, hypertension
Metoprolol Tartrate	Lopressor	angina, hypertension, myocardial infarction
Metronidazole Tabs	Flagyl, Flagyl ER	Flagyl: cervicitis; endocarditis; infections (bacterial/bone, bacterial/endocervical, bacterial/respiratory tract, bacterial/skin, bacterial/systemic, gynecological, intra-abdominal, urinary tract); meningitis; peritonitis; pneumonia, bacterial; septicemia; vaginosis, bacterial Flagyl ER: vaginosis, bacterial
Minocycline	Arestin, Dynacin, Minocin, Solodyn	Arestin: periodontitis Dynacin: acne, anthrax, bartonellosis, brucellosis, chancroid, cholera, conjunctivitis, gonorrhea, infections (bacterial/endocervical, bacterial/rectal, bacterial/respiratory tract, bacterial/skin/systemic, gynecological, urinary tract), listeriosis, meningitis, plague, psittacosis, Rocky Mountain spotted fever, syphilis, trachoma, tularemia, typhus, urethritis, yaws Minocin: acne, actinomycosis, anthrax, bartonellosis, brucellosis, chancroid, cholera, conjunctivitis, fever, gonorrhea, infections (bacterial/endocervical, bacterial/rectal, bacterial/respiratory tract, bacterial/skin, bacterial/systemic, gynecological, urinary tract), listeriosis, meningitis, plague, psittacosis, Rocky Mountain spotted fever, syphilis, trachoma, tularemia, typhus, urethritis, yaws Solodyn: acne
Mirtazapine	**Remeron, RemeronSolTab**	depression, major depressive disorder
Montelukast	**Singulair**	allergy, asthma, rhinitis
Morphine Sulfate ER	Avinza, Kadian, MS Contin, Oramorph SR	pain
Mupirocin	**Bactroban**	impetigo, infections (bacterial/skin)
Nabumetone	Nabumetone (generic)	osteoarthritis, rheumatoid arthritis

Naproxen	Naprosyn, EC-Naprosyn	Naprosyn: ankylosing spondylitis, bursitis, dysmenorrhea, gout, osteoarthritis, pain, rheumatoid arthritis, tendinitis EC-Naprosyn: ankylosing spondylitis, osteoarthritis, rheumatoid arthritis
Nifedipine ER	Adalat CC, Afeditab CR	hypertension
Nitrofurantoin Monohydrate	Macrobid	infections (urinary tract)
Nortriptyline	Pamelor	depression
Nystatin Topical	Nystatin Topical, Nystop	infections (fungal/topical)
Olanzapine	Zyprexa	bipolar disorder, depression, mania, schizophrenia
Omeprazole	Prilosec, Prilosec OTC	Prilosec: erosive esophagitis; GERD; heartburn; *Helicobacter pylori* eradication; hypersecretory conditions; mastocytosis; ulcer, gastrointestinal; Zollinger-Ellison syndrome Prilosec OTC: heartburn
Ondansetron HCl	**Zofran**	chemotherapy adjunct, nausea, radiotherapy adjunct, vomiting
Ondansetron ODT	**Zofran ODT**	chemotherapy adjunct, nausea, vomiting
Oxcarbazepine	Trileptal	seizures
Oxybutynin Chloride	Ditropan, Gelnique	Ditropan: bladder, neurogenic; bladder, overactive; urinary incontinence Gelnique: bladder, overactive; urinary incontinence
Oxycodone	Oxycodone (generic), Oxecta	pain
Oxycodone/Acetaminophen	Endocet, Percocet, Roxicet, Tylox	pain
Pantoprazole	Protonix, Protonix IV	erosive esophagitis, GERD, heartburn, hypersecretory conditions, Zollinger-Ellison syndrome
Paroxetine	Paxil, Paxil CR	Paxil: anxiety, depression, major depressive disorder, obsessive-compulsive disorder, panic disorder, posttraumatic stress disorder Paxil CR: anxiety, depression, major depressive disorder, panic disorder, premenstrual dysphoric disorder
Penicillin VK	Penicillin VK (generic), Veetids	chorea, endocarditis, gingivitis, infections (bacterial/respiratory tract, bacterial/skin, bacterial/systemic), pharyngitis, rheumatic fever
Phenazopyridine HCl	Phenazopyridine (generic)	urinary tract dysuria/pain
Phentermine	**Adipex-P**, Phentermine HCl (generic)	obesity
Phenytoin Sodium ER	Dilantin, Dilantin Kapseals, Phenytek	seizures
Pioglitazone	Actos	diabetes
Polyethylene Glycol	Miralax	constipation
Potassium Chloride	Klor-Con, Klor-Con M, K-Dur, K-Lor, K-Lyte/Cl, K-Lyte/Cl 50, K-Tab, Micro-K	Klor-Co, Klor-Con M, K-Dur, K-Lor, K-Tab, Micro-K: digitalis toxicity, hypokalemia K-Lyte/Cl, K-Lyte/Cl 50: digitalis toxicity, hypochloremia, hypokalemia
Pramipexole Dihydrochloride	Mirapex	Parkinson's disease, restless legs syndrome

Pravastatin Sodium	Pravachol	coronary artery disease; hypercholesterolemia; hyperlipidemia; hypertriglyceridemia; myocardial infarction, reduce risk; revascularization, reduce risk; stroke, reduce risk; TIA, reduce risk
Prednisolone Acetate	Pred Forte, Pred Mild	conjunctivitis; inflammation, ophthalmic
Promethazine DM	Promethazine DM (generic)	allergy; congestion, nasal; cough
Promethazine Tabs	Phenergan, Promethazine HCl (generic)	allergy; anaphylaxis; anxiety; conjunctivitis; motion sickness; nausea; pain; rhinitis; sedation; sedation, preoperative; urticaria; vomiting
Promethazine/Codeine	Promethazine with Codeine (generic)	allergy, cough
Propranolol HCl	Inderal, Innopran XL	Inderal: angina; arrhythmia; hypertension; hypertrophic subaortic stenosis; migraine/tension headache; myocardial infarction, postmanagement; pheochromocytoma; tremor Innopran XL: hypertension
Propranolol HCl ER	Inderal LA	angina, hypertension, hypertrophic subaortic stenosis, migraine/tension headache
Quetiapine	Seroquel	bipolar disorder, schizophrenia
Quinapril	Accupril	heart failure, hypertension
Ramipril	Altace	congestive heart failure; hypertension; myocardial infarction, postmanagement; myocardial infarction, reduce risk; stroke, reduce risk
Ranitidine HCl	**Zantac**, Zantac OTC, Zantac 75, **Zantac 150**	Zantac: erosive esophagitis; GERD; hypersecretory conditions; mastocytosis; ulcer, gastrointestinal; Zollinger-Ellison syndrome Zantac OTC, Zantac 75, Zantac 150: heartburn
Risperidone	Risperdal, Risperdal Consta, Risperdal M-Tab	Risperdal, Risperdal M-Tab: autistic disorder, irritability; bipolar disorder; mania; schizophrenia Risperdal Consta: bipolar disorder, schizophrenia
Ropinirole HCl	**Requip**, **Requip XL**	Requip: Parkinson's disease, restless legs syndrome Requip XL: Parkinson's disease
Sertraline HCl	Zoloft	anxiety, depression, obsessive-compulsive disorder, major depressive disorder, panic disorder, posttraumatic stress disorder, premenstrual dysphoric disorder
Simvastatin	**Zocor**	coronary artery disease; hypercholesterolemia; hyperlipidemia; hypertriglyceridemia; myocardial infarction, reduce risk; revascularization, reduce risk; stroke, reduce risk
Spironolactone	Aldactone	congestive heart failure, edema, hyperaldosteronism, hypertension, hypokalemia
Sucralfate	Carafate	ulcer
Sumatriptan Oral	**Imitrex**	migraine/tension headache
Tamsulosin HCl	Flomax	benign prostatic hypertrophy
Temazepam	Restoril	insomnia
Terazosin	Terazosin HCl (generic)	benign prostatic hypertrophy, hypertension

Terbinafine HCl	Lamisil, Lamisil AT	Lamisil: infections (fungal/topical), onychomycosis Lamisil AT: athlete's foot, infections (fungal/topical)
Timolol Maleate Ophthalmic	Timoptic, Timoptic XE	glaucoma/IOP
Tizanidine HCl	Zanaflex	muscle spasm
Topiramate	Topamax, Topamax Sprinkle Capsules	migraine/tension headache, seizures
Tramadol	Rybix ODT, Ultram, Ultram ER	pain
Tramadol HCl/Acetaminophen	Ultracet	pain
Trazodone HCl	Oleptro, Trazodone (generic)	major depressive disorder
Tretinoin	Atralin, Retin-A, Retin-A micro, Renova, Tretin-X	acne Renova: facial wrinkles
Triamcinolone Acetonide Topical	**Kenalog**	dermatitis; inflammation, topical; pruritus, topical; psoriasis
Triamterene/HCTZ	**Dyazide**, Maxzide, Maxzide-25	edema, hypertension
Trimethoprim/Sulfamethoxazole	Bactrim, Bactrim DS, Septra, Septra DS, Sulfatrim Pediatric	AIDS adjunct, bronchitis, diarrhea, infections (bacterial/respiratory tract, intra-abdominal, otic, urinary tract), otitis media, *Pneumocystis carinii* pneumonia
Valacyclovir HCl	**Valtrex**	AIDS adjunct, chickenpox, herpes, infections (viral/systemic), shingles
Valsartan/HCTZ	**Diovan HCT**	hypertension
Venlafaxine	Effexor	depression, major depressive disorder
Venlafaxine HCl ER	Effexor ER	anxiety, depression, major depressive disorder, panic disorder
Verapamil SR	Calan SR, Covera-HS, Isoptin SR, Verelan, Verelan PM	Calan SR, Isoptin SR, Verelan, Verelan PM: hypertension Covera-HS: angina, hypertension
Warfarin	**Coumadin**, Jantoven	myocardial infarction, postmanagement; myocardial infarction, reduce risk; pulmonary embolism; stroke, reduce risk; thrombosis prevention
Zolpidem Tartrate	Ambien, Ambien CR, Edluar, **Intermezzo**, Zolpimist	insomnia

SECTION 3

PRODUCT CATEGORY INDEX

This index lists products by prescribing category, allowing you to quickly and easily identify all agents with a given therapeutic use or mechanism of action. Categories are based on the latest medical terminology and are comprehensively cross-referenced. Included are all fully described products in the Product Information section of the *PDR*®.

If an entry in the index lists multiple page numbers, the first one shown refers to photographs of the product; the last one to its prescribing information.

PRODUCT CATEGORY INDEX

Key to Controlled Substances Schedule

Products listed with the symbols shown below are subject to the Controlled Substances Act of 1970. These drugs are categorized according to their potential for abuse. The greater the potential, the more severe the limitations on their prescription.

SCHEDULE	INTERPRETATION
C-II	**HIGH POTENTIAL FOR ABUSE.** Use may lead to severe physical or psychological dependence.
C-III	**POTENTIAL FOR ABUSE LESS THAN THE DRUGS OR OTHER SUBSTANCES IN C-II.** Use may lead to low-to-moderate physical dependence or high psychological dependence.
C-IV	**LOW POTENTIAL FOR ABUSE RELATIVE TO DRUGS OR OTHER SUBSTANCES IN C-III.** Use may lead to limited physical or psychological dependence relative to the drugs or other substances in C-III.
C-V	**LOW POTENTIAL FOR ABUSE RELATIVE TO DRUGS OR OTHER SUBSTANCES IN C-IV.** Use may lead to limited physical or psychological dependence relative to the drugs or other substances in C-IV.

Key to FDA Use-in-Pregnancy Ratings

The FDA use-in-pregnancy rating system weighs the degree to which available information has ruled out risk to the fetus against the drug's potential benefit to the patient. The ratings, and their interpretations, are as follows:

SCHEDULE	INTERPRETATION
A	**CONTROLLED STUDIES SHOW NO RISK.** Adequate, well-controlled studies in pregnant women have failed to demonstrate a risk to the fetus in the first trimester of pregnancy (and there is no evidence of a risk in later trimesters).
B	**NO EVIDENCE OF RISK IN HUMANS.** Adequate, well-controlled studies in pregnant women are lacking, and animal studies have not shown increased risk of fetal abnormalities. The chance of fetal harm is remote, but remains a possibility.
C	**RISK CANNOT BE RULED OUT.** Adequate, well-controlled human studies in pregnant women are lacking, and animal studies have shown a risk to the fetus. There is a chance of fetal harm if the drug is administered during pregnancy, but the potential benefits may outweigh the potential risk.
D	**POSITIVE EVIDENCE OF RISK.** Studies in humans, or investigational or postmarketing data, have demonstrated fetal risk. Nevertheless, potential benefits from the use of the drug may outweigh the potential risk. For example, the drug may be acceptable if needed in a life-threatening situation or serious disease for which safer drugs cannot be used or are ineffective.
X	**CONTRAINDICATED IN PREGNANCY.** Studies in animals or humans have demonstrated fetal abnormalities or if there is positive evidence of fetal risk based on adverse reaction reports from investigational or marketing experience, or both, and risk of use clearly outweighs any possible benefit.

U.S. FOOD AND DRUG ADMINISTRATION

Medical Product Reporting Programs

MedWatch (24-hour service) **800-332-1088**
Reporting of problems with drugs, devices, biologics (except vaccines), medical foods, and dietary supplements.

Vaccine Adverse Event Reporting System (24-hour service) **800-822-7967**
Reporting of vaccine-related problems.

Mandatory Medical Device Reporting **800-332-1088**
Reporting required from user facilities regarding device-related deaths and serious injuries.

Veterinary Adverse Drug Reaction Program **888-332-8387**
Reporting of adverse drug events in animals.

Information for Health Professionals

Center for Drug Evaluation and Research Drug Information Hotline **855-543-3784**
Information on human drugs including hormones.

Center for Biologics Office of Communications **800-835-4709**
Information on biological products including vaccines and blood.

Center for Devices and Radiological Health **800-638-2041**
Automated request for information on medical devices and radiation-emitting products.

Office of Prescription Drug Promotion **301-796-1200**
Inquiries from health professionals regarding product promotion.

Emergency Operations **866-300-4374**
Emergencies involving FDA-regulated products, tampering reports, and emergency Investigational New Drug requests.

Office of Orphan Products Development **301-796-8660**
Information on products for rare diseases.

General Information

General Consumer Inquiries **888-463-6332**
Consumer information on regulated products/issues.

Freedom of Information **301-796-8975**
Requests for publicly available FDA documents.

Office of Media Affairs **301 796 4540**
Interviews/press inquiries on FDA activities.

Center for Food Safety and Applied Nutrition **888-723-3366**
Information on food safety, seafood, dietary supplements, women's nutrition, and cosmetics.

Consumer Information Service, Center for Devices and Radiological Health **800-638-2041**
Information on medical devices, mammography facilities, and radiation-emitting products.

POISON ANTIDOTES

Warning: While every effort has been made to ensure the accuracy of this chart, it is not intended to serve as the sole source of information on antidotes. Guidelines may need to be adjusted based on factors such as anticipated usage in the hospital's local area, the nearest alternate sources of antidotes, and distance to tertiary care institutions. Contact your nearest regional poison control center (**1-800-222-1222**) for treatment information regarding any exposure, including indications for use of antidote therapy. Directions in this chart assume that all basic life support and decontamination measures have been initiated as needed.

ANTIDOTE	POISON/DRUG/TOXIN	SUGGESTED MINIMUM STOCK QUANTITY	RATIONALE/COMMENTS
N-Acetylcysteine (NAC) (Mucomyst, Acetadote)	Acetaminophen Carbon tetrachloride Other hepatotoxins	IV: 300mL (60g) Acetadote. PO: 750mL (150mg) of 20% NAC.	Acetaminophen is the most common drug involved in intentional and unintentional poisonings. 750mL (150g) of the oral product provides enough to treat three 100kg adults for 24 hours. Several vials may be stocked in the ED to provide a loading dose and the remaining vials in the pharmacy for the q4h maintenance doses. 300mL (60g) of IV product will treat two 100kg adult patients for the entire 21-hour IV protocol.
Antivenin, *Crotalidae* Polyvalent (Equine origin)	Pit viper envenomation (eg, rattlesnakes, cottonmouths, copperheads)	None.	As of March 31, 2007, this product is no longer available from the manufacturer. However, some supplies may still be available. See **Antivenin, *Crotalidae* Polyvalent Immune Fab – Ovine** in this chart.
Antivenin, *Crotalidae* Polyvalent Immune Fab – Ovine (CroFab)	Pit viper envenomation (eg, rattlesnakes, cottonmouths, copperheads)	12-18 vials.	Advised in geographic areas with endemic populations of copperhead, water moccasin, eastern massasauga, or timber rattlesnakes. In low-risk areas, know nearest alternate source of antivenin. This product has a lower risk of hypersensitivity reaction than previously marketed equine product. 12 vials will cover 8 hours of treatment, while 18 vials will cover 24 hours of treatment. Stock in pharmacy. Store in refrigerator. Equine product was discontinued March 31, 2007 and is no longer available for purchase.
Antivenin, *Latrodectus mactans* (Black widow spider)	Black widow spider envenomation	0 to 1 vial.	This product is only used for severe envenomations. Antivenin must be given in a critical care setting since it is an equine-derived product that may cause anaphylaxis. Stock in pharmacy. Product must be refrigerated at all times. Know the nearest source of antidote.

(Continued)

ANTIDOTE	POISON/DRUG/TOXIN	SUGGESTED MINIMUM STOCK QUANTITY	RATIONALE/COMMENTS
Atropine sulfate	Alpha$_2$ agonists (eg, clonidine, guanabenz, guanfacine) Alzheimer drugs (eg, donepezil, galantamine, rivastigmine, tacrine) Antimyasthenic agents (eg, pyridostigmine) Bradyarrhythmia-producing agents (eg, beta blockers, calcium channel blockers, digitalis glycosides) Cholinergic agonists (eg, bethanechol) Muscarine-containing mushrooms (eg, *Clitocybe*, *Inocybe*) Nerve agents (eg, sarin, soman, tabun, VX) Organophosphate and carbamate insecticides	175mg or greater. Available in various formulations: 0.4mg/mL (1mL, 0.4mg ampules). 0.4mg/mL (20mL, 8mg vials). 0.1mg/mL (10mL, 1mg ampules). Atropine sulfate military-style auto-injectors: (Atropen): 2mg/0.7mL, 1mg/0.7mL, 0.5mg/0.7mL, 0.25mg/0.3mL. (DuoDote): Atropine sulfate 2.1mg/0.7mL with Pralidoxime chloride 600mg/2mL.	The product should be immediately available in the ED. Some also may be stored in the pharmacy or other hospital sites, but should be easily mobilized if a severely poisoned patient needs treatment. Note: Product is necessary to be adequately prepared for WMD incidents; the suggested amount may not be sufficient for mass casualty events. Auto-injectors are available from Bound Tree Medical, Inc (**1-800-533-0523**). Drug stocked in chempack containers is intended only for use in mass casualty events.
Botulinum antitoxin As of March 13, 2010, the only botulinum antitoxin available is HBAT (heptavalent types A-G). This product replaces bivalent antitoxins type AB and antitoxin type E. Baby Botulism Immune Globulin (BIG)	Food-borne botulism Wound botulism Botulism as a biological weapon Note: Heptavalent antitoxin not currently recommended for infant botulism.	None. Product is stored at 9 CDC regional centers (including the Chicago Quarantine). To obtain antitoxin, hospitals must call the Department of Public Health.	Antitoxin must be given in a critical care setting since it is an equine-derived product. Note: Product must be refrigerated at all times. Heptavalent antitoxin is stored in the CDC SNS. BabyBIG is available for infant botulism types A and B, through the Infant Botulism Treatment and Prevention Program, sponsored by the California Department of Public Health, available by telephone at **510-231-7600** or online at **www.infantbotulism.org/physician/obtain.php**.
Calcium disodium EDTA (Versenate)	Lead Zinc salts (eg, zinc chloride)	Two 5mL ampules (200mg/mL).	One ampule provides 1 day of therapy for a child. 2 to 4g per 24 hours may be necessary in adult patients. Stock in pharmacy. Important note: Edetate disodium (Endrate) is not the same as calcium disodium EDTA, and is used primarily as an IV chelator for emergent treatment of hypercalcemia.

ANTIDOTE	POISON/DRUG/TOXIN	SUGGESTED MINIMUM STOCK QUANTITY	RATIONALE/COMMENTS
Calcium chloride and Calcium gluconate	Fluoride salts (eg, NaF) Hydrofluoric acid (HF) Hyperkalemia (not digoxin-induced) Hypermagnesemia	10% calcium chloride: ten 10mL vials. 10% calcium gluconate: thirty 10mL vials.	Many ampules of calcium chloride may be necessary in life-threatening HF poisoning. Stock in ED. More may be stocked in pharmacy. The chloride salt provides 3 times more calcium than the gluconate salt. Calcium chloride is very irritating and administration through a central line is preferable. Topical calcium gluconate or carbonate gels may be extemporaneously prepared by the pharmacy. Calgonate (calcium gluconate 2.5% gel) is not FDA approved but is manufactured in an FDA-GMP approved facility and is distributed by Calgonate Corp in Port St. Lucie, Florida.
Centruroides Immune $F(ab)_2$ – Equine (Anascorp)	Scorpion envenomation	None.	This product is manufactured in Mexico by the Instituto Bioclon. In the U.S., it is marketed by Rare Disease Therapeutics, Inc. in Nashville, Tennessee. It was approved by the FDA in 2011 and can be stored at room temperature. Usual dose: 1 to 3 vials.
Cyanide Antidote: Sodium nitrite and sodium thiosulfate (Nithiodote)	Acetonitrile Acrylonitrile Bromates (thiosulfate only) Chlorates (thiosulfate only) Cyanide (eg, HCN, KCN, NaCN) Cyanogen chloride Cyanogenic glycoside natural sources (eg, apricot pits, peach pits) Hydrogen sulfide (nitrites only) Laetrile Mustard agents (thiosulfate only) Nitroprusside (thiosulfate only) Smoke inhalation (combustion of synthetic materials)	2 to 4 kits. Each kit contains: 1 vial (10mL) sodium nitrite (300mg). 1 vial (50mL) sodium thiosulfate (12.5g).	Stock 2 kits in the ED. Consider also stocking 2 kits in the pharmacy. Note: This kit has a short shelf-life of 24 months. Stocking this kit may be unnecessary if an adequate supply of hydroxocobalamin HCl is available. Significant adverse reactions include methemoglobinemia and hypotension. For smoke inhalation victims, thiosulfate, without the use of nitrites, may be considered. Note: In 2012, the CN kit containing 12 amyl nitrite pearls, two 10mL sodium nitrite vials, and two 50mL sodium thiosulfate vials was discontinued by the manufacturer and is no longer available in the U.S. Amyl nitrite ampules may be ordered separately.
Deferoxamine mesylate (Desferal)	Iron Deferoxamine has also been used for chronic aluminum toxicity in chronic kidney disease patients	12 to 36g (Available in 500mg and 2g vials).	Quantity recommended supplies 8 to 24 hours of therapy for a 100kg adult. Per package insert, the maximum daily dose is 6g (12 vials). However, this dose may be exceeded in serious acute iron poisonings. Stock in pharmacy.

(Continued)

ANTIDOTE	POISON/DRUG/TOXIN	SUGGESTED MINIMUM STOCK QUANTITY	RATIONALE/COMMENTS
Digoxin immune Fab (Digibind, DigiFab)	Cardiac glycoside-containing plants (eg, foxglove, oleander) Digitoxin Digoxin	15 vials. Each vial (38mg) neutralizes 0.5mg of digoxin.	An initial dose of 2 to 3 vials for chronic poisoning or 10 vials for acute poisoning may be given to a digoxin-poisoned patient in whom the digoxin level is unknown. More may be necessary in severe intoxications. 15 vials would effectively neutralize a steady-state digoxin level of 15ng/mL in a 100kg patient. Know nearest source of additional supply. Stock in ED or pharmacy.
Dimercaprol (BAL in oil)	Arsenic Copper Gold Lead Lewisite Mercury	Four 3mL ampules (100mg/mL).	This amount provides 3 doses of 3 to 5mg/kg/dose given q4h to treat 1 seriously poisoned adult (up to 100kg) or provides enough to treat a 15kg child for more than 24 hours. Stock in pharmacy.
DMPS (2,3-dimercaptopropanol-sulfonic acid) (Dimaval, Unithiol)	Arsenic Bismuth Lead Mercury	None. Available as 50mg/mL vials from McGuff Pharmacy.	DMPS is a water soluble analog of BAL. Unlike BAL, it does not have a potential risk of redistributing metals to the CNS. Also has a more favorable side effect profile, though further study is needed to fully elucidate advantages/disadvantages compared to other chelators.
Ethanol	Ethylene glycol Methanol	Consider stocking 180 to 360g in the form of 95% ethanol or equivalents. 10% alcohol in D5W was discontinued in 2004; 5% alcohol in D5W was discontinued in 2007. However, 10% alcohol can be prepared from dehydrated alcohol and D5W. Consult PCC.	180g provides loading and maintenance doses for a 100kg adult for 8 to 24 hours. More alcohol or fomepizole will be needed during dialysis or prolonged treatment. 95% or 40% alcohol diluted in juice may be given PO if IV alcohol is unavailable. Stock in pharmacy. Note: Ethanol is unnecessary if adequate amounts of fomepizole are stocked. See also fomepizole in this chart. Ethanol may cause hypotension or metabolic abnormalities (eg, hypoglycemia) especially in pediatric patients. Since ethanol treatment for toxic alcohol poisoning is not FDA approved and fomepizole offers greater efficacy and safety, fomepizole is the preferred alcohol dehydrogenase inhibitor.
Fat emulsion (Intralipid, Liposyn II, Liposyn III)	Local anesthetics and possibly other cardiac toxins (eg, bupropion, calcium channel blockers, cocaine, beta blockers, tricyclic antidepressants)	Quantity determined by institution. Available in 100mL of 20% emulsion.	Fat emulsion is an experimental therapy showing promise in the reverse of cardiac toxicity induced by local anesthetics and other cardiac toxins. The evidence for the efficacy of fat emulsion therapy is based on animal studies and human case reports, and its safety has not yet been established. Consultation with a regional PCC toxicologist is advised. Initial dose: 1.5mL/kg IV over 1 minute. Follow with infusion of 0.25mL/kg/min over 30 minutes. Loading dose may be repeated once. Rate may be increased to 0.5mL/kg/min for 60 minutes if blood pressure drops. Maximum total dose is 8mL/kg. Consider storage in pharmacy, ED, and possibly surgical units.

ANTIDOTE	POISON/DRUG/TOXIN	SUGGESTED MINIMUM STOCK QUANTITY	RATIONALE/COMMENTS
Flumazenil (Romazicon)	Benzodiazepines	Total 6 to 12mg. Available in 5 and 10mL vials (0.1mg/mL).	Due to risk of seizures, use with extreme caution, if at all, in poisoned patients. More may be stocked in the pharmacy for use in reversal of conscious sedation. Stock in ED, pharmacy, and any unit where procedural sedation is performed.
Folic acid and Folinic acid (Leucovorin)	Formaldehyde/Formic acid Methanol Methotrexate, trimetrexate Pyrimethamine Trimethoprim	Folic acid: three 50mg vials. Folinic acid: one 50mg vial.	For adjunctive treatment of methanol-poisoned patients with an acidosis, give 50mg folinic acid initially, then 50mg of folic acid q4h for 6 doses. For methotrexate-poisoned patients, administer folinic acid only. Stock in pharmacy.
Fomepizole (4-methylpyrazole [4-MP]) (Antizol)	Ethylene glycol Methanol	One to two 1.5g vials. Note: Available in a kit of four 1.5g vials.	One 1.5g vial provides an initial dose of 15mg/kg/12 hours to an adult weighing up to 100kg. Hospitals with critical care and hemodialysis capabilities should consider stocking one kit of 4 vials or more. More frequent dosing (ie, every 4 hours) is required if the patient is dialyzed. Ethanol is unnecessary if adequate supply of fomepizole is stocked. Fomepizole is preferred to ethanol because of ease of use, fewer adverse effects, simplicity of dosing, and less need for close monitoring. Stock in pharmacy. Know where nearest alternate supply is located.
Glucagon HCl	Beta blockers Calcium channel blockers (CCB) Hypoglycemia Hypoglycemic agents	Fifty to ninety 1mg vials.	This quantity provides 4 to 8 hours of maximum dosing, ie, a 10mg IV bolus dose followed by 10mg/h. More may be necessary. Know where nearest alternate supply is located. Stock 30mg in ED and remainder in pharmacy. Note: Insulin/dextrose is more efficacious than glucagon in the setting of severe CCB overdose.
Hydroxocobalamin HCl (Cyanokit)	Acetonitrile Acrylonitrile Cyanide (eg, HCN, KCN, NaCN) Cyanogen chloride Cyanogenic glycoside natural sources (eg, apricot pits, peach pits) Laetrile Nitroprusside Smoke inhalation (combustion of synthetic materials)	Two to four kits. Each kit contains one 5g vial. Note: Diluent is not included in the kit.	Seriously poisoned cyanide patients may require 5 to 10g (1 to 2 kits). Stock two kits in ED. Consider also stocking two kits in the pharmacy. The product has a shelf-life of 30 months post-manufacture.
Hyperbaric oxygen (HBO)	Carbon monoxide and possibly the following: Carbon tetrachloride Cyanide Hydrogen sulfide Methemoglobinemia	Post the location and phone number of nearest HBO chamber in the ED.	Consult PCC to determine if HBO treatment is indicated.

(Continued)

ANTIDOTE	POISON/DRUG/TOXIN	SUGGESTED MINIMUM STOCK QUANTITY	RATIONALE/COMMENTS
Insulin and dextrose	Calcium channel blockers (diltiazem, nifedipine, verapamil)	Quantity determined by institution. Humulin R is available as 100 units/mL in a 1.5mL cartridge and 10mL bottle. Dextrose 50% in water is available in 50mL ampules and syringes. Dextrose 25% is available in 10mL vials and syringes for pediatric use.	High dose insulin and dextrose therapy can reverse cardiovascular toxicity associated with calcium channel blocker overdose. IV Bolus: Recommended starting dose of 1 unit/kg regular insulin (with 1 amp D50). The lowest maintenance dose is 0.5-1 units/kg/hr. Higher doses may be considered under consultation with medical toxicologist. Stock in ED and pharmacy.
Methylene blue	Methemoglobin-inducing agents including: Aniline dyes Dapsone Dinitrophenol Local anesthetics (eg, benzocaine) Metoclopramide Monomethylhydrazine-containing mushrooms (eg, *Gyromitra*) Naphthalene Nitrates and nitrites Nitrobenzene Phenazopyridine	Six 10mL ampules (10mg/mL).	The usual dose is 1 to 2mg/kg IV (0.1 to 0.2mL/kg). A second dose may be given in 1 hour. More may be necessary. 6 ampules provide 3 doses of 2mg/kg for a 100kg adult. Stock in pharmacy.
Naloxone (Narcan)	$Alpha_2$ agonists (eg, clonidine, guanabenz, guanfacine) Unknown poisoning with mental status depression Opioids (eg, codeine, diphenoxylate, fentanyl, heroin, meperidine, morphine, propoxyphene)	Naloxone: total 40mg, any combination of 0.4mg, 1mg, and 2mg ampules.	Stock 20mg naloxone in the ED and 20mg elsewhere in the institution.
Octreotide acetate (Sandostatin)	Sulfonylurea hypoglycemic agents (eg, glipizide, glyburide)	225mcg. Available in 1mL ampules (0.05mg/mL, 0.1mg/mL, and 0.5mg/mL) and 5mL multidose vials (0.2 and 1mg/mL).	Octreotide acetate blocks the release of insulin from pancreatic beta cells that along with IV dextrose can reverse sulfonylurea-induced hypoglycemia. The usual adult dose is 50 to 100mcg IV or SC q6-12h. The usual pediatric dose is 1 to 1.5mcg/kg IV or SC q6-12h. 225mcg provides four 75mcg adult doses. Stock in pharmacy.
D-Penicillamine (Cuprimine)	Arsenic Copper Lead Mercury	None required as an antidote. Available in bottles of 100 capsules (125mg or 250mg/capsule).	D-Penicillamine is no longer considered the drug of choice for heavy metal poisonings. It may be stocked in the pharmacy for other indications such as Wilson's disease or rheumatoid arthritis.

ANTIDOTE	POISON/DRUG/TOXIN	SUGGESTED MINIMUM STOCK QUANTITY	RATIONALE/COMMENTS
Physostigmine salicylate (Antilirium)	Anticholinergic alkaloid-containing plants (eg, deadly nightshade, jimson weed) Antihistamines Atropine and other anticholinergic agents	Two 2mL ampules (1mg/mL).	Usual adult dose is 1 to 2mg slow IV push. Note: Duration of effect is 30 to 60 min. Stock in ED or pharmacy.
Phytonadione (Vitamin K_1) (Aquamephyton, Mephyton)	Indandione derivatives Long-acting anticoagulant rodenticides (eg, brodifacoum, bromadiolone) Warfarin	100mg injectable; 100mg oral. Available as: 0.5mL ampules (2mg/mL) and 1mL ampules (10mg/mL). 5mg tablets in packages of 10, 12, and 100.	Patients who are poisoned by long-acting anticoagulant rodenticides may require 50 to 100mg/day or more for weeks to months to maintain normal INRs. An oral suspension for pediatric patients may be extemporaneously prepared by the pharmacy. Stock in pharmacy.
Pralidoxime chloride (2-PAM) (Protopam)	Organophosphate insecticides (OPI) Nerve agents (eg, sarin, soman, tabun, VX) And possibly: Antimyasthenic agents (eg, pyridostigmine) Tacrine	Eighteen 1g vials. Also available as: Pralidoxime chloride military-style auto-injectors: 600mg/2mL. (DuoDote) Atropine sulfate 2.1mg/0.7mL with Pralidoxime chloride 600mg/2mL.	18g provides an adult dose of 750mg/h for 24 hours. More may be needed in severe poisoning. Healthcare facilities located in agricultural areas where OPIs are used should maintain adequate supplies. Product is necessary to be adequately prepared for WMD incidents; the suggested amount may not be sufficient for mass casualty events. Auto-injectors are available from Bound Tree Medical, Inc (**1-800-533-0523**). The drugs stocked in chempack containers are intended for use in mass casualty events only. Stock in ED or pharmacy.
Protamine sulfate	Heparin Low molecular weight heparins (eg, enoxaparin, dalteparin, tinzaparin)	Variable; consider recommendation of hospital Pharmacy & Therapeutics Committee. Available as 5mL ampules (10mg/mL) and 25mL vials (250mg/25mL).	The usual dose is 1 to 1.5mg for each 100 units of heparin. Stock in pharmacy in refrigerator. Preservative-free formulation does not require refrigeration.
Pyridoxine hydrochloride (Vitamin B_6)	Acrylamide Ethylene glycol Hydrazine Hydrazine MAOIs (isocarboxazid, phenelzine) Isoniazid (INH) Monomethylhydrazine-containing mushrooms (eg, *Gyromitra*)	10g (100 vials). Available as 1mL vials (100mg/mL).	Usual dose is 1g pyridoxine HCl for each g of INH ingested. If amount ingested is unknown, give 5g of pyridoxine. Repeat 5g dose if seizures are uncontrolled. More may be necessary. Know nearest source of additional supply. For ethylene glycol, a dose of 100mg/day may enhance the clearance of toxic metabolite. Stock in ED or pharmacy.

(Continued)

ANTIDOTE	POISON/DRUG/TOXIN	SUGGESTED MINIMUM STOCK QUANTITY	RATIONALE/COMMENTS
Silibinin (Legalon-SIL)	Cyclopeptide-containing mushrooms (eg, *Amanita phalloides*, *Amanita verna*, *Amanita virosa*, *Galerina autumnalis*, *Lepiota josserandi*, and others)	None. 350mg/vial.	Silibinin is a water-soluble preparation of silymarin; a flavolignone extracted from the milk thistle plant. It inhibits uptake of cyclopeptides in hepatocytes. These hepatotoxins are responsible for high morbidity and mortality following ingestion of these mushrooms. Silibinin is manufactured by Madaus, Inc. in Germany, and has been widely used in Europe since 1984. The initial adult loading dose consists of a 1-hour infusion of 5mg/kg followed by the recommended daily dosage of 20mg/kg via continuous IV infusion. Product is now available in the U.S. under an open-treatment investigational new drug. Physicians can obtain the product free-of-charge by contacting the primary investigator at **866-520-4412**.
Sodium bicarbonate	Chlorine gas Hyperkalemia Serum Alkalinization: Agents producing a quinidine-like effect as noted by widened QRS complex on EKG (eg, amantadine, carbamazepine, chloroquine, cocaine, diphenhydramine, flecainide, propafenone, propoxyphene, tricyclic antidepressants, quinidine, and related agents) Urine Alkalinization: Weakly acidic agents (eg, chlorophenoxy herbicides, chlorpropamide, methotrexate, phenobarbital, salicylates)	Twenty to twenty-five 50mL vials of either 8.4% (50mEq/50mL) or 7.5% (44mEq/50mL). Consider stocking 4.2% (5mEq/10mL) for pediatric patients.	Stock twenty vials in ED and remainder in pharmacy. Nebulized 2.5-5% sodium bicarbonate has been demonstrated in anecdotal case reports to provide symptomatic relief for chlorine gas inhalation.
Succimer (dimercaptosuccinic acid [DMSA]) (Chemet)	Arsenic Lead Lewisite Mercury	0 to 10 capsules. Available in bottles of 100 capsules (100mg/capsule).	Initial treatment of severely symptomatic heavy metal poisoning consists of parenterally administered chelators, eg, BAL, Ca Na_2, EDTA. Patients who markedly improve may eventually be started on oral DMSA. Asymptomatic or minimally symptomatic patients do not require parenteral therapy and are often treated as outpatients with an oral chelator. FDA approved only for pediatric lead poisoning, however it has shown efficacy for other heavy metal poisonings. 10 capsules represent an initial dose of 10mg/kg in a 100kg adult. Stock in pharmacy.

ADJUNCTIVE AGENTS

ADJUNCTIVE AGENT	POISON/DRUG/TOXIN	SUGGESTED MINIMUM STOCK QUANTITY	RATIONALE/COMMENTS
Benztropine mesylate (Cogentin)	Medications causing a dystonic reaction or other extrapyramidal symptoms	Quantity determined by institution. Available in tablets of 0.5mg, 1mg, 2mg (bottles of 100 or 1000) and in 2mg/mL injectable ampules.	Maximum daily adult dose is 6mg/d. Stock some in ED and some in pharmacy. See also **Diphenhydramine** in this chart.
L-Carnitine (Carnitor)	Valproic acid	Quantity determined by institution. Available as 330mg and 500mg tablets, 250mg and 300mg capsules, 200mg/mL IV solution, and 100mg/mL PO solution.	L-Carnitine may be considered in valproate intoxication associated with elevated serum ammonia levels and/or hepatotoxicity. Doses of 100mg/kg/d up to 2 grams a day PO divided into 3 doses, or 150-500mg/kg/d IV (maximum 3 grams daily) in 3 or 4 divided doses are recommended for a period of 3 to 4 days or until clinical improvement. Stock in pharmacy.
Cyproheptadine HCl (Periactin)	Medications causing serotonin syndrome	Quantity determined by institution. Available in 4mg tablets (bottles of 100, 250, 500, and 1000) and 2mg/5mL PO solution.	Cyproheptadine HCl is a nonspecific 5-HT antagonist that has been used in the treatment of serotonin syndrome. Adult dose is 12mg PO initially, followed by 2mg every 2 hours if symptoms persist. Maintenance dose is 8mg every 6 hours. Maximum of 32mg/day. Pediatric dose is 0.25mg/kg/day divided every 6 hours, with a max dose of 12mg/day. Stock in pharmacy.
Dantrolene sodium (Dantrium)	Medications causing NMS Medications causing malignant hyperthermia	Quantity determined by institution. Available in 25, 50, and 100mg capsules (bottles of 100 or 500) and injectable 20mg/vial form.	The recommended dose for NMS is 1mg/kg IV; may repeat as needed every 5 to 10 minutes for a maximum of 10mg/kg. Dantrolene sodium inhibits calcium release from the sarcoplasmic reticulum of skeletal muscle and thereby reduces rigidity. Stock in pharmacy. Any hospital using inhalational anesthetics should strongly consider stocking dantrolene for treatment of malignant hyperthermia.

(Continued)

ADJUNCTIVE AGENT	POISON/DRUG/TOXIN	SUGGESTED MINIMUM STOCK QUANTITY	RATIONALE/COMMENTS
Diazepam (Valium)	Chloroquine and related antimalarial drugs NMS Serotonin syndrome Severe agitation from any toxic exposure/overdose (eg, cocaine, PCP, methamphetamine)	Quantity determined by institution. Available as 5mg/mL injectables in 2mL ampules, 2mL disposable syringes, and 10mL multidose vials. Diazepam military-style auto-injectors for nerve agent-induced seizures: 10mg/2mL.	Diazepam is used in conjunction with epinephrine for patients with chloroquine toxicity (seizures, dysrhythmias, hypotension) or if the amount ingested is more than 5g. Intravenous loading dose 2mg/kg over 30 minutes. Maintenance dose of 1 to 2mg/kg per day for 2 to 4 days. Diazepam and other benzodiazepines are also used in poisoned and nonpoisoned patients as an anticonvulsant, muscle relaxant, and antianxiety agent. They are usually the first-line therapy for drug-induced agitation, tachycardia, and hypertension. Benzodiazepines are a mainstay in the treatment of NMS and serotonin syndrome. Stock in ED and pharmacy. Adequate supply is necessary to be prepared for WMD incidents. Auto-injectors are available from Bound Tree Medical, Inc (**1-800-533-0523**).
Diphenhydramine HCl (Benadryl)	Medications causing a dystonic reaction or other extrapyramidal symptoms	Quantity determined by institution. Available in 25 and 50mg capsules (bottles of 30, 100, or 1000). Also in oral liquid formulation of 12.5mg/5mL (4-ounce bottle) and 50mg/mL injectable syringes.	In addition to its use as an anticholinergic agent, diphenhydramine is a widely used antihistamine in the management of minor or severe allergic reactions. Stock in ED and pharmacy.
Glycopyrrolate Bromide (Robinul)	OPIs Nerve agents	Quantity determined by institution. Available as 0.2mg/mL in vials of 1mL, 2mL, 5mL, and 20mL.	The dose of glycopyrrolate for OPI poisoning is 0.01 to 0.02mg/kg IV. Glycopyrrolate is a quaternary ammonium antimuscarinic agent that may assist in the control of hypersecretions caused by acetylcholinesterase inhibition. This agent produces less tachycardia and CNS effects than atropine. Stock in ED and pharmacy.
Phentolamine mesylate (Regitine)	Catecholamine extravasation Intradigital epinephrine injection	Quantity determined by institution. Available as a 5mg/vial powder with 1mL diluent.	Phentolamine is an alpha adrenergic antagonist that will reverse vasoconstriction and peripheral ischemia associated with extravasation of adrenergic agents. When phentolamine is not available, consider using subcutaneous terbutaline sulfate (Brethine). Phentolamine also offers an additional option in the management of drug-induced hypertension. Stock in ED and pharmacy.

ADJUNCTIVE AGENT	POISON/DRUG/TOXIN	SUGGESTED MINIMUM STOCK QUANTITY	RATIONALE/COMMENTS
Sodium nitrite	Hydrogen sulfide (H_2S)	0 to 1 vial. Available as 3% sodium nitrite in 10mL vial.	Nitrite therapy for H_2S poisoning is controversial. Seriously poisoned patients should receive nitrites within 1 hour of exposure. Sodium thiosulfate is not administered in H_2S poisoning. The product is available from Hope Pharmaceuticals in Scottsdale, Arizona. If the amyl nitrite/sodium nitrite/sodium thiosulfate CN antidote kits are stocked, additional sodium nitrite vials may not be necessary. Stock in pharmacy.
Sodium thiosulfate	Bromates Chlorates Mustard agents Nitroprusside Smoke inhalation	Quantity determined by institution. Available in 100mg/mL, 10mL vials and 250mg/mL, 50mL vials.	Sodium thiosulfate (without nitrites) has been advocated in the treatment of smoke inhalation related to CN exposure; however, it would not be necessary if hydroxocobalamin is available. Sodium thiosulfate may be used in conjunction with cisplatin to reduce toxicity of this chemotherapy agent. Sodium thiosulfate is found in the amyl nitrite/sodium nitrite/sodium thiosulfate CN antidote kits; however, additional vials may be stocked. Stock in pharmacy.
Thiamine	Ethanol Ethylene glycol	Quantity determined by institution. Available as 100mg/mL in 2mL vials.	Parenteral thiamine precedes IV dextrose in patients with chronic ethanol abuse. Thiamine 100mg every 6 hours enhances clearance of toxic metabolites of ethylene glycol. Stock in ED and pharmacy.

AGENTS FOR RADIOLOGICAL EXPOSURES

AGENT FOR RADIOLOGICAL EXPOSURES	POISON/DRUG/TOXIN	SUGGESTED MINIMUM STOCK QUANTITY	RATIONALE/COMMENTS
Calcium-diethylenetriamine pentaacetic acid (Ca-DTPA; Pentetate calcium trisodium injection) Zinc-diethylenetriamine pentaacetic acid (Zn-DTPA; Pentetate zinc trisodium injection)	Internal contamination with transuranium elements: americium, curium, plutonium	Quantity determined by institution. Supplied as 200mg/mL, 5mL ampules for IV or inhalation administration. The product is sponsored through Hameln Pharmaceuticals, GmbH, of Hameln, Germany. Distributed in the U.S. by Akorn, Inc.	1 ampule provides the usual adult dose of 1g q24h. More would be necessary in a mass casualty event. Ca-DTPA and Zn-DTPA are available through the SNS and REAC/TS, Oak Ridge, Tennessee at **865-576-3131** (business hours) or **865-576-1005** (after hours).
Potassium Iodide, KI tablets (Iostat, Thyrosafe) KI liquid (Thyroshield, SSKI)	Prevents thyroid uptake of radioactive iodine (I-131)	Quantity determined by institution. Available in 130mg and 65mg tablets, and PO solutions: 65mg/mL (30mL bottle) and 1g/mL (30mL and 240mL bottle).	One 130mg tablet represents the initial daily adult dose. More would be necessary in a mass casualty event. KI tablets and oral solution are OTC.

(Continued)

AGENT FOR RADIOLOGICAL EXPOSURES	POISON/DRUG/TOXIN	SUGGESTED MINIMUM STOCK QUANTITY	RATIONALE/COMMENTS
Prussian blue, ferric hexacyanoferrate (Radiogardase)	Radioactive cesium (Cs-137), radioactive thallium (Tl-201), and non-radioactive thallium	None recommended at the present time. Available in bottles of 30 capsules (500mg/capsule).	The usual oral adult dose is 3g, 3 times a day. The product is manufactured by Haupt Pharma Berlin GmbH for distribution by HEYL Chemisch-pharmazeutische Fabrik GmbH & Co. KG, Berlin, Germany, and is available in the U.S. from Heyltex Corporation. Prussian blue is also available through the SNS and REAC/TS, Oak Ridge, Tennessee at **865-576-3131** (business hours) or **865-576-1005** (after hours).

Abbreviations: BAL = British anti-Lewisite; CDC = Centers for Disease Control and Prevention; ED = emergency department; EDTA = ethylenediaminetetraacetic acid; PCC = poison control center; SNS = Strategic National Stockpile; REAC/TS = radiation emergency assistance center/training site; WMD = weapons of mass destruction.

Note: The suggested antidote stocking levels in this chart were developed from a published consensus guideline panel and consultation with the clinical staff of the Illinois Poison Center. They were designed for guidance for Illinois Hospitals with EDs. Requirements and special circumstances in other areas of the U.S. may justify different stocking quantities (eg, antivenoms for snakes, scorpions, spiders, etc).

DRUGS EXCRETED IN BREAST MILK

The following list is not comprehensive; generic forms and alternate brands of some products may be available. When recommending drugs to pregnant or nursing patients, always check labeling for specific precautions.

Abstral
Accolate
Accupril
Accuretic
Acetaminophen/Codeine
Aclovate
Actiq
Activella
Acyclovir
Adalat CC
Adderall XR
Advicor
Aggrenox
Aldactazide
Aldactone
Allegra-D
Aloprim
Alora
Altace
Ambien
Ambien CR
Amcinonide
Amiloride/HCTZ
Amitriptyline
Amoxapine
Amoxicillin
Ampicillin
Amturnide
Anafranil
Analpram-HC
Angeliq
Ansaid
Anusol-HC Cream
Aplenzin
Apriso
Armour Thyroid
Arthrotec
Asacol
Astramorph PF
Atacand HCT
ATryn
Atuss DS
Augmentin
Augmentin ES-600
Augmentin XR
Avalide
AVC
Avelox
Aviane
Avinza
Aygestin
Azactam
Azasan
Azulfidine
Azulfidine EN
Bactrim
Banzel
Benicar HCT
Bentyl
BenzaClin
Benzamycin
Betamethasone Dipropionate
Betamethasone Valerate
Betapace
Betapace AF
Beyaz
Bicillin C-R
Bicillin L-A
Biltricide
Buprenex
Butisol
Butorphanol
Butrans
Calan
Calan SR
Capex
Carbatrol
Cardene IV
Cardizem
Cardizem CD
Catapres
Cayston
Cefaclor ER
Cefazolin
Cefotetan
Cefoxitin
Cefpodoxime
Cefprozil
Ceftin
Ceftriaxone
Celebrex
Celestone
Celexa
Cenestin
Cephadyn
Cephalexin
Ceredase
Chloral Hydrate
Chlorothiazide
Chlorpromazine
Chlorthalidone
Cipro
Cipro XR
Cisplatin
Claforan
Clarinex
Clarinex-D
Clenia
Cleocin
Cleocin T
Climara
Climara Pro
Clindagel
Clindamax
Clobex
Cloderm
Co-Gesic
Colcrys
CombiPatch
Combivir
Compro
Cordarone
Cordran
Corgard
Cortifoam
Cortisporin
Corzide
Cosopt
Covera-HS
Crinone
Cutivate
Cyclessa
Cyklokapron
Cymbalta
Cytomel
Cytotec
Dantrium IV
Dapsone
Daraprim
Delestrogen
Demeclocycline HCl
Demerol
Depacon
Depakote
Depakote ER
DepoDur
Depo-Estradiol
Depo-Provera
depo-subQ provera 104
Derma-Smoothe/FS
Dermatop
DermOtic Oil
Desonate
Dexamethasone
Dexedrine Spansules
Dexferrum
Dextroamphetamine Sulfate
Diabinese
Diclegis
Dicloxacillin
Didrex
Diethylpropion
Diflorasone
Diflucan
Diflunisal
Dilacor XR
Dilantin
Dilaudid
Diltiazem
Diovan HCT
Dipentum
Diprivan
Diprolene
Dipyridamole
Divigel
Dolophine
Doral
Doryx
Doxorubicin HCl

(Continued)

Droxia
Duac
Duexis
Duragesic
Duramorph
Dyazide
Dynacin
E.E.S.
Edarbyclor
Effexor XR
Elestrin
Elixophyllin
Elocon
Embeda
EMLA
Enalapril/HCTZ
Enalaprilat
Endometrin
Enjuvia
Epifoam
Epivir
Epivir-HBV
Epzicom
Equetro
Ergomar
ERYC
EryPed
Ery-Tab
Erythrocin
Erythrocin Lactobionate
Erythromycin
Erythromycin Ethylsuccinate and Sulfisoxazole Acetyl
Esgic
Esgic-Plus
Estrace
Estraderm
Estradiol
Estrasorb
Estring
EstroGel
Estropipate
Estrostep Fe
Evamist
Evoclin
Exalgo
Exforge HCT
Exparel
Famotidine
Felbatol
Feldene
femhrt
Femring
Femtrace
Fentora
Fioricet
Fioricet w/Codeine
Fiorinal
Fiorinal w/Codeine
Flagyl
Flagyl ER
Flagyl IV
Fleet Enema
Flo-Pred
Fludrocortisone
Fluocinolone Acetonide
Fluocinonide
Fluorescite
Fluoxetine
Fluvoxamine
Folic Acid
Forfivo XL
Fortaz
Fosamax Plus D
Fosinopril/HCTZ
Fragmin
Furosemide
Gablofen
Gadavist
Gengraf Capsules
Gleevec
Glyset
Gralise
Guanidine HCl
Haldol Decanoate
Halog
Haloperidol
Helidac
Hydrea
Hydrochlorothiazide
Hyzaar
Ifex
Imitrex
Implanon
Imuran
Inderal LA
Indomethacin
INFeD
Infumorph
InnoPran XL
Intermezzo
Invanz
Invega
Invega Sustenna
Isoniazid
Isoptin SR
Jenloga
Jentadueto
Kadian
Kapvay ER
Kenalog
Keppra
Keppra XR
Ketoconazole
Ketorolac
Korlym
Labetalol
Lamictal
Lamictal XR
Lamisil
Lanoxin
Lazanda
Levaquin
Levbid
Levoxyl
Levsin
Lexapro
Lialda
Lidocaine Cream
Lidoderm Patch
Lindane
Lioresal
Lipitor
Lithium
Lithium ER
Lo Loestrin Fe
Lo/Ovral
Locoid
Loestrin 21
Loestrin 24 Fe
Loestrin Fe
Lopressor
Lorcet
Lortab
Loseasonique
Lotensin
Lotensin HCT
Lotrel
Lusedra
Luvox CR
Luxiq
Lysteda
Magnevist
Makena
Maprotiline
Marcaine
Marcaine Spinal
Marinol
Maxipime
Maxitrol Ointment
Maxzide
MDP-25
Meclofenamate
Mefloquine
Menest
Menostar
Meperidine
Meprobamate
Meruvax II
Methadone
Methadose
Methotrexate
Methyclothiazide
Methyldopa
Methyldopa/HCTZ
Methyldopate
Metoclopramide
Metoprolol/HCTZ
Metozolv ODT
MetroGel-Vaginal
Mexiletine
Micardis HCT
Microzide
Midazolam
Minipress
Minoxidil
Mircette
Mirena
M-M-R II
Modicon
Monodox
Monopril
Morphine
Moxeza
MS Contin
Myambutol
Myochrysine
Mysoline
Nafcillin Sodium
Nalbuphine
Naprelan
Naprosyn
Natazia
Nature-Throid
Necon 10/11
Nembutal Sodium Solution
Neomycin/Polymyxin B/ Dexamethasone

Neoral
Neurontin
Nexiclon XR
Nexplanon
Nexterone
Niaspan
Nicotrol Nasal Spray
Niravam
Nizatidine
Norco
Nordette-28
Norinyl 1/50
Noritate
Nor-QD
Novacort
Novantrone
NuvaRing
Ofirmev
Ofloxacin
Olux-E
Onfi
Onsolis
Oracea
Orapred
Oraqix
Ortho Evra
Ortho Micronor
Ortho Tri-Cyclen
Ortho Tri-Cyclen Lo
Ortho-Cept
Ortho-Cyclen
Ortho-Novum 1/35
Ortho-Novum 7/7/7
Ovcon-35
Oxecta
Oxistat
Oxycodone IR
OxyContin
Pandel
Paxil
Paxil CR
PCE
Pediapred
Peganone
Penicillin G Potassium
Penicillin G Procaine
Pentasa
Percocet
Percodan
Periostat
Persantine
Pexeva
Pfizerpen
Phenobarbital
Phoslyra
Phrenilin Forte
Plexion
Poly-Pred
Ponstel
Pramosone
Pravachol
Prefest
Premarin
Premphase
Prevpac
Prilosec
Primsol
Prinzide
Pristiq
Proctocort Cream
ProctoFoam-HC
Progesterone
Prograf
Promethazine w/Codeine
Promethazine VC w/Codeine
Prometrium
Propranolol
Propranolol/HCTZ
Propylthiouracil
Proquin XR
Prosed EC
Protonix
Protopic
Provera
Prozac
Pulmicort
Pylera
Pyrazinamide
Qsymia
Qualaquin
Quinidine Gluconate
Quinidine Sulfate
Quixin
Qvar
Rayos
Reserpine
Restasis
Retrovir
Rezira
Rhinocort Aqua
Rifater
Risperdal
Risperdal Consta
Robaxin
Rocaltrol
Rosac
Roxicet
Roxicodone
Rybix ODT
Rythmol SR
Sabril
Safyral
Salsalate
Sandimmune
Sarafem
Seasonale
Seconal Sodium
Sectral
Semprex-D
Sensorcaine-MPF
Septra
Seromycin
Seroquel
Seroquel XR
Silenor
Simcor
Sinemet CR
Solodyn
Solu-Cortef
Solu-Medrol
Soma
Soma Compound
Soma Compound w/Codeine
Soriatane
Spectracef
Sporanox
Sprix
SSKI
St. Joseph 81 mg Aspirin
Stavzor
Stelara
Streptomycin
Stribild
Stromectol
Suboxone Sublingual Film
Subsys
Sumycin
Symbyax
Synthroid
Taclonex
Tambocor
Tapazole
Tarka
Tazicef
Tegretol
Tekturna HCT
Tenoretic
Tenormin
Teveten HCT
Theo-24
Theophylline
Thyrolar
Tiazac
Tilia Fe
Timoptic
Tindamax
Topamax
Toprol-XL
Transderm Scop
Tranxene T-Tab
Trental
Treximet
Triamcinolone
Tribenzor
Trileptal
Tri-Luma
Trimethoprim
Triphasil
Trisenox
Trivora
Trizivir
Tysabri
Tudorza Pressair
Ultane
Ultracet
Ultravate
Unasyn
Uniretic
Unithroid
Urex
Urogesic Blue
UTA
Utira-C
Vagifem
Valium
Valtrex
Vandazole

(Continued)

Vanos
Vascepa
Vasotec
Venlafaxine
Verapamil
Verdeso
Verelan
Verelan PM
Vibramycin
Vicodin
Vigamox
Vimovo
Viramune
Viread
Visudyne
Vivelle-Dot
Vivitrol
Vyvanse
Wellbutrin SR
Wellbutrin XL
Westcort
Westhroid
Xanax
Xanax XR
Ximino
Xylocaine Jelly
Xyzal
Yasmin
YAZ
Zanaflex
Zantac
Zarah
Zarontin
Zebutal
Zegerid
Zestoretic
Zevalin
Ziac
Ziana
Zinacef
Zolpimist
Zonalon
Zonegran
Zosyn
Zovia
Zovirax Oral
Zubsolv
Zyban
Zydone
Zyprexa
Zyprexa Relprevv

Abbreviation: HCTZ = hydrochlorothiazide

SECTION 4

PRODUCT IDENTIFICATION GUIDE

To aid in quick identification, this section provides full-color, actual-sized photographs of tablets and capsules. A variety of other dosage forms and packages are shown at less than actual size.

Products in this section are arranged alphabetically by manufacturer. Late submissions appear alphabetically by manufacturer at the end of the section. In some instances, not all dosage forms and sizes are pictured. If others are available, a † symbol precedes the product's name. Letters or numbers representing the manufacturer's identification code are followed by a * symbol.

For more information on any of the products in this section, please turn to the Product Information section, or check directly with the manufacturer. The page number of each product's text entry appears with its photographs.

While every effort has been made to guarantee faithful reproduction of the photos in this section, changes in size, color, and design are always a possibility. Be sure to confirm a product's identity with the manufacturer or your pharmacist.

INDEX BY MANUFACTURER

This section is made possible through the courtesy of the manufacturers whose products appear on the following pages.

4LIFE

DS 4LIFE P. 2564

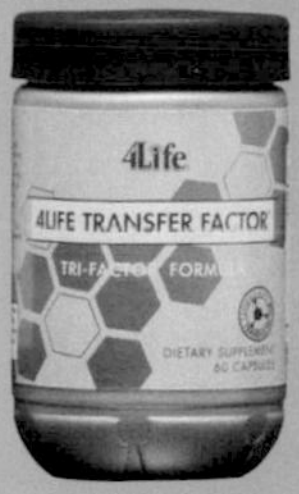

4Life Transfer Factor® Tri-Factor® Formula

While every effort has been made to reproduce products faithfully, this section is to be considered a quick reference identification aid. In cases of suspected overdosing, etc., chemical analysis should be done.

A&Z PHARMACEUTICAL

OTC A&Z PHARMACEUTICAL P. 2565

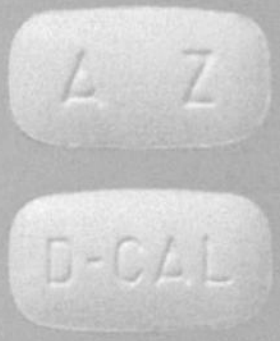

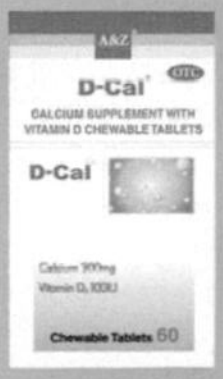

Calcium 300 mg

60 Chewable Tablets

D-Cal®
(calcium carbonate/vitamin D_3)

OTC A&Z PHARMACEUTICAL P. 2565

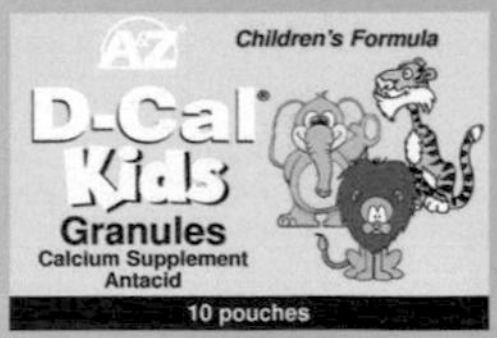

Calcium 300 mg
10 pouches

Granules

D-Cal® Kids
(calcium carbonate)

Products in this section are arranged alphabetically by manufacturer. In some instances, not all dosage forms and/or sizes are pictured. If others are available, a † symbol precedes the product's name. Letters or numbers representing the manufacturer's identification code are followed by a * symbol.

ABBVIE INC.

For description of Abbo-Code Identifications, see Abbo-Code index at the beginning of the AbbVie Information Section.

RX AbbVie Inc. P. 402

500 mg/20 mg

750 mg/20 mg

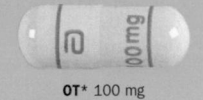

1000 mg/20 mg

1000 mg/40 mg

Advicor®
(niacin extended-release/lovastatin tablets)

C-III AbbVie Inc. P. 409

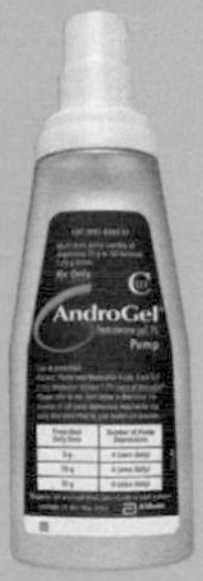

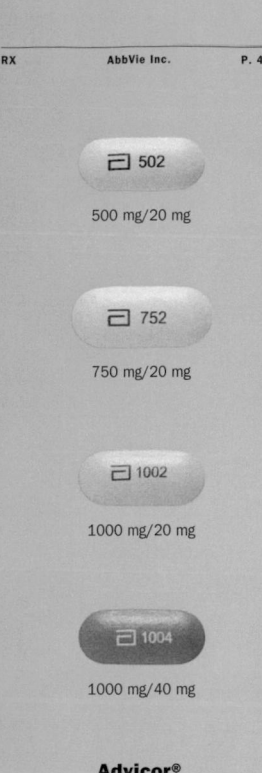

AndroGel® 1%
(testosterone gel)

C-III AbbVie Inc. P. 414

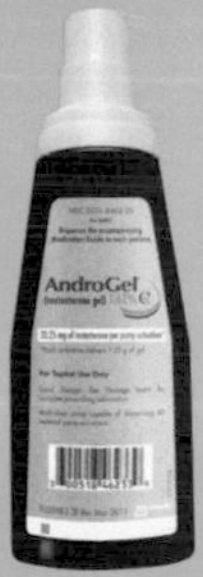

AndroGel® 1.62%
(testosterone gel)

RX AbbVie Inc. P. 420

KJ* 500 mg

Biaxin® XL Filmtab®
(clarithromycin extended-release tablets)

The pictured forms shown in this section may not necessarily be the only dosage forms and/or sizes available. Where a product name is preceded by a † symbol, refer to the description in the Product Information Section for other dosage forms and/or sizes.

RX AbbVie Inc. P. 420

KT* 250 mg

KL* 500 mg

Biaxin® Filmtab®
(clarithromycin tablets, USP)

RX AbbVie Inc. P. 420

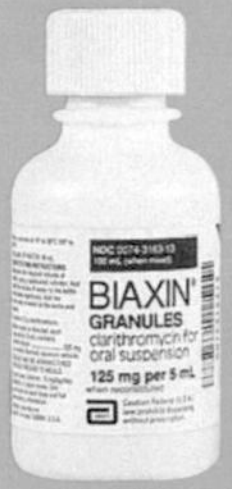

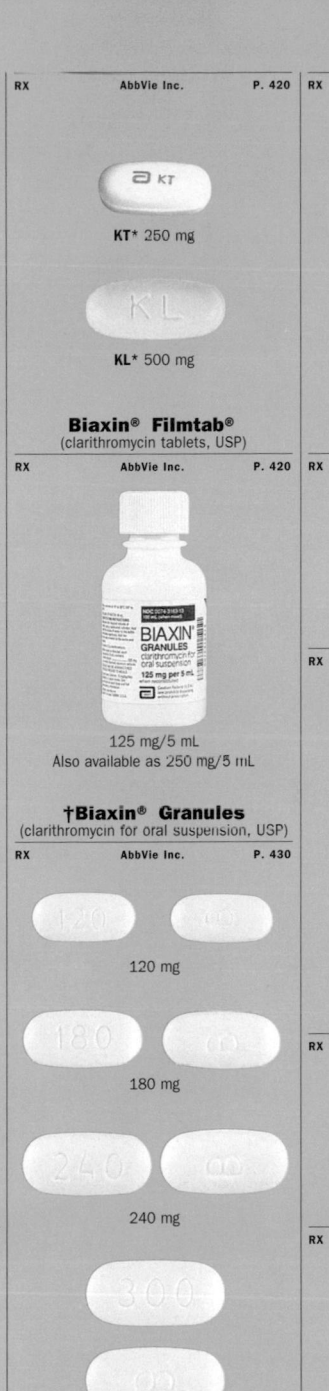

125 mg/5 mL
Also available as 250 mg/5 mL

†Biaxin® Granules
(clarithromycin for oral suspension, USP)

RX AbbVie Inc. P. 430

120 mg

180 mg

240 mg

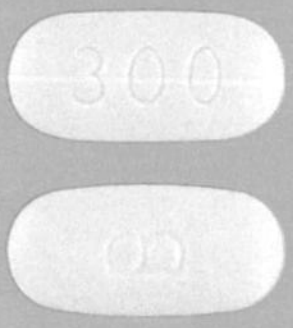

300 mg

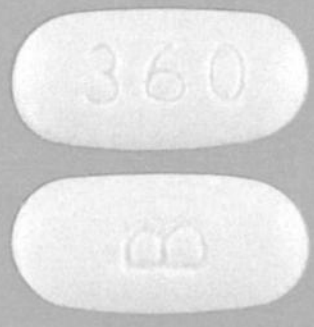

360 mg

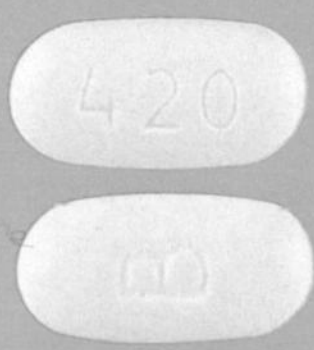

420 mg
Extended-Release Tablets

Cardizem® LA
(diltiazem hydrochloride)
Extended-Release Tablets

RX AbbVie Inc. P. 433

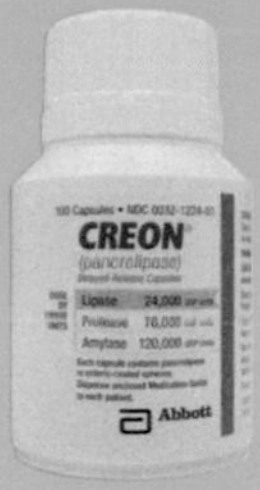

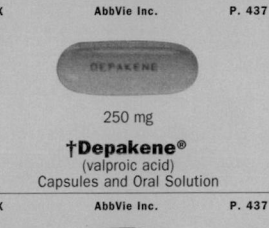

Creon®
(pancrelipase)
Delayed-Release-Capsules

RX AbbVie Inc. P. 437

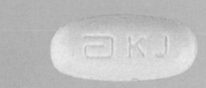

250 mg

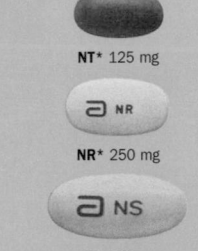

†Depakene®
(valproic acid)
Capsules and Oral Solution

RX AbbVie Inc. P. 437

NT* 125 mg

NR* 250 mg

NS* 500 mg

Depakote®
(divalproex sodium)
Tablets for Oral Use

RX AbbVie Inc. P. 437

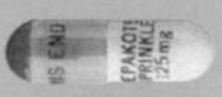

125 mg

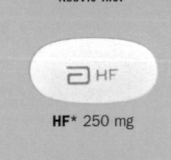

Depakote® Sprinkle Capsules
(divalproex sodium coated particles in capsules)

RX AbbVie Inc. P. 437

HF* 250 mg

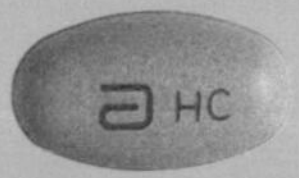

HC* 500 mg

Depakote® ER
(divalproex sodium)
Tablets, Extended-Release for Oral Use

RX AbbVie Inc. P. 448

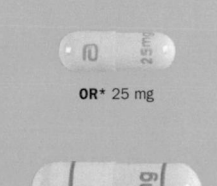

OR* 25 mg

OT* 100 mg

Gengraf® Capsules
(cyclosporine capsules USP [MODIFIED])

RX AbbVie Inc. P. 457

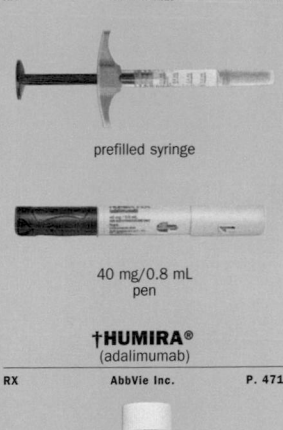

prefilled syringe

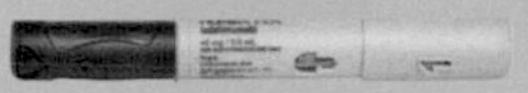

40 mg/0.8 mL
pen

†HUMIRA®
(adalimumab)

RX AbbVie Inc. P. 471

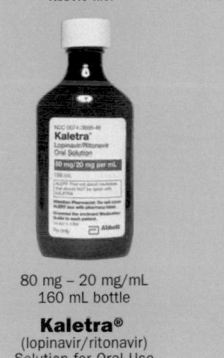

80 mg – 20 mg/mL
160 mL bottle

Kaletra®
(lopinavir/ritonavir)
Solution for Oral Use

RX AbbVie Inc. P. 471

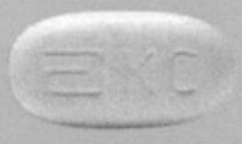

100 mg/25 mg

Kaletra®
(lopinavir/ritonavir)
Tablet Film-Coated for Oral Use

RX AbbVie Inc. P. 471

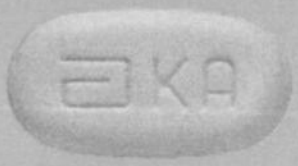

200 mg/50 mg

Kaletra®
(lopinavir/ritonavir)
Tablet Film-Coated for Oral Use

RX AbbVie Inc. P. 500, 508

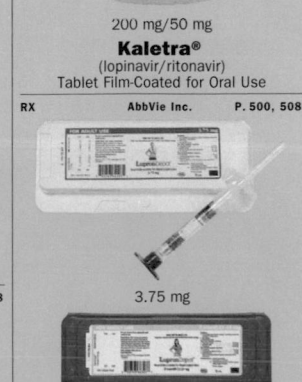

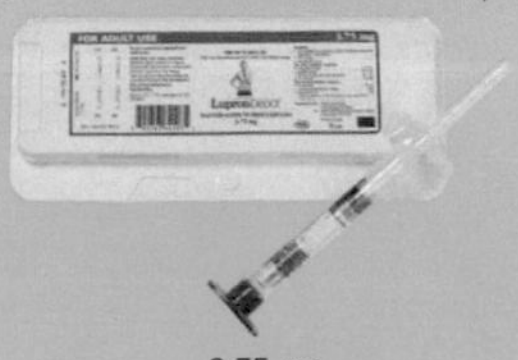

3.75 mg

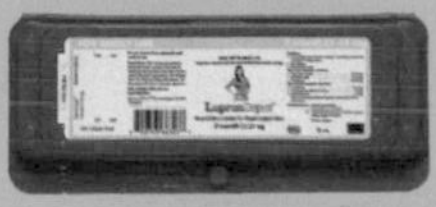

3 Month 11.25 mg

Lupron Depot® GYN
(leuprolide acetate for depot suspension)

While every effort has been made to reproduce products faithfully, this section is to be considered a quick reference identification aid. In cases of suspected overdosing, etc., chemical analysis should be done.

*AbbVie Abbo-Code identification letters. Filmtab® Film-sealed tablets, AbbVie.

†Additional dosage forms and sizes available.

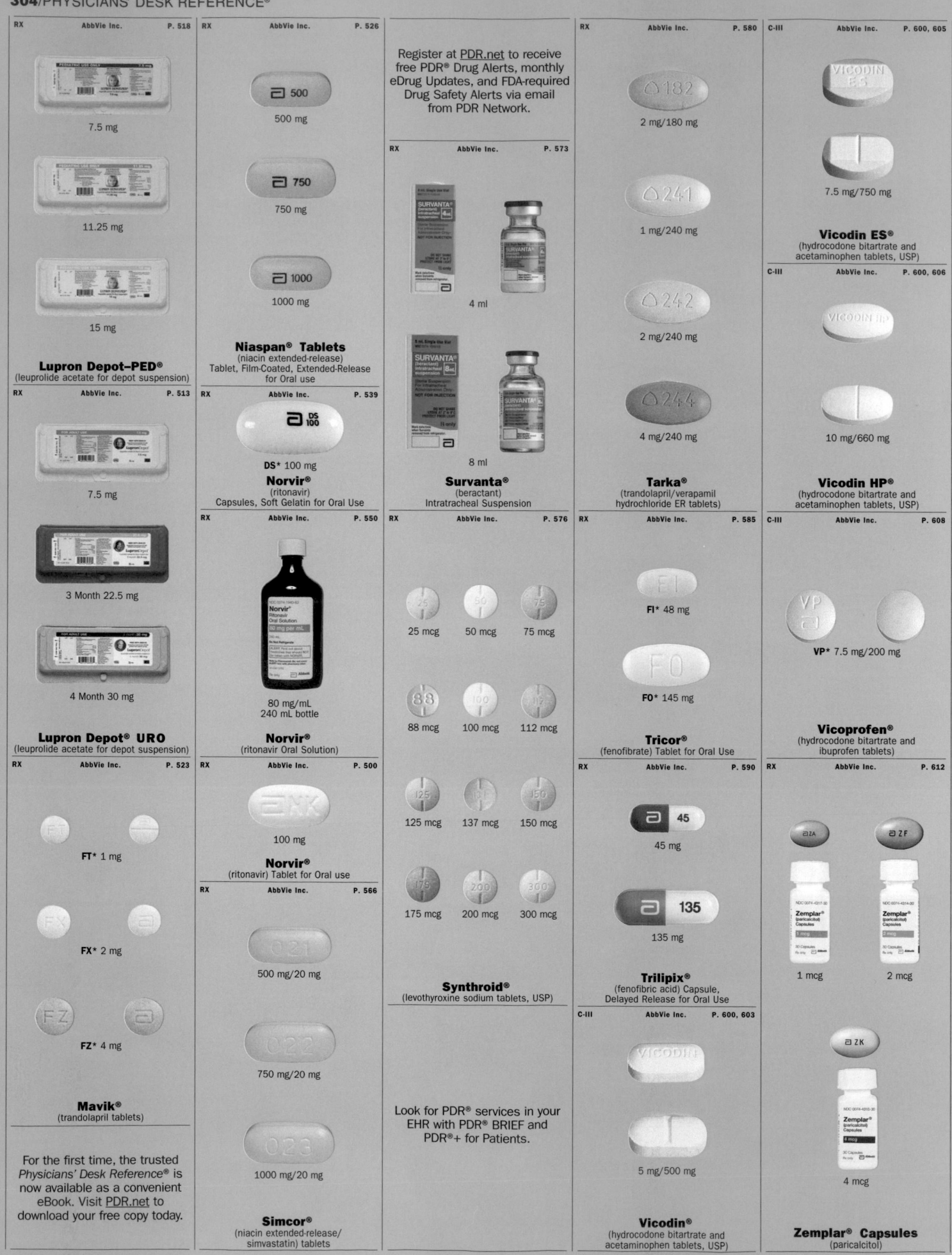

RX AbbVie Inc. P. 518

7.5 mg

11.25 mg

15 mg

Lupron Depot–PED®
(leuprolide acetate for depot suspension)

RX AbbVie Inc. P. 513

7.5 mg

3 Month 22.5 mg

4 Month 30 mg

Lupron Depot® URO
(leuprolide acetate for depot suspension)

RX AbbVie Inc. P. 523

FT* 1 mg

FX* 2 mg

FZ* 4 mg

Mavik®
(trandolapril tablets)

RX AbbVie Inc. P. 526

500 mg

750 mg

1000 mg

Niaspan® Tablets
(niacin extended-release)
Tablet, Film-Coated, Extended-Release for Oral use

RX AbbVie Inc. P. 539

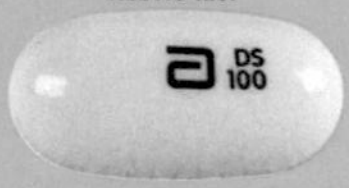

DS* 100 mg

Norvir®
(ritonavir)
Capsules, Soft Gelatin for Oral Use

RX AbbVie Inc. P. 550

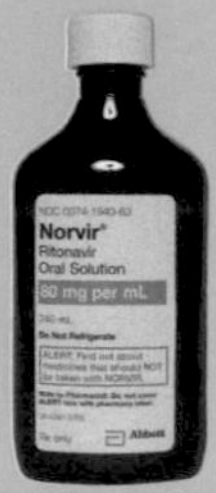

80 mg/mL
240 mL bottle

Norvir®
(ritonavir Oral Solution)

RX AbbVie Inc. P. 500

100 mg

Norvir®
(ritonavir) Tablet for Oral use

RX AbbVie Inc. P. 566

500 mg/20 mg

750 mg/20 mg

1000 mg/20 mg

Simcor®
(niacin extended-release/ simvastatin) tablets

RX AbbVie Inc. P. 573

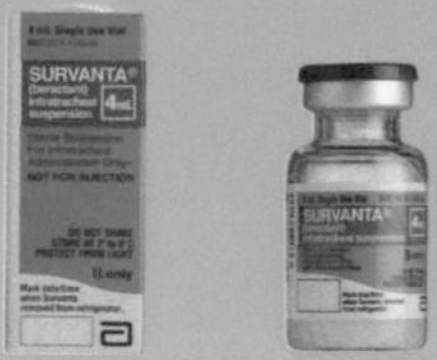

4 ml

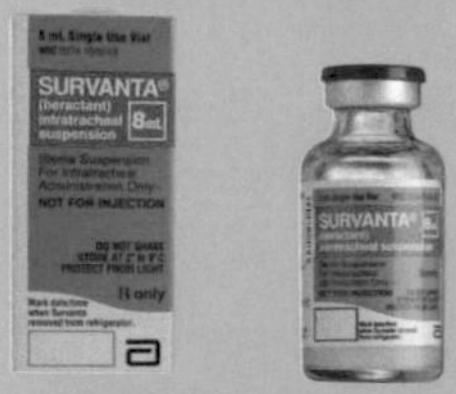

8 ml

Survanta®
(beractant)
Intratracheal Suspension

RX AbbVie Inc. P. 576

25 mcg 50 mcg 75 mcg

88 mcg 100 mcg 112 mcg

125 mcg 137 mcg 150 mcg

175 mcg 200 mcg 300 mcg

Synthroid®
(levothyroxine sodium tablets, USP)

RX AbbVie Inc. P. 580

2 mg/180 mg

1 mg/240 mg

2 mg/240 mg

4 mg/240 mg

Tarka®
(trandolapril/verapamil hydrochloride ER tablets)

RX AbbVie Inc. P. 585

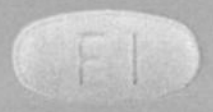

FI* 48 mg

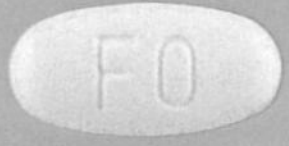

FO* 145 mg

Tricor®
(fenofibrate) Tablet for Oral Use

RX AbbVie Inc. P. 590

45 mg

135 mg

Trilipix®
(fenofibric acid) Capsule, Delayed Release for Oral Use

C-III AbbVie Inc. P. 600, 603

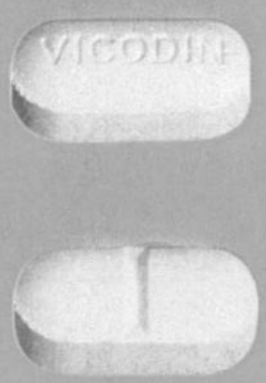

5 mg/500 mg

Vicodin®
(hydrocodone bitartrate and acetaminophen tablets, USP)

C-III AbbVie Inc. P. 600, 605

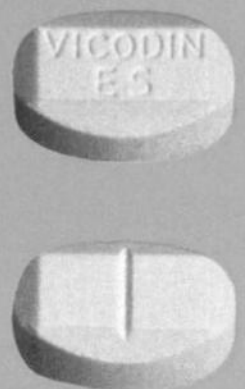

7.5 mg/750 mg

Vicodin ES®
(hydrocodone bitartrate and acetaminophen tablets, USP)

C-III AbbVie Inc. P. 600, 606

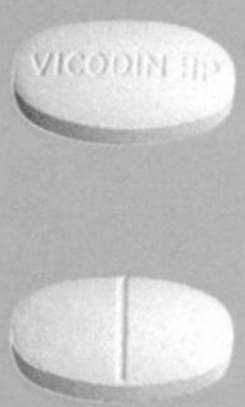

10 mg/660 mg

Vicodin HP®
(hydrocodone bitartrate and acetaminophen tablets, USP)

C-III AbbVie Inc. P. 608

VP* 7.5 mg/200 mg

Vicoprofen®
(hydrocodone bitartrate and ibuprofen tablets)

RX AbbVie Inc. P. 612

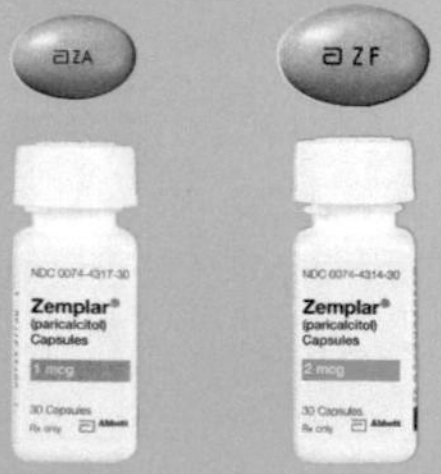

1 mcg 2 mcg

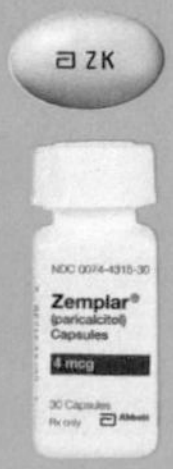

4 mcg

Zemplar® Capsules
(paricalcitol)

*Manufacturer's Identification Code

ALTO

DS ALTO PHARMACEUTICALS, INC. P. 2565

220 mg

Zinc-220®
(zinc sulfate, USP)

AMGEN INC.

RX AMGEN INC. P. 630

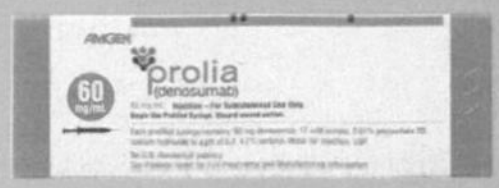

60 mg/1 mL

Prolia®
(denosumab)

While every effort has been made to reproduce products faithfully, this section is to be considered a quick reference identification aid. In cases of suspected overdosing, etc., chemical analysis should be done.

AWARENESSLIFE/ PURETRIM

DS AWARENESSLIFE/PURETRIM P. 2566

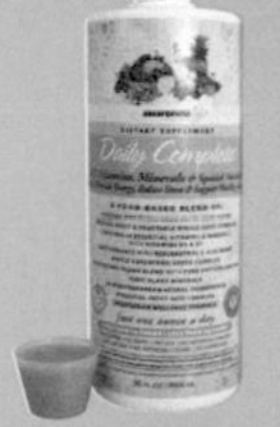

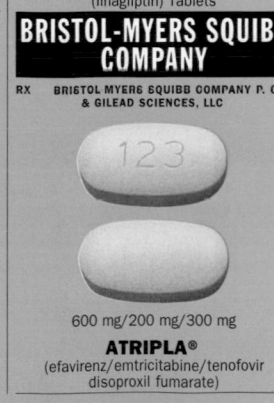

30 fl. oz./886 mL

Liquid Daily Complete®

DS AWARENESSLIFE/PURETRIM P. 2566

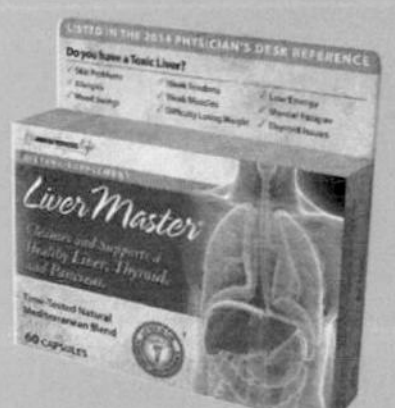

LiverMaster®

DS AWARENESSLIFE/PURETRIM P. 2566

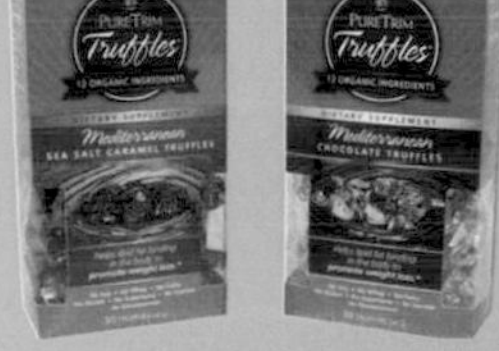

PureTrim Mediterranean Truffles®

DS AWARENESSLIFE/PURETRIM P. 2566

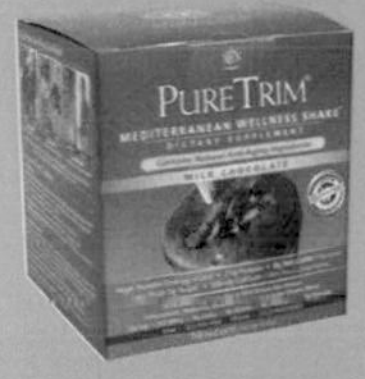

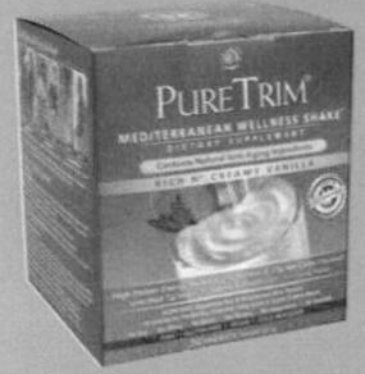

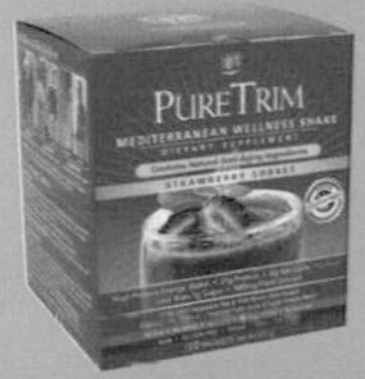

PureTrim® Mediterranean Wellness Shake™

BAYER HEALTHCARE LLC

RX BAYER HEALTHCARE LLC P. 636

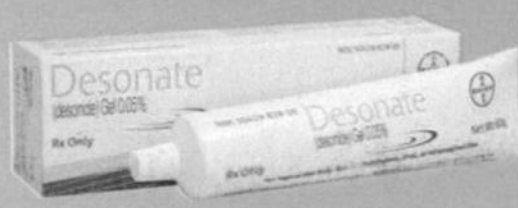

0.5 mg/g
0.05%

Desonate®
(desonide) Gel

RX BAYER HEALTHCARE LLC P. 638

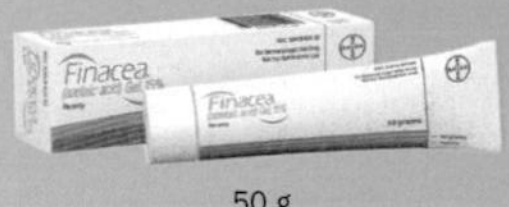

50 g
15%

Finacea® Gel
(azelaic acid)

RX BAYER HEALTHCARE LLC P. 640

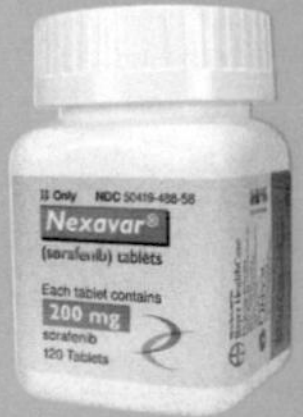

200 mg

Nexavar®
(sorafenib) tablets

RX BAYER HEALTHCARE LLC P. 646

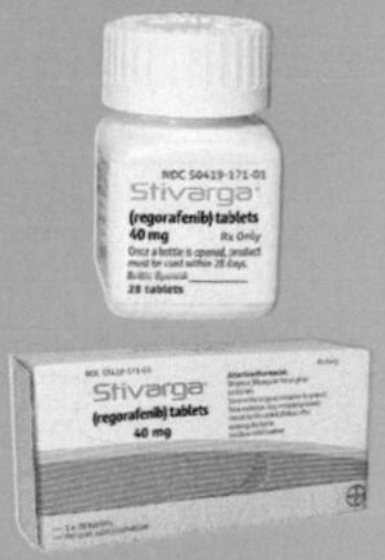

40 mg

Stivarga®
(regorafenib) tablets

RX BAYER HEALTHCARE LLC P. 652

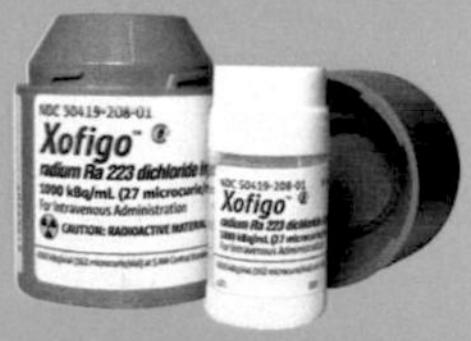

1000 kBq/mL

Xofigo™
(radium Ra 223 dichloride) injection

BOEHRINGER INGELHEIM

RX BOEHRINGER INGELHEIM P. 655

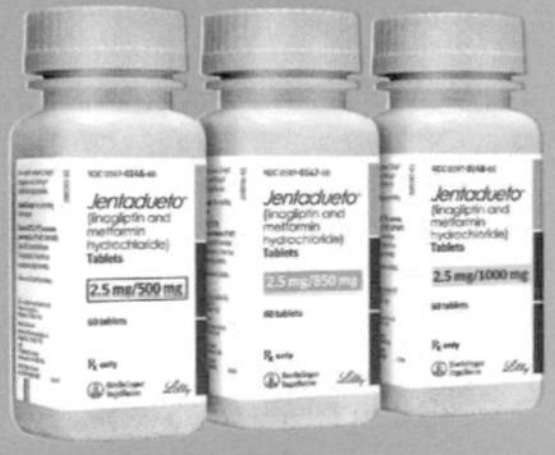

2.5mg/ 500 mg | 2.5mg/ 850 mg | 2.5mg/ 1000 mg

Jentadueto®
(linagliptin and metformin hydrochloride)

RX BOEHRINGER INGELHEIM P. 664

Side One | Side Two

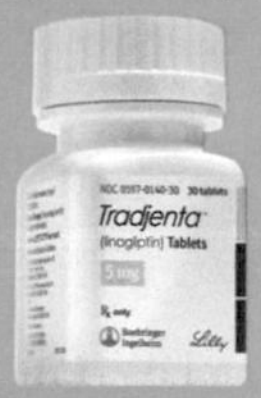

5 mg

Tradjenta®
(linagliptin) Tablets

BRISTOL-MYERS SQUIBB COMPANY

RX BRISTOL MYERS SQUIBB COMPANY P. 672 & GILEAD SCIENCES, LLC

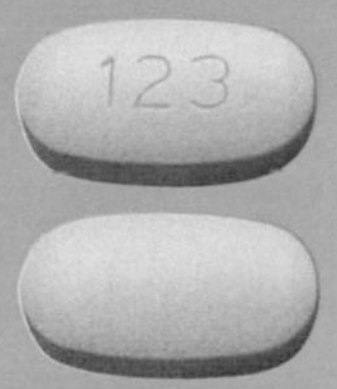

600 mg/200 mg/300 mg

ATRIPLA®
(efavirenz/emtricitabine/tenofovir disoproxil fumarate)

RX BRISTOL-MYERS SQUIBB COMPANY P. 685

0.5 mg

1.0 mg

Also available as 0.05 mg/mL oral solution

Baraclude®
(entecavir) tablets

RX BRISTOL-MYERS SQUIBB COMPANY P. 692

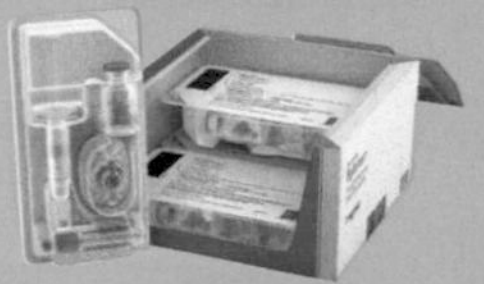

2 mg/vial

Bydureon®
(exenatide extended-release for injectable suspension)

RX BRISTOL-MYERS SQUIBB COMPANY P. 701

5 mcg

10 mcg

Byetta®
(exenatide) injection

RX BRISTOL-MYERS SQUIBB COMPANY P. 712

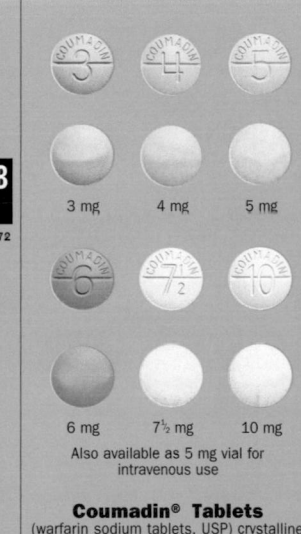

1 mg | 2 mg | 2½ mg

3 mg | 4 mg | 5 mg

6 mg | 7½ mg | 10 mg

Also available as 5 mg vial for intravenous use

Coumadin® Tablets
(warfarin sodium tablets, USP) crystalline

RX BRISTOL-MYERS SQUIBB COMPANY P. 718

2.5 mg

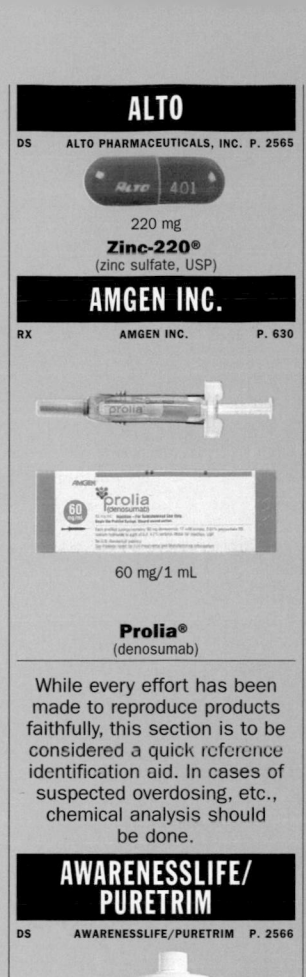

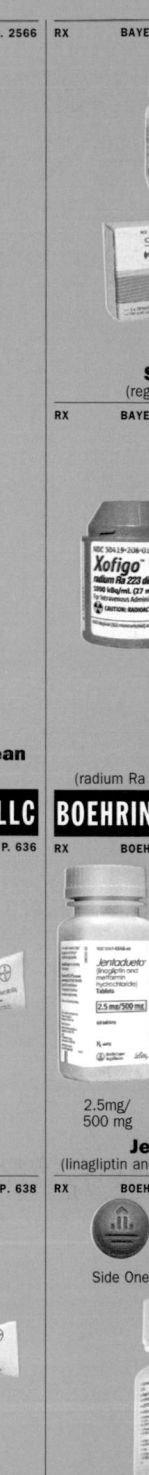

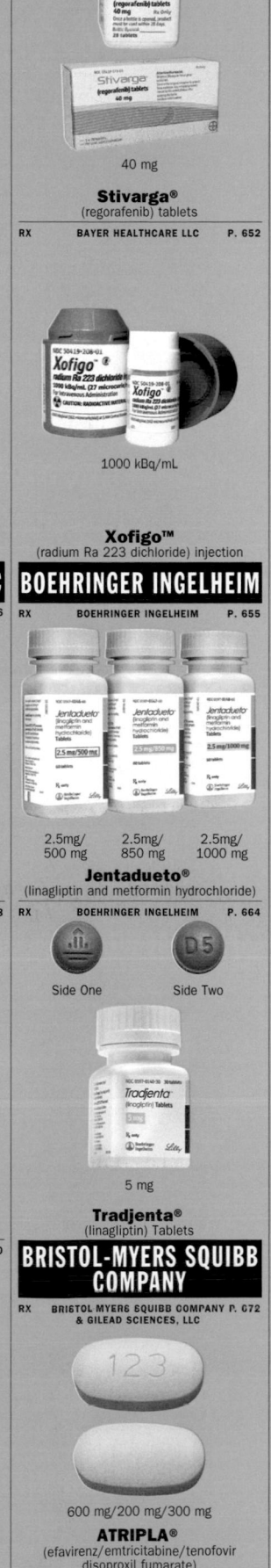

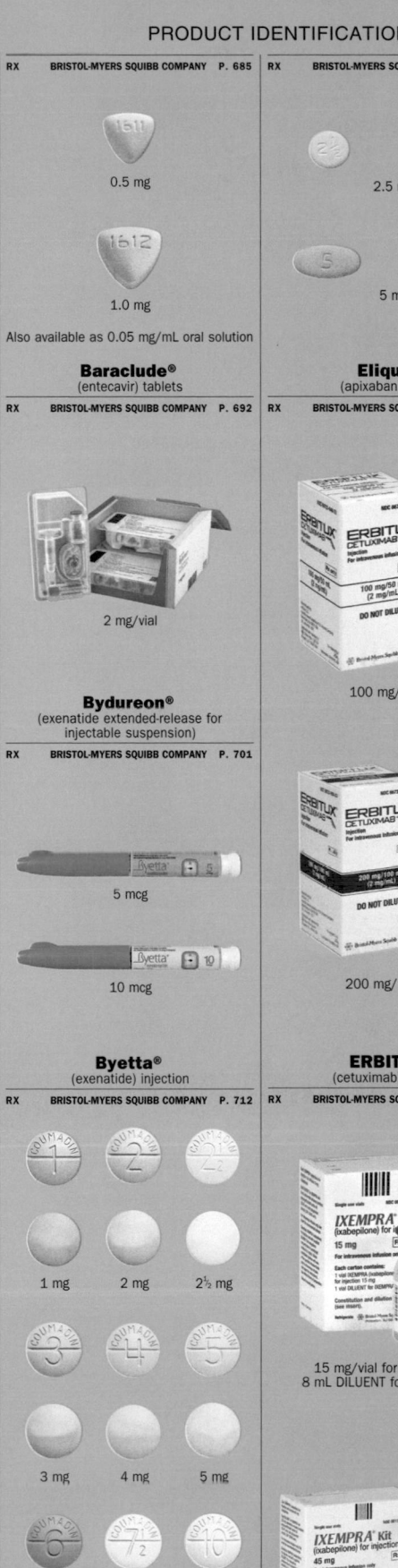

5 mg

Eliquis®
(apixaban) tablets

RX BRISTOL-MYERS SQUIBB COMPANY P. 723

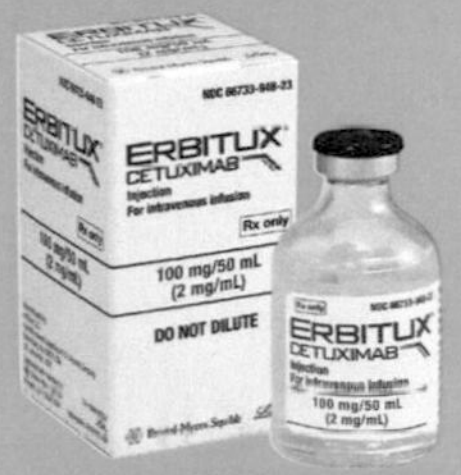

100 mg/50 mL

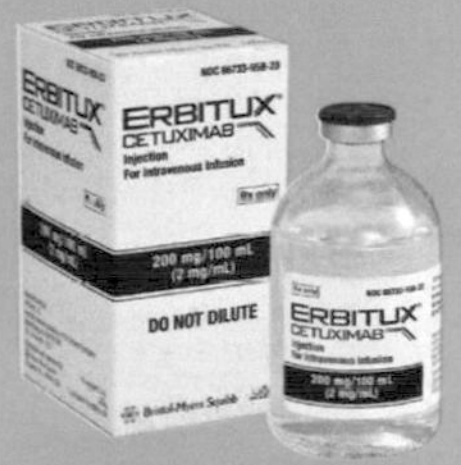

200 mg/100 mL

ERBITUX®
(cetuximab) injection

RX BRISTOL-MYERS SQUIBB COMPANY P. 729

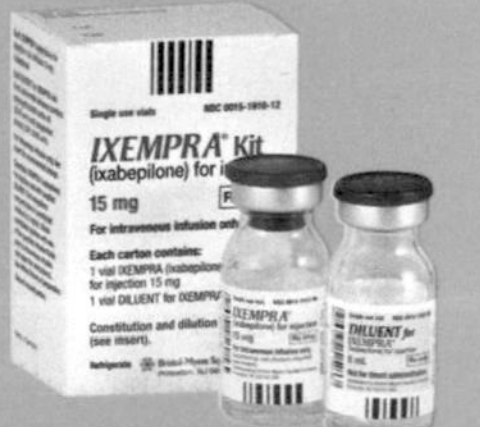

15 mg/vial for injection and 8 mL DILUENT for IXEMPRA/vial

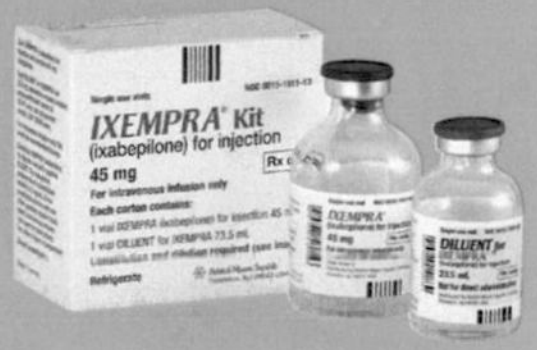

45 mg/vial for injection and 23.5 mL DILUENT for IXEMPRA/vial

IXEMPRA® Kit
(ixabepilone) for injection

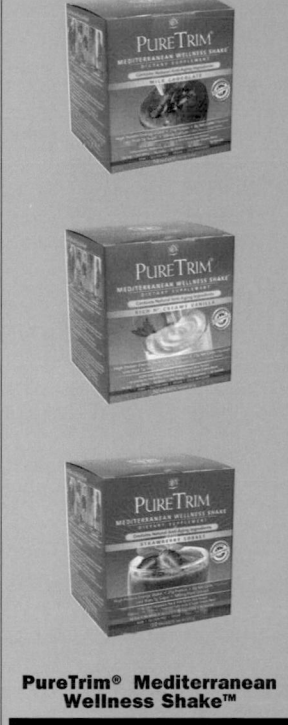

RX BRISTOL-MYERS SQUIBB COMPANY P. 736

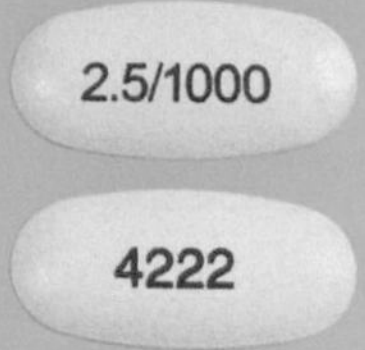

2.5 mg/1000 mg

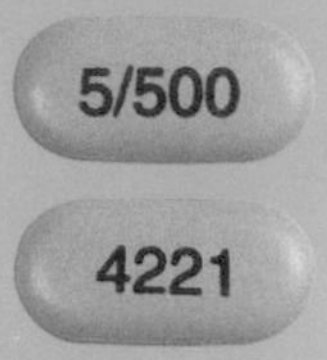

5 mg/500 mg

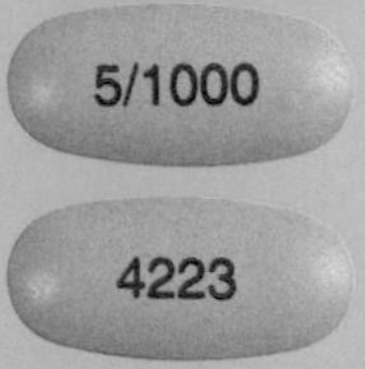

5 mg/1000 mg

Kombiglyze™ XR
(saxagliptin and metformin HCl extended-release) tablets

RX BRISTOL-MYERS SQUIBB COMPANY P. 746

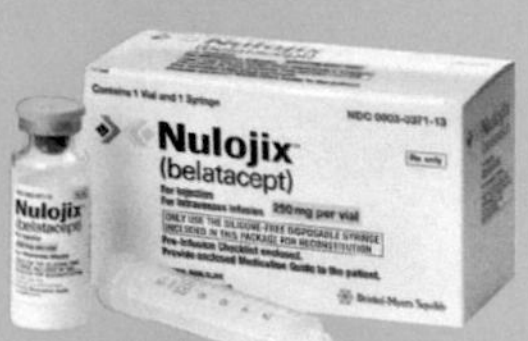

250 mg/vial

Nulojix®
(belatacept) for injection

RX BRISTOL-MYERS SQUIBB COMPANY P. 754

2.5 mg 5 mg

Onglyza®
(saxagliptin) tablets

RX BRISTOL-MYERS SQUIBB COMPANY P. 763

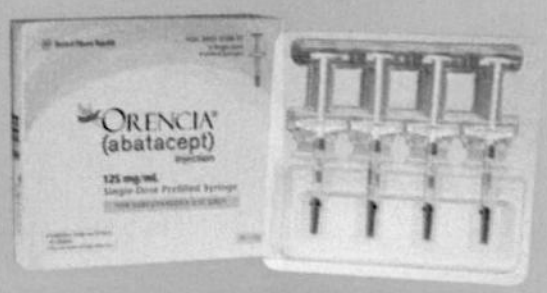

125 mg/mL Prefilled Syringe for subcutaneous use

125 mg/mL Prefilled Syringe with UltraSafe Passive® Needle Guard

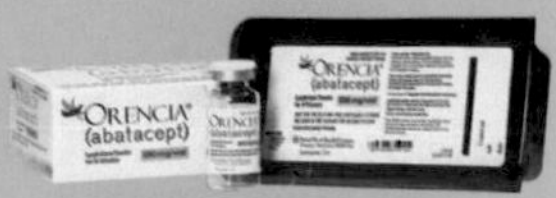

250 mg/vial for intravenous use

Orencia®
(abatacept)

Products in this section are arranged alphabetically by manufacturer. In some instances, not all dosage forms and/or sizes are pictured. If others are available, a † symbol precedes the product's name. Letters or numbers representing the manufacturer's identification code are followed by a * symbol.

RX BRISTOL-MYERS SQUIBB COMPANY P. 772

150 mg

200 mg

300 mg

Reyataz®
(atazanavir sulfate) capsules

RX BRISTOL-MYERS SQUIBB COMPANY P. 789

20 mg 50 mg

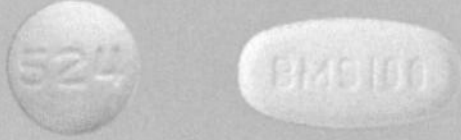

70 mg 100 mg

80 mg 140 mg

Sprycel®
(dasatinib) tablets

RX BRISTOL-MYERS SQUIBB COMPANY P. 795

50 mg

200 mg

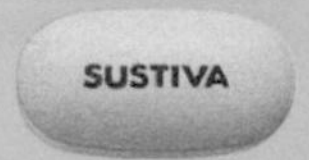

600 mg

SUSTIVA®
(efavirenz) capsules and tablets

RX BRISTOL-MYERS SQUIBB COMPANY P. 808

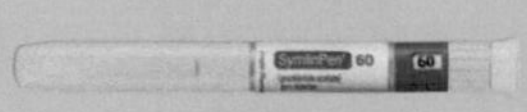

1.5 mL-1000 mcg/mL

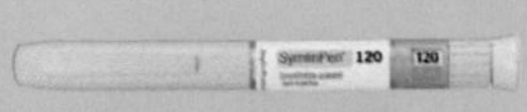

2.7 mL-1000 mcg/mL

SymlinPen®
(pramlintide acetate) pen-injector

The pictured forms shown in this section may not necessarily be the only dosage forms and/or sizes available. Where a product name is preceded by a † symbol, refer to the description in the Product Information Section for other dosage forms and/or sizes.

RX BRISTOL-MYERS SQUIBB COMPANY P. 816

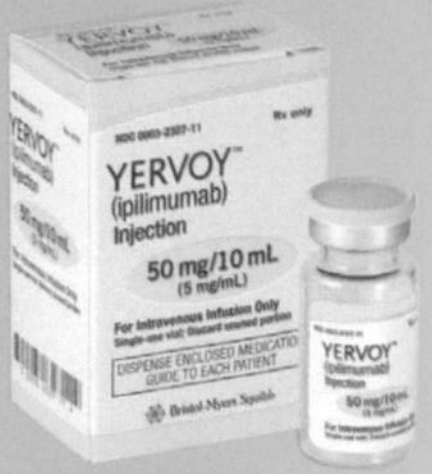

50 mg/10 mL

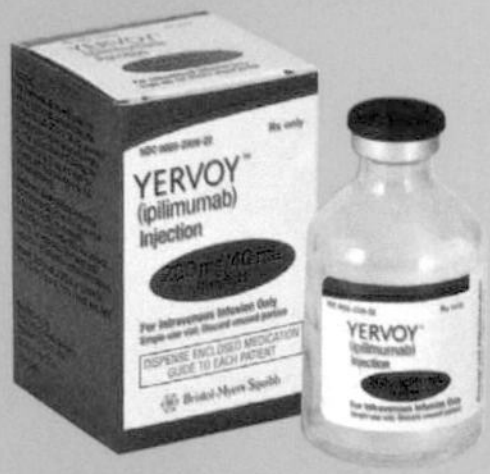

200 mg/40 mL

Yervoy®
(ipilimumab) injection for intravenous infusion

CARLSON LABORATORIES

DS CARLSON LABORATORIES P. 2566

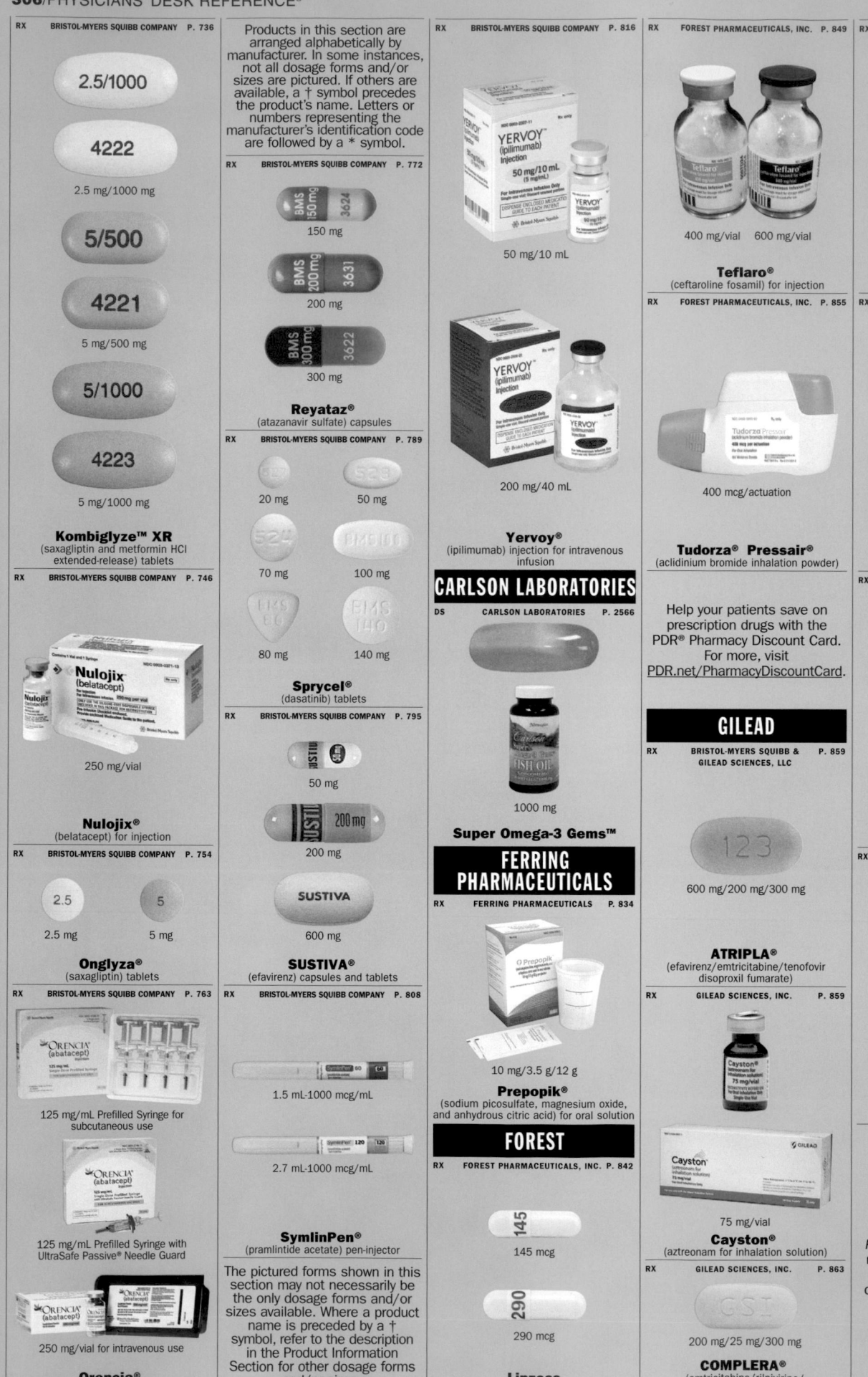

1000 mg

Super Omega-3 Gems™

FERRING PHARMACEUTICALS

RX FERRING PHARMACEUTICALS P. 834

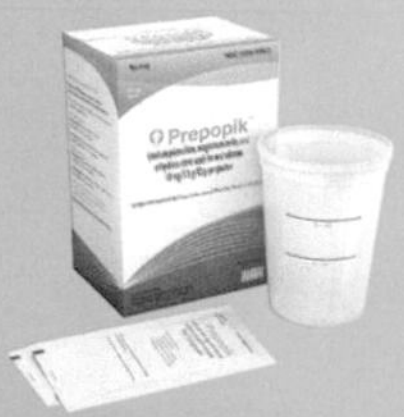

10 mg/3.5 g/12 g

Prepopik®
(sodium picosulfate, magnesium oxide, and anhydrous citric acid) for oral solution

FOREST

RX FOREST PHARMACEUTICALS, INC. P. 842

145 mcg

290 mcg

Linzess
(linaclotide) capsules

RX FOREST PHARMACEUTICALS, INC. P. 849

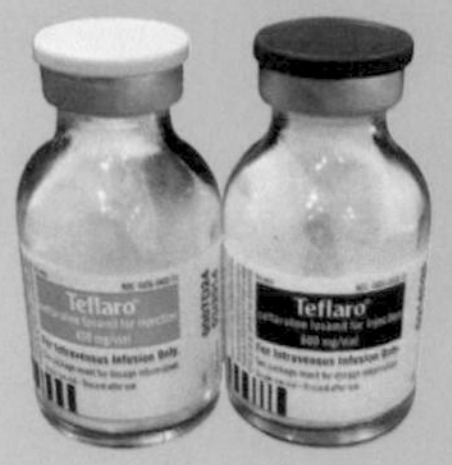

400 mg/vial 600 mg/vial

Teflaro®
(ceftaroline fosamil) for injection

RX FOREST PHARMACEUTICALS, INC. P. 855

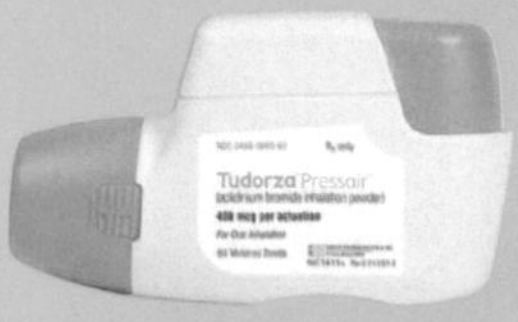

400 mcg/actuation

Tudorza® Pressair®
(aclidinium bromide inhalation powder)

Help your patients save on prescription drugs with the PDR® Pharmacy Discount Card. For more, visit PDR.net/PharmacyDiscountCard.

GILEAD

RX BRISTOL-MYERS SQUIBB & GILEAD SCIENCES, LLC P. 859

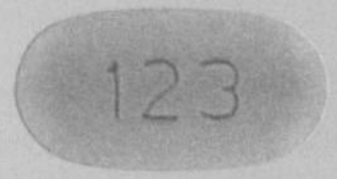

600 mg/200 mg/300 mg

ATRIPLA®
(efavirenz/emtricitabine/tenofovir disoproxil fumarate)

RX GILEAD SCIENCES, INC. P. 859

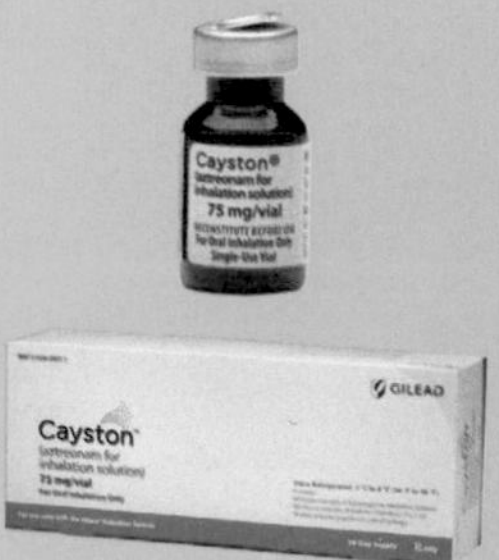

75 mg/vial

Cayston®
(aztreonam for inhalation solution)

RX GILEAD SCIENCES, INC. P. 863

200 mg/25 mg/300 mg

COMPLERA®
(emtricitabine/rilpivirine/tenofovir disoproxil fumarate)

RX GILEAD SCIENCES, INC. P. 873

5 mg

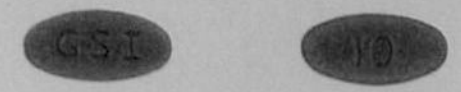

10 mg

Letairis®
(ambrisentan)

RX GILEAD SCIENCES, INC. P. 878

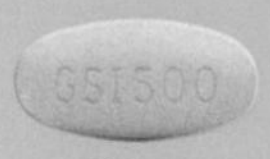

500 mg

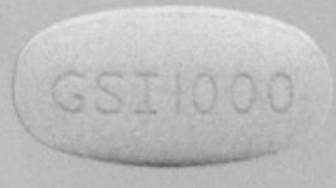

1000 mg

Ranexa®
(ranolazine) extended-release tablets

RX GILEAD SCIENCES, INC. P. 881

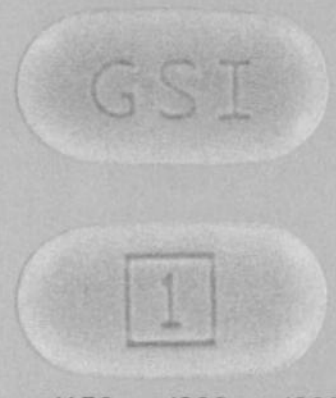

150 mg/150 mg/200 mg/300 mg

Stribild™
(elvitegravir/cobicistat/emtricitabine/tenofovir disoproxil fumarate)

RX GILEAD SCIENCES, INC. P. 892

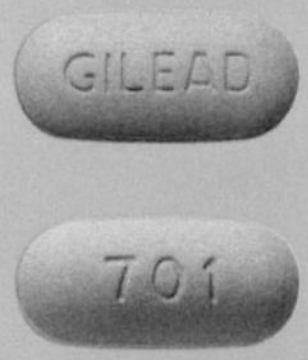

200 mg/300 mg

Truvada®
(emtricitabine/tenofovir disoproxil fumarate)

RX GILEAD SCIENCES, INC. P. 902

150 mg

200 mg

250 mg

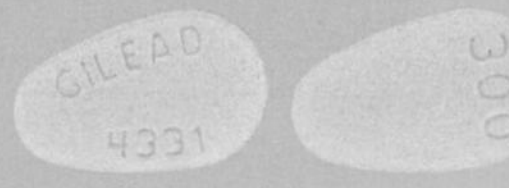

300 mg

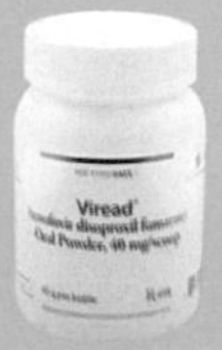

40 mg/scoop

Viread®
(tenofovir disoproxil fumarate)

GLENWOOD

RX GLENWOOD P. 1324

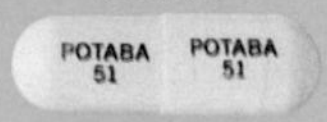

500 mg

Potaba®
(aminobenzoate potassium, USP)

GORDON LABORATORIES

RX GORDON LABORATORIES P. 1324

10%
Available in 60 mL and 120 mL

Formadon
(formaldehyde solution)

OTC GORDON LABORATORIES P. 1325

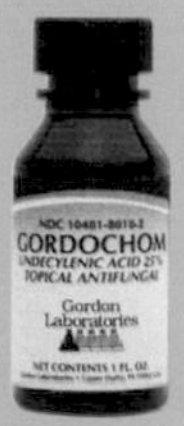

25%
30 mL

Gordochom
(undecylenic acid)

Register at PDR.net to receive free PDR® Drug Alerts, monthly eDrug Updates, and FDA-required Drug Safety Alerts via email from PDR Network.

HALOZYME THERAPEUTICS, INC.

RX HALOZYME THERAPEUTICS, INC. P. 1325

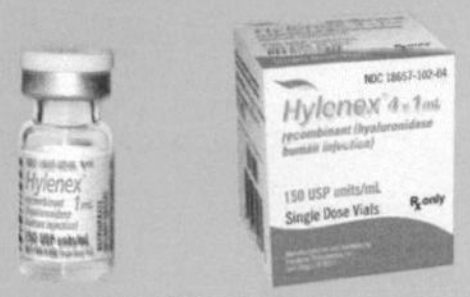

150 USP units/mL
4 x 1 mL single dose vials

Hylenex® recombinant
(hyaluronidase human injection)

Look for PDR® services in your EHR with PDR® BRIEF and PDR®+ for Patients.

HIGH CHEMICAL

RX HIGH CHEMICAL P. 1327

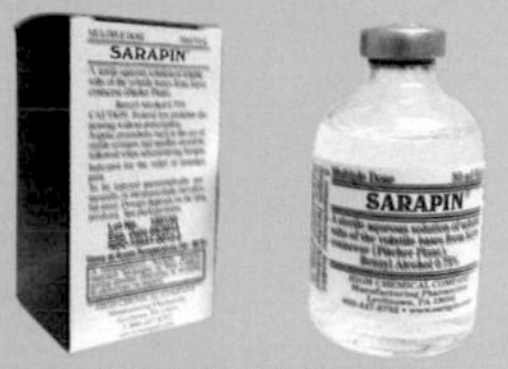

50 mL Multiple Dose Vial

SARAPIN®
(sarraceniaceae)

While every effort has been made to reproduce products faithfully, this section is to be considered a quick reference identification aid. In cases of suspected overdosing, etc., chemical analysis should be done.

JANSSEN PHARMACEUTICALS, INC.

C-II JANSSEN PHARMACEUTICALS, INC. P. 1334

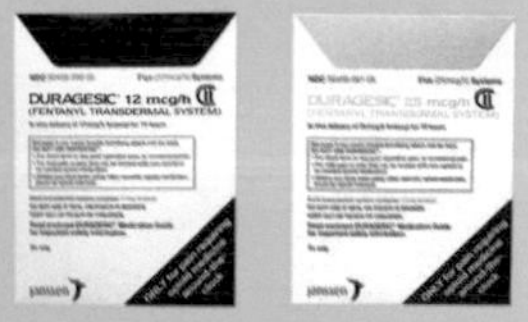

12 mcg/h 25 mcg/h

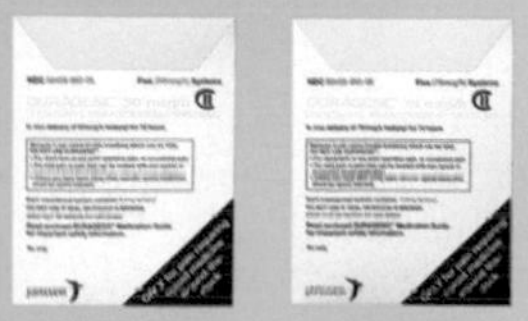

50 mcg/h 75 mcg/h

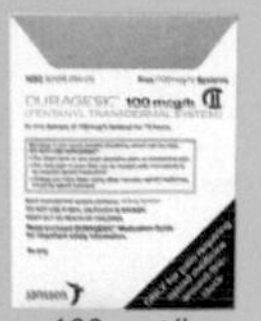

100 mcg/h

DURAGESIC®
(fentanyl transdermal system)

C-II JANSSEN PHARMACEUTICALS, INC. P. 1342

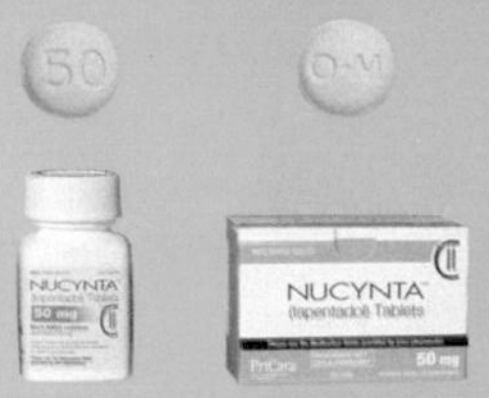

50 mg

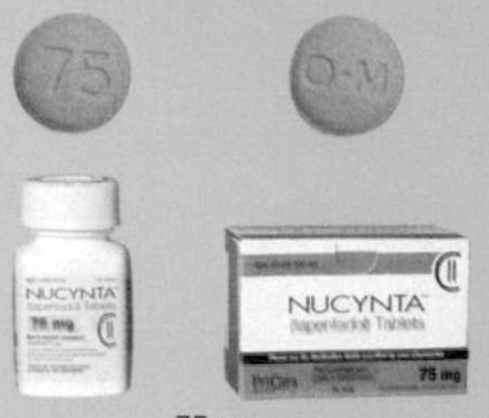

75 mg

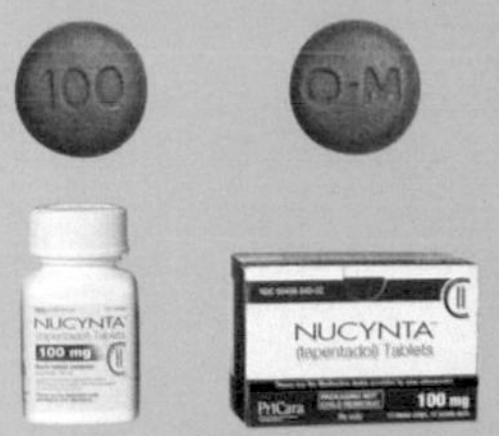

100 mg

NUCYNTA®
(tapentadol)
Immediate-Release Tablets

C-II JANSSEN PHARMACEUTICALS, INC. P. 1347

50 mg

100 mg

150 mg

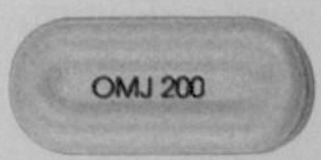

200 mg

250 mg

NUCYNTA® ER
(tapentadol)
Extended-Release Tablets

Products in this section are arranged alphabetically by manufacturer. In some instances, not all dosage forms and/or sizes are pictured. If others are available, a † symbol precedes the product's name. Letters or numbers representing the manufacturer's identification code are followed by a * symbol.

LEGACY FOR LIFE

LEGACY FOR LIFE P. 2568

Dietary Supplement

i26 Powder

MERCK

RX MERCK P. 1391

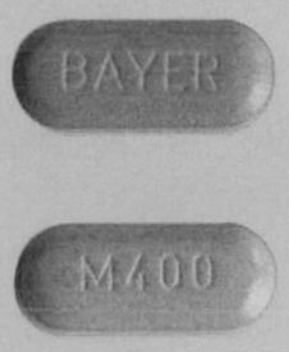

400 mg

Avelox®
(moxifloxacin HCl)

RX MERCK P. 1401

2.5 mL

AzaSite®
(azithromycin ophthalmic solution) 1%

RX MERCK P. 1403

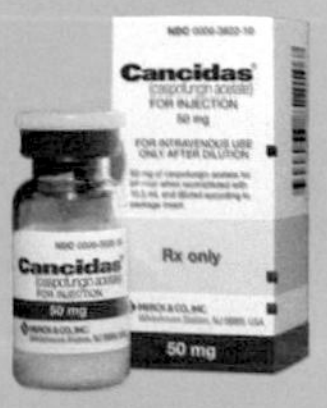

50 mg

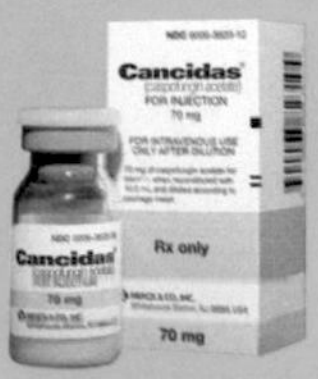

70 mg

Cancidas®
(caspofungin acetate) for Injection

RX MERCK P. 1415

5 mg
Also available in 0.5 mg/1 mL oral solution

Clarinex®
(desloratadine)

RX MERCK P. 1419

2.5 mg/120 mg

Clarinex-D® 12 Hour
(desloratadine/pseudoephedrine sulfate)

RX MERCK P. 1433

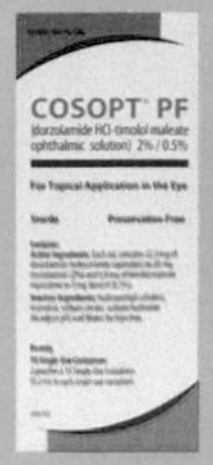

2%/0.5%
0.2 mL

Cosopt® PF
(dorzolamide HCl - timolol maleate ophthalmic solution)

RX MERCK P. 1436

100 mg

200 mg

400 mg

Crixivan®
(indinavir sulfate)

RX MERCK P. 1449

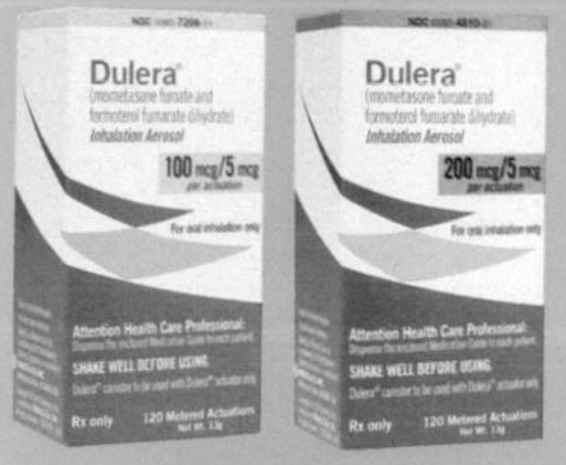

100 mcg/5 mcg 200 mcg/5 mcg

Dulera®
(mometasone furoate and formoterol fumarate dihydrate) Inhalation Aerosol

RX MERCK P. 1463

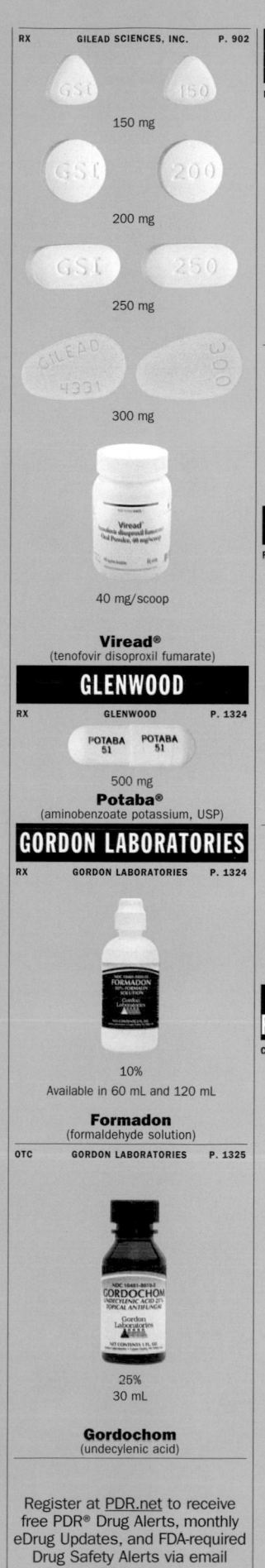

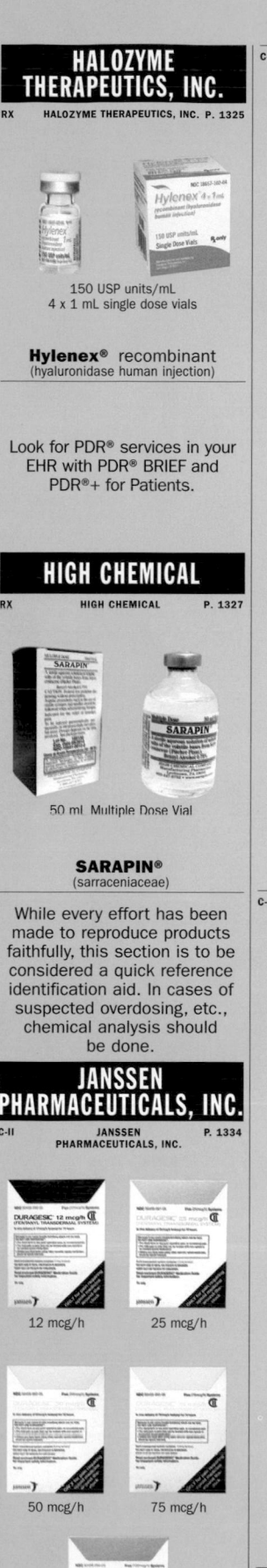

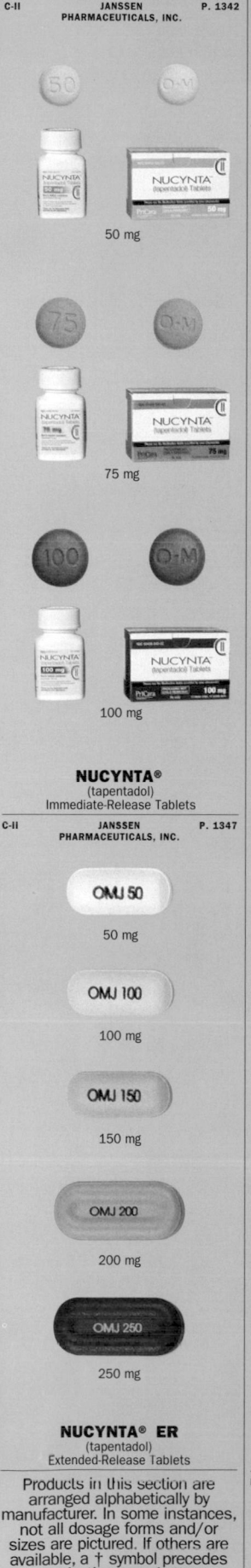

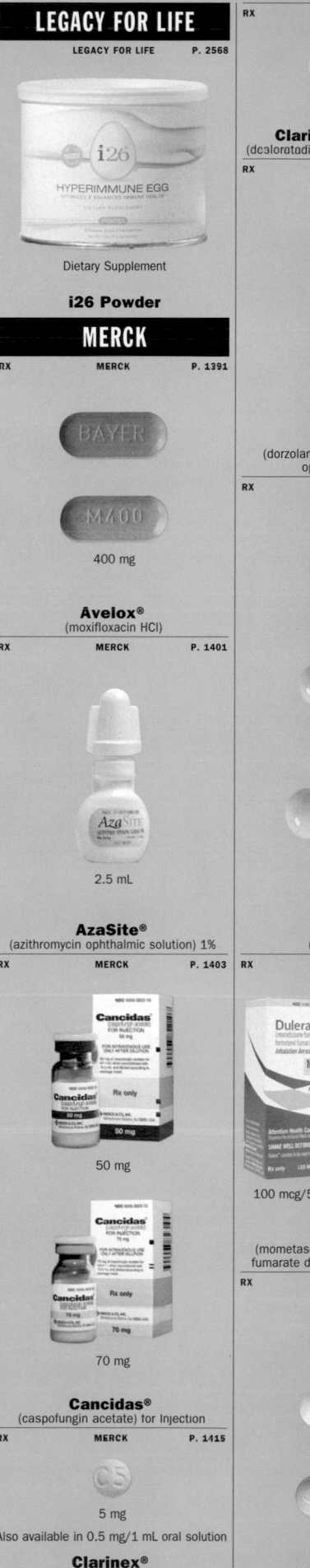

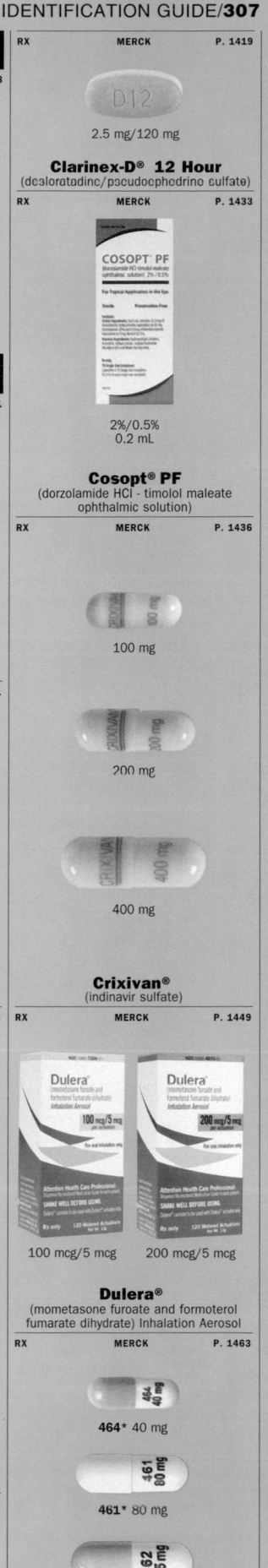

464* 40 mg

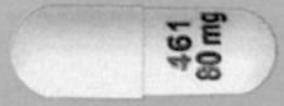

461* 80 mg

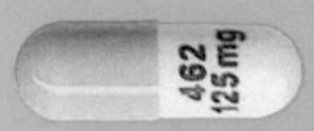

462* 125 mg

†Emend®
(aprepitant)

*Manufacturer's Identification Code

†Additional dosage forms and sizes available

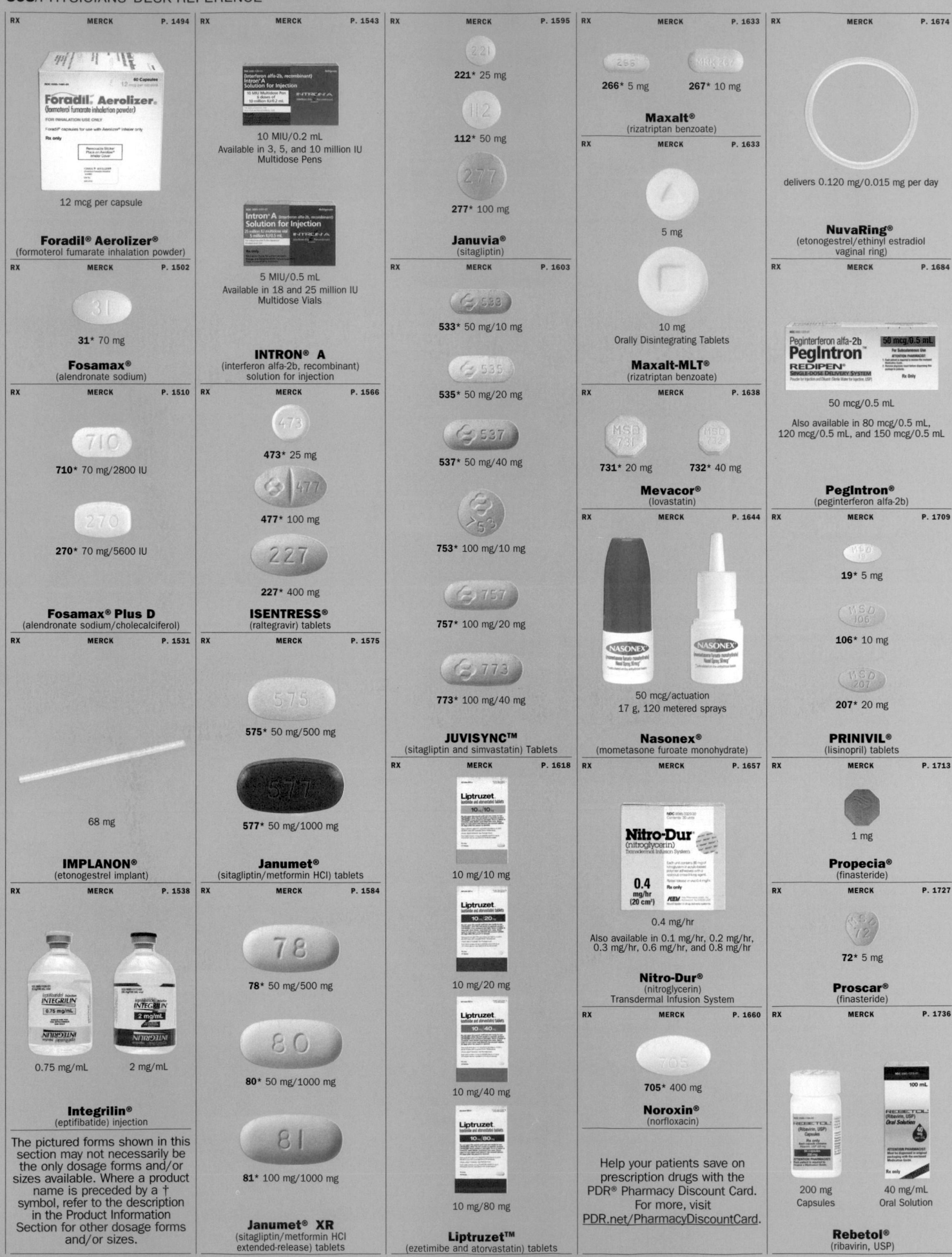

RX MERCK P. 1494

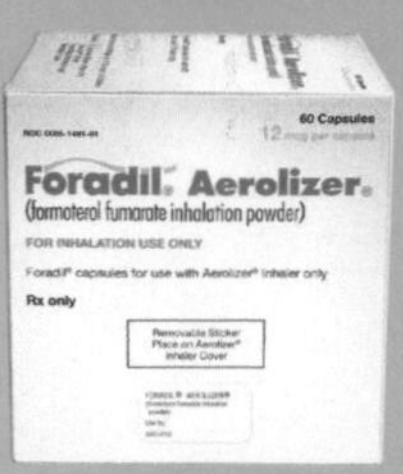

12 mcg per capsule

Foradil® Aerolizer®
(formoterol fumarate inhalation powder)

RX MERCK P. 1502

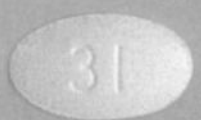

31* 70 mg

Fosamax®
(alendronate sodium)

RX MERCK P. 1510

710* 70 mg/2800 IU

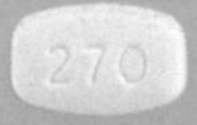

270* 70 mg/5600 IU

Fosamax® Plus D
(alendronate sodium/cholecalciferol)

RX MERCK P. 1531

68 mg

IMPLANON®
(etonogestrel implant)

RX MERCK P. 1538

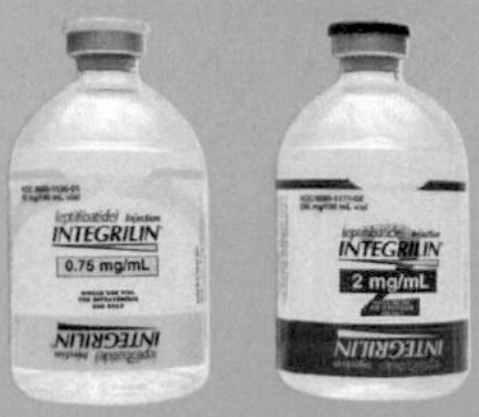

0.75 mg/mL 2 mg/mL

Integrilin®
(eptifibatide) injection

The pictured forms shown in this section may not necessarily be the only dosage forms and/or sizes available. Where a product name is preceded by a † symbol, refer to the description in the Product Information Section for other dosage forms and/or sizes.

RX MERCK P. 1543

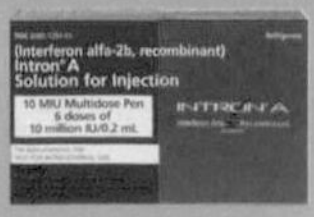

10 MIU/0.2 mL
Available in 3, 5, and 10 million IU Multidose Pens

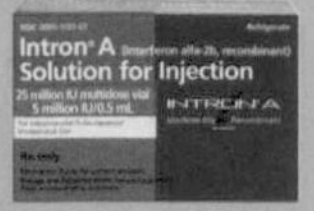

5 MIU/0.5 mL
Available in 18 and 25 million IU Multidose Vials

INTRON® A
(interferon alfa-2b, recombinant) solution for injection

RX MERCK P. 1566

473* 25 mg

477* 100 mg

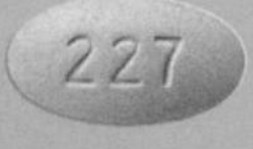

227* 400 mg

ISENTRESS®
(raltegravir) tablets

RX MERCK P. 1575

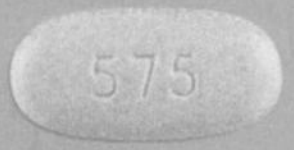

575* 50 mg/500 mg

577* 50 mg/1000 mg

Janumet®
(sitagliptin/metformin HCl) tablets

RX MERCK P. 1584

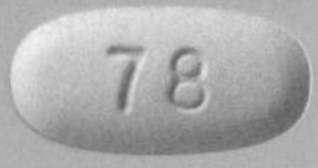

78* 50 mg/500 mg

80* 50 mg/1000 mg

81* 100 mg/1000 mg

Janumet® XR
(sitagliptin/metformin HCl extended-release) tablets

RX MERCK P. 1595

221* 25 mg

112* 50 mg

277* 100 mg

Januvia®
(sitagliptin)

RX MERCK P. 1603

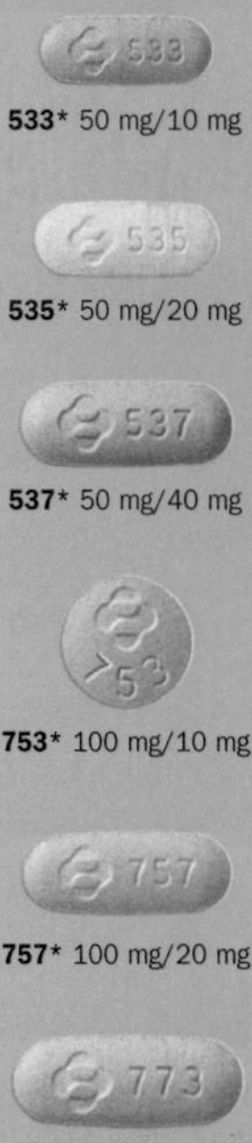

533* 50 mg/10 mg

535* 50 mg/20 mg

537* 50 mg/40 mg

753* 100 mg/10 mg

757* 100 mg/20 mg

773* 100 mg/40 mg

JUVISYNC™
(sitagliptin and simvastatin) Tablets

RX MERCK P. 1618

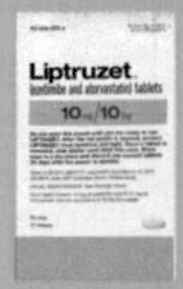

10 mg/10 mg

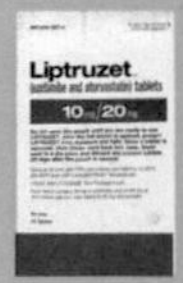

10 mg/20 mg

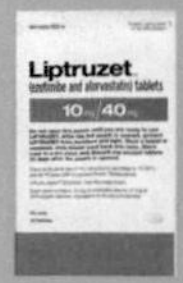

10 mg/40 mg

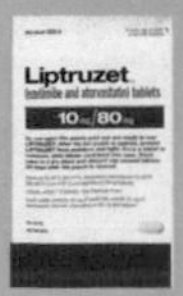

10 mg/80 mg

Liptruzet™
(ezetimibe and atorvastatin) tablets

RX MERCK P. 1633

266* 5 mg **267*** 10 mg

Maxalt®
(rizatriptan benzoate)

RX MERCK P. 1633

5 mg

10 mg
Orally Disintegrating Tablets

Maxalt-MLT®
(rizatriptan benzoate)

RX MERCK P. 1638

731* 20 mg **732*** 40 mg

Mevacor®
(lovastatin)

RX MERCK P. 1644

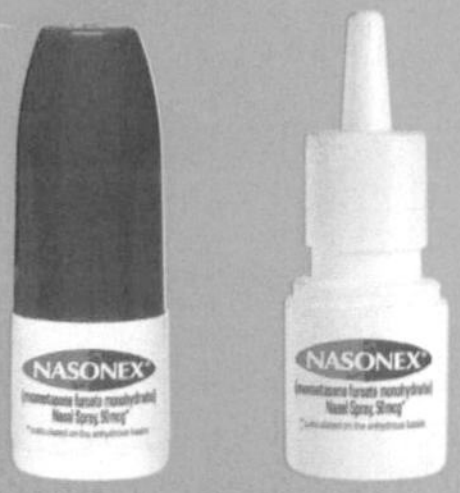

50 mcg/actuation
17 g, 120 metered sprays

Nasonex®
(mometasone furoate monohydrate)

RX MERCK P. 1657

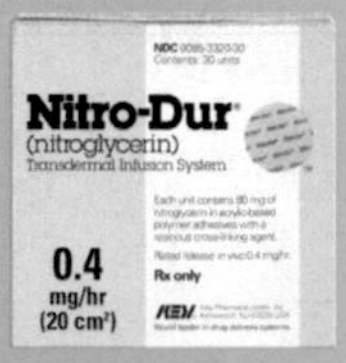

0.4 mg/hr

Also available in 0.1 mg/hr, 0.2 mg/hr, 0.3 mg/hr, 0.6 mg/hr, and 0.8 mg/hr

Nitro-Dur®
(nitroglycerin)
Transdermal Infusion System

RX MERCK P. 1660

705* 400 mg

Noroxin®
(norfloxacin)

RX MERCK P. 1674

delivers 0.120 mg/0.015 mg per day

NuvaRing®
(etonogestrel/ethinyl estradiol vaginal ring)

RX MERCK P. 1684

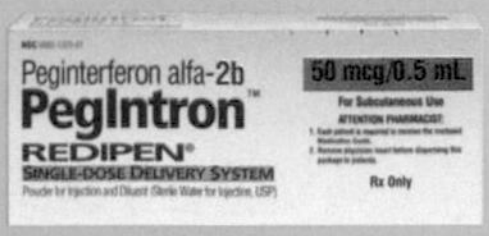

50 mcg/0.5 mL

Also available in 80 mcg/0.5 mL, 120 mcg/0.5 mL, and 150 mcg/0.5 mL

PegIntron®
(peginterferon alfa-2b)

RX MERCK P. 1709

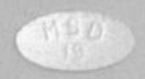

19* 5 mg

106* 10 mg

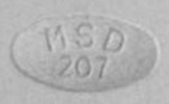

207* 20 mg

PRINIVIL®
(lisinopril) tablets

RX MERCK P. 1713

1 mg

Propecia®
(finasteride)

RX MERCK P. 1727

72* 5 mg

Proscar®
(finasteride)

RX MERCK P. 1736

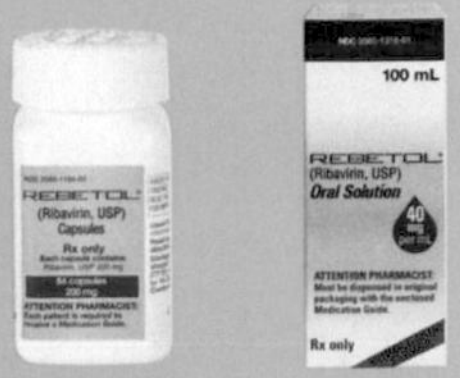

200 mg Capsules 40 mg/mL Oral Solution

Rebetol®
(ribavirin, USP)

*Manufacturer's Identification Code

RX MERCK P. 1752

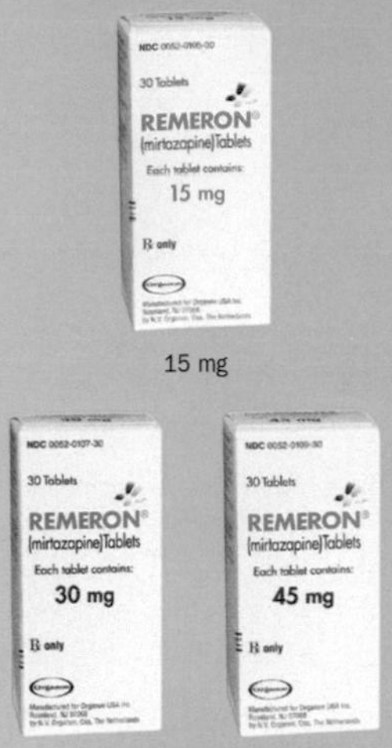

15 mg

30 mg 45 mg

REMERON®
(mirtazapine) Tablets

RX MERCK P. 1758

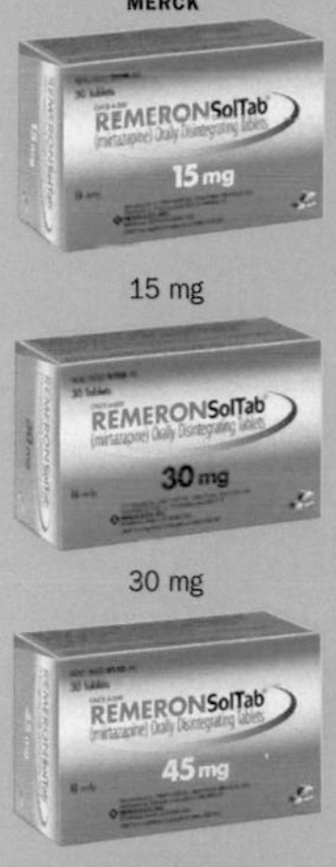

15 mg

30 mg

45 mg
Orally Disintegrating Tablets

REMERONSolTab®
(mirtazapine)

RX MERCK P. 1768

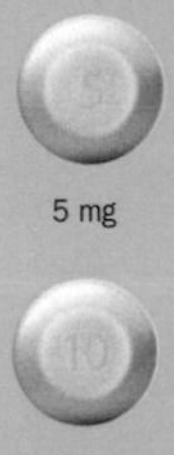

5 mg

10 mg

Saphris®
(asenapine) sublingual tablets

RX MERCK P. 1781

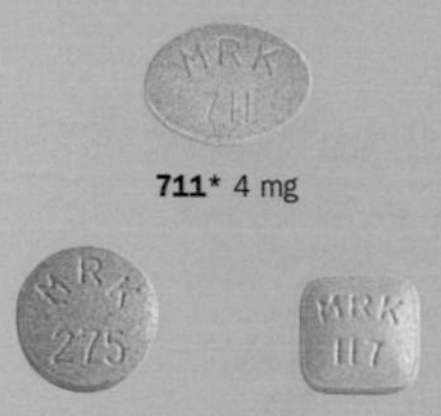

711* 4 mg

275* 5 mg **117*** 10 mg
Also available in 4 mg oral granules

†Singulair®
(montelukast sodium)

RX MERCK P. 1788

32* 3 mg

Stromectol®
(ivermectin)

RX MERCK P. 1796

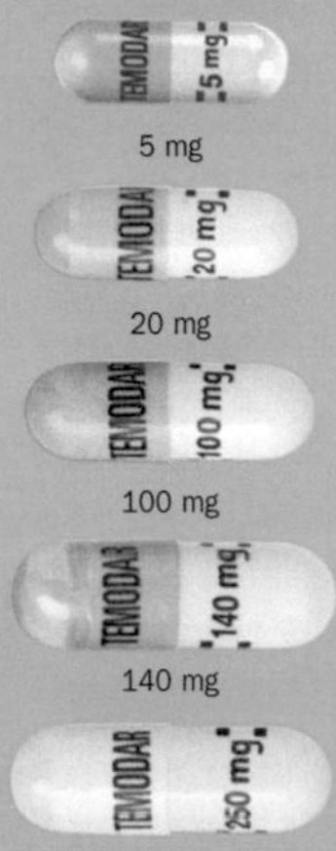

5 mg

20 mg

100 mg

140 mg

250 mg
Also available as 180 mg capsules and 100 mg vials for injection

Temodar®
(temozolomide)

RX MERCK P. 1805

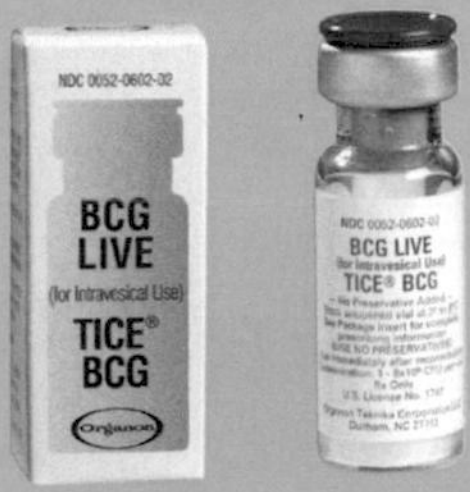

50 mL preservative-free saline

BCG LIVE
TICE® BCG
(for Intravesical Use)

RX MERCK P. 1819

200 mg

VICTRELIS®
(boceprevir) Capsules

RX MERCK P. 1831

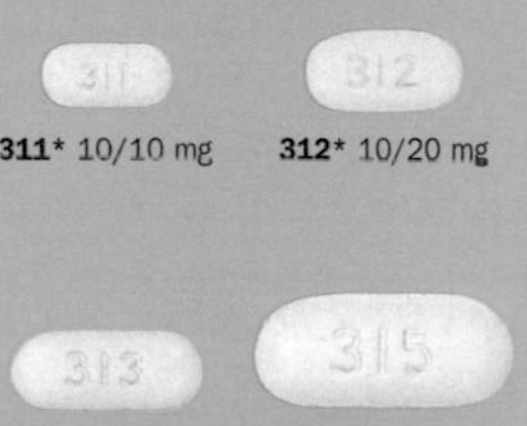

311* 10/10 mg **312*** 10/20 mg

313* 10/40 mg **315*** 10/80 mg

Vytorin®
(ezetimibe/simvastatin)

For the first time, the trusted *Physicians' Desk Reference®* is now available as a convenient eBook. Visit PDR.net to download your free copy today.

Register at PDR.net to receive free PDR® Drug Alerts, monthly eDrug Updates, and FDA-required Drug Safety Alerts via email from PDR Network.

RX MERCK P. 1842

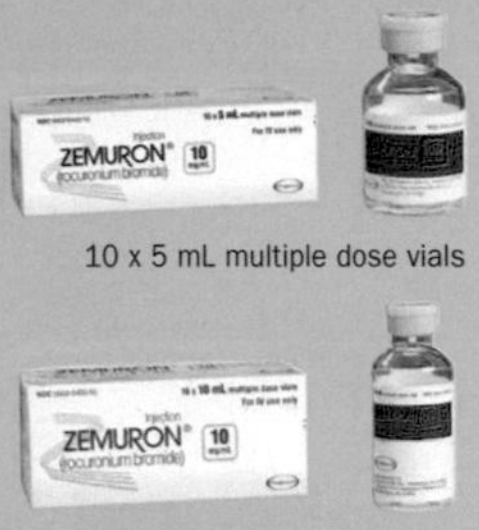

10 x 5 mL multiple dose vials

10 x 10 mL multiple dose vials
10 mg/mL

Zemuron® Injection
(rocuronium bromide)

RX MERCK P. 1848

414* 10 mg

Zetia®
(ezetimibe)

RX MERCK P. 1854

0.0015%
0.3 mL

ZIOPTAN™
(tafluprost ophthalmic solution)

RX MERCK P. 1857

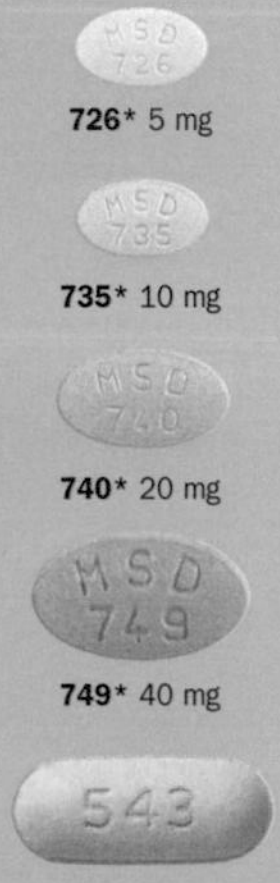

726* 5 mg

735* 10 mg

740* 20 mg

749* 40 mg

543* 80 mg

Zocor®
(simvastatin)

RX MERCK P. 1864

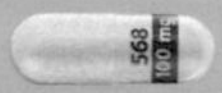

100 mg

Zolinza®
(vorinostat)

NEOPHARM CO., LTD

OTC NEOPHARM CO., LTD P. 1892

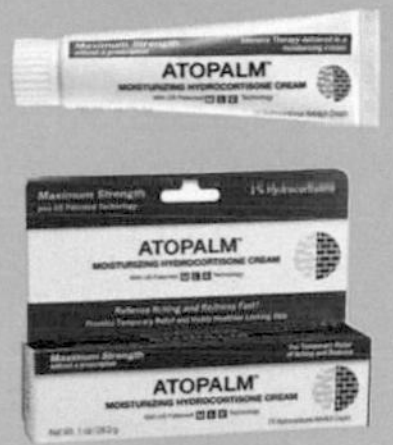

1%

ATOPALM™
(hydrocortisone)

OTC NEOPHARM CO., LTD P. 1893

2%

PSORIAPALM
(salicylic acid)

NOVARTIS PHARMACEUTICALS CORPORATION

RX NOVARTIS PHARMACEUTICALS CORPORATION P. 1893

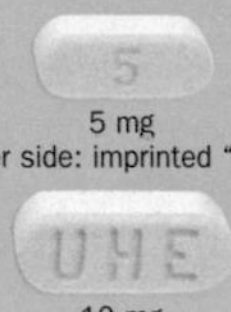

5 mg
Other side: imprinted "NVR"

10 mg
Other side: imprinted "NVR"
Also available in 2.5 mg and 7.5 mg

Afinitor®
(everolimus) Tablets

RX NOVARTIS PHARMACEUTICALS CORPORATION P. 1905

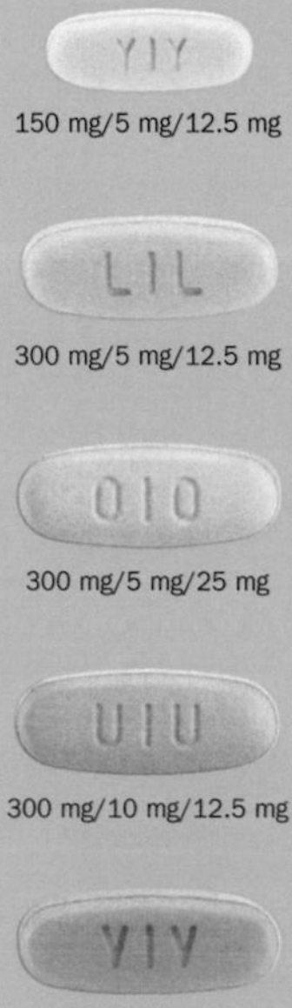

150 mg/5 mg/12.5 mg

300 mg/5 mg/12.5 mg

300 mg/5 mg/25 mg

300 mg/10 mg/12.5 mg

300 mg/10 mg/25 mg

Amturnide™
(aliskiren/amlodipine/
hydrochlorothiazide) Tablets

RX NOVARTIS PHARMACEUTICALS CORPORATION P. 1913

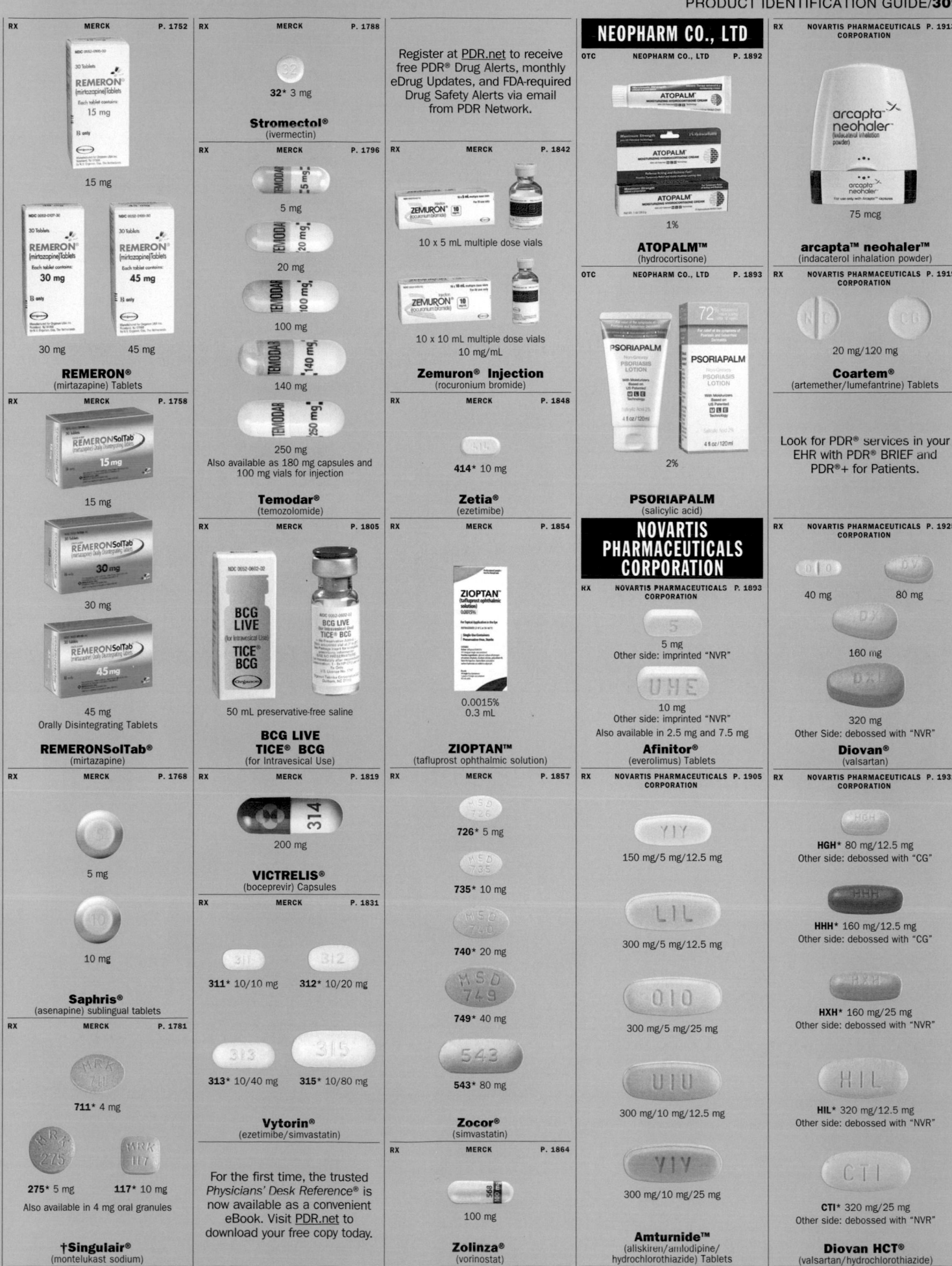

75 mcg

arcapta™ neohaler™
(indacaterol inhalation powder)

RX NOVARTIS PHARMACEUTICALS CORPORATION P. 1919

20 mg/120 mg

Coartem®
(artemether/lumefantrine) Tablets

Look for PDR® services in your EHR with PDR® BRIEF and PDR®+ for Patients.

RX NOVARTIS PHARMACEUTICALS CORPORATION P. 1925

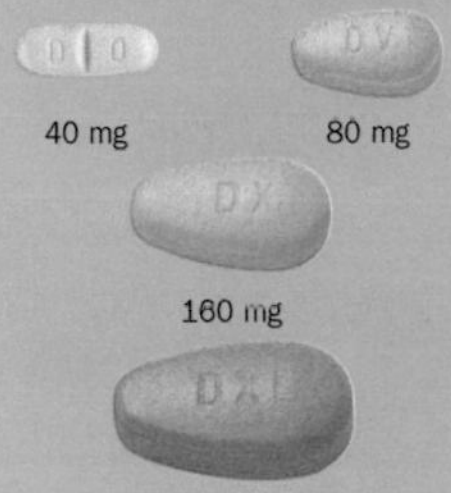

40 mg 80 mg

160 mg

320 mg
Other Side: debossed with "NVR"

Diovan®
(valsartan)

RX NOVARTIS PHARMACEUTICALS CORPORATION P. 1931

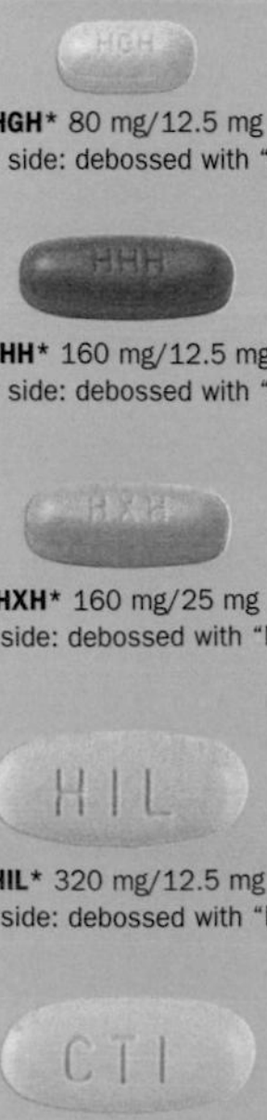

HGH* 80 mg/12.5 mg
Other side: debossed with "CG"

HHH* 160 mg/12.5 mg
Other side: debossed with "CG"

HXH* 160 mg/25 mg
Other side: debossed with "NVR"

HIL* 320 mg/12.5 mg
Other side: debossed with "NVR"

CTI* 320 mg/25 mg
Other side: debossed with "NVR"

Diovan HCT®
(valsartan/hydrochlorothiazide)

*Manufacturer's Identification Code

†Additional dosage forms and sizes available

RX NOVARTIS PHARMACEUTICALS CORPORATION P. 1937

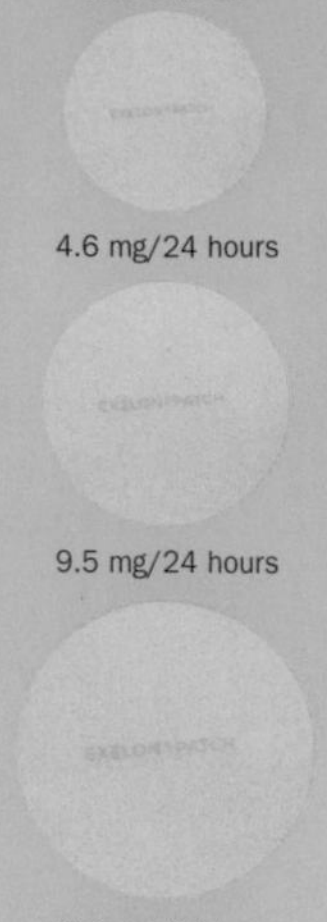

4.6 mg/24 hours

9.5 mg/24 hours

13.3 mg/24 hours

Patches not actual size

Exelon® Patch
(rivastigmine transdermal system)

RX NOVARTIS PHARMACEUTICALS CORPORATION P. 1944

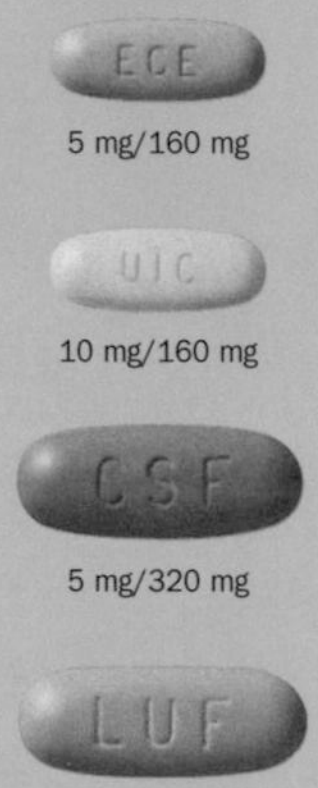

5 mg/160 mg

10 mg/160 mg

5 mg/320 mg

10 mg/320 mg

Exforge®
(amlodipine/valsartan) Tablets

RX NOVARTIS PHARMACEUTICALS CORPORATION P. 1951

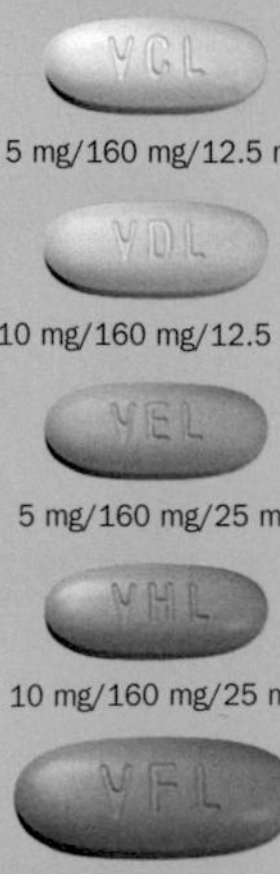

5 mg/160 mg/12.5 mg

10 mg/160 mg/12.5 mg

5 mg/160 mg/25 mg

10 mg/160 mg/25 mg

10 mg/320 mg/25 mg

Exforge HCT®
(amlodipine/valsartan/hydrochlorothiazide) Tablets

While every effort has been made to reproduce products faithfully, this section is to be considered a quick reference identification aid. In cases of suspected overdosing, etc., chemical analysis should be done.

RX NOVARTIS PHARMACEUTICALS CORPORATION P. 1958

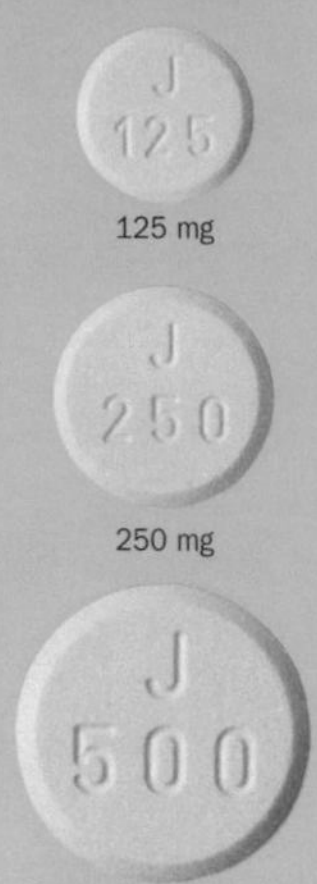

125 mg

250 mg

500 mg

Exjade®
(deferasirox)
Tablets for Oral Suspension

RX NOVARTIS PHARMACEUTICALS CORPORATION P. 1971

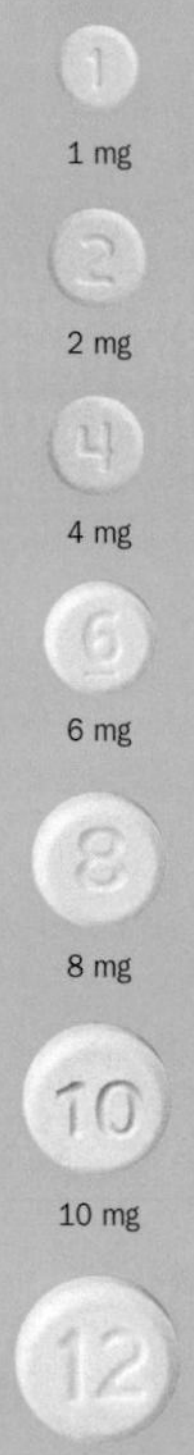

1 mg

2 mg

4 mg

6 mg

8 mg

10 mg

12 mg

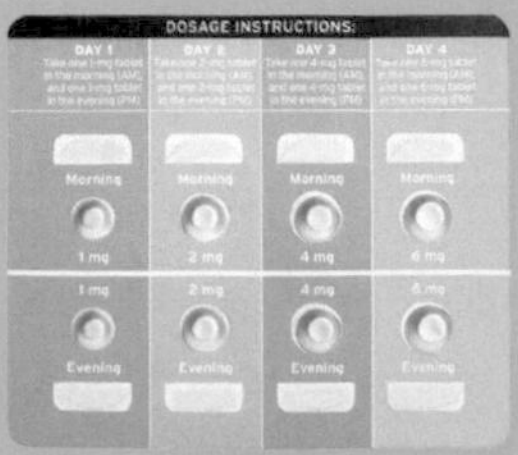

Titration Pack

Fanapt®
(iloperidone) Tablets

RX NOVARTIS PHARMACEUTICALS CORPORATION P. 1977

FV* 2.5 mg
Other side: imprinted "CG"

Femara®
(letrozole)

Products in this section are arranged alphabetically by manufacturer. In some instances, not all dosage forms and/or sizes are pictured. If others are available, a † symbol precedes the product's name. Letters or numbers representing the manufacturer's identification code are followed by a * symbol.

C-II NOVARTIS PHARMACEUTICALS CORPORATION P. 1984

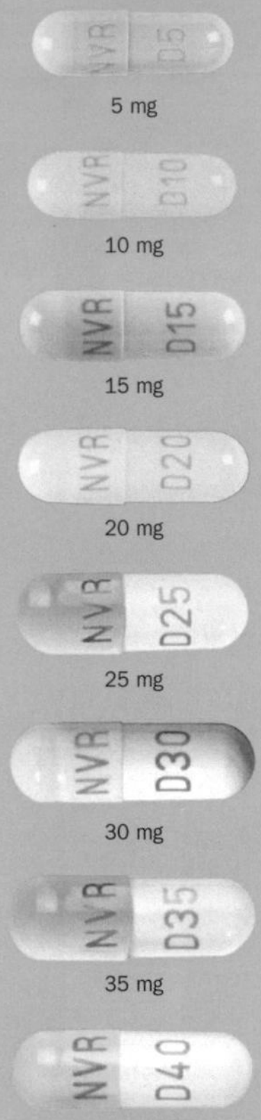

5 mg

10 mg

15 mg

20 mg

25 mg

30 mg

35 mg

40 mg

Extended-Release Capsules

Focalin® XR
(dexmethylphenidate HCl)

RX NOVARTIS PHARMACEUTICALS CORPORATION P. 1989

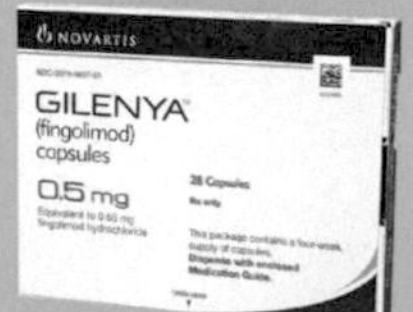

0.5 mg

Gilenya™
(fingolimod) Capsules

RX NOVARTIS PHARMACEUTICALS CORPORATION P. 1995

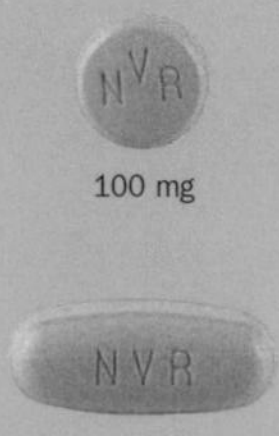

100 mg

400 mg

Gleevec®
(imatinib mesylate)

RX NOVARTIS PHARMACEUTICALS CORPORATION P. 2007

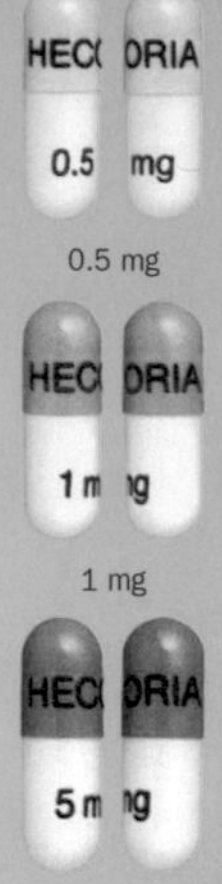

0.5 mg

1 mg

5 mg

Hecoria™
(tacrolimus capsules, USP)

RX NOVARTIS PHARMACEUTICALS CORPORATION P. 2019

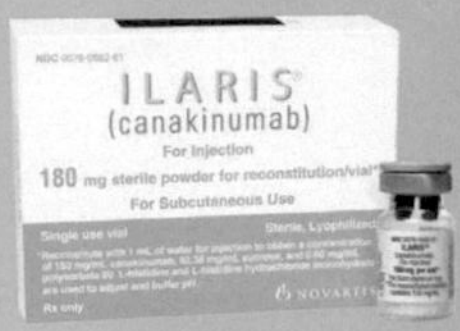

180 mg

Ilaris®
(canakinumab)

RX NOVARTIS PHARMACEUTICALS CORPORATION P. 2024

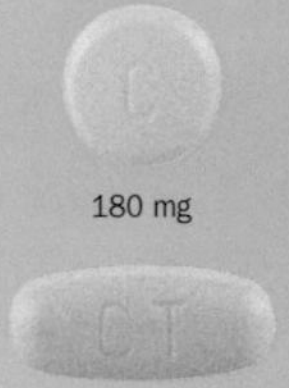

180 mg

360 mg

Myfortic®
(mycophenolic acid*)
delayed-release tablets
*as mycophenolate sodium

The pictured forms shown in this section may not necessarily be the only dosage forms and/or sizes available. Where a product name is preceded by a † symbol, refer to the description in the Product Information Section for other dosage forms and/or sizes.

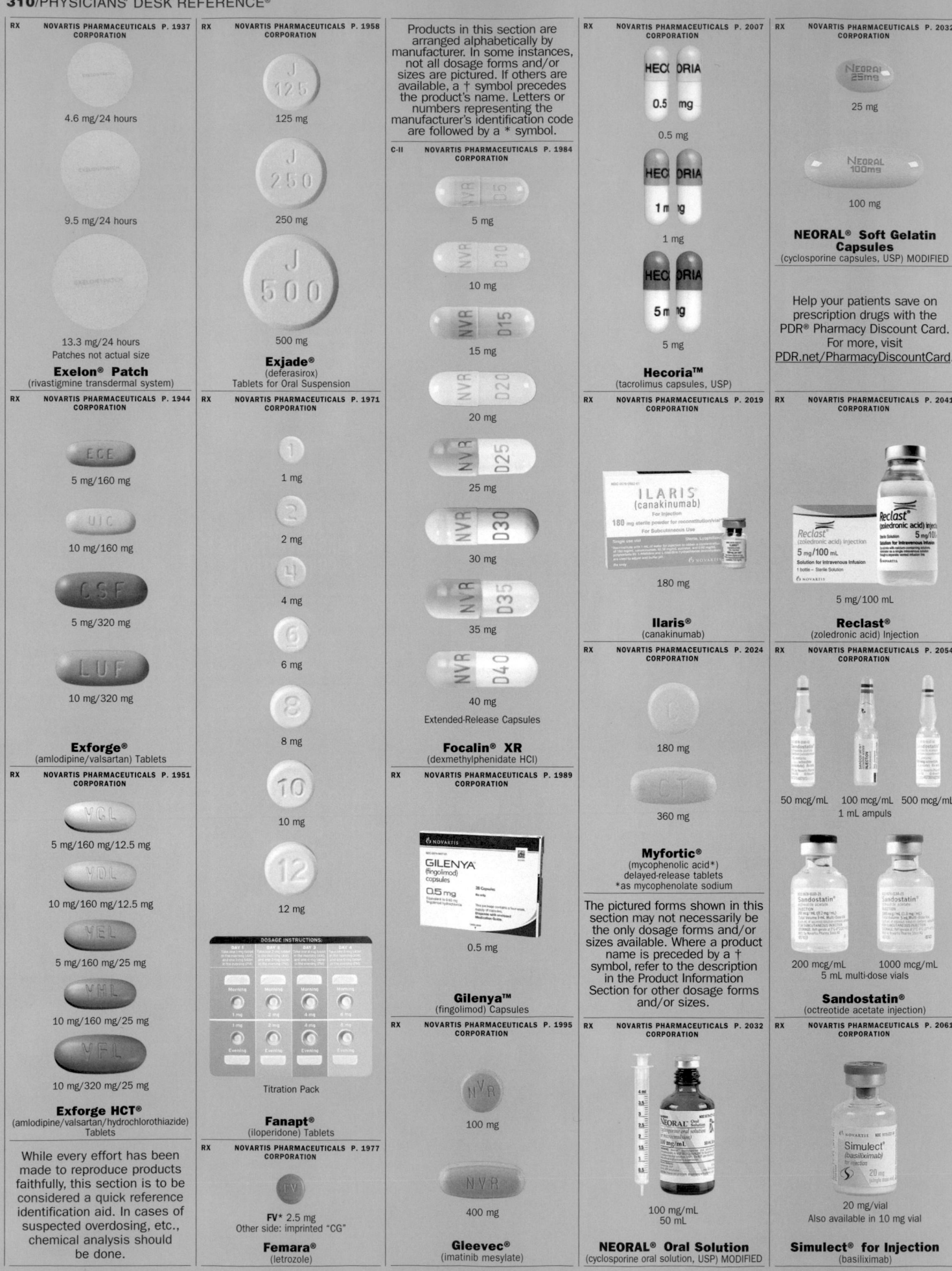

RX NOVARTIS PHARMACEUTICALS CORPORATION P. 2032

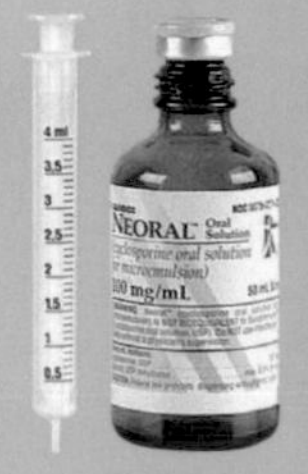

100 mg/mL
50 mL

NEORAL® Oral Solution
(cyclosporine oral solution, USP) MODIFIED

RX NOVARTIS PHARMACEUTICALS CORPORATION P. 2032

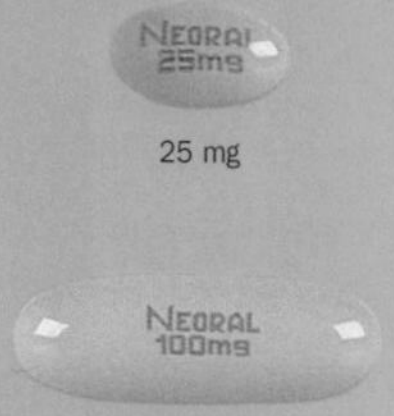

25 mg

100 mg

NEORAL® Soft Gelatin Capsules
(cyclosporine capsules, USP) MODIFIED

Help your patients save on prescription drugs with the PDR® Pharmacy Discount Card. For more, visit PDR.net/PharmacyDiscountCard.

RX NOVARTIS PHARMACEUTICALS CORPORATION P. 2041

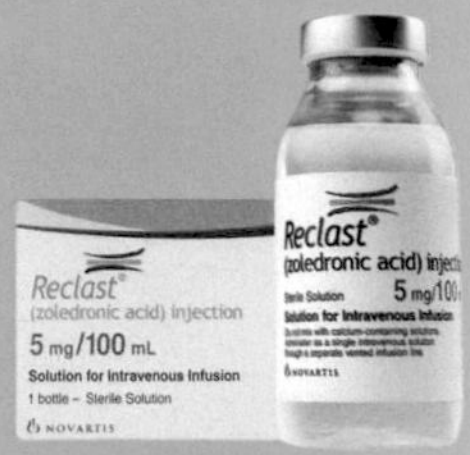

5 mg/100 mL

Reclast®
(zoledronic acid) Injection

RX NOVARTIS PHARMACEUTICALS CORPORATION P. 2054

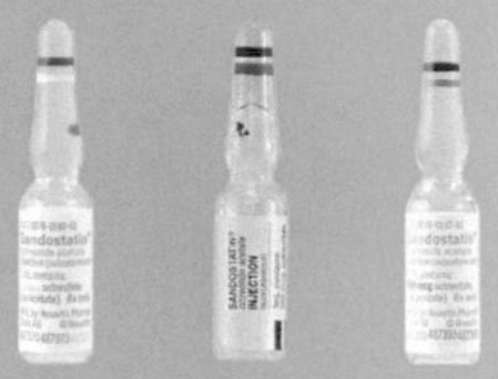

50 mcg/mL 100 mcg/mL 500 mcg/mL
1 mL ampuls

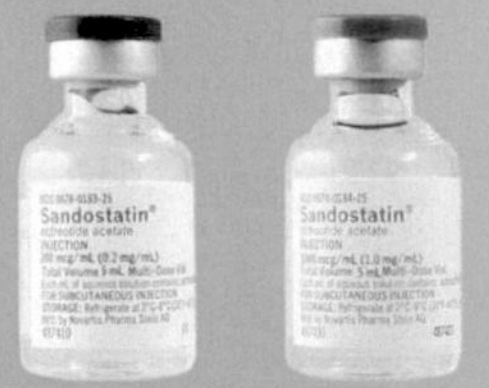

200 mcg/mL 1000 mcg/mL
5 mL multi-dose vials

Sandostatin®
(octreotide acetate injection)

RX NOVARTIS PHARMACEUTICALS CORPORATION P. 2061

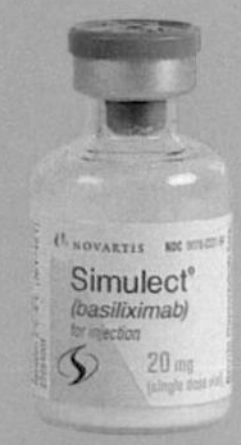

20 mg/vial
Also available in 10 mg vial

Simulect® for Injection
(basiliximab)

RX NOVARTIS PHARMACEUTICALS CORPORATION P. 2056

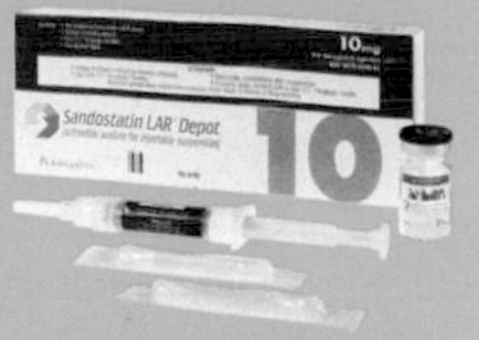

10 mg/vial

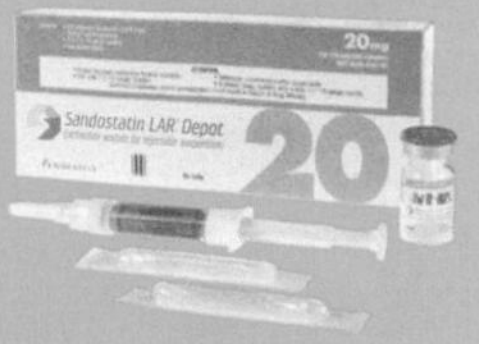

20 mg/vial

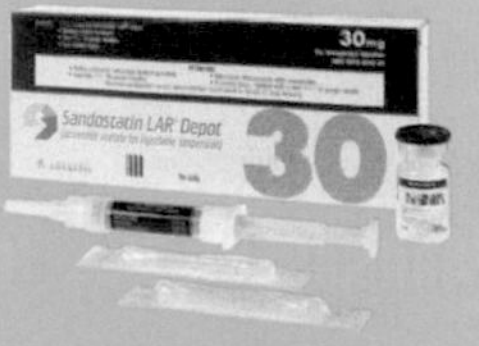

30 mg/vial

Sandostatin® LAR Depot
(octreotide acetate for injectable suspension)

RX NOVARTIS PHARMACEUTICALS CORPORATION P. 2064

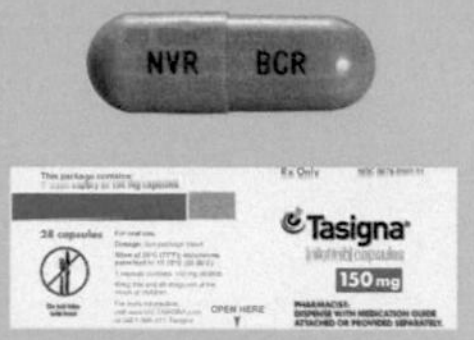

150 mg

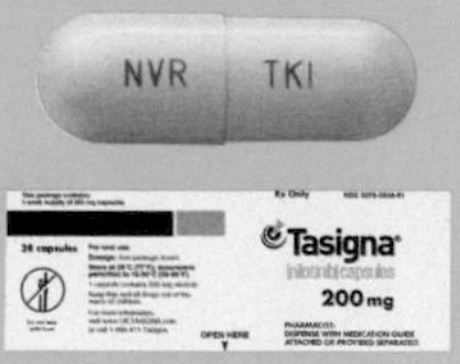

200 mg

Tasigna®
(nilotinib) Capsules

RX NOVARTIS PHARMACEUTICALS CORPORATION P. 2071

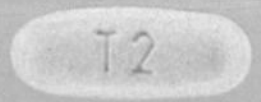

150 mg/5 mg

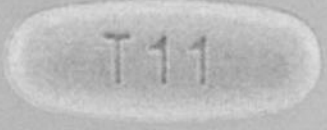

300 mg/5 mg

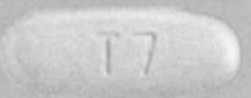

150 mg/10 mg

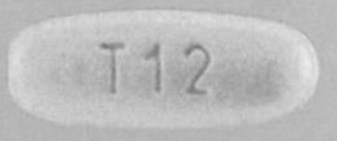

300 mg/10 mg

Tekamlo™
(aliskiren/amlodipine) Tablets

RX NOVARTIS PHARMACEUTICALS CORPORATION P. 2078

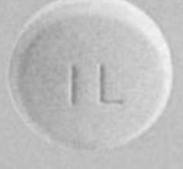

150 mg

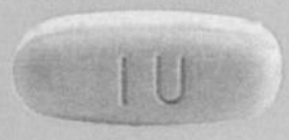

300 mg

Tekturna®
(aliskiren) Tablets

RX NOVARTIS PHARMACEUTICALS CORPORATION P. 2083

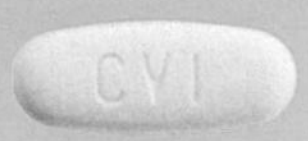

300 mg/12.5 mg

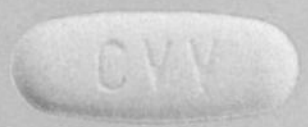

300 mg/25 mg

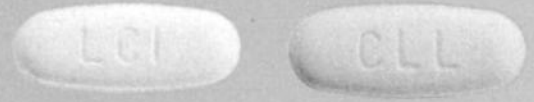

150 mg/12.5 mg 150 mg/25 mg

Tekturna HCT®
(aliskiren/hydrochlorothiazide) Tablets

RX NOVARTIS PHARMACEUTICALS CORPORATION P. 2090

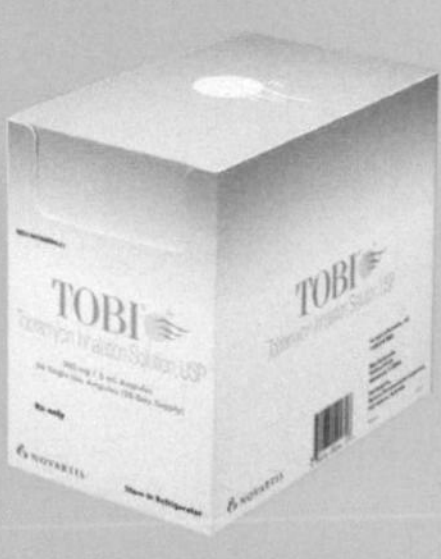

300 mg/5 mL ampules

TOBI®
(tobramycin inhalation solution)

RX NOVARTIS PHARMACEUTICALS CORPORATION P. 2093

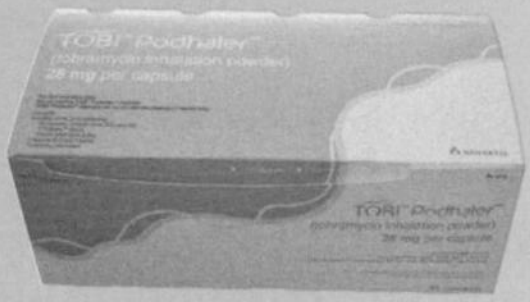

28 mg per capsule
112 mg per dose

TOBI® Podhaler™
(tobramycin inhalation powder)

RX NOVARTIS PHARMACEUTICALS CORPORATION/ GENENTECH USA P. 2098

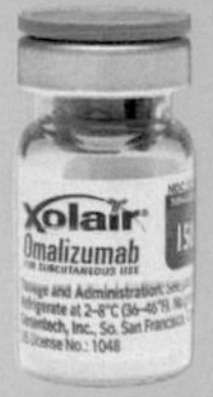

150 mg/5 mL single-use vial

XOLAIR®
(omalizumab) Injection

RX NOVARTIS PHARMACEUTICALS CORPORATION P. 2103

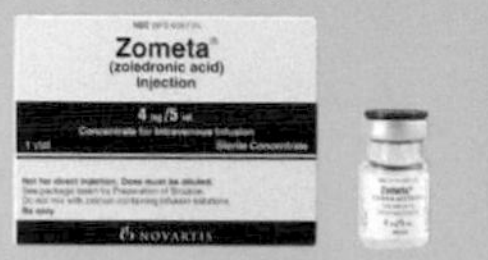

4 mg/5 mL single-use vial of concentrate

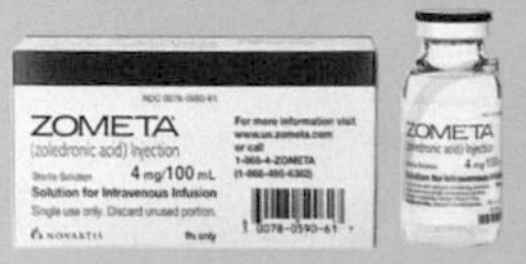

4 mg/100 mL single-use ready-to-use bottle

ZOMETA®
(zoledronic acid) Injection

RX NOVARTIS PHARMACEUTICALS CORPORATION P. 2109

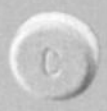

0.25 mg

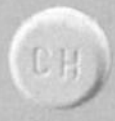

0.5 mg

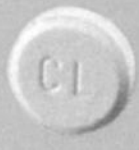

0.75 mg

Zortress®
(everolimus) Tablets

NOVO NORDISK

RX NOVO NORDISK P. 2145

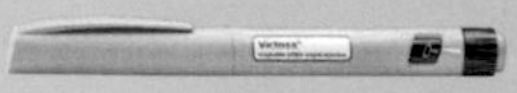

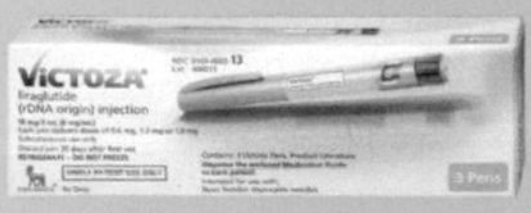

6 mg/mL

Victoza®
(liraglutide [rDNA origin] injection)

ONYX PHARMACEUTICALS, INC.

RX ONYX PHARMACEUTICALS, INC P. 2156

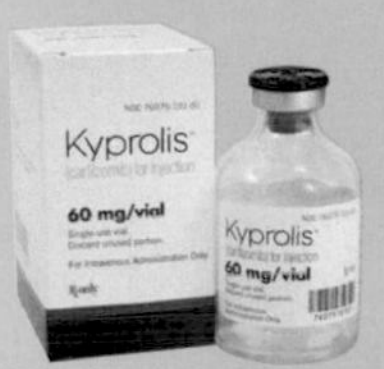

60 mg/vial

Kyprolis™
(carfilzomib) for Injection

OTSUKA AMERICA PHARMACEUTICAL, INC.

RX OTSUKA AMERICA PHARMACEUTICAL, INC. P. 2184

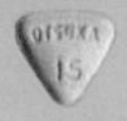

15 mg

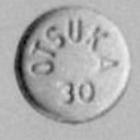

30 mg

SAMSCA®
(tolvaptan) tablets

PBM PHARMACEUTICALS

RX PBM PHARMACEUTICALS P. 2189

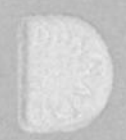

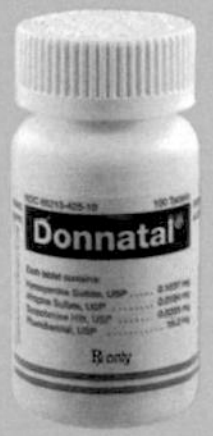

0.1037 mg/0.0194 mg/
0.0065 mg/16.2 mg

Donnatal®
(hyoscyamine sulfate/atropine sulfate/ scopolamine HBr/phenobarbital) tablets

PIVOTAL THERAPEUTICS INC.

RX PIVOTAL THERAPEUTICS INC. P. 2202

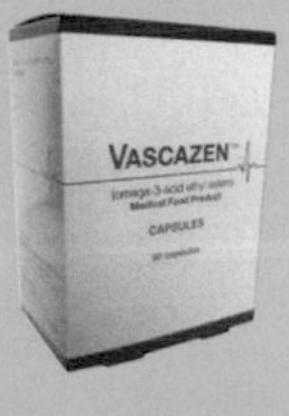

VASCAZEN®
(omega-3-acid ethyl esters) capsules

PRESTIUM PHARMA, INC.

RX PRESTIUM PHARMA, INC. P. 2203

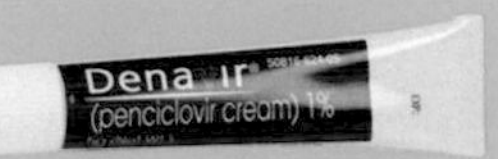

10 mg/g
1%
Available in 1.5 g and 5 g tubes

Denavir®
(penciclovir) cream

RX PRESTIUM PHARMA, INC. P. 2204

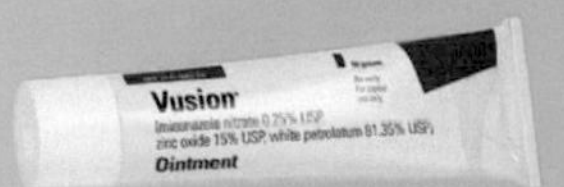

50 g
0.25%/15%/81.35%

Vusion®
(miconazole nitrate/zinc oxide/ white petrolatum) ointment

PURDUE PHARMA L.P.

C-III PURDUE PHARMA L.P. P. 2206

5 mcg/hour

10 mcg/hour

15 mcg/hour

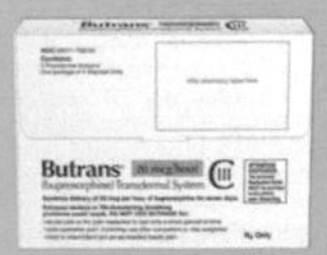

20 mcg/hour

Butrans®
(buprenorphine) Transdermal System

C-II PURDUE PHARMA L.P. P. 2215

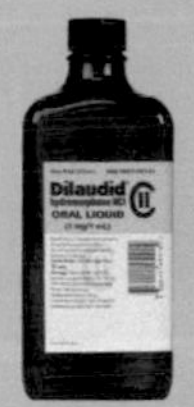

1 mg/1 mL

Dilaudid® Oral Liquid
(hydromorphone HCl)

C-II PURDUE PHARMA L.P. P. 2215

2 mg

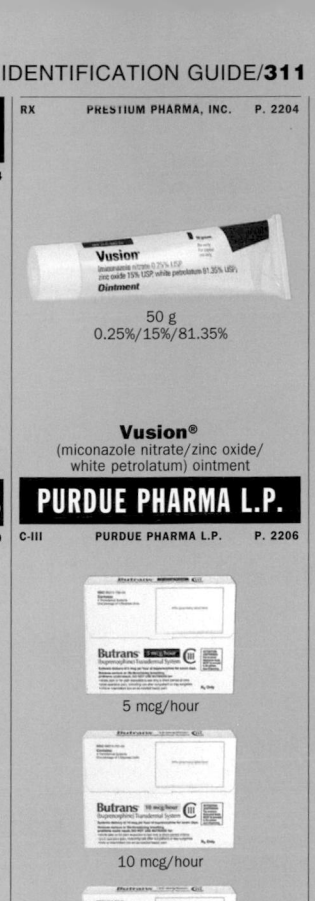

4 mg

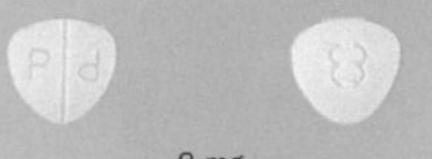

8 mg

Dilaudid® Tablets
(hydromorphone HCl)

C-II PURDUE PHARMA L.P. P. 2217

1 mg/mL

2 mg/mL

4 mg/mL

Dilaudid® Injection
(hydromorphone HCl)

C-II PURDUE PHARMA L.P. P. 2217

10 mg/mL

50 mg/5 mL

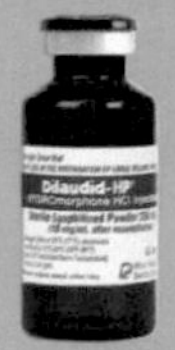

250 mg

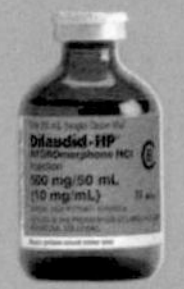

500 mg/50 mL

Dilaudid-HP® Injection
(hydromorphone HCl)

C-IV PURDUE PHARMA L.P. P. 2222

1.75 mg

3.5 mg

Intermezzo®
(zolpidem tartrate) sublingual tablet

While every effort has been made to reproduce products faithfully, this section is to be considered a quick reference identification aid. In cases of suspected overdosing, etc., chemical analysis should be done.

C-II PURDUE PHARMA L.P. P. 2227

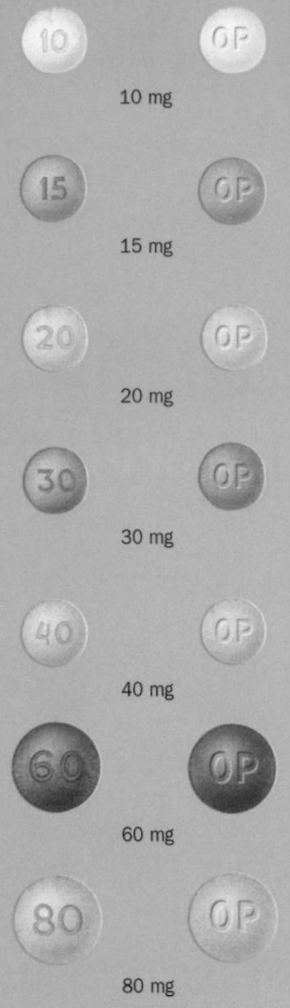

10 mg

15 mg

20 mg

30 mg

40 mg

60 mg

80 mg

Controlled-Release Tablets

OxyContin®
(oxycodone HCl controlled-release) Tablets

RANBAXY LABORATORIES INC.

RX RANBAXY LABORATORIES INC. P. 2234

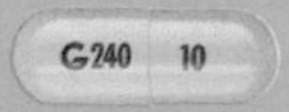

10 mg

20 mg

30 mg

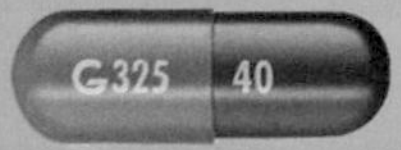

40 mg

ABSORICA™
(isotretinoin) capsules

RECORDATI RARE DISEASES INC.

RX RECORDATI RARE DISEASES INC. P. 2243

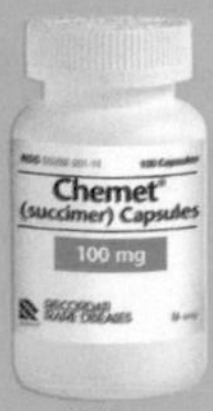

100 mg

Chemet®
(succimer) capsules

RX RECORDATI RARE DISEASES INC. P. 2244

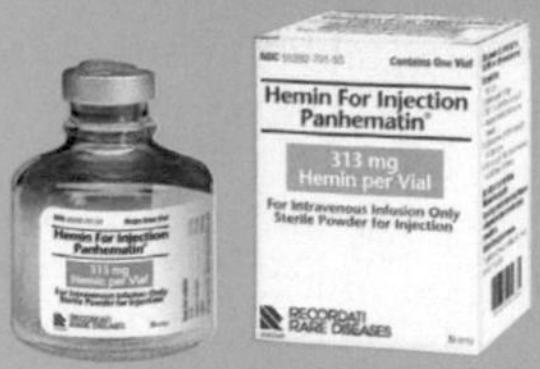

313 mg
Hemin per Vial

Panhematin®
(hemin for injection)

RLC LABS, INC.

RX RLC LABS, INC. P. 2255

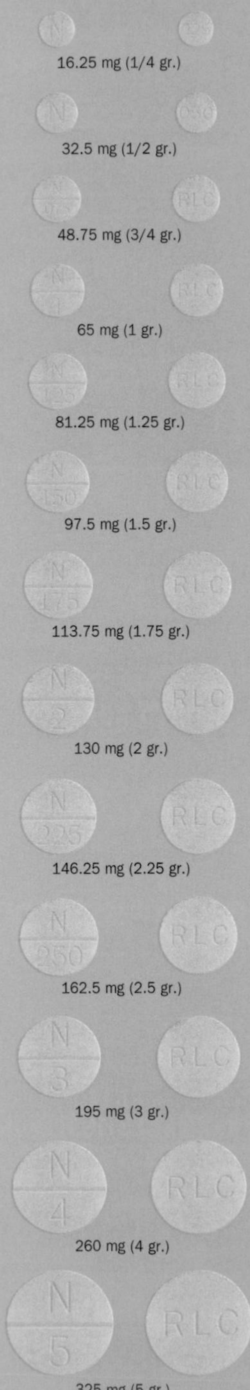

16.25 mg (1/4 gr.)

32.5 mg (1/2 gr.)

48.75 mg (3/4 gr.)

65 mg (1 gr.)

81.25 mg (1.25 gr.)

97.5 mg (1.5 gr.)

113.75 mg (1.75 gr.)

130 mg (2 gr.)

146.25 mg (2.25 gr.)

162.5 mg (2.5 gr.)

195 mg (3 gr.)

260 mg (4 gr.)

325 mg (5 gr.)

Nature-Throid®
(Thyroid USP) tablets

RX RLC LABS, INC. P. 2257

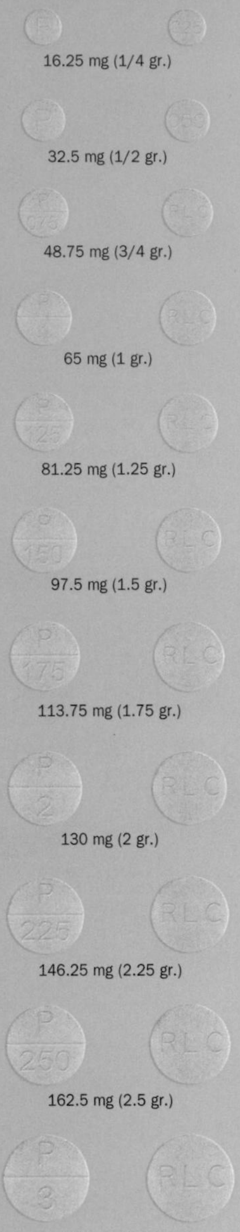

16.25 mg (1/4 gr.)

32.5 mg (1/2 gr.)

48.75 mg (3/4 gr.)

65 mg (1 gr.)

81.25 mg (1.25 gr.)

97.5 mg (1.5 gr.)

113.75 mg (1.75 gr.)

130 mg (2 gr.)

146.25 mg (2.25 gr.)

162.5 mg (2.5 gr.)

195 mg (3 gr.)

WP Thyroid®
(Thyroid USP) tablets

Products in this section are arranged alphabetically by manufacturer. In some instances, not all dosage forms and/or sizes are pictured. If others are available, a † symbol precedes the product's name. Letters or numbers representing the manufacturer's identification code are followed by a * symbol.

REGENERON PHARMACEUTICALS, INC.

RX REGENERON PHARMACEUTICALS, INC. P. 2245

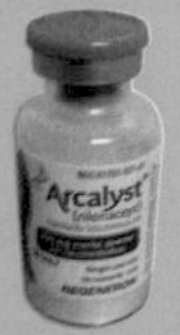

220 mg/20 mL vial
Single-Use Vial

ARCALYST®
(rilonacept) Injection
for Subcutaneous Use

RX REGENERON PHARMACEUTICALS, INC. P. 2251

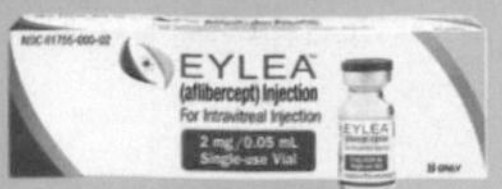

2 mg/0.05 mL vial
Single-Use Vial

EYLEA®
(aflibercept) Injection
for Intravitreal Injection

The pictured forms shown in this section may not necessarily be the only dosage forms and/or sizes available. Where a product name is preceded by a † symbol, refer to the description in the Product Information Section for other dosage forms and/or sizes.

SALIX PHARMACEUTICALS, INC.

RX SALIX PHARMACEUTICALS, INC. P. 2259

0.375 g

Apriso™
(mesalamine)
Extended-Release Capsules

RX SALIX PHARMACEUTICALS, INC. P. 2261

125 mg

Fulyzaq™
(crofelemer)
Delayed-Release Tablets

RX SALIX PHARMACEUTICALS, INC. P. 2263

MoviPrep®
(PEG-3350, sodium sulfate, sodium chloride, potassium chloride, sodium ascorbate and ascorbic acid for oral solution)

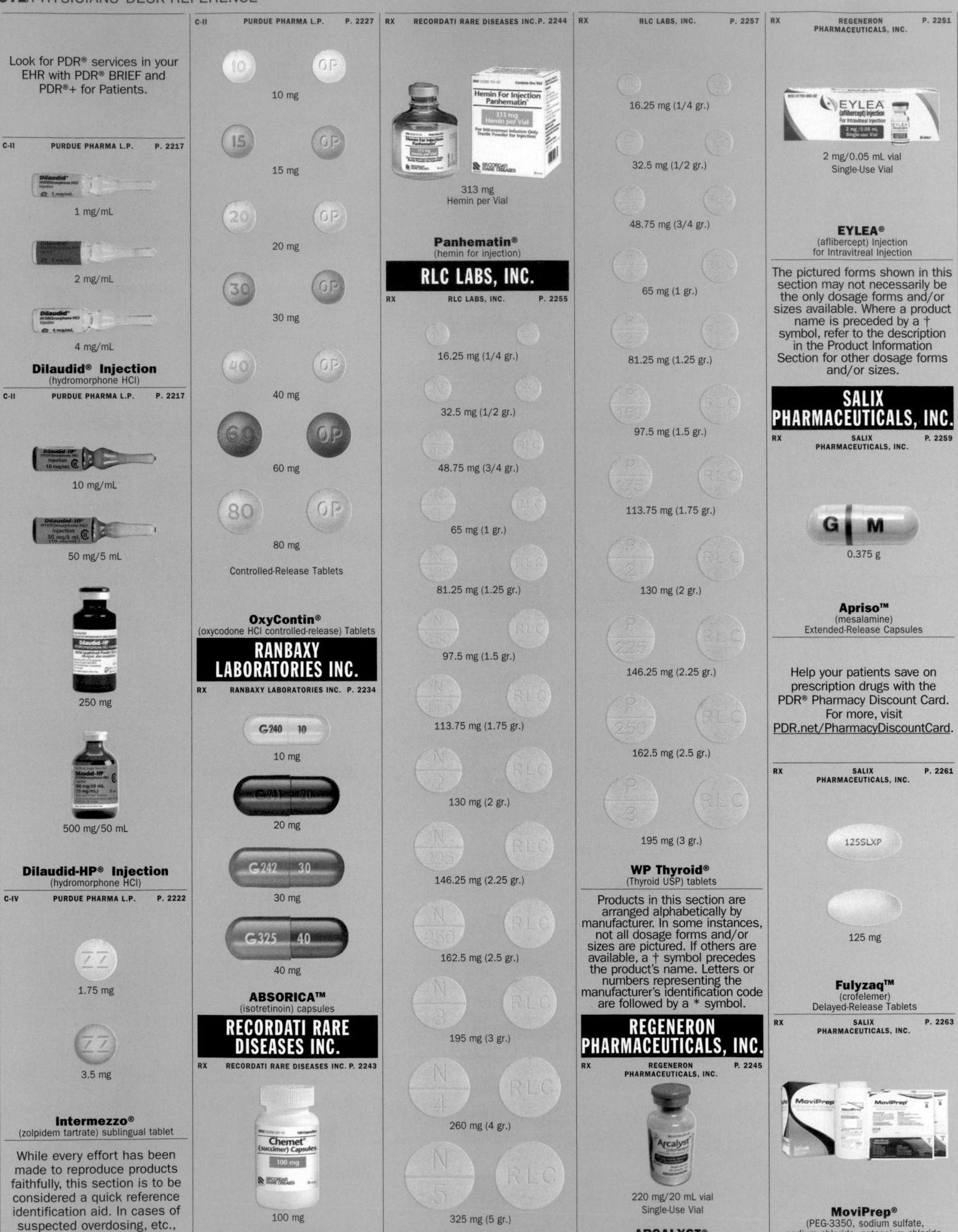

RX SALIX PHARMACEUTICALS, INC. P. 2266

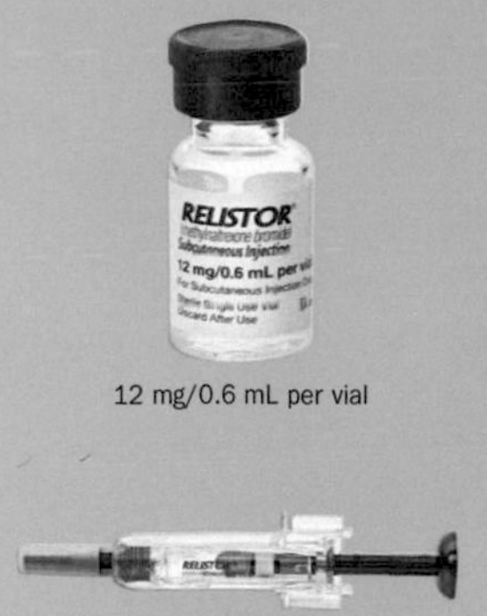

12 mg/0.6 mL per vial

12 mg/0.6 mL per syringe

Also available in 8 mg/0.4 mL per syringe

Relistor®
(methylnaltrexone bromide)
Subcutaneous Injection

RX SALIX PHARMACEUTICALS, INC. P. 2279

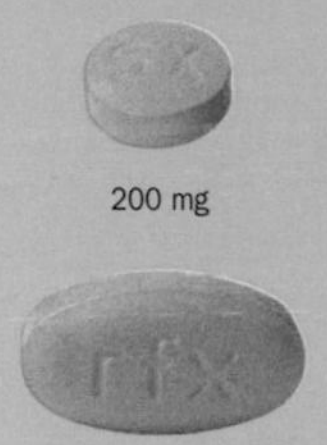

200 mg

550 mg

Xifaxan®
(rifaximin) Tablets

SMITH & NEPHEW

RX SMITH & NEPHEW P. 2283

0.01 %

REGRANEX® Gel
(becaplermin)

RX SMITH & NEPHEW P. 2283

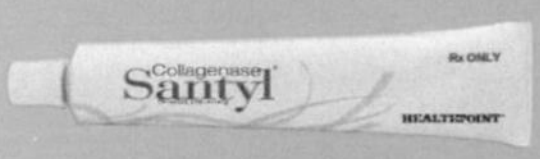

30 g

SANTYL® Ointment
(collagenase)

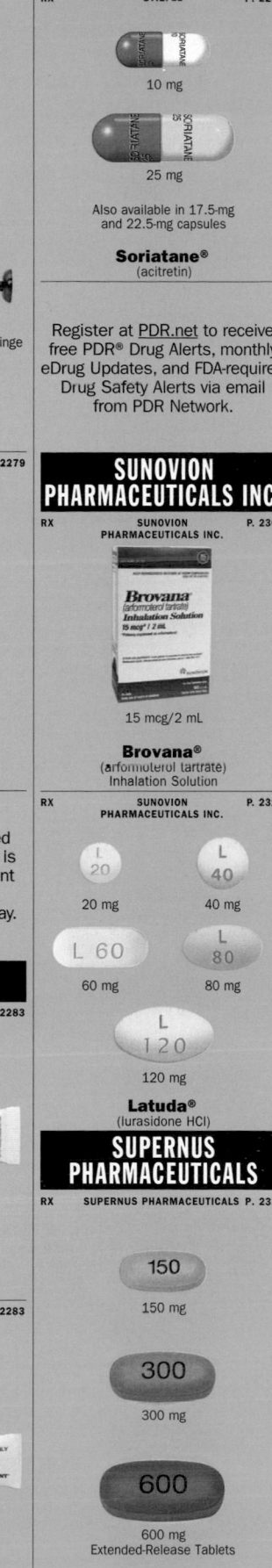

STIEFEL

RX STIEFEL P. 2296

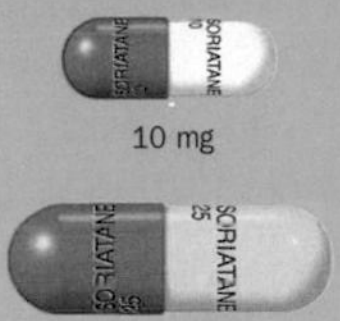

10 mg

25 mg

Also available in 17.5-mg and 22.5-mg capsules

Soriatane®
(acitretin)

SUNOVION PHARMACEUTICALS INC.

RX SUNOVION PHARMACEUTICALS INC. P. 2309

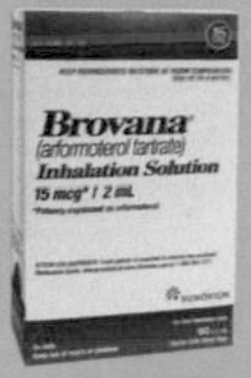

15 mcg/2 mL

Brovana®
(arformoterol tartrate)
Inhalation Solution

RX SUNOVION PHARMACEUTICALS INC. P. 2315

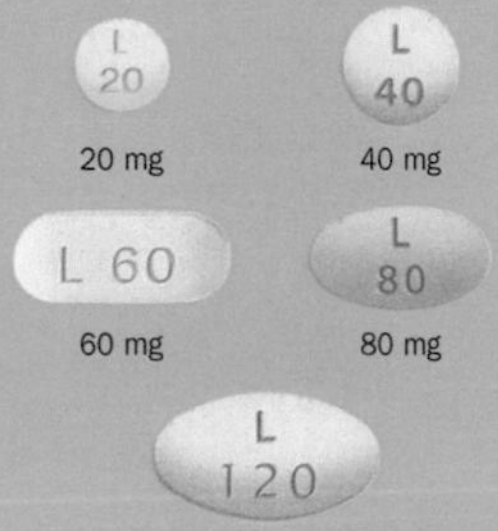

20 mg 40 mg

60 mg 80 mg

120 mg

Latuda®
(lurasidone HCl)

SUPERNUS PHARMACEUTICALS

RX SUPERNUS PHARMACEUTICALS P. 2327

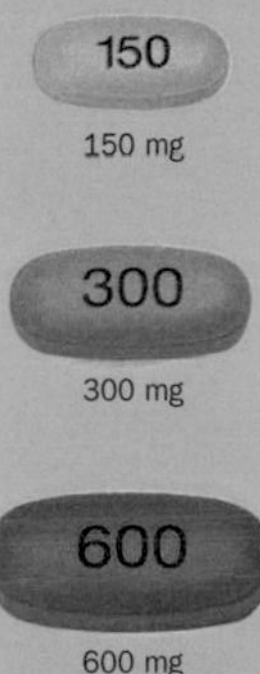

150 mg

300 mg

600 mg
Extended-Release Tablets

Oxtellar XR™
(oxcarbazepine)

RX SUPERNUS PHARMACEUTICALS P. 2334

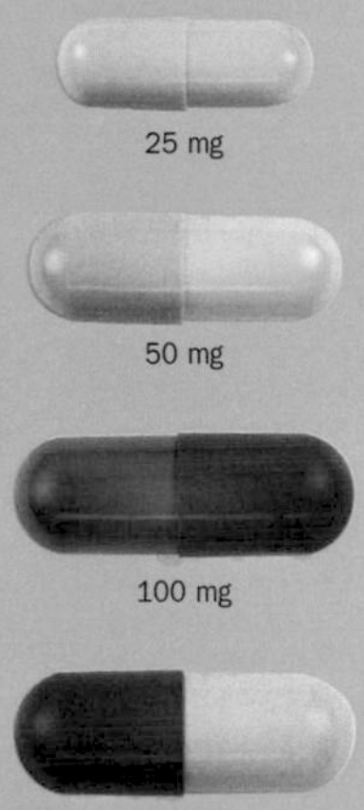

25 mg

50 mg

100 mg

200 mg
Extended-Release Capsules

Trokendi XR™
(topiramate)

SYNERGY WORLDWIDE, INC.

DS SYNERGY WORLDWIDE, INC. P. 2571

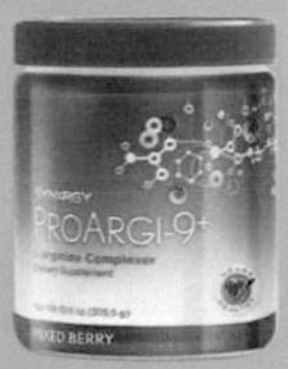

ProArgi-9+
(l-arginine complexer)

TAKEDA PHARMACEUTICALS

RX TAKEDA PHARMACEUTICALS P. 2347

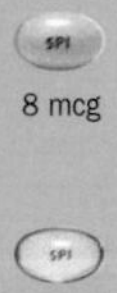

8 mcg

24 mcg

Amitiza®
(lubiprostone)

RX TAKEDA PHARMACEUTICALS P. 2359

0.6 mg

Colcrys®
(colchicine, USP) tablets

While every effort has been made to reproduce products faithfully, this section is to be considered a quick reference identification aid. In cases of suspected overdosing, etc., chemical analysis should be done.

RX TAKEDA PHARMACEUTICALS P. 2365

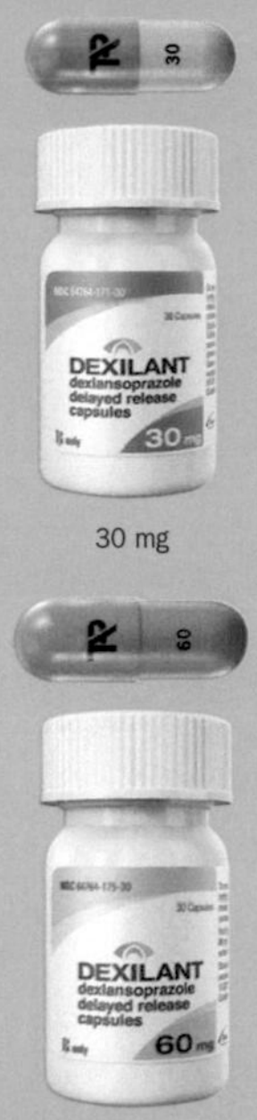

30 mg

60 mg
Delayed-Release Capsules

DEXILANT™
(dexlansoprazole)

RX TAKEDA PHARMACEUTICALS P. 2370

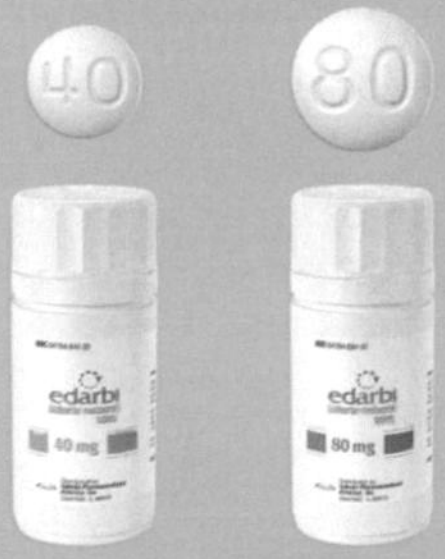

40 mg 80 mg

edarbi®
(azilsartan medoxomil) tablets

RX TAKEDA PHARMACEUTICALS P. 2374

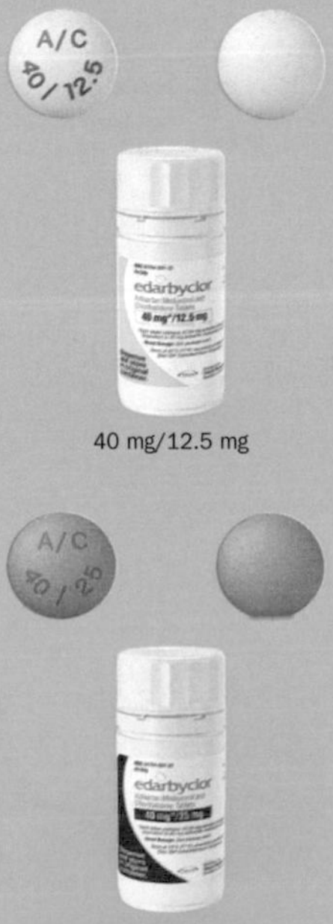

40 mg/12.5 mg

40 mg/25 mg

edarbyclor
(azilsartan medoxomil and chlorthalidone) tablets

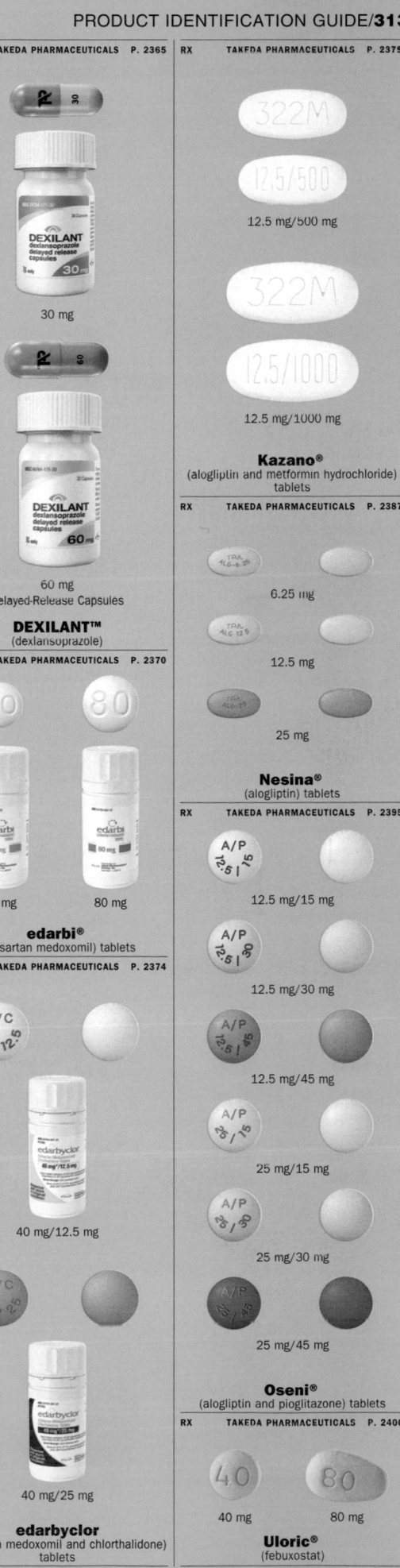

RX TAKEDA PHARMACEUTICALS P. 2379

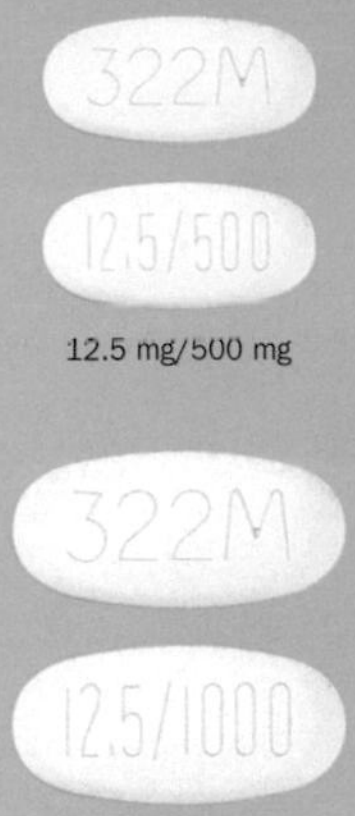

12.5 mg/500 mg

12.5 mg/1000 mg

Kazano®
(alogliptin and metformin hydrochloride) tablets

RX TAKEDA PHARMACEUTICALS P. 2387

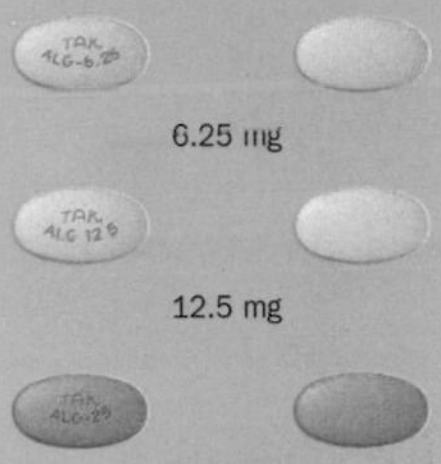

6.25 mg

12.5 mg

25 mg

Nesina®
(alogliptin) tablets

RX TAKEDA PHARMACEUTICALS P. 2395

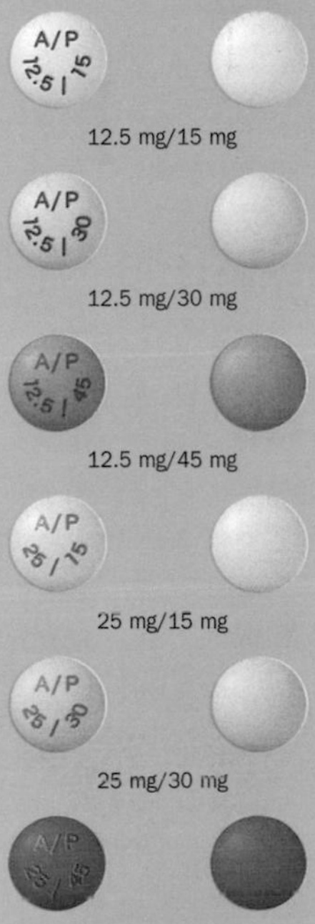

12.5 mg/15 mg

12.5 mg/30 mg

12.5 mg/45 mg

25 mg/15 mg

25 mg/30 mg

25 mg/45 mg

Oseni®
(alogliptin and pioglitazone) tablets

RX TAKEDA PHARMACEUTICALS P. 2406

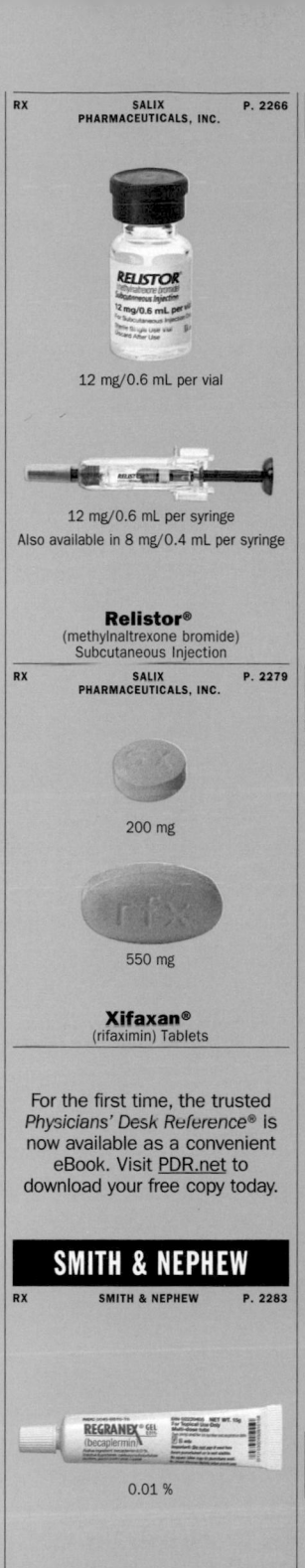

40 mg 80 mg

Uloric®
(febuxostat)

TEVA NEUROSCIENCE

RX TEVA NEUROSCIENCE P. 2411

0.5 mg

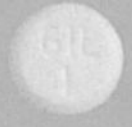

1 mg

Azilect®
(rasagiline mesylate)

RX TEVA NEUROSCIENCE P. 2417

20 mg/1 mL

Copaxone®
(glatiramer acetate injection)

TEVA RESPIRATORY, LLC

RX TEVA RESPIRATORY, LLC P. 2421

90 mcg/inh
8.5 g canister
200 actuations

ProAir® HFA
(albuterol sulfate)

Products in this section are arranged alphabetically by manufacturer. In some instances, not all dosage forms and/or sizes are pictured. If others are available, a † symbol precedes the product's name. Letters or numbers representing the manufacturer's identification code are followed by a * symbol.

TEVA SELECT BRANDS

C-IV TEVA SELECT BRANDS P. 2430

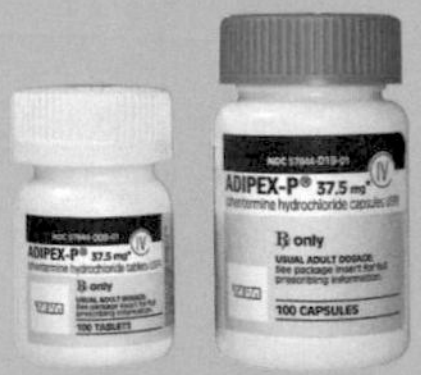

37.5 mg

ADIPEX-P®
(phentermine hydrochloride USP)
capsules and tablets

RX TEVA SELECT BRANDS P. 2432

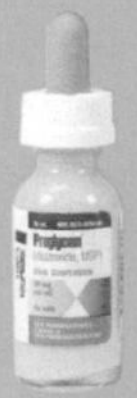

50 mg per mL

Proglycem®
(diazoxide, USP) Oral Suspension

TOPICAL BIOMEDICS, INC.

OTC TOPICAL BIOMEDICS, INC. P. 2437

Topricin Pain Relief Cream
Available: 2oz tube, 4oz jar, 8oz bottle
Professional Size: 16oz & 32oz pump bottles
Topricin Foot Therapy Cream
2oz tube, 4oz jar, & 8oz bottle
Topricin for Children
1.5oz tube

Topricin®

TRIVITA, INC.

DS TRIVITA, INC. P. 2571

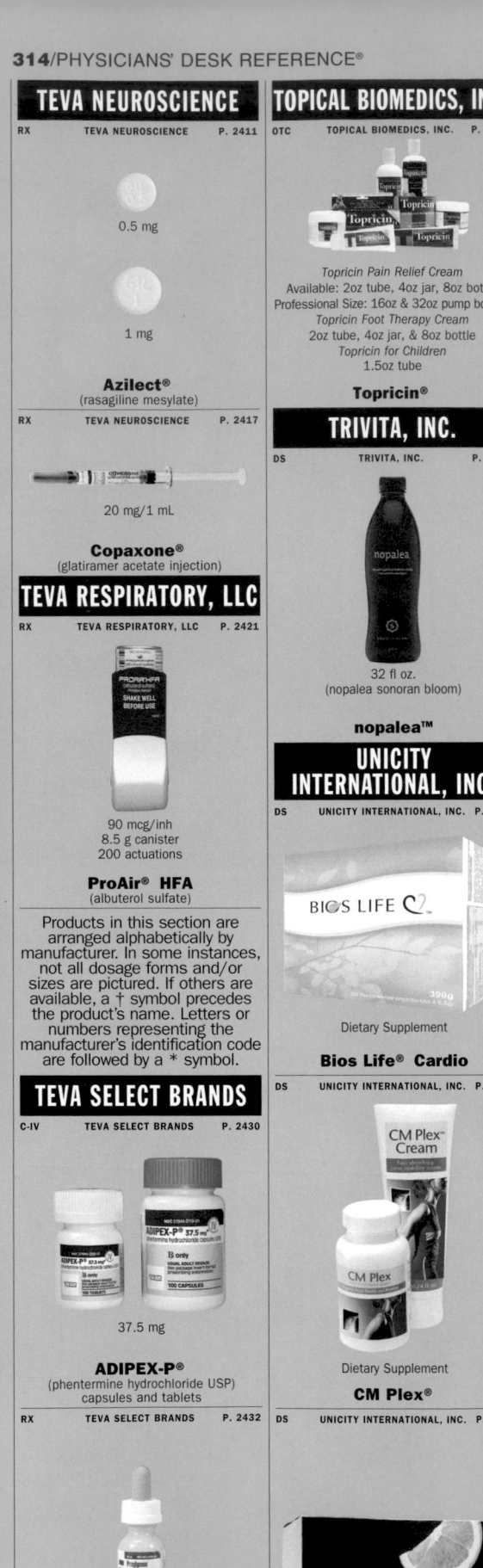

32 fl oz.
(nopalea sonoran bloom)

nopalea™

UNICITY INTERNATIONAL, INC.

DS UNICITY INTERNATIONAL, INC. P. 2572

Dietary Supplement

Bios Life® Cardio

DS UNICITY INTERNATIONAL, INC. P. 2573

Dietary Supplement

CM Plex®

DS UNICITY INTERNATIONAL, INC. P. 2574

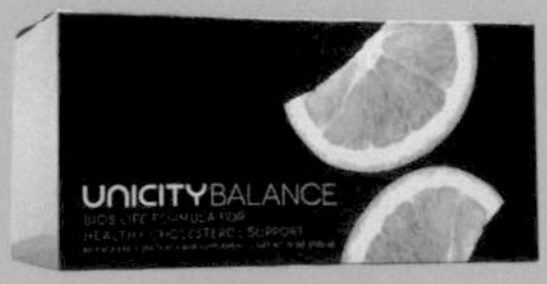

Dietary Supplement

Unicity Balance™

WELLSPRING

RX WELLSPRING PHARMACEUTICAL CORP P. 2532

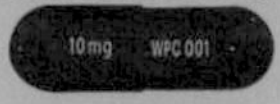

10 mg

Dibenzyline®
(phenoxybenzamine HCl)

RX WELLSPRING PHARMACEUTICAL CORP P. 2533

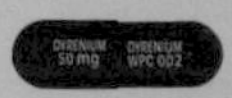

50 mg

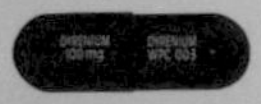

100 mg

Dyrenium®
(triamterene)

Look for PDR in your EHR

PDR® BRIEF gives you the critical drug information you need and the patient support resources you want. Right within your EHR workflow. No more clutter, no more searching multiple resources and no more wondering if the drug information you rely upon is complete or current.

Current drug and drug safety information

Drug alerts, Boxed Warnings & REMS

Melavin
(melavinus)

☎ ✕

Recent Major Change: Aug 2013
Full Prescribing Information

Patient
Drug Info

Updated Aug 2013
Boxed WARNING

Alerts

REMS

Melavin – new 5mg dose available

Important Safety Information

Patient coupon available.
Eligible patient pay no more than $15

Important Safety Information

Terms of Service

✓ **PDR® BRIEF**

Printable PDR+ patient drug education guides. Helps meet MU2.

Provider & patient support resources

With PDR BRIEF, key drug and safety information, as well as pertinent patient resources, are delivered on-screen when you select a medication.

Don't have PDR in your EHR? Tell us at EHR@pdr.net.

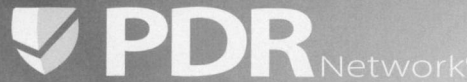

for Patients

Here

Start your patient's drug education...

So They Get Here

FREE Patient Drug Education from PDR

PDR+ helps you educate your patients about their prescriptions. Now in your EHR.

Cost/co-pay*

Unmanaged or unacceptable side effects

Doesn't think the drug works

PDR+

Lack of productive family involvement

Doesn't think that he/she needs the drug

Lack of motivation or self confidence

Doesn't understand how to use or administer the drug

PDR+ is different.

Using the principles of adherence*, **PDR+** has been designed specifically to improve patients' understanding of their medication including:

- How the medication may benefit them
- When they may see results
- How their progress will be measured
- Side effects and ways to manage them

Designed for use with patients.

Unlike pharmacy handouts, PDR+ is designed to be given during the exam to proactively address patients' questions and concerns and to help them commit to therapy.

- Print from PDR BRIEF
- Or send direct to the patient portal

See a sample:
www.pdr.net/PatientSample

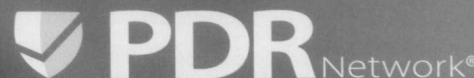

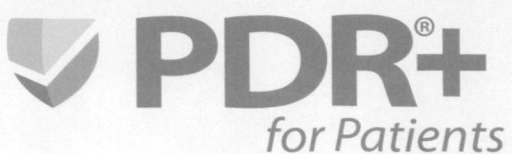

PDR+ supports your workflow.

PDR+ is made available at no cost to you.

- Convenient access via **PDR® BRIEF** in your EHR
- Optimized for print-on-demand
- Better informed patients = fewer calls

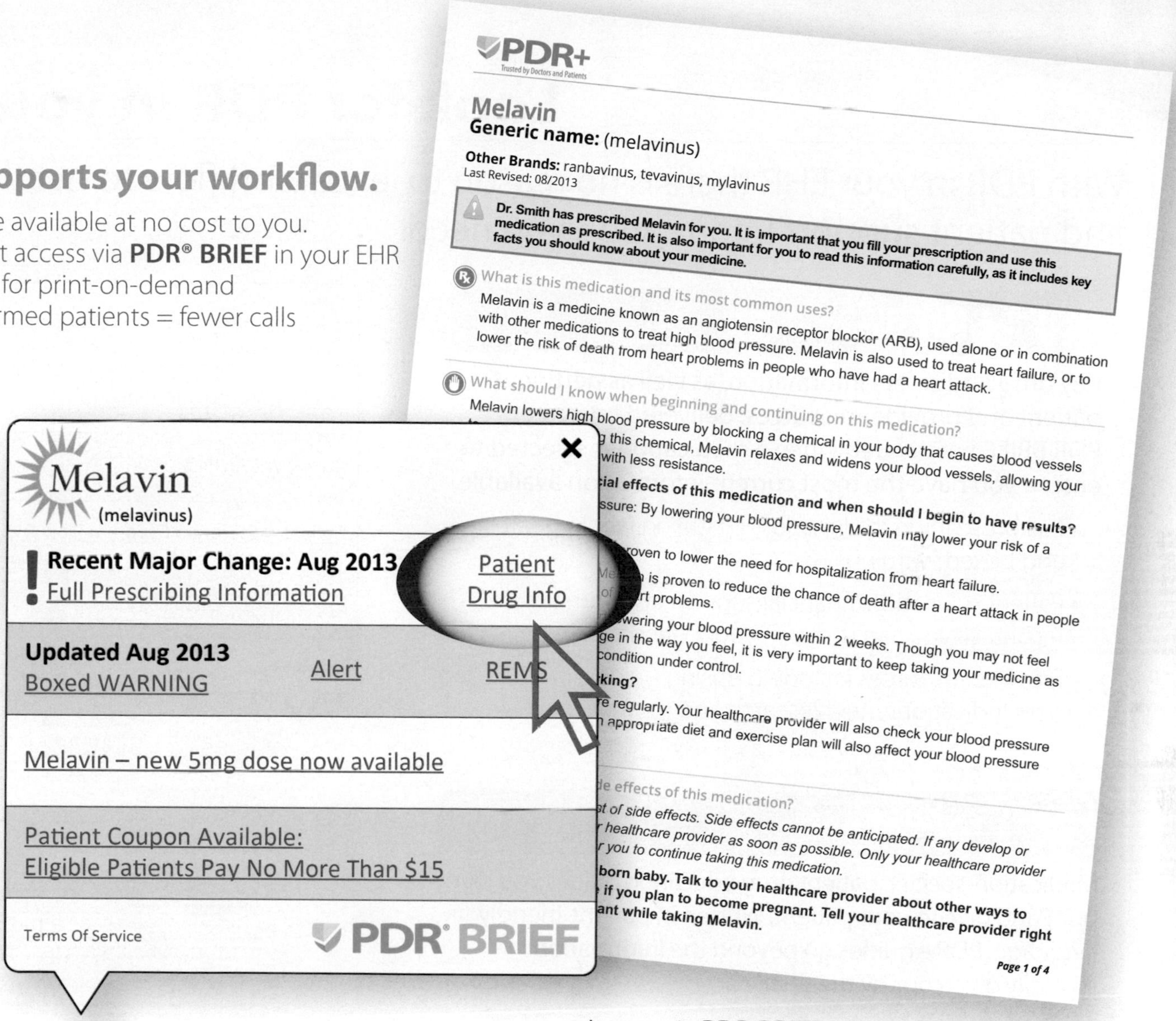

Access via **PDR BRIEF**.
Click on **PATIENT DRUG INFO** to print.

Patients prefer PDR+.

"[PDR+] would make me feel more comfortable about my medicine."

"If I'm not afraid of my medication I will stay on it."

"...if the doctor tells me everything I need to know about my medication, it shows he really cares about me and my health."

70% of patients have never received printed drug information from their physician, but two out three said they wish they'd had.

Source: PDR Patient Research, July 2013.

*Source: American Society of Consultant Pharmacists Foundation "Adult Meducation—Improving Medication Adherence in Older Adults"
**When PDR+ includes a co-pay discount or coupon

PDR Network®

Look for PDR in your EHR

With PDR in your EHR there is no reason to leave workflow to get the drug and patient support information you need.

PDR® BRIEF

Key drug and safety information, as well as pertinent patient and provider resources, delivered on-screen. PDR BRIEF is activated when a medication is selected to ensure you have the most current information available.

- Full prescribing information, including label updates and boxed warnings
- Patient education, financial support, and adherence resources you can use with your patients
- Provider resources including dosing guides, new indications, new research and more

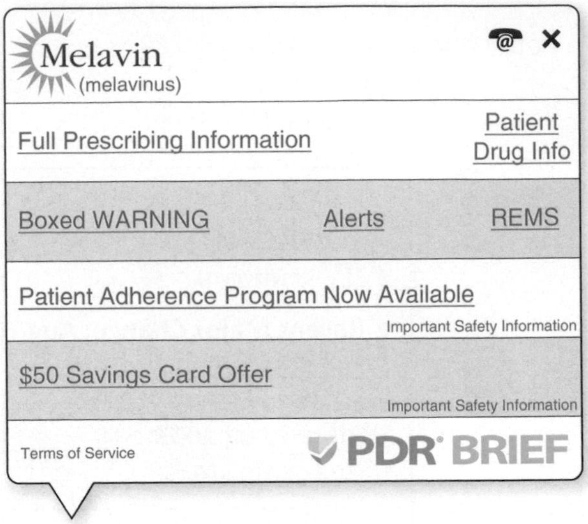

PDR®+ for Patients

Medication-specific patient drug education guides you can print and give to your patient. Written in patient-friendly language, PDR+ guides go beyond the information typically given out by the pharmacy.

- Helps patients better understand their medications
- Conveniently accessed via PDR BRIEF
- Helps meet Meaningful Use

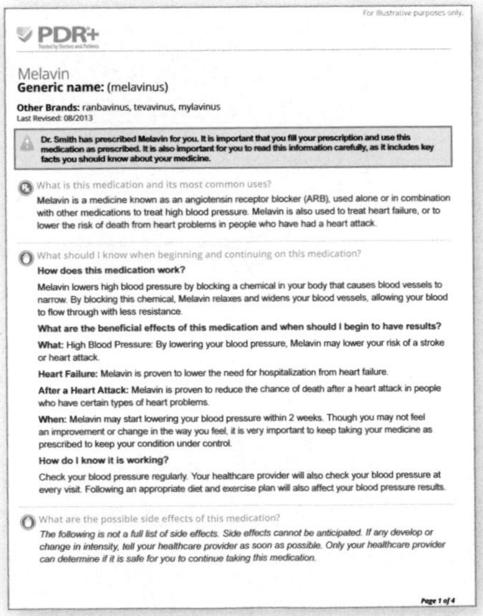

For illustrative purposes only.

PDR+

Melavin
Generic name: (melavinus)

Other Brands: ranbavinus, tevavinus, mylavinus
Last Revised: 08/2013

Dr. Smith has prescribed Melavin for you. It is important that you fill your prescription and use this medication as prescribed. It is also important for you to read this information carefully, as it includes key facts you should know about your medicine.

What is this medication and its most common uses?

Melavin is a medicine known as an angiotensin receptor blocker (ARB), used alone or in combination with other medications to treat high blood pressure. Melavin is also used to treat heart failure, or to lower the risk of death from heart problems in people who have had a heart attack.

What should I know when beginning and continuing on this medication?

How does this medication work?

Melavin lowers high blood pressure by blocking a chemical in your body that causes blood vessels to narrow. By blocking this chemical, Melavin relaxes and widens your blood vessels, allowing your blood to flow through with less resistance.

What are the beneficial effects of this medication and when should I begin to have results?

What: High Blood Pressure: By lowering your blood pressure, Melavin may lower your risk of a stroke or heart attack.

Heart Failure: Melavin is proven to lower the need for hospitalization from heart failure.

After a Heart Attack: Melavin is proven to reduce the chance of death after a heart attack in people who have certain types of heart problems.

When: Melavin may start lowering your blood pressure within 2 weeks. Though you may not feel an improvement or change in the way you feel, it is very important to keep taking your medicine as prescribed to keep your condition under control.

How do I know it is working?

Check your blood pressure regularly. Your healthcare provider will also check your blood pressure at every visit. Following an appropriate diet and exercise plan will also affect your blood pressure results.

What are the possible side effects of this medication?

The following is not a full list of side effects. Side effects cannot be anticipated. If any develop or change in intensity, tell your healthcare provider as soon as possible. Only your healthcare provider can determine if it is safe for you to continue taking this medication.

Page 1 of 4

PDR® Search

Interactive and searchable drug label and safety database

- Full FDA-approved prescribing information and prescribing summaries
- FDA and PDR Drug Safety Alerts

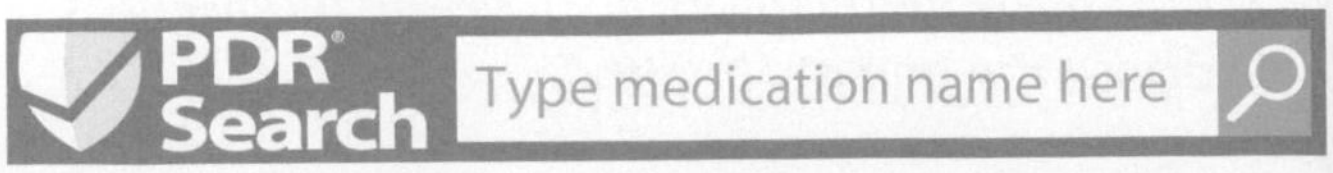

Don't have PDR in your EHR? Tell us at EHR@pdr.net.

PDR Network®

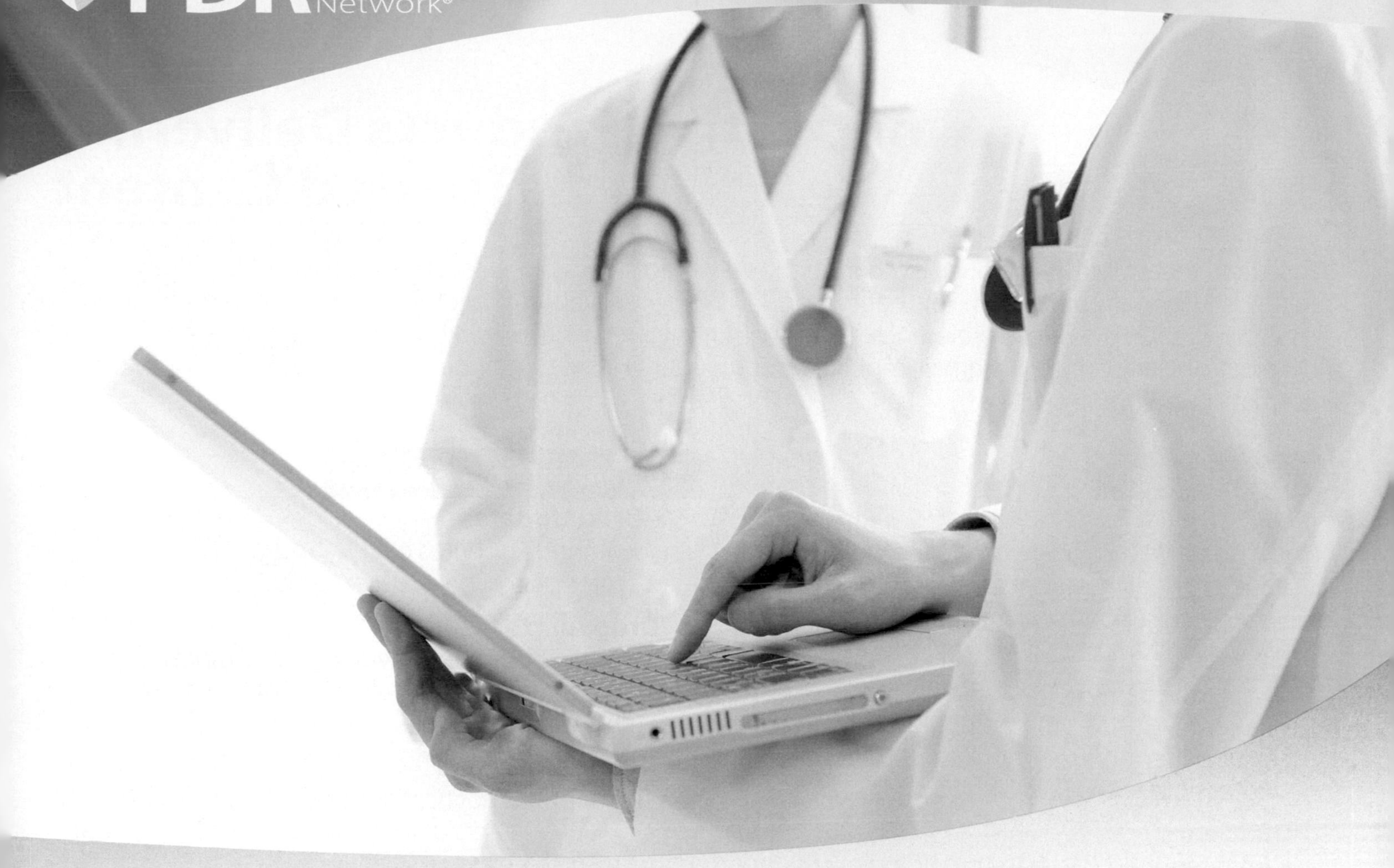

Today's Physicians' Desk Reference®

Innovation to Meet Healthcare Providers' Needs

As a healthcare provider today, you face more challenges than ever. Increasing responsibilities call for more of your time, forcing you to be more efficient to continue providing optimal patient care. You need tools that support you throughout your day, to save you more time for what's most important – your patients. PDR Network® understands those demands and has developed innovative new resources to meet your needs.

As a company, PDR® has always been committed to providers like you, pioneering new ways to deliver our trusted prescribing and patient safety information to support your ever-changing needs. Our latest digital innovations deliver critical information within your workflow to efficiently offer the tools you need to provide the best care for your patients. Whether online, via email, mobile, through your EHR, or our new eBook, PDR provides resources that you can rely on to help you and your patients.

PDR Network®

Innovative Products Delivering Trusted Content

While new technology continues to change the way medicine is practiced, the need for critical drug reference information remains. For that reason, PDR® now delivers critical drug information in multiple ways to suit each provider's preference and fit within their respective workflow. Whether you access PDR electronically online, via email, mobile, through your EHR system or our new eBook, PDR puts that information at your fingertips.

EHR Innovations

PDR® BRIEF

- An intuitive dashboard of full labeling information and provider resources surfacing within your EHR system to support your treatment decisions within your workflow.

PDR®+ for Patients

- Patient-focused prescribing information to help your patient better understand their treatment, accessible with a click when prescribing.

PDR® Search

- An integrated database providing access to detailed drug information on-demand directly through your EHR application.

Digital Properties

Physicians' Desk Reference® eBook

- Trusted FDA-approved full prescribing information, now available in a convenient eBook format for all desktop and tablet platforms.

*mobile*PDR®

- The single, go-to source for trusted drug information available anywhere, anytime that you have access to a mobile device, and available across platforms.

PDR.net®

- PDR's physician-focused portal providing enhanced search capabilities and drug indexing to quickly and easily deliver critical drug information online.

Communications Services

eDrug Updates

- Monthly updates of FDA-approved labeling information delivered via email.

Drug Alerts

- Critical, time-sensitive updates on prescription drugs delivered via email as information becomes available.

Dear HCP Letters

- Important notifications from bio/pharmaceutical manufacturers detailing new information about their products.

REMS Communications

- Detailed Risk Evaluation and Mitigation Strategies (REMS) plans to support patient safety when prescribing designated medications.

Recalls, Withdrawals, and other Notifications

- Timely communications to keep you up-to-date on changing prescribing information, product availability, and other key issues that may impact your prescribing decisions.

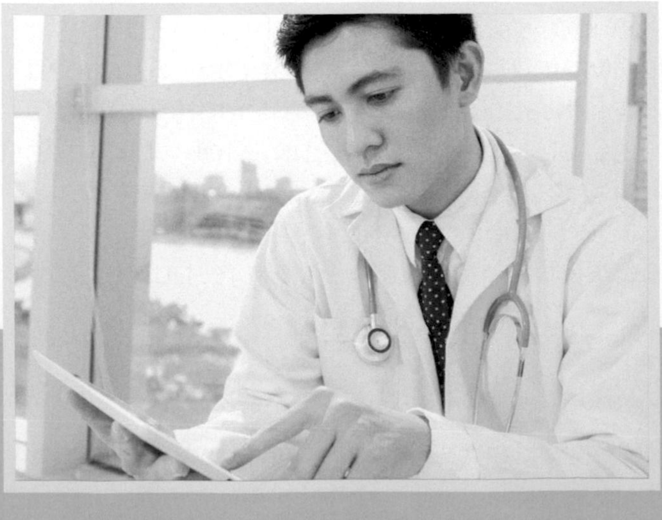

Feedback

As a member of the PDR Network, we welcome any feedback that you may have to shape our products. Please feel free to share your suggestions with us via email at Provider Feedback@PDR.net.

PDR®
Physicians' Desk Reference®

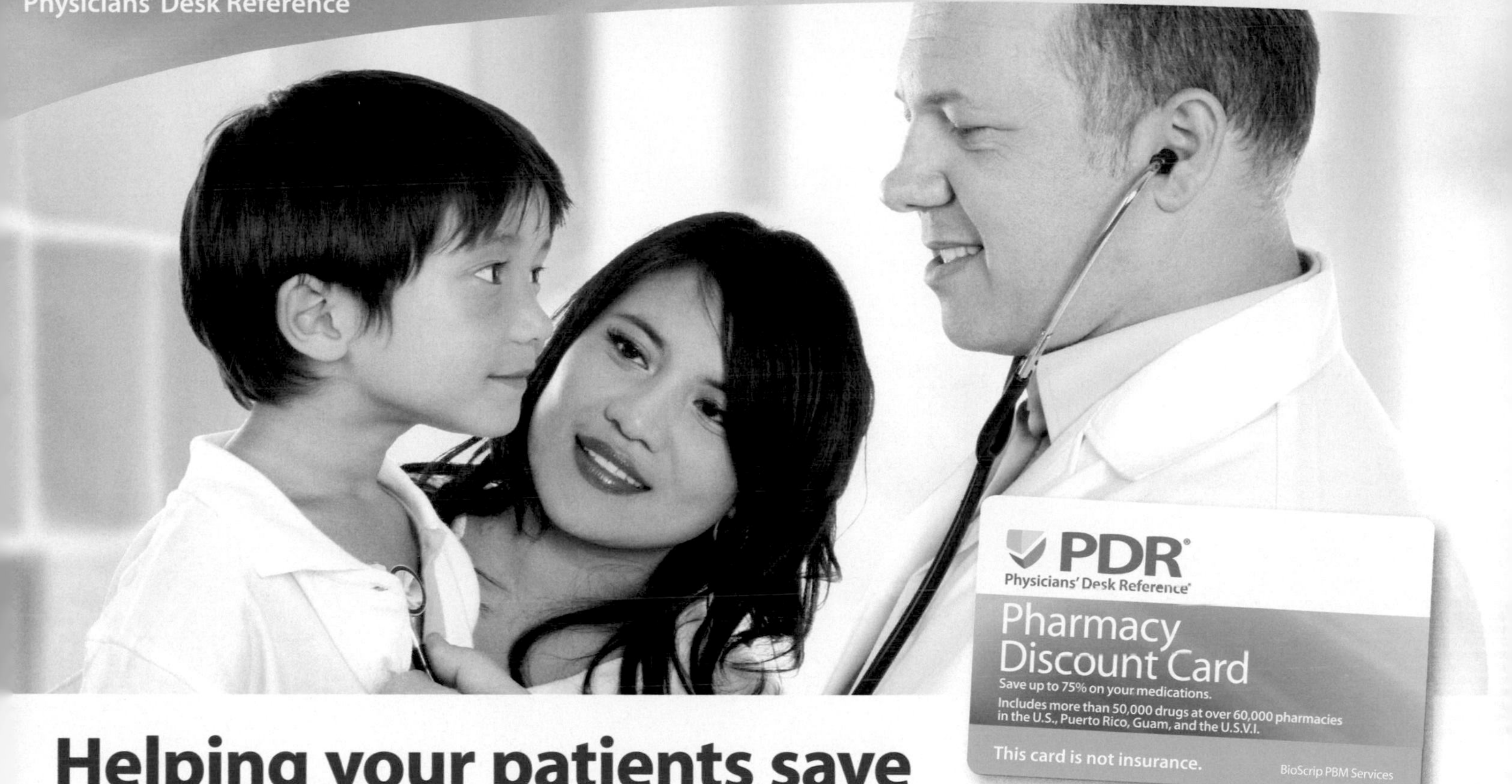
PDR®
Physicians' Desk Reference®
Pharmacy Discount Card
Save up to 75% on your medications.
Includes more than 50,000 drugs at over 60,000 pharmacies in the U.S., Puerto Rico, Guam, and the U.S.V.I.
This card is not insurance.
BioScrip PBM Services

Helping your patients save money on medications is just a few steps away.

Step 1: Enroll in this FREE program

Step 2: Receive your complete program kit

Step 3: Encourage your patients to use their pre-activated PDR® Pharmacy Discount Cards on a regular basis for maximum savings

Benefits of the PDR® Pharmacy Discount Card Program:

- Everyone is eligible
- Patients save up to 75% on prescriptions
- Includes over 50,000 drugs at 60,000 pharmacies nationwide
- Kits available in English or Spanish

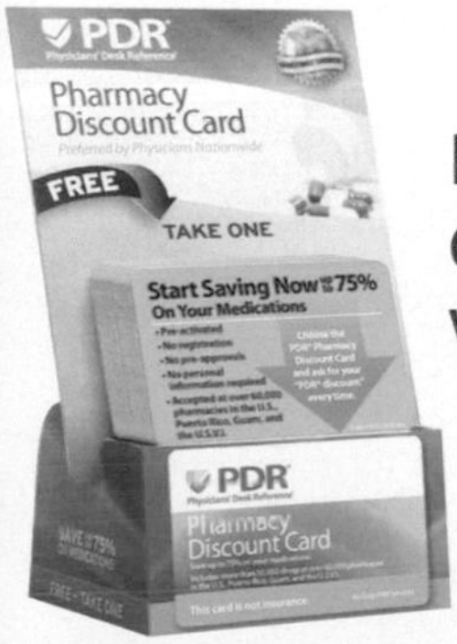
PDR
Pharmacy Discount Card
FREE
TAKE ONE
Start Saving Now up to 75% On Your Medications
PDR
Pharmacy Discount Card

Enrolling is easy.
Call: **800-232-7379**
Visit: **pdr.net/PharmacyDiscountCard**

In a recent survey, **94% of physicians** indicated they prefer a pharmacy discount card from PDR®.

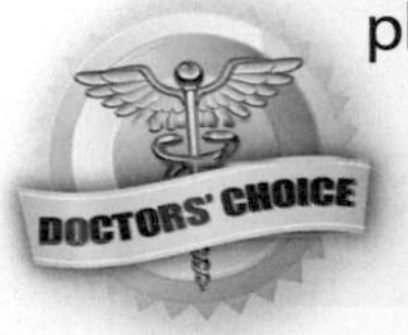
DOCTORS' CHOICE

(PDR Research: Feb 2013; N= 1,772)

This discount plan is NOT insurance or a Medicare prescription drug plan. The plan is not intended as a substitute for insurance and does not meet creditable coverage requirements under state or federal law. The plan provides discounts at participating pharmacies on certain pharmaceutical supplies, prescription drugs, or medical equipment and supplies. The range of discounts will vary depending on the products received. Members are obligated to pay the pharmacy the entire amount of the discounted rate for such products at the point of sale. The plan does not pay pharmacies for products provided to members. No enrollment or periodic fees apply. The pharmacy may pay the plan a fee from amounts the pharmacy collects from the member. The discount plan organization is BioScrip PBM Services, LLC, 100 Clearbrook Road, Elmsford, NY 10523, 1-888-299-5383. Customer service is provided by PDR Network, LLC., 5 Paragon Drive, Montvale, NJ, 07645, 1-800-232-7379, www.pdr.net/PharmacyDiscountCard, customerservice@pdr.net.

SECTION 5

PRODUCT INFORMATION

This edition of the *PDR®* contains the latest full label product information available when the book went to press. Listings are arranged alphabetically by manufacturer; late submissions appear alphabetically by manufacturer at the end of this section. As new drugs are released, and new research data, clinical findings, and safety information emerge throughout the year, it is the responsibility of the manufacturer to provide that information to the medical community and revise that information in the PDR database accordingly.

These revisions are published six times annually in the *PDR Updates*, more regularly on PDR.net® and *mobile*PDR®, as well as emailed via the *PDR® eDrug Update* and *PDR® Drug Alerts*. These updates can also be found in the Electronic Health Record (EHR) of PDR's growing network of EHR partners. To be certain that you have the most current information, always consult PDR.net, *mobile*PDR, *PDR eDrug Update*, *PDR Updates*, or PDR drug information within your EHR before prescribing or administering any product described in the following pages.

AbbVie Inc.
1 North Waukegan Road
North Chicago, IL 60064

Direct Inquiries to:
Customer Service:
(800) 255-5162
Patient Access Program:
(800) 441-4987
For Medical Information Contact:
(800) 633-9110 or www.abbviemedinfo.com
Adverse experiences or side effects
(for all AbbVie drug products):
(800) 633-9110 or www.abbviemedinfo.com
Sales and Ordering:
(800) 255-5162

ABBO-CODE™ INDEX

The Abbo-Code identification system provides positive identification of a drug and dosage strength. The following AbbVie products are imprinted or debossed with an Abbo-Code designation:

PRODUCT	*ABBO-CODE*
Advicor® Tablet (niacin extended-release/lovastatin tablets)	
1000 mg/20 mg	a 1002
1000 mg/40 mg	a 1004
750 mg/20 mg	a 752
500 mg/20 mg	a 502
Biaxin® Filmtab® Tablets (clarithromycin tablets, USP)	
250 mg	KT
500 mg	KL
Biaxin® XL Filmtab® Tablets (clarithromycin extended-release tablets)	
500 mg	KJ
Cardizem LA (Dilitiazem Hydrochloride) Extended-Release Tablets)	
120 mg	b 120
180 mg	b 180
240 mg	b 240
300 mg	b 300
360 mg	b 360
400 mg	b 400
Creon (pancrelipase) delayed-release capsules for oral use	
CREON 3000	Creon 1203
CREON 6000	Creon 1206
CREON 12000	Creon 1212
CREON 24000	Creon 1224
CREON 36000	Creon 1236
Depakene® Capsules (valproic acid capsules, USP)	
250 mg	DEPAKENE
Depakote® ER Tablets (divalproex sodium EXTENDED-RELEASE tablets)	
500 mg	HC
250 mg	HF
Depakote® Sprinkle Capsules (divalproex sodium coated particles in capsules)	
125 mg	↑THIS END UP DEPAKOTE SPRINKLE 125 mg
Depakote® Tablets (divalproex sodium delayed-release tablets)	
125 mg	NT
250 mg	NR
500 mg	NS
Ery-Tab® Enteric-Coated Tablets (erythromycin delayed-release tablets, USP)	
250 mg	EC
333 mg	EH
500 mg	ED
Erythrocin® Stearate Filmtab® Tablets (erythromycin stearate tablets, USP)	
250 mg erythromycin activity	ES
500 mg erythromycin activity	ET
Erythromycin Base Filmtab® Tablets (erythromycin tablets, USP)	
250 mg	EB
500 mg	EA
Erythromycin Delayed-release Capsules, USP	
250 mg	ER
Erythromycin Ethylsuccinate Tablets, USP	
400 mg erythromycin activity	74 ZE
Gengraf® Capsules (cyclosporine capsules, USP [MODIFIED])	
25 mg	OR 25 mg
100 mg	OT 100 mg
Kaletra® (lopinavir/ritonavir)	
133.3 mg lopinavir/33.3 mg ritonavir	PK
Kaletra® Tablet (lopinavir/ritonavir)	
100 mg lopinavir/25 mg ritonavir	KC
200 mg lopinavir/50 mg ritonavir	KA
K-Tab® Filmtab® Tablets (potassium chloride extended-release tablets, USP)	
10 mEq (750 mg)	K-TAB
Marinol® (dronabinal capsules)	
2.5 mg	UM
5 mg	UM
10 mg	UM
Mavik® Tablets (trandolapril)	
1 mg	FT
2 mg	FX
4 mg	FZ
Meridia® Capsules C-IV (sibutramine hydrochloride monohydrate)	
5 mg	MERIDIA 5
10 mg	MERIDIA 10
15 mg	MERIDIA 15
Niaspan® (niacin extended-release tablets) [film-coated]	
500 mg	Niaspan 500
750 mg	Niaspan 750
1000 mg	Niaspan 1000
Norvir® (ritonavir capsules) Soft Gelatin	
100 mg	DS 100
PCE® Dispertab® Tablets (erythromycin particles in tablets)	
333 mg	PCE
500 mg	EK
Prometrium®: (progesterone capsules, USP)	
100 mg	SV
200 mg	SV2
Simcor® Tablet (niacin extended-release/simvastatin tablets)	
500 mg/20 mg	a 500-20
500 mg/40 mg	a 500-40
750 mg/20 mg	a 750-20
1000 mg/20 mg	a 1000-20
1000 mg/40 mg	a 1000-40
Synthroid® Tablets (levothyroxine sodium tablets, USP)	
25 mcg (0.025 mg)	SYNTHROID 25
50 mcg (0.05 mg)	SYNTHROID 50
75 mcg (0.075 mg)	SYNTHROID 75
88 mcg (0.088 mg)	SYNTHROID 88
100 mcg (0.1 mg)	SYNTHROID 100
112 mcg (0.112 mg)	SYNTHROID 112
125 mcg (0.125 mg)	SYNTHROID 125
137 mcg (0.137 mg)	SYNTHROID 137
150 mcg (0.15 mg)	SYNTHROID 150
175 mcg (0.175 mg)	SYNTHROID 175
200 mcg (0.2 mg)	SYNTHROID 200
300 mcg (0.3 mg)	SYNTHROID 300
Tarka® Tablets (trandolapril/verapamil hydrochloride ER)	
2 mg/180 mg	182Δ
1 mg/240 mg	241Δ
2 mg/240 mg	242Δ
4 mg/240 mg	244Δ
Tricor® (fenofibrate tablets)	
48 mg	FI
54 mg	TA
145 mg	FO
160 mg	TC
Trilipix™ Capsules (fenofibric acid delayed release capsules)	
45 mg	a 45
135 mg	a 135
Vicodin® Tablet C-III	**VICODIN**
(hydrocodone bitartrate and acetaminophen tablets, USP)	
hydrocodone bitartrate	5 mg
acetaminophen	500 mg
Vicodin ES® Tablet C-III	**VICODIN ES**
(hydrocodone bitartrate and acetaminophen tablets, USP)	
hydrocodone bitartrate	7.5 mg
acetaminophen	750 mg
Vicodin HP® Tablet C-III	**VICODIN HP**
(hydrocodone bitartrate and acetaminophen tablets, USP)	
hydrocodone bitartrate	10 mg
acetaminophen	660 mg
Vicoprofen® Tablet C-III	**VP**
(hydrocodone bitartrate and ibuprofen tablets)	
hydrocodone bitartrate	7.5 mg
ibuprofen	200 mg
Zemplar® Capsules (paricalcitol)	
1 mcg	ZA
2 mcg	ZF
4 mcg	ZK

ADVICOR® ℞
[ăd-vĭ-kŏr]
(niacin extended-release/lovastatin tablets)

DESCRIPTION

ADVICOR® (niacin extended-release and lovastatin) is intended to facilitate the daily administration of its individual components, Niaspan® and lovastatin, when used together for the intended patient population (see INDICATIONS AND USAGE and DOSAGE AND ADMINISTRATION).

ADVICOR contains niacin extended-release and lovastatin in combination. Lovastatin, an inhibitor of 3-hydroxy-3-methylglutaryl-coenzyme A (HMG-CoA) reductase, and niacin are both lipid-altering agents.

Niacin is nicotinic acid, or 3-pyridinecarboxylic acid. Niacin is a white, nonhygroscopic crystalline powder that is very soluble in water, boiling ethanol and propylene glycol. It is insoluble in ethyl ether. The empirical formula of niacin is $C_6H_5NO_2$ and its molecular weight is 123.11. Niacin has the following structural formula:

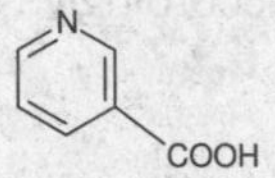

Lovastatin is [1S -[1(alpha)(R *), 3(alpha), 7(beta), 8(beta)(2S *, 4S *), 8a(beta)]]-1,2,3, 7,8,8a-hexahydro-3,7-dimethyl-8-[2-(tetrahydro-4-hydroxy-6-oxo-2H-pyran-2-yl) ethyl]-1-naphthalenyl 2-methylbutanoate. Lovastatin is a white, nonhygroscopic crystalline powder that is insoluble in water and sparingly soluble in ethanol, methanol, and acetonitrile. The empirical formula of lovastatin is $C_{24}H_{36}O_5$ and its molecular weight is 404.55. Lovastatin has the following structural formula:

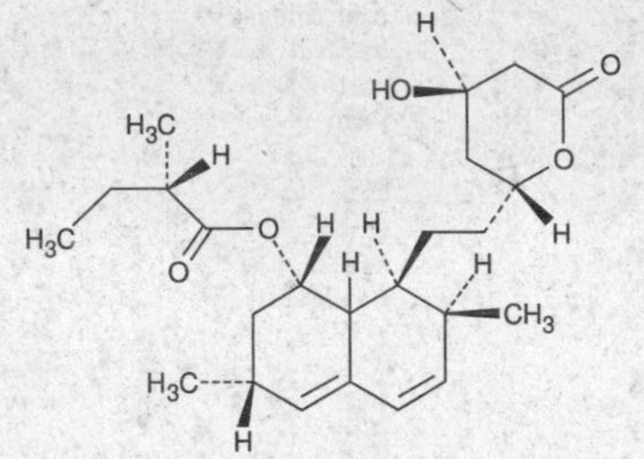

ADVICOR tablets contain the labeled amount of niacin and lovastatin and have the following inactive ingredients: hypromellose, povidone, stearic acid, polyethylene glycol, titanium dioxide, polysorbate 80.

The individual tablet strengths (expressed in terms of mg niacin/mg lovastatin) contain the following coloring agents:
ADVICOR 500 mg/20 mg - Iron Oxide Yellow, Iron Oxide Red.
ADVICOR 750 mg/20 mg - FD&C Yellow #6/Sunset Yellow FCF Aluminum Lake.
ADVICOR 1000 mg/20 mg - Iron Oxide Red, Iron Oxide Yellow, Iron Oxide Black.
ADVICOR 1000 mg/40 mg - Iron Oxide Red.

CLINICAL PHARMACOLOGY

A variety of clinical studies have demonstrated that elevated levels of total cholesterol (TC), low-density lipoprotein cholesterol (LDL-C), and apolipoprotein B-100 (Apo B) promote human atherosclerosis. Similarly, decreased levels of high-density lipoprotein cholesterol (HDL-C) are associated with the development of atherosclerosis. Epidemiological investigations have established that cardiovascular morbidity and mortality vary directly with the level of TC and LDL-C, and inversely with the level of HDL-C.

Cholesterol-enriched triglyceride-rich lipoproteins, including very low-density lipoproteins (VLDL), intermediate-density lipoproteins (IDL), and their remnants, can also promote atherosclerosis. Elevated plasma triglycerides (TG) are frequently found in a triad with low HDL-C levels and small LDL particles, as well as in association with non-lipid metabolic risk factors for coronary heart disease (CHD). As such, total plasma TG have not consistently been shown to be an independent risk factor for CHD.

As an adjunct to diet, the efficacy of niacin and lovastatin in improving lipid profiles (either individually, or in combination with each other, or niacin in combination with other statins) for the treatment of dyslipidemia has been well documented. The effect of combined therapy with niacin and lovastatin on cardiovascular morbidity and mortality has not been determined.

Effects on lipids

ADVICOR

ADVICOR reduces LDL-C, TC, and TG, and increases HDL-C due to the individual actions of niacin and lovastatin. The magnitude of individual lipid and lipoprotein responses may be influenced by the severity and type of underlying lipid abnormality.

Niacin

Niacin functions in the body after conversion to nicotinamide adenine dinucleotide (NAD) in the NAD coenzyme system. Niacin (but not nicotinamide) in gram doses reduces LDL-C, Apo B, Lp(a), TG, and TC, and increases HDL-C. The increase in HDL-C is associated with an increase in apolipoprotein A-I (Apo A-I) and a shift in the distribution of HDL subfractions. These shifts include an increase in the HDL_2:HDL_3 ratio, and an elevation in lipoprotein A-I (Lp A-I, an HDL-C particle containing only Apo A-I). In addition, preliminary reports suggest that niacin causes favorable LDL particle size transformations, although the clinical relevance of this effect is not yet clear.

Lovastatin

Lovastatin has been shown to reduce both normal and elevated LDL-C concentrations. Apo B also falls substantially during treatment with lovastatin. Since each LDL-C particle contains one molecule of Apo B, and since little Apo B is found in other lipoproteins, this strongly suggests that lovastatin does not merely cause cholesterol to be lost from LDL-C, but also reduces the concentration of circulating LDL particles. In addition, lovastatin can produce increases of variable magnitude in HDL-C, and modestly reduces VLDL-C and plasma TG. The effects of lovastatin on Lp(a), fibrinogen, and certain other independent biochemical risk markers for coronary heart disease are not well characterized.

Mechanism of Action

Niacin

The mechanism by which niacin alters lipid profiles is not completely understood and may involve several actions, including partial inhibition of release of free fatty acids from adipose tissue, and increased lipoprotein lipase activity (which may increase the rate of chylomicron triglyceride removal from plasma). Niacin decreases the rate of hepatic synthesis of VLDL-C and LDL-C, and does not appear to affect fecal excretion of fats, sterols, or bile acids.

Lovastatin

Lovastatin is a specific inhibitor of 3-hydroxy-3-methylglutaryl-coenzyme A (HMG-CoA) reductase, the enzyme that catalyzes the conversion of HMG-CoA to mevalonate. The conversion of HMG-CoA to mevalonate is an early step in the biosynthetic pathway for cholesterol. Lovastatin is a prodrug and has little, if any, activity until hydrolyzed to its active beta-hydroxyacid form, lovastatin acid. The mechanism of the LDL-lowering effect of lovastatin may involve both reduction of VLDL-C concentration and induction of the LDL receptor, leading to reduced production and/or increased catabolism of LDL-C.

Pharmacokinetics

Absorption and Bioavailability

ADVICOR

In single-dose studies of ADVICOR, rate and extent of niacin and lovastatin absorption were bioequivalent under fed conditions to that from NIASPAN® (niacin extended-release tablets) and Mevacor® (lovastatin) tablets, respectively. After administration of two ADVICOR 1000 mg/20 mg tablets, peak niacin concentrations averaged about 18 mcg/mL and occurred about 5 hours after dosing; about 72% of the niacin dose was absorbed according to the urinary excretion data. Peak lovastatin concentrations averaged about 11 ng/mL and occurred about 2 hours after dosing.

The extent of niacin absorption from ADVICOR was increased by administration with food. The administration of two ADVICOR 1000 mg/20 mg tablets under low-fat or high-fat conditions resulted in a 22 to 30% increase in niacin bioavailability relative to dosing under fasting conditions. Lovastatin bioavailability is affected by food. Lovastatin C_{max} was increased 48% and 21% after a high- and a low-fat meal, respectively, but the lovastatin AUC was decreased 26% and 24% after a high- and a low-fat meal, respectively, compared to those under fasting conditions.

A relative bioavailability study results indicated that ADVICOR tablet strengths (i.e., two tablets of 500 mg/20 mg and one tablet of 1000 mg/40 mg) are not interchangeable.

Niacin

Due to extensive and saturable first-pass metabolism, niacin concentrations in the general circulation are dose dependent and highly variable. Peak steady-state niacin concentrations were 0.6, 4.9, and 15.5 mcg/mL after doses of 1000, 1500, and 2000 mg NIASPAN once daily (given as two 500 mg, two 750 mg, and two 1000 mg tablets, respectively).

Lovastatin

Lovastatin appears to be incompletely absorbed after oral administration. Because of extensive hepatic extraction, the amount of lovastatin reaching the systemic circulation as active inhibitors after oral administration is low (<5%) and shows considerable inter-individual variation. Peak concentrations of active and total inhibitors occur within 2 to 4 hours after Mevacor® administration.

Lovastatin absorption appears to be increased by at least 30% by grapefruit juice; however, the effect is dependent on the amount of grapefruit juice consumed and the interval between grapefruit juice and lovastatin ingestion. With a once-a-day dosing regimen, plasma concentrations of total inhibitors over a dosing interval achieved a steady-state between the second and third days of therapy and were about 1.5 times those following a single dose of Mevacor®.

Although the mechanism is not fully understood, cyclosporine has been shown to increase the AUC of HMG-CoA reductase inhibitors. The increase in AUC for lovastatin and lovastatin acid is presumably due, in part, to inhibition of CYP3A4.

Distribution

Niacin

Niacin is less than 20% bound to human serum proteins and distributes into milk. Studies using radiolabeled niacin in mice show that niacin and its metabolites concentrate in the liver, kidney, and adipose tissue.

Lovastatin

Both lovastatin and its beta-hydroxyacid metabolite are highly bound (>95%) to human plasma proteins. Distribution of lovastatin or its metabolites into human milk is unknown; however, lovastatin distributes into milk in rats. In animal studies, lovastatin concentrated in the liver, and crossed the blood-brain and placental barriers.

Metabolism

Niacin

Niacin undergoes rapid and extensive first-pass metabolism that is dose-rate specific and, at the doses used to treat dyslipidemia, saturable. In humans, one pathway is through a simple conjugation step with glycine to form nicotinuric acid (NUA). NUA is then excreted, although there may be a small amount of reversible metabolism back to niacin. The other pathway results in the formation of NAD. It is unclear whether nicotinamide is formed as a precursor to, or following the synthesis of, NAD. Nicotinamide is further metabolized to at least N-methylnicotinamide (MNA) and nicotinamide-N-oxide (NNO). MNA is further metabolized to two other compounds, N-methyl-2-pyridone-5-carboxamide (2PY) and N-methyl-4-pyridone-5-carboxamide (4PY). The formation of 2PY appears to predominate over 4PY in humans.

Lovastatin

Lovastatin undergoes extensive first-pass extraction and metabolism by cytochrome P450 3A4 in the liver, its primary site of action. The major active metabolites present in human plasma are the beta-hydroxyacid of lovastatin (lovastatin acid), its 6′-hydroxy derivative, and two additional metabolites.

Elimination

ADVICOR

Niacin is primarily excreted in urine mainly as metabolites. After a single dose of ADVICOR, at least 60% of the niacin dose was recovered in urine as unchanged niacin and its metabolites. The plasma half-life for lovastatin was about 4.5 hours in single-dose studies.

Niacin

The plasma half-life for niacin is about 20 to 48 minutes after oral administration and dependent on dose administered. Following multiple oral doses of NIASPAN, up to 12% of the dose was recovered in urine as unchanged niacin depending on dose administered. The ratio of metabolites recovered in the urine was also dependent on the dose administered.

Lovastatin

Lovastatin is excreted in urine and bile, based on studies of Mevacor®. Following an oral dose of radiolabeled lovastatin in man, 10% of the dose was excreted in urine and 83% in feces. The latter represents absorbed drug equivalents excreted in bile, as well as any unabsorbed drug.

Special Populations

Hepatic

No pharmacokinetic studies have been conducted in patients with hepatic insufficiency for either niacin or lovastatin (see WARNINGS, Liver Dysfunction).

Renal

No information is available on the pharmacokinetics of niacin in patients with renal insufficiency.

In a study of patients with severe renal insufficiency (creatinine clearance 10 to 30 mL/min), the plasma concentrations of total inhibitors after a single dose of lovastatin were approximately two-fold higher than those in healthy volunteers.

ADVICOR should be used with caution in patients with renal disease.

Gender

Plasma concentrations of niacin and metabolites after single- or multiple-dose administration of niacin are generally higher in women than in men, with the magnitude of the difference varying with dose and metabolite. Recovery of niacin and metabolites in urine, however, is generally similar for men and women, indicating similar absorption for both genders. The gender differences observed in plasma niacin and metabolite levels may be due to gender-specific differences in metabolic rate or volume of distribution. Data from clinical trials suggest that women have a greater hypolipidemic response than men at equivalent doses of NIASPAN and ADVICOR.

In a multiple-dose study, plasma concentrations of active and total HMG-CoA reductase inhibitors were 20 to 50% higher in women than in men. In two single-dose studies with ADVICOR, lovastatin concentrations were about 30% higher in women than men, and total HMG-CoA reductase inhibitor concentrations were about 20 to 25% greater in women.

In a multi-center, randomized, double-blind, active-comparator study in patients with Type IIa and IIb hyperlipidemia, ADVICOR was compared to single-agent treatment (NIASPAN and lovastatin). The treatment effects of ADVICOR compared to lovastatin and NIASPAN differed for males and females with a significantly larger treatment effect seen for females. The mean percent change from baseline at endpoint for LDL-C, TG, and HDL-C by gender are as follows (Table 1):

[See table 1 above]

Table 1. Mean percent change from baseline at endpoint for LDL-C, HDL-C and TG by gender

	ADVICOR 2000 mg/40 mg		NIASPAN 2000 mg		Lovastatin 40 mg	
	Women (n=22)	Men (n=30)	Women (n=28)	Men (n=28)	Women (n=21)	Men (n=38)
LDL-C	-47%	-34%	-12%	-9%	-31%	-31%
HDL-C	+33%	+24%	+22%	+15%	+3%	+7%
TG	-48%	-35%	-25%	-15%	-15%	-23%

Drug-drug Interactions

[See table 2 at top of next page]

Clinical Studies

In a multi-center, randomized, double-blind, parallel, 28-week, active-comparator study in patients with Type IIa and IIb hyperlipidemia, ADVICOR was compared to each of its components (NIASPAN and lovastatin). Using a forced dose-escalation study design, patients received each dose for at least 4 weeks. Patients randomized to treatment with ADVICOR initially received 500 mg/20 mg. The dose was increased at 4-week intervals to a maximum of 1000 mg/20 mg in one-half of the patients and 2000 mg/40 mg in the other half. The NIASPAN monotherapy group underwent a similar titration from 500 mg to 2000 mg. The patients randomized to lovastatin monotherapy received 20 mg for 12 weeks titrated to 40 mg for up to 16 weeks. Up to a third of the patients randomized to ADVICOR or NIASPAN discontinued prior to Week 28. In this study, ADVICOR decreased

Information on the AbbVie, Inc. products listed on these pages is from the prescribing information in use as of July 31, 2013. For more information, please visit rxabbvie.com or call 1-800-633-9110.

Table 2. The Effects of Other Drugs on Lovastatin Exposure When Both Were Co-administered

Drug	N	Dose of Co-administered Drug or Grapefruit Juice	Dosing of Lovastatin	AUC Ratio* (with / without co-administered drug)	
				Lovastatin	Lovastatin Acid
Gemfibrozil	11	600 mg BID for 3 days	40 mg	0.96	2.80
Itraconazole‡	12	200 mg QD for 4 days	40 mg on Day 4	> 36§	22
	10	100 mg QD for 4 days	40 mg on Day 4	> 14.8§	15.4
Grapefruit Juice¶ (high dose)	10	200 mL of double-strength TID#	80 mg single dose	15.3	5.0
Grapefruit Juice¶ (low dose)	16	8 oz (about 250 mL) of single-strength[Þ] for 4 days	40 mg single dose	1.94	1.57
Cyclosporine	16	Not described[ß]	10 mg QD for 10 days	5- to 8-fold	ND[à]
	Number of Subjects	Dosing of Coadministered Drug or Grapefruit Juice	Dosing of Lovastatin	AUC Ratio* (with / without co-administered drug) No Effect = 1.00	
				Total Lovastatin Acid[è]	
Diltiazem	10	120 mg BID for 14 days	20 mg	3.57[è]	

* Results based on a chemical assay.
† Lovastatin acid refers to the β-hydroxyacid of lovastatin.
‡ The mean total AUC of lovastatin without itraconazole phase could not be determined accurately. Results could be representative of strong CYP3A4 inhibitors such as ketoconazole, posaconazole, clarithromycin, telithromycin, HIV protease inhibitors, and nefazodone.
§ Estimated minimum change.
¶ The effect of amounts of grapefruit juice between those used in these two studies on lovastatin pharmacokinetics has not been studied.
\# Double-strength: one can of frozen concentrate diluted with one can of water. Grapefruit juice was administered TID for 2 days, and 200 mL together with single dose lovastatin and 30 and 90 minutes following single dose lovastatin on Day 3.
Þ Single-strength: one can of frozen concentrate diluted with 3 cans of water. Grapefruit juice was administered with breakfast for 3 days, and lovastatin was administered in the evening on Day 3.
ß Cyclosporine-treated patients with psoriasis or post kidney or heart transplant patients with stable graft function, transplanted at least 9 months prior to study.
à ND = Analyte not determined.
è Lactone converted to acid by hydrolysis prior to analysis. Figure represents total unmetabolized acid and lactone.

Table 3. LDL-C mean percent change from baseline

Week	ADVICOR			NIASPAN			Lovastatin		
	n*	Dose (mg/mg)	LDL	n*	Dose (mg)	LDL	n*	Dose (mg)	LDL
Baseline	57	-	190.9 mg/dL	61	-	189.7 mg/dL	61	-	185.6 mg/dL
12	47	1000/20	-30%	46	1000	-3%	56	20	-29%
16	45	1000/40	-36%	44	1000	-6%	56	40	-31%
20	42	1500/40	-37%	43	1500	-12%	54	40	-34%
28	42	2000/40	-42%	41	2000	-14%	53	40	-32%

*n = number of patients remaining in the trial at each timepoint

Table 4. HDL-C mean percent change from baseline

Week	ADVICOR			NIASPAN			Lovastatin		
	n*	Dose (mg/mg)	HDL	n*	Dose (mg)	HDL	n*	Dose (mg)	HDL
Baseline	57	-	45 mg/dL	61	-	47 mg/dL	61	-	43 mg/dL
12	47	1000/20	+20%	46	1000	+14%	56	20	+3%
16	45	1000/40	+20%	44	1000	+15%	56	40	+5%
20	42	1500/40	+27%	43	1500	+22%	54	40	+6%
28	42	2000/40	+30%	41	2000	+24%	53	40	+6%

*n = number of patients remaining in the trial at each timepoint

LDL-C, TG and Lp(a), and increased HDL-C in a dose-dependent fashion (Tables 3, 4, 5 and 6 below). Results from this study for LDL-C mean percent change from baseline (the primary efficacy variable) showed that:

1. LDL-lowering with ADVICOR was significantly greater than that achieved with lovastatin 40 mg only after 28 weeks of titration to a dose of 2000 mg/40 mg ($p<.0001$)
2. ADVICOR at doses of 1000 mg/20 mg or higher achieved greater LDL-lowering than NIASPAN ($p<.0001$) The LDL-C results are summarized in Table 3.

[See table 3 above]

ADVICOR achieved significantly greater HDL-raising compared to lovastatin and NIASPAN monotherapy at all doses (Table 4).

[See table 4 above]

In addition, ADVICOR achieved significantly greater TG-lowering at doses of 1000 mg/20 mg or greater compared to lovastatin and NIASPAN monotherapy (Table 5).

[See table 5 at top of next page]

The Lp(a) lowering effects of ADVICOR and NIASPAN were similar, and both were superior to lovastatin (Table 6). The independent effect of lowering Lp(a) with NIASPAN or ADVICOR on the risk of coronary and cardiovascular morbidity and mortality has not been determined.

[See table 6 at top of next page]

ADVICOR Long-Term Study

A total of 814 patients were enrolled in a long-term (52-week), open-label, single-arm study of ADVICOR. Patients were force dose-titrated to 2000 mg/40 mg over 16 weeks. After titration, patients were maintained on the maximum tolerated dose of ADVICOR for a total of 52 weeks. Five hundred-fifty (550) patients (68%) completed the study, and fifty-six percent (56%) of all patients were able to maintain a dose of 2000 mg/40 mg for the 52 weeks of treatment. The lipid-altering effects of ADVICOR peaked after 4 weeks on the maximum tolerated dose, and were maintained for the duration of treatment. These effects were comparable to what was observed in the double-blind study of ADVICOR (Tables 3-5).

INDICATIONS AND USAGE

Therapy with lipid-altering agents should be only one component of multiple risk-factor intervention in individuals at significantly increased risk for atherosclerotic vascular disease due to hypercholesterolemia. Drug therapy is indicated as an adjunct to diet when the response to a diet restricted in saturated fat and cholesterol and other nonpharmacologic measures alone has been inadequate (see also Table 8 and the NCEP treatment guidelines[1]).

ADVICOR

ADVICOR (niacin extended-release and lovastatin) is indicated for use when treatment with both NIASPAN and lovastatin is appropriate. As described in the labeling for Niaspan and lovastatin below, the components of ADVICOR are both indicated for the treatment of hypercholesterolemia. Patients receiving treatment with ADVICOR should be on a standard cholesterol-lowering diet and should continue on this diet during treatment.

NIASPAN (niacin extended-release)

Hypercholesterolemia

NIASPAN is indicated as an adjunct to diet for reduction of elevated TC, LDL-C, Apo B and TG levels, and to increase HDL-C in patients with primary hypercholesterolemia (heterozygous familial and nonfamilial) and mixed dyslipidemia (Table 7), when the response to an appropriate diet has been inadequate.

Secondary Prevention of Cardiovascular Events

In patients with a history of myocardial infarction and hypercholesterolemia, niacin is indicated to reduce the risk of recurrent nonfatal myocardial infarction.

Hypertriglyceridemia

Niacin is also indicated as adjunctive therapy for treatment of adult patients with very high serum triglyceride levels (Table 7) who present a risk of pancreatitis and who do not respond adequately to a determined dietary effort to control them. Such patients typically have serum TG levels over 2000 mg/dL and have elevations of VLDL-C as well as fasting chylomicrons (Table 7). Patients who consistently have total serum or plasma TG below 1000 mg/dL are unlikely to develop pancreatitis. Therapy with niacin may be considered for those patients with TG elevations between 1000 and 2000 mg/dL who have a history of pancreatitis or of recurrent abdominal pain typical of pancreatitis. Some patients with TG under 1000 mg/dL may, through dietary or alcohol indiscretion, convert to a pattern with massive TG elevations accompanying fasting chylomicronemia, but the influence of niacin therapy on risk of pancreatitis in such situations has not been adequately studied. Drug therapy is not indicated for patients with hyperlipoproteinemia, who have elevations of chylomicrons and plasma TG, but who have normal levels of VLDL-C.

Lovastatin

Hypercholesterolemia

Lovastatin is indicated as an adjunct to diet for the reduction of elevated TC and LDL-C levels in patients with primary hypercholesterolemia (Table 7), when the response to diet restricted in saturated fat and cholesterol and to other nonpharmacological measures alone has been inadequate.

Primary Prevention of Cardiovascular Events

In individuals without symptomatic cardiovascular disease, average to moderately elevated TC and LDL-C, and below average HDL-C, lovastatin is indicated to reduce the risk of:

- Myocardial infarction
- Unstable angina
- Coronary revascularization procedures

Secondary Prevention of Cardiovascular Events

Lovastatin is also indicated to slow the progression of coronary atherosclerosis in patients with coronary heart disease as part of a treatment strategy to lower TC and LDL-C to target levels.

The National Cholesterol Education Program (NCEP) Treatment Guidelines are summarized below:

Table 7. Classification of Hyperlipoproteinemias

Type	Lipoproteins Elevated	Lipid Elevations	
I (rare)	Chylomicrons	Major	Minor
IIa	LDL	TG	↑→TC
IIb	LDL,VLDL	TC	-
III (rare)	IDL	TC	TG
IV	VLDL	TC/TG	
V (rare)	Chylomicrons, VLDL	TG	↑→TC

TC = total cholesterol; TG = triglycerides; LDL = low-density lipoprotein; VLDL = very low-density lipoprotein; IDL = intermediate-density lipoprotein ↑→ = increased or no change

General Recommendations

Prior to initiating therapy with a lipid-lowering agent, secondary causes for hypercholesterolemia (e.g., poorly controlled diabetes mellitus, hypothyroidism, nephrotic syndrome, dysproteinemias, obstructive liver disease, other drug therapy, alcoholism) should be excluded, and a lipid profile performed to measure TC, HDL-C, and TG. For patients with TG < 400 mg/dL, LDL-C can be estimated using the following equation:

LDL-C = TC - [(0.20 × TG) + HDL-C]

For TG levels > 400 mg/dL, this equation is less accurate and LDL-C concentrations should be determined by ultracentrifugation. Lipid determinations should be performed at intervals of no less than 4 weeks and dosage adjusted according to the patient's response to therapy. The NCEP Treatment Guidelines are summarized in Table 8.

[See table 8 above]

After the LDL-C goal has been achieved, if the TG is still ≥200 mg/dL, non-HDL-C (TC minus HDL-C) becomes a secondary target of therapy. Non-HDL-C goals are set 30 mg/dL higher than LDL-C goals for each risk category.

Table 5. TG median percent change from baseline

Week	ADVICOR			NIASPAN			Lovastatin		
	n*	Dose (mg/mg)	TG	n*	Dose (mg)	TG	n*	Dose (mg)	TG
Baseline	57	-	174 mg/dL	61	-	186 mg/dL	61	-	171 mg/dL
12	47	1000/20	-32%	46	1000	-22%	56	20	-20%
16	45	1000/40	-39%	44	1000	-23%	56	40	-17%
20	42	1500/40	-44%	43	1500	-31%	54	40	-21%
28	42	2000/40	-44%	41	2000	-31%	53	40	-20%

*n = number of patients remaining in the trial at each timepoint

Table 6. Lp(a) median percent change from baseline

Week	ADVICOR			NIASPAN			Lovastatin		
	n*	Dose (mg/mg)	Lp(a)	n*	Dose (mg)	Lp(a)	n*	Dose (mg)	Lp(a)
Baseline	57	-	34 mg/dL	61	-	41 mg/dL	60	-	42 mg/dL
12	47	1000/20	-9%	46	1000	-8%	55	20	+8%
16	45	1000/40	-9%	44	1000	-12%	55	40	+8%
20	42	1500/40	-17%	43	1500	-22%	53	40	+6%
28	42	2000/40	-22%	41	2000	-32%	52	40	0%

*n = number of patients remaining in the trial at each timepoint

Table 8. NCEP Treatment Guidelines: LDL-C Goals and Cutpoints for Therapeutic Lifestyle Changes and Drug Therapy in Different Risk Categories

Risk Category	LDL Goal (mg/dL)	LDL Level at Which to Initiate Therapeutic Lifestyle Changes (mg/dL)	LDL Level at Which to Consider Drug Therapy (mg/dL)
CHD† or CHD risk equivalents (10-year risk >20%)	<100	≥ 100	≥ 130 (100-129:drug optional) ††
2+ Risk factors (10-year risk ≤20%)	<130	≥ 130	10-year risk 10%-20%: ≥ 130 10-year risk <10%: ≥ 160
0-1 Risk factor †††	<160	≥ 160	≥ 190 (160-189:LDL-lowering drug optional)

† CHD, coronary heart disease

†† Some authorities recommend use of LDL-lowering drugs in this category if an LDL-C level of <100 mg/dL cannot be achieved by therapeutic lifestyle changes. Others prefer use of drugs that primarily modify triglycerides and HDL-C, e.g., nicotinic acid or fibrate. Clinical judgement also may call for deferring drug therapy in this subcategory.

††† Almost all people with 0-1 risk factor have 10-year risk <10%; thus, 10-year risk assessment in people with 0-1 risk factor is not necessary.

CONTRAINDICATIONS

ADVICOR is contraindicated in patients with a known hypersensitivity to niacin, lovastatin or any component of this medication, active liver disease or unexplained persistent elevations in serum transaminases (see WARNINGS), active peptic ulcer disease, or arterial bleeding.

Concomitant administration with strong CYP3A4 inhibitors (e.g., itraconazole, ketoconazole, posaconazole, HIV protease inhibitors, boceprevir, telaprevir, erythromycin, clarithromycin, telithromycin and nefazodone) (see WARNINGS, Myopathy/Rhabdomyolysis).

Pregnancy and lactation - Atherosclerosis is a chronic process and the discontinuation of lipid-lowering drugs during pregnancy should have little impact on the outcome of long-term therapy of primary hypercholesterolemia. Moreover, cholesterol and other products of the cholesterol biosynthesis pathway are essential components for fetal development, including synthesis of steroids and cell membranes. Because of the ability of inhibitors of HMG-CoA reductase, such as lovastatin, to decrease the synthesis of cholesterol and possibly other products of the cholesterol biosynthesis pathway, ADVICOR is contraindicated in women who are pregnant and in lactating mothers. ADVICOR may cause fetal harm when administered to pregnant women. **ADVICOR should be administered to women of childbearing age only when such patients are highly unlikely to conceive.** If the patient becomes pregnant while taking this drug, ADVICOR should be discontinued immediately and the patient should be apprised of the potential hazard to the fetus (see PRECAUTIONS, Pregnancy).

WARNINGS

ADVICOR should not be substituted for equivalent doses of immediate-release (crystalline) niacin. For patients switching from immediate-release niacin to NIASPAN, therapy with NIASPAN should be initiated with low doses (i.e., 500 mg once daily at bedtime) and the NIASPAN dose should then be titrated to the desired therapeutic response (see DOSAGE AND ADMINISTRATION).

Liver Dysfunction

Cases of severe hepatic toxicity, including fulminant hepatic necrosis, have occurred in patients who have substituted sustained-release (modified-release, timed-release) niacin products for immediate-release (crystalline) niacin at equivalent doses.

ADVICOR should be used with caution in patients who consume substantial quantities of alcohol and/or have a past history of liver disease. Active liver disease or unexplained transaminase elevations are contraindications to the use of ADVICOR.

Niacin preparations and lovastatin preparations have been associated with abnormal liver tests. In studies using NIASPAN alone, 0.8% of patients were discontinued for transaminase elevations. In studies using lovastatin alone, 0.2% of patients were discontinued for transaminase elevations.[2] In three safety and efficacy studies involving titration to final daily ADVICOR doses ranging from 500 mg/10 mg to 2500 mg/40 mg, ten of 1028 patients (1.0%) experienced reversible elevations in AST/ALT to more than 3 times the upper limit of normal (ULN). Three of ten elevations occurred at doses outside the recommended dosing limit of 2000 mg/40 mg; no patient receiving 1000 mg/20 mg had 3-fold elevations in AST/ALT.

In clinical studies with ADVICOR, elevations in transaminases did not appear to be related to treatment duration; elevations in AST and ALT levels did appear to be dose related. Transaminase elevations were reversible upon discontinuation of ADVICOR.

It is recommended that liver enzyme tests be obtained prior to initiating therapy with ADVICOR and repeated as clinically indicated.

There have been rare postmarketing reports of fatal and non-fatal hepatic failure in patients taking statins, including lovastatin. If serious liver injury with clinical symptoms and/or hyperbilirubinemia or jaundice occurs during treatment with ADVICOR, promptly interrupt therapy. If an alternate etiology is not found do not restart ADVICOR.

Myopathy/Rhabdomyolysis

Lovastatin and other inhibitors of HMG-CoA reductase occasionally cause myopathy, which is manifested as muscle pain or weakness associated with grossly elevated creatine kinase (> 10 times ULN). **Rhabdomyolysis, with or without acute renal failure secondary to myoglobinuria, has been reported rarely and can occur at any time.** In a large, long-term, clinical safety and efficacy study (the EXCEL study)[3,4] with lovastatin, myopathy occurred in up to 0.2% of patients treated with lovastatin 20 to 80 mg for up to 2 years. When drug treatment was interrupted or discontinued in these patients, muscle symptoms and creatine kinase (CK) increases promptly resolved. The risk of myopathy is increased by concomitant therapy with certain drugs, some of which were excluded by the EXCEL study design.

The risk of myopathy/rhabdomyolysis is increased by concomitant use of lovastatin with the following:

Strong inhibitors of CYP3A4: The risk of myopathy appears to be increased by high levels of HMG-CoA reductase inhibitory activity in plasma. Lovastatin is metabolized by the cytochrome P450 isoform 3A4. Certain drugs which share this metabolic pathway can raise the plasma levels of lovastatin and may increase the risk of myopathy. These include itraconazole, ketoconazole, and posaconazole, the macrolide antibiotics erythromycin and clarithromycin, and the ketolide antibiotic telithromycin, HIV protease inhibitors, boceprevir, telaprevir, the antidepressant nefazodone, or large quantities of grapefruit juice (>1 quart daily). Combination of these drugs with lovastatin is contraindicated. If treatment with itraconazole, ketoconazole, erythromycin, clarithromycin or telithromycin is unavoidable, therapy with lovastatin should be suspended during the course of treatment.

Information on the AbbVie, Inc. products listed on these pages is from the prescribing information in use as of July 31, 2013. For more information, please visit rxabbvie.com or call 1-800-633-9110.

Although not studied clinically, voriconazole has been shown to inhibit lovastatin metabolism *in vitro* (human liver microsomes). Therefore, voriconazole is likely to increase the plasma concentration of lovastatin. It is recommended that dose adjustment of lovastatin be considered during coadministration. Increased lovastatin concentration in plasma has been associated with an increased risk of myopathy/rhabdomyolysis.

Gemfibrozil: **The combined use of lovastatin with gemfibrozil should be avoided.**

Other fibrates: Caution should be used when prescribing other fibrates with lovastatin, as these agents can cause myopathy when given alone. **The benefit of further alterations in lipid levels by the combined use of lovastatin with other fibrates should be carefully weighed against the potential risks of this combination.**

Cyclosporine: **The use of lovastatin with cyclosporine should be avoided.**

Danazol, diltiazem or verapamil with higher doses of lovastatin: **In patients taking concomitant danazol, diltiazem or verapamil, the dose of lovastatin should not exceed 20 mg** (see DOSAGE AND ADMINISTRATION), **as the risk of myopathy increases at higher doses.** The benefits of the use of lovastatin in patients receiving danazol, diltiazem, or verapamil should be carefully weighed against the risks of these combinations.

Amiodarone: **In patients taking concomitant amiodarone, the dose of lovastatin should not exceed 40 mg (see DOSAGE AND ADMINISTRATION), as the risk of myopathy increases at higher doses.**

Colchicine: Cases of myopathy, including rhabdomyolysis, have been reported with lovastatin coadministered with colchicine, and caution should be exercised when prescribing lovastatin with colchicine.

Ranolazine: The risk of myopathy, including rhabdomyolysis, may be increased by concomitant administration of ranolazine. Dose adjustment of lovastatin may be considered during co-administration with ranolazine.

Prescribing recommendations for interacting agents are summarized in Table 9.

Table 9.
Drug Interactions Associated with Increased Risk of Myopathy/Rhabdomyolysis

Interacting Agents	Prescribing Recommendations
Strong CYP3A4 inhibitors, e.g.: Ketoconazole Itraconazole Posaconazole Erythromycin Clarithromycin Telithromycin HIV protease inhibitors Boceprevir Telaprevir Nefazodone	Contraindicated with lovastatin
Gemfibrozil Cyclosporine	Avoid with lovastatin
Danazol Diltiazem Verapamil	Do not exceed 20 mg lovastatin daily
Amiodarone	Do not exceed 40 mg lovastatin daily
Grapefruit juice	Avoid large quantities of grapefruit juice (>1 quart daily)

ADVICOR

Myopathy and/or rhabdomyolysis have been reported when lovastatin is used in combination with lipid-altering doses (≥1g/day) of niacin. Physicians contemplating the use of ADVICOR, a combination of lovastatin and niacin, should weigh the potential benefits and risks, and should carefully monitor patients for any signs and symptoms of muscle pain, tenderness, or weakness, particularly during the initial month of treatment or during any period of upward dosage titration of either drug. Periodic CK determinations may be considered in such situations, but there is no assurance that such monitoring will prevent myopathy.

In clinical studies, no cases of rhabdomyolysis and one suspected case of myopathy have been reported in 1079 patients who were treated with ADVICOR at doses up to 2000 mg/40 mg for periods up to 2 years.

There have been rare reports of immune-mediated necrotizing myopathy (IMNM), an autoimmune myopathy, associated with statin use. IMNM is characterized by: proximal muscle weakness and elevated serum creatine kinase, which persist despite discontinuation of statin treatment; muscle biopsy showing necotizing myopathy without significant inflammation; improvement with immunosuppressive agents.

All patients starting therapy with ADVICOR, or whose dose of ADVICOR is being increased, should be advised of the risk of myopathy, and told to report promptly unexplained muscle pain, tenderness, or weakness particularly if accompanied by malaise or fever or if muscle signs and symptoms persist after discontinuing ADVICOR. A CK level above 10 times ULN in a patient with unexplained muscle symptoms indicates myopathy. ADVICOR therapy should be discontinued immediately if myopathy is diagnosed or suspected.

In patients with complicated medical histories predisposing to rhabdomyolysis, such as preexisting renal insufficiency, dose escalation requires caution. ADVICOR therapy should be discontinued if markedly elevated CPK levels occur or myopathy is diagnosed or suspected. ADVICOR therapy should also be temporarily withheld in any patient experiencing an acute or serious condition predisposing to the development of renal failure secondary to rhabdomyolysis, e.g., sepsis; hypotension; major surgery; trauma; severe metabolic, endocrine, or electrolyte disorders; or uncontrolled epilepsy.

PRECAUTIONS

General

Before instituting therapy with a lipid-altering medication, an attempt should be made to control dyslipidemia with appropriate diet, exercise, and weight reduction in obese patients, and to treat other underlying medical problems (see INDICATIONS AND USAGE).

Patients with a past history of jaundice, hepatobiliary disease, or peptic ulcer should be observed closely during ADVICOR therapy. Frequent monitoring of liver function tests and blood glucose should be performed to ascertain that the drug is producing no adverse effects on these organ systems.

Diabetic patients may experience a dose-related rise in fasting blood sugar (FBS). In three clinical studies, which included 1028 patients exposed to ADVICOR (6 to 22% of whom had diabetes type II at baseline), increases in FBS above normal occurred in 46 to 65% of patients at any time during study treatment with ADVICOR. Fourteen patients (1.4%) were discontinued from study treatment: 3 patients for worsening diabetes, 10 patients for hyperglycemia and 1 patient for a new diagnosis of diabetes. In the studies in which lovastatin and NIASPAN were used as active controls, 24 to 41% of patients receiving lovastatin and 43 to 58% of patients receiving NIASPAN also had increases in FBS above normal. One patient (1.1%) receiving lovastatin was discontinued for hyperglycemia. Diabetic or potentially diabetic patients should be observed closely during treatment with ADVICOR, and adjustment of diet and/or hypoglycemic therapy may be necessary.

In one long-term study of 106 patients treated with ADVICOR, elevations in prothrombin time (PT) >3 times ULN occurred in 2 patients (2%) during study drug treatment. In a long-term study of 814 patients treated with ADVICOR, 7 patients were noted to have platelet counts <100,000 during study drug treatment. Four of these patients were discontinued, and one patient with a platelet count <100,000 had prolonged bleeding after a tooth extraction. Prior studies have shown that NIASPAN can be associated with dose-related reductions in platelet count (mean of -11% with 2000 mg) and increases of PT (mean of approximately +4%). Accordingly, patients undergoing surgery should be carefully evaluated. In controlled studies, ADVICOR has been associated with small but statistically significant dose-related reductions in phosphorus levels (mean of -10% with 2000 mg/40 mg). Phosphorus levels should be monitored periodically in patients at risk for hypophosphatemia. In clinical studies with ADVICOR, hypophosphatemia was more common in males than in females. The clinical relevance of hypophosphatemia in this population is not known.

Niacin

Caution should also be used when ADVICOR is used in patients with unstable angina or in the acute phase of MI, particularly when such patients are also receiving vasoactive drugs such as nitrates, calcium channel blockers, or adrenergic blocking agents.

Elevated uric acid levels have occurred with niacin therapy; therefore, in patients predisposed to gout, niacin therapy should be used with caution. Niacin is rapidly metabolized by the liver, and excreted through the kidneys. ADVICOR is contraindicated in patients with significant or unexplained hepatic dysfunction (see CONTRAINDICATIONS and WARNINGS) and should be used with caution in patients with renal dysfunction.

Lovastatin

Lovastatin may elevate creatine phosphokinase and transaminase levels (see WARNINGS and ADVERSE REACTIONS). This should be considered in the differential diagnosis of chest pain in a patient on therapy with lovastatin.

Endocrine function - Increases in HbA1c and fasting serum glucose levels have been reported with HMG-CoA reductase inhibitors, including lovastatin.

HMG-CoA reductase inhibitors interfere with cholesterol synthesis and as such might theoretically blunt adrenal and/or gonadal steroid production. Results of clinical studies with drugs in this class have been inconsistent with regard to drug effects on basal and reserve steroid levels. However, clinical studies have shown that lovastatin does not reduce basal plasma cortisol concentration or impair adrenal reserve, and does not reduce basal plasma testosterone concentration. Another HMG-CoA reductase inhibitor has been shown to reduce the plasma testosterone response to human chorionic gonadotropin (HCG). In the same study, the mean testosterone response to HCG was slightly but not significantly reduced after treatment with lovastatin 40 mg daily for 16 weeks in 21 men. The effects of HMG-CoA reductase inhibitors on male fertility have not been studied in adequate numbers of male patients. The effects, if any, on the pituitary-gonadal axis in premenopausal women are unknown. Patients treated with lovastatin who develop clinical evidence of endocrine dysfunction should be evaluated appropriately. Caution should also be exercised if an HMG-CoA reductase inhibitor or other agent used to lower cholesterol levels is administered to patients also receiving other drugs (e.g., spironolactone, cimetidine) that may decrease the levels or activity of endogenous steroid hormones.

CNS toxicity - Lovastatin produced optic nerve degeneration (Wallerian degeneration of retinogeniculate fibers) in clinically normal dogs in a dose-dependent fashion starting at 60 mg/kg/day, a dose that produced mean plasma drug levels about 30 times higher than the mean drug level in humans taking the highest recommended dose (as measured by total enzyme inhibitory activity). Vestibulocochlear Wallerian-like degeneration and retinal ganglion cell chromatolysis were also seen in dogs treated for 14 weeks at 180 mg/kg/day, a dose which resulted in a mean plasma drug level (C_{max}) similar to that seen with the 60 mg/kg/day dose.

CNS vascular lesions, characterized by perivascular hemorrhage and edema, mononuclear cell infiltration of perivascular spaces, perivascular fibrin deposits and necrosis of small vessels, were seen in dogs treated with lovastatin at a dose of 180 mg/kg/day, a dose which produced plasma drug levels (C_{max}) which were about 30 times higher than the mean values in humans taking 80 mg/day.

Similar optic nerve and CNS vascular lesions have been observed with other drugs of this class.

Cataracts were seen in dogs treated with lovastatin for 11 and 28 weeks at 180 mg/kg/day and 1 year at 60 mg/kg/day.

Information for Patients

Patients should be advised of the following:

- to report promptly unexplained muscle pain, tenderness, or weakness particularly if accompanied by malaise or fever or if muscle signs and symptoms persist after discontinuing ADVICOR (see WARNINGS, Myopathy/Rhabdomyolysis);
- to report promptly any symptoms that may indicate liver injury, including fatigue, anorexia, right upper abdominal discomfort, dark urine or jaundice (see WARNINGS, Liver Dysfunction);
- to take ADVICOR at bedtime, with a low-fat snack. Administration on an empty stomach is not recommended;
- to carefully follow the prescribed dosing regimen (see DOSAGE AND ADMINISTRATION);
- that flushing is a common side effect of niacin therapy that usually subsides after several weeks of consistent niacin use. Flushing may last for several hours after dosing, may vary in severity, and will, by taking ADVICOR at bedtime, most likely occur during sleep. If awakened by flushing, especially if taking antihypertensives, rise slowly to minimize the potential for dizziness and/or syncope;
- that taking aspirin (up to approximately 30 minutes before taking ADVICOR) may minimize flushing;
- to avoid ingestion of alcohol, hot beverages and spicy foods around the time of ADVICOR administration, to minimize flushing;
- should not be administered with grapefruit juice;
- that if ADVICOR therapy is discontinued for an extended length of time, their physician should be contacted prior to re-starting therapy; re-titration is recommended (see DOSAGE AND ADMINISTRATION);
- to notify their physician if they are taking vitamins or other nutritional supplements containing niacin or related compounds such as nicotinamide (see Drug Interactions);
- to notify their physician if symptoms of dizziness occur;
- if diabetic, to notify their physician of changes in blood glucose;
- that ADVICOR tablets should not be broken, crushed, or chewed, but should be swallowed whole.

Drug Interactions

Niacin

Antihypertensive Therapy - Niacin may potentiate the effects of ganglionic blocking agents and vasoactive drugs resulting in postural hypotension.

Aspirin - Concomitant aspirin may decrease the metabolic clearance of niacin. The clinical relevance of this finding is unclear.

Bile Acid Sequestrants - An *in vitro* study was carried out investigating the niacin-binding capacity of colestipol and cholestyramine. About 98% of available niacin was bound to colestipol, with 10 to 30% binding to cholestyramine. These results suggest that 4 to 6 hours, or as great an interval as possible, should elapse between the ingestion of bile acid-binding resins and the administration of ADVICOR.

Other - Concomitant alcohol or hot drinks may increase the side effects of flushing and pruritus and should be avoided around the time of ADVICOR ingestion. Vitamins or other nutritional supplements containing large doses of niacin or related compounds such as nicotinamide may potentiate the adverse effects of ADVICOR.

Lovastatin

Lovastatin is metabolized by CYP3A4 but has no CYP3A4 inhibitory activity; therefore it is not expected to affect the plasma concentrations of other drugs metabolized by CYP3A4. Strong inhibitors of CYP3A4 (e.g., itraconazole, ketoconazole, posaconazole, clarithromycin, telithromycin, HIV protease inhibitors, boceprevir, telaprevir, nefazodone, and erythromycin), and large quantities of grapefruit juice (>1 quart daily) increase the risk of myopathy by reducing the elimination of lovastatin (see WARNINGS, Myopathy/Rhabdomyolysis).

In vitro studies have demonstrated that voriconazole inhibits the metabolism of lovastatin. Adjustment of the lovastatin dose may be needed to reduce the risk of myopathy, including rhabdomyolysis, if voriconazole must be used concomitantly with lovastatin.

Interactions With Lipid-Lowering Drugs That Can Cause Myopathy When Given Alone

The risk of myopathy is also increased by the following lipid-lowering drugs that are not strong CYP3A4 inhibitors, but which can cause myopathy when given alone (see WARNINGS, Myopathy/Rhabdomyolysis).

Gemfibrozil

Other fibrates

Other Drug Interactions

Cyclosporine: The risk of myopathy/rhabdomyolysis is increased by concomitant administration of cyclosporine (see WARNINGS, Myopathy/Rhabdomyolysis).

Danazol, Diltiazem, or Verapamil: The risk of myopathy/rhabdomyolysis is increased by concomitant administration of danazol, diltiazem, or verapamil particularly with higher doses of lovastatin (see WARNINGS, Myopathy/Rhabdomyolysis and CLINICAL PHARMACOLOGY, Pharmacokinetics).

Amiodarone: The risk of myopathy/rhabdomyolysis is increased when amiodarone is used concomitantly with a closely related member of the HMGCoA reductase inhibitor class (see WARNINGS, Myopathy/Rhabdomyolysis).

Coumarin Anticoagulants - In a small clinical study in which lovastatin was administered to warfarin-treated patients, no effect on PT was detected. However, another HMG-CoA reductase inhibitor has been found to produce a less than two seconds increase in PT in healthy volunteers receiving low doses of warfarin. Also, bleeding and/or increased PT have been reported in a few patients taking coumarin anticoagulants concomitantly with lovastatin. It is recommended that in patients taking anticoagulants, PT be determined before starting ADVICOR and frequently enough during early therapy to insure that no significant alteration of PT occurs. Once a stable PT has been documented, PT can be monitored at the intervals usually recommended for patients on coumarin anticoagulants. If the dose of ADVICOR is changed, the same procedure should be repeated.

Colchicine - Cases of myopathy, including rhabdomyolysis, have been reported with lovastatin coadministered with colchicine.

Ranolazine - The risk of myopathy, including rhabdomyolysis, may be increased by concomitant administration of ranolazine.

Propranolol - In normal volunteers, there was no clinically significant pharmacokinetic or pharmacodynamic interaction with concomitant administration of single doses of lovastatin and propranolol.

Digoxin - In patients with hypercholesterolemia, concomitant administration of lovastatin and digoxin resulted in no effect on digoxin plasma concentrations.

Oral Hypoglycemic Agents - In pharmacokinetic studies of lovastatin in hypercholesterolemic, non-insulin dependent diabetic patients, there was no drug interaction with glipizide or with chlorpropamide.

Drug/Laboratory Test Interactions

Niacin may produce false elevations in some fluorometric determinations of plasma or urinary catecholamines. Niacin may also give false-positive reactions with cupric sulfate solution (Benedict's reagent) in urine glucose tests.

Carcinogenesis, Mutagenesis, Impairment of Fertility

No studies have been conducted with ADVICOR regarding carcinogenesis, mutagenesis, or impairment of fertility.

Niacin

Niacin, administered to mice for a lifetime as a 1% solution in drinking water, was not carcinogenic. The mice in this study received approximately 6 to 8 times a human dose of 3000 mg/day as determined on a mg/m^2 basis. Niacin was negative for mutagenicity in the Ames test. No studies on impairment of fertility have been performed.

Lovastatin

In a 21-month carcinogenic study in mice, there was a statistically significant increase in the incidence of hepatocellular carcinomas and adenomas in both males and females at 500 mg/kg/day. This dose produced a total plasma drug exposure 3 to 4 times that of humans given the highest recommended dose of lovastatin (drug exposure was measured as total HMG-CoA reductase inhibitory activity in extracted plasma). Tumor increases were not seen at 20 and 100 mg/kg/day, doses that produced drug exposures of 0.3 to 2 times that of humans at the 80 mg/day dose. A statistically significant increase in pulmonary adenomas was seen in female mice at approximately 4 times the human drug exposure. (Although mice were given 300 times the human dose on a mg/kg body weight basis, plasma levels of total inhibitory activity were only 4 times higher in mice than in humans given 80 mg of lovastatin.)

There was an increase in incidence of papilloma in the non-glandular mucosa of the stomach of mice beginning at exposures of 1 to 2 times that of humans. The glandular mucosa was not affected. The human stomach contains only glandular mucosa.

In a 24-month carcinogenicity study in rats, there was a positive dose-response relationship for hepatocellular carcinogenicity in males at drug exposures between 2 to 7 times that of human exposure at 80 mg/day (doses in rats were 5, 30, and 180 mg/kg/day).

An increased incidence of thyroid neoplasms in rats appears to be a response that has been seen with other HMG-CoA reductase inhibitors.

A drug in this class chemically similar to lovastatin was administered to mice for 72 weeks at 25, 100, and 400 mg/kg body weight, which resulted in mean serum drug levels approximately 3, 15, and 33 times higher than the mean human serum drug concentration (as total inhibitory activity) after a 40 mg oral dose. Liver carcinomas were significantly increased in high-dose females and mid- and high-dose males, with a maximum incidence of 90% in males. The incidence of adenomas of the liver was significantly increased in mid- and high-dose females. Drug treatment also significantly increased the incidence of lung adenomas in mid- and high-dose males and females. Adenomas of the Harderian gland (a gland of the eye of rodents) were significantly higher in high-dose mice than in controls.

No evidence of mutagenicity was observed in a microbial mutagen test using mutant strains of *Salmonella typhimurium* with or without rat or mouse liver metabolic activation. In addition, no evidence of damage to genetic material was noted in an *in vitro* alkaline elution assay using rat or mouse hepatocytes, a V-79 mammalian cell forward mutation study, an *in vitro* chromosome aberration study in CHO cells, or an *in vivo* chromosomal aberration assay in mouse bone marrow.

Drug-related testicular atrophy, decreased spermatogenesis, spermatocytic degeneration and giant cell formation were seen in dogs starting at 20 mg/kg/day. Similar findings were seen with another drug in this class. No drug-related effects on fertility were found in studies with lovastatin in rats. However, in studies with a similar drug in this class, there was decreased fertility in male rats treated for 34 weeks at 25 mg/kg body weight, although this effect was not observed in a subsequent fertility study when this same dose was administered for 11 weeks (the entire cycle of spermatogenesis, including epididymal maturation). In rats treated with this same reductase inhibitor at 180 mg/kg/day, seminiferous tubule degeneration (necrosis and loss of spermatogenic epithelium) was observed. No microscopic changes were observed in the testes from rats of either study. The clinical significance of these findings is unclear.

Pregnancy

Pregnancy Category X — See CONTRAINDICATIONS.

ADVICOR should be administered to women of childbearing potential only when such patients are highly unlikely to conceive and have been informed of the potential hazard. Safety in pregnant women has not been established and there is no apparent benefit to therapy with ADVICOR during pregnancy (see CONTRAINDICATIONS). Treatment should be immediately discontinued as soon as pregnancy is recognized.

Niacin

Animal reproduction studies have not been conducted with niacin or with ADVICOR. It is also not known whether niacin at doses typically used for lipid disorders can cause fetal harm when administered to pregnant women or whether it can affect reproductive capacity. If a woman receiving niacin or ADVICOR for primary hypercholesterolemia becomes pregnant, the drug should be discontinued.

Lovastatin

Rare reports of congenital anomalies have been received following intrauterine exposure to HMG-CoA reductase inhibitors. In a review[5] of approximately 100 prospectively followed pregnancies in women exposed to lovastatin or another structurally related HMG-CoA reductase inhibitor, the incidences of congenital anomalies, spontaneous abortions and fetal deaths/stillbirths did not exceed what would be expected in the general population. The number of cases is adequate only to exclude a 3- to 4-fold increase in congenital anomalies over the background incidence. In 89% of the prospectively followed pregnancies, drug treatment was initiated prior to pregnancy and was discontinued at some point in the first trimester when pregnancy was identified.

Lovastatin has been shown to produce skeletal malformations at plasma levels 40 times the human exposure (for mouse fetus) and 80 times the human exposure (for rat fetus) based on mg/m^2 surface area (doses were 800 mg/kg/day). No drug-induced changes were seen in either species at multiples of 8 times (rat) or 4 times (mouse) based on surface area. No evidence of malformations was noted in rabbits at exposures up to 3 times the human exposure (dose of 15 mg/kg/day, highest tolerated dose).

Labor and Delivery

No studies have been conducted on the effect of ADVICOR, niacin or lovastatin on the mother or the fetus during labor or delivery, on the duration of labor or delivery, or on the growth, development, and functional maturation of the child.

Nursing Mothers

No studies have been conducted with ADVICOR in nursing mothers.

Because of the potential for serious adverse reactions in nursing infants from lipid-altering doses of niacin and lovastatin (see CONTRAINDICATIONS), ADVICOR should not be taken while a woman is breastfeeding.

Niacin has been reported to be excreted in human milk. It is not known whether lovastatin is excreted in human milk. A small amount of another drug in this class is excreted in human breast milk.

Pediatric Use

No studies in patients under 18 years-of-age have been conducted with ADVICOR. Because pediatric patients are not likely to benefit from cholesterol lowering for at least a decade and because experience with this drug or its active ingredients is limited, treatment of pediatric patients with ADVICOR is not recommended at this time.

Geriatric Use

Of the 214 patients who received ADVICOR in double-blind clinical studies, 37.4% were 65 years-of-age and older, and of the 814 patients who received ADVICOR in open-label clinical studies, 36.2% were 65 years-of-age and older. Responses in LDL-C, HDL-C, and TG were similar in geriatric patients. No overall differences in the percentage of patients with adverse events were observed between older and younger patients. No overall differences were observed in selected chemistry values between the two groups except for amylase which was higher in older patients.

ADVERSE REACTIONS

Overview

In controlled clinical studies, 40/214 (19%) of patients randomized to ADVICOR discontinued therapy prior to study completion. Of the 214 patients enrolled 18 (8%) discontinued due to flushing. In the same controlled studies, 9/94 (10%) of patients randomized to lovastatin and 19/92 (21%) of patients randomized to NIASPAN also discontinued treatment prior to study completion secondary to adverse events. Flushing episodes (i.e., warmth, redness, itching and/or tingling) were the most common treatment-emergent adverse events, and occurred in 53% to 83% of patients treated with ADVICOR. Spontaneous reports with NIASPAN and clinical studies with ADVICOR suggest that flushing may also be accompanied by symptoms of dizziness or syncope, tachycardia, palpitations, shortness of breath, sweating, burning sensation/skin burning sensation, chills, and/or edema.

Adverse Reactions Information

Because clinical studies are conducted under widely varying conditions, adverse reaction rates observed in clinical stud-

Information on the AbbVie, Inc. products listed on these pages is from the prescribing information in use as of July 31, 2013. For more information, please visit rxabbvie.com or call 1-800-633-9110.

ies of a drug cannot be directly compared to rates in the clinical studies of another drug and may not reflect the rates observed in clinical practice. The adverse reaction information from clinical studies does, however provide a basis for identifying the adverse events that appear to be related to drug use and for approximating rates.

The data described in this section reflect the exposure to ADVICOR in two double-blind, controlled clinical studies of 400 patients. The population was 28 to 86 years-of-age, 54% male, 85% Caucasian, 9% Black, and 7% Other, and had mixed dyslipidemia.

In addition to flushing, other adverse events occurring in 5% or greater of patients treated with ADVICOR are shown in Table 10 below.

Table 10. Treatment-Emergent Adverse Events in ≥ 5% of Patients (Events Irrespective of Causality; Data from Controlled, Double-Blind Studies)

Adverse Event	ADVICOR	NIASPAN	Lovastatin
Total Number of Patients	214	92	94
Cardiovascular	**163 (76%)**	**66 (72%)**	**24 (26%)**
Flushing	152 (71%)	60 (65%)	17 (18%)
Body as a Whole	**104 (49%)**	**50 (54%)**	**42 (45%)**
Asthenia	10 (5%)	6 (7%)	5 (5%)
Flu Syndrome	12 (6%)	7 (8%)	4 (4%)
Headache	20 (9%)	12 (13%)	5 (5%)
Infection	43 (20%)	14 (15%)	19 (20%)
Pain	18 (8%)	3 (3%)	9 (10%)
Pain, Abdominal	9 (4%)	1 (1%)	6 (6%)
Pain, Back	10 (5%)	5 (5%)	5 (5%)
Digestive System	**51 (24%)**	**26 (28%)**	**16 (17%)**
Diarrhea	13 (6%)	8 (9%)	2 (2%)
Dyspepsia	6 (3%)	5 (5%)	4 (4%)
Nausea	14 (7%)	11 (12%)	2 (2%)
Vomiting	7 (3%)	5 (5%)	0
Metabolic and Nutrit. System	**37 (17%)**	**18 (20%)**	**13 (14%)**
Hyperglycemia	8 (4%)	6 (7%)	6 (6%)
Musculoskeletal System	**19 (9%)**	**9 (10%)**	**17 (18%)**
Myalgia	6 (3%)	5 (5%)	8 (9%)
Skin and Appendages	**38 (18%)**	**19 (21%)**	**11 (12%)**
Pruritus	14 (7%)	7 (8%)	3 (3%)
Rash	11 (5%)	11 (12%)	3 (3%)

Note: Percentages are calculated from the total number of patients in each column.

See also the full prescribing information for niacin extended release (Niaspan) and lovastatin products.

The following adverse events have also been reported with niacin, lovastatin, and/or other HMG-CoA reductase inhibitors, but not necessarily with ADVICOR, either during clinical studies or in routine patient management.

Body as a Whole:	chest pain; abdominal pain; edema; chills; malaise
Cardiovascular:	atrial fibrillation; tachycardia; palpitations, and other cardiac arrhythmias; postural hypotension, orthostasis; hypotension; syncope
Eye:	toxic amblyopia; cystoid macular edema; ophthalmoplegia; eye irritation, blurred vision, progression of cataracts
Gastrointestinal:	activation of peptic ulcers and peptic ulceration; dyspepsia; vomiting; anorexia; constipation; flatulence, pancreatitis; hepatitis; fatty change in liver; jaundice; and rarely, cirrhosis, fulminant hepatic necrosis, and hepatoma, eructation, fatal and non-fatal hepatic failure
Metabolic:	gout, decreased glucose tolerance
Musculoskeletal:	muscle cramps; myopathy; rhabdomyolysis; arthralgia, myalgia. There have been rare reports of immune-mediated necrotizing myopathy with statin use (see WARNINGS).
Nervous:	dizziness; insomnia; dry mouth; paresthesia; anxiety; tremor; vertigo; peripheral neuropathy; psychic disturbances; dysfunction of certain cranial nerves, nervousness, burning sensation/skin burning sensation, peripheral nerve palsy
Psychiatric	depression
Skin:	hyper-pigmentation; acanthosis nigricans; urticaria; alopecia; dry skin; sweating; and a variety of skin changes (e.g., nodules, discoloration, dryness of mucous membranes, changes to hair/nails), vesiculobullous rash, maculopapular rash
Respiratory:	dyspnea; rhinitis
Urogenital:	gynecomastia; loss of libido; erectile dysfunction
Hypersensitivity reactions:	An apparent hypersensitivity syndrome has been reported rarely, which has included one or more of the following features: anaphylaxis, angioedema, tongue edema, larynx edema, face edema, peripheral edema, laryngismus, lupus erythematous-like syndrome, polymyalgia rheumatica, vasculitis, purpura, thrombocytopenia, leukopenia, hemolytic anemia, positive ANA, ESR increase, eosinophilia, arthritis, arthralgia, urticaria, asthenia, photosensitivity, fever, chills, flushing, malaise, dyspnea, toxic epidermal necrolysis, erythema multiforme, including Stevens-Johnson syndrome, dermatomyositis
Other:	migraine

There have been rare postmarketing reports of cognitive impairment (e.g., memory loss, forgetfulness, amnesia, memory impairment, confusion) associated with statin use. These cognitive issues have been reported for all statins. The reports are generally nonserious, and reversible upon statin discontinuation, with variable times to symptom onset (1 day to years) and symptom resolution (median of 3 weeks).

Clinical Laboratory Abnormalities

Chemistry

Elevations in serum transaminases (see WARNINGS - Liver Dysfunction), CPK and fasting glucose, and reductions in phosphorus. Niacin extended-release tablets have been associated with slight elevations in LDH, uric acid, total bilirubin, amylase and creatine kinase. Lovastatin and/or HMG-CoA reductase inhibitors have been associated with elevations in alkaline phosphatase, γ-glutamyl transpeptidase and bilirubin, and thyroid function abnormalities.

Hematology

Niacin extended-release tablets have been associated with slight reductions in platelet counts and prolongation in PT (see WARNINGS).

DRUG ABUSE AND DEPENDENCE

Neither niacin nor lovastatin is a narcotic drug. ADVICOR has no known addiction potential in humans.

OVERDOSAGE

Information on acute overdose with ADVICOR in humans is limited. Until further experience is obtained, no specific treatment of overdose with ADVICOR can be recommended. The patient should be carefully observed and given supportive treatment.

Niacin

The s.c. LD50 of niacin is 5 g/kg in rats.

The signs and symptoms of an acute overdose of niacin can be anticipated to be those of excessive pharmacologic effect: severe flushing, nausea/vomiting, diarrhea, dyspepsia, dizziness, syncope, hypotension, possibly cardiac arrhythmias and clinical laboratory abnormalities. Insufficient information is available on the potential for the dialyzability of niacin.

Lovastatin

After oral administration of lovastatin to mice the median lethal dose observed was >15 g/m^2.

Five healthy human volunteers have received up to 200 mg of lovastatin as a single dose without clinically significant adverse experiences. A few cases of accidental overdose have been reported; no patients had any specific symptoms, and all patients recovered without sequelae. The maximum dose taken was 5 to 6 g. The dialyzability of lovastatin and its metabolites in man is not known at present.

DOSAGE AND ADMINISTRATION

The patient should be placed on a standard cholesterol-lowering diet before receiving ADVICOR or its individual active components and should continue on this diet during treatment with lipid-altering therapy (see NCEP Treatment Guidelines for details on dietary therapy).

ADVICOR

ADVICOR should be taken at bedtime, with a low-fat snack. ADVICOR tablets should be taken whole and should not be broken, crushed, or chewed before swallowing. Patients not currently on NIASPAN must start ADVICOR at the lowest initial ADVICOR dose, a single 500 mg/20 mg tablet once daily at bedtime. The dose of ADVICOR should not be increased by more than 500 mg daily (based on the NIASPAN component) every 4 weeks. The dose of ADVICOR should be individualized based on targeted goals for cholesterol and triglycerides, and on patient response. Doses of ADVICOR greater than 2000 mg/40 mg daily are not recommended. **If ADVICOR therapy is discontinued for an extended period (>7 days), reinstitution of therapy should begin with the lowest dose of ADVICOR.**

Flushing of the skin (see ADVERSE REACTIONS) may be reduced in frequency or severity by pretreatment with aspirin up to the recommended dose of 325 mg (taken up to approximately 30 minutes prior to ADVICOR dose). Flushing, pruritus, and gastrointestinal distress are also greatly reduced by slowly increasing the dose of niacin and avoiding administration on an empty stomach.

Equivalent doses of ADVICOR may be substituted for equivalent doses of NIASPAN but should not be substituted for other modified-release (sustained-release or time-release) niacin preparations or immediate-release (crystalline) niacin preparations (see WARNINGS). Patients previously receiving niacin products other than NIASPAN should be started on NIASPAN with the recommended NIASPAN titration schedule, and the dose should subsequently be individualized based on patient response. A relative bioavailability study results indicated that ADVICOR tablet strengths (i.e. two tablets of 500 mg/20 mg and one tablet of 1000 mg/40 mg) are not interchangeable.

NIASPAN

NIASPAN should be taken at bedtime, after a low-fat snack, and doses should be individualized according to patient response. Therapy with NIASPAN must be initiated at 500 mg at bedtime in order to reduce the incidence and severity of side effects which may occur during early therapy. NIASPAN must be titrated and the dose should not be increased by more than 500 mg every 4 weeks up to a maximum dose of 2000 mg a day. The recommended dose escalation is shown in Table 11 below. Patients already receiving a stable dose of NIASPAN may be switched directly to a niacin-equivalent dose of ADVICOR.

Table 11. Recommended Dosing

	Week(s)	Daily dose	NIASPAN Dosage
INITIAL TITRATION SCHEDULE	1 to 4	500 mg	1 NIASPAN 500 mg tablet at bedtime
	5 to 8	1000 mg	2 NIASPAN 500 mg tablets at bedtime
	*	1500 mg	2 NIASPAN 750 mg tablets or 3 NIASPAN 500 mg tablets at bedtime
	*	2000 mg	2 NIASPAN 1000 mg tablets or 4 NIASPAN 500 mg tablets at bedtime

* After Week 8, titrate to patient response and tolerance. If response to 1000 mg daily is inadequate, increase dose to 1500 mg daily; may subsequently increase dose to 2000 mg daily. Daily dose should not be increased more than 500 mg in a 4-week period, and doses above 2000 mg daily are not recommended. Women may respond at lower doses than men.

Maintenance Dose:

The daily dosage of NIASPAN should not be increased by more than 500 mg in any 4-week period. The recommended maintenance dose is 1000 mg (two 500 mg tablets) to 2000 mg (two 1000 mg tablets or four 500 mg tablets) once daily at bedtime. Doses greater than 2000 mg daily are not recommended. Women may respond at lower NIASPAN doses than men.

Flushing of the skin (see ADVERSE REACTIONS) may be reduced in frequency or severity by pretreatment with aspirin up to the recommended dose of 325 mg (taken 30 minutes prior to NIASPAN dose). Tolerance to this flushing develops rapidly over the course of several weeks. Flushing, pruritus, and gastrointestinal distress are also greatly reduced by slowly increasing the dose of niacin and avoiding administration on an empty stomach. Concomitant alcoholic, hot drinks or spicy foods may increase the side effects of flushing and pruritus and should be avoided around the time of ADVICOR ingestion.

Equivalent doses of NIASPAN should **not** be substituted for sustained-release (modified-release, timed-release) niacin preparations or immediate-release (crystalline) niacin (see WARNINGS). Patients previously receiving other niacin products should be started with the recommended NIASPAN titration schedule (see Table 11), and the dose should subsequently be individualized based on patient response. Single-dose bioavailability studies have demonstrated that NIASPAN tablet strengths are not interchangeable.

If NIASPAN therapy is discontinued for an extended period, reinstitution of therapy should include a titration phase (see Table 11).

NIASPAN tablets should be taken whole and should not be broken, crushed or chewed before swallowing.

Concomitant Therapy

Concomitant Therapy with Lovastatin

Patients already receiving a stable dose of lovastatin who require further TG-lowering or HDL-raising (e.g., to achieve NCEP non-HDL-C goals), may receive concomitant dosage titration with NIASPAN per NIASPAN recommended initial titration schedule (see Table 10, DOSAGE AND ADMINISTRATION section). For patients already receiving a stable dose of NIASPAN who require further LDL-lowering (e.g., to achieve NCEP LDL-C goals; Table 8), the usual recommended starting dose of lovastatin is 20 mg once a day. Dose adjustments should be made at intervals of 4 weeks or more. Combination therapy with NIASPAN and lovastatin should not exceed doses of 2000 mg and 40 mg daily, respectively.

Dosage in Patients with Renal or Hepatic Insufficiency

Use of NIASPAN in patients with renal or hepatic insufficiency has not been studied. NIASPAN is contraindicated in patients with significant or unexplained hepatic dysfunction (see WARNINGS, PRECAUTIONS). NIASPAN should be used with caution in patients with renal insufficiency (see CLINICAL PHARMACOLOGY).

Lovastatin

The usual recommended starting dose is 20 mg once a day given with the evening meal. The recommended dosing range is 10-80 mg/day in single or two divided doses; the maximum recommended dose is 80 mg/day. Doses should be individualized according to the recommended goal of therapy (see NCEP Guidelines and CLINICAL PHARMACOLOGY). Patients requiring reductions in LDL cholesterol of 20% or more to achieve their goal (see INDICATIONS AND USAGE) should be started on 20 mg/day of lovastatin. A starting dose of 10 mg may be considered for patients requiring smaller reductions. Adjustments should be made at intervals of 4 weeks or more.

Cholesterol levels should be monitored periodically and consideration should be given to reducing the dosage of lovastatin if cholesterol levels fall significantly below the targeted range.

Dosage in Patients taking Danazol, Diltiazem or Verapamil

In patients taking danazol, diltiazem, or verapamil concomitantly with lovastatin (see WARNINGS, Myopathy/Rhabdomyolysis), therapy should begin with 10 mg of lovastatin and should not exceed 20 mg/day.

Dosage in Patients taking Amiodarone

In patients taking amiodarone concomitantly with lovastatin, the dose should not exceed 40 mg/day (see WARNINGS, Myopathy/Rhabdomyolysis and PRECAUTIONS, Drug Interactions, Other drug interactions).

Concomitant Lipid-Lowering Therapy

Use of lovastatin with gemfibrozil should be avoided.

Caution should be used when prescribing other fibrates with lovastatin, as fibrates can cause myopathy when given alone.

Dosage in Patients with Renal Insufficiency

In patients with severe renal insufficiency (creatinine clearance <30 mL/min), dosage increases above 20 mg/day should be carefully considered and, if deemed necessary, implemented cautiously (see CLINICAL PHARMACOLOGY and WARNINGS, Myopathy/Rhabdomyolysis).

HOW SUPPLIED

ADVICOR is an unscored capsule-shaped tablet containing either 500, 750, or 1000 mg of extended-release niacin, and 20 mg of immediate-release lovastatin (ADVICOR 500 mg/20 mg, 750 mg/20 mg, 1000 mg/20 mg), or 1000 mg of extended-release niacin and 40 mg of immediate-release lovastatin (ADVICOR 1000 mg/40 mg). Tablets are color-coated and printed with the "a" logo and a code number specific to the tablet strength on the same side. ADVICOR 500 mg/20 mg tablets are light yellow, code "502". ADVICOR 750 mg/20 mg tablets are light orange, code "752". ADVICOR 1000 mg/20 mg tablets are dark pink/light purple, code "1002". ADVICOR 1000 mg/40 mg tablets are reddish brown, code "1004." Tablets are supplied in bottles of 90 tablets as shown below.

500 mg/20 mg tablets: bottles of 90 - NDC# 0074-3005-90
750 mg/20 mg tablets: bottles of 90 - NDC# 0074-3072-90
1000 mg/20 mg tablets: bottles of 90 - NDC# 0074-3007-90
1000 mg/40 mg tablets: bottles of 90 - NDC# 0074-3010-90

Store at room temperature (20° to 25°C or 68° to 77°F).

NIASPAN is a registered trademark of AbbVie Inc., and Mevacor is a registered trademark of Merck & Co., Inc.

REFERENCES

1. Executive Summary of the Third Report of the National Cholesterol Education Program (NCEP) Expert Panel on Detection, Evaluation, and Treatment of High Blood Cholesterol in Adults (Adult Treatment Panel III). *JAMA* 2001; 285:2486-2497.
2. Downs JR, et al. *JAMA* 1998; 279:1615-1622.
3. Bradford RH, et al. *Arch Intern Med* 1991;151:43-49.
4. Bradford RH, et al. *Am J Cardiol* 1994; 74:667-673.
5. Manson JM, et al. *Reprod Toxicol* 1996; 10(6): 439-446.

Manufactured by AbbVie LTD, Barceloneta, PR 00617
for AbbVie Inc., North Chicago, IL 60064, U.S.A.

Ref: 03-A745-R8-Revised February, 2013

Shown in Product Identification Guide, page 303

ANDROGEL® 1% CIII

[*ăn drō-jĕl*]

(testosterone gel) for topical use

HIGHLIGHTS OF PRESCRIBING INFORMATION

These highlights do not include all the information needed to use AndroGel 1% safely and effectively. See full prescribing information for AndroGel 1%.

AndroGel® (testosterone gel) 1% for topical use CIII

Initial U.S. Approval: 1953

> **WARNING: SECONDARY EXPOSURE TO TESTOSTERONE**
>
> ***See full prescribing information for complete boxed warning.***
>
> - **Virilization has been reported in children who were secondarily exposed to testosterone gel. (5.2, 6.2)**
> - **Children should avoid contact with unwashed or unclothed application sites in men using testosterone gel. (2.2, 5.2)**
> - **Healthcare providers should advise patients to strictly adhere to recommended instructions for use. (2.2, 5.2, 17)**

RECENT MAJOR CHANGES

Indications and Usage. (1) 09/2012

INDICATIONS AND USAGE

AndroGel 1% is an androgen indicated for replacement therapy in males for conditions associated with a deficiency or absence of endogenous testosterone:

- Primary hypogonadism (congenital or acquired). (1)
- Hypogonadotropic hypogonadism (congenital or acquired). (1)

Important limitations of use:

- Safety and efficacy of AndroGel 1% in males less than 18 years old have not been established. (8.4)
- Topical testosterone products may have different doses, strengths or application instructions that may result in different systemic exposure. (1, 12.3)

DOSAGE AND ADMINISTRATION

- **Dosage and Administration for AndroGel 1% differs from AndroGel 1.62 %. For dosage and administration of AndroGel 1.62% refer to its full prescribing information. (2)**
- Starting dose of AndroGel 1% is 50 mg of testosterone (4 pump actuations, two 25 mg packets, or one 50 mg packet), applied once daily in the morning. (2.1)
- Apply to clean, dry, intact skin of shoulders and upper arms and/or abdomen. Do NOT apply AndroGel 1% to any other parts of the body including the genitals, chest or back. (2.2)
- Dose adjustment: AndroGel 1% can be dose adjusted using 50 mg, 75 mg, or 100 mg of testosterone on the basis of total serum testosterone concentration. The dose should be titrated based on the serum testosterone concentration. Additionally, serum testosterone concentration should be assessed periodically. (2.1)
- Patients should wash hands immediately with soap and water after applying AndroGel 1% and cover the application site(s) with clothing after the gel has dried. Wash the application site thoroughly with soap and water prior to any situation where skin-to-skin contact of the application site with another person is anticipated. (2.2)

DOSAGE FORMS AND STRENGTHS

AndroGel (testosterone gel) 1% for topical use is available as follows:

- Metered-dose pump that delivers 12.5 mg of testosterone per actuation. (3)
- Packets containing 25 mg of testosterone. (3)
- Packets containing 50 mg of testosterone. (3)

CONTRAINDICATIONS

- Men with carcinoma of the breast or known or suspected prostate cancer. (4, 5.1)
- Pregnant or breastfeeding women. Testosterone may cause fetal harm. (4, 8.1, 8.3)

WARNINGS AND PRECAUTIONS

- Monitor patients with benign prostatic hyperplasia (BPH) for worsening of signs and symptoms of BPH. (5.1)
- Avoid unintentional exposure of women or children to AndroGel 1%. Secondary exposure to testosterone can produce signs of virilization. AndroGel 1% should be discontinued until the cause of virilization is identified. (5.2)
- Exogenous administration of androgens may lead to azoospermia. (5.5)
- Edema, with or without congestive heart failure (CHF), may be a complication in patients with preexisting cardiac, renal, or hepatic disease. (5.7, 6.2)
- Sleep apnea may occur in those with risk factors. (5.9)
- Monitor serum testosterone, prostate specific antigen (PSA), hemoglobin, hematocrit, liver function tests, and lipid concentrations periodically. (5.1, 5.3, 5.6, 5.10)
- AndroGel 1% is flammable until dry. (5.13)

ADVERSE REACTIONS

Most common adverse reactions (incidence ≥ 5%) are acne, application site reaction, abnormal lab tests, and prostatic disorders. (6.1)

To report SUSPECTED ADVERSE REACTIONS, contact AbbVie Inc. at 1-800-633-9110 or FDA at 1-800-FDA-1088 or *www.fda.gov/medwatch.*

DRUG INTERACTIONS

- Androgens may decrease blood glucose and therefore may decrease insulin requirements in diabetic patients. (7.1)
- Changes in anticoagulant activity may be seen with androgens. More frequent monitoring of INR and prothrombin time is recommended. (7.2)
- Use of testosterone with adrenocorticotrophic hormone (ACTH) or corticosteroids may result in increased fluid retention. Use with caution, particularly in patients with cardiac, renal, or hepatic disease. (7.3)

USE IN SPECIFIC POPULATIONS

- There are insufficient long-term safety data in geriatric patients using AndroGel 1% to assess the potential risks of cardiovascular disease and prostate cancer. (8.5)

See 17 for PATIENT COUNSELING INFORMATION and Medication Guide

Revised: 05/2013

FULL PRESCRIBING INFORMATION: CONTENTS*

Information on the AbbVie, Inc. products listed on these pages is from the prescribing information in use as of July 31, 2013. For more information, please visit rxabbvie.com or call 1-800-633-9110.

* Sections or subsections omitted from the full prescribing information are not listed

FULL PRESCRIBING INFORMATION

WARNING: SECONDARY EXPOSURE TO TESTOSTERONE

- **Virilization has been reported in children who were secondarily exposed to testosterone gel *[see Warnings and Precautions (5.2) and Adverse Reactions (6.2)].***
- **Children should avoid contact with unwashed or unclothed application sites in men using testosterone gel *[see Dosage and Administration (2.2) and Warnings and Precautions (5.2)].***
- **Healthcare providers should advise patients to strictly adhere to recommended instructions for use *[see Dosage and Administration (2.2), Warnings and Precautions (5.2) and Patient Counseling Information (17)].***

1 INDICATIONS AND USAGE

AndroGel 1% is an androgen indicated for replacement therapy in adult males for conditions associated with a deficiency or absence of endogenous testosterone:

- Primary hypogonadism (congenital or acquired): testicular failure due to conditions such as cryptorchidism, bilateral torsion, orchitis, vanishing testis syndrome, orchiectomy, Klinefelter's syndrome, chemotherapy, or toxic damage from alcohol or heavy metals. These men usually have low serum testosterone concentrations and gonadotropins (follicle-stimulating hormone [FSH], luteinizing hormone [LH]) above the normal range.
- Hypogonadotropic hypogonadism (congenital or acquired): idiopathic gonadotropin or luteinizing hormone-releasing hormone (LHRH) deficiency or pituitary-hypothalamic injury from tumors, trauma, or radiation. These men have low testosterone serum concentrations, but have gonadotropins in the normal or low range.

Important limitations of use:

- Safety and efficacy of AndroGel 1% in males less than 18 years old have not been established *[see Use in Specific Populations (8.4)]*.
- Topical testosterone products may have different doses, strengths or application instructions that may result in different systemic exposure (1, 12.3).

2 DOSAGE AND ADMINISTRATION

Dosage and Administration for AndroGel 1% differs from AndroGel 1.62%. For dosage and administration of AndroGel 1.62% refer to its full prescribing information. (2)

2.1 Dosing and Dose Adjustment

The recommended starting dose of AndroGel 1% is 50 mg of testosterone (4 pump actuations, two 25 mg packets, or one 50 mg packet), applied topically once daily in the morning to the shoulders and upper arms and/or abdomen area (preferably at the same time every day).

Dose Adjustment

To ensure proper dosing, serum testosterone concentrations should be measured at intervals. If the serum testosterone concentration is below the normal range, the daily AndroGel 1% dose may be increased from 50 mg to 75 mg and from 75 mg to 100 mg for adult males as instructed by the physician (see Table 1, Dosing Information for AndroGel 1%). If the serum testosterone concentration exceeds the normal range, the daily AndroGel 1% dose may be decreased. If the serum testosterone concentration consistently exceeds the normal range at a daily dose of 50 mg, AndroGel 1% therapy should be discontinued. In addition, serum testosterone concentrations should be assessed periodically.

The application site and dose of AndroGel 1% are not interchangeable with other topical testosterone products.

2.2 Administration Instructions

AndroGel 1% should be applied to clean, dry, healthy, intact skin of the right and left upper arms/shoulders and/or right and left abdomen. Area of application should be limited to the area that will be covered by the patient's short sleeve T-shirt. Do not apply AndroGel 1% to any other part of the body including the genitals, chest or back. AndroGel 1% should be evenly distributed between the right and left upper arms/shoulders or both sides of the abdomen.

The prescribed daily dose of AndroGel 1% should be applied to the right and left upper arms/shoulders and/or right/left abdomen as shown in the shaded areas in the figure below.

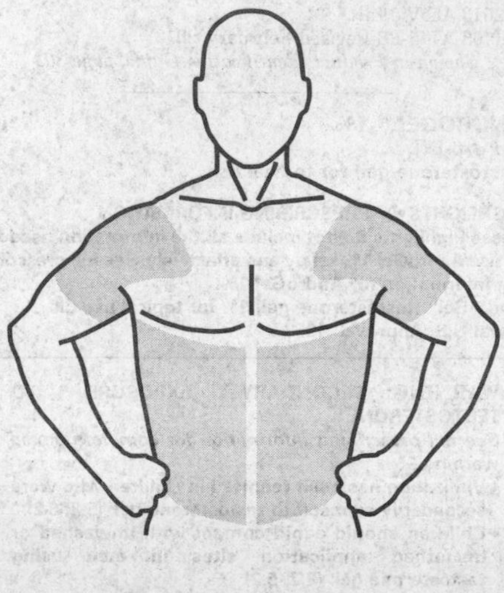

After applying the gel, the application site should be allowed to dry prior to dressing. Hands should be washed thoroughly with soap and water after application. Avoid fire, flames or smoking until the gel has dried since alcohol based products, including AndroGel 1%, are flammable.

The patient should be advised to avoid swimming or showering for at least 5 hours after the application of AndroGel 1%.

Multi-Dose Pump

To obtain a full first dose, it is necessary to prime the canister pump. To do so, with the canister in the upright position, slowly and fully depress the actuator three times. Safely discard the gel from the first three actuations. It is only necessary to prime the pump before the first dose. After the priming procedure, patients should completely depress the pump one time actuation for every 12.5 mg of testosterone required to achieve the daily prescribed dosage. The product should be delivered directly into the palm of the hand and then applied to the desired application sites. Alternatively, AndroGel 1% can be applied directly to the application sites. Table 1 provides dosing information for adult males.

Table 1: Dosing Information for AndroGel 1%

Amount of Testosterone	Number of Pump Actuations
50 mg	4 (once daily)
75 mg	6 (once daily)
100 mg	8 (once daily)

Packets

The entire contents should be squeezed into the palm of the hand and immediately applied to the application sites. Alternately, patients may squeeze a portion of the gel from the packet into the palm of the hand and apply to application sites. Repeat until entire contents have been applied.

Strict adherence to the following precautions is advised in order to minimize the potential for secondary exposure to testosterone from AndroGel 1%-treated skin:

- Children and women should avoid contact with unwashed or unclothed application site(s) of men using AndroGel 1%.
- Patients should wash hands with soap and water immediately after application of AndroGel 1%.
- Patients should cover the application site(s) with clothing (e.g., a T-shirt) after the gel has dried.
- Prior to situation in which direct skin-to-skin contact is anticipated, patients should wash the application site thoroughly with soap and water to remove any testosterone residue.
- In the event that unwashed or unclothed skin to which AndroGel 1% has been applied comes in direct contact with the skin of another person, the general area of contact on the other person should be washed with soap and water as soon as possible.

3 DOSAGE FORMS AND STRENGTHS

AndroGel (testosterone gel) 1% for topical use is available as follows:

- A metered-dose pump. Each pump actuation delivers 12.5 mg of testosterone in 1.25 g of gel.
- A unit dose packet containing 25 mg of testosterone provided in 2.5 g of gel.
- A unit dose packet containing 50 mg of testosterone provided in 5 g of gel.

4 CONTRAINDICATIONS

- AndroGel 1% is contraindicated in men with carcinoma of the breast or known or suspected carcinoma of the prostate *[see Warnings and Precautions (5.1), Adverse Reactions (6.1),* and *Nonclinical Toxicology (13.1)]*.
- AndroGel 1% is contraindicated in women who are or may become pregnant, or who are breastfeeding. AndroGel 1% may cause fetal harm when administered to a pregnant woman. AndroGel 1% may cause serious adverse reactions in nursing infants. Exposure of a female fetus or nursing infant to androgens may result in varying degrees of virilization. Pregnant women or those who may become pregnant need to be aware of the potential for transfer of testosterone from men treated with AndroGel 1%. If a pregnant woman is exposed to AndroGel 1%, she should be apprised of the potential hazard to the fetus *[see Warnings and Precautions (5.2)* and *Use in Specific Populations (8.1, 8.3)]*.

5 WARNINGS AND PRECAUTIONS

5.1 Worsening of Benign Prostatic Hyperplasia (BPH) and Potential Risk of Prostate Cancer

- Patients with BPH treated with androgens are at an increased risk for worsening of signs and symptoms of BPH. Monitor patients with BPH for worsening signs and symptoms.
- Patients treated with androgens may be at increased risk for prostate cancer. Evaluate patients for prostate cancer prior to initiating and during treatment with androgens *[see Contraindications (4), Adverse Reactions (6.1)* and *Nonclinical Toxicology (13.1)]*.

5.2 Potential for Secondary Exposure to Testosterone

Cases of secondary exposure resulting in virilization of children have been reported in postmarketing surveillance. Signs and symptoms have included enlargement of the penis or clitoris, development of pubic hair, increased erections and libido, aggressive behavior, and advanced bone age. In most cases, these signs and symptoms regressed with removal of the exposure to testosterone gel. In a few cases, however, enlarged genitalia did not fully return to age-appropriate normal size, and bone age remained modestly greater than chronological age. The risk of transfer was increased in some of these cases by not adhering to precautions for the appropriate use of the topical testosterone product. Children and women should avoid contact with unwashed or unclothed application sites in men using AndroGel 1% *[see Dosage and Administration (2.2), Use in Specific Populations (8.1)* and *Clinical Pharmacology (12.3)]*.

Inappropriate changes in genital size or development of pubic hair or libido in children, or changes in body hair distribution, significant increase in acne, or other signs of virilization in adult women should be brought to the attention of a physician and the possibility of secondary exposure to testosterone gel should also be brought to the attention of a physician. Testosterone gel should be promptly discontinued until the cause of virilization has been identified.

5.3 Polycythemia

Increases in hematocrit, reflective of increases in red blood cell mass, may require lowering or discontinuation of testosterone. Check hematocrit prior to initiating treatment. It would also be appropriate to re-evaluate the hematocrit 3 to 6 months after starting treatment, and then annually. If hematocrit becomes elevated, stop therapy until hematocrit decreases to an acceptable concentration. An increase in red blood cell mass may increase the risk of thromboembolic events.

5.4 Use in Women

Due to lack of controlled evaluations in women and potential virilizing effects, AndroGel 1% is not indicated for use in women *[see Contraindications (4)* and *Use in Specific Populations (8.1, 8.3)]*.

5.5 Potential for Adverse Effects on Spermatogenesis

With large doses of exogenous androgens, including AndroGel 1%, spermatogenesis may be suppressed through feedback inhibition of pituitary follicle-stimulating hormone (FSH) which could possibly lead to adverse effects on semen parameters including sperm count.

5.6 Hepatic Adverse Effects

Prolonged use of high doses of orally active 17-alpha-alkyl androgens (e.g., methyltestosterone) has been associated with serious hepatic adverse effects (peliosis hepatis, hepatic neoplasms, cholestatic hepatitis, and jaundice). Peliosis hepatis can be a life-threatening or fatal complication. Long-term therapy with intramuscular testosterone enanthate has produced multiple hepatic adenomas. AndroGel 1% is not known to cause these adverse effects.

5.7 Edema

Androgens, including AndroGel 1%, may promote retention of sodium and water. Edema, with or without congestive heart failure, may be a serious complication in patients with preexisting cardiac, renal, or hepatic disease *[see Adverse Reactions (6.2)]*.

5.8 Gynecomastia

Gynecomastia may develop and persist in patients being treated with androgens, including AndroGel 1%, for hypogonadism.

5.9 Sleep Apnea

The treatment of hypogonadal men with testosterone may potentiate sleep apnea in some patients, especially those with risk factors such as obesity or chronic lung diseases *[see Adverse Reactions (6.2)]*.

5.10 Lipids

Changes in serum lipid profile may require dose adjustment or discontinuation of testosterone therapy.

5.11 Hypercalcemia

Androgens, including AndroGel 1%, should be used with caution in cancer patients at risk of hypercalcemia (and associated hypercalciuria). Regular monitoring of serum calcium concentrations is recommended in these patients.

5.12 Decreased Thyroxine-binding Globulin

Androgens, including AndroGel 1%, may decrease concentrations of thyroxin-binding globulins, resulting in decreased total T4 serum concentrations and increased resin uptake of T3 and T4. Free thyroid hormone concentrations remain unchanged, however, and there is no clinical evidence of thyroid dysfunction.

5.13 Flammability

Alcohol based products, including AndroGel 1%, are flammable; therefore, patients should be advised to avoid fire, flame or smoking until the AndroGel 1% has dried.

6 ADVERSE REACTIONS

6.1 Clinical Trial Experience

Because clinical trials are conducted under widely varying conditions, adverse reaction rates observed in the clinical trials of a drug cannot be directly compared to rates in the clinical trials of another drug and may not reflect the rates observed in practice.

Clinical Trials in Hypogonadal Men

Table 2 shows the incidence of all adverse events judged by the investigator to be at least possibly related to treatment with AndroGel 1% and reported by >1% of patients in a 180 Day, Phase 3 study.

Table 2: Adverse Events Possibly, Probably or Definitely Related to Use of AndroGel 1% in the 180-Day Controlled Clinical Trial

Adverse Event	Dose of AndroGel 1%		
	50 mg	75 mg	100 mg
	N = 77	N = 40	N = 78
Acne	1%	3%	8%
Alopecia	1%	0%	1%
Application Site Reaction	5%	3%	4%
Asthenia	0%	3%	1%
Depression	1%	0%	1%
Emotional Lability	0%	3%	3%
Gynecomastia	1%	0%	3%
Headache	4%	3%	0%
Hypertension	3%	0%	3%
Lab Test Abnormal*	6%	5%	3%
Libido Decreased	0%	3%	1%
Nervousness	0%	3%	1%
Pain Breast	1%	3%	1%
Prostate Disorder**	3%	3%	5%
Testis Disorder***	3%	0%	0%

**Lab test abnormal* occurred in nine patients with one or more of the following events reported: elevated hemoglobin or hematocrit, hyperlipidemia, elevated triglycerides, hypokalemia, decreased HDL, elevated glucose, elevated creatinine, elevated total bilirubin.

***Prostate disorders* included five patients with enlarged prostate, one with BPH, and one with elevated PSA results.

****Testis disorders* were reported in two patients: one with left varicocele and one with slight sensitivity of left testis.

Other less common adverse reactions, reported in fewer than 1% of patients included: amnesia, anxiety, discolored hair, dizziness, dry skin, hirsutism, hostility, impaired urination, paresthesia, penis disorder, peripheral edema, sweating, and vasodilation.

In this 180 day clinical trial, skin reactions at the site of application were reported with AndroGel 1%, but none was severe enough to require treatment or discontinuation of drug.

Six patients (4%) in this trial had adverse events that led to discontinuation of AndroGel 1%. These events included: cerebral hemorrhage, convulsion (neither of which were considered related to AndroGel 1% administration), depression, sadness, memory loss, elevated prostate specific antigen, and hypertension. No AndroGel 1% patient discontinued due to skin reactions.

In a separate uncontrolled pharmacokinetic study of 10 patients, two had adverse events associated with AndroGel 1%; these were asthenia and depression in one patient and increased libido and hyperkinesia in the other.

In a 3 year, flexible dose, extension study, the incidence of all adverse events judged by the investigator to be at least possibly related to treatment with AndroGel 1% and reported by > 1% of patients is shown in Table 3.

Table 3: Adverse Events Possibly, Probably or Definitely Related to Use of AndroGel 1% in the 3 Year, Flexible Dose, Extension Study

Adverse Event	Percent of Subjects
	(N = 162)
Lab Test Abnormal+	9.3
Skin dry	1.9
Application Site Reaction	5.6
Acne	3.1
Pruritus	1.9
Enlarged Prostate	11.7
Carcinoma of Prostate	1.2
Urinary Symptoms*	3.7
Testis Disorder**	1.9
Gynecomastia	2.5
Anemia	2.5

+*Lab test abnormal* occurred in 15 patients with one or more of the following events reported: elevated AST, elevated ALT, elevated testosterone, elevated hemoglobin or hematocrit, elevated cholesterol, elevated cholesterol/LDL ratio, elevated triglycerides, elevated HDL, elevated serum creatinine.

**Urinary symptoms* included nocturia, urinary hesitancy, urinary incontinence, urinary retention, urinary urgency and weak urinary stream.

***Testis disorders* included three patients. There were two with a non-palpable testis and one with slight right testicular tenderness.

Two patients reported serious adverse events considered possibly related to treatment: deep vein thrombosis (DVT) and prostate disorder requiring a transurethral resection of the prostate (TURP).

Discontinuation for adverse events in this study included: two patients with application site reactions, one with kidney failure, and five with prostate disorders (including increase in serum PSA in 4 patients, and increase in PSA with prostate enlargement in a fifth patient).

Increases in Serum PSA Observed in Clinical Trials of Hypogonadal Men

During the initial 6-month study, the mean change in PSA values had a statistically significant increase of 0.26 ng/mL. Serum PSA was measured every 6 months thereafter in the 162 hypogonadal men on AndroGel 1% in the 3-year extension study. There was no additional statistically significant increase observed in mean PSA from 6 months through 36 months. However, there were increases in serum PSA observed in approximately 18% of individual patients. The overall mean change from baseline in serum PSA values for the entire group from month 6 to 36 was 0.11 ng/mL.

Twenty-nine patients (18%) met the per-protocol criterion for increase in serum PSA, defined as >2X the baseline or any single serum PSA >6 ng/mL. Most of these (25/29) met this criterion by at least doubling of their PSA from baseline. In most cases where PSA at least doubled (22/25), the maximum serum PSA value was still <2 ng/mL. The first occurrence of a pre-specified, post-baseline increase in serum PSA was seen at or prior to Month 12 in most of the patients who met this criterion (23 of 29; 79%).

Four patients met this criterion by having a serum PSA >6 ng/mL and in these, maximum serum PSA values were 6.2 ng/mL, 6.6 ng/mL, 6.7 ng/mL, and 10.7 ng/mL. In two of these patients, prostate cancer was detected on biopsy. The first patient's PSA levels were 4.7 ng/mL and 6.2 ng/mL at baseline and at Month 6/Final, respectively. The second patient's PSA levels were 4.2 ng/mL, 5.2 ng/mL, 5.8 ng/mL, and 6.6 ng/mL at baseline, Month 6, Month 12, and Final, respectively.

6.2 Postmarketing Experience

The following adverse reactions have been identified during post approval use of AndroGel 1%. Because the reactions are reported voluntarily from a population of uncertain size, it is not always possible to reliably estimate their frequency or establish a causal relationship to drug exposure (Table 4).

Table 4: Adverse Drug Reactions from Postmarketing Experience of AndroGel 1% by MedDRA System Organ Class

Blood and the lymphatic system disorders:	Elevated Hgb, Hct (polycythemia)
Endocrine disorders:	Hirsutism
Gastrointestinal disorders:	Nausea
General disorders and administration site reactions:	Asthenia, edema, malaise
Genitourinary disorders:	Impaired urination
Hepatobiliary disorders:	Abnormal liver function tests (e.g. transaminases, elevated GGTP, bilirubin)
Investigations:	Elevated PSA, electrolyte changes (nitrogen, calcium, potassium, phosphorus, sodium), changes in serum lipids (hyperlipidemia, elevated triglycerides, decreased HDL), impaired glucose tolerance, fluctuating testosterone concentrations, weight increase
Neoplasms benign, malignant and unspecified (cysts and polyps):	Prostate cancer
Nervous system:	Headache, dizziness, sleep apnea, insomnia
Psychiatric disorders:	Depression, emotional lability, decreased libido, nervousness, hostility, amnesia, anxiety
Reproductive system and breast disorders:	Gynecomastia, mastodynia, prostatic enlargement, testicular atrophy, oligospermia, priapism (frequent or prolonged erections)
Respiratory disorders:	Dyspnea
Skin and subcutaneous tissue disorders:	Acne, alopecia, application site reaction (pruritus, dry skin, erythema, rash, discolored hair, paresthesia), sweating
Vascular disorders:	Hypertension, vasodilation (hot flushes)

Secondary Exposure to Testosterone in Children

Cases of secondary exposure to testosterone resulting in virilization of children have been reported in postmarket surveillance. Signs and symptoms of these reported cases have included enlargement of the clitoris (with surgical intervention) or the penis, development of pubic hair, increased erections and libido, aggressive behavior, and advanced bone age. In most cases with a reported outcome, these signs and symptoms were reported to have regressed with removal of the testosterone gel exposure. In a few cases, however, enlarged genitalia did not fully return to age appropriate normal size, and bone age remained modestly greater than chronological age. In some of the cases, direct contact with the sites of application on the skin of men using testosterone gel was reported. In at least one reported case, the reporter considered the possibility of secondary expo-

Information on the AbbVie, Inc. products listed on these pages is from the prescribing information in use as of July 31, 2013. For more information, please visit rxabbvie.com or call 1-800-633-9110.

sure from items such as the testosterone gel user's shirts and/or other fabric, such as towels and sheets *[see Warnings and Precautions (5.2)]*.

7 DRUG INTERACTIONS

7.1 Insulin

Changes in insulin sensitivity or glycemic control may occur in patients treated with androgens. In diabetic patients, the metabolic effects of androgens may decrease blood glucose and, therefore, may decrease insulin requirements.

7.2 Oral Anticoagulants

Changes in anticoagulant activity may be seen with androgens, therefore more frequent monitoring of international normalized ratio (INR) and prothrombin time are recommended in patients taking anticoagulants, especially at the initiation and termination of androgen therapy.

7.3 Corticosteroids

The concurrent use of testosterone with adrenocorticotropic hormone (ACTH) or corticosteroids may result in increased fluid retention and requires careful monitoring particularly in patients with cardiac, renal or hepatic disease.

8 USE IN SPECIFIC POPULATIONS

8.1 Pregnancy

Pregnancy Category X *[see Contraindications (4)]*: AndroGel 1% is contraindicated during pregnancy or in women who may become pregnant. Testosterone is teratogenic and may cause fetal harm. Exposure of a female fetus to androgens may result in varying degrees of virilization. If this drug is used during pregnancy, or if the patient becomes pregnant while taking this drug, the patient should be apprised of the potential hazard to a fetus.

8.3 Nursing Mothers

Although it is not known how much testosterone transfers into human milk, AndroGel 1% is contraindicated in nursing women because of the potential for serious adverse reactions in nursing infants. Testosterone and other androgens may adversely affect lactation *[see Contraindications (4)]*.

8.4 Pediatric Use

The safety and efficacy of AndroGel 1% in pediatric patients less than 18 years old has not been established. Improper use may result in acceleration of bone age and premature closure of epiphyses.

8.5 Geriatric Use

There have not been sufficient numbers of geriatric patients involved in controlled clinical studies utilizing AndroGel 1% to determine whether efficacy in those over 65 years of age differs from younger subjects. Additionally, there is insufficient long-term safety data in geriatric patients to assess the potential risks of cardiovascular disease and prostate cancer.

Geriatric patients treated with androgens may also be at risk for worsening of signs and symptoms of BPH.

8.6 Renal Impairment

No studies were conducted in patients with renal impairment.

8.7 Hepatic Impairment

No studies were conducted in patients with hepatic impairment.

9 DRUG ABUSE AND DEPENDENCE

9.1 Controlled Substance

AndroGel 1% contains testosterone, a Schedule III controlled substance in the Controlled Substances Act.

9.2 Abuse

Anabolic steroids, such as testosterone, are abused. Abuse is often associated with adverse physical and psychological effects.

9.3 Dependence

Although drug dependence is not documented in individuals using therapeutic doses of anabolic steroids for approved indications, dependence is observed in some individuals abusing high doses of anabolic steroids. In general, anabolic steroid dependence is characterized by any three of the following:

- Taking more drug than intended
- Continued drug use despite medical and social problems
- Significant time spent in obtaining adequate amounts of drug
- Desire for anabolic steroids when supplies of the drugs are interrupted
- Difficulty in discontinuing use of the drug despite desires and attempts to do so
- Experience of a withdrawal syndrome upon discontinuation of anabolic steroid use

10 OVERDOSAGE

There is one report of acute overdosage with use of an approved injectable testosterone product: this subject had serum testosterone concentrations of up to 11,400 ng/dL with a cerebrovascular accident.

Treatment of overdosage would consist of discontinuation of AndroGel 1%, washing the application site with soap and water, and appropriate symptomatic and supportive care.

11 DESCRIPTION

AndroGel (testosterone gel) 1% is a clear, colorless hydroalcoholic gel containing testosterone.

The active pharmacologic ingredient in AndroGel 1% is testosterone, an androgen. Testosterone USP is a white to practically white crystalline powder chemically described as 17-beta hydroxyandrost-4-en-3-one. The structural formula is:

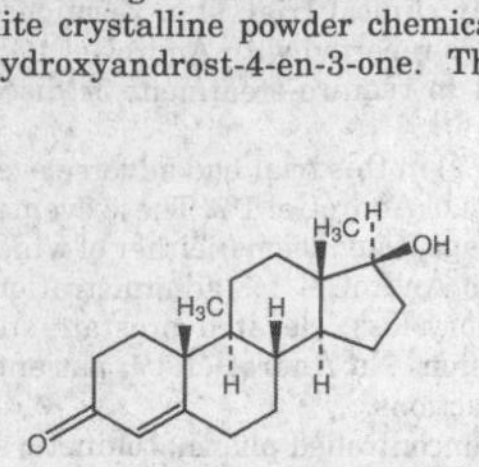

Testosterone

$C_{19}H_{28}O_2$ MW 288.42

Pharmacologically inactive ingredients in AndroGel 1% are carbomer 980, ethanol 67.0%, isopropyl myristate, purified water, and sodium hydroxide. These ingredients are not pharmacologically active.

12 CLINICAL PHARMACOLOGY

12.1 Mechanism of Action

Endogenous androgens, including testosterone and dihydrotestosterone (DHT), are responsible for the normal growth and development of the male sex organs and for maintenance of secondary sex characteristics. These effects include the growth and maturation of prostate, seminal vesicles, penis and scrotum; the development of male hair distribution, such as facial, pubic, chest and axillary hair; laryngeal enlargement, vocal chord thickening, alterations in body musculature and fat distribution. Testosterone and DHT are necessary for the normal development of secondary sex characteristics. Male hypogonadism results from insufficient secretion of testosterone and is characterized by low serum testosterone concentrations. Signs/symptoms associated with male hypogonadism include erectile dysfunction and decreased sexual desire, fatigue and loss of energy, mood depression, regression of secondary sexual characteristics and osteoporosis.

Male hypogonadism can present as primary hypogonadism caused by defects of the gonads, such as Klinefelter's Syndrome or Leydig cell aplasia while secondary hypogonadism is the failure of the hypothalamus or pituitary to produce sufficient gonadotropins (FSH, LH).

12.2 Pharmacodynamics

No specific pharmacodynamic studies were conducted using AndroGel 1%.

12.3 Pharmacokinetics

Absorption

AndroGel 1% delivers physiologic amounts of testosterone, producing circulating testosterone concentrations that approximate normal concentrations (298 - 1043 ng/dL) seen in healthy men. AndroGel 1% provides continuous transdermal delivery of testosterone for 24 hours following a single application to intact, clean, dry skin of the shoulders, upper arms and/or abdomen.

AndroGel 1% is a hydroalcoholic formulation that dries quickly when applied to the skin surface. The skin serves as a reservoir for the sustained release of testosterone into the systemic circulation. Approximately 10% of the testosterone dose applied on the skin surface from AndroGel is absorbed into systemic circulation. In a study with AndroGel 1% 100 mg , all patients showed an increase in serum testosterone within 30 minutes, and eight of nine patients had a serum testosterone concentration within normal range by 4 hours after the initial application. Absorption of testosterone into the blood continues for the entire 24-hour dosing interval. Serum concentrations approximate the steady-state concentration by the end of the first 24 hours and are at steady state by the second or third day of dosing.

With single daily applications of AndroGel 1%, follow-up measurements 30, 90 and 180 days after starting treatment have confirmed that serum testosterone concentrations are generally maintained within the eugonadal range. Figure 1 summarizes the 24-hour pharmacokinetic profiles of testosterone for hypogonadal men (less than 300 ng/dL) maintained on AndroGel 1% 50 mg or 100 mg for 30 days. The average (± SD) daily testosterone concentration produced by AndroGel 1% 100 mg on Day 30 was 792 (± 294) ng/dL and by AndroGel 1% 50 mg 566 (± 262) ng/dL.

[See figure 1 at top of next column]

Distribution

Circulating testosterone is primarily bound in the serum to sex hormone-binding globulin (SHBG) and albumin. Approximately 40% of testosterone in plasma is bound to SHBG, 2% remains unbound (free) and the rest is bound to albumin and other proteins.

Figure 1: Mean (± SD) Steady-State Serum Testosterone Concentrations on Day 30 in Patients Applying AndroGel 1% Once Daily

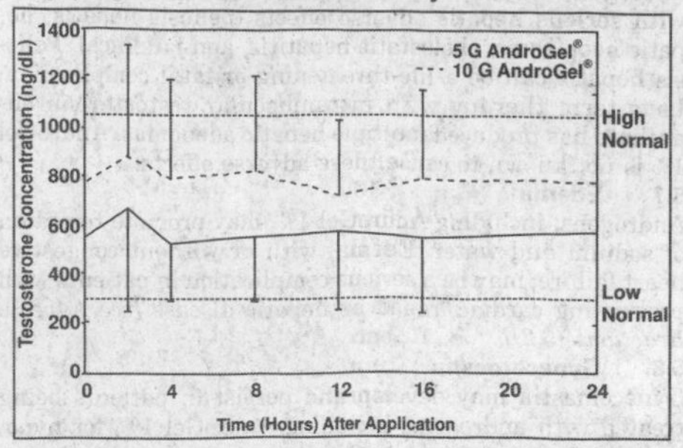

Metabolism

Testosterone is metabolized to various 17-keto steroids through two different pathways. The major active metabolites of testosterone are estradiol and dihydrotestosterone (DHT).

DHT concentrations increased in parallel with testosterone concentrations during AndroGel 1% treatment. The mean steady-state DHT/T ratio during 180 days of AndroGel treatment ranged from 0.23 to 0.29 (50 mg of AndroGel 1%/day) and from 0.27 to 0.33 (100 mg of AndroGel 1%/day).

Excretion

There is considerable variation in the half-life of testosterone concentration as reported in the literature, ranging from 10 to 100 minutes. About 90% of a dose of testosterone given intramuscularly is excreted in the urine as glucuronic and sulfuric acid conjugates of testosterone and its metabolites. About 6% of a dose is excreted in the feces, mostly in the unconjugated form. Inactivation of testosterone occurs primarily in the liver.

When AndroGel 1% treatment is discontinued after achieving steady state, serum testosterone concentrations remain in the normal range for 24 to 48 hours but return to their pretreatment concentrations by the fifth day after the last application.

Testosterone Transfer from Male Patients to Female Partners

The potential for dermal testosterone transfer following AndroGel 1% use was evaluated in a clinical study between males dosed with AndroGel 1% and their untreated female partners. Two (2) to 12 hours after application of 100 mg of testosterone administered as AndroGel 1% by the male subjects, the couples (N = 38 couples) engaged in daily, 15-minute sessions of vigorous skin-to-skin contact so that the female partners gained maximum exposure to the AndroGel 1% application sites. Under these study conditions, all unprotected female partners had a serum testosterone concentration >2 times the baseline value at some time during the study. When a shirt covered the application site(s), the transfer of testosterone from the males to the female partners was completely prevented.

13 NONCLINICAL TOXICOLOGY

13.1 Carcinogenesis, Mutagenesis, Impairment of Fertility

Testosterone has been tested by subcutaneous injection and implantation in mice and rats. In mice, the implant induced cervical-uterine tumors which metastasized in some cases. There is suggestive evidence that injection of testosterone into some strains of female mice increases their susceptibility to hepatoma. Testosterone is also known to increase the number of tumors and decrease the degree of differentiation of chemically induced carcinomas of the liver in rats. Testosterone was negative in the *in vitro* Ames and in the *in vivo* mouse micronucleus assays. The administration of exogenous testosterone has been reported to suppress spermatogenesis in the rat, dog and non-human primates, which was reversible on cessation of the treatment.

14 CLINICAL STUDIES

14.1 Clinical Trials in Adult Hypogonadal Males

AndroGel 1% was evaluated in a multi-center, randomized, parallel-group, active-controlled, 180-day trial in 227 hypogonadal men. The study was conducted in 2 phases. During the Initial Treatment Period (Days 1-90), 73 patients were randomized to AndroGel 1% 50 mg daily, 78 patients to AndroGel 1% 100 mg daily, and 76 patients to a non-scrotal testosterone transdermal system. The study was double-blind for dose of AndroGel 1% but open-label for active control. Patients who were originally randomized to AndroGel 1% and who had single-sample serum testosterone concentrations above or below the normal range on Day 60 were titrated to 75 mg daily on Day 91. During the Extended Treatment Period (Days 91-180), 51 patients continued on AndroGel 1% 50 mg daily, 52 patients continued on AndroGel 1% 100 mg daily, 41 patients continued on a non-scrotal testosterone transdermal system (5 mg daily), and 40 patients received AndroGel 1% 75 mg daily. Upon completion of the initial study, 163 enrolled and 162 patients received treatment in an open-label extension study of AndroGel 1% for an additional period of up to 3 years.

Mean peak, trough and average serum testosterone concentrations within the normal range (298-1043 ng/dL) were achieved on the first day of treatment with doses of 50 mg and 100 mg of AndroGel 1%. In patients continuing on AndroGel 1% 50 mg and 100 mg, these mean testosterone concentrations were maintained within the normal range for the 180-day duration of the original study. Figure 2 summarizes the 24-hour pharmacokinetic profiles of testosterone administered as AndroGel 1% for 30, 90 and 180 days. Testosterone concentrations were maintained as long as the patient continued to properly apply the prescribed AndroGel 1% treatment.

Figure 2: Mean Steady-State Testosterone Concentrations in Patients with Once-Daily AndroGel 1% Therapy

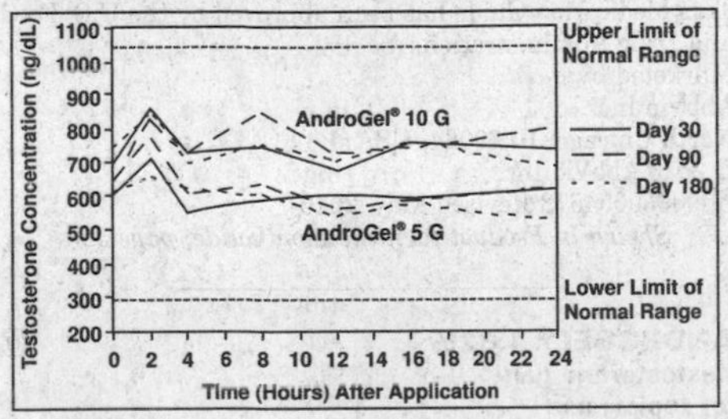

Table 5 summarizes the mean testosterone concentrations on Treatment Day 180 for patients receiving 50 mg, 75 mg, or 100 mg of AndroGel 1%. The 75 mg dose produced mean concentrations intermediate to those produced by 50 mg and 100 mg of AndroGel 1%.

Table 5: Mean (± SD) Steady-State Serum Testosterone Concentrations During Therapy (Day 180)

	50 mg N = 44	75 mg N = 37	100 mg N = 48
C_{avg}	555 ± 225	601 ± 309	713 ± 209
C_{max}	830 ± 347	901 ± 471	1083 ± 434
C_{min}	371 ± 165	406 ± 220	485 ± 156

Of 129 hypogonadal men who were appropriately titrated with AndroGel 1% and who had sufficient data for analysis, 87% achieved an average serum testosterone concentration within the normal range on Treatment Day 180.

In patients treated with AndroGel 1%, there were no observed differences in the average daily serum testosterone concentrations at steady-state based on age, cause of hypogonadism, or body mass index.

AndroGel 1% 50 mg/day and 100 mg/day resulted in significant increases over time in total body mass and total body lean mass, while total body fat mass and the percent body fat decreased significantly. These changes were maintained for 180 days of treatment during the original study. Changes in the 75 mg dose group were similar. Bone mineral density in both hip and spine increased significantly from Baseline to Day 180 with AndroGel 1% 100 mg.

AndroGel 1% treatment at 50 mg/day and 100 mg/day for 90 days produced significant improvement in libido (measured by sexual motivation, sexual activity and enjoyment of sexual activity as assessed by patient responses to a questionnaire). The degree of penile erection as subjectively estimated by the patients, increased with AndroGel 1% treatment, as did the subjective score for "satisfactory duration of erection." AndroGel 1% treatment at 50 mg/day and 100 mg/day produced positive effects on mood and fatigue. Similar changes were seen after 180 days of treatment and in the group treated with the 75 mg dose. DHT concentrations increased in parallel with testosterone concentrations at AndroGel 1% doses of 50 mg/day and 100 mg/day, but the DHT/T ratio stayed within the normal range, indicating enhanced availability of the major physiologically active androgen. Serum estradiol (E2) concentrations increased significantly within 30 days of starting treatment with AndroGel 1% 50 or 100 mg/day and remained elevated throughout the treatment period but remained within the normal range for eugonadal men. Serum levels of SHBG decreased very slightly (1 to 11%) during AndroGel 1% treatment. In men with hypergonadotropic hypogonadism, serum levels of LH and FSH fell in a dose- and time-dependent manner during treatment with AndroGel 1%.

14.2 Phototoxicity in Humans

The phototoxic potential of AndroGel 1% was evaluated in a double-blind, single-dose study in 27 subjects with photosensitive skin types. The Minimal Erythema Dose (MED) of ultraviolet radiation was determined for each subject. A single 24 (+1) hour application of duplicate patches containing test articles (placebo gel, testosterone gel, or saline) was made to naive skin sites on Day 1. On Day 2, each subject received five exposure times of ultraviolet radiation, each exposure being 25% greater than the previous one. Skin evaluations were made on Days 2 to 5. Exposure of test and control article application sites to ultraviolet light did not produce increased inflammation relative to non-irradiated sites, indicating no phototoxic effect.

16 HOW SUPPLIED/STORAGE AND HANDLING

AndroGel 1% is supplied in non-aerosol, metered-dose pumps that deliver 12.5 mg of testosterone per complete pump actuation. The pumps are composed of plastic and stainless steel and an LDPE/aluminum foil inner liner encased in rigid plastic with a polypropylene cap. Each 88 g metered-dose pump is capable of dispensing 75 g of gel or 60-metered pump actuations; each pump actuation dispenses 1.25 g of gel.

AndroGel 1% is also supplied in unit-dose aluminum foil packets in cartons of 30. Each packet of 2.5 g or 5 g gel contains 25 mg or 50 mg testosterone, respectively.

NDC Number	Package Size
0051-8488-88	2 × 75 g pump (each pump dispenses 60 metered pump actuations with each pump actuation containing 12.5 mg of testosterone in 1.25 g of gel)
0051-8425-30	30 packets (a unit dose packet containing 25 mg of testosterone provided in 2.5 g of gel)
0051-8450-30	30 packets (a unit dose packet containing 50 mg of testosterone provided in 5 g of gel)

Storage

Store at 25°C (77°F); excursions permitted to 15° to 30°C (59° to 86°F) [see USP Controlled Room Temperature].

Disposal

Used AndroGel 1% pumps or used AndroGel 1% packets should be discarded in household trash in a manner that prevents accidental application or ingestion by children or pets.

17 PATIENT COUNSELING INFORMATION

See FDA-Approved Patient Labeling (Medication Guide)

Patients should be informed of the following:

17.1 Use in Men with Known or Suspected Prostate or Breast Cancer

Men with known or suspected prostate or breast cancer should not use AndroGel 1% *[see Contraindications (4) and Warnings and Precautions (5.1)]*.

17.2 Potential for Secondary Exposure to Testosterone and Steps to Prevent Secondary Exposure

Secondary exposure to testosterone in children and women can occur with the use of testosterone gel in men. Cases of secondary exposure to testosterone have been reported in children.

Physicians should advise patients of the reported signs and symptoms of secondary exposure which may include the following:

- In children; unexpected sexual development including inappropriate enlargement of the penis or clitoris, premature development of pubic hair, increased erections, and aggressive behavior
- In women; changes in hair distribution, increase in acne, or other signs of testosterone effects
- The possibility of secondary exposure to testosterone gel should be brought to the attention of a healthcare provider
- AndroGel 1% should be promptly discontinued until the cause of virilization is identified

Strict adherence to the following precautions is advised to minimize the potential for secondary exposure to testosterone from testosterone gel in men *[see Medication Guide]*:

- **Children and women should avoid contact with unwashed or unclothed application site(s)** of men using testosterone gel
- Patients using AndroGel 1% should apply the product as directed and strictly adhere to the following:
  - **Wash hands** with soap and water after application
  - **Cover the application site(s)** with clothing after the gel has dried
  - **Wash the application site(s) thoroughly** with soap and water prior to any situation where skin-to-skin contact of the application site with another person is anticipated
  - In the event that unwashed or unclothed skin to which AndroGel 1% has been applied comes in contact with the skin of another person, the general area of contact on the other person should be washed with soap and water as soon as possible *[see Dosage and Administration (2.2), Warnings and Precautions (5.2) and Clinical Pharmacology (12.3)]*.

17.3 Potential Adverse Reactions with Androgens

Patients should be informed that treatment with androgens may lead to adverse reactions which include:

- Changes in urinary habits such as increased urination at night, trouble starting your urine stream, passing urine many times during the day, having an urge that you have to go to the bathroom right away, having a urine accident, being unable to pass urine and weak urine flow.
- Breathing disturbances, including those associated with sleep, or excessive daytime sleepiness.
- Too frequent or persistent erections of the penis.
- Nausea, vomiting, changes in skin color, or ankle swelling.

17.4 Patients Should Be Advised of the Following Instructions for Use:

- **Read the Medication Guide before starting AndroGel 1% therapy and to reread it each time the prescription is renewed**
- **AndroGel 1% should be applied and used appropriately to maximize the benefits and to minimize the risk of secondary exposure in children and women**
- **Keep AndroGel 1% out of the reach of children**
- **AndroGel 1% is an alcohol based product and is flammable; therefore avoid fire, flame or smoking until the gel has dried**
- **It is important to adhere to all recommended monitoring**
- **Report any changes in their state of health, such as changes in urinary habits, breathing, sleep, and mood**
- AndroGel 1% is prescribed to meet the patient's specific needs; therefore, the patient should never share AndroGel 1% with anyone.
- Wait 5 hours before swimming or washing following application of AndroGel 1%. This will ensure that the greatest amount of AndroGel 1% is absorbed into their system.

Medication Guide

ANDROGEL® (AN DROW JEL) CIII

(testosterone gel) 1%

Read this Medication Guide that comes with ANDROGEL 1% before you start taking it and each time you get a refill. There may be new information. This Medication Guide does not take the place of talking to your healthcare provider about your medical condition or your treatment.

What is the most important information I should know about ANDROGEL 1%?

1. **Early signs and symptoms of puberty have happened in young children who were accidentally exposed to testosterone through contact with men using ANDROGEL 1%.**

   Signs and symptoms of early puberty in a child may include:
   - enlarged penis or clitoris
   - early development of pubic hair
   - increased erections or sex drive
   - aggressive behavior

   ANDROGEL 1% can transfer from your body to others.

2. **Women and children should avoid contact with the unwashed or unclothed area where ANDROGEL 1% has been applied to your skin.**

   Stop using ANDROGEL 1% and call your healthcare provider right away if you see any signs and symptoms in a child or a woman that may have occurred through accidental exposure to ANDROGEL 1%.

   Signs and symptoms of exposure to ANDROGEL 1% in children may include:
   - enlarged penis or clitoris
   - early development of pubic hair
   - increased erections or sex drive
   - aggressive behavior

   Signs and symptoms of exposure to ANDROGEL 1% in women may include:
   - changes in body hair
   - a large increase in acne

- **To lower the risk of transfer of ANDROGEL 1% from your body to others, you should follow these important instructions:**
  - Apply ANDROGEL 1% **only** to areas that will be covered by a short sleeve T-shirt. These areas are your shoulders and upper arms, or stomach area (abdomen), or shoulders, upper arms and stomach area.
  - Wash your hands **right away** with soap and water after applying ANDROGEL 1%.
  - After the gel has dried, **cover the application area with clothing.** Keep the area covered until you have washed the application area well or have showered.
  - **If you expect to have skin-to-skin contact with another person, first wash the application area well with soap and water.**

Information on the AbbVie, Inc. products listed on these pages is from the prescribing information in use as of July 31, 2013. For more information, please visit rxabbvie.com or call 1-800-633-9110.

◦ **If a woman or child makes contact with the ANDROGEL 1% application area, that area on the woman or child should be washed well with soap and water right away.**

What is ANDROGEL 1%?

ANDROGEL 1% is a prescription medicine that contains testosterone. ANDROGEL 1% is used to treat adult males who have low or no testosterone.

Your healthcare provider will test your blood before you start and while you are taking ANDROGEL 1%.

It is not known if ANDROGEL 1% is safe or effective in children younger than 18 years old. Improper use of ANDROGEL 1% may affect bone growth in children.

ANDROGEL 1% is a controlled substance (CIII) because it contains testosterone that can be a target for people who abuse prescription medicines. Keep your ANDROGEL 1% in a safe place to protect it. Never give your ANDROGEL 1% to anyone else, even if they have the same symptoms you have. Selling or giving away this medicine may harm others and is against the law.

ANDROGEL 1% is not meant for use in women.

Who should not use ANDROGEL 1%?

Do not use ANDROGEL 1% if you:

- have breast cancer
- have or might have prostate cancer
- are pregnant or may become pregnant or breast-feeding. ANDROGEL 1% may harm your unborn or breast-feeding baby.
  Women who are pregnant or who may become pregnant should avoid contact with the area of skin where ANDROGEL 1% has been applied.

Talk to your healthcare provider before taking this medicine if you have any of the above conditions.

What should I tell my healthcare provider before using ANDROGEL 1%?

Before you use ANDROGEL 1%, tell your healthcare provider if you:

- have breast cancer
- have or might have prostate cancer
- have urinary problems due to an enlarged prostate
- have heart problems
- have liver or kidney problems
- have problems breathing while you sleep (sleep apnea)
- have any other medical conditions

Tell your healthcare provider about all the medicines you take, including prescription and non-prescription medicines, vitamins, and herbal supplements.

Using ANDROGEL 1% with certain other medicines can affect each other.

Especially, tell your healthcare provider if you take:

- insulin
- corticosteroids
- medicines that decrease blood clotting

Know the medicines you take. Ask your healthcare provider or pharmacist for a list of these medicines, if you are not sure. Keep a list of them and show it to your healthcare provider and pharmacist when you get a new medicine.

How should I use ANDROGEL 1%?

- It is important that you apply ANDROGEL 1% exactly as your healthcare provider tells you to.
- Your healthcare provider will tell you how much ANDROGEL 1% to apply and when to apply it.
- Your healthcare provider may change your ANDROGEL 1% dose. **Do not** change your ANDROGEL 1% dose without talking to your healthcare provider.
- **ANDROGEL 1% is to be applied to the area of your shoulders, upper arms, or abdomen that will be covered by a short sleeve t-shirt. Do not** apply ANDROGEL 1% to any other parts of your body such as your penis, scrotum, chest, or back.
- Apply AndroGel 1% at the same time each morning. ANDROGEL 1% should be applied after showering or bathing.
- **Wash your hands right away** with soap and water after applying ANDROGEL 1%.
- Avoid showering, swimming, or bathing for at least 5 hours after you apply ANDROGEL 1%.
- ANDROGEL 1% is flammable until dry. Let ANDROGEL 1% dry before smoking or going near an open flame.
- Let the application areas dry completely before putting on a t-shirt.

Applying ANDROGEL 1%:

ANDROGEL 1% comes in a pump or in packets.

- **Before applying ANDROGEL 1%, make sure that your shoulders, upper arms, and abdomen are clean, dry, and there is no broken skin.**
- The application sites for ANDROGEL 1% are the shoulders, upper arms, or abdomen that will be covered by a short sleeve t-shirt (See Figure A).

[See figure A at top of next column]

If you are using the ANDROGEL 1% pump:

- Before using a new bottle of ANDROGEL 1% for the first time, you will need to prime the pump. To prime the ANDROGEL 1% pump, slowly push the pump all the way down 3 times. **Do not** use any ANDROGEL 1% that came

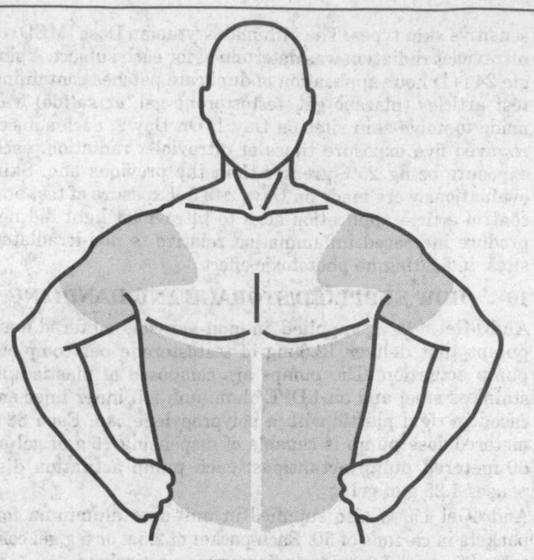

(Figure A)

out while priming. Wash it down the sink to avoid accidental exposure to others. Your ANDROGEL 1% pump is ready to use.

- Remove the cap from the pump. Then, position the nozzle over the palm of your hand and slowly push the pump all the way down. Apply ANDROGEL 1% to the application site. You may also apply ANDROGEL 1% directly to the application site.
- **Wash your hands with soap and water right away.**
- Your healthcare provider will tell you the number of times to press the pump for each dose.

If you are using ANDROGEL 1% packets:

- Tear open the packet completely at the dotted line. Squeeze from the bottom of the packet to the top.
- Squeeze all of the ANDROGEL 1% out of the packet into the palm of your hand. Apply ANDROGEL 1% to the application site. You may also apply ANDROGEL 1% from the packet directly to the application site.
- ANDROGEL 1% should be applied right away.
- **Wash your hands with soap and water right away.**

What are the possible side effects of ANDROGEL 1%?

See **"What is the most important information I should know about ANDROGEL 1%?"**

ANDROGEL 1% can cause serious side effects including:

- **If you already have enlargement of your prostate gland your signs and symptoms can get worse while using ANDROGEL 1%.** This can include:
  - ◦ increased urination at night
  - ◦ trouble starting your urine stream
  - ◦ having to pass urine many times during the day
  - ◦ having an urge that you have to go to the bathroom right away
  - ◦ having a urine accident
  - ◦ being unable to pass urine or weak urine flow
- **Possible increased risk of prostate cancer.** Your healthcare provider should check you for prostate cancer or any other prostate problems before you start and while you use ANDROGEL 1%.
- **In large doses ANDROGEL 1% may lower your sperm count.**
- **Swelling of your ankles, feet, or body, with or without heart failure.**
- **Enlarged or painful breasts.**
- **Have problems breathing while you sleep (sleep apnea).**
- **Blood clots in the legs.** This can include pain, swelling or redness of your legs.

Call your healthcare provider right away if you have any of the serious side effects listed above.

The most common side effects of ANDROGEL 1% include:

- acne
- skin irritation where ANDROGEL 1% is applied
- lab test changes
- increased prostate specific antigen (a test used to screen for prostate cancer)

Other side effects include more erections than are normal for you or erections that last a long time.

Tell your healthcare provider if you have any side effect that bothers you or that does not go away.

These are not all the possible side effects of ANDROGEL 1%. For more information, ask your healthcare provider or pharmacist.

Call your doctor for medical advice about side effects. You may report side effects to FDA at 1-800-FDA-1088.

How should I store ANDROGEL 1%?

- Store ANDROGEL 1% between 59°F to 86°F (15°C to 30°C).
- Safely throw away used ANDROGEL 1% in household trash. Be careful to prevent accidental exposure of children or pets.
- Keep ANDROGEL 1% away from fire.

Keep ANDROGEL 1% and all medicines out of the reach of children.

General information about the safe and effective use of ANDROGEL 1%

Medicines are sometimes prescribed for purposes other than those listed in a Medication Guide. Do not use ANDROGEL 1% for a condition for which it was not prescribed. Do not give ANDROGEL 1% to other people, even if they have the same symptoms you have. It may harm them.

This Medication Guide summarizes the most important information about ANDROGEL 1%. If you would like more information, talk to your healthcare provider. You can ask your pharmacist or healthcare provider for information about ANDROGEL 1% that is written for health professionals.

For more information, go to www.ANDROGEL.com or call 1-800-633-9110.

What are the ingredients in ANDROGEL 1%?

Active ingredient: testosterone

Inactive ingredients: carbomer 980, ethyl alcohol 67.0%, isopropyl myristate, purified water and sodium hydroxide.

This Medication Guide has been approved by the U.S. Food and Drug Administration.

Marketed by:
AbbVie Inc.
North Chicago, IL 60064, USA

A090630054573 Revised May, 2013

Shown in Product Identification Guide, page 303

ANDROGEL® 1.62% ⒸⅢ

(testosterone gel)
for topical use

HIGHLIGHTS OF PRESCRIBING INFORMATION

These highlights do not include all the information needed to use ANDROGEL 1.62% safely and effectively. See full prescribing information for ANDROGEL 1.62%.

AndroGel® (testosterone gel) 1.62% for topical use CIII

Initial U.S. Approval: 1953

WARNING: SECONDARY EXPOSURE TO TESTOSTERONE

See full prescribing information for complete boxed warning.

- **Virilization has been reported in children who were secondarily exposed to testosterone gel (5.2, 6.2).**
- **Children should avoid contact with unwashed or unclothed application sites in men using testosterone gel (2.2, 5.2).**
- **Healthcare providers should advise patients to strictly adhere to recommended instructions for use (2.2, 5.2, 17).**

RECENT MAJOR CHANGES

Indications and Usage. (1) 09/2012

INDICATIONS AND USAGE

AndroGel 1.62% is an androgen indicated for replacement therapy in males for conditions associated with a deficiency or absence of endogenous testosterone:

- Primary hypogonadism (congenital or acquired) (1)
- Hypogonadotropic hypogonadism (congenital or acquired) (1)

Important limitations of use:

- Safety and efficacy of AndroGel 1.62% in males less than 18 years old have not been established. (1, 8.4)
- Topical testosterone products may have different doses, strengths, or application instructions that may result in different systemic exposure. (1, 12.3)

DOSAGE AND ADMINISTRATION

- **Dosage and Administration for AndroGel 1.62% differs from AndroGel 1%. For dosage and administration of AndroGel 1% refer to its full prescribing information. (2)**
- Starting dose of AndroGel 1.62% is 40.5 mg of testosterone (2 pump actuations or a single 40.5 mg packet), applied topically once daily in the morning. (2.1)
- Apply to clean, dry, intact skin of the shoulders and upper arms. Do not apply AndroGel 1.62% to any other parts of the body including the abdomen or genitals. (2.2, 12.3)
- Dose adjustment: AndroGel 1.62% can be dose adjusted between a minimum of 20.25 mg of testosterone (1 pump actuation or a single 20.25 mg packet) and a maximum of 81 mg of testosterone (4 pump actuations or two 40.5 mg packets). The dose should be titrated based on the predose morning serum testosterone concentration at approximately 14 days and 28 days after starting treatment or following dose adjustment. Additionally, serum testosterone concentration should be assessed periodically thereafter. (2.1)
- Patients should wash hands immediately with soap and water after applying AndroGel 1.62% and cover the appli-

cation site(s) with clothing after the gel has dried. Wash the application site thoroughly with soap and water prior to any situation where skin-to-skin contact of the application site with another person is anticipated. (2.2)

DOSAGE FORMS AND STRENGTHS

AndroGel (testosterone gel) 1.62% for topical use is available as follows:

- a metered-dose pump that delivers 20.25 mg testosterone per actuation. (3)
- packets containing 20.25 mg testosterone. (3)
- packets containing 40.5 mg testosterone. (3)

CONTRAINDICATIONS

- Men with carcinoma of the breast or known or suspected prostate cancer (4, 5.1)
- Pregnant or breast-feeding women. Testosterone may cause fetal harm (4, 8.1, 8.3)

WARNINGS AND PRECAUTIONS

- Monitor patients with benign prostatic hyperplasia (BPH) for worsening of signs and symptoms of BPH (5.1)
- Avoid unintentional exposure of women or children to AndroGel 1.62%. Secondary exposure to testosterone can produce signs of virilization. AndroGel 1.62% should be discontinued until the cause of virilization is identified (5.2)
- Exogenous administration of androgens may lead to azoospermia (5.5)
- Edema with or without congestive heart failure (CHF) may be a complication in patients with preexisting cardiac, renal, or hepatic disease (5.7)
- Sleep apnea may occur in those with risk factors (5.9)
- Monitor serum testosterone, prostate specific antigen (PSA), hemoglobin, hematocrit, liver function tests and lipid concentrations periodically (5.1, 5.3, 5.6, 5.10)
- AndroGel 1.62% is flammable until dry (5.13)

ADVERSE REACTIONS

The most common adverse reaction (incidence ≥ 5%) is an increase in prostate specific antigen (PSA). (6.1)

To report SUSPECTED ADVERSE REACTIONS, contact AbbVie Inc. at 1-800-633-9110 or FDA at 1-800-FDA-1088 or *www.fda.gov/medwatch*.

DRUG INTERACTIONS

- Androgens may decrease blood glucose and therefore may decrease insulin requirements in diabetic patients (7.1)
- Changes in anticoagulant activity may be seen with androgens. More frequent monitoring of International Normalized Ratio (INR) and prothrombin time is recommended (7.2)
- Use of testosterone with adrenocorticotrophic hormone (ACTH) or corticosteroids may result in increased fluid retention. Use with caution, particularly in patients with cardiac, renal, or hepatic disease (7.3)

USE IN SPECIFIC POPULATIONS

There are insufficient long-term safety data in geriatric patients using AndroGel 1.62% to assess the potential risks of cardiovascular disease and prostate cancer. (8.5)

See 17 for PATIENT COUNSELING INFORMATION and Medication Guide

Revised: 05/2013

FULL PRESCRIBING INFORMATION: CONTENTS*

* Sections or subsections omitted from the full prescribing information are not listed

FULL PRESCRIBING INFORMATION

WARNING: SECONDARY EXPOSURE TO TESTOSTERONE

- **Virilization has been reported in children who were secondarily exposed to testosterone gel *[see Warnings and Precautions (5.2) and Adverse Reactions (6.2)]*.**
- **Children should avoid contact with unwashed or unclothed application sites in men using testosterone gel *[see Dosage and Administration (2.2) and Warnings and Precautions (5.2)]*.**
- **Healthcare providers should advise patients to strictly adhere to recommended instructions for use *[see Dosage and Administration (2.2), Warnings and Precautions (5.2) and Patient Counseling Information (17)]*.**

1 INDICATIONS AND USAGE

AndroGel 1.62% is an androgen indicated for replacement therapy in adult males for conditions associated with a deficiency or absence of endogenous testosterone:

- Primary hypogonadism (congenital or acquired): testicular failure due to conditions such as cryptorchidism, bilateral torsion, orchitis, vanishing testis syndrome, orchiectomy, Klinefelter's syndrome, chemotherapy, or toxic damage from alcohol or heavy metals. These men usually have low serum testosterone concentrations and gonadotropins (follicle-stimulating hormone [FSH], luteinizing hormone [LH]) above the normal range.
- Hypogonadotropic hypogonadism (congenital or acquired): idiopathic gonadotropin or luteinizing hormone-releasing hormone (LHRH) deficiency or pituitary-hypothalamic injury from tumors, trauma, or radiation. These men have low testosterone serum concentrations, but have gonadotropins in the normal or low range.

Important limitations of use:

- Safety and efficacy of AndroGel 1.62% in males less than 18 years old have not been established *[see Use in Specific Populations (8.4)]*.
- Topical testosterone products may have different doses, strengths, or application instructions that may result in different systemic exposure *[see Indications and Usage (1), and Clinical Pharmacology (12.3)]*.

2 DOSAGE AND ADMINISTRATION

Dosage and Administration for AndroGel 1.62% differs from AndroGel 1%. For dosage and administration of AndroGel 1% refer to its full prescribing information. (2)

2.1 Dosing and Dose Adjustment

The recommended starting dose of AndroGel 1.62% is 40.5 mg of testosterone (2 pump actuations or a single 40.5 mg packet) applied topically once daily in the morning to the shoulders and upper arms.

The dose can be adjusted between a minimum of 20.25 mg of testosterone (1 pump actuation or a single 20.25 mg packet) and a maximum of 81 mg of testosterone (4 pump actuations or two 40.5 mg packets). To ensure proper dosing, the dose should be titrated based on the pre-dose morning serum testosterone concentration from a single blood draw at approximately 14 days and 28 days after starting treatment or following dose adjustment. In addition, serum testosterone concentration should be assessed periodically thereafter. Table 1 describes the dose adjustments required at each titration step.

Table 1: Dose Adjustment Criteria

Pre-Dose Morning Total Serum Testosterone Concentration	Dose Titration
Greater than 750 ng/dL	Decrease daily dose by 20.25 mg (1 pump actuation or the equivalent of one 20.25 mg packet)
Equal to or greater than 350 and equal to or less than 750 ng/dL	No change: continue on current dose
Less than 350 ng/dL	Increase daily dose by 20.25 mg (1 pump actuation or the equivalent of one 20.25 mg packet)

The application site and dose of AndroGel 1.62% are not interchangeable with other topical testosterone products.

2.2 Administration Instructions

AndroGel 1.62% should be applied to clean, dry, intact skin of the upper arms and shoulders. Do not apply AndroGel 1.62% to any other parts of the body, including the abdomen or genitals *[see Clinical Pharmacology (12.3)]*. Area of application should be limited to the area that will be covered by the patient's short sleeve t-shirt. Patients should be instructed to use the palm of the hand to apply AndroGel 1.62% and spread across the maximum surface area as directed in Table 2 (for pump) and Table 3 (for packets) and in Figure 1.

Table 2: Application Sites for AndroGel 1.62%, Pump

Total Dose of Testosterone	Total Pump Actuations	Pump Actuations Per Upper Arm and Shoulder	
		Upper Arm and Shoulder #1	Upper Arm and Shoulder #2
20.25 mg	1	1	0
40.5 mg	2	1	1
60.75 mg	3	2	1
81 mg	4	2	2

Table 3: Application Sites for AndroGel 1.62%, Packets

Total Dose of Testosterone	Total packets	Gel Applications Per Upper Arm and Shoulder	
		Upper Arm and Shoulder #1	Upper Arm and Shoulder #2
20.25 mg	One 20.25 mg packet	One 20.25 mg packet	0
40.5 mg	One 40.5 mg packet	Half of contents of One 40.5 mg packet	Half of contents of One 40.5 mg packet
60.75 mg	One 20.25 mg packet AND One 40.5 mg packet	One 40.5 mg packet	One 20.25 mg packet
81 mg	Two 40.5 mg packets	One 40.5 mg packet	One 40.5 mg packet

The prescribed daily dose of AndroGel 1.62% should be applied to the right and left upper arms and shoulders as shown in the shaded areas in Figure 1.

Information on the AbbVie, Inc. products listed on these pages is from the prescribing information in use as of July 31, 2013. For more information, please visit rxabbvie.com or call 1-800-633-9110.

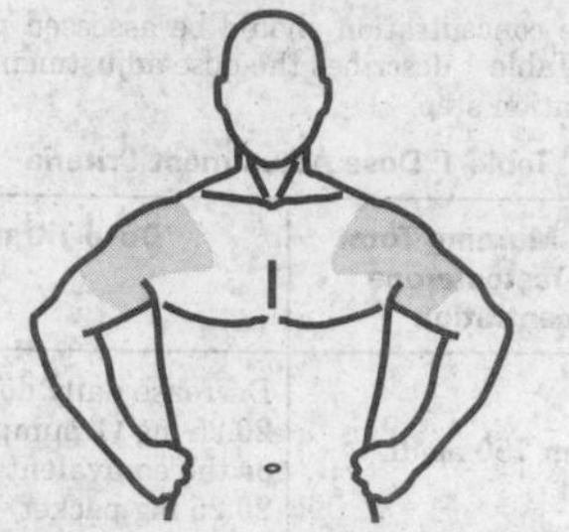

Figure 1. Application Sites for AndroGel 1.62%

Once the application site is dry, the site should be covered with clothing *[see Clinical Pharmacology (12.3)]*. Wash hands thoroughly with soap and water. Avoid fire, flames or smoking until the gel has dried since alcohol based products, including AndroGel 1.62%, are flammable.

The patient should avoid swimming or showering or washing the administration site for a minimum of 2 hours after application *[see Clinical Pharmacology (12.3)]*.

To obtain a full first dose, it is necessary to prime the canister pump. To do so, with the canister in the upright position, slowly and fully depress the actuator three times. Safely discard the gel from the first three actuations. It is only necessary to prime the pump before the first dose.

After the priming procedure, fully depress the actuator once for every 20.25 mg of AndroGel 1.62%. AndroGel 1.62% should be delivered directly into the palm of the hand and then applied to the application sites.

When using packets, the entire contents should be squeezed into the palm of the hand and immediately applied to the application sites. When 40.5 mg packets need to be split between the left and right shoulder, patients may squeeze a portion of the gel from the packet into the palm of the hand and apply to application sites. Repeat until entire contents have been applied. Alternatively, AndroGel 1.62% can be applied directly to the application sites from the pump or packets.

Strict adherence to the following precautions is advised in order to minimize the potential for secondary exposure to testosterone from AndroGel 1.62%-treated skin:

- Children and women should avoid contact with unwashed or unclothed application site(s) of men using AndroGel 1.62%.
- AndroGel 1.62% should only be applied to the upper arms and shoulders. The area of application should be limited to the area that will be covered by a short sleeve t-shirt.
- Patients should wash their hands with soap and water immediately after applying AndroGel 1.62%.
- Patients should cover the application site(s) with clothing (e.g., a t-shirt) after the gel has dried.
- Prior to situations in which direct skin-to-skin contact is anticipated, patients should wash the application site(s) thoroughly with soap and water to remove any testosterone residue.
- In the event that unwashed or unclothed skin to which AndroGel 1.62% has been applied comes in direct contact with the skin of another person, the general area of contact on the other person should be washed with soap and water as soon as possible.

3 DOSAGE FORMS AND STRENGTHS

AndroGel (testosterone gel) 1.62% for topical use only, is available as follows:

- A metered-dose pump. Each pump actuation delivers 20.25 mg of testosterone in 1.25 g of gel.
- A unit dose packet containing 20.25 mg of testosterone in 1.25 g of gel.
- A unit dose packet containing 40.5 mg of testosterone in 2.5 g of gel.

4 CONTRAINDICATIONS

- AndroGel 1.62% is contraindicated in men with carcinoma of the breast or known or suspected carcinoma of the prostate *[see Warnings and Precautions (5.1) and Adverse Reactions (6.1)]*.
- AndroGel 1.62% is contraindicated in women who are or may become pregnant, or who are breastfeeding. AndroGel 1.62% may cause fetal harm when administered to a pregnant woman. AndroGel 1.62% may cause serious adverse reactions in nursing infants. Exposure of a fetus or nursing infant to androgens may result in varying degrees of virilization. Pregnant women or those who may become pregnant need to be aware of the potential for transfer of testosterone from men treated with AndroGel 1.62%. If a pregnant woman is exposed to AndroGel 1.62%, she should be apprised of the potential hazard to the fetus *[see Warnings and Precautions (5.2) and Use in Specific Populations (8.1, 8.3)]*.

5 WARNINGS AND PRECAUTIONS

5.1 Worsening of Benign Prostatic Hyperplasia (BPH) and Potential Risk of Prostate Cancer

- Patients with BPH treated with androgens are at an increased risk for worsening of signs and symptoms of BPH. Monitor patients with BPH for worsening signs and symptoms.
- Patients treated with androgens may be at increased risk for prostate cancer. Evaluation of patients for prostate cancer prior to initiating and during treatment with androgens is appropriate *[see Contraindications (4)]*.

5.2 Potential for Secondary Exposure to Testosterone

Cases of secondary exposure resulting in virilization of children have been reported in postmarketing surveillance of testosterone gel products. Signs and symptoms have included enlargement of the penis or clitoris, development of pubic hair, increased erections and libido, aggressive behavior, and advanced bone age. In most cases, these signs and symptoms regressed with removal of the exposure to testosterone gel. In a few cases, however, enlarged genitalia did not fully return to age-appropriate normal size, and bone age remained modestly greater than chronological age. The risk of transfer was increased in some of these cases by not adhering to precautions for the appropriate use of the topical testosterone product. Children and women should avoid contact with unwashed or unclothed application sites in men using AndroGel 1.62% *[see Dosage and Administration (2.2), Use in Specific Populations (8.1) and Clinical Pharmacology (12.3)]*.

Inappropriate changes in genital size or development of pubic hair or libido in children, or changes in body hair distribution, significant increase in acne, or other signs of virilization in adult women should be brought to the attention of a physician and the possibility of secondary exposure to testosterone gel should also be brought to the attention of a physician. Testosterone gel should be promptly discontinued until the cause of virilization has been identified.

5.3 Polycythemia

Increases in hematocrit, reflective of increases in red blood cell mass, may require lowering or discontinuation of testosterone. Check hematocrit prior to initiating treatment. It would also be appropriate to re-evaluate the hematocrit 3 to 6 months after starting treatment, and then annually. If hematocrit becomes elevated, stop therapy until hematocrit decreases to an acceptable concentration. An increase in red blood cell mass may increase the risk of thromboembolic events.

5.4 Use in Women

Due to the lack of controlled evaluations in women and potential virilizing effects, AndroGel 1.62% is not indicated for use in women *[see Contraindications (4) and Use in Specific Populations (8.1, 8.3)]*.

5.5 Potential for Adverse Effects on Spermatogenesis

With large doses of exogenous androgens, including AndroGel 1.62%, spermatogenesis may be suppressed through feedback inhibition of pituitary FSH possibly leading to adverse effects on semen parameters including sperm count.

5.6 Hepatic Adverse Effects

Prolonged use of high doses of orally active 17-alpha-alkyl androgens (e.g., methyltestosterone) has been associated with serious hepatic adverse effects (peliosis hepatis, hepatic neoplasms, cholestatic hepatitis, and jaundice). Peliosis hepatis can be a life-threatening or fatal complication. Long-term therapy with intramuscular testosterone enanthate has produced multiple hepatic adenomas. AndroGel 1.62% is not known to cause these adverse effects.

5.7 Edema

Androgens, including AndroGel 1.62%, may promote retention of sodium and water. Edema, with or without congestive heart failure, may be a serious complication in patients with preexisting cardiac, renal, or hepatic disease *[see Adverse Reactions (6.2)]*.

5.8 Gynecomastia

Gynecomastia may develop and persist in patients being treated with androgens, including AndroGel 1.62%, for hypogonadism.

5.9 Sleep Apnea

The treatment of hypogonadal men with testosterone may potentiate sleep apnea in some patients, especially those with risk factors such as obesity or chronic lung diseases.

5.10 Lipids

Changes in serum lipid profile may require dose adjustment or discontinuation of testosterone therapy.

5.11 Hypercalcemia

Androgens, including AndroGel 1.62 %, should be used with caution in cancer patients at risk of hypercalcemia (and associated hypercalciuria). Regular monitoring of serum calcium concentrations is recommended in these patients.

5.12 Decreased Thyroxine-binding Globulin

Androgens, including AndroGel 1.62%, may decrease concentrations of thyroxin-binding globulins, resulting in decreased total T4 serum concentrations and increased resin uptake of T3 and T4. Free thyroid hormone concentrations remain unchanged, however, and there is no clinical evidence of thyroid dysfunction.

5.13 Flammability

Alcohol based products, including AndroGel 1.62%, are flammable; therefore, patients should be advised to avoid fire, flame or smoking until the AndroGel 1.62% has dried.

6 ADVERSE REACTIONS

6.1 Clinical Trial Experience

Because clinical trials are conducted under widely varying conditions, adverse reaction rates observed in the clinical trials of a drug cannot be directly compared to rates in the clinical trials of another drug and may not reflect the rates observed in practice.

AndroGel 1.62% was evaluated in a two-phase, 364-day, controlled clinical study. The first phase was a multi-center, randomized, double-blind, parallel-group, placebo-controlled period of 182 days, in which 234 hypogonadal men were treated with AndroGel 1.62% and 40 received placebo. Patients could continue in an open-label, non-comparative, maintenance period for an additional 182 days *[see Clinical Studies (14.1)]*.

The most common adverse reaction reported in the double-blind period was increased prostate specific antigen (PSA) reported in 26 AndroGel 1.62%-treated patients (11.1%). In 17 patients, increased PSA was considered an adverse event by meeting one of the two pre-specified criteria for abnormal PSA values, defined as (1) average serum PSA >4 ng/mL based on two separate determinations, or (2) an average change from baseline in serum PSA of greater than 0.75 ng/mL on two determinations.

During the 182-day, double-blind period of the clinical trial, the mean change in serum PSA value was 0.14 ng/mL for patients receiving AndroGel 1.62% and -0.12 ng/mL for the patients in the placebo group. During the double-blind period, seven patients had a PSA value >4.0 ng/mL, four of these seven patients had PSA less than or equal to 4.0 ng/mL upon repeat testing. The other three patients did not undergo repeat PSA testing.

During the 182-day, open-label period of the study, the mean change in serum PSA values was 0.10 ng/mL for both patients continuing on active therapy and patients transitioning onto active from placebo. During the open-label period, three patients had a serum PSA value > 4.0 ng/mL, two of whom had a serum PSA less than or equal to 4.0 ng/mL upon repeated testing. The other patient did not undergo repeat PSA testing. Among previous placebo patients, 3 of 28 (10.7%), had increased PSA as an adverse event in the open-label period.

Table 4 shows adverse reactions reported by >2% of patients in the 182-day, double-blind period of the AndroGel 1.62% clinical trial and more frequent in the AndroGel 1.62% treated group versus placebo.

Table 4: Adverse Reactions Reported in >2% of Patients in the 182-Day, Double-Blind Period of AndroGel 1.62% Clinical Trial

Adverse Reaction	Number (%) of Patients	
	AndroGel 1.62% N=234	Placebo N= 40
PSA increased*	26 (11.1%)	0%
Emotional lability**	6 (2.6%)	0%
Hypertension	5 (2.1%)	0%
Hematocrit or hemoglobin increased	5 (2.1%)	0%
Contact dermatitis***	5 (2.1%)	0%

******PSA increased*** includes: PSA values that met pre-specified criteria for abnormal PSA values (an average change from baseline > 0.75 ng/mL and/or an average PSA value >4.0 ng/mL based on two measurements) as well as those reported as adverse events.

*****Emotional lability*** includes: mood swings, affective disorder, impatience, anger, and aggression.

******Contact dermatitis*** includes: 4 patients with dermatitis at non-application sites.

Other adverse reactions occurring in less than or equal to 2% of AndroGel 1.62%-treated patients and more frequently than placebo included: frequent urination, and hyperlipidemia.

In the open-label period of the study (N=191), the most commonly reported adverse reaction (experienced by greater than 2% of patients) was increased PSA (n=13; 6.2%) and sinusitis. Other adverse reactions reported by less than or equal to 2% of patients included increased hemoglobin or hematocrit, hypertension, acne, libido decreased, insomnia, and benign prostatic hypertrophy.

During the 182-day, double-blind period of the clinical trial, 25 AndroGel 1.62%-treated patients (10.7%) discontinued treatment because of adverse reactions. These adverse reactions included 17 patients with PSA increased and 1 report each of: hematocrit increased, blood pressure increased, frequent urination, diarrhea, fatigue, pituitary tumor, dizziness, skin erythema and skin nodule (same patient – neither at application site), vasovagal syncope, and diabetes mellitus. During the 182-day, open-label period, 9 patients discontinued treatment because of adverse reactions. These adverse reactions included 6 reports of PSA increased, 2 of hematocrit increased, and 1 each of triglycerides increased and prostate cancer.

Application Site Reactions

In the 182-day double-blind period of the study, application site reactions were reported in two (2/234; 0.9%) patients receiving AndroGel 1.62%, both of which resolved. Neither of these patients discontinued the study due to application site adverse reactions. In the open-label period of the study, application site reactions were reported in three (3/219; 1.4%) additional patients that were treated with AndroGel 1.62%. None of these subjects were discontinued from the study due to application site reactions.

6.2 Postmarketing Experience

The following adverse reactions have been identified during post approval use of AndroGel 1%. Because the reactions are reported voluntarily from a population of uncertain size, it is not always possible to reliably estimate their frequency or establish a causal relationship to drug exposure (Table 5).

Table 5: Adverse Reactions from Post Approval Experience of AndroGel 1% by System Organ Class

System Organ Class	Adverse Reaction
Blood and lymphatic system disorders:	Elevated hemoglobin or hematocrit, polycythemia, anemia
Endocrine disorders:	Hirsutism
Gastrointestinal disorders:	Nausea
General disorders:	Asthenia, edema, malaise
Genitourinary disorders:	Impaired urination*
Hepatobiliary disorders:	Abnormal liver function tests
Investigations:	Lab test abnormal**, elevated PSA, electrolyte changes (nitrogen, calcium, potassium [includes hypokalemia], phosphorus, sodium), impaired glucose tolerance, hyperlipidemia, HDL, fluctuating testosterone levels, weight increase
Neoplasms:	Prostate cancer
Nervous system disorders:	Dizziness, headache, insomnia, sleep apnea
Psychiatric disorders:	Amnesia, anxiety, depression, hostility, emotional lability, decreased libido, nervousness
Reproductive system and breast disorders:	Gynecomastia, mastodynia, oligospermia, priapism (frequent or prolonged erections), prostate enlargement, BPH, testis disorder***
Respiratory disorders:	Dyspnea
Skin and subcutaneous tissue disorders:	Acne, alopecia, application site reaction (discolored hair, dry skin, erythema, paresthesia, pruritus, rash), skin dry, pruritus, sweating
Vascular disorders:	Hypertension, vasodilation (hot flushes)

* ***Impaired urination*** **includes** nocturia, urinary hesitancy, urinary incontinence, urinary retention, urinary urgency and weak urinary stream

** ***Lab test abnormal*** **includes** elevated AST, elevated ALT, elevated testosterone, elevated hemoglobin or hematocrit, elevated cholesterol, elevated cholesterol/LDL ratio, elevated triglycerides, or elevated serum creatinine

*** ***Testis disorder*** **includes** atrophy or non-palpable testis, varicocele, testis sensitivity or tenderness

Secondary Exposure to Testosterone in Children

Cases of secondary exposure to testosterone resulting in virilization of children have been reported in postmarketing surveillance of testosterone gel products. Signs and symptoms of these reported cases have included enlargement of the clitoris (with surgical intervention) or the penis, development of pubic hair, increased erections and libido, aggressive behavior, and advanced bone age. In most cases with a reported outcome, these signs and symptoms were reported to have regressed with removal of the testosterone gel exposure. In a few cases, however, enlarged genitalia did not fully return to age appropriate normal size, and bone age remained modestly greater than chronological age. In some of the cases, direct contact with the sites of application on the skin of men using testosterone gel was reported. In at least one reported case, the reporter considered the possibility of secondary exposure from items such as the testosterone gel user's shirts and/or other fabric, such as towels and sheets *[see Warnings and Precautions (5.2)]*.

7 DRUG INTERACTIONS

7.1 Insulin

Changes in insulin sensitivity or glycemic control may occur in patients treated with androgens. In diabetic patients, the metabolic effects of androgens may decrease blood glucose and, therefore, may decrease insulin requirements.

7.2 Oral Anticoagulants

Changes in anticoagulant activity may be seen with androgens, therefore more frequent monitoring of international normalized ratio (INR) and prothrombin time are recommended in patients taking anticoagulants, especially at the initiation and termination of androgen therapy.

7.3 Corticosteroids

The concurrent use of testosterone with adrenocorticotropic hormone (ACTH) or corticosteroids may result in increased fluid retention and requires careful monitoring particularly in patients with cardiac, renal or hepatic disease.

8 USE IN SPECIFIC POPULATIONS

8.1 Pregnancy

Pregnancy Category X *[see Contraindications (4)]*: AndroGel 1.62% is contraindicated during pregnancy or in women who may become pregnant. Testosterone is teratogenic and may cause fetal harm. Exposure of a fetus to androgens may result in varying degrees of virilization. If this drug is used during pregnancy, or if the patient becomes pregnant while taking this drug, the patient should be made aware of the potential hazard to the fetus.

8.3 Nursing Mothers

Although it is not known how much testosterone transfers into human milk, AndroGel 1.62% is contraindicated in nursing women because of the potential for serious adverse reactions in nursing infants. Testosterone and other androgens may adversely affect lactation *[see Contraindications (4)]*.

8.4 Pediatric Use

The safety and effectiveness of AndroGel 1.62% in pediatric patients less than 18 years old has not been established. Improper use may result in acceleration of bone age and premature closure of epiphyses.

8.5 Geriatric Use

There have not been sufficient numbers of geriatric patients involved in controlled clinical studies utilizing AndroGel 1.62% to determine whether efficacy in those over 65 years of age differs from younger subjects. Of the 234 patients enrolled in the clinical trial utilizing AndroGel 1.62%, 21 were over 65 years of age. Additionally, there is insufficient long-term safety data in geriatric patients to assess the potentially increased risks of cardiovascular disease and prostate cancer.

Geriatric patients treated with androgens may also be at risk for worsening of signs and symptoms of BPH.

8.6 Renal Impairment

No studies were conducted involving patients with renal impairment.

8.7 Hepatic Impairment

No studies were conducted in patients with hepatic impairment.

9 DRUG ABUSE AND DEPENDENCE

9.1 Controlled Substance

AndroGel 1.62% contains testosterone, a Schedule III controlled substance in the Controlled Substances Act.

9.2 Abuse

Anabolic steroids, such as testosterone, are abused. Abuse is often associated with adverse physical and psychological effects.

9.3 Dependence

Although drug dependence is not documented in individuals using therapeutic doses of anabolic steroids for approved indications, dependence is observed in some individuals abusing high doses of anabolic steroids. In general, anabolic steroid dependence is characterized by any three of the following:

- Taking more drug than intended
- Continued drug use despite medical and social problems
- Significant time spent in obtaining adequate amounts of drug
- Desire for anabolic steroids when supplies of the drugs are interrupted
- Difficulty in discontinuing use of the drug despite desires and attempts to do so
- Experience of a withdrawal syndrome upon discontinuation of anabolic steroid use

10 OVERDOSAGE

There is a single report of acute overdosage after parenteral administration of an approved testosterone product in the literature. This subject had serum testosterone concentrations of up to 11,400 ng/dL, which were implicated in a cerebrovascular accident. There were no reports of overdosage in the AndroGel 1.62% clinical trial.

Treatment of overdosage would consist of discontinuation of AndroGel 1.62%, washing the application site with soap and water, and appropriate symptomatic and supportive care.

11 DESCRIPTION

AndroGel 1.62% for topical use is a clear, colorless gel containing testosterone. Testosterone is an androgen. AndroGel 1.62% is available in a metered-dose pump or unit dose packets.

The active pharmacologic ingredient in AndroGel 1.62% is testosterone. Testosterone USP is a white to almost white powder chemically described as 17-beta hydroxyandrost-4-en-3-one. The structural formula is:

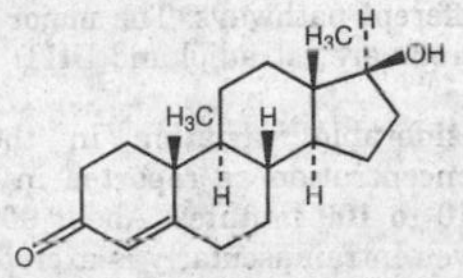

Testosterone

$C_{19}H_{28}O_2$ MW 288.42

The inactive ingredients in AndroGel 1.62% are: carbopol 980, ethyl alcohol, isopropyl myristate, purified water, and sodium hydroxide.

12 CLINICAL PHARMACOLOGY

12.1 Mechanism of Action

Endogenous androgens, including testosterone and dihydrotestosterone (DHT), are responsible for the normal growth and development of the male sex organs and for maintenance of secondary sex characteristics. These effects include the growth and maturation of prostate, seminal vesicles, penis and scrotum; the development of male hair distribution, such as facial, pubic, chest and axillary hair; laryngeal enlargement; vocal chord thickening; and alterations in body musculature and fat distribution. Testosterone and DHT are necessary for the normal development of secondary sex characteristics. Male hypogonadism results from insufficient secretion of testosterone and is characterized by low serum testosterone concentrations. Signs/symptoms associated with male hypogonadism include erectile dysfunction and decreased sexual desire, fatigue and loss of energy, mood depression, regression of secondary sexual characteristics and osteoporosis.

Male hypogonadism can present as primary hypogonadism caused by defects of the gonads, such as Klinefelter's Syndrome or Leydig cell aplasia while secondary hypogonadism is the failure of the hypothalamus or pituitary to produce sufficient gonadotropins (FSH, LH).

12.2 Pharmacodynamics

No specific pharmacodynamic studies were conducted using AndroGel 1.62%.

12.3 Pharmacokinetics

Absorption

AndroGel 1.62% delivers physiologic amounts of testosterone, producing circulating testosterone concentrations that approximate normal levels (300 – 1000 ng/dL) seen in healthy men. AndroGel 1.62% provides continuous transdermal delivery of testosterone for 24 hours following once daily application to clean, dry, intact skin of the shoulders and upper arms. Average serum testosterone concentrations over 24 hours (C_{avg}) observed when AndroGel 1.62% was applied to the upper arms/shoulders were comparable to average serum testosterone concentrations (C_{avg}) when AndroGel 1.62% was applied using a rotation method utilizing the abdomen and upper arms/shoulders. The rota-

Information on the AbbVie, Inc. products listed on these pages is from the prescribing information in use as of July 31, 2013. For more information, please visit rxabbvie.com or call 1-800-633-9110.

tion of abdomen and upper arms/shoulders was a method used in the pivotal clinical trial *[see Clinical Studies (14.1)]*.

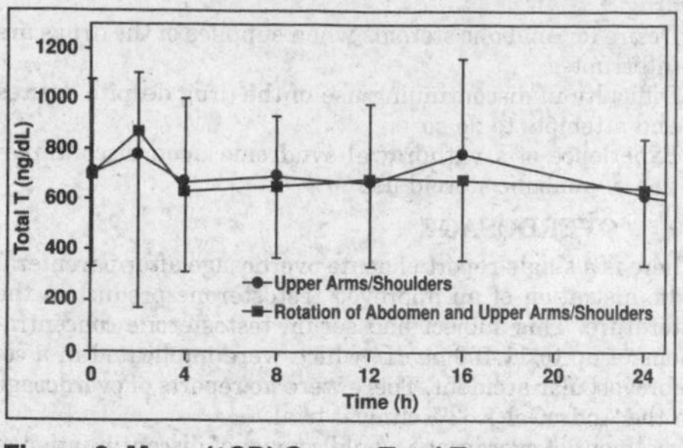

Figure 2: Mean (±SD) Serum Total Testosterone Concentrations on Day 7 in Patients Following AndroGel 1.62% Once-Daily Application of 81 mg of Testosterone (N=33) for 7 Days

Distribution

Circulating testosterone is primarily bound in the serum to sex hormone-binding globulin (SHBG) and albumin. Approximately 40% of testosterone in plasma is bound to SHBG, 2% remains unbound (free) and the rest is loosely bound to albumin and other proteins.

Metabolism

Testosterone is metabolized to various 17-keto steroids through two different pathways. The major active metabolites of testosterone are estradiol and DHT.

Excretion

There is considerable variation in the half-life of testosterone concentration as reported in the literature, ranging from 10 to 100 minutes. About 90% of a dose of testosterone given intramuscularly is excreted in the urine as glucuronic acid and sulfuric acid conjugates of testosterone and its metabolites. About 6% of a dose is excreted in the feces, mostly in the unconjugated form. Inactivation of testosterone occurs primarily in the liver.

When AndroGel 1.62% treatment is discontinued, serum testosterone concentrations return to approximately baseline concentrations within 48-72 hours after administration of the last dose.

Potential for testosterone transfer

The potential for testosterone transfer following administration of AndroGel 1.62% when it was applied only to upper arms/shoulders was evaluated in two clinical studies of males dosed with AndroGel 1.62% and their untreated female partners. In one study, 8 male subjects applied a single dose of AndroGel 1.62% 81 mg to their shoulders and upper arms. Two (2) hours after application, female subjects rubbed their hands, wrists, arms, and shoulders to the application site of the male subjects for 15 minutes. Serum concentrations of testosterone were monitored in female subjects for 24 hours after contact occurred. After direct skin-to-skin contact with the site of application, mean testosterone C_{avg} and C_{max} in female subjects increased by 280% and 267%, respectively, compared to mean baseline testosterone concentrations. In a second study evaluating transfer of testosterone, 12 male subjects applied a single dose of AndroGel 1.62% 81 mg to their shoulders and upper arms. Two (2) hours after application, female subjects rubbed their hands, wrists, arms, and shoulders to the application site of the male subjects for 15 minutes while the site of application was covered by a t-shirt. When a t-shirt was used to cover the site of application, mean testosterone C_{avg} and C_{max} in female subjects increased by 6% and 11%, respectively, compared to mean baseline testosterone concentrations.

A separate study was conducted to evaluate the potential for testosterone transfer from 16 males dosed with AndroGel 1.62% 81 mg when it was applied to abdomen only for 7 days, a site of application not approved for AndroGel 1.62%. Two (2) hours after application to the males on each day, the female subjects rubbed their abdomens for 15 minutes to the abdomen of the males. The males had covered the application area with a T-shirt. The mean testosterone C_{avg} and C_{max} in female subjects on day 1 increased by 43% and 47%, respectively, compared to mean baseline testosterone concentrations. The mean testosterone C_{avg} and C_{max} in female subjects on day 7 increased by 60% and 58%, respectively, compared to mean baseline testosterone concentrations.

Effect of showering

In a randomized, 3-way (3 treatment periods without washout period) crossover study in 24 hypogonadal men, the effect of showering on testosterone exposure was assessed after once daily application of AndroGel 1.62% 81 mg to upper arms/shoulders for 7 days in each treatment period. On the 7th day of each treatment period, hypogonadal men took a shower with soap and water at either 2, 6, or 10 hours after drug application. The effect of showering at 2 or 6 hours post-dose on Day 7 resulted in 13% and 12% decreases in mean C_{avg}, respectively, compared to Day 6 when no shower was taken after drug application. Showering at 10 hours after drug application had no effect on bioavailability. The amount of testosterone remaining in the outer layers of the skin at the application site on the 7th day was assessed using a tape stripping procedure and was reduced by at least 80% after showering 2-10 hours post-dose compared to on the 6th day when no shower was taken after drug application.

Effect of sunscreen or moisturizing lotion on absorption of testosterone

In a randomized, 3-way (3 treatment periods without washout period) crossover study in 18 hypogonadal males, the effect of applying a moisturizing lotion or a sunscreen on the absorption of testosterone was evaluated with the upper arms/shoulders as application sites. For 7 days, moisturizing lotion or sunscreen (SPF 50) was applied daily to the AndroGel 1.62% application site 1 hour after the application of AndroGel 1.62% 40.5 mg. Application of moisturizing lotion increased mean testosterone C_{avg} and C_{max} by 14% and 17%, respectively, compared to AndroGel 1.62% administered alone. Application of sunscreen increased mean testosterone C_{avg} and C_{max} by 8% and 13%, respectively, compared to AndroGel 1.62% applied alone.

13 NONCLINICAL TOXICOLOGY

13.1 Carcinogenesis, Mutagenesis, Impairment of Fertility

Testosterone has been tested by subcutaneous injection and implantation in mice and rats. In mice, the implant induced cervical-uterine tumors which metastasized in some cases. There is suggestive evidence that injection of testosterone into some strains of female mice increases their susceptibility to hepatoma. Testosterone is also known to increase the number of tumors and decrease the degree of differentiation of chemically induced carcinomas of the liver in rats. Testosterone was negative in the *in vitro* Ames and in the *in vivo* mouse micronucleus assays. The administration of exogenous testosterone has been reported to suppress spermatogenesis in the rat, dog and non-human primates, which was reversible on cessation of the treatment.

14 CLINICAL STUDIES

14.1 Clinical Trials in Hypogonadal Males

AndroGel 1.62% was evaluated in a multi-center, randomized, double-blind, parallel-group, placebo-controlled study (182-day double-blind period) in 274 hypogonadal men with body mass index (BMI) 18-40 kg/m^2 and 18-80 years of age (mean age 53.8 years). The patients had an average serum testosterone concentration of <300 ng/dL, as determined by two morning samples collected on the same visit. Patients were Caucasian 83%, Black 13%, Asian or Native American 4%. 7.5% of patients were Hispanic.

Patients were randomized to receive active treatment or placebo using a rotation method utilizing the abdomen and upper arms/shoulders for 182 days. All patients were started at a daily dose of 40.5 mg (two pump actuations) AndroGel 1.62% or matching placebo on Day 1 of the study. Patients returned to the clinic on Day 14, Day 28, and Day 42 for predose serum total testosterone assessments. The patient's daily dose was titrated up or down in 20.25 mg increments if the predose serum testosterone value was outside the range of 350-750 ng/dL. The study included four active AndroGel 1.62% doses: 20.25 mg, 40.5 mg, 60.75 mg, and 81 mg daily.

The primary endpoint was the percentage of patients with C_{avg} within the normal range of 300-1000 ng/dL on Day 112. In patients treated with AndroGel 1.62%, 81.6% (146/179) had C_{avg} within the normal range at Day 112. The secondary endpoint was the percentage of patients, with C_{max} above three pre-determined limits. The percentages of patients with C_{max} greater than 1500 ng/dL, and between 1800 and 2499 ng/dL on Day 112 were 11.2% and 5.5%, respectively. Two patients had a C_{max} >2500 ng/dL on Day 112 (2510 ng/dL and 2550 ng/dL, respectively); neither of these 2 patients demonstrated an abnormal C_{max} on prior or subsequent assessments at the same dose.

Patients could agree to continue in an open-label, active treatment maintenance period of the study for an additional 182 days.

Dose titrations on Days 14, 28, and 42 resulted in final doses of 20.25 mg – 81 mg on Day 112 as shown in Table 6. [See table 6 below]

Figure 3 summarizes the pharmacokinetic profile of total testosterone in patients completing 112 days of AndroGel 1.62% treatment administered as a starting dose of 40.5 mg of testosterone (2 pump actuations) for the initial 14 days followed by possible titration according to the follow-up testosterone measurements.

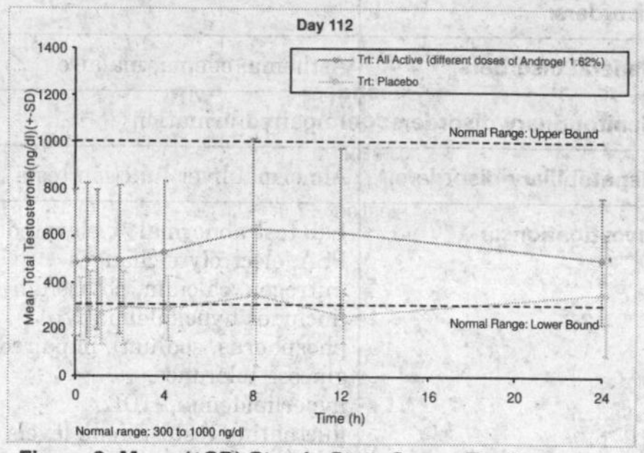

Figure 3: Mean (±SD) Steady-State Serum Total Testosterone Concentrations on Day 112

Efficacy was maintained in the group of men that received AndroGel 1.62% for one full year. In that group, 78% (106/136) had average serum testosterone concentrations in the normal range at Day 364. Figure 4 summarizes the mean total testosterone profile for these patients on Day 364.

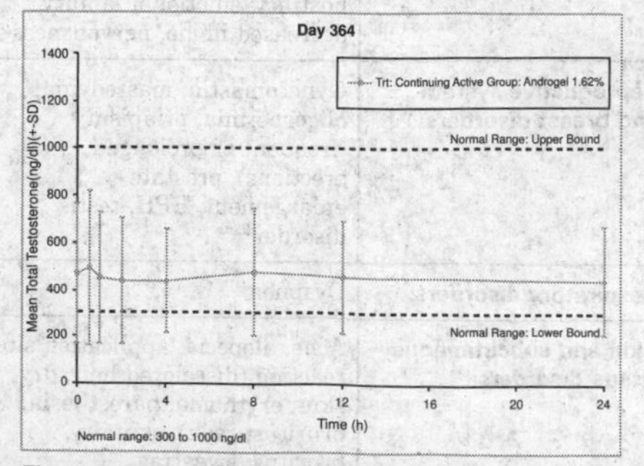

Figure 4: Mean (±SD) Steady-State Serum Total Testosterone Concentrations on Day 364

The mean estradiol and DHT concentration profiles paralleled the changes observed in testosterone. The levels of LH and FSH decreased with testosterone treatment. The decreases in levels of LH and FSH are consistent with reports published in the literature of long-term treatment with testosterone.

16 HOW SUPPLIED/STORAGE AND HANDLING

AndroGel 1.62% is supplied in non-aerosol, metered-dose pumps that deliver 20.25 mg of testosterone per complete pump actuation. The pumps are composed of plastic and

Table 6: Mean (SD) Testosterone Concentrations (C_{avg} and C_{max}) by final dose on Days 112 and 364

Parameter	Final Dose on Day 112					
	Placebo (n=27)	20.25 mg (n=12)	40.5 mg (n=34)	60.75 mg (n=54)	81 mg (n=79)	All Active (n=179)
C_{avg} (ng/dL)	303 (135)	457 (275)	524 (228)	643 (285)	537 (240)	561 (259)
C_{max} (ng/dL)	450 (349)	663 (473)	798 (439)	958 (497)	813 (479)	845 (480)
	Final Dose on Day 364					
		20.25 mg (n=7)	40.5 mg (n=26)	60.75 mg (n=29)	81 mg (n=74)	Continuing Active (n=136)
C_{avg} (ng/dL)		386 (130)	474 (176)	513 (222)	432 (186)	455 (192)
C_{max} (ng/dL)		562 (187)	715 (306)	839 (568)	649 (329)	697 (389)

stainless steel and an LDPE/aluminum foil inner liner encased in rigid plastic with a polypropylene cap. Each 88 g metered-dose pump is capable of dispensing 75 g of gel or 60-metered pump actuations; each pump actuation dispenses 1.25 g of gel.

AndroGel 1.62% is also supplied in unit-dose aluminum foil packets in cartons of 30. Each packet of 1.25 g or 2.5 g gel contains 20.25 mg or 40.5 mg testosterone, respectively.

NDC Number	Package Size
0051-8462-33	88 g pump (each pump dispenses 60 metered pump actuations with each pump actuation containing 20.25 mg of testosterone in 1.25 g of gel)
0051-8462-12	Each unit dose packet contains 20.25 mg of testosterone provided in 1.25 g of gel
0051-8462-31	30 packets (each unit dose packet contains 20.25 mg of testosterone provided in 1.25 g of gel)
0051-8462-01	Each unit dose packet contains 40.5 mg of testosterone provided in 2.5 g of gel
0051-8462-30	30 packets (each unit dose packet contains 40.5 mg of testosterone provided in 2.5 g of gel)

Store at controlled room temperature 20°-25°C (68°-77°F); excursions permitted to 15°- 30°C (59°- 86°F) [see USP Controlled Room Temperature].

Used AndroGel 1.62% pumps or used AndroGel 1.62% packets should be discarded in household trash in a manner that prevents accidental application or ingestion by children or pets.

17 PATIENT COUNSELING INFORMATION

See FDA-Approved Medication Guide

Patients should be informed of the following:

17.1 Use in Men with Known or Suspected Prostate or Breast Cancer

Men with known or suspected prostate or breast cancer should not use AndroGel 1.62% *[see Contraindications (4) and Warnings and Precautions (5.1)]*.

17.2 Potential for Secondary Exposure to Testosterone and Steps to Prevent Secondary Exposure

Secondary exposure to testosterone in children and women can occur with the use of testosterone gel in men. Cases of secondary exposure to testosterone have been reported in children.

Physicians should advise patients of the reported signs and symptoms of secondary exposure, which may include the following:

- In children: unexpected sexual development including inappropriate enlargement of the penis or clitoris, premature development of pubic hair, increased erections, and aggressive behavior.
- In women: changes in hair distribution, increase in acne, or other signs of testosterone effects.
- The possibility of secondary exposure to testosterone gel should be brought to the attention of a healthcare provider.
- AndroGel 1.62% should be promptly discontinued until the cause of virilization is identified.

Strict adherence to the following precautions is advised to minimize the potential for secondary exposure to testosterone from AndroGel 1.62% in men *[see Medication Guide]*:

- **Children and women should avoid contact with unwashed or unclothed application site(s)** of men using AndroGel 1.62%.
- Patients using AndroGel 1.62% should apply the product as directed and strictly adhere to the following:
  - **Wash hands** with soap and water immediately after application.
  - **Cover the application site(s)** with clothing after the gel has dried.
  - **Wash the application site(s) thoroughly** with soap and water prior to any situation where skin-to-skin contact of the application site with another person is anticipated.
- In the event that unwashed or unclothed skin to which AndroGel 1.62% has been applied comes in contact with the skin of another person, the general area of contact on the other person should be washed with soap and water as soon as possible *[see Dosage and Administration (2.2), Warnings and Precautions (5.2) and Clinical Pharmacology (12.3)]*.

17.3 Potential Adverse Reactions with Androgens

Patients should be informed that treatment with androgens may lead to adverse reactions which include:

- Changes in urinary habits such as increased urination at night, trouble starting the urine stream, passing urine many times during the day, having an urge to go to the bathroom right away, having a urine accident, being unable to pass urine and weak urine flow.
- Breathing disturbances, including those associated with sleep, or excessive daytime sleepiness.
- Too frequent or persistent erections of the penis.
- Nausea, vomiting, changes in skin color, or ankle swelling.

17.4 Patients Should Be Advised of the Following Instructions for Use

- **Read the Medication Guide before starting AndroGel 1.62% therapy and to reread it each time the prescription is renewed.**
- **AndroGel 1.62% should be applied and used appropriately to maximize the benefits and to minimize the risk of secondary exposure in children and women.**
- Keep AndroGel 1.62% out of the reach of children.
- **AndroGel 1.62% is an alcohol based product and is flammable; therefore avoid fire, flame or smoking until the gel has dried.**
- It is important to adhere to all recommended monitoring.
- Report any changes in their state of health, such as changes in urinary habits, breathing, sleep, and mood.
- AndroGel 1.62% is prescribed to meet the patient's specific needs; therefore, the patient should never share AndroGel 1.62% with anyone.
- Wait 2 hours before swimming or washing following application of AndroGel 1.62%. This will ensure that the greatest amount of AndroGel 1.62% is absorbed into their system.

Medication Guide
ANDROGEL® (AN DROW JEL) CIII
(testosterone gel) 1.62%

Read this Medication Guide before you start using ANDROGEL 1.62% and each time you get a refill. There may be new information. This information does not take the place of talking with your healthcare provider about your medical condition or treatment.

What is the most important information I should know about ANDROGEL 1.62%?

1. **Early signs and symptoms of puberty have happened in young children who were accidentally exposed to testosterone through contact with men using ANDROGEL 1.62%.**
   Signs and symptoms of early puberty in a child may include:
   - enlarged penis or clitoris
   - early development of pubic hair
   - increased erections or sex drive
   - aggressive behavior

   ANDROGEL 1.62% can transfer from your body to others.
2. **Women and children should avoid contact with the unwashed or unclothed area where ANDROGEL 1.62% has been applied to your skin.**
   Stop using ANDROGEL 1.62% and call your healthcare provider right away if you see any signs and symptoms in a child or a woman that may have occurred through accidental exposure to ANDROGEL 1.62%.
   Signs and symptoms of exposure to ANDROGEL 1.62% in children may include:
   - enlarged penis or clitoris
   - early development of pubic hair
   - increased erections or sex drive
   - aggressive behavior

   Signs and symptoms of exposure to ANDROGEL 1.62% in women may include:
   - changes in body hair
   - a large increase in acne

- **To lower the risk of transfer of ANDROGEL 1.62% from your body to others, you should follow these important instructions:**
  - Apply ANDROGEL 1.62% **only** to your shoulders and upper arms that will be covered by a short sleeve t-shirt.
  - Wash your hands **right away** with soap and water after applying ANDROGEL 1.62%.
  - After the gel has dried, **cover the application area with clothing**. Keep the area covered until you have washed the application area well or have showered.
  - **If you expect to have skin-to-skin contact with another person, first wash the application area well with soap and water.**
  - **If a woman or child makes contact with the ANDROGEL 1.62% application area, that area on the woman or child should be washed well with soap and water right away.**

What is ANDROGEL 1.62%?

ANDROGEL 1.62% is a prescription medicine that contains testosterone. ANDROGEL 1.62% is used to treat adult males who have low or no testosterone.

Your healthcare provider will test your blood before you start and while you are taking ANDROGEL 1.62%.

It is not known if ANDROGEL 1.62% is safe or effective in children younger than 18 years old. Improper use of ANDROGEL 1.62% may affect bone growth in children.

ANDROGEL 1.62% is a controlled substance (CIII) because it contains testosterone that can be a target for people who abuse prescription medicines. Keep your ANDROGEL 1.62% in a safe place to protect it. Never give your ANDROGEL 1.62% to anyone else, even if they have the same symptoms you have. Selling or giving away this medicine may harm others and is against the law.

ANDROGEL 1.62% is not meant for use in women.

Who should not use ANDROGEL 1.62%?

Do not use ANDROGEL 1.62% if you:

- have breast cancer
- have or might have prostate cancer
- are pregnant or may become pregnant or are breast-feeding. ANDROGEL 1.62% may harm your unborn or breast-feeding baby.
  Women who are pregnant or who may become pregnant should avoid contact with the area of skin where ANDROGEL 1.62% has been applied.

Talk to your healthcare provider before taking this medicine if you have any of the above conditions.

What should I tell my healthcare provider before using ANDROGEL 1.62%?

Before you use ANDROGEL 1.62%, tell your healthcare provider if you:

- have breast cancer
- have or might have prostate cancer
- have urinary problems due to an enlarged prostate
- have heart problems
- have kidney or liver problems
- have problems breathing while you sleep (sleep apnea)
- have any other medical conditions

Tell your healthcare provider about all the medicines you take, including prescription and non-prescription medicines, vitamins, and herbal supplements.

Using ANDROGEL 1.62% with certain other medicines can affect each other.

Especially, tell your healthcare provider if you take:

- insulin
- medicines that decrease blood clotting
- corticosteroids

Know the medicines you take. Ask your healthcare provider or pharmacist for a list of all of your medicines, if you are not sure. Keep a list of them and show it to your healthcare provider and pharmacist when you get a new medicine.

How should I use ANDROGEL 1.62%?

- It is important that you apply ANDROGEL 1.62% exactly as your healthcare provider tells you to.
- Your healthcare provider will tell you how much ANDROGEL 1.62% to apply and when to apply it.
- Your healthcare provider may change your ANDROGEL 1.62% dose. **Do not** change your ANDROGEL 1.62% dose without talking to your healthcare provider.
- **ANDROGEL 1.62% is to be applied to the area of your shoulders and upper arms that will be covered by a short sleeve t-shirt. Do not** apply ANDROGEL 1.62% to any other parts of your body such as your stomach area (abdomen), penis, or scrotum.
- Apply ANDROGEL 1.62% at the same time each morning. ANDROGEL 1.62% should be applied after showering or bathing.
- **Wash your hands right away** with soap and water after applying ANDROGEL 1.62%.
- Avoid showering, swimming or bathing for at least 2 hours after you apply ANDROGEL 1.62%.
- ANDROGEL 1.62% is flammable until dry. Let ANDROGEL 1.62% dry before smoking or going near an open flame.
- Let the application site dry completely before putting on a t-shirt.

Applying ANDROGEL 1.62%:

ANDROGEL 1.62% comes in a pump or in packets.

- **Before applying ANDROGEL 1.62% make sure that your shoulders and upper arms are clean, dry, and that there is no broken skin.**
- The application sites for ANDROGEL 1.62% are the upper arms and shoulders that will be covered by a short sleeve t-shirt (See Figure A).

[See figure A at top of next column]

If you are using ANDROGEL 1.62% pump:

- Before using a new bottle of ANDROGEL 1.62 % for the first time, you will need to prime the pump. To prime the ANDROGEL 1.62% pump, slowly push the pump all the way down 3 times. **Do not** use any ANDROGEL 1.62% that came out while priming. Wash it down the sink to avoid accidental exposure to others. Your ANDROGEL 1.62% pump is now ready to use.
- Remove the cap from the pump. Then, position the nozzle over the palm of your hand and slowly push the pump all the way down. Apply ANDROGEL 1.62% to the application site. You may also apply ANDROGEL 1.62% directly to the application site.

Information on the AbbVie, Inc. products listed on these pages is from the prescribing information in use as of July 31, 2013. For more information, please visit rxabbvie.com or call 1-800-633-9110.

Find Your Dose as Prescribed by Your Healthcare Provider		Application Method
1 PUMP DEPRESSION	20.25 mg	Apply 1 pump depression of ANDROGEL 1.62% to 1 upper arm and shoulder.
2 PUMP DEPRESSIONS	40.5 mg	Apply 1 pump depression of ANDROGEL 1.62% to 1 upper arm and shoulder and then apply 1 pump depression of ANDROGEL 1.62% to the opposite upper arm and shoulder.
3 PUMP DEPRESSIONS	60.75 mg	Apply 2 pump depressions of ANDROGEL 1.62% to 1 upper arm and shoulder and then apply 1 pump depression of ANDROGEL 1.62% to the opposite upper arm and shoulder.
4 PUMP DEPRESSIONS	81 mg	Apply 2 pump depressions of ANDROGEL 1.62% to 1 upper arm and shoulder and then apply 2 pump depressions of ANDROGEL 1.62% to the opposite upper arm and shoulder.

Find Your Dose as Prescribed by Your Healthcare Provider		Application Method
One 20.25 mg packet	20.25 mg	Apply 1 packet of ANDROGEL 1.62% to 1 upper arm and shoulder.
One 40.5 mg packet	40.5 mg	Apply half of the 40.5 mg packet of ANDROGEL 1.62% to 1 upper arm and shoulder and then apply the remaining packet contents to the opposite upper arm and shoulder.
One 40.5 mg packet and one 20.25 mg packet	60.75 mg	Apply one 40.5 mg packet of ANDROGEL 1.62% to 1 upper arm and shoulder and then apply one 20.25 mg packet of ANDROGEL 1.62% to the opposite upper arm and shoulder.
Two 40.5 mg packets	81 mg	Apply one 40.5 mg packet of ANDROGEL 1.62% to 1 upper arm and shoulder and then apply one 40.5 mg packet of ANDROGEL 1.62% to the opposite upper arm and shoulder.

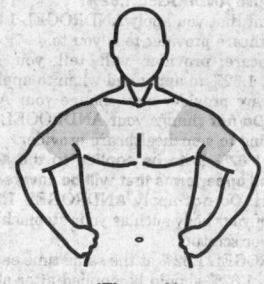

(Figure A)

- **Wash your hands with soap and water right away.**

[See first table above]

If you are using ANDROGEL 1.62% packets:

- Tear open the packet completely at the dotted line. Squeeze from the bottom of the packet to the top.
- Squeeze all of the ANDROGEL 1.62% out of the packet into the palm of your hand. Apply ANDROGEL 1.62% to the application site. You may also apply ANDROGEL 1.62% directly to the application site.
- ANDROGEL 1.62% should be applied right away.
- **Wash your hands with soap and water right away.**

[See second table above]

What are the possible side effects of ANDROGEL 1.62%?

See "What is the most important information I should know about ANDROGEL 1.62%?"

ANDROGEL 1.62% can cause serious side effects including:

- **If you already have enlargement of your prostate gland your signs and symptoms can get worse while using ANDROGEL 1.62%.** This can include:
  - increased urination at night
  - trouble starting your urine stream
  - having to pass urine many times during the day
  - having an urge that you have to go to the bathroom right away
  - having a urine accident
  - being unable to pass urine or weak urine flow
- **Possible increased risk of prostate cancer.** Your healthcare provider should check you for prostate cancer or any other prostate problems before you start and while you use ANDROGEL 1.62%.
- **In large doses ANDROGEL 1.62% may lower your sperm count.**
- **Swelling of your ankles, feet, or body, with or without heart failure.**
- **Enlarged or painful breasts.**
- **Have problems breathing while you sleep (sleep apnea).**
- **Blood clots in the legs.** This can include pain, swelling, or redness of your legs.

Call your healthcare provider right away if you have any of the serious side effects listed above.

The most common side effects of ANDROGEL 1.62% include:

- increased prostate specific antigen (a test used to screen for prostate cancer)
- mood swings
- hypertension
- increased red blood cell count
- skin irritation where ANDROGEL 1.62% is applied

Other side effects include more erections than are normal for you or erections that last a long time.

Tell your healthcare provider if you have any side effect that bothers you or that does not go away.

These are not all the possible side effects of ANDROGEL 1.62%. For more information, ask your healthcare provider or pharmacist.

Call your doctor for medical advice about side effects. You may report side effects to FDA at 1-800-FDA-1088.

How should I store ANDROGEL 1.62%?

- Store ANDROGEL 1.62% at 59°F to 86°F (15°C to 30°C).
- When it is time to throw away the pump or packets, safely throw away used ANDROGEL 1.62% in household trash. Be careful to prevent accidental exposure of children or pets.
- Keep ANDROGEL 1.62% away from fire.

Keep ANDROGEL 1.62% and all medicines out of the reach of children.

General information about the safe and effective use of ANDROGEL 1.62%

Medicines are sometimes prescribed for purposes other than those listed in a Medication Guide. Do not use ANDROGEL 1.62% for a condition for which it was not prescribed. Do not give ANDROGEL 1.62% to other people, even if they have the same symptoms you have. It may harm them.

This Medication Guide summarizes the most important information about ANDROGEL 1.62%. If you would like more information, talk to your healthcare provider. You can ask your pharmacist or healthcare provider for information about ANDROGEL 1.62% that is written for health professionals.

For more information, go to www.androgel.com or call 1-800-633-9110.

What are the ingredients in ANDROGEL 1.62%?

Active ingredient: testosterone

Inactive ingredients: carbopol 980, ethyl alcohol, isopropyl myristate, purified water and sodium hydroxide.

This Medication Guide has been approved by the U.S. Food and Drug Administration.

Marketed by:
AbbVie Inc.
North Chicago, IL 60064, USA
© 2013 AbbVie Inc.
A090630054574 Revised May, 2013

Shown in Product Identification Guide, page 303

BIAXIN® FILMTAB® ℞

[*bī ax ən*]

(clarithromycin tablets, USP)

BIAXIN® XL FILMTAB®

(clarithromycin extended-release tablets)

BIAXIN® GRANULES

(clarithromycin for oral suspension, USP)

To reduce the development of drug-resistant bacteria and maintain the effectiveness of BIAXIN and other antibacterial drugs, BIAXIN should be used only to treat or prevent infections that are proven or strongly suspected to be caused by bacteria.

DESCRIPTION

Clarithromycin is a semi-synthetic macrolide antibiotic. Chemically, it is 6-*0*-methylerythromycin. The molecular formula is $C_{38}H_{69}NO_{13}$, and the molecular weight is 747.96. The structural formula is:

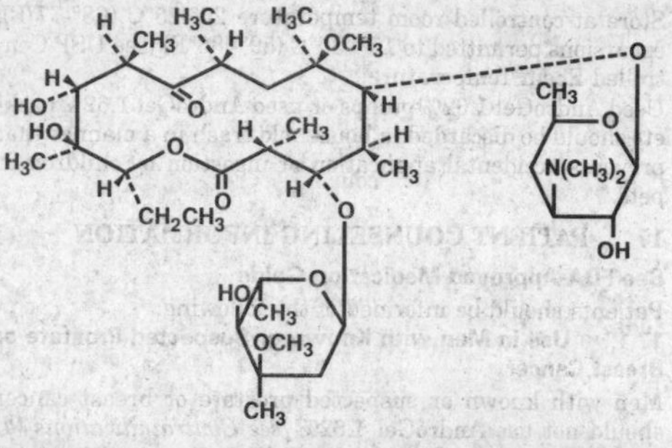

Clarithromycin is a white to off-white crystalline powder. It is soluble in acetone, slightly soluble in methanol, ethanol, and acetonitrile, and practically insoluble in water.

BIAXIN is available as immediate-release tablets, extended-release tablets, and granules for oral suspension.

Each yellow oval film-coated immediate-release BIAXIN tablet (clarithromycin tablets, USP) contains 250 mg or 500 mg of clarithromycin and the following inactive ingredients:

250 mg tablets: hypromellose, hydroxypropyl cellulose, croscarmellose sodium, D&C Yellow No. 10, FD&C Blue No. 1, magnesium stearate, microcrystalline cellulose, povidone, pregelatinized starch, propylene glycol, silicon dioxide, sorbic acid, sorbitan monooleate, stearic acid, talc, titanium dioxide, and vanillin.

500 mg tablets: hypromellose, hydroxypropyl cellulose, colloidal silicon dioxide, croscarmellose sodium, D&C Yellow No. 10, magnesium stearate, microcrystalline cellulose, povidone, propylene glycol, sorbic acid, sorbitan monooleate, titanium dioxide, and vanillin.

Each yellow oval film-coated BIAXIN XL tablet (clarithromycin extended-release tablets) contains 500 mg of clarithromycin and the following inactive ingredients: cellulosic polymers, D&C Yellow No. 10, lactose monohydrate, magnesium stearate, propylene glycol, sorbic acid, sorbitan monooleate, talc, titanium dioxide, and vanillin.

After constitution, each 5 mL of BIAXIN suspension (clarithromycin for oral suspension, USP) contains 125 mg or 250 mg of clarithromycin. Each bottle of BIAXIN granules contains 1250 mg (50 mL size), 2500 mg (50 and 100 mL sizes) or 5000 mg (100 mL size) of clarithromycin and the following inactive ingredients: carbomer, castor oil, citric acid, hypromellose phthalate, maltodextrin, potassium sorbate, povidone, silicon dioxide, sucrose, xanthan gum, titanium dioxide and fruit punch flavor.

CLINICAL PHARMACOLOGY

Pharmacokinetics

Clarithromycin is rapidly absorbed from the gastrointestinal tract after oral administration. The absolute bioavailability of 250 mg clarithromycin tablets was approximately 50%. For a single 500 mg dose of clarithromycin, food slightly delays the onset of clarithromycin absorption, increasing the peak time from approximately 2 to 2.5 hours. Food also increases the clarithromycin peak plasma concentration by about 24%, but does not affect the extent of clarithromycin bioavailability. Food does not affect the onset of formation of the antimicrobially active metabolite, 14-OH clarithromycin or its peak plasma concentration but does slightly decrease the extent of metabolite formation, indicated by an 11% decrease in area under the plasma concentration-time curve (AUC). Therefore, BIAXIN tablets may be given without regard to food.

In nonfasting healthy human subjects (males and females), peak plasma concentrations were attained within 2 to 3 hours after oral dosing. Steady-state peak plasma clarithromycin concentrations were attained within 3 days and were approximately 1 to 2 mcg/mL with a 250 mg dose administered every 12 hours and 3 to 4 mcg/mL with a 500 mg dose administered every 8 to 12 hours. The elimination half-life of clarithromycin was about 3 to 4 hours with 250 mg administered every 12 hours but increased to 5 to 7 hours with 500 mg administered every 8 to 12 hours. The nonlinearity of clarithromycin pharmacokinetics is slight at the recommended doses of 250 mg and 500 mg administered every 8 to 12 hours. With a 250 mg every 12 hours dosing, the principal metabolite, 14-OH clarithromycin, attains a peak steady-state concentration of about 0.6 mcg/mL and has an elimination half-life of 5 to 6 hours. With a 500 mg every 8 to 12 hours dosing, the peak steady-state concentration of 14-OH clarithromycin is slightly higher (up to 1 mcg/mL), and its elimination half-life is about 7 to 9 hours. With any of these dosing regimens, the steady-state concentration of this metabolite is generally attained within 3 to 4 days.

After a 250 mg tablet every 12 hours, approximately 20% of the dose is excreted in the urine as clarithromycin, while after a 500 mg tablet every 12 hours, the urinary excretion of clarithromycin is somewhat greater, approximately 30%. In comparison, after an oral dose of 250 mg (125 mg/5 mL) suspension every 12 hours, approximately 40% is excreted in urine as clarithromycin. The renal clearance of clarithromycin is, however, relatively independent of the dose size and approximates the normal glomerular filtration rate. The major metabolite found in urine is 14-OH clarithromycin, which accounts for an additional 10% to 15% of the dose with either a 250 mg or a 500 mg tablet administered every 12 hours.

Steady-state concentrations of clarithromycin and 14-OH clarithromycin observed following administration of 500 mg doses of clarithromycin every 12 hours to adult patients with HIV infection were similar to those observed in healthy volunteers. In adult HIV-infected patients taking 500- or 1000-mg doses of clarithromycin every 12 hours, steady-state clarithromycin C_{max} values ranged from 2 to 4 mcg/mL and 5 to 10 mcg/mL, respectively.

The steady-state concentrations of clarithromycin in subjects with impaired hepatic function did not differ from those in normal subjects; however, the 14-OH clarithromycin concentrations were lower in the hepatically impaired subjects. The decreased formation of 14-OH clarithromycin was at least partially offset by an increase in renal clearance of clarithromycin in the subjects with impaired hepatic function when compared to healthy subjects.

The pharmacokinetics of clarithromycin was also altered in subjects with impaired renal function. (See **PRECAUTIONS** and **DOSAGE AND ADMINISTRATION**.)

Clarithromycin and the 14-OH clarithromycin metabolite distribute readily into body tissues and fluids. There are no data available on cerebrospinal fluid penetration. Because of high intracellular concentrations, tissue concentrations are higher than serum concentrations. Examples of tissue and serum concentrations are presented below.

CONCENTRATION (after 250 mg q12h)

Tissue Type	Tissue (mcg/g)	Serum (mcg/mL)
Tonsil	1.6	0.8
Lung	8.8	1.7

Clarithromycin extended-release tablets provide extended absorption of clarithromycin from the gastrointestinal tract after oral administration. Relative to an equal total daily dose of immediate-release clarithromycin tablets, clarithromycin extended-release tablets provide lower and later steady-state peak plasma concentrations but equivalent 24-hour AUC's for both clarithromycin and its microbiologically-active metabolite, 14-OH clarithromycin. While the extent of formation of 14-OH clarithromycin following administration of BIAXIN XL tablets (2 × 500 mg once daily) is not affected by food, administration under fasting conditions is associated with approximately 30% lower clarithromycin AUC relative to administration with food. Therefore, BIAXIN XL tablets should be taken with food.

[See figure at top of next column]

In healthy human subjects, steady-state peak plasma clarithromycin concentrations of approximately 2 to 3 mcg/mL were achieved about 5 to 8 hours after oral administration of 2 × 500 mg BIAXIN XL tablets once daily; for 14-OH clarithromycin, steady-state peak plasma concentrations of approximately 0.8 mcg/mL were attained about 6 to 9 hours after dosing. Steady-state peak plasma clarithromycin concentrations of approximately 1 to 2 mcg/mL were achieved about 5 to 6 hours after oral administration of a single 500 mg BIAXIN XL tablet once daily; for 14-OH clarithromycin, steady-state peak plasma concentrations of approximately 0.6 mcg/mL were attained about 6 hours after dosing.

Clarithromycin Tissue Concentrations 2 hours after Dose (mcg/mL)/(mcg/g)

Treatment	N	antrum	fundus	N	mucus
Clarithromycin	5	10.48 ± 2.01	20.81 ± 7.64	4	4.15 ± 7.74
Clarithromycin + Omeprazole	5	19.96 ± 4.71	24.25 ± 6.37	4	39.29 ± 32.79

Steady-State Clarithromycin Plasma Concentration-Time Profiles

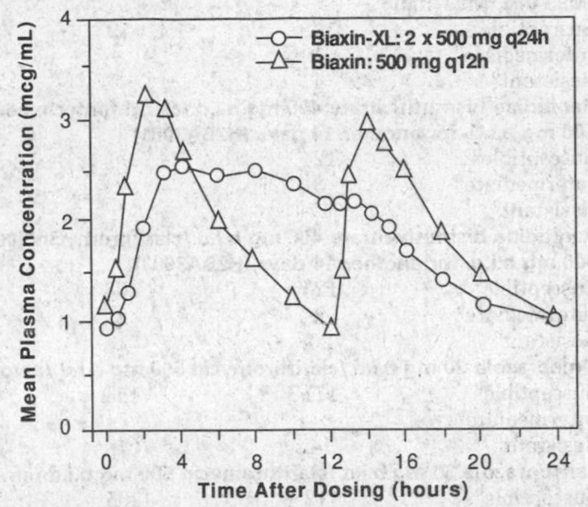

When 250 mg doses of clarithromycin as BIAXIN suspension were administered to fasting healthy adult subjects, peak plasma concentrations were attained around 3 hours after dosing. Steady-state peak plasma concentrations were attained in 2 to 3 days and were approximately 2 mcg/mL for clarithromycin and 0.7 mcg/mL for 14-OH clarithromycin when 250-mg doses of the clarithromycin suspension were administered every 12 hours. Elimination half-life of clarithromycin (3 to 4 hours) and that of 14-OH clarithromycin (5 to 7 hours) were similar to those observed at steady state following administration of equivalent doses of BIAXIN tablets.

For adult patients, the bioavailability of 10 mL of the 125 mg/5 mL suspension or 10 mL of the 250 mg/5 mL suspension is similar to a 250 mg or 500 mg tablet, respectively.

In children requiring antibiotic therapy, administration of 7.5 mg/kg q12h doses of clarithromycin as the suspension generally resulted in steady-state peak plasma concentrations of 3 to 7 mcg/mL for clarithromycin and 1 to 2 mcg/mL for 14-OH clarithromycin.

In HIV-infected children taking 15 mg/kg every 12 hours, steady-state clarithromycin peak concentrations generally ranged from 6 to 15 mcg/mL.

Clarithromycin penetrates into the middle ear fluid of children with secretory otitis media.

CONCENTRATION (after 7.5 mg/kg q12h for 5 doses)

Analyte	Middle Ear Fluid (mcg/mL)	Serum (mcg/mL)
Clarithromycin	2.5	1.7
14-OH Clarithromycin	1.3	0.8

In adults given 250 mg clarithromycin as suspension (n = 22), food appeared to decrease mean peak plasma clarithromycin concentrations from 1.2 (± 0.4) mcg/mL to 1.0 (± 0.4) mcg/mL and the extent of absorption from 7.2 (± 2.5) hr•mcg/mL to 6.5 (± 3.7) hr•mcg/mL.

When children (n = 10) were administered a single oral dose of 7.5 mg/kg suspension, food increased mean peak plasma clarithromycin concentrations from 3.6 (± 1.5) mcg/mL to 4.6 (± 2.8) mcg/mL and the extent of absorption from 10.0 (± 5.5) hr•mcg/mL to 14.2 (± 9.4) hr•mcg/mL.

Clarithromycin 500 mg every 8 hours was given in combination with omeprazole 40 mg daily to healthy adult males. The plasma levels of clarithromycin and 14-hydroxy-clarithromycin were increased by the concomitant administration of omeprazole. For clarithromycin, the mean C_{max} was 10% greater, the mean C_{min} was 27% greater, and the mean AUC_{0-8} was 15% greater when clarithromycin was administered with omeprazole than when clarithromycin was administered alone. Similar results were seen for 14-hydroxy-clarithromycin, the mean C_{max} was 45% greater, the mean C_{min} was 57% greater, and the mean AUC_{0-8} was 45% greater. Clarithromycin concentrations in the gastric tissue and mucus were also increased by concomitant administration of omeprazole.

[See table above]

For information about other drugs indicated in combination with BIAXIN, refer to the **CLINICAL PHARMACOLOGY** section of their package inserts.

Microbiology

Clarithromycin exerts its antibacterial action by binding to the 50S ribosomal subunit of susceptible bacteria resulting in inhibition of protein synthesis.

Clarithromycin is active *in vitro* against a variety of aerobic and anaerobic Gram-positive and Gram-negative bacteria as well as most *Mycobacterium avium* complex (MAC) bacteria.

Additionally, the 14-OH clarithromycin metabolite also has clinically significant antimicrobial activity. The 14-OH clarithromycin is twice as active against *Haemophilus influenzae* microorganisms as the parent compound. However, for *Mycobacterium avium* complex (MAC) isolates the 14-OH metabolite is 4 to 7 times less active than clarithromycin. The clinical significance of this activity against *Mycobacterium avium* complex is unknown.

Clarithromycin has been shown to be active against most strains of the following microorganisms both *in vitro* and in clinical infections as described in the **INDICATIONS AND USAGE** section:

Gram-Positive Microorganisms
Staphylococcus aureus
Streptococcus pneumoniae
Streptococcus pyogenes
Gram-Negative Microorganisms
Haemophilus influenzae
Haemophilus parainfluenzae
Moraxella catarrhalis
Other Microorganisms
Mycoplasma pneumoniae
Chlamydia pneumoniae (TWAR)
Mycobacteria
Mycobacterium avium complex (MAC) consisting of:
Mycobacterium avium
Mycobacterium intracellulare

Beta-lactamase production should have no effect on clarithromycin activity.

NOTE: Most isolates of methicillin-resistant and oxacillin-resistant staphylococci are resistant to clarithromycin.

Omeprazole/clarithromycin dual therapy; ranitidine bismuth citrate/clarithromycin dual therapy; omeprazole/clarithromycin/amoxicillin triple therapy; and lansoprazole/clarithromycin/amoxicillin triple therapy have been shown to be active against most strains of *Helicobacter pylori in vitro* and in clinical infections as described in the **INDICATIONS AND USAGE** section.

Helicobacter
Helicobacter pylori
Pretreatment Resistance

Clarithromycin pretreatment resistance rates were 3.5% (4/113) in the omeprazole/clarithromycin dual therapy studies (M93-067, M93-100) and 9.3% (41/439) in the omeprazole/clarithromycin/amoxicillin triple therapy studies (126, 127, M96-446). Clarithromycin pretreatment resistance was 12.6% (44/348) in the ranitidine bismuth citrate/clarithromycin b.i.d. versus t.i.d. clinical study (H2BA3001). Clarithromycin pretreatment resistance rates were 9.5% (91/960) by E-test and 11.3% (12/106) by agar dilution in the lansoprazole/clarithromycin/amoxicillin triple therapy clinical trials (M93-125, M93-130, M93-131, M95-392, and M95-399).

Amoxicillin pretreatment susceptible isolates (< 0.25 mcg/mL) were found in 99.3% (436/439) of the patients in the omeprazole/clarithromycin/amoxicillin clinical studies (126, 127, M96-446). Amoxicillin pretreatment minimum inhibitory concentrations (MICs) > 0.25 mcg/mL occurred in 0.7% (3/439) of the patients, all of whom were in the clarithromycin/amoxicillin study arm. Amoxicillin pretreatment susceptible isolates (< 0.25 mcg/mL) occurred in 97.8% (936/957) and 98.0% (98/100) of the patients in the lansoprazole/

Information on the AbbVie, Inc. products listed on these pages is from the prescribing information in use as of July 31, 2013. For more information, please visit rxabbvie.com or call 1-800-633-9110.

clarithromycin/amoxicillin triple-therapy clinical trials by E-test and agar dilution, respectively. Twenty-one of the 957 patients (2.2%) by E-test and 2 of 100 patients (2.0%) by agar dilution had amoxicillin pretreatment MICs of > 0.25 mcg/mL. Two patients had an unconfirmed pretreatment amoxicillin minimum inhibitory concentration (MIC) of > 256 mcg/mL by E-test.

[See table above]

Patients not eradicated of *H. pylori* following omeprazole/clarithromycin, ranitidine bismuth citrate/clarithromycin, omeprazole/clarithromycin/amoxicillin, or lansoprazole/clarithromycin/amoxicillin therapy would likely have clarithromycin resistant *H. pylori* isolates. Therefore, for patients who fail therapy, clarithromycin susceptibility testing should be done, if possible. Patients with clarithromycin resistant *H. pylori* should not be treated with any of the following: omeprazole/clarithromycin dual therapy; ranitidine bismuth citrate/clarithromycin dual therapy; omeprazole/clarithromycin/amoxicillin triple therapy; lansoprazole/clarithromycin/amoxicillin triple therapy; or other regimens which include clarithromycin as the sole antimicrobial agent.

Amoxicillin Susceptibility Test Results and Clinical/Bacteriological Outcomes

In the omeprazole/clarithromycin/amoxicillin triple-therapy clinical trials, 84.9% (157/185) of the patients who had pretreatment amoxicillin susceptible MICs (< 0.25 mcg/mL) were eradicated of *H. pylori* and 15.1% (28/185) failed therapy. Of the 28 patients who failed triple therapy, 11 had no post-treatment susceptibility test results, and 17 had post-treatment *H. pylori* isolates with amoxicillin susceptible MICs. Eleven of the patients who failed triple therapy also had post-treatment *H. pylori* isolates with clarithromycin resistant MICs.

In the lansoprazole/clarithromycin/amoxicillin triple-therapy clinical trials, 82.6% (195/236) of the patients that had pretreatment amoxicillin susceptible MICs (< 0.25 mcg/mL) were eradicated of *H. pylori*. Of those with pretreatment amoxicillin MICs of > 0.25 mcg/mL, three of six had the *H. pylori* eradicated. A total of 12.8% (22/172) of the patients failed the 10- and 14-day triple-therapy regimens. Post-treatment susceptibility results were not obtained on 11 of the patients who failed therapy. Nine of the 11 patients with amoxicillin post-treatment MICs that failed the triple-therapy regimen also had clarithromycin resistant *H. pylori* isolates.

The following *in vitro* data are available, **but their clinical significance is unknown**. Clarithromycin exhibits *in vitro* activity against most isolates of the following bacteria; however, the safety and effectiveness of clarithromycin in treating clinical infections due to these bacteria have not been established in adequate and well-controlled clinical trials.

Gram-Positive Bacteria

Streptococcus agalactiae

Streptococci (Groups C, F, G)

Viridans group streptococci

Gram-Negative Bacteria

Bordetella pertussis

Legionella pneumophila

Pasteurella multocida

Gram-Positive Bacteria

Clostridium perfringens

Peptococcus niger

Propionibacterium acnes

Gram-Negative Anaerobic Bacteria

Prevotella melaninogenica (formerly *Bacteriodes melaninogenicus*)

Susceptibility Testing Methods (Excluding Mycobacteria and Helicobacter)

Dilution Techniques

Quantitative methods are used to determine antimicrobial minimum inhibitory concentrations (MICs). These MICs provide estimates of the susceptibility of bacteria to antimicrobial compounds. The MICs should be determined using a standardized procedure. Standardized procedures are based on a dilution method[1] (broth or agar) or equivalent with standardized inoculum concentrations and standardized concentrations of clarithromycin powder. The MIC values should be interpreted according to the following criteria[2]:

Susceptibility Test Interpretive Criteria for *Staphylococcus aureus*

MIC (mcg/mL)	Interpretation
≤ 2.0	Susceptible (S)
4.0	Intermediate (I)
≥ 8.0	Resistant (R)

Clarithromycin Susceptibility Test Results and Clinical/Bacteriological Outcomes[a]

Clarithromycin Pretreatment Results		Clarithromycin Post-treatment Results				
		H. pylori negative - eradicated	*H. pylori* positive - not eradicated Post-treatment susceptibility results			
			S[b]	I[b]	R[b]	No MIC
Omeprazole 40 mg q.d./clarithromycin 500 mg t.i.d. for 14 days followed by omeprazole 20 mg q.d. for another 14 days (M93-067, M93-100)						
Susceptible[b]	108	72	1		26	9
Intermediate[b]	1				1	
Resistant[b]	4				4	
Ranitidine bismuth citrate 400 mg b.i.d./clarithromycin 500 mg t.i.d. for 14 days followed by ranitidine bismuth citrate 400 mg b.i.d. for another 14 days (H2BA3001)						
Susceptible[b]	124	98	4		14	8
Intermediate[b]	3	2				1
Resistant[b]	17	1			15	1
Ranitidine bismuth citrate 400 mg b.i.d./clarithromycin 500 mg b.i.d. for 14 days followed by ranitidine bismuth citrate 400 mg b.i.d. for another 14 days (H2BA3001)						
Susceptible[b]	125	106	1	1	12	5
Intermediate[b]	2	2				
Resistant[b]	20	1			19	
Omeprazole 20 mg b.i.d./clarithromycin 500 mg b.i.d./amoxicillin 1 g b.i.d. for 10 days (126, 127, M96-446)						
Susceptible[b]	171	153	7		3	8
Intermediate[b]						
Resistant[b]	14	4	1		6	3
Lansoprazole 30 mg b.i.d./clarithromycin 500 mg b.i.d./amoxicillin 1 g b.i.d. for 14 days (M95-399, M93-131, M95-392)						
Susceptible[b]	112	105				7
Intermediate[b]	3	3				
Resistant[b]	17	6			7	4
Lansoprazole 30 mg b.i.d./clarithromycin 500 mg b.i.d./amoxicillin 1 g b.i.d. for 10 days (M95-399)						
Susceptible[b]	42	40	1		1	
Intermediate[b]						
Resistant[b]	4	1			3	

[a] Includes only patients with pretreatment clarithromycin susceptibility tests

[b] Breakpoints for antimicrobial susceptibility testing at the time of studies were: Susceptible (S) MIC < 0.25 mcg/mL, Intermediate (I) MIC 0.5-1.0 mcg/mL, Resistant (R) MIC > 2 mcg/mL. For current antimicrobial susceptibility testing guidelines see reference 4. For current susceptibility test interpretive criteria, see Susceptibility Test for *Helicobacter pylori* below.

Susceptibility Test Interpretive Criteria for *Streptococcus pyogenes* and *Streptococcus pneumoniae*[a]

MIC (mcg/mL)	Interpretation
≤ 0.25	Susceptible (S)
0.5	Intermediate (I)
≥ 1.0	Resistant (R)

[a] These interpretive standards are applicable only to broth microdilution susceptibility tests using cation-adjusted Mueller-Hinton broth with 2-5% lysed horse blood.

For testing *Haemophilus spp.*[b]

MIC (mcg/mL)	Interpretation
≤ 8.0	Susceptible (S)
16.0	Intermediate (I)
≥ 32.0	Resistant (R)

[b] These interpretive standards are applicable only to broth microdilution susceptibility tests with *Haemophilus* spp. using Haemophilus Testing Medium (HTM).[1]

Note: When testing *Streptococcus pyogenes* and *Streptococcus pneumoniae*, susceptibility and resistance to clarithromycin can be predicted using erythromycin.

A report of "Susceptible" indicates that the pathogen is likely to be inhibited if the antimicrobial compound in the blood reaches the concentrations usually achievable. A report of "Intermediate" indicates that the result should be considered equivocal, and, if the microorganism is not fully susceptible to alternative, clinically feasible drugs, the test should be repeated. This category implies possible clinical applicability in body sites where the drug is physiologically concentrated or in situations where high dosage of drug can be used. This category also provides a buffer zone which prevents small uncontrolled technical factors from causing major discrepancies in interpretation. A report of "Resistant" indicates that the pathogen is not likely to be inhibited if the antimicrobial compound in the blood reaches the concentrations usually achievable; other therapy should be selected.

Quality Control

Standardized susceptibility test procedures require the use of laboratory control bacteria to monitor and ensure the accuracy and precision of supplies and reagents in the assay, and the techniques of the individual performing the test.[1,2] Standard clarithromycin powder should provide the following MIC ranges.

QC Strain		MIC (mcg/mL)
S. aureus	ATCC® 29213[c]	0.12 to 0.5
S. pneumoniae[d]	ATCC 49619	0.03 to 0.12
Haemophilus influenzae[e]	ATCC 49247	4 to 16

[c] ATCC is a registered trademark of the American Type Culture Collection.

[d] This quality control range is applicable only to *S. pneumoniae* ATCC 49619 tested by a microdilution procedure using cation-adjusted Mueller-Hinton broth with 2-5% lysed horse blood.

[e] This quality control range is applicable only to *H. influenzae* ATCC 49247 tested by a microdilution procedure using HTM[1].

Diffusion Techniques

Quantitative methods that require measurement of zone diameters also provide reproducible estimates of the susceptibility of bacteria to antimicrobial compounds. The zone size provides an estimate of the susceptibility of bacteria to antimicrobial compounds. The zone size should be determined using a standardized method.[2,3] The procedure uses paper disks impregnated with 15 mcg of clarithromycin to test the susceptibility of bacteria. The disk diffusion interpretive criteria are provided below.

Susceptibility Test Interpretive Criteria for *Staphylococcus aureus*

Zone diameter (mm)	Interpretation
≥ 18	Susceptible (S)
14 to 17	Intermediate (I)
≤ 13	Resistant (R)

Susceptibility Test Interpretive Criteria for *Streptococcus pyogenes* and *Streptococcus pneumoniae*[f]

Zone diameter (mm)	Interpretation
≥ 21	Susceptible (S)
17 to 20	Intermediate (I)
≤ 16	Resistant (R)

[f] These zone diameter standards only apply to tests performed using Mueller-Hinton agar supplemented with 5% sheep blood incubated in 5% CO_2.

For testing *Haemophilus spp.*[g]

Zone diameter (mm)	Interpretation
≥ 13	Susceptible (S)
11 to 12	Intermediate (I)
≤ 10	Resistant (R)

[g] These zone diameter standards are applicable only to tests with *Haemophilus* spp. using HTM[2].

Note: When testing *Streptococcus pyogenes* and *Streptococcus pneumoniae*, susceptibility and resistance to clarithromycin can be predicted using erythromycin.

Quality Control

Standardized susceptibility test procedures require the use of laboratory control bacteria to monitor and ensure the accuracy and precision of supplies and reagents in the assay, and the techniques of the individual performing the test.[2,3] For the diffusion technique using the 15 mcg disk, the criteria in the following table should be achieved.

Acceptable Quality Control Ranges for Clarithromycin

QC Strain		Zone diameter (mm)
S. aureus	ATCC 25923	26 to 32
S. pneumoniae[h]	ATCC 49619	25 to 31
Haemophilus influenzae[i]	ATCC 49247	11 to 17

[h] This quality control range is applicable only to tests performed by disk diffusion using Mueller-Hinton agar supplemented with 5% defibrinated sheep blood.

[i] This quality control limit applies to tests conducted with *Haemophilus influenzae* ATCC 49247 using HTM[2].

In vitro Activity of Clarithromycin against Mycobacteria

Clarithromycin has demonstrated *in vitro* activity against *Mycobacterium avium* complex (MAC) microorganisms isolated from both AIDS and non-AIDS patients. While gene probe techniques may be used to distinguish *M. avium* species from *M. intracellulare*, many studies only reported results on *M. avium* complex (MAC) isolates.

Various *in vitro* methodologies employing broth or solid media at different pH's, with and without oleic acid-albumin-dextrose-catalase (OADC), have been used to determine clarithromycin MIC values for mycobacterial species. In general, MIC values decrease more than 16-fold as the pH of Middlebrook 7H12 broth media increases from 5.0 to 7.4. At pH 7.4, MIC values determined with Mueller-Hinton agar were 4- to 8-fold higher than those observed with Middlebrook 7H12 media. Utilization of oleic acid-albumin-dextrose-catalase (OADC) in these assays has been shown to further alter MIC values.

Clarithromycin activity against 80 MAC isolates from AIDS patients and 211 MAC isolates from non-AIDS patients was evaluated using a microdilution method with Middlebrook 7H9 broth. Results showed an MIC value of ≤ 4.0 mcg/mL in 81% and 89% of the AIDS and non-AIDS MAC isolates, respectively. Twelve percent of the non-AIDS isolates had an MIC value ≤ 0.5 mcg/mL. Clarithromycin was also shown to be active against phagocytized *M. avium* complex (MAC) in mouse and human macrophage cell cultures as well as in the beige mouse infection model.

Clarithromycin activity was evaluated against *Mycobacterium tuberculosis* microorganisms. In one study utilizing the agar dilution method with Middlebrook 7H10 media, 3 of 30 clinical isolates had an MIC of 2.5 mcg/mL. Clarithromycin inhibited all isolates at > 10.0 mcg/mL.

Susceptibility Testing for *Mycobacterium avium* Complex (MAC)

The disk diffusion and dilution techniques for susceptibility testing against gram-positive and gram-negative bacteria should not be used for determining clarithromycin MIC values against mycobacteria. *In vitro* susceptibility testing methods and diagnostic products currently available for determining minimum inhibitory concentration (MIC) values against *Mycobacterium avium* complex (MAC) organisms have not been standardized or validated. Clarithromycin MIC values will vary depending on the susceptibility testing method employed, composition and pH of the media, and the utilization of nutritional supplements. Breakpoints to determine whether clinical isolates of *M. avium* or *M. intracellulare* are susceptible or resistant to clarithromycin have not been established.

Susceptibility Test for *Helicobacter pylori*

The reference methodology for susceptibility testing of *H. pylori* is agar dilution MICs.[4] One to three microliters of an inoculum equivalent to a No. 2 McFarland standard (1 x 10^7-1 × 10^8 CFU/mL for *H. pylori*) are inoculated directly onto freshly prepared antimicrobial containing Mueller-Hinton agar plates with 5% aged defibrinated sheep blood (> 2-weeks old). The agar dilution plates are incubated at 35°C in a microaerobic environment produced by a gas generating system suitable for *Campylobacter* species. After 3 days of incubation, the MICs are recorded as the lowest concentration of antimicrobial agent required to inhibit growth of the organism. The clarithromycin and amoxicillin MIC values should be interpreted according to the following criteria:

Susceptibility Test Interpretive Criteria for *H. pylori*

Clarithromycin MIC (mcg/mL)[j]	Interpretation
≤ 0.25	Susceptible (S)
0.5	Intermediate (I)
≥ 1.0	Resistant (R)

Susceptibility Test Interpretive Criteria for *H. pylori*

Amoxicillin MIC (mcg/mL)[j,k]	Interpretation
< 0.25	Susceptible (S)

[j] These are tentative breakpoints for the agar dilution methodology, and should not be used to interpret results obtained using alternative methods.

[k] There were not enough organisms with MICs > 0.25 mcg/mL to determine a resistance breakpoint.

Standardized susceptibility test procedures require the use of laboratory control bacteria to monitor and ensure the accuracy and precision of supplies and reagents in the assay, and the techniques of the individual performing the test. Standard clarithromycin or amoxicillin powder should provide the following MIC ranges.

Acceptable Quality Control Ranges		Antimicrobial Agent	MIC (mcg/mL)[l]
H. pylori	ATCC 43504	Clarithromycin	0.015-0.12 mcg/mL
H. pylori	ATCC 43504	Amoxicillin	0.015-0.12 mcg/mL

[l] These are quality control ranges for the agar dilution methodology and should not be used to control test results obtained using alternative methods.

INDICATIONS AND USAGE

BIAXIN Filmtab (clarithromycin tablets, USP) and BIAXIN Granules (clarithromycin for oral suspension, USP) are indicated for the treatment of mild to moderate infections caused by susceptible isolates of the designated bacteria in the conditions as listed below:

Adults (BIAXIN Filmtab Tablets and Granules for Oral Suspension)

Pharyngitis/Tonsillitis due to *Streptococcus pyogenes* (The usual drug of choice in the treatment and prevention of streptococcal infections and the prophylaxis of rheumatic fever is penicillin administered by either the intramuscular or the oral route. Clarithromycin is generally effective in the eradication of *S. pyogenes* from the nasopharynx; however, data establishing the efficacy of clarithromycin in the subsequent prevention of rheumatic fever are not available at present).

Acute maxillary sinusitis due to *Haemophilus influenzae*, *Moraxella catarrhalis*, or *Streptococcus pneumoniae*.

Acute bacterial exacerbation of chronic bronchitis due to *Haemophilus influenzae*, *Haemophilus parainfluenzae*, *Moraxella catarrhalis*, or *Streptococcus pneumoniae*.

Community-Acquired Pneumonia due to *Haemophilus influenzae*, *Mycoplasma pneumoniae*, *Streptococcus pneumoniae*, or *Chlamydia pneumoniae* (TWAR).

Uncomplicated skin and skin structure infections due to *Staphylococcus aureus*, or *Streptococcus pyogenes* (Abscesses usually require surgical drainage).

Disseminated mycobacterial infections due to *Mycobacterium avium*, or *Mycobacterium intracellulare*

BIAXIN (clarithromycin) Filmtab tablets in combination with amoxicillin and PREVACID (lansoprazole) or PRILOSEC (omeprazole) Delayed-Release Capsules, as triple therapy, are indicated for the treatment of patients with *H. pylori* infection and duodenal ulcer disease (active or five-year history of duodenal ulcer) to eradicate *H. pylori*.

BIAXIN Filmtab tablets in combination with PRILOSEC (omeprazole) capsules or TRITEC (ranitidine bismuth citrate) tablets are also indicated for the treatment of patients with an active duodenal ulcer associated with *H. pylori* infection. However, regimens which contain clarithromycin as the single antimicrobial agent are more likely to be associated with the development of clarithromycin resistance among patients who fail therapy. Clarithromycin-containing regimens should not be used in patients with known or suspected clarithromycin resistant isolates because the efficacy of treatment is reduced in this setting.

In patients who fail therapy, susceptibility testing should be done if possible. If resistance to clarithromycin is demonstrated, a non-clarithromycin-containing therapy is recommended. (For information on development of resistance see **Microbiology** section.) The eradication of *H. pylori* has been demonstrated to reduce the risk of duodenal ulcer recurrence.

Children (BIAXIN Filmtab Tablets and Granules for Oral Suspension)

Pharyngitis/Tonsillitis due to *Streptococcus pyogenes*.

Community-Acquired Pneumonia due to *Mycoplasma pneumoniae*, *Streptococcus pneumoniae*, or *Chlamydia pneumoniae* (TWAR)

Acute maxillary sinusitis due to *Haemophilus influenzae*, *Moraxella catarrhalis*, or *Streptococcus pneumoniae*

Acute otitis media due to *Haemophilus influenzae*, *Moraxella catarrhalis*, or *Streptococcus pneumoniae*

NOTE: For information on otitis media, see **CLINICAL STUDIES - Otitis Media.**

Uncomplicated skin and skin structure infections due to *Staphylococcus aureus*, or *Streptococcus pyogenes* (Abscesses usually require surgical drainage.)

Disseminated mycobacterial infections due to *Mycobacterium avium*, or *Mycobacterium intracellulare*

Adults (BIAXIN XL Filmtab Tablets)

BIAXIN XL Filmtab (clarithromycin extended-release tablets) are indicated for the treatment of adults with mild to moderate infection caused by susceptible strains of the designated microorganisms in the conditions listed below:

Acute maxillary sinusitis due to *Haemophilus influenzae*, *Moraxella catarrhalis*, or *Streptococcus pneumoniae*

Acute bacterial exacerbation of chronic bronchitis due to *Haemophilus influenzae*, *Haemophilus parainfluenzae*, *Moraxella catarrhalis*, or *Streptococcus pneumoniae*

Community-Acquired Pneumonia due to *Haemophilus influenzae*, *Haemophilus parainfluenzae*, *Moraxella catarrhalis*, *Streptococcus pneumoniae*, *Chlamydia pneumoniae* (TWAR), or *Mycoplasma pneumoniae*

THE EFFICACY AND SAFETY OF BIAXIN XL IN TREATING OTHER INFECTIONS FOR WHICH OTHER FORMULATIONS OF BIAXIN ARE APPROVED HAVE NOT BEEN ESTABLISHED.

Prophylaxis

BIAXIN Filmtab tablets and BIAXIN Granules for oral suspension are indicated for the prevention of disseminated *Mycobacterium avium* complex (MAC) disease in patients with advanced HIV infection.

To reduce the development of drug-resistant bacteria and maintain the effectiveness of BIAXIN and other antibacterial drugs, BIAXIN should be used only to treat or prevent infections that are proven or strongly suspected to be caused by susceptible bacteria. When culture and susceptibility information are available, they should be considered in selecting or modifying antibacterial therapy. In the absence of such data, local epidemiology and susceptibility patterns may contribute to the empiric selection of therapy.

CONTRAINDICATIONS

Clarithromycin is contraindicated in patients with a known hypersensitivity to clarithromycin or any of its excipients, erythromycin, or any of the macrolide antibiotics.

Clarithromycin is contraindicated in patients with a history of cholestatic jaundice/hepatic dysfunction associated with prior use of clarithromycin.

Information on the AbbVie, Inc. products listed on these pages is from the prescribing information in use as of July 31, 2013. For more information, please visit rxabbvie.com or call 1-800-633-9110.

Concomitant administration of clarithromycin and any of the following drugs is contraindicated: cisapride, pimozide, astemizole, terfenadine, and ergotamine or dihydroergotamine (see **Drug Interactions**). There have been postmarketing reports of drug interactions when clarithromycin and/or erythromycin are coadministered with cisapride, pimozide, astemizole, or terfenadine resulting in cardiac arrhythmias (QT prolongation, ventricular tachycardia, ventricular fibrillation, and torsades de pointes) most likely due to inhibition of metabolism of these drugs by erythromycin and clarithromycin. Fatalities have been reported.

Concomitant administration of clarithromycin and colchicine is contraindicated in patients with renal or hepatic impairment.

Clarithromycin should not be given to patients with history of QT prolongation or ventricular cardiac arrhythmia, including *torsades de pointes*.

Clarithromycin should not be used concomitantly with HMG-CoA reductase inhibitors (statins) that are extensively metabolized by CYP3A4 (lovastatin or simvastatin), due to the increased risk of myopathy, including rhabdomyolysis. (see **WARNINGS**).

For information about contraindications of other drugs indicated in combination with BIAXIN, refer to the **CONTRAINDICATIONS** section of their package inserts.

WARNINGS

Use In Pregnancy

CLARITHROMYCIN SHOULD NOT BE USED IN PREGNANT WOMEN EXCEPT IN CLINICAL CIRCUMSTANCES WHERE NO ALTERNATIVE THERAPY IS APPROPRIATE. IF PREGNANCY OCCURS WHILE TAKING THIS DRUG, THE PATIENT SHOULD BE APPRISED OF THE POTENTIAL HAZARD TO THE FETUS. CLARITHROMYCIN HAS DEMONSTRATED ADVERSE EFFECTS OF PREGNANCY OUTCOME AND/OR EMBRYO-FETAL DEVELOPMENT IN MONKEYS, RATS, MICE, AND RABBITS AT DOSES THAT PRODUCED PLASMA LEVELS 2 TO 17 TIMES THE SERUM LEVELS ACHIEVED IN HUMANS TREATED AT THE MAXIMUM RECOMMENDED HUMAN DOSES (See PRECAUTIONS - *Pregnancy*).

Hepatotoxicity

Hepatic dysfunction, including increased liver enzymes, and hepatocellular and/or cholestatic hepatitis, with or without jaundice, has been reported with clarithromycin. This hepatic dysfunction may be severe and is usually reversible. In some instances, hepatic failure with fatal outcome has been reported and generally has been associated with serious underlying diseases and/or concomitant medications. Discontinue clarithromycin immediately if signs and symptoms of hepatitis occur.

QT Prolongation

Clarithromycin has been associated with prolongation of the QT interval and infrequent cases of arrhythmia. Cases of *torsades de pointes* have been spontaneously reported during postmarketing surveillance in patients receiving clarithromycin. Fatalities have been reported. Clarithromycin should be avoided in patients with ongoing proarrhythmic conditions such as uncorrected hypokalemia or hypomagnesemia, clinically significant bradycardia (see **CONTRAINDICATIONS**) and in patients receiving Class IA (quinidine, procainamide) or Class III (dofetilide, amiodarone, sotalol) antiarrhythmic agents. Elderly patients may be more susceptible to drug-associated effects on the QT interval.

Drug Interactions

Serious adverse reactions have been reported in patients taking clarithromycin concomitantly with CYP3A4 substrates. These include colchicine toxicity with colchicine; rhabdomyolysis with simvastatin, lovastatin, and atorvastatin; and hypotension with calcium channel blockers metabolized by CYP3A4 (e.g., verapamil, amlodipine, diltiazem) (see **CONTRAINDICATIONS** and **PRECAUTIONS – Drug Interactions**).

Life-threatening and fatal drug interactions have been reported in patients treated with clarithromycin and colchicine. Clarithromycin is a strong CYP3A4 inhibitor and this interaction may occur while using both drugs at their recommended doses. If co-administration of clarithromycin and colchicine is necessary in patients with normal renal and hepatic function, the dose of colchicine should be reduced. Patients should be monitored for clinical symptoms of colchicine toxicity. Concomitant administration of clarithromycin and colchicine is contraindicated in patients with renal or hepatic impairment (see **CONTRAINDICATIONS** and **PRECAUTIONS – Drug Interactions**).

Clostridium difficile Associated Diarrhea

Clostridium difficile associated diarrhea (CDAD) has been reported with use of nearly all antibacterial agents, including BIAXIN, and may range in severity from mild diarrhea to fatal colitis. Treatment with antibacterial agents alters the normal flora of the colon leading to overgrowth of *C. difficile*.

C. difficile produces toxins A and B which contribute to the development of CDAD. Hypertoxin producing strains of *C. difficile* cause increased morbidity and mortality, as these infections can be refractory to antimicrobial therapy and may require colectomy. CDAD must be considered in all patients who present with diarrhea following antibiotic use. Careful medical history is necessary since CDAD has been reported to occur over two months after the administration of antibacterial agents.

If CDAD is suspected or confirmed, ongoing antibiotic use not directed against *C. difficile* may need to be discontinued. Appropriate fluid and electrolyte management, protein supplementation, antibiotic treatment of *C. difficile*, and surgical evaluation should be instituted as clinically indicated.

For information about warnings of other drugs indicated in combination with BIAXIN, refer to the **WARNINGS** section of their package inserts.

Acute Hypersensitivity Reactions

In the event of severe acute hypersensitivity reactions, such as anaphylaxis, Stevens-Johnson Syndrome, toxic epidermal necrolysis, drug rash with eosinophilia and systemic symptoms (DRESS), and Henoch-Schonlein purpura clarithromycin therapy should be discontinued immediately and appropriate treatment should be urgently initiated.

Oral Hypoglycemic Agents/Insulin

The concomitant use of clarithromycin and oral hypoglycemic agents and/or insulin can result in significant hypoglycemia. With certain hypoglycemic drugs such as nateglinide, pioglitazone, repaglinide and rosiglitazone, inhibition of CYP3A enzyme by clarithromycin may be involved and could cause hypolgycemia when used concomitantly. Careful monitoring of glucose is recommended.

Oral Anticoagulants

There is a risk of serious hemorrhage and significant elevations in INR and prothrombin time when clarithromycin is co-administered with warfarin. INR and prothrombin times should be frequently monitored while patients are receiving clarithromycin and oral anticoagulants concurrently.

HMG-CoA Reductase Inhibitors (statins)

Concomitant use of clarithromycin with lovastatin or simvastatin is contraindicated (see **CONTRAINDICATIONS**) as these statins are extensively metabolized by CYP3A4, and concomitant treatment with clarithromycin increases their plasma concentration, which increases the risk of myopathy, including rhabdomyolysis. Cases of rhabdomyolysis have been reported in patients taking clarithromycin concomitantly with these statins. If treatment with clarithromycin cannot be avoided, therapy with lovastatin or simvastatin must be suspended during the course of treatment.

Caution should be exercised when prescribing clarithromycin with statins. In situations where the concomitant use of clarithromycin with atorvastatin or pravastatin cannot be avoided, atorvastatin dose should not exceed 20 mg daily and pravastatin dose should not exceed 40 mg daily. Use of a statin that is not dependent on CYP3A metabolism (e.g.fluvastatin) can be considered. It is recommended to prescribe the lowest registered dose if concomitant use cannot be avoided.

PRECAUTIONS

General

Prescribing BIAXIN in the absence of a proven or strongly suspected bacterial infection or a prophylactic indication is unlikely to provide benefit to the patient and increases the risk of the development of drug-resistant bacteria.

Clarithromycin is principally excreted via the liver and kidney. Clarithromycin may be administered without dosage adjustment to patients with hepatic impairment and normal renal function. However, in the presence of severe renal impairment with or without coexisting hepatic impairment, decreased dosage or prolonged dosing intervals may be appropriate.

Clarithromycin in combination with ranitidine bismuth citrate therapy is not recommended in patients with creatinine clearance less than 25 mL/min (See **DOSAGE AND ADMINISTRATION**).

Clarithromycin in combination with ranitidine bismuth citrate should not be used in patients with a history of acute porphyria.

Exacerbation of symptoms of myasthenia gravis and new onset of symptoms of myasthenic syndrome has been reported in patients receiving clarithromycin therapy.

For information about precautions of other drugs indicated in combination with BIAXIN, refer to the **PRECAUTIONS** section of their package inserts.

Information to Patients

Patients should be counseled that antibacterial drugs including BIAXIN should only be used to treat bacterial infections. They do not treat viral infections (e.g., the common cold). When BIAXIN is prescribed to treat a bacterial infection, patients should be told that although it is common to feel better early in the course of therapy, the medication should be taken exactly as directed. Skipping doses or not completing the full course of therapy may (1) decrease the effectiveness of the immediate treatment and (2) increase the likelihood that bacteria will develop resistance and will not be treatable by BIAXIN or other antibacterial drugs in the future.

Diarrhea is a common problem caused by antibiotics which usually ends when the antibiotic is discontinued. Sometimes after starting treatment with antibiotics, patients can develop watery and bloody stools (with or without stomach cramps and fever) even as late as two or more months after having taken the last dose of the antibiotic. If this occurs, patients should contact their physician as soon as possible.

BIAXIN may interact with some drugs; therefore patients should be advised to report to their doctor the use of any other medications.

BIAXIN tablets and oral suspension can be taken with or without food and can be taken with milk; however, BIAXIN XL tablets should be taken with food. Do **NOT** refrigerate the suspension.

Drug Interactions

Clarithromycin use in patients who are receiving theophylline may be associated with an increase of serum theophylline concentrations. Monitoring of serum theophylline concentrations should be considered for patients receiving high doses of theophylline or with baseline concentrations in the upper therapeutic range. In two studies in which theophylline was administered with clarithromycin (a theophylline sustained-release formulation was dosed at either 6.5 mg/kg or 12 mg/kg together with 250 or 500 mg q12h clarithromycin), the steady-state levels of C_{max}, C_{min}, and the area under the serum concentration time curve (AUC) of theophylline increased about 20%.

Hypotension, bradyarrhythmias, and lactic acidosis have been observed in patients receiving concurrent verapamil, belonging to the calcium channel blockers drug class.

Concomitant administration of single doses of clarithromycin and carbamazepine has been shown to result in increased plasma concentrations of carbamazepine. Blood level monitoring of carbamazepine may be considered.

When clarithromycin and terfenadine were coadministered, plasma concentrations of the active acid metabolite of terfenadine were threefold higher, on average, than the values observed when terfenadine was administered alone. The pharmacokinetics of clarithromycin and the 14-OH-clarithromycin were not significantly affected by coadministration of terfenadine once clarithromycin reached steady-state conditions. Concomitant administration of clarithromycin with terfenadine is contraindicated (See **CONTRAINDICATIONS**).

Clarithromycin 500 mg every 8 hours was given in combination with omeprazole 40 mg daily to healthy adult subjects. The steady-state plasma concentrations of omeprazole were increased (C_{max}, AUC_{0-24}, and $t_{1/2}$ increases of 30%, 89%, and 34%, respectively), by the concomitant administration of clarithromycin. The mean 24-hour gastric pH value was 5.2 when omeprazole was administered alone and 5.7 when coadministered with clarithromycin.

Coadministration of clarithromycin with ranitidine bismuth citrate resulted in increased plasma ranitidine concentrations (57%), increased plasma bismuth trough concentrations (48%), and increased 14-hydroxy-clarithromycin plasma concentrations (31%). These effects are clinically insignificant.

Simultaneous oral administration of BIAXIN tablets and zidovudine to HIV-infected adult patients may result in decreased steady-state zidovudine concentrations. Following administration of clarithromycin 500 mg tablets twice daily with zidovudine 100 mg every 4 hours, the steady-state zidovudine AUC decreased 12% compared to administration of zidovudine alone (n=4). Individual values ranged from a decrease of 34% to an increase of 14%. When clarithromycin tablets were administered two to four hours prior to zidovudine, the steady-state zidovudine C_{max} increased 100% whereas the AUC was unaffected (n=24). Administration of clarithromycin and zidovudine should be separated by at least two hours. The impact of co-administration of clarithromycin extended-release tablets and zidovudine has not been evaluated.

Simultaneous administration of BIAXIN tablets and didanosine to 12 HIV-infected adult patients resulted in no statistically significant change in didanosine pharmacokinetics.

Following administration of fluconazole 200 mg daily and clarithromycin 500 mg twice daily to 21 healthy volunteers, the steady-state clarithromycin C_{min} and AUC increased 33% and 18%, respectively. Steady-state concentrations of 14-OH clarithromycin were not significantly affected by concomitant administration of fluconazole. No dosage adjustment of clarithromycin is necessary when co-administered with fluconazole.

Ritonavir

Concomitant administration of clarithromycin and ritonavir (n = 22) resulted in a 77% increase in clarithromycin AUC and a 100% decrease in the AUC of 14-OH clarithromycin. Clarithromycin may be administered without dosage adjustment to patients with normal renal function taking ritonavir. Since concentrations of 14-OH clarithromycin are significantly reduced when clarithromycin is co-administered with ritonavir, alternative antibacterial therapy should be considered for indications other than infections due to *Mycobacterium avium* complex (see **PRECAUTIONS – Drug Interactions**). Doses of clarithromycin greater than 1000 mg per day should not be co-administered with protease inhibitors.

Spontaneous reports in the post-marketing period suggest that concomitant administration of clarithromycin and oral anticoagulants may potentiate the effects of the oral anticoagulants. Prothrombin times should be carefully monitored while patients are receiving clarithromycin and oral anticoagulants simultaneously.

Digoxin is a substrate for P-glycoprotein (Pgp) and clarithromycin is known to inhibit Pgp. When clarithromycin and digoxin are co-administered, inhibition of Pgp by clarithromycin may lead to increased exposure of digoxin. Elevated digoxin serum concentrations in patients receiving clarithromycin and digoxin concomitantly have been reported in post-marketing surveillance. Some patients have shown clinical signs consistent with digoxin toxicity, including potentially fatal arrhythmias. Monitoring of serum digoxin concentrations should be considered, especially for patients with digoxin concentrations in the upper therapeutic range.

Co-administration of clarithromycin, known to inhibit CYP3A, and a drug primarily metabolized by CYP3A may be associated with elevations in drug concentrations that could increase or prolong both therapeutic and adverse effects of the concomitant drug.

Clarithromycin should be used with caution in patients receiving treatment with other drugs known to be CYP3A enzyme substrates, especially if the CYP3A substrate has a narrow safety margin (e.g., carbamazepine) and/or the substrate is extensively metabolized by this enzyme. Dosage adjustments may be considered, and when possible, serum concentrations of drugs primarily metabolized by CYP3A should be monitored closely in patients concurrently receiving clarithromycin.

The following are examples of some clinically significant CYP3A based drug interactions. Interactions with other drugs metabolized by the CYP3A isoform are also possible.

Carbamazepine and Terfenadine

Increased serum concentrations of carbamazepine and the active acid metabolite of terfenadine were observed in clinical trials with clarithromycin.

Colchicine

Colchicine is a substrate for both CYP3A and the efflux transporter, P-glycoprotein (Pgp). Clarithromycin and other macrolides are known to inhibit CYP3A and Pgp. When a single dose of colchicine 0.6 mg was administered with clarithromycin 250 mg BID for 7 days, the colchicine C_{max} increased 197% and the $AUC_{0-\infty}$ increased 239% compared to administration of colchicine alone. The dose of colchicine should be reduced when co-administered with clarithromycin in patients with normal renal and hepatic function. Concomitant use of clarithromycin and colchicine is contraindicated in patients with renal or hepatic impairment (See **WARNINGS**).

Efavirenz, Nevirapine, Rifampicin, Rifabutin, and Rifapentine

Inducers of CYP3A enzymes, such as efavirenz, nevirapine, rifampicin, rifabutin, and rifapentine will increase the metabolism of clarithromycin, thus decreasing plasma concentrations of clarithromycin, while increasing those of 14-OH-clarithromycin. Since the microbiological activities of clarithromycin and 14-OH-clarithromycin are different for different bacteria, the intended therapeutic effect could be impaired during concomitant administration of clarithromycin and enzyme inducers. Alternative antibacterial treatment should be considered when treating patients receiving inducers of CYP3A.

Sildenafil, Tadalafil, and Vardenafil

Each of these phosphodiesterase inhibitors is primarily metabolized by CYP3A, and CYP3A will be inhibited by concomitant administration of clarithromycin. Co-administration of clarithromycin with sildenafil, tadalafil, or vardenafil will result in increased exposure of these phosphodiesterase inhibitors. Co-administration of these phosphodiesterase inhibitors with clarithromycin is not recommended.

Tolterodine

The primary route of metabolism for tolterodine is via CYP2D6. However, in a subset of the population devoid of CYP2D6, the identified pathway of metabolism is via CYP3A. In this population subset, inhibition of CYP3A results in significantly higher serum concentrations of tolterodine. Tolterodine 1 mg twice daily is recommended in patients deficient in CYP2D6 activity (poor metabolizers) when co-administered with clarithromycin.

Triazolobenzodiazepines (e.g., alprazolam, midazolam, triazolam)

When a single dose of midazolam was co-administered with clarithromycin tablets (500 mg twice daily for 7 days), midazolam AUC increased 174% after intravenous administration of midazolam and 600% after oral administration. When oral midazolam is co-administered with clarithromycin, dose adjustments may be necessary and possible prolongation and intensity of effect should be anticipated. Caution and appropriate dose adjustments should be considered when triazolam or alprazolam is co-administered with clarithromycin. For benzodiazepines which are not metabolized by CYP3A (e.g., temazepam, nitrazepam, lorazepam), a clinically important interaction with clarithromycin is unlikely.

There have been post-marketing reports of drug interactions and central nervous system (CNS) effects (e.g., somnolence and confusion) with the concomitant use of clarithromycin and triazolam. Monitoring the patient for increased CNS pharmacological effects is suggested.

Atazanavir

Both clarithromycin and atazanavir are substrates and inhibitors of CYP3A, and there is evidence of a bi-directional drug interaction. Following administration of clarithromycin (500 mg twice daily) with atazanavir (400 mg once daily), the clarithromycin AUC increased 94%, the 14-OH clarithromycin AUC decreased 70% and the atazanavir AUC increased 28%. When clarithromycin is co-administered with atazanavir, the dose of clarithromycin should be decreased by 50%. Since concentrations of 14-OH clarithromycin are significantly reduced when clarithromycin is co-administered with atazanavir, alternative antibacterial therapy should be considered for indications other than infections due to *Mycobacterium avium* complex (see **PRECAUTIONS – Drug Interactions**). Doses of clarithromycin greater than 1000 mg per day should not be co-administered with protease inhibitors.

Itraconazole

Both clarithromycin and itraconazole are substrates and inhibitors of CYP3A, potentially leading to a bi-directional drug interaction when administered concomitantly. Clarithromycin may increase the plasma concentrations of itraconazole, while itraconazole may increase the plasma concentrations of clarithromycin. Patients taking itraconazole and clarithromycin concomitantly should be monitored closely for signs or symptoms of increased or prolonged adverse reactions.

Saquinavir

Both clarithromycin and saquinavir are substrates and inhibitors of CYP3A and there is evidence of a bi-directional drug interaction. Following administration of clarithromycin (500 mg bid) and saquinavir (soft gelatin capsules, 1200 mg tid) to 12 healthy volunteers, the steady-state saquinavir AUC and C_{max} increased 177% and 187% respectively compared to administration of saquinavir alone. Clarithromycin AUC and C_{max} increased 45% and 39% respectively, whereas the 14–OH clarithromycin AUC and C_{max} decreased 24% and 34% respectively, compared to administration with clarithromycin alone. No dose adjustment of clarithromycin is necessary when clarithromycin is co-administered with saquinavir in patients with normal renal function. When saquinavir is co-administered with ritonavir, consideration should be given to the potential effects of ritonavir on clarithromycin (refer to interaction between clarithromycin and ritonavir) (see **PRECAUTIONS – Drug Interactions**).

The following CYP3A based drug interactions have been observed with erythromycin products and/or with clarithromycin in post-marketing experience:

Antiarrhythmics

There have been post-marketing reports of torsades de pointes occurring with concurrent use of clarithromycin and quinidine or disopyramide. Electrocardiograms should be monitored for QTc prolongation during coadministration of clarithromycin with these drugs. Serum concentrations of these medications should also be monitored.

Ergotamine/Dihydroergotamine

Post-marketing reports indicate that coadministration of clarithromycin with ergotamine or dihydroergotamine has been associated with acute ergot toxicity characterized by vasospasm and ischemia of the extremities and other tissues including the central nervous system. Concomitant administration of clarithromycin with ergotamine or dihydroergotamine is contraindicated (see **CONTRAINDICATIONS**).

Triazolobenzodiazepines (Such as Triazolam and Alprazolam) and Related Benzodiazepines (Such as Midazolam)

Erythromycin has been reported to decrease the clearance of triazolam and midazolam, and thus, may increase the pharmacologic effect of these benzodiazepines. There have been post-marketing reports of drug interactions and CNS effects (e.g., somnolence and confusion) with the concomitant use of clarithromycin and triazolam.

Sildenafil (Viagra)

Erythromycin has been reported to increase the systemic exposure (AUC) of sildenafil. A similar interaction may occur with clarithromycin; reduction of sildenafil dosage should be considered. (See Viagra package insert.)

There have been spontaneous or published reports of CYP3A based interactions of erythromycin and/or clarithromycin with cyclosporine, carbamazepine, tacrolimus, alfentanil, disopyramide, rifabutin, quinidine, methylprednisolone, cilostazol, bromocriptine and vinblastine.

Concomitant administration of clarithromycin with cisapride, pimozide, astemizole, or terfenadine is contraindicated (see **CONTRAINDICATIONS**).

In addition, there have been reports of interactions of erythromycin or clarithromycin with drugs not thought to be metabolized by CYP3A, including hexobarbital, phenytoin, and valproate.

Carcinogenesis, Mutagenesis, Impairment of Fertility

The following *in vitro* mutagenicity tests have been conducted with clarithromycin:

Salmonella/Mammalian Microsomes Test

Bacterial Induced Mutation Frequency Test

In Vitro Chromosome Aberration Test

Rat Hepatocyte DNA Synthesis Assay

Mouse Lymphoma Assay

Mouse Dominant Lethal Study

Mouse Micronucleus Test

All tests had negative results except the *In Vitro* Chromosome Aberration Test which was weakly positive in one test and negative in another.

In addition, a Bacterial Reverse-Mutation Test (Ames Test) has been performed on clarithromycin metabolites with negative results.

Fertility and reproduction studies have shown that daily doses of up to 160 mg/kg/day (1.3 times the recommended maximum human dose based on mg/m^2) to male and female rats caused no adverse effects on the estrous cycle, fertility, parturition, or number and viability of offspring. Plasma levels in rats after 150 mg/kg/day were 2 times the human serum levels.

In the 150 mg/kg/day monkey studies, plasma levels were 3 times the human serum levels. When given orally at 150 mg/kg/day (2.4 times the recommended maximum human dose based on mg/m^2), clarithromycin was shown to produce embryonic loss in monkeys. This effect has been attributed to marked maternal toxicity of the drug at this high dose.

In rabbits, *in utero* fetal loss occurred at an intravenous dose of 33 mg/m^2, which is 17 times less than the maximum proposed human oral daily dose of 618 mg/m^2.

Long-term studies in animals have not been performed to evaluate the carcinogenic potential of clarithromycin.

Pregnancy

Teratogenic Effects

Pregnancy Category C

Four teratogenicity studies in rats (three with oral doses and one with intravenous doses up to 160 mg/kg/day administered during the period of major organogenesis) and two in rabbits at oral doses up to 125 mg/kg/day (approximately 2 times the recommended maximum human dose based on mg/m^2) or intravenous doses of 30 mg/kg/day administered during gestation days 6 to 18 failed to demonstrate any teratogenicity from clarithromycin. Two additional oral studies in a different rat strain at similar doses and similar conditions demonstrated a low incidence of cardiovascular anomalies at doses of 150 mg/kg/day administered during gestation days 6 to 15. Plasma levels after 150 mg/kg/day were 2 times the human serum levels. Four studies in mice revealed a variable incidence of cleft palate following oral doses of 1000 mg/kg/day (2 and 4 times the recommended maximum human dose based on mg/m^2, respectively) during gestation days 6 to 15. Cleft palate was also seen at 500 mg/kg/day. The 1000 mg/kg/day exposure resulted in plasma levels 17 times the human serum levels. In monkeys, an oral dose of 70 mg/kg/day (an approximate equidose of the recommended maximum human dose based on mg/m^2) produced fetal growth retardation at plasma levels that were 2 times the human serum levels.

There are no adequate and well-controlled studies in pregnant women. Clarithromycin should be used during pregnancy only if the potential benefit justifies the potential risk to the fetus (See **WARNINGS**).

Nursing Mothers

It is not known whether clarithromycin is excreted in human milk. Because many drugs are excreted in human milk, caution should be exercised when clarithromycin is administered to a nursing woman. It is known that clarithromycin is excreted in the milk of lactating animals and that other drugs of this class are excreted in human milk. Preweaned rats, exposed indirectly via consumption of

Information on the AbbVie, Inc. products listed on these pages is from the prescribing information in use as of July 31, 2013. For more information, please visit rxabbvie.com or call 1-800-633-9110.

ADULT DOSAGE GUIDELINES

Infection	BIAXIN Tablets Dosage (q12h)	BIAXIN Tablets Duration (days)	BIAXIN XL Tablets Dosage (q24h)	BIAXIN XL Tablets Duration (days)
Pharyngitis/Tonsillitis due to				
S. pyogenes	250 mg	10	-	-
Acute maxillary sinusitis due to	500 mg	14	2 × 500 mg	14
H. influenzae				
M. catarrhalis				
S. pneumoniae				
Acute exacerbation of chronic bronchitis due to				
H. influenzae	500 mg	7-14	2 × 500 mg	7
H. parainfluenzae	500 mg	7	2 × 500 mg	7
M. catarrhalis	250 mg	7-14	2 × 500 mg	7
S. pneumoniae	250 mg	7-14	2 × 500 mg	7
Community-Acquired Pneumonia due to				
H. influenzae	250 mg	7	2 × 500 mg	7
H. parainfluenzae	-	-	2 × 500 mg	7
M. catarrhalis	-	-	2 × 500 mg	7
S. pneumoniae	250 mg	7-14	2 × 500 mg	7
C. pneumoniae	250 mg	7-14	2 × 500 mg	7
M. pneumoniae	250 mg	7-14	2 × 500 mg	7
Uncomplicated skin and skin structure	250 mg	7-14	-	-
S. aureus				
S. pyogenes				

milk from dams treated with 150 mg/kg/day for 3 weeks, were not adversely affected, despite data indicating higher drug levels in milk than in plasma.

Pediatric Use

Safety and effectiveness of clarithromycin in pediatric patients under 6 months of age have not been established. The safety of clarithromycin has not been studied in MAC patients under the age of 20 months. Neonatal and juvenile animals tolerated clarithromycin in a manner similar to adult animals. Young animals were slightly more intolerant to acute overdosage and to subtle reductions in erythrocytes, platelets and leukocytes but were less sensitive to toxicity in the liver, kidney, thymus, and genitalia.

Geriatric Use

In a steady-state study in which healthy elderly subjects (age 65 to 81 years old) were given 500 mg every 12 hours, the maximum serum concentrations and area under the curves of clarithromycin and 14-OH clarithromycin were increased compared to those achieved in healthy young adults. These changes in pharmacokinetics parallel known age-related decreases in renal function. In clinical trials, elderly patients did not have an increased incidence of adverse events when compared to younger patients. Dosage adjustment should be considered in elderly patients with severe renal impairment. Elderly patients may be more susceptible to development of *torsades de pointes* arrhythmias than younger patients (See **WARNINGS** and **PRECAUTIONS**).

ADVERSE REACTIONS

The majority of side effects observed in clinical trials were of a mild and transient nature. Fewer than 3% of adult patients without mycobacterial infections and fewer than 2% of pediatric patients without mycobacterial infections discontinued therapy because of drug-related side effects. Fewer than 2% of adult patients taking BIAXIN XL tablets discontinued therapy because of drug-related side effects.

The most frequently reported events in adults taking BIAXIN tablets (clarithromycin tablets, USP) were diarrhea (3%), nausea (3%), abnormal taste (3%), dyspepsia (2%), abdominal pain/discomfort (2%), and headache (2%). In pediatric patients, the most frequently reported events were diarrhea (6%), vomiting (6%), abdominal pain (3%), rash (3%), and headache (2%). Most of these events were described as mild or moderate in severity. Of the reported adverse events, only 1% was described as severe.

The most frequently reported events in adults taking BIAXIN XL (Clarithromycin extended-release tablets) were diarrhea (6%), abnormal taste (7%), and nausea (3%). Most of these events were described as mild or moderate in severity. Of the reported adverse events, less than 1% were described as severe.

In the acute exacerbation of chronic bronchitis and acute maxillary sinusitis studies overall gastrointestinal adverse events were reported by a similar proportion of patients taking either BIAXIN tablets or BIAXIN XL tablets; however, patients taking BIAXIN XL tablets reported significantly less severe gastrointestinal symptoms compared to patients taking BIAXIN tablets. In addition, patients taking BIAXIN XL tablets had significantly fewer premature discontinuations for drug-related gastrointestinal or abnormal taste adverse events compared to BIAXIN tablets.

In community-acquired pneumonia studies conducted in adults comparing clarithromycin to erythromycin base or erythromycin stearate, there were fewer adverse events involving the digestive system in clarithromycin-treated patients compared to erythromycin-treated patients (13% vs 32%; p < 0.01). Twenty percent of erythromycin-treated patients discontinued therapy due to adverse events compared to 4% of clarithromycin-treated patients.

In two U.S. studies of acute otitis media comparing clarithromycin to amoxicillin/potassium clavulanate in pediatric patients, there were fewer adverse events involving the digestive system in clarithromycin-treated patients compared to amoxicillin/potassium clavulanate-treated patients (21% vs. 40%, p < 0.001). One-third as many clarithromycin-treated patients reported diarrhea as did amoxicillin/potassium clavulanate-treated patients.

Post-Marketing Experience

Allergic reactions ranging from urticaria and mild skin eruptions to rare cases of anaphylaxis, Stevens-Johnson syndrome, drug rash with eosinophilia and systemic symptoms (DRESS), Henoch-Schonlein Purpura and toxic epidermal necrolysis have occurred. Other spontaneously reported adverse events include glossitis, stomatitis, oral moniliasis, anorexia, vomiting, pancreatitis, tongue discoloration, thrombocytopenia, leukopenia, neutropenia, dizziness, myalgia and hemorrhage. There have been reports of tooth discoloration in patients treated with BIAXIN. Tooth discoloration is usually reversible with professional dental cleaning. There have been isolated reports of hearing loss, which is usually reversible, occurring chiefly in elderly women. Reports of alterations of the sense of smell including smell loss, usually in conjunction with taste perversion or taste loss, have also been reported.

Transient CNS events including anxiety, behavioral changes, confusional states, convulsions, depersonalization, disorientation, hallucinations, insomnia, depression, manic behavior, nightmares, psychosis, tinnitus, tremor, and vertigo have been reported during post-marketing surveillance. Events usually resolve with discontinuation of the drug.

Adverse reactions related to hepatic dysfunction have been reported in postmarketing experience with clarithromycin (See **WARNINGS – Hepatotoxicity**).

There have been rare reports of hypoglycemia, some of which have occurred in patients taking oral hypoglycemic agents or insulin.

There have been post-marketing reports of BIAXIN XL tablets in the stool, many of which have occurred in patients with anatomic (including ileostomy or colostomy) or functional gastrointestinal disorders with shortened GI transit times.

As with other macrolides, clarithromycin has been associated with QT prolongation and ventricular arrhythmias, including ventricular tachycardia and torsades de pointes.

There have been reports of interstitial nephritis coincident with clarithromycin use.

There have been post-marketing reports of colchicine toxicity with concomitant use of clarithromycin and colchicine, especially in the elderly, some of which occurred in patients with renal insufficiency. Deaths have been reported in some such patients (See **WARNINGS** and **PRECAUTIONS**).

There have been cases of rhabdomyolysis reported with clarithromycin use. In some cases, clarithromycin was administered concomitantly with other drugs known to be associated with rhabdomyolysis (such as statins, fibrates, colchicine or allopurinol).

Changes in Laboratory Values

Changes in laboratory values with possible clinical significance were as follows:

Hepatic
Elevated SGPT (ALT) < 1%; SGOT (AST) < 1%; GGT < 1%; alkaline phosphatase < 1%; LDH < 1%; total bilirubin < 1%

Hematologic
Decreased WBC < 1%; elevated prothrombin time 1%

Renal
Elevated BUN 4%; elevated serum creatinine < 1%

GGT, alkaline phosphatase, and prothrombin time data are from adult studies only.

OVERDOSAGE

Overdosage of clarithromycin can cause gastrointestinal symptoms such as abdominal pain, vomiting, nausea, and diarrhea.

Adverse reactions accompanying overdosage should be treated by the prompt elimination of unabsorbed drug and supportive measures. As with other macrolides, clarithromycin serum concentrations are not expected to be appreciably affected by hemodialysis or peritoneal dialysis.

DOSAGE AND ADMINISTRATION

BIAXIN® Filmtab® (clarithromycin tablets, USP) and BIAXIN® Granules (clarithromycin for oral suspension, USP) may be given with or without food. BIAXIN® XL Filmtab® (clarithromycin extended-release tablets) should be taken with food. BIAXIN XL tablets should be swallowed whole and not chewed, broken or crushed.

Clarithromycin may be administered without dosage adjustment in the presence of hepatic impairment if there is normal renal function. In patients with severe renal impairment (CL_{CR} < 30 mL/min), the dose of clarithromycin should be reduced by 50%. However, when patients with moderate or severe renal impairment are taking clarithromycin concomitantly with atazanavir or ritonavir, the dose of clarithromycin should be reduced by 50% or 75% for patients with CL_{CR} of 30 to 60 mL/min or < 30 mL/min, respectively.

[See table above]

H. pylori **Eradication to Reduce the Risk of Duodenal Ulcer Recurrence**

Triple therapy: BIAXIN/lansoprazole/amoxicillin

The recommended adult dose is 500 mg BIAXIN, 30 mg lansoprazole, and 1 gram amoxicillin, all given twice daily (q12h) for 10 or 14 days (See **INDICATIONS AND USAGE** and **CLINICAL STUDIES** sections).

Triple therapy: BIAXIN/omeprazole/amoxicillin

The recommended adult dose is 500 mg BIAXIN, 20 mg omeprazole, and 1 gram amoxicillin, all given twice daily (q12h) for 10 days (See **INDICATIONS AND USAGE** and **CLINICAL STUDIES** sections). In patients with an ulcer present at the time of initiation of therapy, an additional 18 days of omeprazole 20 mg once daily is recommended for ulcer healing and symptom relief.

Dual therapy: BIAXIN/omeprazole

The recommended adult dose is 500 mg BIAXIN given three times daily (q8h) and 40 mg omeprazole given once daily (qAM) for 14 days (See **INDICATIONS AND USAGE** and **CLINICAL STUDIES** sections). An additional 14 days of omeprazole 20 mg once daily is recommended for ulcer healing and symptom relief.

Dual therapy: BIAXIN/ranitidine bismuth citrate

The recommended adult dose is 500 mg BIAXIN given twice daily (q12h) or three times daily (q8h) and 400 mg ranitidine bismuth citrate given twice daily (q12h) for 14 days. An additional 14 days of 400 mg twice daily is recommended for ulcer healing and symptom relief. BIAXIN and ranitidine bismuth citrate combination therapy is not recommended in patients with creatinine clearance less than 25 mL/min (See **INDICATIONS AND USAGE** and **CLINICAL STUDIES** sections).

Children

The usual recommended daily dosage is 15 mg/kg/day divided q12h for 10 days.

PEDIATRIC DOSAGE GUIDELINES

Based on Body Weight
Dosing Calculated on 7.5 mg/kg q12h

Weight Kg	Weight lbs	Dose (q12h)	125 mg/5 mL	250 mg/5 mL
9	20	62.5 mg	2.5 mL q12h	1.25 mL q12h
17	37	125 mg	5 mL q12h	2.5 mL q12h
25	55	187.5 mg	7.5 mL q12h	3.75 mL q12h
33	73	250 mg	10 mL q12h	5 mL q12h

Mycobacterial Infections

Prophylaxis

The recommended dose of BIAXIN for the prevention of disseminated *Mycobacterium avium* disease is 500 mg b.i.d. In children, the recommended dose is 7.5 mg/kg b.i.d. up to 500 mg b.i.d. No studies of clarithromycin for MAC prophylaxis have been performed in pediatric populations and the doses recommended for prophylaxis are derived from MAC treatment studies in children. Dosing recommendations for children are in the table above.

Treatment

Clarithromycin is recommended as the primary agent for the treatment of disseminated infection due to *Mycobacterium avium* complex. Clarithromycin should be used in combination with other antimycobacterial drugs that have shown *in vitro* activity against MAC or clinical benefit in MAC treatment (See **CLINICAL STUDIES**). The recommended dose for mycobacterial infections in adults is 500 mg b.i.d. In children, the recommended dose is 7.5 mg/kg b.i.d. up to 500 mg b.i.d. Dosing recommendations for children are in the table above.

Clarithromycin therapy should continue for life if clinical and mycobacterial improvements are observed.

Constituting Instructions

The table below indicates the volume of water to be added when constituting:

Total Volume After Constitution	Clarithromycin Concentration After Constitution	Amount of Water to be Added*
50 mL	125 mg/5 mL	27 mL
100 mL	125 mg/5 mL	55 mL
50 mL	250 mg/5 mL	27 mL
100 mL	250 mg/5 mL	55 mL

* see instructions below.

Add half the volume of water to the bottle and shake vigorously. Add the remainder of water to the bottle and shake. Shake well before each use. Oversize bottle provides shake space. Keep tightly closed. Do not refrigerate. After mixing, store at 15° to 30°C (59° to 86°F) and use within 14 days.

HOW SUPPLIED

BIAXIN® Filmtab® (clarithromycin tablets, USP) are supplied as yellow oval film-coated tablets in the following packaging sizes:

250 mg tablets: (imprinted in blue with the "a" logo and code KT)

Bottles of 60 (**NDC** 0074-3368-60) and unit dose strip packages of 100 (**NDC** 0074-3368-11).

Store BIAXIN 250 mg tablets at controlled room temperature 15° to 30°C (59° to 86°F) in a well-closed container. Protect from light.

500 mg tablets: (debossed with the "a" logo on one side and code KL on the opposite side)

Bottles of 60 (**NDC** 0074-2586-60) and unit dose strip packages of 100 (**NDC** 0074-2586-11).

Store BIAXIN 500 mg tablets at controlled room temperature 20° to 25°C (68° to 77°F) in a well-closed container.

BIAXIN® XL Filmtab® (clarithromycin extended-release tablets) are supplied as yellow oval film-coated 500 mg tablets debossed (on one side) with the "a" logo and a two-letter code designation, KJ in the following packaging sizes:

500 mg tablets:

Bottles of 60 (**NDC** 0074-3165-60), unit dose strip packages of 100 (**NDC** 0074-3165-11), and BIAXIN® XL PAC carton of 4 blister packages 14 tablets each (**NDC** 0074-3165-41).

Store BIAXIN XL tablets at 20° to 25°C (68° to 77°F). Excursions permitted to 15° to 30°C (59° to 86°F). [See USP Controlled Room Temperature.]

BIAXIN® Granules (clarithromycin for oral suspension, USP) is supplied in the following strengths and sizes:

[See table above]

Store BIAXIN granules for oral suspension at controlled room temperature 15° to 30°C (59° to 86°F) in a well-closed container. Do not refrigerate BIAXIN suspension.

Total Volume After Constitution	Clarithromycin Concentration After Constitution	Clarithromycin Contents Per Bottle	NDC
50 mL	125 mg/5 mL	1250 mg	0074-3163-50
100 mL	125 mg/5 mL	2500 mg	0074-3163-13
50 mL	250 mg/5 mL	2500 mg	0074-3188-50
100 mL	250 mg/5 mL	5000 mg	0074-3188-13

CLINICAL STUDIES

Mycobacterial Infections

Prophylaxis

A randomized, double-blind study (561) compared clarithromycin 500 mg b.i.d. to placebo in patients with CDC-defined AIDS and CD_4 counts < 100 cells/µL. This study accrued 682 patients from November 1992 to January 1994, with a median CD_4 cell count at study entry of 30 cells/µL. Median duration of clarithromycin was 10.6 months vs. 8.2 months for placebo. More patients in the placebo arm than the clarithromycin arm discontinued prematurely from the study (75.6% and 67.4%, respectively). However, if premature discontinuations due to MAC or death are excluded, approximately equal percentages of patients on each arm (54.8% on clarithromycin and 52.5% on placebo) discontinued study drug early for other reasons. The study was designed to evaluate the following endpoints:

1. MAC bacteremia, defined as at least one positive culture for *M. avium* complex bacteria from blood or another normally sterile site.
2. Survival.
3. Clinically significant disseminated MAC disease, defined as MAC bacteremia accompanied by signs or symptoms of serious MAC infection, including fever, night sweats, weight loss, anemia, or elevations in liver function tests.

MAC Bacteremia

In patients randomized to clarithromycin, the risk of MAC bacteremia was reduced by 69% compared to placebo. The difference between groups was statistically significant ($p < 0.001$). On an intent-to-treat basis, the one-year cumulative incidence of MAC bacteremia was 5.0% for patients randomized to clarithromycin and 19.4% for patients randomized to placebo. While only 19 of the 341 patients randomized to clarithromycin developed MAC, 11 of these cases were resistant to clarithromycin. The patients with resistant MAC bacteremia had a median baseline CD_4 count of 10 cells/mm^3 (range 2 to 25 cells/mm^3). Information regarding the clinical course and response to treatment of the patients with resistant MAC bacteremia is limited. The 8 patients who received clarithromycin and developed susceptible MAC bacteremia had a median baseline CD_4 count of 25 cells/mm^3 (range 10 to 80 cells/mm^3). Comparatively, 53 of the 341 placebo patients developed MAC; none of these isolates were resistant to clarithromycin. The median baseline CD_4 count was 15 cells/mm^3 (range 2 to 130 cells/mm^3) for placebo patients that developed MAC.

Survival

A statistically significant survival benefit was observed.

Survival All Randomized Patients

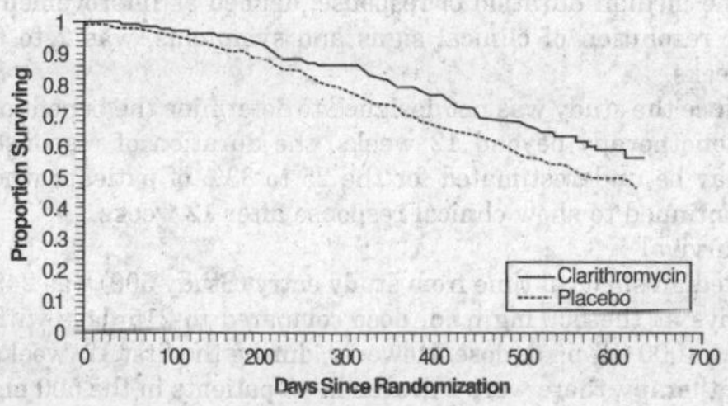

	Mortality		Reduction in Mortality on
	Placebo	Clarithromycin	Clarithromycin
6 month	9.4%	6.5%	31%
12 month	29.7%	20.5%	31%
18 month	46.4%	37.5%	20%

Since the analysis at 18 months includes patients no longer receiving prophylaxis the survival benefit of clarithromycin may be underestimated.

Clinically Significant Disseminated MAC Disease

In association with the decreased incidence of bacteremia, patients in the group randomized to clarithromycin showed reductions in the signs and symptoms of disseminated MAC disease, including fever, night sweats, weight loss, and anemia.

Safety

In AIDS patients treated with clarithromycin over long periods of time for prophylaxis against *M. avium*, it was often difficult to distinguish adverse events possibly associated with clarithromycin administration from underlying HIV disease or intercurrent illness. Median duration of treatment was 10.6 months for the clarithromycin group and 8.2 months for the placebo group.

Treatment-related* Adverse Event Incidence Rates (%) in Immunocompromised Adult Patients Receiving Prophylaxis Against *M. avium* Complex

Body System† Adverse Event	Clarithromycin (n = 339) %	Placebo (n = 339) %
Body as a Whole		
Abdominal pain	5.0%	3.5%
Headache	2.7%	0.9%
Digestive		
Diarrhea	7.7%	4.1%
Dyspepsia	3.8%	2.7%
Flatulence	2.4%	0.9%
Nausea	11.2%	7.1%
Vomiting	5.9%	3.2%
Skin & Appendages		
Rash	3.2%	3.5%
Special Senses		
Taste Perversion	8.0%	0.3%

* Includes those events possibly or probably related to study drug and excludes concurrent conditions.

‡ > 2% Adverse Event Incidence Rates for either treatment group.

Among these events, taste perversion was the only event that had significantly higher incidence in the clarithromycin-treated group compared to the placebo-treated group.

Discontinuation due to adverse events was required in 18% of patients receiving clarithromycin compared to 17% of patients receiving placebo in this trial. Primary reasons for discontinuation in clarithromycin treated patients include headache, nausea, vomiting, depression and taste perversion.

Changes in Laboratory Values of Potential Clinical Importance

In immunocompromised patients receiving prophylaxis against *M. avium*, evaluations of laboratory values were made by analyzing those values outside the seriously abnormal value (i.e., the extreme high or low limit) for the specified test.

Percentage of Patients[a] Exceeding Extreme Laboratory Value in Patients Receiving Prophylaxis Against *M. avium* Complex

		Clarithromycin 500 mg b.i.d.	Placebo
Hemoglobin	< 8 g/dL	4/118 3%	5/103 5%
Platelet Count	$< 50 \times 10^9$/L	11/249 4%	12/250 5%
WBC Count	$< 1 \times 10^9$/L	2/103 4%	0/95 0%
SGOT	> 5 × ULN[b]	7/196 4%	5/208 2%
SGPT	> 5 × ULN[b]	6/217 3%	4/232 2%
Alk. Phos.	> 5 × ULN[b]	5/220 2%	5/218 2%

[a] Includes only patients with baseline values within the normal range or borderline high (hematology variables) and within the normal range or borderline low (chemistry variables).

[b] ULN = Upper Limit of Normal

Treatment

Three randomized studies (500, 577, and 521) compared different dosages of clarithromycin in patients with CDC-defined AIDS and CD_4 counts < 100 cells/µL. These studies accrued patients from May 1991 to March 1992. Study 500 was randomized, double-blind; Study 577 was open-label compassionate use. Both studies used 500 and 1000 mg b.i.d. doses; Study 500 also had a 2000 mg b.i.d. group. Study 521 was a pediatric study at 3.75, 7.5, and 15 mg/kg b.i.d. Study 500 enrolled 154 adult patients, Study 577 enrolled 469 adult patients, and Study 521 enrolled 25 patients between the ages of 1 to 20. The majority of patients had CD_4 cell counts < 50/µL at study entry. The studies were designed to evaluate the following end points:

1. Change in MAC bacteremia or blood cultures negative for *M. avium*.
2. Change in clinical signs and symptoms of MAC infection including one or more of the following: fever, night sweats, weight loss, diarrhea, splenomegaly, and hepatomegaly.

The results for the 500 study are described below. The 577 study results were similar to the results of the 500 study. Results with the 7.5 mg/kg b.i.d. dose in the pediatric study were comparable to those for the 500 mg b.i.d. regimen in the adult studies.

Information on the AbbVie, Inc. products listed on these pages is from the prescribing information in use as of July 31, 2013. For more information, please visit rxabbvie.com or call 1-800-633-9110.

Resolution of Fever

b.i.d. dose (mg)	% ever afebrile	% afebrile ≥ 6 weeks
500	67%	23%
1000	67%	12%
2000	62%	22%

Resolution of Night Sweats

b.i.d. dose (mg)	% ever resolving	% resolving ≥ 6 weeks
500	85%	42%
1000	70%	33%
2000	72%	36%

Weight Gain > 3%

b.i.d. dose (mg)	% ever gaining	% gaining ≥ 6 weeks
500	33%	14%
1000	26%	17%
2000	26%	12%

Hemoglobin Increase > 1 gm

b.i.d. dose (mg)	% ever increasing	% increasing ≥ 6 weeks
500	58%	26%
1000	37%	6%
2000	62%	18%

Study 069 compared the safety and efficacy of clarithromycin in combination with ethambutol versus clarithromycin in combination with ethambutol and clofazimine for the treatment of disseminated MAC (dMAC) infection.[4,5] This 24-week study enrolled 106 patients with AIDS and dMAC, with 55 patients randomized to receive clarithromycin and ethambutol, and 51 patients randomized to receive clarithromycin, ethambutol, and clofazimine. Baseline characteristics between study arms were similar with the exception of median CFU counts being at least 1 log higher in the clarithromycin, ethambutol, and clofazimine arm.

Compared to prior experience with clarithromycin monotherapy, the two-drug regimen of clarithromycin and ethambutol was well tolerated and extended the time to microbiologic relapse, largely through suppressing the emergence of clarithromycin resistant strains. However, the addition of clofazimine to the regimen added no additional microbiologic or clinical benefit. Tolerability of both multidrug regimens was comparable with the most common adverse events being gastrointestinal in nature. Patients receiving the clofazimine-containing regimen had reduced survival rates; however, their baseline mycobacterial colony counts were higher. The results of this trial support the addition of ethambutol to clarithromycin for the treatment of initial dMAC infections but do not support adding clofazimine as a third agent.

MAC Bacteremia

Decreases in MAC bacteremia or negative blood cultures were seen in the majority of patients in all dose groups. Mean reductions in colony forming units (CFU) are shown below. Included in the table are results from a separate study with a four drug regimen[6] (ciprofloxacin, ethambutol, rifampicin, and clofazimine). Since patient populations and study procedures may vary between these two studies, comparisons between the clarithromycin results and the combination therapy results should be interpreted cautiously.

Mean Reductions in Log CFU from Baseline (After 4 Weeks of Therapy)

500 mg b.i.d. (N = 35)	1000 mg b.i.d. (N = 32)	2000 mg b.i.d. (N = 26)	Four Drug Regimen (N = 24)
1.5	2.3	2.3	1.4

Although the 1000 mg and 2000 mg b.i.d. doses showed significantly better control of bacteremia during the first four weeks of therapy, no significant differences were seen beyond that point. The percent of patients whose blood was sterilized as shown by one or more negative cultures at any time during acute therapy was 61% (30/49) for the 500 mg b.i.d. group and 59% (29/49) and 52% (25/48) for the 1000 and 2000 mg b.i.d. groups, respectively. The percent of patients who had 2 or more negative cultures during acute therapy that were sustained through study Day 84 was 25% (12/49) in both the 500 and 1000 mg b.i.d. groups and 8% (4/48) for the 2000 mg b.i.d. group. By Day 84, 23% (11/49), 37% (18/49), and 56% (27/48) of patients had died or discontinued from the study, and 14% (7/49), 12% (6/49), and 13% (6/48) of patients had relapsed in the 500, 1000, and 2000 mg b.i.d. dose groups, respectively. All of the isolates had an MIC < 8 mcg/mL at pre-treatment. Relapse was almost always accompanied by an increase in MIC. The median time to first negative culture was 54, 41, and 29 days for the 500, 1000, and 2000 mg b.i.d. groups, respectively. The time to first decrease of at least 1 log in CFU count was significantly shorter with the 1000 and 2000 mg b.i.d. doses (median equal to 16 and 15 days, respectively) in comparison to the 500 mg b.i.d. group (median equal to 29 days). The median time to first positive culture or study discontinuation following the first negative culture was 43, 59 and 43 days for the 500, 1000, and 2000 mg b.i.d. groups, respectively.

Clinically Significant Disseminated MAC Disease

Among patients experiencing night sweats prior to therapy, 84% showed resolution or improvement at some point during the 12 weeks of clarithromycin at 500 to 2000 mg b.i.d. doses. Similarly, 77% of patients reported resolution or improvement in fevers at some point. Response rates for clinical signs of MAC are given below:

[See first table above]

[See second table above]

The median duration of response, defined as improvement or resolution of clinical signs and symptoms, was 2 to 6 weeks.

Since the study was not designed to determine the benefit of monotherapy beyond 12 weeks, the duration of response may be underestimated for the 25 to 33% of patients who continued to show clinical response after 12 weeks.

Survival

Median survival time from study entry (Study 500) was 249 days at the 500 mg b.i.d. dose compared to 215 days with the 1000 mg b.i.d. dose. However, during the first 12 weeks of therapy, there were 2 deaths in 53 patients in the 500 mg b.i.d. group versus 13 deaths in 51 patients in the 1000 mg b.i.d. group. The reason for this apparent mortality difference is not known. Survival in the two groups was similar beyond 12 weeks. The median survival times for these dosages were similar to recent historical controls with MAC when treated with combination therapies.[6]

Median survival time from study entry in Study 577 was 199 days for the 500 mg b.i.d. dose and 179 days for the 1000 mg b.i.d. dose. During the first four weeks of therapy, while patients were maintained on their originally assigned dose, there were 11 deaths in 255 patients taking 500 mg b.i.d. and 18 deaths in 214 patients taking 1000 mg b.i.d.

Safety

The adverse event profiles showed that both the 500 and 1000 mg b.i.d. doses were well tolerated. The 2000 mg b.i.d. dose was poorly tolerated and resulted in a higher proportion of premature discontinuations.

In AIDS patients and other immunocompromised patients treated with the higher doses of clarithromycin over long periods of time for mycobacterial infections, it was often difficult to distinguish adverse events possibly associated with clarithromycin administration from underlying signs of HIV disease or intercurrent illness.

The following analyses summarize experience during the first 12 weeks of therapy with clarithromycin. Data are reported separately for Study 500 (randomized, double-blind) and Study 577 (open-label, compassionate use) and also combined. Adverse events were reported less frequently in Study 577, which may be due in part to differences in monitoring between the two studies. In adult patients receiving clarithromycin 500 mg b.i.d., the most frequently reported adverse events, considered possibly or probably related to study drug, with an incidence of 5% or greater, are listed below. Most of these events were mild to moderate in severity, although 5% (Study 500: 8%; Study 577: 4%) of patients receiving 500 mg b.i.d. and 5% (Study 500: 4%; Study 577: 6%) of patients receiving 1000 mg b.i.d. reported severe adverse events. Excluding those patients who discontinued therapy or died due to complications of their underlying non-mycobacterial disease, approximately 8% (Study 500: 15%; Study 577: 7%) of the patients who received 500 mg b.i.d. and 12% (Study 500: 14%; Study 577: 12%) of the patients who received 1000 mg b.i.d. discontinued therapy due to drug-related events during the first 12 weeks of therapy. Overall, the 500 and 1000 mg b.i.d. doses had similar adverse event profiles.

Treatment-related* Adverse Event Incidence Rates (%) in Immunocompromised Adult Patients During the First 12 Weeks of Therapy with 500 mg b.i.d. Clarithromycin Dose

Adverse Event	Study 500 (n = 53)	Study 577 (n = 255)	Combined (n = 308)
Abdominal Pain	7.5	2.4	3.2
Diarrhea	9.4	1.6	2.9
Flatulence	7.5	0.0	1.3
Headache	7.5	0.4	1.6
Nausea	28.3	9.0	12.3
Rash	9.4	2.0	3.2
Taste Perversion	18.9	0.4	3.6
Vomiting	24.5	3.9	7.5

* Includes those events possibly or probably related to study drug and excludes concurrent conditions.

A limited number of pediatric AIDS patients have been treated with clarithromycin suspension for mycobacterial infections. The most frequently reported adverse events, excluding those due to the patient's concurrent condition, were consistent with those observed in adult patients.

Changes in Laboratory Values

In immunocompromised patients treated with clarithromycin for mycobacterial infections, evaluations of laboratory values were made by analyzing those values outside the seriously abnormal level (i.e., the extreme high or low limit) for the specified test.

Percentage of Patients[a] Exceeding Extreme Laboratory Value Limits During First 12 Weeks of Treatment 500 mg b.i.d. Dose[b]

		Study 500	Study 577	Combined
BUN	> 50 mg/dL	0%	< 1%	< 1%
Platelet Count	< 50×10^9/L	0%	< 1%	< 1%
SGOT	> 5 × ULN[c]	0%	3%	2%
SGPT	> 5 × ULN[c]	0%	2%	1%
WBC	< 1×10^9/L	0%	1%	1%

[a] Includes only patients with baseline values within the normal range or borderline high (hematology variables) and within the normal range or borderline low (chemistry variables)

[b] Includes all values within the first 12 weeks for patients who start on 500 mg b.i.d.

[c] ULN = Upper Limit of Normal

Otitis Media

In a controlled clinical study of acute otitis media performed in the United States, where significant rates of beta-lactamase producing organisms were found, clarithromycin was compared to an oral cephalosporin. In this study, very strict evaluability criteria were used to determine clinical response. For the 223 patients who were evaluated for clinical efficacy, the clinical success rate (i.e., cure plus improvement) at the post-therapy visit was 88% for clarithromycin and 91% for the cephalosporin.

In a smaller number of patients, microbiologic determinations were made at the pre-treatment visit. The following presumptive bacterial eradication/clinical cure outcomes (i.e., clinical success) were obtained:

U.S. Acute Otitis Media Study Clarithromycin vs. Oral Cephalosporin EFFICACY RESULTS

PATHOGEN	OUTCOME
S. pneumoniae	clarithromycin success rate, 13/15 (87%), control 4/5
*H. influenzae**	clarithromycin success rate, 10/14 (71%), control 3/4
M. catarrhalis	clarithromycin success rate, 4/5,control 1/1
S. pyogenes	clarithromycin success rate, 3/3,control 0/1
Overall	clarithromycin success rate, 30/37 (81%), control 8/11 (73%)

* None of the *H. influenzae* isolated pre-treatment was resistant to clarithromycin; 6% were resistant to the control agent.

Safety

The incidence of adverse events in all patients treated, primarily diarrhea and vomiting, did not differ clinically or statistically for the two agents.

In two other controlled clinical trials of acute otitis media performed in the United States, where significant rates of beta-lactamase producing organisms were found, clarithromycin was compared to an oral antimicrobial agent that contained a specific beta-lactamase inhibitor. In these studies, very strict evaluability criteria were used to determine the clinical responses. In the 233 patients who were evaluated for clinical efficacy, the combined clinical success rate (i.e., cure and improvement) at the post-therapy visit was 91% for both clarithromycin and the control.

For the patients who had microbiologic determinations at the pre-treatment visit, the following presumptive bacterial eradication/clinical cure outcomes (i.e., clinical success) were obtained:

Two U.S. Acute Otitis Media Studies Clarithromycin vs. Antimicrobial/Beta-lactamase Inhibitor EFFICACY RESULTS

PATHOGEN	OUTCOME
S. pneumoniae	clarithromycin success rate, 43/51 (84%), control 55/56 (98%)
*H. influenzae**	clarithromycin success rate, 36/45 (80%), control 31/33 (94%)
M. catarrhalis	clarithromycin success rate, 9/10 (90%), control 6/6
S. pyogenes	clarithromycin success rate, 3/3, control 5/5
Overall	clarithromycin success rate, 91/109 (83%), control 97/100 (97%)

* Of the *H. influenzae* isolated pre-treatment, 3% were resistant to clarithromycin and 10% were resistant to the control agent.

Safety

The incidence of adverse events in all patients treated, primarily diarrhea (15% vs. 38%) and diaper rash (3% vs. 11%) in young children, was clinically and statistically lower in the clarithromycin arm versus the control arm.

Duodenal Ulcer Associated with *H. pylori* Infection

Clarithromycin + Lansoprazole and Amoxicillin

H. pylori Eradication for Reducing the Risk of Duodenal Ulcer Recurrence

Two U.S. randomized, double-blind clinical studies in patients with *H. pylori* and duodenal ulcer disease (defined as an active ulcer or history of an active ulcer within one year) evaluated the efficacy of clarithromycin in combination with lansoprazole and amoxicillin capsules as triple 14-day therapy for eradication of *H. pylori*. Based on the results of these studies, the safety and efficacy of the following eradication regimen were established:

Triple therapy: BIAXIN (clarithromycin) 500 mg b.i.d. + lansoprazole 30 mg b.i.d. + amoxicillin 1 gm b.i.d.

Treatment was for 14 days. *H. pylori* eradication was defined as two negative tests (culture and histology) at 4 to 6 weeks following the end of treatment.

The combination of BIAXIN plus lansoprazole and amoxicillin as triple therapy was effective in eradicating *H. pylori*. Eradication of *H. pylori* has been shown to reduce the risk of duodenal ulcer recurrence.

A randomized, double-blind clinical study performed in the U.S. in patients with *H. pylori* and duodenal ulcer disease (defined as an active ulcer or history of an ulcer within one year) compared the efficacy of clarithromycin in combination with lansoprazole and amoxicillin as triple therapy for 10 and 14 days. This study established that the 10-day triple therapy was equivalent to the 14-day triple therapy in eradicating *H. pylori*.

***H. pylori* Eradication Rates-Triple Therapy (BIAXIN/lansoprazole/amoxicillin) Percent of Patients Cured [95% Confidence Interval] (number of patients)**

Study	Duration	Triple Therapy Evaluable Analysis*	Triple Therapy Intent-to-Treat Analysis#
M93-131	14 days	92† [80.0-97.7] (n = 48)	86† [73.3-93.5] (n = 55)
M95-392	14 days	86‡ [75.7-93.6] (n = 66)	83‡ [72.0-90.8] (n = 70)
M95-399¶	14 days	85 [77.0-91.0] (N = 113)	82 [73.9-88.1] (N = 126)
	10 days	84 [76.0-89.8] (N = 123)	81 [73.9-87.6] (N = 135)

* Based on evaluable patients with confirmed duodenal ulcer (active or within one year) and *H. pylori* infection at baseline defined as at least two of three positive endoscopic tests from CLOtest (Delta West LTD., Bentley, Australia), histology, and/or culture. Patients were included in the analysis if they completed the study. Additionally, if patients were dropped out of the study due to an adverse event related to the study drug, they were included in the analysis as evaluable failures of therapy.

\# Patients were included in the analysis if they had documented *H. pylori* infection at baseline as defined above and had a confirmed duodenal ulcer (active or within one year). All dropouts were included as failures of therapy.

† ($p < 0.05$) versus BIAXIN/lansoprazole and lansoprazole/amoxicillin dual therapy.

‡ ($p < 0.05$) versus BIAXIN/amoxicillin dual therapy.

¶ The 95% confidence interval for the difference in eradication rates, 10-day minus 14-day, is (-10.5, 8.1) in the evaluable analysis and (-9.7, 9.1) in the intent-to-treat analysis.

Per-Protocol and Intent-to-Treat H. pylori Eradication Rates % of Patients Cured [95% Confidence Interval]

	Clarithromycin + omeprazole + amoxicillin		Clarithromycin + amoxicillin	
	Per-Protocol †	Intent-to-Treat ‡	Per-Protocol †	Intent-to-Treat ‡
Study 126	*77 [64, 86] (n = 64)	69 [57, 79] (n = 80)	43 [31, 56] (n = 67)	37 [27, 48] (n = 84)
Study 127	*78 [67, 88] (n = 65)	73 [61, 82] (n = 77)	41 [29, 54] (n = 68)	36 [26, 47] (n = 84)
Study M96-446	*90 [80, 96] (n = 69)	83 [74, 91] (n = 84)	33 [24, 44] (n = 93)	32 [23, 42] (n = 99)

† Patients were included in the analysis if they had confirmed duodenal ulcer disease (active ulcer studies 126 and 127; history of ulcer within 5 years, study M96-446) and *H. pylori* infection at baseline defined as at least two of three positive endoscopic tests from CLOtest®, histology, and/or culture. Patients were included in the analysis if they completed the study. Additionally, if patients dropped out of the study due to an adverse event related to the study drug, they were included in the analysis as failures of therapy. The impact of eradication on ulcer recurrence has not been assessed in patients with a past history of ulcer.

‡ Patients were included in the analysis if they had documented *H. pylori* infection at baseline and had confirmed duodenal ulcer disease. All dropouts were included as failures of therapy.

* $p < 0.05$ versus clarithromycin plus amoxicillin.

Clarithromycin + Omeprazole and Amoxicillin Therapy

H. pylori Eradication for Reducing the Risk of Duodenal Ulcer Recurrence

Three U.S., randomized, double-blind clinical studies in patients with *H. pylori* infection and duodenal ulcer disease (n = 558) compared clarithromycin plus omeprazole and amoxicillin to clarithromycin plus amoxicillin. Two studies (Studies 126 and 127) were conducted in patients with an active duodenal ulcer, and the third study (Study 446) was conducted in patients with a duodenal ulcer in the past 5 years, but without an ulcer present at the time of enrollment. The dosage regimen in the studies was clarithromycin 500 mg b.i.d. plus omeprazole 20 mg b.i.d. plus amoxicillin 1 gram b.i.d. for 10 days. In Studies 126 and 127, patients who took the omeprazole regimen also received an additional 18 days of omeprazole 20 mg q.d. Endpoints studied were eradication of *H. pylori* and duodenal ulcer healing (studies 126 and 127 only). *H. pylori* status was determined by CLOtest®, histology, and culture in all three studies. For a given patient, *H. pylori* was considered eradicated if at least two of these tests were negative, and none was positive. The combination of clarithromycin plus omeprazole and amoxicillin was effective in eradicating *H. pylori*.

[See table above]

Safety

In clinical trials using combination therapy with clarithromycin plus omeprazole and amoxicillin, no adverse reactions peculiar to the combination of these drugs have been observed. Adverse reactions that have occurred have been limited to those that have been previously reported with clarithromycin, omeprazole, or amoxicillin.

The most frequent adverse experiences observed in clinical trials using combination therapy with clarithromycin plus omeprazole and amoxicillin (n = 274) were diarrhea (14%), taste perversion (10%), and headache (7%).

For information about adverse reactions with omeprazole or amoxicillin, refer to the **ADVERSE REACTIONS** section of their package inserts.

Clarithromycin + Omeprazole Therapy

Four randomized, double-blind, multi-center studies (067, 100, 812b, and 058) evaluated clarithromycin 500 mg t.i.d. plus omeprazole 40 mg q.d. for 14 days, followed by omeprazole 20 mg q.d. (067, 100, and 058) or by omeprazole 40 mg q.d. (812b) for an additional 14 days in patients with active duodenal ulcer associated with *H. pylori*. Studies 067 and 100 were conducted in the U.S. and Canada and enrolled 242 and 256 patients, respectively. *H. pylori* infection and duodenal ulcer were confirmed in 219 patients in Study 067 and 228 patients in Study 100. These studies compared the combination regimen to omeprazole and clarithromycin monotherapies. Studies 812b and 058 were conducted in Europe and enrolled 154 and 215 patients, respectively. *H. pylori* infection and duodenal ulcer were confirmed in 148 patients in Study 812b and 208 patients in Study 058. These studies compared the combination regimen to omeprazole monotherapy. The results for the efficacy analyses for these studies are described below.

Duodenal Ulcer Healing

The combination of clarithromycin and omeprazole was as effective as omeprazole alone for healing duodenal ulcer.

End-of-Treatment Ulcer Healing Rates Percent of Patients Healed (n/N)

Study	Clarithromycin + Omeprazole	Omeprazole	Clarithromycin
U.S. Studies			
Study 100	94% (58/62)†	88% (60/68)	71% (49/69)
Study 067	88% (56/64)†	85% (55/65)	64% (44/69)
Non-U.S. Studies			
Study 058	99% (84/85)	95% (82/86)	N/A
Study 812b[1]	100% (64/64)	99% (71/72)	N/A

† $p < 0.05$ for clarithromycin + omeprazole versus clarithromycin monotherapy.

1 In Study 812b patients received omeprazole 40 mg daily for days 15 to 28.

Eradication of *H. pylori* Associated with Duodenal Ulcer

The combination of clarithromycin and omeprazole was effective in eradicating *H. pylori*.

***H. pylori* Eradication Rates (Per-Protocol Analysis) at 4 to 6 weeks Percent of Patients Cured (n/N)**

Study	Clarithromycin + Omeprazole	Omeprazole	Clarithromycin
U.S. Studies			
Study 100	64% (39/61)†‡	0% (0/59)	39% (17/44)
Study 067	74% (39/53)†‡	0% (0/54)	31% (13/42)
Non-U.S. Studies			
Study 058	74% (64/86)‡	1% (1/90)	N/A
Study 812b	83% (50/60)‡	1% (1/74)	N/A

† Statistically significantly higher than clarithromycin monotherapy ($p < 0.05$).

‡ Statistically significantly higher than omeprazole monotherapy ($p < 0.05$).

H. pylori eradication was defined as no positive test (culture or histology) at 4 weeks following the end of treatment, and two negative tests were required to be considered eradicated. In the per-protocol analysis, the following patients were excluded: dropouts, patients with major protocol violations, patients with missing *H. pylori* tests post-treatment,

Information on the AbbVie, Inc. products listed on these pages is from the prescribing information in use as of July 31, 2013. For more information, please visit rxabbvie.com or call 1-800-633-9110.

***H. pylori* Eradication Rates in Study H2BA-3001**

Analysis	RBC 400 mg + Clarithromycin 500 mg b.i.d.	RBC 400 mg + Clarithromycin 500 mg t.i.d.	95% CI Rate Difference
ITT	65% (122/188) [58%, 72%]	63% (122/195) [55%, 69%]	(-8%, 12%)
Per-Protocol	72% (117/162) [65%, 79%]	71% (120/170) [63%, 77%]	(-9%, 12%)

and patients that were not assessed for *H. pylori* eradication at 4 weeks after the end of treatment because they were found to have an unhealed ulcer at the end of treatment.
Ulcer recurrence at 6-months following the end of treatment was assessed for patients in whom ulcers were healed post-treatment.

Ulcer Recurrence at 6 months by *H. pylori* Status at 4-6 Weeks

	H. pylori Negative	*H. pylori* Positive
U.S. Studies		
Study 100		
Clarithromycin + Omeprazole	6% (2/34)	56% (9/16)
Omeprazole	- (0/0)	71% (35/49)
Clarithromycin	12% (2/17)	32% (7/22)
Study 067		
Clarithromycin + Omeprazole	38% (11/29)	50% (6/12)
Omeprazole	- (0/0)	67% (31/46)
Clarithromycin	18% (2/11)	52% (14/27)
Non-U.S. Studies		
Study 058		
Clarithromycin + Omeprazole	6% (3/53)	24% (4/17)
Omeprazole	0% (0/3)	55% (39/71)
Study 812b*		
Clarithromycin + Omeprazole	5% (2/42)	0% (0/7)
Omeprazole	0% (0/1)	54% (32/59)
***12-month recurrence rates:**		
Clarithromycin + Omeprazole	3% (1/40)	0% (0/6)
Omeprazole	0% (0/1)	67% (29/43)

Thus, in patients with duodenal ulcer associated with *H. pylori* infection, eradication of *H. pylori* reduced ulcer recurrence.
Safety
The adverse event profiles for the four studies showed that the combination of clarithromycin 500 mg t.i.d. and omeprazole 40 mg q.d. for 14 days, followed by omeprazole 20 mg q.d. (067, 100, and 058) or 40 mg q.d. (812b) for an additional 14 days was well tolerated. Of the 346 patients who received the combination, 12 (3.5%) patients discontinued study drug due to adverse events.

Adverse Events with an Incidence of 3% or Greater

Adverse Event	Clarithromycin + Omeprazole (N = 346) % of Patients	Omeprazole (N = 355) % of Patients	Clarithromycin (N = 166) % of Patients*
Taste Perversion	15%	1%	16%
Nausea	5%	1%	3%
Headache	5%	6%	9%
Diarrhea	4%	3%	7%
Vomiting	4%	< 1%	1%
Abdominal Pain	3%	2%	1%
Infection	3%	4%	2%

* Studies 067 and 100, only.

Most of these events were mild to moderate in severity.
Changes in Laboratory Values
Changes in laboratory values with possible clinical significance in patients taking clarithromycin and omeprazole were as follows:
Hepatic - elevated direct bilirubin < 1%; GGT < 1%; SGOT (AST) < 1%; SGPT (ALT) < 1%.
Renal - elevated serum creatinine < 1%.
For information on omeprazole, refer to the **ADVERSE REACTIONS** section of the PRILOSEC package insert.

Clarithromycin + Ranitidine Bismuth Citrate Therapy
In a U.S. double-blind, randomized, multicenter, dose-comparison trial, ranitidine bismuth citrate 400 mg b.i.d. for 4 weeks plus clarithromycin 500 mg b.i.d. for the first 2 weeks was found to have an equivalent *H. pylori* eradication rate (based on culture and histology) when compared to ranitidine bismuth citrate 400 mg b.i.d. for 4 weeks plus clarithromycin 500 mg t.i.d. for the first 2 weeks. The intent-to-treat *H. pylori* eradication rates are shown below:
[See table above]
H. pylori eradication was defined as no positive test at 4 weeks following the end of treatment. Patients must have had two tests performed, and these must have been negative to be considered eradicated of *H. pylori*. The following patients were excluded from the per-protocol analysis: patients not infected with *H. pylori* prestudy, dropouts, patients with major protocol violations, patients with missing *H. pylori* tests. Patients excluded from the intent-to-treat analysis included those not infected with *H. pylori* prestudy and those with missing *H. pylori* tests prestudy. Patients were assessed for *H. pylori* eradication (4 weeks following treatment) regardless of their healing status (at the end of treatment).
The relationship between *H. pylori* eradication and duodenal ulcer recurrence was assessed in a combined analysis of six U.S. randomized, double-blind, multicenter, placebo-controlled trials using ranitidine bismuth citrate with or without antibiotics. The results from approximately 650 U.S. patients showed that the risk of ulcer recurrence within 6 months of completing treatment was two times less likely in patients whose *H. pylori* infection was eradicated compared to patients in whom *H. pylori* infection was not eradicated.
Safety
In clinical trials using combination therapy with clarithromycin plus ranitidine bismuth citrate, no adverse reactions peculiar to the combination of these drugs (using clarithromycin twice daily or three times a day) were observed. Adverse reactions that have occurred have been limited to those reported with clarithromycin or ranitidine bismuth citrate. (See **ADVERSE REACTIONS** section of the Tritec package insert.) The most frequent adverse experiences observed in clinical trials using combination therapy with clarithromycin (500 mg three times a day) with ranitidine bismuth citrate (n = 329) were taste disturbance (11%), diarrhea (5%), nausea and vomiting (3%). The most frequent adverse experiences observed in clinical trials using combination therapy with clarithromycin (500 mg twice daily) with ranitidine bismuth citrate (n = 196) were taste disturbance (8%), nausea and vomiting (5%), and diarrhea (4%).

ANIMAL PHARMACOLOGY AND TOXICOLOGY

Clarithromycin is rapidly and well-absorbed with dose-linear kinetics, low protein binding, and a high volume of distribution. Plasma half-life ranged from 1 to 6 hours and was species dependent. High tissue concentrations were achieved, but negligible accumulation was observed. Fecal clearance predominated. Hepatotoxicity occurred in all species tested (i.e., in rats and monkeys at doses 2 times greater than and in dogs at doses comparable to the maximum human daily dose, based on mg/m^2). Renal tubular degeneration (calculated on a mg/m^2 basis) occurred in rats at doses 2 times, in monkeys at doses 8 times, and in dogs at doses 12 times greater than the maximum human daily dose. Testicular atrophy (on a mg/m^2 basis) occurred in rats at doses 7 times, in dogs at doses 3 times, and in monkeys at doses 8 times greater than the maximum human daily dose. Corneal opacity (on a mg/m^2 basis) occurred in dogs at doses 12 times and in monkeys at doses 8 times greater than the maximum human daily dose. Lymphoid depletion (on a mg/m^2 basis) occurred in dogs at doses 3 times greater than and in monkeys at doses 2 times greater than the maximum human daily dose. These adverse events were absent during clinical trials.

REFERENCES

1. Clinical and Laboratory Standards Institute (CLSI). Methods for Dilution Antimicrobial Susceptibility Tests for Bacteria that Grow Aerobically - 9th edition. Approved Standard. CLSI Document M07-A9, CLSI. 950 West Valley Rd, Suite 2500, Wayne, PA 19087, 2012.
2. CLSI. Performance Standards for Antimicrobial Susceptibility Testing, 22nd Informational Supplement, CLSI Document M100-S22, 2012.
3. CLSI. Performance Standards for Antimicrobial Disk Susceptibility Tests, 11th edition. Approved Standard CLSI Document M02-A11, 2012.
4. CLSI. Methods for Antimicrobial Dilution and Disk Diffusion Susceptibility Testing of Infrequently Isolated or Fastidious Bacteria - 2nd edition. CLSI document M45-A2, 2010.
5. Chaisson RE, et al. Clarithromycin and Ethambutol with or without Clofazimine for the Treatment of Bacteremic *Mycobacterium avium* Complex Disease in Patients with HIV Infection. AIDS. 1997;11:311-317.
6. Kemper CA, et al. Treatment of *Mycobacterium avium* Complex Bacteremia in AIDS with a Four-Drug Oral Regimen. *Ann Intern Med*. 1992;116:466-472.

Filmtab® - Film-sealed tablets, AbbVie Inc.
Biaxin Filmtab 250 mg and 500 mg and Biaxin XL 500 mg
Mfd. by AbbVie LTD, Barceloneta, PR 00617
Biaxin Granules for Oral Suspension, 125 mg/5 mL and 250 mg/5 mL
Mfd. by AbbVie Inc., North Chicago, IL 60064
For AbbVie Inc., North Chicago, IL 60064, U.S.A.
03-A639 January, 2013
Shown in Product Identification Guide, page 303

CARDIZEM® LA ℞

[*kăr-dĭ-zĕm LA*]
(Diltiazem Hydrochloride)
Extended-Release Tablets
℞ only
Once-a-Day Dosage

DESCRIPTION

CARDIZEM® LA (diltiazem hydrochloride) is a calcium ion cellular influx inhibitor (slow channel blocker or calcium antagonist). Chemically, diltiazem hydrochloride is 1,5-benzothiazepin-4(5*H*)-one, 3-(acetyloxy)-5-[2-(dimethylamino)ethyl]-2,3-dihydro-2-(4-methoxyphenyl)-, monohydrochloride, (+)-*cis*-. The structural formula is:

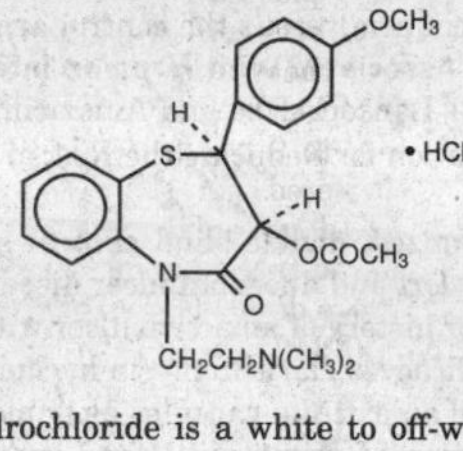

Diltiazem hydrochloride is a white to off-white crystalline powder with a bitter taste. It is soluble in water, methanol and chloroform. It has a molecular weight of 450.99. CARDIZEM LA Tablets, for oral administration are formulated as a once-a-day extended-release tablet containing 120 mg, 180 mg, 240 mg, 300 mg, 360 mg or 420 mg of diltiazem hydrochloride.
Also contains: carnauba wax, colloidal silicon dioxide, croscarmellose sodium, ethyl acrylate and methyl methacrylate copolymer dispersion, hydrogenated vegetable oil, hypromellose, magnesium stearate, microcrystalline cellulose, microcrystalline wax, polydextrose, polyethylene glycol, polysorbate, povidone, pregelatinized starch, simethicone, sodium starch glycolate, sucrose stearate, talc, and titanium dioxide.

CLINICAL PHARMACOLOGY

The therapeutic effects of diltiazem are believed to be related to its ability to inhibit the cellular influx of calcium ions during membrane depolarization of cardiac and vascular smooth muscle.

Mechanisms of Action

Hypertension. Diltiazem produces its antihypertensive effect primarily by relaxation of vascular smooth muscle and the resultant decrease in peripheral vascular resistance. The magnitude of blood pressure reduction is related to the degree of hypertension; thus hypertensive individuals experience an antihypertensive effect, whereas there is only a modest fall in blood pressure in normotensives.
Angina. Diltiazem has been shown to produce increases in exercise tolerance, probably due to its ability to reduce myocardial oxygen demand. This is accomplished via reductions in heart rate and systemic blood pressure at submaximal and maximal work loads. Diltiazem has been shown to be a potent dilator of coronary arteries, both epicardial and subendocardial. Spontaneous and ergonovine-induced coronary artery spasm are inhibited by diltiazem.
In animal models, diltiazem interferes with the slow inward (depolarizing) current in excitable tissue. It causes excitation-contraction uncoupling in various myocardial tissues without changes in the configuration of the action po-

tential. Diltiazem produces relaxation of coronary vascular smooth muscle and dilation of both large and small coronary arteries at drug levels which cause little or no negative inotropic effect. The resultant increases in coronary blood flow (epicardial and subendocardial) occur in ischemic and nonischemic models and are accompanied by dose-dependent decreases in systemic blood pressure and decreases in peripheral resistance.

Pharmacokinetics and Metabolism

Diltiazem is well absorbed from the gastrointestinal tract and is subject to an extensive first-pass effect, giving an absolute bioavailability (compared to intravenous administration) of about 40%. Diltiazem undergoes extensive metabolism in which only 2% to 4% of the unchanged drug appears in the urine. Drugs which induce or inhibit hepatic microsomal enzymes may alter diltiazem disposition.

Total radioactivity measurement following short IV administration in healthy volunteers suggests the presence of other unidentified metabolites, which attain higher concentrations than those of diltiazem and are more slowly eliminated; half-life of total radioactivity is about 20 hours compared to 2 to 5 hours for diltiazem.

In vitro binding studies show diltiazem is 70% to 80% bound to plasma proteins. Competitive *in vitro* ligand binding studies have also shown diltiazem hydrochloride binding is not altered by therapeutic concentrations of digoxin, hydrochlorothiazide, phenylbutazone, propranolol, salicylic acid, or warfarin. The plasma elimination half-life following single or multiple drug administration is approximately 3.0 to 4.5 hours. Desacetyl diltiazem is also present in the plasma at levels of 10% to 20% of the parent drug and is 25% to 50% as potent as a coronary vasodilator as diltiazem. Minimum therapeutic plasma diltiazem concentrations appear to be in the range of 50 to 200 ng/mL. There is a departure from linearity when dose strengths are increased; the half-life is slightly increased with dose. A study that compared patients with normal hepatic function to patients with cirrhosis found an increase in half-life and a 69% increase in bioavailability in the hepatically impaired patients. A single study in nine patients with severely impaired renal function showed no difference in the pharmacokinetic profile of diltiazem compared to patients with normal renal function.

CARDIZEM LA Tablets. A single 360 mg dose of CARDIZEM LA results in detectable plasma levels within 3 to 4 hours and peak plasma levels between 11 and 18 hours; absorption occurs throughout the dosing interval. The apparent elimination half-life for CARDIZEM LA Tablets after single or multiple dosing is 6 to 9 hours. When CARDIZEM LA Tablets were coadministered with a high fat content breakfast, diltiazem peak and systemic exposures were not affected indicating that the tablet can be administered without regard to food. As the dose of CARDIZEM LA Tablets is increased from 120 to 240 mg, area-under-the-curve increases 2.5-fold.

Pharmacodynamics and Clinical Studies

Like other calcium channel antagonists, diltiazem decreases sinoatrial and atrioventricular conduction in isolated tissues and has a negative inotropic effect in isolated preparations. In the intact animal, prolongation of the AH interval can be seen at higher doses.

In man, diltiazem prevents spontaneous and ergonovine-provoked coronary artery spasm. It causes a decrease in peripheral vascular resistance and a modest fall in blood pressure in normotensive individuals and, in exercise tolerance studies in patients with ischemic heart disease, reduces the heart rate-blood pressure product for any given work load. Studies to date, primarily in patients with good ventricular function, have not revealed evidence of a negative inotropic effect; cardiac output, ejection fraction, and left ventricular end diastolic pressure have not been affected. Such data has no predictive value with respect to effects in patients with poor ventricular function, and increased heart failure has been reported in patients with preexisting impairment of ventricular function. There are as yet few data on the interaction of diltiazem and beta-blockers in patients with poor ventricular function. Resting heart rate is usually slightly reduced by diltiazem. Diltiazem decreases vascular resistance, increases cardiac output (by increasing stroke volume), and produces a slight decrease or no change in heart rate.

During dynamic exercise, increases in diastolic pressure are inhibited, while maximum achievable systolic pressure is usually reduced. Chronic therapy with diltiazem produces no change or an increase in plasma catecholamines. No increased activity of the renin-angiotensin-aldosterone axis has been observed. Diltiazem reduces the renal and peripheral effects of angiotensin II. Hypertensive animal models respond to diltiazem with reductions in blood pressure and increased urinary output and natriuresis without a change in urinary sodium/potassium ratio.

Intravenous diltiazem hydrochloride in doses of 20 mg prolongs AH conduction time and AV node functional and effective refractory periods by approximately 20%. In a study involving single oral doses of 300 mg of diltiazem hydrochloride in six normal volunteers, the average maximum PR prolongation was 14% with no instances of greater than first-degree AV block. Diltiazem associated prolongation of the AH interval is not more pronounced in patients with first-degree heart block. In patients with sick sinus syndrome, diltiazem significantly prolongs sinus cycle length (up to 50% in some cases).

Chronic oral administration of diltiazem hydrochloride to patients in doses of up to 540 mg/day has resulted in small increases in PR interval, and on occasion produces abnormal prolongation (see **WARNINGS**).

Hypertension. In a randomized, double-blind, parallel-group, dose-response study involving 478 patients with essential hypertension, evening doses of CARDIZEM LA 120, 240, 360, and 540 mg were compared to placebo and to 360 mg administered in the morning. The mean reductions in diastolic blood pressure by ABPM at roughly 24 hours after the morning (4 AM to 8 AM) or evening (6 PM to 10 PM) administration (i.e., the time corresponding to expected trough serum concentrations) are shown in the table below:

Mean Change in Trough Diastolic Pressure by ABPM

Evening Dosing				Morning Dosing
120 mg	240 mg	360 mg	540 mg	360 mg
-2.0	-4.4	-4.4	-8.1	-6.4

A second randomized, double-blind, parallel-group, dose-response study (N=258) evaluated CARDIZEM LA following morning doses of placebo or 120, 180, 300, or 540 mg. Diastolic blood pressure measured by supine office cuff sphygmomanometer at trough (7 AM to 9 AM) decreased in an apparently linear manner over the dosage range studied. Group mean changes for placebo, 120 mg, 180 mg, 300 mg and 540 mg were -2.6, -1.9, -5.4, -6.1, and -8.6 mm Hg, respectively.

Whether the time of administration impacts the clinical benefits of antihypertensive treatment is not known.

Postural hypotension is infrequently noted upon suddenly assuming an upright position. No reflex tachycardia is associated with the chronic antihypertensive effects.

Angina. The effects of Cardizem LA on angina were evaluated in a randomized, double blind, parallel-group, dose-response trial of 311 patients with chronic stable angina. Evening doses of 180, 360, and 420 mg were compared to placebo and to 360 mg administered in the morning. All doses of Cardizem LA administered at night increased exercise tolerance when compared with placebo after 21 hours. The mean effect, placebo-subtracted, was 20 to 28 seconds for all three doses, and no dose-response was demonstrated. Cardizem LA, 360 mg, given in the morning, also improved exercise tolerance when measured 25 hours later. As expected, the effect was smaller than the effects measured only 21 hours following nighttime administration. Cardizem LA had a larger effect to increase exercise tolerance at peak serum concentrations than at trough.

INDICATIONS AND USAGE

CARDIZEM LA is indicated for the treatment of hypertension. It may be used alone or in combination with other antihypertensive medications.

CARDIZEM LA is indicated for the management of chronic stable angina.

CONTRAINDICATIONS

Diltiazem is contraindicated in (1) patients with sick sinus syndrome except in the presence of a functioning ventricular pacemaker, (2) patients with second- or third-degree AV block except in the presence of a functioning ventricular pacemaker, (3) patients with hypotension (less than 90 mm Hg systolic), (4) patients who have demonstrated hypersensitivity to the drug, and (5) patients with acute myocardial infarction and pulmonary congestion documented by x-ray on admission.

WARNINGS

1. **Cardiac Conduction.** Diltiazem prolongs AV node refractory periods without significantly prolonging sinus node recovery time, except in patients with sick sinus syndrome. This effect may rarely result in abnormally slow heart rates (particularly in patients with sick sinus syndrome) or second- or third-degree AV block (13 of 3290 patients or 0.40%). Concomitant use of diltiazem with beta-blockers or digitalis may result in additive effects on cardiac conduction. A patient with Prinzmetal's angina developed periods of asystole (2 to 5 seconds) after a single dose of 60 mg of diltiazem (see **ADVERSE REACTIONS**).
2. **Congestive Heart Failure.** Although diltiazem has a negative inotropic effect in isolated animal tissue preparations, hemodynamic studies in humans with normal ventricular function have not shown a reduction in cardiac index nor consistent negative effects on contractility (dp/dt). An acute study of oral diltiazem in patients with impaired ventricular function (ejection fraction 24% ± 6%) showed improvement in indices of ventricular function without significant decrease in contractile function (dp/dt). Worsening of congestive heart failure has been reported in patients with preexisting impairment of ventricular function. Experience with the use of diltiazem in combination with beta-blockers in patients with impaired ventricular function is limited. Caution should be exercised when using this combination.
3. **Hypotension.** Decreases in blood pressure associated with diltiazem therapy may occasionally result in symptomatic hypotension.
4. **Acute Hepatic Injury.** Mild elevations of transaminases with and without concomitant elevation in alkaline phosphatase and bilirubin have been observed in clinical studies. Such elevations were usually transient and frequently resolved even with continued diltiazem treatment. In rare instances, significant elevations in enzymes such as alkaline phosphatase, LDH, SGOT, SGPT, and other phenomena consistent with acute hepatic injury have been noted. These reactions tended to occur early after therapy initiation (1 to 8 weeks) and have been reversible upon discontinuation of drug therapy. The relationship to diltiazem is uncertain in some cases, but probable in some (see **PRECAUTIONS**).

PRECAUTIONS

General

Diltiazem hydrochloride is extensively metabolized by the liver and excreted by the kidneys and in bile. As with any drug given over prolonged periods, laboratory parameters of renal and hepatic function should be monitored at regular intervals. The drug should be used with caution in patients with impaired renal or hepatic function.

In subacute and chronic dog and rat studies designed to produce toxicity, high doses of diltiazem were associated with hepatic damage. In special subacute hepatic studies, oral doses of 125 mg/kg and higher in rats were associated with histological changes in the liver which were reversible when the drug was discontinued. In dogs, doses of 20 mg/kg were also associated with hepatic changes; however, these changes were reversible with continued dosing.

Dermatological events (see **ADVERSE REACTIONS**) may be transient and may disappear despite continued use of diltiazem. However, skin eruptions progressing to erythema multiforme and/or exfoliative dermatitis have also been infrequently reported. Should a dermatologic reaction persist, the drug should be discontinued.

Drug Interactions

Due to the potential for additive effects, caution and careful titration are warranted in patients receiving diltiazem concomitantly with other agents known to affect cardiac contractility and/or conduction (see **WARNINGS**). Pharmacologic studies indicate that there may be additive effects in prolonging AV conduction when using beta-blockers or digitalis concomitantly with diltiazem (see **WARNINGS**).

As with all drugs, care should be exercised when treating patients with multiple medications. Diltiazem is both a substrate and an inhibitor of the cytochrome P-450 3A4 enzyme system. Other drugs that are specific substrates, inhibitors, or inducers of this enzyme system may have a significant impact on the efficacy and side effect profile of diltiazem. Patients taking other drugs that are substrates of CYP450 3A4, especially patients with renal and/or hepatic impairment, may require dosage adjustment when starting or stopping concomitantly administered diltiazem in order to maintain optimum therapeutic blood levels.

Anesthetics. The depression of cardiac contractility, conductivity, and automaticity as well as the vascular dilation associated with anesthetics may be potentiated by calcium channel blockers. When used concomitantly, anesthetics and calcium blockers should be titrated carefully.

Benzodiazepines. Studies showed that diltiazem increased the AUC of midazolam and triazolam by 3- to 4-fold and the C_{max} by 2-fold, compared to placebo. The elimination half-life of midazolam and triazolam also increased (1.5- to 2.5-fold) during coadministration with diltiazem. These pharmacokinetic effects seen during diltiazem coadministration can result in increased clinical effects (e.g., prolonged sedation) of both midazolam and triazolam.

Beta-blockers. Controlled and uncontrolled domestic studies suggest that concomitant use of diltiazem and beta-blockers is usually well tolerated, but available data are not sufficient to predict the effects of concomitant treatment in patients with left ventricular dysfunction or cardiac conduction abnormalities.

Information on the AbbVie, Inc. products listed on these pages is from the prescribing information in use as of July 31, 2013. For more information, please visit rxabbvie.com or call 1-800-633-9110.

Administration of diltiazem concomitantly with propranolol in five normal volunteers resulted in increased propranolol levels in all subjects and bioavailability of propranolol was increased approximately 50%. *In vitro*, propranolol appears to be displaced from its binding sites by diltiazem. If combination therapy is initiated or withdrawn in conjunction with propranolol, an adjustment in the propranolol dose may be warranted (see **WARNINGS**).

Buspirone. In nine healthy subjects, diltiazem significantly increased the mean buspirone AUC 5.5-fold and C_{max} 4.1-fold compared to placebo. The $T_{1/2}$ and T_{max} of buspirone were not significantly affected by diltiazem. Enhanced effects and increased toxicity of buspirone may be possible during concomitant administration with diltiazem. Subsequent dose adjustments may be necessary during coadministration, and should be based on clinical assessment.

Carbamazepine. Concomitant administration of diltiazem with carbamazepine has been reported to result in elevated serum levels of carbamazepine (40% to 72% increase), resulting in toxicity in some cases. Patients receiving these drugs concurrently should be monitored for a potential drug interaction.

Cimetidine. A study in six healthy volunteers has shown a significant increase in peak diltiazem plasma levels (58%) and area-under-the-curve (53%) after a 1-week course of cimetidine at 1200 mg per day and a single dose of diltiazem 60 mg. Ranitidine produced smaller, nonsignificant increases. The effect may be mediated by cimetidine's known inhibition of hepatic cytochrome P-450, the enzyme system responsible for the first-pass metabolism of diltiazem. Patients currently receiving diltiazem therapy should be carefully monitored for a change in pharmacological effect when initiating and discontinuing therapy with cimetidine. An adjustment in the diltiazem dose may be warranted.

Clonidine. Sinus bradycardia resulting in hospitalization and pacemaker insertion has been reported in association with the use of clonidine concurrently with diltiazem. Monitor heart rate in patients receiving concomitant diltiazem and clonidine.

Cyclosporine. A pharmacokinetic interaction between diltiazem and cyclosporine has been observed during studies involving renal and cardiac transplant patients. In renal and cardiac transplant recipients, a reduction of cyclosporine dose ranging from 15% to 48% was necessary to maintain cyclosporine trough concentrations similar to those seen prior to the addition of diltiazem. If these agents are to be administered concurrently, cyclosporine concentrations should be monitored, especially when diltiazem therapy is initiated, adjusted, or discontinued.

The effect of cyclosporine on diltiazem plasma concentrations has not been evaluated.

Digitalis. Administration of diltiazem with digoxin in 24 healthy male subjects increased plasma digoxin concentrations approximately 20%. Another investigator found no increase in digoxin levels in 12 patients with coronary artery disease. Since there have been conflicting results regarding the effect of digoxin levels, it is recommended that digoxin levels be monitored when initiating, adjusting, and discontinuing diltiazem therapy to avoid possible over- or under-digitalization (see **WARNINGS**).

Quinidine. Diltiazem significantly increases the AUC $_{(0\rightarrow\infty)}$ of quinidine by 51%, $T_{1/2}$ by 36%, and decreases its CL_{oral} by 33%. Monitoring for quinidine adverse effects may be warranted and the dose adjusted accordingly.

Rifampin. Coadministration of rifampin with diltiazem lowered the diltiazem plasma concentrations to undetectable levels. Coadministration of diltiazem with rifampin or any known CYP3A4 inducer should be avoided when possible, and alternative therapy considered.

Statins. Diltiazem is an inhibitor of CYP3A4 and has been shown to increase significantly the AUC of some statins. The risk of myopathy and rhabdomyolysis with statins metabolized by CYP3A4 may be increased with concomitant use of diltiazem. When possible, use a non-CYP3A4-metabolized statin together with diltiazem; otherwise, dose adjustments for both diltiazem and the statin should be considered along with close monitoring for signs and symptoms of any statin related adverse events.

In a healthy volunteer cross-over study (N=10), co-administration of a single 20 mg dose of simvastatin at the end of a 14 day regimen with 120 mg BID diltiazem SR resulted in a 5-fold increase in mean simvastatin AUC versus simvastatin alone. Subjects with increased average steady-state exposures of diltiazem showed a greater fold increase in simvastatin exposure. Computer-based simulations showed that at a daily dose of 480 mg of diltiazem, an 8- to 9-fold mean increase in simvastatin AUC can be expected. If co-administration of simvastatin with diltiazem is required, limit the daily doses of simvastatin to 10 mg and diltiazem to 240 mg.

In a ten-subject randomized, open label, 4-way cross-over study, co-administration of diltiazem (120 mg BID diltiazem SR for 2 weeks) with a single 20 mg dose of lovastatin resulted in 3- to 4-fold increase in mean lovastatin AUC and C_{max} versus lovastatin alone. In the same study, there was no significant change in 20 mg single dose pravastatin AUC and C_{max} during diltiazem coadministration. Diltiazem plasma levels were not significantly affected by lovastatin or pravastatin.

Carcinogenesis, Mutagenesis, Impairment of Fertility

A 24-month study in rats at oral dosage levels of up to 100 mg/kg/day, and a 21-month study in mice at oral dosage levels of up to 30 mg/kg/day showed no evidence of carcinogenicity. There was also no mutagenic response *in vitro* or *in vivo* in mammalian cell assays or *in vitro* in bacteria. No evidence of impaired fertility was observed in a study performed in male and female rats at oral dosages of up to 100 mg/kg/day.

Pregnancy

Category C. Reproduction studies have been conducted in mice, rats, and rabbits. Administration of doses ranging from five to ten times greater (on a mg/kg basis) than the daily recommended therapeutic dose has resulted in embryo and fetal lethality. These doses, in some studies, have been reported to cause skeletal abnormalities. In the perinatal/postnatal studies, there was an increased incidence of stillbirths at doses of 20 times the human dose or greater.

There are no well-controlled studies in pregnant women; therefore, use diltiazem in pregnant women only if the potential benefit justifies the potential risk to the fetus.

Nursing Mothers

Diltiazem is excreted in human milk. One report suggests that concentrations in breast milk may approximate serum levels. If use of diltiazem is deemed essential, an alternative method of infant feeding should be instituted.

Pediatric Use

Safety and effectiveness in pediatric patients have not been established.

Geriatric Use

Clinical studies of diltiazem did not include sufficient numbers of subjects aged 65 and over to determine whether they respond differently from younger subjects. Other reported clinical experience has not identified differences in responses between the elderly and younger patients. In general, dose selection for an elderly patient should be cautious, usually starting at the low end of the dosing range, reflecting the greater frequency of decreased hepatic, renal, or cardiac function, and of concomitant disease or other drug therapy.

ADVERSE REACTIONS

Serious adverse reactions have been rare in studies carried out to date, but it should be recognized that patients with impaired ventricular function and cardiac conduction abnormalities have usually been excluded from these studies.

In the hypertension study, the following table presents adverse reactions more common on diltiazem than on placebo (but excluding events with no plausible relationship to treatment), as reported in placebo-controlled hypertension trials in patients receiving a diltiazem hydrochloride extended-release formulation (once-a-day dosing) up to 540 mg.

	Placebo	Diltiazem hydrochloride extended-release	
Adverse Reactions (MedDRA Term)	n= 120 # pts (%)	120-360 mg n= 501 # pts (%)	540 mg n= 123 # pts (%)
Edema lower limb	4 (3)	24 (5)	10 (8)
Sinus congestion	0 (0)	2 (1)	2 (2)
Rash NOS	0 (0)	3 (1)	2 (2)

In the angina study, the adverse event profile of CARDIZEM LA was consistent with what has been previously described for CARDIZEM LA and other formulations of diltiazem HCl. The most frequent adverse effects experienced by CARDIZEM LA-treated patients were edema lower-limb (6.8%), dizziness (6.4%), fatigue (4.8%), bradycardia (3.6%), first-degree atrioventricular block (3.2%), and cough (2%).

In clinical trials of other diltiazem formulations involving over 3200 patients, the most common events (i.e., greater than 1%) were edema (4.6%), headache (4.6%), dizziness (3.5%), asthenia (2.6%), first-degree AV block (2.4%), bradycardia (1.7%), flushing (1.4%), nausea (1.4%), and rash (1.2%).

In addition, the following events have been reported infrequently (less than 1%) in angina or hypertension trials:

Cardiovascular: Angina, arrhythmia, AV block (second- or third-degree), bundle branch block, congestive heart failure, ECG abnormalities, hypotension, palpitations, syncope, tachycardia, ventricular extrasystoles.

Nervous System: Abnormal dreams, amnesia, depression, gait abnormality, hallucinations, insomnia, nervousness, paresthesia, personality change, somnolence, tinnitus, tremor.

Gastrointestinal: Anorexia, constipation, diarrhea, dry mouth, dysgeusia, dyspepsia, mild elevations of SGOT, SGPT, LDH, and alkaline phosphatase (see **WARNINGS, Acute Hepatic Injury**), thirst, vomiting, weight increase.

Dermatological: Petechiae, photosensitivity, pruritus, urticaria.

Other: Amblyopia, CPK increase, dyspnea, epistaxis, eye irritation, hyperglycemia, hyperuricemia, impotence, muscle cramps, nasal congestion, nocturia, osteoarticular pain, polyuria, sexual difficulties.

The following postmarketing events have been reported infrequently in patients receiving Cardizem: acute generalized exanthematous pustulosis, allergic reactions, alopecia, angioedema (including facial or periorbital edema), asystole, erythema multiforme (including Stevens-Johnson syndrome, toxic epidermal necrolysis), exfoliative dermatitis, extrapyramidal symptoms, gingival hyperplasia, hemolytic anemia, increased bleeding time, leukopenia, photosensitivity (including lichenoid keratosis and hyperpigmentation at sun-exposed skin areas), purpura, retinopathy, myopathy, and thrombocytopenia. In addition, events such as myocardial infarction have been observed which are not readily distinguishable from the natural history of the disease in these patients. A number of well-documented cases of generalized rash, some characterized as leukocytoclastic vasculitis, have been reported. However, a definitive cause and effect relationship between these events and Cardizem therapy is yet to be established.

OVERDOSAGE

The oral LD_{50}'s in mice and rats range from 415 to 740 mg/kg and from 560 to 810 mg/kg, respectively. The intravenous LD_{50}'s in these species were 60 and 38 mg/kg, respectively. The oral LD_{50} in dogs is considered to be in excess of 50 mg/kg, while lethality was seen in monkeys at 360 mg/kg.

The toxic dose in man is not known. Due to extensive metabolism, blood levels after a standard dose of diltiazem can vary over tenfold, limiting the usefulness of blood levels in overdose cases.

There have been 29 reports of diltiazem overdose in doses ranging from less than 1 g to 18 g. Sixteen of these reports involved multiple drug ingestions.

Twenty-two reports indicated patients had recovered from diltiazem overdose ranging from less than 1 g to 10.8 g. There were seven reports with a fatal outcome; although the amount of diltiazem ingested was unknown, multiple drug ingestions were confirmed in six of the seven reports.

Events observed following diltiazem overdose included bradycardia, hypotension, heart block, and cardiac failure. Most reports of overdose described some supportive medical measure and/or drug treatment. Bradycardia frequently responded favorably to atropine as did heart block, although cardiac pacing was also frequently utilized to treat heart block. Fluids and vasopressors were used to maintain blood pressure and in cases of cardiac failure, inotropic agents were administered. In addition, some patients received treatment with ventilatory support, gastric lavage, activated charcoal, and/or intravenous calcium. Evidence of the effectiveness of intravenous calcium administration to reverse the pharmacological effects of diltiazem overdose was conflicting.

In the event of overdose or exaggerated response, appropriate supportive measures should be employed in addition to gastrointestinal decontamination. Diltiazem does not appear to be removed by peritoneal or hemodialysis. Limited data suggest that plasmapheresis or charcoal hemoperfusion may hasten diltiazem elimination following overdose. Based on the known pharmacological effects of diltiazem and/or reported clinical experiences, the following measures may be considered:

Bradycardia: Administer atropine (0.60 to 1.0 mg). If there is no response to vagal blockage, administer isoproterenol cautiously.

High-degree AV Block: Treat as for bradycardia above. Fixed high-degree AV block should be treated with cardiac pacing.

Cardiac Failure: Administer inotropic agents (isoproterenol, dopamine, or dobutamine) and diuretics.

Hypotension: Vasopressors (e.g., dopamine or norepinephrine).

Actual treatment and dosage should depend on the severity of the clinical situation and the judgment and experience of the treating physician.

DOSAGE AND ADMINISTRATION

CARDIZEM LA Tablets are an extended-release formulation intended for once-a-day administration.

Patients controlled on diltiazem alone or in combination with other medications may be switched to CARDIZEM LA Tablets once-a-day at the nearest equivalent total daily dose. Higher doses of CARDIZEM LA Tablets once-a-day dosage may be needed in some patients. Patients should be closely monitored. Subsequent titration to higher or lower

doses may be necessary and should be initiated as clinically warranted. There is limited general clinical experience with doses above 360 mg, but the safety and efficacy of doses as high as 540 mg have been studied in clinical trials. The incidence of side effects increases as the dose increases with first-degree AV block, dizziness, and sinus bradycardia bearing the strongest relationship to dose.
The tablet should be swallowed whole and not chewed or crushed.

Hypertension.
Dosage needs to be adjusted by titration to individual patient needs. When used as monotherapy, reasonable starting doses are 180 to 240 mg once daily, although some patients may respond to lower doses. Maximum antihypertensive effect is usually observed by 14 days of chronic therapy; therefore, dosage adjustments should be scheduled accordingly. The dosage range studied in clinical trials was 120 to 540 mg once daily. The dosage may be titrated to a maximum of 540 mg daily.
CARDIZEM LA Tablets should be taken about the same time once each day either in the morning or at bedtime. The time of dosing should be considered when making dose adjustments based on trough effects.

Angina.
Dosage for the treatment of angina should be individualized based on response. The initial dose of 180 mg once daily may be increased at intervals of 7 to 14 days if adequate response is not obtained. CARDIZEM LA doses above 360 mg appear to confer no additional benefit.
CARDIZEM LA can be given once daily, either in the evening or in the morning.

Concomitant Use with Other Cardiovascular Agents
1. Sublingual NTG. May be taken as required to abort acute anginal attacks during Diltiazem Hydrochloride Extended-Release therapy.
2. Prophylactic Nitrate Therapy. Diltiazem Hydrochloride Extended-Release Tablets may be safely coadministered with short-and long-acting nitrates.
3. Beta-blockers (see **WARNINGS** and **PRECAUTIONS**).
4. Antihypertensives. CARDIZEM LA has an additive antihypertensive effect when used with other antihypertensive agents. Therefore, the dosage of Diltiazem Hydrochloride Extended-Release Tablets or the concomitant antihypertensives may need to be adjusted when adding one to the other.

HOW SUPPLIED
CARDIZEM® LA is supplied as white, capsule-shaped tablets debossed with "B" on one side and the diltiazem content (mg) on the other.

Strength	NDC # Bottles of 30	NDC # Bottles of 90
120 mg	NDC-0074-3045-30	NDC-0074-3045-90
180 mg	NDC-0074-3061-30	NDC-0074-3061-90
240 mg	NDC-0074-3062-30	NDC-0074-3062-90
300 mg	NDC-0074-3063-30	NDC-0074-3063-90
360 mg	NDC-0074-3064-30	NDC-0074-3064-90
420 mg	NDC-0074-3069-30	NDC-0074-3069-90

Storage conditions: Store at 25°C (77°F); excursions permitted to 15-30°C (59-86°F) [see USP Controlled Room Temperature].
Avoid excessive humidity and temperatures above 30°C (86°F).
Dispense in tight, light resistant container as defined in USP.
Unless otherwise indicated, all trademarks are property of the Valeant family of companies.
Manufactured by:
Valeant Pharmaceuticals International, Inc.
Steinbach, MB
R5G 1Z7
Canada
Manufactured for:
AbbVie Inc.
North Chicago, IL. 60064
USA
LB0024-09 Rev. 03/13
Shown in Product Identification Guide, page 303

CREON® ℞
[*krē'ŏn*]
(pancrelipase)
delayed release capsules for oral use

HIGHLIGHTS OF PRESCRIBING INFORMATION
These highlights do not include all the information needed to use CREON safely and effectively. See full prescribing information for CREON.
CREON (pancrelipase) delayed-release capsules for oral use
Initial U.S. Approval: 2009

INDICATIONS AND USAGE
CREON is a combination of porcine-derived lipases, proteases, and amylases indicated for the treatment of exocrine pancreatic insufficiency due to cystic fibrosis, chronic pancreatitis, pancreatectomy, or other conditions. (1)

DOSAGE AND ADMINISTRATION
CREON is not interchangeable with any other pancrelipase product. (2.1)
Do not crush or chew capsules and capsule contents. For infants or patients unable to swallow intact capsules, the contents may be sprinkled on soft acidic food, e.g., applesauce. (2.1) Dosing should not exceed the recommended maximum dosage set forth by the Cystic Fibrosis Foundation Consensus Conferences Guidelines. (2.2)
Infants (up to 12 months)
- Prior to each feeding, infants may be given 3,000 lipase units (one capsule) per 120 mL of formula or per breast-feeding. (2.1)
- Do not mix CREON capsule contents directly into formula or breast milk prior to administration. (2.1)

Children Older than 12 Months and Younger than 4 Years
- Begin with 1,000 lipase units/kg of body weight per meal for children less than age 4 years to a maximum of 2,500 lipase units/kg of body weight per meal (or less than or equal to 10,000 lipase units/kg of body weight per day), or less than 4,000 lipase units/g fat ingested per day. (2.2)

Children 4 Years and Older and Adults
- Begin with 500 lipase units/kg of body weight per meal for those older than age 4 years to a maximum of 2,500 lipase units/kg of body weight per meal (or less than or equal to 10,000 lipase units/kg of body weight per day), or less than 4,000 lipase units/g fat ingested per day. (2.2)

Adults with Exocrine Pancreatic Insufficiency Due to Chronic Pancreatitis or Pancreatectomy
- Individualize dosage based on clinical symptoms, the degree of steatorrhea present and the fat content of the diet. (2.2)

DOSAGE FORMS AND STRENGTHS
- Delayed-Release Capsules: 3,000 USP units of lipase; 9,500 USP units of protease; 15,000 USP units of amylase (3)
- Delayed-Release Capsules: 6,000 USP units of lipase; 19,000 USP units of protease; 30,000 USP units of amylase (3)
- Delayed-Release Capsules: 12,000 USP units of lipase; 38,000 USP units of protease; 60,000 USP units of amylase (3)
- Delayed-Release Capsules: 24,000 USP units of lipase; 76,000 USP units of protease; 120,000 USP units of amylase (3)
- Delayed-Release Capsules: 36,000 USP units of lipase; 114,000 USP units of protease; 180,000 USP units of amylase (3)

CONTRAINDICATIONS
None (4)

WARNINGS AND PRECAUTIONS
- Fibrosing colonopathy is associated with high-dose use of pancreatic enzyme replacement in the treatment of cystic fibrosis patients. Exercise caution when doses of CREON exceed 2,500 lipase units/kg of body weight per meal (or greater than 10,000 lipase units/kg of body weight per day). (5.1)
- To avoid irritation of oral mucosa, do not chew CREON or retain in the mouth. (5.2)
- Exercise caution when prescribing CREON to patients with gout, renal impairment, or hyperuricemia. (5.3)
- There is theoretical risk of viral transmission with all pancreatic enzyme products including CREON. (5.4)
- Exercise caution when administering pancrelipase to a patient with a known allergy to proteins of porcine origin. (5.5)

ADVERSE REACTIONS
- Adverse reactions occurring in at least 2 cystic fibrosis patients (greater than or equal to 4%) receiving CREON are vomiting, dizziness, and cough. (6.1)
- Adverse reactions that occurred in at least 1 chronic pancreatitis or pancreatectomy patient (greater than or equal to 4%) receiving CREON are hyperglycemia, hypoglycemia, abdominal pain, abnormal feces, flatulence, frequent bowel movements, and nasopharyngitis. (6.1)

To report SUSPECTED ADVERSE REACTIONS, contact AbbVie Inc. at 1-800-633-9110 or FDA at 1-800-FDA-1088 or www.fda.gov/medwatch.
See 17 for PATIENT COUNSELING INFORMATION and Medication Guide
Revised: 03/2013

FULL PRESCRIBING INFORMATION: CONTENTS*

* Sections or subsections omitted from the full prescribing information are not listed

FULL PRESCRIBING INFORMATION

1 INDICATIONS AND USAGE
CREON® (pancrelipase) is indicated for the treatment of exocrine pancreatic insufficiency due to cystic fibrosis, chronic pancreatitis, pancreatectomy, or other conditions.

2 DOSAGE AND ADMINISTRATION
CREON is not interchangeable with other pancrelipase products.
CREON is orally administered. Therapy should be initiated at the lowest recommended dose and gradually increased. The dosage of CREON should be individualized based on clinical symptoms, the degree of steatorrhea present, and the fat content of the diet as described in the Limitations on Dosing below [*see Dosage and Administration (2.2) and Warnings and Precautions (5.1)*].

2.1 Administration
Infants (up to 12 months)
CREON should be administered to infants immediately prior to each feeding, using a dosage of 3,000 lipase units per 120 mL of formula or prior to breast-feeding. Contents of the capsule may be administered directly to the mouth or with a small amount of applesauce. Administration should be followed by breast milk or formula. Contents of the capsule should not be mixed directly into formula or breast milk as this may diminish efficacy. Care should be taken to ensure that CREON is not crushed or chewed or retained in the mouth, to avoid irritation of the oral mucosa.
Children and Adults
CREON should be taken during meals or snacks, with sufficient fluid. CREON capsules and capsule contents should not be crushed or chewed. Capsules should be swallowed whole.
For patients who are unable to swallow intact capsules, the capsules may be carefully opened and the contents added to a small amount of acidic soft food with a pH of 4.5 or less, such as applesauce, at room temperature. The CREON-soft food mixture should be swallowed immediately without crushing or chewing, and followed with water or juice to ensure complete ingestion. Care should be taken to ensure that no drug is retained in the mouth.

2.2 Dosage
Dosage recommendations for pancreatic enzyme replacement therapy were published following the Cystic Fibrosis Foundation Consensus Conferences.[1, 2, 3] CREON should be administered in a manner consistent with the recommendations of the Cystic Fibrosis Foundation Consensus Conferences (also known as Conferences) provided in the following paragraphs, except for infants. Although the Conferences recommend doses of 2,000 to 4,000 lipase units in infants up to 12 months, CREON is available in a 3,000 lipase unit capsule. Therefore, the recommended dose of CREON in infants up to 12 months is 3,000 lipase units per 120 mL of

Information on the AbbVie, Inc. products listed on these pages is from the prescribing information in use as of July 31, 2013. For more information, please visit rxabbvie.com or call 1-800-633-9110.

formula or per breast-feeding. Patients may be dosed on a fat ingestion-based or actual body weight-based dosing scheme.

Additional recommendations for pancreatic enzyme therapy in patients with exocrine pancreatic insufficiency due to chronic pancreatitis or pancreatectomy are based on a clinical trial conducted in these populations.

Infants (up to 12 months)

CREON is available in the strength of 3,000 USP units of lipase thus infants may be given 3,000 lipase units (one capsule) per 120 mL of formula or per breast-feeding. Do not mix CREON capsule contents directly into formula or breast milk prior to administration *[see Administration (2.1)]*.

Children Older than 12 Months and Younger than 4 Years

Enzyme dosing should begin with 1,000 lipase units/kg of body weight per meal for children less than age 4 years to a maximum of 2,500 lipase units/kg of body weight per meal (or less than or equal to 10,000 lipase units/kg of body weight per day), or less than 4,000 lipase units/g fat ingested per day.

Children 4 Years and Older and Adults

Enzyme dosing should begin with 500 lipase units/kg of body weight per meal for those older than age 4 years to a maximum of 2,500 lipase units/kg of body weight per meal (or less than or equal to 10,000 lipase units/kg of body weight per day), or less than 4,000 lipase units/g fat ingested per day.

Usually, half of the prescribed CREON dose for an individualized full meal should be given with each snack. The total daily dose should reflect approximately three meals plus two or three snacks per day.

Enzyme doses expressed as lipase units/kg of body weight per meal should be decreased in older patients because they weigh more but tend to ingest less fat per kilogram of body weight.

Adults with Exocrine Pancreatic Insufficiency Due to Chronic Pancreatitis or Pancreatectomy

The initial starting dose and increases in the dose per meal should be individualized based on clinical symptoms, the degree of steatorrhea present, and the fat content of the diet.

In one clinical trial, patients received CREON at a dose of 72,000 lipase units per meal while consuming at least 100 g of fat per day *[see Clinical Studies (14.2)]*. Lower starting doses recommended in the literature are consistent with the 500 lipase units/kg of body weight per meal lowest starting dose recommended for adults in the Cystic Fibrosis Foundation Consensus Conferences Guidelines.[1, 2, 3, 4] Usually, half of the prescribed CREON dose for an individualized full meal should be given with each snack.

Limitations on Dosing

Dosing should not exceed the recommended maximum dosage set forth by the Cystic Fibrosis Foundation Consensus Conferences Guidelines.[1, 2, 3] If symptoms and signs of steatorrhea persist, the dosage may be increased by the healthcare professional. Patients should be instructed not to increase the dosage on their own. There is great inter-individual variation in response to enzymes; thus, a range of doses is recommended. Changes in dosage may require an adjustment period of several days. If doses are to exceed 2,500 lipase units/kg of body weight per meal, further investigation is warranted. Doses greater than 2,500 lipase units/kg of body weight per meal (or greater than 10,000 lipase units/kg of body weight per day) should be used with caution and only if they are documented to be effective by 3-day fecal fat measures that indicate a significantly improved coefficient of fat absorption. Doses greater than 6,000 lipase units/kg of body weight per meal have been associated with colonic stricture, indicative of fibrosing colonopathy, in children less than 12 years of age *[see Warnings and Precautions (5.1)]*. Patients currently receiving higher doses than 6,000 lipase units/kg of body weight per meal should be examined and the dosage either immediately decreased or titrated downward to a lower range.

3 DOSAGE FORMS AND STRENGTHS

The active ingredient in CREON evaluated in clinical trials is lipase. CREON is dosed by lipase units.

Other active ingredients include protease and amylase. Each CREON delayed-release capsule strength contains the specified amounts of lipase, protease, and amylase as follows:

- 3,000 USP units of lipase; 9,500 USP units of protease; 15,000 USP units of amylase delayed-release capsules have a white opaque cap with imprint "CREON 1203" and a white opaque body.
- 6,000 USP units of lipase; 19,000 USP units of protease; 30,000 USP units of amylase delayed-release capsules have an orange opaque cap with imprint "CREON 1206" and a blue opaque body.
- 12,000 USP units of lipase; 38,000 USP units of protease; 60,000 USP units of amylase delayed-release capsules have a brown opaque cap with imprint "CREON 1212" and a colorless transparent body.
- 24,000 USP units of lipase; 76,000 USP units of protease; 120,000 USP units of amylase delayed-release capsules have an orange opaque cap with imprint "CREON 1224" and a colorless transparent body.
- 36,000 USP units of lipase; 114,000 USP units of protease; 180,000 USP units of amylase delayed-release capsules have a blue opaque cap with imprint "CREON 1236" and a colorless transparent body.

4 CONTRAINDICATIONS

None.

5 WARNINGS AND PRECAUTIONS

5.1 Fibrosing Colonopathy

Fibrosing colonopathy has been reported following treatment with different pancreatic enzyme products.[5, 6] Fibrosing colonopathy is a rare, serious adverse reaction initially described in association with high-dose pancreatic enzyme use, usually over a prolonged period of time and most commonly reported in pediatric patients with cystic fibrosis. The underlying mechanism of fibrosing colonopathy remains unknown. Doses of pancreatic enzyme products exceeding 6,000 lipase units/kg of body weight per meal have been associated with colonic stricture in children less than 12 years of age.[1] Patients with fibrosing colonopathy should be closely monitored because some patients may be at risk of progressing to stricture formation. It is uncertain whether regression of fibrosing colonopathy occurs.[1] It is generally recommended, unless clinically indicated, that enzyme doses should be less than 2,500 lipase units/kg of body weight per meal (or less than 10,000 lipase units/kg of body weight per day) or less than 4,000 lipase units/g fat ingested per day *[see Dosage and Administration (2.1)]*.

Doses greater than 2,500 lipase units/kg of body weight per meal (or greater than 10,000 lipase units/kg of body weight per day) should be used with caution and only if they are documented to be effective by 3-day fecal fat measures that indicate a significantly improved coefficient of fat absorption. Patients receiving higher doses than 6,000 lipase units/kg of body weight per meal should be examined and the dosage either immediately decreased or titrated downward to a lower range.

5.2 Potential for Irritation to Oral Mucosa

Care should be taken to ensure that no drug is retained in the mouth. CREON should not be crushed or chewed or mixed in foods having a pH greater than 4.5. These actions can disrupt the protective enteric coating resulting in early release of enzymes, irritation of oral mucosa, and/or loss of enzyme activity *[see Dosage and Administration (2.2) and Patient Counseling Information (17.1)]*. For patients who are unable to swallow intact capsules, the capsules may be carefully opened and the contents added to a small amount of acidic soft food with a pH of 4.5 or less, such as applesauce, at room temperature. The CREON-soft food mixture should be swallowed immediately and followed with water or juice to ensure complete ingestion.

5.3 Potential for Risk of Hyperuricemia

Caution should be exercised when prescribing CREON to patients with gout, renal impairment, or hyperuricemia. Porcine-derived pancreatic enzyme products contain purines that may increase blood uric acid levels.

5.4 Potential Viral Exposure from the Product Source

CREON is sourced from pancreatic tissue from swine used for food consumption. Although the risk that CREON will transmit an infectious agent to humans has been reduced by testing for certain viruses during manufacturing and by inactivating certain viruses during manufacturing, there is a theoretical risk for transmission of viral disease, including diseases caused by novel or unidentified viruses. Thus, the presence of porcine viruses that might infect humans cannot be definitely excluded. However, no cases of transmission of an infectious illness associated with the use of porcine pancreatic extracts have been reported.

5.5 Allergic Reactions

Caution should be exercised when administering pancrelipase to a patient with a known allergy to proteins of porcine origin. Rarely, severe allergic reactions including anaphylaxis, asthma, hives, and pruritus, have been reported with other pancreatic enzyme products with different formulations of the same active ingredient (pancrelipase). The risks and benefits of continued CREON treatment in patients with severe allergy should be taken into consideration with the overall clinical needs of the patient.

6 ADVERSE REACTIONS

The most serious adverse reactions reported with different pancreatic enzyme products of the same active ingredient (pancrelipase) that are described elsewhere in the label include fibrosing colonopathy, hyperuricemia and allergic reactions *[see Warnings and Precautions (5)]*.

6.1 Clinical Trials Experience

Because clinical trials are conducted under widely varying conditions, adverse reaction rates observed in the clinical trials of a drug cannot be directly compared to the rates in the clinical trials of another drug and may not reflect the rates observed in practice.

The short-term safety of CREON was assessed in clinical trials conducted in 121 patients with exocrine pancreatic insufficiency (EPI): 67 patients with EPI due to cystic fibrosis (CF) and 25 patients with EPI due to chronic pancreatitis or pancreatectomy were treated with CREON.

Cystic Fibrosis

Studies 1 and 2 were randomized, double-blind, placebo-controlled, crossover studies of 49 patients, ages 7 to 43 years, with EPI due to CF. Study 1 included 32 patients ages 12 to 43 years and Study 2 included 17 patients ages 7 to 11 years. In these studies, patients were randomized to receive CREON at a dose of 4,000 lipase units/g fat ingested per day or matching placebo for 5 to 6 days of treatment, followed by crossover to the alternate treatment for an additional 5 to 6 days. The mean exposure to CREON during these studies was 5 days.

In Study 1, one patient experienced duodenitis and gastritis of moderate severity 16 days after completing treatment with CREON. Transient neutropenia without clinical sequelae was observed as an abnormal laboratory finding in one patient receiving CREON and a macrolide antibiotic.

In Study 2, adverse reactions that occurred in at least 2 patients (greater than or equal to 12%) treated with CREON were vomiting and headache. Vomiting occurred in 2 patients treated with CREON and did not occur in patients treated with placebo; headache occurred in 2 patients treated with CREON and did not occur in patients treated with placebo.

The most common adverse reactions (greater than or equal to 4%) in Studies 1 and 2 were vomiting, dizziness, and cough. Table 1 enumerates adverse reactions that occurred in at least 2 patients (greater than or equal to 4%) treated with CREON at a higher rate than with placebo in Studies 1 and 2.

Table 1: Adverse Reactions Occurring in at Least 2 Patients (greater than or equal to 4%) in Cystic Fibrosis (Studies 1 and 2)

Adverse Reaction	CREON Capsules n = 49 (%)	Placebo n = 47 (%)
Vomiting	3 (6)	1 (2)
Dizziness	2 (4)	1 (2)
Cough	2 (4)	0

An additional open-label, single-arm study assessed the short-term safety and tolerability of CREON in 18 infants and children, ages 4 months to 6 years, with EPI due to cystic fibrosis. Patients received their usual pancreatic enzyme replacement therapy (mean dose of 7,000 lipase units/kg/day for a mean duration of 18.2 days) followed by CREON (mean dose of 7,500 lipase units/kg/day for a mean duration of 12.6 days). There were no serious adverse reactions. Adverse reactions that occurred in patients during treatment with CREON were vomiting, irritability, and decreased appetite, each occurring in 6% of patients.

Chronic Pancreatitis or Pancreatectomy

A randomized, double-blind, placebo-controlled, parallel group study was conducted in 54 adult patients, ages 32 to 75 years, with EPI due to chronic pancreatitis or pancreatectomy. Patients received single-blind placebo treatment during a 5-day run-in period followed by an intervening period of up to 16 days of investigator-directed treatment with no restrictions on pancreatic enzyme replacement therapy. Patients were then randomized to receive CREON or matching placebo for 7 days. The CREON dose was 72,000 lipase units per main meal (3 main meals) and 36,000 lipase units per snack (2 snacks). The mean exposure to CREON during this study was 6.8 days in the 25 patients that received CREON.

The most common adverse reactions reported during the study were related to glycemic control and were reported more commonly during CREON treatment than during placebo treatment.

Table 2 enumerates adverse reactions that occurred in at least 1 patient (greater than or equal to 4%) treated with CREON at a higher rate than with placebo.

Table 2: Adverse Reactions in at Least 1 Patient (greater than or equal to 4%) in the Chronic Pancreatitis or Pancreatectomy Trial

Adverse Reaction	CREON Capsules n = 25 (%)	Placebo n = 29 (%)
Hyperglycemia	2 (8)	2 (7)
Hypoglycemia	1 (4)	1 (3)
Abdominal Pain	1 (4)	1 (3)

Abnormal Feces	1 (4)	0
Flatulence	1 (4)	0
Frequent Bowel Movements	1 (4)	0
Nasopharyngitis	1 (4)	0

6.2 Postmarketing Experience

Postmarketing data from this formulation of CREON have been available since 2009. The following adverse reactions have been identified during post approval use of this formulation of CREON. Because these reactions are reported voluntarily from a population of uncertain size, it is not always possible to reliably estimate their frequency or establish a causal relationship to drug exposure.

Gastrointestinal disorders (including abdominal pain, diarrhea, flatulence, constipation and nausea), skin disorders (including pruritus, urticaria and rash), blurred vision, myalgia, muscle spasm, and asymptomatic elevations of liver enzymes have been reported with this formulation of CREON.

Delayed- and immediate-release pancreatic enzyme products with different formulations of the same active ingredient (pancrelipase) have been used for the treatment of patients with exocrine pancreatic insufficiency due to cystic fibrosis and other conditions, such as chronic pancreatitis. The long-term safety profile of these products has been described in the medical literature. The most serious adverse reactions included fibrosing colonopathy, distal intestinal obstruction syndrome (DIOS), recurrence of pre-existing carcinoma, and severe allergic reactions including anaphylaxis, asthma, hives, and pruritus.

7 DRUG INTERACTIONS

No drug interactions have been identified. No formal interaction studies have been conducted.

8 USE IN SPECIFIC POPULATIONS

8.1 Pregnancy

Teratogenic effects

Pregnancy Category C: Animal reproduction studies have not been conducted with pancrelipase. It is also not known whether pancrelipase can cause fetal harm when administered to a pregnant woman or can affect reproduction capacity. CREON should be given to a pregnant woman only if clearly needed. The risk and benefit of pancrelipase should be considered in the context of the need to provide adequate nutritional support to a pregnant woman with exocrine pancreatic insufficiency. Adequate caloric intake during pregnancy is important for normal maternal weight gain and fetal growth. Reduced maternal weight gain and malnutrition can be associated with adverse pregnancy outcomes.

8.3 Nursing Mothers

It is not known whether this drug is excreted in human milk. Because many drugs are excreted in human milk, caution should be exercised when CREON is administered to a nursing woman. The risk and benefit of pancrelipase should be considered in the context of the need to provide adequate nutritional support to a nursing mother with exocrine pancreatic insufficiency.

8.4 Pediatric Use

The short-term safety and effectiveness of CREON were assessed in two randomized, double-blind, placebo-controlled, crossover studies of 49 patients with EPI due to cystic fibrosis, 25 of whom were pediatric patients. Study 1 included 8 adolescents between 12 and 17 years of age. Study 2 included 17 children between 7 and 11 years of age. The safety and efficacy in pediatric patients in these studies were similar to adult patients *[see Adverse Reactions (6.1) and Clinical Studies (14)]*.

An open-label, single-arm, short-term study of CREON was conducted in 18 infants and children, ages 4 months to six years of age, with EPI due to cystic fibrosis. Patients received their usual pancreatic enzyme replacement therapy (mean dose of 7,000 lipase units/kg/day for a mean duration of 18.2 days) followed by CREON (mean dose of 7,500 lipase units/kg/day for a mean duration of 12.6 days). The mean daily fat intake was 48 grams during treatment with usual pancreatic enzyme replacement therapy and 47 grams during treatment with CREON. When patients were switched from their usual pancreatic enzyme replacement therapy to CREON, they demonstrated similar spot fecal fat testing results; the clinical relevance of spot fecal fat testing has not been demonstrated. Adverse reactions that occurred in patients during treatment with CREON were vomiting, irritability, and decreased appetite *[see Adverse Reactions (6.1)]*.

The safety and efficacy of pancreatic enzyme products with different formulations of pancrelipase consisting of the same active ingredient (lipases, proteases, and amylases) for treatment of children with exocrine pancreatic insufficiency due to cystic fibrosis have been described in the medical literature and through clinical experience.

Dosing of pediatric patients should be in accordance with recommended guidance from the Cystic Fibrosis Foundation Consensus Conferences *[see Dosage and Administration (2.1)]*. Doses of other pancreatic enzyme products exceeding 6,000 lipase units/kg of body weight per meal have been associated with fibrosing colonopathy and colonic strictures in children less than 12 years of age *[see Warnings and Precautions (5.1)]*.

8.5 Geriatric Use

Clinical studies of CREON did not include sufficient numbers of subjects aged 65 and over to determine whether they respond differently from younger subjects. Other reported clinical experience has not identified differences in responses between the elderly and younger patients.

10 OVERDOSAGE

There have been no reports of overdose in clinical trials or postmarketing surveillance with this formulation of CREON. Chronic high doses of pancreatic enzyme products have been associated with fibrosing colonopathy and colonic strictures *[see Dosage and Administration (2.2) and Warnings and Precautions (5.1)]*. High doses of pancreatic enzyme products have been associated with hyperuricosuria and hyperuricemia, and should be used with caution in patients with a history of hyperuricemia, gout, or renal impairment *[see Warnings and Precautions (5.3)]*.

11 DESCRIPTION

CREON is a pancreatic enzyme preparation consisting of pancrelipase, an extract derived from porcine pancreatic glands. Pancrelipase contains multiple enzyme classes, including porcine-derived lipases, proteases, and amylases.

Pancrelipase is a beige-white amorphous powder. It is miscible in water and practically insoluble or insoluble in alcohol and ether.

Each delayed-release capsule for oral administration contains enteric-coated spheres (0.71–1.60 mm in diameter).

The active ingredient evaluated in clinical trials is lipase. CREON is dosed by lipase units.

Other active ingredients include protease and amylase.

CREON contains the following inactive ingredients: cetyl alcohol, dimethicone, hypromellose phthalate, polyethylene glycol, and triethyl citrate.

<u>3,000 USP units of lipase;</u> 9,500 USP units of protease; 15,000 USP units of amylase delayed-release capsules have a white opaque cap with imprint "CREON 1203" and a white opaque body. The shells contain titanium dioxide and hypromellose.

<u>6,000 USP units of lipase;</u> 19,000 USP units of protease; 30,000 USP units of amylase delayed-release capsules have a Swedish-orange opaque cap with imprint "CREON 1206" and a blue opaque body. The shells contain FD&C Blue No. 2, gelatin, red iron oxide, sodium lauryl sulfate, titanium dioxide, and yellow iron oxide.

<u>12,000 USP units of lipase;</u> 38,000 USP units of protease; 60,000 USP units of amylase delayed-release capsules have a brown opaque cap with imprint "CREON 1212" and a colorless transparent body. The shells contain black iron oxide, gelatin, red iron oxide, sodium lauryl sulfate, titanium dioxide, and yellow iron oxide.

<u>24,000 USP units of lipase;</u> 76,000 USP units of protease; 120,000 USP units of amylase delayed-release capsules have a Swedish-orange opaque cap with imprint "CREON 1224" and a colorless transparent body. The shells contain gelatin, red iron oxide, sodium lauryl sulfate, titanium dioxide, and yellow iron oxide.

<u>36,000 USP units of lipase;</u> 114,000 USP units of protease; 180,000 USP units of amylase delayed-release capsules have a blue opaque cap with imprint "CREON 1236" and a colorless transparent body. The shells contain gelatin, titanium dioxide, FD&C Blue No. 2 and sodium lauryl sulfate.

12 CLINICAL PHARMACOLOGY

12.1 Mechanism of Action

The pancreatic enzymes in CREON® (pancrelipase) catalyze the hydrolysis of fats to monoglyceride, glycerol and free fatty acids, proteins into peptides and amino acids, and starches into dextrins and short chain sugars such as maltose and maltriose in the duodenum and proximal small intestine, thereby acting like digestive enzymes physiologically secreted by the pancreas.

12.3 Pharmacokinetics

The pancreatic enzymes in CREON are enteric-coated to minimize destruction or inactivation in gastric acid. CREON is designed to release most of the enzymes *in vivo* at an approximate pH of 5.5 or greater. Pancreatic enzymes are not absorbed from the gastrointestinal tract in appreciable amounts.

13 NONCLINICAL TOXICOLOGY

13.1 Carcinogenesis, Mutagenesis, Impairment of Fertility

Carcinogenicity, genetic toxicology, and animal fertility studies have not been performed with pancrelipase.

14 CLINICAL STUDIES

The short-term efficacy of CREON was evaluated in three studies conducted in 103 patients with exocrine pancreatic insufficiency (EPI). Two studies were conducted in 49 patients with EPI due to cystic fibrosis (CF); one study was conducted in 54 patients with EPI due to chronic pancreatitis or pancreatectomy.

14.1 Cystic Fibrosis

Studies 1 and 2 were randomized, double-blind, placebo-controlled, crossover studies in 49 patients, ages 7 to 43 years, with exocrine pancreatic insufficiency due to cystic fibrosis. Study 1 included patients aged 12 to 43 years (n = 32). The final analysis population was limited to 29 patients; 3 patients were excluded due to protocol deviations. Study 2 included patients aged 7 to 11 years (n = 17). The final analysis population was limited to 16 patients; 1 patient withdrew consent prior to stool collection during treatment with CREON. In each study, patients were randomized to receive CREON at a dose of 4,000 lipase units/g fat ingested per day or matching placebo for 5 to 6 days of treatment, followed by crossover to the alternate treatment for an additional 5 to 6 days. All patients consumed a high-fat diet (greater than or equal to 90 grams of fat per day, 40% of daily calories derived from fat) during the treatment periods.

The coefficient of fat absorption (CFA) was determined by a 72-hour stool collection during both treatments, when both fat excretion and fat ingestion were measured. Each patient's CFA during placebo treatment was used as their no-treatment CFA value.

In Study 1, mean CFA was 89% with CREON treatment compared to 49% with placebo treatment. The mean difference in CFA was 41 percentage points in favor of CREON treatment with 95% CI: (34, 47) and $p<0.001$.

In Study 2, mean CFA was 83% with CREON treatment compared to 47% with placebo treatment. The mean difference in CFA was 35 percentage points in favor of CREON treatment with 95% CI: (27, 44) and $p<0.001$.

Subgroup analyses of the CFA results in Studies 1 and 2 showed that mean change in CFA with CREON treatment was greater in patients with lower no-treatment (placebo) CFA values than in patients with higher no-treatment (placebo) CFA values. There were no differences in response to CREON by age or gender, with similar responses to CREON observed in male and female patients, and in younger (under 18 years of age) and older patients.

The coefficient of nitrogen absorption (CNA) was determined by a 72-hour stool collection during both treatments, when nitrogen excretion was measured and nitrogen ingestion from a controlled diet was estimated (based on the assumption that proteins contain 16% nitrogen). Each patient's CNA during placebo treatment was used as their no-treatment CNA value.

In Study 1, mean CNA was 86% with CREON treatment compared to 49% with placebo treatment. The mean difference in CNA was 37 percentage points in favor of CREON treatment with 95% CI: (31, 42) and $p<0.001$.

In Study 2, mean CNA was 80% with CREON treatment compared to 45% with placebo treatment. The mean difference in CNA was 35 percentage points in favor of CREON treatment with 95% CI: (26, 45) and $p<0.001$.

14.2 Chronic Pancreatitis or Pancreatectomy

A randomized, double-blind, placebo-controlled, parallel group study was conducted in 54 adult patients, ages 32 to 75 years, with EPI due to chronic pancreatitis or pancreatectomy. The final analysis population was limited to 52 patients; 2 patients were excluded due to protocol violations. Ten patients had a history of pancreatectomy (7 were treated with CREON). In this study, patients received placebo for 5 days (run-in period), followed by pancreatic enzyme replacement therapy as directed by the investigator for 16 days; this was followed by randomization to CREON or matching placebo for 7 days of treatment (double-blind period). Only patients with CFA less than 80% in the run-in period were randomized to the double-blind period. The dose of CREON during the double-blind period was 72,000 lipase units per main meal (3 main meals) and 36,000 lipase units per snack (2 snacks). All patients consumed a high-fat diet (greater than or equal to 100 grams of fat per day) during the treatment period.

The CFA was determined by a 72-hour stool collection during the run-in and double-blind treatment periods, when both fat excretion and fat ingestion were measured. The mean change in CFA from the run-in period to the end of the double-blind period in the CREON and Placebo groups is shown in Table 3.

Table 3: Change in CFA in the Chronic Pancreatitis and Pancreatectomy Trial (Run-in Period to End of Double-Blind Period)

	CREON n = 24	Placebo n = 28
CFA [%]		
Run-in Period (Mean, SD)	54 (19)	57 (21)
End of Double-Blind Period (Mean, SD)	86 (6)	66 (20)
Change in CFA * [%]		
Run-in Period to End of Double-Blind Period (Mean, SD)	32 (18)	9 (13)
Treatment Difference (95% CI)	21 (14, 28)	

*p<0.0001

Subgroup analyses of the CFA results showed that mean change in CFA was greater in patients with lower run-in period CFA values than in patients with higher run-in period CFA values. Only 1 of the patients with a history of total pancreatectomy was treated with CREON in the study. That patient had a CFA of 26% during the run-in period and a CFA of 73% at the end of the double-blind period. The remaining 6 patients with a history of partial pancreatectomy treated with CREON on the study had a mean CFA of 42% during the run-in period and a mean CFA of 84% at the end of the double-blind period.

15 REFERENCES

[1] Borowitz DS, Grand RJ, Durie PR, et al. Use of pancreatic enzyme supplements for patients with cystic fibrosis in the context of fibrosing colonopathy. *Journal of Pediatrics.* 1995; 127: 681-684.

[2] Borowitz DS, Baker RD, Stallings V. Consensus report on nutrition for pediatric patients with cystic fibrosis. *Journal of Pediatric Gastroenterology Nutrition.* 2002 Sep; 35: 246-259.

[3] Stallings VA, Stark LJ, Robinson KA, et al. Evidence-based practice recommendations for nutrition-related management of children and adults with cystic fibrosis and pancreatic insufficiency: results of a systematic review. *Journal of the American Dietetic Association*. 2008; 108: 832-839.

[4] Dominguez-Munoz JE. Pancreatic enzyme therapy for pancreatic exocrine insufficiency. *Current Gastroenterology Reports.* 2007; 9: 116-122.

[5] Smyth RL, Ashby D, O'Hea U, et al. Fibrosing colonopathy in cystic fibrosis: results of a case-control study. *Lancet.* 1995; 346: 1247-1251.

[6] FitzSimmons SC, Burkhart GA, Borowitz DS, et al. High-dose pancreatic-enzyme supplements and fibrosing colonopathy in children with cystic fibrosis. *New England Journal of Medicine.* 1997; 336: 1283-1289.

16 HOW SUPPLIED/STORAGE AND HANDLING

CREON® (pancrelipase) Delayed-Release Capsules
3,000 USP units of lipase; 9,500 USP units of protease; 15,000 USP units of amylase
Each CREON capsule is available as a two piece hypromellose capsule with a white opaque cap with imprint "CREON 1203" and a white opaque body that contains tan colored, delayed-release pancrelipase supplied in bottles of:
- 70 capsules (NDC 0032-1203-70)

CREON (pancrelipase) Delayed-Release Capsules
6,000 USP units of lipase; 19,000 USP units of protease; 30,000 USP units of amylase
Each CREON capsule is available as a two-piece gelatin capsule with orange opaque cap with imprint "CREON 1206" and a blue opaque body that contains tan-colored, delayed-release pancrelipase supplied in bottles of:
- 100 capsules (NDC 0032-1206-01)
- 250 capsules (NDC 0032-1206-07)

CREON (pancrelipase) Delayed-Release Capsules
12,000 USP units of lipase; 38,000 USP units of protease; 60,000 USP units of amylase
Each CREON capsule is available as a two-piece gelatin capsule with a brown opaque cap with imprint "CREON 1212" and a colorless transparent body that contains tan-colored, delayed-release pancrelipase supplied in bottles of:
- 100 capsules (NDC 0032-1212-01)
- 250 capsules (NDC 0032-1212-07)

CREON (pancrelipase) Delayed-Release Capsules
24,000 USP units of lipase; 76,000 USP units of protease; 120,000 USP units of amylase
Each CREON capsule is available as a two-piece gelatin capsule with orange opaque cap with imprint "CREON 1224" and a colorless transparent body that contains tan-colored, delayed-release pancrelipase supplied in bottles of:
- 100 capsules (NDC 0032-1224-01)
- 250 capsules (NDC 0032-1224-07)

CREON (pancrelipase) Delayed-Release Capsules
36,000 USP units of lipase; 114,000 USP units of protease; 180,000 USP units of amylase
Each CREON capsule is available as a two-piece gelatin capsule with blue opaque cap with imprint "CREON 1236" and a colorless transparent body that contains tan-colored, delayed-release pancrelipase supplied in bottles of:
- 100 capsules (NDC 0032-3016-13)
- 250 capsules (NDC 0032-3016-28)

Storage and Handling
CREON must be stored at room temperature up to 25°C (77°F) and protected from moisture. Temperature excursions are permitted between 25°C to 40°C (77°F and 104°F) for up to 30 days. Product should be discarded if exposed to higher temperature and moisture conditions higher than 70%. After opening, keep bottle tightly closed between uses to protect from moisture.
Bottles of CREON 3,000 USP units of lipase must be stored and dispensed in the original container.
Do not crush CREON delayed-release capsules or the capsule contents.

17 PATIENT COUNSELING INFORMATION

See FDA-approved patient labeling (Medication Guide)

17.1 Dosing and Administration

- Instruct patients and caregivers that CREON should only be taken as directed by their healthcare professional. Patients should be advised that the total daily dose should not exceed 10,000 lipase units/kg body weight/day unless clinically indicated. This needs to be especially emphasized for patients eating multiple snacks and meals per day. Patients should be informed that if a dose is missed, the next dose should be taken with the next meal or snack as directed. Doses should not be doubled *[see Dosage and Administration (2)]*.
- Instruct patients and caregivers that CREON should always be taken with food. Patients should be advised that CREON delayed-release capsules and the capsule contents must not be crushed or chewed as doing so could cause early release of enzymes and/or loss of enzymatic activity. Patients should swallow the intact capsules with adequate amounts of liquid at mealtimes. If necessary, the capsule contents can also be sprinkled on soft acidic foods *[see Dosage and Administration (2)]*.

17.2 Fibrosing Colonopathy

Advise patients and caregivers to follow dosing instructions carefully, as doses of pancreatic enzyme products exceeding 6,000 lipase units/kg of body weight per meal have been associated with colonic strictures in children below the age of 12 years *[see Dosage and Administration (2)]*.

17.3 Allergic Reactions

Advise patients and caregivers to contact their healthcare professional immediately if allergic reactions to CREON develop *[see Warnings and Precautions (5.5)]*.

17.4 Pregnancy and Breast Feeding

- Instruct patients to notify their healthcare professional if they are pregnant or are thinking of becoming pregnant during treatment with CREON *[see Use in Specific Populations (8.1)]*.
- Instruct patients to notify their healthcare professional if they are breast feeding or are thinking of breast feeding during treatment with CREON *[see Use in Specific Populations (8.3)]*.

Manufactured by:
Abbott Laboratories GmbH
Hannover, Germany
Marketed by:
AbbVie Inc.
North Chicago, IL 60064, U.S.A.

1083531 March, 2013

MEDICATION GUIDE
CREON® (krē 'ŏn)
(pancrelipase)
Delayed-Release Capsules

Read this Medication Guide before you start taking CREON and each time you get a refill. There may be new information. This information does not take the place of talking to your doctor about your medical condition or treatment.

What is the most important information I should know about CREON?

CREON may increase your chance of having a rare bowel disorder called fibrosing colonopathy. This condition is serious and may require surgery. The risk of having this condition may be reduced by following the dosing instructions that your doctor gave you. **Call your doctor right away if you have any unusual or severe:**
- stomach area (abdominal) pain
- bloating
- trouble passing stool (having bowel movements)
- nausea, vomiting, or diarrhea

Take CREON exactly as prescribed. Do not take more or less CREON than directed by your doctor.

What is CREON?

CREON is a prescription medicine used to treat people who cannot digest food normally because their pancreas does not make enough enzymes due to cystic fibrosis, swelling of the pancreas that lasts a long time (chronic pancreatitis), removal of some or all of the pancreas (pancreatectomy), or other conditions. CREON may help your body use fats, proteins, and sugars from food.
CREON contains a mixture of digestive enzymes including lipases, proteases, and amylases from pig pancreas.

What should I tell my doctor before taking CREON?

Before taking CREON, tell your doctor about all your medical conditions, including if you:
- are allergic to pork (pig) products
- have a history of intestinal blockage of your intestines, or scarring or thickening of your bowel wall (fibrosing colonopathy)
- have gout, kidney disease, or high blood uric acid (hyperuricemia)
- have trouble swallowing capsules
- have any other medical condition
- are pregnant or plan to become pregnant. It is not known if CREON will harm your unborn baby.
- are breast-feeding or plan to breast-feed. It is not known if CREON passes into your breast milk.

Tell your doctor about all the medicines you take, including prescription and nonprescription medicines, vitamins, and herbal supplements.
Know the medicines you take. Keep a list of them and show it to your doctor and pharmacist when you get a new medicine.

How should I take CREON?
- **Take CREON exactly as your doctor tells you.**
- You should not switch CREON with any other pancreatic enzyme product without first talking to your doctor.
- Do not take more capsules in a day than the number your doctor tells you to take (total daily dose).
- Always take CREON with a meal or snack and enough liquid to swallow CREON completely. If you eat a lot of meals or snacks in a day, be careful not to go over your total daily dose.
- Your doctor may change your dose based on the amount of fatty foods you eat or based on your weight.
- **Do not crush or chew CREON capsules or its contents, and do not hold the capsule or capsule contents in your mouth.** Crushing, chewing or holding the CREON capsules in your mouth may cause irritation in your mouth or change the way CREON works in your body.

Giving CREON to infants (children up to 12 months)
1. Give CREON right before each feeding of formula or breast milk.
2. Do not mix CREON capsule contents directly into formula or breast milk.
3. Open the capsules and sprinkle the contents directly into your infant's mouth or mix the contents in a small amount of room temperature acidic soft food such as applesauce. These foods should be the kind found in baby food jars that you buy at the store, or other food recommended by your doctor.
4. If you sprinkle the CREON on food, give the CREON and food mixture to your child right away. Do not store CREON that is mixed with food.
5. Give your child enough liquid to completely swallow the CREON contents or the CREON and food mixture.
6. Look in your child's mouth to make sure that all of the medicine has been swallowed.

Giving CREON to children and adults
1. Swallow CREON capsules whole and take them with enough liquid to swallow them right away.
2. If you have trouble swallowing capsules, open the capsules and sprinkle the contents on a small amount of room temperature acidic food such as applesauce. Ask your doctor about other foods you can mix with CREON.
3. If you sprinkle CREON on food, swallow it right after you mix it and drink enough water or juice to make sure the medicine is swallowed completely. Do not store CREON that is mixed with food.
4. If you forget to take CREON, call your doctor or wait until your next meal and take your usual number of capsules. Take your next dose at your usual time. **Do not make up for missed doses.**

What are the possible side effects of CREON?

CREON may cause serious side effects, including:
- See " **What is the most important information I should know about CREON?** "
- **Irritation of the inside of your mouth.** This can happen if CREON is not swallowed completely.
- **Increase in blood uric acid levels. This may cause worsening of swollen, painful joints (gout) caused by an increase in your blood uric acid levels.**
- **Allergic reactions, including trouble with breathing, skin rashes, or swollen lips.**

Call your doctor right away if you have any of these symptoms.

The most common side effects of CREON include:
- Blood sugar increase (hyperglycemia) or decrease (hypoglycemia)
- Pain in your stomach (abdominal area)
- Frequent or abnormal bowel movements
- Gas
- Vomiting
- Dizziness
- Sore throat and cough

Other Possible Side Effects:
CREON and other pancreatic enzyme products are made from the pancreas of pigs, the same pigs people eat as pork. These pigs may carry viruses. Although it has never been reported, it may be possible for a person to get a viral infection from taking pancreatic enzyme products that come from pigs.
Tell your doctor if you have any side effect that bothers you or that does not go away.
These are not all the side effects of CREON. For more information, ask your doctor or pharmacist.
Call your doctor for medical advice about side effects. You may report side effects to the FDA at 1-800-FDA-1088.
You may also report side effects to AbbVie Inc. at 1-800-633-9110.

How should I store CREON?
- Store CREON® (pancrelipase) at room temperature below 77°F (25°C). Avoid heat.
- You may store CREON at a temperature between 77°F to 104°F (25°C to 40°C) for up to 30 days. Throw away any CREON stored at these temperatures for more than 30 days.
- Keep CREON in a dry place and in the original container.
- After opening the bottle, keep it closed tightly between uses to protect from moisture.

Keep CREON and all medicines out of the reach of children.
General information about CREON
Medicines are sometimes prescribed for purposes other than those listed in a Medication Guide. Do not use CREON for a condition for which it was not prescribed. Do not give CREON to other people to take, even if they have the same symptoms you have. It may harm them.
This Medication Guide summarizes the most important information about CREON. If you would like more information, talk to your doctor. You can ask your doctor or pharmacist for information about CREON that is written for healthcare professionals. For more information, go to www.creon-us.com or call toll-free [1-800-633-9110].

What are the ingredients in CREON?
Active Ingredient: lipase, protease, amylase
Inactive Ingredients: cetyl alcohol, dimethicone, hypromellose phthalate, polyethylene glycol, and triethyl citrate.
The shells of the CREON 6,000 USP units of lipase, 12,000 USP units of lipase, and 24,000 USP units of lipase strengths contain: gelatin, red iron oxide, sodium lauryl sulfate, titanium dioxide, and yellow iron oxide.
In addition:
The shells for the CREON 3,000 USP units of lipase strength capsules contain titanium dioxide and hypromellose.
The shells of the CREON 6,000 USP units of lipase strength capsules contain FD&C Blue No. 2.
The shells of the CREON 12,000 USP units of lipase strength capsules contain black iron oxide.
The shells of the CREON 36,000 USP units of lipase strength capsules contain gelatin, titanium dioxide, sodium lauryl sulfate and FD&C Blue No. 2.
This Medication Guide has been approved by the U.S. Food and Drug Administration.
Manufactured for:
AbbVie Inc.
North Chicago, IL 60064, U.S.A.

1083531 March, 2013
Shown in Product Identification Guide, page 303

DEPAKOTE ER ℞
[*dĕp'ă-kōte*]
(divalproex sodium)
Extended Release Tablets

HIGHLIGHTS OF PRESCRIBING INFORMATION
These highlights do not include all the information needed to use Depakote ER safely and effectively. See full prescribing information for Depakote ER.
Depakote ER (divalproex sodium) Tablet, Extended Release for Oral use
Initial U.S. Approval: 2000

WARNING: LIFE THREATENING ADVERSE REACTIONS
See full prescribing information for complete boxed warning.
- **Hepatotoxicity, including fatalities, usually during first 6 months of treatment. Children under the age of two years and patients with mitochondrial disorders are at higher risk. Monitor patients closely, and perform serum liver testing prior to therapy and at frequent intervals thereafter (5.1)**
- **Fetal Risk, particularly neural tube defects, other major malformations, and decreased IQ (5.2, 5.3, 5.4)**
- **Pancreatitis, including fatal hemorrhagic cases (5.5)**

RECENT MAJOR CHANGES
Boxed Warning, Hepatotoxicity 05/2013
Boxed Warning, Fetal Risk 05/2013
Indications and Usage, Important Limitations (1.4) 05/2013
Contraindications, Known or Suspected Mitochondrial Disorders (4) 05/2013
Contraindications, Prophylaxis of Migraines in Pregnancy (4) 05/2013
Warnings and Precautions, Hepatotoxicity (5.1) 05/2013
Warnings and Precautions, Birth Defects (5.2) 05/2013
Warnings and Precautions, Decreased IQ (5.3) 05/2013
Warnings and Precautions, Use in Women of Childbearing Potential (5.4) 05/2013
Warnings and Precautions, Brain Atrophy (5.7) 05/2013
Warning and Precautions, Medication Residue in the Stool (5.19) 02/2013

INDICATIONS AND USAGE
Depakote ER is an anti-epileptic drug indicated for:
- Acute treatment of manic or mixed episodes associated with bipolar disorder, with or without psychotic features (1.1)
- Monotherapy and adjunctive therapy of complex partial seizures and simple and complex absence seizures; adjunctive therapy in patients with multiple seizure types that include absence seizures (1.2)
- Prophylaxis of migraine headaches (1.3)

DOSAGE AND ADMINISTRATION
- Depakote ER is intended for once-a-day oral administration. Depakote ER should be swallowed whole and should not be crushed or chewed (2.1, 2.2).
- Mania: Initial dose is 25 mg/kg/day, increasing as rapidly as possible to achieve therapeutic response or desired plasma level (2.1). The maximum recommended dosage is 60 mg/kg/day (2.1, 2.2).
- Complex Partial Seizures: Start at 10 to 15 mg/kg/day, increasing at 1 week intervals by 5 to 10 mg/kg/day to achieve optimal clinical response; if response is not satisfactory, check valproate plasma level; see full prescribing information for conversion to monotherapy (2.2). The maximum recommended dosage is 60 mg/kg/day (2.1, 2.2).
- Absence Seizures: Start at 15 mg/kg/day, increasing at 1 week intervals by 5 to 10 mg/kg/day until seizure control or limiting side effects (2.2). The maximum recommended dosage is 60 mg/kg/day (2.1, 2.2).
- Migraine: The recommended starting dose is 500 mg/day for 1 week, thereafter increasing to 1000 mg/day (2.3).

DOSAGE FORMS AND STRENGTHS
Tablets: 250 mg and 500 mg (3)

CONTRAINDICATIONS
- Hepatic disease or significant hepatic dysfunction (4, 5.1)
- Known mitochondrial disorders caused by mutations in mitochondrial DNA polymerase γ (POLG) (4, 5.1)
- Suspected POLG-related disorder in children under two years of age (4, 5.1)
- Known hypersensitivity to the drug (4, 5.12)
- Urea cycle disorders (4, 5.6)
- Pregnant patients treated for prophylaxis of migraine headaches (4, 8.1)

WARNINGS AND PRECAUTIONS
- Hepatotoxicity; evaluate high risk populations and monitor serum liver tests (5.1)
- Birth defects and decreased IQ following *in utero* exposure; only use to treat pregnant women with epilepsy or bipolar disorder if other medications are unacceptable; should not be administered to a woman of childbearing potential unless essential (5.2, 5.3, 5.4)
- Pancreatitis; Depakote ER should ordinarily be discontinued (5.5)
- Brain Atrophy; evaluate for continued use in the presence of suspected or apparent signs of reversible or irreversible cerebral and cerebellar atrophy (5.7)
- Suicidal behavior or ideation; Antiepileptic drugs, including Depakote ER, increase the risk of suicidal thoughts or behavior (5.8)
- Thrombocytopenia; monitor platelet counts and coagulation tests (5.9)
- Hyperammonemia and hyperammonemic encephalopathy; measure ammonia level if unexplained lethargy and vomiting or changes in mental status, and also with concomitant topiramate use; consider discontinuation of valproate therapy (5.6, 5.10, 5.11)
- Hypothermia; Hypothermia has been reported during valproate therapy with or without associated hyperammonemia. This adverse reaction can also occur in patients using concomitant topiramate (5.12)
- Multi-organ hypersensitivity reaction; discontinue Depakote ER (5.13)
- Somnolence in the elderly can occur. Depakote ER dosage should be increased slowly and with regular monitoring for fluid and nutritional intake (5.15)

ADVERSE REACTIONS
- Most common adverse reactions (reported >5%) reported in adult studies are nausea, somnolence, dizziness, vomiting, asthenia, abdominal pain, dyspepsia, rash, diarrhea, increased appetite, tremor, weight gain, back pain, alopecia, headache, fever, anorexia, constipation, diplopia, amblyopia/blurred, ataxia, nystagmus, emotional lability, thinking abnormal, amnesia, flu syndrome, infection, bronchitis, rhinitis, ecchymosis, peripheral edema, insomnia, nervousness, depression, pharyngitis, dyspnea, tinnitus (6.1, 6.2, 6.3, 6.4).
- The safety and tolerability of valproate in pediatric patients were shown to be comparable to those in adults (8.4).

To report SUSPECTED ADVERSE REACTIONS, contact AbbVie Inc. at 1-800-633-9110 or FDA at 1-800-FDA-1088 or www.fda.gov/medwatch

DRUG INTERACTIONS
- Hepatic enzyme-inducing drugs (e.g., phenytoin, carbamazepine, primidone, phenobarbital, rifampin) can increase valproate clearance, while enzyme inhibitors (e.g., felbamate) can decrease valproate clearance. Therefore increased monitoring of valproate and concomitant drug concentrations and dose adjustment is indicated whenever enzyme-inducing or inhibiting drugs are introduced or withdrawn (7.1)
- Aspirin, carbapenem antibiotics: Monitoring of valproate concentrations are recommended (7.1)
- Co-administration of valproate can affect the pharmacokinetics of other drugs (e.g. diazepam, ethosuximide, lamotrigine, phenytoin) by inhibiting their metabolism or protein binding displacement (7.2)
- Dosage adjustment of amitryptyline/nortryptyline, warfarin, and zidovudine may be necessary if used concomitantly with Depakote ER (7.2)
- Topiramate: Hyperammonemia and encephalopathy (5.11, 7.3)

USE IN SPECIFIC POPULATIONS
- Pregnancy: Depakote ER can cause congenital malformations including neural tube defects and decreased IQ. (5.2, 5.3, 8.1)
- Pediatric: Children under the age of two years are at considerably higher risk of fatal hepatotoxicity (5.1, 8.4)
- Geriatric: Reduce starting dose; increase dosage more slowly; monitor fluid and nutritional intake, and somnolence (5.15, 8.5)

See 17 for PATIENT COUNSELING INFORMATION and Medication Guide

Revised: 05/2013

FULL PRESCRIBING INFORMATION: CONTENTS*

Information on the AbbVie, Inc. products listed on these pages is from the prescribing information in use as of July 31, 2013. For more information, please visit rxabbvie.com or call 1-800-633-9110.

*** Sections or subsections omitted from the full prescribing information are not listed**

FULL PRESCRIBING INFORMATION

WARNING: LIFE THREATENING ADVERSE REACTIONS

Hepatotoxicity

General Population: **Hepatic failure resulting in fatalities has occurred in patients receiving valproate and its derivatives. These incidents usually have occurred during the first six months of treatment. Serious or fatal hepatotoxicity may be preceded by non-specific symptoms such as malaise, weakness, lethargy, facial edema, anorexia, and vomiting. In patients with epilepsy, a loss of seizure control may also occur. Patients should be monitored closely for appearance of these symptoms. Serum liver tests should be performed prior to therapy and at frequent intervals thereafter, especially during the first six months *[see Warnings and Precautions (5.1)]*.**

Children under the age of two years are at a considerably increased risk of developing fatal hepatotoxicity, especially those on multiple anticonvulsants, those with congenital metabolic disorders, those with severe seizure disorders accompanied by mental retardation, and those with organic brain disease. When Depakote ER is used in this patient group, it should be used with extreme caution and as a sole agent. The benefits of therapy should be weighed against the risks. The incidence of fatal hepatotoxicity decreases considerably in progressively older patient groups.

Patients with Mitochondrial Disease: **There is an increased risk of valproate-induced acute liver failure and resultant deaths in patients with hereditary neurometabolic syndromes caused by DNA mutations of the mitochondrial DNA Polymerase γ (POLG) gene (e.g. Alpers Huttenlocher Syndrome). Depakote ER is contraindicated in patients known to have mitochondrial disorders caused by POLG mutations and children under two years of age who are clinically suspected of having a mitochondrial disorder *[see Contraindications (4)]*. In patients over two years of age who are clinically suspected of having a hereditary mitochondrial disease, Depakote ER should only be used after other anticonvulsants have failed. This older group of patients should be closely monitored during treatment with Depakote ER for the development of acute liver injury with regular clinical assessments and serum liver testing. POLG mutation screening should be performed in accordance with current clinical practice *[see Warnings and Precautions (5.1)]*.**

Fetal Risk

Valproate can cause major congenital malformations, particularly neural tube defects (e.g., spina bifida). In addition, valproate can cause decreased IQ scores following *in utero* exposure.

Valproate is therefore contraindicated in pregnant women treated for prophylaxis of migraine *[see Contraindications (4)]*. Valproate should only be used to treat pregnant women with epilepsy or bipolar disorder if other medications have failed to control their symptoms or are otherwise unacceptable.

Valproate should not be administered to a woman of childbearing potential unless the drug is essential to the management of her medical condition. This is especially important when valproate use is considered for a condition not usually associated with permanent injury or death (e.g., migraine). Women should use effective contraception while using valproate *[see Warnings and Precautions (5.2, 5.3, 5.4)]*.

A Medication Guide describing the risks of valproate is available for patients *[see Patient Counseling Information (17)]*.

Pancreatitis

Cases of life-threatening pancreatitis have been reported in both children and adults receiving valproate. Some of the cases have been described as hemorrhagic with a rapid progression from initial symptoms to death. Cases have been reported shortly after initial use as well as after several years of use. Patients and guardians should be warned that abdominal pain, nausea, vomiting and/or anorexia can be symptoms of pancreatitis that require prompt medical evaluation. If pancreatitis is diagnosed, valproate should ordinarily be discontinued. Alternative treatment for the underlying medical condition should be initiated as clinically indicated *[see Warnings and Precautions (5.5)]*.

1 INDICATIONS AND USAGE

1.1 Mania

Depakote ER is a valproate and is indicated for the treatment of acute manic or mixed episodes associated with bipolar disorder, with or without psychotic features. A manic episode is a distinct period of abnormally and persistently elevated, expansive, or irritable mood. Typical symptoms of mania include pressure of speech, motor hyperactivity, reduced need for sleep, flight of ideas, grandiosity, poor judgment, aggressiveness, and possible hostility. A mixed episode is characterized by the criteria for a manic episode in conjunction with those for a major depressive episode (depressed mood, loss of interest or pleasure in nearly all activities).

The efficacy of Depakote ER is based in part on studies of Depakote (divalproex sodium delayed release tablets) in this indication, and was confirmed in a 3-week trial with patients meeting DSM-IV TR criteria for bipolar I disorder, manic or mixed type, who were hospitalized for acute mania *[see Clinical Studies (14.1)]*.

The effectiveness of valproate for long-term use in mania, i.e., more than 3 weeks, has not been demonstrated in controlled clinical trials. Therefore, healthcare providers who elect to use Depakote ER for extended periods should continually reevaluate the long-term risk-benefits of the drug for the individual patient.

1.2 Epilepsy

Depakote ER is indicated as monotherapy and adjunctive therapy in the treatment of adult patients and pediatric patients down to the age of 10 years with complex partial seizures that occur either in isolation or in association with other types of seizures. Depakote ER is also indicated for use as sole and adjunctive therapy in the treatment of simple and complex absence seizures in adults and children 10 years of age or older, and adjunctively in adults and children 10 years of age or older with multiple seizure types that include absence seizures.

Simple absence is defined as very brief clouding of the sensorium or loss of consciousness accompanied by certain generalized epileptic discharges without other detectable clinical signs. Complex absence is the term used when other signs are also present.

1.3 Migraine

Depakote ER is indicated for prophylaxis of migraine headaches. There is no evidence that Depakote ER is useful in the acute treatment of migraine headaches.

1.4 Important Limitations

Because of the risk to the fetus of decreased IQ, neural tube defects, and other major congenital malformations, which may occur very early in pregnancy, valproate should not be administered to a woman of childbearing potential unless the drug is essential to the management of her medical condition *[see Warnings and Precautions (5.2, 5.3, 5.4), Use in Specific Populations (8.1), and Patient Counseling Information (17.3)]*.

Depakote ER is contraindicated for prophylaxis of migraine headaches in women who are pregnant.

2 DOSAGE AND ADMINISTRATION

Depakote ER is an extended-release product intended for once-a-day oral administration. Depakote ER tablets should be swallowed whole and should not be crushed or chewed.

2.1 Mania

Depakote ER tablets are administered orally. The recommended initial dose is 25 mg/kg/day given once daily. The dose should be increased as rapidly as possible to achieve the lowest therapeutic dose which produces the desired clinical effect or the desired range of plasma concentrations. In a placebo-controlled clinical trial of acute mania or mixed type, patients were dosed to a clinical response with a trough plasma concentration between 85 and 125 mcg/mL. The maximum recommended dosage is 60 mg/kg/day.

There is no body of evidence available from controlled trials to guide a clinician in the longer term management of a patient who improves during Depakote ER treatment of an acute manic episode. While it is generally agreed that pharmacological treatment beyond an acute response in mania is desirable, both for maintenance of the initial response and for prevention of new manic episodes, there are no data to support the benefits of Depakote ER in such longer-term treatment (i.e., beyond 3 weeks).

2.2 Epilepsy

Depakote ER (divalproex sodium) extended release tablets are administered orally, and must be swallowed whole. As Depakote ER dosage is titrated upward, concentrations of clonazepam, diazepam, ethosuximide, lamotrigine, tolbutamide, phenobarbital, carbamazepine, and/or phenytoin may be affected *[see Drug Interactions (7.2)]*.

Complex Partial Seizures

For adults and children 10 years of age or older.

Monotherapy (Initial Therapy)

Depakote ER has not been systematically studied as initial therapy. Patients should initiate therapy at 10 to 15 mg/kg/day. The dosage should be increased by 5 to 10 mg/kg/week to achieve optimal clinical response. Ordinarily, optimal clinical response is achieved at daily doses below 60 mg/kg/day. If satisfactory clinical response has not been achieved, plasma levels should be measured to determine whether or not they are in the usually accepted therapeutic range (50 to 100 mcg/mL). No recommendation regarding the safety of valproate for use at doses above 60 mg/kg/day can be made. The probability of thrombocytopenia increases significantly at total trough valproate plasma concentrations above 110 mcg/mL in females and 135 mcg/mL in males. The benefit of improved seizure control with higher doses should be weighed against the possibility of a greater incidence of adverse reactions.

Conversion to Monotherapy

Patients should initiate therapy at 10 to 15 mg/kg/day. The dosage should be increased by 5 to 10 mg/kg/week to achieve optimal clinical response. Ordinarily, optimal clinical response is achieved at daily doses below 60 mg/kg/day. If satisfactory clinical response has not been achieved, plasma levels should be measured to determine whether or not they are in the usually accepted therapeutic range (50 - 100 mcg/mL). No recommendation regarding the safety of valproate for use at doses above 60 mg/kg/day can be made.

Concomitant antiepilepsy drug (AED) dosage can ordinarily be reduced by approximately 25% every 2 weeks. This reduction may be started at initiation of Depakote ER therapy, or delayed by 1 to 2 weeks if there is a concern that seizures are likely to occur with a reduction. The speed and duration of withdrawal of the concomitant AED can be highly variable, and patients should be monitored closely during this period for increased seizure frequency.

Adjunctive Therapy

Depakote ER may be added to the patient's regimen at a dosage of 10 to 15 mg/kg/day. The dosage may be increased by 5 to 10 mg/kg/week to achieve optimal clinical response. Ordinarily, optimal clinical response is achieved at daily doses below 60 mg/kg/day. If satisfactory clinical response has not been achieved, plasma levels should be measured to determine whether or not they are in the usually accepted therapeutic range (50 to 100 mcg/mL). No recommendation regarding the safety of valproate for use at doses above 60 mg/kg/day can be made.

In a study of adjunctive therapy for complex partial seizures in which patients were receiving either carbamazepine or phenytoin in addition to valproate, no adjustment of carbamazepine or phenytoin dosage was needed *[see Clinical Studies (14.2)]*. However, since valproate may interact with these or other concurrently administered AEDs as well as other drugs, periodic plasma concentration determinations of concomitant AEDs are recommended during the early course of therapy *[see Drug Interactions (7)]*.

Simple and Complex Absence Seizures

The recommended initial dose is 15 mg/kg/day, increasing at one week intervals by 5 to 10 mg/kg/day until seizures are controlled or side effects preclude further increases. The maximum recommended dosage is 60 mg/kg/day.

A good correlation has not been established between daily dose, serum concentrations, and therapeutic effect. However, therapeutic valproate serum concentration for most patients with absence seizures is considered to range from 50 to 100 mcg/mL. Some patients may be controlled with lower or higher serum concentrations *[see Clinical Pharmacology (12.3)]*.

As Depakote ER dosage is titrated upward, blood concentrations of phenobarbital and/or phenytoin may be affected *[see Drug Interactions (7.2)]*.

Antiepilepsy drugs should not be abruptly discontinued in patients in whom the drug is administered to prevent major seizures because of the strong possibility of precipitating status epilepticus with attendant hypoxia and threat to life.

2.3 Migraine

Depakote ER is indicated for prophylaxis of migraine headaches in adults.

The recommended starting dose is 500 mg once daily for 1 week, thereafter increasing to 1000 mg once daily. Although doses other than 1000 mg once daily of Depakote ER have not been evaluated in patients with migraine, the effective dose range of Depakote (divalproex sodium delayed-release tablets) in these patients is 500-1000 mg/day. As with other valproate products, doses of Depakote ER should be individualized and dose adjustment may be necessary. If a patient requires smaller dose adjustments than that available with Depakote ER, Depakote should be used instead.

2.4 Conversion from Depakote to Depakote ER

In adult patients and pediatric patients 10 years of age or older with epilepsy previously receiving Depakote, Depakote ER should be administered once-daily using a dose 8 to 20% higher than the total daily dose of Depakote (Table 1). For patients whose Depakote total daily dose cannot be directly converted to Depakote ER, consideration may be given at the clinician's discretion to increase the patient's Depakote total daily dose to the next higher dosage before converting to the appropriate total daily dose of Depakote ER.

Table 1. Dose Conversion

Depakote Total Daily Dose (mg)	Depakote ER (mg)
500* - 625	750
750* - 875	1000
1000*-1125	1250
1250-1375	1500
1500-1625	1750
1750	2000
1875-2000	2250
2125-2250	2500
2375	2750
2500-2750	3000
2875	3250
3000-3125	3500

* These total daily doses of Depakote cannot be directly converted to an 8 to 20% higher total daily dose of Depakote ER because the required dosing strengths of Depakote ER are not available. Consideration may be given at the clinician's discretion to increase the patient's Depakote total daily dose to the next higher dosage before converting to the appropriate total daily dose of Depakote ER.

There is insufficient data to allow a conversion factor recommendation for patients with DEPAKOTE doses above 3125 mg/day. Plasma valproate C_{min} concentrations for DEPAKOTE ER on average are equivalent to DEPAKOTE, but may vary across patients after conversion. If satisfactory clinical response has not been achieved, plasma levels should be measured to determine whether or not they are in the usually accepted therapeutic range (50 to 100 mcg/mL) *[see Clinical Pharmacology (12.2)]*.

2.5 General Dosing Advice

Dosing in Elderly Patients

Due to a decrease in unbound clearance of valproate and possibly a greater sensitivity to somnolence in the elderly, the starting dose should be reduced in these patients. Starting doses in the elderly lower than 250 mg can only be achieved by the use of Depakote. Dosage should be increased more slowly and with regular monitoring for fluid and nutritional intake, dehydration, somnolence, and other adverse reactions. Dose reductions or discontinuation of valproate should be considered in patients with decreased food or fluid intake and in patients with excessive somnolence. The ultimate therapeutic dose should be achieved on the basis of both tolerability and clinical response *[see Warnings and Precautions (5.15), Use in Specific Populations (8.5) and Clinical Pharmacology (12.3)]*.

Dose-Related Adverse Reactions

The frequency of adverse effects (particularly elevated liver enzymes and thrombocytopenia) may be dose-related. The probability of thrombocytopenia appears to increase significantly at total valproate concentrations of ≥ 110 mcg/mL (females) or ≥ 135 mcg/mL (males) *[see Warnings and Precautions (5.9)]*. The benefit of improved therapeutic effect with higher doses should be weighed against the possibility of a greater incidence of adverse reactions.

G.I. Irritation

Patients who experience G.I. irritation may benefit from administration of the drug with food or by slowly building up the dose from an initial low level.

Compliance

Patients should be informed to take Depakote ER every day as prescribed. If a dose is missed it should be taken as soon as possible, unless it is almost time for the next dose. If a dose is skipped, the patient should not double the next dose.

3 DOSAGE FORMS AND STRENGTHS

Depakote ER 250 mg is available as white ovaloid tablets with the "a" logo and the code (HF). Each Depakote ER tablet contains divalproex sodium equivalent to 250 mg of valproic acid.

Depakote ER 500 mg is available as gray ovaloid tablets with the "a" logo and the code HC. Each Depakote ER tablet contains divalproex sodium equivalent to 500 mg of valproic acid.

4 CONTRAINDICATIONS

- Depakote ER should not be administered to patients with hepatic disease or significant hepatic dysfunction *[see Warnings and Precautions (5.1)]*.
- Depakote ER is contraindicated in patients known to have mitochondrial disorders caused by mutations in mitochondrial DNA polymerase γ (POLG; e.g., Alpers-Huttenlocher Syndrome) and children under two years of age who are suspected of having a POLG-related disorder *[see Warnings and Precautions (5.1)]*.
- Depakote ER is contraindicated in patients with known hypersensitivity to the drug *[see Warnings and Precautions (5.13)]*.
- Depakote ER is contraindicated in patients with known urea cycle disorders *[see Warnings and Precautions (5.6)]*.
- Depakote ER is contraindicated for use in prophylaxis of migraine headaches in pregnant women *[see Warnings and Precautions (5.3) and Use in Specific Populations (8.1)]*.

5 WARNINGS AND PRECAUTIONS

5.1 Hepatotoxicity

General Information on Hepatotoxicity

Hepatic failure resulting in fatalities has occurred in patients receiving valproate. These incidents usually have occurred during the first six months of treatment. Serious or fatal hepatotoxicity may be preceded by non-specific symptoms such as malaise, weakness, lethargy, facial edema, anorexia, and vomiting. In patients with epilepsy, a loss of seizure control may also occur. Patients should be monitored closely for appearance of these symptoms. Serum liver tests should be performed prior to therapy and at frequent intervals thereafter, especially during the first six months. However, healthcare providers should not rely totally on serum biochemistry since these tests may not be abnormal in all instances, but should also consider the results of careful interim medical history and physical examination.

Caution should be observed when administering valproate products to patients with a prior history of hepatic disease. Patients on multiple anticonvulsants, children, those with congenital metabolic disorders, those with severe seizure disorders accompanied by mental retardation, and those with organic brain disease may be at particular risk. See below, "Patients with Known or Suspected Mitochondrial Disease."

Experience has indicated that children under the age of two years are at a considerably increased risk of developing fatal hepatotoxicity, especially those with the aforementioned conditions. When Depakote ER is used in this patient group, it should be used with extreme caution and as a sole agent. The benefits of therapy should be weighed against the risks. In progressively older patient groups experience in epilepsy has indicated that the incidence of fatal hepatotoxicity decreases considerably.

Patients with Known or Suspected Mitochondrial Disease

Depakote ER is contraindicated in patients known to have mitochondrial disorders caused by POLG mutations and children under two years of age who are clinically suspected of having a mitochondrial disorder *[see Contraindications (4)]*. Valproate-induced acute liver failure and liver-related deaths have been reported in patients with hereditary neurometabolic syndromes caused by mutations in the gene for mitochondrial DNA polymerase γ (POLG) (e.g., Alpers-Huttenlocher Syndrome) at a higher rate than those without these syndromes. Most of the reported cases of liver failure in patients with these syndromes have been identified in children and adolescents.

POLG-related disorders should be suspected in patients with a family history or suggestive symptoms of a POLG-related disorder, including but not limited to unexplained encephalopathy, refractory epilepsy (focal, myoclonic), status epilepticus at presentation, developmental delays, psychomotor regression, axonal sensorimotor neuropathy, myopathy cerebellar ataxia, opthalmoplegia, or complicated migraine with occipital aura. POLG mutation testing should be performed in accordance with current clinical practice for the diagnostic evaluation of such disorders. The A467T and W748S mutations are present in approximately 2/3 of patients with autosomal recessive POLG-related disorders.

In patients over two years of age who are clinically suspected of having a hereditary mitochondrial disease, Depakote ER should only be used after other anticonvulsants have failed. This older group of patients should be closely monitored during treatment with Depakote ER for the development of acute liver injury with regular clinical assessments and serum liver test monitoring.

The drug should be discontinued immediately in the presence of significant hepatic dysfunction, suspected or apparent. In some cases, hepatic dysfunction has progressed in spite of discontinuation of drug *[see Boxed Warning and Contraindications (4)]*.

5.2 Birth Defects

Valproate can cause fetal harm when administered to a pregnant woman. Pregnancy registry data show that maternal valproate use can cause neural tube defects and other structural abnormalities (e.g., craniofacial defects, cardiovascular malformations and malformations involving various body systems). The rate of congenital malformations among babies born to mothers using valproate is about four times higher than the rate among babies born to epileptic mothers using other anti-seizure monotherapies. Evidence suggests that folic acid supplementation prior to conception and during the first trimester of pregnancy decreases the risk for congenital neural tube defects in the general population.

5.3 Decreased IQ Following *in utero* Exposure

Valproate can cause decreased IQ scores following *in utero* exposure. Published epidemiological studies have indicated that children exposed to valproate *in utero* have lower cognitive test scores than children exposed *in utero* to either another antiepileptic drug or to no antiepileptic drugs. The largest of these studies[1] is a prospective cohort study conducted in the United States and United Kingdom that found that children with prenatal exposure to valproate (n=62) had lower IQ scores at age 6 (97 [95% C.I. 94-101]) than children with prenatal exposure to the other antiepileptic drug monotherapy treatments evaluated: lamotrigine (108 [95% C.I. 105–110]), carbamazepine (105 [95% C.I. 102–108]), and phenytoin (108 [95% C.I. 104–112]). It is not known when during pregnancy cognitive effects in valproate-exposed children occur. Because the women in this study were exposed to antiepileptic drugs throughout pregnancy, whether the risk for decreased IQ was related to a particular time period during pregnancy could not be assessed.

Although all of the available studies have methodological limitations, the weight of the evidence supports the conclusion that valproate exposure *in utero* can cause decreased IQ in children.

In animal studies, offspring with prenatal exposure to valproate had malformations similar to those seen in humans and demonstrated neurobehavioral deficits *[see Use in Specific Populations (8.1)]*.

Valproate use is contraindicated during pregnancy in women being treated for prophylaxis of migraine headaches. Women with epilepsy or bipolar disorder who are

Information on the AbbVie, Inc. products listed on these pages is from the prescribing information in use as of July 31, 2013. For more information, please visit rxabbvie.com or call 1-800-633-9110.

Table 2. Risk by indication for antiepileptic drugs in the pooled analysis

Indication	Placebo Patients with Events Per 1000 Patients	Drug Patients with Events Per 1000 Patients	Relative Risk: Incidence of Events in Drug Patients/ Incidence in Placebo Patients	Risk Difference: Additional Drug Patients with Events Per 1000 Patients
Epilepsy	1.0	3.4	3.5	2.4
Psychiatric	5.7	8.5	1.5	2.9
Other	1.0	1.8	1.9	0.9
Total	2.4	4.3	1.8	1.9

pregnant or who plan to become pregnant should not be treated with valproate unless other treatments have failed to provide adequate symptom control or are otherwise unacceptable. In such women, the benefits of treatment with valproate during pregnancy may still outweigh the risks.

5.4 Use in Women of Childbearing Potential

Because of the risk to the fetus of decreased IQ and major congenital malformations (including neural tube defects), which may occur very early in pregnancy, valproate should not be administered to a woman of childbearing potential unless the drug is essential to the management of her medical condition. This is especially important when valproate use is considered for a condition not usually associated with permanent injury or death (e.g., migraine). Women should use effective contraception while using valproate. Women who are planning a pregnancy should be counseled regarding the relative risks and benefits of valproate use during pregnancy, and alternative therapeutic options should be considered for these patients *[see Boxed Warning and Use in Specific Populations (8.1)]*.

To prevent major seizures, valproate should not be discontinued abruptly, as this can precipitate status epilepticus with resulting maternal and fetal hypoxia and threat to life. Evidence suggests that folic acid supplementation prior to conception and during the first trimester of pregnancy decreases the risk for congenital neural tube defects in the general population. It is not known whether the risk of neural tube defects or decreased IQ in the offspring of women receiving valproate is reduced by folic acid supplementation. Dietary folic acid supplementation both prior to conception and during pregnancy should be routinely recommended for patients using valproate.

5.5 Pancreatitis

Cases of life-threatening pancreatitis have been reported in both children and adults receiving valproate. Some of the cases have been described as hemorrhagic with rapid progression from initial symptoms to death. Some cases have occurred shortly after initial use as well as after several years of use. The rate based upon the reported cases exceeds that expected in the general population and there have been cases in which pancreatitis recurred after rechallenge with valproate. In clinical trials, there were 2 cases of pancreatitis without alternative etiology in 2416 patients, representing 1044 patient-years experience. Patients and guardians should be warned that abdominal pain, nausea, vomiting, and/or anorexia can be symptoms of pancreatitis that require prompt medical evaluation. If pancreatitis is diagnosed, Depakote ER should ordinarily be discontinued. Alternative treatment for the underlying medical condition should be initiated as clinically indicated *[see Boxed Warning]*.

5.6 Urea Cycle Disorders

Depakote ER is contraindicated in patients with known urea cycle disorders (UCD). Hyperammonemic encephalopathy, sometimes fatal, has been reported following initiation of valproate therapy in patients with urea cycle disorders, a group of uncommon genetic abnormalities, particularly ornithine transcarbamylase deficiency. Prior to the initiation of Depakote ER therapy, evaluation for UCD should be considered in the following patients: 1) those with a history of unexplained encephalopathy or coma, encephalopathy associated with a protein load, pregnancy-related or postpartum encephalopathy, unexplained mental retardation, or history of elevated plasma ammonia or glutamine; 2) those with cyclical vomiting and lethargy, episodic extreme irritability, ataxia, low BUN, or protein avoidance; 3) those with a family history of UCD or a family history of unexplained infant deaths (particularly males); 4) those with other signs or symptoms of UCD. Patients who develop symptoms of unexplained hyperammonemic encephalopathy while receiving valproate therapy should receive prompt treatment (including discontinuation of valproate therapy) and be evaluated for underlying urea cycle disorders *[see Contraindications (4) and Warnings and Precautions (5.11)]*.

5.7 Brain Atrophy

There have been postmarketing reports of reversible and irreversible cerebral and cerebellar atrophy temporally associated with the use valproate products; in some cases, patients recovered with permanent sequelae *[see Adverse Reactions (6.4)]*. The motor and cognitive functions of patients on valproate should be routinely monitored and drug should be evaluated for continued use in the presence of suspected or apparent signs of brain atrophy.

Reports of cerebral atrophy have also been reported in children who were exposed *in utero* to valproate products *[see Use in Specific Populations (8.1)]*.

5.8 Suicidal Behavior and Ideation

Antiepileptic drugs (AEDs), including Depakote ER, increase the risk of suicidal thoughts or behavior in patients taking these drugs for any indication. Patients treated with any AED for any indication should be monitored for the emergence or worsening of depression, suicidal thoughts or behavior, and/or any unusual changes in mood or behavior.

Pooled analyses of 199 placebo-controlled clinical trials (mono- and adjunctive therapy) of 11 different AEDs showed that patients randomized to one of the AEDs had approximately twice the risk (adjusted Relative Risk 1.8, 95% CI:1.2, 2.7) of suicidal thinking or behavior compared to patients randomized to placebo. In these trials, which had a median treatment duration of 12 weeks, the estimated incidence rate of suicidal behavior or ideation among 27,863 AED-treated patients was 0.43%, compared to 0.24% among 16,029 placebo-treated patients, representing an increase of approximately one case of suicidal thinking or behavior for every 530 patients treated. There were four suicides in drug-treated patients in the trials and none in placebo-treated patients, but the number is too small to allow any conclusion about drug effect on suicide.

The increased risk of suicidal thoughts or behavior with AEDs was observed as early as one week after starting drug treatment with AEDs and persisted for the duration of treatment assessed. Because most trials included in the analysis did not extend beyond 24 weeks, the risk of suicidal thoughts or behavior beyond 24 weeks could not be assessed.

The risk of suicidal thoughts or behavior was generally consistent among drugs in the data analyzed. The finding of increased risk with AEDs of varying mechanisms of action and across a range of indications suggests that the risk applies to all AEDs used for any indication. The risk did not vary substantially by age (5-100 years) in the clinical trials analyzed.

Table 2 shows absolute and relative risk by indication for all evaluated AEDs.

[See table 2 above]

The relative risk for suicidal thoughts or behavior was higher in clinical trials for epilepsy than in clinical trials for psychiatric or other conditions, but the absolute risk differences were similar for the epilepsy and psychiatric indications.

Anyone considering prescribing Depakote ER or any other AED must balance the risk of suicidal thoughts or behavior with the risk of untreated illness. Epilepsy and many other illnesses for which AEDs are prescribed are themselves associated with morbidity and mortality and an increased risk of suicidal thoughts and behavior. Should suicidal thoughts and behavior emerge during treatment, the prescriber needs to consider whether the emergence of these symptoms in any given patient may be related to the illness being treated.

Patients, their caregivers, and families should be informed that AEDs increase the risk of suicidal thoughts and behavior and should be advised of the need to be alert for the emergence or worsening of the signs and symptoms of depression, any unusual changes in mood or behavior, or the emergence of suicidal thoughts, behavior, or thoughts about self-harm. Behaviors of concern should be reported immediately to healthcare providers.

5.9 Thrombocytopenia

The frequency of adverse effects (particularly elevated liver enzymes and thrombocytopenia) may be dose-related. In a clinical trial of valproate as monotherapy in patients with epilepsy, 34/126 patients (27%) receiving approximately 50 mg/kg/day on average, had at least one value of platelets $\leq 75 \times 10^9$/L. Approximately half of these patients had treatment discontinued, with return of platelet counts to normal. In the remaining patients, platelet counts normalized with continued treatment. In this study, the probability of thrombocytopenia appeared to increase significantly at total valproate concentrations of $\geq$ 110 mcg/mL (females) or $\geq$ 135 mcg/mL (males). The therapeutic benefit which may accompany the higher doses should therefore be weighed against the possibility of a greater incidence of adverse effects.

Because of reports of thrombocytopenia, inhibition of the secondary phase of platelet aggregation, and abnormal coagulation parameters, (e.g., low fibrinogen), platelet counts and coagulation tests are recommended before initiating therapy and at periodic intervals. It is recommended that patients receiving Depakote ER be monitored for platelet count and coagulation parameters prior to planned surgery. Evidence of hemorrhage, bruising, or a disorder of hemostasis/coagulation is an indication for reduction of the dosage or withdrawal of therapy.

5.10 Hyperammonemia

Hyperammonemia has been reported in association with valproate therapy and may be present despite normal liver function tests. In patients who develop unexplained lethargy and vomiting or changes in mental status, hyperammonemic encephalopathy should be considered and an ammonia level should be measured. Hyperammonemia should also be considered in patients who present with hypothermia *[see Warnings and Precautions (5.12)]*. If ammonia is increased, valproate therapy should be discontinued. Appropriate interventions for treatment of hyperammonemia should be initiated, and such patients should undergo investigation for underlying urea cycle disorders *[see Contraindications (4) and Warnings and Precautions (5.6, 5.11)]*.

During the placebo controlled pediatric mania trial, one (1) in twenty (20) adolescents (5%) treated with valproate developed increased plasma ammonia levels compared to no (0) patients treated with placebo.

Asymptomatic elevations of ammonia are more common and when present, require close monitoring of plasma ammonia levels. If the elevation persists, discontinuation of valproate therapy should be considered.

5.11 Hyperammonemia and Encephalopathy associated with Concomitant Topiramate Use

Concomitant administration of topiramate and valproate has been associated with hyperammonemia with or without encephalopathy in patients who have tolerated either drug alone. Clinical symptoms of hyperammonemic encephalopathy often include acute alterations in level of consciousness and/or cognitive function with lethargy or vomiting. Hypothermia can also be a manifestation of hyperammonemia *[see Warnings and Precautions (5.12)]*. In most cases, symptoms and signs abated with discontinuation of either drug. This adverse event is not due to a pharmacokinetic interaction. It is not known if topiramate monotherapy is associated with hyperammonemia. Patients with inborn errors of metabolism or reduced hepatic mitochondrial activity may be at an increased risk for hyperammonemia with or without encephalopathy. Although not studied, an interaction of topiramate and valproate may exacerbate existing defects or unmask deficiencies in susceptible persons. In patients who develop unexplained lethargy, vomiting, or changes in mental status, hyperammonemic encephalopathy should be considered and an ammonia level should be measured *[see Contraindications (4) and Warnings and Precautions (5.6, 5.10)]*.

5.12 Hypothermia

Hypothermia, defined as an unintentional drop in body core temperature to < 35°C (95°F), has been reported in association with valproate therapy both in conjunction with and in the absence of hyperammonemia. This adverse reaction can also occur in patients using concomitant topiramate with valproate after starting topiramate treatment or after increasing the daily dose of topiramate *[see Drug Interactions (7.3)]*. Consideration should be given to stopping valproate in patients who develop hypothermia, which may be manifested by a variety of clinical abnormalities including lethargy, confusion, coma, and significant alterations in other major organ systems such as the cardiovascular and respiratory systems. Clinical management and assessment should include examination of blood ammonia levels.

5.13 Multi-Organ Hypersensitivity Reactions

Multi-organ hypersensitivity reactions have been rarely reported in close temporal association to the initiation of valproate therapy in adult and pediatric patients (median time to detection 21 days: range 1 to 40 days). Although there have been a limited number of reports, many of these cases resulted in hospitalization and at least one death has been reported. Signs and symptoms of this disorder were diverse; however, patients typically, although not exclusively, presented with fever and rash associated with other organ system involvement. Other associated manifestations may include lymphadenopathy, hepatitis, liver function test abnormalities, hematologic abnormalities (e.g., eosinophilia, thrombocytopenia, neutropenia), pruritus, nephritis, oliguria, hepato-renal syndrome, arthralgia, and asthenia. Because the disorder is variable in its expression, other organ system symptoms and signs, not noted here, may occur.

If this reaction is suspected, valproate should be discontinued and an alternative treatment started. Although the existence of cross sensitivity with other drugs that produce this syndrome is unclear, the experience amongst drugs associated with multi-organ hypersensitivity would indicate this to be a possibility.

5.14 Interaction with Carbapenem Antibiotics

Carbapenem antibiotics (for example, ertapenem, imipenem, meropenem; this is not a complete list) may reduce serum valproate concentrations to subtherapeutic levels, resulting in loss of seizure control. Serum valproate concentrations should be monitored frequently after initiating carbapenem therapy. Alternative antibacterial or anticonvulsant therapy should be considered if serum valproate concentrations drop significantly or seizure control deteriorates *[see Drug Interactions (7.1)]*.

5.15 Somnolence in the Elderly

In a double-blind, multicenter trial of valproate in elderly patients with dementia (mean age = 83 years), doses were increased by 125 mg/day to a target dose of 20 mg/kg/day. A significantly higher proportion of valproate patients had somnolence compared to placebo, and although not statistically significant, there was a higher proportion of patients with dehydration. Discontinuations for somnolence were also significantly higher than with placebo. In some patients with somnolence (approximately one-half), there was associated reduced nutritional intake and weight loss. There was a trend for the patients who experienced these events to have a lower baseline albumin concentration, lower valproate clearance, and a higher BUN. In elderly patients, dosage should be increased more slowly and with regular monitoring for fluid and nutritional intake, dehydration, somnolence, and other adverse reactions. Dose reductions or discontinuation of valproate should be considered in patients with decreased food or fluid intake and in patients with excessive somnolence *[see Dosage and Administration (2.4)]*.

5.16 Monitoring: Drug Plasma Concentration

Since valproate may interact with concurrently administered drugs which are capable of enzyme induction, periodic plasma concentration determinations of valproate and concomitant drugs are recommended during the early course of therapy *[see Drug Interactions (7)]*.

5.17 Effect on Ketone and Thyroid Function Tests

Valproate is partially eliminated in the urine as a keto-metabolite which may lead to a false interpretation of the urine ketone test.

There have been reports of altered thyroid function tests associated with valproate. The clinical significance of these is unknown.

5.18 Effect on HIV and CMV Viruses Replication

There are *in vitro* studies that suggest valproate stimulates the replication of the HIV and CMV viruses under certain experimental conditions. The clinical consequence, if any, is not known. Additionally, the relevance of these *in vitro* findings is uncertain for patients receiving maximally suppressive antiretroviral therapy. Nevertheless, these data should be borne in mind when interpreting the results from regular monitoring of the viral load in HIV infected patients receiving valproate or when following CMV infected patients clinically.

5.19 Medication Residue in the Stool

There have been rare reports of medication residue in the stool. Some patients have had anatomic (including ileostomy or colostomy) or functional gastrointestinal disorders with shortened GI transit times. In some reports, medication residues have occurred in the context of diarrhea. It is recommended that plasma valproate levels be checked in patients who experience medication residue in the stool, and patients' clinical condition should be monitored. If clinically indicated, alternative treatment may be considered.

6 ADVERSE REACTIONS

The following adverse reactions are discussed in greater detail in other sections of the labeling:

Hepatic failure (5.1)
Birth defects (5.2)
Decreased IQ following *in utero* exposure (5.3)
Pancreatitis (5.5)
Thrombocytopenia (5.9)
Hyperammonemic encephalopathy (5.10, 5.11)
Multi-organ hypersensitivity reactions (5.13)
Somnolence in the elderly (5.15)

Because clinical studies are conducted under widely varying conditions, adverse reaction rates observed in the clinical studies of a drug cannot be directly compared to rates in the clinical studies of another drug and may not reflect the rates observed in practice.

Information on pediatric adverse reactions is presented in section 8.

6.1 Mania

The incidence of treatment-emergent events has been ascertained based on combined data from two three week placebo-controlled clinical trials of Depakote ER in the treatment of manic episodes associated with bipolar disorder.

Table 3 summarizes those adverse reactions reported for patients in these trials where the incidence rate in the Depakote ER-treated group was greater than 5% and greater than the placebo incidence.

Table 3. Adverse Reactions Reported by > 5% of Depakote-Treated Patients During Placebo-Controlled Trials of Acute Mania[1]

Adverse Event	Depakote ER (n=338)	Placebo (n=263)
Somnolence	26%	14%
Dyspepsia	23%	11%
Nausea	19%	13%
Vomiting	13%	5%
Diarrhea	12%	8%
Dizziness	12%	7%
Pain	11%	10%
Abdominal pain	10%	5%
Accidental injury	6%	5%
Asthenia	6%	5%
Pharyngitis	6%	5%

1. The following adverse reactions/event occurred at an equal or greater incidence for placebo than for Depakote ER: headache

The following additional adverse reactions were reported by greater than 1% but not more than 5% of the Depakote ER-treated patients in controlled clinical trials:

Body as a Whole: Back Pain, Flu Syndrome, Infection, Infection Fungal
Cardiovascular System: Hypertension
Digestive System: Constipation, Dry Mouth, Flatulence
Hemic and Lymphatic System: Ecchymosis
Metabolic and Nutritional Disorders: Peripheral Edema
Musculoskeletal System: Myalgia
Nervous System: Abnormal Gait, Hypertonia, Tremor
Respiratory System: Rhinitis
Skin and Appendages: Pruritus, Rash
Special Senses: Conjunctivitis
Urogenital System: Urinary Tract Infection, Vaginitis

6.2 Epilepsy

Based on a placebo-controlled trial of adjunctive therapy for treatment of complex partial seizures, Depakote was generally well tolerated with most adverse reactions rated as mild to moderate in severity. Intolerance was the primary reason for discontinuation in the Depakote-treated patients (6%), compared to 1% of placebo-treated patients.

Table 4 lists treatment-emergent adverse reactions which were reported by ≥ 5% of Depakote-treated patients and for which the incidence was greater than in the placebo group, in the placebo-controlled trial of adjunctive therapy for treatment of complex partial seizures. Since patients were also treated with other antiepilepsy drugs, it is not possible, in most cases, to determine whether the following adverse reactions can be ascribed to Depakote alone, or the combination of Depakote and other antiepilepsy drugs.

Table 4. Adverse Reactions Reported by ≥ 5% of Patients Treated with Valproate During Placebo-Controlled Trial of Adjunctive Therapy for Complex Partial Seizures

Body System/Event	Depakote (%) (N=77)	Placebo (%) (N=70)
Body as a Whole		
Headache	31	21
Asthenia	27	7
Fever	6	4
Gastrointestinal System		
Nausea	48	14
Vomiting	27	7
Abdominal pain	23	6
Diarrhea	13	6
Anorexia	12	0
Dyspepsia	8	4
Constipation	5	1
Nervous System		
Somnolence	27	11
Tremor	25	6
Dizziness	25	13
Diplopia	16	9
Amblyopia/Blurred Vision	12	9
Ataxia	8	1
Nystagmus	8	1
Emotional Lability	6	4
Thinking Abnormal	6	0
Amnesia	5	1
Respiratory System		
Flu Syndrome	12	9
Infection	12	6
Bronchitis	5	1
Rhinitis	5	4
Other		
Alopecia	6	1
Weight Loss	6	0

Table 5 lists treatment-emergent adverse reactions which were reported by ≥ 5% of patients in the high dose valproate group, and for which the incidence was greater than in the low dose group, in a controlled trial of Depakote monotherapy treatment of complex partial seizures. Since patients were being titrated off another antiepilepsy drug during the first portion of the trial, it is not possible, in many cases, to determine whether the following adverse reactions can be ascribed to Depakote alone, or the combination of valproate and other antiepilepsy drugs.

Table 5. Adverse Reactions Reported by ≥ 5% of Patients in the High Dose Group in the Controlled Trial of Valproate Monotherapy for Complex Partial Seizures[1]

Body System/Event	High Dose (%) (n=131)	Low Dose (%) (n=134)
Body as a Whole		
Asthenia	21	10
Digestive System		
Nausea	34	26
Diarrhea	23	19
Vomiting	23	15
Abdominal pain	12	9
Anorexia	11	4
Dyspepsia	11	10
Hemic/Lymphatic System		
Thrombocytopenia	24	1
Ecchymosis	5	4
Metabolic/Nutritional		
Weight Gain	9	4
Peripheral Edema	8	3
Nervous System		
Tremor	57	19
Somnolence	30	18
Dizziness	18	13
Insomnia	15	9
Nervousness	11	7
Amnesia	7	4
Nystagmus	7	1
Depression	5	4
Respiratory System		
Infection	20	13
Pharyngitis	8	2
Dyspnea	5	1
Skin and Appendages		
Alopecia	24	13
Special Senses		
Amblyopia/Blurred Vision	8	4
Tinnitus	7	1

1. Headache was the only adverse event that occurred in ≥5% of patients in the high dose group and at an equal or greater incidence in the low dose group.

The following additional adverse reactions were reported by greater than 1% but less than 5% of the 358 patients treated with valproate in the controlled trials of complex partial seizures:

Body as a Whole: Back pain, chest pain, malaise.
Cardiovascular System: Tachycardia, hypertension, palpitation.
Digestive System: Increased appetite, flatulence, hematemesis, eructation, pancreatitis, periodontal abscess.

Information on the AbbVie, Inc. products listed on these pages is from the prescribing information in use as of July 31, 2013. For more information, please visit rxabbvie.com or call 1-800-633-9110.

Hemic and Lymphatic System: Petechia.
Metabolic and Nutritional Disorders: SGOT increased, SGPT increased.
Musculoskeletal System: Myalgia, twitching, arthralgia, leg cramps, myasthenia.
Nervous System: Anxiety, confusion, abnormal gait, paresthesia, hypertonia, incoordination, abnormal dreams, personality disorder.
Respiratory System: Sinusitis, cough increased, pneumonia, epistaxis.
Skin and Appendages: Rash, pruritus, dry skin.
Special Senses: Taste perversion, abnormal vision, deafness, otitis media.
Urogenital System: Urinary incontinence, vaginitis, dysmenorrhea, amenorrhea, urinary frequency.

6.3 Migraine

Based on two placebo-controlled clinical trials and their long term extension, valproate was generally well tolerated with most adverse reactions rated as mild to moderate in severity. Of the 202 patients exposed to valproate in the placebo-controlled trials, 17% discontinued for intolerance. This is compared to a rate of 5% for the 81 placebo patients. Including the long term extension study, the adverse reactions reported as the primary reason for discontinuation by ≥ 1% of 248 valproate-treated patients were alopecia (6%), nausea and/or vomiting (5%), weight gain (2%), tremor (2%), somnolence (1%), elevated SGOT and/or SGPT (1%), and depression (1%).

Table 6 includes those adverse reactions reported for patients in the placebo-controlled trial where the incidence rate in the Depakote ER-treated group was greater than 5% and was greater than that for placebo patients.

Table 6. Adverse Reactions Reported by >5% of Depakote ER-Treated Patients During the Migraine Placebo-Controlled Trial with a Greater Incidence than Patients Taking Placebo[1]

Body System Event	Depakote ER (n=122)	Placebo (n=115)
Gastrointestinal System		
Nausea	15%	9%
Dyspepsia	7%	4%
Diarrhea	7%	3%
Vomiting	7%	2%
Abdominal Pain	7%	5%
Nervous System		
Somnolence	7%	2%
Other		
Infection	15%	14%

1. The following adverse reactions occurred in greater than 5% of Depakote ER-treated patients and at a greater incidence for placebo than for Depakote ER: asthenia and flu syndrome.

The following additional adverse reactions were reported by greater than 1% but not more than 5% of Depakote ER-treated patients and with a greater incidence than placebo in the placebo-controlled clinical trial for migraine prophylaxis:
Body as a Whole: Accidental injury, viral infection.
Digestive System: Increased appetite, tooth disorder.
Metabolic and Nutritional Disorders: Edema, weight gain.
Nervous System: Abnormal gait, dizziness, hypertonia, insomnia, nervousness, tremor, vertigo.
Respiratory System: Pharyngitis, rhinitis.
Skin and Appendages: Rash.
Special Senses: Tinnitus.

Table 7 includes those adverse reactions reported for patients in the placebo-controlled trials where the incidence rate in the valproate-treated group was greater than 5% and was greater than that for placebo patients.

Table 7. Adverse Reactions Reported by > 5% of Valproate-Treated Patients During Migraine Placebo-Controlled Trials with a Greater Incidence than Patients Taking Placebo[1]

Body System Reaction	Depakote (n=202)	Placebo (n=81)
Gastrointestinal System		
Nausea	31%	10%
Dyspepsia	13%	9%
Diarrhea	12%	7%
Vomiting	11%	1%
Abdominal pain	9%	4%
Increased appetite	6%	4%
Nervous System		
Asthenia	20%	9%
Somnolence	17%	5%
Dizziness	12%	6%
Tremor	9%	0%
Other		
Weight gain	8%	2%
Back pain	8%	6%
Alopecia	7%	1%

1. The following adverse reactions occurred in greater than 5% of Depakote-treated patients and at a greater incidence for placebo than for Depakote: flu syndrome and pharyngitis.

The following additional adverse reactions were reported by greater than 1% but not more than 5% of the 202 valproate-treated patients in the controlled clinical trials:
Body as a Whole: Chest pain.
Cardiovascular System: Vasodilatation.
Digestive System: Constipation, dry mouth, flatulence, and stomatitis.
Hemic and Lymphatic System: Ecchymosis.
Metabolic and Nutritional Disorders: Peripheral edema.
Musculoskeletal System: Leg cramps.
Nervous System: Abnormal dreams, confusion, paresthesia, speech disorder, and thinking abnormalities.
Respiratory System: Dyspnea, and sinusitis.
Skin and Appendages: Pruritus.
Urogenital System: Metrorrhagia.

6.4 Other Patient Populations

Mania

The following adverse reactions not listed previously were reported by greater than 1% of Depakote-treated patients and with a greater incidence than placebo in placebo-controlled trials of manic episodes associated with bipolar disorder:
Body as a Whole: Chills, chills and fever, drug level increased, neck rigidity.
Cardiovascular System: Arrhythmia, hypotension, postural hypotension.
Digestive System: Dysphagia, fecal incontinence, gastroenteritis, glossitis, gum hemorrhage, mouth ulceration.
Hemic and Lymphatic System: Anemia, bleeding time increased, leucopenia.
Metabolic and Nutritional Disorders: Hypoproteinemia.
Musculoskeletal System: Arthrosis.
Nervous System: Agitation, catatonic reaction, dysarthria, hallucinations, hypokinesia, psychosis, reflexes increased, sleep disorder, tardive dyskinesia.
Respiratory System: Hiccup.
Skin and Appendages: Discoid lupus erythematosus, erythema nodosum, furunculosis, maculopapular rash, seborrhea, sweating, vesiculobullous rash.
Special Senses: Conjunctivitis, dry eyes, eye disorder, eye pain, photophobia, taste perversion.
Urogenital System: Cystitis, menstrual disorder.

Epilepsy

Adverse reactions that have been reported with all dosage forms of valproate from epilepsy trials, spontaneous reports, and other sources are listed below by body system.

Gastrointestinal

The most commonly reported side effects at the initiation of therapy are nausea, vomiting, and indigestion. These effects are usually transient and rarely require discontinuation of therapy. Diarrhea, abdominal cramps, and constipation have been reported. Both anorexia with some weight loss and increased appetite with weight gain have also been reported. The administration of delayed-release divalproex sodium may result in reduction of gastrointestinal side effects in some patients.

CNS Effects

Sedative effects have occurred in patients receiving valproate alone but occur most often in patients receiving combination therapy. Sedation usually abates upon reduction of other antiepileptic medication. Tremor (may be dose-related), hallucinations, ataxia, headache, nystagmus, diplopia, asterixis, "spots before eyes", dysarthria, dizziness, confusion, hypesthesia, vertigo, incoordination, and parkinsonism have been reported with the use of valproate. Rare cases of coma have occurred in patients receiving valproate alone or in conjunction with phenobarbital. In rare instances encephalopathy with or without fever has developed shortly after the introduction of valproate monotherapy without evidence of hepatic dysfunction or inappropriately high plasma valproate levels. Although recovery has been described following drug withdrawal, there have been fatalities in patients with hyperammonemic encephalopathy, particularly in patients with underlying urea cycle disorders *[see Warnings and Precautions (5.6)]*.

There have been postmarketing reports of reversible and irreversible cerebral and cerebellar atrophy temporally associated with the use of valproate products. In some cases the patients recovered with permanent sequelae *[see Warnings and Precautions (5.7)]*. Cerebral atrophy has been reported in children exposed to valproate *in utero [see Use in Specific Populations (8.1)]*.

Dermatologic

Transient hair loss, skin rash, photosensitivity, generalized pruritus, erythema multiforme, and Stevens-Johnson syndrome. Rare cases of toxic epidermal necrolysis have been reported including a fatal case in a 6 month old infant taking valproate and several other concomitant medications. An additional case of toxic epidermal necrosis resulting in death was reported in a 35 year old patient with AIDS taking several concomitant medications and with a history of multiple cutaneous drug reactions. Serious skin reactions have been reported with concomitant administration of lamotrigine and valproate *[see Drug Interactions (7.2)]*.

Psychiatric

Emotional upset, depression, psychosis, aggression, hyperactivity, hostility, and behavioral deterioration.

Musculoskeletal

Weakness.

Hematologic

Thrombocytopenia and inhibition of the secondary phase of platelet aggregation may be reflected in altered bleeding time, petechiae, bruising, hematoma formation, epistaxis, and frank hemorrhage *[see Warnings and Precautions (5.9) and Drug Interactions (7)]*. Relative lymphocytosis, macrocytosis, hypofibrinogenemia, leukopenia, eosinophilia, anemia including macrocytic with or without folate deficiency, bone marrow suppression, pancytopenia, aplastic anemia, agranulocytosis, and acute intermittent porphyria.

Hepatic

Minor elevations of transaminases (e.g., SGOT and SGPT) and LDH are frequent and appear to be dose-related. Occasionally, laboratory test results include increases in serum bilirubin and abnormal changes in other liver function tests. These results may reflect potentially serious hepatotoxicity *[see Warnings and Precautions (5.1)]*.

Endocrine

Irregular menses, secondary amenorrhea, breast enlargement, galactorrhea, and parotid gland swelling. Abnormal thyroid function tests *[see Warnings and Precautions (5.17)]*. There have been rare spontaneous reports of polycystic ovary disease. A cause and effect relationship has not been established.

Pancreatic

Acute pancreatitis including fatalities *[see Warnings and Precautions (5.5)]*.

Metabolic

Hyperammonemia *[see Warnings and Precautions (5.10, 5.11)]*, hyponatremia, and inappropriate ADH secretion.
There have been rare reports of Fanconi's syndrome occurring chiefly in children.
Decreased carnitine concentrations have been reported although the clinical relevance is undetermined.
Hyperglycinemia has occurred and was associated with a fatal outcome in a patient with preexistent nonketotic hyperglycinemia.

Genitourinary

Enuresis and urinary tract infection.

Special Senses

Hearing loss, either reversible or irreversible, has been reported; however, a cause and effect relationship has not been established. Ear pain has also been reported.

Other

Allergic reaction, anaphylaxis, edema of the extremities, lupus erythematosus, bone pain, cough increased, pneumonia, otitis media, bradycardia, cutaneous vasculitis, fever, and hypothermia *[see Warnings and Precautions (5.12)]*.
There have been reports of developmental delay, autism and/or autism spectrum disorder in the offspring of women exposed to valproate during pregnancy.

7 DRUG INTERACTIONS

7.1 Effects of Co-Administered Drugs on Valproate Clearance

Drugs that affect the level of expression of hepatic enzymes, particularly those that elevate levels of glucuronosyltransferases, may increase the clearance of valproate. For example, phenytoin, carbamazepine, and phenobarbital (or primidone) can double the clearance of valproate. Thus, patients on monotherapy will generally have longer half-lives and higher concentrations than patients receiving polytherapy with antiepilepsy drugs.

In contrast, drugs that are inhibitors of cytochrome P450 isozymes, e.g., antidepressants, may be expected to have little effect on valproate clearance because cytochrome P450 microsomal mediated oxidation is a relatively minor secondary metabolic pathway compared to glucuronidation and beta-oxidation.

Because of these changes in valproate clearance, monitoring of valproate and concomitant drug concentrations should be increased whenever enzyme inducing drugs are introduced or withdrawn.

The following list provides information about the potential for an influence of several commonly prescribed medications on valproate pharmacokinetics. The list is not exhaustive nor could it be, since new interactions are continuously being reported.

Drugs for which a potentially important interaction has been observed

Aspirin

A study involving the co-administration of aspirin at antipyretic doses (11 to 16 mg/kg) with valproate to pediatric patients (n=6) revealed a decrease in protein binding and an inhibition of metabolism of valproate. Valproate free fraction was increased 4-fold in the presence of aspirin compared to valproate alone. The β-oxidation pathway consisting of 2-E-valproic acid, 3-OH-valproic acid, and 3-keto valproic acid was decreased from 25% of total metabolites excreted on valproate alone to 8.3% in the presence of aspirin. Whether or not the interaction observed in this study applies to adults is unknown, but caution should be observed if valproate and aspirin are to be co-administered.

Carbapenem Antibiotics

A clinically significant reduction in serum valproic acid concentration has been reported in patients receiving carbapenem antibiotics (for example, ertapenem, imipenem, meropenem; this is not a complete list) and may result in loss of seizure control. The mechanism of this interaction in not well understood. Serum valproic acid concentrations should be monitored frequently after initiating carbapenem therapy. Alternative antibacterial or anticonvulsant therapy should be considered if serum valproic acid concentrations drop significantly or seizure control deteriorates *[see Warnings and Precautions (5.14)]*.

Felbamate

A study involving the co-administration of 1200 mg/day of felbamate with valproate to patients with epilepsy (n=10) revealed an increase in mean valproate peak concentration by 35% (from 86 to 115 mcg/mL) compared to valproate alone. Increasing the felbamate dose to 2400 mg/day increased the mean valproate peak concentration to 133 mcg/mL (another 16% increase). A decrease in valproate dosage may be necessary when felbamate therapy is initiated.

Rifampin

A study involving the administration of a single dose of valproate (7 mg/kg) 36 hours after 5 nights of daily dosing with rifampin (600 mg) revealed a 40% increase in the oral clearance of valproate. Valproate dosage adjustment may be necessary when it is co-administered with rifampin.

Drugs for which either no interaction or a likely clinically unimportant interaction has been observed

Antacids

A study involving the co-administration of valproate 500 mg with commonly administered antacids (Maalox, Trisogel, and Titralac - 160 mEq doses) did not reveal any effect on the extent of absorption of valproate.

Chlorpromazine

A study involving the administration of 100 to 300 mg/day of chlorpromazine to schizophrenic patients already receiving valproate (200 mg BID) revealed a 15% increase in trough plasma levels of valproate.

Haloperidol

A study involving the administration of 6 to 10 mg/day of haloperidol to schizophrenic patients already receiving valproate (200 mg BID) revealed no significant changes in valproate trough plasma levels.

Cimetidine and Ranitidine

Cimetidine and ranitidine do not affect the clearance of valproate.

7.2 Effects of Valproate on Other Drugs

Valproate has been found to be a weak inhibitor of some P450 isozymes, epoxide hydrase, and glucuronosyltransferases.

The following list provides information about the potential for an influence of valproate co-administration on the pharmacokinetics or pharmacodynamics of several commonly prescribed medications. The list is not exhaustive, since new interactions are continuously being reported.

Drugs for which a potentially important valproate interaction has been observed

Amitriptyline/Nortriptyline

Administration of a single oral 50 mg dose of amitriptyline to 15 normal volunteers (10 males and 5 females) who received valproate (500 mg BID) resulted in a 21% decrease in plasma clearance of amitriptyline and a 34% decrease in the net clearance of nortriptyline. Rare postmarketing reports of concurrent use of valproate and amitriptyline resulting in an increased amitriptyline level have been received. Concurrent use of valproate and amitriptyline has rarely been associated with toxicity. Monitoring of amitriptyline levels should be considered for patients taking valproate concomitantly with amitriptyline. Consideration should be given to lowering the dose of amitriptyline/nortriptyline in the presence of valproate.

Carbamazepine/carbamazepine-10,11-Epoxide

Serum levels of carbamazepine (CBZ) decreased 17% while that of carbamazepine-10,11-epoxide (CBZ-E) increased by 45% upon co-administration of valproate and CBZ to epileptic patients.

Clonazepam

The concomitant use of valproate and clonazepam may induce absence status in patients with a history of absence type seizures.

Diazepam

Valproate displaces diazepam from its plasma albumin binding sites and inhibits its metabolism. Co-administration of valproate (1500 mg daily) increased the free fraction of diazepam (10 mg) by 90% in healthy volunteers (n=6). Plasma clearance and volume of distribution for free diazepam were reduced by 25% and 20%, respectively, in the presence of valproate. The elimination half-life of diazepam remained unchanged upon addition of valproate.

Ethosuximide

Valproate inhibits the metabolism of ethosuximide. Administration of a single ethosuximide dose of 500 mg with valproate (800 to 1600 mg/day) to healthy volunteers (n=6) was accompanied by a 25% increase in elimination half-life of ethosuximide and a 15% decrease in its total clearance as compared to ethosuximide alone. Patients receiving valproate and ethosuximide, especially along with other anticonvulsants, should be monitored for alterations in serum concentrations of both drugs.

Lamotrigine

In a steady-state study involving 10 healthy volunteers, the elimination half-life of lamotrigine increased from 26 to 70 hours with valproate co-administration (a 165% increase). The dose of lamotrigine should be reduced when co-administered with valproate. Serious skin reactions (such as Stevens-Johnson syndrome and toxic epidermal necrolysis) have been reported with concomitant lamotrigine and valproate administration. See lamotrigine package insert for details on lamotrigine dosing with concomitant valproate administration.

Phenobarbital

Valproate was found to inhibit the metabolism of phenobarbital. Co-administration of valproate (250 mg BID for 14 days) with phenobarbital to normal subjects (n=6) resulted in a 50% increase in half-life and a 30% decrease in plasma clearance of phenobarbital (60 mg single-dose). The fraction of phenobarbital dose excreted unchanged increased by 50% in presence of valproate.

There is evidence for severe CNS depression, with or without significant elevations of barbiturate or valproate serum concentrations. All patients receiving concomitant barbiturate therapy should be closely monitored for neurological toxicity. Serum barbiturate concentrations should be obtained, if possible, and the barbiturate dosage decreased, if appropriate.

Primidone, which is metabolized to a barbiturate, may be involved in a similar interaction with valproate.

Phenytoin

Valproate displaces phenytoin from its plasma albumin binding sites and inhibits its hepatic metabolism. Co-administration of valproate (400 mg TID) with phenytoin (250 mg) in normal volunteers (n=7) was associated with a 60% increase in the free fraction of phenytoin. Total plasma clearance and apparent volume of distribution of phenytoin increased 30% in the presence of valproate. Both the clearance and apparent volume of distribution of free phenytoin were reduced by 25%.

In patients with epilepsy, there have been reports of breakthrough seizures occurring with the combination of valproate and phenytoin. The dosage of phenytoin should be adjusted as required by the clinical situation.

Tolbutamide

From *in vitro* experiments, the unbound fraction of tolbutamide was increased from 20% to 50% when added to plasma samples taken from patients treated with valproate. The clinical relevance of this displacement is unknown.

Warfarin

In an *in vitro* study, valproate increased the unbound fraction of warfarin by up to 32.6%. The therapeutic relevance of this is unknown; however, coagulation tests should be monitored if valproate therapy is instituted in patients taking anticoagulants.

Zidovudine

In six patients who were seropositive for HIV, the clearance of zidovudine (100 mg q8h) was decreased by 38% after administration of valproate (250 or 500 mg q8h); the half-life of zidovudine was unaffected.

Drugs for which either no interaction or a likely clinically unimportant interaction has been observed

Acetaminophen

Valproate had no effect on any of the pharmacokinetic parameters of acetaminophen when it was concurrently administered to three epileptic patients.

Clozapine

In psychotic patients (n=11), no interaction was observed when valproate was co-administered with clozapine.

Lithium

Co-administration of valproate (500 mg BID) and lithium carbonate (300 mg TID) to normal male volunteers (n=16) had no effect on the steady-state kinetics of lithium.

Lorazepam

Concomitant administration of valproate (500 mg BID) and lorazepam (1 mg BID) in normal male volunteers (n=9) was accompanied by a 17% decrease in the plasma clearance of lorazepam.

Oral Contraceptive Steroids

Administration of a single-dose of ethinyloestradiol (50 mcg)/levonorgestrel (250 mcg) to 6 women on valproate (200 mg BID) therapy for 2 months did not reveal any pharmacokinetic interaction.

7.3 Topiramate

Concomitant administration of valproate and topiramate has been associated with hyperammonemia with and without encephalopathy *[see Contraindications (4) and Warnings and Precautions (5.10, 5.11)]*. Concomitant administration of topiramate with valproate has also been associated with hypothermia in patients who have tolerated either drug alone. It may be prudent to examine blood ammonia levels in patients in whom the onset of hypothermia has been reported *[see Warnings and Precautions (5.10, 5.12)]*.

8 USE IN SPECIFIC POPULATIONS

8.1 Pregnancy

Pregnancy Category D for epilepsy and for manic episodes associated with bipolar disorder *[see Warnings and Precautions (5.2, 5.3)]*.

Pregnancy Category X for prophylaxis of migraine headaches *[see Contraindications (4)]*.

Pregnancy Registry

To collect information on the effects of *in utero* exposure to Depakote, physicians should encourage pregnant patients taking Depakote to enroll in the North American Antiepileptic Drug (NAAED) Pregnancy Registry. This can be done by calling toll free 1-888-233-2334, and must be done by the patients themselves. Information on the registry can be found at the website, http://www.aedpregnancyregistry.org/.

Fetal Risk Summary

All pregnancies have a background risk of birth defects (about 3%), pregnancy loss (about 15%), or other adverse outcomes regardless of drug exposure. Maternal valproate use during pregnancy for any indication increases the risk of congenital malformations, particularly neural tube defects, but also malformations involving other body systems (e.g., craniofacial defects, cardiovascular malformations). The risk of major structural abnormalities is greatest during the first trimester; however, other serious developmental effects can occur with valproate use throughout pregnancy. The rate of congenital malformations among babies born to epileptic mothers who used valproate during pregnancy has been shown to be about four times higher than the rate among babies born to epileptic mothers who used other anti-seizure monotherapies *[see Warnings and Precautions (5.3)]*.

Exposure *in utero* to valproate products has been associated with cerebral atrophy *[see Warnings and Precautions (5.7) and Adverse Reactions (6.4)]*.

Several published epidemiological studies have indicated that children exposed to valproate *in utero* have lower IQ scores than children exposed to either another antiepileptic drug *in utero* or to no antiepileptic drugs *in utero [see Warnings and Precautions (5.3)]*.

In animal studies, offspring with prenatal exposure to valproate had structural malformations similar to those seen in humans and demonstrated neurobehavioral deficits.

Clinical Considerations

- Neural tube defects are the congenital malformation most strongly associated with maternal valproate use. The risk of spina bifida following *in utero* valproate exposure is generally estimated as 1-2%, compared to an estimated general population risk for spina bifida of about 0.06 to 0.07% (6 to 7 in 10,000 births).
- Valproate can cause decreased IQ scores in children whose mothers were treated with valproate during pregnancy.
- Because of the risks of decreased IQ, neural tube defects, and other fetal adverse events, which may occur very early in pregnancy:
  - Valproate should not be administered to a woman of childbearing potential unless the drug is essential to the management of her medical condition. This is especially important when valproate use is considered for a condition not usually associated with permanent injury or death (e.g., migraine).
- Valproate is contraindicated during pregnancy in women being treated for prophylaxis of migraine headaches.

Information on the AbbVie, Inc. products listed on these pages is from the prescribing information in use as of July 31, 2013. For more information, please visit rxabbvie.com or call 1-800-633-9110.

- Valproate should not be used to treat women with epilepsy or bipolar disorder who are pregnant or who plan to become pregnant unless other treatments have failed to provide adequate symptom control or are otherwise unacceptable. In such women, the benefits of treatment with valproate during pregnancy may still outweigh the risks. When treating a pregnant woman or a woman of childbearing potential, carefully consider both the potential risks and benefits of treatment and provide appropriate counseling.
- To prevent major seizures, women with epilepsy should not discontinue valproate abruptly, as this can precipitate status epilepticus with resulting maternal and fetal hypoxia and threat to life. Even minor seizures may pose some hazard to the developing embryo or fetus. However, discontinuation of the drug may be considered prior to and during pregnancy in individual cases if the seizure disorder severity and frequency do not pose a serious threat to the patient.
- Available prenatal diagnostic testing to detect neural tube and other defects should be offered to pregnant women using valproate.
- Evidence suggests that folic acid supplementation prior to conception and during the first trimester of pregnancy decreases the risk for congenital neural tube defects in the general population. It is not known whether the risk of neural tube defects or decreased IQ in the offspring of women receiving valproate is reduced by folic acid supplementation. Dietary folic acid supplementation both prior to conception and during pregnancy should be routinely recommended for patients using valproate.
- Patients taking valproate may develop clotting abnormalities *[see Warnings and Precautions (5.9)]*. A patient who had low fibrinogen when taking multiple anticonvulsants including valproate gave birth to an infant with afibrinogenemia who subsequently died of hemorrhage. If valproate is used in pregnancy, the clotting parameters should be monitored carefully.
- Patients taking valproate may develop hepatic failure *[see Boxed Warning and Warnings and Precautions (5.1)]*. Fatal cases of hepatic failure in infants exposed to valproate *in utero* have also been reported following maternal use of valproate during pregnancy.

Data

Human

There is an extensive body of evidence demonstrating that exposure to valproate *in utero* increases the risk of neural tube defects and other structural abnormalities. Based on published data from the CDC's National Birth Defects Prevention Network, the risk of spina bifida in the general population is about 0.06 to 0.07%. The risk of spina bifida following *in utero* valproate exposure has been estimated to be approximately 1 to 2%.

In one study using NAAED Pregnancy Registry data, 16 cases of major malformations following prenatal valproate exposure were reported among offspring of 149 enrolled women who used valproate during pregnancy. Three of the 16 cases were neural tube defects; the remaining cases included craniofacial defects, cardiovascular malformations and malformations of varying severity involving other body systems. The NAAED Pregnancy Registry has reported a major malformation rate of 10.7% (95% C.I. 6.3% – 16.9%) in the offspring of women exposed to an average of 1,000 mg/day of valproate monotherapy during pregnancy (dose range 500 – 2000 mg/day). The major malformation rate among the internal comparison group of 1,048 epileptic women who received any other antiepileptic drug monotherapy during pregnancy was 2.9% (95% CI 2.0% to 4.1%). These data show a four-fold increased risk for any major malformation (Odds Ratio 4.0; 95% CI 2.1 to 7.4) following valproate exposure *in utero* compared to the risk following exposure *in utero* to any other antiepileptic drug monotherapy.

Published epidemiological studies have indicated that children exposed to valproate *in utero* have lower IQ scores than children exposed to either another antiepileptic drug *in utero* or to no antiepileptic drugs *in utero*. The largest of these studies is a prospective cohort study conducted in the United States and United Kingdom that found that children with prenatal exposure to valproate (n=62) had lower IQ scores at age 6 (97 [95% C.I. 94-101]) than children with prenatal exposure to the other anti-epileptic drug monotherapy treatments evaluated: lamotrigine (108 [95% C.I. 105–110]), carbamazepine (105 [95% C.I. 102–108]) and phenytoin (108 [95% C.I. 104–112]). It is not known when during pregnancy cognitive effects in valproate-exposed children occur. Because the women in this study were exposed to antiepileptic drugs throughout pregnancy, whether the risk for decreased IQ was related to a particular time period during pregnancy could not be assessed.

Although all of the available studies have methodological limitations, the weight of the evidence supports a causal association between valproate exposure *in utero* and subsequent adverse effects on cognitive development.

There are published case reports of fatal hepatic failure in offspring of women who used valproate during pregnancy.

Animal

In developmental toxicity studies conducted in mice, rats, rabbits, and monkeys, increased rates of fetal structural abnormalities, intrauterine growth retardation, and embryo-fetal death occurred following treatment of pregnant animals with valproate during organogenesis at clinically relevant doses (calculated on a body surface area basis). Valproate induced malformations of multiple organ systems, including skeletal, cardiac, and urogenital defects. In mice, in addition to other malformations, fetal neural tube defects have been reported following valproate administration during critical periods of organogenesis, and the teratogenic response correlated with peak maternal drug levels. Behavioral abnormalities (including cognitive, locomotor, and social interaction deficits) and brain histopathological changes have also been reported in mice and rat offspring exposed prenatally to clinically relevant doses of valproate.

8.3 Nursing Mothers

Valproate is excreted in human milk. Caution should be exercised when valproate is administered to a nursing woman.

8.4 Pediatric Use

Experience has indicated that pediatric patients under the age of two years are at a considerably increased risk of developing fatal hepatotoxicity, especially those with the aforementioned conditions *[see Boxed Warning and Warnings and Precautions (5.1)]*. When valproate is used in this patient group, it should be used with extreme caution and as a sole agent. The benefits of therapy should be weighed against the risks. Above the age of 2 years, experience in epilepsy has indicated that the incidence of fatal hepatotoxicity decreases considerably in progressively older patient groups.

Younger children, especially those receiving enzyme inducing drugs, will require larger maintenance doses to attain targeted total and unbound valproate concentrations. Pediatric patients (i.e., between 3 months and 10 years) have 50% higher clearances expressed on weight (i.e., mL/min/kg) than do adults. Over the age of 10 years, children have pharmacokinetic parameters that approximate those of adults.

The variability in free fraction limits the clinical usefulness of monitoring total serum valproic acid concentration. Interpretation of valproic acid concentrations in children should include consideration of factors that affect hepatic metabolism and protein binding.

Pediatric Clinical Trials

Depakote was studied in seven pediatric clinical trials.

Two of the pediatric studies were double-blinded placebo-controlled trials to evaluate the efficacy of Depakote ER for the indications of mania (150 patients aged 10 to 17 years, 76 of whom were on Depakote ER) and migraine (304 patients aged 12 to 17 years, 231 of whom were on Depakote ER). Efficacy was not established for either the treatment of migraine or the treatment of mania. The most common drug-related adverse reactions (reported >5% and twice the rate of placebo) reported in the controlled pediatric mania study were nausea, upper abdominal pain, somnolence, increased ammonia, gastritis and rash.

The remaining five trials were long term safety studies. Two six-month pediatric studies were conducted to evaluate the long-term safety of Depakote ER for the indication of mania (292 patients aged 10 to 17 years). Two twelve-month pediatric studies were conducted to evaluate the long-term safety of Depakote ER for the indication of migraine (353 patients aged 12 to 17 years). One twelve-month study was conducted to evaluate the safety of Depakote Sprinkle Capsules in the indication of partial seizures (169 patients aged 3 to 10 years).

In these seven clinical trials, the safety and tolerability of Depakote in pediatric patients were shown to be comparable to those in adults *[see Adverse Reactions (6)]*.

Juvenile Animal Toxicology

In studies of valproate in immature animals, toxic effects not observed in adult animals included retinal dysplasia in rats treated during the neonatal period (from postnatal day 4) and nephrotoxicity in rats treated during the neonatal and juvenile (from postnatal day 14) periods. The no-effect dose for these findings was less than the maximum recommended human dose on a mg/m^2 basis.

8.5 Geriatric Use

No patients above the age of 65 years were enrolled in double-blind prospective clinical trials of mania associated with bipolar illness. In a case review study of 583 patients, 72 patients (12%) were greater than 65 years of age. A higher percentage of patients above 65 years of age reported accidental injury, infection, pain, somnolence, and tremor. Discontinuation of valproate was occasionally associated with the latter two events. It is not clear whether these events indicate additional risk or whether they result from preexisting medical illness and concomitant medication use among these patients.

A study of elderly patients with dementia revealed drug related somnolence and discontinuation for somnolence *[see Warnings and Precautions (5.15)]*. The starting dose should be reduced in these patients, and dosage reductions or discontinuation should be considered in patients with excessive somnolence *[see Dosage and Administration (2.5)]*.

There is insufficient information available to discern the safety and effectiveness of valproate for the prophylaxis of migraines in patients over 65.

The capacity of elderly patients (age range: 68 to 89 years) to eliminate valproate has been shown to be reduced compared to younger adults (age range: 22 to 26 years) *[see Clinical Pharmacology (12.3)]*.

8.6 Effect of Disease

Liver Disease

[(See Boxed Warning, Contraindications (4), Warnings and Precautions (5), and Clinical Pharmacology (12.3)]. Liver disease impairs the capacity to eliminate valproate.

10 OVERDOSAGE

Over dosage with valproate may result in somnolence, heart block, and deep coma. Fatalities have been reported; however patients have recovered from valproate levels as high as 2120 mcg/mL.

In overdose situations, the fraction of drug not bound to protein is high and hemodialysis or tandem hemodialysis plus hemoperfusion may result in significant removal of drug. The benefit of gastric lavage or emesis will vary with the time since ingestion. General supportive measures should be applied with particular attention to the maintenance of adequate urinary output.

Naloxone has been reported to reverse the CNS depressant effects of valproate over dosage. Because naloxone could theoretically also reverse the antiepileptic effects of valproate, it should be used with caution in patients with epilepsy.

11 DESCRIPTION

Divalproex sodium is a stable co-ordination compound comprised of sodium valproate and valproic acid in a 1:1 molar relationship and formed during the partial neutralization of valproic acid with 0.5 equivalent of sodium hydroxide. Chemically it is designated as sodium hydrogen bis(2-propylpentanoate). Divalproex sodium has the following structure:

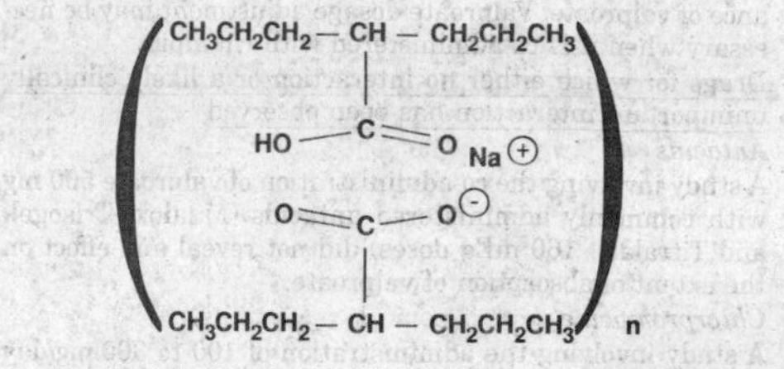

Divalproex sodium occurs as a white powder with a characteristic odor.

Depakote ER 250 and 500 mg tablets are for oral administration. Depakote ER tablets contain divalproex sodium in a once-a-day extended-release formulation equivalent to 250 and 500 mg of valproic acid.

Inactive Ingredients

Depakote ER 250 and 500 mg tablets: FD&C Blue No. 1, hypromellose, lactose, microcrystalline cellulose, polyethylene glycol, potassium sorbate, propylene glycol, silicon dioxide, titanium dioxide, and triacetin.

In addition, 500 mg tablets contain iron oxide and polydextrose.

12 CLINICAL PHARMACOLOGY

12.1 Mechanism of Action

Divalproex sodium dissociates to the valproate ion in the gastrointestinal tract. The mechanisms by which valproate exerts its therapeutic effects have not been established. It has been suggested that its activity in epilepsy is related to increased brain concentrations of gamma-aminobutyric acid (GABA).

12.2 Pharmacodynamics

The relationship between plasma concentration and clinical response is not well documented. One contributing factor is the nonlinear, concentration dependent protein binding of valproate which affects the clearance of the drug. Thus, monitoring of total serum valproate may not provide a reliable index of the bioactive valproate species.

For example, because the plasma protein binding of valproate is concentration dependent, the free fraction increases from approximately 10% at 40 mcg/mL to 18.5% at 130 mcg/mL. Higher than expected free fractions occur in the elderly, in hyperlipidemic patients, and in patients with hepatic and renal diseases.

Epilepsy
The therapeutic range in epilepsy is commonly considered to be 50 to 100 mcg/mL of total valproate, although some patients may be controlled with lower or higher plasma concentrations.
Mania
In placebo-controlled clinical trials of acute mania, patients were dosed to clinical response with trough plasma concentrations between 85 and 125 mcg/mL *[see Dosage and Administration (2.1)]*.

12.3 Pharmacokinetics
Absorption/Bioavailability
The absolute bioavailability of Depakote ER tablets administered as a single dose after a meal was approximately 90% relative to intravenous infusion.
When given in equal total daily doses, the bioavailability of Depakote ER is less than that of Depakote (divalproex sodium delayed-release tablets). In five multiple-dose studies in healthy subjects (N=82) and in subjects with epilepsy (N=86), when administered under fasting and nonfasting conditions, Depakote ER given once daily produced an average bioavailability of 89% relative to an equal total daily dose of Depakote given BID, TID, or QID. The median time to maximum plasma valproate concentrations (C_{max}) after Depakote ER administration ranged from 4 to 17 hours. After multiple once-daily dosing of Depakote ER, the peak-to-trough fluctuation in plasma valproate concentrations was 10-20% lower than that of regular Depakote given BID, TID, or QID.

Conversion from Depakote to Depakote ER
When Depakote ER is given in doses 8 to 20% higher than the total daily dose of Depakote, the two formulations are bioequivalent. In two randomized, crossover studies, multiple daily doses of Depakote were compared to 8 to 20% higher once-daily doses of Depakote ER. In these two studies, Depakote ER and Depakote regimens were equivalent with respect to area under the curve (AUC; a measure of the extent of bioavailability). Additionally, valproate C_{max} was lower, and C_{min} was either higher or not different, for Depakote ER relative to Depakote regimens (see Table 9).
[See table 9 above]

Table 9. Bioavailability of Depakote ER Tablets Relative to Depakote When Depakote ER Dose is 8 to 20% Higher

Study Population	Regimens	Relative Bioavailability		
	Depakote ER vs. Depakote	AUC_{24}	C_{max}	C_{min}
Healthy Volunteers (N=35)	1000 & 1500 mg Depakote ER vs. 875 & 1250 mg Depakote	1.059	0.882	1.173
Patients with epilepsy on concomitant enzyme-inducing antiepilepsy drugs (N = 64)	1000 to 5000 mg Depakote ER vs. 875 to 4250 mg Depakote	1.008	0.899	1.022

Concomitant antiepilepsy drugs (topiramate, phenobarbital, carbamazepine, phenytoin, and lamotrigine were evaluated) that induce the cytochrome P450 isozyme system did not significantly alter valproate bioavailability when converting between Depakote and Depakote ER.
Distribution
Protein Binding
The plasma protein binding of valproate is concentration dependent and the free fraction increases from approximately 10% at 40 mcg/mL to 18.5% at 130 mcg/mL. Protein binding of valproate is reduced in the elderly, in patients with chronic hepatic diseases, in patients with renal impairment, and in the presence of other drugs (e.g., aspirin). Conversely, valproate may displace certain protein-bound drugs (e.g., phenytoin, carbamazepine, warfarin, and tolbutamide) *[see Drug Interactions (7.2)* for more detailed information on the pharmacokinetic interactions of valproate with other drugs*]*.
CNS Distribution
Valproate concentrations in cerebrospinal fluid (CSF) approximate unbound concentrations in plasma (about 10% of total concentration).
Metabolism
Valproate is metabolized almost entirely by the liver. In adult patients on monotherapy, 30-50% of an administered dose appears in urine as a glucuronide conjugate. Mitochondrial β-oxidation is the other major metabolic pathway, typically accounting for over 40% of the dose. Usually, less than 15-20% of the dose is eliminated by other oxidative mechanisms. Less than 3% of an administered dose is excreted unchanged in urine.
The relationship between dose and total valproate concentration is nonlinear; concentration does not increase proportionally with the dose, but rather, increases to a lesser extent due to saturable plasma protein binding. The kinetics of unbound drug are linear.
Elimination
Mean plasma clearance and volume of distribution for total valproate are 0.56 L/hr/1.73 m^2 and 11 L/1.73 m^2, respectively. Mean plasma clearance and volume of distribution for free valproate are 4.6 L/hr/1.73 m^2 and 92 L/1.73 m^2. Mean terminal half-life for valproate monotherapy ranged from 9 to 16 hours following oral dosing regimens of 250 to 1000 mg.
The estimates cited apply primarily to patients who are not taking drugs that affect hepatic metabolizing enzyme systems. For example, patients taking enzyme-inducing antiepileptic drugs (carbamazepine, phenytoin, and phenobarbital) will clear valproate more rapidly. Because of these changes in valproate clearance, monitoring of antiepileptic concentrations should be intensified whenever concomitant antiepileptics are introduced or withdrawn.

Special Populations
Effect of Age
Pediatric
The valproate pharmacokinetic profile following administration of Depakote ER was characterized in a multiple-dose, non-fasting, open label, multi-center study in children and adolescents. Depakote ER once daily doses ranged from 250-1750 mg. Once daily administration of Depakote ER in pediatric patients (10-17 years) produced plasma VPA concentration-time profiles similar to those that have been observed in adults.
Elderly
The capacity of elderly patients (age range: 68 to 89 years) to eliminate valproate has been shown to be reduced compared to younger adults (age range: 22 to 26). Intrinsic clearance is reduced by 39%; the free fraction is increased by 44%. Accordingly, the initial dosage should be reduced in the elderly *[see Dosage and Administration (2.4)]*.
Effect of Sex
There are no differences in the body surface area adjusted unbound clearance between males and females (4.8±0.17 and 4.7±0.07 L/hr per 1.73 m^2, respectively).
Effect of Race
The effects of race on the kinetics of valproate have not been studied.
Effect of Disease
Liver Disease
Liver disease impairs the capacity to eliminate valproate. In one study, the clearance of free valproate was decreased by 50% in 7 patients with cirrhosis and by 16% in 4 patients with acute hepatitis, compared with 6 healthy subjects. In that study, the half-life of valproate was increased from 12 to 18 hours. Liver disease is also associated with decreased albumin concentrations and larger unbound fractions (2 to 2.6 fold increase) of valproate. Accordingly, monitoring of total concentrations may be misleading since free concentrations may be substantially elevated in patients with hepatic disease whereas total concentrations may appear to be normal *[see Boxed Warning, Contraindications (4), and Warnings and Precautions (5.1)]*.
Renal Disease
A slight reduction (27%) in the unbound clearance of valproate has been reported in patients with renal failure (creatinine clearance < 10 mL/minute); however, hemodialysis typically reduces valproate concentrations by about 20%. Therefore, no dosage adjustment appears to be necessary in patients with renal failure. Protein binding in these patients is substantially reduced; thus, monitoring total concentrations may be misleading.

13 NONCLINICAL TOXICOLOGY

13.1 Carcinogenesis, Mutagenesis, and Impairment of Fertility
Carcinogenesis
Valproate was administered orally to rats and mice at doses of 80 and 170 mg/kg/day (less than the maximum recommended human dose on a mg/m^2 basis) for two years. The primary findings were an increase in the incidence of subcutaneous fibrosarcomas in high-dose male rats receiving valproate and a dose-related trend for benign pulmonary adenomas in male mice receiving valproate. The significance of these findings for humans is unknown.
Mutagenesis
Valproate was not mutagenic in an *in vitro* bacterial assay (Ames test), did not produce dominant lethal effects in mice, and did not increase chromosome aberration frequency in an *in vivo* cytogenetic study in rats. Increased frequencies of sister chromatid exchange (SCE) have been reported in a study of epileptic children taking valproate, but this association was not observed in another study conducted in adults. There is some evidence that increased SCE frequencies may be associated with epilepsy. The biological significance of an increase in SCE frequency is not known.
Fertility
Chronic toxicity studies of valproate in juvenile and adult rats and dogs demonstrated reduced spermatogenesis and testicular atrophy at oral doses of 400 mg/kg/day or greater in rats (approximately equivalent to or greater than the maximum recommended human dose (MRHD) on a mg/m^2 basis) and 150 mg/kg/day or greater in dogs (approximately 1.4 times the MRHD or greater on a mg/m^2 basis). Fertility studies in rats have shown no effect on fertility at oral doses of valproate up to 350 mg/kg/day (approximately equal to the MRHD on a mg/m^2 basis) for 60 days. The effect of valproate on testicular development and on sperm production and fertility in humans is unknown.

14 CLINICAL STUDIES

14.1 Mania
The effectiveness of Depakote ER for the treatment of acute mania is based in part on studies establishing the effectiveness of Depakote (divalproex sodium delayed release tablets) for this indication. Depakote ER's effectiveness was confirmed in one randomized, double-blind, placebo-controlled, parallel group, 3-week, multicenter study. The study was designed to evaluate the safety and efficacy of Depakote ER in the treatment of bipolar I disorder, manic or mixed type, in adults. Adult male and female patients who had a current DSM-IV TR primary diagnosis of bipolar I disorder, manic or mixed type, and who were hospitalized for acute mania, were enrolled into this study. Depakote ER was initiated at a dose of 25 mg/kg/day given once daily, increased by 500 mg/day on Day 3, then adjusted to achieve plasma valproate concentrations in the range of 85-125 mcg/mL. Mean daily Depakote ER doses for observed cases were 2362 mg (range: 500-4000), 2874 mg (range: 1500-4500), 2993 mg (range: 1500-4500), 3181 mg (range: 1500-5000), and 3353 mg (range: 1500-5500) at Days 1, 5, 10, 15, and 21, respectively. Mean valproate concentrations were 96.5 mcg/mL, 102.1 mcg/mL, 98.5 mcg/mL, 89.5 mcg/mL at Days 5, 10, 15 and 21, respectively. Patients were assessed on the Mania Rating Scale (MRS; score ranges from 0-52).
Depakote ER was significantly more effective than placebo in reduction of the MRS total score.

14.2 Epilepsy
The efficacy of valproate in reducing the incidence of complex partial seizures (CPS) that occur in isolation or in association with other seizure types was established in two controlled trials.
In one, multi-clinic, placebo controlled study employing an add-on design, (adjunctive therapy) 144 patients who continued to suffer eight or more CPS per 8 weeks during an 8 week period of monotherapy with doses of either carbamazepine or phenytoin sufficient to assure plasma concentrations within the "therapeutic range" were randomized to receive, in addition to their original antiepilepsy drug (AED), either Depakote or placebo. Randomized patients were to be followed for a total of 16 weeks. The following Table presents the findings.

Table 10. Adjunctive Therapy Study Median Incidence of CPS per 8 Weeks

Add-on Treatment	Number of Patients	Baseline Incidence	Experimental Incidence
Depakote	75	16.0	8.9*
Placebo	69	14.5	11.5

* Reduction from baseline statistically significantly greater for valproate than placebo at $p \leq 0.05$ level.

Figure 1 presents the proportion of patients (X axis) whose percentage reduction from baseline in complex partial seizure rates was at least as great as that indicated on the Y axis in the adjunctive therapy study. A positive percent reduction indicates an improvement (i.e., a decrease in seizure frequency), while a negative percent reduction indicates worsening. Thus, in a display of this type, the curve for an effective treatment is shifted to the left of the curve

Information on the AbbVie, Inc. products listed on these pages is from the prescribing information in use as of July 31, 2013. For more information, please visit rxabbvie.com or call 1-800-633-9110.

for placebo. This Figure shows that the proportion of patients achieving any particular level of improvement was consistently higher for valproate than for placebo. For example, 45% of patients treated with valproate had a ≥ 50% reduction in complex partial seizure rate compared to 23% of patients treated with placebo.

Figure 1

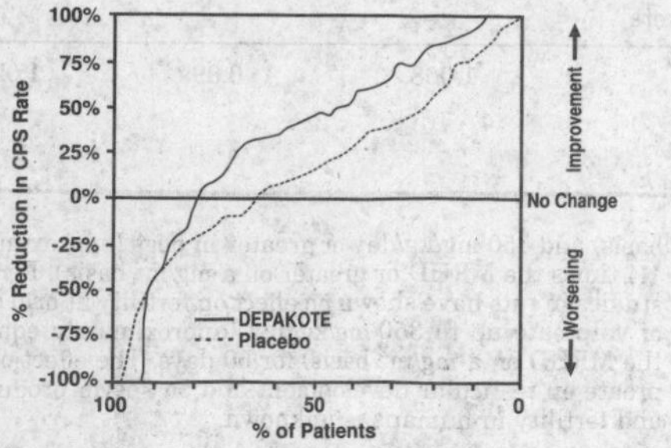

The second study assessed the capacity of valproate to reduce the incidence of CPS when administered as the sole AED. The study compared the incidence of CPS among patients randomized to either a high or low dose treatment arm. Patients qualified for entry into the randomized comparison phase of this study only if 1) they continued to experience 2 or more CPS per 4 weeks during an 8 to 12 week long period of monotherapy with adequate doses of an AED (i.e., phenytoin, carbamazepine, phenobarbital, or primidone) and 2) they made a successful transition over a two week interval to valproate. Patients entering the randomized phase were then brought to their assigned target dose, gradually tapered off their concomitant AED and followed for an interval as long as 22 weeks. Less than 50% of the patients randomized, however, completed the study. In patients converted to Depakote monotherapy, the mean total valproate concentrations during monotherapy were 71 and 123 mcg/mL in the low dose and high dose groups, respectively.

The following Table presents the findings for all patients randomized who had at least one post-randomization assessment.

Table 11. Monotherapy Study Median Incidence of CPS per 8 Weeks

Treatment	Number of Patients	Baseline Incidence	Randomized Phase Incidence
High dose Valproate	131	13.2	10.7*
Low dose Valproate	134	14.2	13.8

* Reduction from baseline statistically significantly greater for high dose than low dose at p ≤ 0.05 level.

Figure 2 presents the proportion of patients (X axis) whose percentage reduction from baseline in complex partial seizure rates was at least as great as that indicated on the Y axis in the monotherapy study. A positive percent reduction indicates an improvement (i.e., a decrease in seizure frequency), while a negative percent reduction indicates worsening. Thus, in a display of this type, the curve for a more effective treatment is shifted to the left of the curve for a less effective treatment. This Figure shows that the proportion of patients achieving any particular level of reduction was consistently higher for high dose valproate than for low dose valproate. For example, when switching from carbamazepine, phenytoin, phenobarbital or primidone monotherapy to high dose valproate monotherapy, 63% of patients experienced no change or a reduction in complex partial seizure rates compared to 54% of patients receiving low dose valproate.

[See figure 2 at top of next column]

Information on pediatric studies are presented in section 8.

14.3 Migraine

The results of a multicenter, randomized, double-blind, placebo-controlled, parallel-group clinical trial demonstrated the effectiveness of Depakote ER in the prophylactic treatment of migraine headache. This trial recruited patients with a history of migraine headaches with or without aura occurring on average twice or more a month for the preceding three months. Patients with cluster or chronic daily headaches were excluded. Women of childbearing potential were allowed in the trial if they were deemed to be practicing an effective method of contraception.

Patients who experienced ≥ 2 migraine headaches in the 4-week baseline period were randomized in a 1:1 ratio to

Figure 2

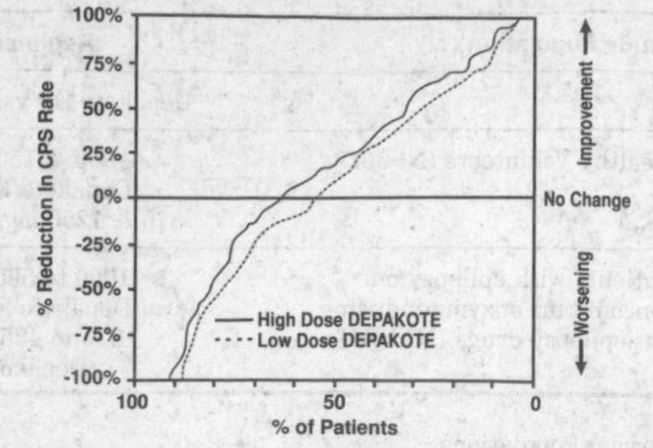

Depakote ER or placebo and treated for 12 weeks. Patients initiated treatment on 500 mg once daily for one week, and were then increased to 1000 mg once daily with an option to permanently decrease the dose back to 500 mg once daily during the second week of treatment if intolerance occurred. Ninety-eight of 114 Depakote ER-treated patients (86%) and 100 of 110 placebo-treated patients (91%) treated at least two weeks maintained the 1000 mg once daily dose for the duration of their treatment periods. Treatment outcome was assessed on the basis of reduction in 4-week migraine headache rate in the treatment period compared to the baseline period.

Patients (50 male, 187 female) ranging in age from 16 to 69 were treated with Depakote ER (N=122) or placebo (N=115). Four patients were below the age of 18 and 3 were above the age of 65. Two hundred and two patients (101 in each treatment group) completed the treatment period. The mean reduction in 4-week migraine headache rate was 1.2 from a baseline mean of 4.4 in the Depakote ER group, versus 0.6 from a baseline mean of 4.2 in the placebo group. The treatment difference was statistically significant (see Figure 3).

Figure 3 Mean Reduction In 4-Week Migraine Headache Rates

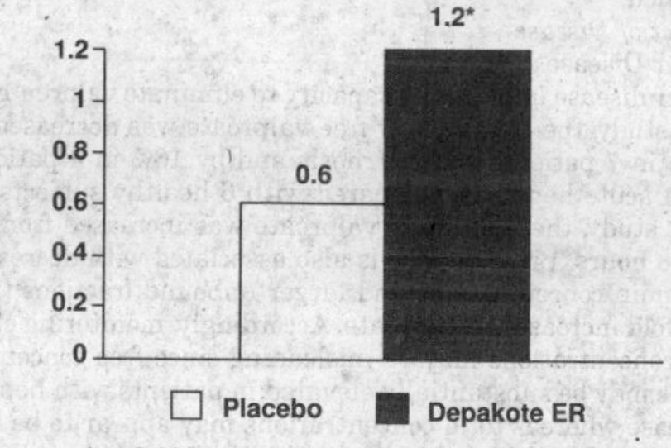

* p=0.006

15 REFERENCES

1. Meador KJ, Baker GA, Browning N, et al. Fetal antiepileptic drug exposure and cognitive outcomes at age 6 years (NEAD study): a prospective observational study. Lancet Neurology 2013; 12 (3):244-252.

16 HOW SUPPLIED/STORAGE AND HANDLING

Depakote ER 250 mg is available as white ovaloid tablets with the "a" logo and the code (HF). Each Depakote ER tablet contains divalproex sodium equivalent to 250 mg of valproic acid in the following package sizes:

Bottles of 60 ....(NDC 0074-3826-60).
Bottles of 100 ....(NDC 0074-3826-13).
Bottles of 500 ....(NDC 0074-3826-53).
Unit Dose Packages of 100..................(NDC 0074-3826-11).

Depakote ER 500 mg is available as gray ovaloid tablets with the "a" logo and the code HC. Each Depakote ER tablet contains divalproex sodium equivalent to 500 mg of valproic acid in the following packaging sizes:

Bottles of 100 ....(NDC 0074-7126-13).
Bottles of 500 ....(NDC 0074-7126-53).
Unit Dose Packages of 100..................(NDC 0074-7126-11).

Recommended Storage

Store tablets at 25°C (77°F); excursions permitted to 15-30°C (59-86°F) [see USP Controlled Room Temperature].

17 PATIENT COUNSELING INFORMATION

See FDA-Approved Medication Guide

17.1 Hepatotoxicity

Warn patients and guardians that nausea, vomiting, abdominal pain, anorexia, diarrhea, asthenia, and/or jaundice can be symptoms of hepatotoxicity and, therefore, require further medical evaluation promptly *[see Warnings and Precautions (5.1)]*.

17.2 Pancreatitis

Warn patients and guardians that abdominal pain, nausea, vomiting, and/or anorexia can be symptoms of pancreatitis and, therefore, require further medical evaluation promptly *[see Warnings and Precautions (5.5)]*.

17.3 Birth Defects and Decreased IQ

Inform pregnant women and women of childbearing potential that use of valproate during pregnancy increases the risk of birth defects and decreased IQ in children who were exposed. Advise women to use effective contraception while using valproate. When appropriate, counsel these patients about alternative therapeutic options. This is particularly important when valproate use is considered for a condition not usually associated with permanent injury or death. Advise patients to read the Medication Guide, which appears as the last section of the labeling *[see Warnings and Precautions (5.2, 5.3, 5.4) and Use in Specific Populations (8.1)]*.

Advise women of childbearing potential to discuss pregnancy planning with their doctor and to contact their doctor immediately if they think they are pregnant.

Encourage patients to enroll in the NAAED Pregnancy Registry if they become pregnant. This registry is collecting information about the safety of antiepileptic drugs during pregnancy. To enroll, patients can call the toll free number 1-888-233-2334 *[see Use in Specific Populations (8.1)]*.

17.4 Suicidal Thinking and Behavior

Counsel patients, their caregivers, and families that AEDs, including Depakote ER, may increase the risk of suicidal thoughts and behavior and should be advised of the need to be alert for the emergence or worsening of symptoms of depression, any unusual changes in mood or behavior, or the emergence of suicidal thoughts, behavior, or thoughts about self-harm. Instruct patients, caregivers, and families to report behaviors of concern immediately to the healthcare providers *[see Warnings and Precautions (5.8)]*.

17.5 Hyperammonemia

Inform patients of the signs and symptoms associated with hyperammonemic encephalopathy and be told to inform the prescriber if any of these symptoms occur *[see Warnings and Precautions (5.10, 5.11)]*.

17.6 CNS Depression

Since valproate products may produce CNS depression, especially when combined with another CNS depressant (e.g., alcohol), advise patients not to engage in hazardous activities, such as driving an automobile or operating dangerous machinery, until it is known that they do not become drowsy from the drug.

17.7 Multi-organ Hypersensitivity Reaction

Instruct patients that a fever associated with other organ system involvement (rash, lymphadenopathy, etc.) may be drug-related and should be reported to the physician immediately *[see Warnings and Precautions (5.13)]*.

17.8 Medication Residue in the Stool

Instruct patients to notify their healthcare provider if they notice a medication residue in the stool *[see Warnings and Precautions (5.19)]*.

250 mg is Mfd. by AbbVie LTD, Barceloneta, PR 00617
500 mg is Mfd. by AbbVie Inc., North Chicago, IL 60064 U.S.A. or
AbbVie LTD, Barceloneta, PR 00617
For AbbVie Inc., North Chicago, IL 60064 U.S.A.

MEDICATION GUIDE

DEPAKOTE ER (dep-a-kOte)
(divalproex sodium)
Extended Release Tablets
DEPAKOTE (dep-a-kOte)
(divalproex sodium)
Tablets
DEPAKOTE (dep-a-kOte)
(divalproex sodium coated particles in capsules)
Sprinkle Capsules
DEPAKENE (dep-a-keen)
(valproic acid)
Capsules and Oral Solution

Read this Medication Guide before you start taking Depakote or Depakene and each time you get a refill. There may be new information. This information does not take the place of talking to your healthcare provider about your medical condition or treatment.

What is the most important information I should know about Depakote and Depakene?

Do not stop taking Depakote or Depakene without first talking to your healthcare provider.

Stopping Depakote or Depakene suddenly can cause serious problems.

Depakote and Depakene can cause serious side effects, including:

1. **Serious liver damage that can cause death, especially in children younger than 2 years old.** The risk of getting this serious liver damage is more likely to happen within the first 6 months of treatment.

   Call your healthcare provider right away if you get any of the following symptoms:

   - nausea or vomiting that does not go away
   - loss of appetite
   - pain on the right side of your stomach (abdomen)
   - dark urine
   - swelling of your face
   - yellowing of your skin or the whites of your eyes

In some cases, liver damage may continue despite stopping the drug.

2. **Depakote or Depakene may harm your unborn baby.**
   - If you take Depakote or Depakene during pregnancy for any medical condition, your baby is at risk for serious birth defects. The most common birth defects with Depakote or Depakene affect the brain and spinal cord and are called spina bifida or neural tube defects. These defects occur in 1 to 2 out of every 100 babies born to mothers who use this medicine during pregnancy. These defects can begin in the first month, even before you know you are pregnant. Other birth defects can happen.
   - Birth defects may occur even in children born to women who are not taking any medicines and do not have other risk factors.
   - Taking folic acid supplements before getting pregnant and during early pregnancy can lower the chance of having a baby with a neural tube defect.
   - If you take Depakote or Depakene during pregnancy for any medical condition, your child is at risk for having a lower IQ.
   - There may be other medicines to treat your condition that have a lower chance of causing birth defects and decreased IQ in your child.
   - Women who are pregnant must not take Depakote or Depakene to prevent migraine headaches.
   - **All women of child-bearing age should talk to their healthcare provider about using other possible treatments instead of Depakote or Depakene. If the decision is made to use Depakote or Depakene, you should use effective birth control (contraception).**
   - Tell your healthcare provider right away if you become pregnant while taking Depakote or Depakene. You and your healthcare provider should decide if you will continue to take Depakote or Depakene while you are pregnant.

   Pregnancy Registry: If you become pregnant while taking Depakote or Depakene, talk to your healthcare provider about registering with the North American Antiepileptic Drug Pregnancy Registry. You can enroll in this registry by calling 1-888-233-2334. The purpose of this registry is to collect information about the safety of antiepileptic drugs during pregnancy.
3. **Inflammation of your pancreas that can cause death.**

   Call your healthcare provider right away if you have any of these symptoms:
   - severe stomach pain that you may also feel in your back
   - nausea or vomiting that does not go away
4. **Like other antiepileptic drugs, Depakote or Depakene may cause suicidal thoughts or actions in a very small number of people, about 1 in 500.**

   Call a healthcare provider right away if you have any of these symptoms, especially if they are new, worse, or worry you:
   - thoughts about suicide or dying
   - attempts to commit suicide
   - new or worse depression
   - new or worse anxiety
   - feeling agitated or restless
   - panic attacks
   - trouble sleeping (insomnia)
   - new or worse irritability
   - acting aggressive, being angry, or violent
   - acting on dangerous impulses
   - an extreme increase in activity and talking (mania)
   - other unusual changes in behavior or mood

   How can I watch for early symptoms of suicidal thoughts and actions?
   - Pay attention to any changes, especially sudden changes in mood, behaviors, thoughts, or feelings.
   - Keep all follow-up visits with your healthcare provider as scheduled.

   Call your healthcare provider between visits as needed, especially if you are worried about symptoms.

   Do not stop Depakote or Depakene without first talking to a healthcare provider. Stopping Depakote or Depakene suddenly can cause serious problems. Stopping a seizure medicine suddenly in a patient who has epilepsy can cause seizures that do not stop (status epilepticus).

   Suicidal thoughts or actions can be caused by things other than medicines. If you have suicidal thoughts or actions, your healthcare provider may check for other causes.

What are Depakote and Depakene?

Depakote and Depakene come in different dosage forms with different usages.

Depakote Tablets and Depakote Extended Release Tablets are prescription medicines used:
- to treat manic episodes associated with bipolar disorder.
- alone or with other medicines to treat:
  - complex partial seizures in adults and children 10 years of age and older
  - simple and complex absence seizures, with or without other seizure types
- to prevent migraine headaches

Depakene (solution and liquid capsules) and Depakote Sprinkles are prescription medicines used alone or with other medicines, to treat:
- complex partial seizures in adults and children 10 years of age and older
- simple and complex absence seizures, with or without other seizure types

Who should not take Depakote or Depakene?

Do not take Depakote or Depakene if you:
- have liver problems
- have or think you have a genetic liver problem caused by a mitochondrial disorder (e.g. Alpers-Huttenlocher syndrome)
- are allergic to divalproex sodium, valproic acid, sodium valproate, or any of the ingredients in Depakote or Depakene. See the end of this leaflet for a complete list of ingredients in Depakote and Depakene.
- have a genetic problem called urea cycle disorder
- are pregnant for the prevention of migraine headaches

What should I tell my healthcare provider before taking Depakote or Depakene?

Before you take Depakote or Depakene, tell your healthcare provider if you:
- have a genetic liver problem caused by a mitochondrial disorder (e.g. Alpers-Huttenlocher syndrome)
- drink alcohol
- are pregnant or breastfeeding. Depakote or Depakene can pass into breast milk. Talk to your healthcare provider about the best way to feed your baby if you take Depakote or Depakene.
- have or have had depression, mood problems, or suicidal thoughts or behavior
- have any other medical conditions

Tell your healthcare provider about all the medicines you take, including prescription and non-prescription medicines, vitamins, herbal supplements and medicines that you take for a short period of time.

Taking Depakote or Depakene with certain other medicines can cause side effects or affect how well they work. Do not start or stop other medicines without talking to your healthcare provider.

Know the medicines you take. Keep a list of them and show it to your healthcare provider and pharmacist each time you get a new medicine.

How should I take Depakote or Depakene?
- Take Depakote or Depakene exactly as your healthcare provider tells you. Your healthcare provider will tell you how much Depakote or Depakene to take and when to take it.
- Your healthcare provider may change your dose.
- Do not change your dose of Depakote or Depakene without talking to your healthcare provider.
- **Do not stop taking Depakote or Depakene without first talking to your healthcare provider.** Stopping Depakote or Depakene suddenly can cause serious problems.
- Swallow Depakote tablets, Depakote ER tablets or Depakene capsules whole. Do not crush or chew Depakote tablets, Depakote ER tablets, or Depakene capsules. Tell your healthcare provider if you can not swallow Depakote or Depakene whole. You may need a different medicine.
- Depakote Sprinkle Capsules may be swallowed whole, or they may be opened and the contents may be sprinkled on a small amount of soft food, such as applesauce or pudding. See the Patient Instructions for Use at the end of this Medication Guide for detailed instructions on how to use Depakote Sprinkle Capsules.
- If you take too much Depakote or Depakene, call your healthcare provider or local Poison Control Center right away.

What should I avoid while taking Depakote or Depakene?
- Depakote and Depakene can cause drowsiness and dizziness. Do not drink alcohol or take other medicines that make you sleepy or dizzy while taking Depakote or Depakene, until you talk with your doctor. Taking Depakote or Depakene with alcohol or drugs that cause sleepiness or dizziness may make your sleepiness or dizziness worse.
- Do not drive a car or operate dangerous machinery until you know how Depakote or Depakene affect you. Depakote and Depakene can slow your thinking and motor skills

What are the possible side effects of Depakote or Depakene?
- See **"What is the most important information I should know about Depakote or Depakene?"**

Depakote or Depakene may cause other serious side effects including:
- **Low blood count:** red or purple spots on your skin, bruising, bleeding from your mouth, teeth or nose.
- **High ammonia levels in your blood:** feeling tired, vomiting, changes in mental status.
- **Low body temperature (hypothermia):** drop in your body temperature to less than 95°F, feeling tired, confusion, coma.
- **Allergic (hypersensitivity) reactions:** fever, skin rash, hives, sores in your mouth, blistering and peeling of your skin, swelling of your lymph nodes, swelling of your face, eyes, lips, tongue, or throat, trouble swallowing or breathing.
- **Drowsiness or sleepiness in the elderly.** This extreme drowsiness may cause you to eat or drink less than you normally would. Tell your doctor if you are not able to eat or drink as you normally do. Your doctor may start you at a lower dose of Depakote or Depakene.

Call your healthcare provider right away, if you have any of the symptoms listed above.

The common side effects of Depakote and Depakene include:
- nausea
- headache
- sleepiness
- vomiting
- weakness
- tremor
- dizziness
- stomach pain
- blurry vision
- double vision
- diarrhea
- increased appetite
- weight gain
- hair loss
- loss of appetite
- problems with walking or coordination

These are not all of the possible side effects of **Depakote or Depakene**. For more information, ask your healthcare provider or pharmacist.

Tell your healthcare provider if you have any side effect that bothers you or that does not go away.

Call your doctor for medical advice about side effects. You may report side effects to FDA at 1-800-FDA-1088.

How should I store Depakote or Depakene?
- Store Depakote Extended Release Tablets between 59°F to 86°F (15°C to 30°C).
- Store Depakote Delayed Release Tablets below 86°F (30°C).
- Store Depakote Sprinkle Capsules below 77°F (25°C).
- Store Depakene Capsules at 59°F to 77°F (15°C to 25°C).
- Store Depakene Oral Solution below 86°F (30°C).

Keep Depakote or Depakene and all medicines out of the reach of children.

General information about the safe and effective use of Depakote or Depakene

Medicines are sometimes prescribed for purposes other than those listed in a Medication Guide. Do not use Depakote or Depakene for a condition for which it was not prescribed. Do not give Depakote or Depakene to other people, even if they have the same symptoms that you have. It may harm them. This Medication Guide summarizes the most important information about Depakote or Depakene. If you would like more information, talk with your healthcare provider. You can ask your pharmacist or healthcare provider for information about Depakote or Depakene that is written for health professionals.

For more information, go to www.rxabbvie.com or call 1-800-633-9110.

What are the ingredients in Depakote or Depakene?

Depakote

Active ingredient: divalproex sodium

Inactive ingredients:
- **Depakote Extended Release Tablets:** FD&C Blue No. 1, hypromellose, lactose, microcrystalline cellulose, polyethylene glycol, potassium sorbate, propylene glycol, silicon dioxide, titanium dioxide, and triacetin. The 500 mg tablets also contain iron oxide and polydextrose.
- **Depakote Tablets:** cellulosic polymers, diacetylated monoglycerides, povidone, pregelatinized starch (contains corn starch), silica gel, talc, titanium dioxide, and vanillin. Individual tablets also contain:

  125 mg tablets: FD&C Blue No. 1 and FD&C Red No. 40,

  250 mg tablets: FD&C Yellow No. 6 and iron oxide,

  500 mg tablets: D&C Red No. 30, FD&C Blue No. 2, and iron oxide.
- **Depakote Sprinkle Capsules:** cellulosic polymers, D&C Red No. 28, FD&C Blue No. 1 gelatin, iron oxide, magnesium stearate, silica gel, titanium dioxide, and triethyl citrate.

Information on the AbbVie, Inc. products listed on these pages is from the prescribing information in use as of July 31, 2013. For more information, please visit rxabbvie.com or call 1-800-633-9110.

Depakene
Active ingredient: valproic acid
Inactive ingredients:
- **Depakene Capsules:** corn oil, FD&C Yellow No. 6, gelatin, glycerin, iron oxide, methylparaben, propylparaben, and titanium dioxide.
- **Depakene Oral Solution:** FD&C Red No. 40, glycerin, methylparaben, propylparaben, sorbitol, sucrose, water, and natural and artificial flavors.

Depakote ER
250 mg is Mfd. by AbbVie LTD, Barceloneta, PR 00617
500 mg is Mfd. by AbbVie Inc., North Chicago, IL 60064 U.S.A. or
AbbVie LTD, Barceloneta, PR 00617
For AbbVie Inc., North Chicago, IL 60064 U.S.A.
Depakote Tablets
Mfd. by AbbVie LTD, Barceloneta, PR 00617
For AbbVie Inc., North Chicago, IL 60064, U.S.A.
Depakote Sprinkle Capsules
AbbVie Inc., North Chicago, IL 60064, U.S.A.
Depakene Capsules
Mfd. by Banner Pharmacaps, Inc., High Point, NC 27265 U.S.A.
For AbbVie Inc., North Chicago, IL 60064, U.S.A.
Depakene Oral solution
Mfd. by AbbVie Inc., North Chicago, IL 60064, U.S.A.
OR by DPT Laboratories, Ltd., San Antonio, TX 78215, U.S.A.
For AbbVie Inc., North Chicago, IL 60064, U.S.A.
This Medication Guide has been approved by the U.S. Food and Drug Administration.
03-A837-R16-Revised May, 2013
Shown in Product Identification Guide, page 303

GENGRAF® CAPSULES ℞
[jen-graf]
(cyclosporine capsules USP [MODIFIED])

WARNING
Only physicians experienced in the management of systemic immunosuppressive therapy for the indicated disease should prescribe Gengraf® Capsules (cyclosporine capsules, USP [**MODIFIED**]). At doses used in solid organ transplantation, only physicians experienced in immunosuppressive therapy and management of organ transplant recipients should prescribe Gengraf®. Patients receiving the drug should be managed in facilities equipped and staffed with adequate laboratory and supportive medical resources. The physician responsible for maintenance therapy should have complete information requisite for the follow-up of the patient.
Gengraf®, a systemic immunosuppressant, may increase the susceptibility to infection and the development of neoplasia. In kidney, liver, and heart transplant patients Gengraf® may be administered with other immunosuppressive agents. Increased susceptibility to infection and the possible development of lymphoma and other neoplasms may result from the increase in the degree of immunosuppression in transplant patients.
Gengraf® Capsules (cyclosporine capsules, USP [**MODIFIED**]) has increased bioavailability in comparison to Sandimmune® Soft Gelatin Capsules (cyclosporine capsules, USP). Gengraf® and Sandimmune® are not bioequivalent and cannot be used interchangeably without physician supervision. For a given trough concentration, cyclosporine exposure will be greater with Gengraf® than with Sandimmune®. If a patient who is receiving exceptionally high doses of Sandimmune® is converted to Gengraf®, particular caution should be exercised. Cyclosporine blood concentrations should be monitored in transplant and rheumatoid arthritis patients taking Gengraf® to avoid toxicity due to high concentrations. Dose adjustments should be made in transplant patients to minimize possible organ rejection due to low concentrations. Comparison of blood concentrations in the published literature with blood concentrations obtained using current assays must be done with detailed knowledge of the assay methods employed.
For Psoriasis Patients (see also Boxed WARNINGS above)
Psoriasis patients previously treated with PUVA and to a lesser extent, methotrexate or other immunosuppressive agents, UVB, coal tar, or radiation therapy, are at an increased risk of developing skin malignancies when taking Gengraf® Capsules (cyclosporine capsules, USP [**MODIFIED**]).
Cyclosporine, the active ingredient in Gengraf®, in recommended dosages, can cause systemic hypertension and nephrotoxicity. The risk increases with increasing dose and duration of cyclosporine therapy. Renal dysfunction, including structural kidney damage, is a potential consequence of cyclosporine, and therefore, renal function must be monitored during therapy.

DESCRIPTION
Gengraf® Capsules (cyclosporine capsules, USP [**MODIFIED**]) is a modified oral formulation of cyclosporine that forms an aqueous dispersion in an aqueous environment.
Cyclosporine, the active principle in Gengraf®, is a cyclic polypeptide immunosuppressant agent consisting of 11 amino acids. It is produced as a metabolite by the fungus species *Aphanocladium album*.
Chemically, cyclosporine is designated as [R-[R*,R*-(E)]]-cyclic-(L-alanyl-D-alanyl-*N*-methyl-L-leucyl-*N* -methyl-L-leucyl-*N*-methyl-L-valyl-3-hydroxy-*N*,4-dimethyl- L-2-amino-6-octenoyl-L-α-amino-butyryl-*N*-methylglycyl-*N* -methyl-L-leucyl-L-valyl-*N*-methyl-L-leucyl).
Gengraf® Capsules (cyclosporine capsules, USP [**MODIFIED**]) are available in 25 mg and 100 mg strengths.
Each 25 mg capsule contains
cyclosporine, 25 mg, alcohol, USP, absolute, 12.8% v/v (10.1% wt/vol.).
Each 100 mg capsule contains
cyclosporine, 100 mg, alcohol, USP, absolute, 12.8% v/v (10.1% wt/vol.).
Inactive Ingredients
FD&C Blue No. 2, gelatin NF, polyethylene glycol NF, polyoxyl 35 castor oil NF, polysorbate 80 NF, propylene glycol USP, sorbitan monooleate NF, titanium dioxide.
The chemical structure for cyclosporine USP is:

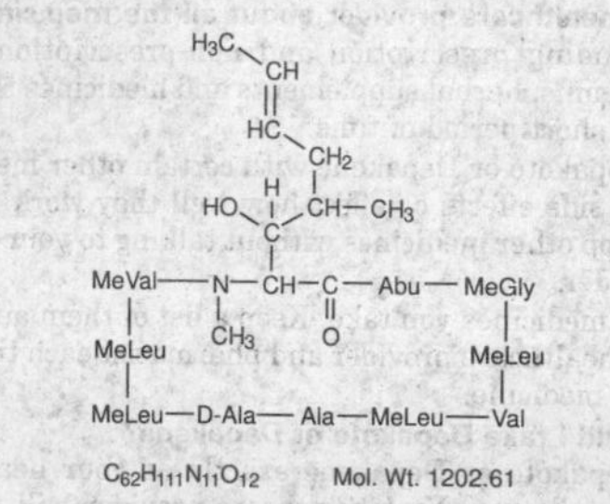

$C_{62}H_{111}N_{11}O_{12}$ Mol. Wt. 1202.61

CLINICAL PHARMACOLOGY
Cyclosporine is a potent immunosuppressive agent that in animals prolongs survival of allogeneic transplants involving skin, kidney, liver, heart, pancreas, bone marrow, small intestine, and lung. Cyclosporine has been demonstrated to suppress some humoral immunity and to a greater extent, cell-mediated immune reactions such as allograft rejection, delayed hypersensitivity, experimental allergic encephalomyelitis, Freund's adjuvant arthritis, and graft vs. host disease in many animal species for a variety of organs.
The effectiveness of cyclosporine results from specific and reversible inhibition of immunocompetent lymphocytes in the G_0- and G_1-phase of the cell cycle. T-lymphocytes are preferentially inhibited. The T-helper cell is the main target, although the T-suppressor cell may also be suppressed. Cyclosporine also inhibits lymphokine production and release including interleukin-2.
No effects on phagocytic function (changes in enzyme secretions, chemotactic migration of granulocytes, macrophage migration, carbon clearance *in vivo*) have been detected in animals. Cyclosporine does not cause bone marrow suppression in animal models or man.
Pharmacokinetics
The immunosuppressive activity of cyclosporine is primarily due to parent drug. Following oral administration, absorption of cyclosporine is incomplete. The extent of absorption of cyclosporine is dependent on the individual patient, the patient population, and the formulation. Elimination of cyclosporine is primarily biliary with only 6% of the dose (parent drug and metabolites) excreted in urine. The disposition of cyclosporine from blood is generally biphasic, with a terminal half-life of approximately 8.4 hours (range 5 to 18 hours). Following intravenous administration, the blood clearance of cyclosporine (assay: HPLC) is approximately 5 to 7 mL/min/kg in adult recipients of renal or liver allografts. Blood cyclosporine clearance appears to be slightly slower in cardiac transplant patients.
The Gengraf® Capsules (cyclosporine capsules, USP [**MODIFIED**]) and Gengraf® Oral Solution (cyclosporine oral solution, USP [**MODIFIED**]) are bioequivalent.
The relationship between administered dose and exposure (area under the concentration versus time curve, AUC) is linear within the therapeutic dose range. The intersubject variability (total, % CV) of cyclosporine exposure (AUC) when cyclosporine (**MODIFIED**) or Sandimmune® is administered ranges from approximately 20% to 50% in renal transplant patients. This intersubject variability contributes to the need for individualization of the dosing regimen for optimal therapy (see **DOSAGE AND ADMINISTRATION**). Intrasubject variability of AUC in renal transplant recipients (% CV) was 9% to 21% for cyclosporine (**MODIFIED**) and 19% to 26% for Sandimmune®. In the same studies, intrasubject variability of trough concentrations (% CV) was 17% to 30% for cyclosporine (**MODIFIED**) and 16% to 38% for Sandimmune®.
Absorption
Cyclosporine (**MODIFIED**) has increased bioavailability compared to Sandimmune®. The absolute bioavailability of cyclosporine administered as Sandimmune® is dependent on the patient population, estimated to be less than 10% in liver transplant patients and as great as 89% in some renal transplant patients. The absolute bioavailability of cyclosporine administered as cyclosporine (**MODIFIED**) has not been determined in adults. In studies of renal transplant, rheumatoid arthritis and psoriasis patients, the mean cyclosporine AUC was approximately 20% to 50% greater and the peak blood cyclosporine concentration (C_{max}) was approximately 40% to 106% greater following administration of cyclosporine (**MODIFIED**) compared to following administration of Sandimmune®. The dose normalized AUC in *de novo* liver transplant patients administered cyclosporine (**MODIFIED**) 28 days after transplantation was 50% greater and C_{max} was 90% greater than in those patients administered Sandimmune®. AUC and C_{max} are also increased (cyclosporine [**MODIFIED**] relative to Sandimmune®) in heart transplant patients, but data are very limited. Although the AUC and C_{max} values are higher on cyclosporine (**MODIFIED**) relative to Sandimmune®, the pre-dose trough concentrations (dose-normalized) are similar for the two formulations.
Following oral administration of cyclosporine (**MODIFIED**), the time to peak blood cyclosporine concentrations (T_{max}) ranged from 1.5 to 2.0 hours. The administration of food with cyclosporine (**MODIFIED**) decreases the cyclosporine AUC and C_{max}. A high fat meal (669 kcal, 45 grams fat) consumed within one-half hour before cyclosporine (**MODIFIED**) administration decreased the AUC by 13% and C_{max} by 33%. The effects of a low fat meal (667 kcal, 15 grams fat) were similar.
The effect of T-tube diversion of bile on the absorption of cyclosporine from cyclosporine (**MODIFIED**) was investigated in eleven *de novo* liver transplant patients. When the patients were administered cyclosporine (**MODIFIED**) with and without T-tube diversion of bile, very little difference in absorption was observed, as measured by the change in maximal cyclosporine blood concentrations from pre-dose values with the T-tube closed relative to when it was open: 6.9 ± 41% (range -55% to 68%).
[See first table at top of next page]
Distribution
Cyclosporine is distributed largely outside the blood volume. The steady state volume of distribution during intravenous dosing has been reported as 3 to 5 L/kg in solid organ transplant recipients. In blood, the distribution is concentration dependent. Approximately 33% to 47% is in plasma, 4% to 9% in lymphocytes, 5% to 12% in granulocytes, and 41% to 58% in erythrocytes. At high concentrations, the binding capacity of leukocytes and erythrocytes becomes saturated. In plasma, approximately 90% is bound to proteins, primarily lipoproteins. Cyclosporine is excreted in human milk (see **PRECAUTIONS - Nursing Mothers**).
Metabolism
Cyclosporine is extensively metabolized by the cytochrome P-450 III-A enzyme system in the liver, and to a lesser degree in the gastrointestinal tract, and the kidney. The metabolism of cyclosporine can be altered by the coadministration of a variety of agents (see **PRECAUTIONS - Drug Interactions**). At least 25 metabolites have been identified from human bile, feces, blood, and urine. The biological activity of the metabolites and their contributions to toxicity are considerably less than those of the parent compound. The major metabolites (M1, M9, and M4N) result from oxidation at the 1-beta, 9-gamma, and 4-N-demethylated positions, respectively. At steady state following the oral administration of Sandimmune®, the mean AUCs for blood concentrations of M1, M9 and M4N are about 70%, 21%, and 7.5% of the AUC for blood cyclosporine concentrations, respectively. Based on blood concentration data from stable renal transplant patients (13 patients administered cyclosporine [**MODIFIED**] and Sandimmune® in a crossover study), and bile concentration data from *de novo* liver transplant patients (4 administered cyclosporine [**MODIFIED**], 3 administered Sandimmune®), the percentage of dose present as M1, M9, and M4N metabolites is similar when either cyclosporine (**MODIFIED**) or Sandimmune® is administered.
Excretion
Only 0.1% of a cyclosporine dose is excreted unchanged in the urine. Elimination is primarily biliary with only 6% of the dose (parent drug and metabolites) excreted in the urine. Neither dialysis nor renal failure alter cyclosporine clearance significantly.

Drug Interactions
(See **PRECAUTIONS - Drug Interactions**). When diclofenac or methotrexate was coadministered with cyclosporine in rheumatoid arthritis patients, the AUC of diclofenac and methotrexate, each was significantly increased (see **PRECAUTIONS - Drug Interactions**). No clinically significant pharmacokinetic interactions occurred between cyclosporine and aspirin, ketoprofen, piroxicam, or indomethacin.

Specific Populationa

Renal Impairment

In a study performed in 4 subjects with end-stage renal disease (creatinine clearance <5 mL/min), an intravenous infusion of 3.5 mg/kg of cyclosporine over 4 hours administered at the end of a hemodialysis session resulted in a mean volume of distribution (Vdss) of 3.49 L/kg and systemic clearance (CL) of 0.369 L/hr/kg. This systemic CL (0.369 L/hr/kg) was approximately two thirds of the mean systemic CL (0.56 L/hr/kg) of cyclosporine in historical control subjects with normal renal function. In 5 liver transplant patients, the mean clearance of cyclosporine on and off hemodialysis was 463 mL/min and 398 mL/min, respectively. Less than 1% of the dose of cyclosporine was recovered in the dialysate.

Hepatic Impairment

Cyclosporine is extensively metabolized by the liver. Since severe hepatic impairment may result in significantly increased cyclosporine exposures, the dosage of cyclosporine may need to be reduced in these patients.

Pediatric Population

Pharmacokinetic data from pediatric patients administered cyclosporine (**MODIFIED**) or Sandimmune® are very limited. In 15 renal transplant patients aged 3 to 16 years, cyclosporine whole blood clearance after IV administration of Sandimmune® was 10.6 ± 3.7 mL/min/kg (assay: Cyclo-trac specific RIA). In a study of 7 renal transplant patients aged 2 to 16, the cyclosporine clearance ranged from 9.8 to 15.5 mL/min/kg. In 9 liver transplant patients aged 0.6 to 5.6 years, clearance was 9.3 ± 5.4 mL/min/kg (assay: HPLC).

In the pediatric population, cyclosporine (**MODIFIED**) also demonstrates an increased bioavailability as compared to Sandimmune®. In 7 liver *de novo* transplant patients aged 1.4 to 10 years, the absolute bioavailability of cyclosporine (**MODIFIED**) was 43% (range 30% to 68%) and for Sandimmune® in the same individuals absolute bioavailability was 28% (range 17% to 42%).

[See second table at right]

Geriatric Population

Comparison of single dose data from both normal elderly volunteers (N = 18, mean age 69 years) and elderly rheumatoid arthritis patients (N = 16, mean age 68 years) to single dose data in young adult volunteers (N = 16, mean age 26 years) showed no significant difference in the pharmacokinetic parameters.

Pharmacokinetic Parameters (mean± SD)

Patient Population	Dose/day[1] (mg/d)	Dose/ weight (mg/kg/d)	AUC[2] (ng•hr/mL)	C_{max} (ng/mL)	Trough[3] (ng/mL)	CL/F (mL/min)	CL/F (mL/min/kg)
De novo renal transplant[4] Week 4 (N = 37)	597 ± 174	7.95 ± 2.81	8772 ± 2089	1802 ± 428	361 ± 129	593 ± 204	7.8 ± 2.9
Stable renal transplant[4] (N = 55)	344 ± 122	4.10 ± 1.58	6035 ± 2194	1333 ± 469	251 ± 116	492 ± 140	5.9 ± 2.1
De novo liver transplant[5] Week 4 (N = 18)	458 ± 190	6.89 ± 3.68	7187 ± 2816	1555 ± 740	268 ± 101	577 ± 309	8.6 ± 5.7
De novo rheumatoid arthritis[6] (N = 23)	182 ± 55.6	2.37 ± 0.36	2641 ± 877	728 ± 263	96.4 ± 37.7	613 ± 196	8.3 ± 2.8
De novo psoriasis[6] Week 4 (N = 18)	189 ± 69.8	2.48 ± 0.65	2324 ± 1048	655 ± 186	74.9 ± 46.7	723 ± 186	10.2 ± 3.9

[1] Total daily dose was divided into two doses administered every 12 hours.
[2] AUC was measured over one dosing interval.
[3] Trough concentration was measured just prior to the morning cyclosporine (**MODIFIED**) dose, approximately 12 hours after the previous dose.
[4] Assay: TDx specific monoclonal fluorescence polarization immunoassay.
[5] Assay: Cyclo-trac specific monoclonal radioimmunoassay.
[6] Assay: INCSTAR specific monoclonal radioimmunoassay.

Pediatric Pharmacokinetic Parameters (mean ± SD)

Patient Population	Dose/ day (mg/d)	Dose/ weight (mg/kg/d)	AUC[1] (ng•hr/mL)	C_{max} (ng/mL)	CL/F (mL/min)	CL/F (mL/min/kg)
Stable liver transplant [2]						
Age 2-8, Dosed TID (N = 9)	101 ± 25	5.95 ± 1.32	2163 ± 801	629 ± 219	285 ± 94	16.6 ± 4.3
Age 8-15, Dosed BID (N = 8)	188 ± 55	4.96 ± 2.09	4272 ± 1462	975 ± 281	378 ± 80	10.2 ± 4.0
Stable liver transplant [3]						
Age 3, Dosed BID (N = 1)	120	8.33	5832	1050	171	11.9
Age 8-15, Dosed BID (N = 5)	158 ± 55	5.51 ± 1.91	4452 ± 2475	1013 ± 635	328 ± 121	11.0 ± 1.9
Stable renal transplant [3]						
Age 7-15, Dosed BID (N = 5)	328 ± 83	7.37 ± 4.11	6922 ± 1988	1827 ± 487	418 ± 143	8.7 ± 2.9

[1] AUC was measured over one dosing interval.
[2] Assay: Cyclo-trac specific monoclonal radioimmunoassay.
[3] Assay: TDx specific monoclonal fluorescence polarization immunoassay.

CLINICAL TRIALS

Rheumatoid Arthritis

The effectiveness of Sandimmune® and cyclosporine (**MODIFIED**) in the treatment of severe rheumatoid arthritis was evaluated in five clinical studies involving a total of 728 cyclosporine treated patients and 273 placebo treated patients.

A summary of the results is presented for the "responder" rates per treatment group, with a responder being defined as a patient having *completed* the trial with a 20% improvement in the tender and the swollen joint count and a 20% improvement in 2 of 4 of investigator global, patient global, disability, and erythrocyte sedimentation rates (ESR) for the Studies 651 and 652 and 3 of 5 of investigator global, patient global, disability, visual analog pain, and ESR for Studies 2008, 654, and 302.

Study 651 enrolled 264 patients with active rheumatoid arthritis with at least 20 involved joints, who had failed at least one major RA drug, using a 3:3:2 randomization to one of the following three groups: (1) cyclosporine dosed at 2.5 to 5 mg/kg/day, (2) methotrexate at 7.5 to 15 mg/week, or (3) placebo. Treatment duration was 24 weeks. The mean cyclosporine dose at the last visit was 3.1 mg/kg/day. See Graph below.

Study 652 enrolled 250 patients with active RA with > 6 active painful or tender joints who had failed at least one major RA drug. Patients were randomized using a 3:3:2 randomization to 1 of 3 treatment arms: (1) 1.5 to 5 mg/kg/day of cyclosporine, (2) 2.5 to 5 mg/kg/day of cyclosporine, and (3) placebo. Treatment duration was 16 weeks. The mean cyclosporine dose for group 2 at the last visit was 2.92 mg/kg/day. See Graph below.

Study 2008 enrolled 144 patients with active RA and > 6 active joints who had unsuccessful treatment courses of aspirin and gold or Penicillamine. Patients were randomized to one of two treatment groups: (1) cyclosporine 2.5 to 5 mg/kg/day with adjustments after the first month to achieve a target trough level and (2) placebo. Treatment duration was 24 weeks. The mean cyclosporine dose at the last visit was 3.63 mg/kg/day. See Graph below.

Study 654 enrolled 148 patients who remained with active joint counts of 6 or more despite treatment with maximally tolerated methotrexate doses for at least three months. Patients continued to take their current dose of methotrexate and were randomized to receive, in addition, one of the following medications: (1) cyclosporine 2.5 mg/kg/day with dose increases of 0.5 mg/kg/day at Weeks 2 and 4 if there was no evidence of toxicity and further increases of 0.5 mg/kg/day at Weeks 8 and 16 if a < 30% decrease in active joint count occurred without any significant toxicity; dose decreases could be made at any time for toxicity or (2) placebo. Treatment duration was 24 weeks. The mean cyclosporine dose at the last visit was 2.8 mg/kg/day (range: 1.3 to 4.1). See Graph below.

Study 302 enrolled 299 patients with severe active RA, 99% of whom were unresponsive or intolerant to at least one prior major RA drug. Patients were randomized to 1 of 2 treatment groups (1) cyclosporine (**MODIFIED**) and (2) Sandimmune® both of which were started at 2.5 mg/kg/day and increased after 4 weeks for inefficacy in increments of 0.5 mg/kg/day to a maximum of 5 mg/kg/day and decreased at any time for toxicity. Treatment duration was 24 weeks. The mean cyclosporine dose at the last visit was 2.91 mg/kg/day (range: 0.72 to 5.17) for cyclosporine (**MODIFIED**) and 3.27 mg/kg/day (range: 0.73 to 5.68) for Sandimmune®. See Graph below.

[See figure at top of next column]

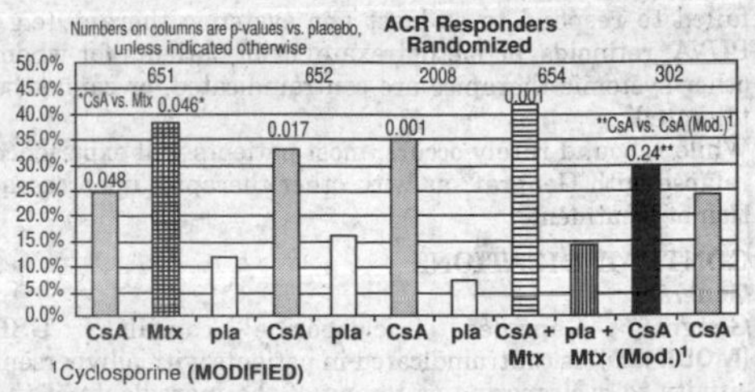

INDICATIONS AND USAGE

Kidney, Liver and Heart Transplantation

Gengraf® Capsules (cyclosporine capsules, USP [**MODIFIED**]) is indicated for the prophylaxis of organ rejection in kidney, liver, and heart allogeneic transplants. Cyclosporine (**MODIFIED**) has been used in combination with azathioprine and corticosteroids.

Rheumatoid Arthritis

Gengraf® Capsules (cyclosporine capsules, USP [**MODIFIED**]) is indicated for the treatment of patients with severe active, rheumatoid arthritis where the disease has not adequately responded to methotrexate. Gengraf® can be used in combination with methotrexate in rheumatoid arthritis patients who do not respond adequately to methotrexate alone.

Psoriasis

Gengraf® Capsules (cyclosporine capsules, USP [**MODIFIED**]) is indicated for the treatment of *adult, nonim-*

Information on the AbbVie, Inc. products listed on these pages is from the prescribing information in use as of July 31, 2013. For more information, please visit rxabbvie.com or call 1-800-633-9110.

Nephrotoxicity vs. Rejection

Parameter	Nephrotoxicity	Rejection
History	Donor > 50 years old or hypotensive Prolonged kidney preservation Prolonged anastomosis time Concomitant nephrotoxic drugs	Anti-donor immune response Retransplant patient
Clinical	Often > 6 weeks postop[b] Prolonged initial nonfunction (acute tubular necrosis)	Often < 4 weeks postop[b] Fever > 37.5°C Weight gain > 0.5 kg Graft swelling and tenderness Decrease in daily urine volume > 500 mL (or 50%)
Laboratory	CyA serum trough level > 200 ng/mL Gradual rise in Cr (< 0.15 mg/dL/day)[a] Cr plateau < 25% above baseline BUN/Cr ≥ 20	CyA serum trough level < 150 ng/mL Rapid rise in Cr (> 0.3 mg/dL/day)[a] Cr > 25% above baseline BUN/Cr < 20
Biopsy	Arteriolopathy (medial hypertrophy[a], hyalinosis, nodular deposits, intimal thickening, endothelial vacuolization, progressive scarring) Tubular atrophy, isometric vacuolization, isolated calcifications Minimal edema Mild focal infiltrates[c] Diffuse interstitial fibrosis, often striped form	Endovasculitis[c] (proliferation[a], intimal arteritis[b], necrosis, sclerosis) Tubulitis with RBC[b] and WBC[b] casts, some irregular vacuolization Interstitial edema[c] and hemorrhage[b] Diffuse moderate to severe mononuclear infiltrates[d] Glomerulitis (mononuclear cells)[c]
Aspiration Cytology	CyA deposits in tubular and endothelial cells Fine isometric vacuolization of tubular cells	Inflammatory infiltrate with mononuclear phagocytes, macrophages, lymphoblastoid cells, and activated T-cells These strongly express HLA-DR antigens
Urine Cytology	Tubular cells with vacuolization and granularization	Degenerative tubular cells, plasma cells, and lymphocyturia > 20% of sediment
Manometry Ultrasonography	Intracapsular pressure < 40 mm Hg[b] Unchanged graft cross sectional area	Intracapsular pressure > 40 mm Hg[b] Increase in graft cross sectional area AP diameter ≥ Transverse diameter
Magnetic Resonance Imagery	Normal appearance	Loss of distinct corticomedullary junction, swelling image intensity of parachyma approaching that of psoas, loss of hilar fat
Radionuclide Scan	Normal or generally decreased perfusion Decrease in tubular function (^{131} I-hippuran) > decrease in perfusion (^{99m} Tc DTPA)	Patchy arterial flow Decrease in perfusion > decrease in tubular function Increased uptake of Indium 111 labeled platelets or Tc-99m in colloid
Therapy	Responds to decreased cyclosporine	Responds to increased steroids or antilymphocyte globulin

[a] $p < 0.05$, [b] $p < 0.01$, [c] $p < 0.001$, [d] $p < 0.0001$

munocompromised patients with severe (i.e., extensive and/or disabling), recalcitrant, plaque psoriasis who have failed to respond to at least one systemic therapy (e.g., PUVA, retinoids, or methotrexate) or in patients for whom other systemic therapies are contraindicated, or cannot be tolerated.

While rebound rarely occurs, most patients will experience relapse with Gengraf® as with other therapies upon cessation of treatment.

CONTRAINDICATIONS

General

Gengraf® Capsules (cyclosporine capsules, USP [**MODIFIED**]) is contraindicated in patients with a hypersensitivity to cyclosporine or to any of the ingredients of the formulation.

Rheumatoid Arthritis

Rheumatoid arthritis patients with abnormal renal function, uncontrolled hypertension or malignancies should not receive Gengraf® Capsules (cyclosporine capsules, USP [**MODIFIED**]).

Psoriasis

Psoriasis patients who are treated with Gengraf® Capsules (cyclosporine capsules, USP [**MODIFIED**]) should not receive concomitant PUVA or UVB therapy, methotrexate or other immunosuppressive agents, coal tar or radiation therapy. Psoriasis patients with abnormal renal function, uncontrolled hypertension, or malignancies should not receive Gengraf®.

WARNINGS

(See also **Boxed WARNINGS**).

All Patients

Cyclosporine, the active ingredient of Gengraf® Capsules (cyclosporine capsules, USP [**MODIFIED**]), can cause nephrotoxicity and hepatotoxicity. The risk increases with increasing doses of cyclosporine. Renal dysfunction including structural kidney damage is a potential consequence of Gengraf® and therefore renal function must be monitored during therapy. **Care should be taken in using cyclosporine with nephrotoxic drugs (see PRECAUTIONS).**

Patients receiving Gengraf® require frequent monitoring of serum creatinine (see Special Monitoring under **DOSAGE AND ADMINISTRATION**). Elderly patients should be monitored with particular care, since decreases in renal function also occur with age. If patients are not properly monitored and doses are not properly adjusted, cyclosporine therapy can be associated with the occurrence of structural kidney damage and persistent renal dysfunction.

An increase in serum creatinine and BUN may occur during Gengraf® therapy and reflect a reduction in the glomerular filtration rate. Impaired renal function at any time requires close monitoring, and frequent dosage adjustment may be indicated. The frequency and severity of serum creatinine elevations increase with dose and duration of cyclosporine therapy. These elevations are likely to become more pronounced without dose reduction or discontinuation.

Because Gengraf® Capsules (cyclosporine capsules, USP [MODIFIED]) is not bioequivalent to Sandimmune® Soft Gelatin Capsules (cyclosporine capsules, USP), conversion from Gengraf® to Sandimmune® using a 1:1 ratio (mg/kg/day) may result in lower cyclosporine blood concentrations. Conversion from Gengraf® to Sandimmune® should be made with increased monitoring to avoid the potential of underdosing.

Kidney, Liver, and Heart Transplant

Nephrotoxicity

Cyclosporine, the active ingredient of Gengraf® Capsules (cyclosporine capsules, USP [**MODIFIED**]), can cause nephrotoxicity and hepatotoxicity when used in high doses. It is not unusual for serum creatinine and BUN levels to be elevated during cyclosporine therapy. These elevations in renal transplant patients do not necessarily indicate rejection, and each patient must be fully evaluated before dosage adjustment is initiated.

Based on the historical Sandimmune® experience with oral solution, nephrotoxicity associated with cyclosporine had been noted in 25% of cases of renal transplantation, 38% of cases of cardiac transplantation, and 37% of cases of liver transplantation. Mild nephrotoxicity was generally noted 2 to 3 months after renal transplant and consisted of an arrest in the fall of the pre-operative elevations of BUN and creatinine at a range of 35 to 45 mg/dL and 2.0 to 2.5 mg/dL respectively. These elevations were often responsive to cyclosporine dosage reduction.

More overt nephrotoxicity was seen early after transplantation and was characterized by a rapidly rising BUN and creatinine. Since these events are similar to renal rejection episodes, care must be taken to differentiate between them. This form of nephrotoxicity is usually responsive to cyclosporine dosage reduction.

Although specific diagnostic criteria which reliably differentiate renal graft rejection from drug toxicity have not been found, a number of parameters have been significantly associated with one or the other. It should be noted however, that up to 20% of patients may have simultaneous nephrotoxicity and rejection.

[See table above]

A form of a cyclosporine-associated nephropathy is characterized by serial deterioration in renal function and morphologic changes in the kidneys. From 5% to 15% of transplant recipients who have received cyclosporine will fail to show a reduction in rising serum creatinine despite a decrease or discontinuation of cyclosporine therapy. Renal biopsies from these patients will demonstrate one or several of the following alterations: tubular vacuolization, tubular microcalcifications, peritubular capillary congestion, arteriolopathy, and a striped form of interstitial fibrosis with tubular atrophy. Though none of these morphologic changes is entirely specific, a diagnosis of cyclosporine-associated structural nephrotoxicity requires evidence of these findings.

When considering the development of cyclosporine-associated nephropathy, it is noteworthy that several authors have reported an association between the appearance of interstitial fibrosis and higher cumulative doses or persistently high circulating trough concentrations of cyclosporine. This is particularly true during the first 6 post-transplant months when the dosage tends to be highest and when, in kidney recipients, the organ appears to be most vulnerable to the toxic effects of cyclosporine. Among other contributing factors to the development of interstitial fibrosis in these patients are prolonged perfusion time, warm ischemia time, as well as episodes of acute toxicity, and acute and chronic rejection. The reversibility of interstitial fibrosis and its correlation to renal function have not yet been determined. Reversibility of arteriolopathy has been reported after stopping cyclosporine or lowering the dosage.

Impaired renal function at any time requires close monitoring, and frequent dosage adjustment may be indicated.

In the event of severe and unremitting rejection, when rescue therapy with pulse steroids and monoclonal antibodies fail to reverse the rejection episode, it may be preferable to switch to alternative immunosuppressive therapy rather than increase the Gengraf® dose to excessive blood concentrations.

Due to the potential for additive or synergistic impairment of renal function, caution should be exercised when coadministering Gengraf® with other drugs that may impair renal function (see **PRECAUTIONS - Drug Interactions**).

Thrombotic Microangiopathy

Occasionally patients have developed a syndrome of thrombocytopenia and microangiopathic hemolytic anemia which may result in graft failure. The vasculopathy can occur in the absence of rejection and is accompanied by avid platelet consumption within the graft as demonstrated by Indium 111 labeled platelet studies. Neither the pathogenesis nor the management of this syndrome is clear. Though resolution has occurred after reduction or discontinuation of cyclosporine and 1) administration of streptokinase and heparin or 2) plasmapheresis, this appears to depend upon early detection with Indium 111 labeled platelet scans (see **ADVERSE REACTIONS**).

Hyperkalemia

Significant hyperkalemia (sometimes associated with hyperchloremic metabolic acidosis) and hyperuricemia have been seen occasionally in individual patients.

Hepatotoxicity

Cases of hepatotoxicity and liver injury including cholestasis, jaundice, hepatitis and liver failure have been reported in patients treated with cyclosporine. Most reports included patients with significant co-morbidities, underlying conditions and other confounding factors including infectious complications and comedications with hepatotoxic potential. In some cases, mainly in transplant patients, fatal outcomes have been reported (see **ADVERSE REACTIONS, Postmarketing Experience, Kidney, Liver and Heart Transplantation**).

Hepatotoxicity usually manifested by elevations of hepatic enzymes and bilirubin, was reported in patients treated with cyclosporine in clinical trials: 4% in renal transplantation, 7% in cardiac transplantation, and 4% in liver transplantation. This was usually noted during the first month of therapy when high doses of cyclosporine were used. The chemistry elevations usually decreased with a reduction in dosage.

Malignancies

As in patients receiving other immunosuppressants, those patients receiving cyclosporine are at increased risk for development of lymphomas and other malignancies, particularly those of the skin. Patients taking cyclosporine should be warned to avoid excess ultraviolet light exposure. The increased risk appears related to the intensity and duration of immunosuppression rather than to the use of specific agents. Because of the danger of oversuppression of the immune system resulting in increased risk of infection or malignancy, a treatment regimen containing multiple immunosuppressants should be used with caution. Some malignancies may be fatal. Transplant patients receiving cyclosporine are at increased risk for serious infection with fatal outcome.

Serious Infections

Patients receiving immunosuppressants, including Gengraf®, are at increased risk of developing bacterial, viral, fungal, and protozoal infections, including opportunistic infections. These infections may lead to serious, including fatal, outcomes (see **Boxed WARNING** and **ADVERSE REACTIONS**).

Polyoma Virus Infections

Patients receiving immunosuppressants including Gengraf® are at increased risk for opportunistic infections, including polyoma virus infections. Polyoma virus infections in transplant patients may have serious, and sometimes, fatal outcomes. These include cases of JC virus-associated progressive multifocal leukoencephalopathy (PML) and polyoma virus-associated nephropathy (PVAN) especially due to BK virus infection which have been observed in patients receiving cyclosporine. PVAN is associated with serious outcomes, including deteriorating renal function and renal graft loss, (see **ADVERSE REACTIONS/Postmarketing Experience, Kidney, Liver and Heart Transplantation**). Patient monitoring may help detect patients at risk for PVAN.

Cases of PML have been reported in patients treated with Gengraf®. PML, which is sometimes fatal, commonly presents with hemiparesis, apathy, confusion, cognitive deficiencies and ataxia. Risk factors for PML include treatment with immunosuppressant therapies and impairment of immune function. In immunosuppressed patients, physicians should consider PML in the differential diagnosis in patients reporting neurological symptoms and consultation with a neurologist should be considered as clinically indicated.

Consideration should be given to reducing the total immunosuppression in transplant patients who develop PML or PVAN. However, reduced immunosuppression may place the graft at risk.

Neurotoxicity

There have been reports of convulsions in adult and pediatric patients receiving cyclosporine, particularly in combination with high dose methylprednisolone.

Encephalopathy, including Posterior Reversible Encephalopathy Syndrome (PRES), has been described both in postmarketing reports and in the literature. Manifestations include impaired consciousness, convulsions, visual disturbances (including blindness), loss of motor function, movement disorders and psychiatric disturbances. In many cases, changes in the white matter have been detected using imaging techniques and pathologic specimens. Predisposing factors such as hypertension, hypomagnesemia, hypocholesterolemia, high-dose corticosteroids, high cyclosporine blood concentrations, and graft-versus-host disease have been noted in many but not all of the reported cases. The changes in most cases have been reversible upon discontinuation of cyclosporine, and in some cases improvement was noted after reduction of dose. It appears that patients receiving liver transplant are more susceptible to encephalopathy than those receiving kidney transplant. Another rare manifestation of cyclosporine-induced neurotoxicity, occurring in transplant patients more frequently than in other indications, is optic disc edema including papilloedema, with possible visual impairment, secondary to benign intracranial hypertension.

Care should be taken in using cyclosporine with nephrotoxic drugs (see **PRECAUTIONS**).

Rheumatoid Arthritis

Cyclosporine nephropathy was detected in renal biopsies of six out of 60 (10%) rheumatoid arthritis patients after the average treatment duration of 19 months. Only one patient, out of these 6 patients, was treated with a dose ≤ 4 mg/kg/day. Serum creatinine improved in all but one patient after discontinuation of cyclosporine. The "maximal creatinine increase" appears to be a factor in predicting cyclosporine nephropathy.

There is a potential, as with other immunosuppressive agents, for an increase in the occurrence of malignant lymphomas with cyclosporine. It is not clear whether the risk with cyclosporine is greater than that in rheumatoid arthritis patients or in rheumatoid arthritis patients on cytotoxic treatment for this indication. Five cases of lymphoma were detected: four in a survey of approximately 2,300 patients treated with cyclosporine for rheumatoid arthritis, and another case of lymphoma was reported in a clinical trial. Although other tumors (12 skin cancers, 24 solid tumors of diverse types, and 1 multiple myeloma) were also reported in this survey, epidemiologic analyses did not support a relationship to cyclosporine other than for malignant lymphomas.

Patients should be thoroughly evaluated before and during Gengraf® Capsules (cyclosporine capsules, USP [**MODIFIED**]) treatment for the development of malignancies. Moreover, use of Gengraf® therapy with other immunosuppressive agents may induce an excessive immunosuppression which is known to increase the risk of malignancy.

Psoriasis

(See also **Boxed WARNINGS** for Psoriasis)

Since cyclosporine is a potent immunosuppressive agent with a number of potentially serious side effects, the risks and benefits of using Gengraf® Capsules (cyclosporine capsules, USP [**MODIFIED**]) should be considered before treatment of patients with psoriasis. Cyclosporine, the active ingredient in Gengraf®, can cause nephrotoxicity and hypertension (see **PRECAUTIONS**) and the risk increases with increasing dose and duration of therapy. Patients who may be at increased risk such as those with abnormal renal function, uncontrolled hypertension or malignancies, should not receive Gengraf®.

Renal dysfunction is a potential consequence of Gengraf®, therefore renal function must be monitored during therapy. Patients receiving Gengraf® require frequent monitoring of serum creatinine (see Special Monitoring under **DOSAGE AND ADMINISTRATION**). Elderly patients should be monitored with particular care, since decreases in renal function also occur with age. If patients are not properly monitored and doses are not properly adjusted, cyclosporine therapy can cause structural kidney damage and persistent renal dysfunction.

An increase in serum creatinine and BUN may occur during Gengraf® therapy and reflects a reduction in the glomerular filtration rate.

Kidney biopsies from 86 psoriasis patients treated for a mean duration of 23 months with 1.2 to 7.6 mg/kg/day of cyclosporine showed evidence of cyclosporine nephropathy in 18/86 (21%) of the patients. The pathology consisted of renal tubular atrophy and interstitial fibrosis. On repeat biopsy of 13 of these patients maintained on various dosages of cyclosporine for a mean of 2 additional years, the number with cyclosporine induced nephropathy rose to 26/86 (30%). The majority of patients (19/26) were on a dose of ≥ 5 mg/kg/day (the highest recommended dose is 4 mg/kg/day). The patients were also on cyclosporine for greater than 15 months (18/26) and/or had a clinically significant increase in serum creatinine for greater than 1 month (21/26). Creatinine levels returned to normal range in 7 of 11 patients in whom cyclosporine therapy was discontinued.

There is an increased risk for the development of skin and lymphoproliferative malignancies in cyclosporine-treated psoriasis patients. The relative risk of malignancies is comparable to that observed in psoriasis patients treated with other immunosuppressive agents.

Tumors were reported in 32 (2.2%) of 1439 psoriasis patients treated with cyclosporine worldwide from clinical trials. Additional tumors have been reported in 7 patients in cyclosporine postmarketing experience. Skin malignancies were reported in 16 (1.1%) of these patients; all but 2 of them had previously received PUVA therapy. Methotrexate was received by 7 patients. UVB and coal tar had been used by 2 and 3 patients, respectively. Seven patients had either a history of previous skin cancer or a potentially predisposing lesion was present prior to cyclosporine exposure. Of the 16 patients with skin cancer, 11 patients had 18 squamous cell carcinomas and 7 patients had 10 basal cell carcinomas. There were two lymphoproliferative malignancies; one case of non-Hodgkin's lymphoma which required chemotherapy, and one case of mycosis fungoides which regressed spontaneously upon discontinuation of cyclosporine. There were four cases of benign lymphocytic infiltration: 3 regressed spontaneously upon discontinuation of cyclosporine, while the fourth regressed despite continuation of the drug. The remainder of the malignancies, 13 cases (0.9%), involved various organs.

Patients should not be treated concurrently with cyclosporine and PUVA or UVB, other radiation therapy, or other immunosuppressive agents, because of the possibility of excessive immunosuppression and the subsequent risk of malignancies (see CONTRAINDICATIONS). Patients should also be warned to protect themselves appropriately when in the sun, and to avoid excessive sun exposure. Patients should be thoroughly evaluated before and during treatment for the presence of malignancies remembering that malignant lesions may be hidden by psoriatic plaques. Skin lesions not typical of psoriasis should be biopsied before starting treatment. Patients should be treated with Gengraf® Capsules (cyclosporine capsules, USP [**MODIFIED**]) only after complete resolution of suspicious lesions, and only if there are no other treatment options (see **Special Monitoring for Psoriasis Patients**).

Special Excipients

Alcohol (ethanol)

The alcohol content (see **DESCRIPTION**) of Gengraf® should be taken into account when given to patients in whom alcohol intake should be avoided or minimized, e.g., pregnant or breastfeeding women, in patients presenting with liver disease or epilepsy, in alcoholic patients, or pediatric patients. For an adult weighing 70 kg, the maximum daily oral dose would deliver about 1 gram of alcohol which is approximately 6% of the amount of alcohol contained in a standard drink.

PRECAUTIONS

General

Hypertension

Cyclosporine is the active ingredient of Gengraf® Capsules (cyclosporine capsules, USP [**MODIFIED**]). Hypertension is a common side effect of cyclosporine therapy which may persist (see **ADVERSE REACTIONS** and **DOSAGE AND ADMINISTRATION** for monitoring recommendations). Mild or moderate hypertension is encountered more frequently than severe hypertension and the incidence decreases over time. In recipients of kidney, liver, and heart allografts treated with cyclosporine, antihypertensive therapy may be required (see **Special Monitoring of Rheumatoid Arthritis and Psoriasis Patients**). However, since cyclosporine may cause hyperkalemia, potassium-sparing diuretics should not be used. While calcium antagonists can be effective agents in treating cyclosporine-associated hypertension, they can interfere with cyclosporine metabolism (see **PRECAUTIONS - Drug Interactions**).

Vaccination

During treatment with cyclosporine, vaccination may be less effective; and the use of live attenuated vaccines should be avoided.

Special Monitoring of Rheumatoid Arthritis Patients

Before initiating treatment, a careful physical examination, including blood pressure measurements (on at least two occasions) and two creatinine levels to estimate baseline should be performed. Blood pressure and serum creatinine should be evaluated every 2 weeks during the initial 3 months and then monthly if the patient is stable. It is advisable to monitor serum creatinine and blood pressure always after an increase of the dose of nonsteroidal anti-inflammatory drugs and after initiation of new nonsteroidal anti-inflammatory drug therapy during Gengraf® Capsules (cyclosporine capsules, USP [**MODIFIED**]) treatment. If coadministered with methotrexate, CBC and liver function tests are recommended to be monitored monthly (see also **PRECAUTIONS - General, Hypertension**).

In patients who are receiving cyclosporine, the dose of Gengraf® should be decreased by 25% to 50% if hypertension occurs. If hypertension persists, the dose of Gengraf® should be further reduced or blood pressure should be controlled with antihypertensive agents. In most cases, blood pressure has returned to baseline when cyclosporine was discontinued.

In placebo-controlled trials of rheumatoid arthritis patients, systolic hypertension (defined as an occurrence of two systolic blood pressure readings > 140 mmHg) and diastolic hypertension (defined as two diastolic blood pressure readings > 90 mmHg) occurred in 33% and 19% of patients treated with cyclosporine, respectively. The corresponding placebo rates were 22% and 8%.

Special Monitoring for Psoriasis Patients

Before initiating treatment, a careful dermatological and physical examination, including blood pressure measurements (on at least two occasions) should be performed. Since Gengraf® (cyclosporine capsules, USP [**MODIFIED**]) is an immunosuppressive agent, patients should be evaluated for the presence of occult infection on their first physical examination and for the presence of tumors initially, and throughout treatment with Gengraf®. Skin lesions not typical for psoriasis should be biopsied before starting Gengraf®. Patients with malignant or premalignant changes of the skin should be treated with Gengraf® only after appropriate treatment of such lesions and if no other treatment option exists.

Baseline laboratories should include serum creatinine (on two occasions), BUN, CBC, serum magnesium, potassium, uric acid, and lipids.

Information on the AbbVie, Inc. products listed on these pages is from the prescribing information in use as of July 31, 2013. For more information, please visit rxabbvie.com or call 1-800-633-9110.

Drugs That May Potentiate Renal Dysfunction

Antibiotics	Antineoplastics	Anti-inflammatory Drugs	Gastrointestinal Agents
ciprofloxacin	melphalan	azapropazon	cimetidine
gentamicin		colchicine	ranitidine
tobramycin	**Antifungals**	diclofenac	
vancomycin	amphotericin B	naproxen	**Immunosuppressives**
trimethoprim with sulfamethoxazole	ketoconazole	sulindac	tacrolimus
			Other Drugs
			fibric acid derivatives (e.g., bezafibrate, fenofibrate)
			methotrexate

1. Drugs That Increase Cyclosporine Concentrations

Calcium Channel Blockers	Antifungals	Antibiotics	Glucocorticoids	Other Drugs
diltiazem	fluconazole	azithromycin	methylprednisolone	allopurinol
nicardipine	itraconazole	clarithromycin		amiodarone
verapamil	ketoconazole	erythromycin		bromocriptine
	voriconazole	quinupristin/dalfopristin		colchicine
				danazol
				imatinib
				metoclopramide
				nefazodone
				oral contraceptives

The risk of cyclosporine nephropathy is reduced when the starting dose is low (2.5 mg/kg/day), the maximum dose does not exceed 4 mg/kg/day, serum creatinine is monitored regularly while cyclosporine is administered, and the dose of Gengraf® is decreased when the rise in creatinine is greater than or equal to 25% above the patients pretreatment level. The increase in creatinine is generally reversible upon timely decrease of the dose of Gengraf® or its discontinuation.

Serum creatinine and BUN should be evaluated every 2 weeks during the initial 3 months of therapy and then monthly if the patient is stable. If the serum creatinine is greater than or equal to 25% above the patient's pretreatment level, serum creatinine should be repeated within two weeks. If the change in serum creatinine remains greater than or equal to 25% above baseline, Gengraf® should be reduced by 25% to 50%. If at **any time** the serum creatinine increases by greater than or equal to 50% above pretreatment level, Gengraf® should be reduced by 25% to 50%. Gengraf® should be discontinued if reversibility (within 25% of baseline) of serum creatinine is not achievable after two dosage modifications. It is advisable to monitor serum creatinine after an increase of the dose of nonsteroidal anti-inflammatory drug and after initiation of new nonsteroidal anti-inflammatory therapy during Gengraf® treatment.

Blood pressure should be evaluated every 2 weeks during the initial 3 months of therapy and then monthly if the patient is stable, or more frequently when dosage adjustments are made. Patients without a history of previous hypertension before initiation of treatment with Gengraf®, should have the drug reduced by 25% to 50% if found to have sustained hypertension. If the patient continues to be hypertensive despite multiple reductions of Gengraf®, then Gengraf® should be discontinued. For patients with treated hypertension, before the initiation of Gengraf® therapy, their medication should be adjusted to control hypertension while on Gengraf®. Gengraf® should be discontinued if a change in hypertension management is not effective or tolerable.

CBC, uric acid, potassium, lipids, and magnesium should also be monitored every 2 weeks for the first 3 months of therapy, and then monthly if the patient is stable or more frequently when dosage adjustments are made. Gengraf® dosage should be reduced by 25% to 50% for any abnormality of clinical concern.

In controlled trials of cyclosporine in psoriasis patients, cyclosporine blood concentrations did not correlate well with either improvement or with side effects such as renal dysfunction.

Information for Patients

Patients should be advised that any change of cyclosporine formulation should be made cautiously and only under physician supervision because it may result in the need for a change in dosage.

Patients should be informed of the necessity of repeated laboratory tests while they are receiving cyclosporine. Patients should be advised of the potential risks during pregnancy and informed of the increased risk of neoplasia. Patients should also be informed of the risk of hypertension and renal dysfunction.

Patients should be advised that during treatment with cyclosporine, vaccination may be less effective and the use of live attenuated vaccines should be avoided.

Patients should be advised to take Gengraf® on a consistent schedule with regard to time of day and relation to meals. Grapefruit and grapefruit juice affect metabolism, increasing blood concentration of cyclosporine, thus should be avoided.

Laboratory Tests

In all patients treated with cyclosporine, renal and liver functions should be assessed repeatedly by measurement of serum creatinine, BUN, serum bilirubin, and liver enzymes. Serum lipids, magnesium, and potassium should also be monitored. Cyclosporine blood concentrations should be routinely monitored in transplant patients (see **DOSAGE AND ADMINISTRATION - Blood Concentration Monitoring in Transplant Patients**), and periodically monitored in rheumatoid arthritis patients.

Drug Interactions

A. Effect of Drugs and Other Agents on Cyclosporine Pharmacokinetics and/or Safety

All of the individual drugs cited below are well substantiated to interact with cyclosporine. In addition, concomitant use of non-steroidal anti-inflammatory drugs with cyclosporine, particularly in the setting of dehydration, may potentiate renal dysfunction. Caution should be exercised when using other drugs which are known to impair renal function (see **WARNINGS - Nephrotoxicity**).

[See first table above]

During the concomitant use of a drug that may exhibit additive or synergistic renal impairment with cyclosporine, close monitoring of renal function (in particular serum creatinine) should be performed. If a significant impairment of renal function occurs, the dosage of the coadministered drug should be reduced or an alternative treatment considered.

Cyclosporine is extensively metabolized by CYP 3A isoenzymes, in particular CYP3A4, and is a substrate of the multidrug efflux transporter P-glycoprotein. Various agents are known to either increase or decrease plasma or whole blood concentrations of cyclosporine usually by inhibition or induction of CYP3A4 or P-glycoprotein transporter or both. Compounds that decrease cyclosporine absorption such as orlistat should be avoided. Appropriate Gengraf® dosage adjustment to achieve the desired cyclosporine concentrations is essential when drugs that significantly alter cyclosporine concentrations are used concomitantly (see **DOSAGE AND ADMINISTRATION - Blood Concentration Monitoring**).

[See second table above]

HIV protease inhibitors

The HIV protease inhibitors (e.g., indinavir, nelfinavir, ritonavir, and saquinavir) are known to inhibit cytochrome P-450 III-A and thus could potentially increase the concentrations of cyclosporine, however no formal studies of the interaction are available. Care should be exercised when these drugs are administered concomitantly.

Grapefruit Juice

Grapefruit and grapefruit juice affect metabolism, increasing blood concentrations of cyclosporine, thus should be avoided.

2. Drugs/Dietary Supplements That Decrease Cyclosporine Concentrations

Antibiotics	Anticonvulsants	Other Drugs/Dietary Supplements
nafcillin	carbamazepine	bosentan
rifampin	oxcarbazepine	octreotide
	phenobarbital	orlistat
	phenytoin	sulfinpyrazone
		St. John's Wort
		terbinafine
		ticlopidine

Bosentan

Coadministration of bosentan (250-1000 mg every 12 hours based on tolerability) and cyclosporine (300 mg every 12 hours for 2 days then dosing to achieve a C_{min} of 200-250 ng/mL) for 7 days in healthy subjects resulted in decreases in the cyclosporine mean dose-normalized AUC, C_{max}, and trough concentration of approximately 50%, 30%, and 60%, respectively, compared to when cyclosporine was given alone (see also *Effect of Cyclosporine on the Pharmacokinetics and/or Safety of Other Drugs or Agents*).

Boceprevir

Coadministration of boceprevir (800 mg three times daily for 7 days) and cyclosporine (100 mg single dose) in healthy subjects resulted in increases in the mean AUC and C_{max} of cyclosporine approximately 2.7-fold and 2-fold, respectively, compared to when cyclosporine was given alone.

Telaprevir

Coadministration of telaprevir (750 mg every 8 hours for 11 days) with cyclosporine (10 mg on day 8) in healthy subjects resulted in increases in the mean dose-normalized AUC and C_{max} of cyclosporine approximately 4.5-fold and 1.3-fold, respectively, compared to when cyclosporine (100 mg single dose) was given alone.

St. John's Wort

There have been reports of a serious drug interaction between cyclosporine and the herbal dietary supplement, St. John's Wort. This interaction has been reported to produce a marked reduction in the blood concentrations of cyclosporine, resulting in subtherapeutic levels, rejection of transplanted organs, and graft loss.

Rifabutin

Rifabutin is known to increase the metabolism of other drugs metabolized by the cytochrome P-450 system. The interaction between rifabutin and cyclosporine has not been studied. Care should be exercised when these two drugs are administered concomitantly.

B. Effect of Cyclosporine on the Pharmacokinetics and/or Safety of Other Drugs or Agents

Cyclosporine is an inhibitor of CYP3A4 and of the multidrug efflux transporter P-glycoprotein and may increase plasma concentrations of comedications that are substrates of CYP3A4 or P-glycoprotein or both.

Cyclosporine may reduce the clearance of digoxin, colchicine, prednisolone, and HMG-CoA reductase inhibitors (statins) and, aliskiren, repaglinide, NSAIDs, sirolimus, etoposide, and other drugs. See the full prescribing information of the other drug for further information and specific recommendations. The decision on co-administration of cyclosporine with other drugs or agents should be made by the physician following the careful assessment of benefits and risks.

Digoxin

Severe digitalis toxicity has been seen within days of starting cyclosporine in several patients taking digoxin. If digoxin is used concurrently with cyclosporine, serum digoxin concentrations should be monitored.

Colchicine

There are reports on the potential of cyclosporine to enhance the toxic effects of colchicine such as myopathy and neuropathy, especially in patients with renal dysfunction. Concomitant administration of cyclosporine and colchicine results in significant increases in colchicine plasma concentrations. If colchicine is used concurrently with cyclosporine, a reduction in the dosage of colchicine is recommended.

HMG-CoA reductase inhibitors (statins)

Literature and postmarketing cases of myotoxicity, including muscle pain and weakness, myositis, and rhabdomyolysis, have been reported with concomitant administration of cyclosporine with lovastatin, simvastatin, atorvastatin, pravastatin, and, rarely, fluvastatin. When concurrently administered with cyclosporine, the dosage of these statins should be reduced according to label recommendations. Statin therapy needs to be temporarily withheld or discontinued in patients with signs and symptoms of myopathy or those with risk factors predisposing to severe renal injury, including renal failure, secondary to rhabdomyolysis.

Repaglinide

Cyclosporine may increase the plasma concentrations of repaglinide and thereby increase the risk of hypoglycemia. In 12 healthy male subjects who received two doses of 100 mg cyclosporine capsule orally 12 hours apart with a single dose of 0.25 mg repaglinide tablet (one half of a 0.5 mg tablet) orally 13 hours after the cyclosporine initial dose, the repaglinide mean C_{max} and AUC were increased 1.8 fold (range: 0.6 to 3.7 fold) and 2.4 fold (range 1.2 to 5.3 fold), respectively. Close monitoring of blood glucose level is advisable for a patient taking cyclosporine and repaglinide concomitantly.

Ambrisentan

Coadministration of ambrisentan (5 mg daily) and cyclosporine (100-150 mg twice daily initially, then dosing to achieve C_{min} 150-200 ng/mL) for 8 days in healthy subjects resulted in mean increases in ambrisentan AUC and C_{max} of approximately 2-fold and 1.5-fold, respectively, compared to ambrisentan alone.

Anthracycline antibiotics

High doses of cyclosporine (e.g., at starting intravenous dose of 16 mg/kg/day) may increase the exposure to anthracycline antibiotics (e.g., doxorubicin, mitoxantrone, daunorubicin) in cancer patients.

Aliskiren

Cyclosporine alters the pharmacokinetics of aliskiren, a substrate of P-glycoprotein and CYP3A4. In 14 healthy subjects who received concomitantly single doses of cyclosporine (200 mg) and reduced dose aliskiren (75 mg), the mean C_{max} of aliskiren was increased by approximately 2.5 fold (90% CI: 1.96 to 3.17) and the mean AUC by approximately 4.3 fold (90% CI: 3.52 to 5.21), compared to when these subjects received aliskiren alone. The concomitant administration of aliskiren with cyclosporine prolonged the median aliskiren elimination half-life (26 hours versus 43 to 45 hours) and the T_{max} (0.5 hours versus 1.5 to 2.0 hours). The mean AUC and C_{max} of cyclosporine were comparable to reported literature values. Co-administration of cyclosporine and aliskiren in these subjects also resulted in an increase in the number and/or intensity of adverse events, mainly headache, hot flush, nausea, vomiting, and somnolence. The co-administration of cyclosporine with aliskiren is not recommended.

Bosentan

In healthy subjects, coadministration of bosentan and cyclosporine resulted in mean increases in dose-normalized bosentan trough concentrations on day 1 and day 8 of approximately 21-fold and 2-fold , respectively, compared to when bosentan was given alone as a single dose on day 1 (see also *Effect of Drugs and Other Agents on Cyclosporine Pharmacokinetics and/or Safety*).

Potassium-Sparing Diuretics

Cyclosporine should not be used with potassium sparing diuretics because hyperkalemia can occur. Caution is also required when cyclosporine is coadministered with potassium sparing drugs (e.g. angiotensin converting enzyme inhibitors, angiotensin II receptor antagonists), potassium containing drugs as well as in patients on a potassium rich diet. Control of potassium levels in these situations is advisable.

Nonsteroidal Anti-Inflammatory Drugs (NSAIDs)

Clinical status and serum creatinine should be closely monitored when cyclosporine is used with nonsteroidal anti-inflammatory agents in rheumatoid arthritis patients (see **WARNINGS**).

Pharmacodynamic interactions have been reported to occur between cyclosporine and both naproxen and sulindac, in that concomitant use is associated with additive decreases in renal function, as determined by ^{99m}Tc-diethylenetriaminepentaacetic acid (DTPA) and (ρ-aminohippuric acid) PAH clearances. Although concomitant administration of diclofenac does not affect blood concentrations of cyclosporine, it has been associated with approximate doubling of diclofenac blood concentrations and occasional reports of reversible decreases in renal function. Consequently, the dose of diclofenac should be in the lower end of the therapeutic range.

Methotrexate Interaction

Preliminary data indicate that when methotrexate and cyclosporine were co-administered to rheumatoid arthritis patients (N=20), methotrexate concentrations (AUCs) were increased approximately 30% and the concentrations (AUCs) of its metabolite, 7-hydroxy methotrexate, were decreased by approximately 80%. The clinical significance of this interaction is not known. Cyclosporine concentrations do not appear to have been altered (N=6).

Sirolimus

Elevations in serum creatinine were observed in studies using sirolimus in combination with full-dose cyclosporine. This effect is often reversible with cyclosporine dose reduction. Simultaneous coadministration of cyclosporine significantly increases blood levels of sirolimus. To minimize increases in sirolimus blood concentrations, it is recommended that sirolimus be given 4 hours after cyclosporine administration.

Nifedipine

Frequent gingival hyperplasia when nifedipine is given concurrently with cyclosporine have been reported. The concomitant use of nifedipine should be avoided in patients in whom gingival hyperplasia develops as a side effect of cyclosporine.

Body System	Adverse Reactions	Randomized Kidney Patients		Cyclosporine Patients (Sandimmune®)		
		Sandimmune® (N = 227) %	Azathioprine (N = 228) %	Kidney (N = 705) %	Heart (N = 112) %	Liver (N = 75) %
Genitourinary						
	Renal Dysfunction	32	6	25	38	37
Cardiovascular						
	Hypertension	26	18	13	53	27
	Cramps	4	< 1	2	< 1	0
Skin						
	Hirsutism	21	< 1	21	28	45
	Acne	6	8	2	2	1
Central Nervous System						
	Tremor	12	0	21	31	55
	Convulsions	3	1	1	4	5
	Headache	2	<1	2	15	4
Gastrointestinal						
	Gum Hyperplasia	4	0	9	5	16
	Diarrhea	3	< 1	3	4	8
	Nausea/Vomiting	2	< 1	4	10	4
	Hepatotoxicity	< 1	< 1	4	7	4
	Abdominal Discomfort	< 1	0	<1	7	0
Autonomic Nervous System						
	Paresthesia	3	0	1	2	1
	Flushing	< 1	0	4	0	4
Hematopoietic						
	Leukopenia	2	19	< 1	6	0
	Lymphoma	< 1	0	1	6	1
Respiratory						
	Sinusitis	< 1	0	4	3	7
Miscellaneous						
	Gynecomastia	< 1	0	< 1	4	3

Methyprednisolone

Convulsions when high dose methylprednisolone is given concomitantly with cyclosporine have been reported.

Other Immunosuppressive Drugs and Agents

Psoriasis patients receiving other immunosuppressive agents or radiation therapy (including PUVA and UVB) should not receive concurrent cyclosporine because of the possibility of excessive immunosuppression.

C. Effect of Cyclosporine on the Efficacy of Live Vaccines

During treatment with cyclosporine, vaccination may be less effective. The use of live vaccines should be avoided.

For additional information on Cyclosporine Drug Interactions please contact AbbVie Inc. Medical Information Department at 1-800-633-9110.

Carcinogenesis, Mutagenesis, and Impairment of Fertility

Carcinogenicity studies were carried out in male and female rats and mice. In the 78-week mouse study, evidence of a statistically significant trend was found for lymphocytic lymphomas in females, and the incidence of hepatocellular carcinomas in mid-dose males significantly exceeded the control value. In the 24-month rat study, pancreatic islet cell adenomas significantly exceeded the control rate in the low dose level. Doses used in the mouse and rat studies were 0.01 to 0.16 times the clinical maintenance dose (6 mg/kg). The hepatocellular carcinomas and pancreatic islet cell adenomas were not dose related. Published reports indicate the co-treatment of hairless mice with UV irradiation and cyclosporine or other immunosuppressive agents shorten the time to skin tumor formation compared to UV irradiation alone.

Cyclosporine was not mutagenic in appropriate test systems. Cyclosporine has not been found to be mutagenic/genotoxic in the Ames Test, the V79-HGPRT Test, the micronucleus test in mice and Chinese hamsters, the chromosome-aberration tests in Chinese hamster bone-marrow, the mouse dominant lethal assay, and the DNA-repair test in sperm from treated mice. A recent study analyzing sister chromatid exchange (SCE) induction by cyclosporine using human lymphocytes *in vitro* gave indication of a positive effect (i.e., induction of SCE), at high concentrations in this system. In two published research studies, rabbits exposed to cyclosporine *in utero* (10 mg/kg/day subcutaneously) demonstrated reduced numbers of nephrons, renal hypertrophy, systemic hypertension and progressive renal insufficiency up to 35 weeks of age. Pregnant rats which received 12 mg/kg/day of cyclosporine intravenously (twice the recommended human intravenous dose) had fetuses with an increased incidence of ventricular septal defect. These findings have not been demonstrated in other species and their relevance for humans is unknown. No impairment in fertility was demonstrated in studies in male and female rats.

Widely distributed papillomatosis of the skin was observed after chronic treatment of dogs with cyclosporine at 9 times the human initial psoriasis treatment dose of 2.5 mg/kg, where doses are expressed on a body surface area basis. This papillomatosis showed a spontaneous regression upon discontinuation of cyclosporine.

An increased incidence of malignancy is a recognized complication of immunosuppression in recipients of organ transplants and patients with rheumatoid arthritis and psoriasis. The most common forms of neoplasms are non-Hodgkin's lymphoma and carcinomas of the skin. The risk of malignancies in cyclosporine recipients is higher than in the normal, healthy population but similar to that in patients receiving other immunosuppressive therapies. Reduction or discontinuance of immunosuppression may cause the lesions to regress.

In psoriasis patients on cyclosporine, development of malignancies, especially those of the skin has been reported (see **WARNINGS**). Skin lesions not typical for psoriasis should be biopsied before starting cyclosporine treatment. Patients with malignant or premalignant changes of the skin should be treated with cyclosporine only after appropriate treatment of such lesions and if no other treatment option exists.

Pregnancy

Pregnancy Category C

Animal studies have shown reproductive toxicity in rats and rabbits. Cyclosporine gave no evidence of mutagenic or teratogenic effects in the standard test systems with oral application (rats up to 17 mg/kg and rabbits up to 30 mg/kg per day orally). Only at dose levels toxic to dams, were adverse effects seen in reproduction studies in rats. Cyclosporine has been shown to be embryo- and fetotoxic in rats and rabbits following oral administration at maternally toxic doses. Fetal toxicity was noted in rats at 0.8 and rabbits at 5.4 times the transplant doses in humans of 6 mg/kg, where dose corrections are based on body surface area. Cyclosporine was embryo- and fetotoxic as indicated by increased pre- and postnatal mortality and reduced fetal weight together with related skeletal retardation.

There are no adequate and well-controlled studies in pregnant women and, therefore, Gengraf® Capsules (cyclosporine capsules, USP [**MODIFIED**]) should not be used during pregnancy unless the potential benefit to the mother justifies the potential risk to the fetus.

In pregnant transplant recipients who are being treated with immunosuppressants the risk of premature births is increased. The following data represent the reported outcomes of 116 pregnancies in women receiving cyclosporine

Information on the AbbVie, Inc. products listed on these pages is from the prescribing information in use as of July 31, 2013. For more information, please visit rxabbvie.com or call 1-800-633-9110.

Cyclosporine (MODIFIED)/Sandimmune® Rheumatoid Arthritis Percentage of Patients with Adverse Events ≥ 3% in any Cyclosporine Treated Group

Body System	Preferred Term	Studies 651+652+2008 Sandimmune®† (N = 269)	Study 302 Sandimmune® (N = 155)	Study 654 Methotrexate & Sandimmune® (N = 74)	Study 654 Methotrexate & Placebo (N = 73)	Study 302 Cyclosporine (MODIFIED) (N = 143)	Studies 651+652 +2008 Placebo (N = 201)
Autonomic Nervous System Disorders							
	Flushing	2%	2%	3%	0%	5%	2%
Body As A Whole - General Disorders							
	Accidental Trauma	0%	1%	10%	4%	4%	0%
	Edema NOS*	5%	14%	12%	4%	10%	< 1%
	Fatigue	6%	3%	8%	12%	3%	7%
	Fever	2%	3%	0%	0%	2%	4%
	Influenza-like symptoms	< 1%	6%	1%	0%	3%	2%
	Pain	6%	9%	10%	15%	13%	4%
	Rigors	1%	1%	4%	0%	3%	1%
Cardiovascular Disorders							
	Arrhythmia	2%	5%	5%	6%	2%	1%
	Chest Pain	4%	5%	1%	1%	6%	1%
	Hypertension	8%	26%	16%	12%	25%	2%
Central and Peripheral Nervous System Disorders							
	Dizziness	8%	6%	7%	3%	8%	3%
	Headache	17%	23%	22%	11%	25%	9%
	Migraine	2%	3%	0%	0%	3%	1%
	Paresthesia	8%	7%	8%	4%	11%	1%
	Tremor	8%	7%	7%	3%	13%	4%
Gastrointestinal System Disorders							
	Abdominal Pain	15%	15%	15%	7%	15%	10%
	Anorexia	3%	3%	1%	0%	3%	3%
	Diarrhea	12%	12%	18%	15%	13%	8%
	Dyspepsia	12%	12%	10%	8%	8%	4%
	Flatulence	5%	5%	5%	4%	4%	1%
	Gastrointestinal Disorder NOS*	0%	2%	1%	4%	4%	0%
	Gingivitis	4%	3%	0%	0%	0%	1%
	Gum Hyperplasia	2%	4%	1%	3%	4%	1%
	Nausea	23%	14%	24%	15%	18%	14%
	Rectal Hemorrhage	0%	3%	0%	0%	1%	1%
	Stomatitis	7%	5%	16%	12%	6%	8%
	Vomiting	9%	8%	14%	7%	6%	5%
Hearing and Vestibular Disorders							
	Ear Disorders NOS*	0%	5%	0%	0%	1%	0%
Metabolic and Nutritional Disorders							
	Hypomagnesemia	0%	4%	0%	0%	6%	0%
Musculoskeletal System Disorders							
	Arthropathy	0%	5%	0%	1%	4%	0%
	Leg Cramps/ Involuntary Muscle Contractions	2%	11%	11%	3%	12%	1%
Psychiatric Disorders							
	Depression	3%	6%	3%	1%	1%	2%
	Insomnia	4%	1%	1%	0%	3%	2%
Renal							
	Creatinine elevations ≥ 30%	43%	39%	55%	19%	48%	13%
	Creatinine elevations ≥ 50%	24%	18%	26%	8%	18%	3%
Reproductive Disorders, Female							
	Leukorrhea	1%	0%	4%	0%	1%	0%
	Menstrual Disorder	3%	2%	1%	0%	1%	1%
Respiratory System Disorders							
	Bronchitis	1%	3%	1%	0%	1%	3%
	Coughing	5%	3%	5%	7%	4%	4%
	Dyspnea	5%	1%	3%	3%	1%	2%
	Infection NOS*	9%	5%	0%	7%	3%	10%
	Pharyngitis	3%	5%	5%	6%	4%	4%
	Pneumonia	1%	0%	4%	0%	1%	1%
	Rhinitis	0%	3%	11%	10%	1%	0%
	Sinusitis	4%	4%	8%	4%	3%	3%
	Upper Respiratory Tract	0%	14%	23%	15%	13%	0%
Skin and Appendages Disorders							
	Alopecia	3%	0%	1%	1%	4%	4%
	Bullous Eruption	1%	0%	4%	1%	1%	1%
	Hypertrichosis	19%	17%	12%	0%	15%	3%
	Rash	7%	12%	10%	7%	8%	10%
	Skin Ulceration	1%	1%	3%	4%	0%	2%
Urinary System Disorders							
	Dysuria	0%	0%	11%	3%	1%	2%
	Micturition Frequency	2%	4%	3%	1%	2%	2%
	NPN, Increased	0%	19%	12%	0%	18%	0%
	Urinary Tract Infection	0%	3%	5%	4%	3%	0%
Vascular (Extracardiac) Disorders							
	Purpura	3%	4%	1%	1%	2%	0%

† Includes patients in 2.5 mg/kg/day dose group only.
* NOS = Not Otherwise Specified.

during pregnancy, 90% of whom were transplant patients, and most of whom received cyclosporine throughout the entire gestational period. The only consistent patterns of abnormality were premature birth (gestational period of 28 to 36 weeks) and low birth weight for gestational age. Sixteen fetal losses occurred. Most of the pregnancies (85 of 100) were complicated by disorders; including, pre-eclampsia, eclampsia, premature labor, abruptio placentae, oligohydramnios, Rh incompatibility and fetoplacental dysfunction. Pre-term delivery occurred in 47%. Seven malformations were reported in 5 viable infants and in 2 cases of fetal loss. Twenty-eight percent of the infants were small for gestational age. Neonatal complications occurred in 27%. Therefore, the risks and benefits of using Gengraf® during pregnancy should be carefully weighed.

A limited number of observations in children exposed to cyclosporine *in utero* is available, up to an age of approximately 7 years. Renal function and blood pressure in these children were normal.

Because of the possible disruption of maternal-fetal interaction, the risk/benefit ratio of using Gengraf® in psoriasis patients during pregnancy should carefully be weighed with serious consideration for discontinuation of Gengraf®.

The alcohol content of the Gengraf® formulations should also be taken into account in pregnant women (see **WARNINGS - Special Excipients**).

Nursing Mothers

Cyclosporine is present in breast milk. Because of the potential for serious adverse drug reactions in nursing infants from Gengraf®, a decision should be made whether to discontinue nursing or to discontinue the drug, taking into account the importance of the drug to the mother. Gengraf® contains ethanol. Ethanol will be present in human milk at levels similar to that found in maternal serum and if present in breast milk will be orally absorbed by a nursing infant (see **WARNINGS**).

Pediatric Use

Although no adequate and well-controlled studies have been completed in children, transplant recipients as young as one year of age have received cyclosporine (**MODIFIED**) with no unusual adverse effects. The safety and efficacy of cyclosporine (**MODIFIED**) treatment in children with juvenile rheumatoid arthritis or psoriasis below the age of 18 have not been established.

Geriatric Use

In rheumatoid arthritis clinical trials with cyclosporine, 17.5% of patients were age 65 or older. These patients were more likely to develop systolic hypertension on therapy, and more likely to show serum creatinine rises ≥ 50% above the baseline after 3 to 4 months of therapy.

Clinical studies of cyclosporine oral solution (modified) in transplant and psoriasis patients did not include a sufficient number of subjects aged 65 and over to determine whether they respond differently from younger subjects. Other reported clinical experiences have not identified differences in response between the elderly and younger patients. In general, dose selection for an elderly patient should be cautious, usually starting at the low end of the dosing range, reflecting the greater frequency of decreased hepatic, renal, or cardiac function, and of concomitant disease or other drug therapy.

ADVERSE REACTIONS

Kidney, Liver, and Heart Transplantation

The principal adverse reactions of cyclosporine therapy are renal dysfunction, tremor, hirsutism, hypertension, and gum hyperplasia.

Hypertension

Hypertension, which is usually mild to moderate, may occur in approximately 50% of patients following renal transplantation and in most cardiac transplant patients.

Glomerular Capillary Thrombosis

Glomerular capillary thrombosis has been found in patients treated with cyclosporine and may progress to graft failure. The pathologic changes resembled those seen in the hemolytic-uremic syndrome and include thrombosis of the renal microvasculature, with platelet-fibrin thrombi occluding glomerular capillaries and afferent arterioles, microangiopathic hemolytic anemia, thrombocytopenia, and decreased renal function. Similar findings have been observed when other immunosuppressives have been employed post-transplantation.

Hypomagnesemia

Hypomagnesemia has been reported in some, but not all, patients exhibiting convulsions while on cyclosporine therapy. Although magnesium-depletion studies in normal subjects suggest that hypomagnesemia is associated with neurologic disorders, multiple factors, including hypertension, high dose methylprednisolone, hypocholesterolemia, and nephrotoxicity associated with high plasma concentrations of cyclosporine appear to be related to the neurological manifestations of cyclosporine toxicity.

Clinical Studies

In controlled studies, the nature, severity and incidence of the adverse events that were observed in 493 transplanted patients treated with cyclosporine (**MODIFIED**) were comparable with those observed in 208 transplanted patients who received Sandimmune® Soft Gelatin Capsules (cyclosporine capsules, USP) in these same studies when the dosage of the two drugs was adjusted to achieve the same cyclosporine blood trough concentrations.

Based on the historical experience with Sandimmune®, the following reactions occurred in 3% or greater of 892 patients involved in clinical trials of kidney, heart, and liver transplants.

[See table at top of page 453]

Among 705 kidney transplant patients treated with cyclosporine oral solution (Sandimmune®) in clinical trials, the reason for treatment discontinuation was renal toxicity in 5.4%, infection in 0.9%, lack of efficacy in 1.4%, acute tubular necrosis in 1.0%, lymphoproliferative disorders in 0.3%, hypertension in 0.3%, and other reasons in 0.7% of the patients.

The following reactions occurred in 2% or less of cyclosporine-treated patients: allergic reactions, anemia, anorexia, confusion, conjunctivitis, edema, fever, brittle fingernails, gastritis, hearing loss, hiccups, hyperglycemia, migraine (Gengraf®), muscle pain, peptic ulcer, thrombocytopenia, tinnitus.

The following reactions occurred rarely: anxiety, chest pain, constipation, depression, hair breaking, hematuria, joint pain, lethargy, mouth sores, myocardial infarction, night sweats, pancreatitis, pruritus, swallowing difficulty, tingling, upper GI bleeding, visual disturbance, weakness, weight loss.

Patients receiving immunosuppressive therapies, including cyclosporine and cyclosporine-containing regimens, are at increased risk of infections (viral, bacterial, fungal, parasitic). Both generalized and localized infections can occur. Pre-existing infections may also be aggravated. Fatal outcomes have been reported (see **WARNINGS**).

Infectious Complications in Historical Randomized Studies in Renal Transplant Patients Using Sandimmune®

Complication	Cyclosporine Treatment (N = 227) % of Complications	Azathioprine with Steroids* (N = 228) % of Complications
Septicemia	5.3	4.8
Abscesses	4.4	5.3
Systemic Fungal Infection	2.2	3.9
Local Fungal Infection	7.5	9.6
Cytomegalovirus	4.8	12.3
Other Viral Infections	15.9	18.4
Urinary Tract Infections	21.1	20.2
Wound and Skin Infections	7.0	10.1
Pneumonia	6.2	9.2

* Some patients also received ALG.

Postmarketing Experience, Kidney, Liver and Heart Transplantation

Hepatotoxicity

Cases of hepatotoxicity and liver injury including cholestasis, jaundice, hepatitis and liver failure; serious and/or fatal outcomes have been reported. [See **WARNINGS, Hepatotoxicity**]

Increased Risk of Infections

Cases of JC virus-associated progressive multifocal leukoencephalopathy (PML), sometimes fatal; and polyoma virus-associated nephropathy (PVAN), especially BK virus resulting in graft loss have been reported. [See **WARNINGS, Polyoma Virus Infection**]

Headache, including Migraine

Cases of migraine have been reported. In some cases, patients have been unable to continue cyclosporine, however the final decision on treatment discontinuation should be made by the treating physician following the careful assessment of benefits versus risks.

Rheumatoid Arthritis

The principal adverse reactions associated with the use of cyclosporine in rheumatoid arthritis are renal dysfunction (see **WARNINGS**), hypertension (see **PRECAUTIONS**), headache, gastrointestinal disturbances and hirsutism/hypertrichosis.

In rheumatoid arthritis patients treated in clinical trials within the recommended dose range, cyclosporine therapy was discontinued in 5.3% of the patients because of hypertension and in 7% of the patients because of increased creatinine. These changes are usually reversible with timely dose decrease or drug discontinuation. The frequency and severity of serum creatinine elevations increase with dose and duration of cyclosporine therapy. These elevations are likely to become more pronounced without dose reduction or discontinuation.

The following adverse events occurred in controlled clinical trials

[See table on page 454]

In addition, the following adverse events have been reported in 1% to < 3% of the rheumatoid arthritis patients in the cyclosporine treatment group in controlled clinical trials.

Autonomic Nervous System

dry mouth, increased sweating

Body as a Whole

allergy, asthenia, hot flushes, malaise, overdose, procedure NOS*, tumor NOS*, weight decrease, weight increase

Cardiovascular

abnormal heart sounds, cardiac failure, myocardial infarction, peripheral ischemia

Central and Peripheral Nervous System

hypoesthesia, neuropathy, vertigo

Endocrine

goiter

Gastrointestinal

constipation, dysphagia, enanthema, eructation, esophagitis, gastric ulcer, gastritis, gastroenteritis, gingival bleeding, glossitis, peptic ulcer, salivary gland enlargement, tongue disorder, tooth disorder

Infection

abscess, bacterial infection, cellulitis, folliculitis, fungal infection, herpes simplex, herpes zoster, renal abscess, moniliasis, tonsillitis, viral infection

Hematologic

anemia, epistaxis, leukopenia, lymphadenopathy

Liver and Biliary System

bilirubinemia

Metabolic and Nutritional

diabetes mellitus, hyperkalemia, hyperuricemia, hypoglycemia

Musculoskeletal System

arthralgia, bone fracture, bursitis, joint dislocation, myalgia, stiffness, synovial cyst, tendon disorder

Neoplasms

breast fibroadenosis, carcinoma

Psychiatric

anxiety, confusion, decreased libido, emotional lability, impaired concentration, increased libido, nervousness, paroniria, somnolence

Reproductive (Female)

breast pain, uterine hemorrhage

Respiratory System

abnormal chest sounds, bronchospasm

Skin and Appendages

abnormal pigmentation, angioedema, dermatitis, dry skin, eczema, nail disorder, pruritus, skin disorder, urticaria

Special Senses

abnormal vision, cataract, conjunctivitis, deafness, eye pain, taste perversion, tinnitus, vestibular disorder

Urinary System

abnormal urine, hematuria, increased BUN, micturition urgency, nocturia, polyuria, pyelonephritis, urinary incontinence

* NOS = Not Otherwise Specified.

Psoriasis

The principal adverse reactions associated with the use of cyclosporine in patients with psoriasis are renal dysfunction, headache, hypertension, hypertriglyceridemia, hirsutism/hypertrichosis, paresthesia or hyperesthesia, influenza-like symptoms, nausea/vomiting, diarrhea, abdominal discomfort, lethargy, and musculoskeletal or joint pain.

In psoriasis patients treated in U.S. controlled clinical studies within the recommended dose range, cyclosporine therapy was discontinued in 1.0% of the patients because of hypertension and in 5.4% of the patients because of increased creatinine. In the majority of cases, these changes were reversible after dose reduction or discontinuation of cyclosporine.

Information on the AbbVie, Inc. products listed on these pages is from the prescribing information in use as of July 31, 2013. For more information, please visit rxabbvie.com or call 1-800-633-9110.

Adverse Events Occurring in 3% or More of Psoriasis Patients in Controlled Clinical Trials

Body System*	Preferred Term	Cyclosporine (MODIFIED) (N = 182)	Sandimmune® (N = 185)
Infection or Potential Infection		24.7%	24.3%
	Influenza-like Symptoms	9.9%	8.1%
	Upper Respiratory Tract Infections	7.7%	11.3%
Cardiovascular System		28.0%	25.4%
	Hypertension**	27.5%	25.4%
Urinary System		24.2%	16.2%
	Increased Creatinine	19.8%	15.7%
Central and Peripheral Nervous System		26.4%	20.5%
	Headache	15.9%	14.0%
	Paresthesia	7.1%	4.8%
Musculoskeletal System		13.2%	8.7%
	Arthralgia	6.0%	1.1%
Body As a Whole – General		29.1%	22.2%
	Pain	4.4%	3.2%
Metabolic and Nutritional		9.3%	9.7%
Reproductive, Female		8.5% (4 of 47 females)	11.5% (6 of 52 females)
Resistance Mechanism		18.7%	21.1%
Skin and Appendages		17.6%	15.1%
	Hypertrichosis	6.6%	5.4%
Respiratory System		5.0%	6.5%
	Bronchospasm, Coughing, Dyspnea, Rhinitis	5.0%	4.9%
Psychiatric		5.0%	3.8%
Gastrointestinal System		19.8%	28.7%
	Abdominal Pain	2.7%	6.0%
	Diarrhea	5.0%	5.9%
	Dyspepsia	2.2%	3.2%
	Gum Hyperplasia	3.8%	6.0%
	Nausea	5.5%	5.9%
White cell and RES		4.4%	2.7%

* Total percentage of events within the system.
** Newly occurring hypertension = SBP ≥160 mm Hg and/or DBP ≥90 mm Hg.

There has been one reported death associated with the use of cyclosporine in psoriasis. A 27 year old male developed renal deterioration and was continued on cyclosporine. He had progressive renal failure leading to death.

Frequency and severity of serum creatinine increases with dose and duration of cyclosporine therapy. These elevations are likely to become more pronounced and may result in irreversible renal damage without dose reduction or discontinuation.

[See table above]

The following events occurred in 1% to less than 3% of psoriasis patients treated with cyclosporine:

Body as a Whole
fever, flushes, hot flushes
Cardiovascular
chest pain
Central and Peripheral Nervous System
appetite increased, insomnia, dizziness, nervousness, vertigo
Gastrointestinal
abdominal distention, constipation, gingival bleeding
Liver and Biliary System
hyperbilirubinemia
Neoplasms
skin malignancies [squamous cell (0.9%) and basal cell (0.4%) carcinomas]
Reticuloendothelial
platelet, bleeding, and clotting disorders, red blood cell disorder
Respiratory
infection, viral and other infection
Skin and Appendages
acne, folliculitis, keratosis, pruritus, rash, dry skin
Urinary System
micturition frequency
Vision
abnormal vision.

Mild hypomagnesemia and hyperkalemia may occur but are asymptomatic. Increases in uric acid may occur and attacks of gout have been rarely reported. A minor and dose related hyperbilirubinemia has been observed in the absence of hepatocellular damage. Cyclosporine therapy may be associated with a modest increase of serum triglycerides or cholesterol. Elevations of triglycerides (> 750 mg/dL) occur in about 15% of psoriasis patients; elevations of cholesterol (> 300 mg/dL) are observed in less than 3% of psoriasis patients. Generally these laboratory abnormalities are reversible upon dose reduction or discontinuation of cyclosporine.

Postmarketing Experience, Psoriasis

Cases of transformation to erythrodermic psoriasis or generalized pustular psoriasis upon either withdrawal or reduction of cyclosporine in patients with chronic plaque psoriasis have been reported.

OVERDOSAGE

There is a minimal experience with cyclosporine overdosage. Forced emesis and gastric lavage can be of value up to 2 hours after administration of Gengraf® Capsules (cyclosporine capsules, USP [MODIFIED]). Transient hepatotoxicity and nephrotoxicity may occur which should resolve following drug withdrawal. Oral doses of cyclosporine up to 10 g (about 150 mg/kg) have been tolerated with relatively minor clinical consequences, such as vomiting, drowsiness, headache, tachycardia and, in a few patients, moderately severe, reversible impairment of renal function. However, serious symptoms of intoxication have been reported following accidental parenteral overdosage with cyclosporine in premature neonates. General supportive measures and symptomatic treatment should be followed in all cases of overdosage. Cyclosporine is not dialyzable to any great extent, nor is it cleared well by charcoal hemoperfusion. The oral dosage at which half of experimental animals are estimated to die is 31 times, 39 times and > 54 times the human maintenance dose for transplant patients (6 mg/kg; corrections based on body surface area) in mice, rats, and rabbits.

DOSAGE AND ADMINISTRATION

Gengraf® Capsules (cyclosporine capsules, USP [MODIFIED]) has increased bioavailability in comparison to Sandimmune® Soft Gelatin Capsules (cyclosporine capsules, USP). Gengraf® and Sandimmune® are not bioequivalent and cannot be used interchangeably without physician supervision.

The daily dose of Gengraf® Capsules (cyclosporine capsules, USP [MODIFIED]) should always be given in two divided doses (BID). It is recommended that Gengraf® be administered on a consistent schedule with regard to time of day and relation to meals. Grapefruit and grapefruit juice affect metabolism, increasing blood concentration of cyclosporine, thus should be avoided.

Specific Populations

Renal Impairment in Kidney, Liver, and Heart Transplantation

Cyclosporine undergoes minimal renal elimination and its pharmacokinetics do not appear to be significantly altered in patients with end-stage renal disease who receive routine hemodialysis treatments (see **CLINICAL PHARMACOLOGY**). However, due to its nephrotoxic potential (see **WARNINGS**), careful monitoring of renal function is recommended; cyclosporine dosage should be reduced if indicated (see **WARNINGS** and **PRECAUTIONS**).

Renal Impairment in Rheumatoid Arthritis and Psoriasis

Patients with impaired renal function should not receive cyclosporine (see **CONTRAINDICATIONS, WARNINGS** and **PRECAUTIONS**).

Hepatic Impairment

The clearance of cyclosporine may be significantly reduced in severe liver disease patients (see **CLINICAL PHARMACOLOGY**). Dose reduction may be necessary in patients with severe liver impairment to maintain blood concentrations within the recommended target range (see **WARNINGS** and **PRECAUTIONS**).

Newly Transplanted Patients

The initial oral dose of Gengraf® Capsules (cyclosporine capsules, USP [**MODIFIED**]) can be given 4 to 12 hours prior to transplantation or be given postoperatively. The initial dose of Gengraf® varies depending on the transplanted organ and the other immunosuppressive agents included in the immunosuppressive protocol. In newly transplanted patients, the initial oral dose of Gengraf® is the same as the initial oral dose of Sandimmune®. Suggested initial doses are available from the results of a 1994 survey of the use of Sandimmune® in U.S. transplant centers. The mean ± SD initial doses were 9 ± 3 mg/kg/day for renal transplant patients (75 centers), 8 ± 4 mg/kg/day for liver transplant patients (30 centers), and 7 ± 3 mg/kg/day for heart transplant patients (24 centers). Total daily doses were divided into two equal daily doses. The Gengraf® dose is subsequently adjusted to achieve a pre-defined cyclosporine blood concentration (see **DOSAGE AND ADMINISTRATION - Blood Concentration Monitoring in Transplant Patients**, below). If cyclosporine trough blood concentrations are used, the target range is the same for Gengraf® as for Sandimmune®. Using the same trough concentration target range for Gengraf® as for Sandimmune® results in greater cyclosporine exposure when Gengraf® is administered (see **CLINICAL PHARMACOLOGY - Pharmacokinetics**, Absorption). Dosing should be titrated based on clinical assessments of rejection and tolerability. Lower Gengraf® doses may be sufficient as maintenance therapy.

Adjunct therapy with adrenal corticosteroids is recommended initially. Different tapering dosage schedules of prednisone appear to achieve similar results. A representative dosage schedule based on the patient's weight started with 2 mg/kg/day for the first 4 days tapered to 1 mg/kg/day by 1 week, 0.6 mg/kg/day by 2 weeks, 0.3 mg/kg/day by 1 month, and 0.15 mg/kg/day by 2 months and thereafter as a maintenance dose. Steroid doses may be further tapered on an individualized basis depending on status of patient and function of graft. Adjustments in dosage of prednisone must be made according to the clinical situation.

Conversion from Sandimmune® (Cyclosporine) to Gengraf® Capsules (Cyclosporine Capsules, USP [MODIFIED]) in Transplant Patients

In transplanted patients who are considered for conversion to Gengraf® from Sandimmune® (cyclosporine), Gengraf® should be started with the same daily dose as was previously used with Sandimmune® (cyclosporine) (1:1 dose conversion). The Gengraf® dose should subsequently be adjusted to attain the pre-conversion cyclosporine blood trough concentration. Using the same trough concentration target range for Gengraf® as for Sandimmune® (cyclosporine) results in greater cyclosporine exposure when Gengraf® is administered (see **CLINICAL PHARMACOLOGY - Pharmacokinetics**, Absorption). Patients with suspected poor absorption of Sandimmune® (cyclosporine) require different dosing strategies (see **DOSAGE AND ADMINISTRATION - Transplant Patients with Poor Absorption of Sandimmune®** (cyclosporine), below). In some patients, the increase in blood trough concentration is more pronounced and may be of clinical significance.

Until the blood trough concentration attains the pre-conversion value, it is strongly recommended that the cyclosporine blood trough concentration be monitored every 4 to 7 days after conversion to Gengraf®. In addition, clinical safety parameters such as serum creatinine and blood pressure should be monitored every two weeks during the first two months after conversion. If the blood trough concentrations are outside the desired range and/or if the clinical safety parameters worsen, the dosage of Gengraf® must be adjusted accordingly.

Transplant Patients with Poor Absorption of Sandimmune® (Cyclosporine)

Patients with lower than expected cyclosporine blood trough concentrations in relation to the oral dose of Sandimmune® (cyclosporine) may have poor or inconsistent absorption of cyclosporine from Sandimmune® (cyclosporine). After conversion to Gengraf® Capsules (cyclosporine capsules, USP [**MODIFIED**]), patients tend to have higher cyclosporine con centrations. **Due to the increase in bioavailability of cyclosporine following conversion to Gengraf®, the cyclosporine blood trough concentration may exceed the target range. Particular caution should be exercised when converting patients to Gengraf® at doses greater than 10 mg/kg/day.** The dose of Gengraf® should be titrated individually based on cyclosporine trough concentrations, tolerability, and clinical response. In this population the cyclosporine blood trough concentration should be measured more frequently, at least twice a week (daily, if initial dose exceeds 10 mg/kg/day) until the concentration stabilizes within the desired range.

Rheumatoid Arthritis

The initial dose of Gengraf® Capsules (cyclosporine capsules, USP [**MODIFIED**]) is 2.5 mg/kg/day, taken twice daily as a divided (BID) oral dose. Salicylates, nonsteroidal anti-inflammatory agents, and oral corticosteroids may be continued (see **WARNINGS** and **PRECAUTIONS - Drug Interactions**). Onset of action generally occurs between 4 and 8 weeks. If insufficient clinical benefit is seen and tolerability is good (including serum creatinine less than 30% above baseline), the dose may be increased by 0.5 to 0.75 mg/kg/day after 8 weeks and again after 12 weeks to a maximum of 4 mg/kg/day. If no benefit is seen by 16 weeks of therapy, Gengraf® therapy should be discontinued.

Dose decreases by 25% to 50% should be made at any time to control adverse events, e.g., hypertension elevations in serum creatinine (30% above patient's pretreatment level) or clinically significant laboratory abnormalities (see **WARNINGS** and **PRECAUTIONS**).

If dose reduction is not effective in controlling abnormalities or if the adverse event or abnormality is severe, Gengraf® should be discontinued. The same initial dose and dosage range should be used if Gengraf® is combined with the recommended dose of methotrexate. Most patients can be treated with Gengraf® doses of 3 mg/kg/day or below when combined with methotrexate doses of up to 15 mg/week (see **CLINICAL PHARMACOLOGY - Clinical Trials**).

There is limited long-term treatment data. Recurrence of rheumatoid arthritis disease activity is generally apparent within four weeks after stopping cyclosporine.

Psoriasis

The initial dose of Gengraf® Capsules (cyclosporine capsules, USP [**MODIFIED**]) should be 2.5 mg/kg/day. Gengraf® should be taken twice daily, as a divided (1.25 mg/kg BID) oral dose. Patients should be kept at that dose for at least 4 weeks, barring adverse events. If significant clinical improvement has not occurred in patients by that time, the patient's dosage should be increased at 2 week intervals. Based on patient response, dose increases of approximately 0.5 mg/kg/day should be made to a maximum of 4 mg/kg/day.

Dose decreases by 25% to 50% should be made at any time to control adverse events, e.g., hypertension, elevations in serum creatinine (≥ 25% above the patient's pretreatment level), or clinically significant laboratory abnormalities.

If dose reduction is not effective in controlling abnormalities, or if the adverse event or abnormality is severe, Gengraf® should be discontinued (see **PRECAUTIONS - Special Monitoring of Psoriasis Patients**).

Patients generally show some improvement in the clinical manifestations of psoriasis in 2 weeks. Satisfactory control and stabilization of the disease may take 12 to 16 weeks to achieve. Results of a dose-titration clinical trial with Gengraf® indicate that an improvement of psoriasis by 75% or more (based on PASI) was achieved in 51% of the patients after 8 weeks and in 79% of the patients after 16 weeks. Treatment should be discontinued if satisfactory response cannot be achieved after 6 weeks at 4 mg/kg/day or the patient's maximum tolerated dose. Once a patient is adequately controlled and appears stable the dose of Gengraf® should be lowered, and the patient treated with the lowest dose that maintains an adequate response (this should not necessarily be total clearing of the patient). In clinical trials, cyclosporine doses at the lower end of the recommended dosage range were effective in maintaining a satisfactory response in 60% of the patients. Doses below 2.5 mg/kg/day may also be equally effective.

Upon stopping treatment with cyclosporine, relapse will occur in approximately six weeks (50% of the patients) to 16 weeks (75% of the patients). In the majority of patients rebound does not occur after cessation of treatment with cyclosporine. Thirteen cases of transformation of chronic plaque psoriasis to more severe forms of psoriasis have been reported. There were 9 cases of pustular and 4 cases of erythrodermic psoriasis. Long term experience with Gengraf® in psoriasis patients is limited and continuous treatment for extended periods greater than one year is not recommended. Alternation with other forms of treatment should be considered in the long term management of patients with this life long disease.

Blood Concentration Monitoring in Transplant Patients

Transplant centers have found blood concentration monitoring of cyclosporine to be an essential component of patient management. Of importance to blood concentration analysis are the type of assay used, the transplanted organ, and other immunosuppressant agents being administered. While no fixed relationship has been established, blood concentration monitoring may assist in the clinical evaluation of rejection and toxicity, dose adjustments, and the assessment of compliance.

Various assays have been used to measure blood concentrations of cyclosporine. Older studies using a non-specific assay often cited concentrations that were roughly twice those of the specific assays. Therefore, comparison between concentrations in the published literature and an individual patient concentration using current assays must be made with detailed knowledge of the assay methods employed. Current assay results are also not interchangeable and their use should be guided by their approved labeling. A discussion of the different assay methods is contained in Annals of Clinical Biochemistry 1994;31:420-446. While several assays and assay matrices are available, there is a consensus that parent-compound-specific assays correlate best with clinical events. Of these, HPLC is the standard reference, but the monoclonal antibody RIAs and the monoclonal antibody FPIA offer sensitivity, reproducibility, and convenience. Most clinicians base their monitoring on trough cyclosporine concentrations. Applied Pharmacokinetics, Principles of Therapeutic Drug Monitoring (1992) contains a broad discussion of cyclosporine pharmacokinetics and drug monitoring techniques. Blood concentration monitoring is not a replacement for renal function monitoring or tissue biopsies.

HOW SUPPLIED

Gengraf® Capsules (Cyclosporine Capsules, USP [MODIFIED])

25 mg

Oval, white imprinted in blue, the "a" logo, 25 mg, and the code OR. Packages of 30 unit-dose blisters. (**NDC** 0074-6463-32).

100 mg

Oval, white, with two blue stripes, imprinted in blue, the "a" logo, 100 mg, and the code OT. Packages of 30 unit-dose blisters. (**NDC** 0074-6479-32).

Store and Dispense

In the original unit-dose container at controlled room temperature

68°-77°F (20°-25°C). (See USP Controlled Room Temperature).

Sandimmune® is a registered trademark of Novartis Pharmaceuticals Corporation.

AbbVie Inc., North Chicago, IL 60064, U.S.A.

03-A831-R15-Revised July, 2013

Shown in Product Identification Guide, page 303

HUMIRA® ℞

[hu-mare-ah]
(adalimumab)

HIGHLIGHTS OF PRESCRIBING INFORMATION

These highlights do not include all the information needed to use HUMIRA safely and effectively. See full prescribing information for HUMIRA.

HUMIRA (adalimumab) injection, for subcutaneous use
Initial U.S. Approval: 2002

WARNING: SERIOUS INFECTIONS AND MALIGNANCY

See full prescribing information for complete boxed warning.

SERIOUS INFECTIONS (5.1, 6.1):

- **Increased risk of serious infections leading to hospitalization or death, including tuberculosis (TB), bacterial sepsis, invasive fungal infections (such as histoplasmosis), and infections due to other opportunistic pathogens.**
- **Discontinue HUMIRA if a patient develops a serious infection or sepsis during treatment.**
- **Perform test for latent TB; if positive, start treatment for TB prior to starting HUMIRA.**
- **Monitor all patients for active TB during treatment, even if initial latent TB test is negative.**

MALIGNANCY (5.2):

- **Lymphoma and other malignancies, some fatal, have been reported in children and adolescent patients treated with TNF blockers including HUMIRA.**
- **Post-marketing cases of hepatosplenic T-cell lymphoma (HSTCL), a rare type of T-cell lymphoma, have occurred in adolescent and young adults with inflammatory bowel disease treated with TNF blockers including HUMIRA.**

RECENT MAJOR CHANGES

Indications and Usage, Ulcerative Colitis (1.6)	9/2012
Dosage and Administration, Ulcerative Colitis (2.4)	9/2012
Dosage and Administration, General Considerations for Administration (2.7)	4/2013
Warnings and Precautions, Serious Infections (5.1)	5/2013
Warnings and Precautions, Malignancies (5.2)	5/2013
Warnings and Precautions, Hypersensitivity Reactions (5.3)	5/2013

INDICATIONS AND USAGE

HUMIRA is a tumor necrosis factor (TNF) blocker indicated for treatment of:

Rheumatoid Arthritis (RA) (1.1):

- Reducing signs and symptoms, inducing major clinical response, inhibiting the progression of structural damage, and improving physical function in adult patients with moderately to severely active RA.

Juvenile Idiopathic Arthritis (JIA) (1.2):

- Reducing signs and symptoms of moderately to severely active polyarticular JIA in pediatric patients 4 years of age and older.

Psoriatic Arthritis (PsA) (1.3):

- Reducing signs and symptoms, inhibiting the progression of structural damage, and improving physical function in adult patients with active PsA.

Ankylosing Spondylitis (AS) (1.4):

- Reducing signs and symptoms in adult patients with active AS.

Crohn's Disease (CD) (1.5):

- Reducing signs and symptoms and inducing and maintaining clinical remission in adult patients with moderately to severely active Crohn's disease who have had an inadequate response to conventional therapy. Reducing signs and symptoms and inducing clinical remission in these patients if they have also lost response to or are intolerant to infliximab.

Ulcerative Colitis (UC) (1.6):

- Inducing and sustaining clinical remission in adult patients with moderately to severely active ulcerative colitis who have had an inadequate response to immunosuppressants such as corticosteroids, azathioprine or 6-mercaptopurine (6-MP). The effectiveness of HUMIRA has not been established in patients who have lost response to or were intolerant to TNF blockers.

Plaque Psoriasis (Ps) (1.7):

- The treatment of adult patients with moderate to severe chronic plaque psoriasis who are candidates for systemic therapy or phototherapy, and when other systemic therapies are medically less appropriate.

DOSAGE AND ADMINISTRATION

- Administered by subcutaneous injection (2)

Rheumatoid Arthritis, Psoriatic Arthritis, Ankylosing Spondylitis (2.1):

- 40 mg every other week.
  - Some patients with RA not receiving methotrexate may benefit from increasing the frequency to 40 mg every week.

Juvenile Idiopathic Arthritis (2.2):

- *15 kg (33 lbs) to < 30 kg (66 lbs):* 20 mg every other week
- *≥ 30 kg (66 lbs):* 40 mg every other week

Crohn's Disease and Ulcerative Colitis (2.3, 2.4):

- Initial dose (Day 1): 160 mg (four 40 mg injections in one day or two 40 mg injections per day for two consecutive days)
- Second dose two weeks later (Day 15): 80 mg
  - Two weeks later (Day 29): Begin a maintenance dose of 40 mg every other week.
- For patients with Ulcerative Colitis only: Only continue HUMIRA in patients who have shown evidence of clinical remission by eight weeks (Day 57) of therapy.

Plaque Psoriasis (2.5):

- 80 mg initial dose, followed by 40 mg every other week starting one week after initial dose.

DOSAGE FORMS AND STRENGTHS

- Injection: 40 mg/0.8 mL in a single-use prefilled pen (HUMIRA Pen) (3)
- Injection: 40 mg/0.8 mL in a single-use prefilled glass syringe (3)
- Injection: 20 mg/0.4 mL in a single-use prefilled glass syringe (3)
- Injection: 40 mg/0.8 mL in a single-use glass vial for institutional use only (3)

Information on the AbbVie, Inc. products listed on these pages is from the prescribing information in use as of July 31, 2013. For more information, please visit rxabbvie.com or call 1-800-633-9110.

CONTRAINDICATIONS

None (4)

WARNINGS AND PRECAUTIONS

- *Serious infections:* Do not start HUMIRA during an active infection. If an infection develops, monitor carefully, and stop HUMIRA if infection becomes serious (5.1)
- *Invasive fungal infections:* For patients who develop a systemic illness on HUMIRA, consider empiric antifungal therapy for those who reside or travel to regions where mycoses are endemic (5.1)
- *Malignancies:* Incidence of malignancies was greater in HUMIRA-treated patients than in controls (5.2)
- *Anaphylaxis or serious allergic reactions* may occur (5.3)
- *Hepatitis B virus reactivation:* Monitor HBV carriers during and several months after therapy. If reactivation occurs, stop HUMIRA and begin anti-viral therapy (5.4)
- *Demyelinating disease:* Exacerbation or new onset, may occur (5.5)
- *Cytopenias, pancytopenia:* Advise patients to seek immediate medical attention if symptoms develop, and consider stopping HUMIRA (5.6)
- *Heart failure:* Worsening or new onset, may occur (5.8)
- *Lupus-like syndrome:* Stop HUMIRA if syndrome develops (5.9)

ADVERSE REACTIONS

Most common adverse reactions (incidence >10%): infections (e.g. upper respiratory, sinusitis), injection site reactions, headache and rash (6.1)

To report SUSPECTED ADVERSE REACTIONS, contact AbbVie Inc. at 1-800-633-9110 or FDA at 1-800-FDA-1088 or www.fda.gov/medwatch

DRUG INTERACTIONS

- *Abatacept:* Increased risk of serious infection (5.1, 5.11, 7.2)
- *Anakinra:* Increased risk of serious infection (5.1, 5.7, 7.2)
- *Live vaccines:* Avoid use with HUMIRA (5.10, 7.3)

See 17 for PATIENT COUNSELING INFORMATION and Medication Guide

Revised: 06/2013

FULL PRESCRIBING INFORMATION: CONTENTS*

* Sections or subsections omitted from the full prescribing information are not listed

FULL PRESCRIBING INFORMATION

WARNING: SERIOUS INFECTIONS AND MALIGNANCY

SERIOUS INFECTIONS

Patients treated with HUMIRA are at increased risk for developing serious infections that may lead to hospitalization or death *[see Warnings and Precautions (5.1)]*. Most patients who developed these infections were taking concomitant immunosuppressants such as methotrexate or corticosteroids.

Discontinue HUMIRA if a patient develops a serious infection or sepsis.

Reported infections include:

- **Active tuberculosis (TB), including reactivation of latent TB. Patients with TB have frequently presented with disseminated or extrapulmonary disease. Test patients for latent TB before HUMIRA use and during therapy. Initiate treatment for latent TB prior to HUMIRA use.**
- **Invasive fungal infections, including histoplasmosis, coccidioidomycosis, candidiasis, aspergillosis, blastomycosis, and pneumocystosis. Patients with histoplasmosis or other invasive fungal infections may present with disseminated, rather than localized, disease. Antigen and antibody testing for histoplasmosis may be negative in some patients with active infection. Consider empiric anti-fungal therapy in patients at risk for invasive fungal infections who develop severe systemic illness.**
- **Bacterial, viral and other infections due to opportunistic pathogens, including Legionella and Listeria.**

Carefully consider the risks and benefits of treatment with HUMIRA prior to initiating therapy in patients with chronic or recurrent infection.

Monitor patients closely for the development of signs and symptoms of infection during and after treatment with HUMIRA, including the possible development of TB in patients who tested negative for latent TB infection prior to initiating therapy *[see Warnings and Precautions (5.1) and Adverse Reactions (6.1)]*.

MALIGNANCY

Lymphoma and other malignancies, some fatal, have been reported in children and adolescent patients treated with TNF blockers including HUMIRA *[see Warnings and Precautions (5.2)]*. Post-marketing cases of hepatosplenic T-cell lymphoma (HSTCL), a rare type of T-cell lymphoma, have been reported in patients treated with TNF blockers including HUMIRA. These cases have had a very aggressive disease course and have been fatal. The majority of reported TNF blocker cases have occurred in patients with Crohn's disease or ulcerative colitis and the majority were in adolescent and young adult males. Almost all these patients had received treatment with azathioprine or 6-mercaptopurine (6–MP) concomitantly with a TNF blocker at or prior to diagnosis. It is uncertain whether the occurrence of HSTCL is related to use of a TNF blocker or a TNF blocker in combination with these other immunosuppressants *[see Warnings and Precautions (5.2)]*.

1 INDICATIONS AND USAGE

1.1 Rheumatoid Arthritis

HUMIRA is indicated for reducing signs and symptoms, inducing major clinical response, inhibiting the progression of structural damage, and improving physical function in adult patients with moderately to severely active rheumatoid arthritis. HUMIRA can be used alone or in combination with methotrexate or other non-biologic disease-modifying anti-rheumatic drugs (DMARDs).

1.2 Juvenile Idiopathic Arthritis

HUMIRA is indicated for reducing signs and symptoms of moderately to severely active polyarticular juvenile idiopathic arthritis in pediatric patients 4 years of age and older. HUMIRA can be used alone or in combination with methotrexate.

1.3 Psoriatic Arthritis

HUMIRA is indicated for reducing signs and symptoms, inhibiting the progression of structural damage, and improving physical function in adult patients with active psoriatic arthritis. HUMIRA can be used alone or in combination with non-biologic DMARDs.

1.4 Ankylosing Spondylitis

HUMIRA is indicated for reducing signs and symptoms in adult patients with active ankylosing spondylitis.

1.5 Crohn's Disease

HUMIRA is indicated for reducing signs and symptoms and inducing and maintaining clinical remission in adult patients with moderately to severely active Crohn's disease who have had an inadequate response to conventional therapy. HUMIRA is indicated for reducing signs and symptoms and inducing clinical remission in these patients if they have also lost response to or are intolerant to infliximab.

1.6 Ulcerative Colitis

HUMIRA is indicated for inducing and sustaining clinical remission in adult patients with moderately to severely active ulcerative colitis who have had an inadequate response to immunosuppressants such as corticosteroids, azathioprine or 6-mercaptopurine (6-MP). The effectiveness of HUMIRA has not been established in patients who have lost response to or were intolerant to TNF blockers *[see Clinical Studies (14.6)]*.

1.7 Plaque Psoriasis

HUMIRA is indicated for the treatment of adult patients with moderate to severe chronic plaque psoriasis who are candidates for systemic therapy or phototherapy, and when other systemic therapies are medically less appropriate. HUMIRA should only be administered to patients who will be closely monitored and have regular follow-up visits with a physician *[see Boxed Warning and Warnings and Precautions (5)]*.

2 DOSAGE AND ADMINISTRATION

HUMIRA is administered by subcutaneous injection.

2.1 Rheumatoid Arthritis, Psoriatic Arthritis, and Ankylosing Spondylitis

The recommended dose of HUMIRA for adult patients with rheumatoid arthritis (RA), psoriatic arthritis (PsA), or ankylosing spondylitis (AS) is 40 mg administered every other week. Methotrexate (MTX), other non-biologic DMARDS, glucocorticoids, nonsteroidal anti-inflammatory drugs (NSAIDs), and/or analgesics may be continued during treatment with HUMIRA. In the treatment of RA, some patients not taking concomitant MTX may derive additional benefit from increasing the dosing frequency of HUMIRA to 40 mg every week.

2.2 Juvenile Idiopathic Arthritis

The recommended dose of HUMIRA for pediatric patients 4 to 17 years of age with polyarticular juvenile idiopathic arthritis (JIA) is based on weight as shown below. MTX, glucocorticoids, NSAIDs, and/or analgesics may be continued during treatment with HUMIRA.

Pediatric Patients (4 to 17 years)	Dose
15 kg (33 lbs) to <30 kg (66 lbs)	20 mg every other week (20 mg Prefilled Syringe)
≥30 kg (66 lbs)	40 mg every other week (HUMIRA Pen or 40 mg Prefilled Syringe)

Limited data are available for HUMIRA treatment in pediatric patients with a weight below 15 kg.

2.3 Crohn's Disease

The recommended HUMIRA dose regimen for adult patients with Crohn's disease (CD) is 160 mg initially on Day 1 (given as four 40 mg injections in one day or as two 40 mg injections per day for two consecutive days), followed by 80 mg two weeks later (Day 15). Two weeks later (Day 29) begin a maintenance dose of 40 mg every other week. Aminosalicylates and/or corticosteroids may be continued during treatment with HUMIRA. Azathioprine, 6-mercaptopurine (6-MP) *[see Warnings and Precautions (5.2)]* or MTX may be continued during treatment with HUMIRA if necessary. The use of HUMIRA in CD beyond one year has not been evaluated in controlled clinical studies.

2.4 Ulcerative Colitis

The recommended HUMIRA dose regimen for adult patients with ulcerative colitis (UC) is 160 mg initially on Day 1 (given as four 40 mg injections in one day or as two 40 mg injections per day for two consecutive days), followed by 80 mg two weeks later (Day 15). Two weeks later (Day 29) continue with a dose of 40 mg every other week.

Only continue HUMIRA in patients who have shown evidence of clinical remission by eight weeks (Day 57) of therapy. Aminosalicylates and/or corticosteroids may be continued during treatment with HUMIRA. Azathioprine and 6-mercaptopurine (6-MP) *[see Warnings and Precautions (5.2)]* may be continued during treatment with HUMIRA if necessary.

2.5 Plaque Psoriasis

The recommended dose of HUMIRA for adult patients with plaque psoriasis (Ps) is an initial dose of 80 mg, followed by 40 mg given every other week starting one week after the initial dose. The use of HUMIRA in moderate to severe chronic Ps beyond one year has not been evaluated in controlled clinical studies.

2.6 Monitoring to Assess Safety

Prior to initiating HUMIRA and periodically during therapy, evaluate patients for active tuberculosis and test for latent infection *[see Warnings and Precautions (5.1)]*.

2.7 General Considerations for Administration

HUMIRA is intended for use under the guidance and supervision of a physician. A patient may self-inject HUMIRA if a physician determines that it is appropriate, and with medical follow-up, as necessary, after proper training in subcutaneous injection technique.

Carefully inspect the solution in the HUMIRA Pen or prefilled syringe for particulate matter and discoloration prior to subcutaneous administration. If particulates and discolorations are noted, do not use the product. HUMIRA does not contain preservatives; therefore, discard unused portions of drug remaining from the syringe. NOTE: Instruct patients sensitive to latex not to handle the needle cover of the syringe because it contains dry rubber (latex).

Instruct patients using the HUMIRA Pen or prefilled syringe to inject the full amount in the syringe (0.8 mL), which provides 40 mg of HUMIRA, according to the directions provided in the Instructions for Use *[see Instructions for Use]*.

Instruct patients (15 kg to <30 kg) using the pediatric prefilled syringe, or their caregivers, to inject the full amount in the syringe (0.4 mL), which provides 20 mg of HUMIRA, according to the directions provided in the Instructions for Use.

Rotate injection sites and do not give injections into areas where the skin is tender, bruised, red or hard.

The HUMIRA institutional use vial is for use and administration within an institutional setting only, such as a hospital, physician's office or clinic. Withdraw the dose using a sterile needle and syringe and administer promptly by a healthcare provider within an institutional setting. Only administer one dose per vial. The vial does not contain preservatives; therefore, discard unused portions.

3 DOSAGE FORMS AND STRENGTHS

• Pen

Injection: A single-use pen (HUMIRA Pen), containing a 1 mL prefilled glass syringe with a fixed 27 gauge ½ inch needle, providing 40 mg (0.8 mL) of HUMIRA.

• Prefilled Syringe

Injection: A single-use, 1 mL prefilled glass syringe with a fixed 27 gauge ½ inch needle, providing 40 mg (0.8 mL) of HUMIRA.

Injection: A single-use, 1 mL prefilled glass syringe with a fixed 27 gauge ½ inch needle, providing 20 mg (0.4 mL) of HUMIRA.

• Institutional Use Vial

Injection: A single-use, glass vial, providing 40 mg (0.8 mL) of HUMIRA for institutional use only.

4 CONTRAINDICATIONS

None.

5 WARNINGS AND PRECAUTIONS

5.1 Serious Infections

Patients treated with HUMIRA are at increased risk for developing serious infections involving various organ systems and sites that may lead to hospitalization or death *[see Boxed Warning]*. Opportunistic infections due to bacterial, mycobacterial, invasive fungal, viral, parasitic, or other opportunistic pathogens including aspergillosis, blastomycosis, candidiasis, coccidioidomycosis, histoplasmosis, legionellosis, listeriosis, pneumocystosis and tuberculosis have been reported with TNF blockers. Patients have frequently presented with disseminated rather than localized disease.

The concomitant use of a TNF blocker and abatacept or anakinra was associated with a higher risk of serious infections in patients with rheumatoid arthritis (RA); therefore, the concomitant use of HUMIRA and these biologic products is not recommended in the treatment of patients with RA *[see Warnings and Precautions (5.7, 5.11) and Drug Interactions (7.2)]*.

Treatment with HUMIRA should not be initiated in patients with an active infection, including localized infections. Patients greater than 65 years of age, patients with co-morbid conditions and/or patients taking concomitant immunosuppressants (such as corticosteroids or methotrexate), may be at greater risk of infection. Consider the risks and benefits of treatment prior to initiating therapy in patients:

- with chronic or recurrent infection;
- who have been exposed to tuberculosis;
- with a history of an opportunistic infection;
- who have resided or traveled in areas of endemic tuberculosis or endemic mycoses, such as histoplasmosis, coccidioidomycosis, or blastomycosis; or
- with underlying conditions that may predispose them to infection.

Tuberculosis

Cases of reactivation of tuberculosis and new onset tuberculosis infections have been reported in patients receiving HUMIRA, including patients who have previously received treatment for latent or active tuberculosis. Reports included cases of pulmonary and extrapulmonary (i.e., disseminated) tuberculosis. Evaluate patients for tuberculosis risk factors and test for latent infection prior to initiating HUMIRA and periodically during therapy.

Treatment of latent tuberculosis infection prior to therapy with TNF blocking agents has been shown to reduce the risk of tuberculosis reactivation during therapy. Prior to initiating HUMIRA, assess if treatment for latent tuberculosis is needed; and consider an induration of ≥ 5 mm a positive tuberculin skin test result, even for patients previously vaccinated with Bacille Calmette-Guerin (BCG).

Consider anti-tuberculosis therapy prior to initiation of HUMIRA in patients with a past history of latent or active tuberculosis in whom an adequate course of treatment cannot be confirmed, and for patients with a negative test for latent tuberculosis but having risk factors for tuberculosis infection. Despite prophylactic treatment for tuberculosis, cases of reactivated tuberculosis have occurred in patients treated with HUMIRA. Consultation with a physician with expertise in the treatment of tuberculosis is recommended to aid in the decision whether initiating anti-tuberculosis therapy is appropriate for an individual patient.

Strongly consider tuberculosis in the differential diagnosis in patients who develop a new infection during HUMIRA treatment, especially in patients who have previously or recently traveled to countries with a high prevalence of tuberculosis, or who have had close contact with a person with active tuberculosis.

Monitoring

Closely monitor patients for the development of signs and symptoms of infection during and after treatment with HUMIRA, including the development of tuberculosis in patients who tested negative for latent tuberculosis infection prior to initiating therapy. Tests for latent tuberculosis infection may also be falsely negative while on therapy with HUMIRA.

Discontinue HUMIRA if a patient develops a serious infection or sepsis. For a patient who develops a new infection during treatment with HUMIRA, closely monitor them, perform a prompt and complete diagnostic workup appropriate for an immunocompromised patient, and initiate appropriate antimicrobial therapy.

Invasive Fungal Infections

If patients develop a serious systemic illness and they reside or travel in regions where mycoses are endemic, consider invasive fungal infection in the differential diagnosis. Antigen and antibody testing for histoplasmosis may be negative in some patients with active infection. Consider appropriate empiric antifungal therapy, taking into account both the risk for severe fungal infection and the risks of antifungal therapy, while a diagnostic workup is being performed. To aid in the management of such patients, consider consultation with a physician with expertise in the diagnosis and treatment of invasive fungal infections.

5.2 Malignancies

Consider the risks and benefits of TNF-blocker treatment including HUMIRA prior to initiating therapy in patients with a known malignancy other than a successfully treated non-melanoma skin cancer (NMSC) or when considering continuing a TNF blocker in patients who develop a malignancy.

Malignancies in Adults

In the controlled portions of clinical trials of some TNF-blockers, including HUMIRA, more cases of malignancies have been observed among TNF-blocker treated adult patients compared to control-treated adult patients. During the controlled portions of 34 global HUMIRA clinical trials in adult patients with rheumatoid arthritis (RA), psoriatic arthritis (PsA), ankylosing spondylitis (AS), Crohn's disease (CD), ulcerative colitis (UC) and plaque psoriasis (Ps), malignancies, other than non-melanoma (basal cell and squamous cell) skin cancer, were observed at a rate (95% confidence interval) of 0.6 (0.38, 0.91) per 100 patient-years among 7304 HUMIRA-treated patients versus a rate of 0.6 (0.30, 1.03) per 100 patient-years among 4232 control-treated patients (median duration of treatment of 4 months for HUMIRA-treated patients and 4 months for control-treated patients). In 47 global controlled and uncontrolled clinical trials of HUMIRA in adult patients with RA, PsA, AS, CD, UC, and Ps, the most frequently observed malignancies, other than lymphoma and NMSC, were breast, colon, prostate, lung, and melanoma. The malignancies in HUMIRA-treated patients in the controlled and uncontrolled portions of the studies were similar in type and number to what would be expected in the general U.S. population according to the SEER database (adjusted for age, gender, and race).[1]

In controlled trials of other TNF blockers in adult patients at higher risk for malignancies (i.e., patients with COPD with a significant smoking history and cyclophosphamide-treated patients with Wegener's granulomatosis), a greater portion of malignancies occurred in the TNF blocker group compared to the control group.

Non-Melanoma Skin Cancer

During the controlled portions of 34 global HUMIRA clinical trials in adult patients with RA, PsA, AS, CD, UC, and Ps, the rate (95% confidence interval) of NMSC was 0.7 (0.49, 1.08) per 100 patient-years among HUMIRA-treated patients and 0.2 (0.08, 0.59) per 100 patient-years among control-treated patients. Examine all patients, and in particular patients with a medical history of prior prolonged immunosuppressant therapy or psoriasis patients with a history of PUVA treatment for the presence of NMSC prior to and during treatment with HUMIRA.

Lymphoma and Leukemia

In the controlled portions of clinical trials of all the TNF-blockers in adults, more cases of lymphoma have been observed among TNF-blocker-treated patients compared to control-treated patients. In the controlled portions of 34 global HUMIRA clinical trials in adult patients with RA, PsA, AS, CD, UC and Ps, 3 lymphomas occurred among 7304 HUMIRA-treated patients versus 1 among 4232 control-treated patients. In 47 global controlled and uncontrolled clinical trials of HUMIRA in adult patients with RA, PsA, AS, CD, UC and Ps with a median duration of approximately 0.6 years, including 23,036 patients and over 34,000 patient-years of HUMIRA, the observed rate of lymphomas was approximately 0.11 per 100 patient-years. This is approximately 3-fold higher than expected in the general U.S. population according to the SEER database (adjusted for age, gender, and race).[1] Rates of lymphoma in clinical trials of HUMIRA cannot be compared to rates of lymphoma in clinical trials of other TNF blockers and may not predict the rates observed in a broader patient population. Patients with RA and other chronic inflammatory diseases, particularly those with highly active disease and/or chronic exposure to immunosuppressant therapies, may be at a higher risk (up to several fold) than the general population for the development of lymphoma, even in the absence of TNF blockers. Post-marketing cases of acute and chronic leukemia have been reported in association with TNF-blocker use in RA and other indications. Even in the absence of TNF-blocker therapy, patients with RA may be at a higher risk (approximately 2-fold) than the general population for the development of leukemia.

Malignancies in Pediatric Patients and Young Adults

Malignancies, some fatal, have been reported among children, adolescents, and young adults who received treatment with TNF-blockers (initiation of therapy ≤ 18 years of age), of which HUMIRA is a member *[see Boxed Warning]*. Approximately half the cases were lymphomas, including Hodgkin's and non-Hodgkin's lymphoma. The other cases represented a variety of different malignancies and included rare malignancies usually associated with immunosuppression and malignancies that are not usually observed in children and adolescents. The malignancies occurred after a median of 30 months of therapy (range 1 to 84 months). Most of the patients were receiving concomitant immunosuppressants. These cases were reported post-marketing and are derived from a variety of sources including registries and spontaneous postmarketing reports.

Postmarketing cases of hepatosplenic T-cell lymphoma (HSTCL), a rare type of T-cell lymphoma, have been reported in patients treated with TNF blockers including HUMIRA *[see Boxed Warning]*. These cases have had a very aggressive disease course and have been fatal. The majority of reported TNF blocker cases have occurred in patients with Crohn's disease or ulcerative colitis and the majority were in adolescent and young adult males. Almost all of these patients had received treatment with the immunosuppressants azathioprine or 6-mercaptopurine (6–MP) concomitantly with a TNF blocker at or prior to diagnosis. It is uncertain whether the occurrence of HSTCL is related to use of a TNF blocker or a TNF blocker in combination with these other immunosuppressants. The potential risk with the combination of azathioprine or 6-mercaptopurine and HUMIRA should be carefully considered.

Information on the AbbVie, Inc. products listed on these pages is from the prescribing information in use as of July 31, 2013. For more information, please visit rxabbvie.com or call 1-800-633-9110.

5.3 Hypersensitivity Reactions
Anaphylaxis and angioneurotic edema have been reported following HUMIRA administration. If an anaphylactic or other serious allergic reaction occurs, immediately discontinue administration of HUMIRA and institute appropriate therapy. In clinical trials of HUMIRA in adults, allergic reactions (e.g., allergic rash, anaphylactoid reaction, fixed drug reaction, non-specified drug reaction, urticaria) have been observed.

5.4 Hepatitis B Virus Reactivation
Use of TNF blockers, including HUMIRA, may increase the risk of reactivation of hepatitis B virus (HBV) in patients who are chronic carriers of this virus. In some instances, HBV reactivation occurring in conjunction with TNF blocker therapy has been fatal. The majority of these reports have occurred in patients concomitantly receiving other medications that suppress the immune system, which may also contribute to HBV reactivation. Evaluate patients at risk for HBV infection for prior evidence of HBV infection before initiating TNF blocker therapy. Exercise caution in prescribing TNF blockers for patients identified as carriers of HBV. Adequate data are not available on the safety or efficacy of treating patients who are carriers of HBV with anti-viral therapy in conjunction with TNF blocker therapy to prevent HBV reactivation. For patients who are carriers of HBV and require treatment with TNF blockers, closely monitor such patients for clinical and laboratory signs of active HBV infection throughout therapy and for several months following termination of therapy. In patients who develop HBV reactivation, stop HUMIRA and initiate effective anti-viral therapy with appropriate supportive treatment. The safety of resuming TNF blocker therapy after HBV reactivation is controlled is not known. Therefore, exercise caution when considering resumption of HUMIRA therapy in this situation and monitor patients closely.

5.5 Neurologic Reactions
Use of TNF blocking agents, including HUMIRA, has been associated with rare cases of new onset or exacerbation of clinical symptoms and/or radiographic evidence of central nervous system demyelinating disease, including multiple sclerosis (MS) and optic neuritis, and peripheral demyelinating disease, including Guillain-Barré syndrome. Exercise caution in considering the use of HUMIRA in patients with preexisting or recent-onset central or peripheral nervous system demyelinating disorders.

5.6 Hematological Reactions
Rare reports of pancytopenia including aplastic anemia have been reported with TNF blocking agents. Adverse reactions of the hematologic system, including medically significant cytopenia (e.g., thrombocytopenia, leukopenia) have been infrequently reported with HUMIRA. The causal relationship of these reports to HUMIRA remains unclear. Advise all patients to seek immediate medical attention if they develop signs and symptoms suggestive of blood dyscrasias or infection (e.g., persistent fever, bruising, bleeding, pallor) while on HUMIRA. Consider discontinuation of HUMIRA therapy in patients with confirmed significant hematologic abnormalities.

5.7 Use with Anakinra
Concurrent use of anakinra (an interleukin-1 antagonist) and another TNF-blocker, was associated with a greater proportion of serious infections and neutropenia and no added benefit compared with the TNF-blocker alone in patients with RA. Therefore, the combination of HUMIRA and anakinra is not recommended *[see Drug Interactions (7.2)]*.

5.8 Heart Failure
Cases of worsening congestive heart failure (CHF) and new onset CHF have been reported with TNF blockers. Cases of worsening CHF have also been observed with HUMIRA. HUMIRA has not been formally studied in patients with CHF; however, in clinical trials of another TNF blocker, a higher rate of serious CHF-related adverse reactions was observed. Exercise caution when using HUMIRA in patients who have heart failure and monitor them carefully.

5.9 Autoimmunity
Treatment with HUMIRA may result in the formation of autoantibodies and, rarely, in the development of a lupus-like syndrome. If a patient develops symptoms suggestive of a lupus-like syndrome following treatment with HUMIRA, discontinue treatment *[see Adverse Reactions (6.1)]*.

5.10 Immunizations
In a placebo-controlled clinical trial of patients with RA, no difference was detected in anti-pneumococcal antibody response between HUMIRA and placebo treatment groups when the pneumococcal polysaccharide vaccine and influenza vaccine were administered concurrently with HUMIRA. Similar proportions of patients developed protective levels of anti-influenza antibodies between HUMIRA and placebo treatment groups; however, titers in aggregate to influenza antigens were moderately lower in patients receiving HUMIRA. The clinical significance of this is unknown. Patients on HUMIRA may receive concurrent vaccinations, except for live vaccines. No data are available on the secondary transmission of infection by live vaccines in patients receiving HUMIRA.

It is recommended that JIA patients, if possible, be brought up to date with all immunizations in agreement with current immunization guidelines prior to initiating HUMIRA therapy. Patients on HUMIRA may receive concurrent vaccinations, except for live vaccines.

5.11 Use with Abatacept
In controlled trials, the concurrent administration of TNF-blockers and abatacept was associated with a greater proportion of serious infections than the use of a TNF-blocker alone; the combination therapy, compared to the use of a TNF-blocker alone, has not demonstrated improved clinical benefit in the treatment of RA. Therefore, the combination of abatacept with TNF-blockers including HUMIRA is not recommended *[see Drug Interactions (7.2)]*.

6 ADVERSE REACTIONS
The most serious adverse reactions described elsewhere in the labeling include the following:
- Serious Infections *[see Warnings and Precautions (5.1)]*
- Malignancies *[see Warnings and Precautions (5.2)]*

6.1 Clinical Trials Experience
Because clinical trials are conducted under widely varying and controlled conditions, adverse reaction rates observed in clinical trials of a drug cannot be directly compared to rates in the clinical trials of another drug and may not predict the rates observed in a broader patient population in clinical practice.
The most common adverse reaction with HUMIRA was injection site reactions. In placebo-controlled trials, 20% of patients treated with HUMIRA developed injection site reactions (erythema and/or itching, hemorrhage, pain or swelling), compared to 14% of patients receiving placebo. Most injection site reactions were described as mild and generally did not necessitate drug discontinuation.
The proportion of patients who discontinued treatment due to adverse reactions during the double-blind, placebo-controlled portion of studies in patients with RA (i.e., Studies RA-I, RA-II, RA-III and RA-IV) was 7% for patients taking HUMIRA and 4% for placebo-treated patients. The most common adverse reactions leading to discontinuation of HUMIRA in these RA studies were clinical flare reaction (0.7%), rash (0.3%) and pneumonia (0.3%).

Infections
In the controlled portions of the 34 global HUMIRA clinical trials in adult patients with RA, PsA, AS, CD, UC and Ps, the rate of serious infections was 4.6 per 100 patient-years in 7304 HUMIRA-treated patients versus a rate of 3.1 per 100 patient-years in 4232 control-treated patients. Serious infections observed included pneumonia, septic arthritis, prosthetic and post-surgical infections, erysipelas, cellulitis, diverticulitis, and pyelonephritis *[see Warnings and Precautions (5.1)]*.

Tuberculosis and Opportunistic Infections
In 47 global controlled and uncontrolled clinical trials in RA, PsA, AS, CD, UC and Ps that included 23,036 HUMIRA-treated patients, the rate of reported active tuberculosis was 0.22 per 100 patient-years and the rate of positive PPD conversion was 0.08 per 100 patient-years. In a subgroup of 9396 U.S. and Canadian HUMIRA-treated patients, the rate of reported active TB was 0.07 per 100 patient-years and the rate of positive PPD conversion was 0.08 per 100 patient-years. These trials included reports of miliary, lymphatic, peritoneal, and pulmonary TB. Most of the TB cases occurred within the first eight months after initiation of therapy and may reflect recrudescence of latent disease. In these global clinical trials, cases of serious opportunistic infections have been reported at an overall rate of 0.08 per 100 patient-years. Some cases of serious opportunistic infections and TB have been fatal *[see Warnings and Precautions (5.1)]*.

Autoantibodies
In the rheumatoid arthritis controlled trials, 12% of patients treated with HUMIRA and 7% of placebo-treated patients that had negative baseline ANA titers developed positive titers at week 24. Two patients out of 3046 treated with HUMIRA developed clinical signs suggestive of new-onset lupus-like syndrome. The patients improved following discontinuation of therapy. No patients developed lupus nephritis or central nervous system symptoms. The impact of long-term treatment with HUMIRA on the development of autoimmune diseases is unknown.

Liver Enzyme Elevations
There have been reports of severe hepatic reactions including acute liver failure in patients receiving TNF-blockers. In controlled Phase 3 trials of HUMIRA (40 mg SC every other week) in patients with RA, PsA, and AS with control period duration ranging from 4 to 104 weeks, ALT elevations ≥ 3 × ULN occurred in 3.5% of HUMIRA-treated patients and 1.5% of control-treated patients. Since many of these patients in these trials were also taking medications that cause liver enzyme elevations (e.g., NSAIDS, MTX), the relationship between HUMIRA and the liver enzyme elevations is not clear. In controlled Phase 3 trials of HUMIRA (initial doses of 160 mg and 80 mg, or 80 mg and 40 mg on Days 1 and 15, respectively, followed by 40 mg every other week) in patients with CD with control period duration ranging from 4 to 52 weeks, ALT elevations ≥ 3 × ULN occurred in 0.9% of HUMIRA-treated patients and 0.9% of control-treated patients. In controlled Phase 3 trials of HUMIRA (initial doses of 160 mg and 80 mg on Days 1 and 15 respectively, followed by 40 mg every other week) in patients with UC with control period duration ranging from 1 to 52 weeks, ALT elevations ≥3 × ULN occurred in 1.5% of HUMIRA-treated patients and 1.0% of control-treated patients. In controlled Phase 3 trials of HUMIRA (initial dose of 80 mg then 40 mg every other week) in patients with Ps with control period duration ranging from 12 to 24 weeks, ALT elevations ≥ 3 × ULN occurred in 1.8% of HUMIRA-treated patients and 1.8% of control-treated patients.

Immunogenicity
Patients in Studies RA-I, RA-II, and RA-III were tested at multiple time points for antibodies to adalimumab during the 6- to 12-month period. Approximately 5% (58 of 1062) of adult RA patients receiving HUMIRA developed low-titer antibodies to adalimumab at least once during treatment, which were neutralizing *in vitro*. Patients treated with concomitant methotrexate (MTX) had a lower rate of antibody development than patients on HUMIRA monotherapy (1% versus 12%). No apparent correlation of antibody development to adverse reactions was observed. With monotherapy, patients receiving every other week dosing may develop antibodies more frequently than those receiving weekly dosing. In patients receiving the recommended dosage of 40 mg every other week as monotherapy, the ACR 20 response was lower among antibody-positive patients than among antibody-negative patients. The long-term immunogenicity of HUMIRA is unknown.
In patients with JIA, adalimumab antibodies were identified in 16% of HUMIRA-treated patients. In patients receiving concomitant MTX, the incidence was 6% compared to 26% with HUMIRA monotherapy.
In patients with AS, the rate of development of antibodies to adalimumab in HUMIRA-treated patients was comparable to patients with RA.
In patients with PsA, the rate of antibody development in patients receiving HUMIRA monotherapy was comparable to patients with RA; however, in patients receiving concomitant MTX the rate was 7% compared to 1% in RA.
In patients with CD, the rate of antibody development was 3%.
In patients with moderately to severely active UC, the rate of antibody development in patients receiving HUMIRA was 5%. However, due to the limitation of the assay conditions, antibodies to adalimumab could be detected only when serum adalimumab levels were < 2 ug/ml. Among the patients whose serum adalimumab levels were < 2 ug/ml (approximately 25% of total patients studied), the immunogenicity rate was 20.7%.
In patients with Ps, the rate of antibody development with HUMIRA monotherapy was 8%. However, due to the limitation of the assay conditions, antibodies to adalimumab could be detected only when serum adalimumab levels were < 2 ug/ml. Among the patients whose serum adalimumab levels were < 2 ug/ml (approximately 40% of total patients studied), the immunogenicity rate was 20.7%. In Ps patients who were on HUMIRA monotherapy and subsequently withdrawn from the treatment, the rate of antibodies to adalimumab after retreatment was similar to the rate observed prior to withdrawal.
The data reflect the percentage of patients whose test results were considered positive for antibodies to adalimumab in an ELISA assay, and are highly dependent on the sensitivity and specificity of the assay. The observed incidence of antibody (including neutralizing antibody) positivity in an assay is highly dependent on several factors including assay sensitivity and specificity, assay methodology, sample handling, timing of sample collection, concomitant medications, and underlying disease. For these reasons, comparison of the incidence of antibodies to adalimumab with the incidence of antibodies to other products may be misleading.

Other Adverse Reactions

Rheumatoid Arthritis Clinical Studies
The data described below reflect exposure to HUMIRA in 2468 patients, including 2073 exposed for 6 months, 1497 exposed for greater than one year and 1380 in adequate and well-controlled studies (Studies RA-I, RA-II, RA-III, and RA-IV). HUMIRA was studied primarily in placebo-controlled trials and in long-term follow up studies for up to 36 months duration. The population had a mean age of 54 years, 77% were female, 91% were Caucasian and had moderately to severely active rheumatoid arthritis. Most patients received 40 mg HUMIRA every other week.
Table 1 summarizes reactions reported at a rate of at least 5% in patients treated with HUMIRA 40 mg every other week compared to placebo and with an incidence higher than placebo. In Study RA-III, the types and frequencies of adverse reactions in the second year open-label extension were similar to those observed in the one-year double-blind portion.

Table 1. Adverse Reactions Reported by ≥5% of Patients Treated with HUMIRA During Placebo-Controlled Period of Pooled RA Studies (Studies RA-I, RA-II, RA-III, and RA-IV)

	HUMIRA 40 mg subcutaneous Every Other Week (N=705)	Placebo (N=690)
Adverse Reaction (Preferred Term)		
Respiratory		
Upper respiratory infection	17%	13%
Sinusitis	11%	9%
Flu syndrome	7%	6%
Gastrointestinal		
Nausea	9%	8%
Abdominal pain	7%	4%
Laboratory Tests*		
Laboratory test abnormal	8%	7%
Hypercholesterolemia	6%	4%
Hyperlipidemia	7%	5%
Hematuria	5%	4%
Alkaline phosphatase increased	5%	3%
Other		
Headache	12%	8%
Rash	12%	6%
Accidental injury	10%	8%
Injection site reaction **	8%	1%
Back pain	6%	4%
Urinary tract infection	8%	5%
Hypertension	5%	3%

* Laboratory test abnormalities were reported as adverse reactions in European trials

** Does not include injection site erythema, itching, hemorrhage, pain or swelling

Less Common Adverse Reactions in Rheumatoid Arthritis Clinical Studies

Other infrequent serious adverse reactions that do not appear in the Warnings and Precautions or Adverse Reaction sections that occurred at an incidence of less than 5% in HUMIRA-treated patients in RA studies were:

Body As A Whole: Pain in extremity, pelvic pain, surgery, thorax pain

Cardiovascular System: Arrhythmia, atrial fibrillation, chest pain, coronary artery disorder, heart arrest, hypertensive encephalopathy, myocardial infarct, palpitation, pericardial effusion, pericarditis, syncope, tachycardia

Digestive System: Cholecystitis, cholelithiasis, esophagitis, gastroenteritis, gastrointestinal hemorrhage, hepatic necrosis, vomiting

Endocrine System: Parathyroid disorder

Hemic And Lymphatic System: Agranulocytosis, polycythemia

Metabolic And Nutritional Disorders: Dehydration, healing abnormal, ketosis, paraproteinemia, peripheral edema

Musculo-Skeletal System: Arthritis, bone disorder, bone fracture (not spontaneous), bone necrosis, joint disorder, muscle cramps, myasthenia, pyogenic arthritis, synovitis, tendon disorder

Neoplasia: Adenoma

Nervous System: Confusion, paresthesia, subdural hematoma, tremor

Respiratory System: Asthma, bronchospasm, dyspnea, lung function decreased, pleural effusion

Special Senses: Cataract

Thrombosis: Thrombosis leg

Urogenital System: Cystitis, kidney calculus, menstrual disorder

Juvenile Idiopathic Arthritis Clinical Studies

In general, the adverse reactions in the HUMIRA-treated pediatric patients in the juvenile idiopathic arthritis (JIA) trial were similar in frequency and type to those seen in adult patients *[see Warnings and Precautions (5), Adverse Reactions (6)]*. Important findings and differences from adults are discussed in the following paragraphs.

HUMIRA was studied in 171 pediatric patients, 4 to 17 years of age, with polyarticular JIA. Severe adverse reactions reported in the study included neutropenia, streptococcal pharyngitis, increased aminotransferases, herpes zoster, myositis, metrorrhagia, appendicitis. Serious infections were observed in 4% of patients within approximately 2 years of initiation of treatment with HUMIRA and included cases of herpes simplex, pneumonia, urinary tract infection, pharyngitis, and herpes zoster.

A total of 45% of children experienced an infection while receiving HUMIRA with or without concomitant MTX in the first 16 weeks of treatment. The types of infections reported in HUMIRA-treated patients were generally similar to those commonly seen in JIA patients who are not treated with TNF blockers. Upon initiation of treatment, the most common adverse reactions occurring in the pediatric population treated with HUMIRA were injection site pain and injection site reaction (19% and 16%, respectively). A less commonly reported adverse event in children receiving HUMIRA was granuloma annulare which did not lead to discontinuation of HUMIRA treatment.

In the first 48 weeks of treatment, non-serious hypersensitivity reactions were seen in approximately 6% of children and included primarily localized allergic hypersensitivity reactions and allergic rash.

Isolated mild to moderate elevations of liver aminotransferases (ALT more common than AST) were observed in children with JIA exposed to HUMIRA alone; liver enzyme test elevations were more frequent among those treated with the combination of HUMIRA and MTX than those treated with HUMIRA alone. In general, these elevations did not lead to discontinuation of HUMIRA treatment.

In the JIA trial, 10% of patients treated with HUMIRA who had negative baseline anti-dsDNA antibodies developed positive titers after 48 weeks of treatment. No patient developed clinical signs of autoimmunity during the clinical trial.

Approximately 15% of children treated with HUMIRA developed mild-to-moderate elevations of creatine phosphokinase (CPK). Elevations exceeding 5 times the upper limit of normal were observed in several patients. CPK levels decreased or returned to normal in all patients. Most patients were able to continue HUMIRA without interruption.

Psoriatic Arthritis and Ankylosing Spondylitis Clinical Studies

HUMIRA has been studied in 395 patients with psoriatic arthritis (PsA) in two placebo-controlled trials and in an open label study and in 393 patients with ankylosing spondylitis (AS) in two placebo-controlled studies. The safety profile for patients with PsA and AS treated with HUMIRA 40 mg every other week was similar to the safety profile seen in patients with RA, HUMIRA Studies RA-I through IV.

Crohn's Disease Clinical Studies

HUMIRA has been studied in 1478 patients with Crohn's disease (CD) in four placebo-controlled and two open-label extension studies. The safety profile for patients with CD treated with HUMIRA was similar to the safety profile seen in patients with RA.

Ulcerative Colitis Clinical Studies

HUMIRA has been studied in 1010 patients with ulcerative colitis (UC) in two placebo-controlled studies and one open-label extension study. The safety profile for patients with UC treated with HUMIRA was similar to the safety profile seen in patients with RA.

Plaque Psoriasis Clinical Studies

HUMIRA has been studied in 1696 patients with plaque psoriasis (Ps) in placebo-controlled and open-label extension studies. The safety profile for patients with Ps treated with HUMIRA was similar to the safety profile seen in patients with RA with the following exceptions. In the placebo-controlled portions of the clinical trials in Ps patients, HUMIRA-treated patients had a higher incidence of arthralgia when compared to controls (3% *vs.* 1%).

6.2 Postmarketing Experience

The following adverse reactions have been identified during post-approval use of HUMIRA. Because these reactions are reported voluntarily from a population of uncertain size, it is not always possible to reliably estimate their frequency or establish a causal relationship to HUMIRA exposure.

Gastrointestinal disorders: Diverticulitis, large bowel perforations including perforations associated with diverticulitis and appendiceal perforations associated with appendicitis, pancreatitis

General disorders and administration site conditions: Pyrexia

Hepato-biliary disorders: Liver failure

Immune system disorders: Sarcoidosis

Neoplasms benign, malignant and unspecified (incl cysts and polyps): Merkel Cell Carcinoma (neuroendocrine carcinoma of the skin)

Nervous system disorders: Demyelinating disorders (e.g., optic neuritis, Guillain-Barré syndrome), cerebrovascular accident

Respiratory disorders: Interstitial lung disease, including pulmonary fibrosis, pulmonary embolism

Skin reactions: Stevens Johnson Syndrome, cutaneous vasculitis, erythema multiforme, new or worsening psoriasis (all sub-types including pustular and palmoplantar), alopecia

Vascular disorders: Systemic vasculitis, deep vein thrombosis

7 DRUG INTERACTIONS

7.1 Methotrexate

HUMIRA has been studied in rheumatoid arthritis (RA) patients taking concomitant methotrexate (MTX). Although MTX reduced the apparent adalimumab clearance, the data do not suggest the need for dose adjustment of either HUMIRA or MTX *[see Clinical Pharmacology (12.3)]*.

7.2 Biological Products

In clinical studies in patients with RA, an increased risk of serious infections has been seen with the combination of TNF blockers with anakinra or abatacept, with no added benefit; therefore, use of HUMIRA with abatacept or anakinra is not recommended in patients with RA *[see Warnings and Precautions (5.7 and 5.11)]*. A higher rate of serious infections has also been observed in patients with RA treated with rituximab who received subsequent treatment with a TNF blocker. There is insufficient information regarding the concomitant use of HUMIRA and other biologic products for the treatment of RA, PsA, AS, CD, UC, and Ps. Concomitant administration of HUMIRA with other biologic DMARDS (e.g., anakinra and abatacept) or other TNF blockers is not recommended based upon the possible increased risk for infections and other potential pharmacological interactions.

7.3 Live Vaccines

Avoid the use of live vaccines with HUMIRA *[see Warnings and Precautions (5.10)]*.

7.4 Cytochrome P450 Substrates

The formation of CYP450 enzymes may be suppressed by increased levels of cytokines (e.g., TNFα, IL-6) during chronic inflammation. It is possible for a molecule that antagonizes cytokine activity, such as adalimumab, to influence the formation of CYP450 enzymes. Upon initiation or discontinuation of HUMIRA in patients being treated with CYP450 substrates with a narrow therapeutic index, monitoring of the effect (e.g., warfarin) or drug concentration (e.g., cyclosporine or theophylline) is recommended and the individual dose of the drug product may be adjusted as needed.

8 USE IN SPECIFIC POPULATIONS

8.1 Pregnancy

Pregnancy Category B

Risk Summary

Adequate and well controlled studies with HUMIRA have not been conducted in pregnant women. Adalimumab is an IgG1 monoclonal antibody and IgG1 is actively transferred across the placenta during the third trimester of pregnancy. Adalimumab serum levels were obtained from ten women treated with HUMIRA during pregnancy and eight newborn infants suggest active placental transfer of adalimumab. No fetal harm was observed in reproductive studies performed in cynomolgus monkeys. Because animal reproductive studies are not always predictive of human response, this drug should be used during pregnancy only if clearly needed.

Clinical Considerations

In general, monoclonal antibodies are transported across the placenta in a linear fashion as pregnancy progresses, with the largest amount transferred during the third trimester.

Human Data

In an independent clinical study conducted in ten pregnant women with inflammatory bowel disease treated with HUMIRA, adalimumab concentrations were measured in maternal blood as well as in cord (n=10) and infant blood (n=8) on the day of birth. The last dose of HUMIRA was given between 1 and 56 days prior to delivery. Adalimumab concentrations were 0.16-19.7 μg/mL in cord blood, 4.28-17.7 μg/mL in infant blood, and 0-16.1 μg/mL in maternal blood. In all but one case, the cord blood level of adalimumab was higher than the maternal level, suggesting adalimumab actively crosses the placenta. In addition, one infant had levels at each of the following: 6 weeks (1.94 μg/mL), 7 weeks (1.31 μg/mL), 8 weeks (0.93 μg/mL), and 11 weeks (0.53 μg/mL), suggesting adalimumab can be detected in the serum of infants exposed in utero for at least 3 months from birth.

Animal Data

An embryo-fetal perinatal developmental toxicity study has been performed in cynomolgus monkeys at dosages up to 100 mg/kg (266 times human AUC when given 40 mg subcutaneously with methotrexate every week or 373 times human AUC when given 40 mg subcutaneously without methotrexate) and has revealed no evidence of harm to the fetuses due to adalimumab.

8.3 Nursing Mothers

Limited data from published literature indicate that adalimumab is present in low levels in human milk and is not likely to be absorbed by a breastfed infant. However, no data is available on the absorption of adalimumab from breastmilk in newborn or preterm infants. Caution should be exercised when HUMIRA is administered to a nursing woman.

Information on the AbbVie, Inc. products listed on these pages is from the prescribing information in use as of July 31, 2013. For more information, please visit rxabbvie.com or call 1-800-633-9110.

Table 2. ACR Responses in Studies RA-II and RA-III (Percent of Patients)

	Study RA-II Monotherapy (26 weeks)			Study RA-III Methotrexate Combination (24 and 52 weeks)	
Response	Placebo N=110	HUMIRA 40 mg every other week N=113	HUMIRA 40 mg weekly N=103	Placebo/MTX N=200	HUMIRA/MTX 40 mg every other week N=207
ACR20					
Month 6	19%	46%*	53%*	30%	63%*
Month 12	NA	NA	NA	24%	59%*
ACR50					
Month 6	8%	22%*	35%*	10%	39%*
Month 12	NA	NA	NA	10%	42%*
ACR70					
Month 6	2%	12%*	18%*	3%	21%*
Month 12	NA	NA	NA	5%	23%*

* p<0.01, HUMIRA *vs.* placebo

8.4 Pediatric Use

Safety and efficacy of HUMIRA in pediatric patients for uses other than juvenile idiopathic arthritis (JIA) have not been established. Due to its inhibition of TNFα, HUMIRA administered during pregnancy could affect immune response in the *in utero*-exposed newborn and infant. Data from eight infants exposed to HUMIRA *in utero*, suggest adalimumab crosses the placenta *[see Use in Specific Populations (8.1)]*. The clinical significance of elevated adalimumab levels in infants is unknown. The safety of administering live or live-attenuated vaccines in exposed infants is unknown. Risks and benefits should be considered prior to vaccinating (live or live-attenuated) exposed infants.

Juvenile Idiopathic Arthritis

In the JIA trial, HUMIRA was shown to reduce signs and symptoms of active polyarticular JIA in patients 4 to 17 years of age *[see Clinical Studies (14.2)]*. HUMIRA has not been studied in children less than 4 years of age, and there are limited data on HUMIRA treatment in children with weight <15 kg.

The safety of HUMIRA in pediatric patients in the JIA trial was generally similar to that observed in adults with certain exceptions *[see Adverse Reactions (6.1)]*.

Post-marketing cases of malignancies, some fatal, have been reported among children, adolescents, and young adults who received treatment with TNF-blockers including HUMIRA *[see Warnings and Precautions (5.2)]*.

8.5 Geriatric Use

A total of 519 RA patients 65 years of age and older, including 107 patients 75 years of age and older, received HUMIRA in clinical studies RA-I through IV. No overall difference in effectiveness was observed between these subjects and younger subjects. The frequency of serious infection and malignancy among HUMIRA treated subjects over 65 years of age was higher than for those under 65 years of age. Because there is a higher incidence of infections and malignancies in the elderly population, use caution when treating the elderly.

10 OVERDOSAGE

Doses up to 10 mg/kg have been administered to patients in clinical trials without evidence of dose-limiting toxicities. In case of overdosage, it is recommended that the patient be monitored for any signs or symptoms of adverse reactions or effects and appropriate symptomatic treatment instituted immediately.

11 DESCRIPTION

HUMIRA® (adalimumab) is a recombinant human IgG1 monoclonal antibody specific for human tumor necrosis factor (TNF). HUMIRA was created using phage display technology resulting in an antibody with human derived heavy and light chain variable regions and human IgG1:k constant regions. Adalimumab is produced by recombinant DNA technology in a mammalian cell expression system and is purified by a process that includes specific viral inactivation and removal steps. It consists of 1330 amino acids and has a molecular weight of approximately 148 kilodaltons.

HUMIRA is supplied as a sterile, preservative-free solution of adalimumab for subcutaneous administration. The drug product is supplied as either a single-use, prefilled pen (HUMIRA Pen) or as a single-use, 1 mL prefilled glass syringe. Enclosed within the pen is a single-use, 1 mL prefilled glass syringe. The solution of HUMIRA is clear and colorless, with a pH of about 5.2.

Each prefilled syringe delivers 0.8 mL (40 mg) of drug product. Each 0.8 mL of HUMIRA contains 40 mg adalimumab, 4.93 mg sodium chloride, 0.69 mg monobasic sodium phosphate dihydrate, 1.22 mg dibasic sodium phosphate dihydrate, 0.24 mg sodium citrate, 1.04 mg citric acid monohydrate, 9.6 mg mannitol, 0.8 mg polysorbate 80, and Water for Injection, USP. Sodium hydroxide added as necessary to adjust pH.

Each pediatric prefilled syringe delivers 0.4 mL (20 mg) of drug product. Each 0.4 mL of HUMIRA contains 20 mg adalimumab, 2.47 mg sodium chloride, 0.34 mg monobasic sodium phosphate dihydrate, 0.61 mg dibasic sodium phosphate dihydrate, 0.12 mg sodium citrate, 0.52 mg citric acid monohydrate, 4.8 mg mannitol, 0.4 mg polysorbate 80, and Water for Injection, USP. Sodium hydroxide added as necessary to adjust pH.

12 CLINICAL PHARMACOLOGY

12.1 Mechanism of Action

Adalimumab binds specifically to TNF-alpha and blocks its interaction with the p55 and p75 cell surface TNF receptors. Adalimumab also lyses surface TNF expressing cells *in vitro* in the presence of complement. Adalimumab does not bind or inactivate lymphotoxin (TNF-beta). TNF is a naturally occurring cytokine that is involved in normal inflammatory and immune responses. Elevated levels of TNF are found in the synovial fluid of patients with RA, JIA, PsA, and AS and play an important role in both the pathologic inflammation and the joint destruction that are hallmarks of these diseases. Increased levels of TNF are also found in psoriasis plaques. In Ps, treatment with HUMIRA may reduce the epidermal thickness and infiltration of inflammatory cells. The relationship between these pharmacodynamic activities and the mechanism(s) by which HUMIRA exerts its clinical effects is unknown.

Adalimumab also modulates biological responses that are induced or regulated by TNF, including changes in the levels of adhesion molecules responsible for leukocyte migration (ELAM-1, VCAM-1, and ICAM-1 with an IC_{50} of 1-2 × 10^{-10}M).

12.2 Pharmacodynamics

After treatment with HUMIRA, a decrease in levels of acute phase reactants of inflammation (C-reactive protein [CRP] and erythrocyte sedimentation rate [ESR]) and serum cytokines (IL-6) was observed compared to baseline in patients with rheumatoid arthritis. A decrease in CRP levels was also observed in patients with Crohn's disease and ulcerative colitis. Serum levels of matrix metalloproteinases (MMP-1 and MMP-3) that produce tissue remodeling responsible for cartilage destruction were also decreased after HUMIRA administration.

12.3 Pharmacokinetics

The maximum serum concentration (C_{max}) and the time to reach the maximum concentration (T_{max}) were 4.7 ± 1.6 μg/mL and 131 ± 56 hours respectively, following a single 40 mg subcutaneous administration of HUMIRA to healthy adult subjects. The average absolute bioavailability of adalimumab estimated from three studies following a single 40 mg subcutaneous dose was 64%. The pharmacokinetics of adalimumab were linear over the dose range of 0.5 to 10.0 mg/kg following a single intravenous dose.

The single dose pharmacokinetics of adalimumab in RA patients were determined in several studies with intravenous doses ranging from 0.25 to 10 mg/kg. The distribution volume (V_{ss}) ranged from 4.7 to 6.0 L. The systemic clearance of adalimumab is approximately 12 mL/hr. The mean terminal half-life was approximately 2 weeks, ranging from 10 to 20 days across studies. Adalimumab concentrations in the synovial fluid from five rheumatoid arthritis patients ranged from 31 to 96% of those in serum.

In RA patients receiving 40 mg HUMIRA every other week, adalimumab mean steady-state trough concentrations of approximately 5 μg/mL and 8 to 9 μg/mL, were observed without and with methotrexate (MTX), respectively. MTX reduced adalimumab apparent clearance after single and multiple dosing by 29% and 44% respectively, in patients with RA. Mean serum adalimumab trough levels at steady state increased approximately proportionally with dose following 20, 40, and 80 mg every other week and every week subcutaneous dosing. In long-term studies with dosing more than two years, there was no evidence of changes in clearance over time.

Adalimumab mean steady-state trough concentrations were slightly higher in psoriatic arthritis patients treated with 40 mg HUMIRA every other week (6 to 10 μg/mL and 8.5 to 12 μg/mL, without and with MTX, respectively) compared to the concentrations in RA patients treated with the same dose.

The pharmacokinetics of adalimumab in patients with AS were similar to those in patients with RA.

In patients with CD, the loading dose of 160 mg HUMIRA on Week 0 followed by 80 mg HUMIRA on Week 2 achieves mean serum adalimumab trough levels of approximately 12 μg/mL at Week 2 and Week 4. Mean steady-state trough levels of approximately 7 μg/mL were observed at Week 24 and Week 56 in CD patients after receiving a maintenance dose of 40 mg HUMIRA every other week.

In patients with UC, the loading dose of 160 mg HUMIRA on Week 0 followed by 80 mg HUMIRA on Week 2 achieves mean serum adalimumab trough levels of approximately 12 μg/mL at Week 2 and Week 4. Mean steady-state trough level of approximately 8 μg/mL was observed at Week 52 in UC patients after receiving a dose of 40 mg HUMIRA every other week, and approximately 15 μg/mL at Week 52 in UC patients who increased to a dose of 40 mg HUMIRA every week.

In patients with Ps, the mean steady-state trough concentration was approximately 5 to 6 μg/mL during HUMIRA 40 mg every other week monotherapy treatment.

Population pharmacokinetic analyses in patients with RA revealed that there was a trend toward higher apparent clearance of adalimumab in the presence of anti-adalimumab antibodies, and lower clearance with increasing age in patients aged 40 to >75 years.

Minor increases in apparent clearance were also predicted in RA patients receiving doses lower than the recommended dose and in RA patients with high rheumatoid factor or CRP concentrations. These increases are not likely to be clinically important.

No gender-related pharmacokinetic differences were observed after correction for a patient's body weight. Healthy volunteers and patients with rheumatoid arthritis displayed similar adalimumab pharmacokinetics.

No pharmacokinetic data are available in patients with hepatic or renal impairment.

In subjects with JIA (4 to 17 years of age), the mean steady-state trough serum adalimumab concentrations for subjects weighing <30 kg receiving 20 mg HUMIRA subcutaneously every other week as monotherapy or with concomitant methotrexate were 6.8 μg/mL and 10.9 μg/mL, respectively. The mean steady-state trough serum adalimumab concentrations for subjects weighing ≥30 kg receiving 40 mg HUMIRA subcutaneously every other week as monotherapy or with concomitant methotrexate were 6.6 μg/mL and 8.1 μg/mL, respectively.

13 NONCLINICAL TOXICOLOGY

13.1 Carcinogenesis, Mutagenesis, Impairment of Fertility

Long-term animal studies of HUMIRA have not been conducted to evaluate the carcinogenic potential or its effect on fertility. No clastogenic or mutagenic effects of HUMIRA were observed in the *in vivo* mouse micronucleus test or the *Salmonella-Escherichia coli* (Ames) assay, respectively.

14 CLINICAL STUDIES

14.1 Rheumatoid Arthritis

The efficacy and safety of HUMIRA were assessed in five randomized, double-blind studies in patients ≥18 years of age with active rheumatoid arthritis (RA) diagnosed according to American College of Rheumatology (ACR) criteria. Patients had at least 6 swollen and 9 tender joints. HUMIRA was administered subcutaneously in combination with methotrexate (MTX) (12.5 to 25 mg, Studies RA-I, RA-III and RA-V) or as monotherapy (Studies RA-II and RA-V) or with other disease-modifying anti-rheumatic drugs (DMARDs) (Study RA-IV).

Study RA-I evaluated 271 patients who had failed therapy with at least one but no more than four DMARDs and had inadequate response to MTX. Doses of 20, 40 or 80 mg of HUMIRA or placebo were given every other week for 24 weeks.

Study RA-II evaluated 544 patients who had failed therapy with at least one DMARD. Doses of placebo, 20 or 40 mg of HUMIRA were given as monotherapy every other week or weekly for 26 weeks.

Study RA-III evaluated 619 patients who had an inadequate response to MTX. Patients received placebo, 40 mg of HUMIRA every other week with placebo injections on alternate weeks, or 20 mg of HUMIRA weekly for up to 52 weeks.

Study RA-III had an additional primary endpoint at 52 weeks of inhibition of disease progression (as detected by X-ray results). Upon completion of the first 52 weeks, 457 patients enrolled in an open-label extension phase in which 40 mg of HUMIRA was administered every other week for up to 5 years.

Study RA-IV assessed safety in 636 patients who were either DMARD-naive or were permitted to remain on their pre-existing rheumatologic therapy provided that therapy was stable for a minimum of 28 days. Patients were randomized to 40 mg of HUMIRA or placebo every other week for 24 weeks.

Study RA-V evaluated 799 patients with moderately to severely active RA of less than 3 years duration who were ≥18 years old and MTX naïve. Patients were randomized to receive either MTX (optimized to 20 mg/week by week 8), HUMIRA 40 mg every other week or HUMIRA/MTX combination therapy for 104 weeks. Patients were evaluated for signs and symptoms, and for radiographic progression of joint damage. The median disease duration among patients enrolled in the study was 5 months. The median MTX dose achieved was 20 mg.

Clinical Response

The percent of HUMIRA treated patients achieving ACR 20, 50 and 70 responses in Studies RA-II and III are shown in Table 2.

[See table 2 at top of previous page]

The results of Study RA-I were similar to Study RA-III; patients receiving HUMIRA 40 mg every other week in Study RA-I also achieved ACR 20, 50 and 70 response rates of 65%, 52% and 24%, respectively, compared to placebo responses of 13%, 7% and 3% respectively, at 6 months (p<0.01).

The results of the components of the ACR response criteria for Studies RA-II and RA-III are shown in Table 3. ACR response rates and improvement in all components of ACR response were maintained to week 104. Over the 2 years in Study RA-III, 20% of HUMIRA patients receiving 40 mg every other week (EOW) achieved a major clinical response, defined as maintenance of an ACR 70 response over a 6-month period. ACR responses were maintained in similar proportions of patients for up to 5 years with continuous HUMIRA treatment in the open-label portion of Study RA-III.

[See table 3 above]

The time course of ACR 20 response for Study RA-III is shown in Figure 1.

In Study RA-III, 85% of patients with ACR 20 responses at week 24 maintained the response at 52 weeks. The time course of ACR 20 response for Study RA-I and Study RA-II were similar.

Figure 1. Study RA-III ACR 20 Responses over 52 Weeks

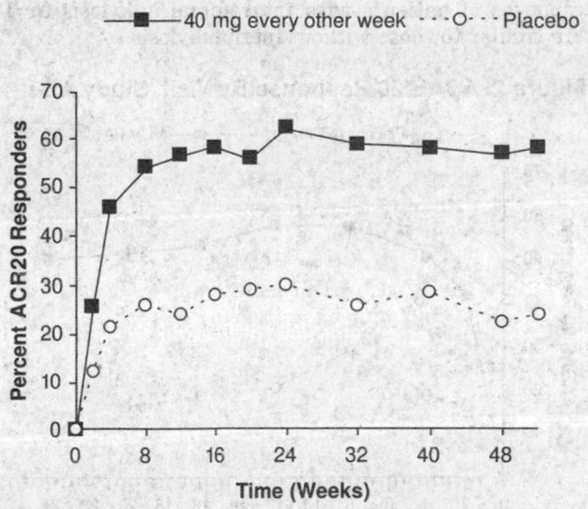

In Study RA-IV, 53% of patients treated with HUMIRA 40 mg every other week plus standard of care had an ACR 20 response at week 24 compared to 35% on placebo plus standard of care (p<0.001). No unique adverse reactions related to the combination of HUMIRA (adalimumab) and other DMARDs were observed.

In Study RA-V with MTX naïve patients with recent onset RA, the combination treatment with HUMIRA plus MTX led to greater percentages of patients achieving ACR responses than either MTX monotherapy or HUMIRA monotherapy at Week 52 and responses were sustained at Week 104 (see Table 4).

[See table 4 above]

At Week 52, all individual components of the ACR response criteria for Study RA-V improved in the HUMIRA/MTX group and improvements were maintained to Week 104.

Radiographic Response

In Study RA-III, structural joint damage was assessed radiographically and expressed as change in Total Sharp Score (TSS) and its components, the erosion score and Joint Space Narrowing (JSN) score, at month 12 compared to baseline. At baseline, the median TSS was approximately 55 in the placebo and 40 mg every other week groups. The results are shown in Table 5. HUMIRA/MTX treated patients demonstrated less radiographic progression than patients receiving MTX alone at 52 weeks.

[See table 5 above]

In the open-label extension of Study RA-III, 77% of the original patients treated with any dose of HUMIRA were evaluated radiographically at 2 years. Patients maintained inhibition of structural damage, as measured by the TSS. Fifty-four percent had no progression of structural damage as defined by a change in the TSS of zero or less. Fifty-five percent (55%) of patients originally treated with 40 mg HUMIRA every other week have been evaluated radiographically at 5 years. Patients had continued inhibition of structural damage with 50% showing no progression of structural damage defined by a change in the TSS of zero or less.

In Study RA-V, structural joint damage was assessed as in Study RA-III. Greater inhibition of radiographic progression, as assessed by changes in TSS, erosion score and JSN was observed in the HUMIRA/MTX combination group as compared to either the MTX or HUMIRA monotherapy group at Week 52 as well as at Week 104 (see Table 6).

[See table 6 above]

Physical Function Response

In studies RA-I through IV, HUMIRA showed significantly greater improvement than placebo in the disability index of Health Assessment Questionnaire (HAQ-DI) from baseline to the end of study, and significantly greater improvement

Table 3. Components of ACR Response in Studies RA-II and RA-III

Parameter (median)	Study RA-II Placebo N=110 Baseline	Wk 26	HUMIRA[a] N=113 Baseline	Wk 26	Study RA-III Placebo/MTX N=200 Baseline	Wk 24	HUMIRA[a]/MTX N=207 Baseline	Wk 24
Number of tender joints (0-68)	35	26	31	16*	26	15	24	8*
Number of swollen joints (0-66)	19	16	18	10*	17	11	18	5*
Physician global assessment[b]	7.0	6.1	6.6	3.7*	6.3	3.5	6.5	2.0*
Patient global assessment[b]	7.5	6.3	7.5	4.5*	5.4	3.9	5.2	2.0*
Pain[b]	7.3	6.1	7.3	4.1*	6.0	3.8	5.8	2.1*
Disability index (HAQ)[c]	2.0	1.9	1.9	1.5*	1.5	1.3	1.5	0.8*
CRP (mg/dL)	3.9	4.3	4.6	1.8*	1.0	0.9	1.0	0.4*

[a] 40 mg HUMIRA administered every other week
[b] Visual analogue scale; 0 = best, 10 = worst
[c] Disability Index of the Health Assessment Questionnaire; 0 = best, 3 = worst, measures the patient's ability to perform the following: dress/groom, arise, eat, walk, reach, grip, maintain hygiene, and maintain daily activity
* p<0.001, HUMIRA *vs.* placebo, based on mean change from baseline

Table 4. ACR Response in Study RA-V (Percent of Patients)

Response	MTX[b] N=257	HUMIRA[c] N=274	HUMIRA/MTX N=268
ACR20			
Week 52	63%	54%	73%
Week 104	56%	49%	69%
ACR50			
Week 52	46%	41%	62%
Week 104	43%	37%	59%
ACR70			
Week 52	27%	26%	46%
Week 104	28%	28%	47%
Major Clinical Response [a]	28%	25%	49%

[a] Major clinical response is defined as achieving an ACR70 response for a continuous six month period
[b] p<0.05, HUMIRA/MTX *vs.* MTX for ACR 20
p<0.001, HUMIRA/MTX *vs.* MTX for ACR 50 and 70, and Major Clinical Response
[c] p<0.001, HUMIRA/MTX *vs.* HUMIRA

Table 5. Radiographic Mean Changes Over 12 Months in Study RA-III

	Placebo/MTX	HUMIRA/MTX 40 mg every other week	Placebo/MTX-HUMIRA/MTX (95% Confidence Interval*)	P-value**
Total Sharp score	2.7	0.1	2.6 (1.4, 3.8)	<0.001
Erosion score	1.6	0.0	1.6 (0.9, 2.2)	<0.001
JSN score	1.0	0.1	0.9 (0.3, 1.4)	0.002

*95% confidence intervals for the differences in change scores between MTX and HUMIRA.
**Based on rank analysis

Table 6. Radiographic Mean Change* in Study RA-V

		MTX[a] N=257	HUMIRA[a,b] N=274	HUMIRA/MTX N=268
52 Weeks	Total Sharp score	5.7 (4.2, 7.3)	3.0 (1.7, 4.3)	1.3 (0.5, 2.1)
	Erosion score	3.7 (2.7, 4.8)	1.7 (1.0, 2.4)	0.8 (0.4, 1.2)
	JSN score	2.0 (1.2, 2.8)	1.3 (0.5, 2.1)	0.5 (0.0, 1.0)
104 Weeks	Total Sharp score	10.4 (7.7, 13.2)	5.5 (3.6, 7.4)	1.9 (0.9, 2.9)
	Erosion score	6.4 (4.6, 8.2)	3.0 (2.0, 4.0)	1.0 (0.4, 1.6)
	JSN score	4.1 (2.7, 5.4)	2.6 (1.5, 3.7)	0.9 (0.3, 1.5)

* mean (95% confidence interval)
[a] p<0.001, HUMIRA/MTX *vs.* MTX at 52 and 104 weeks and for HUMIRA/MTX *vs.* HUMIRA at 104 weeks
[b] p<0.01, for HUMIRA/MTX *vs.* HUMIRA at 52 weeks

Information on the AbbVie, Inc. products listed on these pages is from the prescribing information in use as of July 31, 2013. For more information, please visit rxabbvie.com or call 1-800-633-9110.

Table 8. Components of Disease Activity in Study PsA-I

	Placebo N=162		HUMIRA* N=151	
Parameter: median	Baseline	24 weeks	Baseline	24 weeks
Number of tender joints[a]	23.0	17.0	20.0	5.0
Number of swollen joints[b]	11.0	9.0	11.0	3.0
Physician global assessment[c]	53.0	49.0	55.0	16.0
Patient global assessment[c]	49.5	49.0	48.0	20.0
Pain[c]	49.0	49.0	54.0	20.0
Disability index (HAQ)[d]	1.0	0.9	1.0	0.4
CRP (mg/dL)[e]	0.8	0.7	0.8	0.2

* p<0.001 for HUMIRA *vs.* placebo comparisons based on median changes
[a] Scale 0-78
[b] Scale 0-76
[c] Visual analog scale; 0=best, 100=worst
[d] Disability Index of the Health Assessment Questionnaire; 0=best, 3=worst; measures the patient's ability to perform the following: dress/groom, arise, eat, walk, reach, grip, maintain hygiene, and maintain daily activity.
[e] Normal range: 0-0.287 mg/dL

than placebo in the health-outcomes as assessed by The Short Form Health Survey (SF 36). Improvement was seen in both the Physical Component Summary (PCS) and the Mental Component Summary (MCS).

In Study RA-III, the mean (95% CI) improvement in HAQ-DI from baseline at week 52 was 0.60 (0.55, 0.65) for the HUMIRA patients and 0.25 (0.17, 0.33) for placebo/MTX (p<0.001) patients. Sixty-three percent of HUMIRA-treated patients achieved a 0.5 or greater improvement in HAQ-DI at week 52 in the double-blind portion of the study. Eighty-two percent of these patients maintained that improvement through week 104 and a similar proportion of patients maintained this response through week 260 (5 years) of open-label treatment. Mean improvement in the SF-36 was maintained through the end of measurement at week 156 (3 years).

In Study RA-V, the HAQ-DI and the physical component of the SF-36 showed greater improvement (p<0.001) for the HUMIRA/MTX combination therapy group versus either the MTX monotherapy or the HUMIRA monotherapy group at Week 52, which was maintained through Week 104.

14.2 Juvenile Idiopathic Arthritis

The safety and efficacy of HUMIRA were assessed in a multicenter, randomized, withdrawal, double-blind, parallel-group study in 171 children (4 to 17 years of age) with polyarticular juvenile idiopathic arthritis (JIA). In the study, the patients were stratified into two groups: MTX-treated or non-MTX-treated. All subjects had to show signs of active moderate or severe disease despite previous treatment with NSAIDs, analgesics, corticosteroids, or DMARDS. Subjects who received prior treatment with any biologic DMARDS were excluded from the study.

The study included four phases: an open-label lead in phase (OL-LI; 16 weeks), a double-blind randomized withdrawal phase (DB; 32 weeks), an open-label extension phase (OLE-BSA; up to 136 weeks), and an open-label fixed dose phase (OLE-FD; 16 weeks). In the first three phases of the study, HUMIRA was administered based on body surface area at a dose of 24 mg/m^2 up to a maximum total body dose of 40 mg subcutaneously (SC) every other week. In the OLE-FD phase, the patients were treated with 20 mg of HUMIRA SC every other week if their weight was less than 30 kg and with 40 mg of HUMIRA SC every other week if their weight was 30 kg or greater. Patients remained on stable doses of NSAIDs and or prednisone (≤0.2 mg/kg/day or 10 mg/day maximum).

Patients demonstrating a Pediatric ACR 30 response at the end of OL-LI phase were randomized into the double blind (DB) phase of the study and received either HUMIRA or placebo every other week for 32 weeks or until disease flare. Disease flare was defined as a worsening of ≥30% from baseline in ≥3 of 6 Pediatric ACR core criteria, ≥2 active joints, and improvement of >30% in no more than 1 of the 6 criteria. After 32 weeks or at the time of disease flare during the DB phase, patients were treated in the open-label extension phase based on the BSA regimen (OLE-BSA), before converting to a fixed dose regimen based on body weight (OLE-FD phase).

Clinical Response

At the end of the 16-week OL-LI phase, 94% of the patients in the MTX stratum and 74% of the patients in the non-MTX stratum were Pediatric ACR 30 responders. In the DB phase significantly fewer patients who received HUMIRA experienced disease flare compared to placebo, both without MTX (43% *vs.* 71%) and with MTX (37% *vs.* 65%). More patients treated with HUMIRA continued to show pediatric ACR 30/50/70 responses at Week 48 compared to patients treated with placebo. Pediatric ACR responses were maintained for up to two years in the OLE phase in patients who received HUMIRA throughout the study.

14.3 Psoriatic Arthritis

The safety and efficacy of HUMIRA was assessed in two randomized, double-blind, placebo controlled studies in 413 patients with psoriatic arthritis (PsA). Upon completion of both studies, 383 patients enrolled in an open-label extension study, in which 40 mg HUMIRA was administered every other week.

Study PsA-I enrolled 313 adult patients with moderately to severely active PsA (>3 swollen and >3 tender joints) who had an inadequate response to NSAID therapy in one of the following forms: (1) distal interphalangeal (DIP) involvement (N=23); (2) polyarticular arthritis (absence of rheumatoid nodules and presence of plaque psoriasis) (N=210); (3) arthritis mutilans (N=1); (4) asymmetric PsA (N=77); or (5) AS-like (N=2). Patients on MTX therapy (158 of 313 patients) at enrollment (stable dose of ≤30 mg/week for >1 month) could continue MTX at the same dose. Doses of HUMIRA 40 mg or placebo every other week were administered during the 24-week double-blind period of the study.

Compared to placebo, treatment with HUMIRA resulted in improvements in the measures of disease activity (see Tables 7 and 8). Among patients with PsA who received HUMIRA, the clinical responses were apparent in some patients at the time of the first visit (two weeks) and were maintained up to 88 weeks in the ongoing open-label study. Similar responses were seen in patients with each of the subtypes of psoriatic arthritis, although few patients were enrolled with the arthritis mutilans and ankylosing spondylitis-like subtypes. Responses were similar in patients who were or were not receiving concomitant MTX therapy at baseline.

Patients with psoriatic involvement of at least three percent body surface area (BSA) were evaluated for Psoriatic Area and Severity Index (PASI) responses. At 24 weeks, the proportions of patients achieving a 75% or 90% improvement in the PASI were 59% and 42% respectively, in the HUMIRA group (N=69), compared to 1% and 0% respectively, in the placebo group (N=69) (p<0.001). PASI responses were apparent in some patients at the time of the first visit (two weeks). Responses were similar in patients who were or were not receiving concomitant MTX therapy at baseline.

Table 7. ACR Response in Study PsA-I (Percent of Patients)

	Placebo N=162	HUMIRA* N=151
ACR20		
Week 12	14%	58%
Week 24	15%	57%
ACR50		
Week 12	4%	36%
Week 24	6%	39%
ACR70		
Week 12	1%	20%
Week 24	1%	23%

* p<0.001 for all comparisons between HUMIRA and placebo

[See table 8 above]

Similar results were seen in an additional, 12-week study in 100 patients with moderate to severe psoriatic arthritis who had suboptimal response to DMARD therapy as manifested by ≥3 tender joints and ≥3 swollen joints at enrollment.

Radiographic Response

Radiographic changes were assessed in the PsA studies. Radiographs of hands, wrists, and feet were obtained at baseline and Week 24 during the double-blind period when patients were on HUMIRA or placebo and at Week 48 when all patients were on open-label HUMIRA. A modified Total Sharp Score (mTSS), which included distal interphalangeal joints (i.e., not identical to the TSS used for rheumatoid arthritis), was used by readers blinded to treatment group to assess the radiographs.

HUMIRA-treated patients demonstrated greater inhibition of radiographic progression compared to placebo-treated patients and this effect was maintained at 48 weeks (see Table 9).

Table 9. Change in Modified Total Sharp Score in Psoriatic Arthritis

	Placebo N=141	HUMIRA N=133	
	Week 24	Week 24	Week 48
Baseline mean	22.1	23.4	23.4
Mean Change ± SD	0.9 ± 3.1	-0.1 ± 1.7	-0.2 ± 4.9*

* <0.001 for the difference between HUMIRA, Week 48 and Placebo, Week 24 (primary analysis)

Physical Function Response

In Study PsA-I, physical function and disability were assessed using the HAQ Disability Index (HAQ-DI) and the SF-36 Health Survey. Patients treated with 40 mg of HUMIRA every other week showed greater improvement from baseline in the HAQ-DI score (mean decreases of 47% and 49% at Weeks 12 and 24 respectively) in comparison to placebo (mean decreases of 1% and 3% at Weeks 12 and 24 respectively). At Weeks 12 and 24, patients treated with HUMIRA showed greater improvement from baseline in the SF-36 Physical Component Summary score compared to patients treated with placebo, and no worsening in the SF-36 Mental Component Summary score. Improvement in physical function based on the HAQ-DI was maintained for up to 84 weeks through the open-label portion of the study.

14.4 Ankylosing Spondylitis

The safety and efficacy of HUMIRA 40 mg every other week was assessed in 315 adult patients in a randomized, 24 week double-blind, placebo-controlled study in patients with active ankylosing spondylitis (AS) who had an inadequate response to glucocorticoids, NSAIDs, analgesics, methotrexate or sulfasalazine. Active AS was defined as patients who fulfilled at least two of the following three criteria: (1) a Bath AS disease activity index (BASDAI) score ≥4 cm, (2) a visual analog score (VAS) for total back pain ≥ 40 mm, and (3) morning stiffness ≥ 1 hour. The blinded period was followed by an open-label period during which patients received HUMIRA 40 mg every other week subcutaneously for up to an additional 28 weeks.

Improvement in measures of disease activity was first observed at Week 2 and maintained through 24 weeks as shown in Figure 2 and Table 10.

Responses of patients with total spinal ankylosis (n=11) were similar to those without total ankylosis.

Figure 2. ASAS 20 Response By Visit, Study AS-I

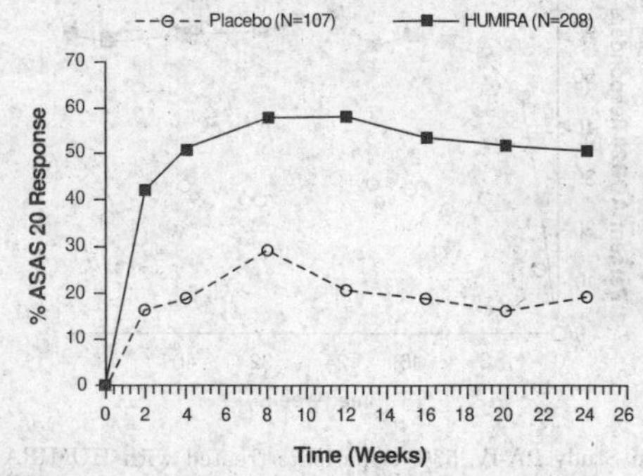

At 12 weeks, the ASAS 20/50/70 responses were achieved by 58%, 38%, and 23%, respectively, of patients receiving HUMIRA, compared to 21%, 10%, and 5% respectively, of patients receiving placebo (p <0.001). Similar responses were seen at Week 24 and were sustained in patients receiving open-label HUMIRA for up to 52 weeks.

A greater proportion of patients treated with HUMIRA (22%) achieved a low level of disease activity at 24 weeks (defined as a value <20 [on a scale of 0 to 100 mm] in each of the four ASAS response parameters) compared to patients treated with placebo (6%).

[See table 10 at top of next page]

A second randomized, multicenter, double-blind, placebo-controlled study of 82 patients with ankylosing spondylitis showed similar results.

Patients treated with HUMIRA achieved improvement from baseline in the Ankylosing Spondylitis Quality of Life Questionnaire (ASQoL) score (-3.6 *vs.* -1.1) and in the Short Form

Health Survey (SF-36) Physical Component Summary (PCS) score (7.4 *vs.* 1.9) compared to placebo-treated patients at Week 24.

14.5 Crohn's Disease

The safety and efficacy of multiple doses of HUMIRA were assessed in adult patients with moderately to severely active Crohn's disease, CD, (Crohn's Disease Activity Index (CDAI) ≥ 220 and ≤ 450) in randomized, double-blind, placebo-controlled studies. Concomitant stable doses of aminosalicylates, corticosteroids, and/or immunomodulatory agents were permitted, and 79% of patients continued to receive at least one of these medications.

Induction of clinical remission (defined as CDAI < 150) was evaluated in two studies. In Study CD-I, 299 TNF-blocker naïve patients were randomized to one of four treatment groups: the placebo group received placebo at Weeks 0 and 2, the 160/80 group received 160 mg HUMIRA at Week 0 and 80 mg at Week 2, the 80/40 group received 80 mg at Week 0 and 40 mg at Week 2, and the 40/20 group received 40 mg at Week 0 and 20 mg at Week 2. Clinical results were assessed at Week 4.

In the second induction study, Study CD-II, 325 patients who had lost response to, or were intolerant to, previous infliximab therapy were randomized to receive either 160 mg HUMIRA at Week 0 and 80 mg at Week 2, or placebo at Weeks 0 and 2. Clinical results were assessed at Week 4.

Maintenance of clinical remission was evaluated in Study CD-III. In this study, 854 patients with active disease received open-label HUMIRA, 80 mg at week 0 and 40 mg at Week 2. Patients were then randomized at Week 4 to 40 mg HUMIRA every other week, 40 mg HUMIRA every week, or placebo. The total study duration was 56 weeks. Patients in clinical response (decrease in CDAI ≥70) at Week 4 were stratified and analyzed separately from those not in clinical response at Week 4.

Induction of Clinical Remission

A greater percentage of the patients treated with 160/80 mg HUMIRA achieved induction of clinical remission versus placebo at Week 4 regardless of whether the patients were TNF blocker naïve (CD-I), or had lost response to or were intolerant to infliximab (CD-II) (see Table 11).

[See table 11 at right]

Maintenance of Clinical Remission

In Study CD-III at Week 4, 58% (499/854) of patients were in clinical response and were assessed in the primary analysis. At Weeks 26 and 56, greater proportions of patients who were in clinical response at Week 4 achieved clinical remission in the HUMIRA 40 mg every other week maintenance group compared to patients in the placebo maintenance group (see Table 12). The group that received HUMIRA therapy every week did not demonstrate significantly higher remission rates compared to the group that received HUMIRA every other week.

Table 12. Maintenance of Clinical Remission in CD-III (Percent of Patients)

	Placebo N=170	40 mg HUMIRA every other week N=172
Week 26		
Clinical remission	17%	40%*
Clinical response	28%	54%*
Week 56		
Clinical remission	12%	36%*
Clinical response	18%	43%*

Clinical remission is CDAI score < 150; clinical response is decrease in CDAI of at least 70 points.
*p<0.001 for HUMIRA vs. placebo pairwise comparisons of proportions

Of those in response at Week 4 who attained remission during the study, patients in the HUMIRA every other week group maintained remission for a longer time than patients in the placebo maintenance group. Among patients who were not in response by Week 12, therapy continued beyond 12 weeks did not result in significantly more responses.

14.6 Ulcerative Colitis

The safety and efficacy of HUMIRA were assessed in adult patients with moderately to severely active ulcerative colitis (Mayo score 6 to 12 on a 12 point scale, with an endoscopy subscore of 2 to 3 on a scale of 0 to 3) despite concurrent or prior treatment with immunosuppressants such as corticosteroids, azathioprine, or 6-MP in two randomized, double-blind, placebo-controlled clinical studies (Studies UC-I and UC-II). Both studies enrolled TNF-blocker naïve patients, but Study UC-II also allowed entry of patients who lost response to or were intolerant to TNF-blockers. Forty percent (40%) of patients enrolled in Study UC-II had previously used another TNF-blocker.

Concomitant stable doses of aminosalicylates and immunosuppressants were permitted. In Studies UC-I and II, patients were receiving aminosalicylates (69%), corticosteroids (59%) and/or azathioprine or 6-MP (37%) at baseline. In both studies, 92% of patients received at least one of these medications.

Induction of clinical remission (defined as Mayo score ≤ 2 with no individual subscores > 1) at Week 8 was evaluated in both studies. Clinical remission at Week 52 and sustained clinical remission (defined as clinical remission at both Weeks 8 and 52) were evaluated in Study UC-II.

In Study UC-I, 390 TNF-blocker naïve patients were randomized to one of three treatment groups for the primary efficacy analysis. The placebo group received placebo at Weeks 0, 2, 4 and 6. The 160/80 group received 160 mg HUMIRA at Week 0 and 80 mg at Week 2, and the 80/40 group received 80 mg HUMIRA at Week 0 and 40 mg at Week 2. After Week 2, patients in both HUMIRA treatment groups received 40 mg every other week (eow).

In Study UC-II, 518 patients were randomized to receive either HUMIRA 160 mg at Week 0, 80 mg at Week 2, and 40 mg eow starting at Week 4 through Week 50, or placebo starting at Week 0 and eow through Week 50. Corticosteroid taper was permitted starting at Week 8.

In both Studies UC-I and UC-II, a greater percentage of the patients treated with 160/80 mg of HUMIRA compared to patients treated with placebo achieved induction of clinical remission. In Study UC-II, a greater percentage of the patients treated with 160/80 mg of HUMIRA compared to patients treated with placebo achieved sustained clinical remission (clinical remission at both Weeks 8 and 52) (Table 13).

[See table 13 above]

In Study UC-I, there was no statistically significant difference in clinical remission observed between the HUMIRA 80/40 mg group and the placebo group at Week 8.

In Study UC-II, 17.3% (43/248) in the HUMIRA group were in clinical remission at Week 52 compared to 8.5% (21/246) in the placebo group (treatment difference: 8.8%; 95% confidence interval (CI): [2.8%, 14.5%]; p<0.05).

In the subgroup of patients in Study UC-II with prior TNF-blocker use, the treatment difference for induction of clinical remission appeared to be lower than that seen in the whole study population, and the treatment differences for sustained clinical remission and clinical remission at Week 52

Table 10. Components of Ankylosing Spondylitis Disease Activity

	Placebo N=107 Baseline mean	Placebo N=107 Week 24 mean	HUMIRA N=208 Baseline mean	HUMIRA N=208 Week 24 mean
ASAS 20 Response Criteria*				
Patient's Global Assessment of Disease Activity[a]*	65	60	63	38
Total back pain*	67	58	65	37
Inflammation[b]*	6.7	5.6	6.7	3.6
BASFI[c]*	56	51	52	34
BASDAI[d] score*	6.3	5.5	6.3	3.7
BASMI[e] score*	4.2	4.1	3.8	3.3
Tragus to wall (cm)	15.9	15.8	15.8	15.4
Lumbar flexion (cm)	4.1	4.0	4.2	4.4
Cervical rotation (degrees)	42.2	42.1	48.4	51.6
Lumbar side flexion (cm)	8.9	9.0	9.7	11.7
Intermalleolar distance (cm)	92.9	94.0	93.5	100.8
CRP[f]*	2.2	2.0	1.8	0.6

[a] Percent of subjects with at least a 20% and 10-unit improvement measured on a Visual Analog Scale (VAS) with 0 = "none" and 100 = "severe"
[b] mean of questions 5 and 6 of BASDAI (defined in 'd')
[c] Bath Ankylosing Spondylitis Functional Index
[d] Bath Ankylosing Spondylitis Disease Activity Index
[e] Bath Ankylosing Spondylitis Metrology Index
[f] C-Reactive Protein (mg/dL)
* statistically significant for comparisons between HUMIRA and placebo at Week 24

Table 11. Induction of Clinical Remission in Studies CD-I and CD-II (Percent of Patients)

	CD-I Placebo N=74	CD-I HUMIRA 160/80 mg N=76	CD-II Placebo N=166	CD-II HUMIRA 160/80 mg N=159
Week 4				
Clinical remission	12%	36%*	7%	21%*
Clinical response	34%	58%**	34%	52%**

Clinical remission is CDAI score < 150; clinical response is decrease in CDAI of at least 70 points.
* p<0.001 for HUMIRA *vs.* placebo pairwise comparison of proportions
** p<0.01 for HUMIRA *vs.* placebo pairwise comparison of proportions

Table 13. Induction of Clinical Remission in Studies UC-I and UC-II and Sustained Clinical Remission in Study UC-II (Percent of Patients)

	Study UC-I Placebo N=130	Study UC-I HUMIRA 160/80 mg N=130	Study UC-I Treatment Difference (95% CI)	Study UC-II Placebo N=246	Study UC-II HUMIRA 160/80 mg N=248	Study UC-II Treatment Difference (95% CI)
Induction of Clinical Remission (Clinical Remission at Week 8)	9.2%	18.5%	9.3%* (0.9%, 17.6%)	9.3%	16.5%	7.2%* (1.2%, 12.9%)
Sustained Clinical Remission (Clinical Remission at both Weeks 8 and 52)	N/A	N/A	N/A	4.1%	8.5%	4.4%* (0.1%, 8.6%)

Clinical remission is defined as Mayo score ≤ 2 with no individual subscores > 1.
CI=Confidence interval
* p<0.05 for HUMIRA *vs.* placebo pairwise comparison of proportions

Information on the AbbVie, Inc. products listed on these pages is from the prescribing information in use as of July 31, 2013. For more information, please visit rxabbvie.com or call 1-800-633-9110.

appeared to be similar to those seen in the whole study population. The subgroup of patients with prior TNF-blocker use achieved induction of clinical remission at 9% (9/98) in the HUMIRA group versus 7% (7/101) in the placebo group, and sustained clinical remission at 5% (5/98) in the HUMIRA group versus 1% (1/101) in the placebo group. In the subgroup of patients with prior TNF-blocker use, 10% (10/98) were in clinical remission at Week 52 in the HUMIRA group versus 3% (3/101) in the placebo group.

14.7 Plaque Psoriasis

The safety and efficacy of HUMIRA were assessed in randomized, double-blind, placebo-controlled studies in 1696 adult patients with moderate to severe chronic plaque psoriasis (Ps) who were candidates for systemic therapy or phototherapy.

Study Ps-I evaluated 1212 patients with chronic Ps with ≥10% body surface area (BSA) involvement, Physician's Global Assessment (PGA) of at least moderate disease severity, and Psoriasis Area and Severity Index (PASI) ≥12 within three treatment periods. In period A, patients received placebo or HUMIRA at an initial dose of 80 mg at Week 0 followed by a dose of 40 mg every other week starting at Week 1. After 16 weeks of therapy, patients who achieved at least a PASI 75 response at Week 16, defined as a PASI score improvement of at least 75% relative to baseline, entered period B and received open-label 40 mg HUMIRA every other week. After 17 weeks of open label therapy, patients who maintained at least a PASI 75 response at Week 33 and were originally randomized to active therapy in period A were re-randomized in period C to receive 40 mg HUMIRA every other week or placebo for an additional 19 weeks. Across all treatment groups the mean baseline PASI score was 19 and the baseline Physician's Global Assessment score ranged from "moderate" (53%) to "severe" (41%) to "very severe" (6%).

Study Ps-II evaluated 99 patients randomized to HUMIRA and 48 patients randomized to placebo with chronic plaque psoriasis with ≥10% BSA involvement and PASI ≥12. Patients received placebo, or an initial dose of 80 mg HUMIRA at Week 0 followed by 40 mg every other week starting at Week 1 for 16 weeks. Across all treatment groups the mean baseline PASI score was 21 and the baseline PGA score ranged from "moderate" (41%) to "severe" (51%) to "very severe" (8%).

Studies Ps-I and II evaluated the proportion of patients who achieved "clear" or "minimal" disease on the 6-point PGA scale and the proportion of patients who achieved a reduction in PASI score of at least 75% (PASI 75) from baseline at Week 16 (see Table 14 and 15).

Additionally, Study Ps-I evaluated the proportion of subjects who maintained a PGA of "clear" or "minimal" disease or a PASI 75 response after Week 33 and on or before Week 52.

Table 14. Efficacy Results at 16 Weeks in Study Ps-I Number of Patients (%)

	HUMIRA 40 mg every other week N = 814	Placebo N = 398
PGA: Clear or minimal*	506 (62%)	17 (4%)
PASI 75	578 (71%)	26 (7%)

* Clear = no plaque elevation, no scale, plus or minus hyperpigmentation or diffuse pink or red coloration
Minimal = possible but difficult to ascertain whether there is slight elevation of plaque above normal skin, plus or minus surface dryness with some white coloration, plus or minus up to red coloration

Table 15. Efficacy Results at 16 Weeks in Study Ps-II Number of Patients (%)

	HUMIRA 40 mg every other week N = 99	Placebo N = 48
PGA: Clear or minimal*	70 (71%)	5 (10%)
PASI 75	77 (78%)	9 (19%)

* Clear = no plaque elevation, no scale, plus or minus hyperpigmentation or diffuse pink or red coloration
Minimal = possible but difficult to ascertain whether there is slight elevation of plaque above normal skin, plus or minus surface dryness with some white coloration, plus or minus up to red coloration

Additionally, in Study Ps-I, subjects on HUMIRA who maintained a PASI 75 were re-randomized to HUMIRA (N = 250) or placebo (N = 240) at Week 33. After 52 weeks of treatment with HUMIRA, more patients on HUMIRA maintained efficacy when compared to subjects who were re-randomized to placebo based on maintenance of PGA of "clear" or "minimal" disease (68% *vs.* 28%) or a PASI 75 (79% *vs.* 43%).

A total of 347 stable responders participated in a withdrawal and retreatment evaluation in an open-label extension study. Median time to relapse (decline to PGA "moderate" or worse) was approximately 5 months. During the withdrawal period, no subject experienced transformation to either pustular or erythrodermic psoriasis. A total of 178 subjects who relapsed re-initiated treatment with 80 mg of HUMIRA, then 40 mg eow beginning at week 1. At week 16, 69% (123/178) of subjects had a response of PGA "clear" or "minimal".

15 REFERENCES

1. National Cancer Institute. Surveillance, Epidemiology, and End Results Database (SEER) Program. SEER Incidence Crude Rates, 11 Registries, 1993-2001.

16 HOW SUPPLIED/STORAGE AND HANDLING

HUMIRA® (adalimumab) is supplied as a preservative-free, sterile solution for subcutaneous administration. The following packaging configurations are available.

• HUMIRA Pen Carton

HUMIRA is dispensed in a carton containing two alcohol preps and two dose trays. Each dose tray consists of a single-use pen, containing a 1 mL prefilled glass syringe with a fixed 27 gauge ½ inch needle, providing 40 mg (0.8 mL) of HUMIRA. The NDC number is 0074-4339-02.

• HUMIRA Pen – Crohn's Disease/Ulcerative Colitis Starter Package

HUMIRA is dispensed in a carton containing 6 alcohol preps and 6 dose trays (Crohn's Disease/Ulcerative Colitis Starter Package). Each dose tray consists of a single-use pen, containing a 1 mL prefilled glass syringe with a fixed 27 gauge ½ inch needle, providing 40 mg (0.8 mL) of HUMIRA. The NDC number is 0074-4339-06.

• HUMIRA Pen – Psoriasis Starter Package

HUMIRA is dispensed in a carton containing 4 alcohol preps and 4 dose trays (Psoriasis Starter Package). Each dose tray consists of a single-use pen, containing a 1 mL prefilled glass syringe with a fixed 27 gauge ½ inch needle, providing 40 mg (0.8 mL) of HUMIRA. The NDC number is 0074-4339-07.

• Prefilled Syringe Carton – 40 mg

HUMIRA is dispensed in a carton containing two alcohol preps and two dose trays. Each dose tray consists of a single-use, 1 mL prefilled glass syringe with a fixed 27 gauge ½ inch needle, providing 40 mg (0.8 mL) of HUMIRA. The NDC number is 0074-3799-02.

• Pediatric Prefilled Syringe Carton – 20 mg

HUMIRA is supplied for pediatric use only in a carton containing two alcohol preps and two dose trays. Each dose tray consists of a single-use, 1 mL pre-filled glass syringe with a fixed 27 gauge ½ inch needle, providing 20 mg (0.4 mL) of HUMIRA. The NDC number is 0074-9374-02.

• Institutional Use Vial Carton – 40 mg

HUMIRA is supplied for institutional use only in a carton containing a single-use, glass vial, providing 40 mg (0.8 mL) of HUMIRA. The NDC number is 0074-3797-01.

Storage and Stability

Do not use beyond the expiration date on the container. HUMIRA must be refrigerated at 36°F to 46°F (2°C to 8°C). DO NOT FREEZE. Do not use if frozen even if it has been thawed. When traveling, store HUMIRA in a cool carrier with an ice pack. Protect the prefilled syringe from exposure to light. Store in original carton until time of administration.

17 PATIENT COUNSELING INFORMATION

See FDA-approved patient labeling (Medication Guide and Instructions for Use).

17.1 Patient Counseling

Provide the HUMIRA "Medication Guide" to patients or their caregivers, and provide them an opportunity to read it and ask questions prior to initiation of therapy and prior to each time the prescription is renewed. If patients develop signs and symptoms of infection, instruct them to seek medical evaluation immediately.

Advise patients of the potential benefits and risks of HUMIRA.

• Infections

Inform patients that HUMIRA may lower the ability of their immune system to fight infections. Instruct patients of the importance of contacting their doctor if they develop any symptoms of infection, including tuberculosis, invasive fungal infections, and reactivation of hepatitis B virus infections.

• Malignancies

Counsel patients about the risk of malignancies while receiving HUMIRA.

• Allergic Reactions

Advise patients to seek immediate medical attention if they experience any symptoms of severe allergic reactions. Advise latex-sensitive patients that the needle cap of the prefilled syringe contains latex.

• Other Medical Conditions

Advise patients to report any signs of new or worsening medical conditions such as congestive heart failure, neurological disease, autoimmune disorders, or cytopenias. Advise patients to report any symptoms suggestive of a cytopenia such as bruising, bleeding, or persistent fever.

17.2 Instruction on Injection Technique

Inform patients that the first injection is to be performed under the supervision of a qualified health care professional. If a patient or caregiver is to administer HUMIRA, instruct them in injection techniques and assess their ability to inject subcutaneously to ensure the proper administration of HUMIRA *[see Instructions for Use]*.

For patients who will use the HUMIRA Pen, tell them that they:

- Will hear a **loud 'click'** when the plum-colored activator button is pressed. The loud click means the **start** of the injection.
- Must keep holding the HUMIRA Pen against their squeezed, raised skin until all of the medicine is injected. This can take up to 10 seconds.
- Will know that the injection has finished when the yellow marker fully appears in the window view and stops moving.

Instruct patients to dispose of their used needles and syringes or used Pen in a FDA-cleared sharps disposal container immediately after use. **Instruct patients not to dispose of loose needles and syringes or Pen in their household trash.** Instruct patients that if they do not have a FDA-cleared sharps disposal container, they may use a household container that is made of a heavy-duty plastic, can be closed with a tight-fitting and puncture-resistant lid without sharps being able to come out, upright and stable during use, leak-resistant, and properly labeled to warn of hazardous waste inside the container.

Instruct patients that when their sharps disposal container is almost full, they will need to follow their community guidelines for the correct way to dispose of their sharps disposal container. Instruct patients that there may be state or local laws regarding disposal of used needles and syringes. Refer patients to the FDA's website at http://www.fda.gov/safesharpsdisposal for more information about safe sharps disposal, and for specific information about sharps disposal in the state that they live in.

Instruct patients not to dispose of their used sharps disposal container in their household trash unless their community guidelines permit this. Instruct patients not to recycle their used sharps disposal container.

AbbVie Inc.
North Chicago, IL 60064, U.S.A.
03-A829 May 2013

MEDICATION GUIDE
HUMIRA® (Hu-MARE-ah)
(adalimumab)
injection

Read the Medication Guide that comes with HUMIRA before you start taking it and each time you get a refill. There may be new information. This Medication Guide does not take the place of talking with your doctor about your medical condition or treatment.

What is the most important information I should know about HUMIRA?

HUMIRA is a medicine that affects your immune system. HUMIRA can lower the ability of your immune system to fight infections. **Serious infections have happened in people taking HUMIRA. These serious infections include tuberculosis (TB) and infections caused by viruses, fungi or bacteria that have spread throughout the body. Some people have died from these infections.**

- Your doctor should test you for TB before starting HUMIRA.
- Your doctor should check you closely for signs and symptoms of TB during treatment with HUMIRA.

You should not start taking HUMIRA if you have any kind of infection unless your doctor says it is okay.

Before starting HUMIRA, tell your doctor if you:

- think you have an infection or have symptoms of infection such as:

• fever, sweats, or chills	• warm, red, or painful skin or sores on your body
• muscle aches	• diarrhea or stomach pain
• cough	• burning when you urinate or urinate more often than normal
• shortness of breath	• feel very tired
• blood in phlegm	
• weight loss	

- are being treated for an infection
- get a lot of infections or have infections that keep coming back
- have diabetes
- have TB, or have been in close contact with someone with TB
- were born in, lived in, or traveled to countries where there is more risk for getting TB. Ask your doctor if you are not sure.
- live or have lived in certain parts of the country (such as the Ohio and Mississippi River valleys) where there is an increased risk for getting certain kinds of fungal infections (histoplasmosis, coccidioidomycosis, or blastomycosis). These infections may happen or become more severe if you use HUMIRA. Ask your doctor if you do not know if you have lived in an area where these infections are common.
- have or have had hepatitis B
- use the medicine ORENCIA® (abatacept), KINERET® (anakinra), RITUXAN® (rituximab), IMURAN® (azathioprine), or PURINETHOL® (6–mercaptopurine, 6-MP).
- are scheduled to have major surgery

After starting HUMIRA, call your doctor right away if you have an infection, or any sign of an infection.

HUMIRA can make you more likely to get infections or make any infection that you may have worse.

Cancer

- For children and adults taking TNF-blockers, including HUMIRA, the chances of getting cancer may increase.
- There have been cases of unusual cancers in children, teenagers, and young adults using TNF-blockers.
- People with RA, especially more serious RA, may have a higher chance for getting a kind of cancer called lymphoma.
- If you use TNF blockers including HUMIRA your chance of getting two types of skin cancer may increase (basal cell cancer and squamous cell cancer of the skin). These types of cancer are generally not life-threatening if treated. Tell your doctor if you have a bump or open sore that doesn't heal.
- Some people receiving TNF blockers including HUMIRA developed a rare type of cancer called hepatosplenic T-cell lymphoma. This type of cancer often results in death. Most of these people were male teenagers or young men. Also, most people were being treated for Crohn's disease or ulcerative colitis with another medicine called IMURAN® (azathioprine) or PURINETHOL® (6-mercaptopurine, 6–MP).

See the "What are the possible side effects of HUMIRA?" section.

What is HUMIRA?

HUMIRA is a medicine called a Tumor Necrosis Factor (TNF) blocker. HUMIRA is used:

- To reduce the signs and symptoms of:
  - **moderate to severe rheumatoid arthritis (RA) in adults.** HUMIRA can be used alone, with methotrexate, or with certain other medicines.
  - **moderate to severe polyarticular juvenile idiopathic arthritis (JIA) in children** 4 years and older. HUMIRA can be used alone, with methotrexate, or with certain other medicines.
  - **psoriatic arthritis (PsA) in adults.** HUMIRA can be used alone or with certain other medicines.
  - **ankylosing spondylitis (AS) in adults.**
  - **moderate to severe Crohn's disease (CD) in adults** when other treatments have not worked well enough.
- In adults, to help get **moderate to severe ulcerative colitis (UC)** under control (induce remission) and keep it under control (sustain remission) when certain other medicines have not worked well enough. It is not known if HUMIRA is effective in people who stopped responding to or could not tolerate TNF-blocker medicines.
- **To treat moderate to severe chronic (lasting a long time) plaque psoriasis (Ps) in adults** who have the condition in many areas of their body and who may benefit from taking injections or pills (systemic therapy) or phototherapy (treatment using ultraviolet light alone or with pills).

What should I tell my doctor before taking HUMIRA?

HUMIRA may not be right for you. Before starting HUMIRA, tell your doctor about all of your health conditions, including if you:

- have an infection. See **"What is the most important information I should know about HUMIRA?"**
- have or have had cancer.
- have any numbness or tingling or have a disease that affects your nervous system such as multiple sclerosis or Guillain-Barré syndrome.
- have or had heart failure.
- have recently received or are scheduled to receive a vaccine. You may receive vaccines, except for live vaccines while using HUMIRA. Children with juvenile idiopathic arthritis should be brought up to date with all vaccines before starting HUMIRA.
- are allergic to rubber or latex. The needle cover on the prefilled syringe contains dry natural rubber. Tell your doctor if you have any allergies to rubber or latex.
- are allergic to HUMIRA or to any of its ingredients. See the end of this Medication Guide for a list of ingredients in HUMIRA.
- are pregnant or planning to become pregnant. It is not known if HUMIRA will harm your unborn baby. HUMIRA should only be used during a pregnancy if needed.
- breastfeeding or plan to breastfeed. You and your doctor should decide if you will breastfeed or use HUMIRA. You should not do both.

Tell your doctor about all the medicines you take, including prescription and non-prescription medicines, vitamins, and herbal supplements.

Especially tell your doctor if you use:

- ORENCIA® (abatacept), KINERET® (anakinra), REMICADE® (infliximab), ENBREL® (etanercept), CIMZIA® (certolizumab pegol) or SIMPONI® (golimumab), because you should not use HUMIRA while you are also taking one of these medicines.
- RITUXAN® (rituximab). Your doctor may not want to give you HUMIRA if you have received RITUXAN® (rituximab) recently.
- IMURAN® (azathioprine) or PURINETHOL® (6–mercaptopurine, 6-MP).

Keep a list of your medicines with you to show your doctor and pharmacist each time you get a new medicine.

How should I take HUMIRA?

- HUMIRA is given by an injection under the skin. Your doctor will tell you how often to take an injection of HUMIRA. This is based on your condition to be treated. **Do not inject HUMIRA more often than you were prescribed.**
- See the **Instructions for Use** inside the carton for complete instructions for the right way to prepare and inject HUMIRA.
- Make sure you have been shown how to inject HUMIRA before you do it yourself. You can call your doctor or 1-800-4HUMIRA (1-800-448-6472) if you have any questions about giving yourself an injection. Someone you know can also help you with your injection after he/she has been shown how to prepare and inject HUMIRA.
- **Do not** try to inject HUMIRA yourself until you have been shown the right way to give the injections. If your doctor decides that you or a caregiver may be able to give your injections of HUMIRA at home, you should receive training on the right way to prepare and inject HUMIRA.
- Do not miss any doses of HUMIRA unless your doctor says it is okay. If you forget to take HUMIRA, inject a dose as soon as you remember. Then, take your next dose at your regular scheduled time. This will put you back on schedule. In case you are not sure when to inject HUMIRA, call your doctor or pharmacist.
- If you take more HUMIRA than you were told to take, call your doctor.

What are the possible side effects of HUMIRA?

HUMIRA can cause serious side effects, including:

See "What is the most important information I should know about HUMIRA?"

- **Serious Infections.**

  Your doctor will examine you for TB and perform a test to see if you have TB. If your doctor feels that you are at risk for TB, you may be treated with medicine for TB before you begin treatment with HUMIRA and during treatment with HUMIRA. Even if your TB test is negative your doctor should carefully monitor you for TB infections while you are taking HUMIRA. People who had a negative TB skin test before receiving HUMIRA have developed active TB. Tell your doctor if you have any of the following symptoms while taking or after taking HUMIRA:
  - cough that does not go away
  - low grade fever
  - weight loss
  - loss of body fat and muscle (wasting)
- **Hepatitis B infection in people who carry the virus in their blood.**

  If you are a carrier of the hepatitis B virus (a virus that affects the liver), the virus can become active while you use HUMIRA. Your doctor should do blood tests before you start treatment, while you are using HUMIRA, and for several months after you stop treatment with HUMIRA. Tell your doctor if you have any of the following symptoms of a possible hepatitis B infection:

• muscle aches	• clay-colored bowel movements
• feel very tired	• fever
• dark urine	• chills
• skin or eyes look yellow	• stomach discomfort
• little or no appetite	• skin rash
	• vomiting

- **Allergic reactions.** Allergic reactions can happen in people who use HUMIRA. Call your doctor or get medical help right away if you have any of these symptoms of a serious allergic reaction:
  - hives
  - swelling of your face, eyes, lips or mouth
  - trouble breathing
- **Nervous system problems.** Signs and symptoms of a nervous system problem include: numbness or tingling, problems with your vision, weakness in your arms or legs, and dizziness.
- **Blood problems.** Your body may not make enough of the blood cells that help fight infections or help to stop bleeding. Symptoms include a fever that does not go away, bruising or bleeding very easily, or looking very pale.
- **New heart failure or worsening of heart failure you already have. Call your doctor right away** if you get new worsening symptoms of heart failure while taking HUMIRA, including:
  - shortness of breath
  - swelling of your ankles or feet
  - sudden weight gain.
- **Immune reactions including a lupus-like syndrome.** Symptoms include chest discomfort or pain that does not go away, shortness of breath, joint pain, or a rash on your cheeks or arms that gets worse in the sun. Symptoms may improve when you stop HUMIRA.
- **Liver Problems.** Liver problems can happen in people who use TNF-blocker medicines. These problems can lead to liver failure and death. Call your doctor right away if you have any of these symptoms:
  - feel very tired
  - skin or eyes look yellow
  - poor appetite or vomiting
  - pain on the right side of your stomach (abdomen)
- **Psoriasis.** Some people using HUMIRA had new psoriasis or worsening of psoriasis they already had. Tell your doctor if you develop red scaly patches or raised bumps that are filled with pus. Your doctor may decide to stop your treatment with HUMIRA.

Call your doctor or get medical care right away if you develop any of the above symptoms. Your treatment with HUMIRA may be stopped.

Common side effects with HUMIRA include:

- injection site reactions: redness, rash, swelling, itching, or bruising. These symptoms usually will go away within a few days. Call your doctor right away if you have pain, redness or swelling around the injection site that does not go away within a few days or gets worse.
- upper respiratory infections (including sinus infections)
- headaches
- rash
- nausea

These are not all the possible side effects with HUMIRA. Tell your doctor if you have any side effect that bothers you or that does not go away. Ask your doctor or pharmacist for more information.

Call your doctor for medical advice about side effects. You may report side effects to the FDA at 1-800-FDA-1088.

How should I store HUMIRA?

- Store HUMIRA in a refrigerator at 36°F to 46°F (2°C to 8°C) in the original container until it is used. Protect from light.
- When traveling, HUMIRA should be stored in a cool carrier with an ice pack.
- **Do not freeze HUMIRA.** Do not use HUMIRA if frozen, even if it has been thawed.
- Refrigerated HUMIRA may be used until the expiration date printed on the HUMIRA carton, dose tray, Pen or prefilled syringe.
- Do not use a Pen or prefilled syringe if the liquid is cloudy, discolored, or has flakes or particles in it.
- Do not drop or crush HUMIRA. The prefilled syringe is glass.
- **Keep HUMIRA, injection supplies, and all other medicines out of the reach of children.**

General information about HUMIRA

Medicines are sometimes prescribed for purposes other than those listed in a Medication Guide. Do not use HUMIRA for a condition for which it was not prescribed. Do not give HUMIRA to other people, even if they have the same condition. It may harm them.

This Medication Guide summarizes the most important information about HUMIRA. If you would like more information, talk with your doctor. You can ask your doctor or pharmacist for information about HUMIRA that was written for healthcare professionals.

For more information go to www.HUMIRA.com or you can enroll in a patient support program by calling 1-800-4HUMIRA (1-800-448-6472).

What are the ingredients in HUMIRA?

Active ingredient: adalimumab

Inactive ingredients: sodium chloride, monobasic sodium phosphate dihydrate, dibasic sodium phosphate dihydrate,

Information on the AbbVie, Inc. products listed on these pages is from the prescribing information in use as of July 31, 2013. For more information, please visit rxabbvie.com or call 1-800-633-9110.

sodium citrate, citric acid monohydrate, mannitol, polysorbate 80, and Water for Injection. Sodium hydroxide is added as necessary to adjust pH.

This Medication Guide has been approved by the U.S. Food and Drug Administration.

AbbVie Inc.
North Chicago, IL 60064, U.S.A.
Content revised 05/2013

INSTRUCTIONS FOR USE
HUMIRA® (Hu-MARE-ah)
(adalimumab)
SINGLE-USE PEN

Do not try to inject HUMIRA yourself until you have been shown the right way to give the injections. If your doctor decides that you or a caregiver may be able to give your injections of HUMIRA at home, you should receive training on the right way to prepare and inject HUMIRA. It is important that you read, understand, and follow these instructions so that you inject HUMIRA the right way. Call your healthcare provider if you or your caregiver has any questions about the right way to inject HUMIRA.

IMPORTANT:
- Do not use HUMIRA if frozen, even if it has been thawed.
- The HUMIRA Pen contains glass. Do not drop or crush the Pen because the glass inside may break.
- Do not remove the gray cap or the plum-colored cap until right before your injection.
- When the plum-colored button on the HUMIRA Pen is pressed to give your dose of HUMIRA, you will hear a loud "click" sound.
  - You must practice injecting HUMIRA with your doctor or nurse so that you are not startled by this click when you start giving yourself the injections at home.
  - The loud click sound means the start of the injection.
  - You will know that the injection has finished when the yellow marker appears fully in the window view and stops moving.

See the section below called **"Prepare the HUMIRA Pen"**.

How should I store HUMIRA?
- Store HUMIRA in a refrigerator at 36°F to 46°F (2°C to 8°C) in the original container until it is used. Protect from light.
- When traveling, HUMIRA should be stored in a cool carrier with an ice pack.
- **Do not freeze HUMIRA**. Do not use HUMIRA if frozen, even if it has been thawed.
- Refrigerated HUMIRA may be used until the expiration date printed on the HUMIRA carton, dose tray, and Pen.
- Do not use a Pen if the liquid is cloudy, discolored, or has flakes or particles in it.
- Do not drop or crush HUMIRA.
- **Keep HUMIRA, injection supplies, and all other medicines out of the reach of children.**

Gather the Supplies for Your Injection
- You will need the following supplies for your injection of HUMIRA.
  Find a clean, flat surface to place the supplies on.
  - 1 alcohol swab
  - 1 cotton ball or gauze pad (not included in your HUMIRA carton)
  - 1 HUMIRA Pen (See Figure A)
  - 1 FDA-cleared sharps disposal container for HUMIRA Pen disposal (not included in your HUMIRA carton)

If you do not have all of the supplies you need to give yourself an injection, go to a pharmacy or call your pharmacist. The diagram below shows what the HUMIRA Pen looks like. See Figure A.

Figure A

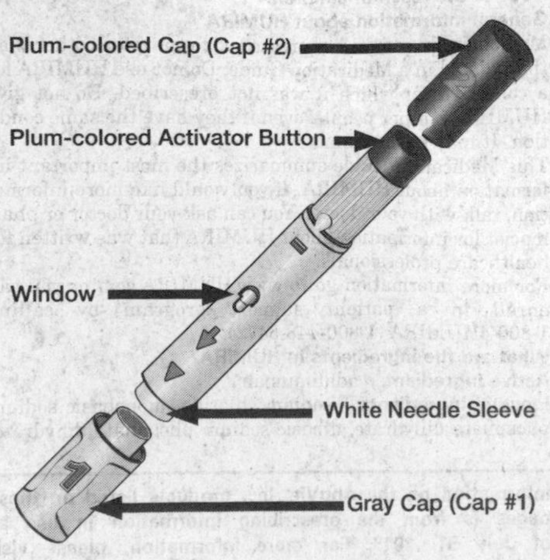

Check the carton, dose tray, and HUMIRA Pen.

1. Make sure the name HUMIRA appears on the carton, dose tray, and HUMIRA Pen label.
2. **Do not** use and call your doctor or pharmacist if:
- you drop or crush your HUMIRA Pen.
- the seals on the top or bottom of the carton are broken or missing.
- the expiration date on the carton, dose tray, and Pen has passed.
- the HUMIRA Pen has been frozen or left in direct sunlight. See the section: **"How should I store HUMIRA?"** at the beginning of these Instructions For Use.

3. Hold the Pen with the gray cap (Cap # 1) pointed down.
4. Make sure the amount of liquid in the Pen is at the fill line or close to the fill line seen through the window. This is the full dose of HUMIRA that you will inject. See Figure B.
5. If the Pen does not have the full amount of liquid, **do not use that Pen**. Call your pharmacist.

Figure B

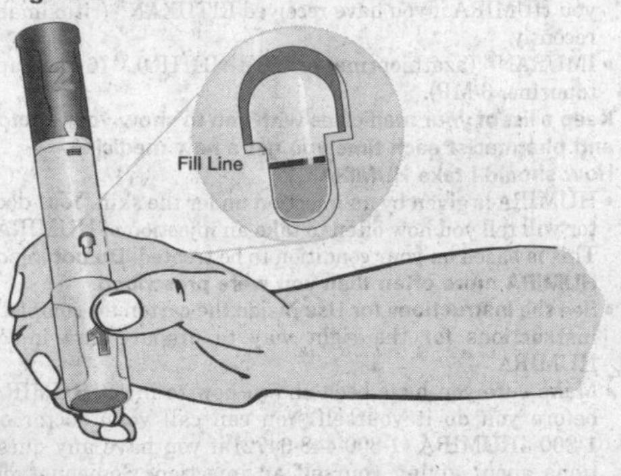

6. Turn the Pen over and hold the Pen with the gray cap (Cap # 1) pointed up. See Figure C.
7. Check the solution through the windows on the side of the Pen to make sure the liquid is clear and colorless. **Do not use** your HUMIRA Pen if the liquid is cloudy, discolored, or if it has flakes or particles in it. Call your pharmacist. It is normal to see one or more bubbles in the window.

Figure C

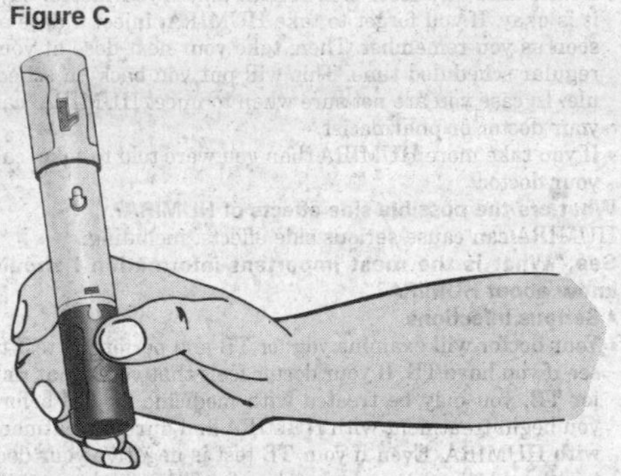

Choose the Injection Site
8. Wash and dry your hands well.
9. Choose an injection site on:
- the front of your thighs or
- your lower abdomen (belly). If you choose your abdomen, do not use the area 2 inches around your belly button (navel). See Figure D.

Figure D

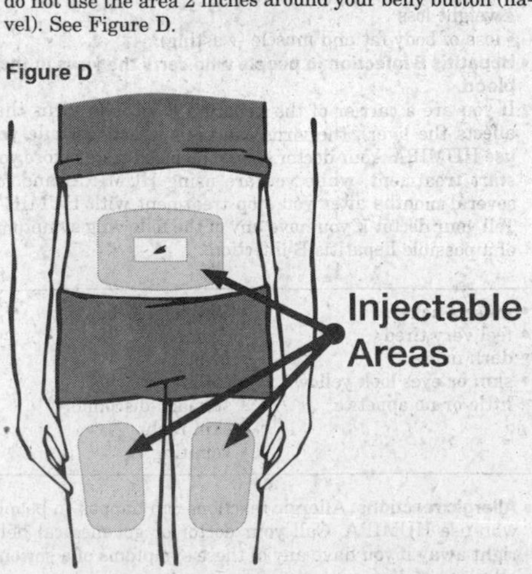

- Choose a different site each time you give yourself an injection. Each new injection should be given at least one inch from a site you used before.
- **Do not** inject HUMIRA into skin that is:
  - sore (tender)
  - bruised
  - red
  - hard
  - scarred or where you have stretch marks
- If you have psoriasis, **do not** inject directly into any raised, thick, red or scaly skin patches or lesions on your skin.
- Do not inject through your clothes.

Prepare the Injection Site
10. Wipe the injection site with an alcohol prep (swab) using a circular motion.
- **Do not** touch this area again before giving the injection. Allow the skin to dry before injecting. **Do not** fan or blow on the clean area.

Preparing the HUMIRA Pen
11. **Do not remove the gray cap (Cap # 1) or the plum-colored cap (Cap # 2) until right before your injection.**
12. Hold the middle of the Pen (gray body) with one hand so that you are not touching the gray cap (Cap # 1) or the plum-colored cap (Cap # 2). Turn the Pen so that the gray cap (Cap # 1) is pointing up. See Figure E.

Figure E

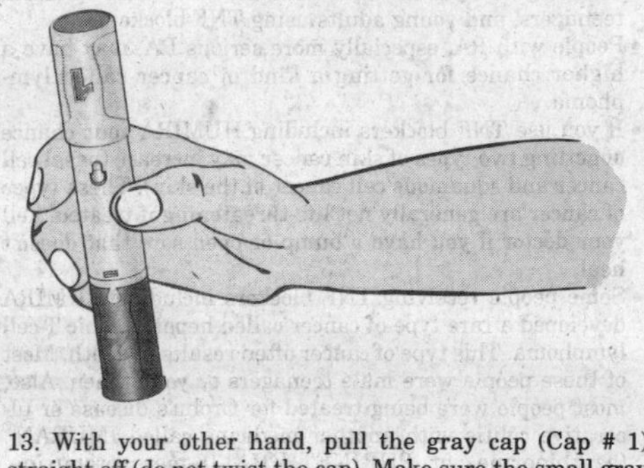

13. With your other hand, pull the gray cap (Cap # 1) straight off (do not twist the cap). Make sure the small gray needle cover of the syringe has come off with the gray cap (Cap # 1). See Figure F.
14. Throw away the gray cap (Cap # 1).

Figure F

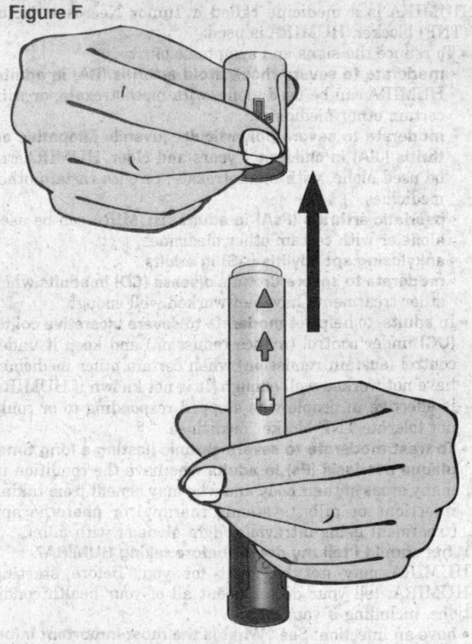

- **Do not** put the gray cap (Cap # 1) back on the Pen. Putting the gray cap (Cap # 1) back on may damage the needle.
- The white needle sleeve, which covers the needle, can now be seen.
- **Do not** touch the needle with your fingers or let the needle touch anything.
- You may see a few drops of liquid come out of the needle. This is normal.

15. Remove the plum-colored cap (Cap # 2) from the bottom of the Pen by pulling it straight off (do not twist the cap). The Pen is now activated. Throw away the plum-colored cap.
- Do not put the plum-colored cap (Cap # 2) back on the Pen because it could cause medicine to come out of the syringe.

The plum-colored activator button:

- Turn the Pen so the plum-colored activator button is pointed up. See Figure G.

Figure G

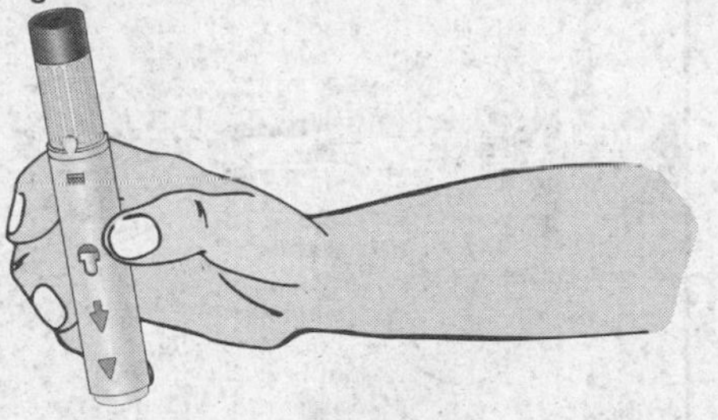

- **Do not** press the plum-colored activator button until you are ready to inject HUMIRA. Pressing the plum-colored activator button will release the medicine from the Pen.
- Hold the Pen so that you can see the window. See Figure H. It is normal to see one or more bubbles in the window.

Figure H

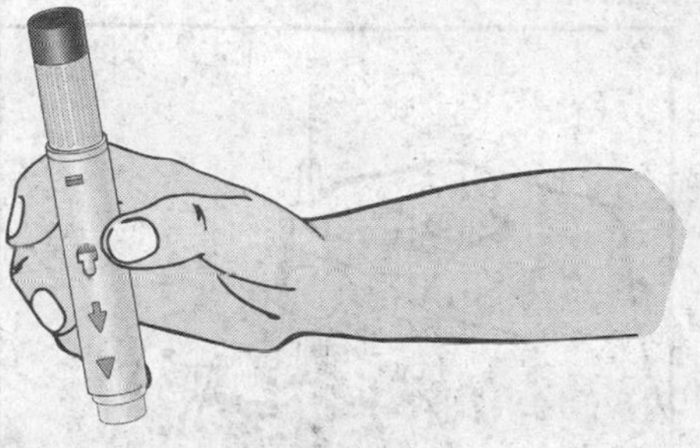

Position the Pen and Inject HUMIRA

16. Position the Pen:

- Gently squeeze the area of the cleaned skin and hold it firmly. See Figure I. You will inject into this raised area of skin.

Figure I

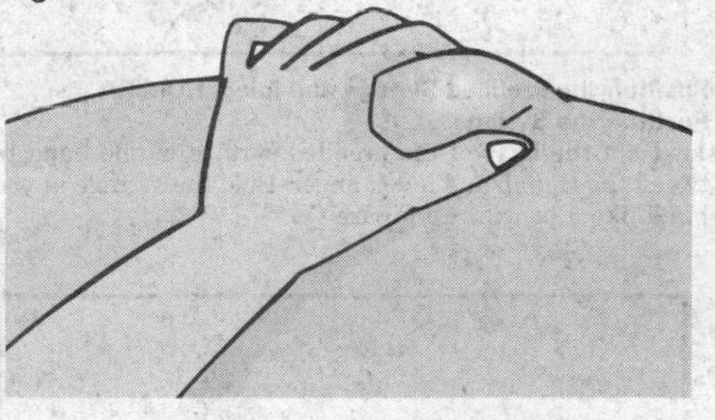

17. Place the white end of the Pen straight (at a 90° angle) and flat against the raised area of your skin that you are squeezing. Place the Pen so that it will not inject the needle into your fingers that are holding the raised skin. See Figure J.

Figure J

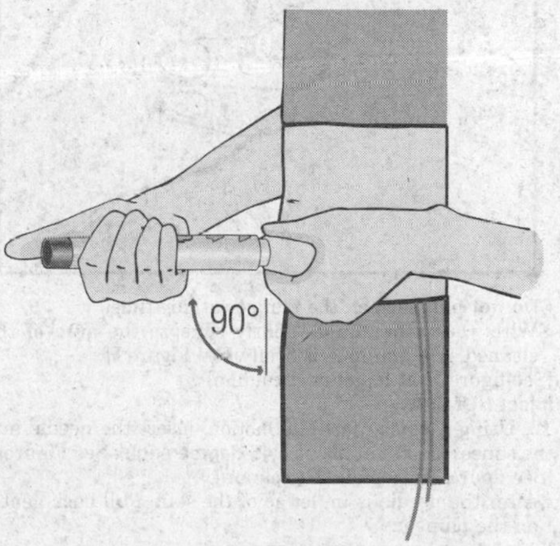

18. Inject HUMIRA

- With your index finger or your thumb, press the plum-colored activator button to begin the injection. Try not to cover the window. See Figure K.

Figure K

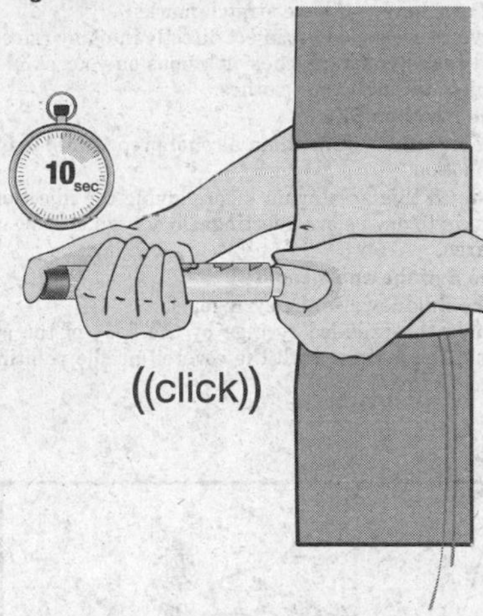

- You will hear a loud 'click' when you press the plum-colored activator button. The loud click means the start of the injection.
- Keep pressing the plum-colored activator button and continue to hold the Pen against your squeezed, raised skin until all of the medicine is injected. This can take up to 10 seconds, so count slowly to ten. Keep holding the Pen against the squeezed, raised skin of your injection site for the whole time so you get the full dose of medicine.
- You will know that the injection has finished when the yellow marker fully appears in the window view and stops moving. See Figure L.

Figure L

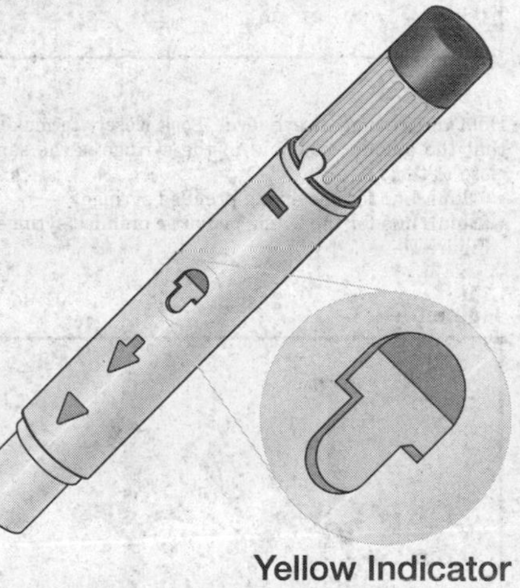

19. When the injection is finished, slowly pull the Pen from your skin. The white needle sleeve will move to cover the needle tip. See Figure M.

- Do not touch the needle. The white needle sleeve is there to prevent you from touching the needle.

Figure M

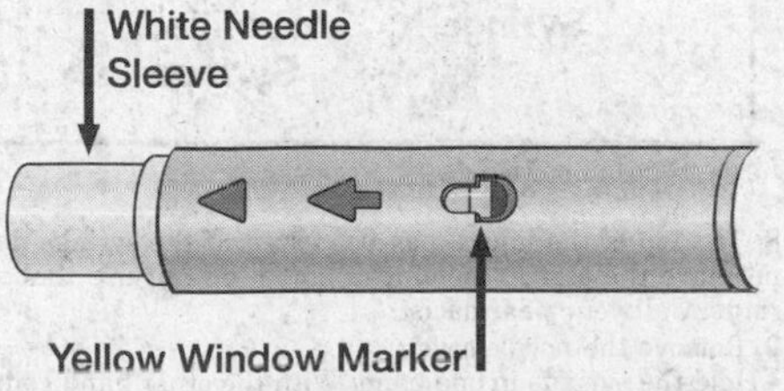

- Press a cotton ball or gauze pad over the injection site and hold it for 10 seconds. Do **not** rub the injection site. You may have slight bleeding. This is normal.

20. Dispose of your used HUMIRA Pen. See the section **"How should I dispose of the used HUMIRA Pen?"**

21. Keep a record of the dates and location of your injection sites. To help you remember when to take HUMIRA, you can mark your calendar ahead of time.

How should I dispose of the used HUMIRA Pen?

- Put your Pen in a FDA-cleared sharps disposal container right away after use. See Figure N. **Do not throw away (dispose of) the Pen in your household trash.**
- Do not try to touch the needle. The white needle sleeve is there to prevent you from touching the needle.

Figure N

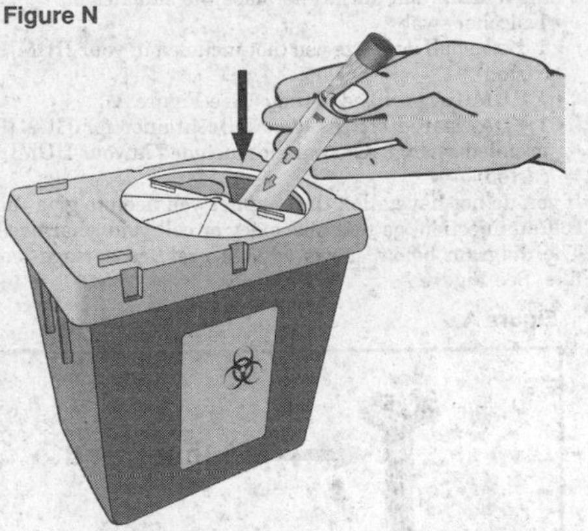

- If you do not have a FDA-cleared sharps disposal container, you may use a household container that is:
  - made of a heavy-duty plastic,
  - can be closed with a tight-fitting, puncture-resistant lid, without sharps being able to come out,
  - upright and stable during use,
  - leak-resistant, and
  - properly labeled to warn of hazardous waste inside the container.
- When your sharps disposal container is almost full, you will need to follow your community guidelines for the right way to dispose of your sharps disposal container. There may be state or local laws about how you should throw away used needles and syringes. For more information about safe sharps disposal, and for specific information about sharps disposal in the state that you live in, go to the FDA's website at: http://www.fda.gov/safesharpsdisposal.
- For the safety and health of you and others, never re-use your HUMIRA Pens.
- The used alcohol pads, cotton balls, dose trays and packaging may be placed in your household trash.
- **Do not dispose of your used sharps disposal container in your household trash unless your community guidelines permit this. Do not recycle your used sharps disposal container.**
- **Always keep the sharps container out of the reach of children.**

This Instructions for Use has been approved by the U.S. Food and Drug Administration.

AbbVie Inc.
North Chicago, IL 60064, U.S.A.
Content revised 01/2013

INSTRUCTIONS FOR USE
HUMIRA® (Hu-MARE-ah)
(adalimumab)
SINGLE-USE PREFILLED SYRINGE

Do not try to inject HUMIRA yourself until you have been shown the right way to give the injections. If your doctor decides that you or a caregiver may be able to give your injections of HUMIRA at home, you should receive training on the right way to prepare and inject HUMIRA. It is important that you read, understand, and follow these instructions so that you inject HUMIRA the right way. Call your healthcare provider if you or your caregiver has any questions about the right way to inject HUMIRA.

How should I store HUMIRA?

- Store HUMIRA in a refrigerator at 36°F to 46°F (2°C to 8°C) in the original container until it is used. Protect from light.
- When traveling, HUMIRA should be stored in a cool carrier with an ice pack.
- **Do not freeze HUMIRA.** Do not use HUMIRA if frozen, even if it has been thawed.
- Refrigerated HUMIRA may be used until the expiration date printed on the HUMIRA carton, dose tray and prefilled syringe.
- Do not use a prefilled syringe if the liquid is cloudy, discolored, or has flakes or particles in it.
- Do not drop or crush HUMIRA. The prefilled syringe is glass.
- **Keep HUMIRA, injection supplies, and all other medicines out of the reach of children.**

Information on the AbbVie, Inc. products listed on these pages is from the prescribing information in use as of July 31, 2013. For more information, please visit rxabbvie.com or call 1-800-633-9110.

Gather the Supplies for Your Injection

- You will need the following supplies for your injection of HUMIRA.
  Find a clean, flat surface to place the supplies on.
  - 1 alcohol swab
  - 1 cotton ball or gauze pad (not included in your HUMIRA carton)
  - 1 HUMIRA prefilled syringe (See Figure A)
  - 1 FDA-cleared sharps disposal container for HUMIRA prefilled syringe disposal (not included in your HUMIRA carton)

If you do not have all of the supplies you need to give yourself an injection, go to a pharmacy or call your pharmacist. The diagram below shows what a prefilled syringe looks like. See Figure A.

Figure A

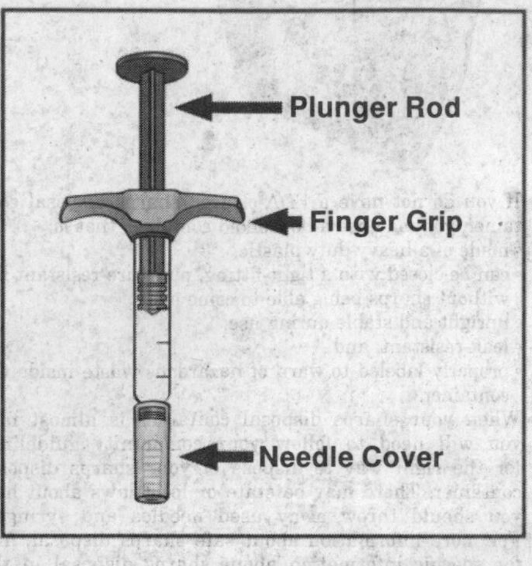

Check the carton, dose tray, and prefilled syringe

1. Make sure the name HUMIRA appears on the dose tray and prefilled syringe label.
2. **Do not use** and call your doctor or pharmacist if:
- the seals on top and bottom of the carton are broken or missing.
- the HUMIRA labeling has an expired date. Check the expiration date on your HUMIRA carton and do not use if the date has passed.
- the prefilled syringe that has been frozen or left in direct sunlight. See the section: **"How should I store HUMIRA?"** at the beginning of these Instructions for Use.
- the liquid in the prefilled syringe is cloudy, discolored or has flakes or particles in it. Make sure the liquid is clear and colorless.

Choose the Injection Site

3. Wash and dry your hands well.
4. Choose an injection site on:
- the front of your thighs or
- your lower abdomen (belly). If you choose your abdomen, do not use the area 2 inches around your belly button (navel). See Figure B.

Figure B

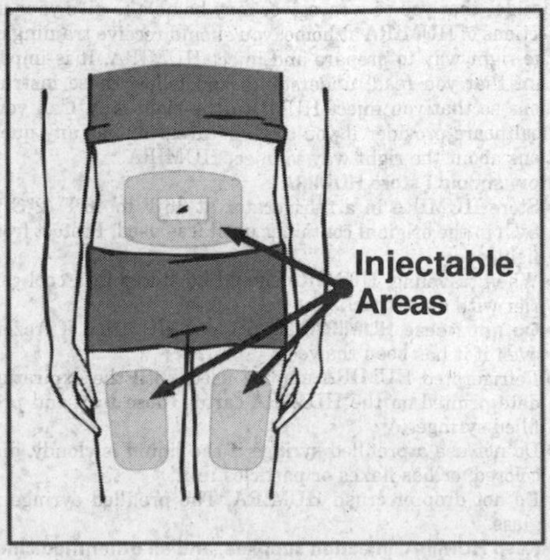

- Choose a different site each time you give yourself an injection. Each new injection should be given at least one inch from a site you used before.
- **Do not** inject into skin that is:
  - sore (tender)
  - bruised
  - red
  - hard
  - scarred or where you have stretch marks
- If you have psoriasis, do not inject directly into any raised, thick, red or scaly skin patches or lesions on your skin.
- Do not inject through your clothes.

Prepare the Injection Site

5. Wipe the injection site with an alcohol prep (swab) using a circular motion.
6. Do **not** touch this area again before giving the injection. Allow the skin to dry before injecting. Do not fan or blow on the clean area.

Prepare the Syringe and Needle

7. Check the fluid level in the syringe:
- Always hold the prefilled syringe by the body of the syringe. Hold the syringe with the covered needle pointing down. See Figure C.

Figure C

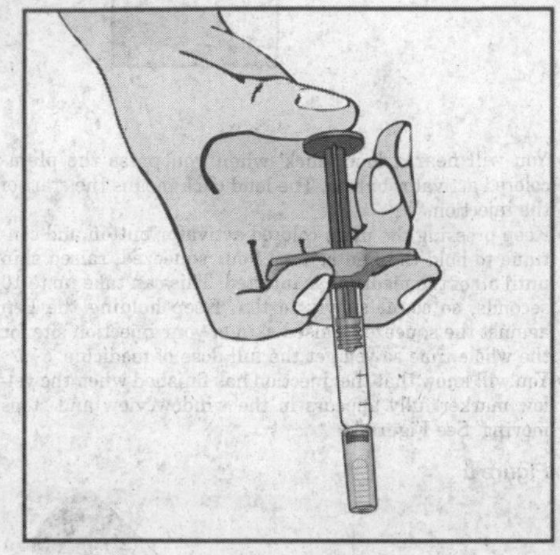

- Hold the syringe at eye level. Look closely to make sure that the amount of liquid in the syringe is the same or close to the:
  - 0.8 mL line for the 40 mg prefilled syringe
  - 0.4 mL line for the 20 mg pediatric prefilled syringe. See Figure D.

Figure D

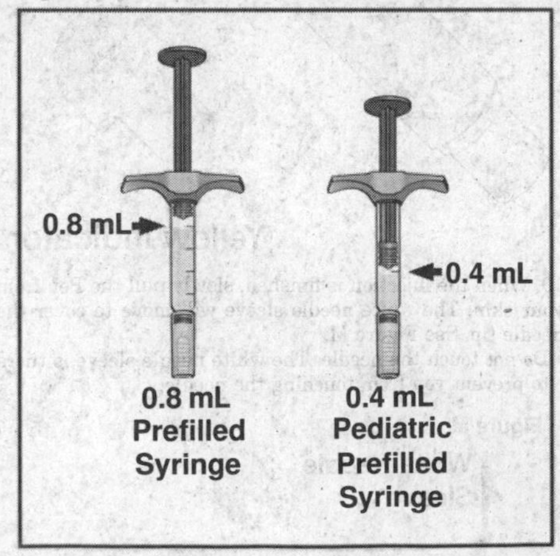

8. The top of the liquid may be curved. If the syringe does not have the correct amount of liquid, **do not use that syringe**. Call your pharmacist.
9. Remove the needle cover:
- Hold the syringe in one hand. With the other hand gently remove the needle cover. See Figure E.
- Throw away the needle cover.

[See figure E at top of next column]

- Do not touch the needle with your fingers or let the needle touch anything.

10. Turn the syringe so the needle is facing up and hold the syringe at eye level with one hand so you can see the air in the syringe. Using your other hand, slowly push the plunger in to push the air out through the needle. See Figure F.

[See figure F at top of next column]

- You may see a drop of liquid at the end of the needle. This is normal.

Figure E

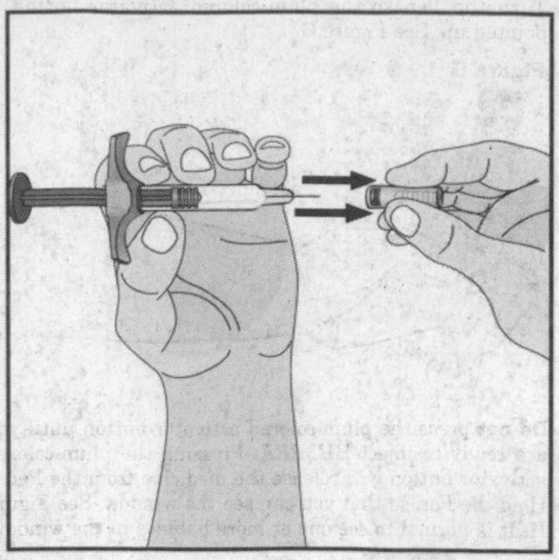

Figure F

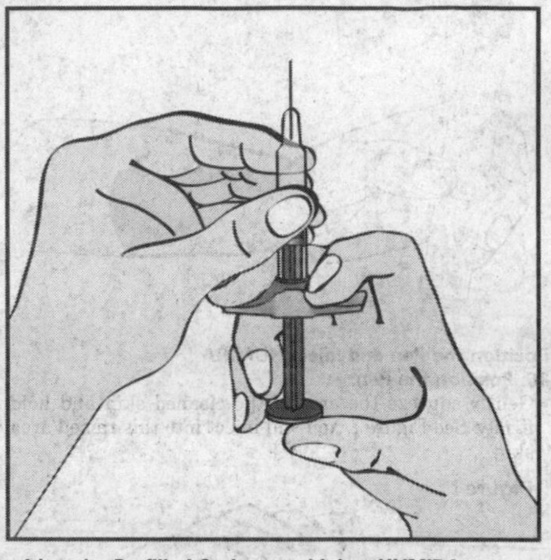

Position the Prefilled Syringe and Inject HUMIRA

Position the Syringe

11. Hold the body of the prefilled syringe in one hand between the thumb and index finger. Hold the syringe in your hand like a pencil. See Figure G.

Figure G

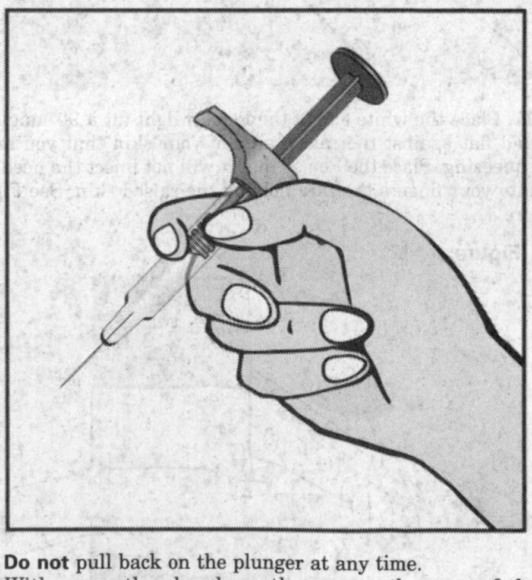

- **Do not** pull back on the plunger at any time.
- With your other hand, gently squeeze the area of the cleaned skin and hold it firmly. See Figure H.

[See figure H at top of next column]

Inject HUMIRA

12. Using a quick, dart-like motion, insert the needle into the squeezed skin at about a **45-degree angle**. See Figure I.

[See figure I at top of next column]

- After the needle is in, let go of the skin. Pull back gently on the plunger.

If blood appears in the syringe:

- It means that you have entered a blood vessel.
- **Do not inject HUMIRA.**
- Pull the needle out of the skin while keeping the syringe at the same angle.

Figure H

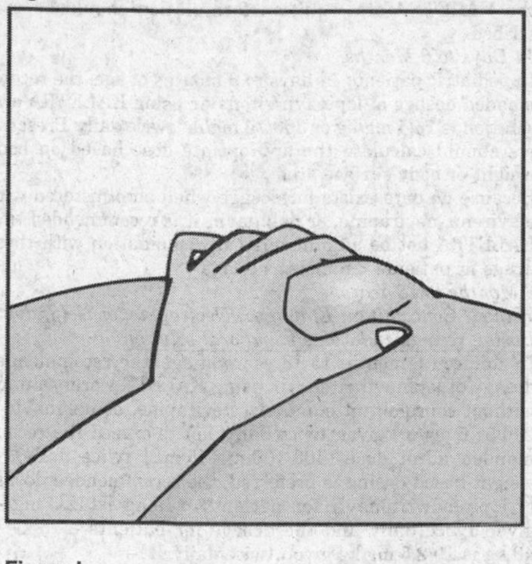

Figure I

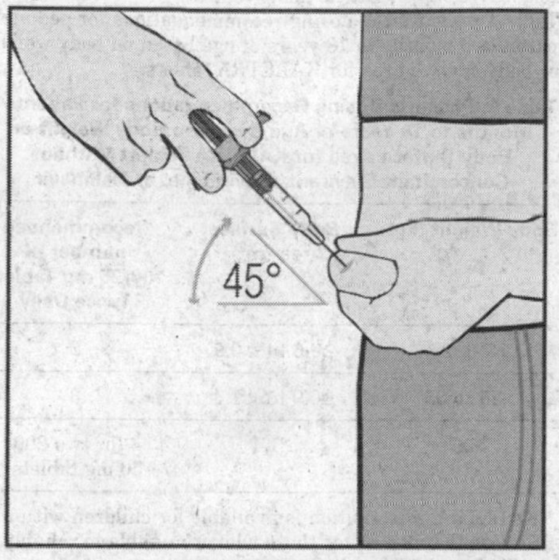

- Press a cotton ball or gauze pad over the injection site and hold it for 10 seconds. See Figure J.

Figure J

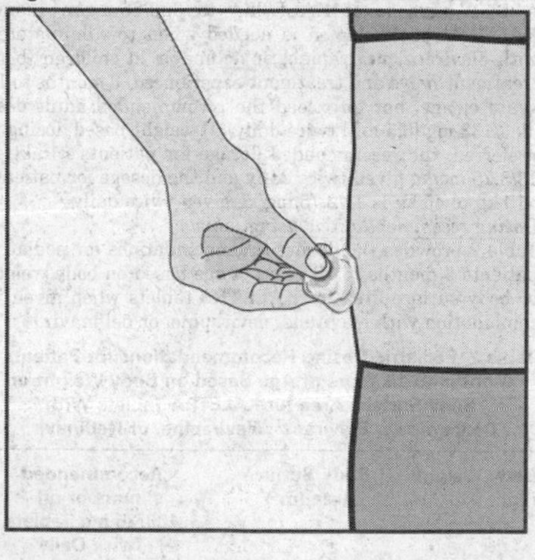

- **Do not** use the same syringe and needle again. Throw away the needle and syringe in your special sharps container.
- **Do not** rub the injection site. You may have slight bleeding. This is normal.
- Repeat Steps 1 through 12 with a new prefilled syringe.

If no blood appears in the syringe:

- Slowly push the plunger all the way in until all of the liquid is injected and the syringe is empty.
- Pull the needle out of the skin while keeping the syringe at the same angle.
- Press a cotton ball or gauze pad over the injection site and hold it for 10 seconds. Do **not** rub the injection site. You may have slight bleeding. This is normal.

13. Throw away the used prefilled syringe and needle. See **"How should I dispose of used prefilled syringes and needles?"**

14. Keep a record of the dates and location of your injection sites. To help you remember when to take HUMIRA, you can mark your calendar ahead of time.

How should I dispose of used prefilled syringes and needles?

- **Put your used needles and syringes in a FDA-cleared sharps disposal container right away after use.** See Figure K. **Do not throw away (dispose of) loose needles and syringes in your household trash.**
- Do not try to touch the needle.

Figure K

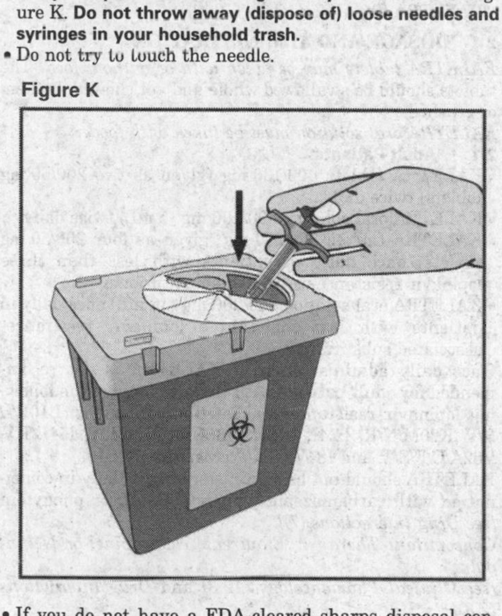

- If you do not have a FDA-cleared sharps disposal container, you may use a household container that is:
  - made of a heavy-duty plastic,
  - can be closed with a tight-fitting, puncture-resistant lid, without sharps being able to come out,
  - upright and stable during use,
  - leak-resistant, and
  - properly labeled to warn of hazardous waste inside the container.
- When your sharps disposal container is almost full, you will need to follow your community guidelines for the right way to dispose of your sharps disposal container. There may be state or local laws about how you should throw away used needles and syringes. For more information about safe sharps disposal, and for specific information about sharps disposal in the state that you live in, go to the FDA's website at: http://www.fda.gov/safesharpsdisposal.
- For the safety and health of you and others, needles and used syringes **must never** be re-used.
- The used alcohol pads, cotton balls, dose trays and packaging may be placed in your household trash.
- **Do not dispose of your used sharps disposal container in your household trash unless your community guidelines permit this. Do not recycle your used sharps disposal container.**
- **Always keep the sharps container out of the reach of children.**

This Instructions for Use has been approved by the U.S. Food and Drug Administration.

AbbVie Inc.
North Chicago, IL 60064, U.S.A.
Content revised 01/2013

Shown in Product Identification Guide, page 303

KALETRA ℞

[*kuh-LEE-tra*]
(lopinavir/ritonavir)
Tablet, Film Coated for Oral use

KALETRA

(lopinavir/ritonavir)
Solution for Oral use

HIGHLIGHTS OF PRESCRIBING INFORMATION

These highlights do not include all the information needed to use KALETRA safely and effectively. See full prescribing information for KALETRA.

KALETRA (lopinavir/ritonavir) Tablet, Film Coated for Oral use

KALETRA (lopinavir/ritonavir) Solution for Oral use

Initial U.S. Approval: 2000

RECENT MAJOR CHANGES

Warnings and Precautions, Immune Reconstitution Syndrome. (5.8)	02/2012
Indications and Usage. (1)	01/2013

INDICATIONS AND USAGE

KALETRA is an HIV-1 protease inhibitor indicated in combination with other antiretroviral agents for the treatment of HIV-1 infection in adults and pediatric patients (14 days and older). (1)

DOSAGE AND ADMINISTRATION

Tablets: May be taken with or without food, swallowed whole and not chewed, broken, or crushed. (2)

Oral solution: must be taken with food. (2)

Do not use once daily administration of KALETRA in:

- HIV-1 infected patients with three or more of the following lopinavir resistance-associated substitutions: L10F/I/R/V, K20M/N/R, L24I, L33F, M36I, I47V, G48V, I54L/T/V, V82A/C/F/S/T, and I84V. (2.1)
- Combination with efavirenz, nevirapine, nelfinavir, carbamazepine, phenobarbital, or phenytoin. (2.1, 7.3)
- Pediatric patients. (2.2)

<u>Adult Patients:</u>

- 400/100 mg (two 200/50 mg tablets or 5 mL oral solution) twice daily.

  or
- 800/200 mg (four 200/50 mg tablets or 10 mL oral solution) once daily in patients with less than three lopinavir resistance-associated substitutions. (2.1)

<u>Pediatric Patients (14 days and older):</u>

- Twice daily dose is based on body weight or body surface area. (2.2)

<u>Concomitant Therapy in Adults and Pediatric Patients:</u>

- Dose adjustments of KALETRA may be needed when coadministering with efavirenz, nevirapine, or nelfinavir. (2.1, 2.2, 7.3)

KALETRA oral solution should not be administered to neonates before a postmenstrual age (first day of the mother's last menstrual period to birth plus the time elapsed after birth) of 42 weeks and a postnatal age of at least 14 days has been attained (2.2, 5.2)

DOSAGE FORMS AND STRENGTHS

- Film-coated tablets: 200 mg lopinavir and 50 mg ritonavir (3)
- Film-coated tablets: 100 mg lopinavir and 25 mg ritonavir (3)
- Oral solution: 80 mg lopinavir and 20 mg ritonavir per milliliter (3)

CONTRAINDICATIONS

Hypersensitivity to KALETRA (e.g., toxic epidermal necrolysis, Stevens-Johnson syndrome, erythema multiforme) or any of its ingredients, including ritonavir. (4)

Co-administration with:

- drugs highly dependent on CYP3A for clearance and for which elevated plasma levels may result in serious and/or life-threatening events. (4)
- potent CYP3A inducers where significantly reduced lopinavir plasma concentrations may be associated with the potential for loss of virologic response and possible resistance and cross resistance. (4)

WARNINGS AND PRECAUTIONS

The following have been observed in patients receiving KALETRA:

- Drug Interactions: Higher plasma concentrations of concomitant medications may occur; consider drug-drug interaction potential to reduce risk of serious or life-threatening adverse reactions. (5.1)
- Toxicity in preterm neonates: KALETRA oral solution should not be used in preterm neonates in the immediate postnatal period because of possible toxicities. A safe and effective dose of KALETRA oral solution in this patient population has not been established. (2.2, 5.2).
- Pancreatitis: Fatalities have occurred; suspend therapy as clinically appropriate. (5.3)
- Hepatotoxicity: Fatalities have occurred. Monitor liver function before and during therapy, especially in patients with underlying hepatic disease, including hepatitis B and hepatitis C, or marked transaminase elevations. (5.4, 8.6)
- QT interval prolongation and isolated cases of torsade de pointes have been reported although causality could not be established. Avoid use in patients with congenital long QT syndrome, those with hypokalemia, and with other drugs that prolong the QT interval. (5.1, 5.5, 12.3)
- PR interval prolongation may occur in some patients. Cases of second and third degree heart block have been reported. Use with caution in patients with pre-existing conduction system disease, ischemic heart disease, cardiomyopathy, underlying structural heart disease or when administering with other drugs that may prolong the PR interval. (5.1, 5.6, 12.3)
- Patients may develop new onset or exacerbations of diabetes mellitus, hyperglycemia (5.7), immune reconstitution syndrome (5.8), redistribution/accumulation of body fat. (5.10)

Information on the AbbVie, Inc. products listed on these pages is from the prescribing information in use as of July 31, 2013. For more information, please visit rxabbvie.com or call 1-800-633-9110.

- Total cholesterol and triglycerides elevations. Monitor prior to therapy and periodically thereafter. (5.9)
- Hemophilia: Spontaneous bleeding may occur, and additional factor VIII may be required. (5.11)

ADVERSE REACTIONS

The most common adverse reactions (greater than 5%) were diarrhea, nausea, abdominal pain, asthenia, vomiting, headache, and dyspepsia. (6.1, 6.2)

To report SUSPECTED ADVERSE REACTIONS, contact AbbVie Inc. at 1-800-633-9110 or FDA at 1-800-FDA-1088 or www.fda.gov/medwatch

DRUG INTERACTIONS

Co-administration of KALETRA can alter the plasma concentrations of other drugs and other drugs may alter the plasma concentrations of lopinavir. The potential for drug-drug interactions must be considered prior to and during therapy. (4, 5.1, 7, 12.3)

See 17 for PATIENT COUNSELING INFORMATION and Medication Guide

Revised: 01/2013

FULL PRESCRIBING INFORMATION: CONTENTS*

* Sections or subsections omitted from the full prescribing information are not listed

FULL PRESCRIBING INFORMATION

1 INDICATIONS AND USAGE

KALETRA is indicated in combination with other antiretroviral agents for the treatment of HIV-1 infection in adults and pediatric patients (14 days and older).

The following points should be considered when initiating therapy with KALETRA:

- The use of other active agents with KALETRA is associated with a greater likelihood of treatment response *[see Microbiology (12.4) and Clinical Studies (14)]*.
- Genotypic or phenotypic testing and/or treatment history should guide the use of KALETRA *[see Microbiology (12.4)]*. The number of baseline lopinavir resistance-associated substitutions affects the virologic response to KALETRA *[see Microbiology (12.4)]*.

2 DOSAGE AND ADMINISTRATION

KALETRA tablets may be taken with or without food. The tablets should be swallowed whole and not chewed, broken, or crushed.

KALETRA oral solution must be taken with food.

2.1 Adult Patients

- KALETRA tablets 400/100 mg (given as two 200/50 mg tablets) twice daily.
- KALETRA oral solution 400/100 mg (5 mL) twice daily.
- KALETRA tablets 800/200 mg (given as four 200/50 mg tablets) once daily in patients with less than three lopinavir resistance-associated substitutions.
- KALETRA oral solution 800/200 mg (10 mL) once daily in patients with less than three lopinavir resistance-associated substitutions.

Once daily administration of KALETRA is not recommended for adult patients with three or more of the following lopinavir resistance-associated substitutions: L10F/I/R/V, K20M/N/R, L24I, L33F, M36I, I47V, G48V, I54L/T/V, V82A/C/F/S/T, and I84V *[see Microbiology (12.4)]*.

KALETRA should not be administered once daily in combination with carbamazepine, phenobarbital, or phenytoin *[see Drug Interactions (7)]*.

Concomitant Therapy: Efavirenz, Nevirapine, or Nelfinavir

[see Clinical Pharmacology (12.3) and Drug Interactions (7.3)]

KALETRA tablets and oral solution should not be administered as a once daily regimen in combination with efavirenz, nevirapine, or nelfinavir.

- A dose increase is recommended for all patients who use KALETRA tablets. The recommended dose of KALETRA tablets is 500/125 mg (such as two 200/50 tablets and one 100/25 mg tablet) twice daily in combination with efavirenz, nevirapine, or nelfinavir.
- A dose increase is recommended for all patients who use KALETRA oral solution. The recommended dose of KALETRA oral solution is 533/133 mg (6.5 mL) twice daily when used in combination with efavirenz, nevirapine, or nelfinavir.

2.2 Pediatric Patients

KALETRA tablets and oral solution should not be administered once daily in pediatric patients < 18 years of age.

KALETRA oral solution should not be administered to neonates before a postmenstrual age (first day of the mother's last menstrual period to birth plus the time elapsed after birth) of 42 weeks and a postnatal age of at least 14 days has been attained *[see Warnings and Precautions (5.2)]*.

KALETRA oral solution contains 42.4% (v/v) alcohol and 15.3% (w/v) propylene glycol. Special attention should be given to accurate calculation of the dose of KALETRA, transcription of the medication order, dispensing information and dosing instructions to minimize the risk for medication errors, and overdose. This is especially important for infants and young children. Total amounts of alcohol and propylene glycol from all medicines that are to be given to pediatric patients 14 days to 6 months of age should be taken into account in order to avoid toxicity from these excipients *[see Warnings and Precautions (5.2) and Overdosage (10)]*.

Prescribers should calculate the appropriate dose of KALETRA for each individual child based on body weight (kg) or body surface area (BSA) to avoid underdosing or exceeding the recommended adult dose.

Body surface area (BSA) can be calculated as follows:

$$^{*}\ \text{BSA (m}^2\text{)} = \sqrt{\frac{\text{Ht (Cm)} \times \text{Wt (kg)}}{3600}}$$

The KALETRA dose can be calculated based on weight or BSA:

Based on Weight:

Patient Weight (kg) × Prescribed lopinavir dose (mg/kg) = Administered lopinavir dose (mg)

Based on BSA:

Patient BSA (m^2) × Prescribed lopinavir dose (mg/m^2) = Administered lopinavir dose (mg)

If KALETRA oral solution is used, the volume (mL) of KALETRA solution can be determined as follows:

Volume of KALETRA solution (mL) = Administered lopinavir dose (mg) ÷ 80 (mg/mL)

The dose of the oral solution should be administered using a calibrated dosing syringe.

Before prescribing KALETRA 100/25 mg tablets, children should be assessed for the ability to swallow intact tablets. If a child is unable to reliably swallow a KALETRA tablet, the KALETRA oral solution formulation should be prescribed.

14 Days to 6 Months:

In pediatric patients 14 days to 6 months of age, the recommended dosage of lopinavir/ritonavir using KALETRA oral solution is 16/4 mg/kg or 300/75 mg/m^2 twice daily. Prescribers should calculate the appropriate dose based on body weight or body surface area.

Because no data exists for dosage when administered with efavirenz, nevirapine, or nelfinavir, it is recommended that KALETRA not be administered in combination with these drugs in patients < 6 months of age.

6 Months to 18 Years:

Without Concomitant Efavirenz, Nevirapine, or Nelfinavir

Dosing recommendations using oral solution

In children 6 months to 18 years of age, the recommended dosage of lopinavir/ritonavir using KALETRA oral solution without concomitant efavirenz, nevirapine, or nelfinavir is 230/57.5 mg/m^2 given twice daily, not to exceed the recommended adult dose (400/100 mg [5 mL] twice daily). If weight-based dosing is preferred, the recommended dosage of lopinavir/ritonavir for patients < 15 kg is 12/3 mg/kg given twice daily and the dosage for patients ≥ 15 kg to 40 kg is 10/2.5 mg/kg given twice daily.

Dosing recommendations using tablets

Table 1 provides the dosing recommendations for pediatric patients 6 months to 18 years of age based on body weight or body surface area for KALETRA tablets.

Table 1. Pediatric Dosing Recommendations for Patients 6 Months to 18 Years of Age Based on Body Weight or Body Surface Area for KALETRA Tablets Without Concomitant Efavirenz, Nevirapine, or Nelfinavir

Body Weight (kg)	Body Surface Area (m^2)*	Recommended number of 100/25 mg Tablets Twice Daily
15 to 25	≥0.6 to < 0.9	2
>25 to 35	≥0.9 to < 1.4	3
>35	≥1.4	4 (or two 200/50 mg tablets)

* KALETRA oral solution is available for children with a BSA less than 0.6 m^2 or those who are unable to reliably swallow a tablet.

Concomitant Therapy: Efavirenz, Nevirapine, or Nelfinavir

Dosing recommendations using oral solution

A dose increase of KALETRA to 300/75 mg/m^2 using KALETRA oral solution is needed when co-administered with efavirenz, nevirapine, or nelfinavir in children (both treatment-naïve and treatment-experienced) 6 months to 18 years of age, not to exceed the recommended adult dose (533/133 mg [6.5 mL] twice daily). If weight-based dosing is preferred, the recommended dosage for patients <15 kg is 13/3.25 mg/kg given twice daily and the dosage for patients >15 kg to 45 kg is 11/2.75 mg/kg given twice daily.

Dosing recommendations using tablets

Table 2 provides the dosing recommendations for pediatric patients 6 months to 18 years of age based on body weight or body surface area for KALETRA tablets when given in combination with efavirenz, nevirapine, or nelfinavir.

Table 2. Pediatric Dosing Recommendations for Patients 6 Months to 18 Years of Age Based on Body Weight or Body Surface Area for KALETRA Tablets With Concomitant Efavirenz†, Nevirapine, or Nelfinavir†

Body Weight (kg)	Body Surface Area (m^2)*	Recommended number of 100/25 mg Tablets Twice Daily
15 to 20	≥0.6 to < 0.8	2
>20 to 30	≥0.8 to < 1.2	3
>30 to 45	≥1.2 to <1.7	4 (or two 200/50 mg tablets)
>45	≥1.7	5 *[see Dosage and Administration*, Adult Patients (2.1)]

* KALETRA oral solution is available for children with a BSA less than 0.6 m^2 or those who are unable to reliably swallow a tablet.

† Please refer to the individual product labels for appropriate dosing in children.

3 DOSAGE FORMS AND STRENGTHS

- **KALETRA Tablets, 200 mg lopinavir/50 mg ritonavir**
  Yellow, film-coated, ovaloid tablets debossed with the "a" logo and the code KA providing 200 mg lopinavir/50 mg ritonavir.
- **KALETRA Tablets, 100 mg lopinavir/25 mg ritonavir**
  Pale yellow, film-coated, ovaloid tablets debossed with the "a" logo and the code KC providing 100 mg lopinavir/25 mg ritonavir.
- **KALETRA Oral Solution**
  Light yellow to orange colored liquid containing 400 mg lopinavir/100 mg ritonavir per 5 mL (80 mg lopinavir/20 mg ritonavir per mL).

4 CONTRAINDICATIONS

- KALETRA® (lopinavir/ritonavir) is contraindicated in patients with previously demonstrated clinically significant hypersensitivity (e.g., toxic epidermal necrolysis, Stevens-Johnson syndrome, erythema multiforme) to any of its ingredients, including ritonavir.
- Co-administration of KALETRA is contraindicated with drugs that are highly dependent on CYP3A for clearance and for which elevated plasma concentrations are associated with serious and/or life-threatening reactions.
- Co-administration of KALETRA is contraindicated with potent CYP3A inducers where significantly reduced lopinavir plasma concentrations may be associated with the potential for loss of virologic response and possible resistance and cross-resistance. These drugs are listed in Table 3.

[See table 3 above]

Table 3. Drugs That are Contraindicated with KALETRA

Drug Class	Drugs Within Class That are Contraindicated with KALETRA	Clinical Comments
Alpha 1- Adrenoreceptor Antagonist	Alfuzosin	Potentially increased alfuzosin concentrations can result in hypotension.
Antimycobacterial	Rifampin	May lead to loss of virologic response and possible resistance to KALETRA or to the class of protease inhibitors or other co-administered antiretroviral agents *[see Drug Interactions (7)]*.
Ergot Derivatives	Dihydroergotamine, ergotamine, methylergonovine	Potential for acute ergot toxicity characterized by peripheral vasospasm and ischemia of the extremities and other tissues.
GI Motility Agent	Cisapride	Potential for cardiac arrhythmias.
Herbal Products	St. John's Wort (hypericum perforatum)	May lead to loss of virologic response and possible resistance to KALETRA or to the class of protease inhibitors.
HMG-CoA Reductase Inhibitors	Lovastatin, simvastatin	Potential for myopathy including rhabdomyolysis.
PDE5 Enzyme Inhibitor	Sildenafil[a] (Revatio®) when used for the treatment of pulmonary arterial hypertension	A safe and effective dose has not been established when used with KALETRA. There is an increased potential for sildenafil-associated adverse events, including visual abnormalities, hypotension, prolonged erection, and syncope *[see Drug Interactions (7)]*.
Neuroleptic	Pimozide	Potential for cardiac arrhythmias.
Sedative/Hypnotics	Triazolam; orally administered midazolam[b]	Prolonged or increased sedation or respiratory depression.

[a] see *Drug Interactions (7)*, *Table 9* for co-administration of sildenafil in patients with erectile dysfunction.
[b] see *Drug Interactions (7)*, *Table 9* for parenterally administered midazolam.

5 WARNINGS AND PRECAUTIONS

5.1 Drug Interactions - CYP3A Enzyme Inhibition

KALETRA is a CYP3A inhibitor. Initiating treatment with KALETRA in patients receiving medications metabolized by CYP3A or initiating medications metabolized by CYP3A in patients already maintained on KALETRA may result in increased plasma concentrations of concomitant medications. Higher plasma concentrations of concomitant medications can result in increased or prolonged therapeutic or adverse effects, potentially leading to severe, life-threatening or fatal events. The potential for drug-drug interactions must be considered prior to and during therapy with KALETRA. Review of other medications taken by patients and monitoring of patients for adverse effects is recommended during therapy with KALETRA.

See Tables 3 and 9 for listing of drugs that are contraindicated for use with KALETRA due to potentially life-threatening adverse events, significant drug interactions, or loss of virologic activity *[see Contraindications (4)* and *Drug Interactions (7)]*.

5.2 Toxicity in Preterm Neonates

KALETRA oral solution contains the excipients alcohol (42.4% v/v) and propylene glycol (15.3% w/v). When administered concomitantly with propylene glycol, ethanol competitively inhibits the metabolism of propylene glycol, which may lead to elevated concentrations. Preterm neonates may be at increased risk of propylene glycol-associated adverse events due to diminished ability to metabolize propylene glycol, thereby leading to accumulation and potential adverse events. Postmarketing life-threatening cases of cardiac toxicity (including complete AV block, bradycardia, and cardiomyopathy), lactic acidosis, acute renal failure, CNS depression and respiratory complications leading to death have been reported, predominantly in preterm neonates receiving KALETRA oral solution.

KALETRA oral solution should not be used in preterm neonates in the immediate postnatal period because of possible toxicities. A safe and effective dose of KALETRA oral solution in this patient population has not been established. However, if the benefit of using KALETRA oral solution to treat HIV infection in infants immediately after birth outweighs the potential risks, infants should be monitored closely for increases in serum osmolality and serum creatinine, and for toxicity related to KALETRA oral solution including: hyperosmolality, with or without lactic acidosis, renal toxicity, CNS depression (including stupor, coma, and apnea), seizures, hypotonia, cardiac arrhythmias and ECG changes, and hemolysis. Total amounts of alcohol and propylene glycol from all medicines that are to be given to infants should be taken into account in order to avoid toxicity from these excipients *[see Dosage and Administration (2.2)* and *Overdosage (10)]*.

5.3 Pancreatitis

Pancreatitis has been observed in patients receiving KALETRA® (lopinavir/ritonavir) therapy, including those who developed marked triglyceride elevations. In some cases, fatalities have been observed. Although a causal relationship to KALETRA has not been established, marked triglyceride elevations are a risk factor for development of pancreatitis *[see Warnings and Precautions (5.9)]*. Patients with advanced HIV-1 disease may be at increased risk of elevated triglycerides and pancreatitis, and patients with a history of pancreatitis may be at increased risk for recurrence during KALETRA therapy.

Pancreatitis should be considered if clinical symptoms (nausea, vomiting, abdominal pain) or abnormalities in laboratory values (such as increased serum lipase or amylase values) suggestive of pancreatitis occur. Patients who exhibit these signs or symptoms should be evaluated and KALETRA and/or other antiretroviral therapy should be suspended as clinically appropriate.

5.4 Hepatotoxicity

Patients with underlying hepatitis B or C or marked elevations in transaminase prior to treatment may be at increased risk for developing or worsening of transaminase elevations or hepatic decompensation with use of KALETRA.

There have been postmarketing reports of hepatic dysfunction, including some fatalities. These have generally occurred in patients with advanced HIV-1 disease taking multiple concomitant medications in the setting of underlying chronic hepatitis or cirrhosis. A causal relationship with KALETRA therapy has not been established.

Elevated transaminases with or without elevated bilirubin levels have been reported in HIV-1 mono-infected and uninfected patients as early as 7 days after the initiation of KALETRA in conjunction with other antiretroviral agents. In some cases, the hepatic dysfunction was serious; however, a definitive causal relationship with KALETRA therapy has not been established.

Appropriate laboratory testing should be conducted prior to initiating therapy with KALETRA and patients should be monitored closely during treatment. Increased AST/ALT monitoring should be considered in the patients with underlying chronic hepatitis or cirrhosis, especially during the first several months of KALETRA treatment *[see Use in Specific Populations (8.6)]*.

5.5 QT Interval Prolongation

Postmarketing cases of QT interval prolongation and torsade de pointes have been reported although causality of KALETRA could not be established. Avoid use in patients with congenital long QT syndrome, those with hypokalemia, and with other drugs that prolong the QT interval *[see Clinical Pharmacology (12.3)]*.

5.6 PR Interval Prolongation

Lopinavir/ritonavir prolongs the PR interval in some patients. Cases of second or third degree atrioventricular block have been reported. KALETRA should be used with caution in patients with underlying structural heart disease, preexisting conduction system abnormalities, ischemic heart disease or cardiomyopathies, as these patients may be at increased risk for developing cardiac conduction abnormalities.

The impact on the PR interval of co-administration of KALETRA with other drugs that prolong the PR interval (including calcium channel blockers, beta-adrenergic blockers, digoxin and atazanavir) has not been evaluated. As a result, co-administration of KALETRA with these drugs should be undertaken with caution, particularly with those drugs metabolized by CYP3A. Clinical monitoring is recommended *[see Clinical Pharmacology (12.3)]*.

5.7 Diabetes Mellitus/Hyperglycemia

New onset diabetes mellitus, exacerbation of pre-existing diabetes mellitus, and hyperglycemia have been reported during post-marketing surveillance in HIV-1 infected patients receiving protease inhibitor therapy. Some patients required either initiation or dose adjustments of insulin or oral hypoglycemic agents for treatment of these events. In some cases, diabetic ketoacidosis has occurred. In those patients who discontinued protease inhibitor therapy, hyperglycemia persisted in some cases. Because these events have been reported voluntarily during clinical practice, estimates of frequency cannot be made and a causal relationship between protease inhibitor therapy and these events has not been established.

5.8 Immune Reconstitution Syndrome

Immune reconstitution syndrome has been reported in patients treated with combination antiretroviral therapy, including KALETRA. During the initial phase of combination antiretroviral treatment, patients whose immune system responds may develop an inflammatory response to indolent or residual opportunistic infections (such as *Mycobacterium avium* infection, cytomegalovirus, *Pneumocystis jirovecii* pneumonia [PCP], or tuberculosis) which may necessitate further evaluation and treatment.

Autoimmune disorders (such as Graves' disease, polymyositis, and Guillain-Barré syndrome) have also been reported to occur in the setting of immune reconstitution, however, the time to onset is more variable, and can occur many months after initiation of treatment.

5.9 Lipid Elevations

Treatment with KALETRA has resulted in large increases in the concentration of total cholesterol and triglycerides *[see Adverse Reactions (6.1)]*. Triglyceride and cholesterol testing should be performed prior to initiating KALETRA therapy and at periodic intervals during therapy. Lipid disorders should be managed as clinically appropriate, taking

Information on the AbbVie, Inc. products listed on these pages is from the prescribing information in use as of July 31, 2013. For more information, please visit rxabbvie.com or call 1-800-633-9110.

into account any potential drug-drug interactions with KALETRA and HMG-CoA reductase inhibitors *[see Contraindications (4) and Drug Interactions (7.3)]*.

5.10 Fat Redistribution

Redistribution/accumulation of body fat including central obesity, dorsocervical fat enlargement (buffalo hump), peripheral wasting, facial wasting, breast enlargement, and "cushingoid appearance" have been observed in patients receiving antiretroviral therapy. The mechanism and long-term consequences of these events are currently unknown. A causal relationship has not been established.

5.11 Patients with Hemophilia

Increased bleeding, including spontaneous skin hematomas and hemarthrosis have been reported in patients with hemophilia type A and B treated with protease inhibitors. In some patients additional factor VIII was given. In more than half of the reported cases, treatment with protease inhibitors was continued or reintroduced. A causal relationship between protease inhibitor therapy and these events has not been established.

5.12 Resistance/Cross-resistance

Because the potential for HIV cross-resistance among protease inhibitors has not been fully explored in KALETRA-treated patients, it is unknown what effect therapy with KALETRA will have on the activity of subsequently administered protease inhibitors *[see Microbiology (12.4)]*.

6 ADVERSE REACTIONS

The following adverse reactions are discussed in greater detail in other sections of the labeling.

- QT Interval Prolongation, PR Interval Prolongation *[see Warnings and Precautions (5.5, 5.6)]*
- Drug Interactions *[see Warnings and Precautions (5.1)]*
- Pancreatitis *[see Warnings and Precautions (5.3)]*
- Hepatotoxicity *[see Warnings and Precautions (5.4)]*

Because clinical trials are conducted under widely varying conditions, adverse reactions rates observed in the clinical trials of a drug cannot be directly compared to rates in the clinical trials of another drug and may not reflect the rates observed in clinical practice.

6.1 Adult Clinical Trial Experience

The safety profile of KALETRA in adults is primarily based on 1,964 HIV-1 infected patients in clinical trials.

The most common adverse reaction was diarrhea, which was generally of mild to moderate severity.

In study 730, the incidence of diarrhea of any severity during 48 weeks of therapy was 60% in patients receiving KALETRA tablets once daily compared to 57% in patients receiving KALETRA tablets twice daily. More patients receiving KALETRA tablets once daily (14, 4.2%) had ongoing diarrhea at the time of discontinuation as compared to patients receiving KALETRA tablets twice daily (6, 1.8%). In study 730, discontinuations due to any adverse reaction were 4.8% in patients receiving KALETRA tablets once daily as compared to 3% in patients receiving KALETRA tablets twice daily. In study 802, the incidence of diarrhea of any severity during 48 weeks of therapy was 50% in patients receiving KALETRA tablets once daily compared to 39% in patients receiving KALETRA tablets twice daily. Moderate or severe drug-related diarrhea occurred in 14% of patients receiving KALETRA tablets once daily as compared to 11% in patients receiving KALETRA tablets twice daily. At the time of discontinuation, 19 (6.3%) patients receiving KALETRA tablets once daily had ongoing diarrhea, as compared to 11 (3.7%) patients receiving KALETRA tablets twice daily. Discontinuations due to any adverse reaction occurred in 4.3% of patients receiving KALETRA tablets once daily compared to 7.0% in patients receiving KALETRA tablets twice daily. In study 863, discontinuations of randomized therapy due to adverse reactions were 3.4% in KALETRA-treated and 3.7% in nelfinavir-treated patients.

Treatment-emergent clinical adverse reactions of moderate or severe intensity in ≥ 2% of patients treated with combination therapy for up to 48 weeks (Studies 863 and 730) and for up to 360 weeks (Study 720) are presented in Table 4 (treatment-naïve patients); and for up to 48 weeks (Studies 888 and 802), 84 weeks (Study 957) and 144 weeks (Study 765) in Table 5 (protease inhibitor-experienced patients).

[See table 4 above]

[See table 5 at top of next page]

Less Common Adverse Reactions

Treatment-emergent adverse reactions occurring in less than 2% of adult patients receiving KALETRA in the clinical trials supporting approval and of at least moderate intensity are listed below by system organ class.

Blood and Lymphatic System Disorders

Anemia, leukopenia, lymphadenopathy, neutropenia, and splenomegaly.

Table 4. Percentage of Adult Patients with Selected Treatment-Emergent[1] Adverse Reactions of Moderate or Severe Intensity Reported in ≥ 2% of Adult Antiretroviral-Naïve Patients

	Study 863 (48 Weeks)		Study 720 (360 Weeks)	Study 730 (48 Weeks)	
	KALETRA 400/100 mg Twice Daily + d4T + 3TC (N = 326)	Nelfinavir 750 mg Three Times Daily + d4T + 3TC (N = 327)	KALETRA Twice Daily[2] + d4T + 3TC (N = 100)	KALETRA 800/200 mg Once Daily + TDF +FTC (N=333)	KALETRA 400/100 mg Twice Daily + TDF +FTC (N=331)
Endocrine Disorders					
Hypogonadism	0%	0%	2%	0%	0%
Gastrointestinal Disorders					
Diarrhea	16%	17%	28%	17%	15%
Nausea	7%	5%	16%	7%	5%
Vomiting	2%	2%	6%	3%	4%
Abdominal Pain	4%	3%	11%	1%	1%
Dyspepsia	2%	<1%	6%	0%	0%
Flatulence	2%	1%	4%	1%	1%
General Disorders and Administration Site Conditions					
Asthenia	4%	3%	9%	<1%	<1%
Infections and Infestations					
Bronchitis	0%	0%	2%	0%	<1%
Investigations					
Weight Decreased	1%	<1%	2%	0%	<1%
Metabolism and Nutrition Disorders					
Anorexia	1%	<1%	2%	<1%	1%
Musculoskeletal and Connective Tissue Disorders					
Myalgia	1%	1%	2%	0%	0%
Nervous System Disorders					
Headache	2%	2%	6%	2%	2%
Paresthesia	1%	1%	2%	0%	0%
Psychiatric Disorders					
Insomnia	2%	1%	3%	1%	0%
Depression	1%	2%	0%	0%	0%
Libido Decreased	<1%	<1%	2%	0%	<1%
Skin and Subcutaneous Tissue Disorders					
Rash	1%	2%	5%	<1%	1%
Vascular Disorders					
Vasodilation	0%	0%	3%	0%	0%

[1] Includes adverse reactions of possible or probable relationship to study drug.

[2] Includes adverse reaction data from dose group I (200/100 mg twice daily [N = 16] and 400/100 mg twice daily [N = 16]) and dose group II (400/100 mg twice daily [N = 35] and 400/200 mg twice daily [N = 33]). Within dosing groups, moderate to severe nausea of probable/possible relationship to KALETRA occurred at a higher rate in the 400/200 mg dose arm compared to the 400/100 mg dose arm in group II.

Definitions: d4T = Stavudine; 3TC = Lamivudine; TDF = Tenofovir Disoproxil Fumarate; FTC = Emtricitabine

Cardiac Disorders

Angina pectoris, atrial fibrillation, atrioventricular block, myocardial infarction, palpitations, and tricuspid valve incompetence.

Ear and Labyrinth Disorders

Hyperacusis, tinnitus, and vertigo.

Endocrine Disorders

Cushing's syndrome and hypothyroidism.

Table 5. Percentage of Adult Patients with Selected Treatment-Emergent[1] Adverse Reactions of Moderate or Severe Intensity Reported in ≥ 2% of Adult Protease Inhibitor-Experienced Patients

	Study 888 (48 Weeks)		Study 957[2] and Study 765[3] (84-144 Weeks)	Study 802 (48 Weeks)	
	KALETRA 400/ 100 mg Twice Daily + NVP + NRTIs (N = 148)	Investigator-Selected Protease Inhibitor(s) + NVP + NRTIs (N = 140)	KALETRA Twice Daily + NNRTI + NRTIs (N = 127)	KALETRA 800/ 200 mg Once Daily +NRTIs (N=300)	KALETRA 400/100 mg Twice Daily + NRTIs (N=299)
Gastrointestinal Disorders					
Diarrhea	7%	9%	23%	14%	11%
Nausea	7%	16%	5%	3%	7%
Vomiting	4%	12%	2%	2%	3%
Abdominal Pain	2%	2%	4%	2%	<1%
Abdominal Pain Upper	N/A	N/A	N/A	1%	2%
Dyspepsia	1%	1%	2%	1%	<1%
Flatulence	1%	2%	2%	1%	1%
Dysphasia	2%	1%	0%	0%	0%
General Disorders and Administration Site Conditions					
Asthenia	3%	6%	9%	<1%	<1%
Pyrexia	2%	1%	2%	0%	<1%
Chills	2%	0%	0%	0%	0%
Investigations					
Weight Decreased	0%	1%	3%	<1%	<1%
Metabolism and Nutrition Disorders					
Anorexia	1%	3%	0%	0%	1%
Musculoskeletal and Connective Tissue Disorders					
Myalgia	1%	1%	2%	0%	0%
Nervous System Disorders					
Headache	2%	3%	2%	<1%	0%
Paresthesia	0%	1%	2%	0%	0%
Psychiatric Disorders					
Depression	1%	2%	3%	<1%	0%
Insomnia	0%	2%	2%	0%	<1%
Skin and Subcutaneous Tissue Disorders					
Rash	2%	1%	2%	0%	0%
Vascular Disorders					
Hypertension	0%	0%	2%	0%	0%

[1] Includes adverse reactions of possible or probable relationship to study drug.
[2] Includes adverse reaction data from patients receiving 400/100 mg twice daily (n = 29) or 533/133 mg twice daily (n = 28) for 84 weeks. Patients received KALETRA in combination with NRTIs and efavirenz.
[3] Includes adverse reaction data from patients receiving 400/100 mg twice daily (n = 36) or 400/200 mg twice daily (n = 34) for 144 weeks. Patients received KALETRA in combination with NRTIs and nevirapine.
Definitions: NVP = Nevirapine; NRTI = Nucleoside Reverse Transcriptase Inhibitors; NNRTI = Non-nucleoside Reverse Transcriptase Inhibitors

Eye Disorders
Eye disorder and visual disturbance.
Gastrointestinal Disorders
Abdominal discomfort, abdominal distension, abdomen pain lower, constipation, duodenitis, dry mouth, enteritis, enterocolitis, enterocolitis hemorrhagic, eructation, esophagitis, fecal incontinence, gastric disorder, gastric ulcer, gastritis, gastroesophageal reflux disease, hemorrhoids, mouth ulceration, pancreatitis, periodontitis, rectal hemorrhage, stomach discomfort, and stomatitis.
General Disorders and Administration Site Conditions
Chest pain, cyst, drug interaction, edema, edema peripheral, face edema, fatigue, hypertrophy, and malaise.
Hepatobiliary Disorders
Cholangitis, cholecystitis, cytolytic hepatitis, hepatic steatosis, hepatitis, hepatomegaly, jaundice, and liver tenderness.
Immune System Disorders
Drug hypersensitivity, hypersensitivity, and immune reconstitution syndrome.
Infections and Infestations
Bacterial infection, bronchopneumonia, cellulitis, folliculitis, furuncle, gastroenteritis, influenza, otitis media, perineal abscess, pharyngitis, rhinitis, sialoadenitis, sinusitis, and viral infection.
Investigations
Drug level increased, glucose tolerance decreased, and weight increased.
Metabolism and Nutrition Disorders
Decreased appetite, dehydration, diabetes mellitus, hypovitaminosis, increased appetite, lactic acidosis, lipomatosis, and obesity.
Musculoskeletal and Connective Tissue Disorders
Arthralgia, arthropathy, back pain, muscular weakness, osteoarthritis, osteonecrosis, and pain in extremity.
Neoplasms Benign, Malignant and Unspecified (incl Cysts and Polyps)
Benign neoplasm of skin, lipoma, and neoplasm.
Nervous System Disorders
Ageusia, amnesia, ataxia, balance disorder, cerebral infarction, convulsion, dizziness, dysgeusia, dyskinesia, encephalopathy, extrapyramidal disorder, facial palsy, hypertonia, migraine, neuropathy, neuropathy peripheral, somnolence, and tremor.
Psychiatric Disorders
Abnormal dreams, affect lability, agitation, anxiety, apathy, confusional state, disorientation, mood swings, nervousness, and thinking abnormal.
Renal and Urinary Disorders
Hematuria, nephritis, nephrolithiasis, renal disorder, urine abnormality, and urine odor abnormal.
Reproductive System and Breast Disorders
Breast enlargement, ejaculation disorder, erectile dysfunction, gynecomastia, and menorrhagia.
Respiratory, Thoracic and Mediastinal Disorders
Asthma, cough, dyspnea, and pulmonary edema.
Skin and Subcutaneous Tissue Disorders
Acne, alopecia, dermatitis acneiform, dermatitis allergic, dermatitis exfoliative, dry skin, eczema, hyperhidrosis, idiopathic capillaritis, nail disorder, pruritis, rash generalized, rash maculo-papular, seborrhea, skin discoloration, skin hypertrophy, skin striae, skin ulcer, and swelling face.
Vascular Disorders
Deep vein thrombosis, orthostatic hypotension, thrombophlebitis, varicose vein, and vasculitis.
Laboratory Abnormalities
The percentages of adult patients treated with combination therapy with Grade 3-4 laboratory abnormalities are presented in Table 6 (treatment-naïve patients) and Table 7 (treatment-experienced patients).
[See table 6 at top of next page]
[See table 7 on pages 476 and 477]

6.2 Pediatric Clinical Trial Experience

KALETRA oral solution dosed up to 300/75 mg/m^2 has been studied in 100 pediatric patients 6 months to 12 years of age. The adverse reaction profile seen during Study 940 was similar to that for adult patients.

Dysgeusia (22%), vomiting (21%), and diarrhea (12%) were the most common adverse reactions of any severity reported in pediatric patients treated with combination therapy for up to 48 weeks in Study 940. A total of 8 patients experienced adverse reactions of moderate to severe intensity. The adverse reactions meeting these criteria and reported for the 8 subjects include: hypersensitivity (characterized by fever, rash and jaundice), pyrexia, viral infection, constipation, hepatomegaly, pancreatitis, vomiting, alanine aminotransferase increased, dry skin, rash, and dysgeusia. Rash was the only event of those listed that occurred in 2 or more subjects (N = 3).

KALETRA oral solution dosed at 300/75 mg/m^2 has been studied in 31 pediatric patients 14 days to 6 months of age. The adverse reaction profile in Study 1030 was similar to that observed in older children and adults. No adverse reaction was reported in greater than 10% of subjects. Adverse drug reactions of moderate to severe intensity occurring in 2 or more subjects included decreased neutrophil count (N=3), anemia (N=2), high potassium (N=2), and low sodium (N=2).

Information on the AbbVie, Inc. products listed on these pages is from the prescribing information in use as of July 31, 2013. For more information, please visit rxabbvie.com or call 1-800-633-9110.

Table 6. Grade 3-4 Laboratory Abnormalities Reported in ≥ 2% of Adult Antiretroviral-Naïve Patients

		Study 863 (48 Weeks)		Study 720 (360 Weeks)	Study 730 (48 Weeks)	
Variable	**Limit[1]**	**KALETRA 400/100 mg Twice Daily + d4T +3TC (N = 326)**	**Nelfinavir 750 mg Three Times Daily + d4T + 3TC (N = 327)**	**KALETRA Twice Daily + d4T + 3TC (N = 100)**	**KALETRA Once Daily + TDF +FTC (N=333)**	**KALETRA Twice Daily + TDF +FTC (N=331)**
Chemistry	**High**					
Glucose	> 250 mg/dL	2%	2%	4%	0%	<1%
Uric Acid	> 12 mg/dL	2%	2%	5%	<1%	1%
SGOT/AST[2]	> 180 U/L	2%	4%	10%	1%	2%
SGPT/ALT[2]	>215 U/L	4%	4%	11%	1%	1%
GGT	>300 U/L	N/A	N/A	10%	N/A	N/A
Total Cholesterol	>300 mg/dL	9%	5%	27%	4%	3%
Triglycerides	>750 mg/dL	9%	1%	29%	3%	6%
Amylase	>2 × ULN	3%	2%	4%	N/A	N/A
Lipase	>2 × ULN	N/A	N/A	N/A	3%	5%
Chemistry	**Low**					
Calculated Creatinine Clearance	<50 mL/min	N/A	N/A	N/A	2%	2%
Hematology	**Low**					
Neutrophils	<0.75 × 10^9/L	1%	3%	5%	2%	1%

[1] ULN = upper limit of the normal range; N/A = Not Applicable.
[2] Criterion for Study 730 was >5x ULN (AST/ALT).

Table 7. Grade 3-4 Laboratory Abnormalities Reported in ≥ 2% of Adult Protease Inhibitor-Experienced Patients

		Study 888 (48 Weeks)		Study 957[2] and Study 765[3] (84-144 Weeks)	Study 802 (48 Weeks)	
Variable	**Limit[1]**	**KALETRA 400/100 mg Twice Daily + NVP + NRTIs (N = 148)**	**Investigator-Selected Protease Inhibitor(s) + NVP + NRTIs (N = 140)**	**KALETRA Twice Daily + NNRTI + NRTIs (N = 127)**	**KALETRA 800/200 mg Once Daily +NRTIs (N=300)**	**KALETRA 400/100 mg Twice Daily +NRTIs (N=299)**
Chemistry	**High**					
Glucose	>250 mg/dL	1%	2%	5%	2%	2%
Total Bilirubin	>3.48 mg/dL	1%	3%	1%	1%	1%
SGOT/AST[4]	>180 U/L	5%	11%	8%	3%	2%
SGPT/ALT[4]	>215 U/L	6%	13%	10%	2%	2%
GGT	>300 U/L	N/A	N/A	29%	N/A	N/A
Total Cholesterol	>300 mg/dL	20%	21%	39%	6%	7%
Triglycerides	>750 mg/dL	25%	21%	36%	5%	6%
Amylase	>2 × ULN	4%	8%	8%	4%	4%
Lipase	>2 × ULN	N/A	N/A	N/A	4%	1%
Creatine Phosphokinase	>4 × ULN	N/A	N/A	N/A	4%	5%
Chemistry	**Low**					
Calculated Creatinine Clearance	<50 mL/min	N/A	N/A	N/A	3%	3%

(Table continued on next page)

KALETRA oral solution and soft gelatin capsules dosed at higher than recommended doses including 400/100 mg/m² (without concomitant NNRTI) and 480/120 mg/m² (with concomitant NNRTI) have been studied in 26 pediatric patients 7 to 18 years of age in Study 1038. Patients also had saquinavir mesylate added to their regimen at Week 4. Rash (12%), blood cholesterol abnormal (12%) and blood triglycerides abnormal (12%) were the only adverse reactions reported in greater than 10% of subjects. Adverse drug reactions of moderate to severe intensity occurring in 2 or more subjects included rash (N=3), blood triglycerides abnormal (N=3), and electrocardiogram QT prolonged (N=2). Both subjects with QT prolongation had additional predisposing conditions such as electrolyte abnormalities, concomitant medications, or pre-existing cardiac abnormalities.

Laboratory Abnormalities

The percentages of pediatric patients treated with combination therapy including KALETRA with Grade 3-4 laboratory abnormalities are presented in Table 8.

Table 8. Grade 3-4 Laboratory Abnormalities Reported in ≥ 2% Pediatric Patients in Study 940

Variable	**Limit[1]**	**KALETRA Twice Daily + RTIs (N = 100)**
Chemistry	**High**	
Sodium	> 149 mEq/L	3%
Total Bilirubin	≥ 3.0 × ULN	3%
SGOT/AST	> 180 U/L	8%
SGPT/ALT	> 215 U/L	7%
Total Cholesterol	> 300 mg/dL	3%
Amylase	> 2.5 × ULN	7%[2]
Chemistry	**Low**	
Sodium	< 130 mEq/L	3%
Hematology	**Low**	
Platelet Count	< 50 × 10^9/L	4%
Neutrophils	< 0.40 × 10^9/L	2%

[1] ULN = upper limit of the normal range.
[2] Subjects with Grade 3-4 amylase confirmed by elevations in pancreatic amylase.

6.3 Postmarketing Experience

The following adverse reactions have been reported during postmarketing use of KALETRA® (lopinavir/ritonavir). Because these reactions are reported voluntarily from a population of unknown size, it is not possible to reliably estimate their frequency or establish a causal relationship to KALETRA exposure.

Body as a Whole

Redistribution/accumulation of body fat has been reported *[see Warnings and Precautions (5.10)].*

Cardiovascular

Bradyarrhythmias. First-degree AV block, second-degree AV block, third-degree AV block, QTc interval prolongation, torsades (torsade) de pointes *[see Warnings and Precautions (5.5, 5.6)].*

Skin and Appendages

Toxic epidermal necrolysis (TEN), Stevens-Johnson syndrome and erythema multiforme.

7 DRUG INTERACTIONS

See also Contraindications (4), Warnings and Precautions (5.1), Clinical Pharmacology (12.3)

7.1 Potential for KALETRA to Affect Other Drugs

Lopinavir/ritonavir is an inhibitor of CYP3A and may increase plasma concentrations of agents that are primarily metabolized by CYP3A. Agents that are extensively metabolized by CYP3A and have high first pass metabolism appear to be the most susceptible to large increases in AUC (> 3-fold) when co-administered with KALETRA. Thus, coadministration of KALETRA with drugs highly dependent on CYP3A for clearance and for which elevated plasma concentrations are associated with serious and/or life-threatening events is contraindicated. Co-administration with other CYP3A substrates may require a dose adjustment or additional monitoring as shown in Table 9.

Additionally, KALETRA induces glucuronidation.

7.2 Potential for Other Drugs to Affect Lopinavir

Lopinavir/ritonavir is a CYP3A substrate; therefore, drugs that induce CYP3A may decrease lopinavir plasma concentrations and reduce KALETRA's therapeutic effect. Although not observed in the KALETRA/ketoconazole drug interaction study, co-administration of KALETRA and other drugs that inhibit CYP3A may increase lopinavir plasma concentrations.

7.3 Established and Other Potentially Significant Drug Interactions

Table 9 provides a listing of established or potentially clinically significant drug interactions. Alteration in dose or

Table 7 *(cont.)*. Grade 3-4 Laboratory Abnormalities Reported in ≥ 2% of Adult Protease Inhibitor-Experienced Patients

		Study 888 (48 Weeks)		Study 957[2] and Study 765[3] (84-144 Weeks)	Study 802 (48 Weeks)	
Variable	**Limit[1]**	**KALETRA 400/100 mg Twice Daily + NVP + NRTIs (N = 148)**	**Investigator-Selected Protease Inhibitor(s) + NVP + NRTIs (N = 140)**	**KALETRA Twice Daily + NNRTI + NRTIs (N = 127)**	**KALETRA 800/200 mg Once Daily +NRTIs (N=300)**	**KALETRA 400/100 mg Twice Daily +NRTIs (N=299)**
Inorganic Phosphorus	<1.5 mg/dL	1%	0%	2%	1%	<1%
Hematology	**Low**					
Neutrophils	<0.75 × 10^9/L	1%	2%	4%	3%	4%
Hemoglobin	<80 g/L	1%	1%	1%	1%	2%

[1] ULN = upper limit of the normal range; N/A = Not Applicable.
[2] Includes clinical laboratory data from patients receiving 400/100 mg twice daily (n = 29) or 533/133 mg twice daily (n = 28) for 84 weeks. Patients received KALETRA in combination with NRTIs and efavirenz.
[3] Includes clinical laboratory data from patients receiving 400/100 mg twice daily (n = 36) or 400/200 mg twice daily (n = 34) for 144 weeks. Patients received KALETRA in combination with NRTIs and nevirapine.
[4] Criterion for Study 802 was >5x ULN (AST/ALT).

Table 9. Established and Other Potentially Significant Drug Interactions

Concomitant Drug Class: Drug Name	Effect on Concentration of Lopinavir or Concomitant Drug	Clinical Comments
	HIV-1 Antiviral Agents	
HIV-1 Protease Inhibitor: fosamprenavir/ritonavir	↓ amprenavir ↓ lopinavir	An increased rate of adverse reactions has been observed with co-administration of these medications. Appropriate doses of the combinations with respect to safety and efficacy have not been established.
HIV-1 Protease Inhibitor: indinavir*	↑ indinavir	Decrease indinavir dose to 600 mg twice daily, when co-administered with KALETRA 400/100 mg twice daily *[see Clinical Pharmacology (12.3)]*. KALETRA once daily has not been studied in combination with indinavir.
HIV-1 Protease Inhibitor: nelfinavir*	↑ nelfinavir ↑ M8 metabolite of nelfinavir ↓ lopinavir	KALETRA should not be administered once daily in combination with nelfinavir *[see Dosage and Administration (2.1) and Clinical Pharmacology (12.3)]*.
HIV-1 Protease Inhibitor: ritonavir*	↑ lopinavir	Appropriate doses of additional ritonavir in combination with KALETRA with respect to safety and efficacy have not been established.
HIV-1 Protease Inhibitor: saquinavir*	↑ saquinavir	The saquinavir dose is 1000 mg twice daily, when co-administered with KALETRA 400/100 mg twice daily. KALETRA once daily has not been studied in combination with saquinavir.
HIV-1 Protease Inhibitor: tipranavir	↓ lopinavir AUC and C_{min}	KALETRA should not be administered with tipranavir (500 mg twice daily) co-administered with ritonavir (200 mg twice daily).
HIV CCR5 – Antagonist: maraviroc	↑ maraviroc	Concurrent administration of maraviroc with KALETRA will increase plasma levels of maraviroc. When co-administered, patients should receive 150 mg twice daily of maraviroc. For further details see complete prescribing information for Selzentry® (maraviroc).
Non-nucleoside Reverse Transcriptase Inhibitors: efavirenz*, nevirapine*	↓ lopinavir	KALETRA dose increase is recommended in all patients *[see Dosage and Administration (2.1) and Clinical Pharmacology (12.3)]*. Increasing the dose of KALETRA tablets to 500/125 mg (given as two 200/50 mg tablets and one 100/25 mg tablet) twice daily co-administered with efavirenz resulted in similar lopinavir concentrations compared to KALETRA tablets 400/100 mg (given as two 200/50 mg tablets) twice daily without efavirenz. Increasing the dose of KALETRA tablets to 600/150 mg (given as three 200/50 mg tablets) twice daily co-administered with efavirenz resulted in significantly higher lopinavir plasma concentrations compared to KALETRA tablets 400/100 mg twice daily without efavirenz. KALETRA should not be administered once daily in combination with efavirenz or nevirapine *[see Dosage and Administration (2.1) and Clinical Pharmacology (12.3)]*.

(Table continued on next page)

regimen may be recommended based on drug interaction studies or predicted interaction *[see Clinical Pharmacology (12.3) for magnitude of interaction]*.
[See table 9 below and on pages 478 through 481]

7.4 Drugs with No Observed or Predicted Interactions with KALETRA

Drug interaction or clinical studies reveal no clinically significant interaction between KALETRA and desipramine (CYP2D6 probe), pitavastatin, pravastatin, stavudine, lamivudine, omeprazole, raltegravir, or ranitidine.

Based on known metabolic profiles, clinically significant drug interactions are not expected between KALETRA and dapsone, trimethoprim/sulfamethoxazole, azithromycin, erythromycin, or fluconazole.

8 USE IN SPECIFIC POPULATIONS

8.1 Pregnancy

Pregnancy Category C.

Antiretroviral Pregnancy Registry: To monitor maternal-fetal outcomes of pregnant women exposed to KALETRA, an Antiretroviral Pregnancy Registry has been established. Physicians are encouraged to register patients by calling 1-800-258-4263.

Human Data:

There are no adequate and well-controlled studies in pregnant women. KALETRA should be used during pregnancy only if the potential benefit justifies the potential risk to the fetus.

Antiretroviral Pregnancy Registry: As of January 2011, the Antiretroviral Pregnancy Registry (APR) has received prospective reports of 2458 exposures to lopinavir containing regimens (738 exposed in the first trimester and 1720 exposed in the second and third trimester). Birth defects occurred in 16 of the 738 (2.2%) live births (first trimester exposure) and 41 of the 1720 (2.4%) live births (second/third trimester exposure). Among pregnant women in the U.S. reference population, the background rate of birth defects is 2.7%. There was no association between lopinavir and overall birth defects observed in the APR.

Animal Data:

No treatment-related malformations were observed when lopinavir in combination with ritonavir was administered to pregnant rats or rabbits. Embryonic and fetal developmental toxicities (early resorption, decreased fetal viability, decreased fetal body weight, increased incidence of skeletal variations and skeletal ossification delays) occurred in rats at a maternally toxic dosage. Based on AUC measurements, the drug exposures in rats at the toxic doses were approximately 0.7-fold for lopinavir and 1.8-fold for ritonavir for males and females that of the exposures in humans at the recommended therapeutic dose (400/100 mg twice daily). In a peri- and postnatal study in rats, a developmental toxicity (a decrease in survival in pups between birth and postnatal Day 21) occurred.

No embryonic and fetal developmental toxicities were observed in rabbits at a maternally toxic dosage. Based on AUC measurements, the drug exposures in rabbits at the toxic doses were approximately 0.6-fold for lopinavir and 1.0-fold for ritonavir that of the exposures in humans at the recommended therapeutic dose (400/100 mg twice daily).

8.3 Nursing Mothers

The Centers for Disease Control and Prevention recommend that HIV-1 infected mothers not breastfeed their infants to avoid risking postnatal transmission of HIV-1. Studies in rats have demonstrated that lopinavir is secreted in milk. It is not known whether lopinavir is secreted in human milk. Because of both the potential for HIV-1 transmission and the potential for serious adverse reactions in nursing infants, mothers should be instructed not to breastfeed if they are receiving KALETRA.

8.4 Pediatric Use

The safety, efficacy, and pharmacokinetic profiles of KALETRA in pediatric patients below the age of 14 days have not been established. KALETRA once daily has not been evaluated in pediatric patients.

An open-label, multi-center, dose-finding trial was performed to evaluate the pharmacokinetic profile, tolerability, safety and efficacy of KALETRA oral solution containing lopinavir 80 mg/mL and ritonavir 20 mg/mL at a dose of 300/75 mg/m^2 twice daily plus two NRTIs in HIV-infected infants ≥14 days and < 6 months of age. Results revealed that infants younger than 6 months of age generally had lower lopinavir AUC_{12} than older children (6 months to 12 years of age), however, despite the lower lopinavir drug exposure observed, antiviral activity was demonstrated as reflected in the proportion of subjects who achieved HIV-1 RNA <400 copies/mL at Week 24 *[see Adverse Reactions (6.2), Clinical Pharmacology (12.3), Clinical Studies (14.4)]*.

Information on the AbbVie, Inc. products listed on these pages is from the prescribing information in use as of July 31, 2013. For more information, please visit rxabbvie.com or call 1-800-633-9110.

Table 9 *(cont.)*. Established and Other Potentially Significant Drug Interactions

Concomitant Drug Class: Drug Name	Effect on Concentration of Lopinavir or Concomitant Drug	Clinical Comments
Non-nucleoside Reverse Transcriptase Inhibitor: delavirdine	↑ lopinavir	Appropriate doses of the combination with respect to safety and efficacy have not been established.
Nucleoside Reverse Transcriptase Inhibitor: didanosine		KALETRA tablets can be administered simultaneously with didanosine without food. For KALETRA oral solution, it is recommended that didanosine be administered on an empty stomach; therefore, didanosine should be given one hour before or two hours after KALETRA oral solution (given with food).
Nucleoside Reverse Transcriptase Inhibitor: tenofovir	↑ tenofovir	KALETRA increases tenofovir concentrations. The mechanism of this interaction is unknown. Patients receiving KALETRA and tenofovir should be monitored for adverse reactions associated with tenofovir.
Nucleoside Reverse Transcriptase Inhibitor: abacavir zidovudine	↓ abacavir ↓ zidovudine	KALETRA induces glucuronidation; therefore, KALETRA has the potential to reduce zidovudine and abacavir plasma concentrations. The clinical significance of this potential interaction is unknown.
		Other Agents
Antiarrhythmics e.g.: amiodarone, bepridil, lidocaine (systemic), quinidine	↑ antiarrhythmics	Caution is warranted and therapeutic concentration monitoring (if available) is recommended for antiarrhythmics when co-administered with KALETRA.
Anticancer Agents: vincristine, vinblastine, dasatinib, nilotinib	↑ anticancer agents	Concentrations of these drugs may be increased when co-administered with KALETRA resulting in the potential for increased adverse events usually associated with these anticancer agents. For vincristine and vinblastine, consideration should be given to temporarily withholding the ritonavir-containing antiretroviral regimen in patients who develop significant hematologic or gastrointestinal side effects when KALETRA is administered concurrently with vincristine or vinblastine. If the antiretroviral regimen must be withheld for a prolonged period, consideration should be given to initiating a revised regimen that does not include a CYP3A or P-gp inhibitor. A decrease in the dosage or an adjustment of the dosing interval of nilotinib and dasatinib may be necessary for patients requiring co-administration with strong CYP3A inhibitors such as KALETRA. Please refer to the nilotinib and dasatinib prescribing information for dosing instructions.
Anticoagulants: warfarin, rivaroxaban	↑ rivaroxaban	Concentrations of warfarin may be affected. It is recommended that INR (international normalized ratio) be monitored. Avoid concomitant use of rivaroxaban and KALETRA. Co-administration of KALETRA and rivaroxaban is expected to result in increased exposure of rivaroxaban which may lead to risk of increased bleeding.
Anticonvulsants: carbamazepine, phenobarbital, phenytoin	↓ lopinavir ↓ phenytoin	KALETRA may be less effective due to decreased lopinavir plasma concentrations in patients taking these agents concomitantly and should be used with caution. KALETRA should not be administered once daily in combination with carbamazepine, phenobarbital, or phenytoin. In addition, co-administration of phenytoin and KALETRA may cause decreases in steady-state phenytoin concentrations. Phenytoin levels should be monitored when co-administering with KALETRA.
Anticonvulsants: lamotrigine, valproate	↓ lamotrigine ↓ or ↔ valproate	Co-administration of KALETRA and lamotrigine or valproate may decrease the exposure of lamotrigine or valproate. A dose increase of lamotrigine or valproate may be needed when co-administered with KALETRA and therapeutic concentration monitoring for lamotrigine may be indicated; particularly during dosage adjustments *[see Clinical Pharmacology (12.3)]*.
Antidepressant: bupropion	↓ bupropion ↓ active metabolite, hydroxybupropion	Concurrent administration of bupropion with KALETRA may decrease plasma levels of both bupropion and its active metabolite (hydroxybupropion). Patients receiving KALETRA and bupropion concurrently should be monitored for an adequate clinical response to bupropion.

(Table continued on next page)

Safety and efficacy in pediatric patients > 6 months of age was demonstrated in a clinical trial in 100 patients. The clinical trial was an open-label, multicenter trial evaluating the pharmacokinetic profile, tolerability, safety, and efficacy of KALETRA oral solution containing lopinavir 80 mg/mL and ritonavir 20 mg/mL in 100 antiretroviral naïve and experienced pediatric patients ages 6 months to 12 years. Dose selection for patients 6 months to 12 years of age was based on the following results. The 230/57.5 mg/m^2 oral solution twice daily regimen without nevirapine and the 300/75 mg/m^2 oral solution twice daily regimen with nevirapine provided lopinavir plasma concentrations similar to those obtained in adult patients receiving the 400/100 mg twice daily regimen (without nevirapine) *[see Adverse Reactions (6.2), Clinical Pharmacology (12.3), Clinical Studies (14.4)]*.

A prospective multicenter, open-label trial evaluated the pharmacokinetic profile, tolerability, safety and efficacy of high-dose KALETRA with or without concurrent NNRTI therapy (Group 1: 400/100 mg/m^2 twice daily + ≥ 2 NRTIs; Group 2: 480/120 mg/m^2 twice daily + ≥ 1 NRTI + 1 NNRTI) in 26 children and adolescents ≥ 2 years to < 18 years of age who had failed prior therapy. Patients also had saquinavir mesylate added to their regimen. This strategy was intended to assess whether higher than approved doses of KALETRA could overcome protease inhibitor cross-resistance. High doses of KALETRA exhibited a safety profile similar to those observed in previous trials; changes in HIV-1 RNA were less than anticipated; three patients had HIV-1 RNA <400 copies/mL at Week 48. CD4+ cell count increases were noted in the eight patients who remained on treatment for 48 weeks *[see Adverse Reactions (6.2), Clinical Pharmacology (12.3)]*.

8.5 Geriatric Use

Clinical studies of KALETRA did not include sufficient numbers of subjects aged 65 and over to determine whether they respond differently from younger subjects. In general, appropriate caution should be exercised in the administration and monitoring of KALETRA in elderly patients reflecting the greater frequency of decreased hepatic, renal, or cardiac function, and of concomitant disease or other drug therapy.

8.6 Hepatic Impairment

KALETRA is principally metabolized by the liver; therefore, caution should be exercised when administering this drug to patients with hepatic impairment, because lopinavir concentrations may be increased *[see Warnings and Precautions (5.4)* and *Clinical Pharmacology (12.3)]*.

10 OVERDOSAGE

Overdoses with KALETRA oral solution have been reported. One of these reports described fatal cardiogenic shock in a 2.1 kg infant who received a single dose of 6.5 mL of KALETRA oral solution (520 mg lopinavir, approximately 10-fold above the recommended lopinavir dose) nine days prior. The following events have been reported in association with unintended overdoses in preterm neonates: complete AV block, cardiomyopathy, lactic acidosis, and acute renal failure *[see Warnings and Precautions (5.2)]*. Healthcare professionals should be aware that KALETRA oral solution is highly concentrated and therefore, should pay special attention to accurate calculation of the dose of KALETRA, transcription of the medication order, dispensing information and dosing instructions to minimize the risk for medication errors and overdose. This is especially important for infants and young children.

KALETRA oral solution contains 42.4% alcohol (v/v) and 15.3% propylene glycol (w/v). Ingestion of the product over the recommended dose by an infant or a young child could result in significant toxicity and could potentially be lethal. Human experience of acute overdosage with KALETRA is limited. Treatment of overdose with KALETRA should consist of general supportive measures including monitoring of vital signs and observation of the clinical status of the patient. There is no specific antidote for overdose with KALETRA. If indicated, elimination of unabsorbed drug should be achieved by gastric lavage. Administration of activated charcoal may also be used to aid in removal of unabsorbed drug. Since lopinavir is highly protein bound, dialysis is unlikely to be beneficial in significant removal of the drug. However, dialysis can remove both alcohol and propylene glycol in the case of overdose with KALETRA oral solution.

11 DESCRIPTION

KALETRA® (lopinavir/ritonavir) is a co-formulation of lopinavir and ritonavir. Lopinavir is an inhibitor of the HIV-1 protease. As co-formulated in KALETRA, ritonavir inhibits the CYP3A-mediated metabolism of lopinavir, thereby providing increased plasma levels of lopinavir.

Lopinavir is chemically designated as [1*S*-[1*R**,(*R**), 3*R**, 4*R**]]-*N*-[4-[[(2,6-dimethylphenoxy)acetyl]amino]-3-hydroxy-5-phenyl-1-(phenylmethyl)pentyl]tetrahydro-alpha-(1-methylethyl)-2-oxo-1(2*H*)-pyrimidineacetamide. Its molecular formula is $C_{37}H_{48}N_4O_5$, and its molecular weight is 628.80. Lopinavir is a white to light tan powder. It is freely soluble in methanol and ethanol, soluble in isopropanol and practically insoluble in water. Lopinavir has the following structural formula:

[See figure at top of third column on next page]

Ritonavir is chemically designated as 10-hydroxy-2-methyl-5-(1-methylethyl)-1- [2-(1-methylethyl)-4-thiazolyl]-3,6-dioxo-8,11-bis(phenylmethyl)-2,4,7,12-tetraazatridecan-13-oic

Table 9 *(cont.)*. Established and Other Potentially Significant Drug Interactions

Concomitant Drug Class: Drug Name	Effect on Concentration of Lopinavir or Concomitant Drug	Clinical Comments
Antidepressant: trazodone	↑ trazodone	Concomitant use of trazodone and KALETRA may increase concentrations of trazodone. Adverse reactions of nausea, dizziness, hypotension and syncope have been observed following co-administration of trazodone and ritonavir. If trazodone is used with a CYP3A4 inhibitor such as ritonavir, the combination should be used with caution and a lower dose of trazodone should be considered.
Anti-infective: clarithromycin	↑ clarithromycin	For patients with renal impairment, the following dosage adjustments should be considered: • For patients with CL_{CR} 30 to 60 mL/min the dose of clarithromycin should be reduced by 50%. • For patients with CL_{CR} < 30 mL/min the dose of clarithromycin should be decreased by 75%. No dose adjustment for patients with normal renal function is necessary.
Antifungals: ketoconazole*, itraconazole, voriconazole	↑ ketoconazole ↑ itraconazole ↓ voriconazole	High doses of ketoconazole (>200 mg/day) or itraconazole (> 200 mg/day) are not recommended. Co-administration of voriconazole with KALETRA has not been studied. However, a study has been shown that administration of voriconazole with ritonavir 100 mg every 12 hours decreased voriconazole steady-state AUC by an average of 39%; therefore, co-administration of KALETRA and voriconazole may result in decreased voriconazole concentrations and the potential for decreased voriconazole effectiveness and should be avoided, unless an assessment of the benefit/risk to the patient justifies the use of voriconazole. Otherwise, alternative antifungal therapies should be considered in these patients.
Anti-gout: colchicine	↑ colchicine	Patients with renal or hepatic impairment should not be given colchicine with KALETRA. <u>Treatment of gout flares-co-administration of colchicine in patients on KALETRA:</u> 0.6 mg (1 tablet) × 1 dose, followed by 0.3 mg (half tablet) 1 hour later. Dose to be repeated no earlier than 3 days. <u>Prophylaxis of gout flares-co-administration of colchicine in patients on KALETRA:</u> If the original colchicine regimen was 0.6 mg twice a day, the regimen should be adjusted to 0.3 mg once a day. If the original colchicine regimen was 0.6 mg once a day, the regimen should be adjusted to 0.3 mg once every other day. <u>Treatment of familial Mediterranean fever (FMF)-co-administration of colchicine in patients on KALETRA:</u> Maximum daily dose of 0.6 mg (may be given as 0.3 mg twice a day).
Antimycobacterial: rifabutin*	↑ rifabutin and rifabutin metabolite	Dosage reduction of rifabutin by at least 75% of the usual dose of 300 mg/day is recommended (i.e., a maximum dose of 150 mg every other day or three times per week). Increased monitoring for adverse reactions is warranted in patients receiving the combination. Further dosage reduction of rifabutin may be necessary.
Antimycobacterial: rifampin	↓ lopinavir	May lead to loss of virologic response and possible resistance to KALETRA or to the class of protease inhibitors or other co-administered antiretroviral agents. A study evaluated combination of rifampin 600 mg once daily, with KALETRA 800/200 mg twice daily or KALETRA 400/100 mg + ritonavir 300 mg twice daily. Pharmacokinetic and safety results from this study do not allow for a dose recommendation. Nine subjects (28%) experienced a ≥ grade 2 increase in ALT/AST, of which seven (21%) prematurely discontinued study per protocol. Based on the study design, it is not possible to determine whether the frequency or magnitude of the ALT/AST elevations observed is higher than what would be seen with rifampin alone *[see Clinical Pharmacology (12.3)* for magnitude of interaction*]*.
Antiparasitic: atovaquone	↓ atovaquone	Clinical significance is unknown; however, increase in atovaquone doses may be needed.
Benzodiazepines: parenterally administered midazolam	↑ midazolam	Midazolam is extensively metabolized by CYP3A4. Increases in the concentration of midazolam are expected to be significantly higher with oral than parenteral administration. Therefore, KALETRA should not be given with orally administered midazolam *[see Contraindications (4)]*. If KALETRA is co-administered with parenteral midazolam, close clinical monitoring for respiratory depression and/or prolonged sedation should be exercised and dosage adjustment should be considered.

(Table continued on next page)

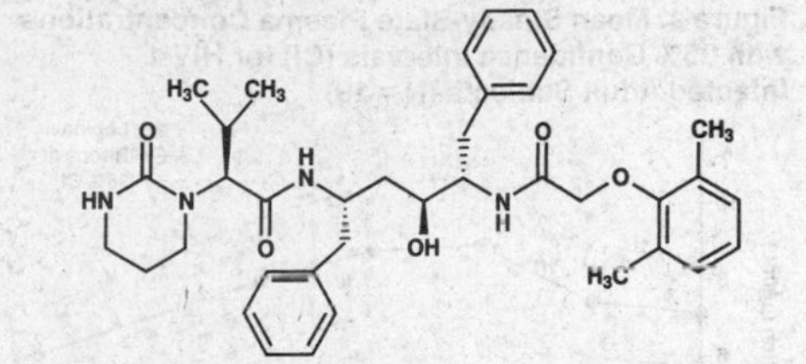

acid, 5-thiazolylmethyl ester, [5*S*-(5*R**,8*R**,10*R**,11*R**)]. Its molecular formula is $C_{37}H_{48}N_6O_5S_2$, and its molecular weight is 720.95. Ritonavir is a white to light tan powder. It is freely soluble in methanol and ethanol, soluble in isopropanol and practically insoluble in water. Ritonavir has the following structural formula:

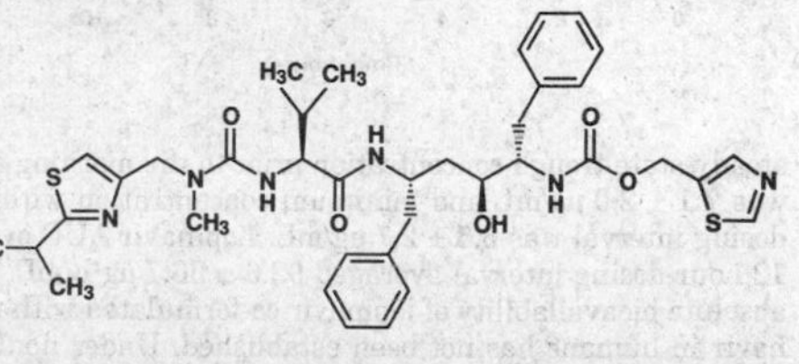

KALETRA film-coated tablets are available for oral administration in two strengths:

- Yellow tablets containing 200 mg of lopinavir and 50 mg of ritonavir
- Pale yellow tablets containing 100 mg of lopinavir and 25 mg of ritonavir.

The yellow, 200 mg lopinavir/50 mg ritonavir, tablets contain the following inactive ingredients: copovidone, sorbitan monolaurate, colloidal silicon dioxide, and sodium stearyl fumarate. The following are the ingredients in the film coating: hypromellose, titanium dioxide, polyethylene glycol 400, hydroxypropyl cellulose, talc, colloidal silicon dioxide, polyethylene glycol 3350, yellow ferric oxide E172, and polysorbate 80.

The pale yellow, 100 mg lopinavir/25 mg ritonavir, tablets contain the following inactive ingredients: copovidone, sorbitan monolaurate, colloidal silicon dioxide, and sodium stearyl fumarate. The following are the ingredients in the film coating: polyvinyl alcohol, titanium dioxide, talc, polyethylene glycol 3350, and yellow ferric oxide E172.

KALETRA oral solution is available for oral administration as 80 mg lopinavir and 20 mg ritonavir per milliliter with the following inactive ingredients: acesulfame potassium, alcohol, artificial cotton candy flavor, citric acid, glycerin, high fructose corn syrup, Magnasweet-110 flavor, menthol, natural & artificial vanilla flavor, peppermint oil, polyoxyl 40 hydrogenated castor oil, povidone, propylene glycol, saccharin sodium, sodium chloride, sodium citrate, and water. <u>KALETRA oral solution contains 42.4% alcohol (v/v).</u>

12 CLINICAL PHARMACOLOGY

12.1 Mechanism of Action

Lopinavir is an antiviral drug *[see Microbiology (12.4)]*.

12.3 Pharmacokinetics

The pharmacokinetic properties of lopinavir co-administered with ritonavir have been evaluated in healthy adult volunteers and in HIV-1 infected patients; no substantial differences were observed between the two groups. Lopinavir is essentially completely metabolized by CYP3A. Ritonavir inhibits the metabolism of lopinavir, thereby increasing the plasma levels of lopinavir. Across studies, administration of KALETRA 400/100 mg twice daily yields mean steady-state lopinavir plasma concentrations 15- to 20-fold higher than those of ritonavir in HIV-1 infected patients. The plasma levels of ritonavir are less than 7% of those obtained after the ritonavir dose of 600 mg twice daily. The *in vitro* antiviral EC_{50} of lopinavir is approximately 10-fold lower than that of ritonavir. Therefore, the antiviral activity of KALETRA is due to lopinavir.

Figure 1 displays the mean steady-state plasma concentrations of lopinavir and ritonavir after KALETRA 400/100 mg twice daily with food for 3 weeks from a pharmacokinetic study in HIV-1 infected adult subjects (n = 19).

[See figure 1 at top of next column]

Absorption

In a pharmacokinetic study in HIV-1 positive subjects (n = 19), multiple dosing with 400/100 mg KALETRA twice daily with food for 3 weeks produced a mean ± SD lopinavir peak plasma concentration (C_{max}) of 9.8 ± 3.7 μg/mL, occurring approximately 4 hours after administration. The mean

Information on the AbbVie, Inc. products listed on these pages is from the prescribing information in use as of July 31, 2013. For more information, please visit rxabbvie.com or call 1-800-633-9110.

Figure 1. Mean Steady-State Plasma Concentrations with 95% Confidence Intervals (CI) for HIV-1 Infected Adult Subjects (N = 19)

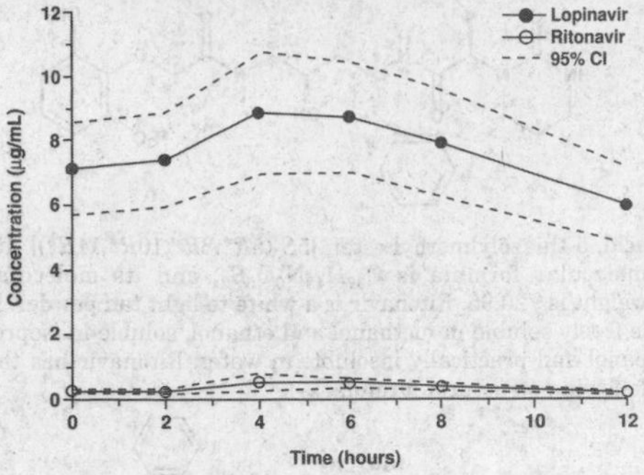

steady-state trough concentration prior to the morning dose was 7.1 ± 2.9 µg/mL and minimum concentration within a dosing interval was 5.5 ± 2.7 µg/mL. Lopinavir AUC over a 12 hour dosing interval averaged 92.6 ± 36.7 µg•h/mL. The absolute bioavailability of lopinavir co-formulated with ritonavir in humans has not been established. Under nonfasting conditions (500 kcal, 25% from fat), lopinavir concentrations were similar following administration of KALETRA co-formulated capsules and oral solution. When administered under fasting conditions, both the mean AUC and C_{max} of lopinavir were 22% lower for the KALETRA oral solution relative to the capsule formulation.

Plasma concentrations of lopinavir and ritonavir after administration of two 200/50 mg KALETRA tablets are similar to three 133.3/33.3 mg KALETRA capsules under fed conditions with less pharmacokinetic variability.

Effects of Food on Oral Absorption

KALETRA Tablets

No clinically significant changes in C_{max} and AUC were observed following administration of KALETRA tablets under fed conditions compared to fasted conditions. Relative to fasting, administration of KALETRA tablets with a moderate fat meal (500 - 682 Kcal, 23 to 25% calories from fat) increased lopinavir AUC and C_{max} by 26.9% and 17.6%, respectively. Relative to fasting, administration of KALETRA tablets with a high fat meal (872 Kcal, 56% from fat) increased lopinavir AUC by 18.9% but not C_{max}. Therefore, KALETRA tablets may be taken with or without food.

KALETRA Oral Solution

Relative to fasting, administration of KALETRA oral solution with a moderate fat meal (500 - 682 Kcal, 23 to 25% calories from fat) increased lopinavir AUC and C_{max} by 80 and 54%, respectively. Relative to fasting, administration of KALETRA oral solution with a high fat meal (872 Kcal, 56% from fat) increased lopinavir AUC and C_{max} by 130% and 56%, respectively. To enhance bioavailability and minimize pharmacokinetic variability KALETRA oral solution should be taken with food.

Distribution

At steady state, lopinavir is approximately 98-99% bound to plasma proteins. Lopinavir binds to both alpha-1-acid glycoprotein (AAG) and albumin; however, it has a higher affinity for AAG. At steady state, lopinavir protein binding remains constant over the range of observed concentrations after 400/100 mg KALETRA twice daily, and is similar between healthy volunteers and HIV-1 positive patients.

Metabolism

In vitro experiments with human hepatic microsomes indicate that lopinavir primarily undergoes oxidative metabolism. Lopinavir is extensively metabolized by the hepatic cytochrome P450 system, almost exclusively by the CYP3A isozyme. Ritonavir is a potent CYP3A inhibitor which inhibits the metabolism of lopinavir, and therefore increases plasma levels of lopinavir. A ^{14}C-lopinavir study in humans showed that 89% of the plasma radioactivity after a single 400/100 mg KALETRA dose was due to parent drug. At least 13 lopinavir oxidative metabolites have been identified in man. Ritonavir has been shown to induce metabolic enzymes, resulting in the induction of its own metabolism. Pre-dose lopinavir concentrations decline with time during multiple dosing, stabilizing after approximately 10 to 16 days.

Elimination

Following a 400/100 mg ^{14}C-lopinavir/ritonavir dose, approximately 10.4 ± 2.3% and 82.6 ± 2.5% of an administered dose of ^{14}C-lopinavir can be accounted for in urine and feces, respectively, after 8 days. Unchanged lopinavir accounted for approximately 2.2 and 19.8% of the administered dose in urine and feces, respectively. After multiple dosing, less than 3% of the lopinavir dose is excreted unchanged in the urine. The apparent oral clearance (CL/F) of lopinavir is 5.98 ± 5.75 L/hr (mean ± SD, n = 19).

Table 9 *(cont.)*. Established and Other Potentially Significant Drug Interactions

Concomitant Drug Class: Drug Name	Effect on Concentration of Lopinavir or Concomitant Drug	Clinical Comments
Contraceptive: ethinyl estradiol*	↓ ethinyl estradiol	Because contraceptive steroid concentrations may be altered when KALETRA is co-administered with oral contraceptives or with the contraceptive patch, alternative methods of nonhormonal contraception are recommended.
Corticosteroids (systemic): e.g. budesonide, dexamethasone, prednisone	↓ lopinavir ↑ glucocorticoids	Use with caution. KALETRA may be less effective due to decreased lopinavir plasma concentrations in patients taking these agents concomitantly. Concomitant use may result in increased steroid concentrations and reduced serum cortisol concentrations. Concomitant use of glucocorticoids that are metabolized by CYP3A, particularly for long-term use, should consider the potential benefit of treatment versus the risk of systemic corticosteroid effects. Concomitant use may increase the risk for development of systemic corticosteroid effects including Cushing's syndrome and adrenal suppression.
Dihydropyridine Calcium Channel Blockers: e.g. felodipine, nifedipine, nicardipine	↑ dihydropyridine calcium channel blockers	Caution is warranted and clinical monitoring of patients is recommended.
Disulfiram/metronidazole		KALETRA oral solution contains alcohol, which can produce disulfiram-like reactions when co-administered with disulfiram or other drugs that produce this reaction (e.g., metronidazole).
Endothelin Receptor Antagonists: bosentan	↑ bosentan	Co-administration of bosentan in patients on KALETRA: In patients who have been receiving KALETRA for at least 10 days, start bosentan at 62.5 mg once daily or every other day based upon individual tolerability. Co-administration of KALETRA in patients on bosentan: Discontinue use of bosentan at least 36 hours prior to initiation of KALETRA. After at least 10 days following the initiation of KALETRA, resume bosentan at 62.5 mg once daily or every other day based upon individual tolerability.
HCV-Protease Inhibitor: boceprevir	↓ lopinavir ↓ boceprevir ↓ ritonavir	It is not recommended to co-administer KALETRA and boceprevir. Concomitant administration of KALETRA and boceprevir reduced boceprevir, lopinavir and ritonavir steady-state exposures *[see Clinical Pharmacology (12.3)]*.
HCV-Protease Inhibitor: telaprevir	↓ telaprevir ↔ lopinavir	It is not recommended to co-administer KALETRA and telaprevir. Concomitant administration of KALETRA and telaprevir reduced steady-state telaprevir exposure, while the steady-state lopinavir exposure was not affected *[see Clinical Pharmacology (12.3)]*.
HMG-CoA Reductase Inhibitors: atorvastatin rosuvastatin	↑ atorvastatin ↑ rosuvastatin	Use atorvastatin with caution and at the lowest necessary dose. Titrate rosuvastatin dose carefully and use the lowest necessary dose; do not exceed rosuvastatin 10 mg/day. See Drugs with No Observed or Predicted Interactions with KALETRA *(7.4)* and Clinical Pharmacology *(12.3)* for drug interaction data with other HMG-CoA reductase inhibitors.
Immunosuppressants: e.g. cyclosporine, tacrolimus, sirolimus	↑ immunosuppressants	Therapeutic concentration monitoring is recommended for immunosuppressant agents when co-administered with KALETRA.
Inhaled or Intranasal Steroids e.g.: fluticasone, budesonide	↑ glucocorticoids	Concomitant use of KALETRA and fluticasone or other glucocorticoids that are metabolized by CYP3A is not recommended unless the potential benefit of treatment outweighs the risk of systemic corticosteroid effects. Concomitant use may result in increased steroid concentrations and reduce serum cortisol concentrations. Systemic corticosteroid effects including Cushing's syndrome and adrenal suppression have been reported during postmarketing use in patients when certain ritonavir-containing products have been co-administered with fluticasone propionate or budesonide.
Long-acting beta-adrenoceptor Agonist: salmeterol	↑ salmeterol	Concurrent administration of salmeterol and KALETRA is not recommended. The combination may result in increased risk of cardiovascular adverse events associated with salmeterol, including QT prolongation, palpitations and sinus tachycardia.

(Table continued on next page)

Once Daily Dosing

The pharmacokinetics of once daily KALETRA have been evaluated in HIV-1 infected subjects naïve to antiretroviral treatment. KALETRA 800/200 mg was administered in combination with emtricitabine 200 mg and tenofovir DF 300 mg as part of a once daily regimen. Multiple dosing of 800/200 mg KALETRA once daily for 4 weeks with food (n = 24) produced a mean ± SD lopinavir peak plasma concentration (C_{max}) of 11.8 ± 3.7 µg/mL, occurring approximately 6 hours after administration. The mean steady-state lopinavir trough concentration prior to the morning dose was 3.2 ± 2.1 µg/mL and minimum concentration within a dosing interval was 1.7 ± 1.6 µg/mL. Lopinavir AUC over a 24 hour dosing interval averaged 154.1 ± 61.4 µg• h/mL.

The pharmacokinetics of once daily KALETRA has also been evaluated in treatment experienced HIV-1 infected subjects. Lopinavir exposure (C_{max}, $AUC_{[0\text{-}24h]}$, C_{trough}) with once daily KALETRA administration in treatment experienced subjects is comparable to the once daily lopinavir exposure in treatment naïve subjects.

Effects on Electrocardiogram

QTcF interval was evaluated in a randomized, placebo and active (moxifloxacin 400 mg once daily) controlled crossover study in 39 healthy adults, with 10 measurements over 12 hours on Day 3. The maximum mean time-matched (95% upper confidence bound) differences in QTcF interval from placebo after baseline-correction were 5.3 (8.1) and 15.2 (18.0) mseconds (msec) for 400/100 mg twice daily and supratherapeutic 800/200 mg twice daily KALETRA, respectively. KALETRA 800/200 mg twice daily resulted in a Day 3 mean C_{max} approximately 2-fold higher than the mean C_{max} observed with the approved once daily and twice daily KALETRA doses at steady state.

PR interval prolongation was also noted in subjects receiving KALETRA in the same study on Day 3. The maximum mean (95% upper confidence bound) difference from placebo in the PR interval after baseline-correction were 24.9 (21.5, 28.3) and 31.9 (28.5, 35.3) msec for 400/100 mg twice daily and supratherapeutic 800/200 mg twice daily KALETRA, respectively *[see Warnings and Precautions (5.5, 5.6)]*.

Special Populations

Gender, Race and Age

No gender related pharmacokinetic differences have been observed in adult patients. No clinically important pharmacokinetic differences due to race have been identified. Lopinavir pharmacokinetics have not been studied in elderly patients.

Pediatric Patients

The pharmacokinetics of KALETRA oral solution 300/75 mg/m^2 twice daily and 230/57.5 mg/m^2 twice daily have been studied in a total of 53 pediatric patients in Study 940, ranging in age from 6 months to 12 years *[see Clinical Studies (14.4)]*. The 230/57.5 mg/m^2 twice daily regimen without nevirapine and the 300/75 mg/m^2 twice daily regimen with nevirapine provided lopinavir plasma concentrations similar to those obtained in adult patients receiving the 400/100 mg twice daily regimen (without nevirapine).

The mean steady-state lopinavir AUC, C_{max}, and C_{min} were 72.6 ± 31.1 µg•h/mL, 8.2 ± 2.9 and 3.4 ± 2.1 µg/mL, respectively after KALETRA oral solution 230/57.5 mg/m^2 twice daily without nevirapine (n = 12), and were 85.8 ± 36.9 µg•h/mL, 10.0 ± 3.3 and 3.6 ± 3.5 µg/mL, respectively, after 300/75 mg/m^2 twice daily with nevirapine (n = 12). The nevirapine regimen was 7 mg/kg twice daily (6 months to 8 years) or 4 mg/kg twice daily (> 8 years).

The pharmacokinetics of KALETRA oral solution at approximately 300/75 mg/m^2 twice daily have also been evaluated in infants at approximately 6 weeks of age (n = 9) and between 6 weeks and 6 months of age (n = 18) in Study 1030. The mean steady-state lopinavir AUC_{12}, C_{max}, and C_{12} were 43.4 ± 14.8 µg• h/mL, 5.2 ± 1.8 µg/mL and 1.9 ± 1.1 µg/mL, respectively, in infants at approximately 6 weeks of age, and 74.5 ± 37.9 µg• h/mL, 9.4 ± 4.9 and 3.1 ± 1.8 µg/mL, respectively, in infants between 6 weeks and 6 months of age after KALETRA oral solution was administered at approximately 300/75 mg/m^2 twice daily without concomitant NNRTI therapy.

The pharmacokinetics of KALETRA soft gelatin capsule and oral solution (Group 1: 400/100 mg/m^2 twice daily + 2 NRTIs; Group 2: 480/120 mg/m^2 twice daily + ≥ 1 NRTI + 1 NNRTI) have been evaluated in children and adolescents age ≥ 2 years to < 18 years of age who had failed prior therapy (n=26) in Study 1038. KALETRA doses of 400/100 and 480/120 mg/m^2 resulted in high lopinavir exposure, as almost all subjects had lopinavir AUC_{12} above 100 µg•h/mL. Both groups of subjects also achieved relatively high average minimum lopinavir concentrations.

KALETRA once daily has not been evaluated in pediatric patients.

Renal Impairment

Lopinavir pharmacokinetics have not been studied in patients with renal impairment; however, since the renal clearance of lopinavir is negligible, a decrease in total body clearance is not expected in patients with renal impairment.

Hepatic Impairment

Lopinavir is principally metabolized and eliminated by the liver. Multiple dosing of KALETRA 400/100 mg twice daily to HIV-1 and HCV co-infected patients with mild to moderate hepatic impairment (n = 12) resulted in a 30% increase in lopinavir AUC and 20% increase in C_{max} compared to HIV-1 infected subjects with normal hepatic function (n = 12). Additionally, the plasma protein binding of lopinavir was statistically significantly lower in both mild and moderate hepatic impairment compared to controls (99.09 vs. 99.31%, respectively). Caution should be exercised when administering KALETRA to subjects with hepatic impairment. KALETRA has not been studied in patients with severe hepatic impairment *[see Warnings and Precautions (5.4) and Use in Specific Populations (8.6)]*.

Drug Interactions

KALETRA is an inhibitor of the P450 isoform CYP3A *in vitro*. Co-administration of KALETRA and drugs primarily metabolized by CYP3A may result in increased plasma concentrations of the other drug, which could increase or prolong its therapeutic and adverse effects *[see Contraindications (4) and Drug Interactions (7)]*.

KALETRA does not inhibit CYP2D6, CYP2C9, CYP2C19, CYP2E1, CYP2B6 or CYP1A2 at clinically relevant concentrations.

KALETRA has been shown *in vivo* to induce its own metabolism and to increase the biotransformation of some drugs metabolized by cytochrome P450 enzymes and by glucuronidation.

KALETRA is metabolized by CYP3A. Drugs that induce CYP3A activity would be expected to increase the clearance of lopinavir, resulting in lowered plasma concentrations of lopinavir. Although not noted with concurrent ketoconazole, co-administration of KALETRA and other drugs that inhibit CYP3A may increase lopinavir plasma concentrations.

Drug interaction studies were performed with KALETRA and other drugs likely to be co-administered and some drugs commonly used as probes for pharmacokinetic interactions. The effects of co-administration of KALETRA on the AUC, C_{max} and C_{min} are summarized in Table 10 (effect of other drugs on lopinavir) and Table 11 (effect of KALETRA on other drugs). The effects of other drugs on ritonavir are not shown since they generally correlate with those observed with lopinavir (if lopinavir concentrations are decreased, ritonavir concentrations are decreased) unless otherwise indicated in the table footnotes. For information regarding clinical recommendations, see Table 9 in *Drug Interactions (7)*.

[See table 10 on pages 482 and 483]
[See table 11 on pages 483 and 484]

Table 9 *(cont.)*. Established and Other Potentially Significant Drug Interactions

Concomitant Drug Class: Drug Name	Effect on Concentration of Lopinavir or Concomitant Drug	Clinical Comments
Narcotic Analgesics: methadone,* fentanyl	↓ methadone ↑ fentanyl	Dosage of methadone may need to be increased when co-administered with KALETRA. Concentrations of fentanyl are expected to increase. Careful monitoring of therapeutic and adverse effects (including potentially fatal respiratory depression) is recommended when fentanyl is concomitantly administered with KALETRA.
PDE5 inhibitors: avanafil, sildenafil, tadalafil, vardenafil	↑ avanafil ↑ sildenafil ↑ tadalafil ↑ vardenafil	Do not use KALETRA with avanafil because a safe and effective avanafil dosage regimen has not been established. Particular caution should be used when prescribing sildenafil, tadalafil, or vardenafil in patients receiving KALETRA. Co-administration of KALETRA with these drugs is expected to substantially increase their concentrations and may result in an increase in PDE5 inhibitor associated adverse reactions including hypotension, syncope, visual changes and prolonged erection. Use of PDE5 inhibitors for pulmonary arterial hypertension (PAH): Sildenafil (Revatio®) is contraindicated when used for the treatment of pulmonary arterial hypertension (PAH) because a safe and effective dose has not been established when used with KALETRA *[see Contraindications (4)]*. The following dose adjustments are recommended for use of tadalafil (Adcirca®) with KALETRA: Co-administration of ADCIRCA in patients on KALETRA: In patients receiving KALETRA for at least one week, start ADCIRCA at 20 mg once daily. Increase to 40 mg once daily based upon individual tolerability. Co-administration of KALETRA in patients on ADCIRCA: Avoid use of ADCIRCA during the initiation of KALETRA. Stop ADCIRCA at least 24 hours prior to starting KALETRA. After at least one week following the initiation of KALETRA, resume ADCIRCA at 20 mg once daily. Increase to 40 mg once daily based upon individual tolerability. Use of PDE5 inhibitors for erectile dysfunction: It is recommended not to exceed the following doses: • Sildenafil: 25 mg every 48 hours • Tadalafil: 10 mg every 72 hours • Vardenafil: 2.5 mg every 72 hours Use with increased monitoring for adverse events.

* *see Clinical Pharmacology (12.3)* for magnitude of interaction.

12.4 Microbiology

Mechanism of Action

Lopinavir, an inhibitor of the HIV-1 protease, prevents cleavage of the Gag-Pol polyprotein, resulting in the production of immature, non-infectious viral particles.

Antiviral Activity

The antiviral activity of lopinavir against laboratory HIV strains and clinical HIV-1 isolates was evaluated in acutely infected lymphoblastic cell lines and peripheral blood lymphocytes, respectively. In the absence of human serum, the mean 50% effective concentration (EC_{50}) values of lopinavir against five different HIV-1 subtype B laboratory strains ranged from 10-27 nM (0.006-0.017 µg/mL, 1 µg/mL = 1.6 µM) and ranged from 4-11 nM (0.003-0.007 µg/mL) against several HIV-1 subtype B clinical isolates (n = 6). In the presence of 50% human serum, the mean EC_{50} values of lopinavir against these five HIV-1 laboratory strains ranged from 65-289 nM (0.04-0.18 µg/mL), representing a 7 to 11-fold attenuation. Combination antiviral drug activity studies with lopinavir in cell cultures demonstrated additive to antagonistic activity with nelfinavir and additive to synergistic activity with amprenavir, atazanavir, indinavir, saquinavir and tipranavir. The EC_{50} values of lopinavir against three different HIV-2 strains ranged from 12-180 nM (0.008-113 µg/mL).

Resistance

HIV-1 isolates with reduced susceptibility to lopinavir have been selected in cell culture. The presence of ritonavir does not appear to influence the selection of lopinavir-resistant viruses in cell culture.

The selection of resistance to KALETRA in antiretroviral treatment naïve patients has not yet been characterized. In a study of 653 antiretroviral treatment naïve patients (Study 863), plasma viral isolates from each patient on

Information on the AbbVie, Inc. products listed on these pages is from the prescribing information in use as of July 31, 2013. For more information, please visit rxabbvie.com or call 1-800-633-9110.

Table 10. Drug Interactions: Pharmacokinetic Parameters for Lopinavir in the Presence of the Co-administered Drug for Recommended Alterations in Dose or Regimen

Co-administered Drug	Dose of Co-administered Drug (mg)	Dose of KALETRA (mg)	n	Ratio (in combination with Co-administered drug/ alone) of Lopinavir Pharmacokinetic Parameters (90% CI); No Effect = 1.00		
				C_{max}	AUC	C_{min}
Boceprevir	800 q8h, 6 d	400/100 tablet twice daily, 22 d	13	0.70 (0.65, 0.77)	0.66[12] (0.60, 0.72)	0.57 (0.49, 0.65)
Efavirenz[1,2]	600 at bedtime, 9 d	400/100 capsule twice daily, 9 d	11, 7*	0.97 (0.78, 1.22)	0.81 (0.64, 1.03)	0.61 (0.38, 0.97)
	600 at bedtime, 9 d	500/125 tablet twice daily, 10 d	19	1.12 (1.02, 1.23)	1.06 (0.96, 1.17)	0.90 (0.78, 1.04)
	600 at bedtime, 9 d	600/150 tablet twice daily, 10 d	23	1.36 (1.28, 1.44)	1.36 (1.28, 1.44)	1.32 (1.21, 1.44)
Fosamprenavir[3]	700 twice daily plus ritonavir 100 twice daily, 14 d	400/100 capsule twice daily, 14 d	18	1.30 (0.85, 1.47)	1.37 (0.80, 1.55)	1.52 (0.72, 1.82)
Ketoconazole	200 single dose	400/100 capsule twice daily, 16 d	12	0.89 (0.80, 0.99)	0.87 (0.75, 1.00)	0.75 (0.55, 1.00)
Nelfinavir	1000 twice daily, 10 d	400/100 capsule twice daily, 21 d	13	0.79 (0.70, 0.89)	0.73 (0.63, 0.85)	0.62 (0.49, 0.78)
Nevirapine	200 twice daily, steady-state (> 1 yr)[4#]	400/100 capsule twice daily, steady-state	22, 19*	0.81 (0.62, 1.05)	0.73 (0.53, 0.98)	0.49 (0.28, 0.74)
	7 mg/kg or 4 mg/kg once daily, 2 wk; twice daily 1 wk[5]	(> 1 yr) 300/ $75\ mg/m^2$ oral solution twice daily, 3 wk	12, 15*	0.86 (0.64, 1.16)	0.78 (0.56, 1.09)	0.45 (0.25, 0.81)
Omeprazole	40 once daily, 5 d	400/100 tablet twice daily, 10 d	12	1.08 (0.99, 1.17)	1.07 (0.99, 1.15)	1.03 (0.90, 1.18)
	40 once daily, 5 d	800/200 tablet once daily, 10 d	12	0.94 (0.88, 1.00)	0.92 (0.86, 0.99)	0.71 (0.57, 0.89)
Pitavastatin[6]	4 mg once daily, 5 d	400/100 tablet twice daily, 16 d	23	0.93 (0.88-0.98)	0.91 (0.86-0.97)	NA
Pravastatin	20 once daily, 4 d	400/100 capsule twice daily, 14 d	12	0.98 (0.89, 1.08)	0.95 (0.85, 1.05)	0.88 (0.77, 1.02)
Rifabutin	150 once daily, 10 d	400/100 capsule twice daily, 20 d	14	1.08 (0.97, 1.19)	1.17 (1.04, 1.31)	1.20 (0.96, 1.65)
Ranitidine	150 single dose	400/100 tablet twice daily, 10 d	12	0.99 (0.95, 1.03)	0.97 (0.93, 1.01)	0.90 (0.85, 0.95)
	150 single dose	800/200 tablet once daily, 10 d	10	0.97 (0.95, 1.00)	0.95 (0.91, 0.99)	0.82 (0.74, 0.91)
Rifampin	600 once daily, 10 d	400/100 capsule twice daily, 20 d	22	0.45 (0.40, 0.51)	0.25 (0.21, 0.29)	0.01 (0.01, 0.02)
	600 once daily, 14 d	800/200 capsule twice daily, 9 d[7]	10	1.02 (0.85, 1.23)	0.84 (0.64, 1.10)	0.43 (0.19, 0.96)
	600 once daily, 14 d	400/400 capsule twice daily, 9 d[8]	9	0.93 (0.81, 1.07)	0.98 (0.81, 1.17)	1.03 (0.68, 1.56)

(Table continued on next page)

treatment with plasma HIV-1 RNA > 400 copies/mL at Week 24, 32, 40 and/or 48 were analyzed. No evidence of resistance to KALETRA was observed in 37 evaluable KALETRA-treated patients (0%). Evidence of genotypic resistance to nelfinavir, defined as the presence of the D30N and/or L90M substitution in HIV-1 protease, was observed in 25/76 (33%) of evaluable nelfinavir-treated patients. The selection of resistance to KALETRA in antiretroviral treatment naïve pediatric patients (Study 940) appears to be consistent with that seen in adult patients (Study 863).

Resistance to KALETRA has been noted to emerge in patients treated with other protease inhibitors prior to KALETRA therapy. In studies of 227 antiretroviral treatment naïve and protease inhibitor experienced patients, isolates from 4 of 23 patients with quantifiable (> 400 copies/ mL) viral RNA following treatment with KALETRA for 12 to 100 weeks displayed significantly reduced susceptibility to lopinavir compared to the corresponding baseline viral isolates. Three of these patients had previously received treatment with a single protease inhibitor (indinavir, nelfinavir, or saquinavir) and one patient had received treatment with multiple protease inhibitors (indinavir, ritonavir, and saquinavir). All four of these patients had at least 4 substitutions associated with protease inhibitor resistance immediately prior to KALETRA therapy. Following viral rebound, isolates from these patients all contained additional substitutions, some of which are recognized to be associated with protease inhibitor resistance. However, there are insufficient data at this time to identify patterns of lopinavir resistance-associated substitutions in isolates from patients on KALETRA therapy. The assessment of these patterns is under study.

Cross-resistance - Preclinical Studies

Varying degrees of cross-resistance have been observed among HIV-1 protease inhibitors. Little information is available on the cross-resistance of viruses that developed decreased susceptibility to lopinavir during KALETRA® (lopinavir/ritonavir) therapy.

The antiviral activity in cell culture of lopinavir against clinical isolates from patients previously treated with a single protease inhibitor was determined. Isolates that displayed > 4-fold reduced susceptibility to nelfinavir (n = 13) and saquinavir (n = 4), displayed < 4-fold reduced susceptibility to lopinavir. Isolates with > 4-fold reduced susceptibility to indinavir (n = 16) and ritonavir (n = 3) displayed a mean of 5.7- and 8.3-fold reduced susceptibility to lopinavir, respectively. Isolates from patients previously treated with two or more protease inhibitors showed greater reductions in susceptibility to lopinavir, as described in the following paragraph.

Clinical Studies - Antiviral Activity of KALETRA in Patients with Previous Protease Inhibitor Therapies

The clinical relevance of reduced susceptibility in cell culture to lopinavir has been examined by assessing the virologic response to KALETRA therapy in treatment-experienced patients, with respect to baseline viral genotype in three studies and baseline viral phenotype in one study.

Virologic response to KALETRA has been shown to be affected by the presence of three or more of the following amino acid substitutions in protease at baseline: L10F/I/R/V, K20M/N/R, L24I, L33F, M36I, I47V, G48V, I54L/T/V, V82A/C/F/S/T, and I84V. Table 12 shows the 48-week virologic response (HIV-1 RNA <400 copies/mL) according to the number of the above protease inhibitor resistance-associated substitutions at baseline in studies 888 and 765 *[see Clinical Studies (14.2) and (14.3)]* and study 957 (see below). Once daily administration of KALETRA for adult patients with three or more of the above substitutions is not recommended.

[See table 12 at top of page 485]

Virologic response to KALETRA therapy with respect to phenotypic susceptibility to lopinavir at baseline was examined in Study 957. In this study 56 NNRTI-naïve patients with HIV-1 RNA >1,000 copies/mL despite previous therapy with at least two protease inhibitors selected from indinavir, nelfinavir, ritonavir, and saquinavir were randomized to receive one of two doses of KALETRA in combination with efavirenz and nucleoside reverse transcriptase inhibitors (NRTIs). The EC_{50} values of lopinavir against the 56 baseline viral isolates ranged from 0.5- to 96-fold the wild-type EC_{50} value. Fifty-five percent (31/56) of these baseline isolates displayed >4-fold reduced susceptibility to lopinavir. These 31 isolates had a median reduction in lopinavir susceptibility of 18-fold. Response to therapy by baseline lopinavir susceptibility is shown in Table 13.

Table 13. HIV-1 RNA Response at Week 48 by Baseline Lopinavir Susceptibility[1]

Lopinavir susceptibility[2] at baseline	HIV-1 RNA <400 copies/mL (%)	HIV-1 RNA <50 copies/mL (%)
< 10 fold	25/27 (93%)	22/27 (81%)
> 10 and < 40 fold	11/15 (73%)	9/15 (60%)
≥ 40 fold	2/8 (25%)	2/8 (25%)

[1] Lopinavir susceptibility was determined by recombinant phenotypic technology performed by Virologic.
[2] Fold change in susceptibility from wild type.

13 NONCLINICAL TOXICOLOGY

13.1 Carcinogenesis, Mutagenesis, Impairment of Fertility

Carcinogenesis

Lopinavir/ritonavir combination was evaluated for carcinogenic potential by oral gavage administration to mice and rats for up to 104 weeks. Results showed an increase in the incidence of benign hepatocellular adenomas and an increase in the combined incidence of hepatocellular adenomas plus carcinoma in both males and females in mice and males in rats at doses that produced approximately 1.6-2.2 times (mice) and 0.5 times (rats) the human exposure (based on $AUC_{0\text{-}24hr}$ measurement) at the recommended dose of 400/100 mg KALETRA twice daily. Administration of lopinavir/ritonavir did not cause a statistically significant increase in the incidence of any other benign or malignant neoplasm in mice or rats.

Carcinogenicity studies in mice and rats have been carried out on ritonavir. In male mice, there was a dose dependent increase in the incidence of both adenomas and combined adenomas and carcinomas in the liver. Based on AUC measurements, the exposure at the high dose was approximately 4-fold for males that of the exposure in humans with the recommended therapeutic dose (400/100 mg KALETRA twice daily). There were no carcinogenic effects seen in females at the dosages tested. The exposure at the high dose was approximately 9-fold for the females that of the exposure in humans. There were no carcinogenic effects in rats. In this study, the exposure at the high dose was approximately 0.7-fold that of the exposure in humans with the 400/100 mg KALETRA twice daily regimen. Based on the exposures achieved in the animal studies, the significance of the observed effects is not known.

Table 10 *(cont.)*. Drug Interactions: Pharmacokinetic Parameters for Lopinavir in the Presence of the Co-administered Drug for Recommended Alterations in Dose or Regimen

Co-administered Drug	Dose of Co-administered Drug (mg)	Dose of KALETRA (mg)	n	Ratio (in combination with Co-administered drug/alone) of Lopinavir Pharmacokinetic Parameters (90% CI); No Effect = 1.00		
				C_{max}	AUC	C_{min}
Ritonavir[4]	100 twice daily, 3-4 wk#	400/100 capsule twice daily, 3-4 wk	8, 21*	1.28 (0.94, 1.76)	1.46 (1.04, 2.06)	2.16 (1.29, 3.62)
Telaprevir	750 q8h, 10 days	400/100 tablet twice daily, 20 days	12[13]	0.96 (0.87, 1.05)	1.06 (0.96, 1.17)	1.14 (0.96, 1.36)
Tenofovir[9]	300 mg once daily, 14 d	400/100 capsule twice daily, 14 d	24	NC†	NC†	NC†
Tipranavir/ritonavir[4]	500/200 mg twice daily (28 doses)#	400/100 capsule twice daily (27 doses)	21	0.53 (0.40, 0.69)[10]	0.45 (0.32, 0.63)[10]	0.30 (0.17, 0.51)[10]
			69			0.48 (0.40, 0.58)[11]

All interaction studies conducted in healthy, HIV-1 negative subjects unless otherwise indicated.
1 The pharmacokinetics of ritonavir are unaffected by concurrent efavirenz.
2 Reference for comparison is lopinavir/ritonavir 400/100 mg twice daily without efavirenz.
3 Data extracted from the fosamprenavir package insert.
4 Study conducted in HIV-1 positive adult subjects.
5 Study conducted in HIV-1 positive pediatric subjects ranging in age from 6 months to 12 years.
6 Data extracted from the pitavastatin package insert and results presented at the 2011 International AIDS Society Conference on HIV Pathogenesis, Treatment and Prevention (Morgan, *et al, poster #MOPE170*).
7 Titrated to 800/200 twice daily as 533/133 twice daily × 1 d, 667/167 twice daily × 1 d, then 800/200 twice daily × 7 d, compared to 400/100 twice daily × 10 days alone.
8 Titrated to 400/400 twice daily as 400/200 twice daily × 1 d, 400/300 twice daily × 1 d, then 400/400 twice daily × 7 d, compared to 400/100 twice daily × 10 days alone.
9 Data extracted from the tenofovir package insert.
10 Intensive PK analysis.
11 Drug levels obtained at 8-16 hrs post-dose.
12 AUC parameter is $AUC_{(0\text{-last})}$
13 N=12 for test arm, 19 for reference arm
* Parallel group design; n for KALETRA + co-administered drug, n for KALETRA alone.
† NC = No change.
\# For the nevirapine 200 mg twice daily study, ritonavir, and tipranavir/ritonavir studies, KALETRA was administered with or without food. For all other studies, KALETRA was administered with food.

Table 11. Drug Interactions: Pharmacokinetic Parameters for Co-administered Drug in the Presence of KALETRA for Recommended Alterations in Dose or Regimen

Co-administered Drug	Dose of Co-administered Drug (mg)	Dose of KALETRA (mg)	n	Ratio (in combination with KALETRA/alone) of Co-administered Drug Pharmacokinetic Parameters (90% CI); No Effect = 1.00		
				C_{max}	AUC	C_{min}
Boceprevir	800 q8h, 6 d	400/100 tablet twice daily, 22 d	13[8]	0.50 (0.45, 0.55)	0.55 (0.49, 0.61)	0.43 (0.36, 0.53)
Desipramine[2]	100 single dose	400/100 capsule twice daily, 10 d	15	0.91 (0.84, 0.97)	1.05 (0.96, 1.16)	N/A
Efavirenz	600 at bedtime, 9 d	400/100 capsule twice daily, 9 d	11, 12*	0.91 (0.72, 1.15)	0.84 (0.62, 1.15)	0.84 (0.58, 1.20)
Ethinyl Estradiol	35 µg once daily, 21 d (Ortho Novum®)	400/100 capsule twice daily, 14 d	12	0.59 (0.52, 0.66)	0.58 (0.54, 0.62)	0.42 (0.36, 0.49)
Fosamprenavir[3]	700 twice daily plus ritonavir 100 twice daily, 14 d	400/100 capsule twice daily, 14 d	18	0.42 (0.30, 0.58)	0.37 (0.28, 0.49)	0.35 (0.27, 0.46)
Indinavir[1]	600 twice daily, 10 d combo nonfasting vs. 800 three times daily, 5 d alone fasting	400/100 capsule twice daily, 15 d	13	0.71 (0.63, 0.81)	0.91 (0.75, 1.10)	3.47 (2.60, 4.64)
Ketoconazole	200 single dose	400/100 capsule twice daily, 16 d	12	1.13 (0.91, 1.40)	3.04 (2.44, 3.79)	N/A
Methadone	5 single dose	400/100 capsule twice daily, 10 d	11	0.55 (0.48, 0.64)	0.47 (0.42, 0.53)	N/A

(Table continued on next page)

Mutagenesis
Neither lopinavir nor ritonavir was found to be mutagenic or clastogenic in a battery of *in vitro* and *in vivo* assays including the Ames bacterial reverse mutation assay using *S. typhimurium* and *E. coli*, the mouse lymphoma assay, the mouse micronucleus test and chromosomal aberration assays in human lymphocytes.

Impairment of Fertility
Lopinavir in combination with ritonavir at a 2:1 ratio produced no effects on fertility in male and female rats at levels of 10/5, 30/15 or 100/50 mg/kg/day. Based on AUC measurements, the exposures in rats at the high doses were approximately 0.7-fold for lopinavir and 1.8-fold for ritonavir of the exposures in humans at the recommended therapeutic dose (400/100 mg twice daily).

14 CLINICAL STUDIES

14.1 Adult Patients without Prior Antiretroviral Therapy

Study 863: KALETRA Capsules twice daily + stavudine + lamivudine compared to nelfinavir three times daily + stavudine + lamivudine

Study 863 was a randomized, double-blind, multicenter trial comparing treatment with KALETRA capsules (400/100 mg twice daily) plus stavudine and lamivudine versus nelfinavir (750 mg three times daily) plus stavudine and lamivudine in 653 antiretroviral treatment naïve patients. Patients had a mean age of 38 years (range: 19 to 84), 57% were Caucasian, and 80% were male. Mean baseline CD4+ cell count was 259 cells/mm^3 (range: 2 to 949 cells/mm^3) and mean baseline plasma HIV-1 RNA was 4.9 $\log_{10}$ copies/mL (range: 2.6 to 6.8 $\log_{10}$ copies/mL).

Treatment response and outcomes of randomized treatment are presented in Table 14.

Table 14. Outcomes of Randomized Treatment Through Week 48 (Study 863)

Outcome	KALETRA+ d4T+3TC (N = 326)	Nelfinavir+ d4T+3TC (N = 327)
Responder[1]	75%	62%
Virologic failure[2]	9%	25%
Rebound	7%	15%
Never suppressed through Week 48	2%	9%
Death	2%	1%
Discontinued due to adverse events	4%	4%
Discontinued for other reasons[3]	10%	8%

1 Patients achieved and maintained confirmed HIV-1 RNA < 400 copies/mL through Week 48.
2 Includes confirmed viral rebound and failure to achieve confirmed < 400 copies/mL through Week 48.
3 Includes lost to follow-up, patient's withdrawal, non-compliance, protocol violation and other reasons. Overall discontinuation through Week 48, including patients who discontinued subsequent to virologic failure, was 17% in the KALETRA arm and 24% in the nelfinavir arm.

Through 48 weeks of therapy, there was a statistically significantly higher proportion of patients in the KALETRA arm compared to the nelfinavir arm with HIV-1 RNA < 400 copies/mL (75% vs. 62%, respectively) and HIV-1 RNA < 50 copies/mL (67% vs. 52%, respectively). Treatment response by baseline HIV-1 RNA level subgroups is presented in Table 15.

[See table 15 at top of page 485]

Through 48 weeks of therapy, the mean increase from baseline in CD4+ cell count was 207 cells/mm^3 for the KALETRA arm and 195 cells/mm^3 for the nelfinavir arm.

Study 730: KALETRA Tablets once daily + tenofovir DF + emtricitabine compared to KALETRA Tablets twice daily + tenofovir DF + emtricitabine.

Study 730 was a randomized, open-label, multicenter trial comparing treatment with KALETRA 800/200 mg once

Information on the AbbVie, Inc. products listed on these pages is from the prescribing information in use as of July 31, 2013. For more information, please visit rxabbvie.com or call 1-800-633-9110.

daily plus tenofovir DF and emtricitabine versus KALETRA 400/100 mg twice daily plus tenofovir DF and emtricitabine in 664 antiretroviral treatment-naïve patients. Patients were randomized in a 1:1 ratio to receive either KALETRA 800/200 mg once daily (n = 333) or KALETRA 400/100 mg twice daily (n = 331). Further stratification within each group was 1:1 (tablet vs. capsule). Patients administered the capsule were switched to the tablet formulation at Week 8 and maintained on their randomized dosing schedule. Patients were administered emtricitabine 200 mg once daily and tenofovir DF 300 mg once daily. Mean age of patients enrolled was 39 years (range: 19 to 71); 75% were Caucasian, and 78% were male. Mean baseline CD4+ cell count was 216 cells/mm^3 (range: 20 to 775 cells/mm^3) and mean baseline plasma HIV-1 RNA was 5.0 $\log_{10}$ copies/mL (range: 1.7 to 7.0 $\log_{10}$ copies/mL).

Treatment response and outcomes of randomized treatment through Week 48 are presented in Table 16.

Table 16. Outcomes of Randomized Treatment Through Week 48 (Study 730)

Outcome	KALETRA Once Daily + TDF + FTC (n = 333)	KALETRA Twice Daily + TDF + FTC (n = 331)
Responder[1]	78%	77%
Virologic failure[2]	10%	8%
Rebound	5%	5%
Never suppressed through Week 48	5%	3%
Death	1%	<1%
Discontinued due to adverse events	4%	3%
Discontinued for other reasons[3]	8%	11%

[1] Patients achieved and maintained confirmed HIV-1 RNA < 50 copies/mL through Week 48.
[2] Includes confirmed viral rebound and failure to achieve confirmed < 50 copies/mL through Week 48.
[3] Includes lost to follow-up, patient's withdrawal, non-compliance, protocol violation and other reasons.

Through 48 weeks of therapy, 78% in the KALETRA once daily arm and 77% in the KALETRA twice daily arm achieved and maintained HIV-1 RNA < 50 copies/mL (95% confidence interval for the difference, -5.9% to 6.8%). Mean CD4+ cell count increases at Week 48 were 186 cells/mm^3 for the KALETRA once daily arm and 198 cells/mm^3 for the KALETRA twice daily arm.

14.2 Adult Patients with Prior Antiretroviral Therapy

Study 888: KALETRA Capsules twice daily + nevirapine + NRTIs compared to investigator-selected protease inhibitor(s) + nevirapine + NRTIs

Study 888 was a randomized, open-label, multicenter trial comparing treatment with KALETRA capsules (400/100 mg twice daily) plus nevirapine and nucleoside reverse transcriptase inhibitors versus investigator-selected protease inhibitor(s) plus nevirapine and nucleoside reverse transcriptase inhibitors in 288 single protease inhibitor-experienced, non-nucleoside reverse transcriptase inhibitor (NNRTI)-naïve patients. Patients had a mean age of 40 years (range: 18 to 74), 68% were Caucasian, and 86% were male. Mean baseline CD4+ cell count was 322 cells/mm^3 (range: 10 to 1059 cells/mm^3) and mean baseline plasma HIV-1 RNA was 4.1 $\log_{10}$ copies/mL (range: 2.6 to 6.0 $\log_{10}$ copies/mL).

Treatment response and outcomes of randomized treatment through Week 48 are presented in Table 17.

Table 17. Outcomes of Randomized Treatment Through Week 48 (Study 888)

Outcome	KALETRA + nevirapine + NRTIs (n = 148)	Investigator-Selected Protease Inhibitor(s) + nevirapine + NRTIs (n = 140)
Responder[1]	57%	33%
Virologic failure[2]	24%	41%
Rebound	11%	19%
Never suppressed through Week 48	13%	23%
Death	1%	2%
Discontinued due to adverse events	5%	11%
Discontinued for other reasons[3]	14%	13%

[1] Patients achieved and maintained confirmed HIV-1 RNA < 400 copies/mL through Week 48.
[2] Includes confirmed viral rebound and failure to achieve confirmed < 400 copies/mL through Week 48.
[3] Includes lost to follow-up, patient's withdrawal, non-compliance, protocol violation and other reasons.

Through 48 weeks of therapy, there was a statistically significantly higher proportion of patients in the KALETRA arm compared to the investigator-selected protease inhibitor(s) arm with HIV-1 RNA < 400 copies/mL (57% vs. 33%, respectively).

Through 48 weeks of therapy, the mean increase from baseline in CD4+ cell count was 111 cells/mm^3 for the KALETRA arm and 112 cells/mm^3 for the investigator-selected protease inhibitor(s) arm.

Study 802: KALETRA Tablets 800/200 mg Once Daily Versus 400/100 mg Twice Daily when Co-administered with Nucleoside/Nucleotide Reverse Transcriptase Inhibitors in Antiretroviral-Experienced, HIV-1 Infected Subjects

M06-802 was a randomized open-label study comparing the safety, tolerability, and antiviral activity of once daily and twice daily dosing of KALETRA tablets in 599 subjects with detectable viral loads while receiving their current antiviral therapy. Of the enrolled subjects, 55% on both treatment arms had not been previously treated with a protease inhibitor and 81 – 88% had received prior NNRTIs as part of their anti-HIV treatment regimen. Patients were randomized in a 1:1 ratio to receive either KALETRA 800/200 mg once daily (n = 300) or KALETRA 400/100 mg twice daily (n = 299). Patients were administered at least two nucleoside/nucleotide reverse transcriptase inhibitors selected by theinvestigator. Mean age of patients enrolled was 41 years (range: 21 to 73); 51% were Caucasian, and 66% were male. Mean baseline CD4+ cell count was 254 cells/mm^3 (range: 4 to 952 cells/mm^3) and mean baseline plasma HIV-1 RNA was 4.3 $\log_{10}$ copies/mL (range: 1.7 to 6.6 $\log_{10}$ copies/mL). Treatment response and outcomes of randomized treatment through Week 48 are presented in Table 18.

Table 11 *(cont.)*. Drug Interactions: Pharmacokinetic Parameters for Co-administered Drug in the Presence of KALETRA for Recommended Alterations in Dose or Regimen

Co-administered Drug	Dose of Co-administered Drug (mg)	Dose of KALETRA (mg)	n	Ratio (in combination with KALETRA/alone) of Co-administered Drug Pharmacokinetic Parameters (90% CI); No Effect = 1.00		
				C_{max}	AUC	C_{min}
Nelfinavir[1]	1000 twice daily, 10 d combo vs. 1250 twice daily 14 d alone	400/100 capsule twice daily, 21 d	13	0.93 (0.82, 1.05)	1.07 (0.95, 1.19)	1.86 (1.57, 2.22)
M8 metabolite				2.36 (1.91, 2.91)	3.46 (2.78, 4.31)	7.49 (5.85, 9.58)
Nevirapine	200 once daily, 14 d; twice daily, 6 d	400/100 capsule twice daily, 20 d	5, 6*	1.05 (0.72, 1.52)	1.08 (0.72, 1.64)	1.15 (0.71, 1.86)
Norethindrone	1 once daily, 21 d (Ortho Novum®)	400/100 capsule twice daily, 14 d	12	0.84 (0.75, 0.94)	0.83 (0.73, 0.94)	0.68 (0.54, 0.85)
Pitavastatin[4]	4 mg once daily, 5 d	400/100 tablet twice daily, 16 d	23	0.96 (0.84-1.10)	0.80 (0.73-0.87)	N/A
Pravastatin	20 once daily, 4 d	400/100 capsule twice daily, 14 d	12	1.26 (0.87, 1.83)	1.33 (0.91, 1.94)	N/A
Rifabutin	150 once daily, 10 d; combo vs. 300 once daily, 10 d; alone	400/100 capsule twice daily, 10 d	12	2.12 (1.89, 2.38)	3.03 (2.79, 3.30)	4.90 (3.18, 5.76)
25-*O*-desacetyl rifabutin				23.6 (13.7, 25.3)	47.5 (29.3, 51.8)	94.9 (74.0, 122)
Rifabutin + 25-*O*-desacetyl rifabutin[5]				3.46 (3.07, 3.91)	5.73 (5.08, 6.46)	9.53 (7.56, 12.01)
Rosuvastatin[6]	20 mg once daily, 7 d	400/100 tablet twice daily, 7 d	15	4.66 (3.4, 6.4)	2.08 (1.66, 2.6)	1.04 (0.9, 1.2)
Telaprevir	750 q8h, 10 days	400/100 tablet twice daily, 20 days	12[9]	0.47 (0.41, 0.52)	0.46 (0.41, 0.52)	0.48 (0.40, 0.56)
Tenofovir[7]	300 mg once daily, 14 d	400/100 capsule twice daily, 14 d	24	NC†	1.32 (1.26, 1.38)	1.51 (1.32, 1.66)

All interaction studies conducted in healthy, HIV-1 negative subjects unless otherwise indicated.
[1] Ratio of parameters for indinavir, and nelfinavir, are not normalized for dose.
[2] Desipramine is a probe substrate for assessing effects on CYP2D6-mediated metabolism.
[3] Data extracted from the fosamprenavir package insert.
[4] Data extracted from the pitavastatin package insert and results presented at the 2011 International AIDS Society Conference on HIV Pathogenesis, Treatment and Prevention (Morgan, *et al, poster #MOPE170*).
[5] Effect on the dose-normalized sum of rifabutin parent and 25-*O*-desacetyl rifabutin active metabolite.
[6] Kiser, et al. J Acquir Immune Defic Syndr. 2008 Apr 15;47(5):570-8.
[7] Data extracted from the tenofovir package insert.
[8] N=12 for C_{min} (test arm)
[9] N=12 for the test arm, 14 for reference arm
* Parallel group design; n for KALETRA + co-administered drug, n for co-administered drug alone.
N/A = Not available.
† NC = No change.

Table 12. Virologic Response (HIV-1 RNA <400 copies/mL) at Week 48 by Baseline KALETRA Susceptibility and by Number of Protease Substitutions Associated with Reduced Response to KALETRA[1]

Number of protease inhibitor substitutions at baseline[1]	Study 888 (Single protease inhibitor-experienced[2], NNRTI-naïve) n=130	Study 765 (Single protease inhibitor-experienced[3], NNRTI-naïve) n=56	Study 957 (Multiple protease inhibitor-experienced[4], NNRTI-naïve) n=50
0-2	76/103 (74%)	34/45 (76%)	19/20 (95%)
3-5	13/26 (50%)	8/11 (73%)	18/26 (69%)
6 or more	0/1 (0%)	N/A	1/4 (25%)

[1] Substitutions considered in the analysis included L10F/I/R/V, K20M/N/R, L24I, L33F, M36I, I47V, G48V, I54L/T/V, V82A/C/F/S/T, and I84V.
[2] 43% indinavir, 42% nelfinavir, 10% ritonavir, 15% saquinavir.
[3] 41% indinavir, 38% nelfinavir, 4% ritonavir, 16% saquinavir.
[4] 86% indinavir, 54% nelfinavir, 80% ritonavir, 70% saquinavir.

Table 15. Proportion of Responders Through Week 48 by Baseline Viral Load (Study 863)

Baseline Viral Load (HIV-1 RNA copies/mL)	KALETRA +d4T+3TC			Nelfinavir +d4T+3TC		
	<400 copies/mL[1]	<50 copies/mL[2]	n	<400 copies/mL[1]	<50 copies/mL[2]	n
< 30,000	74%	71%	82	79%	72%	87
≥ 30,000 to < 100,000	81%	73%	79	67%	54%	79
≥ 100,000 to < 250,000	75%	64%	83	60%	47%	72
≥ 250,000	72%	60%	82	44%	33%	89

[1] Patients achieved and maintained confirmed HIV-1 RNA < 400 copies/mL through Week 48.
[2] Patients achieved HIV-1 RNA < 50 copies/mL at Week 48.

Table 18. Outcomes of Randomized Treatment Through Week 48 (Study 802)

Outcome	KALETRA Once Daily + NRTIs (n = 300)	KALETRA Twice Daily + NRTIs (n = 299)
Virologic Success (HIV-1 RNA <50 copies/mL)	57%	54%
Virologic failure[1]	22%	24%
No virologic data in Week 48 window		
Discontinued study due to adverse event or death[2]	5%	7%
Discontinued study for other reasons[3]	13%	12%
Missing data during window but on study	3%	3%

[1] Includes patients who discontinued prior to Week 48 for lack or loss of efficacy and patients with HIV-1 RNA ≥ 50 copies/mL at Week 48.
[2] Includes patients who discontinued due to adverse events or death at any time from Day 1 through Week 48 if this resulted in no virologic data on treatment at Week 48.
[3] Includes withdrawal of consent, loss to follow-up, non-compliance, protocol violation and other reasons.

Through 48 weeks of treatment, the mean change from baseline for CD4 + cell count was 135 cells/mm^3 for the once daily group and 122 cells/mm^3 for the twice daily group.

14.3 Other Studies Supporting Approval in Adult Patients

Study 720: KALETRA twice daily + stavudine + lamivudine

Study 765: KALETRA twice daily + nevirapine + NRTIs

Study 720 (patients without prior antiretroviral therapy) and study 765 (patients with prior protease inhibitor therapy) were randomized, blinded, multi-center trials evaluating treatment with KALETRA at up to three dose levels (200/100 mg twice daily [720 only], 400/100 mg twice daily, and 400/200 mg twice daily). In Study 720, all patients switched to 400/100 mg twice daily between Weeks 48-72. Patients in study 720 had a mean age of 35 years, 70% were Caucasian, and 96% were male, while patients in study 765 had a mean age of 40 years, 73% were Caucasian, and 90% were male. Mean (range) baseline CD4+ cell counts for patients in study 720 and study 765 were 338 (3-918) and 372 (72-807) cells/mm^3, respectively. Mean (range) baseline plasma HIV-1 RNA levels for patients in study 720 and study 765 were 4.9 (3.3 to 6.3) and 4.0 (2.9 to 5.8) $\log_{10}$ copies/mL, respectively.

Through 360 weeks of treatment in study 720, the proportion of patients with HIV-1 RNA < 400 (< 50) copies/mL was 61% (59%) [n = 100]. Among patients completing 360 weeks of treatment with CD4+ cell count measurements [n=60], the mean (median) increase in CD4+ cell count was 501 (457) cells/mm^3. Thirty-nine patients (39%) discontinued the study, including 13 (13%) discontinuations due to adverse reactions and 1 (1%) death.

Through 144 weeks of treatment in study 765, the proportion of patients with HIV-1 RNA < 400 (< 50) copies/mL was 54% (50%) [n = 70], and the corresponding mean increase in CD4+ cell count was 212 cells/mm^3. Twenty-seven patients (39%) discontinued the study, including 5 (7%) discontinuations secondary to adverse reactions and 2 (3%) deaths.

14.4 Pediatric Studies

Study 1030 was an open-label, multicenter, dose-finding trial evaluating the pharmacokinetic profile, tolerability, safety and efficacy of KALETRA oral solution containing lopinavir 80 mg/mL and ritonavir 20 mg/mL at a dose of 300/75 mg/m^2 twice daily plus 2 NRTIs in HIV-1 infected infants ≥14 days and <6 months of age.

Ten infants, ≥14 days and <6 wks of age, were enrolled at a median (range) age of 5.7 (3.6-6.0) weeks and all completed 24 weeks. At entry, median (range) HIV-1 RNA was 6.0 (4.7-7.2) $\log_{10}$ copies/mL. Seven of 10 infants had HIV-1 RNA <400 copies/mL at Week 24. At entry, median (range) CD4+ percentage was 41 (16-59) with a median decrease of 1% (95% CI: -10, 18) from baseline to week 24 in 6 infants with available data.

Twenty-one infants, between 6 weeks and 6 months of age, were enrolled at a median (range) age of 14.7 (6.9-25.7) weeks and 19 of 21 infants completed 24 weeks. At entry, median (range) HIV RNA level was 5.8 (3.7-6.9) $\log_{10}$ copies/mL. Ten of 21 infants had HIV RNA <400 copies/mL at Week 24. At entry, the median (range) CD4+ percentage was 32 (11-54) with a median increase of 4% (95% CI: -1, 9) from baseline to week 24 in 19 infants with available data.

See Clinical Pharmacology (12.3) for pharmacokinetic results.

Study 940 was an open-label, multicenter trial evaluating the pharmacokinetic profile, tolerability, safety and efficacy of KALETRA oral solution containing lopinavir 80 mg/mL and ritonavir 20 mg/mL in 100 antiretroviral naïve (44%) and experienced (56%) pediatric patients. All patients were non-nucleoside reverse transcriptase inhibitor naïve. Patients were randomized to either 230 mg lopinavir/57.5 mg ritonavir per m^2 or 300 mg lopinavir/75 mg ritonavir per m^2. Naïve patients also received lamivudine and stavudine. Experienced patients received nevirapine plus up to two nucleoside reverse transcriptase inhibitors.

Safety, efficacy and pharmacokinetic profiles of the two dose regimens were assessed after three weeks of therapy in each patient. After analysis of these data, all patients were continued on the 300 mg lopinavir/75 mg ritonavir per m^2 dose. Patients had a mean age of 5 years (range 6 months to 12 years) with 14% less than 2 years. Mean baseline CD4+ cell count was 838 cells/mm^3 and mean baseline plasma HIV-1 RNA was 4.7 $\log_{10}$ copies/mL.

Through 48 weeks of therapy, the proportion of patients who achieved and sustained an HIV-1 RNA < 400 copies/mL was 80% for antiretroviral naïve patients and 71% for antiretroviral experienced patients. The mean increase from baseline in CD4+ cell count was 404 cells/mm^3 for antiretroviral naïve and 284 cells/mm^3 for antiretroviral experienced patients treated through 48 weeks. At 48 weeks, two patients (2%) had prematurely discontinued the study. One antiretroviral naïve patient prematurely discontinued secondary to an adverse reaction, while one antiretroviral experienced patient prematurely discontinued secondary to an HIV-1 related event.

Dose selection in pediatric patients was based on the following:

- Among patients 14 days to 6 months of age receiving 300/75 mg/m^2 twice daily without nevirapine, plasma concentrations were lower than those observed in adults or in older children. This dose resulted in HIV-1 RNA < 400 copies/mL in 55% of patients (70% in those initiating treatment at <6 weeks of age).
- Among patients 6 months to 12 years of age, the 230/57.5 mg/m^2 oral solution twice daily regimen without nevirapine and the 300/75 mg/m^2 oral solution twice daily regimen with nevirapine provided lopinavir plasma concentrations similar to those obtained in adult patients receiving the 400/100 mg twice daily regimen (without nevirapine). These doses resulted in treatment benefit (proportion of patients with HIV-1 RNA < 400 copies/mL) similar to that seen in the adult clinical trials.
- Among patients 12 to 18 years of age receiving 400/100 mg/m^2 or 480/120 mg/m^2 (with efavirenz) twice daily, plasma concentrations were 60-100% higher than among 6 to 12 year old patients receiving 230/57.5 mg/m^2. Mean apparent clearance was similar to that observed in adult patients receiving standard dose and in patients 6 to 12 years of age. Although changes in HIV-1 RNA in patients with prior treatment failure were less than anticipated, the pharmacokinetic data supports use of similar dosing as in patients 6 to 12 years of age, not to exceed the recommended adult dose.
- For all age groups, the body surface area dosing was converted to body weight dosing using the patient's prescribed lopinavir dose.

16 HOW SUPPLIED/STORAGE AND HANDLING

KALETRA® (lopinavir/ritonavir) Film-Coated tablets and Oral Solution are available in the following strengths and package sizes:

16.1 KALETRA Tablets, 200 mg lopinavir/50 mg ritonavir

Yellow film-coated ovaloid tablets debossed with the "a" logo and the code KA:

Bottles of 120 tablets .... (NDC 0074-6799-22)

Recommended Storage

Store KALETRA film-coated tablets at 20°-25°C (68°-77°F); excursions permitted to 15°-30°C (59° to 86°F)[see USP controlled room temperature]. Dispense in original container or USP equivalent tight container (250 mL or less).

For patient use: exposure of this product to high humidity outside the original container or USP equivalent tight container (250 mL or less) for longer than 2 weeks is not recommended.

16.2 KALETRA Tablets, 100 mg lopinavir/25 mg ritonavir

Pale yellow film-coated ovaloid tablets debossed with the "a" logo and the code KC:

Bottles of 60 tablets .... (NDC 0074-0522-60)

Recommended Storage

Store KALETRA film-coated tablets at 20°-25°C (68°-77°F); excursions permitted to 15°-30°C (59° to 86°F)[see USP controlled room temperature]. Dispense in original container or USP equivalent tight container (100 mL or less). For patient use: exposure of this product to high humidity outside the original container or USP equivalent tight container (100 mL or less) for longer than 2 weeks is not recommended.

Information on the AbbVie, Inc. products listed on these pages is from the prescribing information in use as of July 31, 2013. For more information, please visit rxabbvie.com or call 1-800-633-9110.

16.3 KALETRA Oral Solution

KALETRA (lopinavir/ritonavir) oral solution is a light yellow to orange colored liquid supplied in amber-colored multiple-dose bottles containing 400 mg lopinavir/100 mg ritonavir per 5 mL (80 mg lopinavir/20 mg ritonavir per mL) packaged with a marked dosing cup in the following size:

160 mL bottle .... (NDC 0074-3956-46)

Recommended Storage

Store KALETRA oral solution at 2°-8°C (36°-46°F) until dispensed. Avoid exposure to excessive heat. For patient use, refrigerated KALETRA oral solution remains stable until the expiration date printed on the label. If stored at room temperature up to 25°C (77°F), oral solution should be used within 2 months.

17 PATIENT COUNSELING INFORMATION

See FDA-approved patient labeling (Medication Guide)

Information For Patients

Patients or parents of patients should be informed that:

General Information

☐ They should pay special attention to accurate administration of their dose to minimize the risk of accidental overdose or underdose of KALETRA.

☐ They should inform their healthcare provider if their children's weight changes in order to make sure that the child's KALETRA dose is the correct one.

☐ They should take the prescribed dose of KALETRA as directed and to set up a daily routine in order to do so.

☐ KALETRA tablets may be taken with or without food. KALETRA oral solution should be taken with food to enhance absorption.

☐ Sustained decreases in plasma HIV-1 RNA have been associated with a reduced risk of progression to AIDS and death. Patients should remain under the care of a physician while using KALETRA. Patients should be advised to take KALETRA and other concomitant antiretroviral therapy every day as prescribed. KALETRA must always be used in combination with other antiretroviral drugs. Patients should not alter the dose or discontinue therapy without consulting with their doctor. If a dose of KALETRA is missed patients should take the dose as soon as possible and then return to their normal schedule. However, if a dose is skipped the patient should not double the next dose. The amount of HIV-1 virus in their blood may increase if the medicine is stopped for even a short time. The virus may become resistant to KALETRA and become harder to treat.

☐ KALETRA is not a cure for HIV-1 infection and patients may continue to experience illnesses associated with HIV-1 infection, including opportunistic infections. Patients should remain under the care of a physician when using KALETRA.

Patients should be advised to avoid doing things that can spread HIV-1 infection to others.

- **Do not share needles or other injection equipment.**
- **Do not share personal items that can have blood or body fluids on them, like toothbrushes and razor blades.**
- **Do not have any kind of sex without protection.** Always practice safe sex by using a latex or polyurethane condom to lower the chance of sexual contact with semen, vaginal secretions, or blood.
- **Do not breastfeed.** We do not know if KALETRA can be passed to the baby through breast milk and whether it could harm the baby. Also, mothers with HIV-1 should not breastfeed because HIV-1 can be passed to the baby in the breast milk.

Drug Interactions

☐ KALETRA may interact with some drugs; therefore, patients should be advised to report to their doctor the use of any other prescription, non-prescription medication or herbal products, particularly St. John's Wort.

☐ KALETRA tablets can be taken at the same time as didanosine without food. Patients taking didanosine should take didanosine one hour before or two hours after KALETRA oral solution.

☐ If they are receiving avanafil, sildenafil, tadalafil, or vardenafil for the treatment of erectile dysfunction, there may be an increased risk of associated adverse reactions including hypotension, visual changes, and sustained erection, and should promptly report any symptoms to their doctor. If they are currently using or planning to use avanafil or tadalafil (for the treatment of pulmonary arterial hypertension) they should ask their doctor about potential adverse reactions these medications may cause when taken with KALETRA. The doctor may choose not to keep them on avanafil, or may adjust the dose of tadalafil while initiating treatment with KALETRA.

☐ If they are receiving estrogen-based hormonal contraceptives, additional or alternate contraceptive measures should be used during therapy with KALETRA.

☐ If they are taking or before they begin using Serevent® (salmeterol) and KALETRA, they should talk to their doctor about problems these two medications may cause when taken together. The doctor may choose not to keep someone on Serevent® (salmeterol).

☐ If they are taking or before they begin taking Advair® (salmeterol in combination with fluticasone propionate) and KALETRA, they should talk to their doctor about problems these two medications may cause when taken together. The doctor may choose not to keep someone on Advair® (salmeterol in combination with fluticasone propionate).

Potential Adverse Effects

☐ Skin rashes ranging in severity from mild to toxic epidermal necrolysis (TEN), Stevens-Johnson syndrome and Erythema multiforme have been reported in patients receiving KALETRA or its components lopinavir and/or ritonavir. Patients should be advised to contact their healthcare provider if they develop a rash while taking KALETRA. The healthcare provider will determine if treatment should be continued or an alternative antiretroviral regimen used.

☐ Patients should be advised that appropriate liver function testing will be conducted prior to initiating and during therapy with KALETRA. Pre-existing liver disease including Hepatitis B or C can worsen with use of KALETRA. This can be seen as worsening of transaminase elevations or hepatic decompensation. Patients should be advised that their liver function tests will need to be monitored closely especially during the first several months of KALETRA treatment and that they should notify their healthcare provider if they develop the signs and symptoms of worsening liver disease including loss of appetite, abdominal pain, jaundice, and itchy skin.

☐ New onset of diabetes or exacerbation of pre-existing diabetes mellitus, and hyperglycemia have been reported during KALETRA use. Patients should be advised to notify their healthcare provider if they develop the signs and symptoms of diabetes mellitus including frequent urination, excessive thirst, extreme hunger or unusual weight loss and/or an increased blood sugar while on KALETRA as they may require a change in their diabetes treatment or new treatment.

☐ KALETRA might produce changes in the electrocardiogram (e.g., PR and/or QT prolongation). Patients should consult their physician if they experience symptoms such as dizziness, lightheadedness, abnormal heart rhythm or loss of consciousness.

☐ They should seek medical assistance immediately if they develop a sustained penile erection lasting more than 4 hours while taking KALETRA and a PDE 5 Inhibitor such as Viagra, Cialis or Levitra.

☐ Redistribution or accumulation of body fat may occur in patients receiving antiretroviral therapy and that the cause and long term health effects of these conditions are not known at this time.

☐ Patients should be informed that there may be a greater chance of developing diarrhea with the once daily regimen as compared with the twice daily regimen.

KALETRA Tablets, 200 mg lopinavir/50 mg ritonavir
Manufactured by AbbVie LTD, Barceloneta, PR 00617
for AbbVie Inc., North Chicago, IL 60064 USA
KALETRA Tablets, 100 mg lopinavir/25 mg ritonavir and KALETRA Oral Solution
AbbVie Inc., North Chicago, IL 60064 USA
03-A625 - R16 - Rev. January, 2013

MEDICATION GUIDE
KALETRA® (kuh-LEE-tra)
(lopinavir/ritonavir)
Tablets
KALETRA® (kuh-LEE-tra)
(lopinavir/ritonavir)
Oral Solution

Read this Medication Guide before you start taking KALETRA and each time you get a refill. There may be new information. This information does not take the place of talking with your doctor about your medical condition or treatment. You and your doctor should talk about your treatment with KALETRA before you start taking it and at regular check-ups. You should stay under your doctor's care when taking KALETRA.

What is the most important information I should know about KALETRA?

KALETRA may cause serious side effects, including:

- **Interactions with other medicines. It is important to know the medicines that should not be taken with KALETRA.** For more information, see "Who should not take KALETRA?"
- **Changes in your heart rhythm and the electrical activity of your heart.** These changes may be seen on an EKG (electrocardiogram) and can lead to serious heart problems. Your risk for these problems may be higher if you:
  - already have a history of abnormal heart rhythm or other types of heart disease.
  - take other medicines that can affect your heart rhythm while you take KALETRA.

Tell your doctor right away if you have any of these symptoms while taking KALETRA:

- dizziness
- lightheadedness
- fainting
- sensation of abnormal heartbeats

See "What are the possible side effects of KALETRA?" for more information about serious side effects.

What is KALETRA?

KALETRA is a prescription HIV-1 medicine that is used with other HIV medicines to treat HIV-1 (Human Immunodeficiency Virus) infection in adults and children 14 days of age and older. HIV is the virus that causes AIDS (Acquired Immune Deficiency Syndrome). KALETRA is a type of HIV medicine called a protease inhibitor. KALETRA contains two medicines: lopinavir and ritonavir.

When used with other HIV medicines, KALETRA may help to reduce the amount of HIV in your blood (called "viral load"). KALETRA may also help to increase the number of white blood cells called CD4 (T) cell which help fight off other infections. Reducing the amount of HIV and increasing the CD4 (T) cell count may improve your immune system. This may reduce your risk of death or infections that can happen when your immune system is weak (opportunistic infections).

It is not known if KALETRA is safe and effective in children under 14 days old.

KALETRA does not cure HIV infection or AIDS. People taking KALETRA may develop infections or other conditions associated with HIV infection, including opportunistic infections (for example, pneumonia and herpes virus infections).

Avoid doing things that can spread HIV-1 infection to others:

- **Do not share needles or other injection equipment.**
- **Do not share personal items that can have blood or body fluids on them, like toothbrushes and razor blades.**
- **Do not have any kind of sex without protection.** Always practice safe sex by using a latex or polyurethane condom to lower the chance of sexual contact with semen, vaginal secretions, or blood.

Ask your doctor if you have any questions on how to prevent passing HIV to other people.

Who should not take KALETRA?

Do not take KALETRA if you take any of the following medicines:

- alfuzosin (Uroxatral®)
- cisapride (Propulsid®, Quicksolv®)
- ergot containing medicines including
  - ergotamine tartrate (Cafergot®, Migergot®, Ergomar®, Ergostat®, Medihaler®, Ergotamine, Wigraine®, Wigrettes®)
  - dihydroergotamine mesylate (D.H.E. 45®, Migranal®)
  - methylergonovine (Methergine®)
- lovastatin (Advicor®, Altoprev®, Mevacor®)
- midazolam oral syrup
- pimozide (Orap®)
- rifampin (Rifadin®, Rifamate®, Rifater®, Rimactane®)
- sildenafil (Revatio®), when used for the treatment of pulmonary arterial hypertension
- simvastatin (Zocor®, Vytorin®, Simcor®)
- St. John's Wort (Hypericum perforatum)
- triazolam (Halcion®)

Serious problems can happen if you or your child take any of the medicines listed above with KALETRA.

- **Do not take KALETRA if you are allergic to** lopinavir, ritonavir or any of the ingredients in KALETRA. See the end of this Medication Guide for a complete list of ingredients in KALETRA.

What should I tell my doctor before taking KALETRA?

KALETRA may not be right for you. Tell your doctor about all your medical conditions, including if you:

- have any heart problems, including if you have a condition called Congenital Long QT Syndrome.
- have or had pancreas problems.
- have liver problems, including Hepatitis B or Hepatitis C.
- have diabetes.
- have hemophilia. People who take KALETRA may have increased bleeding.
- have low potassium in your blood.
- are pregnant or plan to become pregnant. It is not known if KALETRA will harm your unborn baby.
  Pregnancy Registry. There is a pregnancy registry for women who take antiretroviral medicines during pregnancy. The purpose of the pregnancy registry is to collect information about the health of you and your baby. Talk to your doctor about how you can take part in this registry.
- **Do not breastfeed.** We do not know if KALETRA can be passed to the baby through your breast milk and whether it could harm your baby. Also, mothers with HIV-1 should not breastfeed because HIV-1 can be passed to the baby in the breast milk.

Tell your doctor about all the medicines you take, including prescription and non-prescription medicines, vitamins, and herbal supplements. Many medicines interact with KALETRA. Do not start taking a new medicine without telling your doctor or pharmacist. Your doctor can tell you if it is safe to take KALETRA with other medicines. Your doctor may need to change the dose of other medicines while you take KALETRA.

Especially tell your doctor if you take:

- medicine to treat HIV
- estrogen-based contraceptives (birth control pills and patches). KALETRA may reduce the effectiveness of estrogen-based contraceptives. During treatment with KALETRA, you should use a different type or an extra form of birth control. Talk to your doctor about what types of birth control you can use to prevent pregnancy while taking KALETRA.
- medicines to prevent organ transplant rejection
- medicines to treat cancer
- amiodarone (Cordarone®, Pacerone®)
- atorvastatin (Lipitor®)
- atovaquone (Marlarone®, Mepron®)
- avanafil (Stendra®), sildenafil (Viagra®), tadalafil (Cialis®), or vardenafil (Levitra®) for the treatment of erectile dysfunction (ED). If you get dizzy or faint (low blood pressure), have vision changes or have an erection that last longer than 4 hours, call your doctor or get medical help right away
- bepridil (Bepadin®, Vascor®)
- boceprevir (Victrelis®)
- bosentan (Tracleer®)
- budesonide (Rhinocort®, Symbicort®, Pulmicort®, Entocort EC®)
- bupropion (Aplenzin®, Forfivo XL®, Wellbutrin®, Zyban®)
- carbamazepine (Carbatrol®, Epitol®, Equetro®, Tegretol®)
- clarithromycin (Biaxin®, Prevpac®)
- colchicine (Colcrys®)
- dexamethasone (Maxidex®, Ozurdex®)
- disulfiram
- felodipine
- fentanyl (Abstral®, Actiq®, Duragesic®, Fentora®, Lazanda®, Onsolis®, Subsys®)
- fluticasone (Cutivate®, Flonase®, Flovent®, Flovent Diskus®, Flovent HFA®, Veramyst®)
- itraconazole (Onmel®, Sporanox®)
- ketoconazole (Extina®, Ketozole®, Nizoral®, Xolegel®)
- lamotrigine (Lamictal®)
- lidocaine
- methadone hydrochloride (Dolphine hydrochloride, Methadose®)
- metronidazole
- nicardipine (Cardene®)
- nifedipine (Adalat CC®, Afeditab CR®, Procardia®)
- phenobarbital
- phenytoin (Dilantin®, Phenytek®)
- prednisone
- quinidine (Quinidex®)
- rifabutin (Mycobutin®)
- rivaroxaban (Xarelto®)
- rosuvastatin (Crestor®)
- salmeterol (Serevent®) or salmeterol when taken in combination with fluticasone (Advair Diskus®, Advair HFA®)
- tadalafil (Adcirca®) for the treatment of pulmonary arterial hypertension
- telaprevir (Incivek®)
- trazodone (Oleptro®)
- valproate (Depakote®, Depakene®, Depacon®)
- voriconazole (Vfend®)
- warfarin (Coumadin®, Jantoven®)

KALETRA should not be administered once daily in combination with carbamazepine (Carbatrol®, Epitol®, Equetro®, Tegretol®), phenobarbital, or phenytoin (Dilantin®, Phenytek®)

Ask your doctor or pharmacist if you are not sure if your medicine is one that is listed above.

Know all the medicines that you take. Keep a list of them with you to show doctors and pharmacists when you get a new medicine.

If you are not sure if you are taking a medicine above, ask your doctor.

How should I take KALETRA?

- Take KALETRA every day exactly as prescribed by your doctor.
- It is very important to set up a dosing schedule and follow it every day.
- Do not change your treatment or stop treatment without first talking with your doctor.
- Swallow KALETRA tablets whole. Do not chew, break, or crush KALETRA tablets.
- KALETRA tablets can be taken with or without food.
- If you are taking both didanosine (Videx®) and KALETRA:
  - didanosine can be taken at the same time as KALETRA tablets, without food.
  - take didanosine either one hour before or two hours after taking KALETRA oral solution.
- Do not miss a dose of KALETRA. This could make the virus harder to treat. If you forget to take KALETRA, take the missed dose right away. If it is almost time for your next dose, do not take the missed dose. Instead, follow your regular dosing schedule by taking your next dose at its regular time. Do not take more than one dose of KALETRA at one time.
- If you take more than the prescribed dose of KALETRA, call your doctor or go to the nearest emergency room right away.
- Take KALETRA oral solution with food to help it work better.
- If your child is prescribed KALETRA , tell your doctor if your child's weight changes.
- KALETRA **should not** be given one time each day in children. When giving KALETRA to your child, give KALETRA exactly as prescribed.
- KALETRA oral solution contains propylene glycol and a large amount of alcohol. KALETRA oral solution **should not** be given to babies younger than 14 days of age unless your doctor thinks it is right for your baby.
  - If a young child drinks more than the recommended dose, it could make them sick. Contact your local poison control center or emergency room right away.
  - Talk with your doctor if you take or plan to take metronidazole or disulfiram. You can have severe nausea and vomiting if you take these medicines with KALETRA.
- When your KALETRA supply starts to run low, get more from your doctor or pharmacy. It is important not to run out of KALETRA. The amount of HIV-1 virus in your blood may increase if the medicine is stopped for even a short time. The virus may become resistant to KALETRA and become harder to treat.

What are the possible side effects of KALETRA?

KALETRA can cause serious side effects, including:

- See **"What is the most important information I should know about KALETRA?"**
- **Inflammation of the pancreas (pancreatitis).** Some people who take KALETRA get inflammation of the pancreas which may be serious and cause death. You have a higher chance of getting pancreatitis if you have had it before. Tell your doctor if you have nausea, vomiting, or abdominal pain while taking KALETRA. These may be signs of pancreatitis.
- **Liver problems.** Liver problems, including death, can happen in people who take KALETRA. Your doctor should do blood tests before and during your treatment with KALETRA to check your liver function. Some people with liver disease such as Hepatitis B and Hepatitis C who take KALETRA may have worsening liver disease. Tell your doctor right away if you have any of these signs and symptoms of liver problems:
  - loss of appetite
  - yellow skin and whites of eyes (jaundice)
  - dark-colored urine
  - pale colored stools
  - itchy skin
  - stomach area (abdominal) pain.
- **Diabetes and high blood sugar (hyperglycemia).** Some people who take protease inhibitors including KALETRA get new or more serious diabetes, or high blood sugar. Tell your doctor if you notice an increase in thirst or urinate often while taking KALETRA.
- **Changes in you immune system (Immune Reconstitution Syndrome)** can happen when you start taking HIV medicines. Your immune system may get stronger and begin to fight infections that have been hidden in your body for a long time. Call your doctor right away if you start having new symptoms after starting your HIV medicine.
- **Increases in certain fat (triglycerides and cholesterol) levels in your blood.** Large increases of triglycerides and cholesterol can be seen in blood test results of some people who take KALETRA. Your doctor should do blood tests to check your cholesterol and triglyceride levels before you start taking KALETRA and during your treatment.
- **Changes in body fat.** Changes in body fat in some people who take antiretroviral therapy. These changes may include increased amount of fat in the upper back and neck ("buffalo hump"), breast, and around the trunk. Loss of fat from the legs, arms and face may also happen. The cause and long-term health effects of these conditions are not known at this time.
- **Increased bleeding for hemophiliacs.** Some people with hemophilia have increased bleeding with protease inhibitors including KALETRA.
- **Allergic reactions.** Skin rashes, some of them severe, can occur in people who take KALETRA. Tell your healthcare provider if you had a rash when you took another medicine for your HIV-1 infection or if you notice any skin rash when you take KALETRA.
- **Babies taking KALETRA oral solution may have side effects.** KALETRA oral solution contains alcohol and propylene glycol. Call your doctor right away if your baby appears too sleepy or their breathing has changed.

Common side effects of KALETRA include:

- diarrhea
- nausea
- stomach area (abdominal) pain
- feeling weak
- vomiting
- headache
- upset stomach

Tell your doctor about any side effect that bothers you or that does not go away.

These are not all of the possible side effects of KALETRA. For more information, ask your doctor or pharmacist.

Call your doctor for medical advice about side effects. You may report side effects to FDA at 1-800-FDA-1088.

How should I store KALETRA?

KALETRA tablets:

- Store KALETRA tablets at room temperature, between 59°F to 86°F (15°C to 30°C).
- Do not keep KALETRA tablets out of the container it comes in for longer than 2 weeks, especially in areas where there is a lot of humidity. Keep the container closed tightly.

KALETRA oral solution:

- Store KALETRA oral solution in a refrigerator, between 36°F to 46°F (2°C to 8°C). KALETRA oral solution that is kept refrigerated may be used until the expiration date printed on the label.
- KALETRA oral solution that is stored at room temperature (less than 77°F or 25°C) should be used within 2 months.
- Keep KALETRA away from high heat.

Throw away any medicine that is out of date or that you no longer need.

Keep KALETRA and all medicines out of the reach of children.

General information about KALETRA

Medicines are sometimes prescribed for purposes other than those listed in a Medication Guide. Do not use KALETRA for a condition for which it was not prescribed. Do not give KALETRA to other people, even if they have the same condition you have. It may harm them.

This Medication Guide summarizes the most important information about KALETRA. If you would like more information, talk with your doctor. You can ask your pharmacist or doctor for information about KALETRA that is written for health professionals. For more information about KALETRA call 1-800-633-9110 or go to www.KALETRA.com.

What are the ingredients in KALETRA?

Active ingredients: lopinavir and ritonavir

Inactive ingredients:

KALETRA 200 mg lopinavir and 50 mg ritonavir tablets: copovidone, sorbitan monolaurate, colloidal silicon dioxide, and sodium stearyl fumarate. The film coating contains: hypromellose, titanium dioxide, polyethylene glycol 400, hydroxypropyl cellulose, talc, colloidal silicon dioxide, polyethylene glycol 3350, yellow ferric oxide 172, and polysorbate 80.

KALETRA 100 mg lopinavir and 25 mg ritonavir tablets: copovidone, sorbitan monolaurate, colloidal silicon dioxide, and sodium stearyl fumarate. The film coating contains: polyvinyl alcohol, titanium dioxide, talc, polytheylene glycol 3350, and yellow ferric oxide E172.

KALETRA oral solution: acesulfame potassium, alcohol, artificial cotton candy flavor, citric acid, glycerin, high fructose corn syrup, Magnasweet-110 flavor, menthol, natural and artificial vanilla flavor, peppermint oil, polyoxyl 40 hydrogenated castor oil, povidone, propylene glycol, saccharin sodium, sodium chloride, sodium citrate, and water.

KALETRA oral solution contains 42.4% alcohol (v/v). "See How should I take KALETRA?".

This Medication Guide has been approved by the U.S. Food and Drug Administration.

* The brands listed are trademarks of their respective owners and are not trademarks of AbbVie Inc. The makers of these brands are not affiliated with and do not endorse AbbVie Inc. or its products.

KALETRA Tablets, 200 mg lopinavir/50 mg ritonavir
Manufactured by AbbVie LTD, Barceloneta, PR 00617
for AbbVie Inc., North Chicago, IL 60064 USA
KALETRA Tablets, 100 mg lopinavir/25 mg ritonavir and KALETRA Oral Solution
AbbVie Inc., North Chicago, IL 60064 USA
Ref.: 03-A625-R16-Rev. January 2013

Shown in Product Identification Guide, page 303

Information on the AbbVie, Inc. products listed on these pages is from the prescribing information in use as of July 31, 2013. For more information, please visit rxabbvie.com or call 1-800-633-9110.

LUPANETA PACK™ ℞

Leuprolide Acetate for Depot Suspension 3.75 mg for intramuscular injection only and Norethindrone Acetate tablets, 5 mg for oral administration

HIGHLIGHTS OF PRESCRIBING INFORMATION

These highlights do not include all the information needed to use LUPANETA PACK safely and effectively. See full prescribing information for LUPANETA PACK.

LUPANETA PACK (leuprolide acetate for depot suspension; norethindrone acetate tablets), co-packaged for intramuscular use and for oral use, respectively

Initial U.S. Approval: 2012

INDICATIONS AND USAGE

LUPANETA PACK contains leuprolide acetate, a gonadotropin-releasing hormone (GnRH) agonist and norethindrone acetate, a progestin, indicated for

- Initial management of the painful symptoms of endometriosis (1)
- Management of recurrence of symptoms (1)

Limitations of Use: Initial treatment course is limited to 6 months and use is not recommended longer than a total of 12 months due to concerns about adverse impact on bone mineral density. (1, 2.1, 5.1)

DOSAGE AND ADMINISTRATION

- Leuprolide acetate for depot suspension 3.75 mg given by a healthcare provider as a single intramuscular injection every month for up to six injections (6 months of therapy) (2.1)
- Norethindrone acetate 5 mg tablets taken orally by the patient once per day for up to 6 months (2.1)
- If endometriosis symptoms recur after initial course of therapy, consider retreatment for up to another six months (2.1)
- Assess bone density before retreatment begins (2.1, 5.1)
- Reconstitute leuprolide acetate prior to use, see important administration instructions (2.3)

DOSAGE FORMS AND STRENGTHS

- Leuprolide acetate for depot suspension 3.75 mg syringe (3)
- Norethindrone acetate 5 mg tablets; 30 count bottle (3)

CONTRAINDICATIONS

- Hypersensitivity to GnRH, GnRH agonist or any of the excipients in leuprolide acetate for depot suspension or norethindrone acetate (4)
- Undiagnosed abnormal uterine bleeding (4)
- Pregnancy or suspected pregnancy (4, 8.1)
- Women who are breast-feeding (4)
- Known, suspected or history of breast or other hormone-sensitive cancer (4)
- Thrombotic or thromboembolic disorders (4)
- Liver tumors or liver disease (4)

WARNINGS AND PRECAUTIONS

- Loss of bone mineral density: do not use for more than two six-month treatment courses. (1, 2.1, 5.1)
- Exclude pregnancy before starting treatment and discontinue use if pregnancy occurs; use non-hormonal methods of contraception only. (5.2)
- Discontinue in case of sudden loss of vision or onset of proptosis, diplopia or migraine. (5.3)
- Carefully observe patients with history of depression and discontinue the drug if the depression recurs to a serious degree. (5.4)
- Assess and manage risk factors for cardiovascular disease before starting LUPANETA PACK. (5.6)

ADVERSE REACTIONS

Leuprolide acetate for depot suspension: Most common related adverse reactions (>10%) were hot flashes/sweats, headache/migraine, depression/emotional lability, nausea/vomiting, nervousness/anxiety, insomnia, pain, acne, asthenia, vaginitis, weight gain, constipation/diarrhea (6.1)

Progestins: breakthrough bleeding, spotting (6.1)

To report SUSPECTED ADVERSE REACTIONS, contact AbbVie Inc. at 1-800-633-9110 or FDA at 1-800-FDA-1088 or www.fda.gov/medwatch

USE IN SPECIFIC POPULATIONS

Pediatric: Safety and effectiveness of LUPANETA PACK has not been established in pediatric patients. (8.4)

Geriatric: LUPANETA PACK has not been studied in women over 65 years of age and is not indicated in this population. (8.5)

See 17 for PATIENT COUNSELING INFORMATION and FDA-approved patient labeling

Revised: 03/2013

FULL PRESCRIBING INFORMATION: CONTENTS*

* Sections or subsections omitted from the full prescribing information are not listed

FULL PRESCRIBING INFORMATION

1 INDICATIONS AND USAGE

LUPANETA PACK (leuprolide acetate for depot suspension and norethindrone acetate tablets) is indicated for initial management of the painful symptoms of endometriosis and for management of recurrence of symptoms.

Limitation of Use: Duration of use is limited due to concerns about adverse impact on bone mineral density *[see Warnings and Precautions (5.1)]*. The initial treatment course of LUPANETA PACK is limited to six months. A single retreatment course of not more than six months may be administered after the initial course of treatment if symptoms recur. Use of LUPANETA PACK for longer than a total of 12 months is not recommended.

2 DOSAGE AND ADMINISTRATION

2.1 Dosing Information

LUPANETA PACK is a co-packaging of leuprolide acetate for depot suspension for intramuscular use and norethindrone acetate tablets for oral use. Administer as follows:

- 3.75 mg of leuprolide acetate by intramuscular injection once a month for up to six injections (6 months of therapy); to be administered by a healthcare provider
- 5 mg of norethindrone acetate orally once daily for up to 6 months of therapy

The initial course of treatment with leuprolide acetate for depot suspension 3.75 mg in combination with norethindrone acetate 5 mg daily is not to exceed six months.

If the symptoms of endometriosis recur after the initial course of therapy, consider retreatment with LUPANETA PACK for up to another six months. It is recommended that bone density be assessed before retreatment begins *[see Warnings and Precautions (5.1)]*.

Treatment beyond two six-month courses has not been studied and is not recommended due to concerns about adverse impact on bone mineral density.

2.2 Different Formulations of Leuprolide Acetate

Due to the specific release characteristics of the 1-month depot formulation, HCPs should not administer 3 doses of the 3.75 mg 1-month formulation simultaneously to mimic the pharmacological profile of the 11.25 mg 3-month formulation.

2.3 Reconstitution and Administration for Injection of Leuprolide Acetate

- Reconstitute and administer the lyophilized microspheres as a single intramuscular injection.
- Inject the suspension immediately or discard if not used within two hours, because leuprolide acetate for depot suspension does not contain a preservative.

1. Visually inspect the leuprolide acetate for depot suspension powder. DO NOT USE the syringe if clumping or caking is evident. A thin layer of powder on the wall of the syringe is considered normal prior to mixing with the diluent. The diluent should appear clear.
2. To prepare for injection, screw the white plunger into the end stopper until the stopper begins to turn (see Figure 1 and Figure 2).

[See figure 1 above]

Figure 1:

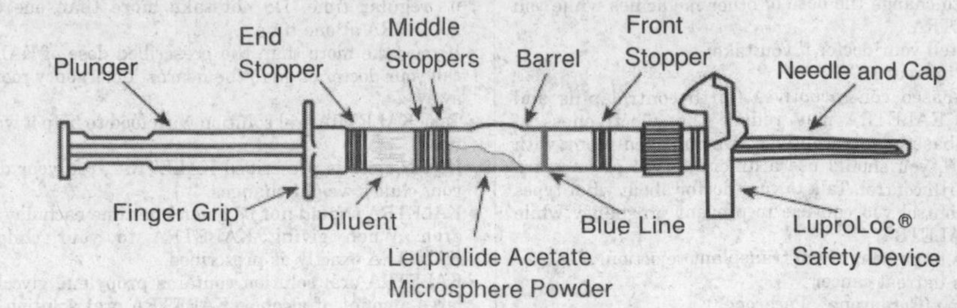

Figure 2:

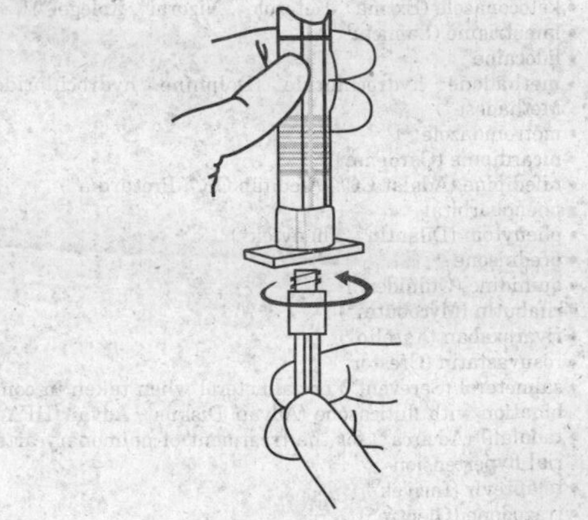

3. Hold the syringe UPRIGHT. Release the diluent by SLOWLY PUSHING (6 to 8 seconds) the plunger until the first middle stopper is at the blue line in the middle of the barrel (see Figure 3).

Figure 3:

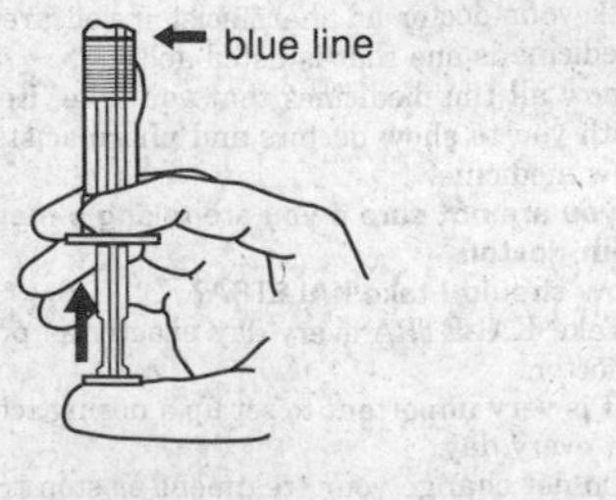

4. Keep the syringe UPRIGHT. Mix the microspheres (powder) thoroughly by gently shaking the syringe until the powder forms a uniform suspension. The suspension will appear milky. If the powder adheres to the stopper or caking/clumping is present, tap the syringe with your finger to disperse. DO NOT USE if any of the powder has not gone into suspension (see Figure 4).

[See figure 4 at top of next column]

5. Keep the syringe UPRIGHT. With the opposite hand pull the needle cap upward without twisting.
6. Keep the syringe UPRIGHT. Advance the plunger to expel the air from the syringe. Now the syringe is ready for injection.

Figure 4:

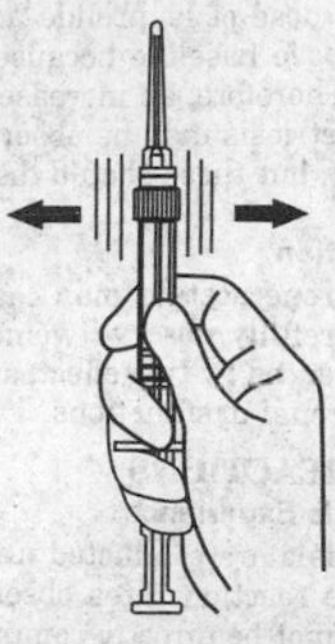

7. After cleaning the injection site with an alcohol swab, administer the intramuscular injection by inserting the needle at a 90 degree angle into the gluteal area, anterior thigh, or deltoid (see Figure 5). Alternate injection sites.

Figure 5:

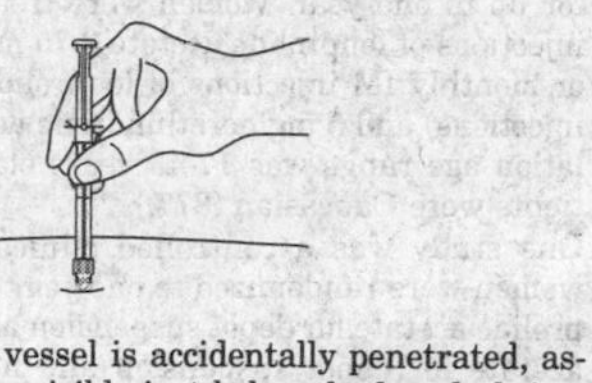

NOTE: If a blood vessel is accidentally penetrated, aspirated blood will be visible just below the luer lock (see Figure 6) and can be seen through the transparent LuproLoc safety device. If blood is present, remove the needle immediately. Do not inject the medication.

Figure 6:

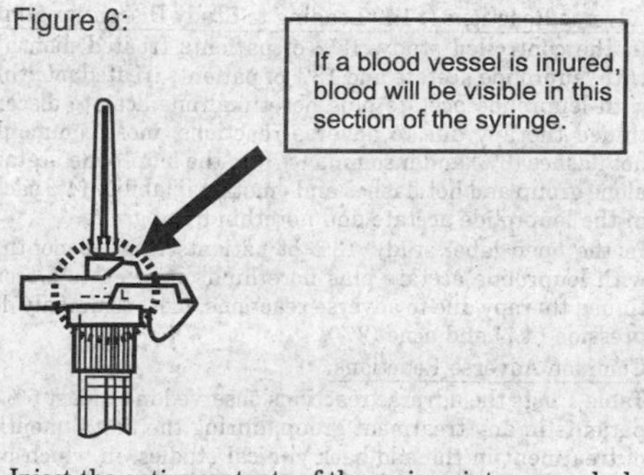

If a blood vessel is injured, blood will be visible in this section of the syringe.

8. Inject the entire contents of the syringe intramuscularly.
9. Withdraw the needle. Once the syringe has been withdrawn, immediately activate the LuproLoc® safety device by pushing the arrow on the lock upward towards the needle tip with the thumb or finger, as illustrated, until the needle cover of the safety device over the needle is fully extended and a CLICK is heard or felt (see Figure 7).

Figure 7:

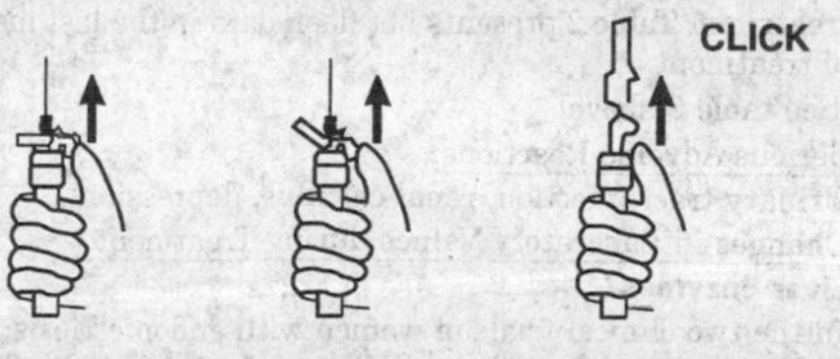

10. Dispose of the syringe according to local regulations/procedures *[see References (15)]*.

3 DOSAGE FORMS AND STRENGTHS

LUPANETA PACK 1-month copackaged kit contains two separate components:

- Leuprolide acetate for depot suspension 3.75 mg for 1-month administration: Leuprolide acetate lyophilized powder for reconstitution with supplied diluent in a prefilled dual chamber syringe
- Norethindrone acetate 5 mg tablets: White to off-white oval, flat-faced beveled edged, uncoated debossed with 'G with breakline' on one side and 304 on other side

4 CONTRAINDICATIONS

LUPANETA PACK is contraindicated in women with the following:

- Hypersensitivity to gonadotropin-releasing hormone (GnRH), GnRH agonist analogs, any of the excipients in leuprolide acetate for depot suspension, or norethindrone acetate
- Undiagnosed abnormal uterine bleeding
- Known, suspected or planned pregnancy during the course of therapy *[see Use in Specific Populations (8.1)]*
- Lactating women *[see Use in Specific Populations (8.3)]*
- Known, suspected or history of breast cancer or other hormone-sensitive cancer
- Current or history of thrombotic or thromboembolic disorder
- Liver tumors or liver disease

Table 1. Adverse Reactions Occurring in the First Six Months of Treatment in ≥ 5% of Patients with Endometriosis

	Controlled Study				Open Label Study	
	LA-Only*		LA/N†		LA/N†	
	N=51		N=55		N=136	
Adverse Reactions	**N**	**%**	**N**	**%**	**N**	**%**
Any Adverse Reaction	50	98	53	96	126	93
Body as a Whole						
Asthenia		18		18		11
Headache/Migraine		65		51		46
Injection Site Reaction		2		9		3
Pain		24		29		21
Cardiovascular System						
Hot flashes/Sweats		98		87		57
Digestive System						
Altered Bowel Function (constipation, diarrhea)		14		15		10
Changes in Appetite		4		0		6
GI Disturbance (dyspepsia, flatulence)		4		7		4
Nausea/Vomiting		25		29		13
Metabolic and Nutritional Disorders						
Edema		0		9		7
Weight Gain		12		13		4
Nervous System						
Depression/Emotional Lability		31		27		34
Dizziness/Vertigo		16		11		7
Insomnia/Sleep Disorder		31		13		15
Decreased Libido		10		4		7
Memory Disorder		6		2		4
Nervousness/Anxiety		8		4		11
Neuromuscular Disorder (leg cramps, paresthesia)		2		9		3
Skin and Appendages						
Androgen-Like Effects (acne, alopecia)		4		5		18
Skin/Mucous Membrane Reaction		4		9		11
Urogenital System						
Breast Changes/Pain/Tenderness		6		13		8
Menstrual Disorders		2		0		5
Vaginitis		20		15		8

* LA-Only = leuprolide acetate 3.75 mg
† LA/N = leuprolide acetate 3.75 mg plus norethindrone acetate 5 mg

5 WARNINGS AND PRECAUTIONS

5.1 Loss of Bone Mineral Density

Leuprolide acetate for depot suspension induces a hypoestrogenic state that results in loss of bone mineral density (BMD), some of which may not be reversible. Concurrent use of norethindrone acetate is effective in reducing the loss of BMD that occurs with leuprolide acetate *[see Clinical Studies (14)]*. Nonetheless, duration of use of LUPANETA PACK is limited to two six-month courses of treatment due to concerns about the adverse impact on BMD. It is recommended that BMD be assessed before retreatment. Retreatment with leuprolide acetate for depot suspension alone is not recommended.

In women with major risk factors for decreased BMD such as chronic alcohol (> 3 units per day) or tobacco use, strong family history of osteoporosis, or chronic use of drugs that can decrease BMD, such as anticonvulsants or corticosteroids, use of LUPANETA PACK may pose an additional risk, and the risks and benefits should be weighed carefully.

5.2 Pregnancy Risk

Leuprolide acetate for depot suspension may cause fetal harm if administered to a pregnant woman. Exclude preg-

Information on the AbbVie, Inc. products listed on these pages is from the prescribing information in use as of July 31, 2013. For more information, please visit rxabbvie.com or call 1-800-633-9110.

Table 2. Hot Flashes in the Month Prior to the Assessment Visit (Controlled Study)

Assessment Visit	Treatment Group	Number of Patients Reporting Hot Flashes		Number of Days with Hot Flashes		Maximum Number of Hot Flashes in 24 Hours	
		N	(%)	N[2]	Mean	N[2]	Mean
Week 24	LA-Only*	32/37	86	37	19	36	5.8
	LA/N†	22/38	58[1]	38	7[1]	38	1.9[1]

* LA-Only = leuprolide acetate 3.75 mg
† LA/N = leuprolide acetate 3.75 mg plus norethindrone acetate 5 mg
[1]Statistically significantly less than the LA-Only group (p<0.01)
[2]Number of patients assessed.

Table 3. Serum Lipids: Mean Percent Changes from Baseline Values at Treatment Week 24

	leuprolide acetate 3.75 mg		leuprolide acetate for depot suspension 3.75 mg plus norethindrone acetate 5 mg daily			
	Controlled Study (n=39)		Controlled Study (n=41)		Open Label Study (n=117)	
	Baseline Value*	Wk 24% Change	Baseline Value*	Wk 24% Change	Baseline Value*	Wk 24% Change
Total Cholesterol	170.5	9.2%	179.3	0.2%	181.2	2.8%
HDL Cholesterol	52.4	7.4%	51.8	-18.8%	51.0	-14.6%
LDL Cholesterol	96.6	10.9%	101.5	14.1%	109.1	13.1%
LDL/HDL Ratio	2.0†	5.0%	2.1†	43.4%	2.3†	39.4%
Triglycerides	107.8	17.5%	130.2	9.5%	105.4	13.8%

* mg/dL
† ratio

Table 4. Percent of Patients with Serum Lipid Values Outside of the Normal Range

	leuprolide acetate for depot suspension 3.75 mg plus norethindrone acetate 5 mg daily			
	Controlled Study (n=41)		Open Label Study (n=117)	
	Baseline	Wk 24*	Baseline	Wk 24*
Total Cholesterol (>240 mg/dL)	15%	20%	6%	7%
HDL Cholesterol (<40 mg/dL)	15%	44%	15%	41%
LDL Cholesterol (>160 mg/dL)	5%	7%	9%	11%
LDL/HDL Ratio (>4.0)	2%	15%	7%	21%
Triglycerides (>200 mg/dL)	12%	10%	5%	9%

* Includes all patients regardless of baseline value.

nancy before initiating treatment with LUPANETA PACK. When used at the recommended dose and dosing interval, leuprolide acetate for depot suspension usually inhibits ovulation and stops menstruation. Contraception, however, is not ensured by taking leuprolide acetate for depot suspension. Therefore, patients should use nonhormonal methods of contraception. Advise patients to notify their healthcare provider if they believe they may be pregnant. Discontinue LUPANETA PACK if a patient becomes pregnant during treatment and inform the patient of potential risk to the fetus *[see Contraindications (4) and Use in Specific Populations (8.1)]*.

5.3 Visual Abnormalities

Discontinue norethindrone acetate tablets in the LUPANETA PACK pending examination if there is a sudden partial or complete loss of vision or if there is sudden onset of proptosis, diplopia, or migraine. Discontinue LUPANETA PACK if examination reveals papilledema or retinal vascular lesions.

5.4 Clinical Depression

Depression may occur or worsen during treatment with LUPANETA PACK. Carefully observe patients with a history of clinical depression and discontinue LUPANETA PACK if the depression recurs to a serious degree.

5.5 Serious Allergic Reactions

In clinical trials of LUPANETA PACK, adverse events of asthma were reported in women with pre-existing histories of asthma, sinusitis and environmental or drug allergies. Symptoms consistent with an anaphylactoid or asthmatic process have been reported postmarketing.

5.6 Cardiovascular and Metabolic Disorders

Assess and manage risk factors for cardiovascular disease before starting LUPANETA PACK. Closely monitor women on norethindrone acetate who have risk factors for arterial vascular disease (e.g., hypertension, diabetes mellitus, tobacco use, hypercholesterolemia, and obesity) and/or venous thromboembolism (e.g., family history of VTE, obesity, and smoking) when using LUPANETA PACK. *[see Contraindications (4)]*.

5.7 Initial Flare of Symptoms

Following the first dose of leuprolide acetate, sex steroids temporarily rise above baseline because of the physiologic effect of the drug. Therefore, an increase in symptoms associated with endometriosis may be observed during the initial days of therapy, but these should dissipate with continued therapy.

5.8 Fluid Retention

Because norethindrone acetate may cause some degree of fluid retention, carefully observe women with conditions that might be influenced by this effect, such as epilepsy, migraine, cardiac or renal dysfunctions.

6 ADVERSE REACTIONS

6.1 Clinical Trials Experience

Because clinical trials are conducted under widely varying conditions, adverse reaction rates observed in the clinical trials of a drug cannot be directly compared to rates in the clinical trials of another drug and may not reflect the rates observed in clinical practice.

The safety of co-administering leuprolide acetate for depot suspension and norethindrone acetate was evaluated in two clinical studies in which a total of 242 women were treated for up to one year. Women were treated with monthly IM injections of leuprolide acetate 3.75 mg (13 injections) alone or monthly IM injections of leuprolide acetate 3.75 mg (13 injections) and 5 mg norethindrone acetate daily. The population age range was 17-43 years old. The majority of patients were Caucasian (87%).

One study was a controlled clinical trial in which 106 women were randomized to one year of treatment with leuprolide acetate for depot suspension alone or with leuprolide acetate for depot suspension and norethindrone acetate. The other study was an open-label single arm clinical study in 136 women of one year of treatment with leuprolide acetate for depot suspension and norethindrone acetate, with follow-up for up to 12 months after completing treatment.

Adverse Reactions (>1%) Leading to Study Discontinuation:

In the controlled study, 18% of patients treated monthly with leuprolide acetate and 18% of patients treated monthly with leuprolide acetate plus norethindrone acetate discontinued therapy due to adverse reactions, most commonly hot flashes (6%) and insomnia (4%) in the leuprolide acetate alone group and hot flashes and emotional lability (4% each) in the leuprolide acetate and norethindrone group.

In the open label study, 13% of patients treated monthly with leuprolide acetate plus norethindrone acetate discontinued therapy due to adverse reactions, most commonly depression (4%) and acne (2%).

Common Adverse Reactions:

Table 1 lists the adverse reactions observed in at least 5% of patients in any treatment group, during the first 6 months of treatment in the add-back clinical studies, in which patients were treated with monthly leuprolide acetate for depot suspension 3.75 mg with or without norethindrone acetate co-treatment. The most frequently-occurring adverse reactions observed in these studies were hot flashes and headaches.

[See table 1 at top of previous page]

In the controlled clinical trial, 50 of 51 (98%) patients in the leuprolide acetate alone group and 48 of 55 (87%) patients in the leuprolide acetate and norethindrone group reported experiencing hot flashes on one or more occasions during treatment. Table 2 presents hot flash data in the last month of treatment.

[See table 2 above]

Serious Adverse Reactions:

Urinary tract infection, renal calculus, depression

Changes in Laboratory Values during Treatment:

Liver Enzymes

In the two clinical trials of women with endometriosis, 4 of 191 patients receiving leuprolide acetate and norethindrone acetate for up to 12 months developed an elevated (at least twice the upper limit of normal) SGPT and 2 of 136 developed an elevated GGT. Five of the 6 increases were observed beyond 6 months of treatment. None was associated with an elevated bilirubin concentration.

Lipids

Percent changes from baseline for serum lipids and percentages of patients with serum lipid values outside of the normal range in the two studies of leuprolide acetate and norethindrone acetate are summarized in the tables below. The major impact of adding norethindrone acetate to treatment with leuprolide acetate for depot suspension was a decrease in serum HDL cholesterol and an increase in the LDL/HDL ratio.

[See table 3 above]

Changes from baseline tended to be greater at Week 52. After treatment, mean serum lipid levels from patients with follow up data (105 of 158 patients) returned to pretreatment values.

[See table 4 above]

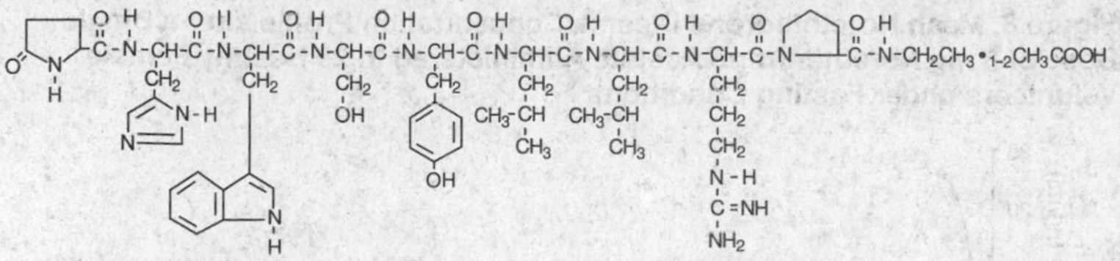

6.2 Postmarketing Experience

The following adverse reactions have been identified during postapproval use of leuprolide acetate for depot suspension or norethindrone acetate. Because these reactions are reported voluntarily from a population of uncertain size, it is not always possible to reliably estimate their frequency or establish a causal relationship to drug exposure.

Leuprolide Acetate for Depot Suspension

During postmarketing surveillance with other dosage forms and in the same or different populations, the following adverse reactions were reported:

- Allergic reactions (anaphylactic, rash, urticaria, and photosensitivity reactions)
- Mood swings, including depression
- Suicidal ideation and attempt
- Symptoms consistent with an anaphylactoid or asthmatic process
- Localized reactions including induration and abscess at the site of injection
- Symptoms consistent with fibromyalgia (e.g., joint and muscle pain, headaches, sleep disorders, gastrointestinal distress, and shortness of breath), individually and collectively

Other adverse reactions reported are:

Hepato-biliary disorder - Serious liver injury

Injury, poisoning and procedural complications - Spinal fracture

Investigations - Decreased white blood count

Musculoskeletal and connective tissue disorder - Tenosynovitis-like symptoms

Nervous System disorder - Convulsion, peripheral neuropathy, paralysis

Vascular disorder - Hypotension, Hypertension

Serious venous and arterial thrombotic and thromboembolic events, including deep vein thrombosis, pulmonary embolism, myocardial infarction, stroke, and transient ischemic attack

Pituitary apoplexy

During post-marketing surveillance, cases of pituitary apoplexy (a clinical syndrome secondary to infarction of the pituitary gland) have been reported after the administration of leuprolide acetate and other GnRH agonists. In a majority of these cases, a pituitary adenoma was diagnosed, with a majority of pituitary apoplexy cases occurring within 2 weeks of the first dose, and some within the first hour. In these cases, pituitary apoplexy has presented as sudden headache, vomiting, visual changes, ophthalmoplegia, altered mental status, and sometimes cardiovascular collapse. Immediate medical attention has been required.

7 DRUG INTERACTIONS

7.1 Drug-Drug Interactions

Leuprolide Acetate for Depot Suspension

No pharmacokinetic-based drug-drug interaction studies have been conducted with leuprolide acetate for depot suspension. However, drug interactions associated with cytochrome P-450 enzymes or protein binding would not be expected to occur *[see Clinical Pharmacology (12.3)]*.

Norethindrone Acetate

No pharmacokinetic drug interaction studies investigating any drug-drug interactions with norethindrone acetate have been conducted. Drugs or herbal products that induce or inhibit certain enzymes, including CYP3A4, may decrease or increase the serum concentrations of norethindrone.

7.2 Drug/Laboratory Test Interactions

Leuprolide Acetate for Depot Suspension

Administration of leuprolide acetate for depot suspension in therapeutic doses results in suppression of the pituitary-gonadal system. Normal function is usually restored within three months after treatment is discontinued. Therefore, diagnostic tests of pituitary gonadotropic and gonadal functions conducted during treatment and for up to three months after discontinuation of leuprolide acetate for depot suspension may be affected.

8 USE IN SPECIFIC POPULATIONS

8.1 Pregnancy

Pregnancy Category X – *[See Contraindications (4)]*

Teratogenic Effects

LUPANETA PACK is contraindicated in women who are or may become pregnant while receiving the drug *[see Contraindications (4)]*. Before starting and during treatment with leuprolide acetate for depot suspension, establish whether the patient is pregnant. Leuprolide acetate for depot suspension is not a contraceptive. In reproductively capable women, a non-hormonal method of contraception should be used *[see Warnings and Precautions (5.4)]*.

Leuprolide acetate for depot suspension may cause fetal harm when administered to a pregnant woman.

When administered on day 6 of pregnancy at test dosages of 0.00024, 0.0024, and 0.024 mg/kg (1/300 to 1/3 of the human dose) to rabbits, leuprolide acetate for depot suspension produced a dose-related increase in major fetal abnormalities. Similar studies in rats failed to demonstrate an increase in fetal malformations. There was increased fetal mortality and decreased fetal weights with the two higher doses of leuprolide acetate for depot suspension in rabbits and with the highest dose (0.024 mg/kg) in rats.

8.3 Nursing Mothers

Do not use LUPANETA PACK in nursing mothers because the effects of leuprolide acetate for depot suspension on lactation and/or the breast-fed child have not been determined. It is not known whether leuprolide acetate for depot suspension is excreted in human milk.

Detectable amounts of progestins have been identified in the milk of mothers receiving them *[see Contraindications (4)]*.

8.4 Pediatric Use

LUPANETA PACK is not indicated in premenarcheal adolescents. Safety and effectiveness of LUPANETA PACK have not been established in pediatric patients. Experience with LUPANETA PACK for treatment of endometriosis has been limited to women 18 years of age and older.

8.5 Geriatric Use

LUPANETA PACK is not indicated in postmenopausal women and has not been studied in women over 65 years of age.

11 DESCRIPTION

LUPANETA PACK (leuprolide acetate for depot suspension; norethindrone acetate tablets) 1-month contains one dual chamber syringe with leuprolide acetate for depot suspension 3.75 mg and norethindrone acetate tablets USP: 5 mg (bottle of 30 tablets).

Leuprolide Acetate for Depot Suspension

Leuprolide acetate for depot suspension is a synthetic nonapeptide analog of gonadotropin-releasing hormone (GnRH or LH-RH), a GnRH agonist. The chemical name is 5- oxo-L-prolyl-L-histidyl-L-tryptophyl-L-seryl-L-tyrosyl-D-leucyl-L-leucyl-L-arginyl-N-ethyl-L-prolinamide acetate (salt) with the following structural formula:

[See chemical structure above]

Leuprolide acetate for depot suspension 3.75 mg is available in a prefilled dual-chamber syringe containing sterile lyophilized microspheres which, when mixed with diluent, become a suspension intended as an intramuscular injection.

The front chamber of leuprolide acetate for depot suspension 3.75 mg prefilled dual-chamber syringe contains leuprolide acetate for depot suspension (3.75 mg), purified gelatin (0.65 mg), DL-lactic and glycolic acids copolymer (33.1 mg), and D-mannitol (6.6 mg). The second chamber of diluent contains carboxymethylcellulose sodium (5 mg), D-mannitol (50 mg), polysorbate 80 (1 mg), water for injection, USP, and glacial acetic acid, USP to control pH.

During the manufacture of leuprolide acetate for depot suspension, acetic acid is lost, leaving the peptide.

Norethindrone Acetate

Norethindrone acetate tablets USP - 5 mg oral tablets.

Norethindrone acetate USP, (17-hydroxy-19-nor-17α-pregn-4-en-20-yn-3-one acetate), a synthetic, orally active progestin, is the acetic acid ester of norethindrone. It is a white, or creamy white, crystalline powder.

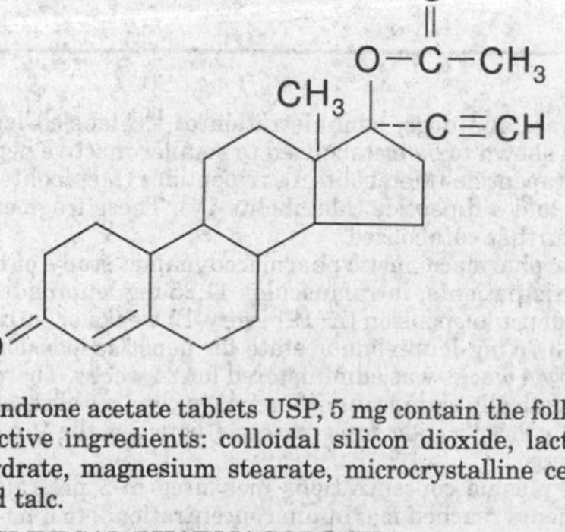

Norethindrone acetate tablets USP, 5 mg contain the following inactive ingredients: colloidal silicon dioxide, lactose monohydrate, magnesium stearate, microcrystalline cellulose and talc.

12 CLINICAL PHARMACOLOGY

12.1 Mechanism of Action

Leuprolide Acetate for Depot Suspension

Leuprolide acetate for depot suspension is a long-acting GnRH analog. A single injection of leuprolide acetate for depot suspension results in an initial elevation followed by a prolonged suppression of pituitary gonadotropins. Repeated dosing at quarterly intervals results in decreased secretion of gonadal steroids; consequently, tissues and functions that depend on gonadal steroids for their maintenance become quiescent. This effect is reversible on discontinuation of drug therapy.

Leuprolide acetate is not active when given orally.

Norethindrone Acetate

Norethindrone acetate induces secretory changes in an estrogen-primed endometrium.

12.2 Pharmacodynamics

In a pharmacokinetic/pharmacodynamic study of leuprolide acetate 11.25 mg for 3-month administration in healthy female subjects (N=20), the onset of estradiol suppression was observed for individual subjects between day 4 and week 4 after dosing. By the third week following the injection, the mean estradiol concentration (8 pg/mL) was in the menopausal range. Throughout the remainder of the dosing period, mean serum estradiol levels ranged from the menopausal to the early follicular range.

Serum estradiol was suppressed to ≤20 pg/mL in all subjects within four weeks and remained suppressed (≤40 pg/mL) in 80% of subjects until the end of the 12-week dosing interval, at which time two of these subjects had a value between 40 and 50 pg/mL. Four additional subjects had at least two consecutive elevations of estradiol (range 43-240 pg/mL) levels during the 12-week dosing interval, but there was no indication of luteal function for any of the subjects during this period.

12.3 Pharmacokinetics

Absorption

Leuprolide Acetate for Depot Suspension

Following a single injection of the three month formulation of leuprolide acetate for depot suspension (11.25 mg) in female subjects, a mean plasma leuprolide concentration of 36.3 ng/mL was observed at 4 hours. Leuprolide appeared to be released at a constant rate following the onset of steady-state levels during the third week after dosing and mean levels then declined gradually to near the lower limit of detection by 12 weeks. The mean (± standard deviation) leuprolide concentration from 3 to 12 weeks was 0.23 ± 0.09 ng/mL. However, intact leuprolide and an inactive major metabolite could not be distinguished by the assay which was employed in the study. The initial burst, followed by the rapid decline to a steady-state level, was similar to the release pattern seen with the monthly formulation.

Norethindrone Acetate

Norethindrone acetate is deacetylated to norethindrone after oral administration, and the disposition of norethindrone acetate is indistinguishable from that of orally administered norethindrone. Norethindrone acetate is absorbed from norethindrone acetate tablets, with maximum plasma concentration of norethindrone generally occurring at about 2 hours post-dose (see Figure 8). The pharmacokinetic parameters of norethindrone following single oral administration of 5 mg norethindrone acetate under fasting conditions in 29 healthy female volunteers are summarized in Table 5.

Table 5. Pharmacokinetic Parameters after a Single Dose of Norethindrone Acetate in Healthy Women

Norethindrone Acetate (n=29) Arithmetic Mean ± SD	
Norethindrone	
AUC (0-inf) (ng/ml*h)	166.90 ± 56.28
C_{max} (ng/ml)	26.19 ± 6.19
t_{max} (h)	1.83 ± 0.58
$t_{1/2}$ (h)	8.51 ± 2.19

AUC = area under the curve,
C_{max} = maximum plasma concentration,
t_{max} = time at maximum plasma concentration,
$t_{1/2}$ = half-life,
SD = standard deviation

Information on the AbbVie, Inc. products listed on these pages is from the prescribing information in use as of July 31, 2013. For more information, please visit rxabbvie.com or call 1-800-633-9110.

Figure 8. Mean Norethindrone Plasma Concentration Profile after a Single Dose of 5 mg Norethindrone Acetate Administered to 29 Healthy Female Volunteers under Fasting Conditions

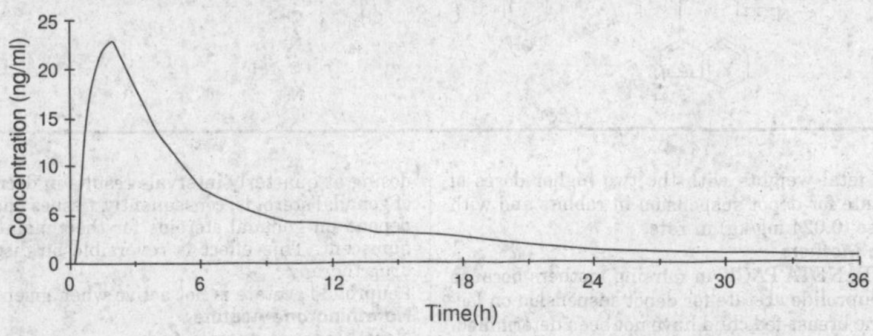

Table 6. Percentages of Patients with Symptoms of Endometriosis and Mean Clinical Severity Scores

			Percent of Patients with Symptom			Clinical Pain Severity Score		
			Baseline		Final	Baseline		Final
Variable	Study	Group	N[1]	(%)[2]	(%)	N[1]	Value[3]	Change
Dysmenorrhea	Controlled Study	LA*	51	(100)	(4)	50	3.2	-2.0
		LA/N†	55	(100)	(4)	54	3.1	-2.0
	Open Label Study	LA/N	136	(99)	(9)	134	3.3	-2.1
Pelvic Pain	Controlled Study	LA	51	(100)	(66)	50	2.9	-1.1
		LA/N	55	(96)	(56)	54	3.1	-1.1
	Open Label Study	LA/N	136	(99)	(63)	134	3.2	-1.2
Deep Dyspareunia	Controlled Study	LA	42	(83)	(37)	25	2.4	-1.0
		LA/N	43	(84)	(45)	30	2.7	-0.8
	Open Label Study	LA/N	102	(91)	(53)	94	2.7	-1.0
Pelvic Tenderness	Controlled Study	LA	51	(94)	(34)	50	2.5	-1.0
		LA/N	54	(91)	(34)	52	2.6	-0.9
	Open Label Study	LA/N	136	(99)	(39)	134	2.9	-1.4
Pelvic Induration	Controlled Study	LA	51	(51)	(12)	50	1.9	-0.4
		LA/N	54	(46)	(17)	52	1.6	-0.4
	Open Label Study	LA/N	136	(75)	(21)	134	2.2	-0.9

* LA = leuprolide acetate 3.75 mg
† LA/N = leuprolide acetate 3.75 mg plus norethindrone acetate 5 mg
[1] Number of patients that were included in the assessment
[2] Percentage of patients with the symptom/sign
[3] Value description: 1=none; 2= mild; 3= moderate; 4= severe

[See figure 8 above]

Effect of Food:

The effect of food administration on the pharmacokinetics of norethindrone acetate has not been studied.

Distribution

Leuprolide Acetate for Depot Suspension

The mean steady-state volume of distribution of leuprolide following intravenous bolus administration to healthy male volunteers was 27 L. *In vitro* binding to human plasma proteins ranged from 43% to 49%.

Norethindrone Acetate

Norethindrone is 36% bound to sex hormone-binding globulin (SHBG) and 61% bound to albumin. Volume of distribution of norethindrone is about 4 L/kg.

Metabolism

Leuprolide Acetate for Depot Suspension

In healthy male volunteers, a 1 mg bolus of leuprolide administered intravenously revealed that the mean systemic clearance was 7.6 L/h, with a terminal elimination half-life of approximately 3 hours based on a two compartment model.

In rats and dogs, administration of ^{14}C-labeled leuprolide was shown to be metabolized to smaller inactive peptides, a pentapeptide (Metabolite I), tripeptides (Metabolites II and III) and a dipeptide (Metabolite IV). These fragments may be further catabolized.

In a pharmacokinetic/pharmacodynamic study of endometriosis patients, intramuscular 11.25 mg leuprolide acetate for depot suspension (n=19) every 12 weeks or intramuscular 3.75 mg leuprolide acetate for depot suspension (n=15) every 4 weeks was administered for 24 weeks. There was no statistically significant difference in changes of serum estradiol concentration from baseline between the 2 treatment groups.

M-I plasma concentrations measured in 5 prostate cancer patients reached maximum concentration 2 to 6 hours after dosing and were approximately 6% of the peak parent drug concentration. One week after dosing, mean plasma M-I concentrations were approximately 20% of mean leuprolide concentrations.

Norethindrone Acetate

Norethindrone undergoes extensive biotransformation, primarily via reduction, followed by sulfate and glucuronide conjugation. The majority of metabolites in the circulation are sulfates, with glucuronides accounting for most of the urinary metabolites.

Excretion

Leuprolide Acetate for Depot Suspension

Following administration of leuprolide acetate for depot suspension 3.75 mg for 1-month administration to 3 patients, less than 5% of the dose was recovered as parent and M-I metabolite in the urine.

Norethindrone Acetate

Plasma clearance value for norethindrone is approximately 0.4 L/hr/kg. Norethindrone is excreted in both urine and feces, primarily as metabolites. The mean terminal elimination half-life of norethindrone following a single dose administration of norethindrone acetate is approximately 9 hours.

Specific Populations

Hepatic Impairment

The effect of hepatic disease on the disposition of norethindrone after norethindrone acetate administration has not been evaluated. However, norethindrone acetate is contraindicated in markedly impaired liver function or liver disease *[see Contraindications (4)]*.

The pharmacokinetics of the leuprolide acetate for depot suspension in hepatically impaired patients has not been determined.

Renal Impairment

The effect of renal disease on the disposition of norethindrone after norethindrone acetate administration has not been evaluated. In pre-menopausal women with chronic renal failure undergoing peritoneal dialysis who received multiple doses of an oral contraceptive containing ethinyl estradiol and norethindrone, plasma norethindrone concentration was unchanged compared to concentrations in pre-menopausal women with normal renal function.

The pharmacokinetics of the leuprolide acetate for depot suspension in renally impaired patients has not been determined.

Race

The effect of race on the disposition of norethindrone after norethindrone acetate administration has not been evaluated.

Drug Interactions

Leuprolide Acetate for Depot Suspension

Leuprolide acetate for depot suspension is a peptide that is primarily degraded by peptidase and not by cytochrome P-450 enzymes as noted in specific studies, and the drug is only about 46% bound to plasma proteins, drug interactions would not be expected to occur.

13 NONCLINICAL TOXICOLOGY

13.1 Carcinogenesis, Mutagenesis, Impairment of Fertility

Leuprolide Acetate for Depot Suspension

A two-year carcinogenicity study was conducted in rats and mice. In rats, a dose-related increase of benign pituitary hyperplasia and benign pituitary adenomas was noted at 24 months when the drug was administered subcutaneously at high daily doses (0.6 to 4 mg/kg). There was a significant but not dose-related increase of pancreatic islet-cell adenomas in females and of testicular interstitial cell adenomas in males (highest incidence in the low dose group). In mice, no leuprolide acetate-induced tumors or pituitary abnormalities were observed at a dose as high as 60 mg/kg for two years. Patients have been treated with leuprolide acetate for up to three years with doses as high as 10 mg/day and for two years with doses as high as 20 mg/day without demonstrable pituitary abnormalities.

Mutagenicity studies have been performed with leuprolide acetate using bacterial and mammalian systems. These studies provided no evidence of a mutagenic potential.

Clinical and pharmacologic studies in adults (>18 years) with leuprolide acetate and similar analogs have shown reversibility of fertility suppression when the drug is discontinued after continuous administration for periods of up to 24 weeks. Although no clinical studies have been completed in children to assess the full reversibility of fertility suppression, animal studies (prepubertal and adult rats and monkeys) with leuprolide acetate and other GnRH analogs have shown functional recovery.

14 CLINICAL STUDIES

Leuprolide Acetate for Depot Suspension

Initial endometriosis efficacy data for leuprolide acetate for depot suspension were based on the 3.75 mg dose administered once monthly.

A pharmacokinetic/pharmacodynamic study in 41 women that included both the 3.75 mg dose administered once monthly and the 11.25 mg dose administered once every three months did not reveal clinically significant differences in terms of efficacy in reducing painful symptoms of endometriosis or magnitude of the decrease in bone mineral density (BMD) associated with use of leuprolide acetate.

Leuprolide Acetate for Depot Suspension Plus Norethindrone Acetate

Two clinical studies with treatment duration of 12 months were conducted to evaluate the effect of coadministration of leuprolide acetate for depot suspension and norethindrone acetate on the loss of bone mineral density (BMD) associated with leuprolide acetate for depot suspension and on the efficacy of leuprolide acetate for depot suspension in relieving symptoms of endometriosis. (All patients in these studies received calcium supplementation with 1000 mg elemental calcium). A total of 242 women were treated with monthly administration of leuprolide acetate 3.75 mg (13 injections) and with 5 mg norethindrone acetate taken daily. The population age range was 17-43 years old. The majority of patients were Caucasian (87%).

One coadministration study was a controlled, randomized and double-blind study included 51 women treated monthly with leuprolide acetate for depot suspension alone and 55 women treated monthly with leuprolide acetate for depot suspension plus norethindrone acetate daily. Women in this trial were followed for up to 24 months after completing one year of treatment. The other study was an open-label single arm clinical study in 136 women of one year of treatment with leuprolide acetate for depot suspension and norethindrone acetate, with follow-up for up to 12 months after completing treatment.

The second study was an open label, single arm study in which 136 women were treated monthly with leuprolide acetate for depot suspension plus norethindrone acetate daily, with follow-up for up to 12 months after completing treatment.

The assessment of efficacy was based on the investigator's or the patient's monthly assessment of five signs or symptoms of endometriosis (dysmenorrhea, pelvic pain, deep dyspareunia, pelvic tenderness and pelvic induration).

Table 6 below provides detailed efficacy data regarding relief of symptoms of endometriosis based on the two studies of coadministration of leuprolide acetate and norethindrone acetate.

[See table 6 at top of previous page]

Suppression of menses (menses was defined as three or more consecutive days of menstrual bleeding) was maintained throughout treatment in 84% and 73% of patients receiving leuprolide acetate and norethindrone acetate, in the controlled study and open label study, respectively. The median time for menses resumption after treatment with leuprolide acetate and norethindrone acetate was 8 weeks.

Changes in Bone Density

The effect of leuprolide acetate for depot suspension and norethindrone acetate on bone mineral density was evaluated by dual energy x-ray absorptiometry (DXA) scan in the two clinical trials. For the open-label study, success in mitigating BMD loss was defined as the lower bound of the 95% confidence interval around the change from baseline at one year of treatment not to exceed –2.2%. The bone mineral density data of the lumbar spine from these two studies are presented in Table 7.

[See table 7 above]

The change in BMD following discontinuation of treatment is shown in Table 8.

[See table 8 above]

These clinical studies demonstrated that coadministration of leuprolide acetate and norethindrone acetate 5 mg daily is effective in significantly reducing the loss of bone mineral density that occurs with leuprolide acetate for depot suspension treatment, and in relieving symptoms of endometriosis.

Table 7. Mean Percent Change from Baseline in BMD of Lumbar Spine

	leuprolide acetate for depot suspension 3.75 mg		leuprolide acetate for depot suspension 3.75 mg plus norethindrone acetate 5 mg daily			
	Controlled Study		Controlled Study		Open Label Study	
	N	Change (Mean, 95% CI)#	N	Change (Mean, 95% CI)#	N	Change (Mean, 95% CI)#
Week 24*	41	-3.2% (-3.8, -2.6)	42	-0.3% (-0.8, 0.3)	115	-0.2% (-0.6, 0.2)
Week 52†	29	-6.3% (-7.1, -5.4)	32	-1.0% (-1.9, -0.1)	84	-1.1% (-1.6, -0.5)

* Includes on-treatment measurements that fell within 2-252 days after the first day of treatment.
† Includes on-treatment measurements >252 days after the first day of treatment.
# 95% CI: 95% Confidence Interval

Table 8. Mean Percent Change from Baseline in BMD of Lumbar Spine in Post-Treatment Follow-up Period

Post Treatment Measurement	Controlled Study						Open Label Study		
	LA-Only			LA/N			LA/N		
	N	Mean % Change	95% CI (%)	N	Mean % Change	95% CI (%)	N	Mean % Change	95% CI (%)[2]
Month 8	19	-3.3	(-4.9, -1.8)	23	-0.9	(-2.1, 0.4)	89	-0.6	(-1.2, 0.0)
Month 12	16	-2.2	(-3.3, -1.1)	12	-0.7	(-2.1, 0.6)	65	0.1	(-0.6, 0.7)

[1] Patients with post treatment measurements
[2] 95% CI (2-sided) of percent change in BMD values from baseline

15 REFERENCES

Leuprolide Acetate for Depot Suspension

1. NIOSH Alert: Preventing occupational exposures to antineoplastic and other hazardous drugs in healthcare settings. 2004. U.S. Department of Health and Human Services, Public Health Service, Centers for Disease Control and Prevention, National Institute for Occupational Safety and Health, DHHS (NIOSH) Publication No. 2004-165.
2. OSHA Technical Manual, TED 1-0.15A, Section VI: Chapter 2. Controlling Occupational Exposure to Hazardous Drugs. OSHA, 1999. http://www.osha.gov/dts/osta/otm/otm_vi/otm_vi_2.html
3. American Society of Health-System Pharmacists. ASHP guidelines on handling hazardous drugs. *Am J Health-Syst Pharm.* 2006; 63; 1172-1193.
4. Polovich, M., White, J.M., & Kelleher, L.O. (eds.) 2005. Chemotherapy and biotherapy guidelines and recommendations for practice (2nd. Ed.) Pittsburgh, PA: Oncology Nursing Society.

16 HOW SUPPLIED/STORAGE AND HANDLING

LUPANETA PACK for 1-month copackaged kit (NDC 0074-1052-05) is available in

cartons containing: leuprolide acetate for depot suspension 3.75 mg for 1-month administration Kit (NDC 0074-3641-04)

norethindrone acetate 5 mg tablets; 30 count bottle (NDC 0074-1049-02)

1. Leuprolide acetate for depot suspension 3.75 mg for 1-month administration kit contains:
   - one prefilled dual-chamber syringe
   - one plunger
   - two alcohol swab

   Each syringe contains sterile lyophilized microspheres of leuprolide acetate incorporated in a biodegradable copolymer of lactic and glycolic acids. When mixed with diluent, leuprolide acetate for depot suspension 3.75 mg for 1-month administration is administered as a single intramuscular injection.
2. Norethindrone acetate 5 mg 30 count bottle

   White to off-white oval, flat faced beveled edged, uncoated tablets debossed with 'G with breakline' on one side and 304 on other side.

Store at 25°C (77°F); excursions permitted to 15 to 30°C (59 to 86°F) [See USP Controlled Room Temperature]

17 PATIENT COUNSELING INFORMATION

See FDA-approved patient labeling (Patient Information)

Counsel patients about the Warnings and Precautions for LUPANETA PACK, including:

- Do not use this drug if they have experienced an allergic reaction to GnRH agonists or progestins
- Do not use this drug if they are pregnant or planning a pregnancy, suspect they may be pregnant, or are breast-feeding
- Risk of loss of bone mineral density and limitation of treatment to two six-month courses of treatment
- Risk to an exposed fetus and need to use nonhormonal contraception
- Discontinue norethindrone if they develop sudden loss of vision, double vision or sudden migraine
- The possibility of development or worsening of depression during treatment with leuprolide acetate for depot suspension
- Need for close monitoring if they have cardiovascular risk factors, or conditions like epilepsy, migraine or renal dysfunction
- Notify their healthcare provider if they develop new or worsened symptoms after beginning treatment

PATIENT INFORMATION

LUPANETA PACK™ *(loo-pan e-tə pæk)*

(leuprolide acetate for depot suspension and norethindrone acetate tablets)

Read this Patient Information before you start taking LUPANETA PACK and each time you get a refill. There may be new information. This information does not take the place of talking with your doctor about your medical condition or your treatment.

What is LUPANETA PACK?

LUPANETA PACK contains 2 different prescription medicines:

- **leuprolide acetate for depot suspension** is a medicine injected into your muscle and used to treat pain due to endometriosis.
- **norethindrone acetate tablets** is a medicine taken by mouth and used to help lower the side effect of bone thinning that is caused by leuprolide acetate for depot suspension.

LUPANETA PACK should not be used longer than 6 months at a time after you first start treatment for your endometriosis symptoms. LUPANETA PACK should not be used for more than a total of 12 months during your treatment.

It is not known if LUPANETA PACK is safe and effective in children under 18 years of age.

Who should not take LUPANETA PACK?

Do not take LUPANETA PACK if you:

- have had an allergic reaction to medicines like leuprolide acetate for depot suspension or norethindrone acetate tablets. See the end of this leaflet for a complete list of ingredients in LUPANETA PACK.
- have uterine bleeding for which a cause has not been found.
- are pregnant or may be pregnant. LUPANETA PACK may harm your unborn baby.
- are breast-feeding or plan to breast-feed. It is not known if LUPANETA PACK passes into your breast milk.
- had or have breast cancer or other cancers that are sensitive to hormones.
- have problems with blood clots, a stroke or a heart attack.
- have liver problems.

What should I tell my doctor before taking LUPANETA PACK?

Before you take LUPANETA PACK, tell your doctor if you:

• drink alcohol	• smoke
• have a family history of bone loss (osteoporosis)	• have depression
• have high cholesterol	• have had blood clots, a stroke or a heart attack
• have migraine headaches	• have diabetes
• have epilepsy	• have kidney problems

Tell your doctor about all the medicines you take, including prescription and non-prescription medicines, vitamins, and herbal supplements.

Especially tell your doctor if you take anticonvulsant (seizure) or corticosteroid medicines.

Ask your doctor for a list of these medicines if you are not sure.

Know the medicines you take. Keep a list of them to show your doctor and pharmacist when you get a new medicine.

Information on the AbbVie, Inc. products listed on these pages is from the prescribing information in use as of July 31, 2013. For more information, please visit rxabbvie.com or call 1-800-633-9110.

How should I take LUPANETA PACK?

- **Leuprolide acetate for depot suspension** for 1 month administration is injected into your muscle 1 time every month by a healthcare professional in your doctor's office.
- **Take norethindrone acetate tablets** exactly as your doctor tells you to take them. Take 1 norethindrone acetate tablet by mouth every day for 1 month after you receive your injection.
- Talk to your doctor about the birth control method that is right for you before you start taking LUPANETA PACK. You will need to use a form of birth control that does not contain hormones, such as:
  - a diaphragm with spermicide
  - condoms with spermicide
  - a copper IUD
- If you become pregnant while taking LUPANETA PACK, stop taking the norethindrone acetate tablets and call your doctor right away.

How well does LUPANETA PACK work?

LUPANETA PACK is used to treat pain due to endometriosis. The pain from endometriosis can happen when you have your period, during other times of the month, or during intercourse (sex). Most women feel some relief from their endometriosis pain after taking both drugs in LUPANETA PACK.

The tablets in LUPANETA PACK help lower the side effect of bone thinning that is caused by leuprolide acetate for depot suspension. Women taking both drugs in LUPANETA PACK lost an average of 1% of their bone density after about 1 year of treatment. Women regained some of their bone density about 1 year after they stopped treatment with LUPANETA PACK.

What are the possible side effects of LUPANETA PACK?

LUPANETA PACK may cause serious side effects, including:

- **bone thinning (decreased bone mineral density)**
- **harm to your unborn baby**
- **vision problems.** Call your doctor right away if you have sudden loss of vision, double vision, bulging eyes, or migraine headaches.
- **depression or worsening depression**
- **allergic reactions.** Get medical help right away if you have any of these symptoms of a serious allergic reaction:
  - swelling of your face, lips, mouth, or tongue
  - trouble breathing
  - wheezing
  - severe itching
  - skin rash, redness, or swelling
  - dizziness or fainting
  - fast heartbeat or pounding in your chest (tachycardia)
  - sweating
- **worsening endometriosis symptoms when you start taking LUPANETA PACK**
- **swelling (fluid retention)**

The most common side effects of LUPANETA PACK include:

- hot flashes and sweats
- headaches or migraine headaches
- depression and mood swings
- nausea and vomiting
- problems sleeping
- nervousness or feeling anxious
- pain
- acne
- weakness
- vaginal infection or inflammation
- weight gain
- constipation or diarrhea

Tell your doctor if you have any side effect that bothers you or that does not go away.

These are not all the possible side effects of LUPANETA PACK. For more information, ask your doctor or pharmacist.

Call your doctor for medical advice about side effects. You may report side effects to FDA at 1-800-FDA-1088.

How should I store norethindrone acetate tablets in the LUPANETA PACK?

- Store norethindrone acetate tablets at room temperature between 68°F to 77°F (20°C to 25°C).

Keep LUPANETA PACK and all medicines out of the reach of children.

General information about the safe and effective use of LUPANETA PACK.

Medicines are sometimes prescribed for purposes other than those listed in a Patient Information leaflet. Do not use LUPANETA PACK for a condition for which it was not prescribed. Do not give LUPANETA PACK to other people, even if they have the same symptoms that you have. It may harm them.

This Patient Information leaflet summarizes the most important information about LUPANETA PACK. If you would like more information, talk with your doctor. You can ask your pharmacist or doctor for information about LUPANETA PACK that is written for health professionals. For more information, go to www.lupanetapack.com or call 1-800-633-9110.

What are the ingredients in LUPANETA PACK?

leuprolide acetate for depot suspension:

Active Ingredients: leuprolide acetate for depot suspension

Inactive Ingredients: purified gelatin, DL-lactic and glycolic acids copolymer, D-mannitol, carboxymethylcellulose sodium, polysorbate 80, water for injection, USP,
and glacial acetic acid, USP to control pH.

norethindrone acetate tablets:

Active Ingredients: norethindrone acetate USP

Inactive Ingredients: colloidal silicon dioxide, lactose monohydrate,
magnesium stearate, microcrystalline cellulose and talc.

This Patient Information has been approved by the U.S. Food and Drug Administration.

Leuprolide Acetate for Depot Suspension:

Manufactured for
AbbVie Inc.
North Chicago, IL 60064
By Takeda Pharmaceutical Company Limited
Osaka, Japan 540-8645

Norethindrone Acetate:

Manufactured for
AbbVie Inc.
North Chicago, IL 60064
By Glenmark Generics Ltd.
Colvale-Bardez, Goa
403 513, India

LUPANETA PACK
Packaged by:
AbbVie Inc.
North Chicago, IL 60064

™ - Trademark
® - Registered Trademark

03-A586 March, 2013

LUPANETA PACK™ ℞

Leuprolide Acetate for Depot Suspension, 11.25 mg for intramuscular injection only and Norethindrone Acetate tablets, 5 mg for oral administration

HIGHLIGHTS OF PRESCRIBING INFORMATION

These highlights do not include all the information needed to use LUPANETA PACK safely and effectively. See full prescribing information for LUPANETA PACK.

LUPANETA PACK (leuprolide acetate for depot suspension; norethindrone acetate tablets), co-packaged for intramuscular use and for oral use, respectively

Initial U.S. Approval: 2012

INDICATIONS AND USAGE

LUPANETA PACK contains leuprolide acetate, a gonadotropin-releasing hormone (GnRH) agonist and norethindrone acetate, a progestin, indicated for

- Initial management of the painful symptoms of endometriosis (1)
- Management of recurrence of symptoms (1)

Limitations of Use: Initial treatment course is limited to 6 months and use is not recommended longer than a total of 12 months due to concerns about adverse impact on bone mineral density. (1, 2.1, 5.1)

DOSAGE AND ADMINISTRATION

- Leuprolide acetate for depot suspension 11.25 mg given by a healthcare provider as a single intramuscular injection every 3 months for up to two injections (6 months of therapy) (2.1)
- Norethindrone acetate 5 mg tablets taken orally by the patient once per day for up to 6 months (2.1)
- If endometriosis symptoms recur after initial course of therapy, consider retreatment for up to another six months (2.1)
- Assess bone density before retreatment begins (2.1, 5.1)
- Reconstitute leuprolide acetate prior to use, see important administration instructions (2.3)

DOSAGE FORMS AND STRENGTHS

- Leuprolide acetate for depot suspension 11.25 mg syringe (3)
- Norethindrone acetate 5 mg tablets; 90 count bottle (3)

CONTRAINDICATIONS

- Hypersensitivity to GnRH, GnRH agonist or any of the excipients in leuprolide acetate for depot suspension or norethindrone acetate (4)
- Undiagnosed abnormal uterine bleeding (4)
- Pregnancy or suspected pregnancy (4, 8.1)
- Women who are breast-feeding (4)
- Known, suspected or history of breast or other hormone-sensitive cancer (4)
- Thrombotic or thromboembolic disorders (4)
- Liver tumors or liver disease (4)

WARNINGS AND PRECAUTIONS

- Loss of bone mineral density: do not use for more than two six-month treatment courses. (1, 2.1, 5.1)
- Exclude pregnancy before starting treatment and discontinue use if pregnancy occurs; use non-hormonal methods of contraception only. (5.2)
- Discontinue in case of sudden loss of vision or onset of proptosis, diplopia or migraine. (5.3)
- Carefully observe patients with history of depression and discontinue the drug if the depression recurs to a serious degree. (5.4)
- Assess and manage risk factors for cardiovascular disease before starting LUPANETA PACK. (5.6)

ADVERSE REACTIONS

Leuprolide acetate for depot suspension: Most common related adverse reactions (>10%) were hot flashes/sweats, headache/migraine, depression/emotional lability, nausea/vomiting, nervousness/anxiety, insomnia, pain, acne, asthenia, vaginitis, weight gain, constipation/diarrhea (6.1)

Progestins: breakthrough bleeding, spotting (6.1)

To report SUSPECTED ADVERSE REACTIONS, contact AbbVie Inc. at 1-800-633-9110 or FDA at 1-800-FDA-1088 or www.fda.gov/medwatch

USE IN SPECIFIC POPULATIONS

Pediatric: Safety and effectiveness of LUPANETA PACK has not been established in pediatric patients. (8.4)

Geriatric: LUPANETA PACK has not been studied in women over 65 years of age and is not indicated in this population. (8.5)

See 17 for PATIENT COUNSELING INFORMATION and FDA-approved patient labeling

Revised: 03/2013

FULL PRESCRIBING INFORMATION: CONTENTS*

* Sections or subsections omitted from the full prescribing information are not listed

FULL PRESCRIBING INFORMATION

1 INDICATIONS AND USAGE

LUPANETA PACK (leuprolide acetate for depot suspension and norethindrone acetate tablets) is indicated for initial management of the painful symptoms of endometriosis and for management of recurrence of symptoms.

Limitation of Use: Duration of use is limited due to concerns about adverse impact on bone mineral density *[see Warnings and Precautions (5.1)]*. The initial treatment course of LUPANETA PACK is limited to six months. A single retreatment course of not more than six months may be administered after the initial course of treatment if symptoms recur. Use of LUPANETA PACK for longer than a total of 12 months is not recommended.

2 DOSAGE AND ADMINISTRATION

2.1 Dosing Information

LUPANETA PACK is a co-packaging of leuprolide acetate for depot suspension for intramuscular use and norethindrone acetate tablets for oral use. Administer as follows:

- 11.25 mg of leuprolide acetate by intramuscular injection once every three months for up to two injections (6 months of therapy); to be administered by a healthcare provider
- 5 mg of norethindrone acetate orally once daily for up to 6 months of therapy

The initial course of treatment with leuprolide acetate for depot suspension 11.25 mg in combination with norethindrone acetate 5 mg daily is not to exceed six months.

If the symptoms of endometriosis recur after the initial course of therapy, consider retreatment with LUPANETA PACK for up to another six months. It is recommended that bone density be assessed before retreatment begins *[see Warnings and Precautions (5.1)]*.

Treatment beyond two six-month courses has not been studied and is not recommended due to concerns about adverse impact on bone mineral density.

2.2 Different Formulations of Leuprolide Acetate

Due to different release characteristics, a fractional dose of the leuprolide acetate for depot suspension 3-month depot formulation is not equivalent to the same dose of the monthly formulation and should not be given.

2.3 Reconstitution and Administration for Injection of Leuprolide Acetate

- Reconstitute and administer the lyophilized microspheres as a single intramuscular injection.
- Inject the suspension immediately or discard if not used within two hours, because leuprolide acetate for depot suspension does not contain a preservative.

1. Visually inspect the leuprolide acetate for depot suspension powder. DO NOT USE the syringe if clumping or caking is evident. A thin layer of powder on the wall of the syringe is considered normal prior to mixing with the diluent. The diluent should appear clear.
2. To prepare for injection, screw the white plunger into the end stopper until the stopper begins to turn (see Figure 1 and Figure 2).

[See figure 1 above]

Figure 1:

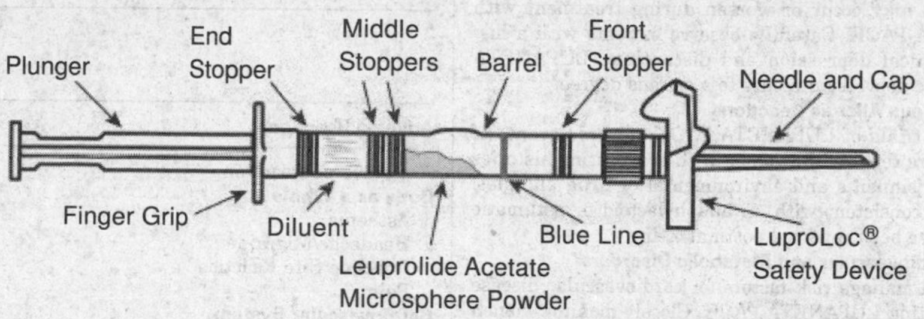

Figure 2:

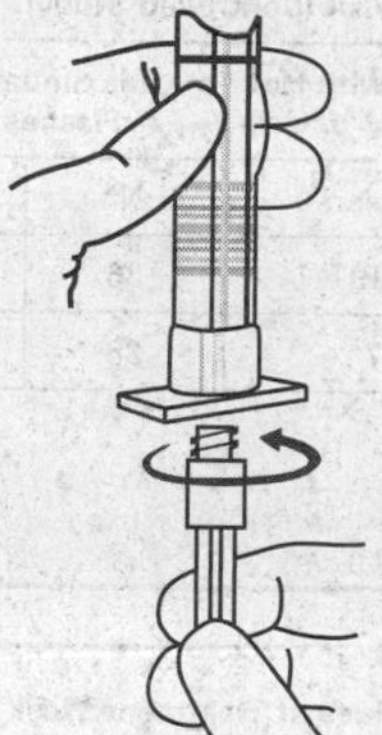

3. Hold the syringe UPRIGHT. Release the diluent by SLOWLY PUSHING (6 to 8 seconds) the plunger until the first middle stopper is at the blue line in the middle of the barrel (see Figure 3).

Figure 3:

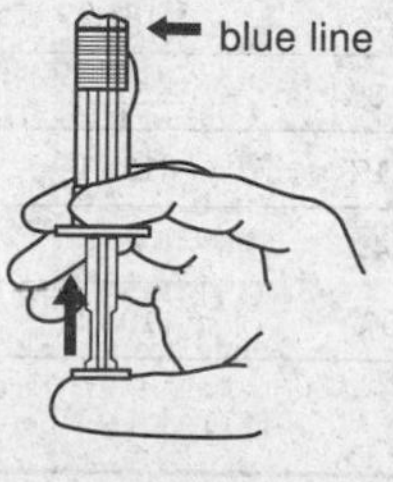

4. Keep the syringe UPRIGHT. Mix the microspheres (powder) thoroughly by gently shaking the syringe until the powder forms a uniform suspension. The suspension will appear milky. If the powder adheres to the stopper or caking/clumping is present, tap the syringe with your finger to disperse. DO NOT USE if any of the powder has not gone into suspension (see Figure 4).

Figure 4:

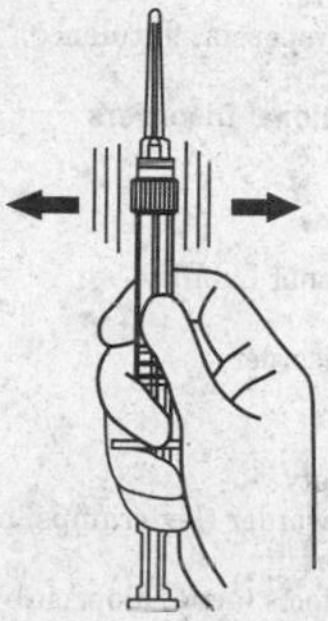

5. Keep the syringe UPRIGHT. With the opposite hand pull the needle cap upward without twisting.
6. Keep the syringe UPRIGHT. Advance the plunger to expel the air from the syringe. Now the syringe is ready for injection.
7. After cleaning the injection site with an alcohol swab, administer the intramuscular injection by inserting the needle at a 90 degree angle into the gluteal area, anterior thigh, or deltoid (see Figure 5).

Figure 5:

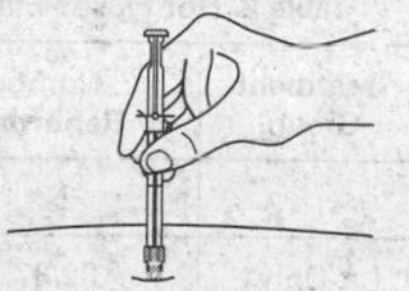

NOTE: If a blood vessel is accidentally penetrated, aspirated blood will be visible just below the luer lock (see Figure 6) and can be seen through the transparent LuproLoc safety device. If blood is present, remove the needle immediately. Do not inject the medication.

Figure 6:

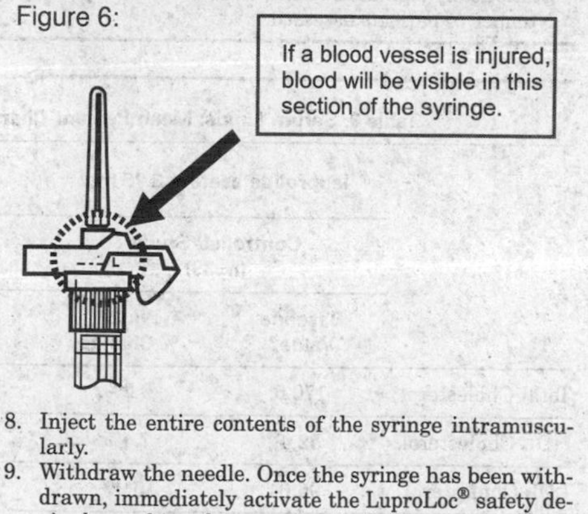

8. Inject the entire contents of the syringe intramuscularly.
9. Withdraw the needle. Once the syringe has been withdrawn, immediately activate the LuproLoc® safety device by pushing the arrow on the lock upward towards the needle tip with the thumb or finger, as illustrated, until the needle cover of the safety device over the needle is fully extended and a CLICK is heard or felt (see Figure 7).

Figure 7:

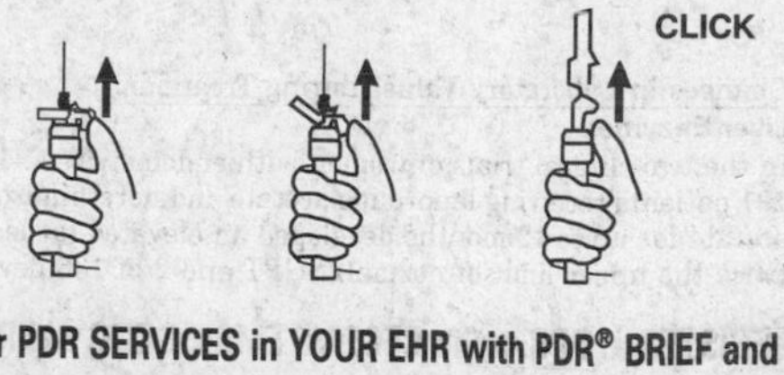

10. Dispose of the syringe according to local regulations/procedures *[see References (15)]*.

3 DOSAGE FORMS AND STRENGTHS

LUPANETA PACK 3-month copackaged kit contains two separate components:

- Leuprolide acetate for depot suspension 11.25 mg for 3-month administration: Leuprolide acetate lyophilized powder for reconstitution with supplied diluent in a prefilled dual chamber syringe
- Norethindrone acetate 5 mg tablets: White to off-white oval, flat-faced beveled edged, uncoated debossed with 'G with breakline' on one side and 304 on other side

4 CONTRAINDICATIONS

LUPANETA PACK is contraindicated in women with the following:

- Hypersensitivity to gonadotropin-releasing hormone (GnRH), GnRH agonist analogs, any of the excipients in leuprolide acetate for depot suspension, or norethindrone acetate
- Undiagnosed abnormal uterine bleeding
- Known, suspected or planned pregnancy during the course of therapy *[see Use in Specific Populations (8.1)]*
- Lactating women *[see Use in Specific Populations (8.3)]*
- Known, suspected or history of breast cancer or other hormone-sensitive cancer
- Current or history of thrombotic or thromboembolic disorder
- Liver tumors or liver disease

5 WARNINGS AND PRECAUTIONS

5.1 Loss of Bone Mineral Density

Leuprolide acetate for depot suspension induces a hypoestrogenic state that results in loss of bone mineral density (BMD), some of which may not be reversible. Concurrent use of norethindrone acetate is effective in reducing the loss of BMD that occurs with leuprolide acetate *[see Clinical Studies (14)]*. Nonetheless, duration of use of LUPANETA PACK is limited to two six-month courses of treatment due to concerns about the adverse impact on BMD. It is recommended that BMD be assessed before retreatment. Retreatment with leuprolide acetate for depot suspension alone is not recommended.

In women with major risk factors for decreased BMD such as chronic alcohol (> 3 units per day) or tobacco use, strong family history of osteoporosis, or chronic use of drugs that can decrease BMD, such as anticonvulsants or corticosteroids, use of LUPANETA PACK may pose an additional risk, and the risks and benefits should be weighed carefully.

5.2 Pregnancy Risk

Leuprolide acetate for depot suspension may cause fetal harm if administered to a pregnant woman. Exclude pregnancy before initiating treatment with LUPANETA PACK. When used at the recommended dose and dosing interval, leuprolide acetate for depot suspension usually inhibits ovulation and stops menstruation. Contraception, however, is not ensured by taking leuprolide acetate for depot suspension. Therefore, patients should use nonhormonal methods of contraception. Advise patients to notify their healthcare provider if they believe they may be pregnant. Discontinue LUPANETA PACK if a patient becomes pregnant during treatment and inform the patient of potential risk to the fetus *[see Contraindications (4) and Use in Specific Populations (8.1)]*.

5.3 Visual Abnormalities

Discontinue norethindrone acetate tablets in the LUPANETA PACK pending examination if there is a sudden partial or complete loss of vision or if there is sudden onset of proptosis, diplopia, or migraine. Discontinue LUPANETA PACK if examination reveals papilledema or retinal vascular lesions.

Information on the AbbVie, Inc. products listed on these pages is from the prescribing information in use as of July 31, 2013. For more information, please visit rxabbvie.com or call 1-800-633-9110.

5.4 Clinical Depression

Depression may occur or worsen during treatment with LUPANETA PACK. Carefully observe patients with a history of clinical depression and discontinue LUPANETA PACK if the depression recurs to a serious degree.

5.5 Serious Allergic Reactions

In clinical trials of LUPANETA PACK, adverse events of asthma were reported in women with pre-existing histories of asthma, sinusitis and environmental or drug allergies. Symptoms consistent with an anaphylactoid or asthmatic process have been reported postmarketing.

5.6 Cardiovascular and Metabolic Disorders

Assess and manage risk factors for cardiovascular disease before starting LUPANETA PACK. Closely monitor women on norethindrone acetate who have risk factors for arterial vascular disease (e.g., hypertension, diabetes mellitus, tobacco use, hypercholesterolemia, and obesity) and/or venous thromboembolism (e.g., family history of VTE, obesity, and smoking) when using LUPANETA PACK *[see Contraindications (4)]*.

5.7 Initial Flare of Symptoms

Following the first dose of leuprolide acetate, sex steroids temporarily rise above baseline because of the physiologic effect of the drug. Therefore, an increase in symptoms associated with endometriosis may be observed during the initial days of therapy, but these should dissipate with continued therapy.

5.8 Fluid Retention

Because norethindrone acetate may cause some degree of fluid retention, carefully observe women with conditions that might be influenced by this effect, such as epilepsy, migraine, cardiac or renal dysfunctions.

6 ADVERSE REACTIONS

6.1 Clinical Trials Experience

Because clinical trials are conducted under widely varying conditions, adverse reaction rates observed in the clinical trials of a drug cannot be directly compared to rates in the clinical trials of another drug and may not reflect the rates observed in clinical practice.

The safety of co-administering leuprolide acetate for depot suspension and norethindrone acetate was evaluated in two clinical studies in which a total of 242 women were treated for up to one year. Women were treated with monthly IM injections of leuprolide acetate 3.75 mg (13 injections) alone or monthly IM injections of leuprolide acetate 3.75 mg (13 injections) and 5 mg norethindrone acetate daily. The population age range was 17-43 years old. The majority of patients were Caucasian (87%).

One study was a controlled clinical trial in which 106 women were randomized to one year of treatment with leuprolide acetate for depot suspension alone or with leuprolide acetate for depot suspension and norethindrone acetate. The other study was an open-label single arm clinical study in 136 women of one year of treatment with leuprolide acetate for depot suspension and norethindrone acetate, with follow-up for up to 12 months after completing treatment.

Adverse Reactions (>1%) Leading to Study Discontinuation:

In the controlled study, 18% of patients treated monthly with leuprolide acetate and 18% of patients treated monthly with leuprolide acetate plus norethindrone acetate discontinued therapy due to adverse reactions, most commonly hot flashes (6%) and insomnia (4%) in the leuprolide acetate alone group and hot flashes and emotional lability (4% each) in the leuprolide acetate and norethindrone group.

In the open label study, 13% of patients treated monthly with leuprolide acetate plus norethindrone acetate discontinued therapy due to adverse reactions, most commonly depression (4%) and acne (2%).

Common Adverse Reactions:

Table 1 lists the adverse reactions observed in at least 5% of patients in any treatment group, during the first 6 months of treatment in the add-back clinical studies, in which patients were treated with monthly leuprolide acetate for depot suspension 3.75 mg with or without norethindrone acetate co-treatment. The most frequently-occurring adverse reactions observed in these studies were hot flashes and headaches.

[See table 1 above]

In the controlled clinical trial, 50 of 51 (98%) patients in the leuprolide acetate alone group and 48 of 55 (87%) patients in the leuprolide acetate and norethindrone group reported experiencing hot flashes on one or more occasions during treatment. Table 2 presents hot flash data in the last month of treatment.

[See table 2 above]

Serious Adverse Reactions:

Urinary tract infection, renal calculus, depression

Table 1. Adverse Reactions Occurring in the First Six Months of Treatment in ≥5% of Patients with Endometriosis

	Controlled Study LA-Only* N=51		Controlled Study LA/N† N=55		Open Label Study LA/N† N=136	
Adverse Reactions	**N**	**%**	**N**	**%**	**N**	**%**
Any Adverse Reaction	50	98	53	96	126	93
Body as a Whole						
Asthenia		18		18		11
Headache/Migraine		65		51		46
Injection Site Reaction		2		9		3
Pain		24		29		21
Cardiovascular System						
Hot flashes/Sweats		98		87		57
Digestive System						
Altered Bowel Function (constipation, diarrhea)		14		15		10
Changes in Appetite		4		0		6
GI Disturbance (dyspepsia, flatulence)		4		7		4
Nausea/Vomiting		25		29		13
Metabolic and Nutritional Disorders						
Edema		0		9		7
Weight Gain		12		13		4
Nervous System						
Depression/Emotional Lability		31		27		34
Dizziness/Vertigo		16		11		7
Insomnia/Sleep Disorder		31		13		15
Decreased Libido		10		4		7
Memory Disorder		6		2		4
Nervousness/Anxiety		8		4		11
Neuromuscular Disorder (leg cramps, paresthesia)		2		9		3
Skin and Appendages						
Androgen-Like Effects (acne, alopecia)		4		5		18
Skin/Mucous Membrane Reaction		4		9		11
Urogenital System						
Breast Changes/Pain/Tenderness		6		13		8
Menstrual Disorders		2		0		5
Vaginitis		20		15		8

* LA-Only = leuprolide acetate 3.75 mg
† LA/N = leuprolide acetate 3.75 mg plus norethindrone acetate 5 mg

Table 2. Hot Flashes in the Month Prior to the Assessment Visit (Controlled Study)

Assessment Visit	Treatment Group	Number of Patients Reporting Hot Flashes		Number of Days with Hot Flashes		Maximum Number Hot Flashes in 24 Hours	
		N	(%)	N[2]	Mean	N[2]	Mean
Week 24	LA-Only*	32/37	86	37	19	36	5.8
	LA/N†	22/38	58[1]	38	7[1]	38	1.9[1]

* LA-Only = leuprolide acetate 3.75 mg
† LA/N = leuprolide acetate 3.75 mg plus norethindrone acetate 5 mg
[1] Statistically significantly less than the LA-Only group (p<0.01)
[2] Number of patients assessed.

Table 3. Serum Lipids: Mean Percent Changes from Baseline Values at Treatment Week 24

	leuprolide acetate 3.75 mg		leuprolide acetate for depot suspension 3.75 mg plus norethindrone acetate 5 mg daily			
	Controlled Study (n=39)		Controlled Study (n=41)		Open Label Study (n=117)	
	Baseline Value*	Wk 24 % Change	Baseline Value*	Wk 24 % Change	Baseline Value*	Wk 24 % Change
Total Cholesterol	170.5	9.2%	179.3	0.2%	181.2	2.8%
HDL Cholesterol	52.4	7.4%	51.8	-18.8%	51.0	-14.6%
LDL Cholesterol	96.6	10.9%	101.5	14.1%	109.1	13.1%
LDL/HDL Ratio	2.0†	5.0%	2.1†	43.4%	2.3†	39.4%
Triglycerides	107.8	17.5%	130.2	9.5%	105.4	13.8%

* mg/dL
† ratio

Changes in Laboratory Values during Treatment:

Liver Enzymes

In the two clinical trials of women with endometriosis, 4 of 191 patients receiving leuprolide acetate and norethindrone acetate for up to 12 months developed an elevated (at least twice the upper limit of normal) SGPT and 2 of 136 developed an elevated GGT. Five of the 6 increases were observed beyond 6 months of treatment. None was associated with an elevated bilirubin concentration.

Lipids

Percent changes from baseline for serum lipids and percentages of patients with serum lipid values outside of the normal range in the two studies of leuprolide acetate and norethindrone acetate are summarized in the tables below. The major impact of adding norethindrone acetate to treatment with leuprolide acetate for depot suspension was a decrease in serum HDL cholesterol and an increase in the LDL/HDL ratio.

[See table 3 at top of previous page]

Changes from baseline tended to be greater at Week 52. After treatment, mean serum lipid levels from patients with follow up data (105 of 158 patients) returned to pretreatment values.

Table 4. Percent of Patients with Serum Lipid Values Outside of the Normal Range

	leuprolide acetate for depot suspension 3.75 mg plus norethindrone acetate 5 mg daily			
	Controlled Study (n=41)		Open Label Study (n=117)	
	Baseline	Wk 24*	Baseline	Wk 24*
Total Cholesterol (>240 mg/dL)	15%	20%	6%	7%
HDL Cholesterol (<40 mg/dL)	15%	44%	15%	41%
LDL Cholesterol (>160 mg/dL)	5%	7%	9%	11%
LDL/HDL Ratio (>4.0)	2%	15%	7%	21%
Triglycerides (>200 mg/dL)	12%	10%	5%	9%

* Includes all patients regardless of baseline value.

6.2 Postmarketing Experience

The following adverse reactions have been identified during postapproval use of leuprolide acetate for depot suspension or norethindrone acetate. Because these reactions are reported voluntarily from a population of uncertain size, it is not always possible to reliably estimate their frequency or establish a causal relationship to drug exposure.

Leuprolide Acetate for Depot Suspension

During postmarketing surveillance with other dosage forms and in the same or different populations, the following adverse reactions were reported:

- Allergic reactions (anaphylactic, rash, urticaria, and photosensitivity reactions)
- Mood swings, including depression
- Suicidal ideation and attempt
- Symptoms consistent with an anaphylactoid or asthmatic process
- Localized reactions including induration and abscess at the site of injection
- Symptoms consistent with fibromyalgia (e.g., joint and muscle pain, headaches, sleep disorders, gastrointestinal distress, and shortness of breath), individually and collectively

Other adverse reactions reported are:

Hepato-biliary disorder - Serious liver injury

Injury, poisoning and procedural complications - Spinal fracture

Investigations - Decreased white blood count

Musculoskeletal and connective tissue disorder - Tenosynovitis-like symptoms

Nervous System disorder - Convulsion, peripheral neuropathy, paralysis

Vascular disorder - Hypotension, Hypertension

Serious venous and arterial thrombotic and thromboembolic events, including deep vein thrombosis, pulmonary embolism, myocardial infarction, stroke, and transient ischemic attack

Pituitary apoplexy

During post-marketing surveillance, cases of pituitary apoplexy (a clinical syndrome secondary to infarction of the pituitary gland) have been reported after the administration of leuprolide acetate and other GnRH agonists. In a majority of these cases, a pituitary adenoma was diagnosed, with a majority of pituitary apoplexy cases occurring within 2 weeks of the first dose, and some within the first hour. In these cases, pituitary apoplexy has presented as sudden headache, vomiting, visual changes, ophthalmoplegia, altered mental status, and sometimes cardiovascular collapse. Immediate medical attention has been required.

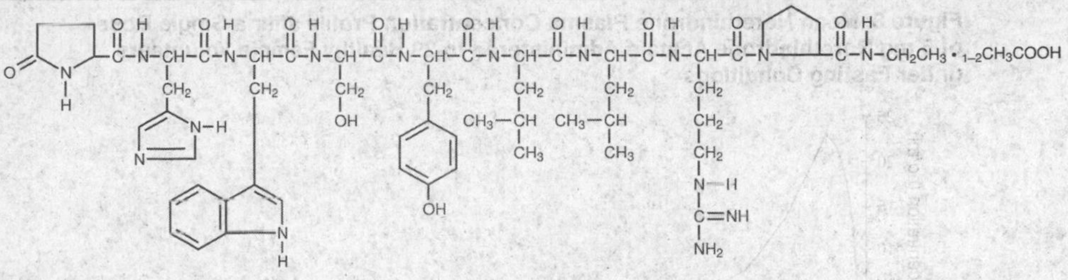

7 DRUG INTERACTIONS

7.1 Drug-Drug Interactions

Leuprolide Acetate for Depot Suspension

No pharmacokinetic-based drug-drug interaction studies have been conducted with leuprolide acetate for depot suspension. However, drug interactions associated with cytochrome P-450 enzymes or protein binding would not be expected to occur *[see Clinical Pharmacology (12.3)]*.

Norethindrone Acetate

No pharmacokinetic drug interaction studies investigating any drug-drug interactions with norethindrone acetate have been conducted. Drugs or herbal products that induce or inhibit certain enzymes, including CYP3A4, may decrease or increase the serum concentrations of norethindrone.

7.2 Drug/Laboratory Test Interactions

Leuprolide Acetate for Depot Suspension

Administration of leuprolide acetate for depot suspension in therapeutic doses results in suppression of the pituitary-gonadal system. Normal function is usually restored within three months after treatment is discontinued. Therefore, diagnostic tests of pituitary gonadotropic and gonadal functions conducted during treatment and for up to three months after discontinuation of leuprolide acetate for depot suspension may be affected.

8 USE IN SPECIFIC POPULATIONS

8.1 Pregnancy

Pregnancy Category X – *[See Contraindications (4)]*

Teratogenic Effects

LUPANETA PACK is contraindicated in women who are or may become pregnant while receiving the drug *[see Contraindications (4)]*. Before starting and during treatment with leuprolide acetate for depot suspension, establish whether the patient is pregnant. Leuprolide acetate for depot suspension is not a contraceptive. In reproductively capable women, a non-hormonal method of contraception should be used *[see Warnings and Precautions (5.4)]*.

Leuprolide acetate for depot suspension may cause fetal harm when administered to a pregnant woman.

When administered on day 6 of pregnancy at test dosages of 0.00024, 0.0024, and 0.024 mg/kg (1/300 to 1/3 of the human dose) to rabbits, leuprolide acetate for depot suspension produced a dose-related increase in major fetal abnormalities. Similar studies in rats failed to demonstrate an increase in fetal malformations. There was increased fetal mortality and decreased fetal weights with the two higher doses of leuprolide acetate for depot suspension in rabbits and with the highest dose (0.024 mg/kg) in rats.

8.3 Nursing Mothers

Do not use LUPANETA PACK in nursing mothers because the effects of leuprolide acetate for depot suspension on lactation and/or the breast-fed child have not been determined. It is not known whether leuprolide acetate for depot suspension is excreted in human milk.

Detectable amounts of progestins have been identified in the milk of mothers receiving them *[see Contraindications (4)]*.

8.4 Pediatric Use

LUPANETA PACK is not indicated in premenarcheal adolescents. Safety and effectiveness of LUPANETA PACK have not been established in pediatric patients. Experience with LUPANETA PACK for treatment of endometriosis has been limited to women 18 years of age and older.

8.5 Geriatric Use

LUPANETA PACK is not indicated in postmenopausal women and has not been studied in women over 65 years of age.

11 DESCRIPTION

LUPANETA PACK (leuprolide acetate for depot suspension; norethindrone acetate tablets) 3-month contains one dual chamber syringe with leuprolide acetate for depot suspension 11.25 mg and norethindrone acetate tablets USP: 5 mg (bottle of 90 tablets).

Leuprolide Acetate for Depot Suspension

Leuprolide acetate for depot suspension is a synthetic nonapeptide analog of gonadotropin-releasing hormone (GnRH or LH-RH), a GnRH agonist. The chemical name is 5-oxo-L-prolyl-L-histidyl-L-tryptophyl-L-seryl-L-tyrosyl-D-leucyl-L-leucyl-L-arginyl-N-ethyl-L-prolinamide acetate (salt) with the following structural formula:

[See chemical structure above]

Leuprolide acetate for depot suspension 11.25 mg is available in a prefilled dual-chamber syringe containing sterile lyophilized microspheres which, when mixed with diluent, become a suspension intended as an intramuscular injection.

The front chamber of leuprolide acetate for depot suspension 11.25 mg for 3-month administration prefilled dual-chamber syringe contains leuprolide acetate for depot suspension (11.25 mg), polylactic acid (99.3 mg) and D-mannitol (19.45 mg). The second chamber of diluent contains carboxymethylcellulose sodium (7.5 mg), D-mannitol (75 mg), polysorbate 80 (1.5 mg), water for injection, USP, and glacial acetic acid, USP to control pH.

During the manufacture of leuprolide acetate for depot suspension, acetic acid is lost, leaving the peptide.

Norethindrone Acetate

Norethindrone acetate tablets USP - 5 mg oral tablets.

Norethindrone acetate USP, (17-hydroxy-19-nor-17α-pregn-4-en-20-yn-3-one acetate), a synthetic, orally active progestin, is the acetic acid ester of norethindrone. It is a white, or creamy white, crystalline powder.

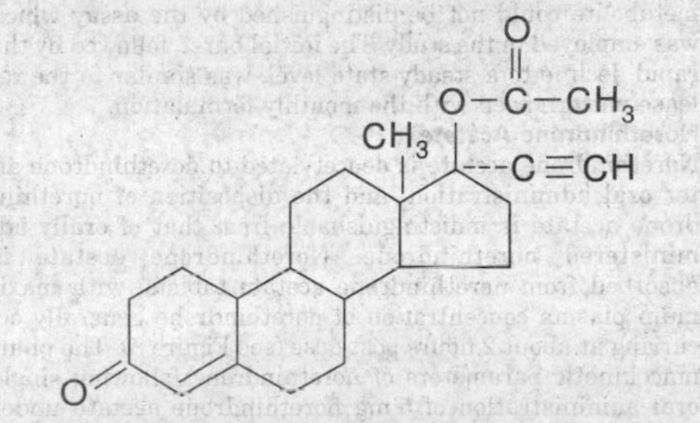

Norethindrone acetate tablets USP, 5 mg contain the following inactive ingredients: colloidal silicon dioxide, lactose monohydrate, magnesium stearate, microcrystalline cellulose and talc.

12 CLINICAL PHARMACOLOGY

12.1 Mechanism of Action

Leuprolide Acetate for Depot Suspension

Leuprolide acetate for depot suspension is a long-acting GnRH analog. A single injection of leuprolide acetate for depot suspension results in an initial elevation followed by a prolonged suppression of pituitary gonadotropins. Repeated dosing at quarterly intervals results in decreased secretion of gonadal steroids; consequently, tissues and functions that depend on gonadal steroids for their maintenance become quiescent. This effect is reversible on discontinuation of drug therapy.

Leuprolide acetate is not active when given orally.

Norethindrone Acetate

Norethindrone acetate induces secretory changes in an estrogen-primed endometrium.

12.2 Pharmacodynamics

In a pharmacokinetic/pharmacodynamic study of leuprolide acetate 11.25 mg for 3-month administration in healthy female subjects (N=20), the onset of estradiol suppression was observed for individual subjects between day 4 and week 4 after dosing. By the third week following the injection, the mean estradiol concentration (8 pg/mL) was in the menopausal range. Throughout the remainder of the dosing period, mean serum estradiol levels ranged from the menopausal to the early follicular range.

Serum estradiol was suppressed to ≤20 pg/mL in all subjects within four weeks and remained suppressed (≤40 pg/mL) in 80% of subjects until the end of the 12-week dosing interval, at which time two of these subjects had a value between 40 and 50 pg/mL. Four additional subjects had at least two consecutive elevations of estradiol (range

Information on the AbbVie, Inc. products listed on these pages is from the prescribing information in use as of July 31, 2013. For more information, please visit rxabbvie.com or call 1-800-633-9110.

Figure 8. Mean Norethindrone Plasma Concentration Profile after a Single Dose of 5 mg Norethindrone Acetate Administered to 29 Healthy Female Volunteers under Fasting Conditions

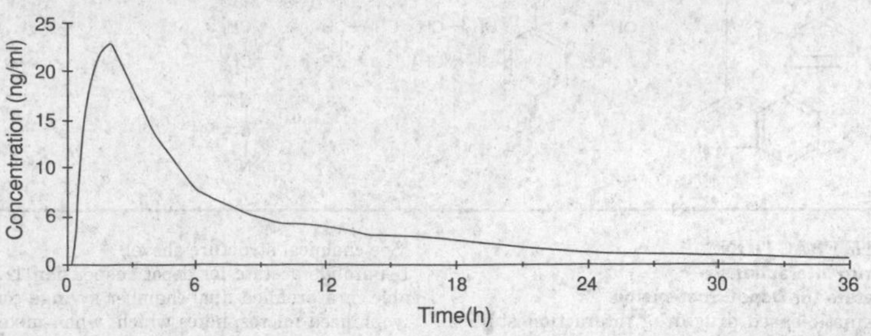

43-240 pg/mL) levels during the 12-week dosing interval, but there was no indication of luteal function for any of the subjects during this period.

12.3 Pharmacokinetics

Absorption

Leuprolide Acetate for Depot Suspension

Following a single injection of the three month formulation of leuprolide acetate for depot suspension (11.25 mg) in female subjects, a mean plasma leuprolide concentration of 36.3 ng/mL was observed at 4 hours. Leuprolide appeared to be released at a constant rate following the onset of steady-state levels during the third week after dosing and mean levels then declined gradually to near the lower limit of detection by 12 weeks. The mean (± standard deviation) leuprolide concentration from 3 to 12 weeks was 0.23 ± 0.09 ng/mL. However, intact leuprolide and an inactive major metabolite could not be distinguished by the assay which was employed in the study. The initial burst, followed by the rapid decline to a steady-state level, was similar to the release pattern seen with the monthly formulation.

Norethindrone Acetate

Norethindrone acetate is deacetylated to norethindrone after oral administration, and the disposition of norethindrone acetate is indistinguishable from that of orally administered norethindrone. Norethindrone acetate is absorbed from norethindrone acetate tablets, with maximum plasma concentration of norethindrone generally occurring at about 2 hours post-dose (see Figure 8). The pharmacokinetic parameters of norethindrone following single oral administration of 5 mg norethindrone acetate under fasting conditions in 29 healthy female volunteers are summarized in Table 5.

Table 5. Pharmacokinetic Parameters after a Single Dose of Norethindrone Acetate in Healthy Women

Norethindrone Acetate (n=29)	Arithmetic Mean ± SD
Norethindrone	
AUC (0-inf) (ng/ml*h)	166.90 ± 56.28
C_{max} (ng/ml)	26.19 ± 6.19
t_{max} (h)	1.83 ± 0.58
$t_{1/2}$ (h)	8.51 ± 2.19

AUC = area under the curve,
C_{max} = maximum plasma concentration,
t_{max} = time at maximum plasma concentration,
$t_{1/2}$ = half-life,
SD = standard deviation

[See figure 8 above]

Effect of Food:

The effect of food administration on the pharmacokinetics of norethindrone acetate has not been studied.

Distribution

Leuprolide Acetate for Depot Suspension

The mean steady-state volume of distribution of leuprolide following intravenous bolus administration to healthy male volunteers was 27 L. *In vitro* binding to human plasma proteins ranged from 43% to 49%.

Norethindrone Acetate

Norethindrone is 36% bound to sex hormone-binding globulin (SHBG) and 61% bound to albumin. Volume of distribution of norethindrone is about 4 L/kg.

Metabolism

Leuprolide Acetate for Depot Suspension

In healthy male volunteers, a 1 mg bolus of leuprolide administered intravenously revealed that the mean systemic clearance was 7.6 L/h, with a terminal elimination half-life of approximately 3 hours based on a two compartment model.

In rats and dogs, administration of ^{14}C-labeled leuprolide was shown to be metabolized to smaller inactive peptides, a pentapeptide (Metabolite I), tripeptides (Metabolites II and III) and a dipeptide (Metabolite IV). These fragments may be further catabolized.

In a pharmacokinetic/pharmacodynamic study of endometriosis patients, intramuscular 11.25 mg leuprolide acetate for depot suspension (n=19) every 12 weeks or intramuscular 3.75 mg leuprolide acetate for depot suspension (n=15) every 4 weeks was administered for 24 weeks. There was no statistically significant difference in changes of serum estradiol concentration from baseline between the 2 treatment groups.

M-I plasma concentrations measured in 5 prostate cancer patients reached maximum concentration 2 to 6 hours after dosing and were approximately 6% of the peak parent drug concentration. One week after dosing, mean plasma M-I concentrations were approximately 20% of mean leuprolide concentrations.

Norethindrone Acetate

Norethindrone undergoes extensive biotransformation, primarily via reduction, followed by sulfate and glucuronide conjugation. The majority of metabolites in the circulation are sulfates, with glucuronides accounting for most of the urinary metabolites.

Excretion

Leuprolide Acetate for Depot Suspension

Following administration of leuprolide acetate for depot suspension 3.75 mg for 1-month administration to 3 patients, less than 5% of the dose was recovered as parent and M-I metabolite in the urine.

Norethindrone Acetate

Plasma clearance value for norethindrone is approximately 0.4 L/hr/kg. Norethindrone is excreted in both urine and feces, primarily as metabolites. The mean terminal elimination half-life of norethindrone following a single dose administration of norethindrone acetate is approximately 9 hours.

Specific Populations

Hepatic Impairment

The effect of hepatic disease on the disposition of norethindrone after norethindrone acetate administration has not been evaluated. However, norethindrone acetate is contraindicated in markedly impaired liver function or liver disease *[see Contraindications (4)]*.

The pharmacokinetics of the leuprolide acetate for depot suspension in hepatically impaired patients has not been determined.

Renal Impairment

The effect of renal disease on the disposition of norethindrone after norethindrone acetate administration has not been evaluated. In pre-menopausal women with chronic renal failure undergoing peritoneal dialysis who received multiple doses of an oral contraceptive containing ethinyl estradiol and norethindrone, plasma norethindrone concentration was unchanged compared to concentrations in pre-menopausal women with normal renal function.

The pharmacokinetics of the leuprolide acetate for depot suspension in renally impaired patients has not been determined.

Race

The effect of race on the disposition of norethindrone after norethindrone acetate administration has not been evaluated.

Drug Interactions

Leuprolide Acetate for Depot Suspension

Leuprolide acetate for depot suspension is a peptide that is primarily degraded by peptidase and not by cytochrome P-450 enzymes as noted in specific studies, and the drug is only about 46% bound to plasma proteins, drug interactions would not be expected to occur.

13 NONCLINICAL TOXICOLOGY

13.1 Carcinogenesis, Mutagenesis, Impairment of Fertility

Leuprolide Acetate for Depot Suspension

A two-year carcinogenicity study was conducted in rats and mice. In rats, a dose-related increase of benign pituitary hyperplasia and benign pituitary adenomas was noted at 24 months when the drug was administered subcutaneously at high daily doses (0.6 to 4 mg/kg). There was a significant but not dose-related increase of pancreatic islet-cell adenomas in females and of testicular interstitial cell adenomas in males (highest incidence in the low dose group). In mice, no leuprolide acetate-induced tumors or pituitary abnormalities were observed at a dose as high as 60 mg/kg for two years. Patients have been treated with leuprolide acetate for up to three years with doses as high as 10 mg/day and for two years with doses as high as 20 mg/day without demonstrable pituitary abnormalities.

Mutagenicity studies have been performed with leuprolide acetate using bacterial and mammalian systems. These studies provided no evidence of a mutagenic potential.

Clinical and pharmacologic studies in adults (> 18 years) with leuprolide acetate and similar analogs have shown reversibility of fertility suppression when the drug is discontinued after continuous administration for periods of up to 24 weeks. Although no clinical studies have been completed in children to assess the full reversibility of fertility suppression, animal studies (prepubertal and adult rats and monkeys) with leuprolide acetate and other GnRH analogs have shown functional recovery.

14 CLINICAL STUDIES

Leuprolide Acetate for Depot Suspension

Initial endometriosis efficacy data for leuprolide acetate for depot suspension were based on the 3.75 mg dose administered once monthly.

A pharmacokinetic/pharmacodynamic study in 41 women that included both the 3.75 mg dose administered once monthly and the 11.25 mg dose administered once every three months did not reveal clinically significant differences in terms of efficacy in reducing painful symptoms of endometriosis or magnitude of the decrease in bone mineral density (BMD) associated with use of leuprolide acetate.

Leuprolide Acetate for Depot Suspension Plus Norethindrone Acetate

Two clinical studies with treatment duration of 12 months were conducted to evaluate the effect of coadministration of leuprolide acetate for depot suspension and norethindrone acetate on the loss of bone mineral density (BMD) associated with leuprolide acetate for depot suspension and on the efficacy of leuprolide acetate for depot suspension in relieving symptoms of endometriosis. (All patients in these studies received calcium supplementation with 1000 mg elemental calcium). A total of 242 women were treated with monthly administration of leuprolide acetate 3.75 mg (13 injections) and with 5 mg norethindrone acetate taken daily. The population age range was 17-43 years old. The majority of patients were Caucasian (87%).

One coadministration study was a controlled, randomized and double-blind study included 51 women treated monthly with leuprolide acetate for depot suspension alone and 55 women treated monthly with leuprolide acetate for depot suspension plus norethindrone acetate daily. Women in this trial were followed for up to 24 months after completing one year of treatment. The other study was an open-label single arm clinical study in 136 women of one year of treatment with leuprolide acetate for depot suspension and norethindrone acetate, with follow-up for up to 12 months after completing treatment.

The second study was an open label, single arm study in which 136 women were treated monthly with leuprolide acetate for depot suspension plus norethindrone acetate daily, with follow-up for up to 12 months after completing treatment.

The assessment of efficacy was based on the investigator's or the patient's monthly assessment of five signs or symptoms of endometriosis (dysmenorrhea, pelvic pain, deep dyspareunia, pelvic tenderness and pelvic induration).

Table 6 below provides detailed efficacy data regarding relief of symptoms of endometriosis based on the two studies of coadministration of leuprolide acetate and norethindrone acetate.

[See table 6 at top of next page]

Suppression of menses (menses was defined as three or more consecutive days of menstrual bleeding) was maintained throughout treatment in 84% and 73% of patients receiving leuprolide acetate and norethindrone acetate, in the controlled study and open label study, respectively. The me-

Table 6. Percentages of Patients with Symptoms of Endometriosis and Mean Clinical Severity Scores

Variable	Study	Group	Percent of Patients with Symptom: Baseline N[1]	(%)[2]	Final (%)	Clinical Pain Severity Score: Baseline N[1]	Value[3]	Final Change
Dysmenorrhea	Controlled Study	LA*	51	(100)	(4)	50	3.2	-2.0
		LA/N†	55	(100)	(4)	54	3.1	-2.0
	Open Label Study	LA/N	136	(99)	(9)	134	3.3	-2.1
Pelvic Pain	Controlled Study	LA	51	(100)	(66)	50	2.9	-1.1
		LA/N	55	(96)	(56)	54	3.1	-1.1
	Open Label Study	LA/N	136	(99)	(63)	134	3.2	-1.2
Deep Dyspareunia	Controlled Study	LA	42	(83)	(37)	25	2.4	-1.0
		LA/N	43	(84)	(45)	30	2.7	-0.8
	Open Label Study	LA/N	102	(91)	(53)	94	2.7	-1.0
Pelvic Tenderness	Controlled Study	LA	51	(94)	(34)	50	2.5	-1.0
		LA/N	54	(91)	(34)	52	2.6	-0.9
	Open Label Study	LA/N	136	(99)	(39)	134	2.9	-1.4
Pelvic Induration	Controlled Study	LA	51	(51)	(12)	50	1.9	-0.4
		LA/N	54	(46)	(17)	52	1.6	-0.4
	Open Label Study	LA/N	136	(75)	(21)	131	2.2	-0.9

* LA = leuprolide acetate 3.75 mg assessment
† LA/N = leuprolide acetate 3.75 mg plus norethindrone acetate 5 mg
[1] Number of patients that were included in the assessment
[2] Percentage of patients with the symptom/sign
[3] Value description: 1=none; 2= mild; 3= moderate; 4= severe

Table 7. Mean Percent Change from Baseline In BMD of Lumbar Spine

	leuprolide acetate for depot suspension 3.75 mg: Controlled Study N	Change (Mean, 95% CI)#	leuprolide acetate for depot suspension 3.75 mg plus norethindrone acetate 5 mg daily: Controlled Study N	Change (Mean, 95% CI)#	Open Label Study N	Change (Mean, 95% CI)#
Week 24*	41	-3.2% (-3.8, -2.6)	42	-0.3% (-0.8, 0.3)	115	-0.2% (-0.6, 0.2)
Week 52†	29	-6.3% (-7.1, -5.4)	32	-1.0% (-1.9, -0.1)	84	-1.1% (-1.6, -0.5)

* Includes on-treatment measurements that fell within 2-252 days after the first day of treatment.
† Includes on-treatment measurements >252 days after the first day of treatment.
\# 95% CI: 95% Confidence Interval

Table 8. Mean Percent Change from Baseline in BMD of Lumbar Spine in Post-Treatment Follow-up Period

Post Treatment Measurement	Controlled Study LA-Only N	Mean % Change	95% CI (%)	Controlled Study LA/N N	Mean % Change	95% CI (%)	Open Label Study LA/N N	Mean % Change	95% CI (%)[2]
Month 8	19	-3.3	(-4.9, -1.8)	23	-0.9	(-2.1, 0.4)	89	-0.6	(-1.2, 0.0)
Month 12	16	-2.2	(-3.3, -1.1)	12	-0.7	(-2.1, 0.6)	65	0.1	(-0.6, 0.7)

[1] Patients with post treatment measurements
[2] 95% CI (2-sided) of percent change in BMD values from baseline

dian time for menses resumption after treatment with leuprolide acetate and norethindrone acetate was 8 weeks.

Changes in Bone Density

The effect of leuprolide acetate for depot suspension and norethindrone acetate on bone mineral density was evaluated by dual energy x-ray absorptiometry (DXA) scan in the two clinical trials. For the open-label study, success in mitigating BMD loss was defined as the lower bound of the 95% confidence interval around the change from baseline at one year of treatment not to exceed -2.2%. The bone mineral density data of the lumbar spine from these two studies are presented in Table 7.

[See table 7 above]

The change in BMD following discontinuation of treatment is shown in Table 8.

[See table 8 above]

These clinical studies demonstrated that coadministration of leuprolide acetate and norethindrone acetate 5 mg daily is effective in significantly reducing the loss of bone mineral density that occurs with leuprolide acetate for depot suspension treatment, and in relieving symptoms of endometriosis.

15 REFERENCES

Leuprolide Acetate for Depot Suspension

1. NIOSH Alert: Preventing occupational exposures to antineoplastic and other hazardous drugs in healthcare settings. 2004. U.S. Department of Health and Human Services, Public Health Service, Centers for Disease Control and Prevention, National Institute for Occupational Safety and Health, DHHS (NIOSH) Publication No. 2004-165.
2. OSHA Technical Manual, TED 1-0.15A, Section VI: Chapter 2. Controlling Occupational Exposure to Hazardous Drugs. OSHA, 1999. http://www.osha.gov/dts/osta/otm/otm_vi/otm_vi_2.html
3. American Society of Health-System Pharmacists. ASHP guidelines on handling hazardous drugs. *Am J Health-Syst Pharm.* 2006; 63; 1172-1193.
4. Polovich, M., White, J.M., & Kelleher, L.O. (eds.) 2005. Chemotherapy and biotherapy guidelines and recommendations for practice (2nd. Ed.) Pittsburgh, PA: Oncology Nursing Society.

16 HOW SUPPLIED/STORAGE AND HANDLING

LUPANETA PACK for 3-month copackaged kit (NDC 0074-1053-05) is available in cartons containing:

leuprolide acetate for depot suspension 11.25 mg for 3-month administration Kit (NDC 0074-3663-04)

norethindrone acetate 5 mg tablets; 90 count bottle (NDC 0074-1049-04)

1. Leuprolide acetate for depot suspension 11.25 mg for 3-month administration kit contains:
   - one prefilled dual-chamber syringe
   - one plunger
   - two alcohol swabs

   Each syringe contains sterile lyophilized microspheres of leuprolide acetate incorporated in a biodegradable polymer of polylactic acid. When mixed with 1.5 mL of the diluent, leuprolide acetate for depot suspension 11.25 mg for 3-month administration is administered as a single intramuscular injection.
2. Norethindrone acetate 5 mg 90 count bottle

   White to off-white oval, flat faced beveled edged, uncoated tablets debossed with 'G with breakline' on one side and 304 on other side.

Store at 25°C (77°F); excursions permitted to 15 to 30°C (59 to 86°F) [See USP Controlled Room Temperature]

17 PATIENT COUNSELING INFORMATION

See FDA-approved patient labeling (Patient Information)

Counsel patients about the Warnings and Precautions for LUPANETA PACK, including:

- Do not use this drug if they have experienced an allergic reaction to GnRH agonists or progestins
- Do not use this drug if they are pregnant or planning a pregnancy, suspect they may be pregnant, or are breast-feeding
- Risk of loss of bone mineral density and limitation of treatment to two six-month courses of treatment
- Risk to an exposed fetus and need to use nonhormonal contraception
- Discontinue norethindrone if they develop sudden loss of vision, double vision or sudden migraine
- The possibility of development or worsening of depression during treatment with leuprolide acetate for depot suspension
- Need for close monitoring if they have cardiovascular risk factors, or conditions like epilepsy, migraine or renal dysfunction
- Notify their healthcare provider if they develop new or worsened symptoms after beginning treatment

Information on the AbbVie, Inc. products listed on these pages is from the prescribing information in use as of July 31, 2013. For more information, please visit rxabbvie.com or call 1-800-633-9110.

PATIENT INFORMATION
LUPANETA PACK™ *(loo-pan-e-tə pæk)*
(leuprolide acetate for depot suspension and norethindrone acetate tablets)

Read this Patient Information before you start taking LUPANETA PACK and each time you get a refill. There may be new information. This information does not take the place of talking with your doctor about your medical condition or your treatment.

What is LUPANETA PACK?

LUPANETA PACK contains 2 different prescription medicines:

- **leuprolide acetate for depot suspension** is a medicine injected into your muscle and used to treat pain due to endometriosis.
- **norethindrone acetate tablets** is a medicine taken by mouth and used to help lower the side effect of bone thinning that is caused by leuprolide acetate for depot suspension.

LUPANETA PACK should not be used longer than 6 months at a time after you first start treatment for your endometriosis symptoms. LUPANETA PACK should not be used for more than a total of 12 months during your treatment.

It is not known if LUPANETA PACK is safe and effective in children under 18 years of age.

Who should not take LUPANETA PACK?

Do not take LUPANETA PACK if you:

- have had an allergic reaction to medicines like leuprolide acetate for depot suspension or norethindrone acetate tablets. See the end of this leaflet for a complete list of ingredients in LUPANETA PACK.
- have uterine bleeding for which a cause has not been found
- are pregnant or may be pregnant. LUPANETA PACK may harm your unborn baby.
- are breastfeeding or plan to breastfeed. It is not known if LUPANETA PACK passes into your breast milk.
- had or have breast cancer or other cancers that are sensitive to hormones
- have problems with blood clots, a stroke or a heart attack.
- have liver problems

What should I tell my doctor before taking LUPANETA PACK?

Before you take LUPANETA PACK, tell your doctor if you:

• drink alcohol	• smoke
• have a family history of bone loss (osteoporosis)	• have depression
• have high cholesterol	• have had blood clots, a stroke or a heart attack
• have migraine headaches	• have diabetes
• have epilepsy	• have kidney problems

Tell your doctor about all the medicines you take, including prescription and non-prescription medicines, vitamins, and herbal supplements.

Especially tell your doctor if you take anticonvulsant (seizure) or corticosteroid medicines.

Ask your doctor for a list of these medicines if you are not sure.

Know the medicines you take. Keep a list of them to show your doctor and pharmacist when you get a new medicine.

How should I take LUPANETA PACK?

- **Leuprolide acetate for depot suspension** for 3–month administration is injected into your muscle 1 time every 3 months by a healthcare professional in your doctor's office.
- **Take norethindrone acetate tablets** exactly as your doctor tells you to take them. Take 1 norethindrone acetate tablet by mouth every day for 3 months after you receive your injection.
- Talk to your doctor about the birth control method that is right for you before you start taking LUPANETA PACK. You will need to use a form of birth control that does not contain hormones, such as:
  - ◦ a diaphragm with spermicide
  - ◦ condoms with spermicide
  - ◦ a copper IUD
- If you become pregnant while taking LUPANETA PACK, stop taking the norethindrone acetate tablets and call your doctor right away.

How well does LUPANETA PACK work?

LUPANETA PACK is used to treat pain due to endometriosis. The pain from endometriosis can happen when you have your period, during other times of the month, or during intercourse (sex). Most women feel some relief from their endometriosis pain after taking both drugs in LUPANETA PACK.

The tablets in LUPANETA PACK help lower the side effect of bone thinning that is caused by leuprolide acetate for depot suspension. Women taking both drugs in LUPANETA PACK lost an average of 1% of their bone density after about 1 year of treatment. Women regained some of their bone density about 1 year after they stopped treatment with LUPANETA PACK.

What are the possible side effects of LUPANETA PACK?

LUPANETA PACK may cause serious side effects, including:

- **bone thinning (decreased bone mineral density)**
- **harm to your unborn baby**
- **vision problems.** Call your doctor right away if you have sudden loss of vision, double vision, bulging eyes, or migraine headaches.
- **depression or worsening depression**
- **allergic reactions.** Get medical help right away if you have any of these symptoms of a serious allergic reaction:
  - ◦ swelling of your face, lips, mouth, or tongue
  - ◦ trouble breathing
  - ◦ wheezing
  - ◦ severe itching
  - ◦ skin rash, redness, or swelling
  - ◦ dizziness or fainting
  - ◦ fast heartbeat or pounding in your chest (tachycardia)
  - ◦ sweating
- **worsening endometriosis symptoms when you start taking LUPANETA PACK**
- **swelling (fluid retention)**

The most common side effects of LUPANETA PACK include:

- hot flashes and sweats
- headaches or migraine headaches
- depression and mood swings
- nausea and vomiting
- problems sleeping
- nervousness or feeling anxious
- pain
- acne
- weakness
- vaginal infection or inflammation
- weight gain
- constipation or diarrhea

Tell your doctor if you have any side effect that bothers you or that does not go away.

These are not all the possible side effects of LUPANETA PACK. For more information, ask your doctor or pharmacist.

Call your doctor for medical advice about side effects. You may report side effects to FDA at 1-800-FDA-1088.

How should I store norethindrone acetate tablets in the LUPANETA PACK?

- Store norethindrone acetate tablets at room temperature between 68°F to 77°F (20°C to 25°C).

Keep LUPANETA PACK and all medicines out of the reach of children.

General information about the safe and effective use of LUPANETA PACK.

Medicines are sometimes prescribed for purposes other than those listed in a Patient Information leaflet. Do not use LUPANETA PACK for a condition for which it was not prescribed. Do not give LUPANETA PACK to other people, even if they have the same symptoms that you have. It may harm them.

This Patient Information leaflet summarizes the most important information about LUPANETA PACK. If you would like more information, talk with your doctor. You can ask your pharmacist or doctor for information about LUPANETA PACK that is written for health professionals.

For more information, go to www.lupanetapack.com or call 1-800-633-9110.

What are the ingredients in LUPANETA PACK?

leuprolide acetate for depot suspension:

Active Ingredients: leuprolide acetate for depot suspension

Inactive Ingredients: polylactic acid, D-mannitol, carboxymethylcellulose sodium, polysorbate 80, water for injection, USP, and glacial acetic acid, USP

norethindrone acetate tablets:

Active Ingredients: norethindrone acetate USP

Inactive Ingredients: colloidal silicon dioxide, lactose monohydrate, magnesium stearate, microcrystalline cellulose and talc.

This Patient Information has been approved by the U.S. Food and Drug Administration.

Leuprolide Acetate for Depot Suspension:
Manufactured for
AbbVie Inc.
North Chicago, IL 60064
By Takeda Pharmaceutical Company Limited
Osaka, Japan 540-8645

Norethindrone Acetate:
Manufactured for
AbbVie Inc.
North Chicago, IL 60064
By Glenmark Generics Ltd.
Colvale-Bardez, Goa
403 513, India

LUPANETA PACK
Packaged by:
AbbVie Inc.
North Chicago, IL 60064
™ - Trademark
® - Registered Trademark

03-A587 March, 2013

LUPRON DEPOT® 3.75 mg ℞

[lew-prŏn]
(leuprolide acetate for depot suspension)
Rx only

This is combined labeling. Examples of different fonts and colors appear below.

- General information
- Information on endometriosis
- Information on uterine fibroids

DESCRIPTION

Leuprolide acetate is a synthetic nonapeptide analog of naturally occurring gonadotropin-releasing hormone (GnRH or LH-RH). The analog possesses greater potency than the natural hormone. The chemical name is 5-oxo-L-prolyl-L-histidyl-L-tryptophyl-L-seryl-L-tyrosyl-D-leucyl-L-leucyl-L-arginyl-N-ethyl-L-prolinamide acetate (salt) with the following structural formula:

[See chemical structure at top of next page]

LUPRON DEPOT is available in a prefilled dual-chamber syringe containing sterile lyophilized microspheres which, when mixed with diluent, become a suspension intended as a monthly intramuscular injection.

The front chamber of LUPRON DEPOT 3.75 mg prefilled dual-chamber syringe contains leuprolide acetate (3.75 mg), purified gelatin (0.65 mg), DL-lactic and glycolic acids copolymer (33.1 mg), and D-mannitol (6.6 mg). The second chamber of diluent contains carboxymethylcellulose sodium (5 mg), D-mannitol (50 mg), polysorbate 80 (1 mg), water for injection, USP, and glacial acetic acid, USP to control pH.

During the manufacture of LUPRON DEPOT 3.75 mg, acetic acid is lost, leaving the peptide.

CLINICAL PHARMACOLOGY

Leuprolide acetate is a long-acting GnRH analog. A single monthly injection of LUPRON DEPOT 3.75 mg results in an initial stimulation followed by a prolonged suppression of pituitary gonadotropins.

Repeated dosing at monthly intervals results in decreased secretion of gonadal steroids; consequently, tissues and functions that depend on gonadal steroids for their maintenance become quiescent. This effect is reversible on discontinuation of drug therapy.

Leuprolide acetate is not active when given orally. Intramuscular injection of the depot formulation provides plasma concentrations of leuprolide over a period of one month.

Pharmacokinetics

Absorption

A single dose of LUPRON DEPOT 3.75 mg was administered by intramuscular injection to healthy female volunteers. The absorption of leuprolide was characterized by an initial increase in plasma concentration, with peak concentration ranging from 4.6 to 10.2 ng/mL at four hours post-dosing. However, intact leuprolide and an inactive metabolite could not be distinguished by the assay used in the study. Following the initial rise, leuprolide concentrations started to plateau within two days after dosing and remained relatively stable for about four to five weeks with plasma concentrations of about 0.30 ng/mL.

Distribution

The mean steady-state volume of distribution of leuprolide following intravenous bolus administration to healthy male volunteers was 27 L. *In vitro* binding to human plasma proteins ranged from 43% to 49%.

Metabolism

In healthy male volunteers, a 1 mg bolus of leuprolide administered intravenously revealed that the mean systemic clearance was 7.6 L/h, with a terminal elimination half-life of approximately 3 hours based on a two compartment model.

In rats and dogs, administration of ^{14}C-labeled leuprolide was shown to be metabolized to smaller inactive peptides, a pentapeptide (Metabolite I), tripeptides (Metabolites II and III) and a dipeptide (Metabolite IV). These fragments may be further catabolized.

The major metabolite (M-I) plasma concentrations measured in 5 prostate cancer patients reached maximum concentration 2 to 6 hours after dosing and were approximately 6% of the peak parent drug concentration. One week after dosing, mean plasma M-I concentrations were approximately 20% of mean leuprolide concentrations.

Excretion
Following administration of LUPRON DEPOT 3.75 mg to 3 patients, less than 5% of the dose was recovered as parent and M-I metabolite in the urine.
Special Populations
The pharmacokinetics of the drug in hepatically and renally impaired patients have not been determined.
Drug Interactions
No pharmacokinetic-based drug-drug interaction studies have been conducted with LUPRON DEPOT. However, because leuprolide acetate is a peptide that is primarily degraded by peptidase and not by cytochrome P-450 enzymes as noted in specific studies, and the drug is only about 46% bound to plasma proteins, drug interactions would not be expected to occur.

CLINICAL STUDIES
Endometriosis
In controlled clinical studies, LUPRON DEPOT 3.75 mg monthly for six months was shown to be comparable to danazol 800 mg/day in relieving the clinical sign/symptoms of endometriosis (pelvic pain, dysmenorrhea, dyspareunia, pelvic tenderness, and induration) and in reducing the size of endometrial implants as evidenced by laparoscopy. The clinical significance of a decrease in endometriotic lesions is not known at this time, and in addition laparoscopic staging of endometriosis does not necessarily correlate with the severity of symptoms.
LUPRON DEPOT 3.75 mg monthly induced amenorrhea in 74% and 98% of the patients after the first and second treatment months respectively. Most of the remaining patients reported episodes of only light bleeding or spotting. In the first, second and third post-treatment months, normal menstrual cycles resumed in 7%, 71% and 95% of patients, respectively, excluding those who became pregnant.
Figure 1 illustrates the percent of patients with symptoms at baseline, final treatment visit and sustained relief at 6 and 12 months following discontinuation of treatment for the various symptoms evaluated during two controlled clinical studies. This included all patients at end of treatment and those who elected to participate in the follow-up period. This might provide a slight bias in the results at follow-up as 75% of the original patients entered the follow-up study, and 36% were evaluated at 6 months and 26% at 12 months.
[See 1 figure above]
Hormonal replacement therapy
Two clinical studies with a treatment duration of 12 months indicate that concurrent hormonal therapy (norethindrone acetate 5 mg daily) is effective in significantly reducing the loss of bone mineral density associated with LUPRON, without compromising the efficacy of LUPRON in relieving symptoms of endometriosis. (All patients in these studies received calcium supplementation with 1000 mg elemental calcium). One controlled, randomized and double-blind study included 51 women treated with LUPRON DEPOT alone and 55 women treated with LUPRON plus norethindrone acetate 5 mg daily. The second study was an open label study in which 136 women were treated with LUPRON plus norethindrone acetate 5 mg daily. This study confirmed the reduction in loss of bone mineral density that was observed in the controlled study. Suppression of menses was maintained throughout treatment in 84% and 73% of patients receiving LD/N in the controlled study and open label study, respectively. The median time for menses resumption after treatment with LD/N was 8 weeks.
Figure 2 illustrates the mean pain scores for the LD/N group from the controlled study.
[See figure 2 at top of next page]
Uterine Leiomyomata (Fibroids)
In controlled clinical trials, administration of LUPRON DEPOT 3.75 mg for a period of three or six months was shown to decrease uterine and fibroid volume, thus allowing for relief of clinical symptoms (abdominal bloating, pelvic pain, and pressure). Excessive vaginal bleeding (menorrhagia and menometrorrhagia) decreased, resulting in improvement in hematologic parameters.
In three clinical trials, enrollment was not based on hematologic status. Mean uterine volume decreased by 41% and myoma volume decreased by 37% at final visit as evidenced by ultrasound or MRI. These patients also experienced a decrease in symptoms including excessive vaginal bleeding and pelvic discomfort. Benefit occurred by three months of therapy, but additional gain was observed with an additional three months of LUPRON DEPOT 3.75 mg. Ninety-five percent of these patients became amenorrheic with 61%, 25%, and 4% experiencing amenorrhea during the first, second, and third treatment months respectively.
Post-treatment follow-up was carried out for a small percentage of LUPRON DEPOT 3.75 mg patients among the 77% who demonstrated a ≥ 25% decrease in uterine volume while on therapy. Menses usually returned within two months of cessation of therapy. Mean time to return to pretreatment uterine size was 8.3 months. Regrowth did not appear to be related to pretreatment uterine volume.

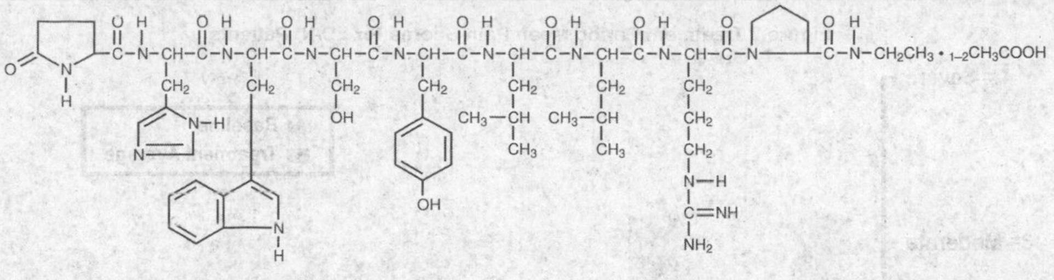

FIGURE 1–PERCENT OF PATIENTS WITH SIGN/SYMPTOMS AT BASELINE, FINAL TREATMENT VISIT, AND AFTER 6 AND 12 MONTHS OF FOLLOW-UP

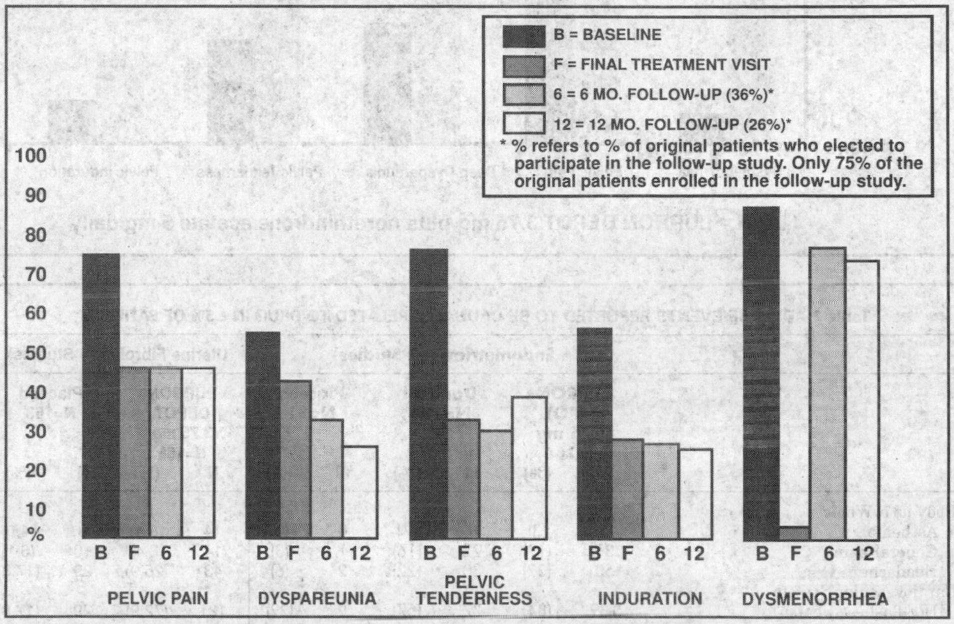

In another controlled clinical study, enrollment was based on hematocrit ≤ 30% and/or hemoglobin ≤ 10.2 g/dL. Administration of LUPRON DEPOT 3.75 mg, concomitantly with iron, produced an increase of ≥ 6% hematocrit and ≥ 2 g/dL hemoglobin in 77% of patients at three months of therapy. The mean change in hematocrit was 10.1% and the mean change in hemoglobin was 4.2 g/dL. Clinical response was judged to be a hematocrit of ≥ 36% and hemoglobin of ≥ 12 g/dL, thus allowing for autologous blood donation prior to surgery. At three months, 75% of patients met this criterion.
At three months, 80% of patients experienced relief from either menorrhagia or menometrorrhagia. As with the previous studies, episodes of spotting and menstrual-like bleeding were noted in some patients.
In this same study, a decrease of ≥ 25% was seen in uterine and myoma volumes in 60% and 54% of patients respectively. LUPRON DEPOT 3.75 mg was found to relieve symptoms of bloating, pelvic pain, and pressure.
There is no evidence that pregnancy rates are enhanced or adversely affected by the use of LUPRON DEPOT 3.75 mg.

INDICATIONS AND USAGE
Endometriosis
LUPRON DEPOT 3.75 mg is indicated for management of endometriosis, including pain relief and reduction of endometriotic lesions. LUPRON DEPOT monthly with norethindrone acetate 5 mg daily is also indicated for initial management of endometriosis and for management of recurrence of symptoms. (Refer also to norethindrone acetate prescribing information for WARNINGS, PRECAUTIONS, CONTRAINDICATIONS and ADVERSE REACTIONS associated with norethindrone acetate). Duration of initial treatment or retreatment should be limited to 6 months.
Uterine Leiomyomata (Fibroids)
LUPRON DEPOT 3.75 mg concomitantly with iron therapy is indicated for the preoperative hematologic improvement of patients with anemia caused by uterine leiomyomata. The clinician may wish to consider a one-month trial period on iron alone inasmuch as some of the patients will respond to iron alone. (See **Table 1**.) LUPRON may be added if the response to iron alone is considered inadequate. Recommended duration of therapy with LUPRON DEPOT 3.75 mg is **up to** three months.
Experience with LUPRON DEPOT in females has been limited to women 18 years of age and older.

Table 1 PERCENT OF PATIENTS ACHIEVING HEMOGLOBIN ≥ 12 GM/DL

Treatment Group	Week 4	Week 8	Week 12
LUPRON DEPOT 3.75 mg with Iron	41*	71†	79*
Iron Alone	17	40	56

* P-Value < 0.01
† P-Value < 0.001

CONTRAINDICATIONS
1. Hypersensitivity to GnRH, GnRH agonist analogs or any of the excipients in LUPRON DEPOT.
2. Undiagnosed abnormal vaginal bleeding.
3. LUPRON DEPOT is contraindicated in women who are or may become pregnant while receiving the drug. LUPRON DEPOT may cause fetal harm when administered to a pregnant woman. Major fetal abnormalities were observed in rabbits but not in rats after administration of LUPRON DEPOT throughout gestation. There was increased fetal mortality and decreased fetal weights in rats and rabbits. (See **Pregnancy** section.) The effects on fetal mortality are expected consequences of the alterations in hormonal levels brought about by the drug. If this drug is used during pregnancy, or if the patient becomes pregnant while taking this drug, the patient should be apprised of the potential hazard to the fetus.

Information on the AbbVie, Inc. products listed on these pages is from the prescribing information in use as of July 31, 2013. For more information, please visit rxabbvie.com or call 1-800-633-9110.

Figure 2 Treatment Period Mean Pain Scores for LD/N* Patients

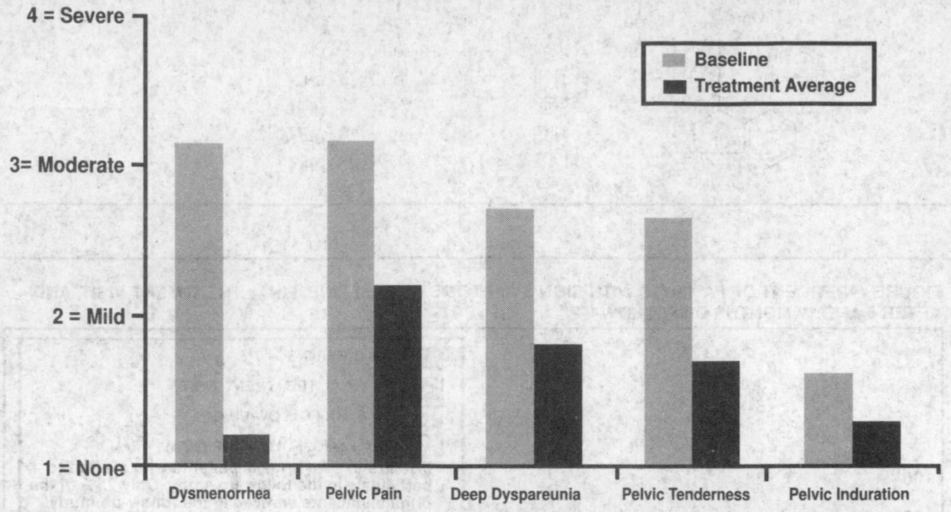

* LD/N = LUPRON DEPOT 3.75 mg plus norethindrone acetate 5 mg daily

Table 2 ADVERSE EVENTS REPORTED TO BE CAUSALLY RELATED TO DRUG IN ≥ 5% OF PATIENTS

	Endometriosis (2 Studies)						Uterine Fibroids (4 Studies)			
	LUPRON DEPOT 3.75 mg N=166		Danazol N=136		Placebo N=31		LUPRON DEPOT 3.75 mg N=166		Placebo N=163	
	N	(%)	N	(%)	N	(%)	N	(%)	N	(%)
Body as a Whole										
Asthenia	5	(3)	9	(7)	0	(0)	14	(8.4)	8	(4.9)
General pain	31	(19)	22	(16)	1	(3)	14	(8.4)	10	(6.1)
Headache*	53	(32)	30	(22)	2	(6)	43	(25.9)	29	(17.8)
Cardiovascular System										
Hot flashes/sweats*	139	(84)	77	(57)	9	(29)	121	(72.9)	29	(17.8)
Gastrointestinal System										
Nausea/vomiting	21	(13)	17	(13)	1	(3)	8	(4.8)	6	(3.7)
GI disturbances*	11	(7)	8	(6)	1	(3)	5	(3.0)	2	(1.2)
Metabolic and Nutritional Disorders										
Edema	12	(7)	17	(13)	1	(3)	9	(5.4)	2	(1.2)
Weight gain/loss	22	(13)	36	(26)	0	(0)	5	(3.0)	2	(1.2)
Endocrine System										
Acne	17	(10)	27	(20)	0	(0)	0	(0)	0	(0)
Hirsutism	2	(1)	9	(7)	1	(3)	1	(0.6)	0	(0)
Musculoskeletal System										
Joint disorder*	14	(8)	11	(8)	0	(0)	13	(7.8)	5	(3.1)
Myalgia*	1	(1)	7	(5)	0	(0)	1	(0.6)	0	(0)
Nervous System										
Decreased libido*	19	(11)	6	(4)	0	(0)	3	(1.8)	0	(0)
Depression/emotional lability*	36	(22)	27	(20)	1	(3)	18	(10.8)	7	(4.3)
Dizziness	19	(11)	4	(3)	0	(0)	3	(1.8)	6	(3.7)
Nervousness*	8	(5)	11	(8)	0	(0)	8	(4.8)	1	(0.6)
Neuromuscular disorders*	11	(7)	17	(13)	0	(0)	3	(1.8)	0	(0)
Paresthesias	12	(7)	11	(8)	0	(0)	2	(1.2)	1	(0.6)
Skin and Appendages										
Skin reactions	17	(10)	20	(15)	1	(3)	5	(3.0)	2	(1.2)
Urogenital System										
Breast changes/tenderness/pain*	10	(6)	12	(9)	0	(0)	3	(1.8)	7	(4.3)
Vaginitis*	46	(28)	23	(17)	0	(0)	19	(11.4)	3	(1.8)

In these same studies, symptoms reported in <5% of patients included: *Body as a Whole* - Body odor, Flu syndrome, Injection site reactions; *Cardiovascular System* - Palpitations, Syncope, Tachycardia; *Digestive System* - Appetite changes, Dry mouth, Thirst; *Endocrine System* - Androgen-like effects; *Hemic and Lymphatic System* - Ecchymosis, Lymphadenopathy; *Nervous System* – Anxiety*, Insomnia/Sleep disorders*, Delusions, Memory disorder, Personality disorder; *Respiratory System* - Rhinitis; *Skin and Appendages* - Alopecia, Hair disorder, Nail disorder; *Special Senses* - Conjunctivitis, Ophthalmologic disorders*, Taste perversion; *Urogenital System* - Dysuria*, Lactation, Menstrual disorders.

* = Possible effect of decreased estrogen.

4. Use in women who are breast-feeding. (See **Nursing Mothers** section.)
5. Norethindrone acetate is contraindicated in women with the following conditions:
   - Thrombophlebitis, thromboembolic disorders, cerebral apoplexy, or a past history of these conditions
   - Markedly impaired liver function or liver disease
   - Known or suspected carcinoma of the breast

WARNINGS

Safe use of leuprolide acetate or norethindrone acetate in pregnancy has not been established clinically. Before starting treatment with LUPRON DEPOT, pregnancy must be excluded.

When used monthly at the recommended dose, LUPRON DEPOT usually inhibits ovulation and stops menstruation. Contraception is not insured, however, by taking LUPRON DEPOT. Therefore, patients should use non-hormonal methods of contraception.

Patients should be advised to see their physician if they believe they may be pregnant. If a patient becomes pregnant during treatment, the drug must be discontinued and the patient must be apprised of the potential risk to the fetus.

During the early phase of therapy, sex steroids temporarily rise above baseline because of the physiologic effect of the drug. Therefore, an increase in clinical signs and symptoms may be observed during the initial days of therapy, but these will dissipate with continued therapy.

Symptoms consistent with an anaphylactoid or asthmatic process have been rarely reported post-marketing.

The following applies to co-treatment with LUPRON and norethindrone acetate:

Norethindrone acetate treatment should be discontinued if there is a sudden partial or complete loss of vision or if there is sudden onset of proptosis, diplopia, or migraine. If examination reveals papilledema or retinal vascular lesions, medication should be withdrawn.

Because of the occasional occurrence of thrombophlebitis and pulmonary embolism in patients taking progestogens, the physician should be alert to the earliest manifestations of the disease in women taking norethindrone acetate.

Assessment and management of risk factors for cardiovascular disease is recommended prior to initiation of add-back therapy with norethindrone acetate. Norethindrone acetate should be used with caution in women with risk factors, including lipid abnormalities or cigarette smoking.

PRECAUTIONS

Information for Patients

Patients should be aware of the following information:

1. Since menstruation usually stops with effective doses of LUPRON DEPOT, the patient should notify her physician if regular menstruation persists. Patients missing successive doses of LUPRON DEPOT may experience breakthrough bleeding.
2. Patients should not use LUPRON DEPOT if they are pregnant, breast feeding, have undiagnosed abnormal vaginal bleeding, or are allergic to any of the ingredients in LUPRON DEPOT.
3. Safe use of the drug in pregnancy has not been established clinically. Therefore, a non-hormonal method of contraception should be used during treatment. Patients should be advised that if they miss successive doses of LUPRON DEPOT, breakthrough bleeding or ovulation may occur with the potential for conception. If a patient becomes pregnant during treatment, she should discontinue treatment and consult her physician.
4. Adverse events occurring in clinical studies with LUPRON DEPOT that are associated with hypoestrogenism include: hot flashes, headaches, emotional lability, decreased libido, acne, myalgia, reduction in breast size, and vaginal dryness. Estrogen levels returned to normal after treatment was discontinued.
5. Patients should be counseled on the possibility of the development or worsening of depression and the occurrence of memory disorders.
6. The induced hypoestrogenic state **also** results in a loss in bone density over the course of treatment, some of which may not be reversible. Clinical studies show that concurrent hormonal therapy with norethindrone acetate 5 mg daily is effective in reducing loss of bone mineral density that occurs with LUPRON. (All patients received calcium supplementation with 1000 mg elemental calcium.) (See ***Changes in Bone Density*** section).
7. If the symptoms of endometriosis recur after a course of therapy, retreatment with a six-month course of LUPRON DEPOT and norethindrone acetate 5 mg daily may be considered. Retreatment beyond this one six month course cannot be recommended. It is recommended that bone density be assessed before retreatment begins to ensure that values are within normal limits. Retreatment with LUPRON DEPOT alone is not recommended.
8. In patients with major risk factors for decreased bone mineral content such as chronic alcohol and/or tobacco use, strong family history of osteoporosis, or chronic use of drugs that can reduce bone mass such as anticonvulsants or corticosteroids, LUPRON DEPOT therapy may pose an additional risk. In these patients, the risks and benefits must be weighed carefully before therapy with LUPRON DEPOT alone is instituted, and concomitant treatment with norethindrone acetate 5 mg daily should be considered. Retreatment with gonadotropin-releasing hormone analogs, including LUPRON is not advisable in patients with major risk factors for loss of bone mineral content.
9. Because norethindrone acetate may cause some degree of fluid retention, conditions which might be influenced by this factor, such as epilepsy, migraine, asthma, cardiac or renal dysfunctions require careful observation during norethindrone acetate add-back therapy.

10. Patients who have a history of depression should be carefully observed during treatment with norethindrone acetate and norethindrone acetate should be discontinued if severe depression occurs.

Laboratory Tests

See **ADVERSE REACTIONS** section.

Drug Interactions

See **CLINICAL PHARMACOLOGY, Pharmacokinetics.**

Drug/Laboratory Test Interactions

Administration of LUPRON DEPOT in therapeutic doses results in suppression of the pituitary-gonadal system. Normal function is usually restored within three months after treatment is discontinued. Therefore, diagnostic tests of pituitary gonadotropic and gonadal functions conducted during treatment and for up to three months after discontinuation of LUPRON DEPOT may be misleading.

Carcinogenesis, Mutagenesis, Impairment of Fertility

A two-year carcinogenicity study was conducted in rats and mice. In rats, a dose-related increase of benign pituitary hyperplasia and benign pituitary adenomas was noted at 24 months when the drug was administered subcutaneously at high daily doses (0.6 to 4 mg/kg). There was a significant but not dose-related increase of pancreatic islet-cell adenomas in females and of testicular interstitial cell adenomas in males (highest incidence in the low dose group). In mice, no leuprolide acetate-induced tumors or pituitary abnormalities were observed at a dose as high as 60 mg/kg for two years. Patients have been treated with leuprolide acetate for up to three years with doses as high as 10 mg/day and for two years with doses as high as 20 mg/day without demonstrable pituitary abnormalities.

Mutagenicity studies have been performed with leuprolide acetate using bacterial and mammalian systems. These studies provided no evidence of a mutagenic potential.

Clinical and pharmacologic studies in adults (>18 years) with leuprolide acetate and similar analogs have shown reversibility of fertility suppression when the drug is discontinued after continuous administration for periods of up to 24 weeks. Although no clinical studies have been completed in children to assess the full reversibility of fertility suppression, animal studies (prepubertal and adult rats and monkeys) with leuprolide acetate and other GnRH analogs have shown functional recovery.

Pregnancy

Teratogenic Effects

Pregnancy Category X (see **CONTRAINDICATIONS** section).

When administered on day 6 of pregnancy at test dosages of 0.00024, 0.0024, and 0.024 mg/kg (1/300 to 1/3 of the human dose) to rabbits, LUPRON DEPOT produced a dose-related increase in major fetal abnormalities. Similar studies in rats failed to demonstrate an increase in fetal malformations. There was increased fetal mortality and decreased fetal weights with the two higher doses of LUPRON DEPOT in rabbits and with the highest dose (0.024 mg/kg) in rats.

Nursing Mothers

It is not known whether LUPRON DEPOT is excreted in human milk. Because many drugs are excreted in human milk, and because the effects of LUPRON DEPOT on lactation and/or the breast-fed child have not been determined, LUPRON DEPOT should not be used by nursing mothers.

Pediatric Use

Experience with LUPRON DEPOT 3.75 mg for treatment of endometriosis has been limited to women 18 years of age and older. See LUPRON DEPOT-PED® (leuprolide acetate for depot suspension) labeling for the safety and effectiveness in children with central precocious puberty.

Geriatric Use

This product has not been studied in women over 65 years of age and is not indicated in this population.

ADVERSE REACTIONS

Clinical Trials

Estradiol levels may increase during the first weeks following the initial injection of LUPRON, but then decline to menopausal levels. This transient increase in estradiol can be associated with a temporary worsening of signs and symptoms (see **WARNINGS** section).

As would be expected with a drug that lowers serum estradiol levels, the most frequently reported adverse reactions were those related to hypoestrogenism.

The **monthly formulation of LUPRON DEPOT 3.75 mg** was utilized in controlled clinical trials that studied the drug in 166 endometriosis and 166 uterine fibroids patients. Adverse events reported in ≥5% of either of these populations and thought to be potentially related to drug are noted in the following table.

[See table 2 at top of previous page]

In one controlled clinical trial utilizing the monthly formulation of LUPRON DEPOT, patients diagnosed with uterine fibroids received a higher dose (7.5 mg) of LUPRON DEPOT. Events seen with this dose that were thought to be potentially related to drug and were not seen at the lower dose included glossitis, hypesthesia, lactation, pyelonephritis, and urinary disorders. Generally, a higher incidence of hypoestrogenic effects was observed at the higher dose.

Table 3 TREATMENT-RELATED ADVERSE EVENTS OCCURRING IN ≥ 5% OF PATIENTS

	Controlled Study				Open Label Study	
	LD - Only* N=51		LD/N† N=55		LD/N† N=136	
Adverse Events	**N**	**(%)**	**N**	**(%)**	**N**	**(%)**
Any Adverse Event	50	(98)	53	(96)	126	(93)
Body as a Whole						
Asthenia	9	(18)	10	(18)	15	(11)
Headache/Migraine	33	(65)	28	(51)	63	(46)
Injection Site Reaction	1	(2)	5	(9)	4	(3)
Pain	12	(24)	16	(29)	29	(21)
Cardiovascular System						
Hot flashes/sweats	50	(98)	48	(87)	78	(57)
Digestive System						
Altered Bowel Function	7	(14)	8	(15)	14	(10)
Changes in Appetite	2	(4)	0	(0)	8	(6)
GI Disturbance	2	(4)	4	(7)	6	(4)
Nausea/Vomiting	13	(25)	16	(29)	17	(13)
Metabolic and Nutritional Disorders						
Edema	0	(0)	5	(9)	9	(7)
Weight Changes	6	(12)	7	(13)	6	(4)
Nervous System						
Anxiety	3	(6)	0	(0)	11	(8)
Depression/Emotional Lability	16	(31)	15	(27)	46	(34)
Dizziness/Vertigo	8	(16)	6	(11)	10	(7)
Insomnia/Sleep Disorder	16	(31)	7	(13)	20	(15)
Libido Changes	5	(10)	2	(4)	10	(7)
Memory Disorder	3	(6)	1	(2)	6	(4)
Nervousness	4	(8)	2	(4)	15	(11)
Neuromuscular Disorder	1	(2)	5	(9)	4	(3)
Skin and Appendages						
Alopecia	0	(0)	5	(9)	4	(3)
Androgen-Like Effects	2	(4)	3	(5)	24	(18)
Skin/Mucous Membrane Reaction	2	(4)	5	(9)	15	(11)
Urogenital System						
Breast Changes/Pain/Tenderness	3	(6)	7	(13)	11	(8)
Menstrual Disorders	1	(2)	0	(0)	7	(5)
Vaginitis	10	(20)	8	(15)	11	(8)

* LD-Only = Lupron Depot 3.75 mg
† LD/N = Lupron Depot 3.75 mg plus norethindrone acetate 5 mg

Table 3 lists the potentially drug-related adverse events observed in at least 5% of patients in any treatment group during the first 6 months of treatment in the add-back clinical studies.

In the controlled clinical trial, 50 of 51 (98%) patients in the LD group and 48 of 55 (87%) patients in the LD/N group reported experiencing hot flashes on one or more occasions during treatment. During Month 6 of treatment, 32 of 37 (86%) patients in the LD group and 22 of 38 (58%) patients in the LD/N group reported having experienced hot flashes. The mean number of days on which hot flashes were reported during this month of treatment was 19 and 7 in the LD and LD/N treatment groups, respectively. The mean maximum number of hot flashes in a day during this month of treatment was 5.8 and 1.9 in the LD and LD/N treatment groups, respectively.

[See table 3 above]

Changes in Bone Density

In controlled clinical studies, patients with endometriosis (six months of therapy) or uterine fibroids (three months of therapy) were treated with LUPRON DEPOT 3.75 mg. In endometriosis patients, vertebral bone density as measured by dual energy x-ray absorptiometry (DEXA) decreased by an average of 3.2% at six months compared with the pretreatment value. Clinical studies demonstrate that concurrent hormonal therapy (norethindrone acetate 5 mg daily) and calcium supplementation is effective in significantly reducing the loss of bone mineral density that occurs with LUPRON treatment, without compromising the efficacy of LUPRON in relieving symptoms of endometriosis.

LUPRON DEPOT 3.75 mg plus norethindrone acetate 5 mg daily was evaluated in two clinical trials. The results from this regimen were similar in both studies. LUPRON DEPOT 3.75 mg was used as a control group in one study. The bone mineral density data of the lumbar spine from these two studies are presented in Table 4.

[See table 4 at top of next page]

When LUPRON DEPOT 3.75 mg was administered for three months in uterine fibroid patients, vertebral trabecular bone mineral density as assessed by quantitative digital radiography (QDR) revealed a mean decrease of 2.7% compared with baseline. Six months after discontinuation of therapy, a trend toward recovery was observed. Use of LUPRON DEPOT for longer than three months (uterine fibroids) or six months (endometriosis) or in the presence of other known risk factors for decreased bone mineral content may cause additional bone loss **and is not recommended.**

Changes in Laboratory Values During Treatment

Plasma Enzymes

Endometriosis

During early clinical trials with LUPRON DEPOT 3.75 mg, regular laboratory monitoring revealed that AST levels were more than twice the upper limit of normal in only one patient. There was no clinical or other laboratory evidence of abnormal liver function.

In two other clinical trials, 6 of 191 patients receiving LUPRON DEPOT 3.75 mg plus norethindrone acetate 5 mg daily for up to 12 months developed an elevated (at least twice the upper limit of normal) SGPT or GGT. Five of the 6 increases were observed beyond 6 months of treatment. None were associated with elevated bilirubin concentration.

Uterine Leiomyomata (Fibroids)

In clinical trials with LUPRON DEPOT 3.75 mg, five (3%) patients had a post-treatment transaminase value that was at least twice the baseline value and above the upper limit of the normal range. None of the laboratory increases were associated with clinical symptoms.

Lipids

Endometriosis

In earlier clinical studies, 4% of the LUPRON DEPOT 3.75 mg patients and 1% of the danazol patients had total cholesterol values above the normal range at enrollment. These patients also had cholesterol values above the normal range at the end of treatment. Of those patients whose pretreatment cholesterol values were in the normal range, 7% of the LUPRON DEPOT 3.75 mg patients and 9% of the danazol patients had post-treatment values above the normal range.

The mean (±SEM) pretreatment values for total cholesterol from all patients were 178.8 (2.9) mg/dL in the LUPRON DEPOT 3.75 mg groups and 175.3 (3.0) mg/dL in the danazol group. At the end of treatment, the mean values for total cholesterol from all patients were 193.3 mg/dL in the LUPRON DEPOT 3.75 mg group and 194.4 mg/dL in the danazol group. These increases from the pretreatment values were statistically significant (p<0.03) in both groups.

Triglycerides were increased above the upper limit of normal in 12% of the patients who received LUPRON DEPOT 3.75 mg and in 6% of the patients who received danazol.

At the end of treatment, HDL cholesterol fractions decreased below the lower limit of the normal range in 2% of the LUPRON DEPOT

Information on the AbbVie, Inc. products listed on these pages is from the prescribing information in use as of July 31, 2013. For more information, please visit rxabbvie.com or call 1-800-633-9110.

Table 4 MEAN PERCENT CHANGE FROM BASELINE IN BONE MINERAL DENSITY OF LUMBAR SPINE

	LUPRON DEPOT 3.75mg Controlled Study		LUPRON DEPOT 3.75 mg plus norethindrone acetate 5 mg daily Controlled Study		Open Label Study	
	N	Change (Mean, 95% CI)#	N	Change (Mean, 95% CI)#	N	Change (Mean, 95% CI)#
Week 24*	41	-3.2% (-3.8, -2.6)	42	-0.3% (-0.8, 0.3)	115	-0.2% (-0.6, 0.2)
Week 52†	29	-6.3% (-7.1, -5.4)	32	-1.0% (-1.9, -0.1)	84	-1.1% (-1.6, -0.5)

* Includes on-treatment measurements that fell within 2–252 days after the first day of treatment.
† Includes on-treatment measurements >252 days after the first day of treatment.
# 95% CI: 95% Confidence Interval

Table 5 SERUM LIPIDS: MEAN PERCENT CHANGES FROM BASELINE VALUES AT TREATMENT WEEK 24

	LUPRON Controlled Study (n=39)		LUPRON plus norethindrone acetate 5 mg daily Controlled Study (n=41)		Open Label Study (n=117)	
	Baseline Value*	Wk 24 % Change	Baseline Value*	Wk 24 % Change	Baseline Value*	Wk 24 % Change
Total Cholesterol	170.5	9.2%	179.3	0.2%	181.2	2.8%
HDL Cholesterol	52.4	7.4%	51.8	-18.8%	51.0	-14.6%
LDL Cholesterol	96.6	10.9%	101.5	14.1%	109.1	13.1%
LDL/HDL Ratio	2.0†	5.0%	2.1†	43.4%	2.3†	39.4%
Triglycerides	107.8	17.5%	130.2	9.5%	105.4	13.8%

* mg/dL
† ratio

Table 6 PERCENTAGE OF PATIENTS WITH SERUM LIPID VALUES OUTSIDE OF THE NORMAL RANGE

	LUPRON Controlled Study (n=39)		LUPRON plus norethindrone acetate 5 mg daily Controlled Study (n=41)		Open Label Study (n=117)	
	Wk 0	Wk 24*	Wk 0	Wk 24*	Wk 0	Wk 24*
Total Cholesterol (>240 mg/dL)	15%	23%	15%	20%	6%	7%
HDL Cholesterol (<40 mg/dL)	15%	10%	15%	44%	15%	41%
LDL Cholesterol (>160 mg/dL)	0%	8%	5%	7%	9%	11%
LDL/HDL Ratio (>4.0)	0%	3%	2%	15%	7%	21%
Triglycerides (>200 mg/dL)	13%	13%	12%	10%	5%	9%

* Includes all patients regardless of baseline value.

3.75 mg patients compared with 54% of those receiving danazol. LDL cholesterol fractions increased above the upper limit of the normal range in 6% of the patients receiving LUPRON DEPOT 3.75 mg compared with 23% of those receiving danazol. There was no increase in the LDL/HDL ratio in patients receiving LUPRON DEPOT 3.75 mg but there was approximately a two-fold increase in the LDL/HDL ratio in patients receiving danazol.
In two other clinical trials, LUPRON DEPOT 3.75 mg plus norethindrone acetate 5 mg daily was evaluated for 12 months of treatment. LUPRON DEPOT 3.75 mg was used as a control group in one study. Percent changes from baseline for serum lipids and percentages of patients with serum lipid values outside of the normal range in the two studies are summarized in the tables below.
[See table 5 above]
Changes from baseline tended to be greater at Week 52. After treatment, mean serum lipid levels from patients with follow up data returned to pretreatment values.
[See table 6 above]
Low HDL-cholesterol (<40 mg/dL) and elevated LDL-cholesterol (>160 mg/dL) are recognized risk factors for cardiovascular disease. The long-term significance of the observed treatment-related changes in serum lipids in women with endometriosis is unknown. Therefore assessment of cardiovascular risk factors should be considered prior to initiation of concurrent treatment with LUPRON and norethindrone acetate.

Uterine Leiomyomata (Fibroids)
In patients receiving LUPRON DEPOT 3.75 mg, mean changes in cholesterol (+11 mg/dL to +29 mg/dL), LDL cholesterol (+8 mg/dL to +22 mg/dL), HDL cholesterol (0 to +6 mg/dL), and the LDL/HDL ratio (-0.1 to +0.5) were observed across studies. In the one study in which triglycerides were determined, the mean increase from baseline was 32 mg/dL.

Other Changes

Endometriosis
The following changes were seen in approximately 5% to 8% of patients. In the earlier comparative studies, LUPRON DEPOT 3.75 mg was associated with elevations of LDH and phosphorus, and decreases in WBC counts. Danazol therapy was associated with increases in hematocrit, platelet count, and LDH. In the hormonal add-back studies LUPRON DEPOT in combination with norethindrone acetate was associated with elevations of GGT and SGPT.

Uterine Leiomyomata (Fibroids)
Hematology: (see **CLINICAL STUDIES** section) In LUPRON DEPOT 3.75 mg treated patients, although there were statistically significant mean decreases in platelet counts from baseline to final visit, the last mean platelet counts were within the normal range. Decreases in total WBC count and neutrophils were observed, but were not clinically significant.
Chemistry: Slight to moderate mean increases were noted for glucose, uric acid, BUN, creatinine, total protein, albumin, bilirubin, alkaline phosphatase, LDH, calcium, and phosphorus. None of these increases were clinically significant.

Postmarketing
The following adverse reactions have been identified during postapproval use of LUPRON DEPOT. Because these reactions are reported voluntarily from a population of uncertain size, it is not always possible to reliably estimate their frequency or establish a causal relationship to drug exposure.
During postmarketing surveillance, the following adverse events were reported. Like other drugs in this class, mood swings, including depression, have been reported. There have been rare reports of suicidal ideation and attempt. Many, but not all, of these patients had a history of depression or other psychiatric illness. Patients should be counseled on the possibility of development or worsening of depression during treatment with LUPRON.
Symptoms consistent with an anaphylactoid or asthmatic process have been rarely reported. Rash, urticaria, and photosensitivity reactions have also been reported.
Localized reactions including induration and abscess have been reported at the site of injection. Symptoms consistent with fibromyalgia (eg: joint and muscle pain, headaches, sleep disorder, gastrointestinal distress, and shortness of breath) have been reported individually and collectively.
Other events reported are:
Hepato-biliary disorder: Rarely reported serious liver injury
Injury, poisoning and procedural complications: Spinal fracture
Investigations: Decreased WBC
Musculoskeletal and Connective tissue disorder: Tenosynovitis-like symptoms
Nervous System Disorder: Convulsion, peripheral neuropathy, paralysis
Vascular Disorder: Hypotension
Cases of serious venous and arterial thromboembolism have been reported, including deep vein thrombosis, pulmonary embolism, myocardial infarction, stroke, and transient ischemic attack. Although a temporal relationship was reported in some cases, most cases were confounded by risk factors or concomitant medication use. It is unknown if there is a causal association between the use of GnRH analogs and these events.
Pituitary apoplexy
During post-marketing surveillance, rare cases of pituitary apoplexy (a clinical syndrome secondary to infarction of the pituitary gland) have been reported after the administration of gonadotropin-releasing hormone agonists. In a majority of these cases, a pituitary adenoma was diagnosed, with a majority of pituitary apoplexy cases occurring within 2 weeks of the first dose, and some within the first hour. In these cases, pituitary apoplexy has presented as sudden headache, vomiting, visual changes, ophthalmoplegia, altered mental status, and sometimes cardiovascular collapse. Immediate medical attention has been required.
See other LUPRON DEPOT and LUPRON Injection package inserts for other events reported in different patient populations.

OVERDOSAGE

In rats subcutaneous administration of 250 to 500 times the recommended human dose, expressed on a per body weight basis, resulted in dyspnea, decreased activity, and local irritation at the injection site. There is no evidence that there is a clinical counterpart of this phenomenon. In early clinical trials using daily subcutaneous leuprolide acetate in patients with prostate cancer, doses as high as 20 mg/day for up to two years caused no adverse effects differing from those observed with the 1 mg/day dose.

DOSAGE AND ADMINISTRATION

LUPRON DEPOT Must Be Administered Under The Supervision Of A Physician.

Endometriosis
The recommended duration of treatment with LUPRON DEPOT 3.75 mg alone or in combination with norethindrone acetate is six months. The choice of LUPRON DEPOT alone or LUPRON DEPOT plus norethindrone acetate therapy for initial management of the symptoms and signs of endometriosis should be made by the health care professional in consultation with the patient and should take into consideration the risks and benefits of the addition of norethindrone to LUPRON DEPOT alone.
If the symptoms of endometriosis recur after a course of therapy, retreatment with a six-month course of LUPRON DEPOT monthly and norethindrone acetate 5 mg daily may be considered. Retreatment beyond this one six-month course cannot be recommended. It is recommended that bone density be assessed before retreatment begins to ensure that values are within normal limits. LUPRON DEPOT alone is not recommended for retreatment. If norethindrone acetate is contraindicated for the individual patient, then retreatment is not recommended.
An assessment of cardiovascular risk and management of risk factors such as cigarette smoking is recommended before beginning treatment with LUPRON DEPOT and norethindrone acetate.

Uterine Leiomyomata (Fibroids)
*Recommended duration of therapy with LUPRON DEPOT 3.75 mg is **up to** 3 months. The symptoms associated with uterine leiomyomata will recur following discontinuation of therapy. If additional treatment with LUPRON DEPOT 3.75 mg is contemplated, bone density should be assessed prior to initiation of therapy to ensure that values are within normal limits.*
The recommended dose of LUPRON DEPOT is 3.75 mg, incorporated in a depot formulation.
For optimal performance of the prefilled dual chamber syringe (PDS), read and follow the following instructions:
Reconstitution and Administration Instructions
- The lyophilized microspheres are to be reconstituted and administered as a single intramuscular injection.
- Since LUPRON DEPOT does not contain a preservative, the suspension should be injected immediately or discarded if not used within two hours.
- As with other drugs administered by injection, the injection site should be varied periodically.

1. The LUPRON DEPOT powder should be visually inspected and the syringe should NOT BE USED if clumping or caking is evident. A thin layer of powder on the wall of the syringe is considered normal prior to mixing with the diluent. The diluent should appear clear.
2. To prepare for injection, screw the white plunger into the end stopper until the stopper begins to turn.

[See figure at top of next column]

3. Hold the syringe UPRIGHT. Release the diluent by SLOWLY PUSHING (6 to 8 seconds) the plunger until

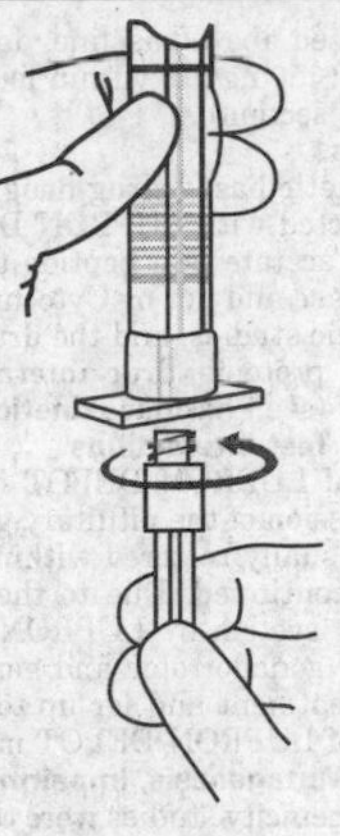

the first stopper is at the blue line in the middle of the barrel.

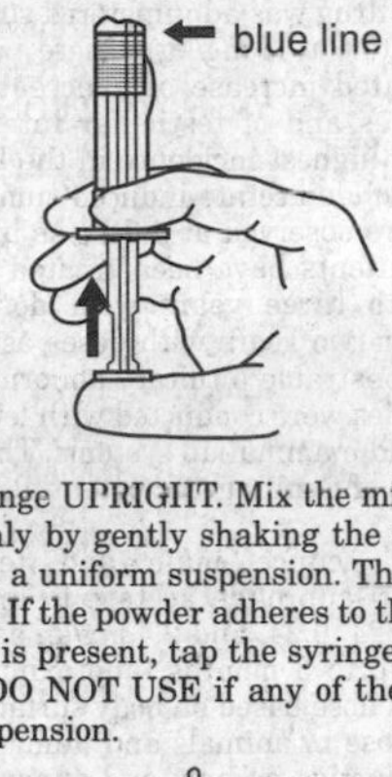

4. Keep the syringe UPRIGHT. Mix the microspheres (powder) thoroughly by gently shaking the syringe until the powder forms a uniform suspension. The suspension will appear milky. If the powder adheres to the stopper or caking/clumping is present, tap the syringe with your finger to disperse. DO NOT USE if any of the powder has not gone into suspension.

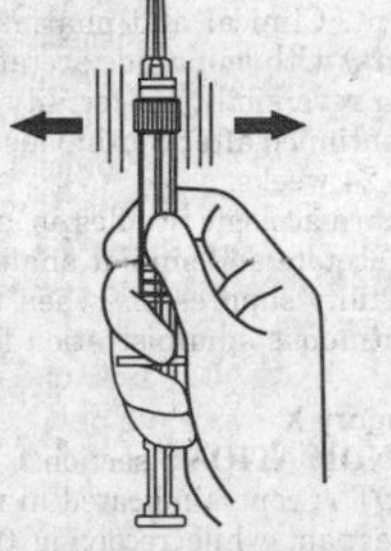

5. Hold the syringe UPRIGHT. With the opposite hand pull the needle cap upward without twisting.
6. Keep the syringe UPRIGHT. Advance the plunger to expel the air from the syringe. Now the syringe is ready for injection.
7. After cleaning the injection site with an alcohol swab, the intramuscular injection should be performed by inserting the needle at a 90 degree angle into the gluteal area, anterior thigh, or deltoid; injection sites should be alternated.

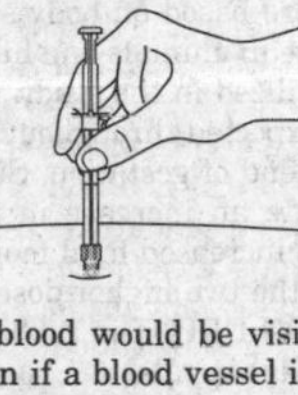

NOTE: Aspirated blood would be visible just below the luer lock connection if a blood vessel is accidentally penetrated. If present, blood can be seen through the transparent LuproLoc® safety device. If blood is present remove the needle immediately. Do not inject the medication.

[See figure at top of next column]

8. Inject the entire contents of the syringe intramuscularly at the time of reconstitution. The suspension settles very quickly following reconstitution; therefore, LUPRON DEPOT should be mixed and used immediately.

AFTER INJECTION

9. Withdraw the needle. Once the syringe has been withdrawn, activate immediately the LuproLoc® safety device by pushing the arrow on the lock upward towards the needle tip with the thumb or finger, as illustrated, until the needle cover of the safety device over the needle is fully extended and a CLICK is heard or felt.

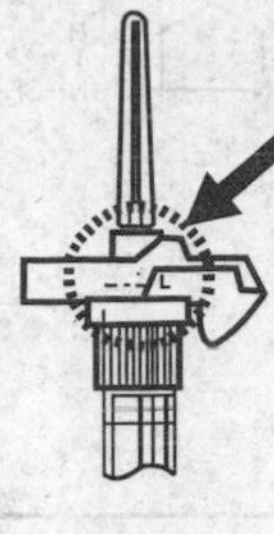

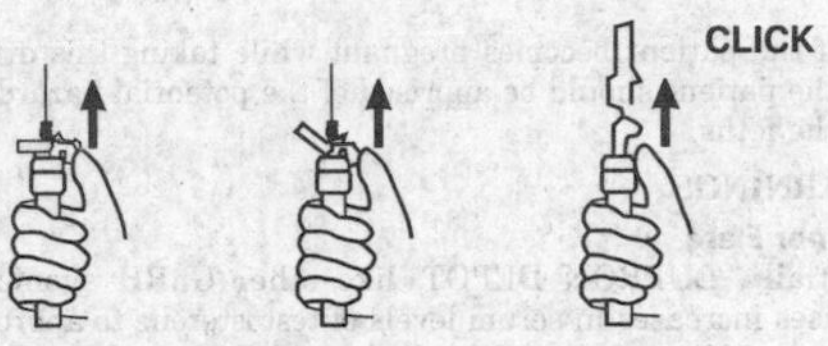

ADDITIONAL INFORMATION

- Dispose of the syringe according to local regulations/procedures.

HOW SUPPLIED

Each LUPRON DEPOT 3.75 mg kit (NDC 0074-3641-03) contains:

- one prefilled dual-chamber syringe
- one plunger
- two alcohol swabs
- a complete prescribing information enclosure

Each syringe contains sterile lyophilized microspheres, which is leuprolide incorporated in a biodegradable copolymer of lactic and glycolic acids. When mixed with diluent, LUPRON DEPOT 3.75 mg is administered as a single monthly IM injection.

Store at 25°C (77°F); excursions permitted to 15-30°C (59-86°F) [See USP Controlled Room Temperature]

REFERENCES

1. NIOSH Alert: Preventing occupational exposures to antineoplastic and other hazardous drugs in healthcare settings. 2004. U.S. Department of Health and Human Services, Public Health Service, Centers for Disease Control and Prevention, National Institute for Occupational Safety and Health, DHHS (NIOSH) Publication No. 2004-165.
2. OSHA Technical Manual, TED 1-0.15A, Section VI: Chapter 2. Controlling Occupational Exposure to Hazardous Drugs. OSHA, 1999. http://www.osha.gov/dts/osta/otm/otm_vi/otm_vi_2.html
3. American Society of Health-System Pharmacists. ASHP guidelines on handling hazardous drugs. *Am J Health-Syst Pharm.* 2006; 63; 1172-1193.
4. Polovich, M., White, J.M., & Kelleher, L.O. (eds.) 2005. Chemotherapy and biotherapy guidelines and recommendations for practice (2nd. Ed.) Pittsburgh, PA: Oncology Nursing Society.

Manufactured for
AbbVie Inc.
North Chicago, IL 60064
by Takeda Pharmaceutical Company Limited
Osaka, Japan 540-8645
™ - Trademark
® - Registered Trademark
(No. 3641)
03-A694 January, 2013

Shown in Product Identification Guide, page 303

LUPRON DEPOT® 7.5 mg for 1-month administration ℞

[lew-prŏn]

(leuprolide acetate for depot suspension)

Rx only

DESCRIPTION

Leuprolide acetate is a synthetic nonapeptide analog of naturally occurring gonadotropin-releasing hormone (GnRH or LH-RH). The analog possesses greater potency than the natural hormone. The chemical name is 5-oxo-L-prolyl-L-histidyl-L-tryptophyl-L-seryl-L-tyrosyl-D-leucyl-L-leucyl-L-arginyl-N-ethyl-L-prolinamide acetate (salt) with the following structural formula:

[See chemical structure at top of next page]

LUPRON DEPOT is available in a prefilled dual-chamber syringe containing sterile lyophilized microspheres which, when mixed with diluent, becomes a suspension intended as a monthly intramuscular injection.

The front chamber of LUPRON DEPOT 7.5 mg for 1-month administration prefilled dual-chamber syringe contains leuprolide acetate (7.5 mg), purified gelatin (1.3 mg), DL-lactic and glycolic acids copolymer (66.2 mg), and D-mannitol (13.2 mg). The second chamber of diluent contains carboxymethylcellulose sodium (5 mg), D-mannitol (50 mg), polysorbate 80 (1 mg), water for injection, USP, and glacial acetic acid, USP to control pH.

During the manufacture of LUPRON DEPOT 7.5 mg for 1-month administration, acetic acid is lost, leaving the peptide.

CLINICAL PHARMACOLOGY

Mechanism of Action

Leuprolide acetate, a GnRH agonist, acts as a potent inhibitor of gonadotropin secretion. Animal studies indicate that following an initial stimulation, chronic administration of leuprolide acetate results in suppression of ovarian and testicular steroidogenesis. This effect is reversible upon discontinuation of drug therapy.

Administration of leuprolide acetate has resulted in inhibition of the growth of certain hormone dependent tumors (prostatic tumors in Noble and Dunning male rats and DMBA-induced mammary tumors in female rats) as well as atrophy of the reproductive organs.

Pharmacodynamics

In humans, administration of leuprolide acetate results in an initial increase in circulating levels of luteinizing hormone (LH) and follicle stimulating hormone (FSH), leading to a transient increase in levels of the gonadal steroids (testosterone and dihydrotestosterone in males, and estrone and estradiol in premenopausal females). However, continuous administration of leuprolide acetate results in decreased levels of LH and FSH. In males, testosterone is reduced to castrate levels. In premenopausal females, estrogens are reduced to postmenopausal levels. These decreases occur within two to four weeks after initiation of treatment, and castrate levels of testosterone in prostatic cancer patients have been demonstrated for more than five years.

Leuprolide acetate is not active when given orally.

Pharmacokinetics

Absorption

Following a single injection of LUPRON DEPOT 7.5 mg for 1-month administration to patients, mean plasma leuprolide concentration was almost 20 ng/mL at 4 hours and 0.36 ng/mL at 4 weeks. However, intact leuprolide and an inactive major metabolite could not be distinguished by the assay which was employed in the study. Nondetectable leuprolide plasma concentrations have been observed during chronic LUPRON DEPOT 7.5 mg administration, but testosterone levels appear to be maintained at castrate levels.

Distribution

The mean steady-state volume of distribution of leuprolide following intravenous bolus administration to healthy male volunteers was 27 L. *In vitro* binding to human plasma proteins ranged from 43% to 49%.

Metabolism

In healthy male volunteers, a 1 mg bolus of leuprolide administered intravenously revealed that the mean systemic clearance was 7.6 L/h, with a terminal elimination half-life of approximately 3 hours based on a two compartment model.

In rats and dogs, administration of ^{14}C-labeled leuprolide was shown to be metabolized to smaller inactive peptides, a pentapeptide (Metabolite I), tripeptides (Metabolites II and III) and a dipeptide (Metabolite IV). These fragments may be further catabolized.

The major metabolite (M-I) plasma concentrations measured in 5 prostate cancer patients reached maximum concentration 2 to 6 hours after dosing and were approximately 6% of the peak parent drug concentration. One week after dosing, mean plasma M-I concentrations were approximately 20% of mean leuprolide concentrations.

Excretion

Following administration of LUPRON DEPOT 3.75 mg to 3 patients, less than 5% of the dose was recovered as parent and M-I metabolite in the urine.

Special Populations

The pharmacokinetics of the drug in hepatically and renally impaired patients have not been determined.

CLINICAL STUDIES

In an open-label, non-comparative, multicenter clinical study of LUPRON DEPOT 7.5 mg for 1-month administration, 56 patients with stage D_2 prostatic adenocarcinoma and no prior systemic treatment were enrolled. The objectives were to determine if a 7.5 mg depot formulation of leuprolide injected once every 4 weeks would reduce and maintain serum testosterone to castrate range (≤50 ng/dL), to evaluate objective clinical response, and to assess the safety of the formulation. During the initial 24 weeks,

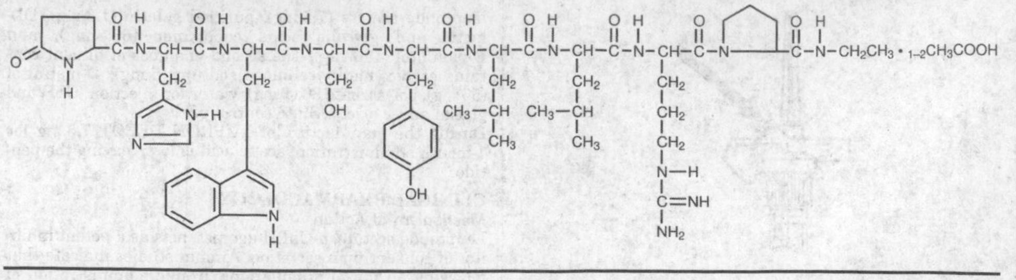

serum testosterone was measured weekly, biweekly, or every four weeks and objective tumor response assessments were performed at Weeks 12 and 24. Once the patient completed the initial 24-week treatment phase, treatment continued at the investigator's discretion. Data from the initial 24-week treatment phase are summarized in this section.

In the majority of patients, serum testosterone increased by 50% or more above baseline during the first week of treatment. Serum testosterone suppressed to the castrate range within 30 days of the initial depot injection in 94% (51/54) of patients for whom testosterone suppression was achieved (2 patients withdrew prior to onset of suppression) and within 66 days in all 54 patients. Mean serum testosterone suppressed to castrate level by Week 3. The median dosing interval between injections was 28 days. One escape from suppression (2 consecutive testosterone values greater than 50 ng/dL after achieving castrate level) was noted at Week 18, associated with a substantial dosing delay. In this patient, serum testosterone returned to the castrate range at the next monthly measurement. Serum testosterone was minimally above the castrate range on a single occasion for 4 other patients. No clinical significance was attributed to these rises in testosterone.

Lupron Depot 7.5 mg
Mean Serum Testosterone Concentrations

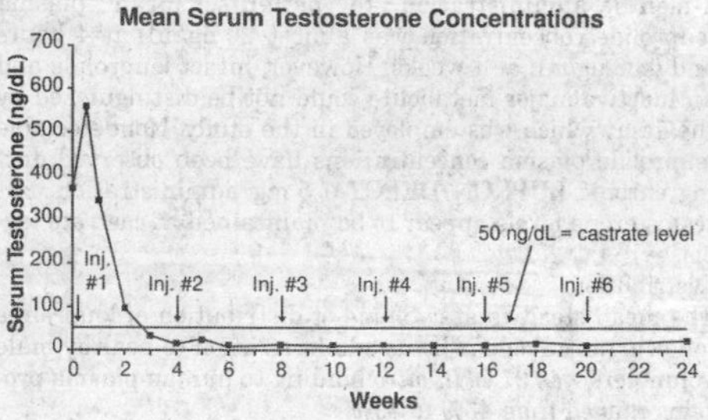

Secondary efficacy endpoints evaluated included objective tumor response, assessed by clinical evaluations of tumor burden (complete response, partial response, objectively stable, and progression), as well as changes in local disease status, assessed by digital rectal examination, and changes in prostatic acid phosphatase (PAP). These evaluations were performed at Weeks 12 and 24. The objective tumor response analysis showed a "no progression" (ie. complete or partial response, or stable disease) in 77% (40/52) of patients at Week 12, and in 84% (42/50) of patients at Week 24. Local disease improved or remained stable in all (42) patients evaluated at Week 12 and in 98% (41/42) of patients elevated at Week 24. PAP normalized or decreased at Week 12 and/or 24 in the majority of patients with elevated baseline PAP.

Periodic monitoring of serum testosterone and PSA levels is recommended, especially if the anticipated clinical or biochemical response to treatment has not been achieved. It should be noted that results of testosterone determinations are dependent on assay methodology. It is advisable to be aware of the type and precision of the assay methodology to make appropriate clinical and therapeutic decisions.

INDICATIONS AND USAGE

LUPRON DEPOT 7.5 mg for 1-month administration is indicated in the palliative treatment of advanced prostatic cancer.

CONTRAINDICATIONS

1. LUPRON DEPOT is contraindicated in individuals with known hypersensitivity to GnRH agonists or any of the excipients in LUPRON DEPOT. Reports of anaphylactic reactions to GnRH agonist analogs have been reported in the medical literature.
2. LUPRON DEPOT may cause fetal harm when administered to a pregnant woman. Expected hormonal changes that occur with LUPRON DEPOT increase the risk for pregnancy loss and fetal harm when administered to a pregnant woman (see **Pregnancy Category X**). LUPRON DEPOT is contraindicated in women who are or may become pregnant. If this drug is used during pregnancy, or if the patient becomes pregnant while taking this drug, the patient should be apprised of the potential hazard to the fetus.

WARNINGS

Tumor Flare

Initially, LUPRON DEPOT, like other GnRH agonists, causes increases in serum levels of testosterone to approximately 50% above baseline during the first week of treatment. Isolated cases of ureteral obstruction and spinal cord compression have been observed, which may contribute to paralysis with or without fatal complications. Transient worsening of symptoms may develop. A small number of patients may experience a temporary increase in bone pain, which can be managed symptomatically.

PRECAUTIONS

Information for Patients

- If they experience an allergic reaction to other drugs like LUPRON DEPOT, they should not use this drug.
- The most common side effects associated with LUPRON DEPOT are hot flashes, pain (especially joint pain and back pain), injection site pain and fatigue.
- LUPRON DEPOT may cause impotence.
- The increase in testosterone that occurs during the first weeks of therapy can cause an increase in urinary symptoms or pain.
- If they have metastatic cancer to the spine or urinary tract, they need close medical attention during the first weeks of therapy.
- They should notify their doctor if they develop new or worsened symptoms after beginning LUPRON DEPOT treatment.

General

Patients with metastatic vertebral lesions and/or with urinary tract obstruction should be closely observed during the first few weeks of therapy (see **WARNINGS** section).

Hyperglycemia and Diabetes

Hyperglycemia and an increased risk of developing diabetes have been reported in men receiving GnRH agonists. Hyperglycemia may represent development of diabetes mellitus or worsening of glycemic control in patients with diabetes. Monitor blood glucose and/or glycosylated hemoglobin (HbA1c) periodically in patients receiving a GnRH agonist and manage with current practice for treatment of hyperglycemia or diabetes.

Cardiovascular Diseases

Increased risk of developing myocardial infarction, sudden cardiac death and stroke has been reported in association with use of GnRH agonists in men. The risk appears low based on the reported odds ratios, and should be evaluated carefully along with cardiovascular risk factors when determining a treatment for patients with prostate cancer. Patients receiving a GnRH agonist should be monitored for symptoms and signs suggestive of development of cardiovascular disease and be managed according to current clinical practice.

Effect on QT/QTc Interval

Long-term androgen deprivation therapy prolongs the QT interval. Physicians should consider whether the benefits of androgen deprivation therapy outweigh the potential risks in patients with congenital long QT syndrome, electrolyte abnormalities, or congestive heart failure and in patients taking class IA (e.g., quinidine, procainamide) or Class III (e.g., amiodarone, sotalol) antiarrhythmic medications.

Convulsions

Postmarketing reports of convulsions have been observed in patients on leuprolide acetate therapy. These included patients with a history of seizures, epilepsy, cerebrovascular disorders, central nervous system anomalies or tumors, and in patients on concomitant medications that have been associated with convulsions such as bupropion and SSRIs. Convulsions have also been reported in patients in the absence of any of the conditions mentioned above. Patients receiving a GnRH agonist who experience convulsions should be managed according to current clinical practice.

Laboratory Tests

Response to LUPRON DEPOT 7.5 mg for 1-month administration should be monitored by measuring serum levels of testosterone. In the majority of patients, testosterone levels increased above baseline, declining thereafter to castration levels (<50 ng/dL) within four weeks (see **CLINICAL STUDIES** section).

Drug Interactions

No pharmacokinetic-based drug-drug interaction studies have been conducted with LUPRON DEPOT. However, because leuprolide acetate is a peptide that is primarily degraded by peptidase and not by Cytochrome P-450 enzymes as noted in specific studies, and the drug is only about 46% bound to plasma proteins, drug interactions would not be expected to occur (see **Pharmacokinetics**).

Drug/Laboratory Test Interactions

Administration of LUPRON DEPOT in therapeutic doses results in suppression of the pituitary-gonadal system. Normal function is usually restored within three months after treatment is discontinued. Due to the suppression of the pituitary-gonadal system by LUPRON DEPOT, diagnostic tests of pituitary gonadotropic and gonadal functions conducted during treatment and for up to three months after discontinuation of LUPRON DEPOT may be affected.

Carcinogenesis, Mutagenesis, Impairment of Fertility

Two-year carcinogenicity studies were conducted in rats and mice. In rats, a dose-related increase of benign pituitary hyperplasia and benign pituitary adenomas was noted at 24 months when the drug was administered subcutaneously at high daily doses (0.6 to 4 mg/kg). There was a significant but not dose-related increase of pancreatic islet-cell adenomas in females and of testicular interstitial cell adenomas in males (highest incidence in the low dose group). In mice, no leuprolide acetate-induced tumors or pituitary abnormalities were observed at a dose as high as 60 mg/kg for two years. Patients have been treated with leuprolide acetate for up to three years with doses as high as 10 mg/day and for two years with doses as high as 20 mg/day without demonstrable pituitary abnormalities.

Genotoxicity studies were conducted with leuprolide acetate using bacterial and mammalian systems. These studies provided no evidence of a mutagenic potential or chromosomal aberrations.

Leuprolide may reduce male and female fertility. Administration of leuprolide acetate to male and female rats at dose of 0.024, 0.24, and 2.4 mg/kg as monthly depot formulation for up to 3 months (approximately as low as 1/30 of the human dose based on body surface area using an estimated daily dose in animals and humans) caused atrophy of the reproductive organs, and suppression of reproductive function. These changes were reversible upon cessation of treatment. Clinical and pharmacologic studies in adults (≥ 18 years) with leuprolide acetate and similar analogs have shown reversibility of fertility suppression when the drug is discontinued after continuous administration for periods of up to 24 weeks.

Clinical and pharmacologic studies in adults (≥ 18 years) with leuprolide acetate and similar analogs have shown reversibility of fertility suppression when the drug is discontinued after continuous administration for periods of up to 24 weeks.

Pregnancy Category X

See **CONTRAINDICATIONS** section.

LUPRON DEPOT is contraindicated in women who are or may become pregnant while receiving the drug. Expected hormonal changes that occur with LUPRON DEPOT treatment increase the risk for pregnancy loss and fetal harm when administered to a pregnant woman. If this drug is used during pregnancy, or if the patient becomes pregnant while taking this drug, the patient should be apprised of the potential hazard to the fetus.

Major fetal abnormalities were observed in rabbits after a single administration of the monthly formulation of LUPRON DEPOT on day 6 of pregnancy at doses of 0.00024, 0.0024, and 0.024 mg/kg (approximately 1/1600 to 1/16 the human dose based on body surface area using an estimated daily dose in animals and humans). Since a depot formulation was utilized in the study, a sustained exposure to leuprolide was expected throughout the period of organogenesis and to the end of gestation. Similar studies in rats did not demonstrate an increase in fetal malformations, however, there was increased fetal mortality and decreased fetal weights with the two higher doses of the monthly formulation of LUPRON DEPOT in rabbits and with the highest dose (0.024 mg/kg) in rats.

Nursing Mothers

LUPRON DEPOT is not indicated for women (see **INDICATIONS AND USAGE** section). It is not known whether leuprolide is excreted in human milk. Because many drugs are excreted in human milk and because of the potential for serious adverse reactions in nursing infants from LUPRON DEPOT, a decision should be made to discontinue nursing or discontinue the drug taking into account the importance of the drug to the mother.

Pediatric Use

See LUPRON DEPOT-PED® (leuprolide acetate for depot suspension) labeling for the safety and effectiveness in children with central precocious puberty.

Geriatric Use

In the clinical trials for LUPRON DEPOT in prostate cancer, the majority (80%) of the subjects studied were at least

65 years of age. Therefore, the labeling reflects the pharmacokinetics, efficacy and safety of LUPRON DEPOT in this population.

ADVERSE REACTIONS

Clinical Trials

In the majority of patients testosterone levels increased above baseline during the first week, declining thereafter to baseline levels or below by the end of the second week of treatment.

Potential exacerbations of signs and symptoms during the first few weeks of treatment is a concern in patients with vertebral metastases and/or urinary obstruction or hematuria which, if aggravated, may lead to neurological problems such as temporary weakness and/or paresthesia of the lower limbs or worsening of urinary symptoms (see **WARNINGS** section).

In a clinical trial of LUPRON DEPOT 7.5 mg for 1-month administration, the following adverse reactions were reported in 5% or more of the patients during the initial 24-week treatment period regardless of causality.

LUPRON DEPOT 7.5 mg for 1-Month Administration (N=56)

	N	(%)
Body as a Whole		
General pain	13	(23.2)
Infection	3	(5.4)
Cardiovascular System		
Hot flashes/sweats*	32	(57.1)
Digestive System		
GI disorders	8	(14.3)
Metabolic and Nutritional Disorders		
Edema	8	(14.3)
Nervous System		
Libido decreased*	3	(5.4)
Respiratory System		
Respiratory disorder	6	(10.7)
Urogenital System		
Urinary disorder	7	(12.5)
Impotence*	3	(5.4)
Testicular atrophy*	3	(5.4)

* Due to the expected physiologic effect of decreased testosterone levels.

In this same study, the following adverse reactions were reported in less than 5% of the patients on LUPRON DEPOT 7.5 mg for 1-month administration.

Body as a Whole - Asthenia, Cellulitis, Fever, Headache, Injection site reaction, Neoplasm; *Cardiovascular System* - Angina, Congestive heart failure; *Digestive System* - Anorexia, Dysphagia, Eructation, Peptic ulcer; *Hemic and Lymphatic System* - Ecchymosis; *Musculoskeletal System* - Myalgia; *Nervous System* - Agitation, Insomnia/sleep disorders, Neuromuscular disorders; *Respiratory System* - Emphysema, Hemoptysis, Lung edema, Sputum increased; *Skin and Appendages* - Hair disorder, Skin reaction; *Urogenital System* - Balanitis, Breast enlargement, Urinary tract infection.

Laboratory: Abnormalities of certain parameters were observed, but their relationship to drug treatment are difficult to assess in this population. The following were recorded in ≥5% of patients at final visit: Decreased albumin, decreased hemoglobin/hematocrit, decreased prostatic acid phosphatase, decreased total protein, decreased urine specific gravity, hyperglycemia, hyperuricemia, increased BUN, increased creatinine, increased liver function tests (AST, LDH), increased phosphorus, increased platelets, increased prostatic acid phosphatase, increased total cholesterol, increased urine specific gravity, leukopenia.

Postmarketing

The following adverse reactions have been identified during postapproval use of LUPRON DEPOT. Because these reactions are reported voluntarily from a population of uncertain size, it is not always possible to reliably estimate their frequency or establish a causal relationship to drug exposure.

During postmarketing surveillance, which includes other dosage forms and other patient populations, the following adverse events were reported.

Like other drugs in this class, mood swings, including depression, have been reported. There have been very rare reports of suicidal ideation and attempt. Many, but not all, of these patients had a history of depression or other psychiatric illness. Patients should be counseled on the possibility of development or worsening of depression during treatment with LUPRON.

Symptoms consistent with an anaphylactoid or asthmatic process have been rarely (incidence rate of about 0.002%) reported. Rash, urticaria, and photosensitivity reactions have also been reported.

Changes in Bone Density: Decreased bone density has been reported in the medical literature in men who have had orchiectomy or who have been treated with an LH-RH agonist analog. In a clinical trial, 25 men with prostate cancer, 12 of whom had been treated previously with leuprolide acetate for at least six months, underwent bone density studies as a result of pain. The leuprolide-treated group had lower bone density scores than the nontreated control group. It can be anticipated that long periods of medical castration in men will have effects on bone density.

Pituitary apoplexy: During post-marketing surveillance, rare cases of pituitary apoplexy (a clinical syndrome secondary to infarction of the pituitary gland) have been reported after the administration of gonadotropin-releasing hormone agonists. In a majority of these cases, a pituitary adenoma was diagnosed, with a majority of pituitary apoplexy cases occurring within 2 weeks of the first dose, and some within the first hour. In these cases, pituitary apoplexy has presented as sudden headache, vomiting, visual changes, ophthalmoplegia, altered mental status, and sometimes cardiovascular collapse. Immediate medical attention has been required.

Localized reactions including induration and abscess have been reported at the site of injection.

Symptoms consistent with fibromyalgia (eg, joint and muscle pain, headaches, sleep disorders, gastrointestinal distress, and shortness of breath) have been reported individually and collectively.

Cardiovascular System – Hypotension, Myocardial infarction, Pulmonary embolism;
Respiratory, thoracic and mediastinal disorder – Interstitial lung disease;
Hepato biliary disorder: Serious drug-induced liver injury
Hemic and Lymphatic System – Decreased WBC;
Central/Peripheral Nervous System – Convulsion, Peripheral neuropathy, Spinal fracture/paralysis;
Endocrine System – Diabetes;
Musculoskeletal System – Tenosynovitis-like symptoms;
Urogenital System – Prostate pain.

See other LUPRON DEPOT and LUPRON Injection package inserts for other events reported in women and pediatric populations.

OVERDOSAGE

There is no experience of overdosage in clinical trials. In rats, a single subcutaneous dose of 100 mg/kg (approximately 4,000 times the estimated daily human dose based on body surface area), resulted in dyspnea, decreased activity, and excessive scratching. In early clinical trials with daily subcutaneous leuprolide acetate, doses as high as 20 mg/day for up to two years caused no adverse effects differing from those observed with the 1 mg/day dose.

DOSAGE AND ADMINISTRATION

LUPRON DEPOT must be administered under the supervision of a physician.

The recommended dose of LUPRON DEPOT is 7.5 mg for 1-month administration, incorporated in a depot formulation. Due to different release characteristics, a fractional dose, or a combination of doses of this depot formulation is not equivalent to the same dose of the monthly formulation and should not be given.

Incorporated in a depot formulation, the lyophilized microspheres are to be reconstituted and administered every 4 weeks as a single intramuscular injection.

For optimal performance of the prefilled dual chamber syringe (PDS), read and follow the following instructions:

- The lyophilized microspheres are to be reconstituted and administered as a single intramuscular injection.
- Since LUPRON DEPOT does not contain a preservative, the suspension should be injected immediately or discarded if not used within two hours.
- As with other drugs administered by injection, the injection site should be varied periodically.

1. The LUPRON DEPOT powder should be visually inspected and the syringe should NOT BE USED if clumping or caking is evident. A thin layer of powder on the wall of the syringe is considered normal prior to mixing with the diluent. The diluent should appear clear.
2. To prepare for injection, screw the white plunger into the end stopper until the stopper begins to turn.

[See first figure at top of next column]

3. Hold the syringe UPRIGHT. Release the diluent by SLOWLY PUSHING (6 to 8 seconds) the plunger until the first stopper is at the blue line in the middle of the barrel.

[See second figure at top of next column]

4. Keep the syringe UPRIGHT. Gently mix the microspheres (powder) thoroughly to form a uniform suspension. The suspension will appear milky. If the powder adheres to the stopper or caking/clumping is present, tap the syringe with your finger to disperse. DO NOT USE if any of the powder has not gone into suspension.

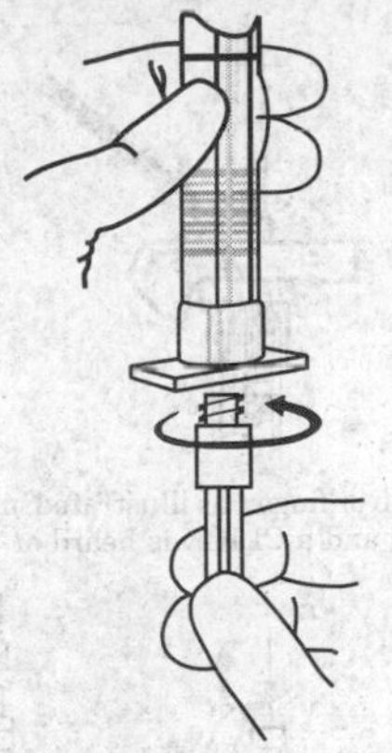

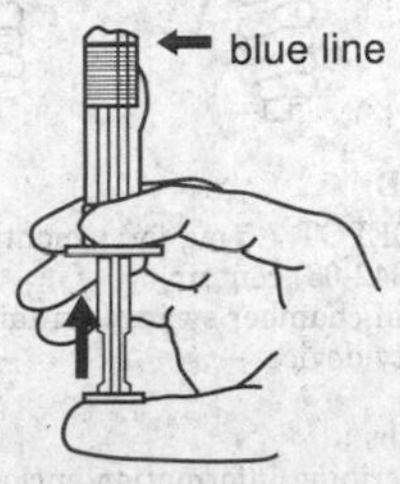

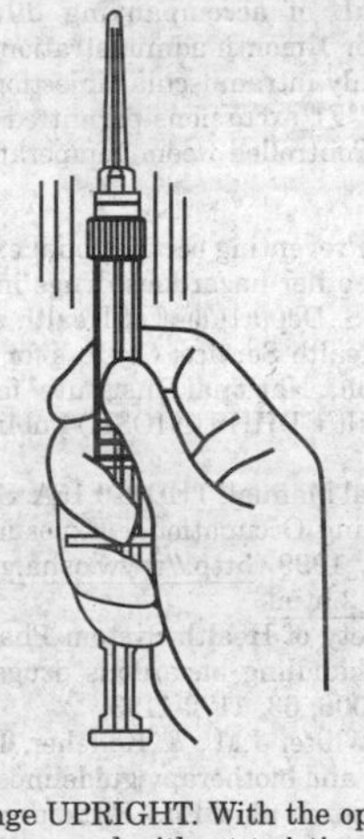

5. Hold the syringe UPRIGHT. With the opposite hand pull the needle cap upward without twisting.
6. Keep the syringe UPRIGHT. Advance the plunger to expel the air from the syringe.
7. After cleaning the injection site with an alcohol swab, insert the needle completely at a 90 degree angle.

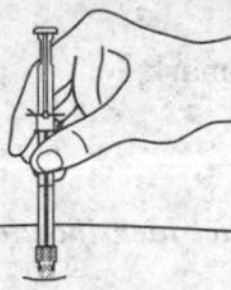

NOTE: Aspirated blood would be visible just below the luer lock connection if a blood vessel is accidentally penetrated. If present, blood can be seen through the transparent LuproLoc® safety device. If blood is present remove the needle immediately. Do not inject the medication.

[See figure at top of next column]

8. Inject the entire contents of the syringe intramuscularly at the time of reconstitution. The suspension settles very quickly following reconstitution; therefore, LUPRON DEPOT should be mixed and used immediately.

AFTER INJECTION

9. Withdraw the needle. Immediately activate the LuproLoc® safety device by pushing the arrow forward

Information on the AbbVie, Inc. products listed on these pages is from the prescribing information in use as of July 31, 2013. For more information, please visit rxabbvie.com or call 1-800-633-9110.

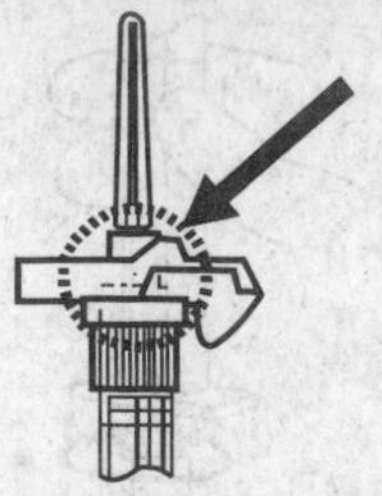

with the thumb or finger, as illustrated, until the device is fully extended and a CLICK is heard or felt.

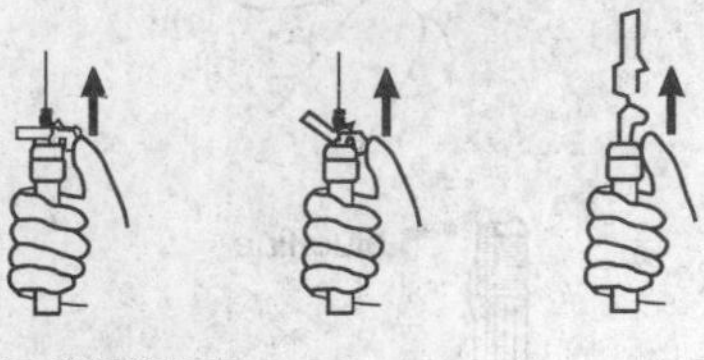

HOW SUPPLIED

Each LUPRON DEPOT 7.5 mg for 1-month administration kit (NDC 0074-3642-03) contains:

- one prefilled dual-chamber syringe containing needle with LuproLoc® safety device
- one plunger
- two alcohol swabs
- a complete prescribing information enclosure

The prefilled dual-chamber syringe contains sterile lyophilized microspheres of leuprolide acetate incorporated in a biodegradable lactic acid/glycolic acid copolymer. When mixed with 1 mL of accompanying diluent, LUPRON DEPOT 7.5 mg for 1-month administration is administered as a single monthly intramuscular injection.

Store at 25°C (77°F); excursions permitted to 15–30°C (59–86°F) [See USP Controlled Room Temperature]

REFERENCES

1. NIOSH Alert: Preventing occupational exposures to antineoplastic and other hazardous drugs in healthcare settings. 2004. U.S. Department of Health and Human Services, Public Health Service, Centers for Disease Control and Prevention, National Institute for Occupational Safety and Health, DHHS (NIOSH) Publication No. 2004-165.
2. OSHA Technical Manual, TED 1-0.15A, Section VI: Chapter 2. Controlling Occupational Exposure to Hazardous Drugs. OSHA, 1999. http://www.osha.gov/dts/osta/otm/otm_vi/otm_vi_2.html
3. American Society of Health-System Pharmacists. ASHP guidelines on handling hazardous drugs. Am J Health-Syst Pharm. 2006; 63; 1172-1193.
4. Polovich, M., White, J.M., & Kelleher, L.O. (eds.) 2005. Chemotherapy and biotherapy guidelines and recommendations for practice (2nd Ed.) Pittsburgh, PA: Oncology Nursing Society.

Manufactured for
AbbVie Inc.
North Chicago, IL 60064
by Takeda Pharmaceutical Company Limited
Osaka, Japan 540-8645
™ - Trademark
® - Registered Trademark
(No. 3642)
03-A852 July, 2013

Shown in Product Identification Guide, page 303

LUPRON DEPOT® -3 MONTH 11.25 MG ℞

[lew-prŏn]
(leuprolide acetate for depot suspension)
3-MONTH FORMULATION

Rx only

This is combined labeling. Examples of different fonts appear below.

- General information
- Information on endometriosis
- Information on uterine fibroids

DESCRIPTION

Leuprolide acetate is a synthetic nonapeptide analog of naturally occurring gonadotropin-releasing hormone (GnRH or LH-RH). The analog possesses greater potency than the natural hormone. The chemical name is 5-oxo-L-prolyl-L-histidyl-L-tryptophyl-L-seryl-L-tyrosyl-D-leucyl-L-leucyl-L-arginyl-N-ethyl-L-prolinamide acetate (salt) with the following structural formula:

[See chemical structure at top of page]

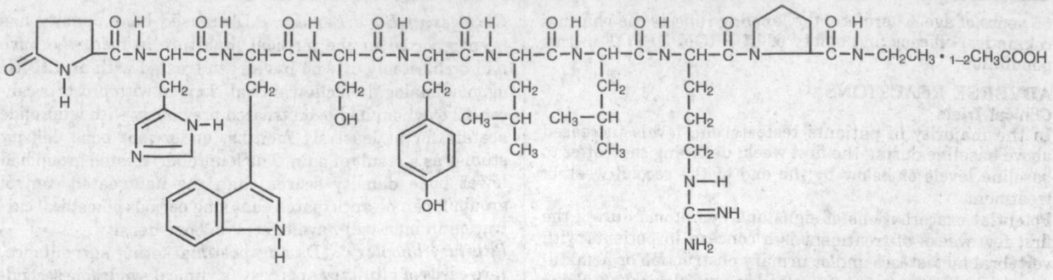

LUPRON DEPOT–3 Month 11.25 mg is available in a prefilled dual-chamber syringe containing sterile lyophilized microspheres which, when mixed with diluent, become a suspension intended as an intramuscular injection to be given **ONCE EVERY THREE MONTHS.**

The front chamber of LUPRON DEPOT–3 Month 11.25 mg prefilled dual-chamber syringe contains leuprolide acetate (11.25 mg), polylactic acid (99.3 mg) and D-mannitol (19.45 mg). The second chamber of diluent contains carboxymethylcellulose sodium (7.5 mg), D-mannitol (75.0 mg), polysorbate 80 (1.5 mg), water for injection, USP, and glacial acetic acid, USP to control pH.

During the manufacture of LUPRON DEPOT–3 Month 11.25 mg, acetic acid is lost, leaving the peptide.

CLINICAL PHARMACOLOGY

Leuprolide acetate is a long-acting GnRH analog. A single injection of LUPRON DEPOT–3 Month 11.25 mg will result in an initial stimulation followed by a prolonged suppression of pituitary gonadotropins. Repeated dosing at quarterly (LUPRON DEPOT–3 Month 11.25 mg) intervals results in decreased secretion of gonadal steroids; consequently, tissues and functions that depend on gonadal steroids for their maintenance become quiescent. This effect is reversible on discontinuation of drug therapy.

Leuprolide acetate is not active when given orally.

Pharmacokinetics

Absorption

Following a single injection of the three month formulation of LUPRON DEPOT–3 Month 11.25 mg in female subjects, a mean plasma leuprolide concentration of 36.3 ng/mL was observed at 4 hours. Leuprolide appeared to be released at a constant rate following the onset of steady-state levels during the third week after dosing and mean levels then declined gradually to near the lower limit of detection by 12 weeks. The mean (± standard deviation) leuprolide concentration from 3 to 12 weeks was 0.23 ± 0.09 ng/mL. However, intact leuprolide and an inactive major metabolite could not be distinguished by the assay which was employed in the study. The initial burst, followed by the rapid decline to a steady-state level, was similar to the release pattern seen with the monthly formulation.

Distribution

The mean steady-state volume of distribution of leuprolide following intravenous bolus administration to healthy male volunteers was 27 L. *In vitro* binding to human plasma proteins ranged from 43% to 49%.

Metabolism

In healthy male volunteers, a 1 mg bolus of leuprolide administered intravenously revealed that the mean systemic clearance was 7.6 L/h, with a terminal elimination half-life of approximately 3 hours based on a two compartment model.

In rats and dogs, administration of ^{14}C-labeled leuprolide was shown to be metabolized to smaller inactive peptides, a pentapeptide (Metabolite I), tripeptides (Metabolites II and III) and a dipeptide (Metabolite IV). These fragments may be further catabolized.

In a pharmacokinetic/pharmacodynamic study of endometriosis patients, intramuscular 11.25 mg LUPRON DEPOT (n=19) every 12 weeks or intramuscular 3.75 mg LUPRON DEPOT (n=15) every 4 weeks was administered for 24 weeks. There was no statistically significant difference in changes of serum estradiol concentration from baseline between the 2 treatment groups.

M-I plasma concentrations measured in 5 prostate cancer patients reached maximum concentration 2 to 6 hours after dosing and were approximately 6% of the peak parent drug concentration. One week after dosing, mean plasma M-I concentrations were approximately 20% of mean leuprolide concentrations.

Excretion

Following administration of LUPRON DEPOT 3.75 mg to 3 patients, less than 5% of the dose was recovered as parent and M-I metabolite in the urine.

Special Populations

The pharmacokinetics of the drug in hepatically and renally impaired patients have not been determined.

Drug Interactions

No pharmacokinetic-based drug-drug interaction studies have been conducted with LUPRON DEPOT. However, because leuprolide acetate is a peptide that is primarily degraded by peptidase and not by cytochrome P-450 enzymes as noted in specific studies, and the drug is only about 46% bound to plasma proteins, drug interactions would not be expected to occur.

CLINICAL STUDIES

In a pharmacokinetic/pharmacodynamic study of healthy female subjects (N=20), the onset of estradiol suppression was observed for individual subjects between day 4 and week 4 after dosing. By the third week following the injection, the mean estradiol concentration (8 pg/mL) was in the menopausal range. Throughout the remainder of the dosing period, mean serum estradiol levels ranged from the menopausal to the early follicular range.

Serum estradiol was suppressed to ≤20 pg/mL in all subjects within four weeks and remained suppressed (≤40 pg/mL) in 80% of subjects until the end of the 12-week dosing interval, at which time two of these subjects had a value between 40 and 50 pg/mL. Four additional subjects had at least two consecutive elevations of estradiol (range 43-240 pg/mL) levels during the 12-week dosing interval, but there was no indication of luteal function for any of the subjects during this period.

LUPRON DEPOT–3 Month 11.25 mg induced amenorrhea in 85% (N=17) of subjects during the initial month and 100% during the second month following the injection. All subjects remained amenorrheic through the remainder of the 12-week dosing interval. Episodes of light bleeding and spotting were reported by a majority of subjects during the first month after the injection and in a few subjects at later time-points. Menses resumed on average 12 weeks (range 2.9 to 20.4 weeks) following the end of the 12-week dosing interval.

LUPRON DEPOT–3 Month 11.25 mg produced similar pharmacodynamic effects in terms of hormonal and menstrual suppression to those achieved with monthly injections of LUPRON DEPOT 3.75 mg during the controlled clinical trials for the management of endometriosis and the anemia caused by uterine fibroids.

Endometriosis

In a Phase IV pharmacokinetic/pharmacodynamic study of patients, LUPRON DEPOT–3 Month 11.25 mg (N=21) was shown to be comparable to monthly LUPRON DEPOT 3.75 mg (N=20) in relieving the clinical signs/symptoms of endometriosis (dysmenorrhea, non-menstrual pelvic pain, pelvic tenderness and pelvic induration). In both treatment groups, suppression of menses was achieved in 100% of the patients who remained in the study for at least 60 days. Suppression is defined as no new menses for at least 60 consecutive days.

In controlled clinical studies, LUPRON DEPOT 3.75 mg monthly for six months was shown to be comparable to danazol 800 mg/day in relieving the clinical sign/symptoms of endometriosis (pelvic pain, dysmenorrhea, dyspareunia, pelvic tenderness, and induration) and in reducing the size of endometrial implants as evidenced by laparoscopy.

The clinical significance of a decrease in endometriotic lesions is not known at this time, and in addition laparoscopic staging of endometriosis does not necessarily correlate with the severity of symptoms.

LUPRON DEPOT 3.75 mg monthly induced amenorrhea in 74% and 98% of the patients after the first and second treatment months respectively. Most of the remaining patients reported episodes of only light bleeding or spotting. In the first, second and third post-treatment months, normal menstrual cycles resumed in 7%, 71% and 95% of patients, respectively, excluding those who became pregnant.

Figure 1 illustrates the percent of patients with symptoms at baseline, final treatment visit and sustained relief at 6 and 12 months following discontinuation of treatment for the various symptoms evaluated during the two controlled clinical studies. A total of 166 patients received LUPRON DEPOT 3.75 mg. Seventy-five percent (N=125) of these elected to participate in the follow-up period. Of these patients, 36% and 24% are included in the 6 month and 12 month follow-up analysis, respectively. All the patients who had a

FIGURE 1 – PERCENT OF PATIENTS WITH SIGN/SYMPTOMS OF ENDOMETRIOSIS AT BASELINE, FINAL TREATMENT VISIT, AND AFTER 6 AND 12 MONTHS OF FOLLOW-UP

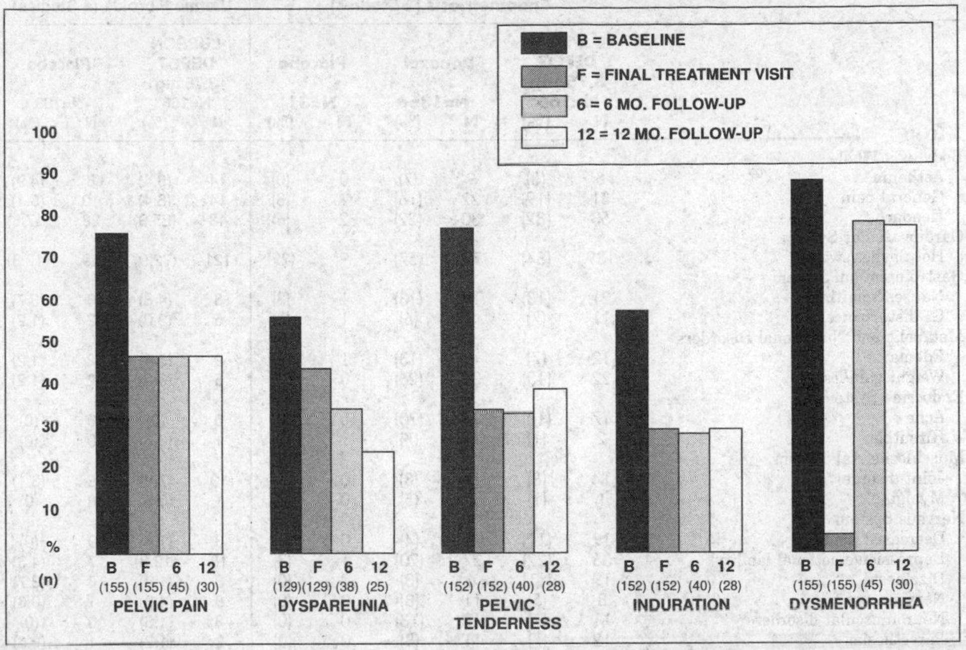

Figure 2
Treatment Period Mean Pain Scores For LD/N* Patients

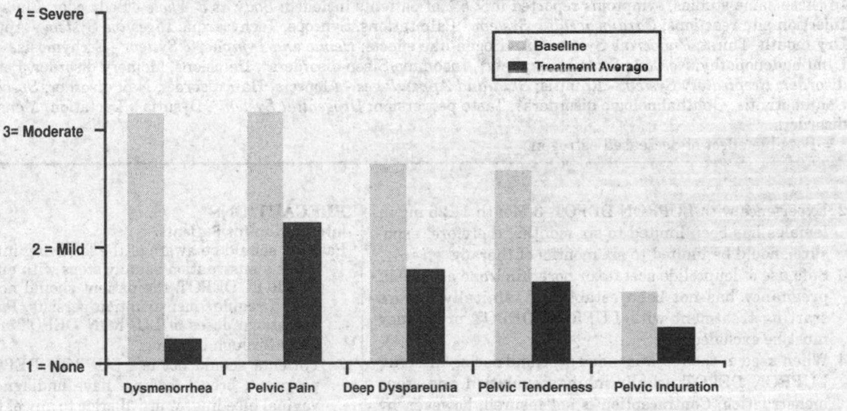

* LD/N = LUPRON DEPOT 3.75 mg plus norethindrone acetate 5 mg daily

pain evaluation at baseline and at a minimum of one treatment visit, are included in the Baseline (B) and final treatment visit (F) analysis.

[See figure 1 above]

Hormonal add-back therapy

Two clinical studies with a treatment duration of 12 months indicate that concurrent hormonal therapy (norethindrone acetate 5 mg daily) is effective in significantly reducing the loss of bone mineral density associated with LUPRON, without compromising the efficacy of LUPRON in relieving symptoms of endometriosis. (All patients in these studies received calcium supplementation with 1000 mg elemental calcium). One controlled, randomized and double-blind study included 51 women treated with LUPRON DEPOT 3.75 mg alone and 55 women treated with LUPRON DEPOT 3.75 mg plus norethindrone acetate 5 mg (LD/N) daily. The second study was an open label study in which 136 women were treated with monthly LUPRON DEPOT 3.75 mg plus norethindrone acetate 5 mg daily. This study confirmed the reduction in loss of bone mineral density that was observed in the controlled study. Suppression of menses was maintained throughout treatment in 84% and 73% of patients receiving LD/N, in the controlled study and open label study, respectively. The median time for menses resumption after treatment with LD/N was 8 weeks.

Figure 2 Illustrates the mean pain scores for the LD/N group from the controlled study.

[See figure 2 above]

Uterine Leiomyomata (Fibroids)

LUPRON DEPOT 3.75 mg for a period of three to six months was studied in four controlled clinical trials.

In one of these clinical studies, enrollment was based on hematocrit ≤ 30% and/or hemoglobin ≤ 10.2 g/dL. Administration of LUPRON DEPOT 3.75 mg, concomitantly with iron, produced an increase of ≥ 6% hematocrit and ≥ 2 g/dL hemoglobin in 77% of patients at three months of therapy. The mean change in hematocrit was 10.1% and the mean change in hemoglobin was 4.2 g/dL. Clinical response was judged to be a hematocrit of ≥ 36% and hemoglobin of ≥ 12 g/dL, thus allowing for autologous blood donation prior to surgery. At two and three months respectively, 71% and 75% of patients met this criterion (Table 1). These data suggest however, that some patients may benefit from iron alone or 1 to 2 months of LUPRON DEPOT 3.75 mg.

Table 1 PERCENT OF PATIENTS ACHIEVING HEMATOCRIT ≥ 36% AND HEMOGLOBIN ≥ 12 GM/DL

Treatment Group	Week 4	Week 8	Week 12
LUPRON DEPOT 3.75 mg with Iron (N=104)	40*	71†	75*
Iron Alone (N=98)	17	39	49

* P-Value < 0.01
† P-Value < 0.001

Excessive vaginal bleeding (menorrhagia or menometrorrhagia) decreased in 80% of patients at three months. Episodes of spotting and menstrual-like bleeding were noted in 16% of patients at final visit.

In this same study, a decrease of ≥ 25% was seen in uterine and myoma volumes in 60% and 54% of patients respectively. The mean fibroid diameter was 6.3 cm at pretreatment and decreased to 5.6 cm at the end of treatment. LUPRON DEPOT 3.75 mg was found to relieve symptoms of bloating, pelvic pain, and pressure.

In three other controlled clinical trials, enrollment was not based on hematologic status. Mean uterine volume decreased by 41% and myoma volume decreased by 37% at final visit as evidenced by ultrasound or MRI. The mean fibroid diameter was 5.6 cm at pretreatment and decreased to 4.7 cm at the end of treatment. These patients also experienced a decrease in symptoms including excessive vaginal bleeding and pelvic discomfort. Ninety-five percent of these patients became amenorrheic with 61%, 25%, and 4% experiencing amenorrhea during the first, second, and third treatment months respectively.

In addition, posttreatment follow-up was carried out in one clinical trial for a small percentage of LUPRON DEPOT 3.75 mg patients (N=46) among the 77% who demonstrated a ≥ 25% decrease in uterine volume while on therapy. Menses usually returned within two months of cessation of therapy. Mean time to return to pretreatment uterine size was 8.3 months. Regrowth did not appear to be related to pretreatment uterine volume.

There is no evidence that pregnancy rates are enhanced or adversely affected by the use of LUPRON DEPOT.

INDICATIONS AND USAGE

Endometriosis

LUPRON DEPOT–3 Month 11.25 mg is indicated for management of endometriosis, including pain relief and reduction of endometriotic lesions. LUPRON DEPOT with norethindrone acetate 5 mg daily is also indicated for initial management of endometriosis and for management of recurrence of symptoms. (Refer also to norethindrone acetate prescribing information for **WARNINGS, PRECAUTIONS, CONTRAINDICATIONS** and **ADVERSE REACTIONS** associated with norethindrone acetate). Duration of initial treatment or retreatment should be limited to 6 months.

Uterine Leiomyomata (Fibroids)

LUPRON DEPOT–3 Month 11.25 mg concomitantly with iron therapy is indicated for the preoperative hematologic improvement of patients with anemia caused by uterine leiomyomata. The clinician may wish to consider a one-month trial period on iron alone inasmuch as some of the patients will respond to iron alone. (See **Table 1, CLINICAL STUDIES** section.) LUPRON may be added if the response to iron alone is considered inadequate. Recommended therapy is a single injection of LUPRON DEPOT–3 Month 11.25 mg. This dosage form is indicated only for women for whom three months of hormonal suppression is deemed necessary.

Experience with LUPRON DEPOT–3 Month 11.25 mg in females has been limited to women 18 years of age and older treated for no more than 6 months.

CONTRAINDICATIONS

1. Hypersensitivity to GnRH, GnRH agonist analogs or any of the excipients in LUPRON DEPOT.
2. Undiagnosed abnormal vaginal bleeding.
3. LUPRON DEPOT is contraindicated in women who are or may become pregnant while receiving the drug. LUPRON DEPOT may cause fetal harm when administered to a pregnant woman. Major fetal abnormalities were observed in rabbits but not in rats after administration of LUPRON DEPOT throughout gestation. There was increased fetal mortality and decreased fetal weights in rats and rabbits. (See **Pregnancy** section.) The effects on fetal mortality are expected consequences of the alterations in hormonal levels brought about by the drug. If this drug is used during pregnancy or if the patient becomes pregnant while taking this drug, the patient should be apprised of the potential hazard to the fetus.
4. Use in women who are breast-feeding. (See **Nursing Mothers** section.)
5. Norethindrone acetate is contraindicated in women with the following conditions:
   - Thrombophlebitis, thromboembolic disorders, cerebral apoplexy, or a past history of these conditions
   - Markedly impaired liver function or liver disease
   - Known or suspected carcinoma of the breast

WARNINGS

1. As the effects of LUPRON DEPOT–3 Month 11.25 mg are present throughout the course of therapy, the drug should only be used in patients who require hormonal suppression for at least three months.

Information on the AbbVie, Inc. products listed on these pages is from the prescribing information in use as of July 31, 2013. For more information, please visit rxabbvie.com or call 1-800-633-9110.

Table 2 ADVERSE EVENTS REPORTED TO BE CAUSALLY RELATED TO DRUG IN ≥ 5% OF PATIENTS

	Endometriosis (2 Studies)						Uterine Fibroids (4 Studies)			
	LUPRON DEPOT 3.75 mg N=166		Danazol N=136		Placebo N=31		LUPRON DEPOT 3.75 mg N=166		Placebo N=163	
	N	(%)	N	(%)	N	(%)	N	(%)	N	(%)
Body as a Whole										
Asthenia	5	(3)	9	(7)	0	(0)	14	(8.4)	8	(4.9)
General pain	31	(19)	22	(16)	1	(3)	14	(8.4)	10	(6.1)
Headache*	53	(32)	30	(22)	2	(6)	43	(25.9)	29	(17.8)
Cardiovascular System										
Hot flashes/sweats*	139	(84)	77	(57)	9	(29)	121	(72.9)	29	(17.8)
Gastrointestinal System										
Nausea/vomiting	21	(13)	17	(13)	1	(3)	8	(4.8)	6	(3.7)
GI disturbances*	11	(7)	8	(6)	1	(3)	5	(3.0)	2	(1.2)
Metabolic and Nutritional Disorders										
Edema	12	(7)	17	(13)	1	(3)	9	(5.4)	2	(1.2)
Weight gain/loss	22	(13)	36	(26)	0	(0)	5	(3.0)	2	(1.2)
Endocrine System										
Acne	17	(10)	27	(20)	0	(0)	0	(0)	0	(0)
Hirsutism	2	(1)	9	(7)	1	(3)	1	(0.6)	0	(0)
Musculoskeletal System										
Joint disorder*	14	(8)	11	(8)	0	(0)	13	(7.8)	5	(3.1)
Myalgia*	1	(1)	7	(5)	0	(0)	1	(0.6)	0	(0)
Nervous System										
Decreased libido*	19	(11)	6	(4)	0	(0)	3	(1.8)	0	(0)
Depression/emotional lability*	36	(22)	27	(20)	1	(3)	18	(10.8)	7	(4.3)
Dizziness	19	(11)	4	(3)	0	(0)	3	(1.8)	6	(3.7)
Nervousness*	8	(5)	11	(8)	0	(0)	8	(4.8)	1	(0.6)
Neuromuscular disorders*	11	(7)	17	(13)	0	(0)	3	(1.8)	0	(0)
Paresthesias	12	(7)	11	(8)	0	(0)	2	(1.2)	1	(0.6)
Skin and Appendages										
Skin reactions	17	(10)	20	(15)	1	(3)	5	(3.0)	2	(1.2)
Urogenital System										
Breast changes/tenderness/pain*	10	(6)	12	(9)	0	(0)	3	(1.8)	7	(4.3)
Vaginitis*	46	(28)	23	(17)	0	(0)	19	(11.4)	3	(1.8)

In these same studies, symptoms reported in < 5% of patients included: *Body as a Whole* - Body odor, Flu syndrome, Injection site reactions; *Cardiovascular System* - Palpitations, Syncope, Tachycardia; *Digestive System* - Appetite changes, Dry mouth, Thirst; *Endocrine System* - Androgen-like effects; *Hemic and Lymphatic System* - Ecchymosis, Lymphadenopathy; *Nervous System* - Anxiety*, Insomnia/Sleep disorders*, Delusions, Memory disorder, Personality disorder; *Respiratory System* - Rhinitis; *Skin and Appendages* - Alopecia, Hair disorder, Nail disorder; *Special Senses* - Conjunctivitis, Ophthalmologic disorders*, Taste perversion; *Urogenital System* - Dysuria*, Lactation, Menstrual disorders.

* = Possible effect of decreased estrogen.

2. Experience with LUPRON DEPOT–3 Month 11.25 mg in females has been limited to six months; therefore, exposure should be limited to six months of therapy.
3. Safe use of leuprolide acetate or norethindrone acetate in pregnancy has not been established clinically. Before starting treatment with LUPRON DEPOT pregnancy must be excluded.
4. When used at the recommended dose and dosing interval, LUPRON DEPOT usually inhibits ovulation and stops menstruation. Contraception is not insured, however, by taking LUPRON DEPOT. Therefore, patients should use non-hormonal methods of contraception. Patients should be advised to see their physician if they believe they may be pregnant. If a patient becomes pregnant during treatment, the drug must be discontinued and the patient must be apprised of the potential risk to the fetus. (See **CONTRAINDICATIONS** section.)
5. During the early phase of therapy, sex steroids temporarily rise above baseline because of the physiologic effect of the drug. Therefore, an increase in clinical signs and symptoms may be observed during the initial days of therapy, but these will dissipate with continued therapy.
6. Symptoms consistent with an anaphylactoid or asthmatic process have been rarely reported post-marketing.
7. The following applies to co-treatment with LUPRON and norethindrone acetate:

Norethindrone acetate treatment should be discontinued if there is a sudden partial or complete loss of vision or if there is sudden onset of proptosis, diplopia, or migraine. If examination reveals papilledema or retinal vascular lesions, medication should be withdrawn.

Because of the occasional occurrence of thrombophlebitis and pulmonary embolism in patients taking progestogens, the physician should be alert to the earliest manifestations of the disease in women taking norethindrone acetate.

Assessment and management of risk factors for cardiovascular disease is recommended prior to initiation of add-back therapy with norethindrone acetate. Norethindrone acetate should be used with caution in women with risk factors, including lipid abnormalities or cigarette smoking.

PRECAUTIONS

Information for Patients

Patients should be aware of the following information:

1. Since menstruation usually stops with effective doses of LUPRON DEPOT, the patient should notify her physician if regular menstruation persists. Patients missing successive doses of LUPRON DEPOT may experience breakthrough bleeding.
2. Patients should not use LUPRON DEPOT if they are pregnant, breast feeding, have undiagnosed abnormal vaginal bleeding, or are allergic to any of the ingredients in LUPRON DEPOT.
3. LUPRON DEPOT is contraindicated for use during pregnancy. Therefore, a non-hormonal method of contraception should be used during treatment. Patients should be advised that if they miss successive doses of LUPRON DEPOT, breakthrough bleeding or ovulation may occur with the potential for conception. If a patient becomes pregnant during treatment, she should discontinue treatment and consult her physician.
4. Adverse events occurring in clinical studies with LUPRON DEPOT that are associated with hypoestrogenism include: hot flashes, headaches, emotional lability, decreased libido, acne, myalgia, reduction in breast size, and vaginal dryness. Estrogen levels returned to normal after treatment was discontinued.
5. Patients should be counseled on the possibility of the development or worsening of depression and the occurrence of memory disorders.
6. The induced hypoestrogenic state **also** results in a loss in bone density over the course of treatment, some of which may not be reversible. Clinical studies show that concurrent hormonal therapy with norethindrone acetate 5 mg daily is effective in reducing loss of bone mineral density that occurs with LUPRON. (All patients received calcium supplementation with 1000 mg elemental calcium.) (See ***Changes in Bone Density*** section).
7. If the symptoms of endometriosis recur after a course of therapy, retreatment with a six-month course of LUPRON DEPOT and norethindrone acetate 5 mg daily may be considered. Retreatment beyond this one six-month course cannot be recommended. It is recommended that bone density be assessed before retreatment begins to ensure that values are within normal limits. Retreatment with LUPRON DEPOT alone is not recommended.
8. In patients with major risk factors for decreased bone mineral content such as chronic alcohol and/or tobacco use, strong family history of osteoporosis, or chronic use of drugs that can reduce bone mass such as anticonvulsants or corticosteroids, LUPRON DEPOT therapy may pose an additional risk. In these patients, the risks and benefits must be weighed carefully before therapy with LUPRON DEPOT alone is instituted, and concomitant treatment with norethindrone acetate 5 mg daily should be considered. Retreatment with gonadotropin-releasing hormone analogs, including LUPRON is not advisable in patients with major risk factors for loss of bone mineral content.
9. Because norethindrone acetate may cause some degree of fluid retention, conditions which might be influenced by this factor, such as epilepsy, migraine, asthma, cardiac or renal dysfunctions require careful observation during norethindrone acetate add-back therapy.
10. Patients who have a history of depression should be carefully observed during treatment with norethindrone acetate and norethindrone acetate should be discontinued if severe depression occurs.

Laboratory Tests

See **ADVERSE REACTIONS** section.

Drug Interactions

See **CLINICAL PHARMACOLOGY, Pharmacokinetics.**

Drug/Laboratory Test Interactions

Administration of LUPRON DEPOT in therapeutic doses results in suppression of the pituitary-gonadal system. Normal function is usually restored within three months after treatment is discontinued. Therefore, diagnostic tests of pituitary gonadotropic and gonadal functions conducted during treatment and for up to three months after discontinuation of LUPRON DEPOT may be misleading.

Carcinogenesis, Mutagenesis, Impairment of Fertility

A two-year carcinogenicity study was conducted in rats and mice. In rats, a dose-related increase of benign pituitary hyperplasia and benign pituitary adenomas was noted at 24 months when the drug was administered subcutaneously at high daily doses (0.6 to 4 mg/kg). There was a significant but not dose-related increase of pancreatic islet-cell adenomas in females and of testicular interstitial cell adenomas in males (highest incidence in the low dose group). In mice, no leuprolide acetate-induced tumors or pituitary abnormalities were observed at a dose as high as 60 mg/kg for two years. Patients have been treated with leuprolide acetate for up to three years with doses as high as 10 mg/day and for two years with doses as high as 20 mg/day without demonstrable pituitary abnormalities.

Mutagenicity studies have been performed with leuprolide acetate using bacterial and mammalian systems. These studies provided no evidence of a mutagenic potential.

Clinical and pharmacologic studies in adults (> 18 years) with leuprolide acetate and similar analogs have shown reversibility of fertility suppression when the drug is discontinued after continuous administration for periods of up to 24 weeks. Although no clinical studies have been completed in children to assess the full reversibility of fertility suppression, animal studies (prepubertal and adult rats and monkeys) with leuprolide acetate and other GnRH analogs have shown functional recovery.

Pregnancy

Teratogenic Effects

Pregnancy Category X (See **CONTRAINDICATIONS** section). When administered on day 6 of pregnancy at test dosages of 0.00024, 0.0024, and 0.024 mg/kg (1/300 to 1/3 of the human dose) to rabbits, LUPRON DEPOT produced a dose-related increase in major fetal abnormalities. Similar studies in rats failed to demonstrate an increase in fetal malformations. There was increased fetal mortality and decreased fetal weights with the two higher doses of LUPRON DEPOT in rabbits and with the highest dose (0.024 mg/kg) in rats.

Nursing Mothers

It is not known whether LUPRON DEPOT is excreted in human milk. Because many drugs are excreted in human milk, and because the effects of LUPRON DEPOT on lactation and/or the breast-fed child have not been determined, LUPRON DEPOT should not be used by nursing mothers.

Pediatric Use

Safety and effectiveness of LUPRON DEPOT–3 Month 11.25 mg have not been established in pediatric patients. Experience with LUPRON DEPOT for treatment of endometriosis has been limited to women 18 years of age and older. See LUPRON DEPOT-PED® (leuprolide acetate for depot suspension) labeling for the safety and effectiveness in children with central precocious puberty.

Geriatric Use

This product has not been studied in women over 65 years of age and is not indicated in this population.

ADVERSE REACTIONS

Clinical Trials

The **monthly formulation of LUPRON DEPOT 3.75 mg** was utilized in controlled clinical trials that studied the drug in 166 endometriosis and 166 uterine fibroids patients. Adverse events reported in ≥ 5% of patients in either of these populations and thought to be potentially related to drug are noted in the following table.

[See table 2 at top of previous page]

In one controlled clinical trial utilizing the monthly formulation of LUPRON DEPOT, patients diagnosed with uterine fibroids received a higher dose (7.5 mg) of LUPRON DEPOT. Events seen with this dose that were thought to be potentially related to drug and were not seen at the lower dose included glossitis, hypesthesia, lactation, pyelonephritis, and urinary disorders. Generally, a higher incidence of hypoestrogenic effects was observed at the higher dose.

In a pharmacokinetic trial involving 20 healthy female subjects receiving LUPRON DEPOT–3 Month 11.25 mg, a few adverse events were reported with this formulation that were not reported previously. These included face edema, agitation, laryngitis, and ear pain.

In a Phase IV study involving endometriosis patients receiving LUPRON DEPOT 3.75 mg (N=20) or LUPRON DEPOT–3 Month 11.25 mg (N=21), similar adverse events were reported by the two groups of patients. In general the safety profiles of the two formulations were comparable in this study.

Table 3 lists the potentially drug-related adverse events observed in at least 5% of patients in any treatment group, during the first 6 months of treatment in the add-back clinical studies, in which patients were treated with monthly LUPRON DEPOT 3.75 mg with or without norethindrone acetate co-treatment.

[See table 3 above]

In the controlled clinical trial, 50 of 51 (98%) patients in the LD group (LUPRON DEPOT 3.75 mg) and 48 of 55 (87%) patients in the LD/N group (LUPRON DEPOT 3.75 mg plus norethindrone acetate 5 mg daily) reported experiencing hot flashes on one or more occasions during treatment. During Month 6 of treatment, 32 of 37 (86%) patients in the LD group and 22 of 38 (58%) patients in the LD/N group reported having experienced hot flashes. The mean number of days on which hot flashes were reported during this month of treatment was 19 and 7 in the LD and LD/N treatment groups, respectively. The mean maximum number of hot flashes in a day during this month of treatment was 5.8 and 1.9 in the LD and LD/N treatment groups, respectively.

Changes in Bone Density

In controlled clinical studies, patients with endometriosis (six months of therapy) or uterine fibroids (three months of therapy) were treated with LUPRON DEPOT 3.75 mg. In endometriosis patients, vertebral bone density as measured by dual energy x-ray absorptiometry (DEXA) decreased by an average of 3.2% at six months compared with the pretreatment value. Clinical studies demonstrate that concurrent hormonal therapy (norethindrone acetate 5 mg daily) and calcium supplementation is effective in significantly reducing the loss of bone mineral density that occurs with LUPRON treatment, without compromising the efficacy of LUPRON in relieving symptoms of endometriosis. LUPRON DEPOT 3.75 mg plus norethindrone acetate 5 mg daily was evaluated in two clinical trials. The results from this regimen were similar in both studies. LUPRON DEPOT 3.75 mg was used as a control group in one study. The bone mineral density data of the lumbar spine from these two studies are presented in Table 4.

[See table 4 above]

In the Phase IV, six-month pharmacokinetic/pharmacodynamic study in endometriosis patients who were treated with LUPRON DEPOT 3.75 mg or LUPRON DEPOT–3 Month 11.25 mg, vertebral bone density measured by DEXA decreased compared with baseline by an average of 3.0% and 2.8% at six months for the two groups, respectively.

When LUPRON DEPOT 3.75 mg was administered for three months in uterine fibroid patients, vertebral trabecular bone mineral density as assessed by quantitative digital radiography (QDR) revealed a mean decrease of 2.7% compared with baseline. Six months after discontinuation of therapy, a trend toward recovery was observed. Use of LUPRON DEPOT for longer than three months (uterine fibroids) or six months (endometriosis) or in the presence of other known risk factors for decreased bone mineral content may cause additional bone loss **and is not recommended.**

Changes in Laboratory Values During Treatment

Liver Enzymes

Three percent of uterine fibroid patients treated with LUPRON DEPOT 3.75 mg, manifested posttreatment transaminase values that were at least twice the baseline value and above the upper limit of the normal range. None of the laboratory increases were associated with clinical symptoms.

In two other clinical trials, 6 of 191 patients receiving LUPRON DEPOT 3.75 mg plus norethindrone acetate 5 mg daily for up to 12 months developed an elevated (at least twice the upper limit of normal) SGPT or GGT. Five of the 6 increases were observed beyond 6 months of treatment. None were associated with an elevated bilirubin concentration.

Lipids

Triglycerides were increased above the upper limit of normal in 12% of the endometriosis patients who received LUPRON DEPOT 3.75 mg and in 32% of the subjects receiving LUPRON DEPOT–3 Month 11.25 mg.

Of those endometriosis and uterine fibroid patients whose pretreatment cholesterol values were in the normal range, mean change following therapy was +16 mg/dL to +17 mg/dL in endometriosis patients and +11 mg/dL to +29 mg/dL in uterine fibroid patients. In the endometriosis treated patients, increases from the pretreatment values were statistically significant ($p<0.03$). There was essentially no increase in the LDL/HDL ratio in patients from either population receiving LUPRON DEPOT 3.75 mg.

In two other clinical trials, LUPRON DEPOT 3.75 mg plus norethindrone acetate 5 mg daily were evaluated for 12 months of treatment. LUPRON DEPOT 3.75 mg was used as a control group in one study. Percent changes from baseline for serum lipids and percentages of patients with serum lipid values outside of the normal range in the two studies are summarized in the tables below.

[See table 5 at top of next page]

Changes from baseline tended to be greater at Week 52. After treatment, mean serum lipid levels from patients with follow up data returned to pretreatment values.

[See table 6 at top of next page]

Low HDL-cholesterol (<40 mg/dL) and elevated LDL-cholesterol (>160 mg/dL) are recognized risk factors for cardiovascular disease. The long-term significance of the observed treatment-related changes in serum lipids in women with endometriosis is unknown. Therefore assessment of cardiovascular risk factors should be considered prior to initiation of concurrent treatment with LUPRON and norethindrone acetate.

Chemistry

Slight to moderate mean increases were noted for glucose, uric acid, BUN, creatinine, total protein, albumin, bilirubin, alkaline phosphatase, LDH, calcium, and phosphorus. None of these increases were clinically significant. In the hormonal add-back studies LUPRON DEPOT in combination with norethindrone acetate was associated with elevations of GGT and SGPT in 6% to 7% of patients.

Postmarketing

The following adverse reactions have been identified during postapproval use of LUPRON DEPOT. Because these reactions are reported voluntarily from a population of uncertain size, it is not always possible to reliably estimate their frequency or establish a causal relationship to drug exposure.

During postmarketing surveillance with other dosage forms and in the same and/or different populations, the following adverse events were reported. Like other drugs in this class,

Table 3 TREATMENT-RELATED ADVERSE EVENTS OCCURRING IN ≥ 5% OF PATIENTS

	Controlled Study				Open Label Study	
	LD - Only* N=51		LD/N† N=55		LD/N† N=136	
Adverse Events	**N**	**(%)**	**N**	**(%)**	**N**	**(%)**
Any Adverse Event	50	(98)	53	(96)	126	(93)
Body as a Whole						
Asthenia	9	(18)	10	(18)	15	(11)
Headache/Migraine	33	(65)	28	(51)	63	(46)
Injection Site Reaction	1	(2)	5	(9)	4	(3)
Pain	12	(24)	16	(29)	29	(21)
Cardiovascular System						
Hot flashes/Sweats	50	(98)	48	(87)	78	(57)
Digestive System						
Altered Bowel Function	7	(14)	8	(15)	14	(10)
Changes in Appetite	2	(4)	0	(0)	8	(6)
GI Disturbance	2	(4)	4	(7)	6	(4)
Nausea/Vomiting	13	(25)	16	(29)	17	(13)
Metabolic and Nutritional Disorders						
Edema	0	(0)	5	(9)	9	(7)
Weight Changes	6	(12)	7	(13)	6	(4)
Nervous System						
Anxiety	3	(6)	0	(0)	11	(8)
Depression/Emotional Lability	16	(31)	15	(27)	46	(34)
Dizziness/Vertigo	8	(16)	6	(11)	10	(7)
Insomnia/Sleep Disorder	16	(31)	7	(13)	20	(15)
Libido Changes	5	(10)	2	(4)	10	(7)
Memory Disorder	3	(6)	1	(2)	6	(4)
Nervousness	4	(8)	2	(4)	15	(11)
Neuromuscular Disorder	1	(2)	5	(9)	4	(3)
Skin and Appendages						
Alopecia	0	(0)	5	(9)	4	(3)
Androgen-Like Effects	2	(4)	3	(5)	24	(18)
Skin/Mucous Membrane Reaction	2	(4)	5	(9)	15	(11)
Urogenital System						
Breast Changes/Pain/Tenderness	3	(6)	7	(13)	11	(8)
Menstrual Disorders	1	(2)	0	(0)	7	(5)
Vaginitis	10	(20)	8	(15)	11	(8)

* LD-Only = LUPRON DEPOT 3.75 mg

† LD/N = LUPRON DEPOT 3.75 mg plus norethindrone acetate 5 mg

Table 4 MEAN PERCENT CHANGE FROM BASELINE IN BONE MINERAL DENSITY OF LUMBAR SPINE

	LUPRON DEPOT 3.75 mg		LUPRON DEPOT 3.75 mg plus norethindrone acetate 5 mg daily			
	Controlled Study		Controlled Study		Open Label Study	
	N	**Change (Mean, 95% CI)#**	**N**	**Change (Mean, 95% CI)#**	**N**	**Change (Mean, 95% CI)#**
Week 24*	41	-3.2% (-3.8, -2.6)	42	-0.3% (-0.8, 0.3)	115	-0.2% (-0.6, 0.2)
Week 52†	29	-6.3% (-7.1, -5.4)	32	-1.0% (-1.9, -0.1)	84	-1.1% (-1.6, -0.5)

* Includes on-treatment measurements that fell within 2-252 days after the first day of treatment.

† Includes on-treatment measurements >252 days after the first day of treatment.

\# 95% CI: 95% Confidence Interval

Information on the AbbVie, Inc. products listed on these pages is from the prescribing information in use as of July 31, 2013. For more information, please visit rxabbvie.com or call 1-800-633-9110.

Table 5 SERUM LIPIDS: MEAN PERCENT CHANGES FROM BASELINE VALUES AT TREATMENT WEEK 24

	LUPRON DEPOT 3.75 mg		LUPRON DEPOT 3.75 mg plus norethindrone acetate 5 mg daily			
	Controlled Study (n=39)		Controlled Study (n=41)		Open Label Study (n=117)	
	Baseline Value*	Wk 24 % Change	Baseline Value*	Wk 24 % Change	Baseline Value*	Wk 24 % Change
Total Cholesterol	170.5	9.2%	179.3	0.2%	181.2	2.8%
HDL Cholesterol	52.4	7.4%	51.8	-18.8%	51.0	-14.6%
LDL Cholesterol	96.6	10.9%	101.5	14.1%	109.1	13.1%
LDL/HDL Ratio	2.0†	5.0%	2.1†	43.4%	2.3†	39.4%
Triglycerides	107.8	17.5%	130.2	9.5%	105.4	13.8%

* mg/dL
† ratio

Table 6 PERCENTAGE OF PATIENTS WITH SERUM LIPID VALUES OUTSIDE OF THE NORMAL RANGE

	LUPRON DEPOT 3.75 mg		LUPRON DEPOT 3.75 mg plus norethindrone acetate 5 mg daily			
	Controlled Study (n=39)		Controlled Study (n=41)		Open Label Study (n=117)	
	Wk 0	Wk 24*	Wk 0	Wk 24*	Wk 0	Wk 24*
Total Cholesterol (>240 mg/dL)	15%	23%	15%	20%	6%	7%
HDL Cholesterol (<40 mg/dL)	15%	10%	15%	44%	15%	41%
LDL Cholesterol (>160 mg/dL)	0%	8%	5%	7%	9%	11%
LDL/HDL Ratio (>4.0)	0%	3%	2%	15%	7%	21%
Triglycerides (>200 mg/dL)	13%	13%	12%	10%	5%	9%

* Includes all patients regardless of baseline value.

mood swings, including depression, have been reported. There have been rare reports of suicidal ideation and attempt. Many, but not all, of these patients had a history of depression or other psychiatric illness. Patients should be counseled on the possibility of development or worsening of depression during treatment with LUPRON.

Symptoms consistent with an anaphylactoid or asthmatic process have been rarely reported. Rash, urticaria, and photosensitivity reactions have also been reported.

Localized reactions including induration and abscess have been reported at the site of injection.

Symptoms consistent with fibromyalgia (eg: joint and muscle pain, headaches, sleep disorders, gastrointestinal distress, and shortness of breath) have been reported individually and collectively.

Other events reported are:

Hepato-biliary disorder: Rarely reported serious liver injury

Injury, poisoning and procedural complications: Spinal fracture

Investigations: Decreased WBC

Musculoskeletal and Connective tissue disorder: Tenosynovitis-like symptoms

Nervous System Disorder: Convulsion, peripheral neuropathy, paralysis

Vascular Disorder: Hypotension

Cases of serious venous and arterial thromboembolism have been reported, including deep vein thrombosis, pulmonary embolism, myocardial infarction, stroke, and transient ischemic attack. Although a temporal relationship was reported in some cases, most cases were confounded by risk factors or concomitant medication use. It is unknown if there is a causal association between the use of GnRH analogs and these events.

Pituitary apoplexy

During post-marketing surveillance, rare cases of pituitary apoplexy (a clinical syndrome secondary to infarction of the pituitary gland) have been reported after the administration of gonadotropin-releasing hormone agonists. In a majority of these cases, a pituitary adenoma was diagnosed, with a majority of pituitary apoplexy cases occurring within 2 weeks of the first dose, and some within the first hour. In these cases, pituitary apoplexy has presented as sudden headache, vomiting, visual changes, ophthalmoplegia, altered mental status, and sometimes cardiovascular collapse. Immediate medical attention has been required.

See other LUPRON DEPOT and LUPRON Injection package inserts for other events reported in the same and different patient populations.

OVERDOSAGE

In clinical trials using daily subcutaneous leuprolide acetate in patients with prostate cancer, doses as high as 20 mg/day for up to two years caused no adverse effects differing from those observed with the 1 mg/day dose.

DOSAGE AND ADMINISTRATION

LUPRON DEPOT Must Be Administered Under the Supervision of a Physician.

Endometriosis

The recommended duration of treatment with LUPRON DEPOT–3 Month 11.25 mg alone or in combination with norethindrone acetate is six months. The choice of LUPRON DEPOT alone or LUPRON DEPOT plus norethindrone acetate therapy for initial management of the symptoms and signs of endometriosis should be made by the health care professional in consultation with the patient and should take into consideration the risks and benefits of the addition of norethindrone to LUPRON DEPOT alone.

If the symptoms of endometriosis recur after a course of therapy, retreatment with a six-month course of LUPRON DEPOT and norethindrone acetate 5 mg daily may be considered. Retreatment beyond this one six-month course cannot be recommended. It is recommended that bone density be assessed before retreatment begins to ensure that values are within normal limits. LUPRON DEPOT alone is not recommended for retreatment. If norethindrone acetate is contraindicated for the individual patient, then retreatment is not recommended.

An assessment of cardiovascular risk and management of risk factors such as cigarette smoking is recommended before beginning treatment with LUPRON DEPOT and norethindrone acetate.

Uterine Leiomyomata (Fibroids)

The recommended dose of LUPRON DEPOT–3 Month 11.25 mg is one injection. The symptoms associated with uterine leiomyomata will recur following discontinuation of therapy. If additional treatment with LUPRON DEPOT–3 Month 11.25 mg is contemplated, bone density should be assessed prior to initiation of therapy to ensure that values are within normal limits.

Due to different release characteristics, a fractional dose of the 3-month depot formulation is not equivalent to the same dose of the monthly formulation and should not be given.

For optimal performance of the prefilled dual chamber syringe (PDS), read and follow the following instructions:

Reconstitution and Administration Instructions

- The lyophilized microspheres are to be reconstituted and administered as a single intramuscular injection.
- Since LUPRON DEPOT does not contain a preservative, the suspension should be injected immediately or discarded if not used within two hours.
- As with other drugs administered by injection, the injection site should be varied periodically.

1. The LUPRON DEPOT powder should be visually inspected and the syringe should NOT BE USED if clumping or caking is evident. A thin layer of powder on the wall of the syringe is considered normal prior to mixing with the diluent. The diluent should appear clear.
2. To prepare for injection, screw the white plunger into the end stopper until the stopper begins to turn.

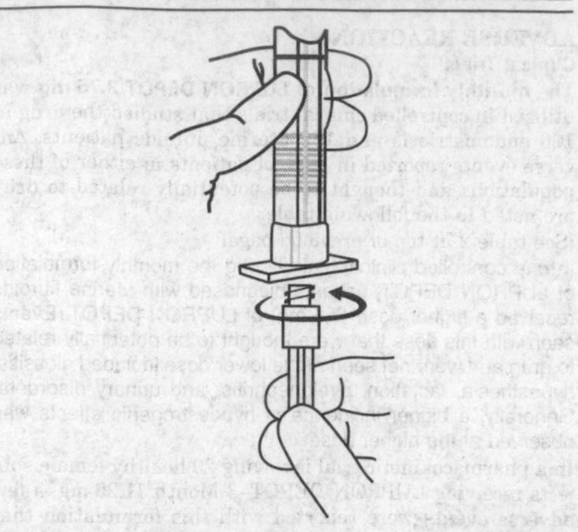

3. Hold the syringe UPRIGHT. Release the diluent by SLOWLY PUSHING (6 to 8 seconds) the plunger until the first stopper is at the blue line in the middle of the barrel.

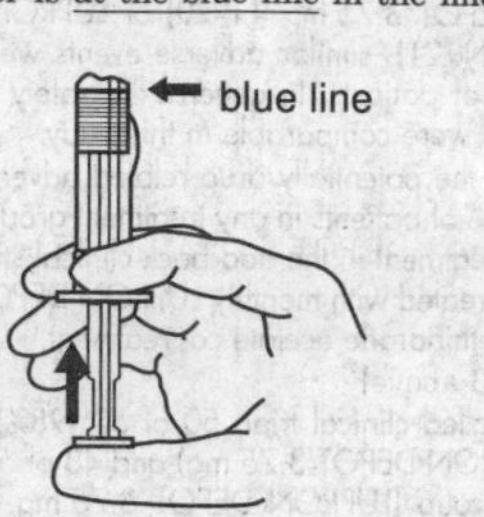

4. Keep the syringe UPRIGHT. Mix the microspheres (powder) thoroughly by gently shaking the syringe until the powder forms a uniform suspension. The suspension will appear milky. If the powder adheres to the stopper or caking/clumping is present, tap the syringe with your finger to disperse. DO NOT USE if any of the powder has not gone into suspension.

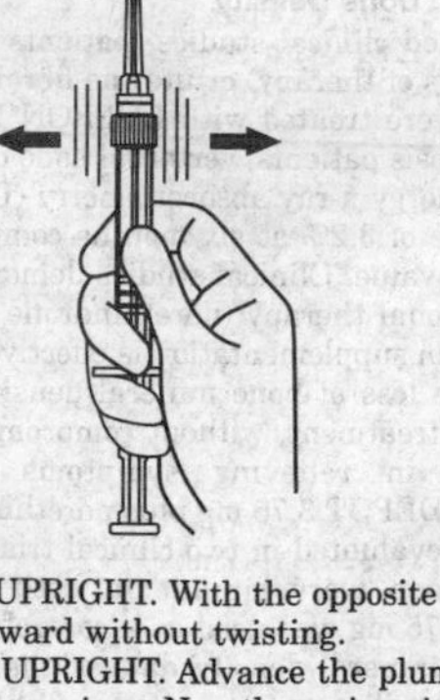

5. Hold the syringe UPRIGHT. With the opposite hand pull the needle cap upward without twisting.
6. Keep the syringe UPRIGHT. Advance the plunger to expel the air from the syringe. Now the syringe is ready for injection.
7. After cleaning the injection site with an alcohol swab, the intramuscular injection should be performed by inserting the needle at a 90 degree angle into the gluteal area, anterior thigh, or deltoid; injection sites should be alternated.

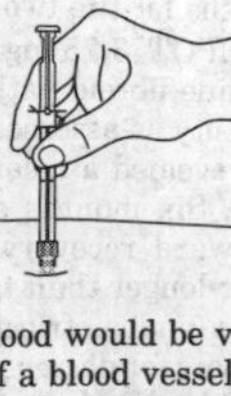

NOTE: Aspirated blood would be visible just below the luer lock connection if a blood vessel is accidentally penetrated. If present, blood can be seen through the transparent LuproLoc® safety device. If blood is present remove the needle immediately. Do not inject the medication.

[See figure at top of next column]

8. Inject the entire contents of the syringe intramuscularly at the time of reconstitution. The suspension settles very quickly following reconstitution; therefore, LUPRON DEPOT should be mixed and used immediately.

AFTER INJECTION

9. Withdraw the needle. Once the syringe has been withdrawn, activate immediately the LuproLoc® safety device by pushing the arrow on the lock upward towards the

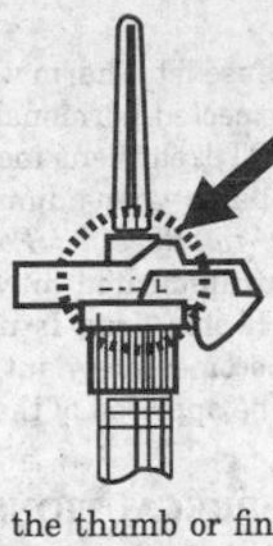

needle tip with the thumb or finger, as illustrated, until the needle cover of the safety device over the needle is fully extended and a CLICK is heard or felt.

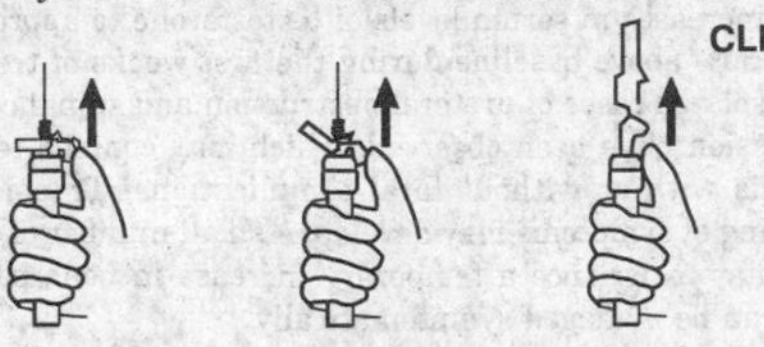

ADDITIONAL INFORMATION

- Dispose of the syringe according to local regulations/procedures.

HOW SUPPLIED

Each LUPRON DEPOT – 3 Month 11.25 mg kit (NDC 0074-3663-03) contains:

- one prefilled dual-chamber syringe
- one plunger
- two alcohol swabs
- a complete prescribing information enclosure

Each syringe contains sterile lyophilized microspheres which are leuprolide acetate incorporated in a biodegradable polymer of polylactic acid. When mixed with 1.5 mL of the diluent, LUPRON DEPOT–3 Month 11.25 mg is administered as a single IM injection **EVERY THREE MONTHS.**

Store at 25°C (77°F); excursions permitted to 15-30°C (59-86°F) [See USP Controlled Room Temperature]

REFERENCES

1. NIOSH Alert: Preventing occupational exposures to antineoplastic and other hazardous drugs in healthcare settings. 2004. U.S. Department of Health and Human Services, Public Health Service, Centers for Disease Control and Prevention, National Institute for Occupational Safety and Health, DHHS (NIOSH) Publication No. 2004-165.
2. OSHA Technical Manual, TED 1-0.15A, Section VI: Chapter 2. Controlling Occupational Exposure to Hazardous Drugs. OSHA, 1999. http://www.osha.gov/dts/osta/otm/otm_vi/otm_vi_2.html
3. American Society of Health-System Pharmacists. ASHP guidelines on handling hazardous drugs. *Am J Health-Syst Pharm.* 2006; 63; 1172-1193.
4. Polovich, M., White, J.M., & Kelleher, L.O. (eds.) 2005. Chemotherapy and biotherapy guidelines and recommendations for practice (2nd. Ed.) Pittsburgh, PA: Oncology Nursing Society.

Manufactured for
AbbVie Inc.
North Chicago, IL 60064
by Takeda Pharmaceutical Company Limited
Osaka, Japan 540-8645
™ - Trademark
® - Registered Trademark
(No. 3663)
Ref: 03-A696 January, 2013

Shown in Product Identification Guide, page 304

LUPRON DEPOT ℞

[lū-prŏn]

(leuprolide acetate for depot suspension)
22.5 mg for 3-Month Administration
30 mg for 4-Month Administration
45 mg for 6-Month Administration

HIGHLIGHTS OF PRESCRIBING INFORMATION

These highlights do not include all the information needed to use Lupron Depot safely and effectively. See full prescribing information for Lupron Depot.

Lupron Depot (leuprolide acetate for depot suspension)
Initial U.S. Approval: 1995

RECENT MAJOR CHANGES

Warnings and Precautions, Convulsions (5.5) 7/2013

INDICATIONS AND USAGE

LUPRON DEPOT is a gonadotropin releasing hormone (GnRH) agonist indicated for:

- palliative treatment of advanced prostatic cancer (1)

Table 1 LUPRON DEPOT Recommended Dosing

Dosage	22.5 mg for 3-Month Administration	30 mg for 4-Month Administration	45 mg for 6-Month Administration
Recommended dose	1 injection every 12 weeks	1 injection every 16 weeks	1 injection every 24 weeks

DOSAGE AND ADMINISTRATION

LUPRON DEPOT must be administered under the supervision of a physician. Due to different release characteristics, the dosage strengths are not additive and must be selected based upon the desired dosing schedule. (2)

- LUPRON DEPOT 22.5 mg for 3–month administration, given as a single intramuscular injection every 12 weeks (2.1)
- LUPRON DEPOT 30 mg for 4–month administration, given as a single intramuscular injection every 16 weeks (2.2)
- LUPRON DEPOT 45 mg for 6–month administration, given as a single intramuscular injection every 24 weeks (2.3)

DOSAGE FORMS AND STRENGTHS

22.5 mg, 30 mg, and 45 mg injections in a kit with prefilled dual chamber syringe (3)

CONTRAINDICATIONS

- Hypersensitivity to GnRH, GnRH agonist or any of the excipients in LUPRON DEPOT (4.1)
- Pregnancy (4.2, 8.1)

WARNINGS AND PRECAUTIONS

- Increased serum testosterone (~ 50% above baseline) during first week of treatment; monitor serum testosterone and PSA (5.1, 5.6)
  - Isolated cases of transient worsening of symptoms, or additional signs and symptoms of prostate cancer during the first few weeks of treatment. (5.1)
  - A small number of patients may experience a temporary increase in bone pain which can be managed symptomatically. (5.1)
  - Isolated cases of ureteral obstruction and spinal cord compression have been reported with GnRH agonists, which may contribute to paralysis with or without fatal complications. (5.1)
- Hyperglycemia and Diabetes: Hyperglycemia and an increased risk of developing diabetes have been reported in men receiving GnRH analogs. Monitor blood glucose level and manage according to current clinical practice. (5.2)
- Cardiovascular Diseases: Increased risk of myocardial infarction, sudden cardiac death and stroke has been reported in association with use of GnRH analogs in men. Monitor for cardiovascular disease and manage according to current clinical practice. (5.3)
- Long-term androgen deprivation therapy prolongs the QT interval. Consider risks and benefits. (5.4)
- Convulsions have been observed in patients with or without a history of predisposing factors. Manage convulsions according to the current clinical practice. (5.5)

ADVERSE REACTIONS

- LUPRON DEPOT 22.5 mg for 3–month administration: The most common related adverse reactions (>10%) were general pain, injection site reaction, hot flashes/sweats, GI disorders, joint disorders, testicular atrophy, urinary disorders. (6.1)
- LUPRON DEPOT 30 mg for 4–month administration: The most common adverse reactions (>10%) were asthenia, flu syndrome, general pain, headache, injection site reaction, hot flashes/sweats, GI disorders, edema, skin reaction, urinary disorders. (6.2)
- LUPRON DEPOT 45 mg for 6–month administration: The most common adverse reactions (>10%) were hot flush, injection site pain, upper respiratory infection, and fatigue. (6.3)

In postmarketing experience, mood swings, depression, rare reports of suicidal ideation and attempt, rare reports of pituitary apoplexy, and rare reports of serious drug-induced liver injury have been reported (6.4).

To report SUSPECTED ADVERSE REACTIONS, contact AbbVie Inc. at 1-800-633-9110 or FDA at 1-800-FDA-1088 or www.fda.gov/medwatch

DRUG INTERACTIONS

- No interactions with LUPRON DEPOT are expected. (7)

USE IN SPECIFIC POPULATIONS

- Pediatric: These LUPRON DEPOT formulations are not indicated for use in children. See the LUPRON DEPOT PED® package insert for the use of leuprolide acetate in children with central precocious puberty.
- Geriatric: This label reflects clinical trials for LUPRON DEPOT in prostate cancer in which the majority of the subjects studied were at least 65 years of age.

See 17 for PATIENT COUNSELING INFORMATION

Revised: 07/2013

FULL PRESCRIBING INFORMATION: CONTENTS*

*** Sections or subsections omitted from the full prescribing information are not listed**

FULL PRESCRIBING INFORMATION

1 INDICATIONS AND USAGE

LUPRON DEPOT 22.5 mg for 3–month administration, 30 mg for 4–month administration, and 45 mg for 6–month administration (leuprolide acetate) are indicated in the palliative treatment of advanced prostatic cancer.

LUPRON DEPOT is a gonadotropin releasing hormone (GnRH) agonist.

2 DOSAGE AND ADMINISTRATION

LUPRON DEPOT must be administered under the supervision of a physician.

[See table 1 above]

2.1 LUPRON DEPOT 22.5 mg for 3-Month Administration

The recommended dose of LUPRON DEPOT 22.5 mg for 3-month administration is one injection every 12 weeks.

Due to different release characteristics, a fractional dose, or a combination of doses of this depot formulation is not equivalent to the same dose of the monthly formulation and should not be given.

Incorporated in a depot formulation, the lyophilized microspheres are to be reconstituted and administered every 12 weeks as a single intramuscular injection.

For optimal performance of the prefilled dual chamber syringe (PDS), read and follow the instructions in Section 2.4.

2.2 LUPRON DEPOT 30 mg for 4-Month Administration

The recommended dose of LUPRON DEPOT 30 mg for 4-month administration is one injection every 16 weeks. Due to different release characteristics, a fractional dose, or a combination of doses of this depot formulation is not equivalent to the same dose of the monthly formulation and should not be given.

Incorporated in a depot formulation, the lyophilized microspheres are to be reconstituted and administered every 16 weeks as a single intramuscular injection.

For optimal performance of the prefilled dual chamber syringe (PDS), read and follow the instructions in Section 2.4.

2.3 LUPRON DEPOT 45 mg for 6-Month Administration

The recommended dose of LUPRON DEPOT 45 mg for 6-month administration is one injection every 24 weeks. Due to different release characteristics, a fractional dose, or a combination of doses of this depot formulation is not equivalent to the same dose of the monthly formulation and should not be given.

Incorporated in a depot formulation, the lyophilized microspheres are to be reconstituted and administered every 24 weeks as a single intramuscular injection.

For optimal performance of the prefilled dual chamber syringe (PDS), read and follow the instructions in Section 2.4.

2.4 Administration of Injection

- The lyophilized microspheres are to be reconstituted and administered as a single intramuscular injection.
- Since LUPRON DEPOT does not contain a preservative, the suspension should be injected immediately or discarded if not used within two hours.
- As with other drugs administered by injection, the injection site should be varied periodically.

1. The LUPRON DEPOT powder should be visually inspected and the syringe should NOT BE USED if clumping or caking is evident. A thin layer of powder on the wall of the syringe is considered normal prior to mixing with the diluent. The diluent should appear clear.
2. To prepare for injection, screw the white plunger into the end stopper until the stopper begins to turn.

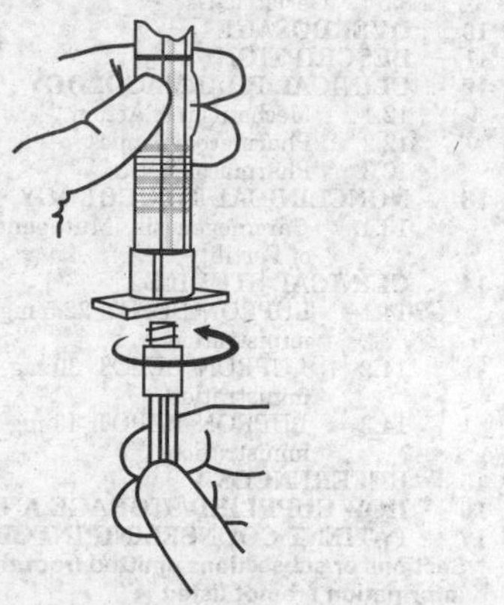

3. Hold the syringe UPRIGHT. Release the diluent by SLOWLY PUSHING (6 to 8 seconds) the plunger until the first stopper is <u>at the blue line</u> in the middle of the barrel.

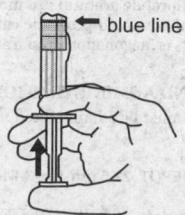

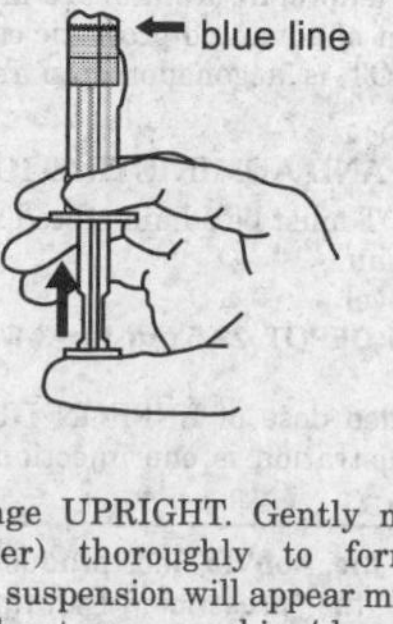

4. Keep the syringe UPRIGHT. Gently mix the microspheres (powder) thoroughly to form a uniform suspension. The suspension will appear milky. If the powder adheres to the stopper or caking/clumping is present, tap the syringe with your finger to disperse. DO NOT USE if any of the powder has not gone into suspension.

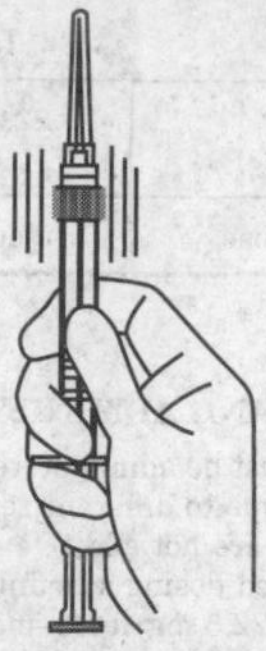

5. Hold the syringe UPRIGHT. With the opposite hand pull the needle cap upward without twisting.
6. Keep the syringe UPRIGHT. Advance the plunger to expel the air from the syringe.
7. After cleaning the injection site with an alcohol swab, insert the needle completely at a 90 degree angle.

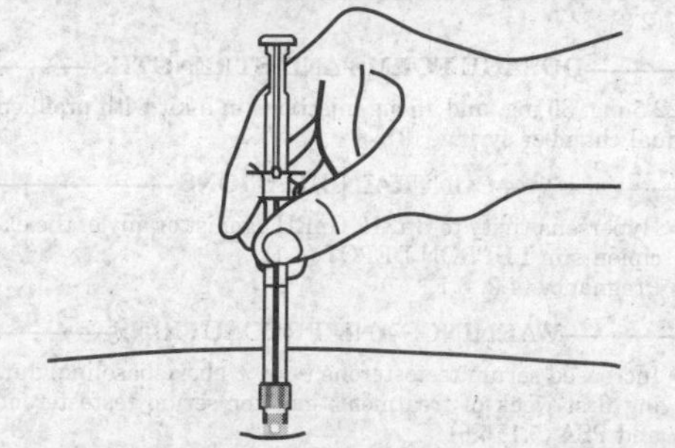

NOTE: Aspirated blood would be visible just below the luer lock connection if a blood vessel is accidentally penetrated. If present, blood can be seen through the transparent LuproLoc® safety device. If blood is present remove the needle immediately. Do not inject the medication

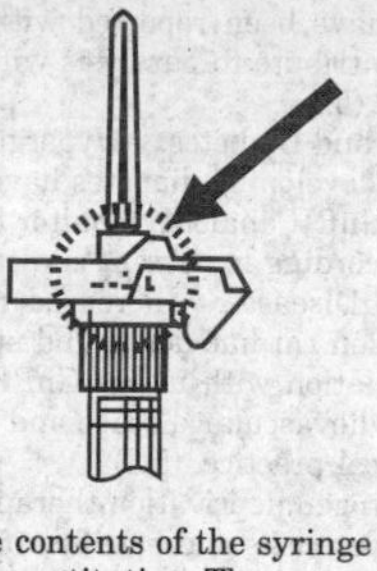

8. Inject the entire contents of the syringe intramuscularly at the time of reconstitution. The suspension settles very quickly following reconstitution; therefore, LUPRON DEPOT should be mixed and used immediately.

AFTER INJECTION

9. Withdraw the needle. Immediately activate the LuproLoc® safety device by pushing the arrow forward with the thumb or finger, as illustrated, until the device is fully extended and a CLICK is heard or felt.

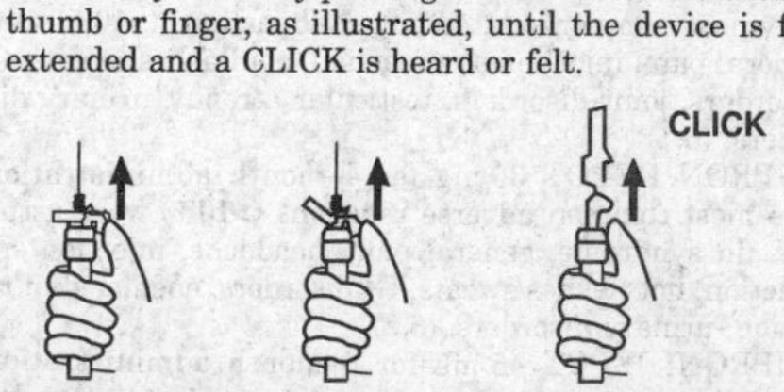

ADDITIONAL INFORMATION

- Please see the handling information in the Reference Section 15.0.
- Dispose of the syringe according to local regulations/procedures.

3 DOSAGE FORMS AND STRENGTHS

LUPRON DEPOT 22.5 mg for 3-month administration, 30 mg for 4-month administration, and 45 mg for 6-month administration are each supplied as a kit with prefilled dual chamber syringe.

4 CONTRAINDICATIONS

4.1 Hypersensitivity

LUPRON DEPOT is contraindicated in individuals with known hypersensitivity to GnRH agonists or any of the excipients in LUPRON DEPOT. Reports of anaphylactic reactions to GnRH agonists have been reported in the medical literature.

4.2 Pregnancy

LUPRON DEPOT may cause fetal harm when administered to a pregnant woman. Expected hormonal changes that occur with LUPRON DEPOT treatment increase the risk for pregnancy loss and fetal harm when administered to a pregnant woman *[see Use in Specific Populations (8.1)]*. LUPRON DEPOT is contraindicated in women who are or may become pregnant. If this drug is used during pregnancy, or if the patient becomes pregnant while taking this drug, the patient should be apprised of the potential hazard to the fetus.

5 WARNINGS AND PRECAUTIONS

5.1 Tumor Flare

Initially, LUPRON DEPOT, like other GnRH agonists, causes increases in serum levels of testosterone to approximately 50% above baseline during the first weeks of treatment. Isolated cases of ureteral obstruction and spinal cord compression have been observed, which may contribute to paralysis with or without fatal complications. Transient worsening of symptoms may develop. A small number of patients may experience a temporary increase in bone pain, which can be managed symptomatically.

Patients with metastatic vertebral lesions and/or with urinary tract obstruction should be closely observed during the first few weeks of therapy.

5.2 Hyperglycemia and Diabetes

Hyperglycemia and an increased risk of developing diabetes have been reported in men receiving GnRH agonists. Hyperglycemia may represent development of diabetes mellitus or worsening of glycemic control in patients with diabetes. Monitor blood glucose and/or glycosylated hemoglobin (HbA1c) periodically in patients receiving a GnRH agonist and manage with current practice for treatment of hyperglycemia or diabetes.

5.3 Cardiovascular Diseases

Increased risk of developing myocardial infarction, sudden cardiac death and stroke has been reported in association with use of GnRH agonists in men. The risk appears low based on the reported odds ratios, and should be evaluated carefully along with cardiovascular risk factors when determining a treatment for patients with prostate cancer. Patients receiving a GnRH agonist should be monitored for symptoms and signs suggestive of development of cardiovascular disease and be managed according to current clinical practice.

5.4 Effect on QT/QTc Interval

Long-term androgen deprivation therapy prolongs the QT interval. Physicians should consider whether the benefits of androgen deprivation therapy outweigh the potential risks in patients with congenital long QT syndrome, electrolyte abnormalities, or congestive heart failure and in patients taking class IA (e.g., quinidine, procainamide) or Class III (e.g., amiodarone, sotalol) antiarrhythmic medications.

5.5 Convulsions

Postmarketing reports of convulsions have been observed in patients on leuprolide acetate therapy. These included patients with a history of seizures, epilepsy, cerebrovascular disorders, central nervous system anomalies or tumors, and in patients on concomitant medications that have been associated with convulsions such as bupropion and SSRIs. Convulsions have also been reported in patients in the absence of any of the conditions mentioned above. Patients receiving a GnRH agonist who experience convulsion should be managed according to current clinical practice.

5.6 Laboratory Tests

Response to LUPRON DEPOT 22.5 mg for 3-month administration, 30 mg for 4-month administration, and 45 mg for 6-month administration should be monitored by measuring serum levels of testosterone. In the majority of patients, testosterone levels increased above baseline, declining thereafter to castrate levels (< 50 ng/dL) within four weeks. *[see Clinical Studies (14) and Adverse Reactions (6)]*.

6 ADVERSE REACTIONS

Because clinical studies are conducted under widely varying conditions, adverse reaction rates observed in the clinical studies of a drug cannot be directly compared to rates in the clinical studies of another drug and may not reflect the rates observed in practice.

6.1 LUPRON DEPOT 22.5 mg for 3-Month Administration

Clinical Trials

In two clinical trials of LUPRON DEPOT 22.5 mg for 3-month administration, the following adverse reactions were reported to have a possible or probable relationship to drug as ascribed by the treating physician in 5% or more of the patients receiving the drug. **Often, causality is difficult to assess in patients with metastatic prostate cancer.** Reactions considered not drug-related are excluded.

Table 2. Adverse Reactions Reported in ≥ 5% of Patients

Body System/Reaction	LUPRON DEPOT 22.5 mg for 3-Month Administration N=94	(%)
Body As A Whole		
Asthenia	7	(7.4)
General Pain	25	(26.6)
Headache	6	(6.4)
Injection Site Reaction	13	(13.8)
Cardiovascular System		
Hot flashes/Sweats	55	(58.5)
Digestive System		
GI Disorders	15	(16.0)
Musculoskeletal System		
Joint Disorders	11	(11.7)
Central/Peripheral Nervous System		
Dizziness/Vertigo	6	(6.4)
Insomnia/Sleep Disorders	8	(8.5)
Neuromuscular Disorders	9	(9.6)
Respiratory System		
Respiratory Disorders	6	(6.4)
Skin and Appendages		
Skin Reaction	8	(8.5)
Urogenital System		
Testicular Atrophy	19	(20.2)
Urinary Disorders	14	(14.9)

In these same studies, the following adverse reactions were reported in less than 5% of the patients on LUPRON DEPOT 22.5 mg for 3-month administration.

Body As A Whole - Enlarged abdomen, Fever

Cardiovascular System - Arrhythmia, Bradycardia, Heart failure, Hypertension, Hypotension, Varicose vein

Digestive System - Anorexia, Duodenal ulcer, Increased appetite, Thirst/dry mouth

Hemic and Lymphatic System - Anemia, Lymphedema

Metabolic and Nutritional Disorders - Dehydration, Edema

Central/Peripheral Nervous System - Anxiety, Delusions, Depression, Hypesthesia, Libido decreased*, Nervousness, Paresthesia

Respiratory System - Epistaxis, Pharyngitis, Pleural effusion, Pneumonia

Special Senses - Abnormal vision, Amblyopia, Dry eyes, Tinnitus

Urogenital System - Gynecomastia, Impotence*, Penis disorders, Testis disorders.

* Physiologic effect of decreased testosterone.

Laboratory

Abnormalities of certain parameters were observed, but are difficult to assess in this population. The following were recorded in ≥5% of patients: Increased BUN, Hyperglycemia, Hyperlipidemia (total cholesterol, LDL-cholesterol, triglycerides), Hyperphosphatemia, Abnormal liver function tests, Increased PT, Increased PTT. Additional laboratory abnormalities reported were: Decreased platelets, Decreased potassium and Increased WBC.

6.2 LUPRON DEPOT 30 mg for 4-Month Administration

Clinical Trials

The 4-month formulation of LUPRON DEPOT 30 mg was utilized in clinical trials that studied the drug in 49 non-orchiectomized prostate cancer patients for 32 weeks or longer and in 24 orchiectomized prostate cancer patients for 20 weeks.

In the above described clinical trials, the following adverse reactions were reported in ≥ 5% of the patients during the treatment period regardless of causality.

[See table 3 above]

In these same studies, the following adverse reactions were reported in less than 5% of the patients on LUPRON DEPOT 30 mg for 4-month administration.

Body As a Whole - Abscess, Accidental injury, Allergic reaction, Cyst, Fever, Generalized edema, Hernia, Neck pain, Neoplasm

Cardiovascular System - Atrial fibrillation, Deep thrombophlebitis, Hypertension

Digestive System - Anorexia, Eructation, Gastrointestinal hemorrhage, Gingivitis, Gum hemorrhage, Hepatomegaly, Increased appetite, Intestinal obstruction, Periodontal abscess

Hemic and Lymphatic System - Lymphadenopathy

Metabolic and Nutritional Disorders - Healing abnormal, Hypoxia, Weight loss

Musculoskeletal System - Leg cramps, Pathological fracture, Ptosis

Nervous System - Abnormal thinking, Amnesia, Confusion, Convulsion, Dementia, Depression, Insomnia/sleep disorders, Libido decreased*, Neuropathy, Paralysis

Respiratory System - Asthma, Bronchitis, Hiccup, Lung disorder, Sinusitis, Voice alteration

Skin and Appendages - Herpes zoster, Melanosis

Table 3. Adverse Events Regardless of Causality Reported in ≥ 5% of Patients

Body System/Events	LUPRON DEPOT 30 mg for 4-Month Administration: Nonorchiectomized Study 013 N=49	(%)	Orchiectomized Study 012 N=24	(%)
Body As a Whole				
Asthenia	6	(12.2)	1	(4.2)
Flu Syndrome	6	(12.2)	0	(0.0)
General Pain	16	(32.7)	1	(4.2)
Headache	5	(10.2)	1	(4.2)
Injection Site Reaction	4	(8.2)	9	(37.5)
Cardiovascular System				
Hot flashes/Sweats	23	(46.9)	2	(8.3)
Digestive System				
GI Disorders	5	(10.2)	3	(12.5)
Metabolic and Nutritional Disorders				
Dehydration	4	(8.2)	0	(0.0)
Edema	4	(8.2)	5	(20.8)
Musculoskeletal System				
Joint Disorder	8	(16.3)	1	(4.2)
Myalgia	4	(8.2)	0	(0.0)
Nervous System				
Dizziness/Vertigo	3	(6.1)	2	(8.3)
Neuromuscular Disorders	3	(6.1)	1	(4.2)
Paresthesia	4	(8.2)	1	(4.2)
Respiratory System				
Respiratory Disorder	4	(8.2)	1	(4.2)
Skin and Appendages				
Skin Reaction	6	(12.2)	0	(0.0)
Urogenital System				
Urinary Disorders	5	(10.2)	4	(16.7)

Table 4. Adverse Events in ≥ 5% of Patients

Adverse Event	LUPRON DEPOT 45 mg for 6-Month Administration: Treatment Emergent N = 151	(%)	Treatment Related N = 151	(%)
Hot Flush/Flushing	89	58.9	88	58.3
Injection Site Pain/Discomfort	29	19.2	16	10.6
Upper Respiratory Tract Infection/Influenza-like Illness[1]	32	21.2	0	0
Fatigue/Lethargy	20	13.2	18	11.9
Constipation	15	9.9	5	3.3
Arthralgia	14	9.3	2	1.3
Insomnia/Sleep Disorder	13	8.6	5	3.3
Headache/Sinus Headache	12	7.9	3	2.0
Musculoskeletal Pain/ Myalgia	12	7.9	3	2.0
Second Primary Neoplasm[2]	11	7.3	0	0
Cough	10	6.6	2	1.3
Hematuria/Hemorrhagic Cystitis	10	6.6	0	0
Hypertension/BP Increased	10	6.6	3	2.0
Rash	9	6.0	3	2.0
Dysuria	9	6.0	1	0.7
Urinary Tract Infection/Cystitis	9	6.0	0	0
Anemia/Hemoglobin Decreased	10	6.6	2	1.3
Back Pain	8	5.3	0	0
COPD	8	5.3	0	0
Dizziness	8	5.3	3	2.0
Dyspnea/Dyspnea on Exertion	8	5.3	2	1.3
Nocturia	8	5.3	2	1.3
Peripheral/Pitting Edema	8	5.3	2	1.3
Coronary Artery Disease/Angina	8	5.3	1	0.7

[1]Includes influenza, nasal congestion, nasopharyngitis, rhinorrhea, upper respiratory tract infection, and viral upper respiratory tract infection

[2]Includes basal cell carcinoma, bladder transitional cell carcinoma, lung neoplasm, malignant melanoma, non-Hodgkin's lymphoma, and squamous cell carcinoma

Urogenital System - Bladder carcinoma, Epididymitis, Impotence*, Prostate disorder, Testicular atrophy*, Urinary incontinence, Urinary tract infection.

* Physiologic effect of decreased testosterone.

Laboratory

Abnormalities of certain parameters were observed, but their relationship to drug treatment is difficult to assess in this population. The following were recorded in ≥ 5% of patients: Decreased bicarbonate, Decreased hemoglobin/hematocrit/RBC, Hyperlipidemia (total cholesterol, LDL-cholesterol, triglycerides), Decreased HDL-cholesterol, Eosinophilia, Increased glucose, Increased liver function tests (ALT, AST, GGTP, LDH), Increased phosphorus. Additional laboratory abnormalities were reported: Increased BUN and PT, Leukopenia, Thrombocytopenia, Uricaciduria.

6.3 LUPRON DEPOT 45 mg for 6-Month Administration

Clinical Trials

One open label, multicenter study was conducted with LUPRON DEPOT 45 mg for 6-month administration in 151 prostate cancer patients. Patients were treated for 48 weeks, with 139/151 receiving two injections 24 weeks apart.

In the above described clinical trial, the following adverse events were reported in ≥ 5% of the patients during the treatment period. The Table 4 includes all adverse events reported in ≥ 5% of patients as well as the incidences of these adverse events that were considered, by the treating physician, to have a definite or possible relationship to LUPRON.

[See table 4 above]

The following adverse events led to discontinuation; fatigue, hot flush, second primary neoplasm, asthenia, coronary artery disease, constipation, hyperkalemia, and sleep disorder. Serious adverse events in ≥ 2% of patients, regardless of causality, included chronic obstructive pulmonary disease, coronary artery disease/angina, cerebrovascular accident/transient ischemic attack, pneumonia, and second primary neoplasms.

Laboratory

At baseline, 13.9% of patients had a CTCAE v4.0 grade 1 or 2 decreased hemoglobin. During the study, 42.4% of subjects

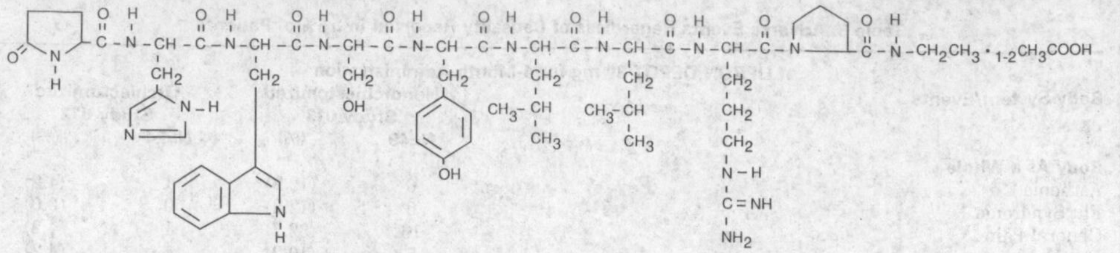

had grade 1 decreased hemoglobin (10 - <12-5 g/dL), 2.0% had grade 2 (8 - <10 g/dL) and 1.3% of subjects had grade 3 or 4 (<8 g/dL). Likewise, 28.5% of patients had a grade 1 or 2 increased cholesterol at baseline while 55.0% had grade 1 increased cholesterol (>199- 300 mg/dL), 3.3% had a grade 2 increase (>300-400 mg/dL), and 0.7% of subjects had grade 3 (>400 mg/dL) during the study.

6.4 Postmarketing

The following adverse reactions have been identified during postapproval use of LUPRON DEPOT. Because these reactions are reported voluntarily from a population of uncertain size, it is not always possible to reliably estimate their frequency or establish a causal relationship to drug exposure.

During postmarketing surveillance, which includes other dosage forms and other patient populations, the following adverse reactions were reported.

Like other drugs in this class, mood swings, including depression, have been reported. There have been very rare reports of suicidal ideation and attempt. Many, but not all, of these patients had a history of depression or other psychiatric illness. Patients should be counseled on the possibility of development or worsening of depression during treatment with LUPRON.

Symptoms consistent with an anaphylactoid or asthmatic process have been rarely (incidence rate of about 0.002%) reported. Rash, urticaria, and photosensitivity reactions have also been reported.

Changes in Bone Density - Decreased bone density has been reported in the medical literature in men who have had orchiectomy or who have been treated with a GnRH agonist analog. In a clinical trial, 25 men with prostate cancer, 12 of whom had been treated previously with leuprolide acetate for at least six months, underwent bone density studies as a result of pain. The leuprolide-treated group had lower bone density scores than the nontreated control group. It can be anticipated that long periods of medical castration in men will have effects on bone density.

Pituitary apoplexy - During post-marketing surveillance, rare cases of pituitary apoplexy (a clinical syndrome secondary to infarction of the pituitary gland) have been reported after the administration of gonadotropin-releasing hormone agonists. In a majority of these cases, a pituitary adenoma was diagnosed, with a majority of pituitary apoplexy cases occurring within 2 weeks of the first dose, and some within the first hour. In these cases, pituitary apoplexy has presented as sudden headache, vomiting, visual changes, ophthalmoplegia, altered mental status, and sometimes cardiovascular collapse. Immediate medical attention has been required.

Localized reactions including induration and abscess have been reported at the site of injection.

Symptoms consistent with fibromyalgia (e.g., joint and muscle pain, headaches, sleep disorders, gastrointestinal distress, and shortness of breath) have been reported individually and collectively.

Cardiovascular System – Hypotension, Myocardial infarction, Pulmonary embolism

Respiratory, thoracic and mediastinal disorder – Interstitial lung disease

Hepato-biliary disorder: Serious drug-induced liver injury

Hemic and Lymphatic System - Decreased WBC

Central/Peripheral Nervous System - Convulsion, Peripheral neuropathy, Spinal fracture/paralysis

Endocrine System – Diabetes

Musculoskeletal System - Tenosynovitis-like symptoms

Urogenital System - Prostate pain

See other LUPRON DEPOT and LUPRON Injection package inserts for other reactions reported in women and pediatric populations.

7 DRUG INTERACTIONS

No pharmacokinetic-based drug-drug interaction studies have been conducted with LUPRON DEPOT. However, because leuprolide acetate is a peptide that is primarily degraded by peptidase and not by Cytochrome P-450 enzymes as noted in specific studies, and the drug is only about 46% bound to plasma proteins, drug interactions would not be expected to occur.

See Clinical Pharmacology (12.3).

7.1 Drug/Laboratory Test Interactions

Administration of LUPRON DEPOT in therapeutic doses results in suppression of the pituitary-gonadal system. Normal function is usually restored within three months after treatment is discontinued. Due to the suppression of the pituitary-gonadal system by LUPRON DEPOT, diagnostic tests of pituitary gonadotropic and gonadal functions conducted during treatment and up to three months after discontinuation of LUPRON DEPOT may be affected.

8 USE IN SPECIFIC POPULATIONS

8.1 Pregnancy

Pregnancy Category X *[see Contraindications (4.2)]*.

LUPRON DEPOT is contraindicated in women who are or may become pregnant while receiving the drug. Expected hormonal changes that occur with LUPRON DEPOT treatment increase the risk for pregnancy loss and fetal harm when administered to a pregnant woman. If this drug is used during pregnancy, or if the patient becomes pregnant while taking this drug, the patient should be apprised of the potential hazard to the fetus.

Major fetal abnormalities were observed in rabbits after a single administration of the monthly formulation of LUPRON DEPOT on day 6 of pregnancy at doses of 0.00024, 0.0024, and 0.024 mg/kg (approximately 1/1600 to 1/16 the human dose based on body surface area using an estimated daily dose in animals and humans). Since a depot formulation was utilized in the study, a sustained exposure to leuprolide was expected throughout the period of organogenesis and to the end of gestation. Similar studies in rats did not demonstrate an increase in fetal malformations, however, there was increased fetal mortality and decreased fetal weights with the two higher doses of the monthly formulation of LUPRON DEPOT in rabbits and with the highest dose (0.024 mg/kg) in rats.

8.3 Nursing Mothers

LUPRON DEPOT is not indicated for women *[see Indications and Usage (1)]*. It is not known whether leuprolide is excreted in human milk. Because many drugs are excreted in human milk and because of the potential for serious adverse reactions in nursing infants from LUPRON DEPOT, a decision should be made to discontinue nursing or discontinue the drug taking into account the importance of the drug to the mother.

8.4 Pediatric Use

See LUPRON DEPOT-PED® (leuprolide acetate for depot suspension) labeling for the safety and effectiveness in children with central precocious puberty.

8.5 Geriatric Use

In the clinical trials for LUPRON DEPOT in prostate cancer, the majority (approximately 80%) of the subjects studied were at least 65 years of age. Therefore, the labeling reflects the pharmacokinetics, efficacy and safety of LUPRON DEPOT in this population.

10 OVERDOSAGE

There is no experience of overdosage in clinical trials. In rats, a single subcutaneous dose of 100 mg/kg (approximately 4,000 times the estimated daily human dose based on body surface area), resulted in dyspnea, decreased activity, and excessive scratching. In early clinical trials with daily subcutaneous leuprolide acetate, doses as high as 20 mg/day for up to two years caused no adverse effects differing from those observed with the 1 mg/day dose.

11 DESCRIPTION

Leuprolide acetate is a synthetic nonapeptide analog of naturally occurring gonadotropin-releasing hormone (GnRH). The analog possesses greater potency than the natural hormone. The chemical name is 5-oxo-L-prolyl-L-histidyl-L-tryptophyl-L-seryl-L-tyrosyl-D-leucyl-L-leucyl-L-arginyl-N-ethyl-L-prolinamide acetate (salt) with the following structural formula:

[See chemical structure above]

LUPRON DEPOT 22.5 mg for 3-month administration is available in a prefilled dual-chamber syringe containing sterile lyophilized microspheres which, when mixed with diluent, become a suspension intended as an intramuscular injection to be given **ONCE EVERY 12 WEEKS**.

The front chamber of LUPRON DEPOT 22.5 mg for 3-month administration prefilled dual-chamber syringe contains leuprolide acetate (22.5 mg), polylactic acid (198.6 mg) and D-mannitol (38.9 mg). The second chamber of diluent contains carboxymethylcellulose sodium (7.5 mg), D-mannitol (75.0 mg), polysorbate 80 (1.5 mg), water for injection, USP, and glacial acetic acid, USP to control pH.

LUPRON DEPOT 30 mg for 4-month administration is available in a prefilled dual-chamber syringe containing sterile lyophilized microspheres which, when mixed with diluent, become a suspension intended as an intramuscular injection to be given **ONCE EVERY 16 WEEKS**.

The front chamber of LUPRON DEPOT 30 mg for 4-month administration prefilled dual-chamber syringe contains leuprolide acetate (30 mg), polylactic acid (264.8 mg) and D-mannitol (51.9 mg). The second chamber of diluent contains carboxymethylcellulose sodium (7.5 mg), D-mannitol (75.0 mg), polysorbate 80 (1.5 mg), water for injection, USP, and glacial acetic acid, USP to control pH.

LUPRON DEPOT 45 mg for 6-month administration is available in a prefilled dual-chamber syringe containing sterile lyophilized microspheres which, when mixed with diluent, become a suspension intended as an intramuscular injection to be given **ONCE EVERY 24 WEEKS**.

The front chamber of LUPRON DEPOT 45 mg for 6-month administration prefilled dual-chamber syringe contains leuprolide acetate (45 mg), polylactic acid (169.9 mg), D-mannitol (39.7 mg), and stearic acid (10.1 mg). The second chamber of diluent contains carboxymethylcellulose sodium (7.5 mg), D-mannitol (75.0 mg), polysorbate 80 (1.5 mg), water for injection, USP, and glacial acetic acid, USP to control pH.

During the manufacture of LUPRON DEPOT 22.5 mg for 3-month administration, 30 mg for 4-month administration, and 45 mg for 6-month administration, acetic acid is lost, leaving the peptide.

12 CLINICAL PHARMACOLOGY

12.1 Mechanism of Action

Leuprolide acetate, a GnRH agonist, acts as an inhibitor of gonadotropin secretion. Animal studies indicate that following an initial stimulation, continuous administration of leuprolide acetate results in suppression of ovarian and testicular steroidogenesis. This effect was reversible upon discontinuation of drug therapy.

Administration of leuprolide acetate has resulted in inhibition of the growth of certain hormone dependent tumors (prostatic tumors in Noble and Dunning male rats and DMBA-induced mammary tumors in female rats) as well as atrophy of the reproductive organs.

12.2 Pharmacodynamics

In humans, administration of leuprolide acetate results in an initial increase in circulating levels of luteinizing hormone (LH) and follicle stimulating hormone (FSH), leading to a transient increase in levels of the gonadal steroids (testosterone and dihydrotestosterone in males, and estrone and estradiol in premenopausal females). However, continuous administration of leuprolide acetate results in decreased levels of LH and FSH. In males, testosterone is reduced to castrate levels. In premenopausal females, estrogens are reduced to postmenopausal levels. These decreases occur within two to four weeks after initiation of treatment, and castrate levels of testosterone in prostatic cancer patients have been demonstrated for more than five years.

Leuprolide acetate is not active when given orally.

12.3 Pharmacokinetics

Absorption

LUPRON DEPOT 22.5 mg for 3-Month Administration

Following a single injection of LUPRON DEPOT 22.5 mg for 3-month administration in patients, mean peak plasma leuprolide concentration of 48.9 ng/mL was observed at 4 hours and then declined to 0.67 ng/mL at 12 weeks. Leuprolide appeared to be released at a constant rate following the onset of steady-state levels during the third week after dosing, providing steady plasma concentrations through the 12-week dosing interval. However, intact leuprolide and an inactive major metabolite could not be distinguished by the assay which was employed in the study. Detectable levels of leuprolide were present at all measurement points in all patients. The initial burst, followed by the rapid decline to a steady-state level, was similar to the release pattern seen with the monthly formulation.

LUPRON DEPOT 30 mg for 4-Month Administration

Following a single injection of LUPRON DEPOT 30 mg for 4-month administration in sixteen orchiectomized prostate cancer patients, mean plasma leuprolide concentration of 59.3 ng/mL was observed at 4 hours and the mean concentration then declined to 0.30 ng/mL at 16 weeks. The mean plasma concentration of leuprolide from weeks 3.5 to 16 was 0.44 ± 0.20 ng/mL (range: 0.20-1.06). Leuprolide appeared to be released at a constant rate following the onset of steady-state levels during the fourth week after dosing, providing steady plasma concentrations throughout the 16-week dosing interval. However, intact leuprolide and an inactive major metabolite could not be distinguished by the assay which was employed in the study. The initial burst, followed by the rapid decline to a steady-state level, was similar to the release pattern seen with the other depot formulations.

LUPRON DEPOT 45 mg for 6-Month Administration

Following a single injection of LUPRON DEPOT 45 mg for 6-month administration in 26 prostate cancer patients, mean peak plasma leuprolide concentration of 6.7 ng/mL was observed at 2 hours and the mean concentration then declined to 0.07 ng/mL at 24 weeks. Leuprolide appeared to be released continuously following the onset of steady-state levels during the third week after dosing providing steady plasma concentrations through the 24-week dosing interval. The initial burst, followed by the rapid decline to a steady-state level, was similar to the release pattern seen with the other depot formulations. In this study, mean leuprolide plasma concentration-time profiles were similar after the first and second dose.

Distribution

The mean steady-state volume of distribution of leuprolide following intravenous bolus administration to healthy male volunteers was 27 L. *In vitro* binding to human plasma proteins ranged from 43% to 49%.

Metabolism

In healthy male volunteers, a 1 mg bolus of leuprolide administered intravenously revealed that the mean systemic clearance was 7.6 L/h, with a terminal elimination half-life of approximately 3 hours based on a two compartment model.

In rats and dogs, administration of ^{14}C-labeled leuprolide was shown to be metabolized to smaller inactive peptides, a pentapeptide (Metabolite I), tripeptides (Metabolites II and III) and a dipeptide (Metabolite IV). These fragments may be further catabolized.

The major metabolite (M-I) plasma concentrations measured in 5 prostate cancer patients reached maximum concentration 2 to 6 hours after dosing and were approximately 6% of the peak parent drug concentration. One week after dosing, mean plasma M-I concentrations were approximately 20% of mean leuprolide concentrations.

Excretion

Following administration of LUPRON DEPOT 3.75 mg to 3 patients, less than 5% of the dose was recovered as parent and M-I metabolite in the urine.

Special Populations

The pharmacokinetics of the drug in hepatically and renally impaired patients have not been determined.

13 NONCLINICAL TOXICOLOGY

13.1 Carcinogenesis, Mutagenesis, Impairment of Fertility

Two-year carcinogenicity studies were conducted in rats and mice. In rats, a dose-related increase of benign pituitary hyperplasia and benign pituitary adenomas was noted at 24 months when the drug was administered subcutaneously at daily doses (0.6 to 4 mg/kg). There was a significant but not dose-related increase of pancreatic islet-cell adenomas in females and of testicular interstitial cell adenomas in males (highest incidence in the low dose group). In mice, no pituitary abnormalities were observed at a dose as high as 60 mg/kg for two years. Patients have been treated with leuprolide acetate for up to three years with doses as high as 10 mg/day and for two years with doses as high as 20 mg/day without demonstrable pituitary abnormalities.

Genotoxicity studies were conducted with leuprolide acetate using bacterial and mammalian systems. These studies provided no evidence of mutagenic effects or chromosomal aberrations.

Leuprolide may reduce male and female fertility. Administration of leuprolide acetate to male and female rats at dose of 0.024, 0.24, and 2.4 mg/kg as monthly depot formulation for up to 3 months (approximately as low as 1/30 of the human dose based on body surface area using an estimated daily dose in animals and humans) caused atrophy of the reproductive organs, and suppression of reproductive function. These changes were reversible upon cessation of treatment. Clinical and pharmacologic studies in adults (≥ 18 years) with leuprolide acetate and similar analogs have shown reversibility of fertility suppression when the drug is discontinued after continuous administration for periods of up to 24 weeks.

Clinical and pharmacologic studies in adults (≥ 18 years) with leuprolide acetate and similar analogs have shown reversibility of fertility suppression when the drug is discontinued after continuous administration for periods of up to 24 weeks.

14 CLINICAL STUDIES

14.1 LUPRON DEPOT 22.5 mg for 3-Month Administration

In clinical studies, serum testosterone was suppressed to castrate within 30 days in 87 of 92 (95%) patients and within an additional two weeks in three patients. Two patients did not suppress for 15 and 28 weeks, respectively.

Figure 3. LUPRON DEPOT 45 mg for 6-Month Administration Serum Testosterone Concentrations (Mean + SE)

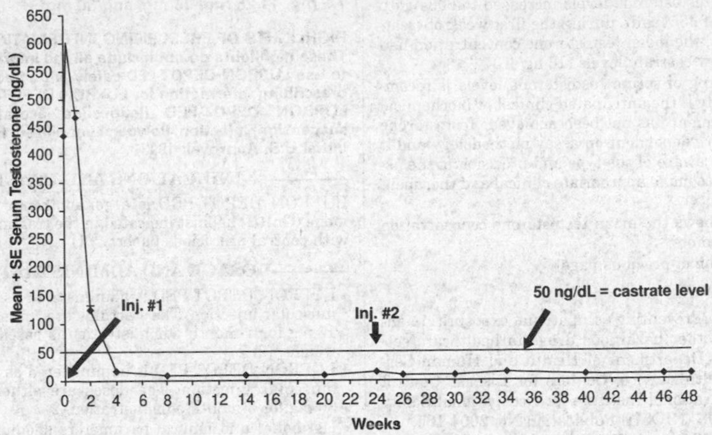

Suppression was maintained in all of these patients with the exception of transient minimal testosterone elevations in one of them, and in another an increase in serum testosterone to above the castrate range was recorded during the 12 hour observation period after a subsequent injection. This represents stimulation of gonadotropin secretion.

Figure 1. LUPRON DEPOT 22.5 mg for 3-Month Administration Mean Serum Testosterone Concentrations

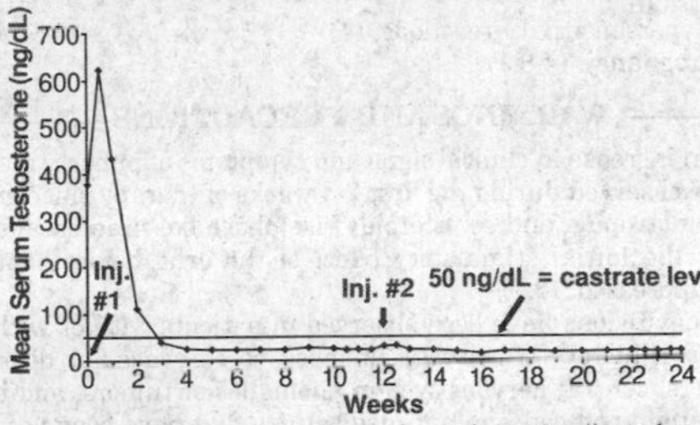

Note: Measurements were taken in a subset of patients from one study at Weeks 10.5, 11.5, 12.5, 22.5 and 23.5

An 85% rate of "no progression" was achieved during the initial 24 weeks of treatment. A decrease from baseline in serum PSA of ≥90% was reported in 71% of the patients and a change to within the normal range (≤3.99 ng/mL) in 63% of the patients.

Periodic monitoring of serum testosterone and PSA levels is recommended, especially if the anticipated clinical or biochemical response to treatment has not been achieved. It should be noted that results of testosterone determinations are dependent on assay methodology. It is advisable to be aware of the type and precision of the assay methodology to make appropriate clinical and therapeutic decisions.

14.2 LUPRON DEPOT 30 mg for 4-Month Administration

In an open-label, noncomparative, multicenter clinical study of LUPRON DEPOT 30 mg for 4-month administration, 49 patients with stage D2 prostatic adenocarcinoma (with no prior treatment) were enrolled. The objectives were to determine whether a 30 mg depot formulation of leuprolide injected once every 16 weeks would reduce and maintain serum testosterone levels at castrate levels (≤ 50 ng/dL), and to assess the safety of the formulation. The study was divided into an initial 32-week treatment phase and a long-term treatment phase. Serum testosterone levels were determined biweekly or weekly during the first 32 weeks of treatment. Once the patient completed the initial 32-week treatment period, treatment continued at the investigator's discretion with serum testosterone levels being done every 4 months prior to the injection.

In the majority of patients, testosterone levels increased 50% or more above the baseline during the first week of treatment. Mean serum testosterone subsequently suppressed to castrate levels within 30 days of the first injection in 94% of patients and within 43 days in all 49 patients during the initial 32-week treatment period. The median dosing interval between injections was 112 days. One escape from suppression (two consecutive testosterone values greater than 50 ng/dL after castrate levels achieved) was noted at Week 16. In this patient, serum testosterone increased to above the castrate range following the second depot injection (Week 16) but returned to the castrate level by Week 18. No adverse reactions were associated with this rise in serum testosterone. A second patient had a rise in testosterone at Week 17, then returned to the castrate level by Week 18 and remained there through Week 32. In the long-term treatment phase two patients experienced testosterone elevations, both at Week 48. Testosterone for one patient returned to the castrate range at Week 52, and one patient discontinued the study at Week 48 due to disease progression.

Secondary efficacy endpoints evaluated in the study were the objective tumor response as assessed by clinical evaluations of tumor burden (complete response, partial response, objectively stable and progression) and evaluations of changes in prostatic involvement and prostate-specific antigen (PSA). These evaluations were performed at Weeks 16 and 32 of the treatment phase. The long-term treatment phase monitored PSA at each visit (every 16 weeks). The objective tumor response analysis showed "no progression" (i.e. complete or partial response, or stable disease) in 86% (37/43) of patients at Week 16, and in 77% (37/48) of patients at Week 32. Local disease improved or remained stable in all patients evaluated at Week 16 and/or 32. For patients with elevated baseline PSA, 50% (23/46) had a normal PSA (less than 4.0 ng/mL) at Week 16, and 51% (19/37) had a normal PSA at Week 32.

Periodic monitoring of serum testosterone and PSA levels is recommended, especially if the anticipated clinical or biochemical response to treatment has not been achieved. It should be noted that results of testosterone determinations are dependent on assay methodology. It is advisable to be aware of the type and precision of the assay methodology to make appropriate clinical and therapeutic decisions.

Using historical comparisons, the safety and efficacy of LUPRON DEPOT 30 mg for 4-month administration appear similar to the other LUPRON DEPOT formulations.

Figure 2. LUPRON DEPOT 30 mg for 4-Month Administration Mean Serum Testosterone Concentrations

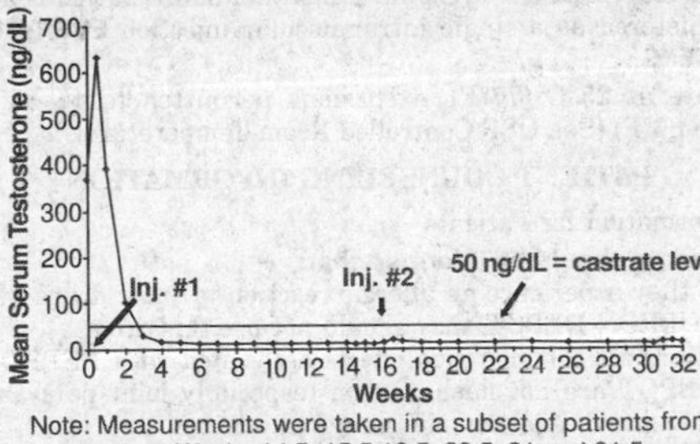

Note: Measurements were taken in a subset of patients from one study at Weeks 14.5, 15.5 16.5, 30.5, 31 and 31.5

14.3 LUPRON DEPOT 45 mg for 6-Month Administration

An open-label, non-comparative, multicenter clinical study of LUPRON DEPOT 45 mg for 6-month administration enrolled 151 patients with prostate cancer. The study drug was administered as two intramuscular injections of LUPRON DEPOT 45 mg at 24 week intervals (139/151 received 2 injections), and patients were followed for a total of 48 weeks.

Among 148 patients who had testosterone value at Week 4, serum testosterone was suppressed to castrate levels (< 50 ng/dL) from Week 4 through Week 48 in an estimated 93.4% (two-sided 95% CI: 89.2%, 97.6%) of patients. One patient failed to achieve testosterone suppression by Week 4,

Information on the AbbVie, Inc. products listed on these pages is from the prescribing information in use as of July 31, 2013. For more information, please visit rxabbvie.com or call 1-800-633-9110.

and eight patients had escapes from suppression (any testosterone value > 50 ng/dL after castrate levels were achieved). Mean testosterone levels increased to 608 ng/dL from a baseline of 435 ng/dL during the first week of treatment. By Week 4, the mean testosterone concentration had decreased to below castrate levels (16 ng/dL).

Periodic monitoring of serum testosterone levels is recommended, especially if the anticipated clinical or biochemical response to treatment has not been achieved. Testosterone determinations are dependent on assay methodology and it is advisable to be aware of the type and precision of the assay methodology to make appropriate clinical and therapeutic decisions.

Figure 3 below shows the mean testosterone concentration at various time points.

[See figure 3 at top of previous page]

15 REFERENCES

1. NIOSH Alert: Preventing occupational exposures to antineoplastic and other hazardous drugs in healthcare settings. 2004. U.S. Department of Health and Human Services, Public Health Service, Centers for Disease Control and Prevention, National Institute for Occupational Safety and Health, DHHS (NIOSH) Publication No. 2004-165.

2. OSHA Technical Manual, TED 1-0.15A, Section VI: Chapter 2. Controlling Occupational Exposure to Hazardous Drugs. OSHA, 1999. http://www.osha.gov/dts/osta/otm/otm_vi/otm_vi_2.html

3. American Society of Health-System Pharmacists. ASHP guidelines on handling hazardous drugs. *Am J Health-Syst Pharm*. 2006; 63; 1172-1193.

4. Polovich, M., White, J.M., & Kelleher, L.O. (eds.) 2005. Chemotherapy and biotherapy guidelines and recommendations for practice (2nd Ed.) Pittsburgh, PA: Oncology Nursing Society.

16 HOW SUPPLIED/STORAGE AND HANDLING

Each LUPRON DEPOT 22.5 mg for 3-month administration (NDC 0074-3346-03), 30 mg for 4-month administration (NDC 0074-3683-03), 45 mg for 6-month administration (NDC 0074-3473-03) contains:

- one prefilled dual-chamber syringe containing needle with LuproLoc® safety device
- one plunger
- two alcohol swabs
- a complete prescribing information enclosure

The prefilled dual-chamber syringe contains sterile lyophilized microspheres of leuprolide acetate incorporated in a biodegradable lactic acid polymer.

When mixed with 1.5 mL of accompanying diluent, LUPRON DEPOT 22.5 mg for 3-month administration is administered as a single intramuscular injection **EVERY 12 WEEKS**.

When mixed with 1.5 mL of accompanying diluent, LUPRON DEPOT 30 mg for 4-month administration is administered as a single intramuscular injection **EVERY 16 WEEKS**.

When mixed with 1.5 mL of accompanying diluent, LUPRON DEPOT 45 mg for 6-month administration is administered as a single intramuscular injection **EVERY 24 WEEKS**.

Store at 25°C (77°F); excursions permitted to 15–30°C (59–86°F) [See USP Controlled Room Temperature].

17 PATIENT COUNSELING INFORMATION

Information for Patients

Patients should be informed that:

- If they experience an allergic reaction to other drugs like LUPRON DEPOT, they should not use this drug.
- The most common side effects associated with LUPRON DEPOT are hot flashes, pain (especially joint pain and back pain), injection site pain and fatigue.
- LUPRON DEPOT may cause impotence.
- The increase in testosterone that occurs during the first weeks of therapy can cause an increase in urinary symptoms or pain.
- If they have metastatic cancer to the spine or urinary tract, they need close medical attention during the first weeks of therapy.
- They should notify their doctor if they develop new or worsened symptoms after beginning LUPRON DEPOT treatment.

Manufactured for
AbbVie Inc.
North Chicago, IL 60064
by Takeda Pharmaceutical Company Limited
Osaka, Japan 540-8645
™-Trademark
®-Registered Trademark
(No. 3346) (No. 3683) (No. 3473)
03-A853-R5 July, 2013

Shown in Product Identification Guide, page 304

LUPRON DEPOT-PED® ℞

(leuprolide acetate for depot suspension)
7.5 mg, 11.25 mg, 15 mg, and 30 mg

HIGHLIGHTS OF PRESCRIBING INFORMATION

These highlights do not include all the information needed to use LUPRON DEPOT-PED safely and effectively. See full prescribing information for LUPRON DEPOT-PED.

LUPRON DEPOT-PED (leuprolide acetate for depot suspension) Injection, Powder, Lyophilized, For Suspension
Initial U.S. Approval: 1993

INDICATIONS AND USAGE

LUPRON DEPOT-PED is a gonadotropin releasing hormone (GnRH) agonist indicated in the treatment of children with central precocious puberty. (1)

DOSAGE AND ADMINISTRATION

- LUPRON DEPOT-PED is administered as a single intramuscular injection. The starting dose 7.5 mg, 11.25 mg, or 15 mg for 1-month administration is based on the child's weight. (2)
- LUPRON DEPOT-PED is administered as a single intramuscular injection. The doses are either 11.25 mg or 30 mg for 3-month administration.(2)
- Hormonal and clinical parameters should be monitored during treatment to ensure adequate suppression. (2)
- The injection site should be varied periodically. (2)

DOSAGE FORMS AND STRENGTHS

LUPRON DEPOT-PED 7.5 mg, 11.25 mg, or 15 mg for 1-month administration and LUPRON DEPOT-PED 11.25 mg or 30 mg for 3-month administration are provided in a prefilled dual chamber syringe for intramuscular injection. (3)

CONTRAINDICATIONS

- Hypersensitivity reactions. (4)
- Pregnancy. (4,8.1)

WARNINGS AND PRECAUTIONS

- An increase in clinical signs and symptoms of puberty may be observed during the first 2-4 weeks of therapy since gonadotropins and sex steroids rise above baseline because of the initial stimulatory effect of the drug before being suppressed. (5.1)
- Convulsions have been observed in patients with or without a history of seizures, epilepsy, cerebrovascular disorders, central nervous system anomalies or tumors, and in patients on concomitant medications that have been associated with convulsions. (5.2)

ADVERSE REACTIONS

- Adverse events related to suppression of endogenous sex steroid secretion may occur with LUPRON DEPOT-PED 7.5 mg, 11.25 mg, or 15 mg for 1-month administration. (6.1, 6.3)
- In clinical studies for LUPRON DEPOT-PED 11.25 mg or 30 mg for 3-month administration, the most frequent (≥ 2 patients) adverse reactions were: injection site pain, weight increased, headache, mood altered, and injection site swelling. (6.2)

To report SUSPECTED ADVERSE REACTIONS, contact AbbVie Inc. at 1-800-633-9110 or FDA at 1-800-FDA-1088 or *www.fda.gov/medwatch*

USE IN SPECIFIC POPULATIONS

- The use of LUPRON DEPOT-PED in children under 2 years is not recommended. (8.4)

See 17 for PATIENT COUNSELING INFORMATION

Revised: 06/2013

FULL PRESCRIBING INFORMATION: CONTENTS*

*** Sections or subsections omitted from the full prescribing information are not listed**

FULL PRESCRIBING INFORMATION

1 INDICATIONS AND USAGE

LUPRON DEPOT-PED is indicated in the treatment of children with central precocious puberty (CPP).

CPP is defined as early onset of secondary sexual characteristics (generally earlier than 8 years of age in girls and 9 years of age in boys) associated with pubertal pituitary gonadotropin activation. It may show a significantly advanced bone age that can result in diminished adult height.

Prior to initiation of treatment a clinical diagnosis of CPP should be confirmed by measurement of blood concentrations of luteinizing hormone (LH) (basal or stimulated with a GnRH analog), sex steroids, and assessment of bone age versus chronological age. Baseline evaluations should include height and weight measurements, diagnostic imaging of the brain (to rule out intracranial tumor), pelvic/testicular/adrenal ultrasound (to rule out steroid secreting tumors), human chorionic gonadotropin levels (to rule out a chorionic gonadotropin secreting tumor), and adrenal steroid measurements to exclude congenital adrenal hyperplasia.

2 DOSAGE AND ADMINISTRATION

2.1 Dose and Principles of Dosing 7.5 mg, 11.25 mg, or 15 mg for 1-month administration

LUPRON DEPOT-PED must be administered under the supervision of a physician.

LUPRON DEPOT-PED is administered as a single intramuscular injection once a month. The starting dose will be dictated by the child's weight, as indicated in the table below.

Table 1. Dosing Recommendations Based on Body Weight for LUPRON DEPOT-PED 1-month Formulations

Body Weight	Recommended Dose
≤ 25 kg	7.5 mg
> 25-37.5 kg	11.25 mg
> 37.5 kg	15 mg

The dose of LUPRON DEPOT-PED must be individualized for each child. If adequate hormonal and clinical suppression is not achieved with the starting dose, it should be increased to the next available higher dose (e.g. 11.25 mg or 15 mg at the next monthly injection). Similarly, the dose may be adjusted with changes in body weight. The injection site should be varied periodically.

The goal of therapy is to suppress pituitary gonadotropins and peripheral sex steroids, and to arrest progression of secondary sexual characteristics. Hormonal and clinical parameters should be monitored after 1–2 months of initiating therapy and with each dose change to ensure adequate pituitary gonadotropin suppression. Once a dose that results in adequate hormonal suppression is found, it can often be maintained for the duration of therapy in most children. It is recommended, however, that adequate hormonal suppression be verified in such patients as weight can increase significantly while on therapy.

Each LUPRON DEPOT-PED strength and formulation has different release characteristics. Do not use partial syringes or a combination of syringes to achieve a particular dose.

LUPRON DEPOT-PED should be discontinued at the appropriate age of onset of puberty at the discretion of the physician.

For optimal performance of the prefilled dual chamber syringe (PDS), read and follow the instructions in Section 2.3.

2.2 Dose and Principles of Dosing 11.25 mg or 30 mg for 3-month administration

LUPRON DEPOT-PED 11.25 mg or 30 mg for 3-month administration must be administered under the supervision of a physician.

LUPRON DEPOT-PED 11.25 mg or 30 mg for 3-month administration should be administered once every three months (12 weeks) as a single intramuscular injection. Regardless of the dose chosen, the goal of therapy is to suppress pituitary gonadotropins and peripheral sex steroids, and to arrest progression of secondary sexual characteristics. Hormonal and clinical parameters should be monitored during treatment, for instance at month 2-3, month 6 and further as judged clinically appropriate, to ensure adequate suppression. In case of inadequate suppression, other available GnRH agonists indicated for the treatment of CPP should be considered.

Each LUPRON DEPOT-PED 11.25 mg or 30 mg for 3-month administration strength and formulation has different release characteristics. Do not use partial syringes or a combination of syringes to achieve a particular dose.

LUPRON DEPOT-PED 11.25 mg or 30 mg for 3-month administration treatment should be discontinued at the appropriate age of onset of puberty at the discretion of the physician.

For optimal performance of the prefilled dual chamber syringe (PDS), read and follow the instructions in Section 2.3.

2.3 Reconstitution and Administration Instructions

- The lyophilized microspheres are to be reconstituted and administered as a single intramuscular injection.
- Since LUPRON DEPOT-PED does not contain a preservative, the suspension should be injected immediately or discarded if not used within two hours.
- As with other drugs administered by injection, the injection site should be varied periodically.

1. The LUPRON DEPOT-PED powder should be visually inspected and the syringe should NOT BE USED if clumping or caking is evident. A thin layer of powder on the wall of the syringe is considered normal prior to mixing with the diluent. The diluent should appear clear.
2. To prepare for injection, screw the white plunger into the end stopper until the stopper begins to turn.

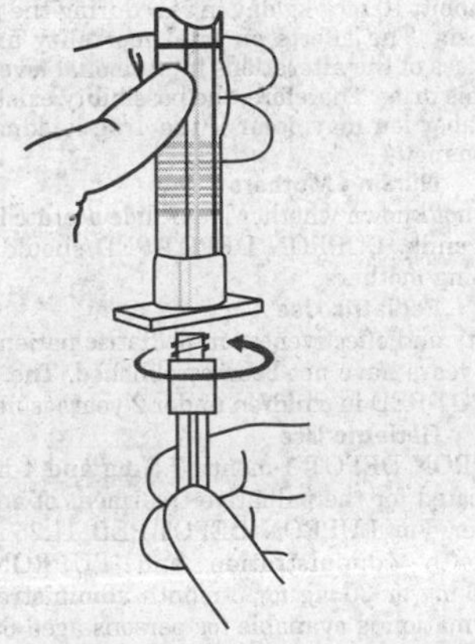

3. Hold the syringe UPRIGHT. Release the diluent by SLOWLY PUSHING (6 to 8 seconds) the plunger until the first stopper is at the blue line in the middle of the barrel.

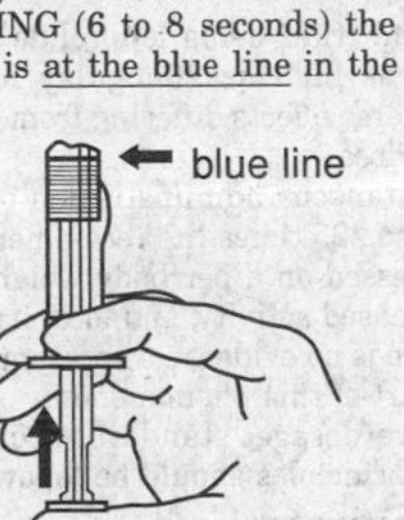

4. Keep the syringe UPRIGHT. Mix the microspheres (powder) thoroughly by gently shaking the syringe until the powder forms a uniform suspension. The suspension will appear milky. If the powder adheres to the stopper or caking/clumping is present, tap the syringe with your finger to disperse. DO NOT USE if any of the powder has not gone into suspension.

[See figure at top of next column]

5. Hold the syringe UPRIGHT. With the opposite hand pull the needle cap upward without twisting.
6. Keep the syringe UPRIGHT. Advance the plunger to expel the air from the syringe.
   Now the syringe is ready for injection.

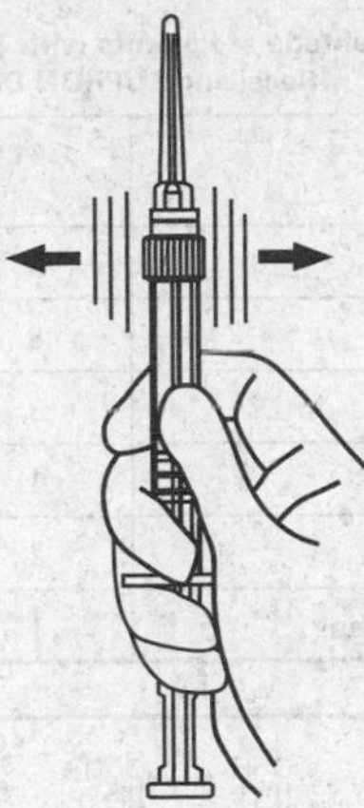

7. After cleaning the injection site with an alcohol swab, the intramuscular injection should be performed by inserting the needle at a 90 degree angle into the gluteal area, anterior thigh, or shoulder; injection sites should be alternated.

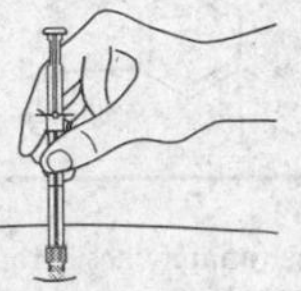

NOTE: Aspirated blood would be visible just below the luer lock connection if a blood vessel is accidentally penetrated. If present, blood can be seen through the transparent LuproLoc® safety device. If blood is present remove the needle immediately. Do not inject the medication.

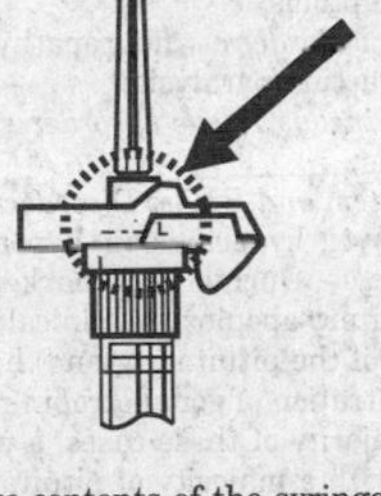

8. Inject the entire contents of the syringe intramuscularly at the time of reconstitution. The suspension settles very quickly following reconstitution; therefore, LUPRON DEPOT-PED should be mixed and used immediately.

AFTER INJECTION

9. Withdraw the needle. Once the syringe has been withdrawn, activate immediately the LuproLoc® safety device by pushing the arrow on the lock upward towards the needle tip with the thumb or finger, as illustrated, until the needle cover of the safety device is fully extended over the needle and a CLICK is heard or felt.

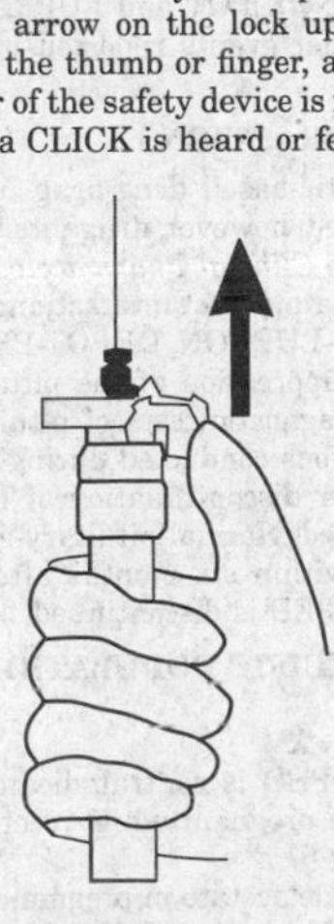

ADDITIONAL INFORMATION

- Dispose of the syringe according to local regulations/procedures.

3 DOSAGE FORMS AND STRENGTHS

LUPRON DEPOT-PED 7.5 mg, 11.25 mg, or 15 mg for 1-month administration and LUPRON DEPOT-PED 11.25 mg or 30 mg for 3-month administration is provided in a prefilled dual chamber syringe for intramuscular injection.

4 CONTRAINDICATIONS

- Hypersensitivity to GnRH, GnRH agonists or any of the excipients in LUPRON DEPOT-PED. Reports of anaphylactic reactions to GnRH agonists have been reported in the medical literature.
- All formulations of LUPRON DEPOT may cause fetal harm if administered to a pregnant woman. When LUPRON DEPOT was administered subcutaneously to rabbits it produced a dose related increase in major fetal abnormalities, and fetal mortality. The possibility exists that spontaneous abortion may occur if the drug is administered during pregnancy. LUPRON DEPOT-PED is contraindicated in women who are or may become pregnant. If this drug is inadvertently used during pregnancy, or if the patient becomes pregnant while taking this drug, the patient should be apprised of the potential hazard to the fetus.

5 WARNINGS AND PRECAUTIONS

5.1 Initial Rise of Gonadotropins and Sex Steroid Levels

During the early phase of therapy, gonadotropins and sex steroids rise above baseline because of the initial stimulatory effect of the drug. Therefore, an increase in clinical signs and symptoms of puberty may be observed *[see Clinical Pharmacology (12.3)]*.

5.2 Convulsions

Postmarketing reports of convulsions have been observed in patients on leuprolide acetate therapy. These included patients with a history of seizures, epilepsy, cerebrovascular disorders, central nervous system anomalies or tumors, and patients on concomitant medications that have been associated with convulsions such as bupropion and SSRIs. Convulsions have also been reported in patients in the absence of any of the conditions mentioned above.

5.3 Monitoring and Laboratory Tests

Response to LUPRON DEPOT-PED 7.5 mg, 11.25 mg, or 15 mg for 1-month administration should be monitored with a GnRHa stimulation test, basal LH or serum concentration of sex steroid levels beginning 1-2 months following initiation of therapy, with changing doses, or potentially during therapy in order to confirm maintenance of efficacy. Measurement of bone age for advancement should be done every 6-12 months.

Response to LUPRON DEPOT-PED 11.25 mg or 30 mg for 3-month administration should be monitored with a GnRHa stimulation test, basal LH or serum concentration of sex steroid levels at months 2-3, month 6 and further as judged clinically appropriate, to ensure adequate suppression. Additionally, height (for calculation of growth rate) and bone age should be assessed every 6-12 months.

Once a therapeutic dose has been established, gonadotropin and sex steroid levels will decline to prepubertal levels. Gonadotropins and/or sex steroids may increase or rise above prepubertal levels if the dose is inadequate. Noncompliance with drug regimen or inadequate dosing may result in inadequate control of the pubertal process with gonadotropins and/or sex steroids increasing above prepubertal levels *[see Clinical Studies (14) and Adverse Reactions (6)]*.

6 ADVERSE REACTIONS

The most common adverse reactions with GnRH agonists including LUPRON DEPOT-PED 7.5 mg, 11.25 mg, or 15 mg for 1-month administration and LUPRON DEPOT-PED 11.25 mg or 30 mg for 3-month administration are injection site reactions/pain including abscess, general pain, headache, emotional lability and hot flushes/sweating.

During the early phase of therapy, gonadotropins and sex steroids rise above baseline because of the initial stimulatory effect of the drug (hormonal flare effect). Therefore, an increase in clinical signs and symptoms of puberty may be observed *[see Warnings and Precautions (5.1)]*.

6.1 LUPRON DEPOT-PED 7.5 mg, 11.25 mg, or 15 mg for 1-month administration - Clinical Trials Experience

Because clinical studies are conducted under widely varying conditions, adverse reaction rates observed in the clinical studies of a drug cannot be directly compared to rates in the clinical studies of another drug and may not reflect the rates observed in practice.

In two studies of children with central precocious puberty, in 2% or more of the patients receiving the drug, the following adverse reactions were reported to have a possible or probable relationship to drug as ascribed by the treating physician. Reactions which are not considered drug-related are excluded.

Information on the AbbVie, Inc. products listed on these pages is from the prescribing information in use as of July 31, 2013. For more information, please visit rxabbvie.com or call 1-800-633-9110.

Table 2. Percentage of Patients with Treatment-Emergent Adverse Reactions Occurring in ≥ 2% of Pediatric Patients Receiving LUPRON DEPOT-PED 1-month

	Number of Patients (N = 421)	
	N	(%)
Body as a Whole		
Injection Site Reactions Including Abscess*	37	(9)
General Pain	12	(3)
Headache	11	(3)
Cardiovascular System		
Vasodilation	9	(2)
Integumentary System (Skin and Appendages)		
Acne/Seborrhea	13	(3)
Rash Including Erythema Multiforme	12	(3)
Nervous System		
Emotional Lability	19	(5)
Urogenital System		
Vaginitis/Vaginal Bleeding/ Vaginal Discharge	13	(3)

* Most events were mild or moderate in severity.

Less Common Adverse Reactions
The following treatment-emergent adverse reactions were reported in less than 2% of the patients and are listed below by body system.
Body as a Whole – aggravation of preexisting tumor and decreased vision, allergic reaction, body odor, fever, flu syndrome, hypertrophy, infection; *Cardiovascular System* – bradycardia, hypertension, peripheral vascular disorder, syncope; *Digestive System* – constipation, dyspepsia, dysphagia, gingivitis, increased appetite, nausea/vomiting; *Endocrine System* – accelerated sexual maturity, feminization, goiter; *Hemic and Lymphatic System* – purpura; *Metabolic and Nutritional Disorders* – growth retarded, peripheral edema, weight gain; *Musculoskeletal System* – arthralgia, joint disorder, myalgia, myopathy; *Nervous System* – depression, hyperkinesia, nervousness, somnolence; *Respiratory System* – asthma, epistaxis, pharyngitis, rhinitis, sinusitis; *Integumentary System (Skin and Appendages)* – alopecia, hair disorder, hirsutism, leukoderma, nail disorder, skin hypertrophy; *Urogenital System* – cervix disorder/ neoplasm, dysmenorrhea, gynecomastia/breast disorders, menstrual disorder, urinary incontinence.
Laboratory: The following laboratory events were reported as adverse reactions: antinuclear antibody present and increased sedimentation rate.

6.2 LUPRON DEPOT-PED 11.25 mg or 30 mg for 3-month administration - Clinical Trials Experience
Because clinical studies are conducted under widely varying conditions, adverse reaction rates observed in the clinical studies of a drug cannot be directly compared to rates in the clinical studies of another drug and may not reflect the rates observed in practice.
[See table 3 above]

Table 3. Percentage of Patients with Treatment-Emergent Adverse Reactions Occurring in ≥ 2 Pediatric Patients Receiving LUPRON DEPOT-PED 11.25 mg or 30 mg for 3-month administration.

	11.25 mg every 3 Months N=42		30 mg every 3 Months N=42		Overall N = 84	
	N	%	N	%	N	%
Injection site pain	8	(19)	9	(21)	17	(20)
Weight increased	3	(7)	3	(7)	6	(7)
Headache	1	(2)	3	(7)	4	(5)
Mood altered	2	(5)	2	(5)	4	(5)
Injection site swelling	1	(2)	1	(2)	2	(2)

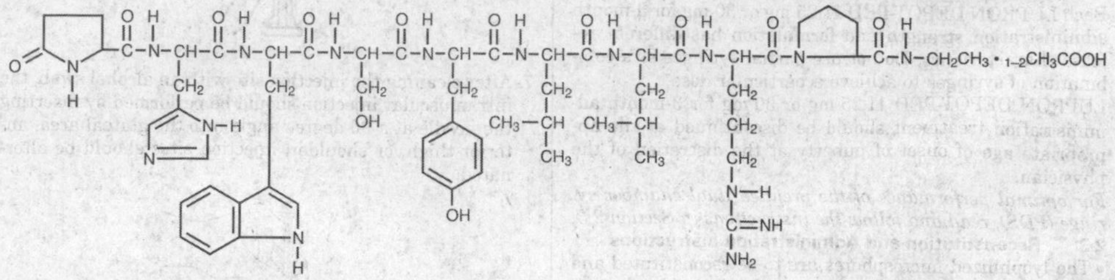

Less Common Adverse Reactions
The following treatment-emergent adverse reactions were reported in one patient and are listed below by system organ class:
Gastrointestinal Disorders – abdominal pain, nausea; *General Disorders and Administration Site Conditions* – asthenia, gait disturbance, injection site abscess sterile, injection site hematoma, injection site induration, injection site warmth, irritability; *Metabolic and Nutritional Disorders* – decreased appetite, obesity; *Musculoskeletal and Connective Tissue Disorders* - musculoskeletal pain, pain in extremity; *Nervous System Disorders* – crying, dizziness; *Psychiatric Disorders* – tearfulness; *Respiratory, Thoracic and Mediastinal Disorders* – cough; *Skin and Subcutaneous Tissue Disorders* – hyperhidrosis; *Vascular Disorders* – pallor.

6.3 Postmarketing
The following adverse events have been observed with this or other formulations of leuprolide acetate injection. As leuprolide has multiple indications, and therefore patient populations, some of these adverse events may not be applicable to every patient.
Allergic reactions (anaphylactic, rash, urticaria, and photosensitivity reactions) have also been reported.
Gastrointestinal Disorders: nausea, abdominal pain, vomiting;
General Disorders and Administration Site Conditions: chest pain, injection site reactions including induration and abscess have been reported;
Investigations: decreased WBC, weight increased;
Metabolism and Nutrition Disorders: diabetes mellitus;
Musculoskeletal and Connective Tissue Disorders: tenosynovitis-like symptoms;
Nervous System Disorders: neuropathy peripheral, convulsion, spinal fracture/paralysis;
Skin and Subcutaneous Tissue Disorders: hot flush, flushing, hyperhidrosis;
Reproductive System and Breast Disorders: prostate pain;
Vascular Disorders: hypertension, hypotension.
Pituitary apoplexy: During post-marketing surveillance, rare cases of pituitary apoplexy (a clinical syndrome secondary to infarction of the pituitary gland) have been reported after the administration of gonadotropin-releasing hormone agonists. In a majority of these cases, a pituitary adenoma was diagnosed, with a majority of pituitary apoplexy cases occurring within 2 weeks of the first dose, and some within the first hour. In these cases, pituitary apoplexy has presented as sudden headache, vomiting, visual changes, ophthalmoplegia, altered mental status, and sometimes cardiovascular collapse. Immediate medical attention has been required.
See other LUPRON DEPOT and LUPRON Injection package inserts for other events reported in different patient populations.

7 DRUG INTERACTIONS

No pharmacokinetic-based drug-drug interaction studies have been conducted; however, drug interactions are not expected to occur *[see Clinical Pharmacology (12.3)]*.

7.1 Drug/Laboratory Test Interactions
Administration of LUPRON DEPOT-PED in therapeutic doses results in suppression of the pituitary-gonadal system. Therefore, diagnostic tests of pituitary gonadotropic and gonadal functions conducted during treatment and up to six months after discontinuation of LUPRON DEPOT-PED may be affected. Normal pituitary-gonadal function is usually restored within six months after treatment with LUPRON DEPOT-PED is discontinued.

8 USE IN SPECIFIC POPULATIONS

8.1 Pregnancy
Pregnancy Category X
LUPRON DEPOT-PED is contraindicated in women who are or may become pregnant while receiving the drug *[see Contraindications (4)]*.
Safe use of leuprolide acetate in pregnancy has not been established in clinical studies. Before starting and during treatment with leuprolide acetate, it is advisable to establish whether the patient is pregnant. Leuprolide acetate is not a contraceptive. If contraception is required, a nonhormonal method of contraception should be used.
When LUPRON DEPOT was administered subcutaneously to groups of rabbits as one time dosing on day 6 of pregnancy at test dosages of 0.00024, 0.0024, and 0.024 mg/kg (1/1900 to 1/19 of the human pediatric dose) it produced a dose-related increase in major fetal abnormalities. Similar studies in rats failed to demonstrate an increase in fetal malformations. There was increased fetal mortality and decreased fetal weights with the two higher doses of LUPRON DEPOT in rabbits and with the highest dose in rats. No fetal malformations but increase in fetal resorptions and mortality were observed in rat and rabbit when the daily injection formulation of leuprolide acetate was dosed subcutaneously once daily at lower doses (0.1-1 mcg/kg/day in rabbit; 10 mcg/kg/day in rat) during the period of organogenesis. The effects on fetal mortality are logical consequences of the alterations in hormonal levels brought about by this drug. Therefore, the possibility exists that spontaneous abortion may occur if the drug is administered during pregnancy.

8.3 Nursing Mothers
It is not known whether leuprolide acetate is excreted in human milk. LUPRON DEPOT-PED should not be used by nursing mothers.

8.4 Pediatric Use
Safety and effectiveness in pediatric patients below the age of 2 years have not been established. The use of LUPRON DEPOT-PED in children under 2 years is not recommended.

8.5 Geriatric Use
LUPRON DEPOT 1-month 7.5 mg and 4-month 30 mg are indicated for the palliative treatment of advanced prostate cancer. For LUPRON DEPOT-PED 11.25 mg or 15 mg for 1-month administration and LUPRON DEPOT-PED 11.25 mg or 30 mg for 3-month administration, no clinical information is available for persons aged 65 and over.

10 OVERDOSAGE

In early clinical trials using leuprolide acetate in adult patients, doses as high as 20 mg/day for up to two years caused no adverse effects differing from those observed with the 1 mg/day dose.
In rats, subcutaneous administration of leuprolide acetate as a single dose 225 times the recommended human pediatric dose, expressed on a per body weight basis, resulted in dyspnea, decreased activity, and local irritation at the injection site. There is no evidence at present that there is a clinical counterpart of this phenomenon.
In cases of overdosage, standard of care monitoring and management principles should be followed.

11 DESCRIPTION

Leuprolide acetate is a synthetic nonapeptide analog of naturally occurring gonadotropin-releasing hormone (GnRH or LH-RH). The analog possesses greater potency than the natural hormone. The chemical name is 5-oxo-L-prolyl-L-histidyl-L-tryptophyl-L-seryl-L-tyrosyl-D-leucyl-L-leucyl-L-arginyl-N-ethyl-L-prolinamide acetate (salt) with the following structural formula:
[See chemical structure above]

LUPRON DEPOT-PED 7.5 mg, 11.25 mg, or 15 mg for 1-month administration
LUPRON DEPOT-PED is available in a prefilled dual-chamber syringe containing sterile lyophilized microspheres which, when mixed with diluent, become a suspension intended as a single intramuscular injection.

The front chamber of LUPRON DEPOT-PED 7.5 mg, 11.25 mg, and 15 mg prefilled dual-chamber syringe contains leuprolide acetate (7.5/11.25/15 mg), purified gelatin (1.3/1.95/2.6 mg), DL-lactic and glycolic acids copolymer (66.2/99.3/132.4 mg), and D-mannitol (13.2/19.8/26.4 mg). The second chamber of diluent contains carboxymethylcellulose sodium (5 mg), D-mannitol (50 mg), polysorbate 80 (1 mg), water for injection, USP, and glacial acetic acid, USP to control pH.

LUPRON DEPOT-PED 11.25 mg or 30 mg for 3-month administration

LUPRON DEPOT-PED 11.25 mg or 30 mg for 3-month administration is available in a prefilled dual-chamber syringe containing sterile lyophilized microspheres which, when mixed with diluent, become a suspension intended as an intramuscular injection to be given **ONCE EVERY THREE MONTHS.**

The front chamber of LUPRON DEPOT-PED 11.25 mg for 3-month administration prefilled dual-chamber syringe contains leuprolide acetate (11.25 mg), polylactic acid (99.3 mg) and D-mannitol (19.45 mg). The second chamber of diluent contains carboxymethylcellulose sodium (7.5 mg), D-mannitol (75.0 mg), polysorbate 80 (1.5 mg), water for injection, USP, and glacial acetic acid, USP to control pH.

The front chamber of LUPRON DEPOT-PED 30 mg for 3-month administration prefilled dual-chamber syringe contains leuprolide acetate (30 mg), polylactic acid (264.8 mg) and D-mannitol (51.9 mg). The second chamber of diluent contains carboxymethylcellulose sodium (7.5 mg), D-mannitol (75.0 mg), polysorbate 80 (1.5 mg), water for injection, USP, and glacial acetic acid, USP to control pH.

12 CLINICAL PHARMACOLOGY

12.1 Mechanism of Action

Leuprolide acetate, a GnRH agonist, acts as a potent inhibitor of gonadotropin secretion when given continuously and in therapeutic doses. Human studies indicate that following an initial stimulation of gonadotropins, chronic stimulation with leuprolide acetate results in suppression or "downregulation" of these hormones and consequent suppression of ovarian and testicular steroidogenesis. These effects are reversible on discontinuation of drug therapy.

Leuprolide acetate is not active when given orally.

12.3 Pharmacokinetics

Absorption

LUPRON DEPOT-PED 7.5 mg, 11.25 mg, or 15 mg for 1-month administration

Following a single LUPRON DEPOT-PED 7.5 mg for 1-month administration to adult patients, mean peak leuprolide plasma concentration was almost 20 ng/mL at 4 hours and then declined to 0.36 ng/mL at 4 weeks. However, intact leuprolide and an inactive major metabolite could not be distinguished by the assay which was employed in the study. Nondetectable leuprolide plasma concentrations have been observed during chronic LUPRON DEPOT-PED 7.5 mg administration, but testosterone levels appear to be maintained at castrate levels.

In a study of 55 children with central precocious puberty, doses of 7.5 mg, 11.25 mg and 15.0 mg of LUPRON DEPOT-PED were given every 4 weeks and in a subset of 22 children, trough leuprolide plasma levels were determined according to weight categories as summarized below:

Patient Weight Range (kg)	Group Weight Average (kg)	Dose (mg)	Trough Plasma Leuprolide Level Mean ±SD (ng/mL)*
20.2 - 27.0	22.7	7.5	0.77±0.033
28.4 - 36.8	32.5	11.25	1.25±1.06
39.3 - 57.5	44.2	15.0	1.59±0.65

* Group average values determined at Week 4 immediately prior to leuprolide injection. Drug levels at 12 and 24 weeks were similar to respective 4 week levels.

LUPRON DEPOT-PED 11.25 mg or 30 mg for 3-month administration

Following a single LUPRON DEPOT-PED 11.25 mg or 30 mg for 3-month administration to children with CPP, leuprolide concentrations increased with increasing dose with mean peak leuprolide plasma concentration of 19.1 and 52.5 ng/mL at 1 hour for the 11.25 and 30 mg dose levels, respectively. The concentrations then declined to 0.08 and 0.25 ng/mL at 2 weeks after dosing for the 11.25 and 30 mg dose levels. Mean leuprolide plasma concentration remained constant from month 1 to month 3 for both 11.25 and 30 mg doses. The mean leuprolide concentrations 3 months after the first and second injections were similar indicating no accumulation of leuprolide from repeated administration.

Distribution

The mean steady-state volume of distribution of leuprolide following intravenous bolus administration to healthy male volunteers was 27 L. *In vitro* binding to human plasma proteins ranged from 43% to 49%.

Metabolism

In healthy male volunteers, a 1 mg bolus of leuprolide administered intravenously revealed that the mean systemic clearance was 7.6 L/h, with a terminal elimination half-life of approximately 3 hours based on a two compartment model.

In rats and dogs, administration of ^{14}C-labeled leuprolide was shown to be metabolized to smaller inactive peptides; a pentapeptide (Metabolite I), tripeptides (Metabolites II and III) and a dipeptide (Metabolite IV). These fragments may be further catabolized.

The major metabolite (M-I) plasma concentrations measured in 5 prostate cancer patients reached maximum concentration 2 to 6 hours after dosing and were approximately 6% of the peak parent drug concentration. One week after dosing, mean plasma M-I concentrations were approximately 20% of mean leuprolide concentrations.

Excretion

Following administration of LUPRON DEPOT 3.75 mg to 3 patients, less than 5% of the dose was recovered as parent and M-I metabolite in the urine.

Specific Populations

The pharmacokinetics of LUPRON DEPOT-PED has not been determined in patients with hepatic or renal impairment.

Drug-Drug Interactions

No pharmacokinetic-based drug-drug interaction studies have been conducted with LUPRON DEPOT-PED. However, because leuprolide acetate is a peptide that is primarily degraded by peptidase and not by cytochrome P-450 enzymes as noted in specific studies, and the drug is only about 46% bound to plasma proteins, drug interactions are not expected to occur.

13 NONCLINICAL TOXICOLOGY

13.1 Carcinogenesis, Mutagenesis, Impairment of Fertility

A two-year carcinogenicity study was conducted in rats and mice. In rats, a dose-related increase of benign pituitary hyperplasia and benign pituitary adenomas was noted at 24 months when the drug was administered subcutaneously at high daily doses (0.6 to 4 mg/kg). There was a significant but not dose-related increase of pancreatic islet-cell adenomas in females and of testicular interstitial cell adenomas in males (highest incidence in the low dose group). In mice, no leuprolide acetate-induced tumors or pituitary abnormalities were observed at a dose as high as 60 mg/kg for two years. Adult patients have been treated with leuprolide acetate for up to three years with doses as high as 10 mg/day and for two years with doses as high as 20 mg/day without demonstrable pituitary abnormalities.

Following subcutaneous administration of LUPRON DEPOT to male and female rats before mating there was atrophy of the reproductive organs and suppression of reproductive performance.

Following a study with leuprolide acetate, immature male rats demonstrated tubular degeneration in the testes even after a recovery period. In spite of the failure to recover histologically, the treated males proved to be as fertile as the controls. Also, no histologic changes were observed in the female rats following the same protocol. In both sexes, the offspring of the treated animals appeared normal. The effect of the treatment of the parents on the reproductive performance of the F1 generation has been evaluated using LUPRON DEPOT formulation to groups of rats as one-time subcutaneous dose of 0.024 mg/kg (1/19 of the pediatric dose) on Day 15 of gestation or dosing on parturition day at doses up to 8 mg/kg (18 fold of the pediatric dose). There was no effect on growth, morphological development and reproductive performance of F1 generation.

14 CLINICAL STUDIES

14.1 LUPRON DEPOT-PED 7.5 mg, 11.25 mg, or 15 mg for 1-month administration

In children with central precocious puberty (CPP), therapeutic doses of LUPRON DEPOT-PED reduce stimulated and basal gonadotropins to prepubertal levels. Testosterone and estradiol are also reduced to prepubertal levels in males and females respectively. Reduction of gonadotropins and sex steroids allow a return to age-appropriate physical and psychological growth and development. The following effects have been noted with the chronic administration of leuprolide: cessation of menses (in girls), normalization and stabilization of linear growth and bone age advancement, stabilization of clinical signs and symptoms of puberty.

55 CPP subjects (49 females and 6 males, naïve to previous GnRHa treatment), were treated with LUPRON DEPOT-PED 1-month formulations until age appropriate for entry into puberty (see treatment period data below) and a subset of 40 subjects were then followed post-treatment (see follow-up period data below).

Treatment Period Data:

During the treatment period, LUPRON DEPOT-PED suppressed gonadotropins and sex steroids to prepubertal levels. Suppression of peak stimulated LH concentrations to < 1.75 mIU/mL was achieved in 96% of subjects by month 1. Five subjects required increased doses of study drug to achieve or retain LH suppression. The number and percentage of subjects with suppression of peak stimulated LH < 1.75 mIU/mL and mean ± SD peak stimulated LH over time is shown in Table 4. The mean ± SD age at the start of treatment was 7 ± 2 years and the duration of treatment was 4 ± 2 years. Six months after the treatment period was finished, the mean peak stimulated LH was 20.6 ± SD 13.7 mIU/mL (n=30).

Table 4. The number and percentage of patients with peak stimulated LH < 1.75 mIU/mL and Mean (SD) peak LH at each clinic visit

Weeks on Study	n with peak stimulated LH < 1.75 mIU/mL/N with a LH measurement for that week		Mean (SD) peak LH
	n/N	%	
Baseline	0/55	0%	35.0 (21.32)
Week 4	53/55	96.4%	0.8 (0.57)
Week 12	48/54	88.9%	1.1 (1.77)
Week 24	48/53	90.6%	0.8 (0.79)
Week 36	51/54	94.4%	0.6 (0.43)
Week 48	51/54	94.4%	0.6 (0.47)
Week 72	52/52	100%	0.5 (0.30)
Week 96	46/46	100%	0.4 (0.33)
Week 120	40/40	100%	0.4 (0.27)
Week 144	36/36	100%	0.4 (0.24)
Week 168	27/28	96.4%	1.2 (4.58)
Week 216	18/19	94.7%	0.5 (0.90)
Week 240	16/17	94.1%	0.4 (0.62)
Week 264	14/15	95.3%	0.4 (0.41)
Week 288	11/11	100%	0.3 (0.22)
Week 312	9/9	100%	0.4 (0.20)
Week 336	6/6	100%	0.3 (0.10)
Week 360	6/6	100%	0.3 (0.13)
Week 384	5/5	100%	0.2 (0.10)
Week 408	3/3	100%	0.2 (0.09)
Week 432	2/2	100%	0.3 (0.04)
Week 456	2/2	100%	0.2 (0.04)
Week 480	1/1	100%	0.2 (NA)
Week 504	1/1	100%	0.2 (NA)

Suppression (defined as regression or no change) of the clinical/physical signs of puberty was achieved in most patients. In females, suppression of breast development ranged from 66.7 to 90.6% of subjects during the first 5 years of treatment. The mean stimulated estradiol was 15.1 pg/mL at baseline, decreased to the lower level of detection (5.0 pg/mL) by Week 4 and was maintained there during the first 5 years of treatment. In males, suppression of genitalia development ranged from 60% to 100% of subjects during the first 5 years of treatment. The mean stimulated testos-

Information on the AbbVie, Inc. products listed on these pages is from the prescribing information in use as of July 31, 2013. For more information, please visit rxabbvie.com or call 1-800-633-9110.

Table 5. Suppression of Peak-Stimulated LH from Month 2 Through Month 6

Parameter	LUPRON DEPOT-PED 11.25 mg every 3 Months			LUPRON DEPOT-PED 30 mg every 3 Months		
	Naïve N = 21	Prev Trt[a] N = 21	Total N = 42	Naïve N = 21	Prev Trt[a] N = 21	Total N = 42
Percent with Suppression	76.2	81.0	78.6	90.5	100	95.2
2-sided 95% CI	52.8, 91.8	58.1, 94.6	63.2, 89.7	69.6, 98.8	83.9, 100	83.8, 99.4

a. Previously treated with GnRHa for at least 6 months prior to enrollment in pivotal Study L-CP07-167.

Figure 1. Mean Peak Stimulated LH for LUPRON DEPOT-PED 11.25 mg for 3-month administration

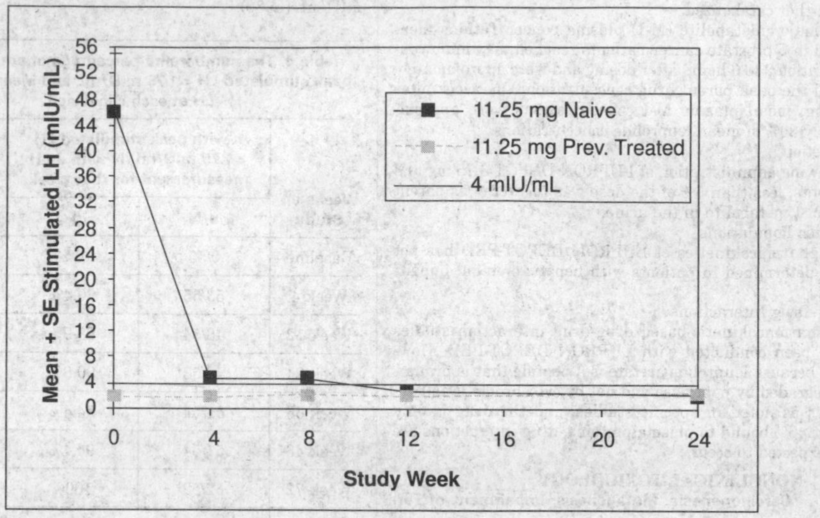

Figure 2. Mean Peak Stimulated LH for LUPRON DEPOT-PED 30 mg for 3-month administration

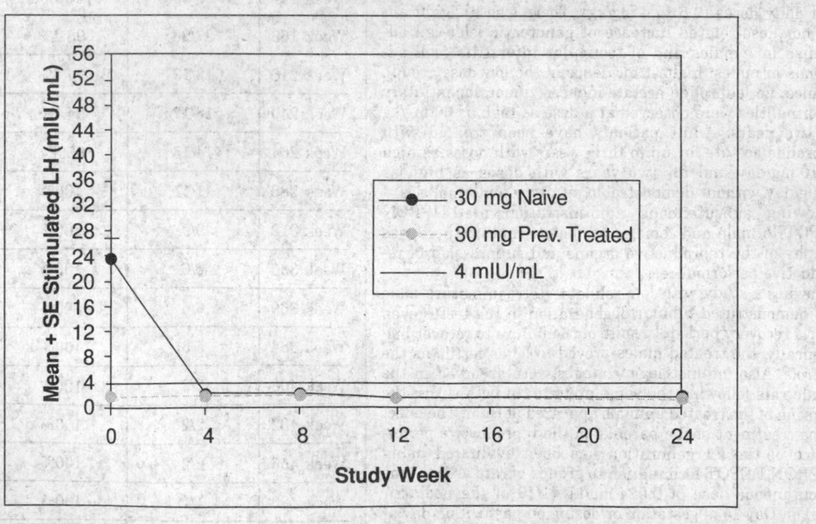

terone was 347.7 ng/dL at baseline and was maintained at levels no greater than 25.3 ng/dL during the first 5 years of treatment.

A "flare effect" of transient bleeding or spotting during the first 4 weeks of treatment was observed in 19.4% (7/36) females who had not reached menarche at baseline. After the first 4 weeks and for the remainder of the treatment period, no subject reported menstrual-like bleeding, and only rare spotting was noted.

In many subjects, growth rate decreased on treatment, as did bone age: chronological age ratio. Through year 5, the mean growth rate ranged between 3.4 and 5.6 cm/yr. The mean ratio of bone age to chronological age decreased from 1.5 at baseline to 1.1 by end of treatment. The mean height standard deviation score changed from 1.6 at baseline to 0.7 at the end of the treatment phase.

Follow-up Period Data:

35 females and 5 males participated in a post-treatment follow-up period to assess reproductive function (in females) and final height. At 6 months post-treatment, most subjects reverted to pubertal levels of LH (87.9%) and clinical signs of resumption of pubertal progression were evident with increase in breast development in girls (66.7%) and increase in genitalia development in boys (80%).

Of the 40 patients evaluated in the follow-up, 33 were observed until they reached final or near-final adult height. These patients had a mean increase in final adult height compared to baseline predicted adult height. The mean final adult height standard deviation score was -0.2.

After stopping treatment, regular menses were reported for all female subjects who reached 12 years of age during follow-up; mean time to menses was approximately 1.5 years; mean age of onset of menstruation after stopping treatment was 12.9 years. Data to assess reproductive function was collected in a post-study survey of 20 girls who reached adulthood (ages 18-26): menstrual cycles were reported to be normal in 80% of women; 12 pregnancies were reported for a total of 7 of the 20 subjects, including multiple pregnancies for 4 subjects.

14.2 LUPRON DEPOT-PED 11.25 mg or 30 mg for 3-month administration

In a randomized, open-label clinical study of LUPRON DEPOT-PED 3-Month formulations, 84 subjects (76 female, 8 male) between 1 and 11 years of age received the LUPRON DEPOT-PED 11.25 mg or 30 mg for 3-month administration formulation. Each dose group had an equal number of treatment-naïve patients who had pubertal LH levels and patients previously treated with GnRHa therapies who had prepubertal LH levels at the time of study entry. The percentage of subjects with suppression of peak-stimulated LH to < 4.0 mIU/mL, as determined by assessments at months 2, 3 and 6 is 78.6% in the 11.25 mg dose and 95.2% in the 30 mg dose as shown in Table 5.

[See table 5 above]

The mean peak stimulated LH levels for all visits are shown by dose and subgroup (naïve vs. previously treated subjects) in Figures 1 and 2.

[See figure 1 above]

[See figure 2 below]

For the LUPRON DEPOT-PED 11.25 mg dose for 3-month administration, 93% (39/42) of subjects and for LUPRON DEPOT-PED 30 mg dose for 3-month administration 100% (42/42) of subjects had sex steroid (estradiol or testosterone) suppressed to prepubertal levels at all visits. Clinical suppression of puberty in female patients was observed in 29 of 32 (90.6%) and 28 of 34 (82.4%) of patients in the 11.25 mg and 30 mg groups, respectively, at month 6. Clinical suppression of puberty in males was observed in 1 of 2 (50.0%) and 2 of 5 (40.0%) patients in the 11.25 mg and 30 mg groups, respectively, at month 6. In subjects with complete data for bone age, 29 of 33 (87.9 %) in the 11.25 mg group and 30 of 40 in the 30 mg group (75.0%) had a decrease in the ratio of bone age to chronological age at month 6 compared to screening.

16 HOW SUPPLIED/STORAGE AND HANDLING

LUPRON DEPOT-PED 7.5 mg, 11.25 mg, or 15 mg for 1-month administration is packaged as follows:

1-month Kit with prefilled dual-chamber syringe	7.5 mg	NDC 0074-2108-03
1-month Kit with prefilled dual-chamber syringe	11.25 mg	NDC 0074-2282-03
1-month Kit with prefilled dual-chamber syringe	15 mg	NDC 0074-2440-03

LUPRON DEPOT-PED 11.25 mg or 30 mg for 3-month administration is packaged as follows:

3-month Kit with prefilled dual-chamber syringe	11.25 mg	NDC 0074-3779-03
3-month Kit with prefilled dual-chamber syringe	30 mg	NDC 0074-9694-03

LUPRON DEPOT-PED prefilled syringe for 1-month administration contains sterile lyophilized microspheres of leuprolide acetate incorporated in a biodegradable lactic acid/glycolic acid copolymer.

LUPRON DEPOT-PED prefilled syringe for 3-month administration contains sterile lyophilized microspheres of leuprolide acetate incorporated in a biodegradable lactic acid polymer.

When mixed with 1 milliliter of accompanying diluent, LUPRON DEPOT-PED for 1-month administration is administered as a single intramuscular injection. When mixed with 1.5 milliliter of accompanying diluent, LUPRON DEPOT-PED for 3-month administration is administered as a single intramuscular injection.

Each kit contains:

- one prefilled dual-chamber syringe containing 1½ inch needle with LuproLoc® safety device
- one plunger
- two alcohol swabs
- population, dose and frequency confirmation insert
- a complete prescribing information enclosure

Store at 25°C (77°F); excursions permitted to 15-30°C (59-86°F) [See USP Controlled Room Temperature]

17 PATIENT COUNSELING INFORMATION

Information for Parents

Prior to starting therapy with LUPRON DEPOT-PED, patients should be informed that:

- All formulations are contraindicated in women who are or may become pregnant. If this drug is used during pregnancy, or if the patient becomes pregnant while taking the drug, the patient should be informed of the potential risk to the fetus.

- Continuous therapy is important and that adherence to the recommended drug administration schedule (monthly for LUPRON DEPOT-PED for 1-month administration and every three months for LUPRON DEPOT-PED for 3-month administration) must be accepted if therapy is to be successful. If the injection schedule is not followed, pubertal development may begin again.
- During the first weeks of treatment, signs of puberty, e.g., vaginal bleeding, may occur. This is a common initial effect of the drug. If these symptoms continue beyond the second month of treatment, the physician should be notified.
- The most common side effects related to treatment with LUPRON DEPOT-PED for 1-month or 3-month administration in clinical studies are: pain, acne/seborrhea, injection site reactions including pain, swelling and abscess, rash including erythema multiforme, vaginitis/bleeding/discharge, increased weight, headache, and altered mood.
- After injection, some pain and irritation is expected; however if more severe symptoms occur, the physician should be contacted. Any unusual signs or symptoms should be reported to the physician.
- The parents should notify the physician if new or worsened symptoms develop after beginning treatment.

Manufactured for
AbbVie Inc.
North Chicago, IL 60064
by Takeda Pharmaceutical Company Limited
Osaka, Japan 540-8645
™ - Trademark
® - Registered Trademark
Ref: 03-A822-R23-Revised: June, 2013

Shown in Product Identification Guide, page 304

MAVIK® ℞

[MAH-vic]
(trandolapril tablets)

> **WARNING: FETAL TOXICITY**
> - **When pregnancy is detected, discontinue MAVIK as soon as possible.**
> - **Drugs that act directly on the renin-angiotensin system can cause injury and death to the developing fetus (See WARNINGS: Fetal Toxicity).**

DESCRIPTION

Trandolapril is the ethyl ester prodrug of a nonsulfhydryl angiotensin converting enzyme (ACE) inhibitor, trandolaprilat. Trandolapril is chemically described as (2S, 3aR, 7aS)-1-[(S)-N-[(S)-1-Carboxy-3-phenylpropyl]alanyl] hexahydro-2-indolinecarboxylic acid, 1-ethyl ester. Its empirical formula is $C_{24}H_{34}N_2O_5$ and its structural formula is

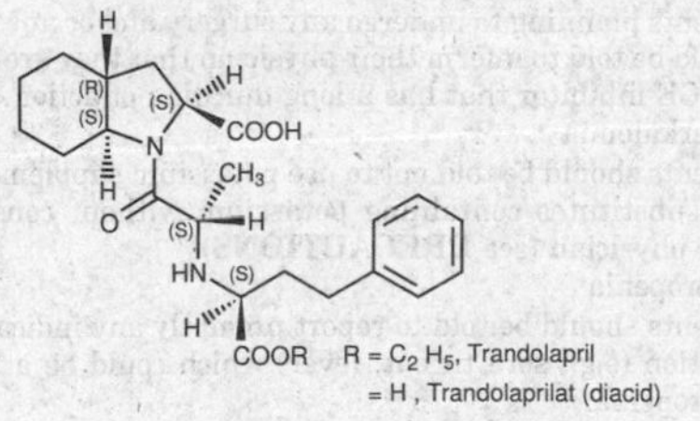

M.W. = 430.54
Melting Point = 125°C
Trandolapril is a white or almost white powder that is soluble (> 100 mg/mL) in chloroform, dichloromethane, and methanol. MAVIK tablets contain 1 mg, 2 mg, or 4 mg of trandolapril for oral administration. Each tablet also contains corn starch, croscarmellose sodium, hypromellose, iron oxide, lactose monohydrate, povidone, sodium stearyl fumarate.

CLINICAL PHARMACOLOGY

Mechanism of Action

Trandolapril is deesterified to the diacid metabolite, trandolaprilat, which is approximately eight times more active as an inhibitor of ACE activity. ACE is a peptidyl dipeptidase that catalyzes the conversion of angiotensin I to the vasoconstrictor, angiotensin II. Angiotensin II is a potent peripheral vasoconstrictor that also stimulates secretion of aldosterone by the adrenal cortex and provides negative feedback for renin secretion. The effect of trandolapril in hypertension appears to result primarily from the inhibition of circulating and tissue ACE activity thereby reducing angiotensin II formation, decreasing vasoconstriction, decreasing aldosterone secretion, and increasing plasma renin. Decreased aldosterone secretion leads to diuresis, natriuresis, and a small increase of serum potassium. In controlled clinical trials, treatment with MAVIK alone resulted in mean increases in potassium of 0.1 mEq/L (see **PRECAUTIONS**.)

ACE is identical to kininase II, an enzyme that degrades bradykinin, a potent peptide vasodilator; whether increased levels of bradykinin play a role in the therapeutic effect of trandolapril remains to be elucidated.

While the principal mechanism of antihypertensive effect is thought to be through the renin-angiotensin-aldosterone system, trandolapril exerts antihypertensive actions even in patients with low-renin hypertension. MAVIK was an effective antihypertensive in all races studied. Both black patients (usually a predominantly low-renin group) and non-black patients responded to 2 to 4 mg of MAVIK.

Pharmacokinetics and Metabolism

Pharmacokinetics

Trandolapril's ACE-inhibiting activity is primarily due to its diacid metabolite, trandolaprilat. Cleavage of the ester group of trandolapril, primarily in the liver, is responsible for conversion. Absolute bioavailability after oral administration of trandolapril is about 10% as trandolapril and 70% as trandolaprilat. After oral trandolapril under fasting conditions, peak trandolapril levels occur at about one hour and peak trandolaprilat levels occur between 4 and 10 hours. The elimination half-life of trandolapril is about 6 hours. At steady state, the effective half-life of trandolaprilat is 22.5 hours. Like all ACE inhibitors, trandolaprilat also has a prolonged terminal elimination phase, involving a small fraction of administered drug, probably representing binding to plasma and tissue ACE. During multiple dosing of trandolapril, there is no significant accumulation of trandolaprilat. Food slows absorption of trandolapril, but does not affect AUC or C_{max} of trandolaprilat or C_{max} of trandolapril.

Metabolism and Excretion

After oral administration of trandolapril, about 33% of parent drug and metabolites are recovered in urine, mostly as trandolaprilat, with about 66% in feces. The extent of the absorbed dose which is biliary excreted has not been determined. Plasma concentrations (C_{max} and AUC of trandolapril and C_{max} of trandolaprilat) are dose proportional over the 1-4 mg range, but the AUC of trandolaprilat is somewhat less than dose proportional. In addition to trandolaprilat, at least 7 other metabolites have been found, principally glucuronides or deesterification products.

Serum protein binding of trandolapril is about 80%, and is independent of concentration. Binding of trandolaprilat is concentration-dependent, varying from 65% at 1000 ng/mL to 94% at 0.1 ng/mL, indicating saturation of binding with increasing concentration.

The volume of distribution of trandolapril is about 18 liters. Total plasma clearances of trandolapril and trandolaprilat after approximately 2 mg IV doses are about 52 liters/hour and 7 liters/hour respectively. Renal clearance of trandolaprilat varies from 1-4 liters/hour, depending on dose.

Special Populations

Pediatric

Trandolapril pharmacokinetics have not been evaluated in patients < 18 years of age.

Geriatric and Gender

Trandolapril pharmacokinetics have been investigated in the elderly (> 65 years) and in both genders. The plasma concentration of trandolapril is increased in elderly hypertensive patients, but the plasma concentration of trandolaprilat and inhibition of ACE activity are similar in elderly and young hypertensive patients. The pharmacokinetics of trandolapril and trandolaprilat and inhibition of ACE activity are similar in male and female elderly hypertensive patients.

Race

Pharmacokinetic differences have not been evaluated in different races.

Renal Insufficiency

Compared to normal subjects, the plasma concentrations of trandolapril and trandolaprilat are approximately 2-fold greater and renal clearance is reduced by about 85% in patients with creatinine clearance below 30 ml/min and in patients on hemodialysis. Dosage adjustment is recommended in renally impaired patients (see **DOSAGE AND ADMINISTRATION**).

Hepatic Insufficiency

Following oral administration in patients with mild to moderate alcoholic cirrhosis, plasma concentrations of trandolapril and trandolaprilat were, respectively, 9-fold and 2-fold greater than in normal subjects, but inhibition of ACE activity was not affected. Lower doses should be considered in patients with hepatic insufficiency (see **DOSAGE AND ADMINISTRATION**).

Drug Interactions

Trandolapril did not affect the plasma concentration (pre-dose and 2 hours post-dose) of oral digoxin (0.25 mg). Coadministration of trandolapril and cimetidine led to an increase of about 44% in C_{max} for trandolapril, but no difference in the pharmacokinetics of trandolaprilat or in ACE inhibition. Coadministration of trandolapril and furosemide led to an increase of about 25% in the renal clearance of trandolaprilat, but no effect was seen on the pharmacokinetics of furosemide or trandolaprilat or on ACE inhibition.

Pharmacodynamics and Clinical Effects

A single 2-mg dose of MAVIK produces 70 to 85% inhibition of plasma ACE activity at 4 hours with about 10% decline at 24 hours and about half the effect manifest at 8 days. Maximum ACE inhibition is achieved with a plasma trandolaprilat concentration of 2 ng/mL. ACE inhibition is a function of trandolaprilat concentration, not trandolapril concentration. The effect of trandolapril on exogenous angiotensin I was not measured.

Hypertension

Four placebo-controlled dose response studies were conducted using once-daily oral dosing of MAVIK in doses from 0.25 to 16 mg per day in 827 black and non-black patients with mild to moderate hypertension. The minimal effective once-daily dose was 1 mg in non-black patients and 2 mg in black patients. Further decreases in trough supine diastolic blood pressure were obtained in non-black patients with higher doses, and no further response was seen with doses above 4 mg (up to 16 mg). The antihypertensive effect diminished somewhat at the end of the dosing interval, but trough/peak ratios are well above 50% for all effective doses. There was a slightly greater effect on the diastolic pressure, but no difference on systolic pressure with b.i.d. dosing. During chronic therapy, the maximum reduction in blood pressure with any dose is achieved within one week. Following 6 weeks of monotherapy in placebo-controlled trials in patients with mild to moderate hypertension, once-daily doses of 2 to 4 mg lowered supine or standing systolic/diastolic blood pressure 24 hours after dosing by an average 7-10/4-5 mmHg below placebo responses in non-black patients. Once-daily doses of 2 to 4 mg lowered blood pressure 4-6/3-4 mmHg in black patients. Trough to peak ratios for effective doses ranged from 0.5 to 0.9. There were no differences in response between men and women, but responses were somewhat greater in patients under 60 than in patients over 60 years old. Abrupt withdrawal of MAVIK has not been associated with a rapid increase in blood pressure. Administration of MAVIK to patients with mild to moderate hypertension results in a reduction of supine, sitting and standing blood pressure to about the same extent without compensatory tachycardia.

Symptomatic hypotension is infrequent, although it can occur in patients who are salt- and/or volume-depleted (see **WARNINGS**). Use of MAVIK in combination with thiazide diuretics gives a blood pressure lowering effect greater than that seen with either agent alone, and the additional effect of trandolapril is similar to the effect of monotherapy.

Heart Failure Post Myocardial Infarction or Left Ventricular Dysfunction Post Myocardial Infarction

The Trandolapril Cardiac Evaluation (TRACE) Trial was a Danish, 27-center, double-blind, placebo controlled, parallel-group study of the effect of trandolapril on all-cause mortality in stable patients with echocardiographic evidence of left ventricular dysfunction 3 to 7 days after a myocardial infarction. Subjects with residual ischemia or overt heart failure were included. Patients tolerant of a test dose of 1 mg trandolapril were randomized to placebo (n=873) or trandolapril (n=876) and followed for 24 months. Among patients randomized to trandolapril, who began treatment on 1 mg, 62% were successfully titrated to a target dose of 4 mg once daily over a period of weeks. The use of trandolapril was associated with a 16% reduction in the risk of all-cause mortality (p=0.042), largely cardiovascular mortality. Trandolapril was also associated with a 20% reduction in the risk of progression of heart failure (p=0.047), defined by a time-to-first-event analysis of death attributed to heart failure, hospitalization for heart failure, or requirement for open-label ACE inhibitor for the treatment of heart failure. There was no significant effect of treatment on other endpoints: subsequent hospitalization, incidence of recurrent myocardial infarction, exercise tolerance, ventricular function, ventricular dimensions, or NYHA class.

The population in TRACE was entirely Caucasian and had less usage than would be typical in a U.S. population of other post-infarction interventions: 42% thrombolysis, 16% beta-adrenergic blockade, and 6.7% PTCA or CABG during the entire period of follow-up. Blood pressure control, especially in the placebo group, was poor: 47 to 53% of patients randomized to placebo and 32 to 40% of patients randomized to trandolapril had blood pressures > 140/95 at 90-day follow up visits.

Information on the AbbVie, Inc. products listed on these pages is from the prescribing information in use as of July 31, 2013. For more information, please visit rxabbvie.com or call 1-800-633-9110.

INDICATIONS AND USAGE

Hypertension

MAVIK is indicated for the treatment of hypertension. It may be used alone or in combination with other antihypertensive medication such as hydrochlorothiazide.

Heart Failure Post Myocardial Infarction or Left-Ventricular Dysfunction Post Myocardial Infarction

MAVIK is indicated in stable patients who have evidence of left-ventricular systolic dysfunction (identified by wall motion abnormalities) or who are symptomatic from congestive heart failure within the first few days after sustaining acute myocardial infarction. Administration of trandolapril to Caucasian patients has been shown to decrease the risk of death (principally cardiovascular death) and to decrease the risk of heart failure-related hospitalization (see **CLINICAL PHARMACOLOGY - Heart Failure or Left-Ventricular Dysfunction Post Myocardial Infarction** for details of the survival trial).

CONTRAINDICATIONS

MAVIK is contraindicated in patients who are hypersensitive to this product, in patients with hereditary/idiopathic angioedema and in patients with a history of angioedema related to previous treatment with an ACE inhibitor.

Do not co-administer aliskiren with MAVIK in patients with diabetes (see **PRECAUTIONS, Drug Interactions**).

WARNINGS

Anaphylactoid and Possibly Related Reactions

Presumably because angiotensin converting enzyme inhibitors affect the metabolism of eicosanoids and polypeptides, including endogenous bradykinin, patients receiving ACE inhibitors, including MAVIK, may be subject to a variety of adverse reactions, some of them serious.

Anaphylactoid Reactions During Desensitization

Two patients undergoing desensitizing treatment with hymenoptera venom while receiving ACE inhibitors sustained life-threatening anaphylactoid reactions. In the same patients, these reactions did not occur when ACE inhibitors were temporarily withheld, but they reappeared when the ACE inhibitors were inadvertently readministered.

Anaphylactoid Reactions During Membrane Exposure

Anaphylactoid reactions have been reported in patients dialyzed with high-flux membranes and treated concomitantly with an ACE inhibitor. Anaphylactoid reactions have also been reported in patients undergoing low-density lipoprotein apheresis with dextran sulfate absorption.

Head and Neck Angioedema

In controlled trials ACE inhibitors (for which adequate data are available) cause a higher rate of angioedema in black than in non-black patients.

Angioedema of the face, extremities, lips, tongue, glottis, and larynx has been reported in patients treated with ACE inhibitors including MAVIK. Symptoms suggestive of angioedema or facial edema occurred in 0.13% of MAVIK-treated patients. Two of the four cases were life-threatening and resolved without treatment or with medication (corticosteroids). Angioedema associated with laryngeal edema can be fatal. If laryngeal stridor or angioedema of the face, tongue or glottis occurs, treatment with MAVIK should be discontinued immediately, the patient treated in accordance with accepted medical care and carefully observed until the swelling disappears. In instances where swelling is confined to the face and lips, the condition generally resolves without treatment; antihistamines may be useful in relieving symptoms. **Where there is involvement of the tongue, glottis, or larynx, likely to cause airway obstruction, emergency therapy, including but not limited to subcutaneous epinephrine solution 1:1,000 (0.3 to 0.5 mL) should be promptly administered** (see **PRECAUTIONS - Information for Patients** and **ADVERSE REACTIONS**).

Intestinal Angioedema

Intestinal angioedema has been reported in patients treated with ACE inhibitors. These patients presented with abdominal pain (with or without nausea or vomiting); in some cases there was no prior history of facial angioedema and C-1 esterase levels were normal. The angioedema was diagnosed by procedures including abdominal CT scan or ultrasound, or at surgery, and symptoms resolved after stopping the ACE inhibitor. Intestinal angioedema should be included in the differential diagnosis of patients on ACE inhibitors presenting with abdominal pain.

Hypotension

MAVIK can cause symptomatic hypotension. Like other ACE inhibitors, MAVIK has only rarely been associated with symptomatic hypotension in uncomplicated hypertensive patients. Symptomatic hypotension is most likely to occur in patients who have been salt- or volume-depleted as a result of prolonged treatment with diuretics, dietary salt restriction, dialysis, diarrhea, or vomiting. Volume and/or salt depletion should be corrected before initiating treatment with MAVIK (see **PRECAUTIONS - Drug Interactions** and **ADVERSE REACTIONS**). In controlled and uncontrolled studies, hypotension was reported as an adverse event in 0.6% of patients and led to discontinuations in 0.1% of patients.

In patients with concomitant congestive heart failure, with or without associated renal insufficiency, ACE inhibitor therapy may cause excessive hypotension, which may be associated with oliguria or azotemia, and rarely, with acute renal failure and death. In such patients, MAVIK therapy should be started at the recommended dose under close medical supervision. These patients should be followed closely during the first 2 weeks of treatment and, thereafter, whenever the dosage of MAVIK or diuretic is increased (see **DOSAGE AND ADMINISTRATION**). Care in avoiding hypotension should also be taken in patients with ischemic heart disease, aortic stenosis, or cerebrovascular disease.

If symptomatic hypotension occurs, the patient should be placed in the supine position and, if necessary, normal saline may be administered intravenously. A transient hypotensive response is not a contraindication to further doses; however, lower doses of MAVIK or reduced concomitant diuretic therapy should be considered.

Neutropenia/Agranulocytosis

Another ACE inhibitor, captopril, has been shown to cause agranulocytosis and bone marrow depression rarely in patients with uncomplicated hypertension, but more frequently in patients with renal impairment, especially if they also have a collagen-vascular disease such as systemic lupus erythematosus or scleroderma. Available data from clinical trials of trandolapril are insufficient to show that trandolapril does not cause agranulocytosis at similar rates. As with other ACE inhibitors, periodic monitoring of white blood cell counts in patients with collagen-vascular disease and/or renal disease should be considered.

Hepatic Failure

ACE inhibitors rarely have been associated with a syndrome of cholestatic jaundice, fulminant hepatic necrosis, and death. The mechanism of this syndrome is not understood. Patients receiving ACE inhibitors who develop jaundice should discontinue the ACE inhibitor and receive appropriate medical follow-up.

Fetal Toxicity

Pregnancy Category D

Use of drugs that act on the renin-angiotensin system during the second and third trimesters of pregnancy reduces fetal renal function and increases fetal and neonatal morbidity and death. Resulting oligohydramnios can be associated with fetal lung hypoplasia and skeletal deformations. Potential neonatal adverse effects include skull hypoplasia, anuria, hypotension, renal failure, and death. When pregnancy is detected, discontinue MAVIK as soon as possible. These adverse outcomes are usually associated with use of these drugs in the second and third trimester of pregnancy. Most epidemiologic studies examining fetal abnormalities after exposure to antihypertensive use in the first trimester have not distinguished drugs affecting the renin-angiotensin system from other antihypertensive agents. Appropriate management of maternal hypertension during pregnancy is important to optimize outcomes for both mother and fetus.

In the unusual case that there is no appropriate alternative to therapy with drugs affecting the renin-angiotensin system for a particular patient, apprise the mother of the potential risk to the fetus. Perform serial ultrasound examinations to assess the intra-amniotic environment. If oligohydramnios is observed, discontinue MAVIK, unless it is considered lifesaving for the mother. Fetal testing may be appropriate, based on the week of pregnancy. Patients and physicians should be aware, however, that oligohydramnios may not appear until after the fetus has sustained irreversible injury. Closely observe infants with histories of *in utero* exposure to MAVIK for hypotension, oliguria, and hyperkalemia (See **PRECAUTIONS, Pediatric Use**).

Doses of 0.8 mg/kg/day (9.4 mg/m^2/day) in rabbits, 1000 mg/kg/day (7000 mg/m^2/day) in rats, and 25 mg/kg/day (295 mg/m^2/day) in cynomolgus monkeys did not produce teratogenic effects. These doses represent 10 and 3 times (rabbits), 1250 and 2564 times (rats), and 312 and 108 times (monkeys) the maximum projected human dose of 4 mg based on body-weight and body-surface-area, respectively assuming a 50 kg woman.

PRECAUTIONS

General

Impaired Renal Function

As a consequence of inhibiting the renin-angiotensin-aldosterone system, changes in renal function may be anticipated in susceptible individuals. In patients with severe heart failure whose renal function may depend on the activity of the renin-angiotensin-aldosterone system, treatment with ACE inhibitors, including MAVIK® (trandolapril), may be associated with oliguria and/or progressive azotemia and rarely with acute renal failure and/or death.

In hypertensive patients with unilateral or bilateral renal artery stenosis, increases in blood urea nitrogen and serum creatinine have been observed in some patients following ACE inhibitor therapy. These increases were almost always reversible upon discontinuation of the ACE inhibitor and/or diuretic therapy. In such patients, renal function should be monitored during the first few weeks of therapy.

Some hypertensive patients with no apparent preexisting renal vascular disease have developed increases in blood urea and serum creatinine, usually minor and transient, especially when ACE inhibitors have been given concomitantly with a diuretic. This is more likely to occur in patients with preexisting renal impairment. Dosage reduction and/or discontinuation of any diuretic and/or the ACE inhibitor may be required. **Evaluation of hypertensive patients should always include assessment of renal function** (see **DOSAGE AND ADMINISTRATION**).

Hyperkalemia and Potassium-sparing Diuretics

In clinical trials, hyperkalemia (serum potassium > 6.00 mEq/L) occurred in approximately 0.4% of hypertensive patients receiving MAVIK. In most cases, elevated serum potassium levels were isolated values, which resolved despite continued therapy. None of these patients were discontinued from the trials because of hyperkalemia. Risk factors for the development of hyperkalemia include renal insufficiency, diabetes mellitus, and the concomitant use of potassium-sparing diuretics, potassium supplements, and/or potassium-containing salt substitutes, which should be used cautiously, if at all, with MAVIK (see **PRECAUTIONS - Drug Interactions**).

Cough

Presumably due to the inhibition of the degradation of endogenous bradykinin, persistent nonproductive cough has been reported with all ACE inhibitors, always resolving after discontinuation of therapy. ACE inhibitor-induced cough should be considered in the differential diagnosis of cough. In controlled trials of trandolapril, cough was present in 2% of trandolapril patients and 0% of patients given placebo. There was no evidence of a relationship to dose.

Surgery/Anesthesia

In patients undergoing major surgery or during anesthesia with agents that produce hypotension, MAVIK will block angiotensin II formation secondary to compensatory renin release. If hypotension occurs and is considered to be due to this mechanism, it can be corrected by volume expansion.

Information for Patients

Angioedema

Angioedema, including laryngeal edema, may occur at any time during treatment with ACE inhibitors, including MAVIK. Patients should be so advised and told to report immediately any signs or symptoms suggesting angioedema (swelling of face, extremities, eyes, lips, tongue, difficulty in swallowing or breathing) and to stop taking the drug until they have consulted with their physician (see **WARNINGS** and **ADVERSE REACTIONS**).

Symptomatic Hypotension

Patients should be cautioned that light-headedness can occur, especially during the first days of MAVIK therapy, and should be reported to a physician. If actual syncope occurs, patients should be told to stop taking the drug until they have consulted with their physician (see **WARNINGS**).

All patients should be cautioned that inadequate fluid intake, excessive perspiration, diarrhea, or vomiting, resulting in reduced fluid volume, may precipitate an excessive fall in blood pressure with the same consequences of light-headedness and possible syncope.

Patients planning to undergo any surgery and/or anesthesia should be told to inform their physician that they are taking an ACE inhibitor that has a long duration of action.

Hyperkalemia

Patients should be told not to use potassium supplements or salt substitutes containing potassium without consulting their physician (see **PRECAUTIONS**).

Neutropenia

Patients should be told to report promptly any indication of infection (e.g., sore throat, fever) which could be a sign of neutropenia.

Pregnancy

Female patients of childbearing age should be told about the consequences of exposure to MAVIK during pregnancy. Discuss treatment options with women planning to become pregnant. Patients should be asked to report pregnancies to their physicians as soon as possible.

NOTE: As with many other drugs, certain advice to patients being treated with MAVIK is warranted. This information is intended to aid in the safe and effective use of this medication. It is not a disclosure of all possible adverse or intended effects.

Drug Interactions

Dual Blockade of the Renin-Angiotensin System (RAS)

Dual blockade of the RAS with angiotensin receptor blockers, ACE inhibitors, or aliskiren is associated with increased risks of hypotension, hyperkalemia, and changes in renal function (including acute renal failure) compared to monotherapy. Closely monitor blood pressure, renal function and electrolytes in patients on MAVIK and other agents that affect the RAS.

Do not co-administer aliskiren with MAVIK in patients with diabetes. Avoid use of aliskiren with MAVIK in patients with renal impairment (GFR <60 ml/min).

Concomitant Diuretic Therapy
As with other ACE inhibitors, patients on diuretics, especially those on recently instituted diuretic therapy, may experience an excessive reduction of blood pressure after initiation of therapy with MAVIK. The possibility of exacerbation of hypotensive effects with MAVIK may be minimized by either discontinuing the diuretic or cautiously increasing salt intake prior to initiation of treatment with MAVIK. If it is not possible to discontinue the diuretic, the starting dose of trandolapril should be reduced (see **DOSAGE AND ADMINISTRATION**).
Agents Increasing Serum Potassium
Trandolapril can attenuate potassium loss caused by thiazide diuretics and increase serum potassium when used alone. Use of potassium-sparing diuretics (spironolactone, triamterene, or amiloride), potassium supplements, or potassium-containing salt substitutes concomitantly with ACE inhibitors can increase the risk of hyperkalemia. If concomitant use of such agents is indicated, they should be used with caution and with appropriate monitoring of serum potassium (see **PRECAUTIONS**).
Antidiabetic Agents
Concomitant use of ACE inhibitors and antidiabetic medicines (insulin or oral hypoglycemic agents) may cause an increased blood glucose lowering effect with greater risk of hypoglycemia.
Lithium
Increased serum lithium levels and symptoms of lithium toxicity have been reported in patients receiving concomitant lithium and ACE inhibitor therapy. These drugs should be coadministered with caution, and frequent monitoring of serum lithium levels is recommended. If a diuretic is also used, the risk of lithium toxicity may be increased.
Non-Steroidal Anti-Inflammatory Agents including Selective Cyclooxygenase-2 Inhibitors (COX-2 Inhibitors)
In patients who are elderly, volume-depleted (including those on diuretic therapy), or with compromised renal function, co-administration of NSAIDs, including selective COX-2 inhibitors, with ACE inhibitors, including trandolapril, may result in deterioration of renal function, including possible acute renal failure. These effects are usually reversible. Monitor renal function periodically in patients receiving trandolapril and NSAID therapy.
The antihypertensive effect of ACE inhibitors, including trandolapril may be attenuated by NSAIDs.
Gold
Nitritoid reactions (symptoms include facial flushing, nausea, vomiting and hypotension) have been reported rarely in patients on therapy with injectable gold (sodium aurothiomalate) and concomitant ACE inhibitor therapy including MAVIK.
Other
No clinically significant pharmacokinetic interaction has been found between trandolaprilat and food, cimetidine, digoxin, or furosemide.
The anticoagulant effect of warfarin was not significantly changed by trandolapril.
The hypotensive effect of certain inhalation anesthetics may be enhanced by ACE inhibitors including trandolapril (see **PRECAUTIONS-Surgery/Anesthesia**).
Carcinogenesis, Mutagenesis, Impairment of Fertility
Long-term studies were conducted with oral trandolapril administered by gavage to mice (78 weeks) and rats (104 and 106 weeks). No evidence of carcinogenic potential was seen in mice dosed up to 25 mg/kg/day (85 mg/m^2/day) or rats dosed up to 8 mg/kg/day (60 mg/m^2/day). These doses are 313 and 32 times (mice), and 100 and 23 times (rats) the maximum recommended human daily dose (MRHDD) of 4 mg based on body-weight and body-surface-area, respectively assuming a 50 kg individual. The genotoxic potential of trandolapril was evaluated in the microbial mutagenicity (Ames) test, the point mutation and chromosome aberration assays in Chinese hamster V79 cells, and the micronucleus test in mice. There was no evidence of mutagenic or clastogenic potential in these *in vitro* and *in vivo* assays.
Reproduction studies in rats did not show any impairment of fertility at doses up to 100 mg/kg/day (710 mg/m^2/day) of trandolapril, or 1250 and 260 times the MRHDD on the basis of body-weight and body-surface-area, respectively.
Nursing Mothers
Radiolabeled trandolapril or its metabolites are secreted in rat milk. MAVIK should not be administered to nursing mothers.
Geriatric Use
In placebo-controlled studies of MAVIK, 31.1% of patients were 60 years and older, 20.1% were 65 years and older, and 2.3% were 75 years and older. No overall differences in effectiveness or safety were observed between these patients and younger patients. (Greater sensitivity of some older individual patients cannot be ruled out).
Pediatric Use
Neonates with a history of *in utero* exposure to MAVIK:
If oliguria or hypotension occurs, direct attention toward support of blood pressure and renal perfusion. Exchange transfusions or dialysis may be required as a means of reversing hypotension and/or substituting for disordered renal function.
The safety and effectiveness of MAVIK in pediatric patients have not been established.

ADVERSE REACTIONS

The safety experience in U.S. placebo-controlled trials included 1069 hypertensive patients, of whom 832 received MAVIK. Nearly 200 hypertensive patients received MAVIK for over one year in open-label trials. In controlled trials, withdrawals for adverse events were 2.1% on placebo and 1.4% on MAVIK. Adverse events considered at least possibly related to treatment occurring in 1% of MAVIK-treated patients and more common on MAVIK than placebo, pooled for all doses, are shown below, together with the frequency of discontinuation of treatment because of these events.

ADVERSE EVENTS IN PLACEBO-CONTROLLED HYPERTENSION TRIALS

	Occurring at 1% or greater MAVIK (N=832) % Incidence (% Discontinuance)	PLACEBO (N=237) % Incidence (% Discontinuance)
Cough	1.9 (0.1)	0.4 (0.4)
Dizziness	1.3 (0.2)	0.4 (0.4)
Diarrhea	1.0 (0.0)	0.4 (0.0)

Headache and fatigue were all seen in more than 1% of MAVIK-treated patients but were more frequently seen on placebo. Adverse events were not usually persistent or difficult to manage.
Left Ventricular Dysfunction Post Myocardial Infarction
Adverse reactions related to MAVIK occurring at a rate greater than that observed in placebo-treated patients with left ventricular dysfunction, are shown below. The incidences represent the experiences from the TRACE study. The follow-up time was between 24 and 50 months for this study.

Percentage of Patients with Adverse Events Greater Than Placebo

Adverse Event	Placebo-Controlled (TRACE) Mortality Study Trandolapril N=876	Placebo N=873
Cough	35	22
Dizziness	23	17
Hypotension	11	6.8
Elevated serum uric acid	15	13
Elevated BUN	9.0	7.6
PICA or CABG	7.3	6.1
Dyspepsia	6.4	6.0
Syncope	5.9	3.3
Hyperkalemia	5.3	2.8
Bradycardia	4.7	4.4
Hypocalcemia	4.7	3.9
Myalgia	4.7	3.1
Elevated creatinine	4.7	2.4
Gastritis	4.2	3.6
Cardiogenic shock	3.8	< 2
Intermittent claudication	3.8	< 2
Stroke	3.3	3.2
Asthenia	3.3	2.6

Clinical adverse experiences possibly or probably related or of uncertain relationship to therapy occurring in 0.3% to 1.0% (except as noted) of the patients treated with MAVIK (with or without concomitant calcium ion antagonist or diuretic) in controlled or uncontrolled trials (N=1134) and less frequent, clinically significant events seen in clinical trials or post-marketing experience include (listed by body system):
General Body Function
Chest pain.
Cardiovascular
AV first degree block, bradycardia, edema, flushing, and palpitations.
Central Nervous System
Drowsiness, insomnia, paresthesia, vertigo.
Dermatologic
Pruritus, rash, pemphigus.
Eye, Ear, Nose, Throat
Epistaxis, throat inflammation, upper respiratory tract infection.
Emotional, Mental, Sexual States
Anxiety, impotence, decreased libido.
Gastrointestinal
Abdominal distention, abdominal pain/cramps, constipation, dyspepsia, diarrhea, vomiting, nausea.
Hemopoietic
Decreased leukocytes, decreased neutrophils.
Metabolism and Endocrine
Increased liver enzymes including SGPT (ALT).
Musculoskeletal System
Extremity pain, muscle cramps, gout.
Pulmonary
Dyspnea.
Postmarketing
The following adverse reactions were identified during post approval use of MAVIK. Because these reactions are reported voluntarily from a population of uncertain size, it is not always possible to reliably estimate their frequency or establish a causal relationship to drug exposure.
General Body Function
Malaise, fever.
Cardiovascular
Myocardial infarction, myocardial ischemia, angina pectoris, cardiac failure, ventricular tachycardia, tachycardia, transient ischemic attack, arrhythmia.
Central Nervous System
Cerebral hemorrhage.
Dermatologic
Alopecia, sweating, Stevens-Johnson syndrome and toxic epidermal necrolysis.
Emotional, Mental, Sexual States
Hallucination, depression.
Gastrointestinal
Dry mouth, pancreatitis, jaundice and hepatitis.
Hemopoietic
Agranulocytosis, pancytopenia.
Metabolism and Endocrine
Increased SGOT (AST).
Pulmonary
Bronchitis.
Renal and Urinary
Renal failure.
Clinical Laboratory Test Findings
Hematology
Thrombocytopenia.
Serum Electrolytes
Hyponatremia.
Creatinine and Blood Urea Nitrogen
Increases in creatinine levels occurred in 1.1% of patients receiving MAVIK alone and 7.3% of patients treated with MAVIK, a calcium ion antagonist and a diuretic. Increases in blood urea nitrogen levels occurred in 0.6% of patients receiving MAVIK alone and 1.4% of patients receiving MAVIK, a calcium ion antagonist, and a diuretic. None of these increases required discontinuation of treatment. Increases in these laboratory values are more likely to occur in patients with renal insufficiency or those pretreated with a diuretic and, based on experience with other ACE inhibitors, would be expected to be especially likely in patients with renal artery stenosis (see **PRECAUTIONS** and **WARNINGS**).
Liver Function Tests
Occasional elevation of transaminases at the rate of 3X upper normals occurred in 0.8% of patients and persistent increase in bilirubin occurred in 0.2% of patients. Discontinuation for elevated liver enzymes occurred in 0.2% of patients.
Other
Another potentially important adverse experience, eosinophilic pneumonitis, has been attributed to other ACE inhibitors.

OVERDOSAGE

No data are available with respect to overdosage in humans. The oral LD_{50} of trandolapril in mice was 4875 mg/Kg in males and 3990 mg/Kg in females. In rats, an oral dose of 5000 mg/Kg caused low mortality (1 male out of 5; 0 females). In dogs, an oral dose of 1000 mg/Kg did not cause mortality and abnormal clinical signs were not observed. In humans, the most likely clinical manifestation would be symptoms attributable to severe hypotension. Symptoms also expected with ACE inhibitors are hypotension, hyperkalemia, and renal failure.
Laboratory determinations of serum levels of trandolapril and its metabolites are not widely available, and such determinations have, in any event, no established role in the management of trandolapril overdose. No data are available to suggest that physiological maneuvers (e.g., maneuvers to change the pH of the urine) might accelerate elimination of trandolapril and its metabolites. Trandolaprilat is removed by hemodialysis. Angiotensin II could presumably serve as a specific antagonist antidote in the setting of trandolapril overdose, but angiotensin II is essentially unavailable outside of scattered research facilities. Because the hypotensive effect of trandolapril is achieved through vasodilation

Information on the AbbVie, Inc. products listed on these pages is from the prescribing information in use as of July 31, 2013. For more information, please visit rxabbvie.com or call 1-800-633-9110.

and effective hypovolemia, it is reasonable to treat trandolapril overdose by infusion of normal saline solution.

DOSAGE AND ADMINISTRATION

Hypertension

The recommended initial dosage of MAVIK for patients not receiving a diuretic is 1 mg once daily in non-black patients and 2 mg in black patients. Dosage should be adjusted according to the blood pressure response. Generally, dosage adjustments should be made at intervals of at least 1 week. Most patients have required dosages of 2 to 4 mg once daily. There is little clinical experience with doses above 8 mg.

Patients inadequately treated with once-daily dosing at 4 mg may be treated with twice-daily dosing. If blood pressure is not adequately controlled with MAVIK monotherapy, a diuretic may be added.

In patients who are currently being treated with a diuretic, symptomatic hypotension occasionally can occur following the initial dose of MAVIK. To reduce the likelihood of hypotension, the diuretic should, if possible, be discontinued two to three days prior to beginning therapy with MAVIK (see **WARNINGS**). Then, if blood pressure is not controlled with MAVIK alone, diuretic therapy should be resumed. If the diuretic cannot be discontinued, an initial dose of 0.5 mg MAVIK should be used with careful medical supervision for several hours until blood pressure has stabilized. The dosage should subsequently be titrated (as described above) to the optimal response (see **WARNINGS, PRECAUTIONS**, and **DRUG INTERACTIONS**).

Concomitant administration of MAVIK with potassium supplements, potassium salt substitutes, or potassium sparing diuretics can lead to increases of serum potassium (see **PRECAUTIONS**).

Heart Failure Post Myocardial Infarction or Left-Ventricular Dysfunction Post Myocardial Infarction

The recommended starting dose is 1 mg, once daily. Following the initial dose, all patients should be titrated (as tolerated) toward a target dose of 4 mg, once daily. If a 4 mg dose is not tolerated, patients can continue therapy with the greatest tolerated dose.

Dosage Adjustment in Renal Impairment or Hepatic Cirrhosis

For patients with a creatinine clearance < 30 mL/min. or with hepatic cirrhosis, the recommended starting dose, based on clinical and pharmacokinetic data, is 0.5 mg daily. Patients should subsequently have their dosage titrated (as described above) to the optimal response.

HOW SUPPLIED

MAVIK® (trandolapril tablets) are supplied as follows:

1 mg tablet - Salmon colored, round shaped, scored, compressed tablets, with the "a" logo on one side and code identification letters FT on the other side. NDC 0074-2278-13 - bottles of 100 NDC 0074-2278-11 - unit dose packs of 100

2 mg tablet - Yellow colored, round shaped, compressed tablets, with the "a" logo on one side and code identification letters FX on the other side. NDC 0074-2279-13 - bottles of 100 NDC 0074-2279-11 - unit dose packs of 100

4 mg tablet - Rose colored, round shaped, compressed tablets, with the "a" logo on one side and code identification letters FZ on the other side. NDC 0074-2280-13 - bottles of 100 NDC 0074-2280-11 - unit dose packs of 100

Dispense in well-closed container with safety closure.

Storage

Store at controlled room temperature: 20-25°C (68-77°F) see USP.

Manufactured by
Halo Pharmaceutical Inc.
Whippany, N.J. 07981, U.S.A.
for
AbbVie Inc.
North Chicago, IL 60064, U.S.A.
03-A670 December 2012

Shown in Product Identification Guide, page 304

NIASPAN® TABLETS ℞

[*ny-a-span*]

(niacin extended-release)

tablet, film coated, extended release for oral use.

HIGHLIGHTS OF PRESCRIBING INFORMATION

These highlights do not include all the information needed to use NIASPAN® safely and effectively. See full prescribing information for NIASPAN.

NIASPAN (niacin extended-release) tablet, film coated, extended release for oral use.

Initial U.S. Approval: 1997

RECENT MAJOR CHANGES

Indications and Usage: Limitations of Use (1)	02/2013
Warnings and Precautions, Mortality and Coronary Heart Disease Morbidity (5.1)	02/2013

INDICATIONS AND USAGE

NIASPAN contains extended-release niacin (nicotinic acid), and is indicated:

- To reduce elevated TC, LDL-C, Apo B and TG, and to increase HDL-C in patients with primary hyperlipidemia and mixed dyslipidemia. (1)
- In combination with simvastatin or lovastatin: to treat primary hyperlipidemia and mixed dyslipidemia when treatment with NIASPAN, simvastatin, or lovastatin monotherapy is considered inadequate. (1)
- To reduce the risk of recurrent nonfatal myocardial infarction in patients with a history of myocardial infarction and hyperlipidemia. (1)
- In combination with a bile acid binding resin:
  - Slows progression or promotes regression of atherosclerotic disease in patients with a history of coronary artery disease (CAD) and hyperlipidemia. (1)
  - As an adjunct to diet to reduce elevated TC and LDL-C in adult patients with primary hyperlipidemia. (1)
- To reduce TG in adult patients with severe hypertriglyceridemia (1)

Limitations of use:

No incremental benefit of NIASPAN coadministered with simvastatin or lovastatin on cardiovascular morbidity and mortality over and above that demonstrated for niacin, simvastatin and lovastatin monotherapy, has been established. NIASPAN, at doses of 1,500-2,000 mg/day, in combination with simvastatin, did not reduce the incidence of cardiovascular events more than simvastatin in a randomized controlled trial of patients with cardiovascular disease and mean baseline LDL-C levels of 74 mg per deciliter (5.1).

DOSAGE AND ADMINISTRATION

- NIASPAN should be taken at bedtime with a low-fat snack. (2)
- Dose range: 500 mg to 2000 mg once daily. (2)
- Therapy with NIASPAN must be initiated at 500 mg at bedtime in order to reduce the incidence and severity of side effects which may occur during early therapy and should not be increased by more than 500 mg in any four week period. (2)
- Maintenance dose: 1000 to 2000 mg once daily. (2)
- Doses greater than 2000 mg daily are not recommended. (2)
- Concomitant therapy with lovastatin: Initial dose of lovastatin is 20 mg once a day; combination therapy with NIASPAN and lovastatin should not exceed doses of 2000 mg and 40 mg daily, respectively. (2)
- Concomitant therapy with simvastatin: Initial dose of simvastatin is 20 mg once a day; combination therapy with NIASPAN and simvastatin should not exceed doses of 2000 mg and 40 mg daily, respectively. (2)

DOSAGE FORMS AND STRENGTHS

Unscored film-coated tablets for oral administration: 500, 750 and 1000 mg niacin extended-release. (3)

CONTRAINDICATIONS

- Active liver disease, which may include unexplained persistent elevations in hepatic transaminase levels. (4, 5.3)
- Active peptic ulcer disease. (4)
- Arterial bleeding. (4)
- Known hypersensitivity to product components. (4, 6.1)

WARNINGS AND PRECAUTIONS

- Severe hepatic toxicity has occurred in patients substituting sustained-release niacin for immediate-release niacin at equivalent doses. (5.3)
- Myopathy has been reported in patients taking NIASPAN. The risk for myopathy and rhabdomyolysis are increased when lovastatin or simvastatin are coadministered with NIASPAN, particularly in elderly patients and patients with diabetes, renal failure, or uncontrolled hypothyroidism. (5.2)
- Liver enzyme abnormalities and monitoring: Persistent elevations in hepatic transaminase can occur. Monitor liver enzymes before and during treatment. (5.3)
- Use with caution in patients with unstable angina or in the acute phase of an MI. (5)
- NIASPAN can increase serum glucose levels. Glucose levels should be closely monitored in diabetic or potentially diabetic patients particularly during the first few months of use or dose adjustment. (5.4)

ADVERSE REACTIONS

Most common adverse reactions (incidence >5% and greater than placebo) are flushing, diarrhea, nausea, vomiting, increased cough, and pruritus. (6.1)

Flushing of the skin may be reduced in frequency or severity by pretreatment with aspirin (up to the recommended dose of 325 mg taken 30 minutes prior to NIASPAN dose). (2)

To report SUSPECTED ADVERSE REACTIONS, contact AbbVie Inc. at 1-800-633-9110 or FDA at 1-800-FDA-1088 or www.fda.gov/medwatch.

DRUG INTERACTIONS

- Statins: Caution should be used when prescribing niacin with statins as these agents can increase risk of myopathy/rhabdomyolysis. (5.2, 7.1)
- Bile Acid Sequestrants: Bile acid sequestrants have a high niacin-binding capacity and should be taken at least 4 - 6 hours before NIASPAN administration. (7.2)

USE IN SPECIFIC POPULATIONS

- Renal impairment: NIASPAN should be used with caution in patients with renal impairment. (5, 8.6)
- Hepatic impairment: NIASPAN is contraindicated in active liver disease or significant or unexplained hepatic dysfunction or unexplained elevations of serum transaminases. (4,5, 5.3, 8.7)

See 17 for PATIENT COUNSELING INFORMATION and FDA-approved patient labeling

Revised: 03/2013

FULL PRESCRIBING INFORMATION: CONTENTS*

* Sections or subsections omitted from the full prescribing information are not listed

FULL PRESCRIBING INFORMATION

1 INDICATIONS AND USAGE

Therapy with lipid-altering agents should be only one component of multiple risk factor intervention in individuals at significantly increased risk for atherosclerotic vascular disease due to hyperlipidemia. Niacin therapy is indicated as an adjunct to diet when the response to a diet restricted in saturated fat and cholesterol and other nonpharmacologic measures alone has been inadequate.

1. NIASPAN is indicated to reduce elevated TC, LDL-C, Apo B and TG levels, and to increase HDL-C in patients with primary hyperlipidemia and mixed dyslipidemia.
2. NIASPAN in combination with simvastatin or lovastatin is indicated for the treatment of primary hyperlipidemia and mixed dyslipidemia when treatment with NIASPAN, simvastatin, or lovastatin monotherapy is considered inadequate.
3. In patients with a history of myocardial infarction and hyperlipidemia, niacin is indicated to reduce the risk of recurrent nonfatal myocardial infarction.
4. In patients with a history of coronary artery disease (CAD) and hyperlipidemia, niacin, in combination with a bile acid binding resin, is indicated to slow progression or promote regression of atherosclerotic disease.
5. NIASPAN in combination with a bile acid binding resin is indicated to reduce elevated TC and LDL-C levels in adult patients with primary hyperlipidemia.
6. Niacin is also indicated as adjunctive therapy for treatment of adult patients with severe hypertriglyceridemia who present a risk of pancreatitis and who do not respond adequately to a determined dietary effort to control them.

Limitations of Use
No incremental benefit of NIASPAN coadministered with simvastatin or lovastatin on cardiovascular morbidity and mortality over and above that demonstrated for niacin, simvastatin, or lovastatin monotherapy has been established.
NIASPAN, at doses of 1,500-2,000 mg/day, in combination with simvastatin, did not reduce the incidence of cardiovascular events more than simvastatin in a randomized controlled trial of patients with cardiovascular disease and mean baseline LDL-C levels of 74 mg per deciliter *[see Warnings and Precautions (5.1)]*.

2 DOSAGE AND ADMINISTRATION

NIASPAN should be taken at bedtime, after a low-fat snack, and doses should be individualized according to patient response. Therapy with NIASPAN must be initiated at 500 mg at bedtime in order to reduce the incidence and severity of side effects which may occur during early therapy. The recommended dose escalation is shown in Table 1 below.

Table 1. Recommended Dosing

	Week(s)	Daily dose	NIASPAN Dosage
INITIAL TITRATION SCHEDULE	1 to 4	500 mg	1 NIASPAN 500 mg tablet at bedtime
	5 to 8	1000 mg	1 NIASPAN 1000 mg tablet or 2 NIASPAN 500 mg tablets at bedtime
	*	1500 mg	2 NIASPAN 750 mg tablets or 3 NIASPAN 500 mg tablets at bedtime
	*	2000 mg	2 NIASPAN 1000 mg tablets or 4 NIASPAN 500 mg tablets at bedtime

* After Week 8, titrate to patient response and tolerance. If response to 1000 mg daily is inadequate, increase dose to 1500 mg daily; may subsequently increase dose to 2000 mg daily. Daily dose should not be increased more than 500 mg in a 4-week period, and doses above 2000 mg daily are not recommended. Women may respond at lower doses than men.

[See table 1 above]

Maintenance Dose

The daily dosage of NIASPAN should not be increased by more than 500 mg in any 4-week period. The recommended maintenance dose is 1000 mg (two 500 mg tablets or one 1000 mg tablet) to 2000 mg (two 1000 mg tablets or four 500 mg tablets) once daily at bedtime. Doses greater than 2000 mg daily are not recommended. Women may respond at lower NIASPAN doses than men *[see Clinical Studies (14.2)]*.
Single-dose bioavailability studies have demonstrated that two of the 500 mg and one of the 1000 mg tablet strengths are interchangeable but three of the 500 mg and two of the 750 mg tablet strengths are not interchangeable.
If lipid response to NIASPAN alone is insufficient or if higher doses of NIASPAN are not well tolerated, some patients may benefit from combination therapy with a bile acid binding resin or statin *[see Drug Interactions (7.3), Concomitant Therapy* below and *Clinical Studies (14.3, 14.4)]*.
Flushing of the skin *[see Adverse Reactions (6.1)]* may be reduced in frequency or severity by pretreatment with aspirin (up to the recommended dose of 325 mg taken 30 minutes prior to NIASPAN dose). Tolerance to this flushing develops rapidly over the course of several weeks. Flushing, pruritus, and gastrointestinal distress are also greatly reduced by slowly increasing the dose of niacin and avoiding administration on an empty stomach. Concomitant alcoholic, hot drinks or spicy foods may increase the side effects of flushing and pruritus and should be avoided around the time of NIASPAN ingestion.
Equivalent doses of NIASPAN should not be substituted for sustained-release (modified-release, timed-release) niacin preparations or immediate-release (crystalline) niacin *[see Warnings and Precautions (5)]*. Patients previously receiving other niacin products should be started with the recommended NIASPAN titration schedule (see Table 1), and the dose should subsequently be individualized based on patient response.
If NIASPAN therapy is discontinued for an extended period, reinstitution of therapy should include a titration phase (see Table 1).
NIASPAN tablets should be taken whole and should not be broken, crushed or chewed before swallowing.

Concomitant Therapy

Concomitant Therapy with Lovastatin or Simvastatin
Patients already receiving a stable dose of lovastatin or simvastatin who require further TG-lowering or HDL-raising (e.g., to achieve NCEP non-HDL-C goals), may receive concomitant dosage titration with NIASPAN per NIASPAN recommended initial titration schedule *[see Dosage and Administration (2)]*. For patients already receiving a stable dose of NIASPAN who require further LDL-lowering (e.g., to achieve NCEP LDL-C goals), the usual recommended starting dose of lovastatin and simvastatin is 20 mg once a day. Dose adjustments should be made at intervals of 4 weeks or more. Combination therapy with NIASPAN and lovastatin or NIASPAN and simvastatin should not exceed doses of 2000 mg NIASPAN and 40 mg lovastatin or simvastatin daily.
Dosage in Patients with Renal or Hepatic Impairment
Use of NIASPAN in patients with renal or hepatic impairment has not been studied. NIASPAN is contraindicated in patients with significant or unexplained hepatic dysfunction. NIASPAN should be used with caution in patients with renal impairment *[see Warnings and Precautions (5)]*.

3 DOSAGE FORMS AND STRENGTHS

- 500 mg unscored, medium-orange, film-coated, capsule-shaped tablets
- 750 mg unscored, medium-orange, film-coated, capsule-shaped tablets
- 1000 mg unscored, medium-orange, film-coated, capsule-shaped tablets

4 CONTRAINDICATIONS

NIASPAN is contraindicated in the following conditions:
- Active liver disease or unexplained persistent elevations in hepatic transaminases *[see Warnings and Precautions (5.3)]*
- Patients with active peptic ulcer disease
- Patients with arterial bleeding
- Hypersensitivity to niacin or any component of this medication *[see Adverse Reactions (6.1)]*

5 WARNINGS AND PRECAUTIONS

NIASPAN preparations should not be substituted for equivalent doses of immediate-release (crystalline) niacin. For patients switching from immediate-release niacin to NIASPAN, therapy with NIASPAN should be initiated with low doses (i.e., 500 mg at bedtime) and the NIASPAN dose should then be titrated to the desired therapeutic response *[see Dosage and Administration (2)]*.
Caution should also be used when NIASPAN is used in patients with unstable angina or in the acute phase of an MI, particularly when such patients are also receiving vasoactive drugs such as nitrates, calcium channel blockers, or adrenergic blocking agents.
Niacin is rapidly metabolized by the liver, and excreted through the kidneys. NIASPAN is contraindicated in patients with significant or unexplained hepatic impairment *[see Contraindications (4) and Warnings and Precautions (5.3)]* and should be used with caution in patients with renal impairment. Patients with a past history of jaundice, hepatobiliary disease, or peptic ulcer should be observed closely during NIASPAN therapy.

5.1 Mortality and Coronary Heart Disease Morbidity

The Atherothrombosis Intervention in Metabolic Syndrome with Low HDL/High Triglycerides: Impact on Global Health Outcomes (AIM-HIGH) trial was a randomized placebo-controlled trial of 3414 patients with stable, previously diagnosed cardiovascular disease. Mean baseline lipid levels were LDL-C 74 mg/dL, HDL-C 35 mg/dL, non-HDL-C 111 mg/dL and median triglyceride level of 163-177 mg/dL. Ninety-four percent of patients were on background statin therapy prior to entering the trial. All participants received simvastatin, 40 to 80 mg per day, plus ezetimibe 10 mg per day if needed, to maintain an LDL-C level of 40-80 mg/dL, and were randomized to receive NIASPAN 1500-2000 mg/day (n=1718) or matching placebo (IR Niacin, 100-150 mg, n=1696). On-treatment lipid changes at two years for LDL-C were -12.0% for the simvastatin plus NIASPAN group and -5.5% for the simvastatin plus placebo group. HDL-C increased by 25.0% to 42 mg/dL in the simvastatin plus NIASPAN group and by 9.8% to 38 mg/dL in the simvastatin plus placebo group (P<0.001). Triglyceride levels decreased by 28.6% in the simvastatin plus NIASPAN group and by 8.1% in the simvastatin plus placebo group. The primary outcome was an ITT composite of the first study occurrence of coronary heart disease death, nonfatal myocardial infarction, ischemic stroke, hospitalization for acute coronary syndrome or symptom-driven coronary or cerebral revascularization procedures. The trial was stopped after a mean follow-up period of 3 years owing to a lack of efficacy. The primary outcome occurred in 282 patients in the simvastatin plus NIASPAN group (16.4%) and in 274 patients in the simvastatin plus placebo group (16.2%) (HR 1.02 [95% CI, 0.87-1.21], P=0.79. In an ITT analysis, there were 42 cases of first occurrence of ischemic stroke reported, 27 (1.6%) in the simvastatin plus NIASPAN group and 15 (0.9%) in the simvastatin plus placebo group, a non-statistically significant result (HR 1.79, [95%CI = 0.95-3.36], p=0.071). The on-treatment ischemic stroke events were 19 for the simvastatin plus NIASPAN group and 15 for the simvastatin plus placebo group *[see Adverse Reactions (6.1)]*.

5.2 Skeletal Muscle

Cases of rhabdomyolysis have been associated with concomitant administration of lipid-altering doses (≥1 g/day) of niacin and statins. Physicians contemplating combined therapy with statins and NIASPAN should carefully weigh the potential benefits and risks and should carefully monitor patients for any signs and symptoms of muscle pain, tenderness, or weakness, particularly during the initial months of therapy and during any periods of upward dosage titration of either drug. Periodic serum creatine phosphokinase (CPK) and potassium determinations should be considered in such situations, but there is no assurance that such monitoring will prevent the occurrence of severe myopathy.
The risk for myopathy and rhabdomyolysis are increased when lovastatin or simvastatin are coadministered with NIASPAN, particularly in elderly patients and patients with diabetes, renal failure, or uncontrolled hypothyroidism.

5.3 Liver Dysfunction

Cases of severe hepatic toxicity, including fulminant hepatic necrosis, have occurred in patients who have substituted sustained-release (modified-release, timed-release) niacin products for immediate-release (crystalline) niacin at equivalent doses.
NIASPAN should be used with caution in patients who consume substantial quantities of alcohol and/or have a past history of liver disease. Active liver diseases or unexplained transaminase elevations are contraindications to the use of NIASPAN.
Niacin preparations have been associated with abnormal liver tests. In three placebo-controlled clinical trials involving titration to final daily NIASPAN doses ranging from 500 to 3000 mg, 245 patients received NIASPAN for a mean duration of 17 weeks. No patient with normal serum transaminase levels (AST, ALT) at baseline experienced elevations to more than 3 times the upper limit of normal (ULN) during treatment with NIASPAN. In these studies, fewer than 1% (2/245) of NIASPAN patients discontinued due to transaminase elevations greater than 2 times the ULN.
In three safety and efficacy studies with a combination tablet of NIASPAN and lovastatin involving titration to final daily doses (expressed as mg of niacin/ mg of lovastatin) 500 mg/10 mg to 2500 mg/40 mg, ten of 1028 patients (1.0%) experienced reversible elevations in AST/ALT to more than 3 times the ULN. Three of ten elevations occurred at doses outside the recommended dosing limit of 2000 mg/40 mg; no patient receiving 1000 mg/20 mg had 3-fold elevations in AST/ALT.
Niacin extended-release and simvastatin can cause abnormal liver tests. In a simvastatin-controlled, 24 week study with a fixed dose combination of NIASPAN and simvastatin in 641 patients, there were no persistent increases (more than 3× the ULN) in serum transaminases. In three placebo-controlled clinical studies of extended-release niacin there were no patients with normal serum transaminase levels at baseline who experienced elevations to more than 3× the ULN. Persistent increases (more than 3× the ULN) in serum transaminases have occurred in approximately 1% of patients who received simvastatin in clinical studies. When drug treatment was interrupted or discontinued in these patients, the transaminases levels usually fell slowly to pretreatment levels. The increases were not associated with jaundice or other clinical signs or symptoms. There was no evidence of hypersensitivity.
In the placebo-controlled clinical trials and the long-term extension study, elevations in transaminases did not appear to be related to treatment duration; elevations in AST levels did appear to be dose related. Transaminase elevations were reversible upon discontinuation of NIASPAN.
Liver function tests should be performed on all patients during therapy with NIASPAN. Serum transaminase levels, including AST and ALT (SGOT and SGPT), should be monitored before treatment begins, every 6 to 12 weeks for the first year, and periodically thereafter (e.g., at approximately

Information on the AbbVie, Inc. products listed on these pages is from the prescribing information in use as of July 31, 2013. For more information, please visit rxabbvie.com or call 1-800-633-9110.

Table 2. Treatment-Emergent Adverse Reactions by Dose Level in ≥ 5% of Patients and at an Incidence Greater than Placebo; Regardless of Causality Assessment in Placebo-Controlled Clinical Trials

		Placebo-Controlled Studies NIASPAN Treatment@			
			Recommended Daily Maintenance Doses †		
	Placebo (n = 157) %	500 mg‡ (n = 87) %	1000 mg (n = 110) %	1500 mg (n = 136) %	2000 mg (n = 95) %
Gastrointestinal Disorders					
Diarrhea	13	7	10	10	14
Nausea	7	5	6	4	11
Vomiting	4	0	2	4	9
Respiratory					
Cough, Increased	6	3	2	< 2	8
Skin and Subcutaneous Tissue Disorders					
Pruritus	2	8	0	3	0
Rash	0	5	5	5	0
Vascular Disorders					
Flushing&	19	68	69	63	55

Note: Percentages are calculated from the total number of patients in each column.
† Adverse reactions are reported at the initial dose where they occur.
@ Pooled results from placebo-controlled studies; for NIASPAN, n = 245 and median treatment duration = 16 weeks. Number of NIASPAN patients (n) are not additive across doses.
‡ The 500 mg/day dose is outside the recommended daily maintenance dosing range *[see Dosage and Administration (2)]*.
& 10 patients discontinued before receiving 500 mg, therefore they were not included.

6-month intervals). Special attention should be paid to patients who develop elevated serum transaminase levels, and in these patients, measurements should be repeated promptly and then performed more frequently. If the transaminase levels show evidence of progression, particularly if they rise to 3 times ULN and are persistent, or if they are associated with symptoms of nausea, fever, and/or malaise, the drug should be discontinued.

5.4 Laboratory Abnormalities

Increase in Blood Glucose: Niacin treatment can increase fasting blood glucose. Frequent monitoring of blood glucose should be performed to ascertain that the drug is producing no adverse effects. Diabetic patients may experience a dose-related increase in glucose intolerance. Diabetic or potentially diabetic patients should be observed closely during treatment with NIASPAN, particularly during the first few months of use or dose adjustment; adjustment of diet and/or hypoglycemic therapy may be necessary.

Reduction in platelet count: NIASPAN has been associated with small but statistically significant dose-related reductions in platelet count (mean of -11% with 2000 mg). Caution should be observed when NIASPAN is administered concomitantly with anticoagulants; platelet counts should be monitored closely in such patients.

Increase in Prothrombin Time (PT): NIASPAN has been associated with small but statistically significant increases in prothrombin time (mean of approximately +4%); accordingly, patients undergoing surgery should be carefully evaluated. Caution should be observed when NIASPAN is administered concomitantly with anticoagulants; prothrombin time should be monitored closely in such patients.

Increase in Uric Acid: Elevated uric acid levels have occurred with niacin therapy, therefore use with caution in patients predisposed to gout.

Decrease in Phosphorus: In placebo-controlled trials, NIASPAN has been associated with small but statistically significant, dose-related reductions in phosphorus levels (mean of -13% with 2000 mg). Although these reductions were transient, phosphorus levels should be monitored periodically in patients at risk for hypophosphatemia.

6 ADVERSE REACTIONS

Because clinical studies are conducted under widely varying conditions, adverse reaction rates observed in the clinical studies of a drug cannot be directly compared to rates in the clinical studies of another drug and may not reflect the rates observed in practice.

6.1 Clinical Studies Experience

In the placebo-controlled clinical trials database of 402 patients (age range 21-75 years, 33% women, 89% Caucasians, 7% Blacks, 3% Hispanics, 1% Asians) with a median treatment duration of 16 weeks, 16% of patients on NIASPAN and 4% of patients on placebo discontinued due to adverse reactions. The most common adverse reactions in the group of patients treated with NIASPAN that led to treatment discontinuation and occurred at a rate greater than placebo were flushing (6% vs. 0%), rash (2% vs. 0%), diarrhea (2% vs. 0%), nausea (1% vs. 0%), and vomiting (1% vs. 0%). The most commonly reported adverse reactions (incidence >5% and greater than placebo) in the NIASPAN controlled clinical trial database of 402 patients were flushing, diarrhea, nausea, vomiting, increased cough and pruritus.

In the placebo-controlled clinical trials, flushing episodes (i.e., warmth, redness, itching and/or tingling) were the most common treatment-emergent adverse reactions (reported by as many as 88% of patients) for NIASPAN. Spontaneous reports suggest that flushing may also be accompanied by symptoms of dizziness, tachycardia, palpitations, shortness of breath, sweating, burning sensation/skin burning sensation, chills, and/or edema, which in rare cases may lead to syncope. In pivotal studies, 6% (14/245) of NIASPAN patients discontinued due to flushing. In comparisons of immediate-release (IR) niacin and NIASPAN, although the proportion of patients who flushed was similar, fewer flushing episodes were reported by patients who received NIASPAN. Following 4 weeks of maintenance therapy at daily doses of 1500 mg, the incidence of flushing over the 4-week period averaged 8.6 events per patient for IR niacin versus 1.9 following NIASPAN.

Other adverse reactions occurring in ≥5% of patients treated with NIASPAN and at an incidence greater than placebo are shown in Table 2 below.

[See table 2 above]

In general, the incidence of adverse events was higher in women compared to men.

Atherothrombosis Intervention in Metabolic Syndrome with Low HDL/ High Triglycerides: Impact on Global Health Outcomes (AIM-HIGH)

In AIM-HIGH involving 3414 patients (mean age of 64 years, 15% women, 92% Caucasians, 34% with diabetes mellitus) with stable, previously diagnosed cardiovascular disease, all patients received simvastatin, 40 to 80 mg per day, plus ezetimibe 10 mg per day if needed, to maintain an LDL-C level of 40-80 mg/dL, and were randomized to receive NIASPAN 1500-2000 mg/day (n=1718) or matching placebo (IR Niacin, 100-150 mg, n=1696). The incidence of the adverse reactions of "blood glucose increased" (6.4% vs. 4.5%) and "diabetes mellitus" (3.6% vs. 2.2%) was significantly higher in the simvastatin plus NIASPAN group as compared to the simvastatin plus placebo group. There were 5 cases of rhabdomyolysis reported, 4 (0.2%) in the simvastatin plus NIASPAN group and one (<0.1%) in the simvastatin plus placebo group *[see Warnings and Precautions (5.1)]*.

6.2 Postmarketing Experience

Because the below reactions are reported voluntarily from a population of uncertain size, it is generally not possible to reliably estimate their frequency or establish a causal relationship to drug exposure.

The following additional adverse reactions have been identified during post-approval use of NIASPAN:

Hypersensitivity reactions, including anaphylaxis, angioedema, urticaria, flushing, dyspnea, tongue edema, larynx edema, face edema, peripheral edema, laryngismus, and vesiculobullous rash; maculopapular rash; dry skin; tachycardia; palpitations; atrial fibrillation; other cardiac arrhythmias; syncope; hypotension; postural hypotension; blurred vision; macular edema; peptic ulcers; eructation; flatulence; hepatitis; jaundice; decreased glucose tolerance; gout; myalgia; myopathy; dizziness; insomnia; asthenia; nervousness; paresthesia; dyspnea; sweating; burning sensation/skin burning sensation; skin discoloration, and migraine.

Clinical Laboratory Abnormalities

Chemistry: Elevations in serum transaminases *[see Warnings and Precautions (5.3)]*, LDH, fasting glucose, uric acid, total bilirubin, amylase and creatine kinase, and reduction in phosphorus.

Hematology: Slight reductions in platelet counts and prolongation in prothrombin time *[see Warnings and Precautions (5.4)]*.

7 DRUG INTERACTIONS

7.1 Statins

Caution should be used when prescribing niacin (≥1 gm/day) with statins as these drugs can increase risk of myopathy/rhabdomyolysis. Combination therapy with NIASPAN and lovastatin or NIASPAN and simvastatin should not exceed doses of 2000 mg NIASPAN and 40 mg lovastatin or simvastatin daily. *[see Warnings and Precautions (5) and Clinical Pharmacology (12.3)]*.

7.2 Bile Acid Sequestrants

An *in vitro* study results suggest that the bile acid-binding resins have high niacin binding capacity. Therefore, 4 to 6 hours, or as great an interval as possible, should elapse between the ingestion of bile acid-binding resins and the administration of NIASPAN *[see Clinical Pharmacology (12.3)]*.

7.3 Aspirin

Concomitant aspirin may decrease the metabolic clearance of nicotinic acid. The clinical relevance of this finding is unclear.

7.4 Antihypertensive Therapy

Niacin may potentiate the effects of ganglionic blocking agents and vasoactive drugs resulting in postural hypotension.

7.5 Other

Vitamins or other nutritional supplements containing large doses of niacin or related compounds such as nicotinamide may potentiate the adverse effects of NIASPAN.

7.6 Laboratory Test Interactions

Niacin may produce false elevations in some fluorometric determinations of plasma or urinary catecholamines. Niacin may also give false-positive reactions with cupric sulfate solution (Benedict's reagent) in urine glucose tests.

8 USE IN SPECIFIC POPULATIONS

8.1 Pregnancy

Pregnancy Category C.

Animal reproduction studies have not been conducted with niacin or with NIASPAN. It is also not known whether niacin at doses typically used for lipid disorders can cause fetal harm when administered to pregnant women or whether it can affect reproductive capacity. If a woman receiving niacin for primary hyperlipidemia becomes pregnant, the drug should be discontinued. If a woman being treated with niacin for hypertriglyceridemia conceives, the benefits and risks of continued therapy should be assessed on an individual basis.

All statins are contraindicated in pregnant and nursing women. When NIASPAN is administered with a statin in a woman of childbearing potential, refer to the pregnancy category and product labeling for the statin.

8.3 Nursing Mothers

Niacin is excreted into human milk but the actual infant dose or infant dose as a percent of the maternal dose is not known. Because of the potential for serious adverse reactions in nursing infants from lipid-altering doses of nicotinic acid, a decision should be made whether to discontinue nursing or to discontinue the drug, taking into account the importance of the drug to the mother. No studies have been conducted with NIASPAN in nursing mothers.

8.4 Pediatric Use

Safety and effectiveness of niacin therapy in pediatric patients (≤16 years) have not been established.

8.5 Geriatric Use

Of 979 patients in clinical studies of NIASPAN, 21% of the patients were age 65 and over. No overall differences in safety and effectiveness were observed between these patients and younger patients, and other reported clinical experience has not identified differences in responses between the elderly and younger patients, but greater sensitivity of some older individuals cannot be ruled out.

8.6 Renal Impairment

No studies have been performed in this population. NIASPAN should be used with caution in patients with renal impairment *[see Warnings and Precautions (5)]*.

8.7 Hepatic Impairment

No studies have been performed in this population. NIASPAN should be used with caution in patients with a past history of liver disease and/or who consume substantial quantities of alcohol. Active liver disease, unexplained transaminase elevations and significant or unexplained hepatic dysfunction are contraindications to the use of NIASPAN *[see Contraindications (4.0) and Warnings and Precautions (5.3)]*.

8.8 Gender

Data from the clinical trials suggest that women have a greater hypolipidemic response than men at equivalent doses of NIASPAN.

10 OVERDOSAGE

Supportive measures should be undertaken in the event of an overdose.

11 DESCRIPTION

NIASPAN (niacin tablet, film-coated extended-release), contains niacin, which at therapeutic doses is an antihyperlipidemic agent. Niacin (nicotinic acid, or 3-pyridinecarboxylic acid) is a white, crystalline powder, very soluble in water, with the following structural formula:

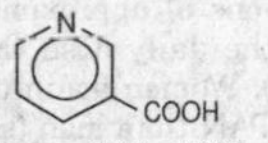

$C_6H_5NO_2$ M.W. = 123.11

NIASPAN is an unscored, medium-orange, film-coated tablet for oral administration and is available in three tablet strengths containing 500, 750, and 1000 mg niacin. NIASPAN tablets also contain the inactive ingredients hypromellose, povidone, stearic acid, and polyethylene glycol, and the following coloring agents: FD&C yellow #6/sunset yellow FCF Aluminum Lake, synthetic red and yellow iron oxides, and titanium dioxide.

12 CLINICAL PHARMACOLOGY

12.1 Mechanism of Action

The mechanism by which niacin alters lipid profiles has not been well defined. It may involve several actions including partial inhibition of release of free fatty acids from adipose tissue, and increased lipoprotein lipase activity, which may increase the rate of chylomicron triglyceride removal from plasma. Niacin decreases the rate of hepatic synthesis of VLDL and LDL, and does not appear to affect fecal excretion of fats, sterols, or bile acids.

12.2 Pharmacodynamics

Niacin functions in the body after conversion to nicotinamide adenine dinucleotide (NAD) in the NAD coenzyme system. Niacin (but not nicotinamide) in gram doses reduces total cholesterol (TC), low density lipoprotein cholesterol (LDL-C), and triglycerides (TG), and increases high-density lipoprotein cholesterol (HDL-C). The magnitude of individual lipid and lipoprotein responses may be influenced by the severity and type of underlying lipid abnormality. The increase in HDL-C is associated with an increase in apolipoprotein A-I (Apo A-I) and a shift in the distribution of HDL subfractions. These shifts include an increase in the HDL_2:HDL_3 ratio, and an elevation in lipoprotein A-I (Lp A-I, an HDL-C particle containing only Apo A-I). Niacin treatment also decreases serum levels of apolipoprotein B-100 (Apo B), the major protein component of the very low-density lipoprotein (VLDL) and LDL fractions, and of Lp(a), a variant form of LDL independently associated with coronary risk. In addition, preliminary reports suggest that niacin causes favorable LDL particle size transformations, although the clinical relevance of this effect requires further investigation. The effect of niacin-induced changes in lipids/proteins on cardiovascular morbidity or mortality in individuals without preexisting coronary disease has not been established.

A variety of clinical studies have demonstrated that elevated levels of TC, LDL-C, and Apo B promote human atherosclerosis. Similarly, decreased levels of HDL-C are associated with the development of atherosclerosis. Epidemiological investigations have established that cardiovascular morbidity and mortality vary directly with the level of Total-C and LDL-C, and inversely with the level of HDL-C.

Like LDL, cholesterol-enriched triglyceride-rich lipoproteins, including VLDL, intermediate-density lipoprotein (IDL), and their remnants, can also promote atherosclerosis. Elevated plasma TG are frequently found in a triad with low HDL-C levels and small LDL particles, as well as in association with non-lipid metabolic risk factors for coronary heart disease (CHD). As such, total plasma TG has not consistently been shown to be an independent risk factor for CHD. Furthermore, the independent effect of raising HDL-C or lowering TG on the risk of coronary and cardiovascular morbidity and mortality has not been determined.

12.3 Pharmacokinetics

Absorption

Due to extensive and saturable first-pass metabolism, niacin concentrations in the general circulation are dose dependent and highly variable. Time to reach the maximum niacin plasma concentrations was about 5 hours following NIASPAN. To reduce the risk of gastrointestinal (GI) upset, administration of NIASPAN with a low-fat meal or snack is recommended.

Single-dose bioavailability studies have demonstrated that the 500 mg and 1000 mg tablet strengths are dosage form equivalent but the 500 mg and 750 mg tablet strengths are not dosage form equivalent.

Metabolism

The pharmacokinetic profile of niacin is complicated due to extensive first-pass metabolism that is dose-rate specific and, at the doses used to treat dyslipidemia, saturable. In humans, one pathway is through a simple conjugation step with glycine to form nicotinuric acid (NUA). NUA is then excreted in the urine, although there may be a small amount of reversible metabolism back to niacin. The other pathway results in the formation of nicotinamide adenine dinucleotide (NAD). It is unclear whether nicotinamide is formed as a precursor to, or following the synthesis of, NAD. Nicotinamide is further metabolized to at least N-methylnicotinamide (MNA) and nicotinamide-N-oxide (NNO). MNA is further metabolized to two other compounds, N-methyl-2-pyridone-5-carboxamide (2PY) and N-methyl-4-pyridone-5-carboxamide (4PY). The formation of 2PY appears to predominate over 4PY in humans. At the doses used to treat hyperlipidemia, these metabolic pathways are saturable, which explains the nonlinear relationship between niacin dose and plasma concentrations following multiple-dose NIASPAN administration.

Nicotinamide does not have hypolipidemic activity; the activity of the other metabolites is unknown.

Elimination

Following single and multiple doses, approximately 60 to 76% of the niacin dose administered as NIASPAN was recovered in urine as niacin and metabolites; up to 12% was recovered as unchanged niacin after multiple dosing. The ratio of metabolites recovered in the urine was dependent on the dose administered.

Pediatric Use

No pharmacokinetic studies have been performed in this population (≤16 years) *[see Use in Specific Populations (8.4)]*.

Geriatric Use

No pharmacokinetic studies have been performed in this population (> 65 years) *[see Use in Specific Populations (8.5)]*.

Renal Impairment

No pharmacokinetic studies have been performed in this population. NIASPAN should be used with caution in patients with renal disease *[see Warnings and Precautions (5)]*.

Hepatic Impairment

No pharmacokinetic studies have been performed in this population. Active liver disease, unexplained transaminase elevations and significant or unexplained hepatic dysfunction are contraindications to the use of NIASPAN *[see Contraindications (4) and Warnings and Precautions (5.3)]*.

Gender

Steady-state plasma concentrations of niacin and metabolites after administration of NIASPAN are generally higher in women than in men, with the magnitude of the difference varying with dose and metabolite. This gender differences observed in plasma levels of niacin and its metabolites may be due to gender-specific differences in metabolic rate or volume of distribution. Recovery of niacin and metabolites in urine, however, is generally similar for men and women, indicating that absorption is similar for both genders *[see Gender (8.8)]*.

Drug interactions

Fluvastatin

Niacin did not affect fluvastatin pharmacokinetics *[see Drug Interactions (7.1)]*.

Lovastatin

When NIASPAN 2000 mg and lovastatin 40 mg were co-administered, NIASPAN increased lovastatin C_{max} and AUC by 2% and 14%, respectively, and decreased lovastatin acid C_{max} and AUC by 22% and 2%, respectively. Lovastatin reduced NIASPAN bioavailability by 2-3% *[see Drug Interactions (7.1)]*.

Simvastatin

When NIASPAN 2000 mg and simvastatin 40 mg were co-administered, NIASPAN increased simvastatin C_{max} and AUC by 1% and 9%, respectively, and simvastatin acid C_{max} and AUC by 2% and 18%, respectively. Simvastatin reduced NIASPAN bioavailability by 2% *[see Drug Interactions (7.1)]*.

Bile Acid Sequestrants

An *in vitro* study was carried out investigating the niacin-binding capacity of colestipol and cholestyramine. About 98% of available niacin was bound to colestipol, with 10 to 30% binding to cholestyramine *[see Drug Interactions (7.2)]*.

Table 3. Lipid Response to NIASPAN Therapy

		Mean Percent Change from Baseline to Week 16*							
Treatment	n	TC	LDL-C	HDL-C	TC/HDL-C	TG	Lp(a)	Apo B	Apo A-I
NIASPAN 1000 mg at bedtime	41	-3	-5	+18	-17	-21	-13	-6	+9
NIASPAN 2000 mg at bedtime	41	-10	-14	+22	-25	-28	-27	-16	+8
Placebo	40	0	-1	+4	-3	0	0	+1	+3
NIASPAN 1500 mg at bedtime	76	-8	-12	+20	-20	-13	-15	-12	+8
Placebo	73	+2	+1	+2	+1	+12	+2	+1	+2

n = number of patients at baseline;
* Mean percent change from baseline for all NIASPAN doses was significantly different (p < 0.05) from placebo for all lipid parameters shown except Apo A-I at 2000 mg.

13 NONCLINICAL TOXICOLOGY

13.1 Carcinogenesis and Mutagenesis and Impairment of Fertility

Niacin administered to mice for a lifetime as a 1% solution in drinking water was not carcinogenic. The mice in this study received approximately 6 to 8 times a human dose of 3000 mg/day as determined on a mg/m^2 basis. Niacin was negative for mutagenicity in the Ames test. No studies on impairment of fertility have been performed. No studies have been conducted with NIASPAN regarding carcinogenesis, mutagenesis, or impairment of fertility.

14 CLINICAL STUDIES

14.1 Niacin Clinical Studies

The role of LDL-C in atherogenesis is supported by pathological observations, clinical studies, and many animal experiments. Observational epidemiological studies have clearly established that high TC or LDL-C and low HDL-C are risk factors for CHD. Additionally, elevated levels of Lp(a) have been shown to be independently associated with CHD risk.

Niacin's ability to reduce mortality and the risk of definite, nonfatal myocardial infarction (MI) has been assessed in long-term studies. The Coronary Drug Project, completed in 1975, was designed to assess the safety and efficacy of niacin and other lipid-altering drugs in men 30 to 64 years old with a history of MI. Over an observation period of 5 years, niacin treatment was associated with a statistically significant reduction in nonfatal, recurrent MI. The incidence of definite, nonfatal MI was 8.9% for the 1,119 patients randomized to nicotinic acid versus 12.2% for the 2,789 patients who received placebo (p<0.004). Total mortality was similar in the two groups at 5 years (24.4% with nicotinic acid versus 25.4% with placebo; p=N.S.). At the time of a 15-year follow-up, there were 11% (69) fewer deaths in the niacin group compared to the placebo cohort (52.0% versus 58.2%; p=0.0004). However, mortality at 15 years was not an original endpoint of the Coronary Drug Project. In addition, patients had not received niacin for approximately 9 years, and confounding variables such as concomitant medication use and medical or surgical treatments were not controlled.

The Cholesterol-Lowering Atherosclerosis Study (CLAS) was a randomized, placebo-controlled, angiographic trial testing combined colestipol and niacin therapy in 162 non-smoking males with previous coronary bypass surgery. The primary, per-subject cardiac endpoint was global coronary artery change score. After 2 years, 61% of patients in the placebo cohort showed disease progression by global change score (n=82), compared with only 38.8% of drug-treated subjects (n=80), when both native arteries and grafts were considered (p<0.005); disease regression also occurred more frequently in the drug-treated group (16.2% versus 2.4%; p=0.002). In a follow-up to this trial in a subgroup of 103 patients treated for 4 years, again, significantly fewer patients in the drug-treated group demonstrated progression than in the placebo cohort (48% versus 85%, respectively; p<0.0001).

The Familial Atherosclerosis Treatment Study (FATS) in 146 men ages 62 and younger with Apo B levels ≥125 mg/dL, established coronary artery disease, and family histories of vascular disease, assessed change in severity

Information on the AbbVie, Inc. products listed on these pages is from the prescribing information in use as of July 31, 2013. For more information, please visit rxabbvie.com or call 1-800-633-9110.

Table 4. Lipid Response in Dose-Escalation Study

		Mean Percent Change from Baseline*							
Treatment	**n**	**TC**	**LDL-C**	**HDL-C**	**TC/HDL-C**	**TG**	**Lp(a)**	**Apo B**	**Apo A-I**
Placebo[‡]	44	-2	-1	+5	-7	-6	-5	-2	+4
NIASPAN	87								
500 mg at bedtime		-2	-3	+10	-10	-5	-3	-2	+5
1000 mg at bedtime		-5	-9	+15	-17	-11	-12	-7	+8
1500 mg at bedtime		-11	-14	+22	-26	-28	-20	-15	+10
2000 mg at bedtime		-12	-17	+26	-29	-35	-24	-16	+12

n = number of patients enrolled;
[‡] Placebo data shown are after 24 weeks of placebo treatment.
* For all NIASPAN doses except 500 mg, mean percent change from baseline was significantly different ($p < 0.05$) from placebo for all lipid parameters shown except Lp(a) and Apo A-I which were significantly different from placebo starting with 1500 mg and 2000 mg, respectively.

Table 5. Selected Lipid Response to NIASPAN in Placebo-Controlled Clinical Studies*

		Mean Baseline and Median Percent Change from Baseline (25th, 75th Percentiles)		
NIASPAN Dose	**n**	**LDL-C**	**HDL-C**	**TG**
1000 mg at bedtime	104			
Baseline (mg/dL)		218	45	172
Percent Change		-7 (-15, 0)	+14 (+7, +23)	-16 (-34, +3)
1500 mg at bedtime	120			
Baseline (mg/dL)		212	46	171
Percent Change		-13 (-21, -4)	+19 (+9, +31)	-25 (-45, -2)
2000 mg at bedtime	85			
Baseline (mg/dL)		220	44	160
Percent Change		-16 (-26, -7)	+22 (+15, +34)	-38 (-52, -14)

* Represents pooled analyses of results; minimum duration on therapy at each dose was 4 weeks.

Table 6. Effect of Gender on NIASPAN Dose Response

		Mean Percent Change from Baseline							
NIASPAN	**n**	**LDL-C**		**HDL-C**		**TG**		**Apo B**	
Dose	(M/F)	M	F	M	F	M	F	M	F
500 mg at bedtime	50/37	-2	-5	+11	+8	-3	-9	-1	-5
1000 mg at bedtime	76/52	-6*	-11*	+14	+20	-10	-20	-5*	-10*
1500 mg at bedtime	104/59	-12	-16	+19	+24	-17	-28	-13	-15
2000 mg at bedtime	75/53	-15	-18	+23	+26	-30	-36	-16	-16

n = number of male/female patients enrolled.
* Percent change significantly different between genders ($p < 0.05$).

Table 7. Lipid Response to NIASPAN in Patients with Low HDL-C

	Mean Baseline and Mean Percent Change from Baseline*									
	n	**TC**	**LDL-C**	**HDL-C**	**TC/HDL-C**	**TG**	**Lp(a)[†]**	**Apo B[†]**	**Apo A-I[†]**	**Lp A-I[††]**
Baseline (mg/dL)	88	190	120	31	6	194	8	106	105	32
Week 19 (% Change)	71	-3	0	+26	-22	-30	-20	-9	+11	+20

n = number of patients
* Mean percent change from baseline was significantly different ($p < 0.05$) for all lipid parameters shown except LDL-C.
[†] n = 72 at baseline and 69 at week 19.
[††] n = 30 at baseline and week 19.

of disease in the proximal coronary arteries by quantitative arteriography. Patients were given dietary counseling and randomized to treatment with either conventional therapy with double placebo (or placebo plus colestipol if the LDL-C was elevated); lovastatin plus colestipol; or niacin plus colestipol. In the conventional therapy group, 46% of patients had disease progression (and no regression) in at least one of nine proximal coronary segments; regression was the only change in 11%. In contrast, progression (as the only change) was seen in only 25% in the niacin plus colestipol group, while regression was observed in 39%. Though not an original endpoint of the trial, clinical events (death, MI, or revascularization for worsening angina) occurred in 10 of 52 patients who received conventional therapy, compared with 2 of 48 who received niacin plus colestipol.

The Harvard Atherosclerosis Reversibility Project (HARP) was a randomized placebo-controlled, 2.5-year study of the effect of a stepped-care antihyperlipidemic drug regimen on 91 patients (80 men and 11 women) with CHD and average baseline TC levels less than 250 mg/dL and ratios of TC to HDL-C greater than 4.0. Drug treatment consisted of an HMG-CoA reductase inhibitor administered alone as initial therapy followed by addition of varying dosages of either a slow-release nicotinic acid, cholestyramine, or gemfibrozil. Addition of nicotinic acid to the HMG-CoA reductase inhibitor resulted in further statistically significant mean reductions in TC, LDL-C, and TG, as well as a further increase in HDL-C in a majority of patients (40 of 44 patients). The ratios of TC to HDL-C and LDL-C to HDL-C were also significantly reduced by this combination drug regimen *[see Warnings and Precautions (5.2)]*.

14.2 NIASPAN Clinical Studies

Placebo-Controlled Clinical Studies in Patients with Primary Hyperlipidemia and Mixed Dyslipidemia: In two randomized, double-blind, parallel, multi-center, placebo-controlled trials, NIASPAN dosed at 1000, 1500 or 2000 mg daily at bedtime with a low-fat snack for 16 weeks (including 4 weeks of dose escalation) favorably altered lipid profiles compared to placebo (Table 3). Women appeared to have a greater response than men at each NIASPAN dose level (see *Gender Effect*, below).

[See table 3 at top of previous page]

In a double-blind, multi-center, forced dose-escalation study, monthly 500 mg increases in NIASPAN dose resulted in incremental reductions of approximately 5% in LDL-C and Apo B levels in the daily dose range of 500 mg through 2000 mg (Table 4). Women again tended to have a greater response to NIASPAN than men (see *Gender Effect*, below).

[See table 4 above]

Pooled results for major lipids from these three placebo-controlled studies are shown below (Table 5).

[See table 5 above]

Gender Effect: Combined data from the three placebo-controlled NIASPAN studies in patients with primary hyperlipidemia and mixed dyslipidemia suggest that, at each NIASPAN dose level studied, changes in lipid concentrations are greater for women than for men (Table 6).

[See table 6 below]

Other Patient Populations: In a double-blind, multi-center, 19-week study the lipid-altering effects of NIASPAN (forced titration to 2000 mg at bedtime) were compared to baseline in patients whose primary lipid abnormality was a low level of HDL-C (HDL-C ≤40 mg/dL, TG ≤400 mg/dL, and LDL-C ≤160, or <130 mg/dL in the presence of CHD). Results are shown below (Table 7).

[See table 7 below]

At NIASPAN 2000 mg/day, median changes from baseline (25th, 75th percentiles) for LDL-C, HDL-C, and TG were -3% (-14, +12%), +27% (+13, +38%), and -33% (-50, -19%), respectively.

14.3 NIASPAN and Lovastatin Clinical Studies

Combination NIASPAN and Lovastatin Study: In a multi-center, randomized, double-blind, parallel, 28-week study, a combination tablet of NIASPAN and lovastatin was compared to each individual component in patients with Type IIa and IIb hyperlipidemia. Using a forced dose-escalation study design, patients received each dose for at least 4 weeks. Patients randomized to treatment with the combination tablet of NIASPAN and lovastatin initially received 500 mg/20 mg (expressed as mg of niacin/mg of lovastatin) once daily before bedtime. The dose was increased by 500 mg at 4-week intervals (based on the NIASPAN component) to a maximum dose of 1000 mg/20 mg in one-half of the patients and 2000 mg/40 mg in the other half. The NIASPAN monotherapy group underwent a similar titration from 500 mg to 2000 mg. The patients randomized to lovastatin monotherapy received 20 mg for 12 weeks titrated to 40 mg for up to 16 weeks. Up to a third of the patients randomized to the combination tablet of NIASPAN and lovastatin or NIASPAN monotherapy discontinued prior to Week 28. Results from this study showed that combination therapy decreased LDL-C, TG and Lp(a), and increased HDL-C in a dose-dependent fashion (Tables 8, 9, 10, and 11). Results from this study for LDL-C mean percent change from baseline (the primary efficacy variable) showed that:

1. LDL-lowering with the combination tablet of NIASPAN and lovastatin was significantly greater than that achieved with lovastatin 40 mg only after 28 weeks of titration to a dose of 2000 mg/40 mg ($p<0.0001$)
2. The combination tablet of NIASPAN and lovastatin at doses of 1000 mg/20 mg or higher achieved greater LDL-lowering than NIASPAN ($p<0.0001$)

The LDL-C results are summarized in Table 8.

[See table 8 at top of next page]

Combination therapy achieved significantly greater HDL-raising compared to lovastatin and NIASPAN monotherapy at all doses (Table 9).

[See table 9 at top of next page]

In addition, combination therapy achieved significantly greater TG lowering at doses of 1000 mg/20 mg or greater compared to lovastatin and NIASPAN monotherapy (Table 10).

[See table 10 at top of next page]

The Lp(a)-lowering effects of combination therapy and NIASPAN monotherapy were similar, and both were superior to lovastatin (Table 11). The independent effect of lowering Lp(a) with NIASPAN or combination therapy on the risk of coronary and cardiovascular morbidity and mortality has not been determined.

[See 11 table at top of next page]

14.4 NIASPAN and Simvastatin Clinical Studies

In a double-blind, randomized, multicenter, multi-national, active-controlled, 24-week study, the lipid effects of a combination tablet of NIASPAN and simvastatin were compared to simvastatin 20 mg and 80 mg in 641 patients with type II hyperlipidemia or mixed dyslipidemia. Following a lipid qualification phase, patients were eligible to enter one

Table 8. LDL-C mean percent change from baseline

Week	Combination Tablet of NIASPAN and Lovastatin			NIASPAN			Lovastatin		
	n*	Dose (mg/mg)	LDL	n*	Dose (mg)	LDL	n*	Dose (mg)	LDL
Baseline	57	–	190.9 mg/dL	61	–	189.7 mg/dL	61	–	185.6 mg/dL
12	47	1000/20	-30%	46	1000	-3%	56	20	-29%
16	45	1000/40	-36%	44	1000	-6%	56	40	-31%
20	42	1500/40	-37%	43	1500	-12%	54	40	-34%
28	42	2000/40	-42%	41	2000	-14%	53	40	-32%

* n = number of patients remaining in trial at each time point

Table 9. HDL-C mean percent change from baseline

Week	Combination Tablet of NIASPAN and Lovastatin			NIASPAN			Lovastatin		
	n*	Dose (mg/mg)	HDL	n*	Dose (mg)	HDL	n*	Dose (mg)	HDL
Baseline	57	–	45 mg/dL	61	–	47 mg/dL	61	–	43 mg/dL
12	47	1000/20	+20%	46	1000	+14%	56	20	+3%
16	45	1000/40	+20%	44	1000	+15%	56	40	+5%
20	42	1500/40	+27%	43	1500	+22%	54	40	+6%
28	42	2000/40	+30%	41	2000	+24%	53	40	+6%

* n = number of patients remaining in trial at each time point

Table 10. TG median percent change from baseline

Week	Combination Tablet of NIASPAN and Lovastatin			NIASPAN			Lovastatin		
	n*	Dose (mg/mg)	TG	n*	Dose (mg)	TG	n*	Dose (mg)	TG
Baseline	57	–	174 mg/dL	61	–	186 mg/dL	61	–	171 mg/dL
12	47	1000/20	-32%	46	1000	-22%	56	20	-20%
16	45	1000/40	-39%	44	1000	-23%	56	40	-17%
20	42	1500/40	-44%	43	1500	-31%	54	40	-21%
28	42	2000/40	-44%	41	2000	-31%	53	40	-20%

* n = number of patients remaining in trial at each time point

Table 11. Lp(a) median percent change from baseline

Week	Combination Tablet of NIASPAN and Lovastatin			NIASPAN			Lovastatin		
	n*	Dose (mg/mg)	Lp(a)	n*	Dose (mg)	Lp(a)	n*	Dose (mg)	Lp(a)
Baseline	57	–	34 mg/dL	61	–	41 mg/dL	60	–	42 mg/dL
12	47	1000/20	-9%	46	1000	-8%	55	20	+8%
16	45	1000/40	-9%	44	1000	-12%	55	40	+8%
20	42	1500/40	-17%	43	1500	-22%	53	40	+6%
28	42	2000/40	-22%	41	2000	-32%	52	40	0%

* n = number of patients remaining in trial at each time point

of two treatment groups. In Group A, patients on simvastatin 20 mg monotherapy, with elevated non-HDL levels and LDL-C levels at goal per the NCEP guidelines, were randomized to one of three treatment arms: combination tablet of NIASPAN and simvastatin 1000/20 mg, combination tablet of NIASPAN and simvastatin 2000/20 mg, or simvastatin 20 mg. In Group B, patients on simvastatin 40 mg monotherapy, with elevated non-HDL levels per the NCEP guidelines regardless of attainment of LDL-C goals, were randomized to one of three treatment arms: combination tablet of NIASPAN and simvastatin 1000/40 mg, combination tablet of NIASPAN and simvastatin 2000/40 mg, or simvastatin 80 mg. Therapy was initiated at the 500 mg dose of combination tablet of NIASPAN and simvastatin and increased by 500 mg every four weeks. Thus patients were titrated to the 1000 mg dose of combination tablet of NIASPAN and simvastatin after four weeks and to the 2000 mg dose of combination tablet of NIASPAN and simvastatin after 12 weeks. All patients randomized to simvastatin monotherapy received 50 mg immediate-release niacin daily in an attempt to keep the study from becoming unblinded due to flushing in the combination tablet of NIASPAN and simvastatin groups. Patients were instructed to take one 325 mg aspirin or 200 mg ibuprofen 30 minutes prior to taking the double-blind medication to help minimize flushing effects.

In Group A, the primary efficacy analysis was a comparison of the mean percent change in non-HDL levels between the combination tablet of NIASPAN and simvastatin 2000/20 mg and simvastatin 20 mg groups, and if statistically significant, then a comparison was conducted between the combination tablet of NIASPAN and simvastatin 1000/20 mg and simvastatin 20 mg groups. In Group B, the primary efficacy analysis was a determination of whether the mean percent change in non-HDL in the combination tablet of NIASPAN and simvastatin 2000/40 mg group was non-inferior to the mean percent change in the simvastatin 80 mg group, and if so, whether the mean percent change in non-HDL in the combination tablet of NIASPAN and simvastatin 1000/40 mg group was non-inferior to the mean percent change in the simvastatin 80 mg group.

In Group A, the non-HDL-C lowering with combination tablet of NIASPAN and simvastatin 2000/20 and combination tablet of NIASPAN and simvastatin 1000/20 was statistically significantly greater than that achieved with simvastatin 20 mg after 24 weeks ($p<0.05$; Table 12). The completion rate after 24 weeks was 72% for the combination tablet of NIASPAN and simvastatin arms and 88% for the simvastatin 20 mg arm. In Group B, the non-HDL-C lowering with combination tablet of NIASPAN and simvastatin 2000/40 and combination tablet of NIASPAN and simvastatin 1000/40 was non-inferior to that achieved with simvastatin 80 mg after 24 weeks (Table 13). The completion rate after 24 weeks was 78% for the combination tablet of NIASPAN and simvastatin arms and 80% for the simvastatin 80 mg arm.

The combination tablet of NIASPAN and simvastatin was not superior to simvastatin in lowering LDL-C in either Group A or Group B. However, the combination tablet of NIASPAN and simvastatin was superior to simvastatin in both groups in lowering TG and raising HDL (Tables 14 and 15).

[See table 12 at top of next page]
[See table 13 at top of next page]
[See table 14 at top of next page]
[See table 15 at top of next page]

16 HOW SUPPLIED/STORAGE AND HANDLING

NIASPAN tablets are supplied as unscored, medium-orange, film-coated, capsule-shaped (containing 500 or 750 mg of niacin) or oval shaped (containing 1000 mg of niacin) tablets, in an extended-release formulation. Tablets are printed with the "a" logo and the tablet strength (500, 750 or 1000). Tablets are supplied in bottles of 30 and 90 as shown below.

500 mg tablets: bottles of 30 - NDC# 0074–3074–30
500 mg tablets: bottles of 90 - NDC# 0074–3074–90
750 mg tablets: bottles of 30 - NDC# 0074–3079–30
750 mg tablets: bottles of 90 - NDC# 0074–3079–90
1000 mg tablets: bottles of 30 - NDC# 0074–3080–30
1000 mg tablets: bottles of 90 - NDC# 0074–3080–90

Storage: Store at room temperature 20° to 25°C (68° to 77°F).

17 PATIENT COUNSELING INFORMATION

17.1 Patient Counseling

Patients should be advised to adhere to their National Cholesterol Education Program (NCEP) recommended diet, a regular exercise program, and periodic testing of a fasting lipid panel.

Patients should be advised to inform other healthcare professionals prescribing a new medication that they are taking NIASPAN.

The patient should be informed of the following:

Dosing Time

NIASPAN tablets should be taken at bedtime, after a low-fat snack. Administration on an empty stomach is not recommended.

Tablet Integrity

NIASPAN tablets should not be broken, crushed or chewed, but should be swallowed whole.

Dosing Interruption

If dosing is interrupted for any length of time, their physician should be contacted prior to restarting therapy; re-titration is recommended.

Muscle Pain

Notify their physician of any unexplained muscle pain, tenderness, or weakness promptly. They should discuss all medication, both prescription and over the counter, with their physician.

Flushing

Flushing (warmth, redness, itching and/or tingling of the skin) is a common side effect of niacin therapy that may subside after several weeks of consistent NIASPAN use. Flushing may vary in severity and is more likely to occur with initiation of therapy, or during dose increases. By dosing at bedtime, flushing will most likely occur during sleep. However, if awakened by flushing at night, the patient should get up slowly, especially if feeling dizzy, feeling faint, or taking blood pressure medications. Advise patients of the symptoms of flushing and how they differ from the symptoms of a myocardial infarction.

Use of Aspirin Medication

Taking aspirin (up to the recommended dose of 325 mg) approximately 30 minutes before dosing can minimize flushing.

Diet

Avoid ingestion of alcohol, hot beverages and spicy foods around the time of taking NIASPAN to minimize flushing.

Supplements

Notify their physician if they are taking vitamins or other nutritional supplements containing niacin or nicotinamide.

Dizziness

Notify their physician if symptoms of dizziness occur.

Diabetics

If diabetic, to notify their physician of changes in blood glucose.

Information on the AbbVie, Inc. products listed on these pages is from the prescribing information in use as of July 31, 2013. For more information, please visit rxabbvie.com or call 1-800-633-9110.

Table 12. Non-HDL Treatment Response Following 24-Week Treatment Mean Percent Change from Simvastatin 20-mg Treated Baseline

Group A	Combination Tablet of NIASPAN and Simvastatin 2000/20			Combination Tablet of NIASPAN and Simvastatin 1000/20			Simvastatin 20		
Week	n[a]	Dose (mg/mg)	Non-HDL[b]	n[a]	Dose (mg/mg)	Non-HDL[b]	n[a]	Dose (mg/mg)	Non-HDL[b]
Baseline	56	–	163.1 mg/dL	108	–	164.8 mg/dL	102	–	163.7 mg/dL
4	52	500/20	-12.9%	86	500/20	-12.8%	91	20	-8.3%
8	46	1000/20	-17.5%	91	1000/20	-15.5%	95	20	-8.3%
12	46	1500/20	-18.9%	90	1000/20	-14.8%	96	20	-6.4%
24	40	2000/20	-19.5%[†]	78	1000/20	-13.6%[†]	90	20	-5.0%
Dropouts by week 24:	28.6%			27.8%			11.8%		

[a] n=number of subjects with values in the analysis window at each timepoint
[b] The percent change from baseline is the model-based mean from a repeated measures mixed model with no imputation for missing data from study dropouts.
[†] significant vs. simvastatin 20 mg at the primary endpoint (Week 24), $p<0.05$

Table 13. Non-HDL Treatment Response Following 24-Week Treatment Mean Percent Change from Simvastatin 40-mg Treated Baseline

Group B	Combination Tablet of NIASPAN and Simvastatin 2000/40			Combination Tablet of NIASPAN and Simvastatin 1000/40			Simvastatin 80		
Week	n[a]	Dose (mg/mg)	Non-HDL[b]	n[a]	Dose (mg/mg)	Non-HDL[b]	n[a]	Dose (mg/mg)	Non-HDL[b]
Baseline	98	–	144.4 mg/dL	111	–	141.2 mg/dL	113	–	134.5 mg/dL
4	96	500/40	-6.0%	108	500/40	-5.9%	110	80	-11.3%
8	93	1000/40	-15.5%	100	1000/40	-16.2%	104	80	-13.7%
12	90	1500/40	-18.4%	97	1000/40	-12.6%	100	80	-9.5%
24	80	2000/40	-7.6%[c]	82	1000/40	-6.7%[d]	90	80	-6.0%
Dropouts by week 24:	18.4%			26.1%			20.4%		

[a] n=number of subjects with values in the analysis window at each timepoint
[b] The percent change from baseline is the model-based mean from a repeated measures mixed model with no imputation for missing data from study dropouts.
[c] non-inferior to simvastatin 80 arm; 95% confidence interval of mean difference in non-HDL for the combination tablet of NIASPAN and simvastatin 2000/40 vs. simvastatin 80 is (-7.7%, 4.5%)
[d] non-inferior to simvastatin 80 arm; 95% confidence interval of mean difference in non-HDL for combination tablet of NIASPAN and simvastatin 1000/40 vs. combination tablet of NIASPAN and simvastatin 80 is (-6.6%, 5.3%)

Table 14. Mean Percent Change from Baseline to Week 24 in Lipoprotein Lipid Levels

Treatment Group A TREATMENT	N	LDL-C	Total-C	HDL-C	TG[a]	Apo B
Baseline (mg/dL)*	266	120	207	43	209	102
Simvastatin 20 mg	102	-6.7%	-4.5%	7.8%	-15.3%	-5.6%
Combination Tablet of NIASPAN and Simvastatin 1000/20	108	-11.9%	-8.8%	20.7%	-26.5%	-13.2%
Combination Tablet of NIASPAN and Simvastatin 2000/20	56	-14.3%	-11.1%	29.0%	-38.0%	-18.5%

* either treatment naive or after receiving simvastatin 20 mg
[a] medians are reported for TG

Table 15. Mean Percent Change from Baseline to Week 24 in Lipoprotein Lipid Levels

Treatment Group B TREATMENT	N	LDL-C	Total-C	HDL-C	TG[a]	Apo B
Baseline (mg/dL)*	322	108	187	47	145	93
Simvastatin 80 mg	113	-11.4%	-6.2%	0.1%	0.3%	-7.5%
Combination Tablet of NIASPAN and Simvastatin 1000/40	111	-7.1%	-3.1%	15.4%	-22.8%	-7.7%
Combination Tablet of NIASPAN and Simvastatin 2000/40	98	-5.1	-1.6%	24.4%	-31.8%	-10.5%

* after receiving simvastatin 40 mg
[a] medians are reported for TG

Pregnancy
Discuss future pregnancy plans with your patients, and discuss when to stop NIASPAN if they are trying to conceive. Patients should be advised that if they become pregnant, they should stop taking NIASPAN and call their healthcare professional.

Breastfeeding
Women who are breastfeeding should be advised to not use NIASPAN. Patients, who have a lipid disorder and are breastfeeding, should be advised to discuss the options with their healthcare professional.

Manufactured for AbbVie Inc., North Chicago, IL 60064, U.S.A.
500 mg tablets
by Norwich Pharmaceuticals, Inc., Norwich, NY 13815
or
500 mg, 750 mg and 1000 mg tablets
by AbbVie LTD, Barceloneta, PR 00617
Ref. 03-A751-R8-Revised March, 2013

PATIENT INFORMATION

NIASPAN® (ny-a-span)
(niacin extended-release) tablets

Read this information carefully before you start taking NIASPAN and each time you get a refill. There may be new information. This information does not take the place of talking with your doctor about your medical condition or your treatment.

What is NIASPAN?
NIASPAN is a prescription medicine used with diet and exercise to increase the good cholesterol (HDL) and lower the bad cholesterol (LDL) and fats (triglycerides) in your blood.
- NIASPAN can be used by itself or with other cholesterol-lowering medicines.
- NIASPAN is also used to lower the risk of heart attack in people who have had a heart attack and have high cholesterol.
- In people with coronary artery disease and high cholesterol, NIASPAN, when used with a bile acid-binding resin (another cholesterol medicine) can slow down or lessen the build-up of plaque (fatty deposits) in your arteries.
- In people with heart problems and well-controlled cholesterol, taking NIASPAN with another cholesterol-lowering medicine (simvastatin) has not been shown to reduce heart attacks or strokes more than taking simvastatin alone.

It is not known if NIASPAN is safe and effective in children 16 years of age and under.

Who should not take NIASPAN?
Do not take NIASPAN if you have:
- liver problems
- a stomach ulcer
- bleeding problems
- an allergy to niacin or any of the ingredients in NIASPAN. See the end of this leaflet for a complete list of ingredients in NIASPAN.

What should I tell my doctor before taking NIASPAN?
Before you take NIASPAN, tell your doctor, if you:
- have diabetes. Tell your doctor if your blood sugar levels change after you take NIASPAN.
- have gout
- have kidney problems
- are pregnant or plan to become pregnant. It is not known if NIASPAN will harm your unborn baby. Talk to your doctor if you are pregnant or plan to become pregnant while taking NIASPAN.
- are breastfeeding or plan to breastfeed. NIASPAN can pass into your breast milk. You and your doctor should decide if you will take NIASPAN or breastfeed. You should not do both. Talk to your doctor about the best way to feed your baby if you take NIASPAN.

Tell your doctor about all the medicines you take, including prescription and non-prescription medicines, vitamins, herbal supplements or other nutritional supplements containing niacin or nicotinamide. NIASPAN and other medicines may affect each other causing side effects. NIASPAN may affect the way other medicines work, and other medicines may affect how NIASPAN works.

Especially tell your doctor if you take:
- other medicines to lower cholesterol or triglycerides
- aspirin
- blood pressure medicines
- blood thinner medicines
- large amounts of alcohol

Know the medicines you take. Keep a list of them to show your doctor and pharmacist when you get a new medicine.

How should I take NIASPAN?
- Take NIASPAN exactly as your doctor tells you to take it.
- Take NIASPAN tablets whole. Do not break, crush or chew NIASPAN tablets before swallowing.
- Take NIASPAN 1 time a day at bedtime after a low-fat snack. NIASPAN should not be taken on an empty stomach.
- All forms of niacin are not the same as NIASPAN. Do not switch between forms of niacin without first talking to your doctor as severe liver damage can occur.
- Do not change your dose or stop taking NIASPAN unless your doctor tells you to.
- If you need to stop taking NIASPAN, call your doctor before you start taking NIASPAN again. Your doctor may need to lower your dose of NIASPAN.
- If you forget to take a dose of NIASPAN, take it as soon as you remember.
- If you take too much NIASPAN, call your doctor right away.
- Medicines used to lower your cholesterol called bile acid resins, such as colestipol and cholestyramine, should not be taken at the same time of day as NIASPAN. You should take NIASPAN and the bile acid resin medicine at least 4 to 6 hours apart.
- Your doctor may do blood tests before you start taking NIASPAN and during your treatment. You should see your doctor regularly to check your cholesterol and triglyceride levels and to check for side effects.

What are the possible side effects of NIASPAN?
NIASPAN may cause serious side effects, including:
- **severe liver problems. Signs of liver problems include:**
  - increased tiredness
  - dark colored urine (tea-colored)
  - loss of appetite
  - light colored stools
  - nausea

- right upper stomach (abdomen) pain
- yellowing of your skin or whites of your eye
- itchy skin

- **unexplained muscle pain, tenderness or weakness**
- **high blood sugar level (glucose)**

Call your doctor right away if you have any of the side effects listed above.

The most common side effects of NIASPAN include:

- flushing
- diarrhea
- nausea
- vomiting
- increased cough
- rash

Flushing is the most common side effect of NIASPAN. Flushing happens when tiny blood vessels near the surface of the skin (especially on the face, neck, chest and/or back) open wider. Symptoms of flushing may include any or all of the following:

- warmth
- redness
- itching
- tingling of the skin

Flushing does not always happen. If it does, it is usually within 2 to 4 hours after taking a dose of NIASPAN. Flushing may last for a few hours. Flushing is more likely to happen when you first start taking NIASPAN or when your dose of NIASPAN is increased. Flushing may get better after several weeks.

If you wake up at night because of flushing, get up slowly, especially if you:

- feel dizzy or faint
- take blood pressure medicines

To lower your chance of flushing:

- Ask your doctor if you can take aspirin to help lower the flushing side effect from NIASPAN. You can take aspirin (up to the recommended dose of 325 mg) about 30 minutes before you take NIASPAN to help lower the flushing side effect.
- Do not drink hot beverages (including coffee), alcohol, or eat spicy foods around the time you take NIASPAN.
- Take NIASPAN with a low-fat snack to lessen upset stomach.

People with high cholesterol and heart disease are at risk for a heart attack. Symptoms of a heart attack may be different from a flushing reaction from NIASPAN. **The following may be symptoms of a heart attack due to heart disease and not a flushing reaction:**

- chest pain
- pain in other areas of your upper body such as one or both arms, back, neck, jaw or stomach
- shortness of breath
- sweating
- nausea
- lightheadedness

The chest pain you have with a heart attack may feel like uncomfortable pressure, squeezing, fullness or pain that lasts more than a few minutes, or that goes away and comes back. Heart attacks may be sudden and intense, but often start slowly, with mild pain or discomfort.

Call your doctor right away if you have any symptoms of a heart attack.

Tell your doctor if you have any side effect that bothers you or does not go away.

These are not all the possible side effects of NIASPAN. For more information, ask your doctor or pharmacist.

Call your doctor for medical advice about side effects. You may report side effects to FDA at 1-800-FDA-1088.

How should I store NIASPAN?

- Store NIASPAN at 68°F to 77°F (20°C to 25°C).

Keep NIASPAN and all medicines out of the reach of children.

General information about the safe and effective use of NIASPAN.

Medicines are sometimes prescribed for purposes other than those listed in a Patient Information leaflet. Do not use NIASPAN for a condition for which it was not prescribed. Do not give NIASPAN to other people, even if they have the same symptoms that you have. It may harm them.

This leaflet summarizes the most important information about NIASPAN. If you would like more information, talk with your doctor. You can ask your pharmacist or doctor for information about NIASPAN that is written for health professionals.

For more information, go to www.NIASPAN.com or call AbbVie Inc. Medical Information at 1-800-633-9110.

What are the ingredients in NIASPAN?

Active ingredient: niacin

Inactive Ingredients: hypromellose, povidone, stearic acid, and polyethylene glycol, and the following coloring agents: FD&C yellow #6/sunset yellow FCF Aluminum Lake, synthetic red and yellow iron oxides, and titanium dioxide.

This Patient Information has been approved by the U.S. Food and Drug Administration.

Manufactured for AbbVie Inc., North Chicago, IL 60064, U.S.A.
500 mg tablets by Norwich Pharmaceuticals, Inc., Norwich, NY 13815
or 500 mg, 750 mg and 1000 mg tablets
by AbbVie LTD, Barceloneta, PR 00617
Ref. 03-A751-R8-Revised March, 2013

Shown in Product Identification Guide, page 304

NIMBEX® ℞
[*nĭm-bĕks*]
(cisatracurium besylate)
Injection

This drug should be administered only by adequately trained individuals familiar with its actions, characteristics, and hazards.

NOT FOR USE IN NEONATES
CONTAINS BENZYL ALCOHOL

DESCRIPTION

NIMBEX® (cisatracurium besylate) is a nondepolarizing skeletal muscle relaxant for intravenous administration. Compared to other neuromuscular blocking agents, it is intermediate in its onset and duration of action. Cisatracurium besylate is one of 10 isomers of atracurium besylate and constitutes approximately 15% of that mixture. Cisatracurium besylate is [1*R*-[1α,2α(1′*R**,2′*R**)]]-2,2′- [1,5-pentanediylbis[oxy(3-oxo-3,1-propanediyl)]]bis[1-[(3,4-dimethoxyphenyl)methyl]-1,2,3,4-tetrahydro-6,7-dimethoxy-2-methylisoquinolinium] dibenzenesulfonate. The molecular formula of the cisatracurium parent bis-cation is $C_{53}H_{72}N_2O_{12}$ and the molecular weight is 929.2. The molecular formula of cisatracurium as the besylate salt is $C_{65}H_{82}N_2O_{18}S_2$ and the molecular weight is 1243.50. The structural formula of cisatracurium besylate is:

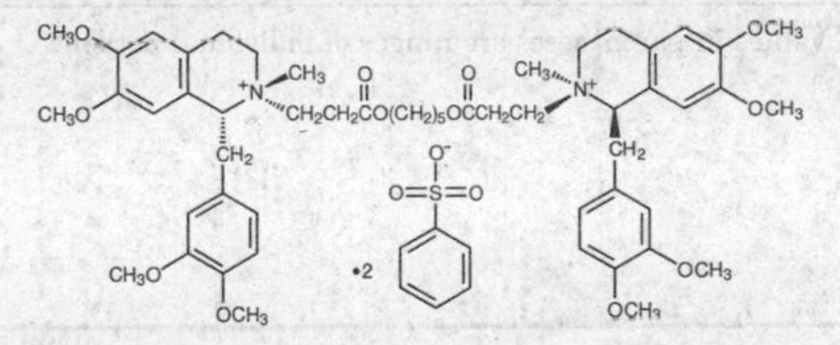

The log of the partition coefficient of cisatracurium besylate is -2.12 in a 1-octanol/distilled water system at 25°C.

NIMBEX Injection is a sterile, non-pyrogenic aqueous solution provided in 5 mL, 10 mL, and 20 mL vials. The pH is adjusted to 3.25 to 3.65 with benzenesulfonic acid. The 5 mL and 10 mL vials each contain cisatracurium besylate, equivalent to 2 mg/mL cisatracurium. The 20 mL vial, **intended for ICU use only**, contains cisatracurium besylate, equivalent to 10 mg/mL cisatracurium. The 10 mL vial, intended for multiple-dose use, contains 0.9% benzyl alcohol as a preservative. The 5 mL and 20 mL vials are single-use vials and do not contain benzyl alcohol.

Cisatracurium besylate slowly loses potency with time at a rate of approximately 5% per year under refrigeration (5°C). NIMBEX should be refrigerated at 2° to 8°C (36° to 46°F) in the carton to preserve potency. The rate of loss in potency increases to approximately 5% per *month* at 25°C (77°F). Upon removal from refrigeration to room temperature storage conditions (25°C/77°F), use NIMBEX within 21 days, even if rerefrigerated.

CLINICAL PHARMACOLOGY

NIMBEX binds competitively to cholinergic receptors on the motor end-plate to antagonize the action of acetylcholine, resulting in block of neuromuscular transmission. This action is antagonized by acetylcholinesterase inhibitors such as neostigmine.

Pharmacodynamics

The neuromuscular blocking potency of NIMBEX is approximately threefold that of atracurium besylate. The time to maximum block is up to 2 minutes longer for equipotent doses of NIMBEX compared to atracurium besylate. The clinically effective duration of action and rate of spontaneous recovery from equipotent doses of NIMBEX and atracurium besylate are similar.

The average ED_{95} (dose required to produce 95% suppression of the adductor pollicis muscle twitch response to ulnar nerve stimulation) of cisatracurium is 0.05 mg/kg (range: 0.048 to 0.053) in adults receiving opioid/nitrous oxide/oxygen anesthesia. For comparison, the average ED_{95} for atracurium when also expressed as the parent bis-cation is 0.17 mg/kg under similar anesthetic conditions.

The pharmacodynamics of 2 × ED_{95} to 8 × ED_{95} doses of cisatracurium administered over 5 to 10 seconds during opioid/nitrous oxide/oxygen anesthesia are summarized in Table 1. When the dose is doubled, the clinically effective duration of block increases by approximately 25 minutes. Once recovery begins, the rate of recovery is independent of dose.

Isoflurane or enflurane administered with nitrous oxide/oxygen to achieve 1.25 MAC [Minimum Alveolar Concentration] may prolong the clinically effective duration of action of initial and maintenance doses, and decrease the average infusion rate requirement of NIMBEX. The magnitude of these effects may depend on the duration of administration of the volatile agents. Fifteen to 30 minutes of exposure to 1.25 MAC isoflurane or enflurane had minimal effects on the duration of action of initial doses of NIMBEX and therefore, no adjustment to the initial dose should be necessary when NIMBEX is administered shortly after initiation of volatile agents. In long surgical procedures during enflurane or isoflurane anesthesia, less frequent maintenance dosing, lower maintenance doses, or reduced infusion rates of NIMBEX may be necessary. The average infusion rate requirement may be decreased by as much as 30% to 40%.

The onset, duration of action, and recovery profiles of NIMBEX during propofol/oxygen or propofol/nitrous oxide/oxygen anesthesia are similar to those during opioid/nitrous oxide/oxygen anesthesia.

[See table 1 at top of next page]

When administered during the induction of adequate anesthesia using propofol, nitrous oxide/oxygen, and co-induction agents (e.g., fentanyl and midazolam), GOOD or EXCELLENT conditions for tracheal intubation occurred in 96/102 (94%) patients in 1.5 to 2.0 minutes following 0.15 mg/kg cisatracurium and in 97/110 (88%) patients in 1.5 minutes following 0.2 mg/kg cisatracurium.

In one intubation study during thiopental anesthesia in which fentanyl and midazolam were administered two minutes prior to induction, intubation conditions were assessed at 120 seconds. Table 2 displays these results in this study of 51 patients.

Table 2. Study of Tracheal Intubation Comparing Two Doses of Cisatracurium (Thiopental Anesthesia)

Intubating Conditions at 120 seconds	3 × ED_{95} 0.15 mg/kg n = 26	4 × ED_{95} 0.20 mg/kg n = 25
Excellent and Good		
Proportion	23/26	24/25
Percent	88%	96%
95% CI	76,100	88,100
Excellent		
Proportion	8/26	15/26
Percent	31%	60%
Good		
Proportion	15/26	9/25
Percent	58%	36%

While GOOD or EXCELLENT intubation conditions were achieved in the majority of patients in this setting, EXCELLENT intubation conditions were more frequently achieved with the 0.2 mg/kg dose (60%) than the 0.15 mg/kg dose (31%) when intubation was attempted 2.0 minutes following cisatracurium.

A second study evaluated intubation conditions after 3 and 4 × ED_{95} (0.15 mg/kg and 0.20 mg/kg) following induction with fentanyl and midazolam and either thiopental or propofol anesthesia. This study compared intubation conditions produced by these doses of cisatracurium after 1.5 minutes. Table 3 displays these results.

[See table 3 at top of next page]

EXCELLENT intubation conditions were more frequently observed with the 0.2 mg/kg dose when intubation was attempted 1.5 minutes following cisatracurium.

A third study in pediatric patients (ages 1 month to 12 years) evaluated intubation conditions at 120 seconds after 0.15 mg/kg NIMBEX following induction with either halothane (with halothane/nitrous oxide/oxygen maintenance) or thiopentone and fentanyl (with thiopentone/fentanyl nitrous oxide/oxygen maintenance). The results are summarized in Table 4.

[See table 4 at top of next page]

EXCELLENT or GOOD intubating conditions were produced 120 seconds following 0.15 mg/kg NIMBEX in 88/90 (98%) of patients induced with halothane and in 85/90 (94%) of patients induced with thiopentone and fentanyl. There were no patients for whom intubation was not possible, but there were 7/120 patients ages 1 12 years for whom intubating conditions were described as poor.

Repeated administration of maintenance doses or a continuous infusion of NIMBEX for up to 3 hours is not associated with development of tachyphylaxis or cumulative neuromuscular blocking effects. The time needed to recover from successive maintenance doses does not change with the

Information on the AbbVie, Inc. products listed on these pages is from the prescribing information in use as of July 31, 2013. For more information, please visit rxabbvie.com or call 1-800-633-9110.

Table 1. Pharmacodynamic Dose Response* of NIMBEX During Opioid/Nitrous Oxide/Oxygen Anesthesia

Initial Dose of NIMBEX (mg/kg)	Time to 90% Block (min)	Time to Maximum Block (min)	Time to Spontaneous Recovery				25%-75% Recovery Index (min)
			5% Recovery (min)	25% Recovery† (min)	95% Recovery (min)	T_4:T_1 Ratio‡≥70% (min)	
Adults							
0.1 (2 × ED_{95}) (n§=98)	3.3 (1.0-8.7)	5.0 (1.2-17.2)	33 (15-51)	42 (22-63)	64 (25-93)	64 (32-91)	13 (5-30)
0.15‖ (3 × ED_{95}) (n=39)	2.6 (1.0-4.4)	3.5 (1.6-6.8)	46 (28-65)	55 (44-74)	76 (60-103)	75 (63-98)	13 (11-16)
0.2 (4 × ED_{95}) (n=30)	2.4 (1.5-4.5)	2.9 (1.9-5.2)	59 (31-103)	65 (43-103)	81 (53-114)	85 (55-114)	12 (2-30)
0.25 (5 × ED_{95}) (n=15)	1.6 (0.8-3.3)	2.0 (1.2-3.7)	70 (58-85)	78 (66-86)	91 (76-109)	97 (82-113)	8 (5-12)
0.4 (8 × ED_{95}) (n=15)	1.5 (1.3-1.8)	1.9 (1.4-2.3)	83 (37-103)	91 (59-107)	121 (110-134)	126 (115-137)	14 (10-18)
Infants (1-23 mos.)							
0.15** (n=18-26)	1.5 (0.7-3.2)	2.0 (1.3-4.3)	36 (28-50)	43 (34-58)	64 (54-84)	59 (49-76)	11.3 (7.3-18.3)
Children (2-12 yr)							
0.08¶ (2 × ED_{95}) (n=60)	2.2 (1.2-6.8)	3.3 (1.7-9.7)	22 (11-38)	29 (20-46)	52 (37-64)	50 (37-62)	11 (7-15)
0.1 (n=16)	1.7 (1.3-2.7)	2.8 (1.8-6.7)	21 (13-31)	28 (21-38)	46 (37-58)	44 (36-58)	10 (7-12)
0.15** (n=23-24)	2.1 (1.3-2.8)	3.0 (1.5-8.0)	29 (19-38)	36 (29-46)	55 (45-72)	54 (44-66)	10.6 (8.5-17.7)

* Values shown are medians of means from individual studies. Values in parentheses are ranges of individual patient values.
† Clinically effective duration of block.
‡ Train-of-four ratio.
§ n=the number of patients with Time to Maximum Block data.
‖ Propofol anesthesia.
¶ Halothane anesthesia.
** Thiopentone, alfentanil, N_2O/O_2 anesthesia

Table 3. Study of Tracheal Intubation Comparing Three Doses of Cisatracurium (Thiopental or Propofol Anesthesia)

Intubating Conditions at 90 seconds	3 × ED_{95} 0.15 mg/kg Propofol n = 31	3 × ED_{95} 0.15 mg/kg Thiopental n = 31	4 × ED_{95} 0.20 mg/kg Propofol n = 30	4 × ED_{95} 0.20 mg/kg Thiopental n = 28
Excellent and Good				
Proportion	29/31	28/31	28/30	27/28
Percent	94%	90%	93%	96%
95% CI	85,100	80,100	84,100	90,100
Excellent				
Proportion	18/31	17/31	22/30	16/28
Percent	58%	55%	70%	57%
Good				
Proportion	11/31	11/31	6/30	11/28
Percent	35%	35%	20%	39%

Table 4. Study of Tracheal Intubation for Pediatrics Stratified by Age Group (0.15 mg/kg NIMBEX with Halothane or Thiopentone/ Fentanyl Anesthesia)

Intubating Conditions at 120 seconds**	NIMBEX 0.15 mg/kg 1-11 mo. n = 30		NIMBEX 0.15 mg/kg 1- 4 years n = 31		NIMBEX 0.15 mg/kg 5-12 years n = 30	
	Halothane Anesthesia	Thiopentone/ Fentanyl Anesthesia	Halothane Anesthesia	Thiopentone/ Fentanyl Anesthesia	Halothane Anesthesia	Thiopentone/ Fentanyl Anesthesia
Excellent and Good						
Proportion	30/30	30/30	29/30	26/30	29/30	29/30
Percent	100%	100%	97%	87%	97%	97%
Excellent						
Proportion	30/30	25/30	27/30	19/30	22/30	21/30
Percent	100%	83%	90%	63%	73%	70%
Good						
Proportion	0	5/30	2/30	7/30	7/30	8/30
Percent	0%	17%	7%	23%	23%	27%
Poor						
Proportion	0/30	0/30	1/30	4/30	1/30	1/30
Percent	0%	0%	3%	13%	3%	3%

** **Excellent:** Easy passage of the tube without coughing. Vocal cords relaxed and abducted.
Good: Passage of tube with slight coughing and/or bucking. Vocal cords relaxed and abducted.
Poor: Passage of tube with moderate coughing and/or bucking. Vocal cords moderately adducted. Response of patient requires adjustment of ventilation pressure and/or rate.

number of doses administered as long as partial recovery is allowed to occur between doses. Maintenance doses can therefore be administered at relatively regular intervals with predictable results. The rate of spontaneous recovery of neuromuscular function after infusion is independent of the duration of infusion and comparable to the rate of recovery following initial doses (Table 1).

Long-term infusion (up to 6 days) of NIMBEX during mechanical ventilation in the ICU has been evaluated in two studies. In a randomized, double-blind study using presence of a single twitch during train-of-four (TOF) monitoring to regulate dosage, patients treated with NIMBEX (n = 19) recovered neuromuscular function (T_4:T_1 ratio ≥ 70%) following termination of infusion in approximately 55 minutes (range: 20 to 270) whereas those treated with vecuronium (n = 12) recovered in 178 minutes (range: 40 minutes to 33 hours). In another study comparing NIMBEX and atracurium, patients recovered neuromuscular function in approximately 50 minutes for both NIMBEX (range: 20 to 175; n = 34) and atracurium (range: 35 to 85; n = 15).

The neuromuscular block produced by NIMBEX is readily antagonized by anticholinesterase agents once recovery has started. As with other nondepolarizing neuromuscular blocking agents, the more profound the neuromuscular block at the time of reversal, the longer the time required for recovery of neuromuscular function.

In children (2 to 12 years) cisatracurium has a lower ED_{95} than in adults (0.04 mg/kg, halothane/nitrous oxide/oxygen anesthesia). At 0.1 mg/kg during opioid anesthesia, cisatracurium had a faster onset and shorter duration of action in children than in adults (Table 1). Recovery following reversal is faster in children than in adults.

At 0.15 mg/kg during opioid anesthesia, cisatracurium had a faster onset and longer clinically effective duration of action in infants aged 1-23 months compared to children aged 2-12 years (Table 1).

Studies were conducted during both opioid-based and halothane-based anesthesia in children aged 1-11 months, 1-4 years, and 5-12 years. Cisatracurium had a faster onset and longer duration of action in infants 1-11 months compared to children 1-4 years, who in turn have a faster onset and longer duration of action for cisatracurium compared to children 5-12 years.

The mean time to onset of maximum T_1 suppression was generally faster for pediatric patients induced with halothane compared to thiopentone/fentanyl and the clinically effective duration (time to 25% recovery) was longer (by up to 15%) for pediatric patients under halothane anesthesia.

Hemodynamics Profile

The cardiovascular profile of NIMBEX allows it to be administered by rapid bolus at higher multiples of the ED_{95} than atracurium. NIMBEX has no dose-related effects on mean arterial blood pressure (MAP) or heart rate (HR) following doses ranging from 2 to 8 × ED_{95} (> 0.1 to > 0.4 mg/kg), administered over 5 to 10 seconds, in healthy adult patients (Figure 1) or in patients with serious cardiovascular disease (Figure 2).

A total of 141 patients undergoing coronary artery bypass grafting (CABG) have been administered NIMBEX in three active controlled clinical trials and have received doses ranging from 2 to 8 × ED_{95}. While the hemodynamic profile was comparable in both the NIMBEX and active control groups, data for doses above 0.3 mg/kg in this population are limited.

Unlike atracurium, NIMBEX® (cisatracurium besylate), at therapeutic doses of 2 × ED_{95} to 8 × ED_{95} (0.1 to 0.4 mg/kg), administered over 5 to 10 seconds, does not cause dose-related elevations in mean plasma histamine concentration.

[See figure 1 at top of next column]
[See figure 2 at top of next column]

No clinically significant changes in MAP or HR were observed following administration of doses up to 0.1 mg/kg NIMBEX over 5 to 10 seconds in 2- to 12-year-old children receiving either halothane/nitrous oxide/oxygen or opioid/nitrous oxide/oxygen anesthesia. Doses of 0.15 mg/kg NIMBEX administered over 5 seconds were not consistently associated with changes in HR and MAP in pediatric patients aged 1 month to 12 years receiving opioid/nitrous oxide/oxygen or halothane/nitrous oxide/oxygen anesthesia.

[See figure 3 in second column on next page]
[See figure 4 in third column on next page]

Pharmacokinetics

General

The neuromuscular blocking activity of NIMBEX is due to parent drug. Cisatracurium plasma concentration-time data following IV bolus administration are best described by a two-compartment open model (with elimination from both compartments) with an elimination half-life ($t_{1/2}\beta$) of 22 minutes, a plasma clearance (CL) of 4.57 mL/min/kg, and a volume of distribution at steady state (V_{ss}) of 145 mL/kg. Cisatracurium undergoes organ-independent Hofmann elimination (a chemical process dependent on pH and temperature) to form the monoquaternary acrylate metabolite and laudanosine, neither of which has any neuromuscular blocking activity (see **Pharmacokinetics** -Metabolism sec-

Figure 1. Maximum Percent Change from Preinjection In Heart Rate (HR) and Mean Arterial Pressure (MAP) During First 5 Minutes after Initial 4 x ED_{95} to 8 x ED_{95} Doses of NIMBEX in Healthy Adult Patients Receiving Opioid/Nitrous Oxide/Oxygen Anesthesia (n = 44)

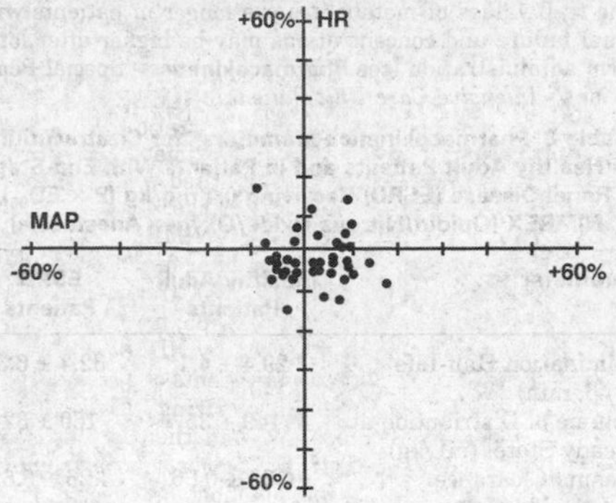

Figure 2. Percent Change from Preinjection in Heart Rate (HR) and Mean Arterial Pressure (MAP) 10 Minutes After an Initial 4 x ED_{95} to 8 x ED_{95} Dose of NIMBEX in Patients Undergoing CABG Surgery Receiving Oxygen/Fentanyl/Midazolam/ Anesthesia (n = 54)

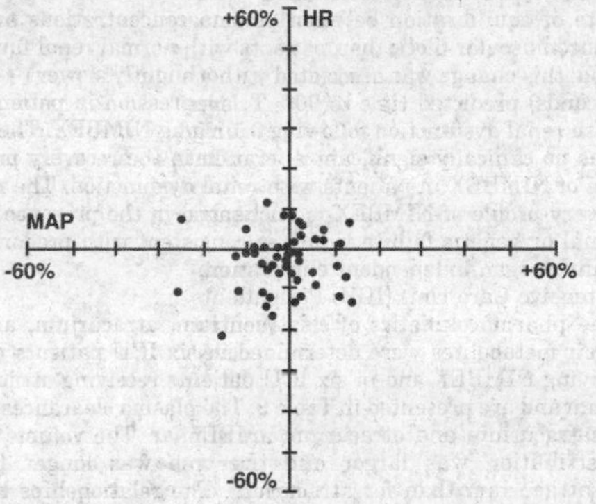

tion). Following administration of radiolabeled cisatracurium, 95% of the dose was recovered in the urine; less than 10% of the dose was excreted as unchanged parent drug. Laudanosine, a metabolite of cisatracurium (and atracurium) has been noted to cause transient hypotension and, in higher doses, cerebral excitatory effects when administered to several animal species. The relationship between CNS excitation and laudanosine concentrations in humans has not been established (see **PRECAUTIONS - Long-term Use in the Intensive Care Unit**). Because cisatracurium is three times more potent than atracurium and lower doses are required, the corresponding laudanosine concentrations following cisatracurium are one third of those that would be expected following an equipotent dose of atracurium (see **Pharmacokinetics** - Special Populations -*Intensive Care Unit Patients*).

Results from population pharmacokinetic/pharmacodynamic (PK/PD) analyses from 241 healthy surgical patients are summarized in Table 5.

Table 5. Key Population PK/PD Parameter Estimates for Cisatracurium in Healthy Surgical Patients* Following 0.1 (2 × ED_{95}) to 0.4 mg/kg (8 × ED_{95}) NIMBEX

Parameter	Estimate†	Magnitude of Interpatient Variability (CV)‡
CL (mL/min/kg)	4.57	16%
V_{ss} (mL/kg)§	145	27%
k_{eo} (min-1)‖	0.0575	61%
EC_{50} (ng/mL)¶	141	52%

* Healthy male non-obese patients 19-64 years of age with creatinine clearance values greater than 70 mL/min who received cisatracurium during opioid anesthesia and had venous samples collected.

† The percent standard error of the mean (%SEM) ranged from 3% to 12% indicating good precision for the PK/PD estimates.

‡ Expressed as a coefficient of variation; the %SEM ranged from 20% to 35% indicating adequate precision for the estimates of interpatient variability.

Figure 3. Heart Rate and MAP Change at 1 Minute After the Initial Dose, By Age Group Treatment Group: NIMBEX 0:3 x ED_{95} Opioid Intubation at 120 Sec.

1-11 Months

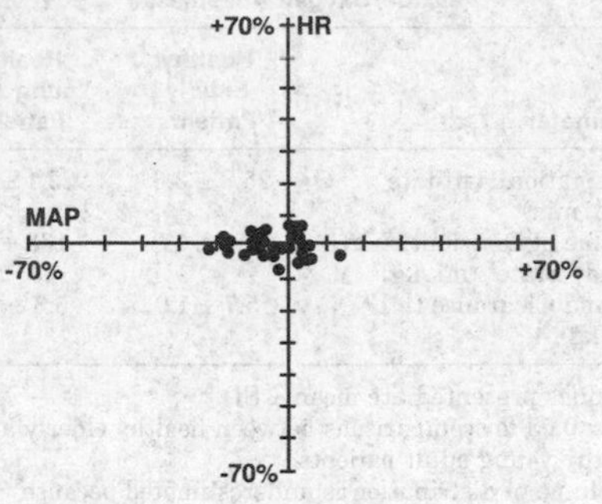

1-5 Years

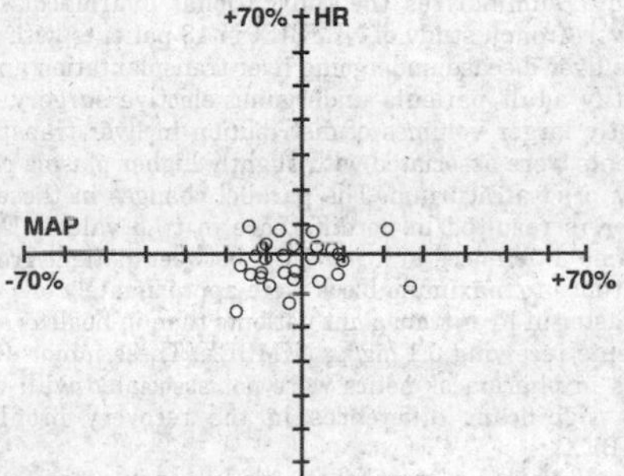

5-13 Years

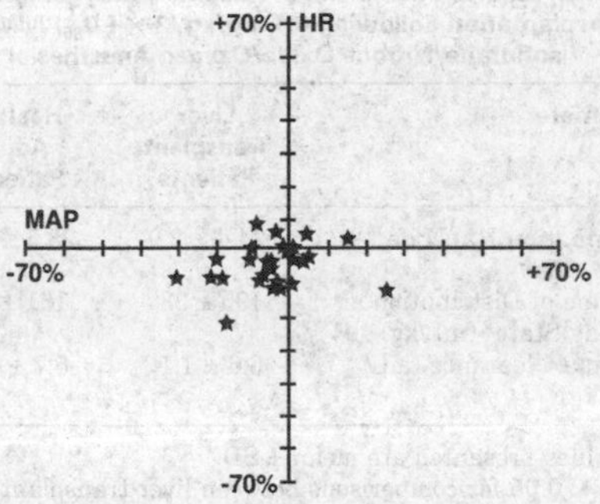

§ V_{ss} is the volume of distribution at steady state estimated using a two-compartment model with elimination from both compartments. V_{ss} is equal to the sum of the volume in the central compartment (V_c) and the volume in the peripheral compartment (Vp); interpatient variability could only be estimated for V_c.

‖ Rate constant describing the equilibration between plasma concentrations and neuromuscular block.

¶ Concentration required to produce 50% T_1 suppression; an index of patient sensitivity.

The magnitude of interpatient variability in CL was low (16%), as expected based on the importance of Hofmann elimination (see **Pharmacokinetics** -Elimination). The magnitudes of interpatient variability in CL and volume of distribution were low in comparison to those for k_{eo} and EC_{50}. This suggests that any alterations in the time course of cisatracurium-induced block are more likely to be due to variability in the pharmacodynamic parameters than in the pharmacokinetic parameters. Parameter estimates from the population pharmacokinetic analyses were supported by noncompartmental pharmacokinetic analyses on data from healthy patients and from special patient populations.

Conventional pharmacokinetic analyses have shown that the pharmacokinetics of cisatracurium are proportional to dose between 0.1 (2 × ED_{95}) and 0.2 (4 × ED_{95}) mg/kg cisatracurium. In addition, population pharmacokinetic

Figure 4. Heart Rate and MAP Change at 1 Minute After the Initial Dose, By Age Group Treatment Group: NIMBEX H:3 x ED_{95} Halothane Intubation at 120 Sec.

1-11 Months

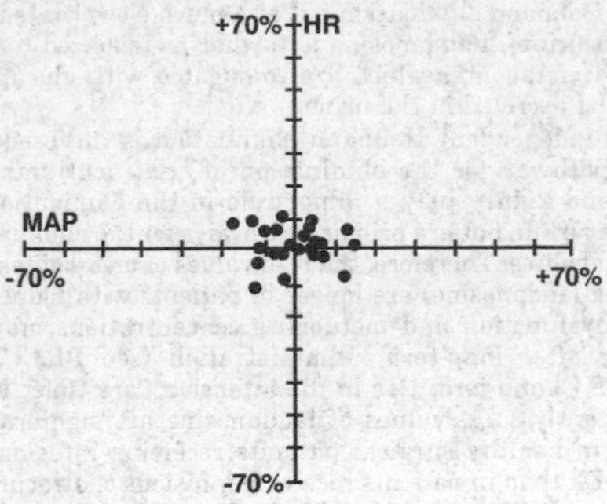

1-5 Years

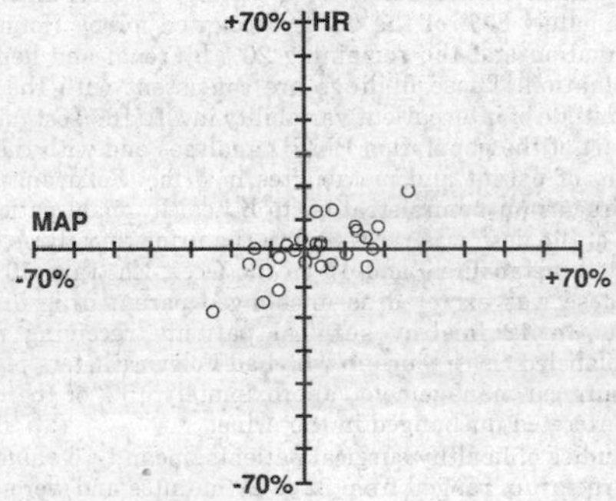

5-13 Years

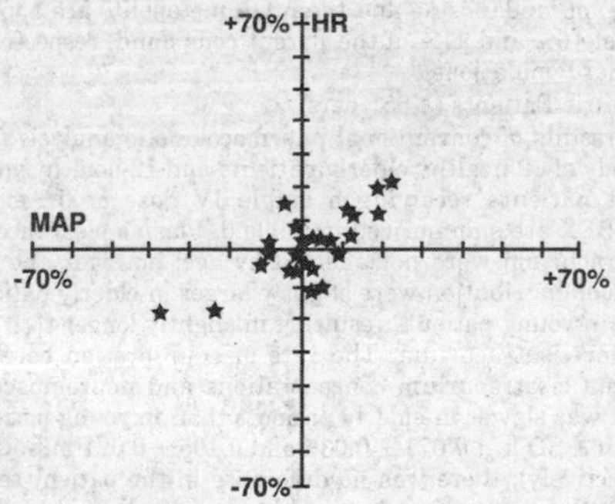

analyses revealed no statistically significant effect of initial dose on CL for doses between 0.1 (2 × ED_{95}) and 0.4 (8 × ED_{95}) mg/kg cisatracurium.

Distribution

The volume of distribution of cisatracurium is limited by its large molecular weight and high polarity. The V_{ss} was equal to 145 mL/kg (Table 4) in healthy 19- to 64-year-old surgical patients receiving opioid anesthesia. The V_{ss} was 21% larger in similar patients receiving inhalation anesthesia (see **Pharmacokinetics** - Special Populations -*Other Patient Factors*).

Protein Binding

The binding of cisatracurium to plasma proteins has not been successfully studied due to its rapid degradation at physiologic pH. Inhibition of degradation requires non-physiological conditions of temperature and pH which are associated with changes in protein binding.

Metabolism

The degradation of cisatracurium is largely independent of liver metabolism. Results from *in vitro* experiments suggest that cisatracurium undergoes Hofmann elimination (a pH

Information on the AbbVie, Inc. products listed on these pages is from the prescribing information in use as of July 31, 2013. For more information, please visit rxabbvie.com or call 1-800-633-9110.

and temperature-dependent chemical process) to form laudanosine (see **PRECAUTIONS - Long-term Use in the Intensive Care Unit**) and the monoquaternary acrylate metabolite. The monoquaternary acrylate undergoes hydrolysis by non-specific plasma esterases to form the monoquaternary alcohol (MQA) metabolite. The MQA metabolite can also undergo Hofmann elimination but at a much slower rate than cisatracurium. Laudanosine is further metabolized to desmethyl metabolites which are conjugated with glucuronic acid and excreted in the urine.

Organ-independent Hofmann elimination is the predominant pathway for the elimination of cisatracurium. The liver and kidney play a minor role in the elimination of cisatracurium but are primary pathways for the elimination of metabolites. Therefore, the $t_{1/2}\beta$ values of metabolites (including laudanosine) are longer in patients with kidney or liver dysfunction and metabolite concentrations may be higher after long-term administration (see **PRECAUTIONS - Long-term Use in the Intensive Care Unit**). Most importantly, C_{max} values of laudanosine are significantly lower in healthy surgical patients receiving infusions of NIMBEX than in patients receiving infusions of atracurium (mean ± SD C_{max}: 60 ± 52 and 342 ± 93 ng/mL, respectively).

Elimination

Clearance and Half-life

Mean CL values for cisatracurium ranged from 4.5 to 5.7 mL/min/kg in studies of healthy surgical patients. Compartmental pharmacokinetic modeling suggests that approximately 80% of the CL is accounted for by Hofmann elimination and the remaining 20% by renal and hepatic elimination. These findings are consistent with the low magnitude of interpatient variability in CL (16%) estimated as part of the population PK/PD analyses and with the recovery of parent and metabolites in urine. Following ^{14}C-cisatracurium administration to 6 healthy male patients, 95% of the dose was recovered in the urine (mostly as conjugated metabolites) and 4% in the feces; less than 10% of the dose was excreted as unchanged parent drug in the urine. In 12 healthy surgical patients receiving non-radiolabeled cisatracurium who had Foley catheters placed for surgical management, approximately 15% of the dose was excreted unchanged in the urine.

In studies of healthy surgical patients, mean $t_{1/2}\beta$ values of cisatracurium ranged from 22 to 29 minutes and were consistent with the $t_{1/2}\beta$ of cisatracurium *in vitro* (29 minutes). The mean ± SD $t_{1/2}\beta$ values of laudanosine were 3.1 ± 0.4 and 3.3 ± 2.1 hours in healthy surgical patients receiving NIMBEX (n = 10) or atracurium (n = 10), respectively. During IV infusions of NIMBEX, peak plasma concentrations (C_{max}) of laudanosine and the MQA metabolite are approximately 6% and 11% of the parent compound, respectively.

Special Populations

Geriatric Patients (≥ 65 years)

The results of conventional pharmacokinetic analysis from a study of 12 healthy elderly patients and 12 healthy young adult patients receiving a single IV dose of 0.1 mg/kg NIMBEX are summarized in Table 6. Plasma clearances of cisatracurium were not affected by age; however, the volumes of distribution were slightly larger in elderly patients than in young patients resulting in slightly longer $t_{1/2}\beta$ values for cisatracurium. The rate of equilibration between plasma cisatracurium concentrations and neuromuscular block was slower in elderly patients than in young patients (mean ± SD k_{eo}: 0.071 ± 0.036 and 0.105 ± 0.021 $minutes^{-1}$, respectively); there was no difference in the patient sensitivity to cisatracurium-induced block, as indicated by EC_{50} values (mean ± SD EC_{50}: 91 ± 22 and 89 ± 23 ng/mL, respectively). These changes were consistent with the 1-minute slower times to maximum block in elderly patients receiving 0.1 mg/kg NIMBEX, when compared to young patients receiving the same dose. The minor differences in PK/PD parameters of cisatracurium between elderly patients and young patients were not associated with clinically significant differences in the recovery profile of NIMBEX® (cisatracurium besylate).

Table 6. Pharmacokinetic Parameters* of Cisatracurium in Healthy Elderly and Young Adult Patients Following 0.1 mg/kg (2 × ED_{95}) NIMBEX (Isoflurane/Nitrous Oxide/Oxygen Anesthesia)

Parameter	Healthy Elderly Patients	Healthy Young Adult Patients
Elimination Half-Life ($t_{1/2}\beta$, min)	25.8 ± 3.6†	22.1 ± 2.5
Volume of Distribution at Steady State‡ (mL/kg)	156 ± 17†	133 ± 15
Plasma Clearance (mL/min/kg)	5.7 ± 1.0	5.3 ± 0.9

* Values presented are mean ± SD.
† P < 0.05 for comparisons between healthy elderly and healthy young adult patients.
‡ Volume of distribution is underestimated because elimination from the peripheral compartment is ignored.

Patients with Hepatic Disease

Table 7 summarizes the conventional pharmacokinetic analysis from a study of NIMBEX in 13 patients with end-stage liver disease undergoing liver transplantation and 11 healthy adult patients undergoing elective surgery. The slightly larger volumes of distribution in liver transplant patients were associated with slightly higher plasma clearances of cisatracurium. The parallel changes in these parameters resulted in no difference in $t_{1/2}\beta$ values. There were no differences in k_{eo} or EC_{50} between patient groups. The times to maximum block were approximately one minute faster in liver transplant patients than in healthy adult patients receiving 0.1 mg/kg NIMBEX. These minor differences in pharmacokinetics were not associated with clinically significant differences in the recovery profile of NIMBEX.

The $t_{1/2}\beta$ values of metabolites are longer in patients with hepatic disease and concentrations may be higher after long-term administration (see **Pharmacokinetics** - Special Populations - *Intensive Care Unit Patients*).

Table 7. Pharmacokinetic Parameters* of Cisatracurium in Healthy Adult Patients and in Patients Undergoing Liver Transplantation Following 0.1 mg/kg (2 × ED_{95}) NIMBEX (Isoflurane/Nitrous Oxide/Oxygen Anesthesia)

Parameter	Liver Transplant Patients	Healthy Adult Patients
Elimination Half-Life ($t_{1/2}\beta$, min)	24.4 ± 2.9	23.5 ± 3.5
Volume of Distribution at Steady State‡ (mL/kg)	195 ± 38†	161 ± 23
Plasma Clearance (mL/min/kg)	6.6 ± 1.1†	5.7 ± 0.8

* Values presented are mean ± SD.
† P < 0.05 for comparisons between liver transplant patients and healthy adult patients.
‡ Volume of distribution is underestimated because elimination from the peripheral compartment is ignored.

Patients with Renal Dysfunction

Results from a conventional pharmacokinetic study of NIMBEX in 13 healthy adult patients and 15 patients with end-stage renal disease (ESRD) undergoing elective surgery are summarized in Table 8. The PK/PD parameters of cisatracurium were similar in healthy adult patients and ESRD patients. The times to 90% block were approximately one minute slower in ESRD patients following 0.1 mg/kg NIMBEX. There were no differences in the durations or rates of recovery of NIMBEX between ESRD and healthy adult patients.

The $t_{1/2}\beta$ values of metabolites are longer in patients with renal failure and concentrations may be higher after long-term administration (see **Pharmacokinetics** - Special Populations - *Intensive Care Unit Patients*).

Table 8. Pharmacokinetic Parameters* for Cisatracurium in Healthy Adult Patients and in Patients With End-Stage Renal Disease (ESRD) Receiving 0.1 mg/kg (2 × ED_{95}) NIMBEX (Opioid/Nitrous Oxide/Oxygen Anesthesia)

Parameter	Healthy Adult Patients	ESRD Patients
Elimination Half-Life ($t_{1/2}\beta$, min)	29.4 ± 4.1	32.3 ± 6.3
Volume of Distribution at Steady State† (mL/kg)	149 ± 35	160 ± 32
Plasma Clearance (mL/min/kg)	4.66 ± 0.86	4.26 ± 0.62

* Values presented are mean ± SD.
† Volume of distribution is underestimated because elimination from the peripheral compartment is ignored.

Population pharmacokinetic analyses revealed that patients with creatinine clearances ≤ 70 mL/min had a slower rate of equilibration between plasma concentrations and neuromuscular block than patients with normal renal function; this change was associated with a slightly slower (~ 40 seconds) predicted time to 90% T_1 suppression in patients with renal dysfunction following 0.1 mg/kg NIMBEX. There was no clinically significant alteration in the recovery profile of NIMBEX in patients with renal dysfunction. The recovery profile of NIMBEX is unchanged in the presence of renal or hepatic failure, which is consistent with predominantly organ-independent elimination.

Intensive Care Unit (ICU) Patients

The pharmacokinetics of cisatracurium, atracurium, and their metabolites were determined in six ICU patients receiving NIMBEX and in six ICU patients receiving atracurium and are presented in Table 9. The plasma clearances of cisatracurium and atracurium are similar. The volume of distribution was larger and the $t_{1/2}\beta$ was longer for cisatracurium than for atracurium. The relationships between plasma cisatracurium or atracurium concentrations and neuromuscular block have not been evaluated in ICU patients. The minor differences in pharmacokinetics were not associated with any differences in the recovery profiles of NIMBEX and atracurium in ICU patients.

[See table 9 below]

Table 9. Parameter Estimates* for Cisatracurium, Atracurium, and Metabolites in ICU Patients After Long-Term (24-48 Hour) Administration of NIMBEX or Atracurium Besylate

	Parameter	Cisatracurium (n = 6)	Atracurium (n = 6)
Parent Compound	CL (mL/min/kg)	7.45 ± 1.02	7.49 ± 0.66†
	$t_{1/2}\beta$ (min)	26.8 ± 11.1	16.5 ± 6.0†
	Vβ (mL/kg)‡	280 ± 103	178 ± 71†
Laudanosine	C_{max} (ng/mL)	707 ± 360	2318 ± 1498
	$t_{1/2}\beta$ (hrs)	6.6 ± 4.1	8.4 ± 7.3
MQA metabolite	C_{max} (ng/mL)	152-181§	943 ± 333‖
	$t_{1/2}\beta$ (min)	26-31§	21-58§

* Presented as mean ± standard deviation.
† n = 5.
‡ Volume of distribution during the terminal elimination phase, an underestimate because elimination from the peripheral compartment is ignored.
§ n = 2, range presented.
‖ n = 3.

Plasma metabolite pharmacokinetics are listed in Table 9. Limited pharmacokinetic data are available for patients with liver/kidney dysfunction receiving NIMBEX. Data from studies of atracurium demonstrate that renal/hepatic failure in ICU patients produces little to no effect on its pharmacokinetics, but decreases the biotransformation and elimination of the metabolites. Following atracurium, $t_{1/2}\beta$ values for laudanosine were longer in ICU patients with renal failure than in ICU patients with normal renal function (15 and 6 hours, respectively). The $t_{1/2}\beta$ values of laudanosine were 39 ± 14 hours in ICU patients with liver failure receiving atracurium after an unsuccessful liver transplantation and 5 ± 2 hours in similar ICU patients after successful liver transplantation. Therefore, relative to ICU patients with normal renal and hepatic function receiving NIMBEX, metabolite concentrations (plasma and tissues) may be higher in ICU patients with renal or hepatic failure (see **Precautions - Long-term Use in the Intensive Care Unit**). Consistent with the decreased infusion rate requirements for NIMBEX, metabolite concentrations were lower in patients receiving NIMBEX than in patients receiving atracurium besylate.

Pediatric Patients

The population PK/PD of cisatracurium were described in 20 healthy pediatric patients during halothane anesthesia, using the same model developed for healthy adult patients. The CL was higher in healthy pediatric patients (5.89 mL/min/kg) than in healthy adult patients (4.57 mL/min/kg) during opioid anesthesia. The rate of equilibration between plasma concentrations and neuromuscular block, as indicated by k_{eo}, was faster in healthy pediatric patients receiving halothane anesthesia (0.1330 $minutes^{-1}$) than in healthy adult patients receiving opioid anesthesia (0.0575 $minutes^{-1}$). The EC_{50} in healthy pediatric patients (125 ng/mL) was similar to the value in healthy adult patients (141 ng/mL) during opioid anesthesia. The minor differences in the PK/PD parameters of cisatracurium were associated with a faster time to onset and a shorter duration of cisatracurium-induced neuromuscular block in pediatric patients.

Other Patient Factors

Population PK/PD analyses revealed that gender and obesity were associated with statistically significant effects on the pharmacokinetics and/or pharmacodynamics of cisatracurium; these factors were not associated with clinically significant alterations in the predicted onset or recovery profile of NIMBEX. The use of inhalation agents was associated with a 21% larger V_{ss}, a 78% larger k_{eo}, and a 15% lower EC_{50} for cisatracurium. These changes resulted in a slightly faster (~45 seconds) predicted time to 90% T_1 suppression in patients receiving 0.1 mg/kg cisatracurium during inhalation anesthesia than in patients receiving the same dose of cisatracurium during opioid anesthesia; however, there were no clinically significant differences in the predicted recovery profile of NIMBEX between patient groups.

Individualization of Dosages

DOSES OF **NIMBEX** SHOULD BE INDIVIDUALIZED AND A PERIPHERAL NERVE STIMULATOR SHOULD BE USED TO MEASURE NEUROMUSCULAR FUNCTION DURING ADMINISTRATION OF **NIMBEX** IN ORDER TO MONITOR DRUG EFFECT, TO DETERMINE THE NEED FOR ADDITIONAL DOSES, AND TO CONFIRM RECOVERY FROM NEUROMUSCULAR BLOCK.

Based on the known action of NIMBEX and other neuromuscular blocking agents, the following factors should be considered when administering NIMBEX.

Renal and Hepatic Disease

See **PRECAUTIONS** section.

Long-Term Use in the Intensive Care Unit (ICU)

The long-term infusion (up to 6 days) of NIMBEX during mechanical ventilation in the ICU has been evaluated in two studies. Average infusion rates of approximately 3 mcg/kg/min (range: 0.5 to 10.2) were required to achieve adequate neuromuscular block. As with other neuromuscular blocking agents, these data indicate the presence of wide interpatient variability in dosage requirements. In addition, dosage requirements may increase or decrease with time (see **PRECAUTIONS**). Use of NIMBEX in the ICU for longer than 6 days has not been studied.

Drugs or Conditions Causing Potentiation of or Resistance to Neuromuscular Block

Persons with certain pre-existing conditions or receiving certain drugs may require individualization of dosing (see **PRECAUTIONS**).

Burns

Patients with burns have been shown to develop resistance to nondepolarizing neuromuscular blocking agents, and may require individualization of dosing (see **PRECAUTIONS**).

INDICATIONS AND USAGE

NIMBEX is an intermediate-onset/intermediate-duration neuromuscular blocking agent indicated for inpatients and outpatients as an adjunct to general anesthesia, to facilitate tracheal intubation, and to provide skeletal muscle relaxation during surgery or mechanical ventilation in the ICU.

CONTRAINDICATIONS

NIMBEX is contraindicated in patients with known hypersensitivity to the product and its components. The 10 mL multiple-dose vials of Nimbex is contraindicated for use in premature infants because the formulation contains benzyl alcohol. (See **WARNINGS** and **PRECAUTIONS – Pediatric Use**).

WARNINGS

Anaphylaxis

Severe anaphylactic reactions to neuromuscular blocking agents, including NIMBEX, have been reported. These reactions have in some cases been life-threatening and fatal. Due to the potential severity of these reactions, the necessary precautions, such as the immediate availability of appropriate emergency treatment, should be taken. Precautions should also be taken in those individuals who have had previous anaphylactic reactions to other neuromuscular blocking agents since cross-reactivity between neuromuscular blocking agents, both depolarizing and non-depolarizing, has been reported in this class of drugs.

Administration

NIMBEX SHOULD BE ADMINISTERED IN CAREFULLY ADJUSTED DOSAGE BY OR UNDER THE SUPERVISION OF EXPERIENCED CLINICIANS WHO ARE FAMILIAR WITH THE DRUG'S ACTIONS AND THE POSSIBLE COMPLICATIONS OF ITS USE. THE DRUG SHOULD NOT BE ADMINISTERED UNLESS PERSONNEL AND FACILITIES FOR RESUSCITATION AND LIFE SUPPORT (TRACHEAL INTUBATION, ARTIFICIAL VENTILATION, OXYGEN THERAPY), AND AN ANTAGONIST OF **NIMBEX** ARE IMMEDIATELY AVAILABLE. IT IS RECOMMENDED THAT A PERIPHERAL NERVE STIMULATOR BE USED TO MEASURE NEUROMUSCULAR FUNCTION DURING THE ADMINISTRATION OF **NIMBEX** IN ORDER TO MONITOR DRUG EFFECT, DETERMINE THE NEED FOR ADDITIONAL DOSES, AND CONFIRM RECOVERY FROM NEUROMUSCULAR BLOCK.

NIMBEX HAS NO KNOWN EFFECT ON CONSCIOUSNESS, PAIN THRESHOLD, OR CEREBRATION. TO AVOID DISTRESS TO THE PATIENT, NEUROMUSCULAR BLOCK SHOULD NOT BE INDUCED BEFORE UNCONSCIOUSNESS.

NIMBEX Injection is acidic (pH 3.25 to 3.65) and may not be compatible with alkaline solutions having a pH greater than 8.5 (e.g., barbiturate solutions).

The 10 mL multiple-dose vials of NIMBEX contain benzyl alcohol, which is potentially toxic when administered locally to neural tissue. Exposure to excessive amounts of benzyl alcohol has been associated with toxicity (hypotension, metabolic acidosis), particularly in neonates, and an increased incidence of kernicterus, particularly in small preterm infants. There have been rare reports of deaths, primarily in preterm infants, associated with exposure to excessive amounts of benzyl alcohol. The amount of benzyl alcohol from medications is usually considered negligible compared to that received in flush solution containing benzyl alcohol. Administration of high dosages of medications containing this preservative must take into account the total amount of benzyl alcohol administered. The amount of benzyl alcohol at which toxicity may occur is not known. If the patient requires more than the recommended dosages or other medications containing this preservative, the practitioner must consider the daily metabolic load of benzyl alcohol from these combined sources. Single-use vials (5 mL and 20 mL) of NIMBEX do not contain benzyl alcohol (see **WARNINGS** and **PRECAUTIONS - Pediatric Use**).

PRECAUTIONS

Because of its intermediate onset of action, NIMBEX is not recommended for rapid sequence endotracheal intubation. Recommended doses of NIMBEX® (cisatracurium besylate) have no clinically significant effects on heart rate; therefore, NIMBEX will not counteract the bradycardia produced by many anesthetic agents or by vagal stimulation.

Neuromuscular blocking agents may have a profound effect in patients with neuromuscular diseases (e.g., myasthenia gravis and the myasthenic syndrome). In these and other conditions in which prolonged neuromuscular block is a possibility (e.g., carcinomatosis), the use of a peripheral nerve stimulator and a dose of not more than 0.02 mg/kg NIMBEX is recommended to assess the level of neuromuscular block and to monitor dosage requirements.

Patients with burns have been shown to develop resistance to nondepolarizing neuromuscular blocking agents, including atracurium. The extent of altered response depends upon the size of the burn and the time elapsed since the burn injury. NIMBEX has not been studied in patients with burns; however, based on its structural similarity to atracurium, the possibility of increased dosing requirements and shortened duration of action must be considered if NIMBEX is administered to burn patients.

Patients with hemiparesis or paraparesis also may demonstrate resistance to nondepolarizing muscle relaxants in the affected limbs. To avoid inaccurate dosing, neuromuscular monitoring should be performed on a non-paretic limb.

Acid-base and/or serum electrolyte abnormalities may potentiate or antagonize the action of neuromuscular blocking agents. No data are available to support the use of NIMBEX by intramuscular injection.

Allergic Reactions

Since allergic cross-reactivity has been reported in this class, request information from your patients about previous anaphylactic reactions to other neuromuscular blocking agents. In addition, inform your patients that severe anaphylactic reactions to neuromuscular blocking agents, including NIMBEX have been reported (see **CONTRAINDICATIONS**).

Renal and Hepatic Disease

No clinically significant alterations in the recovery profile were observed in patients with renal dysfunction or in patients with end-stage liver disease following a 0.1 mg/kg dose of cisatracurium. The onset time was approximately 1 minute faster in patients with end-stage liver disease and approximately 1 minute slower in patients with renal dysfunction than in healthy adult control patients.

Malignant Hyperthermia (MH)

In a study of MH-susceptible pigs, cisatracurium besylate (highest dose 2000 mcg/kg equivalent to 3 × ED_{95} in pigs and 40 × ED_{95} in humans) did not trigger MH. Cisatracurium besylate has not been studied in MH-susceptible patients. Because MH can develop in the absence of established triggering agents, the clinician should be prepared to recognize and treat MH in any patient undergoing general anesthesia.

Long-Term Use in the Intensive Care Unit (ICU)

Long-term infusion (up to 6 days) of NIMBEX during mechanical ventilation in the ICU has been safely used in two studies. Dosage requirements may increase or decrease with time (see **CLINICAL PHARMACOLOGY - Individualization of Doses**).

Little information is available on the plasma levels and clinical consequences of cisatracurium metabolites that may accumulate during days to weeks of cisatracurium administration in ICU patients. Laudanosine, a major, biologically active metabolite of atracurium and cisatracurium without neuromuscular blocking activity, produces transient hypotension and, in higher doses, cerebral excitatory effects (generalized muscle twitching and seizures) when administered to several species of animals. There have been rare spontaneous reports of seizures in ICU patients who have received atracurium or other agents. These patients usually had predisposing causes (such as cranial trauma, cerebral edema, hypoxic encephalopathy, viral encephalitis, uremia). There are insufficient data to determine whether or not laudanosine contributes to seizures in ICU patients. Consistent with the decreased infusion rate requirements for NIMBEX, laudanosine concentrations were lower in patients receiving NIMBEX than in patients receiving atracurium for up to 48 hours (see **Pharmacokinetics** -Special Populations - *Intensive Care Unit Patients*).

In a randomized, double-blind study using train-of-four nerve stimulator monitoring to maintain at least one visible twitch, evaluable patients treated with NIMBEX (n = 19) recovered neuromuscular function (T_4:T_1 ratio ≥ 70%) following termination of infusion in approximately 55 minutes (range: 20 to 270) whereas evaluable vecuronium-treated patients (n = 12) recovered in 178 minutes (range: 40 minutes to 33 hours). In another study comparing NIMBEX and atracurium, patients recovered neuromuscular function in approximately 50 minutes for both NIMBEX (range: 20 to 175; n = 34) and atracurium (range: 35 to 85; n = 15).

WHENEVER THE USE OF **NIMBEX** OR ANY OTHER NEUROMUSCULAR BLOCKING AGENT IN THE ICU IS CONTEMPLATED, IT IS RECOMMENDED THAT NEUROMUSCULAR FUNCTION BE MONITORED DURING ADMINISTRATION WITH A NERVE STIMULATOR. ADDITIONAL DOSES OF **NIMBEX** OR ANY OTHER NEUROMUSCULAR BLOCKING AGENT SHOULD NOT BE GIVEN BEFORE THERE IS A DEFINITE RESPONSE TO NERVE STIMULATION. IF NO RESPONSE IS ELICITED, INFUSION ADMINISTRATION SHOULD BE DISCONTINUED UNTIL A RESPONSE RETURNS.

The effects of hemofiltration, hemodialysis, and hemoperfusion on plasma levels of NIMBEX and its metabolites are unknown.

Drug Interactions

NIMBEX has been used safely following varying degrees of recovery from succinylcholine-induced neuromuscular block. Administration of 0.1 mg/kg (2 × ED_{95}) NIMBEX at 10% or 95% recovery following an intubating dose of succinylcholine (1 mg/kg) produced ≥ 95% neuromuscular block. The time to onset of maximum block following NIMBEX is approximately 2 minutes faster with prior administration of succinylcholine. Prior administration of succinylcholine had no effect on the duration of neuromuscular block following initial or maintenance bolus doses of NIMBEX. Infusion requirements of NIMBEX in patients administered succinylcholine prior to infusions of NIMBEX were comparable to or slightly greater than when succinylcholine was not administered.

The use of NIMBEX before succinylcholine to attenuate some of the side effects of succinylcholine has not been studied.

Although not studied systematically in clinical trials, no drug interactions were observed when vecuronium, pancuronium, or atracurium were administered following varying degrees of recovery from single doses or infusions of NIMBEX.

Isoflurane or enflurane administered with nitrous oxide/oxygen to achieve 1.25 MAC [Minimum Alveolar Concentration] may prolong the clinically effective duration of action of initial and maintenance doses of NIMBEX and decrease the required infusion rate of NIMBEX. The magnitude of these effects may depend on the duration of administration of the volatile agents. Fifteen to 30 minutes of exposure to 1.25 MAC isoflurane or enflurane had minimal effects on the duration of action of initial doses of NIMBEX and therefore, no adjustment to the initial dose should be necessary when NIMBEX is administered shortly after initiation of volatile agents. In long surgical procedures during enflurane or isoflurane anesthesia, less frequent maintenance dosing, lower maintenance doses, or reduced infusion rates of NIMBEX may be necessary. The average infusion rate requirement may be decreased by as much as 30% to 40%.

Information on the AbbVie, Inc. products listed on these pages is from the prescribing information in use as of July 31, 2013. For more information, please visit rxabbvie.com or call 1-800-633-9110.

In clinical studies propofol had no effect on the duration of action or dosing requirements for NIMBEX.

Other drugs which may enhance the neuromuscular blocking action of nondepolarizing agents such as NIMBEX include certain antibiotics (e.g., aminoglycosides, tetracyclines, bacitracin, polymyxins, lincomycin, clindamycin, colistin, and sodium colistemethate), magnesium salts, lithium, local anesthetics, procainamide, and quinidine.

Resistance to the neuromuscular blocking action of nondepolarizing neuromuscular blocking agents has been demonstrated in patients chronically administered phenytoin or carbamazepine. While the effects of chronic phenytoin or carbamazepine therapy on the action of NIMBEX are unknown, slightly shorter durations of neuromuscular block may be anticipated and infusion rate requirements may be higher.

Drug/Laboratory Test Interactions

None known.

Carcinogenesis, Mutagenesis, Impairment of Fertility

Carcinogenesis and fertility studies have not been performed. Cisatracurium besylate was evaluated in a battery of four short-term mutagenicity tests. It was non-mutagenic in the Ames Salmonella assay, a rat bone marrow cytogenetic assay, and an *in vitro* human lymphocyte cytogenetics assay. As was the case with atracurium, the mouse lymphoma assay was positive both in the presence and absence of exogenous metabolic activation (rat liver S-9). In the absence of S-9, cisatracurium besylate was positive at *in vitro* cisatracurium concentrations of 40 mcg/mL and higher. The highest non-mutagenic concentration (30 mcg/mL) and incubation time (4 hours) resulted in an AUC approximately 120 times that noted in clinical studies and approximately 8.5 times the mean peak clinical concentration noted. In the presence of S-9, cisatracurium besylate was positive at a cisatracurium concentration of 300 mcg/mL but not at lower or higher concentrations.

Pregnancy

Teratogenic Effects

Pregnancy Category B

Teratology testing in nonventilated pregnant rats treated subcutaneously with maximum subparalyzing doses (4 mg/kg daily; equivalent to 8 × the human ED_{95} following a bolus dose of 0.2 mg/kg IV) and in ventilated rats treated intravenously with paralyzing doses of NIMBEX at 0.5 and 1.0 mg/kg; equivalent to 10 × and 20 × the human ED_{95} dose, respectively, revealed no maternal or fetal toxicity or teratogenic effects. There are no adequate and well-controlled studies of NIMBEX in pregnant women. Because animal studies are not always predictive of human response, NIMBEX should be used during pregnancy only if clearly needed.

Labor and Delivery

The use of NIMBEX during labor, vaginal delivery, or cesarean section has not been studied in humans and it is not known whether NIMBEX administered to the mother has effects on the fetus. Doses of 0.2 or 0.4 mg/kg cisatracurium given to female beagles undergoing cesarean section resulted in negligible levels of cisatracurium in umbilical vessel blood of neonates and no deleterious effects on the puppies. The action of neuromuscular blocking agents may be enhanced by magnesium salts administered for the management of toxemia of pregnancy.

Nursing Mothers

It is not known whether cisatracurium besylate is excreted in human milk. Because many drugs are excreted in human milk, caution should be exercised following administration of NIMBEX to a nursing woman.

Pediatric Use

NIMBEX has not been studied in pediatric patients below the age of 1 month (see **CLINICAL PHARMACOLOGY** and **DOSAGE AND ADMINISTRATION** for clinical experience and recommendations for use in children 1 month to 12 years of age). Intubation of the trachea in patients 1-4 years old was facilitated more reliably when NIMBEX was used in combination with Halothane than when opioids and nitrous oxide were used for induction of anesthesia.

The 10 mL multiple-dose vials of NIMBEX contain benzyl alcohol as a preservative. Benzyl alcohol, a component of this product, has been associated with serious adverse events and death, particularly in pediatric patients. The "gasping syndrome", (characterized by central nervous system depression, metabolic acidosis, gasping respirations, and high levels of benzyl alcohol and its metabolites found in the blood and urine) has been associated with benzyl alcohol dosages >99 mg/kg/day in neonates and low-birth-weight neonates. Additional symptoms may include gradual neurological deterioration, seizures, intracranial hemorrhage, hematologic abnormalities, skin breakdown, hepatic and renal failure, hypotension, bradycardia, and cardiovascular collapse. Although normal therapeutic doses of this product deliver amounts of benzyl alcohol that are substantially lower than those reported in association with the "gasping syndrome", the minimum amount of benzyl alcohol at which toxicity may occur is not known. Premature and low-birth-weight infants, as well as patients receiving high dosages, may be more likely to develop toxicity. Practitioners administering this and other medications containing benzyl alcohol should consider the combined daily metabolic load of benzyl alcohol from all sources.

Geriatric Use

Of the total number of subjects in clinical studies of NIMBEX, 57 were 65 and over, 63 were 70 and over, and 15 were 80 and over. The geriatric population included a subset of patients with significant cardiovascular disease (see **CLINICAL PHARMACOLOGY - Hemodynamics Profile** and Special Populations - *Geriatric Patients* subsections). No overall differences in safety or effectiveness were observed between these subjects and younger subjects, and other reported clinical experience has not identified differences in responses between elderly and younger subjects, but greater sensitivity of some older individuals to NIMBEX cannot be ruled out.

Minor differences in the pharmacokinetics of cisatracurium between elderly and young adult patients are not associated with clinically significant differences in the recovery profile of NIMBEX following a single 0.1 mg/kg dose; the time to maximum block is approximately 1 minute slower in elderly patients (see **CLINICAL PHARMACOLOGY - Pharmacokinetics**).

ADVERSE REACTIONS

Observed in Clinical Trials of Surgical Patients

Adverse experiences were uncommon among the 945 surgical patients who received NIMBEX in conjunction with other drugs in US and European clinical studies in the course of a wide variety of procedures in patients receiving opioid, propofol, or inhalation anesthesia. The following adverse experiences were judged by investigators during the clinical trials to have a possible causal relationship to administration of NIMBEX:

Incidence Greater than 1%

None.

Incidence Less than 1%

Cardiovascular

bradycardia (0.4%)

hypotension (0.2%)

flushing (0.2%).

Respiratory

bronchospasm (0.2%).

Dermatological

rash (0.1%).

Observed in Clinical Trials of Intensive Care Unit Patients

Adverse experiences were uncommon among the 68 ICU patients who received NIMBEX in conjunction with other drugs in US and European clinical studies. One patient experienced bronchospasm. In one of the two ICU studies, a randomized and double-blind study of ICU patients using TOF neuromuscular monitoring, there were two reports of prolonged recovery (167 and 270 minutes) among 28 patients administered NIMBEX and 13 reports of prolonged recovery (range: 90 minutes to 33 hours) among 30 patients administered vecuronium.

Observed During Clinical Practice

In addition to adverse events reported from clinical trials, the following events have been identified during post-approval use of cisatracurium besylate in conjunction with one or more anesthetic agents in clinical practice. Because they are reported voluntarily from a population of unknown size, estimates of frequency cannot be made. These events have been chosen for inclusion due to a combination of their seriousness, frequency of reporting, or potential causal connection to cisatracurium besylate.

General

Histamine release, hypersensitivity reactions including anaphylactic or anaphylactoid reactions which in some cases have been life threatening and fatal. Because these reactions were reported voluntarily from a population of uncertain size, it is not possible to reliably estimate their frequency (see **WARNINGS** and **PRECAUTIONS**). There are rare reports of wheezing, laryngospasm, bronchospasm, rash and itching following administration of NIMBEX in children. These reported adverse events were not serious and their etiology could not be established with certainty.

Musculoskeletal

Prolonged neuromuscular block, inadequate neuromuscular block, muscle weakness, and myopathy.

OVERDOSAGE

Overdosage with neuromuscular blocking agents may result in neuromuscular block beyond the time needed for surgery and anesthesia. The primary treatment is maintenance of a patent airway and controlled ventilation until recovery of normal neuromuscular function is assured. Once recovery from neuromuscular block begins, further recovery may be facilitated by administration of an anticholinesterase agent (e.g., neostigmine, edrophonium) in conjunction with an appropriate anticholinergic agent (see Antagonism of Neuromuscular Block below).

Antagonism of Neuromuscular Block

ANTAGONISTS (SUCH AS NEOSTIGMINE AND EDROPHONIUM) SHOULD NOT BE ADMINISTERED WHEN COMPLETE NEUROMUSCULAR BLOCK IS EVIDENT OR SUSPECTED. THE USE OF A PERIPHERAL NERVE STIMULATOR TO EVALUATE RECOVERY AND ANTAGONISM OF NEUROMUSCULAR BLOCK IS RECOMMENDED.

Administration of 0.04 to 0.07 mg/kg neostigmine at approximately 10% recovery from neuromuscular block (range: 0 to 15%) produced 95% recovery of the muscle twitch response and a T_4:T_1 ratio ≥ 70% in an average of 9 to 10 minutes. The times from 25% recovery of the muscle twitch response to a T_4:T_1 ratio ≥ 70% following these doses of neostigmine averaged 7 minutes. The mean 25% to 75% recovery index following reversal was 3 to 4 minutes.

Administration of 1.0 mg/kg edrophonium at approximately 25% recovery from neuromuscular block (range: 16% to 30%) produced 95% recovery and a T_4:T_1 ratio ≥ 70% in an average of 3 to 5 minutes.

Patients administered antagonists should be evaluated for evidence of adequate clinical recovery (e.g., 5-second head lift and grip strength). Ventilation must be supported until no longer required.

The onset of antagonism may be delayed in the presence of debilitation, cachexia, carcinomatosis, and the concomitant use of certain broad spectrum antibiotics, or anesthetic agents and other drugs which enhance neuromuscular block or separately cause respiratory depression (see **PRECAUTIONS - Drug Interactions**). Under such circumstances the management is the same as that of prolonged neuromuscular block (see **OVERDOSAGE**).

DOSAGE AND ADMINISTRATION

NOTE: CONTAINS BENZYL ALCOHOL (see **WARNINGS** and **PRECAUTIONS – Pediatric Use**)

NIMBEX SHOULD ONLY BE ADMINISTERED INTRAVENOUSLY.

The dosage information provided below is intended as a guide only. Doses of NIMBEX should be individualized (see CLINICAL PHARMACOLOGY - Individualization of Dosages). The use of a peripheral nerve stimulator will permit the most advantageous use of NIMBEX, minimize the possibility of overdosage or underdosage, and assist in the evaluation of recovery.

Adults

Initial Doses

One of two intubating doses of NIMBEX may be chosen, based on the desired time to tracheal intubation and the anticipated length of surgery. In addition to the dose of neuromuscular blocking agent, the presence of co-induction agents (e.g., fentanyl and midazolam) and the depth of anesthesia are factors that can influence intubation conditions. Doses of 0.15 (3 × ED_{95}) and 0.20 (4 × ED_{95}) mg/kg NIMBEX, as components of a propofol/nitrous oxide/oxygen induction-intubation technique, may produce generally GOOD or EXCELLENT conditions for intubation in 2.0 and 1.5 minutes, respectively. Similar intubation conditions may be expected when these doses of NIMBEX are administered as components of a thiopental/nitrous oxide/oxygen induction-intubation technique. In two intubation studies using thiopental or propofol and midazolam and fentanyl as co-induction agents, EXCELLENT intubation conditions were most frequently achieved with the 0.2 mg/kg compared to 0.15 mg/kg dose of cisatracurium. The clinically effective durations of action for 0.15 and 0.20 mg/kg NIMBEX during propofol anesthesia are 55 minutes (range: 44 to 74 minutes) and 61 minutes (range: 41 to 81 minutes), respectively. Lower doses may result in a longer time for the development of satisfactory intubation conditions. Doses up to 8 × ED_{95} NIMBEX have been safely administered to healthy adult patients and patients with serious cardiovascular disease. These larger doses are associated with longer clinically effective durations of action (see **CLINICAL PHARMACOLOGY**).

Because slower times to onset of complete neuromuscular block were observed in elderly patients and patients with renal dysfunction, extending the interval between administration of NIMBEX and the intubation attempt for these patients may be required to achieve adequate intubation conditions.

A dose of 0.03 mg/kg NIMBEX is recommended for maintenance of neuromuscular block during prolonged surgical procedures. Maintenance doses of 0.03 mg/kg each sustain neuromuscular block for approximately 20 minutes. Maintenance dosing is generally required 40 to 50 minutes following an initial dose of 0.15 mg/kg NIMBEX and 50 to 60 minutes following an initial dose of 0.20 mg/kg NIMBEX, but the need for maintenance doses should be determined by clinical criteria. For shorter or longer durations of action, smaller or larger maintenance doses may be administered. Isoflurane or enflurane administered with nitrous oxide/oxygen to achieve 1.25 MAC (Minimum Alveolar Concentration) may prolong the clinically effective duration of action of initial and maintenance doses. The magnitude of these effects may depend on the duration of administration of the volatile agents. Fifteen to 30 minutes of exposure to 1.25 MAC isoflurane or enflurane had minimal effects on the duration of action of initial doses of NIMBEX and therefore, no adjustment to the initial dose should be necessary when NIMBEX is administered shortly after initiation of volatile agents. In long surgical procedures during enflurane or isoflurane anesthesia, less frequent maintenance dosing or lower maintenance doses of NIMBEX may be necessary. No adjustments to the initial dose of NIMBEX are required when used in patients receiving propofol anesthesia.

Children

Initial Doses

The recommended dose of NIMBEX for children 2 to 12 years of age is 0.10-0.15 mg/kg administered over 5 to 10 seconds during either halothane or opioid anesthesia. When administered during stable opioid/nitrous oxide/oxygen anesthesia, 0.10 mg/kg NIMBEX produces maximum neuromuscular block in an average of 2.8 minutes (range: 1.8 to 6.7 minutes) and clinically effective block for 28 minutes (range: 21 to 38 minutes). When administered during stable opioid/nitrous oxide/oxygen anesthesia, 0.15 mg/kg NIMBEX produces maximum neuromuscular block in about 3.0 minutes (range: 1.5 to 8.0 minutes) and clinically effective block (time to 25% recovery) for 36 minutes (range: 29 to 46 minutes).

Infants

Initial Doses

The recommended dose of NIMBEX for intubation of infants 1 month to 23 months is 0.15 mg/kg administered over 5 to 10 seconds during either halothane or opioid anesthesia. When administered during stable opioid/nitrous oxide/oxygen anesthesia, 0.15 mg/kg NIMBEX produces maximum neuromuscular block in about 2.0 minutes (range: 1.3 to 3.4 minutes) and clinically effective block (time to 25% recovery) for about 43 minutes (range: 34 to 58 minutes).

Use by Continuous Infusion

Infusion in the Operating Room (OR)

After administration of an initial bolus dose of NIMBEX, a diluted solution of NIMBEX can be administered by continuous infusion to adults and children aged 2 or more years for maintenance of neuromuscular block during extended surgical procedures. Infusion of NIMBEX should be individualized for each patient. The rate of administration should be adjusted according to the patient's response as determined by peripheral nerve stimulation. Accurate dosing is best achieved using a precision infusion device.

Infusion of NIMBEX should be initiated only after early evidence of spontaneous recovery from the initial bolus dose. An initial infusion rate of 3 mcg/kg/min may be required to rapidly counteract the spontaneous recovery of neuromuscular function. Thereafter, a rate of 1 to 2 mcg/kg/min should be adequate to maintain continuous neuromuscular block in the range of 89% to 99% in most pediatric and adult patients under opioid/nitrous oxide/oxygen anesthesia.

Reduction of the infusion rate by up to 30% to 40% should be considered when NIMBEX is administered during stable isoflurane or enflurane anesthesia (administered with nitrous oxide/oxygen at the 1.25 MAC level). Greater reductions in the infusion rate of NIMBEX may be required with longer durations of administration of isoflurane or enflurane.

The rate of infusion of atracurium required to maintain adequate surgical relaxation in patients undergoing coronary artery bypass surgery with induced hypothermia (25° to 28°C) is approximately half the rate required during normothermia. Based on the structural similarity between NIMBEX and atracurium, a similar effect on the infusion rate of NIMBEX may be expected.

Spontaneous recovery from neuromuscular block following discontinuation of infusion of NIMBEX may be expected to proceed at a rate comparable to that following administration of a single bolus dose.

Infusion in the Intensive Care Unit (ICU)

The principles for infusion of NIMBEX in the OR are also applicable to use in the ICU. An infusion rate of approximately 3 mcg/kg/min (range: 0.5 to 10.2 mcg/kg/min) should provide adequate neuromuscular block in adult patients in the ICU. There may be wide interpatient variability in dosage requirements and these may increase or decrease with time (see **PRECAUTIONS - Long-Term Use in the Intensive Care Unit [ICU]**). Following recovery from neuromuscular block, readministration of a bolus dose may be necessary to quickly re-establish neuromuscular block prior to reinstitution of the infusion.

Infusion Rate Tables

The amount of infusion solution required per minute will depend upon the concentration of NIMBEX in the infusion solution, the desired dose of NIMBEX, and the patient's weight. The contribution of the infusion solution to the fluid requirements of the patient also must be considered. Tables 10 and 11 provide guidelines for delivery, in mL/hr (equivalent to microdrops/minute when 60 microdrops = 1 mL), of NIMBEX solutions in concentrations of 0.1 mg/mL (10 mg/100 mL) or 0.4 mg/mL (40 mg/100 mL).

Table 10. Infusion Rates of NIMBEX for Maintenance of Neuromuscular Block During Opioid/Nitrous Oxide/Oxygen Anesthesia for a Concentration of 0.1 mg/mL

	Drug Delivery Rate (mcg/kg/min)				
	1.0	1.5	2.0	3.0	5.0
Patient Weight (kg)	Infusion Delivery Rate (mL/hr)				
10	6	9	12	18	30
45	27	41	54	81	135
70	42	63	84	126	210
100	60	90	120	180	300

Table 11. Infusion Rates of NIMBEX for Maintenance of Neuromuscular Block During Opioid/Nitrous Oxide/Oxygen Anesthesia for a Concentration of 0.4 mg/mL

	Drug Delivery Rate (mcg/kg/min)				
	1.0	1.5	2.0	3.0	5.0
Patient Weight (kg)	Infusion Delivery Rate (mL/hr)				
10	1.5	2.3	3.0	4.5	7.5
45	6.8	10.1	13.5	20.3	33.8
70	10.5	15.8	21.0	31.5	52.5
100	15.0	22.5	30.0	45.0	75.0

NIMBEX Injection Compatibility and Admixtures

Y-site Administration

NIMBEX Injection is acidic (pH = 3.25 to 3.65) and may not be compatible with alkaline solution having a pH greater than 8.5 (e.g., barbiturate solutions).

Studies have shown that NIMBEX Injection is compatible with:

- 5% Dextrose Injection, USP
- 0.9% Sodium Chloride Injection, USP
- 5% Dextrose and 0.9% Sodium Chloride Injection, USP
- SUFENTA® (sufentanil citrate) Injection, diluted as directed
- ALFENTA® (alfentanil hydrochloride) Injection, diluted as directed
- SUBLIMAZE® (fentanyl citrate) Injection, diluted as directed
- VERSED® (midazolam hydrochloride) Injection, diluted as directed
- Droperidol Injection, diluted as directed

NIMBEX Injection is not compatible with DIPRIVAN® (propofol) Injection or TORADOL® (ketorolac) Injection for Y-site administration. Studies of other parenteral products have not been conducted.

Dilution Stability

NIMBEX Injection diluted in 5% Dextrose Injection, USP; 0.9% Sodium Chloride Injection, USP; or 5% Dextrose and 0.9% Sodium Chloride Injection, USP to 0.1 mg/mL may be stored either under refrigeration or at room temperature for 24 hours without significant loss of potency. Dilutions to 0.1 mg/mL or 0.2 mg/mL in 5% Dextrose and Lactated Ringer's Injection may be stored under refrigeration for 24 hours.

NIMBEX Injection should not be diluted in Lactated Ringer's Injection, USP due to chemical instability.

NOTE: Parenteral drug products should be inspected visually for particulate matter and discoloration prior to administration whenever solution and container permit. Solutions which are not clear, or contain visible particulates, should not be used. NIMBEX Injection is a colorless to slightly yellow or greenish-yellow solution.

HOW SUPPLIED

NIMBEX Injection, 2 mg cisatracurium per mL, is supplied in the following:

List No.	Container	Size
4378	Single-dose Vial	5 mL
4380	Multiple-dose Vial	10 mL

NOTE: 10 mL Multiple-dose Vials contain 0.9% w/v benzyl alcohol as a preservative (see **WARNINGS** concerning newborn infants).

NIMBEX Injection, 10 mg cisatracurium per mL is supplied in the following:

4382	Single-dose Vial	20 mL

Intended only for use in the ICU.

STORAGE

NIMBEX Injection should be refrigerated at 2° to 8°C (36° to 46°F) in the carton to preserve potency. Protect from light. DO NOT FREEZE. Upon removal from refrigeration to room temperature storage conditions (25°C/77°F), use NIMBEX Injection within 21 days even if rerefrigerated.

Nimbex® is a registered trademark of GlaxoSmithKline, licensed for use by AbbVie Inc.

Mfd By: Hospira, Inc.
Lake Forest, IL 60045 USA
For: AbbVie Inc.
North Chicago, IL 60064 USA
EN-3172 Revised January, 2013

NORVIR ℞

[*nor - veer*]
(ritonavir)
Capsules, Soft Gelatin for Oral use

HIGHLIGHTS OF PRESCRIBING INFORMATION
These highlights do not include all the information needed to use NORVIR safely and effectively. See full prescribing information for NORVIR.
NORVIR (ritonavir) Capsules, Soft Gelatin for Oral use
Initial U.S. Approval: 1996

WARNING: DRUG-DRUG INTERACTIONS LEADING TO POTENTIALLY SERIOUS AND/OR LIFE THREATENING REACTIONS
See full prescribing information for complete boxed warning
Co-administration of NORVIR with several classes of drugs including sedative hypnotics, antiarrhythmics, or ergot alkaloid preparations may result in potentially serious and/or life-threatening adverse events due to possible effects of NORVIR on the hepatic metabolism of certain drugs. Review medications taken by patients prior to prescribing NORVIR or when prescribing other medications to patients already taking NORVIR [see Contraindications (4), Warnings and Precautions (5.1), Drug Interactions (7), and Clinical Pharmacology (12.3)].

RECENT MAJOR CHANGES

Contraindications (4) 12/2011
Warnings and Precautions, Drug Interactions (5.1) 12/2011
Warnings and Precautions, Allergic Reactions (5.4) 12/2011
Warnings and Precautions, Immune Reconstitution Syndrome (5.8) 02/2012

INDICATIONS AND USAGE

NORVIR is an HIV protease inhibitor indicated in combination with other antiretroviral agents for the treatment of HIV-1 infection. (1)

DOSAGE AND ADMINISTRATION

- Dose modification for NORVIR is necessary when used with other protease inhibitors. (2)
- Adult patients: 600 mg twice-daily with meals if possible. (2.1)
- Pediatrics patients: The recommended twice daily dose for children greater than one month of age is based on body surface area and should not exceed 600 mg twice daily with meals if possible. (2.2)

DOSAGE FORMS AND STRENGTHS

- Capsule, Soft Gelatin: 100 mg. (3)

CONTRAINDICATIONS

- NORVIR is contraindicated in patients with known hypersensitivity to ritonavir (e.g., toxic epidermal necrolysis, Stevens-Johnson syndrome) or any of its ingredients. (4)
- Co-administration with drugs highly dependent on CYP3A for clearance and for which elevated plasma concentrations may be associated with serious and/or life-threatening events. (4)
- Co-administration with drugs that significantly reduce ritonavir. (4)

WARNINGS AND PRECAUTIONS

The following have been observed in patients receiving NORVIR:

- Drug Interactions: Consider drug-drug interaction potential to reduce risk of serious or life threatening adverse reactions. (5.1)
- Hepatic Reactions: Fatalities have occurred. Monitor liver function before and during therapy, especially in patients with underlying hepatic disease, including hepatitis B and hepatitis C, or marked transaminase elevations. (5.2, 8.6)

Information on the AbbVie, Inc. products listed on these pages is from the prescribing information in use as of July 31, 2013. For more information, please visit rxabbvie.com or call 1-800-633-9110.

- Pancreatitis: Fatalities have occurred; suspend therapy as clinically appropriate. (5.3)
- Allergic Reactions/Hypersensitivity: Allergic reactions have been reported and include anaphylaxis, toxic epidermal necrolysis, Stevens-Johnson syndrome, bronchospasm and angioedema. Discontinue treatment if severe reactions develop. (5.4, 6.3)
- PR interval prolongation may occur in some patients. Cases of second and third degree heart block have been reported. Use with caution with patients with preexisting conduction system disease, ischemic heart disease, cardiomyopathy, underlying structural heart disease or when administering with other drugs that may prolong the PR interval. (5.5, 12.3)
- Total cholesterol and triglycerides elevations: Monitor prior to therapy and periodically thereafter. (5.6)
- Patients may develop new onset or exacerbations of diabetes mellitus, hyperglycemia. (5.7)
- Patients may develop immune reconstitution syndrome. (5.8)
- Patients may develop redistribution/accumulation of body fat. (5.9)
- Hemophilia: Spontaneous bleeding may occur, and additional factor VIII may be required. (5.10)

ADVERSE REACTIONS

The most common adverse reactions (greater than 5% and of moderate to severe intensity) were abdominal pain, asthenia, headache, malaise, anorexia, diarrhea, dyspepsia, nausea, vomiting, paresthesia, circumoral paresthesia, peripheral paresthesia, dizziness, and taste perversion. (6.1)

To report SUSPECTED ADVERSE REACTIONS, contact AbbVie Inc. at 1-800-633-9110 or FDA at 1-800-FDA-1088 or www.fda.gov/medwatch.

DRUG INTERACTIONS

- Co-administration of NORVIR can alter the concentrations of other drugs. The potential for drug-drug interactions must be considered prior to and during therapy. (4, 5.1, 7, 12.3)

USE IN SPECIFIC POPULATIONS

- Nursing Mothers: Because of both the potential for HIV transmission and the potential for serious adverse reactions in nursing infants, mothers should be instructed not to breastfeed if they are receiving NORVIR. (8.3)

See 17 for PATIENT COUNSELING INFORMATION and FDA-approved patient labeling

Revised: 01/2013

FULL PRESCRIBING INFORMATION: CONTENTS*

* Sections or subsections omitted from the full prescribing information are not listed

Table 1. Drugs that are Contraindicated with NORVIR

Drug Class	Drugs Within Class That Are Contraindicated With NORVIR**	Clinical Comments
Alpha$_1$-adrenoreceptor antagonist	Alfuzosin HCL	Potential for hypotension.
Antiarrhythmics	Amiodarone, flecainide, propafenone, quinidine	Potential for cardiac arrhythmias.
Antifungal	Voriconazole	Co-administration of voriconazole with ritonavir 400 mg every 12 hours significantly decreases voriconazole plasma concentrations and may lead to loss of antifungal response. Voriconazole is contraindicated with ritonavir doses of 400 mg every 12 hours or greater *[see Drug Interactions (7.2)]*.
Ergot Derivatives	Dihydroergotamine, ergonovine, ergotamine, methylergonovine	Potential for acute ergot toxicity characterized by vasospasm and ischemia of the extremities and other tissues including the central nervous system.
GI Motility Agent	Cisapride	Potential for cardiac arrhythmias.
Herbal Products	St. John's Wort (hypericum perforatum)	Co-administration of NORVIR with St. John's Wort may result in decreased ritonavir plasma concentrations and may lead to loss of virologic response and possible resistance to NORVIR or to the class of protease inhibitors.
HMG-CoA Reductase Inhibitors	Lovastatin, simvastatin	Potential for myopathy including rhabdomyolysis.
Neuroleptic	Pimozide	Potential for cardiac arrhythmias.
PDE5 enzyme inhibitor	Sildenafil* (Revatio®) only when used for the treatment of pulmonary arterial hypertension (PAH)	A safe and effective dose has not been established when used with ritonavir. There is an increased potential for sildenafil-associated adverse events, including visual abnormalities, hypotension, prolonged erection, and syncope *[see Drug Interactions (7)]*.
Sedative/hypnotics	Oral midazolam, triazolam	Prolonged or increased sedation or respiratory depression *[see Drug Interactions (7.2)]*.

**see Drug Interactions (7)* for co-administration of sildenafil in patients with erectile dysfunction.
** For additional information for these contraindicated drugs, *see also Drug Interactions (7)*.

FULL PRESCRIBING INFORMATION

WARNING: DRUG-DRUG INTERACTIONS LEADING TO POTENTIALLY SERIOUS AND/OR LIFE THREATENING REACTIONS

Co-administration of NORVIR with several classes of drugs including sedative hypnotics, antiarrhythmics, or ergot alkaloid preparations may result in potentially serious and/or life-threatening adverse events due to possible effects of NORVIR on the hepatic metabolism of certain drugs. Review medications taken by patients prior to prescribing NORVIR or when prescribing other medications to patients already taking NORVIR *[see Contraindications (4), Warnings and Precautions (5.1), Drug Interactions (7), and Clinical Pharmacology (12.3)]*.

1 INDICATIONS AND USAGE

NORVIR is indicated in combination with other antiretroviral agents for the treatment of HIV-1 infection.

2 DOSAGE AND ADMINISTRATION

NORVIR is administered orally in combination with other antiretroviral agents. It is recommended that NORVIR be taken with meals if possible.

General Dosing Guidelines

Patients should be aware that frequently observed adverse events, such as mild to moderate gastrointestinal disturbances and paraesthesias, may diminish as therapy is continued.

Dose modification for NORVIR

Dose reduction of NORVIR is necessary when used with other protease inhibitors: atazanavir, darunavir, fosamprenavir, saquinavir, and tipranavir.

Prescribers should consult the full prescribing information and clinical study information of these protease inhibitors if they are co-administered with a reduced dose of ritonavir *[see Warnings and Precautions (5),* and *Drug Interactions (7)]*.

2.1 Adult Patients

Recommended Dosage for treatment of HIV-1

The recommended dosage of ritonavir is 600 mg twice daily by mouth. Use of a dose titration schedule may help to reduce treatment-emergent adverse events while maintaining appropriate ritonavir plasma levels. Ritonavir should be started at no less than 300 mg twice daily and increased at 2 to 3 day intervals by 100 mg twice daily. The maximum dose of 600 mg twice daily should not be exceeded upon completion of the titration.

2.2 Pediatric Patients

The recommended dosage of ritonavir in children greater than 1 month is 350 to 400 mg per m^2 twice daily by mouth and should not exceed 600 mg twice daily. Ritonavir should be started at 250 mg per m^2 twice daily and increased at 2 to 3 day intervals by 50 mg per m^2 twice daily. If patients do not tolerate 400 mg per m^2 twice daily due to adverse events, the highest tolerated dose may be used for maintenance therapy in combination with other antiretroviral agents, however, alternative therapy should be considered. The use of NORVIR oral solution is recommended for children greater than 1 month who cannot swallow capsules. Please refer to the NORVIR oral solution full prescribing information for pediatric dosage and administration.

3 DOSAGE FORMS AND STRENGTHS

- NORVIR (ritonavir) capsules, soft gelatin

White soft gelatin capsules imprinted with the "a" logo, 100 and the code DS, providing 100 mg of ritonavir.

4 CONTRAINDICATIONS

- When co-administering NORVIR with other protease inhibitors, see the full prescribing information for that protease inhibitor including contraindication information.
- NORVIR is contraindicated in patients with known hypersensitivity (e.g., toxic epidermal necrolysis (TEN) or Stevens-Johnson syndrome) to ritonavir or any of its ingredients.
- Co-administration of NORVIR with several classes of drugs (including sedative hypnotics, antiarrhythmics, or ergot alkaloid preparations) is contraindicated and may result in potentially serious and/or life-threatening adverse events due to possible effects of NORVIR on the hepatic metabolism of these drugs (see Table 1). Voriconazole and St. John's Wort are exceptions in that co-administration of NORVIR and voriconazole results in a significant decrease in plasma concentrations of voriconazole, and co-administration of NORVIR with St. John's Wort may result in decreased ritonavir plasma concentrations.

[See table 1 at top of previous page]

5 WARNINGS AND PRECAUTIONS

When co-administering NORVIR with other protease inhibitors, see the full prescribing information for that protease inhibitor including Warnings and Precautions.

5.1 Drug Interactions

NORVIR is a CYP3A inhibitor. Initiating treatment with NORVIR in patients receiving medications metabolized by CYP3A or initiating medications metabolized by CYP3A in patients already maintained on NORVIR may result in increased plasma concentrations of concomitant medications. Higher plasma concentrations of concomitant medications can result in increased or prolonged therapeutic or adverse effects, potentially leading to severe, life-threatening or fatal events. The potential for drug-drug interactions must be considered prior to and during therapy with NORVIR. Review of other medications taken by patients and monitoring of patients for adverse effects is recommended during therapy with NORVIR.

See Table 1 for a listing of drugs that are contraindicated with NORVIR due to potentially life-threatening adverse events, significant drug interactions, or loss of virologic activity. Also, see Table 4 for a listing of drugs with established and other significant drug interactions *[see Contraindications (4), Drug Interactions (7),* and *Clinical Pharmacology (12.3)]*.

5.2 Hepatic Reactions

Hepatic transaminase elevations exceeding 5 times the upper limit of normal, clinical hepatitis, and jaundice have occurred in patients receiving NORVIR alone or in combination with other antiretroviral drugs (see Table 3). There may be an increased risk for transaminase elevations in patients with underlying hepatitis B or C. Therefore, caution should be exercised when administering NORVIR to patients with pre-existing liver diseases, liver enzyme abnormalities, or hepatitis. Increased AST/ALT monitoring should be considered in these patients, especially during the first three months of NORVIR treatment *[see Use In Specific Populations (8.6)]*.

There have been postmarketing reports of hepatic dysfunction, including some fatalities. These have generally occurred in patients taking multiple concomitant medications and/or with advanced AIDS.

5.3 Pancreatitis

Pancreatitis has been observed in patients receiving NORVIR therapy, including those who developed hypertriglyceridemia. In some cases fatalities have been observed. Patients with advanced HIV-1 disease may be at increased risk of elevated triglycerides and pancreatitis *[see Warnings and Precautions (5.8)]*. Pancreatitis should be considered if clinical symptoms (nausea, vomiting, abdominal pain) or abnormalities in laboratory values (such as increased serum lipase or amylase values) suggestive of pancreatitis should occur. Patients who exhibit these signs or symptoms should be evaluated and NORVIR therapy should be discontinued if a diagnosis of pancreatitis is made.

5.4 Allergic Reactions/Hypersensitivity

Allergic reactions including urticaria, mild skin eruptions, bronchospasm, and angioedema have been reported. Cases of anaphylaxis, toxic epidermal necrolysis (TEN), and Stevens-Johnson syndrome have also been reported. Discontinue treatment if severe reactions develop.

5.5 PR Interval Prolongation

Ritonavir prolongs the PR interval in some patients. Post marketing cases of second or third degree atrioventricular block have been reported in patients.

NORVIR should be used with caution in patients with underlying structural heart disease, preexisting conduction system abnormalities, ischemic heart disease, cardiomyopathies, as these patients may be at increased risk for developing cardiac conduction abnormalities.

The impact on the PR interval of co-administration of ritonavir with other drugs that prolong the PR interval (including calcium channel blockers, beta-adrenergic blockers, digoxin and atazanavir) has not been evaluated. As a result, co-administration of ritonavir with these drugs should be undertaken with caution, particularly with those drugs metabolized by CYP3A. Clinical monitoring is recommended *[see Drug Interactions (7),* and *Clinical Pharmacology (12.3)]*.

5.6 Lipid Disorders

Treatment with NORVIR therapy alone or in combination with saquinavir has resulted in substantial increases in the concentration of total cholesterol and triglycerides *[see Adverse Reactions (6.1)]*. Triglyceride and cholesterol testing should be performed prior to initiating NORVIR therapy and at periodic intervals during therapy. Lipid disorders should be managed as clinically appropriate, taking into account any potential drug-drug interactions with NORVIR and HMG CoA reductase inhibitors *[see Contraindications (4),* and *Drug Interactions (7)]*.

5.7 Diabetes Mellitus/Hyperglycemia

New onset diabetes mellitus, exacerbation of pre-existing diabetes mellitus, and hyperglycemia have been reported during postmarketing surveillance in HIV-1 infected patients receiving protease inhibitor therapy. Some patients required either initiation or dose adjustments of insulin or oral hypoglycemic agents for treatment of these events. In some cases, diabetic ketoacidosis has occurred. In those patients who discontinued protease inhibitor therapy, hyperglycemia persisted in some cases. Because these events have been reported voluntarily during clinical practice, estimates of frequency cannot be made and a causal relationship between protease inhibitor therapy and these events has not been established.

5.8 Immune Reconstitution Syndrome

Immune reconstitution syndrome has been reported in HIV-1 infected patients treated with combination antiretroviral therapy, including NORVIR. During the initial phase of combination antiretroviral treatment, patients whose immune system responds may develop an inflammatory response to indolent or residual opportunistic infections (such as *Mycobacterium avium* infection, cytomegalovirus, *Pneumocystis jiroveci* pneumonia (PCP), or tuberculosis), which may necessitate further evaluation and treatment.

Autoimmune disorders (such as Graves' disease, polymyositis, and Guillain-Barré syndrome) have also been reported to occur in the setting of immune reconstitution, however, the time to onset is more variable, and can occur many months after initiation of treatment.

5.9 Fat Redistribution

Redistribution/accumulation of body fat including central obesity, dorsocervical fat enlargement (buffalo hump), pe-

Table 2. Percentage of Patients with Treatment-emergent Adverse Events[1] of Moderate or Severe Intensity Occurring in greater than or equal to 2% of Adult Patients Receiving NORVIR

Adverse Events	Study 245 Naive Patients[2]			Study 247 Advanced Patients[3]		Study 462 PI-Naive Patients[4]
	NORVIR plus ZDV n = 116	NORVIR n = 117	ZDV n = 119	NORVIR n = 541	Placebo n = 545	NORVIR plus Saquinavir n = 141
Body as a Whole						
Abdominal Pain	5.2	6.0	5.9	8.3	5.1	2.1
Asthenia	28.4	10.3	11.8	15.3	6.4	16.3
Fever	1.7	0.9	1.7	5.0	2.4	0.7
Headache	7.8	6.0	6.7	6.5	5.7	4.3
Malaise	5.2	1.7	3.4	0.7	0.2	2.8
Pain (unspecified)	0.9	1.7	0.8	2.2	1.8	4.3
Cardiovascular						
Syncope	0.9	1.7	0.8	0.6	0.0	2.1
Vasodilation	3.4	1.7	0.8	1.7	0.0	3.5
Digestive						
Anorexia	8.6	1.7	4.2	7.8	4.2	4.3
Constipation	3.4	0.0	0.8	0.2	0.4	1.4
Diarrhea	25.0	15.4	2.5	23.3	7.9	22.7
Dyspepsia	2.6	0.0	1.7	5.9	1.5	0.7
Fecal Incontinence	0.0	0.0	0.0	0.0	0.0	2.8
Flatulence	2.6	0.9	1.7	1.7	0.7	3.5
Local Throat Irritation	0.9	1.7	0.8	2.8	0.4	1.4
Nausea	46.6	25.6	26.1	29.8	8.4	18.4
Vomiting	23.3	13.7	12.6	17.4	4.4	7.1
Metabolic and Nutritional						
Weight Loss	0.0	0.0	0.0	2.4	1.7	0.0
Musculoskeletal						
Arthralgia	0.0	0.0	0.0	1.7	0.7	2.1
Myalgia	1.7	1.7	0.8	2.4	1.1	2.1
Nervous						
Anxiety	0.9	0.0	0.8	1.7	0.9	2.1
Circumoral Paresthesia	5.2	3.4	0.0	6.7	0.4	6.4
Confusion	0.0	0.9	0.0	0.6	0.6	2.1
Depression	1.7	1.7	2.5	1.7	0.7	7.1
Dizziness	5.2	2.6	3.4	3.9	1.1	8.5
Insomnia	3.4	2.6	0.8	2.0	1.8	2.8
Paresthesia	5.2	2.6	0.0	3.0	0.4	2.1
Peripheral Paresthesia	0.0	6.0	0.8	5.0	1.1	5.7
Somnolence	2.6	2.6	0.0	2.4	0.2	0.0
Thinking Abnormal	2.6	0.0	0.8	0.9	0.4	0.7
Respiratory						
Pharyngitis	0.9	2.6	0.0	0.4	0.4	1.4
Skin and Appendages						
Rash	0.9	0.0	0.8	3.5	1.5	0.7
Sweating	3.4	2.6	1.7	1.7	1.1	2.8
Special Senses						
Taste Perversion	17.2	11.1	8.4	7.0	2.2	5.0
Urogenital						
Nocturia	0.0	0.0	0.0	0.2	0.0	2.8

1 Includes those adverse events at least possibly related to study drug or of unknown relationship and excludes concurrent HIV-1 conditions.
2 The median duration of treatment for patients randomized to regimens containing NORVIR in Study 245 was 9.1 months.
3 The median duration of treatment for patients randomized to regimens containing NORVIR in Study 247 was 9.4 months.
4 The median duration of treatment for patients in Study 462 was 48 weeks.

Information on the AbbVie, Inc. products listed on these pages is from the prescribing information in use as of July 31, 2013. For more information, please visit rxabbvie.com or call 1-800-633-9110.

Table 3. Percentage of Adult Patients, by Study and Treatment Group, with Chemistry and Hematology Abnormalities Occurring in greater than 3% of Patients Receiving NORVIR

		Study 245 Naive Patients			Study 247 Advanced Patients		Study 462 PI-Naive Patients
Variable	**Limit**	**NORVIR plus ZDV**	**NORVIR**	**ZDV**	**NORVIR**	**Placebo**	**NORVIR plus Saquinavir**
Chemistry	**High**						
Cholesterol	> 240 mg/dL	30.7	44.8	9.3	36.5	8.0	65.2
CPK	> 1000 IU/L	9.6	12.1	11.0	9.1	6.3	9.9
GGT	> 300 IU/L	1.8	5.2	1.7	19.6	11.3	9.2
SGOT (AST)	> 180 IU/L	5.3	9.5	2.5	6.4	7.0	7.8
SGPT (ALT)	> 215 IU/L	5.3	7.8	3.4	8.5	4.4	9.2
Triglycerides	> 800 mg/dL	9.6	17.2	3.4	33.6	9.4	23.4
Triglycerides	> 1500 mg/dL	1.8	2.6	-	12.6	0.4	11.3
Triglycerides Fasting	> 1500 mg/dL	1.5	1.3	-	9.9	0.3	-
Uric Acid	> 12 mg/dL	-	-	-	3.8	0.2	1.4
Hematology	**Low**						
Hematocrit	< 30%	2.6	-	0.8	17.3	22.0	0.7
Hemoglobin	< 8.0 g/dL	0.9	-	-	3.8	3.9	-
Neutrophils	$\leq 0.5 \times 10^9$/L	-	-	-	6.0	8.3	-
RBC	$< 3.0 \times 10^{12}$/L	1.8	-	5.9	18.6	24.4	-
WBC	$< 2.5 \times 10^9$/L	-	0.9	6.8	36.9	59.4	3.5

- Indicates no events reported.

ripheral wasting, facial wasting, breast enlargement, and "cushingoid appearance" have been observed in patients receiving antiretroviral therapy. The mechanism and long-term consequences of these events are currently unknown. A causal relationship has not been established.

5.10 Patients with Hemophilia

There have been reports of increased bleeding, including spontaneous skin hematomas and hemarthrosis, in patients with hemophilia type A and B treated with protease inhibitors. In some patients additional factor VIII was given. In more than half of the reported cases, treatment with protease inhibitors was continued or reintroduced. A causal relationship between protease inhibitor therapy and these events has not been established.

5.11 Resistance/Cross-resistance

Varying degrees of cross-resistance among protease inhibitors have been observed. Continued administration of ritonavir 600 mg twice daily following loss of viral suppression may increase the likelihood of cross-resistance to other protease inhibitors *[see Microbiology (12.4)]*.

5.12 Laboratory Tests

Ritonavir has been shown to increase triglycerides, cholesterol, SGOT (AST), SGPT (ALT), GGT, CPK, and uric acid. Appropriate laboratory testing should be performed prior to initiating NORVIR therapy and at periodic intervals or if any clinical signs or symptoms occur during therapy.

6 ADVERSE REACTIONS

The following adverse reactions are discussed in greater detail in other sections of the labeling.

- Drug Interactions *[see Warnings and Precautions (5.1)]*
- Hepatotoxicity *[see Warnings and Precautions (5.2)]*
- Pancreatitis *[see Warnings and Precautions (5.3)]*
- Allergic Reactions/Hypersensitivity *[see Warnings and Precautions (5.4)]*

When co-administering NORVIR with other protease inhibitors, see the full prescribing information for that protease inhibitor including adverse reactions.

6.1 Adult Clinical Trial Experience

Because clinical trials are conducted under widely varying conditions, adverse reaction rates observed in the clinical trials of a drug cannot be directly compared to rates in the clinical trials of another drug and may not reflect the rates observed in clinical practice.

The safety of NORVIR alone and in combination with nucleoside reverse transcriptase inhibitors was studied in 1,270 adult patients. Table 2 lists treatment-emergent adverse events (at least possibly related and of at least moderate intensity) that occurred in 2% or greater of adult patients receiving NORVIR alone or in combination with nucleoside reverse transcriptase inhibitors in Study 245 or Study 247 and in combination with saquinavir in study 462. In that study, 141 protease inhibitor-naive, HIV-1 infected patients with mean baseline CD_4 of 300 cells per µL were randomized to one of four regimens of NORVIR plus saquinavir, including NORVIR 400 mg twice-daily plus saquinavir 400 mg twice-daily. Overall the most frequently reported clinical adverse events, other than asthenia, among adult patients receiving NORVIR were gastrointestinal and neurological disturbances including nausea, diarrhea, vomiting, anorexia, abdominal pain, taste perversion, and circumoral and peripheral paresthesias. Similar adverse event profiles were reported in adult patients receiving ritonavir in other trials.

[See table 2 at top of previous page]

Adverse events occurring in less than 2% of adult patients receiving NORVIR in all phase II/phase III studies and considered at least possibly related or of unknown relationship to treatment and of at least moderate intensity are listed below by body system.

Body as a Whole

Abdomen enlarged, accidental injury, allergic reaction, back pain, cachexia, chest pain, chills, facial edema, facial pain, flu syndrome, hormone level altered, hypothermia, kidney pain, neck pain, neck rigidity, pelvic pain, photosensitivity reaction, and substernal chest pain.

Cardiovascular System

Cardiovascular disorder, cerebral ischemia, cerebral venous thrombosis, hypertension, hypotension, migraine, myocardial infarct, palpitation, peripheral vascular disorder, phlebitis, postural hypotension, tachycardia and vasospasm.

Digestive System

Abnormal stools, bloody diarrhea, cheilitis, cholestatic jaundice, colitis, dry mouth, dysphagia, eructation, esophageal ulcer, esophagitis, gastritis, gastroenteritis, gastrointestinal disorder, gastrointestinal hemorrhage, gingivitis, hepatic coma, hepatitis, hepatomegaly, hepatosplenomegaly, ileus, liver damage, melena, mouth ulcer, pancreatitis, pseudomembranous colitis, rectal disorder, rectal hemorrhage, sialadenitis, stomatitis, tenesmus, thirst, tongue edema, and ulcerative colitis.

Endocrine System

Adrenal cortex insufficiency and diabetes mellitus.

Hemic and Lymphatic System

Acute myeloblastic leukemia, anemia, ecchymosis, leukopenia, lymphadenopathy, lymphocytosis, myeloproliferative disorder, and thrombocytopenia.

Metabolic and Nutritional Disorders

Albuminuria, alcohol intolerance, avitaminosis, BUN increased, dehydration, edema, enzymatic abnormality, glycosuria, gout, hypercholesteremia, peripheral edema, and xanthomatosis.

Musculoskeletal System

Arthritis, arthrosis, bone disorder, bone pain, extraocular palsy, joint disorder, leg cramps, muscle cramps, muscle weakness, myositis, and twitching.

Nervous System

Abnormal dreams, abnormal gait, agitation, amnesia, aphasia, ataxia, coma, convulsion, dementia, depersonalization, diplopia, emotional lability, euphoria, grand mal convulsion, hallucinations, hyperesthesia, hyperkinesia, hypesthesia, incoordination, libido decreased, manic reaction, nervousness, neuralgia, neuropathy, paralysis, peripheral neuropathic pain, peripheral neuropathy, peripheral sensory neuropathy, personality disorder, sleep disorder, speech disorder, stupor, subdural hematoma, tremor, urinary retention, vertigo, and vestibular disorder.

Respiratory System

Asthma, bronchitis, dyspnea, epistaxis, hiccup, hypoventilation, increased cough, interstitial pneumonia, larynx edema, lung disorder, rhinitis, and sinusitis.

Skin and Appendages

Acne, contact dermatitis, dry skin, eczema, erythema multiforme, exfoliative dermatitis, folliculitis, fungal dermatitis, furunculosis, maculopapular rash, molluscum contagiosum, onychomycosis, pruritus, psoriasis, pustular rash, seborrhea, skin discoloration, skin disorder, skin hypertrophy, skin melanoma, urticaria, and vesiculobullous rash.

Special Senses

Abnormal electro-oculogram, abnormal electroretinogram, abnormal vision, amblyopia/blurred vision, blepharitis, conjunctivitis, ear pain, eye disorder, eye pain, hearing impairment, increased cerumen, iritis, parosmia, photophobia, taste loss, tinnitus, uveitis, visual field defect, and vitreous disorder.

Urogenital System

Acute kidney failure, breast pain, cystitis, dysuria, hematuria, impotence, kidney calculus, kidney failure, kidney function abnormal, kidney pain, menorrhagia, penis disorder, polyuria, urethritis, urinary frequency, urinary tract infection, and vaginitis.

Laboratory Abnormalities

Table 3 shows the percentage of adult patients who developed marked laboratory abnormalities.

[See table 3 above]

6.2 Pediatric Clinical Trial Experience

NORVIR has been studied in 265 pediatric patients greater than 1 month to 21 years of age. The adverse event profile observed during pediatric clinical trials was similar to that for adult patients.

Vomiting, diarrhea, and skin rash/allergy were the only drug-related clinical adverse events of moderate to severe intensity observed in greater than or equal to 2% of pediatric patients enrolled in NORVIR clinical trials.

Laboratory Abnormalities

The following Grade 3-4 laboratory abnormalities occurred in greater than 3% of pediatric patients who received treatment with NORVIR either alone or in combination with reverse transcriptase inhibitors: neutropenia (9%), hyperamylasemia (7%), thrombocytopenia (5%), anemia (4%), and elevated AST (3%).

6.3 Postmarketing Experience

The following adverse events have been reported during post-marketing use of NORVIR. Because these reactions are reported voluntarily from a population of unknown size, it is not possible to reliably estimate their frequency or establish a causal relationship to NORVIR exposure.

Body as a Whole

Dehydration, usually associated with gastrointestinal symptoms, and sometimes resulting in hypotension, syncope, or renal insufficiency has been reported. Syncope, orthostatic hypotension, and renal insufficiency have also been reported without known dehydration.

Co-administration of ritonavir with ergotamine or dihydroergotamine has been associated with acute ergot toxicity characterized by vasospasm and ischemia of the extremities and other tissues including the central nervous system.

Cardiovascular System

First-degree AV block, second-degree AV block, third-degree AV block, right bundle branch block have been reported *[see Warnings and Precautions (5.5)]*.

Cardiac and neurologic events have been reported when ritonavir has been co-administered with disopyramide, mexiletine, nefazodone, fluoxetine, and beta blockers. The possibility of drug interaction cannot be excluded.

Endocrine System

Cushing's syndrome and adrenal suppression have been reported when ritonavir has been co-administered with fluticasone propionate or budesonide.

Table 4. Established and Other Potentially Significant Drug Interactions

Concomitant Drug Class: Drug Name	Effect on Concentration of Ritonavir or Concomitant Drug	Clinical Comments
		HIV-Antiviral Agents
HIV-1 Protease Inhibitor: atazanavir	When co-administered with reduced doses of atazanavir and ritonavir ↑ atazanavir (↑ AUC, ↑ C_{max}, ↑ C_{min})	Atazanavir plasma concentrations achieved with atazanavir 300 mg once daily and ritonavir 100 mg once daily are higher than those achieved with atazanavir 400 mg once daily. See the complete prescribing information for Reyataz® (atazanavir) for details on co-administration of atazanavir 300 mg once daily with ritonavir 100 mg once daily.
HIV-1 Protease Inhibitor: darunavir	When co-administered with reduced doses of ritonavir ↑ darunavir (↑ AUC, ↑ C_{max}, ↑ C_{min})	See the complete prescribing information for Prezista® (darunavir) for details on co-administration of darunavir 600 mg twice daily with ritonavir 100 mg twice daily or darunavir 800 mg once daily with ritonavir 100 mg once daily.
HIV-1 Protease Inhibitor: fosamprenavir	When co-administered with reduced doses of ritonavir ↑ amprenavir (↑ AUC, ↑ C_{max}, ↑ C_{min})	See the complete prescribing information for Lexiva® (fosamprenavir) for details on co-administration of fosamprenavir 700 mg twice daily with ritonavir 100 mg twice daily, fosamprenavir 1400 mg once daily with ritonavir 200 mg once daily or fosamprenavir 1400 mg once daily with ritonavir 100 mg once daily.
HIV-1 Protease Inhibitor: indinavir	When co-administered with reduced doses of indinavir and ritonavir ↑ indinavir (↔ AUC, ↓ C_{max}, ↑ C_{min})	Alterations in concentrations are noted when reduced doses of indinavir are co-administered with NORVIR. Appropriate doses for this combination, with respect to efficacy and safety, have not been established.
HIV-1 Protease Inhibitor: saquinavir	When co-administered with reduced doses of ritonavir ↑ saquinavir (↑ AUC, ↑ C_{max}, ↑ C_{min})	See the complete prescribing information for Invirase® (saquinavir) for details on co-administration of saquinavir 1000 mg twice daily with ritonavir 100 mg twice daily. Saquinavir/ritonavir should not be given together with rifampin, due to the risk of severe hepatotoxicity (presenting as increased hepatic transaminases) if the three drugs are given together.
HIV-1 Protease Inhibitor: tipranavir	When co-administered with reduced doses of ritonavir ↑ tipranavir (↑ AUC, ↑ C_{max}, ↑ C_{min})	See the complete prescribing information for Aptivus® (tipranavir) for details on co-administration of tipranavir 500 mg twice daily with ritonavir 200 mg twice daily. There have been reports of clinical hepatitis and hepatic decompensation including some fatalities. All patients should be followed closely with clinical and laboratory monitoring, especially those with chronic hepatitis B or C co-infection, as these patients have an increased risk of hepatotoxicity. Liver function tests should be performed prior to initiating therapy with tipranavir/ritonavir, and frequently throughout the duration of treatment.
Non-Nucleoside Reverse Transcriptase Inhibitor: delavirdine	↑ ritonavir (↑AUC, ↑C_{max}, ↑ C_{min})	Appropriate doses of this combination with respect to safety and efficacy have not been established.
HIV-1 CCR5 – antagonist: maraviroc	↑ maraviroc	Concurrent administration of maraviroc with ritonavir will increase plasma levels of maraviroc. For specific dosage adjustment recommendations, please refer to the complete prescribing information for Selzentry® (maraviroc).
Integrase Inhibitor: Raltegravir	↓ raltegravir	The effects of ritonavir on raltegravir with ritonavir dosage regimens greater than 100 mg twice daily have not been evaluated, however raltegravir concentrations may be decreased with ritonavir coadministration.
		Other Agents
Analgesics, Narcotic: tramadol, propoxyphene		A dose decrease may be needed for these drugs when co-administered with ritonavir.
Anesthetic: meperidine	↓ meperidine/ ↑ normeperidine (metabolite)	Dosage increase and long-term use of meperidine with ritonavir are not recommended due to the increased concentrations of the metabolite normeperidine which has both analgesic activity and CNS stimulant activity (e.g., seizures).
Antialcoholics: disulfiram/ metronidazole		Ritonavir formulations contain alcohol, which can produce disulfiram-like reactions when co-administered with disulfiram or other drugs that produce this reaction (e.g., metronidazole).
Antiarrhythmics: disopyramide, lidocaine, mexiletine	↑antiarrhythmics	Caution is warranted and therapeutic concentration monitoring is recommended for antiarrhythmics when co-administered with ritonavir, if available.

(Table continued on next page)

Nervous System
There have been postmarketing reports of seizure. Also, see Cardiovascular System.
Skin and subcutaneous tissue disorders
Toxic epidermal necrolysis (TEN) has been reported.

7 DRUG INTERACTIONS

See also Contraindications (4), Warnings and Precautions (5.1), and Clinical Pharmacology (12.3)

When co-administering NORVIR with other protease inhibitors (atazanavir, darunavir, fosamprenavir, saquinavir, and tipranavir), see the full prescribing information for that protease inhibitor including important information for drug interactions.

7.1 Potential for NORVIR to Affect Other Drugs

Ritonavir has been found to be an inhibitor of cytochrome P450 3A (CYP3A) and may increase plasma concentrations of agents that are primarily metabolized by CYP3A. Agents that are extensively metabolized by CYP3A and have high first pass metabolism appear to be the most susceptible to large increases in AUC (greater than 3-fold) when co-administered with ritonavir. Thus, co-administration of NORVIR with drugs highly dependent on CYP3A for clearance and for which elevated plasma concentrations are associated with serious and/or life-threatening events is contraindicated. Co-administration with other CYP3A substrates may require a dose adjustment or additional monitoring as shown in Table 4.

Ritonavir also inhibits CYP2D6 to a lesser extent. Co-administration of substrates of CYP2D6 with ritonavir could result in increases (up to 2-fold) in the AUC of the other agent, possibly requiring a proportional dosage reduction. Ritonavir also appears to induce CYP3A, CYP1A2, CYP2C9, CYP2C19, and CYP2B6 as well as other enzymes, including glucuronosyl transferase.

7.2 Established and Other Potentially Significant Drug Interactions

Table 4 provides a list of established or potentially clinically significant drug interactions. Alteration in dose or regimen may be recommended based on drug interaction studies or predicted interaction *[see Clinical Pharmacology (12.3) for magnitude of interaction]*.

[See table 4 above and on pages 544 through 546]

8 USE IN SPECIFIC POPULATIONS

When co-administering NORVIR with other protease inhibitors, see the full prescribing information for the co-administered protease inhibitor including important information for use in special populations.

8.1 Pregnancy

Pregnancy Category B

Antiretroviral Pregnancy Registry: To monitor maternal-fetal outcomes of pregnant women exposed to NORVIR, an Antiretroviral Pregnancy Registry has been established. Physicians are encouraged to register patients by calling 1-800-258-4263.

Human Data

There are no adequate and well-controlled studies in pregnant women. NORVIR should be used during pregnancy only if the potential benefit justifies the potential risk to the fetus.

Antiretroviral Pregnancy Registry:

As of January 2012, the Antiretroviral Pregnancy Registry (APR) has received prospective reports of 3860 exposures to ritonavir containing regimens (1567 exposed in the first trimester and 2293 exposed in the second and third trimester). Birth defects occurred in 35 of the 1567 (2.2%) live births (first trimester exposure) and 59 of the 2293 (2.6%) live births (second/third trimester exposure).

Among pregnant women in the U.S. reference population, the background rate of birth defects is 2.7%. There was no association between ritonavir and overall birth defects observed in the APR.

Animal Data

No treatment related malformations were observed when ritonavir was administered to pregnant rats or rabbits. Developmental toxicity observed in rats (early resorptions, decreased fetal body weight and ossification delays and developmental variations) occurred at a maternally toxic dosage at an exposure equivalent to approximately 30% of that achieved with the proposed therapeutic dose. A slight increase in the incidence of cryptorchidism was also noted in rats at an exposure approximately 22% of that achieved with the proposed therapeutic dose.

Developmental toxicity observed in rabbits (resorptions, decreased litter size and decreased fetal weights) also occurred at a maternally toxic dosage equivalent to 1.8 times the proposed therapeutic dose based on a body surface area conversion factor.

8.3 Nursing Mothers

The Centers for Disease Control and Prevention recommend that HIV-infected mothers not breastfeed their infants to avoid risking postnatal transmission of HIV. It is not known whether ritonavir is secreted in human milk. Because of

Information on the AbbVie, Inc. products listed on these pages is from the prescribing information in use as of July 31, 2013. For more information, please visit rxabbvie.com or call 1-800-633-9110.

Table 4 *(cont.)*. Established and Other Potentially Significant Drug Interactions

Concomitant Drug Class: Drug Name	Effect on Concentration of Ritonavir or Concomitant Drug	Clinical Comments
Anticancer Agents: dasatinib, nilotinib, vincristine, vinblastine	↑ anticancer agents	Concentrations of these drugs may be increased when co-administered with ritonavir resulting in the potential for increased adverse events usually associated with these anticancer agents. For vincristine and vinblastine, consideration should be given to temporarily withholding the ritonavir containing antiretroviral regimen in patients who develop significant hematologic or gastrointestinal side effects when ritonavir is administered concurrently with vincristine or vinblastine. Clinicians should be aware that if the ritonavir containing regimen is withheld for a prolonged period, consideration should be given to altering the regimen to not include a CYP3A or P-gp inhibitor in order to control HIV-1 viral load. A decrease in the dosage or an adjustment of the dosing interval of nilotinib and dasatinib may be necessary for patients requiring co-administration with strong CYP3A inhibitors such as NORVIR. Please refer to the nilotinib and dasatinib prescribing information for dosing instructions.
Anticoagulant: warfarin	↓ R-warfarin ↓↑ S-warfarin	Initial frequent monitoring of the INR during ritonavir and warfarin co-administration is indicated.
Anticoagulant: rivaroxaban	↑ rivaroxaban	Avoid concomitant use of rivaroxaban and ritonavir. Co-administration of ritonavir and rivaroxaban is expected to result in increased exposure of rivaroxaban which may lead to risk of increased bleeding.
Anticonvulsants: carbamazepine, clonazepam, ethosuximide	↑anticonvulsants	Use with caution. A dose decrease may be needed for these drugs when co-administered with ritonavir and therapeutic concentration monitoring is recommended for these anticonvulsants, if available.
Anticonvulsants: divalproex, lamotrigine, phenytoin	↓anticonvulsants	Use with caution. A dose increase may be needed for these drugs when co-administered with ritonavir and therapeutic concentration monitoring is recommended for these anticonvulsants, if available.
Antidepressants: nefazodone, selective serotonin reuptake inhibitors (SSRIs): e.g. fluoxetine, paroxetine, tricyclics: e.g. amitriptyline, nortriptyline	↑antidepressants	A dose decrease may be needed for these drugs when co-administered with ritonavir.
Antidepressant: bupropion	↓ bupropion ↓ active metabolite, hydroxybupropion	Concurrent administration of bupropion with ritonavir may decrease plasma levels of both bupropion and its active metabolite (hydroxybupropion). Patients receiving ritonavir and bupropion concurrently should be monitored for an adequate clinical response to bupropion.
Antidepressant: desipramine	↑ desipramine	Dosage reduction and concentration monitoring of desipramine is recommended.
Antidepressant: trazodone	↑ trazodone	Concomitant use of trazodone and NORVIR increases plasma concentrations of trazodone. Adverse events of nausea, dizziness, hypotension and syncope have been observed following co-administration of trazodone and NORVIR. If trazodone is used with a CYP3A4 inhibitor such as ritonavir, the combination should be used with caution and a lower dose of trazodone should be considered.
Antiemetic: dronabinol	↑ dronabinol	A dose decrease of dronabinol may be needed when co-administered with ritonavir.
Antifungal: ketoconazole itraconazole voriconazole	↑ ketoconazole ↑ itraconazole ↓ voriconazole	High doses of ketoconazole or itraconazole (greater than 200 mg per day) are not recommended. Co-administration of voriconazole and ritonavir doses of 400 mg every 12 hours or greater is contraindicated. Co-administration of voriconazole and ritonavir 100 mg should be avoided, unless an assessment of the benefit/risk to the patient justifies the use of voriconazole.

(Table continued on next page)

both the potential for HIV transmission and the potential for serious adverse reactions in nursing infants, mothers should be instructed not to breastfeed if they are receiving NORVIR.

8.4 Pediatric Use

In HIV-1 infected patients age greater than 1 month to 21 years, the antiviral activity and adverse event profile seen during clinical trials and through postmarketing experience were similar to that for adult patients.

8.5 Geriatric Use

Clinical studies of NORVIR did not include sufficient numbers of subjects aged 65 and over to determine whether they respond differently from younger subjects. In general, dose selection for an elderly patient should be cautious, usually starting at the low end of the dosing range, reflecting the greater frequency of decreased hepatic, renal or cardiac function, and of concomitant disease or other drug therapy.

8.6 Hepatic Impairment

No dose adjustment of ritonavir is necessary for patients with either mild (Child-Pugh Class A) or moderate (Child-Pugh Class B) hepatic impairment. No pharmacokinetic or safety data are available regarding the use of ritonavir in subjects with severe hepatic impairment (Child-Pugh Class C), therefore, ritonavir is not recommended for use in patients with severe hepatic impairment *[see Warnings and Precautions (5.2), and Clinical Pharmacology (12.3)]*.

10 OVERDOSAGE

10.1 Acute Overdosage - Human Overdose Experience

Human experience of acute overdose with NORVIR is limited. One patient in clinical trials took NORVIR 1500 mg per day for two days. The patient reported paresthesias which resolved after the dose was decreased. A post-marketing case of renal failure with eosinophilia has been reported with ritonavir overdose.

The approximate lethal dose was found to be greater than 20 times the related human dose in rats and 10 times the related human dose in mice.

10.2 Management of Overdosage

Treatment of overdose with NORVIR consists of general supportive measures including monitoring of vital signs and observation of the clinical status of the patient. There is no specific antidote for overdose with NORVIR. If indicated, elimination of unabsorbed drug should be achieved by emesis or gastric lavage; usual precautions should be observed to maintain the airway. Administration of activated charcoal may also be used to aid in removal of unabsorbed drug. Since ritonavir is extensively metabolized by the liver and is highly protein bound, dialysis is unlikely to be beneficial in significant removal of the drug. A Certified Poison Control Center should be consulted for up-to-date information on the management of overdose with NORVIR.

11 DESCRIPTION

NORVIR (ritonavir) is an inhibitor of HIV-1 protease with activity against the Human Immunodeficiency Virus (HIV) type 1.

Ritonavir is chemically designated as 10-Hydroxy-2-methyl-5-(1-methylethyl)-1- [2-(1-methylethyl)-4-thiazolyl]-3,6-dioxo-8,11-bis(phenylmethyl)-2,4,7,12- tetraazatridecan-13-oic acid, 5-thiazolylmethyl ester, [5S-(5R*,8R*,10R*,11R*)]. Its molecular formula is $C_{37}H_{48}N_6O_5S_2$, and its molecular weight is 720.95. Ritonavir has the following structural formula:

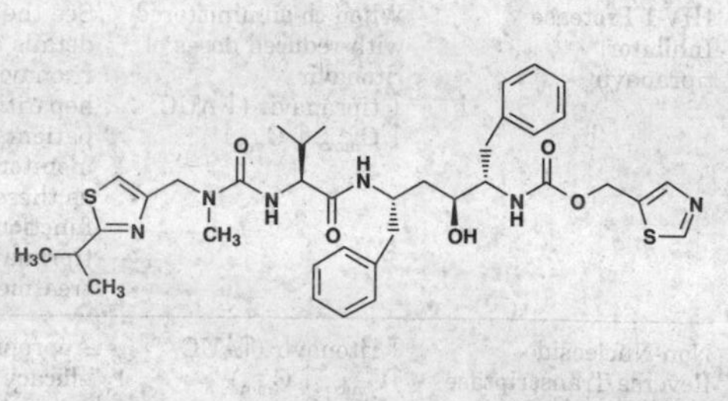

Ritonavir is a white-to-light-tan powder. Ritonavir has a bitter metallic taste. It is freely soluble in methanol and ethanol, soluble in isopropanol and practically insoluble in water.

NORVIR soft gelatin capsules are available for oral administration in a strength of 100 mg ritonavir with the following inactive ingredients: Butylated hydroxytoluene, ethanol, gelatin, iron oxide, oleic acid, polyoxyl 35 castor oil, and titanium dioxide.

12 CLINICAL PHARMACOLOGY

12.1 Mechanism of Action

Ritonavir is an antiviral drug *[see Microbiology (12.4)]*.

12.3 Pharmacokinetics

The pharmacokinetics of ritonavir have been studied in healthy volunteers and HIV-1 infected patients (CD_4 greater than or equal to 50 cells per µL). See Table 5 for ritonavir pharmacokinetic characteristics.

Absorption

The absolute bioavailability of ritonavir has not been determined.

Effect of Food on Oral Absorption

After a single 600 mg dose under non-fasting conditions, in two separate studies, the soft gelatin capsule (n = 57) formulation yielded a mean ± SD area under the plasma concentration-time curve (AUC) of 121.7 ± 53.8. Relative to fasting conditions, the extent of absorption of ritonavir from the soft gelatin capsule formulation was 13% higher when administered with a meal (615 KCal; 14.5% fat, 9% protein, and 76% carbohydrate).

Metabolism

Nearly all of the plasma radioactivity after a single oral 600 mg dose of ^{14}C-ritonavir oral solution (n = 5) was attributed to unchanged ritonavir. Five ritonavir metabolites have been identified in human urine and feces. The isopropylthiazole oxidation metabolite (M-2) is the major metabolite and has antiviral activity similar to that of parent drug; however, the concentrations of this metabolite in plasma are low. *In vitro* studies utilizing human liver microsomes have demonstrated that cytochrome P450 3A (CYP3A) is the ma-

Table 4 *(cont.)*. Established and Other Potentially Significant Drug Interactions

Concomitant Drug Class: Drug Name	Effect on Concentration of Ritonavir or Concomitant Drug	Clinical Comments
Anti-gout: colchicine	↑ colchicine	Patients with renal or hepatic impairment should not be given colchicine with ritonavir. Treatment of gout flares-co-administration of colchicine in patients on ritonavir: 0.6 mg (one tablet) for one dose, followed by 0.3 mg (half tablet) one hour later. Dose to be repeated no earlier than three days. Prophylaxis of gout flares-co-administration of colchicine in patients on ritonavir: If the original colchicine regimen was 0.6 mg twice a day, the regimen should be adjusted to 0.3 mg once a day. If the original colchicine regimen was 0.6 mg once a day, the regimen should be adjusted to 0.3 mg once every other day. Treatment of familial Mediterranean fever (FMF)-co-administration of colchicine in patients on ritonavir: Maximum daily dose of 0.6 mg (may be given as 0.3 mg twice a day).
Anti-infective: clarithromycin	↑ clarithromycin	For patients with renal impairment the following dosage adjustments should be considered: • For patients with CL_{CR} 30 to 60 mL per min the dose of clarithromycin should be reduced by 50%. • For patients with CL_{CR} less than 30 mL per min the dose of clarithromycin should be decreased by 75%. No dose adjustment for patients with normal renal function is necessary.
Antimycobacterial: rifabutin	↑ rifabutin and rifabutin metabolite	Dosage reduction of rifabutin by at least three-quarters of the usual dose of 300 mg per day is recommended (e.g., 150 mg every other day or three times a week). Further dosage reduction may be necessary.
Antimycobacterial: rifampin	↓ ritonavir	May lead to loss of virologic response. Alternate antimycobacterial agents such as rifabutin should be considered (see Antimycobacterial: rifabutin, for dose reduction recommendations).
Antiparasitic: atovaquone	↓ atovaquone	Clinical significance is unknown; however, increase in atovaquone dose may be needed.
Antiparasitic: quinine	↑ quinine	A dose decrease of quinine may be needed when co-administered with ritonavir.
β-Blockers: metoprolol, timolol	↑ Beta-Blockers	Caution is warranted and clinical monitoring of patients is recommended. A dose decrease may be needed for these drugs when co-administered with ritonavir.
Bronchodilator: theophylline	↓ theophylline	Increased dosage of theophylline may be required; therapeutic monitoring should be considered.
Calcium channel blockers: diltiazem, nifedipine, verapamil	↑ calcium channel blockers	Caution is warranted and clinical monitoring of patients is recommended. A dose decrease may be needed for these drugs when co-administered with ritonavir.
Digoxin	↑ digoxin	Concomitant administration of ritonavir with digoxin may increase digoxin levels. Caution should be exercised when co-administering ritonavir with digoxin, with appropriate monitoring of serum digoxin levels.
Endothelin receptor antagonists: bosentan	↑ bosentan	Co-administration of bosentan in patients on ritonavir: In patients who have been receiving ritonavir for at least 10 days, start bosentan at 62.5 mg once daily or every other day based upon individual tolerability Co-administration of ritonavir in patients on bosentan: Discontinue use of bosentan at least 36 hours prior to initiation of ritonavir. After at least 10 days following the initiation of ritonavir, resume bosentan at 62.5 mg once daily or every other day based upon individual tolerability.
HMG-CoA Reductase Inhibitor: atorvastatin rosuvastatin	↑ atorvastatin ↑ rosuvastatin	Titrate atorvastatin and rosuvastatin dose carefully and use the lowest necessary dose. If NORVIR is used with another protease inhibitor, see the complete prescribing information for the concomitant protease inhibitor for details on co-administration with atorvastatin and rosuvastatin.
Immunosuppressants: cyclosporine, tacrolimus, sirolimus (rapamycin)	↑ immunosuppressants	Therapeutic concentration monitoring is recommended for immunosuppressant agents when co-administered with ritonavir.

(Table continued on next page)

jor isoform involved in ritonavir metabolism, although CYP2D6 also contributes to the formation of M-2.

Elimination

In a study of five subjects receiving a 600 mg dose of ^{14}C-ritonavir oral solution, 11.3 ± 2.8% of the dose was excreted into the urine, with 3.5 ± 1.8% of the dose excreted as unchanged parent drug. In that study, 86.4 ± 2.9% of the dose was excreted in the feces with 33.8 ± 10.8% of the dose excreted as unchanged parent drug. Upon multiple dosing, ritonavir accumulation is less than predicted from a single dose possibly due to a time and dose-related increase in clearance.

Table 5. Ritonavir Pharmacokinetic Characteristics

Parameter	n	Values (Mean ± SD)
$V_\beta/F^‡$	91	0.41 ± 0.25 L/kg
t½		3 - 5 h
CL/F SS†	10	8.8 ± 3.2 L/h
CL/F‡	91	4.6 ± 1.6 L/h
CL_R	62	< 0.1 L/h
RBC/Plasma Ratio		0.14
Percent Bound*		98 to 99%

† SS = steady state; patients taking ritonavir 600 mg q12h.
‡ Single ritonavir 600 mg dose.
* Primarily bound to human serum albumin and alpha-1 acid glycoprotein over the ritonavir concentration range of 0.01 to 30 μg/mL.

Effects on Electrocardiogram

QTcF interval was evaluated in a randomized, placebo and active (moxifloxacin 400 mg once-daily) controlled crossover study in 45 healthy adults, with 10 measurements over 12 hours on Day 3. The maximum mean (95% upper confidence bound) time-matched difference in QTcF from placebo after baseline correction was 5.5 (7.6) milliseconds (msec) for 400 mg twice-daily ritonavir. Ritonavir 400 mg twice daily resulted in Day 3 ritonavir exposure that was approximately 1.5 fold higher than observed with ritonavir 600 mg twice-daily dose at steady state.

PR interval prolongation was also noted in subjects receiving ritonavir in the same study on Day 3. The maximum mean (95% confidence interval) difference from placebo in the PR interval after baseline correction was 22 (25) msec for 400 mg twice-daily ritonavir *[see Warnings and Precautions (5.5)]*.

Special Populations

Gender, Race and Age

No age-related pharmacokinetic differences have been observed in adult patients (18 to 63 years). Ritonavir pharmacokinetics have not been studied in older patients.

A study of ritonavir pharmacokinetics in healthy males and females showed no statistically significant differences in the pharmacokinetics of ritonavir. Pharmacokinetic differences due to race have not been identified.

Pediatric Patients

Steady-state pharmacokinetics were evaluated in 37 HIV-1 infected patients ages 2 to 14 years receiving doses ranging from 250 mg per m^2 twice-daily to 400 mg per m^2 twice-daily in PACTG Study 310, and in 41 HIV-1 infected patients ages 1 month to 2 years at doses of 350 and 450 mg per m^2 twice-daily in PACTG Study 345. Across dose groups, ritonavir steady-state oral clearance (CL per F per m^2) was approximately 1.5 to 1.7 times faster in pediatric patients than in adult subjects. Ritonavir concentrations obtained after 350 to 400 mg per m^2 twice-daily in pediatric patients greater than 2 years were comparable to those obtained in adults receiving 600 mg (approximately 330 mg per m^2) twice-daily. The following observations were seen regarding ritonavir concentrations after administration with 350 or 450 mg per m^2 twice-daily in children less than 2 years of age. Higher ritonavir exposures were not evident with 450 mg per m^2 twice-daily compared to the 350 mg per m^2 twice-daily. Ritonavir trough concentrations were somewhat lower than those obtained in adults receiving 600 mg twice-daily. The area under the ritonavir plasma concentration-time curve and trough concentrations obtained after administration with 350 or 450 mg per m^2 twice-daily in children less than 2 years were approximately 16% and 60% lower, respectively, than that obtained in adults receiving 600 mg twice-daily.

Renal Impairment

Ritonavir pharmacokinetics have not been studied in patients with renal impairment, however, since renal clearance is negligible, a decrease in total body clearance is not expected in patients with renal impairment.

Information on the AbbVie, Inc. products listed on these pages is from the prescribing information in use as of July 31, 2013. For more information, please visit rxabbvie.com or call 1-800-633-9110.

Table 4 *(cont.)*. Established and Other Potentially Significant Drug Interactions

Concomitant Drug Class: Drug Name	Effect on Concentration of Ritonavir or Concomitant Drug	Clinical Comments
Inhaled or Intranasal Steroid: e.g. fluticasone budesonide	↑ glucocorticoids	Concomitant use of ritonavir and fluticasone or other glucocorticoids that are metabolized by CYP3A is not recommended unless the potential benefit of treatment outweighs the risk of systemic corticosteroid effects. Concomitant use may result in increased steroid concentrations and reduced serum cortisol concentrations. Systemic corticosteroid effects including Cushing's syndrome and adrenal suppression have been reported during postmarketing use in patients when ritonavir has been coadministered with fluticasone propionate or budesonide.
Long-acting beta-adrenoceptor agonist: salmeterol	↑ salmeterol	Concurrent administration of salmeterol and ritonavir is not recommended. The combination may result in increased risk of cardiovascular adverse events associated with salmeterol, including QT prolongation, palpitations and sinus tachycardia.
Narcotic Analgesic: methadone fentanyl	↓ methadone ↑ fentanyl	Dosage increase of methadone may be considered. Concentrations of fentanyl are expected to increase. Careful monitoring of therapeutic and adverse effects (including potentially fatal respiratory depression) is recommended when fentanyl is concomitantly administered with NORVIR.
Neuroleptics: perphenazine, risperidone, thioridazine	↑ neuroleptics	A dose decrease may be needed for these drugs when co-administered with ritonavir.
Oral Contraceptives or Patch Contraceptives: ethinyl estradiol	↓ ethinyl estradiol	Alternate methods of contraception should be considered.
PDE5 Inhibitors: avanafil sildenafil, tadalafil, vardenafil	↑ avanafil ↑ sildenafil ↑ tadalafil ↑ vardenafil	Do not use ritonavir with avanafil because a safe and effective avanafil dosage regimen has not been established. Particular caution should be used when prescribing sildenafil, tadalafil or vardenafil in patients receiving ritonavir. Coadministration of ritonavir with these drugs is expected to substantially increase their concentrations and may result in an increase in PDE5 inhibitor associated adverse events, including hypotension, syncope, visual changes, and prolonged erection. Use of PDE5 inhibitors for pulmonary arterial hypertension (PAH): Sildenafil (Revatio®) is contraindicated when used for the treatment of pulmonary arterial hypertension (PAH) because a safe and effective dose has not been established when used with ritonavir [see *Contraindications (4)*]. The following dose adjustments are recommended for use of tadalafil (Adcirca™) with ritonavir: <u>Co-administration of ADCIRCA in patients on ritonavir:</u> In patients receiving ritonavir for at least one week, start ADCIRCA at 20 mg once daily. Increase to 40 mg once daily based upon individual tolerability. <u>Co-administration of ritonavir in patients on ADCIRCA:</u> Avoid use of ADCIRCA during the initiation of ritonavir. Stop ADCIRCA at least 24 hours prior to starting ritonavir. After at least one week following the initiation of ritonavir, resume ADCIRCA at 20 mg once daily. Increase to 40 mg once daily based upon individual tolerability. Use of PDE5 inhibitors for the treatment of erectile dysfunction: It is recommended not to exceed the following doses: • Sildenafil: 25 mg every 48 hours • Tadalafil: 10 mg every 72 hours • Vardenafil: 2.5 mg every 72 hours. Use with increased monitoring for adverse events.
Sedative/hypnotics: buspirone, clorazepate, diazepam, estazolam, flurazepam, zolpidem	↑ sedative/hypnotics	A dose decrease may be needed for these drugs when co-administered with ritonavir.
Sedative/hypnotics: Parenteral midazolam	↑ midazolam	Co-administration of oral midazolam with NORVIR is CONTRAINDICATED. Concomitant use of parenteral midazolam with NORVIR may increase plasma concentrations of midazolam. Co-administration should be done in a setting which ensures close clinical monitoring and appropriate medical management in case of respiratory depression and/or prolonged sedation. Dosage reduction for midazolam should be considered, especially if more than a single dose of midazolam is administered.
Steroids (systemic): e.g. budesonide dexamethasone, prednisone	↑ glucocorticoids	Concomitant use of glucocorticoids that are metabolized by CYP3A is not recommended unless the potential benefit of treatment outweighs the risk of systemic corticosteroid effects. Concomitant use may result in increased steroid concentrations and reduced serum cortisol concentrations. This may increase the risk for development of systemic corticosteroid effects including Cushing's syndrome and adrenal suppression.
Stimulant: methamphetamine	↑ methamphetamine	Use with caution. A dose decrease of methamphetamine may be needed when co-administered with ritonavir.

Hepatic Impairment

Dose-normalized steady-state ritonavir concentrations in subjects with mild hepatic impairment (400 mg twice-daily, n = 6) were similar to those in control subjects dosed with 500 mg twice-daily. Dose-normalized steady-state ritonavir exposures in subjects with moderate hepatic impairment (400 mg twice-daily, n= 6) were about 40% lower than those in subjects with normal hepatic function (500 mg twice-daily, n = 6). Protein binding of ritonavir was not statistically significantly affected by mild or moderately impaired hepatic function. No dose adjustment is recommended in patients with mild or moderate hepatic impairment. However, health care providers should be aware of the potential for lower ritonavir concentrations in patients with moderate hepatic impairment and should monitor patient response carefully. Ritonavir has not been studied in patients with severe hepatic impairment.

Drug Interactions

[see also Contraindications (4), Warnings and Precautions (5.1), and Drug Interactions (7)]

Table 6 and Table 7 summarize the effects on AUC and C_{max}, with 95% confidence intervals (95% CI), of co-administration of ritonavir with a variety of drugs. For information about clinical recommendations see Table 4 in *Drug Interactions (7)*.

[See table 6 at top of next page]

[See table 7 at top of pages 548 and 549]

12.4 Microbiology

Mechanism of Action

Ritonavir is a peptidomimetic inhibitor of the HIV-1 protease. Inhibition of HIV protease renders the enzyme incapable of processing the *gag-pol* polyprotein precursor which leads to production of non-infectious immature HIV-1 particles.

Antiviral Activity in Cell Culture

The activity of ritonavir was assessed in acutely infected lymphoblastoid cell lines and in peripheral blood lymphocytes. The concentration of drug that inhibits 50% (EC_{50}) value of viral replication ranged from 3.8 to 153 nM depending upon the HIV-1 isolate and the cells employed. The average EC_{50} for low passage clinical isolates was 22 nM (n = 13). In MT_4 cells, ritonavir demonstrated additive effects against HIV-1 in combination with either didanosine (ddI) or zidovudine (ZDV). Studies which measured cytotoxicity of ritonavir on several cell lines showed that greater than 20 μM was required to inhibit cellular growth by 50% resulting in a cell culture therapeutic index of at least 1,000.

Resistance

HIV-1 isolates with reduced susceptibility to ritonavir have been selected in cell culture. Genotypic analysis of these isolates showed mutations in the HIV-1 protease gene encoding at amino acid substitutions I84V, V82F, A71V, and M46I. Phenotypic (n = 18) and genotypic (n = 48) changes in HIV-1 isolates from selected patients treated with ritonavir were monitored in phase I/II trials over a period of 3 to 32 weeks. Substitutions associated with the HIV-1 viral protease in isolates obtained from 43 patients appeared to occur in a stepwise and ordered fashion; in sequence, these substitutions were position V82A/F/T/S, I54V, A71V/T, and I36L, followed by combinations of substitutions at an additional 5 specific amino acid positions (M46I/L, K20R, I84V, L33F and L90M). Of 18 patients for whom both phenotypic and genotypic analysis were performed on free virus isolated from plasma, 12 showed reduced susceptibility to ritonavir in cell culture. All 18 patients possessed one or more substitutions in the viral protease gene. The V82A/F substitution appeared to be necessary but not sufficient to confer phenotypic resistance. Phenotypic resistance was defined as a greater than or equal to 5-fold decrease in viral sensitivity in cell culture from baseline.

Cross-Resistance to Other Antiretrovirals

Among protease inhibitors variable cross-resistance has been recognized. Serial HIV-1 isolates obtained from six patients during ritonavir therapy showed a decrease in ritonavir susceptibility in cell culture but did not demonstrate a concordant decrease in susceptibility to saquinavir in cell culture when compared to matched baseline isolates. However, isolates from two of these patients demonstrated decreased susceptibility to indinavir in cell culture (8-fold). Isolates from 5 patients were also tested for cross-resistance to amprenavir and nelfinavir; isolates from 3 patients had a decrease in susceptibility to nelfinavir (6- to 14-fold), and none to amprenavir. Cross-resistance between ritonavir and reverse transcriptase inhibitors is unlikely because of the different enzyme targets involved. One ZDV-resistant HIV-1 isolate tested in cell culture retained full susceptibility to ritonavir.

13 NONCLINICAL TOXICOLOGY

13.1 Carcinogenesis, Mutagenesis, Impairment of Fertility

<u>Carcinogenesis</u>

Carcinogenicity studies in mice and rats have been carried out on ritonavir. In male mice, at levels of 50, 100 or 200 mg per kg per day, there was a dose dependent increase in the incidence of both adenomas and combined adenomas and carcinomas in the liver. Based on AUC measurements, the exposure at the high dose was approximately 0.3-fold for males that of the exposure in humans with the recommended therapeutic dose (600 mg twice-daily). There were no carcinogenic effects seen in females at the dosages tested. The exposure at the high dose was approximately 0.6-fold for the females that of the exposure in humans. In rats dosed at levels of 7, 15 or 30 mg per kg per day there were no carcinogenic effects. In this study, the exposure at the high dose was approximately 6% that of the exposure in humans with the recommended therapeutic dose. Based on the exposures achieved in the animal studies, the significance of the observed effects is not known.

Mutagenesis

Ritonavir was found to be negative for mutagenic or clastogenic activity in a battery of *in vitro* and *in vivo* assays including the Ames bacterial reverse mutation assay using *S. typhimurium* and *E. coli*, the mouse lymphoma assay, the mouse micronucleus test and chromosomal aberration assays in human lymphocytes.

Impairment of Fertility

Ritonavir produced no effects on fertility in rats at drug exposures approximately 40% (male) and 60% (female) of that achieved with the proposed therapeutic dose. Higher dosages were not feasible due to hepatic toxicity.

14 CLINICAL STUDIES

The activity of NORVIR as monotherapy or in combination with nucleoside reverse transcriptase inhibitors has been evaluated in 1446 patients enrolled in two double-blind, randomized trials.

14.1 Advanced Patients with Prior Antiretroviral Therapy

Study 247 was a randomized, double-blind trial (with open-label follow-up) conducted in HIV-1 infected patients with at least nine months of prior antiretroviral therapy and baseline CD_4 cell counts less than or equal to 100 cells per μL. NORVIR 600 mg twice-daily or placebo was added to each patient's baseline antiretroviral therapy regimen, which could have consisted of up to two approved antiretroviral agents. The study accrued 1090 patients, with mean baseline CD_4 cell count at study entry of 32 cells per μL. After the clinical benefit of NORVIR therapy was demonstrated, all patients were eligible to switch to open-label NORVIR for the duration of the follow-up period. Median duration of double-blind therapy with NORVIR and placebo was 6 months. The median duration of follow-up through the end of the open-label phase was 13.5 months for patients randomized to NORVIR and 14 months for patients randomized to placebo.

The cumulative incidence of clinical disease progression or death during the double-blind phase of Study 247 was 26% (140/543) for patients initially randomized to NORVIR compared to 42% (229/547) for patients initially randomized to placebo. This difference in rates was statistically significant.

Cumulative mortality through the end of the open-label follow-up phase for patients enrolled in Study 247 was 18% (99/543) for patients initially randomized to NORVIR compared to 26% (142/547) for patients initially randomized to placebo. This difference in rates was statistically significant. However, since the analysis at the end of the open-label phase includes patients in the placebo arm who were switched from placebo to NORVIR therapy, the survival benefit of NORVIR cannot be precisely estimated.

During the double-blind phase of Study 247, CD_4 cell counts increases from baseline for patients randomized to NORVIR at Week 2 and Week 4 were observed. From Week 4 and through Week 24, mean CD_4 cell counts for patients randomized to NORVIR appeared to plateau. In contrast, there was no apparent change in mean CD_4 cell counts for patients randomized to placebo at any visit between baseline and Week 24 of the double-blind phase of Study 247.

14.2 Patients Without Prior Antiretroviral Therapy

In Study 245, 356 antiretroviral-naive HIV-1 infected patients (mean baseline CD_4 = 364 cells/μL) were randomized to receive either NORVIR 600 mg twice-daily, zidovudine 200 mg three-times-daily, or a combination of these drugs. During the double-blind phase of study 245, greater mean CD_4 cell count increases were observed from baseline to Week 12 in the NORVIR-containing arms compared to the zidovudine arms. Mean CD_4 cell count changes subsequently appeared to plateau through Week 24 in the NORVIR arm, whereas mean CD_4 cell counts gradually diminished through Week 24 in the zidovudine and NORVIR plus zidovudine arms.

Greater mean reductions in plasma HIV-1 RNA levels were observed from baseline to Week 2 for the NORVIR-containing arms compared to the zidovudine arm. After Week 2 and through Week 24, mean plasma HIV-1 RNA levels either remained stable in the NORVIR and zidovudine arms or gradually rebounded toward baseline in the NORVIR plus zidovudine arm.

Table 6. Drug Interactions - Pharmacokinetic Parameters for Ritonavir in the Presence of the Co-administered Drug

Co-administered Drug	Dose of Co-administered Drug (mg)	Dose of NORVIR (mg)	n	AUC % (95% CI)	C_{max} (95% CI)	C_{min} (95% CI)
Clarithromycin	500 q12h, 4 d	200 q8h, 4 d	22	↑ 12% (2, 23%)	↑ 15% (2, 28%)	↑ 14% (-3, 36%)
Didanosine	200 q12h, 4 d	600 q12h, 4 d	12	↔	↔	↔
Fluconazole	400 single dose, day 1; 200 daily, 4 d	200 q6h, 4 d	8	↑ 12% (5, 20%)	↑ 15% (7, 22%)	↑ 14% (0, 26%)
Fluoxetine	30 q12h, 8 d	600 single dose, 1 d	16	↑ 19% (7, 34%)	↔	ND
Ketoconazole	200 daily, 7 d	500 q12h, 10 d	12	↑ 18% (-3, 52%)	↑ 10% (-11, 36%)	ND
Rifampin	600 or 300 daily, 10 d	500 q12h, 20 d	7, 9*	↓ 35% (7, 55%)	↓ 25% (-5, 46%)	↓ 49% (-14, 91%)
Voriconazole	400 q12h, 1 d; then 200 q12h, 8 d	400 q12h, 9 d		↔	↔	ND
Zidovudine	200 q8h, 4 d	300 q6h, 4 d	10	↔	↔	↔

15 REFERENCES

1. Sewester CS. Calculations. In: Drug Facts and Comparisons. St. Louis, MO: J.B. Lippincott Co; January, 1997:xix.

16 HOW SUPPLIED/STORAGE AND HANDLING

NORVIR (ritonavir) soft gelatin capsules are white capsules imprinted with the "a" logo, 100 and the code DS, available in the following package size:

Bottles of 120 capsules each (**NDC** 0074-6633-22).

Bottles of 30 capsules each (**NDC** 0074-6633-30).

Recommended Storage

Store NORVIR soft gelatin capsules in the refrigerator between 2°-8°C (36°-46°F) until dispensed. Refrigeration of NORVIR soft gelatin capsules by the patient is recommended, but not required if used within 30 days and stored below 25°C (77°F). Protect from light. Avoid exposure to excessive heat.

Product should be stored and dispensed in the original container.

Keep cap tightly closed.

17 PATIENT COUNSELING INFORMATION

See FDA-approved patient labeling (Patient Information)

Information For Patients

Patients or parents of patients should be informed that:

General Information

☐ They should pay special attention to accurate administration of their dose to minimize the risk of accidental overdose or underdose of NORVIR.

☐ They should inform their healthcare provider if their children's weight changes in order to make sure that the child's NORVIR dose is the correct one.

☐ Take NORVIR with meals.

☐ For adult patients taking NORVIR capsules, the maximum dose of 600 mg twice daily by mouth with meals should not be exceeded.

☐ Patients should remain under the care of a physician while using NORVIR. Patients should be advised to take NORVIR and other concomitant antiretroviral therapy every day as prescribed. NORVIR must always be used in combination with other antiretroviral drugs. Patients should not alter the dose or discontinue therapy without consulting with their doctor. If a dose of NORVIR is missed patients should take the dose as soon as possible and then return to their normal schedule. However, if a dose is skipped the patient should not double the next dose.

☐ NORVIR is not a cure for HIV-1 infection and patients may continue to experience illnesses associated with HIV-1 infection, including opportunistic infections. Patients should remain under the care of a physician when using NORVIR.

Patients should be advised to avoid doing things that can spread HIV-1 infection to others.

- **Do not share needles or other injection equipment.**
- **Do not share personal items that can have blood or body fluids on them, like toothbrushes and razor blades.**
- **Do not have any kind of sex without protection.** Always practice safe sex by using a latex or polyurethane condom to lower the chance of sexual contact with semen, vaginal secretions, or blood.
- **Do not breastfeed.** We do not know if NORVIR can be passed to the baby through breast milk and whether it could harm the baby. Also, mothers with HIV-1 should not breastfeed because HIV-1 can be passed to the baby in the breast milk.

☐ Sustained decreases in plasma HIV-1 RNA have been associated with a reduced risk of progression to AIDS and death.

Drug Interactions

☐ NORVIR may interact with some drugs; therefore, patients should be advised to report to their doctor the use of any other prescription, non-prescription medication or herbal products, particularly St. John's Wort.

☐ If they are receiving estrogen-based hormonal contraceptives, additional or alternate contraceptive measures should be used during therapy with NORVIR.

Potential Adverse Effects

☐ Pre-existing liver disease including Hepatitis B or C can worsen with use of NORVIR. This can be seen as worsening of transaminase elevations or hepatic decompensation. Patients should be advised that their liver function tests will need to be monitored closely especially during the first several months of NORVIR treatment and that they should notify their healthcare provider if they develop the signs and symptoms of worsening liver disease including loss of appetite, abdominal pain, jaundice, and itchy skin.

☐ Pancreatitis, including some fatalities, has been observed in patients receiving NORVIR therapy. Your patients should let you know of signs and symptoms (nausea, vomiting, and abdominal pain) that might be suggestive of pancreatitis.

☐ Skin rashes ranging in severity from mild to Stevens-Johnson syndrome have been reported in patients receiving NORVIR. Patients should be advised to contact their healthcare provider if they develop a rash while taking NORVIR. The healthcare provider will determine if treatment should be continued or an alternative antiretroviral regimen used.

☐ NORVIR may produce changes in the electrocardiogram (e.g., PR prolongation). Patients should consult their physician if they experience symptoms such as dizziness, lightheadedness, abnormal heart rhythm or loss of consciousness.

☐ Treatment with NORVIR therapy can result in substantial increases in the concentration of total cholesterol and triglycerides.

☐ New onset of diabetes or exacerbation of pre-existing diabetes mellitus, and hyperglycemia have been reported. Patients should be advised to notify their healthcare provider if they develop the signs and symptoms of diabetes mellitus including frequent urination, excessive thirst, extreme hunger or unusual weight loss and/or an increased blood sugar while on NORVIR as they may require a change in their diabetes treatment or new treatment.

☐ Immune reconstitution syndrome has been reported in HIV-1 infected patients treated with combination antiretroviral therapy, including NORVIR.

☐ Redistribution or accumulation of body fat may occur in patients receiving antiretroviral therapy and that the cause and long term health effects of these conditions are not known at this time.

☐ Patients with hemophilia may experience increased bleeding when treated with protease inhibitors such as NORVIR.

Information on the AbbVie, Inc. products listed on these pages is from the prescribing information in use as of July 31, 2013. For more information, please visit rxabbvie.com or call 1-800-633-9110.

Table 7. Drug Interactions - Pharmacokinetic Parameters for Co-administered Drug in the Presence of NORVIR

Co-administered Drug	Dose of Co-administered Drug (mg)	Dose of NORVIR (mg)	n	AUC % (95% CI)	C_{max} (95% CI)	C_{min} (95% CI)
Alprazolam	1, single dose	500 q12h, 10 d	12	↓ 12% (-5, 30%)	↓ 16% (5, 27%)	ND
Avanafil	50, single dose	600 q12h	14[6]	↑ 13-fold	↑ 2.4-fold	ND
Clarithromycin	500 q12h, 4 d	200 q8h, 4 d	22	↑ 77% (56, 103%)	↑ 31% (15, 51%)	↑ 2.8-fold (2.4, 3.3×)
14-OH clarithromycin metabolite				↓ 100%	↓ 99%	↓ 100%
Desipramine	100, single dose	500 q12h, 12 d	14	↑ 145% (103, 211%)	↑ 22% (12, 35%)	ND
2-OH desipramine metabolite				↓ 15% (3, 26%)	↓ 67% (62, 72%)	ND
Didanosine	200 q12h, 4 d	600 q12h, 4 d	12	↓ 13% (0, 23%)	↓ 16% (5, 26%)	↔
Ethinyl estradiol	50 µg single dose	500 q12h, 16 d	23	↓ 40% (31, 49%)	↓ 32% (24, 39%)	ND
Fluticasone propionate aqueous nasal spray	200 mcg qd, 7 d	100 mg q12h, 7 d	18	↑ approximately 350-fold[5]	↑ approximately 25-fold[5]	
Indinavir[1]	400 q12h, 15 d	400 q12h, 15 d	10			
Day 14				↑ 6% (-14, 29%)	↓ 51% (40, 61%)	↑ 4-fold (2.8, 6.8×)
Day 15				↓ 7% (-22, 28%)	↓ 62% (52, 70%)	↑ 4-fold (2.5, 6.5×)
Ketoconazole	200 daily, 7 d	500 q12h, 10 d	12	↑ 3.4-fold (2.8, 4.3×)	↑ 55% (40, 72%)	ND
Meperidine	50 oral single dose	500 q12h, 10 d	8	↓ 62% (59, 65%)	↓ 59% (42, 72%)	ND
Normeperidine metabolite			6	↑ 47% (-24, 345%)	↑ 87% (42, 147%)	ND
Methadone[2]	5, single dose	500 q12h, 15 d	11	↓ 36% (16, 52%)	↓ 38% (28, 46%)	ND
Raltegravir	400, single dose	100 q12h, 16 d	10	↓ 16% (-30, 1%)	↓ 24% (-45, 4%)	↓ 1% (-30, 40%)
Rivaroxaban	10, single dose (days 0 and 7)	600 q12h (days 2 to 7)	12	↑ 150% (130-170%)[7]	↑ 60% (40-70%)[7]	ND
Rifabutin	150 daily, 16 d	500 q12h, 10 d	5, 11*	↑ 4-fold (2.8, 6.1×)	↑ 2.5-fold (1.9, 3.4×)	↑ 6-fold (3.5, 18.3×)
25-*O*-desacetyl rifabutin metabolite				↑ 38-fold (28, 56×)	↑ 16-fold (13, 20×)	↑ 181-fold (ND)
Sildenafil	100, single dose	500 twice daily, 8 d	28	↑ 11-fold	↑ 4-fold	ND
Sulfamethoxazole[3]	800, single dose	500 q12h, 12 d	15	↓ 20% (16, 23%)	↔	ND
Tadalafil	20 mg, single dose	200 mg q12h		↑ 124%	↔	ND
Theophylline	3 mg/kg q8h, 15 d	500 q12h, 10 d	13, 11*	↓ 43% (42, 45%)	↓ 32% (29, 34%)	↓ 57% (55, 59%)
Trazodone	50 mg, single dose	200 mg q12h, 4 doses	10	↑ 2.4-fold	↑ 34%	
Trimethoprim[3]	160, single dose	500 q12h, 12 d	15	↑ 20% (3, 43%)	↔	ND
Vardenafil	5 mg	600 q12h		↑ 49-fold	↑ 13-fold	ND

(Table continued on next page)

☐ If they are receiving avanafil, sildenafil, tadalafil, or vardenafil for the treatment of erectile dysfunction, they may be at an increased risk of associated adverse reactions including hypotension, visual changes, and sustained erection, and should promptly report any symptoms to their doctor. They should seek medical assistance immediately if they develop a sustained penile erection lasting more than 4 hours while taking NORVIR and a PDE5 Inhibitor such as Stendra®, Viagra®, Cialis® or Levitra®. If they are currently using or planning to use avanafil or tadalafil (for the treatment of pulmonary arterial hypertension) they should ask their doctor about potential adverse reactions these medications may cause when taken with NORVIR. The doctor may choose not to keep them on avanafil, or may adjust the dose of tadalafil while initiating treatment with NORVIR. Concomitant use of Revatio® (sildenafil) with NORVIR is contraindicated in patients with pulmonary arterial hypertension (PAH).

☐ Continued NORVIR therapy at a dose of 600 mg twice daily following loss of viral suppression may increase the likelihood of cross-resistance to other protease inhibitors.

NORVIR 100 mg soft gelatin capsules are manufactured for:
AbbVie Inc.
North Chicago, IL 60064 USA
Ref. 03-A753-R33-Rev. January, 2013

PATIENT INFORMATION
NORVIR® (NOR - VEER)
(ritonavir)
Capsules Soft Gelatin

Read this Patient Information before you start taking NORVIR and each time you get a refill. There may be new information. This information does not take the place of talking to your doctor about your medical condition or your treatment.

What is the most important information I should know about NORVIR?

- **NORVIR can interact with other medicines and cause serious side effects.** It is important to know the medicines that should not be taken with NORVIR. **See the section "Who should not take NORVIR?"**

What is NORVIR?

NORVIR is a prescription anti-HIV medicine used with other anti-HIV medicines to treat people with human immunodeficiency virus (HIV) infection. NORVIR is a type of anti-HIV medicine called a protease inhibitor. HIV is the virus that causes AIDS (Acquired Immune Deficiency Syndrome).

When used with other HIV medicines, NORVIR may reduce the amount of HIV in your blood (called "viral load"). NORVIR may also help to increase the number of CD_4 (T) cells in your blood which help fight off other infections. Reducing the amount of HIV and increasing the CD_4 (T) cell count may improve your immune system. This may reduce your risk of death or infections that can happen when your immune system is weak (opportunistic infections).

NORVIR does not cure HIV infection or AIDS and you may continue to experience illnesses associated with HIV-1 infection, including opportunistic infections. You should remain under the care of a doctor when using NORVIR.

Avoid doing things that can spread HIV-1 infection:

- **Do not share needles or other injection equipment.**
- **Do not share personal items that can have blood or body fluids on them, like toothbrushes and razor blades.**
- **Do not have any kind of sex without protection.** Always practice safe sex by using a latex or polyurethane condom to lower the chance of sexual contact with semen, vaginal secretions, or blood.

Who should not take NORVIR?

Do not take NORVIR if you are allergic to ritonavir or any of the ingredients in NORVIR. See the end of this leaflet for a complete list of ingredients in NORVIR.

Do not take NORVIR with any of the following medicines:

- alfuzosin (Uroxatral)
- amiodarone (Cordarone, Nexterone, Pacerone), flecainide (Tambocor), propafenone (Rhythmol) or quinidine (Nuedext, Quinaglute, Cardioquin, Quinidex, and others)
- voriconazole (VFend) if NORVIR dose is 400 mg every 12 hours or greater
- dihydroergotamine (D.H.E. 45, Embolex, Migranal), ergonovine, ergotamine (Cafergot, Ergomar) methylergonovine (Methergine)
- cisapride (Propulsid)
- St. John's Wort (Hypericum perforatum)
- the cholesterol lowering medicines lovastatin (Mevacor, Altoprev, Advicor) or simvastatin (Zocor, Simcor, Vytorin)
- pimozide (Orap)
- sildenafil (Revatio) only when used for the treatment of pulmonary arterial hypertension
- oral midazolam or triazolam (Halcion)

Serious problems can happen if you or your child takes any of these medicines with NORVIR.

What should I tell my doctor before taking NORVIR?

Before taking NORVIR, tell your doctor if you:

- have liver problems, including Hepatitis B or Hepatitis C.
- have heart problems.
- have high blood sugar (diabetes).
- have bleeding problems or hemophilia.
- are pregnant or plan to become pregnant. It is not known if NORVIR can harm your unborn baby. **Pregnancy Registry:** You and your doctor will need to decide if taking NORVIR is right for you. If you take NORVIR while you are pregnant, talk to your doctor about how you can take part in the Antiretroviral Pregnancy Registry. The purpose of the registry is to follow the health of you and your baby.
- are breastfeeding: **Do not breastfeed.** We do not know if NORVIR can be passed to the baby through your breast milk and whether it could harm the baby. Also, mothers with HIV-1 should not breastfeed because HIV-1 can be passed to the baby in the breast milk.

Tell your doctor about all the medicines you take including prescription and nonprescription medicines, vitamins, and herbal supplements. Taking NORVIR and certain other medicines may affect each other causing serious side effects. NORVIR may affect the way other medicines work and other medicines may affect how NORVIR works.

Especially tell your doctor if you take:

- medicine to treat HIV
- estrogen-based contraceptives (birth control). NORVIR might reduce the effectiveness of estrogen-based contraceptives. You must take additional precautions for birth control such as a condom
- medicine for pain such as tramadol (Ryzolt, Ultracet, Conzip, Ultram), propoxyphene, or meperidine (Demerol)
- medicine to treat alcohol abuse such as disulfiram (Antabuse)
- medicine for your heart such as disopyramide (Norpace), lidocaine (Xylocaine Viscous), mexiletine, digoxin (Lanoxin), nifedipine (Procardia, Adalat, Afeditab CR), dil-

Table 7 *(cont.)*. Drug Interactions - Pharmacokinetic Parameters for Co-administered Drug in the Presence of NORVIR

Co-administered Drug	Dose of Co-administered Drug (mg)	Dose of NORVIR (mg)	n	AUC % (95% CI)	C_{max} (95% CI)	C_{min} (95% CI)
Voriconazole	400 q12h, 1 d; then 200 q12h, 8 d	400 q12h, 9 d		↓ 82%	↓ 66%	
	400 q12h, 1 d; then 200 q12h, 8 d	100 q12h, 9 d		↓ 39%	↓ 24%	
Warfarin	5, single dose	400 q12h, 12d	12			
S-Warfarin				↑ 9% (-17, 44%)[4]	↓ 9% (-16, -2%)[4]	ND
R-Warfarin				↓ 33% (-38, -27%)[4]	↔	ND
Zidovudine	200 q8h, 4 d	300 q6h, 4 d	9	↓ 25% (15, 34%)	↓ 27% (4, 45%)	ND

1 Ritonavir and indinavir were co-administered for 15 days; Day 14 doses were administered after a 15%-fat breakfast (757 Kcal) and 9%-fat evening snack (236 Kcal), and Day 15 doses were administered after a 15%-fat breakfast (757 Kcal) and 32%-fat dinner (815 Kcal). Indinavir C_{min} was also increased 4-fold. Effects were assessed relative to an indinavir 800 mg q8h regimen under fasting conditions.
2 Effects were assessed on a dose-normalized comparison to a methadone 20 mg single dose.
3 Sulfamethoxazole and trimethoprim taken as single combination tablet.
4 90% CI presented for R- and S-warfarin AUC and C_{max} ratios.
5 This significant increase in plasma fluticasone propionate exposure resulted in a significant decrease (86%) in plasma cortisol AUC.
6 For the reference arm: N=14 for C_{max} and $AUC_{(0-inf)}$, and for the test arm: N=13 for C_{max} and N=4 for $AUC_{(0-inf)}$.
7 90% CI presented for rivaroxaban
↑ Indicates increase.
↓ Indicates decrease.
↔ Indicates no change.
* Parallel group design; entries are subjects receiving combination and control regimens, respectively.

tiazem (Cardizem, Dilacor, Cartia, Diltzac, Dilt, Taztia, Tiazac) or verapamil (Calan, Covera, Isoptin, Tarka, Verelan)
- medicines for panic disorder or anxiety such as buspirone, clorazepate, diazepam, estazolam, flurazepam, and zolpidem
- medicine for cancer such as dasatinib (Sprycel), nilotinib (Tasigna) vincristine, or vinblastine
- warfarin (Coumadin, Jantoven), rivaroxaban (Xarelto)
- medicine for seizures such as carbamazepine (Carbatrol, Equetro, Tegretol, Epitol), clonazepam (Klonopin), ethosuximide (Zarontin, Ethosuximide), divalproex (Depakote, Divalproex Sodium), lamotrigine (Lamictal) or phenytoin (Dilantin, Phenytek)
- medicine for depression such as nefazodone, bupropion (Wellbutrin, Aplenzin, Zyban), desipramine (Norpramin) or trazadone, fluoxetine (Prozac), paroxetine (Paxil), amitriptyline, or nortriptyline
- medicine for nausea and vomiting such as dronabinol (Marinol) or perphenazine
- medicine for fungal infections such as ketoconazole (Nizoral), itraconazole (Sporanox, Onmel) or voriconazole (VFend)
- colchicine (Colcrys, Col-Probenecid, Probenecid and Colchine)
- medicine for infections such as clarithromycin (Prevpac, Biaxin), rifabutin (Mycobutin), rifampin (Rimactane, Rifadin, Rifater, Rifamate), atovaquone (Mepron, Malarone), quinine (Qualaquin) or metronidazole (Flagyl, Helidac, Metrocream)
- medicine used to treat blood pressure, a heart attack, heart failure, or to lower pressure in the eye such as metoprolol (Lopressor, Toprol-XL), timolol (Cosopt, Betimol, Timoptic, Isatolol, Combigan)
- medicine for lung disease such as theophylline and salmeterol (Serevent)
- bosentan (Tracleer)
- medicine to prevent organ transplant failure such as cyclosporine (Gengraf, Sandimmune, Neoral), tacrolimus (Prograf,) sirolimus (Rapamune)
- steroids such as dexamethasone, fluticasone (Advair Diskus, Veramyst, Flovent, Flonase), budesonide (Entocort EC, Pulmicort, Rhinocort), or prednisone
- a narcotic medicine such as methadone (Methadose, Dolophine Hydrochloride) or fentanyl (Abstral, Actiq, Fentora, Lazanda, Onsolis, Duragesic)
- medicine to treat schizophrenia such as risperidone (Risperdal) or thioridazine
- medicine to treat erectile dysfunction or pulmonary hypertension such as avanafil (Stendra), sildenafil (Viagra, Revatio), vardenafil (Levitra, Staxyn), tadalafil (Cialis, Adcirca). If you are taking avanafil (Stendra), your doctor may need to change it to a different medicine
- midazolam by injection
- methamphetamine (Desoxyn)
- cholesterol lowering medicine such as atorvastatin (Lipitor) or rosuvasatin (Crestor)

This is not a complete list of medicines that you should tell your doctor that you are taking. Ask your doctor, provider or pharmacist if you are not sure if your medicine is one that is listed above.

Know the medicines you take. Keep a list of them to show your doctor or pharmacist when you get a new medicine. Do not start any new medicines while you are taking NORVIR without first talking with your doctor.

How should I take NORVIR?
- Take NORVIR exactly as prescribed by your doctor.
- You should stay under a doctor's care when taking NORVIR. Do not change your dose of NORVIR or stop treatment without talking with your doctor first.
- If your child is taking NORVIR, your child's doctor will decide the right dose based on your child's height and weight. Tell your doctor if your child's weight changes. Your child should take NORVIR with food.
- Take NORVIR with food if possible.
- Do not run out of NORVIR. Get your NORVIR prescription refilled from you doctor or pharmacy before you run out.
- If you miss a dose of NORVIR, take it as soon as possible and then take your next scheduled dose at its regular time. If it is almost time for your next dose, wait and take the next dose at the regular time. Do not double the next dose.
- If you take too much NORVIR, call your local poison control center or go to the nearest hospital emergency room right away.

What are the possible side effects of NORVIR?

NORVIR can cause serious side effects including:
- **See "What is the most important information I should know about NORVIR?"**
- **Liver disease.** Some people taking NORVIR in combination with other anti-HIV medicines have developed liver problems which may be life-threatening. Your doctor should do regular blood tests during your combination treatment with NORVIR. If you have chronic hepatitis B or C infection, your doctor should check your blood tests more often because you have an increased chance of developing liver problems. Tell your doctor if you have any of the below signs and symptoms of liver problems:
  - loss of appetite
  - pain or tenderness on your right side below your ribs
  - yellowing of your skin or whites of your eyes
  - itchy skin
- **Swelling of your pancreas (Pancreatitis).** NORVIR can cause serious pancreas problems, which may lead to death. Tell your doctor right away if you have signs or symptoms of pancreatitis such as:
  - nausea
  - vomiting
  - stomach (abdominal) pain
- **Allergic Reactions.** Sometimes these allergic reactions can become severe and require treatment in a hospital. You should call your doctor right away if you develop a rash. Stop taking NORVIR and get medical help right away if you have any of the following symptoms of a severe allergic reaction:
  - trouble breathing
  - wheezing
  - dizziness or fainting
  - throat tightness or hoarseness
  - fast heartbeat or pounding in your chest (tachycardia)
  - sweating
  - swelling of your face, lips or tongue
  - muscle or joint pain
  - blisters or skin lesions
  - mouth sores or ulcers
- **Changes in the electrical activity of your heart called PR prolongation. PR prolongation can cause irregular heartbeats.** Tell your doctor right away if you have symptoms such as:
  - dizziness
  - lightheadedness
  - feeling faint or passing out
  - abnormal heart beat
- **Increase in some fats (cholesterol and triglyceride levels) in your blood.** Treatment with NORVIR may increase your blood levels of cholesterol and triglycerides. Your doctor should do blood tests before you start your treatment with NORVIR and regularly to check for an increase in your cholesterol and triglycerides levels.
- **Diabetes and high blood sugar (hyperglycemia).** Some people who take protease inhibitors including NORVIR can get high blood sugar, develop diabetes, or their diabetes can get worse. Tell your doctor if you notice an increase in thirst or urinate often while taking NORVIR.
- **Changes in your immune system (Immune reconstitution syndrome)** can happen when you start taking HIV medicines. Your immune system may get stronger and begin to fight infections that have been hidden in your body for a long time. Call your doctor right away if you start having new symptoms after starting your HIV medicine.
- **Change in body fat.** These changes can happen in people who take antiretroviral therapy. The changes may include an increase amount of fat in the upper back and neck ("buffalo hump"), breast, and around the back and stomach area. Loss of fat from the legs, arms, and face may also happen. The exact cause and long-term health effects of these conditions are not known.
- **Increased bleeding for hemophiliacs.** Some people with hemophilia have increased bleeding with protease inhibitors including NORVIR.

The most common side effects of NORVIR include:
- feeling weak or tired
- nausea
- vomiting
- diarrhea
- loss of appetite
- abdominal pain
- changes in taste
- tingling feeling or numbness in hands or feet or around the lips
- headache
- dizziness

Tell your doctor if you have any side effect that bothers you or that does not go away.

These are not all of the possible side effects of NORVIR. For more information, ask your doctor or pharmacist.

Call your doctor for medical advice about side effects. You may report side effects to FDA at 1-800-FDA-1088.

How do I Store NORVIR?

Store NORVIR soft gelatin capsules in the refrigerator between 36°F to 46°F (2°C to 8°C) NORVIR soft gelatin capsules may be stored below 77°F (25°C) if used within 30 days.
- Protect NORVIR soft gelatin capsules from light.
- Keep NORVIR soft gelatin capsules away from heat.
- Store NORVIR soft gelatin capsules tightly closed in the original container.
- Use NORVIR soft gelatin capsules by the expiration date on the bottle.

Keep NORVIR and all medicines out of the reach of children.

General information about NORVIR

Medicines are sometimes prescribed for purposes other than those listed in a Patient Information Leaflet. Do not use this medicine for a condition for which it was not prescribed. Do not share this medicine with other people.

This leaflet summarizes the most important information about NORVIR. If you would like more information, talk to your doctor. You can ask your doctor or pharmacist for information about NORVIR that is written for healthcare professionals.

For more information, call 1-800-633-9110.

Information on the AbbVie, Inc. products listed on these pages is from the prescribing information in use as of July 31, 2013. For more information, please visit rxabbvie.com or call 1-800-633-9110.

What are the ingredients in NORVIR?
Active ingredient: ritonavir
Inactive ingredients:
NORVIR soft gelatin capsules: butylated hydroxytoluene, ethanol, gelatin, iron oxide, oleic acid, polyoxyl 35 castor oil, and titanium dioxide
This Patient Information has been approved by the U.S. Food and Drug Administration.
NORVIR 100 mg soft gelatin capsules are manufactured for:
AbbVie Inc.
North Chicago, IL 60064 USA
* The brands listed are trademarks of their respective owners and are not trademarks of AbbVie Inc. The makers of these brands are not affiliated with and do not endorse AbbVie Inc. or its products.
Ref. 03-A753-R33-Rev. January, 2013
Shown in Product Identification Guide, page 304

NORVIR® ℞
[*NOR-VEER*]
(ritonavir)
Tablet for Oral use
NORVIR®
(ritonavir)
Solution for Oral use

HIGHLIGHTS OF PRESCRIBING INFORMATION
These highlights do not include all the information needed to use NORVIR safely and effectively. See full prescribing information for NORVIR.
NORVIR (ritonavir) Tablet for Oral use
NORVIR (ritonavir) Solution for Oral use
Initial U.S. Approval: 1996

> WARNING: DRUG-DRUG INTERACTIONS LEADING TO POTENTIALLY SERIOUS AND/OR LIFE THREATENING REACTIONS
> ***See full prescribing information for complete boxed warning***
> **Co-administration of NORVIR with several classes of drugs including sedative hypnotics, antiarrhythmics, or ergot alkaloid preparations may result in potentially serious and/or life-threatening adverse events due to possible effects of NORVIR on the hepatic metabolism of certain drugs. Review medications taken by patients prior to prescribing NORVIR or when prescribing other medications to patients already taking NORVIR *[see Contraindications (4), Warnings and Precautions (5.1), Drug Interactions (7),* and *Clinical Pharmacology (12.3)]*.**

RECENT MAJOR CHANGES

Dosage and Administration (2.2) 11/2012
Contraindications (4) 12/2011
Warnings and Precautions:
- Drug Interactions (5.1) 12/2011
- Toxicity in Preterm Neonates (5.2) 11/2012
- Allergic Reactions (5.5) 12/2011
- Immune Reconstitution Syndrome (5.9) 02/2012

INDICATIONS AND USAGE

NORVIR is an HIV protease inhibitor indicated in combination with other antiretroviral agents for the treatment of HIV-1 infection (1)

DOSAGE AND ADMINISTRATION

- Dose modification for NORVIR is necessary when used with other protease inhibitors (2)
- Adult patients: 600 mg twice-day with meals (2.1)
- Pediatrics patients: The recommended twice daily dose for children greater than one month of age is based on body surface area and should not exceed 600 mg twice daily with meals (2.2)
- NORVIR oral solution should not be administered to neonates before a postmenstrual age (first day of the mother's last menstrual period to birth plus the time elapsed after birth) of 44 weeks has been attained (2.2, 5.2)

DOSAGE FORMS AND STRENGTHS

- Tablet: 100 mg ritonavir (3)
- Oral solution: 80 mg ritonavir per milliliter (3)

CONTRAINDICATIONS

- NORVIR is contraindicated in patients with known hypersensitivity to ritonavir (e.g., toxic epidermal necrolysis, Stevens-Johnson syndrome) or any of its ingredients (4)
- Co-administration with drugs highly dependent on CYP3A for clearance and for which elevated plasma concentrations may be associated with serious and/or life-threatening events (4)
- Co-administration with drugs that significantly reduce ritonavir (4)

WARNINGS AND PRECAUTIONS

The following have been observed in patients receiving NORVIR:
- Drug Interactions: Consider drug-drug interaction potential to reduce risk of serious or life-threatening adverse reactions (5.1)
- Toxicity in preterm neonates: NORVIR oral solution should not be used in preterm neonates in the immediate postnatal period because of possible toxicities. A safe and effective dose of NORVIR oral solution in this patient population has not been established (2.2, 5.2)
- Hepatic Reactions: Fatalities have occurred. Monitor liver function before and during therapy, especially in patients with underlying hepatic disease, including hepatitis B and hepatitis C, or marked transaminase elevations (5.3, 8.6)
- Pancreatitis: Fatalities have occurred; suspend therapy as clinically appropriate (5.4)
- Allergic Reactions/Hypersensitivity: Allergic reactions have been reported and include anaphylaxis, toxic epidermal necrolysis, Stevens-Johnson syndrome, bronchospasm and angioedema. Discontinue treatment if severe reactions develop (5.5, 6.3)
- PR interval prolongation may occur in some patients. Cases of second and third degree heart block have been reported. Use with caution with patients with preexisting conduction system disease, ischemic heart disease, cardiomyopathy, underlying structural heart disease or when administering with other drugs that may prolong the PR interval (5.6, 12.3)
- Total cholesterol and triglycerides elevations: Monitor prior to therapy and periodically thereafter (5.7)
- Patients may develop new onset or exacerbations of diabetes mellitus, hyperglycemia (5.8)
- Patients may develop immune reconstitution syndrome (5.9)
- Patients may develop redistribution/accumulation of body fat (5.10)
- Hemophilia: Spontaneous bleeding may occur, and additional factor VIII may be required (5.11)

ADVERSE REACTIONS

The most common adverse reactions (greater than 5% and of moderate to severe intensity) were abdominal pain, asthenia, headache, malaise, anorexia, diarrhea, dyspepsia, nausea, vomiting, paresthesia, circumoral paresthesia, peripheral paresthesia, dizziness, and taste perversion (6.1)
To report SUSPECTED ADVERSE REACTIONS, contact AbbVie Inc. at 1-800-633-9110 or FDA at 1-800-FDA-1088 or www.fda.gov/medwatch.

DRUG INTERACTIONS

- Co-administration of NORVIR can alter the concentrations of other drugs. The potential for drug-drug interactions must be considered prior to and during therapy (4, 5.1, 7, 12.3)

USE IN SPECIFIC POPULATIONS

- Nursing Mothers: Because of both the potential for HIV transmission and the potential for serious adverse reactions in nursing infants, mothers should be instructed not to breastfeed if they are receiving NORVIR (8.3)

See 17 for PATIENT COUNSELING INFORMATION and FDA-approved patient labeling

Revised: 01/2013

FULL PRESCRIBING INFORMATION: CONTENTS*

* Sections or subsections omitted from the full prescribing information are not listed

FULL PRESCRIBING INFORMATION

> **WARNING: DRUG-DRUG INTERACTIONS LEADING TO POTENTIALLY SERIOUS AND/OR LIFE THREATENING REACTIONS**
> **Co-administration of NORVIR with several classes of drugs including sedative hypnotics, antiarrhythmics, or ergot alkaloid preparations may result in potentially serious and/or life-threatening adverse events due to possible effects of NORVIR on the hepatic metabolism of certain drugs. Review medications taken by patients prior to prescribing NORVIR or when prescribing other medications to patients already taking NORVIR *[see Contraindications (4), Warnings and Precautions (5.1), Drug Interactions (7),* and *Clinical Pharmacology (12.3)]*.**

1 INDICATIONS AND USAGE

NORVIR is indicated in combination with other antiretroviral agents for the treatment of HIV-1 infection.

2 DOSAGE AND ADMINISTRATION

NORVIR is administered orally. NORVIR tablets should be swallowed whole, and not chewed, broken or crushed. Take NORVIR with meals. Patients may improve the taste of NORVIR oral solution by mixing with chocolate milk, Ensure®, or Advera® within one hour of dosing.

General Dosing Guidelines

Patients who take the 600 mg twice daily soft gel capsule NORVIR dose may experience more gastrointestinal side effects such as nausea, vomiting, abdominal pain or diarrhea when switching from the soft gel capsule to the tablet formulation because of greater maximum plasma concentration (C_{max}) achieved with the tablet formulation relative to the soft gel capsule *[see Clinical Pharmacology (12.3)]*. Patients should also be aware that these adverse events (gastrointestinal or paresthesias) may diminish as therapy is continued.

Dose Modification for NORVIR

Dose reduction of NORVIR is necessary when used with other protease inhibitors: atazanavir, darunavir, fosamprenavir, saquinavir, and tipranavir.

Prescribers should consult the full prescribing information and clinical study information of these protease inhibitors if they are co-administered with a reduced dose of ritonavir *[see Warnings and Precautions (5),* and *Drug Interactions (7)]*.

2.1 Adult Patients

Recommended Dosage for Treatment of HIV-1:

The recommended dosage of ritonavir is 600 mg twice daily by mouth to be taken with meals. Use of a dose titration schedule may help to reduce treatment-emergent adverse events while maintaining appropriate ritonavir plasma levels. Ritonavir should be started at no less than 300 mg twice daily and increased at 2 to 3 day intervals by 100 mg twice daily. The maximum dose of 600 mg twice daily should not be exceeded upon completion of the titration.

2.2 Pediatric Patients

Ritonavir should be used in combination with other antiretroviral agents *[see Dosage and Administration (2)]*. The recommended dosage of ritonavir in children greater than 1 month is 350 to 400 mg per m^2 twice daily by mouth to be taken with meals and should not exceed 600 mg twice daily. Ritonavir should be started at 250 mg per m^2 twice daily and increased at 2 to 3 day intervals by 50 mg per m^2 twice daily. If patients do not tolerate 400 mg per m^2 twice daily due to adverse events, the highest tolerated dose may be used for maintenance therapy in combination with other antiretroviral agents, however, alternative therapy should be considered. When possible, dose should be administered using a calibrated dosing syringe.

NORVIR oral solution should not be administered to neonates before a postmenstrual age (first day of the mother's last menstrual period to birth plus the time elapsed after birth) of 44 weeks has been attained *[see Warnings and Precautions (5.2)]*.

NORVIR oral solution contains 43.2% (v/v) alcohol and 26.57% (w/v) propylene glycol. Special attention should be given to accurate calculation of the dose of NORVIR, transcription of the medication order, dispensing information and dosing instructions to minimize the risk for medication errors, and overdose. This is especially important for young children. Total amounts of alcohol and propylene glycol from all medicines that are to be given to pediatric patients 1 to 6 months of age should be taken into account in order to avoid toxicity from these excipients *[see Warnings and Precautions (5.2)* and *Overdosage (10)]*.

[See table 1 above]

Body surface area (BSA) can be calculated as follows[1]:

$$BSA\ (m^2) = \sqrt{\frac{Ht\ (Cm) \times Wt\ (kg)}{3600}}$$

Table 1. Pediatric Dosage Guidelines

Body Surface Area (m^2)	Twice Daily Dose 250 mg per m^2	Twice Daily Dose 300 mg per m^2	Twice Daily Dose 350 mg per m^2	Twice Daily Dose 400 mg per m^2
0.20	0.6 mL (50 mg)	0.75 mL (60 mg)	0.9 mL (70 mg)	1.0 mL (80 mg)
0.25	0.8 mL (62.5 mg)	0.9 mL (75 mg)	1.1 mL (87.5 mg)	1.25 mL (100 mg)
0.50	1.6 mL (125 mg)	1.9 mL (150 mg)	2.2 mL (175 mg)	2.5 mL (200 mg)
0.75	2.3 mL (187.5 mg)	2.8 mL (225 mg)	3.3 mL (262.5 mg)	3.75 mL (300 mg)
1.00	3.1 mL (250 mg)	3.75 mL (300 mg)	4.4 mL (350 mg)	5 mL (400 mg)
1.25	3.9 mL (312.5 mg)	4.7 mL (375 mg)	5.5 mL (437.5 mg)	6.25 mL (500 mg)
1.50	4.7 mL (375 mg)	5.6 mL (450 mg)	6.6 mL (525 mg)	7.5 mL (600 mg)

3 DOSAGE FORMS AND STRENGTHS

• NORVIR Tablets

White film-coated ovaloid tablets debossed with the "a" logo and the code NK providing 100 mg ritonavir.

• NORVIR Oral Solution

Orange-colored liquid containing 600 mg ritonavir per 7.5 mL marked dosage cup (80 mg per mL).

4 CONTRAINDICATIONS

- When co-administering NORVIR with other protease inhibitors, see the full prescribing information for that protease inhibitor including contraindication information.
- NORVIR is contraindicated in patients with known hypersensitivity (e.g., toxic epidermal necrolysis (TEN) or Stevens-Johnson syndrome) to ritonavir or any of its ingredients.
- Co-administration of NORVIR with several classes of drugs (including sedative hypnotics, antiarrhythmics, or ergot alkaloid preparations) is contraindicated and may result in potentially serious and/or life-threatening adverse events due to possible effects of NORVIR on the hepatic metabolism of these drugs (see Table 2). Voriconazole and St. John's Wort are exceptions in that co-administration of NORVIR and voriconazole results in a significant decrease in plasma concentrations of voriconazole, and co-administration of NORVIR with St. John's Wort may result in decreased ritonavir plasma concentrations.

[See table 2 above]

Table 2. Drugs that are Contraindicated with NORVIR

Drug Class	Drugs Within Class That Are Contraindicated With NORVIR**	Clinical Comments:
Alpha$_1$-adrenoreceptor antagonist	Alfuzosin HCL	Potential for hypotension.
Antiarrhythmics	Amiodarone, flecainide, propafenone, quinidine	Potential for cardiac arrhythmias.
Antifungal	Voriconazole	Co-administration of voriconazole with ritonavir 400 mg every 12 hours significantly decreases voriconazole plasma concentrations and may lead to loss of antifungal response. Voriconazole is contraindicated with ritonavir doses of 400 mg every 12 hours or greater *[see Drug Interactions (7.2)]*.
Ergot Derivatives	Dihydroergotamine, ergonovine, ergotamine, methylergonovine	Potential for acute ergot toxicity characterized by vasospasm and ischemia of the extremities and other tissues including the central nervous system.
GI Motility Agent	Cisapride	Potential for cardiac arrhythmias.
Herbal Products	St. John's Wort (hypericum perforatum)	Co-administration of NORVIR with St. John's Wort may result in decreased ritonavir plasma concentrations and may lead to loss of virologic response and possible resistance to NORVIR or to the class of protease inhibitors.
HMG-CoA Reductase Inhibitors:	Lovastatin, simvastatin	Potential for myopathy including rhabdomyolysis.
Neuroleptic	Pimozide	Potential for cardiac arrhythmias.
PDE5 enzyme inhibitor	Sildenafil* (Revatio®) only when used for the treatment of pulmonary arterial hypertension (PAH)	A safe and effective dose has not been established when used with ritonavir. There is an increased potential for sildenafil-associated adverse events, including visual abnormalities, hypotension, prolonged erection, and syncope *[see Drug Interactions (7.2)]*.
Sedative/hypnotics	Oral midazolam, triazolam	Prolonged or increased sedation or respiratory depression *[see Drug Interactions (7.2)]*.

* *see Drug Interactions (7)* for co-administration of sildenafil in patients with erectile dysfunction.
** For additional information for these contraindicated drugs, *see also Drug Interactions (7)*.

5 WARNINGS AND PRECAUTIONS

When co-administering NORVIR with other protease inhibitors, see the full prescribing information for that protease inhibitor including important Warnings and Precautions.

5.1 Drug Interactions

NORVIR is a CYP3A inhibitor. Initiating treatment with NORVIR in patients receiving medications metabolized by CYP3A or initiating medications metabolized by CYP3A in patients already maintained on NORVIR may result in increased plasma concentrations of concomitant medications. Higher plasma concentrations of concomitant medications can result in increased or prolonged therapeutic or adverse effects, potentially leading to severe, life-threatening or fatal events. The potential for drug-drug interactions must be considered prior to and during therapy with NORVIR. Review of other medications taken by patients and monitoring of patients for adverse effects is recommended during therapy with NORVIR.

See Table 2 for a listing of drugs that are contraindicated with NORVIR due to potentially life-threatening adverse events, significant drug interactions, or loss of virologic activity. Also, see Table 5 for a listing of drugs with established and other significant drug interactions *[see Contraindications (4), Drug Interactions (7),* and *Clinical Pharmacology (12.3)]*.

5.2 Toxicity in Preterm Neonates

NORVIR oral solution contains the excipients alcohol (43.2% v/v) and propylene glycol (26.57% w/v). When administered concomitantly with propylene glycol, ethanol competitively inhibits the metabolism of propylene glycol, which may lead to elevated concentrations. Preterm neonates may be at an increased risk of propylene glycol-associated adverse events due to diminished ability to metabolize propylene glycol, thereby leading to accumulation and potential adverse events. Postmarketing life-threatening cases of cardiac toxicity (including complete AV block, bradycardia, and cardiomyopathy), lactic acidosis, acute renal failure, CNS depression and respiratory complications leading to death have been reported, predominantly in preterm neonates receiving lopinavir/ritonavir oral solution which also contains the excipients alcohol and propylene glycol.

NORVIR oral solution should not be used in preterm neonates in the immediate postnatal period because of possible toxicities. However, if the benefit of using NORVIR oral solution to treat HIV infection in infants immediately after birth outweighs the potential risks, infants should be monitored closely for increases in serum osmolality and serum creatinine, and for toxicity related to NORVIR oral solution including: hyperosmolality, with or without lactic acidosis, renal toxicity, CNS depression (including stupor, coma, and apnea), seizures, hypotonia, cardiac arrhythmias and ECG changes, and hemolysis. Total amounts of alcohol and propylene glycol from all medicines that are to be given to infants should be taken into account in order to avoid toxicity from these excipients *[see Dosage and Administration (2.2)* and *Overdosage (10)]*.

5.3 Hepatic Reactions

Hepatic transaminase elevations exceeding 5 times the upper limit of normal, clinical hepatitis, and jaundice have occurred in patients receiving NORVIR alone or in combination with other antiretroviral drugs (see Table 4). There may be an increased risk for transaminase elevations in patients with underlying hepatitis B or C. Therefore, caution should be exercised when administering NORVIR to patients with pre-existing liver diseases, liver enzyme abnormalities, or hepatitis. Increased AST/ALT monitoring should be considered in these patients, especially during the first three months of NORVIR treatment *[see Use in Specific Populations (8.6)]*.

There have been postmarketing reports of hepatic dysfunction, including some fatalities. These have generally occurred in patients taking multiple concomitant medications and/or with advanced AIDS.

5.4 Pancreatitis

Pancreatitis has been observed in patients receiving NORVIR therapy, including those who developed hypertriglyceridemia. In some cases fatalities have been observed. Patients with advanced HIV disease may be at increased risk of elevated triglycerides and pancreatitis *[see Warnings and Precautions (5.7)]*. Pancreatitis should be considered if clinical symptoms (nausea, vomiting, abdominal pain) or abnormalities in laboratory values (such as increased serum lipase or amylase values) suggestive of pancreatitis should

Information on the AbbVie, Inc. products listed on these pages is from the prescribing information in use as of July 31, 2013. For more information, please visit rxabbvie.com or call 1-800-633-9110.

Table 3. Percentage of Patients with Treatment-emergent Adverse Events[1] of Moderate or Severe Intensity Occurring in ≥ 2% of Adult Patients Receiving NORVIR

Adverse Events	Study 245 Naive Patients[2]			Study 247 Advanced Patients[3]		Study 462 PI-Naive Patients[4]
	NORVIR + ZDV n = 116	NORVIR n = 117	ZDV n = 119	NORVIR n = 541	Placebo n = 545	NORVIR + Saquinavir n= 141
Body as a Whole						
Abdominal Pain	5.2	6.0	5.9	8.3	5.1	2.1
Asthenia	28.4	10.3	11.8	15.3	6.4	16.3
Fever	1.7	0.9	1.7	5.0	2.4	0.7
Headache	7.8	6.0	6.7	6.5	5.7	4.3
Malaise	5.2	1.7	3.4	0.7	0.2	2.8
Pain (unspecified)	0.9	1.7	0.8	2.2	1.8	4.3
Cardiovascular						
Syncope	0.9	1.7	0.8	0.6	0.0	2.1
Vasodilation	3.4	1.7	0.8	1.7	0.0	3.5
Digestive						
Anorexia	8.6	1.7	4.2	7.8	4.2	4.3
Constipation	3.4	0.0	0.8	0.2	0.4	1.4
Diarrhea	25.0	15.4	2.5	23.3	7.9	22.7
Dyspepsia	2.6	0.0	1.7	5.9	1.5	0.7
Fecal Incontinence	0.0	0.0	0.0	0.0	0.0	2.8
Flatulence	2.6	0.9	1.7	1.7	0.7	3.5
Local Throat Irritation	0.9	1.7	0.8	2.8	0.4	1.4
Nausea	46.6	25.6	26.1	29.8	8.4	18.4
Vomiting	23.3	13.7	12.6	17.4	4.4	7.1
Metabolic and Nutritional						
Weight Loss	0.0	0.0	0.0	2.4	1.7	0.0
Musculoskeletal						
Arthralgia	0.0	0.0	0.0	1.7	0.7	2.1
Myalgia	1.7	1.7	0.8	2.4	1.1	2.1
Nervous						
Anxiety	0.9	0.0	0.8	1.7	0.9	2.1
Circumoral Paresthesia	5.2	3.4	0.0	6.7	0.4	6.4
Confusion	0.0	0.9	0.0	0.6	0.6	2.1
Depression	1.7	1.7	2.5	1.7	0.7	7.1
Dizziness	5.2	2.6	3.4	3.9	1.1	8.5
Insomnia	3.4	2.6	0.8	2.0	1.8	2.8
Paresthesia	5.2	2.6	0.0	3.0	0.4	2.1
Peripheral Paresthesia	0.0	6.0	0.8	5.0	1.1	5.7
Somnolence	2.6	2.6	0.0	2.4	0.2	0.0
Thinking Abnormal	2.6	0.0	0.8	0.9	0.4	0.7

(Table continued on next page)

occur. Patients who exhibit these signs or symptoms should be evaluated and NORVIR therapy should be discontinued if a diagnosis of pancreatitis is made.

5.5 Allergic Reactions/Hypersensitivity

Allergic reactions including urticaria, mild skin eruptions, bronchospasm, and angioedema have been reported. Cases of anaphylaxis, toxic epidermal necrolysis (TEN), and Stevens-Johnson syndrome have also been reported. Discontinue treatment if severe reactions develop.

5.6 PR Interval Prolongation

Ritonavir prolongs the PR interval in some patients. Post marketing cases of second or third degree atrioventricular block have been reported in patients.

NORVIR should be used with caution in patients with underlying structural heart disease, preexisting conduction system abnormalities, ischemic heart disease, cardiomyopathies, as these patients may be at increased risk for developing cardiac conduction abnormalities.

The impact on the PR interval of co-administration of ritonavir with other drugs that prolong the PR interval (including calcium channel blockers, beta-adrenergic blockers, digoxin and atazanavir) has not been evaluated. As a result, co-administration of ritonavir with these drugs should be undertaken with caution, particularly with those drugs metabolized by CYP3A. Clinical monitoring is recommended *[see Drug Interactions (7),* and *Clinical Pharmacology (12.3)]*.

5.7 Lipid Disorders

Treatment with NORVIR therapy alone or in combination with saquinavir has resulted in substantial increases in the concentration of total cholesterol and triglycerides *[see Adverse Reactions (6.1)]*. Triglyceride and cholesterol testing should be performed prior to initiating NORVIR therapy and at periodic intervals during therapy. Lipid disorders should be managed as clinically appropriate, taking into account any potential drug-drug interactions with NORVIR and HMG CoA reductase inhibitors *[see Contraindications (4)* and *Drug Interactions (7)]*.

5.8 Diabetes Mellitus/Hyperglycemia

New onset diabetes mellitus, exacerbation of pre-existing diabetes mellitus, and hyperglycemia have been reported during postmarketing surveillance in HIV-infected patients receiving protease inhibitor therapy. Some patients required either initiation or dose adjustments of insulin or oral hypoglycemic agents for treatment of these events. In some cases, diabetic ketoacidosis has occurred. In those patients who discontinued protease inhibitor therapy, hyperglycemia persisted in some cases. Because these events have been reported voluntarily during clinical practice, estimates of frequency cannot be made and a causal relationship between protease inhibitor therapy and these events has not been established.

5.9 Immune Reconstitution Syndrome

Immune reconstitution syndrome has been reported in HIV-infected patients treated with combination antiretroviral therapy, including NORVIR. During the initial phase of combination antiretroviral treatment, patients whose immune system responds may develop an inflammatory response to indolent or residual opportunistic infections (such as *Mycobacterium avium* infection, cytomegalovirus, *Pneumocystis jiroveci* pneumonia, or tuberculosis), which may necessitate further evaluation and treatment.

Autoimmune disorders (such as Graves' disease, polymyositis, and Guillain-Barré syndrome) have also been reported to occur in the setting of immune reconstitution, however, the time to onset is more variable, and can occur many months after initiation of treatment.

5.10 Fat Redistribution

Redistribution/accumulation of body fat including central obesity, dorsocervical fat enlargement (buffalo hump), peripheral wasting, facial wasting, breast enlargement, and "cushingoid appearance" have been observed in patients receiving antiretroviral therapy. The mechanism and long-term consequences of these events are currently unknown. A causal relationship has not been established.

5.11 Patients with Hemophilia

There have been reports of increased bleeding, including spontaneous skin hematomas and hemarthrosis, in patients with hemophilia type A and B treated with protease inhibitors. In some patients additional factor VIII was given. In more than half of the reported cases, treatment with protease inhibitors was continued or reintroduced. A causal relationship between protease inhibitor therapy and these events has not been established.

5.12 Resistance/Cross-resistance

Varying degrees of cross-resistance among protease inhibitors have been observed. Continued administration of ritonavir 600 mg twice daily following loss of viral suppression may increase the likelihood of cross-resistance to other protease inhibitors *[see Microbiology (12.4)]*.

5.13 Laboratory Tests

Ritonavir has been shown to increase triglycerides, cholesterol, SGOT (AST), SGPT (ALT), GGT, CPK, and uric acid. Appropriate laboratory testing should be performed prior to initiating NORVIR therapy and at periodic intervals or if any clinical signs or symptoms occur during therapy.

6 ADVERSE REACTIONS

The following adverse reactions are discussed in greater detail in other sections of the labeling.

- Drug Interactions *[see Warnings and Precautions (5.1)]*
- Hepatotoxicity *[see Warnings and Precautions (5.3)]*
- Pancreatitis *[see Warnings and Precautions (5.4)]*
- Allergic Reactions/Hypersensitivity *[see Warnings and Precautions (5.5)]*

When co-administering NORVIR with other protease inhibitors, see the full prescribing information for that protease inhibitor including adverse reactions.

6.1 Adult Clinical Trial Experience

Because clinical trials are conducted under widely varying conditions, adverse reactions rates observed in the clinical

Table 3 *(cont.)*. Percentage of Patients with Treatment-emergent Adverse Events[1] of Moderate or Severe Intensity Occurring in ≥ 2% of Adult Patients Receiving NORVIR

Adverse Events	Study 245 Naive Patients[2]		Study 247 Advanced Patients[3]			Study 462 PI-Naive Patients[4]
	NORVIR + ZDV n = 116	NORVIR n = 117	ZDV n = 119	NORVIR n = 541	Placebo n = 545	NORVIR + Saquinavir n= 141
Respiratory						
Pharyngitis	0.9	2.6	0.0	0.4	0.4	1.4
Skin and Appendages						
Rash	0.9	0.0	0.8	3.5	1.5	0.7
Sweating	3.4	2.6	1.7	1.7	1.1	2.8
Special Senses						
Taste Perversion	17.2	11.1	8.4	7.0	2.2	5.0
Urogenital						
Nocturia	0.0	0.0	0.0	0.2	0.0	2.8

1 Includes those adverse events at least possibly related to study drug or of unknown relationship and excludes concurrent HIV conditions.
2 The median duration of treatment for patients randomized to regimens containing NORVIR in Study 245 was 9.1 months.
3 The median duration of treatment for patients randomized to regimens containing NORVIR in Study 247 was 9.4 months.
4 The median duration of treatment for patients in Study 462 was 48 weeks.

Table 4. Percentage of Adult Patients, by Study and Treatment Group, with Chemistry and Hematology Abnormalities Occurring in greater than 3% of Patients Receiving NORVIR

Variable	Limit	Study 245 Naive Patients		Study 247 Advanced Patients			Study 462 PI-Naive Patients
		NORVIR plus ZDV	NORVIR	ZDV	NORVIR	Placebo	NORVIR plus Saquinavir
Chemistry	**High**						
Cholesterol	> 240 mg/dL	30.7	44.8	9.3	36.5	8.0	65.2
CPK	> 1000 IU/L	9.6	12.1	11.0	9.1	6.3	9.9
GGT	> 300 IU/L	1.8	5.2	1.7	19.6	11.3	9.2
SGOT (AST)	> 180 IU/L	5.3	9.5	2.5	6.4	7.0	7.8
SGPT (ALT)	> 215 IU/L	5.3	7.8	3.4	8.5	4.4	9.2
Triglycerides	> 800 mg/dL	9.6	17.2	3.4	33.6	9.4	23.4
Triglycerides	> 1500 mg/dL	1.8	2.6	-	12.6	0.4	11.3
Triglycerides Fasting	> 1500 mg/dL	1.5	1.3	-	9.9	0.3	-
Uric Acid	> 12 mg/dL	-	-	-	3.8	0.2	1.4
Hematology	**Low**						
Hematocrit	< 30%	2.6	-	0.8	17.3	22.0	0.7
Hemoglobin	< 8.0 g/dL	0.9	-	-	3.8	3.9	-
Neutrophils	$\leq 0.5 \times 10^9$/L	-	-	-	6.0	8.3	-
RBC	$< 3.0 \times 10^{12}$/L	1.8	-	5.9	18.6	24.4	-
WBC	$< 2.5 \times 10^9$/L	-	0.9	6.8	36.9	59.4	3.5

- Indicates no events reported.

trials of a drug cannot be directly compared to rates in the clinical trials of another drug and may not reflect the rates observed in practice.

The safety of NORVIR alone and in combination with nucleoside reverse transcriptase inhibitors was studied in 1270 adult patients. Table 3 lists treatment-emergent adverse events (at least possibly related and of at least moderate intensity) that occurred in 2% or greater of adult patients receiving NORVIR alone or in combination with nucleoside reverse transcriptase inhibitors in Study 245 or Study 247 and in combination with saquinavir in study 462.

In that study, 141 protease inhibitor-naive, HIV-infected patients with mean baseline CD_4 of 300 cells/μL were randomized to one of four regimens of NORVIR + saquinavir, including NORVIR 400 mg twice-daily + saquinavir 400 mg twice-daily. Overall the most frequently reported clinical adverse events, other than asthenia, among adult patients receiving NORVIR were gastrointestinal and neurological disturbances including nausea, diarrhea, vomiting, anorexia, abdominal pain, taste perversion, and circumoral and peripheral paresthesias. Similar adverse event profiles were reported in adult patients receiving ritonavir in other trials.

[See table 3 on previous page and above]

Adverse events occurring in less than 2% of adult patients receiving NORVIR in all phase II/phase III studies and considered at least possibly related or of unknown relationship to treatment and of at least moderate intensity are listed below by body system.

Body as a Whole
Abdomen enlarged, accidental injury, allergic reaction, back pain, cachexia, chest pain, chills, facial edema, facial pain, flu syndrome, hormone level altered, hypothermia, kidney pain, neck pain, neck rigidity, pelvic pain, photosensitivity reaction, and substernal chest pain.

Cardiovascular System
Cardiovascular disorder, cerebral ischemia, cerebral venous thrombosis, hypertension, hypotension, migraine, myocardial infarct, palpitation, peripheral vascular disorder, phlebitis, postural hypotension, tachycardia and vasospasm.

Digestive System
Abnormal stools, bloody diarrhea, cheilitis, cholestatic jaundice, colitis, dry mouth, dysphagia, eructation, esophageal ulcer, esophagitis, gastritis, gastroenteritis, gastrointestinal disorder, gastrointestinal hemorrhage, gingivitis, hepatic coma, hepatitis, hepatomegaly, hepatosplenomegaly, ileus, liver damage, melena, mouth ulcer, pancreatitis, pseudomembranous colitis, rectal disorder, rectal hemorrhage, sialadenitis, stomatitis, tenesmus, thirst, tongue edema, and ulcerative colitis.

Endocrine System
Adrenal cortex insufficiency and diabetes mellitus.

Hemic and Lymphatic System
Acute myeloblastic leukemia, anemia, ecchymosis, leukopenia, lymphadenopathy, lymphocytosis, myeloproliferative disorder, and thrombocytopenia.

Metabolic and Nutritional Disorders
Albuminuria, alcohol intolerance, avitaminosis, BUN increased, dehydration, edema, enzymatic abnormality, glycosuria, gout, hypercholesteremia, peripheral edema, and xanthomatosis.

Musculoskeletal System
Arthritis, arthrosis, bone disorder, bone pain, extraocular palsy, joint disorder, leg cramps, muscle cramps, muscle weakness, myositis, and twitching.

Nervous System
Abnormal dreams, abnormal gait, agitation, amnesia, aphasia, ataxia, coma, convulsion, dementia, depersonalization, diplopia, emotional lability, euphoria, grand mal convulsion, hallucinations, hyperesthesia, hyperkinesia, hypesthesia, incoordination, libido decreased, manic reaction, nervousness, neuralgia, neuropathy, paralysis, peripheral neuropathic pain, peripheral neuropathy, peripheral sensory neuropathy, personality disorder, sleep disorder, speech disorder, stupor, subdural hematoma, tremor, urinary retention, vertigo, and vestibular disorder.

Respiratory System
Asthma, bronchitis, dyspnea, epistaxis, hiccup, hypoventilation, increased cough, interstitial pneumonia, larynx edema, lung disorder, rhinitis, and sinusitis.

Skin and Appendages
Acne, contact dermatitis, dry skin, eczema, erythema multiforme, exfoliative dermatitis, folliculitis, fungal dermatitis, furunculosis, maculopapular rash, molluscum contagiosum, onychomycosis, pruritus, psoriasis, pustular rash, seborrhea, skin discoloration, skin disorder, skin hypertrophy, skin melanoma, urticaria, and vesiculobullous rash.

Special Senses
Abnormal electro-oculogram, abnormal electroretinogram, abnormal vision, amblyopia/blurred vision, blepharitis, conjunctivitis, ear pain, eye disorder, eye pain, hearing impairment, increased cerumen, iritis, parosmia, photophobia, taste loss, tinnitus, uveitis, visual field defect, and vitreous disorder.

Urogenital System
Acute kidney failure, breast pain, cystitis, dysuria, hematuria, impotence, kidney calculus, kidney failure, kidney function abnormal, kidney pain, menorrhagia, penis disorder, polyuria, urethritis, urinary frequency, urinary tract infection, and vaginitis.

Laboratory Abnormalities
Table 4 shows the percentage of adult patients who developed marked laboratory abnormalities.

[See table 4 above]

6.2 Pediatric Clinical Trial Experience

NORVIR has been studied in 265 pediatric patients greater than 1 month to 21 years of age. The adverse event profile observed during pediatric clinical trials was similar to that for adult patients.

Information on the AbbVie, Inc. products listed on these pages is from the prescribing information in use as of July 31, 2013. For more information, please visit rxabbvie.com or call 1-800-633-9110.

Table 5. Established and Other Potentially Significant Drug Interactions

Concomitant Drug Class: Drug Name	Effect on Concentration of Ritonavir or Concomitant Drug	Clinical Comment
		HIV-Antiviral Agents
HIV Protease Inhibitor: atazanavir	When co-administered with reduced doses of atazanavir and ritonavir ↑ atazanavir (↑ AUC, ↑ C_{max}, ↑ C_{min})	Atazanavir plasma concentrations achieved with atazanavir 300 mg once daily and ritonavir 100 mg once daily are higher than those achieved with atazanavir 400 mg once daily. See the complete prescribing information for Reyataz® (atazanavir) for details on co-administration of atazanavir 300 mg once daily with ritonavir 100 mg once daily.
HIV Protease Inhibitor: darunavir	When co-administered with reduced doses of ritonavir ↑ darunavir (↑ AUC, ↑ C_{max}, ↑ C_{min})	See the complete prescribing information for Prezista® (darunavir) for details on co-administration of darunavir 600 mg twice daily with ritonavir 100 mg twice daily or darunavir 800 mg once daily with ritonavir 100 mg once daily.
HIV Protease Inhibitor: fosamprenavir	When co-administered with reduced doses of ritonavir ↑ amprenavir (↑ AUC, ↑ C_{max}, ↑ C_{min})	See the complete prescribing information for Lexiva® (fosamprenavir) for details on co-administration of fosamprenavir 700 mg twice daily with ritonavir 100 mg twice daily, fosamprenavir 1400 mg once daily with ritonavir 200 mg once daily or fosamprenavir 1400 mg once daily with ritonavir 100 mg once daily.
HIV Protease Inhibitor: indinavir	When co-administered with reduced doses of indinavir and ritonavir ↑ indinavir (↔ AUC, ↓ C_{max}, ↑ C_{min})	Alterations in concentrations are noted when reduced doses of indinavir are co-administered with NORVIR. Appropriate doses for this combination, with respect to efficacy and safety, have not been established.
HIV Protease Inhibitor: saquinavir	When co-administered with reduced doses of ritonavir ↑ saquinavir (↑ AUC, ↑ C_{max}, ↑ C_{min})	See the complete prescribing information for Invirase® (saquinavir) for details on co-administration of saquinavir 1000 mg twice daily with ritonavir 100 mg twice daily. Saquinavir/ritonavir should not be given together with rifampin, due to the risk of severe hepatotoxicity (presenting as increased hepatic transaminases) if the three drugs are given together.
HIV Protease Inhibitor: tipranavir	When co-administered with reduced doses of ritonavir ↑ tipranavir (↑ AUC, ↑ C_{max}, ↑ C_{min})	See the complete prescribing information for Aptivus® (tipranavir) for details on co-administration of tipranavir 500 mg twice daily with ritonavir 200 mg twice daily. There have been reports of clinical hepatitis and hepatic decompensation including some fatalities. All patients should be followed closely with clinical and laboratory monitoring, especially those with chronic hepatitis B or C co-infection, as these patients have an increased risk of hepatotoxicity. Liver function tests should be performed prior to initiating therapy with tipranavir/ritonavir, and frequently throughout the duration of treatment.
Non-Nucleoside Reverse Transcriptase Inhibitor: delavirdine	↑ ritonavir (↑AUC, ↑C_{max}, ↑ C_{min})	Appropriate doses of this combination with respect to safety and efficacy have not been established.
HIV CCR5 – antagonist: maraviroc	↑ maraviroc	Concurrent administration of maraviroc with ritonavir will increase plasma levels of maraviroc. For specific dosage adjustment recommendations, please refer to the complete prescribing information for Selzentry® (maraviroc).
Integrase Inhibitor: Raltegravir	↓ raltegravir	The effects of ritonavir on raltegravir with ritonavir dosage regimens greater than 100 mg twice daily have not been evaluated, however raltegravir concentrations may be decreased with ritonavir coadministration.
		Other Agents
Analgesics, Narcotic: tramadol, propoxyphene		A dose decrease may be needed for these drugs when co-administered with ritonavir.
Anesthetic: meperidine	↓ meperidine/ ↑ normeperidine (metabolite)	Dosage increase and long-term use of meperidine with ritonavir are not recommended due to the increased concentrations of the metabolite normeperidine which has both analgesic activity and CNS stimulant activity (e.g., seizures).
Antialcoholics: disulfiram/ metronidazole		Ritonavir formulations contain alcohol, which can produce disulfiram-like reactions when co-administered with disulfiram or other drugs that produce this reaction (e.g., metronidazole).
Antiarrhythmics: disopyramide, lidocaine, mexiletine	↑ antiarrhythmics	Caution is warranted and therapeutic concentration monitoring is recommended for antiarrhythmics when co-administered with ritonavir, if available.

(Table continued on next page)

Vomiting, diarrhea, and skin rash/allergy were the only drug-related clinical adverse events of moderate to severe intensity observed in greater than or equal to 2% of pediatric patients enrolled in NORVIR clinical trials.

Laboratory Abnormalities

The following Grade 3-4 laboratory abnormalities occurred in greater than 3% of pediatric patients who received treatment with NORVIR either alone or in combination with reverse transcriptase inhibitors: neutropenia (9%), hyperamylasemia (7%), thrombocytopenia (5%), anemia (4%), and elevated AST (3%).

6.3 Postmarketing Experience

The following adverse events (not previously mentioned in the labeling) have been reported during post-marketing use of NORVIR. Because these reactions are reported voluntarily from a population of unknown size, it is not possible to reliably estimate their frequency or establish a causal relationship to NORVIR exposure.

Body as a Whole

Dehydration, usually associated with gastrointestinal symptoms, and sometimes resulting in hypotension, syncope, or renal insufficiency has been reported. Syncope, orthostatic hypotension, and renal insufficiency have also been reported without known dehydration.

Co-administration of ritonavir with ergotamine or dihydroergotamine has been associated with acute ergot toxicity characterized by vasospasm and ischemia of the extremities and other tissues including the central nervous system.

Cardiovascular System

First-degree AV block, second-degree AV block, third-degree AV block, right bundle branch block have been reported *[see Warnings and Precautions (5.6)]*.

Cardiac and neurologic events have been reported when ritonavir has been co-administered with disopyramide, mexiletine, nefazodone, fluoxetine, and beta blockers. The possibility of drug interaction cannot be excluded.

Endocrine System

Cushing's syndrome and adrenal suppression have been reported when ritonavir has been co-administered with fluticasone propionate or budesonide.

Nervous System

There have been postmarketing reports of seizure. Also, see Cardiovascular System.

Skin and subcutaneous tissue disorders

Toxic epidermal necrolysis (TEN) has been reported.

7 DRUG INTERACTIONS

See also Contraindications (4), Warnings and Precautions (5.1), and *Clinical Pharmacology (12.3)*

When co-administering NORVIR with other protease inhibitors (atazanavir, darunavir, fosamprenavir, saquinavir, and tipranavir), see the full prescribing information for that protease inhibitor including important information for drug interactions.

7.1 Potential for NORVIR to Affect Other Drugs

Ritonavir has been found to be an inhibitor of cytochrome P450 3A (CYP3A) and may increase plasma concentrations of agents that are primarily metabolized by CYP3A. Agents that are extensively metabolized by CYP3A and have high first pass metabolism appear to be the most susceptible to large increases in AUC (greater than 3-fold) when co-administered with ritonavir. Thus, co-administration of NORVIR with drugs highly dependent on CYP3A for clearance and for which elevated plasma concentrations are associated with serious and/or life-threatening events is contraindicated. Co-administration with other CYP3A substrates may require a dose adjustment or additional monitoring as shown in Table 5.

Ritonavir also inhibits CYP2D6 to a lesser extent. Co-administration of substrates of CYP2D6 with ritonavir could result in increases (up to 2-fold) in the AUC of the other agent, possibly requiring a proportional dosage reduction. Ritonavir also appears to induce CYP3A, CYP1A2, CYP2C9, CYP2C19, and CYP2B6 as well as other enzymes, including glucuronosyl transferase.

7.2 Established and Other Potentially Significant Drug Interactions

Table 5 provides a list of established or potentially clinically significant drug interactions. Alteration in dose or regimen may be recommended based on drug interaction studies or predicted interaction *[see Clinical Pharmacology (12.3) for magnitude of interaction]*.

[See table 5 above and on pages 555 through 558]

8 USE IN SPECIFIC POPULATIONS

When co-administering NORVIR with other protease inhibitors, see the full prescribing information for the co-administered protease inhibitor including important information for use in special populations.

8.1 Pregnancy

Pregnancy Category B

Antiretroviral Pregnancy Registry: To monitor maternal-fetal outcomes of pregnant women exposed to NORVIR, an Antiretroviral Pregnancy Registry has been established. Physicians are encouraged to register patients by calling 1–800–258–4263.

Human Data:

There are no adequate and well-controlled studies in pregnant women. NORVIR should be used during pregnancy only if the potential benefit justifies the potential risk to the fetus.

Table 5 *(cont.)*. Established and Other Potentially Significant Drug Interactions

Concomitant Drug Class: Drug Name	Effect on Concentration of Ritonavir or Concomitant Drug	Clinical Comment
Anticancer Agents: dasatinib, nilotinib, vincristine, vinblastine	↑ anticancer agents	Concentrations of these drugs may be increased when co-administered with ritonavir resulting in the potential for increased adverse events usually associated with these anticancer agents. For vincristine and vinblastine, consideration should be given to temporarily withholding the ritonavir containing antiretroviral regimen in patients who develop significant hematologic or gastrointestinal side effects when ritonavir is administered concurrently with vincristine or vinblastine. Clinicians should be aware that if the ritonavir containing regimen is withheld for a prolonged period, consideration should be given to altering the regimen to not include a CYP3A or P-gp inhibitor in order to control HIV-1 viral load. A decrease in the dosage or an adjustment of the dosing interval of nilotinib and dasatinib may be necessary for patients requiring co-administration with strong CYP3A inhibitors such as NORVIR. Please refer to the nilotinib and dasatinib prescribing information for dosing instructions.
Anticoagulant: warfarin	↓ R-warfarin ↓↑ S-warfarin	Initial frequent monitoring of the INR during ritonavir and warfarin co-administration is indicated.
Anticoagulant: rivaroxaban	↑ rivaroxaban	Avoid concomitant use of rivaroxaban and ritonavir. Co-administration of ritonavir and rivaroxaban is expected to result in increased exposure of rivaroxaban which may lead to risk of increased bleeding.
Anticonvulsants: carbamazepine, clonazepam, ethosuximide	↑ anticonvulsants	Use with caution. A dose decrease may be needed for these drugs when co-administered with ritonavir and therapeutic concentration monitoring is recommended for these anticonvulsants, if available.
Anticonvulsants: divalproex, lamotrigine, phenytoin	↓ anticonvulsants	Use with caution. A dose increase may be needed for these drugs when co-administered with ritonavir and therapeutic concentration monitoring is recommended for these anticonvulsants, if available.
Antidepressants: nefazodone, selective serotonin reuptake inhibitors (SSRIs): e.g. fluoxetine, paroxetine, tricyclics: e.g. amitriptyline, nortriptyline	↑ antidepressants	A dose decrease may be needed for these drugs when co-administered with ritonavir.
Antidepressant: bupropion	↓ bupropion ↓ active metabolite, hydroxybupropion	Concurrent administration of bupropion with ritonavir may decrease plasma levels of both bupropion and its active metabolite (hydroxybupropion). Patients receiving ritonavir and bupropion concurrently should be monitored for an adequate clinical response to bupropion.
Antidepressant: desipramine	↑ desipramine	Dosage reduction and concentration monitoring of desipramine is recommended.
Antidepressant: trazodone	↑ trazodone	Concomitant use of trazodone and NORVIR increases plasma concentrations of trazodone. Adverse events of nausea, dizziness, hypotension and syncope have been observed following co-administration of trazodone and NORVIR. If trazodone is used with a CYP3A4 inhibitor such as ritonavir, the combination should be used with caution and a lower dose of trazodone should be considered.
Antiemetic: dronabinol	↑ dronabinol	A dose decrease of dronabinol may be needed when co-administered with ritonavir.
Antifungal: ketoconazole itraconazole voriconazole	↑ ketoconazole ↑ itraconazole ↓ voriconazole	High doses of ketoconazole or itraconazole (greater than 200 mg per day) are not recommended. Co-administration of voriconazole and ritonavir doses of 400 mg every 12 hours or greater is contraindicated. Co-administration of voriconazole and ritonavir 100 mg should be avoided, unless an assessment of the benefit/risk to the patient justifies the use of voriconazole.

(Table continued on next page)

Antiretroviral Pregnancy Registry:
As of January 2012, the Antiretroviral Pregnancy Registry (APR) has received prospective reports of 3860 exposures to ritonavir containing regimens (1567 exposed in the first trimester and 2293 exposed in the second and third trimester). Birth defects occurred in 35 of the 1567 (2.2%) live births (first trimester exposure) and 59 of the 2293 (2.6%) live births (second/third trimester exposure).

Among pregnant women in the U.S. reference population, the background rate of birth defects is 2.7%. There was no association between ritonavir and overall birth defects observed in the APR.

Animal Data

No treatment related malformations were observed when ritonavir was administered to pregnant rats or rabbits. Developmental toxicity observed in rats (early resorptions, decreased fetal body weight and ossification delays and developmental variations) occurred at a maternally toxic dosage at an exposure equivalent to approximately 30% of that achieved with the proposed therapeutic dose. A slight increase in the incidence of cryptorchidism was also noted in rats at an exposure approximately 22% of that achieved with the proposed therapeutic dose.

Developmental toxicity observed in rabbits (resorptions, decreased litter size and decreased fetal weights) also occurred at a maternally toxic dosage equivalent to 1.8 times the proposed therapeutic dose based on a body surface area conversion factor.

8.3 Nursing Mothers

The Centers for Disease Control and Prevention recommend that HIV-infected mothers not breastfeed their infants to avoid risking postnatal transmission of HIV. It is not known whether ritonavir is secreted in human milk. Because of both the potential for HIV transmission and the potential for serious adverse reactions in nursing infants, mothers should be instructed not to breastfeed if they are receiving NORVIR.

8.4 Pediatric Use

In HIV-infected patients age greater than 1 month to 21 years, the antiviral activity and adverse event profile seen during clinical trials and through postmarketing experience were similar to that for adult patients.

8.5 Geriatric Use

Clinical studies of NORVIR did not include sufficient numbers of subjects aged 65 and over to determine whether they respond differently from younger subjects. In general, dose selection for an elderly patient should be cautious, usually starting at the low end of the dosing range, reflecting the greater frequency of decreased hepatic, renal or cardiac function, and of concomitant disease or other drug therapy.

8.6 Hepatic Impairment

No dose adjustment of ritonavir is necessary for patients with either mild (Child-Pugh Class A) or moderate (Child-Pugh Class B) hepatic impairment. No pharmacokinetic or safety data are available regarding the use of ritonavir in subjects with severe hepatic impairment (Child-Pugh Class C), therefore, ritonavir is not recommended for use in patients with severe hepatic impairment *[see Warnings and Precautions (5.3), Clinical Pharmacology (12.3)]*.

10 OVERDOSAGE

10.1 Acute Overdosage - Human Overdose Experience

Human experience of acute overdose with NORVIR is limited. One patient in clinical trials took NORVIR 1500 mg per day for two days. The patient reported paresthesias which resolved after the dose was decreased. A postmarketing case of renal failure with eosinophilia has been reported with ritonavir overdose.

The approximate lethal dose was found to be greater than 20 times the related human dose in rats and 10 times the related human dose in mice.

10.2 Management of Overdosage

NORVIR oral solution contains 43.2% (v/v) alcohol and 26.57% (w/v) propylene glycol. Ingestion of the product over the recommended dose by a young child could result in significant toxicity and could potentially be lethal.

Treatment of overdose with NORVIR consists of general supportive measures including monitoring of vital signs and observation of the clinical status of the patient. There is no specific antidote for overdose with NORVIR. If indicated, elimination of unabsorbed drug should be achieved by gastric lavage; usual precautions should be observed to maintain the airway. Administration of activated charcoal may also be used to aid in removal of unabsorbed drug. Since ritonavir is extensively metabolized by the liver and is highly protein bound, dialysis is unlikely to be beneficial in significant removal of the drug. However, dialysis can remove both alcohol and propylene glycol in the case of overdose with ritonavir oral solution. A Certified Poison Control Center should be consulted for up-to-date information on the management of overdose with NORVIR.

11 DESCRIPTION

NORVIR (ritonavir) is an inhibitor of HIV protease with activity against the Human Immunodeficiency Virus (HIV).

Ritonavir is chemically designated as 10-Hydroxy-2-methyl-5-(1-methylethyl)-1- [2-(1-methylethyl)-4-thiazolyl]-3,6-dioxo-8,11-bis(phenylmethyl)-2,4,7,12- tetraazatridecan-13-oic acid, 5-thiazolylmethyl ester, [5S-(5R*,8R*,10R*,11R*)]. Its molecular formula is $C_{37}H_{48}N_6O_5S_2$, and its molecular weight is 720.95. Ritonavir has the following structural formula:

[See chemical structure in third column on next page]

Ritonavir is a white-to-light-tan powder. Ritonavir has a bitter metallic taste. It is freely soluble in methanol and ethanol, soluble in isopropanol and practically insoluble in water.

Information on the AbbVie, Inc. products listed on these pages is from the prescribing information in use as of July 31, 2013. For more information, please visit rxabbvie.com or call 1-800-633-9110.

Table 5 *(cont.)*. Established and Other Potentially Significant Drug Interactions

Concomitant Drug Class: Drug Name	Effect on Concentration of Ritonavir or Concomitant Drug	Clinical Comment
Anti-gout: colchicine	↑ colchicine	Patients with renal or hepatic impairment should not be given colchicine with ritonavir. Treatment of gout flares-co-administration of colchicine in patients on ritonavir: 0.6 mg (one tablet) for one dose, followed by 0.3 mg (half tablet) one hour later. Dose to be repeated no earlier than three days. Prophylaxis of gout flares-co-administration of colchicine in patients on ritonavir: If the original colchicine regimen was 0.6 mg twice a day, the regimen should be adjusted to 0.3 mg once a day. If the original colchicine regimen was 0.6 mg once a day, the regimen should be adjusted to 0.3 mg once every other day. Treatment of familial Mediterranean fever (FMF)-co-administration of colchicine in patients on ritonavir: Maximum daily dose of 0.6 mg (may be given as 0.3 mg twice a day).
Anti-infective: clarithromycin	↑ clarithromycin	For patients with renal impairment the following dosage adjustments should be considered: • For patients with CL_{CR} 30 to 60 mL per min the dose of clarithromycin should be reduced by 50%. • For patients with CL_{CR} less than 30 mL per min the dose of clarithromycin should be decreased by 75%. No dose adjustment for patients with normal renal function is necessary.
Antimycobacterial: rifabutin	↑ rifabutin and rifabutin metabolite	Dosage reduction of rifabutin by at least three-quarters of the usual dose of 300 mg per day is recommended (e.g., 150 mg every other day or three times a week). Further dosage reduction may be necessary.
Antimycobacterial: rifampin	↓ ritonavir	May lead to loss of virologic response. Alternate antimycobacterial agents such as rifabutin should be considered (see Antimycobacterial: rifabutin, for dose reduction recommendations).
Antiparasitic: atovaquone	↓ atovaquone	Clinical significance is unknown; however, increase in atovaquone dose may be needed.
Antiparasitic: quinine	↑ quinine	A dose decrease of quinine may be needed when co-administered with ritonavir.
β-Blockers: metoprolol, timolol	↑ Beta-Blockers	Caution is warranted and clinical monitoring of patients is recommended. A dose decrease may be needed for these drugs when co-administered with ritonavir.
Bronchodilator: theophylline	↓ theophylline	Increased dosage of theophylline may be required; therapeutic monitoring should be considered.
Calcium channel blockers: diltiazem, nifedipine, verapamil	↑ calcium channel blockers	Caution is warranted and clinical monitoring of patients is recommended. A dose decrease may be needed for these drugs when co-administered with ritonavir.
Digoxin	↑ digoxin	Concomitant administration of ritonavir with digoxin may increase digoxin levels. Caution should be exercised when co-administering ritonavir with digoxin, with appropriate monitoring of serum digoxin levels.
Endothelin receptor antagonists: bosentan	↑ bosentan	Co-administration of bosentan in patients on ritonavir: In patients who have been receiving ritonavir for at least 10 days, start bosentan at 62.5 mg once daily or every other day based upon individual tolerability. Co-administration of ritonavir in patients on bosentan: Discontinue use of bosentan at least 36 hours prior to initiation of ritonavir. After at least 10 days following the initiation of ritonavir, resume bosentan at 62.5 mg once daily or every other day based upon individual tolerability.
HMG-CoA Reductase Inhibitor: atorvastatin rosuvastatin	↑ atorvastatin ↑ rosuvastatin	Titrate atorvastatin and rosuvastatin dose carefully and use the lowest necessary dose. If NORVIR is used with another protease inhibitor, see the complete prescribing information for the concomitant protease inhibitor for details on co-administration with atorvastatin and rosuvastatin.
Immunosuppressants: cyclosporine, tacrolimus, sirolimus (rapamycin)	↑ immunosuppressants	Therapeutic concentration monitoring is recommended for immunosuppressant agents when co-administered with ritonavir.

(Table continued on next page)

NORVIR tablets are available for oral administration in a strength of 100 mg ritonavir with the following inactive ingredients: copovidone, anhydrous dibasic calcium phosphate, sorbitan monolaurate, colloidal silicon dioxide, and sodium stearyl fumarate. The following are the ingredients in the film coating: hypromellose, titanium dioxide, polyethylene glycol 400, hydroxypropyl cellulose, talc, polyethylene glycol 3350, colloidal silicon dioxide, and polysorbate 80.

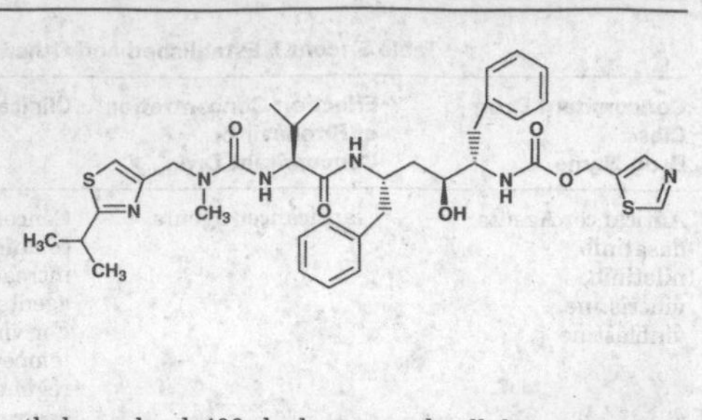

NORVIR oral solution is available for oral administration as 80 mg per mL of ritonavir in a peppermint and caramel flavored vehicle. Each 8-ounce bottle contains 19.2 grams of ritonavir. NORVIR oral solution also contains ethanol, water, polyoxyl 35 castor oil, propylene glycol, anhydrous citric acid to adjust pH, saccharin sodium, peppermint oil, creamy caramel flavoring, and FD&C Yellow No. 6.

12 CLINICAL PHARMACOLOGY

12.1 Mechanism of Action

Ritonavir is an antiviral drug *[see Microbiology (12.4)]*.

12.3 Pharmacokinetics

The pharmacokinetics of ritonavir have been studied in healthy volunteers and HIV-infected patients (CD_4 greater than or equal to 50 cells per µL). See Table 6 for ritonavir pharmacokinetic characteristics.

Absorption

The absolute bioavailability of ritonavir has not been determined. After a 600 mg dose of oral solution, peak concentrations of ritonavir were achieved approximately 2 hours and 4 hours after dosing under fasting and non-fasting (514 KCal; 9% fat, 12% protein, and 79% carbohydrate) conditions, respectively.

NORVIR tablets are not bioequivalent to NORVIR capsules. Under moderate fat conditions (857 kcal; 31% fat, 13% protein, 56% carbohydrates), when a single 100 mg NORVIR dose was administered as a tablet compared with a capsule, $AUC_{(0-\infty)}$ met equivalence criteria but mean C_{max} was increased by 26% (92.8% confidence intervals: ↑15 -↑39%). No information is available comparing NORVIR tablets to NORVIR capsules under fasting conditions.

Effect of Food on Oral Absorption

When the oral solution was given under non-fasting conditions, peak ritonavir concentrations decreased 23% and the extent of absorption decreased 7% relative to fasting conditions. Dilution of the oral solution, within one hour of administration, with 240 mL of chocolate milk, Advera® or Ensure® did not significantly affect the extent and rate of ritonavir absorption. Administration of a single 600 mg dose oral solution under non-fasting conditions yielded mean ± SD areas under the plasma concentration-time curve (AUCs) of 129.0 ± 39.3 mg•h per mL.

A food effect is observed for NORVIR tablets. Food decreased the bioavailability of the ritonavir tablets when a single 100 mg dose of NORVIR was administered. Under high fat conditions (907 kcal; 52% fat, 15% protein, 33% carbohydrates), a 23% decrease in mean AUC(0-∞) [90% confidence intervals: ↓30%-↓15%], and a 23% decrease in mean C_{max} [90% confidence intervals: ↓34%-↓11%]) was observed relative to fasting conditions. Under moderate fat conditions, a 21% decrease in mean AUC(0-∞) [90% confidence intervals: ↓28%-↓13%], and a 22% decrease in mean C_{max} [90% confidence intervals: ↓33%-↓9%]) was observed relative to fasting conditions.

However, the type of meal administered did not change ritonavir tablet bioavailability when high fat was compared to moderate fat meals.

Metabolism

Nearly all of the plasma radioactivity after a single oral 600 mg dose of ^{14}C-ritonavir oral solution (n = 5) was attributed to unchanged ritonavir. Five ritonavir metabolites have been identified in human urine and feces. The isopropylthiazole oxidation metabolite (M-2) is the major metabolite and has antiviral activity similar to that of parent drug; however, the concentrations of this metabolite in plasma are low. *In vitro* studies utilizing human liver microsomes have demonstrated that cytochrome P450 3A (CYP3A) is the major isoform involved in ritonavir metabolism, although CYP2D6 also contributes to the formation of M–2.

Elimination

In a study of five subjects receiving a 600 mg dose of ^{14}C-ritonavir oral solution, 11.3 ± 2.8% of the dose was excreted into the urine, with 3.5 ± 1.8% of the dose excreted as un-

Table 5 (cont.). Established and Other Potentially Significant Drug Interactions

Concomitant Drug Class: Drug Name	Effect on Concentration of Ritonavir or Concomitant Drug	Clinical Comment
Inhaled or Intranasal Steroid e.g.: Fluticasone Budesonide	↑ glucocorticoids	Concomitant use of ritonavir and fluticasone or other glucocorticoids that are metabolized by CYP3A is not recommended unless the potential benefit of treatment outweighs the risk of systemic corticosteroid effects. Concomitant use may result in increased steroid concentrations and reduced serum cortisol concentrations. Systemic corticosteroid effects including Cushing's syndrome and adrenal suppression have been reported during postmarketing use in patients when ritonavir has been coadministered with fluticasone propionate or budesonide.
Long-acting beta-adrenoceptor agonist: salmeterol	↑ salmeterol	Concurrent administration of salmeterol and ritonavir is not recommended. The combination may result in increased risk of cardiovascular adverse events associated with salmeterol, including QT prolongation, palpitations and sinus tachycardia.
Narcotic Analgesic: methadone fentanyl	↓ methadone ↑ fentanyl	Dosage increase of methadone may be considered. Concentrations of fentanyl are expected to increase. Careful monitoring of therapeutic and adverse effects (including potentially fatal respiratory depression) is recommended when fentanyl is concomitantly administered with NORVIR.
Neuroleptics: perphenazine, risperidone, thioridazine	↑ neuroleptics	A dose decrease may be needed for these drugs when co-administered with ritonavir.
Oral Contraceptives or Patch Contraceptives: ethinyl estradiol	↓ ethinyl estradiol	Alternate methods of contraception should be considered.
PDE5 Inhibitors: avanafil sildenafil, tadalafil, vardenafil	↑ avanafil ↑ sildenafil ↑ tadalafil ↑ vardenafil	Do not use ritonavir with avanafil because a safe and effective avanafil dosage regimen has not been established. Particular caution should be used when prescribing sildenafil, tadalafil or vardenafil in patients receiving ritonavir. Co-administration of ritonavir with these drugs is expected to substantially increase their concentrations and may result in an increase in PDE5 inhibitor associated adverse events, including hypotension, syncope, visual changes, and prolonged erection. Use of PDE5 inhibitors for pulmonary arterial hypertension (PAH): Sildenafil (Revatio®) is contraindicated when used for the treatment of pulmonary arterial hypertension (PAH) because a safe and effective dose has not been established when used with ritonavir *[see Contraindications (4)]*. The following dose adjustments are recommended for use of tadalafil (Adcirca™) with ritonavir: Co-administration of ADCIRCA in patients on ritonavir: In patients receiving ritonavir for at least one week, start ADCIRCA at 20 mg once daily. Increase to 40 mg once daily based upon individual tolerability. Co-administration of ritonavir in patients on ADCIRCA: Avoid use of ADCIRCA during the initiation of ritonavir. Stop ADCIRCA at least 24 hours prior to starting ritonavir. After at least one week following the initiation of ritonavir, resume ADCIRCA at 20 mg once daily. Increase to 40 mg once daily based upon individual tolerability. Use of PDE5 inhibitors for the treatment of erectile dysfunction: It is recommended not to exceed the following doses: • Sildenafil: 25 mg every 48 hours • Tadalafil: 10 mg every 72 hours • Vardenafil: 2.5 mg every 72 hours Use with increased monitoring for adverse events.
Sedative/hypnotics: buspirone, clorazepate, diazepam, estazolam, flurazepam, zolpidem	↑ sedative/hypnotics	A dose decrease may be needed for these drugs when co-administered with ritonavir.
Sedative/hypnotics: Parenteral midazolam	↑ midazolam	Co-administration of oral midazolam with NORVIR is CONTRAINDICATED. Concomitant use of parenteral midazolam with NORVIR may increase plasma concentrations of midazolam. Co-administration should be done in a setting which ensures close clinical monitoring and appropriate medical management in case of respiratory depression and/or prolonged sedation. Dosage reduction for midazolam should be considered, especially if more than a single dose of midazolam is administered.

(Table continued on next page)

changed parent drug. In that study, 86.4 ± 2.9% of the dose was excreted in the feces with 33.8 ± 10.8% of the dose excreted as unchanged parent drug. Upon multiple dosing, ritonavir accumulation is less than predicted from a single dose possibly due to a time and dose-related increase in clearance.

Table 6. Ritonavir Pharmacokinetic Characteristics

Parameter	N	Values (Mean ± SD)
$V_\beta/F^‡$	91	0.41 ± 0.25 L/kg
$t_{1/2}$		3 - 5 h
CL/F SS†	10	8.8 ± 3.2 L/h
CL/F‡	91	4.6 ± 1.6 L/h
CL_R	62	< 0.1 L/h
RBC/Plasma Ratio		0.14
Percent Bound*		98 to 99%

† SS = steady state; patients taking ritonavir 600 mg q12h.
‡ Single ritonavir 600 mg dose.
* Primarily bound to human serum albumin and alpha-1 acid glycoprotein over the ritonavir concentration range of 0.01 to 30 μg/mL.

Effects on Electrocardiogram
QTcF interval was evaluated in a randomized, placebo and active (moxifloxacin 400 mg once-daily) controlled crossover study in 45 healthy adults, with 10 measurements over 12 hours on Day 3. The maximum mean (95% upper confidence bound) time-matched difference in QTcF from placebo after baseline correction was 5.5 (7.6) milliseconds (msec) for 400 mg twice-daily ritonavir. Ritonavir 400 mg twice daily resulted in Day 3 ritonavir exposure that was approximately 1.5 fold higher than observed with ritonavir 600 mg twice-daily dose at steady state.

PR interval prolongation was also noted in subjects receiving ritonavir in the same study on Day 3. The maximum mean (95% confidence interval) difference from placebo in the PR interval after baseline correction was 22 (25) msec for 400 mg twice-daily ritonavir *[see Warnings and Precautions (5.6)]*.

Special Populations

Gender, Race and Age

No age-related pharmacokinetic differences have been observed in adult patients (18 to 63 years). Ritonavir pharmacokinetics have not been studied in older patients.

A study of ritonavir pharmacokinetics in healthy males and females showed no statistically significant differences in the pharmacokinetics of ritonavir. Pharmacokinetic differences due to race have not been identified.

Pediatric Patients

Steady-state pharmacokinetics were evaluated in 37 HIV-infected patients ages 2 to 14 years receiving doses ranging from 250 mg per m^2 twice-daily to 400 mg per m^2 twice-daily in PACTG Study 310, and in 41 HIV-infected patients ages 1 month to 2 years at doses of 350 and 450 mg per m^2 twice-daily in PACTG Study 345. Across dose groups, ritonavir steady-state oral clearance ($CL/F/m^2$) was approximately 1.5 to 1.7 times faster in pediatric patients than in adult subjects. Ritonavir concentrations obtained after 350 to 400 mg per m^2 twice-daily in pediatric patients greater than 2 years were comparable to those obtained in adults receiving 600 mg (approximately 330 mg per m^2) twice-daily. The following observations were seen regarding ritonavir concentrations after administration with 350 or 450 mg per m^2 twice-daily in children less than 2 years of age. Higher ritonavir exposures were not evident with 450 mg per m^2 twice-daily compared to the 350 mg per m^2 twice-daily. Ritonavir trough concentrations were somewhat lower than those obtained in adults receiving 600 mg twice-daily. The area under the ritonavir plasma concentration time curve and trough concentrations obtained after administration with 350 or 450 mg per m^2 twice-daily in children less than 2 years were approximately 16% and 60% lower, respectively, than that obtained in adults receiving 600 mg twice daily.

Renal Impairment

Ritonavir pharmacokinetics have not been studied in patients with renal impairment, however, since renal clearance is negligible, a decrease in total body clearance is not expected in patients with renal impairment.

Hepatic Impairment

Dose-normalized steady-state ritonavir concentrations in subjects with mild hepatic impairment (400 mg twice-daily, n = 6) were similar to those in control subjects dosed with 500 mg twice-daily. Dose-normalized steady-state ritonavir

Information on the AbbVie, Inc. products listed on these pages is from the prescribing information in use as of July 31, 2013. For more information, please visit rxabbvie.com or call 1-800-633-9110.

Table 5 *(cont.)*. Established and Other Potentially Significant Drug Interactions

Concomitant Drug Class: Drug Name	Effect on Concentration of Ritonavir or Concomitant Drug	Clinical Comment
Steroids (systemic) e.g.: budesonide, dexamethasone, prednisone	↑ glucocorticoids	Concomitant use of glucocorticoids that are metabolized by CYP3A is not recommended unless the potential benefit of treatment outweighs the risk of systemic corticosteroid effects. Concomitant use may result in increased steroid concentrations and reduced serum cortisol concentrations. This may increase the risk for development of systemic corticosteroid effects including Cushing's syndrome and adrenal suppression.
Stimulant: methamphetamine	↑ methamphetamine	Use with caution. A dose decrease of methamphetamine may be needed when co-administered with ritonavir.

Table 7. Drug Interactions - Pharmacokinetic Parameters for Ritonavir in the Presence of the Co-administered Drug

Co-administered Drug	Dose of Co-administered Drug (mg)	Dose of NORVIR (mg)	N	AUC % (95% CI)	C_{max} (95% CI)	C_{min} (95% CI)
Clarithromycin	500 q12h, 4 d	200 q8h, 4 d	22	↑ 12% (2, 23%)	↑ 15% (2, 28%)	↑ 14% (-3, 36%)
Didanosine	200 q12h, 4 d	600 q12h, 4 d	12	↔	↔	↔
Fluconazole	400 single dose, day 1; 200 daily, 4 d	200 q6h, 4 d	8	↑ 12% (5, 20%)	↑ 15% (7, 22%)	↑ 14% (0, 26%)
Fluoxetine	30 q12h, 8 d	600 single dose, 1 d	16	↑ 19% (7, 34%)	↔	ND
Ketoconazole	200 daily, 7 d	500 q12h, 10 d	12	↑ 18% (-3, 52%)	↑ 10% (-11, 36%)	ND
Rifampin	600 or 300 daily, 10 d	500 q12h, 20 d	7, 9*	↓ 35% (7, 55%)	↓ 25% (-5, 46%)	↓ 49% (-14, 91%)
Voriconazole	400 q12h, 1 d; then 200 q12h, 8 d	400 q12h, 9 d		↔	↔	ND
Zidovudine	200 q8h, 4 d	300 q6h, 4 d	10	↔	↔	↔

exposures in subjects with moderate hepatic impairment (400 mg twice-daily, n= 6) were about 40% lower than those in subjects with normal hepatic function (500 mg twice-daily, n = 6). Protein binding of ritonavir was not statistically significantly affected by mild or moderately impaired hepatic function. No dose adjustment is recommended in patients with mild or moderate hepatic impairment. However, health care providers should be aware of the potential for lower ritonavir concentrations in patients with moderate hepatic impairment and should monitor patient response carefully. Ritonavir has not been studied in patients with severe hepatic impairment.

Drug Interactions

[see also Contraindications (4), Warnings and Precautions (5.1), and Drug Interactions (7)]

Table 7 and Table 8 summarize the effects on AUC and C_{max}, with 95% confidence intervals (95% CI), of co-administration of ritonavir with a variety of drugs. For information about clinical recommendations see Table 5 in *Drug Interactions (7)*.

[See table 7 above]

[See table 8 at top of pages 559 and 560]

12.4 Microbiology

Mechanism of Action

Ritonavir is a peptidomimetic inhibitor of the HIV-1 protease. Inhibition of HIV protease renders the enzyme incapable of processing the *gag-pol* polyprotein precursor which leads to production of non-infectious immature HIV particles.

Antiviral Activity in Cell Culture

The activity of ritonavir was assessed in acutely infected lymphoblastoid cell lines and in peripheral blood lymphocytes. The concentration of drug that inhibits 50% (EC_{50}) value of viral replication ranged from 3.8 to 153 nM depending upon the HIV-1 isolate and the cells employed. The average EC_{50} value for low passage clinical isolates was 22 nM (n = 13). In MT_4 cells, ritonavir demonstrated additive effects against HIV-1 in combination with either didanosine (ddI) or zidovudine (ZDV). Studies which measured cytotoxicity of ritonavir on several cell lines showed that greater than 20 μM was required to inhibit cellular growth by 50% resulting in a cell culture therapeutic index of at least 1000.

Resistance

HIV-1 isolates with reduced susceptibility to ritonavir have been selected in cell culture. Genotypic analysis of these isolates showed mutations in the HIV-1 protease gene leading to amino acid substitutions I84V, V82F, A71V, and M46I. Phenotypic (n = 18) and genotypic (n = 48) changes in HIV-1 isolates from selected patients treated with ritonavir were monitored in phase I/II trials over a period of 3 to 32 weeks. Substitutions associated with the HIV–1 viral protease in isolates obtained from 43 patients appeared to occur in a stepwise and ordered fashion at positions V82A/F/T/S, I54V, A71V/T, and I36L, followed by combinations of substitutions at an additional 5 specific amino acid positions (M46I/L, K20R, I84V, L33F and L90M). Of 18 patients for whom both phenotypic and genotypic analysis were performed on free virus isolated from plasma, 12 showed reduced susceptibility to ritonavir in cell culture. All 18 patients possessed one or more substitutions in the viral protease gene. The V82A/F substitution appeared to be necessary but not sufficient to confer phenotypic resistance. Phenotypic resistance was defined as a greater than or equal to 5-fold decrease in viral sensitivity in cell culture from baseline.

Cross-Resistance to Other Antiretrovirals

Among protease inhibitors variable cross-resistance has been recognized. Serial HIV-1 isolates obtained from six patients during ritonavir therapy showed a decrease in ritonavir susceptibility in cell culture but did not demonstrate a concordant decrease in susceptibility to saquinavir in cell culture when compared to matched baseline isolates. However, isolates from two of these patients demonstrated decreased susceptibility to indinavir in cell culture (8-fold). Isolates from 5 patients were also tested for cross-resistance to amprenavir and nelfinavir; isolates from 3 patients had a decrease in susceptibility to nelfinavir (6- to 14-fold), and none to amprenavir. Cross-resistance between ritonavir and reverse transcriptase inhibitors is unlikely because of the different enzyme targets involved. One ZDV-resistant HIV-1 isolate tested in cell culture retained full susceptibility to ritonavir.

13 NONCLINICAL TOXICOLOGY

13.1 Carcinogenesis, Mutagenesis, Impairment of Fertility

Carcinogenesis

Carcinogenicity studies in mice and rats have been carried out on ritonavir. In male mice, at levels of 50, 100 or 200 mg per kg per day, there was a dose dependent increase in the incidence of both adenomas and combined adenomas and carcinomas in the liver. Based on AUC measurements, the exposure at the high dose was approximately 0.3-fold for males that of the exposure in humans with the recommended therapeutic dose (600 mg twice-daily). There were no carcinogenic effects seen in females at the dosages tested. The exposure at the high dose was approximately 0.6-fold for the females that of the exposure in humans. In rats dosed at levels of 7, 15 or 30 mg per kg per day there were no carcinogenic effects. In this study, the exposure at the high dose was approximately 6% that of the exposure in humans with the recommended therapeutic dose. Based on the exposures achieved in the animal studies, the significance of the observed effects is not known.

Mutagenesis

However, ritonavir was found to be negative for mutagenic or clastogenic activity in a battery of in *in vitro* and *in vivo* assays including the Ames bacterial reverse mutation assay using *S. typhimurium* and *E. coli*, the mouse lymphoma assay, the mouse micronucleus test and chromosomal aberration assays in human lymphocytes.

Impairment of Fertility

Ritonavir produced no effects on fertility in rats at drug exposures approximately 40% (male) and 60% (female) of that achieved with the proposed therapeutic dose. Higher dosages were not feasible due to hepatic toxicity.

14 CLINICAL STUDIES

The activity of NORVIR as monotherapy or in combination with nucleoside reverse transcriptase inhibitors has been evaluated in 1446 patients enrolled in two double-blind, randomized trials.

14.1 Advanced Patients with Prior Antiretroviral Therapy

Study 247 was a randomized, double-blind trial (with open-label follow-up) conducted in HIV-infected patients with at least nine months of prior antiretroviral therapy and baseline CD_4 cell counts less than or equal to 100 cells per μL. NORVIR 600 mg twice-daily or placebo was added to each patient's baseline antiretroviral therapy regimen, which could have consisted of up to two approved antiretroviral agents. The study accrued 1,090 patients, with mean baseline CD_4 cell count at study entry of 32 cells per μL. After the clinical benefit of NORVIR therapy was demonstrated, all patients were eligible to switch to open-label NORVIR for the duration of the follow-up period. Median duration of double-blind therapy with NORVIR and placebo was 6 months. The median duration of follow-up through the end of the open-label phase was 13.5 months for patients randomized to NORVIR and 14 months for patients randomized to placebo.

The cumulative incidence of clinical disease progression or death during the double-blind phase of Study 247 was 26% for patients initially randomized to NORVIR compared to 42% for patients initially randomized to placebo. This difference in rates was statistically significant.

Cumulative mortality through the end of the open-label follow-up phase for patients enrolled in Study 247 was 18% (99/543) for patients initially randomized to NORVIR compared to 26% (142/547) for patients initially randomized to placebo. This difference in rates was statistically significant. However, since the analysis at the end of the open-label phase includes patients in the placebo arm who were switched from placebo to NORVIR therapy, the survival benefit of NORVIR cannot be precisely estimated.

During the double-blind phase of Study 247, CD_4 cell counts increases from baseline for patients randomized to NORVIR at Week 2 and Week 4 were observed. From Week 4 and through Week 24, mean CD_4 cell counts for patients randomized to NORVIR appeared to plateau. In contrast, there was no apparent change in mean CD_4 cell counts for patients randomized to placebo at any visit between baseline and Week 24 of the double-blind phase of Study 247.

14.2 Patients without Prior Antiretroviral Therapy

In Study 245, 356 antiretroviral-naive HIV-infected patients (mean baseline CD_4 = 364 cells per μL) were randomized to receive either NORVIR 600 mg twice-daily, zidovudine 200 mg three-times-daily, or a combination of these drugs.

During the double-blind phase of study 245, greater mean CD_4 cell count increases were observed from baseline to Week 12 in the NORVIR-containing arms compared to the zidovudine arms. Mean CD_4 cell count changes subsequently appeared to plateau through Week 24 in the NORVIR arm, whereas mean CD_4 cell counts gradually diminished through Week 24 in the zidovudine and NORVIR plus zidovudine arms.

Greater mean reductions in plasma HIV-1 RNA levels were observed from baseline to Week 2 for the NORVIR-containing arms compared to the zidovudine arm. After Week 2 and through Week 24, mean plasma HIV-1 RNA levels either remained stable in the NORVIR and zidovudine arms or gradually rebounded toward baseline in the NORVIR plus zidovudine arm.

15 REFERENCES

1. Sewester CS. Calculations. In: Drug Facts and Comparisons. St. Louis, MO: J.B. Lippincott Co; January, 1997:xix.

16 HOW SUPPLIED/STORAGE AND HANDLING

NORVIR (ritonavir) tablets and NORVIR (ritonavir) oral solution are available in the following strengths and package sizes:

16.1 NORVIR Tablets, 100 mg Ritonavir

NORVIR (ritonavir) tablets are white film-coated ovaloid tablets debossed with the "a" logo and the code NK.

Bottles of 30 tablets each (**NDC** 0074 3333-30).

Recommended Storage

Store at or below 30°C (86°F). Exposure to temperatures up to 50°C (122°F) for seven days permitted. Dispense in original container or USP equivalent tight container (60 mL or less). For patient use: exposure of this product to high humidity outside the original or USP equivalent tight container (60 mL or less) for longer than 2 weeks is not recommended.

16.2 NORVIR Oral Solution, 80 mg per mL Ritonavir

NORVIR (ritonavir) oral solution is an orange-colored liquid, supplied in amber-colored, multi-dose bottles containing 600 mg ritonavir per 7.5 mL marked dosage cup (80 mg per mL).

240 mL bottles (**NDC** 0074-1940-63).

Recommended Storage

Store NORVIR oral solution at room temperature 20°-25°C (68°-77°F). Do not refrigerate. Shake well before each use. Use by product expiration date.

Product should be stored and dispensed in the original container.

Avoid exposure to excessive heat. Keep cap tightly closed.

17 PATIENT COUNSELING INFORMATION

See FDA-approved patient labeling (Patient Information)

Information For Patients

Patients or parents of patients should be informed that:

General Information

☐ They should pay special attention to accurate administration of their dose to minimize the risk of accidental overdose or underdose of NORVIR.

☐ They should inform their healthcare provider if their children's weight changes in order to make sure that the child's NORVIR dose is the correct one.

☐ Take NORVIR with meals.

☐ For adult patients taking NORVIR tablets, the maximum dose of 600 mg twice daily by mouth with meals should not be exceeded.

☐ Patients should remain under the care of a physician while using NORVIR. Patients should be advised to take NORVIR and other concomitant antiretroviral therapy every day as prescribed. NORVIR must always be used in combination with other antiretroviral drugs. Patients should not alter the dose or discontinue therapy without consulting with their doctor. If a dose of NORVIR is missed patients should take the dose as soon as possible and then return to their normal schedule. However, if a dose is skipped the patient should not double the next dose.

☐ NORVIR is not a cure for HIV-1 infection and patients may continue to experience illnesses associated with HIV-1 infection, including opportunistic infections. Patients should remain under the care of a physician when using NORVIR.

Patients should be advised to avoid doing things that can spread HIV-1 infection to others.

- **Do not share needles or other injection equipment.**
- **Do not share personal items that can have blood or body fluids on them, like toothbrushes and razor blades.**
- **Do not have any kind of sex without protection.** Always practice safe sex by using a latex or polyurethane condom to lower the chance of sexual contact with semen, vaginal secretions, or blood.
- **Do not breastfeed.** We do not know if NORVIR can be passed to the baby through breast milk and whether it could harm the baby. Also, mothers with HIV-1 should not breastfeed because HIV-1 can be passed to the baby in the breast milk.

☐ Sustained decreases in plasma HIV-1 RNA have been associated with a reduced risk of progression to AIDS and death.

Drug Interactions

☐ NORVIR may interact with some drugs; therefore, patients should be advised to report to their doctor the use of any other prescription, non-prescription medication or herbal products, particularly St. John's Wort.

☐ If they are receiving estrogen-based hormonal contraceptives, additional or alternate contraceptive measures should be used during therapy with NORVIR.

Potential Adverse Effects

☐ Pre-existing liver disease including Hepatitis B or C can worsen with use of NORVIR. This can be seen as worsening of transaminase elevations or hepatic decompensation. Patients should be advised that their liver function tests will need to be monitored closely especially during the first several months of NORVIR treatment and that they should notify their healthcare provider if they develop the signs and symptoms of worsening liver disease including loss of appetite, abdominal pain, jaundice, and itchy skin.

☐ Pancreatitis, including some fatalities, has been observed in patients receiving NORVIR therapy. Your patients should let you know of signs and symptoms (nausea, vomiting, and abdominal pain) that might be suggestive of pancreatitis.

☐ Skin rashes ranging in severity from mild to Stevens-Johnson syndrome have been reported in patients receiving NORVIR. Patients should be advised to contact their healthcare provider if they develop a rash while taking NORVIR. The healthcare provider will determine if treatment should be continued or an alternative antiretroviral regimen used.

☐ NORVIR may produce changes in the electrocardiogram (e.g., PR prolongation). Patients should consult their physician if they experience symptoms such as dizziness, lightheadedness, abnormal heart rhythm or loss of consciousness.

☐ Treatment with NORVIR therapy can result in substantial increases in the concentration of total cholesterol and triglycerides.

☐ New onset of diabetes or exacerbation of pre-existing diabetes mellitus, and hyperglycemia have been reported. Patients should be advised to notify their healthcare provider if they develop the signs and symptoms of diabetes mellitus

Table 8. Drug Interactions - Pharmacokinetic Parameters for Co-administered Drug in the Presence of NORVIR

Co-administered Drug	Dose of Co-administered Drug (mg)	Dose of NORVIR (mg)	N	AUC % (95% CI)	C_{max} (95% CI)	C_{min} (95% CI)
Alprazolam	1, single dose	500 q12h, 10 d	12	↓ 12% (-5, 30%)	↓ 16% (5, 27%)	ND
Avanafil	50, single dose	600 q12h	14[6]	↑ 13-fold	↑ 2.4-fold	ND
Clarithromycin 14-OH clarithromycin metabolite	500 q12h, 4 d	200 q8h, 4 d	22	↑ 77% (56, 103%) ↓ 100%	↑ 31% (15, 51%) ↓ 99%	↑ 2.8-fold (2.4, 3.3×) ↓ 100%
Desipramine 2-OH desipramine metabolite	100, single dose	500 q12h, 12 d	14	↑ 145% (103, 211%) ↓ 15% (3, 26%)	↑ 22% (12, 35%) ↓ 67% (62, 72%)	ND ND
Didanosine	200 q12h, 4 d	600 q12h, 4 d	12	↓ 13% (0, 23%)	↓ 16% (5, 26%)	↔
Ethinyl estradiol	50 µg single dose	500 q12h, 16 d	23	↓ 40% (31, 49%)	↓ 32% (24, 39%)	ND
Fluticasone propionate aqueous nasal spray	200 mcg qd, 7 d	100 mg q12h, 7 d	18	↑ approximately 350-fold[5]	↑ approximately 25-fold[5]	
Indinavir[1] Day 14 Day 15	400 q12h, 15 d	400 q12h, 15 d	10	 ↑ 6% (-14, 29%) ↓ 7% (-22, 28%)	 ↓ 51% (40, 61%) ↓ 62% (52, 70%)	 ↑ 4-fold (2.8, 6.8×) ↑ 4-fold (2.5, 6.5×)
Ketoconazole	200 daily, 7 d	500 q12h, 10 d	12	↑ 3.4-fold (2.8, 4.3×)	↑ 55% (40, 72%)	ND
Meperidine Normeperidine metabolite	50 oral single dose	500 q12h, 10 d	8 6	↓ 62% (59, 65%) ↑ 47% (-24, 345%)	↓ 59% (42, 72%) ↑ 87% (42, 147%)	ND ND
Methadone[2]	5, single dose	500 q12h, 15 d	11	↓ 36% (16, 52%)	↓ 38% (28, 46%)	ND
Raltegravir	400, single dose	100 q12h, 16 d	10	↓ 16% (-30, 1%)	↓ 24% (-45, 4%)	↓ 1% (-30, 40%)
Rivaroxaban	10, single dose (days 0 and 7)	600 q12h (days 2 to 7)	12	↑ 150% (130-170%)[7]	↑ 60% (40-70%)[7]	ND
Rifabutin 25-*O*-desacetyl rifabutin metabolite	150 daily, 16 d	500 q12h, 10 d	5, 11*	↑ 4-fold (2.8, 6.1×) ↑ 38-fold (28, 56×)	↑ 2.5-fold (1.9, 3.4×) ↑ 16-fold (13, 20×)	↑ 6-fold (3.5, 18.3×) ↑ 181-fold (ND)
Sildenafil	100, single dose	500 twice daily, 8 d	28	↑ 11-fold	↑ 4-fold	ND
Sulfamethoxazole[3]	800, single dose	500 q12h, 12 d	15	↓ 20% (16, 23%)	↔	ND
Tadalafil	20 mg, single dose	200 mg q12h		↑ 124%	↔	
Theophylline	3 mg/kg q8h, 15 d	500 q12h, 10 d	13, 11*	↓ 43% (42, 45%)	↓ 32% (29, 34%)	↓ 57% (55, 59%)
Trazodone	50 mg, single dose	200 mg q12h, 4 doses	10	↑ 2.4-fold	↑ 34%	
Trimethoprim[3]	160, single dose	500 q12h, 12 d	15	↑ 20% (3, 43%)	↔	ND
Vardenafil	5 mg	600 q12h		↑ 49-fold	↑ 13-fold	ND

(Table continued on next page)

Information on the AbbVie, Inc. products listed on these pages is from the prescribing information in use as of July 31, 2013. For more information, please visit rxabbvie.com or call 1-800-633-9110.

Table 8 *(cont.)*. Drug Interactions - Pharmacokinetic Parameters for Co-administered Drug in the Presence of NORVIR

Co-administered Drug	Dose of Co-administered Drug (mg)	Dose of NORVIR (mg)	N	AUC % (95% CI)	C_{max} (95% CI)	C_{min} (95% CI)
Voriconazole	400 q12h, 1 d; then 200 q12h, 8 d	400 q12h, 9 d		↓ 82%	↓ 66%	
	400 q12h, 1 d; then 200 q12h, 8 d	100 q12h, 9 d		↓ 39%	↓ 24%	
Warfarin	5, single dose	400 q12h, 12d	12			
S-Warfarin				↑ 9% (-17, 44%)[4]	↓ 9% (-16, -2%)[4]	ND
R-Warfarin				↓ 33% (-38, -27%)[4]	↔	ND
Zidovudine	200 q8h, 4 d	300 q6h, 4 d	9	↓ 25% (15, 34%)	↓ 27% (4, 45%)	ND

1 Ritonavir and indinavir were co-administered for 15 days; Day 14 doses were administered after a 15%-fat breakfast (757 Kcal) and 9%-fat evening snack (236 Kcal), and Day 15 doses were administered after a 15%-fat breakfast (757 Kcal) and 32%-fat dinner (815 Kcal). Indinavir C_{min} was also increased 4-fold. Effects were assessed relative to an indinavir 800 mg q8h regimen under fasting conditions.
2 Effects were assessed on a dose-normalized comparison to a methadone 20 mg single dose.
3 Sulfamethoxazole and trimethoprim taken as single combination tablet.
4 90% CI presented for R- and S-warfarin AUC and C_{max} ratios.
5 This significant increase in plasma fluticasone propionate exposure resulted in a significant decrease (86%) in plasma cortisol AUC.
6 For the reference arm: N=14 for C_{max} and $AUC_{(0\text{-}inf)}$, and for the test arm: N=13 for C_{max} and N=4 for $AUC_{(0\text{-}inf)}$.
7 90% CI presented for rivaroxaban
↑ Indicates increase.
↓ Indicates decrease.
↔ Indicates no change.
* Parallel group design; entries are subjects receiving combination and control regimens, respectively.

including frequent urination, excessive thirst, extreme hunger or unusual weight loss and/or an increased blood sugar while on NORVIR as they may require a change in their diabetes treatment or new treatment.

☐ Immune reconstitution syndrome has been reported in HIV-infected patients treated with combination antiretroviral therapy, including NORVIR.

☐ Redistribution or accumulation of body fat may occur in patients receiving antiretroviral therapy and that the cause and long term health effects of these conditions are not known at this time.

☐ Patients with hemophilia may experience increased bleeding when treated with protease inhibitors such as NORVIR.

☐ If they are receiving avanafil, sildenafil, tadalafil, or vardenafil for the treatment of erectile dysfunction, they may be at an increased risk of associated adverse reactions including hypotension, visual changes, and sustained erection, and should promptly report any symptoms to their doctor. They should seek medical assistance immediately if they develop a sustained penile erection lasting more than 4 hours while taking NORVIR and a PDE 5 Inhibitor such as Stendra®, Viagra®, Cialis® or Levitra®. If they are currently using or planning to use avanafil or tadalafil (for the treatment of pulmonary arterial hypertension) they should ask their doctor about potential adverse reactions these medications may cause when taken with NORVIR. The doctor may choose not to keep them on avanafil, or may adjust the dose of tadalafil while initiating treatment with NORVIR. Concomitant use of Revatio® (sildenafil) with NORVIR is contraindicated in patients with pulmonary arterial hypertension (PAH).

☐ Continued NORVIR therapy at a dose of 600 mg twice daily following loss of viral suppression may increase the likelihood of cross-resistance to other protease inhibitors.

NORVIR tablets and oral solution are manufactured by:
AbbVie Inc.
North Chicago, IL 60064 USA

Patient Information
NORVIR® (NOR-VEER)
(ritonavir) Tablets
(ritonavir) Oral Solution

Read this Patient Information before you start taking NORVIR and each time you get a refill. There may be new information. This information does not take the place of talking to your doctor about your medical condition or your treatment.

What is the most important information I should know about NORVIR?

- NORVIR can interact with other medicines and cause serious side effects. It is important to know the medicines that should not be taken with NORVIR. See the section "Who should not take NORVIR?"

What is NORVIR?

NORVIR is a prescription anti-HIV medicine used with other anti-HIV medicines to treat people with human immunodeficiency virus (HIV) infection. NORVIR is a type of anti-HIV medicine called a protease inhibitor. HIV is the virus that causes AIDS (Acquired Immune Deficiency Syndrome).

When used with other HIV medicines, NORVIR may reduce the amount of HIV in your blood (called "viral load"). NORVIR may also help to increase the number of CD_4 (T) cells in your blood which help fight off other infections. Reducing the amount of HIV and increasing the CD_4 (T) cell count may improve your immune system. This may reduce your risk of death or infections that can happen when your immune system is weak (opportunistic infections). Patients who took NORVIR in clinical studies had significant reductions in both death and AIDS defining diseases; however NORVIR may not have these effects in all patients.

NORVIR does not cure HIV infection or AIDS and you may continue to experience illnesses associated with HIV-1 infection, including opportunistic infections. You should remain under the care of a doctor when using NORVIR.

Avoid doing things that can spread HIV-1 infection.

- **Do not share needles or other injection equipment.**
- **Do not share personal items that can have blood or body fluids on them, like toothbrushes and razor blades.**
- **Do not have any kind of sex without protection.** Always practice safe sex by using a latex or polyurethane condom to lower the chance of sexual contact with semen, vaginal secretions, or blood.

Who should not take NORVIR?

Do not take NORVIR if you are allergic to ritonavir or any of the ingredients in NORVIR. See the end of this leaflet for a complete list of ingredients in NORVIR.

Do not take NORVIR with any of the following medicines:

- alfuzosin (Uroxatral)
- amiodarone (Cordarone, Nexterone, Pacerone), flecainide (Tambocor), propafenone (Rhythmol) or quinidine (Nuedext, Quinaglute, Cardioquin, Quinidex, and others)
- voriconazole (VFend) if NORVIR dose is 400 mg every 12 hours or greater
- dihydroergotamine (D.H.E. 45, Embolex, Migranal), ergonovine, ergotamine (Cafergot, Ergomar) methylergonovine (Methergine)
- cisapride (Propulsid)
- St. John's Wort (Hypericum perforatum)
- the cholesterol lowering medicines lovastatin (Mevacor, Altoprev, Advicor) or simvastatin (Zocor, Simcor, Vytorin)
- pimozide (Orap)
- sildenafil (Revatio) only when used for the treatment of pulmonary arterial hypertension
- oral midazolam or triazolam (Halcion)

Serious problems can happen if you or your child takes any of these medicines with NORVIR.

What should I tell my doctor before taking NORVIR?

Before taking NORVIR, tell your doctor if you:

- have liver problems, including Hepatitis B or Hepatitis C.
- have heart problems.
- have high blood sugar (diabetes).
- have bleeding problems or hemophilia.
- are pregnant or plan to become pregnant. It is not known if NORVIR can harm your unborn baby. **Pregnancy Registry:** You and your doctor will need to decide if taking NORVIR is right for you. If you take NORVIR while you are pregnant, talk to your doctor about how you can take part in the Antiretroviral Pregnancy Registry. The purpose of the registry is to follow the health of you and your baby.
- are breastfeeding. **Do not breastfeed.** We do not know if NORVIR can be passed to the baby through your breast milk and whether it could harm the baby. Also, mothers with HIV-1 should not breastfeed because HIV-1 can be passed to the baby in the breast milk.

Tell your doctor about all the medicines you take including prescription and nonprescription medicines, vitamins, and herbal supplements. Taking NORVIR and certain other medicines may affect each other causing serious side effects. NORVIR may affect the way other medicines work and other medicines may affect how NORVIR works.

Especially tell your doctor if you take:

- medicine to treat HIV
- estrogen-based contraceptives (birth control). NORVIR might reduce the effectiveness of estrogen-based contraceptives. You must take additional precautions for birth control such as a condom
- medicine for pain such as tramadol (Ryzolt, Ultracet, Conzip, Ultram), propoxyphene, or meperidine (Demerol)
- medicine to treat alcohol abuse such as disulfiram (Antabuse)
- medicine for your heart such as disopyramide (Norpace), lidocaine (Xylocaine Viscous), mexiletine, digoxin (Lanoxin), nifedipine (Procardia, Adalat, Afeditab CR), diltiazem (Cardizem, Dilacor, Cartia, Diltzac, Dilt, Taztia, Tiazac) or verapamil (Calan, Covera, Isoptin, Tarka, Verelan)
- medicines for panic disorder or anxiety such as buspirone, clorazepate, diazepam, estazolam, flurazepam, and zolpidem
- medicine for cancer such as dasatinib (Sprycel), nilotinib (Tasigna) vincristine, or vinblastine
- warfarin (Coumadin, Jantoven), rivaroxaban (Xarelto)
- medicine for seizures such as carbamazepine (Carbatrol, Equetro, Tegretol, Epitol), clonazepam (Klonopin), ethosuximide (Zarontin, Ethosuximide), divalproex (Depakote, Divalproex Sodium), lamotrigine (Lamictal) or phenytoin (Dilantin, Phenytek)
- medicine for depression such as nefazodone, bupropion (Wellbutrin, Aplenzin, Zyban), desipramine (Norpramin) or trazadone, fluoxetine (Prozac), paroxetine (Paxil), amitriptyline, or nortriptyline
- medicine for nausea and vomiting such as dronabinol (Marinol) or perphenazine
- medicine for fungal infections such as ketoconazole (Nizoral), itraconazole (Sporanox, Onmel) or voriconazole (VFend)
- colchicine (Colcrys, Col-Probenecid, Probenecid and Colchine)
- medicine for infections such as clarithromycin (Prevpac, Biaxin), rifabutin (Mycobutin), rifampin (Rimactane, Rifadin, Rifater, Rifamate), atovaquone (Mepron, Malarone), quinine (Qualaquin) or metronidazole (Flagyl, Helidac, Metrocream)
- medicine used to treat blood pressure, a heart attack, heart failure, or to lower pressure in the eye such as metoprolol (Lopressor, Toprol-XL), timolol (Cosopt, Betimol, Timoptic, Isatolol, Combigan)
- medicine for lung disease such as theophylline and salmeterol (Serevent)
- bosentan (Tracleer)
- medicine to prevent organ transplant failure such as cyclosporine (Gengraf, Sandimmune, Neoral), tacrolimus (Prograf), sirolimus (Rapamune)
- steroids such as dexamethasone, fluticasone (Advair Diskus, Veramyst, Flovent, Flonase), budesonide (Entocort EC, Pulmicort, Rhinocort), or prednisone
- a narcotic medicine such as methadone (Methadose, Dolophine Hydrochloride) or fentanyl (Abstral, Actiq, Fentora, Lazanda, Onsolis, Duragesic)
- medicine to treat schizophrenia such as risperidone (Risperdal) or thioridazine
- medicine to treat erectile dysfunction or pulmonary hypertension such as avanafil (Stendra), sildenafil (Viagra, Revatio), vardenafil (Levitra, Staxyn), tadalafil (Cialis, Adcirca). If you are taking avanafil (Stendra), your doctor may need to change it to a different medicine.
- midazolam by injection
- methamphetamine (Desoxyn)
- cholesterol lowering medicine such as atorvastatin (Lipitor) or rosuvasatin (Crestor)

This is not a complete list of medicines that you should tell your doctor that you are taking. Ask your doctor, provider or pharmacist if you are not sure if your medicine is one that is listed above.

Know the medicines you take. Keep a list of them to show your doctor or pharmacist when you get a new medicine. Do not start any new medicines while you are taking NORVIR without first talking with your doctor.

How should I take NORVIR?

- Take NORVIR exactly as prescribed by your doctor.
- You should stay under a doctor's care when taking NORVIR. Do not change your dose of NORVIR or stop your treatment without talking with your doctor first.
- If your child is taking NORVIR, your child's doctor will decide the right dose based on your child's height and weight. Tell your doctor if your child's weight changes. Your child should take NORVIR with food. If your child does not tolerate NORVIR Oral Solution, ask your child's doctor for advice.
- Swallow NORVIR tablets whole. Do not chew, break, or crush tablets before swallowing. If you cannot swallow NORVIR tablets whole, tell your doctor. You may need a different medicine.
- Take NORVIR with meals.
- NORVIR Oral Solution is peppermint or caramel flavored. You can take it alone, or may improve the taste by mixing it with 8 ounces of chocolate milk, Ensure®, or Advera®. NORVIR Oral Solution should be taken within 1 hour if mixed with these fluids. Ask your doctor, nurse or pharmacist about other ways to improve the taste of NORVIR Oral Solution.
- Do not run out of NORVIR. Get your NORVIR prescription refilled from you doctor or pharmacy before you run out.
- If you miss a dose of NORVIR, take it as soon as possible and then take your next scheduled dose at its regular time. If it is almost time for your next dose, wait and take the next dose at the regular time. Do not double the next dose.
- If you take too much NORVIR, call your local poison control center or go to the nearest hospital emergency room right away.

What are the possible side effects of NORVIR?

NORVIR can cause serious side effects including:

- See "What is the most important information I should know about NORVIR?"
- **Liver disease.** Some people taking NORVIR in combination with other anti-HIV medicines have developed liver problems which may be life-threatening. Your doctor should do regular blood tests during your combination treatment with NORVIR. If you have chronic hepatitis B or C infection, your doctor should check your blood tests more often because you have an increased chance of developing liver problems. Tell your doctor if you have any of the below signs and symptoms of liver problems:
    - loss of appetite
    - pain or tenderness on your right side below your ribs
    - yellowing of your skin or whites of your eyes
    - itchy skin
- **Swelling of your pancreas (Pancreatitis).** NORVIR can cause serious pancreas problems, which may lead to death. Tell your doctor right away if you have signs or symptoms of pancreatitis such as:
    - nausea
    - vomiting
    - stomach (abdominal) pain
- **Allergic Reactions.** Sometimes these allergic reactions can become severe and require treatment in a hospital. You should call your doctor right away if you develop a rash. Stop taking NORVIR and get medical help right away if you have any of the following symptoms of a severe allergic reaction:
    - trouble breathing
    - wheezing
    - dizziness or fainting
    - throat tightness or hoarseness
    - fast heartbeat or pounding in your chest (tachycardia)
    - sweating
    - swelling of your face, lips or tongue
    - muscle or joint pain
    - blisters or skin lesions
    - mouth sores or ulcers
- **Changes in the electrical activity of your heart called PR prolongation. PR prolongation can cause irregular heart-beats.** Tell your doctor right away if you have symptoms such as:
    - dizziness
    - lightheadedness
    - feel faint or pass out
    - abnormal heart beat
- **Increase in cholesterol and triglyceride levels.** Treatment with NORVIR may increase your blood levels of cholesterol and triglycerides. Your doctor should do blood tests before you start your treatment with NORVIR and regularly to check for an increase in your cholesterol and triglycerides levels.
- **Diabetes and high blood sugar (hyperglycemia).** Some people who take protease inhibitors including NORVIR can get high blood sugar, develop diabetes, or your diabetes can get worse. Tell your doctor if you notice an increase in thirst or urinate often while taking NORVIR.
- **Changes in your immune system (Immune reconstitution syndrome)** can happen when you start taking HIV medicines. Your immune system may get stronger and begin to fight infections that have been hidden in your body for a long time. Call your doctor right away if you start having new symptoms after starting your HIV medicine.
- **Change in body fat.** These changes can happen in people who take antiretroviral therapy. The changes may include an increase amount of fat in the upper back and neck ("buffalo hump"), breast, and around the back and stomach area. Loss of fat from the legs, arms, and face may also happen. The exact cause and long-term health effects of these conditions are not known.
- **Increased bleeding for hemophiliacs.** Some people with hemophilia have increased bleeding with protease inhibitors including NORVIR.

The most common side effects of NORVIR include:

- feeling weak or tired
- nausea
- vomiting
- diarrhea
- loss of appetite
- abdominal pain
- changes in taste
- tingling feeling or numbness in hands or feet or around the lips
- headache
- dizziness

NORVIR liquid contains a large amount of alcohol. If a toddler or young child accidentally drinks more than the recommended dose of NORVIR, it could make him/her sick from too much alcohol. Contact your local poison control center or emergency room immediately if this happens.

Tell your doctor if you have any side effect that bothers you or that does not go away.

These are not all of the possible side effects of NORVIR. For more information, ask your doctor or pharmacist.

Call your doctor for medical advice about side effects. You may report side effects to FDA at 1-800-FDA-1088.

How do I Store NORVIR?

- Store NORVIR Oral Solution at room temperature between 68°F to 77°F (20°C to 25°C).
- Store NORVIR tablets below 30°C (86°F). Exposure to temperatures up to 50°C (122°F) for seven days permitted.
- Do not refrigerate NORVIR Oral Solution.
- Shake NORVIR Oral Solution well before each use.
- Keep NORVIR Oral Solution away from heat.
- Store NORVIR tablets and NORVIR oral solution in the original container given to you by the pharmacist.
- Exposure of NORVIR tablets to high humidity outside the original container for longer than 2 weeks is not recommended.
- Use NORVIR tablets and NORVIR Oral Solution by the expiration date on the bottle.

Keep NORVIR and all medicines out of the reach of children.

General information about NORVIR

Medicines are sometimes prescribed for purposes other than those listed in a Patient Information Leaflet. Do not use this medicine for a condition for which it was not prescribed. Do not share this medicine with other people.

This leaflet summarizes the most important information about NORVIR. If you would like more information, talk to your doctor. You can ask your doctor or pharmacist for information about NORVIR that is written for healthcare professionals.

For more information, call 1-800-633-9110.

What are the ingredients in NORVIR?

Active ingredient: ritonavir

Inactive ingredients:

NORVIR Tablet: copovidone, anhydrous dibasic calcium phosphate, sorbitan monolaurate, colloidal silicon dioxide, and sodium stearyl fumarate. The film coating contains: hypromellose, titanium dioxide, polyethylene glycol 400, hydroxypropyl cellulose, talc, polyethylene glycol 3350, colloidal silicon dioxide, and polysorbate 80.

NORVIR Oral Solution: ethanol, water, polyoxyl 35 castor oil, propylene glycol, anhydrous citric acid to adjust pH, saccharin sodium, peppermint oil, creamy caramel flavoring, and FD&C Yellow No. 6.

This Patient Information has been approved by the U.S. Food and Drug Administration.

* The brands listed are trademarks of their respective owners and are not trademarks of AbbVie Inc. The makers of these brands are not affiliated with and do not endorse AbbVie Inc. or its products.

NORVIR tablets and oral solution are manufactured by:
AbbVie Inc.
North Chicago, IL 60064 USA
Ref: 03-A728-R8-Rev. January, 2013

Shown in Product Identification Guide, page 304

PROMETRIUM® ℞

[pro-mē-trē-um]

(progesterone, USP)
Capsules 100 mg
Capsules 200 mg

WARNING: CARDIOVASCULAR DISORDERS, BREAST CANCER and PROBABLE DEMENTIA FOR ESTROGEN PLUS PROGESTIN THERAPY

Cardiovascular Disorders and Probable Dementia

Estrogens plus progestin therapy should not be used for the prevention of cardiovascular disease or dementia. (See **CLINICAL STUDIES** and **WARNINGS, Cardiovascular disorders** and **Probable dementia.**)

The Women's Health Initiative (WHI) estrogen plus progestin substudy reported increased risks of deep vein thrombosis, pulmonary embolism, stroke and myocardial infarction in postmenopausal women (50 to 79 years of age) during 5.6 years of treatment with daily oral conjugated estrogens (CE) [0.625 mg] combined with medroxyprogesterone acetate (MPA) [2.5 mg], relative to placebo. (See **CLINICAL STUDIES** and **WARNINGS, Cardiovascular disorders.**)

The WHI Memory Study (WHIMS) estrogen plus progestin ancillary study of the WHI reported an increased risk of developing probable dementia in postmenopausal women 65 years of age or older during 4 years of treatment with daily CE (0.625 mg) combined with MPA (2.5 mg), relative to placebo. It is unknown whether this finding applies to younger postmenopausal women. (See **CLINICAL STUDIES** and **WARNINGS, Probable dementia** and **PRECAUTIONS, Geriatric Use.**)

Breast Cancer

The WHI estrogen plus progestin substudy also demonstrated an increased risk of invasive breast cancer. (See **CLINICAL STUDIES** and **WARNINGS, Malignant neoplasms, *Breast Cancer*.**)

In the absence of comparable data, these risks should be assumed to be similar for other doses of CE and MPA, and other combinations and dosage forms of estrogens and progestins.

Progestins with estrogens should be prescribed at the lowest effective doses and for the shortest duration consistent with treatment goals and risks for the individual woman.

DESCRIPTION

PROMETRIUM® (progesterone, USP) Capsules contain micronized progesterone for oral administration. Progesterone has a molecular weight of 314.47 and a molecular formula of $C_{21}H_{30}O_2$. Progesterone (pregn-4-ene-3, 20-dione) is a white or creamy white, odorless, crystalline powder practically insoluble in water, soluble in alcohol, acetone and dioxane and sparingly soluble in vegetable oils, stable in air, melting between 126° and 131°C. The structural formula is:

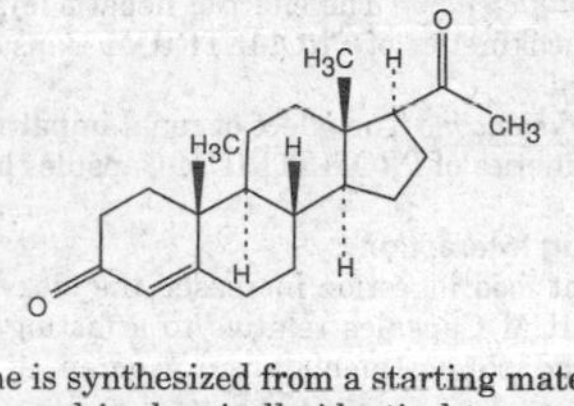

Progesterone is synthesized from a starting material from a plant source and is chemically identical to progesterone of human ovarian origin. PROMETRIUM Capsules are available in multiple strengths to afford dosage flexibility for optimum management. PROMETRIUM Capsules contain 100 mg or 200 mg micronized progesterone.

The inactive ingredients for PROMETRIUM Capsules 100 mg include: peanut oil NF, gelatin NF, glycerin USP, lecithin NF, titanium dioxide USP, D&C Yellow No. 10, and FD&C Red No. 40.

The inactive ingredients for PROMETRIUM Capsules 200 mg include: peanut oil NF, gelatin NF, glycerin USP, lecithin NF, titanium dioxide USP, D&C Yellow No. 10, and FD&C Yellow No. 6.

CLINICAL PHARMACOLOGY

PROMETRIUM Capsules are an oral dosage form of micronized progesterone which is chemically identical to progesterone of ovarian origin. The oral bioavailability of progesterone is increased through micronization.

Information on the AbbVie, Inc. products listed on these pages is from the prescribing information in use as of July 31, 2013. For more information, please visit rxabbvie.com or call 1-800-633-9110.

Pharmacokinetics

A. Absorption

After oral administration of progesterone as a micronized soft-gelatin capsule formulation, maximum serum concentrations were attained within 3 hours. The absolute bioavailability of micronized progesterone is not known. Table 1 summarizes the mean pharmacokinetic parameters in postmenopausal women after five oral daily doses of PROMETRIUM Capsules 100 mg as a micronized soft-gelatin capsule formulation.

TABLE 1. Pharmacokinetic Parameters of PROMETRIUM Capsules

Parameter	PROMETRIUM Capsules Daily Dose		
	100 mg	200 mg	300 mg
Cmax (ng/mL)	17.3 ± 21.9[a]	38.1 ± 37.8	60.6 ± 72.5
Tmax (hr)	1.5 ± 0.8	2.3 ± 1.4	1.7 ± 0.6
AUC (0-10) (ng × hr/mL)	43.3 ± 30.8	101.2 ± 66.0	175.7 ± 170.3

[a] Mean ± S.D.

Serum progesterone concentrations appeared linear and dose proportional following multiple dose administration of PROMETRIUM Capsules 100 mg over the dose range 100 mg per day to 300 mg per day in postmenopausal women. Although doses greater than 300 mg per day were not studied in females, serum concentrations from a study in male volunteers appeared linear and dose proportional between 100 mg per day and 400 mg per day. The pharmacokinetic parameters in male volunteers were generally consistent with those seen in postmenopausal women.

B. Distribution

Progesterone is approximately 96 percent to 99 percent bound to serum proteins, primarily to serum albumin (50 to 54 percent) and transcortin (43 to 48 percent).

C. Metabolism

Progesterone is metabolized primarily by the liver largely to pregnanediols and pregnanolones. Pregnanediols and pregnanolones are conjugated in the liver to glucuronide and sulfate metabolites. Progesterone metabolites which are excreted in the bile may be deconjugated and may be further metabolized in the intestine via reduction, dehydroxylation, and epimerization.

D. Excretion

The glucuronide and sulfate conjugates of pregnanediol and pregnanolone are excreted in the bile and urine. Progesterone metabolites are eliminated mainly by the kidneys. Progesterone metabolites which are excreted in the bile may undergo enterohepatic recycling or may be excreted in the feces.

E. Special Populations

The pharmacokinetics of PROMETRIUM Capsules have not been assessed in low body weight or obese patients.

Hepatic Insufficiency: The effect of hepatic impairment on the pharmacokinetics of PROMETRIUM Capsules has not been studied.

Renal Insufficiency: The effect of renal impairment on the pharmacokinetics of PROMETRIUM Capsules has not been studied.

F. Food–Drug Interaction

Concomitant food ingestion increased the bioavailability of PROMETRIUM Capsules relative to a fasting state when administered to postmenopausal women at a dose of 200 mg.

G. Drug Interactions

The metabolism of progesterone by human liver microsomes was inhibited by ketoconazole ($IC_{50} < 0.1$ µM). Ketoconazole is a known inhibitor of cytochrome P450 3A4, hence these data suggest that ketoconazole or other known inhibitors of this enzyme may increase the bioavailability of progesterone. The clinical relevance of the *in vitro* findings is unknown.

Co administration of conjugated estrogens and PROMETRIUM Capsules to 29 postmenopausal women over a 12-day period resulted in an increase in total estrone concentrations (Cmax 3.68 ng/mL to 4.93 ng/mL) and total equilin concentrations (Cmax 2.27 ng/mL to 3.22 ng/mL) and a decrease in circulating 17β estradiol concentrations (Cmax 0.037 ng/mL to 0.030 ng/mL). The half-life of the conjugated estrogens was similar with coadministration of PROMETRIUM Capsules. Table 2 summarizes the pharmacokinetic parameters.

[See table 2 above]

TABLE 2. Mean (± S.D.) Pharmacokinetic Parameters for Estradiol, Estrone, and Equilin Following Coadministration of Conjugated Estrogens 0.625 mg and PROMETRIUM Capsules 200 mg for 12 Days to Postmenopausal Women

Drug	Conjugated Estrogens			Conjugated Estrogens plus PROMETRIUM Capsules		
	Cmax (ng/mL)	Tmax (hr)	AUC(0-24h) (ng × h/mL)	Cmax (ng/mL)	Tmax (hr)	AUC(0-24h) (ng × h/mL)
Estradiol	0.037 ± 0.048	12.7 ± 9.1	0.676 ± 0.737	0.030 ± 0.032	17.32 ± 1.21	0.561 ± 0.572
Estrone Total [a]	3.68 ± 1.55	10.6 ± 6.8	61.3 ± 26.36	4.93 ± 2.07	7.5 ± 3.8	85.9 ± 41.2
Equilin Total [a]	2.27 ± 0.95	6.0 ± 4.0	28.8 ± 13.0	3.22 ± 1.13	5.3 ± 2.6	38.1 ± 20.2

[a] Total estrogens is the sum of conjugated and unconjugated estrogen.

TABLE 3. Incidence of Endometrial Hyperplasia in Women Receiving 3 Years of Treatment

Endometrial Diagnosis	Treatment Group					
	Conjugated Estrogens 0.625 mg + PROMETRIUM Capsules 200 mg (cyclical)		Conjugated Estrogens 0.625 mg (alone)		Placebo	
	Number of patients	% of patients	Number of patients	% of patients	Number of patients	% of patients
	n=117		n=115		n=116	
HYPERPLASIA [a]	7	6	74	64	3	3
Adenocarcinoma	0	0	0	0	1	1
Atypical hyperplasia	1	1	14	12	0	0
Complex hyperplasia	0	0	27	23	1	1
Simple hyperplasia	6	5	33	29	1	1

[a] Most advanced result to least advanced result:
Adenocarcinoma > atypical hyperplasia > complex hyperplasia > simple hyperplasia

CLINICAL STUDIES

Effects on the endometrium

In a randomized, double-blind clinical trial, 358 postmenopausal women, each with an intact uterus, received treatment for up to 36 months. The treatment groups were: PROMETRIUM® (progesterone, USP) Capsules at the dose of 200 mg per day for 12 days per 28-day cycle in combination with conjugated estrogens 0.625 mg per day (n=120); conjugated estrogens 0.625 mg per day only (n=119); or placebo (n=119). The subjects in all three treatment groups were primarily Caucasian women (87 percent or more of each group). The results for the incidence of endometrial hyperplasia in women receiving up to 3 years of treatment are shown in Table 3. A comparison of the PROMETRIUM Capsules plus conjugated estrogens treatment group to the conjugated estrogens only group showed a significantly lower rate of hyperplasia (6 percent combination product versus 64 percent estrogen alone) in the PROMETRIUM Capsules plus conjugated estrogens treatment group throughout 36 months of treatment.

[See table 3 above]

The times to diagnosis of endometrial hyperplasia over 36 months of treatment are shown in Figure 1. This figure illustrates graphically that the proportion of patients with hyperplasia was significantly greater for the conjugated estrogens group (64 percent) compared to the conjugated estrogens plus PROMETRIUM Capsules group (6 percent).

[See figure 1 at top of next column]

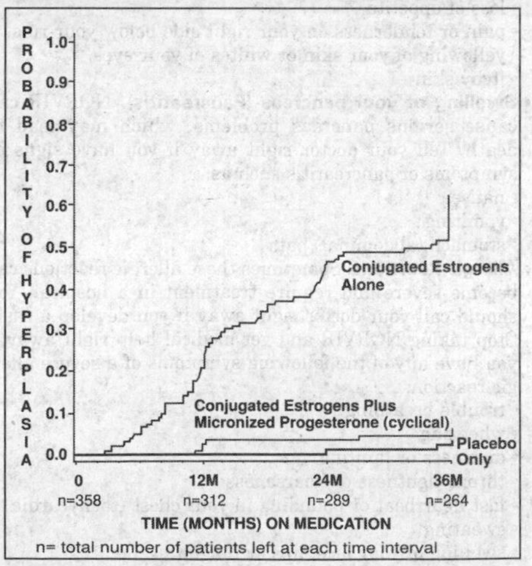

Figure 1. Time to Hyperplasia in Women Receiving up to 36 Months of Treatment

The discontinuation rates due to hyperplasia over the 36 months of treatment are as shown in Table 4. For any degree of hyperplasia, the discontinuation rate for patients who received conjugated estrogens plus PROMETRIUM Capsules was similar to that of the placebo only group, while the discontinuation rate for patients who received conjugated estrogens alone was significantly higher. Women who permanently discontinued treatment due to hyperplasia were similar in demographics to the overall study population.

[See table 4 at top of next page]

Effects on secondary amenorrhea

In a single-center, randomized, double-blind clinical study that included premenopausal women with secondary amenorrhea for at least 90 days, administration of 10 days of PROMETRIUM Capsules therapy resulted in 80 percent of women experiencing withdrawal bleeding within 7 days of the last dose of PROMETRIUM Capsules, 300 mg per day (n=20), compared to 10 percent of women experiencing withdrawal bleeding in the placebo group (n=21).

In a multicenter, parallel-group, open label, postmarketing dosing study that included premenopausal women with secondary amenorrhea for at least 90 days, administration of 10 days of PROMETRIUM Capsules during two 28-day treatment cycles, 300 mg per day (n=107) or 400 mg per day (n=99), resulted in 73.8 percent and 76.8 percent of women, respectively, experiencing withdrawal bleeding.

The rate of secretory transformation was evaluated in a multicenter, randomized, double-blind clinical study in estrogen-primed postmenopausal women. PROMETRIUM Capsules administered orally for 10 days at 400 mg per day (n=22) induced complete secretory changes in the endometrium in 45 percent of women compared to 0 percent in the placebo group (n=23).

A second multicenter, parallel-group, open label post-marketing dosing study in premenopausal women with secondary amenorrhea for at least 90 days also evaluated the rate of secretory transformation. All subjects received daily oral conjugated estrogens over 3 consecutive 28-day treatment cycles and PROMETRIUM Capsules, 300 mg per day (n=107) or 400 mg per day (n=99) for 10 days of each

TABLE 4. Discontinuation Rate Due to Hyperplasia Over 36 Months of Treatment

Most Advanced Biopsy Result Through 36 Months of Treatment	Treatment Group					
	Conjugated Estrogens + PROMETRIUM Capsules (cyclical)		Conjugated Estrogens (alone)		Placebo	
	n=120		n=119		n=119	
	Number of patients	% of patients	Number of patients	% of patients	Number of patients	% of patients
Adenocarcinoma	0	0	0	0	1	1
Atypical hyperplasia	1	1	10	8	0	0
Complex hyperplasia	0	0	21	18	1	1
Simple hyperplasia	1	1	13	11	0	0

TABLE 5. Relative and Absolute Risk Seen in the Estrogen Plus Progestin Substudy of WHI at an Average of 5.6 Years[a, b]

Event	Relative Risk CE/MPA versus Placebo (95% nCI [c])	CE/MPA n = 8,506	Placebo n = 8,102
		Absolute Risk per 10,000 Women-Years	
CHD events	1.23 (0.99-1.53)	41	34
Non-fatal MI	*1.28 (1.00-1.63)*	*31*	*25*
CHD death	*1.10 (0.70-1.75)*	*8*	*8*
All stroke	1.31 (1.03-1.88)	33	25
Ischemic Stroke	*1.44 (1.09-1.90)*	*26*	*18*
Deep vein thrombosis [d]	1.95 (1.43-2.67)	26	13
Pulmonary embolism	2.13 (1.45-3.11)	18	8
Invasive breast cancer [e]	1.24 (1.01-1.54)	41	33
Colorectal cancer	0.61 (0.42-0.87)	10	16
Endometrial cancer [d]	0.81 (0.48-1.36)	6	7
Cervical cancer [d]	1.44 (0.47-4.42)	2	1
Hip fracture	0.67 (0.47-0.96)	11	16
Vertebral fractures [d]	0.65 (0.46-0.92)	11	17
Lower arm/wrist fractures [d]	0.71 (0.59-0.85)	44	62
Total fractures [d]	0.76 (0.69-0.83)	152	199
Overall mortality [f]	1.00 (0.83-1.19)	52	52
Global Index [g]	1.13 (1.02-1.25)	184	165

[a] Adapted from numerous WHI publications. WHI publications can be viewed at www.nhlbi.nih.gov/whi.
[b] Results are based on centrally adjudicated data.
[c] Nominal confidence intervals unadjusted for multiple looks and multiple comparisons.
[d] Not included in Global Index.
[e] Includes metastatic and non-metastatic breast cancer with the exception of *in situ* breast cancer.
[f] All deaths, except from breast or colorectal cancer, definite or probable CHD, PE or cerebrovascular disease.
[g] A subset of the events was combined in a "global index" defined as the earliest occurrence of CHD events, invasive breast cancer, stroke, pulmonary embolism, endometrial cancer, colorectal cancer, hip fracture, or death due to other causes.

treatment cycle. The rate of complete secretory transformation was 21.5 percent and 28.3 percent, respectively.

Women's Health Initiative Studies

The Women's Health Initiative (WHI) enrolled approximately 27,000 predominantly healthy postmenopausal women in two substudies to assess the risks and benefits of daily oral conjugated estrogens (CE) [0.625 mg]-alone or in combination with medroxyprogesterone acetate (MPA) [2.5 mg] compared to placebo in the prevention of certain chronic diseases. The primary endpoint was the incidence of coronary heart disease [(CHD) defined as nonfatal myocardial infarction (MI), silent MI and CHD death], with invasive breast cancer as the primary adverse outcome. A "global index" included the earliest occurrence of CHD, invasive breast cancer, stroke, pulmonary embolism (PE), endometrial cancer (only in the CE plus MPA substudy), colorectal cancer, hip fracture, or death due to other cause. These sub studies did not evaluate the effects of CE–alone or CE plus MPA on menopausal symptoms.

WHI Estrogen Plus Progestin Substudy

The WHI estrogen plus progestin substudy was stopped early. According to the predefined stopping rule, after an average follow-up of 5.6 years of treatment, the increased risk of breast cancer and cardiovascular events exceeded the specified benefits included in the "global index." The absolute excess risk of events in the "global index" was 19 per 10,000 women-years.

For those outcomes included in the WHI "global index" that reached statistical significance after 5.6 years of follow-up, the absolute excess risks per 10,000 women-years in the group treated with CE plus MPA were 7 more CHD events, 8 more strokes, 10 more PEs, and 8 more invasive breast cancers, while the absolute risk reductions per 10,000 women-years were 6 fewer colorectal cancers and 5 fewer hip fractures.

Results of the estrogen plus progestin substudy, which included 16,608 women (average 63 years of age, range 50 to 79; 83.9 percent White, 6.8 percent Black, 5.4 percent Hispanic, 3.9 percent Other) are presented in Table 5. These results reflect centrally adjudicated data after an average follow-up of 5.6 years.

[See table 5 below]

Timing of the initiation of estrogen plus progestin therapy relative to the start of menopause may affect the overall risk benefit profile. The WHI estrogen plus progestin substudy stratified for age showed in women 50 to 59 years of age a non-significant trend toward reducing risk of overall mortality [hazard ratio (HR) 0.69 (95 percent CI, 0.44-1.07)].

Women's Health Initiative Memory Study

The estrogen plus progestin Women's Health Initiative Memory Study (WHIMS), an ancillary study of WHI, enrolled 4,532 predominantly healthy postmenopausal women 65 years of age and older (47 percent were 65 to 69 years of age; 35 percent were 70 to 74 years of age; and 18 percent were 75 years of age and older) to evaluate the effects of daily CE (0.625 mg) plus MPA (2.5 mg) on the incidence of probable dementia (primary outcome) compared to placebo. After an average follow-up of 4 years, the relative risk of probable dementia for CE plus MPA versus placebo was 2.05 (95 percent CI, 1.21 – 3.48). The absolute risk of probable dementia for CE plus MPA versus placebo was 45 versus 22 per 10,000 women-years. Probable dementia as defined in this study included Alzheimer's disease (AD), vascular dementia (VaD) and mixed type (having features of both AD and VaD). The most common classification of probable dementia in the treatment group and the placebo group was AD. Since the ancillary study was conducted in women 65 to 79 years of age, it is unknown whether these findings apply to younger postmenopausal women. (See **WARNINGS, Probable dementia** and **PRECAUTIONS, Geriatric Use**.)

INDICATIONS AND USAGE

PROMETRIUM® (progesterone, USP) Capsules are indicated for use in the prevention of endometrial hyperplasia in nonhysterectomized postmenopausal women who are receiving conjugated estrogens tablets. They are also indicated for use in secondary amenorrhea.

CONTRAINDICATIONS

PROMETRIUM Capsules should not be used in women with any of the following conditions:

1. **PROMETRIUM Capsules should not be used in patients with known hypersensitivity to its ingredients. PROMETRIUM Capsules contain peanut oil and should never be used by patients allergic to peanuts.**
2. Undiagnosed abnormal genital bleeding.
3. Known, suspected, or history of breast cancer.
4. Active deep vein thrombosis, pulmonary embolism or history of these conditions.
5. Active arterial thromboembolic disease (for example, stroke and myocardial infarction), or a history of these conditions.
6. Known liver dysfunction or disease.
7. Known or suspected pregnancy.

WARNINGS

See **BOXED WARNING**.

1. Cardiovascular disorders

An increased risk of pulmonary embolism, deep vein thrombosis (DVT), stroke, and myocardial infarction has been reported with estrogen plus progestin therapy. Should any of these occur or be suspected, estrogen with progestin therapy should be discontinued immediately.

Risk factors for arterial vascular disease (for example, hypertension, diabetes mellitus, tobacco use, hypercholesterolemia, and obesity) and/or venous thromboembolism (for example, personal history or family history of venous thromboembolism [VTE], obesity, and systemic lupus erythematosus) should be managed appropriately.

a. Stroke

In the Women's Health Initiative (WHI) estrogen plus progestin substudy, a statistically significant increased risk of stroke was reported in women 50 to 79 years of age receiving daily CE (0.625 mg) plus MPA (2.5 mg) compared to women in the same age group receiving placebo (33 versus 25 per 10,000 women-years). The increase in risk was demonstrated after the first year and persisted. (See **CLINICAL STUDIES**.) Should a stroke occur or be suspected, estrogen plus progestin therapy should be discontinued immediately.

b. Coronary Heart Disease

In the WHI estrogen plus progestin substudy, there was a statistically non-significant increased risk of coronary heart disease (CHD) events (defined as nonfatal myocardial infarction [MI], silent MI, or CHD death) reported in women

Information on the AbbVie, Inc. products listed on these pages is from the prescribing information in use as of July 31, 2013. For more information, please visit rxabbvie.com or call 1-800-633-9110.

receiving daily CE (0.625 mg) plus MPA (2.5 mg) compared to women receiving placebo (41 versus 34 per 10,000 women-years). An increase in relative risk was demonstrated in year 1 and a trend toward decreasing relative risk was reported in years 2 through 5. (See **CLINICAL STUDIES**.)

In postmenopausal women with documented heart disease (n = 2,763, average age 66.7 years), in a controlled clinical trial of secondary prevention of cardiovascular disease (Heart and Estrogen/Progestin Replacement Study [HERS]), treatment with daily CE (0.625 mg) plus MPA (2.5 mg) demonstrated no cardiovascular benefit. During an average follow-up of 4.1 years, treatment with CE plus MPA did not reduce the overall rate of CHD events in postmenopausal women with established coronary heart disease. There were more CHD events in the CE plus MPA-treated group than in the placebo group in year 1, but not during the subsequent years. Two thousand, three hundred and twenty-one (2,321) women from the original HERS trial agreed to participate in an open-label extension of HERS, HERS II. Average follow-up in HERS II was an additional 2.7 years, for a total of 6.8 years overall. Rates of CHD events were comparable among women in the CE plus MPA group and the placebo group in HERS, HERS II, and overall.

c. Venous Thromboembolism

In the WHI estrogen plus progestin substudy, a statistically significant 2-fold greater rate of VTE (DVT and pulmonary embolism [PE]) was reported in women receiving daily CE (0.625 mg) plus MPA (2.5 mg) compared to women receiving placebo (35 versus 17 per 10,000 women-years). Statistically significant increases in risk for both DVT (26 versus 13 per 10,000 women-years) and PE (18 versus 8 per 10,000 women-years) were also demonstrated. The increase in VTE risk was demonstrated during the first year and persisted. (See **CLINICAL STUDIES**.) Should a VTE occur or be suspected, estrogen plus progestin therapy should be discontinued immediately.

If feasible, estrogens with progestins should be discontinued at least 4 to 6 weeks before surgery of the type associated with an increased risk of thromboembolism, or during periods of prolonged immobilization.

2. Malignant neoplasms

a. Breast Cancer

The most important randomized clinical trial providing information about breast cancer in estrogen plus progestin users is the Women's Health Initiative (WHI) substudy of daily CE (0.625 mg) plus MPA (2.5 mg). After a mean follow-up of 5.6 years, the estrogen plus progestin substudy reported an increased risk of invasive breast cancer in women who took daily CE plus MPA. In this substudy, prior use of estrogen-alone or estrogen plus progestin therapy was reported by 26 percent of the women. The relative risk of invasive breast cancer was 1.24 (95 percent nCI, 1.01-1.54), and the absolute risk was 41 versus 33 cases per 10,000 women-years, for CE plus MPA compared with placebo.

Among women who reported prior use of hormone therapy, the relative risk of invasive breast cancer was 1.86, and the absolute risk was 46 versus 25 cases per 10,000 women-years, for estrogen plus progestin compared with placebo. Among women who reported no prior use of hormone therapy, the relative risk of invasive breast cancer was 1.09, and the absolute risk was 40 versus 36 cases per 10,000 women-years for CE plus MPA compared with placebo. In the same substudy, invasive breast cancers were larger, were more likely to be node positive, and were diagnosed at a more advanced stage in the CE (0.625 mg) plus MPA (2.5 mg) group compared with the placebo group. Metastatic disease was rare, with no apparent difference between the two groups. Other prognostic factors such as histologic subtype, grade and hormone receptor status did not differ between the groups. (See **CLINICAL STUDIES**.)

Consistent with the WHI clinical trials, observational studies have also reported an increased risk of breast cancer for estrogen plus progestin therapy, and a smaller increased risk for estrogen-alone therapy, after several years of use. The risk increased with duration of use, and appeared to return to baseline over about 5 years after stopping treatment (only the observational studies have substantial data on risk after stopping). Observational studies also suggest that the risk of breast cancer was greater, and became apparent earlier, with estrogen plus progestin therapy as compared to estrogen-alone therapy. However, these studies have not generally found significant variation in the risk of breast cancer among different estrogen plus progestin combinations, doses, or routes of administration.

The use of estrogen plus progestin has been reported to result in an increase in abnormal mammograms requiring further evaluation. All women should receive yearly breast examinations by a healthcare provider and perform monthly breast self-examinations. In addition, mammography examinations should be scheduled based on patient age, risk factors, and prior mammogram results.

b. Endometrial Cancer

An increased risk of endometrial cancer has been reported with the use of unopposed estrogen therapy in a woman with a uterus. The reported endometrial cancer risk among unopposed estrogen users is about 2 to 12 times greater than in non-users, and appears dependent on duration of treatment and on estrogen dose. Most studies show no significant increased risk associated with the use of estrogens for less than 1 year. The greatest risk appears associated with prolonged use, with increased risks of 15- to 24-fold for 5 to 10 years or more and this risk has been shown to persist for at least 8 to 15 years after estrogen therapy is discontinued.

Clinical surveillance of all women using estrogen plus progestin therapy is important. Adequate diagnostic measures, including directed or random endometrial sampling when indicated, should be undertaken to rule out malignancy in all cases of undiagnosed persistent or recurring abnormal genital bleeding. There is no evidence that the use of natural estrogens results in a different endometrial risk profile than synthetic estrogens of equivalent estrogen dose. Adding a progestin to estrogen therapy in postmenopausal women has been shown to reduce the risk of endometrial hyperplasia, which may be a precursor to endometrial cancer.

c. Ovarian Cancer

The WHI estrogen plus progestin substudy reported a statistically non-significant increased risk of ovarian cancer. After an average follow-up of 5.6 years, the relative risk for ovarian cancer for CE plus MPA versus placebo was 1.58 (95 percent nCI, 0.77 – 3.24). The absolute risk for CE plus MPA versus placebo was 4 versus 3 cases per 10,000 women-years. In some epidemiologic studies, the use of estrogen plus progestin and estrogen-only products, in particular for 5 or more years, has been associated with an increased risk of ovarian cancer. However, the duration of exposure associated with increased risk is not consistent across all epidemiologic studies and some report no association.

3. Probable dementia

In the estrogen plus progestin Women's Health Initiative Memory Study (WHIMS), an ancillary study of WHI, a population of 4,532 postmenopausal women 65 to 79 years of age was randomized to daily CE (0.625 mg) plus MPA (2.5 mg) or placebo.

In the WHIMS estrogen plus progestin ancillary study, after an average follow-up of 4 years, 40 women in the CE plus MPA group and 21 women in the placebo group were diagnosed with probable dementia. The relative risk of probable dementia for estrogen plus progestin versus placebo was 2.05 (95 percent CI, 1.21-3.48). The absolute risk of probable dementia for CE plus MPA versus placebo was 45 versus 22 cases per 10,000 women-years. It is unknown whether these findings apply to younger postmenopausal women. (See **CLINICAL STUDIES** and **PRECAUTIONS, Geriatric Use**.)

4. Vision abnormalities

Retinal vascular thrombosis has been reported in patients receiving estrogen. Discontinue estrogen plus progestin therapy pending examination if there is sudden partial or complete loss of vision, or if there is a sudden onset of proptosis, diplopia or migraine. If examination reveals papilledema or retinal vascular lesions, estrogen plus progestin therapy should be permanently discontinued.

PRECAUTIONS

A. General

1. Addition of a progestin when a woman has not had a hysterectomy

Studies of the addition of a progestin for 10 or more days of a cycle of estrogen administration, or daily with estrogen in a continuous regimen, have reported a lowered incidence of endometrial hyperplasia than would be induced by estrogen treatment alone. Endometrial hyperplasia may be a precursor to endometrial cancer.

There are, however, possible risks that may be associated with the use of progestins with estrogens compared with estrogen-alone regimens. These include an increased risk of breast cancer.

2. Fluid Retention

Progesterone may cause some degree of fluid retention. Women with conditions that might be influenced by this factor, such as cardiac or renal dysfunction, warrant careful observation.

3. Dizziness and Drowsiness

PROMETRIUM® (progesterone, USP) Capsules may cause transient dizziness and drowsiness and should be used with caution when driving a motor vehicle or operating machinery. PROMETRIUM Capsules should be taken as a single daily dose at bedtime.

B. Patient Information

General: This product contains peanut oil and should not be used if you are allergic to peanuts.

Physicians are advised to discuss the contents of the Patient Information leaflet with patients for whom they prescribe PROMETRIUM Capsules.

C. Drug-Laboratory Test Interactions

The following laboratory results may be altered by the use of estrogen plus progestin therapy:

- Increased sulfobromophthalein retention and other hepatic function tests.
- Coagulation tests: increase in prothrombin factors VII, VIII, IX and X.
- Pregnanediol determination.
- Thyroid function: increase in PBI, and butanol extractable protein bound iodine and decrease in T3 uptake values.

D. Carcinogenesis, Mutagenesis, Impairment of Fertility

Progesterone has not been tested for carcinogenicity in animals by the oral route of administration. When implanted into female mice, progesterone produced mammary carcinomas, ovarian granulosa cell tumors and endometrial stromal sarcomas. In dogs, long-term intramuscular injections produced nodular hyperplasia and benign and malignant mammary tumors. Subcutaneous or intramuscular injections of progesterone decreased the latency period and increased the incidence of mammary tumors in rats previously treated with a chemical carcinogen.

Progesterone did not show evidence of genotoxicity in *in vitro* studies for point mutations or for chromosomal damage. *In vivo* studies for chromosome damage have yielded positive results in mice at oral doses of 1000 mg/kg and 2000 mg/kg. Exogenously administered progesterone has been shown to inhibit ovulation in a number of species and it is expected that high doses given for an extended duration would impair fertility until the cessation of treatment.

E. Pregnancy

PROMETRIUM Capsules should not be used during pregnancy. (See **CONTRAINDICATIONS**).

Pregnancy Category B: Reproductive studies have been performed in mice at doses up to 9 times the human oral dose, in rats at doses up to 44 times the human oral dose, in rabbits at a dose of 10 mcg/day delivered locally within the uterus by an implanted device, in guinea pigs at doses of approximately one-half the human oral dose and in rhesus monkeys at doses approximately the human dose, all based on body surface area, and have revealed little or no evidence of impaired fertility or harm to the fetus due to progesterone.

F. Nursing Women

Detectable amounts of progestin have been identified in the milk of nursing women receiving progestins. Caution should be exercised when PROMETRIUM Capsules are administered to a nursing woman.

G. Pediatric Use

PROMETRIUM Capsules are not indicated in children. Clinical studies have not been conducted in the pediatric population.

H. Geriatric Use

There have not been sufficient numbers of geriatric women involved in clinical studies utilizing PROMETRIUM Capsules to determine whether those over 65 years of age differ from younger subjects in their response to PROMETRIUM Capsules.

The Women's Health Initiative Study

In the Women's Health Initiative (WHI) estrogen plus progestin substudy (daily CE [0.625 mg] plus MPA [2.5 mg] versus placebo), there was a higher relative risk of nonfatal stroke and invasive breast cancer in women greater than 65 years of age. (See **CLINICAL STUDIES** and **WARNINGS, Cardiovascular disorders** and **Malignant neoplasms**.)

The Women's Health Initiative Memory Study

In the Women's Health Initiative Memory Study (WHIMS) of postmenopausal women 65 to 79 years of age, there was an increased risk of developing probable dementia in the estrogen plus progestin ancillary study when compared to placebo. (See **CLINICAL STUDIES** and **WARNINGS, Probable dementia**.)

ADVERSE REACTIONS

See **BOXED WARNING**, **WARNINGS** and **PRECAUTIONS**.

Because clinical trials are conducted under widely varying conditions, adverse reaction rates observed in the clinical trials of a drug cannot be directly compared to rates in the clinical trials of another drug and may not reflect the rates observed in practice.

In a multicenter, randomized, double-blind, placebo-controlled clinical trial, the effects of PROMETRIUM Capsules on the endometrium was studied in a total of 875 postmenopausal women. Table 6 lists adverse reactions greater than or equal to 2 percent of women who received cyclic PROMETRIUM Capsules 200 mg daily (12 days per calendar month cycle) with 0.625 mg conjugated estrogens or placebo.

TABLE 6. Adverse Reactions (≥ 2%) Reported in an 875 Patient Placebo-Controlled Trial in Postmenopausal Women Over a 3-Year Period [Percentage (%) of Patients Reporting]

	PROMETRIUM Capsules 200 mg with Conjugated Estrogens 0.625 mg	Placebo
	(n=178)	(n=174)
Headache	31	27
Breast Tenderness	27	6
Joint Pain	20	29
Depression	19	12
Dizziness	15	9
Abdominal Bloating	12	5
Hot Flashes	11	35
Urinary Problems	11	9
Abdominal Pain	10	10
Vaginal Discharge	10	3
Nausea / Vomiting	8	7
Worry	8	4
Chest Pain	7	5
Diarrhea	7	4
Night Sweats	7	17
Breast Pain	6	2
Swelling of Hands and Feet	6	9
Vaginal Dryness	6	10
Constipation	3	2
Breast Carcinoma	2	<1
Breast Excisional Biopsy	2	<1
Cholecystectomy	2	<1

Effects on Secondary Amenorrhea

In a multicenter, randomized, double-blind, placebo-controlled clinical trial, the effects of PROMETRIUM Capsules on secondary amenorrhea was studied in 49 estrogen-primed postmenopausal women. Table 7 lists adverse reactions greater than or equal to 5 percent of women who received PROMETRIUM Capsules or placebo.

TABLE 7. Adverse Reactions (≥ 5%) Reported in Patients Using 400 mg/day in a Placebo-Controlled Trial in Estrogen-Primed Postmenopausal Women

Adverse Experience	PROMETRIUM Capsules 400 mg	Placebo
	n=25	n=24
	Percentage (%) of Patients	
Fatigue	8	4
Headache	16	8
Dizziness	24	4
Abdominal Distention (Bloating)	8	8
Abdominal Pain (Cramping)	20	13
Diarrhea	8	4
Nausea	8	0
Back Pain	8	8
Musculoskeletal Pain	12	4
Irritability	8	4
Breast Pain	16	8
Infection Viral	12	0
Coughing	8	0

In a multicenter, parallel-group, open label postmarketing dosing study consisting of three consecutive 28-day treatment cycles, 220 premenopausal women with secondary amenorrhea were randomized to receive daily conjugated estrogens therapy (0.625 mg conjugated estrogens) and PROMETRIUM Capsules, 300 mg per day (n=113) or PROMETRIUM Capsules, 400 mg per /day (n=107) for 10 days of each treatment cycle. Overall, the most frequently reported treatment-emergent adverse reactions, reported in greater than or equal to 5 percent of subjects, were nausea, fatigue, vaginal mycosis, nasopharyngitis, upper respiratory tract infection, headache, dizziness, breast tenderness, abdominal distension, acne, dysmenorrhea, mood swing, and urinary tract infection.

Postmarketing Experience:

The following additional adverse reactions have been reported with PROMETRIUM Capsules. Because these reactions are reported voluntarily from a population of uncertain size, it is not always possible to reliably estimate the frequency or establish a causal relationship to drug exposure.

Genitourinary System: endometrial carcinoma, hypospadia, intra-uterine death, menorrhagia, menstrual disorder, metrorrhagia, ovarian cyst, spontaneous abortion.

Cardiovascular: circulatory collapse, congenital heart disease (including ventricular septal defect and patent ductus arteriosus), hypertension, hypotension, tachycardia.

Gastrointestinal: acute pancreatitis, cholestasis, cholestatic hepatitis, dysphagia, hepatic failure, hepatic necrosis, hepatitis, increased liver function tests (including alanine aminotransferase increased, aspartate aminotransferase increased, gamma-glutamyl transferase increased), jaundice, swollen tongue.

Skin: alopecia, pruritus, urticaria.

Eyes: blurred vision, diplopia, visual disturbance.

Central Nervous System: aggression, convulsion, depersonalization, depressed consciousness, disorientation, dysarthria, loss of consciousness, paresthesia, sedation, stupor, syncope (with and without hypotension), transient ischemic attack, suicidal ideation.

During initial therapy, a few women have experienced a constellation of many or all of the following symptoms: extreme dizziness and/or drowsiness, blurred vision, slurred speech, difficulty walking, loss of consciousness, vertigo, confusion, disorientation, feeling drunk, and shortness of breath.

Miscellaneous: abnormal gait, anaphylactic reaction, arthralgia, blood glucose increased, choking, cleft lip, cleft palate, difficulty walking, dyspnea, face edema, feeling abnormal, feeling drunk, hypersensitivity, asthma, muscle cramp, throat tightness, tinnitus, vertigo, weight decreased, weight increased.

OVERDOSAGE

No studies on overdosage have been conducted in humans. In the case of overdosage, PROMETRIUM Capsules should be discontinued and the patient should be treated symptomatically.

DOSAGE AND ADMINISTRATION

Prevention of Endometrial Hyperplasia

PROMETRIUM Capsules should be given as a single daily dose at bedtime, 200 mg orally for 12 days sequentially per 28-day cycle, to a postmenopausal woman with a uterus who is receiving daily conjugated estrogens tablets.

Treatment of Secondary Amenorrhea

PROMETRIUM Capsules may be given as a single daily dose of 400 mg at bedtime for 10 days.

Some women may experience difficulty swallowing PROMETRIUM Capsules. For these women, PROMETRIUM Capsules should be taken with a glass of water while in the standing position.

HOW SUPPLIED

PROMETRIUM (progesterone, USP) Capsules 100 mg are round, peach-colored capsules branded with black imprint "SV."

NDC 0032-1708-01 (Bottle of 100)

PROMETRIUM (progesterone, USP) Capsules 200 mg are oval, pale yellow-colored capsules branded with black imprint "SV2."

NDC 0032-1711-01 (Bottle of 100)

Store at 25°C (77°F); excursions permitted to 15° to 30°C (59° to 86°F) [See USP Controlled Room Temperature].

Protect from excessive moisture.

Dispense in tight, light-resistant container as defined in USP/NF, accompanied by a Patient Insert.

Keep out of reach of children.

Manufactured by:
Catalent Pharma Solutions
St. Petersburg, FL 33716

Marketed by:
AbbVie Inc.
North Chicago, IL 60064, USA

500032 Rev 02/13-Revised: February, 2013

PATIENT INFORMATION

PROMETRIUM® (progesterone, USP)
Capsules 100 mg
Capsules 200 mg

Read this PATIENT INFORMATION before you start taking PROMETRIUM Capsules and read what you get each time you refill your PROMETRIUM Capsules prescription. There may be new information. This information does not take the place of talking to your healthcare provider about your medical condition or your treatment.

WHAT IS THE MOST IMPORTANT INFORMATION I SHOULD KNOW ABOUT PROMETRIUM CAPSULES (A Progesterone Hormone)?

- Progestins with estrogens should not be used to prevent heart disease, heart attacks, strokes, or dementia.
- Using progestins with estrogens may increase your chance of getting heart attacks, strokes, breast cancer, and blood clots.
- Using progestins with estrogens may increase your chance of getting dementia, based on a study of women age 65 and older.
- You and your healthcare provider should talk regularly about whether you still need treatment with PROMETRIUM Capsules.

THIS PRODUCT CONTAINS PEANUT OIL AND SHOULD NOT BE USED IF YOU ARE ALLERGIC TO PEANUTS.

What is PROMETRIUM Capsules?

PROMETRIUM Capsules contain the female hormone called progesterone.

What is PROMETRIUM Capsules used for?

Treatment of Menstrual Irregularities

PROMETRIUM Capsules are used for the treatment of secondary amenorrhea (absence of menstrual periods in women who have previously had a menstrual period) due to a decrease in progesterone. When you do not produce enough progesterone, menstrual irregularities can occur. If your healthcare provider has determined your body does not produce enough progesterone on its own, PROMETRIUM Capsules may be prescribed to provide the progesterone you need.

Protection of the Endometrium (Lining of the Uterus)

PROMETRIUM Capsules are used in combination with estrogen-containing medications in a postmenopausal woman with a uterus (womb). Taking estrogen-alone increases the chance of developing a condition called endometrial hyperplasia that may lead to cancer of the lining of the uterus (womb). The addition of a progestin is generally recommended for a woman with a uterus to reduce the chance of getting cancer of the uterus (womb).

Who should not take PROMETRIUM Capsules?

Do not start taking PROMETRIUM Capsules if you:

- **Are allergic to peanuts**
- **Have unusual vaginal bleeding**
- **Currently have or have had certain cancers**
  Estrogen plus progestin treatment may increase the chance of getting certain types of cancers, including cancer of the breast or uterus. If you have or have had cancer, talk with your healthcare provider about whether you should take PROMETRIUM Capsules.
- **Had a stroke or heart attack**
- **Currently have or have had blood clots**
- **Currently have or have had liver problems**
- **Are allergic to PROMETRIUM Capsules or any of its ingredients**
  See the list of ingredients in PROMETRIUM Capsules at the end of this leaflet.
- **Think you may be pregnant**

Tell your healthcare provider:

- **If you are breastfeeding.** The hormone in PROMETRIUM Capsules can pass into your breast milk.

Information on the AbbVie, Inc. products listed on these pages is from the prescribing information in use as of July 31, 2013. For more information, please visit rxabbvie.com or call 1-800-633-9110.

- **About all of your medical problems.** Your healthcare provider may need to check you more carefully if you have certain conditions, such as asthma (wheezing), epilepsy (seizures), diabetes, migraine, endometriosis, lupus, problems with your heart, liver, thyroid, or kidneys, or have high calcium levels in your blood.
- **About all the medicines you take.** This includes prescription and nonprescription medicines, vitamins, and herbal supplements. Some medicines may affect how PROMETRIUM Capsules work. PROMETRIUM Capsules may also affect how your other medicines work.

How should I take PROMETRIUM Capsules?

1. Prevention of Endometrial Hyperplasia: A postmenopausal woman with a uterus who is taking estrogens should take a single daily dose of 200 mg PROMETRIUM Capsules at bedtime for 12 continuous days per 28-day cycle.
2. Secondary Amenorrhea: PROMETRIUM Capsules may be given as a single daily dose of 400 mg at bedtime for 10 days.
3. **PROMETRIUM Capsules are to be taken at bedtime as some women become very drowsy and/or dizzy after taking PROMETRIUM Capsules. In a few cases, symptoms may include blurred vision, difficulty speaking, difficulty with walking, and feeling abnormal. If you experience these symptoms, discuss them with your healthcare provider right away.**
4. If you experience difficulty in swallowing PROMETRIUM Capsules, it is recommended that you take your daily dose at bedtime with a glass of water while in the standing position.

What are the possible side effects of PROMETRIUM Capsules?

Side effects are grouped by how serious they are and how often they happen when you are treated:

Serious, but less common side effects include:

- ***Risk to the Fetus:*** Cases of cleft palate, cleft lip, hypospadias, ventricular septal defect, patent ductus arteriosus, and other congenital heart defects.
- ***Abnormal Blood Clotting:*** Stroke, heart attack, pulmonary embolus, visual loss or blindness.

Some of the warning signs of serious side effects include:

- Changes in vision or speech
- Sudden new severe headaches
- Severe pains in your chest or legs with or without shortness of breath, weakness and fatigue
- Dizziness and faintness
- Vomiting

Call your healthcare provider right away if you get any of these warning signs, or any other unusual symptoms that concern you.

Less serious, but common side effects include:

- Headaches
- Breast pain
- Irregular vaginal bleeding or spotting
- Stomach or abdominal cramps, bloating
- Nausea and vomiting
- Hair loss
- Fluid retention
- Vaginal yeast infection

These are not all the possible side effects of PROMETRIUM Capsules. For more information, ask your healthcare provider or pharmacist for advice about side effects. You may report side effects to AbbVie Inc. at 1-800-633-9110 or to FDA at 1-800-FDA-1088.

What can I do to lower my chances of getting a serious side effect with PROMETRIUM Capsules?

- Talk with your healthcare provider regularly about whether you should continue taking PROMETRIUM Capsules.
- See your healthcare provider right away if you get unusual vaginal bleeding while taking PROMETRIUM Capsules.
- Have a pelvic exam, breast exam, and mammogram (breast X-ray) every year unless your healthcare provider tells you something else. If members of your family have had breast cancer or if you have ever had breast lumps or an abnormal mammogram, you may need to have breast exams more often.
- If you have high blood pressure, high cholesterol (fat in the blood), diabetes, are overweight, or if you use tobacco, you may have higher chances for getting heart disease. Ask your healthcare provider for ways to lower your chances for getting heart disease.

General information about safe and effective use of PROMETRIUM Capsules

- Medicines are sometimes prescribed for conditions that are not mentioned in patient information leaflets. Do not take PROMETRIUM Capsules for conditions for which it was not prescribed.
- Your healthcare provider has prescribed this drug for you and you alone. Do not give PROMETRIUM Capsules to other people, even if they have the same symptoms you have. It may harm them.
- PROMETRIUM Capsules should be taken as a single daily dose at bedtime. Some women may experience extreme dizziness and/or drowsiness during initial therapy. In a few cases, symptoms may include blurred vision, difficulty speaking, difficulty with walking, and feeling abnormal. If you experience these symptoms, discuss them with your healthcare provider right away.
- Use caution when driving a motor vehicle or operating machinery as dizziness or drowsiness may occur.

Keep PROMETRIUM Capsules out of the reach of children.

This leaflet provides a summary of the most important information about PROMETRIUM Capsules. If you would like more information, talk with your healthcare provider or pharmacist. You can ask for information about PROMETRIUM Capsules that is written for health professionals. You can get more information by calling the toll free number 1-800-633-9110.

What are the ingredients in PROMETRIUM Capsules?

Active ingredient: 100 mg or 200 mg micronized progesterone

The inactive ingredients for PROMETRIUM Capsules 100 mg include: peanut oil NF, gelatin NF, glycerin USP, lecithin NF, titanium dioxide USP, D&C Yellow No. 10, and FD&C Red No. 40.

The inactive ingredients for PROMETRIUM Capsules 200 mg include: peanut oil NF, gelatin NF, glycerin USP, lecithin NF, titanium dioxide USP, D&C Yellow No. 10, and FD&C Yellow No. 6.

HOW SUPPLIED

PROMETRIUM Capsules 100 mg are round, peach-colored capsules branded with black imprint "SV."

PROMETRIUM Capsules 200 mg are oval, pale yellow-colored capsules branded with black imprint "SV2."

Store at 25°C (77°F); excursions permitted to 15° to 30°C (59° to 86°F) [See USP Controlled Room Temperature].

Protect from excessive moisture.

Manufactured by:

Catalent Pharma Solutions
St. Petersburg, FL 33716

Marketed by:

AbbVie Inc.
North Chicago, IL 60064, USA

500033 Rev 02/13 Revised: February, 2013

SIMCOR® ℞

[sĭm-kŏr]

(niacin extended-release/simvastatin) tablets

HIGHLIGHTS OF PRESCRIBING INFORMATION

These highlights do not include all the information needed to use SIMCOR® safely and effectively. See full prescribing information for SIMCOR.

SIMCOR (niacin extended-release/simvastatin) tablet, film coated for oral use.

Initial U.S. Approval: 2008

RECENT MAJOR CHANGES

Warnings and Precautions, Myopathy/ Rhabdomyolysis (5.2)	10/2012
Adverse Reactions, Postmarketing Experience (6.2)	10/2012
Indications and Usage, Limitations of Use (1.1)	02/2013
Warnings and Precautions, Mortality and Coronary Heart Disease Morbidity (5.1)	02/2013
Adverse Reactions, Clinical Studies Experience (6.1)	02/2013

INDICATIONS AND USAGE

SIMCOR is a combination of simvastatin, an HMG-Co-A reductase inhibitor, and niacin extended-release (NIASPAN), nicotinic acid. SIMCOR is indicated to:

- Reduce elevated Total-C, LDL-C, Apo B, non-HDL-C, TG, or to increase HDL-C in patients with primary hypercholesterolemia and mixed dyslipidemia when treatment with simvastatin monotherapy or niacin extended-release monotherapy is considered inadequate. (1.1)
- Reduce TG in patients with hypertriglyceridemia when treatment with simvastatin monotherapy or niacin extended-release monotherapy is considered inadequate. (1.1)

Limitations of use:

No incremental benefit of SIMCOR on cardiovascular morbidity and mortality over and above that demonstrated for simvastatin monotherapy and niacin monotherapy has been established. (1.1)

Niacin extended-release, one of the components of SIMCOR, at doses of 1,500 – 2,000 mg/day, in combination with simvastatin, did not reduce the incidence of cardiovascular events more than simvastatin in a randomized controlled trial of patients with cardiovascular disease and mean baseline LDL-C levels of 74 mg per deciliter (5.1).

DOSAGE AND ADMINISTRATION

- SIMCOR should be taken at bedtime with a low-fat snack. (2)
- Dose range: 500/20 mg to 2000/40 mg once daily. (2)
- Initial dose for patients naïve to or switching from immediate-release niacin: 500/20 mg once daily. (2)
- The initial dose for patients already receiving niacin extended-release should not exceed 2000/40 mg once daily. (2)
- Maintenance dose: 1000/20 mg to 2000/40 mg once daily. (2)
- Doses greater than 2000/40 mg daily are not recommended. (2)

DOSAGE FORMS AND STRENGTHS

- Unscored film-coated tablets:
  500 mg niacin extended-release/20 mg simvastatin (3)
  500 mg niacin extended-release/40 mg simvastatin (3)
  750 mg niacin extended-release/20 mg simvastatin (3)
  1000 mg niacin extended-release/20 mg simvastatin (3)
  1000 mg niacin extended-release/40 mg simvastatin (3)

CONTRAINDICATIONS

- Active liver disease, which may include unexplained persistent elevations in hepatic transaminase levels (4, 5.3)
- Active peptic ulcer disease (4)
- Arterial bleeding (4)
- Concomitant administration of strong CYP3A4 inhibitors (4, 5.2)
- Concomitant administration of gemfibrozil, cyclosporine, or danazol (4, 5.2)
- Concomitant administration of verapamil or diltiazem (4, 5.2)
- Women who are pregnant or may become pregnant (4, 8.1)
- Nursing mothers (4, 8.3)
- Known hypersensitivity to product components (4, 6.1)

WARNINGS AND PRECAUTIONS

- Skeletal muscle effects (e.g., myopathy and rhabdomyolysis): Risks increase with higher doses and concomitant use of certain medicines. Predisposing factors include advanced age (≥ 65), female gender, uncontrolled hypothyroidism, and renal impairment. Patients should be advised to report promptly any unexplained and/or persistent muscle pain, tenderness, or weakness. SIMCOR therapy should be discontinued immediately if myopathy is diagnosed or suspected. (4, 5.2, 8.5, 8.7)
- Liver enzyme abnormalities: Persistent elevations in hepatic transaminases can occur. Check liver enzyme tests before initiating therapy and as clinically indicated thereafter. (5.3)
- Severe hepatic toxicity has occurred in patients substituting sustained-release niacin for immediate-release niacin at equivalent doses. If switching from niacin preparations other than niacin extended-release (NIASPAN), initiate with lowest SIMCOR dose; niacin extended-release can be converted at equivalent doses. (5.3)
- Niacin extended-release can increase serum glucose levels. Glucose levels should be closely monitored in diabetic or potentially diabetic patients particularly during the first few months of use. (5.4)

ADVERSE REACTIONS

The most common (incidence > 3%) adverse reactions with SIMCOR are flushing, headache, back pain, diarrhea, nausea, and pruritus. (6.1)

To report SUSPECTED ADVERSE REACTIONS, contact AbbVie Inc. at 1-800-633-9110 or FDA at 1-800-FDA-1088 or www.fda.gov/medwatch.

DRUG INTERACTIONS

Drug Interactions Associated with Increased Risk of Myopathy/Rhabdomyolysis (2.2, 4, 5.2, 7.1, 7.2, 7.3, 7.4, 12.3)

Interacting Agents	Prescribing Recommendations
Strong CYP3A4 inhibitors (e.g., itraconazole, ketoconazole, posaconazole, erythromycin, clarithromycin, telithromycin, HIV protease inhibitors, boceprevir, telaprevir, nefazodone), gemfibrozil, cyclosporine, danazol, verapamil, diltiazem	Contraindicated with SIMCOR
Amiodarone, amlodipine, ranolazine	Do not exceed 1000/20 mg SIMCOR daily
Grapefruit juice	Avoid large quantities of grapefruit juice (>1 quart daily)

- Fenofibrate: Combination with SIMCOR increases the risk of adverse skeletal muscle effects and should be avoided. (7.3)
- Coumarin anticoagulants: Combination prolongs INR. Achieve stable INR prior to starting SIMCOR. Monitor INR frequently until stable upon initiation or alteration of SIMCOR therapy. (7.7)

USE IN SPECIFIC POPULATIONS

- Severe renal impairment (not on dialysis): SIMCOR should be used with extreme caution. (8.7)

See 17 for PATIENT COUNSELING INFORMATION

Revised: 03/2013

FULL PRESCRIBING INFORMATION: CONTENTS*

* Sections or subsections omitted from the full prescribing information are not listed

FULL PRESCRIBING INFORMATION

1 INDICATIONS AND USAGE

Therapy with lipid-altering agents should be only one component of multiple risk factor intervention in individuals at significantly increased risk for atherosclerotic vascular disease due to hypercholesterolemia. Drug therapy is indicated as an adjunct to diet when the response to a diet restricted in saturated fat and cholesterol and other nonpharmacologic measures alone has been inadequate.

1.1 Patients with Hypercholesterolemia Requiring Modifications of Lipid Profiles

SIMCOR

SIMCOR is indicated to reduce Total-C, LDL-C, Apo B, non-HDL-C, TG, or to increase HDL-C in patients with primary hypercholesterolemia and mixed dyslipidemia when treatment with simvastatin monotherapy or niacin extended-release monotherapy is considered inadequate.

SIMCOR is indicated to reduce TG in patients with hypertriglyceridemia when treatment with simvastatin monotherapy or niacin extended-release monotherapy is considered inadequate.

Limitations of use

No incremental benefit of SIMCOR on cardiovascular morbidity and mortality over and above that demonstrated for simvastatin monotherapy and niacin monotherapy has been established.

Niacin extended-release, one of the components of SIMCOR, at doses of 1,500 – 2,000 mg/day, in combination with simvastatin, did not reduce the incidence of cardiovascular events more than simvastatin in a randomized controlled trial of patients with cardiovascular disease and mean baseline LDL-C levels of 74 mg per deciliter *[see Warnings and Precautions (5.1)]*.

2 DOSAGE AND ADMINISTRATION

2.1 Recommended Dosing

SIMCOR should be taken as a single daily dose at bedtime, with a low fat snack. Patients not currently on niacin extended-release and patients currently on niacin products other than niacin extended-release should start SIMCOR at a single 500/20 mg tablet daily at bedtime. Patients already taking simvastatin 20 to 40 mg who need additional management of their lipid levels may be started on a SIMCOR dose of 500/40 mg once daily at bedtime *[see Warnings and Precautions (5.3)]*. The dose of niacin extended-release should not be increased by more than 500 mg daily every 4 weeks - see Table 1.

Table 1. Recommended niacin extended-release dosing

	Week(s)	Daily dose of niacin extended-release
Initial Titration Schedule	1 to 4	500 mg
	5 to 8	1000 mg
	*	1500 mg
	*	2000 mg

* After Week 8, titrate to patient response and tolerance. If response to 1000 mg daily is inadequate, increase dose to 1500 mg daily; may subsequently increase dose to 2000 mg daily. Daily dose should not be increased more than 500 mg in a 4-week period, and doses above 2000 mg daily are not recommended.

The recommended maintenance dose for SIMCOR is 1000/20 mg to 2000/40 mg (two 1000/20 mg tablets) once daily depending on patient tolerability and lipid levels. **The efficacy and safety of doses of SIMCOR greater than 2000/40 mg daily have not been studied and are therefore not recommended.**

If SIMCOR therapy is discontinued for an extended period of time (> 7 days), re-titration as tolerated is recommended. SIMCOR tablets should be taken whole and should not be broken, crushed, or chewed before swallowing.

Due to the increased risk of hepatotoxicity with other modified-release (sustained-release or time-release) niacin preparations or immediate-release (crystalline) niacin, SIMCOR should only be substituted for equivalent doses of niacin extended-release (NIASPAN).

Flushing *[see Adverse Reactions (6.1)]* may be reduced in frequency or severity by pretreatment with aspirin up to the recommended dose of 325 mg (taken approximately 30 minutes prior to SIMCOR dose). Flushing, pruritus, and gastrointestinal distress are also reduced by gradually increasing the dose of niacin (refer to Table 1) and avoiding administration on an empty stomach. Concomitant alcoholic, hot drinks or spicy foods may increase the side effects of flushing and pruritus and should be avoided around the time of SIMCOR ingestion.

2.2 Coadministration with Other Drugs

Patients taking Amiodarone, Amlodipine or Ranolazine

- The dose of SIMCOR should not exceed 1000/20 mg/day *[see Warnings and Precautions (5.2), Drug Interactions (7.4), and Clinical Pharmacology (12.3)]*.

2.3 Chinese Patients Taking SIMCOR

Because of an increased risk for myopathy in Chinese patients taking simvastatin 40 mg coadministered with lipid-modifying doses (≥1 g/day niacin) of niacin-containing products, caution should be used when prescribing SIMCOR in doses that exceed 1000/20 mg/day to Chinese patients. The cause of the increased risk of myopathy is not known. It is also unknown if the risk for myopathy with coadministration of simvastatin with lipid-modifying doses of niacin-containing products observed in Chinese patients applies to other Asian patients *[see Warnings and Precautions (5.2)]*.

3 DOSAGE FORMS AND STRENGTHS

SIMCOR tablets are formulated for oral administration in the following strength combinations:

[See table 2 above]

Table 2. SIMCOR Tablet Strengths

	500mg/20mg	500mg/40mg	750mg/20mg	1000mg/20mg	1000mg/40mg
Niacin extended-release equivalent (mg)	500	500	750	1000	1000
simvastatin equivalent (mg)	20	40	20	20	40

4 CONTRAINDICATIONS

SIMCOR is contraindicated in the following conditions:

- Active liver disease, which may include unexplained persistent elevations in hepatic transaminase levels *[see Warnings and Precautions (5.3)]*
- Patients with active peptic ulcer disease
- Patients with arterial bleeding
- Concomitant administration of strong CYP3A4 inhibitors (e.g. itraconazole, ketoconazole, posaconazole, HIV protease inhibitors, boceprevir, telaprevir, erythromycin, clarithromycin, telithromycin and nefazodone) *[see Warnings and Precautions (5.2)]*
- Concomitant administration of gemfibrozil, cyclosporine, or danazol *[see Warnings and Precautions (5.2)]*
- Concomitant administration of verapamil or diltiazem *[see Warnings and Precautions (5.2)]*
- Women who are pregnant or may become pregnant. SIMCOR may cause fetal harm when administered to a pregnant woman. Serum cholesterol and triglycerides increase during normal pregnancy, and cholesterol or cholesterol derivatives are essential for fetal development. Atherosclerosis is a chronic process and discontinuation of lipid-lowering drugs during pregnancy should have little impact on long-term outcomes of primary hypercholesterolemia therapy. There are no adequate and well-controlled studies of SIMCOR use during pregnancy; however in rare reports congenital anomalies were observed following intrauterine exposure to HMG-CoA reductase inhibitors. If SIMCOR is used during pregnancy or if the patient becomes pregnant while taking this drug, the patient should be apprised of the potential hazard to the fetus *[see Use In Specific Populations (8.1)]*. In rat and rabbit animal reproduction studies, simvastatin revealed no evidence of teratogenicity. There are no animal reproductive studies conducted with niacin.
- Nursing mothers. SIMCOR contains simvastatin and nicotinic acid. Nicotinic acid is excreted into human milk and it is not known whether simvastatin is excreted into human milk; however a small amount of another drug in this class does pass into breast milk. Because of the potential for serious adverse reactions in nursing infants, women who require SIMCOR treatment should not breastfeed their infants *[see Use In Specific Populations (8.3)]*.
- Patients with a known hypersensitivity to any component of this product. Hypersensitivity reactions including one of more of the following adverse reactions have been reported for simvastatin and/or niacin extended-release: anaphylaxis, angioedema, urticaria, fever, dyspnea, tongue edema, larynx edema, face edema, peripheral edema, laryngismus, and flushing *[see Adverse Reactions (6.1)]*.

5 WARNINGS AND PRECAUTIONS

SIMCOR should not be substituted for equivalent doses of immediate-release (crystalline) niacin. For patients switch-

Information on the AbbVie, Inc. products listed on these pages is from the prescribing information in use as of July 31, 2013. For more information, please visit rxabbvie.com or call 1-800-633-9110.

ing from immediate-release niacin to SIMCOR, therapy with SIMCOR should be initiated at 500/20 mg and appropriately titrated to the desired therapeutic response. Patients already taking simvastatin 20-40 mg who need additional management of their lipid levels may be started on a SIMCOR dose of 500/40 mg once daily at bedtime. Doses of SIMCOR greater than 2000/40 mg are not recommended.

5.1 Mortality and Coronary Heart Disease Morbidity

The Atherothrombosis Intervention in Metabolic Syndrome with Low HDL/High Triglycerides: Impact on Global Health Outcomes (AIM-HIGH) trial was a randomized placebo-controlled trial of 3414 patients with stable, previously diagnosed cardiovascular disease. Mean baseline lipid levels were LDL-C 74 mg/dL, HDL-C 35 mg/dL, non-HDL-C 111 mg/dL and median triglyceride level of 163-177 mg/dL. Ninety-four percent of patients were on background statin therapy prior to entering the trial. All participants received simvastatin, 40 to 80 mg per day, plus ezetimibe 10 mg per day if needed, to maintain an LDL-C level of 40-80 mg/dL, and were randomized to receive niacin extended-release tablets 1500-2000 mg/day (n=1718) or matching placebo (niacin immediate-release tablets, 100-150 mg, n=1696).

On-treatment lipid changes at two years for LDL-C were -12.0% for the simvastatin plus niacin extended-release group and -5.5% for the simvastatin plus placebo group. HDL-C increased by 25.0% to 42 mg/dL in the simvastatin plus niacin extended-release group and by 9.8% to 38 mg/dL in the simvastatin plus placebo group (P<0.001). Triglyceride levels decreased by 28.6% in the simvastatin plus niacin extended-release group and by 8.1% in the simvastatin plus placebo group.

The primary outcome was an ITT composite of the first study occurrence of coronary heart disease death, nonfatal myocardial infarction, ischemic stroke, hospitalization for acute coronary syndrome or symptom-driven coronary or cerebral revascularization procedures. The trial was stopped after a mean follow-up period of 3 years owing to a lack of efficacy. The primary outcome occurred in 282 patients in the simvastatin plus niacin extended-release group (16.4%) and in 274 patients in the simvastatin plus placebo group (16.2%) (HR 1.02 [95% CI, 0.87-1.21], P=0.79.

In an ITT analysis, there were 42 cases of first occurrence of ischemic stroke reported, 27 (1.6%) in the simvastatin plus niacin extended-release group and 15 (0.9%) in the simvastatin plus placebo group, a non-statistically significant result (HR 1.79, [95%CI = 0.95-3.36], p=0.071). The on-treatment ischemic stroke events were 19 for the simvastatin plus niacin extended-release group and 15 for the simvastatin plus placebo group *[see Adverse Reactions (6.1)]*.

5.2 Myopathy/Rhabdomyolysis

Simvastatin

Simvastatin occasionally causes myopathy manifested as muscle pain, tenderness or weakness with creatine kinase (CK) above ten times the upper limit of normal (ULN). Myopathy sometimes takes the form of rhabdomyolysis with or without acute renal failure secondary to myoglobinuria, and rare fatalities have occurred. The risk of myopathy is increased by high levels of HMG-CoA reductase inhibitory activity in plasma. Predisposing factors for myopathy include advanced age (≥65 years), female gender, uncontrolled hypothyroidism, and renal impairment.

The risk of myopathy/rhabdomyolysis is dose related. In a clinical trial database in which 41,413 patients were treated with simvastatin with 24,747 (approximately 60%) of whom were enrolled in studies with a median follow-up of at least 4 years, the incidence of myopathy was approximately 0.03% and 0.08% at 20 and 40 mg/day, respectively. The incidence of myopathy with 80 mg (0.61%) was disproportionately higher than that observed at the lower doses. In these trials, patients were carefully monitored and some interacting medicinal products were excluded.

In a clinical trial in which 12,064 patients with a history of myocardial infarction were treated with ZOCOR (mean follow-up 6.7 years), the incidence of myopathy (defined as unexplained muscle weakness or pain with a serum creatine kinase [CK] >10 times upper limit of normal [ULN]) in patients on 80 mg/day was approximately 0.9% compared with 0.02% for patients on 20 mg/day; the incidence of rhabdomyolysis (defined as myopathy with a CK >40 times ULN) was approximately 0.4% in patients on 80 mg/day compared with 0% for patients on 20 mg/day. The incidence of myopathy, including rhabdomyolysis, was highest during the first year and then notably decreased during the subsequent years of treatment. In this trial, patients were carefully monitored and some interacting medicinal products were excluded.

There have been rare reports of immune-mediated necrotizing myopathy (IMNM), an autoimmune myopathy, associated with statin use. IMNM is characterized by: proximal muscle weakness and elevated serum creatine kinase, which persist despite discontinuation of statin treatment; muscle biopsy showing necrotizing myopathy without significant inflammation; improvement with immunosuppressive agents.

All patients starting therapy with SIMCOR, or whose dose of SIMCOR is being increased, should be advised of the risk of myopathy, including rhabdomyolysis, and told to report promptly any unexplained muscle pain, tenderness or weakness particularly if accompanied by malaise or fever or if muscle signs and symptoms persist after discontinuing SIMCOR. SIMCOR therapy should be discontinued immediately if myopathy is diagnosed or suspected. In most cases, muscle symptoms and CK increases resolved when treatment was promptly discontinued. Periodic CK determinations may be considered in patients starting therapy with SIMCOR or whose dose is being increased, but there is no assurance that such monitoring will prevent myopathy.

Many of the patients who have developed rhabdomyolysis on therapy with simvastatin have had complicated medical histories, including renal insufficiency usually as a consequence of long-standing diabetes mellitus. Such patients merit closer monitoring. SIMCOR therapy should be discontinued if markedly elevated CPK levels occur or myopathy is diagnosed or suspected. SIMCOR therapy should also be temporarily withheld in any patient experiencing an acute or serious condition predisposing to the development of renal failure secondary to rhabdomyolysis, e.g., sepsis; hypotension; major surgery; trauma; severe metabolic, endocrine, or electrolyte disorders; or uncontrolled epilepsy.

Drug Interactions

The risk of myopathy and rhabdomyolysis is increased by high levels of statin activity in plasma. Simvastatin is metabolized by the cytochrome P450 isoform 3A4. Certain drugs which inhibit this metabolic pathway can raise the plasma levels of simvastatin and may increase the risk of myopathy. These include itraconazole, ketoconazole, and posaconazole, the macrolide antibiotics erythromycin and clarithromycin, and the ketolide antibiotic telithromycin, HIV protease inhibitors, boceprevir, telaprevir, the antidepressant nefazodone, or large quantities of grapefruit juice (>1 quart daily), and combination of these drugs with SIMCOR is contraindicated. If treatment with itraconazole, ketoconazole, posaconazole, erythromycin, clarithromycin or telithromycin is unavoidable, therapy with SIMCOR must be suspended during the course of treatment *[see Contraindications (4) and Drug Interactions (7.1)]*. *In vitro* studies have demonstrated a potential for voriconazole to inhibit the metabolism of simvastatin. Adjustment of the SIMCOR dose may be needed to reduce the risk of myopathy/rhabdomyolysis if voriconazole must be used concomitantly with simvastatin *[see Drug Interactions (7.1)]*.

The combined use of SIMCOR with gemfibrozil, cyclosporine, or danazol is contraindicated *[see Contraindications (4) and Drug Interactions (7.1)]*.

The combined use of SIMCOR with verapamil or diltiazem is contraindicated, because dosages of simvastatin are not to exceed 10 mg when these drugs are co-administered and all doses of SIMCOR contain simvastatin in excess of 10 mg *[see Contraindications (4) and Drug Interactions (7.2)]*.

The combined use of SIMCOR with drugs that cause myopathy/rhabdomyolysis when given alone, such as fibrates, should be avoided *[see Drug Interactions (7.3)]*.

Cases of myopathy, including rhabdomyolysis, have been reported with simvastatin coadministered with colchicine, and caution should be exercised when prescribing SIMCOR with colchicine *[see Drug Interactions (7.8)]*.

The benefits of the combined use of SIMCOR with amlodipine or ranolazine should be carefully weighed against the potential risks of combination *[see Drug Interactions (7.4)]*. Periodic CK determinations may be considered in patients starting therapy with or increasing the dose of these agents, but there is no assurance that such monitoring will prevent myopathy.

Cases of myopathy, including rhabdomyolysis, have been observed with simvastatin coadministered with lipid-modifying doses (≥1 g/day niacin) of niacin-containing products. In an ongoing, double-blind, randomized cardiovascular outcomes trial, an independent safety monitoring committee identified that the incidence of myopathy is higher in Chinese compared with non-Chinese patients taking simvastatin 40 mg coadministered with lipid modifying doses of a niacin-containing product. Caution should be used when prescribing SIMCOR in doses that exceed 1000/20 mg/day to Chinese patients. It is unknown if the risk for myopathy with coadministration of simvastatin with lipid modifying doses of niacin-containing products observed in Chinese patients applies to other Asian patients *[see Dosage and Administration (2.3)]*.

Prescribing recommendations for interacting agents are summarized in Table 3 *[see also Dosage and Administration (2.2), Contraindications (4), Drug Interactions (7), Clinical Pharmacology (12.3)]*.

Table 3.
Drug Interactions Associated with Increased Risk of Myopathy/Rhabdomyolysis

Interacting Agents	Prescribing Recommendations
Strong CYP3A4 inhibitors, e.g., Itraconazole Ketoconazole Posaconazole Erythromycin Clarithromycin Telithromycin HIV protease inhibitors Boceprevir Telaprevir Nefazodone Gemfibrozil Cyclosporine Danazol Verapamil Diltiazem	Contraindicated with SIMCOR
Amiodarone Amlodipine Ranolazine	Do not exceed 1000/20 mg SIMCOR daily
Grapefruit juice	Avoid large quantities of grapefruit juice (>1 quart daily)

SIMCOR

Myopathy and/or rhabdomyolysis have been reported when simvastatin is used in combination with lipid-altering doses (≥ 1 gram/day) of niacin. Physicians contemplating the use of SIMCOR, a combination of simvastatin and niacin extended-release (NIASPAN), should weigh the potential benefits and risks, and should carefully monitor for any signs and symptoms of muscle pain, tenderness, or weakness, particularly during the initial month of treatment or during any period of upward dosage titration of either drug. Periodic determination of serum creatine kinase (CK) determinations may be considered in such situations, but there is no assurance that such monitoring will prevent myopathy. Patients starting therapy with SIMCOR should be advised of the risk of myopathy, and told to report promptly unexplained muscle pain, tenderness, or weakness. A CK level above ten times the upper limit of normal (ULN) in a patient with unexplained muscle symptoms indicates myopathy. SIMCOR therapy should be discontinued if myopathy is diagnosed or suspected.

In patients with complicated medical histories predisposing to rhabdomyolysis, such as renal insufficiency, dose escalation requires caution. Also, as there are no known adverse consequences of brief interruption of therapy, treatment with SIMCOR should be stopped for a few days before elective major surgery and when any major acute medical or surgical condition supervenes (e.g., sepsis, hypotension, dehydration, major surgery, trauma, severe metabolic, endocrine, and electrolyte disorders, or uncontrolled seizures).

5.3 Liver Dysfunction

Cases of severe hepatic toxicity, including fulminant hepatic necrosis, have occurred in patients who have substituted sustained-release (modified-release, timed-release) niacin products for immediate-release (crystalline) niacin at equivalent doses. Patients previously receiving niacin products other than niacin extended-release (NIASPAN) should be started on SIMCOR at the lowest recommended starting dose *[see Dosage and Administration (2)]*.

SIMCOR should be used with caution in patients who consume substantial quantities of alcohol and/or have a past history of liver disease. Active liver disease or unexplained transaminase elevations are contraindications to the use of SIMCOR *[see Contraindications (4)]*.

Niacin extended-release (NIASPAN) and simvastatin can cause abnormal liver tests. In a simvastatin-controlled, 24 week study with SIMCOR in 641 patients, there were no persistent increases (to more than 3× the ULN) in serum transaminases. In three placebo-controlled clinical studies of niacin extended-release, patients with normal serum transaminases levels at baseline did not experience any transaminase elevations greater than 3× the ULN. Persistent increases (to more than 3× the ULN) in serum transaminases have occurred in approximately 1% of patients who received simvastatin in clinical studies. When drug treatment was interrupted or discontinued in these patients, the transaminases levels usually fell slowly to pretreatment levels. The increases were not associated with jaundice or other clinical signs or symptoms. There was no evidence of hypersensitivity.

It is recommended that liver enzyme tests be obtained prior to initiating therapy with SIMCOR and repeated as clinically indicated. There have been rare postmarketing reports of fatal and non-fatal hepatic failure in patients taking statins, including simvastatin. If serious liver injury with clinical symptoms and/or hyperbilirubinemia or jaundice occurs during treatment with SIMCOR, promptly interrupt therapy. If an alternate etiology is not found do not restart SIMCOR. Note that ALT may emanate from muscle, therefore ALT rising with CK may indicate myopathy *[see Warnings and Precautions (5.2)]*.

5.4 Laboratory Abnormalities

Increase in Blood Glucose: Niacin treatment can increase fasting blood glucose. In a simvastatin-controlled, 24-week study with SIMCOR the change from baseline in glycosylated hemoglobin levels was 0.2% for SIMCOR-treated patients and 0.2% for simvastatin-treated patients. Diabetic or potentially diabetic patients should be observed closely during treatment with SIMCOR, particularly during the first few months of therapy. Adjustment of diet and/or hypoglycemic therapy or discontinuation of SIMCOR may be necessary.

Reduction in platelet count: Niacin can reduce platelet count. In a simvastatin-controlled, 24-week study with SIMCOR the mean percent change from baseline for patients treated with 2000/40 mg daily was -5.6%.

Increase in ProthrombinTime (PT): Niacin can cause small increases in PT. In a simvastatin-controlled, 24-week study with SIMCOR this effect was not seen.

Increase in Uric Acid: Elevated uric acid levels have occurred with niacin therapy. In a simvastatin-controlled, 24-week study with SIMCOR this effect was not seen. Nevertheless, in patients predisposed to gout, SIMCOR therapy should be used with caution.

Decrease in Phosphorus: Small dose-related reductions in phosphorous levels were seen in clinical studies with niacin. In a simvastatin-controlled, 24-week study with SIMCOR this effect was not seen.

5.5 Endocrine Function

Increases in HbA1c and fasting serum glucose levels have been reported with HMG-CoA reductase inhibitors, including simvastatin.

6 ADVERSE REACTIONS

Overview

In a controlled clinical study, 14% of patients randomized to SIMCOR discontinued therapy due to an adverse event. Flushing episodes (i.e., warmth, redness, itching and/or tingling) were the most common treatment-emergent adverse reactions, occurring in up to 59% of patients treated with SIMCOR. Spontaneous reports with niacin extended-release and clinical studies of SIMCOR suggest that flushing may be accompanied by symptoms of dizziness or syncope, tachycardia, palpitations, shortness of breath, sweating, burning sensation/skin burning sensation, chills, and/or edema.

6.1 Clinical Studies Experience

SIMCOR

Because clinical studies are conducted under widely varying conditions, adverse reaction rates observed in the clinical studies of a drug cannot be directly compared to rates in the clinical studies of another drug and may not reflect the rates observed in practice.

The safety data described below reflect exposure to SIMCOR in 403 patients in a controlled study for a period of 6 months.

Flushing: Flushing (warmth, redness, itching and/or tingling) occurred in up to 59% of patients treated with SIMCOR. Flushing resulted in study discontinuation for 6.0% of patients.

More Common Adverse Reactions: In addition to flushing, adverse reactions occurring in ≥ 3% of patients (irrespective of investigator causality) treated with SIMCOR are shown in Table 4 below:

Table 4. Adverse Reactions Occurring in ≥ 3% of Patients in a Controlled Clinical Trial

Adverse Event	SIMCOR overall *	Simvastatin overall **
Total Number of Patients	N=403	N=238
Headache	18 (4.5%)	11 (4.6%)
Pruritus	13 (3.2%)	0 (0.0%)
Nausea	13 (3.2%)	10 (4.2%)
Back Pain	13 (3.2%)	5 (2.1%)
Diarrhea	12 (3.0%)	7 (2.9%)

* SIMCOR overall included all doses from 500/20 mg to 2000/40 mg

** Simvastatin overall included 20 mg, 40 mg, and 80 mg doses

Atherothrombosis Intervention in Metabolic Syndrome with Low HDL/High Triglycerides: Impact on Global Health Outcomes (AIM-HIGH)

In AIM-HIGH involving 3414 patients (mean age of 64 years, 15% women, 92% Caucasians, 34% with diabetes mellitus) with stable, previously diagnosed cardiovascular disease, all patients received simvastatin, 40 to 80 mg per day, plus ezetimibe 10 mg per day if needed, to maintain an LDL-C level of 40-80 mg/dL, and were randomized to receive NIASPAN 1500-2000 mg/day (n=1718) or matching placebo (IR Niacin, 100-150 mg, n=1696). The incidence of the adverse reactions of "blood glucose increased" (6.4% vs. 4.5%) and "diabetes mellitus" (3.6% vs. 2.2%) was significantly higher in the simvastatin plus NIASPAN group as compared to the simvastatin plus placebo group. There were 5 cases of rhabdomyolysis reported, 4 (0.2%) in the simvastatin plus NIASPAN group and one (<0.1%) in the simvastatin plus placebo group *[see Warnings and Precautions (5.1)]*.

Simvastatin

In pre-marketing controlled clinical studies and their open extensions (2,423 patients with mean duration of follow-up of approximately 18 months) 1.4% of patients discontinued due to adverse reactions. The most commonly reported adverse reactions (incidence > 1%) in simvastatin controlled clinical trials were: headache (3.5%), abdominal pain (3.5%), constipation (2.3%), upper respiratory infection (2.1%), diarrhea (1.9%), and flatulence (1.9%).

Other Clinical Studies

In a clinical trial in which 12,064 patients with a history of myocardial infarction were treated with simvastatin (mean follow-up 6.7 years), the incidence of myopathy (defined as unexplained muscle weakness or pain with a serum creatine kinase [CK] >10 times upper limit of normal [ULN]) in patients on 80 mg/day was approximately 0.9% compared with 0.02% for patients on 20 mg/day. The incidence of rhabdomyolysis (defined as myopathy with a CK >40 times ULN) in patients on 80 mg/day was approximately 0.4% compared with 0% for patients on 20 mg/day. The incidence of myopathy, including rhabdomyolysis, was highest during the first year and then notably decreased during the subsequent years of treatment.

Niacin Extended-Release

In placebo-controlled clinical trials (n=245), flushing episodes were the most common treatment-emergent adverse events (up to 88% of patients) for niacin extended-release. Other adverse events occurring in 5% or greater of patients treated with niacin extended-release are headache (9%), diarrhea (7%), nausea (5%), rhinitis (5%), and dyspepsia (4%) at a maintenance dose of 1000mg daily.

Clinical Laboratory Abnormalities:

SIMCOR

Chemistry

Elevations in serum transaminases *[see Warnings and Precautions (5.3)]*, CK, fasting glucose, uric acid, alkaline phosphatase, LDH, amylase, γ-glutamyl transpeptidase, bilirubin, and reductions in phosphorus, and abnormal thyroid function tests.

Hematology

Reductions in platelet counts and prolongation of PT *[see Warnings and Precautions (5.4)]*.

6.2 Postmarketing Experience

See also the full prescribing information for niacin extended release (Niaspan) and simvastatin products.

Because the below reactions are reported voluntarily from a population of uncertain size, it is generally not possible to reliably estimate their frequency or establish a causal relationship to drug exposure.

Simvastatin

The following additional adverse reactions have been identified during postapproval use of simvastatin. Hypersensitivity reaction including one or more of the following features: anaphylaxis, angioedema, lupus erythematous-like syndrome, vasculitis, purpura, thrombocytopenia, leucopenia, hemolytic anemia, positive ANA, ESR increase, eosinophilia, arthritis, photosensitivity, chills, toxic epidermal necrolysis, erythema multiforme, Stevens-Johnson syndrome, urticaria, fever, dyspnea, and arthralgia; pancreatitis, hepatitis, fatal and non-fatal hepatic failure, pruritus, cataracts, polymyositis, dermatomyositis, polymyalgia rheumatica, tendon rupture, peripheral neuropathy, erectile dysfunction, depression, interstitial lung disease, alopecia, a variety of skin changes (e.g., nodules, discoloration, dryness of skin/mucous membranes, changes to hair/nails), muscle cramps, vomiting, malaise.

There have been rare reports of immune-mediated necrotizing myopathy with statin use *[see Warnings and Precautions (5.2)]*.

There have been rare postmarketing reports of cognitive impairment (e.g., memory loss, forgetfulness, amnesia, memory impairment, confusion) associated with statin use. These cognitive issues have been reported for all statins. The reports are generally nonserious, and reversible upon statin discontinuation, with variable times to symptom onset (1 day to years) and symptom resolution (median of 3 weeks).

NIASPAN

The following additional adverse reactions have been identified during post-approval use of NIASPAN. Hypersensitivity reaction including one or more of the following features: anaphylaxis, dyspnea, angioedema, tongue edema, larynx edema, face edema, laryngismus; tachycardia, atrial fibrillation, other cardiac arrhythmias, palpitations, hypotension, postural hypotension, dizziness, syncope, flushing, burning sensation/skin burning sensation, paresthesia, urticaria, vesiculobullous rash, maculopapular rash, sweating, dry skin, skin discoloration, blurred vision, macular edema, myalgia, myopathy, peptic ulcers, eructation, flatulence, hepatitis, jaundice, peripheral edema, asthenia, nervousness, insomnia, migraine, gout, and decreased glucose tolerance.

7 DRUG INTERACTIONS

No drug interaction studies were conducted with SIMCOR. However, the following interactions have been noted with the individual components of SIMCOR:

Simvastatin

7.1 Strong CYP3A4 Inhibitors, Cyclosporine, or Danazol

Strong CYP3A4 inhibitors: Simvastatin, like several other inhibitors of HMG-CoA reductase, is a substrate of CYP3A4. Simvastatin is metabolized by CYP3A4 but has no CYP3A4 inhibitory activity; therefore it is not expected to affect the plasma concentrations of other drugs metabolized by CYP3A4.

Elevated plasma levels of HMG-CoA reductase inhibitory activity increases the risk of myopathy and rhabdomyolysis, particularly with higher doses of SIMCOR *[see Warnings and Precautions (5.2) and Clinical Pharmacology (12.3)]*. Concomitant use of drugs labeled as having a strong inhibitory effect on CYP3A4 is contraindicated *[see Contraindications (4)]*. If treatment with itraconazole, ketoconazole, posaconazole, erythromycin, clarithromycin or telithromycin is unavoidable, therapy with SIMCOR must be suspended during the course of treatment.

Although not studied clinically, voriconazole has been shown to inhibit lovastatin metabolism *in vitro* (human liver microsomes). Therefore, voriconazole is likely to increase the plasma concentration of simvastatin. It is recommended that dose adjustment of SIMCOR be considered during concomitant use of voriconazole and SIMCOR to reduce the risk of myopathy, including rhabdomyolysis *[see Warnings and Precautions (5.2)]*.

Cyclosporine or Danazol: The risk of myopathy, including rhabdomyolysis is increased by concomitant administration of cyclosporine or danazol. Therefore, concomitant use of these drugs is contraindicated *[see Contraindications (4), Warnings and Precautions (5.2) and Clinical Pharmacology (12.3)]*.

7.2 Verapamil or Diltiazem

The risk of myopathy, including rhabdomyolysis is increased by concomitant administration of verapamil or diltiazem with doses of simvastatin exceeding 10 mg. Because all doses of SIMCOR contain simvastatin in excess of 10 mg, concomitant use of these drugs is contraindicated *[see Contraindications (4), Warnings and Precautions (5.2) and Clinical Pharmacology (12.3)]*.

7.3 Lipid-Lowering Drugs That Can Cause Myopathy When Given Alone

Gemfibrozil: Contraindicated with SIMCOR *[see Contraindications (4) and Warnings and Precautions (5.2)]*. Other fibrates: Combined use with SIMCOR should be avoided *[see Warnings and Precautions (5.2)]*.

7.4 Amlodipine or Ranolazine

The risk of myopathy, including rhabdomyolysis, is increased by concomitant administration of amlodipine or ranolazine *[see Dosage and Administration (2.2) and Warnings and Precautions (5.2) and Table 5 in Clinical Pharmacology (12.3)]*.

7.5 Propranolol

In healthy male volunteers there was a significant decrease in mean C_{max}, but no change in AUC, for simvastatin total and active inhibitors with concomitant administration of single doses of simvastatin and propranolol. The clinical relevance of this finding is unclear. The pharmacokinetics of the enantiomers of propranolol were not affected.

7.6 Digoxin

Concomitant administration of a single dose of digoxin in healthy male volunteers receiving simvastatin resulted in a slight elevation (less than 0.3 ng/mL) in digoxin concentrations in plasma (as measured by a radioimmunoassay) compared to concomitant administration of placebo and digoxin. Patients taking digoxin should be monitored appropriately when SIMCOR is initiated.

7.7 Coumarin Anticoagulants

In normal volunteers and hypercholesterolemic patients, simvastatin 20-40 mg/day modestly potentiated the effect of

Information on the AbbVie, Inc. products listed on these pages is from the prescribing information in use as of July 31, 2013. For more information, please visit rxabbvie.com or call 1-800-633-9110.

coumarin anticoagulants since the prothrombin time, reported as International Normalized Ratio (INR), increased from a baseline of 1.7 to 1.8 and from 2.6 to 3.4 in the volunteers and patients, respectively. With other reductase inhibitors, clinically evident bleeding and/or increased prothrombin time has been reported in a few patients taking coumarin anticoagulants concomitantly. In such patients, prothrombin time should be determined before starting SIMCOR and frequently enough during early therapy to ensure that no significant alteration of prothrombin time occurs. Once a stable prothrombin time has been documented, prothrombin times can be monitored at the intervals usually recommended for patients on coumarin anticoagulants. If the dose of SIMCOR is changed or discontinued, the same procedure should be repeated.

7.8 Colchicine

Cases of myopathy, including rhabdomyolysis, have been reported with simvastatin coadministered with colchicine, and caution should be exercised when prescribing SIMCOR with colchicine *[see Warnings and Precautions (5.2)]*.

Niacin

7.9 Aspirin

Concomitant use of aspirin may decrease the metabolic clearance of niacin. The clinical relevance of this finding is unclear.

7.10 Antihypertensive Therapy

Niacin may potentiate the effects of ganglionic blocking agents and vasoactive drugs resulting in postural hypotension.

7.11 Bile Acid Sequestrants

An *in vitro* study was carried out investigating the niacin-binding capacity of colestipol and cholestyramine. About 98% of available niacin was bound to colestipol, with 10 to 30% binding to cholestyramine. These results suggest that 4 to 6 hours, or as great an interval as possible, should elapse between the ingestion of bile acid-binding resins and the administration of SIMCOR.

7.12 Other

Nutritional supplements containing large doses of niacin or related compounds may potentiate the adverse effects of SIMCOR.

8 USE IN SPECIFIC POPULATIONS

8.1 Pregnancy

Pregnancy Category X – *[see Contraindications (4)]*

SIMCOR is contraindicated in women who are or may become pregnant. Lipid lowering drugs offer no benefit during pregnancy, because cholesterol and cholesterol derivatives are needed for normal fetal development. Serum cholesterol and triglycerides increase during normal pregnancy. Atherosclerosis is a chronic process, and discontinuation of lipid-lowering drugs during pregnancy should have little impact on long-term outcomes of primary hypercholesterolemia therapy. There are no adequate and well-controlled studies of SIMCOR use during pregnancy; however, there are rare reports of congenital anomalies in infants exposed to HMG-CoA reductase inhibitors *in utero*. Animal reproduction studies of simvastatin in rats and rabbits showed no evidence of teratogenicity. SIMCOR may cause fetal harm when administered to a pregnant woman. If SIMCOR is used during pregnancy or if the patient becomes pregnant while taking this drug, the patient should be apprised of the potential hazard to the fetus.

SIMCOR contains simvastatin (a HMG-CoA reductase inhibitor) and niacin (nicotinic acid). There are rare reports of congenital anomalies following intrauterine exposure to HMG-CoA reductase inhibitors. In a review of approximately 100 prospectively followed pregnancies in women exposed to simvastatin or another structurally related HMG-CoA reductase inhibitor, the incidences of congenital anomalies, spontaneous abortions, and fetal deaths/stillbirths did not exceed those expected in the general population. However, the study was only able to exclude a 3- to 4-fold increased risk of congenital anomalies over the background rate. In 89% of these cases, drug treatment was initiated prior to pregnancy and was discontinued during the first trimester when pregnancy was identified. It is not known whether niacin at doses used for lipid disorders can cause fetal harm when administered to a pregnant woman. Simvastatin was not teratogenic in rats or rabbits at doses that resulted in 3 times the human exposure based on mg/m^2 surface area. However, in studies with another structurally-related HMG-CoA reductase inhibitor, skeletal malformations were observed in rats and mice. Animal reproduction studies have not been conducted with niacin.

Women of childbearing potential, who require SIMCOR treatment for a lipid disorder, should use effective contraception. Patients trying to conceive should contact their prescriber to discuss stopping SIMCOR treatment. If pregnancy occurs, SIMCOR should be immediately discontinued.

8.3 Nursing Mothers

It is not known whether simvastatin is excreted into human milk; however, a small amount of another drug in this class does pass into breast milk. Niacin is excreted into human milk but the actual infant dose or infant dose as a percent of the maternal dose is not known. Because of the potential for serious adverse reactions in nursing infants, nursing mothers who require SIMCOR treatment should not breastfeed their infants. A decision should be made whether to discontinue nursing or discontinue drug, taking into account the importance of the drug to the mother *[see Contraindications (4)]*.

8.4 Pediatric Use

The safety and effectiveness of SIMCOR in pediatric patients have not been established.

8.5 Geriatric Use

There were 281 (30.8%) patients aged 65 years and older treated with SIMCOR in Phase III clinical studies. No overall differences in safety and effectiveness were observed between these patients and younger patients, but greater sensitivity of some older individuals cannot be ruled out. A pharmacokinetic study with simvastatin showed the mean plasma level of HMG-CoA reductase inhibitory activity to be approximately 45% higher in elderly patients between 70-78 years of age compared with patients between 18-30 years of age.

Because advanced age (≥65 years) is a predisposing factor for myopathy, including rhabdomyolysis, SIMCOR should be prescribed with caution in the elderly. In a clinical trial of patients treated with simvastatin 80 mg/day, patients ≥65 years of age had an increased risk of myopathy, including rhabdomyolysis, compared to patients <65 years of age *[see Warnings and Precautions (5.2) and Clinical Pharmacology (12.3)]*.

8.6 Gender

Data from the clinical trials suggest that women have a greater hypolipidemic response than men at equivalent doses of niacin extended-release. No consistent gender differences in efficacy and safety were observed in SIMCOR studies.

8.7 Renal Impairment

No pharmacokinetic studies have been conducted in patients with renal impairment for SIMCOR. Caution should be exercised when SIMCOR is administered to patients with renal disease. For patients with severe renal insufficiency, SIMCOR should not be started unless the patient has already tolerated treatment with simvastatin at a dose of 10 mg or higher. Caution should be exercised when SIMCOR is administered to these patients and they should be closely monitored.

8.8 Hepatic Impairment

No pharmacokinetic studies have been conducted in patients with hepatic insufficiency for SIMCOR *[see Warnings and Precautions (5.3)]*.

10 OVERDOSAGE

Supportive measures should be taken in the event of an overdose. The dialyzability of niacin, or of simvastatin and its metabolites, is not known.

A few cases of overdosage with simvastatin have been reported; the maximum dose taken was 3.6 g. All patients recovered without sequelae.

11 DESCRIPTION

SIMCOR tablets contain niacin extended-release (NIASPAN) and simvastatin in combination. Simvastatin, an inhibitor of HMG-CoA reductase, and niacin are both lipid-altering agents.

Niacin Extended-Release

Niacin is nicotinic acid, or 3-pyridinecarboxylic acid. Niacin is a white, nonhygroscopic crystalline powder that is very soluble in water, boiling ethanol, and propylene glycol. It is insoluble in ethyl ether. The empirical formula of niacin is $C_6H_5NO_2$ and its molecular weight is 123.11. Niacin has the following structural formula:

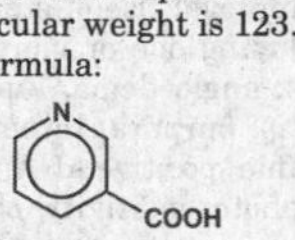

Simvastatin

Simvastatin is butanoic acid, 2,2-dimethyl-,1,2,3,7,8,8a-hexahydro-3-7-dimethyl-8-[2-(tetrahydro-4-hydroxy-6-oxo-2H-pyran-2-yl)-ethyl]-1-naphthalenyl ester, [1S-[1α,3α, 7β,8β(2S*4S*),-8aβ]]. Simvastatin is a white to off-white, nonhygroscopic, crystalline powder that is practically insoluble in water and freely soluble in chloroform, methanol, and ethanol. The empirical formula of simvastatin is $C_{25}H_{38}O_5$ and its molecular weight is 418.57. Simvastatin has the following structural formula:

[See chemical structure at top of next column]

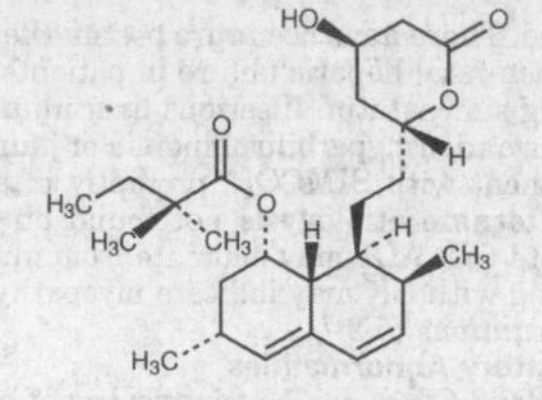

SIMCOR is available for oral administration as tablets containing 500 mg of niacin extended-release (NIASPAN) and 20 mg simvastatin (SIMCOR 500/20 mg), 500 mg of niacin extended-release (NIASPAN) and 40 mg simvastatin (SIMCOR 500/40 mg), 750 mg of niacin extended-release (NIASPAN) and 20 mg simvastatin (SIMCOR 750/20 mg), 1000 mg of niacin extended-release (NIASPAN) and 20 mg simvastatin (SIMCOR 1000/20 mg) and 1000 mg of niacin extended-release (NIASPAN) and 40 mg simvastatin (SIMCOR 1000/40 mg). Each tablet contains the following inactive ingredients: hypromellose, povidone, stearic acid, polyethylene glycol, butylated hydroxyanisole, FD&C Blue #2, lactose monohydrate, titanium dioxide, triacetin. SIMCOR 500/20 mg, SIMCOR 750/20 mg, and SIMCOR 1000/20 mg also contain iron oxide.

12 CLINICAL PHARMACOLOGY

12.1 Mechanism of Action

Niacin

Niacin functions in the body after conversion to nicotinamide adenine dinucleotide (NAD) in the NAD coenzyme system. The mechanism by which niacin alters lipid profiles is not completely understood and may involve several actions, including partial inhibition of release of free fatty acids from adipose tissue, and increased lipoprotein lipase activity (which may increase the rate of chylomicron triglyceride removal from plasma). Niacin decreases the rate of hepatic synthesis of VLDL-C and LDL-C, and does not appear to affect fecal excretion of fats, sterols, or bile acids.

Simvastatin

Simvastatin is a prodrug and is hydrolyzed to its active β-hydroxyacid form, simvastatin acid, after administration. Simvastatin is a specific inhibitor of 3-hydroxy-3-methylglutaryl-coenzyme A (HMG-CoA) reductase, the enzyme that catalyzes the conversion of HMG-CoA to mevalonate, an early and rate-limiting step in the biosynthetic pathway for cholesterol. In addition, simvastatin reduces VLDL and TG and increases HDL-C.

12.2 Pharmacodynamics

A variety of clinical studies have demonstrated that elevated levels of Total-C, LDL-C, and Apo B promote human atherosclerosis. Similarly, decreased levels of HDL-C are associated with the development of atherosclerosis. Epidemiological investigations have established that cardiovascular morbidity and mortality vary directly with the level of Total-C and LDL-C, and inversely with the level of HDL-C. Like LDL, cholesterol-enriched triglyceride-rich lipoproteins, including VLDL, intermediate-density lipoprotein (IDL), and their remnants, can also promote atherosclerosis. Elevated plasma TG are frequently found in a triad with low HDL-C levels and small LDL particles, as well as in association with non-lipid metabolic risk factors for coronary heart disease (CHD). As such, total plasma TG has not consistently been shown to be an independent risk factor for CHD. Furthermore, the independent effect of raising HDL-C or lowering TG on the risk of coronary and cardiovascular morbidity and mortality has not been determined.

SIMCOR

SIMCOR reduces Total-C, LDL-C, non-HDL-C, Apo B, TG, and Lp(a) levels and increases HDL-C in patients with primary hyperlipidemia, mixed dyslipidemia, or hypertriglyceridemia.

Niacin

Niacin (but not nicotinamide) in gram doses reduces LDL-C, Apo B, Lp(a), TG, and Total-C, and increases HDL-C. The magnitude of individual lipid and lipoprotein responses may be influenced by the severity and type of underlying lipid abnormality. The increase in HDL-C is associated with an increase in apolipoprotein A-I (Apo A-I) and a shift in the distribution of HDL subfractions. These shifts include an increase in the HDL2:HDL3 ratio, and an elevation in lipoprotein A-I (Lp A-I, an HDL-C particle containing only Apo A-I). Niacin treatment also decreases serum levels of apolipoprotein B-100 (Apo B), the major protein component of the very low-density lipoprotein (VLDL) and LDL fractions, and of Lp(a), a variant form of LDL independently associated with coronary risk. In addition, preliminary reports suggest that niacin causes favorable LDL particle size transformations, although the clinical relevance of this effect requires further investigation.

Simvastatin

Simvastatin reduces elevated Total-C, LDL-C, Apo B, and TG, and increases HDL-C in patients with primary heterozygous familial and nonfamilial hypercholesterolemia and mixed dyslipidemia. Simvastatin reduces Total-C and LDL-C in patients with homozygous familial hypercholesterolemia. Simvastatin decreases VLDL, Total-C/HDL-C ratio, and LDL-C/HDL-C ratio.

12.3 Pharmacokinetics

Absorption and Bioavailability

SIMCOR

The relative bioavailability of niacin (Nicotinuric acid, NUA, C_{max} and total urinary excretion as the surrogate), simvastatin, and simvastatin acid was evaluated under a light snack conditions in healthy volunteers (n=42), following administration of two 1000/20 mg SIMCOR tablets. Niacin exposure (C_{max} and AUC) after SIMCOR was similar to that of a niacin extended-release formulation. However, simvastatin and simvastatin acid AUC after SIMCOR increased by 23% and 41%, respectively, compared to those of a simvastatin immediate release formulation. The mean time to C_{max} (T_{max}) for niacin ranged from 4.6 to 4.9 hours and simvastatin from 1.9 to 2.0 hours. Following administration of 2 × 1000/20 mg SIMCOR, the mean C_{max}, T_{max} and $AUC_{(0-t)}$ for simvastatin acid, active metabolite of simvastatin, were 3.29 ng/mL, 6.56 hours and 30.81 ng•hr/mL respectively.

Bioequivalence has not been evaluated among different SIMCOR dosage strengths except between 1000/40 and 500/20 mg. SIMCOR tablets 1000/40 mg and 500/20 mg were bioequivalent following a single dose of 2000/80 mg. Therefore, dosage strengths of SIMCOR should not be considered exchangeable except between these two strengths.

Niacin

Due to extensive and saturable first-pass metabolism, niacin concentrations in the general circulation are dose dependent and highly variable. Peak steady-state niacin concentrations were 0.6, 4.9, and 15.5 mcg/mL after doses of 1000, 1500, and 2000 mg NIASPAN once daily (given as two 500 mg, two 750 mg, and two 1000 mg tablets, respectively). To reduce the risk of gastrointestinal upset, administration of niacin extended-release with a low-fat meal or snack is recommended.

Simvastatin

Since simvastatin undergoes extensive first-pass extraction in the liver, the availability of the drug to the general circulation is low (<5%). Peak plasma concentrations of both active and total inhibitors were attained within 1.3 to 2.4 hours postdose. Following an oral dose of ^{14}C-labeled simvastatin in man, plasma concentration of total radioactivity (simvastatin plus ^{14}C-metabolites) peaked at 4 hours and declined rapidly to about 10% of peak by 12 hours postdose. Relative to the fasting state, the plasma profile of inhibitors was not affected when simvastatin was administered immediately before an American Heart Association recommended low-fat meal.

Metabolism

SIMCOR

Following administration of SIMCOR, niacin and simvastatin undergo rapid and extensive first-pass metabolism as described in the following niacin and simvastatin sections. Following administration of 2 × 1000/20 mg SIMCOR in healthy volunteers, 10.2%, 10.7%, and 29.5% of the administered niacin dose was recovered in urine as niacin metabolites, NUA, N-methylnicotinamide (MNA), and N-methyl-2-pyridone-5-carboxamide (2PY), respectively. Following administration of 2 × 1000/20 mg SIMCOR, the mean C_{max}, T_{max}, and $AUC_{(0-t)}$ for the simvastatin metabolite, simvastatin acid were 3.29 ng/mL, 6.56 hours, and 30.81 ng•hr/mL respectively.

Niacin

Niacin undergoes rapid and extensive first-pass metabolism that is dose-rate specific and, at the doses used to treat dyslipidemia, saturable. In humans, one pathway is through a simple conjugation step with glycine to form NUA. NUA is then excreted, although there may be a small amount of reversible metabolism back to niacin. The other pathway results in the formation of nicotinamide adenine dinucleotide (NAD). It is unclear whether nicotinamide is formed as a precursor to, or following the synthesis of, NAD. Nicotinamide is further metabolized to at least MNA and nicotinamide-N-oxide NNO. MNA is further metabolized to two other compounds, 2PY and N-methyl-4-pyridone-5-carboxamide (4PY). The formation of 2PY appears to predominate over 4PY in humans.

Simvastatin

Simvastatin is a substrate of CYP3A4. Simvastatin is a lactone that is readily hydrolyzed *in vivo* to the corresponding β-hydroxyacid, a potent inhibitor of HMG-CoA reductase. The major active metabolites of simvastatin present in human plasma are the β-hydroxyacid of simvastatin and its 6'-hydroxy, 6'-hydroxymethyl, and 6'-exomethylene derivatives.

Elimination

SIMCOR

Following 2 × 1000/20 mg SIMCOR administration, approximately 54% of the niacin dose administered was recovered in urine in 96 hours as niacin and metabolites of which 3.6% was recovered as niacin.

After SIMCOR administration, the mean terminal plasma half-life for simvastatin was 4.2 to 4.9 hours and for simvastatin acid was 4.6 to 5.0 hours.

Niacin

Niacin and its metabolites are rapidly eliminated in the urine. Following single and multiple doses of 1500 to 2000 mg niacin, approximately 53 to 77% of the niacin dose administered as NIASPAN was recovered in urine as niacin and metabolites; up to 7.7% of the dose was recovered in urine as unchanged niacin after multiple dosing with 2 × 1000 mg NIASPAN. The ratio of metabolites recovered in the urine was dependent on the dose administered.

Simvastatin

Simvastatin is excreted in urine, based on studies in humans. Following an oral dose of ^{14}C-labeled simvastatin in man, 13% of the dose was excreted in urine and 60% in feces.

Special Populations

A pharmacokinetic study with simvastatin showed the mean plasma level of HMG-CoA reductase inhibitory activity to be approximately 45% higher in elderly patients between 70-78 years of age compared with patients between 18-30 years of age.

Steady-state plasma concentrations of niacin and metabolites after administration of niacin extended-release are generally higher in women than in men, with the magnitude of the difference varying with dose and metabolite. Recovery of niacin and metabolites in urine, however, is generally similar for men and women, indicating that absorption is similar for both genders. The gender differences observed in plasma levels of niacin and its metabolites may be due to gender-specific differences in metabolic rate or volume of distribution.

Pharmacokinetic studies with a statin having a similar principal route of elimination to that of simvastatin have suggested that for a given dose level, higher systemic exposure may be achieved in patients with severe renal insufficiency (as measured by creatinine clearance).

Drug Interaction

Effect of other drugs on simvastatin:

[See table 5 at top of next page]

Simvastatin effect on other drugs:

In a study of 12 healthy volunteers, simvastatin at the 80-mg dose had no effect on the metabolism of the probe cytochrome P450 isoform 3A4 (CYP3A4) substrates midazolam and erythromycin. This indicates that simvastatin is not an inhibitor of CYP3A4, and, therefore, is not expected to affect the plasma levels of other drugs metabolized by CYP3A4.

Coadministration of simvastatin (40 mg QD for 10 days) resulted in an increase in the maximum mean levels of cardioactive digoxin (given as a single 0.4 mg dose on day 10) by approximately 0.3 ng/mL.

Niacin effect on other drugs:

Niacin did not affect fluvastatin pharmacokinetics.

When NIASPAN 2000 mg and lovastatin 40 mg were coadministered, NIASPAN increased lovastatin C_{max} and AUC by 2% and 14%, respectively, and decreased lovastatin acid C_{max} and AUC by 22% and 2%, respectively. Lovastatin reduced NIASPAN bioavailability by 2-3%.

13 NONCLINICAL TOXICOLOGY

13.1 Carcinogenesis, Mutagenesis, Impairment of Fertility

No studies have been conducted with SIMCOR regarding carcinogenesis, mutagenesis, or impairment of fertility.

Niacin

Niacin, administered to mice for a lifetime as a 1% solution in drinking water, was not carcinogenic. The mice in this study received approximately 6 to 8 times a human dose of 3000 mg/day as determined on a mg/m^2 basis. Niacin was negative for mutagenicity in the Ames test. No studies on impairment of fertility have been performed.

Simvastatin

In a 72-week carcinogenicity study, mice were administered daily doses of simvastatin of 25, 100, and 400 mg/kg body weight, which resulted in mean plasma drug levels approximately 1, 4, and 8 times higher than the mean human plasma drug level, respectively (as total inhibitory activity based on AUC) after an 80-mg oral dose. Liver carcinomas were significantly increased in high-dose females and mid- and high-dose males with a maximum incidence of 90% in males. The incidence of adenomas of the liver was significantly increased in mid- and high-dose females. Drug treatment also significantly increased the incidence of lung adenomas in mid- and high-dose males and females. Adenomas of the Harderian gland (a gland of the eye of rodents) were significantly higher in high-dose mice than in controls. No evidence of a tumorigenic effect was observed at 25 mg/kg/day.

In a separate 92-week carcinogenicity study in mice at doses up to 25 mg/kg/day, no evidence of a tumorigenic effect was observed (mean plasma drug levels were 1 times higher than humans given 80 mg simvastatin as measured by AUC). In a two-year study in rats at 25 mg/kg/day, there was a statistically significant increase in the incidence of thyroid follicular adenomas in female rats exposed to approximately 11 times higher levels of simvastatin than in humans given 80 mg simvastatin (as measured by AUC). A second two-year rat carcinogenicity study with doses of 50 and 100 mg/kg/day produced hepatocellular adenomas and carcinomas (in female rats at both doses and in males at 100 mg/kg/day). Thyroid follicular cell adenomas were increased in males and females at both doses; thyroid follicular cell carcinomas were increased in females at 100 mg/kg/day. The increased incidence of thyroid neoplasms appears to be consistent with findings from other HMG-CoA reductase inhibitors. These treatment levels represented plasma drug levels (AUC) of approximately 7 and 15 times (males) and 22 and 25 times (females) the mean human plasma drug exposure after an 80 milligram daily dose. No evidence of mutagenicity was observed in a microbial mutagenicity (Ames) test with or without rat or mouse liver metabolic activation. In addition, no evidence of damage to genetic material was noted in an *in vitro* alkaline elution assay using rat hepatocytes, a V-79 mammalian cell forward mutation study, an *in vitro* chromosome aberration study in CHO cells, or an *in vivo* chromosomal aberration assay in mouse bone marrow. There was decreased fertility in male rats treated with simvastatin for 34 weeks at 25 mg/kg body weight (4 times the maximum human exposure level, based on AUC, in patients receiving 80 mg/day); however, this effect was not observed during a subsequent fertility study in which simvastatin was administered at this same dose level to male rats for 11 weeks (the entire cycle of spermatogenesis including epididymal maturation). No microscopic changes were observed in the testes of rats from either study. At 180 mg/kg/day, (which produces exposure levels 22 times higher than those in humans taking 80 mg/day based on surface area, mg/m^2), seminiferous tubule degeneration (necrosis and loss of spermatogenic epithelium) was observed. In dogs, there was drug-related testicular atrophy, decreased spermatogenesis, spermatocytic degeneration and giant cell formation at 10 mg/kg/day, (approximately 2 times the human exposure, based on AUC, at 80 mg/day). The clinical significance of these findings is unclear.

13.2 Animal Toxicology and/or Pharmacology

SIMCOR

No animal toxicology or pharmacology studies were done with SIMCOR.

Niacin

No animal toxicology or pharmacology studies were done with niacin extended-release.

Simvastatin

Optic nerve degeneration was seen in clinically normal dogs treated with simvastatin for 14 weeks at 180 mg/kg/day, a dose that produced mean plasma drug levels about 12 times higher than the mean plasma drug level in humans taking 80 mg/day. A chemically similar drug in this class also produced optic nerve degeneration (Wallerian degeneration of retinogeniculate fibers) in clinically normal dogs in a dose-dependent fashion starting at 60 mg/kg/day, a dose that produced mean plasma drug levels about 30 times higher than the mean plasma drug level in humans taking the highest recommended dose (as measured by total enzyme inhibitory activity). This same drug also produced vestibulocochlear Wallerian-like degeneration and retinal ganglion cell chromatolysis in dogs treated for 14 weeks at 180 mg/kg/day, a dose that resulted in a mean plasma drug level similar to that seen with the 60 mg/kg/day dose.

Central Nervous System (CNS) vascular lesions, characterized by perivascular hemorrhage and edema, mononuclear cell infiltration of perivascular spaces, perivascular fibrin deposits and necrosis of small vessels were seen in dogs treated with simvastatin at a dose of 360 mg/kg/day, a dose that produced mean plasma drug levels that were about 14 times higher than the mean plasma drug levels in humans taking 80 mg/day. Similar CNS vascular lesions have been observed with several other drugs of this class.

There were cataracts in female rats after two years of simvastatin treatment with 50 and 100 mg/kg/day (22 and 25 times the human AUC at 80 mg/day, respectively) and in dogs after three months at 90 mg/kg/day (19 times) and at two years at 50 mg/kg/day (5 times).

Reproductive Toxicology Studies

Simvastatin was not teratogenic in rats at doses of 25 mg/kg/day or in rabbits at doses up to 10 mg/kg/day. These doses resulted in 3 times (rat) or 3 times (rabbit) the human exposure based on mg/m^2 surface area. However, in studies with another structurally-related HMG-CoA reductase inhibitor, skeletal malformations were observed in rats and mice.

Information on the AbbVie, Inc. products listed on these pages is from the prescribing information in use as of July 31, 2013. For more information, please visit rxabbvie.com or call 1-800-633-9110.

14 CLINICAL STUDIES

14.1 Modifications of Lipid Profiles

SIMCOR

In a double-blind, randomized, multicenter, multi-national, active-controlled, 24-week study, the lipid effects of SIMCOR were compared to simvastatin 20 mg and 80 mg in 641 patients with type II hyperlipidemia or mixed dyslipidemia. Following a lipid qualification phase, patients were eligible to enter one of two treatment groups. In Group A, patients on simvastatin 20 mg monotherapy with elevated non-HDL levels and LDL-C levels at goal, per the NCEP guidelines, were randomized to one of three treatment arms: SIMCOR 1000/20 mg, SIMCOR 2000/20 mg, or simvastatin 20 mg. In Group B, patients on simvastatin 40 mg monotherapy, with elevated non-HDL levels per the NCEP guidelines regardless of attainment of LDL-C goals, were randomized to one of three treatment arms: SIMCOR 1000/40 mg, SIMCOR 2000/40 mg, or simvastatin 80 mg. Therapy was initiated at the 500 mg dose of SIMCOR and increased by 500 mg every four weeks. Thus patients were titrated to the 1000 mg dose of SIMCOR after four weeks and to the 2000 mg dose of SIMCOR after 12 weeks. All patients randomized to simvastatin monotherapy received 50 mg immediate-release niacin daily in an attempt to keep the study from becoming unblinded due to flushing in the SIMCOR groups. Patients were instructed to take one 325 mg aspirin 30 minutes prior to taking the double-blind medication to help minimize flushing effects.

In Group A, the primary efficacy analysis was a comparison of the mean percent change in non-HDL levels between the SIMCOR 2000/20 mg and simvastatin 20 mg groups, and if statistically significant, then a comparison was conducted between the SIMCOR 1000/20 mg and simvastatin 20 mg groups. In Group B, the primary efficacy analysis was a determination of whether the mean percent change in non-HDL in the SIMCOR 2000/40 mg group was non-inferior to the mean percent change in the simvastatin 80 mg group, and if so, whether the mean percent change in non-HDL in the SIMCOR 1000/40 mg group was non-inferior to the mean percent change in the simvastatin 80 mg group.

In Group A, the non-HDL-C lowering with SIMCOR 2000/20 and SIMCOR 1000/20 was statistically significantly greater than that achieved with simvastatin 20 mg after 24 weeks ($p<0.05$; Table 6). The completion rate after 24 weeks was 72% for the SIMCOR arms and 88% for the simvastatin 20 mg arm. In Group B, the non-HDL-C lowering with SIMCOR 2000/40 and SIMCOR 1000/40 was non-inferior to that achieved with simvastatin 80 mg after 24 weeks (Table 7). The completion rate after 24 weeks was 78% for the SIMCOR arms and 80% for the simvastatin 80 mg arm.

SIMCOR was not superior to simvastatin in lowering LDL-C in either Group A or Group B. However, SIMCOR was superior to simvastatin in both groups in lowering TG and raising HDL (Tables 8 and 9).

[See table 6 at bottom of next page]
[See table 7 at bottom of next page]
[See table 8 at bottom of next page]
[See table 9 at bottom of next page]

16 HOW SUPPLIED/STORAGE AND HANDLING

SIMCOR 500 mg/20 mg, 750 mg/20 mg and 1000 mg/20 mg tablets are available as blue, unscored, tablets, printed with black ink and packaged in bottles of 90 tablets. SIMCOR 500 mg/40 mg and 1000 mg/40 mg tablets are available as dark blue, unscored, tablets, printed with white ink and packaged in bottles of 90 tablets. Each tablet is printed on one side with the "a" logo and a code number specific to the tablet strength. Please see the table below:

SIMCOR Tablet Strength	Printed ID	NDC Number
500 mg/20 mg	a 500-20	0074-3312-90
500 mg/40 mg	a 500-40	0074-3459-90
750 mg/20 mg	a 750-20	0074-3315-90
1000 mg/20 mg	a 1000-20	0074-3455-90
1000 mg/40 mg	a 1000-40	0074-3457-90

Storage: Store at controlled room temperature 20°-25°C (68°-77°F).

17 PATIENT COUNSELING INFORMATION

Patients should be advised to adhere to their National Cholesterol Education Program (NCEP)-recommended diet, a regular exercise program, and periodic testing of a fasting lipid panel.

Patients should be advised about substances they should not take concomitantly with simvastatin *[see Contraindications (4) and Warnings and Precautions (5.2)]*. Patients should also be advised to inform other healthcare professionals prescribing a new medication or increasing the dose of an existing medication that they are taking SIMCOR.

Table 5.
Effect of Coadministered Drugs or Grapefruit Juice on Simvastatin Systemic Exposure

Coadministered Drug or Grapefruit Juice	Dosing of Coadministered Drug or Grapefruit Juice	Dosing of Simvastatin		Geometric Mean Ratio (Ratio* with / without coadministered drug) No Effect = 1.00	
				AUC	C_{max}
Contraindicated with simvastatin *[see Contraindications (4) and Warnings and Precautions (5.2)]*					
Telithromycin[†]	200 mg QD for 4 days	80 mg	simvastatin acid[‡] simvastatin	12 8.9	15 5.3
Nelfinavir[†]	1250 mg BID for 14 days	20 mg QD for 28 days	simvastatin acid[‡] simvastatin	6	6.2
Itraconazole[†]	200 mg QD for 4 days	80 mg	simvastatin acid[‡] simvastatin		13.1 13.1
Posaconazole	100 mg (oral suspension) QD for 13 days	40 mg	simvastatin acid simvastatin	7.3 10.3	9.2 9.4
	200 mg (oral suspension) QD for 13 days	40 mg	simvastatin acid simvastatin	8.5 10.6	9.5 11.4
Gemfibrozil	600 mg BID for 3 days	40 mg	simvastatin acid simvastatin	2.85 1.35	2.18 0.91
Avoid >1 quart of grapefruit juice with simvastatin *[see Warnings and Precautions (5.2)]*					
Grapefruit Juice[§] (high dose)	200 mL of double-strength TID[¶]	60 mg single dose	simvastatin acid simvastatin	7 16	
Grapefruit Juice[§] (low dose)	8 oz (about 237 mL) of single-strength[#]	20 mg single dose	simvastatin acid simvastatin	1.3 1.9	
Avoid taking with >10 mg simvastatin, based on clinical and/or post-marketing experience *[see Warnings and Precautions (5.2)]*					
Verapamil SR	240 mg QD Days 1-7 then 240 mg BID on Days 8-10	80 mg on Day 10	simvastatin acid simvastatin	2.3 2.5	2.4 2.1
Diltiazem	120 mg BID for 10 days	80 mg on Day 10	simvastatin acid simvastatin	2.69 3.10	2.69 2.88
Diltiazem	120 mg BID for 14 days	20 mg on Day 14	simvastatin	4.6	3.6
Avoid taking with >20 mg simvastatin, based on clinical and/or post-marketing experience *[see Warnings and Precautions (5.2)]*					
Amiodarone	400 mg QD for 3 days	40 mg on Day 3	simvastatin acid simvastatin	1.75 1.76	1.72 1.79
Amlodipine	10 mg QD for 10 days	80 mg on Day 10	simvastatin acid simvastatin	1.58 1.77	1.56 1.47
Ranolazine SR	1000 mg BID for 7 days	80 mg on Day 1, and Day 6-9	simvastatin acid simvastatin	2.26 1.86	2.28 1.75
No dosing adjustments required for the following:					
Fenofibrate	160 mg QD for 14 days	80 mg QD on Days 8-14	simvastatin acid simvastatin	0.64 0.89	0.89 0.83
Niacin extended-release[þ]	2 g single dose	20 mg single dose	simvastatin acid simvastatin	1.6 1.4	1.84 1.08
Propranolol	80 mg single dose	80 mg single dose	total inhibitor active inhibitor	0.79 0.79	↓ from 33.6 to 21.1 ng•eq/mL ↓ from 7.0 to 4.7 ng•eq/mL

* Results based on a chemical assay except results with propranolol as indicated.
† Results could be representative of the following CYP3A4 inhibitors: ketoconazole, erythromycin, clarithromycin, HIV protease inhibitors, and nefazodone.
‡ Simvastatin acid refers to the β-hydroxyacid of simvastatin.
§ The effect of amounts of grapefruit juice between those used in these two studies on simvastatin pharmacokinetics has not been studied.

¶ Double-strength: one can of frozen concentrate diluted with one can of water. Grapefruit juice was administered TID for 2 days, and 200 mL together with single dose simvastatin and 30 and 90 minutes following single dose simvastatin on Day 3.
# Single-strength: one can of frozen concentrate diluted with 3 cans of water. Grapefruit juice was administered with breakfast for 3 days, and simvastatin was administered in the evening on Day 3.

þ Because Chinese patients have an increased risk for myopathy with simvastatin coadministered with lipid-modifying doses (≥1 gram/day niacin) of niacin-containing products, and the risk is dose-related, Chinese patients should not receive simvastatin 80 mg coadministered with lipid-modifying doses of niacin-containing products *[see Warnings and Precautions (5.2)]*.

17.1 Muscle Pain
All patients starting therapy with SIMCOR should be advised of the risk of myopathy, including rhabdomyolysis, and told to report promptly any unexplained muscle pain, tenderness or weakness particularly if accompanied by malaise or fever or if these muscle signs or symptoms persist after discontinuing SIMCOR. The risk of myopathy, including rhabdomyolysis, occurring with the use of SIMCOR is increased when taking certain types of medication or consuming larger quantities of grapefruit juice. Patients should discuss all medication, both prescription and over the counter, with their healthcare professional.

17.2 Liver Enzymes
It is recommended that liver enzyme tests be performed before the initiation of SIMCOR, and if signs or symptoms of liver injury occur. All patients treated with SIMCOR should be advised to report promptly any symptoms that may indicate liver injury, including fatigue, anorexia, right upper abdominal discomfort, dark urine or jaundice.

17.3 Dosing Time
SIMCOR tablets should be taken at bedtime, after a low-fat snack. Administration on an empty stomach is not recommended.

17.4 Tablet Integrity
SIMCOR tablets should not be broken, crushed or chewed, but should be swallowed whole.

17.5 Dosing Interruption
If dosing is interrupted for any length of time, their physician should be contacted prior to re-starting therapy; re-titration is recommended.

17.6 Flushing
Flushing is a common side effect of niacin therapy that may subside after several weeks of consistent SIMCOR use. Flushing may vary in severity and is more likely to occur with initiation of therapy, or during dose increases. By dosing at bedtime, flushing will most likely occur during sleep. However, if awakened by flushing at night, the patient should get up slowly, especially if feeling dizzy, feeling faint, or taking blood pressure medications.

17.7 Use of Aspirin
Taking aspirin approximately 30 minutes before dosing can minimize flushing.

17.8 Diet
To avoid ingestion of alcohol, hot beverages and spicy foods around the time of taking SIMCOR to minimize flushing.

17.9 Supplements
To notify their physician if they are taking vitamins or other nutritional supplements containing niacin or nicotinamide.

17.10 Dizziness
To notify their physician if symptoms of dizziness occur.

17.11 Diabetics
If diabetic, to notify their physician of changes in blood glucose.

17.12 Pregnancy
Women of childbearing age should use an effective method of birth control to prevent pregnancy while using SIMCOR. Discuss future pregnancy plans with your healthcare professional, and discuss when to stop SIMCOR if you are trying to conceive. If you are pregnant, stop SIMCOR and call your healthcare professional.

17.13 Breastfeeding
Women who are breastfeeding should not use SIMCOR. If you have a lipid disorder and are breastfeeding, speak with your healthcare professionals about your lipid disorder and whether or not you should breastfeed your infant.

Manufactured by AbbVie LTD, Barceloneta, PR 00617
for AbbVie Inc., North Chicago, IL 60064, U.S.A.
Ref: 03-A744-R10-Revised March, 2013
Shown in Product Identification Guide, page 304

Table 6. Non-HDL Treatment Response Following 24-Week Treatment Mean Percent Change from Simvastatin 20-mg Treated Baseline

Group A

	SIMCOR 2000/20			SIMCOR 1000/20			Simvastatin 20		
Week	n[a]	dose (mg/mg)	non-HDL[b]	n[a]	Dose (mg/mg)	non-HDL[b]	n[a]	Dose (mg/mg)	non-HDL[b]
Baseline	56	---	163.1 mg/dL	108	---	164.8 mg/dL	102	---	163.7 mg/dL
4	52	500/20	-12.9%	86	500/20	-12.8%	91	20	-8.3%
8	46	1000/20	-17.5%	91	1000/20	-15.5%	95	20	-8.3%
12	46	1500/20	-18.9%	90	1000/20	-14.8%	96	20	-6.4%
24	40	2000/20	-19.5%[†]	78	1000/20	-13.6%[†]	90	20	-5.0%
Dropouts by week 24:	28.6%			27.8%			11.8%		

[a] n=number of subjects with values in the analysis window at each timepoint
[b] The percent change from baseline is the model-based mean from a repeated measures mixed model with no imputation for missing data from study dropouts.
[†] significant vs. simvastatin 20 mg at the primary endpoint (Week 24), $p<0.05$

Table 7. Non-HDL Treatment Response Following 24-Week Treatment Mean Percent Change from Simvastatin 40-mg Treated Baseline

Group B

	SIMCOR 2000/40			SIMCOR 1000/40			Simvastatin 80		
Week	n[a]	dose (mg/mg)	non-HDL[b]	n[a]	Dose (mg/mg)	non-HDL[b]	n[a]	Dose (mg/mg)	non-HDL[b]
Baseline	98	---	144.4 mg/dL	111	---	141.2 mg/dL	113	---	134.5 mg/dL
4	96	500/40	-6.0%	108	500/40	-5.9%	110	80	11.3%
8	93	1000/40	-15.5%	100	1000/40	-16.2%	104	80	-13.7%
12	90	1500/40	-18.4%	97	1000/40	-12.6%	100	80	-9.5%
24	80	2000/40	-7.6%[c]	82	1000/40	-6.7%[d]	90	80	-6.0%
Dropouts by week 24:	18.4%			26.1%			20.4%		

[a] n=number of subjects with values in the analysis window at each timepoint
[b] The percent change from baseline is the model-based mean from a repeated measures mixed model with no imputation for missing data from study dropouts.
[c] non-inferior to Simvastatin 80 arm; 95% confidence interval of mean difference in non-HDL for SIMCOR 2000/40 vs. Simvastatin 80 is (-7.7%, 4.5%)
[d] non-inferior to Simvastatin 80 arm; 95% confidence interval of mean difference in non-HDL for SIMCOR 1000/40 vs. SIMCOR 80 is (-6.6%, 5.3%)

Table 8. Mean Percent Change from Baseline to Week 24 in Lipoprotein Lipid Levels

	Treatment Group A					
TREATMENT	N	LDL-C	Total-C	HDL-C	TG[a]	Apo B
Baseline (mg/dL)*	266	120	207	43	209	102
Simvastatin 20 mg	102	-6.7%	-4.5%	7.8%	-15.3%	-5.6%
SIMCOR 1000/20	108	-11.9%	-8.8%	20.7%	-26.5%	-13.2%
SIMCOR 2000/20	56	-14.3%	-11.1%	29.0%	-38.0%	-18.5%

* either treatment naïve or after receiving simvastatin 20 mg
[a] medians are reported for TG

Table 9. Mean Percent Change from Baseline to Week 24 in Lipoprotein Lipid Levels

	Treatment Group B					
TREATMENT	N	LDL-C	Total-C	HDL-C	TG[a]	Apo B
Baseline (mg/dL)*	322	108	187	47	145	93
Simvastatin 80 mg	113	-11.4%	-6.2%	0.1%	0.3%	-7.5%
SIMCOR 1000/40	111	-7.1%	-3.1%	15.4%	-22.8%	-7.7%
SIMCOR 2000/40	98	-5.1%	-1.6%	24.4%	-31.8%	-10.5%

* after receiving simvastatin 40 mg
[a] medians are reported for TG

SURVANTA®
℞

(beractant)
intratracheal suspension
Sterile Suspension
For Intratracheal Administration Only

DESCRIPTION
SURVANTA® (beractant) Intratracheal Suspension is a sterile, non-pyrogenic pulmonary surfactant intended for intratracheal use only. It is a natural bovine lung extract containing phospholipids, neutral lipids, fatty acids, and surfactant-associated proteins to which colfosceril palmitate (dipalmitoylphosphatidylcholine), palmitic acid, and tripalmitin are added to standardize the composition and to mimic surface-tension lowering properties of natural lung surfactant. The resulting composition provides 25 mg/mL phospholipids (including 11.0-15.5 mg/mL disaturated phosphatidylcholine), 0.5-1.75 mg/mL triglycerides, 1.4-3.5 mg/mL free fatty acids, and less than 1.0 mg/mL protein. It is suspended in 0.9% sodium chloride solution, and heat-sterilized. SURVANTA contains no preservatives. Its protein content consists of two hydrophobic, low molecular weight, surfactant-associated proteins commonly known as SP-B and SP-C. It does not contain the hydrophilic, large molecular weight surfactant-associated protein known as SP-A.

Each mL of SURVANTA contains 25 mg of phospholipids. It is an off-white to light brown liquid supplied in single-use glass vials containing 4 mL (100 mg phospholipids) or 8 mL (200 mg phospholipids).

Information on the AbbVie, Inc. products listed on these pages is from the prescribing information in use as of July 31, 2013. For more information, please visit rxabbvie.com or call 1-800-633-9110.

CLINICAL PHARMACOLOGY

Endogenous pulmonary surfactant lowers surface tension on alveolar surfaces during respiration and stabilizes the alveoli against collapse at resting transpulmonary pressures. Deficiency of pulmonary surfactant causes Respiratory Distress Syndrome (RDS) in premature infants. SURVANTA replenishes surfactant and restores surface activity to the lungs of these infants.

Activity

In vitro, SURVANTA reproducibly lowers minimum surface tension to less than 8 dynes/cm as measured by the pulsating bubble surfactometer and Wilhelmy Surface Balance. *In situ,* SURVANTA restores pulmonary compliance to excised rat lungs artificially made surfactant-deficient. *In vivo,* single SURVANTA doses improve lung pressure-volume measurements, lung compliance, and oxygenation in premature rabbits and sheep.

Animal Metabolism

SURVANTA is administered directly to the target organ, the lungs, where biophysical effects occur at the alveolar surface. In surfactant-deficient premature rabbits and lambs, alveolar clearance of radio-labelled lipid components of SURVANTA is rapid. Most of the dose becomes lung-associated within hours of administration, and the lipids enter endogenous surfactant pathways of reutilization and recycling. In surfactant-sufficient adult animals, SURVANTA clearance is more rapid than in premature and young animals. There is less reutilization and recycling of surfactant in adult animals.

Limited animal experiments have not found effects of SURVANTA on endogenous surfactant metabolism. Precursor incorporation and subsequent secretion of saturated phosphatidylcholine in premature sheep are not changed by SURVANTA treatments.

No information is available about the metabolic fate of the surfactant-associated proteins in SURVANTA. The metabolic disposition in humans has not been studied.

Clinical Studies

Clinical effects of SURVANTA were demonstrated in six single-dose and four multiple-dose randomized, multicenter, controlled clinical trials involving approximately 1700 infants. Three open trials, including a Treatment IND, involved more than 8500 infants. Each dose of SURVANTA in all studies was 100 mg phospholipids/kg birth weight and was based on published experience with Surfactant TA, a lyophilized powder dosage form of SURVANTA having the same composition.

Prevention Studies

Infants of 600-1250 g birth weight and 23 to 29 weeks estimated gestational age were enrolled in two *multiple-dose* studies. A dose of SURVANTA was given within 15 minutes of birth to prevent the development of RDS. Up to three additional doses in the first 48 hours, as often as every 6 hours, were given if RDS subsequently developed and infants required mechanical ventilation with an $FiO_2 \geq 0.30$. Results of the studies at 28 days of age are shown in Table 1.

TABLE 1

Study 1

	SURVANTA	Control	P-Value
Number infants studied	119	124	
Incidence of RDS (%)	27.6	63.5	< 0.001
Death due to RDS (%)	2.5	19.5	< 0.001
Death or BPD due to RDS (%)	48.7	52.8	0.536
Death due to any cause (%)	7.6	22.8	0.001
Air Leaks[a] (%)	5.9	21.7	0.001
Pulmonary interstitial emphysema (%)	20.8	40.0	0.001

Study 2[b]

	SURVANTA	Control	P-Value
Number infants studied	91	96	
Incidence of RDS (%)	28.6	48.3	0.007
Death due to RDS (%)	1.1	10.5	0.006
Death or BPD due to RDS (%)	27.5	44.2	0.018
Death due to any cause [c](%)	16.5	13.7	0.633
Air Leaks [a](%)	14.5	19.6	0.374
Pulmonary interstitial emphysema (%)	26.5	33.2	0.298

[a]Pneumothorax or pneumopericardium
[b]Study discontinued when Treatment IND initiated
[c]No cause of death in the SURVANTA group was significantly increased; the higher number of deaths in this group was due to the sum of all causes.

Rescue Studies

Infants of 600-1750 g birth weight with RDS requiring mechanical ventilation and an $FiO_2 \geq 0.40$ were enrolled in two *multiple-dose* rescue studies. The initial dose of SURVANTA was given after RDS developed and before 8 hours of age. Infants could receive up to three additional doses in the first 48 hours, as often as every 6 hours, if they required mechanical ventilation and an $FiO_2 \geq 0.30$. Results of the studies at 28 days of age are shown in Table 2.

TABLE 2

Study 3[a]

	SURVANTA	Control	P-Value
Number infants studied	198	193	
Death due to RDS (%)	11.6	18.1	0.071
Death or BPD due to RDS (%)	59.1	66.8	0.102
Death due to any cause (%)	21.7	26.4	0.285
Air Leaks[b] (%)	11.8	29.5	<0.001
Pulmonary interstitial emphysema (%)	16.3	34.0	<0.001

Study 4

	SURVANTA	Control	P-Value
Number infants studied	204	203	
Death due to RDS (%)	6.4	22.3	< 0.001
Death or BPD due to RDS (%)	43.6	63.4	< 0.001
Death due to any cause (%)	15.2	28.2	0.001
Air Leaks[b] (%)	11.2	22.2	0.005
Pulmonary interstitial emphysema (%)	20.8	44.4	< 0.001

[a]Study discontinued when Treatment IND initiated
[b]Pneumothorax or pneumopericardium

Acute Clinical Effects

Marked improvements in oxygenation may occur within minutes of administration of SURVANTA.

All controlled clinical studies with SURVANTA provided information regarding the acute effects of SURVANTA on the arterial-alveolar oxygen ratio (a/APO_2), FiO_2, and mean airway pressure (MAP) during the first 48 to 72 hours of life. Significant improvements in these variables were sustained for 48-72 hours in SURVANTA-treated infants in four single-dose and two multiple-dose rescue studies and in two multiple-dose prevention studies. In the single-dose prevention studies, the FiO_2 improved significantly.

Indications and Usage

SURVANTA is indicated for prevention and treatment ("rescue") of Respiratory Distress Syndrome (RDS) (hyaline membrane disease) in premature infants. SURVANTA significantly reduces the incidence of RDS, mortality due to RDS and air leak complications.

Prevention

In premature infants less than 1250 g birth weight or with evidence of surfactant deficiency, give SURVANTA as soon as possible, preferably within 15 minutes of birth.

Rescue

To treat infants with RDS confirmed by x-ray and requiring mechanical ventilation, give SURVANTA as soon as possible, preferably by 8 hours of age.

Contraindications

None known.

Warnings

SURVANTA is intended for intratracheal use only.

SURVANTA CAN RAPIDLY AFFECT OXYGENATION AND LUNG COMPLIANCE. Therefore, its use should be restricted to a highly supervised clinical setting with immediate availability of clinicians experienced with intubation, ventilator management, and general care of premature infants. Infants receiving SURVANTA should be frequently monitored with arterial or transcutaneous measurement of systemic oxygen and carbon dioxide.

DURING THE DOSING PROCEDURE, TRANSIENT EPISODES OF BRADYCARDIA AND DECREASED OXYGEN SATURATION HAVE BEEN REPORTED. If these occur, stop the dosing procedure and initiate appropriate measures to alleviate the condition. After stabilization, resume the dosing procedure.

Precautions

General

Rales and moist breath sounds can occur transiently after administration. Endotracheal suctioning or other remedial action is not necessary unless clear-cut signs of airway obstruction are present.

Increased probability of post-treatment nosocomial sepsis in SURVANTA-treated infants was observed in the controlled clinical trials (Table 3). The increased risk for sepsis among SURVANTA-treated infants was not associated with increased mortality among these infants. The causative organisms were similar in treated and control infants. There was no significant difference between groups in the rate of post-treatment infections other than sepsis.

Use of SURVANTA in infants less than 600 g birth weight or greater than 1750 g birth weight has not been evaluated in controlled trials. There is no controlled experience with use of SURVANTA in conjunction with experimental therapies for RDS (eg, high-frequency ventilation or extracorporeal membrane oxygenation).

No information is available on the effects of doses other than 100 mg phospholipids/kg, more than four doses, dosing more frequently than every 6 hours, or administration after 48 hours of age.

Carcinogenesis, Mutagenesis, Impairment of Fertility

Carcinogenicity studies have not been performed with SURVANTA. SURVANTA was negative when tested in the Ames test for mutagenicity. Using the maximum feasible dose volume, SURVANTA up to 500 mg phospholipids/kg/day (approximately one-third the premature infant dose based on $mg/m^2/day$) was administered subcutaneously to newborn rats for 5 days. The rats reproduced normally and there were no observable adverse effects in their offspring.

Adverse Reactions

The most commonly reported adverse experiences were associated with the dosing procedure. In the multiple-dose controlled clinical trials, each dose of SURVANTA was divided into four quarter-doses which were instilled through a catheter inserted into the endotracheal tube by briefly disconnecting the endotracheal tube from the ventilator. Transient bradycardia occurred with 11.9% of *doses*. Oxygen desaturation occurred with 9.8% of *doses*.

Other reactions during the dosing procedure occurred with fewer than 1% of doses and included endotracheal tube reflux, pallor, vasoconstriction, hypotension, endotracheal tube blockage, hypertension, hypocarbia, hypercarbia, and apnea. No deaths occurred during the dosing procedure, and all reactions resolved with symptomatic treatment.

The occurrence of concurrent illnesses common in premature infants was evaluated in the controlled trials. The rates in all controlled studies are in Table 3.

TABLE 3

	All Controlled Studies		
Concurrent Event	**SURVANTA (%)**	**Control (%)**	**P-Value[a]**
Patent ductus arteriosus	46.9	47.1	0.814
Intracranial hemorrhage	48.1	45.2	0.241
Severe intracranial hemorrhage	24.1	23.3	0.693
Pulmonary air leaks	10.9	24.7	< 0.001
Pulmonary interstitial emphysema	20.2	38.4	< 0.001
Necrotizing enterocolitis	6.1	5.3	0.427
Apnea	65.4	59.6	0.283
Severe apnea	46.1	42.5	0.114
Post-treatment sepsis	20.7	16.1	0.019
Post-treatment infection	10.2	9.1	0.345
Pulmonary hemorrhage	7.2	5.3	0.166

[a]*P*-value comparing groups in controlled studies

When all controlled studies were pooled, there was no difference in intracranial hemorrhage. However, in one of the single-dose rescue studies and one of the multiple-dose prevention studies, the rate of intracranial hemorrhage was significantly higher in SURVANTA patients than control patients (63.3% *v* 30.8%, $P = 0.001$; and 48.8% *v* 34.2%, $P = 0.047$, respectively). The rate in a Treatment IND involving approximately 8100 infants was lower than in the controlled trials.

In the controlled clinical trials, there was no effect of SURVANTA on results of common laboratory tests: white blood cell count and serum sodium, potassium, bilirubin, and creatinine.

More than 4300 pretreatment and post-treatment serum samples from approximately 1500 patients were tested by Western Blot Immunoassay for antibodies to surfactant-associated proteins SP-B and SP-C. No IgG or IgM antibodies were detected.

Several other complications are known to occur in premature infants. The following conditions were reported in the controlled clinical studies. The rates of the complications were not different in treated and control infants, and none of the complications were attributed to SURVANTA.

Respiratory
lung consolidation, blood from the endotracheal tube, deterioration after weaning, respiratory decompensation, subglottic stenosis, paralyzed diaphragm, respiratory failure.
Cardiovascular
hypotension, hypertension, tachycardia, ventricular tachycardia, aortic thrombosis, cardiac failure, cardio-respiratory arrest, increased apical pulse, persistent fetal circulation, air embolism, total anomalous pulmonary venous return.
Gastrointestinal
abdominal distention, hemorrhage, intestinal perforations, volvulus, bowel infarct, feeding intolerance, hepatic failure, stress ulcer.
Renal
renal failure, hematuria.
Hematologic
coagulopathy, thrombocytopenia, disseminated intravascular coagulation.
Central Nervous System
seizures.
Endocrine/Metabolic
adrenal hemorrhage, inappropriate ADH secretion, hyperphosphatemia.
Musculoskeletal
inguinal hernia.
Systemic
fever, deterioration.
Follow-Up Evaluations
To date, no long-term complications or sequelae of SURVANTA therapy have been found.
Single-Dose Studies
Six-month adjusted-age follow-up evaluations of 232 infants (115 treated) demonstrated no clinically important differences between treatment groups in pulmonary and neurologic sequelae, incidence or severity of retinopathy of prematurity, rehospitalizations, growth, or allergic manifestations.
Multiple-Dose Studies
Six-month adjusted age follow-up evaluations have been completed in 631 (345 treated) of 916 surviving infants. There were significantly less cerebral palsy and need for supplemental oxygen in SURVANTA infants than controls. Wheezing at the time of examination was significantly more frequent among SURVANTA infants, although there was no difference in bronchodilator therapy.
Final twelve-month follow-up data from the multiple-dose studies are available from 521 (272 treated) of 909 surviving infants. There was significantly less wheezing in SURVANTA infants than controls, in contrast to the six-month results. There was no difference in the incidence of cerebral palsy at twelve months.
Twenty-four month adjusted age evaluations were completed in 429 (226 treated) of 906 surviving infants. There were significantly fewer SURVANTA infants with rhonchi, wheezing, and tachypnea at the time of examination. No other differences were found.

Overdosage

Overdosage with SURVANTA has not been reported. Based on animal data, overdosage might result in acute airway obstruction. Treatment should be symptomatic and supportive.
Rales and moist breath sounds can transiently occur after SURVANTA is given, and do not indicate overdosage. Endotracheal suctioning or other remedial action is not required unless clear-cut signs of airway obstruction are present.

Dosage and Administration

FOR INTRATRACHEAL ADMINISTRATION ONLY.
SURVANTA should be administered by or under the supervision of clinicians experienced in intubation, ventilator management, and general care of premature infants.
Marked improvements in oxygenation may occur within minutes of administration of SURVANTA. Therefore, frequent and careful clinical observation and monitoring of systemic oxygenation are essential to avoid hyperoxia.
Review of audiovisual instructional materials describing dosage and administration procedures is recommended before using SURVANTA. Materials are available upon request from AbbVie Inc.
Dosage
Each dose of SURVANTA is 100 mg of phospholipids/kg birth weight (4 mL/kg). The SURVANTA DOSING CHART shows the total dosage for a range of birth weights.

SURVANTA DOSING CHART

Weight (grams)	Total Dose (mL)	Weight (grams)	Total Dose (mL)
600-650	2.6	1301-1350	5.4
651-700	2.8	1351-1400	5.6
701-750	3.0	1401-1450	5.8
751-800	3.2	1451-1500	6.0
801-850	3.4	1501-1550	6.2
851-900	3.6	1551-1600	6.4
901-950	3.8	1601-1650	6.6
951-1000	4.0	1651-1700	6.8
1001-1050	4.2	1701-1750	7.0
1051-1100	4.4	1751-1800	7.2
1101-1150	4.6	1801-1850	7.4
1151-1200	4.8	1851-1900	7.6
1201-1250	5.0	1901-1950	7.8
1251-1300	5.2	1951-2000	8.0

Four doses of SURVANTA can be administered in the first 48 hours of life. Doses should be given no more frequently than every 6 hours.
Directions for Use
SURVANTA should be inspected visually for discoloration prior to administration. The color of SURVANTA is off-white to light brown. If settling occurs during storage, swirl the vial gently (DO NOT SHAKE) to redisperse. Some foaming at the surface may occur during handling and is inherent in the nature of the product.
SURVANTA is stored refrigerated (2-8°C). Date and time need to be recorded in the box on front of the carton or vial, whenever SURVANTA is removed from the refrigerator. Before administration, SURVANTA should be warmed by standing at room temperature for at least 20 minutes or warmed in the hand for at least 8 minutes. ARTIFICIAL WARMING METHODS SHOULD NOT BE USED. If a prevention dose is to be given, preparation of SURVANTA should begin before the infant's birth.
Unopened, unused vials of SURVANTA that have been warmed to room temperature may be returned to the refrigerator within 24 hours of warming, and stored for future use. SURVANTA SHOULD NOT BE REMOVED FROM THE REFRIGERATOR FOR MORE THAN 24 HOURS. SURVANTA SHOULD NOT BE WARMED AND RETURNED TO THE REFRIGERATOR MORE THAN ONCE. Each single-use vial of SURVANTA should be entered only once. Used vials with residual drug should be discarded.
SURVANTA DOES NOT REQUIRE RECONSTITUTION OR SONICATION BEFORE USE.

Dosing Procedures

General
SURVANTA is administered intratracheally by instillation through a 5 French end-hole catheter. The catheter can be inserted into the infant's endotracheal tube without interrupting ventilation by passing the catheter through a neonatal suction valve attached to the endotracheal tube. Alternatively, SURVANTA can be instilled through the catheter by briefly disconnecting the endotracheal tube from the ventilator.
The neonatal suction valve used for administering SURVANTA should be a type that allows entry of the catheter into the endotracheal tube without interrupting ventilation and also maintains a closed airway circuit system by sealing the valve around the catheter.
If the neonatal suction valve is used, the catheter should be rigid enough to pass easily into the endotracheal tube. A very soft and pliable catheter may twist or curl within the neonatal suction valve. The length of the catheter should be shortened so that the tip of the catheter protrudes just beyond the end of the endotracheal tube above the infant's carina. SURVANTA should not be instilled into a mainstem bronchus.
To ensure homogenous distribution of SURVANTA throughout the lungs, each dose is divided into *four quarter-doses.* Each quarter-dose is administered with the infant in a different position. The recommended positions are:

- Head and body inclined 5-10° down, head turned to the right
- Head and body inclined 5-10° down, head turned to the left
- Head and body inclined 5-10° up, head turned to the right
- Head and body inclined 5-10° up, head turned to the left

The dosing procedure is facilitated if one person administers the dose while another person positions and monitors the infant.
First Dose
Determine the total dose of SURVANTA from the SURVANTA DOSING CHART based on the infant's birth weight. Slowly withdraw the entire contents of the vial into a plastic syringe through a large-gauge needle (eg, at least 20 gauge). DO NOT FILTER SURVANTA AND AVOID SHAKING.
Attach the premeasured 5 French end-hole catheter to the syringe. Fill the catheter with SURVANTA. Discard excess SURVANTA through the catheter so that only the total dose to be given remains in the syringe.
BEFORE ADMINISTERING SURVANTA, assure proper placement and patency of the endotracheal tube. At the discretion of the clinician, the endotracheal tube may be suctioned before administering SURVANTA. The infant should be allowed to stabilize before proceeding with dosing.
In the prevention strategy, weigh, intubate and stabilize the infant. Administer the dose as soon as possible after birth, preferably within 15 minutes. Position the infant appropriately and gently inject the first quarter-dose through the catheter over 2-3 seconds.
After administration of the first quarter-dose, remove the catheter from the endotracheal tube. Manually ventilate with a hand-bag with sufficient oxygen to prevent cyanosis, at a rate of 60 breaths/minute, and sufficient positive pressure to provide adequate air exchange and chest wall excursion.
In the rescue strategy, the first dose should be given as soon as possible after the infant is placed on a ventilator for management of RDS. In the clinical trials, immediately before instilling the first quarter-dose, the infant's ventilator settings were changed to rate 60/minute, inspiratory time 0.5 second, and FiO_2 1.0.
Position the infant appropriately and gently inject the first quarter-dose through the catheter over 2-3 seconds. After administration of the first quarter-dose, remove the catheter from the endotracheal tube and continue mechanical ventilation.
In both strategies, ventilate the infant for at least 30 seconds or until stable. Reposition the infant for instillation of the next quarter-dose.
Instill the remaining quarter-doses using the same procedures. After instillation of each quarter-dose, remove the catheter and ventilate for at least 30 seconds or until the infant is stabilized. After instillation of the final quarter-dose, remove the catheter without flushing it. Do not suction the infant for 1 hour after dosing unless signs of significant airway obstruction occur.
AFTER COMPLETION OF THE DOSING PROCEDURE, RESUME USUAL VENTILATOR MANAGEMENT AND CLINICAL CARE.
Repeat Doses
The dosage of SURVANTA for repeat doses is also 100 mg phospholipids/kg and is based on the infant's birth weight. The infant should not be reweighed for determination of the SURVANTA dosage. Use the SURVANTA DOSING CHART to determine the total dosage.
The need for additional doses of SURVANTA is determined by evidence of continuing respiratory distress. Using the following criteria for redosing, significant reductions in mortality due to RDS were observed in the multiple-dose clinical trials with SURVANTA.

> Dose no sooner than 6 hours after the preceding dose if the infant remains intubated and requires at least 30% inspired oxygen to maintain a PaO_2 less than or equal to 80 torr.
> Radiographic confirmation of RDS should be obtained before administering additional doses to those who received a prevention dose.

Prepare SURVANTA and position the infant for administration of each quarter-dose as previously described. After instillation of each quarter-dose, remove the dosing catheter from the endotracheal tube and ventilate the infant for at least 30 seconds or until stable.
In the clinical studies, ventilator settings used to administer repeat doses were different than those used for the first dose. For repeat doses, the FiO_2 was increased by 0.20 or an amount sufficient to prevent cyanosis. The ventilator delivered a rate of 30/minute with an inspiratory time less than 1.0 second. If the infant's pretreatment rate was 30 or greater, it was left unchanged during SURVANTA instillation.
Manual hand-bag ventilation should not be used to administer repeat doses. DURING THE DOSING PROCEDURE, VENTILATOR SETTINGS MAY BE ADJUSTED AT THE DISCRETION OF THE CLINICIAN TO MAINTAIN APPROPRIATE OXYGENATION AND VENTILATION.
AFTER COMPLETION OF THE DOSING PROCEDURE, RESUME USUAL VENTILATOR MANAGEMENT AND CLINICAL CARE.
Dosing Precautions
If an infant experiences bradycardia or oxygen desaturation during the dosing procedure, stop the dosing procedure and initiate appropriate measures to alleviate the condition. After the infant has stabilized, resume the dosing procedure.
Rales and moist breath sounds can occur transiently after administration of SURVANTA. Endotracheal suctioning or other remedial action is unnecessary unless clear-cut signs of airway obstruction are present.

How Supplied

SURVANTA (beractant) Intratracheal Suspension is supplied in single-use glass vials containing 4 mL (NDC 0074-

Information on the AbbVie, Inc. products listed on these pages is from the prescribing information in use as of July 31, 2013. For more information, please visit rxabbvie.com or call 1-800-633-9110.

1040-04) or 8 mL of SURVANTA (NDC 0074-1040-08). Each milliliter contains 25 mg of phospholipids suspended in 0.9% sodium chloride solution. The color is off-white to light brown.

Store unopened vials at refrigeration temperature (2-8°C). Protect from light. Store vials in carton until ready for use. Vials are for single use only. Upon opening, discard unused drug.

LITHO IN USA

AbbVie Inc.
North Chicago, IL 60064, U.S.A.
03-A683 December, 2012

Shown in Product Identification Guide, page 304

SYNTHROID® ℞

[*sĭn-thrŏid*]

(levothyroxine sodium tablets, USP)

DESCRIPTION

SYNTHROID (levothyroxine sodium tablets, USP) contain synthetic crystalline L-3,3′,5,5′-tetraiodothyronine sodium salt [levothyroxine (T_4) sodium]. Synthetic T_4 is identical to that produced in the human thyroid gland. Levothyroxine (T_4) sodium has an empirical formula of $C_{15}H_{10}I_4N\ NaO_4 \bullet H_2O$, molecular weight of 798.86 g/mol (anhydrous), and structural formula as shown:

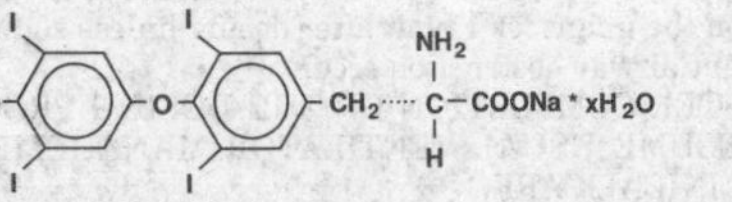

Inactive Ingredients

Acacia, confectioner's sugar (contains corn starch), lactose monohydrate, magnesium stearate, povidone, and talc. The following are the color additives by tablet strength:

Strength (mcg)	Color additive(s)
25	FD&C Yellow No. 6 Aluminum Lake*
50	None
75	FD&C Red No. 40 Aluminum Lake, FD&C Blue No. 2 Aluminum Lake
88	FD&C Blue No. 1 Aluminum Lake, FD&C Yellow No. 6 Aluminum Lake*, D&C Yellow No. 10 Aluminum Lake
100	D&C Yellow No. 10 Aluminum Lake, FD&C Yellow No. 6 Aluminum Lake*
112	D&C Red No. 27 & 30 Aluminum Lake
125	FD&C Yellow No. 6 Aluminum Lake*, FD&C Red No. 40 Aluminum Lake, FD&C Blue No. 1 Aluminum Lake
137	FD&C Blue No. 1 Aluminum Lake
150	FD&C Blue No. 2 Aluminum Lake
175	FD&C Blue No. 1 Aluminum Lake, D&C Red No. 27 & 30 Aluminum Lake
200	FD&C Red No. 40 Aluminum Lake
300	D&C Yellow No. 10 Aluminum Lake, FD&C Yellow No. 6 Aluminum Lake*, FD&C Blue No. 1 Aluminum Lake

*Note – FD&C Yellow No. 6 is orange in color.

Meets USP Dissolution Test 3

CLINICAL PHARMACOLOGY

Thyroid hormone synthesis and secretion is regulated by the hypothalamic-pituitary-thyroid axis. Thyrotropin-releasing hormone (TRH) released from the hypothalamus stimulates secretion of thyrotropin-stimulating hormone, TSH, from the anterior pituitary. TSH, in turn, is the physiologic stimulus for the synthesis and secretion of thyroid hormones, L-thyroxine (T_4) and L-triiodothyronine (T_3), by the thyroid gland. Circulating serum T_3 and T_4 levels exert a feedback effect on both TRH and TSH secretion. When serum T_3 and T_4 levels increase, TRH and TSH secretion decrease. When thyroid hormone levels decrease, TRH and TSH secretion increase.

The mechanisms by which thyroid hormones exert their physiologic actions are not completely understood, but it is thought that their principal effects are exerted through control of DNA transcription and protein synthesis. T_3 and T_4 diffuse into the cell nucleus and bind to thyroid receptor proteins attached to DNA. This hormone nuclear receptor complex activates gene transcription and synthesis of messenger RNA and cytoplasmic proteins.

Thyroid hormones regulate multiple metabolic processes and play an essential role in normal growth and development, and normal maturation of the central nervous system and bone. The metabolic actions of thyroid hormones include augmentation of cellular respiration and thermogenesis, as well as metabolism of proteins, carbohydrates and lipids. The protein anabolic effects of thyroid hormones are essential to normal growth and development.

The physiological actions of thyroid hormones are produced predominantly by T_3, the majority of which (approximately 80%) is derived from T_4 by deiodination in peripheral tissues.

Levothyroxine, at doses individualized according to patient response, is effective as replacement or supplemental therapy in hypothyroidism of any etiology, except transient hypothyroidism during the recovery phase of subacute thyroiditis.

Levothyroxine is also effective in the suppression of pituitary TSH secretion in the treatment or prevention of various types of euthyroid goiters, including thyroid nodules, Hashimoto's thyroiditis, multinodular goiter and, as adjunctive therapy in the management of thyrotropin-dependent well-differentiated thyroid cancer (see **INDICATIONS AND USAGE, PRECAUTIONS**, and **DOSAGE AND ADMINISTRATION**).

Pharmacokinetics

Absorption

Absorption of orally administered T_4 from the gastrointestinal (GI) tract ranges from 40% to 80%. The majority of the levothyroxine dose is absorbed from the jejunum and upper ileum. The relative bioavailability of SYNTHROID tablets, compared to an equal nominal dose of oral levothyroxine sodium solution, is approximately 93%. T_4 absorption is increased by fasting, and decreased in malabsorption syndromes and by certain foods such as soybean infant formula. Dietary fiber decreases bioavailability of T_4. Absorption may also decrease with age. In addition, many drugs and foods affect T_4 absorption (see **PRECAUTIONS - Drug Interactions** and **Drug-Food Interactions**).

Distribution

Circulating thyroid hormones are greater than 99% bound to plasma proteins, including thyroxine-binding globulin (TBG), thyroxine-binding prealbumin (TBPA), and albumin (TBA), whose capacities and affinities vary for each hormone. The higher affinity of both TBG and TBPA for T_4 partially explains the higher serum levels, slower metabolic clearance, and longer half-life of T_4 compared to T_3. Protein-bound thyroid hormones exist in reverse equilibrium with small amounts of free hormone. Only unbound hormone is metabolically active. Many drugs and physiologic conditions affect the binding of thyroid hormones to serum proteins (see **PRECAUTIONS - Drug Interactions** and **Drug-Laboratory Test Interactions**). Thyroid hormones do not readily cross the placental barrier (see **PRECAUTIONS - Pregnancy**).

Metabolism

T_4 is slowly eliminated (see **Table 1**). The major pathway of thyroid hormone metabolism is through sequential deiodination. Approximately eighty-percent of circulating T_3 is derived from peripheral T_4 by monodeiodination. The liver is the major site of degradation for both T_4 and T_3, with T_4 deiodination also occurring at a number of additional sites, including the kidney and other tissues. Approximately 80% of the daily dose of T_4 is deiodinated to yield equal amounts of T_3 and reverse T_3 (rT_3). T_3 and rT_3 are further deiodinated to diiodothyronine. Thyroid hormones are also metabolized via conjugation with glucuronides and sulfates and excreted directly into the bile and gut where they undergo enterohepatic recirculation.

Elimination

Thyroid hormones are primarily eliminated by the kidneys. A portion of the conjugated hormone reaches the colon unchanged and is eliminated in the feces. Approximately 20% of T_4 is eliminated in the stool. Urinary excretion of T_4 decreases with age.

[See table 1 below]

Table 1. Pharmacokinetic Parameters of Thyroid Hormones in Euthyroid Patients

Hormone	Ratio in Thyroglobulin	Biologic Potency	$t_{1/2}$ (days)	Protein Binding (%)[2]
Levothyroxine (T_4)	10 - 20	1	6-7[1]	99.96
Liothyronine (T_3)	1	4	≤ 2	99.5

[1] 3 to 4 days in hyperthyroidism, 9 to 10 days in hypothyroidism
[2] Includes TBG, TBPA, and TBA

INDICATIONS AND USAGE

Levothyroxine sodium is used for the following indications:

Hypothyroidism

As replacement or supplemental therapy in congenital or acquired hypothyroidism of any etiology, except transient hypothyroidism during the recovery phase of subacute thyroiditis. Specific indications include: primary (thyroidal), secondary (pituitary), and tertiary (hypothalamic) hypothyroidism and subclinical hypothyroidism. Primary hypothyroidism may result from functional deficiency, primary atrophy, partial or total congenital absence of the thyroid gland, or from the effects of surgery, radiation, or drugs, with or without the presence of goiter.

Pituitary TSH Suppression

In the treatment or prevention of various types of euthyroid goiters (see **WARNINGS** and **PRECAUTIONS**), including thyroid nodules (see **WARNINGS** and **PRECAUTIONS**), subacute or chronic lymphocytic thyroiditis (Hashimoto's thyroiditis), multinodular goiter (see **WARNINGS** and **PRECAUTIONS**) and, as an adjunct to surgery and radioiodine therapy in the management of thyrotropin-dependent well-differentiated thyroid cancer.

CONTRAINDICATIONS

Levothyroxine is contraindicated in patients with untreated subclinical (suppressed serum TSH level with normal T_3 and T_4 levels) or overt thyrotoxicosis of any etiology and in patients with acute myocardial infarction. Levothyroxine is contraindicated in patients with uncorrected adrenal insufficiency since thyroid hormones may precipitate an acute adrenal crisis by increasing the metabolic clearance of glucocorticoids (see **PRECAUTIONS**). SYNTHROID is contraindicated in patients with hypersensitivity to any of the inactive ingredients in SYNTHROID tablets (See **DESCRIPTION - Inactive Ingredients**).

WARNINGS

Boxed Warning

WARNING: Thyroid hormones, including SYNTHROID, either alone or with other therapeutic agents, should not be used for the treatment of obesity or for weight loss. In euthyroid patients, doses within the range of daily hormonal requirements are ineffective for weight reduction. Larger doses may produce serious or even life threatening manifestations of toxicity, particularly when given in association with sympathomimetic amines such as those used for their anorectic effects.

Levothyroxine sodium should not be used in the treatment of male or female infertility unless this condition is associated with hypothyroidism.

In patients with nontoxic diffuse goiter or nodular thyroid disease, particularly the elderly or those with underlying cardiovascular disease, levothyroxine sodium therapy is contraindicated if the serum TSH level is already suppressed due to the risk of precipitating overt thyrotoxicosis (see **CONTRAINDICATIONS**). If the serum TSH level is not suppressed, SYNTHROID should be used with caution in conjunction with careful monitoring of thyroid function for evidence of hyperthyroidism and clinical monitoring for potential associated adverse cardiovascular signs and symptoms of hyperthyroidism.

PRECAUTIONS

General

Levothyroxine has a narrow therapeutic index. Regardless of the indication for use, careful dosage titration is necessary to avoid the consequences of over- or under-treatment. These consequences include, among others, effects on growth and development, cardiovascular function, bone metabolism, reproductive function, cognitive function, emotional state, gastrointestinal function, and on glucose and lipid metabolism. Many drugs interact with levothyroxine sodium necessitating adjustments in dosing to maintain therapeutic response (see **Drug Interactions**).

Effects on Bone Mineral Density

In women, long-term levothyroxine sodium therapy has been associated with increased bone resorption, thereby decreasing bone mineral density, especially in post-menopausal women on greater than replacement doses or in women who are receiving suppressive doses of levothyroxine sodium. The increased bone resorption may be associated with increased serum levels and urinary excretion of calcium and phosphorous, elevations in bone alkaline phosphatase and suppressed serum parathyroid hormone levels. Therefore, it is recommended that patients receiving levothyroxine sodium be given the minimum dose necessary to achieve the desired clinical and biochemical response.

Patients with Underlying Cardiovascular Disease

Exercise caution when administering levothyroxine to patients with cardiovascular disorders and to the elderly in whom there is an increased risk of occult cardiac disease. In these patients, levothyroxine therapy should be initiated at lower doses than those recommended in younger individuals or in patients without cardiac disease (see **WARNINGS, PRECAUTIONS - Geriatric Use,** and **DOSAGE AND ADMINISTRATION**). If cardiac symptoms develop or worsen, the levothyroxine dose should be reduced or withheld for one week and then cautiously restarted at a lower dose. Overtreatment with levothyroxine sodium may have adverse cardiovascular effects such as an increase in heart rate, cardiac wall thickness, and cardiac contractility and may precipitate angina or arrhythmias. Patients with coronary artery disease who are receiving levothyroxine therapy should be monitored closely during surgical procedures, since the possibility of precipitating cardiac arrhythmias may be greater in those treated with levothyroxine. Concomitant administration of levothyroxine and sympathomimetic agents to patients with coronary artery disease may precipitate coronary insufficiency.

Patients with Nontoxic Diffuse Goiter or Nodular Thyroid Disease

Exercise caution when administering levothyroxine to patients with nontoxic diffuse goiter or nodular thyroid disease in order to prevent precipitation of thyrotoxicosis (see **WARNINGS**). If the serum TSH is already suppressed, levothyroxine sodium should not be administered (see **CONTRAINDICATIONS**).

Associated Endocrine Disorders

Hypothalamic/pituitary hormone deficiencies

In patients with secondary or tertiary hypothyroidism, additional hypothalamic/pituitary hormone deficiencies should be considered, and, if diagnosed, treated (see **PRECAUTIONS - Autoimmune polyglandular syndrome** for adrenal insufficiency).

Autoimmune polyglandular syndrome

Occasionally, chronic autoimmune thyroiditis may occur in association with other autoimmune disorders such as adrenal insufficiency, pernicious anemia, and insulin-dependent diabetes mellitus. Patients with concomitant adrenal insufficiency should be treated with replacement glucocorticoids prior to initiation of treatment with levothyroxine sodium. Failure to do so may precipitate an acute adrenal crisis when thyroid hormone therapy is initiated, due to increased metabolic clearance of glucocorticoids by thyroid hormone. Patients with diabetes mellitus may require upward adjustments of their antidiabetic therapeutic regimens when treated with levothyroxine (see **PRECAUTIONS - Drug Interactions**).

Other associated medical conditions

Infants with congenital hypothyroidism appear to be at increased risk for other congenital anomalies, with cardiovascular anomalies (pulmonary stenosis, atrial septal defect, and ventricular septal defect) being the most common association.

Information for Patients

Patients should be informed of the following information to aid in the safe and effective use of SYNTHROID:

1. Notify your physician if you are allergic to any foods or medicines, are pregnant or intend to become pregnant, are breast-feeding or are taking any other medications, including prescription and over-the-counter preparations.
2. Notify your physician of any other medical conditions you may have, particularly heart disease, diabetes, clotting disorders, and adrenal or pituitary gland problems. Your dose of medications used to control these other conditions may need to be adjusted while you are taking SYNTHROID. If you have diabetes, monitor your blood and/or urinary glucose levels as directed by your physician and immediately report any changes to your physician. If you are taking anticoagulants (blood thinners), your clotting status should be checked frequently.
3. Use SYNTHROID only as prescribed by your physician. Do not discontinue or change the amount you take or how often you take it, unless directed to do so by your physician.
4. The levothyroxine in SYNTHROID is intended to replace a hormone that is normally produced by your thyroid gland. Generally, replacement therapy is to be taken for life, except in cases of transient hypothyroidism, which is usually associated with an inflammation of the thyroid gland (thyroiditis).
5. Take SYNTHROID as a single dose, preferably on an empty stomach, one-half to one hour before breakfast. Levothyroxine absorption is increased on an empty stomach.
6. It may take several weeks before you notice an improvement in your symptoms.
7. Notify your physician if you experience any of the following symptoms: rapid or irregular heartbeat, chest pain, shortness of breath, leg cramps, headache, nervousness, irritability, sleeplessness, tremors, change in appetite, weight gain or loss, vomiting, diarrhea, excessive sweating, heat intolerance, fever, changes in menstrual periods, hives or skin rash, or any other unusual medical event.
8. Notify your physician if you become pregnant while taking SYNTHROID. It is likely that your dose of SYNTHROID will need to be increased while you are pregnant.
9. Notify your physician or dentist that you are taking SYNTHROID prior to any surgery.
10. Partial hair loss may occur rarely during the first few months of SYNTHROID therapy, but this is usually temporary.
11. SYNTHROID should not be used as a primary or adjunctive therapy in a weight control program.
12. Keep SYNTHROID out of the reach of children. Store SYNTHROID away from heat, moisture, and light.
13. Agents such as iron and calcium supplements and antacids can decrease the absorption of levothyroxine sodium tablets. Therefore, levothyroxine sodium tablets should not be administered within 4 hours of these agents.

Laboratory Tests

General

The diagnosis of hypothyroidism is confirmed by measuring TSH levels using a sensitive assay (second generation assay sensitivity ≤ 0.1 mIU/L or third generation assay sensitivity ≤ 0.01 mIU/L) and measurement of free-T_4.

The adequacy of therapy is determined by periodic assessment of appropriate laboratory tests and clinical evaluation. The choice of laboratory tests depends on various factors including the etiology of the underlying thyroid disease, the presence of concomitant medical conditions, including pregnancy, and the use of concomitant medications (see **PRECAUTIONS - Drug Interactions** and **Drug-Laboratory Test Interactions**). Persistent clinical and laboratory evidence of hypothyroidism despite an apparent adequate replacement dose of SYNTHROID may be evidence of inadequate absorption, poor compliance, drug interactions, or decreased T_4 potency of the drug product.

Adults

In adult patients with primary (thyroidal) hypothyroidism, serum TSH levels (using a sensitive assay) alone may be used to monitor therapy. The frequency of TSH monitoring during levothyroxine dose titration depends on the clinical situation but it is generally recommended at 6-8 week intervals until normalization. For patients who have recently initiated levothyroxine therapy and whose serum TSH has normalized or in patients who have had their dosage or brand of levothyroxine changed, the serum TSH concentration should be measured after 8-12 weeks. When the optimum replacement dose has been attained, clinical (physical examination) and biochemical monitoring may be performed every 6-12 months, depending on the clinical situation, and whenever there is a change in the patient's status. It is recommended that a physical examination and a serum TSH measurement be performed at least annually in patients receiving SYNTHROID (see **WARNINGS, PRECAUTIONS,** and **DOSAGE AND ADMINISTRATION**).

Pediatrics

In patients with congenital hypothyroidism, the adequacy of replacement therapy should be assessed by measuring both serum TSH (using a sensitive assay) and total- or free- T_4. During the first three years of life, the serum total- or free-T_4 should be maintained at all times in the upper half of the normal range. While the aim of therapy is to also normalize the serum TSH level, this is not always possible in a small percentage of patients, particularly in the first few months of therapy. TSH may not normalize due to a resetting of the pituitary-thyroid feedback threshold as a result of *in utero* hypothyroidism. Failure of the serum T_4 to increase into the upper half of the normal range within 2 weeks of initiation of SYNTHROID therapy and/or of the serum TSH to decrease below 20 mU/L within 4 weeks should alert the physician to the possibility that the child is not receiving adequate therapy. Careful inquiry should then be made regarding compliance, dose of medication administered, and method of administration prior to raising the dose of SYNTHROID.

The recommended frequency of monitoring of TSH and total or free T_4 in children is as follows: at 2 and 4 weeks after the initiation of treatment; every 1-2 months during the first year of life; every 2-3 months between 1 and 3 years of age; and every 3 to 12 months thereafter until growth is completed. More frequent intervals of monitoring may be necessary if poor compliance is suspected or abnormal values are obtained. It is recommended that TSH and T_4 levels, and a physical examination, if indicated, be performed 2 weeks after any change in SYNTHROID dosage. Routine clinical examination, including assessment of mental and physical growth and development, and bone maturation, should be performed at regular intervals (see **PRECAUTIONS - Pediatric Use** and **DOSAGE AND ADMINISTRATION**).

Secondary (Pituitary) and Tertiary (Hypothalamic) Hypothyroidism

Adequacy of therapy should be assessed by measuring serum free-T_4 levels, which should be maintained in the upper half of the normal range in these patients.

Drug Interactions

Many drugs affect thyroid hormone pharmacokinetics and metabolism (e.g., absorption, synthesis, secretion, catabolism, protein binding, and target tissue response) and may alter the therapeutic response to SYNTHROID. In addition, thyroid hormones and thyroid status have varied effects on the pharmacokinetics and actions of other drugs. A listing of drug-thyroidal axis interactions is contained in Table 2.

The list of drug-thyroidal axis interactions in Table 2 may not be comprehensive due to the introduction of new drugs that interact with the thyroidal axis or the discovery of previously unknown interactions. The prescriber should be aware of this fact and should consult appropriate reference sources (e.g., package inserts of newly approved drugs, medical literature) for additional information if a drug-drug interaction with levothyroxine is suspected.

[See table 2 on pages 578 through 580]

Oral anticoagulants

Levothyroxine increases the response to oral anticoagulant therapy. Therefore, a decrease in the dose of anticoagulant may be warranted with correction of the hypothyroid state or when the SYNTHROID dose is increased. Prothrombin time should be closely monitored to permit appropriate and timely dosage adjustments (see **Table 2**).

Digitalis glycosides

The therapeutic effects of digitalis glycosides may be reduced by levothyroxine. Serum digitalis glycoside levels may be decreased when a hypothyroid patient becomes euthyroid, necessitating an increase in the dose of digitalis glycosides (see **Table 2**).

Drug-Food Interactions

Consumption of certain foods may affect levothyroxine absorption thereby necessitating adjustments in dosing. Soybean flour (infant formula), cotton seed meal, walnuts, and dietary fiber may bind and decrease the absorption of levothyroxine sodium from the GI tract.

Drug-Laboratory Test Interactions

Changes in TBG concentration must be considered when interpreting T_4 and T_3 values, which necessitates measurement and evaluation of unbound (free) hormone and/or determination of the free T_4 index (FT_4I). Pregnancy, infectious hepatitis, estrogens, estrogen-containing oral contraceptives, and acute intermittent porphyria increase TBG concentrations. Decreases in TBG concentrations are observed in nephrosis, severe hypoproteinemia, severe liver disease, acromegaly, and after androgen or corticosteroid therapy (see also **Table 2**). Familial hyper- or hypothyroxine binding globulinemias have been described, with the incidence of TBG deficiency approximating 1 in 9000.

Carcinogenesis, Mutagenesis, and Impairment of Fertility

Animal studies have not been performed to evaluate the carcinogenic potential, mutagenic potential or effects on fertility of levothyroxine. The synthetic T_4 in SYNTHROID is identical to that produced naturally by the human thyroid gland. Although there has been a reported association between prolonged thyroid hormone therapy and breast cancer, this has not been confirmed. Patients receiving SYNTHROID for appropriate clinical indications should be titrated to the lowest effective replacement dose.

Pregnancy

Category A

Studies in women taking levothyroxine sodium during pregnancy have not shown an increased risk of congenital abnormalities. Therefore, the possibility of fetal harm appears remote. SYNTHROID should not be discontinued during pregnancy and hypothyroidism diagnosed during pregnancy should be promptly treated.

Hypothyroidism during pregnancy is associated with a higher rate of complications, including spontaneous abortion, pre-eclampsia, stillbirth and premature delivery. Maternal hypothyroidism may have an adverse effect on fetal and childhood growth and development. During pregnancy, serum T_4 levels may decrease and serum TSH levels increase to values outside the normal range. Since elevations in serum TSH may occur as early as 4 weeks gestation, pregnant women taking SYNTHROID should have their TSH measured during each trimester. An elevated serum TSH level should be corrected by an increase in the dose of SYNTHROID. Since postpartum TSH levels are similar to preconception values, the SYNTHROID dosage should return to the pre-pregnancy dose immediately after delivery. A serum TSH level should be obtained 6-8 weeks postpartum.

Thyroid hormones cross the placental barrier to some extent as evidenced by levels in cord blood of athyreotic fetuses being approximately one-third maternal levels. Transfer of

Information on the AbbVie, Inc. products listed on these pages is from the prescribing information in use as of July 31, 2013. For more information, please visit rxabbvie.com or call 1-800-633-9110.

Table 2. Drug-Thyroidal Axis Interactions

Drug or Drug Class	Effect
Drugs that may reduce TSH secretion – the reduction is not sustained; therefore, hypothyroidism does not occur	
Dopamine/Dopamine Agonists Glucocorticoids Octreotide	Use of these agents may result in a transient reduction in TSH secretion when administered at the following doses: Dopamine (≥ 1 mcg/kg/min); Glucocorticoids (hydrocortisone ≥ 100 mg/day or equivalent); Octreotide (> 100 mcg/day).
Drugs that alter thyroid hormone secretion	
Drugs that may decrease thyroid hormone secretion, which may result in hypothyroidism	
Aminoglutethimide Amiodarone Iodide (including iodine-containing radiographic contrast agents) Lithium Methimazole Propylthiouracil (PTU) Sulfonamides Tolbutamide	Long-term lithium therapy can result in goiter in up to 50% of patients, and either subclinical or overt hypothyroidism, each in up to 20% of patients. The fetus, neonate, elderly and euthyroid patients with underlying thyroid disease (e.g., Hashimoto's thyroiditis or with Grave's disease previously treated with radioiodine or surgery) are among those individuals who are particularly susceptible to iodine-induced hypothyroidism. Oral cholecystographic agents and amiodarone are slowly excreted, producing more prolonged hypothyroidism than parenterally administered iodinated contrast agents. Long-term aminoglutethimide therapy may minimally decrease T_4 and T_3 levels and increase TSH, although all values remain within normal limits in most patients.
Drugs that may increase thyroid hormone secretion, which may result in hyperthyroidism	
Amiodarone Iodide (including iodine-containing radiographic contrast agents)	Iodide and drugs that contain pharmacologic amounts of iodide may cause hyperthyroidism in euthyroid patients with Grave's disease previously treated with antithyroid drugs or in euthyroid patients with thyroid autonomy (e.g., multinodular goiter or hyperfunctioning thyroid adenoma). Hyperthyroidism may develop over several weeks and may persist for several months after therapy discontinuation. Amiodarone may induce hyperthyroidism by causing thyroiditis.
Drugs that may decrease T_4 absorption, which may result in hypothyroidism	
Antacids - Aluminum & Magnesium Hydroxides - Simethicone Bile Acid Sequestrants - Cholestyramine - Colestipol Calcium Carbonate Cation Exchange Resins - Kayexalate Ferrous Sulfate Orlistat Sucralfate	Concurrent use may reduce the efficacy of levothyroxine by binding and delaying or preventing absorption, potentially resulting in hypothyroidism. Calcium carbonate may form an insoluble chelate with levothyroxine, and ferrous sulfate likely forms a ferric-thyroxine complex. Administer levothyroxine at least 4 hours apart from these agents. Patients treated concomitantly with orlistat and levothyroxine should be monitored for changes in thyroid function.
Drugs that may alter T_4 and T_3 serum transport - but FT_4 concentration remains normal; and therefore, the patient remains euthyroid	
Drugs that may increase serum TBG concentration	**Drugs that may decrease serum TBG concentration**
Clofibrate Estrogen-containing oral contraceptives Estrogens (oral) Heroin / Methadone 5-Fluorouracil Mitotane Tamoxifen	Androgens / Anabolic Steroids Asparaginase Glucocorticoids Slow-Release Nicotinic Acid
Drugs that may cause protein-binding site displacement	
Furosemide (> 80 mg IV) Heparin Hydantoins Non Steroidal Anti-Inflammatory Drugs - Fenamates - Phenylbutazone Salicylates (> 2 g/day)	Administration of these agents with levothyroxine results in an initial transient increase in FT_4. Continued administration results in a decrease in serum T_4 and normal FT_4 and TSH concentrations and, therefore, patients are clinically euthyroid. Salicylates inhibit binding of T_4 and T_3 to TBG and transthyretin. An initial increase in serum FT_4 is followed by return of FT_4 to normal levels with sustained therapeutic serum salicylate concentrations, although total-T_4 levels may decrease by as much as 30%.

(Table continued on next page)

thyroid hormone from the mother to the fetus, however, may not be adequate to prevent *in utero* hypothyroidism.

Nursing Mothers

Although thyroid hormones are excreted only minimally in human milk, caution should be exercised when SYNTHROID is administered to a nursing woman. However, adequate replacement doses of levothyroxine are generally needed to maintain normal lactation.

Pediatric Use

General

The goal of treatment in pediatric patients with hypothyroidism is to achieve and maintain normal intellectual and physical growth and development.

The initial dose of levothyroxine varies with age and body weight (see **DOSAGE AND ADMINISTRATION - Table 3**).

Dosing adjustments are based on an assessment of the individual patient's clinical and laboratory parameters (see **PRECAUTIONS - Laboratory Tests**).

In children in whom a diagnosis of permanent hypothyroidism has not been established, it is recommended that levothyroxine administration be discontinued for a 30-day trial period, but only after the child is at least 3 years of age. Serum T_4 and TSH levels should then be obtained. If the T_4 is low and the TSH high, the diagnosis of permanent hypothyroidism is established, and levothyroxine therapy should be reinstituted. If the T_4 and TSH levels are normal, euthyroidism may be assumed and, therefore, the hypothyroidism can be considered to have been transient. In this instance, however, the physician should carefully monitor the child and repeat the thyroid function tests if any signs or symptoms of hypothyroidism develop. In this setting, the clinician should have a high index of suspicion of relapse. If the results of the levothyroxine withdrawal test are inconclusive, careful follow-up and subsequent testing will be necessary.

Since some more severely affected children may become clinically hypothyroid when treatment is discontinued for 30 days, an alternate approach is to reduce the replacement dose of levothyroxine by half during the 30-day trial period. If, after 30 days, the serum TSH is elevated above 20 mU/L, the diagnosis of permanent hypothyroidism is confirmed, and full replacement therapy should be resumed. However, if the serum TSH has not risen to greater than 20 mU/L, levothyroxine treatment should be discontinued for another 30-day trial period followed by repeat serum T_4 and TSH testing.

The presence of concomitant medical conditions should be considered in certain clinical circumstances and, if present, appropriately treated (see **PRECAUTIONS**).

Congenital Hypothyroidism

(see **PRECAUTIONS - Laboratory Tests** and **DOSAGE AND ADMINISTRATION**)

Rapid restoration of normal serum T_4 concentrations is essential for preventing the adverse effects of congenital hypothyroidism on intellectual development as well as on overall physical growth and maturation. Therefore, SYNTHROID therapy should be initiated immediately upon diagnosis and is generally continued for life.

During the first 2 weeks of SYNTHROID therapy, infants should be closely monitored for cardiac overload, arrhythmias, and aspiration from avid suckling.

The patient should be monitored closely to avoid undertreatment or overtreatment. Undertreatment may have deleterious effects on intellectual development and linear growth. Overtreatment has been associated with craniosynostosis in infants, and may adversely affect the tempo of brain maturation and accelerate the bone age with resultant premature closure of the epiphyses and compromised adult stature.

Acquired Hypothyroidism in Pediatric Patients

The patient should be monitored closely to avoid undertreatment and overtreatment. Undertreatment may result in poor school performance due to impaired concentration and slowed mentation and in reduced adult height. Overtreatment may accelerate the bone age and result in premature epiphyseal closure and compromised adult stature.

Treated children may manifest a period of catch-up growth, which may be adequate in some cases to normalize adult height. In children with severe or prolonged hypothyroidism, catch-up growth may not be adequate to normalize adult height.

Geriatric Use

Because of the increased prevalence of cardiovascular disease among the elderly, levothyroxine therapy should not be initiated at the full replacement dose (see **WARNINGS**, **PRECAUTIONS**, and **DOSAGE AND ADMINISTRATION**).

ADVERSE REACTIONS

Adverse reactions associated with levothyroxine therapy are primarily those of hyperthyroidism due to therapeutic overdosage (see **PRECAUTIONS** and **OVERDOSAGE**). They include the following:

General

fatigue, increased appetite, weight loss, heat intolerance, fever, excessive sweating;

Central nervous system

headache, hyperactivity, nervousness, anxiety, irritability, emotional lability, insomnia;

Musculoskeletal

tremors, muscle weakness;

Cardiovascular

palpitations, tachycardia, arrhythmias, increased pulse and blood pressure, heart failure, angina, myocardial infarction, cardiac arrest;

Respiratory
dyspnea;
Gastrointestinal
diarrhea, vomiting, abdominal cramps and elevations in liver function tests;
Dermatologic
hair loss, flushing;
Endocrine
decreased bone mineral density;
Reproductive
menstrual irregularities, impaired fertility.

Pseudotumor cerebri and slipped capital femoral epiphysis have been reported in children receiving levothyroxine therapy. Overtreatment may result in craniosynostosis in infants and premature closure of the epiphyses in children with resultant compromised adult height.

Seizures have been reported rarely with the institution of levothyroxine therapy.

Inadequate levothyroxine dosage will produce or fail to ameliorate the signs and symptoms of hypothyroidism.

Hypersensitivity reactions to inactive ingredients have occurred in patients treated with thyroid hormone products. These include urticaria, pruritus, skin rash, flushing, angioedema, various GI symptoms (abdominal pain, nausea, vomiting and diarrhea), fever, arthralgia, serum sickness and wheezing. Hypersensitivity to levothyroxine itself is not known to occur.

Overdosage

The signs and symptoms of overdosage are those of hyperthyroidism (see **PRECAUTIONS** and **ADVERSE REACTIONS**). In addition, confusion and disorientation may occur. Cerebral embolism, shock, coma, and death have been reported. Seizures have occurred in a child ingesting 18 mg of levothyroxine. Symptoms may not necessarily be evident or may not appear until several days after ingestion of levothyroxine sodium.

Treatment of Overdosage

Levothyroxine sodium should be reduced in dose or temporarily discontinued if signs or symptoms of overdosage occur.

Acute Massive Overdosage

This may be a life-threatening emergency, therefore, symptomatic and supportive therapy should be instituted immediately. If not contraindicated (e.g., by seizures, coma, or loss of the gag reflex), the stomach should be emptied by emesis or gastric lavage to decrease gastrointestinal absorption. Activated charcoal or cholestyramine may also be used to decrease absorption. Central and peripheral increased sympathetic activity may be treated by administering β-receptor antagonists, e.g., propranolol, provided there are no medical contraindications to their use. Provide respiratory support as needed; control congestive heart failure and arrhythmia; control fever, hypoglycemia, and fluid loss as necessary. Large doses of antithyroid drugs (e.g., methimazole or propylthiouracil) followed in one to two hours by large doses of iodine may be given to inhibit synthesis and release of thyroid hormones. Glucocorticoids may be given to inhibit the conversion of T_4 to T_3. Plasmapheresis, charcoal hemoperfusion and exchange transfusion have been reserved for cases in which continued clinical deterioration occurs despite conventional therapy. Because T_4 is highly protein bound, very little drug will be removed by dialysis.

DOSAGE AND ADMINISTRATION

General Principles

The goal of replacement therapy is to achieve and maintain a clinical and biochemical euthyroid state. The goal of suppressive therapy is to inhibit growth and/or function of abnormal thyroid tissue. The dose of SYNTHROID that is adequate to achieve these goals depends on a variety of factors including the patient's age, body weight, cardiovascular status, concomitant medical conditions, including pregnancy, concomitant medications, and the specific nature of the condition being treated (see **WARNINGS** and **PRECAUTIONS**). Hence, the following recommendations serve only as dosing guidelines. Dosing must be individualized and adjustments made based on periodic assessment of the patient's clinical response and laboratory parameters (see **PRECAUTIONS - Laboratory Tests**).

SYNTHROID is administered as a single daily dose, preferably one-half to one-hour before breakfast. SYNTHROID should be taken at least 4 hours apart from drugs that are known to interfere with its absorption (see **PRECAUTIONS - Drug Interactions**).

Due to the long half-life of levothyroxine, the peak therapeutic effect at a given dose of levothyroxine sodium may not be attained for 4-6 weeks.

Caution should be exercised when administering SYNTHROID to patients with underlying cardiovascular disease, to the elderly, and to those with concomitant adrenal insufficiency (see **PRECAUTIONS**).

Table 2 ***(cont.)*****. Drug-Thyroidal Axis Interactions**

Drug or Drug Class	Effect
Drugs that may alter T_4 and T_3 metabolism	
Drugs that may increase hepatic metabolism, which may result in hypothyroidism	
Carbamazepine Hydantoins Phenobarbital Rifampin	Stimulation of hepatic microsomal drug-metabolizing enzyme activity may cause increased hepatic degradation of levothyroxine, resulting in increased levothyroxine requirements. Phenytoin and carbamazepine reduce serum protein binding of levothyroxine, and total- and free- T_4 may be reduced by 20% to 40%, but most patients have normal serum TSH levels and are clinically euthyroid.
Drugs that may decrease T_4 5'-deiodinase activity	
Amiodarone Beta-adrenergic antagonists - (e.g., Propranolol > 160 mg/day) Glucocorticoids - (e.g., Dexamethasone ≥ 4 mg/day) Propylthiouracil (PTU)	Administration of these enzyme inhibitors decreases the peripheral conversion of T_4 to T_3, leading to decreased T_3 levels. However, serum T_4 levels are usually normal but may occasionally be slightly increased. In patients treated with large doses of propranolol (> 160 mg/day), T_3 and T_4 levels change slightly, TSH levels remain normal, and patients are clinically euthyroid. It should be noted that actions of particular beta-adrenergic antagonists may be impaired when the hypothyroid patient is converted to the euthyroid state. Short-term administration of large doses of glucocorticoids may decrease serum T_3 concentrations by 30% with minimal change in serum T_4 levels. However, long-term glucocorticoid therapy may result in slightly decreased T_3 and T_4 levels due to decreased TBG production (see above).
Miscellaneous	
Anticoagulants (oral) - Coumarin Derivatives - Indandione Derivatives	Thyroid hormones appear to increase the catabolism of vitamin K-dependent clotting factors, thereby increasing the anticoagulant activity of oral anticoagulants. Concomitant use of these agents impairs the compensatory increases in clotting factor synthesis. Prothrombin time should be carefully monitored in patients taking levothyroxine and oral anticoagulants and the dose of anticoagulant therapy adjusted accordingly.
Antidepressants - Tricyclics (e.g., Amitriptyline) - Tetracyclics (e.g., Maprotiline) - Selective Serotonin Reuptake Inhibitors (SSRIs; e.g., Sertraline)	Concurrent use of tri/tetracyclic antidepressants and levothyroxine may increase the therapeutic and toxic effects of both drugs, possibly due to increased receptor sensitivity to catecholamines. Toxic effects may include increased risk of cardiac arrhythmias and CNS stimulation; onset of action of tricyclics may be accelerated. Administration of sertraline in patients stabilized on levothyroxine may result in increased levothyroxine requirements.
Antidiabetic Agents - Biguanides - Meglitinides - Sulfonylureas - Thiazolidinediones - Insulin	Addition of levothyroxine to antidiabetic or insulin therapy may result in increased antidiabetic agent or insulin requirements. Careful monitoring of diabetic control is recommended, especially when thyroid therapy is started, changed, or discontinued.
Cardiac Glycosides	Serum digitalis glycoside levels may be reduced in hyperthyroidism or when the hypothyroid patient is converted to the euthyroid state. Therapeutic effect of digitalis glycosides may be reduced.
Cytokines - Interferon-α - Interleukin-2	Therapy with interferon-α has been associated with the development of antithyroid microsomal antibodies in 20% of patients and some have transient hypothyroidism, hyperthyroidism, or both. Patients who have antithyroid antibodies before treatment are at higher risk for thyroid dysfunction during treatment. Interleukin-2 has been associated with transient painless thyroiditis in 20% of patients. Interferon-β and -γ have not been reported to cause thyroid dysfunction.
Growth Hormones - Somatrem - Somatropin	Excessive use of thyroid hormones with growth hormones may accelerate epiphyseal closure. However, untreated hypothyroidism may interfere with growth response to growth hormone.

(Table continued on next page)

Specific Patient Populations

Hypothyroidism in Adults and in Children in Whom Growth and Puberty are Complete

(see **WARNINGS** and **PRECAUTIONS - Laboratory Tests**)

Therapy may begin at full replacement doses in otherwise healthy individuals less than 50 years old and in those older than 50 years who have been recently treated for hyperthyroidism or who have been hypothyroid for only a short time (such as a few months). The average full replacement dose of levothyroxine sodium is approximately 1.7 mcg/kg/day (e.g., **100-125 mcg/day** for a 70 kg adult). Older patients may require less than 1 mcg/kg/day. Levothyroxine sodium doses greater than 200 mcg/day are seldom required. An in-

Information on the AbbVie, Inc. products listed on these pages is from the prescribing information in use as of July 31, 2013. For more information, please visit rxabbvie.com or call 1-800-633-9110.

Table 2 *(cont.)*. Drug-Thyroidal Axis Interactions

Drug or Drug Class	Effect
Ketamine	Concurrent use may produce marked hypertension and tachycardia; cautious administration to patients receiving thyroid hormone therapy is recommended.
Methylxanthine Bronchodilators - (e.g., Theophylline)	Decreased theophylline clearance may occur in hypothyroid patients; clearance returns to normal when the euthyroid state is achieved.
Radiographic Agents	Thyroid hormones may reduce the uptake of ^{123}I, ^{131}I, and ^{99m}Tc.
Sympathomimetics	Concurrent use may increase the effects of sympathomimetics or thyroid hormone. Thyroid hormones may increase the risk of coronary insufficiency when sympathomimetic agents are administered to patients with coronary artery disease.
Chloral Hydrate Diazepam Ethionamide Lovastatin Metoclopramide 6-Mercaptopurine Nitroprusside Para-aminosalicylate sodium Perphenazine Resorcinol (excessive topical use) Thiazide Diuretics	These agents have been associated with thyroid hormone and/or TSH level alterations by various mechanisms.

Strength (mcg)	Color	NDC# for bottles of 90	NDC # for bottles of 100	NDC # for bottles of 1000	NDC # for unit dose cartons of 100
25	orange	0074-4341-90	0074-4341-13	0074-4341-19	--
50	white	0074-4552-90	0074-4552-13	0074-4552-19	0074-4552-11
75	violet	0074-5182-90	0074-5182-13	0074-5182-19	0074-5182-11
88	olive	0074-6594-90	0074-6594-13	0074-6594-19	--
100	yellow	0074-6624-90	0074-6624-13	0074-6624-19	0074-6624-11
112	rose	0074-9296-90	0074-9296-13	0074-9296-19	--
125	brown	0074-7068-90	0074-7068-13	0074-7068-19	0074-7068-11
137	turquoise	0074-3727-90	0074-3727-13	0074-3727-19	--
150	blue	0074-7069-90	0074-7069-13	0074-7069-19	0074-7069-11
175	lilac	0074-7070-90	0074-7070-13	0074-7070-19	--
200	pink	0074-7148-90	0074-7148-13	0074-7148-19	0074-7148-11
300	green	0074-7149-90	0074-7149-13	0074-7149-19	--

adequate response to daily doses ≥ 300 mcg/day is rare and may indicate poor compliance, malabsorption, and/or drug interactions.

For most patients older than 50 years or for patients under 50 years of age with underlying cardiac disease, an initial starting dose of **25-50 mcg/day** of levothyroxine sodium is recommended, with gradual increments in dose at 6-8 week intervals, as needed. The recommended starting dose of levothyroxine sodium in elderly patients with cardiac disease is **12.5-25 mcg/day**, with gradual dose increments at 4-6 week intervals. The levothyroxine sodium dose is generally adjusted in 12.5-25 mcg increments until the patient with primary hypothyroidism is clinically euthyroid and the serum TSH has normalized.

In patients with severe hypothyroidism, the recommended initial levothyroxine sodium dose is **12.5-25 mcg/day** with increases of 25 mcg/day every 2-4 weeks, accompanied by clinical and laboratory assessment, until the TSH level is normalized.

In patients with secondary (pituitary) or tertiary (hypothalamic) hypothyroidism, the levothyroxine sodium dose should be titrated until the patient is clinically euthyroid and the serum free- T_4 level is restored to the upper half of the normal range.

Pediatric Dosage - Congenital or Acquired Hypothyroidism (see **PRECAUTIONS - Laboratory Tests**)

General Principles

In general, levothyroxine therapy should be instituted at full replacement doses as soon as possible. Delays in diagnosis and institution of therapy may have deleterious effects on the child's intellectual and physical growth and development.

Undertreatment and overtreatment should be avoided (see **PRECAUTIONS - Pediatric Use**). SYNTHROID may be administered to infants and children who cannot swallow intact tablets by crushing the tablet and suspending the freshly crushed tablet in a small amount (5-10 mL or 1-2 teaspoons) of water. This suspension can be administered by spoon or by dropper. **DO NOT STORE THE SUSPENSION.** Foods that decrease absorption of levothyroxine, such as soybean infant formula, should not be used for administering levothyroxine sodium tablets (see **PRECAUTIONS - Drug-Food Interactions**).

Newborns

The recommended starting dose of levothyroxine sodium in newborn infants is **10-15 mcg/kg/day** . A lower starting dose (e.g., 25 mcg/day) should be considered in infants at risk for cardiac failure, and the dose should be increased in 4-6 weeks as needed based on clinical and laboratory response to treatment. In infants with very low (< 5 mcg/dL) or undetectable serum T_4 concentrations, the recommended initial starting dose is **50 mcg/day** of levothyroxine sodium.

Infants and Children

Levothyroxine therapy is usually initiated at full replacement doses, with the recommended dose per body weight decreasing with age (see **Table 3**). However, in children with chronic or severe hypothyroidism, an initial dose of **25 mcg/day** of levothyroxine sodium is recommended with increments of 25 mcg every 2-4 weeks until the desired effect is achieved.

Hyperactivity in an older child can be minimized if the starting dose is one-fourth of the recommended full replacement dose, and the dose is then increased on a weekly basis by an amount equal to one-fourth the full-recommended replacement dose until the full recommended replacement dose is reached.

Table 3. Levothyroxine Sodium Dosing Guidelines for Pediatric Hypothyroidism

AGE	Daily Dose Per Kg Body Weight[a]
0-3 months	10-15 mcg/kg/day
3-6 months	8-10 mcg/kg/day
6-12 months	6-8 mcg/kg/day
1-5 years	5-6 mcg/kg/day
6-12 years	4-5 mcg/kg/day
> 12 years but growth and puberty incomplete	2-3 mcg/kg/day
Growth and puberty complete	1.7 mcg/kg/day

[a] The dose should be adjusted based on clinical response and laboratory parameters (see **PRECAUTIONS - Laboratory Tests and Pediatric Use**).

Pregnancy

Pregnancy may increase levothyroxine requirements (see **PREGNANCY**).

Subclinical Hypothyroidism

If this condition is treated, a lower levothyroxine sodium dose (e.g., **1 mcg/kg/day**) than that used for full replacement may be adequate to normalize the serum TSH level. Patients who are not treated should be monitored yearly for changes in clinical status and thyroid laboratory parameters.

TSH Suppression in Well-differentiated Thyroid Cancer and Thyroid Nodules

The target level for TSH suppression in these conditions has not been established with controlled studies. In addition, the efficacy of TSH suppression for benign nodular disease is controversial. Therefore, the dose of SYNTHROID used for TSH suppression should be individualized based on the specific disease and the patient being treated.

In the treatment of well-differentiated (papillary and follicular) thyroid cancer, levothyroxine is used as an adjunct to surgery and radioiodine therapy. Generally, TSH is suppressed to < 0.1 mU/L, and this usually requires a levothyroxine sodium dose of **greater than 2 mcg/kg/day**. However, in patients with high-risk tumors, the target level for TSH suppression may be < 0.01 mU/L.

In the treatment of benign nodules and nontoxic multinodular goiter, TSH is generally suppressed to a higher target (e.g., 0.1 to either 0.5 or 1.0 mU/L) than that used for the treatment of thyroid cancer. Levothyroxine sodium is contraindicated if the serum TSH is already suppressed due to the risk of precipitating overt thyrotoxicosis (see **CONTRAINDICATIONS, WARNINGS** and **PRECAUTIONS**).

Myxedema Coma

Myxedema coma is a life-threatening emergency characterized by poor circulation and hypometabolism, and may result in unpredictable absorption of levothyroxine sodium from the gastrointestinal tract. Therefore, oral thyroid hormone drug products are not recommended to treat this condition. Thyroid hormone products formulated for intravenous administration should be administered.

HOW SUPPLIED

SYNTHROID® (levothyroxine sodium tablets, USP) are round, color coded, scored and debossed with "SYNTHROID" on one side and potency on the other side. They are supplied as follows:

[See second table at right]

Storage Conditions

Store at 25°C (77°F); excursions permitted to 15-30°C (59-86°F) [see USP Controlled Room Temperature]. SYNTHROID tablets should be protected from light and moisture.

(Nos. 4341, 4552, 5182, 6594, 9296, 7068, 3727, 7069, 7070, 7148, 7149)

03-A663-R7-Rev. September, 2012

AbbVie Inc.

North Chicago, IL 60064, U.S.A.

Shown in Product Identification Guide, page 304

TARKA® ℞

(trandolapril/verapamil hydrochloride ER tablets)

> **WARNING: FETAL TOXICITY**
> - **When pregnancy is detected, discontinue TARKA as soon as possible.**
> - **Drugs that act directly on the renin-angiotensin system can cause injury and death to the developing fetus (see WARNINGS: Fetal Toxicity).**

DESCRIPTION

TARKA® (trandolapril/verapamil hydrochloride ER) combines a slow release formulation of a calcium channel blocker, verapamil hydrochloride, and an immediate release formulation of an angiotensin converting enzyme inhibitor, trandolapril.

Verapamil Component

Verapamil hydrochloride is chemically described as benzeneacetonitrile, α[3-[[2-(3,4-dimethoxyphenyl)ethyl] methylamino]propyl]-3, 4-dimethoxy-α-(1-methylethyl) hydrochloride. Its empirical formula is $C_{27}H_{38}N_2O_4$ HCl and its structural formula is:

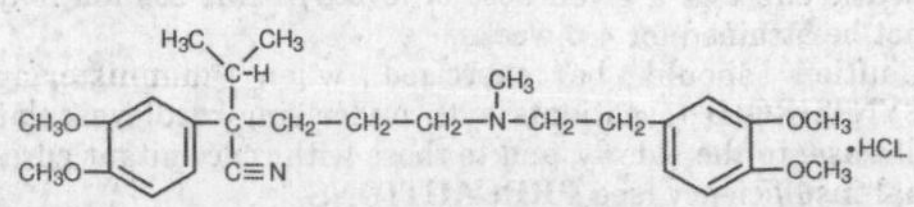

Verapamil hydrochloride is an almost white crystalline powder, with a molecular weight of 491.08. It is soluble in water, chloroform, and methanol. It is practically free of odor, with a bitter taste.

Trandolapril Component

Trandolapril is the ethyl ester prodrug of a nonsulfhydryl angiotensin converting enzyme (ACE) inhibitor, trandolaprilat. It is chemically described as (2S,3aR,7aS)-1-[(S)-N-[(S)-1-Carboxy-3-phenylpropyl]alanyl] hexahydro-2-indolinecarboxylic acid, 1-ethyl ester. Its empirical formula is $C_{24}H_{34}N_2O_5$ and its structural formula is:

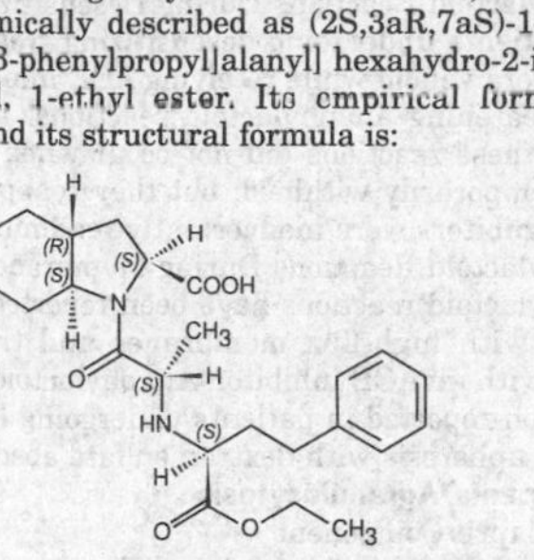

Trandolapril is a white or almost white powder with a molecular weight of 430.54. It is soluble (>100 mg/mL) in chloroform, dichloromethane, and methanol.

TARKA tablets are formulated for oral administration, containing verapamil hydrochloride as a controlled release formulation and trandolapril as an immediate release formulation. The tablet strengths are trandolapril 2 mg/verapamil hydrochloride ER 180 mg, trandolapril 1 mg/verapamil hydrochloride ER 240 mg, trandolapril 2 mg/verapamil hydrochloride ER 240 mg, and trandolapril 4 mg/verapamil hydrochloride ER 240 mg. The tablets also contain the following ingredients: corn starch, dioctyl sodium sulfosuccinate, ethanol, hydroxypropyl cellulose, hypromellose, lactose monohydrate, magnesium stearate, microcrystalline cellulose, polyethylene glycol, povidone, purified water, silicon dioxide, sodium alginate, sodium stearyl fumarate, synthetic iron oxides, talc, and titanium dioxide.

CLINICAL PHARMACOLOGY

Verapamil hydrochloride and trandolapril have been used individually and in combination for the treatment of hypertension. For the four dosing strengths, the antihypertensive effect of the combination is approximately additive to the individual components.

Verapamil Component

Verapamil is a calcium channel blocker that exerts its pharmacologic effects by modulating the influx of ionic calcium across the cell membrane of the arterial smooth muscle as well as in conductile and contractile myocardial cells. Verapamil exerts antihypertensive effects by decreasing systemic vascular resistance, usually without orthostatic decreases in blood pressure or reflex tachycardia. During isometric or dynamic exercise, verapamil does not alter systolic cardiac function in patients with normal ventricular function. Verapamil does not alter total serum calcium levels.

Trandolapril Component

Trandolapril is de-esterified to its diacid metabolite, trandolaprilat. Both inhibit angiotensin-converting enzyme (ACE) in human subjects and in animals. Trandolaprilat is about 8 times more potent than trandolapril. ACE is a peptidyl dipeptidase that catalyzes the conversion of angiotensin I to the vasoconstrictor, angiotensin II. Angiotensin II also stimulates aldosterone secretion by the adrenal cortex. Inhibition of ACE results in decreased plasma angiotensin II, which leads to decreased vasopressor activity and to decreased aldosterone secretion. The latter decrease may result in a small increase of serum potassium. In controlled clinical trials, treatment with TARKA resulted in mean increases in potassium of 0.1 mEq/L (see **PRECAUTIONS**). Removal of angiotensin II negative feedback on renin secretion leads to increased plasma renin activity (PRA).

ACE is identical to kininase II, an enzyme that degrades bradykinin. Whether increased levels of bradykinin, a potent vasodepressor peptide, play a role in the therapeutic effect of TARKA remains to be elucidated.

While the mechanism through which trandolapril lowers blood pressure is believed to be primarily suppression of the renin-angiotensin-aldosterone system, trandolapril has an antihypertensive effect even in patients with low renin hypertension. Trandolapril is an effective antihypertensive in all races studied. Both black patients (usually a predominantly low renin group) and non-black patients respond to 2 to 4 mg of trandolapril.

Pharmacokinetics and Metabolism

TARKA

Following a single oral dose of TARKA in healthy subjects, peak plasma concentrations are reached within 0.5-2 hours for trandolapril and within 4-15 hours for verapamil. Peak plasma concentrations of the active desmethyl metabolite of verapamil, norverapamil, are reached within 5-15 hours. Cleavage of the ester group converts trandolapril to its active diacid metabolite, trandolaprilat, which reaches peak plasma concentrations within 2-12 hours. The pharmacokinetics of trandolapril and trandolaprilat are not altered when trandolapril is administered in combination with verapamil, compared to monotherapy.

The AUC and C_{max} for both verapamil and norverapamil are increased when 240 mg of controlled release verapamil is administered concomitantly with 4 mg trandolapril. The increase in C_{max} is 54 and 30% and the AUC is increased by 65 and 32% for verapamil and norverapamil, respectively. Administration of TARKA 4/240 (4 mg trandolapril and 240 mg verapamil hydrochloride ER) with a high-fat meal does not alter the bioavailability of trandolapril whereas verapamil peak concentrations and area under the curve (AUC) decrease 37% and 28%, respectively. Food thus decreases verapamil bioavailability and the time to peak plasma concentration for both verapamil and norverapamil are delayed by approximately 7 hours. Both optical isomers of verapamil are similarly affected.

The elimination half life of trandolapril is about 6 hours. At steady state, the effective half-life of trandolaprilat is 22.5 hours. Like all ACE inhibitors, trandolaprilat also has a prolonged terminal elimination phase, involving a small fraction of administered drug, probably representing binding to plasma and tissue ACE.

The terminal half-life of verapamil is 6-11 hours. Steady-state plasma concentrations of the two components are achieved after about a week of once-daily dosing of TARKA. At steady-state, plasma concentrations of verapamil and trandolaprilat are up to two-fold higher than those observed after a single oral TARKA dose.

The pharmacokinetics of verapamil and trandolaprilat are significantly different in the elderly (≥65 years) than in younger subjects. The bioavailability of verapamil and norverapamil are increased by 87% and 77%, respectively, and that of trandolapril by approximately 35% in the elderly. AUCs are approximately 80% and 35% higher, respectively.

Verapamil Component

With the immediate release formulation, more than 90% of the orally administered dose is absorbed with peak plasma concentrations of verapamil observed 1 to 2 hours after dosing. A delayed rate but similar extent of absorption is observed for the sustained release formulation when compared to the immediate release formulation. Because of the rapid biotransformation of verapamil during its first pass through the portal circulation, absolute bioavailability ranges from 20% to 35%. A nonlinear correlation exists between verapamil dose and plasma concentrations.

In early dose titration with verapamil, a relationship exists between plasma concentrations of verapamil and prolongation of the PR interval. However, during chronic administration, this relationship may disappear. No relationship has been established between the plasma concentration of verapamil and reduction in blood pressure.

In healthy subjects, orally administered verapamil undergoes extensive metabolism in the liver. Twelve metabolites have been identified in plasma; all except norverapamil are present in trace amounts only. Approximately 70% of an administered dose is excreted as metabolites in the urine and 16% or more in the feces within 5 days. Urinary excretion of unchanged drug is about 3% to 4% of the dose. Verapamil is approximately 90% bound to plasma proteins.

In patients with hepatic insufficiency, verapamil clearance is decreased about 30% and the elimination half-life is prolonged up to 14 to 16 hours (see **PRECAUTIONS**). In patients with liver dysfunction, a dosage adjustment may be required. In the elderly (≥65 years), verapamil clearance is reduced resulting in increases in elimination half-life.

Trandolapril Component

Following oral administration of trandolapril, the absolute bioavailability of trandolapril is approximately 10% as trandolapril and 70% as trandolaprilat. Plasma concentrations of trandolaprilat but not trandolapril increase in proportion with dose. Plasma concentrations of trandolaprilat decline in a triphasic manner. The more prolonged terminal elimination phase probably represents a small fraction of dose saturably bound to ACE.

After an oral radiolabeled dose of trandolapril, excretion of trandolapril and metabolites account for 33% of the dose in the urine and about 66% in the feces. Less than 1% of the dose is excreted in the urine as unchanged drug. Serum protein binding of trandolapril is about 80%, and is independent of concentration. Binding of trandolaprilat is concentration-dependent, varying from 65% at 1000 ng/mL to 94% at 0.1 ng/mL, indicating saturation of binding with increasing concentration.

Compared to normal subjects, the plasma concentrations of trandolapril and trandolaprilat are approximately 2-fold greater and renal clearance is reduced by about 85% in patients with creatinine clearance below 30 mL/min and in patients on hemodialysis. Dosage adjustment is recommended in renally impaired patients (see **DOSAGE AND ADMINISTRATION**).

Following oral administration in patients with mild to moderate alcoholic cirrhosis, plasma concentrations of trandolapril and trandolaprilat were, respectively, 9-fold and 2-fold greater than in normal subjects, but inhibition of ACE activity was not affected. Lower doses should be considered in patients with hepatic insufficiency (see **DOSAGE AND ADMINISTRATION**).

Pharmacodynamics

TARKA

Verapamil does not interfere with ACE inhibition by trandolapril. Trandolapril does not alter the effect of verapamil on intra-cardiac conduction.

Verapamil Component

Verapamil dilates the main coronary arteries and coronary arterioles, both in normal and ischemic regions, and is a potent inhibitor of coronary artery spasm. This property increases myocardial oxygen delivery in patients with coronary artery spasm, and is responsible for the effectiveness of verapamil in vasospastic (Prinzmetal's or variant) as well as unstable angina at rest.

Verapamil regularly reduces the total systemic resistance (afterload) by dilating peripheral arterioles. By decreasing the influx of calcium, verapamil prolongs the effective refractory period within the AV node and slows AV conduction in a rate-related manner.

Normal sinus rhythm is usually not affected, but in patients with sick sinus syndrome, verapamil may interfere with sinus node impulse generation and may induce sinus arrest or sinoatrial block. Atrioventricular block can occur in patients without preexisting conduction defects (see **WARNINGS**).

Verapamil does not alter the normal atrial action potential or intraventricular conduction time, but depresses amplitude, velocity of depolarization and conduction in depressed atrial fibers. Verapamil may shorten the antegrade effective refractory period of accessory bypass tracts. Acceleration of ventricular rate and/or ventricular fibrillation has been reported in patients with atrial flutter or atrial fibrillation and a coexisting accessory AV pathway following administration of verapamil (see **WARNINGS**).

Hemodynamics and Myocardial Metabolism: Verapamil reduces afterload and myocardial contractility. Improved left ventricular diastolic function in patients with idiopathic hypertrophic subaortic stenosis (IHSS) and those with coronary heart disease has also been observed with verapamil therapy. In most patients, including those with organic cardiac disease, the negative inotropic action of verapamil is countered by a reduction of afterload and cardiac index is usually not reduced. However, in patients with severe left ventricular dysfunction (e.g., pulmonary wedge pressure about 20 mmHg or ejection fraction less than 30%), or in patients taking beta-adrenergic blocking agents or other cardio-depressant drugs, deterioration of ventricular function may occur (see **PRECAUTIONS - Drug Interactions**).

Pulmonary Function: Verapamil does not induce bronchoconstriction and hence, does not impair ventilatory function.

Trandolapril Component

After a single 2 mg dose of trandolapril, inhibition of ACE activity reaches a maximum (70-85%) at 4 hours with about 10% decline at 24 hours. Eight days after dosing, ACE inhibition is still 40%.

Four placebo-controlled dose response studies were conducted using once daily oral dosing of trandolapril in doses from 0.25 to 16 mg per day in 827 black and non-black patients with mild to moderate hypertension. The minimal effective once daily dose was 1.0 mg in non-black patients and 2.0 mg in black patients. Further decreases in trough supine diastolic blood pressure were obtained in non-black patients with higher doses, and no further response was seen with doses above 4 mg (up to 16 mg). The antihypertensive effect diminished somewhat at the end of the dosing interval.

During chronic therapy, the maximum reduction in blood pressure with any dose is achieved within one week. Following 6 weeks of monotherapy in placebo-controlled trials in patients with mild to moderate hypertension, once daily doses of 2 to 4 mg lowered supine or standing systolic/diastolic blood pressure 24 hours after dosing by an average 7-10/4-5 mmHg below placebo responses in non-black patients. Once daily doses of 2 to 4 mg lowered blood pressures 4-6/3-4 mmHg below placebo responses in black patients.

CLINICAL STUDIES

In controlled clinical trials, once daily doses of TARKA, trandolapril 4 mg/verapamil HCl ER 240 mg or trandolapril 2 mg/verapamil HCl ER 180 mg, decreased placebo-corrected seated pressure (systolic/diastolic) 24 hours after

Information on the AbbVie, Inc. products listed on these pages is from the prescribing information in use as of July 31, 2013. For more information, please visit rxabbvie.com or call 1-800-633-9110.

dosing by about 7-12/6-8 mmHg. Each of the components of TARKA added to the antihypertensive effect. Treatment effects were consistent across age groups (<65, ≥65 years), and gender (male, female).
Blood pressure reductions were significantly greater for the TARKA 4/240 combination than for either of the components used alone.
The antihypertensive effects of TARKA have continued during therapy for at least 1 year.

INDICATIONS AND USAGE

TARKA is indicated for the treatment of hypertension.
This fixed combination drug is not indicated for the initial therapy of hypertension (see DOSAGE AND ADMINISTRATION).
In using TARKA, consideration should be given to the fact that an angiotensin converting enzyme inhibitor, captopril, has caused agranulocytosis, particularly in patients with renal impairment or collagen vascular disease, and that available data are insufficient to show that trandolapril does not have similar risk (see **WARNINGS - Neutropenia/Agranulocytosis**).

CONTRAINDICATIONS

TARKA is contraindicated in patients who are hypersensitive to any ACE inhibitor or verapamil.
Because of the verapamil component, TARKA is contraindicated in:
1. Severe left ventricular dysfunction (see **WARNINGS**).
2. Hypotension (systolic pressure less than 90 mmHg) or cardiogenic shock.
3. Sick sinus syndrome (except in patients with a functioning artificial ventricular pacemaker).
4. Second- or third-degree AV block (except in patients with a functioning artificial ventricular pacemaker).
5. Patients with atrial flutter or atrial fibrillation and an accessory bypass tract (e.g. Wolff-Parkinson-White, Lown-Ganong-Levine syndromes) (see **WARNINGS**).

Because of the trandolapril component, TARKA is contraindicated in patients with a history of angioedema related to previous treatment with an angiotensin converting enzyme (ACE) inhibitor.
Do not co-administer aliskiren with TARKA in patients with diabetes (see **PRECAUTIONS, Drug Interactions**).

WARNINGS

Heart Failure

Verapamil Component
Verapamil has a negative inotropic effect which, in most patients, is compensated by its afterload reduction (decreased systemic vascular resistance) properties without a net impairment of ventricular performance. In clinical experience with 4,954 patients, 87 (1.8%) developed congestive heart failure or pulmonary edema. Verapamil should be avoided in patients with severe left ventricular dysfunction (e.g., ejection fraction less than 30%, pulmonary wedge pressure above 20 mmHg, or severe symptoms of cardiac failure) and in patients with any degree of ventricular dysfunction if they are receiving a beta adrenergic blocker (see **PRECAUTIONS - Drug Interactions**). Patients with milder ventricular dysfunction should, if possible, be controlled with optimum doses of digitalis and/or diuretics before verapamil treatment (Note interactions with digoxin under: **PRECAUTIONS**).
Trandolapril Component
Trandolapril, as an ACE inhibitor, may cause excessive hypotension in patients with congestive heart failure (see **WARNINGS - Hypotension**).

Hypotension

Verapamil Component
Occasionally, the pharmacologic action of verapamil may produce a decrease in blood pressure below normal levels which may result in dizziness or symptomatic hypotension.
Trandolapril Component
Trandolapril can cause symptomatic hypotension. Like other ACE inhibitors, trandolapril has only rarely been associated with symptomatic hypotension in uncomplicated hypertensive patients. Symptomatic hypotension is most likely to occur in patients who are salt- or volume-depleted as a result of prolonged treatment with diuretics, dietary salt restriction, dialysis, diarrhea, or vomiting. Volume and/or salt depletion should be corrected before initiating treatment with trandolapril (see **PRECAUTIONS - Drug Interactions** and **ADVERSE REACTIONS**).
In controlled studies, hypotension was observed in 0.6% of patients receiving any combination of trandolapril and verapamil HCl ER.
In patients with concomitant congestive heart failure, with or without associated renal insufficiency, ACE inhibitor therapy may cause excessive hypotension, which may be associated with oliguria or azotemia, and, rarely, with acute renal failure and death (see **DOSAGE AND ADMINISTRATION**).
If symptomatic hypotension occurs, the patient should be placed in the supine position and, if necessary, normal saline may be administered intravenously. A transient hypotensive response is not a contraindication to further doses; however, lower doses of verapamil HCl ER and/or trandolapril or reduced concomitant diuretic therapy should be considered.

Elevated Liver Enzymes/Hepatic Failure

Verapamil Component
Elevations of transaminases with and without concomitant elevations in alkaline phosphatase and bilirubin have been reported. Such elevations have sometimes been transient and may disappear even in the face of continued verapamil treatment. Several cases of hepatocellular injury related to verapamil have been proven by rechallenge; half of these had clinical symptoms (malaise, fever, and/or right upper quadrant pain) in addition to elevations of SGOT, SGPT, and alkaline phosphatase.
Trandolapril Component
ACE inhibitors rarely have been associated with a syndrome of cholestatic jaundice, fulminant hepatic necrosis, and death. The mechanism of this syndrome is not understood. Patients receiving ACE inhibitors who develop jaundice should discontinue the ACE inhibitor and receive appropriate medical follow-up.
Liver abnormalities were noted in 3.2% of patients taking any of several combinations of trandolapril/verapamil doses. Periodic monitoring of liver function in patients taking TARKA is therefore prudent.

Accessory Bypass Tract (Wolff-Parkinson-White or Lown-Ganong-Levine Syndromes)

Verapamil Component
Some patients with paroxysmal and/or chronic atrial fibrillation or atrial flutter and a coexisting accessory AV pathway have developed increased antegrade conduction across the accessory pathway bypassing the AV node, producing a very rapid ventricular response or ventricular fibrillation after receiving intravenous verapamil (or digitalis). Although a risk of this occurring with oral verapamil has not been established, such patients receiving oral verapamil may be at risk and its use in these patients is contraindicated (see **CONTRAINDICATIONS**).
Treatment is usually DC-cardioversion. Cardioversion has been used safely and effectively after oral verapamil.

Atrioventricular Block

Verapamil Component
The effect of verapamil on AV conduction and the SA node may lead to asymptomatic first-degree AV block and transient bradycardia, sometimes accompanied by nodal escape rhythms. PR interval prolongation is correlated with verapamil plasma concentrations, especially during the early titration phases of therapy. Higher degrees of AV block, however, were infrequently (0.8%) observed. Marked first-degree block or progressive development to second- or third-degree AV block requires a reduction in dosage or, in rare instances, discontinuation of verapamil HCl and institution of appropriate therapy depending upon the clinical situation.

Patients with Hypertrophic Cardiomyopathy (IHSS)

Verapamil Component
In 120 patients with hypertrophic cardiomyopathy (most of them refractory or intolerant to propranolol) who received therapy with verapamil at doses up to 720 mg/day, a variety of serious adverse effects were seen. Three patients died in pulmonary edema; all had severe left ventricular outflow obstruction and a past history of left ventricular dysfunction. Eight other patients had pulmonary edema and/or severe hypotension; abnormally high (over 20 mmHg) capillary wedge pressure and a marked left ventricular outflow obstruction were present in most of these patients. Sinus bradycardia occurred in 11% of the patients, second-degree AV block in 4% and sinus arrest in 2%. It must be appreciated that this group of patients had a serious disease with a high mortality rate. Most adverse effects responded well to dose reduction and only rarely did verapamil have to be discontinued.

Anaphylactoid and Possibly Related Reactions

Presumably because angiotensin-converting enzyme inhibitors affect the metabolism of eicosanoids and polypeptides, including endogenous bradykinin, patients receiving ACE inhibitors, including trandolapril may be subject to a variety of adverse reactions, some of them serious.
Angioedema
Angioedema of the face, extremities, lips, tongue, glottis, and larynx has been reported in patients treated with ACE inhibitors including trandolapril. Symptoms suggestive of angioedema or facial edema occurred in 0.13% of trandolapril-treated patients. Two of the four cases were life-threatening and resolved without treatment or with medication (corticosteroids). Angioedema associated with laryngeal edema can be fatal. If laryngeal stridor or angioedema of the face, tongue or glottis occurs, treatment with TARKA should be discontinued immediately, the patient treated in accordance with accepted medical care and carefully observed until the swelling disappears. In instances where swelling is confined to the face and lips, the condition generally resolves without treatment; antihistamines may be useful in relieving symptoms. **Where there is involvement of the tongue, glottis, or larynx, likely to cause airway obstruction, emergency therapy, including but not limited to subcutaneous epinephrine solution 1:1,000 (0.3 to 0.5 mL) should be promptly administered** (see **PRECAUTIONS** and **ADVERSE REACTIONS**).
Anaphylactoid Reactions During Desensitization
Two patients undergoing desensitizing treatment with hymenoptera venom while receiving ACE inhibitors sustained life-threatening anaphylactoid reactions. In the same patients, these reactions did not occur when ACE inhibitors were temporarily withheld, but they reappeared when the ACE inhibitors were inadvertently readministered.
Anaphylactoid Reactions During Membrane Exposure
Anaphylactoid reactions have been reported in patients dialyzed with high-flux membranes and treated concomitantly with an ACE inhibitor. Anaphylactoid reactions have also been reported in patients undergoing low-density lipoprotein apheresis with dextran sulfate absorption.

Neutropenia/Agranulocytosis

Trandolapril Component
Another ACE inhibitor, captopril, has been shown to cause agranulocytosis and bone marrow depression rarely in patients with uncomplicated hypertension, but more frequently in patients with renal impairment, especially if they also have a collagen-vascular disease such as systemic lupus erythematosus or scleroderma. Available data from clinical trials of trandolapril or TARKA are insufficient to show that trandolapril does not cause agranulocytosis at similar rates. As with other ACE inhibitors, periodic monitoring of white blood cell counts in patients with collagen-vascular disease and/or renal disease should be considered.

Fetal Toxicity

Pregnancy Category D
Trandolapril Component
Use of drugs that act on the renin-angiotensin system during the second and third trimesters of pregnancy reduces fetal renal function and increases fetal and neonatal morbidity and death. Resulting oligohydramnios can be associated with fetal lung hypoplasia and skeletal deformations. Potential neonatal adverse effects include skull hypoplasia, anuria, hypotension, renal failure, and death. When pregnancy is detected, discontinue TARKA as soon as possible. These adverse outcomes are usually associated with use of these drugs in the second and third trimester of pregnancy. Most epidemiologic studies examining fetal abnormalities after exposure to antihypertensive use in the first trimester have not distinguished drugs affecting the renin-angiotensin system from other antihypertensive agents. Appropriate management of maternal hypertension during pregnancy is important to optimize outcomes for both mother and fetus.
In the unusual case that there is no appropriate alternative to therapy with drugs affecting the renin-angiotensin system for a particular patient, apprise the mother of the potential risk to the fetus. Perform serial ultrasound examinations to assess the intra-amniotic environment. If oligohydramnios is observed, discontinue TARKA, unless it is considered lifesaving for the mother. Fetal testing may be appropriate, based on the week of pregnancy. Patients and physicians should be aware, however, that oligohydramnios may not appear until after the fetus has sustained irreversible injury. Closely observe infants with histories of *in utero* exposure to TARKA for hypotension, oliguria, and hyperkalemia (see **PRECAUTIONS - Pediatric Use**).
Doses of 0.8 mg/kg/day (9.4 mg/m2/day) in rabbits, 1000 mg/kg/day (7000 mg/m2/day) in rats, and 25 mg/kg/day (295 mg/m2/day) in cynomolgus monkeys did not produce teratogenic effects. These doses represent 10 and 3 times (rabbits), 1250 and 2564 times (rats), and 312 and 108 times (monkeys) the maximum projected human dose of 4 mg based on body-weight and body-surface-area, respectively assuming a 50 kg woman.
Trandolapril in doses of 0.8 mg/kg/day in rabbits, 100.0 mg/kg/day in rats, and 25 mg/kg/day in cynomolgus monkeys (10, 1250, and 312 times the maximum projected human dose, respectively, assuming a 50 kg woman) did not produce teratogenic effects.

PRECAUTIONS

Use in Patients with Impaired Hepatic Function

TARKA has not been evaluated in subjects with impaired hepatic function.
Verapamil Component
Since verapamil is highly metabolized by the liver, it should be administered cautiously to patients with impaired hepatic function. Severe liver dysfunction prolongs the elimination half-life of immediate release verapamil to about 14 to 16 hours; hence, approximately 30% of the dose given to patients with normal liver function should be administered to these patients.
Careful monitoring for abnormal prolongation of the PR interval or other signs of excessive pharmacologic effects (see **OVERDOSAGE**) should be carried out.

Trandolapril Component
Trandolapril and trandolaprilat concentrations increase in patients with impaired liver function.

Use in Patients with Impaired Renal Function
TARKA has not been evaluated in patients with impaired renal function.
Verapamil Component
About 70% of an administered dose of verapamil is excreted as metabolites in the urine. Verapamil is not removed by hemodialysis. Until further data are available, verapamil should be administered cautiously to patients with impaired renal function. These patients should be carefully monitored for abnormal prolongation of the PR interval or other signs of overdosage (see **OVERDOSAGE**).
Trandolapril Component
As a consequence of inhibiting the renin-angiotensin-aldosterone system, changes in renal function may be anticipated in susceptible individuals. In patients with severe heart failure whose renal function may depend on the activity of the renin-angiotensin-aldosterone system, treatment with ACE inhibitors, including trandolapril, may be associated with oliguria and/or progressive azotemia and rarely with acute renal failure and/or death.
In hypertensive patients with unilateral or bilateral renal artery stenosis, increases in blood urea nitrogen and serum creatinine have been observed in some patients following ACE inhibitor therapy. These increases were almost always reversible upon discontinuation of the ACE inhibitor and/or diuretic therapy. In such patients, renal function should be monitored during the first few weeks of therapy.
Some hypertensive patients with no apparent pre-existing renal vascular disease have developed increases in blood urea and serum creatinine, usually minor and transient, especially when ACE inhibitors have been given concomitantly with a diuretic. This is more likely to occur in patients with pre-existing renal impairment. Dosage reduction and/or discontinuation of any diuretic and/or the ACE inhibitor may be required.
Evaluation of hypertensive patients should always include assessment of renal function (see **DOSAGE AND ADMINISTRATION**).

Use in Patients with Attenuated (Decreased) Neuromuscular Transmission
Verapamil Component
It has been reported that verapamil decreases neuromuscular transmission in patients with Duchenne's muscular dystrophy, and that verapamil prolongs recovery from the neuromuscular blocking agent vecuronium. It may be necessary to decrease the dosage of verapamil when it is administered to patients with attenuated neuromuscular transmission (see **PRECAUTIONS - Surgery/Anesthesia**).

Hyperkalemia and Potassium-sparing Diuretics
Trandolapril Component
In clinical trials, hyperkalemia (serum potassium > 6.00 mEq/L) occurred in approximately 0.4 percent of hypertensive patients receiving trandolapril and in 0.8% of patients receiving a dose of trandolapril (0.5-8 mg) in combination with a dose of verapamil SR (120-240 mg). In most cases, elevated serum potassium levels were isolated values, which resolved despite continued therapy. None of these patients were discontinued from the trials because of hyperkalemia. Risk factors for the development of hyperkalemia include renal insufficiency, diabetes mellitus, and the concomitant use of potassium-sparing diuretics, potassium supplements, and/or potassium-containing salt substitutes, which should be used cautiously, if at all, with trandolapril (see **PRECAUTIONS - Drug Interactions**).

Cough
Presumably due to the inhibition of the degradation of endogenous bradykinin, persistent nonproductive cough has been reported with all ACE inhibitors, always resolving after discontinuation of therapy. ACE inhibitor-induced cough should be considered in the differential diagnosis of cough. In controlled trials of trandolapril, cough was present in 2% of trandolapril patients and 0% of patients given placebo. There was no evidence of a relationship to dose.

Surgery/anesthesia
Trandolapril Component
In patients undergoing major surgery or during anesthesia with agents that produce hypotension, trandolapril will block angiotensin II formation secondary to compensatory renin release. If hypotension occurs and is considered to be due to this mechanism, it can be corrected by volume expansion (see **PRECAUTIONS - Use in Patients with Attenuated (Decreased) Neuromuscular Transmission**).

Drug Interactions
In vitro metabolic studies indicate that verapamil is metabolized by cytochrome P450 including CYP3A4, CYP1A2, CYP2C8, CYP2C9 and CYP2C18. Verapamil has been shown to be an inhibitor of CYP3A4 enzymes and P-glycoprotein (P-gp).
Clinically significant interactions have been reported with inhibitors of CYP3A4 (e.g. erythromycin, ritonavir) causing elevation of plasma levels of verapamil while inducers of CYP3A4 (e.g. rifampin) have caused a lowering of plasma levels of verapamil. Therefore, patients receiving inhibitors or inducers of the cytochrome P450 system should be monitored for drug interactions.
Digitalis
Clinical use of verapamil in digitalized patients has shown the combination to be well tolerated if digoxin doses are properly adjusted. Chronic verapamil treatment can increase serum digoxin levels by 50 to 75% during the first week of therapy, and this can result in digoxin toxicity. In patients with hepatic cirrhosis, the influence of verapamil on digoxin kinetics is magnified. Verapamil may reduce total body clearance and extrarenal clearance of digitoxin by 27% and 29%, respectively. Maintenance digoxin doses should be reduced when verapamil is administered, and the patient should be carefully monitored to avoid over- or under-digitalization. Whenever overdigitalization is suspected, the daily dose of digoxin should be reduced or temporarily discontinued. Upon discontinuation of any verapamil-containing regime including TARKA® (trandolapril/verapamil hydrochloride ER), the patient should be reassessed to avoid underdigitalization. No clinically significant pharmacokinetic interaction has been found between trandolapril (or its metabolites) and digoxin.
Lithium
Verapamil Component
Increased sensitivity to the effects of lithium (neurotoxicity) has been reported during concomitant verapamil-lithium therapy with either no change or an increase in serum lithium levels. Increased serum lithium levels and symptoms of lithium toxicity have been reported in patients receiving concomitant lithium and ACE inhibitor therapy. TARKA and lithium should be coadministered with caution, and frequent monitoring of serum lithium levels is recommended. If a diuretic is also used, the risk of lithium toxicity may be increased.
Clarithromycin
Hypotension, bradyarrhythmias, and lactic acidosis have been observed in patients receiving concurrent clarithromycin.
Erythromycin
Hypotension, bradyarrhythmias, and lactic acidosis have been observed in patients receiving concurrent erythromycin ethylsuccinate.
Cimetidine
The interaction between cimetidine and chronically administered verapamil has not been studied. Variable results on clearance have been obtained in acute studies of healthy volunteers; clearance of verapamil was either reduced or unchanged. No clinically significant pharmacokinetic interaction has been found between trandolapril (or its metabolites) and cimetidine.
Antiarrhythmic Agents
Verapamil Component
Disopyramide Phosphate
Data on possible interactions between verapamil and disopyramide phosphate are not available. Therefore, disopyramide should not be administered within 48 hours before or 24 hours after verapamil administration.
Flecainide
A study of healthy volunteers showed that the concomitant administration of flecainide and verapamil may have additive effects on myocardial contractility, AV conduction, and repolarization. Concomitant therapy with flecainide and verapamil may result in additive negative inotropic effect and prolongation of atrioventricular conduction.
Quinidine
In a small number of patients with hypertrophic cardiomyopathy (IHSS), concomitant use of verapamil and quinidine resulted in significant hypotension. Until further data are obtained, combined therapy of verapamil and quinidine in patients with hypertrophic cardiomyopathy should probably be avoided.
The electrophysiological effects of quinidine and verapamil on AV conduction were studied in 8 patients. Verapamil significantly counteracted the effects of quinidine on AV conduction. There has been a report of increased quinidine levels during verapamil therapy.
Antihypertensive Agents
Concomitant use of TARKA with other antihypertensive agents including diuretics, vasodilators, beta-adrenergic blockers, and alpha-antagonists may result in additive hypotensive effects. There are reports that verapamil may result in higher concentrations of the alpha-agonists prazosin and terazosin.
Dual Blockade of the Renin-Angiotensin System (RAS)
Trandolapril Component
Dual blockade of the RAS with angiotensin receptor blockers, ACE inhibitors, or aliskiren is associated with increased risks of hypotension, hyperkalemia, and changes in renal function (including acute renal failure) compared to monotherapy. Closely monitor blood pressure, renal function and electrolytes in patients on TARKA and other agents that affect the RAS.
Do not co-administer aliskiren with TARKA in patients with diabetes. Avoid use of aliskiren with TARKA in patients with renal impairment (GFR <60 ml/min).
Beta Blockers
Verapamil Component
Concomitant therapy with beta-adrenergic blockers and verapamil may result in additive negative effects on heart rate, atrioventricular conduction, and/or cardiac contractility. Drug interaction studies have indicated that the maximum concentrations of metoprolol and propanolol are increased after the administration of verapamil. The use of verapamil in combination with a beta-adrenergic blocker should be used only with caution, and close monitoring.
Asymptomatic bradycardia (36 beats/min) with a wandering atrial pacemaker has been observed in a patient receiving concomitant timolol (a beta-adrenergic blocker) eyedrops and oral verapamil.
Concomitant Diuretic Therapy
Trandolapril Component
As with other ACE inhibitors, patients on diuretics, especially those on recently instituted diuretic therapy, may occasionally experience an excessive reduction of blood pressure after initiation of therapy with TARKA. The possibility of exacerbation of hypotensive effects with TARKA may be minimized by either discontinuing the diuretic or cautiously increasing salt intake prior to initiation of treatment with TARKA. If it is not possible to discontinue the diuretic, the starting dose of TARKA should be reduced (see **DOSAGE AND ADMINISTRATION**). No clinically significant pharmacokinetic interaction has been found between trandolapril (or its metabolites) and furosemide.
Agents Increasing Serum Potassium
Trandolapril Component
Trandolapril can attenuate potassium loss caused by thiazide diuretics and increase serum potassium when used alone. Use of potassium-sparing diuretics (spironolactone, triamterene, or amiloride), potassium supplements, or potassium-containing salt substitutes concomitantly with ACE inhibitors can increase the risk of hyperkalemia. If concomitant use of such agents is indicated, they should be used with caution and with appropriate monitoring of serum potassium (see **PRECAUTIONS**).
HMG-CoA Reductase Inhibitors ("Statins")
Verapamil component
The use of HMG-CoA reductase inhibitors that are CYP3A4 substrates in combination with verapamil has been associated with reports of myopathy/rhabdomyolysis.
Co-administration of multiple doses of 10 mg of verapamil with 80 mg simvastatin resulted in exposure to simvastatin 2.5-fold that following simvastatin alone. Limit the dose of simvastatin in patients on verapamil to 10 mg daily. Limit the daily dose of lovastatin to 40 mg. Lower starting and maintenance doses of other CYP3A4 substrates (e.g., atorvastatin) may be required as verapamil may increase the plasma concentration of these drugs.
Non-Steroidal Anti-Inflammatory Agents including Selective Cyclooxygenase-2 Inhibitors (COX-2 Inhibitors)
Trandolapril component
In patients who are elderly, volume-depleted (including those on diuretic therapy), or with compromised renal function, co-administration of NSAIDs, including selective COX-2 inhibitors, with ACE inhibitors, including trandolapril, may result in deterioration of renal function, including possible acute renal failure. These effects are usually reversible. Monitor renal function periodically in patients receiving trandolapril and NSAID therapy.
The antihypertensive effect of ACE inhibitors, including trandolapril may be attenuated by NSAIDs.
Other (Verapamil Component)
Nitrates
Verapamil has been given concomitantly with short- and long-acting nitrates without any undesirable drug interactions. The pharmacologic profile of both drugs and the clinical experience suggest beneficial interactions.
Carbamazepine
Verapamil may increase carbamazepine concentrations during combined therapy. This may produce carbamazepine side effects such as diplopia, headache, ataxia, or dizziness.
Anti-infective Agents
Therapy with rifampin may markedly reduce oral verapamil bioavailability. There have been reports that erythromycin and telithromycin may increase concentrations of verapamil.
Barbiturates
Phenobarbital therapy may increase verapamil clearance.

Information on the AbbVie, Inc. products listed on these pages is from the prescribing information in use as of July 31, 2013. For more information, please visit rxabbvie.com or call 1-800-633-9110.

ADVERSE EVENTS OCCURRING in ≥ 1% of TARKA PATIENTS IN U.S. PLACEBO-CONTROLLED TRIALS

	TARKA (N = 541) % Incidence (% Discontinuance)	PLACEBO (N = 206) % Incidence (% Discontinuance)
AV Block First Degree	3.9 (0.2)	0.5 (0.0)
Bradycardia	1.8 (0.0)	0.0 (0.0)
Bronchitis	1.5 (0.0)	0.5 (0.0)
Chest Pain	2.2 (0.0)	1.0 (0.0)
Constipation	3.3 (0.0)	1.0 (0.0)
Cough	4.6 (0.0)	2.4 (0.0)
Diarrhea	1.5 (0.2)	1.0 (0.0)
Dizziness	3.1 (0.0)	1.9 (0.5)
Dyspnea	1.3 (0.4)	0.0 (0.0)
Edema	1.3 (0.0)	2.4 (0.0)
Fatigue	2.8 (0.4)	2.4 (0.0)
Headache(s)+	8.9 (0.0)	9.7 (0.5)
Increased Liver Enzymes*	2.8 (0.2)	1.0 (0.0)
Nausea	1.5 (0.2)	0.5 (0.0)
Pain Extremity(ies)	1.1 (0.2)	0.5 (0.0)
Pain Back+	2.2 (0.0)	2.4 (0.0)
Pain Joint(s)	1.7 (0.0)	1.0 (0.0)
Upper Respiratory Tract Infection(s)+	5.4 (0.0)	7.8 (0.0)
Upper Respiratory Tract Congestion+	2.4 (0.0)	3.4 (0.0)

* Also includes increase in SGPT, SGOT, Alkaline Phosphatase
\+ Incidence of adverse events is higher in Placebo group than TARKA patients

Immunosuppressive Agents
Verapamil therapy may increase serum levels of cyclosporin, sirolimus and tacrolimus.
Theophylline
Verapamil therapy may inhibit the clearance and increase the plasma levels of theophylline.
Tranquilizers/ Anti-depressants
Due to metabolism via the CYP enzyme system, there have been reports that verapamil may increase the concentrations of buspirone, midazolam, almotriptan and imipramine.
Colchicine
Colchicine is a substrate for both CYP3A and the efflux transporter, P-gp. Verapamil is known to inhibit CYP3A and P-gp. When verapamil and colchicine are administered together, the potential inhibition of P-gp and/or CYP3A by verapamil may lead to increased exposure to colchicine (see **PRECAUTIONS - Drug Interactions**).
Other
Concentrations of verapamil may be increased by the concomitant administration of protease inhibitors such as ritonavir, and reduced by the concomitant administration of sulfinpyrazone, or St John's Wort.
Concentrations of doxorubicin may be increased by the administration of verapamil.
There have been reports that verapamil may elevate the concentrations of the oral anti-diabetic glyburide.
Inhalation Anesthetics
Animal experiments have shown that inhalation anesthetics depress cardiovascular activity by decreasing the inward movement of calcium ions. When used concomitantly, inhalation anesthetics and calcium antagonists, such as verapamil, should be titrated carefully to avoid excessive cardiovascular depression.
Neuromuscular Blocking Agents
Clinical data and animal studies suggest that verapamil may potentiate the activity of neuromuscular blocking agents (curare-like and depolarizing). It may be necessary to decrease the dose of verapamil and/or the dose of the neuromuscular blocking agent when the drugs are used concomitantly.
Gold
Nitritoid reactions (symptoms include facial flushing, nausea, vomiting and hypotension) have been reported rarely in patients on therapy with injectable gold (sodium aurothiomalate) and concomitant ACE inhibitor therapy including TARKA.
Other (Trandolapril Component)
No clinically significant pharmacokinetic interaction has been found between trandolapril (or its metabolites) and nifedipine.
The anticoagulant effect of warfarin was not significantly changed by trandolapril.
Anti-diabetic Agents
The concomitant use of ACE inhibitors such as trandolapril with antidiabetic medications (insulin or oral hypoglycemic agents) may result in increased blood glucose lowering effects.

Carcinogenesis, Mutagenesis, Impairment of Fertility
Verapamil Component
An 18-month toxicity study in rats, at a low multiple (6 fold) of the maximum recommended human dose, and not the maximum tolerated dose, did not suggest a tumorigenic potential. There was no evidence of a carcinogenic potential of verapamil administered in the diet of rats for two years at doses of 10, 35, and 120 mg/kg per day or approximately 1×, 3.5×, and 12×, respectively, the maximum recommended human daily dose (480 mg per day or 9.6 mg/kg/day).
Verapamil was not mutagenic in the Ames test in 5 test strains at 3 mg per plate, with or without metabolic activation.
Studies in female rats at daily dietary doses up to 5.5 times (55 mg/kg/day) the maximum recommended human dose did not show impaired fertility. Effects on male fertility have not been determined.
Long-term studies were conducted with oral trandolapril administered by gavage to mice (78 weeks) and rats (104 and 106 weeks). No evidence of carcinogenic potential was seen in mice dosed up to 25 mg/kg/day (85 mg/m^2/day) or rats dosed up to 8 mg/kg/day (60 mg/m^2/day). These doses are 313 and 32 times (mice), and 100 and 23 times (rats) the maximum recommended human daily dose (MRHDD) of 4 mg based on body-weight and body-surface-area, respectively assuming a 50 kg individual. The genotoxic potential of trandolapril was evaluated in the microbial mutagenicity (Ames) test, the point mutation and chromosome aberration assays in Chinese hamster V79 cells, and the micronucleus test in mice. There was no evidence of mutagenic or clastogenic potential in these *in vitro* and *in vivo* assays.
Reproduction studies in rats did not show any impairment of fertility at doses up to 100 mg/kg/day (710 mg/m^2/day) of trandolapril, or 1250 and 260 times the MRHDD on the basis of body-weight and body-surface-area, respectively.

Pregnancy
Female patients of childbearing age should be told about the consequences of exposure to TARKA during pregnancy. Discuss treatment options with women planning to become pregnant. Patients should be asked to report pregnancies to their physicians as soon as possible.

Nursing Mothers
Verapamil is excreted in human milk. Radiolabeled trandolapril or its metabolites are secreted in rat milk. TARKA should not be administered to nursing mothers.

Geriatric Use
In placebo-controlled studies, where 23% of patients receiving TARKA were 65 years and older, and 2.4% were 75 years and older, no overall differences in effectiveness or safety were observed between these patients and younger patients. However, greater sensitivity of some older individual patients cannot be ruled out.

Pediatric Use
Neonates with a history of *in utero* exposure to TARKA:
If oliguria or hypotension occurs, direct attention toward support of blood pressure and renal perfusion. Exchange transfusions or dialysis may be required as a means of reversing hypotension and/or substituting for disordered renal function.
The safety and effectiveness of TARKA in children below the age of 18 have not been established.

Animal Pharmacology and/or Animal Toxicology
In chronic animal toxicology studies, verapamil caused lenticular and/or suture line changes at 30 mg/kg/day or greater and frank cataracts at 62.5 mg/kg/day or greater in the beagle dog but not the rat. Development of cataracts due to verapamil has not been reported in man.

ADVERSE REACTIONS
TARKA has been evaluated in over 1,957 subjects and patients. Of these, 541 patients, including 23% elderly patients, participated in U.S. controlled clinical trials, and 251 were studied in foreign controlled clinical trials. In clinical trials with TARKA, no adverse experiences peculiar to this combination drug have been observed. Adverse experiences that have occurred have been limited to those that have been previously reported with verapamil or trandolapril. TARKA has been evaluated for long-term safety in 272 patients treated for 1 year or more. Adverse experiences were usually mild and transient.
Discontinuation of therapy because of adverse events in U.S. placebo-controlled hypertension studies was required in 2.6% and 1.9% of patients treated with TARKA and placebo, respectively.
Adverse experiences occurring in 1% or more of the 541 patients in placebo-controlled hypertension trials who were treated with a range of trandolapril (0.5-8 mg) and verapamil (120-240 mg) combinations are shown below.
[See table above]
Other clinical adverse experiences possibly, probably, or definitely related to drug treatment occurring in 0.3% or more of patients treated with trandolapril/verapamil combinations with or without concomitant diuretic in controlled or uncontrolled trials (N = 990) and less frequent, clinically significant events (in italics) include the following:
Cardiovascular
Angina, AV block second degree, bundle branch block, edema, flushing, hypotension, myocardial infarction , palpitations, premature ventricular contractions, nonspecific ST-T changes, near syncope, tachycardia.
Central Nervous System
Drowsiness, hypesthesia, insomnia, loss of balance, paresthesia, vertigo.
Dermatologic
Pruritus, rash.
Emotional, Mental, Sexual States
Anxiety, impotence, abnormal mentation.
Eye, Ear, Nose, Throat
Epistaxis, tinnitus, upper respiratory tract infection, blurred vision.
Gastrointestinal
Diarrhea, dyspepsia, dry mouth, nausea.
General Body Function
Chest pain, malaise, weakness.
Genitourinary
Endometriosis, hematuria, nocturia, polyuria, proteinuria.
Hemopoietic
Decreased leukocytes, decreased neutrophils.
Musculoskeletal System
Arthralgias/myalgias, gout (increased uric acid).
Pulmonary
Dyspnea.
Angioedema
Angioedema has been reported in 3 (0.15%) patients receiving TARKA in U.S. and foreign studies (N = 1,957). Angioedema associated with laryngeal edema may be fatal. If angioedema of the face, extremities, lips, tongue, glottis, and/or larynx occurs, treatment with TARKA should be discontinued and appropriate therapy instituted immediately (see **WARNINGS**).
Hypotension
(See **WARNINGS**). In hypertensive patients, hypotension occurred in 0.6% and near syncope occurred in 0.1%. Hypotension or syncope was a cause for discontinuation of therapy in 0.4% of hypertensive patients.
Treatment of Acute Cardiovascular Adverse Reactions
The frequency of cardiovascular adverse reactions which require therapy is rare, hence, experience with their treatment is limited. Whenever severe hypotension or complete AV block occur following oral administration of TARKA (verapamil component), the appropriate emergency measures should be applied immediately, e.g., intravenously administered isoproterenol HCl, levarterenol bitartrate, atropine (all in the usual doses), or calcium gluconate (10% solution). In patients with hypertrophic cardiomyopathy (IHSS), alpha-adrenergic agents (phenylephrine, metaraminol bitartrate or methoxamine) should be used to maintain blood pressure, and isoproterenol and levarterenol should be avoided. If further support is necessary, inotropic agents (dopamine or dobutamine) may be administered. Actual treatment and dosage should depend on the severity and the clinical situation and the judgment and experience of the treating physician.
Other adverse experiences (in addition to those in table and listed above) that have been reported with the individual components are listed below.
Verapamil Component
Cardiovascular
(See **WARNINGS**). CHF/pulmonary edema, AV block 3°, atrioventricular dissociation, claudication, purpura (vasculitis), syncope.
Digestive System
Gingival hyperplasia. Reversible, (upon discontinuation of verapamil) nonobstructive, paralytic ileus has been infrequently reported in association with the use of verapamil.

Hemic and Lymphatic
Ecchymosis or bruising.
Nervous System
Cerebrovascular accident, confusion, psychotic symptoms, shakiness, somnolence.
Skin
Exanthema, hair loss, hyperkeratosis, maculae, sweating, urticaria, Stevens-Johnson syndrome, erythema multiform.
Urogenital
Gynecomastia, galactorrhea/hyperprolactinemia, increased urination, spotty menstruation.
Trandolapril Component
Emotional, Mental, Sexual States
Decreased libido.
Gastrointestinal
Pancreatitis.

Clinical Laboratory Test Findings

Hematology
(See **WARNINGS**). Low white blood cells, low neutrophils, low lymphocytes, low platelets.
Serum Electrolytes
Hyperkalemia (see **PRECAUTIONS**), hyponatremia.
Renal Function Tests
Increases in creatinine and blood urea nitrogen levels occurred in 1.1 percent and 0.3 percent, respectively, of patients receiving TARKA with or without hydrochlorothiazide therapy. None of these increases required discontinuation of treatment. Increases in these laboratory values are more likely to occur in patients with renal insufficiency or those pretreated with a diuretic and, based on experience with other ACE inhibitors, would be expected to be especially likely in patients with renal artery stenosis (see **PRECAUTIONS** and **WARNINGS**).
Liver Function Tests
Elevations of liver enzymes (SGOT, SGPT, LDH, and alkaline phosphatase) and/or serum bilirubin occurred. Discontinuation for elevated liver enzymes occurred in 0.9 percent of patients (see **WARNINGS**).
Post Marketing Experience
There has been a single postmarketing report of paralysis (tetraparesis) associated with the combined use of verapamil and colchicine. This may have been caused by colchicine crossing the blood-brain barrier due to CYP3A4 and P-gp inhibition by verapamil. Combined use of verapamil and colchicine is not recommended (see **PRECAUTIONS - Drug Interactions**).

OVERDOSAGE

No specific information is available on the treatment of overdosage with TARKA.

Verapamil Component

Overdose with verapamil may lead to pronounced hypotension, bradycardia, and conduction system abnormalities (e.g., junctional rhythm with AV dissociation and high degree AV block, including asystole). Other symptoms secondary to hypoperfusion (e.g., metabolic acidosis, hyperglycemia, hyperkalemia, renal dysfunction, and convulsions) may be evident.

Treat all verapamil overdoses as serious and maintain observation for at least 48 hours, preferably under continuous hospital care. Delayed pharmacodynamic consequences may occur with the sustained release formulation. Verapamil is known to decrease gastrointestinal transit time. In cases of overdose, tablets of ISOPTIN SR have occasionally been reported to form concretions within the stomach or intestines. These concretions have not been visible on plain radiographs of the abdomen, and no medical means of gastrointestinal emptying is of proven efficacy in removing them. Endoscopy might reasonably be considered in cases of overdose when symptoms are unusually prolonged. Verapamil cannot be removed by hemodialysis.

Treatment of overdosage should be supportive. Beta adrenergic stimulation or parenteral administration of calcium solutions may increase calcium ion flux across the slow channel, and have been used effectively in treatment of deliberate overdosage with verapamil. The following measures may be considered:

Bradycardia and Conduction System Abnormalities
Atropine, isoproterenol, and cardiac pacing.
Hypotension
Intravenous fluids, vasopressors (e.g., dopamine, dobutamine), calcium solutions (e.g., 10% calcium chloride solution).
Cardiac Failures
Inotropic agents (e.g., isoproterenol, dopamine, dobutamine), diuretics. Asystole should be handled by the usual measures including cardiopulmonary resuscitation.

Trandolapril Component

The oral LD_{50} of trandolapril in mice was 4875 mg/kg in males and 3990 mg/kg in females. In rats, an oral dose of 5000 mg/kg caused low mortality (1 male out of 5; 0 females). In dogs, an oral dose of 1000 mg/kg did not cause mortality and abnormal clinical signs were not observed.

In humans, the most likely clinical manifestation would be symptoms attributable to severe hypotension. Laboratory determinations of serum levels of trandolapril and its metabolites are not widely available, and such determinations have, in any event, no established role in the management of trandolapril overdose. No data are available to suggest that physiological maneuvers (e.g., maneuvers to change pH of the urine) might accelerate elimination of trandolapril and its metabolites. It is not known if trandolapril or trandolaprilat can be usefully removed from the body by hemodialysis.

Angiotensin II could presumably serve as a specific antagonist antidote in the setting of trandolapril overdose, but angiotensin II is essentially unavailable outside of scattered research facilities. Because the hypotensive effect of trandolapril is achieved through vasodilation and effective hypovolemia, it is reasonable to treat trandolapril overdose by infusion of normal saline solution.

DOSAGE AND ADMINISTRATION

The recommended usual dosage range of trandolapril for hypertension is 1 to 4 mg per day administered in a single dose or two divided doses. The recommended usual dosage range of Isoptin-SR for hypertension is 120 to 480 mg per day administered in a single dose or two divided doses.

The hazards (see **WARNINGS**) of trandolapril are generally independent of dose; those of verapamil are a mixture of dose-dependent phenomena (primarily dizziness, AV block, constipation) and dose-independent phenomena, the former much more common than the latter. Therapy with any combination of trandolapril and verapamil will thus be associated with both sets of dose-independent hazards. The dose-dependent side effects of verapamil have not been shown to be decreased by the addition of trandolapril nor vice versa.

Rarely, the dose-independent hazards of trandolapril are serious. To minimize dose-independent hazards, it is usually appropriate to begin therapy with TARKA only after a patient has either (a) failed to achieve the desired antihypertensive effect with one or the other monotherapy at its respective maximally recommended dose and shortest dosing interval, or (b) the dose of one or the other monotherapy cannot be increased further because of dose-limiting side effects.

Clinical trials with TARKA have explored only once-a-day doses. The antihypertensive effect and or adverse effects of adding 4 mg of trandolapril once-a-day to a dose of 240 mg Isoptin-SR administered twice-a-day has not been studied, nor have the effects of adding as little of 180 mg Isoptin-SR to 2 mg trandolapril administered twice-a-day been evaluated. Over the dose range of Isoptin-SR 120 to 240 mg once-a-day and trandolapril 0.5 to 8 mg once-a-day, the effects of the combination increase with increasing doses of either component.

Replacement Therapy

For convenience, patients receiving trandolapril (up to 8 mg) and verapamil (up to 240 mg) in separate tablets, administered once-a-day, may instead wish to receive tablets of TARKA containing the same component doses.

TARKA should be administered with food.

HOW SUPPLIED

TARKA 2/180 mg tablets are supplied as pink, oval, film-coated tablets containing 2 mg trandolapril in an immediate release form and 180 mg verapamil hydrochloride in a sustained release form. The tablet is debossed with a triangle and 182 on one side and plain on the other side.

NDC 0074-3287-13 - bottles of 100

TARKA 1/240 mg tablets are supplied as white, oval, film-coated tablets containing 1 mg trandolapril in an immediate release form and 240 mg verapamil hydrochloride in a sustained release form. The tablet is debossed with a triangle and 241 on one side and plain on the other side.

NDC 0074-3288-13 - bottles of 100

TARKA 2/240 mg tablets are supplied as gold, oval, film-coated tablets containing 2 mg trandolapril in an immediate release form and 240 mg verapamil hydrochloride in a sustained release form. The tablet is debossed with a triangle and 242 on one side and plain on the other side.

NDC 0074-3289-13 - bottles of 100

TARKA 4/240 mg tablets are supplied as reddish-brown, oval, film-coated tablets containing 4 mg trandolapril in an immediate release form and 240 mg verapamil hydrochloride in a sustained release form. The tablet is debossed with a triangle and 244 on one side and plain on the other side.

NDC 0074-3290-13 - bottles of 100

Dispense in well-closed container with safety closure.

Storage

Store at 15°-25°C (59°-77°F) see USP.

AbbVie Inc.
North Chicago, IL 60064, U.S.A.
03-A778 February, 2013

Shown in Product Identification Guide, page 304

TRICOR® ℞

[tri cŏr]
(fenofibrate)
Tablet for oral use

HIGHLIGHTS OF PRESCRIBING INFORMATION
These highlights do not include all the information needed to use TRICOR safely and effectively. See full prescribing information for TRICOR.
TRICOR (fenofibrate) Tablet for oral use
Initial U.S. Approval: 1993

INDICATIONS AND USAGE

TRICOR is a peroxisome proliferator receptor alpha (PPARα) activator indicated as an adjunct to diet:

- To reduce elevated LDL-C, Total-C, TG and Apo B, and to increase HDL-C in adult patients with primary hypercholesterolemia or mixed dyslipidemia (1.1).
- For treatment of adult patients with severe hypertriglyceridemia (1.2).

Important Limitations of Use: Fenofibrate was not shown to reduce coronary heart disease morbidity and mortality in patients with type 2 diabetes mellitus (5.1).

DOSAGE AND ADMINISTRATION

- Primary hypercholesterolemia or mixed dyslipidemia: Initial dose of 145 mg once daily (2.2).
- Severe hypertriglyceridemia: Initial dose of 48 to 145 mg once daily. Maximum dose is 145 mg (2.3).
- Renally impaired patients: Initial dose of 48 mg once daily (2.4).
- Geriatric patients: Select the dose on the basis of renal function (2.5).
- Maybe taken without regard to meals (2.1).

DOSAGE FORMS AND STRENGTHS

Oral Tablets: 48 mg and 145 mg (3).

CONTRAINDICATIONS

- Severe renal dysfunction, including patients receiving dialysis (4, 8.6, 12.3).
- Active liver disease (4, 5.3).
- Gallbladder disease (4, 5.5).
- Known hypersensitivity to fenofibrate (4).
- Nursing mothers (4, 8.3).

WARNINGS AND PRECAUTIONS

- Myopathy and rhabdomyolysis have been reported in patients taking fenofibrate. The risks for myopathy and rhabdomyolysis are increased when fibrates are co-administered with a statin (with a significantly higher rate observed for gemfibrozil), particularly in elderly patients and patients with diabetes, renal failure, or hypothyroidism (5.2).
- TRICOR can increase serum transaminases. Monitor liver tests, including ALT, periodically during therapy (5.3).
- TRICOR can reversibly increase serum creatinine levels (5.4). Monitor renal function periodically in patients with renal impairment (8.6).
- TRICOR increases cholesterol excretion into the bile, leading to risk of cholelithiasis. If cholelithiasis is suspected, gallbladder studies are indicated (5.5).
- Exercise caution in concomitant treatment with oral coumarin anticoagulants. Adjust the dosage of coumarin anticoagulant to maintain the prothrombin time/INR at the desired level to prevent bleeding complications (5.6).

ADVERSE REACTIONS

The most common adverse reactions (> 2% and at least 1% greater than placebo) are abnormal liver tests, increased AST, increased ALT, increased CPK, and rhinitis (6).

To report SUSPECTED ADVERSE REACTIONS, contact AbbVie Inc. at 1-800-633-9110 or FDA at 1-800-FDA-1088 or www.fda.gov/medwatch

DRUG INTERACTIONS

- Coumarin anticoagulants: (7.1).
- Immunosuppressants: (7.2).
- Bile acid resins: (7.3).

USE IN SPECIFIC POPULATIONS

- Geriatric Use: Determine dose selection based on renal function (8.5).
- Renal Impairment: Avoid use in patients with severe renal impairment. Dose reduction is required in patients with mild to moderate renal impairment (8.6).

See 17 for PATIENT COUNSELING INFORMATION

Revised: 02/2013

FULL PRESCRIBING INFORMATION: CONTENTS*

Information on the AbbVie, Inc. products listed on these pages is from the prescribing information in use as of July 31, 2013. For more information, please visit rxabbvie.com or call 1-800-633-9110.

* Sections or subsections omitted from the full prescribing information are not listed

FULL PRESCRIBING INFORMATION

1 INDICATIONS AND USAGE

1.1 Primary Hypercholesterolemia or Mixed Dyslipidemia

TRICOR is indicated as adjunctive therapy to diet to reduce elevated low-density lipoprotein cholesterol (LDL-C), total cholesterol (Total-C), Triglycerides and apolipoprotein B (Apo B), and to increase high-density lipoprotein cholesterol (HDL-C) in adult patients with primary hypercholesterolemia or mixed dyslipidemia.

1.2 Severe Hypertriglyceridemia

TRICOR is also indicated as adjunctive therapy to diet for treatment of adult patients with severe hypertriglyceridemia. Improving glycemic control in diabetic patients showing fasting chylomicronemia will usually obviate the need for pharmacologic intervention.

Markedly elevated levels of serum triglycerides (e.g. > 2,000 mg/dL) may increase the risk of developing pancreatitis. The effect of fenofibrate therapy on reducing this risk has not been adequately studied.

1.3 Important Limitations of Use

Fenofibrate at a dose equivalent to 145 mg of TRICOR was not shown to reduce coronary heart disease morbidity and mortality in a large, randomized controlled trial of patients with type 2 diabetes mellitus *[see Warnings and Precautions (5.1)]*.

2 DOSAGE AND ADMINISTRATION

2.1 General Considerations

Patients should be placed on an appropriate lipid-lowering diet before receiving TRICOR, and should continue this diet during treatment with TRICOR. TRICOR tablets can be given without regard to meals.

The initial treatment for dyslipidemia is dietary therapy specific for the type of lipoprotein abnormality. Excess body weight and excess alcoholic intake may be important factors in hypertriglyceridemia and should be addressed prior to any drug therapy. Physical exercise can be an important ancillary measure. Diseases contributory to hyperlipidemia, such as hypothyroidism or diabetes mellitus should be looked for and adequately treated. Estrogen therapy, thiazide diuretics and beta-blockers, are sometimes associated with massive rises in plasma triglycerides, especially in subjects with familial hypertriglyceridemia. In such cases, discontinuation of the specific etiologic agent may obviate the need for specific drug therapy of hypertriglyceridemia.

Lipid levels should be monitored periodically and consideration should be given to reducing the dosage of TRICOR if lipid levels fall significantly below the targeted range.

Therapy should be withdrawn in patients who do not have an adequate response after two months of treatment with the maximum recommended dose of 145 mg once daily.

2.2 Primary Hypercholesterolemia or Mixed Dyslipidemia

The initial dose of TRICOR is 145 mg once daily.

2.3 Severe Hypertriglyceridemia

The initial dose is 48 to 145 mg per day. Dosage should be individualized according to patient response, and should be adjusted if necessary following repeat lipid determinations at 4 to 8 week intervals. The maximum dose is 145 mg once daily.

2.4 Impaired Renal Function

Treatment with TRICOR should be initiated at a dose of 48 mg per day in patients having mild to moderately impaired renal function, and increased only after evaluation of the effects on renal function and lipid levels at this dose. The use of TRICOR should be avoided in patients with severe renal impairment *[see Use in Specific Populations (8.6) and Clinical Pharmacology (12.3)]*.

2.5 Geriatric Patients

Dose selection for the elderly should be made on the basis of renal function *[see Use in Specific Populations (8.5)]*.

3 DOSAGE FORMS AND STRENGTHS

- 48 mg yellow tablets, imprinted with the "a" logo and code identification letters "FI".
- 145 mg white tablets, imprinted with the "a" logo and code identification letters "FO".

4 CONTRAINDICATIONS

TRICOR is contraindicated in:

- patients with severe renal impairment, including those receiving dialysis *[see Clinical Pharmacology (12.3)]*.
- patients with active liver disease, including those with primary biliary cirrhosis and unexplained persistent liver function abnormalities *[see Warnings and Precautions (5.3)]*.
- patients with preexisting gallbladder disease *[see Warnings and Precautions (5.5)]*.
- nursing mothers *[see Use in Specific Populations (8.3)]*.
- patients with known hypersensitivity to fenofibrate or fenofibric acid *[see Warnings and Precautions (5.9)]*.

5 WARNINGS AND PRECAUTIONS

5.1 Mortality and Coronary Heart Disease Morbidity

The effect of TRICOR on coronary heart disease morbidity and mortality and non-cardiovascular mortality has not been established.

The Action to Control Cardiovascular Risk in Diabetes Lipid (ACCORD Lipid) trial was a randomized placebo-controlled study of 5518 patients with type 2 diabetes mellitus on background statin therapy treated with fenofibrate. The mean duration of follow-up was 4.7 years. Fenofibrate plus statin combination therapy showed a non-significant 8% relative risk reduction in the primary outcome of major adverse cardiovascular events (MACE), a composite of non-fatal myocardial infarction, non-fatal stroke, and cardiovascular disease death (hazard ratio [HR] 0.92, 95% CI 0.79-1.08) (p=0.32) as compared to statin monotherapy. In a gender subgroup analysis, the hazard ratio for MACE in men receiving combination therapy versus statin monotherapy was 0.82 (95% CI 0.69-0.99), and the hazard ratio for MACE in women receiving combination therapy versus statin monotherapy was 1.38 (95% CI 0.98-1.94) (interaction p=0.01). The clinical significance of this subgroup finding is unclear.

The Fenofibrate Intervention and Event Lowering in Diabetes (FIELD) study was a 5-year randomized, placebo-controlled study of 9795 patients with type 2 diabetes mellitus treated with fenofibrate. Fenofibrate demonstrated a non-significant 11% relative reduction in the primary outcome of coronary heart disease events (hazard ratio [HR] 0.89, 95% CI 0.75-1.05, p=0.16) and a significant 11% reduction in the secondary outcome of total cardiovascular disease events (HR 0.89 [0.80-0.99], p=0.04). There was a non-significant 11% (HR 1.11 [0.95, 1.29], p=0.18) and 19% (HR 1.19 [0.90, 1.57], p=0.22) increase in total and coronary heart disease mortality, respectively, with fenofibrate as compared to placebo.

Because of chemical, pharmacological, and clinical similarities between TRICOR (fenofibrate tablets), clofibrate, and gemfibrozil, the adverse findings in 4 large randomized, placebo-controlled clinical studies with these other fibrate drugs may also apply to TRICOR.

In the Coronary Drug Project, a large study of post myocardial infarction of patients treated for 5 years with clofibrate, there was no difference in mortality seen between the clofibrate group and the placebo group. There was however, a difference in the rate of cholelithiasis and cholecystitis requiring surgery between the two groups (3.0% vs. 1.8%).

In a study conducted by the World Health Organization (WHO), 5000 subjects without known coronary artery disease were treated with placebo or clofibrate for 5 years and followed for an additional one year. There was a statistically significant, higher age - adjusted all-cause mortality in the clofibrate group compared with the placebo group (5.70% vs. 3.96%, p = < 0.01). Excess mortality was due to a 33% increase in non-cardiovascular causes, including malignancy, post-cholecystectomy complications, and pancreatitis. This appeared to confirm the higher risk of gallbladder disease seen in clofibrate-treated patients studied in the Coronary Drug Project.

The Helsinki Heart Study was a large (n=4081) study of middle-aged men without a history of coronary artery disease. Subjects received either placebo or gemfibrozil for 5 years, with a 3.5 year open extension afterward. Total mortality was numerically higher in the gemfibrozil randomization group but did not achieve statistical significance (p = 0.19, 95% confidence interval for relative risk G:P = .91-1.64). Although cancer deaths trended higher in the gemfibrozil group (p = 0.11), cancers (excluding basal cell carcinoma) were diagnosed with equal frequency in both study groups. Due to the limited size of the study, the relative risk of death from any cause was not shown to be different than that seen in the 9 year follow-up data from World Health Organization study (RR=1.29).

A secondary prevention component of the Helsinki Heart Study enrolled middle-aged men excluded from the primary prevention study because of known or suspected coronary heart disease. Subjects received gemfibrozil or placebo for 5 years. Although cardiac deaths trended higher in the gemfibrozil group, this was not statistically significant (hazard ratio 2.2, 95% confidence interval: 0.94-5.05). The rate of gallbladder surgery was not statistically significant between study groups, but did trend higher in the gemfibrozil group, (1.9% vs. 0.3%, p = 0.07).

5.2 Skeletal Muscle

Fibrates increase the risk for myopathy and have been associated with rhabdomyolysis. The risk for serious muscle toxicity appears to be increased in elderly patients and in patients with diabetes, renal insufficiency, or hypothyroidism.

Myopathy should be considered in any patient with diffuse myalgias, muscle tenderness or weakness, and/or marked elevations of creatine phosphokinase (CPK) levels.

Patients should be advised to report promptly unexplained muscle pain, tenderness or weakness, particularly if accompanied by malaise or fever. CPK levels should be assessed in patients reporting these symptoms, and TRICOR therapy should be discontinued if markedly elevated CPK levels occur or myopathy/myositis is suspected or diagnosed.

Data from observational studies indicate that the risk for rhabdomyolysis is increased when fibrates, in particular gemfibrozil, are co-administered with an HMG-CoA reductase inhibitor (statin). The combination should be avoided unless the benefit of further alterations in lipid levels is likely to outweigh the increased risk of this drug combination *[see Clinical Pharmacology (12.3)]*.

Cases of myopathy, including rhabdomyolysis, have been reported with fenofibrates co-administered with colchicine, and caution should be exercised when prescribing fenofibrate with colchicine *[see Drug Interactions (7.4)]*.

5.3 Liver Function

Fenofibrate at doses equivalent to 96 mg to 145 mg TRICOR per day has been associated with increases in serum transaminases [AST (SGOT) or ALT (SGPT)]. In a pooled analysis of 10 placebo-controlled trials, increases to > 3 times the upper limit of normal occurred in 5.3% of patients taking fenofibrate versus 1.1% of patients treated with placebo.

When transaminase determinations were followed either after discontinuation of treatment or during continued treatment, a return to normal limits was usually observed. The incidence of increases in transaminases related to fenofibrate therapy appear to be dose related. In an 8-week dose-ranging study, the incidence of ALT or AST elevations to at least three times the upper limit of normal was 13% in patients receiving dosages equivalent to 96 mg to 145 mg TRICOR per day and was 0% in those receiving dosages equivalent to 48 mg or less TRICOR per day, or placebo. Hepatocellular, chronic active and cholestatic hepatitis associated with fenofibrate therapy have been reported after exposures of weeks to several years. In extremely rare cases, cirrhosis has been reported in association with chronic active hepatitis.

Baseline and regular periodic monitoring of liver function, including serum ALT (SGPT) should be performed for the duration of therapy with TRICOR, and therapy discontinued if enzyme levels persist above three times the normal limit.

5.4 Serum Creatinine

Elevations in serum creatinine have been reported in patients on fenofibrate. These elevations tend to return to baseline following discontinuation of fenofibrate. The clinical significance of these observations is unknown. Monitor renal function in patients with renal impairment taking TRICOR. Renal monitoring should also be considered for patients taking TRICOR at risk for renal insufficiency such as the elderly and patients with diabetes.

5.5 Cholelithiasis

Fenofibrate, like clofibrate and gemfibrozil, may increase cholesterol excretion into the bile, leading to cholelithiasis. If cholelithiasis is suspected, gallbladder studies are indicated. TRICOR therapy should be discontinued if gallstones are found.

5.6 Coumarin Anticoagulants

Caution should be exercised when coumarin anticoagulants are given in conjunction with TRICOR because of the potentiation of coumarin-type anticoagulant effects in prolonging the Prothrombin Time/International Normalized Ratio (PT/INR). To prevent bleeding complications, frequent monitoring of PT/INR and dose adjustment of the anticoagulant are recommended until PT/INR has stabilized *[see Drug Interactions (7.1)]*.

5.7 Pancreatitis

Pancreatitis has been reported in patients taking fenofibrate, gemfibrozil, and clofibrate. This occurrence may represent a failure of efficacy in patients with severe hypertriglyceridemia, a direct drug effect, or a secondary phenomenon mediated through biliary tract stone or sludge formation with obstruction of the common bile duct.

5.8 Hematologic Changes

Mild to moderate hemoglobin, hematocrit, and white blood cell decreases have been observed in patients following initiation of fenofibrate therapy. However, these levels stabilize during long-term administration. Thrombocytopenia and agranulocytosis have been reported in individuals treated with fenofibrate. Periodic monitoring of red and white blood cell counts are recommended during the first 12 months of TRICOR administration.

5.9 Hypersensitivity Reactions

Acute hypersensitivity reactions such as Stevens-Johnson syndrome and toxic epidermal necrolysis requiring patient hospitalization and treatment with steroids have been reported in individuals treated with fenofibrates. Urticaria was seen in 1.1 vs. 0%, and rash in 1.4 vs. 0.8% of fenofibrate and placebo patients respectively in controlled trials.

5.10 Venothromboembolic Disease

In the FIELD trial, pulmonary embolus (PE) and deep vein thrombosis (DVT) were observed at higher rates in the fenofibrate- than the placebo-treated group. Of 9,795 patients enrolled in FIELD, there were 4,900 in the placebo group and 4,895 in the fenofibrate group. For DVT, there were 48 events (1%) in the placebo group and 67 (1%) in the fenofibrate group ($p = 0.074$); and for PE, there were 32 (0.7%) events in the placebo group and 53 (1%) in the fenofibrate group ($p = 0.022$).

In the Coronary Drug Project, a higher proportion of the clofibrate group experienced definite or suspected fatal or nonfatal pulmonary embolism or thrombophlebitis than the placebo group (5.2% vs. 3.3% at five years; $p < 0.01$).

5.11 Paradoxical Decreases in HDL Cholesterol Levels

There have been postmarketing and clinical trial reports of severe decreases in HDL cholesterol levels (as low as 2 mg/dL) occurring in diabetic and non-diabetic patients initiated on fibrate therapy. The decrease in HDL-C is mirrored by a decrease in apolipoprotein A1. This decrease has been reported to occur within 2 weeks to years after initiation of fibrate therapy. The HDL-C levels remain depressed until fibrate therapy has been withdrawn; the response to withdrawal of fibrate therapy is rapid and sustained. The clinical significance of this decrease in HDL-C is unknown. It is recommended that HDL-C levels be checked within the first few months after initiation of fibrate therapy. If a severely depressed HDL-C level is detected, fibrate therapy should be withdrawn, and the HDL-C level monitored until it has returned to baseline, and fibrate therapy should not be re-initiated.

6 ADVERSE REACTIONS

6.1 Clinical Trials Experience

Because clinical studies are conducted under widely varying conditions, adverse reaction rates observed in the clinical studies of a drug cannot be directly compared to rates in the clinical studies of another drug and may not reflect the rates observed in practice.

Adverse events reported by 2% or more of patients treated with fenofibrate (and greater than placebo) during the double-blind, placebo-controlled trials, regardless of causality, are listed in Table 1 below. Adverse events led to discontinuation of treatment in 5.0% of patients treated with fenofibrate and in 3.0% treated with placebo. Increases in liver function tests were the most frequent events, causing discontinuation of fenofibrate treatment in 1.6% of patients in double-blind trials.

Table 1. Adverse Reactions Reported by 2% or More of Patients Treated with Fenofibrate and Greater than Placebo During the Double-Blind, Placebo-Controlled Trials

BODY SYSTEM	Fenofibrate*	Placebo
Adverse Reaction	**(N=439)**	**(N=365)**
BODY AS A WHOLE		
Abdominal Pain	4.6%	4.4%
Back Pain	3.4%	2.5%
Headache	3.2%	2.7%
DIGESTIVE		
Nausea	2.3%	1.9%
Constipation	2.1%	1.4%
METABOLIC AND NUTRITIONAL DISORDERS		
Abnormal Liver Function Tests	7.5%**	1.4%
Increased ALT	3.0%	1.6%
Increased CPK	3.0%	1.4%
Increased AST	3.4%**	0.5%
RESPIRATORY		
Respiratory Disorder	6.2%	5.5%
Rhinitis	2.3%	1.1%

* Dosage equivalent to 145 mg TRICOR.
** Significantly different from Placebo.

6.2 Postmarketing Experience

The following adverse reactions have been identified during postapproval use of fenofibrate: myalgia, rhabdomyolysis, pancreatitis, acute renal failure, muscle spasm, hepatitis, cirrhosis, anemia, arthralgia, decreases in hemoglobin, decreases in hematocrit, white blood cell decreases, asthenia, and severely depressed HDL-cholesterol levels. Because these reactions are reported voluntarily from a population of uncertain size, it is not always possible to reliably estimate their frequency or establish a causal relationship to drug exposure.

7 DRUG INTERACTIONS

7.1 Coumarin Anticoagulants

Potentiation of coumarin-type anticoagulant effects has been observed with prolongation of the PT/INR.

Caution should be exercised when coumarin anticoagulants are given in conjunction with TRICOR. The dosage of the anticoagulants should be reduced to maintain the PT/INR at the desired level to prevent bleeding complications. Frequent PT/INR determinations are advisable until it has been definitely determined that the PT/INR has stabilized *[see Warnings and Precautions (5.6)]*.

7.2 Immunosuppressants

Immunosuppressants such as cyclosporine and tacrolimus can produce nephrotoxicity with decreases in creatinine clearance and rises in serum creatinine, and because renal excretion is the primary elimination route of fibrate drugs including TRICOR, there is a risk that an interaction will lead to deterioration of renal function. The benefits and risks of using TRICOR (fenofibrate tablets) with immunosuppressants and other potentially nephrotoxic agents should be carefully considered, and the lowest effective dose employed and renal function monitored.

7.3 Bile Acid Binding Resins

Since bile acid binding resins may bind other drugs given concurrently, patients should take TRICOR at least 1 hour before or 4 to 6 hours after a bile acid binding resin to avoid impeding its absorption.

7.4 Colchicine

Cases of myopathy, including rhabdomyolysis, have been reported with fenofibrates co-administered with colchicine, and caution should be exercised when prescribing fenofibrate with colchicine.

8 USE IN SPECIFIC POPULATIONS

8.1 Pregnancy

Pregnancy Category C

Safety in pregnant women has not been established. There are no adequate and well controlled studies of fenofibrate in pregnant women. Fenofibrate should be used during pregnancy only if the potential benefit justifies the potential risk to the fetus.

In female rats given oral dietary doses of 15, 75, and 300 mg/kg/day of fenofibrate from 15 days prior to mating through weaning, maternal toxicity was observed at 0.3 times the MRHD, based on body surface area comparisons; mg/m^2.

In pregnant rats given oral dietary doses of 14, 127, and 361 mg/kg/day from gestation day 6-15 during the period of organogenesis, adverse developmental findings were not observed at 14 mg/kg/day (less than 1 times the MRHD, based on body surface area comparisons; mg/m^2). At higher multiples of human doses evidence of maternal toxicity was observed.

In pregnant rabbits given oral gavage doses of 15, 150, and 300 mg/kg/day from gestation day 6-18 during the period of organogenesis and allowed to deliver, aborted litters were observed at 150 mg/kg/day (10 times the MRHD, based on body surface area comparisons: mg/m^2). No developmental findings were observed at 15 mg/kg/day (at less than 1 times the MRHD, based on body surface area comparisons; mg/m^2).

In pregnant rats given oral dietary doses of 15, 75, and 300 mg/kg/day from gestation day 15 through lactation day 21 (weaning), maternal toxicity was observed at less than 1 times the maximum recommended human dose (MRHD), based on body surface area comparisons; mg/m^2.

8.3 Nursing Mothers

Fenofibrate should not be used in nursing mothers. A decision should be made whether to discontinue nursing or to discontinue the drug, taking into account the importance of the drug to the mother.

8.4 Pediatric Use

Safety and effectiveness have not been established in pediatric patients.

8.5 Geriatric Use

Fenofibric acid is known to be substantially excreted by the kidney, and the risk of adverse reactions to this drug may be greater in patients with impaired renal function. Fenofibric acid exposure is not influenced by age. Since elderly patients have a higher incidence of renal impairment, dose selection for the elderly should be made on the basis of renal function *[see Dosage and Administration (2.5) and Clinical Pharmacology (12.3)]*. Elderly patients with normal renal function should require no dose modifications. Consider monitoring renal function in elderly patients taking TRICOR.

8.6 Renal Impairment

The use of TRICOR should be avoided in patients who have severe renal impairment *[see Contraindications (4)]*. Dose reduction is required in patients with mild to moderate renal impairment *[see Dosage and Administration (2.4) and Clinical Pharmacology (12.3)]*. Monitoring renal function in patients with renal impairment is recommended.

8.7 Hepatic Impairment

The use of TRICOR has not been evaluated in subjects with hepatic impairment *[see Contraindications (4) and Clinical Pharmacology (12.3)]*.

10 OVERDOSAGE

There is no specific treatment for overdose with TRICOR. General supportive care of the patient is indicated, including monitoring of vital signs and observation of clinical status, should an overdose occur. If indicated, elimination of unabsorbed drug should be achieved by emesis or gastric lavage; usual precautions should be observed to maintain the airway. Because fenofibric acid is highly bound to plasma proteins, hemodialysis should not be considered.

11 DESCRIPTION

TRICOR (fenofibrate tablets), is a lipid regulating agent available as tablets for oral administration. Each tablet contains 48 mg or 145 mg of fenofibrate. The chemical name for fenofibrate is 2-[4-(4-chlorobenzoyl) phenoxy]-2-methyl-propanoic acid, 1-methylethyl ester with the following structural formula:

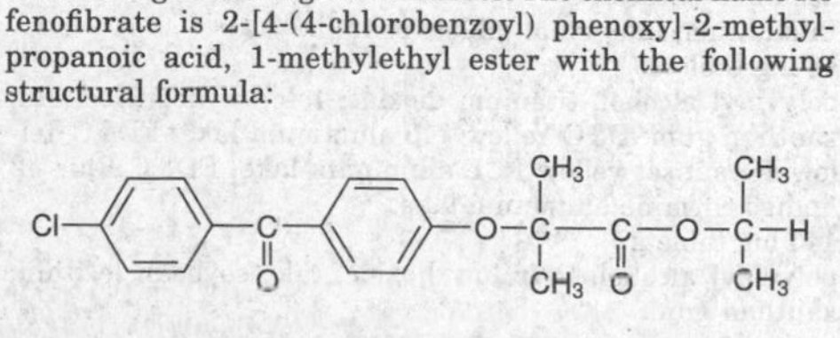

The empirical formula is $C_{20}H_{21}O_4Cl$ and the molecular weight is 360.83; fenofibrate is insoluble in water. The melting point is 79-82°C. Fenofibrate is a white solid which is stable under ordinary conditions.

Inactive Ingredients

Each tablet contains hypromellose 2910 (3 cps), docusate sodium, sucrose, sodium lauryl sulfate, lactose monohydrate,

Information on the AbbVie, Inc. products listed on these pages is from the prescribing information in use as of July 31, 2013. For more information, please visit rxabbvie.com or call 1-800-633-9110.

Table 2. Effects of Co-Administered Drugs on Fenofibric Acid Systemic Exposure from Fenofibrate Administration

Co-Administered Drug	Dosage Regimen of Co-Administered Drug	Dosage Regimen of Fenofibrate	Changes in Fenofibric Acid Exposure	
			AUC	C_{max}
Lipid-lowering agents				
Atorvastatin	20 mg once daily for 10 days	Fenofibrate 160 mg[1] once daily for 10 days	↓2%	↓4%
Pravastatin	40 mg as a single dose	Fenofibrate 3 × 67 mg[2] as a single dose	↓1%	↓2%
Fluvastatin	40 mg as a single dose	Fenofibrate 160 mg[1] as a single dose	↓2%	↓10%
Anti-diabetic agents				
Glimepiride	1 mg as a single dose	Fenofibrate 145 mg[1] once daily for 10 days	↑1%	↓1%
Metformin	850 mg three times daily for 10 days	Fenofibrate 54 mg[1] three times daily for 10 days	↓9%	↓6%
Rosiglitazone	8 mg once daily for 5 days	Fenofibrate 145 mg[1] once daily for 14 days	↑10%	↑3%

[1] TriCor (fenofibrate) oral tablet
[2] TriCor (fenofibrate) oral micronized capsule

Table 3. Effects of Fenofibrate Co-Administration on Systemic Exposure of Other Drugs

Dosage Regimen of Fenofibrate	Dosage Regimen of Co-Administered Drug	Change in Co-Administered Drug Exposure		
		Analyte	AUC	C_{max}
Lipid-lowering agents				
Fenofibrate 160 mg[1] once daily for 10 days	Atorvastatin, 20 mg once daily for 10 days	Atorvastatin	↓17%	0%
Fenofibrate 3 × 67 mg[2] as a single dose	Pravastatin, 40 mg as a single dose	Pravastatin	↑13%	↑13%
		3α-Hydroxyl-iso-pravastatin	↑26%	↑29%
Fenofibrate 160 mg[1] as a single dose	Fluvastatin, 40 mg as a single dose	(+)-3R, 5S-Fluvastatin	↑15%	↑16%
Anti-diabetic agents				
Fenofibrate 145 mg[1] once daily for 10 days	Glimepiride, 1 mg as a single dose	Glimepiride	↑35%	↑18%
Fenofibrate 54 mg[1] three times daily for 10 days	Metformin, 850 mg three times daily for 10 days	Metformin	↑3%	↑6%
Fenofibrate 145 mg[1] once daily for 14 days	Rosiglitazone, 8 mg once daily for 5 days	Rosiglitazone	↑6%	↓1%

[1] TriCor (fenofibrate) oral tablet
[2] TriCor (fenofibrate) oral micronized capsule

silicified microcrystalline cellulose, crospovidone, and magnesium stearate.
In addition, individual tablets contain:
48 mg tablets
polyvinyl alcohol, titanium dioxide, talc, soybean lecithin, xanthan gum, D&C Yellow #10 aluminum lake, FD&C Yellow #6 /sunset yellow FCF aluminum lake, FD&C Blue #2 /indigo carmine aluminum lake.
145 mg tablets
polyvinyl alcohol, titanium dioxide, talc, soybean lecithin, xanthan gum.

12 CLINICAL PHARMACOLOGY

12.1 Mechanism of Action

The active moiety of TRICOR is fenofibric acid. The pharmacological effects of fenofibric acid in both animals and humans have been extensively studied through oral administration of fenofibrate.
The lipid-modifying effects of fenofibric acid seen in clinical practice have been explained *in vivo* in transgenic mice and *in vitro* in human hepatocyte cultures by the activation of peroxisome proliferator activated receptor α (PPARα). Through this mechanism, fenofibrate increases lipolysis and elimination of triglyceride-rich particles from plasma by activating lipoprotein lipase and reducing production of apoprotein C-III (an inhibitor of lipoprotein lipase activity).
The resulting decrease in TG produces an alteration in the size and composition of LDL from small, dense particles (which are thought to be atherogenic due to their susceptibility to oxidation), to large buoyant particles. These larger particles have a greater affinity for cholesterol receptors and are catabolized rapidly. Activation of PPARα also induces an increase in the synthesis of apolipoproteins AI, A-II and HDL-cholesterol.
Fenofibrate also reduces serum uric acid levels in hyperuricemic and normal individuals by increasing the urinary excretion of uric acid.

12.2 Pharmacodynamics

A variety of clinical studies have demonstrated that elevated levels of total-C, LDL-C, and apo B, an LDL membrane complex, are associated with human atherosclerosis. Similarly, decreased levels of HDL-C and its transport complex, apolipoprotein A (apo AI and apo AII) are associated with the development of atherosclerosis. Epidemiologic investigations have established that cardiovascular morbidity and mortality vary directly with the level of total-C, LDL-C, and TG, and inversely with the level of HDL-C. The independent effect of raising HDL-C or lowering triglycerides (TG) on the risk of cardiovascular morbidity and mortality has not been determined.
Fenofibric acid, the active metabolite of fenofibrate, produces reductions in total cholesterol, LDL cholesterol, apolipoprotein B, total triglycerides and triglyceride rich lipoprotein (VLDL) in treated patients. In addition, treatment with fenofibrate results in increases in high density lipoprotein (HDL) and apolipoproteins apoAI and apoAII.

12.3 Pharmacokinetics

Plasma concentrations of fenofibric acid after administration of three 48 mg or one 145 mg tablets are equivalent under fed conditions to one 200 mg micronized fenofibrate capsule.
Fenofibrate is a pro-drug of the active chemical moiety fenofibric acid. Fenofibrate is converted by ester hydrolysis in the body to fenofibric acid which is the active constituent measurable in the circulation.

Absorption

The absolute bioavailability of fenofibrate cannot be determined as the compound is virtually insoluble in aqueous media suitable for injection. However, fenofibrate is well absorbed from the gastrointestinal tract. Following oral administration in healthy volunteers, approximately 60% of a single dose of radiolabelled fenofibrate appeared in urine, primarily as fenofibric acid and its glucuronate conjugate, and 25% was excreted in the feces. Peak plasma levels of fenofibric acid occur within 6 to 8 hours after administration.
Exposure to fenofibric acid in plasma, as measured by C_{max} and AUC, is not significantly different when a single 145 mg dose of fenofibrate is administered under fasting or nonfasting conditions.

Distribution

Upon multiple dosing of fenofibrate, fenofibric acid steady state is achieved within 9 days. Plasma concentrations of fenofibric acid at steady state are approximately double of those following a single dose. Serum protein binding was approximately 99% in normal and hyperlipidemic subjects.

Metabolism

Following oral administration, fenofibrate is rapidly hydrolyzed by esterases to the active metabolite, fenofibric acid; no unchanged fenofibrate is detected in plasma.
Fenofibric acid is primarily conjugated with glucuronic acid and then excreted in urine. A small amount of fenofibric acid is reduced at the carbonyl moiety to a benzhydrol metabolite which is, in turn, conjugated with glucuronic acid and excreted in urine.
In vivo metabolism data indicate that neither fenofibrate nor fenofibric acid undergo oxidative metabolism (e.g., cytochrome P450) to a significant extent.

Elimination

After absorption, fenofibrate is mainly excreted in the urine in the form of metabolites, primarily fenofibric acid and fenofibric acid glucuronide. After administration of radiolabelled fenofibrate, approximately 60% of the dose appeared in the urine and 25% was excreted in the feces.
Fenofibric acid is eliminated with a half-life of 20 hours, allowing once daily dosing.

Special Populations

Geriatrics

In elderly volunteers 77 to 87 years of age, the oral clearance of fenofibric acid following a single oral dose of fenofibrate was 1.2 L/h, which compares to 1.1 L/h in young adults. This indicates that a similar dosage regimen can be used in elderly with normal renal function, without increasing accumulation of the drug or metabolites *[see Dosage and Administration (2.5) and Use in Specific Populations (8.5)]*.

Pediatrics

The pharmacokinetics of TRICOR has not been studied in pediatric populations.

Gender

No pharmacokinetic difference between males and females has been observed for fenofibrate.

Race

The influence of race on the pharmacokinetics of fenofibrate has not been studied, however fenofibrate is not metabolized by enzymes known for exhibiting inter-ethnic variability.

Renal Impairment

The pharmacokinetics of fenofibric acid was examined in patients with mild, moderate, and severe renal impairment. Patients with severe renal impairment (estimated glomerular filtration rate [eGFR] < 30 mL/min/1.73m^2) showed 2.7-fold increase in exposure for fenofibric acid and increased accumulation of fenofibric acid during chronic dosing compared to that of healthy subjects. Patients with mild to moderate renal impairment (eGFR 30-59 mL/min/1.73m^2) had similar exposure but an increase in the half-life for fenofibric acid compared to that of healthy subjects. Based on these findings, the use of TRICOR should be avoided in patients who have severe renal impairment and dose reduction is required in patients having mild to moderate renal impairment *[see Dosage and Administration (2.4)]*.

Hepatic Impairment

No pharmacokinetic studies have been conducted in patients with hepatic impairment.

Drug-drug Interactions
In vitro studies using human liver microsomes indicate that fenofibrate and fenofibric acid are not inhibitors of cytochrome (CYP) P450 isoforms CYP3A4, CYP2D6, CYP2E1, or CYP1A2. They are weak inhibitors of CYP2C8, CYP2C19 and CYP2A6, and mild-to-moderate inhibitors of CYP2C9 at therapeutic concentrations.
Table 2 describes the effects of co-administered drugs on fenofibric acid systemic exposure. Table 3 describes the effects of coadministered fenofibrate or fenofibric acid on other drugs.
[See table 2 at top of previous page]
[See table 3 at top of previous page]

13 NONCLINICAL TOXICOLOGY

13.1 Carcinogenesis and Mutagenesis and Impairment of Fertility

Two dietary carcinogenicity studies have been conducted in rats with fenofibrate. In the first 24-month study, Wistar rats were dosed with fenofibrate at 10, 45, and 200 mg/kg/day, approximately 0.3, 1, and 6 times the maximum recommended human dose (MRHD), based on body surface area comparisons (mg/m^2). At a dose of 200 mg/kg/day (at 6 times the MRHD), the incidence of liver carcinomas was significantly increased in both sexes. A statistically significant increase in pancreatic carcinomas was observed in males at 1 and 6 times the MRHD; an increase in pancreatic adenomas and benign testicular interstitial cell tumors was observed at 6 times the MRHD in males. In a second 24-month rat carcinogenicity study in a different strain of rats (Sprague-Dawley), doses of 10 and 60 mg/kg/day (0.3 and 2 times the MRHD) produced significant increases in the incidence of pancreatic acinar adenomas in both sexes and increases in testicular interstitial cell tumors in males at 2 times the MRHD.
A 117-week carcinogenicity study was conducted in rats comparing three drugs: fenofibrate 10 and 60 mg/kg/day (0.3 and 2 times the MRHD), clofibrate (400 mg/kg/day; 2 times the human dose), and gemfibrozil (250 mg/kg/day; 2 times the human dose, based on mg/m^2 surface area). Fenofibrate increased pancreatic acinar adenomas in both sexes. Clofibrate increased hepatocellular carcinoma and pancreatic acinar adenomas in males and hepatic neoplastic nodules in females. Gemfibrozil increased hepatic neoplastic nodules in males and females, while all three drugs increased testicular interstitial cell tumors in males.
In a 21-month study in CF-1 mice, fenofibrate 10, 45, and 200 mg/kg/day (approximately 0.2, 1, and 3 times the MRHD on the basis of mg/m^2 surface area) significantly increased the liver carcinomas in both sexes at 3 times the MRHD. In a second 18-month study at 10, 60, and 200 mg/kg/day, fenofibrate significantly increased the liver carcinomas in male mice and liver adenomas in female mice at 3 times the MRHD.
Electron microscopy studies have demonstrated peroxisomal proliferation following fenofibrate administration to the rat. An adequate study to test for peroxisome proliferation in humans has not been done, but changes in peroxisome morphology and numbers have been observed in humans after treatment with other members of the fibrate class when liver biopsies were compared before and after treatment in the same individual.
Mutagenesis: Fenofibrate has been demonstrated to be devoid of mutagenic potential in the following tests: Ames, mouse lymphoma, chromosomal aberration and unscheduled DNA synthesis in primary rat hepatocytes.
Impairment of Fertility: In fertility studies rats were given oral dietary doses of fenofibrate, males received 61 days prior to mating and females 15 days prior to mating through weaning which resulted in no adverse effect on fertility at doses up to 300 mg/kg/day (~10 times the MRHD, based on mg/m^2 surface area comparisons).

14 CLINICAL STUDIES

14.1 Primary Hypercholesterolemia (Heterozygous Familial and Nonfamilial) and Mixed Dyslipidemia

The effects of fenofibrate at a dose equivalent to 145 mg TRICOR (fenofibrate tablets) per day were assessed from four randomized, placebo-controlled, double-blind, parallel-group studies including patients with the following mean baseline lipid values: total-C 306.9 mg/dL; LDL-C 213.8 mg/dL; HDL-C 52.3 mg/dL; and triglycerides 191.0 mg/dL. TRICOR therapy lowered LDL-C, Total-C, and the LDL-C/HDL-C ratio. TRICOR therapy also lowered triglycerides and raised HDL-C (see Table 4).
[See table 4 above]

Table 4. Mean Percent Change in Lipid Parameters at End of Treatment†

Treatment Group	Total-C	LDL-C	HDL-C	TG
Pooled Cohort				
Mean baseline lipid values (n=646)	306.9 mg/dL	213.8 mg/dL	52.3 mg/dL	191.0 mg/dL
All FEN (n=361)	-18.7%*	-20.6%*	+11.0%*	-28.9%*
Placebo (n=285)	-0.4%	-2.2%	+0.7%	+7.7%
Baseline LDL-C > 160 mg/dL and TG < 150 mg/dL				
Mean baseline lipid values (n=334)	307.7 mg/dL	227.7 mg/dL	58.1 mg/dL	101.7 mg/dL
All FEN (n=193)	-22.4%*	-31.4%*	+9.8%*	-23.5%*
Placebo (n=141)	+0.2%	-2.2%	+2.6%	+11.7%
Baseline LDL-C >160 mg/dL and TG ≥ 150 mg/dL				
Mean baseline lipid values (n=242)	312.8 mg/dL	219.8 mg/dL	46.7 mg/dL	231.9 mg/dL
All FEN (n=126)	-16.8%*	-20.1%*	+14.6%*	-35.9%*
Placebo (n=116)	-3.0%	-6.6%	+2.3%	+0.9%

† Duration of study treatment was 3 to 6 months.
* p = < 0.05 vs. Placebo

In a subset of the subjects, measurements of apo B were conducted. TRICOR treatment significantly reduced apo B from baseline to endpoint as compared with placebo (-25.1% vs. 2.4%, $p < 0.0001$, n=213 and 143 respectively).

14.2 Severe Hypertriglyceridemia

The effects of fenofibrate on serum triglycerides were studied in two randomized, double-blind, placebo-controlled clinical trials of 147 hypertriglyceridemic patients. Patients were treated for eight weeks under protocols that differed only in that one entered patients with baseline TG levels of 500 to 1500 mg/dL, and the other TG levels of 350 to 500 mg/dL. In patients with hypertriglyceridemia and normal cholesterolemia with or without hyperchylomicronemia, treatment with fenofibrate at dosages equivalent to TRICOR 145 mg per day decreased primarily very low density lipoprotein (VLDL) triglycerides and VLDL cholesterol. Treatment of patients with elevated triglycerides often results in an increase of LDL-C (see Table 5).
[See table 5 above]

Table 5. Effects of TRICOR in Patients With Severe Hypertriglyceridemia

Study 1	Placebo				TRICOR			
Baseline TG levels 350 to 499 mg/dL	**N**	**Baseline (Mean)**	**Endpoint (Mean)**	**% Change (Mean)**	**N**	**Baseline (Mean)**	**Endpoint (Mean)**	**% Change (Mean)**
Triglycerides	28	449	450	-0.5	27	432	223	-46.2*
VLDL Triglycerides	19	367	350	2.7	19	350	178	-44.1*
Total Cholesterol	28	255	261	2.8	27	252	227	-9.1*
HDL Cholesterol	28	35	36	4	27	34	40	19.6*
LDL Cholesterol	28	120	129	12	27	128	137	14.5
VLDL Cholesterol	27	99	99	5.8	27	92	46	-44.7*
Study 2	**Placebo**				**TRICOR**			
Baseline TG levels 500 to 1500 mg/dL	**N**	**Baseline (Mean)**	**Endpoint (Mean)**	**% Change (Mean)**	**N**	**Baseline (Mean)**	**Endpoint (Mean)**	**% Change (Mean)**
Triglycerides	44	710	750	7.2	48	726	308	-54.5*
VLDL Triglycerides	29	537	571	18.7	33	543	205	-50.6*
Total Cholesterol	44	272	271	0.4	48	261	223	-13.8*
HDL Cholesterol	44	27	28	5.0	48	30	36	22.9*
LDL Cholesterol	42	100	90	-4.2	45	103	131	45.0*
VLDL Cholesterol	42	137	142	11.0	45	126	54	-49.4*

* =p < 0.05 vs. Placebo

The effect of TRICOR on cardiovascular morbidity and mortality has not been determined.

16 HOW SUPPLIED/STORAGE AND HANDLING

TRICOR® (fenofibrate tablets) is available in two strengths:
48 mg yellow tablets, imprinted with the "a" logo and code identification letters "FI", available in bottles of 90 (NDC 0074-6122-90).
145 mg white tablets, imprinted with the "a" logo and code identification letters "FO", available in bottles of 90 (NDC 0074-6123-90).

Storage
Store at 25°C (77°F); excursions permitted to 15-30°C (59-86°F).
[See USP Controlled Room Temperature]. Keep out of the reach of children. Protect from moisture.

17 PATIENT COUNSELING INFORMATION

Patients should be advised:
- of the potential benefits and risks of TRICOR.
- not to use TRICOR if there is a known hypersensitivity to fenofibrate or fenofibric acid.
- of medications that should not be taken in combination with TRICOR.

Information on the AbbVie, Inc. products listed on these pages is from the prescribing information in use as of July 31, 2013. For more information, please visit rxabbvie.com or call 1-800-633-9110.

- that if they are taking coumarin anticoagulants, TRICOR may increase their anti-coagulant effect, and increased monitoring may be necessary.
- to continue to follow an appropriate lipid-modifying diet while taking TRICOR.
- to take TRICOR once daily, without regard to food, at the prescribed dose, swallowing each tablet whole.
- to return for routine monitoring.
- to inform their physician of all medications, supplements, and herbal preparations they are taking and any change to their medical condition. Patients should also be advised to inform their physicians prescribing a new medication that they are taking TRICOR.
- to inform their physician of any muscle pain, tenderness, or weakness; onset of abdominal pain; or any other new symptoms.

Manufactured for AbbVie Inc., North Chicago, IL 60064, U.S.A.
by Fournier Laboratories Ireland Limited, Anngrove, Carrigtwohill Co. Cork, Ireland.
03-A774-R8, Revised: February, 2013

Shown in Product Identification Guide, page 304

TRILIPIX® ℞

[try-lip-iks]
(fenofibric acid)
capsule, delayed release for oral use

HIGHLIGHTS OF PRESCRIBING INFORMATION
These highlights do not include all the information needed to use TRILIPIX safely and effectively. See full prescribing information for TRILIPIX.
TRILIPIX (fenofibric acid) capsule, delayed release for oral use
Initial U.S. Approval: 2008

RECENT MAJOR CHANGES

Warnings and Precautions, Skeletal Muscle (5.2) 09/2012
Warnings and Precautions, Paradoxical Decreased in HDL Cholesterol Levels (5.11) 09/2012

INDICATIONS AND USAGE

Trilipix is a peroxisome proliferator receptor alpha (PPARα) activator indicated:

- In combination with a statin to reduce TG and increase HDL-C in patients with mixed dyslipidemia and CHD or a CHD risk equivalent who are on optimal statin therapy to achieve their LDL-C goal (1.1).
- As monotherapy to reduce TG in patients with severe hypertriglyceridemia (1.2).
- As monotherapy to reduce elevated LDL-C, Total-C, TG and Apo B, and to increase HDL-C in patients with primary hyperlipidemia or mixed dyslipidemia (1.3).

Important Limitations of Use: No incremental benefit of Trilipix on cardiovascular morbidity and mortality over and above that demonstrated for statin monotherapy has been established. Fenofibrate at a dose equivalent to 135 mg of Trilipix was not shown to reduce coronary heart disease morbidity and mortality in patients with type 2 diabetes mellitus.

DOSAGE AND ADMINISTRATION

- Mixed dyslipidemia: 135 mg once daily (2.2).
- Hypertriglyceridemia: 45 to 135 mg once daily (2.3).
- Renally impaired patients: 45 mg once daily (2.5).
- Maximum dose: 135 mg once daily (2.1).
- May be taken without regard to food (2.1).
- May be taken at the same time as a statin (2.2).
- Co-administration with the maximum dose of a statin has not been evaluated in clinical studies and should be avoided unless the benefits are expected to outweigh the risks (2.2).

DOSAGE FORMS AND STRENGTHS

Oral Delayed Release Capsules: 45 mg and 135 mg (3).

CONTRAINDICATIONS

- Severe renal dysfunction, including patients receiving dialysis (4, 12.3).
- Active liver disease (4, 5.3).
- Gallbladder disease (4, 5.4).
- Nursing mothers (4, 8.3).
- Known hypersensitivity to fenofibric acid or fenofibrate (4, 5.9)

WARNINGS AND PRECAUTIONS

- Myopathy and rhabdomyolysis have been reported in patients taking fenofibrate. The risks for myopathy and rhabdomyolysis are increased when fibrates are co-administered with a statin (with a significantly higher rate observed for gemfibrozil), particularly in elderly patients and patients with diabetes, renal failure, or hypothyroidism (5.1).
- Trilipix can increase serum transaminases. Liver tests should be monitored periodically (5.3).
- Trilipix can reversibly increase serum creatinine levels (5.2). Renal function should be monitored periodically in patients with renal insufficiency (8.6).
- Trilipix increases cholesterol excretion into the bile, leading to risk of cholelithiasis. If cholelithiasis is suspected, gallbladder studies are indicated (5.4).
- Exercise caution in concomitant treatment with oral coumarin anticoagulants. Adjust the dosage of coumarin anticoagulant to maintain the prothrombin time/INR at the desired level to prevent bleeding complications (5.5).

ADVERSE REACTIONS

The most common adverse events (≥ 3% of patients receiving Trilipix or Trilipix co-administered with statins) are headache, back pain, nasopharyngitis, nausea, myalgia, diarrhea, and upper respiratory tract infection (6.1).
To report SUSPECTED ADVERSE REACTIONS, contact AbbVie Inc. at 1-800-633-9110 or FDA at 1-800-FDA-1088 or www.fda.gov/medwatch

DRUG INTERACTIONS

- Coumarin Anticoagulants: (7.1).
- Bile Acid Binding Resins: (7.2).
- Immunosuppressants: (7.3).

USE IN SPECIFIC POPULATIONS

- Geriatric Use: Dose selection for the elderly should be made on the basis of renal function (8.5).
- Renal Impairment: Trilipix should be avoided in patients with severe renal impairment. Dose adjustment is required in patients with mild to moderate renal impairment (8.6).

See 17 for PATIENT COUNSELING INFORMATION and Medication Guide

Revised: 03/2013

FULL PRESCRIBING INFORMATION: CONTENTS*

* Sections or subsections omitted from the full prescribing information are not listed

FULL PRESCRIBING INFORMATION

1 INDICATIONS AND USAGE

1.1 Co-administration Therapy with Statins for the Treatment of Mixed Dyslipidemia

Trilipix is indicated as an adjunct to diet in combination with a statin to reduce TG and increase HDL-C in patients with mixed dyslipidemia and CHD or a CHD risk equivalent who are on optimal statin therapy to achieve their LDL-C goal.
CHD risk equivalents comprise:

- Other clinical forms of atherosclerotic disease (peripheral arterial disease, abdominal aortic aneurysm, and symptomatic carotid artery disease);
- Diabetes;
- Multiple risk factors that confer a 10-year risk for CHD > 20%

1.2 Treatment of Severe Hypertriglyceridemia

Trilipix is indicated as adjunctive therapy to diet to reduce TG in patients with severe hypertriglyceridemia. Improving glycemic control in diabetic patients showing fasting chylomicronemia will usually obviate the need for pharmacological intervention. Markedly elevated levels of serum triglycerides (e.g. > 2,000 mg/dL) may increase the risk of developing pancreatitis. The effect of Trilipix therapy on reducing this risk has not been adequately studied.

1.3 Treatment of Primary Hypercholesterolemia or Mixed Dyslipidemia

Trilipix is indicated as adjunctive therapy to diet to reduce elevated low-density lipoprotein cholesterol (LDL-C), total cholesterol (Total-C), triglycerides (TG), and apolipoprotein B (Apo B), and to increase high-density lipoprotein cholesterol (HDL-C) in patients with primary hypercholesterolemia or mixed dyslipidemia.

1.4 Important Limitations of Use

No incremental benefit of Trilipix on cardiovascular morbidity and mortality over and above that demonstrated for statin monotherapy has been established. Fenofibrate at a dose equivalent to 135 mg of Trilipix was not shown to reduce coronary heart disease morbidity and mortality in 2 large, randomized controlled trials of patients with type 2 diabetes mellitus.

1.5 General Considerations for Treatment

Laboratory studies should be performed to establish that lipid levels are abnormal before instituting Trilipix therapy. Every reasonable attempt should be made to control serum lipids with non-drug methods including appropriate diet, exercise, weight loss in obese patients, and control of any medical problems such as diabetes mellitus and hypothyroidism that may be contributing to the lipid abnormalities. Medications known to exacerbate hypertriglyceridemia (beta-blockers, thiazides, estrogens) should be discontinued or changed if possible, and excessive alcohol intake should be addressed before triglyceride-lowering drug therapy is considered. If the decision is made to use lipid-altering drugs, the patient should be instructed that this does not reduce the importance of adhering to diet.
Drug therapy is not indicated for patients who have elevations of chylomicrons and plasma triglycerides, but who have normal levels of VLDL.

2 DOSAGE AND ADMINISTRATION

2.1 General Considerations

Patients should be placed on an appropriate lipid-lowering diet before receiving Trilipix as monotherapy or co-administered with a statin, and should continue this diet during treatment. Trilipix delayed release capsules can be taken without regard to meals. Patients should be advised to swallow Trilipix capsules whole. Do not open, crush, dissolve, or chew capsules. Serum lipids should be monitored periodically.

2.2 Co-administration Therapy with Statins for the Treatment of Mixed Dyslipidemia

Trilipix 135 mg may be co-administered with an HMG-CoA reductase inhibitor (statin) in patients with mixed dyslipidemia. For convenience, the daily dose of Trilipix may be taken at the same time as a statin, according to the dosing recommendations for each medication. Co-administration with the maximum dose of a statin has not been evaluated in clinical studies and should be avoided unless the benefits are expected to outweigh the risks.

2.3 Severe Hypertriglyceridemia

The initial dose of Trilipix is 45 to 135 mg once daily. Dosage should be individualized according to patient response, and should be adjusted if necessary following repeat lipid determinations at 4 to 8 week intervals. The maximum dose is 135 mg once daily.

2.4 Primary Hypercholesterolemia or Mixed Dyslipidemia

The dose of Trilipix is 135 mg once daily.

2.5 Impaired Renal Function

Treatment with Trilipix should be initiated at a dose of 45 mg once daily in patients with mild to moderate renal impairment and should only be increased after evaluation of the effects on renal function and lipid levels at this dose. The use of Trilipix should be avoided in patients with severely impaired renal function *[see Use in Specific Populations (8.6) and Clinical Pharmacology (12.3)]*.

2.6 Geriatric Patients

Dose selection for the elderly should be made on the basis of renal function *[see Use in Specific Populations (8.5)]*.

3 DOSAGE FORMS AND STRENGTHS

- 45 mg capsules with a reddish-brown cap imprinted in white ink the "a" logo and a yellow body imprinted in black ink the number "45".
- 135 mg capsules with a blue cap imprinted in white ink the "a" logo and a yellow body imprinted in black ink the number "135".

4 CONTRAINDICATIONS

Trilipix is contraindicated in:

- patients with severe renal impairment, including those receiving dialysis *[see Clinical Pharmacology (12.3)]*.
- patients with active liver disease, including those with primary biliary cirrhosis and unexplained persistent liver function abnormalities *[see Warnings and Precautions (5.3)]*.
- patients with preexisting gallbladder disease *[see Warnings and Precautions (5.5)]*.
- nursing mothers *[see Use in Specific Populations (8.3)]*.
- patients with hypersensitivity to fenofibric acid or fenofibrate *[see Warnings and Precautions (5.9)]*.

When Trilipix is co-administered with a statin, refer to the *Contraindications* section of the respective statin labeling.

5 WARNINGS AND PRECAUTIONS

5.1 Mortality and Coronary Heart Disease Morbidity

The effect of Trilipix on coronary heart disease morbidity and mortality and non-cardiovascular mortality has not been established. Because of similarities between Trilipix and fenofibrate, clofibrate, and gemfibrozil, the findings in the following large randomized, placebo-controlled clinical studies with these fibrate drugs may also apply to Trilipix.

The Action to Control Cardiovascular Risk in Diabetes Lipid (ACCORD Lipid) trial was a randomized placebo-controlled study of 5518 patients with type 2 diabetes mellitus on background statin therapy treated with fenofibrate. The mean duration of follow-up was 4.7 years. Fenofibrate plus statin combination therapy showed a non-significant 8% relative risk reduction in the primary outcome of major adverse cardiovascular events (MACE), a composite of non-fatal myocardial infarction, non-fatal stroke, and cardiovascular disease death (hazard ratio [HR] 0.92, 95% CI 0.79-1.08) (p=0.32) as compared to statin monotherapy. In a gender subgroup analysis, the hazard ratio for MACE in men receiving combination therapy versus statin monotherapy was 0.82 (95% CI 0.69-0.99), and the hazard ratio for MACE in women receiving combination therapy versus statin monotherapy was 1.38 (95% CI 0.98-1.94) (interaction p=0.01). The clinical significance of this subgroup finding is unclear.

The Fenofibrate Intervention and Event Lowering in Diabetes (FIELD) study was a 5-year randomized, placebo-controlled study of 9795 patients with type 2 diabetes mellitus treated with fenofibrate. Fenofibrate demonstrated a non-significant 11% relative reduction in the primary outcome of coronary heart disease events (hazard ratio [HR] 0.89, 95% CI 0.75-1.05, p = 0.16) and a significant 11% reduction in the secondary outcome of total cardiovascular disease events (HR 0.89 [0.80-0.99], p = 0.04). There was a non-significant 11% (HR 1.11 [0.95, 1.29], p = 0.18) and 19% (HR 1.19 [0.90, 1.57], p = 0.22) increase in total and coronary heart disease mortality, respectively, with fenofibrate as compared to placebo.

In the Coronary Drug Project, a large study of post-myocardial infarction patients treated for 5 years with clofibrate, there was no difference in mortality seen between the clofibrate group and the placebo group. There was, however, a difference in the rate of cholelithiasis and cholecystitis requiring surgery between the two groups (3.0% vs. 1.8%).

In a study conducted by the World Health Organization (WHO), 5000 subjects without known coronary artery disease were treated with placebo or clofibrate for 5 years and followed for an additional one year. There was a statistically significant, higher age-adjusted all-cause mortality in the clofibrate group compared with the placebo group (5.70% vs. 3.96%, p = < 0.01). Excess mortality was due to a 33% increase in non-cardiovascular causes, including malignancy, post-cholecystectomy complications, and pancreatitis. This appeared to confirm the higher risk of gallbladder disease seen in clofibrate-treated patients studied in the Coronary Drug Project.

The Helsinki Heart Study was a large (N = 4081) study of middle-aged men without a history of coronary artery disease. Subjects received either placebo or gemfibrozil for 5 years, with a 3.5 year open extension afterward. Total mortality was numerically higher in the gemfibrozil randomization group but did not achieve statistical significance (p = 0.19, 95% confidence interval for relative risk G:P = 0.91-1.64). Although cancer deaths trended higher in the gemfibrozil group (p = 0.11), cancers (excluding basal cell carcinoma) were diagnosed with equal frequency in both study groups. Due to the limited size of the study, the relative risk of death from any cause was not shown to be different than that seen in the 9 year follow-up data from WHO study (RR = 1.29). A secondary prevention component of the Helsinki Heart Study enrolled middle-aged men excluded from the primary prevention study because of known or suspected coronary heart disease. Subjects received gemfibrozil or placebo for 5 years. Although cardiac deaths trended higher in the gemfibrozil group, this was not statistically significant (hazard ratio 2.2, 95% confidence interval: 0.94-5.05).

5.2 Skeletal Muscle

Fibrate and statin monotherapy increase the risk of myositis or myopathy, and have been associated with rhabdomyolysis. Data from observational studies suggest that the risk for rhabdomyolysis is increased when fibrates are co-administered with a statin (with a numerically higher rate observed with gemfibrozil/statin combination use compared to fenofibrate/statin combination use). Refer to the respective statin labeling for important drug-drug interactions that increase statin levels and could increase this risk. The risk for serious muscle toxicity appears to be increased in elderly patients and in patients with diabetes, renal failure, or hypothyroidism.

In phase 3 clinical trials with Trilipix, myalgia was reported in 3.3% of patients treated with Trilipix monotherapy and 3.1% to 3.5% of patients treated with Trilipix co-administered with statins compared to 4.7% to 6.1% of patients treated with statin monotherapy. Increases in creatine phosphokinase (CPK) to > 5 times upper limit of normal occurred in no patients treated with Trilipix monotherapy and 0.2% to 1.2% of patients treated with Trilipix co-administered with statins compared to 0.4% to 1.3% of patients treated with statin monotherapy.

Myopathy should be considered in any patient with diffuse myalgias, muscle tenderness or weakness, and/or marked elevations of CPK levels. Patients should promptly report unexplained muscle pain, tenderness or weakness, particularly if accompanied by malaise or fever. CPK levels should be assessed in patients reporting these symptoms, and Trilipix and statin therapy should be discontinued if markedly elevated CPK levels occur or myopathy or myositis is suspected or diagnosed.

Cases of myopathy, including rhabdomyolysis, have been reported with fenofibrates co-administered with colchicine, and caution should be exercised when prescribing fenofibrate with colchicine *[see Drug Interactions (7.4)]*.

5.3 Liver Function

Trilipix at a dose of 135 mg once daily administered as monotherapy or co-administered with low to moderate doses of statins has been associated with increases in serum transaminases [AST (SGOT) or ALT (SGPT)]. In a pooled analysis of three double-blind controlled studies of Trilipix administered as monotherapy or in combination with statins, increases to > 3 times the upper limit of normal on two consecutive occasions in ALT and AST occurred in 1.9% and 0.2%, respectively, of patients receiving Trilipix monotherapy and in 1.3% and 0.4%, respectively, of patients receiving Trilipix co-administered with statins. Increases to > 3 times the upper limit of normal in ALT and AST occurred in no patients receiving low- to moderate-dose statin monotherapy. Increases to > 3 times the upper limit of normal in ALT and AST occurred in 0.8% and 0.4%, respectively in patients receiving high-dose statin monotherapy. In a long-term study of Trilipix co-administered with statins for up to 52 weeks, increases of > 3 times the upper limit of normal on two consecutive occasions of ALT and AST occurred in 1.2% and 0.5% of patients, respectively. When transaminase determinations were followed either after discontinuation of treatment or during continued treatment, a return to normal limits was usually observed. Increases in ALT and/or AST were not accompanied by increases in bilirubin or clinically significant increases in alkaline phosphatase.

In a pooled analysis of 10 placebo-controlled trials of fenofibrate, increases to > 3 times the upper limit of normal in ALT occurred in 5.3% of patients taking fenofibrate versus 1.1% of patients treated with placebo. The incidence of increases in transaminases observed with fenofibrate therapy may be dose related. In an 8-week dose-ranging study of fenofibrate in hypertriglyceridemia, the incidence of ALT or AST elevations ≥ 3 times the upper limit of normal was 13% in patients receiving dosages equivalent to 90 mg to 135 mg Trilipix once daily and was 0% in those receiving dosages equivalent to 45 mg Trilipix once daily or less, or placebo. Hepatocellular, chronic active, and cholestatic hepatitis observed with fenofibrate therapy have been reported after exposures of weeks to several years. In extremely rare cases, cirrhosis has been reported in association with chronic active hepatitis.

Baseline and regular monitoring of liver function, including serum ALT (SGPT) should be performed for the duration of therapy with Trilipix, and therapy discontinued if enzyme levels persist above 3 times the upper limit of normal.

5.4 Serum Creatinine

Reversible elevations in serum creatinine have been reported in patients receiving Trilipix as monotherapy or co-administered with statins as well as patients receiving fenofibrate. In the pooled analysis of three double-blind controlled studies of Trilipix administered as monotherapy or in combination with statins, increases in creatinine to > 2 mg/dL occurred in 0.8% of patients treated with Trilipix monotherapy and 1.1% to 1.3% of patients treated with Trilipix co-administered with statins compared to 0% to 0.4% of patients treated with statin monotherapy. Elevations in serum creatinine were generally stable over time with no evidence for continued increases in serum creatinine with long-term therapy and tended to return to baseline following discontinuation of treatment. The clinical significance of these observations is unknown. Monitoring renal function in patients with renal impairment taking Trilipix is suggested. Renal monitoring should be considered for patients at risk for renal insufficiency, such as the elderly and those with diabetes.

5.5 Cholelithiasis

Trilipix, like fenofibrate, clofibrate, and gemfibrozil, may increase cholesterol excretion into the bile, potentially leading to cholelithiasis. If cholelithiasis is suspected, gallbladder studies are indicated. Trilipix therapy should be discontinued if gallstones are found.

5.6 Coumarin Anticoagulants

Caution should be exercised when Trilipix is given in conjunction with oral coumarin anticoagulants. Trilipix may potentiate the anticoagulant effects of these agents resulting in prolongation of the prothrombin time/International Normalized Ratio (PT/INR). Frequent monitoring of PT/INR and dose adjustment of the oral anticoagulant are recommended until the PT/INR has stabilized in order to prevent bleeding complications *[see Drug Interactions (7.1)]*.

5.7 Pancreatitis

Pancreatitis has been reported in patients taking drugs of the fibrate class, including Trilipix. This occurrence may represent a failure of efficacy in patients with severe hypertriglyceridemia, a direct drug effect, or a secondary phenomenon mediated through biliary tract stone or sludge formation with obstruction of the common bile duct.

5.8 Hematological Changes

Mild to moderate hemoglobin, hematocrit, and white blood cell decreases have been observed in patients following initiation of Trilipix and fenofibrate therapy. However, these levels stabilize during long-term administration. Thrombocytopenia and agranulocytosis have been reported in individuals treated with fenofibrates. Periodic monitoring of red and white blood cell counts are recommended during the first 12 months of Trilipix administration.

5.9 Hypersensitivity Reactions

Acute hypersensitivity reactions such as Stevens-Johnson syndrome and toxic necrolysis requiring patient hospitalization and treatment with steroids have been reported in individuals treated with fenofibrates.

5.10 Venothromboembolic Disease

In the FIELD trial, pulmonary embolus (PE) and deep vein thrombosis (DVT) were observed at higher rates in the fenofibrate- than the placebo-treated group. Of 9,795 patients enrolled in FIELD, there were 4,900 in the placebo group and 4,895 in the fenofibrate group. For DVT, there were 48 events (1%) in the placebo group and 67 (1%) in the fenofibrate group (p = 0.074); and for PE, there were 32 (0.7%) events in the placebo group and 53 (1%) in the fenofibrate group (p = 0.022).

In the Coronary Drug Project, a higher proportion of the clofibrate group experienced definite or suspected fatal or nonfatal PE or thrombophlebitis than the placebo group (5.2% vs. 3.3% at five years; p < 0.01).

5.11 Paradoxical Decreases in HDL Cholesterol Levels

There have been postmarketing and clinical trial reports of severe decreases in HDL cholesterol levels (as low as 2 mg/dL) occurring in diabetic and non-diabetic patients initiated on fibrate therapy. The decrease in HDL-C is mirrored by a decrease in apolipoprotein A1. This decrease has been reported to occur within 2 weeks to years after initia-

Information on the AbbVie, Inc. products listed on these pages is from the prescribing information in use as of July 31, 2013. For more information, please visit rxabbvie.com or call 1-800-633-9110.

Table 1. Treatment-Emergent Adverse Events Reported in ≥ 3% of Patients Receiving Trilipix or Trilipix Co-Administered with a Statin During Double-Blind Controlled Studies [Number (%)]

Adverse Event	Trilipix (N = 490)	Low-Dose Statin (N = 493)	Trilipix + Low-Dose Statin (N = 490)	Moderate-Dose Statin (N = 491)	Trilipix + Moderate-Dose Statin (N = 489)	High-Dose Statin (N = 245)
Gastrointestinal Disorders						
Constipation	16 (3.3)	11 (2.2)	16 (3.3)	13 (2.6)	15 (3.1)	6 (2.4)
Diarrhea	19 (3.9)	16 (3.2)	15 (3.1)	24 (4.9)	18 (3.7)	17 (6.9)
Dyspepsia	18 (3.7)	13 (2.6)	13 (2.7)	17 (3.5)	23 (4.7)	6 (2.4)
Nausea	21 (4.3)	18 (3.7)	17 (3.5)	22 (4.5)	27 (5.5)	10 (4.1)
General Disorders and Administration Site Conditions						
Fatigue	10 (2.0)	13 (2.6)	13 (2.7)	13 (2.6)	16 (3.3)	5 (2.0)
Pain	17 (3.5)	9 (1.8)	16 (3.3)	8 (1.6)	7 (1.4)	8 (3.3)
Infections and Infestations						
Nasopharyngitis	17 (3.5)	29 (5.9)	23 (4.7)	16 (3.3)	21 (4.3)	9 (3.7)
Sinusitis	16 (3.3)	4 (0.8)	14 (2.9)	8 (1.6)	17 (3.5)	4 (1.6)
Upper Respiratory Tract Infection	26 (5.3)	13 (2.6)	18 (3.7)	23 (4.7)	23 (4.7)	7 (2.9)
Investigations						
ALT Increased	6 (1.2)	2 (0.4)	15 (3.1)	2 (0.4)	12 (2.5)	4 (1.6)
Musculoskeletal and Connective Tissue Disorders						
Arthralgia	19 (3.9)	22 (4.5)	21 (4.3)	21 (4.3)	17 (3.5)	12 (4.9)
Back Pain	31 (6.3)	31 (6.3)	30 (6.1)	32 (6.5)	20 (4.1)	8 (3.3)
Muscle Spasms	8 (1.6)	18 (3.7)	12 (2.4)	24 (4.9)	15 (3.1)	6 (2.4)
Myalgia	16 (3.3)	24 (4.9)	17 (3.5)	23 (4.7)	15 (3.1)	15 (6.1)
Pain in Extremity	22 (4.5)	24 (4.9)	14 (2.9)	21 (4.3)	13 (2.7)	9 (3.7)
Nervous System Disorders						
Dizziness	20 (4.1)	8 (1.6)	19 (3.9)	11 (2.2)	16 (3.3)	2 (0.8)
Headache	62 (12.7)	64 (13.0)	64 (13.1)	82 (16.7)	58 (11.9)	32 (13.1)

Low-dose statin = rosuvastatin 10 mg, simvastatin 20 mg, or atorvastatin 20 mg
Moderate-dose statin = rosuvastatin 20 mg, simvastatin 40 mg, or atorvastatin 40 mg
High-dose statin = rosuvastatin 40 mg, simvastatin 80 mg, or atorvastatin 80 mg

tion of fibrate therapy. The HDL-C levels remain depressed until fibrate therapy has been withdrawn; the response to withdrawal of fibrate therapy is rapid and sustained. The clinical significance of this decrease in HDL-C is unknown. It is recommended that HDL-C levels be checked within the first few months after initiation of fibrate therapy. If a severely depressed HDL-C level is detected, fibrate therapy should be withdrawn, and the HDLC level monitored until it has returned to baseline, and fibrate therapy should not be re-initiated.

6 ADVERSE REACTIONS

6.1 Clinical Trials Experience

Because clinical studies are conducted under widely varying conditions, adverse event rates observed in the clinical studies of a drug cannot be directly compared to rates in the clinical studies of another drug.

Trilipix (fenofibric acid)

<u>Monotherapy</u>

Treatment-emergent adverse events reported in 3% or more of patients treated with Trilipix during the randomized controlled trials are listed in Table 1 below.

<u>Co-Administration Therapy with Statins (Double-blind Controlled Trials)</u>

Treatment-emergent adverse events reported in 3% or more of patients treated with Trilipix co-administered with statins during the randomized controlled trials are listed in Table 1 below.

[See table 1 above]

<u>Co-Administration Therapy with Statins (Long-Term Exposure for up to 64 Weeks)</u>

Patients successfully completing any one of the three double-blind, controlled studies were eligible to participate in a 52-week long-term extension study where they received Trilipix co-administered with the moderate dose statin. A total of 2201 patients received at least one dose of Trilipix co-administered with a statin in the double-blind controlled study or the long-term extension study for up to a total of 64 weeks of treatment. Additional treatment-emergent adverse events (not listed in Table 1 above) reported in 3% or more of patients receiving Trilipix co-administered with a statin in either the double-blind controlled studies or the long-term extension study are provided below.

Infections and Infestations
Bronchitis, influenza, and urinary tract infection.

Investigations
AST increased, blood CPK increased, and hepatic enzyme increased.

Musculoskeletal and Connective Tissue Disorders
Musculoskeletal pain.

Psychiatric Disorders
Insomnia.

Respiratory, Thoracic, and Mediastinal Disorders
Cough and pharyngolaryngeal pain.

Vascular Disorders
Hypertension.

Fenofibrate

Fenofibric acid is the active metabolite of fenofibrate. Adverse events reported by 2% or more of patients treated with fenofibrate and greater than placebo during double-blind, placebo-controlled trials are listed in Table 2. Adverse events led to discontinuation of treatment in 5.0% of patients treated with fenofibrate and in 3.0% treated with placebo. Increases in liver tests were the most frequent events, causing discontinuation of fenofibrate treatment in 1.6% of patients in double-blind trials.

Table 2. Adverse Events Reported by 2% or More of Patients Treated with Fenofibrate and Greater than Placebo During the Double-Blind, Placebo-Controlled Trials

BODY SYSTEM Adverse Event	Fenofibrate* (N = 439)	Placebo (N = 365)
BODY AS A WHOLE		
Abdominal Pain	4.6%	4.4%
Back Pain	3.4%	2.5%
Headache	3.2%	2.7%
DIGESTIVE		
Nausea	2.3%	1.9%
Constipation	2.1%	1.4%
INVESTIGATIONS		
Abnormal Liver Tests	7.5%	1.4%
Increased AST	3.4%	0.5%
Increased ALT	3.0%	1.6%
Increased Creatine Phosphokinase	3.0%	1.4%
RESPIRATORY		
Respiratory Disorder	6.2%	5.5%
Rhinitis	2.3%	1.1%

* Dosage equivalent to 135 mg Trilipix

6.2 Postmarketing Experience

The following adverse events have been identified during postapproval use of fenofibrate: myalgia, rhabdomyolysis, pancreatitis, renal failure, muscle spasms, acute renal failure, hepatitis, cirrhosis, anemia, arthralgia, asthenia, and severely depressed HDL-cholesterol levels.

Because these events are reported voluntarily from a population of uncertain size, it is not always possible to reliably estimate their frequency or establish a casual relationship to drug exposure.

7 DRUG INTERACTIONS

7.1 Coumarin Anticoagulants

Potentiation of coumarin-type anticoagulant effect has been observed with prolongation of the PT/INR.

Caution should be exercised when oral coumarin anticoagulants are given in conjunction with Trilipix. The dosage of the anticoagulant should be reduced to maintain the PT/INR at the desired level to prevent bleeding complications. Frequent PT/INR determinations are advisable until it has been definitely determined that the PT/INR has stabilized *[see Warnings and Precautions (5.6)]*.

7.2 Bile Acid Binding Resins

Since bile acid binding resins may bind other drugs given concurrently, patients should take Trilipix at least 1 hour before or 4 to 6 hours after a bile acid resin to avoid impeding its absorption.

7.3 Immunosuppressants

Immunosuppressants such as cyclosporine and tacrolimus can produce nephrotoxicity with decreases in creatinine clearance and rises in serum creatinine, and because renal excretion is the primary elimination route of drugs of the fibrate class including Trilipix, there is a risk that an interaction will lead to deterioration of renal function. The benefits and risks of using Trilipix with immunosuppressants and other potentially nephrotoxic agents should be carefully considered, and the lowest effective dose employed.

7.4 Colchicine

Cases of myopathy, including rhabdomyolysis, have been reported with fenofibrates co-administered with colchicine, and caution should be exercised when prescribing fenofibrate with colchicine.

8 USE IN SPECIFIC POPULATIONS

8.1 Pregnancy

Pregnancy Category: C

The safety of Trilipix in pregnant women has not been established. There are no adequate and well controlled studies of Trilipix in pregnant women. Trilipix should be used during pregnancy only if the potential benefit justifies the potential risk to the fetus.

When Trilipix is administered with a statin in a woman of childbearing potential, refer to pregnancy category and product labeling for the statin. All statins are contraindicated in pregnant women.

In pregnant rats given oral dietary doses of 14, 127, and 361 mg/kg/day from gestation day 6-15 during the period of organogenesis, adverse developmental findings were not observed at 14 mg/kg/day (less than 1 times the maximum recommended human dose [MRHD], based on body surface area comparisons; mg/m^2). At higher multiples of human doses evidence of maternal toxicity was observed.

In pregnant rabbits given oral gavage doses of 15, 150, and 300 mg/kg/day from gestation day 6-18 during the period of organogenesis and allowed to deliver, aborted litters were observed at 150 mg/kg/day (10 times the MRHD, based on body surface area comparisons; mg/m^2). No developmental findings were observed at 15 mg/kg/day (at less than 1 times the MRHD, based on body surface area comparisons; mg/m^2).

In pregnant rats given oral dietary doses of 15, 75, and 300 mg/kg/day from gestation day 15 through lactation day 21 (weaning), maternal toxicity was observed at less than 1 times the MRHD, based on body surface area comparisons; mg/m^2.

8.3 Nursing Mothers

Trilipix should not be used in nursing mothers. A decision should be made whether to discontinue nursing or to discontinue the drug taking into account the importance of the drug to the mother.

8.4 Pediatric Use

The safety and effectiveness of Trilipix monotherapy or co-administration with a statin in pediatric patients have not been established.

8.5 Geriatric Use

Trilipix is substantially excreted by the kidney as fenofibric acid and fenofibric acid glucuronide, and the risk of adverse reactions to this drug may be greater in patients with impaired renal function. Fenofibric acid exposure is not influenced by age. Since elderly patients have a higher incidence of renal impairment, dose selection for the elderly should be made on the basis of renal function *[see Dosage and Administration (2.6) and Clinical Pharmacology (12.3)]*. Elderly patients with normal renal function should require no dose modifications. Consider monitoring renal function in elderly patients taking Trilipix.

8.6 Renal Impairment

The use of Trilipix should be avoided in patients who have severe renal impairment *[see Contraindications (4)]*. Dose reduction is required in patients with mild to moderate renal impairment *[see Dosage and Administration (2.5) and Clinical Pharmacology (12.3)]*. Monitoring renal function in patients with renal impairment is recommended.

8.7 Hepatic Impairment

The use of Trilipix has not been evaluated in subjects with hepatic impairment *[see Contraindications (4) and Clinical Pharmacology (12.3)]*.

10 OVERDOSAGE

There is no specific treatment for overdose with Trilipix. General supportive care of the patient is indicated, including monitoring of vital signs and observation of clinical status, should an overdose occur. If indicated, elimination of unabsorbed drug should be achieved by emesis or gastric lavage; usual precautions should be observed to maintain the airway. Because Trilipix is highly bound to plasma proteins, hemodialysis should not be considered.

11 DESCRIPTION

Trilipix (fenofibric acid) is a lipid regulating agent available as delayed release capsules for oral administration. Each delayed release capsule contains choline fenofibrate, equivalent to 45 mg or 135 mg of fenofibric acid. The chemical name for choline fenofibrate is ethanaminium, 2-hydroxy-N,N,N-trimethyl, 2-{4-(4-chlorobenzoyl)phenoxy] -2-methylpropanoate (1:1) with the following structural formula:

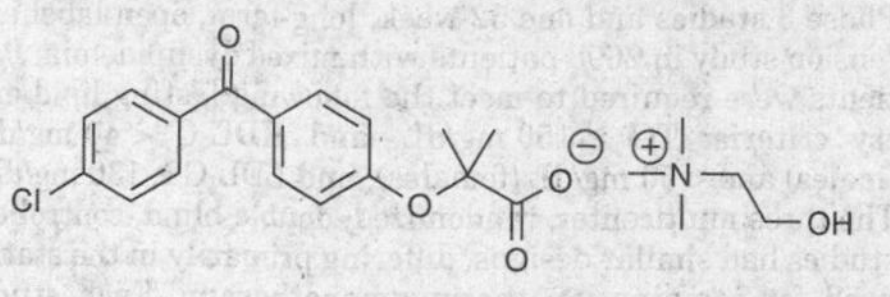

The empirical formula is $C_{22}H_{28}ClNO_5$ and the molecular weight is 421.91. Choline fenofibrate is freely soluble in water. The melting point is approximately 210°C. Choline fenofibrate is a white to yellow powder, which is stable under ordinary conditions.

Each delayed release capsule contains enteric coated mini-tablets comprised of choline fenofibrate and the following inactive ingredients: hypromellose, povidone, water, hydroxylpropyl cellulose, colloidal silicon dioxide, sodium stearyl fumarate, methacrylic acid copolymer, talc, triethyl citrate. The capsule shell of the 45 mg capsule contains the following inactive ingredients: gelatin, titanium dioxide, yellow iron oxide, black iron oxide, and red iron oxide. The capsule shell of the 135 mg capsule contains the following inactive ingredients: gelatin, titanium dioxide, yellow iron oxide, and FD&C Blue #2.

12 CLINICAL PHARMACOLOGY

12.1 Mechanism of Action

The active moiety of Trilipix is fenofibric acid. The pharmacological effects of fenofibric acid in both animals and humans have been extensively studied through oral administration of fenofibrate.

The lipid-modifying effects of fenofibric acid seen in clinical practice have been explained *in vivo* in transgenic mice and *in vitro* in human hepatocyte cultures by the activation of peroxisome proliferator activated receptor α (PPARα). Through this mechanism, fenofibric acid increases lipolysis and elimination of triglyceride-rich particles from plasma by activating lipoprotein lipase and reducing production of Apo CIII (an inhibitor of lipoprotein lipase activity).

The resulting decrease in TG produces an alteration in the size and composition of LDL from small, dense particles (which are thought to be atherogenic due to their susceptibility to oxidation), to large buoyant particles. These larger particles have a greater affinity for cholesterol receptors and are catabolized rapidly. Activation of PPARα also induces an increase in the synthesis of HDL-C and Apo AI and AII.

12.2 Pharmacodynamics

Elevated levels of Total-C, LDL-C, and Apo B, and decreased levels of HDL-C and its transport complex, Apo AI and Apo AII, are risk factors for human atherosclerosis. Epidemiologic studies have established that cardiovascular morbidity and mortality vary directly with the levels of Total-C, LDL-C, and TG, and inversely with the level of HDL-C. The independent effect of raising HDL-C or lowering TG on the risk of cardiovascular morbidity and mortality has not been determined.

Fenofibric acid, the active metabolite of fenofibrate, produces reductions in TC, LDL-C, Apo B, TG, and triglyceride-rich lipoprotein (VLDL) in treated patients. In addition, treatment with fenofibric acid results in increases in HDL-C and Apo AI and Apo AII.

12.3 Pharmacokinetics

Trilipix contains fenofibric acid, which is the only circulating pharmacologically active moiety in plasma after oral administration of Trilipix. Fenofibric acid is also the circulating pharmacologically active moiety in plasma after oral administration of fenofibrate, the ester of fenofibric acid.

Plasma concentrations of fenofibric acid after administration of one 135 mg Trilipix delayed release capsule are equivalent to those after one 200 mg capsule of micronized fenofibrate administered under fed conditions.

Absorption

Fenofibric acid is well absorbed throughout the gastrointestinal tract. The absolute bioavailability of fenofibric acid is approximately 81%.

Peak plasma levels of fenofibric acid occur within 4 to 5 hours after a single dose administration of Trilipix capsule under fasting conditions.

Table 3. Effects of Co-Administered Drugs on Fenofibric Acid Systemic Exposure from Trilipix or Fenofibrate Administration

Co-Administered Drug	Dosage Regimen of Co-Administered Drug	Dosage Regimen of Trilipix or Fenofibrate	Changes in Fenofibric Acid Exposure AUC	C_{max}
Lipid-lowering agents				
Rosuvastatin	40 mg once daily for 10 days	Trilipix 135 mg once daily for 10 days	↓2%	↓2%
Atorvastatin	20 mg once daily for 10 days	Fenofibrate 160 mg[1] once daily for 10 days	↓2%	↓4%
Atorvastatin + ezetimibe	Atorvastatin, 80 mg once daily and ezetimibe, 10 mg once daily for 10 days	Trilipix 135 mg once daily for 10 days	↑5%	↑5%
Pravastatin	40 mg as a single dose	Fenofibrate 3 × 67 mg[2] as a single dose	↓1%	↓2%
Fluvastatin	40 mg as a single dose	Fenofibrate 160 mg[1] as a single dose	↓2%	↓10%
Simvastatin	80 mg once daily for 7 days	Fenofibrate 160 mg[1] once daily for 7 days	↓5%	↓11%
Anti-diabetic agents				
Glimepiride	1 mg as a single dose	Fenofibrate 145 mg[1] once daily for 10 days	↑1%	↓1%
Metformin	850 mg 3 times daily for 10 days	Fenofibrate 54 mg[1] 3 times daily for 10 days	↓9%	↓6%
Rosiglitazone	8 mg once daily for 5 days	Fenofibrate 145 mg[1] once daily for 14 days	↑10%	↑3%
Gastrointestinal agents				
Omeprazole	40 mg once daily for 5 days	Trilipix 135 mg as a single dose fasting	↑6%	↑17%
Omeprazole	40 mg once daily for 5 days	Trilipix 135 mg as a single dose with food	↑4%	↓2%

[1] TriCor (fenofibrate) oral tablet
[2] TriCor (fenofibrate) oral micronized capsule

Fenofibric acid exposure in plasma, as measured by C_{max} and AUC, is not significantly different when a single 135 mg dose of Trilipix is administered under fasting or nonfasting conditions.

Distribution

Upon multiple dosing of Trilipix, fenofibric acid levels reach steady state within 8 days. Plasma concentrations of fenofibric acid at steady state are approximately slightly more than double those following a single dose. Serum protein binding is approximately 99% in normal and dyslipidemic subjects.

Metabolism

Fenofibric acid is primarily conjugated with glucuronic acid and then excreted in urine. A small amount of fenofibric acid is reduced at the carbonyl moiety to a benzhydrol metabolite which is, in turn, conjugated with glucuronic acid and excreted in urine.

In vivo metabolism data after fenofibrate administration indicate that fenofibric acid does not undergo oxidative metabolism (e.g., cytochrome P450) to a significant extent.

Elimination

After absorption, Trilipix is primarily excreted in the urine in the form of fenofibric acid and fenofibric acid glucuronide. Fenofibric acid is eliminated with a half-life of approximately 20 hours, allowing once daily administration of Trilipix.

Specific Populations

Geriatrics

In five elderly volunteers 77 to 87 years of age, the oral clearance of fenofibric acid following a single oral dose of fenofibrate was 1.2 L/h, which compares to 1.1 L/h in young adults. This indicates that an equivalent dose of Trilipix can be used in elderly subjects with normal renal function, without increasing accumulation of the drug or metabolites *[see Use in Specific Populations (8.5)]*.

Pediatrics

The pharmacokinetics of Trilipix has not been studied in pediatric populations.

Gender

No pharmacokinetic difference between males and females has been observed for Trilipix.

Race

The influence of race on the pharmacokinetics of Trilipix has not been studied; however, fenofibric acid is not metabolized by enzymes known for exhibiting inter-ethnic variability.

Renal Impairment

The pharmacokinetics of fenofibric acid was examined in patients with mild, moderate, and severe renal impairment. Patients with severe renal impairment (estimated glomerular filtration rate [eGFR] <30 mL/min/1.73m²) showed a 2.7-fold increase in exposure for fenofibric acid and increased accumulation of fenofibric acid during chronic dosing compared to that of healthy subjects. Patients with mild to moderate renal impairment (eGFR 30-59 mL/min/1.73m²) had similar exposure but an increase in the half-life for fenofibric acid compared to that of healthy subjects. Based on these findings, the use of Trilipix should be avoided in patients who have severe renal impairment and dose reduction is required in patients having mild to moderate renal impairment *[see Dosage and Administration (2.5)]*.

Hepatic Impairment

No pharmacokinetic studies have been conducted in patients with hepatic impairment.

Drug-drug Interactions

In vitro studies using human liver microsomes indicate that fenofibric acid is not an inhibitor of cytochrome (CYP) P450 isoforms CYP3A4, CYP2D6, CYP2E1, or CYP1A2. It is a weak inhibitor of CYP2C8, CYP2C19, and CYP2A6, and mild-to-moderate inhibitor of CYP2C9 at therapeutic concentrations.

Comparison of atorvastatin exposures when atorvastatin (80 mg once daily for 10 days) is given in combination with fenofibric acid (Trilipix 135 mg once daily for 10 days) and ezetimibe (10 mg once daily for 10 days) versus when atorvastatin is given in combination with ezetimibe only (ezetimibe 10 mg once daily and atorvastatin, 80 mg once daily for 10 days): The C_{max} decreased by 1% for atorvastatin and ortho-hydroxy-atorvastatin and increased by 2% for parahydroxy-atorvastatin. The AUC decreased 6% and 9% for atorvastatin and orthohydroxy-atorvastatin, respectively, and did not change for para-hydroxy-atorvastatin.

Comparison of ezetimibe exposures when ezetimibe (10 mg once daily for 10 days) is given in combination with fenofibric acid (Trilipix 135 mg once daily for 10 days) and atorvastatin (80 mg once daily for 10 days) versus when ezetimibe is given in combination with atorvastatin only (ezetimibe 10 mg once daily and atorvastatin, 80 mg once daily for 10 days): The C_{max} increased by 26% and 7% for total and free ezetimibe, respectively. The AUC increased by 27% and 12% for total and free ezetimibe, respectively.

Table 3 describes the effects of co-administered drugs on fenofibric acid systemic exposure. Table 4 describes the effects of co-administered fenofibric acid on other drugs.

[See table 3 above]

[See table 4 at top of next page]

13 NONCLINICAL TOXICOLOGY

13.1 Carcinogenesis, Mutagenesis, Impairment of Fertility

Trilipix (fenofibric acid)

No carcinogenicity and fertility studies have been conducted with choline fenofibrate or fenofibric acid. However, because fenofibrate is rapidly converted to its active metabolite, fenofibric acid, either during or immediately following absorption both in animals and humans, studies conducted with fenofibrate are relevant for the assessment of the tox-

Information on the AbbVie, Inc. products listed on these pages is from the prescribing information in use as of July 31, 2013. For more information, please visit rxabbvie.com or call 1-800-633-9110.

Table 4. Effects of Trilipix or Fenofibrate Co-Administration on Systemic Exposure of Other Drugs

Dosage Regimen of Trilipix or Fenofibrate	Dosage Regimen of Co-Administered Drug	Change in Co-Administered Drug Exposure		
		Analyte	AUC	C_{max}
Lipid-lowering agents				
Trilipix 135 mg once daily for 10 days	Rosuvastatin, 40 mg once daily for 10 days	Rosuvastatin	↑6%	↑20%
Fenofibrate 160 mg[1] once daily for 10 days	Atorvastatin, 20 mg once daily for 10 days	Atorvastatin	↓17%	0%
Fenofibrate 3 × 67 mg[2] as a single dose	Pravastatin, 40 mg as a single dose	Pravastatin	↑13%	↑13%
		3α-Hydroxyl-iso-pravastatin	↑26%	↑29%
Fenofibrate 160 mg[1] as a single dose	Fluvastatin, 40 mg as a single dose	(+)-3R, 5S-Fluvastatin	↑15%	↑16%
Fenofibrate 160 mg[1] once daily for 7 days	Simvastatin, 80 mg once daily for 7 days	Simvastatin acid	↓36%	↓11%
		Simvastatin	↓11%	↓17%
		Active HMG-CoA Inhibitors	↓12%	↓1%
		Total HMG-CoA Inhibitors	↓8%	↓10%
Anti-diabetic agents				
Fenofibrate 145 mg[1] once daily for 10 days	Glimepiride, 1 mg as a single dose	Glimepiride	↑35%	↑18%
Fenofibrate 54 mg[1] 3 times daily for 10 days	Metformin, 850 mg 3 times daily for 10 days	Metformin	↑3%	↑6%
Fenofibrate 145 mg[1] once daily for 14 days	Rosiglitazone, 8 mg once daily for 5 days	Rosiglitazone	↑6%	↓1%

[1] TriCor (fenofibrate) oral tablet
[2] TriCor (fenofibrate) oral micronized capsule

Table 5. Mean Percent Change from Baseline to the Final Value in HDL-C, TG, and LDL-C (Pooled Double-Blind, Controlled Studies)

	Trilipix	Low-Dose Statin	Trilipix + Low-Dose Statin	Between-group Δ (p-value)	Moderate-Dose Statin	Trilipix + Moderate-Dose Statin	Between-group Δ (p-value)	High-Dose Statin
HDL-C (mg/dL)	(N = 420)	(N = 455)	(N = 423)		(N = 430)	(N = 422)		(N = 217)
BL mean	38.4	38.4	38.2		38.4	38.1		38.0
Mean % Δ	16.3%	7.4%	18.1%	10.7%[a] (< 0.001)	8.7%	17.5%	8.8%[a] (< 0.001)	7.9%
TG (mg/dL)	(N = 459)	(N = 477)	(N = 470)		(N = 472)	(N = 462)		(N = 235)
BL mean	280.7	286.1	282.1		287.9	286.1		282.5
Mean % Δ	-31.0%	-16.8%	-43.9%	-27.2%[a] (< 0.001)	-23.7%	-42.0%	-18.3%[a] (< 0.001)	-28.1%
LDL-C (mg/dL)	(N = 427)	(N = 463)	(N = 436)		(N = 439)	(N = 434)		(N = 225)
BL mean	158.4	153.8	155.7		158.0	156.4		156.1
Mean % Δ	-5.1%	-33.9%	-33.1%	-28.0%[b] (< 0.001)	-40.6%	-34.6%	-29.5%[b] (< 0.001)	-47.1%

[a] Combination therapy vs. corresponding statin monotherapy
[b] Combination therapy vs. Trilipix monotherapy
Low-dose statin = rosuvastatin 10 mg, simvastatin 20 mg, or atorvastatin 20 mg
Moderate-dose statin = rosuvastatin 20 mg, simvastatin 40 mg, or atorvastatin 40 mg
High-dose statin = rosuvastatin 40 mg, simvastatin 80 mg, or atorvastatin 80 mg
BL = Baseline
% Δ = Percent change from baseline to final value

icity profile of fenofibric acid. A similar toxicity spectrum is expected after treatment with either Trilipix or fenofibrate.

Fenofibrate

Two dietary carcinogenicity studies have been conducted in rats with fenofibrate. In the first 24-month study, Wistar rats were dosed with fenofibrate at 10, 45, and 200 mg/kg/day, approximately 0.3, 1, and 6 times the maximum recommended human dose (MRHD), based on body surface area comparisons (mg/m^2). At a dose of 200 mg/kg/day (6 times the MRHD), the incidence of liver carcinomas was significantly increased in both sexes. A statistically significant increase in pancreatic carcinomas was observed in males at 1 and 6 times the MRHD; an increase in pancreatic adenomas and benign testicular interstitial cell tumors was observed at 6 times the MRHD in males. In a second 24-month rat carcinogenicity study in a different strain of rats (Sprague-Dawley), (doses of 10 and 60 mg/kg/day (0.3 and 2 times the MRHD), produced significant increases in the incidence of pancreatic acinar adenomas in both sexes and increases in interstitial cell tumors of the testes at 2 times the MRHD.

A 117-week carcinogenicity study was conducted in rats comparing three drugs: fenofibrate 10 and 60 mg/kg/day (0.3 and 2 times the MRHD), clofibrate (400 mg/kg/day; 2 times the human dose), and gemfibrozil (250 mg/kg/day; 2 times the MRHD). Fenofibrate increased pancreatic acinar adenomas in both sexes. Clofibrate increased hepatocellular carcinoma and pancreatic acinar adenomas in males and hepatic neoplastic nodules in females. Gemfibrozil increased hepatic neoplastic nodules in males and females, while all three drugs increased testicular interstitial cell tumors in males.

In a 21-month study in CF-1 mice, fenofibrate 10, 45, and 200 mg/kg/day (approximately 0.2, 1, and 3 times the MRHD on the basis of mg/m^2 surface area) significantly increased the liver carcinomas in both sexes at 3 times the MRHD. In a second 18-month study at 10, 60, and 200 mg/kg/day, fenofibrate significantly increased the liver carcinomas in male and female mice at 3 times the MRHD. Electron microscopy studies have demonstrated peroxisomal proliferation following fenofibrate administration to the rat. An adequate study to test for peroxisome proliferation in humans has not been done, but changes in peroxisome morphology and numbers have been observed in humans after treatment with other members of the fibrate class when liver biopsies were compared before and after treatment in the same individual.

Mutagenesis: Fenofibrate has been demonstrated to be devoid of mutagenic potential in the following tests: Ames, and micronucleus *in vivo*/rat. In addition, fenofibric acid, has been demonstrated to be devoid of mutagenic potential in the following tests: Ames, mouse lymphoma, chromosomal aberration and sister chromatid exchange in human lymphocytes, and unscheduled DNA synthesis in primary rat hepatocytes.

Impairment of Fertility: In a fertility study, rats were given oral dietary doses of fenofibrate. Males received doses for 61 days prior to mating and females for 15 days prior to mating through weaning, which resulted in no adverse effect on fertility at doses up to 300 mg/kg/day (~10 times the MRHD, based on mg/m^2 surface area comparisons).

14 CLINICAL STUDIES

14.1 Co-Administration Therapy with Statins

Efficacy and safety of Trilipix co-administered with statins were assessed in three 12-week, double-blind, controlled Phase 3 studies and one 52-week, long-term, open-label extension study in 2698 patients with mixed dyslipidemia. Patients were required to meet the following fasting lipid entry criteria: TG ≥ 150 mg/dL, and HDL-C < 40 mg/dL (males) and < 50 mg/dL (females), and LDL-C ≥ 130 mg/dL. The three multicenter, randomized, double-blind, controlled studies had similar designs, differing primarily in the statin used for combination therapy/monotherapy. Each study compared the effects of 135 mg Trilipix co-administered with either a low dose or a moderate dose of statin with Trilipix monotherapy and statin monotherapy at the corresponding dose on CHD lipid risk factors. A smaller group of patients received a high dose of statin monotherapy. In study 1, patients received Trilipix co-administered with 10 mg or 20 mg rosuvastatin. In study 2, patients received Trilipix co-administered with 20 mg or 40 mg simvastatin. In study 3, patients received Trilipix co-administered with 20 mg or 40 mg atorvastatin.

Patients were enrolled for a total of approximately 22 weeks, consisting of a 6-week diet run-in/washout period, a 12-week treatment period, and a 30-day safety follow up period. Patients who completed the 12-week treatment period were eligible to participate in the 52-week long-term extension study. Of the 2698 randomized and treated subjects in the controlled studies, 51.6% were female and 48.4% were male; 92.6% of all subjects were White, 4.7% were Black, and 2.8% were of other races. Hispanics comprised 9.9% of the study population. Mean age was 54.9 years.

The primary efficacy endpoints for all three studies were mean percent changes from baseline to final value in HDL-C, TG, and LDL-C. For each statin dose co-administered with Trilipix, there were three primary comparisons. For HDL-C and TG, Trilipix co-administered with each statin dose was compared with statin monotherapy at the corresponding dose. For LDL-C, Trilipix co-administered with each statin dose was compared with Trilipix monotherapy. In order to declare combination therapy successful for a particular statin dose, all three primary comparisons were required to demonstrate superiority of the combination therapy over the corresponding monotherapy. The primary efficacy results were consistent in the three studies and were confirmed by the pooled analysis of the three studies. The results from the individual studies and the pooled analysis demonstrated that Trilipix co-administered with low-dose statins and moderate-dose statins was superior to the corresponding monotherapy. Statistically significant differences were observed for all three primary efficacy comparisons for both doses of combination therapy in all three double-blind, controlled studies as well as the pooled analysis.

In the pooled analysis, Trilipix co-administered with both low-dose statins and moderate-dose statins resulted in mean percent increases (18.1% and 17.5%) in HDL-C and mean percent decreases (-43.9% and -42.0%) in TG that were significantly greater than the corresponding dose of statin monotherapy (7.4% and 8.7% for HDL-C; -16.8% and -23.7% for TG). In addition, both doses of combination therapy resulted in mean percent decreases (-33.1% and -34.6%) in LDL-C that were significantly greater than Trilipix monotherapy (-5.1%). The results of the pooled analysis are described in Table 5.

[See table 5 above]

Secondary efficacy endpoints in all three double-blind, controlled studies were percent changes in non-HDL-C (Trilipix co-administered with statin compared to Trilipix monotherapy and corresponding statin monotherapy), and percent changes in VLDL-C, Total-C, and Apo B (Trilipix co-administered with statin compared to corresponding statin monotherapy). Co-administration of Trilipix with statins resulted in the following changes in secondary parameters (Table 6).

[See table 6 at top of next page]

A total of 1895 patients who completed 12 weeks of treatment in the double-blind, controlled studies were treated in the 52-week, long-term extension study. Patients received Trilipix co-administered with the moderate-dose of the statin that had been used in the double-blind, controlled study in which they were enrolled. Whether combination therapy was initiated during the double-blind, controlled studies or introduced during the long-term extension study, the treatment effect of combination therapy was observed within four weeks, and was sustained over the duration of treatment in the long-term study. A total of 568 patients completed 52 weeks of treatment with Trilipix co-administered with statins. Mean 52-week values and mean percent change from baseline (at time of enrollment in randomized controlled trials) were 91.7 mg/dL (-38.2%) for LDL-C, 47.3 mg/dL (+24.0%) for HDL-C, 135.5 mg/dL (-47.6%) for TG, 117.9 mg/dL (-45.7%) for non-HDL-C, 26.2 mg/dL (-53.1%) for VLDL-C, 165.2 mg/dL (-35.4%) for Total-C, and 81.4 mg/dL (-43.6%) for Apo B.

Table 6. Percent Change from Baseline to the Final Value in Non-HDL-C, VLDL-C, Total-C, and Apo B (Pooled Double-Blind, Controlled Studies)

Secondary Endpoints	Trilipix	Low-Dose Statin	Trilipix + Low-Dose Statin	Between-group Δ	Moderate-Dose Statin	Trilipix + Moderate-Dose Statin	Between-group Δ	High-Dose Statin
Non HDL-C								
(mg/dL)	(N = 420)	(N = 454)	(N = 422)		(N = 431)	(N = 420)		(N = 217)
BL mean	222.5	217.6	219.9		222.4	218.9		220.2
Mean % Δ	-17.3%	-34.9%	-40.4%	-23.1%[a] -5.5%[b]	-42.4%	-42.0%	-24.8%[a] 0.4%[b]	-47.3%
VLDL-C								
(mg/dL)	(N = 449)	(N = 463)	(N = 455)		(N = 458)	(N = 449)		(N = 232)
BL mean	65.0	66.0	65.5		67.8	64.5		66.1
Mean % Δ	-34.2%	-32.1%	-50.0%	-18.0%[b]	-38.9%	-51.2%	-12.3%[b]	-42.1%
Total-C								
(mg/dL)	(N = 459)	(N = 477)	(N = 469)		(N = 472)	(N = 462)		(N = 235)
BL mean	260.9	257.0	258.6		261.3	257.3		258.8
Mean % Δ	-12.4%	-28.7%	-31.5%	-2.8%[b]	-34.7%	-33.3%	1.4%[b]	-39.5%
Apo B								
(mg/dL)	(N = 455)	(N = 470)	(N = 465)		(N = 468)	(N = 455)		(N = 229)
BL mean	146.2	145.0	146.1		147.1	145.0		146.0
Mean % Δ	-15.6%	-31.1%	-36.3%	-5.2%[b]	-36.9%	-36.7%	0.2%[b]	-42.4%

[a] Trilipix + statin vs. Trilipix monotherapy
[b] Trilipix + statin vs. corresponding statin monotherapy
Low-dose statin = rosuvastatin 10 mg, simvastatin 20 mg, or atorvastatin 20 mg
Moderate-dose statin = rosuvastatin 20 mg, simvastatin 40 mg, or atorvastatin 40 mg
High-dose statin = rosuvastatin 40 mg, simvastatin 80 mg, or atorvastatin 80 mg
BL = Baseline
% Δ = Percent change from baseline to final value

14.2 Severe Hypertriglyceridemia

The effects of fenofibrate on serum triglycerides were studied in two randomized, double-blind, placebo-controlled clinical trials of 147 hypertriglyceridemic patients. Patients were treated for eight weeks under protocols that differed only in that one entered patients with baseline TG levels of 500 to 1500 mg/dL, and the other TG levels of 350 to 500 mg/dL. In patients with hypertriglyceridemia and normal cholesterolemia with or without hyperchylomicronemia, treatment with fenofibrate at dosages equivalent to 135 mg once daily of Trilipix decreased primarily VLDL-TG and VLDL-C. Treatment of patients with elevated TG often results in an increase of LDL-C (Table 7).

[See table 7 below]

Table 7. Effects of Fenofibrate in Patients With Severe Hypertriglyceridemia

Study 1 Baseline TG levels 350 to 499 mg/dL	Placebo N	Baseline Mean (mg/dL)	Endpoint Mean (mg/dL)	Mean % Change	Fenofibrate N	Baseline Mean (mg/dL)	Endpoint Mean (mg/dL)	Mean % Change
Triglycerides	28	449	450	-0.5	27	432	223	-46.2*
VLDL Triglycerides	19	367	350	2.7	19	350	178	-44.1*
Total Cholesterol	28	255	261	2.8	27	252	227	-9.1*
HDL Cholesterol	28	35	36	4	27	34	40	19.6*
LDL Cholesterol	28	120	129	12	27	128	137	14.5
VLDL Cholesterol	27	99	99	5.8	27	92	46	-44.7*
Study 2 **Baseline TG levels 500 to 1500 mg/dL**	**Placebo** **N**	**Baseline Mean (mg/dL)**	**Endpoint Mean (mg/dL)**	**Mean % Change**	**Fenofibrate** **N**	**Baseline Mean (mg/dL)**	**Endpoint Mean (mg/dL)**	**Mean % Change**
Triglycerides	44	710	750	7.2	48	726	308	-54.5*
VLDL Triglycerides	29	537	571	18.7	33	543	205	-50.6*
Total Cholesterol	44	272	271	0.4	48	261	223	-13.8*
HDL Cholesterol	44	27	28	5.0	48	30	36	22.9*
LDL Cholesterol	42	100	90	-4.2	45	103	131	45.0*
VLDL Cholesterol	42	137	142	11.0	45	126	54	-49.4*

* = $p < 0.05$ vs. Placebo

14.3 Primary Hypercholesterolemia (Heterozygous Familial and Nonfamilial) and Mixed Dyslipidemia

The effects of fenofibrate at a dose equivalent to Trilipix 135 mg once daily were assessed from four randomized, placebo-controlled, double-blind, parallel-group studies including patients with the following mean baseline lipid values: Total-C 306.9 mg/dL; LDL-C 213.8 mg/dL; HDL-C 52.3 mg/dL; and triglycerides 191.0 mg/dL. Fenofibrate therapy lowered LDL-C, Total-C, and the LDL-C/HDL-C ratio. Fenofibrate therapy also lowered triglycerides and raised HDL-C (Table 8).

[See table 8 at top of next page]

In a subset of the subjects, measurements of Apo B were conducted. Fenofibrate treatment significantly reduced Apo B from baseline to endpoint as compared with placebo (-25.1% vs. 2.4%, p < 0.0001, n = 213 and 143, respectively).

16 HOW SUPPLIED/STORAGE AND HANDLING

Trilipix (fenofibric acid) delayed release capsules 45 mg have a reddish-brown cap imprinted in white ink the "a" logo and a yellow body imprinted in black ink the number "45".

Cartons of 30 (NDC 0074-9642-10) and bottles of 90 (NDC 0074-9642-90).

Trilipix (fenofibric acid) delayed release capsules 135 mg have a blue cap imprinted in white ink the "a" logo and a yellow body imprinted in black ink the number "135".

Cartons of 30 (NDC 0074-9189-10) and bottles of 90 (NDC 0074-9189-90).

Store at 25°C (77°F); excursions permitted to 15°-30°C (59° to 86°F) [See USP controlled room temperature]. Keep out of the reach of children. Protect from moisture.

17 PATIENT COUNSELING INFORMATION

See Medication Guide

17.1 Patient Counseling

Patients should be advised:

- of the potential benefits and risks of Trilipix.
- to read the Medication Guide before starting Trilipix therapy and to reread it each time the prescription is renewed.
- of medications that should not be taken in combination with Trilipix.
- to continue to follow an appropriate lipid-modifying diet while taking Trilipix.
- to take Trilipix once daily, without regard to food, at the prescribed dose, swallowing each capsule whole. If Trilipix is co-administered with a statin, they may be taken together.
- to return for routine monitoring.
- to inform their physician of all medications, supplements, and herbal preparations they are taking and any change to their medical condition. Patients should also be advised to inform their physicians prescribing a new medication that they are taking Trilipix.
- to inform their physician of any muscle pain, tenderness, or weakness; onset of abdominal pain; or any other new symptoms.

Manufactured for AbbVie Inc., North Chicago, IL 60064, U.S.A. by Fournier Laboratories Ireland Limited, Anngrove, Carrigtwohill Co. Cork, Ireland, or AbbVie LTD, Barceloneta, PR 00617.
03-A785 March, 2013

MEDICATION GUIDE

Trilipix®
(try-lip-iks)
(fenofibric acid, delayed release capsules)

Read this Medication Guide before you start taking Trilipix and each time you get a refill. There may be new information. This information does not take the place of talking to your healthcare provider about your medical condition or your treatment.

What is the most important information I should know about Trilipix?

Trilipix can be used with other cholesterol-lowering medicines called statins. Statins include:

- atorvastatin (Lipitor, Caduet)
- fluvastatin (Lescol, Lescol XL)
- lovastatin (Altoprev, Mevacor, Advicor)
- pitavastatin (Livalo)
- pravastatin (Pravachol)
- rosuvastatin (Crestor)
- simvastatin (Zocor, Simcor, Vytorin)

Statins can cause muscle pain, tenderness or weakness, which may be symptoms of a rare but serious muscle condition called rhabdomyolysis. In some cases rhabdomyolysis can cause kidney damage and death. The risk of rhabdomyolysis may be higher when Trilipix is given with statins. If you take a statin, tell your healthcare provider.

Other medicines or large amounts of grapefruit juice (more than a quart) may raise the levels of statins in your body, and could then raise the risk of muscle problems. Tell your healthcare provider if you are taking any medicines listed below.

- Heart medicine
- Stomach medicine
- Antibiotic
- Anti-fungal
- Cholesterol-lowering medicine
- Hormones
- HIV/AIDS medicine
- Antidepressant
- Immunosuppressant
- Anti-seizure medicine

Ask your healthcare provider or pharmacist for a list of these medicines, if you are not sure.

Tell your healthcare provider if you drink grapefruit juice.

What is Trilipix?

Trilipix is a prescription medicine used to treat cholesterol in the blood by lowering the total amount of triglycerides and LDL (bad) cholesterol, and increasing the HDL (good) cholesterol. **Trilipix has not been shown to lower your risk of having heart problems or a stroke.** You should be on a low fat and low cholesterol diet while you take Trilipix.

The safety and effectiveness of Trilipix in children is not known.

Who should not take Trilipix?

Do not take Trilipix if you:

- are allergic to fenofibric acid, or any of the ingredients in Trilipix. See the end of this Medication Guide for a list of all the ingredients in Trilipix.
- have severe kidney disease.

Information on the AbbVie, Inc. products listed on these pages is from the prescribing information in use as of July 31, 2013. For more information, please visit rxabbvie.com or call 1-800-633-9110.

Table 8. Mean Percent Change in Lipid Parameters at End of Treatment†

Treatment Group	Total-C (mg/dL)	LDL-C (mg/dL)	HDL-C (mg/dL)	TG (mg/dL)
Pooled Cohort				
Mean baseline lipid values (n = 646)	306.9	213.8	52.3	191.0
All Fenofibrate (n = 361)	-18.7%*	-20.6%*	+11.0%*	-28.9%*
Placebo (n = 285)	-0.4%	-2.2%	+0.7%	+7.7%
Baseline LDL-C > 160 mg/dL and TG < 150 mg/dL				
Mean baseline lipid values (n = 334)	307.7	227.7	58.1	101.7
All Fenofibrate (n = 193)	-22.4%*	-31.4%*	+9.8%*	-23.5%*
Placebo (n = 141)	+0.2%	-2.2%	+2.6%	+11.7%
Baseline LDL-C > 160 mg/dL and TG ≥ 150 mg/dL				
Mean baseline lipid values (n = 242)	312.8	219.8	46.7	231.9
All Fenofibrate (n = 126)	-16.8%*	-20.1%*	+14.6%*	-35.9%*
Placebo (n = 116)	-3.0%	-6.6%	+2.3%	+0.9%

† Duration of study treatment was 3 to 6 months
* p = < 0.05 vs. Placebo

- have liver disease.
- have gallbladder disease.
- are a nursing mother.

Talk to your healthcare provider before you take Trilipix if you have any of these conditions.

What should I tell my healthcare provider before taking Trilipix?

Before taking Trilipix, tell your healthcare provider about all your medical conditions, including if you:

- are allergic to any medicines.
- have ever had kidney problems.
- have ever had liver problems.
- have ever had gallbladder problems.
- are pregnant or if you plan to become pregnant. It is not known if Trilipix will harm your unborn baby.
- are breastfeeding or plan to breastfeed. It is not known if Trilipix passes into your breast milk. You and your healthcare provider should decide if you will take Trilipix or breastfeed. You should not do both.

Tell your healthcare provider about all the medicines you take, including prescription and non-prescription medicines, vitamins and herbal supplements.

Using Trilipix with certain other medicines can affect the way these medicines work and other medicines may affect how Trilipix works. In some cases, using Trilipix with other medicines can cause serious side effects.

Know all the medicines you take. Keep a list of them and show it to your healthcare provider when you get a new medicine.

It is especially important to tell your healthcare provider if you take any of the medicines mentioned in, "What is the most important information I should know about Trilipix?" or any of the medicines listed below:

- **anticoagulants,** also known as blood thinners (warfarin, Coumadin)
- **bile acid resins**
- **cyclosporine**

Ask your healthcare provider if you are not sure if your medicine is one of these.

How should I take Trilipix?

- You should be on a low fat and low cholesterol diet while you take Trilipix.
- Take Trilipix one time each day as prescribed by your healthcare provider.
- Take Trilipix with or without food.
- Swallow Trilipix capsules whole. Do not break, crush, dissolve, or chew Trilipix capsules before swallowing. If you cannot swallow Trilipix capsules whole, tell your healthcare provider, you may need a different medicine.
- If you take a medicine called a statin, you can take Trilipix and your statin at the same time of day.
- If you miss a dose of Trilipix, take it as soon as you remember. If it is almost time for your next dose, just skip the missed dose. Take the next dose at your regular time. If you are not sure about your dosing, call your healthcare provider. **Do not take more than one dose of Trilipix a day unless your healthcare provider tells you to.**
- If you take too much Trilipix, contact your healthcare provider or your local emergency department.
- Do not change your dose or stop Trilipix unless your healthcare provider tells you to.
- Your healthcare provider may do blood tests before you start taking Trilipix and during treatment. See your healthcare provider regularly to check your cholesterol and triglyceride levels and to check for side effects.

What are the possible side effects with Trilipix?

Trilipix may cause serious side effects, including:

- **muscle pain, tenderness, or weakness.** See "What is the most important information that I should know about Trilipix?"
- **tiredness and fever.**
- **abdominal pain, nausea, or vomiting.** These may be signs of inflammation (swelling) of the gallbladder or pancreas.

Call your healthcare provider right away if you have any of these serious side effects.

The most common side effects with Trilipix include:

- headache
- heartburn (indigestion)
- nausea
- muscle aches
- increases in muscle or liver enzymes that are measured by blood tests

Tell your healthcare provider if you have any side effect that bothers you or that does not go away. These are not all the possible side effects of Trilipix. For more information, ask your healthcare provider or pharmacist.

Call your doctor for medical advice about side effects. You may report side effects to FDA at 1-800-FDA-1088.

How do I store Trilipix?

- Store Trilipix between 59° to 86° F (15° to 30° C).
- Protect Trilipix from moisture.

Keep Trilipix and all medicines out of the reach of children.

General information about the safe and effective use of Trilipix

Medicines are sometimes prescribed for conditions that are not mentioned in the Medication Guide. Do not use Trilipix for a condition for which it was not prescribed. Do not give Trilipix to other people, even if they have the same condition you have. It may harm them.

This Medication Guide summarizes the most important information about Trilipix. If you would like more information, talk to your healthcare provider. You can also ask your pharmacist or healthcare provider for information that is written for health professionals.

For more information go to www.Trilipix.com or call 1-800-633-9110.

What are the ingredients in Trilipix?

Active Ingredient: Fenofibric acid

Inactive Ingredients: Hypromellose, povidone, water, hydroxylpropyl cellulose, colloidal silicon dioxide, sodium stearyl fumarate, methacrylic acid copolymer, talc, triethyl citrate, gelatin, titanium dioxide, and yellow iron oxide. Additionally, the 45 mg capsule shell contains black iron oxide and red iron oxide, and the 135 mg capsule shell contains FD&C Blue #2.

Manufactured for AbbVie Inc., North Chicago, IL 60064, U.S.A. by Fournier Laboratories Ireland Limited, Anngrove, Carrigtwohill Co. Cork, Ireland, or AbbVie LTD, Barceloneta, PR 00617.

Ref: 03-A785 March, 2013

This Medication Guide has been approved by the U.S. Food and Drug Administration.

Shown in Product Identification Guide, page 304

ULTANE® ℞

[*ul-tān*]

(sevoflurane)

volatile liquid for inhalation

DESCRIPTION

ULTANE (sevoflurane), volatile liquid for inhalation, a nonflammable and nonexplosive liquid administered by vaporization, is a halogenated general inhalation anesthetic drug. Sevoflurane is fluoromethyl 2,2,2,-trifluoro-1-(trifluoromethyl) ethyl ether and its structural formula is:

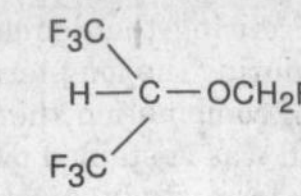

Sevoflurane, Physical Constants are:

Molecular weight	200.05
Boiling point at 760 mm Hg	58.6°C
Specific gravity at 20°C	1.520 - 1.525
Vapor pressure in mm Hg	157 mm Hg at 20°C
	197 mm Hg at 25°C
	317 mm Hg at 36°C

Distribution Partition Coefficients at 37°C:

Blood/Gas	0.63 - 0.69
Water/Gas	0.36
Olive Oil/Gas	47 – 54
Brain/Gas	1.15

Mean Component/Gas Partition Coefficients at 25°C for Polymers Used Commonly in Medical Applications:

Conductive rubber	14.0
Butyl rubber	7.7
Polyvinylchloride	17.4
Polyethylene	1.3

Sevoflurane is nonflammable and nonexplosive as defined by the requirements of International Electrotechnical Commission 601-2-13.

Sevoflurane is a clear, colorless, liquid containing no additives. Sevoflurane is not corrosive to stainless steel, brass, aluminum, nickel-plated brass, chrome-plated brass or copper beryllium. Sevoflurane is nonpungent. It is miscible with ethanol, ether, chloroform, and benzene, and it is slightly soluble in water. Sevoflurane is stable when stored under normal room lighting conditions according to instructions. No discernible degradation of sevoflurane occurs in the presence of strong acids or heat. When in contact with alkaline CO_2 absorbents (e.g Baralyme® and to a lesser extent soda lime) within the anesthesia machine, sevoflurane can undergo degradation under certain conditions. Degradation of sevoflurane is minimal, and degradants are either undetectable or present in non-toxic amounts when used as directed with fresh absorbents. Sevoflurane degradation and subsequent degradant formation are enhanced by increasing absorbent temperature increased sevoflurane concentration, decreased fresh gas flow and desiccated CO_2 absorbents (especially with potassium hydroxide containing absorbents e.g. Baralyme).

Sevoflurane alkaline degradation occurs by two pathways. The first results from the loss of hydrogen fluoride with the formation of pentafluoroisopropenyl fluoromethyl ether, (PIFE, $C_4H_2F_6O$), also known as Compound A, and trace amounts of pentafluoromethoxy isopropyl fluoromethyl ether, (PMFE, $C_5H_6F_6O$), also known as Compound B. The second pathway for degradation of sevoflurane, which occurs primarily in the presence of desiccated CO_2 absorbents, is discussed later.

In the first pathway, the defluorination pathway, the production of degradants in the anesthesia circuit results from the extraction of the acidic proton in the presence of a strong base (KOH and/or NaOH) forming an alkene (Compound A) from sevoflurane similar to formation of 2-bromo-2-chloro-1,1-difluoro ethylene (BCDFE) from halothane. Laboratory simulations have shown that the concentration of these degradants is inversely correlated with the fresh gas flow rate (See Figure 1).

Figure 1. Fresh Gas Flow Rate versus Compound A Levels in a Circle Absorber System

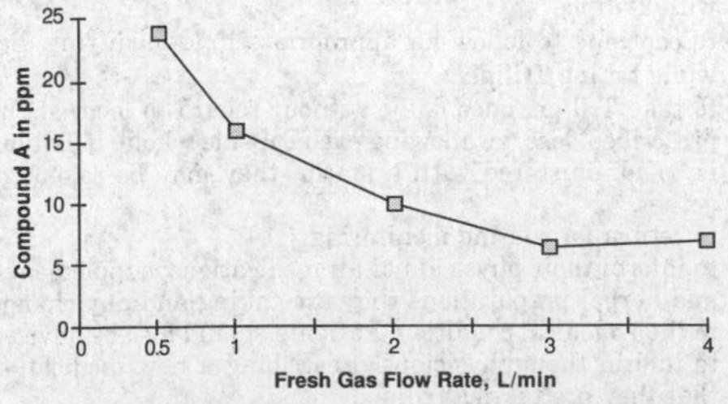

Since the reaction of carbon dioxide with absorbents is exothermic, the temperature increase will be determined by quantities of CO_2 absorbed, which in turn will depend on fresh gas flow in the anesthesia circle system, metabolic status of the patient, and ventilation. The relationship of temperature produced by varying levels of CO_2 and Compound A production is illustrated in the following *in vitro* simulation where CO_2 was added to a circle absorber system.

Figure 2. Carbon Dioxide Flow versus Compound A and Maximum Temperature

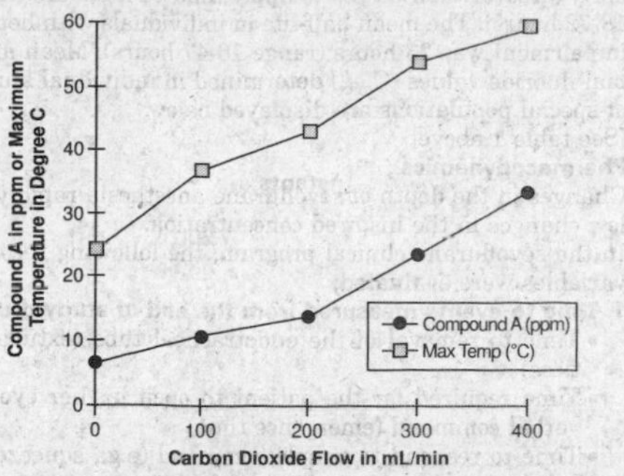

Compound A concentration in a circle absorber system increases as a function of increasing CO_2 absorbent temperature and composition (Baralyme producing higher levels than soda lime), increased body temperature, and increased minute ventilation, and decreasing fresh gas flow rates. It has been reported that the concentration of Compound A increases significantly with prolonged dehydration of Baralyme. Compound A exposure in patients also has been shown to rise with increased sevoflurane concentrations and duration of anesthesia. In a clinical study in which sevoflurane was administered to patients under low flow conditions for ≥2 hours at flow rates of 1 Liter/minute, Compound A levels were measured in an effort to determine the relationship between MAC hours and Compound A levels produced. The relationship between Compound A levels and sevoflurane exposure are shown in Figure 2a.

Figure 2a. ppm·hr versus MAC·hr at Flow Rate of 1 L/min

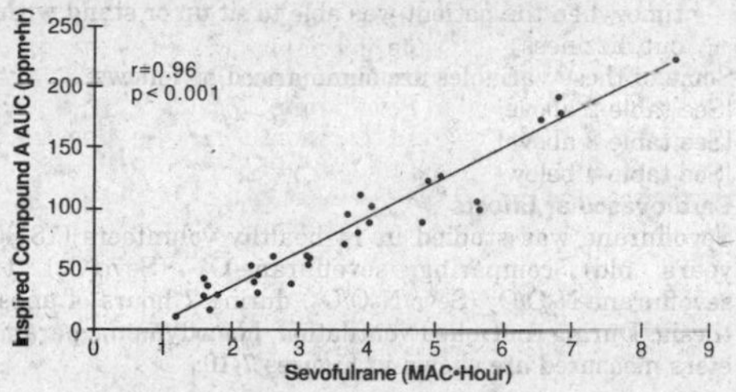

Compound A has been shown to be nephrotoxic in rats after exposures that have varied in duration from one to three hours. No histopathologic change was seen at a concentration of up to 270 ppm for one hour. Sporadic single cell necrosis of proximal tubule cells has been reported at a concentration of 114 ppm after a 3-hour exposure to Compound A in rats. The LC_{50} reported at 1 hour is 1050-1090 ppm (male-female) and, at 3 hours, 350-490 ppm (male-female).

An experiment was performed comparing sevoflurane plus 75 or 100 ppm Compound A with an active control to evaluate the potential nephrotoxicity of Compound A in non-human primates. A single 8-hour exposure of Sevoflurane in the presence of Compound A produced single-cell renal tubular degeneration and single-cell necrosis in cynomolgus monkeys. These changes are consistent with the increased urinary protein, glucose level and enzymic activity noted on days one and three on the clinical pathology evaluation. This nephrotoxicity produced by Compound A is dose and duration of exposure dependent.

At a fresh gas flow rate of 1 L/min, mean maximum concentrations of Compound A in the anesthesia circuit in clinical settings are approximately 20 ppm (0.002%) with soda lime and 30 ppm (0.003%) with Baralyme in adult patients; mean maximum concentrations in pediatric patients with soda lime are about half those found in adults. The highest concentration observed in a single patient with Baralyme was 61 ppm (0.0061%) and 32 ppm (0.0032%) with soda lime. The levels of Compound A at which toxicity occurs in humans is not known.

The second pathway for degradation of sevoflurane occurs primarily in the presence of desiccated CO_2 absorbents and leads to the dissociation of sevoflurane into hexafluoroisopropanol (HFIP) and formaldehyde. HFIP is inactive, non-genotoxic, rapidly glucuronidated and cleared by the liver. Formaldehyde is present during normal metabolic processes. Upon exposure to a highly desiccated absorbent, formaldehyde can further degrade into methanol and formate. Formate can contribute to the formation of carbon monoxide in the presence of high temperature that can be associated with desiccated Baralyme®. Methanol can react with Compound A to form the methoxy addition product Compound B. Compound B can undergo further HF elimination to form Compounds C, D, and E.

Sevoflurane degradants were observed in the respiratory circuit of an experimental anesthesia machine using desiccated CO_2 absorbents and maximum sevoflurane concentrations (8%) for extended periods of time (> 2 hours). Concentrations of formaldehyde observed with desiccated soda lime in this experimental anesthesia respiratory circuit were consistent with levels that could potentially result in respiratory irritation. Although KOH containing CO_2 absorbents are no longer commercially available, in the laboratory experiments, exposure of sevoflurane to the desiccated KOH containing CO_2 absorbent, Baralyme, resulted in the detection of substantially greater degradant levels.

CLINICAL PHARMACOLOGY

Sevoflurane is an inhalational anesthetic agent for use in induction and maintenance of general anesthesia. Minimum alveolar concentration (MAC) of sevoflurane in oxygen for a 40-year-old adult is 2.1%. The MAC of sevoflurane decreases with age (see **DOSAGE AND ADMINISTRATION** for details).

Pharmacokinetics

Uptake and Distribution

Solubility

Because of the low solubility of sevoflurane in blood (blood/gas partition coefficient @ 37°C = 0.63-0.69), a minimal amount of sevoflurane is required to be dissolved in the blood before the alveolar partial pressure is in equilibrium with the arterial partial pressure. Therefore there is a rapid rate of increase in the alveolar (end-tidal) concentration (F_A) toward the inspired concentration (F_I) during induction.

Induction of Anesthesia

In a study in which seven healthy male volunteers were administered 70% N_2O/30%O_2 for 30 minutes followed by 1.0% sevoflurane and 0.6% isoflurane for another 30 minutes the F_A/F_I ratio was greater for sevoflurane than isoflurane at all time points. The time for the concentration in the alveoli to reach 50% of the inspired concentration was 4-8 minutes for isoflurane and approximately 1 minute for sevoflurane.

F_A/F_I data from this study were compared with F_A/F_I data of other halogenated anesthetic agents from another study. When all data were normalized to isoflurane, the uptake and distribution of sevoflurane was shown to be faster than isoflurane and halothane, but slower than desflurane. The results are depicted in Figure 3.

Recovery from Anesthesia

The low solubility of sevoflurane facilitates rapid elimination via the lungs. The rate of elimination is quantified as the rate of change of the alveolar (end-tidal) concentration following termination of anesthesia (F_A), relative to the last alveolar concentration (Fa_0) measured immediately before discontinuance of the anesthetic. In the healthy volunteer study described above, rate of elimination of sevoflurane was similar compared with desflurane, but faster compared with either halothane or isoflurane. These results are depicted in Figure 4.

Figure 3. Ratio of Concentration of Anesthetic in Alveolar Gas to Inspired Gas

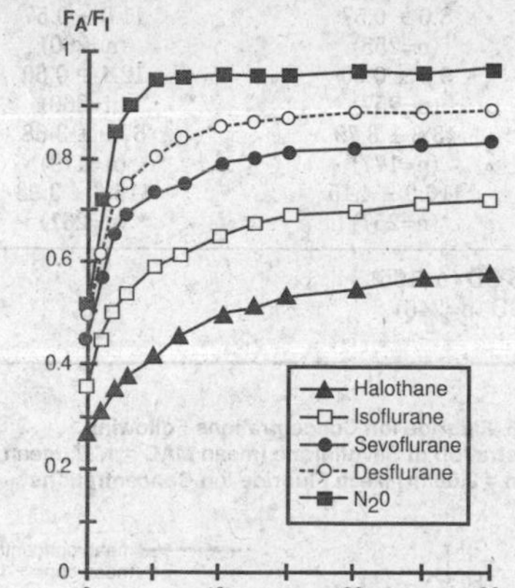

[See figure 4 at top of next column]

Yasuda N, Lockhart S, Eger EI II, et al: Comparison of kinetics of sevoflurane and isoflurane in humans. Anesth Analg 72:316, 1991.

Protein Binding

The effects of sevoflurane on the displacement of drugs from serum and tissue proteins have not been investigated. Other fluorinated volatile anesthetics have been shown to displace drugs from serum and tissue proteins *in vitro*. The clinical significance of this is unknown. Clinical studies have shown no untoward effects when sevoflurane is administered to patients taking drugs that are highly bound and have a small volume of distribution (e.g., phenytoin).

Figure 4. Concentration of Anesthetic in Alveolar Gas Following Termination of Anesthesia

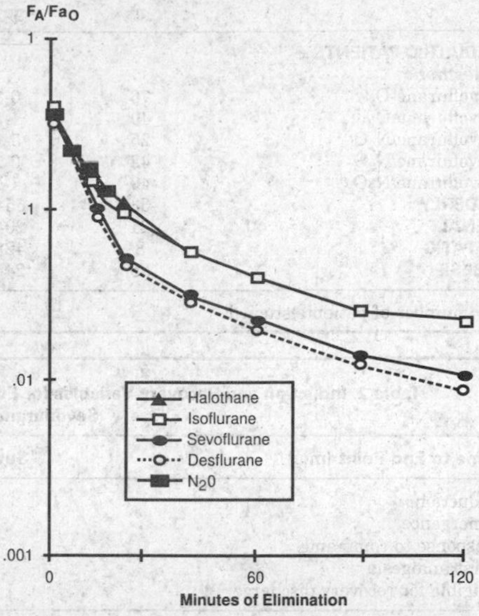

Metabolism

Sevoflurane is metabolized by cytochrome P450 2E1, to hexafluoroisopropanol (HFIP) with release of inorganic fluoride and CO_2. Once formed HFIP is rapidly conjugated with glucuronic acid and eliminated as a urinary metabolite. No other metabolic pathways for sevoflurane have been identified. *In vivo* metabolism studies suggest that approximately 5% of the sevoflurane dose may be metabolized.

Cytochrome P450 2E1 is the principal isoform identified for sevoflurane metabolism and this may be induced by chronic exposure to isoniazid and ethanol. This is similar to the metabolism of isoflurane and enflurane and is distinct from that of methoxyflurane which is metabolized via a variety of cytochrome P450 isoforms. The metabolism of sevoflurane is not inducible by barbiturates. As shown in Figure 5, inorganic fluoride concentrations peak within 2 hours of the end of sevoflurane anesthesia and return to baseline concentrations within 48 hours post-anesthesia in the majority of cases (67%). The rapid and extensive pulmonary elimination of sevoflurane minimizes the amount of anesthetic available for metabolism.

Figure 5. Serum Inorganic Fluoride Concentrations for Sevoflurane and Other Volatile Anesthetics

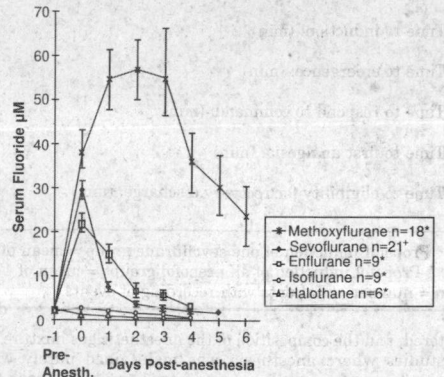

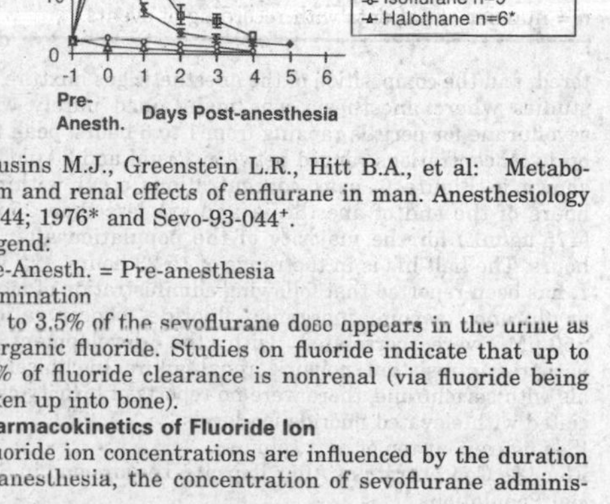

Cousins M.J., Greenstein L.R., Hitt B.A., et al: Metabolism and renal effects of enflurane in man. Anesthesiology 44:44; 1976* and Sevo-93-044+.

Legend:

Pre-Anesth. = Pre-anesthesia

Elimination

Up to 3.5% of the sevoflurane dose appears in the urine as inorganic fluoride. Studies on fluoride indicate that up to 50% of fluoride clearance is nonrenal (via fluoride being taken up into bone).

Pharmacokinetics of Fluoride Ion

Fluoride ion concentrations are influenced by the duration of anesthesia, the concentration of sevoflurane adminis-

Information on the AbbVie, Inc. products listed on these pages is from the prescribing information in use as of July 31, 2013. For more information, please visit rxabbvie.com or call 1-800-633-9110.

Table 1. Fluoride Ion Estimates in Special Populations Following Administration of Sevoflurane

	n	Age (yr)	Duration (hr)	Dose (MAC·hr)	C_{max} (μM)
PEDIATRIC PATIENTS					
Anesthetic					
Sevoflurane-O_2	76	0-11	0.8	1.1	12.6
Sevoflurane-O_2	40	1-11	2.2	3.0	16.0
Sevoflurane/N_2O	25	5-13	1.9	2.4	21.3
Sevoflurane/N_2O	42	0-18	2.4	2.2	18.4
Sevoflurane/N_2O	40	1-11	2.0	2.6	15.5
ELDERLY	33	65-93	2.6	1.4	25.6
RENAL	21	29-83	2.5	1.0	26.1
HEPATIC	8	42-79	3.6	2.2	30.6
OBESE	35	24-73	3.0	1.7	38.0

n = number of patients studied.

Table 2. Induction and Recovery Variables for Evaluable Pediatric Patients in Two Comparative Studies: Sevoflurane versus Halothane

Time to End-Point (min)	Sevoflurane Mean ± SEM	Halothane Mean ± SEM
Induction	2.0 ± 0.2 (n=294)	2.7 ± 0.2 (n=252)
Emergence	11.3 ± 0.7 (n=293)	15.8 ± 0.8 (n=252)
Response to command	13.7 ± 1.0 (n=271)	19.3 ± 1.1 (n=230)
First analgesia	52.2 ± 8.5 (n=216)	67.6 ± 10.6 (n=150)
Eligible for recovery discharge	76.5 ± 2.0 (n=292)	81.1 ± 1.9 (n=246)

n = number of patients with recording of events.

Table 3. Recovery Variables for Evaluable Adult Patients in Two Comparative Studies: Sevoflurane versus Isoflurane

Time to Parameter: (min)	Sevoflurane Mean ± SEM	Isoflurane Mean ± SEM
Emergence	7.7 ± 0.3 (n=395)	9.1 ± 0.3 (n=348)
Response to command	8.1 ± 0.3 (n=395)	9.7 ± 0.3 (n=345)
First analgesia	42.7 ± 3.0 (n=269)	52.9 ± 4.2 (n=228)
Eligible for recovery discharge	87.6 ± 5.3 (n=244)	79.1 ± 5.2 (n=252)

n = number of patients with recording of recovery events.

Table 4. Meta-Analyses for Induction and Emergence Variables for Evaluable Adult Patients in Comparative Studies: Sevoflurane versus Propofol

Parameter	No. of Studies	Sevoflurane Mean ± SEM	Propofol Mean ± SEM
Mean maintenance anesthesia exposure	3	1.0 MAC•hr. ± 0.8 (n=259)	7.2 mg/kg/hr ± 2.6 (n=258)
Time to induction: (min)	1	3.1 ± 0.18* (n=93)	2.2 ± 0.18** (n=93)
Time to emergence: (min)	3	8.6 ± 0.57 (n=255)	11.0 ± 0.57 (n=260)
Time to respond to command: (min)	3	9.9 ± 0.60 (n=257)	12.1 ± 0.60 (n=260)
Time to first analgesia: (min)	3	43.8 ± 3.79 (n=177)	57.9 ± 3.68 (n=179)
Time to eligibility for recovery discharge: (min)	3	116.0 ± 4.15 (n=257)	115.6 ± 3.98 (n=261)

* Propofol induction of one sevoflurane group = mean of 178.8 mg ±72.5 SD (n=165)
** Propofol induction of all propofol groups = mean of 170.2 mg ±60.6 SD (n=245)
n = number of patients with recording of events.

tered, and the composition of the anesthetic gas mixture. In studies where anesthesia was maintained purely with sevoflurane for periods ranging from 1 to 6 hours, peak fluoride concentrations ranged between 12 μM and 90 μM. As shown in Figure 6, peak concentrations occur within 2 hours of the end of anesthesia and are less than 25 μM (475 ng/mL) for the majority of the population after 10 hours. The half-life is in the range of 15-23 hours.

It has been reported that following administration of methoxyflurane, serum inorganic fluoride concentrations >50 μM were correlated with the development of vasopressin-resistant, polyuric, renal failure. In clinical trials with sevoflurane, there were no reports of toxicity associated with elevated fluoride ion levels.

[See figure 6 at top of next column]

Fluoride Concentrations After Repeat Exposure and in Special Populations

Fluoride concentrations have been measured after single, extended, and repeat exposure to sevoflurane in normal surgical and special patient populations, and pharmacokinetic parameters were determined.

Compared with healthy individuals, the fluoride ion half-life was prolonged in patients with renal impairment, but

Figure 6. Fluoride Ion Concentrations Following Administration of Sevoflurane (mean MAC = 1.27, mean duration = 2.06 hr) Mean Fluoride Ion Concentrations (n = 48)

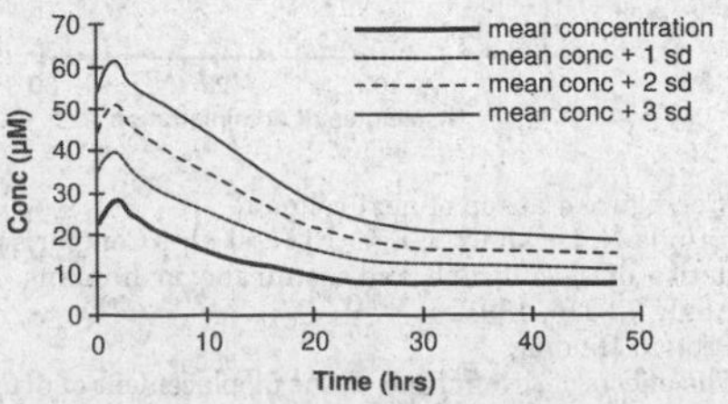

not in the elderly. A study in 8 patients with hepatic impairment suggests a slight prolongation of the half-life. The mean half-life in patients with renal impairment averaged approximately 33 hours (range 21-61 hours) as compared to a mean of approximately 21 hours (range 10-48 hours) in normal healthy individuals. The mean half-life in the elderly (greater than 65 years) approximated 24 hours (range 18-72 hours). The mean half-life in individuals with hepatic impairment was 23 hours (range 16-47 hours). Mean maximal fluoride values (C_{max}) determined in individual studies of special populations are displayed below.

[See table 1 above]

Pharmacodynamics

Changes in the depth of sevoflurane anesthesia rapidly follow changes in the inspired concentration.

In the sevoflurane clinical program, the following recovery variables were evaluated:

1. Time to events measured from the end of study drug:
- Time to removal of the endotracheal tube (extubation time)
- Time required for the patient to open his/her eyes on verbal command (emergence time)
- Time to respond to simple command (e.g., squeeze my hand) or demonstrates purposeful movement (response to command time, orientation time)

2. Recovery of cognitive function and motor coordination was evaluated based on:
- psychomotor performance tests (Digit Symbol Substitution Test [DSST], Treiger Dot Test)
- the results of subjective (Visual Analog Scale [VAS]) and objective (objective pain-discomfort scale [OPDS]) measurements
- time to administration of the first post-anesthesia analgesic medication
- assessments of post-anesthesia patient status

3. Other recovery times were:
- time to achieve an Aldrete Score of ≥ 8
- time required for the patient to be eligible for discharge from the recovery area, per standard criteria at site
- time when the patient was eligible for discharge from the hospital
- time when the patient was able to sit up or stand without dizziness

Some of these variables are summarized as follows:

[See table 2 above]
[See table 3 above]
[See table 4 below]

Cardiovascular Effects

Sevoflurane was studied in 14 healthy volunteers (18-35 years old) comparing sevoflurane-O_2 (Sevo/O_2) to sevoflurane-N_2O/O_2 (Sevo/N_2O/O_2) during 7 hours of anesthesia. During controlled ventilation, hemodynamic parameters measured are shown in Figures 7-10:

Figure 7. Heart Rate

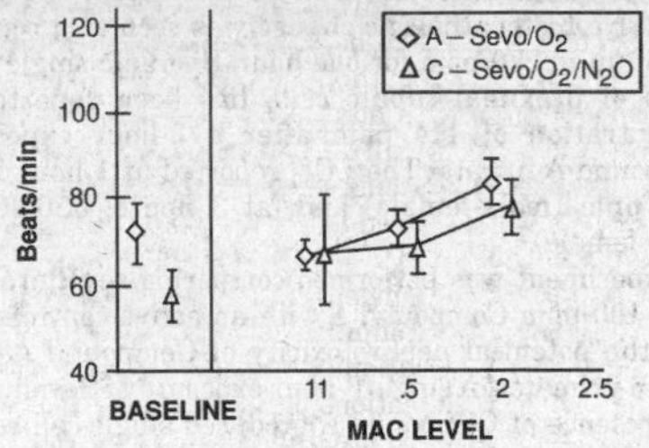

Figure 8. Mean Arterial Pressure

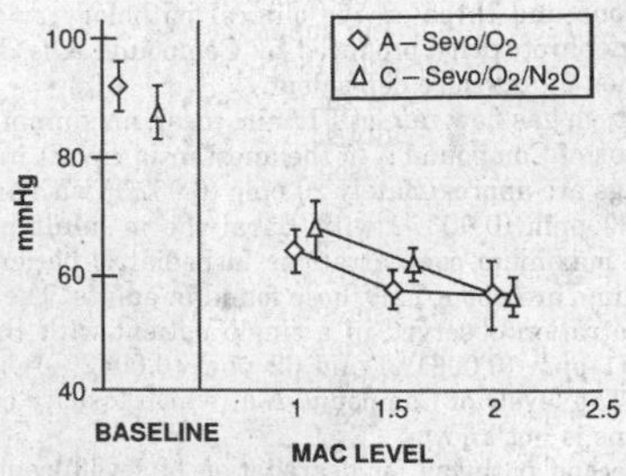

Figure 9. Systemic Vascular Resistance

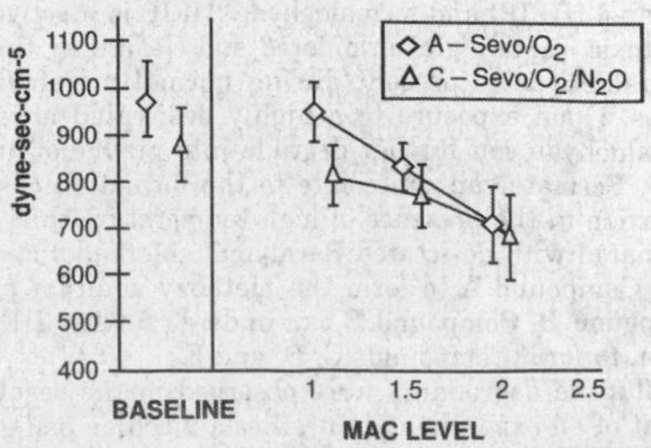

Figure 10. Cardiac Index

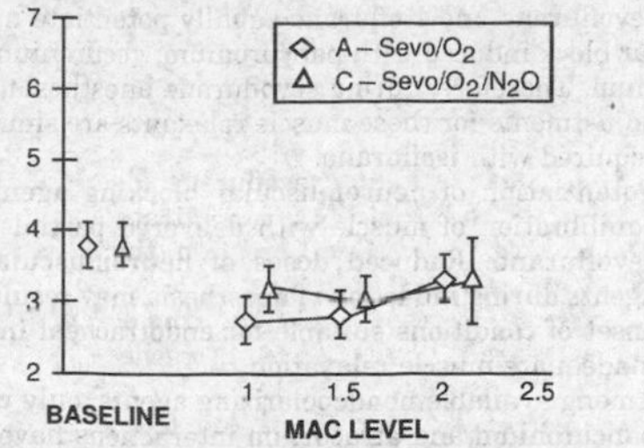

Sevoflurane is a dose-related cardiac depressant. Sevoflurane does not produce increases in heart rate at doses less than 2 MAC.

A study investigating the epinephrine induced arrhythmogenic effect of sevoflurane versus isoflurane in adult patients undergoing transsphenoidal hypophysectomy demonstrated that the threshold dose of epinephrine (i.e., the dose at which the first sign of arrhythmia was observed) producing multiple ventricular arrhythmias was 5 mcg/kg with both sevoflurane and isoflurane. Consequently, the interaction of sevoflurane with epinephrine appears to be equal to that seen with isoflurane.

Clinical Trials

Sevoflurane was administered to a total of 3185 patients prior to sevoflurane NDA submission. The types of patients are summarized as follows:

Table 5. Patients Receiving Sevoflurane in Clinical Trials

Type of Patients	Number Studied
ADULT	2223
Cesarean Delivery	29
Cardiovascular and patients at risk of myocardial ischemia	246
Neurosurgical	22
Hepatic impairment	8
Renal impairment	35
PEDIATRIC	962

Clinical experience with these patients is described below.

Adult Anesthesia

The efficacy of sevoflurane in comparison to isoflurane, enflurane, and propofol was investigated in 3 outpatient and 25 inpatient studies involving 3591 adult patients. Sevoflurane was found to be comparable to isoflurane, enflurane, and propofol for the maintenance of anesthesia in adult patients. Patients administered sevoflurane showed shorter times (statistically significant) to some recovery events (extubation, response to command, and orientation) than patients who received isoflurane or propofol.

Mask Induction

Sevoflurane has a nonpungent odor and does not cause respiratory irritability. Sevoflurane is suitable for mask induction in adults. In 196 patients, mask induction was smooth and rapid, with complications occurring with the following frequencies: cough, 6%; breathholding, 6%; agitation, 6%; laryngospasm, 5%.

Ambulatory Surgery

Sevoflurane was compared to isoflurane and propofol for maintenance of anesthesia supplemented with N_2O in two studies involving 786 adult (18-84 years of age) ASA Class I, II, or III patients. Shorter times to emergence and response to commands (statistically significant) were observed with sevoflurane compared to isoflurane and propofol.

[See table 6 above]

Inpatient Surgery

Sevoflurane was compared to isoflurane and propofol for maintenance of anesthesia supplemented with N_2O in two multicenter studies involving 741 adult ASA Class I, II or III (18-92 years of age) patients. Shorter times to emergence, command response, and first post-anesthesia analgesia (statistically significant) were observed with sevoflurane compared to isoflurane and propofol.

[See table 7 above]

Pediatric Anesthesia

The concentration of sevoflurane required for maintenance of general anesthesia is age-dependent (see **DOSAGE AND ADMINISTRATION**). Sevoflurane or halothane was used to anesthetize 1620 pediatric patients aged 1 day to 18 years, and ASA physical status I or II (948 sevoflurane, 672 halothane). In one study involving 90 infants and children, there were no clinically significant decreases in heart rate compared to awake values at 1 MAC. Systolic blood pressure decreased 15-20% in comparison to awake values following administration of 1 MAC sevoflurane; however, clinically significant hypotension requiring immediate intervention did not occur. Overall incidences of bradycardia [more than 20 beats/min lower than normal (80 beats/min)] in comparative studies was 3% for sevoflurane and 7% for halothane. Patients who received sevoflurane had slightly faster emergence times (12 vs. 19 minutes), and a higher incidence of post-anesthesia agitation (14% vs. 10%).

Sevoflurane (n=91) was compared to halothane (n=89) in a single-center study for elective repair or palliation of congenital heart disease. The patients ranged in age from 9 days to 11.8 years with an ASA physical status of II, III, and IV (18%, 68%, and 13% respectively). No significant differences were demonstrated between treatment groups with respect to the primary outcome measures: cardiovascular decompensation and severe arterial desaturation. Adverse event data was limited to the study outcome variables collected during surgery and before institution of cardiopulmonary bypass.

Mask Induction

Sevoflurane has a nonpungent odor and is suitable for mask induction in pediatric patients. In controlled pediatric studies in which mask induction was performed, the incidence of induction events is shown below (see **ADVERSE REACTIONS**).

Table 6. Recovery Parameters in Two Outpatient Surgery Studies: Least Squares Mean ± SEM

	Sevoflurane/N_2O	Isoflurane/N_2O	Sevoflurane/N_2O	Propofol/N_2O
Mean Maintenance Anesthesia Exposure ± SD	0.64 ± 0.03 MAC•hr. (n=245)	0.66 ± 0.03 MAC•hr. (n=249)	0.8 ± 0.5 MAC•hr. (n=166)	7.3 ± 2.3 mg/kg/hr. (n=166)
Time to Emergence (min)	8.2 ± 0.4 (n=246)	9.3 ± 0.3 (n=251)	8.3 ± 0.7 (n=137)	10.4 ± 0.7 (n=142)
Time to Respond to Commands (min)	8.5 ± 0.4 (n=246)	9.8 ± 0.4 (n=248)	9.1 ± 0.7 (n=139)	11.5 ± 0.7 (n=143)
Time to First Analgesia (min)	45.9 ± 4.7 (n=160)	59.1 ± 6.0 (n=252)	46.1 ± 5.4 (n=83)	60.0 ± 4.7 (n=88)
Time to Eligibility for Discharge from Recovery Area (min)	87.6 ± 5.3 (n=244)	79.1 ± 5.2 (n=252)	103.1 ± 3.8 (n=139)	105.1 ± 3.7 (n=143)

n = number of patients with recording of recovery events.

Table 7. Recovery Parameters in Two Inpatient Surgery Studies: Least Squares Mean ± SEM

	Sevoflurane/N_2O	Isoflurane/N_2O	Sevoflurane/N_2O	Propofol/N_2O
Mean Maintenance Anesthesia Exposure ± SD	1.27 MAC•hr. ±0.05 (n=271)	1.58 MAC•hr. ±0.06 (n=282)	1.43 MAC•hr. ±0.94 (n=93)	7.0 mg/kg/hr ±2.9 (n=92)
Time to Emergence (min)	11.0 ± 0.6 (n=270)	16.4 ± 0.6 (n=281)	8.8 ± 1.2 (n=92)	13.2 ± 1.2 (n=92)
Time to Respond to Commands (min)	12.8 ± 0.7 (n=270)	18.4 ± 0.7 (n=281)	11.0 ± 1.20 (n=92)	14.4 ± 1.21 (n=91)
Time to First Analgesia (min)	46.1 ± 3.0 (n=233)	55.4 ± 3.2 (n=242)	37.8 ± 3.3 (n=82)	49.2 ± 3.3 (n=79)
Time to Eligibility for Discharge from Recovery Area (min)	139.2 ± 15.6 (n=268)	165.9 ± 16.3 (n=282)	148.4 ± 8.9 (n=92)	141.4 ± 8.9 (n=92)

n = number of patients with recording of recovery events.

Table 8. Incidence of Pediatric Induction Events

	Sevoflurane (n=836)	Halothane (n=660)
Agitation	14%	11%
Cough	6%	10%
Breathholding	5%	6%
Secretions	3%	3%
Laryngospasm	2%	2%
Bronchospasm	<1%	0%

n = number of patients.

Ambulatory Surgery

Sevoflurane (n=518) was compared to halothane (n=382) for the maintenance of anesthesia in pediatric outpatients. All patients received N_2O and many received fentanyl, midazolam, bupivacaine, or lidocaine. The time to eligibility for discharge from post-anesthesia care units was similar between agents (see **CLINICAL PHARMACOLOGY** and **ADVERSE REACTIONS**).

Cardiovascular Surgery

Coronary Artery Bypass Graft (CABG) Surgery

Sevoflurane was compared to isoflurane as an adjunct with opioids in a multicenter study of 273 patients undergoing CABG surgery. Anesthesia was induced with midazolam (0.1-0.3 mg/kg); vecuronium (0.1-0.2 mg/kg), and fentanyl (5-15 mcg/kg). Both isoflurane and sevoflurane were administered at loss of consciousness in doses of 1.0 MAC and titrated until the beginning of cardiopulmonary bypass to a maximum of 2.0 MAC. The total dose of fentanyl did not exceed 25 mcg/kg. The average MAC dose was 0.49 for sevoflurane and 0.53 for isoflurane. There were no significant differences in hemodynamics, cardioactive drug use, or ischemia incidence between the two groups. Outcome was also equivalent. In this small multicenter study, sevoflurane appears to be as effective and as safe as isoflurane for supplementation of opioid anesthesia for coronary bypass grafting.

Non-Cardiac Surgery Patients at Risk for Myocardial Ischemia

Sevoflurane-N_2O was compared to isoflurane-N_2O for maintenance of anesthesia in a multicenter study in 214 patients, age 40-87 years who were at mild-to-moderate risk for myocardial ischemia and were undergoing elective noncardiac surgery. Forty-six percent (46%) of the operations were cardiovascular, with the remainder evenly divided between gastrointestinal and musculoskeletal and small numbers of other surgical procedures. The average duration of surgery was less than 2 hours. Anesthesia induction usually was performed with thiopental (2-5 mg/kg) and fentanyl (1-5 mcg/kg). Vecuronium (0.1-0.2 mg/kg) was also administered to facilitate intubation, muscle relaxation or immobility during surgery. The average MAC dose was 0.49 for both anesthetics. There was no significant difference between the anesthetic regimens for intraoperative hemodynamics, cardioactive drug use, or ischemic incidents, although only 83 patients in the sevoflurane group and 85 patients in the isoflurane group were successfully monitored for ischemia. The outcome was also equivalent in terms of adverse events, death, and postoperative myocardial infarction. Within the limits of this small multicenter study in patients at mild-to-moderate risk for myocardial ischemia, sevoflurane was a satisfactory equivalent to isoflurane in providing supplemental inhalation anesthesia to intravenous drugs.

Cesarean Section

Sevoflurane (n=29) was compared to isoflurane (n=27) in ASA Class I or II patients for the maintenance of anesthesia during cesarean section. Newborn evaluations and recovery events were recorded. With both anesthetics, Apgar scores averaged 8 and 9 at 1 and 5 minutes, respectively.

Use of sevoflurane as part of general anesthesia for elective cesarean section produced no untoward effects in mother or neonate. Sevoflurane and isoflurane demonstrated equivalent recovery characteristics. There was no difference between sevoflurane and isoflurane with regard to the effect on the newborn, as assessed by Apgar Score and Neurological and Adaptive Capacity Score (average=29.5). The safety of sevoflurane in labor and vaginal delivery has not been evaluated.

Neurosurgery

Three studies compared sevoflurane to isoflurane for maintenance of anesthesia during neurosurgical procedures. In a

Information on the AbbVie, Inc. products listed on these pages is from the prescribing information in use as of July 31, 2013. For more information, please visit rxabbvie.com or call 1-800-633-9110.

study of 20 patients, there was no difference between sevoflurane and isoflurane with regard to recovery from anesthesia. In 2 studies, a total of 22 patients with intracranial pressure (ICP) monitors received either sevoflurane or isoflurane. There was no difference between sevoflurane and isoflurane with regard to ICP response to inhalation of 0.5, 1.0, and 1.5 MAC inspired concentrations of volatile agent during N_2O-O_2-fentanyl anesthesia. During progressive hyperventilation from $PaCO_2 = 40$ to $PaCO_2 = 30$, ICP response to hypocarbia was preserved with sevoflurane at both 0.5 and 1.0 MAC concentrations. In patients at risk for elevations of ICP, sevoflurane should be administered cautiously in conjunction with ICP-reducing maneuvers such as hyperventilation.

Hepatic Impairment

A multicenter study (2 sites) compared the safety of sevoflurane and isoflurane in 16 patients with mild-to-moderate hepatic impairment utilizing the lidocaine MEGX assay for assessment of hepatocellular function. All patients received intravenous propofol (1-3 mg/kg) or thiopental (2-7 mg/kg) for induction and succinylcholine, vecuronium, or atracurium for intubation. Sevoflurane or isoflurane was administered in either 100% O_2 or up to 70% N_2O/O_2. Neither drug adversely affected hepatic function. No serum inorganic fluoride level exceeded 45 µM/L, but sevoflurane patients had prolonged terminal disposition of fluoride, as evidenced by longer inorganic fluoride half-life than patients with normal hepatic function (23 hours vs. 10-48 hours).

Renal Impairment

Sevoflurane was evaluated in renally impaired patients with baseline serum creatinine >1.5 mg/dL. Fourteen patients who received sevoflurane were compared with 12 patients who received isoflurane. In another study, 21 patients who received sevoflurane were compared with 20 patients who received enflurane. Creatinine levels increased in 7% of patients who received sevoflurane, 8% of patients who received isoflurane, and 10% of patients who received enflurane. Because of the small number of patients with renal insufficiency (baseline serum creatinine greater than 1.5 mg/dL) studied, the safety of sevoflurane administration in this group has not yet been fully established. Therefore, sevoflurane should be used with caution in patients with renal insufficiency (see **WARNINGS**).

INDICATIONS AND USAGE

Sevoflurane is indicated for induction and maintenance of general anesthesia in adult and pediatric patients for inpatient and outpatient surgery.

Sevoflurane should be administered only by persons trained in the administration of general anesthesia. Facilities for maintenance of a patent airway, artificial ventilation, oxygen enrichment, and circulatory resuscitation must be immediately available. Since level of anesthesia may be altered rapidly, only vaporizers producing predictable concentrations of sevoflurane should be used.

CONTRAINDICATIONS

Sevoflurane can cause malignant hyperthermia. It should not be used in patients with known sensitivity to sevoflurane or to other halogenated agents nor in patients with known or suspected susceptibility to malignant hyperthermia.

WARNINGS

Although data from controlled clinical studies at low flow rates are limited, findings taken from patient and animal studies suggest that there is a potential for renal injury which is presumed due to Compound A. Animal and human studies demonstrate that sevoflurane administered for more than 2 MAC•hours and at fresh gas flow rates of <2 L/min may be associated with proteinuria and glycosuria.

While a level of Compound A exposure at which clinical nephrotoxicity might be expected to occur has not been established, it is prudent to consider all of the factors leading to Compound A exposure in humans, especially duration of exposure, fresh gas flow rate, and concentration of sevoflurane. During sevoflurane anesthesia the clinician should adjust inspired concentration and fresh gas flow rate to minimize exposure to Compound A. To minimize exposure to Compound A, sevoflurane exposure should not exceed 2 MAC•hours at flow rates of 1 to <2 L/min. Fresh gas flow rates <1 L/min are not recommended.

Because clinical experience in administering sevoflurane to patients with renal insufficiency (creatinine >1.5 mg/dL) is limited, its safety in these patients has not been established.

Sevoflurane may be associated with glycosuria and proteinuria when used for long procedures at low flow rates. The safety of low flow sevoflurane on renal function was evaluated in patients with normal preoperative renal function. One study compared sevoflurane (N=98) to an active control (N=90) administered for ≥2 hours at a fresh gas flow rate of ≤1 Liter/minute. Per study defined criteria (Hou et al.) one patient in the sevoflurane group developed elevations of creatinine, in addition to glycosuria and proteinuria. This patient received sevoflurane at fresh gas flow rates of ≤800 mL/minute. Using these same criteria, there were no patients in the active control group who developed treatment emergent elevations in serum creatinine.

Sevoflurane may present an increased risk in patients with known sensitivity to volatile halogenated anesthetic agents. KOH containing CO_2 absorbents are not recommended for use with sevoflurane.

Reports of QT prolongation, associated with torsade de pointes (in exceptional cases, fatal), have been received. Caution should be exercised when administering sevoflurane to susceptible patients (e.g. patients with congenital Long QT Syndrome or patients taking drugs that can prolong the QT interval).

Malignant Hyperthermia

In susceptible individuals, potent inhalation anesthetic agents, including sevoflurane, may trigger a skeletal muscle hypermetabolic state leading to high oxygen demand and the clinical syndrome known as malignant hyperthermia. In clinical trials, one case of malignant hyperthermia was reported. In genetically susceptible pigs, sevoflurane induced malignant hyperthermia. The clinical syndrome is signaled by hypercapnia, and may include muscle rigidity, tachycardia, tachypnea, cyanosis, arrhythmias, and/or unstable blood pressure. Some of these nonspecific signs may also appear during light anesthesia, acute hypoxia, hypercapnia, and hypovolemia.

Treatment of malignant hyperthermia includes discontinuation of triggering agents, administration of intravenous dantrolene sodium, and application of supportive therapy. (Consult prescribing information for dantrolene sodium intravenous for additional information on patient management.) Renal failure may appear later, and urine flow should be monitored and sustained if possible.

Perioperative Hyperkalemia

Use of inhaled anesthetic agents has been associated with rare increases in serum potassium levels that have resulted in cardiac arrhythmias and death in pediatric patients during the postoperative period. Patients with latent as well as overt neuromuscular disease, particularly Duchenne muscular dystrophy, appear to be most vulnerable. Concomitant use of succinylcholine has been associated with most, but not all, of these cases. These patients also experienced significant elevations in serum creatine kinase levels and, in some cases, changes in urine consistent with myoglobinuria. Despite the similarity in presentation to malignant hyperthermia, none of these patients exhibited signs or symptoms of muscle rigidity or hypermetabolic state. Early and aggressive intervention to treat the hyperkalemia and resistant arrhythmias is recommended; as is subsequent evaluation for latent neuromuscular disease.

PRECAUTIONS

During the maintenance of anesthesia, increasing the concentration of sevoflurane produces dose-dependent decreases in blood pressure. Due to sevoflurane's insolubility in blood, these hemodynamic changes may occur more rapidly than with other volatile anesthetics. Excessive decreases in blood pressure or respiratory depression may be related to depth of anesthesia and may be corrected by decreasing the inspired concentration of sevoflurane.

Rare cases of seizures have been reported in association with sevoflurane use (see **PRECAUTIONS - Pediatric Use** and **ADVERSE REACTIONS**).

The recovery from general anesthesia should be assessed carefully before a patient is discharged from the post-anesthesia care unit.

Drug Interactions

In clinical trials, no significant adverse reactions occurred with other drugs commonly used in the perioperative period, including: central nervous system depressants, autonomic drugs, skeletal muscle relaxants, anti-infective agents, hormones and synthetic substitutes, blood derivatives, and cardiovascular drugs.

Intravenous Anesthetics

Sevoflurane administration is compatible with barbiturates, propofol, and other commonly used intravenous anesthetics.

Benzodiazepines and Opioids

Benzodiazepines and opioids would be expected to decrease the MAC of sevoflurane in the same manner as with other inhalational anesthetics. Sevoflurane administration is compatible with benzodiazepines and opioids as commonly used in surgical practice.

Nitrous Oxide

As with other halogenated volatile anesthetics, the anesthetic requirement for sevoflurane is decreased when administered in combination with nitrous oxide. Using 50% N_2O, the MAC equivalent dose requirement is reduced approximately 50% in adults, and approximately 25% in pediatric patients (see **DOSAGE AND ADMINISTRATION**).

Neuromuscular Blocking Agents

As is the case with other volatile anesthetics, sevoflurane increases both the intensity and duration of neuromuscular blockade induced by nondepolarizing muscle relaxants. When used to supplement alfentanil-N_2O anesthesia, sevoflurane and isoflurane equally potentiate neuromuscular block induced with pancuronium, vecuronium or atracurium. Therefore, during sevoflurane anesthesia, the dosage adjustments for these muscle relaxants are similar to those required with isoflurane.

Potentiation of neuromuscular blocking agents requires equilibration of muscle with delivered partial pressure of sevoflurane. Reduced doses of neuromuscular blocking agents during induction of anesthesia may result in delayed onset of conditions suitable for endotracheal intubation or inadequate muscle relaxation.

Among available nondepolarizing agents, only vecuronium, pancuronium and atracurium interactions have been studied during sevoflurane anesthesia. In the absence of specific guidelines:

1. For endotracheal intubation, do not reduce the dose of nondepolarizing muscle relaxants.
2. During maintenance of anesthesia, the required dose of nondepolarizing muscle relaxants is likely to be reduced compared to that during N_2O/opioid anesthesia. Administration of supplemental doses of muscle relaxants should be guided by the response to nerve stimulation.

The effect of sevoflurane on the duration of depolarizing neuromuscular blockade induced by succinylcholine has not been studied.

Hepatic Function

Results of evaluations of laboratory parameters (e.g., ALT, AST, alkaline phosphatase, and total bilirubin, etc.), as well as investigator-reported incidence of adverse events relating to liver function, demonstrate that sevoflurane can be administered to patients with normal or mild-to-moderately impaired hepatic function. However, patients with severe hepatic dysfunction were not investigated.

Occasional cases of transient changes in postoperative hepatic function tests were reported with both sevoflurane and reference agents. Sevoflurane was found to be comparable to isoflurane with regard to these changes in hepatic function.

Very rare cases of mild, moderate and severe post-operative hepatic dysfunction or hepatitis with or without jaundice have been reported from postmarketing experiences. Clinical judgement should be exercised when sevoflurane is used in patients with underlying hepatic conditions or under treatment with drugs known to cause hepatic dysfunction (see **ADVERSE REACTIONS**).

It has been reported that previous exposure to halogenated hydrocarbon anesthetics may increase the potential for hepatic injury.

Desiccated CO_2 Absorbents

An exothermic reaction occurs when sevoflurane is exposed to CO_2 absorbents. This reaction is increased when the CO_2 absorbent becomes desiccated, such as after an extended period of dry gas flow through the CO_2 absorbent canisters. Rare cases of extreme heat, smoke, and/or spontaneous fire in the anesthesia breathing circuit have been reported during sevoflurane use in conjunction with the use of desiccated CO_2 absorbent, specifically those containing potassium hydroxide (e.g. Baralyme). KOH containing CO_2 absorbents are not recommended for use with sevoflurane. An unusually delayed rise or unexpected decline of inspired sevoflurane concentration compared to the vaporizer setting may be associated with excessive heating of the CO_2 absorbent and chemical breakdown of sevoflurane.

As with other inhalational anesthetics, degradation and production of degradation products can occur when sevoflurane is exposed to desiccated absorbents. When a clinician suspects that the CO_2 absorbent may be desiccated, it should be replaced. The color indicator of most CO_2 absorbents may not change upon desiccation. Therefore, the lack of significant color change should not be taken as an assurance of adequate hydration. CO_2 absorbents should be replaced routinely regardless of the state of the color indicator.

Carcinogenesis, Mutagenesis, Impairment of Fertility

Studies on carcinogenesis have not been performed for either sevoflurane or Compound A. No mutagenic effect of sevoflurane was noted in the Ames test, mouse micronucleus test, mouse lymphoma mutagenicity assay, human lymphocyte culture assay, mammalian cell transformation assay, ^{32}P DNA adduct assay, and no chromosomal aberrations were induced in cultured mammalian cells.

Similarly, no mutagenic effect of Compound A was noted in the Ames test, the Chinese hamster chromosomal aberration assay and the *in vivo* mouse micronucleus assay. However, positive responses were observed in the human lymphocyte chromosome aberration assay. These responses were seen only at high concentrations and in the absence of metabolic activation (human S-9).

Pregnancy Category B

Reproduction studies have been performed in rats and rabbits at doses up to 1 MAC (minimum alveolar concentration) without CO_2 absorbent and have revealed no evidence of impaired fertility or harm to the fetus due to sevoflurane at 0.3 MAC, the highest nontoxic dose. Developmental and reproductive toxicity studies of sevoflurane in animals in the presence of strong alkalies (i.e., degradation of sevoflurane and production of Compound A) have not been conducted. There are no adequate and well-controlled studies in pregnant women. Because animal reproduction studies are not always predictive of human response, sevoflurane should be used during pregnancy only if clearly needed.

Labor and Delivery

Sevoflurane has been used as part of general anesthesia for elective cesarean section in 29 women. There were no untoward effects in mother or neonate (see **PHARMACODYNAMICS - Clinical Trials**). The safety of sevoflurane in labor and delivery has not been demonstrated.

Nursing Mothers

The concentrations of sevoflurane in milk are probably of no clinical importance 24 hours after anesthesia. Because of rapid washout, sevoflurane concentrations in milk are predicted to be below those found with many other volatile anesthetics.

Geriatric Use

MAC decreases with increasing age. The average concentration of sevoflurane to achieve MAC in an 80 year old is approximately 50% of that required in a 20 year old.

Pediatric Use

Induction and maintenance of general anesthesia with sevoflurane have been established in controlled clinical trials in pediatric patients aged 1 to 18 years (see **PHARMACODYNAMICS - Clinical Trials** and **ADVERSE REACTIONS**). Sevoflurane has a nonpungent odor and is suitable for mask induction in pediatric patients.

The concentration of sevoflurane required for maintenance of general anesthesia is age dependent. When used in combination with nitrous oxide, the MAC equivalent dose of sevoflurane should be reduced in pediatric patients. MAC in premature infants has not been determined (see **PRECAUTIONS - Drug Interactions** and **DOSAGE AND ADMINISTRATION** for recommendations in pediatric patients 1 day of age and older).

The use of sevoflurane has been associated with seizures (see **PRECAUTIONS** and **ADVERSE REACTIONS**). The majority of these have occurred in children and young adults starting from 2 months of age, most of whom had no predisposing risk factors. Clinical judgement should be exercised when using sevoflurane in patients who may be at risk for seizures.

ADVERSE REACTIONS

Adverse events are derived from controlled clinical trials conducted in the United States, Canada, and Europe. The reference drugs were isoflurane, enflurane, and propofol in adults and halothane in pediatric patients. The studies were conducted using a variety of premedications, other anesthetics, and surgical procedures of varying length. Most adverse events reported were mild and transient, and may reflect the surgical procedures, patient characteristics (including disease) and/or medications administered.

Of the 5182 patients enrolled in the clinical trials, 2906 were exposed to sevoflurane, including 118 adults and 507 pediatric patients who underwent mask induction. Each patient was counted once for each type of adverse event. Adverse events reported in patients in clinical trials and considered to be possibly or probably related to sevoflurane are presented within each body system in order of decreasing frequency in the following listings. One case of malignant hyperthermia was reported in pre-registration clinical trials.

Adverse Events During the Induction Period (from Onset of Anesthesia by Mask Induction to Surgical Incision) Incidence > 1%

Adult Patients (N = 118)
Cardiovascular
Bradycardia 5%, Hypotension 4%, Tachycardia 2%
Nervous System
Agitation 7%
Respiratory System
Laryngospasm 8%, Airway obstruction 8%, Breathholding 5%, Cough Increased 5%
Pediatric Patients (N = 507)
Cardiovascular
Tachycardia 6%, Hypotension 4%
Nervous System
Agitation 15%
Respiratory System
Breathholding 5%, Cough Increased 5%, Laryngospasm 3%, Apnea 2%
Digestive System
Increased salivation 2%

Adverse Events During Maintenance and Emergence Periods, Incidence >1% (N = 2906)

Body as a whole
Fever 1%, Shivering 6%, Hypothermia 1%, Movement 1%, Headache 1%
Cardiovascular
Hypotension 11%, Hypertension 2%, Bradycardia 5%, Tachycardia 2%
Nervous System
Somnolence 9%, Agitation 9%, Dizziness 4%, Increased salivation 4%
Digestive System
Nausea 25%, Vomiting 18%
Respiratory System
Cough increased 11%, Breathholding 2%, Laryngospasm 2%

Adverse Events, All Patients in Clinical Trials (N = 2906), All Anesthetic Periods, Incidence <1% (Reported in 3 or More Patients)

Body as a whole
Asthenia, Pain
Cardiovascular
Arrhythmia, Ventricular Extrasystoles, Supraventricular Extrasystoles, Complete AV Block, Bigeminy, Hemorrhage, Inverted T Wave, Atrial Fibrillation, Atrial Arrhythmia, Second Degree AV Block, Syncope, S-T Depressed
Nervous System
Crying, Nervousness, Confusion, Hypertonia, Dry Mouth, Insomnia
Respiratory System
Sputum Increased, Apnea, Hypoxia, Wheezing, Bronchospasm, Hyperventilation, Pharyngitis, Hiccup, Hypoventilation, Dyspnea, Stridor
Metabolism and Nutrition
Increases in LDH, AST, ALT, BUN, Alkaline Phosphatase, Creatinine, Bilirubinemia, Glycosuria, Fluorosis, Albuminuria, Hypophosphatemia, Acidosis, Hyperglycemia
Hemic and Lymphatic System
Leucocytosis, Thrombocytopenia
Skin and Special Senses
Amblyopia, Pruritus, Taste Perversion, Rash, Conjunctivitis
Urogenital
Urination Impaired, Urine Abnormality, Urinary Retention, Oliguria

See **WARNINGS** for information regarding malignant hyperthermia.

Post-Marketing Adverse Events

The following adverse events have been identified during post-approval use of Ultane (sevoflurane USP). Due to the spontaneous nature of these reports, the actual incidence and relationship of Ultane to these events cannot be established with certainty.

CNS

Seizures — Post-marketing reports indicate that sevoflurane use has been associated with seizures. The majority of cases were in children and young adults, most of whom had no medical history of seizures. Several cases reported no concomitant medications, and at least one case was confirmed by EEG. Although many cases were single seizures that resolved spontaneously or after treatment, cases of multiple seizures have also been reported. Seizures have occurred during, or soon after sevoflurane induction, during emergence, and during post-operative recovery up to a day following anesthesia.

Cardiac

Cardiac arrest

Hepatic

- Cases of mild, moderate and severe post-operative hepatic dysfunction or hepatitis with or without jaundice have been reported. Histological evidence was not provided for any of the reported hepatitis cases. In most of these cases, patients had underlying hepatic conditions or were under treatment with drugs known to cause hepatic dysfunction. Most of the reported events were transient and resolved spontaneously (see **PRECAUTIONS**).
- Hepatic necrosis
- Hepatic failure

Other

- Malignant hyperthermia (see **CONTRAINDICATIONS** and **WARNINGS**)
- Allergic reactions, such as rash, urticaria, pruritus, bronchospasm, anaphylactic or anaphylactoid reactions (see **CONTRAINDICATIONS**)
- Reports of hypersensitivity (including contact dermatitis, rash, dyspnea, wheezing, chest discomfort, swelling face, or anaphylactic reaction) have been received, particularly in association with long-term occupational exposure to inhaled anesthetic agents, including sevoflurane (see **OCCUPATIONAL CAUTION**).

Laboratory Findings

- Transient elevations in glucose, liver function tests, and white blood cell count may occur as with use of other anesthetic agents.

OVERDOSAGE

In the event of overdosage, or what may appear to be overdosage, the following action should be taken: discontinue administration of sevoflurane, maintain a patent airway, initiate assisted or controlled ventilation with oxygen, and maintain adequate cardiovascular function.

DOSAGE AND ADMINISTRATION

The concentration of sevoflurane being delivered from a vaporizer during anesthesia should be known. This may be accomplished by using a vaporizer calibrated specifically for sevoflurane. The administration of general anesthesia must be individualized based on the patient's response.

Replacement of Desiccated CO_2 Absorbents

When a clinician suspects that the CO_2 absorbent may be desiccated, it should be replaced. The exothermic reaction that occurs with sevoflurane and CO_2 absorbents is increased when the CO_2 absorbent becomes desiccated, such as after an extended period of dry gas flow through the CO_2 absorbent canisters (see **PRECAUTIONS**).

Pre-anesthetic Medication

No specific premedication is either indicated or contraindicated with sevoflurane. The decision as to whether or not to premedicate and the choice of premedication is left to the discretion of the anesthesiologist.

Induction

Sevoflurane has a nonpungent odor and does not cause respiratory irritability; it is suitable for mask induction in pediatrics and adults.

Maintenance

Surgical levels of anesthesia can usually be achieved with concentrations of 0.5 - 3% sevoflurane with or without the concomitant use of nitrous oxide. Sevoflurane can be administered with any type of anesthesia circuit.

Table 9. MAC Values for Adults and Pediatric Patients According to Age

Age of Patient (years)	Sevoflurane in Oxygen	Sevoflurane in 65% N_2O/35% O_2
0 - 1 months #	3.3%	
1 - < 6 months	3.0%	
6 months - < 3 years	2.8%	2.0%@
3 - 12	2.5%	
25	2.6%	1.4%
40	2.1%	1.1%
60	1.7%	0.9%
80	1.4%	0.7%

\# Neonates are full-term gestational age. MAC in premature infants has not been determined.
@ In 1 - < 3 year old pediatric patients, 60% N_2O/40% O_2 was used.

HOW SUPPLIED

ULTANE (sevoflurane), Volatile Liquid for Inhalation, is packaged in amber colored bottles containing 250 mL sevoflurane, List 4456, NDC # 0074-4456-04 (plastic).

SAFETY AND HANDLING

Occupational Caution

There is no specific work exposure limit established for sevoflurane. However, the National Institute for Occupational Safety and Health has recommended an 8 hour time-weighted average limit of 2 ppm for halogenated anesthetic agents in general (0.5 ppm when coupled with exposure to N_2O) (see **ADVERSE REACTIONS**).

Storage

Store at controlled room temperature, 15° - 30°C (59° - 86°F). See USP.

Product of Japan

Product inquiries should be directed to AbbVie Inc., North Chicago, IL 60064, USA

Manufactured by:
AbbVie Inc., North Chicago, IL 60064, USA under license from Maruishi Pharmaceutical Company LTD. 2-3-5, Fushimi-machi, Chuo-Ku, Osaka, Japan.

Ref. 03-A748-R6-Revised March, 2013

VICODIN®
VICODIN ES®
VICODIN HP®

Ⓒ℞

(hydrocodone bitartrate and acetaminophen) Tablets, USP

WARNING

HEPATOTOXICITY

ACETAMINOPHEN HAS BEEN ASSOCIATED WITH CASES OF ACUTE LIVER FAILURE, AT

Information on the AbbVie, Inc. products listed on these pages is from the prescribing information in use as of July 31, 2013. For more information, please visit rxabbvie.com or call 1-800-633-9110.

TIMES RESULTING IN LIVER TRANSPLANT AND DEATH. MOST OF THE CASES OF LIVER INJURY ARE ASSOCIATED WITH THE USE OF ACETAMINOPHEN AT DOSES THAT EXCEED 4000 MILLIGRAMS PER DAY, AND OFTEN INVOLVE MORE THAN ONE ACETAMINOPHEN-CONTAINING PRODUCT.

DESCRIPTION

Hydrocodone bitartrate and acetaminophen is supplied in tablet form for oral administration.

WARNING: May be habit-forming (see **PRECAUTIONS, Information for Patients/Caregivers**, and **DRUG ABUSE AND DEPENDENCE**).

Hydrocodone bitartrate is an opioid analgesic and antitussive and occurs as fine, white crystals or as a crystalline powder. It is affected by light. The chemical name is 4,5α-epoxy-3-methoxy-17-methylmorphinan-6-one tartrate (1:1) hydrate (2:5). It has the following structural formula:

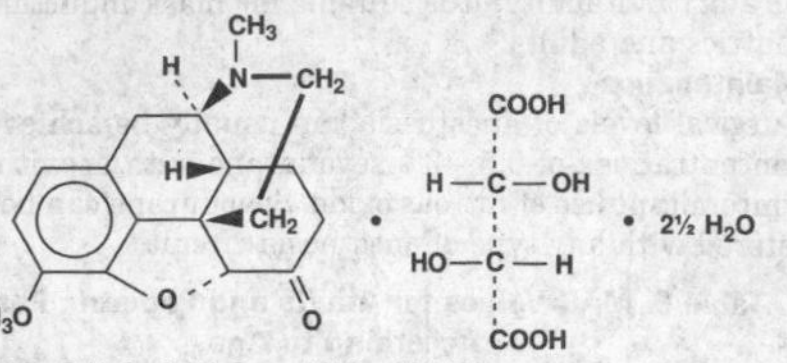

$C_{18}H_{21}NO_3 \cdot C_4H_6O_6 \cdot 2\frac{1}{2}H_2O$ M.W. = 494.490

Acetaminophen, 4′-hydroxyacetanilide, a slightly bitter, white, odorless, crystalline powder, is a non-opiate, non-salicylate analgesic and antipyretic. It has the following structural formula:

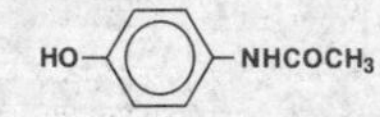

$C_8H_9NO_2$ M.W. = 151.16

Hydrocodone Bitartrate Acetaminophen Tablets, USP is available in the following strengths:

VICODIN®: Hydrocodone Bitartrate............5 mg
WARNING: May be habit-forming.
Acetaminophen..300 mg
VICODIN ES®: Hydrocodone Bitartrate.......7.5 mg
WARNING: May be habit-forming.
Acetaminophen..300 mg
VICODIN HP®: Hydrocodone Bitartrate......10 mg
WARNING: May be habit-forming.
Acetaminophen..300 mg

In addition each tablet contains the following inactive ingredients: colloidal silicon dioxide, crospovidone, magnesium stearate, microcrystalline cellulose, povidone, pregelatinized starch, and stearic acid.

This product complies with USP dissolution test 2.

CLINICAL PHARMACOLOGY

Hydrocodone is a semisynthetic narcotic analgesic and antitussive with multiple actions qualitatively similar to those of codeine. Most of these involve the central nervous system and smooth muscle. The precise mechanism of action of hydrocodone and other opiates is not known, although it is believed to relate to the existence of opiate receptors in the central nervous system. In addition to analgesia, narcotics may produce drowsiness, changes in mood and mental clouding.

The analgesic action of acetaminophen involves peripheral influences, but the specific mechanism is as yet undetermined. Antipyretic activity is mediated through hypothalamic heat regulating centers. Acetaminophen inhibits prostaglandin synthetase. Therapeutic doses of acetaminophen have negligible effects on the cardiovascular or respiratory systems; however, toxic doses may cause circulatory failure and rapid, shallow breathing.

Pharmacokinetics

The behavior of the individual components is described below.

Hydrocodone

Following a 10 mg oral dose of hydrocodone administered to five adult male subjects, the mean peak concentration was 23.6 ± 5.2 ng/mL. Maximum serum levels were achieved at 1.3 ± 0.3 hours and the half-life was determined to be 3.8 ± 0.3 hours. Hydrocodone exhibits a complex pattern of metabolism including O-demethylation, N-demethylation and 6-keto reduction to the corresponding 6-α- and 6-β-hydroxymetabolites. See **OVERDOSAGE** for toxicity information.

Acetaminophen

Acetaminophen is rapidly absorbed from the gastrointestinal tract and is distributed throughout most body tissues. The plasma half-life is 1.25 to 3 hours, but may be increased by liver damage and following overdosage. Elimination of acetaminophen is principally by liver metabolism (conjugation) and subsequent renal excretion of metabolites. Approximately 85% of an oral dose appears in the urine within 24 hours of administration, most as the glucuronide conjugate, with small amounts of other conjugates and unchanged drug. See **OVERDOSAGE** for toxicity information.

INDICATIONS AND USAGE

Hydrocodone bitartrate and acetaminophen tablets are indicated for the relief of moderate to moderately severe pain.

CONTRAINDICATIONS

This product should not be administered to patients who have previously exhibited hypersensitivity to hydrocodone or acetaminophen.

Patients known to be hypersensitive to other opioids may exhibit cross sensitivity to hydrocodone.

WARNINGS

Hepatotoxicity

Acetaminophen has been associated with cases of acute liver failure, at times resulting in liver transplant and death. Most of the cases of liver injury are associated with the use of acetaminophen at doses that exceed 4000 milligrams per day, and often involve more than one acetaminophen-containing product. The excessive intake of acetaminophen may be intentional to cause self-harm or unintentional as patients attempt to obtain more pain relief or unknowingly take other acetaminophen-containing products.

The risk of acute liver failure is higher in individuals with underlying liver disease and in individuals who ingest alcohol while taking acetaminophen.

Instruct patients to look for acetaminophen or APAP on package labels and not to use more than one product that contains acetaminophen. Instruct patients to seek medical attention immediately upon ingestion of more than 4000 milligrams of acetaminophen per day, even if they feel well.

Hypersensitivity/anaphylaxis

There have been post-marketing reports of hypersensitivity and anaphylaxis associated with use of acetaminophen. Clinical signs included swelling of the face, mouth and throat, respiratory distress, urticaria, rash, pruritus, and vomiting. There were infrequent reports of life-threatening anaphylaxis requiring emergency medical attention. Instruct patients to discontinue hydrocodone bitartrate and acetaminophen tablets immediately and seek medical care if they experience these symptoms. Do not prescribe hydrocodone bitartrate and acetaminophen tablets for patients with acetaminophen allergy.

Respiratory Depression

At high doses or in sensitive patients, hydrocodone may produce dose-related respiratory depression by acting directly on the brain stem respiratory center. Hydrocodone also affects the center that controls respiratory rhythm, and may produce irregular and periodic breathing.

Head Injury and Increased Intracranial Pressure

The respiratory depressant effects of narcotics and their capacity to elevate cerebrospinal fluid pressure may be markedly exaggerated in the presence of head injury, other intracranial lesions or a preexisting increase in intracranial pressure. Furthermore, narcotics produce adverse reactions which may obscure the clinical course of patients with head injuries.

Acute Abdominal Conditions

The administration of narcotics may obscure the diagnosis or clinical course of patients with acute abdominal conditions.

PRECAUTIONS

General

Special Risk Patients

As with any narcotic analgesic agent, hydrocodone bitartrate and acetaminophen tablets should be used with caution in elderly or debilitated patients and those with severe impairment of hepatic or renal function, hypothyroidism, Addison's disease, prostatic hypertrophy or urethral stricture. The usual precautions should be observed and the possibility of respiratory depression should be kept in mind.

Cough Reflex

Hydrocodone suppresses the cough reflex; as with all narcotics, caution should be exercised when hydrocodone bitartrate and acetaminophen tablets are used postoperatively and in patients with pulmonary disease.

Information for Patients/Caregivers

- Do not take hydrocodone bitartrate and acetaminophen tablets if you are allergic to any of its ingredients.
- If you develop signs of allergy such as a rash or difficulty breathing stop taking hydrocodone bitartrate and acetaminophen tablets and contact your healthcare provider immediately.
- Do not take more than 4000 milligrams of acetaminophen per day. Call your doctor if you took more than the recommended dose.

Hydrocodone, like all narcotics, may impair the mental and/or physical abilities required for the performance of potentially hazardous tasks such as driving a car or operating machinery; patients should be cautioned accordingly.

Alcohol and other CNS depressants may produce an additive CNS depression, when taken with this combination product, and should be avoided.

Hydrocodone may be habit forming. Patients should take the drug only for as long as it is prescribed, in the amounts prescribed, and no more frequently than prescribed.

Laboratory Tests

In patients with severe hepatic or renal disease, effects of therapy should be monitored with serial liver and/or renal function tests.

Drug Interactions

Patients receiving other narcotics, antihistamines, antipsychotics, antianxiety agents, or other CNS depressants (including alcohol) concomitantly with hydrocodone bitartrate and acetaminophen tablets may exhibit an additive CNS depression. When combined therapy is contemplated, the dose of one or both agents should be reduced.

The use of MAO inhibitors or tricyclic antidepressants with hydrocodone preparations may increase the effect of either the antidepressant or hydrocodone.

Drug/Laboratory Test Interactions

Acetaminophen may produce false-positive test results for urinary 5-hydroxyindoleacetic acid.

Carcinogenesis, Mutagenesis, Impairment of Fertility

No adequate studies have been conducted in animals to determine whether hydrocodone or acetaminophen have a potential for carcinogenesis, mutagenesis, or impairment of fertility.

Pregnancy

Teratogenic Effects

Pregnancy Category C

There are no adequate and well-controlled studies in pregnant women. Hydrocodone bitartrate and acetaminophen tablets should be used during pregnancy only if the potential benefit justifies the potential risk to the fetus.

Nonteratogenic Effects

Babies born to mothers who have been taking opioids regularly prior to delivery will be physically dependent. The withdrawal signs include irritability and excessive crying, tremors, hyperactive reflexes, increased respiratory rate, increased stools, sneezing, yawning, vomiting, and fever. The intensity of the syndrome does not always correlate with the duration of maternal opioid use or dose. There is no consensus on the best method of managing withdrawal.

Labor and Delivery

As with all narcotics, administration of this product to the mother shortly before delivery may result in some degree of respiratory depression in the newborn, especially if higher doses are used.

Nursing Mothers

Acetaminophen is excreted in breast milk in small amounts, but the significance of its effects on nursing infants is not known. It is not known whether hydrocodone is excreted in human milk. Because many drugs are excreted in human milk and because of the potential for serious adverse reactions in nursing infants from hydrocodone and acetaminophen, a decision should be made whether to discontinue nursing or to discontinue the drug, taking into account the importance of the drug to the mother.

Pediatric Use

Safety and effectiveness in pediatric patients have not been established.

Geriatric Use

Clinical studies of hydrocodone bitartrate and acetaminophen tablets did not include sufficient numbers of subjects aged 65 and over to determine whether they respond differently from younger subjects. Other reported clinical experience has not identified differences in responses between the elderly and younger patients. In general, dose selection for an elderly patient should be cautious, usually starting at the low end of the dosing range, reflecting the greater frequency of decreased hepatic, renal, or cardiac function, and of concomitant disease or other drug therapy.

Hydrocodone and the major metabolites of acetaminophen are known to be substantially excreted by the kidney. Thus the risk of toxic reactions may be greater in patients with impaired renal function due to accumulation of the parent compound and/or metabolites in the plasma. Because elderly patients are more likely to have decreased renal function, care should be taken in dose selection, and it may be useful to monitor renal function.

Hydrocodone may cause confusion and over-sedation in the elderly; elderly patients generally should be started on low doses of hydrocodone bitartrate and acetaminophen tablets and observed closely.

ADVERSE REACTIONS

The most frequently reported adverse reactions are lightheadedness, dizziness, sedation, nausea and vomiting.

These effects seem to be more prominent in ambulatory than in nonambulatory patients, and some of these adverse reactions may be alleviated if the patient lies down.

Other adverse reactions include:

Central Nervous System

Drowsiness, mental clouding, lethargy, impairment of mental and physical performance, anxiety, fear, dysphoria, psychic dependence, mood changes.

Gastrointestinal System

Prolonged administration of hydrocodone bitartrate and acetaminophen tablets may produce constipation.

Genitourinary System

Ureteral spasm, spasm of vesical sphincters and urinary retention have been reported with opiates.

Respiratory Depression

Hydrocodone bitartrate may produce dose-related respiratory depression by acting directly on the brain stem respiratory centers (see **OVERDOSAGE**).

Special Senses

Cases of hearing impairment or permanent loss have been reported predominantly in patients with chronic overdose.

Dermatological

Skin rash, pruritus.

The following adverse drug events may be borne in mind as potential effects of acetaminophen: allergic reactions, rash, thrombocytopenia, agranulocytosis, Stevens-Johnson syndrome, toxic epidermal necrolysis.

Potential effects of high dosage are listed in the **OVERDOSAGE** section.

DRUG ABUSE AND DEPENDENCE

Controlled Substance

Hydrocone bitartrate and acetaminophen tablets is classified as a Schedule III controlled substance.

Abuse and Dependence

Psychic dependence, physical dependence, and tolerance may develop upon repeated administration of narcotics; therefore, this product should be prescribed and administered with caution. However, psychic dependence is unlikely to develop when hydrocodone bitartrate and acetaminophen tablets are used for a short time for the treatment of pain.

Physical dependence, the condition in which continued administration of the drug is required to prevent the appearance of a withdrawal syndrome, assumes clinically significant proportions only after several weeks of continued narcotic use, although some mild degree of physical dependence may develop after a few days of narcotic therapy. Tolerance, in which increasingly large doses are required in order to produce the same degree of analgesia, is manifested initially by a shortened duration of analgesic effect, and subsequently by decreases in the intensity of analgesia. The rate of development of tolerance varies among patients.

OVERDOSAGE

Following an acute overdosage, toxicity may result from hydrocodone or acetaminophen.

Signs and Symptoms

Hydrocodone: Serious overdose with hydrocodone is characterized by respiratory depression (a decrease in respiratory rate and/or tidal volume, Cheyne-Stokes respiration, cyanosis), extreme somnolence progressing to stupor or coma, skeletal muscle flaccidity, cold and clammy skin, and sometimes bradycardia and hypotension. In severe overdosage, apnea, circulatory collapse, cardiac arrest and death may occur.

Acetaminophen: In acetaminophen overdosage: dose-dependent, potentially fatal hepatic necrosis is the most serious adverse effect. Renal tubular necrosis, hypoglycemic coma, and coagulation defects may also occur.

Early symptoms following a potentially hepatotoxic overdose may include: nausea, vomiting, diaphoresis and general malaise. Clinical and laboratory evidence of hepatic toxicity may not be apparent until 48 to 72 hours post-ingestion.

Treatment

A single or multiple drug overdose with hydrocodone and acetaminophen is a potentially lethal polydrug overdose, and consultation with a regional poison control center is recommended.

Immediate treatment includes support of cardiorespiratory function and measures to reduce drug absorption.

Oxygen, intravenous fluids, vasopressors, and other supportive measures should be employed as indicated. Assisted or controlled ventilation should also be considered.

For hydrocodone overdose, primary attention should be given to the reestablishment of adequate respiratory exchange through provision of a patent airway and the institution of assisted or controlled ventilation. The narcotic antagonist naloxone hydrochloride is a specific antidote against respiratory depression which may result from overdosage or unusual sensitivity to narcotics, including hydrocodone. Since the duration of action of hydrocodone may exceed that of the antagonist, the patient should be kept under continued surveillance, and repeated doses of the antagonist should be administered as needed to maintain adequate respiration. A narcotic antagonist should not be administered in the absence of clinically significant respiratory or cardiovascular depression.

Gastric decontamination with activated charcoal should be administered just prior to N-acetylcysteine (NAC) to decrease systemic absorption if acetaminophen ingestion is known or suspected to have occurred within a few hours of presentation. Serum acetaminophen levels should be obtained immediately if the patient presents 4 hours or more after ingestion to assess potential risk of hepatotoxicity; acetaminophen levels drawn less than 4 hours post-ingestion may be misleading. To obtain the best possible outcome, NAC should be administered as soon as possible where impending or evolving liver injury is suspected. Intravenous NAC may be administered when circumstances preclude oral administration.

Vigorous supportive therapy is required in severe intoxication. Procedures to limit the continuing absorption of the drug must be readily performed since the hepatic injury is dose dependent and occurs early in the course of intoxication.

DOSAGE AND ADMINISTRATION

Dosage should be adjusted according to the severity of the pain and the response of the patient. However, it should be kept in mind that tolerance to hydrocodone can develop with continued use and that the incidence of untoward effects is dose related.

VICODIN® (Hydrocodone Bitartrate and Acetaminophen Tablets, USP 5 mg/300 mg): The usual adult dosage is one or two tablets every four to six hours as needed for pain. The total daily dosage should not exceed 8 tablets.

VICODIN ES® (Hydrocodone Bitartrate and Acetaminophen Tablets, USP 7.5 mg/300 mg): The usual adult dosage is one tablet every four to six hours as needed for pain. The total daily dosage should not exceed 6 tablets.

VICODIN HP® (Hydrocodone Bitartrate and Acetaminophen Tablets, USP 10 mg/300 mg): The usual adult dosage is one tablet every four to six hours as needed for pain. The total daily dosage should not exceed 6 tablets.

HOW SUPPLIED

VICODIN®, VICODIN ES® and VICODIN HP® (Hydrocodone Bitartrate and Acetaminophen) Tablets, USP are supplied as follows:

VICODIN® 5 mg/300 mg

White, capsule-shaped, bisected tablets, debossed "5" score "300"on one side and "VICODIN" on the other side in bottles of 100 and 500 tablets:

Bottles of 100 - NDC 0074-3041-13
Bottles of 500 - NDC 0074-3041-53

VICODIN ES® 7.5 mg/300 mg

White, capsule-shaped, bisected tablets, debossed "7.5" score "300" on one side and "VICODIN ES" on the other side in bottles of 100 and 500 tablets:

Bottles of 100 - NDC 0074-3043-13
Bottles of 500 - NDC 0074-3043-53

VICODIN HP® 10 mg/300 mg

White, capsule-shaped, bisected tablets, debossed "10" score "300" on one side and "VICODIN HP" on the other side in bottles of 100 and 500 tablets:

Bottles of 100 - NDC 0074-3054-13
Bottles of 500 - NDC 0074-3054-53

STORAGE

Store at 20° to 25°C (68° to 77°F). [See USP Controlled Room Temperature].

PHARMACIST: Dispense in a tight, light-resistant container with a child-resistant closure.

A Schedule III Narcotic

Manufactured for
AbbVie Inc.
North Chicago, IL 60064 U.S.A.
Manufactured by:
Mikart, Inc.
Atlanta, GA 30318
Ref: 1122F00 Rev. 03/13 - Revised March, 2013

Shown in Product Identification Guide, page 304

VICODIN® ℂⅢ

(hydrocodone bitartrate and acetaminophen tablets, USP)
5 mg/500 mg

> **BOXED WARNING**
>
> **Hepatotoxicity**
>
> Acetaminophen has been associated with cases of acute liver failure, at times resulting in liver transplant and death. Most of the cases of liver injury are associated with the use of acetaminophen at doses that exceed 4000 milligrams per day, and often involve more than one acetaminophen-containing product.

DESCRIPTION

Hydrocodone bitartrate and acetaminophen is supplied in tablet form for oral administration.

Hydrocodone bitartrate is an opioid analgesic and antitussive and occurs as fine, white crystals or as a crystalline powder. It is affected by light. The chemical name is: 4,5α-epoxy-3-methoxy-17-methylmorphinan-6-one tartrate (1:1) hydrate (2:5). It has the following structural formula:

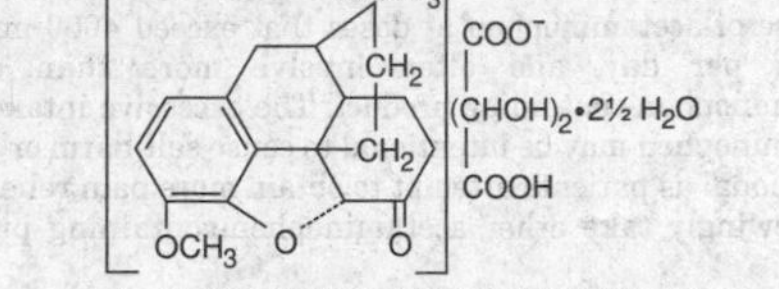

$C_{18}H_{21}NO_3 \cdot C_4H_6O_6 \cdot 2\frac{1}{2}H_2O$ M.W. 494.50

Acetaminophen, 4′-hydroxyacetanilide, a slightly bitter, white, odorless, crystalline powder, is a non-opiate, non-salicylate analgesic and antipyretic. It has the following structural formula:

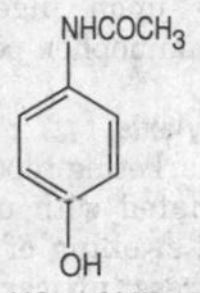

$C_8H_9NO_2$ M.W. 151.16

Each VICODIN tablet contains:
Hydrocodone Bitartrate 5 mg
Acetaminophen 500 mg

In addition each tablet contains the following inactive ingredients: colloidal silicon dioxide, starch, croscarmellose sodium, dibasic calcium phosphate, magnesium stearate, microcrystalline cellulose, povidone, and stearic acid.

Meets USP Dissolution Test 2.

CLINICAL PHARMACOLOGY

Hydrocodone is a semisynthetic narcotic analgesic and antitussive with multiple actions qualitatively similar to those of codeine. Most of these involve the central nervous system and smooth muscle. The precise mechanism of action of hydrocodone and other opiates is not known, although it is believed to relate to the existence of opiate receptors in the central nervous system. In addition to analgesia, narcotics may produce drowsiness, changes in mood and mental clouding.

The analgesic action of acetaminophen involves peripheral influences, but the specific mechanism is as yet undetermined. Antipyretic activity is mediated through hypothalamic heat regulating centers. Acetaminophen inhibits prostaglandin synthetase. Therapeutic doses of acetaminophen have negligible effects on the cardiovascular or respiratory systems; however, toxic doses may cause circulatory failure and rapid, shallow breathing.

Pharmacokinetics

The behavior of the individual components is described below.

Hydrocodone

Following a 10 mg oral dose of hydrocodone administered to five adult male subjects, the mean peak concentration was 23.6 ± 5.2 ng/mL. Maximum serum levels were achieved at 1.3 ± 0.3 hours and the half-life was determined to be 3.8 ± 0.3 hours. Hydrocodone exhibits a complex pattern of metabolism including O-demethylation, N-demethylation and 6-keto reduction to the corresponding 6-α- and 6-β-hydroxymetabolites. See **OVERDOSAGE** for toxicity information.

Acetaminophen

Acetaminophen is rapidly absorbed from the gastrointestinal tract and is distributed throughout most body tissues. The plasma half-life is 1.25 to 3 hours, but may be increased by liver damage and following overdosage. Elimination of acetaminophen is principally by liver metabolism (conjugation) and subsequent renal excretion of metabolites. Approximately 85% of an oral dose appears in the urine within 24 hours of administration, most as the glucuronide conjugate, with small amounts of other conjugates and unchanged drug. See OVERDOSAGE for toxicity information.

Information on the AbbVie, Inc. products listed on these pages is from the prescribing information in use as of July 31, 2013. For more information, please visit rxabbvie.com or call 1-800-633-9110.

INDICATIONS AND USAGE

VICODIN tablets are indicated for the relief of moderate to moderately severe pain.

CONTRAINDICATIONS

This product should not be administered to patients who have previously exhibited hypersensitivity to hydrocodone or acetaminophen.

Patients known to be hypersensitive to other opioids may exhibit cross-sensitivity to hydrocodone.

WARNINGS

Hepatotoxicity

Acetaminophen has been associated with cases of acute liver failure, at times resulting in liver transplant and death. Most of the cases of liver injury are associated with the use of acetaminophen at doses that exceed 4000 milligrams per day, and often involve more than one acetaminophen-containing product. The excessive intake of acetaminophen may be intentional to cause self-harm or unintentional as patients attempt to obtain more pain relief or unknowingly take other acetaminophen-containing products.

The risk of acute liver failure is higher in individuals with underlying liver disease and in individuals who ingest alcohol while taking acetaminophen.

Instruct patients to look for acetaminophen or APAP on package labels and not to use more than one product that contains acetaminophen. Instruct patients to seek medical attention immediately upon ingestion of more than 4000 milligrams of acetaminophen per day, even if they feel well.

Hypersensitivity/anaphylaxis

There have been post-marketing reports of hypersensitivity and anaphylaxis associated with use of acetaminophen. Clinical signs included swelling of the face, mouth, and throat, respiratory distress, urticaria, rash, pruritis, and vomiting. There were infrequent reports of life-threatening anaphylaxis requiring emergency medical attention. Instruct patients to discontinue VICODIN Tablets immediately and seek medical care if they experience these symptoms. Do not prescribe VICODIN Tablets for patients with acetaminophen allergy.

Respiratory Depression

At high doses or in sensitive patients, hydrocodone may produce dose-related respiratory depression by acting directly on the brain stem respiratory center. Hydrocodone also affects the center that controls respiratory rhythm, and may produce irregular and periodic breathing.

Head Injury and Increased Intracranial Pressure

The respiratory depressant effects of narcotics and their capacity to elevate cerebrospinal fluid pressure may be markedly exaggerated in the presence of head injury, other intracranial lesions or a preexisting increase in intracranial pressure. Furthermore, narcotics produce adverse reactions which may obscure the clinical course of patients with head injuries.

Acute Abdominal Conditions

The administration of narcotics may obscure the diagnosis or clinical course of patients with acute abdominal conditions.

Misuse, Abuse, and Diversion of Opioids

VICODIN tablets contains hydrocodone an opioid agonist, and is a Schedule III controlled substance. Opioid agonists have the potential for being abused and are sought by abusers and people with addiction disorders, and are subject to diversion.

VICODIN tablets can be abused in a manner similar to other opioid agonists, legal or illicit. This should be considered when prescribing or dispensing VICODIN tablets in situations where the physician or pharmacist is concerned about an increased risk of misuse, abuse or diversion (see **DRUG ABUSE AND DEPENDENCE**).

PRECAUTIONS

General

Special Risk Patients

As with any narcotic analgesic agent, VICODIN Tablets should be used with caution in elderly or debilitated patients and those with severe impairment of hepatic or renal function, hypothyroidism, Addison's disease, prostatic hypertrophy or urethral stricture. The usual precautions should be observed and the possibility of respiratory depression should be kept in mind.

Cough Reflex

Hydrocodone suppresses the cough reflex; as with all narcotics, caution should be exercised when VICODIN Tablets are used postoperatively and in patients with pulmonary disease.

Information for Patients/Caregivers

- Do not take VICODIN Tablets if you are allergic to any of its ingredients.
- If you develop signs of allergy such as a rash or difficulty breathing stop taking VICODIN Tablets and contact your healthcare provider immediately.
- Do not take more than 4000 milligrams of acetaminophen per day. Call your doctor if you took more than the recommended dose.

Hydrocodone, like all narcotics, may impair the mental and/or physical abilities required for the performance of potentially hazardous tasks such as driving a car or operating machinery; patients should be cautioned accordingly. Alcohol and other CNS depressants may produce an additive CNS depression, when taken with this combination product, and should be avoided.

Hydrocodone may be habit forming. Patients should take the drug only for as long as it is prescribed, in the amounts prescribed, and no more frequently than prescribed.

Laboratory Tests

In patients with severe hepatic or renal disease, effects of therapy should be monitored with serial liver and/or renal function tests.

Drug Interactions

Patients receiving other narcotic analgesics, antihistamines, antipsychotics, antianxiety agents, or other CNS depressants (including alcohol) concomitantly with VICODIN Tablets may exhibit an additive CNS depression. When combined therapy is contemplated, the dose of one or both agents should be reduced.

The use of MAO inhibitors or tricyclic antidepressants with hydrocodone preparations may increase the effect of either the antidepressant or hydrocodone.

Drug/Laboratory Test Interactions

Acetaminophen may produce false-positive test results for urinary 5-hydroxyindoleacetic acid.

Carcinogenesis, Mutagenesis, Impairment of Fertility

No adequate studies have been conducted in animals to determine whether hydrocodone or acetaminophen have a potential for carcinogenesis, mutagenesis, or impairment of fertility.

Pregnancy

Teratogenic Effects

Pregnancy Category C

There are no adequate and well-controlled studies in pregnant women. VICODIN Tablets should be used during pregnancy only if the potential benefit justifies the potential risk to the fetus.

Nonteratogenic Effects

Babies born to mothers who have been taking opioids regularly prior to delivery will be physically dependent. The withdrawal signs include irritability and excessive crying, tremors, hyperactive reflexes, increased respiratory rate, increased stools, sneezing, yawning, vomiting, and fever. The intensity of the syndrome does not always correlate with the duration of maternal opioid use or dose. There is no consensus on the best method of managing withdrawal.

Labor and Delivery

As with all narcotics, administration of VICODIN Tablets to the mother shortly before delivery may result in some degree of respiratory depression in the newborn, especially if higher doses are used.

Nursing Mothers

Acetaminophen is excreted in breast milk in small amounts, but the significance of its effects on nursing infants is not known. It is not known whether hydrocodone is excreted in human milk. Because many drugs are excreted in human milk and because of the potential for serious adverse reactions in nursing infants from hydrocodone and acetaminophen, a decision should be made whether to discontinue nursing or to discontinue the drug, taking into account the importance of the drug to the mother.

Pediatric Use

Safety and effectiveness in the pediatric population have not been established.

Geriatric Use

Clinical studies of VICODIN® (hydrocodone bitartrate 5 mg and acetaminophen 500 mg) did not include sufficient numbers of subjects aged 65 and over to determine whether they respond differently from younger subjects. Other reported clinical experience has not identified differences in responses between the elderly and younger patients. In general, dose selection for an elderly patient should be cautious, usually starting at the low end of the dosing range, reflecting the greater frequency of decreased hepatic, renal, or cardiac function, and of concomitant disease or other drug therapy.

Hydrocodone and the major metabolites of acetaminophen are known to be substantially excreted by the kidney. Thus the risk of toxic reactions may be greater in patients with impaired renal function due to accumulation of the parent compound and/or metabolites in the plasma. Because elderly patients are more likely to have decreased renal function, care should be taken in dose selection, and it may be useful to monitor renal function.

Hydrocodone may cause confusion and over-sedation in the elderly; elderly patients generally should be started on low doses of hydrocodone bitartrate and acetaminophen tablets and observed closely.

ADVERSE REACTIONS

The most frequently reported adverse reactions include: lightheadedness, dizziness, sedation, nausea and vomiting. These effects seem to be more prominent in ambulatory than in nonambulatory patients and some of these adverse reactions may be alleviated if the patient lies down.

Other adverse reactions include:

Central Nervous System

Drowsiness, mental clouding, lethargy, impairment of mental and physical performance, anxiety, fear, dysphoria, psychic dependence, mood changes.

Gastrointestinal System

Prolonged administration of VICODIN Tablets may produce constipation.

Genitourinary System

Ureteral spasm, spasm of vesical sphincters and urinary retention have been reported with opiates.

Respiratory Depression

Hydrocodone bitartrate may produce dose-related respiratory depression by acting directly on the brain stem respiratory center. (see **OVERDOSAGE**).

Special Senses

Cases of hearing impairment or permanent loss have been reported predominantly in patients with chronic overdose.

Dermatological

Skin rash, pruritus.

The following adverse drug events may be borne in mind as potential effects of acetaminophen: allergic reactions, rash, thrombocytopenia, agranulocytosis, Stevens-Johnson syndrome, toxic epidermal necrolysis.

Potential effects of high dosage are listed in the **OVERDOSAGE** section.

DRUG ABUSE AND DEPENDENCE

Misuse, Abuse, and Diversion of Opioids

VICODIN contains hydrocodone, an opioid agonist, and is a Schedule III controlled substance. VICODIN, and other opioids used in analgesia can be abused and are subject to criminal diversion.

Addiction is a primary, chronic, neurobiologic disease, with genetic, psychosocial, and environmental factors influencing its development and manifestations. It is characterized by behaviors that include one or more of the following: impaired control over drug use, compulsive use, continued use despite harm, and craving. Drug addiction is a treatable disease utilizing a multidisciplinary approach, but relapse is common.

"Drug seeking" behavior is very common in addicts and drug abusers. Drug-seeking tactics include emergency calls or visits near the end of office hours, refusal to undergo appropriate examination, testing or referral, repeated "loss" of prescriptions, tampering with prescriptions and reluctance to provide prior medical records or contact information for other treating physician(s). "Doctor shopping" to obtain additional prescriptions is common among drug abusers and people suffering from untreated addiction.

Abuse and addiction are separate and distinct from physical dependence and tolerance. Physical dependence usually assumes clinically significant dimensions only after several weeks of continued opioid use, although a mild degree of physical dependence may develop after a few days of opioid therapy. Tolerance, in which increasingly large doses are required in order to produce the same degree of analgesia, is manifested initially by a shortened duration of analgesic effect, and subsequently by decreases in the intensity of analgesia. The rate of development of tolerance varies among patients. Physicians should be aware that abuse of opioids can occur in the absence of true addiction and is characterized by misuse for non-medical purposes, often in combination with other psychoactive substances. VICODIN, like other opioids, may be diverted for non-medical use. Record-keeping of prescribing information, including quantity, frequency, and renewal requests is strongly advised.

Proper assessment of the patient, proper prescribing practices, periodic re-evaluation of therapy, and proper dispensing and storage are appropriate measures that help to limit abuse of opioid drugs.

OVERDOSAGE

Following an acute overdosage, toxicity may result from hydrocodone or acetaminophen.

Signs and Symptoms

Hydrocodone: Serious overdose with hydrocodone is characterized by respiratory depression (a decrease in respiratory rate and/or tidal volume, Cheyne-Stokes respiration, cyanosis), extreme somnolence progressing to stupor or coma, skeletal muscle flaccidity, cold and clammy skin, and sometimes bradycardia and hypotension. In severe overdosage, apnea, circulatory collapse, cardiac arrest and death may occur.

Acetaminophen: In acetaminophen overdosage: dose-dependent, potentially fatal hepatic necrosis is the most serious adverse effect. Renal tubular necrosis, hypoglycemic coma, and coagulation defects may also occur.

Early symptoms following a potentially hepatotoxic overdose may include: nausea, vomiting, diaphoresis and general malaise. Clinical and laboratory evidence of hepatic toxicity may not be apparent until 48 to 72 hours post-ingestion.

Treatment

A single or multiple drug overdose with hydrocodone and acetaminophen is a potentially lethal polydrug overdose, and consultation with a regional poison control center is recommended.

Immediate treatment includes support of cardiorespiratory function and measures to reduce drug absorption.

Oxygen, intravenous fluids, vasopressors, and other supportive measures should be employed as indicated. Assisted or controlled ventilation should also be considered.

For hydrocodone overdose, primary attention should be given to the reestablishment of adequate respiratory exchange through provision of a patent airway and the institution of assisted or controlled ventilation. The narcotic antagonist naloxone hydrochloride is a specific antidote against respiratory depression which may result from overdosage or unusual sensitivity to narcotics, including hydrocodone. Since the duration of action of hydrocodone may exceed that of the antagonist, the patient should be kept under continued surveillance, and repeated doses of the antagonist should be administered as needed to maintain adequate respiration. A narcotic antagonist should not be administered in the absence of clinically significant respiratory or cardiovascular depression.

Gastric decontamination with activated charcoal should be administered just prior to N-acetylcysteine (NAC) to decrease systemic absorption if acetaminophen ingestion is known or suspected to have occurred within a few hours of presentation. Serum acetaminophen levels should be obtained immediately if the patient presents 4 hours or more after ingestion to assess potential risk of hepatotoxicity; acetaminophen levels drawn less than 4 hours post-ingestion may be misleading. To obtain the best possible outcome, NAC should be administered as soon as possible where impending or evolving liver injury is suspected. Intravenous NAC may be administered when circumstances preclude oral administration.

Vigorous supportive therapy is required in severe intoxication. Procedures to limit the continuing absorption of the drug must be readily performed since the hepatic injury is dose dependent and occurs early in the course of intoxication.

DOSAGE AND ADMINISTRATION

Dosage should be adjusted according to the severity of the pain and the response of the patient. However, it should be kept in mind that tolerance to hydrocodone can develop with continued use and that the incidence of untoward effects is dose related.

The usual adult dosage is one or two tablets every four to six hours as needed for pain. The total daily dosage should not exceed 8 tablets.

HOW SUPPLIED

VICODIN is supplied as white, capsule-shaped tablets containing 5 mg hydrocodone bitartrate and 500 mg acetaminophen, bisected on one side and debossed with "VICODIN" on the other.

Bottles of 100-NDC 0074-1949-14.
Bottles of 500-NDC 0074-1949-54.
Hospital Unit Dose Package-100 tablets (4 × 25 tablets)-NDC 0074-1949-12.

Storage

Store at 25°C (77°F); excursions permitted to 15°-30°C (59°-86°F). [See USP Controlled Room Temperature].

Dispense in a tight, light-resistant container as defined in the USP.

A Schedule CIII controlled drug substance.

©Abbott

Manufactured for
Abbott Laboratories
North Chicago, IL 60064 U.S.A.
by Halo Pharmaceutical Inc.
Whippany, NJ 07981 U.S.A.
Ref. 03-A540-R8-Rev. September, 2011

Shown in Product Identification Guide, page 304

VICODIN ES® CIII

(hydrocodone bitartrate and acetaminophen tablets, USP)
7.5 mg/750 mg

BOXED WARNING

Hepatotoxicity

Acetaminophen has been associated with cases of acute liver failure, at times resulting in liver transplant and death. Most of the cases of liver injury are associated with the use of acetaminophen at doses that exceed 4000 milligrams per day, and often involve more than one acetaminophen-containing product.

DESCRIPTION

Hydrocodone bitartrate and acetaminophen is supplied in tablet form for oral administration.

Hydrocodone bitartrate is an opioid analgesic and antitussive and occurs as fine, white crystals or as a crystalline powder. It is affected by light. The chemical name is: 4,5α-epoxy-3-methoxy-17-methylmorphinan-6-one tartrate (1:1) hydrate (2:5). It has the following structural formula:

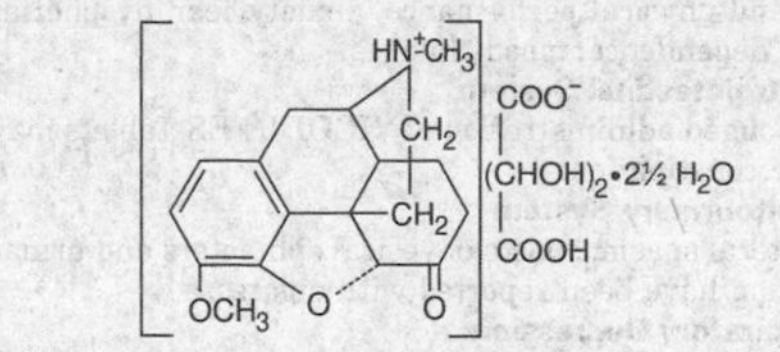

$C_{18}H_{21}NO_3 \cdot C_4H_6O_6 \cdot 2½H_2O$ M.W. – 494.50

Acetaminophen, 4′-hydroxyacetanilide, a slightly bitter, white, odorless, crystalline powder, is a non-opiate, non-salicylate analgesic and antipyretic. It has the following structural formula:

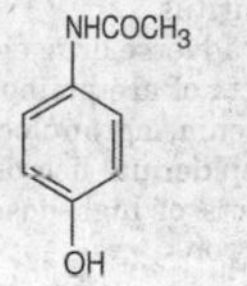

$C_8H_9NO_2$ M.W.151.16

Each VICODIN ES Tablet contains:
Hydrocodone Bitartrate 7.5 mg
Acetaminophen 750 mg

In addition each tablet contains the following inactive ingredients: Colloidal silicon dioxide, pregelatinized starch, magnesium stearate, croscarmellose sodium povidone, and stearic acid.

Meets USP Dissolution Test 2.

CLINICAL PHARMACOLOGY

Hydrocodone is a semisynthetic narcotic analgesic and antitussive with multiple actions qualitatively similar to those of codeine. Most of these involve the central nervous system and smooth muscle. The precise mechanism of action of hydrocodone and other opiates is not known, although it is believed to relate to the existence of opiate receptors in the central nervous system. In addition to analgesia, narcotics may produce drowsiness, changes in mood and mental clouding.

The analgesic action of acetaminophen involves peripheral influences, but the specific mechanism is as yet undetermined. Antipyretic activity is mediated through hypothalamic heat regulating centers. Acetaminophen inhibits prostaglandin synthetase. Therapeutic doses of acetaminophen have negligible effects on the cardiovascular or respiratory systems; however, toxic doses may cause circulatory failure and rapid, shallow breathing.

Pharmacokinetics

The behavior of the individual components is described below.

Hydrocodone

Following a 10 mg oral dose of hydrocodone administered to five adult male subjects, the mean peak concentration was 23.6 ± 5.2 ng/mL. Maximum serum levels were achieved at 1.3 ± 0.3 hours and the half-life was determined to be 3.8 ± 0.3 hours. Hydrocodone exhibits a complex pattern of metabolism including O-demethylation, N-demethylation and 6-keto reduction to the corresponding 6-α- and 6-β- hydroxymetabolites. See **OVERDOSAGE** for toxicity information.

Acetaminophen

Acetaminophen is rapidly absorbed from the gastrointestinal tract and is distributed throughout most body tissues. The plasma half-life is 1.25 to 3 hours, but may be increased by liver damage and following overdosage. Elimination of acetaminophen is principally by liver metabolism (conjugation) and subsequent renal excretion of metabolites. Approximately 85% of an oral dose appears in the urine within 24 hours of administration, most as the glucuronide conjugate, with small amounts of other conjugates and unchanged drug. See **OVERDOSAGE** for toxicity information.

INDICATIONS AND USAGE

VICODIN ES Tablets are indicated for the relief of moderate to moderately severe pain.

CONTRAINDICATIONS

This product should not be administered to patients who have previously exhibited hypersensitivity to hydrocodone or acetaminophen.

Patients known to be hypersensitive to other opioids may exhibit cross-sensitivity to hydrocodone.

WARNINGS

Hepatotoxicity

Acetaminophen has been associated with cases of acute liver failure, at times resulting in liver transplant and death. Most of the cases of liver injury are associated with the use of acetaminophen at doses that exceed 4000 milligrams per day, and often involve more than one acetaminophen-containing product. The excessive intake of acetaminophen may be intentional to cause self-harm or unintentional as patients attempt to obtain more pain relief or unknowingly take other acetaminophen-containing products.

The risk of acute liver failure is higher in individuals with underlying liver disease and in individuals who ingest alcohol while taking acetaminophen.

Instruct patients to look for acetaminophen or APAP on package labels and not to use more than one product that contains acetaminophen. Instruct patients to seek medical attention immediately upon ingestion of more than 4000 milligrams of acetaminophen per day, even if they feel well.

Hypersensitivity/anaphylaxis

There have been post-marketing reports of hypersensitivity and anaphylaxis associated with use of acetaminophen. Clinical signs included swelling of the face, mouth, and throat, respiratory distress, urticaria, rash, pruritis, and vomiting. There were infrequent reports of life-threatening anaphylaxis requiring emergency medical attention. Instruct patients to discontinue VICODIN ES Tablets immediately and seek medical care if they experience these symptoms. Do not prescribe VICODIN ES Tablets for patients with acetaminophen allergy.

Respiratory Depression

At high doses or in sensitive patients, hydrocodone may produce dose-related respiratory depression by acting directly on the brain stem respiratory center. Hydrocodone also affects the center that controls respiratory rhythm, and may produce irregular and periodic breathing.

Head Injury and Increased Intracranial Pressure

The respiratory depressant effects of narcotics and their capacity to elevate cerebrospinal fluid pressure may be markedly exaggerated in the presence of head injury, other intracranial lesions or a preexisting increase in intracranial pressure. Furthermore, narcotics produce adverse reactions, which may obscure the clinical course of patients with head injuries.

Acute Abdominal Conditions

The administration of narcotics may obscure the diagnosis or clinical course of patients with acute abdominal conditions.

Misuse Abuse and Diversion of Opioids

VICODIN ES contains hydrocodone an opioid agonist, and is a Schedule III controlled substance. Opioid agonists have the potential for being abused and are sought by abusers and people with addiction disorders, and are subject to diversion.

VICODIN ES can be abused in a manner similar to other opioid agonists, legal or illicit. This should be considered when prescribing or dispensing VICODIN ES in situations where the physician or pharmacist is concerned about an increased risk of misuse, abuse or diversion (see **DRUG ABUSE AND DEPENDENCE**).

PRECAUTIONS

General

Special Risk Patients

As with any narcotic analgesic agent, VICODIN ES Tablets should be used with caution in elderly or debilitated patients and those with severe impairment of hepatic or renal function, hypothyroidism, Addison's disease, prostatic hypertrophy or urethral stricture. The usual precautions should be observed and the possibility of respiratory depression should be kept in mind.

Cough Reflex

Hydrocodone suppresses the cough reflex; as with all narcotics, caution should be exercised when VICODIN ES Tablets are used postoperatively and in patients with pulmonary disease.

Information for Patients/Caregivers

- Do not take VICODIN ES Tablets if you are allergic to any of its ingredients.

Information on the AbbVie, Inc. products listed on these pages is from the prescribing information in use as of July 31, 2013. For more information, please visit rxabbvie.com or call 1-800-633-9110.

- If you develop signs of allergy such as a rash or difficulty breathing stop taking VICODIN ES Tablets and contact your healthcare provider immediately.
- Do not take more than 4000 milligrams of acetaminophen per day. Call your doctor if you took more than the recommended dose.

Hydrocodone, like all narcotics, may impair the mental and/or physical abilities required for the performance of potentially hazardous tasks such as driving a car or operating machinery; patients should be cautioned accordingly.

Alcohol and other CNS depressants may produce an additive CNS depression, when taken with this combination product, and should be avoided.

Hydrocodone may be habit forming. Patients should take the drug only for as long as it is prescribed, in the amounts prescribed, and no more frequently than prescribed.

Laboratory Tests

In patients with severe hepatic or renal disease, effects of therapy should be monitored with serial liver and/or renal function tests.

Drug Interactions

Patients receiving other narcotic analgesics, antihistamines, antipsychotics, antianxiety agents, or other CNS depressants (including alcohol) concomitantly with VICODIN ES Tablets may exhibit an additive CNS depression. When combined therapy is contemplated, the dose of one or both agents should be reduced.

The use of MAO inhibitors or tricyclic antidepressants with hydrocodone preparations may increase the effect of either the antidepressant or hydrocodone.

Drug/Laboratory Test Interactions

Acetaminophen may produce false-positive test results for urinary 5-hydroxyindoleacetic acid.

Carcinogenesis, Mutagenesis, Impairment of Fertility

No adequate studies have been conducted in animals to determine whether hydrocodone or acetaminophen have a potential for carcinogenesis, mutagenesis, or impairment of fertility.

Pregnancy

Teratogenic Effects

Pregnancy Category C

There are no adequate and well-controlled studies in pregnant women. VICODIN ES Tablets should be used during pregnancy only if the potential benefit justifies the potential risk to the fetus.

Nonteratogenic Effects

Babies born to mothers who have been taking opioids regularly prior to delivery will be physically dependent. The withdrawal signs include irritability and excessive crying, tremors, hyperactive reflexes, increased respiratory rate, increased stools, sneezing, yawning, vomiting, and fever. The intensity of the syndrome does not always correlate with the duration of maternal opioid use or dose. There is no consensus on the best method of managing withdrawal.

Labor and Delivery

As with all narcotics, administration of VICODIN ES Tablets to the mother shortly before delivery may result in some degree of respiratory depression in the newborn, especially if higher doses are used.

Nursing Mothers

Acetaminophen is excreted in breast milk in small amounts, but the significance of its effects on nursing infants is not known. It is not known whether hydrocodone is excreted in human milk. Because many drugs are excreted in human milk and because of the potential for serious adverse reactions in nursing infants from hydrocodone and acetaminophen, a decision should be made whether to discontinue nursing or to discontinue the drug, taking into account the importance of the drug to the mother.

Pediatric Use

Safety and effectiveness in the pediatric population have not been established.

Geriatric Use

Clinical studies of VICODIN ES® (hydrocodone bitartrate 7.5 mg and acetaminophen 750 mg) did not include sufficient numbers of subjects aged 65 and over to determine whether they respond differently from younger subjects. Other reported clinical experience has not identified differences in responses between the elderly and younger patients. In general, dose selection for an elderly patient should be cautious, usually starting at the low end of the dosing range, reflecting the greater frequency of decreased hepatic, renal, or cardiac function, and of concomitant disease or other drug therapy.

Hydrocodone and the major metabolites of acetaminophen are known to be substantially excreted by the kidney. Thus the risk of toxic reactions may be greater in patients with impaired renal function due to accumulation of the parent compound and/or metabolites in the plasma. Because elderly patients are more likely to have decreased renal function, care should be taken in dose selection, and it may be useful to monitor renal function.

Hydrocodone may cause confusion and over-sedation in the elderly; elderly patients generally should be started on low doses of hydrocodone bitartrate and acetaminophen tablets and observed closely.

ADVERSE REACTIONS

The most frequently reported adverse reactions include: lightheadedness, dizziness, sedation, nausea and vomiting. These effects seem to be more prominent in ambulatory than in nonambulatory patients and some of these adverse reactions may be alleviated if the patient lies down.

Other adverse reactions include:

Central Nervous System

Drowsiness, mental clouding, lethargy, impairment of mental and physical performance, anxiety, fear, dysphoria, psychic dependence, mood changes.

Gastrointestinal System

Prolonged administration of VICODIN ES Tablets may produce constipation.

Genitourinary System

Ureteral spasm, spasm of vesical sphincters and urinary retention have been reported with opiates.

Respiratory Depression

Hydrocodone bitartrate may produce dose-related respiratory depression by acting directly on the brain stem respiratory center. (see **OVERDOSAGE**).

Special Senses

Cases of hearing impairment or permanent loss have been reported predominantly in patients with chronic overdose.

Dermatological

Skin rash, pruritus.

The following adverse drug events may be borne in mind as potential effects of acetaminophen: allergic reactions, rash, thrombocytopenia, agranulocytosis, Stevens-Johnson syndrome, toxic epidermal necrolysis.

Potential effects of high dosage are listed in the **OVERDOSAGE** section.

DRUG ABUSE AND DEPENDENCE

Misuse Abuse and Diversion of Opioids

VICODIN ES contains hydrocodone, an opioid agonist, and is a Schedule III controlled substance. VICODIN ES, and other opioids used in analgesia can be abused and are subject to criminal diversion.

Addiction is a primary, chronic, neurobiologic disease, with genetic, psychosocial, and environmental factors influencing its development and manifestations. It is characterized by behaviors that include one or more of the following: impaired control over drug use, compulsive use, continued use despite harm, and craving. Drug addiction is a treatable disease utilizing a multidisciplinary approach, but relapse is common.

"Drug seeking" behavior is very common in addicts and drug abusers. Drug-seeking tactics include emergency calls or visits near the end of office hours, refusal to undergo appropriate examination, testing or referral, repeated "loss" of prescriptions, tampering with prescriptions and reluctance to provide prior medical records or contact information for other treating physician(s). "Doctor shopping" to obtain additional prescriptions is common among drug abusers and people suffering from untreated addiction.

Abuse and addiction are separate and distinct from physical dependence and tolerance. Physical dependence usually assumes clinically significant dimensions only after several weeks of continued opioid use, although a mild degree of physical dependence may develop after a few days of opioid therapy. Tolerance, in which increasingly large doses are required in order to produce the same degree of analgesia, is manifested initially by a shortened duration of analgesic effect, and subsequently by decreases in the intensity of analgesia. The rate of development of tolerance varies among patients. Physicians should be aware that abuse of opioids can occur in the absence of true addiction and is characterized by misuse for non-medical purposes, often in combination with other psychoactive substances. VICODIN ES, like other opioids, may be diverted for non-medical use. Record-keeping of prescribing information, including quantity, frequency, and renewal requests is strongly advised.

Proper assessment of the patient, proper prescribing practices, periodic re-evaluation of therapy, and proper dispensing and storage are appropriate measures that help to limit abuse of opioid drugs.

OVERDOSAGE

Following an acute overdosage, toxicity may result from hydrocodone or acetaminophen.

Signs and Symptoms

Hydrocodone: Serious overdose with hydrocodone is characterized by respiratory depression (a decrease in respiratory rate and/or tidal volume, Cheyne-Stokes respiration, cyanosis), extreme somnolence progressing to stupor or coma, skeletal muscle flaccidity, cold and clammy skin, and sometimes bradycardia and hypotension. In severe overdosage, apnea, circulatory collapse, cardiac arrest and death may occur.

Acetaminophen: In acetaminophen overdosage: dose-dependent, potentially fatal hepatic necrosis is the most serious adverse effect. Renal tubular necrosis, hypoglycemic coma, and coagulation defects may also occur.

Early symptoms following a potentially hepatotoxic overdose may include: nausea, vomiting, diaphoresis and general malaise. Clinical and laboratory evidence of hepatic toxicity may not be apparent until 48 to 72 hours post-ingestion.

Treatment

A single or multiple drug overdose with hydrocodone and acetaminophen is a potentially lethal polydrug overdose, and consultation with a regional poison control center is recommended.

Immediate treatment includes support of cardiorespiratory function and measures to reduce drug absorption.

Oxygen, intravenous fluids, vasopressors, and other supportive measures should be employed as indicated. Assisted or controlled ventilation should also be considered.

For hydrocodone overdose, primary attention should be given to the reestablishment of adequate respiratory exchange through provision of a patent airway and the institution of assisted or controlled ventilation. The narcotic antagonist naloxone hydrochloride is a specific antidote against respiratory depression which may result from overdosage or unusual sensitivity to narcotics, including hydrocodone. Since the duration of action of hydrocodone may exceed that of the antagonist, the patient should be kept under continued surveillance, and repeated doses of the antagonist should be administered as needed to maintain adequate respiration. A narcotic antagonist should not be administered in the absence of clinically significant respiratory or cardiovascular depression.

Gastric decontamination with activated charcoal should be administered just prior to N-acetylcysteine (NAC) to decrease systemic absorption if acetaminophen ingestion is known or suspected to have occurred within a few hours of presentation. Serum acetaminophen levels should be obtained immediately if the patient presents 4 hours or more after ingestion to assess potential risk of hepatotoxicity; acetaminophen levels drawn less than 4 hours post-ingestion may be misleading. To obtain the best possible outcome, NAC should be administered as soon as possible where impending or evolving liver injury is suspected. Intravenous NAC may be administered when circumstances preclude oral administration.

Vigorous supportive therapy is required in severe intoxication. Procedures to limit the continuing absorption of the drug must be readily performed since the hepatic injury is dose dependent and occurs early in the course of intoxication.

DOSAGE AND ADMINISTRATION

Dosage should be adjusted according to the severity of the pain and the response of the patient. However, it should be kept in mind that tolerance to hydrocodone can develop with continued use and that the incidence of untoward effects is dose related. The usual adult dosage is one tablet every four to six hours as needed for pain. The total daily dosage should not exceed 5 tablets.

HOW SUPPLIED

White, oval-shaped, faceted edged tablet bisected on one side and imprinted with "VICODIN ES" on the other side.

Bottles of 100-NDC #0074-1973-14

Bottles of 500-NDC #0074-1973-54

Hospital Unit Dosage Package-100 tablets (4 × 25 tablets)-NDC #0074-1973-12.

Storage

Store at 25°C (77°F); excursions permitted to 15°-30°C (59°-86°F). [See USP Controlled Room Temperature].

Dispense in a tight, light-resistant container as defined in the USP.

A Schedule (CIII) Controlled Drug Substance.

Manufactured for
Abbott Laboratories
North Chicago, IL 60064 U.S.A.
by Halo Pharmaceutical Inc.
Whippany, NJ 07981 U.S.A.
Ref. 03-A541-R8-Rev. September, 2011

Shown in Product Identification Guide, page 304

VICODIN HP® (CIII)

[*vīkō-dĭn*]

(hydrocodone bitartrate and acetaminophen tablets, USP)

10 mg/660 mg

BOXED WARNING

Hepatotoxicity

Acetaminophen has been associated with cases of acute liver failure, at times resulting in liver transplant and death. Most of the cases of liver injury are associated with the use of acetaminophen at doses that exceed 4000 milligrams per day, and often involve more than one acetaminophen-containing product.

DESCRIPTION

Hydrocodone bitartrate and acetaminophen is supplied in tablet form for oral administration.

Hydrocodone bitartrate is an opioid analgesic and antitussive and occurs as fine, white crystals or as a crystalline powder. It is affected by light. The chemical name is 4,5α-epoxy-3-methoxy-17-methylmorphinan-6-one tartrate (1:1) hydrate (2:5). It has the following structural formula:

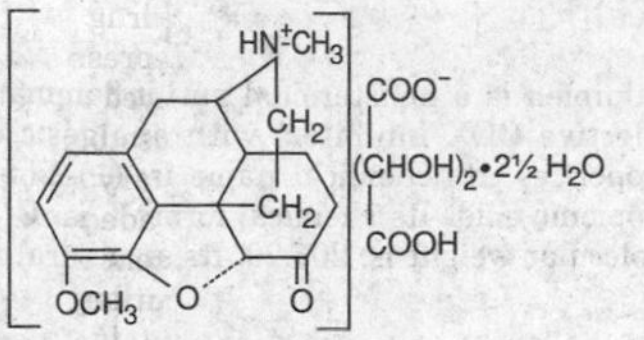

$C_{18}H_{21}NO_3 \cdot C_4H_6O_6 \cdot 2\frac{1}{2}H_2O$ M.W. = 494.50

Acetaminophen, 4′-hydroxyacetanilide, a slightly bitter, white, odorless, crystalline powder, is a non-opiate, non-salicylate analgesic and antipyretic. It has the following structural formula:

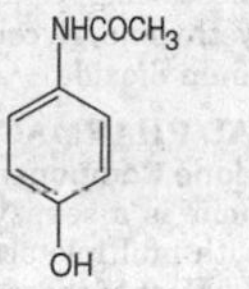

$C_8H_9NO_2$ M.W. = 151.17

Each VICODIN HP Tablet contains:
Hydrocodone Bitartrate 10 mg
Acetaminophen 660 mg

In addition each tablet contains the following inactive ingredients: colloidal silicon dioxide, croscarmellose sodium, magnesium stearate, microcrystalline cellulose, povidone, pregelatinized starch, and stearic acid.

Meets USP Dissolution Test 2.

CLINICAL PHARMACOLOGY

Hydrocodone is a semisynthetic narcotic analgesic and antitussive with multiple actions qualitatively similar to those of codeine. Most of these involve the central nervous system and smooth muscle. The precise mechanism of action of hydrocodone and other opiates is not known, although it is believed to relate to the existence of opiate receptors in the central nervous system. In addition to analgesia, narcotics may produce drowsiness, changes in mood and mental clouding.

The analgesic action of acetaminophen involves peripheral influences, but the specific mechanism is as yet undetermined. Antipyretic activity is mediated through hypothalamic heat regulating centers. Acetaminophen inhibits prostaglandin synthetase. Therapeutic doses of acetaminophen have negligible effects on the cardiovascular or respiratory systems; however, toxic doses may cause circulatory failure and rapid, shallow breathing.

Pharmacokinetics

The behavior of the individual components is described below.

Hydrocodone

Following a 10 mg oral dose of hydrocodone administered to five adult male subjects, the mean peak concentration was 23.6 ± 5.2 ng/mL. Maximum serum levels were achieved at 1.3 ± 0.3 hours and the half-life was determined to be 3.8 ± 0.3 hours. Hydrocodone exhibits a complex pattern of metabolism including O-demethylation, N-demethylation and 6-keto reduction to the corresponding 6-α- and 6-β-hydroxy-metabolites. See **OVERDOSAGE** for toxicity information.

Acetaminophen

Acetaminophen is rapidly absorbed from the gastrointestinal tract and is distributed throughout most body tissues. The plasma half-life is 1.25 to 3 hours, but may be increased by liver damage and following overdosage. Elimination of acetaminophen is principally by liver metabolism (conjugation) and subsequent renal excretion of metabolites. Approximately 85% of an oral dose appears in the urine within 24 hours of administration, most as the glucuronide conjugate, with small amounts of other conjugates and unchanged drug. See **OVERDOSAGE** for toxicity information.

INDICATIONS AND USAGE

VICODIN HP Tablets are indicated for the relief of moderate to moderately severe pain.

CONTRAINDICATIONS

This product should not be administered to patients who have previously exhibited hypersensitivity to hydrocodone or acetaminophen.

Patients known to be hypersensitive to other opioids may exhibit cross-sensitivity to hydrocodone.

WARNINGS

Hepatotoxicity

Acetaminophen has been associated with cases of acute liver failure, at times resulting in liver transplant and death. Most of the cases of liver injury are associated with the use of acetaminophen at doses that exceed 4000 milligrams per day, and often involve more than one acetaminophen-containing product. The excessive intake of acetaminophen may be intentional to cause self-harm or unintentional as patients attempt to obtain more pain relief or unknowingly take other acetaminophen-containing products.

The risk of acute liver failure is higher in individuals with underlying liver disease and in individuals who ingest alcohol while taking acetaminophen.

Instruct patients to look for acetaminophen or APAP on package labels and not to use more than one product that contains acetaminophen. Instruct patients to seek medical attention immediately upon ingestion of more than 4000 milligrams of acetaminophen per day, even if they feel well.

Hypersensitivity/anaphylaxis

There have been post-marketing reports of hypersensitivity and anaphylaxis associated with use of acetaminophen. Clinical signs included swelling of the face, mouth and throat, respiratory distress, urticaria, rash, pruritus, and vomiting. There were infrequent reports of life-threatening anaphylaxis requiring emergency medical attention. Instruct patients to discontinue VICODIN HP Tablets immediately and seek medical care if they experience these symptoms. Do not prescribe VICODIN HP Tablets for patients with acetaminophen allergy.

Respiratory Depression

At high doses or in sensitive patients, hydrocodone may produce dose-related respiratory depression by acting directly on the brain stem respiratory center. Hydrocodone also affects the center that controls respiratory rhythm, and may produce irregular and periodic breathing.

Head Injury and Increased Intracranial Pressure

The respiratory depressant effects of narcotics and their capacity to elevate cerebrospinal fluid pressure may be markedly exaggerated in the presence of head injury, other intracranial lesions or a preexisting increase in intracranial pressure. Furthermore, narcotics produce adverse reactions which may obscure the clinical course of patients with head injuries.

Acute Abdominal Conditions

The administration of narcotics may obscure the diagnosis or clinical course of patients with acute abdominal conditions.

Misuse Abuse and Diversion of Opioids

VICODIN HP contains hydrocodone an opioid agonist, and is a Schedule III controlled substance. Opioid agonists have the potential for being abused and are sought by abusers and people with addiction disorders, and are subject to diversion.

VICODIN HP can be abused in a manner similar to other opioid agonists, legal or illicit. This should be considered when prescribing or dispensing VICODIN HP in situations where the physician or pharmacist is concerned about an increased risk of misuse, abuse or diversion (see DRUG ABUSE AND DEPENDENCE).

PRECAUTIONS

General

Special Risk Patients

As with any narcotic analgesic agent, VICODIN HP Tablets should be used with caution in elderly or debilitated patients, and those with severe impairment of hepatic or renal function, hypothyroidism, Addison's disease, prostatic hypertrophy or urethral stricture. The usual precautions should be observed and the possibility of respiratory depression should be kept in mind.

Cough Reflex

Hydrocodone suppresses the cough reflex; as with all narcotics, caution should be exercised when VICODIN HP Tablets are used postoperatively and in patients with pulmonary disease.

Information for Patients/Caregivers

- Do not take VICODIN HP Tablets if you are allergic to any of its ingredients.
- If you develop signs of allergy such as a rash or difficulty breathing stop taking VICODIN HP Tablets and contact your healthcare provider immediately.
- Do not take more than 4000 milligrams of acetaminophen per day. Call your doctor if you took more than the recommended dose.

Hydrocodone, like all narcotics, may impair the mental and/or physical abilities required for the performance of potentially hazardous tasks such as driving a car or operating machinery; patients should be cautioned accordingly. Alcohol and other CNS depressants may produce an additive CNS depression, when taken with this combination product, and should be avoided.

Hydrocodone may be habit forming. Patients should take the drug only for as long as it is prescribed, in the amounts prescribed, and no more frequently than prescribed.

Laboratory Tests

In patients with severe hepatic or renal disease, effects of therapy should be monitored with serial liver and/or renal function tests.

Drug Interactions

Patients receiving narcotics, antihistamines, antipsychotics, antianxiety agents, or other CNS depressants (including alcohol) concomitantly with VICODIN HP Tablets may exhibit an additive CNS depression. When combined therapy is contemplated, the dose of one or both agents should be reduced.

The use of MAO inhibitors or tricyclic antidepressants with hydrocodone preparations may increase the effect of either the antidepressant or hydrocodone.

Drug/Laboratory Test Interactions

Acetaminophen may produce false-positive test results for urinary 5-hydroxyindoleacetic acid.

Carcinogenesis, Mutagenesis, Impairment of Fertility

No adequate studies have been conducted in animals to determine whether hydrocodone or acetaminophen have a potential for carcinogenesis, mutagenesis, or impairment of fertility.

Pregnancy

Teratogenic Effects

Pregnancy Category C

There are no adequate and well-controlled studies in pregnant women. VICODIN HP Tablets should be used during pregnancy only if the potential benefit justifies the potential risk to the fetus.

Nonteratogenic Effects

Babies born to mothers who have been taking opioids regularly prior to delivery will be physically dependent. The withdrawal signs include irritability and excessive crying, tremors, hyperactive reflexes, increased respiratory rate, increased stools, sneezing, yawning, vomiting, and fever. The intensity of the syndrome does not always correlate with the duration of maternal opioid use or dose. There is no consensus on the best method of managing withdrawal.

Labor and Delivery

As with all narcotics, administration of VICODIN HP Tablets to the mother shortly before delivery may result in some degree of respiratory depression in the newborn, especially if higher doses are used.

Nursing Mothers

Acetaminophen is excreted in breast milk in small amounts, but the significance of its effects on nursing infants is not known. It is not known whether hydrocodone is excreted in human milk. Because many drugs are excreted in human milk and because of the potential for serious adverse reactions in nursing infants from hydrocodone and acetaminophen, a decision should be made whether to discontinue nursing or to discontinue the drug, taking into account the importance of the drug to the mother.

Pediatric Use

Safety and effectiveness in the pediatric population have not been established.

Geriatric Use

Clinical studies of VICODIN HP® (hydrocodone bitartrate and acetaminophen 10 mg/660 mg) did not include sufficient numbers of subjects aged 65 and over to determine whether they respond differently from younger subjects. Other reported clinical experience has not identified differences in responses between the elderly and younger patients. In general, dose selection for an elderly patient should be cautious, usually starting at the low end of the dosing range, reflecting the greater frequency of decreased hepatic, renal, or cardiac function, and of concomitant disease or other drug therapy.

Hydrocodone and the major metabolites of acetaminophen are known to be substantially excreted by the kidney. Thus the risk of toxic reactions may be greater in patients with impaired renal function due to accumulation of the parent compound and/or metabolites in the plasma. Because elderly patients are more likely to have decreased renal function, care should be taken in dose selection, and it may be useful to monitor renal function.

Information on the AbbVie, Inc. products listed on these pages is from the prescribing information in use as of July 31, 2013. For more information, please visit rxabbvie.com or call 1-800-633-9110.

Hydrocodone may cause confusion and over-sedation in the elderly; elderly patients generally should be started on low doses of hydrocodone bitartrate and acetaminophen tablets and observed closely.

ADVERSE REACTIONS

The most frequently reported adverse reactions are lightheadedness, dizziness, sedation, nausea and vomiting. These effects seem to be more prominent in ambulatory than in nonambulatory patients, and some of these adverse reactions may be alleviated if the patient lies down.
Other adverse reactions include:

Central Nervous System
Drowsiness, mental clouding, lethargy, impairment of mental and physical performance, anxiety, fear, dysphoria, psychic dependence, mood changes.

Gastrointestinal System
Prolonged administration of VICODIN HP Tablets may produce constipation.

Genitourinary System
Ureteral spasm, spasm of vesical sphincters and urinary retention have been reported with opiates.

Respiratory Depression
Hydrocodone bitartrate may produce dose-related respiratory depression by acting directly on the brain stem respiratory centers (see **OVERDOSAGE**).

Special Senses
Cases of hearing impairment or permanent loss have been reported predominantly in patients with chronic overdose.

Dermatological
Skin rash, pruritus.

The following adverse drug events may be borne in mind as potential effects of acetaminophen: allergic reactions, rash, thrombocytopenia, agranulocytosis, Stevens-Johnson syndrome, toxic epidermal necrolysis.

Potential effects of high dosage are listed in the **OVERDOSAGE** section.

DRUG ABUSE AND DEPENDENCE

Misuse Abuse and Diversion of Opioids
VICODIN HP contains hydrocodone, an opioid agonist, and is a Schedule III controlled substance. VICODIN HP, and other opioids used in analgesia can be abused and are subject to criminal diversion.

Addiction is a primary, chronic, neurobiologic disease, with genetic, psychosocial, and environmental factors influencing its development and manifestations. It is characterized by behaviors that include one or more of the following: impaired control over drug use, compulsive use, continued use despite harm, and craving. Drug addiction is a treatable disease utilizing a multidisciplinary approach, but relapse is common.

"Drug seeking" behavior is very common in addicts and drug abusers. Drug-seeking tactics include emergency calls or visits near the end of office hours, refusal to undergo appropriate examination, testing or referral, repeated "loss" of prescriptions, tampering with prescriptions and reluctance to provide prior medical records or contact information for other treating physician(s). "Doctor shopping" to obtain additional prescriptions is common among drug abusers and people suffering from untreated addiction.

Abuse and addiction are separate and distinct from physical dependence and tolerance. Physical dependence usually assumes clinically significant dimensions only after several weeks of continued opioid use, although a mild degree of physical dependence may develop after a few days of opioid therapy. Tolerance, in which increasingly large doses are required in order to produce the same degree of analgesia, is manifested initially by a shortened duration of analgesic effect, and subsequently by decreases in the intensity of analgesia. The rate of development of tolerance varies among patients. Physicians should be aware that abuse of opioids can occur in the absence of true addiction and is characterized by misuse for non-medical purposes, often in combination with other psychoactive substances. VICODIN HP, like other opioids, may be diverted for non-medical use. Recordkeeping of prescribing information, including quantity, frequency, and renewal requests is strongly advised.

Proper assessment of the patient, proper prescribing practices, periodic re-evaluation of therapy, and proper dispensing and storage are appropriate measures that help to limit abuse of opioid drugs.

OVERDOSAGE

Following an acute overdosage, toxicity may result from hydrocodone or acetaminophen.

Signs and Symptoms
Hydrocodone: Serious overdose with hydrocodone is characterized by respiratory depression (a decrease in respiratory rate and/or tidal volume, Cheyne-Stokes respiration, cyanosis), extreme somnolence progressing to stupor or coma, skeletal muscle flaccidity, cold and clammy skin, and sometimes bradycardia and hypotension. In severe overdosage, apnea, circulatory collapse, cardiac arrest and death may occur.

Acetaminophen: In acetaminophen overdosage: dose-dependent, potentially fatal hepatic necrosis is the most serious adverse effect. Renal tubular necrosis, hypoglycemic coma, and coagulation defects may also occur.

Early symptoms following a potentially hepatotoxic overdose may include: nausea, vomiting, diaphoresis and general malaise. Clinical and laboratory evidence of hepatic toxicity may not be apparent until 48 to 72 hours post-ingestion.

Treatment
A single or multiple drug overdose with hydrocodone and acetaminophen is a potentially lethal polydrug overdose, and consultation with a regional poison control center is recommended.

Immediate treatment includes support of cardiorespiratory function and measures to reduce drug absorption.

Oxygen, intravenous fluids, vasopressors, and other supportive measures should be employed as indicated. Assisted or controlled ventilation should also be considered.

For hydrocodone overdose, primary attention should be given to the reestablishment of adequate respiratory exchange through provision of a patent airway and the institution of assisted or controlled ventilation. The narcotic antagonist naloxone hydrochloride is a specific antidote against respiratory depression which may result from overdosage or unusual sensitivity to narcotics, including hydrocodone. Since the duration of action of hydrocodone may exceed that of the antagonist, the patient should be kept under continued surveillance, and repeated doses of the antagonist should be administered as needed to maintain adequate respiration. A narcotic antagonist should not be administered in the absence of clinically significant respiratory or cardiovascular depression.

Gastric decontamination with activated charcoal should be administered just prior to N-acetylcysteine (NAC) to decrease systemic absorption if acetaminophen ingestion is known or suspected to have occurred within a few hours of presentation. Serum acetaminophen levels should be obtained immediately if the patient presents 4 hours or more after ingestion to assess potential risk of hepatotoxicity; acetaminophen levels drawn less than 4 hours post-ingestion may be misleading. To obtain the best possible outcome, NAC should be administered as soon as possible where impending or evolving liver injury is suspected. Intravenous NAC may be administered when circumstances preclude oral administration.

Vigorous supportive therapy is required in severe intoxication. Procedures to limit the continuing absorption of the drug must be readily performed since the hepatic injury is dose dependent and occurs early in the course of intoxication.

DOSAGE AND ADMINISTRATION

Dosage should be adjusted according to severity of pain and the response of the patient. However, it should be kept in mind that tolerance to hydrocodone can develop with continued use and that the incidence of untoward effects is dose related.

The usual adult dosage is one tablet every four to six hours as needed for pain. The total daily dosage should not exceed 6 tablets.

HOW SUPPLIED

VICODIN HP (hydrocodone bitartrate and acetaminophen, 10 mg/660 mg) is supplied as a white, oval-shaped, tablet bisected on one side and debossed with "VICODIN HP" on the other side.

Bottles of 100-NDC #0074-2274-14
Bottles of 500-NDC #0074-2274-54

Storage
Store at 25°C (77°F); excursions permitted to 15°-30°C (59°-86°F). [see USP Controlled Room Temperature]. Dispense in a tight, light-resistant container as defined in the USP.

A Schedule Ⓒ III Controlled Drug Substance.

Manufactured for
Abbott Laboratories
North Chicago, IL 60064 U.S.A.
by Halo Pharmaceutical Inc.
Whippany, NJ 07981 U.S.A.
Ref: 03-A542-R7- Rev. September, 2011

Shown in Product Identification Guide, page 304

VICOPROFEN® Ⓒ III

(hydrocodone bitartrate and ibuprofen tablets)
7.5 mg/200 mg

DESCRIPTION

Each VICOPROFEN tablet contains:
Hydrocodone Bitartrate, USP 7.5 mg
Ibuprofen, USP 200 mg

VICOPROFEN is supplied in a fixed combination tablet form for oral administration. VICOPROFEN combines the opioid analgesic agent, hydrocodone bitartrate, with the nonsteroidal anti-inflammatory (NSAID) agent, ibuprofen. Hydrocodone bitartrate is a semisynthetic and centrally acting opioid analgesic. Its chemical name is: 4,5 α-epoxy-3-methoxy-17-methylmorphinan-6-one tartrate (1:1) hydrate (2:5). Its chemical formula is: $C_{18}H_{21}NO_3 \bullet C_4H_6O_6 \bullet 2\frac{1}{2}H_2O$, and the molecular weight is 494.50. Its structural formula is:

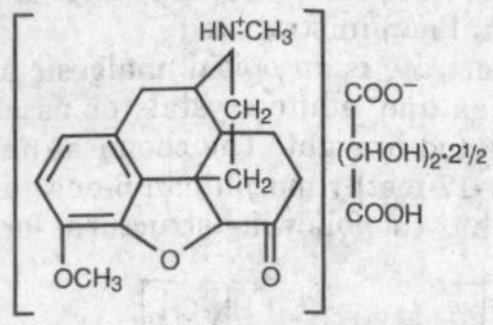

Ibuprofen is a nonsteroidal anti-inflammatory agent [non-selective COX inhibitor] with analgesic and antipyretic properties. Its chemical name is: (±)-2-(*p*-isobutylphenyl) propionic acid. Its chemical formula is: $C_{13}H_{18}O_2$, and the molecular weight is: 206.29. Its structural formula is:

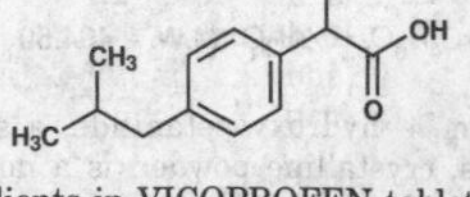

Inactive ingredients in VICOPROFEN tablets include: colloidal silicon dioxide, corn starch, croscarmellose sodium, hypromellose, magnesium stearate, microcrystalline cellulose, polyethylene glycol, polysorbate 80, propylene glycol and titanium dioxide.

CLINICAL PHARMACOLOGY

Hydrocodone Component
Hydrocodone is a semisynthetic opioid analgesic and antitussive with multiple actions qualitatively similar to those of codeine. Most of these involve the central nervous system and smooth muscle. The precise mechanism of action of hydrocodone and other opioids is not known, although it is believed to relate to the existence of opiate receptors in the central nervous system. In addition to analgesia, opioids may produce drowsiness, changes in mood, and mental clouding.

Ibuprofen Component
Ibuprofen is a non-steroidal anti-inflammatory agent that possesses analgesic and antipyretic activities. Its mode of action, like that of other NSAIDs, is not completely understood, but may be related to inhibition of cyclooxygenase activity and prostaglandin synthesis. Ibuprofen is a peripherally acting analgesic. Ibuprofen does not have any known effects on opiate receptors.

Pharmacokinetics

Absorption
After oral dosing with the VICOPROFEN tablet, a peak hydrocodone plasma level of 27 ng/mL is achieved at 1.7 hours, and a peak ibuprofen plasma level of 30 mcg/mL is achieved at 1.8 hours. The effect of food on the absorption of either component from the VICOPROFEN tablet has not been established.

Distribution
Ibuprofen is highly protein-bound (99%) like most other non-steroidal anti-inflammatory agents. Although the extent of protein binding of hydrocodone in human plasma has not been definitely determined, structural similarities to related opioid analgesics suggest that hydrocodone is not extensively protein bound. As most agents in the 5-ring morphinan group of semi-synthetic opioids bind plasma protein to a similar degree (range 19% [hydromorphone] to 45% [oxycodone]), hydrocodone is expected to fall within this range.

Metabolism
Hydrocodone exhibits a complex pattern of metabolism, including *O*-demethylation, *N*-demethylation, and 6-keto reduction to the corresponding 6-α-and 6-β-hydroxy metabolites. Hydromorphone, a potent opioid, is formed from the *O*-demethylation of hydrocodone and contributes to the total analgesic effect of hydrocodone. The *O*- and *N*- demethylation processes are mediated by separate P-450 isoenzymes: CYP2D6 and CYP3A4, respectively.

Ibuprofen is present in this product as a racemate, and following absorption it undergoes interconversion in the plasma from the R-isomer to the S-isomer. Both the R- and S- isomers are metabolized to two primary metabolites: (+)-2-4′-(2hydroxy-2-methyl-propyl) phenyl propionic acid and (+)-2-4′-(2carboxypropyl) phenyl propionic acid, both of which circulate in the plasma at low levels relative to the parent.

Elimination
Hydrocodone and its metabolites are eliminated primarily in the kidneys, with a mean plasma half-life of 4.5 hours. Ibuprofen is excreted in the urine, 50% to 60% as metabolites and approximately 15% as unchanged drug and conjugate. The plasma half-life is 2.2 hours.

Special Populations
No significant pharmacokinetic differences based on age or gender have been demonstrated. The pharmacokinetics of hydrocodone and ibuprofen from VICOPROFEN has not been evaluated in children.
Renal Impairment
The effect of renal insufficiency on the pharmacokinetics of the VICOPROFEN dosage form has not been determined.

CLINICAL STUDIES

In single-dose studies of post surgical pain (abdominal, gynecological, orthopedic), 940 patients were studied at doses of one or two tablets. VICOPROFEN produced greater efficacy than placebo and each of its individual components given at the same dose. No advantage was demonstrated for the two-tablet dose.

INDICATIONS AND USAGE

Carefully consider the potential benefits and risks of VICOPROFEN and other treatment options before deciding to use VICOPROFEN. Use the lowest effective dose for the shortest duration consistent with individual patient treatment goals (see **WARNINGS**).
VICOPROFEN tablets are indicated for the short-term (generally less than 10 days) management of acute pain. VICOPROFEN is not indicated for the treatment of such conditions as osteoarthritis or rheumatoid arthritis.

CONTRAINDICATIONS

VICOPROFEN is contraindicated in patients with known hypersensitivity to hydrocodone or ibuprofen. Patients known to be hypersensitive to other opioids may exhibit cross-sensitivity to hydrocodone.
VICOPROFEN should not be given to patients who have experienced asthma, urticaria, or allergic-type reactions after taking aspirin or other NSAIDs. Severe, rarely fatal, anaphylactic-like reactions to NSAIDs have been reported in such patients (see **WARNINGS – Anaphylactoid Reactions**, and **PRECAUTIONS - Preexisting Asthma**).
VICOPROFEN is contraindicated for the treatment of perioperative pain in the setting of coronary artery bypass graft (CABG) surgery (see **WARNINGS**).

WARNINGS

CARDIOVASCULAR EFFECTS

Cardiovascular Thrombotic Events
Clinical trials of several COX-2 selective and nonselective NSAIDs of up to three years duration have shown an increased risk of serious cardiovascular (CV) thrombotic events, myocardial infarction, and stroke, which can be fatal. All NSAIDs, both COX-2 selective and nonselective, may have a similar risk. Patients with known CV disease or risk factors for CV disease may be at greater risk. To minimize the potential risk for an adverse CV event in patients treated with an NSAID, the lowest effective dose should be used for the shortest duration possible. Physicians and patients should remain alert for the development of such events, even in the absence of previous CV symptoms. Patients should be informed about the signs and/or symptoms of serious CV events and the steps to take if they occur.
There is no consistent evidence that concurrent use of aspirin mitigates the increased risk of serious CV thrombotic events associated with NSAID use. The concurrent use of aspirin and an NSAID does increase the risk of serious GI events (see **GI WARNINGS**).
Two large, controlled, clinical trials of a COX-2 selective NSAID for the treatment of pain in the first 10-14 days following CABG surgery found an increased incidence of myocardial infarction and stroke (see **CONTRAINDICATIONS**).
Hypertension
NSAID-containing products, including VICOPROFEN, can lead to onset of new hypertension or worsening of preexisting hypertension, either of which may contribute to the increased incidence of CV events. Patients taking thiazides or loop diuretics may have impaired response to these therapies when taking NSAIDs. NSAID-containing products, including VICOPROFEN, should be used with caution in patients with hypertension. Blood pressure (BP) should be monitored closely during the initiation of NSAID treatment and throughout the course of therapy.
Congestive Heart Failure and Edema
Fluid retention and edema have been observed in some patients taking NSAIDs. VICOPROFEN should be used with caution in patients with fluid retention or heart failure.

Misuse Abuse and Diversion of Opioids
VICOPROFEN contains hydrocodone an opioid agonist, and is a Schedule III controlled substance. Opioid agonists have the potential for being abused and are sought by abusers and people with addiction disorders, and are subject to diversion.
VICOPROFEN can be abused in a manner similar to other opioid agonists, legal or illicit. This should be considered when prescribing or dispensing VICOPROFEN in situations where the physician or pharmacist is concerned about an increased risk of misuse, abuse or diversion (see **DRUG ABUSE AND DEPENDENCE**).

Respiratory Depression
At high doses or in opioid-sensitive patients, hydrocodone may produce dose-related respiratory depression by acting directly on the brain stem respiratory centers. Hydrocodone also affects the center that controls respiratory rhythm, and may produce irregular and periodic breathing.

Head Injury and Increased Intracranial Pressure
The respiratory depressant effects of opioids and their capacity to elevate cerebrospinal fluid pressure may be markedly exaggerated in the presence of head injury, intracranial lesions or a pre-existing increase in intracranial pressure. Furthermore, opioids produce adverse reactions, which may obscure the clinical course of patients with head injuries.

Acute Abdominal Conditions
The administration of opioids may obscure the diagnosis or clinical course of patients with acute abdominal conditions.

Gastrointestinal (GI) Effects - Risk of GI Ulceration, Bleeding and Perforation
NSAIDs, including VICOPROFEN, can cause serious gastrointestinal (GI) adverse events including inflammation, bleeding, ulceration, and perforation of the stomach, small intestine, or large intestine, which can be fatal. These serious adverse events can occur at any time, with or without warning symptoms, in patients treated with NSAIDs. Only one in five patients who develops a serious upper GI adverse event on NSAID therapy, is symptomatic. Upper GI ulcers, gross bleeding, or perforation caused by NSAIDs occur in approximately 1% of patients treated for 3-6 months, and in about 2-4% of patients treated for one year. These trends continue with longer duration of use, increasing the likelihood of developing a serious GI event at some time during the course of therapy. However, even short-term therapy is not without risk.
NSAIDs should be prescribed with extreme caution in those with a prior history of ulcer disease or gastrointestinal bleeding. Patients with a *prior history of peptic ulcer disease and/or gastrointestinal bleeding who* use NSAIDs have a greater than 10-fold increased risk for developing a GI bleed compared to patients with neither of these risk factors. Other factors that increase the risk for GI bleeding in patients treated with NSAIDs include concomitant use of oral corticosteroids or anticoagulants, longer duration of NSAID therapy, smoking, use of alcohol, older age, and poor general health status. Most spontaneous reports of fatal GI events are in elderly or debilitated patients and therefore, special care should be taken in treating this population.
To minimize the potential risk for an adverse GI event in patients treated with an NSAID, the lowest effective dose should be used for the shortest possible duration. Patients and physicians should remain alert for signs and symptoms of GI ulceration and bleeding during NSAID therapy and promptly initiate additional evaluation and treatment if a serious GI adverse event is suspected. This should include discontinuation of the NSAID until a serious GI adverse event is ruled out. For high-risk patients, alternate therapies that do not involve NSAIDs should be considered.

Renal Effects
Long-term administration of NSAIDs has resulted in renal papillary necrosis and other renal injury. Renal toxicity has also been seen in patients in whom renal prostaglandins have a compensatory role in the maintenance of renal perfusion. In these patients, administration of a nonsteroidal anti-inflammatory drug may cause a dose-dependent reduction in prostaglandin formation and, secondarily, in renal blood flow, which may precipitate overt renal decompensation. Patients at greatest risk of this reaction are those with impaired renal function, heart failure, liver dysfunction, those taking diuretics and ACE inhibitors, and the elderly. Discontinuation of NSAID therapy is usually followed by recovery to the pretreatment state.

Advanced Renal Disease
No information is available from controlled clinical studies regarding the use of VICOPROFEN in patients with advanced renal disease. Therefore, treatment with VICOPROFEN is not recommended in patients with advanced renal disease. If VICOPROFEN therapy must be initiated, close monitoring of the patient's renal function is advisable.

Anaphylactoid Reactions
As with other NSAID-containing products, anaphylactoid reactions may occur in patients without known prior exposure to VICOPROFEN. VICOPROFEN should not be given to patients with the aspirin triad. This symptom complex typically occurs in asthmatic patients who experience rhinitis with or without nasal polyps, or who exhibit severe, potentially fatal bronchospasm after taking aspirin or other NSAIDs. Fatal reactions to NSAIDs have been reported in such patients (see **CONTRAINDICATIONS** and **PRECAUTIONS** - Pre-existing Asthma). Emergency help should be sought in cases where an anaphylactoid reaction occurs.

Skin Reactions
Products containing NSAIDs, including VICOPROFEN, can cause serious skin adverse events such as exfoliative dermatitis, Stevens-Johnson Syndrome (SJS), and toxic epidermal necrolysis (TEN), which can be fatal. These serious events may occur without warning. Patients should be informed about the signs and symptoms of serious skin manifestations and use of the drug should be discontinued at the first appearance of skin rash or any other sign of hypersensitivity.

Pregnancy
As with other NSAID-containing products, VICOPROFEN should be avoided in late pregnancy because it may cause premature closure of the ductus arteriosus.

PRECAUTIONS

General

VICOPROFEN cannot be expected to substitute for corticosteroids or to treat corticosteroid insufficiency. Abrupt discontinuation of corticosteroids may lead to disease exacerbation. Patients on prolonged corticosteroid therapy should have their therapy tapered slowly if a decision is made to discontinue corticosteroids.
The pharmacological activity of VICOPROFEN in reducing fever and inflammation may diminish the utility of these diagnostic signs in detecting complications of presumed noninfectious, painful conditions.
Special Risk Patients
As with any opioid analgesic agent, VICOPROFEN tablets should be used with caution in elderly or debilitated patients, and those with severe impairment of hepatic or renal function, hypothyroidism, Addison's disease, prostatic hypertrophy or urethral stricture. The usual precautions should be observed and the possibility of respiratory depression should be kept in mind.
Cough Reflex
Hydrocodone suppresses the cough reflex; as with opioids, caution should be exercised when VICOPROFEN is used postoperatively and in patients with pulmonary disease.
Hepatic Effects
Borderline elevations of one or more liver enzymes may occur in up to 15% of patients taking NSAIDs including ibuprofen as found in VICOPROFEN. These laboratory abnormalities may progress, may remain essentially unchanged, or may be transient with continued therapy. Notable elevations of SGPT (ALT) or SGOT (AST) (approximately three or more times the upper limit of normal) have been reported in approximately 1% of patients in clinical trials with NSAIDS. In addition, rare cases of severe hepatic reactions, including jaundice and fatal fulminant hepatitis, liver necrosis and hepatic failure, some of them with fatal outcomes have been reported.
A patient with symptoms and/or signs suggesting liver dysfunction, or in whom an abnormal liver test has occurred, should be evaluated for evidence of the development of more severe hepatic reactions while on VICOPROFEN therapy. If clinical signs and symptoms consistent with liver disease develop, or if systemic manifestations occur (e.g., eosinophilia, rash, etc.), VICOPROFEN should be discontinued.
Hematological Effects
Anemia is sometimes seen in patients receiving NSAIDs including ibuprofen as found in VICOPROFEN. This may be due to fluid retention, occult or gross GI blood loss, or an incompletely described effect upon erythropoiesis. Patients on long-term treatment with NSAIDs including ibuprofen, should have their hemoglobin or hematocrit checked if they exhibit any signs or symptoms of anemia.
NSAIDs inhibit platelet aggregation and have been shown to prolong bleeding time in some patients. Unlike aspirin, their effect on platelet function is quantitatively less, of shorter duration, and reversible. Patients receiving VICOPROFEN who may be adversely affected by alterations in platelet function, such as those with coagulation disorders or patients receiving anticoagulants, should be carefully monitored.
Pre-existing Asthma
Patients with asthma may have aspirin-sensitive asthma. The use of aspirin in patients with aspirin-sensitive asthma has been associated with severe bronchospasm, which may be fatal. Since cross-reactivity between aspirin and other NSAIDs has been reported in such aspirin-sensitive patients, VICOPROFEN should not be administered to patients with this form of aspirin sensitivity and should be used with caution in patients with pre-existing asthma.
Aseptic Meningitis
Aseptic meningitis with fever and coma has been observed on rare occasions in patients on ibuprofen therapy as found in VICOPROFEN. Although it is probably more likely to oc-

Information on the AbbVie, Inc. products listed on these pages is from the prescribing information in use as of July 31, 2013. For more information, please visit rxabbvie.com or call 1-800-633-9110.

cur in patients with systemic lupus erythematosus and related connective tissue diseases, it has been reported in patients who do not have an underlying chronic disease. If signs or symptoms of meningitis develop in a patient on VICOPROFEN, the possibility of its being related to ibuprofen should be considered.

Information for Patients

Patients should be informed of the following information before initiating therapy with an NSAID and periodically during the course of ongoing therapy. Patients should also be encouraged to read the NSAID Medication Guide that accompanies each prescription dispensed.

1. VICOPROFEN® (hydrocodone bitartrate 7.5 mg and ibuprofen 200 mg), like other opioid-containing analgesics, may impair mental and/or physical abilities required for the performance of potentially hazardous tasks such as driving a car or operating machinery; patients should be cautioned accordingly.
2. Alcohol and other CNS depressants may produce an additive CNS depression, when taken with this combination product, and should be avoided.
3. VICOPROFEN can be abused in a manner similar to other opioid agonists, legal or illicit. VICOPROFEN may be habit-forming. Patients should take the drug only for as long as it is prescribed, in the amounts prescribed, and no more frequently than prescribed.
4. VICOPROFEN, like other NSAID-containing products, may cause serious CV side effects, such as MI or stroke, which may result in hospitalization and even death. Although serious CV events can occur without warning symptoms, patients should be alert for the signs and symptoms of chest pain, shortness of breath, weakness, slurring of speech, and should ask for medical advice when observing any indicative sign or symptoms. Patients should be apprised of the importance of this follow-up (see **WARNINGS, Cardiovascular Effects**).
5. VICOPROFEN, like other NSAID-containing products, can cause GI discomfort and serious GI side effects, such as ulcers and bleeding, which may result in hospitalization and even death. Although serious GI tract ulcerations and bleeding can occur without warning symptoms, patients should be alert for the signs and symptoms of ulcerations and bleeding, and should ask for medical advice when observing any indicative sign or symptoms including epigastric pain, dyspepsia, melena, and hematemesis. Patients should be apprised of the importance of this follow-up (see **WARNINGS, Gastrointestinal Effects: Risk of Ulceration, Bleeding, and Perforation**).
6. VICOPROFEN, like other NSAID-containing products, can cause serious skin side effects such as exfoliative dermatitis, SJS, and TEN, which may result in hospitalizations and even death. Although serious skin reactions may occur without warning, patients should be alert for the signs and symptoms of skin rash and blisters, fever, or other signs of hypersensitivity such as itching, and should ask for medical advice when observing any indicative signs or symptoms. Patients should be advised to stop the drug immediately if they develop any type of rash and contact their physicians as soon as possible.
7. Patients should promptly report signs or symptoms of unexplained weight gain or edema to their physicians.
8. Patients should be informed of the warning signs and symptoms of hepatotoxicity (e.g., nausea, fatigue, lethargy, pruritus, jaundice, right upper quadrant tenderness, and "flu-like" symptoms). If these occur, patients should be instructed to stop therapy and seek immediate medical therapy.
9. Patients should be informed of the signs of an anaphylactoid reaction (e.g., difficulty breathing, swelling of the face or throat). If these occur, patients should be instructed to seek immediate emergency help (see **WARNINGS**).
10. In late pregnancy, as with other NSAIDs, VICOPROFEN should be avoided because it may cause premature closure of the ductus arteriosus.
11. Patients should be instructed to report any signs of blurred vision or other eye symptoms.

Laboratory Tests

Because serious GI tract ulcerations and bleeding can occur without warning symptoms, physicians should monitor for signs or symptoms of GI bleeding. Patients on long-term treatment with NSAIDs should have their CBC and a chemistry profile checked periodically. If clinical signs and symptoms consistent with liver or renal disease develop, systemic manifestations occur (e.g., eosinophilia, rash, etc.) or if abnormal liver tests persist or worsen, VICOPROFEN should be discontinued.

Drug Interactions

ACE-inhibitors

Reports suggest that NSAIDs may diminish the antihypertensive effect of ACE-inhibitors. This interaction should be given consideration in patients taking VICOPROFEN concomitantly with ACE-inhibitors.

Anticholinergics

The concurrent use of anticholinergics with hydrocodone preparations may produce paralytic ileus.

Antidepressants

The use of Monoamine Oxidase Inhibitors (MAOIs) or tricyclic antidepressants with VICOPROFEN may increase the effect of either the antidepressant or hydrocodone.

MAOIs have been reported to intensify the effects of at least one opioid drug causing anxiety, confusion and significant depression of respiration or coma. The use of hydrocodone is not recommended for patients taking MAOIs or within 14 days of stopping such treatment.

Aspirin

When VICOPROFEN is administered with aspirin, the protein binding of aspirin is reduced, although the clearance of free VICOPROFEN is not altered. The clinical significance of this interaction is not known; however, as with other NSAID-containing products, concomitant administration of VICOPROFEN and aspirin is not generally recommended because of the potential of increased adverse effects.

CNS Depressants

Patients receiving other opioids, antihistamines, antipsychotics, antianxiety agents, or other CNS depressants (including alcohol) concomitantly with VICOPROFEN may exhibit an additive CNS depression. When combined therapy is contemplated, the dose of one or both agents should be reduced.

Diuretics

Ibuprofen has been shown to reduce the natriuretic effect of furosemide and thiazides in some patients. This response has been attributed to inhibition of renal prostaglandin synthesis. During concomitant therapy with VICOPROFEN the patient should be observed closely for signs of renal failure (see **WARNINGS** - Renal Effects), as well as diuretic efficacy.

Lithium

Ibuprofen has been shown to elevate plasma lithium concentration and reduce renal lithium clearance. The mean minimum lithium concentration increased 15% and the renal clearance was decreased by approximately 20%. This effect has been attributed to inhibition of renal prostaglandin synthesis by ibuprofen. Thus, when VICOPROFEN and lithium are administered concurrently, patients should be observed for signs of lithium toxicity.

Methotrexate

Ibuprofen, as well as other NSAIDs, has been reported to competitively inhibit methotrexate accumulation in rabbit kidney slices. This may indicate that ibuprofen could enhance the toxicity of methotrexate. Caution should be used when VICOPROFEN is administered concomitantly with methotrexate.

Mixed Agonist/Antagonist Opioid Analgesics

Agonist/antagonist analgesics (i.e., pentazocine, nalbuphine, butorphanol and buprenorphine) should be administered with caution to patients who have received or are receiving a course of therapy with a pure opioid agonist analgesic such as hydrocodone. In this situation, mixed agonist/antagonist analgesics may reduce the analgesic effect of hydrocodone and/or may precipitate withdrawal symptoms in these patients.

Neuromuscular Blocking Agents

Hydrocodone, as well as other opioid analgesics, may enhance the neuromuscular blocking action of skeletal muscle relaxants and produce an increased degree of respiratory depression.

Warfarin

The effects of warfarin and NSAIDs on GI bleeding are synergistic, such that users of both drugs together have a risk of serious GI bleeding higher than users of either drug alone.

Carcinogenicity, Mutagenicity, and Impairment of Fertility

The carcinogenic and mutagenic potential of VICOPROFEN has not been investigated. The ability of VICOPROFEN to impair fertility has not been assessed.

Pregnancy

Pregnancy Category C.

Teratogenic Effects

Reproductive studies conducted in rats and rabbits have not demonstrated evidence of developmental abnormalities.

VICOPROFEN, administered to rabbits at 95 mg/kg (5.72 and 1.9 times the maximum clinical dose based on body weight and surface area, respectively), a maternally toxic dose, resulted in an increase in the percentage of litters and fetuses with any major abnormality and an increase in the number of litters and fetuses with one or more nonossified metacarpals (a minor abnormality). VICOPROFEN, administered to rats at 166 mg/kg (10.0 and 1.66 times the maximum clinical dose based on body weight and surface area, respectively), a maternally toxic dose, did not result in any reproductive toxicity. However, animal reproduction studies are not always predictive of human response. There are no adequate and well-controlled studies in pregnant women. VICOPROFEN should be used during pregnancy only if the potential benefit justifies the potential risk to the fetus.

Nonteratogenic Effects

Because of the known effects of nonsteroidal anti-inflammatory drugs on the fetal cardiovascular system (closure of the ductus arteriosus), use during pregnancy (particularly late pregnancy) should be avoided. Babies born to mothers who have been taking opioids regularly prior to delivery will be physically dependent. The withdrawal signs include irritability and excessive crying, tremors, hyperactive reflexes, increased respiratory rate, increased stools, sneezing, yawning, vomiting, and fever. The intensity of the syndrome does not always correlate with the duration of maternal opioid use or dose. There is no consensus on the best method of managing withdrawal.

Labor and Delivery

As with other drugs known to inhibit prostaglandin synthesis, an increased incidence of dystocia and delayed parturition occurred in rats. Administration of VICOPROFEN is not recommended during labor and delivery. The effects of VICOPROFEN on labor and delivery in pregnant women are unknown.

Nursing Mothers

It is not known whether hydrocodone is excreted in human milk. In limited studies, an assay capable of detecting 1 mcg/mL did not demonstrate ibuprofen in the milk of lactating mothers. However, because of the limited nature of the studies, and because of the potential for serious adverse reactions in nursing infants from VICOPROFEN, a decision should be made whether to discontinue nursing or to discontinue the drug, taking into account the importance of the drug to the mother.

Pediatric Use

The safety and effectiveness of VICOPROFEN in pediatric patients below the age of 16 have not been established.

Geriatric Use

In controlled clinical trials there was no difference in tolerability between patients < 65 years of age and those ≥ 65, apart from an increased tendency of the elderly to develop constipation. However, because the elderly may be more sensitive to the renal and gastrointestinal effects of nonsteroidal anti-inflammatory agents as well as possible increased risk of respiratory depression with opioids, extra caution and reduced dosages should be used when treating the elderly with VICOPROFEN.

ADVERSE REACTIONS

VICOPROFEN was administered to approximately 300 pain patients in a safety study that employed dosages and a duration of treatment sufficient to encompass the recommended usage (see **DOSAGE AND ADMINISTRATION**). Adverse event rates generally increased with increasing daily dose. The event rates reported below are from approximately 150 patients who were in a group that received one tablet of VICOPROFEN an average of three to four times daily. The overall incidence rates of adverse experiences in the trials were fairly similar for this patient group and those who received the comparison treatment, acetaminophen 600 mg with codeine 60 mg.

The following lists adverse events that occurred with an incidence of 1% or greater in clinical trials of VICOPROFEN, without regard to the causal relationship of the events to the drug. To distinguish different rates of occurrence in clinical studies, the adverse events are listed as follows:

name of adverse event = less than 3%

*adverse events marked with an asterisk * = 3% to 9%*

adverse event rates over 9% are in parentheses.

Body as a Whole

Abdominal pain*; Asthenia*; Fever; Flu syndrome; Headache (27%); Infection*; Pain.

Cardiovascular

Palpitations; Vasodilation.

Central Nervous System

Anxiety*; Confusion; Dizziness (14%); Hypertonia; Insomnia*; Nervousness*; Paresthesia; Somnolence (22%); Thinking abnormalities.

Digestive

Anorexia; Constipation (22%); Diarrhea*; Dry mouth*; Dyspepsia (12%); Flatulence*; Gastritis; Melena; Mouth ulcers (21%); Nausea (21%); Thirst; Vomiting*.

Metabolic and Nutritional Disorders

Edema*.

Respiratory

Dyspnea; Hiccups; Pharyngitis; Rhinitis.

Skin and Appendages

Pruritus*; Sweating*.

Special Senses

Tinnitus.

Urogenital

Urinary frequency.

Incidence less than 1%

Body as a Whole

Allergic reaction.

Cardiovascular

Arrhythmia; Hypotension; Tachycardia.

Central Nervous System
Agitation; Abnormal dreams; Decreased libido; Depression; Euphoria; Mood changes; Neuralgia; Slurred speech; Tremor, Vertigo.
Digestive
Chalky stool; "Clenching teeth"; Dysphagia; Esophageal spasm; Esophagitis; Gastroenteritis; Glossitis; Liver enzyme elevation.
Metabolic and Nutritional
Weight decrease.
Musculoskeletal
Arthralgia; Myalgia.
Respiratory
Asthma; Bronchitis; Hoarseness; Increased cough; Pulmonary congestion; Pneumonia; Shallow breathing; Sinusitis.
Skin and Appendages
Rash; Urticaria.
Special Senses
Altered vision; Bad taste; Dry eyes.
Urogenital
Cystitis; Glycosuria; Impotence; Urinary incontinence; Urinary retention.

DRUG ABUSE AND DEPENDENCE

Misuse Abuse and Diversion of Opioids

VICOPROFEN contains hydrocodone, an opioid agonist, and is a Schedule III controlled substance. VICOPROFEN, and other opioids used in analgesia can be abused and are subject to criminal diversion.

Addiction is a primary, chronic, neurobiologic disease, with genetic, psychosocial, and environmental factors influencing its development and manifestations. It is characterized by behaviors that include one or more of the following: impaired control over drug use, compulsive use, continued use despite harm, and craving. Drug addiction is a treatable disease utilizing a multidisciplinary approach, but relapse is common.

"Drug seeking" behavior is very common in addicts and drug abusers. Drug-seeking tactics include emergency calls or visits near the end of office hours, refusal to undergo appropriate examination, testing or referral, repeated "loss" of prescriptions, tampering with prescriptions and reluctance to provide prior medical records or contact information for other treating physician(s). "Doctor shopping" to obtain additional prescriptions is common among drug abusers and people suffering from untreated addiction.

Abuse and addiction are separate and distinct from physical dependence and tolerance. Physical dependence usually assumes clinically significant dimensions only after several weeks of continued opioid use, although a mild degree of physical dependence may develop after a few days of opioid therapy. Tolerance, in which increasingly large doses are required in order to produce the same degree of analgesia, is manifested initially by a shortened duration of analgesic effect, and subsequently by decreases in the intensity of analgesia. The rate of development of tolerance varies among patients. Physicians should be aware that abuse of opioids can occur in the absence of true addiction and is characterized by misuse for non-medical purposes, often in combination with other psychoactive substances. VICOPROFEN, like other opioids, may be diverted for non-medical use. Record-keeping of prescribing information, including quantity, frequency, and renewal requests is strongly advised.

Proper assessment of the patient, proper prescribing practices, periodic re-evaluation of therapy, and proper dispensing and storage are appropriate measures that help to limit abuse of opioid drugs.

OVERDOSAGE

Following an acute overdosage, toxicity may result from hydrocodone and/or ibuprofen.

Signs and Symptoms

Hydrocodone Component

Serious overdose with hydrocodone is characterized by respiratory depression (a decrease in respiratory rate and/or tidal volume, Cheyne-Stokes respiration, cyanosis) extreme somnolence progressing to stupor or coma, skeletal muscle flaccidity, cold and clammy skin, and sometimes bradycardia and hypotension. In severe overdosage, apnea, circulatory collapse, cardiac arrest and death may occur.

Ibuprofen Component

Symptoms include gastrointestinal irritation with erosion and hemorrhage or perforation, kidney damage, liver damage, heart damage, hemolytic anemia, agranulocytosis, thrombocytopenia, aplastic anemia, and meningitis. Other symptoms may include headache, dizziness, tinnitus, confusion, blurred vision, mental disturbances, skin rash, stomatitis, edema, reduced retinal sensitivity, corneal deposits, and hyperkalemia.

Treatment

Primary attention should be given to the re-establishment of adequate respiratory exchange through provision of a patent airway and the institution of assisted or controlled ventilation. Naloxone, a narcotic antagonist, can reverse respiratory depression and coma associated with opioid overdose or unusual sensitivity to opioids, including hydrocodone. Therefore, an appropriate dose of naloxone hydrochloride should be administered intravenously with simultaneous efforts at respiratory resuscitation. Since the duration of action of hydrocodone may exceed that of the naloxone, the patient should be kept under continuous surveillance and repeated doses of the antagonist should be administered as needed to maintain adequate respiration. Supportive measures should be employed as indicated. Gastric emptying may be useful in removing unabsorbed drug. In cases where consciousness is impaired it may be inadvisable to perform gastric lavage. If gastric lavage is performed, little drug will likely be recovered if more than an hour has elapsed since ingestion. Ibuprofen is acidic and is excreted in the urine; therefore, it may be beneficial to administer alkali and induce diuresis. In addition to supportive measures the use of oral activated charcoal may help to reduce the absorption and reabsorption of ibuprofen. Dialysis is not likely to be effective for removal of ibuprofen because it is very highly bound to plasma proteins.

DOSAGE AND ADMINISTRATION

Carefully consider the potential benefits and risks of VICOPROFEN and other treatment options before deciding to use VICOPROFEN. Use the lowest effective dose for the shortest duration consistent with individual patient treatment goals (see **WARNINGS**).

After observing the response to initial therapy with VICOPROFEN, the dose and frequency should be adjusted to suit an individual patient's needs.

For the short-term (generally less than 10 days) management of acute pain, the recommended dose of VICOPROFEN is one tablet every 4 to 6 hours, as necessary. Dosage should not exceed 5 tablets in a 24-hour period. It should be kept in mind that tolerance to hydrocodone can develop with continued use and that the incidence of untoward effects is dose related.

The lowest effective dose or the longest dosing interval should be sought for each patient (see **WARNINGS**), especially in the elderly. After observing the initial response to therapy with VICOPROFEN, the dose and frequency of dosing should be adjusted to suit the individual patient's need, without exceeding the total daily dose recommended.

HOW SUPPLIED

VICOPROFEN tablets are available as:
White film-coated round convex tablets, engraved with "VP" over "a" logo on one side and plain on the other side.
Bottles of 100-NDC 0074-2277-14
Bottles of 500-NDC 0074-2277-54
Hospital Unit Dosage Package-100 tablets
(4 × 25 tablets)-NDC 0074-2277-12

Storage

Store at 25°C (77°F); excursions permitted to 15°-30°C (59°-86°F). [See USP Controlled Room Temperature].
Dispense in a tight, light-resistant container.
A Schedule CS-III Controlled Substance.

Manufactured by Halo Pharmaceutical Inc.
Whippany, NJ 07981 U.S.A.
for AbbVie Inc.
North Chicago, IL 60064 U.S.A.
Ref. 03-A691-R5-Revised April, 2013

Medication Guide
for
Non-Steroidal Anti-Inflammatory Drugs (NSAIDs)
(See the end of this Medication Guide for a list of prescription NSAID medicines.)

What is the most important information I should know about medicines called Non-Steroidal Anti-Inflammatory Drugs (NSAIDs)?

NSAID medicines may increase the chance of a heart attack or stroke that can lead to death.

This chance increases:
- with longer use of NSAID medicines
- in people who have heart disease

NSAID medicines should never be used right before or after a heart surgery called a "coronary artery bypass graft (CABG)."

NSAID medicines can cause ulcers and bleeding in the stomach and intestines at any time during treatment. Ulcers and bleeding:
- can happen without warning symptoms
- may cause death

The chance of a person getting an ulcer or bleeding increases with:
- taking medicines called "corticosteroids" and "anticoagulants"
- longer use
- smoking
- drinking alcohol
- older age
- having poor health

NSAID medicines should only be used:
- exactly as prescribed
- at the lowest dose possible for your treatment
- for the shortest time needed

What are Non-Steroidal Anti-Inflammatory Drugs (NSAIDs)?

NSAID medicines are used to treat pain and redness, swelling, and heat (inflammation) from medical conditions such as:
- different types of arthritis
- menstrual cramps and other types of short-term pain

Who should not take a Non-Steroidal Anti-Inflammatory Drug (NSAID)?

Do not take an NSAID medicine:
- if you had an asthma attack, hives, or other allergic reaction with aspirin or any other NSAID medicine
- for pain right before or after heart bypass surgery

Tell your healthcare provider:
- about all your medical conditions.
- about all of the medicines you take. NSAIDs and some other medicines can interact with each other and cause serious side effects. **Keep a list of your medicines to show to your healthcare provider and pharmacist.**
- if you are pregnant. **NSAID medicines should not be used by pregnant women late in their pregnancy.**
- if you are breastfeeding. **Talk to your doctor.**

What are the possible side effects of Non-Steroidal Anti-Inflammatory Drugs (NSAIDs)?

Serious side effects include:	Other side effects include:
• heart attack	• stomach pain
• stroke	• constipation
• high blood pressure	• diarrhea
• heart failure from body swelling (fluid retention)	• gas
• kidney problems including kidney failure	• heartburn
• bleeding and ulcers in the stomach and intestine	• nausea
• low red blood cells (anemia)	• vomiting
• life-threatening skin reactions	• dizziness
• life-threatening allergic reactions	
• liver problems including liver failure	
• asthma attacks in people who have asthma	

Get emergency help right away if you have any of the following symptoms:
- shortness of breath or trouble breathing
- chest pain
- weakness in one part or side of your body
- slurred speech
- swelling of the face or throat

Stop your NSAID medicine and call your healthcare provider right away if you have any of the following symptoms:
- nausea
- more tired or weaker than usual
- itching
- your skin or eyes look yellow
- stomach pain
- flu-like symptoms
- vomit blood
- there is blood in your bowel movement or it is black and sticky like tar
- unusual weight gain
- skin rash or blisters with fever
- swelling of the arms and legs, hands and feet

These are not all the side effects with NSAID medicines. Talk to your healthcare provider or pharmacist for more information about NSAID medicines. Call your doctor for medical advice about side effects. You may report side effects to FDA at 1–800–FDA-1088.

Other information about Non-Steroidal Anti-Inflammatory Drugs (NSAIDs)
- Aspirin is an NSAID medicine but it does not increase the chance of a heart attack. Aspirin can cause bleeding in the brain, stomach, and intestines. Aspirin can also cause ulcers in the stomach and intestines.
- Some of these NSAID medicines are sold in lower doses without a prescription (over the counter). Talk to your healthcare provider before using over the counter NSAIDs for more than 10 days.

Information on the AbbVie, Inc. products listed on these pages is from the prescribing information in use as of July 31, 2013. For more information, please visit rxabbvie.com or call 1-800-633-9110.

NSAID medicines that need a prescription

Generic Name	Tradename
Celecoxib	Celebrex
Diclofenac	Cataflam, Voltaren, Arthrotec (combined with misoprostol)
Diflunisal	Dolobid
Etodolac	Lodine, Lodine XL
Fenoprofen	Nalfon, Nalfon 200
Flurbirofen	Ansaid
Ibuprofen	Motrin, Tab-Profen, Vicoprofen* (combined with hydrocodone), Combunox (combined with oxycodone)
Indomethacin	Indocin, Indocin SR, Indo-Lemmon, Indomethagan
Ketoprofen	Oruvail
Ketorolac	Toradol
Mefenamic Acid	Ponstel
Meloxicam	Mobic
Nabumetone	Relafen
Naproxen	Naprosyn, Anaprox, Anaprox DS, EC-Naproxyn, Naprelan, Naprapac (copackaged with lansoprazole)
Oxaprozin	Daypro
Piroxicam	Feldene
Sulindac	Clinoril
Tolmetin	Tolectin, Tolectin DS, Tolectin 600

* Vicoprofen contains the same dose of ibuprofen as over-the-counter (OTC) NSAIDs, and is usually used for less than 10 days to treat pain. The OTC NSAID label warns that long term continuous use may increase the risk of heart attack or stroke.

Manufactured by Halo Pharmaceutical Inc.
Whippany, NJ 07981 U.S.A.
for AbbVie Inc.
North Chicago, IL 60064 U.S.A.
Ref. 03-A691-R5-Revised April, 2013
This Medication Guide has been approved by the U.S. Food and Drug Administration.

Shown in Product Identification Guide, page 304

ZEMPLAR® ℞
[zĕm-plər]
(paricalcitol) capsules

HIGHLIGHTS OF PRESCRIBING INFORMATION
These highlights do not include all the information needed to use ZEMPLAR safely and effectively.
See full prescribing information for ZEMPLAR.
ZEMPLAR (paricalcitol) capsules
Initial U.S. Approval: 1998

INDICATIONS AND USAGE

Zemplar is a vitamin D analog indicated for the prevention and treatment of secondary hyperparathyroidism associated with
- Chronic kidney disease (CKD) Stages 3 and 4 (1.1).
- CKD Stage 5 in patients on hemodialysis (HD) or peritoneal dialysis (PD) (1.2).

DOSAGE AND ADMINISTRATION

- CKD Stages 3 and 4: Zemplar Capsules may be administered once daily or every other day, three times a week (2.1).
- CKD Stage 5: Zemplar Capsules are dosed every other day, three times a week (2.2). To minimize the risk of hypercalcemia patients should be treated only after their baseline serum calcium has been reduced to 9.5 mg/dL or lower.

[See first table above]
[See second table above]

DOSAGE FORMS AND STRENGTHS

Capsules: 1 mcg, 2 mcg, and 4 mcg (3).

Initial Dosage

CKD Stages 3, 4		CKD Stage 5
Baseline intact parathyroid (iPTH) Level	Starting Dose	
≤ 500 pg/mL	1 mcg daily or 2 mcg three times a week (e.g. every other day)	Dose in micrograms is based on baseline iPTH level (pg/mL)/80. Dose three times a week (e.g. every other day).
> 500 pg/mL	2 mcg daily or 4 mcg three times a week (e.g. every other day)	

Dose Titration

CKD Stages 3, 4		CKD Stage 5
iPTH Level Relative to Baseline	Dosing Recommendation	
Decreased by < 30%	Increase dose by 1 mcg daily or 2 mcg three times a week (e.g. every other day)	Dose in micrograms is based on most recent iPTH level (pg/mL)/80 with adjustments based on serum calcium and phosphorous levels.
Decreased by ≥ 30% and ≤ 60%	Maintain dose	Dose three times a week (e.g. every other day).
Decreased by > 60% or iPTH < 60 pg/mL	Decrease dose by 1 mcg daily or 2 mcg three times a week (e.g. every other day)	

CONTRAINDICATIONS

Evidence of hypercalcemia or vitamin D toxicity (4).

WARNINGS AND PRECAUTIONS

- Hypercalcemia: Excessive administration of Zemplar Capsules can cause over suppression of PTH, hypercalcemia, hypercalciuria, hyperphosphatemia, and adynamic bone disease. Prescription-based doses of vitamin D and its derivatives should be withheld during Zemplar treatment (5.1).
- Digitalis toxicity: Potentiated by hypercalcemia of any cause. Use caution when Zemplar Capsules are prescribed concomitantly with digitalis compounds (5.2).
- Laboratory tests: Monitor serum calcium, serum phosphorus, and serum or plasma iPTH during initial dosing or following any dose adjustment (5.3).
- Aluminum overload and toxicity: Avoid excessive use of aluminum containing compounds (5.4).

ADVERSE REACTIONS

The most common adverse reactions (> 5% and more frequent than placebo) include diarrhea, hypertension, dizziness and vomiting.

To report SUSPECTED ADVERSE REACTIONS, contact AbbVie Inc. at 1-800-633-9110 or FDA at 1-800-FDA-1088 or www.fda.gov/medwatch

DRUG INTERACTIONS

- Strong CYP3A inhibitors (e.g. ketoconazole) will increase the exposure of paricalcitol. Use with caution (7.1).
- Cholestyramine, Mineral Oil: Intestinal absorption of Zemplar may be reduced if administered simultaneously with mineral oil or cholestyramine (7.2,7.3).

See 17 for PATIENT COUNSELING INFORMATION

Revised: 01/2013

FULL PRESCRIBING INFORMATION: CONTENTS*

*** Sections or subsections omitted from the full prescribing information are not listed**

FULL PRESCRIBING INFORMATION

1 INDICATIONS AND USAGE

1.1 Chronic Kidney Disease Stages 3 and 4

Zemplar Capsules are indicated for the prevention and treatment of secondary hyperparathyroidism associated with Chronic Kidney Disease (CKD) Stages 3 and 4.

1.2 Chronic Kidney Disease Stage 5

Zemplar Capsules are indicated for the prevention and treatment of secondary hyperparathyroidism associated with CKD Stage 5 in patients on hemodialysis (HD) or peritoneal dialysis (PD).

2 DOSAGE AND ADMINISTRATION

2.1 Chronic Kidney Disease Stages 3 and 4

Zemplar Capsules may be administered daily or three times a week. When dosing three times weekly, the dose should be administered not more frequently than every other day. The total weekly doses for both daily and three times a week dosage regimens are similar [*see Clinical Studies (14.1)*].

Zemplar Capsules may be taken without regard to food. No dosing adjustment is required in patients with mild and moderate hepatic impairment.

Initial Dose

The initial dose of Zemplar Capsules for CKD Stages 3 and 4 patients is based on baseline intact parathyroid hormone (iPTH) levels.

Baseline iPTH Level	Daily Dose	Three Times a Week Dose*
≤ 500 pg/mL	1 mcg	2 mcg
> 500 pg/mL	2 mcg	4 mcg

* To be administered not more often than every other day

Dose Titration

Dosing must be individualized and based on serum or plasma iPTH levels, with monitoring of serum calcium and serum phosphorus. The following is a suggested approach to dose titration.

iPTH Level Relative to Baseline	Zemplar Capsule Dose	Dose Adjustment at 2 to 4 Week Intervals	
		Daily Dosage	Three Times a Week Dosage*
The same, increased or decreased by < 30%	Increase dose by	1 mcg	2 mcg
Decreased by ≥ 30% and ≤ 60%	Maintain dose	-	-
Decreased by > 60% or iPTH < 60 pg/mL	Decrease dose by	1 mcg	2 mcg

* To be administered not more often than every other day

If a patient is taking the lowest dose, 1 mcg, on the daily regimen and a dose reduction is needed, the dose can be decreased to 1 mcg three times a week. If a further dose reduction is required, the drug should be withheld as needed and restarted at a lower dosing frequency. If a patient is on a calcium-based phosphate binder, the phosphate-binder dose may be decreased or withheld, or the patient may be switched to a non-calcium-based phosphate binder. If hypercalcemia or an elevated Ca × P is observed, the dose of Zemplar should be reduced or withheld until these parameters are normalized.

Serum calcium and phosphorus levels should be closely monitored after initiation of Zemplar Capsules, during dose titration periods and during co-administration with strong CYP3A inhibitors [see *Warnings and Precautions (5.3)*, *Drug Interactions (7)* and *Clinical Pharmacology (12.3)*].

2.2 Chronic Kidney Disease Stage 5

Zemplar Capsules are to be administered three times a week, not more frequently than every other day.

Zemplar Capsules may be taken without regard to food. No dosing adjustment is required in patients with mild and moderate hepatic impairment.

Initial Dose

The initial dose of Zemplar Capsules in micrograms is based on a baseline iPTH level (pg/mL)/80. To minimize the risk of hypercalcemia patients should be treated only after their baseline serum calcium has been adjusted to 9.5 mg/dL or lower [see *Clinical Pharmacology (12.2)* and *Clinical Studies (14.2)*].

Dose Titration

Subsequent dosing should be individualized and based on iPTH, serum calcium and phosphorus levels. A suggested dose titration of Zemplar Capsules is based on the following formula:

Titration dose (micrograms) = most recent iPTH level (pg/ml)/80

Serum calcium and phosphorus levels should be closely monitored after initiation, during dose titration periods, and with co-administration of strong P450 3A inhibitors. If an elevated serum calcium or elevated Ca × P is observed and the patient is on a calcium-based phosphate binder, the binder dose may be decreased or withheld, or the patient may be switched to a non-calcium-based phosphate binder. If serum calcium or Ca × P are elevated, the dose should be decreased by 2 to 4 micrograms lower than that calculated by the most recent iPTH/80. If further adjustment is required, the dose of paricalcitol capsules should be reduced or withheld until these parameters are normalized.

As iPTH approaches the target range, small, individualized dose adjustments may be necessary in order to achieve a stable iPTH. In situations where monitoring of iPTH, Ca or P occurs less frequently than once per week, a more modest initial and dose titration ratio (e.g., iPTH/100) may be warranted.

3 DOSAGE FORMS AND STRENGTHS

Zemplar Capsules are available as 1 mcg, 2 mcg, and 4 mcg soft gelatin capsules.

- 1 mcg: oval, gray capsule imprinted with the "a" logo and "ZA"
- 2 mcg: oval, orange-brown capsule imprinted with the "a" logo and "ZF"
- 4 mcg. oval, gold capsule imprinted with the "a" logo and "ZK"

4 CONTRAINDICATIONS

Zemplar Capsules should not be given to patients with evidence of

- hypercalcemia or
- vitamin D toxicity [see *Warnings and Precautions (5.1)*].

5 WARNINGS AND PRECAUTIONS

Excessive administration of vitamin D compounds, including Zemplar Capsules, can cause over suppression of PTH, hypercalcemia, hypercalciuria, hyperphosphatemia, and adynamic bone disease.

5.1 Hypercalcemia

Progressive hypercalcemia due to overdosage of vitamin D and its metabolites may be so severe as to require emergency attention [see *Overdosage (10)*]. Acute hypercalcemia may exacerbate tendencies for cardiac arrhythmias and seizures and may potentiate the action of digitalis. Chronic hypercalcemia can lead to generalized vascular calcification and other soft-tissue calcification. Concomitant administration of high doses of calcium-containing preparations or thiazide diuretics with Zemplar may increase the risk of hypercalcemia. High intake of calcium and phosphate concomitant with vitamin D compounds may lead to serum abnormalities requiring more frequent patient monitoring and individualized dose titration. Patients also should be informed about the symptoms of elevated calcium, which include feeling tired, difficulty thinking clearly, loss of appetite, nausea, vomiting, constipation, increased thirst, increased urination and weight loss.

Prescription-based doses of vitamin D and its derivatives should be withheld during Zemplar treatment to avoid hypercalcemia.

5.2 Digitalis Toxicity

Digitalis toxicity is potentiated by hypercalcemia of any cause. Use caution when Zemplar Capsules are prescribed concomitantly with digitalis compounds.

5.3 Laboratory Tests

During the initial dosing or following any dose adjustment of medication, serum calcium, serum phosphorus, and serum or plasma iPTH should be monitored at least every two weeks for 3 months, then monthly for 3 months, and every 3 months thereafter.

5.4 Aluminum Overload and Toxicity

Aluminum-containing preparations (e.g., antacids, phosphate binders) should not be administered chronically with Zemplar, as increased blood levels of aluminum and aluminum bone toxicity may occur.

6 ADVERSE REACTIONS

Because clinical studies are conducted under widely varying conditions, adverse reaction rates observed in the clinical studies of a drug cannot be directly compared to rates in the clinical studies of another drug and may not reflect the rates observed in practice.

6.1 Clinical Trials Experience

CKD Stages 3 and 4

The safety of Zemplar Capsules has been evaluated in three 24-week (approximately six-month), double-blind, placebo-controlled, multicenter clinical studies involving 220 CKD Stages 3 and 4 patients. Six percent (6%) of Zemplar Capsules treated patients and 4% of placebo treated patients discontinued from clinical studies due to an adverse event. Adverse events occurring in the Zemplar Capsules group at a frequency of 2% or greater and more frequently than in the placebo group are presented in Table 1:

Table 1. Treatment-Emergent Adverse Events by Body System Occurring in ≥ 2% of Subjects in the Zemplar-Treated Group of Three, Double-Blind, Placebo-Controlled, Phase 3, CKD Stages 3 and 4 Studies; All Treated Patients

Adverse Event[a]	Number (%) of Subjects			
	Zemplar Capsules (n = 107)		Placebo (n = 113)	
Overall	**88**	**(82%)**	**86**	**(76%)**
Ear and Labyrinth Disorders				
Vertigo	5	(4.7%)	0	(0.0%)
Gastrointestinal Disorders				
Abdominal Discomfort	4	(3.7%)	1	(0.9%)
Constipation	4	(3.7%)	4	(3.5%)
Diarrhea	7	(6.5%)	5	(4.4%)
Nausea	6	(5.6%)	4	(3.5%)
Vomiting	5	(4.7%)	5	(4.4%)
General Disorders and Administration Site Conditions				
Chest Pain	3	(2.8%)	1	(0.9%)
Edema	6	(5.6%)	5	(4.4%)
Pain	4	(3.7%)	4	(3.5%)
Immune System Disorders				
Hypersensitivity	6	(5.6%)	2	(1.8%)
Infections and Infestations				
Fungal Infection	3	(2.8%)	0	(0.0%)
Gastroenteritis	3	(2.8%)	3	(2.7%)
Infection	3	(2.8%)	3	(2.7%)
Sinusitis	3	(2.8%)	1	(0.9%)
Urinary Tract Infection	3	(2.8%)	1	(0.9%)
Viral Infection	8	(7.5%)	8	(7.1%)
Metabolism and Nutrition Disorders				
Dehydration	3	(2.8%)	1	(0.9%)
Musculoskeletal and Connective Tissue Disorders				
Arthritis	5	(4.7%)	0	(0.0%)
Back Pain	3	(2.8%)	1	(0.9%)
Muscle Spasms	3	(2.8%)	0	(0.0%)
Nervous System Disorders				
Dizziness	5	(4.7%)	5	(4.4%)
Headache	5	(4.7%)	5	(4.4%)
Syncope	3	(2.8%)	1	(0.9%)
Psychiatric Disorders				
Depression	3	(2.8%)	0	(0.0%)
Respiratory, Thoracic and Mediastinal Disorders				
Cough	3	(2.8%)	2	(1.8%)
Oropharyngeal Pain	4	(3.7%)	0	(0.0%)
Skin and Subcutaneous Tissue Disorders				
Pruritus	3	(2.8%)	3	(2.7%)
Rash	4	(3.7%)	1	(0.9%)
Skin Ulcer	3	(2.8%)	0	(0.0%)
Vascular Disorders				
Hypertension	7	(6.5%)	4	(3.5%)
Hypotension	5	(4.7%)	3	(2.7%)

a. Includes only events more common in the Zemplar treatment group.

The following adverse reactions, with a causal relationship to Zemplar, occurred in <2% of the Zemplar treated patients in the above double-blind, placebo-controlled clinical trial data set.

Gastrointestinal Disorders: Dry mouth
Investigations: Hepatic enzyme abnormal
Nervous System Disorders: Dysgeusia
Skin and Subcutaneous Tissue Disorders: Urticaria

CKD Stage 5

The safety of Zemplar Capsules has been evaluated in one 12-week, double-blind, placebo-controlled, multicenter clin-

Information on the AbbVie, Inc. products listed on these pages is from the prescribing information in use as of July 31, 2013. For more information, please visit rxabbvie.com or call 1-800-633-9110.

ical study involving 88 CKD Stage 5 patients. Sixty-one patients received Zemplar Capsules and 27 patients received placebo.

The proportion of patients who terminated prematurely from the study due to adverse events was 7% for Zemplar Capsules treated patients and 7% for placebo patients.

Adverse events occurring in the Zemplar Capsules group at a frequency of 2% or greater and more frequently than in the placebo group are as follows:

Table 2. Treatment-Emergent Adverse Events by Body System Occurring in ≥ 2% of Subjects in the Zemplar-Treated Group, Double-Blind, Placebo-Controlled, Phase 3, CKD Stage 5 Study; All Treated Patients

	Number (%) of Subjects			
Adverse Events[a]	**Zemplar Capsules (n=61)**		**Placebo (n = 27)**	
Overall	**43**	**(70%)**	**19**	**(70%)**
Gastrointestinal Disorders				
Constipation	3	(4.9%)	0	(0.0%)
Diarrhea	7	(11.5%)	3	(11.1%)
Vomiting	4	(6.6%)	0	(0.0%)
General Disorders and Administration Site Conditions				
Fatigue	2	(3.3%)	0	(0.0%)
Edema Peripheral	2	(3.3%)	0	(0.0%)
Infections and Infestations				
Nasopharyngitis	5	(8.2%)	2	(7.4%)
Peritonitis	3	(4.9%)	0	(0.0%)
Sinusitis	2	(3.3%)	0	(0.0%)
Urinary Tract Infection	2	(3.3%)	0	(0.0%)
Metabolism and Nutrition Disorders				
Fluid Overload	3	(4.9%)	0	(0.0%)
Hypoglycemia	2	(3.3%)	0	(0.0%)
Nervous System Disorders				
Dizziness	4	(6.6%)	0	(0.0%)
Headache	2	(3.3%)	0	(0.0%)
Psychiatric Disorders				
Anxiety	2	(3.3%)	0	(0.0%)
Insomnia	3	(4.9%)	0	(0.0%)
Renal and Urinary Disorders				
Renal Failure Chronic	2	(3.3%)	0	(0.0%)

a. Includes only events more common in the Zemplar treatment group.

The following adverse reactions, with a causal relationship to Zemplar, occurred in <2% of the Zemplar treated patients in the above double-blind, placebo-controlled clinical trial data set.

Gastrointestinal Disorders: Gastroesophageal reflux disease

Metabolism and Nutrition Disorders: Decreased appetite, hypercalcemia, hypocalcemia

Reproductive System and Breast Disorders: Breast tenderness

Skin and Subcutaneous Tissue Disorders: Acne

6.2 Postmarketing Experience

The following additional adverse reactions have been reported during post-approval use with the active ingredient in Zemplar capsules: angioedema (including laryngeal edema).

7 DRUG INTERACTIONS

7.1 CYP3A Inhibitors

Since paricalcitol is partially metabolized by CYP3A, exposure of paricalcitol will be increased while paricalcitol is coadministered with strong CYP3A inhibitors including the following drugs but not limited to: ketoconazole, atazanavir, clarithromycin, indinavir, itraconazole, nefazodone, nelfinavir, ritonavir, saquinavir, telithromycin or voriconazole. Dose adjustment of Zemplar Capsules may be required, and iPTH and serum calcium concentrations should be closely monitored if a patient initiates or discontinues therapy with a strong CYP3A4 inhibitor [see *Clinical Pharmacology (12.3)*].

7.2 Cholestyramine

Drugs that impair intestinal absorption of fat-soluble vitamins, such as cholestyramine, may interfere with the absorption of Zemplar Capsules.

7.3 Mineral Oil

The use of mineral oil or other substances that may affect absorption of fat may influence the absorption of Zemplar Capsules.

8 USE IN SPECIFIC POPULATIONS

8.1 Pregnancy

Pregnancy Category C.

Paricalcitol has been shown to cause minimal decreases in fetal viability (5%) when administered daily to rabbits at a dose 0.5 times a human dose of 14 mcg or 0.24 mcg/kg (based on body surface area, mcg/m^2), and when administered to rats at a dose two times the 0.24 mcg/kg human dose (based on body surface area, mcg/m^2). At the highest dose tested, 20 mcg/kg administered three times per week in rats (13 times the 14 mcg human dose based on surface area, mcg/m^2), there was a significant increase in the mortality of newborn rats at doses that were maternally toxic and are known to produce hypercalcemia in rats. No other effects on offspring development were observed.

Paricalcitol was not teratogenic at the doses tested.

Paricalcitol (20 mcg/kg) has been shown to cross the placental barrier in rats. There are no adequate and well-controlled clinical studies in pregnant women. Zemplar Capsules should be used during pregnancy only if the potential benefit to the mother justifies the potential risk to the fetus.

8.3 Nursing Mothers

Studies in rats have shown that paricalcitol is present in the milk. It is not known whether paricalcitol is excreted in human milk. In the nursing patient, a decision should be made whether to discontinue nursing or to discontinue the drug, taking into account the importance of the drug to the mother.

8.4 Pediatric Use

Safety and efficacy of Zemplar Capsules in pediatric patients have not been established.

8.5 Geriatric Use

Of the total number (n = 220) of CKD Stages 3 and 4 patients in clinical studies of Zemplar Capsules, 49% were age 65 and over, while 17% were age 75 and over. Of the total number (n = 88) of CKD Stage 5 patients in the pivotal study of Zemplar Capsules, 28% were age 65 and over, while 6% were age 75 and over. No overall differences in safety and effectiveness were observed between these patients and younger patients, and other reported clinical experience has not identified differences in responses between the elderly and younger patients, but greater sensitivity of some older individuals cannot be ruled out.

10 OVERDOSAGE

Excessive administration of Zemplar Capsules can cause hypercalcemia, hypercalciuria, and hyperphosphatemia, and over suppression of PTH [see *Warnings and Precautions (5.1)*].

Treatment of Overdosage

The treatment of acute overdosage of Zemplar Capsules should consist of general supportive measures. If drug ingestion is discovered within a relatively short time, induction of emesis or gastric lavage may be of benefit in preventing further absorption. If the drug has passed through the stomach, the administration of mineral oil may promote its fecal elimination. Serial serum electrolyte determinations (especially calcium), rate of urinary calcium excretion, and assessment of electrocardiographic abnormalities due to hypercalcemia should be obtained. Such monitoring is critical in patients receiving digitalis. Discontinuation of supplemental calcium and institution of a low-calcium diet are also indicated in accidental overdosage. Due to the relatively short duration of the pharmacological action of paricalcitol, further measures are probably unnecessary. If persistent and markedly elevated serum calcium levels occur, there are a variety of therapeutic alternatives that may be considered depending on the patient's underlying condition. These include the use of drugs such as phosphates and corticosteroids, as well as measures to induce an appropriate forced diuresis.

Zemplar is not significantly removed by dialysis.

11 DESCRIPTION

Paricalcitol, USP, the active ingredient in Zemplar Capsules, is a synthetically manufactured, metabolically active vitamin D analog of calcitriol with modifications to the side chain (D_2) and the A (19-nor) ring. Zemplar is indicated for the prevention and treatment of secondary hyperparathyroidism in chronic kidney disease. Zemplar is available as soft gelatin capsules for oral administration containing 1 microgram, 2 micrograms or 4 micrograms of paricalcitol. Each capsule also contains medium chain triglycerides, alcohol, and butylated hydroxytoluene. The medium chain triglycerides are fractionated from coconut oil or palm kernel oil. The capsule shell is composed of gelatin, glycerin, titanium dioxide, iron oxide red (2 microgram capsules only), iron oxide yellow (2 microgram and 4 microgram capsules), iron oxide black (1 microgram capsules only), and water.

Paricalcitol is a white, crystalline powder with the empirical formula of $C_{27}H_{44}O_3$, which corresponds to a molecular weight of 416.64. Paricalcitol is chemically designated as 19-nor-1α,3β,25-trihydroxy-9,10-secoergosta-5(Z),7(E),22(E)-triene and has the following structural formula:

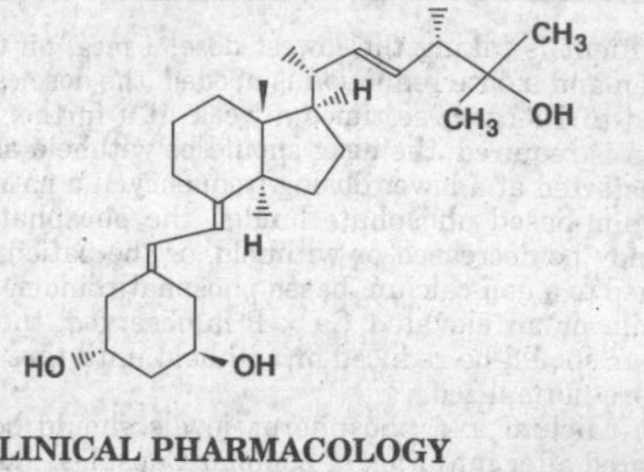

12 CLINICAL PHARMACOLOGY

Secondary hyperparathyroidism is characterized by an elevation in parathyroid hormone (PTH) associated with inadequate levels of active vitamin D hormone. The source of vitamin D in the body is from synthesis in the skin as vitamin D_3 and from dietary intake as either vitamin D_2 or D_3. Both vitamin D_2 and D_3 require two sequential hydroxylations in the liver and the kidney to bind to and to activate the vitamin D receptor (VDR). The endogenous VDR activator, calcitriol [$1,25(OH)_2D_3$], is a hormone that binds to VDRs that are present in the parathyroid gland, intestine, kidney, and bone to maintain parathyroid function and calcium and phosphorus homeostasis, and to VDRs found in many other tissues, including prostate, endothelium and immune cells. VDR activation is essential for the proper formation and maintenance of normal bone. In the diseased kidney, the activation of vitamin D is diminished, resulting in a rise of PTH, subsequently leading to secondary hyperparathyroidism and disturbances in the calcium and phosphorus homeostasis. Decreased levels of $1,25(OH)_2D_3$ have been observed in early stages of chronic kidney disease. The decreased levels of $1,25(OH)_2D_3$ and resultant elevated PTH levels, both of which often precede abnormalities in serum calcium and phosphorus, affect bone turnover rate and may result in renal osteodystrophy.

12.1 Mechanism of Action

Paricalcitol is a synthetic, biologically active vitamin D_2 analog of calcitriol. Preclinical and *in vitro* studies have demonstrated that paricalcitol's biological actions are mediated through binding of the VDR, which results in the selective activation of vitamin D responsive pathways. Vitamin D and paricalcitol have been shown to reduce parathyroid hormone levels by inhibiting PTH synthesis and secretion.

12.2 Pharmacodynamics

Paricalcitol decreases serum intact parathyroid hormone (iPTH) and increases serum calcium and serum phosphorous in both HD and PD patients. This observed relationship was quantified using a mathematical model for HD and PD patient populations separately. Computer-based simulations of 100 trials in HD or PD patients (N = 100) using these relationships predict slightly lower efficacy (at least two consecutive ≥ 30% reductions from baseline iPTH) with lower hypercalcemia rates (at least two consecutive serum calcium ≥ 10.5 mg/dL) for lower iPTH-based dosing regimens. Further lowering of hypercalcemia rates was predicted if the treatment with paricalcitol is initiated in patients with lower serum calcium levels at screening.

Based on these simulations, a dosing regimen of iPTH/80 with a screening serum calcium ≤ 9.5 mg/dL, approximately 76.5% (95% CI: 75.6% – 77.3%) of HD patients are predicted to achieve at least two consecutive weekly ≥ 30% reductions from baseline iPTH over a duration of 12 weeks. The predicted incidence of hypercalcemia is 0.8% (95% CI: 0.7% – 1.0%). In PD patients, with this dosing regimen, approximately 83.3% (95% CI: 82.6% – 84.0%) of patients are predicted to achieve at least two consecutive weekly ≥ 30% reductions from baseline iPTH. The predicted incidence of hypercalcemia is 12.4% (95% CI: 11.7% - 13.0%) [*see Clinical Studies (14.2) and Dosage and Administration (2.2)*].

12.3 Pharmacokinetics

Absorption

The mean absolute bioavailability of Zemplar Capsules under low-fat fed condition ranged from 72% to 86% in healthy subjects, CKD Stage 5 patients on HD, and CKD Stage 5 patients on PD. A food effect study in healthy subjects indicated that the C_{max} and $AUC_{0-\infty}$ were unchanged when paricalcitol was administered with a high fat meal compared to fasting. Food delayed T_{max} by about 2 hours. The $AUC_{0-\infty}$ of paricalcitol increased proportionally over the dose range of 0.06 to 0.48 mcg/kg in healthy subjects.

Distribution

Paricalcitol is extensively bound to plasma proteins (≥ 99.8%). The mean apparent volume of distribution following a 0.24 mcg/kg dose of paricalcitol in healthy subjects was 34 L. The mean apparent volume of distribution following a 4 mcg dose of paricalcitol in CKD Stage 3 and a 3 mcg dose in CKD Stage 4 patients is between 44 and 46 L.

Metabolism

After oral administration of a 0.48 mcg/kg dose of ^3H-paricalcitol, parent drug was extensively metabolized, with only about 2% of the dose eliminated unchanged in the feces, and no parent drug was found in the urine. Several metabolites were detected in both the urine and feces. Most of the systemic exposure was from the parent drug. Two minor metabolites, relative to paricalcitol, were detected in human plasma. One metabolite was identified as 24(R)-hydroxy paricalcitol, while the other metabolite was unidentified. The 24(R)-hydroxy paricalcitol is less active than paricalcitol in an *in vivo* rat model of PTH suppression.

In vitro data suggest that paricalcitol is metabolized by multiple hepatic and non-hepatic enzymes, including mitochondrial CYP24, as well as CYP3A4 and UGT1A4. The identified metabolites include the product of 24(R)-hydroxylation, 24,26- and 24,28-dihydroxylation and direct glucuronidation.

Elimination

Paricalcitol is eliminated primarily via hepatobiliary excretion; approximately 70% of the radiolabeled dose is recovered in the feces and 18% is recovered in the urine. While the mean elimination half-life of paricalcitol is 4 to 6 hours in healthy subjects, the mean elimination half-life of paricalcitol in CKD Stages 3, 4, and 5 (on HD and PD) patients ranged from 14 to 20 hours.

[See table 3 above]

Table 3. Paricalcitol Capsule Pharmacokinetic Characteristics in CKD Stages 3, 4, and 5 Patients

Pharmacokinetic Parameters	CKD Stage 3 n = 15*	CKD Stage 4 n = 14*	CKD Stage 5 HD** n = 14	CKD Stage 5 PD** n = 8
C_{max} (ng/mL)	0.11 ± 0.04	0.06 ± 0.01	0.575 ± 0.17	0.413 ± 0.06
$AUC_{0-\infty}$ (ng•h/mL)	2.42 ± 0.61	2.13 ± 0.73	11.67 ± 3.23	13.41 ± 5.48
CL/F (L/h)	1.77 ± 0.50	1.52 ± 0.36	1.82 ± 0.75	1.76 ± 0.77
V/F (L)	43.7 ± 14.4	46.4 ± 12.4	38 ± 16.4	48.7 ± 15.6
$t_{1/2}$	16.8 ± 2.65	19.7 ± 7.2	13.9 ± 5.1	17.7 ± 9.6

* Four mcg paricalcitol capsules were given to CKD Stage 3 patients; three mcg paricalcitol capsules were given to CKD Stage 4 patients.

** CKD Stage 5 HD and PD patients received a 0.24 mcg/kg dose of paricalcitol as capsules.

Specific Populations

Geriatric

The pharmacokinetics of paricalcitol has not been investigated in geriatric patients greater than 65 years [*see Use in Specific Populations (8.5)*].

Pediatric

The pharmacokinetics of paricalcitol has not been investigated in patients less than 18 years of age.

Gender

The pharmacokinetics of paricalcitol following single doses over the 0.06 to 0.48 mcg/kg dose range was gender independent.

Hepatic Impairment

The disposition of paricalcitol (0.24 mcg/kg) was compared in patients with mild (n = 5) and moderate (n = 5) hepatic impairment (as indicated by the Child-Pugh method) and subjects with normal hepatic function (n = 10). The pharmacokinetics of unbound paricalcitol was similar across the range of hepatic function evaluated in this study. No dose adjustment is required in patients with mild and moderate hepatic impairment. The influence of severe hepatic impairment on the pharmacokinetics of paricalcitol has not been evaluated.

Renal Impairment

Following administration of Zemplar Capsules, the pharmacokinetic profile of paricalcitol for CKD Stage 5 on HD or PD was comparable to that in CKD 3 or 4 patients. Therefore, no special dose adjustments are required other than those recommended in the Dosage and Administration section [*see Dosage and Administration (2)*].

Drug Interactions

An *in vitro* study indicates that paricalcitol is neither an inhibitor of CYP1A2, CYP2A6, CYP2B6, CYP2C8, CYP2C9, CYP2C19, CYP2D6, CYP2E1 or CYP3A nor an inducer of CYP2B6, CYP2C9 or CYP3A. Hence, paricalcitol is neither expected to inhibit nor induce the clearance of drugs metabolized by these enzymes.

Omeprazole

The effect of omeprazole (40 mg capsule), a strong inhibitor of CYP2C19, on paricalcitol (four 4 mcg capsules) pharmacokinetics was investigated in a single dose, crossover study in healthy subjects. The pharmacokinetics of paricalcitol was not affected when omeprazole was administered approximately 2 hours prior to the paricalcitol dose.

Ketoconazole

The effect of multiple doses of ketoconazole, a strong inhibitor of CYP3A, administered as 200 mg BID for 5 days on the pharmacokinetics of paricalcitol (4 mcg capsule) has been studied in healthy subjects. The C_{max} of paricalcitol was minimally affected, but $AUC_{0-\infty}$ approximately doubled in the presence of ketoconazole. The mean half-life of paricalcitol was 17.0 hours in the presence of ketoconazole as compared to 9.8 hours, when paricalcitol was administered alone [*see Drug Interactions (7)*].

13 NONCLINICAL TOXICOLOGY

13.1 Carcinogenesis, Mutagenesis and Impairment of Fertility

In a 104-week carcinogenicity study in CD-1 mice, an increased incidence of uterine leiomyoma and leiomyosarcoma was observed at subcutaneous doses of 1, 3, 10 mcg/kg given three times weekly (2 to 15 times the AUC at a human dose of 14 mcg, equivalent to 0.24 mcg/kg based on AUC). The incidence rate of uterine leiomyoma was significantly different than the control group at the highest dose of 10 mcg/kg. In a 104-week carcinogenicity study in rats, there was an increased incidence of benign adrenal pheochromocytoma at subcutaneous doses of 0.15, 0.5, 1.5 mcg/kg (< 1 to 7 times the exposure following a human dose of 14 mcg, equivalent to 0.24 mcg/kg based on AUC). The increased incidence of pheochromocytomas in rats may be related to the alteration of calcium homeostasis by paricalcitol. Paricalcitol did not exhibit genetic toxicity *in vitro* with or without metabolic activation in the microbial mutagenesis assay (Ames Assay), mouse lymphoma mutagenesis assay (L5178Y), or a human lymphocyte cell chromosomal aberration assay. There was also no evidence of genetic toxicity in an *in vivo* mouse micronucleus assay. Paricalcitol had no effect on fertility (male or female) in rats at intravenous doses up to 20 mcg/kg/dose (equivalent to 13 times a human dose of 14 mcg based on surface area, mcg/m^2).

14 CLINICAL STUDIES

14.1 Chronic Kidney Disease Stages 3 and 4

The safety and efficacy of Zemplar Capsules were evaluated in three, 24-week, double blind, placebo-controlled, randomized, multicenter, Phase 3 clinical studies in CKD Stages 3 and 4 patients. Two studies used an identical three times a week dosing design, and one study used a daily dosing design. A total of 107 patients received Zemplar Capsules and 113 patients received placebo. The mean age of the patients was 63 years, 68% were male, 71% were Caucasian, and 26% were African-American. The average baseline iPTH was 274 pg/mL (range: 145-856 pg/mL). The average duration of CKD prior to study entry was 5.7 years. At study entry 22% were receiving calcium based phosphate binders and/or calcium supplements. Baseline 25-hydroxyvitamin D levels were not measured.

The initial dose of Zemplar Capsules was based on baseline iPTH. If iPTH was ≤ 500 pg/mL, Zemplar Capsules were administered 1 mcg daily or 2 mcg three times a week, not more than every other day. If iPTH was > 500 pg/mL, Zemplar Capsules were administered 2 mcg daily or 4 mcg three times a week, not more than every other day. The dose was increased by 1 mcg daily or 2 mcg three times a week every 2 to 4 weeks until iPTH levels were reduced by at least 30% from baseline. The overall average weekly dose of Zemplar Capsules was 9.6 mcg/week in the daily regimen and 9.5 mcg/week in the three times a week regimen.

In the clinical studies, doses were titrated for any of the following reasons: if iPTH fell to < 60 pg/mL, or decreased > 60% from baseline, the dose was reduced or temporarily withheld; if iPTH decreased < 30% from baseline and serum calcium was ≤ 10.3 mg/dL and serum phosphorus was ≤ 5.5 mg/dL, the dose was increased; and if iPTH decreased between 30 to 60% from baseline and serum calcium and phosphorus were ≤ 10.3 mg/dL and ≤ 5.5 mg/dL, respectively, the dose was maintained. Additionally, if serum calcium was between 10.4 to 11.0 mg/dL, the dose was reduced irrespective of iPTH, and the dose was withheld if serum calcium was > 11.0 mg/dL. If serum phosphorus was > 5.5 mg/dL, dietary counseling was provided, and phosphate binders could have been initiated or increased. If the elevation persisted, the Zemplar Capsules dose was decreased. Seventy-seven percent (77%) of the Zemplar Capsules treated patients and 82% of the placebo treated patients completed the 24-week treatment. The primary efficacy endpoint of at least two consecutive ≥ 30% reductions from baseline iPTH was achieved by 91% of Zemplar Capsules treated patients and 13% of the placebo treated patients ($p < 0.001$). The proportion of Zemplar Capsules treated patients achieving two consecutive ≥ 30% reductions was similar between the daily and the three times a week regimens (daily: 30/33, 91%; three times a week: 62/68, 91%).

The incidence of hypercalcemia (defined as two consecutive serum calcium values > 10.5 mg/dL), hyperphosphatemia and elevated Ca × P product in Zemplar Capsules treated patients was similar to placebo. There were no treatment related adverse events associated with hypercalcemia or hyperphosphatemia in the Zemplar Capsules group. No increases in urinary calcium or phosphorous were detected in Zemplar Capsules treated patients compared to placebo.

The pattern of change in the mean values for serum iPTH during the studies is shown in Figure 1.

Figure 1. Mean Values for Serum iPTH Over Time in the Three Double-Blind, Placebo-Controlled, Phase 3, CKD Stages 3 and 4 Studies Combined

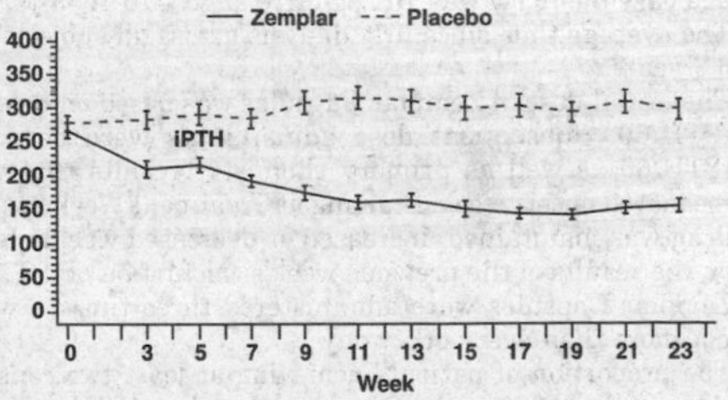

The mean changes from baseline to final treatment visit in serum iPTH, calcium, phosphorus, calcium-phosphorus product (Ca × P), and bone-specific alkaline phosphatase are shown in Table 4.

Table 4. Mean Changes from Baseline to Final Treatment Visit in Serum iPTH, Bone Specific Alkaline Phosphatase, Calcium, Phosphorus, and Calcium × Phosphorus Product in Three Combined Double-Blind, Placebo-Controlled, Phase 3, CKD Stages 3 and 4 Studies

	Zemplar Capsules	Placebo
iPTH (pg/mL)	n = 104	n = 110
Mean Baseline Value	266	279
Mean Final Treatment Value	162	315
Mean Change from Baseline (SE)	-104 (9.2)	+35 (9.0)
Bone Specific Alkaline Phosphatase (mcg/L)	n = 101	n = 107
Mean Baseline	17.1	18.8

Information on the AbbVie, Inc. products listed on these pages is from the prescribing information in use as of July 31, 2013. For more information, please visit rxabbvie.com or call 1-800-633-9110.

Mean Final Treatment Value	9.2	17.4
Mean Change from Baseline (SE)	-7.9 (0.76)	-1.4 (0.74)
Calcium (mg/dL)	n = 104	n = 110
Mean Baseline	9.3	9.4
Mean Final Treatment Value	9.5	9.3
Mean Change from Baseline (SE)	+0.2 (0.04)	-0.1 (0.04)
Phosphorus (mg/dL)	n = 104	n = 110
Mean Baseline	4.0	4.0
Mean Final Treatment Value	4.3	4.3
Mean Change from Baseline (SE)	+0.3 (0.08)	+0.3 (0.08)
Calcium × Phosphorus Product (mg^2/dL^2)	n = 104	n = 110
Mean Baseline	36.7	36.9
Mean Final Treatment Value	40.7	39.7
Mean Change from Baseline (SE)	+4.0 (0.74)	+2.9 (0.72)

14.2 Chronic Kidney Disease Stage 5

The safety and efficacy of Zemplar Capsules were evaluated in a Phase 3, 12-week, double blind, placebo-controlled, randomized, multicenter study in patients with CKD Stage 5 on HD or PD. The study used a three times a week dosing design. A total of 61 patients received Zemplar Capsules and 27 patients received placebo. The mean age of the patients was 57 years, 67% were male, 50% were Caucasian, 45% were African- American, and 53% were diabetic. The average baseline iPTH was 701 pg/mL (range: 216-1933 pg/mL). The average time since first dialysis across all subjects was 3.3 years.

The initial dose of Zemplar Capsules was based on baseline iPTH/60. Subsequent dose adjustments were based on iPTH/60 as well as primary chemistry results that were measured once a week. Starting at Treatment Week 2, study drug was maintained, increased or decreased weekly based on the results of the previous week's calculation of iPTH/60. Zemplar Capsules were administered three times a week, not more than every other day.

The proportion of patients achieving at least two consecutive weekly ≥ 30% reductions from baseline iPTH was 88% of Zemplar Capsules treated patients and 13% of the placebo treated patients. The proportion of patients achieving at least two consecutive weekly ≥ 30% reductions from baseline iPTH was similar for HD and PD patients.

The incidence of hypercalcemia (defined as two consecutive serum calcium values > 10.5 mg/dL) in patients treated with Zemplar Capsules was 6.6% as compared to 0% for patients given placebo. In PD patients the incidence of hypercalcemia in patients treated with Zemplar Capsules was 21% as compared to 0% for patients given placebo. The patterns of change in the mean values for serum iPTH are shown in Figure 2. The rate of hypercalcemia with Zemplar Capsules may be reduced with a lower dosing regimen based on the iPTH/80 formula as shown by computer simulations. The hypercalcemia rate can be further predicted to decrease, if the treatment is initiated in only those with baseline serum calcium ≤ 9.5 mg/dL [*see Clinical Pharmacology (12.2) and Dosage and Administration (2.2)*].

[See figure 2 at top of next column]

16 HOW SUPPLIED/STORAGE AND HANDLING

Zemplar Capsules are available as 1 mcg, 2 mcg, and 4 mcg capsules.

The 1 mcg capsule is an oval, gray, soft gelatin capsule imprinted with the "a" logo and ZA, and is available in the following package size:

Bottles of 30 (NDC 0074-4317-30)

The 2 mcg capsule is an oval, orange-brown, soft gelatin capsule imprinted with the "a" logo and ZF, and is available in the following package size:

Bottles of 30 (NDC 0074-4314-30)

The 4 mcg capsule is an oval, gold soft gelatin capsule imprinted with the "a" logo and ZK, and is available in the following package size:

Bottles of 30 (NDC 0074-4315-30)

Figure 2. Mean Values for Serum iPTH Over Time in a Phase 3, Double-Blind, Placebo-Controlled CKD Stage 5 Study

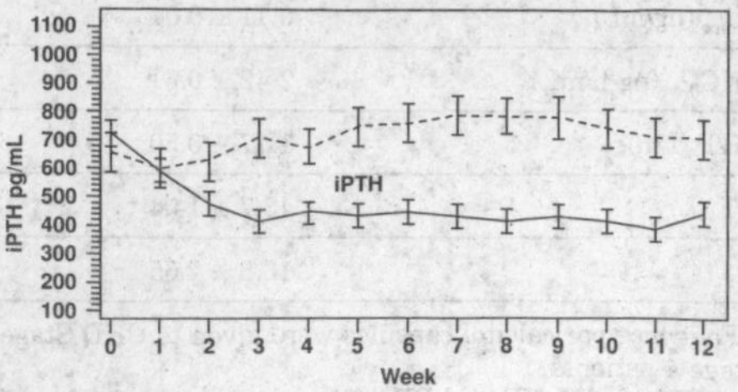

Storage

Store Zemplar Capsules at 25°C (77°F). Excursions permitted between 15°- 30°C (59°- 86°F). See USP Controlled Room Temperature.

17 PATIENT COUNSELING INFORMATION

Patients should be advised:

- of the most common adverse reactions with use of Zemplar Capsules, which include diarrhea, hypertension, dizziness and vomiting.
- to adhere to instructions regarding diet and phosphorus restriction.
- to contact a health care provider if you develop symptoms of elevated calcium, (e.g. feeling tired, difficulty thinking clearly, loss of appetite, nausea, vomiting, constipation, increased thirst, increased urination and weight loss).
- to return to the physician's office for routine monitoring. More frequent monitoring is necessary during the initiation of therapy, following dose changes or when potentially interacting medications are started or discontinued.
- to inform their physician of all medications, including prescription and nonprescription drugs, supplements, and herbal preparations they are taking and any change to their medical condition. Patients should also be advised to inform their physicians prescribing a new medication that they are taking Zemplar Capsules.

Manufactured for
AbbVie Inc.
North Chicago, IL 60064, U.S.A.
03-A689-R8-Revised January, 2013

Shown in Product Identification Guide, page 304

ZEMPLAR® ℞
[*zĕm-plar*]
(paricalcitol) Injection
Fliptop Vial

DESCRIPTION

Paricalcitol, USP, the active ingredient in Zemplar Injection, is a synthetically manufactured analog of calcitriol, the metabolically active form of vitamin D indicated for the prevention and treatment of secondary hyperparathyroidism associated with chronic kidney disease (CKD) Stage 5. Zemplar is available as a sterile, clear, colorless, aqueous solution for intravenous injection. Each mL contains paricalcitol, 2 mcg or 5 mcg and the following inactive ingredients: alcohol, 20% (v/v) and propylene glycol, 30% (v/v).

Paricalcitol is a white powder chemically designated as 19-nor-1α,3β,25-trihydroxy-9,10-secoergosta-5(Z),7(E),22(E)-triene and has the following structural formula:

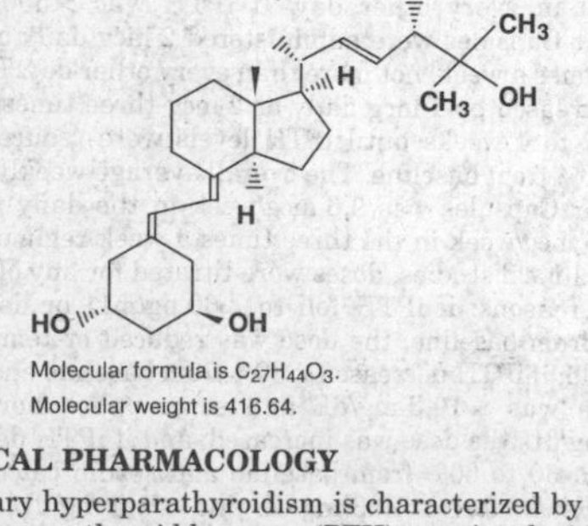

Molecular formula is $C_{27}H_{44}O_3$.
Molecular weight is 416.64.

CLINICAL PHARMACOLOGY

Secondary hyperparathyroidism is characterized by an elevation in parathyroid hormone (PTH) associated with inadequate levels of active vitamin D hormone. The source of vitamin D in the body is from synthesis in the skin and from dietary intake. Vitamin D requires two sequential hydroxylations in the liver and the kidney to bind to and to activate the vitamin D receptor (VDR). The endogenous VDR activator, calcitriol [1,25$(OH)_2$ D_3], is a hormone that binds to VDRs that are present in the parathyroid gland, intestine, kidney, and bone to maintain parathyroid function and calcium and phosphorus homeostasis, and to VDRs found in many other tissues, including prostate, endothelium and immune cells. VDR activation is essential for the proper formation and maintenance of normal bone. In the diseased kidney, the activation of vitamin D is diminished, resulting in a rise of PTH, subsequently leading to secondary hyperparathyroidism, and disturbances in the calcium and phosphorus homeostasis. The decreased levels of 1,25$(OH)_2$ D_3 and resultant elevated PTH levels, both of which often precede abnormalities in serum calcium and phosphorus, affect bone turnover rate and may result in renal osteodystrophy.

Mechanism of Action

Paricalcitol is a synthetic, biologically active vitamin D analog of calcitriol with modifications to the side chain (D_2) and the A (19-nor) ring. Preclinical and *in vitro* studies have demonstrated that paricalcitol's biological actions are mediated through binding of the VDR, which results in the selective activation of vitamin D responsive pathways. Vitamin D and paricalcitol have been shown to reduce parathyroid hormone levels by inhibiting PTH synthesis and secretion.

Pharmacokinetics

Within two hours after administering Zemplar intravenous doses ranging from 0.04 to 0.24 mcg/kg, concentrations of paricalcitol decreased rapidly; thereafter, concentrations of paricalcitol declined log-linearly. No accumulation of paricalcitol was observed with three times a week dosing.

Distribution

Paricalcitol is extensively bound to plasma proteins (≥99.8%). In healthy subjects, the steady state volume of distribution is approximately 23.8 L. The mean volume of distribution following a 0.24 mcg/kg dose of paricalcitol in CKD Stage 5 subjects requiring hemodialysis (HD) and peritoneal dialysis (PD) is between 31 and 35 L.

Metabolism

After IV administration of a 0.48 mcg/kg dose of ^{3}H-paricalcitol, parent drug was extensively metabolized, with only about 2% of the dose eliminated unchanged in the feces and no parent drug found in the urine. Several metabolites were detected in both the urine and feces. Most of the systemic exposure was from the parent drug. Two minor metabolites, relative to paricalcitol, were detected in human plasma. One metabolite was identified as 24(R)-hydroxy paricalcitol, while the other metabolite was unidentified. The 24(R)-hydroxy paricalcitol is less active than paricalcitol in an *in vivo* rat model of PTH suppression.

In vitro data suggest that paricalcitol is metabolized by multiple hepatic and non-hepatic enzymes, including mitochondrial CYP24, as well as CYP3A4 and UGT1A4. The identified metabolites include the product of 24(R)-hydroxylation (present at low levels in plasma), as well as 24,26- and 24,28-dihydroxylation and direct glucuronidation.

Elimination

Paricalcitol is excreted primarily by hepatobiliary excretion. Approximately 63% of the radioactivity was eliminated in the feces and 19% was recovered in the urine in healthy subjects. In healthy subjects, the mean elimination half-life of paricalcitol is about five to seven hours over the studied dose range of 0.04 to 0.16 mcg/kg. The pharmacokinetics of paricalcitol has been studied in CKD Stage 5 subjects requiring hemodialysis (HD) and peritoneal dialysis (PD). The mean elimination half-life of paricalcitol after administration of 0.24 mcg/kg paricalcitol IV bolus dose in CKD Stage 5 HD and PD patients is 13.9 and 15.4 hours, respectively (Table 1).

Table 1 Mean ± SD Paricalcitol Pharmacokinetic Parameters in CKD Stage 5 Subjects Following Single 0.24 mcg/kg IV Bolus Dose

	CKD Stage 5-HD (n=14)	CKD Stage 5-PD (n=8)
C_{max} (ng/mL)	1.680 ± 0.511	1.832 ± 0.315
$AUC_{0-\infty}$ (ng•h/mL)	14.51 ± 4.12	16.01 ± 5.98
β (1/h)	0.050 ± 0.023	0.045 ± 0.026
$t_{1/2}$ (h)†	13.9 ± 7.3	15.4 ± 10.5
CL (L/h)	1.49 ± 0.60	1.54 ± 0.95
$Vd_β$ (L)	30.8 ± 7.5	34.9 ± 9.5

† harmonic mean ± pseudo standard deviation, HD: hemodialysis, PD: peritoneal dialysis

No accumulation of paricalcitol was observed with three times a week dosing which is consistent with the observed half-life.

Special Populations

Geriatric

The pharmacokinetics of paricalcitol have not been investigated in geriatric patients greater than 65 years.

Pediatrics

The pharmacokinetics of paricalcitol have not been investigated in patients less than 18 years of age.

Gender
The pharmacokinetics of paricalcitol were gender independent.

Hepatic Impairment
The disposition of paricalcitol (0.24 mcg/kg) was compared in patients with mild (n=5) and moderate (n=5) hepatic impairment (as indicated by the Child-Pugh method) and subjects with normal hepatic function (n=10). The pharmacokinetics of unbound paricalcitol were similar across the range of hepatic function evaluated in this study. No dose adjustment is required in patients with mild and moderate hepatic impairment. The influence of severe hepatic impairment on the pharmacokinetics of paricalcitol has not been evaluated.

Renal Impairment
The pharmacokinetics of paricalcitol have been studied in CKD Stage 5 subjects requiring hemodialysis (HD) and peritoneal dialysis (PD). Hemodialysis procedure has essentially no effect on paricalcitol elimination. However, compared to healthy subjects, CKD Stage 5 subjects showed a decreased CL and increased half-life (see **Pharmacokinetics**-Elimination).

Drug Interactions
An *in vitro* study indicates that paricalcitol is not an inhibitor of CYP1A2, CYP2A6, CYP2B6, CYP2C8, CYP2C9, CYP2C19, CYP2D6, CYP2E1, or CYP3A at concentrations up to 50 nM (21 ng/mL) (approximately 20-fold greater than that obtained after highest tested dose). In fresh primary cultured hepatocytes, the induction observed at paricalcitol concentrations up to 50 nM was less than two-fold for CYP2B6, CYP2C9 or CYP3A, where the positive controls rendered a six- to nineteen-fold induction. Hence, paricalcitol is not expected to inhibit or induce the clearance of drugs metabolized by these enzymes.
Drug interactions with paricalcitol injection have not been studied.

Omeprazole
The pharmacokinetic interaction between paricalcitol capsule (16 mcg) and omeprazole (40 mg; oral), a strong inhibitor of CYP2C19, was investigated in a single dose, crossover study in healthy subjects. The pharmacokinetics of paricalcitol were unaffected when omeprazole was administrated approximately 2 hours prior to the paricalcitol dose.

Ketoconazole
Although no data are available for the drug interaction between paricalcitol injection and ketoconazole, a strong inhibitor of CYP3A, the effect of multiple doses of ketoconazole administered as 200 mg BID for 5 days on the pharmacokinetics of paricalcitol capsule has been studied in healthy subjects. The C_{max} of paricalcitol was minimally affected, but $AUC_{0-\infty}$ approximately doubled in the presence of ketoconazole. The mean half-life of paricalcitol was 17.0 hours in the presence of ketoconazole as compared to 9.8 hours, when paricalcitol was administered alone (See **PRECAUTIONS**).

CLINICAL STUDIES

In three 12-week, placebo-controlled, phase 3 studies in chronic kidney disease Stage 5 patients on dialysis, the dose of Zemplar was started at 0.04 mcg/kg 3 times per week. The dose was increased by 0.04 mcg/kg every 2 weeks until intact parathyroid hormone (iPTH) levels were decreased at least 30% from baseline or a fifth escalation brought the dose to 0.24 mcg/kg, or iPTH fell to less than 100 pg/mL, or the Ca × P product was greater than 75 within any 2 week period, or serum calcium became greater than 11.5 mg/dL at any time.
Patients treated with Zemplar achieved a mean iPTH reduction of 30% within 6 weeks. In these studies, there was no significant difference in the incidence of hypercalcemia or hyperphosphatemia between Zemplar and placebo-treated patients. The results from these studies are as follows:
[See table above]
A long-term, open-label safety study of 164 CKD Stage 5 patients (mean dose of 7.5 mcg three times per week), demonstrated that mean serum Ca, P, and Ca × P remained within clinically appropriate ranges with PTH reduction (mean decrease of 319 pg/mL at 13 months).
[See figure at top of next column]

INDICATIONS AND USAGE

Zemplar is indicated for the prevention and treatment of secondary hyperparathyroidism associated with chronic kidney disease Stage 5.

CONTRAINDICATIONS

Zemplar should not be given to patients with evidence of vitamin D toxicity, hypercalcemia, or hypersensitivity to any ingredient in this product (see **WARNINGS**).

WARNINGS

Acute overdose of Zemplar may cause hypercalcemia, and require emergency attention (see **OVERDOSAGE**). During dose adjustment, serum calcium and phosphorus levels should be monitored closely (e.g., twice weekly). If clinically significant hypercalcemia develops, the dose should be reduced or interrupted. Chronic administration of Zemplar may place patients at risk of hypercalcemia, elevated Ca × P product, and metastatic calcification. Chronic hypercalcemia can lead to generalized vascular calcification and other soft-tissue calcification.
Concomitant administration of high doses of calcium-containing preparations or thiazide diuretics with Zemplar may increase the risk of hypercalcemia. High intake of calcium and phosphate concomitant with vitamin D compounds may lead to serum abnormalities requiring more frequent patient monitoring and individualized dose titration. Patients also should be informed about the symptoms of elevated calcium, which include feeling tired, difficulty thinking clearly, loss of appetite, nausea, vomiting, constipation, increased thirst, increased urination and weight loss.
Prescription-based doses of vitamin D and its derivatives should be withheld during Zemplar treatment to avoid hypercalcemia.
Aluminum-containing preparations (e.g., antacids, phosphate binders) should not be administered chronically with Zemplar, as increased blood levels of aluminum and aluminum bone toxicity may occur.

Group (No. of Pts.)		Baseline Mean (Range)	Mean (SE) Change From Baseline to Final Evaluation
PTH (pg/mL)	Zemplar (n = 40)	783 (291 – 2076)	-379 (43.7)
	placebo (n = 38)	745 (320 –1671)	-69.6 (44.8)
Alkaline	Zemplar (n = 31)	150 (40 – 600)	-41.5 (10.6)
Phosphatase (U/L)	placebo (n = 34)	169 (56 – 911)	+2.6 (10.1)
Calcium (mg/dL)	Zemplar (n = 40)	9.3 (7.2 – 10.4)	+0.47 (0.1)
	placebo (n = 38)	9.1 (7.8 – 10.7)	+0.02 (0.1)
Phosphorus (mg/dL)	Zemplar (n = 40)	5.8 (3.7 – 10.2)	+0.47 (0.3)
	placebo (n = 38)	6.0 (2.8 – 8.8)	-0.47 (0.3)
Calcium ×	Zemplar (n = 40)	54 (32 – 106)	+7.9 (2.2)
Phosphorus Product	placebo (n = 38)	54 (26 – 77)	-3.9 (2.3)

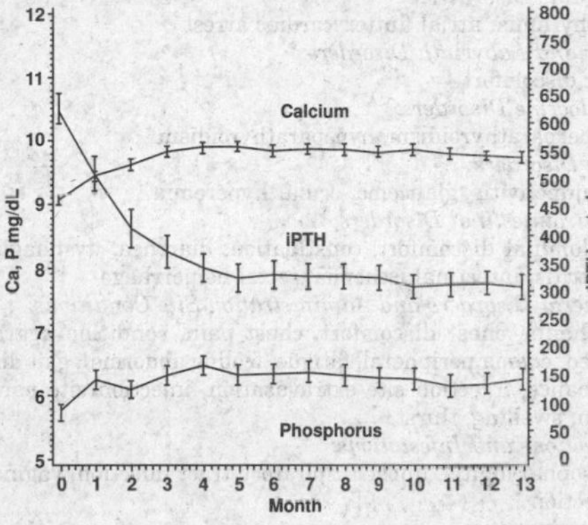

PRECAUTIONS

General
Digitalis toxicity is potentiated by hypercalcemia of any cause, so caution should be applied when digitalis compounds are prescribed concomitantly with Zemplar. Adynamic bone lesions may develop if PTH levels are suppressed to abnormal levels.

Information for the Patient
The patient should be instructed that, to ensure effectiveness of Zemplar therapy, it is important to adhere to a dietary regimen of calcium supplementation and phosphorus restriction. Appropriate types of phosphate-binding compounds may be needed to control serum phosphorus levels in patients with chronic kidney disease (CKD) Stage 5, but excessive use of aluminum containing compounds should be avoided (see **WARNINGS**). Patients should also be carefully informed about the symptoms of elevated calcium (see **WARNINGS**).

Laboratory Tests
During the initial phase of medication, serum calcium and phosphorus should be determined frequently (e.g., twice weekly). Once dosage has been established, serum calcium and phosphorus should be measured at least monthly. Measurements of serum or plasma PTH are recommended every 3 months. During dose adjustment of Zemplar, laboratory tests may be required more frequently.

Drug Interactions
Specific interaction studies were not performed with Zemplar Injection. Paricalcitol is not expected to inhibit the clearance of drugs metabolized by cytochrome P450 enzymes CYP1A2, CYP2A6, CYP2B6, CYP2C8, CYP2C9, CYP2C19, CYP2D6, CYP2E1, or CYP3A nor induce the clearance of drug metabolized by CYP2B6, CYP2C9 or CYP3A.
A multiple dose drug-drug interaction study with ketoconazole and paricalcitol capsule demonstrated that ketoconazole approximately doubled paricalcitol $AUC_{0-\infty}$ (see **CLINICAL PHARMACOLOGY**). Since paricalcitol is partially metabolized by CYP3A and ketoconazole is known to be a strong inhibitor of cytochrome P450 3A enzyme, care should be taken while paricalcitol is co-administered with ketoconazole and other strong P450 3A inhibitors including the following drugs but not limited to: atazanavir, clarithromycin, indinavir, itraconazole, nefazodone, nelfinavir, ritonavir, saquinavir, telithromycin or voriconazole.
Digitalis toxicity is potentiated by hypercalcemia of any cause, so caution should be applied when digitalis compounds are prescribed concomitantly with Zemplar.

Carcinogenesis, Mutagenesis, Impairment of Fertility
In a 104-week carcinogenicity study in CD-1 mice, an increased incidence of uterine leiomyoma and leiomyosarcoma was observed at subcutaneous doses of 1, 3, 10 mcg/kg (2 to 15 times the AUC at a human dose of 14 mcg, equivalent to 0.24 mcg/kg based on AUC). The incidence rate of uterine leiomyoma was significantly different than the control group at the highest dose of 10 mcg/kg.
In a 104-week carcinogenicity study in rats, there was an increased incidence of benign adrenal pheochromocytoma at subcutaneous doses of 0.15, 0.5, 1.5 mcg/kg (< 1 to 7 times the exposure following a human dose of 14 mcg, equivalent to 0.24 mcg/kg based on AUC). The increased incidence of pheochromocytomas in rats may be related to the alteration of calcium homeostasis by paricalcitol.
Paricalcitol did not exhibit genetic toxicity *in vitro* with or without metabolic activation in the microbial mutagenesis assay (Ames Assay), mouse lymphoma mutagenesis assay (L5178Y), or a human lymphocyte cell chromosomal aberration assay. There was also no evidence of genetic toxicity in an *in vivo* mouse micronucleus assay. Zemplar had no effect on fertility (male or female) in rats at intravenous doses up to 20 mcg/kg/dose [equivalent to 13 times the highest recommended human dose (0.24 mcg/kg) based on surface area, mg/m^2].

Pregnancy
Pregnancy Category C
Paricalcitol has been shown to cause minimal decreases in fetal viability (5%) when administered daily to rabbits at a dose 0.5 times the 0.24 mcg/kg human dose (based on surface area, mg/m^2) and when administered to rats at a dose 2 times the 0.24 mcg/kg human dose (based on plasma levels of exposure). At the highest dose tested (20 mcg/kg 3 times per week in rats, 13 times the 0.24 mcg/kg human dose based on surface area), there was a significant increase of the mortality of newborn rats at doses that were maternally toxic (hypercalcemia). No other effects on offspring development were observed. Paricalcitol was not teratogenic at the doses tested.
There are no adequate and well-controlled studies in pregnant women. Zemplar should be used during pregnancy only if the potential benefit to the mother justifies the potential risk to the fetus.

Nursing Mothers
Studies in rats have shown that paricalcitol is present in the milk. It is not known whether paricalcitol is excreted in human milk. In the nursing patient, a decision should be made whether to discontinue nursing or to discontinue the drug, taking into account the importance of the drug to the mother.

Pediatric Use
The safety and effectiveness of Zemplar were examined in a 12-week randomized, double-blind, placebo-controlled study of 29 pediatric patients, aged 5-19 years, with end-stage renal disease on hemodialysis and nearly all had received some form of vitamin D prior to the study. Seventy-six percent of the patients were male, 52% were Caucasian and 45% were African-American. The initial dose of Zemplar was 0.04 mcg/kg 3 times per week based on baseline iPTH level of less than 500 pg/mL, or 0.08 mcg/kg 3 times a week,

Information on the AbbVie, Inc. products listed on these pages is from the prescribing information in use as of July 31, 2013. For more information, please visit rxabbvie.com or call 1-800-633-9110.

List No.	Volume/Container	Concentration	Total Content	Vial Type
4637-01	1 mL/Fliptop Vial	2 mcg/mL	2 mcg	Single-dose
1658-01	1 mL/Fliptop Vial	5 mcg/mL	5 mcg	Single-dose
1658-05	2 mL/Fliptop Vial	5 mcg/mL	10 mcg	Multi-dose

based on baseline iPTH level of ≥ 500 pg/mL, respectively. The dose of Zemplar was adjusted in 0.04 mcg/kg increments based on the levels of serum iPTH, calcium and Ca × P. The mean baseline levels of iPTH were 841 pg/mL for the 15 Zemplar-treated patients and 740 pg/mL for the 14 placebo-treated subjects. The mean dose of Zemplar administered was 4.6 mcg (range: 0.8 mcg – 9.6 mcg). Ten of the 15 (67%) Zemplar-treated patients and 2 of the 14 (14%) placebo-treated patients completed the trial. Ten of the placebo patients (71%) were discontinued due to excessive elevations in iPTH levels as defined by 2 consecutive iPTH levels > 700 pg/mL and greater than baseline after 4 weeks of treatment.

In the primary efficacy analysis, 9 of 15 (60%) subjects in the Zemplar group had 2 consecutive 30% decreases from baseline iPTH compared with 3 of 14 (21%) patients in the placebo group (95% CI for the difference between groups –1%, 63%). Twenty-three percent of Zemplar vs. 31% of placebo patients had at least one serum calcium level > 10.3 mg/dL, and 40% vs. 14% of Zemplar vs. placebo subjects had at least one Ca × P ion product > 72 $(mg/dL)^2$. The overall percentage of serum calcium measurements > 10.3 mg/dL was 7% in the Zemplar group and 7% in the placebo group; the overall percentage of patients with Ca × P product > 72 $(mg/dL)^2$ was 8% in the Zemplar group and 7% in the placebo group. No subjects in either the Zemplar group or placebo group developed hypercalcemia (defined as at least one calcium value > 11.2 mg/dL) during the study.

Geriatric Use

Of the 40 patients receiving Zemplar in the three phase 3 placebo-controlled CKD Stage 5 studies, 10 patients were 65 years or over. In these studies, no overall differences in efficacy or safety were observed between patients 65 years or older and younger patients.

ADVERSE REACTIONS

Zemplar has been evaluated for safety in clinical studies in 609 CKD Stage 5 patients. In four, placebo-controlled, double-blind, multicenter studies, discontinuation of therapy due to any adverse event occurred in 6.5% of 62 patients treated with Zemplar (dosage titrated as tolerated, see **CLINICAL PHARMACOLOGY - Clinical Studies**) and 2.0% of 51 patients treated with placebo for 1 to 3 months. Adverse events occurring in the Zemplar group at a frequency of 2% or greater and with an incidence greater than that in the placebo group, regardless of causality, are presented in the following table:

Adverse Event Incidence Rates for All Treated Patients In All Placebo-Controlled Studies

Adverse Event	Zemplar (n = 62) %	Placebo (n = 51) %
Overall	**71**	**78**
Cardiac Disorders		
Palpitations	3.2	0.0
Gastrointestinal Disorders		
Dry Mouth	3.2	2.0
Gastrointestinal Hemorrhage	4.8	2.0
Nausea	12.9	7.8
Vomiting	8.1	5.9
General Disorders and Administration Site Conditions		
Chills	4.8	2.0
Edema	6.5	0.0
Malaise	3.2	0.0
Pyrexia	4.8	2.0
Infections and Infestations		
Influenza	4.8	3.9
Pneumonia	4.8	0.0
Sepsis	4.8	2.0
Musculoskeletal and Connective Tissue Disorders		
Arthralgia	4.8	3.9

A patient who reported the same medical term more than once was counted only once for that medical term.

Safety parameters (changes in mean Ca, P, Ca × P) in an open-label safety study up to 13 months in duration support the long-term safety of Zemplar in this patient population (see **CLINICAL STUDIES**).

Other Adverse Reactions Observed During Clinical Evaluation of Zemplar Injection

The following adverse reactions, with a causal relationship to Zemplar, occurred in <2% of the Zemplar treated patients in the above double-blind, placebo-controlled clinical trial data set. In addition, the following also includes adverse reactions reported in Zemplar-treated patients who participated in other studies (non placebo-controlled), including double-blind, active-controlled and open-label studies:

Blood and Lymphatic System Disorders:
Anemia, lymphadenopathy
Cardiac Disorders:
Arrhythmia, atrial flutter, cardiac arrest
Ear and Labyrinth Disorders:
Ear discomfort
Endocrine Disorders:
Hyperparathyroidism, hypoparathyroidism
Eye Disorders:
Conjunctivitis, glaucoma, ocular hyperemia
Gastrointestinal Disorders:
Abdominal discomfort, constipation, diarrhea, dysphagia, gastritis, intestinal ischemia, rectal hemorrhage
General Disorders and Administration Site Conditions:
Asthenia, chest discomfort, chest pain, condition aggravated, edema peripheral, fatigue, feeling abnormal, gait disturbance, injection site extravasation, injection site pain, pain, swelling, thirst
Infections and Infestations:
Nasopharyngitis, upper respiratory tract infection, vaginal infection
Investigations:
Aspartate aminotransferase increased, bleeding time prolonged, heart rate irregular, laboratory test abnormal, weight decreased
Metabolism and Nutrition Disorders:
Decreased appetite, hypercalcemia, hyperkalemia, hyperphosphatemia, hypocalcemia
Musculoskeletal and Connective Tissue Disorders:
Joint stiffness, muscle twitching, myalgia
Neoplasms Benign, Malignant and Unspecified:
Breast cancer
Nervous System Disorders:
Cerebrovascular accident, dizziness, dysgeusia, headache, hypoesthesia, myoclonus, paresthesia, syncope, unresponsive to stimuli
Psychiatric Disorders:
Agitation, confusional state, delirium, insomnia, nervousness, restlessness
Reproductive System and Breast Disorders:
Breast pain, erectile dysfunction
Respiratory, Thoracic and Mediastinal Disorders:
Cough, dyspnea, orthopnea, pulmonary edema, wheezing
Skin and Subcutaneous Tissue Disorders:
Alopecia, blister, hirsutism, night sweats, rash pruritic, pruritus, skin burning sensation
Vascular Disorders:
Hypertension, hypotension

Additional Adverse Events Reported During Post-marketing Experience

Allergic reactions, such as rash, urticaria, and angioedema (including laryngeal edema) have been reported.

OVERDOSAGE

Overdosage of Zemplar may lead to hypercalcemia, hypercalciuria, hyperphosphatemia, and over suppression of PTH. (see **WARNINGS**).

Treatment of Overdosage and Hypercalcemia

The treatment of acute overdosage should consist of general supportive measures. Serial serum electrolyte determinations (especially calcium), rate of urinary calcium excretion, and assessment of electrocardiographic abnormalities due to hypercalcemia should be obtained. Such monitoring is critical in patients receiving digitalis. Discontinuation of supplemental calcium and institution of a low calcium diet are also indicated in acute overdosage.

General treatment of hypercalcemia due to overdosage consists of immediate dose reduction or suspension of Zemplar therapy, institution of a low calcium diet, withdrawal of calcium supplements, patient mobilization, and attention to fluid and electrolyte imbalances. Serum calcium levels should be determined at least weekly until normocalcemia ensues. When serum calcium levels have returned to within normal limits, Zemplar may be reinitiated at a lower dose. If persistent and markedly elevated serum calcium levels occur, there are a variety of therapeutic alternatives that may be considered. These include the use of drugs such as phosphates and corticosteroids as well as measures to induce diuresis. Also, one may consider dialysis against a calcium-free dialysate.

Zemplar is not significantly removed by dialysis.

DOSAGE AND ADMINISTRATION

The currently accepted target range for iPTH levels in CKD Stage 5 patients is no more than 1.5 to 3 times the non-uremic upper limit of normal.

The recommended initial dose of Zemplar is 0.04 mcg/kg to 0.1 mcg/kg (2.8 – 7 mcg) administered as a bolus dose no more frequently than every other day at any time during dialysis.

If a satisfactory response is not observed, the dose may be increased by 2 to 4 mcg at 2- to 4-week intervals. During any dose adjustment period, serum calcium and phosphorus levels should be monitored more frequently, and if an elevated calcium level or a Ca × P product greater than 75 is noted, the drug dosage should be immediately reduced or interrupted until these parameters are normalized. Then, Zemplar should be reinitiated at a lower dose. If a patient is on a calcium-based phosphate binder, the dose may be decreased or withheld, or the patient may be switched to a non-calcium-based phosphate binder. Zemplar doses may need to be decreased as the PTH levels decrease in response to therapy. Thus, incremental dosing must be individualized.

The following table is a suggested approach in dose titration:

Suggested Dosing Guidelines

PTH Level	Zemplar Dose
the same or increasing	increase
decreasing by < 30%	increase
decreasing by > 30%, < 60%	maintain
decreasing by > 60%	decrease
one and one-half to three times upper limit of normal	maintain

The influence of mild to moderately impaired hepatic function on paricalcitol pharmacokinetics is sufficiently small that no dosing adjustment is required.

Parenteral drug products should be inspected visually for particulate matter and discoloration prior to administration whenever solution and container permit.

After initial vial use, the contents of the multi-dose vial remain stable up to seven days when stored at controlled room temperature (see **HOW SUPPLIED**). Discard unused portion of the single-dose vial.

HOW SUPPLIED

Zemplar Injection is available as 2 mcg/mL (**NDC** 0074-4637-01) and 5 mcg/mL (**NDC** 0074-1658-01 and **NDC** 0074–1658–05) in trays of 25 vials.

[See table above]

Store at 25°C (77°F). Excursions permitted between 15° - 30°C (59° - 86°F).

Manufactured for
AbbVie Inc.
North Chicago, IL 60064, U.S.A.
Ref. EN-2945-Rev. January, 2013

Alcon Laboratories, Inc.

AND ITS AFFILIATES
CORPORATE HEADQUARTERS
6201 SOUTH FREEWAY
FORT WORTH, TX 76134

Address Inquiries to:
6201 South Freeway
Fort Worth, TX 76134
(800) 757-9195
Outside the U.S. call (817) 568-6725
alcon.medinfo@alcon.com

CIPRODEX® ℞

[*sĭ-prō-dĕks*]
(ciprofloxacin 0.3% and dexamethasone 0.1%)
Sterile Otic Suspension

DESCRIPTION

CIPRODEX® (ciprofloxacin 0.3% and dexamethasone 0.1%) Sterile Otic Suspension contains the synthetic broad-spectrum antibacterial agent, ciprofloxacin hydrochloride, combined with the anti-inflammatory corticosteroid, dexamethasone, in a sterile, preserved suspension for otic use. Each mL of CIPRODEX® Otic contains ciprofloxacin hydrochloride (equivalent to 3 mg ciprofloxacin base), 1 mg dexamethasone, and 0.1 mg benzalkonium chloride as a preservative. The inactive ingredients are boric acid, sodium chloride, hydroxyethyl cellulose, tyloxapol, acetic acid, sodium acetate, edetate disodium, and purified water. Sodium hydroxide or hydrochloric acid may be added for adjustment of pH.

Ciprofloxacin, a fluoroquinolone is available as the monohydrochloride monohydrate salt of 1-cyclopropyl-6-fluoro-1,4-dihydro-4-oxo-7-(1-piperazinyl)-3-quinolinecarboxylic acid. The empirical formula is $C_{17}H_{18}FN_3O_3 \cdot HCl \cdot H_2O$ and the structural formula is:

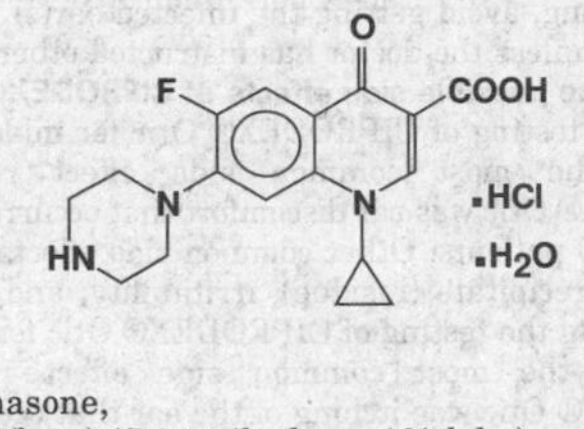

Dexamethasone, 9-fluoro-11(beta),17,21-trihydroxy-16(alpha)-methylpregna-1,4-diene-3,20-dione, is an anti-inflammatory corticosteroid. The empirical formula is $C_{22}H_{29}FO_5$ and the structural formula is:

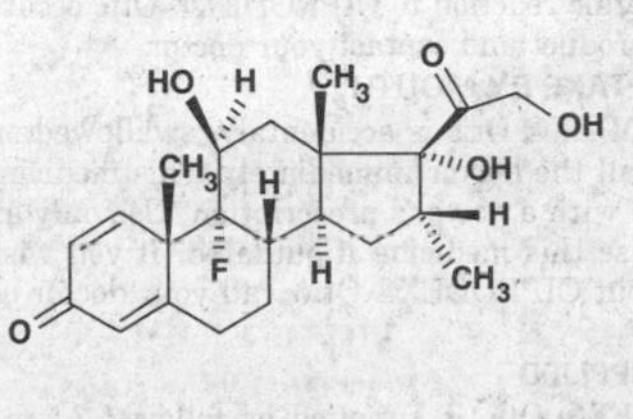

CLINICAL PHARMACOLOGY

Pharmacokinetics: Following a single bilateral 4-drop (total dose = 0.28 mL, 0.84 mg ciprofloxacin, 0.28 mg dexamethasone) topical otic dose of CIPRODEX® Otic to pediatric patients after tympanostomy tube insertion, measurable plasma concentrations of ciprofloxacin and dexamethasone were observed at 6 hours following administration in 2 of 9 patients and 5 of 9 patients, respectively.

Mean ± SD peak plasma concentrations of ciprofloxacin were 1.39 ± 0.880 ng/mL (n=9). Peak plasma concentrations ranged from 0.543 ng/mL to 3.45 ng/mL and were on average approximately 0.1% of peak plasma concentrations achieved with an oral dose of 250-mg [1]. Peak plasma concentrations of ciprofloxacin were observed within 15 minutes to 2 hours post dose application.

Mean ± SD peak plasma concentrations of dexamethasone were 1.14 ± 1.54 ng/mL (n=9). Peak plasma concentrations ranged from 0.135 ng/mL to 5.10 ng/mL and were on average approximately 14% of peak concentrations reported in the literature following an oral 0.5-mg tablet dose[2]. Peak plasma concentrations of dexamethasone were observed within 15 minutes to 2 hours post dose application.

Dexamethasone has been added to aid in the resolution of the inflammatory response accompanying bacterial infection (such as otorrhea in pediatric patients with AOM with tympanostomy tubes).

Microbiology: Ciprofloxacin has *in vitro* activity against a wide range of gram-positive and gram-negative microorganisms. The bactericidal action of ciprofloxacin results from interference with the enzyme, DNA gyrase, which is needed for the synthesis of bacterial DNA. Cross-resistance has been observed between ciprofloxacin and other fluoroquinolones. There is generally no cross-resistance between ciprofloxacin and other classes of antibacterial agents such as beta-lactams or aminoglycosides.

Ciprofloxacin has been shown to be active against most isolates of the following microorganisms, both *in vitro* and clinically in otic infections as described in the **INDICATIONS AND USAGE** section.

Aerobic and facultative gram-positive microorganisms

Staphylococcus aureus
Streptococcus pneumoniae

Aerobic and facultative gram-negative microorganisms

Haemophilus influenzae
Moraxella catarrhalis
Pseudomonas aeruginosa

INDICATIONS AND USAGE

CIPRODEX® Otic is indicated for the treatment of infections caused by susceptible isolates of the designated microorganisms in the specific conditions listed below:

Acute Otitis Media in pediatric patients (age 6 months and older) with tympanostomy tubes due to *Staphylococcus aureus, Streptococcus pneumoniae, Haemophilus influenzae, Moraxella catarrhalis*, and *Pseudomonas aeruginosa*.

Acute Otitis Externa in pediatric (age 6 months and older), adult and elderly patients due to *Staphylococcus aureus* and *Pseudomonas aeruginosa*.

CONTRAINDICATIONS

CIPRODEX® Otic is contraindicated in patients with a history of hypersensitivity to ciprofloxacin, to other quinolones, or to any of the components in this medication. Use of this product is contraindicated in viral infections of the external canal including herpes simplex infections.

WARNINGS

FOR OTIC USE ONLY

(This product is not approved for ophthalmic use.)

NOT FOR INJECTION

CIPRODEX® Otic should be discontinued at the first appearance of a skin rash or any other sign of hypersensitivity. Serious and occasionally fatal hypersensitivity (anaphylactic) reactions, some following the first dose, have been reported in patients receiving systemic quinolones. Serious acute hypersensitivity reactions may require immediate emergency treatment.

PRECAUTIONS

General: As with other antibacterial preparations, use of this product may result in overgrowth of nonsusceptible organisms, including yeast and fungi. If the infection is not improved after one week of treatment, cultures should be obtained to guide further treatment. If otorrhea persists after a full course of therapy, or if two or more episodes of otorrhea occur within six months, further evaluation is recommended to exclude an underlying condition such as cholesteatoma, foreign body, or a tumor.

The systemic administration of quinolones, including ciprofloxacin at doses much higher than given or absorbed by the otic route, has led to lesions or erosions of the cartilage in weight-bearing joints and other signs of arthropathy in immature animals of various species.

Guinea pigs dosed in the middle ear with CIPRODEX® Otic for one month exhibited no drug-related structural or functional changes of the cochlear hair cells and no lesions in the ossicles. CIPRODEX® Otic was also shown to lack dermal sensitizing potential in the guinea pig when tested according to the method of Buehler.

No signs of local irritation were found when CIPRODEX® Otic was applied topically in the rabbit eye.

Information for Patients

For otic use only. (This product is not approved for use in the eye.) Warm the bottle in your hand for one to two minutes prior to use and shake well immediately before using.

Avoid contaminating the tip with material from the ear, fingers, or other sources.

Protect from light.

If rash or allergic reaction occurs, discontinue use immediately and contact your physician.

It is very important to use the ear drops for as long as the doctor has instructed, **even if the symptoms improve**. Discard unused portion after therapy is completed.

Acute Otitis Media in pediatric patients with tympanostomy tubes Prior to administration of CIPRODEX® Otic in patients (6 months and older) with acute otitis media through tympanostomy tubes, the suspension should be warmed by holding the bottle in the hand for one or two minutes to avoid dizziness which may result from the instillation of a cold suspension. The patient should lie with the affected ear upward, and then the drops should be instilled. The tragus should then be pumped 5 times by pushing inward to facilitate penetration of the drops into the middle ear. This position should be maintained for 60 seconds. Repeat, if necessary, for the opposite ear (see **DOSAGE AND ADMINISTRATION**).

Acute Otitis Externa

Prior to administration of CIPRODEX® Otic in patients with acute otitis externa, the suspension should be warmed by holding the bottle in the hand for one or two minutes to avoid dizziness which may result from the instillation of a cold suspension. The patient should lie with the affected ear upward, and then the drops should be instilled. This position should be maintained for 60 seconds to facilitate penetration of the drops into the ear canal. Repeat, if necessary, for the opposite ear (see **DOSAGE AND ADMINISTRATION**).

Drug Interactions

Specific drug interaction studies have not been conducted with CIPRODEX® Otic.

Carcinogenesis, Mutagenesis, Impairment of Fertility

Long-term carcinogenicity studies in mice and rats have been completed for ciprofloxacin. After daily oral doses of 750 mg/kg (mice) and 250 mg/kg (rats) were administered for up to 2 years, there was no evidence that ciprofloxacin had any carcinogenic or tumorigenic effects in these species. No long term studies of CIPRODEX® Otic have been performed to evaluate carcinogenic potential.

Eight *in vitro* mutagenicity tests have been conducted with ciprofloxacin, and the test results are listed below:

Salmonella/Microsome Test (Negative)
E. coli DNA Repair Assay (Negative)
Mouse Lymphoma Cell Forward Mutation Assay (Positive)
Chinese Hamster V_{79} Cell HGPRT Test (Negative)
Syrian Hamster Embryo Cell Transformation Assay (Negative)
Saccharomyces cerevisiae Point Mutation Assay (Negative)
Saccharomyces cerevisiae Mitotic Crossover and Gene Conversion Assay (Negative)
Rat Hepatocyte DNA Repair Assay (Positive)

Thus, 2 of the 8 tests were positive, but results of the following 3 *in vivo* test systems gave negative results:

Rat Hepatocyte DNA Repair Assay
Micronucleus Test (Mice)
Dominant Lethal Test (Mice)

Fertility studies performed in rats at oral doses of ciprofloxacin up to 100 mg/kg/day revealed no evidence of impairment. This would be over 100 times the maximum recommended clinical dose of ototopical ciprofloxacin based upon body surface area, assuming total absorption of ciprofloxacin from the ear of a patient treated with CIPRODEX® Otic twice per day according to label directions.

Long term studies have not been performed to evaluate the carcinogenic potential of topical otic dexamethasone. Dexamethasone has been tested for *in vitro* and *in vivo* genotoxic potential and shown to be positive in the following assays; chromosomal aberrations, sister-chromatid exchange in human lymphocytes and micronuclei and sister-chromatid exchanges in mouse bone marrow. However, the Ames/Salmonella assay, both with and without S9 mix, did not show any increase in His+ revertants.

The effect of dexamethasone on fertility has not been investigated following topical otic application. However, the lowest toxic dose of dexamethasone identified following topical dermal application was 1.802 mg/kg in a 26-week study in male rats and resulted in changes to the testes, epididymis, sperm duct, prostate, seminal vessicle, Cowper's gland and accessory glands. The relevance of this study for short term topical otic use is unknown.

Pregnancy

Teratogenic Effects. Pregnancy Category C:

Reproduction studies have been performed in rats and mice using oral doses of up to 100 mg/kg and IV doses up to 30 mg/kg and have revealed no evidence of harm to the fetus as a result of ciprofloxacin. In rabbits, ciprofloxacin (30 and 100 mg/kg orally) produced gastrointestinal disturbances resulting in maternal weight loss and an increased incidence of abortion, but no teratogenicity was observed at either dose. After intravenous administration of doses up to 20 mg/kg, no maternal toxicity was produced in the rabbit, and no embryotoxicity or teratogenicity was observed.

Corticosteroids are generally teratogenic in laboratory animals when administered systemically at relatively low dosage levels. The more potent corticosteroids have been shown to be teratogenic after dermal application in laboratory animals.

Animal reproduction studies have not been conducted with CIPRODEX® Otic. No adequate and well controlled studies have been performed in pregnant women. Caution should be exercised when CIPRODEX® Otic is used by a pregnant woman.

Nursing Mothers:

Ciprofloxacin and corticosteroids, as a class, appear in milk following oral administration. Dexamethasone in breast milk could suppress growth, interfere with endogenous corticosteroid production, or cause other untoward effects. It is not known whether topical otic administration of ciprofloxacin or dexamethasone could result in sufficient systemic absorption to produce detectable quantities in human milk. Because of the potential for unwanted effects in nursing infants, a decision should be made whether to discontinue nursing or to discontinue the drug, taking into account the importance of the drug to the mother.

Pediatric Use:

The safety and efficacy of CIPRODEX® Otic have been established in pediatric patients 6 months and older (937 patients) in adequate and well-controlled clinical trials. Although no data are available on patients less than age 6 months, there are no known safety concerns or differences in the disease process in this population that would preclude use of this product. (See **DOSAGE AND ADMINISTRATION**.)

No clinically relevant changes in hearing function were observed in 69 pediatric patients (age 4 to 12 years) treated with CIPRODEX® Otic and tested for audiometric parameters.

ADVERSE REACTIONS

In Phases II and III clinical trials, a total of 937 patients were treated with CIPRODEX® Otic. This included 400 patients with acute otitis media with tympanostomy tubes and 537 patients with acute otitis externa. The reported treatment-related adverse events are listed below:

Acute Otitis Media in pediatric patients with tympanostomy tubes

The following treatment-related adverse events occurred in 0.5% or more of the patients with non-intact tympanic membranes.

Adverse Event	Incidence (N=400)
Ear discomfort	3.0%
Ear pain	2.3%
Ear precipitate (residue)	0.5%
Irritability	0.5%
Taste perversion	0.5%

The following treatment-related adverse events were each reported in a single patient: tympanostomy tube blockage; ear pruritus; tinnitus; oral moniliasis; crying; dizziness; and erythema.

Acute Otitis Externa

The following treatment-related adverse events occurred in 0.4% or more of the patients with intact tympanic membranes.

Adverse Event	Incidence (N=537)
Ear pruritus	1.5%
Ear debris	0.6%
Superimposed ear infection	0.6%
Ear congestion	0.4%
Ear pain	0.4%
Erythema	0.4%

The following treatment-related adverse events were each reported in a single patient: ear discomfort; decreased hearing; and ear disorder (tingling).

DOSAGE AND ADMINISTRATION

CIPRODEX® OTIC SHOULD BE SHAKEN WELL IMMEDIATELY BEFORE USE

CIPRODEX® Otic contains 3 mg (3000 µg/mL) ciprofloxacin and 1 mg/mL dexamethasone.

Acute Otitis Media in pediatric patients with tympanostomy tubes: The recommended dosage regimen for the treatment of acute otitis media in pediatric patients (age 6 months and older) through tympanostomy tubes is:

Four drops (0.14 mL, 0.42 mg ciprofloxacin, 0.14 mg dexamethasone) instilled into the affected ear twice daily for seven days. The suspension should be warmed by holding the bottle in the hand for one or two minutes to avoid dizziness, which may result from the instillation of a cold suspension. The patient should lie with the affected ear upward, and then the drops should be instilled. The tragus should then be pumped 5 times by pushing inward to facilitate penetration of the drops into the middle ear. This position should be maintained for 60 seconds. Repeat, if necessary, for the opposite ear. Discard unused portion after therapy is completed.

Acute Otitis Externa: The recommended dosage regimen for the treatment of acute otitis externa is: For patients (age 6 months and older): Four drops (0.14 mL, 0.42 mg ciprofloxacin, 0.14 mg dexamethasone) instilled into the affected ear twice daily for seven days. The suspension should be warmed by holding the bottle in the hand for one or two minutes to avoid dizziness, which may result from the instillation of a cold suspension. The patient should lie with the affected ear upward, and then the drops should be instilled. This position should be maintained for 60 seconds to facilitate penetration of the drops into the ear canal. Repeat, if necessary, for the opposite ear. Discard unused portion after therapy is completed.

HOW SUPPLIED

CIPRODEX® (ciprofloxacin 0.3% and dexamethasone 0.1%) Sterile Otic Suspension is supplied as follows: 7.5 mL fill in a DROP-TAINER® system. The DROP-TAINER® system consists of a natural polyethylene bottle and natural plug, with a white polypropylene closure. Tamper evidence is provided with a shrink band around the closure and neck area of the package.

NDC 0065-8533-02, 7.5 mL fill

Storage:

Store at 20°-25°C (68° - 77°F); excursions permitted to 15°-30°C (59° - 86°F) [see USP Controlled Room Temperature]. Avoid freezing. Protect from light.

CLINICAL STUDIES

In a randomized, multicenter, controlled clinical trial, CIPRODEX® Otic dosed 2 times per day for 7 days demonstrated clinical cures in the per protocol analysis in 86% of AOMT patients compared to 79% for ofloxacin solution, 0.3%, dosed 2 times per day for 10 days. Among culture positive patients, clinical cures were 90% for CIPRODEX® Otic compared to 79% for ofloxacin solution, 0.3%. Microbiological eradication rates for these patients in the same clinical trial were 91% for CIPRODEX® Otic compared to 82% for ofloxacin solution, 0.3%. In 2 randomized multicenter, controlled clinical trials, CIPRODEX® Otic dosed 2 times per day for 7 days demonstrated clinical cures in 87% and 94% of per protocol evaluable AOE patients, respectively, compared to 84% and 89%, respectively, for otic suspension containing neomycin 0.35%, polymyxin B 10,000 IU/mL, and hydrocortisone 1.0% (neo/poly/HC). Among culture positive patients clinical cures were 86% and 92% for CIPRODEX® Otic compared to 84% and 89%, respectively, for neo/poly/HC. Microbiological eradication rates for these patients in the same clinical trials were 86% and 92% for CIPRODEX® Otic compared to 85% and 85%, respectively, for neo/poly/HC.

REFERENCES:

1. Campoli-Richards DM, Monk JP, Price A, Benfield P, Todd PA, Ward A. Ciprofloxacin: A review of its antibacterial activity, pharmacokinetic properties and therapeutic use. Drugs 1988;35:373-447.
2. Loew D, Schuster O, and Graul E. Dose-dependent pharmacokinetics of dexamethasone. Eur J Clin Pharmacol 1986;30:225-230.

U.S. Patent Nos. 6,284,804; 6,359,016

Licensed to Alcon, Inc. by Bayer Schering Pharma AG.

CIPRODEX is a registered trademark of Bayer AG, licensed to Alcon, Inc by Bayer AG.

Rx Only

Revision date: 19 November 2012

PATIENT INFORMATION

CIPRODEX® (CI-PRO-DEX)
(ciprofloxacin 0.3% and dexamethasone 0.1%)
Sterile Otic Suspension

IMPORTANT PATIENT INFORMATION AND INSTRUCTIONS. READ BEFORE USE.

What is CIPRODEX® Otic?

CIPRODEX® Otic is an antibiotic/steroid combination product in a sterile suspension used to treat:

- **Middle Ear Infection with Drainage Through a Tube in Children 6 months and older:** A middle ear infection is a bacterial infection behind the eardrum. People with a tube in the eardrum may notice drainage from the ear canal.
- **Outer Ear Canal Infection in Patients 6 months and older:** An outer ear canal infection, also known as "Swimmer's Ear", is a bacterial infection of the outer ear canal. The ear canal and the outer part of the ear may swell, turn red, and be painful. Also, a fluid discharge may appear in the ear canal.

Who should NOT use CIPRODEX® Otic?

- Do not use this product if allergic to ciprofloxacin or to other quinolone antibiotics.
- Do not use this product if allergic to dexamethasone or to other steroids.
- Do not give this product to pediatric patients who are less than 6 months old.

How often should CIPRODEX® Otic be given?

CIPRODEX® Otic ear drops should be given 2 times each day (about 12 hours apart, for example, 8 AM and 8 PM) in each infected ear unless the doctor has instructed otherwise. The best times to use the ear drops are in the morning and at night. It is very important to use the ear drops for as long as the doctor has instructed, **even if the symptoms improve.** If CIPRODEX® Otic ear drops are not used for as long as the doctor has instructed, the infection may return.

What if a dose is missed?

If a dose of CIPRODEX® Otic is missed, it should be given as soon as possible. If it is almost time for the next dose, skip the missed dose and go back to the regular dosing schedule. Do not use a double dose unless the doctor has instructed you to do so. If the infection is not improved after one week, you should consult your doctor. If you have two or more episodes of drainage within six months, it is recommended you see your doctor for further evaluation.

What activities should be avoided while using CIPRODEX® Otic?

It is important that the infected ear(s) remain clean and dry. When bathing, avoid getting the infected ear(s) wet. Avoid swimming unless the doctor has instructed otherwise.

What are the possible side effects of CIPRODEX® Otic?

During the testing of CIPRODEX® Otic for middle ear infections, the most common side effect related to CIPRODEX® Otic was ear discomfort that occurred in up to 3 out of 100 patients. Other common side effects were: ear pain; ear precipitate (residue); irritability; and abnormal taste. During the testing of CIPRODEX® Otic for ear canal infections, the most common side effect related to CIPRODEX® Otic was itching of the ear that occurred in 1 to 2 out of 100 patients. Other common side effects were: ear debris; ear infection in the treated ear; ear congestion; ear pain; and rash.

If any of these side effects persist, call the doctor.

If an allergic reaction to CIPRODEX® Otic occurs, stop using the product and contact your doctor.

DO NOT TAKE BY MOUTH

If CIPRODEX® Otic is accidentally swallowed or overdose occurs, call the doctor immediately. This medicine is available only with a doctor's prescription. Use only as directed. Do not use this medicine if outdated. If you wish to learn more about CIPRODEX® Otic, call your doctor or pharmacist.

HOW SUPPLIED

CIPRODEX® Otic is supplied as follows: 7.5 mL fill in a DROP-TAINER® system. The DROP-TAINER® system consists of a natural polyethylene bottle and natural plug, with a white polypropylene closure. Tamper evidence is provided with a shrink band around the closure and neck area of the package. NDC 0065-8533-02, 7.5 mL fill

Storage:

Store at 20°-25°C (68° - 77°F); excursions permitted to 15°-30°C (59° - 86°F) [see USP Controlled Room Temperature]. Avoid freezing. Protect from light.

U.S. Patent Nos. 6,284,804; 6,359,016

Licensed to Alcon by Bayer Pharma AG. CIPRODEX is a registered trademark of Bayer AG. Licensed to Alcon by Bayer AG.

Rx Only

How should CIPRODEX® Otic be given?

1. Wash hands

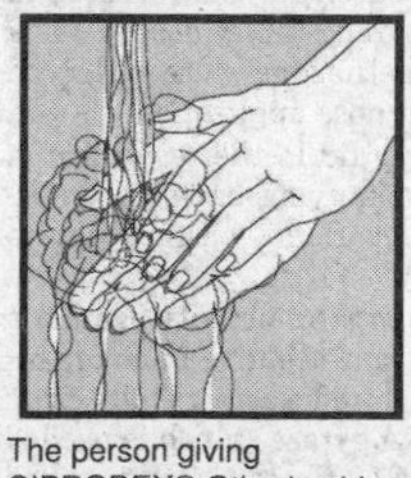

The person giving CIPRODEX® Otic should wash his/her hands with soap and water.

2. Warm & shake bottle

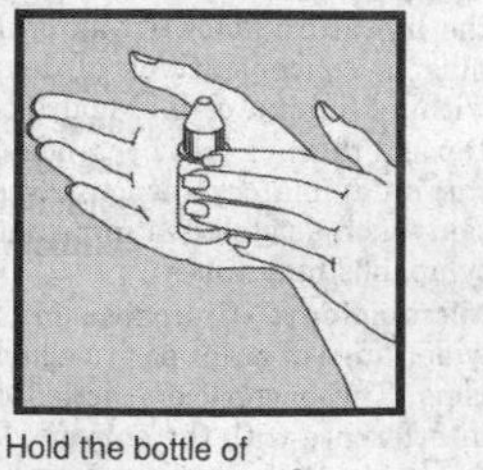

Hold the bottle of CIPRODEX® Otic in the hand for one or two minutes to warm the suspension, then shake well.

3. Add drops

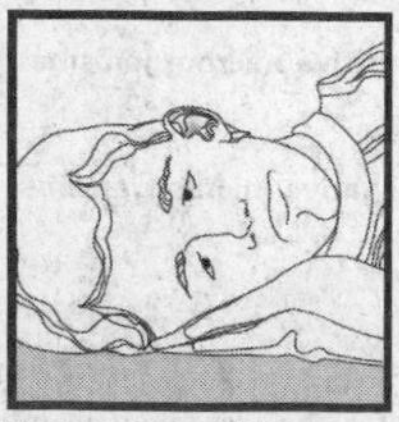

The person receiving CIPRODEX® Otic should lie on his/her side with the infected ear up.

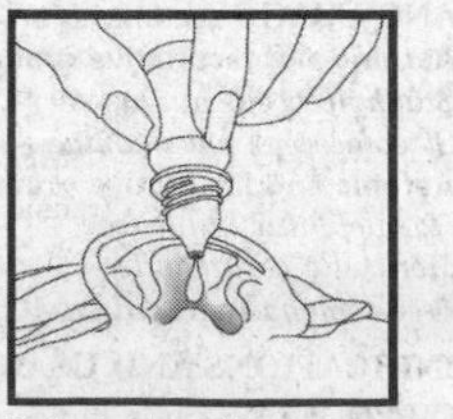

Patients should have 4 drops of CIPRODEX® Otic put into the infected ear. The tip of the bottle should not touch the fingers, or the ear, or any other surfaces.

BE SURE TO FOLLOW INSTRUCTIONS BELOW FOR THE PATIENT'S SPECIFIC EAR INFECTION.

4. For Patients with Middle Ear Infection with Tubes:

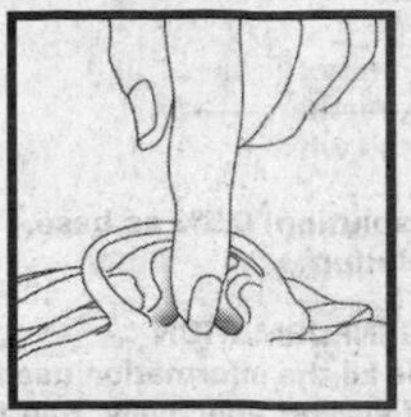

While the person receiving CIPRODEX® Otic lies on his/her side, the person giving the drops should gently press the tragus (see diagram) 5 times in a pumping motion. This will allow the drops to pass through the tube in the eardrum and into the middle ear.

5. For Patients with Outer Ear Infection ("Swimmer's Ear"):

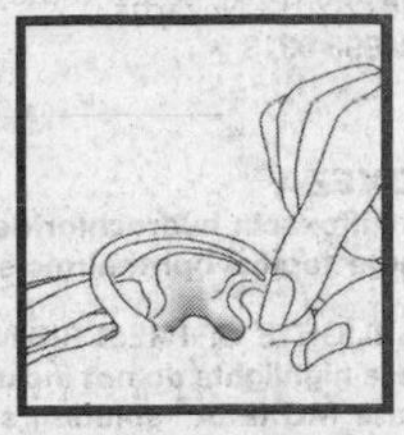

While the person receiving the drops lies on his/her side, the person giving the drops should gently pull the outer ear lobe upward and backward. This will allow the ear drops to flow down into the ear canal.

6. Stay on side

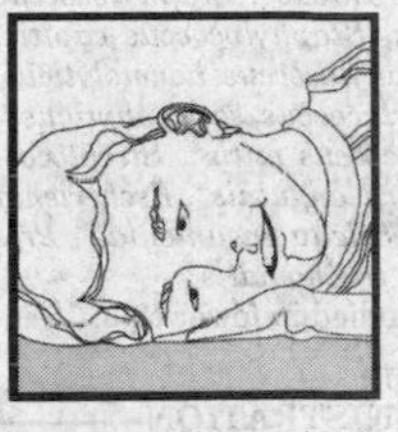

The person who received the ear drops should remain on his/her side for at least 60 seconds. Repeat Steps 2-5 for the other ear if both ears are infected.

9008833-1112

ILEVRO™ ℞

(nepafenac ophthalmic suspension), 0.3%
topical ophthalmic

HIGHLIGHTS OF PRESCRIBING INFORMATION
These highlights do not include all the information needed to use ILEVRO™ (nepafenac ophthalmic suspension), 0.3% safely and effectively. See full prescribing information for ILEVRO™ (nepafenac ophthalmic suspension), 0.3%.
ILEVRO™ (nepafenac ophthalmic suspension), 0.3%, topical ophthalmic
Initial U.S. Approval: 2005

INDICATIONS AND USAGE

ILEVRO™ (nepafenac ophthalmic suspension), 0.3% is a nonsteroidal, anti-inflammatory prodrug indicated for the treatment of pain and inflammation associated with cataract surgery (1).

DOSAGE AND ADMINISTRATION

One drop of ILEVRO™ (nepafenac ophthalmic suspension), 0.3% should be applied to the affected eye one-time-daily beginning 1 day prior to cataract surgery, continued on the day of surgery and through the first 2 weeks of the postoperative period. An additional drop should be administered 30 to 120 minutes prior to surgery. (2)

DOSAGE FORMS AND STRENGTHS

Sterile ophthalmic suspension 0.3%: 1.7 mL in a 4 mL bottle. (3)

CONTRAINDICATIONS

Hypersensitivity to any of the ingredients in the formula or to other NSAIDS.(4)

WARNINGS AND PRECAUTIONS

Increased bleeding time due to interference with thrombocyte aggregation (5.1)
Delayed healing (5.2)
Corneal effects including keratitis (5.3)

ADVERSE REACTIONS

Most common adverse reactions (5 to 10%) are capsular opacity, decreased visual acuity, foreign body sensation, increased intraocular pressure, and sticky sensation. (6.1)
To report SUSPECTED ADVERSE REACTIONS, contact Alcon Laboratories, Inc. at 1-800-757-9195 or FDA at 1-800-FDA-1088 or www.fda.gov/medwatch.
See 17 for PATIENT COUNSELING INFORMATION
Revised: 10/2012

FULL PRESCRIBING INFORMATION: CONTENTS*

*** Sections or subsections omitted from the full prescribing information are not listed**

FULL PRESCRIBING INFORMATION

1 INDICATIONS AND USAGE

ILEVRO™ (nepafenac ophthalmic suspension), 0.3% is indicated for the treatment of pain and inflammation associated with cataract surgery.

2 DOSAGE AND ADMINISTRATION

2.1 Recommended Dosing

One drop of ILEVRO™ (nepafenac ophthalmic suspension), 0.3% should be applied to the affected eye one-time-daily beginning 1 day prior to cataract surgery, continued on the day of surgery and through the first 2 weeks of the postoperative period. An additional drop should be administered 30 to 120 minutes prior to surgery.

2.2 Use with Other Topical Ophthalmic Medications

ILEVRO™ (nepafenac ophthalmic suspension), 0.3% may be administered in conjunction with other topical ophthalmic medications such as beta-blockers, carbonic anhydrase inhibitors, alpha-agonists, cycloplegics, and mydriatics.

If more than one topical ophthalmic medication is being used, the medicines must be administered at least 5 minutes apart.

3 DOSAGE FORMS AND STRENGTHS

Sterile ophthalmic suspension 0.3%
1.7 mL in a 4 mL bottle

4 CONTRAINDICATIONS

ILEVRO™ (nepafenac ophthalmic suspension), 0.3% is contraindicated in patients with previously demonstrated hypersensitivity to any of the ingredients in the formula or to other NSAIDs.

5 WARNINGS AND PRECAUTIONS

5.1 Increased Bleeding Time

With some nonsteroidal anti-inflammatory drugs including ILEVRO™ (nepafenac ophthalmic suspension), 0.3%, there exists the potential for increased bleeding time due to interference with thrombocyte aggregation. There have been reports that ocularly applied nonsteroidal anti-inflammatory drugs may cause increased bleeding of ocular tissues (including hyphema) in conjunction with ocular surgery.

It is recommended that ILEVRO™ (nepafenac ophthalmic suspension), 0.3% be used with caution in patients with known bleeding tendencies or who are receiving other medications which may prolong bleeding time.

5.2 Delayed Healing

Topical nonsteroidal anti-inflammatory drugs (NSAIDs) including ILEVRO™ (nepafenac ophthalmic suspension), 0.3%, may slow or delay healing. Topical corticosteroids are also known to slow or delay healing. Concomitant use of topical NSAIDs and topical steroids may increase the potential for healing problems.

5.3 Corneal Effects

Use of topical NSAIDs may result in keratitis. In some susceptible patients, continued use of topical NSAIDs may result in epithelial breakdown, corneal thinning, corneal erosion, corneal ulceration or corneal perforation. These events may be sight threatening. Patients with evidence of corneal epithelial breakdown should immediately discontinue use of topical NSAIDs including ILEVRO™ (nepafenac ophthalmic suspension), 0.3% and should be closely monitored for corneal health.

Postmarketing experience with topical NSAIDs suggests that patients with complicated ocular surgeries, corneal denervation, corneal epithelial defects, diabetes mellitus, ocular surface diseases (e.g., dry eye syndrome), rheumatoid arthritis, or repeat ocular surgeries within a short period of time may be at increased risk for corneal adverse events which may become sight threatening. Topical NSAIDs should be used with caution in these patients.

Postmarketing experience with topical NSAIDs also suggests that use more than 1 day prior to surgery or use beyond 14 days post-surgery may increase patient risk and severity of corneal adverse events.

5.4 Contact Lens Wear

ILEVRO™ (nepafenac ophthalmic suspension), 0.3% should not be administered while using contact lenses.

6 ADVERSE REACTIONS

Because clinical studies are conducted under widely varying conditions, adverse reaction rates observed in the clinical studies of a drug cannot be directly compared to the rates in the clinical studies of another drug and may not reflect the rates observed in practice.

6.1 Serious and Otherwise Important Adverse Reactions

The following adverse reactions are discussed in greater detail in other sections of labeling.
- Increased Bleeding Time (*Warnings and Precautions 5.1*)
- Delayed Healing (*Warnings and Precautions 5.2*)
- Corneal Effects (*Warnings and Precautions 5.3*)

6.2 Ocular Adverse Reactions

The most frequently reported ocular adverse reactions following cataract surgery were capsular opacity, decreased visual acuity, foreign body sensation, increased intraocular pressure, and sticky sensation. These reactions occurred in approximately 5 to 10% of patients.

Other ocular adverse reactions occurring at an incidence of approximately 1 to 5% included conjunctival edema, corneal edema, dry eye, lid margin crusting, ocular discomfort, ocular hyperemia, ocular pain, ocular pruritus, photophobia, tearing and vitreous detachment.

Some of these reactions may be the consequence of the cataract surgical procedure.

6.3 Non-Ocular Adverse Reactions

Non-ocular adverse reactions reported at an incidence of 1 to 4% included headache, hypertension, nausea/vomiting, and sinusitis.

8 USE IN SPECIFIC POPULATIONS

8.1 Pregnancy

Teratogenic Effects.

Pregnancy Category C: Reproduction studies performed with nepafenac in rabbits and rats at oral doses up to 10 mg/kg/day have revealed no evidence of teratogenicity due to nepafenac, despite the induction of maternal toxicity. At this dose, the animal plasma exposure to nepafenac and amfenac was approximately 70 and 630 times human plasma exposure at the recommended human topical ophthalmic dose for rats and 20 and 180 times human plasma exposure for rabbits, respectively. In rats, maternally toxic doses ≥ 10 mg/kg were associated with dystocia, increased postimplantation loss, reduced fetal weights and growth, and reduced fetal survival.

Nepafenac has been shown to cross the placental barrier in rats. There are no adequate and well-controlled studies in pregnant women. Because animal reproduction studies are not always predictive of human response, ILEVRO™ (nepafenac ophthalmic suspension), 0.3% should be used during pregnancy only if the potential benefit justifies the potential risk to the fetus.

Non-teratogenic Effects.

Because of the known effects of prostaglandin biosynthesis inhibiting drugs on the fetal cardiovascular system (closure of the ductus arteriosus), the use of ILEVRO™ (nepafenac ophthalmic suspension), 0.3% during late pregnancy should be avoided.

8.3 Nursing Mothers

Nepafenac is excreted in the milk of lactating rats. It is not known whether this drug is excreted in human milk. Because many drugs are excreted in human milk, caution should be exercised when ILEVRO™ (nepafenac ophthalmic suspension), 0.3% is administered to a nursing woman.

8.4 Pediatric Use

The safety and effectiveness of ILEVRO™ (nepafenac ophthalmic suspension), 0.3% in pediatric patients below the age of 10 years have not been established.

8.5 Geriatric Use

No overall differences in safety and effectiveness have been observed between elderly and younger patients.

11 DESCRIPTION

ILEVRO™ (nepafenac ophthalmic suspension), 0.3% is a sterile, topical, nonsteroidal anti-inflammatory (NSAID) prodrug for ophthalmic use. Each mL of ILEVRO™ (nepafenac ophthalmic suspension), 0.3% contains 3 mg of nepafenac. Nepafenac is designated chemically as 2-amino-3-benzoylbenzeneacetamide with an empirical formula of $C_{15}H_{14}N_2O_2$. The structural formula of nepafenac is:

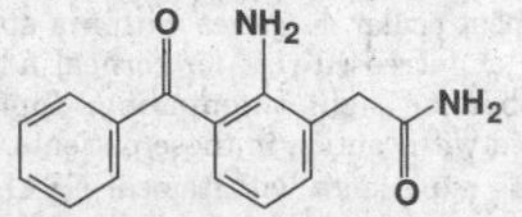

Nepafenac is a yellow crystalline powder. The molecular weight of nepafenac is 254.28. ILEVRO™ (nepafenac ophthalmic suspension), 0.3% is supplied as a sterile, aqueous suspension with a pH approximately of 6.8.

The osmolality of ILEVRO™ (nepafenac ophthalmic suspension), 0.3% is approximately 300 mOsm/kg.

Each mL of ILEVRO™ (nepafenac ophthalmic suspension), 0.3% contains: Active: nepafenac 0.3% Inactives: boric acid, propylene glycol, carbomer 974P, sodium chloride, guar gum, carboxymethylcellulose sodium, edetate disodium, benzalkonium chloride 0.005% (preservative), sodium hydroxide and/or hydrochloric acid to adjust pH and purified water, USP.

12 CLINICAL PHARMACOLOGY

12.1 Mechanism of Action

After topical ocular dosing, nepafenac penetrates the cornea and is converted by ocular tissue hydrolases to amfenac, a nonsteroidal anti-inflammatory drug. Nepafenac and amfenac are thought to inhibit the action of prostaglandin H synthase (cyclooxygenase), an enzyme required for prostaglandin production.

12.3 Pharmacokinetics

Following bilateral topical ocular once-daily dosing of ILEVRO™ (nepafenac ophthalmic suspension), 0.3%, the concentrations of nepafenac and amfenac peaked at a median time of 0.5 hour and 0.75 hour, respectively on both Day 1 and Day 4. The mean steady-state C_{max} for nepafenac and for amfenac were 0.847 ± 0.269 ng/mL and 1.13 ± 0.491 ng/mL, respectively.

Nepafenac at concentrations up to 3000 ng/mL and amfenac at concentrations up to 1000 ng/mL did not inhibit the *in vitro* metabolism of 6 specific marker substrates of cytochrome P450 (CYP) isozymes (CYP1A2, CYP2C9, CYP2C19, CYP2D6, CYP2E1, and CYP3A4). Therefore, drug-drug interactions involving CYP mediated metabolism of concomitantly administered drugs are unlikely.

13 NONCLINICAL TOXICOLOGY

13.1 Carcinogenesis, Mutagenesis, Impairment of Fertility

Nepafenac has not been evaluated in long-term carcinogenicity studies. Increased chromosomal aberrations were observed in Chinese hamster ovary cells exposed *in vitro* to nepafenac suspension. Nepafenac was not mutagenic in the Ames assay or in the mouse lymphoma forward mutation assay. Oral doses up to 5,000 mg/kg did not result in an increase in the formation of micronucleated polychromatic erythrocytes *in vivo* in the mouse micronucleus assay in the bone marrow of mice.

Nepafenac did not impair fertility when administered orally to male and female rats at 3 mg/kg.

14 CLINICAL STUDIES

In two double masked, randomized clinical trials in which patients were dosed daily beginning one day prior to cataract surgery, continued on the day of surgery and for the first two weeks of the postoperative period, ILEVRO™ (nepafenac ophthalmic suspension), 0.3% demonstrated superior clinical efficacy compared to its vehicle in treating postoperative pain and inflammation.

Treatment effect over vehicle for resolution of ocular pain occurred as early as day 1 post-surgery. Treatment effect over vehicle for resolution of inflammation was significantly better than vehicle in both studies at day 7 and day 14 post-surgery.

[See table below]

16 HOW SUPPLIED/STORAGE AND HANDLING

ILEVRO™ (nepafenac ophthalmic suspension), 0.3% is supplied in a white, oval, low density polyethylene DROP-TAINER® dispenser with a natural low density polyethylene dispensing plug and gray polypropylene cap presented in an overwrap. Tamper evidence is provided with a shrink band around the closure and neck area of the package.

1.7 mL in 4 mL bottle NDC 0065-1750-07

Storage: Store at 2 - 25°C (36 - 77°F).

Protect from light.

17 PATIENT COUNSELING INFORMATION

17.1 Slow or Delayed Healing

Patients should be informed of the possibility that slow or delayed healing may occur while using nonsteroidal anti-inflammatory drugs (NSAIDs).

17.2 Avoiding Contamination of the Product

Patients should be instructed to avoid allowing the tip of the dispensing container to contact the eye or surrounding structures because this could cause the tip to become contaminated by common bacteria known to cause ocular infections. Serious damage to the eye and subsequent loss of vision may result from using contaminated solutions.

Use of the same bottle for both eyes is not recommended with topical eye drops that are used in association with surgery.

17.3 Contact Lens Wear

ILEVRO™ (nepafenac ophthalmic suspension), 0.3% should not be administered while wearing contact lens.

17.4 Intercurrent Ocular Conditions

Patients should be advised that if they develop an intercurrent ocular condition (e.g., trauma, or infection) or have ocular surgery, they should immediately seek their physician's advice concerning the continued use of the multi-dose container.

17.5 Concomitant Topical Ocular Therapy

If more than one topical ophthalmic medication is being used, the medicines must be administered at least 5 minutes apart.

Inflammation and Ocular Pain Resolution Results of Nepafenac ophthalmic suspension, 0.3% versus Vehicle at Day 14 Post-surgery (All-Randomized Population)

Studies	Treatment	Inflammation Resolution at Postop Day 14	Ocular Pain Resolution at Postop Day 14
Study 1	Nepafenac ophthalmic suspension, 0.3% (n/N) (1)	552/851 (65%)	734/851 (86%)
	NEVANAC (n/N) (1)	568/845 (67%)	737/845 (87%)
	Vehicle (n/N) (1)	67/211 (32%)	98/211 (46%)
	Difference (95% CI) (2)	33% (26%, 40%)	40% (32%, 47%)
Study 2	Nepafenac ophthalmic suspension, 0.3% (n/N) (1)	331/540 (61%)	456/540 (84%)
	Vehicle (n/N) (1)	63/268 (24%)	101/268 (38%)
	Difference (95% CI) (2)	38% (31%, 45%)	47% (40%, 54%)

(1) n/N is the ratio of those with complete resolution of anterior chamber cell and flare by the postoperative day 14 visit over all randomized subjects.

(2) Difference is Nepafenac ophthalmic suspension, 0.3% (n/N) – vehicle. The 95% confidence interval is derived using asymptotic approximation.

17.6 Shake Well Before Use

Patients should be instructed to shake well before each use.

U.S. Patent Nos. 5,475,034; 6,403,609; and 7,169,767

ALCON®

ALCON LABORATORIES, INC.
Fort Worth, Texas 76134 USA

9008996-0313

MOXEZA® ℞

(moxifloxacin hydrochloride solution) 0.5% as base
Sterile topical ophthalmic solution

HIGHLIGHTS OF PRESCRIBING INFORMATION
These highlights do not include all the information needed to use MOXEZA® solution safely and effectively. See full prescribing information for MOXEZA®.
MOXEZA® (moxifloxacin hydrochloride ophthalmic solution) 0.5% as base
Sterile topical ophthalmic solution
Initial U.S. Approval: 1999

INDICATIONS AND USAGE

MOXEZA® solution is a topical fluoroquinolone anti-infective indicated for the treatment of bacterial conjunctivitis caused by susceptible strains of the following organisms:

Aerococcus viridans, Corynebacterium macginleyi*, Enterococcus faecalis*, Micrococcus luteus*, Staphylococcus arlettae*, Staphylococcus aureus, Staphylococcus capitis, Staphylococcus epidermidis, Staphylococcus haemolyticus, Staphylococcus hominis, Staphylococcus saprophyticus*, Staphylococcus warneri*, Streptococcus mitis*, Streptococcus pneumoniae, Streptococcus parasanguinis*, Escherichia coli*, Haemophilus influenzae, Klebsiella pneumoniae*, Propionibacterium acnes, Chlamydia trachomatis**

*Efficacy for this organism was studied in fewer than 10 infections. (1)

DOSAGE AND ADMINISTRATION

Instill 1 drop in the affected eye(s) 2 times daily for 7 days. (2)

DOSAGE FORMS AND STRENGTHS

4 mL bottle filled with 3 mL sterile ophthalmic solution of moxifloxacin hydrochloride, 0.5% as base. (3)

CONTRAINDICATIONS

None. (4)

WARNINGS AND PRECAUTIONS

- Topical ophthalmic use only. (5.1)
- Hypersensitivity and anaphylaxis have been reported with systemic use of moxifloxacin. (5.2)
- Prolonged use may result in overgrowth of non-susceptible organisms, including fungi. (5.3)
- Patients should not wear contact lenses if they have signs or symptoms of bacterial conjunctivitis. (5.4)

ADVERSE REACTIONS

The most common adverse reactions reported in 1-2% of patients were eye irritation, pyrexia, and conjunctivitis. (6)

To report SUSPECTED ADVERSE REACTIONS, contact Alcon Laboratories, Inc. at 1-800-757-9195 or FDA at 1-800-FDA-1088 or www.fda.gov/medwatch.

See 17 for PATIENT COUNSELING INFORMATION

Revised: 09/2012

FULL PRESCRIBING INFORMATION: CONTENTS*

*** Sections or subsections omitted from the full prescribing information are not listed**

FULL PRESCRIBING INFORMATION

1 INDICATIONS AND USAGE

MOXEZA® solution is indicated for the treatment of bacterial conjunctivitis caused by susceptible strains of the following organisms:

*Aerococcus viridans**
*Corynebacterium macginleyi**
*Enterococcus faecalis**
*Micrococcus luteus**
*Staphylococcus arlettae**
Staphylococcus aureus
Staphylococcus capitis
Staphylococcus epidermidis
Staphylococcus haemolyticus
Staphylococcus hominis
*Staphylococcus saprophyticus**
*Staphylococcus warneri**
*Streptococcus mitis**
Streptococcus pneumoniae
*Streptococcus parasanguinis**
*Escherichia coli**
Haemophilus influenzae
*Klebsiella pneumoniae**
Propionibacterium acnes
*Chlamydia trachomatis**

*Efficacy for this organism was studied in fewer than 10 infections.

2 DOSAGE AND ADMINISTRATION

Instill 1 drop in the affected eye(s) 2 times daily for 7 days.

3 DOSAGE FORMS AND STRENGTHS

4 mL bottle filled with 3 mL of sterile ophthalmic solution of moxifloxacin hydrochloride, 0.5% as base.

4 CONTRAINDICATIONS

None.

5 WARNINGS AND PRECAUTIONS

5.1 Topical Ophthalmic Use Only

NOT FOR INJECTION. MOXEZA® solution is for topical ophthalmic use only and should not be injected subconjunctivally or introduced directly into the anterior chamber of the eye.

5.2 Hypersensitivity Reactions

In patients receiving systemically administered quinolones, including moxifloxacin, serious and occasionally fatal hypersensitivity (anaphylactic) reactions have been reported, some following the first dose. Some reactions were accompanied by cardiovascular collapse, loss of consciousness, angioedema (including laryngeal, pharyngeal or facial edema), airway obstruction, dyspnea, urticaria, and itching. If an allergic reaction to moxifloxacin occurs, discontinue use of the drug. Serious acute hypersensitivity reactions may require immediate emergency treatment. Oxygen and airway management should be administered as clinically indicated.

5.3 Growth of Resistant Organisms with Prolonged Use

As with other anti-infectives, prolonged use may result in overgrowth of non-susceptible organisms, including fungi. If superinfection occurs, discontinue use and institute alternative therapy. Whenever clinical judgment dictates, the patient should be examined with the aid of magnification, such as slit-lamp biomicroscopy, and, where appropriate, fluorescein staining.

5.4 Avoidance of Contact Lens Wear

Patients should be advised not to wear contact lenses if they have signs or symptoms of bacterial conjunctivitis.

6 ADVERSE REACTIONS

Because clinical trials are conducted under widely varying conditions, adverse reaction rates observed in the clinical trials of a drug cannot be directly compared to the rates in the clinical trials of another drug and may not reflect the rates observed in practice.

The data described below reflect exposure to MOXEZA® solution in 1263 patients, between 4 months and 92 years of age, with signs and symptoms of bacterial conjunctivitis. The most frequently reported adverse reactions were eye irritation, pyrexia and conjunctivitis, reported in 1-2% of patients.

8 USE IN SPECIFIC POPULATIONS

8.1 Pregnancy

Pregnancy Category C. Moxifloxacin was not teratogenic when administered to pregnant rats during organogenesis at oral doses as high as 500 mg/kg/day (approximately 25,000 times the highest recommended total daily human ophthalmic dose); however, decreased fetal body weights and slightly delayed fetal skeletal development were observed. There was no evidence of teratogenicity when pregnant Cynomolgus monkeys were given oral doses as high as 100 mg/kg/day (approximately 5,000 times the highest recommended total daily human ophthalmic dose). An increased incidence of smaller fetuses was observed at 100 mg/kg/day.

Since there are no adequate and well-controlled studies in pregnant women, MOXEZA® solution should be used during pregnancy only if the potential benefit justifies the potential risk to the fetus.

8.3 Nursing Mothers

Moxifloxacin has not been measured in human milk, although it can be presumed to be excreted in human milk. Caution should be exercised when MOXEZA® solution is administered to a nursing mother.

8.4 Pediatric Use

The safety and effectiveness of MOXEZA® solution in infants below 4 months of age have not been established.

There is no evidence that the ophthalmic administration of moxifloxacin has any effect on weight bearing joints, even though oral administration of some quinolones has been shown to cause arthropathy in immature animals.

8.5 Geriatric Use

No overall differences in safety and effectiveness have been observed between elderly and younger patients.

11 DESCRIPTION

MOXEZA® is a sterile solution for topical ophthalmic use. Moxifloxacin hydrochloride is an 8-methoxy fluoroquinolone anti-infective, with a diazabicyclononyl ring at the C7 position.

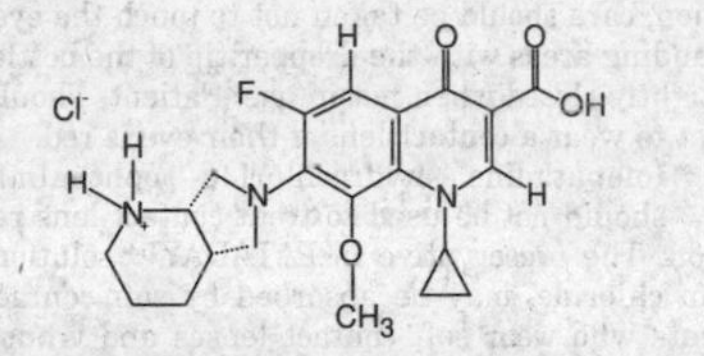

$C_{21}H_{24}FN_3O_4$•HCl Mol Wt 437.9

Chemical Name:
1-Cyclopropyl-6-fluoro-1,4-dihydro-8-methoxy-7-[(4aS,7aS)-octahydro-6H-pyrrolol[3,4-b]pyridin-6-yl]-4-oxo-3-quinolinecarboxylic acid, monohydrochloride.

Each mL of MOXEZA® solution contains 5.45 mg moxifloxacin hydrochloride, equivalent to 5 mg moxifloxacin base.

Inactives: Sodium chloride, xanthan gum, boric acid, sorbitol, tyloxapol, purified water, and hydrochloric acid and/or sodium hydroxide to adjust pH.

MOXEZA® is a greenish-yellow, isotonic solution with an osmolality of 300-370 mOsm/kg and a pH of approximately 7.4. Moxifloxacin hydrochloride is a slightly yellow to yellow crystalline powder.

12 CLINICAL PHARMACOLOGY

12.1 Mechanism of Action

Moxifloxacin is a member of the fluoroquinolone class of anti-infective drugs. [*see Clinical Pharmacology (12.4)*].

12.3 Pharmacokinetics

Moxifloxacin steady-state plasma pharmacokinetics were evaluated in healthy adult male and female subjects who were administered multiple, bilateral, topical ocular doses of MOXEZA® solution two times daily for four days with a final dose on day 5. The average steady-state AUC_{0-12} was 8.17 ± 5.31 ng*h/mL. Moxifloxacin C_{max} following twice-daily bilateral ophthalmic administration of moxifloxacin 0.5% for 5 days is approximately 0.02% of that achieved with the oral formulation of moxifloxacin hydrochloride (C_{max} following oral dosing of 400 mg AVELOX*, 4.5 ± 0.5 mcg/mL).

12.4 Microbiology

The antibacterial action of moxifloxacin results from inhibition of the topoisomerase II (DNA gyrase) and topoisomerase IV. DNA gyrase is an essential enzyme that is involved in the replication, transcription and repair of bacterial DNA. Topoisomerase IV is an enzyme known to play a key role in the partitioning of the chromosomal DNA during bacterial cell division.

The mechanism of action for quinolones, including moxifloxacin, is different from that of macrolides, aminoglycosides, or tetracyclines. Therefore, moxifloxacin may be active against pathogens that are resistant to these antibiotics and these antibiotics may be active against pathogens that are resistant to moxifloxacin. There is no cross-resistance between moxifloxacin and the aforementioned classes of antibiotics. Cross resistance has been observed between systemic moxifloxacin and some other quinolones. *In vitro* resistance to moxifloxacin develops via multiple-step mutations. Resistance to moxifloxacin occurs *in vitro* at a general frequency of between 1.8×10^{-9} to $< 1 \times 10^{-11}$ for Gram-positive bacteria.

Moxifloxacin has been shown to be active against most strains of the following microorganisms, both *in vitro* and in clinical infections as described in the INDICATIONS AND USAGE section:

*Aerococcus viridans**
*Corynebacterium macginleyi**
*Enterococcus faecalis**
*Micrococcus luteus**
*Staphylococcus arlettae**
Staphylococcus aureus
Staphylococcus capitis
Staphylococcus epidermidis
Staphylococcus haemolyticus
Staphylococcus hominis
*Staphylococcus saprophyticus**
*Staphylococcus warneri**
*Streptococcus mitis**
Streptococcus pneumoniae
*Streptococcus parasanguinis**
*Escherichia coli**
Haemophilus influenzae
*Klebsiella pneumoniae**
Propionibacterium acnes
*Chlamydia trachomatis**

*Efficacy for this organism was studied in fewer than 10 infections.

The following *in vitro* data are available, but their clinical significance in ophthalmic infections is unknown. The safety and effectiveness of MOXEZA® solution in treating ophthalmic infections due to these organisms have not been established in adequate and well-controlled trials.

Moxifloxacin has been shown to be active *in vitro* against most strains of the microorganisms listed below. These organisms are considered susceptible when evaluated using systemic breakpoints; however, a correlation between the *in vitro* systemic breakpoint and ophthalmologic efficacy has not been established. The list of organisms is provided as guidance only in assessing the potential treatment of conjunctival infections. Moxifloxacin exhibits *in vitro* minimal inhibitory concentrations (MICs) of 2 mcg/mL or less (systemic susceptible breakpoint) against most (≥ 90%) strains of the following ocular pathogens.

<u>Aerobic Gram-positive microorganisms:</u>
Staphylococcus caprae
Staphylococcus cohnii
Staphylococcus lugdunensis
Staphylococcus pasteuri
Streptococcus agalactiae
Streptococcus milleri group
Streptococcus oralis
Streptococcus pyogenes
Streptococcus salivarius
Streptococcus sanguis

<u>Aerobic Gram-negative microorganisms:</u>
Acinetobacter baumannii
Acinetobacter calcoaceticus
Acinetobacter junii
Enterobacter aerogenes
Enterobacter cloacae
Haemophilus parainfluenzae
Klebsiella oxytoca
Moraxella catarrhalis
Moraxella osloensis
Morganella morganii
Neisseria gonorrhoeae
Neisseria meningitidis
Pantoea agglomerans
Proteus vulgaris
Pseudomonas stutzeri
Serratia liquefaciens
Serratia marcescens
Stenotrophomonas maltophilia

<u>Anaerobic microorganisms:</u>
Clostridium perfringens
Peptostreptococcus anaerobius
Peptostreptococcus magnus
Peptostreptococcus micros
Peptostreptococcus prevotii

<u>Other microorganisms:</u>
Mycobacterium tuberculosis
Mycobacterium avium
Mycobacterium kansasii
Mycobacterium marinum

13 NONCLINICAL TOXICOLOGY

13.1 Carcinogenesis, Mutagenesis, Impairment of Fertility

Long-term studies in animals to determine the carcinogenic potential of moxifloxacin have not been performed.

Moxifloxacin was not mutagenic in four bacterial strains used in the Ames *Salmonella* reversion assay. As with other quinolones, the positive response observed with moxifloxacin in strain TA 102 using the same assay may be due to the inhibition of DNA gyrase. Moxifloxacin was not

mutagenic in the CHO/HGPRT mammalian cell gene mutation assay. An equivocal result was obtained in the same assay when v79 cells were used. Moxifloxacin was clastogenic in the v79 chromosome aberration assay, but it did not induce unscheduled DNA synthesis in cultured rat hepatocytes. There was no evidence of genotoxicity *in vivo* in a micronucleus test or a dominant lethal test in mice.
Moxifloxacin had no effect on fertility in male and female rats at oral doses as high as 500 mg/kg/day, approximately 25,000 times the highest recommended total daily human ophthalmic dose. At 500 mg/kg orally there were slight effects on sperm morphology (head-tail separation) in male rats and on the estrous cycle in female rats.

14 CLINICAL STUDIES

In one randomized, double-masked, multicenter, vehicle-controlled clinical trial in which patients with bacterial conjunctivitis were dosed with MOXEZA® solution 2 times a day, MOXEZA® was superior to its vehicle for both clinical and microbiological outcomes. Clinical cure achieved on Day 4 was 63% (265/424) in MOXEZA® solution treated patients, versus 51% (214/423) in vehicle treated patients. Microbiologic success (eradication of baseline pathogens) was achieved on Day 4 in 75% (316/424) of MOXEZA® solution treated patients versus 56% (237/423) of vehicle treated patients. Microbiologic eradication does not always correlate with clinical outcome in anti-infective trials.

16 HOW SUPPLIED/STORAGE AND HANDLING

MOXEZA® solution is supplied as a sterile ophthalmic solution in the Alcon DROP-TAINER® dispensing system consisting of a natural low density polyethylene bottle and dispensing plug and tan polypropylene closure. Tamper evidence is provided with a shrink band around the closure and neck area of the package.
3 mL in a 4 mL bottle - NDC 0065-0006-03
Storage: Store at 2°C- 25°C (36°F - 77°F).

17 PATIENT COUNSELING INFORMATION

17.1 Avoid Contamination of the Product
Patients should be advised not to touch the dropper tip to any surface to avoid contaminating the contents.
17.2 Avoid Contact Lens Wear
Patients should be advised not to wear contact lenses if they have signs and symptoms of bacterial conjunctivitis.
17.3 Hypersensitivity Reactions
Systemically administered quinolones, including moxifloxacin, have been associated with hypersensitivity reactions, even following a single dose. Patients should be told to discontinue use immediately and contact their physician at the first sign of a rash or allergic reaction.
Licensed to Alcon by Bayer Pharma AG.
U.S. PAT. NO. 5,607,942; 6,716,830; 7,671,070

*AVELOX is a registered trademark of Bayer AG.
Alcon®
ALCON LABORATORIES, INC.
6201 South Freeway
Fort Worth, Texas 76134 USA
MedInfo@AlconLabs.com
9008566-1112

PATADAY™ ℞

(olopatadine hydrochloride ophthalmic solution) 0.2%

DESCRIPTION

PATADAY™ (olopatadine hydrochloride ophthalmic solution) 0.2% is a sterile ophthalmic solution containing olopatadine for topical administration to the eyes. Olopatadine hydrochloride is a white, crystalline, water-soluble powder with a molecular weight of 373.88 and a molecular formula of $C_{21}H_{23}NO_3 \cdot HCl$.
Chemical Name: 11-[(Z)-3-(Dimethylamino) propylidene]-6-11-dihydrodibenz[b,e] oxepin-2-acetic acid, hydrochloride.
Each mL of PATADAY™ solution contains: **Active:** 2.22 mg olopatadine hydrochloride equivalent to 2 mg olopatadine. **Inactives:** povidone; dibasic sodium phosphate; sodium chloride; edetate disodium; benzalkonium chloride 0.01% **(preservative)** hydrochloric acid / sodium hydroxide (adjust pH); and purified water.
It has a pH of approximately 7 and an osmolality of approximately 300 mOsm/kg.

CLINICAL PHARMACOLOGY

Olopatadine is a relatively selective histamine H_1 antagonist and an inhibitor of the release of histamine from the mast cells. Decreased chemotaxis and inhibition of eosinophil activation has also been demonstrated. Olopatadine is devoid of effects on alpha-adrenergic, dopaminergic, and muscarinic type 1 and 2 receptors.
Systemic bioavailability data upon topical ocular administration of PATADAY™ solution are not available. Following topical ocular administration of olopatadine 0.15% ophthalmic solution in man, olopatadine was shown to have a low systemic exposure. Two studies in normal volunteers (totaling 24 subjects) dosed bilaterally with olopatadine 0.15% ophthalmic solution once every 12 hours for 2 weeks demonstrated plasma concentrations to be generally below the quantitation limit of the assay (< 0.5 ng/mL). Samples in which olopatadine was quantifiable were typically found within 2 hours of dosing and ranged from 0.5 to 1.3 ng/mL. The elimination half-life in plasma following oral dosing was 8 to 12 hours, and elimination was predominantly through renal excretion. Approximately 60–70% of the dose was recovered in the urine as parent drug. Two metabolites, the mono-desmethyl and the N-oxide, were detected at low concentrations in the urine.

CLINICAL STUDIES

Results from clinical studies of up to 12 weeks duration demonstrate that PATADAY™ solution when dosed once a day is effective in the treatment of ocular itching associated with allergic conjunctivitis.

INDICATIONS AND USAGE

PATADAY™ solution is indicated for the treatment of ocular itching associated with allergic conjunctivitis.

CONTRAINDICATIONS

Hypersensitivity to any components of this product.

WARNINGS

For topical ocular use only. Not for injection or oral use.

PRECAUTIONS

Information for Patients
As with any eye drop, to prevent contaminating the dropper tip and solution, care should be taken not to touch the eyelids or surrounding areas with the dropper tip of the bottle. Keep bottle tightly closed when not in use. Patients should be advised not to wear a contact lens if their eye is red.
PATADAY™ (olopatadine hydrochloride ophthalmic solution) 0.2% should not be used to treat contact lens related irritation. The preservative in PATADAY™ solution, benzalkonium chloride, may be absorbed by soft contact lenses. Patients who wear soft contact lenses and **whose eyes are not red**, should be instructed to wait at least ten minutes after instilling PATADAY™ (olopatadine hydrochloride ophthalmic solution) 0.2% before they insert their contact lenses.
Carcinogenesis, Mutagenesis, Impairment of Fertility
Olopatadine administered orally was not carcinogenic in mice and rats in doses up to 500 mg/kg/day and 200 mg/kg/day, respectively. Based on a 40 µL drop size and a 50 kg person, these doses were approximately 150,000 and 50,000 times higher than the maximum recommended ocular human dose (MROHD). No mutagenic potential was observed when olopatadine was tested in an *in vitro* bacterial reverse mutation (Ames) test, an *in vitro* mammalian chromosome aberration assay or an *in vivo* mouse micronucleus test. Olopatadine administered to male and female rats at oral doses of approximately 100,000 times MROHD level resulted in a slight decrease in the fertility index and reduced implantation rate; no effects on reproductive function were observed at doses of approximately 15,000 times the MROHD level.
Pregnancy:
Teratogenic effects: Pregnancy Category C
Olopatadine was found not to be teratogenic in rats and rabbits. However, rats treated at 600 mg/kg/day, or 150,000 times the MROHD and rabbits treated at 400 mg/kg/day, or approximately 100,000 times the MROHD, during organogenesis showed a decrease in live fetuses. In addition, rats treated with 600 mg/kg/day of olopatadine during organogenesis showed a decrease in fetal weight. Further, rats treated with 600 mg/kg/day of olopatadine during late gestation through the lactation period showed a decrease in neonatal survival and body weight.
There are, however, no adequate and well-controlled studies in pregnant women. Because animal studies are not always predictive of human responses, this drug should be used in pregnant women only if the potential benefit to the mother justifies the potential risk to the embryo or fetus.
Nursing Mothers:
Olopatadine has been identified in the milk of nursing rats following oral administration. It is not known whether topical ocular administration could result in sufficient systemic absorption to produce detectable quantities in the human breast milk. Nevertheless, caution should be exercised when PATADAY™ (olopatadine hydrochloride ophthalmic solution) 0.2% is administered to a nursing mother.
Pediatric Use:
Safety and effectiveness in pediatric patients below the age of 3 years have not been established.
Geriatric Use:
No overall differences in safety and effectiveness have been observed between elderly and younger patients.

ADVERSE REACTIONS

Symptoms similar to cold syndrome and pharyngitis were reported at an incidence of approximately 10%.
The following adverse experiences have been reported in 5% or less of patients:
Ocular: blurred vision, burning or stinging, conjunctivitis, dry eye, foreign body sensation, hyperemia, hypersensitivity, keratitis, lid edema, pain and ocular pruritus.
Non-ocular: asthenia, back pain, flu syndrome, headache, increased cough, infection, nausea, rhinitis, sinusitis and taste perversion.
Some of these events were similar to the underlying disease being studied.

DOSAGE AND ADMINISTRATION

The recommended dose is one drop in each affected eye once a day.

HOW SUPPLIED

PATADAY™ (olopatadine hydrochloride ophthalmic solution) 0.2% is supplied in a white, oval, low density polyethylene DROP-TAINER® dispenser with a natural low density polyethylene dispensing plug and a white polypropylene cap. Tamper evidence is provided with a shrink band around the closure and neck area of the package.
NDC 0065-0272-25 2.5 mL fill in 4 mL oval bottle
Storage:
Store at 2°C to 25°C (36°F to 77°F)
U.S. Patents Nos. 5,116,863; 5,641,805; 6,995,186; 7,402,609
Rx Only
ALCON LABORATORIES, INC.
Fort Worth, Texas 76134 USA

SIMBRINZA™ ℞

(brinzolamide/brimonidine tartrate ophthalmic suspension)
1%/0.2%

HIGHLIGHTS OF PRESCRIBING INFORMATION
These highlights do not include all the information needed to use SIMBRINZA™ safely and effectively. See full prescribing information for SIMBRINZA™.
SIMBRINZA™ (brinzolamide/brimonidine tartrate ophthalmic suspension) 1%/0.2%
Initial U.S. Approval: 2013

INDICATIONS AND USAGE

SIMBRINZA™ is a fixed combination of a carbonic anhydrase inhibitor and an alpha 2 adrenergic receptor agonist indicated for the reduction of elevated intraocular pressure in patients with open-angle glaucoma or ocular hypertension. (1)

DOSAGE AND ADMINISTRATION

Shake well before use. Instill one drop in the affected eye(s) three times daily. If more than one topical ophthalmic drug is being used, the drugs should be administered at least five (5) minutes apart. (2)

DOSAGE FORMS AND STRENGTHS

Suspension containing 10 mg/mL brinzolamide and 2 mg/mL brimonidine tartrate. (3)

CONTRAINDICATIONS

- Hypersensitivity to any component of this product. (4.1)
- Neonates and infants (under the age of 2 years). (4.2)

WARNINGS AND PRECAUTIONS

- Potential for sulfonamide hypersensitivity reactions because of the brinzolamide tartrate component (5.1)
- Potential for corneal endothelium cell loss (5.2)
- Severe renal impairment may limit the metabolism of the brinzolamide tartrate component (5.3)

ADVERSE REACTIONS

Most common adverse reactions occurring in approximately 3 to 5% of patients included blurred vision, eye irritation, dysgeusia (bad taste), dry mouth, eye allergy. (6.1)
To report SUSPECTED ADVERSE REACTIONS, contact Alcon Laboratories, Inc. at 1-800-757-9195 or FDA at 1-800-FDA-1088 or www.fda.gov/medwatch.

DRUG INTERACTIONS

- Oral Carbonic Anhydrase Inhibitors (7.1)
- High-dose Salicylate Therapy (7.2)
- CNS Depressants (7.3)
- Antihypertensives/Cardiac Glycosides (7.4)
- Tricyclic Antidepressants (7.5)
- Monoamine Oxidase Inhibitors (7.6)

See 17 for PATIENT COUNSELING INFORMATION
Revised: 04/2013

FULL PRESCRIBING INFORMATION: CONTENTS*

*** Sections or subsections omitted from the full prescribing information are not listed**

FULL PRESCRIBING INFORMATION

1 INDICATIONS AND USAGE

SIMBRINZA™ (brinzolamide/brimonidine tartrate ophthalmic suspension) 1%/0.2% is a fixed combination of a carbonic anhydrase inhibitor and an alpha 2 adrenergic receptor agonist indicated for the reduction of elevated intraocular pressure (IOP) in patients with open-angle glaucoma or ocular hypertension.

2 DOSAGE AND ADMINISTRATION

The recommended dose is one drop of SIMBRINZA™ in the affected eye(s) three times daily. Shake well before use. SIMBRINZA™ ophthalmic suspension may be used concomitantly with other topical ophthalmic drug products to lower intraocular pressure. If more than one topical ophthalmic drug is being used, the drugs should be administered at least five (5) minutes apart.

3 DOSAGE FORMS AND STRENGTHS

Suspension containing 10 mg/mL brinzolamide and 2 mg/mL brimonidine tartrate.

4 CONTRAINDICATIONS

4.1 Hypersensitivity

SIMBRINZA™ is contraindicated in patients who are hypersensitive to any component of this product.

4.2 Neonates and Infants (under the age of 2 years)

SIMBRINZA™ is contraindicated in neonates and infants (under the age of 2 years) *[see Use in Specific Populations (8.4)]*.

5 WARNINGS AND PRECAUTIONS

5.1 Sulfonamide Hypersensitivity Reactions

SIMBRINZA™ contains brinzolamide, a sulfonamide, and although administered topically is absorbed systemically. Therefore, the same types of adverse reactions that are attributable to sulfonamides may occur with topical administration of SIMBRINZA™. Fatalities have occurred due to severe reactions to sulfonamides including Stevens-Johnson syndrome, toxic epidermal necrolysis, fulminant hepatic necrosis, agranulocytosis, aplastic anemia, and other blood dyscrasias. Sensitization may recur when a sulfonamide is re-administered irrespective of the route of administration. If signs of serious reactions or hypersensitivity occur, discontinue the use of this preparation *[see Patient Counseling Information (17.1)]*.

5.2 Corneal Endothelium

Carbonic anhydrase activity has been observed in both the cytoplasm and around the plasma membranes of the corneal endothelium. There is an increased potential for developing corneal edema in patients with low endothelial cell counts. Caution should be used when prescribing SIMBRINZA™ to this group of patients.

5.3 Severe Renal Impairment

SIMBRINZA™ has not been specifically studied in patients with severe renal impairment (CrCl < 30 mL/min). Since brinzolamide and its metabolite are excreted predominantly by the kidney, SIMBRINZA™ is not recommended in such patients.

5.4 Acute Angle-Closure Glaucoma

The management of patients with acute angle-closure glaucoma requires therapeutic interventions in addition to ocular hypotensive agents. SIMBRINZA™ has not been studied in patients with acute angle-closure glaucoma.

5.5 Contact Lens Wear

The preservative in SIMBRINZA™, benzalkonium chloride, may be absorbed by soft contact lenses. Contact lenses should be removed during instillation of SIMBRINZA™ but may be reinserted 15 minutes after instillation *[see Patient Counseling Information (17.7)]*.

5.6 Severe Cardiovascular Disease

Brimonidine tartrate, a component of SIMBRINZA™, has a less than 5% mean decrease in blood pressure 2 hours after dosing in clinical studies; caution should be exercised in treating patients with severe cardiovascular disease.

5.7 Severe Hepatic Impairment

Because brimonidine tartrate, a component of SIMBRINZA™, has not been studied in patients with hepatic impairment, caution should be exercised in such patients.

5.8 Potentiation of Vascular Insufficiency

Brimonidine tartrate, a component of SIMBRINZA™, may potentiate syndromes associated with vascular insufficiency. SIMBRINZA™ should be used with caution in patients with depression, cerebral or coronary insufficiency, Raynaud's phenomenon, orthostatic hypotension, or thromboangitis obliterans.

5.9 Contamination of Topical Ophthalmic Products After Use

There have been reports of bacterial keratitis associated with the use of multiple-dose containers of topical ophthalmic products. These containers have been inadvertently contaminated by patients who, in most cases, had a concurrent corneal disease or a disruption of the ocular epithelial surface *[see Patient Counseling Information (17.4)]*.

6 ADVERSE REACTIONS

6.1 Clinical Studies Experience

Because clinical studies are conducted under widely varying conditions, adverse reaction rates observed in the clinical studies of a drug cannot be directly compared to the rates in the clinical studies of another drug and may not reflect the rates observed in practice.

SIMBRINZA™ In two clinical trials of 3 months duration 435 patients were treated with SIMBRINZA™, and 915 were treated with the two individual components. The most frequently reported adverse reactions in patients treated with SIMBRINZA™ occurring in approximately 3 to 5% of patients in descending order of incidence were blurred vision, eye irritation, dysgeusia (bad taste), dry mouth, and eye allergy. Rates of adverse reactions reported with the individual components were comparable. Treatment discontinuation, mainly due to adverse reactions, was reported in 11% of SIMBRINZA™ patients.

Other adverse reactions that have been reported with the individual components during clinical trials are listed below.

Brinzolamide 1%

In clinical studies of brinzolamide ophthalmic suspension 1%, the most frequently reported adverse reactions reported in 5 to 10% of patients were blurred vision and bitter, sour or unusual taste. Adverse reactions occurring in 1 to 5% of patients were blepharitis, dermatitis, dry eye, foreign body sensation, headache, hyperemia, ocular discharge, ocular discomfort, ocular keratitis, ocular pain, ocular pruritus and rhinitis.

The following adverse reactions were reported at an incidence below 1%: allergic reactions, alopecia, chest pain, conjunctivitis, diarrhea, diplopia, dizziness, dry mouth, dyspnea, dyspepsia, eye fatigue, hypertonia, keratoconjunctivitis, keratopathy, kidney pain, lid margin crusting or sticky sensation, nausea, pharyngitis, tearing and urticaria.

Brimonidine Tartrate 0.2%

In clinical studies of brimonidine tartrate 0.2%, adverse reactions occurring in approximately 10 to 30% of the subjects, in descending order of incidence, included oral dryness, ocular hyperemia, burning and stinging, headache, blurring, foreign body sensation, fatigue/drowsiness, conjunctival follicles, ocular allergic reactions, and ocular pruritus.

Reactions occurring in approximately 3 to 9% of the subjects, in descending order included corneal staining/erosion, photophobia, eyelid erythema, ocular ache/pain, ocular dryness, tearing, upper respiratory symptoms, eyelid edema, conjunctival edema, dizziness, blepharitis, ocular irritation, gastrointestinal symptoms, asthenia, conjunctival blanching, abnormal vision and muscular pain.

The following adverse reactions were reported in less than 3% of the patients: lid crusting, conjunctival hemorrhage, abnormal taste, insomnia, conjunctival discharge, depression, hypertension, anxiety, palpitations/arrhythmias, nasal dryness and syncope.

6.2 Postmarketing Experience

The following reactions have been identified during postmarketing use of brimonidine tartrate ophthalmic solutions in clinical practice. Because they are reported voluntarily from a population of unknown size, estimates of frequency cannot be made. The reactions, which have been chosen for inclusion due to either their seriousness, frequency of reporting, possible causal connection to brimonidine tartrate ophthalmic solutions, or a combination of these factors, include: bradycardia, hypersensitivity, iritis, keratoconjunctivitis sicca, miosis, nausea, skin reactions (including erythema, eyelid pruritus, rash, and vasodilation), and tachycardia.

Apnea, bradycardia, coma, hypotension, hypothermia, hypotonia, lethargy, pallor, respiratory depression, and somnolence have been reported in infants receiving brimonidine tartrate ophthalmic solutions *[see Contraindications (4.3)]*.

7 DRUG INTERACTIONS

7.1 Oral Carbonic Anhydrase Inhibitors

There is a potential for an additive effect on the known systemic effects of carbonic anhydrase inhibition in patients receiving an oral carbonic anhydrase inhibitor and brinzolamide ophthalmic suspension 1%, a component of SIMBRINZA™. The concomitant administration of SIMBRINZA™ and oral carbonic anhydrase inhibitors is not recommended.

7.2 High-Dose Salicylate Therapy

Carbonic anhydrase inhibitors may produce acid-base and electrolyte alterations. These alterations were not reported in the clinical trials with brinzolamide ophthalmic suspension 1%. However, in patients treated with oral carbonic anhydrase inhibitors, rare instances of acid-base alterations have occurred with high-dose salicylate therapy. Therefore, the potential for such drug interactions should be considered in patients receiving SIMBRINZA™.

7.3 CNS Depressants

Although specific drug interaction studies have not been conducted with SIMBRINZA™, the possibility of an additive or potentiating effect with CNS depressants (alcohol, opiates, barbiturates, sedatives, or anesthetics) should be considered.

7.4 Antihypertensives/Cardiac Glycosides

Because brimonidine tartrate, a component of SIMBRINZA™, may reduce blood pressure, caution in using drugs such as antihypertensives and/or cardiac glycosides with SIMBRINZA™ is advised.

7.5 Tricyclic Antidepressants

Tricyclic antidepressants have been reported to blunt the hypotensive effect of systemic clonidine. It is not known whether the concurrent use of these agents with SIMBRINZA™ in humans can lead to resulting interference with the IOP lowering effect. Caution is advised in patients taking tricyclic antidepressants which can affect the metabolism and uptake of circulating amines.

7.6 Monoamine Oxidase Inhibitors

Monoamine oxidase (MAO) inhibitors may theoretically interfere with the metabolism of brimonidine tartrate and potentially result in an increased systemic side-effect such as hypotension. Caution is advised in patients taking MAO inhibitors which can affect the metabolism and uptake of circulating amines.

8 USE IN SPECIFIC POPULATIONS

8.1 Pregnancy

Pregnancy Category C: Developmental toxicity studies with brinzolamide in rabbits at oral doses of 1, 3, and 6 mg/kg/day (20, 60, and 120 times the recommended human ophthalmic dose) produced maternal toxicity at 6 mg/kg/day and a significant increase in the number of fetal variations, such as accessory skull bones, which was only slightly higher than the historic value at 1 and 6 mg/kg. In rats, statistically decreased body weights of fetuses from dams receiving oral doses of 18 mg/kg/day (180 times the recommended human ophthalmic dose) during gestation were

Table 1. Mean (SD) IOP values at baseline

		SIMBRINZA™	Brinzolamide	Brimonidine
Study 1		(n=209)	(n=224)	(n=216)
	8 AM	26.9 (2.63)	27.1 (2.64)	27.0 (2.56)
	10 AM	25.3 (2.76)	25.4 (2.74)	25.4 (2.78)
	3 PM	23.7 (2.98)	23.8 (3.24)	24.0 (3.27)
	5 PM	23.2 (3.08)	23.6 (3.39)	23.7 (3.30)
Study 2		(n=218)	(n=229)	(n=232)
	8 AM	27.2 (2.75)	27.2 (2.72)	27.3 (2.73)
	10 AM	25.8 (3.09)	26.0 (3.20)	25.8 (3.02)
	3 PM	24.4 (3.67)	24.4 (3.58)	24.0 (3.39)
	5 PM	24.1 (3.71)	24.2 (3.86)	23.7 (3.58)

Table 2 Mean IOP (mmHg) by Treatment Group and Treatment Difference in Mean IOP

	SIMBRINZA™	Brinzolamide		Brimonidine	
Study 1	(N=209)	(N=224)		(N=216)	
	Mean	Mean	Difference (95%CI)**	Mean	Difference (95%CI)**
Week 2					
8 AM	20.4	22.0	-1.6 (-2.3, -0.9)	22.4	-2.0 (-2.7, -1.3)
10 AM	17.1	20.5	-3.4 (-4.1, -2.7)	19.4	-2.3 (-3.0, -1.6)
3 PM	18.4	20.4	-1.9 (-2.6, -1.3)	20.6	-2.2 (-2.9, -1.5)
5 PM	16.6	19.7	-3.2 (-3.9, -2.5)	18.4	-1.9 (-2.6, -1.2)
Week 6					
8 AM	20.4	21.9	-1.5 (-2.2, -0.8)	22.6	-2.3 (-3.0, -1.6)
10 AM	17.5	20.2	-2.7 (-3.4, -2.0)	19.5	-2.0 (-2.7, -1.3)
3 PM	18.9	20.2	-1.2 (-1.9, -0.5)	21.1	-2.1 (-2.8, -1.4)
5 PM	17.0	19.7	-2.6 (-3.3, -1.9)	18.6	-1.5 (-2.2, -0.8)
Month 3					
8 AM	20.5	21.6	-1.1 (-1.8, -0.4)	23.3	-2.8 (-3.5, -2.1)
10 AM	17.2	20.4	-3.2 (-3.9, -2.5)	19.7	-2.5 (-3.2, -1.8)
3 PM	18.7	20.4	-1.8 (-2.5, -1.1)	21.3	-2.6 (-3.3, -1.9)
5 PM	17.0	20.0	-3.0 (-3.7, -2.3)	18.8	-1.8 (-2.5, -1.1)

(Table continued on next page)

proportional to the reduced maternal weight gain, with no statistically significant effects on organ or tissue development. Increases in unossified sternebrae, reduced ossification of the skull, and unossified hyoid that occurred at 6 and 18 mg/kg were not statistically significant. No treatment-related malformations were seen. Following oral administration of ^{14}C-brinzolamide to pregnant rats, radioactivity was found to cross the placenta and was present in the fetal tissues and blood.

Developmental toxicity studies performed in rats with oral doses of 0.66 mg brimonidine base/kg revealed no evidence of harm to the fetus. Dosing at this level resulted in a plasma drug concentration approximately 100 times higher than that seen in humans at the recommended human ophthalmic dose. In animal studies, brimonidine crossed the placenta and entered into the fetal circulation to a limited extent.

There are no adequate and well-controlled studies in pregnant women. SIMBRINZA™ should be used during pregnancy only if the potential benefit justifies the potential risk to the fetus.

8.3 Nursing Mothers

In a study of brinzolamide in lactating rats, decreases in body weight gain in offspring at an oral dose of 15 mg/kg/day (150 times the recommended human ophthalmic dose) were observed during lactation. No other effects were observed. However, following oral administration of ^{14}C-brinzolamide to lactating rats, radioactivity was found in milk at concentrations below those in the blood and plasma. In animal studies, brimonidine was excreted in breast milk. It is not known whether brinzolamide and brimonidine tartrate are excreted in human milk following topical ocular administration. Because many drugs are excreted in human milk and because of the potential for serious adverse reactions in nursing infants from SIMBRINZA™ (brinzolamide/brimonidine tartrate ophthalmic suspension) 1%/0.2%, a decision should be made whether to discontinue nursing or to discontinue the drug, taking into account the importance of the drug to the mother.

8.4 Pediatric Use

The individual component, brinzolamide, has been studied in pediatric glaucoma patients 4 weeks to 5 years of age. The individual component, brimonidine tartrate, has been studied in pediatric patients 2 to 7 years old. Somnolence (50-83%) and decreased alertness was seen in patients 2 to 6 years old. SIMBRINZA™ is contraindicated in children under the age of 2 years *[see Contraindications (4.3)]*.

8.5 Geriatric Use

No overall differences in safety or effectiveness have been observed between elderly and adult patients.

10 OVERDOSAGE

Although no human data are available, electrolyte imbalance, development of an acidotic state, and possible nervous system effects may occur following an oral overdose of brinzolamide. Serum electrolyte levels (particularly potassium) and blood pH levels should be monitored.

Very limited information exists on accidental ingestion of brimonidine in adults; the only adverse event reported to date has been hypotension. Symptoms of brimonidine overdose have been reported in neonates, infants, and children receiving brimonidine as part of medical treatment of congenital glaucoma or by accidental oral ingestion. Treatment of an oral overdose includes supportive and symptomatic therapy; a patent airway should be maintained.

11 DESCRIPTION

SIMBRINZA™ (brinzolamide/brimonidine tartrate ophthalmic suspension) 1%/0.2% is a fixed combination of a carbonic anhydrase inhibitor and an alpha 2 adrenergic receptor agonist.

Brinzolamide is described chemically as: (R)-(+)-4-Ethylamino-2-(3-methoxypropyl)-3,4-dihydro-2H-thieno [3,2-e]-1,2-thiazine-6-sulfonamide-1,1- dioxide. Its empirical formula is $C_{12}H_{21}N_3O_5S_3$, and its structural formula is:

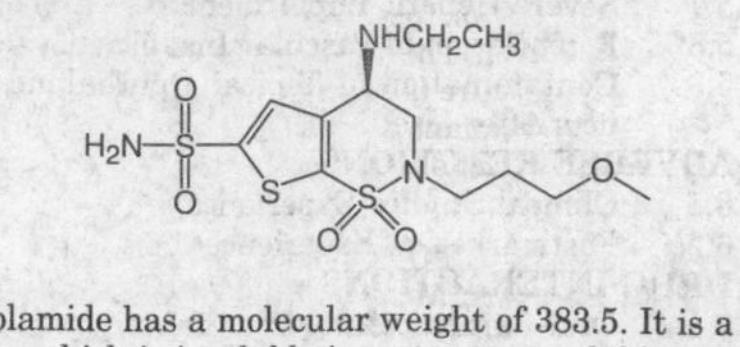

Brinzolamide has a molecular weight of 383.5. It is a white powder, which is insoluble in water, very soluble in methanol and soluble in ethanol.

Brimonidine tartrate is described chemically as: 5-bromo-6-(2-imidazolidinylideneamino) quinoxaline L-tartrate. Its empirical formula of $C_{11}H_{10}BrN_5 - C_4H_6O_6$ and its structural formula is:

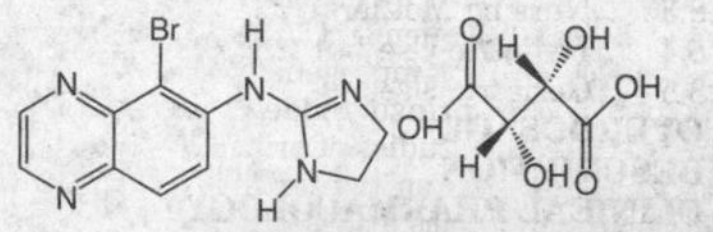

Brimonidine tartrate has a molecular weight of 442.2. It is a white to yellow powder that is soluble in water (34 mg/mL) at pH 6.5.

SIMBRINZA™ (brinzolamide/brimonidine tartrate ophthalmic suspension) 1%/0.2% is supplied as a sterile, aqueous suspension which has been formulated to be readily suspended following shaking. It has a pH of approximately 6.5 and an osmolality of approximately 270 mOsm/kg.

Each mL of SIMBRINZA™ (brinzolamide/brimonidine tartrate ophthalmic suspension) 1%/0.2% contains: **Active ingredients:** brinzolamide 10 mg, brimonidine tartrate 2 mg (equivalent to 1.32 mg as brimonidine free base); **Preservative:** benzalkonium chloride 0.03 mg; **Inactive ingredients:** propylene glycol, carbomer 974P, boric acid, mannitol, sodium chloride, tyloxapol and purified water. Hydrochloric acid and/or sodium hydroxide may be added to adjust pH.

12 CLINICAL PHARMACOLOGY

12.1 Mechanism of Action

SIMBRINZA™ is comprised of two components: brinzolamide (carbonic anhydrase inhibitor) and brimonidine tartrate (alpha 2 adrenergic receptor agonist). Each of these two components decreases elevated intraocular pressure. Elevated intraocular pressure is a major risk factor in the pathogenesis of optic nerve damage and glaucomatous visual field loss. The higher the level of intraocular pressure, the greater the likelihood of glaucomatous field loss and optic nerve damage.

Brinzolamide inhibits carbonic anhydrase in the ciliary processes of the eye to decrease aqueous humor secretion, presumably by slowing the formation of bicarbonate ions with subsequent reduction in sodium and fluid transport. Brinzolamide has a peak ocular hypotensive effect occurring at 2 to 3 hours post-dosing. Fluorophotometric studies in animals and humans suggest that brimonidine tartrate has a dual mechanism of action by reducing aqueous humor production and increasing uveoscleral outflow. Brimonidine tartrate has a peak ocular hypotensive effect occurring at two hours post-dosing. The result is a reduction in intraocular pressure (IOP).

12.3 Pharmacokinetics

Following topical ocular administration, brinzolamide is absorbed into the systemic circulation. Due to its affinity for CA-II, brinzolamide distributes extensively into the RBCs and exhibits a long half-life in whole blood (approximately 111 days). In humans, the metabolite N-desethyl brinzolamide is formed, which also binds to CA and accumulates in RBCs. This metabolite binds mainly to CA-I in the presence of brinzolamide. In plasma, both parent brinzolamide and N-desethyl brinzolamide concentrations are <10 ng/mL. Binding to plasma proteins is approximately 60%. Brinzolamide is eliminated predominantly in the urine as unchanged drug. N-Desethyl brinzolamide is also found in the urine along with lower concentrations of the N-desmethoxypropyl and O-desmethyl metabolites.

After ocular administration of a 0.2% solution of brimonidine tartrate, plasma concentrations peaked within 1 to 4 hours and declined with a systemic half-life of approximately 3 hours. In humans, systemic metabolism of brimonidine is extensive. It is metabolized primarily by the liver. Urinary excretion is the major route of elimination of the drug and its metabolites. Approximately 87% of an orally-administered radioactive dose was eliminated within 120 hours, with 74% found in the urine.

In humans, a study was conducted to evaluate the pharmacokinetics of the fixed combination of brinzolamide / brimonidine tartrate 1%/ 0.2% ophthalmic suspension. Healthy volunteers were randomly assigned to receive twice or three times a day either the fixed combination, or either of its individual components, brinzolamide or brimonidine. Subjects who were assigned to the brinzolamide alone or combination arms were administered oral brinzolamide capsules for two weeks prior to beginning dosing with the topical ocular suspension. The results demonstrate that the systemic plasma exposure (AUC and Cmax) to brinzolamide and brimonidine in humans is similar after dosing with the fixed combination to that observed following dosing with the individual components.

13 NONCLINICAL TOXICOLOGY

13.1 Carcinogenesis, Mutagenesis, Impairment of Fertility

The following tests for mutagenic potential of brinzolamide were negative: (1) *in vivo* mouse micronucleus assay; (2) *in vivo* sister chromatid exchange assay; and (3) Ames *E. coli* test. The *in vitro* mouse lymphoma forward mutation assay was negative in the absence of activation, but positive in the presence of microsomal activation. In this assay, there was no consistent dose-response relationship to the increased mutation frequency and cytotoxicity likely contributed to the high mutation frequency. Carbonic anhydrase inhibitors, as a class, are not mutagenic and the weight of evidence supports that brinzolamide is consistent with the class. In reproduction studies of brinzolamide in rats, there were no adverse effects on the fertility or reproductive capacity of males or females at doses up to 18 mg/kg/day (180 times the recommended human ophthalmic dose).

Brimonidine tartrate was not carcinogenic in either a 21-month mouse or 24-month rat study. In these studies, dietary administration of brimonidine tartrate at doses up to 2.5 mg/kg/day in mice and 1 mg/kg/day in rats resulted in plasma drug concentrations 80 and 120 times higher than the human plasma drug level at the recommended clinical dose, respectively. Brimonidine tartrate was not mutagenic or cytogenic in a series of *in vitro* and *in vivo* studies including the Ames test, chromosomal aberration assay in Chinese Hamster Ovary (CHO) cells, a host-mediated assay and cytogenic studies in mice, and a dominant lethal assay. In reproductive studies performed in rats with oral doses of 0.66 mg brimonidine base/kg (approximately 100 times the plasma drug concentration level seen in humans following multiple ophthalmic doses), fertility was not impaired.

14 CLINICAL STUDIES

Two clinical trials of 3 months duration were conducted in patients with open-angle glaucoma or ocular hypertension to compare the IOP-lowering effect of SIMBRINZA™ (brinzolamide/brimonidine tartrate ophthalmic suspension) 1%/0.2% dosed three times daily (TID) to individually administered 1% brinzolamide three times daily and 0.2% brimonidine tartrate three times daily. Mean IOP values at baseline are presented in Table 1.

[See table 1 at top of previous page]

The IOP-lowering effect of SIMBRINZA™ was 1 to 3 mmHg greater than monotherapy with either 1% brinzolamide or 0.2% brimonidine tartrate throughout the duration of the trials. Least Square Mean IOP (mmHg) and the results at Week 2, Week 6 and Month 3 for each study are provided in Table 2.

[See table 2 on previous page and above]

Figures 1 and 2 present the mean of individual subject IOP changes from baseline at week 2, week 6, and at month 3 based on the observed data for the intent-to-treat population.

[See figures 1 and 2 above]

16 HOW SUPPLIED/STORAGE AND HANDLING

SIMBRINZA™ (brinzolamide/brimonidine tartrate ophthalmic suspension) 1%/0.2% is supplied in white low density polyethylene (LDPE) DROP-TAINER® bottles with a natural LDPE dispensing-tip and white polypropylene cap as follows:

8 mL in a 10 mL bottle NDC 0065-4147-27

Storage and Handling

Store SIMBRINZA™ at 2 - 25°C (36 - 77°F).

17 PATIENT COUNSELING INFORMATION

17.1 Sulfonamide Reactions

Advise patients that if serious or unusual ocular or systemic reactions or signs of hypersensitivity occur, they should discontinue the use of the product and consult their physician.

17.2 Temporary Blurred Vision

Vision may be temporarily blurred following dosing with SIMBRINZA™. Care should be exercised in operating machinery or driving a motor vehicle.

Table 2 *(cont.)* Mean IOP (mmHg) by Treatment Group and Treatment Difference in Mean IOP

Study 2	SIMBRINZA™ (N=218)	Brinzolamide (N=229)		Brimonidine (N=232)	
Week 2					
8 AM	20.5	22.2	-1.7 (-2.4, -1.0)	22.8	-2.4 (-3.1, -1.7)
10 AM	17.4	20.7	-3.3 (-4.0, -2.6)	19.2	-1.8 (-2.5, -1.2)
3 PM	18.7	20.5	-1.7 (-2.4, -1.1)	21.1	-2.3 (-3.0, -1.6)
5 PM	16.5	20.1	-3.6 (-4.3, -2.9)	18.3	-1.8 (-2.4, -1.1)
Week 6					
8 AM	20.7	21.9	-1.2 (-1.9, -0.5)	23.2	-2.5 (-3.2, -1.8)
10 AM	17.4	20.5	-3.1 (-3.8, -2.4)	19.7	-2.3 (-3.0, -1.6)
3 PM	19.3	20.2	-0.8 (-1.5, -0.2)	21.2	-1.9 (-2.6, -1.2)
5 PM	16.9	19.9	-3.0 (-3.7, -2.3)	18.5	-1.7 (-2.4, -1.0)
Month 3					
8 AM	21.1	22.0	-1.0 (-1.7, -0.3)	23.2	-2.2 (-2.9, -1.5)
10 AM	18.0	20.8	-2.8 (-3.5, -2.1)	19.9	-1.9 (-2.6, -1.2)
3 PM	19.5	20.7	-1.2 (-1.9, -0.5)	21.5	-2.0 (-2.7, -1.3)
5 PM	17.2	20.4	-3.2 (-3.9, -2.5)	18.9	-1.7 (-2.4, -1.0)

*Based on the Intent-to-Treat Population defined as all patients who received study drug and completed at least 1 on-therapy study visit. **The estimates are based on least square means derived from a linear mixed model that accounts for correlated IOP measurements within patient; Treatment difference is SIMBRINZA minus individual component. CI=95% Confidence Interval

Figure 1. Mean IOP Change from Baseline (Study 1)

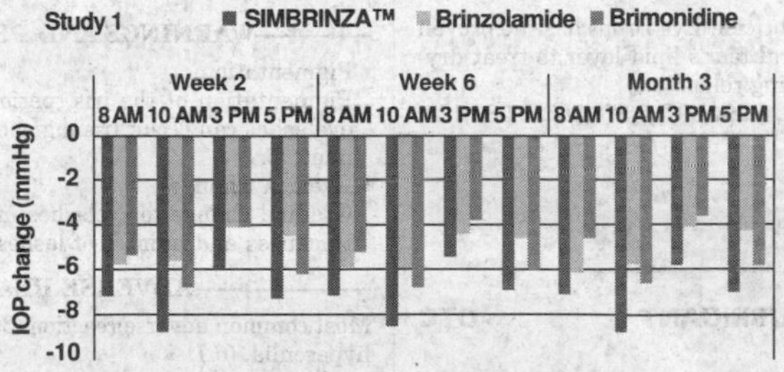

Figure 2. Mean IOP Change from Baseline (Study 2)

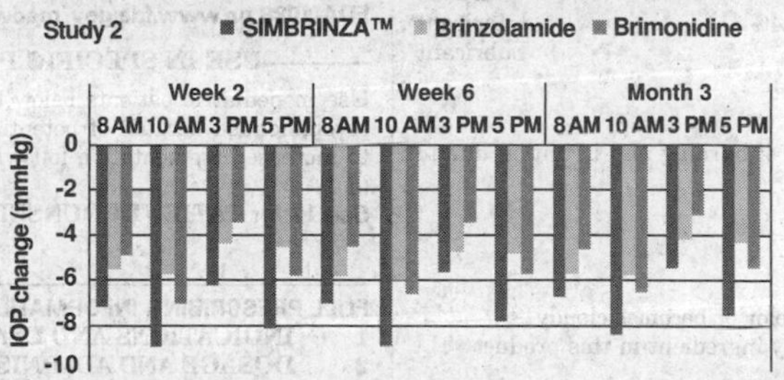

17.3 Effect on Ability to Drive and Use Machinery

As with other drugs in this class, SIMBRINZA™ may cause fatigue and/or drowsiness in some patients. Caution patients who engage in hazardous activities of the potential for a decrease in mental alertness.

17.4 Avoiding Contamination of the Product

Instruct patients that ocular solutions, if handled improperly or if the tip of the dispensing container contacts the eye or surrounding structures, can become contaminated by common bacteria known to cause ocular infections. Serious damage to the eye and subsequent loss of vision may result from using contaminated solutions *[see Warnings and Precautions (5.9)]*. Always replace the cap after using. If solution changes color or becomes cloudy, do not use. Do not use the product after the expiration date marked on the bottle.

17.5 Intercurrent Ocular Conditions

Advise patients that if they have ocular surgery or develop an intercurrent ocular condition (e.g., trauma or infection), they should immediately seek their physician's advice concerning the continued use of the present multidose container.

17.6 Concomitant Topical Ocular Therapy

If more than one topical ophthalmic drug is being used, the drugs should be administered at least five minutes apart.

17.7 Contact Lens Wear

The preservative in SIMBRINZA™, benzalkonium chloride, may be absorbed by soft contact lenses. Contact lenses should be removed during instillation of SIMBRINZA™, but may be reinserted 15 minutes after instillation.

U.S. Patent No: 6,316,441

Alcon®
ALCON LABORATORIES, INC.
Fort Worth, Texas 76134 USA
1-800-757-9195
alcon.medinfo@alcon.com
9008066-0213

SYSTANE® BALANCE LUBRICANT EYE DROPS — OTC

Drug Facts

Active Ingredients	***Purpose***
Propylene Glycol 0.6%	Lubricant

USES

- For the temporary relief of burning and irritation due to dryness of the eye

WARNINGS

For external use only.

Do not use

- if this product changes color
- if you are sensitive to any ingredient in this product

When using this product

- do not touch tip of container to any surface to avoid contamination
- replace cap after each use

Stop use and ask a doctor if

- you feel eye pain
- changes in vision occur
- redness or irritation of the eye(s) gets worse, persists or lasts more than 72 hours

Keep out of reach of children.

If swallowed, get medical help or contact a Poison Control Center right away.

DIRECTIONS

- Shake well before using.
- Instill 1 or 2 drops in the affected eye(s) as needed.

Other Information

- Store at room temperature.

Inactive Ingredients:

Boric acid, dimyristoyl phosphatidylglycerol, edetate disodium, hydroxypropyl guar, mineral oil, polyoxyl 40 stearate, POLYQUAD® (polyquaternium-1) 0.001% preservative, sorbitan tristearate, sorbitol and purified water. May contain hydrochloric acid and/or sodium hydroxide to adjust pH.

Questions:

In the U.S. call **1-800-757-9195**

www.systane.com

MedInfo@AlconLabs.com

SYSTANE®BALANCE Lubricant Eye Drops has the proven power to restore the natural tear's lipid layer to treat dryness and provide long lasting relief.

U.S. Patent Nos. 5,278,151; 5,294,607; 5,578,586; 6,583,124; 6,838,449; 6,849,253

©2010 Alcon, Inc.

Alcon Laboratories, Inc.
Fort Worth, TX 76134 USA

SYSTANE® ULTRA LUBRICANT EYE DROPS — OTC

DRUG FACTS

Active Ingredients	***Purpose***
Polyethylene Glycol 400 0.4%	Lubricant
Propylene Glycol 0.3%	Lubricant

USES

- For the temporary relief of burning and irritation due to dryness of the eye

WARNINGS

For external use only.

Do not use

- if this product changes color or becomes cloudy
- if you are sensitive to any ingredient in this product

When using this product

- do not touch tip of container to any surface to avoid contamination
- replace cap after each use

Stop use and ask a doctor if

- you feel eye pain
- changes in vision occur
- redness or irritation of the eye(s) gets worse, persists or lasts more than 72 hours

Keep out of reach of children.

If swallowed, get medical help or contact a Poison Control Center right away.

DIRECTIONS

- Shake well before using.
- Instill 1 or 2 drops in the affected eye(s) as needed.

Other Information

- Store at room temperature.

Inactive Ingredients:

Aminomethylpropanol, boric acid, hydroxypropyl guar, POLYQUAD® (polyquaternium-1) 0.001% preservative, potassium chloride, purified water, sodium chloride, sorbitol. May contain hydrochloric acid and/or sodium hydroxide to adjust pH.

Questions:

In the U.S. call **1-800-757-9195**

www.systane.com

MedInfo@AlconLabs.com

TAMPER EVIDENT: For your protection, this bottle has an imprinted seal around the neck. Do not use if seal is damaged or missing at time of purchase.

Open your eyes to a breakthrough in comfort with SYSTANE® ULTRA Lubricant Eye Drops. SYSTANE® ULTRA elevates the science of dry eye therapy to a new level. From first blink, eyes feel lubricated and refreshed. Feel the difference in dry eye relief with SYSTANE® ULTRA.

U.S. Patent Nos. 6,403,609, 6,583,124 and 6,838,449.

©2008-2011 Alcon, Inc.

Alcon Laboratories, Inc.
Fort Worth, TX 76134 USA

TRAVATAN Z® — ℞

[tra-va-tan]

(travoprost ophthalmic solution) 0.004%
OPHTHALMIC SOLUTION

HIGHLIGHTS OF PRESCRIBING INFORMATION

These highlights do not include all the information needed to use TRAVATAN Z® (travoprost ophthalmic solution) 0.004% safely and effectively. See full prescribing information for TRAVATAN Z®.

TRAVATAN Z® (travoprost ophthalmic solution) 0.004%
Initial U.S. Approval: 2001

INDICATIONS AND USAGE

TRAVATAN Z® is a prostaglandin analog indicated for the reduction of elevated intraocular pressure in patients with open-angle glaucoma or ocular hypertension. *(1)*

DOSAGE AND ADMINISTRATION

One drop in the affected eye(s) once daily in the evening. *(2)*

DOSAGE FORMS AND STRENGTHS

Solution containing 0.04 mg/mL travoprost ophthalmic solution. *(3)*

WARNINGS AND PRECAUTIONS

- Pigmentation.
  Pigmentation of the iris, periorbital tissue (eyelid) and eyelashes can occur. Iris pigmentation likely to be permanent. *(5.1)*
- Eyelash Changes.
  Gradual change to eyelashes including increased length, thickness and number of lashes. Usually reversible. *(5.2)*

ADVERSE REACTIONS

Most common adverse reaction (30% to 50%) is conjunctival hyperemia. *(6.1)*

To report SUSPECTED ADVERSE REACTIONS, contact Alcon Laboratories Inc. at 1-800-757-9195 or FDA at 1-800-FDA-1088 or www.fda.gov/medwatch.

USE IN SPECIFIC POPULATIONS

Use in pediatric patients below the age of 16 years is not recommended because of potential safety concerns related to increased pigmentation following long-term chronic use. *(8.4)*

See 17 for PATIENT COUNSELING INFORMATION

Revised: 09/2010

FULL PRESCRIBING INFORMATION: CONTENTS*

*** Sections or subsections omitted from the full prescribing information are not listed**

FULL PRESCRIBING INFORMATION

1 INDICATIONS AND USAGE

TRAVATAN Z® (travoprost ophthalmic solution) 0.004% is indicated for the reduction of elevated intraocular pressure in patients with open-angle glaucoma or ocular hypertension.

2 DOSAGE AND ADMINISTRATION

The recommended dosage is one drop in the affected eye(s) once daily in the evening. TRAVATAN Z® (travoprost ophthalmic solution) should not be administered more than once daily since it has been shown that more frequent administration of prostaglandin analogs may decrease the intraocular pressure lowering effect.

Reduction of the intraocular pressure starts approximately 2 hours after the first administration with maximum effect reached after 12 hours.

TRAVATAN Z® may be used concomitantly with other topical ophthalmic drug products to lower intraocular pressure. If more than one topical ophthalmic drug is being used, the drugs should be administered at least five (5) minutes apart.

3 DOSAGE FORMS AND STRENGTHS

Ophthalmic solution containing travoprost 0.04 mg/mL.

4 CONTRAINDICATIONS

None

5 WARNINGS AND PRECAUTIONS

5.1 Pigmentation

Travoprost ophthalmic solution has been reported to cause changes to pigmented tissues. The most frequently reported changes have been increased pigmentation of the iris, periorbital tissue (eyelid) and eyelashes. Pigmentation is expected to increase as long as travoprost is administered. The pigmentation change is due to increased melanin content in the melanocytes rather than to an increase in the number of melanocytes. After discontinuation of travoprost, pigmentation of the iris is likely to be permanent, while pigmentation of the periorbital tissue and eyelash changes have been reported to be reversible in some patients. Patients who receive treatment should be informed of the possibility of increased pigmentation. The long term effects of increased pigmentation are not known.

Iris color change may not be noticeable for several months to years. Typically, the brown pigmentation around the pupil spreads concentrically towards the periphery of the iris and the entire iris or parts of the iris become more brownish. Neither nevi nor freckles of the iris appear to be affected by treatment. While treatment with TRAVATAN Z® (travoprost ophthalmic solution) 0.004% can be continued in patients who develop noticeably increased iris pigmentation, these patients should be examined regularly. *(see PATIENT COUNSELING INFORMATION, 17.1).*

5.2 Eyelash Changes

TRAVATAN Z® may gradually change eyelashes and vellus hair in the treated eye. These changes include increased length, thickness, and number of lashes. Eyelash changes are usually reversible upon discontinuation of treatment.

5.3 Intraocular Inflammation

TRAVATAN Z® should be used with caution in patients with active intraocular inflammation (e.g., uveitis) because the inflammation may be exacerbated.

5.4 Macular Edema

Macular edema, including cystoid macular edema, has been reported during treatment with travoprost ophthalmic solution. TRAVATAN Z® should be used with caution in aphakic patients, in pseudophakic patients with a torn posterior lens capsule, or in patients with known risk factors for macular edema.

5.5 Angle-closure, Inflammatory or Neovascular Glaucoma

TRAVATAN Z® has not been evaluated for the treatment of angle-closure, inflammatory or neovascular glaucoma.

5.6 Bacterial Keratitis

There have been reports of bacterial keratitis associated with the use of multiple-dose containers of topical ophthalmic products. These containers had been inadvertently contaminated by patients who, in most cases, had a concurrent corneal disease or a disruption of the ocular epithelial surface *(see PATIENT COUNSELING INFORMATION, 17.3)*.

5.7 Use with Contact Lenses

Contact lenses should be removed prior to instillation of TRAVATAN Z® and may be reinserted 15 minutes following its administration.

6 ADVERSE REACTIONS

6.1 Clinical Studies Experience

Because clinical studies are conducted under widely varying conditions, adverse reaction rates observed in the clinical studies of a drug cannot be directly compared to rates in the clinical studies of another drug and may not reflect the rates observed in practice.

The most common adverse reaction observed in controlled clinical studies with TRAVATAN® (travoprost ophthalmic solution) 0.004% and TRAVATAN Z® (travoprost ophthalmic solution) 0.004% was ocular hyperemia which was reported in 30 to 50% of patients. Up to 3% of patients discontinued therapy due to conjunctival hyperemia. Ocular adverse reactions reported at an incidence of 5 to 10% in these clinical studies included decreased visual acuity, eye discomfort, foreign body sensation, pain and pruritus.

Ocular adverse reactions reported at an incidence of 1 to 4% in clinical studies with TRAVATAN® or TRAVATAN Z® included abnormal vision, blepharitis, blurred vision, cataract, conjunctivitis, corneal staining, dry eye, iris discoloration, keratitis, lid margin crusting, ocular inflammation, photophobia, subconjunctival hemorrhage and tearing.

Nonocular adverse reactions reported at an incidence of 1 to 5% in these clinical studies were allergy, angina pectoris, anxiety, arthritis, back pain, bradycardia, bronchitis, chest pain, cold/flu syndrome, depression, dyspepsia, gastrointestinal disorder, headache, hypercholesterolemia, hypertension, hypotension, infection, pain, prostate disorder, sinusitis, urinary incontinence and urinary tract infections.

8 USE IN SPECIFIC POPULATIONS

8.1 Pregnancy

Pregnancy Category C

Teratogenic effects: Travoprost was teratogenic in rats, at an intravenous (IV) dose up to 10 mcg/kg/day (250 times the maximal recommended human ocular dose (MRHOD), evidenced by an increase in the incidence of skeletal malformations as well as external and visceral malformations, such as fused sternebrae, domed head and hydrocephaly. Travoprost was not teratogenic in rats at IV doses up to 3 mcg/kg/day (75 times the MRHOD), or in mice at subcutaneous doses up to 1 mcg/kg/day (25 times the MRHOD). Travoprost produced an increase in post-implantation losses and a decrease in fetal viability in rats at IV doses > 3 mcg/kg/day (75 times the MRHOD) and in mice at subcutaneous doses > 0.3 mcg/kg/day (7.5 times the MRHOD).

In the offspring of female rats that received travoprost subcutaneously from Day 7 of pregnancy to lactation Day 21 at doses of ≥ 0.12 mcg/kg/day (3 times the MRHOD), the incidence of postnatal mortality was increased, and neonatal body weight gain was decreased. Neonatal development was also affected, evidenced by delayed eye opening, pinna detachment and preputial separation, and by decreased motor activity.

There are no adequate and well-controlled studies of TRAVATAN Z® (travoprost ophthalmic solution) 0.004% administration in pregnant women. Because animal reproductive studies are not always predictive of human response, TRAVATAN Z® should be administered during pregnancy only if the potential benefit justifies the potential risk to the fetus.

8.3 Nursing Mothers

A study in lactating rats demonstrated that radiolabeled travoprost and/or its metabolites were excreted in milk. It is not known whether this drug or its metabolites are excreted in human milk. Because many drugs are excreted in human milk, caution should be exercised when TRAVATAN Z® is administered to a nursing woman.

8.4 Pediatric Use

Use in pediatric patients below the age of 16 years is not recommended because of potential safety concerns related to increased pigmentation following long-term chronic use.

8.5 Geriatric Use

No overall clinical differences in safety or effectiveness have been observed between elderly and other adult patients.

8.6 Hepatic and Renal Impairment

Travoprost ophthalmic solution 0.004% has been studied in patients with hepatic impairment and also in patients with renal impairment. No clinically relevant changes in hematology, blood chemistry, or urinalysis laboratory data were observed in these patients.

11 DESCRIPTION

Travoprost is a synthetic prostaglandin F analogue. Its chemical name is [1*R*-[1α(*Z*) ,2β(1*E*,3*R**),3α,5α]]-7-[3,5-Dihydroxy-2-[3-hydroxy-4-[3-(trifluoromethyl) phenoxy]-1-butenyl]cyclopentyl]-5-heptenoic acid, 1-methylethylester. It has a molecular formula of $C_{26}H_{35}F_3O_6$ and a molecular weight of 500.55. The chemical structure of travoprost is:

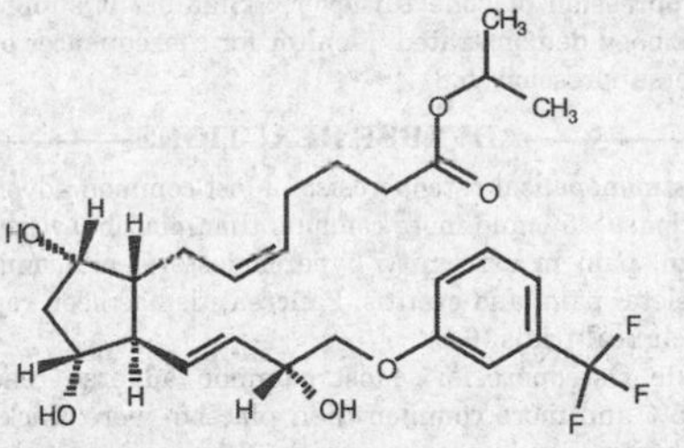

Travoprost is a clear, colorless to slightly yellow oil that is very soluble in acetonitrile, methanol, octanol, and chloroform. It is practically insoluble in water.

TRAVATAN Z® (travoprost ophthalmic solution) 0.004% is supplied as sterile, buffered aqueous solution of travoprost with a pH of approximately 5.7 and an osmolality of approximately 290 mOsmol/kg.

TRAVATAN Z® contains Active: travoprost 0.04 mg/mL; Inactives: polyoxyl 40 hydrogenated castor oil, *sof*Zia® (boric acid, propylene glycol, sorbitol, zinc chloride), sodium hydroxide and/or hydrochloric acid (to adjust pH) and purified water, USP. Preserved in the bottle with an ionic buffered system, *sof*Zia®.

12 CLINICAL PHARMACOLOGY

12.1 Mechanism of Action

Travoprost free acid, a prostaglandin analog is a selective FP prostanoid receptor agonist which is believed to reduce intraocular pressure by increasing uveoscleral outflow. The exact mechanism of action is unknown at this time.

12.3 Pharmacokinetics

Travoprost is absorbed through the cornea and is hydrolyzed to the active free acid. Data from four multiple dose pharmacokinetic studies (totaling 107 subjects) have shown that plasma concentrations of the free acid are below 0.01 ng/ml (the quantitation limit of the assay) in two-thirds of the subjects. In those individuals with quantifiable plasma concentrations (N=38), the mean plasma C_{max} was 0.018 ± 0.007 ng/ml (ranged 0.01 to 0.052 ng/mL) and was reached within 30 minutes. From these studies, travoprost is estimated to have a plasma half-life of 45 minutes. There was no difference in plasma concentrations between Days 1 and 7, indicating steady-state was reached early and that there was no significant accumulation.

Travoprost, an isopropyl ester prodrug, is hydrolyzed by esterases in the cornea to its biologically active free acid. Systemically, travoprost free acid is metabolized to inactive metabolites via beta-oxidation of the α(carboxylic acid) chain to give the 1,2-dinor and 1,2,3,4-tetranor analogs, via oxidation of the 15-hydroxyl moiety, as well as via reduction of the 13,14 double bond.

The elimination of travoprost free acid from plasma was rapid and levels were generally below the limit of quantification within one hour after dosing. The terminal elimination half-life of travoprost free acid was estimated from fourteen subjects and ranged from 17 minutes to 86 minutes with the mean half-life of 45 minutes. Less than 2% of the topical ocular dose of travoprost was excreted in the urine within 4 hours as the travoprost free acid.

13 NONCLINICAL TOXICOLOGY

13.1 Carcinogenesis, Mutagenesis, Impairment of Fertility

Two-year carcinogenicity studies in mice and rats at subcutaneous doses of 10, 30, or 100 mcg/kg/day did not show any evidence of carcinogenic potential. However, at 100 mcg/kg/day, male rats were only treated for 82 weeks, and the maximum tolerated dose (MTD) was not reached in the mouse study. The high dose (100 mcg/kg) corresponds to exposure levels over 400 times the human exposure at the maximum recommended human ocular dose (MRHOD) of 0.04 mcg/kg, based on plasma active drug levels.

Travoprost was not mutagenic in the Ames test, mouse micronucleus test or rat chromosome aberration assay. A slight increase in the mutant frequency was observed in one of two mouse lymphoma assays in the presence of rat S-9 activation enzymes.

Travoprost did not affect mating or fertility indices in male or female rats at subcutaneous doses up to 10 mcg/kg/day [250 times the maximum recommended human ocular dose of 0.04 mcg/kg/day on a mcg/kg basis (MRHOD)]. At 10 mcg/kg/day, the mean number of corpora lutea was reduced, and the post-implantation losses were increased. These effects were not observed at 3 mcg/kg/day (75 times the MRHOD).

14 CLINICAL STUDIES

In clinical studies, patients with open-angle glaucoma or ocular hypertension and baseline pressure of 25-27 mmHg who were treated with TRAVATAN® (travoprost ophthalmic solution) 0.004% or TRAVATAN Z® (travoprost ophthalmic solution) 0.004% dosed once-daily in the evening demonstrated 7-8 mmHg reductions in intraocular pressure. In subgroup analyses of these studies, mean IOP reduction in black patients was up to 1.8 mmHg greater than in non-black patients. It is not known at this time whether this difference is attributed to race or to heavily pigmented irides. In a multi-center, randomized, controlled trial, patients with mean baseline intraocular pressure of 24-26 mmHg on TIMOPTIC[1] 0.5% BID who were treated with TRAVATAN® (travoprost ophthalmic solution) 0.004% dosed QD adjunctively to TIMOPTIC[1] 0.5% BID demonstrated 6-7 mmHg reductions in intraocular pressure.

[1]TIMOPTIC is a registered trademark of Merck & Co., Inc.

16 HOW SUPPLIED/STORAGE AND HANDLING

TRAVATAN Z® (travoprost ophthalmic solution) 0.004% is a sterile, isotonic, buffered, preserved, aqueous solution of travoprost (0.04 mg/mL) supplied in Alcon's oval DROP-TAINER® package system.

TRAVATAN Z® is supplied as a 2.5 mL solution in a 4 mL and a 5 mL solution in a 7.5 mL natural polypropylene dispenser bottle with a natural polypropylene dropper tip and a turquoise polypropylene or high density polyethylene overcap. Tamper evidence is provided with a shrink band around the closure and neck area of the package.

2.5 mL fill	NDC 0065-0260-25
5 mL fill	NDC 0065-0260-05

Storage: Store at 2° - 25°C (36° - 77°F).

17 PATIENT COUNSELING INFORMATION

17.1 Potential for Pigmentation

Patients should be advised about the potential for increased brown pigmentation of the iris, which may be permanent. Patients should also be informed about the possibility of eyelid skin darkening, which may be reversible after discontinuation of TRAVATAN Z® (travoprost ophthalmic solution) 0.004%.

17.2 Potential for Eyelash Changes

Patients should also be informed of the possibility of eyelash and vellus hair changes in the treated eye during treatment with TRAVATAN Z®. These changes may result in a disparity between eyes in length, thickness, pigmentation, number of eyelashes or vellus hairs, and/or direction of eyelash growth. Eyelash changes are usually reversible upon discontinuation of treatment.

17.3 Handling the Container

Patients should be instructed to avoid allowing the tip of the dispensing container to contact the eye, surrounding structures, fingers, or any other surface in order to avoid contamination of the solution by common bacteria known to cause ocular infections. Serious damage to the eye and subsequent loss of vision may result from using contaminated solutions.

17.4 When to Seek Physician Advice

Patients should also be advised that if they develop an intercurrent ocular condition (e.g., trauma or infection), have ocular surgery, or develop any ocular reactions, particularly conjunctivitis and eyelid reactions, they should immediately seek their physician's advice concerning the continued use of TRAVATAN Z®.

17.5 Use with Contact Lenses

Contact lenses should be removed prior to instillation of TRAVATAN® and may be reinserted 15 minutes following its administration.

17.6 Use with Other Ophthalmic Drugs

If more than one topical ophthalmic drug is being used, the drugs should be administered at least five (5) minutes between applications.

Rx Only

U.S. Patent Nos. 5,631,287; 5,889,052, 6,011,062; 6,235,781; 6,503,497; and 6,849,253

Alcon®

ALCON LABORATORIES, INC.
Fort Worth, Texas 76134 USA

Amgen
ONE AMGEN CENTER DRIVE
THOUSAND OAKS, CA 91320-1799

For Product Inquiries and Adverse Event Reporting Contact:
Amgen Medical Information
(800) 772-6436
FAX: (866) 292-6436
Sales and Ordering:
Amgen Trade Operations
(800) 282-6436
FAX: (866) 292-6436

PROLIA® ℞
[PRŌ-lee-a]
(denosumab)
Injection, for subcutaneous use

HIGHLIGHTS OF PRESCRIBING INFORMATION
These highlights do not include all the information needed to use PROLIA safely and effectively. See full prescribing information for PROLIA.
Prolia® (denosumab)
Injection, for subcutaneous use
Initial U.S. Approval: 2010

RECENT MAJOR CHANGES

Indications and Usage (1.2)	09/2012
Dosage and Administration (2.2)	09/2012
Contraindications (4.3)	07/2013
Warnings and Precautions (5.2)	07/2013
Warnings and Precautions (5.7)	09/2012

INDICATIONS AND USAGE

Prolia is a RANK ligand (RANKL) inhibitor indicated for:
- Treatment of postmenopausal women with osteoporosis at high risk for fracture (1.1)
- Treatment to increase bone mass in men with osteoporosis at high risk for fracture (1.2)
- Treatment to increase bone mass in men at high risk for fracture receiving androgen deprivation therapy for nonmetastatic prostate cancer (1.3)
- Treatment to increase bone mass in women at high risk for fracture receiving adjuvant aromatase inhibitor therapy for breast cancer (1.4)

DOSAGE AND ADMINISTRATION

- Prolia should be administered by a healthcare professional (2.1)
- Administer 60 mg every 6 months as a subcutaneous injection in the upper arm, upper thigh, or abdomen (2.1)
- Instruct patients to take calcium 1000 mg daily and at least 400 IU vitamin D daily (2.1)

DOSAGE FORMS AND STRENGTHS

- Single-use prefilled syringe containing 60 mg in a 1 mL solution (3)
- Single-use vial containing 60 mg in a 1 mL solution (3)

CONTRAINDICATIONS

- Hypocalcemia (4.1, 5.3)
- Pregnancy (4.2, 8.1)
- Known hypersensitivity to Prolia (4.3, 5.2)

WARNINGS AND PRECAUTIONS

- Same Active Ingredient: Patients receiving Prolia should not receive XGEVA® (5.1)
- Hypersensitivity including anaphylactic reactions may occur. Discontinue permanently if a clinically significant reaction occurs (5.2)
- Hypocalcemia: Must be corrected before initiating Prolia. May worsen, especially in patients with renal impairment. Adequately supplement patients with calcium and vitamin D (5.3)
- Serious infections including skin infections: May occur, including those leading to hospitalization. Advise patients to seek prompt medical attention if they develop signs or symptoms of infection, including cellulitis (5.4)
- Dermatologic reactions: Dermatitis, rashes, and eczema have been reported. Consider discontinuing Prolia if severe symptoms develop (5.5)
- Osteonecrosis of the jaw: Has been reported with Prolia. Monitor for symptoms (5.6)
- Atypical femoral fractures: Have been reported. Evaluate patients with thigh or groin pain to rule out a femoral fracture (5.7)
- Suppression of bone turnover: Significant suppression has been demonstrated. Monitor for consequences of bone oversuppression (5.8)

ADVERSE REACTIONS

- Postmenopausal osteoporosis: Most common adverse reactions (> 5% and more common than placebo) were: back pain, pain in extremity, hypercholesterolemia, musculoskeletal pain, and cystitis. Pancreatitis has been reported in clinical trials (6.1)
- Male Osteoporosis: Most common adverse reactions (> 5% and more common than placebo) were: back pain, arthralgia, and nasopharyngitis (6.1)
- Bone loss due to hormone ablation for cancer: Most common adverse reactions (≥ 10% and more common than placebo) were: arthralgia and back pain. Pain in extremity and musculoskeletal pain have also been reported in clinical trials (6.1)

To report SUSPECTED ADVERSE REACTIONS, contact Amgen Inc. at 1-800-77-AMGEN (1-800-772-6436) or FDA at 1-800-FDA-1088 or www.fda.gov/medwatch.

USE IN SPECIFIC POPULATIONS

- Nursing mothers: Discontinue drug or nursing taking into consideration importance of drug to mother (8.3)
- Pediatric patients: Safety and efficacy not established (8.4)
- Renal impairment: No dose adjustment is necessary in patients with renal impairment. Patients with creatinine clearance < 30 mL/min or receiving dialysis are at risk for hypocalcemia. Supplement with calcium and vitamin D, and consider monitoring serum calcium (8.6)

See 17 for PATIENT COUNSELING INFORMATION and Medication Guide

Revised: 07/2013

FULL PRESCRIBING INFORMATION: CONTENTS*

*** Sections or subsections omitted from the full prescribing information are not listed**

FULL PRESCRIBING INFORMATION

1 INDICATIONS AND USAGE

1.1 Treatment of Postmenopausal Women with Osteoporosis at High Risk for Fracture

Prolia is indicated for the treatment of postmenopausal women with osteoporosis at high risk for fracture, defined as a history of osteoporotic fracture, or multiple risk factors for fracture; or patients who have failed or are intolerant to other available osteoporosis therapy. In postmenopausal women with osteoporosis, Prolia reduces the incidence of vertebral, nonvertebral, and hip fractures *[see Clinical Studies (14.1)]*.

1.2 Treatment to Increase Bone Mass in Men with Osteoporosis

Prolia is indicated for treatment to increase bone mass in men with osteoporosis at high risk for fracture, defined as a history of osteoporotic fracture, or multiple risk factors for fracture; or patients who have failed or are intolerant to other available osteoporosis therapy *[see Clinical Studies (14.2)]*.

1.3 Treatment of Bone Loss in Men Receiving Androgen Deprivation Therapy for Prostate Cancer

Prolia is indicated as a treatment to increase bone mass in men at high risk for fracture receiving androgen deprivation therapy for nonmetastatic prostate cancer. In these patients Prolia also reduced the incidence of vertebral fractures *[see Clinical Studies (14.3)]*.

1.4 Treatment of Bone Loss in Women Receiving Adjuvant Aromatase Inhibitor Therapy for Breast Cancer

Prolia is indicated as a treatment to increase bone mass in women at high risk for fracture receiving adjuvant aromatase inhibitor therapy for breast cancer *[see Clinical Studies (14.4)]*.

2 DOSAGE AND ADMINISTRATION

2.1 Recommended Dosage

Prolia should be administered by a healthcare professional.
The recommended dose of Prolia is 60 mg administered as a single subcutaneous injection once every 6 months. Administer Prolia via subcutaneous injection in the upper arm, the upper thigh, or the abdomen. All patients should receive calcium 1000 mg daily and at least 400 IU vitamin D daily *[see Warnings and Precautions (5.3)]*.
If a dose of Prolia is missed, administer the injection as soon as the patient is available. Thereafter, schedule injections every 6 months from the date of the last injection.

2.2 Preparation and Administration

Visually inspect Prolia for particulate matter and discoloration prior to administration whenever solution and container permit. Prolia is a clear, colorless to pale yellow solution that may contain trace amounts of translucent to white proteinaceous particles. Do not use if the solution is discolored or cloudy or if the solution contains many particles or foreign particulate matter.
Latex Allergy: People sensitive to latex should not handle the grey needle cap on the single-use prefilled syringe, which contains dry natural rubber (a derivative of latex).
Prior to administration, Prolia may be removed from the refrigerator and brought to room temperature (up to 25°C/77°F) by standing in the original container. This generally takes 15 to 30 minutes. Do not warm Prolia in any other way *[see How Supplied/Storage and Handling (16)]*.
Instructions for Prefilled Syringe with Needle Safety Guard
IMPORTANT: In order to minimize accidental needlesticks, the Prolia single-use prefilled syringe will have a green safety guard; manually activate the safety guard after the injection is given.
DO NOT slide the green safety guard forward over the needle before administering the injection; it will lock in place and prevent injection.

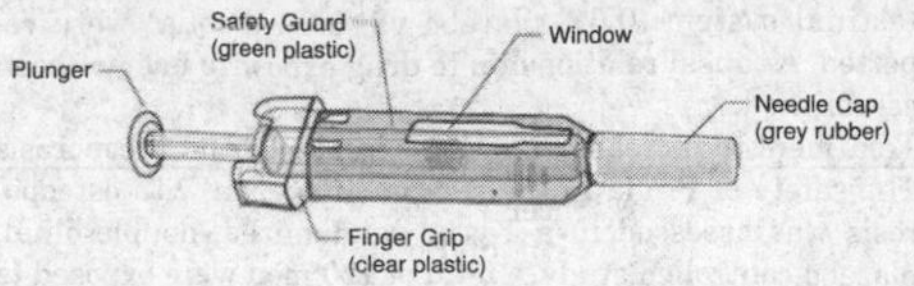

Activate the green safety guard (slide over the needle) after the injection.

The grey needle cap on the single-use prefilled syringe contains dry natural rubber (a derivative of latex); people sensitive to latex should not handle the cap.

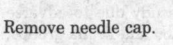

Step 1: Remove Grey Needle Cap

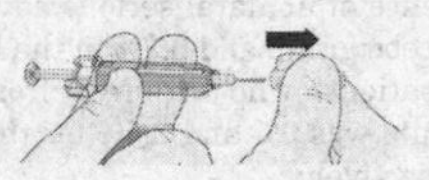

Remove needle cap.

Step 2: Administer Subcutaneous Injection

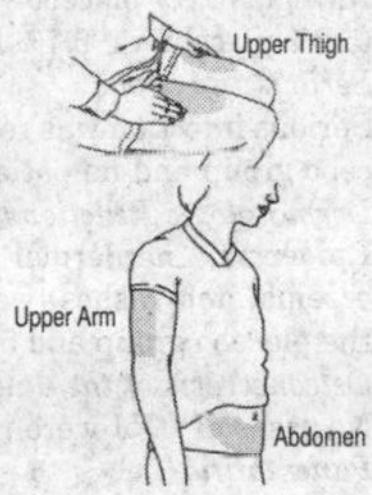

Choose an injection site. The recommended injection sites for Prolia include: the upper arm OR the upper thigh OR the abdomen.

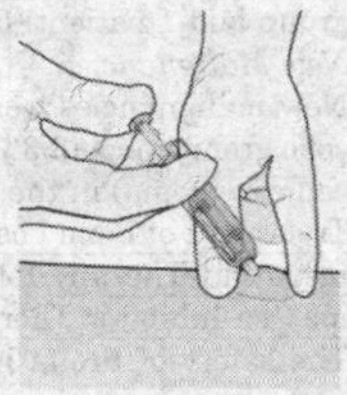

Insert needle and inject all the liquid subcutaneously. Do not administer into muscle or blood vessel.

DO NOT put grey needle cap back on needle.

Step 3: Immediately Slide Green Safety Guard Over Needle

With the *needle pointing away from you...*

Hold the prefilled syringe by the clear plastic finger grip with one hand. Then, with the other hand, grasp the green safety guard by its base and gently slide it towards the needle until the green safety guard locks securely in place and/or you hear a "click." **DO NOT** grip the green safety guard too firmly – it will move easily if you hold and slide it gently.

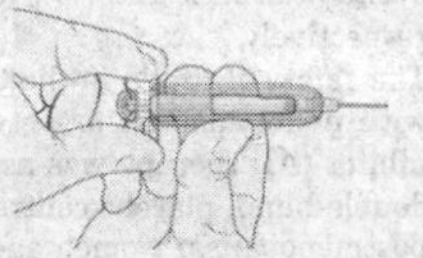

Hold clear finger grip.

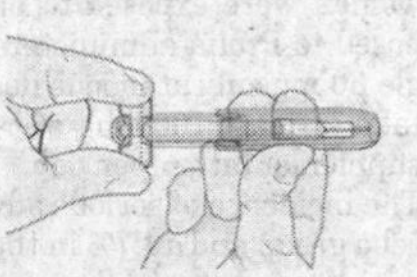

Gently slide green safety guard over needle and lock securely in place. Do not grip green safety guard too firmly when sliding over needle.

Immediately dispose of the syringe and needle cap in the nearest sharps container. **DO NOT** put the needle cap back on the used syringe.

Instructions for Single-use Vial

For administration of Prolia from the single-use vial, use a 27-gauge needle to withdraw and inject the 1 mL dose. Do not re-enter the vial. Discard vial and any liquid remaining in the vial.

3 DOSAGE FORMS AND STRENGTHS

- 1 mL of a 60 mg/mL solution in a single-use prefilled syringe
- 1 mL of a 60 mg/mL solution in a single-use vial

4 CONTRAINDICATIONS

4.1 Hypocalcemia

Pre-existing hypocalcemia must be corrected prior to initiating therapy with Prolia *[see Warnings and Precautions (5.3)]*.

4.2 Pregnancy

Prolia may cause fetal harm when administered to a pregnant woman. In utero denosumab exposure in cynomolgus monkeys resulted in increased fetal loss, stillbirths, and postnatal mortality, along with evidence of absent lymph nodes, abnormal bone growth and decreased neonatal growth. Prolia is contraindicated in women who are pregnant. If this drug is used during pregnancy, or if the patient becomes pregnant while taking this drug, the patient should be apprised of the potential hazard to a fetus *[see Use in Specific Populations (8.1)]*.

4.3 Hypersensitivity

Prolia is contraindicated in patients with a history of systemic hypersensitivity to any component of the product. Reactions have included anaphylaxis, facial swelling and urticaria *[see Warnings and Precautions (5.2), Adverse Reactions (6.2)]*.

5 WARNINGS AND PRECAUTIONS

5.1 Drug Products with Same Active Ingredient

Prolia contains the same active ingredient (denosumab) found in Xgeva. Patients receiving Prolia should not receive Xgeva.

5.2 Hypersensitivity

Clinically significant hypersensitivity including anaphylaxis has been reported with Prolia. Symptoms have included hypotension, dyspnea, throat tightness, facial and upper airway edema, pruritis, and urticaria. If an anaphylactic or other clinically significant allergic reaction occurs, initiate appropriate therapy and discontinue further use of Prolia. *[see Contraindications (4.3), Adverse Reactions (6.2)]*.

5.3 Hypocalcemia and Mineral Metabolism

Hypocalcemia may be exacerbated by the use of Prolia. Pre-existing hypocalcemia must be corrected prior to initiating therapy with Prolia. In patients predisposed to hypocalcemia and disturbances of mineral metabolism (e.g. history of hypoparathyroidism, thyroid surgery, parathyroid surgery, malabsorption syndromes, excision of small intestine, severe renal impairment [creatinine clearance < 30 mL/min] or receiving dialysis), clinical monitoring of calcium and mineral levels (phosphorus and magnesium) is highly recommended.

Hypocalcemia following Prolia administration is a significant risk in patients with severe renal impairment [creatinine clearance < 30 mL/min] or receiving dialysis. Instruct all patients with severe renal impairment, including those receiving dialysis, about the symptoms of hypocalcemia and the importance of maintaining calcium levels with adequate calcium and vitamin D supplementation.

Adequately supplement all patients with calcium and vitamin D *[see Dosage and Administration (2.1), Contraindications (4.1), Adverse Reactions (6.1), and Patient Counseling Information (17.2)]*.

5.4 Serious Infections

In a clinical trial of over 7800 women with postmenopausal osteoporosis, serious infections leading to hospitalization were reported more frequently in the Prolia group than in the placebo group *[see Adverse Reactions (6.1)]*. Serious skin infections, as well as infections of the abdomen, urinary tract, and ear, were more frequent in patients treated with Prolia. Endocarditis was also reported more frequently in Prolia-treated patients. The incidence of opportunistic infections was similar between placebo and Prolia groups, and the overall incidence of infections was similar between the treatment groups. Advise patients to seek prompt medical attention if they develop signs or symptoms of severe infection, including cellulitis.

Patients on concomitant immunosuppressant agents or with impaired immune systems may be at increased risk for serious infections. Consider the benefit-risk profile in such patients before treating with Prolia. In patients who develop serious infections while on Prolia, prescribers should assess the need for continued Prolia therapy.

5.5 Dermatologic Adverse Reactions

In a large clinical trial of over 7800 women with postmenopausal osteoporosis, epidermal and dermal adverse events such as dermatitis, eczema, and rashes occurred at a significantly higher rate in the Prolia group compared to the placebo group. Most of these events were not specific to the injection site *[see Adverse Reactions (6.1)]*. Consider discontinuing Prolia if severe symptoms develop.

5.6 Osteonecrosis of the Jaw

Osteonecrosis of the jaw (ONJ), which can occur spontaneously, is generally associated with tooth extraction and/or local infection with delayed healing. ONJ has been reported in patients receiving denosumab *[see Adverse Reactions (6.1)]*. A routine oral exam should be performed by the prescriber prior to initiation of Prolia treatment. A dental examination with appropriate preventive dentistry should be considered prior to treatment with Prolia in patients with risk factors for ONJ such as invasive dental procedures (e.g. tooth extraction, dental implants, oral surgery), diagnosis of cancer, concomitant therapies (e.g. chemotherapy, corticosteroids), poor oral hygiene, and co-morbid disorders (e.g. periodontal and/or other pre-existing dental disease, anemia, coagulopathy, infection, ill-fitting dentures). Good oral hygiene practices should be maintained during treatment with Prolia.

For patients requiring invasive dental procedures, clinical judgment of the treating physician and/or oral surgeon should guide the management plan of each patient based on individual benefit-risk assessment.

Patients who are suspected of having or who develop ONJ while on Prolia should receive care by a dentist or an oral surgeon. In these patients, extensive dental surgery to treat ONJ may exacerbate the condition. Discontinuation of Prolia therapy should be considered based on individual benefit-risk assessment.

5.7 Atypical Subtrochanteric and Diaphyseal Femoral Fractures

Atypical low-energy or low trauma fractures of the shaft have been reported in patients receiving Prolia *[see Adverse Reactions (6.1)]*. These fractures can occur anywhere in the femoral shaft from just below the lesser trochanter to above the supracondylar flare and are transverse or short oblique in orientation without evidence of comminution. Causality has not been established as these fractures also occur in osteoporotic patients who have not been treated with antiresorptive agents.

Atypical femoral fractures most commonly occur with minimal or no trauma to the affected area. They may be bilateral and many patients report prodromal pain in the affected area, usually presenting as dull, aching thigh pain, weeks to months before a complete fracture occurs. A number of reports note that patients were also receiving treatment with glucocorticoids (e.g. prednisone) at the time of fracture.

During Prolia treatment, patients should be advised to report new or unusual thigh, hip, or groin pain. Any patient who presents with thigh or groin pain should be suspected of having an atypical fracture and should be evaluated to rule out an incomplete femur fracture. Patient presenting with an atypical femur fracture should also be assessed for symptoms and signs of fracture in the contralateral limb. Interruption of Prolia therapy should be considered, pending a risk/benefit assessment, on an individual basis.

5.8 Suppression of Bone Turnover

In clinical trials in women with postmenopausal osteoporosis, treatment with Prolia resulted in significant suppression of bone remodeling as evidenced by markers of bone turnover and bone histomorphometry *[see Clinical Pharmacology (12.2) and Clinical Studies (14.1)]*. The significance of these findings and the effect of long-term treatment with Prolia are unknown. The long-term consequences of the degree of suppression of bone remodeling observed with Prolia may contribute to adverse outcomes such as osteonecrosis of the jaw, atypical fractures, and delayed fracture healing. Monitor patients for these consequences.

6 ADVERSE REACTIONS

The following serious adverse reactions are discussed below and also elsewhere in the labeling:

- Hypocalcemia *[see Warnings and Precautions (5.3)]*
- Serious Infections *[see Warnings and Precautions (5.4)]*
- Dermatologic Adverse Reactions *[see Warnings and Precautions (5.5)]*
- Osteonecrosis of the Jaw *[see Warnings and Precautions (5.6)]*
- Atypical Subtrochanteric and Diaphyseal Femoral Fractures *[see Warnings and Precautions (5.7)]*

The most common adverse reactions reported with Prolia in patients with postmenopausal osteoporosis are back pain, pain in extremity, musculoskeletal pain, hypercholesterolemia, and cystitis.

The most common adverse reactions reported with Prolia in men with osteoporosis are back pain, arthralgia, and nasopharyngitis.

The most common (per patient incidence ≥ 10%) adverse reactions reported with Prolia in patients with bone loss receiving androgen deprivation therapy for prostate cancer or adjuvant aromatase inhibitor therapy for breast cancer are arthralgia and back pain. Pain in extremity and musculoskeletal pain have also been reported in clinical trials.

The most common adverse reactions leading to discontinuation of Prolia in patients with postmenopausal osteoporosis are back pain and constipation.

The Prolia Postmarketing Active Safety Surveillance Program is available to collect information from prescribers on specific adverse events. Please see www.proliasafety.com or call 1-800-772-6436 for more information about this program.

6.1 Clinical Trials Experience

Because clinical studies are conducted under widely varying conditions, adverse reaction rates observed in the clinical studies of a drug cannot be directly compared to rates in the clinical studies of another drug and may not reflect the rates observed in clinical practice.

Table 1. Adverse Reactions Occurring in ≥ 2% of Patients with Osteoporosis and More Frequently than in Placebo-treated Patients

SYSTEM ORGAN CLASS Preferred Term	Prolia (N = 3886) n (%)	Placebo (N = 3876) n (%)
BLOOD AND LYMPHATIC SYSTEM DISORDERS		
Anemia	129 (3.3)	107 (2.8)
CARDIAC DISORDERS		
Angina pectoris	101 (2.6)	87 (2.2)
Atrial fibrillation	79 (2.0)	77 (2.0)
EAR AND LABYRINTH DISORDERS		
Vertigo	195 (5.0)	187 (4.8)
GASTROINTESTINAL DISORDERS		
Abdominal pain upper	129 (3.3)	111 (2.9)
Flatulence	84 (2.2)	53 (1.4)
Gastroesophageal reflux disease	80 (2.1)	66 (1.7)
GENERAL DISORDERS AND ADMINISTRATION SITE CONDITIONS		
Edema peripheral	189 (4.9)	155 (4.0)
Asthenia	90 (2.3)	73 (1.9)
INFECTIONS AND INFESTATIONS		
Cystitis	228 (5.9)	225 (5.8)
Upper respiratory tract infection	190 (4.9)	167 (4.3)
Pneumonia	152 (3.9)	150 (3.9)
Pharyngitis	91 (2.3)	78 (2.0)
Herpes zoster	79 (2.0)	72 (1.9)
METABOLISM AND NUTRITION DISORDERS		
Hypercholesterolemia	280 (7.2)	236 (6.1)
MUSCULOSKELETAL AND CONNECTIVE TISSUE DISORDERS		
Back pain	1347 (34.7)	1340 (34.6)
Pain in extremity	453 (11.7)	430 (11.1)
Musculoskeletal pain	297 (7.6)	291 (7.5)
Bone pain	142 (3.7)	117 (3.0)
Myalgia	114 (2.9)	94 (2.4)
Spinal osteoarthritis	82 (2.1)	64 (1.7)
NERVOUS SYSTEM DISORDERS		
Sciatica	178 (4.6)	149 (3.8)
PSYCHIATRIC DISORDERS		
Insomnia	126 (3.2)	122 (3.1)
SKIN AND SUBCUTANEOUS TISSUE DISORDERS		
Rash	96 (2.5)	79 (2.0)
Pruritus	87 (2.2)	82 (2.1)

Treatment of Postmenopausal Women with Osteoporosis

The safety of Prolia in the treatment of postmenopausal osteoporosis was assessed in a 3-year, randomized, double-blind, placebo-controlled, multinational study of 7808 postmenopausal women aged 60 to 91 years. A total of 3876 women were exposed to placebo and 3886 women were exposed to Prolia administered subcutaneously once every 6 months as a single 60 mg dose. All women were instructed to take at least 1000 mg of calcium and 400 IU of vitamin D supplementation per day.

The incidence of all-cause mortality was 2.3% (n = 90) in the placebo group and 1.8% (n = 70) in the Prolia group. The incidence of nonfatal serious adverse events was 24.2% in the placebo group and 25.0% in the Prolia group. The percentage of patients who withdrew from the study due to adverse events was 2.1% and 2.4% for the placebo and Prolia groups, respectively.

Adverse reactions reported in ≥ 2% of postmenopausal women with osteoporosis and more frequently in the Prolia-treated women than in the placebo-treated women are shown in the table below.

[See table 1 above]

Hypocalcemia

Decreases in serum calcium levels to less than 8.5 mg/dL at any visit were reported in 0.4% women in the placebo group and 1.7% women in the Prolia group. The nadir in serum calcium level occurs at approximately day 10 after Prolia dosing in subjects with normal renal function.

In clinical studies, subjects with impaired renal function were more likely to have greater reductions in serum calcium levels compared to subjects with normal renal function. In a study of 55 subjects with varying degrees of renal function, serum calcium levels < 7.5 mg/dL or symptomatic hypocalcemia were observed in 5 subjects. These included no subjects in the normal renal function group, 10% of subjects in the creatinine clearance 50 to 80 mL/min group, 29% of subjects in the creatinine clearance < 30 mL/min group, and 29% of subjects in the hemodialysis group. These subjects did not receive calcium and vitamin D supplementation. In a study of 4550 postmenopausal women with osteoporosis, the mean change from baseline in serum calcium level 10 days after Prolia dosing was -5.5% in subjects with creatinine clearance < 30 mL/min vs. -3.1% in subjects with creatinine clearance ≥ 30 mL/min.

Serious Infections

Receptor activator of nuclear factor kappa-B ligand (RANKL) is expressed on activated T and B lymphocytes and in lymph nodes. Therefore, a RANKL inhibitor such as Prolia may increase the risk of infection.

In the clinical study of 7808 postmenopausal women with osteoporosis, the incidence of infections resulting in death was 0.2% in both placebo and Prolia treatment groups. However, the incidence of nonfatal serious infections was 3.3% in the placebo and 4.0% in the Prolia groups. Hospitalizations due to serious infections in the abdomen (0.7% placebo vs. 0.9% Prolia), urinary tract (0.5% placebo vs. 0.7% Prolia), and ear (0.0% placebo vs. 0.1% Prolia) were reported. Endocarditis was reported in no placebo patients and 3 patients receiving Prolia.

Skin infections, including erysipelas and cellulitis, leading to hospitalization were reported more frequently in patients treated with Prolia (< 0.1% placebo vs. 0.4% Prolia).

The incidence of opportunistic infections was similar to that reported with placebo.

Dermatologic Reactions

A significantly higher number of patients treated with Prolia developed epidermal and dermal adverse events (such as dermatitis, eczema, and rashes), with these events reported in 8.2% of the placebo and 10.8% of the Prolia groups (p < 0.0001). Most of these events were not specific to the injection site *[see Warnings and Precautions (5.5)]*.

Osteonecrosis of the Jaw

ONJ has been reported in the osteoporosis clinical trial program in patients treated with Prolia *[see Warnings and Precautions (5.6)]*.

Atypical Subtrochanteric and Diaphyseal Fractures

In the osteoporosis clinical trial program, atypical femoral fractures were reported in patients treated with Prolia. The duration of Prolia exposure to time of atypical femoral fracture diagnosis was as early as 2½ years *[see Warnings and Precautions (5.7)]*.

Pancreatitis

Pancreatitis was reported in 4 patients (0.1%) in the placebo and 8 patients (0.2%) in the Prolia groups. Of these reports, 1 patient in the placebo group and all 8 patients in the Prolia group had serious events, including one death in the Prolia group. Several patients had a prior history of pancreatitis. The time from product administration to event occurrence was variable.

New Malignancies

The overall incidence of new malignancies was 4.3% in the placebo and 4.8% in the Prolia groups. New malignancies related to the breast (0.7% placebo vs. 0.9% Prolia), reproductive system (0.2% placebo vs. 0.5% Prolia), and gastrointestinal system (0.6% placebo vs. 0.9% Prolia) were reported. A causal relationship to drug exposure has not been established.

Treatment to Increase Bone Mass in Men with Osteoporosis

The safety of Prolia in the treatment of men with osteoporosis was assessed in a 1-year randomized, double-blind, placebo-controlled study. A total of 120 men were exposed to placebo and 120 men were exposed to Prolia administered subcutaneously once every 6 months as a single 60 mg dose. All men were instructed to take at least 1000 mg of calcium and 800 IU of vitamin D supplementation per day.

The incidence of all-cause mortality was 0.8% (n = 1) in the placebo group and 0.8% (n = 1) in the Prolia group. The incidence of nonfatal serious adverse events was 7.5% in the placebo group and 8.3% in the Prolia group. The percentage of patients who withdrew from the study due to adverse events was 0% and 2.5% for the placebo and Prolia groups, respectively.

Adverse reactions reported in ≥ 5% of men with osteoporosis and more frequently with Prolia than in the placebo-treated patients were: back pain (6.7% placebo vs. 8.3% Prolia), arthralgia (5.8% placebo vs. 6.7% Prolia), and nasopharyngitis (5.8% placebo vs. 6.7% Prolia).

Serious Infections

Serious infection was reported in 1 patient (0.8%) in the placebo group and no patients in the Prolia group.

Dermatologic Reactions

Epidermal and dermal adverse events (such as dermatitis, eczema, and rashes) were reported in 4 patients (3.3%) in the placebo group and 5 patients (4.2%) in the Prolia group.

Osteonecrosis of the Jaw

No cases of ONJ were reported.

Pancreatitis

Pancreatitis was reported in 1 patient (0.8%) in the placebo group and 1 patient (0.8%) in the Prolia group.

New Malignancies

New malignancies were reported in no patients in the placebo group and 4 (3.3%) patients (3 prostate cancers, 1 basal cell carcinoma) in the Prolia group.

Treatment of Bone Loss in Patients Receiving Androgen Deprivation Therapy for Prostate Cancer or Adjuvant Aromatase Inhibitor Therapy for Breast Cancer

The safety of Prolia in the treatment of bone loss in men with nonmetastatic prostate cancer receiving androgen deprivation therapy (ADT) was assessed in a 3–year, randomized, double-blind, placebo-controlled, multinational study of 1468 men aged 48 to 97 years. A total of 725 men were exposed to placebo and 731 men were exposed to Prolia administered once every 6 months as a single 60 mg subcutaneous dose. All men were instructed to take at least 1000 mg of calcium and 400 IU of vitamin D supplementation per day.

The incidence of serious adverse events was 30.6% in the placebo group and 34.6% in the Prolia group. The percentage of patients who withdrew from the study due to adverse events was 6.1% and 7.0% for the placebo and Prolia groups, respectively.

The safety of Prolia in the treatment of bone loss in women with nonmetastatic breast cancer receiving aromatase inhibitor (AI) therapy was assessed in a 2–year, randomized, double-blind, placebo-controlled, multinational study of 252 postmenopausal women aged 35 to 84 years. A total of 120 women were exposed to placebo and 129 women were exposed to Prolia administered once every 6 months as a single 60 mg subcutaneous dose. All women were instructed to take at least 1000 mg of calcium and 400 IU of vitamin D supplementation per day.

The incidence of serious adverse events was 9.2% in the placebo group and 14.7% in the Prolia group. The percentage of patients who withdrew from the study due to adverse events was 4.2% and 0.8% for the placebo and Prolia groups, respectively.

Adverse reactions reported in ≥ 10% of Prolia-treated patients receiving ADT for prostate cancer or adjuvant AI therapy for breast cancer, and more frequently than in the placebo-treated patients were: arthralgia (13.0% placebo vs. 14.3% Prolia) and back pain (10.5% placebo vs. 11.5% Prolia). Pain in extremity (7.7% placebo vs. 9.9% Prolia) and musculoskeletal pain (3.8% placebo vs. 6.0% Prolia) have also been reported in clinical trials. Additionally in Prolia-treated men with nonmetastatic prostate cancer receiving ADT, a greater incidence of cataracts was observed (1.2% placebo vs. 4.7% Prolia). Hypocalcemia (serum calcium < 8.4 mg/dL) was reported only in Prolia-treated patients (2.4% vs. 0%) at the month 1 visit.

6.2 Postmarketing Experience

Because postmarketing reactions are reported voluntarily from a population of uncertain size, it is not always possible to reliably estimate their frequency or establish a causal relationship to drug exposure.

The following adverse reactions have been identified during post approval use of Prolia:

- Drug-related hypersensitivity reactions: anaphylaxis, rash, urticaria, facial swelling, and erythema.
- Hypocalcemia: severe symptomatic hypocalcemia

6.3 Immunogenicity

Denosumab is a human monoclonal antibody. As with all therapeutic proteins, there is potential for immunogenicity. Using an electrochemiluminescent bridging immunoassay, less than 1% (55 out of 8113) of patients treated with Prolia for up to 5 years tested positive for binding antibodies (including pre-existing, transient, and developing antibodies). None of the patients tested positive for neutralizing antibodies, as was assessed using a chemiluminescent cell-based in vitro biological assay. No evidence of altered pharmacokinetic profile, toxicity profile, or clinical response was associated with binding antibody development.

The incidence of antibody formation is highly dependent on the sensitivity and specificity of the assay. Additionally, the observed incidence of a positive antibody (including neutralizing antibody) test result may be influenced by several factors, including assay methodology, sample handling, timing of sample collection, concomitant medications, and underlying disease. For these reasons, comparison of antibodies to denosumab with the incidence of antibodies to other products may be misleading.

7 DRUG INTERACTIONS

In subjects with postmenopausal osteoporosis, Prolia (60 mg subcutaneous injection) did not affect the pharmacokinetics of midazolam, which is metabolized by cytochrome P450 3A4 (CYP3A4), indicating that it should not affect the pharmacokinetics of drugs metabolized by this enzyme in this population *[see Clinical Pharmacology (12.3)]*.

8 USE IN SPECIFIC POPULATIONS

8.1 Pregnancy

Pregnancy Category X

Risk Summary

Prolia may cause fetal harm when administered to a pregnant woman based on findings in animals. In utero denosumab exposure in cynomolgus monkeys resulted in increased fetal loss, stillbirths, and postnatal mortality, along with evidence of absent lymph nodes, abnormal bone growth and decreased neonatal growth. Prolia is contraindicated in women who are pregnant. If this drug is used during pregnancy, or if the patient becomes pregnant while taking this drug, the patient should be apprised of the potential hazard to a fetus.

Women who become pregnant during Prolia treatment are encouraged to enroll in Amgen's Pregnancy Surveillance Program. Patients or their physicians should call 1-800-77-AMGEN (1-800-772-6436) to enroll.

Clinical Considerations

The effects of Prolia on the fetus are likely to be greater during the second and third trimesters of pregnancy. Monoclonal antibodies, such as denosumab, are transported across the placenta in a linear fashion as pregnancy progresses, with the largest amount transferred during the third trimester. If the patient becomes pregnant during Prolia therapy, treatment should be discontinued and the patient should consult their physician.

Animal Data

The effects of denosumab on prenatal development have been studied in both cynomolgus monkeys and genetically engineered mice in which RANK ligand (RANKL) expression was turned off by gene removal (a "knockout mouse"). In cynomolgus monkeys dosed subcutaneously with denosumab throughout pregnancy at a pharmacologically active dose, there was increased fetal loss during gestation, stillbirths, and postnatal mortality. Other findings in offspring included absence of axillary, inguinal, mandibular, and mesenteric lymph nodes; abnormal bone growth, reduced bone strength, reduced hematopoiesis, dental dysplasia and tooth malalignment; and decreased neonatal growth. At birth out to 1 month of age, infants had measurable blood levels of denosumab (22-621% of maternal levels).

Following a recovery period from birth out to 6 months of age, the effects on bone quality and strength returned to normal; there were no adverse effects on tooth eruption, though dental dysplasia was still apparent; axillary and inguinal lymph nodes remained absent, while mandibular and mesenteric lymph nodes were present, though small; and minimal to moderate mineralization in multiple tissues was seen in one recovery animal. There was no evidence of maternal harm prior to labor; adverse maternal effects occurred infrequently during labor. Maternal mammary gland development was normal. There was no fetal NOAEL (no observable adverse effect level) established for this study because only one dose of 50 mg/kg was evaluated.

In RANKL knockout mice, absence of RANKL (the target of denosumab) also caused fetal lymph node agenesis and led to postnatal impairment of dentition and bone growth. Pregnant RANKL knockout mice showed altered maturation of the maternal mammary gland, leading to impaired lactation *[see Use in Specific Populations (8.3) and Nonclinical Toxicology (13.2)]*.

8.3 Nursing Mothers

It is not known whether Prolia is excreted into human milk. Measurable concentrations of denosumab were present in the maternal milk of cynomolgus monkeys up to 1 month after the last dose of denosumab (≤ 0.5% milk:serum ratio). Because many drugs are excreted in human milk and because of the potential for serious adverse reactions in nursing infants from Prolia, a decision should be made whether to discontinue nursing or discontinue the drug, taking into account the importance of the drug to the mother.

Maternal exposure to Prolia during pregnancy may impair mammary gland development and lactation based on animal studies in pregnant mice lacking the RANK/RANKL signaling pathway that have shown altered maturation of the maternal mammary gland, leading to impaired lactation postpartum. However in cynomolgus monkeys treated with denosumab throughout pregnancy, maternal mammary gland development was normal, with no impaired lactation. Mammary gland histopathology at 6 months of age was normal in female offspring exposed to denosumab in utero; however, development and lactation have not been fully evaluated *[see Use in Specific Populations (8.1) and Nonclinical Toxicology (13.2)]*.

8.4 Pediatric Use

Prolia is not recommended in pediatric patients. The safety and effectiveness of Prolia in pediatric patients have not been established.

Treatment with Prolia may impair bone growth in children with open growth plates and may inhibit eruption of dentition. In neonatal rats, inhibition of RANKL (the target of Prolia therapy) with a construct of osteoprotegerin bound to Fc (OPG-Fc) at doses ≤ 10 mg/kg was associated with inhibition of bone growth and tooth eruption. Adolescent primates treated with denosumab at doses 10 and 50 times (10 and 50 mg/kg dose) higher than the recommended human dose of 60 mg administered every 6 months, based on body weight (mg/kg), had abnormal growth plates, considered to be consistent with the pharmacological activity of denosumab.

Cynomolgus monkeys exposed in utero to denosumab exhibited bone abnormalities, an absence of axillary, inguinal, mandibular, and mesenteric lymph nodes, reduced hematopoiesis, tooth malalignment, and decreased neonatal growth. Some bone abnormalities recovered once exposure was ceased following birth; however, axillary and inguinal lymph nodes remained absent 6 months post-birth *[see Use in Specific Populations (8.1)]*.

8.5 Geriatric Use

Of the total number of patients in clinical studies of Prolia, 9943 patients (76%) were ≥ 65 years old, while 3576 (27%) were ≥ 75 years old. Of the patients in the osteoporosis study in men, 133 patients (55%) were ≥ 65 years old, while 39 patients (16%) were ≥ 75 years old. No overall differences in safety or efficacy were observed between these patients and younger patients and other reported clinical experience has not identified differences in responses between the elderly and younger patients, but greater sensitivity of some older individuals cannot be ruled out.

8.6 Renal Impairment

No dose adjustment is necessary in patients with renal impairment.

In clinical studies, patients with severe renal impairment (creatinine clearance < 30 mL/min) or receiving dialysis were at greater risk of developing hypocalcemia. Consider the benefit-risk profile when administering Prolia to patients with severe renal impairment or receiving dialysis. Clinical monitoring of calcium and mineral levels (phosphorus and magnesium) is highly recommended. Adequate intake of calcium and vitamin D is important in patients with severe renal impairment or receiving dialysis *[see Warnings and Precautions (5.3), Adverse Reactions (6.1),* and Clinical Pharmacology (12.3)].

8.7 Hepatic Impairment

No clinical studies have been conducted to evaluate the effect of hepatic impairment on the pharmacokinetics of Prolia.

8.8 Males

Prolia may cause fetal harm *[see Use in Specific Populations (8.1)]*.

The extent to which denosumab is present in seminal fluid is unknown. There is a potential for fetal exposure to denosumab when a man treated with Prolia has unprotected sexual intercourse with a pregnant partner. The risk of fetal harm is likely to be low. Advise men being treated with Prolia who have a pregnant partner of this potential risk.

10 OVERDOSAGE

There is no experience with overdosage with Prolia.

11 DESCRIPTION

Prolia (denosumab) is a human IgG2 monoclonal antibody with affinity and specificity for human RANKL (receptor activator of nuclear factor kappa-B ligand). Denosumab has an approximate molecular weight of 147 kDa and is produced in genetically engineered mammalian (Chinese hamster ovary) cells.

Prolia is a sterile, preservative-free, clear, colorless to pale yellow solution.

Each 1 mL single-use prefilled syringe of Prolia contains 60 mg denosumab (60 mg/mL solution), 4.7% sorbitol, 17 mM acetate, 0.01% polysorbate 20, Water for Injection (USP), and sodium hydroxide to a pH of 5.2.

Each 1 mL single-use vial of Prolia contains 60 mg denosumab (60 mg/mL solution), 4.7% sorbitol, 17 mM acetate, Water for Injection (USP), and sodium hydroxide to a pH of 5.2.

12 CLINICAL PHARMACOLOGY

12.1 Mechanism of Action

Prolia binds to RANKL, a transmembrane or soluble protein essential for the formation, function, and survival of osteoclasts, the cells responsible for bone resorption. Prolia prevents RANKL from activating its receptor, RANK, on the surface of osteoclasts and their precursors. Prevention of the RANKL/RANK interaction inhibits osteoclast formation, function, and survival, thereby decreasing bone resorption and increasing bone mass and strength in both cortical and trabecular bone.

12.2 Pharmacodynamics

In clinical studies, treatment with 60 mg of Prolia resulted in reduction in the bone resorption marker serum type 1 C-telopeptide (CTX) by approximately 85% by 3 days, with maximal reductions occurring by 1 month. CTX levels were below the limit of assay quantitation (0.049 ng/mL) in 39% to 68% of patients 1 to 3 months after dosing of Prolia. At the end of each dosing interval, CTX reductions were partially attenuated from a maximal reduction of ≥ 87% to ≥ 45% (range: 45% to 80%), as serum denosumab levels diminished, reflecting the reversibility of the effects of Prolia on bone remodeling. These effects were sustained with continued treatment. Upon reinitiation, the degree of inhibition of CTX by Prolia was similar to that observed in patients initiating Prolia treatment.

Consistent with the physiological coupling of bone formation and resorption in skeletal remodeling, subsequent reductions in bone formation markers (i.e. osteocalcin and procollagen type 1 N-terminal peptide [PlNP]) were observed starting 1 month after the first dose of Prolia. After discontinuation of Prolia therapy, markers of bone resorption increased to levels 40% to 60% above pretreatment values but returned to baseline levels within 12 months.

12.3 Pharmacokinetics

In a study conducted in healthy male and female volunteers (n = 73, age range: 18 to 64 years) following a single subcutaneously administered Prolia dose of 60 mg after fasting (at least for 12 hours), the mean maximum denosumab concentration (C_{max}) was 6.75 mcg/mL (standard deviation [SD] = 1.89 mcg/mL). The median time to maximum denosumab concentration (T_{max}) was 10 days (range: 3 to 21 days). After C_{max}, serum denosumab concentrations declined over a period of 4 to 5 months with a mean half-life of 25.4 days (SD = 8.5 days; n = 46). The mean area-under-the-concentration-time curve up to 16 weeks ($AUC_{0\text{-}16\ weeks}$) of denosumab was 316 mcg•day/mL (SD = 101 mcg•day/mL).

No accumulation or change in denosumab pharmacokinetics with time was observed upon multiple dosing of 60 mg subcutaneously administered once every 6 months.

Prolia pharmacokinetics were not affected by the formation of binding antibodies.

A population pharmacokinetic analysis was performed to evaluate the effects of demographic characteristics. This analysis showed no notable differences in pharmacokinetics with age (in postmenopausal women), race, or body weight (36 to 140 kg).

Drug Interactions

In a study of 17 postmenopausal women with osteoporosis, midazolam (2 mg oral) was administered two weeks after a single dose of denosumab (60 mg subcutaneous injection), which approximates the T_{max} of denosumab. Denosumab did not affect the pharmacokinetics of midazolam, which is metabolized by cytochrome P450 3A4 (CYP3A4). This indicates that denosumab should not alter the pharmacokinetics of drugs metabolized by CYP3A4 in postmenopausal women with osteoporosis.

Table 2. The Effect of Prolia on the Incidence of New Vertebral Fractures in Postmenopausal Women

	Proportion of Women With Fracture (%)*		Absolute Risk Reduction (%)† (95% CI)	Relative Risk Reduction (%)† (95% CI)
	Placebo N = 3691 (%)	Prolia N = 3702 (%)		
0-1 Year	2.2	0.9	1.4 (0.8, 1.9)	61 (42, 74)
0-2 Years	5.0	1.4	3.5 (2.7, 4.3)	71 (61, 79)
0-3 Years	7.2	2.3	4.8 (3.9, 5.8)	68 (59, 74)

* Event rates based on crude rates in each interval.
† Absolute risk reduction and relative risk reduction based on Mantel-Haenszel method adjusting for age group variable.

Table 3. The Effect of Prolia on the Incidence of Nonvertebral Fractures at Year 3

	Proportion of Women With Fracture (%)*		Absolute Risk Reduction (%) (95% CI)	Relative Risk Reduction (%) (95% CI)
	Placebo N = 3906 (%)	Prolia N = 3902 (%)		
Nonvertebral fracture†	8.0	6.5	1.5 (0.3, 2.7)	20 (5, 33)‡

* Event rates based on Kaplan-Meier estimates at 3 years.
† Excluding those of the vertebrae (cervical, thoracic, and lumbar), skull, facial, mandible, metacarpus, and finger and toe phalanges.
‡ p-value = 0.01.

Specific Populations

Gender: Mean serum denosumab concentration-time profiles observed in a study conducted in healthy men ≥ 50 years were similar to those observed in a study conducted in postmenopausal women using the same dose regimen.

Age: The pharmacokinetics of denosumab were not affected by age across all populations studied whose ages ranged from 28 to 87 years.

Race: The pharmacokinetics of denosumab were not affected by race.

Renal Impairment: In a study of 55 patients with varying degrees of renal function, including patients on dialysis, the degree of renal impairment had no effect on the pharmacokinetics of denosumab; thus, dose adjustment for renal impairment is not necessary.

Hepatic Impairment: No clinical studies have been conducted to evaluate the effect of hepatic impairment on the pharmacokinetics of denosumab.

13 NONCLINICAL TOXICOLOGY

13.1 Carcinogenesis, Mutagenesis, Impairment of Fertility

Carcinogenicity

The carcinogenic potential of denosumab has not been evaluated in long-term animal studies.

Mutagenicity

The genotoxic potential of denosumab has not been evaluated.

Impairment of Fertility

Denosumab had no effect on female fertility or male reproductive organs in monkeys at doses that were 13- to 50-fold higher than the recommended human dose of 60 mg subcutaneously administered once every 6 months, based on body weight (mg/kg).

13.2 Animal Toxicology and/or Pharmacology

Denosumab is an inhibitor of osteoclastic bone resorption via inhibition of RANKL.

In ovariectomized monkeys, once-monthly treatment with denosumab suppressed bone turnover and increased bone mineral density (BMD) and strength of cancellous and cortical bone at doses 50-fold higher than the recommended human dose of 60 mg administered once every 6 months, based on body weight (mg/kg). Bone tissue was normal with no evidence of mineralization defects, accumulation of osteoid, or woven bone.

Because the biological activity of denosumab in animals is specific to nonhuman primates, evaluation of genetically engineered ("knockout") mice or use of other biological inhibitors of the RANK/RANKL pathway, namely OPG-Fc, provided additional information on the pharmacodynamic properties of denosumab. RANK/RANKL knockout mice exhibited absence of lymph node formation, as well as an absence of lactation due to inhibition of mammary gland maturation (lobulo-alveolar gland development during pregnancy). Neonatal RANK/RANKL knockout mice exhibited reduced bone growth and lack of tooth eruption. A corroborative study in 2-week-old rats given the RANKL inhibitor OPG-Fc also showed reduced bone growth, altered growth plates, and impaired tooth eruption. These changes were partially reversible in this model when dosing with the RANKL inhibitors was discontinued.

14 CLINICAL STUDIES

14.1 Postmenopausal Women with Osteoporosis

The efficacy and safety of Prolia in the treatment of postmenopausal osteoporosis was demonstrated in a 3-year, randomized, double-blind, placebo-controlled trial. Enrolled women had a baseline BMD T–score between -2.5 and -4.0 at either the lumbar spine or total hip. Women with other diseases (such as rheumatoid arthritis, osteogenesis imperfecta, and Paget's disease) or on therapies that affect bone were excluded from this study. The 7808 enrolled women were aged 60 to 91 years with a mean age of 72 years. Overall, the mean baseline lumbar spine BMD T-score was -2.8, and 23% of women had a vertebral fracture at baseline. Women were randomized to receive subcutaneous injections of either placebo (N = 3906) or Prolia 60 mg (N = 3902) once every 6 months. All women received at least 1000 mg calcium and 400 IU vitamin D supplementation daily.

The primary efficacy variable was the incidence of new morphometric (radiologically-diagnosed) vertebral fractures at 3 years. Vertebral fractures were diagnosed based on lateral spine radiographs (T4-L4) using a semiquantitative scoring method. Secondary efficacy variables included the incidence of hip fracture and nonvertebral fracture, assessed at 3 years.

Effect on Vertebral Fractures

Prolia significantly reduced the incidence of new morphometric vertebral fractures at 1, 2, and 3 years ($p < 0.0001$), as shown in Table 2. The incidence of new vertebral fractures at year 3 was 7.2% in the placebo-treated women compared to 2.3% for the Prolia-treated women. The absolute risk reduction was 4.8% and relative risk reduction was 68% for new morphometric vertebral fractures at year 3.
[See table 2 above]

Prolia was effective in reducing the risk for new morphometric vertebral fractures regardless of age, baseline rate of bone turnover, baseline BMD, baseline history of fracture, or prior use of a drug for osteoporosis.

Effect on Hip Fractures

The incidence of hip fracture was 1.2% for placebo-treated women compared to 0.7% for Prolia-treated women at year 3. The age-adjusted absolute risk reduction of hip fractures was 0.3% with a relative risk reduction of 40% at 3 years ($p = 0.04$) (Figure 1).
[See figure 1 at top of next column]

Effect on Nonvertebral Fractures

Treatment with Prolia resulted in a significant reduction in the incidence of nonvertebral fractures (Table 3).
[See table 3 above]

Figure 1. Cumulative Incidence of Hip Fractures Over 3 Years

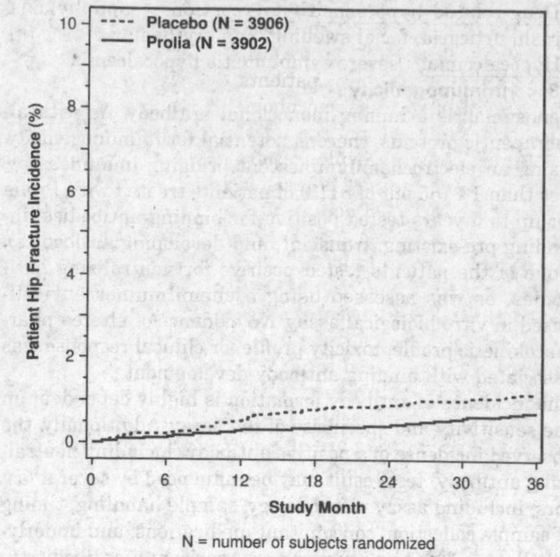

Effect on Bone Mineral Density (BMD)

Treatment with Prolia significantly increased BMD at all anatomic sites measured at 3 years. The treatment differences in BMD at 3 years were 8.8% at the lumbar spine, 6.4% at the total hip, and 5.2% at the femoral neck. Consistent effects on BMD were observed at the lumbar spine, regardless of baseline age, race, weight/body mass index (BMI), baseline BMD, and level of bone turnover.

After Prolia discontinuation, BMD returned to approximately baseline levels within 12 months.

Bone Histology and Histomorphometry

A total of 115 transiliac crest bone biopsy specimens were obtained from 92 postmenopausal women with osteoporosis at either month 24 and/or month 36 (53 specimens in Prolia group, 62 specimens in placebo group). Of the biopsies obtained, 115 (100%) were adequate for qualitative histology and 7 (6%) were adequate for full quantitative histomorphometry assessment.

Qualitative histology assessments showed normal architecture and quality with no evidence of mineralization defects, woven bone, or marrow fibrosis in patients treated with Prolia.

The presence of double tetracycline labeling in a biopsy specimen provides an indication of active bone remodeling, while the absence of tetracycline label suggests suppressed bone formation. In patients treated with Prolia, 35% had no tetracycline label present at the month 24 biopsy and 38% had no tetracycline label present at the month 36 biopsy, while 100% of placebo-treated patients had double label present at both time points. When compared to placebo, treatment with Prolia resulted in virtually absent activation frequency and markedly reduced bone formation rates. However, the long-term consequences of this degree of suppression of bone remodeling are unknown.

14.2 Treatment to Increase Bone Mass in Men with Osteoporosis

The efficacy and safety of Prolia in the treatment to increase bone mass in men with osteoporosis was demonstrated in a 1-year, randomized, double-blind, placebo-controlled trial. Enrolled men had a baseline BMD T-score between -2.0 and -3.5 at the lumbar spine or femoral neck. Men with a BMD T-score between -1.0 and -3.5 at the lumbar spine or femoral neck were also enrolled if there was a history of prior fragility fracture. Men with other diseases (such as rheumatoid arthritis, osteogenesis imperfecta, and Paget's disease) or on therapies that may affect bone were excluded from this study. The 242 men enrolled in the study ranged in age from 31 to 84 years with a mean age of 65 years. Men were randomized to receive SC injections of either placebo (n = 121) or Prolia 60 mg (n = 121) once every 6 months. All men received at least 1000 mg calcium and at least 800 IU vitamin D supplementation daily.

Effect on Bone Mineral Density (BMD)

The primary efficacy variable was percent change in lumbar spine BMD from baseline to 1 year. Secondary efficacy variables included percent change in total hip, and femoral neck BMD from baseline to 1 year.

Treatment with Prolia significantly increased BMD at 1 year. The treatment differences in BMD at 1 year were 4.8% (+0.9% placebo, +5.7% Prolia; (95% CI: 4.0, 5.6); $p < 0.0001$) at the lumbar spine, 2.0% (+0.3% placebo, +2.4% Prolia) at the total hip, and 2.2% (0.0% placebo, +2.1% Prolia) at femoral neck. Consistent effects on BMD were observed at the lumbar spine regardless of baseline age, race, BMD, testosterone concentrations and level of bone turnover.

Bone Histology and Histomorphometry
A total of 29 transiliac crest bone biopsy specimens were obtained from men with osteoporosis at 12 months (17 specimens in Prolia group, 12 specimens in placebo group). Of the biopsies obtained, 29 (100%) were adequate for qualitative histology and, in Prolia patients, 6 (35%) were adequate for full quantitative histomorphometry assessment. Qualitative histology assessments showed normal architecture and quality with no evidence of mineralization defects, woven bone, or marrow fibrosis in patients treated with Prolia. The presence of double tetracycline labeling in a biopsy specimen provides an indication of active bone remodeling, while the absence of tetracycline label suggests suppressed bone formation. In patients treated with Prolia, 6% had no tetracycline label present at the month 12 biopsy, while 100% of placebo-treated patients had double label present. When compared to placebo, treatment with Prolia resulted in markedly reduced bone formation rates. However, the long-term consequences of this degree of suppression of bone remodeling are unknown.

14.3 Treatment of Bone Loss in Men with Prostate Cancer
The efficacy and safety of Prolia in the treatment of bone loss in men with nonmetastatic prostate cancer receiving androgen deprivation therapy (ADT) were demonstrated in a 3–year, randomized (1:1), double-blind, placebo-controlled, multinational study. Men less than 70 years of age had either a BMD T–score at the lumbar spine, total hip, or femoral neck between –1.0 and -4.0, or a history of an osteoporotic fracture. The mean baseline lumbar spine BMD T-score was -0.4, and 22% of men had a vertebral fracture at baseline. The 1468 men enrolled ranged in age from 48 to 97 years (median 76 years). Men were randomized to receive subcutaneous injections of either placebo (n = 734) or Prolia 60 mg (n = 734) once every 6 months for a total of 6 doses. Randomization was stratified by age (< 70 years vs. ≥ 70 years) and duration of ADT at trial entry (≤ 6 months vs. > 6 months). Seventy-nine percent of patients received ADT for more than 6 months at study entry. All men received at least 1000 mg calcium and 400 IU vitamin D supplementation daily.

Effect on Bone Mineral Density (BMD)
The primary efficacy variable was percent change in lumbar spine BMD from baseline to month 24. An additional key secondary efficacy variable was the incidence of new vertebral fracture through month 36 diagnosed based on x-ray evaluation by two independent radiologists. Lumbar spine BMD was higher at 2 years in Prolia-treated patients as compared to placebo-treated patients [-1.0% placebo, +5.6% Prolia; treatment difference 6.7% (95% CI: 6.2, 7.1); $p < 0.0001$].
With approximately 62% of patients followed for 3 years, treatment differences in BMD at 3 years were 7.9% (-1.2% placebo, +6.8% Prolia) at the lumbar spine, 5.7% (-2.6% placebo, +3.2% Prolia) at the total hip, and 4.9% (-1.8% placebo, +3.0% Prolia) at the femoral neck. Consistent effects on BMD were observed at the lumbar spine in relevant subgroups defined by baseline age, BMD, and baseline history of vertebral fracture.

Effect on Vertebral Fractures
Prolia significantly reduced the incidence of new vertebral fractures at 3 years ($p = 0.0125$), as shown in Table 4.
[See table 4 above]

Table 4. The Effect of Prolia on the Incidence of New Vertebral Fractures in Men with Nonmetastatic Prostate Cancer

	Proportion of Men With Fracture (%)*		Absolute Risk Reduction (%)† (95% CI)	Relative Risk Reduction (%)† (95% CI)
	Placebo N = 673 (%)	Prolia N = 679 (%)		
0-1 Year	1.9	0.3	1.6 (0.5, 2.8)	85 (33, 97)
0-2 Years	3.3	1.0	2.2 (0.7, 3.8)	69 (27, 86)
0-3 Years	3.9	1.5	2.4 (0.7, 4.1)	62 (22, 81)

* Event rates based on crude rates in each interval.
† Absolute risk reduction and relative risk reduction based on Mantel-Haenszel method adjusting for age group and ADT duration variables.

14.4 Treatment of Bone Loss in Women with Breast Cancer
The efficacy and safety of Prolia in the treatment of bone loss in women receiving adjuvant aromatase inhibitor (AI) therapy for breast cancer was assessed in a 2–year, randomized (1:1), double-blind, placebo-controlled, multinational study. Women had baseline BMD T-scores between –1.0 to –2.5 at the lumbar spine, total hip, or femoral neck, and had not experienced fracture after age 25. The mean baseline lumbar spine BMD T-score was -1.1, and 2.0% of women had a vertebral fracture at baseline. The 252 women enrolled ranged in age from 35 to 84 years (median 59 years). Women were randomized to receive subcutaneous injections of either placebo (n = 125) or Prolia 60 mg (n = 127) once every 6 months for a total of 4 doses. Randomization was stratified by duration of adjuvant AI therapy at trial entry (≤ 6 months vs. > 6 months). Sixty-two percent of patients received adjuvant AI therapy for more than 6 months at study entry. All women received at least 1000 mg calcium and 400 IU vitamin D supplementation daily.

Effect on Bone Mineral Density (BMD)
The primary efficacy variable was percent change in lumbar spine BMD from baseline to month 12. Lumbar spine BMD was higher at 12 months in Prolia-treated patients as compared to placebo-treated patients [-0.7% placebo, +4.8% Prolia; treatment difference 5.5% (95% CI: 4.8, 6.3); $p < 0.0001$].
With approximately 81% of patients followed for 2 years, treatment differences in BMD at 2 years were 7.6% (-1.4% placebo, +6.2% Prolia) at the lumbar spine, 4.7 % (-1.0% placebo, +3.8% Prolia) at the total hip, and 3.6% (-0.8% placebo, +2.8% Prolia) at the femoral neck.

16 HOW SUPPLIED/STORAGE AND HANDLING
Prolia is supplied in a single-use prefilled syringe with a safety guard or in a single-use vial. The grey needle cap on the single-use prefilled syringe contains dry natural rubber (a derivative of latex).

60 mg/1 mL in a single-use prefilled syringe	1 per carton	NDC 55513-710-01
60 mg/1 mL in a single-use vial	1 per carton	NDC 55513-720-01

Store Prolia in a refrigerator at 2°C to 8°C (36°F to 46°F) in the original carton. Do not freeze. Prior to administration, Prolia may be allowed to reach room temperature (up to 25°C/77°F) in the original container. Once removed from the refrigerator, Prolia must not be exposed to temperatures above 25°C/77°F and must be used within 14 days. If not used within the 14 days, Prolia should be discarded. Do not use Prolia after the expiry date printed on the label.
Protect Prolia from direct light and heat.
Avoid vigorous shaking of Prolia.

17 PATIENT COUNSELING INFORMATION
See FDA-approved patient labeling (Medication Guide).

17.1 Drug Products with Same Active Ingredient
Advise patients that denosumab is also marketed as Xgeva, and if taking Prolia, they should not receive Xgeva *[see Warnings and Precautions (5.1)]*.

17.2 Hypocalcemia
Adequately supplement patients with calcium and vitamin D and instruct them on the importance of maintaining serum calcium levels while receiving Prolia *[see Warnings and Precautions (5.3) and Use in Specific Populations (8.6)]*.
Advise patients to seek prompt medical attention if they develop signs or symptoms of hypocalcemia.

17.3 Serious Infections
Advise patients to seek prompt medical attention if they develop signs or symptoms of infections, including cellulitis *[see Warnings and Precautions (5.4)]*.

17.4 Dermatologic Reactions
Advise patients to seek prompt medical attention if they develop signs or symptoms of dermatological reactions (dermatitis, rashes, and eczema) *[see Warnings and Precautions (5.5)]*.

17.5 Osteonecrosis of the Jaw
Advise patients to maintain good oral hygiene during treatment with Prolia and to inform their dentist prior to dental procedures that they are receiving Prolia. Patients should inform their physician or dentist if they experience persistent pain and/or slow healing of the mouth or jaw after dental surgery *[see Warnings and Precautions (5.6)]*.

17.6 Atypical Subtrochanteric and Diaphyseal Femoral Fractures
Advise patients to report new or unusual thigh, hip, or groin pain *[see Warnings and Precautions (5.7)]*.

17.7 Hypersensitivity
Advise patients to seek prompt medical attention if signs or symptoms of hypersensitivity reactions occur. Advise patients who have had signs or symptoms of systemic hypersensitivity reactions that they should not receive denosumab (Prolia or Xgeva) *[see Warnings & Precautions (5.2), Contraindications (4.3)]*.

17.8 Embryo-Fetal Toxicity
Pregnancy
Advise patients that Prolia is contraindicated in women who are pregnant and may cause fetal harm *[see Contraindications (4.2), Use in Specific Populations (8.1)]*.
Males
Advise patients of a potential for fetal exposure to denosumab when a man treated with Prolia has unprotected sexual intercourse with a pregnant partner *[see Use in Specific Populations (8.8)]*.

17.9 Nursing Mothers
Advise patients that because many drugs are excreted in human milk and because of the potential for serious adverse reactions in nursing infants from Prolia, a decision should be made whether to discontinue nursing or discontinue the drug, taking into account the importance of the drug to the mother *[see Use in Specific Populations (8.3)]*.

17.10 Schedule of Administration
If a dose of Prolia is missed, administer the injection as soon as convenient. Thereafter, schedule injections every 6 months from the date of the last injection.

Manufactured by:
Amgen Manufacturing Limited, a subsidiary of Amgen Inc.
One Amgen Center Drive
Thousand Oaks, California 91320-1799
This product, its production, and/or its use may be covered by one or more U.S. Patents, including U.S. Patent Nos. 6,740,522; 7,097,834; 7,364,736; and 7,411,050, as well as other patents or patents pending.

1xxxxxx - v6
PMV6

MEDICATION GUIDE
Prolia® (PRÓ-lee-a)
(denosumab)
Injection, for subcutaneous use
Read the Medication Guide that comes with Prolia before you start taking it and each time you get a refill. There may be new information. This Medication Guide does not take the place of talking with your doctor about your medical condition or treatment. Talk to your doctor if you have any questions about Prolia.

What is the most important information I should know about Prolia?
If you receive Prolia, you should not receive XGEVA®. Prolia contains the same medicine as Xgeva (denosumab).
Prolia can cause serious side effects including:

- **Low calcium levels in your blood (hypocalcemia).**
  Prolia may lower the calcium levels in your blood. If you have low blood calcium before you start receiving Prolia, it may get worse during treatment. Your low blood calcium must be treated before you receive Prolia. Most people with low blood calcium levels do not have symptoms, but some people may have symptoms. Call your doctor right away if you have symptoms of low blood calcium such as:
  - Spasms, twitches, or cramps in your muscles
  - Numbness or tingling in your fingers, toes, or around your mouth

  Your doctor may prescribe calcium and vitamin D to help prevent low calcium levels in your blood while you take Prolia. Take calcium and vitamin D as your doctor tells you to.
- **Serious allergic reactions.**
  Serious allergic reactions have happened in people who take Prolia. Call your doctor or go to your nearest emergency room right away if you have any symptoms of a serious allergic reactions. Symptoms of a serious allergic reaction may include:
  - low blood pressure (hypotension)
  - trouble breathing
  - throat tightness
  - swelling of your face, lips, or tongue
  - rash
  - itching
  - hives
- **Serious infections.**
  Serious infections in your skin, lower stomach area (abdomen), bladder, or ear may happen if you take Prolia. Inflammation of the inner lining of the heart (endocarditis) due to an infection also may happen more often in people who take Prolia. You may need to go to the hospital for treatment if you develop an infection.
  Prolia is a medicine that may affect your immune system. People who have weakened immune system or take medi-

cines that affect the immune system may have an increased risk for developing serious infections.

Call your doctor right away if you have any of the following symptoms of infection:
- Fever or chills
- Skin that looks red or swollen and is hot or tender to touch
- Severe abdominal pain
- Frequent or urgent need to urinate or burning feeling when you urinate

- **Skin problems.** Skin problems such as inflammation of your skin (dermatitis), rash, and eczema may happen if you take Prolia. Call your doctor if you have any of the following symptoms of skin problems that do not go away or get worse:
  - Redness
  - Itching
  - Small bumps or patches (rash)
  - Your skin is dry or feels like leather
  - Blisters that ooze or become crusty
  - Skin peeling
- **Severe jaw bone problems (osteonecrosis).** Severe jaw bone problems may happen when you take Prolia. Your doctor should examine your mouth before you start Prolia. Your doctor may tell you to see your dentist before you start Prolia. It is important for you to practice good mouth care during treatment with Prolia.
- **Unusual thigh bone fractures.** Some people have developed unusual fractures in their thigh bone. Symptoms of a fracture include new or unusual pain in your hip, groin, or thigh.

Call your doctor right away if you have any of these side effects.

What is Prolia?

Prolia is a prescription medicine used to:
- Treat osteoporosis (thinning and weakening of bone) in women after menopause ("change of life") who:
  - are at high risk for fracture (broken bone)
  - cannot use another osteoporosis medicine or other osteoporosis medicines did not work well
- Increase bone mass in men with osteoporosis who are at high risk for fracture
- Treat bone loss in men who are at high risk for fracture receiving certain treatments for prostate cancer that has not spread to other parts of the body
- Treat bone loss in women who are at high risk for fracture receiving certain treatments for breast cancer that has not spread to other parts of the body

It is not known if Prolia is safe and effective in children.

Who should not take Prolia?

Do not take Prolia if you:
- have been told by your doctor that your blood calcium level is too low.
- are pregnant or plan to become pregnant
- are allergic to denosumab or any of the ingredients in Prolia. See the end of this leaflet for a complete list of ingredients in Prolia.

What should I tell my doctor before taking Prolia?

Before taking Prolia, tell your doctor if you:
- Are taking a medicine called Xgeva (denosumab). Xgeva contains the same medicine as Prolia.
- Have low blood calcium
- Cannot take daily calcium and vitamin D
- Had parathyroid or thyroid surgery (glands located in your neck)
- Have been told you have trouble absorbing minerals in your stomach or intestines (malabsorption syndrome)
- Have kidney problems or are on kidney dialysis
- Plan to have dental surgery or teeth removed.
- Are pregnant or plan to become pregnant. Prolia may harm your unborn baby. Tell your doctor right away if you become pregnant while taking Prolia.
  - **Pregnancy Surveillance Program:** Prolia is not intended for use in pregnant women. If you become pregnant while taking Prolia, talk to your doctor about enrolling in Amgen's Pregnancy Surveillance Program or call 1-800-772-6436 (1-800-77-AMGEN). The purpose of this program is to collect information about women who have become pregnant while taking Prolia.
  - **If you are a man and you receive Prolia:** Small amounts of Prolia may be in semen. If your sexual partner is pregnant, some Prolia from your semen may reach the unborn baby. While the risk is likely to be low, it is important to talk to your doctor if your partner becomes pregnant while you are taking Prolia.
- Are breastfeeding or plan to breastfeed. It is not known if Prolia passes into your breast milk. You and your doctor should decide if you will take Prolia or breastfeed. You should not do both.

Tell your doctor about all the medicines you take, including prescription and nonprescription drugs, vitamins, and herbal supplements.

Know the medicines you take. Keep a list of medicines with you to show to your doctor or pharmacist when you get a new medicine.

How will I receive Prolia?
- Prolia is an injection that will be given to you by a healthcare professional. Prolia is injected under your skin (subcutaneous).
- You will receive Prolia 1 time every 6 months.
- You should take calcium and vitamin D as your doctor tells you to while you receive Prolia.
- If you miss a dose of Prolia, you should receive your injection as soon as you can.
- Take good care of your teeth and gums while you receive Prolia. Brush and floss your teeth regularly.
- Tell your dentist that you are receiving Prolia before you have dental work.

What are the possible side effects of Prolia?

Prolia may cause serious side effects.
- See **"What is the most important information I should know about Prolia?"**
- It is not known if the use of Prolia over a long period of time may cause slow healing of broken bones.

The most common side effects of Prolia in women who are being treated for osteoporosis after menopause are:
- back pain
- pain in your arms and legs
- high cholesterol
- muscle pain
- bladder infection

The most common side effects of Prolia in men with osteoporosis are:
- back pain
- joint pain
- common cold (runny nose or sore throat)

The most common side effects of Prolia in patients receiving certain treatments for prostate or breast cancer are:
- joint pain
- back pain
- pain in your arms and legs
- muscle pain

Tell your doctor if you have any side effect that bothers you or that does not go away.

These are not all the possible side effects of Prolia. For more information, ask your doctor or pharmacist.

Call your doctor for medical advice about side effects. You may report side effects to FDA at 1-800-FDA-1088.

How should I store Prolia if I need to pick it up from a pharmacy?
- Keep Prolia in a refrigerator at 36°F to 46°F (2°C to 8°C) in the original carton.
- Do not freeze Prolia.
- When you remove Prolia from the refrigerator, Prolia must be kept at room temperature [up to 77°F (25°C)] in the original carton and must be used within 14 days.
- Do not keep Prolia at temperatures above 77°F (25°C). Warm temperatures will affect how Prolia works.
- Do not shake Prolia.
- Keep Prolia in the original carton to protect from light.

Keep Prolia and all medicines out of reach of children.

General information about Prolia.

Do not give Prolia to other people even if they have the same symptoms that you have. It may harm them.

This Medication Guide summarizes the most important information about Prolia. If you would like more information, talk with your doctor. You can ask your doctor or pharmacist for information about Prolia that is written for health professionals.

For more information, go to www.Prolia.com or call Amgen at 1-800-772-6436.

What are the ingredients in Prolia?

Active ingredient: denosumab

Inactive ingredients: sorbitol, acetate, polysorbate 20 (prefilled syringe only), Water for Injection (USP), and sodium hydroxide

Amgen Manufacturing Limited, a subsidiary of Amgen Inc.
One Amgen Center Drive
Thousand Oaks, California 91320-1799

This Medication Guide has been approved by the U.S. Food and Drug Administration.

1xxxxxx - v6
Revised: 07/2013
PMV6

Shown in Product Identification Guide, page 305

Bayer HealthCare LLC

100 Bayer Boulevard
Whippany, NJ 07981

Direct Inquiries to:
Phone: 1-888-84-BAYER
(1-888-842-2937)
http//www.bayerhealthcare.com

For Medical Information contact:
Vice President, Medical Communications
1-888-84-Bayer (1-888-842-2937)

DESONATE® ℞

[de-son-ate]
(desonide) Gel 0.05%
for topical use only

HIGHLIGHTS OF PRESCRIBING INFORMATION

These highlights do not include all the information needed to use DESONATE® Gel safely and effectively. See full prescribing information for DESONATE® Gel.
DESONATE® (desonide) Gel 0.05% for topical use only
Initial U.S. Approval: 1972

INDICATIONS AND USAGE

Desonate® is a corticosteroid indicated for the topical treatment of mild to moderate atopic dermatitis in patients 3 months of age and older. (1)

DOSAGE AND ADMINISTRATION

- Apply as a thin layer to the affected areas two times daily and rub in gently. (2)
- Therapy should be discontinued when control is achieved. (2)
- If no improvement is seen within 4 weeks, reassessment of diagnosis may be necessary. (2)
- Should not be used with occlusive dressings. (2)
- Treatment beyond 4 consecutive weeks is not recommended. (2)
- For topical use only. Not for oral, ophthalmic, or intravaginal use. (2)

DOSAGE FORMS AND STRENGTHS

Gel, 0.05%; (0.5mg/g) desonide in a translucent to opaque gel (3)

CONTRAINDICATIONS

History of hypersensitivity to any of the components of the preparation. (4)

WARNINGS AND PRECAUTIONS

- Topical corticosteroids can produce reversible hypothalamic pituitary adrenal (HPA) axis suppression, Cushing's syndrome and unmask latent diabetes. (5.1)
- Systemic absorption may require evaluation for HPA axis suppression (5.1).
- Modify use should HPA axis suppression develop (5.1)
- Potent corticosteroids, use on large areas, prolonged use or occlusive use may increase systemic absorption (5.1)
- Local adverse reactions may include atrophy, striae, irritation, acneiform eruptions, hypopigmentation, and allergic contact dermatitis and may be more likely with occlusive use or more potent corticosteroids. (5.2, 5.4, 6)
- Children may be more susceptible to systemic toxicity when treated with topical corticosteroids. (5.1, 8.4)

ADVERSE REACTIONS

The most common adverse reactions (incidence ≥ 1%) are headache and application site burning. (6)

To report SUSPECTED ADVERSE REACTIONS, contact Bayer HealthCare Pharmaceuticals Inc. at 1-888-842-2937 or FDA at 1-800-FDA-1088 or www.fda.gov/medwatch

USE IN SPECIFIC POPULATIONS

Safety and effectiveness of Desonate in pediatric patients less than 3 months of age have not been evaluated, and therefore its use in this age group is not recommended. (8.4)

See 17 for PATIENT COUNSELING INFORMATION

Revised: 05/2012

FULL PRESCRIBING INFORMATION: CONTENTS*

*** Sections or subsections omitted from the full prescribing information are not listed**

FULL PRESCRIBING INFORMATION

1 INDICATIONS AND USAGE

Desonate® is indicated for the treatment of mild to moderate atopic dermatitis in patients 3 months of age and older. Patients should be instructed to use Desonate for the minimum amount of time as necessary to achieve the desired results because of the potential for Desonate to suppress the hypothalamic-pituitary-adrenal (HPA) axis *[see Warnings and Precautions (5.1)]*. Treatment should not exceed 4 consecutive weeks *[see Dosage and Administration (2)]*.

2 DOSAGE AND ADMINISTRATION

Apply a thin layer to the affected areas two times daily and rub in gently. Discontinue use when control is achieved. If no improvement is seen within 4 weeks, reassessment of diagnosis may be necessary. Treatment beyond 4 consecutive weeks is not recommended. Do not use with occlusive dressings. Avoid contact with eyes or other mucous membranes. For topical use only. Not for oral, ophthalmic, or intravaginal use.

3 DOSAGE FORMS AND STRENGTHS

Gel, 0.05%; (0.5mg/g) desonide in a translucent to opaque gel

4 CONTRAINDICATIONS

Desonate is contraindicated in those patients with a history of hypersensitivity to any of the components of the preparation.

5 WARNINGS AND PRECAUTIONS

5.1 Effects on Endocrine System

Systemic absorption of topical corticosteroids can produce reversible hypothalamic-pituitary-adrenal (HPA) axis suppression with the potential for clinical glucocorticosteroid insufficiency. This may occur during treatment or upon withdrawal of the topical corticosteroid.

The effect of Desonate on HPA axis function was investigated in pediatric subjects, 6 months to 6 years old, with atopic dermatitis covering at least 35% of their body, who were treated with Desonate twice daily for 4 weeks. One of 37 subjects (3%) displayed adrenal suppression after 4 weeks of use, based on the cosyntropin stimulation test. As follow-up evaluation of the subject's adrenal axis was not performed, it is unknown whether the suppression was reversible *[see Use In Specific Populations (8.4) and Clinical Pharmacology (12.2)]*.

Pediatric patients may be more susceptible than adults to systemic toxicity from equivalent doses of Desonate due to their larger skin surface-to-body mass ratios *[see Use In Specific Populations (8.4)]*.

Because of the potential for systemic absorption, use of topical corticosteroids may require that patients be periodically evaluated for HPA axis suppression. Factors that predispose a patient using a topical corticosteroid to HPA axis suppression include the use of more potent steroids, use over large surface areas, use over prolonged periods, use under occlusion, use on an altered skin barrier, and use in patients with liver failure.

An ACTH stimulation test may be helpful in evaluating patients for HPA axis suppression. If HPA axis suppression is documented, an attempt should be made to gradually withdraw the drug, to reduce the frequency of application, or to substitute a less potent steroid. Manifestations of adrenal insufficiency may require supplemental systemic corticosteroids. Recovery of HPA axis function is generally prompt and complete upon discontinuation of topical corticosteroids.

Cushing's syndrome, hyperglycemia, and unmasking of latent diabetes mellitus can also result from systemic absorption of topical corticosteroids.

Use of more than one corticosteroid-containing product at the same time may increase the total systemic corticosteroid exposure.

5.2 Local Adverse Reactions with Topical Corticosteroids

Local adverse reactions may be more likely to occur with occlusive use, prolonged use or use of higher potency corticosteroids. Reactions may include skin atrophy, striae, telangiectasias, burning, itching, irritation, dryness, folliculitis, acneiform eruptions, hypopigmentation, perioral dermatitis, allergic contact dermatitis, secondary infection, and miliaria. Some local adverse reactions may be irreversible.

5.3 Concomitant Skin Infections

If concomitant skin infections are present or develop during treatment, an appropriate antifungal or antibacterial agent should be used. If a favorable response does not occur promptly, use of Desonate should be discontinued until the infection is adequately controlled.

5.4 Skin Irritation

If irritation develops, Desonate should be discontinued and appropriate therapy instituted. Allergic contact dermatitis with corticosteroids is usually diagnosed by observing failure to heal rather than noting a clinical exacerbation as with most topical products not containing corticosteroids. Such an observation should be corroborated with appropriate diagnostic patch testing.

6 ADVERSE REACTIONS

Because clinical trials are conducted under widely varying conditions, adverse reaction rates observed in the clinical trials of a drug cannot be directly compared to rates in the clinical trials of another drug and may not reflect the rates observed in practice.

In controlled clinical studies of 425 Desonate treated subjects and 157 Vehicle-treated subjects, adverse events occurred at the application site in 3% of subjects treated with Desonate and the incidence rate was not higher compared with vehicle-treated subjects. The most common local adverse events in Desonate treated subjects were application site burning in 1% (4/425) and rash in 1% (3/425) followed by application site pruritus in <1% (2/425).

Adverse events that resulted in premature discontinuation of study drug in Desonate treated subjects were telangiectasia and worsening of atopic dermatitis in one subject each. Additional adverse events observed during clinical trials for patients treated with Desonate included headache in 2% (8/425) compared with 1% (2/157) in those treated with vehicle.

The following additional local adverse reactions have been reported infrequently with topical corticosteroids. They may occur more frequently with the use of occlusive dressings, especially with higher potency corticosteroids. These reactions are listed in an approximate decreasing order of occurrence: folliculitis, acneiform eruptions, hypopigmentation, perioral dermatitis, secondary infection, skin atrophy, striae, and miliaria.

8 USE IN SPECIFIC POPULATIONS

8.1 Pregnancy

Teratogenic effects: Pregnancy Category C:

There are no adequate and well-controlled studies in pregnant women. Therefore, Desonate should be used during pregnancy only if the potential benefit justifies the potential risk to the fetus.

Corticosteroids have been shown to be teratogenic in laboratory animals when administered systemically at relatively low dosage levels. Some corticosteroids have been shown to be teratogenic after dermal application in laboratory animals.

No reproductive studies in animals have been performed with Desonate. Dermal embryofetal development studies were conducted in rats and rabbits with a desonide cream, 0.05% formulation. Topical doses of 0.2, 0.6, and 2.0 g cream/kg/day of a desonide cream, 0.05% formulation or 2.0 g/kg of the cream base were administered topically to pregnant rats (gestational days 6-15) and pregnant rabbits (gestational days 6-18). Maternal body weight loss was noted at all dose levels of the desonide cream, 0.05% formulation in rats and rabbits. Teratogenic effects characteristic of corticosteroids were noted in both species. The desonide cream, 0.05% formulation was teratogenic in rats at topical doses of 0.6 and 2.0 g cream/kg/day and in rabbits at a topical dose of 2.0 g cream/kg/day. No teratogenic effects were noted for the desonide cream, 0.05% formulation at a topical dose of 0.2 g cream/kg/day in rats and 0.6 g cream/kg/day in rabbits. These doses (0.2 g cream/kg/day and 0.6 g cream/kg/day) are similar to the maximum recommended human dose based on body surface area comparisons.

8.3 Nursing Mothers

Systemically administered corticosteroids appear in human milk and could suppress growth, interfere with endogenous corticosteroid production, or cause other untoward effects. It is not known whether topical administration of corticosteroids could result in sufficient systemic absorption to produce detectable quantities in human milk. Because many drugs are excreted in human milk, caution should be exercised when Desonate is administered to a nursing woman.

8.4 Pediatric Use

Safety and effectiveness of Desonate in pediatric patients less than 3 months of age have not been evaluated, and therefore its use in this age group is not recommended.

The effect of Desonate on HPA axis function was investigated in pediatric subjects, with atopic dermatitis covering at least 35% of their body, who were treated with Desonate twice daily for 4 weeks. One of 37 subjects (3%) displayed adrenal suppression after 4 weeks of use, based on the cosyntropin stimulation test *[see Warnings and Precautions (5.1)]*.

In controlled clinical studies in subjects 3 months to 18 years of age, 425 subjects were treated with Desonate and 157 subjects were treated with vehicle *[see Adverse Reactions (6) and Clinical Studies (14)]*.

Because of a higher ratio of skin surface area to body mass, pediatric patients are at a greater risk than adults of HPA axis suppression when they are treated with topical corticosteroids. They are therefore also at greater risk of glucocorticosteroid insufficiency after withdrawal of treatment and of Cushing's syndrome while on treatment.

Adverse effects, including striae, have been reported with inappropriate use of topical corticosteroids in infants and children. HPA axis suppression, Cushing's syndrome, linear growth retardation, delayed weight gain and intracranial hypertension have been reported in children receiving topical corticosteroids. Manifestations of adrenal suppression in children include low plasma cortisol levels and absence of response to ACTH stimulation. Manifestations of intracranial hypertension include bulging fontanelles, headaches, and bilateral papilledema.

8.5 Geriatric Use

Clinical studies of Desonate did not include patients aged 65 and older to determine if they respond differently than younger patients. Treatment of this patient population should reflect the greater frequency of decreased hepatic, renal, or cardiac function, and of concomitant disease or other drug therapy.

10 OVERDOSAGE

Topically applied Desonate can be absorbed in sufficient amounts to produce systemic effects *[see Warnings and Precautions (5.1)]*.

11 DESCRIPTION

Desonate contains desonide [(pregna-1, 4-diene-3, 20-dione, 11, 21-dihydroxy-16, 17-[(1-methylethylidene) bis(oxy)]-, (11β,16α)]- a synthetic nonfluorinated corticosteroid for topical dermatologic use. Chemically, desonide is $C_{24}H_{32}O_6$. It has the following structural formula:

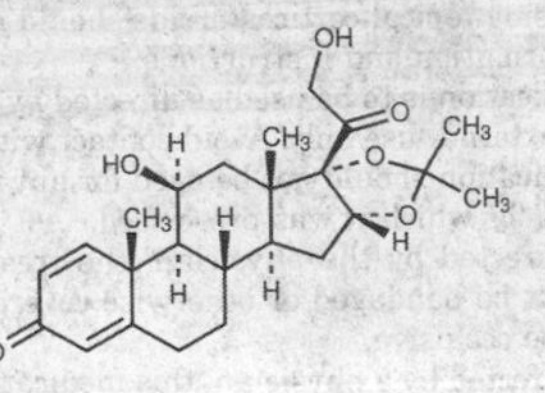

Desonide has the molecular weight of 416.52. It is a white to off-white odorless powder which is soluble in methanol and practically insoluble in water. Each gram of Desonate contains 0.5 mg of desonide in an aqueous gel base of purified water, glycerin, propylene glycol, edetate disodium dihydrate, methylparaben, propylparaben, sodium hydroxide, and Carbopol® 981.

12 CLINICAL PHARMACOLOGY

12.1 Mechanism of Action

The mechanism of action of desonide is unknown.

12.2 Pharmacodynamics

In an HPA axis suppression study, one of 37 (3%) pediatric subjects, 6 months to 6 years old, with moderate to severe atopic dermatitis covering at least 35% body surface area who applied Desonate experienced suppression of the adrenal glands following 4 weeks of therapy *[see Warnings And Precautions (5.1) and Use In Specific Populations (8.4)]*. A follow-up evaluation of the subject's adrenal axis was not performed, it is unknown whether the suppression was reversible.

12.3 Pharmacokinetics

The extent of percutaneous absorption of topical corticosteroids is determined by many factors, including product formulation and the integrity of the epidermal barrier. Occlusion, inflammation and/or other disease processes in the skin may also increase percutaneous absorption. Once absorbed through the skin, topical corticosteroids are handled through pharmacokinetic pathways similar to systemically administered corticosteroids. They are metabolized primarily in the liver and then are excreted by the kidneys. Some corticosteroids and their metabolites are also excreted in the bile.

13 NONCLINICAL TOXICOLOGY

13.1 Carcinogenesis, Mutagenesis, Impairment of Fertility

Long-term animal studies have not been performed to evaluate the carcinogenic or photoco-carcinogenic potential of Desonate or the effect of desonide on fertility. Desonide revealed no evidence of mutagenic potential based on the results of an *in vitro* genotoxicity test (Ames assay) and an *in vivo* genotoxicity test (mouse micronucleus assay). Desonide was positive without S9 activation and was equivocal with S9 activation in an in vitro mammalian cell mutagenesis assay (L5178YITK+ mouse lymphoma assay). A dose response trend was not noted in this assay.

14 CLINICAL STUDIES

In two randomized vehicle-controlled clinical studies, subjects 3 months to 18 years of age with mild to moderate atopic dermatitis were treated twice daily for 4 weeks with either Desonate or vehicle. Treatment success was defined as achieving clear or almost clear on the Investigator's Global Severity Score (IGSS) with at least a 2-point change (decrease) from the subject's baseline IGSS when compared to the Week 4 IGSS. The results of the 2 clinical trials are summarized in Table 1:

Table 1: Subjects Achieving Treatment Success

Clinical Trial 1	
Desonate N = 289	Vehicle N = 92
128 (44%)	13 (14%)
Clinical Trial 2	
Desonate N = 136	Vehicle N = 65
38 (28%)	4 (6%)

16 HOW SUPPLIED/STORAGE AND HANDLING

Desonate is a translucent to opaque gel supplied in 60g tubes in cartons containing 1× 60g tube (NDC 50419-828-06), or a 2 × 60g tube Twin Pack (NDC 50419-828-12).

Storage:

Store at 25°C (77°F); excursions permitted to15-30°C (59-86°F). *[See USP Controlled Room Temperature].*

Keep out of reach of children.

17 PATIENT COUNSELING INFORMATION

Patients using topical corticosteroids should receive the following information and instructions:

- This medication is to be used as directed by the physician. It is for external use only. Avoid contact with the eyes.
- This medication should not be used for any disorder other than that for which it was prescribed.
- Unless directed by the physician, the treated skin area should not be bandaged or otherwise covered or wrapped so as to be occlusive.
- Unless directed by a physician, this medication should not be used on the underarm or groin areas of pediatric patients.
- Parents of pediatric patients should be advised not to use Desonate in the treatment of diaper dermatitis. Desonate should not be applied in the diaper area, as diapers or plastic pants may constitute occlusive dressing *[see Dosage and Administration (2)].*
- Patients should report to their physician any signs of local adverse reactions.
- Other corticosteroid-containing products should not be used with Desonate without first consulting with the physician.
- As with other corticosteroids, therapy should be discontinued when control is achieved. If no improvement is seen within 4 weeks, contact the physician.

Manufactured for:
Bayer HealthCare Pharmaceuticals Inc.
Wayne, NJ 07470
Manufactured in Canada
6706905

Shown in Product Identification Guide, page 305

FINACEA®

[fī′nā-shē-ə] ℞

(azelaic acid) Gel, 15%
for topical use

HIGHLIGHTS OF PRESCRIBING INFORMATION

These highlights do not include all the information needed to use FINACEA® Gel safely and effectively. See full prescribing information for FINACEA Gel.

FINACEA (azelaic acid) Gel, 15% for topical use
Initial U.S. Approval: 1995

INDICATIONS AND USAGE

FINACEA Gel is indicated for the topical treatment of inflammatory papules and pustules of mild to moderate rosacea. Efficacy for treatment of erythema in rosacea in the absence of papules and pustules has not been evaluated. (1)

DOSAGE AND ADMINISTRATION

- Not for oral, ophthalmic or intravaginal use. (2)
- Apply a thin layer of FINACEA Gel twice daily to affected area(s). (2)
- Use only very mild soaps or soapless cleansing lotion before applying FINACEA Gel. (2)
- Cosmetics may be applied after the application of FINACEA Gel has dried. (2)
- Avoid spicy foods, thermally hot foods and drinks, alcoholic beverages. (2)

DOSAGE FORMS AND STRENGTHS

Gel, 15% (3)

CONTRAINDICATIONS

None (4)

WARNINGS AND PRECAUTIONS

- Skin irritation (i.e. pruritus, burning or stinging) may occur, usually during the first few weeks of treatment with FINACEA Gel. If sensitivity or severe irritation develops and persists, discontinue treatment and institute appropriate therapy. (5.1)
- There have been isolated reports of hypopigmentation after the use of azelaic acid. Since azelaic acid has not been well-studied in patients with dark complexion, monitor these patients for early signs of hypopigmentation (5.1)
- FINACEA Gel has been reported to cause irritation of the eyes. Therefore, avoid contact with the eyes and mucous membranes. (5.2)

ADVERSE REACTIONS

The most common adverse reactions are burning/stinging/tingling (29%), pruritus (11%), scaling/dry skin/xerosis (8%) and erythema/irritation (4%). (6)

To report SUSPECTED ADVERSE REACTIONS, contact Bayer HealthCare at 1-866-463-3634 or FDA at 1-800-FDA-1088 or www.fda.gov/medwatch

See 17 for PATIENT COUNSELING INFORMATION

Revised: 12/2012

FULL PRESCRIBING INFORMATION: CONTENTS*

*** Sections or subsections omitted from the full prescribing information are not listed**

FULL PRESCRIBING INFORMATION

1 INDICATIONS AND USAGE

FINACEA® Gel is indicated for topical treatment of the inflammatory papules and pustules of mild to moderate rosacea. Although some reduction of erythema which was present in patients with papules and pustules of rosacea occurred in clinical studies, efficacy for treatment of erythema in rosacea in the absence of papules and pustules has not been evaluated.

2 DOSAGE AND ADMINISTRATION

- Apply and gently massage a thin layer of FINACEA Gel into the affected areas on the face twice daily (morning and evening).
- Use only very mild soaps or soapless cleansing lotion before application of FINACEA Gel.
- Cosmetics may be applied after the application of FINACEA Gel has dried.
- Avoid the use of occlusive dressings or wrappings.
- Not for oral, ophthalmic or intravaginal use.
- Patients should be reassessed if no improvement is observed upon completing 12 weeks of therapy.
- Instruct patients to avoid spicy foods, thermally hot foods and drinks, alcoholic beverages.

3 DOSAGE FORMS AND STRENGTHS

FINACEA Gel is a clear, colorless aqueous gel. Each gram of FINACEA Gel contains 0.15 gm of azelaic acid (15% w/w).

4 CONTRAINDICATIONS

None

5 WARNINGS AND PRECAUTIONS

5.1 Skin Reactions

Skin irritation (i.e. pruritus, burning or stinging) may occur during use of FINACEA Gel, usually during the first few weeks of treatment. If sensitivity or severe irritation develops and persists, discontinue treatment and institute appropriate therapy.

There have been isolated reports of hypopigmentation after use of azelaic acid. Since azelaic acid has not been well studied in patients with dark complexion, monitor these patients for early signs of hypopigmentation.

5.2 Eye and Mucous Membrane Irritation

Avoid contact with the eyes, mouth and other mucous membranes. If FINACEA Gel does come in contact with the eyes, wash the eyes with large amounts of water and consult a physician if eye irritation persists *[see Adverse Reactions (6.2)].*

6 ADVERSE REACTIONS

6.1 Clinical Trials Experience

Because clinical trials are conducted under widely varying conditions, adverse reaction rates observed in the clinical trials of a drug cannot be directly compared to rates in the clinical trials of another drug and may not reflect the rates observed in practice.

In two vehicle-controlled and one active-controlled U.S. clinical trials, treatment safety was monitored in 788 subjects who used twice-daily FINACEA Gel for 12 weeks (N=333) or 15 weeks (N=124), or the gel vehicle (N=331) for 12 weeks. In all three trials, the most common treatment-related adverse events were: burning/stinging/tingling (29%), pruritus (11%), scaling/dry skin/xerosis (8%) and erythema/irritation (4%). In the active-controlled trial, overall adverse reactions (including burning, stinging/tingling, dryness/tightness/scaling, itching, and erythema/irritation/redness) were 19.4% (24/124) for FINACEA Gel compared to 7.1% (9/127) for the active comparator gel at 15 weeks.

[See table 1 at top of next page]

In patients using azelaic acid formulations, the following adverse events have been reported: worsening of asthma, vitiligo, depigmentation, small depigmented spots, hypertrichosis, reddening (signs of keratosis pilaris) and exacerbation of recurrent herpes labialis.

Local Tolerability Studies

FINACEA Gel and its vehicle caused irritant reactions at the application site in human dermal safety studies. FINACEA Gel caused significantly more irritation than its vehicle in a cumulative irritation study. Some improvement in irritation was demonstrated over the course of the clinical trials, but this improvement might be attributed to subject dropouts. No phototoxicity or photoallergenicity were reported in human dermal safety studies.

6.2 Post-Marketing Experience

The following adverse reactions have been identified post approval of FINACEA Gel. Because these reactions are reported voluntarily from a population of uncertain size, it is not always possible to reliably estimate the frequency or establish a causal relationship to drug exposure:

Eyes: iridocyclitis upon accidental exposure of the eyes to FINACEA Gel

7 DRUG INTERACTIONS

There have been no formal studies of the interaction of FINACEA Gel with other drugs.

8 USE IN SPECIFIC POPULATIONS

8.1 Pregnancy

Teratogenic Effects: Pregnancy Category B

There are no adequate and well-controlled studies in pregnant women. Therefore, FINACEA Gel should be used during pregnancy only if the potential benefit justifies the potential risk to the fetus.

Dermal embryofetal developmental toxicology studies have not been performed with azelaic acid, 15% gel. Oral embryofetal developmental studies were conducted with azelaic acid in rats, rabbits, and cynomolgus monkeys. Azelaic acid was administered during the period of organogenesis in all three animal species. Embryotoxicity was observed in rats, rabbits, and monkeys at oral doses of azelaic acid that generated some maternal toxicity. Embryotoxicity was observed in rats given 2500 mg/kg/day [162 times the maximum recommended human dose (MRHD) based on body surface area (BSA)], rabbits given 150 or 500 mg/kg/day (19 or 65 times the MRHD based on BSA) and cynomolgus monkeys given 500 mg/kg/day (65 times the MRHD based on BSA) azelaic acid. No teratogenic effects were observed in the oral embryofetal developmental studies conducted in rats, rabbits and cynomolgus monkeys.

An oral peri- and post-natal developmental study was conducted in rats. Azelaic acid was administered from gestational day 15 through day 21 postpartum up to a dose level of 2500 mg/kg/day. Embryotoxicity was observed in rats at an oral dose of 2500 mg/kg/day (162 times the MRHD based on BSA) that generated some maternal toxicity. In addition, slight disturbances in the post-natal development of fetuses was noted in rats at oral doses that generated some maternal toxicity (500 and 2500 mg/kg/day; 32 and 162 times the MRHD based on BSA). No effects on sexual maturation of the fetuses were noted in this study.

8.3 Nursing Mothers

It is not known whether azelaic acid is excreted in human milk; however, *in vitro* studies using equilibrium dialysis were conducted to assess the potential for human milk partitioning. The studies demonstrated that, at an azelaic acid concentration of 25 µg/mL, the milk/plasma distribution coefficient was 0.7 and the milk/buffer distribution was 1.0. These data indicate that passage of drug into maternal milk may occur. Since less than 4% of a topically applied dose of 20% azelaic acid cream is systemically absorbed, the uptake of azelaic acid into maternal milk is not expected to cause a significant change from baseline azelaic acid levels in the milk. Nevertheless, a decision should be made to discontinue nursing or to discontinue the drug, taking into account the importance of the drug to the mother.

8.4 Pediatric Use

Safety and effectiveness of FINACEA Gel in pediatric patients have not been established.

8.5 Geriatric Use

Clinical studies of FINACEA Gel did not include sufficient numbers of subjects aged 65 and over to determine whether they respond differently from younger subjects.

10 OVERDOSAGE

There are no reported human experiences with overdosage of FINACEA Gel.

11 DESCRIPTION

FINACEA (azelaic acid) Gel, 15%, is an aqueous gel which contains azelaic acid, a naturally-occurring saturated dicarboxylic acid. Chemically, azelaic acid is 1,7-heptanedicarboxylic acid. The molecular formula for azelaic acid is $C_9H_{16}O_4$. It has the following structure:

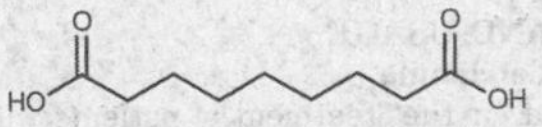

$[HOOC-(CH_2)_7-COOH]$

Azelaic acid has a molecular weight of 188.22. It is a white, odorless crystalline solid. It is poorly soluble in water at 20°C (0.24%) but freely soluble in boiling water and in ethanol.

FINACEA Gel is a clear, colorless aqueous gel for topical use; each gram contains 0.15 gm azelaic acid (15%w/w) in an aqueous gel base containing benzoic acid (as a preservative), disodium EDTA, lecithin, medium-chain triglycerides, polyacrylic acid, polysorbate 80, propylene glycol, purified water, and sodium hydroxide to adjust pH.

12 CLINICAL PHARMACOLOGY

12.1 Mechanism of Action

The mechanism(s) by which azelaic acid interferes with the pathogenic events in rosacea are unknown.

12.2 Pharmacodynamics

The pharmacodynamics of azelaic acid in association with the treatment of rosacea are unknown.

12.3 Pharmacokinetics

The percutaneous absorption of azelaic acid after topical application of FINACEA Gel could not be reliably determined. Mean plasma azelaic acid concentrations in rosacea subjects treated with FINACEA Gel twice daily for at least 8 weeks are in the range of 42 to 63.1 ng/mL. These values are within the maximum concentration range of 24.0 to 90.5 ng/mL observed in rosacea subjects treated with vehicle only. This indicates that FINACEA Gel does not increase plasma azelaic acid concentration beyond the range derived from nutrition and endogenous metabolism.

In vitro and human data suggest negligible cutaneous metabolism of ^{3}H-azelaic acid after topical application of 20% azelaic acid cream. Azelaic acid is mainly excreted unchanged in the urine, but undergoes some ß oxidation to shorter chain dicarboxylic acids.

Table 1: Adverse Events Occurring in ≥1% of Subjects in the Rosacea Trials by Treatment Group and Maximum Intensity*

	FINACEA Gel, 15% N=457 (100%)			Vehicle N=331 (100%)		
	Mild n=99 (22%)	Moderate n=61 (13%)	Severe n=27 (6%)	Mild n=46 (14%)	Moderate n=30 (9%)	Severe n=5 (2%)
Burning/stinging/tingling	71 (16%)	42 (9%)	17 (4%)	8 (2%)	6 (2%)	2 (1%)
Pruritus	29 (6%)	18 (4%)	5 (1%)	9 (3%)	6 (2%)	0 (0%)
Scaling/dry skin/xerosis	21 (5%)	10 (2%)	5 (1%)	31 (9%)	14 (4%)	1 (<1%)
Erythema/irritation	6 (1%)	7 (2%)	2 (<1%)	8 (2%)	4 (1%)	2 (1%)
Contact dermatitis	2 (<1%)	3 (1%)	0 (0%)	1 (<1%)	0 (0%)	0 (0%)
Edema	3 (1%)	2 (<1%)	0 (0%)	3 (1%)	0 (0%)	0 (0%)
Acne	3 (1%)	1 (<1%)	0 (0%)	1 (<1%)	0 (0%)	0 (0%)

* Subjects may have >1 cutaneous adverse event; thus, the sum of the frequencies of preferred terms may exceed the number of subjects with at least 1 cutaneous adverse event.

Table 2: Inflammatory Papules and Pustules (ITT population)*

	Study One FINACEA Gel,15% N = 164	Study One VEHICLE N = 165	Study Two FINACEA Gel, 15% N = 167	Study Two VEHICLE N = 166
Mean Lesion Count Baseline	17.5	17.6	17.9	18.5
End of Treatment[1]	6.8	10.5	9.0	12.1
Mean Percent Reduction End of Treatment[1]	57.9%	39.9%	50.0%	38.2%

** ITT population with last observation carried forward (LOCF)*

13 NONCLINICAL TOXICOLOGY

13.1 Carcinogenesis, Mutagenesis, Impairment of Fertility

Systemic long-term animal studies have not been performed to evaluate the carcinogenic potential of azelaic acid. In a 26-week dermal carcinogenicity study using transgenic (Tg.AC) mice, FINACEA Gel and the gel vehicle, when applied once or twice daily, did not increase the number of female Tg.AC animals with papillomas at the treatment site. No statistically significant increase in the number of animals with papillomas at the treatment site was observed in male Tg.AC animals after once daily application. After twice daily application, FINACEA Gel and the gel vehicle induced a statistically significant increase in the number of male animals with papillomas at the treatment site when compared to untreated males. This suggests that the positive effect may be associated with the vehicle application. The clinical relevance of the findings in animals to humans is not clear.

Azelaic acid was not mutagenic or clastogenic in a battery of *in vitro* [Ames assay, HGPRT in V79 cells (Chinese hamster lung cells), and chromosomal aberration assay in human lymphocytes] and *in vivo* (dominant lethal assay in mice and mouse micronucleus assay) genotoxicity tests.

Oral administration of azelaic acid at dose levels up to 2500 mg/kg/day (162 times the MRHD based on BSA) did not affect fertility or reproductive performance in male or female rats.

14 CLINICAL STUDIES

FINACEA Gel was evaluated for the treatment of mild to moderate papulopustular rosacea in two multicenter, randomized, double-blind, vehicle-controlled, 12-week clinical trials having identical protocols and involving a total of 664 (active: 333; vehicle: 331) subjects aged 21 to 86 years (mean age = 49). Overall, 92.5% of subjects were Caucasian and 73% of subjects were female. Enrolled subjects had mild to moderate rosacea with a mean lesion count of 18 (range 8 to 60) inflammatory papules and pustules. The following subjects were excluded: a) those without papules and pustules; b) those with nodules, rhinophyma, or ocular involvement and c) those with a history of hypersensitivity to propylene glycol or to any other ingredients of the study drug. FINACEA Gel or its vehicle were to be applied twice daily for 12 weeks; no other topical or systemic medication affecting the course of rosacea and/or evaluability was to be used during the studies. Subjects were instructed to avoid spicy foods, thermally hot food/drink and alcoholic beverages during the study. Subjects were also instructed to use only very mild soaps or soapless cleansing lotion for facial cleansing.

The primary efficacy endpoints included both 1) change from baseline in inflammatory lesion counts as well as 2) success defined as a score of "clear" or "minimal" with at least a 2-step reduction from baseline on the Investigator's Global Assessment (IGA), defined as follows below:

CLEAR:
No papules and/or pustules; no or residual erythema; no or mild to moderate telangiectasia

MINIMAL:
Rare papules and/or pustules; residual to mild erythema; mild to moderate telangiectasia

MILD:
Few papules and/or pustules; mild erythema; mild to moderate telangiectasia

MILD TO MODERATE:
Distinct number of papules and/or pustules; mild to moderate erythema; mild to moderate telangiectasia

MODERATE:
Pronounced number of papules and/or pustules; moderate erythema; mild to moderate telangiectasia

MODERATE TO SEVERE:
Many papules and/or pustules, occasionally with large inflamed lesions; moderate erythema; moderate degree of telangiectasia

SEVERE:
Numerous papules and/or pustules, occasionally with confluent areas of inflamed lesions; moderate or severe erythema; moderate or severe telangiectasia

Primary efficacy assessment was based on the "intent-to-treat" (ITT) population with the "last observation carried forward" (LOCF).

Both trials demonstrated a statistically significant difference in favor of FINACEA Gel over its vehicle in both reducing the number of inflammatory papules and pustules associated with rosacea (Table 2) as well as demonstrating success on the IGA in the ITT-LOCF population at the end of treatment.

[See table 2 above]

Although some reduction of erythema which was present in subjects with papules and pustules of rosacea occurred in clinical trials, efficacy for treatment of erythema in rosacea in the absence of papules and pustules has not been evaluated.

FINACEA Gel was superior to the vehicle with regard to success based on the IGA of rosacea on a 7-point static score at the end of treatment (ITT population; Table 3).

Table 3: Investigator's Global Assessment at the End of Treatment*

	Study One FINACEA Gel, 15% N = 164	Study One VEHICLE N = 165	Study Two FINACEA Gel, 15% N = 167	Study Two VEHICLE N = 166
Clear, Minimal or Mild at End of Treatment (% of Subjects)	61%	40%	61%	48%

*ITT population with last observation carried forward (LOCF)

[See table 3 above]

16 HOW SUPPLIED/STORAGE AND HANDLING

How Supplied

FINACEA Gel, a clear, colorless aqueous gel, is supplied in 50 g tubes (NDC 50419-825-02).

Storage and Handling

Store at 25°C (77°F); excursions permitted between 15–30°C (59–86°F) *[See USP Controlled Room Temperature]*.

17 PATIENT COUNSELING INFORMATION

Inform patients using FINACEA Gel, 15% of the following information and instructions:

Use only as directed by your physician.

- For external use only.
- Before applying FINACEA Gel, cleanse affected area(s) with a very mild soap or a soapless cleansing lotion and pat dry with a soft towel.
- Avoid use of alcoholic cleansers, tinctures and astringents, abrasives and peeling agents.
- Avoid contact with the eyes, mouth and other mucous membranes. If FINACEA Gel does come in contact with the eyes, wash the eyes with large amounts of water and consult your physician if eye irritation persists.
- Wash hands immediately following application of FINACEA Gel.
- Cosmetics may be applied after the application of FINACEA Gel has dried.
- Avoid the use of occlusive dressings or wrappings.
- Skin irritation (e.g., pruritus, burning, or stinging) may occur during use of FINACEA Gel, usually during the first few weeks of treatment. If irritation is excessive or persists, discontinue use and consult your physician.
- Report abnormal changes in skin color to your physician.
- To help manage rosacea, avoid any triggers that may provoke erythema, flushing, and blushing. These triggers can include spicy and thermally hot food and drinks such as hot coffee, tea, or alcoholic beverages.

Manufactured for:
Bayer HealthCare Pharmaceuticals Inc.
Wayne, NJ 07470
Manufactured in Italy
670685

Shown in Product Identification Guide, page 305

NEXAVAR ℞
(sorafenib)
tablets, oral

HIGHLIGHTS OF PRESCRIBING INFORMATION
These highlights do not include all the information needed to use NEXAVAR safely and effectively.
See full prescribing information for NEXAVAR.
NEXAVAR (sorafenib) tablets, oral
Initial U.S. Approval: 2005

RECENT MAJOR CHANGES

Warnings and Precautions
- Risk of Dermatologic Toxicities (5.4) 08/2012
- Drug-Induced Hepatitis (5.10) 08/2012

INDICATIONS AND USAGE

NEXAVAR is a kinase inhibitor indicated for the treatment of
- Unresectable hepatocellular carcinoma (1.1)
- Advanced renal cell carcinoma (1.2)

DOSAGE AND ADMINISTRATION

- 400 mg (2 tablets) orally twice daily without food. (2)
- Treatment interruption and/or dose reduction may be needed to manage suspected adverse drug reactions. Dose may be reduced to 400 mg once daily or to 400 mg every other day. (2)

DOSAGE FORMS AND STRENGTHS

200 mg Tablets (3)

CONTRAINDICATIONS

- NEXAVAR is contraindicated in patients with known severe hypersensitivity to sorafenib or any other component of NEXAVAR. (4)
- NEXAVAR in combination with carboplatin and paclitaxel is contraindicated in patients with squamous cell lung cancer. (4)

WARNINGS AND PRECAUTIONS

- Cardiac ischemia and/or infarction may occur. Consider temporary or permanent discontinuation of NEXAVAR. (5.1)
- Bleeding may occur. If bleeding necessitates medical intervention, consider discontinuation of NEXAVAR. (5.2)
- Hypertension usually occurred early in the course of treatment and was managed with antihypertensive therapy. Monitor blood pressure weekly during the first 6 weeks and periodically thereafter and treat, as required. (5.3)
- Hand-foot skin reaction and rash are common. Management may include topical therapies for symptomatic relief, temporary treatment interruption and/or dose modification, or in severe or persistent cases, permanent discontinuation. Stevens-Johnson syndrome and toxic epidermal necrolysis have also occurred. Discontinue if suspected. (5.4)
- Gastrointestinal perforation is an uncommon adverse reaction. In the event of a gastrointestinal perforation, NEXAVAR should be discontinued. (5.5)
- Temporary interruption of NEXAVAR is recommended in patients undergoing major surgical procedures. (5.7)
- QT Prolongation: Monitor for prolonged QT intervals in patients with congestive heart failure, bradyarrhythmias, drugs known to prolong the QT interval, and electrolyte abnormalities. Avoid in patients with congenital long QT syndrome. (5.9, 12.2)
- Drug-induced hepatitis characterized by a hepatocellular pattern may result in hepatic failure and death. Monitor liver function tests regularly and discontinue if there is no alternative explanation for transaminase elevations. (5.10)
- NEXAVAR may cause fetal harm when administered to a pregnant woman. Advise women of childbearing potential to avoid becoming pregnant while on NEXAVAR. (5.11, 8.1)

ADVERSE REACTIONS

The most common adverse reactions (≥20%), which were considered to be related to NEXAVAR, are fatigue, weight loss, rash/desquamation, hand-foot skin reaction, alopecia, diarrhea, anorexia, nausea and abdominal pain. (6)

To report SUSPECTED ADVERSE REACTIONS, contact Bayer HealthCare Pharmaceuticals Inc. at 1-888-842-2937, or FDA at 1-800-FDA-1088 or www.fda.gov/medwatch

DRUG INTERACTIONS

- CYP3A4 inducers: Can increase the metabolism of sorafenib and decrease the AUC of sorafenib. (2, 7.1)

USE IN SPECIFIC POPULATIONS

- Hepatic impairment: No dose adjustment is necessary for patients with mild (Child-Pugh A) or moderate (Child-Pugh B) hepatic impairment. NEXAVAR has not been studied in patients with severe (Child-Pugh C) hepatic impairment. (8.6)
- Renal impairment: No dose adjustment is necessary for patients with mild (CrCl 50-80 mL/min), moderate (CrCl 30 - <50 mL/min), or severe (CrCl < 30 mL/min) renal impairment. NEXAVAR has not been studied in patients who are on dialysis. (8.7)

See 17 for PATIENT COUNSELING INFORMATION and FDA-approved patient labeling

Revised: 06/2013

FULL PRESCRIBING INFORMATION: CONTENTS*

*** Sections or subsections omitted from the full prescribing information are not listed**

FULL PRESCRIBING INFORMATION

1 INDICATIONS AND USAGE

1.1 Hepatocellular Carcinoma

NEXAVAR® is indicated for the treatment of patients with unresectable hepatocellular carcinoma (HCC).

1.2 Renal Cell Carcinoma

NEXAVAR is indicated for the treatment of patients with advanced renal cell carcinoma (RCC).

2 DOSAGE AND ADMINISTRATION

The recommended daily dose of NEXAVAR is 400 mg (2 × 200 mg tablets) taken twice daily without food (at least 1 hour before or 2 hours after a meal). Treatment should continue until the patient is no longer clinically benefiting from therapy or until unacceptable toxicity occurs.

Management of suspected adverse drug reactions may require temporary interruption and/or dose reduction of NEXAVAR. When dose reduction is necessary, the NEXAVAR dose may be reduced to 400 mg once daily. If additional dose reduction is required, NEXAVAR may be reduced to a single 400 mg dose every other day *[see Warnings and Precautions (5)]*.

Suggested dose modifications for skin toxicity are outlined in Table 1.

[See table 1 at top of next page]

No dose adjustment is required on the basis of patient age, gender, or body weight.

Concomitant strong CYP3A4 inducers: Avoid concomitant use of strong CYP3A4 inducers (such as, carbamazepine, dexamethasone, phenobarbital, phenytoin, rifampin, rifabutin, St. John's wort), when possible, because inducers can decrease the systemic exposure to sorafenib *[seeDrug Interactions (7.1)]*.

3 DOSAGE FORMS AND STRENGTHS

Tablets containing sorafenib tosylate (274 mg) equivalent to 200 mg of sorafenib.

NEXAVAR tablets are round, biconvex, red film-coated tablets, debossed with the "Bayer cross" on one side and "200" on the other side.

4 CONTRAINDICATIONS

- NEXAVAR is contraindicated in patients with known severe hypersensitivity to sorafenib or any other component of NEXAVAR.
- NEXAVAR in combination with carboplatin and paclitaxel is contraindicated in patients with squamous cell lung cancer *[see Warnings and Precautions (5.8)]*.

5 WARNINGS AND PRECAUTIONS

5.1 Risk of Cardiac Ischemia and/or Infarction

In the HCC study, the incidence of cardiac ischemia/infarction was 2.7% in NEXAVAR-treated patients compared with 1.3% in the placebo-treated group and in RCC Study 1, the incidence of cardiac ischemia/infarction was higher in the NEXAVAR-treated group (2.9%) compared with the placebo-treated group (0.4%). Patients with unstable coronary artery disease or recent myocardial infarction were excluded from this study. Temporary or permanent discontinuation of NEXAVAR should be considered in patients who develop cardiac ischemia and/or infarction.

5.2 Risk of Hemorrhage

An increased risk of bleeding may occur following NEXAVAR administration. In the HCC study, an excess of bleeding regardless of causality was not apparent and the rate of bleeding from esophageal varices was 2.4% in NEXAVAR-treated patients and 4% in placebo-treated patients. Bleeding with a fatal outcome from any site was reported in 2.4% of NEXAVAR-treated patients and 4% in placebo-treated patients. In RCC Study 1, bleeding regardless of causality was reported in 15.3% of patients in the NEXAVAR-treated group and 8.2% of patients in the placebo-treated group. The incidence of CTCAE Grade 3 and 4 bleeding was 2% and 0%, respectively, in NEXAVAR-treated patients, and 1.3% and 0.2%, respectively, in placebo-treated patients. There was one fatal hemorrhage in each treatment group in RCC Study 1. If any bleeding necessitates medical intervention, permanent discontinuation of NEXAVAR should be considered.

5.3 Risk of Hypertension

Monitor blood pressure weekly during the first 6 weeks of NEXAVAR. Thereafter, monitor blood pressure and treat hypertension, if required, in accordance with standard medical practice. In the HCC study, hypertension was reported in approximately 9.4% of NEXAVAR-treated patients and 4.3% of patients in the placebo-treated group. In RCC Study 1, hypertension was reported in approximately 16.9% of NEXAVAR-treated patients and 1.8% of patients in the placebo-treated group. Hypertension was usually mild to moderate, occurred early in the course of treatment, and was managed with standard antihypertensive therapy. In cases of severe or persistent hypertension despite institution of antihypertensive therapy, consider temporary or permanent discontinuation of NEXAVAR. Permanent discontinuation due to hypertension occurred in 1 of 297 NEXAVAR-treated patients in the HCC study and 1 of 451 NEXAVAR-treated patients in RCC Study 1.

5.4 Risk of Dermatologic Toxicities

Hand-foot skin reaction and rash represent the most common adverse reactions attributed to NEXAVAR. Rash and hand-foot skin reaction are usually CTCAE Grade 1 and 2 and generally appear during the first six weeks of treatment with NEXAVAR. Management of dermatologic toxicities may include topical therapies for symptomatic relief, temporary treatment interruption and/or dose modification of NEXAVAR, or in severe or persistent cases, permanent discontinuation of NEXAVAR. Permanent discontinuation of therapy due to hand-foot skin reaction occurred in 4 of 297 NEXAVAR-treated patients with HCC and 3 of 451 NEXAVAR-treated patients with RCC.

There have been reports of severe dermatologic toxicities, including Stevens-Johnson syndrome (SJS) and toxic epidermal necrolysis (TEN). These cases may be life-threatening. Discontinue NEXAVAR if SJS or TEN are suspected.

5.5 Risk of Gastrointestinal Perforation

Gastrointestinal perforation is an uncommon adverse reaction and has been reported in less than 1% of patients taking NEXAVAR. In some cases this was not associated with apparent intra-abdominal tumor. In the event of a gastrointestinal perforation, discontinue NEXAVAR.

5.6 Warfarin

Infrequent bleeding or elevations in the International Normalized Ratio (INR) have been reported in some patients taking warfarin while on NEXAVAR. Monitor patients taking concomitant warfarin regularly for changes in prothrombin time (PT), INR or clinical bleeding episodes.

5.7 Wound Healing Complications

No formal studies of the effect of NEXAVAR on wound healing have been conducted. Temporary interruption of NEXAVAR is recommended in patients undergoing major surgical procedures. There is limited clinical experience regarding the timing of reinitiation of NEXAVAR following major surgical intervention. Therefore, the decision to resume NEXAVAR following a major surgical intervention should be based on clinical judgment of adequate wound healing.

Table 1: Suggested Dose Modifications for Skin Toxicity

Skin Toxicity Grade	Occurrence	Suggested Dose Modification
Grade 1: Numbness, dysesthesia, paresthesia, tingling, painless swelling, erythema or discomfort of the hands or feet which does not disrupt the patient's normal activities	Any occurrence	Continue treatment with NEXAVAR and consider topical therapy for symptomatic relief
Grade 2: Painful erythema and swelling of the hands or feet and/or discomfort affecting the patient's normal activities	1st occurrence	Continue treatment with NEXAVAR and consider topical therapy for symptomatic relief If no improvement within 7 days, see below
	No improvement within 7 days or 2nd or 3rd occurrence	Interrupt NEXAVAR treatment until toxicity resolves to Grade 0–1 When resuming treatment, decrease NEXAVAR dose by one dose level (400 mg daily or 400 mg every other day)
	4th occurrence	Discontinue NEXAVAR treatment
Grade 3: Moist desquamation, ulceration, blistering or severe pain of the hands or feet, or severe discomfort that causes the patient to be unable to work or perform activities of daily living	1st or 2nd occurrence	Interrupt NEXAVAR treatment until toxicity resolves to Grade 0–1 When resuming treatment, decrease NEXAVAR dose by one dose level (400 mg daily or 400 mg every other day)
	3rd occurrence	Discontinue NEXAVAR treatment

5.8 Increased Mortality Observed with NEXAVAR Administered in Combination with Carboplatin/Paclitaxel and Gemcitabine/Cisplatin in Squamous Cell Lung Cancer

In a subset analysis of two randomized controlled trials in chemo-naive patients with Stage IIIB-IV non-small cell lung cancer, patients with squamous cell carcinoma experienced higher mortality with the addition of sorafenib compared to those treated with carboplatin/paclitaxel alone (HR 1.81, 95% CI 1.19–2.74) and gemcitabine/cisplatin alone (HR 1.22, 95% CI 0.82-1.80). The use of sorafenib in combination with carboplatin/paclitaxel is contraindicated in patients with squamous cell lung cancer. Sorafenib in combination with gemcitabine/cisplatin is not recommended in patients with squamous cell lung cancer. The safety and effectiveness of NEXAVAR has not been established in patients with non-small cell lung cancer.

5.9 Risk of QT Interval Prolongation

NEXAVAR can prolong the QT/QTc interval. QT/QTc interval prolongation increases the risk for ventricular arrhythmias. Avoid NEXAVAR in patients with congenital long QT syndrome. Monitor patients with congestive heart failure, bradyarrhythmias, drugs known to prolong the QT interval, including Class Ia and III antiarrhythmics, and electrolyte abnormalities with on-treatment electrocardiograms and electrolytes (magnesium, potassium, calcium) *[see Clinical Pharmacology (12.2)]*.

5.10 Drug-Induced Hepatitis

Sorafenib-induced hepatitis is characterized by a hepatocellular pattern of liver damage with significant increases of transaminases which may result in hepatic failure and death. Increases in bilirubin and INR may also occur. Monitor liver function tests regularly. In case of significantly increased transaminases without alternative explanation such as viral hepatitis or progressing underlying malignancy, discontinue NEXAVAR.

5.11 Risk of Fetal Harm

There are no adequate and well-controlled studies in pregnant women using NEXAVAR. However, based on its mechanism of action and findings in animals, NEXAVAR may cause fetal harm when administered to a pregnant woman. Sorafenib caused embryo-fetal toxicities in animals at maternal exposures that were significantly lower than the human exposures at the recommended dose of 400 mg twice daily. Advise women of childbearing potential to avoid becoming pregnant while on NEXAVAR because of the potential hazard to the fetus *[see Use in Specific Populations (8.1)]*.

6 ADVERSE REACTIONS

The following serious adverse reactions are discussed elsewhere in the labeling:

- Cardiac ischemia, infarction *[see Warnings and Precautions (5.1)]*
- Hemorrhage *[see Warnings and Precautions (5.2)]*
- Hypertension *[see Warnings and Precautions (5.3)]*
- Hand-foot skin reaction, rash, Stevens-Johnson syndrome, and toxic epidermal necrolysis *[seeWarnings and Precautions (5.4)]*
- Gastrointestinal perforation *[see Warnings and Precautions (5.5)]*
- QT Interval Prolongation *[see Warnings and Precautions (5.9) and Clinical Pharmacology (12.2)]*
- Drug-Induced Hepatitis *[see Warnings and Precautions (5.10)]*

Because clinical trials are conducted under widely varying conditions, adverse reaction rates observed in the clinical trials of a drug cannot be directly compared to rates in the clinical trials of another drug and may not reflect the rates observed in practice.

The data described in sections 6.1 and 6.2 reflect exposure to NEXAVAR in 748 patients who participated in placebo controlled studies in hepatocellular carcinoma (N=297) or advanced renal cell carcinoma (N=451).

The most common adverse reactions (≥20%), which were considered to be related to NEXAVAR, in patients with HCC or RCC are fatigue, weight loss, rash/desquamation, hand-foot skin reaction, alopecia, diarrhea, anorexia, nausea and abdominal pain.

6.1 Adverse Reactions in HCC Study

Table 2 shows the percentage of patients with HCC experiencing adverse reactions that were reported in at least 10% of patients and at a higher rate in the NEXAVAR arm than the placebo arm. CTCAE Grade 3 adverse reactions were reported in 39% of patients receiving NEXAVAR compared to 24% of patients receiving placebo. CTCAE Grade 4 adverse reactions were reported in 6% of patients receiving NEXAVAR compared to 8% of patients receiving placebo.

[See table 2 at top of next page]

Hypertension was reported in 9% of patients treated with NEXAVAR and 4% of those treated with placebo. CTCAE Grade 3 hypertension was reported in 4% of NEXAVAR-treated patients and 1% of placebo-treated patients. No patients were reported with CTCAE Grade 4 reactions in either treatment group.

Hemorrhage/bleeding was reported in 18% of those receiving NEXAVAR and 20% of placebo-treated patients. The rates of CTCAE Grade 3 and 4 bleeding were also higher in the placebo-treated group (CTCAE Grade 3 – 3% NEXAVAR and 5% placebo and CTCAE Grade 4 – 2% NEXAVAR and 4% placebo). Bleeding from esophageal varices was reported in 2.4% in NEXAVAR-treated patients and 4% of placebo-treated patients.

Renal failure was reported in <1% of patients treated with NEXAVAR and 3% of placebo-treated patients.

The rate of adverse reactions (including those associated with progressive disease) resulting in permanent discontinuation was similar in both the NEXAVAR and placebo-treated groups (32% of NEXAVAR-treated patients and 35% of placebo-treated patients).

Laboratory Abnormalities

The following laboratory abnormalities were observed in patients with HCC:

Hypophosphatemia was a common laboratory finding, observed in 35% of NEXAVAR-treated patients compared to 11% of placebo-treated patients; CTCAE Grade 3 hypophosphatemia (1–2 mg/dL) occurred in 11% of NEXAVAR-treated patients and 2% of patients in the placebo-treated group; there was 1 case of CTCAE Grade 4 hypophosphatemia (<1 mg/dL) reported in the placebo-treated group. The etiology of hypophosphatemia associated with NEXAVAR is not known.

Elevated lipase was observed in 40% of patients treated with NEXAVAR compared to 37% of patients in the placebo-treated group. CTCAE Grade 3 or 4 lipase elevations occurred in 9% of patients in each group. Elevated amylase was observed in 34% of patients treated with NEXAVAR compared to 29% of patients in the placebo-treated group.

Table 2: Adverse Reactions Reported in at Least 10% of Patients and at a Higher Rate in NEXAVAR Arm than the Placebo Arm – HCC Study

	NEXAVAR N=297			Placebo N=302		
Adverse Reaction NCI- CTCAE v3 Category/Term	All Grades %	Grade 3 %	Grade 4 %	All Grades %	Grade 3 %	Grade 4 %
Any Adverse Reaction	98	39	6	96	24	8
Constitutional symptoms						
Fatigue	46	9	1	45	12	2
Weight loss	30	2	0	10	1	0
Dermatology/skin						
Rash/desquamation	19	1	0	14	0	0
Pruritus	14	<1	0	11	<1	0
Hand-foot skin reaction	21	8	0	3	<1	0
Dry skin	10	0	0	6	0	0
Alopecia	14	0	0	2	0	0
Gastrointestinal						
Diarrhea	55	10	<1	25	2	0
Anorexia	29	3	0	18	3	<1
Nausea	24	1	0	20	3	0
Vomiting	15	2	0	11	2	0
Constipation	14	0	0	10	0	0
Hepatobiliary/pancreas						
Liver dysfunction	11	2	1	8	2	1
Pain						
Pain, abdomen	31	9	0	26	5	1

CTCAE Grade 3 or 4 amylase elevations were reported in 2% of patients in each group. Many of the lipase and amylase elevations were transient, and in the majority of cases NEXAVAR treatment was not interrupted. Clinical pancreatitis was reported in 1 of 297 NEXAVAR-treated patients (CTCAE Grade 2).

Elevations in liver function tests were comparable between the 2 arms of the study. Hypoalbuminemia was observed in 59% of NEXAVAR-treated patients and 47% of placebo-treated patients; no CTCAE Grade 3 or 4 hypoalbuminemia was observed in either group.

INR elevations were observed in 42% of NEXAVAR-treated patients and 34% of placebo-treated patients; CTCAE Grade 3 INR elevations were reported in 4% of NEXAVAR-treated patients and 2% of placebo-treated patients; there was no CTCAE Grade 4 INR elevation in either group.

Lymphopenia was observed in 47% of NEXAVAR-treated patients and 42% of placebo-treated patients.

Thrombocytopenia was observed in 46% of NEXAVAR-treated patients and 41% of placebo-treated patients; CTCAE Grade 3 or 4 thrombocytopenia was reported in 4% of NEXAVAR-treated patients and less than 1% of placebo-treated patients.

Hypocalcemia was reported in 27% of NEXAVAR-treated patients and 15% of placebo-treated patients. CTCAE Grade 3 hypocalcemia (6–7 mg /dL) occurred in 2% of NEXAVAR-treated patients and 1% of placebo-treated patients. CTCAE Grade 4 hypocalcemia (<6 mg/dL) occurred in 0.4% of NEXAVAR-treated patients and in no placebo-treated patients.

Hypokalemia was reported in 9.4% of NEXAVAR- treated patients compared to 5.9% of placebo-treated patients. Most reports of hypokalemia were low grade (CTCAE Grade 1). CTCAE Grade 3 hypokalemia occurred in 0.3% of NEXAVAR-treated patients and 0.7% of placebo-treated patients. There were no reports of Grade 4 hypokalemia.

6.2 Adverse Reactions in RCC Study 1

Table 3 shows the percentage of patients with RCC experiencing adverse reactions that were reported in at least 10% of patients and at a higher rate in the NEXAVAR arm than the placebo arm. CTCAE Grade 3 adverse reactions were reported in 31% of patients receiving NEXAVAR compared to 22% of patients receiving placebo. CTCAE Grade 4 adverse reactions were reported in 7% of patients receiving NEXAVAR compared to 6% of patients receiving placebo.

[See table 3 at top of next page]

The rate of adverse reactions (including those associated with progressive disease) resulting in permanent discontinuation was similar in both the NEXAVAR and placebo-treated groups (10% of NEXAVAR-treated patients and 8% of placebo-treated patients).

Laboratory Abnormalities

The following laboratory abnormalities were observed in patients with RCC in Study 1:

Hypophosphatemia was a common laboratory finding, observed in 45% of NEXAVAR-treated patients compared to 11% of placebo-treated patients. CTCAE Grade 3 hypophosphatemia (1–2 mg/dL) occurred in 13% of NEXAVAR-treated patients and 3% of patients in the placebo-treated group. There were no cases of CTCAE Grade 4 hypophosphatemia (<1 mg/dL) reported in either NEXAVAR or placebo-treated patients. The etiology of hypophosphatemia associated with NEXAVAR is not known.

Elevated lipase was observed in 41% of patients treated with NEXAVAR compared to 30% of patients in the placebo-treated group. CTCAE Grade 3 or 4 lipase elevations occurred in 12% of patients in the NEXAVAR-treated group compared to 7% of patients in the placebo-treated group. Elevated amylase was observed in 30% of patients treated with NEXAVAR compared to 23% of patients in the placebo-treated group. CTCAE Grade 3 or 4 amylase elevations were reported in 1% of patients in the NEXAVAR-treated group compared to 3% of patients in the placebo-treated group. Many of the lipase and amylase elevations were transient, and in the majority of cases NEXAVAR treatment was not interrupted. Clinical pancreatitis was reported in 3 of 451 NEXAVAR-treated patients (one CTCAE Grade 2 and two Grade 4) and 1 of 451 patients (CTCAE Grade 2) in the placebo-treated group.

Lymphopenia was observed in 23% of NEXAVAR-treated patients and 13% of placebo-treated patients. CTCAE Grade 3 or 4 lymphopenia was reported in 13% of NEXAVAR-treated patients and 7% of placebo-treated patients. Neutropenia was observed in 18% of NEXAVAR-treated patients and 10% of placebo-treated patients. CTCAE Grade 3 or 4 neutropenia was reported in 5% of NEXAVAR-treated patients and 2% of placebo-treated patients.

Anemia was observed in 44% of NEXAVAR-treated patients and 49% of placebo-treated patients. CTCAE Grade 3 or 4 anemia was reported in 2% of NEXAVAR-treated patients and 4% of placebo-treated patients.

Thrombocytopenia was observed in 12% of NEXAVAR-treated patients and 5% of placebo-treated patients. CTCAE Grade 3 or 4 thrombocytopenia was reported in 1% of NEXAVAR-treated patients and in no placebo-treated patients.

Hypocalcemia was reported in 12% of NEXAVAR-treated patients and 8% of placebo-treated patients. CTCAE Grade 3 hypocalcemia (6–7 mg/dL) occurred in 1% of NEXAVAR-treated patients and 0.2% of placebo-treated patients, and CTCAE Grade 4 hypocalcemia (<6 mg/dL) occurred in 1% of NEXAVAR-treated patients and 0.5% of placebo-treated patients.

Hypokalemia was reported in 5.4% of NEXAVAR-treated patients compared to 0.7% of placebo-treated patients. Most reports of hypokalemia were low grade (CTCAE Grade 1). CTCAE Grade 3 hypokalemia occurred in 1.3% of NEXAVAR-treated patients and 0.2% of placebo-treated patients. There were no reports of Grade 4 hypokalemia.

6.3 Additional Data from Multiple Clinical Trials

The following additional drug-related adverse reactions and laboratory abnormalities were reported from clinical trials of NEXAVAR (*very common* 10% or greater, *common* 1 to less than 10%, *uncommon* 0.1% to less than 1%):

Cardiovascular: *Common:* congestive heart failure[1,2], myocardial ischemia and/or infarction *Uncommon:* hypertensive crisis[1] *Rare:* QT prolongation[1]

Dermatologic: *Very common:* erythema *Common:* exfoliative dermatitis, acne, flushing *Uncommon:* folliculitis, eczema, erythema multiforme, keratoacanthomas/squamous cell cancer of the skin

Digestive: *Very common:* increased lipase, increased amylase *Common:* mucositis, stomatitis (including dry mouth and glossodynia), dyspepsia, dysphagia *Uncommon:* pancreatitis, gastrointestinal reflux, gastritis, gastrointestinal perforations[1], cholecystitis, cholangitis

Note that elevations in lipase are very common (41%, see below); a diagnosis of pancreatitis should not be made solely on the basis of abnormal laboratory values

General Disorders: *Very common:* hemorrhage (including gastrointestinal[1] & respiratory tract[1] and uncommon cases of cerebral hemorrhage[1]), asthenia, pain (including mouth, bone, and tumor pain) *Common:* decreased appetite, influenza-like illness, pyrexia *Uncommon:* infection

Hematologic: *Very common:* leukopenia, lymphopenia *Common:* anemia, neutropenia, thrombocytopenia *Uncommon:* INR abnormal

Hypersensitivity: *Uncommon:* hypersensitivity reactions (including skin reactions and urticaria)

Metabolic and Nutritional: *Very common:* hypophosphatemia *Common:* transient increases in transaminases, hypocalcemia, hypokalemia *Uncommon:* dehydration, hyponatremia, transient increases in alkaline phosphatase, increased bilirubin (including jaundice), hypothyroidism, hyperthyroidism

Musculoskeletal: *Common:* arthralgia, myalgia

Nervous System and Psychiatric: *Common:* depression *Uncommon:* tinnitus, reversible posterior leukoencephalopathy[1]

Renal and Genitourinary: *Common:* renal failure, proteinuria *Rare:* Nephrotic syndrome

Reproductive: *Common:* erectile dysfunction *Uncommon:* gynecomastia

Respiratory: *Common:* hoarseness *Uncommon:* rhinorrhea, interstitial lung disease-like events (includes reports of pneumonitis, radiation pneumonitis, acute respiratory distress, interstitial pneumonia, pulmonitis and lung inflammation)

In addition, the following medically significant adverse reactions were uncommon during clinical trials of NEXAVAR: transient ischemic attack, arrhythmia, thromboembolism. For these adverse reactions, the causal relationship to NEXAVAR has not been established.

[1]adverse reactions may have a life-threatening or fatal outcome.

[2]reported in 1.9% of patients treated with sorafenib (N= 2276).

6.4 Postmarketing Experience

The following adverse drug reactions have been identified during post-approval use of NEXAVAR. Because these reactions are reported voluntarily from a population of uncertain size, it is not always possible to reliably estimate their frequency or establish a causal relationship to drug exposure.

Dermatologic: Stevens-Johnson syndrome and toxic epidermal necrolysis (TEN)

Hepatobiliary disorders: Drug-induced hepatitis, including reports of hepatic failure and death

Hypersensitivity: Angioedema, anaphylactic reaction

Musculoskeletal: Rhabdomyolysis, osteonecrosis of the jaw

Respiratory: Interstitial lung disease-like events (which may have a life-threatening or fatal outcome)

7 DRUG INTERACTIONS

7.1 Drug Metabolism

Effect of Cytochrome P450 Inducers on Sorafenib

Rifampin, a strong CYP3A4 inducer, administered at a dose of 600 mg once daily for 5 days with a single oral dose of NEXAVAR 400 mg in healthy volunteers resulted in a 37% decrease in the mean AUC of sorafenib. Other inducers of CYP3A4 activity (such as, carbamazepine, dexamethasone, phenobarbital, phenytoin, rifabutin, rifampin, St. John's wort) can increase the metabolism of sorafenib and thus, decrease systemic exposure of sorafenib *[see Dosage and Administration (2) and Clinical Pharmacology (12.3)]*.

Effect of Cytochrome P450 Inhibitors on Sorafenib

Ketoconazole, a strong inhibitor of CYP3A4 and P-glycoprotein, administered at a dose of 400 mg once daily for 7 days did not alter the mean AUC of a single oral dose of NEXAVAR 50 mg in healthy volunteers.

Effect of Sorafenib on Other Drugs

NEXAVAR 400 mg twice daily for 28 days did not increase the systemic exposure of concomitantly administered midazolam (CYP3A4 substrate), dextromethorphan (CYP2D6 substrate), and omeprazole (CYP2C19 substrate). *[see Clinical Pharmacology (12.3)]*.

7.2 Neomycin

Neomycin administered as an oral dose of 1 g three times daily for 5 days decreased the mean AUC of sorafenib by 54% in healthy volunteers administered a single oral dose of NEXAVAR 400 mg. The effects of other antibiotics on the pharmacokinetics of sorafenib have not been studied *[see Clinical Pharmacology (12.3)]*.

7.3 Drugs that Increase Gastric pH

The aqueous solubility of sorafenib is pH dependent, with higher pH resulting in lower solubility. However, omeprazole, a proton pump inhibitor, administered at a dose of 40 mg once daily for 5 days, did not result in a clinically meaningful change in sorafenib single dose exposure. No dose adjustment for NEXAVAR is necessary.

8 USE IN SPECIFIC POPULATIONS

8.1 Pregnancy

Pregnancy Category D *[see Warnings and Precautions (5.11)]*.

Based on its mechanism of action and findings in animals, NEXAVAR may cause fetal harm when administered to a pregnant woman. Sorafenib caused embryo-fetal toxicities in animals at maternal exposures that were significantly lower than the human exposures at the recommended dose of 400 mg twice daily. There are no adequate and well-controlled studies in pregnant women using NEXAVAR. Inform patients of childbearing potential that NEXAVAR can cause birth defects or fetal loss. Instruct both men and women of childbearing potential to use effective birth control during treatment with NEXAVAR and for at least 2 weeks after stopping treatment. Counsel female patients to contact their healthcare provider if they become pregnant while taking NEXAVAR.

When administered to rats and rabbits during the period of organogenesis, sorafenib was teratogenic and induced embryo-fetal toxicity (including increased post-implantation loss, resorptions, skeletal retardations, and retarded fetal weight). The effects occurred at doses considerably below the recommended human dose of 400 mg twice daily (approximately 500 mg/m^2/day on a body surface area basis). Adverse intrauterine development effects were seen at doses ≥0.2 mg/kg/day (1.2 mg/m^2/day) in rats and 0.3 mg/kg/day (3.6 mg/m^2/day) in rabbits. These doses result in exposures (AUC) approximately 0.008 times the AUC seen in patients at the recommended human dose. A NOAEL (no observed adverse effect level) was not defined for either species, since lower doses were not tested.

8.3 Nursing Mothers

It is not known whether sorafenib is excreted in human milk. Because many drugs are excreted in human milk and because of the potential for serious adverse reactions in nursing infants from NEXAVAR, a decision should be made whether to discontinue nursing or to discontinue the drug, taking into account the importance of the drug to the mother.

Following administration of radiolabeled sorafenib to lactating Wistar rats, approximately 27% of the radioactivity was secreted into the milk. The milk to plasma AUC ratio was approximately 5:1.

8.4 Pediatric Use

The safety and effectiveness of NEXAVAR in pediatric patients have not been studied.

Repeat dosing of sorafenib to young and growing dogs resulted in irregular thickening of the femoral growth plate at daily sorafenib doses ≥ 600 mg/m^2 (approximately 0.3 times the AUC at the recommended human dose), hypocellularity of the bone marrow adjoining the growth plate at 200 mg/m^2/day (approximately 0.1 times the AUC at the recommended human dose), and alterations of the dentin composition at 600 mg/m^2/day. Similar effects were not observed in adult dogs when dosed for 4 weeks or less.

Table 3: Adverse Reactions Reported in at Least 10% of Patients and at a Higher Rate in NEXAVAR Arm than the Placebo Arm – RCC Study 1

Adverse Reactions NCI- CTCAE v3 Category/Term	NEXAVAR N=451			Placebo N=451		
	All Grades %	Grade 3 %	Grade 4 %	All Grades %	Grade 3 %	Grade 4 %
Any Adverse Reactions	95	31	7	86	22	6
Cardiovascular, General						
Hypertension	17	3	<1	2	<1	0
Constitutional symptoms						
Fatigue	37	5	<1	28	3	<1
Weight loss	10	<1	0	6	0	0
Dermatology/skin						
Rash/desquamation	40	<1	0	16	<1	0
Hand-foot skin reaction	30	6	0	7	0	0
Alopecia	27	<1	0	3	0	0
Pruritus	19	<1	0	6	0	0
Dry skin	11	0	0	4	0	0
Gastrointestinal symptoms						
Diarrhea	43	2	0	13	<1	0
Nausea	23	<1	0	19	<1	0
Anorexia	16	<1	0	13	1	0
Vomiting	16	<1	0	12	1	0
Constipation	15	<1	0	11	<1	0
Hemorrhage/bleeding						
Hemorrhage – all sites	15	2	0	8	1	<1
Neurology						
Neuropathy-sensory	13	<1	0	6	<1	0
Pain						
Pain, abdomen	11	2	0	9	2	0
Pain, joint	10	2	0	6	<1	0
Pain, headache	10	<1	0	6	<1	0
Pulmonary						
Dyspnea	14	3	<1	12	2	<1

8.5 Geriatric Use

In total, 59% of HCC patients treated with NEXAVAR were age 65 years or older, and 19% were 75 and older. In total, 32% of RCC patients treated with NEXAVAR were age 65 years or older, and 4% were 75 and older. No differences in safety or efficacy were observed between older and younger patients, and other reported clinical experience has not identified differences in responses between the elderly and younger patients, but greater sensitivity of some older individuals cannot be ruled out.

8.6 Patients with Hepatic Impairment

In a trial of HCC patients with mild (Child-Pugh A) or moderate (Child-Pugh B) hepatic impairment, the systemic exposure (AUC) of sorafenib was within the range observed in patients without hepatic impairment. In another trial in subjects without HCC, the mean AUC was similar for subjects with mild (n=15) and moderate (n=14) hepatic impairment compared to subjects (n=15) with normal hepatic function. No dose adjustment is necessary for patients with mild or moderate hepatic impairment. The pharmacokinetics of sorafenib have not been studied in patients with severe (Child-Pugh C) hepatic impairment *[see Clinical Pharmacology (12.3)]*.

8.7 Patients with Renal Impairment

No correlation between sorafenib exposure and renal function was observed following administration of a single oral dose of NEXAVAR 400 mg to subjects with normal renal function and subjects with mild (CrCl 50–80 mL/min), moderate (CrCl 30–<50 mL/min), or severe (CrCl <30 mL/min) renal impairment who are not on dialysis. No dose adjustment is necessary for patients with mild, moderate or severe renal impairment who are not on dialysis. The pharmacokinetics of sorafenib have not been studied in patients who are on dialysis *[see Clinical Pharmacology (12.3)]*.

10 OVERDOSAGE

There is no specific treatment for NEXAVAR overdose.

The highest dose of NEXAVAR studied clinically is 800 mg twice daily. The adverse reactions observed at this dose were primarily diarrhea and dermatologic. No information is available on symptoms of acute overdose in animals because of the saturation of absorption in oral acute toxicity studies conducted in animals.

In cases of suspected overdose, NEXAVAR should be withheld and supportive care instituted.

11 DESCRIPTION

NEXAVAR, a kinase inhibitor, is the tosylate salt of sorafenib.

Table 4: Efficacy Results from HCC Study

Efficacy Parameter	NEXAVAR (N=299)	Placebo (N=303)	Hazard Ratio* (95% CI)	P-value (log-rank test)†
Overall Survival Median, months (95% CI) No. of events	10.7 (9.4, 13.3) 143	7.9 (6.8, 9.1) 178	0.69 (0.55, 0.87)	0.00058
Time to Progression‡ Median, months (95% CI) No. of events	5.5 (4.1, 6.9) 107	2.8 (2.7, 3.9) 156	0.58 (0.45, 0.74)	0.000007

* Hazard ratio, sorafenib/placebo, stratified Cox model
† Stratified log rank (for the interim analysis of survival, the stopping boundary one-sided alpha = 0.0077)
‡ The time-to-progression (TTP) analysis, based on independent radiologic review, was based on data from an earlier time point than the survival analysis

Sorafenib tosylate has the chemical name 4-(4-{3-[4-Chloro-3-(trifluoromethyl)phenyl]ureido}phenoxy)N2-methylpyridine-2-carboxamide 4-methylbenzenesulfonate and its structural formula is:

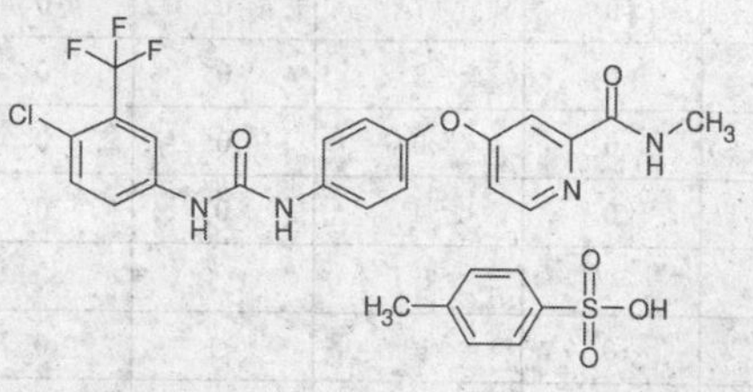

Sorafenib tosylate is a white to yellowish or brownish solid with a molecular formula of $C_{21}H_{16}ClF_3N_4O_3 \times C_7H_8O_3S$ and a molecular weight of 637.0 g/mole. Sorafenib tosylate is practically insoluble in aqueous media, slightly soluble in ethanol and soluble in PEG 400.

Each red, round NEXAVAR film-coated tablet contains sorafenib tosylate (274 mg) equivalent to 200 mg of sorafenib and the following inactive ingredients: croscarmellose sodium, microcrystalline cellulose, hypromellose, sodium lauryl sulphate, magnesium stearate, polyethylene glycol, titanium dioxide and ferric oxide red.

12 CLINICAL PHARMACOLOGY

12.1 Mechanism of Action

Sorafenib is a kinase inhibitor that decreases tumor cell proliferation *in vitro*. Sorafenib was shown to inhibit multiple intracellular (CRAF, BRAF and mutant BRAF) and cell surface kinases (KIT, FLT-3, RET, VEGFR-1, VEGFR-2, VEGFR-3, and PDGFR-ß). Several of these kinases are thought to be involved in tumor cell signaling, angiogenesis, and apoptosis. Sorafenib inhibited tumor growth and angiogenesis of human hepatocellular carcinoma and renal cell carcinoma, and several other human tumor xenografts in immunocompromised mice.

12.2 Pharmacodynamics

Cardiac Electrophysiology

The effect of NEXAVAR 400 mg twice daily on the QTc interval was evaluated in a multi-center, open-label, nonrandomized trial in 53 patients with advanced cancer. No large changes in the mean QTc intervals (that is, >20 ms) from baseline were detected in the trial. After one 28-day treatment cycle, the largest mean QTc interval change of 8.5 ms (upper bound of two-sided 90% confidence interval, 13.3 ms) was observed at 6 hours post-dose on day 1 of cycle 2 *[see Warnings and Precautions (5.9)]*.

12.3 Pharmacokinetics

After administration of NEXAVAR tablets, the mean relative bioavailability was 38–49% when compared to an oral solution. The mean elimination half-life of sorafenib was approximately 25 to 48 hours. Multiple doses of NEXAVAR for 7 days resulted in a 2.5- to 7-fold accumulation compared to a single dose. Steady-state plasma sorafenib concentrations were achieved within 7 days, with a peak-to-trough ratio of mean concentrations of less than 2.

Absorption and Distribution: Following oral administration, sorafenib reached peak plasma levels in approximately 3 hours. With a moderate-fat meal (30% fat; 700 calories), bioavailability was similar to that in the fasted state. With a high-fat meal (50% fat; 900 calories), bioavailability was reduced by 29% compared to that in the fasted state. It is recommended that NEXAVAR be administered without food *[see Dosage and Administration (2)]*.

Mean C_{max} and AUC increased less than proportionally beyond oral doses of 400 mg administered twice daily. *In vitro* binding of sorafenib to human plasma proteins was 99.5%.

Metabolism and Elimination: Sorafenib undergoes oxidative metabolism by hepatic CYP3A4, as well as glucuronidation by UGT1A9. Inducers of CYP3A4 activity can decrease the systemic exposure of sorafenib *[see Dosage and Administration (2) and Drug Interactions (7.1)]*.

Sorafenib accounted for approximately 70–85% of the circulating analytes in plasma at steady-state. Eight metabolites of sorafenib have been identified, of which 5 have been detected in plasma. The main circulating metabolite of sorafenib, the pyridine N-oxide that comprises approximately 9–16% of circulating analytes at steady-state, showed *in vitro* potency similar to that of sorafenib.

Following oral administration of a 100 mg dose of a solution formulation of sorafenib, 96% of the dose was recovered within 14 days, with 77% of the dose excreted in feces and 19% of the dose excreted in urine as glucuronidated metabolites. Unchanged sorafenib, accounting for 51% of the dose, was found in feces but not in urine.

Effects of Age, Gender and Race: A study of the pharmacokinetics of sorafenib indicated that the mean AUC of sorafenib in Asians (N=78) was 30% lower than in Caucasians (N=40). Gender and age do not have a clinically meaningful effect on the pharmacokinetics of sorafenib.

Renal Impairment: Mild (CrCl 50-80 mL/min), moderate (CrCl 30 - <50 mL/min), and severe (CrCl <30 mL/min) renal impairment do not affect the pharmacokinetics of sorafenib.No dose adjustment is necessary *[see Use in Specific Populations (8.7)]*.

Hepatic Impairment: Mild (Child-Pugh A) and moderate (Child-Pugh B) hepatic impairment do not affect the pharmacokinetics of sorafenib. No dose adjustment is necessary *[see Use in Specific Populations (8.6)]*.

Drug-Drug Interactions: Studies in human liver microsomes demonstrated that sorafenib competitively inhibited CYP2B6, CYP2C8, CYP2C9, CYP2C19, CYP2D6, and CYP3A4. However, NEXAVAR 400 mg twice daily for 28 days with substrates of CYP3A4, CYP2D6 and CYP2C19 did not increase the systemic exposure of these substrates *[see Drug Interactions (7.1)]*.

Studies with cultured human hepatocytes demonstrated that sorafenib did not increase CYP1A2 and CYP3A4 activities, suggesting that sorafenib is unlikely to induce CYP1A2 or CYP3A4 in humans.

Sorafenib inhibits glucuronidation by UGT1A1 and UGT1A9 *in vitro*. NEXAVAR could increase the systemic exposure of concomitantly administered drugs that are UGT1A1 or UGT1A9 substrates.

Sorafenib inhibited P-glycoprotein *in vitro*. NEXAVAR could increase the concentrations of concomitantly administered drugs that are P-glycoprotein substrates.

13 NONCLINICAL TOXICOLOGY

13.1 Carcinogenesis, Mutagenesis, Impairment of Fertility

Carcinogenicity studies have not been performed with sorafenib.

Sorafenib was clastogenic when tested in an *in vitro* mammalian cell assay (Chinese hamster ovary) in the presence of metabolic activation. Sorafenib was not mutagenic in the *in vitro* Ames bacterial cell assay or clastogenic in an *in vivo* mouse micronucleus assay. One intermediate in the manufacturing process, which is also present in the final drug substance (<0.15%), was positive for mutagenesis in an *in vitro* bacterial cell assay (Ames test) when tested independently.

No specific studies with sorafenib have been conducted in animals to evaluate the effect on fertility. However, results from the repeat-dose toxicity studies suggest there is a potential for sorafenib to impair reproductive function and fertility. Multiple adverse effects were observed in male and female reproductive organs, with the rat being more susceptible than mice or dogs. Typical changes in rats consisted of testicular atrophy or degeneration, degeneration of epididymis, prostate, and seminal vesicles, central necrosis of the corpora lutea and arrested follicular development. Sorafenib-related effects on the reproductive organs of rats were manifested at daily oral doses ≥ 5 mg/kg (30 mg/m²). This dose results in an exposure (AUC) that is approximately 0.5 times the AUC in patients at the recommended human dose. Dogs showed tubular degeneration in the testes at 30 mg/kg/day (600 mg/m²/day).This dose results in an exposure that is approximately 0.3 times the AUC at the recommended human dose. Oligospermia was observed in dogs at 60 mg/kg/day (1200 mg/m²/day) of sorafenib.

Adequate contraception should be used during therapy and for at least 2 weeks after completing therapy.

14 CLINICAL STUDIES

The clinical safety and efficacy of NEXAVAR have been studied in patients with hepatocellular carcinoma (HCC) and renal cell carcinoma (RCC).

14.1 Hepatocellular Carcinoma

The **HCC Study** was a Phase 3, international, multicenter, randomized, double blind, placebo-controlled trial in patients with unresectable hepatocellular carcinoma. Overall survival was the primary endpoint. A total of 602 patients were randomized; 299 to NEXAVAR 400 mg twice daily and 303 to matching placebo.

Demographics and baseline disease characteristics were similar between the NEXAVAR and placebo-treated groups with regard to age, gender, race, performance status, etiology (including hepatitis B, hepatitis C and alcoholic liver disease), TNM stage (stage I: <1% vs. <1%; stage II: 10.4% vs. 8.3%; stage III: 37.8% vs. 43.6%; stage IV: 50.8% vs. 46.9%), absence of both macroscopic vascular invasion and extrahepatic tumor spread (30.1% vs. 30.0%), and Barcelona Clinic Liver Cancer stage (stage B: 18.1% vs. 16.8%; stage C: 81.6% vs. 83.2%; stage D: <1% vs. 0%). Liver impairment by Child-Pugh score was comparable between the NEXAVAR and placebo-treated groups (Class A: 95% vs. 98%; B: 5% vs. 2%). Only one patient with Child-Pugh class C was entered. Prior treatments included surgical resection procedures (19.1% vs. 20.5%), locoregional therapies (including radiofrequency ablation, percutaneous ethanol injection and transarterial chemoembolization; 38.8% vs. 40.6%), radiotherapy (4.3% vs. 5.0%) and systemic therapy (3.0% vs. 5.0%).

The trial was stopped for efficacy following a pre-specified second interim analysis for survival showing a statistically significant advantage for NEXAVAR over placebo for overall survival (HR: 0.69, p= 0.00058) (see Table 4 and Figure 1). This advantage was consistent across all subsets analyzed. Final analysis of time to tumor progression (TTP) based on data from an earlier time point (by independent radiologic review) also was significantly longer in the NEXAVAR arm (HR: 0.58, p=0.000007) (see Table 4).

[See table 4 above]

Figure 1: Kaplan-Meier Curve of Overall Survival in HCC Study (Intent-to-Treat Population)

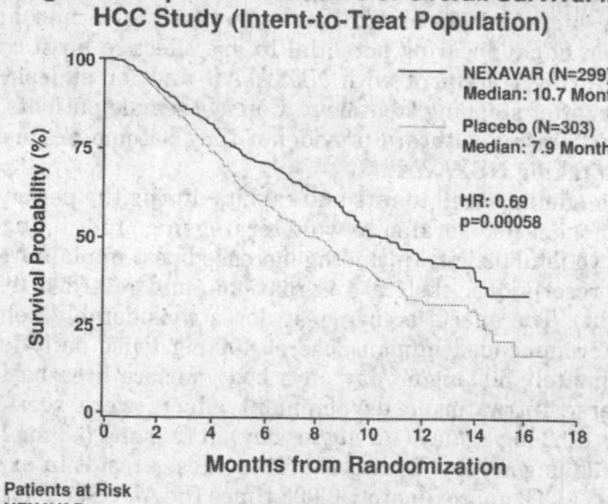

Patients at Risk									
NEXAVAR	270	234	200	140	89	48	24	1	0
Placebo	272	217	174	108	69	31	14	3	0

14.2 Renal Cell Carcinoma

The safety and efficacy of NEXAVAR in the treatment of advanced renal cell carcinoma (RCC) were studied in the following two randomized controlled clinical trials.

RCC Study 1 was a Phase 3, international, multicenter, randomized, double blind, placebo-controlled trial in patients with advanced renal cell carcinoma who had received one prior systemic therapy. Primary study endpoints included overall survival and progression-free survival (PFS). Tumor response rate was a secondary endpoint. The PFS analysis included 769 patients stratified by MSKCC (Memorial Sloan Kettering Cancer Center) prognostic risk category (low or intermediate) and country and randomized to NEXAVAR 400 mg twice daily (N=384) or to placebo (N=385).

Table 5 summarizes the demographic and disease characteristics of the study population analyzed. Baseline demographics and disease characteristics were well balanced for both treatment groups. The median time from initial diagnosis of RCC to randomization was 1.6 and 1.9 years for the NEXAVAR and placebo-treated groups, respectively.

Table 5: Demographic and Disease Characteristics – RCC Study 1

Characteristics	NEXAVAR N=384		Placebo N=385	
	n	(%)	n	(%)
Gender				
Male	267	(70)	287	(75)
Female	116	(30)	98	(25)
Race				
White	276	(72)	278	(73)
Black/Asian/Hispanic/ Other	11	(3)	10	(2)
Not reported *	97	(25)	97	(25)
Age group				
< 65 years	255	(67)	280	(73)
≥ 65 years	127	(33)	103	(27)
ECOG performance status at baseline				
0	184	(48)	180	(47)
1	191	(50)	201	(52)
2	6	(2)	1	(<1)
Not reported	3	(<1)	3	(<1)
MSKCC prognostic risk category				
Low	200	(52)	194	(50)
Intermediate	184	(48)	191	(50)
Prior IL-2 and/or interferon				
Yes	319	(83)	313	(81)
No	65	(17)	72	(19)

* Race was not collected from the 186 patients enrolled in France due to local regulations. In 8 other patients, race was not available at the time of analysis.

Progression-free survival, defined as the time from randomization to progression or death from any cause, whichever occurred earlier, was evaluated by blinded independent radiological review using RECIST criteria.

Figure 2 depicts Kaplan-Meier curves for PFS. The PFS analysis was based on a two-sided Log-Rank test stratified by MSKCC prognostic risk category and country.

Figure 2: Kaplan-Meier Curves for Progression-free Survival – RCC Study 1

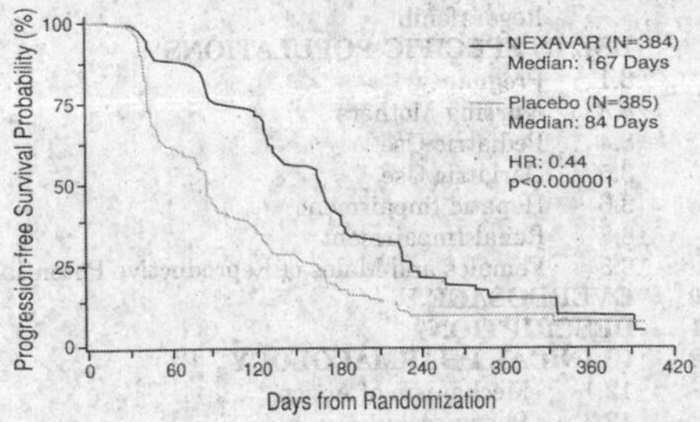

NOTE: HR is from Cox regression model with the following covariates: MSKCC prognostic risk category and country. P-value is from two-sided Log-Rank test stratified by MSKCC prognostic risk category and country.

The median PFS for patients randomized to NEXAVAR was 167 days compared to 84 days for patients randomized to placebo. The estimated hazard ratio (risk of progression with NEXAVAR compared to placebo) was 0.44 (95% CI: 0.35, 0.55).

A series of patient subsets were examined in exploratory univariate analyses of PFS. The subsets included age above or below 65 years, ECOG PS 0 or 1, MSKCC prognostic risk category, whether the prior therapy was for progressive metastatic disease or for an earlier disease setting and time from diagnosis of less than or greater than 1.5 years. The effect of NEXAVAR on PFS was consistent across these subsets, including patients with no prior IL-2 or interferon therapy (N=137; 65 patients receiving NEXAVAR and 72 placebo), for whom the median PFS was 172 days on NEXAVAR compared to 85 days on placebo.

Tumor response was determined by independent radiologic review according to RECIST criteria. Overall, of 672 patients who were evaluable for response, 7 (2%) NEXAVAR-treated patients and 0 (0%) placebo-treated patients had a confirmed partial response. Thus the gain in PFS in NEXAVAR-treated patients primarily reflects the stable disease population.

At the time of a planned interim survival analysis, based on 220 deaths, overall survival was longer for NEXAVAR than placebo with a hazard ratio (NEXAVAR over placebo) of 0.72. This analysis did not meet the prespecified criteria for statistical significance. Additional analyses are planned as the survival data mature.

RCC Study 2 was a Phase 2 randomized discontinuation trial in patients with metastatic malignancies, including RCC. The primary endpoint was the percentage of randomized patients remaining progression-free at 24 weeks. All patients received NEXAVAR for the first 12 weeks. Radiologic assessment was repeated at week 12. Patients with <25% change in bi-dimensional tumor measurements from baseline were randomized to NEXAVAR or placebo for a further 12 weeks. Patients who were randomized to placebo were permitted to cross over to open-label NEXAVAR upon progression. Patients with tumor shrinkage ≥25% continued NEXAVAR, whereas patients with tumor growth ≥25% discontinued treatment.

Two hundred and two patients with advanced RCC were enrolled into RCC Study 2, including patients who had received no prior therapy and patients with tumor histology other than clear cell carcinoma. After the initial 12 weeks of NEXAVAR, 79 patients with RCC continued on open-label NEXAVAR, and 65 patients were randomized to NEXAVAR or placebo. After an additional 12 weeks, at week 24, for the 65 randomized patients, the progression-free rate was significantly higher in patients randomized to NEXAVAR (16/32, 50%) than in patients randomized to placebo (6/33, 18%) (p=0.0077). Progression-free survival was significantly longer in the NEXAVAR-treated group (163 days) than in the placebo-treated group (41 days) (p=0.0001, HR=0.29).

16 HOW SUPPLIED/STORAGE AND HANDLING

NEXAVAR tablets are supplied as round, biconvex, red film-coated tablets, debossed with the "Bayer cross" on one side and "200" on the other side, each containing sorafenib tosylate equivalent to 200 mg of sorafenib.

Bottles of 120 tablets NDC 50419-488-58

Storage

Store at 25°C (77°F); excursions permitted to 15–30°C (59–86°F) (see USP controlled room temperature). Store in a dry place.

17 PATIENT COUNSELING INFORMATION

See FDA-approved Patient Labeling

17.1 Cardiac Ischemia; Infarction

Discuss with patients that cardiac ischemia and/or infarction has been reported during NEXAVAR treatment, and that they should immediately report any episodes of chest pain or other symptoms of cardiac ischemia *[see Warnings and Precautions (5.1)]*.

17.2 Bleeding

Inform patients that NEXAVAR can increase the risk of bleeding and that they should promptly report any episodes of *bleeding [see Warnings and Precautions (5.2)]*.

Inform patients that bleeding or elevations in the International Normalized Ratio (INR) have been reported in some patients taking warfarin while on NEXAVAR and that their INR should be monitored regularly *[see Warnings and Precautions (5.6)]*.

17.3 Hypertension

Inform patients that hypertension can develop during NEXAVAR treatment, especially during the first six weeks of therapy, and that blood pressure should be monitored regularly during treatment *[see Warnings and Precautions (5.3)]*.

17.4 Skin Reactions

Advise patients of the possible occurrence of hand-foot skin reaction and rash during NEXAVAR treatment and appropriate countermeasures *[see Warnings and Precautions (5.4)]*.

17.5 Gastrointestinal Perforation

Advise patients that cases of gastrointestinal perforation have been reported in patients taking NEXAVAR *[see Warnings and Precautions (5.5)]*.

17.6 Wound Healing Complications

Inform patients that temporary interruption of NEXAVAR is recommended in patients undergoing major surgical procedures *[see Warnings and Precautions (5.7)]*.

17.7 QT Interval Prolongation

Inform patients with a history of prolonged QT interval that NEXAVAR can worsen the condition *[see Warnings and Precautions (5.9) and Clinical Pharmacology (12.2)]*.

17.8 Drug-Induced Hepatitis

Inform patients that NEXAVAR can cause hepatitis which may result in hepatic failure and death. Advise patients that liver function tests should be monitored regularly during treatment and to report signs and symptoms of hepatitis *[see Warnings and Precautions (5.10)]*.

17.9 Birth Defects and Fetal Loss

Inform patients that NEXAVAR can cause birth defects or fetal loss. Counsel both male and female patients to use effective birth control during treatment with NEXAVAR and for at least 2 weeks after stopping treatment. Inform female patients to contact their healthcare provider if they become pregnant while taking NEXAVAR *[see Warnings and Precautions (5.11), Use in Specific Populations (8.1)]*.

17.10 Nursing Mothers

Advise mothers not to breast-feed while taking NEXAVAR *[see Use in Specific Populations (8.3)]*.

17.11 Missed Doses

Instruct patients that if a dose of NEXAVAR is missed, to take the next dose at the regularly scheduled time, and not double the dose. Instruct patients to contact their healthcare provider immediately if they take too much NEXAVAR.

Patient Information

NEXAVAR® (NEX-A-VAR)

(sorafenib)

tablets, oral

Read this Patient Information before you start taking NEXAVAR and each time you get a refill. There may be new information. This information does not take the place of talking with your doctor about your medical condition or your treatment.

What is NEXAVAR?

NEXAVAR is an anticancer medicine used to treat a certain type of liver or kidney cancer called:

- Hepatocellular carcinoma (HCC, a type of liver cancer), when it can not be treated with surgery
- Renal cell carcinoma (RCC, a type of kidney cancer)

NEXAVAR has not been studied in children.

Who should not take NEXAVAR?

Do not take NEXAVAR if you:

- are allergic to sorafenib or any of the other ingredients of NEXAVAR. See the end of this leaflet for a complete list of ingredients in NEXAVAR.
- have a specific type of lung cancer (squamous cell) and receive carboplatin and paclitaxel.

What should I tell my doctor before taking NEXAVAR?

Before you take NEXAVAR, tell your doctor if you:

- have any allergies
- have heart problems, including a problem called "congenital long QT syndrome"
- have chest pain
- have bleeding problems
- have high blood pressure
- plan to have any surgical procedures
- have lung cancer or are being treated for lung cancer
- have kidney problems in addition to kidney cancer
- have liver problems in addition to liver cancer
- are pregnant or plan to become pregnant. See **"What are the possible side effects of NEXAVAR?"**
- are breast-feedingorplanning to breast-feed. It is not known if NEXAVAR passes into your breast milk. You and your doctor should decide if you will take NEXAVAR or breast-feed. You should not do both.

Tell your doctor about all the medicines you take, including prescription and non-prescription medicines, vitamins, and herbal supplements.

NEXAVAR and certain other medicines can interact with each other and cause serious side effects.

Especially tell your doctor if you are taking the following medicines:

- **warfarin (Coumadin, Jantoven®)**
- **neomycin**
- **St. Johns Wort**
- **dexamethasone**
- **phenytoin (Fosphenytoin sodium, Dilantin, Phenytek)**
- **carbamazepine (Carbatrol, Equetro, Tegretol. Teril, Epitol)**
- **rifampin (Rifater, Rifamate, Rifadin, Rimactane)**
- **rifabutin (Mycobutin)**
- **phenobarbital**

Know the medicines you take. Keep a list of your medicines and show it to your doctor and pharmacist when you get a new medicine. Do not take other medicines with NEXAVAR until you have talked with your doctor.

How should I take NEXAVAR?

- Take NEXAVAR exactly as prescribed by your doctor.
- The usual dose of NEXAVAR is 2 tablets taken two times a day (for a total of 4 tablets each day). Your doctor may change your dose during treatment or stop treatment for some time if you have side effects.

- Take NEXAVAR without food (at least 1 hour before or 2 hours after a meal).
- If you miss a dose of NEXAVAR, skip the missed dose, and take your next dose at your regular time. Do not double your dose of NEXAVAR.
- If you take too much NEXAVAR call your doctor or go to the nearest hospital emergency room right away.

What are the possible side effects of NEXAVAR?

NEXAVAR may cause serious side effects, including:

- **decreased blood flow to the heart and heart attack.** Get emergency help right away and call your doctor if you get symptoms such as chest pain, shortness of breath, feel lightheaded or faint, nausea, vomiting, sweating a lot.
- **bleeding problems.** NEXAVAR can cause bleeding which can be serious and sometimes lead to death. Tell your doctor if you have any bleeding while taking NEXAVAR.
- **high-blood pressure.** Your blood pressure should be checked every week during the first 6 weeks of starting NEXAVAR. Your blood pressure should be checked regularly and any high blood pressure should be treated while you are receiving NEXAVAR.
- **a skin problem called hand-foot skin reaction.** This causes redness, pain, swelling, or blisters on the palms of your hands or soles of your feet. If you get this side effect, your doctor may change your dose or stop treatment for some time.
- **serious skin and mouth reactions.** NEXAVAR can cause serious skin reactions which can be life-threatening. Tell your doctor if you have any of the following symptoms:
  - skin rash
  - blistering and peeling of the skin
  - blistering and peeling on the inside of your mouth
- **an opening in the wall of your stomach or intestines (perforation of the bowel).** Tell your doctor right away if you get high fever, nausea, vomiting, severe stomach or abdominal pain.
- **possible wound healing problems.** If you need to have a surgical procedure, tell your doctor that you are taking NEXAVAR. NEXAVAR may need to be stopped until your wound heals after some types of surgery.
- **changes in the electrical activity of your heart called QT prolongation.** QT prolongation can cause irregular heartbeats that can be life-threatening. Your doctor may do tests during your treatment with NEXAVAR to check the levels of potassium, magnesium, and calcium in your blood, and check the electrical activity of your heart with an ECG. Tell your doctor right away if you feel faint, lightheaded, dizzy or feel your heart beating irregularly or fast while taking NEXAVAR.
- **inflammation of your liver (drug-induced hepatitis).** NEXAVAR may cause liver problems that may lead to liver failure and death. Your doctor may stop your treatment with NEXAVAR if you develop changes in certain liver function tests. Call your doctor right away if you develop any of the following symptoms:
  - your skin or the white part of your eyes turns yellow (jaundice)
  - dark "tea-colored" urine
  - light-colored bowel movements (stools)
  - worsening nausea
  - worsening vomiting
  - abdominal pain
- **birth defects or death of an unborn baby.** Women should not get pregnant during treatment with NEXAVAR and for at least 2 weeks after stopping treatment. Men and women should use effective birth control during treatment with NEXAVAR and for at least 2 weeks after stopping treatment. Talk with your doctor about effective birth control methods.Call your doctor right away if you become pregnant during treatment with NEXAVAR.

The most common side effects of NEXAVAR include:

- rash, redness, itching or peeling of your skin
- hairthinning or patchy hair loss
- diarrhea(frequent or loose bowel movements)
- nausea or vomiting
- lossof appetite
- abdominalpain
- tiredness
- weightloss

Tell your doctor if you have any side effect that bothers you or that does not go away. These are not all the possible side effects of NEXAVAR. Ask your doctor or pharmacist for more information.

Call your doctor for medical advice about side effects. You may report side effects to FDA at 1-800-FDA-1088.

How should I store NEXAVAR?

- Store NEXAVAR tablets at room temperature between 68° F to 77° F (20° C to 25° C).
- Store NEXAVAR tablets in a dry place.

Keep NEXAVAR and all medicines out of the reach of children.

General information about NEXAVAR

Medicines are sometimes prescribed for purposes other than those listed in the Patient Information leaflet. Do not use NEXAVAR for a condition for which it is not prescribed. Do not give NEXAVAR to other people even if they have the same symptoms you have. It may harm them.

This Patient Information leaflet summarizes the most important information about NEXAVAR. If you would like more information, talk with your doctor. You can ask your doctor or pharmacist for information about NEXAVAR that is written for healthcare professionals.

For more information, go to www.NEXAVAR.com, or call (1-866-639-2827).

What are the ingredients in NEXAVAR?

Active Ingredient: sorafenib tosylate

Inactive Ingredients: croscarmellose sodium, microcrystalline cellulose, hypromellose, sodium lauryl sulphate, magnesium stearate, polyethylene glycol, titanium dioxide and ferric oxide red.

This Patient Information has been approved by the U.S. Food and Drug Administration.

Manufactured for:
Bayer HealthCare Pharmaceuticals Inc.,
Wayne, NJ 07470
Manufactured in Germany
Onyx Pharmaceuticals, Inc.,
249 East Grand Avenue, South San Francisco, CA 94080
Distributed and marketed by:
Bayer HealthCare Pharmaceuticals Inc.,
Wayne, NJ 07470
Marketed by:
Onyx Pharmaceuticals, Inc.
249 East Grand Avenue, South San Francisco, CA 94080

Revised: 06/13
80771372, R.9

Shown in Product Identification Guide, page 305

STIVARGA ℞
(regorafenib)
tablets, for oral use

HIGHLIGHTS OF PRESCRIBING INFORMATION
These highlights do not include all the information needed to use STIVARGA safely and effectively. See full prescribing information for STIVARGA.
STIVARGA (regorafenib) tablets, for oral use
Initial U.S. Approval: 2012

WARNING: HEPATOTOXICITY
See full prescribing information for complete boxed warning.
- **Severe and sometimes fatal hepatotoxicity has been observed in clinical trials. (5.1)**
- **Monitor hepatic function prior to and during treatment. (5.1)**
- **Interrupt and then reduce or discontinue Stivarga for hepatotoxicity as manifested by elevated liver function tests or hepatocellular necrosis, depending upon severity and persistence. (2.2)**

RECENT MAJOR CHANGES

Indications and Usage (1.2)	02/2013
Warnings and Precautions (5.1, 5.2, 5.3, 5.4, 5.5)	02/2013

INDICATIONS AND USAGE

Stivarga is a kinase inhibitor indicated for the treatment of patients with:

- Metastatic colorectal cancer (CRC) who have been previously treated with fluoropyrimidine-, oxaliplatin- and irinotecan-based chemotherapy, an anti-VEGF therapy, and, if KRAS wild type, an anti-EGFR therapy. (1.1)
- Locally advanced, unresectable or metastatic gastrointestinal stromal tumor (GIST) who have been previously treated with imatinib mesylate and sunitinib malate. (1.2)

DOSAGE AND ADMINISTRATION

- Recommended Dose: 160 mg orally, once daily for the first 21 days of each 28-day cycle. (2.1)
- Take Stivarga with food (a low-fat breakfast). (2.1, 12.3)

DOSAGE FORMS AND STRENGTHS

40 mg film-coated tablets (3)

CONTRAINDICATIONS

None. (4)

WARNINGS AND PRECAUTIONS

- Hemorrhage: Permanently discontinue Stivarga for severe or life-threatening hemorrhage. (5.2)
- Dermatological toxicity: Interrupt and then reduce or discontinue Stivarga depending on severity and persistence of dermatologic toxicity. (5.3)
- Hypertension: Temporarily or permanently discontinue Stivarga for severe or uncontrolled hypertension. (5.4)
- Cardiac ischemia and infarction: Withhold Stivarga for new or acute cardiac ischemia/infarction and resume only after resolution of acute ischemic events. (5.5)
- Reversible Posterior Leukoencephalopathy Syndrome (RPLS): Discontinue Stivarga. (5.6)
- Gastrointestinal perforation or fistulae: Discontinue Stivarga. (5.7)
- Wound healing complications: Stop Stivarga before surgery. Discontinue in patients with wound dehiscence. (5.8)
- Embryofetal toxicity: Can cause fetal harm. Advise women of potential risk to a fetus. (5.9, 8.1)

ADVERSE REACTIONS

The most common adverse reactions (≥20%) are asthenia/fatigue, HFSR, diarrhea, decreased appetite/food intake, hypertension, mucositis, dysphonia, and infection, pain (not otherwise specified), decreased weight, gastrointestinal and abdominal pain, rash, fever, and nausea. (6)

To report SUSPECTED ADVERSE REACTIONS, contact Bayer HealthCare Pharmaceuticals Inc. at 1-888-842-2937 or FDA at 1-800-FDA-1088 or www.fda.gov/medwatch

DRUG INTERACTIONS

- Strong CYP3A4 inducers: Avoid strong CYP3A4 inducers. (7.1)
- Strong CYP3A4 inhibitors: Avoid strong CYP3A4 inhibitors. (7.2)

USE IN SPECIFIC POPULATIONS

Nursing Mothers: Discontinue drug or nursing, taking into consideration the importance of the drug to the mother. (8.3)

See 17 for PATIENT COUNSELING INFORMATION and FDA-approved patient labeling

Revised: 08/2013

FULL PRESCRIBING INFORMATION: CONTENTS*

*** Sections or subsections omitted from the full prescribing information are not listed**

FULL PRESCRIBING INFORMATION

WARNING: HEPATOTOXICITY
- **Severe and sometimes fatal hepatotoxicity has been observed in clinical trials** ***[see Warnings and Precautions (5.1)].***
- **Monitor hepatic function prior to and during treatment** ***[see Warnings and Precautions (5.1)].***
- **Interrupt and then reduce or discontinue Stivarga for hepatotoxicity as manifested by elevated liver function tests or hepatocellular necrosis, depending upon severity and persistence** ***[see Dosage and Administration (2.2)].***

1 INDICATIONS AND USAGE

1.1 Colorectal Cancer

Stivarga® is indicated for the treatment of patients with metastatic colorectal cancer (CRC) who have been previously treated with fluoropyrimidine-, oxaliplatin- and irinotecan-based chemotherapy, an anti-VEGF therapy, and, if KRAS wild type, an anti-EGFR therapy.

1.2 Gastrointestinal Stromal Tumors

Stivarga is indicated for the treatment of patients with locally advanced, unresectable or metastatic gastrointestinal stromal tumor (GIST) who have been previously treated with imatinib mesylate and sunitinib malate.

2 DOSAGE AND ADMINISTRATION

2.1 Recommended Dose

The recommended dose is 160 mg regorafenib (four 40 mg tablets) taken orally once daily for the first 21 days of each 28-day cycle. Continue treatment until disease progression or unacceptable toxicity.

Take Stivarga at the same time each day. Swallow tablet whole with a low-fat breakfast that contains less than 30% fat *[see Clinical Pharmacology (12.3)]*. Examples of a low-fat breakfast include 2 slices of white toast with 1 tablespoon of low fat margarine and 1 tablespoon of jelly, and 8 ounces of skim milk (319 calories and 8.2 g fat); or 1 cup of cereal, 8 ounces of skim milk, 1 slice of toast with jam, apple juice, and 1 cup of coffee or tea (520 calories and 2 g fat). Do not take two doses of Stivarga on the same day to make up for a missed dose from the previous day.

2.2 Dose Modifications

Interrupt Stivarga for the following:
- NCI CTCAE Grade 2 hand-foot skin reaction (HFSR) [palmar-plantar erythrodysesthesia (PPE)] that is recurrent or does not improve within 7 days despite dose reduction; interrupt therapy for a minimum of 7 days for Grade 3 HFSR
- Symptomatic Grade 2 hypertension
- Any NCI CTCAE Grade 3 or 4 adverse reaction

Reduce the dose of Stivarga to 120 mg:
- For the first occurrence of Grade 2 HFSR of any duration
- After recovery of any Grade 3 or 4 adverse reaction
- For Grade 3 aspartate aminotransferase (AST)/alanine aminotransferase (ALT) elevation; only resume if the potential benefit outweighs the risk of hepatotoxicity

Reduce the dose of Stivarga to 80 mg:
- For re-occurrence of Grade 2 HFSR at the 120 mg dose
- After recovery of any Grade 3 or 4 adverse reaction at the 120 mg dose (except hepatotoxicity)

Discontinue Stivarga permanently for the following:
- Failure to tolerate 80 mg dose
- Any occurrence of AST or ALT more than 20 times the upper limit of normal (ULN)
- Any occurrence of AST or ALT more than 3 times ULN with concurrent bilirubin more than 2 times ULN
- Re-occurrence of AST or ALT more than 5 times ULN despite dose reduction to 120 mg
- For any Grade 4 adverse reaction; only resume if the potential benefit outweighs the risks

3 DOSAGE FORMS AND STRENGTHS

Stivarga is a 40 mg, light pink, oval shaped, film-coated tablet, debossed with 'BAYER' on one side and '40' on the other side.

4 CONTRAINDICATIONS

None

5 WARNINGS AND PRECAUTIONS

5.1 Hepatotoxicity

Severe drug induced liver injury with fatal outcome occurred in 0.3% of 1200 Stivarga-treated patients across all clinical trials. Liver biopsy results, when available, showed hepatocyte necrosis with lymphocyte infiltration. In Study 1, fatal hepatic failure occurred in 1.6% of patients in the regorafenib arm and in 0.4% of patients in the placebo arm; all the patients with hepatic failure had metastatic disease in the liver. In Study 2, fatal hepatic failure occurred in 0.8% of patients in the regorafenib arm *[see Adverse Reactions (6.1)]*.

Obtain liver function tests (ALT, AST and bilirubin) before initiation of Stivarga and monitor at least every two weeks during the first 2 months of treatment. Thereafter, monitor monthly or more frequently as clinically indicated. Monitor liver function tests weekly in patients experiencing elevated liver function tests until improvement to less than 3 times the ULN or baseline.

Temporarily hold and then reduce or permanently discontinue Stivarga depending on the severity and persistence of hepatotoxicity as manifested by elevated liver function tests or hepatocellular necrosis *[see Dosage and Administration (2.2)]*.

Table 1 Adverse drug reactions (≥10%) reported in patients treated with Stivarga in Study 1 and reported more commonly than in patients receiving placebo

Adverse Reactions	Stivarga (N=500)		Placebo (N=253)	
	Grade		Grade	
	All %	≥ 3 %	All %	≥ 3 %
General disorders and administration site conditions				
Asthenia/fatigue	64	15	46	9
Pain	29	3	21	2
Fever	28	2	15	0
Metabolism and nutrition disorders				
Decreased appetite and food intake	47	5	28	4
Skin and subcutaneous tissue disorders				
HFSR/PPE	45	17	7	0
Rash [a]	26	6	4	<1
Gastrointestinal disorders				
Diarrhea	43	8	17	2
Mucositis	33	4	5	0
Investigations				
Weight loss	32	<1	10	0
Infections and infestations				
Infection	31	9	17	6
Vascular disorders				
Hypertension	30	8	8	<1
Hemorrhage [b]	21	2	8	<1
Respiratory, thoracic and mediastinal disorders				
Dysphonia	30	0	6	0
Nervous system disorders				
Headache	10	<1	7	0

[a] The term rash represents reports of events of drug eruption, rash, erythematous rash, generalized rash, macular rash, maculo-papular rash, papular rash, and pruritic rash.
[b] Fatal outcomes observed.

Table 2 Laboratory test abnormalities reported in Study 1

Laboratory Parameter	Stivarga (N=500 [a])			Placebo (N=253 [a])		
	Grade [b]			Grade [b]		
	All %	3 %	4 %	All %	3 %	4 %
Blood and lymphatic system disorders						
Anemia	79	5	1	66	3	0
Thrombocytopenia	41	2	<1	17	<1	0
Neutropenia	3	1	0	0	0	0
Lymphopenia	54	9	0	34	3	0
Metabolism and nutrition disorders						
Hypocalcemia	59	1	<1	18	1	0
Hypokalemia	26	4	0	8	<1	0
Hyponatremia	30	7	1	22	4	0
Hypophosphatemia	57	31	1	11	4	0
Hepatobiliary disorders						
Hyperbilirubinemia	45	10	3	17	5	3
Increased AST	65	5	1	46	4	1
Increased ALT	45	5	1	30	3	<1
Renal and urinary disorders						
Proteinuria	60	<1	0	34	<1	0
Investigations						
Increased INR [c]	24	4	N/A	17	2	N/A
Increased Lipase	46	9	2	19	3	2
Increased Amylase	26	2	<1	17	2	<1

[a] % based on number of patients with post-baseline samples which may be less than 500 (regorafenib) or 253 (placebo).
[b] Common Terminology Criteria for Adverse Events (CTCAE), v3.0.
[c] International normalized ratio: No Grade 4 denoted in CTCAE, v3.0.

Table 3 Adverse reactions (≥10%) reported in patients treated with Stivarga in Study 2 and reported more commonly than in patients receiving placebo

Adverse Reactions	Stivarga (N=132)		Placebo (N=66)	
	Grade		Grade	
	All %	≥ 3 %	All %	≥ 3 %
Skin and subcutaneous tissue disorders				
HFSR/PPE	67	22	15	2
Rash [a]	30	7	3	0
Alopecia	24	2	2	0
General disorders and administration site conditions				
Asthenia/Fatigue	52	4	39	2
Fever	21	0	11	2
Vascular disorders				
Hypertension	59	28	27	5
Hemorrhage	11	4	3	0
Gastrointestinal disorders				
Diarrhea	47	8	9	0
Mucositis	40	2	8	2
Nausea	20	2	12	2
Vomiting	17	<1	8	0
Respiratory, thoracic and mediastinal disorders				
Dysphonia	39	0	9	0
Infections and infestations				
Infection	32	5	5	0
Metabolism and nutrition disorders				
Decreased appetite and food intake	31	<1	21	3
Hypothyroidism [b]	18	0	6	0
Nervous system disorders				
Headache	16	0	9	0
Investigations				
Weight loss	14	0	8	0
Musculoskeletal and connective tissue disorders				
Musculoskeletal stiffness	14	0	3	0

[a] The term rash represents reports of events of rash, erythematous rash, macular rash, maculo-papular rash, papular rash and pruritic rash.
[b] Hypothyroidism incidence based on subset of patients with normal TSH and no thyroid supplementation at baseline.

5.2 Hemorrhage

Stivarga caused an increased incidence of hemorrhage. The overall incidence (Grades 1-5) was 21% and 11% in Stivarga-treated patients compared to 8% and 3% in placebo-treated patients in Studies 1 and 2. Fatal hemorrhage occurred in 4 of 632 (0.6%) of Stivarga-treated patients in Studies 1 and 2 and involved the respiratory, gastrointestinal, or genitourinary tracts.

Permanently discontinue Stivarga in patients with severe or life-threatening hemorrhage. Monitor INR levels more frequently in patients receiving warfarin *[see Clinical Pharmacology (12.3)]*.

5.3 Dermatological Toxicity

Stivarga caused increased incidences of adverse reactions involving the skin and subcutaneous tissues (72% versus 24% in Study 1 and 78% versus 24% in Study 2), including hand-foot skin reaction (HFSR) also known as palmar-plantar erythrodysesthesia (PPE), and severe rash requiring dose modification.

The overall incidence of HFSR was higher in Stivarga-treated patients, (45% versus 7% in Study 1 and 67% versus 12% in Study 2), than in the placebo-treated patients. Most cases of HFSR in Stivarga-treated patients appeared during the first cycle of treatment (69% and 71% of patients who developed HFSR in Study 1 and Study 2, respectively). The incidence of Grade 3 HFSR (17% versus 0% in Study 1 and 22% versus 0% in Study 2), Grade 3 rash (6% versus <1% in Study 1 and 7% versus 0% in Study 2), serious adverse reactions of erythema multiforme (0.2% vs. 0% in Study 1) and Stevens Johnson Syndrome (0.2% vs. 0% in Study 1) was higher in Stivarga-treated patients *[see Adverse Reactions (6.1)]*.

Toxic epidermal necrolysis occurred in 0.17% of 1200 Stivarga-treated patients across all clinical trials.

Withhold Stivarga, reduce the dose, or permanently discontinue Stivarga depending on the severity and persistence of dermatologic toxicity *[see Dosage and Administration (2.2)]*. Institute supportive measures for symptomatic relief.

5.4 Hypertension

Stivarga caused an increased incidence of hypertension (30% versus 8% in Study 1 and 59% versus 27% in Study 2) *[see Adverse Reactions (6.1)]*. Hypertensive crisis occurred in 0.25% of 1200 Stivarga-treated patients across all clinical trials. The onset of hypertension occurred during the first cycle of treatment in most patients who developed hypertension (72% in Study 1 and Study 2).

Do not initiate Stivarga unless blood pressure is adequately controlled. Monitor blood pressure weekly for the first 6 weeks of treatment and then every cycle, or more frequently, as clinically indicated. Temporarily or permanently withhold Stivarga for severe or uncontrolled hypertension *[see Dosage and Administration (2.2)]*.

5.5 Cardiac Ischemia and Infarction

Stivarga increased the incidence of myocardial ischemia and infarction in Study 1 (1.2% versus 0.4%) *[see Adverse Reactions (6.1)]*. Withhold Stivarga in patients who develop new or acute onset cardiac ischemia or infarction. Resume Stivarga only after resolution of acute cardiac ischemic events, if the potential benefits outweigh the risks of further cardiac ischemia.

5.6 Reversible Posterior Leukoencephalopathy Syndrome (RPLS)

Reversible Posterior Leukoencephalopathy Syndrome (RPLS), a syndrome of subcortical vasogenic edema diagnosed by characteristic finding on MRI, occurred in one of 1200 Stivarga-treated patients across all clinical trials. Perform an evaluation for RPLS in any patient presenting with seizures, headache, visual disturbances, confusion or altered mental function. Discontinue Stivarga in patients who develop RPLS.

5.7 Gastrointestinal Perforation or Fistula

Gastrointestinal perforation or fistula occurred in 0.6% of 1200 patients treated with Stivarga across all clinical trials; this included four fatal events. In Study 2, 2.1 % (4/188) of Stivarga-treated patients who were treated during the blinded or open-label portion of the study developed gastrointestinal fistula or perforation; of these, two cases of gastrointestinal perforation were fatal. Permanently discontinue Stivarga in patients who develop gastrointestinal perforation or fistula.

5.8 Wound Healing Complications

No formal studies of the effect of regorafenib on wound healing have been conducted. Since vascular endothelial growth factor receptor (VEGFR) inhibitors such as regorafenib can impair wound healing, treatment with regorafenib should be stopped at least 2 weeks prior to scheduled surgery. The decision to resume regorafenib after surgery should be based on clinical judgment of adequate wound healing. Regorafenib should be discontinued in patients with wound dehiscence.

5.9 Embryo-Fetal Toxicity

Stivarga can cause fetal harm when administered to a pregnant woman. Regorafenib was embryolethal and teratogenic in rats and rabbits at exposures lower than human exposures at the recommended dose, with increased incidences of cardiovascular, genitourinary, and skeletal malformations. If this drug is used during pregnancy, or if the patient becomes pregnant while taking this drug, the patient should be apprised of the potential hazard to a fetus *[see Use in Specific Populations (8.1)]*.

6 ADVERSE REACTIONS

The following serious adverse reactions are discussed elsewhere in the labeling:

- Hepatotoxicity *[See Warnings and Precautions (5.1)]*
- Hemorrhage *[See Warnings and Precautions (5.2)]*
- Dermatological Toxicity *[See Warnings and Precautions (5.3)]*
- Hypertension *[See Warnings and Precautions (5.4)]*
- Cardiac Ischemia and Infarction *[See Warnings and Precautions (5.5)]*
- Reversible Posterior Leukoencephalopathy Syndrome (RPLS) *[See Warnings and Precautions (5.6)]*
- Gastrointestinal Perforation or Fistula *[See Warnings and Precautions (5.7)]*

Because clinical trials are conducted under widely varying conditions, adverse reaction rates observed in the clinical trials of a drug cannot be directly compared to rates in the clinical trials of another drug and may not reflect the rate observed in practice.

The most frequently observed adverse drug reactions (≥20%) in patients receiving Stivarga are asthenia/fatigue, HFSR, diarrhea, decreased appetite/food intake, hypertension, mucositis, dysphonia, infection, pain (not otherwise specified), decreased weight, gastrointestinal and abdominal pain, rash, fever, and nausea.

The most serious adverse drug reactions in patients receiving Stivarga are hepatotoxicity, hemorrhage, and gastrointestinal perforation.

6.1 Clinical Trials Experience

Colorectal Cancer

The safety data described below, except where noted, are derived from a randomized (2:1), double-blind, placebo-controlled trial (Study 1) in which 500 patients (median age 61 years; 61% men) with previously treated metastatic colorectal cancer received Stivarga as a single agent at the dose of 160 mg daily for the first 3 weeks of each 4 week treatment cycle and 253 patients (median age 61 years; 60% men) received placebo. The median duration of therapy was 7.3 (range 0.3, 47.0) weeks for patients receiving Stivarga. Due to adverse reactions, 61% of the patients receiving Stivarga required a dose interruption and 38% of the patients had their dose reduced. Drug-related adverse reactions that resulted in treatment discontinuation were reported in 8.2% of Stivarga-treated patients compared to 1.2% of patients who received placebo. Hand-foot skin reaction (HFSR) and rash were the most common reasons for permanent discontinuation of Stivarga.

Table 1 compares the incidence of adverse reactions (≥10%) in patients receiving Stivarga and reported more commonly than in patients receiving placebo (Study 1).

[See table 1 at top of previous page]

Laboratory Abnormalities

Laboratory abnormalities observed in Study 1 are shown in Table 2.

[See table 2 at top of previous page]

Gastrointestinal Stromal Tumors

The safety data described below are derived from a randomized (2:1), double-blind, placebo-controlled trial (Study 2) in which 132 patients (median age 60 years; 64% men) with previously treated GIST received Stivarga as a single agent at a dose of 160 mg daily for the first 3 weeks of each 4 week treatment cycle and 66 patients (median age 61 years; 64% men) received placebo. The median duration of therapy was 22.9 (range 0.1, 50.9) weeks for patients receiving Stivarga. Dose interruptions for adverse events were required in 58% of patients receiving Stivarga and 50% of patients had their dose reduced. Drug-related adverse reactions that resulted in treatment discontinuation were reported in 2.3% of Stivarga-treated patients compared to 1.5% of patients who received placebo.

Table 3 compares the incidence of adverse reactions (≥10%) in GIST patients receiving Stivarga and reported more commonly than in patients receiving placebo (Study 2).

[See table 3 at top of previous page]

Laboratory Abnormalities

Laboratory abnormalities observed in Study 2 are shown in Table 4.

[See table 4 above]

Table 4 Laboratory test abnormalities reported in Study 2

Laboratory Parameter	Stivarga (N=132 [a]) Grade [b]			Placebo (N=66 [a]) Grade [b]		
	All %	3 %	4 %	All %	3 %	4 %
Blood and lymphatic system disorders						
Thrombocytopenia	13	1	0	2	0	2
Neutropenia	16	2	0	12	3	0
Lymphopenia	30	8	0	24	3	0
Metabolism and nutrition disorders						
Hypocalcemia	17	2	0	5	0	0
Hypokalemia	21	3	0	3	0	0
Hypophosphatemia	55	20	2	3	2	0
Hepatobiliary disorders						
Hyperbilirubinemia	33	3	1	12	2	0
Increased AST	58	3	1	47	3	0
Increased ALT	39	4	1	39	2	0
Renal and urinary disorders						
Proteinuria	33	3	- [c]	30	3	- [c]
Investigations						
Increased Lipase	14	0	1	5	0	0

[a] % based on number of patients with post-baseline samples which may be less than 132 (regorafenib) or 66 (placebo).
[b] CTCAE, v4.0.
[c] No Grade 4 denoted in CTCAE, v4.0.

7 DRUG INTERACTIONS

7.1 Effect of Strong CYP3A4 Inducers on Regorafenib

Co-administration of a strong CYP3A4 inducer (rifampin) with a single 160 mg dose of Stivarga decreased the mean exposure of regorafenib, increased the mean exposure of the active metabolite M-5, and resulted in no change in the mean exposure of the active metabolite M-2. Avoid concomitant use of Stivarga with strong CYP3A4 inducers (e.g. rifampin, phenytoin, carbamazepine, phenobarbital, and St. John's Wort) *[see Clinical Pharmacology (12.3)]*.

7.2 Effect of Strong CYP3A4 Inhibitors on Regorafenib

Co-administration of a strong CYP3A4 inhibitor (ketoconazole) with a single 160 mg dose of Stivarga increased the mean exposure of regorafenib and decreased the mean exposure of the active metabolites M-2 and M-5. Avoid concomitant use of Stivarga with strong inhibitors of CYP3A4 activity (e.g. clarithromycin, grapefruit juice, itraconazole, ketoconazole, nefazadone, posaconazole, telithromycin, and voriconazole) *[see Clinical Pharmacology (12.3)]*.

8 USE IN SPECIFIC POPULATIONS

8.1 Pregnancy

Pregnancy Category D *[see Warnings and Precautions (5.9)]*

Risk Summary

Based on its mechanism of action, Stivarga can cause fetal harm when administered to a pregnant woman. There are no adequate and well-controlled studies with Stivarga in pregnant women. Regorafenib was embryolethal and teratogenic in rats and rabbits at exposures lower than human exposures at the recommended dose, with increased incidences of cardiovascular, genitourinary, and skeletal malformations. If this drug is used during pregnancy or if the patient becomes pregnant while taking this drug, the patient should be apprised of the potential hazard to a fetus.

Animal Data

In embryo-fetal development studies, a total loss of pregnancy (100% resorption of litter) was observed in rats at doses as low as 1 mg/kg (approximately 6% of the recommended human dose, based on body surface area) and in rabbits at doses as low as 1.6 mg/kg (approximately 25% of the human exposure at the clinically recommended dose measured by AUC).

In a single dose distribution study in pregnant rats, there was increased penetration of regorafenib across the blood-brain barrier in fetuses compared to dams. In a repeat dose study with daily administration of regorafenib to pregnant rats during organogenesis, findings included delayed ossification in fetuses at doses ≥ 0.8 mg/kg (approximately 5% of the recommended human dose based on body surface area) with dose-dependent increases in skeletal malformations including cleft palate and enlarged fontanelle at doses ≥ 1 mg/kg (approximately 10% of the clinical exposure based on AUC). At doses ≥ 1.6 mg/kg (approximately 11% of the recommended human dose based on body surface area), there were dose-dependent increases in the incidence of cardiovascular malformations, external abnormalities, diaphragmatic hernia, and dilation of the renal pelvis.

In pregnant rabbits administered regorafenib daily during organogenesis, there were findings of ventricular septal defects evident at the lowest tested dose of 0.4 mg/kg (approximately 7% of the AUC in patients at the recommended dose). At doses of ≥ 0.8 mg/kg (approximately 15% of the human exposure at the recommended human dose based on AUC), administration of regorafenib resulted in dose-dependent increases in the incidence of additional cardiovascular malformations and skeletal anomalies as well as significant adverse effects on the urinary system including missing kidney/ureter; small, deformed and malpositioned kidney; and hydronephrosis. The proportion of viable fetuses that were male decreased with increasing dose in two rabbit embryo-fetal toxicity studies.

8.3 Nursing Mothers

It is unknown whether regorafenib or its metabolites are excreted in human milk. In rats, regorafenib and its metabolites are excreted in milk. Because many drugs are excreted in human milk and because of the potential for serious adverse reactions in nursing infants from Stivarga, a decision should be made whether to discontinue nursing or discontinue the drug, taking into account the importance of the drug to the mother.

8.4 Pediatric Use

The safety and efficacy of Stivarga in pediatric patients less than 18 years of age have not been established.

In 28 day repeat dose studies in rats there were dose-dependent findings of dentin alteration and angiectasis. These findings were observed at regorafenib doses as low as 4 mg/kg (approximately 25% of the AUC in humans at the recommended dose). In 13-week repeat dose studies in dogs there were similar findings of dentin alteration at doses as low as 20 mg/kg (approximately 43% of the AUC in humans at the recommended dose). Administration of regorafenib in these animals also led to persistent growth and thickening of the femoral epiphyseal growth plate.

8.5 Geriatric Use

Of the 632 Stivarga-treated patients enrolled in Studies 1 and 2, 37% were 65 years of age or older and over, while 8% were 75 and over. No overall differences in safety or efficacy were observed between these patients and younger patients.

8.6 Hepatic Impairment

No clinically important differences in the mean exposure of regorafenib or the active metabolites M-2 and M-5 were observed in patients with hepatocellular carcinoma and mild (Child-Pugh A) or moderate (Child-Pugh B) hepatic impairment compared to patients with normal hepatic function *[see Clinical Pharmacology (12.3)]*. No dose adjustment is recommended in patients with mild or moderate hepatic impairment. Closely monitor patients with hepatic impairment for adverse reactions *[see Warnings and Precautions (5.1)]*.

Stivarga is not recommended for use in patients with severe hepatic impairment (Child-Pugh Class C), as it has not been studied in this population.

8.7 Renal Impairment

No clinically relevant differences in the mean exposure of regorafenib and the active metabolites M-2 and M-5 were observed in patients with mild renal impairment (CLcr 60-89 mL/min) compared to patients with normal renal function following regorafenib 160 mg daily for 21 days *[see Clinical Pharmacology (12.3)]*. No dose adjustment is recommended for patients with mild renal impairment. Limited pharmacokinetic data are available from patients with moderate renal impairment (CLcr 30-59 mL/min). Stivarga has not been studied in patients with severe renal impairment or end-stage renal disease.

8.8 Females and Males of Reproductive Potential

Contraception

Use effective contraception during treatment and up to 2 months after completion of therapy.

Infertility

There are no data on the effect of Stivarga on human fertility. Results from animal studies indicate that regorafenib can impair male and female fertility *[see Nonclinical Toxicology (13.1)]*.

10 OVERDOSAGE

The highest dose of Stivarga studied clinically is 220 mg per day. In the event of suspected overdose, interrupt Stivarga, institute supportive care, and observe until clinical stabilization.

11 DESCRIPTION

Stivarga (regorafenib) has the chemical name 4-[4-({[4-chloro-3-(trifluoromethyl) phenyl] carbamoyl} amino)-3-fluorophenoxy]-N-methylpyridine-2-carboxamide monohydrate. Regorafenib has the following structural formula:

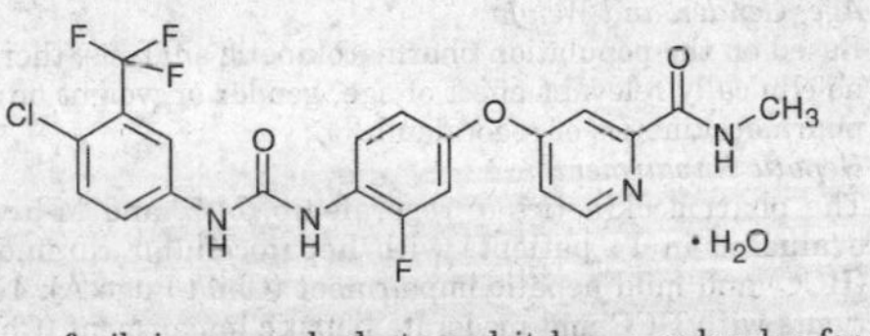

Regorafenib is a monohydrate and it has a molecular formula $C_{21}H_{15}ClF_4N_4O_3 \cdot H_2O$ and a molecular weight of 500.83. Regorafenib is practically insoluble in water, slightly soluble in acetonitrile, methanol, ethanol, and ethyl acetate and sparingly soluble in acetone.

Stivarga tablets for oral administration are formulated as light pink oval shaped tablets debossed with "BAYER" on one side and "40" on the other. Each tablet contains 40 mg of regorafenib in the anhydrous state, which corresponds to 41.49 mg of regorafenib monohydrate, and the following inactive ingredients: cellulose microcrystalline, croscarmellose sodium, magnesium stearate, povidone, and colloidal silicon dioxide. The film-coating contains the following inactive ingredients: ferric oxide red, ferric oxide yellow, lecithin (soy), polyethylene glycol 3350, polyvinyl alcohol, talc, and titanium dioxide.

12 CLINICAL PHARMACOLOGY

12.1 Mechanism of Action

Regorafenib is a small molecule inhibitor of multiple membrane-bound and intracellular kinases involved in normal cellular functions and in pathologic processes such as oncogenesis, tumor angiogenesis, and maintenance of the tumor microenvironment. In *in vitro* biochemical or cellular assays, regorafenib or its major human active metabolites M-2 and M-5 inhibited the activity of RET, VEGFR1, VEGFR2, VEGFR3, KIT, PDGFR-alpha, PDGFR-beta, FGFR1, FGFR2, TIE2, DDR2, TrkA, Eph2A, RAF-1, BRAF, $BRAF^{V600E}$, SAPK2, PTK5, and Abl at concentrations of regorafenib that have been achieved clinically. In *in vivo* models, regorafenib demonstrated anti-angiogenic activity in a rat tumor model, and inhibition of tumor growth as well as anti-metastatic activity in several mouse xenograft models including some for human colorectal carcinoma.

12.3 Pharmacokinetics

Absorption

Following a single 160 mg dose of Stivarga in patients with advanced solid tumors, regorafenib reaches a geometric mean peak plasma level (C_{max}) of 2.5 μg/mL at a median time of 4 hours and a geometric mean area under the plasma concentration vs. time curve (AUC) of 70.4 μg*h/mL. The AUC of regorafenib at steady-state increases less than dose proportionally at doses greater than 60 mg. At steady-state, regorafenib reaches a geometric mean C_{max} of

3.9 μg/mL and a geometric mean AUC of 58.3 μg*h/mL. The coefficient of variation of AUC and C_{max} is between 35% and 44%.

The mean relative bioavailability of tablets compared to an oral solution is 69% to 83%.

In a food-effect study, 24 healthy men received a single 160 mg dose of Stivarga on three separate occasions: under a fasted state, with a high-fat meal and with a low-fat meal. A high-fat meal (945 calories and 54.6 g fat) increased the mean AUC of regorafenib by 48% and decreased the mean AUC of the M-2 and M-5 metabolites by 20% and 51%, respectively, as compared to the fasted state. A low-fat meal (319 calories and 8.2 g fat) increased the mean AUC of regorafenib, M-2 and M-5 by 36%, 40% and 23%, respectively as compared to fasted conditions. Stivarga was administered with a low-fat meal in Studies 1 and 2 *[see Dosage and Administration (2.1), Clinical Studies (14)]*.

Distribution

Regorafenib undergoes enterohepatic circulation with multiple plasma concentration peaks observed across the 24-hour dosing interval. Regorafenib is highly bound (99.5%) to human plasma proteins.

Metabolism

Regorafenib is metabolized by CYP3A4 and UGT1A9. The main circulating metabolites of regorafenib measured at steady-state in human plasma are M-2 (N-oxide) and M-5 (N-oxide and N-desmethyl), both of them having similar *in vitro* pharmacological activity and steady-state concentrations as regorafenib. M-2 and M-5 are highly protein bound (99.8% and 99.95%, respectively).

Elimination

Following a single 160 mg oral dose of Stivarga, the geometric mean (range) elimination half-lives for regorafenib and the M-2 metabolite in plasma are 28 hours (14 to 58 hours) and 25 hours (14 to 32 hours), respectively. M-5 has a longer mean (range) elimination half-life of 51 hours (32 to 70 hours).

Approximately 71% of a radiolabeled dose was excreted in feces (47% as parent compound, 24% as metabolites) and 19% of the dose was excreted in urine (17% as glucuronides) within 12 days after administration of a radiolabeled oral solution at a dose of 120 mg.

Age, Gender, and Weight

Based on the population pharmacokinetic analysis, there is no clinically relevant effect of age, gender or weight on the pharmacokinetics of regorafenib.

Hepatic Impairment

The pharmacokinetics of regorafenib, M-2, and M-5 was evaluated in 14 patients with hepatocellular carcinoma (HCC) and mild hepatic impairment (Child-Pugh A); 4 patients with HCC and moderate hepatic impairment (Child-Pugh B); and 10 patients with solid tumors and normal hepatic function after the administration of a single 100 mg dose of Stivarga. No clinically important differences in the mean exposure of regorafenib, M-2, or M-5 were observed in patients with mild or moderate hepatic impairment compared to the patients with normal hepatic function. The pharmacokinetics of regorafenib has not been studied in patients with severe hepatic impairment (Child-Pugh C).

Renal Impairment

The pharmacokinetics of regorafenib, M-2, and M-5 was evaluated in 10 patients with mild renal impairment (CLcr 60-89 mL/min) and 18 patients with normal renal function following the administration of Stivarga at a dose of 160 mg daily for 21 days. No differences in the mean steady-state exposure of regorafenib, M-2, or M-5 were observed in patients with mild renal impairment compared to patients with normal renal function. Limited pharmacokinetic data are available from patients with moderate renal impairment (CLcr 30-59 mL/min). The pharmacokinetics of regorafenib has not been studied in patients with severe renal impairment or end-stage renal disease.

Drug-Drug Interactions

Effect of Regorafenib on Cytochrome P450 Substrates: In vitro studies suggested that regorafenib is an inhibitor of CYP2C8, CYP2C9, CYP2B6, CYP3A4 and CYP2C19; M-2 metabolite is an inhibitor of CYP2C9, CYP2C8, CYP3A4 and CYP2D6, and M-5 metabolite is an inhibitor of CYP2C8. *In vitro* studies suggested that regorafenib is not an inducer of CYP1A2, CYP2B6, CYP2C19, and CYP3A4 enzyme activity.

Patients with advanced solid tumors received single oral doses of CYP substrates, 2 mg of midazolam (CYP3A4), 40 mg of omeprazole (CYP2C19) and 10 mg of warfarin (CYP2C9) or 4 mg of rosiglitazone (CYP2C8) one week before and two weeks after Stivarga at a dose of 160 mg once daily. No clinically relevant change was observed in the mean AUC of rosiglitazone (N=12) or the mean omeprazole (N=11) plasma concentrations measured 6 hours after dosing or the mean AUC of midazolam (N=15). The mean AUC of warfarin (N=8) increased by 25% *[see Warnings and Precautions (5.2)]*.

Effect of CYP3A4 Strong Inducers on Regorafenib: Twenty-two healthy men received a single 160 mg dose of Stivarga alone and then 7 days after starting rifampin. Rifampin, a strong CYP3A4 inducer, was administered at a dose of 600 mg daily for 9 days. The mean AUC of regorafenib decreased by 50% and mean AUC of M-5 increased by 264%. No change in the mean AUC of M-2 was observed *[see Drug Interactions (7.1)]*.

Effect of CYP3A4 Strong Inhibitors on Regorafenib: Eighteen healthy men received a single 160 mg dose of Stivarga alone and then 5 days after starting ketoconazole. Ketoconazole, a strong CYP3A4 inhibitor, was administered at a dose of 400 mg daily for 18 days. The mean AUC of regorafenib increased by 33% and the mean AUC of M-2 and M-5 both decreased by 93% *[see Drug Interactions (7.2)]*.

Effect of Regorafenib on UGT1A1 Substrates: In vitro studies showed that regorafenib, M-2, and M-5 competitively inhibit UGT1A9 and UGT1A1 at therapeutically relevant concentrations. Eleven patients received irinotecan-containing combination chemotherapy with Stivarga at a dose of 160 mg. The mean AUC of irinotecan increased 28% and the mean AUC of SN-38 increased by 44% when irinotecan was administered 5 days after the last of 7 daily doses of Stivarga.

In vitro screening of transporters: In vitro data suggested that regorafenib is an inhibitor of ABCG2 (Breast Cancer Resistance Protein) and ABCB1 (P-glycoprotein).

12.6 Cardiac Electrophysiology

The effect of multiple doses of Stivarga (160 mg once daily for 21 days) on the QTc interval was evaluated in an open label, single arm study in 25 patients with advanced solid tumors. No large changes in the mean QTc interval (i.e., > 20 msec) were detected in the study.

13 NONCLINICAL TOXICOLOGY

13.1 Carcinogenesis, Mutagenesis, Impairment of Fertility

Studies examining the carcinogenic potential of regorafenib have not been conducted. Regorafenib itself did not demonstrate genotoxicity in *in vitro* or *in vivo* assays; however, a major human active metabolite of regorafenib, (M-2), was positive for clastogenicity, causing chromosome aberration in Chinese hamster V79 cells.

Dedicated studies to examine the effects of regorafenib on fertility have not been conducted; however, there were histological findings of tubular atrophy and degeneration in the testes, atrophy in the seminal vesicle, and cellular debris and oligospermia in the epididymides in male rats at doses similar to those in human at the clinical recommended dose based on AUC. In female rats, there were increased findings of necrotic corpora lutea in the ovaries at the same exposures. There were similar findings in dogs of both sexes in repeat dose studies at exposures approximately 83% of the human exposure at the recommended human dose based on AUC. These findings suggest that regorafenib may adversely affect fertility in humans.

13.2 Animal Toxicology and/or Pharmacology

In a chronic 26 week repeat dose study in rats there was a dose-dependent increase in the finding of thickening of the atrioventricular valve. At a dose that resulted in an exposure of approximately 12% of the human exposure at the recommended dose, this finding was present in half of the examined animals.

14 CLINICAL STUDIES

14.1 Colorectal Cancer

The clinical efficacy and safety of Stivarga were evaluated in an international, multi-center, randomized (2:1), double-blind, placebo-controlled trial (Study 1) in 760 patients with previously treated metastatic colorectal cancer. The major efficacy outcome measure was overall survival (OS); supportive efficacy outcome measures included progression-free survival (PFS) and objective tumor response rate.

Patients were randomized to receive 160 mg regorafenib orally once daily (N=505) plus Best Supportive Care (BSC) or placebo (N=255) plus BSC for the first 21 days of each 28-day cycle. Stivarga was administered with a low-fat breakfast that contains less than 30% fat *[see Dosage and Administration (2.1), Clinical Pharmacology (12.3)]*. Treatment continued until disease progression or unacceptable toxicity.

In the all-randomized population, median age was 61 years, 61% were men, 78% were White, and all patients had baseline ECOG performance status of 0 or 1. The primary site of disease was colon (65%), rectum (29%), or both (6%). History of KRAS evaluation was reported for 729 (96%) patients; 430 (59%) of these patients were reported to have KRAS mutation. The median number of prior lines of therapy for metastatic disease was 3. All patients received prior treatment with fluoropyrimidine-, oxaliplatin-, and irinotecan-based chemotherapy, and with bevacizumab. All but one patient with KRAS mutation-negative tumors received panitumumab or cetuximab.

The addition of Stivarga to BSC resulted in a statistically significant improvement in survival compared to placebo plus BSC (see Table 5 and Figure 1).

Table 5 Efficacy Results from Study 1

	Stivarga (N=505)	Placebo (N=255)
Overall Survival		
Number of deaths, N (%)	275 (55%)	157 (62%)
Median Overall Survival (months)	6.4	5.0
95% CI	(5.8, 7.3)	(4.4, 5.8)
HR (95% CI)	0.77 (0.64, 0.94)	
Stratified Log-Rank Test P-value [a, b]	0.0102	
Progression-free Survival		
Number of Death or Progression, N (%)	417 (83%)	231 (91%)
Median Progression-free Survival (months)	2.0	1.7
95% CI	(1.9, 2.3)	(1.7, 1.8)
HR (95% CI)	0.49 (0.42, 0.58)	
Stratified Log-Rank Test P-value [a]	<0.0001	
Overall Response Rate		
Overall response, N (%)	5 (1%)	1 (0.4%)
95% CI	0.3%, 2.3%	0%, 2.2%

[a] Stratified by geographic region and time from diagnosis of metastatic disease.

[b] Crossed the O'Brien-Fleming boundary (two-sided p-value < 0.018) at second interim analysis.

Figure 1 Kaplan-Meier Curves of Overall Survival

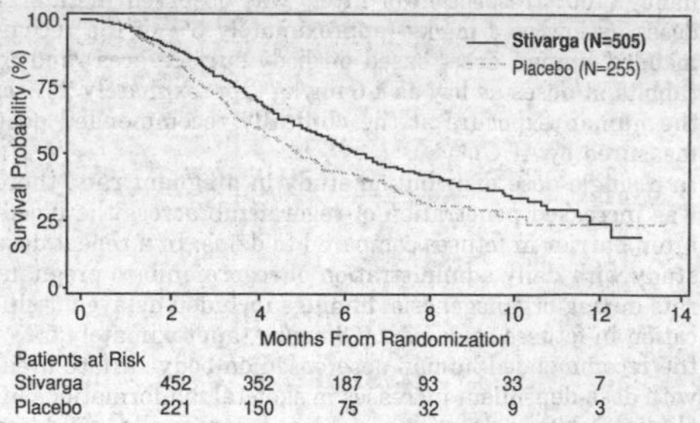

14.2 Gastrointestinal Stromal Tumors

The efficacy and safety of Stivarga were evaluated in an international, multi-center, randomized (2:1), double-blind, placebo-controlled trial (Study 2) in 199 patients with unresectable, locally advanced or metastatic gastrointestinal stromal tumor (GIST), who had been previously treated with imatinib mesylate and sunitinib malate. Randomization was stratified by line of therapy (third vs. four or more) and geographic region (Asia vs. rest of the world).

The major efficacy outcome measure of Study 2 was progression-free survival (PFS) based on disease assessment by independent radiological review using modified RECIST 1.1 criteria, in which lymph nodes and bone lesions were not target lesions and progressively growing new tumor nodule within a pre-existing tumor mass was progression. The key secondary outcome measure was overall survival.

Patients were randomized to receive 160 mg regorafenib orally once daily (N=133) plus best supportive care (BSC) or placebo (N=66) plus BSC for the first 21 days of each 28-day cycle. Treatment continued until disease progression or unacceptable toxicity. In Study 2, the median age of patients was 60 years, 64% were men, 68% were White, and all patients had baseline ECOG performance status of 0 (55%) or 1 (45%). At the time of disease progression as assessed by central review, the study blind was broken and all patients were offered the opportunity to take Stivarga at the investigator's discretion. Fifty-six (85%) patients randomized to placebo and 41 (31%) patients randomized to Stivarga received open-label Stivarga.

A statistically significant improvement in PFS was demonstrated among patients treated with Stivarga compared to placebo (see Table 6 and Figure 2). There was no statistically significant difference in overall survival at the time of the planned interim analysis based on 29% of the total events for the final analysis.

Table 6 Efficacy Results for Study 2

	Stivarga (N=133)	Placebo (N=66)
Progression-free Survival		
Number of Death or Progression, N (%)	82 (62%)	63 (96%)
Median Progression-free Survival (months)	4.8	0.9
95% CI	(3.9, 5.7)	(0.9, 1.1)
HR (95% CI)	0.27 (0.19, 0.39)	
Stratified Log-Rank Test P-value [a]	<0.0001	
Overall Survival		
Number of Deaths, N (%)	29 (22%)	17 (26%)
Median Overall Survival (months)	NR[b]	NR[b]
HR (95% CI)	0.77 (0.42, 1.41)	
Stratified Log-Rank Test P-value [a, b]	0.2	

[a] Stratified by line of treatment and geographical region.
[b] NR: Not Reached.

Figure 2 Kaplan-Meier Curves of Progression-free Survival for Study 2

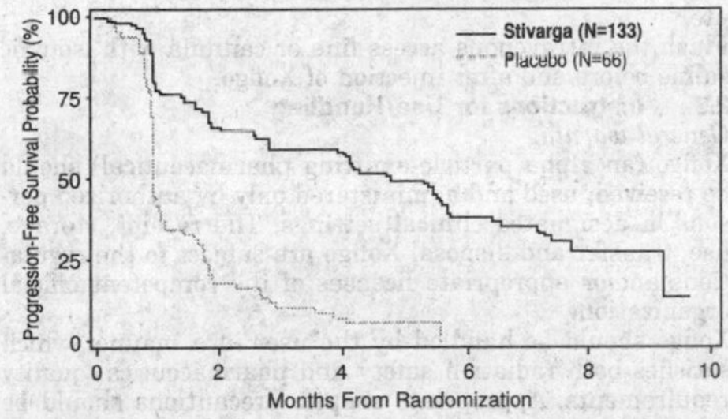

Patients at Risk				
Stivarga	82	72	27	9
Placebo	12	5	0	0

16 HOW SUPPLIED/STORAGE AND HANDLING

16.1 How Supplied

Stivarga tablets are supplied in packages containing three bottles, with each bottle containing 28 tablets, for a total of 84 tablets per package (NDC 50419-171-03).

16.2 Storage and Handling

Store Stivarga at 25°C (77°F); excursions are permitted from 15 to 30°C (59 to 86°F) [See USP Controlled Room Temperature].

Store tablets in the original bottle and do not remove the desiccant. Keep the bottle tightly closed after first opening. Discard any unused tablets 28 days after opening the bottle. Dispose of unused tablets in accordance with local requirements.

17 PATIENT COUNSELING INFORMATION

See FDA-Approved Patient Labeling (Patient Information).

Inform your patients of the following:

- Stivarga may cause severe or life-threatening liver damage. Inform patients that they will need to undergo monitoring for liver damage and to immediately report any signs or symptoms of severe liver damage to their health care provider.
- Stivarga can cause severe bleeding. Advise patients to contact their health care provider for any episode of bleeding.
- Stivarga can cause hand-foot skin reactions or rash elsewhere. Advise patients to contact their health care provider if they experience skin changes associated with redness, pain, blisters, bleeding, or swelling.
- Stivarga can cause or exacerbate existing hypertension. Advise patients they will need to undergo blood pressure monitoring and to contact their health care provider if blood pressure is elevated or if symptoms from hypertension occur including severe headache, lightheadedness, or neurologic symptoms.
- Stivarga increased the risk for myocardial ischemia and infarction. Advise patients to seek immediate emergency help if they experience chest pain, shortness of breath, or feel dizzy or like passing out.
- Contact a healthcare provider immediately if they experience severe pains in their abdomen, persistent swelling of the abdomen, high fever, chills, nausea, vomiting, severe diarrhea (frequent or loose bowel movements), or dehydration.
- Stivarga may complicate wound healing. Advise patients to inform their health care provider if they plan to undergo a surgical procedure or had recent surgery.
- Inform patients that regorafenib can cause fetal harm. Advise women of reproductive potential and men of the need for effective contraception during Stivarga treatment and for up to 2 months after completion of treatment. Instruct women of reproductive potential to immediately contact her health care provider if pregnancy is suspected or confirmed during or within 2 months of completing treatment with Stivarga.
- Advise nursing mothers that it is not known whether regorafenib is present in breast milk and discuss whether to discontinue nursing or to discontinue regorafenib.
- Inform patients to take any missed dose on the same day, as soon as they remember, and that they must not take two doses on the same day to make up for a dose missed on the previous day.
- Inform patients to store medicine in the original container. Do not place medication in daily or weekly pill boxes. Any remaining tablets should be discarded 28 days after opening the bottle. Tightly close bottle after each opening and keep the desiccant in the bottle.

Patient Information
Stivarga (sti-VAR-gah)
(regorafenib)
tablets

Read this Patient Information before you start taking Stivarga and each time you get a refill. There may be new information. This information does not take the place of talking to your healthcare provider about your medical condition or treatment.

What is the most important information I should know about Stivarga?

Stivarga can cause serious side effects, including:

Liver problems. Stivarga can cause liver problems which can be serious and sometimes lead to death. Your healthcare provider will do blood tests to check your liver function before you start taking Stivarga and during your treatment with Stivarga to check for liver problems. Tell your healthcare provider right away if you get any of these symptoms of liver problems during treatment:

- yellowing of your skin or the white part of your eyes (jaundice)
- nausea or vomiting
- dark "tea-colored" urine
- change in sleep pattern

What is Stivarga?

Stivarga is a prescription medicine used to treat people with:

- colon or rectal cancer that has spread to other parts of the body and for which they have received previous treatment with certain chemotherapy medicines
- a rare stomach, bowel, or esophagus cancer called GIST (gastrointestinal stromal tumors) that cannot be treated with surgery or that has spread to other parts of the body and for which they have received previous treatment with certain medicines

Stivarga has not been used to treat children less than 18 years of age.

What should I tell my healthcare provider before taking Stivarga?

Before you take Stivarga, tell your healthcare provider if you:

- have liver problems
- have bleeding problems
- have high blood pressure
- have heart problems or chest pain
- plan to have any surgical procedures
- have any other medical conditions
- are pregnant or plan to become pregnant. Stivarga can harm your unborn baby. Females and males should use effective birth control during treatment with Stivarga and for 2 months after your last dose of Stivarga. Tell your healthcare provider right away if you or your partner becomes pregnant either while taking Stivarga or within 2 months after your last dose of Stivarga.
- are breastfeeding or plan to breastfeed. It is not known if Stivarga passes into your breast milk. You and your healthcare provider should decide if you will take Stivarga or breastfeed.

Tell your healthcare provider about all the medicines you take, including prescription and non-prescription medicines, vitamins and herbal supplements. Stivarga may affect the way other medicines work, and other medicines may affect how Stivarga works.

Know the medicines you take. Keep a list of your medicines and show it to your healthcare provider and pharmacist when you get a new medicine.

How should I take Stivarga?

- Take Stivarga exactly as your healthcare provider tells you.
- You will usually take Stivarga 1 time a day for 21 days (3 weeks) and then stop for 7 days (1 week). This is 1 cycle of treatment. Repeat this cycle for as long as your healthcare provider tells you to.
- Swallow Stivarga tablets whole.
- Take Stivarga at the same time each day with a low-fat breakfast.

  Examples of a low-fat breakfast include:
- 2 slices of white toast with 1 tablespoon of low-fat margarine and 1 tablespoon of jelly, and 8 ounces of skim milk (319 calories and 8.2 grams fat), **or**
- 1 cup of cereal, 8 ounces of skim milk, 1 slice of toast with jelly, apple juice, and 1 cup of coffee or tea (520 calories and 2 grams fat).
- Your healthcare provider may stop your treatment or change the dose of your treatment if you get side effects.
- If you miss a dose, take it as soon as you remember on that day. Do not take two doses on the same day to make up for a missed dose.
- If you take too much Stivarga call your healthcare provider or go to the nearest emergency room right away.

What should I avoid while taking Stivarga?

- Avoid drinking grapefruit juice and taking St. John's Wort while taking Stivarga. These can affect the way Stivarga works.

What are the possible side effects of Stivarga?

Stivarga can cause serious side effects including:

- See **"What is the most important information I should know about Stivarga?"**
- **severe bleeding.** Stivarga can cause bleeding which can be serious and sometimes lead to death. Tell your healthcare provider if you have any signs of bleeding while taking Stivarga including:
  - vomiting blood or if your vomit looks like coffee-grounds
  - pink or brown urine
  - red or black (looks like tar) stools
  - coughing up blood or blood clots
  - menstrual bleeding that is heavier than normal
  - unusual vaginal bleeding
  - nose bleeds that happen often
- **a skin problem called hand-foot skin reaction and severe skin rash.** Hand-foot skin reactions can cause redness, pain, blisters, bleeding, or swelling on the palms of your hands or soles of your feet. If you get this side effect or a severe skin rash, your healthcare provider may stop your treatment for some time.
- **high blood pressure.** Your blood pressure should be checked every week for the first 6 weeks of starting Stivarga. Your blood pressure should be checked regularly and any high blood pressure should be treated while you are receiving Stivarga. Tell your healthcare provider if you have severe headaches, lightheadedness, or changes in your vision.
- **decreased blood flow to the heart and heart attack.** Get emergency help right away and call your healthcare provider if you get symptoms such as chest pain, shortness of breath, feel dizzy or feel like passing out.
- **a condition called Reversible Posterior Leukoencephalopathy Syndrome (RPLS).** Call your healthcare provider right away if you get: severe headaches, seizure, confusion, change in vision, or problems thinking.
- **a tear in your stomach or intestinal wall (bowel perforation).** Stivarga may cause a tear in your stomach or bowel perforation that can be serious and sometimes lead to death. Tell your healthcare provider right away if you get:
  - severe pain in your stomach-area (abdomen)
  - swelling of the abdomen
  - high fever
- **wound healing problems.** If you need to have a surgical procedure, tell your healthcare provider that you are taking Stivarga. You should stop taking Stivarga at least 2 weeks before any planned surgery.

The most common side effects of Stivarga include:

- tiredness, weakness, fatigue
- frequent or loose bowel movements (diarrhea)
- loss of appetite
- swelling, pain and redness of the lining in your mouth, throat, stomach and bowel (mucositis)
- voice changes or hoarseness
- infection
- pain in other parts of your body
- weight loss
- nausea

Tell your healthcare provider if you have any side effect that bothers you or that does not go away.

These are not all of the possible side effects of Stivarga. For more information, ask your healthcare provider or pharmacist.

Call your doctor for medical advice about side effects. You may report side effects to FDA at 1-800-FDA-1088.

How do I store Stivarga?

- Store Stivarga tablets at room temperature between 68° F to 77° F (20° C to 25° C).
- Keep Stivarga in the bottle that it comes in. Do not put Stivarga tablets in a daily or weekly pill box.
- The Stivarga bottle contains a desiccant to help keep your medicine dry. Keep the desiccant in the bottle.
- Keep the bottle of Stivarga tightly closed.
- Safely throw away (discard) any unused Stivarga tablets after 28 days of opening the bottle.

Keep Stivarga and all medicines out of the reach of children.

General information about Stivarga.

Medicines are sometimes prescribed for purposes other than those listed in a Patient Information leaflet. Do not use Stivarga for a condition for which it was not prescribed. Do not give Stivarga to other people even if they have the same symptoms you have. It may harm them.

This leaflet summarizes the most important information about Stivarga. If you would like more information, talk with your healthcare provider. You can ask your healthcare provider or pharmacist for information about Stivarga this is written for health professionals.

For more information, go to www.STIVARGA-US.com or call 1-888-842-2937.

What are the ingredients in Stivarga?

Active ingredient: regorafenib

Inactive ingredients: cellulose microcrystalline, croscarmellose sodium, magnesium stearate, povidone and colloidal silicon dioxide.

Film coat: ferric oxide red, ferric oxide yellow, lecithin (soy), polyethylene glycol 3350, polyvinyl alcohol, talc and titanium dioxide.

This Patient Information has been approved by the U.S. Food and Drug Administration.

Manufactured in Germany

Distributed and marketed by:

Bayer HealthCare Pharmaceuticals Inc.

Wayne, NJ 07470

Revised: 8/2013

Shown in Product Identification Guide, page 305

XOFIGO ℞

(radium Ra 223 dichloride)

Injection, for intravenous use

HIGHLIGHTS OF PRESCRIBING INFORMATION

These highlights do not include all the information needed to use XOFIGO safely and effectively. See full prescribing information for XOFIGO.

Xofigo (radium Ra 223 dichloride) Injection, for intravenous use

Initial U.S. Approval: 2013

INDICATIONS AND USAGE

Xofigo is an alpha particle-emitting radioactive therapeutic agent indicated for the treatment of patients with castration-resistant prostate cancer, symptomatic bone metastases and no known visceral metastatic disease. (1)

DOSAGE AND ADMINISTRATION

The dose regimen of Xofigo is 50 kBq (1.35 microcurie) per kg body weight, given at 4 week intervals for 6 injections. (2.1)

DOSAGE FORMS AND STRENGTHS

Single-use vial at a concentration of 1,000 kBq/mL (27 microcurie/mL) at the reference date with a total radioactivity of 6,000 kBq/vial (162 microcurie/vial) at the reference date (3)

CONTRAINDICATIONS

Pregnancy (4, 8.1)

WARNINGS AND PRECAUTIONS

Bone Marrow Suppression: Measure blood counts prior to treatment initiation and before every dose of Xofigo. Discontinue Xofigo if hematologic values do not recover within 6 to 8 weeks after treatment. Monitor patients with compromised bone marrow reserve closely. Discontinue Xofigo in patients who experience life-threatening complications despite supportive care measures. (5.1)

ADVERSE REACTIONS

The most common adverse drug reactions (≥ 10%) in patients receiving Xofigo were nausea, diarrhea, vomiting, and peripheral edema.

The most common hematologic laboratory abnormalities (≥ 10%) were anemia, lymphocytopenia, leukopenia, thrombocytopenia, and neutropenia (6.1).

To report SUSPECTED ADVERSE REACTIONS, contact Bayer HealthCare Pharmaceuticals Inc. at 1-888-842-2937 or FDA at 1-800-FDA-1088 or www.fda.gov/medwatch

See 17 for PATIENT COUNSELING INFORMATION

Revised: 05/2013

FULL PRESCRIBING INFORMATION: CONTENTS*

*** Sections or subsections omitted from the full prescribing information are not listed**

FULL PRESCRIBING INFORMATION

1 INDICATIONS AND USAGE

Xofigo is indicated for the treatment of patients with castration-resistant prostate cancer, symptomatic bone metastases and no known visceral metastatic disease.

2 DOSAGE AND ADMINISTRATION

2.1 Recommended Dosage

The dose regimen of Xofigo is 50 kBq (1.35 microcurie) per kg body weight, given at 4 week intervals for 6 injections. Safety and efficacy beyond 6 injections with Xofigo have not been studied.

The volume to be administered to a given patient should be calculated using the:

- Patient's body weight (kg)
- Dosage level 50 kBq/kg body weight or 1.35 microcurie/kg body weight
- Radioactivity concentration of the product (1,000 kBq/mL; 27 microcurie/mL) at the reference date
- Decay correction factor to correct for physical decay of radium-223.

The total volume to be administered to a patient is calculated as follows:

$$\text{Volume to be administered (mL)} = \frac{\text{Body weight in kg} \times 50\ \text{kBq/kg body weight}}{\text{Decay factor} \times 1{,}000\ \text{kBq/mL}}$$

or

$$\text{Volume to be administered (mL)} = \frac{\text{Body weight in kg} \times 1.35\ \text{microcurie/kg body weight}}{\text{Decay factor} \times 27\ \text{microcurie/mL}}$$

Table 1: Decay Correction Factor Table

Days from Reference Date	Decay Factor	Days from Reference Date	Decay Factor
-14	2.296	0	0.982
-13	2.161	1	0.925
-12	2.034	2	0.870
-11	1.914	3	0.819
-10	1.802	4	0.771
-9	1.696	5	0.725
-8	1.596	6	0.683
-7	1.502	7	0.643
-6	1.414	8	0.605
-5	1.330	9	0.569
-4	1.252	10	0.536
-3	1.178	11	0.504
-2	1.109	12	0.475
-1	1.044	13	0.447
		14	0.420

The Decay Correction Factor Table is corrected to 12 noon Central Standard Time (CST). To determine the decay correction factor, count the number of days before or after the reference date. The Decay Correction Factor Table includes a correction to account for the 7 hour time difference between 12 noon Central European Time (CET) at the site of manufacture and 12 noon US CST, which is 7 hours earlier than CET.

Immediately before and after administration, the net patient dose of administered Xofigo should be determined by measurement in an appropriate radioisotope dose calibrator that has been calibrated with a National Institute of Standards and Technology (NIST) traceable radium-223 standard (available upon request from Bayer) and corrected for decay using the date and time of calibration. The dose calibrator must be calibrated with nationally recognized standards, carried out at the time of commissioning, after any maintenance procedure that could affect the dosimetry and at intervals not to exceed one year.

2.2 Administration

Administer Xofigo by slow intravenous injection over 1 minute.

Flush the intravenous access line or cannula with isotonic saline before and after injection of Xofigo.

2.3 Instructions for Use/Handling

General warning

Xofigo (an alpha particle-emitting pharmaceutical) should be received, used and administered only by authorized persons in designated clinical settings. The receipt, storage, use, transfer and disposal Xofigo are subject to the regulations and/or appropriate licenses of the competent official organization.

Xofigo should be handled by the user in a manner which satisfies both radiation safety and pharmaceutical quality requirements. Appropriate aseptic precautions should be taken.

Radiation protection

The administration of Xofigo is associated with potential risks to other persons (e.g., medical staff, caregivers and patient's household members) from radiation or contamination from spills of bodily fluids such as urine, feces, or vomit. Therefore, radiation protection precautions must be taken in accordance with national and local regulations.

For drug handling

Follow the normal working procedures for the handling of radiopharmaceuticals and use universal precautions for handling and administration such as gloves and barrier gowns when handling blood and bodily fluids to avoid contamination. In case of contact with skin or eyes, the affected area should be flushed immediately with water. In the event of spillage of Xofigo, the local radiation safety officer should be contacted immediately to initiate the necessary measurements and required procedures to decontaminate the area. A complexing agent such as 0.01 M ethylene-diamine-tetraacetic acid (EDTA) solution is recommended to remove contamination.

For patient care

Whenever possible, patients should use a toilet and the toilet should be flushed several times after each use. When handling bodily fluids, simply wearing gloves and hand washing will protect caregivers. Clothing soiled with Xofigo or patient fecal matter or urine should be washed promptly and separately from other clothing.

Radium-223 is primarily an alpha emitter, with a 95.3% fraction of energy emitted as alpha-particles. The fraction emitted as beta-particles is 3.6%, and the fraction emitted as gamma-radiation is 1.1%. The external radiation exposure associated with handling of patient doses is expected to be low, because the typical treatment activity will be below 8,000 kBq (216 microcurie). In keeping with the **A**s **L**ow **A**s **R**easonably **A**chievable (ALARA) principle for minimization of radiation exposure, it is recommended to minimize the time spent in radiation areas, to maximize the distance to

radiation sources, and to use adequate shielding. Any unused product or materials used in connection with the preparation or administration are to be treated as radioactive waste and should be disposed of in accordance with local regulations.
The gamma radiation associated with the decay of radium-223 and its daughters allows for the radioactivity measurement of Xofigo and the detection of contamination with standard instruments.
Instructions for preparation
Parenteral drug products should be inspected visually for particulate matter and discoloration prior to administration, whenever solution and container permit.
Xofigo is a ready-to-use solution and should not be diluted or mixed with any solutions. Each vial is for single use only.
Dosimetry
The absorbed radiation doses in major organs were calculated based on clinical biodistribution data in five patients with castration-resistant prostate cancer. Calculations of absorbed radiation doses were performed using OLINDA/EXM (**O**rgan **L**evel **IN**ternal **D**ose **A**ssessment/**EX**ponential **M**odeling), a software program based on the Medical Internal Radiation Dose (MIRD) algorithm, which is widely used for established beta and gamma emitting radionuclides. For radium-223, which is primarily an alpha particle-emitter, assumptions were made for intestine, red marrow and bone/osteogenic cells to provide the best possible absorbed radiation dose calculations for Xofigo, considering its observed biodistribution and specific characteristics.
The calculated absorbed radiation doses to different organs are listed in Table 2. The organs with highest absorbed radiation doses were bone (osteogenic cells), red marrow, upper large intestine wall, and lower large intestine wall. The calculated absorbed doses to other organs are lower.

Table 2: Calculated Absorbed Radiation Doses to Organs

Target Organ	Mean (Gy/MBq)	Mean (rad/mCi)	Coefficient of Variation (%)
Adrenals	0.00012	0.44	56
Brain	0.00010	0.37	80
Breasts	0.00005	0.18	120
Gallbladder wall	0.00023	0.85	14
LLI[1] Wall	0.04645	171.88	83
Small intestine wall	0.00726	26.87	45
Stomach wall	0.00014	0.51	22
ULI[2] wall	0.03232	119.58	50
Heart wall	0.00173	6.40	42
Kidneys	0.00320	11.86	36
Liver	0.00298	11.01	36
Lungs	0.00007	0.27	90
Muscle	0.00012	0.44	41
Ovaries	0.00049	1.80	40
Pancreas	0.00011	0.41	43
Red marrow	0.13879	513.51	41
Osteogenic cells	1.15206	4262.60	41
Skin	0.00007	0.27	79
Spleen	0.00009	0.33	54
Testes	0.00008	0.31	59
Thymus	0.00006	0.21	109
Thyroid	0.00007	0.26	96
Urinary bladder wall	0.00403	14.90	63
Uterus	0.00026	0.94	28
Whole body	0.02311	85.50	16

[1]LLI: lower large intestine
[2]ULI: upper large intestine

Table 3: Adverse Reactions in the Randomized Trial

System/Organ Class Preferred Term	Xofigo (n=600)		Placebo (n=301)	
	Grades 1-4 %	Grades 3-4 %	Grades 1-4 %	Grades 3-4 %
Blood and lymphatic system disorders				
Pancytopenia	2	1	0	0
Gastrointestinal disorders				
Nausea	36	2	35	2
Diarrhea	25	2	15	2
Vomiting	19	2	14	2
General disorders and administration site conditions				
Peripheral edema	13	2	10	1
Renal and urinary disorders				
Renal failure and impairment	3	1	1	1

3 DOSAGE FORMS AND STRENGTHS

Xofigo (radium Ra 223 dichloride injection) is available in single-use vials containing 6 mL of solution at a concentration of 1,000 kBq/mL (27 microcurie/mL) at the reference date with a total radioactivity of 6,000 kBq/vial (162 microcurie/vial) at the reference date.

4 CONTRAINDICATIONS

Xofigo is contraindicated in pregnancy.
Xofigo can cause fetal harm when administered to a pregnant woman based on its mechanism of action. Xofigo is not indicated for use in women. Xofigo is contraindicated in women who are or may become pregnant. If this drug is used during pregnancy, or if the patient becomes pregnant while taking this drug, apprise the patient of the potential hazard to the fetus *[see Use in Specific Populations (8.1)]*.

5 WARNINGS AND PRECAUTIONS

5.1 Bone Marrow Suppression

In the randomized trial, 2% of patients on the Xofigo arm experienced bone marrow failure or ongoing pancytopenia compared to no patients treated with placebo. There were two deaths due to bone marrow failure and for 7 of 13 patients treated with Xofigo, bone marrow failure was ongoing at the time of death. Among the 13 patients who experienced bone marrow failure, 54% required blood transfusions. Four percent (4%) of patients on the Xofigo arm and 2% on the placebo arm permanently discontinued therapy due to bone marrow suppression.
In the randomized trial, deaths related to vascular hemorrhage in association with myelosuppression were observed in 1% of Xofigo-treated patients compared to 0.3% of patients treated with placebo. The incidence of infection-related deaths (2%), serious infections (10%), and febrile neutropenia (<1%) were similar for patients treated with Xofigo and placebo. Myelosuppression; notably thrombocytopenia, neutropenia, pancytopenia, and leukopenia; has been reported in patients treated with Xofigo. In the randomized trial, complete blood counts (CBCs) were obtained every 4 weeks prior to each dose and the nadir CBCs and times of recovery were not well characterized. In a separate single-dose phase 1 study of Xofigo, neutrophil and platelet count nadirs occurred 2 to 3 weeks after Xofigo administration at doses that were up to 1 to 5 times the recommended dose, and most patients recovered approximately 6 to 8 weeks after administration *[see Adverse Reactions (6)]*.
Hematologic evaluation of patients must be performed at baseline and prior to every dose of Xofigo. Before the first administration of Xofigo, the absolute neutrophil count (ANC) should be $\geq 1.5 \times 10^9$/L, the platelet count $\geq 100 \times 10^9$/L and hemoglobin ≥ 10 g/dL. Before subsequent administrations of Xofigo, the ANC should be $\geq 1 \times 10^9$/L and the platelet count $\geq 50 \times 10^9$/L. If there is no recovery to these values within 6 to 8 weeks after the last administration of Xofigo, despite receiving supportive care, further treatment with Xofigo should be discontinued. Patients with evidence of compromised bone marrow reserve should be monitored closely and provided with supportive care measures when clinically indicated. Discontinue Xofigo in patients who experience life-threatening complications despite supportive care for bone marrow failure.
The safety and efficacy of concomitant chemotherapy with Xofigo have not been established. Outside of a clinical trial, concomitant use with chemotherapy is not recommended due to the potential for additive myelosuppression. If chemotherapy, other systemic radioisotopes or hemibody external radiotherapy are administered during the treatment period, Xofigo should be discontinued.

6 ADVERSE REACTIONS

The following serious adverse reactions are discussed in greater detail in another section of the label:
• Bone Marrow Suppression *[see Warnings and Precautions (5.1)]*

6.1 Clinical Trials Experience

Because clinical trials are conducted under widely varying conditions, adverse reaction rates observed in the clinical trials of a drug cannot be directly compared to rates in the clinical trials of another drug and may not reflect the rates observed in practice.
In the randomized clinical trial in patients with metastatic castration-resistant prostate cancer with bone metastases, 600 patients received intravenous injections of 50 kBq/kg (1.35 microcurie/kg) of Xofigo and best standard of care and 301 patients received placebo and best standard of care once every 4 weeks for up to 6 injections. Prior to randomization, 58% and 57% of patients had received docetaxel in the Xofigo and placebo arms, respectively. The median duration of treatment was 20 weeks (6 cycles) for Xofigo and 18 weeks (5 cycles) for placebo.
The most common adverse reactions (≥ 10%) in patients receiving Xofigo were nausea, diarrhea, vomiting, and peripheral edema (Table 3). Grade 3 and 4 adverse events were reported among 57% of Xofigo-treated patients and 63% of placebo-treated patients. The most common hematologic laboratory abnormalities in Xofigo-treated patients (≥ 10%) were anemia, lymphocytopenia, leukopenia, thrombocytopenia, and neutropenia (Table 4).
Treatment discontinuations due to adverse events occurred in 17% of patients who received Xofigo and 21% of patients who received placebo. The most common hematologic laboratory abnormalities leading to discontinuation for Xofigo were anemia (2%) and thrombocytopenia (2%).
Table 3 shows adverse reactions occurring in ≥ 2% of patients and for which the incidence for Xofigo exceeds the incidence for placebo.
[See table 3 above]
Laboratory Abnormalities
Table 4 shows hematologic laboratory abnormalities occurring in ≥ 10% of patients and for which the incidence for Xofigo exceeds the incidence for placebo.
[See table 4 at top of next page]
As an adverse reaction, grade 3-4 thrombocytopenia was reported in 6% of patients on Xofigo and in 2% of patients on placebo. Among patients who received Xofigo, the laboratory abnormality grade 3-4 thrombocytopenia occurred in 1% of docetaxel naïve patients and in 4% of patients who had received prior docetaxel. Grade 3-4 neutropenia occurred in 1% of docetaxel naïve patients and in 3% of patients who have received prior docetaxel.
Fluid Status
Dehydration occurred in 3% of patients on Xofigo and 1% of patients on placebo. Xofigo increases adverse reactions such as diarrhea, nausea, and vomiting which may result in dehydration. Monitor patients' oral intake and fluid status carefully and promptly treat patients who display signs or symptoms of dehydration or hypovolemia.
Injection Site Reactions
Erythema, pain, and edema at the injection site were reported in 1% of patients on Xofigo.

Table 4: Hematologic Laboratory Abnormalities

Hematologic Laboratory Abnormalities	Xofigo (n=600)		Placebo (n=301)	
	Grades 1-4 %	Grades 3-4 %	Grades 1-4 %	Grades 3-4 %
Anemia	93	6	88	6
Lymphocytopenia	72	20	53	7
Leukopenia	35	3	10	<1
Thrombocytopenia	31	3	22	<1
Neutropenia	18	2	5	<1

Laboratory values were obtained at baseline and prior to each 4-week cycle.

Secondary Malignant Neoplasms

Xofigo contributes to a patient's overall long-term cumulative radiation exposure. Long-term cumulative radiation exposure may be associated with an increased risk of cancer and hereditary defects. Due to its mechanism of action and neoplastic changes, including osteosarcomas, in rats following administration of radium-223 dichloride, Xofigo may increase the risk of osteosarcoma or other secondary malignant neoplasms *[see Nonclinical Toxicology (13.1)]*. However, the overall incidence of new malignancies in the randomized trial was lower on the Xofigo arm compared to placebo (<1% vs. 2%; respectively), but the expected latency period for the development of secondary malignancies exceeds the duration of follow up for patients on the trial.

Subsequent Treatment with Cytotoxic Chemotherapy

In the randomized clinical trial, 16% patients in the Xofigo group and 18% patients in the placebo group received cytotoxic chemotherapy after completion of study treatments. Adequate safety monitoring and laboratory testing was not performed to assess how patients treated with Xofigo will tolerate subsequent cytotoxic chemotherapy.

7 DRUG INTERACTIONS

No formal clinical drug interaction studies have been performed.

Subgroup analyses indicated that the concurrent use of bisphosphonates or calcium channel blockers did not affect the safety and efficacy of Xofigo in the randomized clinical trial.

8 USE IN SPECIFIC POPULATIONS

8.1 Pregnancy

Category X *[see Contraindications (4)]*

Xofigo can cause fetal harm when administered to a pregnant woman based on its mechanism of action. While there are no human or animal data on the use of Xofigo in pregnancy and Xofigo is not indicated for use in women, maternal use of a radioactive therapeutic agent could affect development of a fetus. Xofigo is contraindicated in women who are or may become pregnant while receiving the drug. If this drug is used during pregnancy, or if the patient becomes pregnant while taking this drug, apprise the patient of the potential hazard to the fetus and the potential risk for pregnancy loss. Advise females of reproductive potential to avoid becoming pregnant during treatment with Xofigo.

8.3 Nursing Mothers

Xofigo is not indicated for use in women. It is not known whether radium-223 dichloride is excreted in human milk. Because many drugs are excreted in human milk, and because of potential for serious adverse reactions in nursing infants from Xofigo, a decision should be made whether to discontinue nursing, or discontinue the drug taking into account the importance of the drug to the mother.

8.4 Pediatric Use

The safety and efficacy of Xofigo in pediatric patients have not been established.

In single- and repeat-dose toxicity studies in rats, findings in the bones (depletion of osteocytes, osteoblasts, osteoclasts, fibro-osseous lesions, disruption/disorganization of the physis/growth line) and teeth (missing, irregular growth, fibro-osseous lesions in bone socket) correlated with a reduction of osteogenesis that occurred at clinically relevant doses beginning in the range of 20 – 80 kBq (0.541 - 2.16 microcurie) per kg body weight.

8.5 Geriatric Use

Of the 600 patients treated with Xofigo in the randomized trial, 75% were 65 years of age and over and while 33% were 75 years of age and over. No dosage adjustment is considered necessary in elderly patients. No overall differences in safety or effectiveness were observed between these subjects and younger subjects, and other reported clinical experience has not identified differences in responses between the elderly and younger patients, but greater sensitivity of some older individuals cannot be ruled out.

8.6 Patients with Hepatic Impairment

No dedicated hepatic impairment trial for Xofigo has been conducted. Since radium-223 is neither metabolized by the liver nor eliminated via the bile, hepatic impairment is unlikely to affect the pharmacokinetics of radium-223 dichloride *[see Clinical Pharmacology (12.3)]*. Based on subgroup analyses in the randomized clinical trial, dose adjustment is not needed in patients with mild hepatic impairment. No dose adjustments can be recommended for patients with moderate or severe hepatic impairment due to lack of clinical data.

8.7 Patients with Renal Impairment

No dedicated renal impairment trial for Xofigo has been conducted. Based on subgroup analyses in the randomized clinical trial, dose adjustment is not needed in patients with existing mild (creatinine clearance [CrCl] 60 to 89 mL/min) or moderate (CrCl 30 to 59 mL/min) renal impairment. No dose adjustment can be recommended for patients with severe renal impairment (CrCl less than 30 mL/min) due to limited data available (n = 2) *[see Clinical Pharmacology (12.3)]*.

8.8 Males of Reproductive Potential

Contraception

Because of potential effects on spermatogenesis associated with radiation, advise men who are sexually active to use condoms and their female partners of reproductive potential to use a highly effective contraceptive method during and for 6 months after completing treatment with Xofigo.

Infertility

There are no data on the effects of Xofigo on human fertility. There is a potential risk that radiation by Xofigo could impair human fertility *[see Nonclinical Toxicology (13.1)]*.

10 OVERDOSAGE

There have been no reports of inadvertent overdosing of Xofigo during clinical studies.

There is no specific antidote. In the event of an inadvertent overdose of Xofigo, utilize general supportive measures, including monitoring for potential hematological and gastrointestinal toxicity, and consider using medical countermeasures such as aluminum hydroxide, barium sulfate, calcium carbonate, calcium gluconate, calcium phosphate, or sodium alginate.[1]

Single Xofigo doses up to 250 kBq (6.76 microcurie) per kg body weight were evaluated in a phase 1 clinical trial and no dose-limiting toxicities were observed.

11 DESCRIPTION

Radium Ra 223 dichloride, an alpha particle-emitting pharmaceutical, is a radiotherapeutic drug.

Xofigo is supplied as a clear, colorless, isotonic, and sterile solution to be administered intravenously with pH between 6 and 8.

Each milliliter of solution contains 1,000 kBq radium-223 dichloride (27 microcurie), corresponding to 0.53 ng radium-223, at the reference date. Radium is present in the solution as a free divalent cation.

Each vial contains 6 mL of solution (6,000 kBq (162 microcurie) radium-223 dichloride at the reference date). The inactive ingredients are 6.3 mg/mL sodium chloride USP (tonicity agent), 7.2 mg/mL sodium citrate USP (for pH adjustment), 0.2 mg/mL hydrochloric acid USP (for pH adjustment), and water for injection USP.

The molecular weight of radium-223 dichloride, $^{223}RaCl_2$, is 293.9 g/mol.

Radium-223 has a half-life of 11.4 days. The specific activity of radium-223 is 1.9 MBq (51.4 microcurie)/ng.

The six-stage-decay of radium-223 to stable lead-207 occurs via short-lived daughters, and is accompanied predominantly by alpha emissions. There are also beta and gamma emissions with different energies and emission probabilities. The fraction of energy emitted from radium-223 and its daughters as alpha-particles is 95.3% (energy range of 5 - 7.5 MeV). The fraction emitted as beta-particles is 3.6% (average energies are 0.445 MeV and 0.492 MeV), and the fraction emitted as gamma-radiation is 1.1% (energy range of 0.01 - 1.27 MeV).

12 CLINICAL PHARMACOLOGY

12.1 Mechanism of Action

The active moiety of Xofigo is the alpha particle-emitting isotope radium-223 (as radium Ra 223 dichloride), which mimics calcium and forms complexes with the bone mineral hydroxyapatite at areas of increased bone turnover, such as bone metastases (see Table 2). The high linear energy transfer of alpha emitters (80 keV/micrometer) leads to a high frequency of double-strand DNA breaks in adjacent cells, resulting in an anti-tumor effect on bone metastases. The alpha particle range from radium-223 dichloride is less than 100 micrometers (less than 10 cell diameters) which limits damage to the surrounding normal tissue.

12.2 Pharmacodynamics

Compared with placebo, there was a significant difference in favor of Xofigo for all five serum biomarkers for bone turnover studied in a phase 2 randomized study (bone formation markers: bone alkaline phosphatase [ALP], total ALP and procollagen I N propeptide [PINP], bone resorption markers: C-terminal crosslinking telopeptide of type I collagen [S-CTX-I] and type I collagen crosslinked C-telopeptide [ICTP]).

12.3 Pharmacokinetics

The pharmacokinetics of radium-223 dichloride in blood was linear in terms of dose proportionality and time independence in the dose range investigated (46 to 250 kBq [1.24 to 6.76 microcurie] per kg body weight).

Distribution

After intravenous injection, radium-223 is rapidly cleared from the blood and is distributed primarily into bone or is excreted into intestine. Fifteen minutes post-injection, about 20% of the injected radioactivity remained in blood. At 4 hours, about 4% of the injected radioactivity remained in blood, decreasing to less than 1% at 24 hours after the injection. At 10 minutes post-injection, radioactivity was observed in bone and in intestine. At 4 hours post-injection, the percentage of the radioactive dose present in bone and intestine was approximately 61% and 49%, respectively. No significant uptake was seen in other organs such as heart, liver, kidneys, urinary bladder, and spleen at 4 hours post-injection *[see Dosage and Administration (2.3)]*.

Metabolism

Radium-223 is an isotope that decays and is not metabolized.

Elimination

The whole body measurements indicated that approximately 63% of the administered radioactivity was excreted from the body within 7 days after injection (after correcting for decay). Fecal excretion is the major route of elimination from the body. At 48 hours after injection, the cumulative fecal excretion was 13% (range 0 - 34%), and the cumulative urine excretion was 2% (range 1 - 5%). There was no evidence of hepato-biliary excretion based on imaging data.

The rate of elimination of radium-223 dichloride from the gastrointestinal tract is influenced by the high variability in intestinal transit rates across the population. Patients with a slower intestinal transit rate could potentially receive a higher intestinal radiation exposure. It is not known whether this will result in increased gastrointestinal toxicity.

Special Populations

Pediatric patients

Safety and effectiveness of Xofigo have not been established in children and adolescents below 18 years of age.

Patients with hepatic impairment

No dedicated pharmacokinetic study in patients with hepatic impairment has been conducted. However, since radium-223 is not metabolized and there is no evidence of hepato-biliary excretion based on imaging data, hepatic impairment is not expected to affect the pharmacokinetics of radium-223 dichloride.

Patients with renal impairment

No dedicated pharmacokinetic study in patients with renal impairment has been conducted. However, since excretion in urine is minimal and the major route of elimination is via the feces, renal impairment is not expected to affect the pharmacokinetics of radium-223 dichloride.

12.6 Cardiac Electrophysiology

The effect of a single dose of 50 kBq/kg of radium-223 dichloride on the QTc interval was evaluated in a subgroup of 29 patients (21 received Xofigo and 8 received placebo) in the randomized clinical trial. No large changes in the mean QTc interval (i.e., greater than 20 ms) were detected up to 6 hours post-dose. The potential for delayed effects on the QT interval after 6 hours was not evaluated.

13 NONCLINICAL TOXICOLOGY

13.1 Carcinogenesis, Mutagenesis, Impairment of Fertility

Animal studies have not been conducted to evaluate the carcinogenic potential of radium-223 dichloride. However, in repeat-dose toxicity studies in rats, osteosarcomas, a known effect of bone-seeking radionuclides, were observed at clinically relevant doses 7 to 12 months after the start of treatment. The presence of other neoplastic changes, including lymphoma and mammary gland carcinoma, was also reported in 12- to 15-month repeat-dose toxicity studies in rats.

Genetic toxicology studies have not been conducted with radium-223 dichloride. However, the mechanism of action of radium-223 dichloride involves induction of double-strand DNA breaks, which is a known effect of radiation.

Animal studies have not been conducted to evaluate the effects of radium-223 dichloride on male or female fertility or reproductive function. Xofigo may impair fertility and reproductive function in humans based on its mechanism of action.

14 CLINICAL STUDIES

The efficacy and safety of Xofigo were evaluated in a double-blind, randomized, placebo-controlled phase 3 clinical trial of patients with castration-resistant prostate cancer with symptomatic bone metastases. Patients with visceral metastases and malignant lymphadenopathy exceeding 3 cm were excluded. The primary efficacy endpoint was overall survival. A key secondary efficacy endpoint was time to first symptomatic skeletal event (SSE) defined as external beam radiation therapy (EBRT) to relieve skeletal symptoms, new symptomatic pathologic bone fracture, occurrence of spinal cord compression, or tumor-related orthopedic surgical intervention. There were no scheduled radiographic assessments performed on study. All patients were to continue androgen deprivation therapy. At the cut-off date of the preplanned interim analysis, a total of 809 patients had been randomized 2:1 to receive Xofigo 50 kBq (1.35 microcurie)/kg intravenously every 4 weeks for 6 cycles (n = 541) plus best standard of care or matching placebo plus best standard of care (n = 268). Best standard of care included local EBRT, corticosteroids, antiandrogens, estrogens, estramustine or ketoconazole. Therapy was continued until unacceptable toxicity or initiation of cytotoxic chemotherapy, other systemic radioisotope, hemi-body EBRT or other investigational drug. Patients with Crohn's disease, ulcerative colitis, prior hemibody radiation or untreated imminent spinal cord compression were excluded from the study. In patients with bone fractures, orthopedic stabilization was performed before starting or resuming treatment with Xofigo.

The following patient demographics and baseline disease characteristics were balanced between the arms. The median age was 71 (range 44-94) with a racial distribution of 94% Caucasian, 4% Asian, 2% Black and <1% Other. Patients were enrolled predominantly from Europe (85%) with 4% of patients enrolled from North America. ECOG performance status was 0-1 in 86% of patients. Eighty-five percent of patients had 6 or more bone scan lesions and of those 40% had > 20 lesions or a superscan. Opiate pain medications were used for cancer-related pain in 54% of patients, non-opiate pain medications in 44% of patients and no pain medications in 2% of patients. Patients were stratified by baseline ALP, bisphosphonate use, and prior docetaxel exposure. Prior bisphosphonates were used by 41% of patients and 58% had received prior docetaxel. During the treatment period, 83% of Xofigo patients and 82% of placebo patients received gonadotropin-releasing hormone agonists and 21% of Xofigo patients and 34% of placebo patients received concomitant antiandrogens. Use of systemic steroids (41%) and bisphosphonates (40%) was balanced between the arms.

The pre-specified interim analysis of overall survival revealed a statistically significant improvement in patients receiving XOFIGO plus best standard of care compared with patients receiving placebo plus best standard of care. An exploratory updated overall survival analysis performed before patient crossover with an additional 214 events resulted in findings consistent with the interim analysis (Table 5).

Table 5: Overall Survival Results from the Phase 3 Clinical Trial

	Xofigo	Placebo
Interim Analysis		
Subjects randomized	541	268
Number of deaths	191 (35.3%)	123 (45.9%)
Censored	350 (64.7%)	145 (54.1%)
Median survival (months)[a]	14.0	11.2
(95% CI)	(12.1, 15.8)	(9.0, 13.2)
p-value[b]	0.00185	
Hazard ratio (95% CI)[c]	0.695 (0.552, 0.875)	
Updated Analysis		
Subjects randomized	614	307
Number of deaths	333 (54.2%)	195 (63.5%)
Censored	281 (45.8%)	112 (36.5%)
Median survival (months)[a]	14.9	11.3
(95% CI)	(13.9, 16.1)	(10.4, 12.8)
Hazard ratio (95% CI)[c]	0.695 (0.581, 0.832)	

[a] Survival time is calculated as months from date of randomization to date of death from any cause. Subjects who are not deceased at time of analysis are censored on the last date subject was known to be alive or lost to follow-up.

[b] p-value is from a log-rank test stratified by total ALP, current use of bisphosphonates, and prior use of docetaxel.

[c] Hazard ratio is from a Cox proportional hazards model adjusted for total ALP, current use of bisphosphonates, and prior use of docetaxel. Hazard ratio < 1 favors radium-223 dichloride.

The Kaplan-Meier curves for overall survival based on the updated survival results are shown in Figure 1.

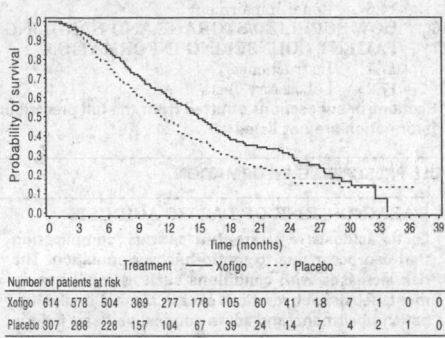

Figure 1: Kaplan-Meier Overall Survival Curves from the Phase 3 Clinical Trial

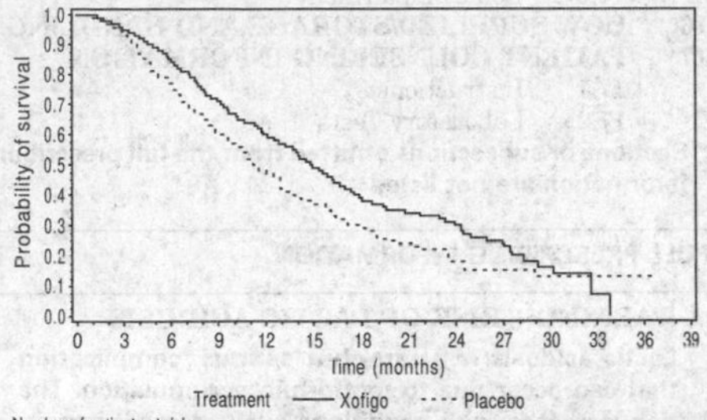

Number of patients at risk

	0	3	6	9	12	15	18	21	24	27	30	33	36	39
Xofigo	614	578	504	369	277	178	105	60	41	18	7	1	0	0
Placebo	307	288	228	157	104	67	39	24	14	7	4	2	1	0

The survival results were supported by a delay in the time to first SSE favoring the Xofigo arm. The majority of events consisted of external beam radiotherapy to bone metastases.

15 REFERENCES

1. Radiation Emergency Medical Management. [REMM/ National Library of Medicine Website.] http://www.remm.nlm.gov/ int_contamination.htm#blockingagents

16 HOW SUPPLIED/STORAGE AND HANDLING

Xofigo (radium Ra 223 dichloride injection) is supplied in single-use vials containing 6 mL of solution at a concentration of 1,000 kBq/mL (27 microcurie/mL) with a total radioactivity of 6,000 kBq/vial (162 microcurie/vial) at the reference date (NDC 50419-208-01).

Store at room temperature, below 40° C (104° F). Store Xofigo in the original container or equivalent radiation shielding.

This preparation is approved for use by persons under license by the Nuclear Regulatory Commission or the relevant regulatory authority of an Agreement State.

Follow procedures for proper handling and disposal of radioactive pharmaceuticals *[see Dosage and Administration (2.3)]*.

17 PATIENT COUNSELING INFORMATION

Advise patients:

- To be compliant with blood cell count monitoring appointments while receiving Xofigo. Explain the importance of routine blood cell counts. Instruct patients to report signs of bleeding or infections.
- To stay well hydrated and to monitor oral intake, fluid status, and urine output while being treated with Xofigo. Instruct patients to report signs of dehydration, hypovolemia, urinary retention, or renal failure / insufficiency.
- There are no restrictions regarding contact with other people after receiving Xofigo. Follow good hygiene practices while receiving Xofigo and for at least 1 week after the last injection in order to minimize radiation exposure from bodily fluids to household members and caregivers. Whenever possible, patients should use a toilet and the toilet should be flushed several times after each use. Clothing soiled with patient fecal matter or urine should be washed promptly and separately from other clothing. Caregivers should use universal precautions for patient care such as gloves and barrier gowns when handling bodily fluids to avoid contamination. When handling bodily fluids, wearing gloves and hand washing will protect caregivers.
- Who are sexually active to use condoms and their female partners of reproductive potential to use a highly effective method of birth control during treatment and for 6 months following completion of Xofigo treatment.

Manufactured for:
Bayer HealthCare Pharmaceuticals Inc.
Wayne, NJ 07470
Manufactured in Norway
Xofigo is a trademark of Bayer Aktiengesellschaft.

Revised: 05/2013

Boehringer Ingelheim Pharmaceuticals, Inc.
900 RIDGEBURY ROAD
P.O. BOX 368
RIDGEFIELD, CT 06877-0368

Direct inquiries to:
(800) 243-0127
TTY (800) 246-6196

For medical information or to report an adverse drug experience contact:
(800) 542-6257
TTY (800) 459-9906
(option 4)
http://us.boehringer-ingelheim.com

JENTADUETO® ℞

(linagliptin and metformin hydrochloride) tablets

HIGHLIGHTS OF PRESCRIBING INFORMATION
These highlights do not include all the information needed to use JENTADUETO safely and effectively. See full prescribing information for JENTADUETO.
Jentadueto® (linagliptin and metformin hydrochloride) tablets
Initial U.S. Approval: 2012

WARNING: RISK OF LACTIC ACIDOSIS
See full prescribing information for complete boxed warning.

- **Lactic acidosis can occur due to metformin accumulation. The risk increases with conditions such as renal impairment, sepsis, dehydration, excess alcohol intake, hepatic impairment, and acute congestive heart failure. (5.1)**
- **Symptoms include malaise, myalgias, respiratory distress, increasing somnolence, and nonspecific abdominal distress. Laboratory abnormalities include low pH, increased anion gap, and elevated blood lactate. (5.1)**
- **If acidosis is suspected, discontinue JENTADUETO and hospitalize the patient immediately (5.1)**

RECENT MAJOR CHANGES

Indications and Usage	
Important Limitations of Use (1.2)	6/2013
Dosage and Administration	
Concomitant Use with an Insulin Secretagogue (e.g., Sulfonylurea) or with Insulin (2.2)	9/2013
Warnings and Precautions	
Pancreatitis (5.2)	6/2013
Use with Medications Known to Cause Hypoglycemia (5.5)	9/2013

INDICATIONS AND USAGE

JENTADUETO is a dipeptidyl peptidase-4 (DPP-4) inhibitor and biguanide combination product indicated as an adjunct to diet and exercise to improve glycemic control in adults with type 2 diabetes mellitus when treatment with both linagliptin and metformin is appropriate (1.1)

Important limitations of use:

- Not for treatment of type 1 diabetes or diabetic ketoacidosis (1.2)
- Has not been studied in patients with a history of pancreatitis (1.2)

DOSAGE AND ADMINISTRATION

- Individualize the starting dose of JENTADUETO based on the patient's current regimen (2.1)
- The maximum recommended dose is 2.5 mg linagliptin/ 1000 mg metformin twice daily (2.1)
- Should be given twice daily with meals, with gradual dose escalation to reduce the gastrointestinal side effects due to metformin (2.1)

DOSAGE FORMS AND STRENGTHS

Tablets:
2.5 mg linagliptin/500 mg metformin hydrochloride
2.5 mg linagliptin/850 mg metformin hydrochloride
2.5 mg linagliptin/1000 mg metformin hydrochloride (3)

CONTRAINDICATIONS

- Renal impairment (4)
- Metabolic acidosis, including diabetic ketoacidosis (4)
- Hypersensitivity to linagliptin or metformin (4)

WARNINGS AND PRECAUTIONS

- Lactic acidosis: Warn against excessive alcohol use. JENTADUETO is not recommended in hepatic impairment or hypoxic states and is contraindicated in renal im-

pairment. Ensure normal renal function before initiating and at least annually thereafter. (5.1, 5.3, 5.4, 5.7, 5.8)
- There have been postmarketing reports of acute pancreatitis, including fatal pancreatitis. If pancreatitis is suspected, promptly discontinue JENTADUETO. (5.2)
- Temporarily discontinue JENTADUETO in patients undergoing radiologic studies with intravascular administration of iodinated contrast materials or any surgical procedures necessitating restricted intake of food and fluids (5.3)
- Hypoglycemia: When used with an insulin secretagogue (e.g., sulfonylurea (SU) or insulin, consider lowering the dose of the insulin secretagogue or insulin to reduce the risk of hypoglycemia (2.2, 5.5)
- Vitamin B_{12} deficiency: Metformin may lower vitamin B_{12} levels. Monitor hematologic parameters annually. (5.6)
- Macrovascular outcomes: No conclusive evidence of macrovascular risk reduction with JENTADUETO or any other antidiabetic drug (5.9)

ADVERSE REACTIONS

- Adverse reactions reported in ≥5% of patients treated with JENTADUETO and more commonly than in patients treated with placebo are nasopharyngitis and diarrhea (6.1)
- Hypoglycemia was more commonly reported in patients treated with the combination of JENTADUETO and SU compared with those treated with the combination of SU and metformin (6.1)

To report SUSPECTED ADVERSE REACTIONS, contact Boehringer Ingelheim Pharmaceuticals, Inc. at 1-800-542-6257 or 1-800-459-9906 TTY, or FDA at 1-800-FDA-1088 or www.fda.gov/medwatch.

DRUG INTERACTIONS

- Cationic drugs eliminated by renal tubular secretion: May reduce metformin elimination. Use with caution. (7.1)
- P-glycoprotein/CYP3A4 inducer: The efficacy of JENTADUETO may be reduced when administered in combination (e.g., rifampin). Use of alternative treatments is strongly recommended. (7.2)

USE IN SPECIFIC POPULATIONS

- Pregnancy: There are no adequate and well-controlled studies in pregnant women. JENTADUETO tablets should be used during pregnancy only if clearly needed. (8.1)
- Nursing mothers: Caution should be exercised when JENTADUETO is administered to a nursing woman (8.3)
- Pediatric patients: Safety and effectiveness of JENTADUETO in patients below the age of 18 have not been established (8.4)

See 17 for PATIENT COUNSELING INFORMATION and Medication Guide

Revised: 09/2013

FULL PRESCRIBING INFORMATION: CONTENTS*

*** Sections or subsections omitted from the full prescribing information are not listed**

FULL PRESCRIBING INFORMATION

WARNING: RISK OF LACTIC ACIDOSIS

Lactic acidosis is a rare, but serious, complication that can occur due to metformin accumulation. The risk increases with conditions such as renal impairment, sepsis, dehydration, excess alcohol intake, hepatic impairment, and acute congestive heart failure.

The onset is often subtle, accompanied only by nonspecific symptoms such as malaise, myalgias, respiratory distress, increasing somnolence, and nonspecific abdominal distress.

Laboratory abnormalities include low pH, increased anion gap, and elevated blood lactate.

If acidosis is suspected, JENTADUETO should be discontinued and the patient hospitalized immediately *[see Warnings and Precautions (5.1)]*.

1 INDICATIONS AND USAGE

1.1 Indication

JENTADUETO tablets are indicated as an adjunct to diet and exercise to improve glycemic control in adults with type 2 diabetes mellitus when treatment with both linagliptin and metformin is appropriate *[see Dosage and Administration (2.1) and Clinical Studies (14.1)]*.

1.2 Important Limitations of Use

JENTADUETO should not be used in patients with type 1 diabetes or for the treatment of diabetic ketoacidosis, as it would not be effective in these settings.

JENTADUETO has not been studied in patients with a history of pancreatitis. It is unknown whether patients with a history of pancreatitis are at an increased risk for the development of pancreatitis while using JENTADUETO *[see Warnings and Precautions (5.2)]*.

2 DOSAGE AND ADMINISTRATION

2.1 Recommended Dosing

The dosage of JENTADUETO should be individualized on the basis of both effectiveness and tolerability, while not exceeding the maximum recommended dose of 2.5 mg linagliptin/1000 mg metformin hydrochloride twice daily. JENTADUETO should be given twice daily with meals. Dose escalation should be gradual to reduce the gastrointestinal (GI) side effects associated with metformin use. For available dosage forms and strengths see *[Dosage Forms and Strengths (3)]*.

Recommended starting dose:

- In patients currently not treated with metformin, initiate treatment with 2.5 mg linagliptin/500 mg metformin hydrochloride twice daily
- In patients already treated with metformin, start with 2.5 mg linagliptin and the current dose of metformin taken at each of the two daily meals (e.g., a patient on metformin 1000 mg twice daily would be started on 2.5 mg linagliptin/1000 mg metformin hydrochloride twice daily with meals).
- Patients already treated with linagliptin and metformin individual components may be switched to JENTADUETO containing the same doses of each component.

No studies have been performed specifically examining the safety and efficacy of JENTADUETO in patients previously treated with other oral antihyperglycemic agents and switched to JENTADUETO. Any change in therapy of type 2 diabetes mellitus should be undertaken with care and appropriate monitoring as changes in glycemic control can occur.

2.2 Concomitant Use with an Insulin Secretagogue (e.g., Sulfonylurea) or with Insulin

When JENTADUETO is used in combination with an insulin secretagogue (e.g., sulfonylurea) or with insulin, a lower dose of the insulin secretagogue or insulin may be required to reduce the risk of hypoglycemia *[see Warnings and Precautions (5.5)]*.

3 DOSAGE FORMS AND STRENGTHS

JENTADUETO is a combination of linagliptin and metformin hydrochloride. JENTADUETO tablets are available in the following dosage forms and strengths:

- 2.5 mg linagliptin/500 mg metformin hydrochloride tablets are light yellow, oval, biconvex tablets debossed with "D2/500" on one side and the Boehringer Ingelheim logo on the other side
- 2.5 mg linagliptin/850 mg metformin hydrochloride tablets are light orange, oval, biconvex tablets debossed with "D2/850" on one side and the Boehringer Ingelheim logo on the other side
- 2.5 mg linagliptin/1000 mg metformin hydrochloride tablets are light pink, oval, biconvex tablets debossed with "D2/1000" on one side and the Boehringer Ingelheim logo on the other side

4 CONTRAINDICATIONS

JENTADUETO is contraindicated in patients with:

- Renal impairment (e.g., serum creatinine ≥1.5 mg/dL for men, ≥1.4 mg/dL for women, or abnormal creatinine clearance) which may also result from conditions such as cardiovascular collapse (shock), acute myocardial infarction, and septicemia *[see Warnings and Precautions (5.1, 5.3)]*
- Acute or chronic metabolic acidosis, including diabetic ketoacidosis. Diabetic ketoacidosis should be treated with insulin *[see Warnings and Precautions (5.1)]*
- A history of hypersensitivity reaction to linagliptin (such as urticaria, angioedema, or bronchial hyperreactivity) or metformin *[see Adverse Reactions (6.1)]*

5 WARNINGS AND PRECAUTIONS

5.1 Lactic Acidosis

Metformin

Lactic acidosis is a serious, metabolic complication that can occur due to metformin accumulation during treatment with JENTADUETO and is fatal in approximately 50% of cases. Lactic acidosis may also occur in association with a number of pathophysiologic conditions, including diabetes mellitus, and whenever there is significant tissue hypoperfusion and hypoxemia. Lactic acidosis is characterized by elevated blood lactate levels (>5 mmol/L), decreased blood pH, electrolyte disturbances with an increased anion gap, and an increased lactate/pyruvate ratio. When metformin is implicated as the cause of lactic acidosis, metformin plasma levels of >5 µg/mL are generally found.

The reported incidence of lactic acidosis in patients receiving metformin is approximately 0.03 cases/1000 patient-years, (with approximately 0.015 fatal cases/1000 patient-years). In more than 20,000 patient-years exposure to metformin in clinical trials, there were no reports of lactic acidosis. Reported cases have occurred primarily in diabetic patients with significant renal impairment, including both intrinsic renal disease and renal hypoperfusion, often in the setting of multiple concomitant medical/surgical problems and multiple concomitant medications. Patients with congestive heart failure requiring pharmacologic management, particularly when accompanied by hypoperfusion and hypoxemia due to unstable or acute failure, are at increased risk of lactic acidosis. The risk of lactic acidosis increases with the degree of renal impairment and the patient's age. The risk of lactic acidosis may, therefore, be significantly decreased by regular monitoring of renal function in patients taking metformin. In particular, treatment of the elderly should be accompanied by careful monitoring of renal function. Metformin treatment should not be initiated in any patient unless measurement of creatinine clearance demonstrates that renal function is not reduced. In addition, metformin should be promptly withheld in the presence of any condition associated with hypoxemia, dehydration, or sepsis. Because impaired hepatic function may significantly limit the ability to clear lactate, metformin should be avoided in patients with clinical or laboratory evidence of hepatic impairment. Patients should be cautioned against excessive alcohol intake when taking metformin, since alcohol potentiates the effects of metformin on lactate metabolism. In addition, metformin should be temporarily discontinued prior to any intravascular radiocontrast study and for any surgical procedure necessitating restricted intake of food or fluids. Use of topiramate, a carbonic anhydrase inhibitor, in epilepsy and migraine prophylaxis may cause dose-dependent metabolic acidosis and may exacerbate the risk of metformin-induced lactic acidosis *[see Drug Interactions (7.1) and Clinical Pharmacology (12.3)]*.

The onset of lactic acidosis is often subtle, and accompanied by nonspecific symptoms such as malaise, myalgias, respiratory distress, increasing somnolence, and nonspecific abdominal distress. More severe acidosis may be associated with signs such as hypothermia, hypotension, and resistant bradyarrhythmias. Patients should be educated to recognize and promptly report these symptoms. If present,

JENTADUETO should be discontinued until lactic acidosis is ruled out. Gastrointestinal symptoms, which are commonly reported during initiation of metformin therapy are less frequently observed in subjects on a chronic, stable, dose of metformin. Gastrointestinal symptoms in subjects on chronic, stable, dose of metformin could be caused by lactic acidosis or other serious disease.

To rule out lactic acidosis, serum electrolytes, ketones, blood glucose, blood pH, lactate levels, and blood metformin levels may be useful. Levels of fasting venous plasma lactate above the upper limit of normal but less than 5 mmol/L in patients taking metformin do not necessarily indicate impending lactic acidosis and may be due to other mechanisms, such as poorly-controlled diabetes or obesity, vigorous physical activity, or technical problems in sample handling.

Lactic acidosis should be suspected in any diabetic patient with metabolic acidosis lacking evidence of ketoacidosis (ketonuria and ketonemia). Lactic acidosis is a medical emergency that must be treated in a hospital setting. In a patient with lactic acidosis who is taking metformin, the drug should be discontinued immediately and supportive measures promptly instituted. Metformin is dialyzable (clearance of up to 170 mL/min under good hemodynamic conditions) and prompt hemodialysis is recommended to remove the accumulated metformin and correct the metabolic acidosis. Such management often results in prompt reversal of symptoms and recovery *[see Boxed Warning]*.

5.2 Pancreatitis

There have been postmarketing reports of acute pancreatitis, including fatal pancreatitis, in patients taking linagliptin. Take careful notice of potential signs and symptoms of pancreatitis. If pancreatitis is suspected, promptly discontinue JENTADUETO and initiate appropriate management. It is unknown whether patients with a history of pancreatitis are at increased risk for the development of pancreatitis while using JENTADUETO.

5.3 Monitoring of Renal Function

Although linagliptin undergoes minimal renal excretion, metformin is known to be substantially excreted by the kidney. The risk of metformin accumulation and lactic acidosis increases with the degree of renal impairment. Therefore, JENTADUETO is contraindicated in patients with renal impairment.

Before initiation of therapy with JENTADUETO and at least annually thereafter, renal function should be assessed and verified to be normal. In patients in whom development of renal impairment is anticipated (e.g., elderly), renal function should be assessed more frequently and JENTADUETO discontinued if evidence of renal impairment is present.

Linagliptin may be continued as a single entity tablet at the same total daily dose of 5 mg if JENTADUETO is discontinued due to evidence of renal impairment. No dose adjustment of linagliptin is recommended in patients with renal impairment.

***Use of concomitant medications that may affect renal function or metformin disposition*:**

Concomitant medication(s) that may affect renal function or result in significant hemodynamic change or interfere with the disposition of metformin should be used with caution *[see Drug Interactions (7.1) and Clinical Pharmacology (12.3)]*.

Radiological studies and surgical procedures:

Radiologic studies involving the use of intravascular iodinated contrast materials (e.g., intravenous urogram, intravenous cholangiography, angiography, and computed tomography) can lead to acute alteration of renal function and have been associated with lactic acidosis in patients receiving metformin. Therefore, in patients in whom any such study is planned, JENTADUETO should be temporarily discontinued at the time of or prior to the procedure, and withheld for 48 hours subsequent to the procedure and reinstituted only after renal function has been confirmed to be normal.

JENTADUETO should be temporarily discontinued for any surgical procedure (except minor procedures not associated with restricted intake of food and fluids) and should not be restarted until the patient's oral intake has resumed and renal function has been evaluated as normal.

5.4 Impaired Hepatic Function

Because impaired hepatic function has been associated with some cases of lactic acidosis with metformin therapy, JENTADUETO should generally be avoided in patients with clinical or laboratory evidence of hepatic disease *[see Warnings and Precautions (5.1)]*.

5.5 Use with Medications Known to Cause Hypoglycemia

Linagliptin

Insulin secretagogues and insulin are known to cause hypoglycemia. The use of linagliptin in combination with an insulin secretagogue (e.g., sulfonylurea) was associated with a higher rate of hypoglycemia compared with placebo in a clinical trial *[see Adverse Reactions (6.1)]*. The use of linagliptin in combination with insulin in subjects with severe renal impairment was associated with a higher rate of hypoglycemia *[see Adverse Reactions (6.1)]*. Therefore, a lower dose of the insulin secretagogue or insulin may be required to reduce the risk of hypoglycemia when used in combination with JENTADUETO *[see Dosage and Administration (2.2)]*.

Metformin

Hypoglycemia does not occur in patients receiving metformin alone under usual circumstances of use, but could occur when caloric intake is deficient, when strenuous exercise is not compensated by caloric supplementation, or during concomitant use with other glucose-lowering agents (such as SUs and insulin) or ethanol. Elderly, debilitated, or malnourished patients, and those with adrenal or pituitary insufficiency or alcohol intoxication are particularly susceptible to hypoglycemic effects. Hypoglycemia may be difficult to recognize in the elderly, and in people who are taking β-adrenergic blocking drugs.

5.6 Vitamin B_{12} Levels

In controlled, 29-week clinical trials of metformin, a decrease to subnormal levels of previously normal serum vitamin B_{12} levels, without clinical manifestations, was observed in approximately 7% of metformin-treated patients. Such decrease, possibly due to interference with B_{12} absorption from the B_{12}-intrinsic factor complex, is, however, very rarely associated with anemia or neurologic manifestations due to the short duration (<1 year) of the clinical trials. This risk may be more relevant to patients receiving long-term treatment with metformin, and adverse hematologic and neurologic reactions have been reported postmarketing. The decrease in vitamin B_{12} levels appears to be rapidly reversible with discontinuation of metformin or vitamin B_{12} supplementation. Measurement of hematologic parameters on an annual basis is advised in patients on JENTADUETO and any apparent abnormalities should be appropriately investigated and managed. Certain individuals (those with inadequate vitamin B_{12} or calcium intake or absorption) appear to be predisposed to developing subnormal vitamin B_{12} levels. In these patients, routine serum vitamin B_{12} measurement at 2- to 3-year intervals may be useful.

5.7 Alcohol Intake

Alcohol is known to potentiate the effect of metformin on lactate metabolism. Patients, therefore, should be warned against excessive alcohol intake while receiving JENTADUETO *[see Warnings and Precautions (5.1)]*.

5.8 Hypoxic States

Cardiovascular collapse (shock) from whatever cause (e.g., acute congestive heart failure, acute myocardial infarction, and other conditions characterized by hypoxemia) have been associated with lactic acidosis and may also cause prerenal azotemia. When such events occur in patients on JENTADUETO therapy, the drug should be promptly discontinued *[see Warnings and Precautions (5.1)]*.

5.9 Macrovascular Outcomes

There have been no clinical studies establishing conclusive evidence of macrovascular risk reduction with linagliptin or metformin or any other antidiabetic drug.

6 ADVERSE REACTIONS

6.1 Clinical Trials Experience

Because clinical trials are conducted under widely varying conditions, adverse reaction rates observed in the clinical trials of a drug cannot be directly compared to rates in the clinical trials of another drug and may not reflect the rates observed in practice.

Linagliptin/Metformin

The safety of concomitantly administered linagliptin (daily dose 5 mg) and metformin (mean daily dose of approximately 1800 mg) has been evaluated in 2816 patients with type 2 diabetes mellitus treated for ≥12 weeks in clinical trials.

Three placebo-controlled studies with linagliptin + metformin were conducted: 2 studies were 24 weeks in duration, 1 study was 12 weeks in duration. In the 3 placebo-controlled clinical studies, adverse events which occurred in ≥5% of patients receiving linagliptin + metformin (n=875) and were more common than in patients given placebo + metformin (n=539) included nasopharyngitis (5.7% vs 4.3%).

In a 24-week factorial design study, adverse events reported in ≥5% of patients receiving linagliptin + metformin and were more common than in patients given placebo are shown in Table 1.

Table 1 Adverse Reactions Reported in ≥5% of Patients Treated with Linagliptin + Metformin and Greater than with Placebo in a 24-week Factorial-Design Study

	Placebo n=72	Linagliptin Monotherapy n=142	Metformin Monotherapy n=291	Combination of Linagliptin with Metformin n=286
	n (%)	n (%)	n (%)	n (%)
Nasopharyngitis	1 (1.4)	8 (5.6)	8 (2.7)	18 (6.3)
Diarrhea	2 (2.8)	5 (3.5)	11 (3.8)	18 (6.3)

[See table 1 above]

Other adverse reactions reported in clinical studies with treatment of linagliptin + metformin were hypersensitivity (e.g., urticaria, angioedema, or bronchial hyperreactivity), cough, decreased appetite, nausea, vomiting, pruritus, and pancreatitis.

Linagliptin

Adverse reactions reported in ≥2% of patients treated with linagliptin 5 mg and more commonly than in patients treated with placebo included: nasopharyngitis (7.0% vs 6.1%), diarrhea (3.3% vs 3.0%), and cough (2.1% vs 1.4%).

Rates for other adverse reactions for linagliptin 5 mg vs placebo when linagliptin was used in combination with specific anti-diabetic agents were: urinary tract infection (3.1% vs 0%) and hypertriglyceridemia (2.4% vs 0%) when linagliptin was used as add-on to sulfonylurea; hyperlipidemia (2.7% vs 0.8%) and weight increased (2.3% vs 0.8%) when linagliptin was used as add-on to pioglitazone; and constipation (2.1% vs 1%) when linagliptin was used as add-on to basal insulin therapy.

Other adverse reactions reported in clinical studies with treatment of linagliptin monotherapy were hypersensitivity (e.g., urticaria, angioedema, localized skin exfoliation, or bronchial hyperreactivity) and myalgia. In the clinical trial program, pancreatitis was reported in 15.2 cases per 10,000 patient year exposure while being treated with linagliptin compared with 3.7 cases per 10,000 patient year exposure while being treated with comparator (placebo and active comparator, sulfonylurea). Three additional cases of pancreatitis were reported following the last administered dose of linagliptin.

Metformin

The most common adverse reactions due to initiation of metformin are diarrhea, nausea/vomiting, flatulence, asthenia, indigestion, abdominal discomfort, and headache.

Long-term treatment with metformin has been associated with a decrease in vitamin B_{12} absorption which may very rarely result in clinically significant vitamin B_{12} deficiency (e.g., megaloblastic anemia) *[see Warnings and Precautions (5.5)]*.

Hypoglycemia

Linagliptin/Metformin

In a 24-week factorial design study, hypoglycemia was reported in 4 (1.4%) of 286 subjects treated with linagliptin + metformin, 6 (2.1%) of 291 subjects treated with metformin, and 1 (1.4%) of 72 subjects treated with placebo. When linagliptin was administered in combination with metformin and a sulfonylurea, 181 (22.9%) of 792 patients reported hypoglycemia compared with 39 (14.8%) of 263 patients administered placebo in combination with metformin and sulfonylurea. Adverse reactions of hypoglycemia were based on all reports of hypoglycemia. A concurrent glucose measurement was not required or was normal in some patients. Therefore, it is not possible to conclusively determine that all these reports reflect true hypoglycemia.

Linagliptin

In the study of patients receiving linagliptin as add-on therapy to a stable dose of insulin for up to 52 weeks (n=1261), no significant difference in the incidence of investigator reported hypoglycemia, defined as all symptomatic or asymptomatic episodes with a self measured blood glucose ≤70 mg/dL, was noted between the linagliptin- (31.4%) and placebo- (32.9%) treated groups.

Use in Renal Impairment

Linagliptin was compared to placebo as add-on to pre-existing antidiabetic therapy over 52 weeks in 133 patients with severe renal impairment (estimated GFR <30 mL/min). For the initial 12 weeks of the study, background antidiabetic therapy was kept stable and included insulin, sulfonylurea, glinides, and pioglitazone. For the remainder of the trial, dose adjustments in antidiabetic background therapy were allowed.

In general, the incidence of adverse events including severe hypoglycemia was similar to those reported in other linagliptin trials. The observed incidence of hypoglycemia was higher (linagliptin, 63% compared to placebo, 49%) due to an increase in asymptomatic hypoglycemic events especially during the first 12 weeks when background glycemic therapies were kept stable. Ten linagliptin-treated patients (15%) and 11 placebo-treated patients (17%) reported at least one episode of confirmed symptomatic hypoglycemia (accompanying finger stick glucose ≤54 mg/dL). During the same time period, severe hypoglycemic events, defined as an event requiring the assistance of another person to actively administer carbohydrate, glucagon or other resuscitative actions, were reported in 3 (4.4%) linagliptin-treated patients and 3 (4.6%) placebo-treated patients. Events that were considered life-threatening or required hospitalization were reported in 2 (2.9%) patients on linagliptin and 1 (1.5%) patient on placebo.

Renal function as measured by mean eGFR and creatinine clearance did not change over 52 weeks' treatment compared to placebo.

Laboratory Tests

Changes in laboratory findings were similar in patients treated with linagliptin + metformin compared to patients treated with placebo + metformin. Changes in laboratory values that occurred more frequently in the linagliptin + metformin group and ≥1% more than in the placebo group were not detected.

No clinically meaningful changes in vital signs were observed in patients treated with linagliptin.

6.2 Postmarketing Experience

Additional adverse reactions have been identified during postapproval use of linagliptin. Because these reactions are reported voluntarily from a population of uncertain size, it is generally not possible to reliably estimate their frequency or establish a causal relationship to drug exposure.

- Acute pancreatitis, including fatal pancreatitis *[see Indications and Usage (1.2) and Warnings and Precautions (5.2)]*
- Rash

7 DRUG INTERACTIONS

7.1 Drug Interactions with Metformin

Cationic Drugs

Cationic drugs (e.g., amiloride, digoxin, morphine, procainamide, quinidine, quinine, ranitidine, triamterene, trimethoprim, or vancomycin) that are eliminated by renal tubular secretion theoretically have the potential for interaction with metformin by competing for common renal tubular transport systems. Although such interactions remain theoretical (except for cimetidine), careful patient monitoring and dose adjustment of JENTADUETO and/or the interfering drug is recommended in patients who are taking cationic medications that are excreted via the proximal renal tubular secretory system *[see Warnings and Precautions (5.3) and Clinical Pharmacology (12.3)]*.

Carbonic Anhydrase Inhibitors

Topiramate or other carbonic anhydrase inhibitors (e.g., zonisamide, acetazolamide or dichlorphenamide) frequently decrease serum bicarbonate and induce non-anion gap, hyperchloremic metabolic acidosis. Concomitant use of these drugs may induce metabolic acidosis. Use these drugs with caution in patients treated with JENTADUETO, as the risk of lactic acidosis may increase *[see Warnings and Precautions (5.1) and Clinical Pharmacology (12.3)]*.

7.2 Drug Interactions with Linagliptin

Inducers of P-glycoprotein and CYP3A4 Enzymes

Rifampin decreased linagliptin exposure, suggesting that the efficacy of linagliptin may be reduced when administered in combination with a strong P-gp inducer or CYP 3A4 inducer. As JENTADUETO is a fixed-dose combination of linagliptin and metformin, use of alternative treatments (not containing linagliptin) is strongly recommended when concomitant treatment with a strong P-gp or CYP 3A4 inducer is necessary *[see Clinical Pharmacology (12.3)]*.

7.3 Drugs Affecting Glycemic Control

Certain drugs tend to produce hyperglycemia and may lead to loss of glycemic control. These drugs include the thiazides and other diuretics, corticosteroids, phenothiazines, thyroid products, estrogens, oral contraceptives, phenytoin, nicotinic acid, sympathomimetics, calcium channel blocking drugs, and isoniazid. When such drugs are administered to a patient receiving JENTADUETO, the patient should be closely observed to maintain adequate glycemic control *[see Clinical Pharmacology (12.3)]*. When such drugs are withdrawn from a patient receiving JENTADUETO, the patient should be observed closely for hypoglycemia.

8 USE IN SPECIFIC POPULATIONS

8.1 Pregnancy

Pregnancy Category B

JENTADUETO

There are no adequate and well controlled studies in pregnant women with JENTADUETO or its individual components, and some clinical data is available for metformin which indicate that the risk for major malformations was not increased when metformin is taken during the first trimester in pregnancy. In addition, metformin was not associated with increased perinatal complications. Nevertheless, because these clinical data cannot rule out the possibility of harm, JENTADUETO should be used during pregnancy only if clearly needed.

JENTADUETO was not teratogenic when administered to Wistar Han rats during the period of organogenesis at doses similar to clinical exposure. At higher maternally toxic doses (9 and 23 times the clinical dose based on exposure), the metformin component of the combination was associated with an increased incidence of fetal rib and scapula malformations.

Linagliptin

Linagliptin was not teratogenic when administered to pregnant Wistar Han rats and Himalayan rabbits during the period of organogenesis at doses up to 240 mg/kg and 150 mg/kg, respectively. These doses represent approximately 943 times the clinical dose in rats and 1943 times the clinical dose in rabbits, based on exposure. No functional, behavioral, or reproductive toxicity was observed in offspring of female Wistar Han rats when administered linagliptin from gestation day 6 to lactation day 21 at a dose 49 times the maximum recommended human dose, based on exposure.

Linagliptin crosses the placenta into the fetus following oral dosing in pregnant rats and rabbits.

Metformin Hydrochloride

Metformin has been studied for embryofetal effects in 2 rat strains and in rabbits. Metformin was not teratogenic in Sprague Dawley rats up to 600 mg/kg or in Wistar Han rats up to 200 mg/kg (2-3 times the clinical dose based on body surface area or exposure, respectively). At higher maternally toxic doses (9 and 23 times the clinical dose based on exposure), an increased incidence of rib and scapula skeletal malformations was observed in the Wistar Han strain. Metformin was not teratogenic in rabbits at doses up to 140 mg/kg (similar to clinical dose based on body surface area).

Metformin administered to female Sprague Dawley rats from gestation day 6 to lactation day 21 up to 600 mg/kg/day (2 times the maximum clinical dose based on body surface area) had no effect on prenatal or postnatal development of offspring.

Metformin crosses the placenta into the fetus in rats and humans.

8.3 Nursing Mothers

No studies in lactating animals have been conducted with the combined components of JENTADUETO. In studies performed with the individual components, both linagliptin and metformin were secreted in the milk of lactating rats. It is not known whether linagliptin is excreted in human milk. Metformin is excreted in human milk in low concentrations. Because the potential for hypoglycemia in nursing infants may exist, a decision should be made whether to discontinue nursing or to discontinue the drug, taking into account the importance of the drug to the mother.

8.4 Pediatric Use

Safety and effectiveness of JENTADUETO in pediatric patients under 18 years of age have not been established.

8.5 Geriatric Use

Linagliptin is minimally excreted by the kidney; however, metformin is substantially excreted by the kidney. Considering that aging can be associated with reduced renal function, JENTADUETO should be used with caution as age increases *[see Warnings and Precautions (5.1, 5.3) and Clinical Pharmacology (12.3)]*.

Linagliptin

There were 4040 type 2 diabetes patients treated with linagliptin 5 mg from 15 clinical trials of linagliptin; 1085 (27%) patients were 65 years and over, while 131 (3%) were 75 years and over. Of these patients, 2566 were enrolled in 12 double-blind placebo-controlled studies; 591 (23%) were 65 years and over, while 82 (3%) were 75 years and over. No overall differences in safety or effectiveness were observed between patients 65 years and over and younger patients. Therefore, no dose adjustment is recommended in the elderly population. While clinical studies of linagliptin have not identified differences in response between the elderly and younger patients, greater sensitivity of some older individuals cannot be ruled out.

Metformin

Controlled clinical studies of metformin did not include sufficient numbers of elderly patients to determine whether they respond differently from younger patients, although other reported clinical experience has not identified differences in responses between the elderly and young patients. The initial and maintenance dosing of metformin should be conservative in patients with advanced age, due to the potential for decreased renal function in this population. Any dose adjustment should be based on a careful assessment of renal function *[see Contraindications (4), Warnings and Precautions (5.3), and Clinical Pharmacology (12.3)]*.

10 OVERDOSAGE

In the event of an overdose with JENTADUETO, contact the Poison Control Center. Employ the usual supportive measures (e.g., remove unabsorbed material from the gastrointestinal tract, employ clinical monitoring, and institute supportive treatment) as dictated by the patient's clinical status. Removal of linagliptin by hemodialysis or peritoneal dialysis is unlikely. However, metformin is dialyzable with a clearance of up to 170 mL/min under good hemodynamic conditions. Therefore, hemodialysis may be useful partly for removal of accumulated metformin from patients in whom JENTADUETO overdosage is suspected.

Linagliptin

During controlled clinical trials in healthy subjects, with single doses of up to 600 mg of linagliptin (equivalent to 120 times the recommended daily dose), there were no dose-related clinical adverse drug reactions. There is no experience with doses above 600 mg in humans.

Metformin

Overdose of metformin has occurred, including ingestion of amounts greater than 50 grams. Hypoglycemia was reported in approximately 10% of cases, but no causal association with metformin has been established. Lactic acidosis has been reported in approximately 32% of metformin overdose cases *[see Boxed Warning and Warnings and Precautions (5.1)]*.

11 DESCRIPTION

JENTADUETO tablets contain 2 oral antihyperglycemic drugs used in the management of type 2 diabetes mellitus: linagliptin and metformin hydrochloride.

Linagliptin

Linagliptin is an orally-active inhibitor of the dipeptidyl peptidase-4 (DPP-4) enzyme.

Linagliptin is described chemically as 1H-Purine-2,6-dione, 8-[(3R)-3-amino-1-piperidinyl]-7-(2-butyn-1-yl)-3,7-dihydro-3-methyl-1-[(4-methyl-2-quinazolinyl)methyl]-

The empirical formula is $C_{25}H_{28}N_8O_2$ and the molecular weight is 472.54 g/mol. The structural formula is:

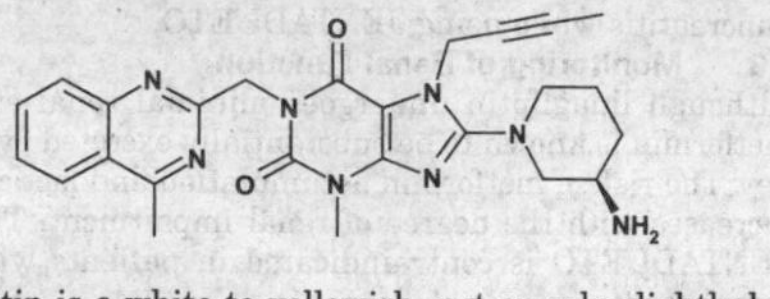

Linagliptin is a white to yellowish, not or only slightly hygroscopic solid substance. It is very slightly soluble in water (0.9 mg/mL). Linagliptin is soluble in methanol (ca. 60 mg/mL), sparingly soluble in ethanol (ca. 10 mg/mL), very slightly soluble in isopropanol (<1 mg/mL), and very slightly soluble in acetone (ca. 1 mg/mL).

Metformin Hydrochloride

Metformin hydrochloride (*N,N*-dimethylimidodicarbonimidic diamide hydrochloride) is not chemically or pharmacologically related to any other classes of oral antihyperglycemic agents. Metformin hydrochloride is a white to off-white crystalline compound with a molecular formula of $C_4H_{11}N_5$•HCl and a molecular weight of 165.63. Metformin hydrochloride is freely soluble in water and is practically insoluble in acetone, ether, and chloroform. The pKa of metformin is 12.4. The pH of a 1% aqueous solution of metformin hydrochloride is 6.68. The structural formula is:

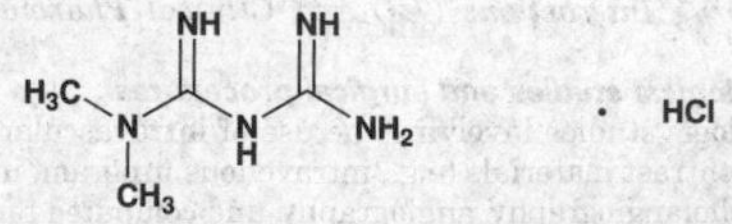

JENTADUETO

JENTADUETO is available for oral administration as tablets containing 2.5 mg linagliptin and 500 mg metformin hydrochloride (JENTADUETO 2.5 mg/500 mg), 850 mg metformin hydrochloride (JENTADUETO 2.5 mg/850 mg) or 1000 mg metformin hydrochloride (JENTADUETO 2.5 mg/1000 mg). Each film-coated tablet of JENTADUETO contains the following inactive ingredients: arginine, corn starch, copovidone, colloidal silicon dioxide, magnesium stearate, titanium dioxide, propylene glycol, hypromellose, talc, yellow ferric oxide (2.5 mg/500 mg; 2.5 mg/850 mg) and/or red ferric oxide (2.5 mg/850 mg; 2.5 mg/1000 mg).

12 CLINICAL PHARMACOLOGY

12.1 Mechanism of Action

JENTADUETO

JENTADUETO combines 2 antihyperglycemic agents with complementary mechanisms of action to improve glycemic control in patients with type 2 diabetes mellitus: linagliptin, a dipeptidyl peptidase-4 (DPP-4) inhibitor, and metformin, a member of the biguanide class.

Linagliptin

Linagliptin is an inhibitor of DPP-4, an enzyme that degrades the incretin hormones glucagon-like peptide-1 (GLP-1) and glucose-dependent insulinotropic polypeptide (GIP). Thus, linagliptin increases the concentrations of active incretin hormones, stimulating the release of insulin in a glucose-dependent manner and decreasing the levels of glucagon in the circulation. Both incretin hormones are involved in the physiological regulation of glucose homeostasis. Incretin hormones are secreted at a low basal level throughout the day and levels rise immediately after meal intake. GLP-1 and GIP increase insulin biosynthesis and secretion from pancreatic beta cells in the presence of normal and elevated blood glucose levels. Furthermore, GLP-1 also reduces glucagon secretion from pancreatic alpha cells, resulting in a reduction in hepatic glucose output.

Metformin

Metformin is an antihyperglycemic agent which improves glucose tolerance in patients with type 2 diabetes mellitus, lowering both basal and postprandial plasma glucose. Its pharmacologic mechanisms of action are different from other classes of oral antihyperglycemic agents. Metformin decreases hepatic glucose production, decreases intestinal absorption of glucose, and improves insulin sensitivity by increasing peripheral glucose uptake and utilization. Unlike SUs, metformin does not produce hypoglycemia in either patients with type 2 diabetes mellitus or normal subjects (except in special circumstances) *[see Warnings and Precautions (5.9)]* and does not cause hyperinsulinemia. With metformin therapy, insulin secretion remains unchanged while fasting insulin levels and day-long plasma insulin response may actually decrease.

12.2 Pharmacodynamics

Linagliptin

Linagliptin binds to DPP-4 in a reversible manner and increases the concentrations of incretin hormones. Linagliptin glucose-dependently increases insulin secretion and lowers glucagon secretion, thus resulting in a better regulation of the glucose homeostasis. Linagliptin binds selectively to DPP-4 and selectively inhibits DPP-4, but not DPP-8 or DPP-9 activity *in vitro* at concentrations approximating therapeutic exposures.

Cardiac Electrophysiology

In a randomized, placebo-controlled, active-comparator, 4-way crossover study, 36 healthy subjects were administered a single oral dose of linagliptin 5 mg, linagliptin 100 mg (20 times the recommended dose), moxifloxacin, and placebo. No increase in QTc was observed with either the recommended dose of 5 mg or the 100-mg dose. At the 100-mg dose, peak linagliptin plasma concentrations were approximately 38-fold higher than the peak concentrations following a 5-mg dose.

12.3 Pharmacokinetics

JENTADUETO

The results of a bioequivalence study in healthy subjects demonstrated that JENTADUETO (linagliptin/metformin hydrochloride) 2.5 mg/500 mg, 2.5 mg/850 mg, and 2.5 mg/1000 mg combination tablets are bioequivalent to coadministration of corresponding doses of linagliptin and metformin as individual tablets. Administration of linagliptin 2.5 mg/metformin hydrochloride 1000 mg fixed-dose combination with food resulted in no change in overall exposure of linagliptin. There was no change in metformin AUC; however, mean peak serum concentration of metformin was decreased by 18% when administered with food. A delayed time-to-peak serum concentrations by 2 hours was observed for metformin under fed conditions. These changes are not likely to be clinically significant.

Absorption

Linagliptin

The absolute bioavailability of linagliptin is approximately 30%. Following oral administration, plasma concentrations of linagliptin decline in at least a biphasic manner with a long terminal half-life (>100 hours), related to the saturable binding of linagliptin to DPP-4. However, the prolonged elimination does not contribute to the accumulation of the drug. The effective half-life for accumulation of linagliptin, as determined from oral administration of multiple doses of linagliptin 5 mg, is approximately 12 hours. After once-daily dosing, steady state plasma concentrations of linagliptin 5 mg are reached by the third dose, and C_{max} and AUC increased by a factor of 1.3 at steady-state compared with the first dose. Plasma AUC of linagliptin increased in a less than dose-proportional manner in the dose range of 1 to 10 mg. The pharmacokinetics of linagliptin is similar in healthy subjects and in patients with type 2 diabetes.

Metformin

The absolute bioavailability of a metformin hydrochloride 500-mg tablet given under fasting conditions is approximately 50% to 60%. Studies using single oral doses of metformin tablets 500 mg to 1500 mg, and 850 mg to 2550 mg, indicate that there is a lack of dose proportionality with increasing doses, which is due to decreased absorption rather than an alteration in elimination.

Distribution

Linagliptin

The mean apparent volume of distribution at steady state following a single intravenous dose of linagliptin 5 mg to healthy subjects is approximately 1110 L, indicating that linagliptin extensively distributes to the tissues. Plasma protein binding of linagliptin is concentration-dependent decreasing from about 99% at 1 nmol/L to 75% to 89% at ≥30 nmol/L, reflecting saturation of binding to DPP-4 with increasing concentration of linagliptin. At high concentrations, where DPP-4 is fully saturated, 70% to 80% of linagliptin remains bound to plasma proteins and 20% to 30% is unbound in plasma. Plasma binding is not altered in patients with renal or hepatic impairment.

Table 2 Effect of Coadministered Drugs on Systemic Exposure of Linagliptin

Coadministered Drug	Dosing of Coadministered Drug*	Dosing of Linagliptin*	Geometric Mean Ratio (ratio with/without coadministered drug) No effect=1.0	
			AUC†	C_{max}
No dosing adjustments required for linagliptin when given with the following coadministered drugs:				
Metformin	850 mg TID	10 mg QD	1.20	1.03
Glyburide	1.75 mg#	5 mg QD	1.02	1.01
Pioglitazone	45 mg QD	10 mg QD	1.13	1.07
Ritonavir	200 mg BID	5 mg#	2.01	2.96
The efficacy of JENTADUETO may be reduced when administered in combination with strong inducers of CYP3A4 or P-gp (e.g., rifampin). Use of alternative treatments is strongly recommended *[see Drug Interactions (7.2)]*.				
Rifampin	600 mg QD	5 mg QD	0.60	0.56

*Multiple dose (steady state) unless otherwise noted

Single dose

†AUC = AUC(0 to 24 hours) for single-dose treatments and AUC = AUC(TAU) for multiple-dose treatments

QD = once daily

BID = twice daily

TID = three times daily

Metformin

The apparent volume of distribution (V/F) of metformin following single oral doses of immediate-release metformin hydrochloride tablets 850 mg averaged 654±358 L. Metformin is negligibly bound to plasma proteins, in contrast to SUs, which are more than 90% protein bound. Metformin partitions into erythrocytes, most likely as a function of time. At usual clinical doses and dosing schedules of metformin tablets, steady-state plasma concentrations of metformin are reached within 24 to 48 hours and are generally <1 mcg/mL. During controlled clinical trials of metformin, maximum metformin plasma levels did not exceed 5 mcg/mL, even at maximum doses.

Metabolism

Linagliptin

Following oral administration, the majority (about 90%) of linagliptin is excreted unchanged, indicating that metabolism represents a minor elimination pathway. A small fraction of absorbed linagliptin is metabolized to a pharmacologically inactive metabolite, which shows a steady-state exposure of 13.3% relative to linagliptin.

Metformin

Intravenous single-dose studies in normal subjects demonstrate that metformin is excreted unchanged in the urine and does not undergo hepatic metabolism (no metabolites have been identified in humans) nor biliary excretion.

Excretion

Linagliptin

Following administration of an oral [^{14}C]linagliptin dose to healthy subjects, approximately 85% of the administered radioactivity was eliminated via the enterohepatic system (80%) or urine (5%) within 4 days of dosing. Renal clearance at steady state was approximately 70 mL/min.

Metformin

Renal clearance is approximately 3.5 times greater than creatinine clearance, which indicates that tubular secretion is the major route of metformin elimination. Following oral administration, approximately 90% of the absorbed drug is eliminated via the renal route within the first 24 hours, with a plasma elimination half-life of approximately 6.2 hours. In blood, the elimination half-life is approximately 17.6 hours, suggesting that the erythrocyte mass may be a compartment of distribution.

Specific Populations

Renal Impairment

JENTADUETO: Studies characterizing the pharmacokinetics of linagliptin and metformin after administration of JENTADUETO in renally impaired patients have not been performed. Since metformin is contraindicated in patients with renal impairment, use of JENTADUETO is also contraindicated in patients with renal impairment (e.g., serum creatinine ≥1.5 mg/dL [males] or ≥1.4 mg/dL [females], or abnormal creatinine clearance) *[see Contraindications (4) and Warnings and Precautions (5.3)]*.

Linagliptin: Under steady-state conditions, linagliptin exposure in patients with mild renal impairment was comparable to healthy subjects. In patients with moderate renal impairment under steady-state conditions, mean exposure of linagliptin increased ($AUC_{\tau,ss}$ by 71% and C_{max} by 46%) compared with healthy subjects. This increase was not associated with a prolonged accumulation half-life, terminal half-life, or an increased accumulation factor. Renal excretion of linagliptin was below 5% of the administered dose and was not affected by decreased renal function.

Patients with type 2 diabetes mellitus and severe renal impairment showed steady-state exposure approximately 40% higher than that of patients with type 2 diabetes mellitus and normal renal function (increase in AUC by 42% and C_{max} by 35%). For both type 2 diabetes mellitus groups, renal excretion was below 7% of the administered dose.

Metformin: In patients with decreased renal function (based on measured creatinine clearance), the plasma and blood half-life of metformin is prolonged and the renal clearance is decreased in proportion to the decrease in creatinine clearance *[see Contraindications (4) and Warnings and Precautions (5.3)]*.

Hepatic Impairment

JENTADUETO: Studies characterizing the pharmacokinetics of linagliptin and metformin after administration of JENTADUETO in hepatically impaired patients have not been performed. However, use of metformin alone in patients with hepatic impairment has been associated with some cases of lactic acidosis. Therefore, use of JENTADUETO is not recommended in patients with hepatic impairment *[see Warnings and Precautions (5.4)]*.

Linagliptin: In patients with mild hepatic impairment (Child-Pugh class A) steady-state exposure ($AUC_{\tau,ss}$) of linagliptin was approximately 25% lower and $C_{max,ss}$ was approximately 36% lower than in healthy subjects. In patients with moderate hepatic impairment (Child-Pugh class B), AUC_{ss}, of linagliptin was about 14% lower and $C_{max,ss}$ was approximately 8% lower than in healthy subjects. Patients with severe hepatic impairment (Child-Pugh class C) had comparable exposure of linagliptin in terms of AUC_{0-24} and approximately 23% lower C_{max} compared with healthy subjects. Reductions in the pharmacokinetic parameters seen in patients with hepatic impairment did not result in reductions in DPP-4 inhibition.

Metformin hydrochloride: No pharmacokinetic studies of metformin have been conducted in patients with hepatic impairment.

Body Mass Index (BMI)/Weight

Linagliptin: BMI/Weight had no clinically meaningful effect on the pharmacokinetics of linagliptin based on a population pharmacokinetic analysis.

Gender

Linagliptin: Gender had no clinically meaningful effect on the pharmacokinetics of linagliptin based on a population pharmacokinetic analysis.

Metformin hydrochloride: Metformin pharmacokinetic parameters did not differ significantly between normal subjects and patients with type 2 diabetes mellitus when analyzed according to gender. Similarly, in controlled clinical studies in patients with type 2 diabetes mellitus, the antihyperglycemic effect of metformin was comparable in males and females.

Table 3 Effect of Linagliptin on Systemic Exposure of Coadministered Drugs

Coadministered Drug	Dosing of Coadministered Drug*	Dosing of Linagliptin*	Geometric Mean Ratio (ratio with/without coadministered drug) No effect=1.0		
				AUC†	C_{max}
No dosing adjustments required for the following coadministered drugs:					
Metformin	850 mg TID	10 mg QD	metformin	1.01	0.89
Glyburide	1.75 mg#	5 mg QD	glyburide	0.86	0.86
Pioglitazone	45 mg QD	10 mg QD	pioglitazone metabolite M-III metabolite M-IV	0.94 0.98 1.04	0.86 0.96 1.05
Digoxin	0.25 mg QD	5 mg QD	digoxin	1.02	0.94
Simvastatin	40 mg QD	10 mg QD	simvastatin simvastatin acid	1.34 1.33	1.10 1.21
Warfarin	10 mg#	5 mg QD	R-warfarin S-warfarin INR PT	0.99 1.03 0.93** 1.03**	1.00 1.01 1.04** 1.15**
Ethinylestradiol and levonorgestrel	ethinylestradiol 0.03 mg and levonorgestrel 0.150 mg QD	5 mg QD	ethinylestradiol levonorgestrel	1.01 1.09	1.08 1.13

* Multiple dose (steady state) unless otherwise noted
\# Single dose
†AUC = AUC(INF) for single-dose treatments and AUC = AUC(TAU) for multiple-dose treatments
**AUC=AUC(0-168) and C_{max}=E_{max} for pharmacodynamic end points
INR = International Normalized Ratio
PT = Prothrombin Time
QD = once daily
TID = three times daily

Table 4 Effect of Coadministered Drug on Plasma Metformin Systemic Exposure

Coadministered Drug	Dosing of Coadministered Drug*	Dose of Metformin*	Geometric Mean Ratio (ratio with/without coadministered drug) No effect=1.0		
				AUC†	C_{max}
No dosing adjustments required for the following coadministered drugs:					
Furosemide	40 mg	850 mg	metformin	1.09‡	1.22‡
Nifedipine	10 mg	850 mg	metformin	1.16	1.21
Propranolol	40 mg	850 mg	metformin	0.90	0.94
Ibuprofen	400 mg	850 mg	metformin	1.05‡	1.07‡
Cationic drugs eliminated by renal tubular secretion may reduce metformin elimination: use with caution *[see Warnings and Precautions (5.3) and Drug Interactions (7.1)].*					
Cimetidine	400 mg	850 mg	metformin	1.40	1.61
Carbonic anhydrase inhibitors may cause metabolic acidosis: use with caution *[see Warnings and Precautions (5.1) and Drug Interactions (7.1)].*					
Topiramate**	100 mg	500 mg	metformin	1.25	1.17

* All metformin and coadministered drugs were given as single doses
† AUC = AUC(INF)
‡ Ratio of arithmetic means
**At steady state with topiramate 100 mg every 12 hours and metformin 500 mg every 12 hours; AUC = AUC0-12h

Geriatric
JENTADUETO: Studies characterizing the pharmacokinetics of linagliptin and metformin after administration of JENTADUETO in geriatric patients have not been performed. Based on the metformin component, JENTADUETO treatment should not be initiated in patients ≥80 years of age unless measurement of creatinine clearance demonstrates that renal function is not reduced *[see Warnings and Precautions (5.1, 5.3) and Use in Specific Populations (8.5)].*
Linagliptin: Age did not have a clinically meaningful impact on the pharmacokinetics of linagliptin based on a population pharmacokinetic analysis.
Metformin hydrochloride: Limited data from controlled pharmacokinetic studies of metformin in healthy elderly subjects suggest that total plasma clearance of metformin is decreased, the half-life is prolonged, and C_{max} is increased, compared with healthy young subjects. From these data, it appears that the change in metformin pharmacokinetics with aging is primarily accounted for by a change in renal function.
Pediatric
Studies characterizing the pharmacokinetics of linagliptin and metformin after administration of JENTADUETO in pediatric patients have not yet been performed.
Race
Linagliptin: Race had no clinically meaningful effect on the pharmacokinetics of linagliptin based on available pharmacokinetic data, including subjects of White, Hispanic, Black, and Asian racial groups.
Metformin hydrochloride: No studies of metformin pharmacokinetic parameters according to race have been performed. In controlled clinical studies of metformin in patients with type 2 diabetes mellitus, the antihyperglycemic effect was comparable in Caucasians (n=249), Blacks (n=51), and Hispanics (n=24).

Drug Interactions
Pharmacokinetic drug interaction studies with JENTADUETO have not been performed; however, such studies have been conducted with the individual components of JENTADUETO (linagliptin and metformin hydrochloride).
Linagliptin
In vitro Assessment of Drug Interactions
Linagliptin is a weak to moderate inhibitor of CYP isozyme CYP3A4, but does not inhibit other CYP isozymes and is not an inducer of CYP isozymes, including CYP1A2, 2A6, 2B6, 2C8, 2C9, 2C19, 2D6, 2E1, and 4A11.
Linagliptin is a P-glycoprotein (P-gp) substrate, and inhibits P-gp mediated transport of digoxin at high concentrations. Based on these results and *in vivo* drug interaction studies, linagliptin is considered unlikely to cause interactions with other P-gp substrates at therapeutic concentrations.
In vivo Assessment of Drug Interactions
Inducers of CYP3A4 or P-gp (e.g., rifampin) decrease exposure to linagliptin to subtherapeutic and likely ineffective concentrations. For patients requiring use of such drugs, an alternative to linagliptin is strongly recommended. *In vivo* studies indicated evidence of a low propensity for causing drug interactions with substrates of CYP3A4, CYP2C9, CYP2C8, P-gp, and OCT. No dose adjustment of linagliptin is recommended based on results of the described pharmacokinetic studies.
[See table 2 at top of previous page]
[See table 3 above]
Metformin hydrochloride
[See table 4 below]
[See table 5 at top of next page]

13 NONCLINICAL TOXICOLOGY

13.1 Carcinogenesis, Mutagenesis, Impairment of Fertility

JENTADUETO
No animal studies have been conducted with the combined products in JENTADUETO to evaluate carcinogenesis, mutagenesis, or impairment of fertility. General toxicity studies in rats up to 13 weeks were performed with JENTADUETO.
The following data are based on the findings in studies with linagliptin and metformin individually.
Linagliptin
Linagliptin did not increase the incidence of tumors in male and female rats in a 2-year study at doses of 6, 18, and 60 mg/kg. The highest dose of 60 mg/kg is approximately 418 times the clinical dose of 5 mg/day based on AUC exposure. Linagliptin did not increase the incidence of tumors in mice in a 2-year study at doses up to 80 mg/kg (males) and 25 mg/kg (females), or approximately 35 and 270 times the clinical dose based on AUC exposure. Higher doses of linagliptin in female mice (80 mg/kg) increased the incidence of lymphoma at approximately 215 times the clinical dose based on AUC exposure.
Linagliptin was not mutagenic or clastogenic with or without metabolic activation in the Ames bacterial mutagenicity assay, a chromosomal aberration test in human lymphocytes, and an *in vivo* micronucleus assay.
In fertility studies in rats, linagliptin had no adverse effects on early embryonic development, mating, fertility, or bearing live young up to the highest dose of 240 mg/kg (approximately 943 times the clinical dose based on AUC exposure).
Metformin Hydrochloride
Long-term carcinogenicity studies have been performed in rats (dosing duration of 104 weeks) and mice (dosing duration of 91 weeks) at doses up to and including 900 mg/kg/day and 1500 mg/kg/day, respectively. These doses are both approximately 4 times the maximum recommended human daily dose of 2000 mg/kg/day based on body surface area comparisons. No evidence of carcinogenicity with metformin was found in either male or female mice. Similarly, there was no tumorigenic potential observed with metformin in male rats. There was, however, an increased incidence of benign stromal uterine polyps in female rats treated with 900 mg/kg/day.
There was no evidence of a mutagenic potential of metformin in the following *in vitro* tests: Ames test (*Salmonella typhimurium*), gene mutation test (mouse lymphoma cells), or chromosomal aberrations test (human lymphocytes). Results in the *in vivo* mouse micronucleus test were also negative.
Fertility of male or female rats was unaffected by metformin when administered at doses as high as 600 mg/kg/day, which is approximately 2 times the MRHD based on body surface area comparisons.

14 CLINICAL STUDIES

The coadministration of linagliptin and metformin has been studied in patients with type 2 diabetes mellitus inadequately controlled on diet and exercise and in combination with sulfonylurea.

Table 5 Effect of Metformin on Coadministered Drug Systemic Exposure

Coadministered Drug	Dosing of Coadministered Drug*	Dose of Metformin*	Geometric Mean Ratio (ratio with/without metformin) No effect=1.0		
				AUC†	C_{max}
No dosing adjustments required for the following coadministered drugs:					
Glyburide	5 mg	500 mg§	glyburide	0.78‡	0.63‡
Furosemide	40 mg	850 mg	furosemide	0.87‡	0.69‡
Nifedipine	10 mg	850 mg	nifedipine	1.10§	1.08
Propranolol	40 mg	850 mg	propranolol	1.01§	0.94
Ibuprofen	400 mg	850 mg	ibuprofen	0.97¶	1.01¶

* All metformin and coadministered drugs were given as single doses
† AUC = AUC(INF) unless otherwise noted
‡ Ratio of arithmetic means, p-value of difference <0.05
§ AUC(0-24 hr) reported
¶ Ratio of arithmetic means

Table 6 Glycemic Parameters at Final Visit (24-Week Study) for Linagliptin and Metformin, Alone and in Combination in Randomized Patients with Type 2 Diabetes Mellitus Inadequately Controlled on Diet and Exercise**

	Placebo	Linagliptin 5 mg Once Daily*	Metformin 500 mg Twice Daily	Linagliptin 2.5 mg Twice Daily* + Metformin 500 mg Twice Daily	Metformin 1000 mg Twice Daily	Linagliptin 2.5 mg Twice Daily* + Metformin 1000 mg Twice Daily
A1C (%)						
Number of patients	n=65	n=135	n=141	n=137	n=138	n=140
Baseline (mean)	8.7	8.7	8.7	8.7	8.5	8.7
Change from baseline (adjusted mean****)	0.1	-0.5	-0.6	-1.2	-1.1	-1.6
Difference from placebo (adjusted mean) (95% CI)	--	-0.6 (-0.9, -0.3)	-0.8 (-1.0, -0.5)	-1.3 (-1.6, -1.1)	-1.2 (-1.5, -0.9)	-1.7 (-2.0, -1.4)
Patients [n (%)] achieving A1C <7%***	7 (10.8)	14 (10.4)	26 (18.6)	41 (30.1)	42 (30.7)	74 (53.6)
Patients (%) receiving rescue medication	29.2	11.1	13.5	7.3	8.0	4.3
FPG (mg/dL)						
Number of patients	n=61	n=134	n=136	n=135	n=132	n=136
Baseline (mean)	203	195	191	199	191	196
Change from baseline (adjusted mean****)	10	-9	-16	-33	-32	-49
Difference from placebo (adjusted mean) (95% CI)	--	-19 (-31, -6)	-26 (-38, -14)	-43 (-56, -31)	-42 (-55, -30)	-60 (-72, -47)

*Total daily dose of linagliptin is equal to 5 mg
**Full analysis population using last observation on study
***Metformin 500 mg twice daily, n=140; Linagliptin 2.5 mg twice daily + Metformin 500 twice daily, n=136; Metformin 1000 mg twice daily, n=137; Linagliptin 2.5 mg twice daily + Metformin 1000 mg twice daily, n=138.
****HbA1c: ANCOVA model included treatment and number of prior OADs as class-effects, as well as baseline HbA1c as continuous covariates. FPG: ANCOVA model included treatment and number of prior OADs as class-effects, as well as baseline HbA1c and baseline FPG as continuous covariates.

There have been no clinical efficacy studies conducted with JENTADUETO; however, bioequivalence of JENTADUETO to linagliptin and metformin coadministered as individual tablets was demonstrated in healthy subjects.

14.1 Initial Combination Therapy with Metformin

A total of 791 patients with type 2 diabetes mellitus and inadequate glycemic control on diet and exercise participated in the 24-week, randomized, double-blind, portion of this placebo-controlled factorial study designed to assess the efficacy of linagliptin as initial therapy with metformin. Patients on an antihyperglycemic agent (52%) underwent a drug washout period of 4 weeks' duration. After the washout period and after completing a 2-week single-blind placebo run-in period, patients with inadequate glycemic control (A1C ≥7.0% to ≤10.5%) were randomized. Patients with inadequate glycemic control (A1C ≥7.5% to <11.0%) not on antihyperglycemic agents at study entry (48%) immediately entered the 2-week single-blind placebo run-in period and then were randomized. Randomization was stratified by baseline A1C (<8.5% vs ≥8.5%) and use of a prior oral antidiabetic drug (none vs monotherapy). Patients were randomized in a 1:2:2:2:2:2 ratio to either placebo or one of 5 active-treatment arms. Approximately equal numbers of patients were randomized to receive initial therapy with 5 mg of linagliptin once daily, 500 mg or 1000 mg of metformin twice daily, or 2.5 mg of linagliptin twice daily in combination with 500 mg or 1000 mg of metformin twice daily. Patients who failed to meet specific glycemic goals during the study were treated with sulfonylurea, thiazolidinedione, or insulin rescue therapy.

Initial therapy with the combination of linagliptin and metformin provided significant improvements in A1C, and fasting plasma glucose (FPG) compared to placebo, to metformin alone, and to linagliptin alone (Table 6, Figure 1). The adjusted mean treatment difference in A1C from baseline to week 24 (LOCF) was -0.5% (95% CI -0.7, -0.3; p<0.0001) for linagliptin 2.5 mg/metformin 1000 mg twice daily compared to metformin 1000 mg twice daily; -1.1% (95% CI -1.4, -0.9; p<0.0001) for linagliptin 2.5 mg/metformin 1000 mg twice daily compared to linagliptin 5 mg once daily; -0.6% (95% CI -0.8, -0.4; p<0.0001) for linagliptin 2.5 mg/metformin 500 mg twice daily compared to metformin 500 mg twice daily; and 0.8% (95% CI -1.0, -0.6; p<0.0001) for linagliptin 2.5 mg/metformin 500 mg twice daily compared to linagliptin 5 mg once daily.

Lipid effects were generally neutral. No meaningful change in body weight was noted in any of the 6 treatment groups. [See table 6 below]

Figure 1 Adjusted Mean Change from Baseline for A1C (%) over 24 Weeks with Linagliptin and Metformin, Alone and in Combination in Patients with Type 2 Diabetes Mellitus Inadequately Controlled with Diet and Exercise - FAS completers

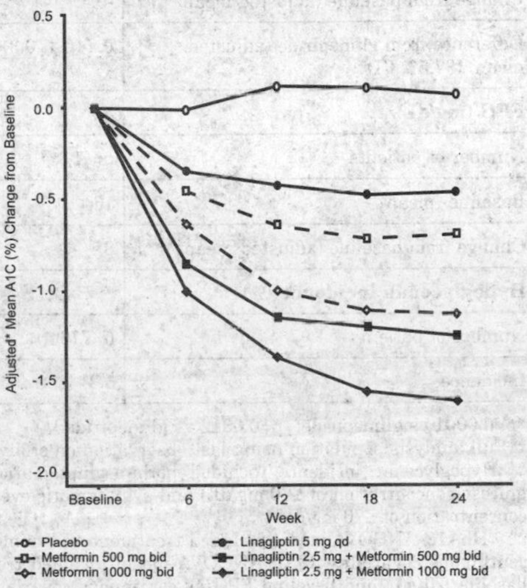

*Variables used in adjustment: Baseline A1C and prior use of OADs

14.2 Add-On Combination Therapy with Metformin

A total of 701 patients with type 2 diabetes participated in a 24-week, randomized, double-blind, placebo-controlled study designed to assess the efficacy of linagliptin in combination with metformin. Patients already on metformin (n=491) at a dose of at least 1500 mg per day were randomized after completing a 2-week open-label placebo run-in period. Patients on metformin and another antihyperglycemic agent (n=207) were randomized after a run-in period of approximately 6 weeks on metformin (at a dose of at least 1500 mg per day) in monotherapy. Patients were randomized to the addition of either linagliptin 5 mg or placebo, administered once daily. Patients who failed to meet specific glycemic goals during the studies were treated with glimepiride rescue.

In combination with metformin, linagliptin provided statistically significant improvements in A1C, FPG, and 2-hour PPG compared with placebo (Table 7). Rescue glycemic therapy was used in 7.8% of patients treated with linagliptin 5 mg and in 18.9% of patients treated with placebo. A similar decrease in body weight was observed for both treatment groups.

Table 7 Glycemic Parameters in Placebo-Controlled Study for Linagliptin in Combination with Metformin*

	Linagliptin 5 mg + Metformin	Placebo + Metformin
A1C (%)		
Number of patients	n=513	n=175
Baseline (mean)	8.1	8.0
Change from baseline (adjusted mean***)	-0.5	0.15
Difference from placebo + metformin (adjusted mean) (95% CI)	-0.6 (-0.8, -0.5)	--
Patients [n (%)] achieving A1C <7% **	127 (26.2)	15 (9.2)
FPG (mg/dL)		
Number of patients	n=495	n=159

Table 8 Glycemic Parameters at 52 and 104 Weeks in Study Comparing Linagliptin to Glimepiride as Add-On Therapy in Patients Inadequately Controlled on Metformin**

	Week 52		Week 104	
	Linagliptin 5 mg + Metformin	**Glimepiride + Metformin (mean glimepiride dose 3 mg)**	**TRADJENTA 5 mg + Metformin**	**Glimepiride + Metformin (mean glimepiride dose 3 mg)**
A1C (%)				
Number of patients	n=764	n=755	n=764	n=755
Baseline (mean)	7.7	7.7	7.7	7.7
Change from baseline (adjusted mean****)	-0.4	-0.6	-0.2	-0.4
Difference from glimepiride (adjusted mean) (97.5% CI)	0.2 (0.1, 0.3)	--	0.2 (0.1, 0.3)	--
FPG (mg/dL)				
Number of patients	n=733	n=725	n=733	n=725
Baseline (mean)	164	166	164	166
Change from baseline (adjusted mean****)	8*	-15	-2†	-9
Hypoglycemia incidence (%)***				
Number of patients	n=776	n=775	n=776	n=775
Incidence	5.3*	31.1	7.5 *	36.1

*p<0.0001 vs glimepiride; †p=0.0012 vs glimepiride
**Full analysis population using last observation on study
***Hypoglycemic incidence included both asymptomatic events (not accompanied by typical symptoms and plasma glucose concentration of ≤70 mg/dL) and symptomatic events with typical symptoms of hypoglycemia and plasma glucose concentration of ≤70 mg/dL.
****HbA1c: ANCOVA model included treatment and number of prior OADs as class-effects, as well as baseline HbA1c as continuous covariates. FPG: ANCOVA model included treatment and number of prior OADs as class-effects, as well as baseline HbA1c and baseline FPG as continuous covariates. Hypoglycemia incidence (%): Cochran-Mantel-Haenszel test was performed on the patient population contained in the treated set, to compare the proportion of patients with hypoglycemic events between patients treated with linagliptin and patients treated with glimepiride.

Baseline (mean)	169	164
Change from baseline (adjusted mean***)	-11	11
Difference from placebo + metformin (adjusted mean) (95% CI)	-21 (-27, -15)	--
2-hour PPG (mg/dL)		
Number of patients	n=78	n=21
Baseline (mean)	270	274
Change from baseline (adjusted mean***)	-49	18
Difference from placebo + metformin (adjusted mean) (95% CI)	-67 (-95, -40)	--

* Full analysis population using last observation on study
**Linagliptin 5 mg + Metformin, n=485; Placebo + Metformin, n=163.
***HbA1c: ANCOVA model included treatment and number of prior oral OADs as class-effects, as well as baseline HbA1c as continuous covariates. FPG: ANCOVA model included treatment and number of prior OADs as class-effects, as well as baseline HbA1c and baseline FPG as continuous covariates. PPG: ANCOVA model included treatment and number of prior OADs as class-effects, as well as baseline HbA1c and baseline postprandial glucose after two hours as covariate.

14.3 Active-Controlled Study vs Glimepiride in Combination with Metformin

The efficacy of linagliptin was evaluated in a 104-week double-blind, glimepiride-controlled non-inferiority study in type 2 diabetic patients with insufficient glycemic control despite metformin therapy. Patients being treated with metformin only entered a run-in period of 2 weeks' duration, whereas patients pretreated with metformin and one additional antihyperglycemic agent entered a run-in treatment period of 6 weeks' duration with metformin monotherapy (dose of ≥1500 mg per day) and washout of the other agent. After an additional 2-week placebo run-in period, those with inadequate glycemic control (A1C 6.5% to 10%) were randomized 1:1 to the addition of linagliptin 5 mg once daily or glimepiride. Randomization was stratified by baseline HbA1c (<8.5% vs ≥8.5%), and the previous use of antidiabetic drugs (metformin alone vs metformin plus one other OAD). Patients receiving glimepiride were given an initial dose of 1 mg/day and then electively titrated over the next 12 weeks to a maximum dose of 4 mg/day as needed to optimize glycemic control. Thereafter, the glimepiride dose was to be kept constant, except for down-titration to prevent hypoglycemia.

After 52 weeks and 104 weeks, linagliptin and glimepiride both had reductions from baseline in A1C (52 weeks: -0.4% for linagliptin, -0.6% for glimepiride; 104 weeks: -0.2% for TRADJENTA, -0.4% for glimepiride) from a baseline mean of 7.7% (Table 8). The mean difference between groups in A1C change from baseline was 0.2% with 2-sided 97.5% confidence interval (0.1%, 0.3%) for the intent-to-treat population using last observation carried forward. These results were consistent with the completers analysis.

[See table 8 above]

Patients treated with linagliptin had a mean baseline body weight of 86 kg and were observed to have an adjusted mean decrease in body weight of 1.1 kg at 52 weeks and 1.4 kg at 104 weeks. Patients on glimepiride had a mean baseline body weight of 87 kg and were observed to have an adjusted mean increase from baseline in body weight of 1.4 kg at 52 weeks and 1.3 kg at 104 weeks (treatment difference p<0.0001 for both timepoints).

14.4 Add-On Combination Therapy with Metformin and a Sulfonylurea

A total of 1058 patients with type 2 diabetes mellitus participated in a 24-week, randomized, double-blind, placebo-controlled study designed to assess the efficacy of linagliptin in combination with a sulfonylurea and metformin. The most common sulfonylureas used by patients in the study were glimepiride (31%), glibenclamide (26%), and gliclazide (26% [not available in the United States]). Patients on a sulfonylurea and metformin were randomized to receive linagliptin 5 mg or placebo, each administered once daily. Patients who failed to meet specific glycemic goals during the study were treated with pioglitazone rescue. Glycemic end points measured included A1C and FPG.

In combination with a sulfonylurea and metformin, linagliptin provided statistically significant improvements in A1C and FPG compared with placebo (Table 9). In the entire study population (patients on linagliptin in combination with a sulfonylurea and metformin), a mean reduction from baseline relative to placebo in A1C of -0.6% and in FPG of -13 mg/dL was seen. Rescue therapy was used in 5.4% of patients treated with linagliptin 5 mg and in 13% of patients treated with placebo. Change from baseline in body weight did not differ significantly between the groups.

Table 9 Glycemic Parameters at Final Visit (24-Week Study) for Linagliptin in Combination with Metformin and Sulfonylurea*

	Linagliptin 5 mg + Metformin + SU	**Placebo + Metformin + SU**
A1C (%)		
Number of patients	n=778	n=262
Baseline (mean)	8.2	8.1
Change from baseline (adjusted mean***)	-0.7	-0.1
Difference from placebo (adjusted mean) (95% CI)	-0.6 (-0.7, -0.5)	--
Patients [n (%)] achieving A1C <7%**	217 (29.2)	20 (8.1)
FPG (mg/dL)		
Number of patients	n=739	n=248
Baseline (mean)	159	163
Change from baseline (adjusted mean***)	-5	8
Difference from placebo (adjusted mean) (95% CI)	-13 (-18, -7)	--

SU=sulfonylurea
*Full analysis population using last observation on study
**Linagliptin 5 mg + Metformin + SU, n=742; Placebo + Metformin + SU, n=247
***HbA1c: ANCOVA model included treatment as class-effects and baseline HbA1c as continuous covariates. FPG: ANCOVA model included treatment as class-effects, as well as baseline HbA1c and baseline FPG as continuous covariates.

14.5 Add-On Combination Therapy with Insulin

A total of 1261 patients with type 2 diabetes inadequately controlled on basal insulin alone or basal insulin in combination with oral drugs participated in a randomized, double-blind placebo-controlled trial designed to evaluate the efficacy of linagliptin as add-on therapy to basal insulin over 24 weeks. Randomization was stratified by baseline HbA1c (<8.5% vs ≥8.5%), renal function impairment status (based on baseline eGFR), and concomitant use of oral antidiabetic drugs (none, metformin only, pioglitazone only, metformin + pioglitazone). Patients with a baseline A1C of ≥7% and ≤10% were included in the study including 709 patients with renal impairment (eGFR <90 mL/min), most of whom (n=575) were categorized as mild renal impairment (eGFR 60 to <90 mL/min). Patients entered a 2-week placebo run-in period on basal insulin (e.g., insulin glargine, insulin detemir, or NPH insulin) with or without metformin and/or pioglitazone background therapy. Following the run-in period, patients with inadequate glycemic control were randomized to the addition of either 5 mg of linagliptin or placebo, administered once daily. Patients were maintained on a stable dose of insulin prior to enrollment, during the run-in period, and during the first 24 weeks of treatment. Patients who failed to meet specific glycemic goals during the double-blind treatment period were rescued by increasing background insulin dose.

Linagliptin used in combination with insulin (with or without metformin and/or pioglitazone), provided statistically significant improvements in A1C and FPG compared to placebo (Table 10) after 24 weeks of treatment. The mean total daily insulin dose at baseline was 42 units for patients treated with linagliptin and 40 units for patients treated with placebo. Background baseline diabetes therapy included use of: insulin alone (16.1%), insulin combined with metformin only (75.5%), insulin combined with metformin and pioglitazone (7.4%), and insulin combined with pioglitazone only (1%). The mean change from baseline to Week 24 in the daily dose of insulin was +1.3 IU in the placebo group and +0.6 IU in the linagliptin group. The mean change in body weight from baseline to Week 24 was similar in the two treatment groups. The rate of hypoglycemia, defined as all symptomatic or asymptomatic episodes with a self measured blood glucose was also similar in both groups (21.4% linagliptin; 22.9% placebo) in the first 24 weeks of the study.

Table 10 Glycemic Parameters in Placebo-Controlled Study for Linagliptin in Combination with Insulin*

	Linagliptin 5 mg + Insulin	Placebo + Insulin
A1C (%)		
Number of patients	n=618	n=617
Baseline (mean)	8.3	8.3
Change from baseline (adjusted mean***)	-0.6	0.1
Difference from placebo (adjusted mean) (95% CI)	-0.7 (-0.7, -0.6)	--
Patients [n (%)] achieving A1C <7%**	116 (19.5)	48 (8.1)
FPG (mg/dL)		
Number of patients	n=613	n=608
Baseline (mean)	147	151
Change from baseline (adjusted mean***)	-8	3
Difference from placebo (adjusted mean) (95% CI)	-11 (-16, -6)	--

*Full analysis population using last observation carried forward (LOCF) method on study
**Linagliptin + Insulin, n=595; Placebo + Insulin, n=593
***HbA1c: ANCOVA model included treatment, categorical renal function impairment status and concomitant OADs as class-effects, as well as baseline HbA1c as continuous covariates. FPG: ANCOVA model included treatment, categorical renal function impairment status and concomitant OADs as class-effects, as well as baseline HbA1c and baseline FPG as continuous covariates.

The difference between treatment with linagliptin and placebo in terms of adjusted mean change from baseline in HbA1c after 24 weeks was comparable for patients with no renal impairment (eGRF ≥90 mL/min, n=539), with mild renal impairment (eGFR 60 to <90 mL/min, n=565), or with moderate renal impairment (eGFR 30 to <60 mL/min, n=124).

14.6 Renal Impairment

A total of 133 patients with type 2 diabetes participated in a 52 week, double-blind, randomized, placebo-controlled trial designed to evaluate the efficacy and safety of linagliptin in patients with both type 2 diabetes and severe chronic renal impairment. Participants with an estimated (based on the four variables modified diet in renal disease [MDRD] equation) GFR value of <30 mL/min were eligible to participate in the study. Randomization was stratified by baseline HbA1c (≤8% and >8%) and background antidiabetic therapy (insulin or any combination with insulin, SU or glinides as monotherapy and pioglitazone or any other antidiabetics excluding any other DPP-4 inhibitors). For the initial 12 weeks of the study, background antidiabetic therapy was kept stable and included insulin, sulfonylurea, glinides, and pioglitazone. For the remainder of the trial, dose adjustments in antidiabetic background therapy were allowed. At baseline in this trial, 62.5% of patients were receiving insulin alone as background diabetes therapy, and 12.5% were receiving sulfonylurea alone.

After 12 weeks of treatment, linagliptin 5 mg provided statistically significant improvement in A1C compared to placebo, with an adjusted mean change of -0.6% compared to placebo (95% confidence interval -0.9, -0.3) based on the analysis using last observation carried forward (LOCF). With adjustments in antidiabetic background therapy after the initial 12 weeks, efficacy was maintained for 52 weeks, with an adjusted mean change from baseline in A1C of -0.7% compared to placebo (95% confidence interval -1.0, -0.4) based on analysis using LOCF.

16 HOW SUPPLIED/STORAGE AND HANDLING

JENTADUETO (linagliptin and metformin hydrochloride) tablets 2.5 mg/500 mg are supplied as follows:
Bottles of 60 (NDC 0597-0146-60)
Bottles of 180 (NDC 0597-0146-18)
JENTADUETO (linagliptin and metformin hydrochloride) tablets 2.5 mg/850 mg are supplied as follows:
Bottles of 60 (NDC 0597-0147-60)
Bottles of 180 (NDC 0597-0147-18)
JENTADUETO (linagliptin and metformin hydrochloride) tablets 2.5 mg/1000 mg are supplied as follows:
Bottles of 60 (NDC 0597-0148-60)
Bottles of 180 (NDC 0597-0148-18)

Storage

Store at 25°C (77°F); excursions permitted to 15°-30°C (59°-86°F) [see USP Controlled Room Temperature]. Protect from exposure to high humidity. Store in a safe place out of reach of children.

17 PATIENT COUNSELING INFORMATION

See FDA-approved patient labeling (Medication Guide)

17.1 Instructions

Inform patients of the potential risks and benefits of JENTADUETO and of alternative modes of therapy. Also inform patients about the importance of adherence to dietary instructions, regular physical activity, periodic blood glucose monitoring and A1C testing, recognition and management of hypoglycemia and hyperglycemia, and assessment for diabetes complications. Advise patients to seek medical advice promptly during periods of stress such as fever, trauma, infection, or surgery, as medication requirements may change.

Inform patients of the risks of lactic acidosis due to the metformin component, its symptoms, and conditions that predispose to its development *[see Warnings and Precautions (5.1)]*. Advise patients to discontinue JENTADUETO immediately and to notify their doctor promptly if unexplained hyperventilation, malaise, myalgia, unusual somnolence, slow or irregular heart beat, sensation of feeling cold (especially in the extremities), or other nonspecific symptoms occur. GI symptoms are common during initiation of metformin treatment and may occur during initiation of JENTADUETO therapy; however, advise patients to consult their doctor if they develop unexplained symptoms. Although GI symptoms that occur after stabilization are unlikely to be drug related, such an occurrence of symptoms should be evaluated to determine if it may be due to metformin-induced lactic acidosis or other serious disease.

Inform patients that the risk of hypoglycemia is increased when JENTADUETO is used in combination with an insulin secretagogue (e.g., sulfonylurea), and that a lower dose of the insulin secretagogue may be required to reduce the risk of hypoglycemia.

Inform patients that acute pancreatitis has been reported during postmarketing use of linagliptin. Inform patients that persistent severe abdominal pain, sometimes radiating to the back, which may or may not be accompanied by vomiting, is the hallmark symptom of acute pancreatitis. Instruct patients to discontinue JENTADUETO promptly and contact their physician if persistent severe abdominal pain occurs *[see Warnings and Precautions (5.2)]*.

Instruct patients to take JENTADUETO only as prescribed. If a dose is missed, advise patients not to double their next dose.

Warn patients against excessive alcohol intake, either acute or chronic, while receiving JENTADUETO *[see Warnings and Precautions (5.6)]*.

Inform patients about the importance of regular testing of renal function and hematological parameters when receiving treatment with JENTADUETO.

Instruct patients to read the Medication Guide before starting JENTADUETO therapy and to reread each time the prescription is renewed. Instruct patients to inform their doctor if they develop any bothersome or unusual symptom, or if any symptom persists or worsens.

17.2 Laboratory Tests

Inform patients that response to all diabetic therapies should be monitored by periodic measurements of blood glucose and A1C levels, with a goal of decreasing these levels toward the normal range. A1C monitoring is especially useful for evaluating long-term glycemic control.

Initial and periodic monitoring of hematologic parameters (e.g., hemoglobin/hematocrit and red blood cell indices) and renal function (serum creatinine) should be performed, at least on an annual basis. While megaloblastic anemia has rarely been seen with metformin therapy, if this is suspected, Vitamin B_{12} deficiency should be excluded.

Distributed by:
Boehringer Ingelheim Pharmaceuticals, Inc.
Ridgefield, CT 06877 USA
Marketed by:
Boehringer Ingelheim Pharmaceuticals, Inc.
Ridgefield, CT 06877 USA
and
Eli Lilly and Company
Indianapolis, IN 46285 USA
Licensed from:
Boehringer Ingelheim International GmbH, Ingelheim, Germany

IT5571EI102013
300661-03

IT5645D
302118-02

MEDICATION GUIDE
JENTADUETO (JEN ta doo e' toe)
(linagliptin and metformin hydrochloride)
Tablets

Read this Medication Guide carefully before you start taking JENTADUETO and each time you get a refill. There may be new information. This information does not take the place of talking to your doctor about your medical condition or your treatment. If you have any questions about JENTADUETO, ask your doctor or pharmacist.

What is the most important information I should know about JENTADUETO?

Serious side effects can happen in people taking JENTADUETO, including:

1. **Lactic Acidosis.** Metformin, one of the medicines in JENTADUETO, can cause a rare but serious condition called lactic acidosis (a build-up of lactic acid in the blood) that can cause death. Lactic acidosis is a medical emergency and must be treated in the hospital.
   Stop taking JENTADUETO and call your doctor right away if you get any of the following symptoms of lactic acidosis:
   - feel very weak or tired
   - have unusual (not normal) muscle pain
   - have trouble breathing
   - have unusual sleepiness or sleep longer than usual
   - have sudden stomach or intestinal problems with nausea and vomiting or diarrhea
   - feel cold, especially in your arms and legs
   - feel dizzy or lightheaded
   - have a slow or irregular heartbeat

   You have a higher chance of getting lactic acidosis if you:
   - have kidney problems. People whose kidneys are not working properly should not take JENTADUETO.
   - have liver problems
   - have congestive heart failure that requires treatment with medicines
   - drink alcohol very often, or drink a lot of alcohol in short-term ("binge" drinking)
   - get dehydrated (lose a large amount of body fluids). This can happen if you are sick with a fever, vomiting, or diarrhea. Dehydration can also happen when you sweat a lot with activity or exercise and do not drink enough fluids.
   - have certain x-ray tests with dyes or contrast agents that are injected into your body
   - have surgery
   - have a heart attack, severe infection, or stroke
   - are 80 years of age or older and have not had your kidneys tested
2. **Inflammation of the pancreas (pancreatitis)** which may be severe and lead to death.
   Certain medical problems make you more likely to get pancreatitis.
   Before you start taking JENTADUETO:
   Tell your doctor if you have ever had:
   - inflammation of your pancreas (pancreatitis)
   - stones in your gallbladder (gallstones)
   - a history of alcoholism
   - high blood triglyceride levels

   Stop taking JENTADUETO and call your doctor right away if you have pain in your stomach area (abdomen) that is severe and will not go away. The pain may be felt going from your abdomen through to your back. The pain may happen with or without vomiting. These may be symptoms of pancreatitis.

What is JENTADUETO?

- JENTADUETO is a prescription medicine that contains 2 diabetes medicines, linagliptin and metformin. JENTADUETO can be used along with diet and exercise to lower blood sugar in adults with type 2 diabetes when treatment with both linagliptin and metformin is appropriate.
- JENTADUETO is not for people with type 1 diabetes.
- JENTADUETO is not for people with diabetic ketoacidosis (increased ketones in the blood or urine).
- If you have had pancreatitis in the past, it is not known if you have a higher chance of getting pancreatitis while you take JENTADUETO.
- It is not known if JENTADUETO is safe and effective in children under 18 years of age.

Who should not take JENTADUETO?

Do not take JENTADUETO if you:
- have kidney problems
- have a condition called metabolic acidosis or diabetic ketoacidosis (increased ketones in the blood or urine).
- are allergic to linagliptin, metformin, or any of the ingredients in JENTADUETO. See the end of this Medication Guide for a complete list of ingredients in JENTADUETO.

  Symptoms of a serious allergic reaction to JENTADUETO may include:

- skin rash, itching, flaking or peeling
- raised red patches on your skin (hives)
- swelling of your face, lips, tongue and throat that may cause difficulty in breathing or swallowing
- difficulty with swallowing or breathing

If you have any of these symptoms, stop taking JENTADUETO and contact your doctor or go to the nearest hospital emergency room right away.

What should I tell my doctor before using JENTADUETO?

Before you take JENTADUETO, tell your doctor if you:

- have or have had inflammation of your pancreas (pancreatitis).
- have kidney problems
- have liver problems
- have heart problems, including congestive heart failure
- drink alcohol very often, or drink a lot of alcohol in short term "binge" drinking
- are 80 years of age or older, you should not take JENTADUETO unless your kidneys have been checked and they are normal
- are going to get an injection of dye or contrast agents for an x-ray procedure. JENTADUETO will need to be stopped for a short time. Talk to your doctor about when you should stop JENTADUETO and when you should start JENTADUETO again. See "**What is the most important information I should know about JENTADUETO?**"
- have type 1 diabetes. JENTADUETO should not be used to treat people with type 1 diabetes.
- have any other medical conditions
- are pregnant or plan to become pregnant. It is not known if JENTADUETO will harm your unborn baby. If you are pregnant, talk with your doctor about the best way to control your blood sugar while you are pregnant.
- are breastfeeding or plan to breastfeed. It is not known if JENTADUETO passes into your breast milk. Talk with your doctor about the best way to feed your baby if you take JENTADUETO.

Tell your doctor about all the medicines you take, including prescription and non-prescription medicines, vitamins, and herbal supplements. JENTADUETO may affect the way other medicines work, and other medicines may affect how JENTADUETO works.

Especially tell your doctor if you take:

- other medicines that can lower your blood sugar
- rifampin* (Rifadin®, Rimactane®, Rifater®, Rifamate®), an antibiotic that is used to treat tuberculosis

Ask your doctor or pharmacist for a list of these medicines if you are not sure if your medicine is one that is listed above.

Know the medicines you take. Keep a list of them and show it to your doctor and pharmacist when you get a new medicine.

How should I take JENTADUETO?

- Take JENTADUETO exactly as your doctor tells you to take it.
- Take JENTADUETO 2 times each day with meals. Taking JENTADUETO with meals may lower your chance of having an upset stomach.
- If you miss a dose, take it with food as soon as you remember. If you do not remember until it is time for your next dose, skip the missed dose and go back to your regular schedule. Do not take 2 doses of JENTADUETO at the same time.
- If you take too much JENTADUETO, call your doctor or Poison Control Center at 1-800-222-1222 or go to the nearest hospital emergency room right away.
- Your doctor may tell you to take JENTADUETO along with other diabetes medicines. Low blood sugar can happen more often when JENTADUETO is taken with certain other diabetes medicines. See "**What are the possible side effects of JENTADUETO?**"
- You may need to stop taking JENTADUETO for a short time. Call your doctor for instructions if you:
  - are dehydrated (have lost too much body fluid). Dehydration can occur if you are sick with severe vomiting, diarrhea, or fever, or if you drink a lot less fluid than normal.
  - plan to have surgery
  - are going to get an injection of dye or contrast agent for an x-ray procedure. See "**What is the most important information I should know about JENTADUETO?**" and "**Who should not take JENTADUETO?**".
- When your body is under some types of stress, such as fever, trauma (such as a car accident), infection, or surgery, the amount of diabetes medicine that you need may change. Tell your doctor right away if you have any of these conditions and follow your doctor's instructions.
- Check your blood sugar as your doctor tells you to.
- Stay on your prescribed diet and exercise program while taking JENTADUETO.
- Your doctor will check your diabetes with regular blood tests, including your blood sugar levels and your hemoglobin A1C.
- Your doctor will do blood tests to check how well your kidneys are working before and during your treatment with JENTADUETO.

What are the possible side effects of JENTADUETO tablets?

JENTADUETO may cause serious side effects, including:

- See "**What is the most important information I should know about JENTADUETO?**"
- **low blood sugar (hypoglycemia).** If you take JENTADUETO with another medication that can cause low blood sugar, such as sulfonylurea or insulin, your risk of getting low blood sugar is higher. The dose of your sulfonylurea medicine or insulin may need to be lowered while you take JENTADUETO. Signs and symptoms of low blood sugar may include:

• headache	• irritability
• hunger	• drowsiness
• fast heart beat	• weakness
• sweating	• dizziness
• feeling jittery	• confusion

The most common side effects of JENTADUETO include:

- stuffy or runny nose and sore throat
- diarrhea

These are not all the possible side effects of JENTADUETO. For more information, ask your doctor or pharmacist.

Tell your doctor if you have any side effects that bother you or that do not go away.

Call your doctor for medical advice about side effects. You may report side effects to FDA at 1-800-FDA-1088.

How should I store JENTADUETO tablets?

- Store JENTADUETO between 68°F and 77°F (20°C and 25°C).
- Keep tablets dry.

Keep JENTADUETO and all medicines out of the reach of children.

General information about the safe and effective use of JENTADUETO

Medicines are sometimes prescribed for purposes other than those listed in Medication Guides. Do not use JENTADUETO for a condition for which it was not prescribed. Do not give JENTADUETO to other people, even if they have the same symptoms you have. It may harm them. This Medication Guide summarizes the most important information about JENTADUETO. If you would like more information, talk with your doctor. You can ask your pharmacist or doctor for information about JENTADUETO that is written for health professionals.

For more information, go to www.jentadueto.com or call Boehringer Ingelheim Pharmaceuticals, Inc. at 1-800-542-6257, or (TTY) 1-800-459-9906.

What are the ingredients in JENTADUETO?

Active Ingredients: linagliptin and metformin hydrochloride

Inactive Ingredients: arginine, corn starch, copovidone, colloidal silicon dioxide, magnesium stearate, titanium dioxide, propylene glycol, hypromellose, talc.

2.5 mg/500 mg and 2.5 mg/850 mg tablets also contain yellow ferric oxide.

2.5 mg/850 mg and 2.5 mg/1000 mg tablets also contain red ferric oxide.

What is type 2 diabetes?

Type 2 diabetes is a condition in which your body does not make enough insulin, and/or the insulin that your body produces does not work as well as it should. Your body can also make too much sugar. When this happens, sugar (glucose) builds up in the blood. This can lead to serious medical problems.

The main goal of treating diabetes is to lower your blood sugar to a normal level. High blood sugar can be lowered by diet and exercise, and by certain medicines when necessary. Talk to your doctor about how to prevent, recognize, and take care of low blood sugar (hypoglycemia), high blood sugar (hyperglycemia), and other problems you have because of your diabetes.

This Medication Guide has been approved by the U. S. Food and Drug Administration.

Distributed by:
Boehringer Ingelheim Pharmaceuticals, Inc.
Ridgefield, CT 06877 USA
Marketed by:
Boehringer Ingelheim Pharmaceuticals, Inc.
Ridgefield, CT 06877 USA
and
Eli Lilly and Company
Indianapolis, IN 46285 USA
Licensed from:
Boehringer Ingelheim International GmbH
Ingelheim, Germany
Revised: September 2013

*The brands listed are trademarks of their respective owners and are not trademarks of Boehringer Ingelheim Pharmaceuticals, Inc. The makers of these brands are not affiliated with and do not endorse Boehringer Ingelheim Pharmaceuticals, Inc., or its products.

IT5571EI102013
300661-03
IT5645D
302118-02

Shown in Product Identification Guide, page 305

TRADJENTA® ℞
(linagliptin)
tablets

HIGHLIGHTS OF PRESCRIBING INFORMATION

These highlights do not include all the information needed to use TRADJENTA safely and effectively. See full prescribing information for TRADJENTA.

Tradjenta® (linagliptin) tablets

Initial U.S. Approval: 2011

RECENT MAJOR CHANGES

Indications and Usage	
Important Limitations of Use (1.2)	6/2013
Dosage and Administration	
Concomitant Use with an Insulin Secretagogue (e.g., Sulfonylurea) or with Insulin (2.2)	8/2012
Warnings and Precautions	
Pancreatitis (5.1)	6/2013
Use with Medications Known to Cause Hypoglycemia (5.2)	8/2012

INDICATIONS AND USAGE

TRADJENTA is a dipeptidyl peptidase-4 (DPP-4) inhibitor indicated as an adjunct to diet and exercise to improve glycemic control in adults with type 2 diabetes mellitus (1.1)

Important limitations of use:

- Should not be used in patients with type 1 diabetes or for the treatment of diabetic ketoacidosis (1.2)
- Has not been studied in patients with a history of pancreatitis (1.2)

DOSAGE AND ADMINISTRATION

- The recommended dose of TRADJENTA is 5 mg once daily. (2.1)
- TRADJENTA can be taken with or without food. (2.1)

DOSAGE FORMS AND STRENGTHS

Tablets: 5 mg (3)

CONTRAINDICATIONS

History of hypersensitivity reaction to linagliptin, such as urticaria, angioedema, or bronchial hyperreactivity (4)

WARNINGS AND PRECAUTIONS

- There have been postmarketing reports of acute pancreatitis, including fatal pancreatitis. If pancreatitis is suspected, promptly discontinue TRADJENTA. (5.1)
- When used with an insulin secretagogue (e.g., sulfonylurea) or insulin, consider lowering the dose of the insulin secretagogue or insulin to reduce the risk of hypoglycemia (5.2)
- There have been no clinical studies establishing conclusive evidence of macrovascular risk reduction with TRADJENTA or any other antidiabetic drug (5.3)

ADVERSE REACTIONS

- Adverse reactions reported in ≥5% of patients treated with TRADJENTA and more commonly than in patients treated with placebo included nasopharyngitis (6.1)
- Hypoglycemia was more commonly reported in patients treated with the combination of TRADJENTA and sulfonylurea compared with those treated with the combination of placebo and sulfonylurea (6.1)

To report SUSPECTED ADVERSE REACTIONS, contact Boehringer Ingelheim Pharmaceuticals, Inc. at 1-800-542-6257 or 1-800-459-9906 TTY, or FDA at 1-800-FDA-1088 or www.fda.gov/medwatch.

DRUG INTERACTIONS

P-glycoprotein/CYP3A4 inducer: The efficacy of TRADJENTA may be reduced when administered in combination (e.g., with rifampin). Use of alternative treatments is strongly recommended. (7.1)

USE IN SPECIFIC POPULATIONS

- Pregnancy: There are no adequate and well-controlled studies in pregnant women. TRADJENTA tablets should be used during pregnancy only if clearly needed. (8.1)
- Nursing mothers: Caution should be exercised when TRADJENTA is administered to a nursing woman (8.3)
- Pediatric patients: Safety and effectiveness of TRADJENTA in patients below the age of 18 have not been established (8.4)
- Renal or hepatic impairment: No dose adjustment recommended (8.6, 8.7)

See 17 for PATIENT COUNSELING INFORMATION and Medication Guide

Revised: 06/2013

FULL PRESCRIBING INFORMATION: CONTENTS*

*** Sections or subsections omitted from the full prescribing information are not listed**

FULL PRESCRIBING INFORMATION

1 INDICATIONS AND USAGE

1.1 Monotherapy and Combination Therapy

TRADJENTA tablets are indicated as an adjunct to diet and exercise to improve glycemic control in adults with type 2 diabetes mellitus *[see Clinical Studies (14.1)]*.

1.2 Important Limitations of Use

TRADJENTA should not be used in patients with type 1 diabetes or for the treatment of diabetic ketoacidosis, as it would not be effective in these settings.

TRADJENTA has not been studied in patients with a history of pancreatitis. It is unknown whether patients with a history of pancreatitis are at an increased risk for the development of pancreatitis while using TRADJENTA *[see Warnings and Precautions (5.1)]*.

2 DOSAGE AND ADMINISTRATION

2.1 Recommended Dosing

The recommended dose of TRADJENTA is 5 mg once daily. TRADJENTA tablets can be taken with or without food.

2.2 Concomitant Use with an Insulin Secretagogue (e.g., Sulfonylurea) or with Insulin

When TRADJENTA is used in combination with an insulin secretagogue (e.g., sulfonylurea) or with insulin, a lower dose of the insulin secretagogue or insulin may be required to reduce the risk of hypoglycemia *[see Warnings and Precautions (5.1)]*.

3 DOSAGE FORMS AND STRENGTHS

TRADJENTA (linagliptin) 5 mg tablets are light red, round, biconvex, bevel-edged, film-coated tablets with "D5" debossed on one side and the Boehringer Ingelheim logo debossed on the other side.

4 CONTRAINDICATIONS

TRADJENTA is contraindicated in patients with a history of a hypersensitivity reaction to linagliptin, such as urticaria, angioedema, or bronchial hyperreactivity *[see Adverse Reactions (6.1)]*.

5 WARNINGS AND PRECAUTIONS

5.1 Pancreatitis

There have been postmarketing reports of acute pancreatitis, including fatal pancreatitis, in patients taking TRADJENTA. Take careful notice of potential signs and symptoms of pancreatitis. If pancreatitis is suspected, promptly discontinue TRADJENTA and initiate appropriate management. It is unknown whether patients with a history of pancreatitis are at increased risk for the development of pancreatitis while using TRADJENTA.

5.2 Use with Medications Known to Cause Hypoglycemia

Insulin secretagogues and insulin are known to cause hypoglycemia. The use of TRADJENTA in combination with an insulin secretagogue (e.g., sulfonylurea) was associated with a higher rate of hypoglycemia compared with placebo in a clinical trial *[see Adverse Reactions (6.1)]*. The use of TRADJENTA in combination with insulin in subjects with severe renal impairment was associated with a higher rate of hypoglycemia *[see Adverse Reactions (6.1)]*. Therefore, a lower dose of the insulin secretagogue or insulin may be required to reduce the risk of hypoglycemia when used in combination with TRADJENTA.

5.3 Macrovascular Outcomes

There have been no clinical studies establishing conclusive evidence of macrovascular risk reduction with TRADJENTA tablets or any other antidiabetic drug.

6 ADVERSE REACTIONS

6.1 Clinical Trials Experience

Because clinical trials are conducted under widely varying conditions, adverse reaction rates observed in the clinical trials of a drug cannot be directly compared to rates in the clinical trials of another drug and may not reflect the rates observed in practice.

The safety evaluation of TRADJENTA 5 mg once daily in patients with type 2 diabetes is based on 14 placebo-controlled trials, 1 active-controlled study, and one study in patients with severe renal impairment. In the 14 placebo-controlled studies, a total of 3625 patients were randomized and treated with TRADJENTA 5 mg daily and 2176 with placebo. The mean exposure in patients treated with TRADJENTA across studies was 29.6 weeks. The maximum follow-up was 78 weeks.

TRADJENTA 5 mg once daily was studied as monotherapy in three placebo-controlled trials of 18 and 24 weeks' duration and in five additional placebo-controlled studies lasting ≤ 18 weeks. The use of TRADJENTA in combination with other antihyperglycemic agents was studied in six placebo-controlled trials: two with metformin (12 and 24 weeks' treatment duration); one with a sulfonylurea (18 weeks' treatment duration); one with metformin and sulfonylurea (24 weeks' treatment duration); one with pioglitazone (24 weeks' treatment duration); and one with insulin (primary endpoint at 24 weeks).

In a pooled dataset of 14 placebo-controlled clinical trials, adverse reactions that occurred in ≥2% of patients receiving TRADJENTA (n = 3625) and more commonly than in patients given placebo (n = 2176), are shown in Table 1. The overall incidence of adverse events with TRADJENTA were similar to placebo.

Table 1 Adverse Reactions Reported in ≥2% of Patients Treated with TRADJENTA and Greater than Placebo in Placebo-Controlled Clinical Studies of TRADJENTA Monotherapy or Combination Therapy

	Number (%) of Patients	
	TRADJENTA 5 mg n = 3625	Placebo n = 2176
Nasopharyngitis	254 (7.0)	132 (6.1)
Diarrhea	119 (3.3)	65 (3.0)
Cough	76 (2.1)	30 (1.4)

Rates for other adverse reactions for TRADJENTA 5 mg versus placebo when TRADJENTA was used in combination with specific anti-diabetic agents were: urinary tract infection (3.1% vs 0%) and hypertriglyceridemia (2.4% vs 0%) when TRADJENTA was used as add-on to sulfonylurea; hyperlipidemia (2.7% vs 0.8%) and weight increased (2.3% vs 0.8%) when TRADJENTA was used as add-on to pioglitazone; and constipation (2.1% vs 1%) when TRADJENTA was used as add-on to basal insulin therapy.

Following 104 weeks' treatment in a controlled study comparing TRADJENTA with glimepiride in which all patients were also receiving metformin, adverse reactions reported in ≥5% of patients treated with TRADJENTA (n = 776) and more frequently than in patients treated with a sulfonylurea (n = 775) were back pain (9.1% vs 8.4%), arthralgia (8.1% vs 6.1%), upper respiratory tract infection (8.0% vs 7.6%), headache (6.4% vs 5.2%), cough (6.1% vs 4.9%), and pain in extremity (5.3% vs 3.9%).

Other adverse reactions reported in clinical studies with treatment of TRADJENTA were hypersensitivity (e.g., urticaria, angioedema, localized skin exfoliation, or bronchial hyperreactivity), and myalgia. In the clinical trial program, pancreatitis was reported in 15.2 cases per 10,000 patient year exposure while being treated with TRADJENTA compared with 3.7 cases per 10,000 patient year exposure while being treated with comparator (placebo and active comparator, sulfonylurea). Three additional cases of pancreatitis were reported following the last administered dose of linagliptin.

Hypoglycemia

In the placebo-controlled studies, 199 (6.6%) of the total 2994 patients treated with TRADJENTA 5 mg reported hypoglycemia compared to 56 patients (3.6%) of 1546 placebo-treated patients. The incidence of hypoglycemia was similar to placebo when TRADJENTA was administered as monotherapy or in combination with metformin, or with pioglitazone. When TRADJENTA was administered in combination with metformin and a sulfonylurea, 181 of 792 (22.9%) patients reported hypoglycemia compared with 39 of 263 (14.8%) patients administered placebo in combination with metformin and a sulfonylurea. Adverse reactions of hypoglycemia were based on all reports of hypoglycemia. A concurrent glucose measurement was not required or was normal in some patients. Therefore, it is not possible to conclusively determine that all these reports reflect true hypoglycemia.

In the study of patients receiving TRADJENTA as add-on therapy to a stable dose of insulin for up to 52 weeks (n=1261), no significant difference in the incidence of investigator reported hypoglycemia, defined as all symptomatic or asymptomatic episodes with a self measured blood glucose ≤70 mg/dL, was noted between the TRADJENTA (31.4%) and placebo (32.9%) treated groups. During the same time period, severe hypoglycemic events, defined as requiring the assistance of another person to actively administer carbohydrate, glucagon or other resuscitative actions, were reported in 11 (1.7%) of TRADJENTA treated patients and 7 (1.1%) of placebo treated patients. Events that were considered life-threatening or required hospitalization were reported in 3 (0.5%) patients on TRADJENTA and 1 (0.2%) on placebo.

Use in Renal Impairment

TRADJENTA was compared to placebo as add-on to pre-existing antidiabetic therapy over 52 weeks in 133 patients with severe renal impairment (estimated GFR <30 mL/min). For the initial 12 weeks of the study, background antidiabetic therapy was kept stable and included insulin, sulfonylurea, glinides, and pioglitazone. For the remainder of the trial, dose adjustments in antidiabetic background therapy were allowed.

In general, the incidence of adverse events including severe hypoglycemia was similar to those reported in other TRADJENTA trials. The observed incidence of hypoglycemia was higher (TRADJENTA, 63% compared to placebo, 49%) due to an increase in asymptomatic hypoglycemic events especially during the first 12 weeks when background glycemic therapies were kept stable. Ten TRADJENTA-treated patients (15%) and 11 placebo-treated patients (17%) reported at least one episode of confirmed symptomatic hypoglycemia (accompanying finger stick glucose ≤54 mg/dL). During the same time period, severe hypoglycemic events, defined as an event requiring the assistance of another person to actively administer carbohydrate, glucagon or other resuscitative actions, were reported in 3 (4.4%) TRADJENTA-treated patients and 3 (4.6%) placebo-treated patients. Events that were considered life-threatening or required hospitalization were reported in 2 (2.9%) patients on TRADJENTA and 1 (1.5%) on placebo.

Renal function as measured by mean eGFR and creatinine clearance did not change over 52 weeks treatment compared to placebo.

Laboratory Tests

Changes in laboratory findings were similar in patients treated with TRADJENTA 5 mg compared to patients treated with placebo. Changes in laboratory values that occurred more frequently in the TRADJENTA group and ≥1% more than in the placebo group were increases in uric acid (1.3% in the placebo group, 2.7% in the TRADJENTA group).

No clinically meaningful changes in vital signs were observed in patients treated with TRADJENTA.

6.2 Postmarketing Experience

Additional adverse reactions have been identified during postapproval use of TRADJENTA. Because these reactions are reported voluntarily from a population of uncertain size, it is generally not possible to reliably estimate their frequency or establish a causal relationship to drug exposure.

- Acute pancreatitis, including fatal pancreatitis *[see Indications and Usage (1.2) and Warnings and Precautions (5.1)]*
- Rash

7 DRUG INTERACTIONS

7.1 Inducers of P-glycoprotein or CYP3A4 Enzymes

Rifampin decreased linagliptin exposure, suggesting that the efficacy of TRADJENTA may be reduced when administered in combination with a strong P-gp or CYP3A4 inducer. Therefore, use of alternative treatments is strongly recommended when linagliptin is to be administered with a strong P-gp or CYP3A4 inducer *[see Clinical Pharmacology (12.3)]*.

8 USE IN SPECIFIC POPULATIONS

8.1 Pregnancy

Pregnancy Category B

Reproduction studies have been performed in rats and rabbits. There are, however, no adequate and well-controlled studies in pregnant women. Because animal reproduction studies are not always predictive of human response, this drug should be used during pregnancy only if clearly needed.

Linagliptin administered during the period of organogenesis was not teratogenic at doses up to 30 mg/kg in the rat and 150 mg/kg in the rabbit, or approximately 49 and 1943 times the clinical dose based on AUC exposure. Doses of linagliptin causing maternal toxicity in the rat and the rabbit also caused developmental delays in skeletal ossification and slightly increased embryofetal loss in the rat (1000 times the clinical dose) and increased fetal resorptions and visceral and skeletal variations in the rabbit (1943 times the clinical dose).

Linagliptin administered to female rats from gestation day 6 to lactation day 21 resulted in decreased body weight and delays in physical and behavioral development in male and female offspring at maternally toxic doses (exposures >1000 times the clinical dose). No functional, behavioral, or reproductive toxicity was observed in offspring of rats exposed to 49 times the clinical dose.

Linagliptin crossed the placenta into the fetus following oral dosing in pregnant rats and rabbits.

8.3 Nursing Mothers

Available animal data have shown excretion of linagliptin in milk at a milk-to-plasma ratio of 4:1. It is not known whether this drug is excreted in human milk. Because many drugs are excreted in human milk, caution should be exercised when TRADJENTA is administered to a nursing woman.

8.4 Pediatric Use

Safety and effectiveness of TRADJENTA in pediatric patients under 18 years of age have not been established.

8.5 Geriatric Use

There were 4040 type 2 diabetes patients treated with linagliptin 5 mg from 15 clinical trials of TRADJENTA; 1085 (27%) were 65 years and over, while 131 (3%) were 75 years and over. Of these patients, 2566 were enrolled in 12 double-blind placebo-controlled studies; 591 (23%) were 65 years and over, while 82 (3%) were 75 years and over. No overall differences in safety or effectiveness were observed between patients 65 years and over and younger patients. Therefore, no dose adjustment is recommended in the elderly population. While clinical studies of linagliptin have not identified differences in response between the elderly and younger patients, greater sensitivity of some older individuals cannot be ruled out.

8.6 Renal Impairment

No dose adjustment is recommended for patients with renal impairment *[see Clinical Pharmacology (12.3)]*.

8.7 Hepatic Impairment

No dose adjustment is recommended for patients with hepatic impairment *[see Clinical Pharmacology (12.3)]*.

10 OVERDOSAGE

In the event of an overdose with TRADJENTA, contact the Poison Control Center. Employ the usual supportive measures (e.g., remove unabsorbed material from the gastrointestinal tract, employ clinical monitoring, and institute supportive treatment) as dictated by the patient's clinical status. Removal of linagliptin by hemodialysis or peritoneal dialysis is unlikely.

During controlled clinical trials in healthy subjects, with single doses of up to 600 mg of TRADJENTA (equivalent to 120 times the recommended daily dose) there were no dose-related clinical adverse drug reactions. There is no experience with doses above 600 mg in humans.

11 DESCRIPTION

TRADJENTA (linagliptin) tablets contain, as the active ingredient, an orally-active inhibitor of the dipeptidyl peptidase-4 (DPP-4) enzyme.

Linagliptin is described chemically as 1H-Purine-2,6-dione, 8-[(3R)-3-amino-1-piperidinyl]-7-(2-butyn-1-yl)-3,7-dihydro-3-methyl-1-[(4-methyl-2-quinazolinyl)methyl]-

The empirical formula is $C_{25}H_{28}N_8O_2$ and the molecular weight is 472.54 g/mol. The structural formula is:

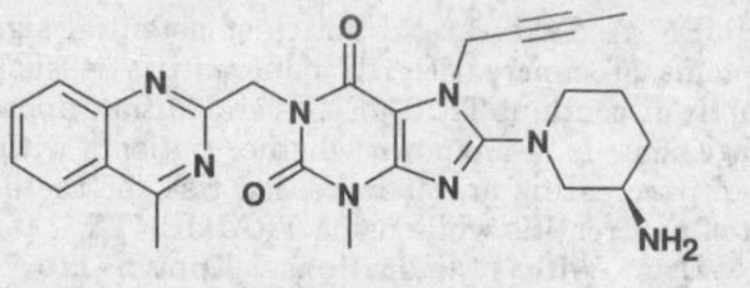

Linagliptin is a white to yellowish, not or only slightly hygroscopic solid substance. It is very slightly soluble in water (0.9 mg/mL). Linagliptin is soluble in methanol (ca. 60 mg/mL), sparingly soluble in ethanol (ca. 10 mg/mL), very slightly soluble in isopropanol (<1 mg/mL), and very slightly soluble in acetone (ca. 1 mg/mL).

Each film-coated tablet of TRADJENTA contains 5 mg of linagliptin free base and the following inactive ingredients: mannitol, pregelatinized starch, corn starch, copovidone, and magnesium stearate. In addition, the film coating contains the following inactive ingredients: hypromellose, titanium dioxide, talc, polyethylene glycol, and red ferric oxide.

12 CLINICAL PHARMACOLOGY

12.1 Mechanism of Action

Linagliptin is an inhibitor of DPP-4, an enzyme that degrades the incretin hormones glucagon-like peptide-1 (GLP-1) and glucose-dependent insulinotropic polypeptide (GIP). Thus, linagliptin increases the concentrations of active incretin hormones, stimulating the release of insulin in a glucose-dependent manner and decreasing the levels of glucagon in the circulation. Both incretin hormones are involved in the physiological regulation of glucose homeostasis. Incretin hormones are secreted at a low basal level throughout the day and levels rise immediately after meal intake. GLP-1 and GIP increase insulin biosynthesis and secretion from pancreatic beta-cells in the presence of normal and elevated blood glucose levels. Furthermore, GLP-1 also reduces glucagon secretion from pancreatic alpha-cells, resulting in a reduction in hepatic glucose output.

12.2 Pharmacodynamics

Linagliptin binds to DPP-4 in a reversible manner and thus increases the concentrations of incretin hormones. Linagliptin glucose dependently increases insulin secretion and lowers glucagon secretion, thus resulting in better regulation of glucose homeostasis. Linagliptin binds selectively to DPP-4, and selectively inhibits DPP-4 but not DPP-8 or DPP-9 activity *in vitro* at concentrations approximating therapeutic exposures.

Cardiac Electrophysiology

In a randomized, placebo-controlled, active-comparator, 4-way crossover study, 36 healthy subjects were administered a single oral dose of linagliptin 5 mg, linagliptin 100 mg (20 times the recommended dose), moxifloxacin, and placebo. No increase in QTc was observed with either the recommended dose of 5 mg or the 100-mg dose. At the 100-mg dose, peak linagliptin plasma concentrations were approximately 38-fold higher than the peak concentrations following a 5-mg dose.

12.3 Pharmacokinetics

The pharmacokinetics of linagliptin has been characterized in healthy subjects and patients with type 2 diabetes. After oral administration of a single 5-mg dose to healthy subjects, peak plasma concentrations of linagliptin occurred at approximately 1.5 hours post dose (T_{max}); the mean plasma area under the curve (AUC) was 139 nmol*h/L and maximum concentration (C_{max}) was 8.9 nmol/L.

Plasma concentrations of linagliptin decline in at least a biphasic manner with a long terminal half-life (>100 hours), related to the saturable binding of linagliptin to DPP-4. The prolonged elimination phase does not contribute to the accumulation of the drug. The effective half-life for accumulation of linagliptin, as determined from oral administration of multiple doses of linagliptin 5 mg, is approximately 12 hours. After once-daily dosing, steady-state plasma concentrations of linagliptin 5 mg are reached by the third dose, and C_{max} and AUC increased by a factor of 1.3 at steady state compared with the first dose. The intra-subject and inter-subject coefficients of variation for linagliptin AUC were small (12.6% and 28.5%, respectively). Plasma AUC of linagliptin increased in a less than dose-proportional manner in the dose range of 1 to 10 mg. The pharmacokinetics of linagliptin is similar in healthy subjects and in patients with type 2 diabetes.

Absorption

The absolute bioavailability of linagliptin is approximately 30%. High-fat meal reduced C_{max} by 15% and increased AUC by 4%; this effect is not clinically relevant. TRADJENTA may be administered with or without food.

Distribution

The mean apparent volume of distribution at steady state following a single intravenous dose of linagliptin 5 mg to healthy subjects is approximately 1110 L, indicating that linagliptin extensively distributes to the tissues. Plasma protein binding of linagliptin is concentration-dependent, decreasing from about 99% at 1 nmol/L to 75%-89% at ≥30 nmol/L, reflecting saturation of binding to DPP-4 with increasing concentration of linagliptin. At high concentrations, where DPP-4 is fully saturated, 70% to 80% of linagliptin remains bound to plasma proteins and 20% to 30% is unbound in plasma. Plasma binding is not altered in patients with renal or hepatic impairment.

Metabolism

Following oral administration, the majority (about 90%) of linagliptin is excreted unchanged, indicating that metabolism represents a minor elimination pathway. A small fraction of absorbed linagliptin is metabolized to a pharmacologically inactive metabolite, which shows a steady-state exposure of 13.3% relative to linagliptin.

Excretion

Following administration of an oral [^{14}C]-linagliptin dose to healthy subjects, approximately 85% of the administered radioactivity was eliminated via the enterohepatic system (80%) or urine (5%) within 4 days of dosing. Renal clearance at steady state was approximately 70 mL/min.

Specific Populations

Renal Impairment

An open-label pharmacokinetic study evaluated the pharmacokinetics of linagliptin 5 mg in male and female patients with varying degrees of chronic renal impairment. The study included 6 healthy subjects with normal renal function (creatinine clearance [CrCl] ≥80 mL/min), 6 patients with mild renal impairment (CrCl 50 to <80 mL/min), 6 patients with moderate renal impairment (CrCl 30 to <50 mL/min), 10 patients with type 2 diabetes mellitus and severe renal impairment (CrCl <30 mL/min), and 11 patients with type 2 diabetes mellitus and normal renal function. Creatinine clearance was measured by 24-hour urinary creatinine clearance measurements or estimated from serum creatinine based on the Cockcroft-Gault formula.

Under steady-state conditions, linagliptin exposure in patients with mild renal impairment was comparable to healthy subjects.

In patients with moderate renal impairment under steady-state conditions, mean exposure of linagliptin increased ($AUC_{\tau,ss}$ by 71% and C_{max} by 46%) compared with healthy subjects. This increase was not associated with a prolonged accumulation half-life, terminal half-life, or an increased accumulation factor. Renal excretion of linagliptin was below 5% of the administered dose and was not affected by decreased renal function.

Patients with type 2 diabetes mellitus and severe renal impairment showed steady-state exposure approximately 40% higher than that of patients with type 2 diabetes mellitus and normal renal function (increase in $AUC_{\tau,ss}$ by 42% and C_{max} by 35%). For both type 2 diabetes mellitus groups, renal excretion was below 7% of the administered dose.

These findings were further supported by the results of population pharmacokinetic analyses.

Hepatic Impairment

In patients with mild hepatic impairment (Child-Pugh class A), steady-state exposure ($AUC_{\tau,ss}$) of linagliptin was approximately 25% lower and $C_{max,ss}$ was approximately 36% lower than in healthy subjects. In patients with moderate hepatic impairment (Child-Pugh class B), AUC_{ss} of linagliptin was about 14% lower and $C_{max,ss}$ was approximately 8% lower than in healthy subjects. Patients with severe hepatic impairment (Child-Pugh class C) had comparable exposure of linagliptin in terms of $AUC_{0\text{-}24}$ and approximately 23% lower C_{max} compared with healthy subjects. Reductions in the pharmacokinetic parameters seen in patients with hepatic impairment did not result in reductions in DPP-4 inhibition.

Body Mass Index (BMI)/Weight

No dose adjustment is necessary based on BMI/weight. BMI/weight had no clinically meaningful effect on the pharmacokinetics of linagliptin based on a population pharmacokinetic analysis.

Gender

No dose adjustment is necessary based on gender. Gender had no clinically meaningful effect on the pharmacokinetics of linagliptin based on a population pharmacokinetic analysis.

Geriatric

Age did not have a clinically meaningful impact on the pharmacokinetics of linagliptin based on a population pharmacokinetic analysis.

Pediatric

Studies characterizing the pharmacokinetics of linagliptin in pediatric patients have not yet been performed.

Race

No dose adjustment is necessary based on race. Race had no clinically meaningful effect on the pharmacokinetics of linagliptin based on available pharmacokinetic data, including subjects of White, Hispanic, Black, and Asian racial groups.

Drug Interactions

In vitro Assessment of Drug Interactions

Linagliptin is a weak to moderate inhibitor of CYP isozyme CYP3A4, but does not inhibit other CYP isozymes and is not an inducer of CYP isozymes, including CYP1A2, 2A6, 2B6, 2C8, 2C9, 2C19, 2D6, 2E1, and 4A11.

Linagliptin is a P-glycoprotein (P-gp) substrate, and inhibits P-gp mediated transport of digoxin at high concentrations. Based on these results and *in vivo* drug interaction studies, linagliptin is considered unlikely to cause interactions with other P-gp substrates at therapeutic concentrations.

In vivo Assessment of Drug Interactions

Inducers of CYP3A4 or P-gp (e.g., rifampin) decrease exposure to linagliptin to subtherapeutic and likely ineffective concentrations. For patients requiring use of such drugs, an alternative to linagliptin is strongly recommended. *In vivo* studies indicated evidence of a low propensity for causing drug interactions with substrates of CYP3A4, CYP2C9, CYP2C8, P-gp and organic cationic transporter (OCT). No dose adjustment of TRADJENTA is recommended based on results of the described pharmacokinetic studies.

[See table 2 above]

[See table 3 above]

Table 2 Effect of Coadministered Drugs on Systemic Exposure of Linagliptin

Coadministered Drug	Dosing of Coadministered Drug*	Dosing of Linagliptin*	Geometric Mean Ratio (ratio with/without coadministered drug) No effect = 1.0	
			AUC†	Cmax
No dosing adjustments required for TRADJENTA when given with following coadministered drugs:				
Metformin	850 mg TID	10 mg QD	1.20	1.03
Glyburide	1.75 mg#	5 mg QD	1.02	1.01
Pioglitazone	45 mg QD	10 mg QD	1.13	1.07
Ritonavir	200 mg BID	5 mg#	2.01	2.96
The efficacy of TRADJENTA may be reduced when administered in combination with strong inducers of CYP3A4 or P-gp (e.g., rifampin). Use of alternative treatments is strongly recommended *[see Drug Interactions (7.1)]*.				
Rifampin	600 mg QD	5 mg QD	0.60	0.56

*Multiple dose (steady state) unless otherwise noted
#Single dose
†AUC = AUC(0 to 24 hours) for single dose treatments and AUC = AUC(TAU) for multiple dose treatments
QD = once daily
BID = twice daily
TID = three times daily

Table 3 Effect of Linagliptin on Systemic Exposure of Coadministered Drugs

Coadministered Drug	Dosing of Coadministered Drug*	Dosing of Linagliptin*	Geometric Mean Ratio (ratio with/without coadministered drug) No effect = 1.0		
				AUC†	Cmax
No dosing adjustments required for the following coadministered drugs:					
Metformin	850 mg TID	10 mg QD	metformin	1.01	0.89
Glyburide	1.75 mg#	5 mg QD	glyburide	0.86	0.86
Pioglitazone	45 mg QD	10 mg QD	pioglitazone metabolite M-III metabolite M-IV	0.94 0.98 1.04	0.86 0.96 1.05
Digoxin	0.25 mg QD	5 mg QD	digoxin	1.02	0.94
Simvastatin	40 mg QD	10 mg QD	simvastatin simvastatin acid	1.34 1.33	1.10 1.21
Warfarin	10 mg#	5 mg QD	R-warfarin S-warfarin INR PT	0.99 1.03 0.93** 1.03**	1.00 1.01 1.04** 1.15**
Ethinylestradiol and levonorgestrel	ethinylestradiol 0.03 mg and levonorgestrel 0.150 mg QD	5 mg QD	ethinylestradiol levonorgestrel	1.01 1.09	1.08 1.13

*Multiple dose (steady state) unless otherwise noted
#Single dose
†AUC = AUC(INF) for single dose treatments and AUC = AUC(TAU) for multiple dose treatments
**AUC=AUC(0-168) and Cmax=Emax for pharmacodynamic end points
INR = International Normalized Ratio
PT = Prothrombin Time
QD = once daily
TID = three times daily

13 NONCLINICAL TOXICOLOGY

13.1 Carcinogenesis, Mutagenesis, Impairment of Fertility

Linagliptin did not increase the incidence of tumors in male and female rats in a 2-year study at doses of 6, 18, and 60 mg/kg. The highest dose of 60 mg/kg is approximately 418 times the clinical dose of 5 mg/day based on AUC exposure. Linagliptin did not increase the incidence of tumors in mice in a 2-year study at doses up to 80 mg/kg (males) and 25 mg/kg (females), or approximately 35- and 270-times the clinical dose based on AUC exposure. Higher doses of linagliptin in female mice (80 mg/kg) increased the incidence of lymphoma at approximately 215-times the clinical dose based on AUC exposure.

Linagliptin was not mutagenic or clastogenic with or without metabolic activation in the Ames bacterial mutagenicity assay, a chromosomal aberration test in human lymphocytes, and an *in vivo* micronucleus assay.

In fertility studies in rats, linagliptin had no adverse effects on early embryonic development, mating, fertility, or bearing live young up to the highest dose of 240 mg/kg (approximately 943-times the clinical dose based on AUC exposure).

14 CLINICAL STUDIES

TRADJENTA has been studied as monotherapy and in combination with metformin, glimepiride, pioglitazone, and insulin.

A total of 3648 patients with type 2 diabetes were randomized and exposed to linagliptin for at least 12 weeks in 10 double-blind, placebo-controlled clinical efficacy studies evaluating the effects of TRADJENTA on glycemic control. The overall ethnic/racial distribution in these studies was 69% White, 29% Asian, and 2.5% Black, and included 16% Hispanic/Latino patients. Fifty two percent of patients were male. Patients had an overall mean age of 57 years (range 20 to 91 years). In addition, an active (glimepiride)-controlled study of 104 weeks' duration was conducted in 1551 patients with type 2 diabetes who had inadequate glycemic control on metformin, and a placebo-controlled study of 52 weeks' duration was conducted in 133 patients with type 2 diabetes and severe chronic renal impairment (eGFR <30 mL/min).

In patients with type 2 diabetes, treatment with TRADJENTA produced clinically significant improvements in hemoglobin A1c (A1C), fasting plasma glucose (FPG), and 2-hour post-prandial glucose (PPG) compared with placebo.

14.1 Monotherapy

A total of 730 patients with type 2 diabetes participated in 2 double-blind, placebo-controlled studies, one of 18 weeks' and another of 24 weeks' duration, to evaluate the efficacy and safety of TRADJENTA monotherapy. In both monotherapy studies, patients currently on an antihyperglycemic agent discontinued the agent and underwent a diet, exercise, and drug washout period of about 6 weeks that included an open-label placebo run-in during the last 2 weeks. Patients with inadequate glycemic control (A1C 7% to 10%) after the washout period were randomized; patients not currently on antihyperglycemic agents (off therapy for at least 8 weeks) with inadequate glycemic control (A1C 7% to 10%) were randomized after completing the 2-week, open-label, placebo run in period. In the 18-week study, only patients ineligible for metformin were recruited. In the 18-week study, 76 patients were randomized to placebo and 151 to TRADJENTA 5 mg; in the 24-week study, 167 patients were randomized to placebo and 336 to TRADJENTA 5 mg. Patients who failed to meet specific glycemic goals during the 18-week study received rescue therapy with pioglitazone and/or insulin; metformin rescue therapy was used in the 24-week trial.

Treatment with TRADJENTA 5 mg daily provided statistically significant improvements in A1C, FPG, and 2-hour PPG compared with placebo (Table 4). In the 18-week study, 12% of patients receiving TRADJENTA 5 mg and 18% who received placebo required rescue therapy. In the 24-week study, 10.2% of patients receiving TRADJENTA 5 mg and 20.9% of patients receiving placebo required rescue therapy. The improvement in A1C compared with placebo was not affected by gender, age, race, prior antihyperglycemic therapy, baseline BMI, or a standard index of insulin resistance (HOMA-IR). As is typical for trials of agents to treat type 2 diabetes, the mean reduction in A1C with TRADJENTA appears to be related to the degree of A1C elevation at baseline. In these 18- and 24-week studies, the changes from baseline in A1C were -0.4% and -0.4%, respectively, for those given TRADJENTA, and 0.1% and 0.3%, respectively, for those given placebo. Change from baseline in body weight did not differ significantly between the groups.

[See table 4 at top of next page]

14.2 Combination Therapy

Add-on Combination Therapy with Metformin

A total of 701 patients with type 2 diabetes participated in a 24-week, randomized, double-blind, placebo-controlled study designed to assess the efficacy of TRADJENTA in combination with metformin. Patients already on metformin (n = 491) at a dose of at least 1500 mg per day were randomized after completing a 2-week, open-label, placebo run-in period. Patients on metformin and another antihyperglycemic agent (n = 207) were randomized after a run-in period of approximately 6 weeks on metformin (at a dose of at least 1500 mg per day) in monotherapy. Patients were randomized to the addition of either TRADJENTA 5 mg or placebo, administered once daily. Patients who failed to meet specific glycemic goals during the studies were treated with glimepiride rescue.

In combination with metformin, TRADJENTA provided statistically significant improvements in A1C, FPG, and 2-hour PPG compared with placebo (Table 5). Rescue glycemic therapy was used in 7.8% of patients treated with TRADJENTA 5 mg and in 18.9% of patients treated with placebo. A similar decrease in body weight was observed for both treatment groups.

Table 4 Glycemic Parameters in Placebo-Controlled Monotherapy Studies of TRADJENTA*

	18-Week Study		24-Week Study	
	TRADJENTA 5 mg	Placebo	TRADJENTA 5 mg	Placebo
A1C (%)				
Number of patients	n = 147	n = 73	n = 333	n = 163
Baseline (mean)	8.1	8.1	8.0	8.0
Change from baseline (adjusted mean)***	-0.4	0.1	-0.4	0.3
Difference from placebo (adjusted mean) (95% CI)	-0.6 (-0.9, -0.3)	--	-0.7 (-0.9, -0.5)	--
Patients [n (%)] achieving A1C <7%**	32 (23.5)	8 (11.8)	77 (25)	17 (12)
FPG (mg/dL)				
Number of patients	n = 138	n = 66	n = 318	n = 149
Baseline (mean)	178	176	164	166
Change from baseline (adjusted mean)***	-13	7	-9	15
Difference from placebo (adjusted mean) (95% CI)	-21 (-31, -10)	--	-23 (-30, -16)	--
2-hour PPG (mg/dL)				
Number of patients	Data not available	Data not available	n = 67	n = 24
Baseline (mean)	--	--	258	244
Change from baseline (adjusted mean)***	--	--	-34	25
Difference from placebo (adjusted mean) (95% CI)	--	--	-58 (-82, -34)	--

*Full analysis population using last observation on study
**18-week study: Placebo, n=68; TRADJENTA, n=136
24-week study: Placebo, n=147; TRADJENTA, n=306
***18-week study. HbA1c; ANCOVA model included treatment, reason for metformin intolerance and number of prior oral anti-diabetic medicine(s) (OADs) as class-effects, as well as baseline HbA1c as continuous covariates. FPG: ANCOVA model included treatment, reason for metformin intolerance and number of prior OADs as class-effects, as well as baseline HbA1c and baseline FPG as continuous covariates.
24-week study. HbA1c: ANCOVA model included treatment and number of prior OADs as class-effects, as well as baseline HbA1c as continuous covariates. FPG: ANCOVA model included treatment and number of prior OADs as class-effects, as well as baseline HbA1c and baseline FPG as continuous covariates. PPG: ANCOVA model included treatment and number of prior OADs as class-effects, as well as baseline HbA1c and baseline postprandial glucose after two hours as covariate.

Table 5 Glycemic Parameters in Placebo-Controlled Study for TRADJENTA in Combination with Metformin*

	TRADJENTA 5 mg + Metformin	Placebo + Metformin
A1C (%)		
Number of patients	n = 513	n = 175
Baseline (mean)	8.1	8.0
Change from baseline (adjusted mean)***	-0.5	0.15
Difference from placebo + metformin (adjusted mean) (95% CI)	-0.6 (-0.8, -0.5)	--
Patients [n (%)] achieving A1C <7%**	127 (26.2)	15 (9.2)
FPG (mg/dL)		
Number of patients	n = 495	n = 159
Baseline (mean)	169	164
Change from baseline (adjusted mean)***	-11	11
Difference from placebo + metformin (adjusted mean) (95% CI)	-21 (-27, -15)	--
2-hour PPG (mg/dL)		
Number of patients	n = 78	n = 21
Baseline (mean)	270	274
Change from baseline (adjusted mean)***	-49	18
Difference from placebo + metformin (adjusted mean) (95% CI)	-67 (-95, -40)	--

*Full analysis population using last observation on study
**TRADJENTA 5 mg + Metformin, n=485; Placebo + Metformin, n=163.
***HbA1c: ANCOVA model included treatment and number of prior oral OADs as class-effects, as well as baseline HbA1c as continuous covariates. FPG: ANCOVA model included treatment and number of prior OADs as class-effects, as well as baseline HbA1c and baseline FPG as continuous covariates. PPG: ANCOVA model included treatment and number of prior OADs as class-effects, as well as baseline HbA1c and baseline postprandial glucose after two hours as covariate.

Initial Combination Therapy with Metformin
A total of 791 patients with type 2 diabetes mellitus and inadequate glycemic control on diet and exercise participated in the 24-week, randomized, double-blind, portion of this placebo-controlled factorial study designed to assess the efficacy of TRADJENTA as initial therapy with metformin. Patients on an antihyperglycemic agent (52%) underwent a drug washout period of 4 weeks' duration. After the washout period and after completing a 2-week single-blind placebo run-in period, patients with inadequate glycemic control (A1C ≥7.0% to ≤10.5%) were randomized. Patients with inadequate glycemic control (A1C ≥7.5% to <11.0%) not on antihyperglycemic agents at study entry (48%) immediately entered the 2-week, single-blind, placebo run-in period and then were randomized. Randomization was stratified by baseline A1C (<8.5% vs ≥8.5%) and use of a prior oral antidiabetic drug (none vs monotherapy). Patients were randomized in a 1:2:2:2:2:2 ratio to either placebo or one of 5 active-treatment arms. Approximately equal numbers of patients were randomized to receive initial therapy with 5 mg of TRADJENTA once daily, 500 mg or 1000 mg of metformin twice daily, or 2.5 mg of linagliptin twice daily in combination with 500 mg or 1000 mg of metformin twice daily. Patients who failed to meet specific glycemic goals during the study were treated with sulfonylurea, thiazolidinedione, or insulin rescue therapy.
Initial therapy with the combination of linagliptin and metformin provided significant improvements in A1C and fasting plasma glucose (FPG) compared to placebo, to metformin alone, and to linagliptin alone (Table 6).
The adjusted mean treatment difference in A1C from baseline to week 24 (LOCF) was -0.5% (95% CI -0.7, -0.3; p<0.0001) for linagliptin 2.5 mg/metformin 1000 mg twice daily compared to metformin 1000 twice daily; -1.1% (95% CI -1.4, -0.9; p<0.0001) for linagliptin 2.5 mg/metformin 1000 mg twice daily compared to TRADJENTA 5 mg once daily; -0.6% (95% CI -0.8, -0.4; p<0.0001) for linagliptin 2.5 mg/metformin 500 mg twice daily compared to metformin 500 mg twice daily; and -0.8% (95% CI -1.0, -0.6; p<0.0001) for linagliptin 2.5 mg/metformin 500 mg twice daily compared to TRADJENTA 5 mg once daily.
Lipid effects were generally neutral. No meaningful change in body weight was noted in any of the 6 treatment groups.
[See table 6 at top of next page]

Active-Controlled Study vs Glimepiride in Combination with Metformin
The efficacy of TRADJENTA was evaluated in a 104-week, double-blind, glimepiride-controlled, non-inferiority study in patients with type 2 diabetes with insufficient glycemic control despite metformin therapy. Patients being treated with metformin only entered a run-in period of 2 weeks' duration, whereas patients pretreated with metformin and one additional antihyperglycemic agent entered a run-in treatment period of 6 weeks' duration with metformin monotherapy (dose of ≥1500 mg/day) and washout of the other agent. After an additional 2-week placebo run-in period, those with inadequate glycemic control (A1C 6.5% to 10%) were randomized 1:1 to the addition of TRADJENTA 5 mg once daily or glimepiride. Randomization was stratified by baseline HbA1c (<8.5% versus ≥8.5%), and the previous use of antidiabetic drugs (metformin alone vs metformin plus one other OAD). Patients receiving glimepiride were given an initial dose of 1 mg/day and then electively titrated over the next 12 weeks to a maximum dose of 4 mg/day as needed to optimize glycemic control. Thereafter, the glimepiride dose was to be kept constant, except for down-titration to prevent hypoglycemia.
After 52 and 104 weeks, TRADJENTA and glimepiride both had reductions from baseline in A1C (52 weeks: -0.4% for TRADJENTA, -0.6% for glimepiride; 104 weeks: -0.2% for TRADJENTA, -0.4% for glimepiride) from a baseline mean of 7.7% (Table 7). The mean difference between groups in A1C change from baseline was 0.2% with 2-sided 97.5% confidence interval (0.1%, 0.3%) for the intent-to-treat population using last observation carried forward. These results were consistent with the completers analysis.
[See table 7 on pages 669 and 670]
Patients treated with linagliptin had a mean baseline body weight of 86 kg and were observed to have an adjusted mean decrease in body weight of 1.1 kg at 52 weeks and 1.4 kg at 104 weeks. Patients on glimepiride had a mean baseline body weight of 87 kg and were observed to have an adjusted mean increase from baseline in body weight of 1.4 kg at 52 weeks and 1.3 kg at 104 weeks (treatment difference p<0.0001 for both timepoints).

Add-On Combination Therapy with Pioglitazone
A total of 389 patients with type 2 diabetes participated in a 24-week, randomized, double-blind, placebo-controlled study designed to assess the efficacy of TRADJENTA in combination with pioglitazone. Therapy was stopped in patients on oral antihyperglycemic therapy for a period of 6 weeks (4 weeks followed by a 2-week, open-label, placebo run-in period). Drug-naïve patients entered directly into the 2-week placebo run-in period. After the run-in period, patients were randomized to receive either TRADJENTA 5 mg or placebo, both in addition to pioglitazone 30 mg daily. Patients who failed to meet specific glycemic goals during the studies were treated with metformin rescue. Glycemic endpoints measured were A1C and FPG.
In initial combination with pioglitazone 30 mg, TRADJENTA 5 mg provided statistically significant improvements in A1C and FPG compared to placebo with pioglitazone (Table 8). Rescue therapy was used in 7.9% of patients treated with TRADJENTA 5 mg/pioglitazone 30 mg and 14.1% of patients treated with placebo/pioglitazone 30 mg. Patient weight increased in both groups during the study with an adjusted mean change from baseline of 2.3 kg and 1.2 kg in the TRADJENTA 5 mg/pioglitazone 30 mg and placebo/pioglitazone 30 mg groups, respectively (p = 0.0141).

Table 8 Glycemic Parameters in Placebo-Controlled Study for TRADJENTA in Combination Therapy with Pioglitazone*

	TRADJENTA 5 mg + Pioglitazone	Placebo + Pioglitazone
A1C (%)		
Number of patients	n = 252	n = 128
Baseline (mean)	8.6	8.6
Change from baseline (adjusted mean)**	-1.1	-0.6
Difference from placebo + pioglitazone (adjusted mean) (95% CI)	-0.5 (-0.7, -0.3)	--
Patients [n (%)] achieving A1C <7%	108 (42.9)	39 (30.5)
FPG (mg/dL)		
Number of patients	n = 243	n = 122
Baseline (mean)	188	186
Change from baseline (adjusted mean)**	-33	-18
Difference from placebo + pioglitazone (adjusted mean) (95% CI)	-14 (-21, -7)	--

*Full analysis population using last observation on study
**HbA1c: ANCOVA model included treatment and number of prior OADs as class-effects, as well as baseline HbA1c as continuous covariates. FPG: ANCOVA model included treatment and number of prior OADs as class-effects, as well as baseline HbA1c and baseline FPG as continuous covariates.

Table 6 Glycemic Parameters at Final Visit (24-Week Study) for Linagliptin and Metformin, Alone and in Combination in Randomized Patients with Type 2 Diabetes Mellitus Inadequately Controlled on Diet and Exercise**

	Placebo	TRADJENTA 5 mg Once Daily	Metformin 500 mg Twice Daily	Linagliptin 2.5 mg Twice Daily* + Metformin 500 mg Twice Daily	Metformin 1000 mg Twice Daily	Linagliptin 2.5 mg Twice Daily* + Metformin 1000 mg Twice Daily
A1C (%)						
Number of patients	n = 65	n = 135	n = 141	n = 137	n = 138	n = 140
Baseline (mean)	8.7	8.7	8.7	8.7	8.5	8.7
Change from baseline (adjusted mean)****	0.1	-0.5	-0.6	-1.2	-1.1	-1.6
Difference from placebo (adjusted mean) (95% CI)	--	-0.6 (-0.9, -0.3)	-0.8 (-1.0, -0.5)	-1.3 (-1.6, -1.1)	-1.2 (-1.5, -0.9)	-1.7 (-2.0, -1.4)
Patients [n (%)] achieving A1C <7%***	7 (10.8)	14 (10.4)	26 (18.6)	41 (30.1)	42 (30.7)	74 (53.6)
Patients (%) receiving rescue medication	29.2	11.1	13.5	7.3	8.0	4.3
FPG (mg/dL)						
Number of patients	n = 61	n = 134	n = 136	n = 135	n = 132	n = 136
Baseline (mean)	203	195	191	199	191	196
Change from baseline (adjusted mean)****	10	-9	-16	-33	-32	-49
Difference from placebo (adjusted mean) (95% CI)	--	-19 (-31, -6)	-26 (-38, -14)	-43 (-56, -31)	-42 (-55, -30)	-60 (-72, -47)

*Total daily dose of TRADJENTA is equal to 5 mg
**Full analysis population using last observation on study
***Metformin 500 mg twice daily, n=140; Linagliptin 2.5 mg twice daily + met 500 twice daily, n=136; Metformin 1000 mg twice daily, n=137; Linagliptin 2.5 mg twice daily and Metformin 1000 mg twice daily, n=138.
****HbA1c: ANCOVA model included treatment and number of prior OADs as class-effects, as well as baseline HbA1c as continuous covariates. FPG: ANCOVA model included treatment and number of prior OADs as class-effects, as well as baseline HbA1c and baseline FPG as continuous covariates.

Table 7 Glycemic Parameters at 52 and 104 Weeks in Study Comparing TRADJENTA to Glimepiride as Add-On Therapy in Patients Inadequately Controlled on Metformin**

	Week 52		Week 104	
	TRADJENTA 5 mg + Metformin	Glimepiride + Metformin (mean Glimepiride dose 3 mg)	TRADJENTA 5 mg + Metformin	Glimepiride + Metformin (mean Glimepiride dose 3 mg)
A1C (%)				
Number of patients	n = 764	n = 755	n = 764	n = 755
Baseline (mean)	7.7	7.7	7.7	7.7
Change from baseline (adjusted mean)****	-0.4	-0.6	-0.2	-0.4
Difference from glimepiride (adjusted mean) (97.5% CI)	0.2 (0.1, 0.3)	--	0.2 (0.1, 0.3)	--

(Table continued on next page)

Add-On Combination with Sulfonylureas
A total of 245 patients with type 2 diabetes participated in an 18-week, randomized, double-blind, placebo-controlled study designed to assess the efficacy of TRADJENTA in combination with sulfonylurea (SU). Patients on sulfonylurea monotherapy (n = 142) were randomized after completing a 2-week, single-blind, placebo run-in period. Patients on a sulfonylurea plus one additional oral antihyperglycemic agent (n = 103) were randomized after a wash-out period of 4 weeks and a 2-week, single-blind, placebo run-in period. Patients were randomized to the addition of TRADJENTA 5 mg or to placebo, each administered once daily. Patients who failed to meet specific glycemic goals during the studies were treated with metformin rescue. Glycemic endpoints measured included A1C and FPG.
In combination with a sulfonylurea, TRADJENTA provided statistically significant improvements in A1C compared with placebo following 18 weeks' treatment; the improvements in FPG observed with TRADJENTA were not statistically significant compared with placebo (Table 9). Rescue therapy was used in 7.6% of patients treated with TRADJENTA 5 mg and 15.9% of patients treated with placebo. There was no significant difference between TRADJENTA and placebo in body weight.

Table 9 Glycemic Parameters in Placebo-Controlled Study for TRADJENTA in Combination with Sulfonylurea*

	TRADJENTA 5 mg + SU	Placebo + SU
A1C (%)		
Number of patients	n = 158	n = 82
Baseline (mean)	8.6	8.6
Change from baseline (adjusted mean)***	-0.5	-0.1
Difference from placebo + SU (adjusted mean) (95% CI)	-0.5 (-0.7, -0.2)	--
Patients [n (%)] achieving A1C <7%**	23 (14.7)	3 (3.7)
FPG (mg/dL)		
Number of patients	n = 155	n = 78
Baseline (mean)	180	171
Change from baseline (adjusted mean)***	-8	-2
Difference from placebo + SU (adjusted mean) (95% CI)	-6 (-17, 4)	--

SU = sulfonylurea
*Full analysis population using last observation on study
**TRADJENTA 5 mg+SU, n=156; Placebo + SU, n=82.
***HbA1c: ANCOVA model included treatment and number of prior OADs as class-effects, as well as baseline HbA1c as continuous covariates. FPG: ANCOVA model included treatment and number of prior OADs as class-effects, as well as baseline HbA1c and baseline FPG as continuous covariates

Add-On Combination Therapy with Metformin and a Sulfonylurea
A total of 1058 patients with type 2 diabetes participated in a 24-week, randomized, double-blind, placebo-controlled study designed to assess the efficacy of TRADJENTA in combination with a sulfonylurea and metformin. The most common sulfonylureas used by patients in the study were: glimepiride (31%), glibenclamide (26%), and gliclazide (26%, not available in the United States). Patients on a sulfonylurea and metformin were randomized to receive TRADJENTA 5 mg or placebo, each administered once daily. Patients who failed to meet specific glycemic goals during the study were treated with pioglitazone rescue. Glycemic endpoints measured included A1C and FPG.
In combination with a sulfonylurea and metformin, TRADJENTA provided statistically significant improvements in A1C and FPG compared with placebo (Table 10). In the entire study population (patients on TRADJENTA in combination with sulfonylurea and metformin), a mean reduction from baseline relative to placebo in A1C of -0.6% and in FPG of -13 mg/dL was seen. Rescue therapy was used in 5.4% of patients treated with TRADJENTA 5 mg and in 13% of patients treated with placebo. Change from baseline in body weight did not differ significantly between the groups.

Table 7 *(cont.)* Glycemic Parameters at 52 and 104 Weeks in Study Comparing TRADJENTA to Glimepiride as Add-On Therapy in Patients Inadequately Controlled on Metformin**

	Week 52		Week 104	
	TRADJENTA 5 mg + Metformin	**Glimepiride + Metformin (mean Glimepiride dose 3 mg)**	**TRADJENTA 5 mg + Metformin**	**Glimepiride + Metformin (mean Glimepiride dose 3 mg)**
FPG (mg/dL)				
Number of patients	n = 733	n = 725	n = 733	n = 725
Baseline (mean)	164	166	164	166
Change from baseline (adjusted mean)****	-8*	-15	-2†	-9
Hypoglycemia incidence (%)***				
Number of patients	n = 776	n = 775	n = 776	n = 775
Incidence****	5.3*	31.1	7.5*	36.1

*p<0.0001 vs glimepiride; †p=0.0012 vs glimepiride
**Full analysis population using last observation on study
***Hypoglycemic incidence included both asymptomatic events (not accompanied by typical symptoms and plasma glucose concentration of ≤70 mg/dL) and symptomatic events with typical symptoms of hypoglycemia and plasma glucose concentration of ≤70 mg/dL.
****HbA1c: ANCOVA model included treatment and number of prior OADs as class-effects, as well as baseline HbA1c as continuous covariates. FPG: ANCOVA model included treatment and number of prior OADs as class-effects, as well as baseline HbA1c and baseline FPG as continuous covariates. Hypoglycemia incidence (%): Cochran-Mantel-Haenszel test was performed on the patient population contained in the treated set, to compare the proportion of patients with hypoglycemic events between patients treated with linagliptin and patients treated with glimepiride.

Table 10 Glycemic Parameters in Placebo-Controlled Study for TRADJENTA in Combination with Metformin and Sulfonylurea*

	TRADJENTA 5 mg + Metformin + SU	**Placebo + Metformin + SU**
A1C (%)		
Number of patients	n = 778	n = 262
Baseline (mean)	8.2	8.1
Change from baseline (adjusted mean)***	-0.7	-0.1
Difference from placebo (adjusted mean) (95% CI)	-0.6 (-0.7, -0.5)	--
Patients [n (%)] achieving A1C <7%**	217 (29.2)	20 (8.1)
FPG (mg/dL)		
Number of patients	n = 739	n = 248
Baseline (mean)	159	163
Change from baseline (adjusted mean)***	-5	8
Difference from placebo (adjusted mean) (95% CI)	-13 (-18, -7)	--

SU = sulfonylurea
*Full analysis population using last observation on study
**TRADJENTA 5 mg+Metformin+SU, n=742; Placebo + Metformin+ SU, n=247
***HbA1c: ANCOVA model included treatment as class-effects and baseline HbA1c as continuous covariates. FPG; ANCOVA model included treatment as class-effects, as well as baseline HbA1c and baseline FPG as continuous covariates.

Add-On Combination Therapy with Insulin

A total of 1261 patients with type 2 diabetes inadequately controlled on basal insulin alone or basal insulin in combination with oral drugs participated in a randomized, double-blind placebo controlled trial designed to evaluate the efficacy of TRADJENTA as add-on therapy to basal insulin over 24-weeks. Randomization was stratified by baseline HbA1c (<8.5% versus ≥8.5%), renal function impairment status (based on baseline eGFR), and concomitant use of oral antidiabetic drugs (none, metformin only, pioglitazone only, metformin + pioglitazone). Patients with a baseline A1C of ≥7% and ≤10% were included in the study including 709 patients with renal impairment (eGFR <90 mL/min), most of whom (n=575) were categorized as mild renal impairment (eGFR 60 to <90 mL/min). Patients entered a 2-week placebo run-in period on basal insulin (e.g., insulin glargine, insulin detemir, or NPH insulin) with or without metformin and/or pioglitazone background therapy. Following the run-in period, patients with inadequate glycemic control were randomized to the addition of either 5 mg of TRADJENTA or placebo, administered once daily. Patients were maintained on a stable dose of insulin prior to enrollment, during the run-in period and during the first 24 weeks of treatment. Patients who failed to meet specific glycemic goals during the double-blind treatment period were rescued by increasing background insulin dose.

TRADJENTA used in combination with insulin (with or without metformin and/or pioglitazone), provided statistically significant improvements in A1C and FPG compared to placebo (Table 11) after 24 weeks of treatment. The mean total daily insulin dose at baseline was 42 units for patients treated with TRADJENTA and 40 units for patients treated with placebo. Background baseline diabetes therapy included use of: insulin alone (16.1%), insulin combined with metformin only (75.5%), insulin combined with metformin and pioglitazone (7.4%), and insulin combined with pioglitazone only (1%). The mean change from baseline to Week 24 in the daily dose of insulin was +1.3 IU in the placebo group and +0.6 IU in the TRADJENTA group. The mean change in body weight from baseline to Week 24 was similar in the two treatment groups. The rate of hypoglycemia, defined as all symptomatic or asymptomatic episodes with a self measured blood glucose was also similar in both groups (21.4% TRADJENTA; 22.9% placebo) in the first 24-weeks of the study.

Table 11 Glycemic Parameters in Placebo-Controlled Study for TRADJENTA in Combination with Insulin*

	TRADJENTA 5 mg + Insulin	**Placebo + Insulin**
A1C (%)		
Number of patients	n = 618	n = 617
Baseline (mean)	8.3	8.3
Change from baseline (adjusted mean***)	-0.6	0.1
Difference from placebo (adjusted mean***) (95% CI)	-0.7 (-0.7, -0.6)	--
Patients [n (%)] achieving A1C <7%**	116 (19.5)	48 (8.1)
FPG (mg/dL)		
Number of patients	n = 613	n = 608
Baseline (mean)	147	151
Change from baseline (adjusted mean***)	-8	3
Difference from placebo (adjusted mean***) (95% CI)	-11 (-16, -6)	--

*Full analysis population using last observation carried forward (LOCF) method on study
**TRADJENTA+Insulin, N=595; Placebo+Insulin, N=593
***HbA1c: ANCOVA model included treatment, categorical renal function impairment status and concomitant OADs as class-effects, as well as baseline HbA1c as continuous covariates. FPG: ANCOVA model included treatment, categorical renal function impairment status and concomitant OADs as class-effects, as well as baseline HbA1c and baseline FPG as continuous covariates.

The difference between treatment with linagliptin and placebo in terms of adjusted mean change from baseline in HbA1c after 24 weeks was comparable for patients with no renal impairment (eGFR ≥ 90 mL/min, n=539), with mild renal impairment (eGFR 60 to <90 mL/min, n= 565), or with moderate renal impairment (eGFR 30 to <60 mL/min, n=124).

14.3 Renal Impairment

A total of 133 patients with type 2 diabetes participated in a 52 week, double-blind, randomized, placebo-controlled trial designed to evaluate the efficacy and safety of TRADJENTA in patients with both type 2 diabetes and severe chronic renal impairment. Participants with an estimated [based on the four variables modified diet in renal disease (MDRD) equation] GFR value of <30 mL/min were eligible to participate in the study. Randomization was stratified by baseline HbA1c (≤8% and >8%) and background antidiabetic therapy (insulin or any combination with insulin, SU or glinides as monotherapy and pioglitazone or any other antidiabetics excluding any other DPP-4 inhibitors). For the initial 12 weeks of the study, background antidiabetic therapy was kept stable and included insulin, sulfonylurea, glinides, and pioglitazone. For the remainder of the trial, dose adjustments in antidiabetic background therapy were allowed. At baseline in this trial, 62.5% of patients were receiving insulin alone as background diabetes therapy, and 12.5% were receiving sulfonylurea alone.

After 12 weeks of treatment, TRADJENTA 5 mg provided statistically significant improvement in A1C compared to placebo, with an adjusted mean change of -0.6% compared to placebo (95% Confidence Interval -0.9, -0.3) based on the analysis using last observation carried forward (LOCF). With adjustments in antidiabetic background therapy after the initial 12 weeks, efficacy was maintained for 52 weeks, with an adjusted mean change from baseline in A1C of -0.7% compared to placebo (95% Confidence Interval -1.0, -0.4) based on analysis using LOCF.

16 HOW SUPPLIED/STORAGE AND HANDLING

TRADJENTA tablets are available as light red, round, biconvex, bevel-edged, film-coated tablets containing 5 mg of linagliptin. TRADJENTA tablets are debossed with "D5" on one side and the Boehringer Ingelheim logo on the other side.

They are supplied as follows:
Bottles of 30 (NDC 0597-0140-30)
Bottles of 90 (NDC 0597-0140-90)
Cartons containing 10 blister cards of 10 tablets each (10 × 10) (NDC 0597-0140-61)

If repackaging is required, dispense in a tight container as defined in USP.

Storage

Store at 25°C (77°F); excursions permitted to 15°-30°C (59°-86°F) [see USP Controlled Room Temperature]. Store in a safe place out of reach of children.

17 PATIENT COUNSELING INFORMATION

See FDA-approved patient labeling (Medication Guide)

17.1 Instructions

Inform patients of the potential risks and benefits of TRADJENTA and of alternative modes of therapy. Also inform patients about the importance of adherence to dietary instructions, regular physical activity, periodic blood glucose monitoring and A1C testing, recognition and management of hypoglycemia and hyperglycemia, and assessment for diabetes complications. Advise patients to seek medical advice promptly during periods of stress such as fever, trauma, infection, or surgery, as medication requirements may change.

Inform patients that acute pancreatitis has been reported during postmarketing use of TRADJENTA. Inform patients that persistent severe abdominal pain, sometimes radiating to the back, which may or may not be accompanied by vomiting, is the hallmark symptom of acute pancreatitis. Instruct patients to discontinue TRADJENTA promptly and contact their physician if persistent severe abdominal pain occurs [*see Warnings and Precautions (5.1)*].

Inform patients that the incidence of hypoglycemia is increased when TRADJENTA is added to a sulfonylurea or insulin and that a lower dose of the sulfonylurea or insulin may be required to reduce the risk of hypoglycemia.

Instruct patients to take TRADJENTA only as prescribed. If a dose is missed, advise patients not to double their next dose.

Instruct patients to read the Medication Guide before starting TRADJENTA therapy and to reread it each time the prescription is renewed. Instruct patients to inform their doctor or pharmacist if they develop any unusual symptom, or if any known symptom persists or worsens.

17.2 Laboratory Tests

Inform patients that response to all diabetic therapies should be monitored by periodic measurements of blood glucose and A1C levels, with a goal of decreasing these levels toward the normal range. A1C monitoring is especially useful for evaluating long-term glycemic control.

Distributed by:
Boehringer Ingelheim Pharmaceuticals, Inc.
Ridgefield, CT 06877 USA
Marketed by:
Boehringer Ingelheim Pharmaceuticals, Inc.
Ridgefield, CT 06877 USA
and
Eli Lilly and Company
Indianapolis, IN 46285 USA
Licensed from:
Boehringer Ingelheim International GmbH, Ingelheim, Germany

IT5253NF192013
10007261/07
IT5437K
10007237/07

MEDICATION GUIDE
TRADJENTA® (TRAD gen ta)
(linagliptin)
Tablets

Read this Medication Guide carefully before you start taking TRADJENTA and each time you get a refill. There may be new information. This information does not take the place of talking to your doctor about your medical condition or your treatment. If you have any questions about TRADJENTA, ask your doctor or pharmacist.

What is the most important information I should know about TRADJENTA?

Serious side effects can happen to people taking TRADJENTA, including inflammation of the pancreas (pancreatitis) which may be severe and lead to death.

Certain medical problems make you more likely to get pancreatitis.

Before you start taking TRADJENTA:

Tell your doctor if you have ever had:
- inflammation of your pancreas (pancreatitis)
- stones in your gallbladder (gallstones)
- a history of alcoholism
- high blood triglyceride levels

Stop taking TRADJENTA and call your doctor right away if you have pain in your stomach area (abdomen) that is severe and will not go away. The pain may be felt going from your abdomen through to your back. The pain may happen with or without vomiting. These may be symptoms of pancreatitis.

What is TRADJENTA?
- TRADJENTA is a prescription medicine used along with diet and exercise to lower blood sugar in adults with type 2 diabetes.
- TRADJENTA is not for people with type 1 diabetes.
- TRADJENTA is not for people with diabetic ketoacidosis (increased ketones in the blood or urine).
- If you have had pancreatitis in the past, it is not known if you have a higher chance of getting pancreatitis while you take TRADJENTA.

It is not known if TRADJENTA is safe and effective in children under 18 years of age.

Who should not take TRADJENTA?

Do not take TRADJENTA if you:
- are allergic to linagliptin or any of the ingredients in TRADJENTA. See the end of this Medication Guide for a complete list of ingredients in TRADJENTA.

Symptoms of a serious allergic reaction to TRADJENTA may include:
- skin rash, itching, flaking or peeling
- raised red patches on your skin (hives)
- swelling of your face, lips, tongue and throat that may cause difficulty in breathing or swallowing
- difficulty with swallowing or breathing

If you have any of these symptoms, stop taking TRADJENTA and contact your doctor or go to the nearest hospital emergency room right away.

What should I tell my doctor before using TRADJENTA?

Before you take TRADJENTA, tell your doctor if you:
- have or have had inflammation of your pancreas (pancreatitis).
- have any other medical conditions
- are pregnant or plan to become pregnant. It is not known if TRADJENTA will harm your unborn baby. If you are pregnant, talk with your doctor about the best way to control your blood sugar while you are pregnant.
- are breastfeeding or plan to breastfeed. It is not known if TRADJENTA passes into your breast milk. Talk with your doctor about the best way to feed your baby if you take TRADJENTA.

Tell your doctor about all the medicines you take, including prescription and non-prescription medicines, vitamins, and herbal supplements.

TRADJENTA may affect the way other medicines work, and other medicines may affect how TRADJENTA works.

Especially tell your doctor if you take
- other medicines that can lower your blood sugar
- rifampin (Rifadin®, Rimactane®, Rifater®, Rifamate®)*, an antibiotic that is used to treat tuberculosis

Ask your doctor or pharmacist for a list of these medicines if you are not sure if your medicine is one that is listed above.

Know the medicines you take. Keep a list of them and show it to your doctor and pharmacist when you get a new medicine.

How should I take TRADJENTA?
- Take 1 tablet 1 time each day with or without food.
- Your doctor will tell you when to take TRADJENTA.
- Talk with your doctor if you do not understand how to take TRADJENTA.
- If you miss a dose, take it as soon as you remember. If you do not remember until it is time for your next dose, skip the missed dose and go back to your regular schedule. Do not take two doses of TRADJENTA at the same time.
- Your doctor may tell you to take TRADJENTA along with other diabetes medicines. Low blood sugar can happen more often when TRADJENTA is taken with certain other diabetes medicines. See "What are the possible side effects of TRADJENTA?"
- If you take too much TRADJENTA, call your doctor or Poison Control Center at 1-800-222-1222 or go to the nearest hospital emergency room right away.
- When your body is under some types of stress, such as fever, trauma (such as a car accident), infection, or surgery, the amount of diabetes medicine that you need may change. Tell your doctor right away if you have any of these conditions and follow your doctor's instructions.
- Check your blood sugar as your doctor tells you to.
- Stay on your prescribed diet and exercise program while taking TRADJENTA.
- Your doctor will check your diabetes with regular blood tests, including your blood sugar levels and your hemoglobin A1C.

What are the possible side effects of TRADJENTA?

TRADJENTA may cause serious side effects, including:
- See **"What is the most important information I should know about TRADJENTA?"**.
- **low blood sugar (hypoglycemia).** If you take TRADJENTA with another medicine that can cause low blood sugar, such as a sulfonylurea or insulin, your risk of getting low blood sugar is higher. The dose of your sulfonylurea medicine or insulin may need to be lowered while you take TRADJENTA. Signs and symptoms of low blood sugar may include:
  - headache
  - drowsiness
  - weakness
  - dizziness
  - confusion
  - irritability
  - hunger
  - fast heart beat
  - sweating
  - feeling jittery

The most common side effects of TRADJENTA include:
- stuffy or runny nose and sore throat
- cough
- diarrhea

These are not all the possible side effects of TRADJENTA. For more information, ask your doctor or pharmacist.

Tell your doctor if you have any side effect that bothers you or that does not go away.

Call your doctor for medical advice about side effects. You may report side effects to FDA at 1-800-FDA-1088.

How should I store TRADJENTA?
- Store TRADJENTA between 68°F and 77°F (20°C and 25°C).

Keep TRADJENTA and all medicines out of the reach of children.

General information about the safe and effective use of TRADJENTA.

Medicines are sometimes prescribed for purposes other than those listed in Medication Guides. Do not use TRADJENTA for a condition for which it was not prescribed. Do not give TRADJENTA to other people, even if they have the same symptoms you have. It may harm them.

This Medication Guide summarizes the most important information about TRADJENTA. If you would like more information, talk with your doctor. You can ask your pharmacist or doctor for information about TRADJENTA that is written for health professionals.

For more information, go to www.TRADJENTA.com or call Boehringer Ingelheim Pharmaceuticals, Inc. at 1-800-542-6257, or (TTY) 1-800-459-9906.

What are the ingredients in TRADJENTA?

Active Ingredient: linagliptin

Inactive Ingredients: mannitol, pregelatinized starch, corn starch, copovidone, and magnesium stearate. The film coating contains the following inactive ingredients: hypromellose, titanium dioxide, talc, polyethylene glycol, and red ferric oxide.

What is type 2 diabetes?

Type 2 diabetes is a condition in which your body does not make enough insulin, and/or the insulin that your body produces does not work as well as it should. Your body can also make too much sugar. When this happens, sugar (glucose) builds up in the blood. This can lead to serious medical problems.

The main goal of treating diabetes is to lower your blood sugar to a normal level. High blood sugar can be lowered by diet and exercise, and by certain medicines when necessary.

Talk to your doctor about how to prevent, recognize, and take care of low blood sugar (hypoglycemia), high blood sugar (hyperglycemia), and other problems you have because of your diabetes.

This Medication Guide has been approved by the U. S. Food and Drug Administration.

Distributed by:
Boehringer Ingelheim Pharmaceuticals, Inc.
Ridgefield, CT 06877 USA
Marketed by:
Boehringer Ingelheim Pharmaceuticals, Inc.
Ridgefield, CT 06877 USA
and
Eli Lilly and Company
Indianapolis, IN 46285 USA
Licensed from:
Boehringer Ingelheim International GmbH
Ingelheim, Germany

*The brands listed are trademarks of their respective owners and are not trademarks of Boehringer Ingelheim Pharmaceuticals, Inc. The makers of these brands are not affiliated with and do not endorse Boehringer Ingelheim Pharmaceuticals, Inc., or its products.

IT5253NF192013
10007261/07
IT5437K
10007237/07
Revised: June 2013

Shown in Product Identification Guide, page 305

Bristol-Myers Squibb Company

P.O. BOX 4500
PRINCETON, NJ 08543-4500

For Medical Information Contact:
Generally:
Bristol-Myers Squibb Medical Information Department
P.O. Box 4500
Princeton, NJ 08543-4500
(800) 321-1335 between 8:00 AM-8:00 PM EST
To report SUSPECTED ADVERSE REACTIONS,
Contact Bristol-Myers Squibb Company at
(800) 721-5072 between 8:00 AM-8:00 PM EST
Sales and Ordering:
Orders may be placed by:
Calling your purchase orders in toll-free between
9:00 AM-5:00 PM EST:
(800) 631-5244
E-mailing your purchase orders to:
customerserviceoperations@BMS.com
Faxing your purchase orders in:
(800) 277-0988

ATRIPLA® ℞

[uh TRIP luh]
(efavirenz/emtricitabine/tenofovir disoproxil fumarate) tablets, for oral use

HIGHLIGHTS OF PRESCRIBING INFORMATION
These highlights do not include all the information needed to use ATRIPLA safely and effectively. See full prescribing information for ATRIPLA.
ATRIPLA® (efavirenz/emtricitabine/tenofovir disoproxil fumarate) tablets, for oral use
Initial U.S. Approval: 2006

WARNING: LACTIC ACIDOSIS/SEVERE HEPATOMEGALY WITH STEATOSIS and POST-TREATMENT EXACERBATION OF HEPATITIS B
See full prescribing information for complete boxed warning.
- **Lactic acidosis and severe hepatomegaly with steatosis, including fatal cases, have been reported with the use of nucleoside analogs, including tenofovir disoproxil fumarate, a component of ATRIPLA. (5.1)**
- **ATRIPLA is not approved for the treatment of chronic hepatitis B virus (HBV) infection. Severe acute exacerbations of hepatitis B have been reported in patients coinfected with HBV and HIV-1 who have discontinued EMTRIVA or VIREAD, two of the components of ATRIPLA. Hepatic function should be monitored closely in these patients. If appropriate, initiation of anti-hepatitis B therapy may be warranted. (5.2)**

RECENT MAJOR CHANGES

Indications and Usage (1)	06/2012
Dosage and Administration (2)	06/2012
Warnings and Precautions	
Drug Interactions (5.3)	06/2012
Coadministration with Related Products (5.4)	04/2013
Rash (5.9)	04/2013
Decreases in Bone Mineral Density (5.11)	06/2012
Immune Reconstitution Syndrome (5.13)	06/2012

INDICATIONS AND USAGE

ATRIPLA, a combination of 2 nucleoside analog HIV-1 reverse transcriptase inhibitors and 1 non-nucleoside HIV-1 reverse transcriptase inhibitor, is indicated for use alone as a complete regimen or in combination with other antiretroviral agents for the treatment of HIV-1 infection in adults and pediatric patients 12 years of age and older. (1)

DOSAGE AND ADMINISTRATION

- Recommended dose in adults and pediatric patients (12 years of age and older and weighing at least 40 kg): One tablet once daily taken orally on an empty stomach, preferably at bedtime. (2)
- Dose in renal impairment: Should not be administered in patients with creatinine clearance below 50 mL/min. (2)
- With rifampin coadministration, an additional 200 mg/day of efavirenz is recommended for patients weighing 50 kg or more. (2)

DOSAGE FORMS AND STRENGTHS

Tablet containing 600 mg of efavirenz, 200 mg of emtricitabine and 300 mg of tenofovir disoproxil fumarate. (3)

CONTRAINDICATIONS

- Previously demonstrated hypersensitivity (e.g., Stevens-Johnson syndrome, erythema multiforme, or toxic skin eruptions) to efavirenz, a component of ATRIPLA. (4.1)
- For some drugs, competition for CYP3A by efavirenz could result in inhibition of their metabolism and create the potential for serious and/or life-threatening adverse reactions (e.g., cardiac arrhythmias, prolonged sedation, or respiratory depression). (4.2)

WARNINGS AND PRECAUTIONS

- Serious psychiatric symptoms: Immediate medical evaluation is recommended. (5.5, 6.1)
- Nervous system symptoms (NSS): NSS are frequent, usually begin 1–2 days after initiating therapy and resolve in 2–4 weeks. Dosing at bedtime may improve tolerability. NSS are not predictive of onset of psychiatric symptoms. (2, 5.6)
- New onset or worsening renal impairment: Can include acute renal failure and Fanconi syndrome. Assess creatinine clearance (CrCl) before initiating treatment with ATRIPLA (efavirenz/emtricitabine/tenofovir disoproxil fumarate). Monitor CrCl and serum phosphorus in patients at risk. Avoid administering ATRIPLA with concurrent or recent use of nephrotoxic drugs. (5.7)
- Pregnancy: Fetal harm can occur when administered to a pregnant woman during the first trimester. Women should be apprised of the potential harm to the fetus. A pregnancy registry is available. (5.8, 8.1)
- Rash: Discontinue if severe rash develops. (5.9, 6.1)
- Hepatotoxicity: Monitor liver function tests before and during treatment in patients with underlying hepatic disease, including hepatitis B or C coinfection, marked transaminase elevations, or who are taking medications associated with liver toxicity. Among reported cases of hepatic failure, a few occurred in patients with no pre-existing hepatic disease. (5.10, 6.3, 8.6)
- Decreases in bone mineral density (BMD): Consider assessment of BMD in patients with a history of pathological fracture or other risk factors for osteoporosis or bone loss. (5.11)
- Convulsions: Use caution in patients with a history of seizures. (5.12)
- Immune reconstitution syndrome: May necessitate further evaluation and treatment. (5.13)
- Redistribution/accumulation of body fat: Observed in patients receiving antiretroviral therapy. (5.14)
- Coadministration with other products: Do not use with drugs containing emtricitabine or tenofovir disoproxil fumarate including COMPLERA, EMTRIVA, STRIBILD, TRUVADA, or VIREAD; or with drugs containing lamivudine. SUSTIVA (efavirenz) should not be coadministered with ATRIPLA unless required for dose-adjustment when coadministered with rifampin. (5.4) Do not administer in combination with HEPSERA. (5.2)

ADVERSE REACTIONS

Most common adverse reactions (incidence greater than or equal to 10%) observed in an active-controlled clinical trial of efavirenz, emtricitabine, and tenofovir DF are diarrhea, nausea, fatigue, headache, dizziness, depression, insomnia, abnormal dreams, and rash. (6)

To report SUSPECTED ADVERSE REACTIONS, contact Gilead Sciences, Inc. at 1-800-GILEAD-5 or FDA at 1-800-FDA-1088 or www.fda.gov/medwatch

DRUG INTERACTIONS

- Efavirenz: Coadministration of efavirenz can alter the concentrations of other drugs and other drugs may alter the concentrations of efavirenz. The potential for drug-drug interactions must be considered before and during therapy. (4.2, 7.1, 12.3)
- Didanosine: Tenofovir disoproxil fumarate increases didanosine concentrations. Use with caution and monitor for evidence of didanosine toxicity (e.g., pancreatitis, neuropathy) when coadministered. Consider dose reductions or discontinuations of didanosine if warranted. (7.2)
- Atazanavir: Coadministration of ATRIPLA and atazanavir or atazanavir/ritonavir is not recommended. (7.3)
- Lopinavir/ritonavir: Coadministration increases tenofovir concentrations. Monitor for evidence of tenofovir toxicity. (7.3)

USE IN SPECIFIC POPULATIONS

- Pregnancy: Women should avoid pregnancy while receiving ATRIPLA and for 12 weeks after discontinuation. (5.8)
- Nursing mothers: Women infected with HIV should be instructed not to breastfeed. (8.3)
- Hepatic impairment: ATRIPLA is not recommended for patients with moderate or severe hepatic impairment. Use caution in patients with mild hepatic impairment. (5.10, 8.6)
- Pediatrics: The incidence of rash was higher than in adults. (5.9, 6.1)

See 17 for PATIENT COUNSELING INFORMATION and FDA-approved patient labeling

Revised: 06/2013

FULL PRESCRIBING INFORMATION: CONTENTS*

*** Sections or subsections omitted from the full prescribing information are not listed**

FULL PRESCRIBING INFORMATION

WARNING: LACTIC ACIDOSIS/SEVERE HEPATOMEGALY WITH STEATOSIS and POST-TREATMENT EXACERBATION OF HEPATITIS B

Lactic acidosis and severe hepatomegaly with steatosis, including fatal cases, have been reported with the use of nucleoside analogs, including tenofovir disoproxil fumarate, a component of ATRIPLA (efavirenz/emtricitabine/tenofovir disoproxil fumarate), in combination with other antiretrovirals *[See Warnings and Precautions (5.1)]*.

ATRIPLA is not approved for the treatment of chronic hepatitis B virus (HBV) infection and the safety and efficacy of ATRIPLA have not been established in patients coinfected with HBV and HIV-1. Severe acute exacerbations of hepatitis B have been reported in patients who have discontinued EMTRIVA or VIREAD, which are components of ATRIPLA. Hepatic function should be monitored closely with both clinical and laboratory follow-up for at least several months in patients who are coinfected with HIV-1 and HBV and

discontinue ATRIPLA (efavirenz/emtricitabine/tenofovir disoproxil fumarate). If appropriate, initiation of anti-hepatitis B therapy may be warranted *[See Warnings and Precautions (5.2)]*.

1 INDICATIONS AND USAGE

ATRIPLA® is indicated for use alone as a complete regimen or in combination with other antiretroviral agents for the treatment of HIV-1 infection in adults and pediatric patients 12 years of age and older.

2 DOSAGE AND ADMINISTRATION

Adults and pediatric patients 12 years of age and older with body weight at least 40 kg (at least 88 lbs): The dose of ATRIPLA is one tablet once daily taken orally on an empty stomach. Dosing at bedtime may improve the tolerability of nervous system symptoms.

Renal Impairment: Because ATRIPLA is a fixed-dose combination, it should not be prescribed for patients requiring dosage adjustment such as those with moderate or severe renal impairment (creatinine clearance below 50 mL/min).

Rifampin Coadministration: When ATRIPLA is administered with rifampin to patients weighing 50 kg or more, an additional 200 mg/day of efavirenz is recommended *[See Drug Interactions (7.3), Table 4, and Clinical Pharmacology (12.3), Table 5]*.

3 DOSAGE FORMS AND STRENGTHS

ATRIPLA is available as tablets. Each tablet contains 600 mg of efavirenz, 200 mg of emtricitabine and 300 mg of tenofovir disoproxil fumarate (tenofovir DF, which is equivalent to 245 mg of tenofovir disoproxil). The tablets are pink, capsule-shaped, film-coated, debossed with "123" on one side and plain-faced on the other side.

4 CONTRAINDICATIONS

4.1 Hypersensitivity

ATRIPLA is contraindicated in patients with previously demonstrated clinically significant hypersensitivity (e.g., Stevens-Johnson syndrome, erythema multiforme, or toxic skin eruptions) to efavirenz, a component of ATRIPLA.

4.2 Contraindicated Drugs

For some drugs, competition for CYP3A by efavirenz could result in inhibition of their metabolism and create the potential for serious and/or life-threatening adverse reactions (e.g., cardiac arrhythmias, prolonged sedation, or respiratory depression). Drugs that are contraindicated with ATRIPLA are listed in Table 1.

[See table 1 above]

Table 1: Drugs That Are Contraindicated or Not Recommended for Use With ATRIPLA

Drug Class: Drug Name	Clinical Comment
Antifungal: voriconazole	Efavirenz significantly decreases voriconazole plasma concentrations, and coadministration may decrease the therapeutic effectiveness of voriconazole. Also, voriconazole significantly increases efavirenz plasma concentrations, which may increase the risk of efavirenz-associated side effects. Because ATRIPLA is a fixed-dose combination product, the dose of efavirenz cannot be altered. *[See Clinical Pharmacology (12.3) Tables 5 and 6]*
Ergot derivatives (dihydroergotamine, ergonovine, ergotamine, methylergonovine)	Potential for serious and/or life-threatening reactions such as acute ergot toxicity characterized by peripheral vasospasm and ischemia of the extremities and other tissues.
Benzodiazepines: midazolam, triazolam	Potential for serious and/or life-threatening reactions such as prolonged or increased sedation or respiratory depression.
Calcium channel blocker: bepridil	Potential for serious and/or life-threatening reactions such as cardiac arrhythmias.
GI motility agent: cisapride	Potential for serious and/or life-threatening reactions such as cardiac arrhythmias.
Neuroleptic: pimozide	Potential for serious and/or life-threatening reactions such as cardiac arrhythmias.
St. John's wort (*Hypericum perforatum*)	May lead to loss of virologic response and possible resistance to efavirenz or to the class of non-nucleoside reverse transcriptase inhibitors (NNRTIs).

5 WARNINGS AND PRECAUTIONS

5.1 Lactic Acidosis/Severe Hepatomegaly with Steatosis

Lactic acidosis and severe hepatomegaly with steatosis, including fatal cases, have been reported with the use of nucleoside analogs including tenofovir DF, a component of ATRIPLA, in combination with other antiretrovirals. A majority of these cases have been in women. Obesity and prolonged nucleoside exposure may be risk factors. Particular caution should be exercised when administering nucleoside analogs to any patient with known risk factors for liver disease; however, cases have also been reported in patients with no known risk factors. Treatment with ATRIPLA should be suspended in any patient who develops clinical or laboratory findings suggestive of lactic acidosis or pronounced hepatotoxicity (which may include hepatomegaly and steatosis even in the absence of marked transaminase elevations).

5.2 Patients Coinfected with HIV-1 and HBV

It is recommended that all patients with HIV-1 be tested for the presence of chronic HBV before initiating antiretroviral therapy. ATRIPLA is not approved for the treatment of chronic HBV infection, and the safety and efficacy of ATRIPLA have not been established in patients coinfected with HBV and HIV-1. Severe acute exacerbations of hepatitis B have been reported in patients who are coinfected with HBV and HIV-1 and have discontinued emtricitabine or tenofovir DF, two of the components of ATRIPLA. In some patients infected with HBV and treated with emtricitabine, the exacerbations of hepatitis B were associated with liver decompensation and liver failure. Patients who are coinfected with HIV-1 and HBV should be closely monitored with both clinical and laboratory follow-up for at least several months after stopping treatment with ATRIPLA. If appropriate, initiation of anti-hepatitis B therapy may be warranted.

ATRIPLA should not be administered with HEPSERA® (adefovir dipivoxil) *[See Drug Interactions (7.2)]*.

5.3 Drug Interactions

Efavirenz plasma concentrations may be altered by substrates, inhibitors, or inducers of CYP3A. Likewise, efavirenz may alter plasma concentrations of drugs metabolized by CYP3A or CYP2B6 *[See Contraindications (4.2), Drug Interactions (7.1)]*.

5.4 Coadministration with Related Products

Related drugs not for coadministration with ATRIPLA (efavirenz/emtricitabine/tenofovir disoproxil fumarate) include COMPLERA® (emtricitabine/rilpivirine/tenofovir DF), EMTRIVA® (emtricitabine), STRIBILD® (elvitegravir/cobicistat/emtricitabine/tenofovir DF), TRUVADA® (emtricitabine/tenofovir DF), and VIREAD® (tenofovir DF), which contain the same active components as ATRIPLA. SUSTIVA® (efavirenz) should not be coadministered with ATRIPLA unless needed for dose-adjustment (e.g., with rifampin) *[See Dosage and Administration (2), Drug Interactions (7.1)]*. Due to similarities between emtricitabine and lamivudine, ATRIPLA should not be coadministered with drugs containing lamivudine, including Combivir (lamivudine/zidovudine), Epivir, or Epivir-HBV (lamivudine), Epzicom (abacavir sulfate/lamivudine), or Trizivir (abacavir sulfate/lamivudine/zidovudine).

5.5 Psychiatric Symptoms

Serious psychiatric adverse experiences have been reported in patients treated with efavirenz. In controlled trials of 1008 subjects treated with regimens containing efavirenz for a mean of 2.1 years and 635 subjects treated with control regimens for a mean of 1.5 years, the frequency (regardless of causality) of specific serious psychiatric events among subjects who received efavirenz or control regimens, respectively, were: severe depression (2.4%, 0.9%), suicidal ideation (0.7%, 0.3%), nonfatal suicide attempts (0.5%, 0%), aggressive behavior (0.4%, 0.5%), paranoid reactions (0.4%, 0.3%), and manic reactions (0.2%, 0.3%). When psychiatric symptoms similar to those noted above were combined and evaluated as a group in a multifactorial analysis of data from Study AI266006 (006), treatment with efavirenz was associated with an increase in the occurrence of these selected psychiatric symptoms. Other factors associated with an increase in the occurrence of these psychiatric symptoms were history of injection drug use, psychiatric history, and receipt of psychiatric medication at trial entry; similar associations were observed in both the efavirenz and control treatment groups. In Study 006, onset of new serious psychiatric symptoms occurred throughout the trial for both efavirenz-treated and control-treated subjects. One percent of efavirenz-treated subjects discontinued or interrupted treatment because of one or more of these selected psychiatric symptoms. There have also been occasional postmarketing reports of death by suicide, delusions, and psychosis-like behavior, although a causal relationship to the use of efavirenz cannot be determined from these reports. Patients with serious psychiatric adverse experiences should seek immediate medical evaluation to assess the possibility that the symptoms may be related to the use of efavirenz, and if so, to determine whether the risks of continued therapy outweigh the benefits *[See Adverse Reactions (6)]*.

5.6 Nervous System Symptoms

Fifty-three percent (531/1008) of subjects receiving efavirenz in controlled trials reported central nervous system symptoms (any grade, regardless of causality) compared to 25% (156/635) of subjects receiving control regimens. These symptoms included dizziness (28.1% of the 1008 subjects), insomnia (16.3%), impaired concentration (8.3%), somnolence (7.0%), abnormal dreams (6.2%), and hallucinations (1.2%). Other reported symptoms were euphoria, confusion, agitation, amnesia, stupor, abnormal thinking, and depersonalization. The majority of these symptoms were mild-to-moderate (50.7%); symptoms were severe in 2.0% of subjects. Overall, 2.1% of subjects discontinued therapy as a result. These symptoms usually begin during the first or second day of therapy and generally resolve after the first 2–4 weeks of therapy. After 4 weeks of therapy, the prevalence of nervous system symptoms of at least moderate severity ranged from 5% to 9% in subjects treated with regimens containing efavirenz and from 3% to 5% in subjects treated with a control regimen. Patients should be informed that these common symptoms were likely to improve with continued therapy and were not predictive of subsequent onset of the less frequent psychiatric symptoms *[See Warnings and Precautions (5.5)]*. Dosing at bedtime may improve the tolerability of these nervous system symptoms *[See Dosage and Administration (2)]*.

Analysis of long-term data from Study 006 (median follow-up 180 weeks, 102 weeks, and 76 weeks for subjects treated with efavirenz + zidovudine + lamivudine, efavirenz + indinavir, and indinavir + zidovudine + lamivudine, respectively) showed that, beyond 24 weeks of therapy, the incidences of new-onset nervous system symptoms among efavirenz-treated subjects were generally similar to those in the indinavir-containing control arm.

Patients receiving ATRIPLA (efavirenz/emtricitabine/tenofovir disoproxil fumarate) should be alerted to the potential for additive central nervous system effects when ATRIPLA is used concomitantly with alcohol or psychoactive drugs.

Patients who experience central nervous system symptoms such as dizziness, impaired concentration, and/or drowsiness should avoid potentially hazardous tasks such as driving or operating machinery.

5.7 New Onset or Worsening Renal Impairment

Emtricitabine and tenofovir are principally eliminated by the kidney; however, efavirenz is not. Since ATRIPLA is a combination product and the dose of the individual components cannot be altered, patients with creatinine clearance below 50 mL/min should not receive ATRIPLA.

Renal impairment, including cases of acute renal failure and Fanconi syndrome (renal tubular injury with severe hypophosphatemia), has been reported with the use of tenofovir DF *[See Adverse Reactions (6.3)]*.

It is recommended that creatinine clearance be calculated in all patients prior to initiating therapy and as clinically appropriate during therapy with ATRIPLA. Routine monitoring of calculated creatinine clearance and serum phosphorus should be performed in patients at risk for renal impairment, including patients who have previously experienced renal events while receiving HEPSERA.

ATRIPLA should be avoided with concurrent or recent use of a nephrotoxic agent.

5.8 Reproductive Risk Potential

Pregnancy Category D: Efavirenz may cause fetal harm when administered during the first trimester to a pregnant woman. Pregnancy should be avoided in women receiving ATRIPLA. Barrier contraception must always be used in combination with other methods of contraception (e.g., oral or other hormonal contraceptives). Because of the long half-life of efavirenz, use of adequate contraceptive measures for 12 weeks after discontinuation of ATRIPLA is recommended. Women of childbearing potential should undergo pregnancy testing before initiation of ATRIPLA (efavirenz/emtricitabine/tenofovir disoproxil fumarate). If this drug is used during the first trimester of pregnancy, or if the patient becomes pregnant while taking this drug, the patient should be apprised of the potential harm to the fetus.

There are no adequate and well-controlled trials of ATRIPLA in pregnant women. ATRIPLA should be used during pregnancy only if the potential benefit justifies the potential risk to the fetus, such as in pregnant women without other therapeutic options *[See Use in Specific Populations (8.1)]*.

5.9 Rash

In controlled clinical trials, 26% (266/1008) of subjects treated with 600 mg efavirenz experienced new-onset skin rash compared with 17% (111/635) of subjects treated in control groups. Rash associated with blistering, moist desquamation, or ulceration occurred in 0.9% (9/1008) of subjects treated with efavirenz. The incidence of Grade 4 rash (e.g., erythema multiforme, Stevens-Johnson syndrome) in subjects treated with efavirenz in all trials and expanded access was 0.1%. Rashes are usually mild-to-moderate maculopapular skin eruptions that occur within the first 2 weeks of initiating therapy with efavirenz (median time to onset of rash in adults was 11 days) and, in most subjects continuing therapy with efavirenz, rash resolves within 1 month (median duration, 16 days). The discontinuation rate for rash in clinical trials was 1.7% (17/1008). ATRIPLA can be reinitiated in patients interrupting therapy because of rash. ATRIPLA should be discontinued in patients developing severe rash associated with blistering, desquamation, mucosal involvement, or fever. Appropriate antihistamines and/or corticosteroids may improve the tolerability and hasten the resolution of rash. For patients who have had a life-threatening cutaneous reaction (e.g., Stevens-Johnson syndrome), alternative therapy should be considered *[See also Contraindications (4.1)]*.

Experience with efavirenz in subjects who discontinued other antiretroviral agents of the NNRTI class is limited. Nineteen subjects who discontinued nevirapine because of rash have been treated with efavirenz. Nine of these subjects developed mild-to-moderate rash while receiving therapy with efavirenz, and two of these subjects discontinued because of rash.

Rash was reported in 26 of 57 pediatric subjects (46%) treated with efavirenz *[See Adverse Reactions (6.1)]*. One pediatric subject experienced Grade 3 rash (confluent rash with fever), and two subjects had Grade 4 rash (erythema multiforme). The median time to onset of rash in pediatric subjects was 8 days. Prophylaxis with appropriate antihistamines before initiating therapy with ATRIPLA in pediatric patients should be considered.

5.10 Hepatotoxicity

Monitoring of liver enzymes before and during treatment is recommended for patients with underlying hepatic disease, including hepatitis B or C infection; patients with marked transaminase elevations; and patients treated with other medications associated with liver toxicity *[See also Warnings and Precautions (5.2)]*. A few of the postmarketing reports of hepatic failure occurred in patients with no pre-existing hepatic disease or other identifiable risk factors *[See Adverse Reactions (6.3)]*. Liver enzyme monitoring should also be considered for patients without pre-existing hepatic dysfunction or other risk factors. In patients with persistent elevations of serum transaminases to greater than five times the upper limit of the normal range, the benefit of continued therapy with ATRIPLA needs to be weighed against the unknown risks of significant liver toxicity *[See Adverse Reactions (6.2)]*.

5.11 Decreases in Bone Mineral Density

Assessment of bone mineral density (BMD) should be considered for patients who have a history of pathologic bone fracture or other risk factors for osteoporosis or bone loss. Although the effect of supplementation with calcium and vitamin D was not studied, such supplementation may be beneficial for all patients. If bone abnormalities are suspected then appropriate consultation should be obtained.

In a 144-week trial of treatment-naive adult subjects receiving tenofovir DF, decreases in BMD were seen at the lumbar spine and hip in both arms of the trial. At Week 144, there was a significantly greater mean percentage decrease from baseline in BMD at the lumbar spine in subjects receiving tenofovir DF + lamivudine + efavirenz compared with subjects receiving stavudine + lamivudine + efavirenz. Changes in BMD at the hip were similar between the two treatment groups. In both groups, the majority of the reduction in BMD occurred in the first 24–48 weeks of the trial and this reduction was sustained through 144 weeks. Twenty-eight percent of tenofovir DF-treated subjects vs. 21% of the comparator subjects lost at least 5% of BMD at the spine or 7% of BMD at the hip. Clinically relevant fractures (excluding fingers and toes) were reported in 4 subjects in the tenofovir DF group and 6 subjects in the comparator group. Tenofovir DF was associated with significant increases in biochemical markers of bone metabolism (serum bone-specific alkaline phosphatase, serum osteocalcin, serum C-telopeptide, and urinary N-telopeptide), suggesting increased bone turnover. Serum parathyroid hormone levels and 1,25 Vitamin D levels were also higher in subjects receiving tenofovir DF.

In a clinical trial of HIV-1 infected pediatric subjects 12 years of age and older (Study 321), bone effects were similar to adult subjects. Under normal circumstances BMD increases rapidly in this age group. In this trial, the mean rate of bone gain was less in the tenofovir DF-treated group compared to the placebo group. Six tenofovir DF-treated subjects and one placebo-treated subject had significant (greater than 4%) lumbar spine BMD loss at 48 weeks. Among 28 subjects receiving 96 weeks of tenofovir DF, Z-scores declined by -0.341 for lumbar spine and -0.458 for total body. Skeletal growth (height) appeared to be unaffected. Markers of bone turnover in tenofovir DF-treated pediatric subjects 12 years of age and older suggest increased bone turnover, consistent with the effects observed in adults.

The effects of tenofovir DF-associated changes in BMD and biochemical markers on long-term bone health and future fracture risk are unknown. For additional information, consult the VIREAD prescribing information.

Cases of osteomalacia (associated with proximal renal tubulopathy and which may contribute to fractures) have been reported in association with the use of tenofovir DF *[See Adverse Reactions (6.3)]*.

5.12 Convulsions

Convulsions have been observed in patients receiving efavirenz, generally in the presence of known medical history of seizures. Caution must be taken in any patient with a history of seizures.

Patients who are receiving concomitant anticonvulsant medications primarily metabolized by the liver, such as phenytoin and phenobarbital, may require periodic monitoring of plasma levels *[See Drug Interactions (7.3)]*.

5.13 Immune Reconstitution Syndrome

Immune reconstitution syndrome has been reported in patients treated with combination antiretroviral therapy, including the components of ATRIPLA (efavirenz/emtricitabine/tenofovir disoproxil fumarate). During the initial phase of combination antiretroviral treatment, patients whose immune system responds may develop an inflammatory response to indolent or residual opportunistic infections [such as *Mycobacterium avium* infection, cytomegalovirus, *Pneumocystis jirovecii* pneumonia (PCP), or tuberculosis], which may necessitate further evaluation and treatment.

Autoimmune disorders (such as Graves' disease, polymyositis, and Guillain-Barré syndrome) have also been reported to occur in the setting of immune reconstitution, however, the time to onset is more variable, and can occur many months after initiation of treatment.

5.14 Fat Redistribution

Redistribution/accumulation of body fat including central obesity, dorsocervical fat enlargement (buffalo hump), peripheral wasting, facial wasting, breast enlargement, and "cushingoid appearance" have been observed in patients receiving antiretroviral therapy. The mechanism and long-term consequences of these events are currently unknown. A causal relationship has not been established.

6 ADVERSE REACTIONS

Efavirenz, Emtricitabine and Tenofovir Disoproxil Fumarate: The following adverse reactions are discussed in other sections of the labeling:

- Lactic Acidosis/Severe Hepatomegaly with Steatosis *[See Boxed Warning, Warnings and Precautions (5.1)]*.
- Severe Acute Exacerbations of Hepatitis B *[See Boxed Warning, Warnings and Precautions (5.2)]*.
- Psychiatric Symptoms *[See Warnings and Precautions (5.5)]*.
- Nervous System Symptoms *[See Warnings and Precautions (5.6)]*.
- New Onset or Worsening Renal Impairment *[See Warnings and Precautions (5.7)]*.
- Rash *[See Warnings and Precautions (5.9)]*.
- Hepatotoxicity *[See Warnings and Precautions (5.10)]*.
- Decreases in Bone Mineral Density *[See Warnings and Precautions (5.11)]*.
- Immune Reconstitution Syndrome *[See Warnings and Precautions (5.13)]*.
- Drug Interactions *[See Contraindications (4.2), Warnings and Precautions (5.3) and Drug Interactions (7)]*.

For additional safety information about SUSTIVA (efavirenz), EMTRIVA (emtricitabine), or VIREAD (tenofovir DF) in combination with other antiretroviral agents, consult the prescribing information for these products.

6.1 Adverse Reactions from Clinical Trials Experience

Because clinical trials are conducted under widely varying conditions, adverse reaction rates observed in the clinical trials of a drug cannot be directly compared to rates in the clinical trials of another drug and may not reflect the rates observed in practice.

Clinical Trials in Adult Subjects

Study 934

Study 934 was an open-label active-controlled trial in which 511 antiretroviral-naive subjects received either emtricitabine + tenofovir DF administered in combination with efavirenz (N=257) or zidovudine/lamivudine administered in combination with efavirenz (N=254).

The most common adverse reactions (incidence greater than or equal to 10%, any severity) occurring in Study 934 include diarrhea, nausea, fatigue, headache, dizziness, depression, insomnia, abnormal dreams, and rash. Adverse reactions observed in Study 934 were generally consistent with those seen in previous trials of the individual components (Table 2).

Table 2: Selected Treatment-Emergent Adverse Reactions* (Grades 2–4) Reported in ≥5% in Either Treatment Group in Study 934 (0–144 Weeks)

	FTC + TDF + EFV† N=257	AZT/3TC + EFV N=254
Gastrointestinal Disorder		
Diarrhea	9%	5%
Nausea	9%	7%
Vomiting	2%	5%
General Disorders and Administration Site Condition		
Fatigue	9%	8%
Infections and Infestations		
Sinusitis	8%	4%
Upper respiratory tract infections	8%	5%
Nasopharyngitis	5%	3%
Nervous System Disorders		
Headache	6%	5%
Dizziness	8%	7%
Psychiatric Disorders		
Anxiety	5%	4%
Depression	9%	7%
Insomnia	5%	7%
Skin and Subcutaneous Tissue Disorders		
Rash Event‡	7%	9%

* Frequencies of adverse reactions are based on all treatment-emergent adverse events, regardless of relationship to study drug.

† From Weeks 96 to 144 of the trial, subjects received emtricitabine/tenofovir DF administered in combination with efavirenz in place of emtricitabine + tenofovir DF with efavirenz.

‡ Rash event includes rash, exfoliative rash, rash generalized, rash macular, rash maculopapular, rash pruritic, and rash vesicular.

Study 073

In Study 073, subjects with stable, virologic suppression on antiretroviral therapy and no history of virologic failure were randomized to receive ATRIPLA (efavirenz/emtricitabine/tenofovir disoproxil fumarate) or to stay on their baseline regimen. The adverse reactions observed in Study 073 were generally consistent with those seen in Study 934 and those seen with the individual components of ATRIPLA when each was administered in combination with other antiretroviral agents.

Efavirenz, Emtricitabine, or Tenofovir Disoproxil Fumarate

In addition to the adverse reactions in Study 934 and Study 073, the following adverse reactions were observed in clinical trials of efavirenz, emtricitabine, or tenofovir DF in combination with other antiretroviral agents.

Efavirenz: The most significant adverse reactions observed in subjects treated with efavirenz are nervous system symptoms *[See Warnings and Precautions (5.6)]*, psychiatric symptoms *[See Warnings and Precautions (5.5)]*, and rash *[See Warnings and Precautions (5.9)]*.

Selected adverse reactions of moderate-to-severe intensity observed in greater than or equal to 2% of efavirenz-treated subjects in two controlled clinical trials included pain, impaired concentration, abnormal dreams, somnolence, anorexia, dyspepsia, abdominal pain, nervousness, and pruritus.

Pancreatitis has also been reported, although a causal relationship with efavirenz has not been established. Asymptomatic increases in serum amylase levels were observed in a significantly higher number of subjects treated with efavirenz 600 mg than in control subjects.

Emtricitabine and Tenofovir Disoproxil Fumarate: Adverse reactions that occurred in at least 5% of treatment-experienced or treatment-naive subjects receiving emtricitabine or tenofovir DF with other antiretroviral agents in clinical trials include arthralgia, increased cough, dyspepsia, fever, myalgia, pain, abdominal pain, back pain, paresthesia, peripheral neuropathy (including peripheral neuritis and neuropathy), pneumonia, rhinitis and rash event (including rash, pruritus, maculopapular rash, urticaria, vesiculobullous rash, pustular rash, and allergic reaction).

Skin discoloration has been reported with higher frequency among emtricitabine-treated subjects; it was manifested by hyperpigmentation on the palms and/or soles and was generally mild and asymptomatic. The mechanism and clinical significance are unknown.

Clinical Trials in Pediatric Subjects

Efavirenz: In a pediatric clinical trial in 57 NRTI-experienced subjects aged 3 to 16 years, the type and frequency of adverse experiences was generally similar to that of adult subjects with the exception of a higher incidence of rash, which was reported in 46% (26/57) of pediatric subjects compared to 26% of adults, and a higher frequency of Grade 3 or 4 rash reported in 5% (3/57) of pediatric subjects compared to 0.9% of adults *[See Warnings and Precautions (5.9)]*. For additional information, please consult the SUSTIVA prescribing information.

Emtricitabine: In addition to the adverse reactions reported in adults, anemia and hyperpigmentation were observed in 7% and 32%, respectively, of pediatric subjects (3 months to less than 18 years of age) who received treatment with emtricitabine in the larger of two open-label, uncontrolled pediatric trials (N=116). For additional information, please consult the EMTRIVA prescribing information.

Tenofovir Disoproxil Fumarate: In a pediatric clinical trial conducted in subjects 12 to less than 18 years of age, the adverse reactions observed in pediatric subjects who received treatment with tenofovir DF were consistent with those observed in clinical trials of tenofovir DF in adults *[See Warnings and Precautions (5.11)]*.

6.2 Laboratory Abnormalities

Efavirenz, Emtricitabine and Tenofovir Disoproxil Fumarate: Laboratory abnormalities observed in Study 934 were generally consistent with those seen in previous trials (Table 3).

Table 3: Significant Laboratory Abnormalities Reported in ≥1% of Subjects in Either Treatment Group in Study 934 (0–144 Weeks)

	FTC + TDF + EFV* N=257	AZT/3TC + EFV N=254
Any ≥ Grade 3 Laboratory Abnormality	30%	26%
Fasting Cholesterol (>240 mg/dL)	22%	24%
Creatine Kinase (M: >990 U/L) (F: >845 U/L)	9%	7%
Serum Amylase (>175 U/L)	8%	4%
Alkaline Phosphatase (>550 U/L)	1%	0%
AST (M: >180 U/L) (F: >170 U/L)	3%	3%
ALT (M: >215 U/L) (F: >170 U/L)	2%	3%
Hemoglobin (<8.0 mg/dL)	0%	4%
Hyperglycemia (>250 mg/dL)	2%	1%
Hematuria (>75 RBC/HPF)	3%	2%
Glycosuria (≥3+)	<1%	1%
Neutrophils (<750/mm^3)	3%	5%
Fasting Triglycerides (>750 mg/dL)	4%	2%

* From Weeks 96 to 144 of the trial, subjects received emtricitabine/tenofovir DF administered in combination with efavirenz in place of emtricitabine + tenofovir DF with efavirenz.

Laboratory abnormalities observed in Study 073 were generally consistent with those in Study 934.

In addition to the laboratory abnormalities described for Study 934 (Table 3), Grade 3/4 laboratory abnormalities of increased bilirubin (greater than 2.5 × upper limit of normal (ULN)), increased pancreatic amylase (greater than 2.0 × ULN), increased or decreased serum glucose (less than 40 or greater than 250 mg/dL), and increased serum lipase (greater than 2.0 × ULN) occurred in up to 3% of subjects treated with emtricitabine or tenofovir DF with other antiretroviral agents in clinical trials.

Hepatic Events: In Study 934, 19 subjects treated with efavirenz, emtricitabine, and tenofovir DF and 20 subjects treated with efavirenz and fixed-dose zidovudine/lamivudine were hepatitis B surface antigen or hepatitis C antibody positive. Among these coinfected subjects, one subject (1/19) in the efavirenz, emtricitabine and tenofovir DF arm had elevations in transaminases to greater than five times ULN through 144 weeks. In the fixed-dose zidovudine/lamivudine arm, two subjects (2/20) had elevations in transaminases to greater than five times ULN through 144 weeks. No HBV and/or HCV coinfected subject discontinued from the trial due to hepatobiliary disorders *[See Warnings and Precautions (5.10)]*.

6.3 Postmarketing Experience

The following adverse reactions have been identified during postapproval use of efavirenz, emtricitabine, or tenofovir DF. Because postmarketing reactions are reported voluntarily from a population of uncertain size, it is not always possible to reliably estimate their frequency or establish a causal relationship to drug exposure.

Efavirenz:

Cardiac Disorders
Palpitations

Ear and Labyrinth Disorders
Tinnitus, vertigo

Endocrine Disorders
Gynecomastia

Eye Disorders
Abnormal vision

Gastrointestinal Disorders
Constipation, malabsorption

General Disorders and Administration Site Conditions
Asthenia

Hepatobiliary Disorders
Hepatic enzyme increase, hepatic failure, hepatitis. A few of the postmarketing reports of hepatic failure, including cases in patients with no pre-existing hepatic disease or other identifiable risk factors, were characterized by a fulminant course, progressing in some cases to transplantation or death.

Immune System Disorders
Allergic reactions

Metabolism and Nutrition Disorders
Redistribution/accumulation of body fat *[See Warnings and Precautions (5.14)]*, hypercholesterolemia, hypertriglyceridemia

Musculoskeletal and Connective Tissue Disorders
Arthralgia, myalgia, myopathy

Nervous System Disorders
Abnormal coordination, ataxia, cerebellar coordination and balance disturbances, convulsions, hypoesthesia, paresthesia, neuropathy, tremor

Psychiatric Disorders
Aggressive reactions, agitation, delusions, emotional lability, mania, neurosis, paranoia, psychosis, suicide

Respiratory, Thoracic and Mediastinal Disorders
Dyspnea

Skin and Subcutaneous Tissue Disorders
Flushing, erythema multiforme, photoallergic dermatitis, Stevens-Johnson syndrome

Emtricitabine: No postmarketing adverse reactions have been identified for inclusion in this section.

Tenofovir Disoproxil Fumarate:

Immune System Disorders
Allergic reaction, including angioedema

Metabolism and Nutrition Disorders
Lactic acidosis, hypokalemia, hypophosphatemia

Respiratory, Thoracic, and Mediastinal Disorders
Dyspnea

Gastrointestinal Disorders
Pancreatitis, increased amylase, abdominal pain

Hepatobiliary Disorders
Hepatic steatosis, hepatitis, increased liver enzymes (most commonly AST, ALT, gamma GT)

Skin and Subcutaneous Tissue Disorders
Rash

Musculoskeletal and Connective Tissue Disorders
Rhabdomyolysis, osteomalacia (manifested as bone pain and which may contribute to fractures), muscular weakness, myopathy

Renal and Urinary Disorders
Acute renal failure, renal failure, acute tubular necrosis, Fanconi syndrome, proximal renal tubulopathy, interstitial nephritis (including acute cases), nephrogenic diabetes insipidus, renal insufficiency, increased creatinine, proteinuria, polyuria

General Disorders and Administration Site Conditions
Asthenia

The following adverse reactions, listed under the body system headings above, may occur as a consequence of proximal renal tubulopathy: rhabdomyolysis, osteomalacia, hypokalemia, muscular weakness, myopathy, hypophosphatemia.

7 DRUG INTERACTIONS

This section describes clinically relevant drug interactions with ATRIPLA (efavirenz/emtricitabine/tenofovir disoproxil fumarate). Drug interaction trials are described elsewhere in the labeling *[See Clinical Pharmacology (12.3)]*.

7.1 Efavirenz

Efavirenz has been shown *in vivo* to induce CYP3A and CYP2B6. Other compounds that are substrates of CYP3A or CYP2B6 may have decreased plasma concentrations when coadministered with efavirenz. *In vitro* studies have demonstrated that efavirenz inhibits CYP2C9, 2C19, and 3A4 isozymes in the range of observed efavirenz plasma concentrations. Coadministration of efavirenz with drugs primarily metabolized by these isozymes may result in altered plasma concentrations of the coadministered drug. Therefore, appropriate dose adjustments may be necessary for these drugs.

Drugs that induce CYP3A activity (e.g., phenobarbital, rifampin, rifabutin) would be expected to increase the clearance of efavirenz, resulting in lowered plasma concentrations *[See Dosage and Administration (2)]*.

7.2 Emtricitabine and Tenofovir Disoproxil Fumarate

Since emtricitabine and tenofovir are primarily eliminated by the kidneys, coadministration of ATRIPLA with drugs that reduce renal function or compete for active tubular secretion may increase serum concentrations of emtricitabine, tenofovir, and/or other renally eliminated drugs. Some examples include, but are not limited to, acyclovir, adefovir dipivoxil, cidofovir, ganciclovir, valacyclovir, and valganciclovir.

Coadministration of tenofovir DF and didanosine should be undertaken with caution and patients receiving this combination should be monitored closely for didanosine-associated adverse reactions. Didanosine should be discontinued in patients who develop didanosine-associated adverse reactions [for didanosine dosing adjustment recommendations, see *Table 4*]. Suppression of CD4$^+$ cell counts has been observed in patients receiving tenofovir DF with didanosine 400 mg daily.

Lopinavir/ritonavir has been shown to increase tenofovir concentrations. The mechanism of this interaction is unknown. Patients receiving lopinavir/ritonavir with ATRIPLA should be monitored for tenofovir-associated adverse reactions. ATRIPLA should be discontinued in patients who develop tenofovir-associated adverse reactions *[See Table 4]*.

Coadministration of atazanavir with ATRIPLA is not recommended since coadministration of atazanavir with either efavirenz or tenofovir DF has been shown to decrease plasma concentrations of atazanavir. Also, atazanavir has been shown to increase tenofovir concentrations. There are insufficient data to support dosing recommendations for atazanavir or atazanavir/ritonavir in combination with ATRIPLA *[See Table 4]*.

7.3 Efavirenz, Emtricitabine and Tenofovir Disoproxil Fumarate

Other important drug interaction information for ATRIPLA is summarized in Table 1 and Table 4. The drug interactions described are based on trials conducted with efavirenz, emtricitabine or tenofovir DF as individual agents or are potential drug interactions; no drug interaction trials have been conducted using ATRIPLA [for pharmacokinetics data see *Clinical Pharmacology (12.3)*, Tables 5–8]. The tables include potentially significant interactions, but are not all inclusive.

[See table 4 on pages 676 and 677]

7.4 Efavirenz Assay Interference

Cannabinoid Test Interaction: Efavirenz does not bind to cannabinoid receptors. False-positive urine cannabinoid test results have been observed in non-HIV-infected volunteers receiving efavirenz when the Microgenics Cedia DAU Multi-Level THC assay was used for screening. Negative results were obtained when more specific confirmatory testing was performed with gas chromatography/mass spectrometry. For more information, please consult the SUSTIVA prescribing information.

8 USE IN SPECIFIC POPULATIONS

8.1 Pregnancy

Pregnancy Category D *[See Warnings and Precautions (5.8)]*

Antiretroviral Pregnancy Registry: To monitor fetal outcomes of pregnant women, an Antiretroviral Pregnancy Registry has been established. Physicians are encouraged to register patients who become pregnant by calling (800) 258-4263.

Table 4: Established and Other Potentially Significant* Drug Interactions: Alteration in Dose or Regimen May Be Recommended Based on Drug Interaction Trials or Predicted Interaction

Concomitant Drug Class: Drug Name	Effect	Clinical Comment
HIV antiviral agents		
Protease inhibitor: atazanavir	↓atazanavir ↑ tenofovir	Coadministration of atazanavir with ATRIPLA is not recommended. Coadministration of atazanavir with either efavirenz or tenofovir DF decreases plasma concentrations of atazanavir. The combined effect of efavirenz plus tenofovir DF on atazanavir plasma concentrations is not known. Also, atazanavir has been shown to increase tenofovir concentrations. There are insufficient data to support dosing recommendations for atazanavir or atazanavir/ritonavir in combination with ATRIPLA.
Protease inhibitor: fosamprenavir calcium	↓ amprenavir	Fosamprenavir (unboosted): Appropriate doses of fosamprenavir and ATRIPLA with respect to safety and efficacy have not been established. Fosamprenavir/ritonavir: An additional 100 mg/day (300 mg total) of ritonavir is recommended when ATRIPLA is administered with fosamprenavir/ritonavir once daily. No change in the ritonavir dose is required when ATRIPLA is administered with fosamprenavir plus ritonavir twice daily.
Protease inhibitor: indinavir	↓ indinavir	The optimal dose of indinavir, when given in combination with efavirenz, is not known. Increasing the indinavir dose to 1000 mg every 8 hours does not compensate for the increased indinavir metabolism due to efavirenz.
Protease inhibitor: lopinavir/ritonavir	↓ lopinavir ↑ tenofovir	Do not use once daily administration of lopinavir/ritonavir. Dose adjustment of lopinavir/ritonavir is recommended when coadministered with efavirenz. Refer to the full prescribing information for lopinavir/ritonavir for guidance on coadministration with efavirenz- or tenofovir-containing regimens, such as ATRIPLA. Patients should be monitored for tenofovir-associated adverse reactions.
Protease inhibitor: ritonavir	↑ ritonavir ↑ efavirenz	When ritonavir 500 mg every 12 hours was coadministered with efavirenz 600 mg once daily, the combination was associated with a higher frequency of adverse clinical experiences (e.g., dizziness, nausea, paresthesia) and laboratory abnormalities (elevated liver enzymes). Monitoring of liver enzymes is recommended when ATRIPLA is used in combination with ritonavir.
Protease inhibitor: saquinavir	↓ saquinavir	Appropriate doses of the combination of efavirenz and saquinavir/ritonavir with respect to safety and efficacy have not been established.
CCR5 co-receptor antagonist: maraviroc	↓ maraviroc	Efavirenz decreases plasma concentrations of maraviroc. Refer to the full prescribing information for maraviroc for guidance on coadministration with ATRIPLA.
NRTI: didanosine	↑ didanosine	Coadministration of ATRIPLA and didanosine should be undertaken with caution and patients receiving this combination should be monitored closely for didanosine-associated adverse reactions including pancreatitis, lactic acidosis, and neuropathy. A dose reduction of didanosine is recommended when coadministered with tenofovir DF. For additional information on coadministration with tenofovir DF-containing products, please refer to the didanosine prescribing information.
NNRTI: Other NNRTIs	↑ or ↓ efavirenz and/or NNRTI	Combining two NNRTIs has not been shown to be beneficial. ATRIPLA contains efavirenz and should not be coadministered with other NNRTIs.
Integrase strand transfer inhibitor: raltegravir	↓ raltegravir	Efavirenz reduces plasma concentrations of raltegravir. The clinical significance of this interaction has not been directly assessed.
Hepatitis C antiviral agents		
Protease inhibitor: boceprevir	↓ boceprevir	Plasma trough concentrations of boceprevir were decreased when boceprevir was coadministered with efavirenz, which may result in loss of therapeutic effect. The combination should be avoided.
Protease inhibitor: telaprevir	↓ telaprevir ↓ efavirenz	Concomitant administration of telaprevir and efavirenz resulted in reduced steady-state exposures to telaprevir and efavirenz.
Other agents		
Anticoagulant: warfarin	↑ or ↓ warfarin	Plasma concentrations and effects potentially increased or decreased by efavirenz.

(Table continued on next page)

Efavirenz: As of July 2010, the Antiretroviral Pregnancy Registry has received prospective reports of 792 pregnancies exposed to efavirenz-containing regimens, nearly all of which were first-trimester exposures (718 pregnancies). Birth defects occurred in 17 of 604 live births (first-trimester exposure) and 2 of 69 live births (second/third-trimester exposure). One of these prospectively reported defects with first-trimester exposure was a neural tube defect. A single case of anophthalmia with first-trimester exposure to efavirenz has also been prospectively reported; however, this case included severe oblique facial clefts and amniotic banding, a known association with anophthalmia. There have been six retrospective reports of findings consistent with neural tube defects, including meningomyelocele. All mothers were exposed to efavirenz-containing regimens in the first trimester. Although a causal relationship of these events to the use of efavirenz has not been established, similar defects have been observed in preclinical studies of efavirenz.

Animal Data

Effects of efavirenz on embryo-fetal development have been studied in three nonclinical species (cynomolgus monkeys, rats, and rabbits). In monkeys, efavirenz 60 mg/kg/day was administered to pregnant females throughout pregnancy (gestation Days 20 through 150). The maternal systemic drug exposures (AUC) were 1.3 times the exposure in humans at the recommended clinical dose (600 mg/day), with fetal umbilical venous drug concentrations approximately 0.7 times the maternal values. Three fetuses of 20 fetuses/infants had one or more malformations; there were no malformed fetuses or infants from placebo-treated mothers. The malformations that occurred in these three monkey fetuses included anencephaly and unilateral anophthalmia in one fetus, microophthalmia in a second, and cleft palate in the third. There was no NOAEL (no observable adverse effect level) established for this study because only one dosage was evaluated. In rats, efavirenz was administered either during organogenesis (gestation Days 7 to 18) or from gestation Day 7 through lactation Day 21 at 50, 100, or 200 mg/kg/day. Administration of 200 mg/kg/day in rats was associated with an increase in the incidence of early resorptions, and doses 100 mg/kg/day and greater were associated with early neonatal mortality. The AUC at the NOAEL (50 mg/kg/day) in this rat study was 0.1 times that in humans at the recommended clinical dose. Drug concentrations in the milk on lactation Day 10 were approximately 8 times higher than those in maternal plasma. In pregnant rabbits, efavirenz was neither embryo lethal nor teratogenic when administered at doses of 25, 50, and 75 mg/kg/day over the period of organogenesis (gestation Days 6 through 18). The AUC at the NOAEL (75 mg/kg/day) in rabbits was 0.4 times that in humans at the recommended clinical dose.

8.3 Nursing Mothers

The Centers for Disease Control and Prevention recommend that HIV-1 infected mothers not breastfeed their infants to avoid risking postnatal transmission of HIV-1. Studies in rats have demonstrated that efavirenz is secreted in milk. Studies in humans have shown that both tenofovir and emtricitabine are excreted in human milk. Because the risks of low level exposure to emtricitabine and tenofovir to infants are unknown, and because of the potential for HIV-1 transmission, **mothers should be instructed not to breastfeed if they are receiving ATRIPLA.**

Emtricitabine

Samples of breast milk obtained from five HIV-1 infected mothers show that emtricitabine is secreted in human milk. Breastfeeding infants whose mothers are being treated with emtricitabine may be at risk for developing viral resistance to emtricitabine. Other emtricitabine-associated risks in infants breastfed by mothers being treated with emtricitabine are unknown.

Tenofovir Disoproxil Fumarate

Samples of breast milk obtained from five HIV-1 infected mothers show that tenofovir is secreted in human milk. Tenofovir-associated risks, including the risk of viral resistance to tenofovir, in infants breastfed by mothers being treated with tenofovir disoproxil fumarate are unknown.

8.4 Pediatric Use

ATRIPLA (efavirenz/emtricitabine/tenofovir disoproxil fumarate) should only be administered to pediatric patients 12 years of age and older with a body weight greater than or equal to 40 kg (greater than or equal to 88 lbs). Because ATRIPLA is a fixed-dose combination tablet, the dose adjustments recommended for pediatric patients younger than 12 years of age for each individual component cannot be made with ATRIPLA *[See Warnings and Precautions (5.9, 5.11), Adverse Reactions (6.1) and Clinical Pharmacology (12.3)]*.

8.5 Geriatric Use

Clinical trials of efavirenz, emtricitabine, or tenofovir DF did not include sufficient numbers of subjects aged 65 and over to determine whether they respond differently from younger subjects. In general, dose selection for elderly patients should be cautious, keeping in mind the greater frequency of decreased hepatic, renal, or cardiac function, and of concomitant disease or other drug therapy.

8.6 Hepatic Impairment

ATRIPLA is not recommended for patients with moderate or severe hepatic impairment because there are insufficient data to determine an appropriate dose. Patients with mild hepatic impairment may be treated with ATRIPLA at the approved dose. Because of the extensive cytochrome P450-mediated metabolism of efavirenz and limited clinical experience in patients with hepatic impairment, caution should be exercised in administering ATRIPLA (efavirenz/emtricitabine/tenofovir disoproxil fumarate) to these patients *[See Warnings and Precautions (5.10) and Clinical Pharmacology (12.3)]*.

8.7 Renal Impairment

Because ATRIPLA is a fixed-dose combination, it should not be prescribed for patients requiring dosage adjustment such as those with moderate or severe renal impairment (creatinine clearance below 50 mL/min) *[See Warnings and Precautions (5.7)]*.

10 OVERDOSAGE

If overdose occurs, the patient should be monitored for evidence of toxicity, including monitoring of vital signs and observation of the patient's clinical status; standard supportive treatment should then be applied as necessary. Administration of activated charcoal may be used to aid removal of unabsorbed efavirenz. Hemodialysis can remove both emtricitabine and tenofovir DF (refer to detailed information below), but is unlikely to significantly remove efavirenz from the blood.

Efavirenz: Some patients accidentally taking 600 mg twice daily have reported increased nervous system symptoms. One patient experienced involuntary muscle contractions.

Emtricitabine: Limited clinical experience is available at doses higher than the therapeutic dose of emtricitabine. In one clinical pharmacology trial single doses of emtricitabine 1200 mg were administered to 11 subjects. No severe adverse reactions were reported.

Hemodialysis treatment removes approximately 30% of the emtricitabine dose over a 3-hour dialysis period starting within 1.5 hours of emtricitabine dosing (blood flow rate of 400 mL/min and a dialysate flow rate of 600 mL/min). It is not known whether emtricitabine can be removed by peritoneal dialysis.

Tenofovir Disoproxil Fumarate: Limited clinical experience at doses higher than the therapeutic dose of tenofovir DF 300 mg is available. In one trial, 600 mg tenofovir DF was administered to 8 subjects orally for 28 days, and no severe adverse reactions were reported. The effects of higher doses are not known.

Tenofovir is efficiently removed by hemodialysis with an extraction coefficient of approximately 54%. Following a single 300 mg dose of tenofovir DF, a 4-hour hemodialysis session removed approximately 10% of the administered tenofovir dose.

11 DESCRIPTION

ATRIPLA is a fixed-dose combination tablet containing efavirenz, emtricitabine, and tenofovir disoproxil fumarate (tenofovir DF). SUSTIVA is the brand name for efavirenz, a non-nucleoside reverse transcriptase inhibitor. EMTRIVA is the brand name for emtricitabine, a synthetic nucleoside analog of cytidine. VIREAD is the brand name for tenofovir DF, which is converted *in vivo* to tenofovir, an acyclic nucleoside phosphonate (nucleotide) analog of adenosine 5′-monophosphate. VIREAD and EMTRIVA are the components of TRUVADA.

ATRIPLA tablets are for oral administration. Each tablet contains 600 mg of efavirenz, 200 mg of emtricitabine, and 300 mg of tenofovir DF (which is equivalent to 245 mg of tenofovir disoproxil) as active ingredients. The tablets include the following inactive ingredients: croscarmellose sodium, hydroxypropyl cellulose, magnesium stearate, microcrystalline cellulose, and sodium lauryl sulfate. The tablets are film-coated with a coating material containing black iron oxide, polyethylene glycol, polyvinyl alcohol, red iron oxide, talc, and titanium dioxide.

Efavirenz: Efavirenz is chemically described as (*S*)-6-chloro-4-(cyclopropylethynyl)-1,4-dihydro-4-(trifluoromethyl)-2*H*-3,1-benzoxazin-2-one. Its molecular formula is $C_{14}H_9ClF_3NO_2$ and its structural formula is:

[See first chemical structure at top of next column]

Efavirenz is a white to slightly pink crystalline powder with a molecular mass of 315.68. It is practically insoluble in water (less than 10 µg/mL).

Emtricitabine: The chemical name of emtricitabine is 5-fluoro-1-(2*R*,5*S*)-[2-(hydroxymethyl)-1,3-oxathiolan-5-yl]cytosine. Emtricitabine is the (-) enantiomer of a thio analog of cytidine, which differs from other cytidine analogs in that it has a fluorine in the 5-position.

It has a molecular formula of $C_8H_{10}FN_3O_3S$ and a molecular weight of 247.24. It has the following structural formula:

[See second chemical structure at top of next column]

Emtricitabine is a white to off-white crystalline powder with a solubility of approximately 112 mg/mL in water at 25 °C.

Tenofovir Disoproxil Fumarate: Tenofovir DF is a fumaric acid salt of the *bis*-isopropoxycarbonyloxymethyl ester derivative of tenofovir. The chemical name of tenofovir disoproxil fumarate is 9-[(*R*)-2[[bis[[(isopropoxycarbonyl)-oxy]-methoxy]phosphinyl]methoxy]propyl]adenine fumarate (1:1). It has a molecular formula of $C_{19}H_{30}N_5O_{10}P$ •

Table 4 *(cont.)*: Established and Other Potentially Significant* Drug Interactions: Alteration in Dose or Regimen May Be Recommended Based on Drug Interaction Trials or Predicted Interaction

Concomitant Drug Class: Drug Name	Effect	Clinical Comment
Anticonvulsants: carbamazepine	↓ carbamazepine ↓ efavirenz	There are insufficient data to make a dose recommendation for ATRIPLA. Alternative anticonvulsant treatment should be used.
phenytoin phenobarbital	↓ anticonvulsant ↓ efavirenz	Potential for reduction in anticonvulsant and/or efavirenz plasma levels; periodic monitoring of anticonvulsant plasma levels should be conducted.
Antidepressants: bupropion	↓ buproprion	The effect of efavirenz on bupropion exposure is thought to be due to the induction of bupropion metabolism. Increases in bupropion dosage should be guided by clinical response, but the maximum recommended dose of bupropion should not be exceeded.
sertraline	↓ sertraline	Increases in sertraline dose should be guided by clinical response.
Antifungals: itraconazole ketoconazole	↓ itraconazole ↓ hydroxy-itraconazole ↓ ketoconazole	Since no dose recommendation for itraconazole can be made, alternative antifungal treatment should be considered. Drug interaction trials with ATRIPLA and ketoconazole have not been conducted. Efavirenz has the potential to decrease plasma concentrations of ketoconazole.
posaconazole	↓ posaconazole	Avoid concomitant use unless the benefit outweighs the risks.
Anti-infective: clarithromycin	↓ clarithromycin ↑ 14-OH metabolite	Clinical significance unknown. In uninfected volunteers, 46% developed rash while receiving efavirenz and clarithromycin. No dose adjustment of ATRIPLA is recommended when given with clarithromycin. Alternatives to clarithromycin, such as azithromycin, should be considered. Other macrolide antibiotics, such as erythromycin, have not been studied in combination with ATRIPLA.
Antimycobacterial: rifabutin	↓ rifabutin	Increase daily dose of rifabutin by 50%. Consider doubling the rifabutin dose in regimens where rifabutin is given 2 or 3 times a week.
rifampin	↓ efavirenz	If ATRIPLA is coadministered with rifampin to patients weighing 50 kg or more, an additional 200 mg/day of efavirenz is recommended.
Calcium channel blockers: diltiazem	↓ diltiazem ↓ desacetyl diltiazem ↓ N-monodesmethyl diltiazem	Diltiazem dose adjustments should be guided by clinical response (refer to the full prescribing information for diltiazem). No dose adjustment of ATRIPLA is necessary when administered with diltiazem.
Others (e.g., felodipine, nicardipine, nifedipine, verapamil)	↓ calcium channel blocker	No data are available on the potential interactions of efavirenz with other calcium channel blockers that are substrates of CYP3A. The potential exists for reduction in plasma concentrations of the calcium channel blocker. Dose adjustments should be guided by clinical response (refer to the full prescribing information for the calcium channel blocker).
HMG-CoA reductase inhibitors: atorvastatin pravastatin simvastatin	↓ atorvastatin ↓ pravastatin ↓ simvastatin	Plasma concentrations of atorvastatin, pravastatin, and simvastatin decreased with efavirenz. Consult the full prescribing information for the HMG-CoA reductase inhibitor for guidance on individualizing the dose.
Hormonal contraceptives: Oral: ethinyl estradiol/norgestimate	↓ active metabolites of norgestimate	A reliable method of barrier contraception must be used in addition to hormonal contraceptives. Efavirenz had no effect on ethinyl estradiol concentrations, but progestin levels (norelgestromin and levonorgestrel) were markedly decreased. No effect of ethinyl estradiol/norgestimate on efavirenz plasma concentrations was observed.
Implant: etonogestrel	↓ etonogestrel	A reliable method of barrier contraception must be used in addition to hormonal contraceptives. The interaction between etonogestrel and efavirenz has not been studied. Decreased exposure of etonogestrel may be expected. There have been postmarketing reports of contraceptive failure with etonogestrel in efavirenz-exposed patients.
Immunosuppressants: cyclosporine, tacrolimus, sirolimus, and others metabolized by CYP3A	↓ immunosuppressant	Decreased exposure of the immunosuppressant may be expected due to CYP3A induction by efavirenz. These immunosuppressants are not anticipated to affect exposure of efavirenz. Dose adjustments of the immunosuppressant may be required. Close monitoring of immunosuppressant concentrations for at least 2 weeks (until stable concentrations are reached) is recommended when starting or stopping treatment with ATRIPLA.
Narcotic analgesic: methadone	↓ methadone	Coadministration of efavirenz in HIV-1 infected individuals with a history of injection drug use resulted in decreased plasma levels of methadone and signs of opiate withdrawal. Methadone dose was increased by a mean of 22% to alleviate withdrawal symptoms. Patients should be monitored for signs of withdrawal and their methadone dose increased as required to alleviate withdrawal symptoms.

* This table is not all inclusive.

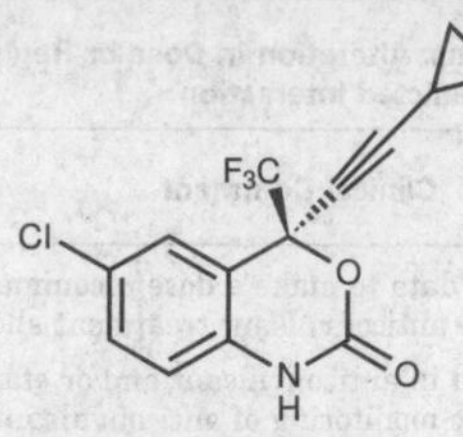

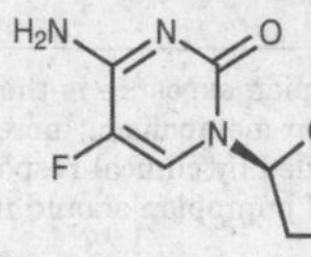

$C_4H_4O_4$ and a molecular weight of 635.52. It has the following structural formula:

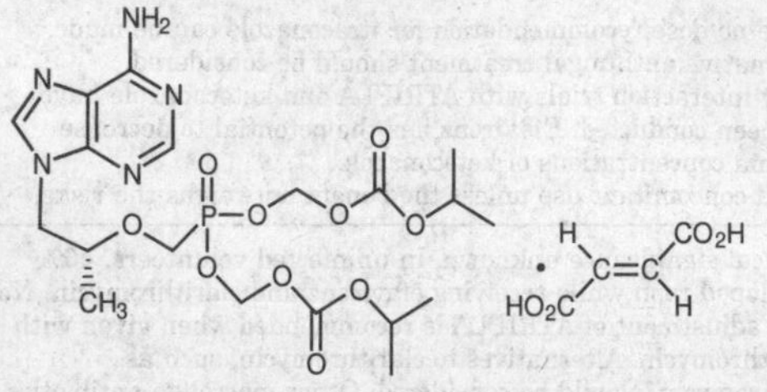

Tenofovir DF is a white to off-white crystalline powder with a solubility of 13.4 mg/mL in water at 25 °C.

12 CLINICAL PHARMACOLOGY

For additional information on Mechanism of Action, Antiviral Activity, Resistance and Cross Resistance, please consult the SUSTIVA, EMTRIVA and VIREAD prescribing information.

12.1 Mechanism of Action

ATRIPLA (efavirenz/emtricitabine/tenofovir disoproxil fumarate) is a fixed-dose combination of antiviral drugs efavirenz, emtricitabine and tenofovir disoproxil fumarate *[See Clinical Pharmacology (12.4)]*.

12.3 Pharmacokinetics

ATRIPLA: One ATRIPLA tablet is bioequivalent to one SUSTIVA tablet (600 mg) plus one EMTRIVA capsule (200 mg) plus one VIREAD tablet (300 mg) following single-dose administration to fasting healthy subjects (N=45).

Efavirenz: In HIV-1 infected subjects time-to-peak plasma concentrations were approximately 3–5 hours and steady-state plasma concentrations were reached in 6–10 days. In 35 HIV-1 infected subjects receiving efavirenz 600 mg once daily, steady-state C_{max} was 12.9 ± 3.7 μM (mean ± SD), C_{min} was 5.6 ± 3.2 μM, and AUC was 184 ± 73 μM•hr. Efavirenz is highly bound (approximately 99.5–99.75%) to human plasma proteins, predominantly albumin. Following administration of ^{14}C-labeled efavirenz, 14–34% of the dose was recovered in the urine (mostly as metabolites) and 16–61% was recovered in feces (mostly as parent drug). *In vitro* studies suggest CYP3A and CYP2B6 are the major isozymes responsible for efavirenz metabolism. Efavirenz has been shown to induce CYP enzymes, resulting in induction of its own metabolism. Efavirenz has a terminal half-life of 52–76 hours after single doses and 40–55 hours after multiple doses.

Emtricitabine: Following oral administration, emtricitabine is rapidly absorbed, with peak plasma concentrations occurring at 1–2 hours post-dose. Following multiple dose oral administration of emtricitabine to 20 HIV-1 infected subjects, the steady-state plasma emtricitabine C_{max} was 1.8 ± 0.7 μg/mL (mean ± SD) and the AUC over a 24-hour dosing interval was 10.0 ± 3.1 μg•hr/mL. The mean steady-state plasma trough concentration at 24 hours post-dose was 0.09 μg/mL. The mean absolute bioavailability of emtricitabine was 93%. Less than 4% of emtricitabine binds to human plasma proteins *in vitro* and the binding is independent of concentration over the range of 0.02–200 μg/mL. Following administration of radiolabelled emtricitabine, approximately 86% is recovered in the urine and 13% is recovered as metabolites. The metabolites of emtricitabine include 3′-sulfoxide diastereomers and their glucuronic acid conjugate. Emtricitabine is eliminated by a combination of glomerular filtration and active tubular secretion with a renal clearance in adults with normal renal function of 213 ± 89 mL/min (mean ± SD). Following a single oral dose, the plasma emtricitabine half-life is approximately 10 hours.

Tenofovir Disoproxil Fumarate: Following oral administration of a single 300 mg dose of tenofovir DF to HIV-1 infected subjects in the fasted state, maximum serum concentrations (C_{max}) were achieved in 1.0 ± 0.4 hrs (mean ± SD) and C_{max} and AUC values were 296 ± 90 ng/mL and 2287 ± 685 ng•hr/mL, respectively. The oral bioavailability of tenofovir from tenofovir DF in fasted subjects is approximately 25%. Less than 0.7% of tenofovir binds to human plasma proteins *in vitro* and the binding is independent of concentration over the range of 0.01–25 μg/mL. Approximately 70–80% of the intravenous dose of tenofovir is recovered as unchanged drug in the urine. Tenofovir is eliminated by a combination of glomerular filtration and active tubular secretion with a renal clearance in adults with normal renal function of 243 ± 33 mL/min (mean ± SD). Following a single oral dose, the terminal elimination half-life of tenofovir is approximately 17 hours.

Table 5: Drug Interactions: Changes in Pharmacokinetic Parameters for Efavirenz in the Presence of the Coadministered Drug

Coadministered Drug	Dose of Coadministered Drug (mg)	Efavirenz Dose (mg)	N	Mean % Change of Efavirenz Pharmacokinetic Parameters* (90% CI)		
				C_{max}	AUC	C_{min}
Indinavir	800 mg q8h × 14 days	200 mg qd × 14 days	11	↔	↔	↔
Lopinavir/ ritonavir	400/100 mg q12h × 9 days	600 mg qd × 9 days	11, 12†	↔	↓ 16 (↓ 38 to ↑ 15)	↓ 16 (↓ 42 to ↑ 20)
Nelfinavir	750 mg q8h × 7 days	600 mg qd × 7 days	10	↓ 12 (↓ 32 to ↑ 13)‡	↓ 12 (↓ 35 to ↑ 18)‡	↓ 21 (↓ 53 to ↑ 33)
Ritonavir	500 mg q12h × 8 days	600 mg qd × 10 days	9	↑ 14 (↑ 4 to ↑ 26)	↑ 21 (↑ 10 to ↑ 34)	↑ 25 (↑ 7 to ↑ 46)‡
Saquinavir SGC§	1200 mg q8h × 10 days	600 mg qd × 10 days	13	↓ 13 (↓ 5 to ↓ 20)	↓ 12 (↓ 4 to ↓ 19)	↓ 14 (↓ 2 to ↓ 24)‡
Boceprevir	800 mg tid × 6 days	600 mg qd × 16 days	NA	↑ 11 (↑ 2 to ↑ 20)	↑ 20 (↑ 15 to ↑ 26)	NA
Telaprevir	750 mg q8h × 10 days	600 mg qd × 20 days	21	↓ 16 (↓ 7 to ↓ 24)	↓ 7 (↓ 2 to ↓ 13)	↓ 2 (↓ 6 to ↑ 2)
Telaprevir, coadministered with tenofovir disoproxil fumarate (TDF)	1125 mg q8h × 7 days	600 mg efavirenz/ 300 mg TDF qd × 7 days	15	↓ 24 (↓ 15 to ↓ 32)	↓ 18 (↓ 10 to ↓ 26)	↓ 10 (↓ 19 to ↑ 1)
	1500 mg q12h × 7 days	600 mg efavirenz/ 300 mg TDF qd × 7 days	16	↓ 20 (↓ 14 to ↓ 26)	↓ 15 (↓ 9 to ↓ 21)	↓ 11 (↓ 4 to ↓ 18)
Clarithromycin	500 mg q12h × 7 days	400 mg qd × 7 days	12	↑ 11 (↑ 3 to ↑ 19)	↔	↔
Itraconazole	200 mg q12h × 14 days	600 mg qd × 28 days	16	↔	↔	↔
Rifabutin	300 mg qd × 14 days	600 mg qd × 14 days	11	↔	↔	↓ 12 (↓ 24 to ↑ 1)
Rifampin	600 mg × 7 days	600 mg qd × 7 days	12	↓ 20 (↓ 11 to ↓ 28)	↓ 26 (↓ 15 to ↓ 36)	↓ 32 (↓ 15 to ↓ 46)
Atorvastatin	10 mg qd × 4 days	600 mg qd × 15 days	14	↔	↔	↔
Pravastatin	40 mg qd × 4 days	600 mg qd × 15 days	11	↔	↔	↔
Simvastatin	40 mg qd × 4 days	600 mg qd × 15 days	14	↓ 12 (↓ 28 to ↑ 8)	↔	↓ 12 (↓ 25 to ↑ 3)
Carbamazepine	200 mg qd × 3 days, 200 mg bid × 3 days, then 400 mg qd × 15 days	600 mg qd × 35 days	14	↓ 21 (↓ 15 to ↓ 26)	↓ 36 (↓ 32 to ↓ 40)	↓ 47 (↓ 41 to ↓ 53)
Diltiazem	240 mg × 14 days	600 mg qd × 28 days	12	↑ 16 (↑ 6 to ↑ 26)	↑ 11 (↑ 5 to ↑ 18)	↑ 13 (↑ 1 to ↑ 26)

(Table continued on next page)

Effects of Food on Oral Absorption

ATRIPLA (efavirenz/emtricitabine/tenofovir disoproxil fumarate) has not been evaluated in the presence of food. Administration of efavirenz tablets with a high fat meal increased the mean AUC and C_{max} of efavirenz by 28% and 79%, respectively, compared to administration in the fasted state. Compared to fasted administration, dosing of tenofovir DF and emtricitabine in combination with either a high fat meal or a light meal increased the mean AUC and C_{max} of tenofovir by 35% and 15%, respectively, without affecting emtricitabine exposures *[See Dosage and Administration (2) and Patient Counseling Information (17.7)].*

Special Populations

Race

Efavirenz: The pharmacokinetics of efavirenz in HIV-1 infected subjects appear to be similar among the racial groups studied.

Emtricitabine: No pharmacokinetic differences due to race have been identified following the administration of emtricitabine.

Tenofovir Disoproxil Fumarate: There were insufficient numbers from racial and ethnic groups other than Caucasian to adequately determine potential pharmacokinetic differences among these populations following the administration of tenofovir DF.

Gender

Efavirenz, Emtricitabine, and Tenofovir Disoproxil Fumarate: Efavirenz, emtricitabine, and tenofovir pharmacokinetics are similar in male and female subjects.

Pediatric Patients

ATRIPLA (efavirenz/emtricitabine/tenofovir disoproxil fumarate) should only be administered to pediatric patients 12 years of age and weighing greater than or equal to 40 kg (greater than or equal to 88 lb).

Efavirenz: In an open-label trial in NRTI-experienced pediatric subjects (mean age 8 years, range 3–16), the pharmacokinetics of efavirenz in pediatric subjects were similar to the pharmacokinetics in adults who received a 600 mg daily dose of efavirenz. In 48 pediatric subjects, receiving the equivalent of a 600 mg dose of efavirenz, mean (± SD) steady-state C_{max} was 14.2 ± 5.8 μM, steady-state C_{min} was 5.6 ± 4.1 μM, and AUC was 218 ± 104 μM•hr.

Emtricitabine: The pharmacokinetics of emtricitabine at steady state were determined in 27 HIV-1-infected pediatric subjects 13 to 17 years of age receiving a daily dose of 6 mg/kg up to a maximum dose of 240 mg oral solution or a 200 mg capsule; 26 of 27 subjects in this age group received the 200 mg EMTRIVA capsule. Mean (± SD) C_{max} and AUC were 2.7 ± 0.9 μg/mL and 12.6 ± 5.4 μg•hr/mL, respectively. Exposures achieved in pediatric subjects 12 to less than 18 years of age were similar to those achieved in adults receiving a once daily dose of 200 mg.

Tenofovir Disoproxil Fumarate: Steady-state pharmacokinetics of tenofovir were evaluated in 8 HIV-1 infected pediatric subjects (12 to less than 18 years). Mean (± SD) C_{max} and AUC_{tau} are 0.38 ± 0.13 μg/mL and 3.39 ± 1.22 μg•hr/mL, respectively. Tenofovir exposure achieved in these pediatric subjects receiving oral daily doses of VIREAD 300 mg was similar to exposures achieved in adults receiving once-daily doses of VIREAD 300 mg.

Geriatric Patients

Pharmacokinetics of efavirenz, emtricitabine and tenofovir have not been fully evaluated in the elderly (65 years of age and older) *[See Use in Specific Populations (8.5)].*

Patients with Impaired Renal Function

Efavirenz: The pharmacokinetics of efavirenz have not been studied in subjects with renal insufficiency; however, less than 1% of efavirenz is excreted unchanged in the urine, so the impact of renal impairment on efavirenz elimination should be minimal.

Emtricitabine and Tenofovir Disoproxil Fumarate: The pharmacokinetics of emtricitabine and tenofovir DF are altered in subjects with renal impairment. In subjects with creatinine clearance below 50 mL/min, C_{max} and $AUC_{0-\infty}$ of emtricitabine and tenofovir were increased *[See Warnings and Precautions (5.7)].*

Patients with Hepatic Impairment

Efavirenz: A multiple-dose trial showed no significant effect on efavirenz pharmacokinetics in subjects with mild hepatic impairment (Child-Pugh Class A) compared with controls. There were insufficient data to determine whether moderate or severe hepatic impairment (Child-Pugh Class B or C) affects efavirenz pharmacokinetics *[See Warnings and Precautions (5.10) and Use in Specific Populations (8.6)].*

Emtricitabine: The pharmacokinetics of emtricitabine have not been studied in subjects with hepatic impairment; however, emtricitabine is not significantly metabolized by liver enzymes, so the impact of liver impairment should be limited.

Tenofovir Disoproxil Fumarate: The pharmacokinetics of tenofovir following a 300 mg dose of tenofovir DF have been studied in non-HIV infected subjects with moderate to severe hepatic impairment. There were no substantial alterations in tenofovir pharmacokinetics in subjects with hepatic impairment compared with unimpaired subjects.

Assessment of Drug Interactions

The drug interaction trials described were conducted with efavirenz, emtricitabine, or tenofovir DF as individual agents; no drug interaction trials have been conducted using ATRIPLA.

Efavirenz: The steady-state pharmacokinetics of efavirenz and tenofovir were unaffected when efavirenz and tenofovir DF were administered together versus each agent dosed alone. Specific drug interaction trials have not been performed with efavirenz and NRTIs other than tenofovir, lamivudine, and zidovudine. Clinically significant interactions would not be expected based on NRTIs elimination pathways.

Efavirenz has been shown *in vivo* to cause hepatic enzyme induction, thus increasing the biotransformation of some drugs metabolized by CYP3A and CYP2B6. *In vitro* studies have shown that efavirenz inhibited CYP isozymes 2C9, 2C19, and 3A4 with K_i values (8.5–17 μM) in the range of observed efavirenz plasma concentrations. In *in vitro* studies, efavirenz did not inhibit CYP2E1 and inhibited CYP2D6 and CYP1A2 (K_i values 82–160 μM) only at concentrations well above those achieved clinically. Coadministration of efavirenz with drugs primarily metabolized by 2C9, 2C19, and 3A4 isozymes may result in altered plasma concentrations of the coadministered drug. Drugs which induce CYP3A activity would be expected to increase the clearance of efavirenz resulting in lowered plasma concentrations.

Drug interaction trials were performed with efavirenz and other drugs likely to be coadministered or drugs commonly used as probes for pharmacokinetic interaction. There was no clinically significant interaction observed between efavirenz and zidovudine, lamivudine, azithromycin, fluconazole, lorazepam, cetirizine, or paroxetine. Single doses of famotidine or an aluminum and magnesium antacid with simethicone had no effects on efavirenz exposures. The effects of coadministration of efavirenz on C_{max}, AUC, and C_{min} are summarized in Table 5 (effect of other drugs on efavirenz) and Table 6 (effect of efavirenz on other drugs). For information regarding clinical recommendations see *Drug Interactions (7).*

[See table 5 on previous page and above]

[See table 6 on pages 680 through 682]

Table 5 *(cont.)*: Drug Interactions: Changes in Pharmacokinetic Parameters for Efavirenz in the Presence of the Coadministered Drug

				Mean % Change of Efavirenz Pharmacokinetic Parameters* (90% CI)		
Coadministered Drug	**Dose of Coadministered Drug (mg)**	**Efavirenz Dose (mg)**	**N**	**C_{max}**	**AUC**	**C_{min}**
Sertraline	50 mg qd × 14 days	600 mg qd × 14 days	13	↑ 11 (↑ 6 to ↑ 16)	↔	↔
Voriconazole	400 mg po q12h × 1 day then 200 mg po q12h × 8 days	400 mg qd × 9 days	NA	↑ 38¶	↑ 44¶	NA
	300 mg po q12h days 2–7	300 mg qd × 7 days	NA	↓ 14# (↓ 7 to ↓ 21)	↔#	NA
	400 mg po q12h days 2–7	300 mg qd × 7 days	NA	↔#	↑ 17# (↑ 6 to ↑ 29)	NA

NA = not available
* Increase = ↑; Decrease = ↓; No Effect = ↔
† Parallel-group design; N for efavirenz + lopinavir/ritonavir, N for efavirenz alone.
‡ 95% CI
§ Soft Gelatin Capsule
¶ 90% CI not available
\# Relative to steady state administration of efavirenz (600 mg once daily for 9 days).

Emtricitabine and Tenofovir Disoproxil Fumarate: The steady-state pharmacokinetics of emtricitabine and tenofovir were unaffected when emtricitabine and tenofovir DF were administered together versus each agent dosed alone.

In vitro and clinical pharmacokinetic drug-drug interaction studies have shown that the potential for CYP mediated interactions involving emtricitabine and tenofovir with other medicinal products is low.

Emtricitabine and tenofovir are primarily excreted by the kidneys by a combination of glomerular filtration and active tubular secretion. No drug-drug interactions due to competition for renal excretion have been observed; however, coadministration of emtricitabine and tenofovir DF with drugs that are eliminated by active tubular secretion may increase concentrations of emtricitabine, tenofovir, and/or the coadministered drug.

Drugs that decrease renal function may increase concentrations of emtricitabine and/or tenofovir.

No clinically significant drug interactions have been observed between emtricitabine and famciclovir, indinavir, stavudine, tenofovir DF and zidovudine. Similarly, no clinically significant drug interactions have been observed between tenofovir DF and abacavir, efavirenz, emtricitabine, entecavir, indinavir, lamivudine, lopinavir/ritonavir, methadone, nelfinavir, oral contraceptives, ribavirin, saquinavir/ritonavir or tacrolimus in trials conducted in healthy volunteers.

Following multiple dosing to HIV-negative subjects receiving either chronic methadone maintenance therapy, oral contraceptives, or single doses of ribavirin, steady-state tenofovir pharmacokinetics were similar to those observed in previous trials, indicating a lack of clinically significant drug interactions between these agents and tenofovir DF.

The effects of coadministered drugs on the C_{max}, AUC, and C_{min} of tenofovir are shown in Table 7. The effects of coadministration of tenofovir DF on C_{max}, AUC, and C_{min} of coadministered drugs are shown in Table 8.

[See table 7 at top of page 682]

[See table 8 at top of page 683]

Coadministration of tenofovir DF with didanosine results in changes in the pharmacokinetics of didanosine that may be of clinical significance. Concomitant dosing of tenofovir DF with didanosine enteric-coated capsules significantly increases the C_{max} and AUC of didanosine. When didanosine 250 mg enteric-coated capsules were administered with tenofovir DF, systemic exposures of didanosine were similar to those seen with the 400 mg enteric-coated capsules alone under fasted conditions. The mechanism of this interaction is unknown [for didanosine dosing adjustment recommendations see *Drug Interactions (7.3)*, Table 4].

12.4 Microbiology

Mechanism of Action

Efavirenz: Efavirenz is a non-nucleoside reverse transcriptase (RT) inhibitor of HIV-1. Efavirenz activity is mediated predominantly by noncompetitive inhibition of HIV-1 reverse transcriptase (RT). HIV-2 RT and human cellular DNA polymerases α, β, γ, and σ are not inhibited by efavirenz.

Emtricitabine: Emtricitabine, a synthetic nucleoside analog of cytidine, is phosphorylated by cellular enzymes to form emtricitabine 5′-triphosphate. Emtricitabine 5′-triphosphate inhibits the activity of the HIV-1 RT by competing with the natural substrate deoxycytidine 5′-triphosphate and by being incorporated into nascent viral DNA which results in chain termination. Emtricitabine 5′-triphosphate is a weak inhibitor of mammalian DNA polymerase α, β, ϵ, and mitochondrial DNA polymerase γ.

Tenofovir Disoproxil Fumarate: Tenofovir DF is an acyclic nucleoside phosphonate diester analog of adenosine monophosphate. Tenofovir DF requires initial diester hydrolysis for conversion to tenofovir and subsequent phosphorylations by cellular enzymes to form tenofovir diphosphate. Tenofovir diphosphate inhibits the activity of HIV-1 RT by competing with the natural substrate deoxyadenosine 5′-triphosphate and, after incorporation into DNA, by DNA chain termination. Tenofovir diphosphate is a weak inhibitor of mammalian DNA polymerases α, β, and mitochondrial DNA polymerase γ.

Table 6: Drug Interactions: Changes in Pharmacokinetic Parameters for Coadministered Drug in the Presence of Efavirenz

Coadministered Drug	Dose of Coadministered Drug (mg)	Efavirenz Dose (mg)	N	Mean % Change of Coadministered Drug Pharmacokinetic Parameters* (90% CI) C_{max}	AUC	C_{min}
Atazanavir	400 mg qd with a light meal d 1–20	600 mg qd with a light meal d 7–20	27	↓ 59 (↓ 49 to ↓ 67)	↓ 74 (↓ 68 to ↓ 78)	↓ 93 (↓ 90 to ↓ 95)
	400 mg qd d 1–6, then 300 mg qd d 7–20 with ritonavir 100 mg qd and a light meal	600 mg qd 2 h after atazanavir and ritonavir d 7–20	13	↑ 14[†] (↓ 17 to ↑ 58)	↑ 39[†] (↑ 2 to ↑ 88)	↑ 48[†] (↑ 24 to ↑ 76)
	300 mg qd/ritonavir 100 mg qd d 1–10 (pm), then 400 mg qd/ritonavir 100 mg qd d 11–24 (pm) (simultaneous with efavirenz)	600 mg qd with a light snack d 11–24 (pm)	14	↑ 17 (↑ 8 to ↑ 27)	↔	↓ 42 (↓ 31 to ↓ 51)
Indinavir	1000 mg q8h × 10 days	600 mg qd × 10 days	20			
	After morning dose			↔[‡]	↓ 33[‡] (↓ 26 to ↓ 39)	↓ 39[‡] (↓ 24 to ↓ 51)
	After afternoon dose			↔[‡]	↓ 37[‡] (↓ 26 to ↓ 46)	↓ 52[‡] (↓ 47 to ↓ 57)
	After evening dose			↓ 29[‡] (↓ 11 to ↓ 43)	↓ 46[‡] (↓ 37 to ↓ 54)	↓ 57[‡] (↓ 50 to ↓ 63)
Lopinavir/ ritonavir	400/100 mg q12h × 9 days	600 mg qd × 9 days	11, 7[§]	↔[¶]	↓ 19[¶] (↓ 36 to ↑ 3)	↓ 39[¶] (↓ 3 to ↓ 62)
Nelfinavir	750 mg q8h × 7 days	600 mg qd × 7 days	10	↑ 21 (↑ 10 to ↑ 33)	↑ 20 (↑ 8 to ↑ 34)	↔
Metabolite AG-1402				↓ 40 (↓ 30 to ↓ 48)	↓ 37 (↓ 25 to ↓ 48)	↓ 43 (↓ 21 to ↓ 59)
Ritonavir	500 mg q12h × 8 days	600 mg qd × 10 days	11			
	After AM dose			↑ 24 (↑ 12 to ↑ 38)	↑ 18 (↑ 6 to ↑ 33)	↑ 42 (↑ 9 to ↑ 86)[#]
	After PM dose			↔	↔	↑ 24 (↑ 3 to ↑ 50)[#]
Saquinavir SGC[b]	1200 mg q8h × 10 days	600 mg qd × 10 days	12	↓ 50 (↓ 28 to ↓ 66)	↓ 62 (↓ 45 to ↓ 74)	↓ 56 (↓ 16 to ↓ 77)[#]
Maraviroc	100 mg bid	600 mg qd	12	↓ 51 (↓ 37 to ↓ 62)	↓ 45 (↓ 38 to ↓ 51)	↓ 45 (↓ 28 to ↓ 57)
Raltegravir	400 mg single dose	600 mg qd	9	↓ 36 (↓ 2 to ↓ 59)	↓ 36 (↓ 20 to ↓ 48)	↓ 21 (↓ 51 to ↑ 28)
Boceprevir	800 mg tid × 6 days	600 mg qd × 16 days	NA	↓ 8 (↓ 22 to ↑ 8)	↓ 19 (↓ 11 to ↓ 25)	↓ 44 (↓ 26 to ↓ 58)
Telaprevir	750 mg q8h × 10 days	600 mg qd × 20 days	21	↓ 9 (↓18 to ↑ 2)	↓ 26 (↓16 to ↓ 35)	↓ 47 (↓ 35 to ↓ 56)

(Table continued on next page)

Antiviral Activity

Efavirenz, Emtricitabine, and Tenofovir Disoproxil Fumarate: In combination studies evaluating the antiviral activity in cell culture of emtricitabine and efavirenz together, efavirenz and tenofovir together, and emtricitabine and tenofovir together, additive to synergistic antiviral effects were observed.

Efavirenz: The concentration of efavirenz inhibiting replication of wild-type laboratory adapted strains and clinical isolates in cell culture by 90–95% (EC_{90-95}) ranged from 1.7–25 nM in lymphoblastoid cell lines, peripheral blood mononuclear cells, and macrophage/monocyte cultures. Efavirenz demonstrated additive antiviral activity against HIV-1 in cell culture when combined with non-nucleoside reverse transcriptase inhibitors (NNRTIs) (delavirdine and nevirapine), nucleoside reverse transcriptase inhibitors (NRTIs) (abacavir, didanosine, lamivudine, stavudine, zalcitabine, and zidovudine), protease inhibitors (PIs) (amprenavir, indinavir, lopinavir, nelfinavir, ritonavir, and saquinavir), and the fusion inhibitor enfuvirtide. Efavirenz demonstrated additive to antagonistic antiviral activity in cell culture with atazanavir. Efavirenz demonstrated antiviral activity against clade B and most non-clade B isolates (subtypes A, AE, AG, C, D, F, G, J, and N), but had reduced antiviral activity against group O viruses. Efavirenz is not active against HIV-2.

Emtricitabine: The antiviral activity in cell culture of emtricitabine against laboratory and clinical isolates of HIV-1 was assessed in lymphoblastoid cell lines, the MAGI-CCR5 cell line, and peripheral blood mononuclear cells. The 50% effective concentration (EC_{50}) values for emtricitabine were in the range of 0.0013–0.64 µM (0.0003–0.158 µg/mL). In drug combination studies of emtricitabine with NRTIs (abacavir, lamivudine, stavudine, zalcitabine, and zidovudine), NNRTIs (delavirdine, efavirenz, and nevirapine), and PIs (amprenavir, nelfinavir, ritonavir, and saquinavir), additive to synergistic effects were observed. Emtricitabine displayed antiviral activity in cell culture against HIV-1 clades A, B, C, D, E, F, and G (EC_{50} values ranged from 0.007–0.075 µM) and showed strain specific activity against HIV-2 (EC_{50} values ranged from 0.007–1.5 µM).

Tenofovir Disoproxil Fumarate: The antiviral activity in cell culture of tenofovir against laboratory and clinical isolates of HIV-1 was assessed in lymphoblastoid cell lines, primary monocyte/macrophage cells and peripheral blood lymphocytes. The EC_{50} values for tenofovir were in the range of 0.04–8.5 µM. In drug combination studies of tenofovir with NRTIs (abacavir, didanosine, lamivudine, stavudine, zalcitabine, and zidovudine), NNRTIs (delavirdine, efavirenz, and nevirapine), and PIs (amprenavir, indinavir, nelfinavir, ritonavir, and saquinavir), additive to synergistic effects were observed. Tenofovir displayed antiviral activity in cell culture against HIV-1 clades A, B, C, D, E, F, G and O (EC_{50} values ranged from 0.5–2.2 µM) and showed strain specific activity against HIV-2 (EC_{50} values ranged from 1.6 µM–5.5 µM).

Resistance

Efavirenz, Emtricitabine, and Tenofovir Disoproxil Fumarate: HIV-1 isolates with reduced susceptibility to the combination of emtricitabine and tenofovir have been selected in cell culture and in clinical trials. Genotypic analysis of these isolates identified the M184V/I and/or K65R amino acid substitutions in the viral RT.

In a clinical trial of treatment-naive subjects *[Study 934, see Clinical Studies (14)]* resistance analysis was performed on HIV-1 isolates from all confirmed virologic failure subjects with greater than 400 copies/mL of HIV-1 RNA at Week 144 or early discontinuations. Genotypic resistance to efavirenz, predominantly the K103N substitution, was the most common form of resistance that developed. Resistance to efavirenz occurred in 13/19 analyzed subjects in the emtricitabine + tenofovir DF group and in 21/29 analyzed subjects in the zidovudine/lamivudine fixed-dose combination group. The M184V amino acid substitution, associated with resistance to emtricitabine and lamivudine, was observed in 2/19 analyzed subject isolates in the emtricitabine + tenofovir DF group and in 10/29 analyzed subject isolates in the zidovudine/lamivudine group. Through 144 weeks of Study 934, no subjects developed a detectable K65R substitution in their HIV-1 as analyzed through standard genotypic analysis.

In a clinical trial of treatment-naive subjects, isolates from 8/47 (17%) analyzed subjects receiving tenofovir DF developed the K65R substitution through 144 weeks of therapy; 7 of these occurred in the first 48 weeks of treatment and one at Week 96. In treatment experienced subjects, 14/304 (5%) of tenofovir DF treated subjects with virologic failure through Week 96 showed greater than 1.4-fold (median 2.7) reduced susceptibility to tenofovir. Genotypic analysis of the resistant isolates showed a substitution in the HIV-1 RT gene resulting in the K65R amino acid substitution.

Efavirenz: Clinical isolates with reduced susceptibility in cell culture to efavirenz have been obtained. The most frequently observed amino acid substitution in clinical trials with efavirenz is K103N (54%). One or more RT substitutions at amino acid positions 98, 100, 101, 103, 106, 108, 188, 190, 225, 227, and 230 were observed in subjects failing treatment with efavirenz in combination with other antiretrovirals. Other resistance substitutions observed to emerge commonly included L100I (7%), K101E/Q/R (14%), V108I (11%), G190S/T/A (7%), P225H (18%), and M230I/L (11%). HIV-1 isolates with reduced susceptibility to efavirenz (greater than 380-fold increase in EC_{90} value) emerged rapidly under selection in cell culture. Genotypic characterization of these viruses identified substitutions resulting in single amino acid substitutions L100I or V179D, double substitutions L100I/V108I, and triple substitutions L100I/V179D/Y181C in RT.

Emtricitabine: Emtricitabine-resistant isolates of HIV-1 have been selected in cell culture and in clinical trials. Genotypic analysis of these isolates showed that the reduced susceptibility to emtricitabine was associated with a substitution in the HIV-1 RT gene at codon 184 which resulted in an amino acid substitution of methionine by valine or isoleucine (M184V/I).

Tenofovir Disoproxil Fumarate: HIV-1 isolates with reduced susceptibility to tenofovir have been selected in cell culture. These viruses expressed a K65R substitution in RT and showed a 2- to 4-fold reduction in susceptibility to tenofovir.

Cross Resistance

Efavirenz, Emtricitabine, and Tenofovir Disoproxil Fumarate: Cross-resistance has been recognized among NNRTIs. Cross resistance has also been recognized among certain NRTIs. The M184V/I and/or K65R substitutions selected in cell culture by the combination of emtricitabine and tenofovir are also observed in some HIV-1 isolates from subjects failing treatment with tenofovir in combination with either lamivudine or emtricitabine, and either abacavir or didanosine. Therefore, cross-resistance among these drugs may occur in patients whose virus harbors either or both of these amino acid substitutions.

Efavirenz: Clinical isolates previously characterized as efavirenz-resistant were also phenotypically resistant in cell culture to delavirdine and nevirapine compared to baseline. Delavirdine- and/or nevirapine-resistant clinical viral isolates with NNRTI resistance-associated substitutions (A98G, L100I, K101E/P, K103N/S, V106A, Y181X, Y188X, G190X, P225H, F227L, or M230L) showed reduced susceptibility to efavirenz in cell culture. Greater than 90% of NRTI-resistant isolates tested in cell culture retained susceptibility to efavirenz.

Emtricitabine: Emtricitabine-resistant isolates (M184V/I) were cross-resistant to lamivudine and zalcitabine but retained susceptibility in cell culture to didanosine, stavudine, tenofovir, zidovudine, and NNRTIs (delavirdine, efavirenz, and nevirapine). HIV-1 isolates containing the K65R substitution, selected *in vivo* by abacavir, didanosine, tenofovir, and zalcitabine, demonstrated reduced susceptibility to inhibition by emtricitabine. Viruses harboring substitutions conferring reduced susceptibility to stavudine and zidovudine (M41L, D67N, K70R, L210W, T215Y/F, and K219Q/E) or didanosine (L74V) remained sensitive to emtricitabine.

Tenofovir Disoproxil Fumarate: The K65R substitution selected by tenofovir is also selected in some HIV-1 infected patients treated with abacavir, didanosine, or zalcitabine. HIV-1 isolates with the K65R substitution also showed reduced susceptibility to emtricitabine and lamivudine. Therefore, cross-resistance among these drugs may occur in patients whose virus harbors the K65R substitution. HIV-1 isolates from subjects (N=20) whose HIV-1 expressed a mean of 3 zidovudine-associated RT amino acid substitutions (M41L, D67N, K70R, L210W, T215Y/F, or K219Q/E/N) showed a 3.1-fold decrease in the susceptibility to tenofovir. Subjects whose virus expressed an L74V substitution without zidovudine resistance associated substitutions (N=8) had reduced response to VIREAD. Limited data are available for patients whose virus expressed a Y115F substitution (N=3), Q151M substitution (N=2), or T69 insertion (N=4), all of whom had a reduced response.

13 NONCLINICAL TOXICOLOGY

13.1 Carcinogenesis, Mutagenesis, Impairment of Fertility

Efavirenz: Long-term carcinogenicity studies in mice and rats were carried out with efavirenz. Mice were dosed with 0, 25, 75, 150, or 300 mg/kg/day for 2 years. Incidences of hepatocellular adenomas and carcinomas and pulmonary alveolar/bronchiolar adenomas were increased above background in females. No increases in tumor incidence above background were seen in males. In studies in which rats were administered efavirenz at doses of 0, 25, 50, or 100 mg/kg/day for 2 years, no increases in tumor incidence above background were observed. The systemic exposure (based on AUCs) in mice was approximately 1.7-fold that in humans receiving the 600-mg/day dose. The exposure in rats was lower than that in humans. The mechanism of the carcinogenic potential is unknown. However, in genetic toxicology assays, efavirenz showed no evidence of mutagenic or clastogenic activity in a battery of *in vitro* and *in vivo* studies. These included bacterial mutation assays in *S. typhimurium* and *E. coli*, mammalian mutation assays in Chinese hamster ovary cells, chromosome aberration assays in human peripheral blood lymphocytes or Chinese hamster ovary cells, and an *in vivo* mouse bone marrow micronucleus assay. Given the lack of genotoxic activity of efavirenz, the relevance to humans of neoplasms in efavirenz-treated mice is not known.

Efavirenz did not impair mating or fertility of male or female rats, and did not affect sperm of treated male rats. The reproductive performance of offspring born to female rats given efavirenz was not affected. As a result of the rapid clearance of efavirenz in rats, systemic drug exposures achieved in these studies were equivalent to or below those achieved in humans given therapeutic doses of efavirenz.

Table 6 *(cont.)*: Drug Interactions: Changes in Pharmacokinetic Parameters for Coadministered Drug in the Presence of Efavirenz

				Mean % Change of Coadministered Drug Pharmacokinetic Parameters* (90% CI)		
Coadministered Drug	**Dose of Coadministered Drug (mg)**	**Efavirenz Dose (mg)**	**N**	**C_{max}**	**AUC**	**C_{min}**
Clarithromycin	500 mg q12h × 7 days	400 mg qd × 7 days	11	↓ 26 (↓ 15 to ↓ 35)	↓ 39 (↓ 30 to ↓ 46)	↓ 53 (↓ 42 to ↓ 63)
14-OH metabolite				↑ 49 (↑ 32 to ↑ 69)	↑ 34 (↑ 18 to ↑ 53)	↑ 26 (↑ 9 to ↑ 45)
Itraconazole	200 mg q12h × 28 days	600 mg qd × 14 days	18	↓ 37 (↓ 20 to ↓ 51)	↓ 39 (↓ 21 to ↓ 53)	↓ 44 (↓ 27 to ↓ 58)
Hydroxy-itraconazole				↓ 35 (↓ 12 to ↓ 52)	↓ 37 (↓ 14 to ↓ 55)	↓ 43 (↓ 18 to ↓ 60)
Posaconazole	400 mg (oral suspension) bid × 10 and 20 days	400 mg qd × 10 and 20 days	11	↓ 45 (↓ 34 to ↓ 53)	↓ 50 (↓ 40 to ↓ 57)	NA
Rifabutin	300 mg qd × 14 days	600 mg qd × 14 days	9	↓ 32 (↓ 15 to ↓ 46)	↓ 38 (↓ 28 to ↓ 47)	↓ 45 (↓ 31 to ↓ 56)
Atorvastatin	10 mg qd × 4 days	600 mg qd × 15 days	14	↓ 14 (↓ 1 to ↓ 26)	↓ 43 (↓ 34 to ↓ 50)	↓ 69 (↓ 49 to ↓ 81)
Total active (including metabolites)				↓ 15 (↓ 2 to ↓ 26)	↓ 32 (↓ 21 to ↓ 41)	↓ 48 (↓ 23 to ↓ 64)
Pravastatin	40 mg qd × 4 days	600 mg qd × 15 days	13	↓ 32 (↓ 59 to ↑ 12)	↓ 44 (↓ 26 to ↓ 57)	↓ 19 (↓ 0 to ↓ 35)
Simvastatin	40 mg qd × 4 days	600 mg qd × 15 days	14	↓ 72 (↓ 63 to ↓ 79)	↓ 68 (↓ 62 to ↓ 73)	↓ 45 (↓ 20 to ↓ 62)
Total active (including metabolites)				↓ 68 (↓ 55 to ↓ 78)	↓ 60 (↓ 52 to ↓ 68)	NA[ß]
Carbamazepine	200 mg qd × 3 days, 200 mg bid × 3 days, then 400 mg qd × 29 days	600 mg qd × 14 days	12	↓ 20 (↓ 15 to ↓ 24)	↓ 27 (↓ 20 to ↓ 33)	↓ 35 (↓ 24 to ↓ 44)
Epoxide metabolite				↔	↔	↓ 13 (↓ 30 to ↑ 7)
Diltiazem	240 mg × 21 days	600 mg qd × 14 days	13	↓ 60 (↓ 50 to ↓ 68)	↓ 69 (↓ 55 to ↓ 79)	↓ 63 (↓ 44 to ↓ 75)
Desacetyl diltiazem				↓ 64 (↓ 57 to ↓ 69)	↓ 75 (↓ 59 to ↓ 84)	↓ 62 (↓ 44 to ↓ 75)
N-monodesmethyl diltiazem				↓ 28 (↓ 7 to ↓ 44)	↓ 37 (↓ 17 to ↓ 52)	↓ 37 (↓ 17 to ↓ 52)
Ethinyl estradiol/ Norgestimate	0.035 mg/0.25 mg × 14 days	600 mg qd × 14 days				
Ethinyl estradiol			21	↔	↔	↔
Norelgestromin			21	↓ 46 (↓39 to ↓ 52)	↓ 64 (↓ 62 to ↓ 67)	↓ 82 (↓ 79 to ↓ 85)
Levonorgestrel			6	↓ 80 (↓77 to ↓ 83)	↓ 83 (↓79 to ↓ 87)	↓ 86 (↓80 to ↓ 90)
Methadone	Stable maintenance 35–100 mg daily	600 mg qd × 14–21 days	11	↓ 45 (↓ 25 to ↓ 59)	↓ 52 (↓ 33 to ↓ 66)	NA

(Table continued on next page)

Emtricitabine: In long-term carcinogenicity studies of emtricitabine, no drug-related increases in tumor incidence were found in mice at doses up to 750 mg/kg/day (26 times the human systemic exposure at the therapeutic dose of 200 mg/day) or in rats at doses up to 600 mg/day (31 times the human systemic exposure at the therapeutic dose).

Emtricitabine was not genotoxic in the reverse mutation bacterial test (Ames test), mouse lymphoma or mouse micronucleus assays.

Emtricitabine did not affect fertility in male rats at approximately 140-fold or in male and female mice at approximately 60-fold higher exposures (AUC) than in humans

Table 6 (*cont.*): Drug Interactions: Changes in Pharmacokinetic Parameters for Coadministered Drug in the Presence of Efavirenz

Coadministered Drug	Dose of Coadministered Drug (mg)	Efavirenz Dose (mg)	N	Mean % Change of Coadministered Drug Pharmacokinetic Parameters* (90% CI)		
				C_{max}	AUC	C_{min}
Bupropion	150 mg single dose (sustained-release)	600 mg qd × 14 days	13	↓ 34 (↓21 to ↓47)	↓ 55 (↓48 to ↓62)	NA
Hydroxybupropion				↑ 50 (↑ 20 to ↑ 80)	↔	NA
Sertraline	50 mg qd × 14 days	600 mg qd × 14 days	13	↓ 29 (↓ 15 to ↓ 40)	↓ 39 (↓ 27 to ↓ 50)	↓ 46 (↓ 31 to ↓ 58)
Voriconazole	400 mg po q12h × 1 day then 200 mg po q12h × 8 days	400 mg qd × 9 days	NA	↓ 61[à]	↓ 77[à]	NA
	300 mg po q12h days 2–7	300 mg qd × 7 days	NA	↓ 36[è] (↓ 21 to ↓ 49)	↓ 55[è] (↓ 45 to ↓ 62)	NA
	400 mg po q12h days 2–7	300 mg qd × 7 days	NA	↑ 23[è] (↓ 1 to ↑ 53	↓ 7[è] (↓ 23 to ↑ 13)	NA

NA = not available
* Increase = ↑; Decrease = ↓; No Effect = ↔
† Compared with atazanavir 400 mg qd alone.
‡ Comparator dose of indinavir was 800 mg q8h × 10 days.
§ Parallel-group design; N for efavirenz + lopinavir/ritonavir, N for lopinavir/ritonavir alone.
¶ Values are for lopinavir. The pharmacokinetics of ritonavir 100 mg q12h are unaffected by concurrent efavirenz.
# 95% CI
Þ Soft Gelatin Capsule
ß Not available because of insufficient data.
à 90% CI not available
è Relative to steady-state administration of voriconazole (400 mg for 1 day, then 200 mg po q12h for 2 days).

Table 7: Drug Interactions: Changes in Pharmacokinetic Parameters for Tenofovir in the Presence of the Coadministered Drug*,†

Coadministered Drug	Dose of Coadministered Drug (mg)	N	Mean % Change of Tenofovir Pharmacokinetic Parameters‡ (90% CI)		
			C_{max}	AUC	C_{min}
Atazanavir[§]	400 once daily × 14 days	33	↑ 14 (↑ 8 to ↑ 20)	↑ 24 (↑ 21 to ↑ 28)	↑ 22 (↑ 15 to ↑ 30)
Didanosine[¶]	250 or 400 once daily × 7 days	14	↔	↔	↔
Lopinavir/ritonavir	400/100 twice daily × 14 days	24	↔	↑ 32 (↑ 25 to ↑ 38)	↑ 51 (↑ 37 to ↑ 66)

* All interaction trials conducted in healthy volunteers.
† Subjects received tenofovir DF 300 mg once daily.
‡ Increase = ↑; Decrease = ↓; No Effect = ↔
§ Reyataz Prescribing Information
¶ Subjects received didanosine buffered tablets.

given the recommended 200 mg daily dose. Fertility was normal in the offspring of mice exposed daily from before birth *(in utero)* through sexual maturity at daily exposures (AUC) of approximately 60-fold higher than human exposures at the recommended 200 mg daily dose.

Tenofovir Disoproxil Fumarate: Long-term oral carcinogenicity studies of tenofovir DF in mice and rats were carried out at exposures up to approximately 16 times (mice) and 5 times (rats) those observed in humans at the therapeutic dose for HIV-1 infection. At the high dose in female mice, liver adenomas were increased at exposures 16 times that in humans. In rats, the study was negative for carcinogenic findings at exposures up to 5 times that observed in humans at the therapeutic dose.

Tenofovir DF was mutagenic in the *in vitro* mouse lymphoma assay and negative in an *in vitro* bacterial mutagenicity test (Ames test). In an *in vivo* mouse micronucleus assay, tenofovir DF was negative when administered to male mice.

There were no effects on fertility, mating performance or early embryonic development when tenofovir DF was administered to male rats at a dose equivalent to 10 times the human dose based on body surface area comparisons for 28 days prior to mating and to female rats for 15 days prior to mating through Day seven of gestation. There was, however, an alteration of the estrous cycle in female rats.

13.2 Animal Toxicology and/or Pharmacology

Efavirenz: Nonsustained convulsions were observed in 6 of 20 monkeys receiving efavirenz at doses yielding plasma AUC values 4- to 13-fold greater than those in humans given the recommended dose.

Tenofovir Disoproxil Fumarate: Tenofovir and tenofovir DF administered in toxicology studies to rats, dogs and monkeys at exposures (based on AUCs) greater than or equal to 6-fold those observed in humans caused bone toxicity. In monkeys the bone toxicity was diagnosed as osteomalacia. Osteomalacia observed in monkeys appeared to be reversible upon dose reduction or discontinuation of tenofovir. In rats and dogs, the bone toxicity manifested as reduced bone mineral density. The mechanism(s) underlying bone toxicity is unknown.

Evidence of renal toxicity was noted in 4 animal species administered tenofovir and tenofovir DF. Increases in serum creatinine, BUN, glycosuria, proteinuria, phosphaturia and/or calciuria and decreases in serum phosphate were observed to varying degrees in these animals. These toxicities were noted at exposures (based on AUCs) 2- to 20-times higher than those observed in humans. The relationship of the renal abnormalities, particularly the phosphaturia, to the bone toxicity is not known.

14 CLINICAL STUDIES

Clinical Study 934 supports the use of ATRIPLA tablets in antiretroviral treatment-naive HIV-1 infected patients. Additional data in support of the use of ATRIPLA in treatment-naive patients can be found in the prescribing information for VIREAD.

Clinical Study 073 provides clinical experience in subjects with stable, virologic suppression and no history of virologic failure who switched from their current regimen to ATRIPLA (efavirenz/emtricitabine/tenofovir disoproxil fumarate).

In antiretroviral treatment-experienced patients, the use of ATRIPLA tablets may be considered for patients with HIV-1 strains that are expected to be susceptible to the components of ATRIPLA as assessed by treatment history or by genotypic or phenotypic testing *[See Clinical Pharmacology (12.4)]*.

Study 934: Data through 144 weeks are reported for Study 934, a randomized, open-label, active-controlled multicenter trial comparing emtricitabine + tenofovir DF administered in combination with efavirenz versus zidovudine/lamivudine fixed-dose combination administered in combination with efavirenz in 511 antiretroviral-naive subjects. From Weeks 96 to 144 of the trial, subjects received emtricitabine/tenofovir DF fixed-dose combination with efavirenz in place of emtricitabine + tenofovir DF with efavirenz. Subjects had a mean age of 38 years (range 18–80), 86% were male, 59% were Caucasian and 23% were Black. The mean baseline $CD4^+$ cell count was 245 cells/mm^3 (range 2–1191) and median baseline plasma HIV-1 RNA was 5.01 log_{10} copies/mL (range 3.56–6.54). Subjects were stratified by baseline $CD4^+$ cell count (< or ≥200 cells/mm^3) and 41% had $CD4^+$ cell counts <200 cells/mm^3. Fifty-one percent (51%) of subjects had baseline viral loads >100,000 copies/mL. Treatment outcomes through 48 and 144 weeks for those subjects who did not have efavirenz resistance at baseline (N=487) are presented in Table 9.

[See table 9 at top of next page]

Through Week 48, 84% and 73% of subjects in the emtricitabine + tenofovir DF group and the zidovudine/lamivudine group, respectively, achieved and maintained HIV-1 RNA <400 copies/mL (71% and 58% through Week 144). The difference in the proportion of subjects who achieved and maintained HIV-1 RNA <400 copies/mL through 48 weeks largely results from the higher number of discontinuations due to adverse events and other reasons in the zidovudine/lamivudine group in this open-label trial. In addition, 80% and 70% of subjects in the emtricitabine + tenofovir DF group and the zidovudine/lamivudine group, respectively, achieved and maintained HIV-1 RNA <50 copies/mL through Week 48 (64% and 56% through Week 144). The mean increase from baseline in $CD4^+$ cell count was 190 cells/mm^3 in the emtricitabine + tenofovir DF group and 158 cells/mm^3 in the zidovudine/lamivudine group at Week 48 (312 and 271 cells/mm^3 at Week 144).

Through 48 weeks, 7 subjects in the emtricitabine + tenofovir DF group and 5 subjects in the zidovudine/lamivudine group experienced a new CDC Class C event (10 and 6 subjects through 144 weeks).

Study 073: Study 073 was a 48-week open-label, randomized clinical trial in subjects with stable virologic suppression on combination antiretroviral therapy consisting of at least two nucleoside reverse transcriptase inhibitors (NRTIs) administered in combination with a protease inhibitor (with or without ritonavir) or a non-nucleoside reverse transcriptase inhibitor (NNRTI).

To be enrolled, subjects were to have HIV-1 RNA <200 copies/mL for at least 12 weeks on their current regimen prior to trial entry with no known HIV-1 substitutions conferring resistance to the components of ATRIPLA and no history of virologic failure.

The trial compared the efficacy of switching to ATRIPLA or staying on the baseline antiretroviral regimen (SBR). Subjects were randomized in a 2:1 ratio to switch to ATRIPLA (N=203) or stay on SBR (N=97). Subjects had a mean age of 43 years (range 22–73 years), 88% were male, 68% were white, 29% were Black or African-American, and 3% were of other races. At baseline, median $CD4^+$ cell count was 516 cells/mm^3 and 96% had HIV-1 RNA <50 copies/mL. The median time since onset of antiretroviral therapy was 3 years and 88% of subjects were receiving their first antiretroviral regimen at trial enrollment.

At Week 48, 89% and 87% of subjects who switched to ATRIPLA maintained HIV RNA <200 copies/mL and <50 copies/mL, respectively, compared to 88% and 85% who remained on SBR; this difference was not statistically significant. No changes in $CD4^+$ cell counts from baseline to Week 48 were observed in either treatment arm.

16 HOW SUPPLIED/STORAGE AND HANDLING

ATRIPLA tablets are pink, capsule-shaped, film-coated, debossed with "123" on one side and plain-faced on the other side. Each bottle contains 30 tablets (NDC 15584-0101-1) and silica gel desiccant, and is closed with a child-resistant closure.

Store at 25 °C (77 °F); excursions permitted to 15–30 °C (59–86 °F) *[See USP Controlled Room Temperature]*.

- Keep container tightly closed.
- Dispense only in original container.
- Do not use if seal over bottle opening is broken or missing.

17 PATIENT COUNSELING INFORMATION

See FDA-approved patient labeling (Patient Information)

17.1 Drug Interactions

A statement to patients and healthcare providers is included on the product's bottle labels: *ALERT: Find out about medicines that should NOT be taken with ATRIPLA.* ATRIPLA (efavirenz/emtricitabine/tenofovir disoproxil fumarate) may interact with some drugs; therefore, patients should be advised to report to their doctor the use of any other prescription, nonprescription medication, or herbal products, particularly St. John's wort.

17.2 General Information for Patients

Patients should be advised that:

- ATRIPLA is not a cure for HIV-1 infection and patients may continue to experience illnesses associated with HIV-1 infection, including opportunistic infections. Patients should remain under the care of a physician when using ATRIPLA.
- Patients should avoid doing things that can spread HIV-1 to others.
  - **Do not share needles or other injection equipment.**
  - **Do not share personal items that can have blood or body fluids on them, like toothbrushes and razor blades.**
  - **Do not have any kind of sex without protection.** Always practice safe sex by using a latex or polyurethane condom to lower the chance of sexual contact with semen, vaginal secretions, or blood.
  - **Do not breastfeed.** Some of the medicines in ATRIPLA can be passed to your baby in your breast milk. We do not know whether it could harm your baby. Also, mothers with HIV-1 should not breastfeed because HIV-1 can be passed to the baby in the breast milk.
- The long-term effects of ATRIPLA are unknown.
- Redistribution or accumulation of body fat may occur in patients receiving antiretroviral therapy and that the cause and long-term health effects of these conditions are not known.
- ATRIPLA should not be coadministered with COMPLERA, EMTRIVA, STRIBILD, TRUVADA, or VIREAD; or drugs containing lamivudine, including Combivir, Epivir, Epivir-HBV, Epzicom, or Trizivir. SUSTIVA should not be coadministered with ATRIPLA unless needed for dose adjustment *[See Warnings and Precautions (5.4)]*.
- ATRIPLA should not be administered with HEPSERA *[See Warnings and Precautions (5.2)]*.

17.3 Lactic Acidosis/Severe Hepatomegaly with Steatosis

Patients should be informed that lactic acidosis and severe hepatomegaly with steatosis, including fatal cases, have been reported. Treatment will be suspended in any patients who develop clinical symptoms suggestive of lactic acidosis or pronounced hepatotoxicity (including nausea, vomiting, unusual or unexpected stomach discomfort, and weakness) *[See Warnings and Precautions (5.1)]*.

17.4 Patients Coinfected with HIV-1 and HBV

Patients with HIV-1 should be tested for hepatitis B virus (HBV) before initiating antiretroviral therapy.

Patients should be advised that severe acute exacerbations of hepatitis B have been reported in patients who are coinfected with HBV and HIV-1 and have discontinued EMTRIVA (emtricitabine) or VIREAD (tenofovir DF), which are components of ATRIPLA.

17.5 New Onset or Worsening Renal Impairment

Renal impairment, including cases of acute renal failure and Fanconi syndrome, has been reported. ATRIPLA should be avoided with concurrent or recent use of a nephrotoxic agent *[See Warnings and Precautions (5.7)]*.

17.6 Decreases in Bone Mineral Density

Patients should be informed that decreases in bone mineral density have been observed with the use of tenofovir DF. Bone mineral density monitoring may be performed in patients who have a history of pathologic bone fracture or other risk factors for osteoporosis or bone loss *[See Warnings and Precautions (5.11)]*.

17.7 Dosing Instructions

Patients should be advised to take ATRIPLA orally on an empty stomach and that it is important to take ATRIPLA on a regular dosing schedule to avoid missing doses.

17.8 Nervous System Symptoms

Patients should be informed that central nervous system symptoms (NSS) including dizziness, insomnia, impaired concentration, drowsiness, and abnormal dreams are commonly reported during the first weeks of therapy with efavirenz. Dosing at bedtime may improve the tolerability of these symptoms, which are likely to improve with continued therapy. Patients should be alerted to the potential for additive effects when ATRIPLA (efavirenz/emtricitabine/tenofovir disoproxil fumarate) is used concomitantly with alcohol or psychoactive drugs. Patients should be instructed that if they experience NSS they should avoid potentially hazardous tasks such as driving or operating machinery *[See Warnings and Precautions (5.6) and Dosage and Administration (2)]*.

17.9 Psychiatric Symptoms

Patients should be informed that serious psychiatric symptoms including severe depression, suicide attempts, aggressive behavior, delusions, paranoia, and psychosis-like symptoms have been reported in patients receiving efavirenz. If they experience severe psychiatric adverse experiences they should seek immediate medical evaluation. Patients should be advised to inform their physician of any history of mental illness or substance abuse *[See Warnings and Precautions (5.5)]*.

17.10 Rash

Patients should be informed that a common side effect is rash. Rashes usually go away without any change in treatment. However, since rash may be serious, patients should be advised to contact their physician promptly if rash occurs.

17.11 Reproductive Risk Potential

Women receiving ATRIPLA (efavirenz/emtricitabine/tenofovir disoproxil fumarate) should be instructed to avoid pregnancy *[See Warnings and Precautions (5.8)]*. A reliable form of barrier contraception must always be used in combination with other methods of contraception, including oral or other hormonal contraception. Because of the long half-life of efavirenz, use of adequate contraceptive measures for 12 weeks after discontinuation of ATRIPLA is recommended. Women should be advised to notify their physician if they become pregnant or plan to become pregnant while taking ATRIPLA. If this drug is used during the first trimester of pregnancy, or if the patient becomes pregnant while taking this drug, she should be apprised of the potential harm to the fetus.

Table 8: Drug Interactions: Changes in Pharmacokinetic Parameters for Coadministered Drug in the Presence of Tenofovir Disoproxil Fumarate*,†

Coadministered Drug	Dose of Coadministered Drug (mg)	N	Mean % Change of Coadministered Drug Pharmacokinetic Parameters‡ (90% CI)		
			C_{max}	AUC	C_{min}
Atazanavir§	400 once daily × 14 days	34	↓ 21 (↓ 27 to ↓ 14)	↓ 25 (↓ 30 to ↓ 19)	↓ 40 (↓ 48 to ↓ 32)
	Atazanavir/ritonavir 300/100 once daily × 42 days	10	↓ 28 (↓ 50 to ↑ 5)	↓ 25¶ (↓ 42 to ↓ 3)	↓ 23¶ (↓ 46 to ↑ 10)
Didanosine#	250 once, simultaneously with tenofovir DF and a light mealÞ	33	↓ 20ß (↓ 32 to ↓ 7)	↔ß	NA
Lopinavir	Lopinavir/ritonavir 400/100 twice daily × 14 days	24	↔	↔	↔
Ritonavir	Lopinavir/ritonavir 400/100 twice daily × 14 days	24	↔	↔	↔

* All interaction trials conducted in healthy volunteers.
† Subjects received tenofovir DF 300 mg once daily.
‡ Increase = ↑; Decrease = ↓; No Effect = ↔
§ Reyataz Prescribing Information.
¶ In HIV-infected patients, addition of tenofovir DF to atazanavir 300 mg plus ritonavir 100 mg, resulted in AUC and C_{min} values of atazanavir that were 2.3- and 4-fold higher than the respective values observed for atazanavir 400 mg when given alone.
# Videx EC Prescribing Information. Subjects received didanosine enteric-coated capsules.
Þ 373 kcal, 8.2 g fat.
ß Compared with didanosine (enteric-coated) 400 mg administered alone under fasting conditions.

Table 9: Outcomes of Randomized Treatment at Weeks 48 and 144 (Study 934)

Outcomes	At Week 48		At Week 144	
	FTC + TDF + EFV (N=244)	AZT/3TC + EFV (N=243)	FTC + TDF + EFV (N=227)*	AZT/3TC + EFV (N=229)*
Responder†	84%	73%	71%	58%
Virologic failure‡	2%	4%	3%	6%
Rebound	1%	3%	2%	5%
Never suppressed	0%	0%	0%	0%
Change in antiretroviral regimen	1%	1%	1%	1%
Death	<1%	1%	1%	1%
Discontinued due to adverse event	4%	9%	5%	12%
Discontinued for other reasons§	10%	14%	20%	22%

* Subjects who were responders at Week 48 or Week 96 (HIV-1 RNA <400 copies/mL) but did not consent to continue trial after Week 48 or Week 96 were excluded from analysis.
† Subjects achieved and maintained confirmed HIV-1 RNA <400 copies/mL through Weeks 48 and 144.
‡ Includes confirmed viral rebound and failure to achieve confirmed HIV-1 RNA <400 copies/mL through Weeks 48 and 144.
§ Includes lost to follow-up, patient withdrawal, noncompliance, protocol violation and other reasons.

Patient Information
ATRIPLA® (uh TRIP luh) Tablets

ALERT: Find out about medicines that should NOT be taken with ATRIPLA (efavirenz/emtricitabine/tenofovir disoproxil fumarate).

Please also read the section **"MEDICINES YOU SHOULD NOT TAKE WITH ATRIPLA."**

Generic name: efavirenz, emtricitabine and tenofovir disoproxil fumarate (eh FAH vih renz, em tri SIT uh bean and te NOE' fo veer dye soe PROX il FYOU mar ate)

Read the Patient Information that comes with ATRIPLA before you start taking it and each time you get a refill since there may be new information. This information does not take the place of talking to your healthcare provider about your medical condition or treatment. You should stay under a healthcare provider's care when taking ATRIPLA. **Do not change or stop your medicine without first talking with your healthcare provider.** Talk to your healthcare provider or pharmacist if you have any questions about ATRIPLA.

What is the most important information I should know about ATRIPLA?

- **Some people who have taken medicine like ATRIPLA (which contains nucleoside analogs) have developed a serious condition called lactic acidosis** (build up of an acid in the blood). Lactic acidosis can be a medical emergency and may need to be treated in the hospital. **Call your healthcare provider right away if you get the following signs or symptoms of lactic acidosis:**
  - You feel very weak or tired.
  - You have unusual (not normal) muscle pain.
  - You have trouble breathing.
  - You have stomach pain with nausea and vomiting.
  - You feel cold, especially in your arms and legs.
  - You feel dizzy or lightheaded.
  - You have a fast or irregular heartbeat.
- **Some people who have taken medicines like ATRIPLA have developed serious liver problems called hepatotoxicity,** with liver enlargement (hepatomegaly) and fat in the liver (steatosis). **Call your healthcare provider right away if you get the following signs or symptoms of liver problems:**
  - Your skin or the white part of your eyes turns yellow (jaundice).
  - Your urine turns dark.
  - Your bowel movements (stools) turn light in color.
  - You don't feel like eating food for several days or longer.
  - You feel sick to your stomach (nausea).
  - You have lower stomach area (abdominal) pain.
- **You may be more likely to get lactic acidosis or liver problems** if you are female, very overweight (obese), or have been taking nucleoside analog-containing medicines, like ATRIPLA, for a long time.
- **If you also have hepatitis B virus (HBV) infection and you stop taking ATRIPLA, you may get a "flare-up" of your hepatitis. A "flare-up" is when the disease suddenly returns in a worse way than before.** Patients with HBV who stop taking ATRIPLA need close medical follow-up for several months, including medical exams and blood tests to check for hepatitis that could be getting worse. ATRIPLA is not approved for the treatment of HBV, so you must discuss your HBV therapy with your healthcare provider.

What is ATRIPLA?

ATRIPLA contains 3 medicines, SUSTIVA® (efavirenz), EMTRIVA® (emtricitabine) and VIREAD® (tenofovir disoproxil fumarate also called tenofovir DF) combined in one pill. EMTRIVA and VIREAD are HIV-1 (human immunodeficiency virus) nucleoside analog reverse transcriptase inhibitors (NRTIs) and SUSTIVA is an HIV-1 non-nucleoside analog reverse transcriptase inhibitor (NNRTI). VIREAD and EMTRIVA are the components of TRUVADA®. ATRIPLA can be used alone as a complete regimen, or in combination with other anti-HIV-1 medicines to treat people with HIV-1 infection. ATRIPLA is for adults and children 12 years of age and older who weigh at least 40 kg (at least 88 lbs). ATRIPLA is not recommended for children younger than 12 years of age. ATRIPLA has not been studied in adults over 65 years of age.

HIV infection destroys $CD4^+$ T cells, which are important to the immune system. The immune system helps fight infection. After a large number of T cells are destroyed, acquired immune deficiency syndrome (AIDS) develops.

ATRIPLA helps block HIV-1 reverse transcriptase, a viral chemical in your body (enzyme) that is needed for HIV-1 to multiply. ATRIPLA lowers the amount of HIV-1 in the blood (viral load). ATRIPLA may also help to increase the number of T cells ($CD4^+$ cells), allowing your immune system to improve. Lowering the amount of HIV-1 in the blood lowers the chance of death or infections that happen when your immune system is weak (opportunistic infections).

Does ATRIPLA cure HIV-1 or AIDS?

ATRIPLA does not cure HIV-1 infection or AIDS and you may continue to experience illnesses associated with HIV-1 infection, including opportunistic infections. You should remain under the care of a doctor when using ATRIPLA.

Who should not take ATRIPLA (efavirenz/emtricitabine/tenofovir disoproxil fumarate)?

Together with your healthcare provider, you need to decide whether ATRIPLA is right for you.

Do not take ATRIPLA if you are allergic to ATRIPLA or any of its ingredients. The active ingredients of ATRIPLA are efavirenz, emtricitabine, and tenofovir DF. See the end of this leaflet for a complete list of ingredients.

What should I tell my healthcare provider before taking ATRIPLA?

Tell your healthcare provider if you:

- **Are pregnant or planning to become pregnant** (see "What should I avoid while taking ATRIPLA?").
- **Are breastfeeding** (see "What should I avoid while taking ATRIPLA?").
- **Have kidney problems or are undergoing kidney dialysis treatment.**
- **Have bone problems.**
- **Have liver problems, including hepatitis B virus infection.** Your healthcare provider may want to do tests to check your liver while you take ATRIPLA or may switch you to another medicine.
- **Have ever had mental illness or are using drugs or alcohol.**
- **Have ever had seizures or are taking medicine for seizures.**

What important information should I know about taking other medicines with ATRIPLA?

ATRIPLA may change the effect of other medicines, including the ones for HIV-1, and may cause serious side effects. Your healthcare provider may change your other medicines or change their doses. Other medicines, including herbal products, may affect ATRIPLA. For this reason, **it is very important to** let all your healthcare providers and pharmacists know what medications, herbal supplements, or vitamins you are taking.

MEDICINES YOU SHOULD NOT TAKE WITH ATRIPLA

- The following medicines may cause serious and life-threatening side effects when taken with ATRIPLA. You should not take any of these medicines while taking ATRIPLA: Vascor (bepridil), Propulsid (cisapride), Versed (midazolam), Orap (pimozide), Halcion (triazolam), ergot medications (for example, Wigraine and Cafergot).
- ATRIPLA also should not be used with Combivir (lamivudine/zidovudine), COMPLERA®, EMTRIVA, Epivir, Epivir-HBV (lamivudine), Epzicom (abacavir sulfate/lamivudine), STRIBILD®, Trizivir (abacavir sulfate/lamivudine/zidovudine), TRUVADA, or VIREAD. ATRIPLA also should not be used with SUSTIVA unless recommended by your healthcare provider.
- Vfend (voriconazole) should not be taken with ATRIPLA since it may lose its effect or may increase the chance of having side effects from ATRIPLA.
- **Do not take St. John's wort (*Hypericum perforatum*), or products containing St. John's wort with ATRIPLA.** St. John's wort is an herbal product sold as a dietary supplement. Talk with your healthcare provider if you are taking or are planning to take St. John's wort. Taking St. John's wort may decrease ATRIPLA levels and lead to increased viral load and possible resistance to ATRIPLA or cross-resistance to other anti-HIV-1 drugs.
- ATRIPLA should not be used with HEPSERA® (adefovir dipivoxil).

It is also important to tell your healthcare provider if you are taking any of the following:

- Fortovase, Invirase (saquinavir), Biaxin (clarithromycin), Noxafil (posaconazole), Sporanox (itraconazole), or Victrelis (boceprevir); **these medicines may need to be replaced with another medicine when taken with ATRIPLA.**
- Calcium channel blockers such as Cardizem or Tiazac (diltiazem), Covera HS or Isoptin (verapamil) and others; Crixivan (indinavir), Selzentry (maraviroc); the immunosuppressant medicines cyclosporine (Gengraf, Neoral, Sandimmune, and others), Prograf (tacrolimus), or Rapamune (sirolimus); Methadone; Mycobutin (rifabutin); Rifampin; cholesterol-lowering medicines such as Lipitor (atorvastatin), Pravachol (pravastatin sodium), and Zocor (simvastatin); or the anti-depressant medications bupropion (Wellbutrin, Wellbutrin SR, Wellbutrin XL, and Zyban) or Zoloft (sertraline); **dose changes may be needed when these drugs are taken with ATRIPLA.**
- Videx, Videx EC (didanosine); tenofovir DF (a component of ATRIPLA) may increase the amount of didanosine in your blood, which could result in more side effects. **You may need to be monitored more carefully** if you are taking ATRIPLA and didanosine together. Also, the dose of didanosine may need to be changed.
- Reyataz (atazanavir sulfate) or Kaletra (lopinavir/ritonavir); these medicines may increase the amount of tenofovir DF (a component of ATRIPLA) in your blood, which could result in more side effects. Reyataz is not recommended with ATRIPLA. **You may need to be monitored more carefully** if you are taking ATRIPLA and Kaletra together. Also, the dose of Kaletra may need to be changed.
- Medicine for seizures [for example, Dilantin (phenytoin), Tegretol (carbamazepine), or phenobarbital]; your healthcare provider may want to switch you to another medicine or check drug levels in your blood from time to time.

These are not all the medicines that may cause problems if you take ATRIPLA (efavirenz/emtricitabine/tenofovir disoproxil fumarate). Be sure to tell your healthcare provider about all medicines that you take.

Keep a complete list of all the prescription and nonprescription medicines as well as any herbal remedies that you are taking, how much you take, and how often you take them. Make a new list when medicines or herbal remedies are added or stopped, or if the dose changes. Give copies of this list to all of your healthcare providers and pharmacists **every** time you visit your healthcare provider or fill a prescription. This will give your healthcare provider a complete picture of the medicines you use. Then he or she can decide the best approach for your situation.

How should I take ATRIPLA?

- Take the exact amount of ATRIPLA your healthcare provider prescribes. Never change the dose on your own. Do not stop this medicine unless your healthcare provider tells you to stop.
- You should take ATRIPLA on an empty stomach.
- Swallow ATRIPLA with water.
- Taking ATRIPLA at bedtime may make some side effects less bothersome.
- Do not miss a dose of ATRIPLA. If you forget to take ATRIPLA, take the missed dose right away, unless it is almost time for your next dose. Do not double the next dose. Carry on with your regular dosing schedule. If you need help in planning the best times to take your medicine, ask your healthcare provider or pharmacist.
- If you believe you took more than the prescribed amount of ATRIPLA, contact your local poison control center or emergency room right away.
- Tell your healthcare provider if you start any new medicine or change how you take old ones. Your doses may need adjustment.
- When your ATRIPLA supply starts to run low, get more from your healthcare provider or pharmacy. This is very important because the amount of virus in your blood may increase if the medicine is stopped for even a short time. The virus may develop resistance to ATRIPLA and become harder to treat.
- Your healthcare provider may want to do blood tests to check for certain side effects while you take ATRIPLA.

What should I avoid while taking ATRIPLA?

- **Women should not become pregnant while taking ATRIPLA and for 12 weeks after stopping it.** Serious birth defects have been seen in the babies of animals and women treated with efavirenz (a component of ATRIPLA) during pregnancy. It is not known whether efavirenz caused these defects. **Tell your healthcare provider right away if you are pregnant.** Also talk with your healthcare provider if you want to become pregnant.
- Women should not rely only on hormone-based birth control, such as pills, injections, or implants, because ATRIPLA may make these contraceptives ineffective. Women must use a reliable form of barrier contraception, such as a condom or diaphragm, even if they also use other methods of birth control. Efavirenz, a component of ATRIPLA, may remain in your blood for a time after therapy is stopped. Therefore, you should continue to use contraceptive measures for 12 weeks after you stop taking ATRIPLA.
- **Do not breastfeed if you are taking ATRIPLA.** Some of the medicines in ATRIPLA can be passed to your baby in your breast milk. We do not know whether it could harm your baby. Also, mothers with HIV-1 should not breastfeed because HIV-1 can be passed to the baby in the breast milk. Talk with your healthcare provider if you are breastfeeding. You should stop breastfeeding or may need to use a different medicine.
- Taking ATRIPLA with alcohol or other medicines causing similar side effects as ATRIPLA, such as drowsiness, may increase those side effects.
- Do not take any other medicines, including prescription and nonprescription medicines and herbal products, without checking with your healthcare provider.
- Avoid doing things that can spread HIV-1 to others.
  - **Do not share needles or other injection equipment.**
  - **Do not share personal items that can have blood or body fluids on them, like toothbrushes and razor blades.**
  - **Do not have any kind of sex without protection.** Always practice safe sex by using a latex or polyurethane condom to lower the chance of sexual contact with semen, vaginal secretions, or blood.

What are the possible side effects of ATRIPLA?

ATRIPLA may cause the following serious side effects:

- **Lactic acidosis** (buildup of an acid in the blood). Lactic acidosis can be a medical emergency and may need to be treated in the hospital. **Call your healthcare provider right away if you get signs of lactic acidosis.** (See "What is the most important information I should know about ATRIPLA?")
- **Serious liver problems (hepatotoxicity),** with liver enlargement (hepatomegaly) and fat in the liver (steatosis).

Call your healthcare provider right away if you get any signs of liver problems. (See "What is the most important information I should know about ATRIPLA?")

- **"Flare-ups" of hepatitis B virus (HBV) infection**, in which the disease suddenly returns in a worse way than before, can occur if you have HBV and you stop taking ATRIPLA (efavirenz/emtricitabine/tenofovir disoproxil fumarate). Your healthcare provider will monitor your condition for several months after stopping ATRIPLA if you have both HIV-1 and HBV infection and may recommend treatment for your HBV. ATRIPLA is not approved for the treatment of hepatitis B virus infection. If you have advanced liver disease and stop treatment with ATRIPLA, the "flare-up" of hepatitis B may cause your liver function to decline.
- **Serious psychiatric problems.** A small number of patients may experience severe depression, strange thoughts, or angry behavior while taking ATRIPLA. Some patients have thoughts of suicide and a few have actually committed suicide. These problems may occur more often in patients who have had mental illness. Contact your healthcare provider right away if you think you are having these psychiatric symptoms, so your healthcare provider can decide if you should continue to take ATRIPLA.
- **Kidney problems** (including decline or failure of kidney function). If you have had kidney problems in the past or take other medicines that can cause kidney problems, your healthcare provider should do regular blood tests to check your kidneys. Symptoms that may be related to kidney problems include a high volume of urine, thirst, muscle pain, and muscle weakness.
- **Other serious liver problems.** Some patients have experienced serious liver problems including liver failure resulting in transplantation or death. Most of these serious side effects occurred in patients with a chronic liver disease such as hepatitis infection, but there have also been a few reports in patients without any existing liver disease.
- **Changes in bone mineral density (thinning bones).** Laboratory tests show changes in the bones of patients treated with tenofovir DF, a component of ATRIPLA. Some HIV patients treated with tenofovir DF developed thinning of the bones (osteopenia) which could lead to fractures. If you have had bone problems in the past, your healthcare provider may need to do tests to check your bone mineral density or may prescribe medicines to help your bone mineral density. Additionally, bone pain and softening of the bone (which may contribute to fractures) may occur as a consequence of kidney problems.

Common side effects:

Patients may have dizziness, headache, trouble sleeping, drowsiness, trouble concentrating, and/or unusual dreams during treatment with ATRIPLA. These side effects may be reduced if you take ATRIPLA at bedtime on an empty stomach. They also tend to go away after you have taken the medicine for a few weeks. If you have these common side effects, such as dizziness, it does not mean that you will also have serious psychiatric problems, such as severe depression, strange thoughts, or angry behavior. Tell your healthcare provider right away if any of these side effects continue or if they bother you. It is possible that these symptoms may be more severe if ATRIPLA is used with alcohol or mood altering (street) drugs.

If you are dizzy, have trouble concentrating, or are drowsy, avoid activities that may be dangerous, such as driving or operating machinery.

Rash may be common. Rashes usually go away without any change in treatment. In a small number of patients, rash may be serious. If you develop a rash, call your healthcare provider right away. **Rash may be a serious problem in some children.** Tell your child's healthcare provider right away if you notice rash or any other side effects while your child is taking ATRIPLA.

Other common side effects include tiredness, upset stomach, vomiting, gas, and diarrhea.

Other possible side effects with ATRIPLA:

- Changes in body fat. Changes in body fat develop in some patients taking anti HIV-1 medicine. These changes may include an increased amount of fat in the upper back and neck ("buffalo hump"), in the breasts, and around the trunk. Loss of fat from the legs, arms, and face may also happen. The cause and long-term health effects of these fat changes are not known.
- Skin discoloration (small spots or freckles) may also happen with ATRIPLA.
- In some patients with advanced HIV infection (AIDS), signs and symptoms of inflammation from previous infections may occur soon after anti-HIV treatment is started. It is believed that these symptoms are due to an improvement in the body's immune response, enabling the body to fight infections that may have been present with no obvious symptoms. If you notice any symptoms of infection, please inform your doctor immediately.
- Additional side effects are inflammation of the pancreas, allergic reaction (including swelling of the face, lips, tongue, or throat), shortness of breath, pain, stomach pain, weakness and indigestion.

Tell your healthcare provider or pharmacist if you notice any side effects while taking ATRIPLA (efavirenz/emtricitabine/tenofovir disoproxil fumarate).

Contact your healthcare provider before stopping ATRIPLA because of side effects or for any other reason.

This is not a complete list of side effects possible with ATRIPLA. Ask your healthcare provider or pharmacist for a more complete list of side effects of ATRIPLA and all the medicines you will take.

How do I store ATRIPLA?

- **Keep ATRIPLA and all other medicines out of reach of children.**
- Store ATRIPLA at room temperature 77 °F (25 °C).
- Keep ATRIPLA in its original container and keep the container tightly closed.
- Do not keep medicine that is out of date or that you no longer need. If you throw any medicines away make sure that children will not find them.

General information about ATRIPLA:

Medicines are sometimes prescribed for conditions that are not mentioned in patient information leaflets. Do not use ATRIPLA for a condition for which it was not prescribed. Do not give ATRIPLA to other people, even if they have the same symptoms you have. It may harm them.

This leaflet summarizes the most important information about ATRIPLA. If you would like more information, talk with your healthcare provider. You can ask your healthcare provider or pharmacist for information about ATRIPLA that is written for health professionals.

Do not use ATRIPLA if the seal over bottle opening is broken or missing.

What are the ingredients of ATRIPLA?

Active Ingredients: efavirenz, emtricitabine, and tenofovir disoproxil fumarate

Inactive Ingredients: croscarmellose sodium, hydroxypropyl cellulose, microcrystalline cellulose, magnesium stearate, sodium lauryl sulfate. The film coating contains black iron oxide, polyethylene glycol, polyvinyl alcohol, red iron oxide, talc, and titanium dioxide.

June 2013

21-937-GS-012

Shown in Product Identification Guide, page 305

BARACLUDE® ℞
[BEAR ah klude]
(entecavir)
Tablets, for oral use
BARACLUDE®
(entecavir)
Oral Solution

HIGHLIGHTS OF PRESCRIBING INFORMATION

These highlights do not include all the information needed to use BARACLUDE safely and effectively. See full prescribing information for BARACLUDE.

BARACLUDE® (entecavir) Tablets, for oral use
BARACLUDE® (entecavir) Oral Solution
Initial U.S. Approval: 2005

WARNING: SEVERE ACUTE EXACERBATIONS OF HEPATITIS B, PATIENTS CO-INFECTED WITH HIV AND HBV, and LACTIC ACIDOSIS AND HEPATOMEGALY

See full prescribing information for complete boxed warning.

- **Severe acute exacerbations of hepatitis B have been reported in patients who have discontinued anti-hepatitis B therapy, including entecavir. Hepatic function should be monitored closely for at least several months after discontinuation. Initiation of anti-hepatitis B therapy may be warranted. (5.1)**
- **BARACLUDE is not recommended for patients co-infected with human immunodeficiency virus (HIV) and hepatitis B virus (HBV) who are not also receiving highly active antiretroviral therapy (HAART), because of the potential for the development of resistance to HIV nucleoside reverse transcriptase inhibitors. (5.2)**
- **Lactic acidosis and severe hepatomegaly with steatosis, including fatal cases, have been reported with the use of nucleoside analogues. (5.3)**

INDICATIONS AND USAGE

BARACLUDE is a nucleoside analogue indicated for the treatment of chronic hepatitis B virus infection in adults with evidence of active viral replication and either evidence of persistent elevations in serum aminotransferases (ALT or AST) or histologically active disease. (1)

DOSAGE AND ADMINISTRATION

- Nucleoside-treatment-naïve with compensated liver disease (greater than or equal to 16 years old): 0.5 mg once daily. (2.1)
- Lamivudine-refractory or known lamivudine or telbivudine resistance mutations (greater than or equal to 16 years old): 1 mg once daily. (2.1)
- Decompensated liver disease (adults): 1 mg once daily. (2.1)
- Renal impairment: Dosage adjustment is recommended if creatinine clearance is less than 50 mL/min. (2.2)
- BARACLUDE should be administered on an empty stomach. (2)

DOSAGE FORMS AND STRENGTHS

- Tablets: 0.5 mg and 1 mg (3, 16)
- Oral solution: 0.05 mg/mL (3, 16)

CONTRAINDICATIONS

- None. (4)

WARNINGS AND PRECAUTIONS

- Severe acute exacerbations of hepatitis B virus infection after discontinuation: Monitor hepatic function closely for at least several months. (5.1, 6.1)
- Co-infection with HIV: BARACLUDE is not recommended unless the patient is also receiving HAART. (5.2)
- Lactic acidosis and severe hepatomegaly with steatosis: If suspected, treatment should be suspended. (5.3)

ADVERSE REACTIONS

- Most common adverse reactions (≥3%, all severity grades) are headache, fatigue, dizziness, and nausea. (6.1)

To report SUSPECTED ADVERSE REACTIONS, contact Bristol-Myers Squibb at 1-800-721-5072 or FDA at 1-800-FDA-1088 or www.fda.gov/medwatch

USE IN SPECIFIC POPULATIONS

- Nursing mothers: Discontinue nursing or BARACLUDE taking into consideration the importance of BARACLUDE to the mother. (8.3)
- Liver transplant recipients: Limited data on safety and efficacy are available. (8.8)

See 17 for PATIENT COUNSELING INFORMATION and FDA-approved patient labeling

Revised: 10/2012

FULL PRESCRIBING INFORMATION: CONTENTS*

Table 1: Recommended Dosage of BARACLUDE in Patients with Renal Impairment

Creatinine Clearance (mL/min)	Usual Dose (0.5 mg)	Lamivudine-Refractory or Decompensated Liver Disease (1 mg)
≥50	0.5 mg once daily	1 mg once daily
30 to <50	0.25 mg once daily[a] **OR** 0.5 mg every 48 hours	0.5 mg once daily **OR** 1 mg every 48 hours
10 to <30	0.15 mg once daily[a] **OR** 0.5 mg every 72 hours	0.3 mg once daily[a] **OR** 1 mg every 72 hours
<10 Hemodialysis[b] or CAPD	0.05 mg once daily[a] **OR** 0.5 mg every 7 days	0.1 mg once daily[a] **OR** 1 mg every 7 days

[a] For doses less than 0.5 mg, BARACLUDE Oral Solution is recommended.
[b] If administered on a hemodialysis day, administer BARACLUDE after the hemodialysis session.

Table 2: Clinical Adverse Reactions[a] of Moderate-Severe Intensity (Grades 2–4) Reported in Four Entecavir Clinical Trials Through 2 Years

	Nucleoside-Naïve[b]		Lamivudine-Refractory[c]	
Body System/ Adverse Reaction	**BARACLUDE 0.5 mg n=679**	**Lamivudine 100 mg n=668**	**BARACLUDE 1 mg n=183**	**Lamivudine 100 mg n=190**
Any Grade 2–4 adverse reaction[a]	15%	18%	22%	23%
Gastrointestinal				
Diarrhea	<1%	0	1%	0
Dyspepsia	<1%	<1%	1%	0
Nausea	<1%	<1%	<1%	2%
Vomiting	<1%	<1%	<1%	0
General				
Fatigue	1%	1%	3%	3%
Nervous System				
Headache	2%	2%	4%	1%
Dizziness	<1%	<1%	0	1%
Somnolence	<1%	<1%	0	0
Psychiatric				
Insomnia	<1%	<1%	0	<1%

[a] Includes events of possible, probable, certain, or unknown relationship to treatment regimen.
[b] Studies AI463022 and AI463027.
[c] Includes Study AI463026 and the BARACLUDE 1 mg and lamivudine treatment arms of Study AI463014, a Phase 2 multinational, randomized, double-blind study of three doses of BARACLUDE (0.1, 0.5, and 1 mg) once daily versus continued lamivudine 100 mg once daily for up to 52 weeks in subjects who experienced recurrent viremia on lamivudine therapy.

* Sections or subsections omitted from the full prescribing information are not listed

FULL PRESCRIBING INFORMATION

WARNING: SEVERE ACUTE EXACERBATIONS OF HEPATITIS B, PATIENTS CO-INFECTED WITH HIV AND HBV, and LACTIC ACIDOSIS AND HEPATOMEGALY

Severe acute exacerbations of hepatitis B have been reported in patients who have discontinued anti-hepatitis B therapy, including entecavir. Hepatic function should be monitored closely with both clinical and laboratory follow-up for at least several months in patients who discontinue anti-hepatitis B therapy. If appropriate, initiation of anti-hepatitis B therapy may be warranted [see *Warnings and Precautions (5.1)*].

Limited clinical experience suggests there is a potential for the development of resistance to HIV (human immunodeficiency virus) nucleoside reverse transcriptase inhibitors if BARACLUDE is used to treat chronic hepatitis B virus (HBV) infection in patients with HIV infection that is not being treated. Therapy with BARACLUDE is not recommended for HIV/HBV co-infected patients who are not also receiving highly active antiretroviral therapy (HAART) [see *Warnings and Precautions (5.2)*].

Lactic acidosis and severe hepatomegaly with steatosis, including fatal cases, have been reported with the use of nucleoside analogues alone or in combination with antiretrovirals [see *Warnings and Precautions (5.3)*].

1 INDICATIONS AND USAGE

BARACLUDE® (entecavir) is indicated for the treatment of chronic hepatitis B virus infection in adults with evidence of active viral replication and either evidence of persistent elevations in serum aminotransferases (ALT or AST) or histologically active disease.

The following points should be considered when initiating therapy with BARACLUDE (entecavir):

- This indication is based on histologic, virologic, biochemical, and serologic responses in nucleoside-treatment-naïve and lamivudine-resistant adult subjects with HBeAg-positive or HBeAg-negative chronic HBV infection and compensated liver disease [see *Clinical Studies (14)*].
- Virologic, biochemical, serologic, and safety data are available from a controlled study in adult subjects with chronic HBV infection and decompensated liver disease [see *Adverse Reactions (6.1)* and *Clinical Studies (14.1)*].
- Virologic, biochemical, serologic, and safety data are available for a limited number of adult subjects with HIV/HBV co-infection who have received prior lamivudine therapy [see *Warnings and Precautions (5.2)* and *Clinical Studies (14.1)*].

2 DOSAGE AND ADMINISTRATION

BARACLUDE should be administered on an empty stomach (at least 2 hours after a meal and 2 hours before the next meal).

2.1 Recommended Dosage

Compensated Liver Disease

The recommended dose of BARACLUDE for chronic hepatitis B virus infection in nucleoside-treatment-naïve adults and adolescents 16 years of age and older is 0.5 mg once daily.

The recommended dose of BARACLUDE in adults and adolescents (at least 16 years of age) with a history of hepatitis B viremia while receiving lamivudine or known lamivudine or telbivudine resistance mutations rtM204I/V with or without rtL180M, rtL80I/V, or rtV173L is 1 mg once daily.

Decompensated Liver Disease

The recommended dose of BARACLUDE for chronic hepatitis B virus infection in adults with decompensated liver disease is 1 mg once daily.

Oral Solution

BARACLUDE (entecavir) Oral Solution contains 0.05 mg of entecavir per milliliter. Therefore, 10 mL of the oral solution provides a 0.5 mg dose and 20 mL provides a 1 mg dose of entecavir.

2.2 Renal Impairment

In subjects with renal impairment, the apparent oral clearance of entecavir decreased as creatinine clearance decreased [see *Clinical Pharmacology (12.3)*]. Dosage adjustment is recommended for patients with creatinine clearance less than 50 mL/min, including patients on hemodialysis or continuous ambulatory peritoneal dialysis (CAPD), as shown in Table 1. The once-daily dosing regimens are preferred.

[See table 1 above]

2.3 Hepatic Impairment

No dosage adjustment is necessary for patients with hepatic impairment.

2.4 Duration of Therapy

The optimal duration of treatment with BARACLUDE for patients with chronic hepatitis B virus infection and the relationship between treatment and long-term outcomes such as cirrhosis and hepatocellular carcinoma are unknown.

3 DOSAGE FORMS AND STRENGTHS

- BARACLUDE 0.5 mg film-coated tablets are white to off-white, triangular-shaped, and debossed with "BMS" on one side and "1611" on the other side.
- BARACLUDE 1 mg film-coated tablets are pink, triangular-shaped, and debossed with "BMS" on one side and "1612" on the other side.
- BARACLUDE oral solution, 0.05 mg/mL, is a ready-to-use, orange-flavored, clear, colorless to pale yellow, aqueous solution.

4 CONTRAINDICATIONS

None.

5 WARNINGS AND PRECAUTIONS

5.1 Severe Acute Exacerbations of Hepatitis B

Severe acute exacerbations of hepatitis B have been reported in patients who have discontinued anti-hepatitis B therapy, including entecavir [see *Adverse Reactions (6.1)*]. Hepatic function should be monitored closely with both clinical and laboratory follow-up for at least several months in patients who discontinue anti-hepatitis B therapy. If appropriate, initiation of anti-hepatitis B therapy may be warranted.

5.2 Patients Co-infected with HIV and HBV

BARACLUDE has not been evaluated in HIV/HBV co-infected patients who were not simultaneously receiving effective HIV treatment. Limited clinical experience suggests there is a potential for the development of resistance to HIV nucleoside reverse transcriptase inhibitors if BARACLUDE is used to treat chronic hepatitis B virus infection in patients with HIV infection that is not being treated [see *Microbiology (12.4)*]. Therefore, therapy with BARACLUDE is not recommended for HIV/HBV co-infected patients who are not also receiving HAART. Before initiating BARACLUDE therapy, HIV antibody testing should be offered to all patients. BARACLUDE has not been studied as a treatment for HIV infection and is not recommended for this use.

5.3 Lactic Acidosis and Severe Hepatomegaly with Steatosis

Lactic acidosis and severe hepatomegaly with steatosis, including fatal cases, have been reported with the use of nucleoside analogues, including BARACLUDE, alone or in combination with antiretrovirals. A majority of these cases have been in women. Obesity and prolonged nucleoside exposure may be risk factors. Particular caution should be exercised when administering nucleoside analogues to any patient with known risk factors for liver disease; however, cases have also been reported in patients with no known risk factors.

Lactic acidosis with BARACLUDE use has been reported, often in association with hepatic decompensation, other serious medical conditions, or drug exposures. Patients with decompensated liver disease may be at higher risk for lactic acidosis. Treatment with BARACLUDE should be suspended in any patient who develops clinical or laboratory findings suggestive of lactic acidosis or pronounced hepatotoxicity (which may include hepatomegaly and steatosis even in the absence of marked transaminase elevations).

6 ADVERSE REACTIONS

The following adverse reactions are discussed in other sections of the labeling:

- Exacerbations of hepatitis after discontinuation of treatment [see *Boxed Warning, Warnings and Precautions (5.1)*].
- Lactic acidosis and severe hepatomegaly with steatosis [see *Boxed Warning, Warnings and Precautions (5.3)*].

6.1 Clinical Trial Experience

Because clinical trials are conducted under widely varying conditions, adverse reaction rates observed in the clinical trials of a drug cannot be directly compared to rates in the clinical trials of another drug and may not reflect the rates observed in practice.

Compensated Liver Disease

Assessment of adverse reactions is based on four studies (AI463014, AI463022, AI463026, and AI463027) in which 1720 subjects with chronic hepatitis B virus infection and compensated liver disease received double-blind treatment with BARACLUDE 0.5 mg/day (n=679), BARACLUDE 1 mg/day (n=183), or lamivudine (n=858) for up to 2 years. Median duration of therapy was 69 weeks for BARACLUDE-treated subjects and 63 weeks for lamivudine-treated subjects in Studies AI463022 and AI463027 and 73 weeks for BARACLUDE-treated subjects and 51 weeks for lamivudine-treated subjects in Studies AI463026 and AI463014. The safety profiles of BARACLUDE (entecavir) and lamivudine were comparable in these studies.

The most common adverse reactions of any severity (≥3%) with at least a possible relation to study drug for BARACLUDE-treated subjects were headache, fatigue, dizziness, and nausea. The most common adverse reactions among lamivudine-treated subjects were headache, fatigue, and dizziness. One percent of BARACLUDE-treated subjects in these four studies compared with 4% of lamivudine-treated subjects discontinued for adverse events or abnormal laboratory test results.

Clinical adverse reactions of moderate-severe intensity and considered at least possibly related to treatment occurring during therapy in four clinical studies in which BARACLUDE was compared with lamivudine are presented in Table 2.

[See table 2 at top of previous page]

Laboratory Abnormalities

Frequencies of selected treatment-emergent laboratory abnormalities reported during therapy in four clinical trials of BARACLUDE compared with lamivudine are listed in Table 3.

[See table 3 above]

Table 3: Selected Treatment-Emergent[a] Laboratory Abnormalities Reported in Four Entecavir Clinical Trials Through 2 Years

Test	Nucleoside-Naïve[b] BARACLUDE 0.5 mg n=679	Nucleoside-Naïve[b] Lamivudine 100 mg n=668	Lamivudine-Refractory[c] BARACLUDE 1 mg n=183	Lamivudine-Refractory[c] Lamivudine 100 mg n=190
Any Grade 3–4 laboratory abnormality[d]	35%	36%	37%	45%
ALT >10 × ULN and >2 × baseline	2%	4%	2%	11%
ALT >5.0 × ULN	11%	16%	12%	24%
Albumin <2.5 g/dL	<1%	<1%	0	2%
Total bilirubin >2.5 × ULN	2%	2%	3%	2%
Lipase ≥2.1 × ULN	7%	6%	7%	7%
Creatinine >3.0 × ULN	0	0	0	0
Confirmed creatinine increase ≥0.5 mg/dL	1%	1%	2%	1%
Hyperglycemia, fasting >250 mg/dL	2%	1%	3%	1%
Glycosuria[e]	4%	3%	4%	6%
Hematuria[f]	9%	10%	9%	6%
Platelets <50,000/mm^3	<1%	<1%	<1%	<1%

[a] On-treatment value worsened from baseline to Grade 3 or Grade 4 for all parameters except albumin (any on-treatment value <2.5 g/dL), confirmed creatinine increase ≥0.5 mg/dL, and ALT >10 × ULN and >2 × baseline.
[b] Studies AI463022 and AI463027.
[c] Includes Study AI463026 and the BARACLUDE 1 mg and lamivudine treatment arms of Study AI463014, a Phase 2 multinational, randomized, double-blind study of three doses of BARACLUDE (0.1, 0.5, and 1 mg) once daily versus continued lamivudine 100 mg once daily for up to 52 weeks in subjects who experienced recurrent viremia on lamivudine therapy.
[d] Includes hematology, routine chemistries, renal and liver function tests, pancreatic enzymes, and urinalysis.
[e] Grade 3 = 3+, large, ≥ 500 mg/dL; Grade 4 = 4+, marked, severe.
[f] Grade 3 = 3+, large; Grade 4 = ≥ 4+, marked, severe, many.
ULN=upper limit of normal.

Among BARACLUDE-treated subjects in these studies, on-treatment ALT elevations greater than 10 times the upper limit of normal (ULN) and greater than 2 times baseline generally resolved with continued treatment. A majority of these exacerbations were associated with a ≥2 $\log_{10}$/mL reduction in viral load that preceded or coincided with the ALT elevation. Periodic monitoring of hepatic function is recommended during treatment.

Exacerbations of Hepatitis after Discontinuation of Treatment

An exacerbation of hepatitis or ALT flare was defined as ALT greater than 10 times ULN and greater than 2 times the subject's reference level (minimum of the baseline or last measurement at end of dosing). For all subjects who discontinued treatment (regardless of reason), Table 4 presents the proportion of subjects in each study who experienced post-treatment ALT flares. In these studies, a subset of subjects was allowed to discontinue treatment at or after 52 weeks if they achieved a protocol-defined response to therapy. If BARACLUDE is discontinued without regard to treatment response, the rate of post-treatment flares could be higher. [See also *Warnings and Precautions (5.1).*]

Table 4: Exacerbations of Hepatitis During Off-Treatment Follow-up, Subjects in Studies AI463022, AI463027, and AI463026

	Subjects with ALT Elevations >10 × ULN and >2 × Reference[a] BARACLUDE	Lamivudine
Nucleoside-naïve		
HBeAg-positive	4/174 (2%)	13/147 (9%)
HBeAg-negative	24/302 (8%)	30/270 (11%)
Lamivudine-refractory	6/52 (12%)	0/16

[a] Reference is the minimum of the baseline or last measurement at end of dosing. Median time to off-treatment exacerbation was 23 weeks for BARACLUDE-treated subjects and 10 weeks for lamivudine-treated subjects.

Decompensated Liver Disease

Study AI463048 was a randomized, open-label study of BARACLUDE 1 mg once daily versus adefovir dipivoxil 10 mg once daily given for up to 48 weeks in adult subjects with chronic HBV infection and evidence of hepatic decompensation, defined as a Child-Turcotte-Pugh (CTP) score of 7 or higher [see *Clinical Studies (14.1)*]. Among the 102 subjects receiving BARACLUDE, the most common treatment-emergent adverse events of any severity, regardless of causality, occurring through Week 48 were peripheral edema (16%), ascites (15%), pyrexia (14%), hepatic encephalopathy (10%), and upper respiratory infection (10%). Clinical adverse reactions not listed in Table 2 that were observed through Week 48 include blood bicarbonate decreased (2%) and renal failure (<1%).

Eighteen of 102 (18%) subjects treated with BARACLUDE (entecavir) and 18/89 (20%) subjects treated with adefovir dipivoxil died during the first 48 weeks of therapy. The majority of deaths (11 in the BARACLUDE group and 16 in the adefovir dipivoxil group) were due to liver-related causes such as hepatic failure, hepatic encephalopathy, hepatorenal syndrome, and upper gastrointestinal hemorrhage. The rate of hepatocellular carcinoma (HCC) through Week 48 was 6% (6/102) for subjects treated with BARACLUDE and 8%
(7/89) for subjects treated with adefovir dipivoxil. Five percent of subjects in either treatment arm discontinued therapy due to an adverse event through Week 48.

No subject in either treatment arm experienced an on-treatment hepatic flare (ALT >2 × baseline and >10 × ULN) through Week 48. Eleven of 102 (11%) subjects treated with BARACLUDE and 11/89 (13%) subjects treated with adefovir dipivoxil had a confirmed increase in serum creatinine of 0.5 mg/dL through Week 48.

HIV/HBV Co-infected

The safety profile of BARACLUDE 1 mg (n=51) in HIV/HBV co-infected subjects enrolled in Study AI463038 was similar to that of placebo (n=17) through 24 weeks of blinded treatment and similar to that seen in non-HIV infected subjects [see *Warnings and Precautions (5.2)*].

Liver Transplant Recipients

Among 65 subjects receiving BARACLUDE in an open-label, post-liver transplant trial [see *Use in Specific Populations (8.8)*], the frequency and nature of adverse events were consistent with those expected in patients who have received a liver transplant and the known safety profile of BARACLUDE.

6.2 Postmarketing Experience

The following adverse reactions have been reported during postmarketing use of BARACLUDE. Because these reactions were reported voluntarily from a population of unknown size, it is not possible to reliably estimate their frequency or establish a causal relationship to BARACLUDE exposure.

Immune system disorders: Anaphylactoid reaction.
Metabolism and nutrition disorders: Lactic acidosis.
Hepatobiliary disorders: Increased transaminases.
Skin and subcutaneous tissue disorders: Alopecia, rash.

7 DRUG INTERACTIONS

Since entecavir is primarily eliminated by the kidneys [see *Clinical Pharmacology (12.3)*], coadministration of BARACLUDE with drugs that reduce renal function or compete for active tubular secretion may increase serum concentrations of either entecavir or the coadministered drug. Coadministration of entecavir with lamivudine, adefovir dipivoxil, or tenofovir disoproxil fumarate did not result in significant drug interactions. The effects of coadministration of BARACLUDE with other drugs that are renally eliminated or are known to affect renal function have not been evaluated, and patients should be monitored closely for adverse events when BARACLUDE is coadministered with such drugs.

8 USE IN SPECIFIC POPULATIONS

8.1 Pregnancy

Pregnancy Category C

There are no adequate and well-controlled studies of BARACLUDE (entecavir) in pregnant women. When pregnant rats and rabbits received entecavir at 28 and 212 times the human exposure at the highest human dose, there were no signs of embryofetal toxicity. Because animal reproduction studies are not always predictive of human response, BARACLUDE should be used during pregnancy only if clearly needed and after careful consideration of the risks and benefits.

Pregnancy Registry: To monitor fetal outcomes of pregnant women exposed to entecavir, a pregnancy registry has been established. Healthcare providers are encouraged to register patients by calling 1-800-258-4263.

Developmental toxicity studies were performed in rats and rabbits. There were no signs of embryofetal or maternal toxicity when pregnant animals received oral entecavir at approximately 28 (rat) and 212 (rabbit) times the human exposure achieved at the highest recommended human dose of 1 mg/day. In rats, maternal toxicity, embryofetal toxicity (resorptions), lower fetal body weights, tail and vertebral malformations, reduced ossification (vertebrae, sternebrae, and phalanges), and extra lumbar vertebrae and ribs were observed at exposures 3100 times those in humans. In rabbits, embryofetal toxicity (resorptions), reduced ossification (hyoid), and an increased incidence of 13th rib were observed at exposures 883 times those in humans. In a peri-postnatal study, no adverse effects on offspring occurred when rats received oral entecavir at exposures greater than 94 times those in humans.

8.2 Labor and Delivery

There are no studies in pregnant women and no data on the effect of BARACLUDE on transmission of HBV from mother to infant. Therefore, appropriate interventions should be used to prevent neonatal acquisition of HBV.

8.3 Nursing Mothers

It is not known whether BARACLUDE is excreted into human milk; however, entecavir is excreted into the milk of rats. Because many drugs are excreted into human milk and because of the potential for serious adverse reactions in nursing infants from BARACLUDE, a decision should be made to discontinue nursing or to discontinue BARACLUDE taking into consideration the importance of continued hepatitis B therapy to the mother and the known benefits of breastfeeding.

8.4 Pediatric Use

Safety and effectiveness of entecavir in pediatric patients below the age of 16 years have not been established.

8.5 Geriatric Use

Clinical studies of BARACLUDE did not include sufficient numbers of subjects aged 65 years and over to determine whether they respond differently from younger subjects. Entecavir is substantially excreted by the kidney, and the risk of toxic reactions to this drug may be greater in patients with impaired renal function. Because elderly patients are more likely to have decreased renal function, care should be taken in dose selection, and it may be useful to monitor renal function [see *Dosage and Administration (2.2)*].

8.6 Racial/Ethnic Groups

There are no significant racial differences in entecavir pharmacokinetics. The safety and efficacy of BARACLUDE (entecavir) 0.5 mg once daily were assessed in a single-arm, open-label trial of HBeAg-positive or -negative, nucleoside-naïve, Black/African American (n=40) and Hispanic (n=6) subjects with chronic HBV infection. In this trial, 76% of subjects were male, the mean age was 42 years, 57% were HBeAg-positive, the mean baseline HBV DNA was 7.0 $\log_{10}$ IU/mL, and the mean baseline ALT was 162 U/L. At Week 48 of treatment, 32 of 46 (70%) subjects had HBV DNA <50 IU/mL (approximately 300 copies/mL), 31 of 46 (67%) subjects had ALT normalization (≤1 × ULN), and 12 of 26 (46%) HBeAg-positive subjects had HBe seroconversion. Safety data were similar to those observed in the larger controlled clinical trials.

Because of low enrollment, safety and efficacy have not been established in the US Hispanic population.

8.7 Renal Impairment

Dosage adjustment of BARACLUDE is recommended for patients with creatinine clearance less than 50 mL/min, including patients on hemodialysis or CAPD [see *Dosage and Administration (2.2)* and *Clinical Pharmacology (12.3)*].

8.8 Liver Transplant Recipients

The safety and efficacy of BARACLUDE were assessed in a single-arm, open-label trial in 65 subjects who received a liver transplant for complications of chronic HBV infection. Eligible subjects who had HBV DNA less than 172 IU/mL (approximately 1000 copies/mL) at the time of transplant were treated with BARACLUDE 1 mg once daily in addition to usual post-transplantation management, including hepatitis B immune globulin. The trial population was 82% male, 39% Caucasian, and 37% Asian, with a mean age of 49 years; 89% of subjects had HBeAg-negative disease at the time of transplant.

Four of the 65 subjects received 4 weeks or less of BARACLUDE (2 deaths, 1 retransplantation, and 1 protocol violation) and were not considered evaluable. Of the 61 subjects who received more than 4 weeks of BARACLUDE, 60 received hepatitis B immune globulin post-transplant. Fifty-three subjects (82% of all 65 subjects treated) completed the trial and had HBV DNA measurements at or after 72 weeks treatment post-transplant. All 53 subjects had HBV DNA <50 IU/mL (approximately 300 copies/mL). Eight evaluable subjects did not have HBV DNA data available at 72 weeks, including 3 subjects who died prior to study completion. No subjects had HBV DNA values ≥50 IU/mL while receiving BARACLUDE (plus hepatitis B immune globulin). All 61 evaluable subjects lost HBsAg post-transplant; 2 of these subjects experienced recurrence of measurable HBsAg without recurrence of HBV viremia. This trial was not designed to determine whether addition of BARACLUDE to hepatitis B immune globulin decreased the proportion of subjects with measurable HBV DNA post-transplant compared to hepatitis B immune globulin alone.

If BARACLUDE treatment is determined to be necessary for a liver transplant recipient who has received or is receiving an immunosuppressant that may affect renal function, such as cyclosporine or tacrolimus, renal function must be carefully monitored both before and during treatment with BARACLUDE [see *Dosage and Administration (2.2)* and *Clinical Pharmacology (12.3)*].

10 OVERDOSAGE

There is limited experience of entecavir overdosage reported in patients. Healthy subjects who received single entecavir doses up to 40 mg or multiple doses up to 20 mg/day for up to 14 days had no increase in or unexpected adverse events. If overdose occurs, the patient must be monitored for evidence of toxicity, and standard supportive treatment applied as necessary.

Following a single 1 mg dose of entecavir, a 4-hour hemodialysis session removed approximately 13% of the entecavir dose.

11 DESCRIPTION

BARACLUDE® (entecavir) is the tradename for entecavir, a guanosine nucleoside analogue with selective activity against HBV. The chemical name for entecavir is 2-amino-1,9-dihydro-9-[(*1S,3R,4S*)-4-hydroxy-3-(hydroxymethyl)-2-methylenecyclopentyl]-*6H*-purin-6-one, monohydrate. Its molecular formula is $C_{12}H_{15}N_5O_3 \cdot H_2O$, which corresponds to a molecular weight of 295.3. Entecavir has the following structural formula:

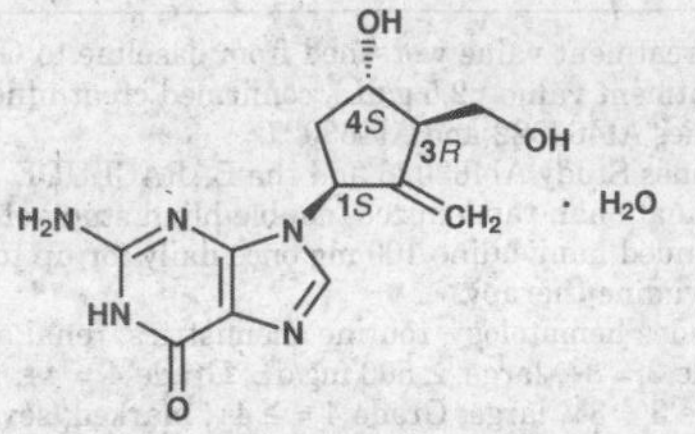

Entecavir is a white to off-white powder. It is slightly soluble in water (2.4 mg/mL), and the pH of the saturated solution in water is 7.9 at 25° C ± 0.5° C.

BARACLUDE film-coated tablets are available for oral administration in strengths of 0.5 mg and 1 mg of entecavir. BARACLUDE 0.5 mg and 1 mg film-coated tablets contain the following inactive ingredients: lactose monohydrate, microcrystalline cellulose, crospovidone, povidone, and magnesium stearate. The tablet coating contains titanium dioxide, hypromellose, polyethylene glycol 400, polysorbate 80 (0.5 mg tablet only), and iron oxide red (1 mg tablet only). BARACLUDE Oral Solution is available for oral administration as a ready-to-use solution containing 0.05 mg of entecavir per milliliter. BARACLUDE Oral Solution contains the following inactive ingredients: maltitol, sodium citrate, citric acid, methylparaben, propylparaben, and orange flavor.

12 CLINICAL PHARMACOLOGY

12.1 Mechanism of Action

Entecavir is an antiviral drug [see *Microbiology (12.4)*].

12.3 Pharmacokinetics

The single- and multiple-dose pharmacokinetics of entecavir were evaluated in healthy subjects and subjects with chronic hepatitis B virus infection.

Absorption

Following oral administration in healthy subjects, entecavir peak plasma concentrations occurred between 0.5 and 1.5 hours. Following multiple daily doses ranging from 0.1 to 1.0 mg, C_{max} and area under the concentration-time curve (AUC) at steady state increased in proportion to dose. Steady state was achieved after 6 to 10 days of once-daily administration with approximately 2-fold accumulation. For a 0.5 mg oral dose, C_{max} at steady state was 4.2 ng/mL and trough plasma concentration (C_{trough}) was 0.3 ng/mL. For a 1 mg oral dose, C_{max} was 8.2 ng/mL and C_{trough} was 0.5 ng/mL.

In healthy subjects, the bioavailability of the tablet was 100% relative to the oral solution. The oral solution and tablet may be used interchangeably.

Effects of food on oral absorption: Oral administration of 0.5 mg of entecavir with a standard high-fat meal (945 kcal, 54.6 g fat) or a light meal (379 kcal, 8.2 g fat) resulted in a delay in absorption (1.0–1.5 hours fed vs. 0.75 hours fasted), a decrease in C_{max} of 44%–46%, and a decrease in AUC of 18%–20% [see *Dosage and Administration (2)*].

Distribution

Based on the pharmacokinetic profile of entecavir after oral dosing, the estimated apparent volume of distribution is in excess of total body water, suggesting that entecavir is extensively distributed into tissues.

Binding of entecavir to human serum proteins *in vitro* was approximately 13%.

Metabolism and Elimination

Following administration of ^{14}C-entecavir in humans and rats, no oxidative or acetylated metabolites were observed. Minor amounts of phase II metabolites (glucuronide and sulfate conjugates) were observed. Entecavir is not a substrate, inhibitor, or inducer of the cytochrome P450 (CYP450) enzyme system [see *Drug Interactions,* below]. After reaching peak concentration, entecavir plasma concentrations decreased in a bi-exponential manner with a terminal elimination half-life of approximately 128–149 hours. The observed drug accumulation index is approximately 2-fold with once-daily dosing, suggesting an effective accumulation half-life of approximately 24 hours.

Entecavir is predominantly eliminated by the kidney with urinary recovery of unchanged drug at steady state ranging from 62% to 73% of the administered dose. Renal clearance is independent of dose and ranges from 360 to 471 mL/min suggesting that entecavir undergoes both glomerular filtration and net tubular secretion [see *Drug Interactions (7)*].

Special Populations

Gender: There are no significant gender differences in entecavir pharmacokinetics.

Race: There are no significant racial differences in entecavir pharmacokinetics.

Elderly: The effect of age on the pharmacokinetics of entecavir was evaluated following administration of a single 1 mg oral dose in healthy young and elderly volunteers. Entecavir AUC was 29.3% greater in elderly subjects compared to young subjects. The disparity in exposure between elderly and young subjects was most likely attributable to differences in renal function. Dosage adjustment of BARACLUDE (entecavir) should be based on the renal function of the patient, rather than age [see *Dosage and Administration (2.2)*].

Pediatrics: Pharmacokinetic studies have not been conducted in children.

Renal impairment: The pharmacokinetics of entecavir following a single 1 mg dose were studied in subjects (without chronic hepatitis B virus infection) with selected degrees of renal impairment, including subjects whose renal impairment was managed by hemodialysis or continuous ambulatory peritoneal dialysis (CAPD). Results are shown in Table 5 [see *Dosage and Administration (2.2)*].

[See table 5 below]

Following a single 1 mg dose of entecavir administered 2 hours before the hemodialysis session, hemodialysis removed approximately 13% of the entecavir dose over 4 hours. CAPD removed approximately 0.3% of the dose over 7 days [see *Dosage and Administration (2.2)*].

Hepatic impairment: The pharmacokinetics of entecavir following a single 1 mg dose were studied in subjects (without chronic hepatitis B virus infection) with moderate or severe hepatic impairment (Child-Turcotte-Pugh Class B or C). The pharmacokinetics of entecavir were similar between hepatically impaired and healthy control subjects; therefore, no dosage adjustment of BARACLUDE is recommended for patients with hepatic impairment.

Post-liver transplant: Limited data are available on the safety and efficacy of BARACLUDE in liver transplant recipients. In a small pilot study of entecavir use in HBV-infected liver transplant recipients on a stable dose of cyclosporine A (n=5) or tacrolimus (n=4), entecavir exposure was approximately 2-fold the exposure in healthy subjects with normal renal function. Altered renal function contributed to the increase in entecavir exposure in these subjects. The potential for pharmacokinetic interactions between entecavir and cyclosporine A or tacrolimus was not formally evaluated [see *Use in Specific Populations (8.8)*].

Drug Interactions

The metabolism of entecavir was evaluated in *in vitro* and *in vivo* studies. Entecavir is not a substrate, inhibitor, or inducer of the cytochrome P450 (CYP450) enzyme system. At concentrations up to approximately 10,000-fold higher than those obtained in humans, entecavir inhibited none of the major human CYP450 enzymes 1A2, 2C9, 2C19, 2D6, 3A4, 2B6, and 2E1. At concentrations up to approximately 340-fold higher than those observed in humans, entecavir did not induce the human CYP450 enzymes 1A2, 2C9, 2C19,

Table 5: Pharmacokinetic Parameters in Subjects with Selected Degrees of Renal Function

	Renal Function Group					
	Baseline Creatinine Clearance (mL/min)					
	Unimpaired >80 n=6	Mild >50–≤80 n=6	Moderate 30–50 n=6	Severe <30 n=6	Severe Managed with Hemodialysis[a] n=6	Severe Managed with CAPD n=4
C_{max} (ng/mL)	8.1	10.4	10.5	15.3	15.4	16.6
(CV%)	(30.7)	(37.2)	(22.7)	(33.8)	(56.4)	(29.7)
$AUC_{(0-T)}$ (ng•h/mL)	27.9	51.5	69.5	145.7	233.9	221.8
(CV)	(25.6)	(22.8)	(22.7)	(31.5)	(28.4)	(11.6)
CLR (mL/min)	383.2	197.9	135.6	40.3	NA	NA
(SD)	(101.8)	(78.1)	(31.6)	(10.1)		
CLT/F (mL/min)	588.1	309.2	226.3	100.6	50.6	35.7
(SD)	(153.7)	(62.6)	(60.1)	(29.1)	(16.5)	(19.6)

[a] Dosed immediately following hemodialysis.

CLR = renal clearance; CLT/F = apparent oral clearance.

3A4, 3A5, and 2B6. The pharmacokinetics of entecavir are unlikely to be affected by coadministration with agents that are either metabolized by, inhibit, or induce the CYP450 system. Likewise, the pharmacokinetics of known CYP substrates are unlikely to be affected by coadministration of entecavir.

The steady-state pharmacokinetics of entecavir and coadministered drug were not altered in interaction studies of entecavir with lamivudine, adefovir dipivoxil, and tenofovir disoproxil fumarate [see *Drug Interactions (7)*].

12.4 Microbiology

Mechanism of Action

Entecavir, a guanosine nucleoside analogue with activity against HBV reverse transcriptase (rt), is efficiently phosphorylated to the active triphosphate form, which has an intracellular half-life of 15 hours. By competing with the natural substrate deoxyguanosine triphosphate, entecavir triphosphate functionally inhibits all three activities of the HBV reverse transcriptase: (1) base priming, (2) reverse transcription of the negative strand from the pregenomic messenger RNA, and (3) synthesis of the positive strand of HBV DNA. Entecavir triphosphate is a weak inhibitor of cellular DNA polymerases α, β, and δ and mitochondrial DNA polymerase γ with K_i values ranging from 18 to >160 μM.

Antiviral Activity

Entecavir inhibited HBV DNA synthesis (50% reduction, EC_{50}) at a concentration of 0.004 μM in human HepG2 cells transfected with wild-type HBV. The median EC_{50} value for entecavir against lamivudine-resistant HBV (rtL180M, rtM204V) was 0.026 μM (range 0.010–0.059 μM).

The coadministration of HIV nucleoside/nucleotide reverse transcriptase inhibitors (NRTIs) with BARACLUDE (entecavir) is unlikely to reduce the antiviral efficacy of BARACLUDE against HBV or of any of these agents against HIV. In HBV combination assays in cell culture, abacavir, didanosine, lamivudine, stavudine, tenofovir, or zidovudine were not antagonistic to the anti-HBV activity of entecavir over a wide range of concentrations. In HIV antiviral assays, entecavir was not antagonistic to the cell culture anti-HIV activity of these six NRTIs or emtricitabine at concentrations greater than 100 times the C_{max} of entecavir using the 1 mg dose.

Antiviral Activity against HIV

A comprehensive analysis of the inhibitory activity of entecavir against a panel of laboratory and clinical HIV type 1 (HIV-1) isolates using a variety of cells and assay conditions yielded EC_{50} values ranging from 0.026 to >10 μM; the lower EC_{50} values were observed when decreased levels of virus were used in the assay. In cell culture, entecavir selected for an M184I substitution in HIV reverse transcriptase at micromolar concentrations, confirming inhibitory pressure at high entecavir concentrations. HIV variants containing the M184V substitution showed loss of susceptibility to entecavir.

Resistance

In Cell Culture

In cell-based assays, 8- to 30-fold reductions in entecavir phenotypic susceptibility were observed for lamivudine-resistant strains. Further reductions (>70-fold) in entecavir phenotypic susceptibility required the presence of amino acid substitutions rtM204I/V with or without rtL180M along with additional substitutions at residues rtT184, rtS202, or rtM250, or a combination of these substitutions with or without an rtI169 substitution in the HBV reverse transcriptase.

Clinical Studies

Nucleoside-naïve subjects: Genotypic evaluations were performed on evaluable samples (>300 copies/mL serum HBV DNA) from 562 subjects who were treated with BARACLUDE for up to 96 weeks in nucleoside-naïve studies (AI463022, AI463027, and rollover study AI463901). By Week 96, evidence of emerging amino acid substitution rtS202G with rtM204V and rtL180M substitutions was detected in the HBV of 2 subjects (2/562=<1%), and 1 of them experienced virologic rebound (≥1 log_{10} increase above nadir). In addition, emerging amino acid substitutions at rtM204I/V and rtL180M, rtL80I, or rtV173L, which conferred decreased phenotypic susceptibility to entecavir in the absence of rtT184, rtS202, or rtM250 changes, were detected in the HBV of 3 subjects (3/562=<1%) who experienced virologic rebound. For subjects who continued treatment beyond 48 weeks, 75% (202/269) had HBV DNA <300 copies/mL at end of dosing (up to 96 weeks).

HBeAg-positive (n=243) and -negative (n=39) treatment-naïve subjects who failed to achieve the study-defined complete response by 96 weeks were offered continued entecavir treatment in a rollover study. Complete response for HBeAg-positive was <0.7 MEq/mL (approximately 7 × 10^5 copies/mL) serum HBV DNA and HBeAg loss and, for HBeAg-negative was <0.7 MEq/mL HBV DNA and ALT normalization. Subjects received 1 mg entecavir once daily for up to an additional 144 weeks. Of these 282 subjects, 141 HBeAg-positive and 8 HBeAg-negative subjects entered the long-term follow-up rollover study and were evaluated for entecavir resistance. Of the 149 subjects entering the rollover study, 88% (131/149), 92% (137/149), and 92% (137/149) attained serum HBV DNA <300 copies/mL by Weeks 144, 192, and 240 (including end of dosing), respectively. No novel entecavir resistance-associated substitutions were identified in a comparison of the genotypes of evaluable isolates with their respective baseline isolates. The cumulative probability of developing rtT184, rtS202, or rtM250 entecavir resistance associated substitutions (in the presence of rtM204V and rtL180M substitutions) at Weeks 48, 96, 144, 192, and 240 was 0.2%, 0.5%, 1.2%, 1.2%, and 1.2%, respectively.

Lamivudine-refractory subjects: Genotypic evaluations were performed on evaluable samples from 190 subjects treated with BARACLUDE (entecavir) for up to 96 weeks in studies of lamivudine-refractory HBV (AI463026, AI463014, AI463015, and rollover study AI463901). By Week 96, resistance-associated amino acid substitutions at rtS202, rtT184, or rtM250, with or without rtI169 changes, in the presence of amino acid substitutions rtM204I/V with or without rtL180M, rtL80V, or rtV173L/M emerged in the HBV from 22 subjects (22/190=12%), 16 of whom experienced virologic rebound (≥1 log_{10} increase above nadir) and 4 of whom were never suppressed <300 copies/mL. The HBV from 4 of these subjects had entecavir resistance substitutions at baseline and acquired further changes on entecavir treatment. In addition to the 22 subjects, 3 subjects experienced virologic rebound with the emergence of rtM204I/V and rtL180M, rtL80V, or rtV173L/M. For isolates from subjects who experienced virologic rebound with the emergence of resistance substitutions (n=19), the median fold-change in entecavir EC_{50} values from reference was 19-fold at baseline and 106-fold at the time of virologic rebound. For subjects who continued treatment beyond 48 weeks, 40% (31/77) had HBV DNA <300 copies/mL at end of dosing (up to 96 weeks).

Lamivudine-refractory subjects (n=157) who failed to achieve the study-defined complete response by Week 96 were offered continued entecavir treatment. Subjects received 1 mg entecavir once daily for up to an additional 144 weeks. Of these subjects, 80 subjects entered the long-term follow-up study and were evaluated for entecavir resistance. By Weeks 144, 192, and 240 (including end of dosing), 34% (27/80), 35% (28/80), and 36% (29/80), respectively, attained HBV DNA <300 copies/mL. The cumulative probability of developing rtT184, rtS202, or rtM250 entecavir resistance-associated substitutions (in the presence of rtM204I/V with or without rtL180M substitutions) at Weeks 48, 96, 144, 192, and 240 was 6.2%, 15%, 36.3%, 46.6%, and 51.5%, respectively. The HBV of 6 subjects developed rtA181C/G/S/T amino acid substitutions while receiving entecavir, and of these, 4 developed entecavir resistance-associated substitutions at rtT184, rtS202, or rtM250 and 1 had an rtT184S substitution at baseline. Of 7 subjects whose HBV had an rtA181 substitution at baseline, 2 also had substitutions at rtT184, rtS202, or rtM250 at baseline and another 2 developed them while on treatment with entecavir.

Cross-resistance

Cross-resistance has been observed among HBV nucleoside analogues. In cell-based assays, entecavir had 8- to 30-fold less inhibition of HBV DNA synthesis for HBV containing lamivudine and telbivudine resistance substitutions rtM204I/V with or without rtL180M than for wild-type HBV. Substitutions rtM204I/V with or without rtL180M, rtL80I/V, or rtV173L, which are associated with lamivudine and telbivudine resistance, also confer decreased phenotypic susceptibility to entecavir. The efficacy of entecavir against HBV harboring adefovir resistance-associated substitutions has not been established in clinical trials. HBV isolates from lamivudine-refractory subjects failing entecavir therapy were susceptible in cell culture to adefovir but remained resistant to lamivudine. Recombinant HBV genomes encoding adefovir resistance-associated substitutions at either rtN236T or rtA181V had 0.3- and 1.1-fold shifts in susceptibility to entecavir in cell culture, respectively.

13 NONCLINICAL TOXICOLOGY

13.1 Carcinogenesis, Mutagenesis, Impairment of Fertility

Long-term oral carcinogenicity studies of entecavir in mice and rats were carried out at exposures up to approximately 42 times (mice) and 35 times (rats) those observed in humans at the highest recommended dose of 1 mg/day. In mouse and rat studies, entecavir was positive for carcinogenic findings.

In mice, lung adenomas were increased in males and females at exposures 3 and 40 times those in humans. Lung carcinomas in both male and female mice were increased at exposures 40 times those in humans. Combined lung adenomas and carcinomas were increased in male mice at exposures 3 times and in female mice at exposures 40 times those in humans. Tumor development was preceded by pneumocyte proliferation in the lung, which was not observed in rats, dogs, or monkeys administered entecavir, supporting the conclusion that lung tumors in mice may be a species-specific event. Hepatocellular carcinomas were increased in males and combined liver adenomas and carcinomas were also increased at exposures 42 times those in humans. Vascular tumors in female mice (hemangiomas of ovaries and uterus and hemangiosarcomas of spleen) were increased at exposures 40 times those in humans. In rats, hepatocellular adenomas were increased in females at exposures 24 times those in humans; combined adenomas and carcinomas were also increased in females at exposures 24 times those in humans. Brain gliomas were induced in both males and females at exposures 35 and 24 times those in humans. Skin fibromas were induced in females at exposures 4 times those in humans.

It is not known how predictive the results of rodent carcinogenicity studies may be for humans.

Entecavir was clastogenic to human lymphocyte cultures. Entecavir was not mutagenic in the Ames bacterial reverse mutation assay using *S. typhimurium* and *E. coli* strains in the presence or absence of metabolic activation, a mammalian-cell gene mutation assay, and a transformation assay with Syrian hamster embryo cells. Entecavir was also negative in an oral micronucleus study and an oral DNA repair study in rats. In reproductive toxicology studies, in which animals were administered entecavir at up to 30 mg/kg for up to 4 weeks, no evidence of impaired fertility was seen in male or female rats at systemic exposures greater than 90 times those achieved in humans at the highest recommended dose of 1 mg/day. In rodent and dog toxicology studies, seminiferous tubular degeneration was observed at exposures 35 times or greater than those achieved in humans. No testicular changes were evident in monkeys.

14 CLINICAL STUDIES

The safety and efficacy of BARACLUDE (entecavir) were evaluated in three Phase 3 active-controlled trials [see *(Clinical Studies 14.1, 14.2)*]. These studies included 1633 subjects 16 years of age or older with chronic hepatitis B virus infection (serum HBsAg-positive for at least 6 months) accompanied by evidence of viral replication (detectable serum HBV DNA, as measured by the bDNA hybridization or PCR assay). Subjects had persistently elevated ALT levels at least 1.3 times ULN and chronic inflammation on liver biopsy compatible with a diagnosis of chronic viral hepatitis. The safety and efficacy of BARACLUDE were also evaluated in a study of 191 HBV-infected subjects with decompensated liver disease and in a study of 68 subjects co-infected with HBV and HIV [see *Clinical Studies (14.1)*].

14.1 Outcomes at 48 Weeks

Nucleoside-naïve Subjects with Compensated Liver Disease

HBeAg-positive: Study AI463022 was a multinational, randomized, double-blind study of BARACLUDE 0.5 mg once daily versus lamivudine 100 mg once daily for a minimum of 52 weeks in 709 (of 715 randomized) nucleoside-naïve subjects with chronic hepatitis B virus infection, compensated liver disease, and detectable HBeAg. The mean age of subjects was 35 years, 75% were male, 57% were Asian, 40% were Caucasian, and 13% had previously received interferon-α. At baseline, subjects had a mean Knodell Necroinflammatory Score of 7.8, mean serum HBV DNA as measured by Roche COBAS Amplicor® PCR assay was 9.66 log_{10} copies/mL, and mean serum ALT level was 143 U/L. Paired, adequate liver biopsy samples were available for 89% of subjects.

HBeAg-negative (anti-HBe-positive/HBV DNA-positive): Study AI463027 was a multinational, randomized, double-blind study of BARACLUDE 0.5 mg once daily versus lamivudine 100 mg once daily for a minimum of 52 weeks in 638 (of 648 randomized) nucleoside-naïve subjects with HBeAg-negative (HBeAb-positive) chronic hepatitis B virus infection and compensated liver disease. The mean age of subjects was 44 years, 76% were male, 39% were Asian, 58% were Caucasian, and 13% had previously received interferon-α. At baseline, subjects had a mean Knodell Necroinflammatory Score of 7.8, mean serum HBV DNA as measured by Roche COBAS Amplicor PCR assay was 7.58 log_{10} copies/mL, and mean serum ALT level was 142 U/L. Paired, adequate liver biopsy samples were available for 88% of subjects.

In Studies AI463022 and AI463027, BARACLUDE was superior to lamivudine on the primary efficacy endpoint of Histologic Improvement, defined as a 2-point or greater reduction in Knodell Necroinflammatory Score with no worsening in Knodell Fibrosis Score at Week 48, and on the secondary efficacy measures of reduction in viral load and ALT normalization. Histologic Improvement and change in Ishak Fibrosis Score are shown in Table 6. Selected virologic, biochemical, and serologic outcome measures are shown in Table 7.

[See table 6 at top of next page]

[See table 7 at top of next page]

Table 6: Histologic Improvement and Change in Ishak Fibrosis Score at Week 48, Nucleoside-Naïve Subjects in Studies AI463022 and AI463027

	Study AI463022 (HBeAg-Positive)		Study AI463027 (HBeAg-Negative)	
	BARACLUDE 0.5 mg n=314[a]	Lamivudine 100 mg n=314[a]	BARACLUDE 0.5 mg n=296[a]	Lamivudine 100 mg n=287[a]
Histologic Improvement (Knodell Scores)				
Improvement[b]	72%	62%	70%	61%
No improvement	21%	24%	19%	26%
Ishak Fibrosis Score				
Improvement[c]	39%	35%	36%	38%
No change	46%	40%	41%	34%
Worsening[c]	8%	10%	12%	15%
Missing Week 48 biopsy	7%	14%	10%	13%

[a] Subjects with evaluable baseline histology (baseline Knodell Necroinflammatory Score ≥2).
[b] ≥2-point decrease in Knodell Necroinflammatory Score from baseline with no worsening of the Knodell Fibrosis Score.
[c] For Ishak Fibrosis Score, improvement = ≥1-point decrease from baseline and worsening = ≥1-point increase from baseline.

Table 7: Selected Virologic, Biochemical, and Serologic Endpoints at Week 48, Nucleoside-Naïve Subjects in Studies AI463022 and AI463027

	Study AI463022 (HBeAg-Positive)		Study AI463027 (HBeAg-Negative)	
	BARACLUDE 0.5 mg n=354	Lamivudine 100 mg n=355	BARACLUDE 0.5 mg n=325	Lamivudine 100 mg n=313
HBV DNA[a]				
Proportion undetectable (<300 copies/mL)	67%	36%	90%	72%
Mean change from baseline (log_{10} copies/mL)	–6.86	–5.39	–5.04	–4.53
ALT normalization (≤1 × ULN)	68%	60%	78%	71%
HBeAg seroconversion	21%	18%	NA	NA

[a] Roche COBAS Amplicor PCR assay [lower limit of quantification (LLOQ) = 300 copies/mL].

Histologic Improvement was independent of baseline levels of HBV DNA or ALT.

Lamivudine-refractory Subjects with Compensated Liver Disease

Study AI463026 was a multinational, randomized, double-blind study of BARACLUDE (entecavir) in 286 (of 293 randomized) subjects with lamivudine-refractory chronic hepatitis B virus infection and compensated liver disease. Subjects receiving lamivudine at study entry either switched to BARACLUDE 1 mg once daily (with neither a washout nor an overlap period) or continued on lamivudine 100 mg for a minimum of 52 weeks. The mean age of subjects was 39 years, 76% were male, 37% were Asian, 62% were Caucasian, and 52% had previously received interferon-α. The mean duration of prior lamivudine therapy was 2.7 years, and 85% had lamivudine resistance mutations at baseline by an investigational line probe assay. At baseline, subjects had a mean Knodell Necroinflammatory Score of 6.5, mean serum HBV DNA as measured by Roche COBAS Amplicor PCR assay was 9.36 log_{10} copies/mL, and mean serum ALT level was 128 U/L. Paired, adequate liver biopsy samples were available for 87% of subjects.

BARACLUDE was superior to lamivudine on a primary endpoint of Histologic Improvement (using the Knodell Score at Week 48). These results and change in Ishak Fibrosis Score are shown in Table 8. Table 9 shows selected virologic, biochemical, and serologic endpoints.

Table 8: Histologic Improvement and Change in Ishak Fibrosis Score at Week 48, Lamivudine-Refractory Subjects in Study AI463026

	BARACLUDE 1 mg n=124[a]	Lamivudine 100 mg n=116[a]
Histologic Improvement (Knodell Scores)		
Improvement[b]	55%	28%
No improvement	34%	57%
Ishak Fibrosis Score		
Improvement[c]	34%	16%
No change	44%	42%
Worsening[c]	11%	26%
Missing Week 48 biopsy	11%	16%

[a] Subjects with evaluable baseline histology (baseline Knodell Necroinflammatory Score ≥2).
[b] ≥2-point decrease in Knodell Necroinflammatory Score from baseline with no worsening of the Knodell Fibrosis Score.
[c] For Ishak Fibrosis Score, improvement = ≥1-point decrease from baseline and worsening = ≥1-point increase from baseline.

Table 9: Selected Virologic, Biochemical, and Serologic Endpoints at Week 48, Lamivudine-Refractory Subjects in Study AI463026

	BARACLUDE 1 mg n=141	Lamivudine 100 mg n=145
HBV DNA[a]		
Proportion undetectable (<300 copies/mL)	19%	1%
Mean change from baseline (log_{10} copies/mL)	–5.11	–0.48
ALT normalization (≤1 × ULN)	61%	15%
HBeAg seroconversion	8%	3%

[a] Roche COBAS Amplicor PCR assay (LLOQ = 300 copies/mL).

Histologic Improvement was independent of baseline levels of HBV DNA or ALT.

Subjects with Decompensated Liver Disease

Study AI463048 was a randomized, open-label study of BARACLUDE (entecavir) 1 mg once daily versus adefovir dipivoxil 10 mg once daily in 191 (of 195 randomized) adult subjects with HBeAg-positive or -negative chronic HBV infection and evidence of hepatic decompensation, defined as a Child-Turcotte-Pugh (CTP) score of 7 or higher. Subjects were either HBV-treatment-naïve or previously treated, predominantly with lamivudine or interferon-α.

In Study AI463048, 100 subjects were randomized to treatment with BARACLUDE and 91 subjects to treatment with adefovir dipivoxil. Two subjects randomized to treatment with adefovir dipivoxil actually received treatment with BARACLUDE (entecavir) for the duration of the study. The mean age of subjects was 52 years, 74% were male, 54% were Asian, 33% were Caucasian, and 5% were Black/African American. At baseline, subjects had a mean serum HBV DNA by PCR of 7.83 log_{10} copies/mL and mean ALT level of 100 U/L; 54% of subjects were HBeAg-positive; 35% had genotypic evidence of lamivudine resistance. The baseline mean CTP score was 8.6. Results for selected study endpoints at Week 48 are shown in Table 10.

Table 10: Selected Endpoints at Week 48, Subjects with Decompensated Liver Disease, Study AI463048

	BARACLUDE 1 mg n=100[a]	Adefovir Dipivoxil 10 mg n=91[a]
HBV DNA[b]		
Proportion undetectable (<300 copies/mL)	57%	20%
Stable or improved CTP score[c]	61%	67%
HBsAg loss	5%	0
Normalization of ALT (≤1 × ULN)[d]	49/78 (63%)	33/71 (46%)

[a] Endpoints were analyzed using intention-to-treat (ITT) method, treated subjects as randomized.
[b] Roche COBAS Amplicor PCR assay (LLOQ = 300 copies/mL).
[c] Defined as decrease or no change from baseline in CTP score.
[d] Denominator is subjects with abnormal values at baseline.
ULN=upper limit of normal.

Subjects Co-infected with HIV and HBV

Study AI463038 was a randomized, double-blind, placebo-controlled study of BARACLUDE versus placebo in 68 subjects co-infected with HIV and HBV who experienced recurrence of HBV viremia while receiving a lamivudine-containing highly active antiretroviral (HAART) regimen. Subjects continued their lamivudine-containing HAART regimen (lamivudine dose 300 mg/day) and were assigned to add either BARACLUDE 1 mg once daily (51 subjects) or placebo (17 subjects) for 24 weeks followed by an open-label phase for an additional 24 weeks where all subjects received BARACLUDE. At baseline, subjects had a mean serum HBV DNA level by PCR of 9.13 log_{10} copies/mL. Ninety-nine percent of subjects were HBeAg-positive at baseline, with a mean baseline ALT level of 71.5 U/L. Median HIV RNA level remained stable at approximately 2 log_{10} copies/mL through 24 weeks of blinded therapy. Virologic and biochemical endpoints at Week 24 are shown in Table 11. There are no data in patients with HIV/HBV co-infection who have not received prior lamivudine therapy. BARACLUDE has not been evaluated in HIV/HBV co-infected patients who were not simultaneously receiving effective HIV treatment [see *Warnings and Precautions (5.2)*].

Table 11: Virologic and Biochemical Endpoints at Week 24, Study AI463038

	BARACLUDE 1 mg[a] n=51	Placebo[a] n=17
HBV DNA[b]		
Proportion undetectable (<300 copies/mL)	6%	0
Mean change from baseline (log_{10} copies/mL)	–3.65	+0.11
ALT normalization (≤1 × ULN)	34%[c]	8%[c]

[a] All subjects also received a lamivudine-containing HAART regimen.
[b] Roche COBAS Amplicor PCR assay (LLOQ = 300 copies/mL).
[c] Percentage of subjects with abnormal ALT (>1 × ULN) at baseline who achieved ALT normalization (n=35 for BARACLUDE and n=12 for placebo).

For subjects originally assigned to BARACLUDE, at the end of the open-label phase (Week 48), 8% of subjects had HBV DNA <300 copies/mL by PCR, the mean change from baseline HBV DNA by PCR was –4.20 log_{10} copies/mL, and 37% of subjects with abnormal ALT at baseline had ALT normalization (≤1 × ULN).

14.2 Outcomes beyond 48 Weeks

The optimal duration of therapy with BARACLUDE is unknown. According to protocol-mandated criteria in the Phase 3 clinical trials, subjects discontinued BARACLUDE or lamivudine treatment after 52 weeks according to a definition of response based on HBV virologic suppression (<0.7 MEq/mL by bDNA assay) and loss of HBeAg (in HBeAg-positive subjects) or ALT <1.25 × ULN (in HBeAg-negative subjects) at Week 48. Subjects who achieved virologic suppression but did not have serologic response (HBeAg-positive) or did not achieve ALT <1.25 × ULN (HBeAg-negative) continued blinded dosing through 96 weeks or until the response criteria were met. These protocol-specified subject management guidelines are not intended as guidance for clinical practice.

Nucleoside-naïve subjects: Among nucleoside-naïve, HBeAg-positive subjects (Study AI463022), 243 (69%) BARACLUDE-treated subjects and 164 (46%) lamivudine-treated subjects continued blinded treatment for up to 96 weeks. Of those continuing blinded treatment in Year 2, 180 (74%) BARACLUDE (entecavir) subjects and 60 (37%) lamivudine subjects achieved HBV DNA <300 copies/mL by PCR at the end of dosing (up to 96 weeks). 193 (79%) BARACLUDE subjects achieved ALT ≤1 × ULN compared to 112 (68%) lamivudine subjects, and HBeAg seroconversion occurred in 26 (11%) BARACLUDE subjects and 20 (12%) lamivudine subjects.

Among nucleoside-naïve, HBeAg-positive subjects, 74 (21%) BARACLUDE subjects and 67 (19%) lamivudine subjects met the definition of response at Week 48, discontinued study drugs, and were followed off treatment for 24 weeks. Among BARACLUDE responders, 26 (35%) subjects had HBV DNA <300 copies/mL, 55 (74%) subjects had ALT ≤1 × ULN, and 56 (76%) subjects sustained HBeAg seroconversion at the end of follow-up. Among lamivudine responders, 20 (30%) subjects had HBV DNA <300 copies/mL, 41 (61%) subjects had ALT ≤1 × ULN, and 47 (70%) subjects sustained HBeAg seroconversion at the end of follow-up.

Among nucleoside-naïve, HBeAg-negative subjects (Study AI463027), 26 (8%) BARACLUDE-treated subjects and 28 (9%) lamivudine-treated subjects continued blinded treatment for up to 96 weeks. In this small cohort continuing treatment in Year 2, 22 BARACLUDE and 16 lamivudine subjects had HBV DNA <300 copies/mL by PCR, and 7 and 6 subjects, respectively, had ALT ≤1 × ULN at the end of dosing (up to 96 weeks).

Among nucleoside-naïve, HBeAg-negative subjects, 275 (85%) BARACLUDE subjects and 245 (78%) lamivudine subjects met the definition of response at Week 48, discontinued study drugs, and were followed off treatment for 24 weeks. In this cohort, very few subjects in each treatment arm had HBV DNA <300 copies/mL by PCR at the end of follow-up. At the end of follow-up, 126 (46%) BARACLUDE subjects and 84 (34%) lamivudine subjects had ALT ≤1 × ULN.

Lamivudine-refractory subjects: Among lamivudine-refractory subjects (Study AI463026), 77 (55%) BARACLUDE-treated subjects and 3 (2%) lamivudine subjects continued blinded treatment for up to 96 weeks. In this cohort of BARACLUDE subjects, 31 (40%) subjects achieved HBV DNA <300 copies/mL, 62 (81%) subjects had ALT ≤1 × ULN, and 8 (10%) subjects demonstrated HBeAg seroconversion at the end of dosing.

16 HOW SUPPLIED/STORAGE AND HANDLING

BARACLUDE® (entecavir) Tablets and Oral Solution are available in the following strengths and configurations of plastic bottles with child-resistant closures:

[See table above]

Product Strength and Dosage Form	Description	Quantity	NDC Number
0.5 mg film-coated tablet	White to off-white, triangular-shaped tablet, debossed with "BMS" on one side and "1611" on the other side.	30 tablets 90 tablets	0003-1611-12 0003-1611-13
1.0 mg film coated tablet	Pink, triangular-shaped tablet, debossed with "BMS" on one side and "1612" on the other side.	30 tablets	0003-1612-12
0.05 mg/mL oral solution	Ready-to-use, orange-flavored, clear, colorless to pale yellow, aqueous solution in a 260 mL bottle.	210 mL	0003-1614-12

BARACLUDE Oral Solution is a ready-to-use product; dilution or mixing with water or any other solvent or liquid product is not recommended. Each bottle of the oral solution is accompanied by a dosing spoon that is calibrated in 1 mL increments up to 10 mL [see *Patient Counseling Information (17.1)*].

Storage

BARACLUDE Tablets should be stored in a tightly closed container at 25° C (77° F); excursions permitted between 15–30° C (59–86° F) [see USP Controlled Room Temperature].

BARACLUDE Oral Solution should be stored in the outer carton at 25° C (77° F); excursions permitted between 15–30° C (59–86° F) [see USP Controlled Room Temperature]. Protect from light. After opening, the oral solution can be used up to the expiration date on the bottle. The bottle and its contents should be discarded after the expiration date.

17 PATIENT COUNSELING INFORMATION

See FDA-approved patient labeling (Patient Information).

17.1 Information about Treatment

Physicians should inform their patients of the following important points when initiating BARACLUDE treatment:

- Patients should remain under the care of a physician while taking BARACLUDE. They should discuss any new symptoms or concurrent medications with their physician.
- Patients should be advised that treatment with BARACLUDE has not been shown to reduce the risk of transmission of HBV to others through sexual contact or blood contamination.
- Patients should be advised to take BARACLUDE (entecavir) on an empty stomach (at least 2 hours after a meal and 2 hours before the next meal).
- Patients using the oral solution should be instructed to hold the dosing spoon in a vertical position and fill it gradually to the mark corresponding to the prescribed dose. Rinsing of the dosing spoon with water is recommended after each daily dose.
- Patients should be advised to take a missed dose as soon as remembered unless it is almost time for the next dose. Patients should not take two doses at the same time.
- Patients should be advised that treatment with BARACLUDE will not cure HBV.
- Patients should be informed that BARACLUDE may lower the amount of HBV in the body, may lower the ability of HBV to multiply and infect new liver cells, and may improve the condition of the liver.
- Patients should be informed that it is not known whether BARACLUDE will reduce their chances of getting liver cancer or cirrhosis.

17.2 Post-treatment Exacerbation of Hepatitis

Patients should be informed that deterioration of liver disease may occur in some cases if treatment is discontinued, and that they should discuss any change in regimen with their physician.

17.3 HIV/HBV Co-infection

Patients should be offered HIV antibody testing before starting BARACLUDE therapy. They should be informed that if they have HIV infection and are not receiving effective HIV treatment, BARACLUDE may increase the chance of HIV resistance to HIV medication.

Patient Information
BARACLUDE® (BEAR ah klude)
(entecavir)
Tablets and Oral Solution

Read this Patient Information before you start taking BARACLUDE and each time you get a refill. There may be new information. This information does not take the place of talking with your healthcare provider about your medical condition or treatment.

What is the most important information I should know about BARACLUDE?

1. Your hepatitis B virus infection may get worse if you stop taking BARACLUDE. This usually happens within 6 months after stopping BARACLUDE.
- Take BARACLUDE exactly as prescribed.
- Do not run out of BARACLUDE.
- Do not stop BARACLUDE without talking to your healthcare provider.
- Your healthcare provider should monitor your health and do regular blood tests to check your liver if you stop taking BARACLUDE.

2. If you have or get HIV that is not being treated with medicines while taking BARACLUDE, the HIV virus may develop resistance to certain HIV medicines and become harder to treat. You should get an HIV test before you start taking BARACLUDE and anytime after that when there is a chance you were exposed to HIV.

BARACLUDE can cause serious side effects including:

3. Lactic acidosis (buildup of acid in the blood). Some people who have taken BARACLUDE or medicines like BARACLUDE (a nucleoside analogue) have developed a serious condition called lactic acidosis. Lactic acidosis is a serious medical emergency that can cause death. Lactic acidosis must be treated in the hospital. Reports of lactic acidosis with BARACLUDE generally involved patients who were seriously ill due to their liver disease or other medical condition.

Call your healthcare provider right away if you get any of the following signs or symptoms of lactic acidosis:
- You feel very weak or tired.
- You have unusual (not normal) muscle pain.
- You have trouble breathing.
- You have stomach pain with nausea and vomiting.
- You feel cold, especially in your arms and legs.
- You feel dizzy or light-headed.
- You have a fast or irregular heartbeat.

4. Serious liver problems. Some people who have taken medicines like BARACLUDE have developed serious liver problems called hepatotoxicity, with liver enlargement (hepatomegaly) and fat in the liver (steatosis). Hepatomegaly with steatosis is a serious medical emergency that can cause death.

Call your healthcare provider right away if you get any of the following signs or symptoms of liver problems:
- Your skin or the white part of your eyes turns yellow (jaundice).
- Your urine turns dark.
- Your bowel movements (stools) turn light in color.
- You don't feel like eating food for several days or longer.
- You feel sick to your stomach (nausea).
- You have lower stomach pain.

You may be more likely to get lactic acidosis or serious liver problems if you are female, very overweight, or have been taking nucleoside analogue medicines, like BARACLUDE, for a long time.

What is BARACLUDE?

BARACLUDE (entecavir) is a prescription medicine used to treat chronic hepatitis B virus (HBV) in adults who have active liver damage.
- BARACLUDE will not cure HBV.
- BARACLUDE may lower the amount of HBV in the body.
- BARACLUDE may lower the ability of HBV to multiply and infect new liver cells.
- BARACLUDE may improve the condition of your liver.
- It is not known whether BARACLUDE will reduce your chances of getting liver cancer or liver damage (cirrhosis), which may be caused by chronic HBV infection.
- It is not known if BARACLUDE is safe and effective for use in children.

What should I tell my healthcare provider before taking BARACLUDE?

Before you take BARACLUDE, tell your healthcare provider if you:
- have kidney problems. Your BARACLUDE dose or schedule may need to be changed.
- have received medicine for HBV before. Some people, especially those who have already been treated with certain other medicines for HBV infection, may develop resistance to BARACLUDE. These people may have less benefit from treatment with BARACLUDE and may have worsening of hepatitis after resistant virus appears. Your healthcare provider will test the level of the hepatitis B virus in your blood regularly.
- have any other medical conditions.
- are pregnant or plan to become pregnant. It is not known if BARACLUDE will harm your unborn baby. Talk to your healthcare provider if you are pregnant or plan to become pregnant.

  Pregnancy Registry. If you take BARACLUDE while you are pregnant, talk to your healthcare provider about how you can take part in the BARACLUDE Pregnancy Registry. The purpose of the pregnancy registry is to collect information about the health of you and your baby.
- are breast-feeding or plan to breast-feed. It is not known if BARACLUDE can pass into your breast milk. You and your healthcare provider should decide if you will take BARACLUDE or breast-feed.

Tell your healthcare provider about all the medicines you take, including prescription and nonprescription medicines, vitamins, and herbal supplements.

Know the medicines you take. Keep a list of your medicines with you to show your healthcare provider and pharmacist when you get a new medicine.

How should I take BARACLUDE?
- Take BARACLUDE exactly as your healthcare provider tells you to.
- Your healthcare provider will tell you how much BARACLUDE to take.
- Your healthcare provider will tell you when and how often to take BARACLUDE.
- **Take BARACLUDE on an empty stomach,** at least 2 hours after a meal and at least 2 hours before the next meal.
- If you are taking BARACLUDE Oral Solution, carefully measure your dose with the spoon provided, as follows:
  - Hold the spoon in a vertical (upright) position and fill it gradually to the mark corresponding to the prescribed dose. Holding the spoon with the volume marks facing you, check that it has been filled to the proper mark.
  - Swallow the medicine directly from the measuring spoon.

- After each use, rinse the spoon with water and allow it to air dry.
- If you lose the spoon, call your pharmacist or healthcare provider for instructions.
- **Do not change your dose or stop taking BARACLUDE without talking to your healthcare provider.**
- **If you forget to take BARACLUDE (entecavir),** take it as soon as you remember and then take your next dose at its regular time. If it is almost time for your next dose, skip the missed dose. Do not take two doses at the same time. Call your healthcare provider or pharmacist if you are not sure what to do.
- When your supply of BARACLUDE starts to run low, call your healthcare provider or pharmacy for a refill. **Do not run out of BARACLUDE** (entecavir).
- **If you take too much BARACLUDE,** call your healthcare provider or go to the nearest emergency room right away.

What are the possible side effects of BARACLUDE?

BARACLUDE may cause serious side effects. See **"What is the most important information I should know about BARACLUDE?"**

The most common side effects of BARACLUDE include:

- headache
- tiredness
- dizziness
- nausea

Tell your healthcare provider if you have any side effect that bothers you or that does not go away.

These are not all the possible side effects of BARACLUDE. For more information, ask your healthcare provider or pharmacist.

Call your doctor for medical advice about side effects. You may report side effects to the FDA at 1-800-FDA-1088.

How should I store BARACLUDE?

- Store BARACLUDE Tablets or Oral Solution at room temperature, between 59° F to 86° F (15° C to 30° C).
- Keep BARACLUDE Tablets in a tightly closed container.
- Do not store BARACLUDE Tablets in a damp place such as a bathroom medicine cabinet or near the kitchen sink.
- Store BARACLUDE Oral Solution in the original carton, and keep BARACLUDE Oral Solution out of the light.
- Safely throw away BARACLUDE that is out of date or no longer needed. Dispose of unused medicines through community take-back disposal programs when available or place BARACLUDE in an unrecognizable closed container in the household trash.

Keep BARACLUDE and all medicines out of the reach of children.

General information about the safe and effective use of BARACLUDE

BARACLUDE does not stop you from spreading the hepatitis B virus (HBV) to others by sex, sharing needles, or being exposed to your blood. Talk with your healthcare provider about safe sexual practices that protect your partner. Never share needles. Do not share personal items that can have blood or body fluids on them, like toothbrushes or razor blades. A shot (vaccine) is available to protect people at risk from becoming infected with HBV.

Medicines are sometimes prescribed for purposes other than those listed in a patient information leaflet. Do not use BARACLUDE for a condition for which it was not prescribed. Do not give BARACLUDE to other people, even if they have the same symptoms you have. It may harm them.

This Patient Information Leaflet summarizes the most important information about BARACLUDE. If you would like more information, talk with your healthcare provider. You can ask your healthcare provider or pharmacist for information about BARACLUDE that is written for healthcare professionals.

For more information, go to *www.Baraclude.com* or call 1-800-321-1335.

What are the ingredients in BARACLUDE?

Active ingredient: entecavir

Inactive ingredients in BARACLUDE Tablets: lactose monohydrate, microcrystalline cellulose, crospovidone, povidone, magnesium stearate.

Tablet film-coat: titanium dioxide, hypromellose, polyethylene glycol 400, polysorbate 80 (0.5 mg tablet only), and iron oxide red (1 mg tablet only).

Inactive ingredients in BARACLUDE Oral Solution: maltitol, sodium citrate, citric acid, methylparaben, propylparaben, and orange flavor.

Bristol-Myers Squibb Company
Princeton, NJ 08543 USA

This Patient Information Leaflet has been approved by the U.S. Food and Drug Administration.

1195459B3
Rev October 2012

Shown in Product Identification Guide, page 305

BYDUREON® ℞

[by-DUR-ee-on]
(exenatide extended-release for injectable suspension)

HIGHLIGHTS OF PRESCRIBING INFORMATION
These highlights do not include all the information needed to use BYDUREON safely and effectively. See full prescribing information for BYDUREON.
BYDUREON® (exenatide extended-release for injectable suspension)
Initial U.S. Approval: 2012

> **WARNING: RISK OF THYROID C-CELL TUMORS**
> ***See full prescribing information for complete boxed warning.***
> - **Exenatide extended-release causes thyroid C-cell tumors at clinically relevant exposures in rats. It is unknown whether BYDUREON causes thyroid C-cell tumors, including medullary thyroid carcinoma (MTC), in humans, as human relevance could not be determined by clinical or nonclinical studies (5.1).**
> - **BYDUREON is contraindicated in patients with a personal or family history of MTC or in patients with Multiple Endocrine Neoplasia syndrome type 2 (MEN 2) (5.1).**

INDICATIONS AND USAGE

BYDUREON is a glucagon-like peptide-1 (GLP-1) receptor agonist indicated as an adjunct to diet and exercise to improve glycemic control in adults with type 2 diabetes mellitus in multiple clinical settings (1.1, 14).

BYDUREON is an extended-release formulation of exenatide. Do not coadminister with BYETTA.

Important Limitations of Use

- Not recommended as first-line therapy for patients inadequately controlled on diet and exercise (5.1).
- Should not be used to treat type 1 diabetes or diabetic ketoacidosis (1.2).
- Use with insulin has not been studied and is not recommended (1.2).
- Has not been studied in patients with a history of pancreatitis. Consider other antidiabetic therapies in patients with a history of pancreatitis (1.2, 5.2).

DOSAGE AND ADMINISTRATION

- Administer 2 mg by subcutaneous injection once every seven days (weekly), at any time of day and with or without meals (2.1).
- Administer immediately after the powder is suspended (2.1).

DOSAGE FORMS AND STRENGTHS

BYDUREON is 2 mg exenatide for extended-release injectable suspension. (3)

CONTRAINDICATIONS

- Do not use if personal or family history of medullary thyroid carcinoma or in patients with Multiple Endocrine Neoplasia syndrome type 2 (4.1).
- Do not use if history of serious hypersensitivity to exenatide or any product components (4.2).

WARNINGS AND PRECAUTIONS

- Thyroid C-cell tumors in animals: Human relevance unknown. Counsel patients regarding the risk of medullary thyroid carcinoma and the symptoms of thyroid tumors (5.1).
- Pancreatitis: Postmarketing reports with exenatide, including fatal and non-fatal hemorrhagic or necrotizing pancreatitis. Discontinue promptly if pancreatitis is suspected. Do not restart if pancreatitis is confirmed. Consider other antidiabetic therapies if history of pancreatitis (5.2).
- Hypoglycemia: Increased risk when BYDUREON is used in combination with a sulfonylurea. Consider reducing the sulfonylurea dose (5.3).
- Renal Impairment: Postmarketing reports with exenatide, sometimes requiring hemodialysis and kidney transplantation. Not recommended if severe renal impairment or end-stage renal disease. Use with caution in patients with renal transplantation or moderate renal impairment (5.4, 8.6, 12.3).
- Severe Gastrointestinal Disease: Not recommended if severe gastrointestinal disease (e.g., gastroparesis) (5.5).
- Hypersensitivity: Postmarketing reports with exenatide of serious hypersensitivity reactions (e.g., anaphylaxis and angioedema). In such cases, patients are to discontinue BYDUREON and other suspect medications and promptly seek medical advice (5.7).
- Macrovascular outcomes: There have been no clinical studies establishing conclusive evidence of macrovascular risk reduction with BYDUREON or any other antidiabetic drug (5.8).

ADVERSE REACTIONS

- Most common (≥5%) and occurring more frequently than comparator in clinical trials: nausea, diarrhea, headache, vomiting, constipation, injection-site pruritus, injection-site nodule, and dyspepsia (5.3, 6.1).

To report SUSPECTED ADVERSE REACTIONS, contact Bristol-Myers Squibb at 1-877-700-7365 and www.bydureon.com or FDA at 1-800-FDA-1088 or *www.fda.gov/medwatch.*

DRUG INTERACTIONS

- May impact absorption of orally administered medications (7.1, 12.3).
- Warfarin: Postmarketing reports with exenatide of increased INR sometimes associated with bleeding. Monitor INR frequently until stable upon initiation of BYDUREON therapy (6.2, 7.2).

USE IN SPECIFIC POPULATIONS

- Pregnancy: Based on animal data, may cause fetal harm. Use during pregnancy only if the potential benefit justifies the potential risk to the fetus. To report drug exposure during pregnancy call 1-800-633-9081 (8.1).
- Nursing Mothers: Use caution when administering to a nursing woman (8.3).

See 17 for PATIENT COUNSELING INFORMATION and Medication Guide

Revised: 02/2013

FULL PRESCRIBING INFORMATION: CONTENTS*

*** Sections or subsections omitted from the full prescribing information are not listed**

FULL PRESCRIBING INFORMATION

> **WARNING: RISK OF THYROID C-CELL TUMORS**
> **Exenatide extended-release causes an increased incidence in thyroid C-cell tumors at clinically**

relevant exposures in rats compared to controls. It is unknown whether BYDUREON causes thyroid C-cell tumors, including medullary thyroid carcinoma (MTC), in humans, as human relevance could not be determined by clinical or nonclinical studies. BYDUREON is contraindicated in patients with a personal or family history of MTC and in patients with Multiple Endocrine Neoplasia syndrome type 2 (MEN 2). Routine serum calcitonin or thyroid ultrasound monitoring is of uncertain value in patients treated with BYDUREON. Patients should be counseled regarding the risk and symptoms of thyroid tumors [see *Contraindications (4.1)*, *Warnings and Precautions (5.1)*, and *Nonclinical Toxicology (13.1)*].

1 INDICATIONS AND USAGE

BYDUREON (exenatide extended-release for injectable suspension) is an extended-release formulation of exenatide, administered as an injection once every 7 days (weekly).

1.1 Type 2 Diabetes Mellitus

BYDUREON is indicated as an adjunct to diet and exercise to improve glycemic control in adults with type 2 diabetes mellitus in multiple clinical settings [see *Clinical Studies (14)*].

1.2 Important Limitations of Use

Because of the uncertain relevance of the rat thyroid C-cell tumor findings to humans, prescribe BYDUREON only to patients for whom the potential benefits are considered to outweigh the potential risk.

BYDUREON is not recommended as first-line therapy for patients who have inadequate glycemic control on diet and exercise.

BYDUREON is not a substitute for insulin. BYDUREON should not be used in patients with type 1 diabetes or for the treatment of diabetic ketoacidosis, as it would not be effective in these settings.

The concurrent use of BYDUREON with insulin has not been studied and cannot be recommended.

BYDUREON and BYETTA® (exenatide) injection both contain the same active ingredient, exenatide, and therefore should not be used together.

Based on postmarketing data, exenatide has been associated with acute pancreatitis, including fatal and non-fatal hemorrhagic or necrotizing pancreatitis. BYDUREON has not been studied in patients with a history of pancreatitis. It is unknown whether patients with a history of pancreatitis are at increased risk for pancreatitis while using BYDUREON. Other antidiabetic therapies should be considered in patients with a history of pancreatitis.

2 DOSAGE AND ADMINISTRATION

2.1 Recommended Dosing

BYDUREON (2 mg per dose) should be administered once every 7 days (weekly). The dose can be administered at any time of day, with or without meals.

Missed Dose

If a dose is missed, it should be administered as soon as noticed, provided the next regularly scheduled dose is due at least 3 days later. Thereafter, patients can resume their usual dosing schedule of once every 7 days (weekly).

If a dose is missed and the next regularly scheduled dose is due 1 or 2 days later, the patient should not administer the missed dose and instead resume BYDUREON with the next regularly scheduled dose.

Changing Weekly Dosing Schedule

The day of weekly administration can be changed if necessary as long as the last dose was administered 3 or more days before.

2.2 Administration

BYDUREON is intended for patient self-administration. BYDUREON is provided in a single-dose tray containing: one vial of 2 mg exenatide, one vial connector, one prefilled diluent syringe, and two needles (one provided as a spare) [see *How Supplied/Storage and Handling (16.1)*]. **Do not substitute needles or any other components in the tray.**

BYDUREON must be injected immediately after the powder is suspended in the diluent and transferred to the syringe. BYDUREON is administered as a subcutaneous (SC) injection in the abdomen, thigh, or upper arm region. Advise patients to use a different injection site each week when injecting in the same region. BYDUREON must not be administered intravenously or intramuscularly.

See the BYDUREON Instructions for Use for complete administration instructions with illustrations. The instructions can also be found at www.bydureon.com.

2.3 Changing from BYETTA to BYDUREON

Prior treatment with BYETTA is not required when initiating BYDUREON therapy. If the decision is made to start BYDUREON in an appropriate patient already taking BYETTA, BYETTA should be discontinued. Patients changing from BYETTA to BYDUREON may experience transient (approximately 2 weeks) elevations in blood glucose concentrations.

3 DOSAGE FORMS AND STRENGTHS

BYDUREON (exenatide extended-release for injectable suspension) is 2 mg exenatide extended-release for injectable suspension for subcutaneous administration once every 7 days (weekly).

4 CONTRAINDICATIONS

4.1 Medullary Thyroid Carcinoma

BYDUREON is contraindicated in patients with a personal or family history of medullary thyroid carcinoma (MTC) or in patients with Multiple Endocrine Neoplasia syndrome type 2 (MEN 2).

4.2 Hypersensitivity

BYDUREON is contraindicated in patients with a prior serious hypersensitivity reaction to exenatide or to any of the product components.

5 WARNINGS AND PRECAUTIONS

5.1 Risk of Thyroid C-cell Tumors

In both genders of rats, exenatide extended-release caused a dose-related and treatment-duration–dependent increase in the incidence of thyroid C-cell tumors (adenomas and/or carcinomas) at clinically relevant exposures compared to controls [see *Nonclinical Toxicology (13.1)*]. A statistically significant increase in malignant thyroid C-cell carcinomas was observed in female rats receiving exenatide extended-release at 25 times clinical exposure compared to controls and higher incidences were noted in males above controls in all treated groups at ≥2-times clinical exposure. The potential of exenatide extended-release to induce C-cell tumors in mice has not been evaluated. Other GLP-1 receptor agonists have also induced thyroid C-cell adenomas and carcinomas in male and female mice and rats at clinically relevant exposures. It is unknown whether BYDUREON will cause thyroid C-cell tumors, including medullary thyroid carcinoma (MTC), in humans as the human relevance of exenatide extended-release–induced rodent thyroid C-cell tumors could not be determined by clinical or nonclinical studies. Serum calcitonin was not assessed in the clinical trials supporting the approval of BYDUREON [see *Boxed Warning* and *Contraindications (4.1)*].

Serum calcitonin is a biological marker of MTC. Patients with MTC usually have calcitonin values >50 ng/L. Patients with thyroid nodules noted on physical examination or neck imaging should be referred to an endocrinologist for further evaluation. Routine monitoring of serum calcitonin or using thyroid ultrasound is of uncertain value for early detection of MTC in patients treated with BYDUREON. Such monitoring may increase the risk of unnecessary procedures, due to the low specificity of serum calcitonin testing for MTC and a high background incidence of thyroid disease. If serum calcitonin is measured and found to be elevated, the patient should be referred to an endocrinologist for further evaluation [see *Patient Counseling Information (17)*].

5.2 Acute Pancreatitis

Based on postmarketing data, exenatide has been associated with acute pancreatitis, including fatal and non-fatal hemorrhagic or necrotizing pancreatitis. After initiation of BYDUREON, observe patients carefully for signs and symptoms of pancreatitis (including persistent severe abdominal pain, sometimes radiating to the back, which may or may not be accompanied by vomiting). If pancreatitis is suspected, BYDUREON should promptly be discontinued and appropriate management should be initiated. If pancreatitis is confirmed, BYDUREON should not be restarted. Consider antidiabetic therapies other than BYDUREON in patients with a history of pancreatitis.

5.3 Hypoglycemia

The risk of hypoglycemia is increased when exenatide is used in combination with a sulfonylurea. Therefore, patients receiving BYDUREON and a sulfonylurea may require a lower dose of the sulfonylurea to minimize the risk of hypoglycemia. It is also possible that the use of BYDUREON with other glucose-independent insulin secretagogues (e.g., meglitinides) could increase the risk of hypoglycemia.

For additional information on glucose-dependent effects see *Clinical Pharmacology (12.1)*.

5.4 Renal Impairment

BYDUREON should not be used in patients with severe renal impairment (creatinine clearance <30 mL/min) or end-stage renal disease and should be used with caution in patients with renal transplantation [see *Use in Specific Populations (8.6)*]. In patients with end-stage renal disease receiving dialysis, single doses of BYETTA 5 mcg were not well tolerated due to gastrointestinal side effects. Because BYDUREON may induce nausea and vomiting with transient hypovolemia, treatment may worsen renal function. Use BYDUREON with caution in patients with moderate renal impairment (creatinine clearance 30-50 mL/min) [see *Use in Specific Populations (8.6)* and *Clinical Pharmacology (12.3)*]. BYDUREON has not been studied in patients with end-stage renal disease or severe renal impairment.

There have been postmarketing reports of altered renal function with exenatide, including increased serum creatinine, renal impairment, worsened chronic renal failure and acute renal failure, sometimes requiring hemodialysis or kidney transplantation. Some of these events occurred in patients receiving one or more pharmacologic agents known to affect renal function or hydration status such as angiotensin converting enzyme inhibitors, nonsteroidal anti-inflammatory drugs, or diuretics. Some events occurred in patients who had been experiencing nausea, vomiting, or diarrhea, with or without dehydration. Reversibility of altered renal function has been observed in many cases with supportive treatment and discontinuation of potentially causative agents, including exenatide. Exenatide has not been found to be directly nephrotoxic in preclinical or clinical studies.

5.5 Gastrointestinal Disease

Exenatide has not been studied in patients with severe gastrointestinal disease, including gastroparesis. Because exenatide is commonly associated with gastrointestinal adverse reactions, including nausea, vomiting, and diarrhea, the use of BYDUREON (exenatide extended-release for injectable suspension) is not recommended in patients with severe gastrointestinal disease.

5.6 Immunogenicity

Patients may develop antibodies to exenatide following treatment with BYDUREON. Anti-exenatide antibodies were measured in all BYDUREON-treated patients in the five comparator-controlled 24- to 30-week studies of BYDUREON. In 6% of BYDUREON-treated patients, antibody formation was associated with an attenuated glycemic response. If there is worsening glycemic control or failure to achieve targeted glycemic control, alternative antidiabetic therapy should be considered [see *Adverse Reactions (6.1)*].

5.7 Hypersensitivity

There have been postmarketing reports of serious hypersensitivity reactions (e.g., anaphylaxis and angioedema) in patients treated with exenatide. If a hypersensitivity reaction occurs, the patient should discontinue BYDUREON and other suspect medications and promptly seek medical advice [see *Adverse Reactions (6.2)*].

5.8 Macrovascular Outcomes

There have been no clinical studies establishing conclusive evidence of macrovascular risk reduction with BYDUREON or any other antidiabetic drug.

6 ADVERSE REACTIONS

6.1 Clinical Trial Experience

Because clinical trials are conducted under widely varying conditions, adverse reaction rates observed in the clinical trials of a drug cannot be directly compared to rates in the clinical trials of another drug and may not reflect the rates observed in practice.

The safety of BYDUREON was assessed in five comparator-controlled trials in patients who entered the studies not achieving adequate glycemic control on their current therapy. In a double-blind 26-week trial, patients on diet and exercise were treated with BYDUREON 2 mg once every 7 days (weekly), sitagliptin 100 mg daily, pioglitazone 45 mg daily, or metformin 2000 mg daily. In a double-blind 26-week trial, patients on metformin were treated with BYDUREON 2 mg once every 7 days (weekly), sitagliptin 100 mg daily, or pioglitazone 45 mg daily. In an open-label 26-week trial, patients on metformin or metformin plus sulfonylurea were treated with BYDUREON 2 mg once every 7 days (weekly) or optimized insulin glargine. In two open-label 24- to 30-week studies, patients on diet and exercise or metformin, a sulfonylurea, a thiazolidinedione, or combination of oral agents were treated with BYDUREON 2 mg once every 7 days (weekly) or BYETTA 10 mcg twice daily.

Withdrawals

The incidence of withdrawal due to adverse events was 4.9% (N=45) for BYDUREON-treated patients, 4.9% (N=13) for BYETTA-treated patients, and 2.0% (N=23) for other comparator-treated patients in the five comparator-controlled 24- to 30-week trials. The most common adverse reactions leading to withdrawal for BYDUREON-treated patients were nausea 0.5% (N=5) versus 1.5% (N=4) for BYETTA and 0.3% (N=3) for other comparators, injection-site nodule 0.5% (N=5) versus 0.0% for BYETTA and 0.0% for other comparators, diarrhea 0.3% (N=3) versus 0.4% (N=1) for BYETTA and 0.3% (N=3) for other comparators, injection-site reaction 0.2% (N=2) versus 0.0% for BYETTA and 0.0% for other comparators, and headache 0.2% (N=2) versus 0.0% for BYETTA and 0.0% for other comparators.

Hypoglycemia

Table 1 summarizes the incidence and rate of minor hypoglycemia in the five comparator-controlled 24- to 30-week trials of BYDUREON used as monotherapy or as add-on to metformin, a sulfonylurea, a thiazolidinedione, or combination of these oral antidiabetic agents. In these trials, an event was classified as minor hypoglycemia if there were symptoms of hypoglycemia with a concomitant glucose <54 mg/dL and the patient was able to self-treat.

Table 1: Incidence (% of Subjects) and Rate (Episodes/ Subject Year) of Minor† Hypoglycemia in the Monotherapy Trial and in the Combination Therapy Trials

26-Week Monotherapy Trial	
BYDUREON 2 mg (N = 248)	2.0% (0.05)
Sitagliptin 100 mg (N = 163)	0.0% (0.00)
Pioglitazone 45 mg (N = 163)	0.0% (0.00)
Metformin 2000 mg QD (N = 246)	0.0% (0.00)
26-Week Add-On to Metformin Trial	
BYDUREON 2 mg (N = 160)	1.3% (0.03)
Sitagliptin 100 mg (N = 166)	3.0% (0.12)
Pioglitazone 45 mg (N = 165)	1.2% (0.03)
26-Week Add-On to Metformin or Metformin + Sulfonylurea Trial	
With Concomitant Sulfonylurea Use (N = 136)	
BYDUREON 2 mg (N = 70)	20.0% (1.11)
Titrated Insulin Glargine (N = 66)	43.9% (2.87)
Without Concomitant Sulfonylurea Use (N = 320)	
BYDUREON 2 mg (N = 163)	3.7% (0.11)
Titrated Insulin Glargine‡ (N = 157)	19.1% (0.64)
24-Week Monotherapy or Add-On to Metformin, a Sulfonylurea, a Thiazolidinedione, or Combination of Oral Agents Trial	
With Concomitant Sulfonylurea Use (N = 74)	
BYDUREON 2 mg (N = 40)	12.5% (0.72)
BYETTA 10 mcg (N = 34)	11.8% (0.31)
Without Concomitant Sulfonylurea Use (N = 178)	
BYDUREON 2 mg (N = 89)	0.0% (0.00)
BYETTA 10 mcg (N = 89)	0.0% (0.00)
30-Week Monotherapy or Add-On to Metformin, a Sulfonylurea, a Thiazolidinedione, or Combination of Oral Agents Trial	
With Concomitant Sulfonylurea Use (N = 107)	
BYDUREON 2 mg (N = 55)	14.5% (0.55)
BYETTA 10 mcg (N = 52)	15.4% (0.37)
Without Concomitant Sulfonylurea Use (N = 186)	
BYDUREON 2 mg (N = 93)	0.0% (0.00)
BYETTA 10 mcg (N = 93)	1.1% (0.02)

N = number of intent-to-treat patients.

Note: Percentages are based on the number of intent-to-treat patients in each treatment group.

† Reported event that has symptoms consistent with hypoglycemia with a concomitant glucose <54 mg/dL and the patient was able to self-treat.

‡ Insulin glargine was dosed to a target fasting glucose concentration of 72 to 100 mg/dL. The mean dose of insulin glargine was 10 Units/day at baseline and 31 Units/day at endpoint.

There were no reported events of major hypoglycemia in these five comparator-controlled 24- to 30-week trials. Major hypoglycemia was defined as loss of consciousness, seizure, or coma (or other mental status change consistent with neuroglycopenia in the judgment of the investigator or physician) which resolved after administration of glucagon or glucose or required third-party assistance to resolve because of severe impairment in consciousness or behavior. Patients were to have a concomitant glucose <54 mg/dL.

Immunogenicity

Anti-exenatide antibodies were measured at prespecified intervals (4-14 weeks) in all BYDUREON-treated patients (N=918) in the five comparator-controlled studies of BYDUREON (exenatide extended-release for injectable suspension). In these five trials, 452 BYDUREON-treated patients (49%) had low titer antibodies (≤125) to exenatide at any time during the trials and 405 BYDUREON-treated patients (45%) had low titer antibodies to exenatide at study endpoint (24-30 weeks). The level of glycemic control in these patients was generally comparable to that observed in the 379 BYDUREON-treated patients (43%) without antibody titers. An additional 107 BYDUREON-treated patients (12%) had higher titer antibodies at endpoint. Of these patients, 50 (6% overall) had an attenuated glycemic response to BYDUREON (<0.7% reduction in HbA_{1c}); the remaining 57 (6% overall) had a glycemic response comparable to that of patients without antibodies [see *Warnings and Precautions (5.6)*]. In the 30-week trial in which anti-exenatide antibody assessments were performed at baseline and at 4-week intervals from week 6 to week 30, the mean anti-exenatide antibody titer in the BYDUREON-treated patients peaked at week 6 then declined by 56% from this peak by week 30.

A total of 246 patients with antibodies to exenatide in the BYETTA and BYDUREON clinical trials were tested for the presence of cross-reactive antibodies to GLP-1 and/or glucagon. No treatment-emergent cross-reactive antibodies were observed across the range of titers.

Other Adverse Reactions

BYDUREON

Tables 2 and 3 summarize adverse reactions with an incidence ≥5% reported in the five comparator-controlled 24- to 30-week trials of BYDUREON used as monotherapy or as add-on to metformin, a sulfonylurea, a thiazolidinedione, or combination of these oral antidiabetic agents.

[See table 2 below]

[See table 3 at top of next page]

Nausea was the most common adverse reaction associated with initiation of treatment with BYDUREON, and usually decreased over time.

Injection-Site Reactions

In the five comparator-controlled 24- to 30-week trials, injection-site reactions were observed more frequently in patients treated with BYDUREON (17.1%) than in patients treated with BYETTA (12.7%), titrated insulin glargine (1.8%), or those patients who received placebo injections (sitagliptin (10.6%), pioglitazone (6.4%), and metformin (13.0%) treatment groups). These reactions for patients treated with BYDUREON were more commonly observed in antibody-positive patients (14.2%) compared with antibody-negative patients (3.1%), with a greater incidence in those with higher titer antibodies [see *Warnings and Precautions (5.6)*]. Incidence of injection-site reactions for patients treated with BYETTA was similar for antibody-positive patients (5.8%) and antibody-negative patients (7.0%). One percent of patients treated with BYDUREON (exenatide extended-release for injectable suspension) withdrew due to injection-site adverse reactions (injection-site mass, injection-site nodule, injection-site pruritus, and injection-site reaction).

Small, asymptomatic subcutaneous injection-site nodules are seen with the use of BYDUREON. In a separate 15-week study in which information on nodules were collected and analyzed, 24 out of 31 subjects (77%) experienced at least 1 injection-site nodule during treatment; 2 subjects (6.5%) reported accompanying localized symptoms. The mean duration of events was 27 days. The formation of nodules is consistent with the known properties of the microspheres used in BYDUREON.

BYETTA

In three 30-week controlled trials of BYETTA (N=963) add-on to metformin and/or sulfonylurea, adverse reactions (excluding hypoglycemia) with an incidence of ≥1% and reported more frequently than with placebo included nausea (44% BYETTA, 18% placebo), vomiting (13% BYETTA, 4% placebo), diarrhea (13% BYETTA, 6% placebo), feeling jittery (9% BYETTA, 4% placebo), dizziness (9% BYETTA, 6% placebo), headache (9% BYETTA, 6% placebo), dyspepsia (6% BYETTA, 3% placebo), asthenia (4% BYETTA, 2% placebo), gastroesophageal reflux (3% BYETTA, 1% placebo), hyperhidrosis (3% BYETTA, 1% placebo), and decreased appetite (1% BYETTA, <1% placebo). Similar types of adverse reactions were observed in 24-week and 16-week controlled trials of BYETTA used as monotherapy or as add-on to a thiazolidinedione, with or without metformin, respectively.

6.2 Postmarketing Experience

BYETTA

The following additional adverse reactions have been reported during postapproval use of BYETTA. Because these events are reported voluntarily from a population of uncertain size, it is generally not possible to reliably estimate their frequency or establish a causal relationship to drug exposure.

Allergy/Hypersensitivity: injection-site reactions, generalized pruritus and/or urticaria, macular or papular rash, angioedema; anaphylactic reaction [see *Warnings and Precautions (5.7)*].

Drug Interactions: increased international normalized ratio (INR), sometimes associated with bleeding, with concomitant warfarin use [see *Drug Interactions (7.2)*].

Gastrointestinal: nausea, vomiting, and/or diarrhea resulting in dehydration; abdominal distension, abdominal pain, eructation, constipation, flatulence, acute pancreatitis, hemorrhagic and necrotizing pancreatitis sometimes resulting in death [see *Indications and Usage (1.2)* and *Warnings and Precautions (5.2)*].

Neurologic: dysgeusia; somnolence

Renal and Urinary Disorders: altered renal function, including increased serum creatinine, renal impairment, worsened chronic renal failure or acute renal failure (sometimes requiring hemodialysis), kidney transplant and kidney transplant dysfunction [see *Warnings and Precautions (5.4)*].

Skin and Subcutaneous Tissue Disorders: alopecia

7 DRUG INTERACTIONS

7.1 Orally Administered Drugs

Exenatide slows gastric emptying. Therefore, BYDUREON has the potential to reduce the rate of absorption of orally administered drugs. Use caution when administering oral medications with BYDUREON [see *Clinical Pharmacology (12.3)*].

In patients with type 2 diabetes, BYDUREON did not affect the absorption of orally administered acetaminophen to any clinically relevant degree.

7.2 Warfarin

BYDUREON has not been studied with warfarin. However, in a drug interaction study, BYETTA did not have a significant effect on INR [see *Clinical Pharmacology (12.3)*]. There have been postmarketing reports for BYETTA of increased INR with concomitant use of warfarin, sometimes associated with bleeding [see *Adverse Reactions (6.2)*]. In patients taking warfarin, the INR should be monitored more frequently after initiating BYDUREON. Once a stable INR has been documented, the INR can be monitored at the intervals usually recommended for patients on warfarin.

8 USE IN SPECIFIC POPULATIONS

8.1 Pregnancy

Pregnancy Category C

There are no adequate and well-controlled studies of BYDUREON use in pregnant women. In rats, exenatide extended-release administered during the major period of organogenesis reduced fetal growth and produced skeletal ossification deficits in association with maternal effects;

Table 2: Treatment-Emergent Adverse Reactions Reported in ≥5% of BYDUREON-Treated Patients in Monotherapy Trial

	26-Week Monotherapy Trial			
	BYDUREON 2 mg N = 248 %	Sitagliptin 100 mg N = 163 %	Pioglitazone 45 mg N = 163 %	Metformin 2000 mg N = 246 %
Nausea	11.3	3.7	4.3	6.9
Diarrhea	10.9	5.5	3.7	12.6
Injection-site nodule†	10.5	6.7	3.7	10.2
Constipation	8.5	2.5	1.8	3.3
Headache	8.1	9.2	8.0	12.2
Dyspepsia	7.3	1.8	4.9	3.3

N = number of intent-to-treat patients.

Note: Percentages are based on the number of intent-to-treat patients in each treatment group.

† Patients in the sitagliptin, pioglitazone, and metformin treatment groups received weekly placebo injections.

exenatide extended-release was not teratogenic in rats. In animal developmental studies, exenatide, the active ingredient of BYDUREON (exenatide extended-release for injectable suspension), caused cleft palate, irregular skeletal ossification, and an increased number of neonatal deaths. BYDUREON should be used during pregnancy only if the potential benefit justifies the potential risk to the fetus.

Fetuses from pregnant rats given subcutaneous doses of exenatide extended-release at 0.3, 1, or 3 mg/kg on gestation days 6, 9, 12, and 15 demonstrated reduced fetal growth at all doses and produced skeletal ossification deficits at 1 and 3 mg/kg in association with maternal effects (decreased food intake and decreased body weight gain). There was no evidence of malformations. Doses of 0.3, 1, and 3 mg/kg correspond to systemic exposures of 3, 7, and 17 times, respectively, the human exposure resulting from the recommended dose of 2 mg/week, based on area under the time-concentration curve (AUC) [see *Nonclinical Toxicology (13.3)*].

Female mice given subcutaneous doses of exenatide, the active ingredient of BYDUREON, at 6, 68, or 760 mcg/kg/day beginning 2 weeks prior to and throughout mating until gestation day 7 had no adverse fetal effects. At the maximal dose, 760 mcg/kg/day, systemic exposures were up to 148 times the human exposure resulting from the recommended dose of 2 mg/week, based on AUC [see *Nonclinical Toxicology (13.3)*].

In developmental toxicity studies, pregnant animals received exenatide, the active ingredient of BYDUREON, subcutaneously during organogenesis. Specifically, fetuses from pregnant rabbits given subcutaneous doses of exenatide at 0.2, 2, 22, 156, or 260 mcg/kg/day from gestation day 6 through 18 experienced irregular skeletal ossifications from exposures 4 times the human exposure resulting from the recommended dose of 2 mg/week, based on AUC. Fetuses from pregnant mice given subcutaneous doses of exenatide at 6, 68, 460, or 760 mcg/kg/day from gestation day 6 through 15 demonstrated reduced fetal and neonatal growth, cleft palate, and skeletal effects at systemic exposure that is equivalent to the human exposure resulting from the recommended dose of 2 mg/week, based on AUC [see *Nonclinical Toxicology (13.3)*].

Lactating mice given subcutaneous doses of exenatide, the active ingredient of BYDUREON, at 6, 68, or 760 mcg/kg/day from gestation day 6 through lactation day 20 (weaning), experienced an increased number of neonatal deaths. Deaths were observed on postpartum days 2 to 4 in dams given 6 mcg/kg/day, a systemic exposure that is equivalent to the human exposure resulting from the recommended dose of 2 mg/week, based on AUC [see *Nonclinical Toxicology (13.3)*].

Pregnancy Registry

A Pregnancy Registry has been implemented to monitor pregnancy outcomes of women exposed to exenatide during pregnancy. Physicians are encouraged to register patients by calling 1-800-633-9081.

8.3 Nursing Mothers

Exenatide is present in the milk of lactating mice at concentrations less than or equal to 2.5% of the concentration in maternal plasma following subcutaneous dosing. It is not known whether exenatide is excreted in human milk. Because many drugs are excreted in human milk and because of the potential for tumorigenicity shown for exenatide extended-release in animal studies, a decision should be made whether to discontinue nursing or to discontinue BYDUREON, taking into account the importance of the drug to the mother.

8.4 Pediatric Use

Safety and effectiveness of BYDUREON have not been established in pediatric patients. BYDUREON is not recommended for use in pediatric patients.

8.5 Geriatric Use

In the five comparator-controlled 24- to 30-week trials, BYDUREON was studied in 132 patients (16.6%) who were at least 65 years old and 20 patients who were at least 75 years old. No differences in safety (N=152) and efficacy (N=52) were observed between these patients and younger patients, but the small sample size for patients ≥75 years old limits conclusions.

In separate trials, BYETTA was studied in 282 patients at least 65 years old and in 16 patients at least 75 years old. No differences in safety and efficacy were observed between these patients and younger patients, but the small sample size for patients ≥75 years old limits conclusions.

Because elderly patients are more likely to have decreased renal function, use caution when initiating BYDUREON in the elderly.

8.6 Renal Impairment

BYDUREON is not recommended for use in patients with end-stage renal disease or severe renal impairment (creatinine clearance <30 mL/min) and should be used with caution in patients with renal transplantation. Use BYDUREON with caution in patients with moderate renal impairment (creatinine clearance 30-50 mL/min) [see *Warn-*

Table 3: Treatment-Emergent Adverse Reactions Reported in ≥5% of BYDUREON-Treated Patients in 24- to 30-Week Add-On Combination Therapy Trials

26-Week Add-On to Metformin Trial

	BYDUREON 2 mg N = 160 %	Sitagliptin 100 mg N = 166 %	Pioglitazone 45 mg N = 165 %
Nausea	24.4	9.6	4.8
Diarrhea	20.0	9.6	7.3
Vomiting	11.3	2.4	3.0
Headache	9.4	9.0	5.5
Constipation	6.3	3.6	1.2
Fatigue	5.6	0.6	3.0
Dyspepsia	5.0	3.6	2.4
Decreased appetite	5.0	1.2	0.0
Injection-site pruritus†	5.0	4.8	1.2

26-Week Add-On to Metformin or Metformin + Sulfonylurea Trial

	BYDUREON 2 mg N = 233 %	Insulin Glargine Titrated N = 223 %
Nausea	12.9	1.3
Headache	9.9	7.6
Diarrhea	9.4	4.0
Injection-site nodule	6.0	0.0

30-Week Monotherapy or as Add-On to Metformin, a Sulfonylurea, a Thiazolidinedione, or Combination of Oral Agents Trial

	BYDUREON 2 mg N = 148 %	BYETTA 10 mcg N = 145 %
Nausea	27.0	33.8
Diarrhea	16.2	12.4
Vomiting	10.8	18.6
Injection-site pruritus	18.2	1.4
Constipation	10.1	6.2
Gastroenteritis viral	8.8	5.5
Gastroesophageal reflux disease	7.4	4.1
Dyspepsia	7.4	2.1
Injection-site erythema	7.4	0.0
Fatigue	6.1	3.4
Headache	6.1	1.4
Injection-site hematoma	5.4	11.0

24-Week Monotherapy or as Add-On to Metformin, a Sulfonylurea, a Thiazolidinedione, or Combination of Oral Agents Trial

	BYDUREON 2 mg N = 129 %	BYETTA 10 mcg N = 123 %
Nausea	14.0	35.0
Diarrhea	9.3	4.1
Injection-site erythema	5.4	2.4

N = number of intent-to-treat patients.
Note: Percentages are based on the number of intent-to-treat patients in each treatment group.
† Patients in the sitagliptin, pioglitazone, and metformin treatment groups received weekly placebo injections.

ings and Precautions (5.4) and *Clinical Pharmacology (12.3)*].

8.7 Hepatic Impairment

No pharmacokinetic study has been performed in patients with a diagnosis of acute or chronic hepatic impairment. Because exenatide is cleared primarily by the kidney, hepatic impairment is not expected to affect blood concentrations of exenatide [see *Clinical Pharmacology (12.3)*].

10 OVERDOSAGE

There were no reports of overdose in the five comparator-controlled 24- to 30-week trials of BYDUREON. Effects of overdoses with BYETTA in clinical studies included severe nausea, severe vomiting, and rapidly declining blood glucose concentrations, including severe hypoglycemia requiring parenteral glucose administration. In the event of overdose, appropriate supportive treatment should be initiated according to the patient's clinical signs and symptoms.

11 DESCRIPTION

BYDUREON (exenatide extended-release for injectable suspension) is supplied as a sterile powder to be suspended in the diluent included in the single-dose tray and administered by subcutaneous injection. Exenatide is a 39-amino acid synthetic peptide amide with an empirical formula of $C_{184}H_{282}N_{50}O_{60}S$ and a molecular weight of 4186.6 Daltons. The amino acid sequence for exenatide is shown below.

H-His-Gly-Glu-Gly-Thr-Phe-Thr-Ser-Asp-Leu-Ser-Lys-Gln-Met-Glu-Glu-Glu-Ala-Val-Arg-Leu-Phe-Ile-Glu-Trp-Leu-Lys-Asn-Gly-Gly-Pro-Ser-Ser-Gly-Ala-Pro-Pro-Pro-Ser-NH_2

BYDUREON is a white to off-white powder that is available in a dosage strength of 2 mg exenatide per vial. Exenatide is incorporated in an extended-release microsphere formulation containing the 50:50 poly(D,L-lactide-co-glycolide) polymer (37.2 mg per vial) along with sucrose (0.8 mg per vial). The powder must be suspended in the diluent prior to injection. The diluent is provided in a prefilled syringe. Each prefilled syringe delivers 0.65 mL of the diluent as a clear, colorless to pale yellow solution composed of carboxymethylcellulose sodium (23 mg), polysorbate 20 (0.77 mg), sodium phosphate monobasic monohydrate (0.74 mg), sodium phosphate dibasic heptahydrate (0.62 mg), sodium chloride (5.0 mg), and water for injection.

12 CLINICAL PHARMACOLOGY

12.1 Mechanism of Action

Incretins, such as glucagon-like peptide-1 (GLP-1), enhance glucose-dependent insulin secretion and exhibit other antihyperglycemic actions following their release into the circulation from the gut. BYDUREON is a GLP-1 receptor agonist that enhances glucose-dependent insulin secretion by the pancreatic beta-cell, suppresses inappropriately elevated glucagon secretion, and slows gastric emptying.

The amino acid sequence of exenatide partially overlaps that of human GLP-1. Exenatide is a GLP-1 receptor agonist that has been shown to bind and activate the human GLP-1 receptor *in vitro*. This leads to an increase in both glucose-dependent synthesis of insulin and *in vivo* secretion of insulin from pancreatic beta cells, by mechanisms involving cyclic AMP and/or other intracellular signaling pathways. Exenatide promotes insulin release from pancreatic beta-cells in the presence of elevated glucose concentrations.

12.2 Pharmacodynamics

Exenatide improves glycemic control by reducing fasting and postprandial glucose concentrations in patients with type 2 diabetes through the actions described below.

Glucose-Dependent Insulin Secretion

The effect of exenatide infusion on glucose-dependent insulin secretion rates (ISR) was investigated in 11 healthy subjects. In these healthy subjects, on average, the ISR response was glucose-dependent (Figure 1). Exenatide did not impair the normal glucagon response to hypoglycemia.

[See figure 1 at top of next column]

Glucagon Secretion

In patients with type 2 diabetes, exenatide moderates glucagon secretion and lowers serum glucagon concentrations during periods of hyperglycemia.

Gastric Emptying

Exenatide slows gastric emptying, thereby reducing the rate at which postprandial glucose appears in the circulation.

Food Intake

Infusion of exenatide in 8 healthy subjects resulted in a 19% decrease in caloric intake following an *ad libitum* meal.

Fasting and Postprandial Glucose

In a separate 15-week controlled study where fasting glucose was assessed on a weekly basis, BYDUREON treatment resulted in a mean reduction in fasting glucose of 17 mg/dL following 2 weeks of therapy with full effect on fasting glucose not observed until approximately 9 weeks.

In a 30-week controlled study of exenatide extended-release compared to BYETTA, postprandial glucose levels were measured during a mixed meal tolerance test in a subset of patients with type 2 diabetes mellitus. Following treatment

Figure 1: Mean (SE) Insulin Secretion Rates During Infusion of Exenatide or Placebo by Treatment, Time, and Glycemic Condition in Healthy Subjects

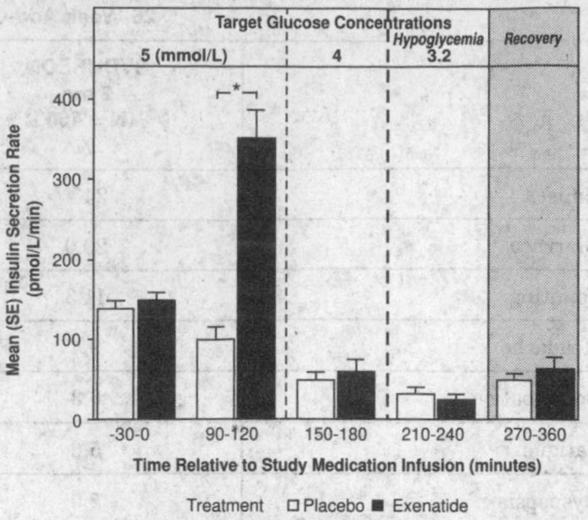

SE = standard error.

Notes: 5 mmol = 90 mg/dL, 4 mmol/L = 72 mg/dL, 3.2 mmol/L = 58 mg/dL;

Study medication infusion was started at time = 0 minutes

Statistical assessments were for the last 30 minutes of each glycemic step, during which the target glucose concentrations were maintained.

*p <0.05, exenatide treatment relative to placebo.

for 14 weeks, when steady-state concentrations had been achieved (approximately 280-310 pg/mL), the LS mean change from baseline was significantly greater with BYETTA (−126 mg/dL) than exenatide extended-release (−96 mg/dL).

Cardiac Electrophysiology

The effect of exenatide at therapeutic (253 pg/mL) and supratherapeutic (627 pg/mL) concentrations, following an intravenous infusion on QTc interval was evaluated in a randomized, placebo- and active-controlled (moxifloxacin 400 mg) three-period crossover thorough QT study in 74 healthy subjects. The upper bound of the one-sided 95% confidence interval for the largest placebo adjusted, baseline-corrected QTc based on population correction method (QTcP) was below 10 ms. Therefore, exenatide was not associated with prolongation of the QTc interval at therapeutic and supratherapeutic concentrations.

12.3 Pharmacokinetics

Absorption

Following a single dose of BYDUREON (exenatide extended-release for injectable suspension), exenatide is released from the microspheres over approximately 10 weeks. There is an initial period of release of surface-bound exenatide followed by a gradual release of exenatide from the microspheres, which results in two subsequent peaks of exenatide in plasma at around week 2 and week 6 to 7, respectively, representing the hydration and erosion of the microspheres.

Following initiation of once every 7 days (weekly) administration of 2 mg BYDUREON, gradual increase in the plasma exenatide concentration is observed over 6 to 7 weeks. After 6 to 7 weeks, mean exenatide concentrations of approximately 300 pg/mL were maintained over once every 7 days (weekly) dosing intervals indicating that steady state was achieved.

Distribution

The mean apparent volume of distribution of exenatide following subcutaneous administration of a single dose of BYETTA is 28.3 L and is expected to remain unchanged for BYDUREON.

Metabolism and Elimination

Nonclinical studies have shown that exenatide is predominantly eliminated by glomerular filtration with subsequent proteolytic degradation. The mean apparent clearance of exenatide in humans is 9.1 L/hour and is independent of the dose. Approximately 10 weeks after discontinuation of BYDUREON therapy, plasma exenatide concentrations generally fall below the minimal detectable concentration of 10 pg/mL.

Drug Interactions

Acetaminophen

When 1000 mg acetaminophen tablets were administered, either with or without a meal, following 14 weeks of BYDUREON therapy (2 mg weekly), no significant changes in acetaminophen AUC were observed compared to the control period. Acetaminophen C_{max} decreased by 16% (fasting) and 5% (fed) and T_{max} was increased from approximately 1 hour in the control period to 1.4 hours (fasting) and 1.3 hours (fed).

The following drug interactions have been studied using BYETTA. The potential for drug-drug interaction with BYDUREON is expected to be similar to that of BYETTA.

Digoxin

Administration of repeated doses of BYETTA 30 minutes before oral digoxin (0.25 mg once daily) decreased the C_{max} of digoxin by 17% and delayed the T_{max} of digoxin by approximately 2.5 hours; however, the overall steady-state pharmacokinetic exposure (e.g., AUC) of digoxin was not changed.

Lovastatin

Administration of BYETTA (10 mcg twice daily) 30 minutes before a single oral dose of lovastatin (40 mg) decreased the AUC and C_{max} of lovastatin by approximately 40% and 28%, respectively, and delayed the T_{max} by about 4 hours compared with lovastatin administered alone. In the 30-week controlled clinical trials of BYETTA, the use of BYETTA in patients already receiving HMG CoA reductase inhibitors was not associated with consistent changes in lipid profiles compared to baseline.

Lisinopril

In patients with mild to moderate hypertension stabilized on lisinopril (5-20 mg/day), BYETTA (10 mcg twice daily) did not alter steady-state C_{max} or AUC of lisinopril. Lisinopril steady-state T_{max} was delayed by 2 hours. There were no changes in 24-hour mean systolic and diastolic blood pressure.

Oral Contraceptives

The effect of BYETTA (10 mcg twice daily) on single and on multiple doses of a combination oral contraceptive (30 mcg ethinyl estradiol plus 150 mcg levonorgestrel) was studied in healthy female subjects. Repeated daily doses of the oral contraceptive (OC) given 30 minutes after BYETTA administration decreased the C_{max} of ethinyl estradiol and levonorgestrel by 45% and 27%, respectively, and delayed the T_{max} of ethinyl estradiol and levonorgestrel by 3.0 hours and 3.5 hours, respectively, as compared to the oral contraceptive administered alone. Administration of repeated daily doses of the OC one hour prior to BYETTA administration decreased the mean C_{max} of ethinyl estradiol by 15%, but the mean C_{max} of levonorgestrel was not significantly changed as compared to when the OC was given alone. BYETTA did not alter the mean trough concentrations of levonorgestrel after repeated daily dosing of the oral contraceptive for both regimens. However, the mean trough concentration of ethinyl estradiol was increased by 20% when the OC was administered 30 minutes after BYETTA administration injection as compared to when the OC was given alone. The effect of BYETTA on OC pharmacokinetics is confounded by the possible food effect on OC in this study [see *Drug Interactions (7.1)*].

Warfarin

Administration of warfarin (25 mg) 35 minutes after repeated doses of BYETTA (5 mcg twice daily on days 1-2 and 10 mcg twice daily on days 3-9) in healthy volunteers delayed warfarin T_{max} by approximately 2 hours. No clinically relevant effects on C_{max} or AUC of *S*- and *R*-enantiomers of warfarin were observed. BYETTA did not significantly alter the pharmacodynamic properties (e.g., international normalized ratio) of warfarin [see *Drug Interactions (7.2)*].

Specific Populations

Renal Impairment

BYDUREON (exenatide extended-release for injectable suspension) has not been studied in patients with severe renal impairment (creatinine clearance <30 mL/min) or end-stage renal disease receiving dialysis. Population pharmacokinetic analysis of renally impaired patients receiving 2 mg BYDUREON indicate that there is a 62% and 33% increase in exposure in moderate (N=10) and mild (N=56) renally impaired patients, respectively, as compared to patients with normal renal function (N=84).

In a study of BYETTA in subjects with end-stage renal disease receiving dialysis, mean exenatide exposure increased by 3.4-fold compared to that of subjects with normal renal function [see *Use in Specific Populations (8.6)*].

Hepatic Impairment

BYDUREON has not been studied in patients with acute or chronic hepatic impairment [see *Use in Specific Populations (8.7)*].

Age

Population pharmacokinetic analysis of patients ranging from 22 to 73 years of age suggests that age does not influence the pharmacokinetic properties of exenatide [see *Use in Specific Populations (8.5)*].

Gender

Population pharmacokinetic analysis suggests that gender does not influence the steady-state concentrations of exenatide following BYDUREON administration.

Race

There were no apparent differences in steady-state concentrations of exenatide among Caucasian, Hispanic, and Black patients following BYDUREON administration.

Body Mass Index

Population pharmacokinetic analysis of patients with body mass indices (BMI) ≥30 kg/m^2 and <30 kg/m^2 suggests that BMI has no significant effect on the pharmacokinetics of exenatide.

Pediatric

BYDUREON has not been studied in pediatric patients [see *Use in Specific Populations (8.4)*].

13 NONCLINICAL TOXICOLOGY

13.1 Carcinogenesis, Mutagenesis, Impairment of Fertility

A 104-week carcinogenicity study was conducted with exenatide extended-release in male and female rats at doses of 0.3, 1.0, and 3.0 mg/kg (2-, 9-, and 26-times human systemic exposure based on AUC, respectively) administered by subcutaneous injection every other week. A statistically significant increase in thyroid C-cell tumor incidence was observed in both males and females. The incidence of C-cell adenomas was statistically significantly increased at all doses (27%-31%) in females and at 1.0 and 3.0 mg/kg (46% and 47%, respectively) in males compared with the control group (13% for males and 7% for females). A statistically significantly higher incidence of C-cell carcinomas occurred in the high-dose group females (6%), while numerically higher incidences of 3%, 7%, and 4% (nonstatistically significant versus controls) were noted in the low-, mid-, and high-dose group males compared with the control group (0% for both males and females). An increase in benign fibromas was seen in the skin subcutis at injection sites of males given 3 mg/kg. No treatment-related injection-site fibrosarcomas were observed at any dose. The human relevance of these findings is currently unknown.

A 104-week carcinogenicity study was conducted with exenatide, the active ingredient in BYDUREON (exenatide extended-release for injectable suspension), in male and female rats at doses of 18, 70, or 250 mcg/kg/day (3-, 6-, and 27-times human systemic exposure based on AUC, respectively) administered by once-daily bolus subcutaneous injection. Benign thyroid C-cell adenomas were observed in female rats at all exenatide doses. The incidences in female rats were 8% and 5% in the two control groups and 14%, 11%, and 23% in the low-, medium-, and high-dose groups.

In a 104-week carcinogenicity study with exenatide, the active ingredient in BYDUREON, in male and female mice at doses of 18, 70, or 250 mcg/kg/day administered by once-daily bolus subcutaneous injection, no evidence of tumors was observed at doses up to 250 mcg/kg/day, a systemic exposure up to 16 times the human exposure resulting from the recommended dose of 2 mg/week, based on AUC. The carcinogenicity of exenatide extended-release has not been evaluated in mice.

BYDUREON and exenatide, the active ingredient in BYDUREON, were not mutagenic or clastogenic, with or without metabolic activation, in the Ames bacterial mutagenicity assay or chromosomal aberration assay in Chinese hamster ovary cells. Exenatide was negative in the *in vivo* mouse micronucleus assay.

In mouse fertility studies with exenatide, the active ingredient in BYDUREON, at twice-daily subcutaneous doses of 6, 68, or 760 mcg/kg/day, males were treated for 4 weeks prior to and throughout mating, and females were treated 2 weeks prior to mating and throughout mating until gestation day 7. No adverse effect on fertility was observed at 760 mcg/kg/day, a systemic exposure 148 times the human exposure resulting from the recommended dose of 2 mg/week, based on AUC.

13.3 Reproductive and Developmental Toxicology

A rat embryo-fetal developmental toxicity study was conducted with exenatide extended-release. A complete reproductive and developmental toxicity program was conducted with exenatide, the active ingredient in BYDUREON.

Fetuses from pregnant rats given subcutaneous doses of exenatide extended-release at 0.3, 1, or 3 mg/kg on gestation days 6, 9, 12, and 15 demonstrated reduced fetal growth at all doses and produced skeletal ossification deficits at 1 and 3 mg/kg in association with maternal effects (decreased food intake and decreased body weight gain). There was no evidence of malformations. Doses of 0.3, 1, and 3 mg/kg correspond to systemic exposures of 3, 7, and 17 times, respectively, the human exposure resulting from the recommended dose of 2 mg/week, based on AUC.

In female mice given twice-daily subcutaneous doses of 6, 68, or 760 mcg/kg/day exenatide, the active ingredient in BYDUREON, beginning 2 weeks prior to and throughout mating until gestation day 7, there were no adverse fetal effects at doses up to 760 mcg/kg/day, systemic exposures up to 148 times the human exposure resulting from the maximum recommended dose of 2 mg/day, based on AUC.

In pregnant mice given twice-daily subcutaneous doses of 6, 68, 460, or 760 mcg/kg/day exenatide, the active ingredient in BYDUREON, from gestation day 6 through 15 (organogenesis), cleft palate (some with holes), and irregular fetal skeletal ossification of rib and skull bones were observed at 6 mcg/kg/day, a systemic exposure equal to the human exposure resulting from the maximum recommended dose of 2 mg/day, based on AUC.

In pregnant rabbits given twice-daily subcutaneous doses of 0.2, 2, 22, 156, or 260 mcg/kg/day exenatide, the active ingredient in BYDUREON, from gestation day 6 through 18 (organogenesis), irregular fetal skeletal ossifications were observed at 2 mcg/kg/day, a systemic exposure 4 times the human exposure resulting from the maximum recommended dose of 2 mg/day, based on AUC.

In pregnant mice given twice-daily subcutaneous doses of 6, 68, or 760 mcg/kg/day exenatide, the active ingredient in BYDUREON (exenatide extended-release for injectable suspension), from gestation day 6 through lactation day 20 (weaning), an increased number of neonatal deaths was observed on postpartum days 2 to 4 in dams given 6 mcg/kg/day, a systemic exposure equal to the human exposure resulting from the maximum recommended dose of 2 mg/day, based on AUC.

14 CLINICAL STUDIES

BYDUREON has been studied as monotherapy and in combination with metformin, a sulfonylurea, a thiazolidinedione, a combination of metformin and a sulfonylurea, or a combination of metformin and a thiazolidinedione.

14.1 24-Week Comparator-Controlled Study

A 24-week, randomized, open-label trial was conducted to compare the safety and efficacy of BYDUREON to BYETTA in patients with type 2 diabetes and inadequate glycemic control with diet and exercise alone or with oral antidiabetic therapy, including metformin, a sulfonylurea, a thiazolidinedione, or combination of two of those therapies.

A total of 252 patients were studied: 149 (59%) were Caucasian, 78 (31%) Hispanic, 15 (6%) Black, and 10 (4%) Asian. Patients were treated with diet and exercise alone (19%), a single oral antidiabetic agent (47%), or combination therapy of oral antidiabetic agents (35%). The mean baseline HbA_{1c} was 8.4%. Patients were randomly assigned to receive BYDUREON 2 mg once every 7 days (weekly) or BYETTA (10 mcg twice daily), in addition to existing oral antidiabetic agents. Patients assigned to BYETTA initiated treatment with 5 mcg twice daily then increased the dose to 10 mcg twice daily after 4 weeks.

The primary endpoint was change in HbA_{1c} from baseline to Week 24 (or the last value at time of early discontinuation). Change in body weight was a secondary endpoint. Twenty-four week study results are summarized in Table 4.

Table 4: Results of 24-Week Trial of BYDUREON

	BYDUREON 2 mg	BYETTA 10 mcg*
Intent-to-Treat Population (N)	129	123
HbA_{1c} (%)		
Mean Baseline	8.5	8.4
Mean Change at Week 24†	−1.6	−0.9
Difference from BYETTA† [95% CI]	−0.7 [−0.9, −0.4]¶	
Percentage Achieving HbA_{1c} <7% at Week 24 (%)	58 ¶	30
Fasting Plasma Glucose (mg/dL)		
Mean Baseline	173	168
Mean Change at Week 24	−25	−5
Difference from BYETTA† [95% CI]	−20 [−31, −10] ¶	

N = number of patients in each treatment group.

Note: mean change is least squares mean change

* BYETTA 5 mcg twice daily before the morning and evening meals for 4 weeks followed by 10 mcg twice daily for 20 weeks.

† Least squares (LS) means are adjusted for baseline HbA_{1c} strata, background antihyperglycemic therapy, and baseline value of the dependent variable (if applicable).

¶ p<0.001, treatment vs comparator.

Reductions from mean baseline (97/94 kg) in body weight were observed in both BYDUREON (−2.3 kg) and BYETTA (−1.4 kg) treatment groups.

BYDUREON did not have adverse effects on blood pressure. An LS mean increase from baseline (74 beats per minute) in heart rate of 4 beats per minute was observed with BYDUREON treatment and 2 beats per minute with BYETTA treatment. The long-term effects of the increase in pulse rate have not been established [see *Warnings and Precautions (5.8)*].

16 HOW SUPPLIED/STORAGE AND HANDLING

16.1 How Supplied

BYDUREON (exenatide extended-release for injectable suspension) for once every 7 days (weekly) subcutaneous administration is supplied in cartons of 4 single-dose trays for use (NDC 66780-219-04).

Each single-dose tray contains:
- One vial containing 2 mg exenatide (as a white to off-white powder)
- One prefilled syringe delivering 0.65 mL diluent
- One vial connector
- Two custom needles (23G, 5/16″) specific to this delivery system (one is a spare needle)

Do **not** substitute needles or any other components in the tray.

16.2 Storage and Handling

- BYDUREON (exenatide extended-release for injectable suspension) should be stored in the refrigerator at 36°F to 46°F (2°C to 8°C), up to the expiration date or until preparing for use. BYDUREON should not be used past the expiration date. The expiration date can be found on the carton and the cover of the single-dose tray.
- Do not freeze the BYDUREON tray. Do not use BYDUREON if it has been frozen. Protect from light.
- Each single-dose tray can be kept at room temperature not to exceed 77°F (25°C) [see USP Controlled Room Temperature] for no more than a total of 4 weeks, if needed.
- Use the diluent only if it is clear and free of particulate matter.
- After suspension, the mixture should be white to off-white and cloudy.
- BYDUREON must be administered immediately after the exenatide powder is suspended in the diluent and transferred to the syringe.
- Use a puncture-resistant container to discard the syringe with the needle still attached. Do not reuse or share needles or syringes.
- Keep out of the reach of children.

17 PATIENT COUNSELING INFORMATION

See FDA-approved Medication Guide.

Inform patients about the potential risks and benefits of BYDUREON and of alternative modes of therapy. Also inform patients about the importance of diabetes self-management practices, such as regular physical activity, adhering to meal planning, periodic blood glucose monitoring and HbA_{1c} testing, recognition and management of hypoglycemia and hyperglycemia, and assessment for diabetes complications.

17.1 Risk of Thyroid C-cell Tumors

Inform patients that exenatide extended-release causes benign and malignant thyroid C-cell tumors in rats and that the human relevance of this finding is unknown. Counsel patients to report symptoms of thyroid tumors (e.g., a lump in the neck, hoarseness, dysphagia, or dyspnea) [see *Warnings and Precautions (5.1)*].

17.2 Risk of Pancreatitis

Inform patients treated with BYDUREON of the potential risk for pancreatitis. Explain that persistent severe abdominal pain that may radiate to the back, and which may or may not be accompanied by vomiting, is the hallmark symptom of acute pancreatitis. Instruct patients to promptly discontinue BYDUREON and contact their healthcare provider if persistent severe abdominal pain occurs [see *Warnings and Precautions (5.2)*].

17.3 Risk of Hypoglycemia

The risk of hypoglycemia is increased when BYDUREON is used in combination with an agent that induces hypoglycemia, such as a sulfonylurea [see *Warnings and Precautions (5.3)*]. Explain the symptoms, treatment, and conditions that predispose to the development of hypoglycemia. While the patient's usual instructions for hypoglycemia management do not need to be changed, these instructions should be reviewed and reinforced when initiating BYDUREON therapy, particularly when concomitantly administered with a sulfonylurea [see *Warnings and Precautions (5.3)*].

17.4 Risk of Renal Impairment

Inform patients treated with BYDUREON of the potential risk for worsening renal function and explain the associated signs and symptoms of renal impairment, as well as the possibility of dialysis as a medical intervention if renal failure occurs [see *Warnings and Precautions (5.4)*].

17.5 Risk of Hypersensitivity Reactions

Inform patients that serious hypersensitivity reactions have been reported during postmarketing use of exenatide. If symptoms of hypersensitivity reactions occur, patients must stop taking BYDUREON and seek medical advice promptly [see *Warnings and Precautions (5.7)*].

17.6 Use in Pregnancy

Advise patients to inform their healthcare provider if they are pregnant or intend to become pregnant [see *Use in Specific Populations (8.1)*].

17.7 Instructions

Each dose of BYDUREON should be administered as a subcutaneous injection at any time on the dosing day, with or without meals. Patients should be informed that the day of once every 7 days (weekly) administration can be changed if necessary as long as the last dose was administered 3 or more days before. If a dose is missed, it should be administered as soon as noticed, provided the next regularly scheduled dose is due at least 3 days later. Thereafter, patients can resume their usual once every 7 days (weekly) dosing schedule. If a dose is missed and the next regularly scheduled dose is due in 1 or 2 days, the patient should not administer the missed dose and instead resume BYDUREON with the next regularly scheduled dose [see *Dosage and Administration (2.1)*].

Counsel patients that they should never share a BYDUREON (exenatide extended-release for injectable suspension) single-dose tray with another person, even if the needle is changed. Sharing of the single-dose trays or needles between patients may pose a risk of transmission of infection.

If a patient is currently taking BYETTA, it should be discontinued upon starting BYDUREON. Patients formerly on BYETTA who start BYDUREON may experience transient elevations in blood glucose concentrations, which generally improve within the first 2 weeks after initiation of therapy [see *Dosage and Administration (2.3)* and *Clinical Studies (14.1)*].

Treatment with BYDUREON may also result in nausea, particularly upon initiation of therapy [see *Adverse Reactions (6)*].

Inform patients about the importance of proper storage of BYDUREON, injection technique, and dosing [see *Dosage and Administration (2)* and *How Supplied/Storage and Handling (16)*].

The patient should read the BYDUREON Medication Guide and the Instructions for Use before starting BYDUREON therapy and review them each time the prescription is refilled.

Manufactured by:
Bristol-Myers Squibb Company
Princeton, NJ 08543 USA
Marketed by:
Bristol-Myers Squibb Company
Princeton, NJ 08543
and
AstraZeneca Pharmaceuticals LP
Wilmington, DE 19850

BYDUREON is a registered trademark of Amylin Pharmaceuticals, LLC.
832001-LL/02
Rev February 2013

MEDICATION GUIDE
BYDUREON® (by-DUR-ee-on)
(exenatide extended-release
for injectable suspension)

Read this Medication Guide and Instructions for Use before you start using BYDUREON and each time you get a refill. There may be new information. This information does not take the place of talking with your healthcare provider about your medical condition or your treatment. If you have questions about BYDUREON after reading this information, ask your healthcare provider or pharmacist.

What is the most important information I should know about BYDUREON?

Serious side effects may happen in people who take BYDUREON, including:

1. **Possible thyroid tumors, including cancer**. During the drug testing process, the medicine in BYDUREON caused rats to develop tumors of the thyroid gland. Some of these tumors were cancers. It is not known if BYDUREON will cause thyroid tumors or a type of thyroid cancer called medullary thyroid cancer in people.
   - Before you start taking BYDUREON, tell your healthcare provider if you or any of your family members have had thyroid cancer, especially medullary thyroid cancer, or Multiple Endocrine Neoplasia syndrome type 2. **Do not** take BYDUREON if you or any of your family members have medullary thyroid cancer, or if you have Multiple Endocrine Neoplasia syndrome type 2. People with these conditions already have a higher chance of developing medullary thyroid cancer in general and should not take BYDUREON.
   - While taking BYDUREON, tell your healthcare provider if you get a lump or swelling in your neck, hoarseness, trouble swallowing, or shortness of breath. These may be symptoms of thyroid cancer.
2. **Inflammation of the pancreas (pancreatitis)**, which may be severe and lead to death.

   Before taking BYDUREON, tell your healthcare provider if you have had:
   - pancreatitis
   - stones in your gallbladder (gallstones)
   - a history of alcoholism
   - high blood triglyceride levels

   These medical conditions can make you more likely to get pancreatitis. It is not known if having these conditions will lead to a higher chance of getting pancreatitis while taking BYDUREON.

   Stop taking BYDUREON and call your healthcare provider right away if you have pain in your stomach area (abdomen) that is severe, and will not go away. The pain may happen with or without vomiting. The pain may be felt going from your abdomen through to your back. This type of pain may be a symptom of pancreatitis.

What is BYDUREON?
- BYDUREON (exenatide extended-release for injectable suspension) is an injectable prescription medicine that may improve blood sugar (glucose) in adults with type 2 diabetes mellitus, and should be used along with diet and exercise.
- BYDUREON is a long-acting form of the medication contained in BYETTA. Do not use BYDUREON and BYETTA together.
- BYDUREON is not recommended as the first choice of medication for treating diabetes.
- BYDUREON is not insulin.
- It is not known if BYDUREON is safe and effective when used with insulin.
- BYDUREON is not for use in people with type 1 diabetes or people with a condition caused by very high blood sugar (diabetic ketoacidosis).
- It is not known if BYDUREON is safe and effective in children. BYDUREON is not recommended for use in children.
- It is not known if BYDUREON is safe and effective in people who have a history of pancreatitis.
- BYDUREON has not been studied in people who have severe kidney problems.

Who should not use BYDUREON?

Do not use BYDUREON if:
- you or any of your family members have a history of medullary thyroid cancer.
- you have Multiple Endocrine Neoplasia syndrome type 2 (MEN 2). This is a disease where people have tumors in more than one gland in their body.
- you are allergic to exenatide or any of the ingredients in BYDUREON. See the end of this Medication Guide for a complete list of ingredients in BYDUREON. Symptoms of a severe allergic reaction may include:
  - swelling of your face, lips, tongue, or throat
  - problems breathing or swallowing
  - severe rash or itching
  - fainting or feeling dizzy
  - very rapid heartbeat

Talk to your healthcare provider before taking this medicine if you have any of these conditions.

What should I tell my healthcare provider before using BYDUREON?

Before using BYDUREON, tell your healthcare provider if you:
- have any of the conditions listed in the section **"What is the most important information I should know about BYDUREON?"**
- have severe problems with your stomach such as slow emptying of your stomach (gastroparesis) or problems digesting food.
- have or have had kidney problems, or have had a kidney transplant.
- have any other medical conditions.
- are pregnant or are planning to become pregnant. It is not known if BYDUREON may harm your unborn baby. Tell your healthcare provider if you become pregnant while taking BYDUREON.

  Pregnancy Registry: A registry has been implemented for women who take BYDUREON during pregnancy. The purpose of this registry is to collect information about the health of you and your baby. If you take BYDUREON at any time during your pregnancy, you may enroll in this registry by calling 1-800-633-9081.
- are breastfeeding or plan to breastfeed. It is not known if BYDUREON passes into your breast milk. You and your healthcare provider should decide if you will take BYDUREON or breastfeed. You should not do both without talking with your healthcare provider first.

Tell your healthcare provider about all of the medicines you take, including prescription and nonprescription medicines, vitamins, and herbal supplements. BYDUREON may affect the way some medicines work and some other medicines may affect the way BYDUREON works.

Especially tell your healthcare provider if you take:
- other diabetes medicines, especially insulin or a sulfonylurea
- any medicine taken by mouth
- warfarin sodium (Coumadin®, Jantoven®)

Know the medicines you take. Keep a list of them to show your healthcare provider and pharmacist each time you get a new medicine.

How should I use BYDUREON?

For detailed instructions, see the Instructions for Use that comes with your BYDUREON.
- Use BYDUREON exactly as your healthcare provider tells you to.
- BYDUREON is injected once every seven days (weekly) any time during the day.
- BYDUREON is a subcutaneous injection. Inject BYDUREON into your skin exactly the way your healthcare provider told you to. You can take the injection in your stomach area (abdomen), your thigh, or the back of your upper arm. Each week you can use the same area of your body. But be sure to choose a different injection site in that area.
- You can take BYDUREON (exenatide extended-release for injectable suspension) with or without food.
- **If you miss a dose of BYDUREON, it should be taken as soon as you remember, provided the next regularly scheduled dose is due at least three days later.**
- **If you miss a dose of BYDUREON and the next regularly scheduled dose is due one or two days later, do not take the missed dose but take BYDUREON on the next regularly scheduled day.**
- **Do not** take 2 doses of BYDUREON less than 3 days apart.
- If you want to change your dosing day, you can. Your new dosing day must be at least 3 days after your last dose.
- Your healthcare provider must teach you how to inject BYDUREON before you use it for the first time. If you have any questions or do not understand the instructions, talk with your healthcare provider or pharmacist.
- BYDUREON must be injected right after you mix it.
- **If you are taking BYETTA and your healthcare provider prescribed BYDUREON, you should follow your healthcare provider's instructions about when to stop taking BYETTA and when to start taking BYDUREON.** BYETTA is a different form of the same medicine that is in BYDUREON, so do not take BYETTA when you are taking BYDUREON. When you first change from BYETTA to BYDUREON, your blood sugar levels may be higher than usual and should get better in about 2 weeks.
- Inject your dose of BYDUREON under the skin (subcutaneous injection), as you are told to by your healthcare provider. **Do not inject BYDUREON into a vein or muscle.**
- **Do not** share your BYDUREON tray with another person even if the needle is changed. Sharing your tray with another person can cause you or someone else to get an infection.
- Follow your healthcare provider's instructions for diet, exercise, how often to test your blood sugar, and when to get your HbA_{1c} checked. If you see your blood sugar increasing during treatment with BYDUREON, talk to your healthcare provider because you may need to adjust your current treatment plan for your diabetes.
- Talk to your healthcare provider about how to manage high blood sugar (hyperglycemia) and low blood sugar (hypoglycemia), and how to recognize problems that can happen with your diabetes.

What are the possible side effects of BYDUREON?

BYDUREON can cause serious side effects, including:
- **See "What is the most important information I should know about BYDUREON?"**
- **Low blood sugar (hypoglycemia)**. Your risk for getting low blood sugar is higher if you take BYDUREON with another medicine that can cause low blood sugar, such as a sulfonylurea. The dose of your sulfonylurea medicine may need to be lowered while you use BYDUREON. Signs and symptoms of low blood sugar may include:
  - shakiness
  - sweating
  - headache
  - drowsiness
  - hunger
  - fast heartbeat
  - weakness
  - dizziness
  - confusion
  - irritability
  - feeling jittery

Talk with your healthcare provider about how to recognize and treat low blood sugar. Make sure that your family and other people around you a lot know how to recognize and treat low blood sugar.
- **Kidney problems (kidney failure)**. BYDUREON may cause nausea, vomiting or diarrhea leading to loss of fluids (dehydration). Dehydration may cause kidney failure, which can lead to the need for dialysis. This can happen in people who have never had kidney problems before. Drinking plenty of fluids may reduce your chance of dehydration. Call your healthcare provider right away if you have nausea, vomiting, or diarrhea that will not go away, or if you cannot drink liquids by mouth.
- **Severe allergic reactions.** Severe allergic reactions can happen with BYDUREON. Stop taking BYDUREON, and get medical help right away if you have any symptom of a severe allergic reaction. See **"Who should not take BYDUREON?"**

The most common side effects of BYDUREON include:
- nausea
- diarrhea
- headache
- vomiting
- constipation
- itching at the injection site
- a small bump (nodule) at the injection site
- indigestion

Nausea is most common when you first start using BYDUREON, but decreases over time in most people as their body gets used to the medicine.

Talk to your healthcare provider about any side effect that bothers you or does not go away.

These are not all the side effects of BYDUREON (exenatide extended-release for injectable suspension). For more information, ask your healthcare provider or pharmacist.

Call your doctor for medical advice about side effects. You may report side effects to FDA at 1-800-FDA-1088.

How should I store BYDUREON?

- Store BYDUREON in the refrigerator at 36°F to 46°F (2°C to 8°C).
- Do not use BYDUREON past the expiration date. The expiration date is labeled *EXP* and can be found on the paper cover of the single-dose tray.
- Do not freeze BYDUREON trays. Do not use BYDUREON if it has been frozen.
- Protect BYDUREON from light until you are ready to prepare and use your dose.
- If needed, you can keep your BYDUREON tray out of the refrigerator at 68°F to 77°F (20°C to 25°C) for up to 4 weeks.
- See the Instructions for Use for information about how to throw away your used BYDUREON parts.

Keep BYDUREON, and all medicines, out of the reach of children.

General information about safe and effective use of BYDUREON

Medicines are sometimes prescribed for purposes other than those listed in a Medication Guide. Do not use BYDUREON for a condition for which it was not prescribed. Do not give your BYDUREON to other people, even if they have the same symptoms you have. It may harm them.

This Medication Guide summarizes the most important information about BYDUREON. If you would like more information, talk with your healthcare provider. You can ask your healthcare provider or pharmacist for information about BYDUREON that is written for healthcare professionals.

For more information about BYDUREON, go to www.BYDUREON.com or call 1-877-700-7365.

What are the ingredients in BYDUREON?

Contents of vial:

Active Ingredient: exenatide

Inactive Ingredients: polylactide-co-glycolide and sucrose

Contents of liquid (diluent) in syringe:

Inactive Ingredients: carboxymethylcellulose sodium, polysorbate 20, sodium phosphate monobasic monohydrate, sodium phosphate dibasic heptahydrate, sodium chloride, water for injection.

This Medication Guide has been approved by the U.S. Food and Drug Administration.

BYDUREON is a registered trademark and BYETTA is a registered trademark of Amylin Pharmaceuticals, LLC. All other marks are the marks of their respective owners.

Manufactured by:
Bristol-Myers Squibb Company
Princeton, NJ 08543 USA
Marketed by:
Bristol-Myers Squibb Company
Princeton, NJ 08543
and
AstraZeneca Pharmaceuticals LP
Wilmington, DE 19850
833001-HH/02 Rev February 2013

Instructions for Use
BYDUREON® (by-DUR-ee-on)
exenatide extended-release
for injectable suspension

Read the BYDUREON Medication Guide for important safety information.

Your Step-by-Step Guide

CAUTION: Keep guide and medicine out of the reach of children.

If you have questions about taking BYDUREON® (exenatide extended-release for injectable suspension)

- Refer to the **Common Questions and Answers** section
- Call **1-877-700-7365**
- Visit **www.BYDUREON.com**

> **IMPORTANT:**
> **Read this Instructions for Use before you start using BYDUREON and each time you get a refill. There may be new information. This information does not take the place of talking to your healthcare provider about your medical condition or your treatment.**

Consider marking your calendar to remind yourself to take your injection once every seven days (weekly).

Your guide to the parts

- Single-dose tray

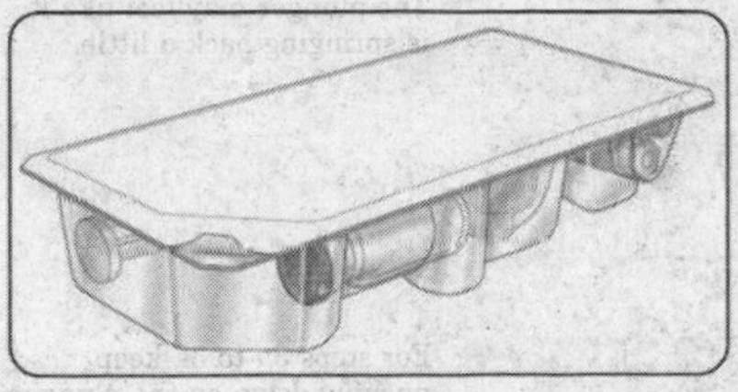

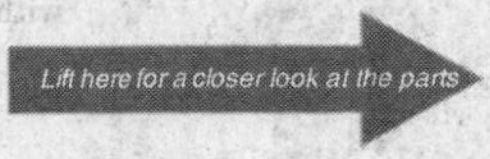

Keep this flap open so you can refer to it as you go through the steps.

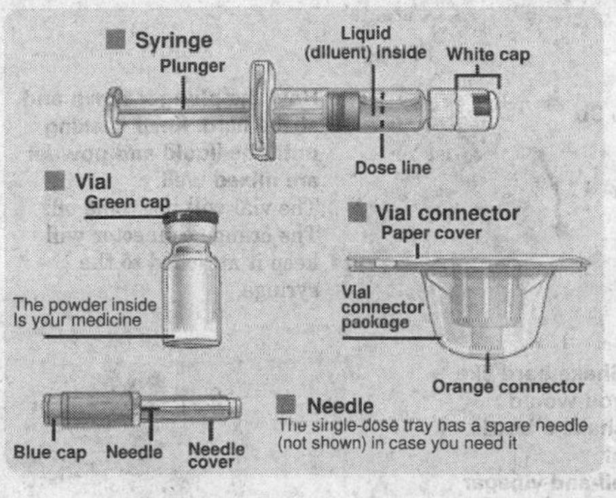

Your guide to the parts

- Single-dose tray

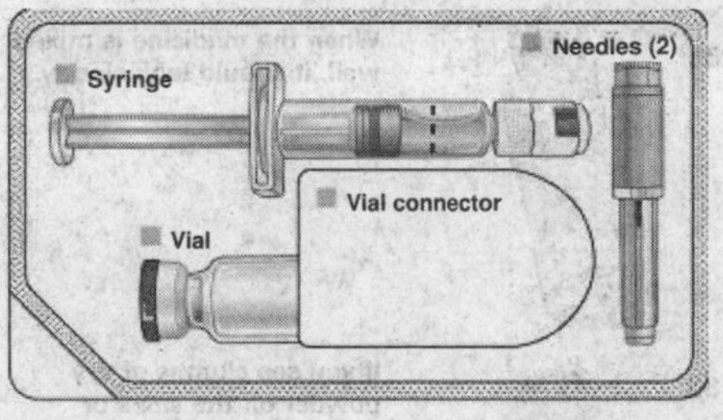

What's Inside

To take the correct dose, read **each** page so that you do **every** step in order.

This step-by-step guide is divided into 4 sections:

- Getting Started
- Connecting the Parts
- Mixing the Medicine and Filling the Syringe
- Injecting the Medicine

For **Common Questions and Answers,** see page 32.

How to store your single-dose trays of BYDUREON

- Store your BYDUREON (exenatide extended-release for injectable suspension) in the refrigerator at 36°F to 46°F (2°C to 8°C).
- If needed, you can keep your BYDUREON tray out of the refrigerator at 68°F to 77°F (20°C to 25°C) for up to 4 weeks.
- Protect BYDUREON from light until you are ready to prepare and use your dose.
- Do not freeze BYDUREON trays.
- Do not use BYDUREON past the expiration date. The expiration date is labeled *EXP* and can be found on the paper cover of each tray.
- Keep BYDUREON, and all medicines, out of the reach of children.

1.
Getting Started

Helpful Hints

- Try to be patient. It can take time to get used to giving yourself injections
- Set aside enough time to complete all the steps without stopping
- As you do the steps, it can be helpful to read the directions aloud

1a) Take a single-dose tray from the refrigerator.

You will also need a puncture-resistant container with a lid to hold used needles and syringes. This is not included in the tray. You may use a red biohazard container, a hard plastic container (such as an empty detergent bottle), or a metal container (such as an empty coffee can). Ask your healthcare provider how to safely throw away used needles and the container. There may be state and local laws about this. Do not throw the container in your household trash or try to recycle it.

1b) Wash your hands. Prepare to clean your injection site with soap and water or an alcohol swab prior to injecting your medicine.

1c

Peel back the paper cover to open.

Remove the syringe. The liquid in the syringe should be clear with no particles in it. It is okay if there are bubbles.

Place the needle, vial connector package, vial, and syringe on a clean, flat surface.

1d

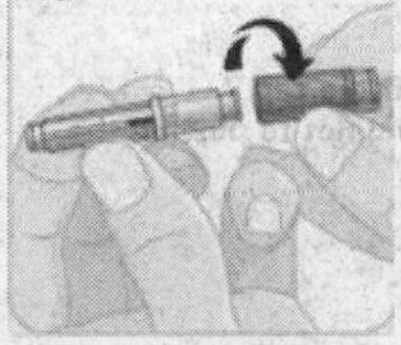

Pick up the needle, and twist off the blue cap.

Set the covered needle aside. You will use it later.

There is a spare needle in the tray if you need it.

1e

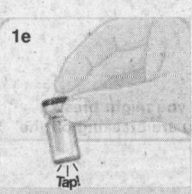

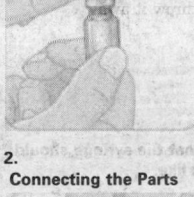

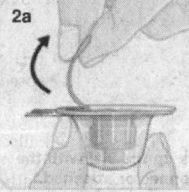

Pick up the vial.

Tap the vial several times against a hard surface to loosen the powder.

1f

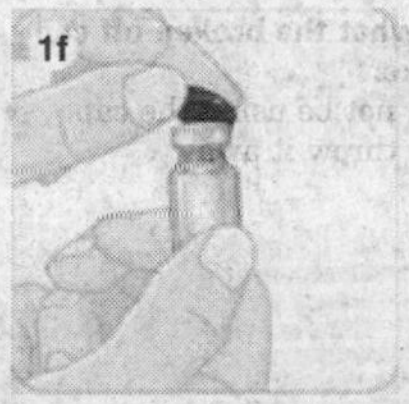

Use your thumb to remove the green cap.

Put the vial aside.

2.
Connecting the Parts

2a

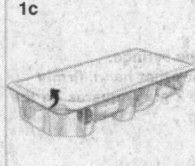

Pick up the vial connector package and peel off the paper cover. Do not touch the orange connector inside.

2b

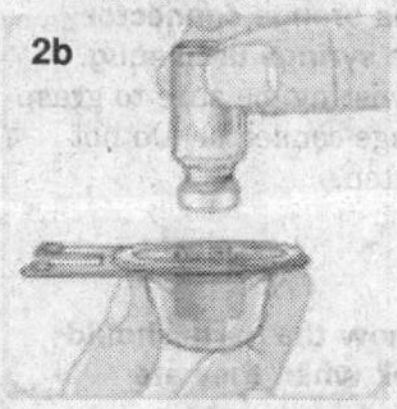

Hold the vial connector package.
In your other hand, hold the vial.

2c

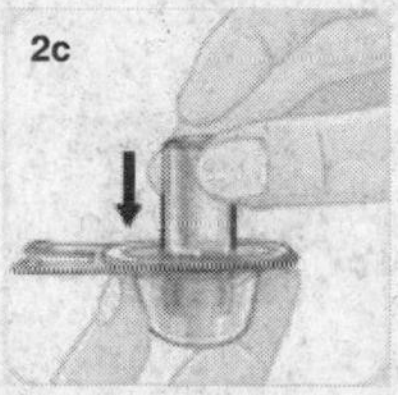

Press the top of the vial firmly into the orange connector.

2d

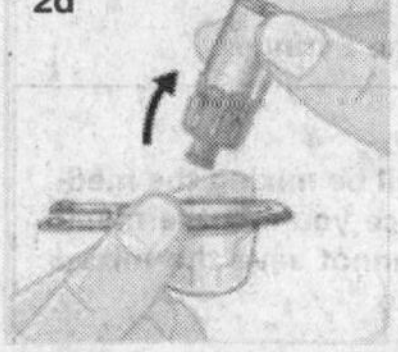

Then lift the vial with the orange connector now attached out of the clear package.

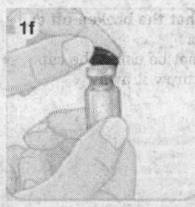

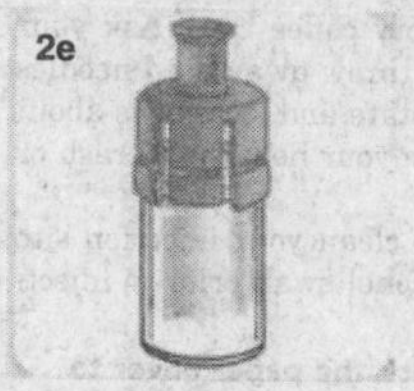

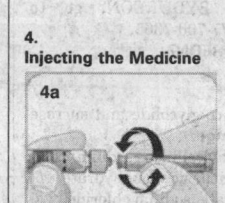

This is what the vial should now look like.
Put it aside for later.

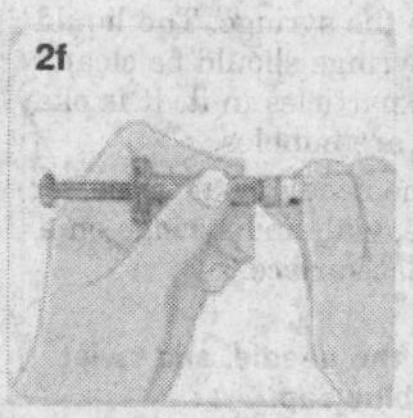

Pick up the syringe.
With your other hand, firmly grasp the 2 gray squares on the white cap.

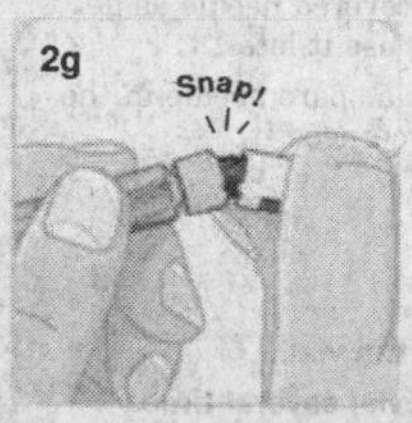

Break off the cap.
Be careful not to push in the plunger.

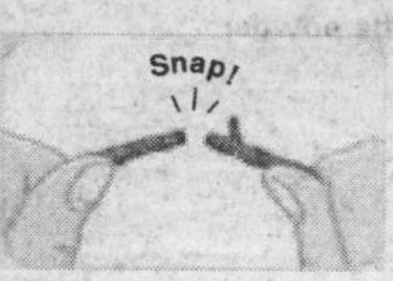

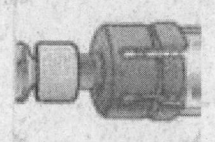

Just like you might break a stick, you are breaking off the cap.

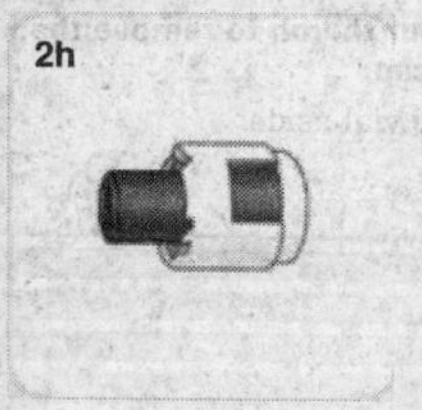

This is what the broken-off cap looks like.
You will not be using the cap and can throw it away.

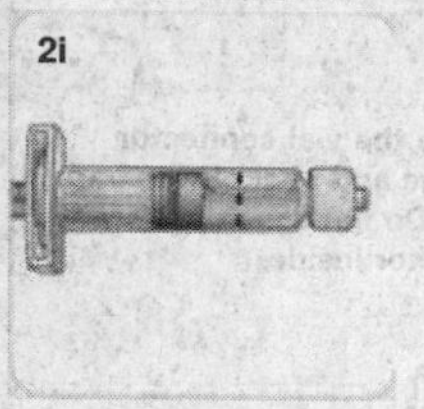

This is what the syringe should now look like.

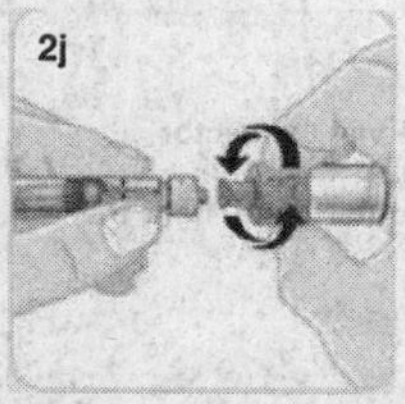

Now, pick up the vial with the orange connector attached. Twist the orange connector onto the syringe until snug.
While twisting, be sure to grasp the orange connector. Do not overtighten.

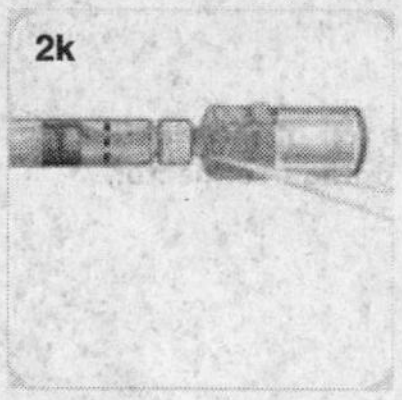

This is how the parts should now look when they are connected.

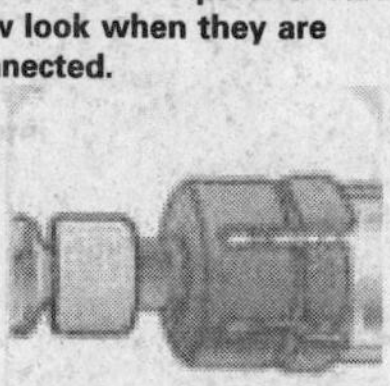

3.
Mixing the Medicine and Filling the Syringe

> **IMPORTANT:**
> **During these next steps, you will be mixing the medicine and filling the syringe. Once you mix the medicine, you must inject it. You cannot save the mixed medicine to inject at a later time.**

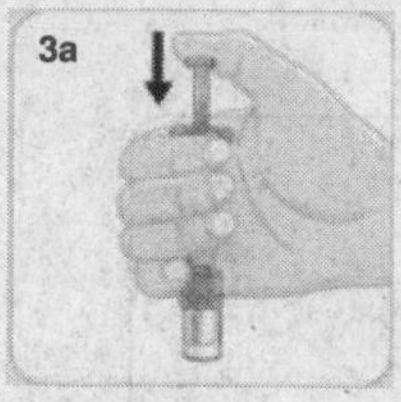

With your thumb, push down the plunger until it stops.
The plunger may feel like it is springing back a little.

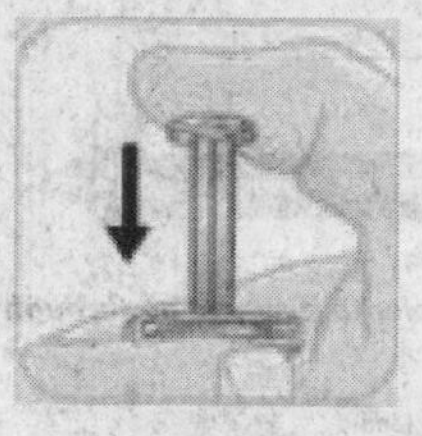

For steps 3a to 3f, keep pushing down on the plunger with your thumb.

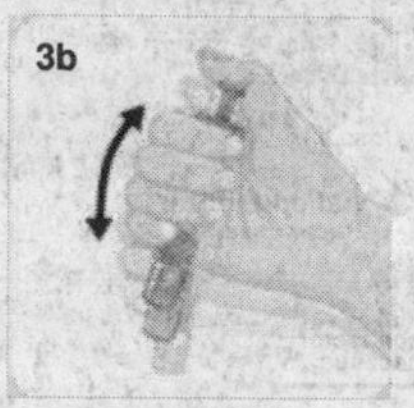

Hold the plunger down and shake hard. Keep shaking until the liquid and powder are mixed well.
The vial will not come off. The orange connector will keep it attached to the syringe.

Shake hard like you would shake a bottle of oil-and-vinegar salad dressing.

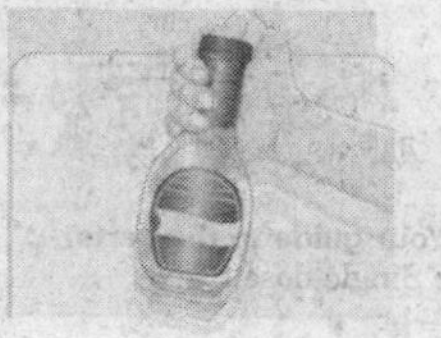

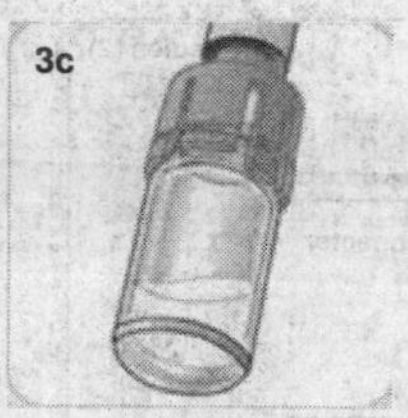

When the medicine is mixed well, it should look cloudy.

If you see clumps of dry powder on the sides or bottom of the vial, the medicine is not mixed well. Shake hard again until well mixed.
Keep pushing down on the plunger while shaking.

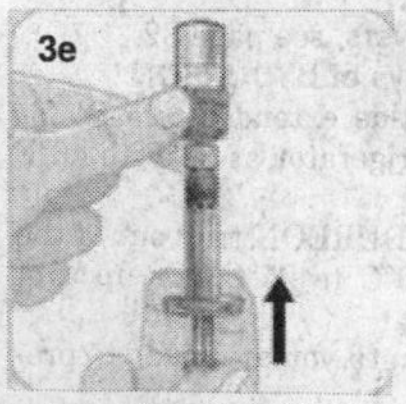

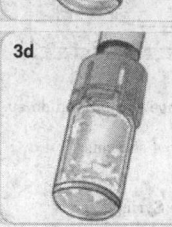

Now, hold the vial upside down so the syringe is pointing up. Continue to hold the plunger in place with your thumb.

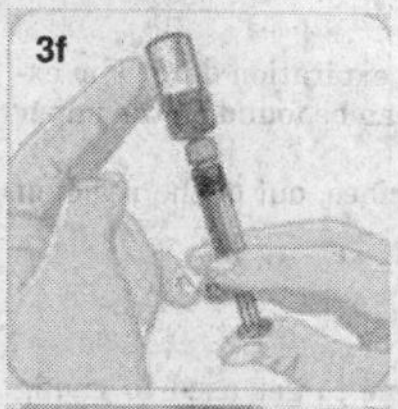

Gently tap the vial with the other hand. Continue to hold the plunger in place.
The tapping helps the medicine drip down. It is okay if there are bubbles.

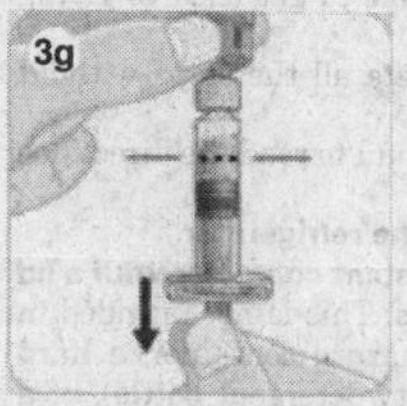

Pull the plunger down beyond the black dashed Dose Line.
This draws the medicine from the vial into the syringe. You may see air bubbles. This is normal.
A little bit of liquid may cling to the sides of the vial.

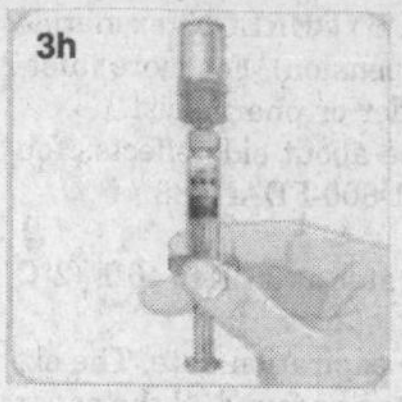

With one hand, hold the plunger in place so it does not move.

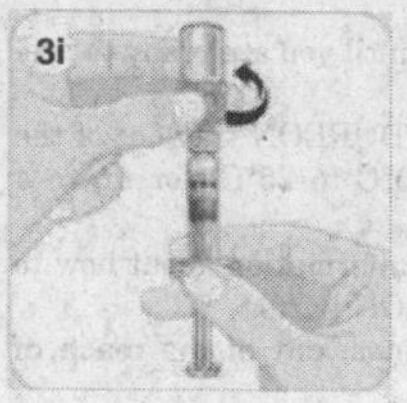

With the other hand, twist the orange connector to remove it from the syringe. Be careful not to push in the plunger.

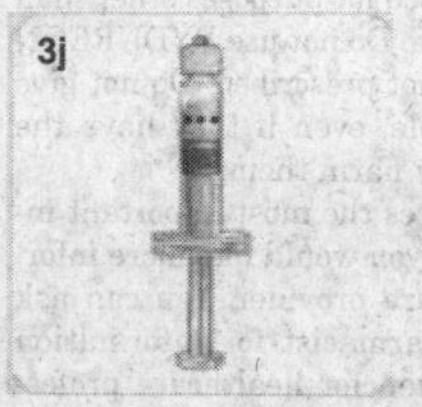

This is what the syringe should now look like.

4.
Injecting the Medicine

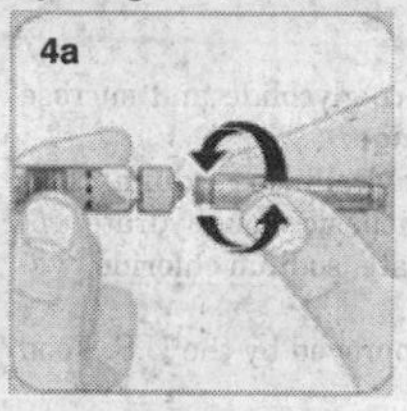

Pick up the needle. Twist the needle onto the syringe until snug. Do not remove the needle cover yet.

> **IMPORTANT:**
> **Read the next steps carefully and look closely at the pictures. This helps you get the correct dose of medicine.**

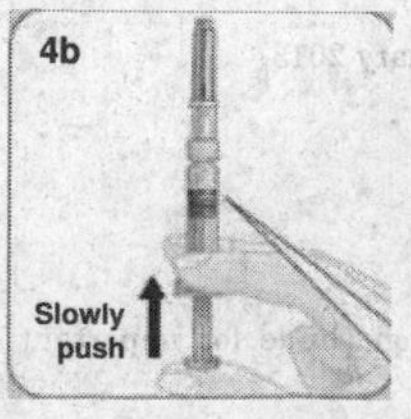

Slowly push in the plunger so the top of the plunger lines up with the black dashed Dose Line.
Then, take your thumb off the plunger.

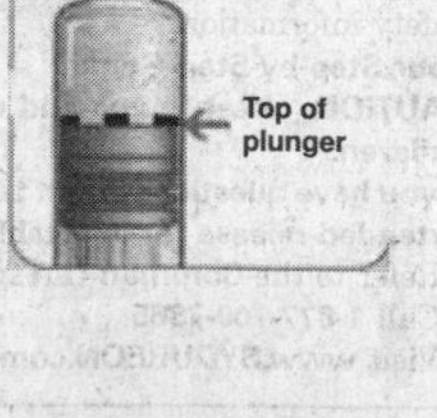

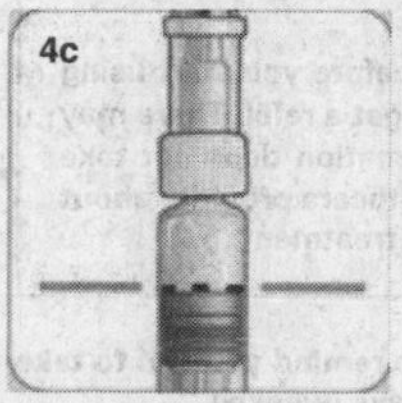

The top of the plunger must stay lined up with the black dashed Dose Line as you go through the next steps. This will help you get the correct dose of medicine.
Put aside the syringe with the needle attached.

IMPORTANT:
It is normal to see a few bubbles in the mixture. The bubbles will not harm you or affect your dose.

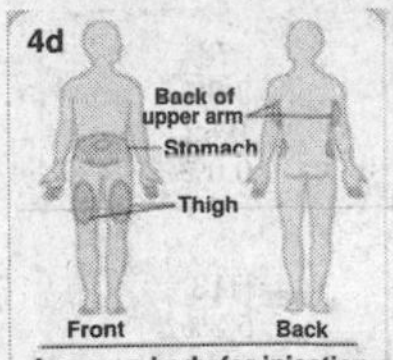

Areas on body for injection

You can inject the medicine in your stomach area (abdomen), your thigh, or the back of your upper arm.
Each week you can use the same area of your body. But be sure to choose a different injection site in that area.
Clean the injection site prior to injecting the medicine (with soap and water or an alcohol swab).

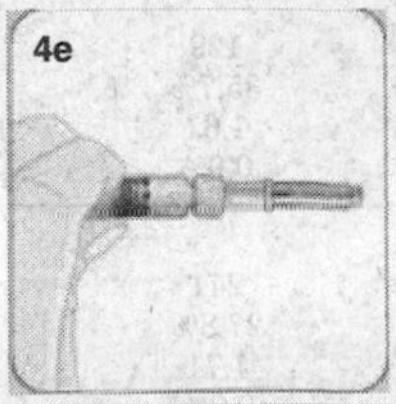

Now, pick up the syringe and hold it near the black dashed Dose Line.

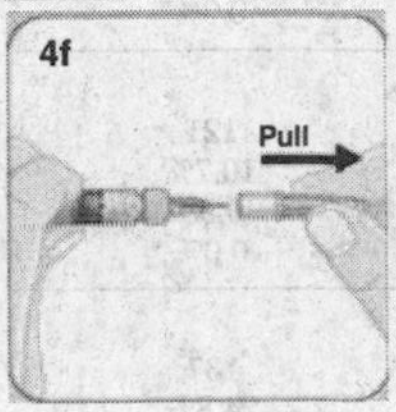

Pull the needle cover straight off. Do not twist.
Be careful not to push in the plunger.
When you remove the cover, you may see 1 or 2 drops of liquid. This is normal.

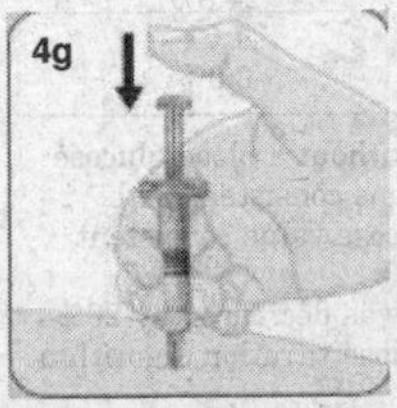

Insert the needle into your skin (subcutaneously). To inject your full dose, push down on the plunger with your thumb until it stops.
Withdraw the needle.
Be sure to use the injection technique recommended by your healthcare provider.

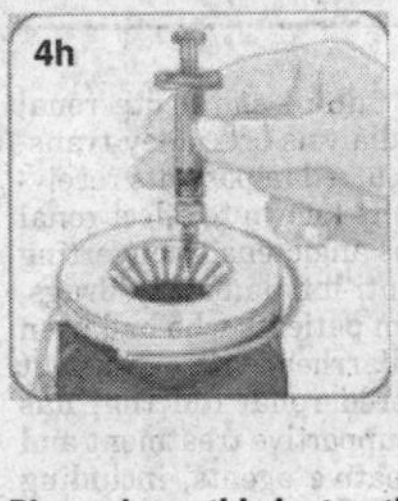

Use the puncture-resistant container to throw away the syringe with the needle still attached. To avoid a needlestick injury, do not put the cover back on the needle.
Throw away all other parts in the trash. You do not have to save them. Each single-dose tray has a new supply of parts to use for your next dose of BYDUREON.

Please keep this Instructions for Use for your next dose.

Common Questions and Answers

If your question is about:	*See question number:*
How soon to inject after mixing	1
Mixing the medicine	2
Air bubbles in syringe	3
Attaching the needle	4
Removing the needle cover	5
Plunger not lining up with black dashed Dose Line	6
Being unable to push the plunger down when injecting	7

1. **After I mix the medicine, how long can I wait before taking the injection?**
You must take your injection of BYDUREON (exenatide extended-release for injectable suspension) right after mixing it. If you do not inject BYDUREON right away, the medicine will start to form small clumps in the syringe. These clumps can clog the needle when you take the injection (see question 7).
2. **How do I know that the medicine is mixed well?**
When the medicine is mixed well, it should look cloudy. There should not be any dry powder on the sides or bottom of the vial. **If you do see any dry powder, shake hard while continuing to push down on the plunger with your thumb.** (This question relates to the steps shown on pages 18 through 20.)
3. **I'm ready to take the injection. What should I do if I see air bubbles in the syringe?**
It is normal for air bubbles to be in the syringe. The air bubbles will not harm you or affect your dose. BYDUREON is injected into your skin (subcutaneously). Air bubbles are not a problem with this type of injection (This question relates to step 3f shown on page 21 and step 4c shown on page 27.).
4. **What should I do if I have trouble attaching the needle?**
First, be sure you have removed the blue cap. Then, **twist** the needle onto the syringe until snug. To prevent losing medicine, do not push in the plunger while attaching the needle. (This question relates to step 4a on page 25.)
5. **What should I do if I have trouble removing the needle cover?**
With one hand, hold the syringe near the black dashed Dose Line. With your other hand, hold the needle cover. **Pull the needle cover straight off.** Do not twist it. (This question relates to step 4f on page 29.)
6. **I am at step 4c. What should I do if the top of the plunger has been pushed past the black dashed Dose Line?**
The black dashed Dose Line shows the correct dose. If the top of the plunger has been pushed past the line, you should continue from step 4d and take the injection. Before your next injection in 1 week, carefully review the instructions on pages 17 through 31.
7. **When I inject, what should I do if I cannot push the plunger all the way down?**
This means the needle has become clogged. Remove the needle from your skin and replace it with the spare needle from your tray. Then choose a different injection site and finish taking the injection.
To review how to:
   - Remove the blue cap of the needle, see page 9
   - Attach the needle, see page 25
   - Remove the needle cover and give the injection, see pages 29 and 30 If you still cannot push the plunger all the way down, remove the needle from your skin. Use a puncture-resistant container to throw away the syringe with the needle still attached. It is important that you then call 1-877-700-7365.

   To help prevent a clogged needle, always mix the medicine very well, and inject right after mixing.

Where to learn more about BYDUREON
- **Talk with your healthcare provider**
- **Read the Medication Guide that came with your BYDUREON.** The Medication Guide can help answer your questions about BYDUREON (exenatide extended-release for injectable suspension), such as what it is used for, possible side effects, and when to take BYDUREON.
- Enroll in BYDUREON Support for FREE ongoing help managing your diabetes. **Visit www.BYDUREON.com or call 1-877-700-7365.**

This Instructions for Use has been approved by the U.S. Food and Drug Administration.
BYDUREON® is a registered trademark of Amylin Pharmaceuticals, LLC.
Manufactured by:
Bristol-Myers Squibb Company
Princeton, NJ 08543 USA
Marketed by:
Bristol-Myers Squibb Company
Princeton, NJ 08543
and
AstraZeneca Pharmaceuticals LP
Wilmington, DE 19850
935001-03 / 735001-03
Rev February 2013

Shown in Product Identification Guide, page 305

BYETTA® ℞
[*bye-A-tuh*]
(exenatide)
Injection

HIGHLIGHTS OF PRESCRIBING INFORMATION
These highlights do not include all the information needed to use BYETTA safely and effectively. See full prescribing information for BYETTA.
BYETTA® (exenatide) Injection
Initial U.S. Approval: 2005

INDICATIONS AND USAGE

BYETTA is a glucagon-like peptide-1 (GLP-1) receptor agonist indicated as an adjunct to diet and exercise to improve glycemic control in adults with type 2 diabetes mellitus (1.1, 14).

Important Limitations of Use
- Not a substitute for insulin. BYETTA should not be used for the treatment of type 1 diabetes or diabetic ketoacidosis (1.2).
- Concurrent use with prandial insulin has not been studied and cannot be recommended (1.2).
- Has not been studied in patients with a history of pancreatitis. Consider other antidiabetic therapies in patients with a history of pancreatitis (1.2).

DOSAGE AND ADMINISTRATION

- Inject subcutaneously within 60 minutes prior to morning and evening meals (or before the two main meals of the day, approximately 6 hours or more apart) (2.1).
- Initiate at 5 mcg per dose twice daily; increase to 10 mcg twice daily after 1 month based on clinical response (2.1).

DOSAGE FORMS AND STRENGTHS

BYETTA is supplied as 250 mcg/mL exenatide in:
- 5 mcg per dose, 60 doses, 1.2 mL prefilled pen
- 10 mcg per dose, 60 doses, 2.4 mL prefilled pen

CONTRAINDICATIONS

- History of severe hypersensitivity to exenatide or any product components (4.1).

WARNINGS AND PRECAUTIONS

- Pancreatitis: Postmarketing reports with exenatide, including fatal and non-fatal hemorrhagic or necrotizing pancreatitis. *Discontinue BYETTA promptly. BYETTA should not be restarted.* Consider other antidiabetic therapies in patients with a history of pancreatitis (5.1).
- Hypoglycemia: Increased risk when BYETTA is used in combination with medications known to cause hypoglycemia (e.g. insulin or insulin secretagogue). Consider reducing the dose of insulin or insulin secretagogue (5.2).
- Renal Impairment: Postmarketing reports with exenatide, sometimes requiring hemodialysis and kidney transplantation. BYETTA (exenatide) should *not* be used in patients with severe renal impairment or end-stage renal disease and should be used with caution in patients with renal transplantation. Caution should be applied when initiating BYETTA or escalating the dose of BYETTA in patients with moderate renal failure (5.3, 8.6, 12.3).
- Severe Gastrointestinal Disease: Use of BYETTA is not recommended in patients with severe gastrointestinal disease (e.g., gastroparesis) (5.4).
- Hypersensitivity: Postmarketing reports with exenatide of hypersensitivity reactions (e.g., anaphylaxis and angioedema). The patient should discontinue BYETTA and other suspect medications and promptly seek medical advice (5.6).
- Macrovascular outcomes: There have been no clinical studies establishing conclusive evidence of macrovascular risk reduction with BYETTA or any other antidiabetic drug (5.7).

ADVERSE REACTIONS

- Most common (≥5%) and occurring more frequently than placebo in clinical trials: nausea, hypoglycemia, vomiting, diarrhea, feeling jittery, dizziness, headache, dyspepsia, constipation, asthenia. Nausea usually decreases over time (5.2, 6).
- Postmarketing reports with exenatide of increased international normalized ratio (INR) with concomitant use of warfarin, sometimes with bleeding (6.2, 7.2).

To report SUSPECTED ADVERSE REACTIONS contact Bristol-Myers Squibb at 1-800-868-1190 and www.byetta.com or FDA at 1-800-FDA-1088 or *www.fda.gov/medwatch*.

DRUG INTERACTIONS

- May impact absorption of orally administered medications (7.1, 12.3).
- Warfarin: Postmarketing reports of increased INR sometimes associated with bleeding. Monitor INR frequently until stable upon initiation or alteration of BYETTA therapy (6.2, 7.2).

USE IN SPECIFIC POPULATIONS

- Pregnancy: Based on animal data, BYETTA may cause fetal harm. BYETTA should be used during pregnancy only if the potential benefit justifies the potential risk to the fetus. To report drug exposure during pregnancy call 1-800-633-9081 (8.1).
- Nursing Mothers: Caution should be exercised when BYETTA is administered to a nursing woman (8.3).

See 17 for PATIENT COUNSELING INFORMATION and Medication Guide

Revised: 02/2013

FULL PRESCRIBING INFORMATION: CONTENTS*

*** Sections or subsections omitted from the full prescribing information are not listed**

FULL PRESCRIBING INFORMATION

1 INDICATIONS AND USAGE

1.1 Type 2 Diabetes Mellitus

BYETTA® (exenatide) is indicated as an adjunct to diet and exercise to improve glycemic control in adults with type 2 diabetes mellitus [see *Clinical Studies (14)*].

1.2 Important Limitations of Use

BYETTA is not a substitute for insulin. BYETTA should not be used for the treatment of type 1 diabetes or diabetic ketoacidosis, as it would not be effective in these settings.

The concurrent use of BYETTA with prandial insulin has not been studied and cannot be recommended.

Based on postmarketing data BYETTA has been associated with acute pancreatitis, including fatal and non-fatal hemorrhagic or necrotizing pancreatitis. BYETTA has not been studied in patients with a history of pancreatitis. It is unknown whether patients with a history of pancreatitis are at increased risk for pancreatitis while using BYETTA. Other antidiabetic therapies should be considered in patients with a history of pancreatitis.

2 DOSAGE AND ADMINISTRATION

2.1 Recommended Dosing

BYETTA should be initiated at 5 mcg administered twice daily (BID) at any time within the 60-minute period before the morning and evening meals (or before the two main meals of the day, approximately 6 hours or more apart). BYETTA should not be administered after a meal. Based on clinical response, the dose of BYETTA can be increased to 10 mcg twice daily after 1 month of therapy. Initiation with 5 mcg reduces the incidence and severity of gastrointestinal side effects. Each dose should be administered as a subcutaneous (SC) injection in the thigh, abdomen, or upper arm. Do not mix BYETTA with insulin. Do not transfer BYETTA from the pen to a syringe or a vial. No data are available on the safety or efficacy of intravenous or intramuscular injection of BYETTA.

Use BYETTA only if it is clear, colorless and contains no particles.

3 DOSAGE FORMS AND STRENGTHS

BYETTA is supplied as a sterile solution for subcutaneous injection containing 250 mcg/mL exenatide in the following packages:

- 5 mcg per dose, 60 doses, 1.2 mL prefilled pen
- 10 mcg per dose, 60 doses, 2.4 mL prefilled pen

4 CONTRAINDICATIONS

4.1 Hypersensitivity

BYETTA is contraindicated in patients with prior severe hypersensitivity reactions to exenatide or to any of the product components.

5 WARNINGS AND PRECAUTIONS

5.1 Acute Pancreatitis

Based on postmarketing data, BYETTA has been associated with acute pancreatitis, including fatal and non-fatal hemorrhagic or necrotizing pancreatitis. After initiation of BYETTA (exenatide), and after dose increases, observe patients carefully for signs and symptoms of pancreatitis (including persistent severe abdominal pain, sometimes radiating to the back, which may or may not be accompanied by vomiting). If pancreatitis is suspected, BYETTA should promptly be discontinued and appropriate management should be initiated. If pancreatitis is confirmed, BYETTA should not be restarted. Consider antidiabetic therapies other than BYETTA in patients with a history of pancreatitis.

Table 1: Incidence (%) and Rate of Hypoglycemia when BYETTA was used as Monotherapy or with Concomitant Antidiabetic Therapy in Six Placebo-Controlled Clinical Trials*

	Placebo BID	BYETTA 5 mcg BID	BYETTA 10 mcg BID
Monotherapy (24 Weeks)			
N	77	77	78
% Overall	1.3%	5.2%	3.8%
Rate (episodes/patient-year)	0.03	0.21	0.52
% Severe	0.0%	0.0%	0.0%
With Metformin (30 Weeks)			
N	113	110	113
% Overall	5.3%	4.5%	5.3%
Rate (episodes/patient-year)	0.12	0.13	0.12
% Severe	0.0%	0.0%	0.0%
With a Sulfonylurea (30 Weeks)			
N	123	125	129
% Overall	3.3%	14.4%	35.7%
Rate (episodes/patient-year)	0.07	0.64	1.61
% Severe	0.0%	0.0%	0.0%
With Metformin and a Sulfonylurea (30 Weeks)			
N	247	245	241
% Overall	12.6%	19.2%	27.8%
Rate (episodes/patient-year)	0.58	0.78	1.71
% Severe	0.0%	0.4%	0.0%
With a Thiazolidinedione (16 Weeks)			
N	112	not evaluated	121
% Overall	7.1%	not evaluated	10.7%
Rate (episodes/patient-years)	0.56	not evaluated	0.98
% Severe	0.0%	not evaluated	0.0%
With Insulin Glargine (30 Weeks)†			
N	122	not evaluated	137
% Overall	29.5%	not evaluated	24.8%
Rate (episodes/patient-years)	1.58	not evaluated	1.61
% Severe	0.8%	not evaluated	0.0%

* A hypoglycemic episode was recorded if a patient reported symptoms of hypoglycemia with or without a blood glucose value consistent with hypoglycemia. Severe hypoglycemia was defined as an event with symptoms consistent with hypoglycemia requiring the assistance of another person and associated with either a blood glucose value consistent with hypoglycemia or prompt recovery after treatment for hypoglycemia.

† When BYETTA was initiated in combination with insulin glargine, the dose of insulin glargine was decreased by 20% in patients with an HbA_{1c} ≤8.0% to minimize the risk of hypoglycemia. See Table 9 for insulin dose titration algorithm.

N = number of Intent-to-Treat subjects in each treatment group.

5.2 Use with Medications Known to Cause Hypoglycemia

The risk of hypoglycemia is increased when BYETTA is used in combination with a sulfonylurea. Therefore, patients receiving BYETTA and a sulfonylurea may require a lower dose of the sulfonylurea to reduce the risk of hypoglycemia.

When BYETTA is used in combination with insulin, the dose of insulin should be evaluated. In patients at increased risk of hypoglycemia consider reducing the dose of insulin [see *Adverse Reactions (6.1)*]. The concurrent use of BYETTA with prandial insulin has not been studied and cannot be recommended. It is also possible that the use of BYETTA with other glucose-independent insulin secretagogues (e.g., meglitinides) could increase the risk of hypoglycemia.

For additional information on glucose-dependent effects see *Mechanism of Action (12.1)*.

5.3 Renal Impairment

BYETTA should not be used in patients with severe renal impairment (creatinine clearance <30 mL/min) or end-stage renal disease and should be used with caution in patients with renal transplantation [see *Use in Specific Populations (8.6)*]. In patients with end-stage renal disease receiving dialysis, single doses of BYETTA 5 mcg were not well tolerated due to gastrointestinal side effects. Because BYETTA may induce nausea and vomiting with transient hypovolemia, treatment may worsen renal function. Caution should be applied when initiating or escalating doses of BYETTA from 5 to 10 mcg in patients with moderate renal impairment (creatinine clearance 30-50 mL/min).

There have been postmarketing reports of altered renal function, including increased serum creatinine, renal impairment, worsened chronic renal failure and acute renal failure, sometimes requiring hemodialysis or kidney transplantation. Some of these events occurred in patients receiving one or more pharmacologic agents known to affect renal function or hydration status, such as angiotensin converting enzyme inhibitors, nonsteroidal anti-inflammatory drugs, or diuretics. Some events occurred in patients who had been experiencing nausea, vomiting, or diarrhea, with or without dehydration. Reversibility of altered renal function has been observed in many cases with supportive treatment and discontinuation of potentially causative agents, including BYETTA. Exenatide has not been found to be directly nephrotoxic in preclinical or clinical studies.

5.4 Gastrointestinal Disease

BYETTA (exenatide) has not been studied in patients with severe gastrointestinal disease, including gastroparesis. Because BYETTA is commonly associated with gastrointestinal adverse reactions, including nausea, vomiting, and diarrhea, the use of BYETTA is not recommended in patients with severe gastrointestinal disease.

5.5 Immunogenicity

Patients may develop antibodies to exenatide following treatment with BYETTA. Antibody levels were measured in 90% of subjects in the 30-week, 24-week, and 16-week studies of BYETTA. In 3%, 4%, and 1% of these patients, respectively, antibody formation was associated with an attenuated glycemic response. If there is worsening glycemic control or failure to achieve targeted glycemic control, alternative antidiabetic therapy should be considered [see *Adverse Reactions (6.1)*].

5.6 Hypersensitivity

There have been postmarketing reports of serious hypersensitivity reactions (e.g., anaphylaxis and angioedema) in patients treated with BYETTA. If a hypersensitivity reaction occurs, the patient should discontinue BYETTA and other suspect medications and promptly seek medical advice [see *Adverse Reactions (6.2)*].

5.7 Macrovascular Outcomes

There have been no clinical studies establishing conclusive evidence of macrovascular risk reduction with BYETTA or any other antidiabetic drug.

6 ADVERSE REACTIONS

6.1 Clinical Trial Experience

Because clinical trials are conducted under widely varying conditions, adverse reaction rates observed in the clinical trials of a drug cannot be directly compared to rates in the clinical trials of another drug and may not reflect the rates observed in practice.

Hypoglycemia

Table 1 summarizes the incidence and rate of hypoglycemia with BYETTA (exenatide) in six placebo-controlled clinical trials.

[See table 1 at top of previous page]

Immunogenicity

Antibodies were assessed in 90% of subjects in the 30-week, 24-week, and 16-week studies of BYETTA. In the 30-week controlled trials of BYETTA add-on to metformin and/or sulfonylurea, antibodies were assessed at 2- to 6-week intervals. The mean antibody titer peaked at week 6 and was reduced by 55% by week 30. Three hundred and sixty patients (38%) had low titer antibodies (<625) to exenatide at 30 weeks. The level of glycemic control (HbA_{1c}) in these patients was generally comparable to that observed in the 534 patients (56%) without antibody titers. An additional 59 patients (6%) had higher titer antibodies (≥625) at 30 weeks. Of these patients, 32 (3% overall) had an attenuated glycemic response to BYETTA; the remaining 27 (3% overall) had a glycemic response comparable to that of patients without antibodies [see *Warnings and Precautions (5.5)*].

In the 16-week trial of BYETTA add-on to thiazolidinediones, with or without metformin, 36 patients (31%) had low titer antibodies to exenatide at 16 weeks. The level of glycemic control in these patients was generally comparable to that observed in the 69 patients (60%) without antibody titer. An additional 10 patients (9%) had higher titer antibodies at 16 weeks. Of these patients, 4 (4% overall) had an attenuated glycemic response to BYETTA; the remaining 6 (5% overall) had a glycemic response comparable to that of patients without antibodies [see *Warnings and Precautions (5.5)*].

In the 24-week trial of BYETTA used as monotherapy, 40 patients (28%) had low titer antibodies to exenatide at 24 weeks. The level of glycemic control in these patients was generally comparable to that observed in the 101 patients (70%) without antibody titers. An additional 3 patients (2%) had higher titer antibodies at 24 weeks. Of these patients, 1 (1% overall) had an attenuated glycemic response to BYETTA; the remaining 2 (1% overall) had a glycemic response comparable to that of patients without antibodies [see *Warnings and Precautions (5.5)*].

Antibodies to exenatide were not assessed in the 30-week trial of BYETTA used in combination with insulin glargine. Two hundred and ten patients with antibodies to exenatide in the BYETTA clinical trials were tested for the presence of cross-reactive antibodies to GLP-1 and/or glucagon. No treatment-emergent cross reactive antibodies were observed across the range of titers.

Other Adverse Reactions

Monotherapy

For the 24-week placebo-controlled study of BYETTA used as a monotherapy, Table 2 summarizes adverse reactions (excluding hypoglycemia) occurring with an incidence ≥2% and occurring more frequently in BYETTA-treated patients compared with placebo-treated patients.

Table 2: Treatment-Emergent Adverse Reactions ≥2% Incidence with BYETTA used as Monotherapy (excluding Hypoglycemia)*

Monotherapy	Placebo BID N = 77 %	All BYETTA BID N = 155 %
Nausea	0	8
Vomiting	0	4
Dyspepsia	0	3

* In a 24-week placebo-controlled trial.
BID = twice daily.

Adverse reactions reported in ≥1.0% to <2.0% of patients receiving BYETTA and reported more frequently than with placebo included decreased appetite, diarrhea, and dizziness. The most frequently reported adverse reaction associated with BYETTA, nausea, occurred in a dose-dependent fashion.

Two of the 155 patients treated with BYETTA withdrew due to adverse reactions of headache and nausea. No placebo-treated patients withdrew due to adverse reactions.

Combination Therapy

Add-On to Metformin and/or Sulfonylurea

In the three 30-week controlled trials of BYETTA add-on to metformin and/or sulfonylurea, adverse reactions (excluding hypoglycemia) with an incidence ≥2% and occurring more frequently in BYETTA-treated patients compared with placebo-treated patients [see *Warnings and Precautions (5.2)*] are summarized in Table 3.

Table 3: Treatment-Emergent Adverse Reactions ≥2% Incidence and Greater Incidence with BYETTA Treatment used with Metformin and/or a Sulfonylurea (excluding Hypoglycemia)*

	Placebo BID N = 483 %	All BYETTA BID N = 963 %
Nausea	18	44
Vomiting	4	13
Diarrhea	6	13
Feeling Jittery	4	9
Dizziness	6	9
Headache	6	9
Dyspepsia	3	6
Asthenia	2	4
Gastroesophageal Reflux Disease	1	3
Hyperhidrosis	1	3

* In three 30-week placebo-controlled clinical trials.
BID = twice daily.

Adverse reactions reported in ≥1.0% to <2.0% of patients receiving BYETTA (exenatide) and reported more frequently than with placebo included decreased appetite. Nausea was the most frequently reported adverse reaction and occurred in a dose-dependent fashion. With continued therapy, the frequency and severity decreased over time in most of the patients who initially experienced nausea. Patients in the long-term uncontrolled open-label extension studies at 52 weeks reported no new types of adverse reactions than those observed in the 30-week controlled trials.

The most common adverse reactions leading to withdrawal for BYETTA-treated patients were nausea (3% of patients) and vomiting (1%). For placebo-treated patients, <1% withdrew due to nausea and none due to vomiting.

Add-On to Thiazolidinedione with or without Metformin

For the 16-week placebo-controlled study of BYETTA add-on to a thiazolidinedione, with or without metformin, Table 4 summarizes the adverse reactions (excluding hypoglycemia) with an incidence of ≥2% and occurring more frequently in BYETTA-treated patients compared with placebo-treated patients.

Table 4: Treatment-Emergent Adverse Reactions ≥2% Incidence with BYETTA used with a Thiazolidinedione (TZD), with or without Metformin (MET) (excluding Hypoglycemia)*

With a TZD or TZD/MET	Placebo N = 112 %	All BYETTA BID N = 121 %
Nausea	15	40
Vomiting	1	13
Dyspepsia	1	7
Diarrhea	3	6
Gastroesophageal Reflux Disease	0	3

* In a 16-week placebo-controlled clinical trial.
BID = twice daily.

Adverse reactions reported in ≥1.0% to <2.0% of patients receiving BYETTA and reported more frequently than with placebo included decreased appetite. Chills (n=4) and injection-site reactions (n=2) occurred only in BYETTA-treated patients. The two patients who reported an injection-site reaction had high titers of antibodies to exenatide. Two serious adverse events (chest pain and chronic hypersensitivity pneumonitis) were reported in the BYETTA arm. No serious adverse events were reported in the placebo arm.

The most common adverse reactions leading to withdrawal for BYETTA-treated patients were nausea (9%) and vomiting (5%). For placebo-treated patients, <1% withdrew due to nausea.

Add-On to Insulin Glargine with or without Metformin and/or Thiazolidinedione

For the 30-week placebo-controlled study of BYETTA as add-on to insulin glargine with or without oral antihyperglycemic medications, Table 5 summarizes adverse reactions (excluding hypoglycemia) occurring with an incidence ≥2% and occurring more frequently in BYETTA-treated patients compared with placebo-treated patients.

Table 5: Treatment-Emergent Adverse Reactions ≥2% Incidence with BYETTA used with Insulin Glargine with or without Oral Antihyperglycemic Medications (excluding Hypoglycemia)*

With Insulin Glargine	Placebo N = 122 %	All BYETTA BID N = 137 %
Nausea	8	41
Vomiting	4	18
Diarrhea	8	18
Headache	4	14
Constipation	2	10
Dyspepsia	2	7
Asthenia	1	5
Abdominal Distension	1	4
Decreased Appetite	0	3
Flatulence	1	2
Gastroesophageal Reflux Disease	1	2

* In a 30-week placebo-controlled clinical trial.
BID = twice daily.

The most frequently reported adverse reactions leading to withdrawal for BYETTA-treated patients were nausea (5.1%) and vomiting (2.9%). No placebo-treated patients withdrew due to nausea or vomiting.

6.2 Postmarketing Experience

The following additional adverse reactions have been reported during postapproval use of BYETTA (exenatide). Because these events are reported voluntarily from a population of uncertain size, it is generally not possible to reliably estimate their frequency or establish a causal relationship to drug exposure.

Allergy/Hypersensitivity: injection-site reactions, generalized pruritus and/or urticaria, macular or papular rash, angioedema, anaphylactic reaction [see *Warnings and Precautions (5.6)*].

Drug Interactions: International normalized ratio (INR) increased with concomitant warfarin use sometimes associated with bleeding [see *Drug Interactions (7.2)*].

Gastrointestinal: nausea, vomiting, and/or diarrhea resulting in dehydration; abdominal distension, abdominal pain, eructation, constipation, flatulence, acute pancreatitis, hemorrhagic and necrotizing pancreatitis sometimes resulting in death [see *Indications and Usage (1.2)* and *Warnings and Precautions (5.1)*].

Neurologic: dysgeusia; somnolence

Renal and Urinary Disorders: altered renal function, including increased serum creatinine, renal impairment, worsened chronic renal failure or acute renal failure (sometimes requiring hemodialysis), kidney transplant and kidney transplant dysfunction [see *Warnings and Precautions (5.3)*].

Skin and Subcutaneous Tissue Disorders: alopecia

7 DRUG INTERACTIONS

7.1 Orally Administered Drugs

The effect of BYETTA to slow gastric emptying can reduce the extent and rate of absorption of orally administered drugs. BYETTA should be used with caution in patients receiving oral medications that have narrow therapeutic index or require rapid gastrointestinal absorption [see *Adverse Reactions (6.2)*]. For oral medications that are dependent on threshold concentrations for efficacy, such as contraceptives and antibiotics, patients should be advised to take those drugs at least 1 hour before BYETTA injection. If such drugs are to be administered with food, patients should be advised to take them with a meal or snack when BYETTA is not administered [see *Clinical Pharmacology (12.3)*].

7.2 Warfarin

There are postmarketing reports of increased INR sometimes associated with bleeding, with concomitant use of warfarin and BYETTA [see *Adverse Reactions (6.2)*]. In a drug interaction study, BYETTA did not have a significant effect on INR [see *Clinical Pharmacology (12.3)*]. In patients taking warfarin, prothrombin time should be monitored more frequently after initiation or alteration of BYETTA therapy. Once a stable prothrombin time has been documented, prothrombin times can be monitored at the intervals usually recommended for patients on warfarin.

8 USE IN SPECIFIC POPULATIONS

8.1 Pregnancy

Pregnancy Category C

There are no adequate and well-controlled studies of BYETTA use in pregnant women. In animal studies, exenatide caused cleft palate, irregular skeletal ossification and an increased number of neonatal deaths. BYETTA should be used during pregnancy only if the potential benefit justifies the potential risk to the fetus.

Female mice given SC doses of 6, 68, or 760 mcg/kg/day beginning 2 weeks prior to and throughout mating until gestation day 7 had no adverse fetal effects. At the maximal dose, 760 mcg/kg/day, systemic exposures were up to 390 times the human exposure resulting from the maximum recommended dose of 20 mcg/day, based on AUC [see *Nonclinical Toxicology (13.3)*].

In developmental toxicity studies, pregnant animals received exenatide subcutaneously during organogenesis. Specifically, fetuses from pregnant rabbits given SC doses of 0.2, 2, 22, 156, or 260 mcg/kg/day from gestation day 6 through 18 experienced irregular skeletal ossifications from exposures 12 times the human exposure resulting from the maximum recommended dose of 20 mcg/day, based on AUC. Moreover, fetuses from pregnant mice given SC doses of 6, 68, 460, or 760 mcg/kg/day from gestation day 6 through 15 demonstrated reduced fetal and neonatal growth, cleft palate and skeletal effects at systemic exposure 3 times the human exposure resulting from the maximum recommended dose of 20 mcg/day, based on AUC [see *Nonclinical Toxicology (13.3)*].

Lactating mice given SC doses of 6, 68, or 760 mcg/kg/day from gestation day 6 through lactation day 20 (weaning), experienced an increased number of neonatal deaths. Deaths were observed on postpartum days 2 to 4 in dams given 6 mcg/kg/day, a systemic exposure 3 times the human exposure resulting from the maximum recommended dose of 20 mcg/day, based on AUC [see *Nonclinical Toxicology (13.3)*].

Pregnancy Registry

A Pregnancy Registry has been implemented to monitor pregnancy outcomes of women exposed to exenatide during pregnancy. Physicians are encouraged to register patients by calling 1-800-633-9081.

8.3 Nursing Mothers

It is not known whether exenatide is excreted in human milk. However, exenatide is present at low concentrations (less than or equal to 2.5% of the concentration in maternal plasma following subcutaneous dosing) in the milk of lactating mice. Many drugs are excreted in human milk and because of the potential for clinically significant adverse reactions in nursing infants from exenatide, a decision should be made whether to discontinue nursing or discontinue the drug, taking into account these potential risks against the glycemic benefits to the lactating woman. Caution should be exercised when BYETTA (exenatide) is administered to a nursing woman.

8.4 Pediatric Use

Safety and effectiveness of BYETTA have not been established in pediatric patients.

8.5 Geriatric Use

Population pharmacokinetic analysis of patients ranging from 22 to 73 years of age suggests that age does not influence the pharmacokinetic properties of exenatide [see *Clinical Pharmacology (12.3)*]. BYETTA was studied in 282 patients 65 years of age or older and in 16 patients 75 years of age or older. No differences in safety or effectiveness were observed between these patients and younger patients. Because elderly patients are more likely to have decreased renal function, care should be taken in dose selection in the elderly based on renal function.

8.6 Renal Impairment

BYETTA is not recommended for use in patients with end-stage renal disease or severe renal impairment (creatinine clearance <30 mL/min) and should be used with caution in patients with renal transplantation. No dosage adjustment of BYETTA is required in patients with mild renal impairment (creatinine clearance 50-80 mL/min). Caution should be applied when initiating or escalating doses of BYETTA from 5 to 10 mcg in patients with moderate renal impairment (creatinine clearance 30-50 mL/min) [see *Clinical Pharmacology (12.3)*].

8.7 Hepatic Impairment

No pharmacokinetic study has been performed in patients with a diagnosis of acute or chronic hepatic impairment. Because exenatide is cleared primarily by the kidney, hepatic dysfunction is not expected to affect blood concentrations of exenatide [see *Clinical Pharmacology (12.3)*].

10 OVERDOSAGE

In a clinical study of BYETTA, three patients with type 2 diabetes each experienced a single overdose of 100 mcg SC (10 times the maximum recommended dose). Effects of the overdoses included severe nausea, severe vomiting, and rapidly declining blood glucose concentrations. One of the three patients experienced severe hypoglycemia requiring parenteral glucose administration. The three patients recovered without complication. In the event of overdose, appropriate supportive treatment should be initiated according to the patient's clinical signs and symptoms.

11 DESCRIPTION

BYETTA (exenatide) is a synthetic peptide that was originally identified in the lizard *Heloderma suspectum*. Exenatide differs in chemical structure and pharmacological action from insulin, sulfonylureas (including D-phenylalanine derivatives and meglitinides), biguanides, thiazolidinediones, alpha-glucosidase inhibitors, amylinomimetics and dipeptidyl peptidase-4 inhibitors.

Exenatide is a 39-amino acid peptide amide. Exenatide has the empirical formula $C_{184}H_{282}N_{50}O_{60}S$ and molecular weight of 4186.6 Daltons. The amino acid sequence for exenatide is shown below.

H-His-Gly-Glu-Gly-Thr-Phe-Thr-Ser-Asp-Leu-Ser-Lys-Gln-Met-Glu-Glu-Glu-Ala-Val-Arg-Leu-Phe-Ile-Glu-Trp-Leu-Lys-Asn-Gly-Gly-Pro-Ser-Ser-Gly-Ala-Pro-Pro-Pro-Ser-NH_2

BYETTA is supplied for SC injection as a sterile, preserved isotonic solution in a glass cartridge that has been assembled in a pen-injector (pen). Each milliliter (mL) contains 250 micrograms (mcg) synthetic exenatide, 2.2 mg metacresol as an antimicrobial preservative, mannitol as a tonicity-adjusting agent, and glacial acetic acid and sodium acetate trihydrate in water for injection as a buffering solution at pH 4.5. Two prefilled pens are available to deliver unit doses of 5 mcg or 10 mcg. Each prefilled pen will deliver 60 doses to provide for 30 days of twice daily administration (BID).

12 CLINICAL PHARMACOLOGY

12.1 Mechanism of Action

Incretins, such as glucagon-like peptide-1 (GLP-1), enhance glucose-dependent insulin secretion and exhibit other antihyperglycemic actions following their release into the circulation from the gut. BYETTA (exenatide) is a GLP-1 receptor agonist that enhances glucose-dependent insulin secretion by the pancreatic beta-cell, suppresses inappropriately elevated glucagon secretion, and slows gastric emptying.

The amino acid sequence of exenatide partially overlaps that of human GLP-1. Exenatide has been shown to bind and activate the human GLP-1 receptor *in vitro*. This leads to an increase in both glucose-dependent synthesis of insulin, and *in vivo* secretion of insulin from pancreatic beta cells, by mechanisms involving cyclic AMP and/or other intracellular signaling pathways.

BYETTA improves glycemic control by reducing fasting and postprandial glucose concentrations in patients with type 2 diabetes through the actions described below.

12.2 Pharmacodynamics

Glucose-Dependent Insulin Secretion

BYETTA has acute effects on pancreatic beta-cell responsiveness to glucose leading to insulin release predominantly in the presence of elevated glucose concentrations. This insulin secretion subsides as blood glucose concentrations decrease and approach euglycemia. However, BYETTA does not impair the normal glucagon response to hypoglycemia.

First-Phase Insulin Response

In healthy individuals, robust insulin secretion occurs during the first 10 minutes following intravenous (IV) glucose administration. This secretion, known as the "first-phase insulin response," is characteristically absent in patients with type 2 diabetes. The loss of the first-phase insulin response is an early beta-cell defect in type 2 diabetes. Administration of BYETTA at therapeutic plasma concentrations restored first-phase insulin response to an IV bolus of glucose in patients with type 2 diabetes (Figure 1). Both first-phase insulin secretion and second-phase insulin secretion were significantly increased in patients with type 2 diabetes treated with BYETTA compared with saline (p<0.001 for both).

Figure 1: Mean (+SEM) Insulin Secretion Rate during Infusion of BYETTA or Saline in Patients with Type 2 Diabetes and during Infusion of Saline in Healthy Subjects

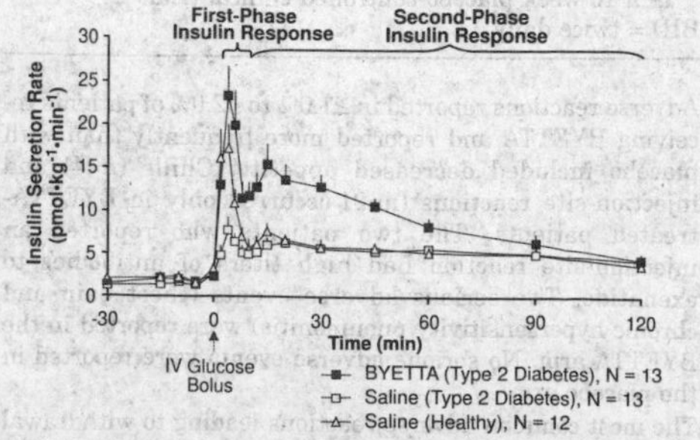

Patients received an IV infusion of insulin for 6.5 h (discontinued at time [t] = -30 min) to normalize plasma glucose concentrations and a continuous IV infusion of either BYETTA or saline for 5 h beginning 3 h prior to an IV bolus of glucose (0.3 g/kg over 30 sec) at t = 0 min.

Glucagon Secretion

In patients with type 2 diabetes, BYETTA moderates glucagon secretion and lowers serum glucagon concentrations during periods of hyperglycemia. Lower glucagon concentrations lead to decreased hepatic glucose output and decreased insulin demand.

Gastric Emptying

BYETTA (exenatide) slows gastric emptying, thereby reducing the rate at which meal-derived glucose appears in the circulation.

Food Intake

In both animals and humans, administration of exenatide has been shown to reduce food intake.

Postprandial Glucose

In patients with type 2 diabetes, BYETTA reduces postprandial plasma glucose concentrations (Figure 2).

Figure 2: Mean (+SEM) Postprandial Plasma Glucose Concentrations on Day 1 of BYETTA[a] Treatment in Patients with Type 2 Diabetes Treated with Metformin, a Sulfonylurea, or Both (N=54)

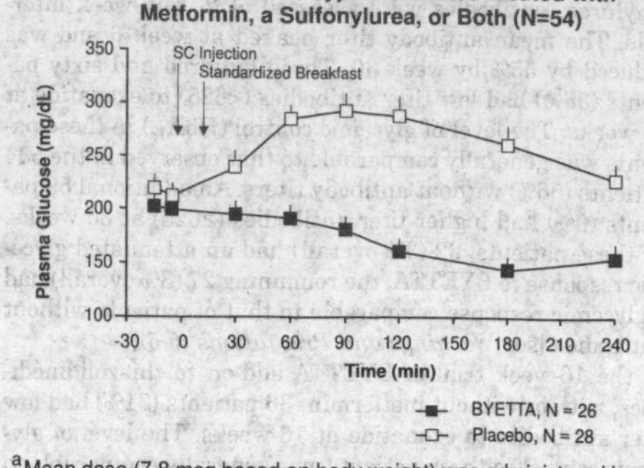

[a]Mean dose (7.8 mcg based on body weight) was administered by subcutaneous (SC) injection.

Fasting Glucose

In a single-dose crossover study in patients with type 2 diabetes and fasting hyperglycemia, immediate insulin release followed injection of BYETTA. Plasma glucose concentrations were significantly reduced with BYETTA compared with placebo (Figure 3).

Figure 3: Mean (+SEM) Serum Insulin and Plasma Glucose Concentrations Following a One-Time Injection of BYETTA[a] or Placebo in Fasting Patients with Type 2 Diabetes (N = 12)

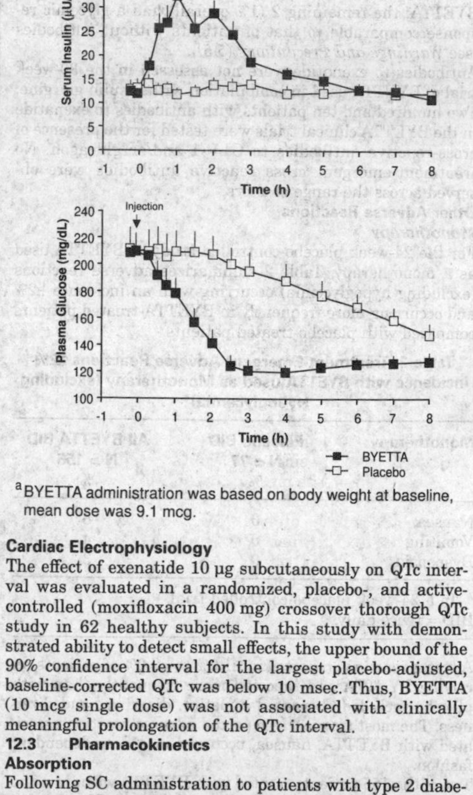

[a]BYETTA administration was based on body weight at baseline, mean dose was 9.1 mcg.

Cardiac Electrophysiology

The effect of exenatide 10 µg subcutaneously on QTc interval was evaluated in a randomized, placebo-, and active-controlled (moxifloxacin 400 mg) crossover thorough QTc study in 62 healthy subjects. In this study with demonstrated ability to detect small effects, the upper bound of the 90% confidence interval for the largest placebo-adjusted, baseline-corrected QTc was below 10 msec. Thus, BYETTA (10 mcg single dose) was not associated with clinically meaningful prolongation of the QTc interval.

12.3 Pharmacokinetics

Absorption

Following SC administration to patients with type 2 diabetes, exenatide reaches median peak plasma concentrations in 2.1 hours. The mean peak exenatide concentration (C_{max}) was 211 pg/mL and overall mean area under the time-concentration curve (AUC_{0-inf}) was 1036 pg•h/mL following SC administration of a 10-mcg dose of BYETTA. Exenatide exposure (AUC) increased proportionally over the therapeutic dose range of 5 to 10 mcg. The C_{max} values increased less than proportionally over the same range. Similar exposure is achieved with SC administration of BYETTA in the abdomen, thigh, or upper arm.

Distribution

The mean apparent volume of distribution of exenatide following SC administration of a single dose of BYETTA (exenatide) is 28.3 L.

Metabolism and Elimination

Nonclinical studies have shown that exenatide is predominantly eliminated by glomerular filtration with subsequent proteolytic degradation. The mean apparent clearance of exenatide in humans is 9.1 L/hour and the mean terminal half-life is 2.4 hours. These pharmacokinetic characteristics of exenatide are independent of the dose. In most individuals, exenatide concentrations are measurable for approximately 10 hours post-dose.

Drug Interactions

Acetaminophen

When 1000 mg acetaminophen elixir was given with 10 mcg BYETTA (0 hour) and 1 hour, 2 hours, and 4 hours after BYETTA injection, acetaminophen AUCs were decreased by 21%, 23%, 24%, and 14%, respectively; C_{max} was decreased by 37%, 56%, 54%, and 41%, respectively; T_{max} was increased from 0.6 hour in the control period to 0.9 hour, 4.2 hours, 3.3 hours, and 1.6 hours, respectively. Acetaminophen AUC, C_{max} and T_{max} were not significantly changed when acetaminophen was given 1 hour before BYETTA injection.

Digoxin

Administration of repeated doses of BYETTA (10 mcg BID) 30 minutes before oral digoxin (0.25 mg once daily) decreased the C_{max} of digoxin by 17% and delayed the T_{max} of digoxin by approximately 2.5 hours; however, the overall steady-state pharmacokinetic exposure (e.g., AUC) of digoxin was not changed.

Lovastatin

Administration of BYETTA (10 mcg BID) 30 minutes before a single oral dose of lovastatin (40 mg) decreased the AUC and C_{max} of lovastatin by approximately 40% and 28%, respectively, and delayed the T_{max} by about 4 hours compared with lovastatin administered alone. In the 30-week controlled clinical trials of BYETTA, the use of BYETTA in patients already receiving HMG CoA reductase inhibitors was not associated with consistent changes in lipid profiles compared to baseline.

Lisinopril

In patients with mild to moderate hypertension stabilized on lisinopril (5-20 mg/day), BYETTA (10 mcg BID) did not alter steady-state C_{max} or AUC of lisinopril. Lisinopril steady-state T_{max} was delayed by 2 hours. There were no changes in 24-hour mean systolic and diastolic blood pressure.

Oral Contraceptives

The effect of BYETTA (10 mcg BID) on single and on multiple doses of a combination oral contraceptive (30 mcg ethinyl estradiol plus 150 mcg levonorgestrel) was studied in healthy female subjects. Repeated daily doses of the oral contraceptive (OC) given 30 minutes after BYETTA administration decreased the C_{max} of ethinyl estradiol and levonorgestrel by 45% and 27%, respectively and delayed the T_{max} of ethinyl estradiol and levonorgestrel by 3.0 hours and 3.5 hours, respectively, as compared to the oral contraceptive administered alone. Administration of repeated daily doses of the OC one hour prior to BYETTA administration decreased the mean C_{max} of ethinyl estradiol by 15% but the mean C_{max} of levonorgestrel was not significantly changed as compared to when the OC was given alone. BYETTA did not alter the mean trough concentrations of levonorgestrel after repeated daily dosing of the oral contraceptive for both regimens. However, the mean trough concentration of ethinyl estradiol was increased by 20% when the OC was administered 30 minutes after BYETTA administration injection as compared to when the OC was given alone. The effect of BYETTA on OC pharmacokinetics is confounded by the possible food effect on OC in this study. Therefore, OC products should be administered at least one hour prior to BYETTA injection.

Warfarin

Administration of warfarin (25 mg) 35 minutes after repeated doses of BYETTA (5 mcg BID on days 1-2 and 10 mcg BID on days 3-9) in healthy volunteers delayed warfarin T_{max} by approximately 2 hours. No clinically relevant effects on C_{max} or AUC of *S*- and *R*-enantiomers of warfarin were observed. BYETTA did not significantly alter the pharmacodynamic properties (e.g., international normalized ratio) of warfarin [see *Drug Interactions (7.2)*].

Specific Populations

Renal Impairment

Pharmacokinetics of exenatide was studied in subjects with normal, mild, or moderate renal impairment and subjects with end-stage renal disease. In subjects with mild to moderate renal impairment (creatinine clearance 30-80 mL/min), exenatide exposure was similar to that of subjects with normal renal function. However, in subjects with end-stage renal disease receiving dialysis, mean exenatide exposure increased by 3.37-fold compared to that of subjects with normal renal function. [see *Use in Specific Populations (8.6)*].

Hepatic Impairment

No pharmacokinetic study has been performed in patients with a diagnosis of acute or chronic hepatic impairment [see *Use in Specific Populations (8.7)*].

Age

Population pharmacokinetic analysis of patients ranging from 22 to 73 years of age suggests that age does not influence the pharmacokinetic properties of exenatide [see *Use in Specific Population (8.5)*].

Gender

Population pharmacokinetic analysis of male and female patients suggests that gender does not influence the distribution and elimination of exenatide.

Race

Population pharmacokinetic analysis of samples from Caucasian, Hispanic, Asian, and Black patients suggests that race has no significant influence on the pharmacokinetics of exenatide.

Body Mass Index

Population pharmacokinetic analysis of patients with body mass indices (BMI) ≥ 30 kg/m^2 and <30 kg/m^2 suggests that BMI has no significant effect on the pharmacokinetics of exenatide.

13 NONCLINICAL TOXICOLOGY

13.1 Carcinogenesis, Mutagenesis, Impairment of Fertility

A 104-week carcinogenicity study was conducted in male and female rats at doses of 18, 70, or 250 mcg/kg/day administered by bolus SC injection. Benign thyroid C-cell adenomas were observed in female rats at all exenatide doses. The incidences in female rats were 8% and 5% in the two control groups and 14%, 11%, and 23% in the low-, medium-, and high-dose groups with systemic exposures of 5, 22, and 130 times, respectively, the human exposure resulting from the maximum recommended dose of 20 mcg/day, based on plasma area under the curve (AUC).

In a 104-week carcinogenicity study in mice at doses of 18, 70, or 250 mcg/kg/day administered by bolus SC injection, no evidence of tumors was observed at doses up to 250 mcg/kg/day, a systemic exposure up to 95 times the human exposure resulting from the maximum recommended dose of 20 mcg/day, based on AUC.

Exenatide was not mutagenic or clastogenic, with or without metabolic activation, in the Ames bacterial mutagenicity assay or chromosomal aberration assay in Chinese hamster ovary cells. Exenatide was negative in the *in vivo* mouse micronucleus assay.

In mouse fertility studies with SC doses of 6, 68, or 760 mcg/kg/day, males were treated for 4 weeks prior to and throughout mating, and females were treated 2 weeks prior to mating and throughout mating until gestation day 7. No adverse effect on fertility was observed at 760 mcg/kg/day, a systemic exposure 390 times the human exposure resulting from the maximum recommended dose of 20 mcg/day, based on AUC.

13.3 Reproductive and Developmental Toxicology

In female mice given SC doses of 6, 68, or 760 mcg/kg/day beginning 2 weeks prior to and throughout mating until gestation day 7, there were no adverse fetal effects at doses up to 760 mcg/kg/day, systemic exposures up to 390 times the human exposure resulting from the maximum recommended dose of 20 mcg/day, based on AUC.

In pregnant mice given SC doses of 6, 68, 460, or 760 mcg/kg/day from gestation day 6 through 15 (organogenesis), cleft palate (some with holes) and irregular fetal skeletal ossification of rib and skull bones were observed at 6 mcg/kg/day, a systemic exposure 3 times the human exposure resulting from the maximum recommended dose of 20 mcg/day, based on AUC.

In pregnant rabbits given SC doses of 0.2, 2, 22, 156, or 260 mcg/kg/day from gestation day 6 through 18 (organogenesis), irregular fetal skeletal ossifications were observed at 2 mcg/kg/day, a systemic exposure 12 times the human exposure resulting from the maximum recommended dose of 20 mcg/day, based on AUC.

In pregnant mice given SC doses of 6, 68, or 760 mcg/kg/day from gestation day 6 through lactation day 20 (weaning), an increased number of neonatal deaths was observed on postpartum days 2-4 in dams given 6 mcg/kg/day, a systemic exposure 3 times the human exposure resulting from the maximum recommended dose of 20 mcg/day, based on AUC.

14 CLINICAL STUDIES

BYETTA (exenatide) has been studied as monotherapy and in combination with metformin, a sulfonylurea, a thiazolidinedione, a combination of metformin and a sulfonylurea, a combination of metformin and a thiazolidinedione, or in combination with insulin glargine with or without metformin and/or thiazolidinedione.

14.1 Monotherapy

In a randomized, double-blind, placebo-controlled trial of 24 weeks duration, BYETTA 5 mcg BID (n=77), BYETTA 10 mcg BID (n=78), or placebo BID (n=77) was used as monotherapy in patients with entry HbA_{1c} ranging from 6.5% to 10%. All patients assigned to BYETTA initially received 5 mcg BID for 4 weeks. After 4 weeks, those patients either continued to receive BYETTA 5 mcg BID or had their dose increased to 10 mcg BID. Patients assigned to placebo received placebo BID throughout the trial. BYETTA or placebo was injected subcutaneously before the morning and evening meals. The majority of patients (68%) were Caucasian, 26% West Asian, 3% Hispanic, 3% Black, and 0.4% East Asian.

The primary endpoint was the change in HbA_{1c} from baseline to Week 24 (or the last value at time of early discontinuation). Compared to placebo, BYETTA 5 mcg BID and 10 mcg BID resulted in statistically significant reductions in HbA_{1c} from baseline at Week 24 (Table 6).

Table 6: Results of 24-Week Placebo-Controlled Trial of BYETTA used as Monotherapy

	Placebo BID	BYETTA 5 mcg BID	BYETTA 10 mcg* BID
Intent-to-Treat Population (N)	77	77	78
HbA_{1c} (%), Mean			
Baseline	7.8	7.9	7.8
Change at Week 24†	−0.2	−0.7	−0.9
Difference from placebo† (95% CI)		−0.5 [−0.9, −0.2]‡	−0.7 [−1.0, −0.3]‡
Proportion Achieving HbA_{1c} <7%	38%	48%	53%
Body Weight (kg), Mean			
Baseline	86.1	85.1	86.2
Change at Week 24†	−1.5	−2.7	−2.9
Difference from placebo† (95% CI)		−1.3 [−2.3, −0.2]	−1.5 [−2.5, −0.4]
Fasting Serum Glucose§ (mg/dL), Mean			
Baseline	159	166	155
Change at Week 24†	−5	−17	−19
Difference from placebo† (95% CI)		−12 [−23.2, −1.3]	−14 [−24.5, −2.5]

* BYETTA 5 mcg twice daily (BID) for 1 month followed by 10 mcg BID for 5 months before the morning and evening meals.

† Least squares means are adjusted for screening HbA_{1c} strata and baseline value of the dependent variable.

‡ $p <0.01$, treatment vs. placebo.

§ Measured using the hexokinase-based glucose method.

BID = twice daily.

[See table 6 above]

On average, there were no adverse effects of exenatide on blood pressure or lipids.

14.2 Combination Therapy with Oral Antihyperglycemic Medicines

Three 30-week, double-blind, placebo-controlled trials were conducted to evaluate the safety and efficacy of BYETTA in patients with type 2 diabetes whose glycemic control was inadequate with metformin alone, a sulfonylurea alone, or metformin in combination with a sulfonylurea. In addition, a 16-week, placebo-controlled trial was conducted where BYETTA was added to existing thiazolidinedione (pioglitazone or rosiglitazone) treatment, with or without metformin, in patients with type 2 diabetes with inadequate glycemic control.

In the 30-week trials, after a 4-week placebo lead-in period, patients were randomly assigned to receive BYETTA 5 mcg BID, BYETTA 10 mcg BID, or placebo BID before the morning and evening meals, in addition to their existing oral an-

Table 7: Results of 30-Week and 16-Week Placebo-Controlled Trials of BYETTA used in Combination with Oral Antidiabetic Agents

	Placebo BID	BYETTA 5 mcg BID	BYETTA 10 mcg* BID
	In Combination with Metformin (30 Weeks)		
Intent-to-Treat Population (N)	113	110	113
HbA_{1c} (%), Mean			
Baseline	8.2	8.3	8.2
Change at Week 30†	–0.0	–0.5	–0.9
Difference from placebo† (95% CI)		–0.5 [–0.7, –0.2]‡	–0.9 [–1.1, –0.6]‡
Proportion Achieving HbA_{1c} <7%	12%	32%	40%
Body Weight (kg), Mean			
Baseline	99.9	100.0	100.9
Change at Week 30†	–0.2	–1.3	–2.6
Difference from placebo† (95% CI)		–1.1 [–2.2, –0.0]	–2.4 [–3.5, –1.3]
Fasting Plasma Glucose§ (mg/dL), Mean			
Baseline	169	176	168
Change at Week 30†	+14	–5	–10
Difference from placebo† (95% CI)		–20 [–32, –7]	–24 [–37, –12]
	In Combination with a Sulfonylurea (30 Weeks)		
Intent-to-Treat Population (N)	123	125	129
HbA_{1c} (%), Mean			
Baseline	8.7	8.5	8.6
Change at Week 30†	+0.1	–0.5	–0.9
Difference from placebo† (95% CI)		–0.6 [–0.9, –0.3]‡	–1.0 [–1.3, –0.7]‡
Proportion Achieving HbA_{1c} <7%	10%	25%	36%
Body Weight (kg), Mean			
Baseline	99.1	94.9	95.2
Change at Week 30†	–0.8	–1.1	–1.6
Difference from placebo† (95% CI)		–0.3 [–1.1, 0.6]	–0.9 [–1.7, –0.0]
Fasting Plasma Glucose§ (mg/dL), Mean			
Baseline	194	180	178
Change at Week 30†	+6	–5	–11
Difference from placebo† (95% CI)		–11 [–25, 3]	–17 [–30, –3]
	In Combination with Metformin and a Sulfonylurea (30 Weeks)		
Intent-to-Treat Population (N)	247	245	241
HbA_{1c} (%), Mean			
Baseline	8.5	8.5	8.5
Change at Week 30†	+0.1	–0.7	–0.9
Difference from placebo† (95% CI)		–0.8 [–1.0, –0.6]‡	–1.0 [–1.2, –0.8]‡
Proportion Achieving HbA_{1c} <7%	8%	25%	31%
Body Weight (kg), Mean			
Baseline	99.1	96.9	98.4
Change at Week 30†	–0.9	–1.6	–1.6
Difference from placebo† (95% CI)		–0.7 [–1.2, –0.2]	–0.7 [–1.3, –0.2]
Fasting Plasma Glucose§ (mg/dL), Mean			
Baseline	181	182	178
Change at Week 30†	+13	–11	–12
Difference from placebo† (95% CI)		–24 [–33, –15]	–25 [–34, –16]
	In Combination with a Thiazolidinedione or a Thiazolidinedione plus Metformin (16 Weeks)		
Intent-to-Treat Population (N)	112	Dose not studied	121
HbA_{1c} (%), Mean			
Baseline	7.9	Dose not studied	7.9
Change at Week 16†	+0.1	Dose not studied	–0.7
Difference from placebo† (95% CI)		Dose not studied	–0.9 [–1.1, –0.7]‡
Proportion Achieving HbA_{1c} <7%	15%	Dose not studied	51%
Body Weight (kg), Mean			
Baseline	96.8	Dose not studied	97.5
Change at Week 16†	–0.0	Dose not studied	–1.5
Difference from placebo† (95% CI)		Dose not studied	–1.5 [–2.2, –0.7]
Fasting Serum Glucose§ (mg/dL), Mean			
Baseline	159	Dose not studied	164
Change at Week 16†	+4	Dose not studied	–21
Difference from placebo† (95% CI)		Dose not studied	–25 [–33, –16]

* BYETTA 5 mcg twice daily for 1 month followed by 10 mcg BID for 6 months for the 30-week trials or 10 mcg BID for 3 months in the 16-week trial before the morning and evening meals.
† Least squares means are adjusted for baseline HbA_{1c} strata or value, investigator site, baseline value of the dependent variable (if applicable), and background antihyperglycemic therapy (if applicable).
‡ p <0.01, treatment vs. placebo.
§ Measured using the hexokinase-based glucose method.
BID = twice daily.

tidiabetic agent. All patients assigned to BYETTA (exenatide) initially received 5 mcg BID for 4 weeks. After 4 weeks, those patients either continued to receive BYETTA 5 mcg BID or had their dose increased to 10 mcg BID. Patients assigned to placebo received placebo BID throughout the study. A total of 1446 patients were randomized in the three 30-week trials: 991 (69%) were Caucasian, 224 (16%) Hispanic, and 174 (12%) Black. Mean HbA_{1c} values at baseline for the trials ranged from 8.2% to 8.7%.

In the placebo-controlled trial of 16 weeks duration, BYETTA (n=121) or placebo (n=112) was added to existing thiazolidinedione (pioglitazone or rosiglitazone) treatment, with or without metformin. Randomization to BYETTA (exenatide) or placebo was stratified based on whether the patients were receiving metformin. BYETTA treatment was initiated at a dose of 5 mcg BID for 4 weeks then increased to 10 mcg BID for 12 more weeks. Patients assigned to placebo received placebo BID throughout the study. BYETTA or placebo was injected subcutaneously before the morning and evening meals. In this trial, 79% of patients were taking a thiazolidinedione and metformin and 21% were taking a thiazolidinedione alone. The majority of patients (84%) were Caucasian, 8% Hispanic, and 3% Black. The mean baseline HbA_{1c} values were 7.9% for BYETTA (exenatide) and placebo.

The primary endpoint in each study was the mean change in HbA_{1c} from baseline to study end (or early discontinuation). Table 7 summarizes the study results for the 30- and 16-week clinical trials.

[See table 7 above]

HbA_{1c}

The addition of BYETTA to a regimen of metformin, a sulfonylurea, or both, resulted in statistically significant reductions from baseline in HbA_{1c} compared with patients receiving placebo added to these agents in the three controlled trials (Table 7).

In the 16-week trial of BYETTA add-on to thiazolidinediones, with or without metformin, BYETTA resulted in statistically significant reductions from baseline in HbA_{1c} compared with patients receiving placebo (Table 7).

Postprandial Glucose

Postprandial glucose was measured after a mixed meal tolerance test in 9.5% of patients participating in the 30-week add-on to metformin, add-on to sulfonylurea, and add-on to metformin in combination with sulfonylurea clinical trials. In this pooled subset of patients, BYETTA reduced postprandial plasma glucose concentrations in a dose-dependent manner. The mean (SD) change in 2-hour postprandial glucose concentration following administration of BYETTA at Week 30 relative to baseline was –63 (65) mg/dL for 5 mcg BID (n=42), –71 (73) mg/dL or 10 mcg BID (n=52), and +11 (69) mg/dL for placebo BID (n=44).

14.3 Combination with Insulin Glargine

A 30-week, double-blind, placebo-controlled trial was conducted to evaluate the efficacy and safety of BYETTA (n=137) versus placebo (n=122) when added to titrated insulin glargine, with or without metformin and/or thiazolidinedione, in patients with type 2 diabetes with inadequate glycemic control.

All patients assigned to BYETTA initially received 5 mcg BID for 4 weeks. After 4 weeks, those patients assigned to BYETTA had their dose increased to 10 mcg BID. Patients assigned to placebo received placebo BID throughout the trial. BYETTA or placebo was injected subcutaneously before the morning and evening meals. Patients with an HbA_{1c} ≤8.0% decreased their prestudy dose of insulin glargine by 20% and patients with an HbA_{1c} ≥8.1% maintained their current dose of insulin glargine. Five weeks after initiating randomized treatment, insulin doses were titrated with guidance from the investigator toward predefined fasting glucose targets according to the dose titration algorithm provided in Table 9. The majority of patients (78%) were Caucasian, 10% American Indian or Alaska Native, 9% Black, 3% Asian, and 0.8% of multiple origins.

The primary endpoint was the change in HbA_{1c} from baseline to Week 30. Compared to placebo, BYETTA 10 mcg BID resulted in statistically significant reductions in HbA_{1c} from baseline at Week 30 (Table 8) in patients receiving titrated insulin glargine.

[See table 8 at top of next page]

Table 9: Dosing Algorithm for Titration of Insulin Glargine*

Fasting Plasma Glucose Values (mg/dL)	Dose Change (U)
<56†	–4
56 to 72†	–2
73 to 99‡	0
100 to 119‡	+2
120 to 139‡	+4
140 to 179‡	+6
≥180‡	+8

Abbreviations: U = units.
* Adapted from Riddle et al. 2003.
† Value for at least 1 fasting plasma glucose measurement since the last assessment.
‡ Based on the average of fasting plasma glucose measurements taken over the prior 3 to 7 days. The increase in the total daily dose should not have exceeded more than 10 units per day or 10% of the current total daily dose, whichever was greater.

16 HOW SUPPLIED/STORAGE AND HANDLING

16.1 How Supplied

BYETTA is supplied as a sterile solution for subcutaneous injection containing 250 mcg/mL exenatide.

The following packages are available:
- 5 mcg per dose, 60 doses, 1.2 mL prefilled pen, NDC 66780-210-07
- 10 mcg per dose, 60 doses, 2.4 mL prefilled pen, NDC 66780-212-01

16.2 Storage and Handling
- Prior to first use, BYETTA (exenatide) must be stored refrigerated at 36°F to 46°F (2°C to 8°C).
- After first use, BYETTA can be kept at a temperature not to exceed 77°F (25°C).
- Do not freeze. Do not use BYETTA if it has been frozen.
- BYETTA should be protected from light.
- The pen should be discarded 30 days after first use, even if some drug remains in the pen.
- Use a puncture-resistant container to discard the needles. Do not reuse or share needles.
- BYETTA should not be used past the expiration date.
- **BYETTA pens are not to be shared with other patients.**

17 PATIENT COUNSELING INFORMATION

See FDA-approved Medication Guide.

Patients should be advised that BYETTA pens are never to be shared with another patient.

Patients should be informed of the potential risks and benefits of BYETTA and of alternative modes of therapy. Patients should also be fully informed about self-management practices, including the importance of proper storage of BYETTA, injection technique, timing of dosage of BYETTA and concomitant oral drugs, adherence to meal planning, regular physical activity, periodic blood glucose monitoring and HbA_{1c} testing, recognition and management of hypoglycemia and hyperglycemia, and assessment for diabetes complications.

17.1 Risk of Pancreatitis

Patients should be informed that persistent severe abdominal pain that may radiate to the back and which may or may not be accompanied by vomiting, is the hallmark symptom of acute pancreatitis. Patients should be instructed to promptly discontinue BYETTA and contact their physician if persistent severe abdominal pain occurs [see *Warnings and Precautions (5.1)*].

17.2 Risk of Hypoglycemia

The risk of hypoglycemia is increased when BYETTA is used in combination with a sulfonylurea. Therefore, patients receiving BYETTA and a sulfonylurea may require a lower dose of the sulfonylurea to reduce the risk of hypoglycemia. Patients should be informed that it is also possible that the use of BYETTA with other glucose-independent insulin secretagogues (e.g., meglitinides) could increase the risk of hypoglycemia.

When BYETTA is used in combination with insulin, evaluate the dose of insulin. Consider reducing the dose of insulin in patients at increased risk of hypoglycemia [see *Adverse Reactions (6.1)*]. Patients treated with BYETTA should be informed that the concurrent use of BYETTA with prandial insulin has not been studied and cannot be recommended.

The symptoms, treatment, and conditions that predispose to development of hypoglycemia should be explained to the patient. The patient's usual instructions for hypoglycemia management should be reviewed and reinforced when initiating BYETTA therapy, particularly when concomitantly administered with a sulfonylurea or insulin [see *Warnings and Precautions (5.2)*].

17.3 Risk of Renal Impairment

Patients treated with BYETTA should be informed of the potential risk for worsening renal function and informed about associated signs and symptoms of renal dysfunction, as well as the possibility of dialysis as a medical intervention if renal failure occurs [see *Warnings and Precautions (5.3)*].

17.4 Risk of Hypersensitivity Reactions

Patients should be informed that serious hypersensitivity reactions have been reported during postmarketing use of BYETTA. If symptoms of hypersensitivity reactions occur, patients must stop taking BYETTA and seek medical advice promptly [see *Warnings and Precautions (5.6)*].

17.5 Use in Pregnancy

Patients should be advised to inform their physicians if they are pregnant or intend to become pregnant.

17.6 Instructions

Each dose of BYETTA should be administered as a SC injection in the thigh, abdomen, or upper arm at any time within the 60-minute period **before** the morning and evening meals (or before the two main meals of the day, approximately 6 hours or more apart). BYETTA **should not** be administered after a meal. If a dose is missed, the treatment regimen should be resumed as prescribed with the next scheduled dose.

Patients should be advised that treatment with BYETTA may result in a reduction in appetite, food intake, and/or body weight, and that there is no need to modify the dosing regimen due to such effects. Treatment with BYETTA may also result in nausea, particularly upon initiation of therapy [see *Adverse Reactions (6)*].

Table 8: 30-Week Placebo-Controlled Trial of BYETTA Used in Combination with Insulin Glargine with or without Metformin and/or Thiazolidinediones

	Placebo BID + Titrated Insulin Glargine	BYETTA 10 mcg* BID + Titrated Insulin Glargine
Intent-to-Treat Population (N)	122	137
HbA_{1c} (%), Mean		
Baseline	8.5	8.3
Change at Week 30†	−1.0	−1.7
Difference from placebo† (95% CI)		−0.7 [−1.0, −0.5]¶
Proportion Achieving HbA_{1c} <7%	30%	57%
Body Weight (kg), Mean		
Baseline	93.8	95.4
Change at Week 30‡	1.0	−1.8
Difference from placebo‡ (95% CI)		−2.7 [−3.7, −1.7]¶
Fasting Serum Glucose§ (mg/dL), Mean		
Baseline	133	132
Change at Week 30‡	−16	−23
Difference from placebo‡ (95% CI)		−7 [−18, 3]

* BYETTA 5 mcg twice daily for 1 month followed by 10 mcg BID for 5 months for the 30-week trial.
† Least squares means are based on a mixed model adjusting for treatment, pooled investigator, visit, baseline HbA_{1c} value, and treatment by visit, where subject is treated as a random effect.
‡ Least squares means are based on a mixed model adjusting for treatment, pooled investigator, visit, baseline HbA_{1c} stratum, baseline value of the dependent variable (where applicable), and treatment by visit, where subject is treated as a random effect.
§ Patients in both groups titrated insulin glargine dose to achieve optimal fasting glucose concentrations.
¶ $p < 0.01$, treatment vs. placebo.
BID = twice daily.

The patient should read the Medication Guide and the Pen User Manual before starting BYETTA (exenatide) therapy and review them each time the prescription is refilled. The patient should be instructed on proper use and storage of the pen, emphasizing how and when to set up a new pen and noting that only one setup step is necessary at initial use. The patient should be advised not to share the pen and needles.

Patients should be informed that pen needles are not included with the pen and must be purchased separately. Patients should be advised which needle length and gauge should be used.

Manufactured for:
Bristol-Myers Squibb Company
Princeton, NJ 08543 USA
Marketed by:
Bristol-Myers Squibb Company
Princeton, NJ 08543
and
AstraZeneca Pharmaceuticals LP
Wilmington, DE 19850
BYETTA is a registered trademark of Amylin Pharmaceuticals, LLC.
822018-BB
Rev February 2013

MEDICATION GUIDE
BYETTA® (bye-A-tuh)
(exenatide)
Injection

Read this Medication Guide and the Pen User Manual that come with BYETTA before you start using it and each time you get a refill. There may be new information. This Medication Guide does not take the place of talking with your healthcare provider about your medical condition or your treatment. If you have questions about BYETTA after reading this information, ask your healthcare provider or pharmacist.

What is the most important information I should know about BYETTA?

Serious side effects can happen in people who take BYETTA, including inflammation of the pancreas (pancreatitis) which may be severe and lead to death.

Before taking BYETTA, tell your healthcare provider if you have had:
- pancreatitis
- stones in your gallbladder (gallstones)
- a history of alcoholism
- high blood triglyceride levels

These medical conditions can make you more likely to get pancreatitis in general. It is not known if having these conditions will lead to a higher chance of getting pancreatitis while taking BYETTA.

While taking BYETTA:

Call your healthcare provider right away if you have pain in your stomach area (abdomen) that is severe, and will not go away. The pain may happen with or without vomiting. The pain may be felt going from your abdomen through to your back. These may be symptoms of pancreatitis.

What is BYETTA?
- BYETTA (exenatide) is an injectable prescription medicine that may improve blood sugar (glucose) control in adults with type 2 diabetes mellitus, when used with a diet and exercise program.
- BYETTA is not insulin.
- You should not take BYETTA instead of insulin.
- The use of BYETTA with short acting insulin is not recommended.
- The use of BYETTA with rapid acting insulin is not recommended.
- BYETTA is not for people with type 1 diabetes or people with diabetic ketoacidosis.
- It is not known if BYETTA is safe and effective in children.
- BYETTA has not been studied in people who have pancreatitis.
- BYETTA should not be used in people who have severe kidney problems.

Who should not use BYETTA?

Do not use BYETTA if:
- you have had an allergic reaction to exenatide or any of the other ingredients in BYETTA. See the end of this Medication Guide for a complete list of ingredients in BYETTA.

Symptoms of a severe allergic reaction with BYETTA may include:
- swelling of your face, lips, tongue, or throat
- problems breathing or swallowing
- severe rash or itching
- fainting or feeling dizzy
- very rapid heartbeat

What should I tell my healthcare provider before using BYETTA?

Before taking BYETTA, tell your healthcare provider if you:
- have or have had pancreatitis, stones in your gallbladder (gallstones), a history of alcoholism, or high blood triglyceride levels.
- have severe problems with your stomach, such as delayed emptying of your stomach (gastroparesis) or problems with digesting food.
- have or have had kidney problems, or have had a kidney transplant.
- have any other medical conditions.
- are pregnant or plan to become pregnant. It is not known if BYETTA will harm your unborn baby.
  Pregnancy Registry: A registry has been implemented for women who take BYETTA during pregnancy. The purpose of this registry is to collect information about the health of you and your baby. If you take BYETTA at any time during pregnancy you may enroll in this registry by calling 1-800-633-9081.
- are breastfeeding or plan to breast-feed. It is not known if BYETTA passes into your breast milk. You and your healthcare provider should decide if you will take BYETTA or breast-feed. You should not do both without talking with your healthcare provider first.

Tell your healthcare provider about all the medicines you take including prescription and nonprescription medicines, vitamins, and herbal supplements. BYETTA slows stomach emptying and can affect medicines that need to pass through the stomach quickly. BYETTA may affect the way some medicines work and some other medicines may affect the way BYETTA works.

Especially tell your healthcare provider if you take:
- other anti-diabetes medicines, especially sulfonylurea medicines or insulin.
- birth control pills that are taken by mouth (oral contraceptives). BYETTA (exenatide) may lower the amount of the medicine in your blood from your birth control pills and they may not work as well to prevent pregnancy. Take your birth control pills at least one hour before your injection of BYETTA. If you must take your birth control pills with food, take it with a meal or snack where you do not also take BYETTA.
- an antibiotic. Take antibiotic medicines at least one hour before taking BYETTA. If you must take your antibiotic with food, take it with a meal or snack where you do not also take BYETTA.
- warfarin sodium (Coumadin®, Jantoven®).
- a blood pressure medicine.
- a water pill (diuretic).
- a pain medicine.
- lovastatin (Altoprev®, Mevacor®, Advicor®).

Ask your healthcare provider if you are not sure if your medicine is listed above.

Know the medicines you take. Keep a list of them with you to show your healthcare provider and pharmacist each time you get a new medicine.

How should I use BYETTA?

See the Pen User Manual that comes with BYETTA for instructions for using the BYETTA Pen and injecting BYETTA.
- Your healthcare provider may prescribe BYETTA alone or with certain other medicines to help control your blood sugar.
- BYETTA comes in a prefilled pen.
- Use BYETTA exactly as prescribed by your healthcare provider. Do not change your dose unless your healthcare provider has told you to change your dose.
- Your healthcare provider must teach you how to inject BYETTA before you use it for the first time. If you have questions or do not understand the instructions, talk to your healthcare provider or pharmacist.
- Pen needles are not included. You may need a prescription to purchase pen needles from your pharmacist. Ask your healthcare provider which needle length and gauge is best for you.
- Inject your dose of BYETTA under the skin (subcutaneous injection) of your upper leg (thigh), stomach area (abdomen), or upper arm as instructed by your healthcare provider. **Do not inject into a vein or muscle.**
- **Do not** mix BYETTA and insulin in the same syringe or vial even if you take them at the same time.
- BYETTA is injected two times each day, at any time within the 60 minutes (1 hour) **before** your morning and evening meals (or **before** the two main meals of the day, approximately 6 hours or more apart). **Do not take BYETTA after your meal.**
- If you miss a dose of BYETTA, skip that dose and take your next dose at the next prescribed time. Do not take an extra dose or increase the amount of your next dose to make up for a missed dose.
- If you use too much BYETTA, call your healthcare provider or poison control center at 1-800-222-1222 right away. Too much BYETTA can cause your blood sugar to drop quickly and you may have symptoms of low blood sugar. You may need medical treatment right away. Too much BYETTA can also cause severe nausea and vomiting.
- Follow your healthcare provider's instructions for diet, exercise, and how often to test your blood sugar. If you see your blood sugar increasing during treatment with BYETTA, talk to your healthcare provider because you may need to adjust your current treatment plan for your diabetes.
- Talk to your healthcare provider about how to manage high blood sugar (hyperglycemia) and low blood sugar (hypoglycemia), and how to recognize problems that can happen with your diabetes.
- Never share your BYETTA pen with another person. You may give an infection to them, or get an infection from them, and BYETTA may harm them.

What are the possible side effects of BYETTA?

BYETTA can cause serious side effects.

See "What is the most important information I should know about BYETTA?"

It is not known whether BYETTA, or other anti-diabetes medications, increase your risk of a heart attack or stroke.
- **Low blood sugar (hypoglycemia).** Your risk for getting low blood sugar is higher if you take BYETTA with another medicine that can cause low blood sugar, such as a sulfonylurea or insulin. The dose of your sulfonylurea or insulin medicine may need to be lowered while you use BYETTA. Signs and symptoms of low blood sugar may include:

• headache	• irritability
• drowsiness	• hunger
• weakness	• fast heart beat
• dizziness	• sweating
• confusion	• feeling jittery

Talk with your healthcare provider about how to treat low blood sugar.
- **Kidney problems.** BYETTA (exenatide) may cause new or worse problems with kidney function, including kidney failure. Dialysis or kidney transplant may be needed.
  - **While taking BYETTA:**
    Call your healthcare provider right away if you have nausea, vomiting, or diarrhea that will not go away, or if you cannot take liquids by mouth. You may be at increased risk for kidney problems.
- **Severe allergic reactions.** Severe allergic reactions can happen with BYETTA. Stop taking BYETTA and get medical help right away if you have any symptom of a severe allergic reaction. See **"Who should not use BYETTA?"**

The most common side effects with BYETTA include:
- nausea. Nausea most commonly happens when first starting BYETTA, but may become less over time

• vomiting	• headache
• diarrhea	• acid stomach
• feeling jittery	• constipation
• dizziness	• weakness

Talk to your healthcare provider about any side effect that bothers you or that does not go away.

These are not all the side effects with BYETTA.

Call your doctor for medical advice about side effects. You may report side effects to FDA at 1-800-FDA-1088.

How should I store BYETTA?
- Store your new, unused BYETTA Pen in the original carton in a refrigerator at 36°F to 46°F (2°C to 8°C).
- After first use, keep your BYETTA Pen at a temperature cooler than 77°F (25°C).
- Do not freeze your BYETTA Pen. Do not use BYETTA if it has been frozen.
- Protect BYETTA from light.
- Use a BYETTA Pen for only 30 days. Throw away a used BYETTA Pen after 30 days, even if there is some medicine left in the pen.
- Do not use BYETTA after the expiration date printed on the label.
- Do not store the BYETTA Pen with the needle attached. If the needle is left on, medicine may leak from the BYETTA Pen or air bubbles may form in the cartridge.
- See the BYETTA Pen User Manual for instructions about the right way to throw away your BYETTA Pen.
- **Keep your BYETTA Pen, pen needles, and all medicines out of the reach of children.**

General information about BYETTA

Medicines are sometimes prescribed for purposes other than those listed in a Medication Guide. Do not use BYETTA for a condition for which it was not prescribed. Do not give BYETTA to other people, even if they have the same symptoms you have. It may harm them.

This Medication Guide includes the most important information you should know about using BYETTA. If you would like more information, talk with your healthcare provider. You can ask your healthcare provider or pharmacist for information about BYETTA that is written for health professionals.

For more information about BYETTA, go to www.BYETTA.com or call BYETTA Customer Service at 1-800-868-1190.

What are the ingredients in BYETTA?

Active Ingredient: exenatide

Inactive Ingredients: metacresol, mannitol, glacial acetic acid, and sodium acetate trihydrate in water for injection.

This Medication Guide has been approved by the U.S. Food and Drug Administration.

BYETTA is a registered trademark of Amylin Pharmaceuticals, LLC. All other trademarks are the trademarks of their respective owners.

Manufactured for:
Bristol-Myers Squibb Company
Princeton, NJ 08543 USA
Marketed by:
Bristol-Myers Squibb Company
Princeton, NJ 08543
and
AstraZeneca Pharmaceuticals LP
Wilmington, DE 19850
823016-BB
Rev February 2013

PEN USER MANUAL
BYETTA® exenatide injection
250 mcg/mL, 1.2 mL
5 mcg
5 mcg PEN USER MANUAL

Section 1 **Read this section completely before you begin. Then, move on to Section 2—Getting Started.**

WHAT YOU NEED TO KNOW ABOUT YOUR BYETTA PEN

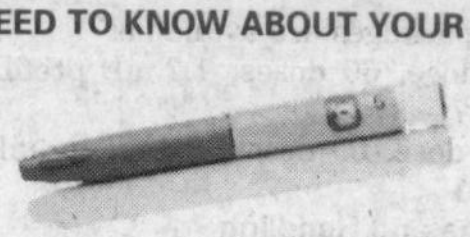

PEN USER MANUAL

Read these instructions carefully BEFORE using your BYETTA Pen. For complete dosing and safety information, also read the BYETTA *Medication Guide* that comes with the BYETTA (exenatide) Pen carton.

It is important that you use your pen correctly. Failure to follow these instructions completely may result in a wrong dose, a broken pen or an infection.

These instructions do not take the place of talking with your healthcare provider about your medical condition or your treatment. If you are having problems using your BYETTA Pen, call toll free 800-868-1190.

IMPORTANT INFORMATION ABOUT YOUR BYETTA PEN
- Each BYETTA Pen contains enough medicine for injection two times each day for 30 days. You do not have to measure any doses, the pen measures each dose for you.
- **Do not transfer the medicine in the BYETTA Pen to a syringe or vial.**
- **Do not** mix BYETTA and insulin in the same syringe or vial even if you take them at the same time.
- If any part of your pen appears broken or damaged, do not use the pen.
- This BYETTA Pen is not recommended for use by people who are blind or have vision problems without the help of a person trained in the proper use of the pen.
- **Follow the injection method explained to you by your healthcare provider.**
- Follow Section 2 only to set up a new pen before first use.
- Section 3 of this manual should be used for every injection.

ABOUT PEN NEEDLES

What kinds of needles can be used with my BYETTA Pen?
- **Pen needles are not included with your pen.** You may need a prescription to get them from your pharmacist.
- Use 29 (thin), 30, or 31 (thinner) gauge disposable pen needles with your BYETTA Pen. Ask your healthcare provider which needle gauge and length is best for you.

Do I use a new needle for each injection?
- Yes. Do not reuse needles.
- Remove the needle from the pen immediately after you complete each injection. This will help prevent leakage of BYETTA, keep out air bubbles, reduce needle clogs, and decrease the risk of infection.
- Do not push the injection button on your pen unless a needle is attached to the pen.

How do I throw away my needles?
- Do not throw away the pen with a needle attached.
- Place used needles in a closeable, puncture-resistant container. You may use a sharps container (such as a red biohazard container), a hard plastic container (such as a detergent bottle), or a metal container (such as an empty coffee can). Ask your healthcare provider for instructions on the right way to throw away (dispose of) your used pens and the container. There may be state and local laws about how you should throw away used pens and needles.
- Do not throw the disposal container in the household trash. Do not recycle.
- Always keep the puncture-proof container out of reach of children.

Never share your BYETTA pen or needles with another person. You may give an infection to them, or get an infection from them, and BYETTA may harm them.

STORING YOUR BYETTA PEN

How do I store my BYETTA Pen?
- Prior to first use, store your unused BYETTA Pen in the original carton in a refrigerator at 36°F to 46°F (2°C to 8°C).
- After first use, your BYETTA Pen can be kept at a temperature not to exceed 77°F (25°C).
- Do not freeze. Do not use BYETTA if it has been frozen. BYETTA should be protected from light.
- When carrying the pen away from home, store the pen at a temperature between 36°F to 77°F (2°C to 25°C) and keep dry.
- Do not store the pen with the needle attached. If the needle is left on the pen, BYETTA may leak from the pen and air bubbles may form in the cartridge.

Keep your pen and needles out of the reach of children.

How long can I use a BYETTA Pen?
- You can use your BYETTA Pen for up to 30 days after setting up a new pen for first use. **After 30 days, throw away the BYETTA Pen, even if it is not completely empty.**
- Mark the date when you first used your pen and the date 30 days later in the spaces below:

Date of First Use ____________

Date to Throw Away Pen ____________
- BYETTA should not be used after the expiration date printed on the pen label.

How do I clean my BYETTA Pen?
- Wipe the outside of the pen with a clean, damp cloth.
- White particles may appear on the outside tip of the cartridge during normal use. You may remove them with an alcohol wipe or alcohol swab.

See the complete BYETTA *Medication Guide* that comes with BYETTA. For more information, call toll free 800-868-1190 or visit www.BYETTA.com

Section 2 Read and follow the directions in this section only after you've read Section 1—What You Need To Know About Your BYETTA Pen.

GETTING STARTED

Set up your new pen just before you use it the first time. For routine use, do not repeat this one-time-only new pen setup. If you do, you will run out of BYETTA (exenatide) before 30 days of use.

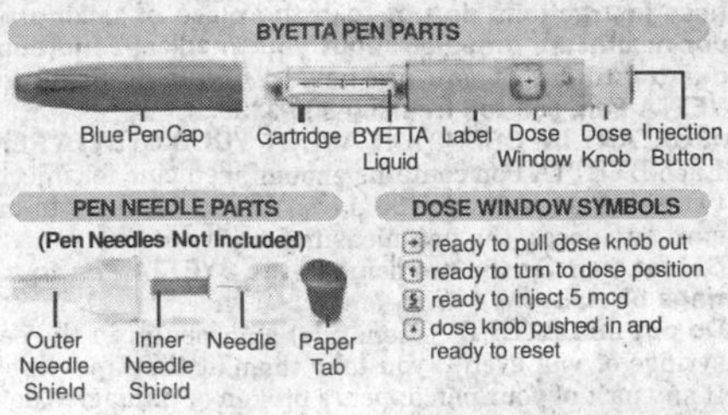

[See table above in next column]

Section 3 Now that you have done the one-time-only new pen setup, follow Section 3 for all of your injections.

[See table at top of next page]

STEP 7 Store Pen for Next Dose
- Replace Blue Pen Cap on pen before storage.
- Store your BYETTA Pen at a temperature between 36°F to 77°F (2°C to 25°C). (See **Storing Your BYETTA Pen** in Section 1 of this user manual for complete storage information.)
- When it is time for your next routine dose, go to **Section 3, Step 1,** and repeat Steps 1–7.

Section 4

COMMONLY ASKED QUESTIONS

1. **Do I need to do the One-Time-Only New Pen Setup before every dose?**
   - No. **The One-Time-Only New Pen Setup is done only once, just before each new pen is used for the first time.**
   - The purpose of the setup is to make sure that your BYETTA Pen is ready to use for the next 30 days.
   - **If you repeat the One-Time-Only New Pen Setup before each routine dose, you will not have enough BYETTA for 30 days.** The small amount of BYETTA used in the new pen setup will not affect the 30-day supply of BYETTA.
2. **Why are there air bubbles in the cartridge?**
   - A small air bubble is normal. It will not harm you or affect your dose.
   - If the pen is stored with a needle attached, air bubbles may form in the cartridge. **Do not** store the pen with the needle attached.
3. **What should I do if BYETTA does not come out of the needle tip after four tries during One-Time-Only New Pen Setup?**
   - Carefully put the outer needle shield back over the needle. Remove the needle by unscrewing it. Throw away the needle properly.
   - Attach a new needle and repeat **One-Time-Only New Pen Setup, Steps B–E,** in Section 2 of this user manual. Once you see several drops or a stream of liquid coming out of the tip of the needle, the setup is complete.
4. **Why do I see BYETTA leaking from my needle after I have finished my injection?**
   It is normal for a single drop to remain on the tip of your needle after your injection is complete. If you see more than one drop:
   - You may not have received your full dose. **Do not inject another dose.** Talk with your healthcare provider about what to do about a partial dose.
   - To make sure that you get your full dose, when you take your injections, **firmly push and hold** the injection button in and **slowly count to 5** (see **Section 3, Step 4: Inject the Dose**).
5. **How can I tell when the injection is complete?**
   The injection is complete when:
   - You have firmly pushed the injection button in all the way **until it stops**
     and
   - **You have slowly counted to 5** while you are still holding the injection button in and the needle is still in your skin
     and
   - The • is in the center of the dose window.

ONE-TIME-ONLY NEW PEN SETUP

STEP A Check the Pen

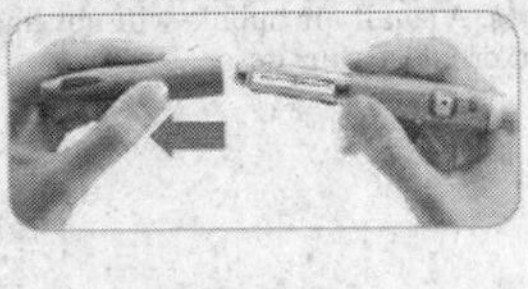

- Wash hands prior to use.
- Check pen label to make sure it is your 5 mcg pen.
- Pull off the blue pen cap.

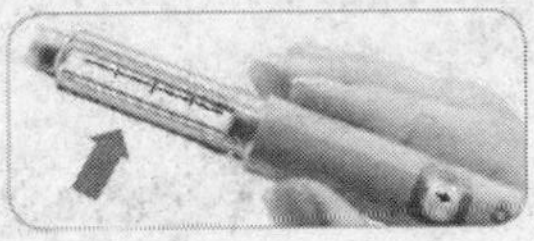

- Check BYETTA in the cartridge. The liquid should be clear, colorless, and free of particles. If not, do not use.

Note: A small air bubble in the cartridge is normal.

STEP B Attach the Needle

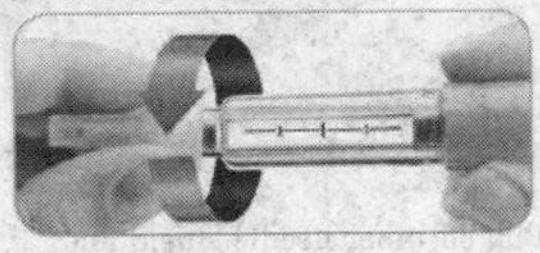

- Remove paper tab from outer needle shield.
- **Push** outer needle shield containing the needle **straight** onto the pen, then **screw** needle on until secure.

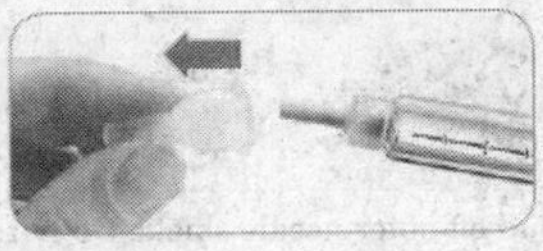

- Pull off outer needle shield. **Do not** throw away.

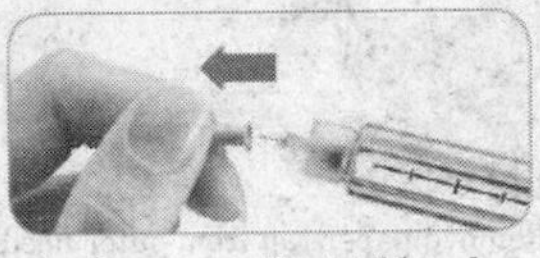

- Pull off inner needle shield and throw away. A small drop of liquid may appear. This is normal.

STEP C Dial the Dose

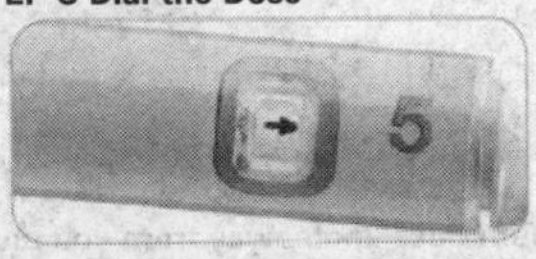

- Check that the → is in the dose window. If not, turn dose knob away from you (clockwise) **until it stops** and the → is in the dose window.

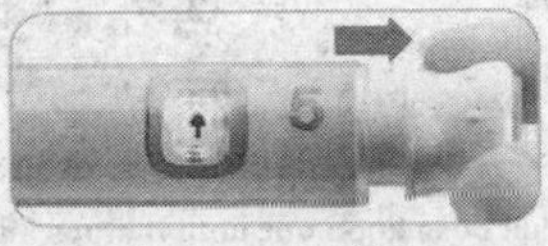

- **Pull dose knob out until it stops** and the ↑ is in the dose window.

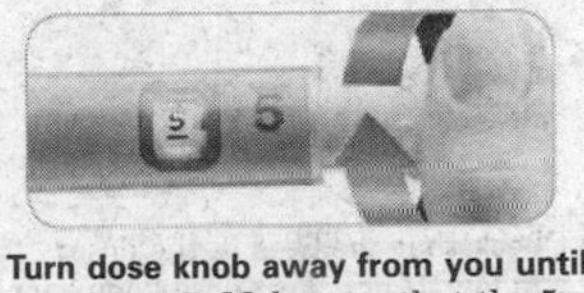

- **Turn dose knob away from you until it stops** at 5. Make sure that the 5 with the line under it is in the center of the dose window.

Note: If you cannot turn the dose knob away from you to the 5, see **Commonly Asked Questions,** number 7, in Section 4 of this user manual.

STEP D Prepare the Pen

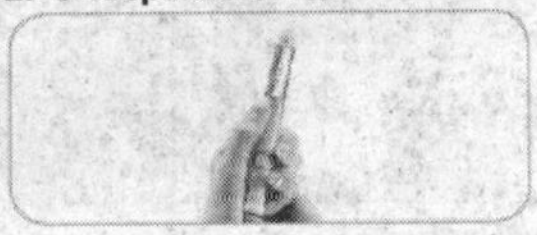

- Point the needle of the pen up and away from you.

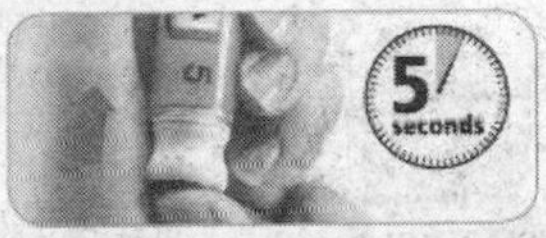

PUSH & HOLD
- **Use thumb to firmly push injection button in until it stops,** then continue holding the injection button in while **slowly counting to 5.**
- **If you do not see a stream or several drops come from the needle tip, repeat Steps C & D.**

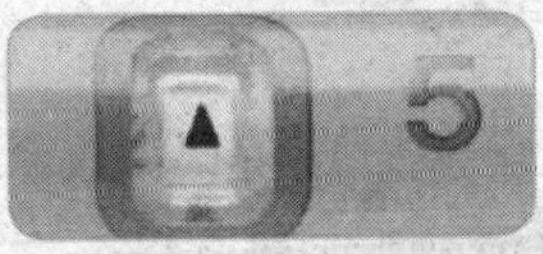

- Pen preparation is complete when the • is in the center of the dose window AND you have seen a stream or several drops come from the needle tip.

Note: If you do not see liquid after 4 times, see **Commonly Asked Questions,** number 3, in Section 4 of this user manual.

STEP E Complete New Pen Setup

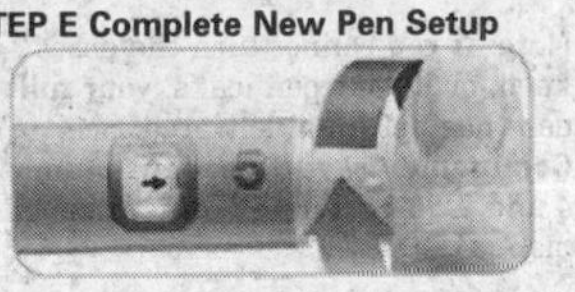

- **Turn dose knob away from you until it stops** and the → is in the dose window.

- **For routine use,** do not repeat this one-time-only new pen setup. If you do, you will run out of BYETTA before 30 days of use.

- You are now ready for your first dose of BYETTA.
- **Go to Section 3, Step 3, for instructions on how to inject your first routine dose.**

Note: If you cannot turn the dose knob, see **Commonly Asked Questions,** number 7, in Section 4 of user manual.

If you hear a click sound from your BYETTA Pen, ignore it. You must follow all the steps listed above to make sure your injection is complete.

6. **Where should I inject BYETTA?**
   Inject BYETTA (exenatide) into your abdomen, thigh, or upper arm using the injection method explained to you by your healthcare provider.

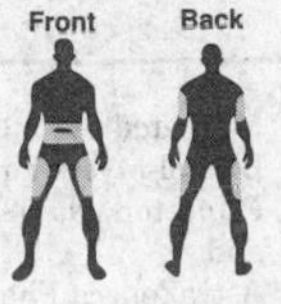

7. **What if I cannot pull, turn, or push the dose knob?**
   Check the symbol in the dose window. Follow the steps next to the matching symbol.

If → is in the dose window:
- Pull the dose knob out until ↑ appears.

If ↑ is in the dose window and the dose knob will not turn:
- The cartridge in your BYETTA Pen may not have enough medicine to deliver a full dose. A small amount of BYETTA will always stay in the cartridge. If the cartridge contains a small amount and the dose knob will not turn, your pen does not have enough BYETTA (exenatide) and will not deliver any more doses. Obtain a new BYETTA Pen.

If ↑ and part of 5 are in the dose window and the dose knob cannot be pushed in:
- The dose knob was not turned all the way. Continue turning the dose knob away from you until 5 is in the center of the dose window.

If part of 5 and part of • are in the dose window and the dose knob cannot be pushed in:
- The needle may be clogged, bent, or incorrectly attached.
- Attach a new needle. Make sure needle is on straight and screwed on all the way.
- Firmly push the injection button in all the way. BYETTA should come from needle tip.

If • is in the dose window and the dose knob will not turn:
- The injection button was not pushed in all the way and a complete dose was not delivered. **Talk with your healthcare provider about what to do about a partial dose.**
- Follow these steps to reset your pen for your next injection:

ROUTINE USE

STEP 1 Check the Pen

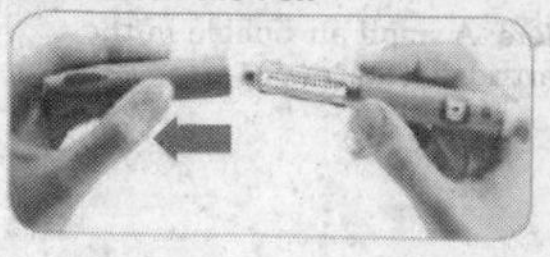

- Wash hands prior to use.
- Check pen label to make sure it is your 5 mcg pen.
- Pull off the blue pen cap.

- Check BYETTA in the cartridge.
- The liquid should be clear, colorless, and free of particles. If it is not, do not use.

Note: A small air bubble will not harm you or affect your dose.

STEP 2 Attach the Needle

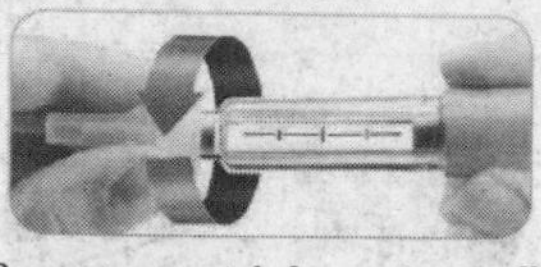

- Remove paper tab from outer needle shield.
- **Push** outer needle shield containing the needle **straight** onto pen, then **screw** needle on until secure.

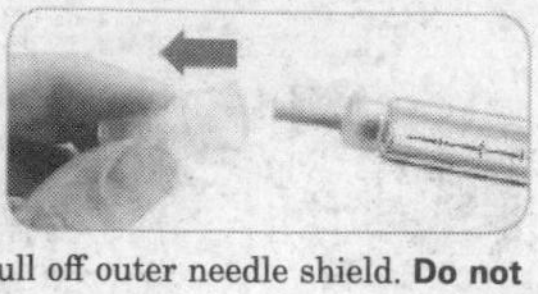

- Pull off outer needle shield. **Do not** throw away.

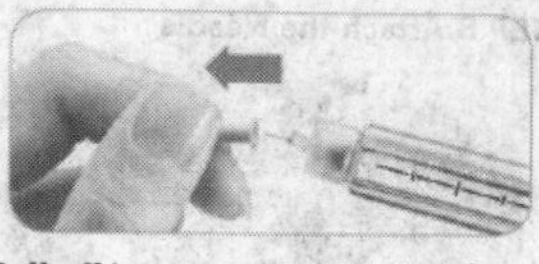

- Pull off inner needle shield and throw away. A small drop of liquid may appear. This is normal.

STEP 3 Dial the Dose

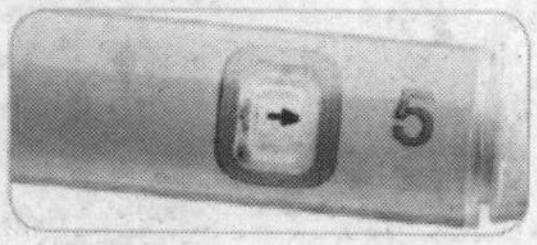

- Check that the ⊖ is in the dose window. If not, turn dose knob away from you (clockwise) **until it stops** and the ⊖ is in the dose window.

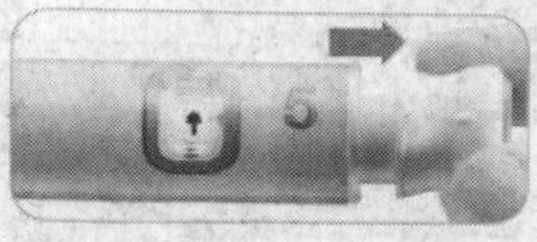

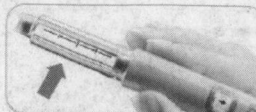

- **Pull dose knob out until it stops** and the ⊕ is in the dose window.

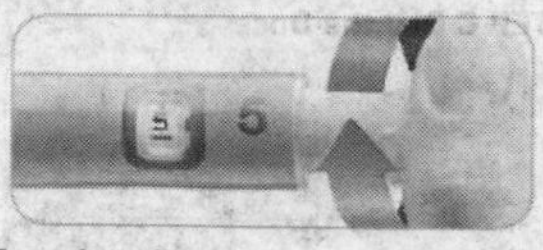

- **Turn dose knob away from you until it stops** at ⊜. Make sure that the 5 with the line under it is in the center of the dose window.

Note: If you cannot turn the dose knob away from you to the ⊜, see **Commonly Asked Questions,** number 7, in Section 4 of this user manual.

STEP 4 Inject the Dose

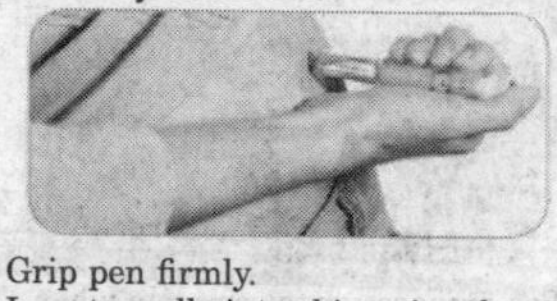

- Grip pen firmly.
- Insert needle into skin using the under-the-skin (subcutaneous) injection method explained by your healthcare provider.

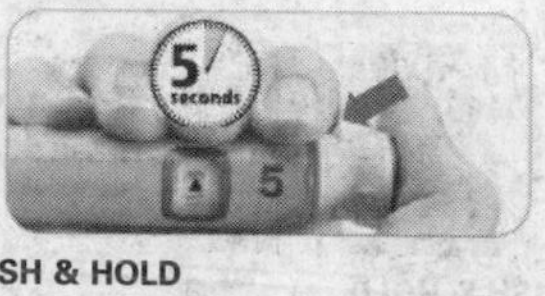

PUSH & HOLD

- **Use thumb to firmly push injection button in until it stops.** Continue holding in the injection button while **slowly counting to 5** to get a full dose.
- Remove needle from skin.

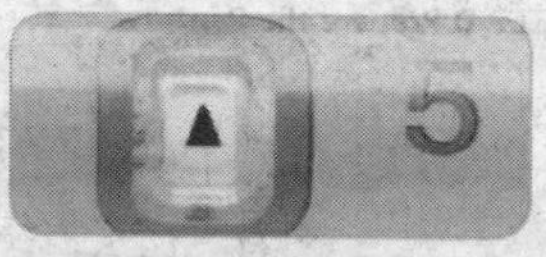

- Injection is complete when the ⊖ is in the center of the dose window.
- The pen is now ready to reset.

Note: If you see several drops of BYETTA leaking from the needle after the injection, you may not have received a complete dose. See **Commonly Asked Questions,** number 4, in Section 4 of this user manual.

STEP 5 Reset the Pen

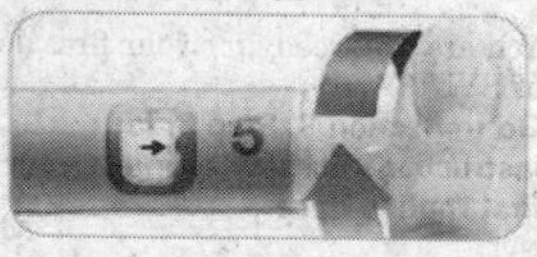

- **Turn dose knob away from you until it stops** and the ⊖ is in the dose window.

Note: If you cannot turn the dose knob, or if your pen leaks, your full dose has not been delivered. See **Commonly Asked Questions,** numbers 4 and 7, in Section 4 of this user manual.

STEP 6 Remove and Dispose of the Needle

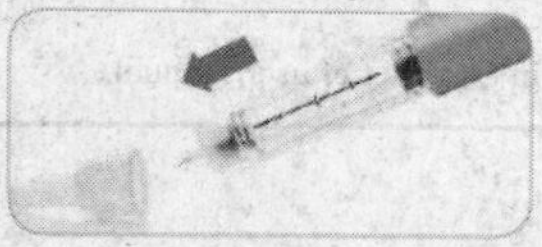

- Carefully put the outer needle shield back over the needle.
- **Remove the needle after each injection.**

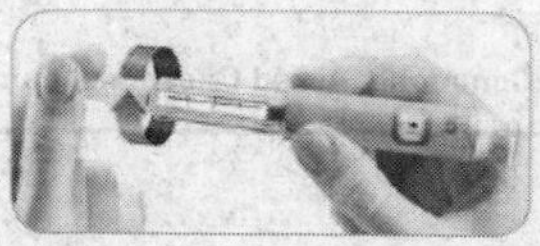

- Unscrew the needle.

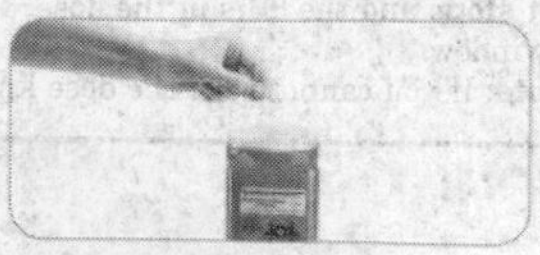

- Throw away needles in a puncture-resistant container or as recommended by your healthcare provider.

- Firmly push the injection button in all the way **until it stops.** Keep holding the injection button in and **slowly count to 5.** Then release the injection button and turn the dose knob away from you until ⊖ appears in the dose window.
- If you cannot turn the dose knob, the needle may be clogged. Replace the needle and repeat the step above.
- For your next dose, be sure to **firmly push and hold** the injection button in and **slowly count to 5** before removing needle from skin.

See the complete BYETTA *Medication Guide* that comes with BYETTA. For more information, call toll free 800-868-1190 or visit www.BYETTA.com

Manufactured for:
Bristol-Myers Squibb Company
Princeton, NJ 08543 USA

Marketed by:
Bristol-Myers Squibb Company
Princeton, NJ 08543
and
AstraZeneca Pharmaceuticals LP
Wilmington, DE 19850
BYETTA is a registered trademark of Amylin Pharmaceuticals, LLC.
825006-BB
Rev February 2013

PEN USER MANUAL
BYETTA® exenatide injection
250 mcg/mL, 2.4 mL
10 mcg
10 mcg PEN USER MANUAL

Section 1 Read this section completely before you begin. Then, move on to Section 2—Getting Started.

WHAT YOU NEED TO KNOW ABOUT YOUR BYETTA PEN

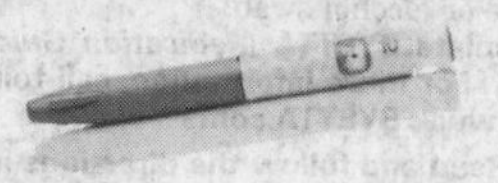

PEN USER MANUAL

Read these instructions carefully BEFORE using your BYETTA Pen. For complete dosing and safety information, also read the BYETTA *Medication Guide* that comes with the BYETTA Pen carton.

It is important that you use your pen correctly. Failure to follow these instructions completely may result in a wrong dose, a broken pen or an infection.

These instructions do not take the place of talking with your healthcare provider about your medical condition or your treatment. If you are having problems using your BYETTA Pen, call toll free 800-868-1190.

IMPORTANT INFORMATION ABOUT YOUR BYETTA PEN

- Each BYETTA Pen contains enough medicine for injection two times each day for 30 days. You do not have to measure any doses, the pen measures each dose for you.
- **Do not transfer the medicine in the BYETTA Pen to a syringe or vial.**
- **Do not** mix BYETTA (exenatide) and insulin in the same syringe or vial even if you take them at the same time.
- If any part of your pen appears broken or damaged, do not use the pen.
- This BYETTA Pen is not recommended for use by people who are blind or have vision problems without the help of a person trained in the proper use of the pen.
- **Follow the injection method explained to you by your healthcare provider.**
- Follow Section 2 only to set up a new pen before first use.
- Section 3 of this manual should be used for every injection.

ABOUT PEN NEEDLES

What kinds of needles can be used with my BYETTA Pen?

- **Pen needles are not included with your pen.** You may need a prescription to get them from your pharmacist.
- Use 29 (thin), 30, or 31 (thinner) gauge disposable pen needles with your BYETTA Pen. Ask your healthcare provider which needle gauge and length is best for you.

Do I use a new needle for each injection?

- Yes. Do not reuse needles.
- Remove the needle from the pen immediately after you complete each injection. This will help prevent leakage of BYETTA, keep out air bubbles, reduce needle clogs, and decrease the risk of infection.
- Do not push the injection button on your pen unless a needle is attached to the pen.

How do I throw away my needles?

- Do not throw away the pen with a needle attached.
- Place used needles in a closeable, puncture-resistant container. You may use a sharps container (such as a red biohazard container), a hard plastic container (such as a detergent bottle), or a metal container (such as an empty coffee can). Ask your healthcare provider for instructions on the right way to throw away (dispose of) your used pens and the container. There may be state and local laws about how you should throw away used pens and needles.
- Do not throw the disposal container in the household trash. Do not recycle.
- Always keep the puncture-proof container out of reach of children.

Never share your BYETTA pen or needles with another person. You may give an infection to them, or get an infection from them, and BYETTA may harm them.

STORING YOUR BYETTA PEN

How do I store my BYETTA Pen?

- Prior to first use, store your unused BYETTA Pen in the original carton in a refrigerator at 36°F to 46°F (2°C to 8°C).
- After first use, your BYETTA Pen can be kept at a temperature not to exceed 77°F (25°C).
- Do not freeze. Do not use BYETTA if it has been frozen. BYETTA should be protected from light.
- When carrying the pen away from home, store the pen at a temperature between 36°F to 77°F (2°C to 25°C) and keep dry.
- Do not store the pen with the needle attached. If the needle is left on the pen, BYETTA may leak from the pen and air bubbles may form in the cartridge.

Keep your pen and needles out of the reach of children.

How long can I use a BYETTA Pen?

- You can use your BYETTA Pen for up to 30 days after setting up a new pen for first use. **After 30 days, throw away the BYETTA Pen, even if it is not completely empty.**
- Mark the date when you first used your pen and the date 30 days later in the spaces below:

Date of First Use ____________

Date to Throw Away Pen ____________

- BYETTA should not be used after the expiration date printed on the pen label.

How do I clean my BYETTA Pen?
- Wipe the outside of the pen with a clean, damp cloth.
- White particles may appear on the outside tip of the cartridge during normal use. You may remove them with an alcohol wipe or alcohol swab.

See the complete BYETTA *Medication Guide* that comes with BYETTA. For more information, call toll free 800-868-1190 or visit www.BYETTA.com

Section 2 Read and follow the directions in this section only after you've read Section 1—What You Need To Know About Your BYETTA Pen.

GETTING STARTED

Set up your new pen just before you use it the first time. For routine use, do not repeat this one-time-only new pen setup. If you do, you will run out of BYETTA (exenatide) before 30 days of use.

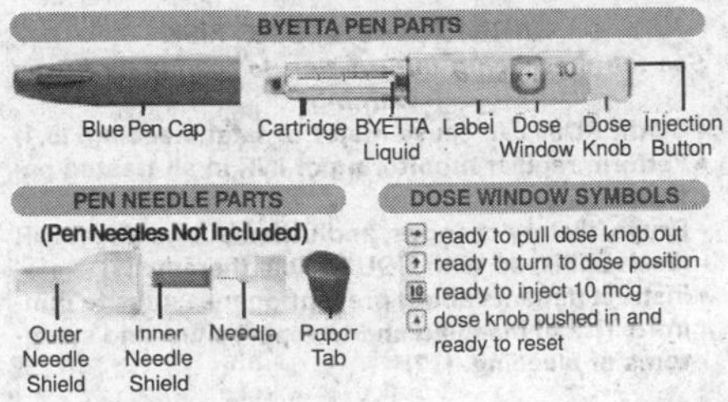

[See table above in next column]

Section 3 Now that you have done the one-time-only new pen setup, follow Section 3 for all of your injections.

[See table at top of next page]

STEP 7 Store Pen for Next Dose
- Replace Blue Pen Cap on pen before storage.
- Store your BYETTA Pen at a temperature between 36°F to 77°F (2°C to 25°C). (See **Storing Your BYETTA Pen** in Section 1 of this user manual for complete storage information.)
- When it is time for your next routine dose, go to **Section 3, Step 1,** and repeat Steps 1–7.

Section 4

COMMONLY ASKED QUESTIONS

1. Do I need to do the One-Time-Only New Pen Setup before every dose?
- No. **The One-Time-Only New Pen Setup is done only once, just before each new pen is used for the first time.**
- The purpose of the setup is to make sure that your BYETTA Pen is ready to use for the next 30 days.
- **If you repeat the One-Time-Only New Pen Setup before each routine dose, you will not have enough BYETTA for 30 days.** The small amount of BYETTA used in the new pen setup will not affect the 30-day supply of BYETTA.

2. Why are there air bubbles in the cartridge?
- A small air bubble is normal. It will not harm you or affect your dose.
- If the pen is stored with a needle attached, air bubbles may form in the cartridge. **Do not** store the pen with the needle attached.

3. What should I do if BYETTA does not come out of the needle tip after four tries during One-Time-Only New Pen Setup?
- Carefully put the outer needle shield back over the needle. Remove the needle by unscrewing it. Throw away the needle properly.
- Attach a new needle and repeat **One-Time-Only New Pen Setup, Steps B–E,** in Section 2 of this user manual. Once you see several drops or a stream of liquid coming out of the tip of the needle, the setup is complete.

4. Why do I see BYETTA leaking from my needle after I have finished my injection?

It is normal for a single drop to remain on the tip of your needle after your injection is complete. If you see more than one drop:
- You may not have received your full dose. **Do not inject another dose.** Talk with your healthcare provider about what to do about a partial dose.
- To make sure that you get your full dose, when you take your injections, **firmly push and hold** the injection button in and **slowly count to 5** (see **Section 3, Step 4: Inject the Dose**).

5. How can I tell when the injection is complete?

The injection is complete when:
- You have firmly pushed the injection button in all the way **until it stops**

  and
- **You have slowly counted to 5** while you are still holding the injection button in and the needle is still in your skin

  and
- The ⊡ is in the center of the dose window.

ONE-TIME-ONLY NEW PEN SETUP

STEP A Check the Pen

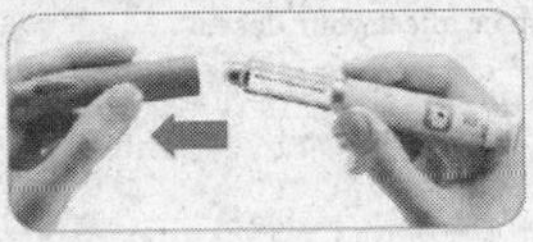

- Wash hands prior to use.
- Check pen label to make sure it is your 10 mcg pen.
- Pull off the blue pen cap.

- Check BYETTA in the cartridge. The liquid should be clear, colorless, and free of particles. If not, do not use.

Note: A small air bubble in the cartridge is normal.

STEP B Attach the Needle

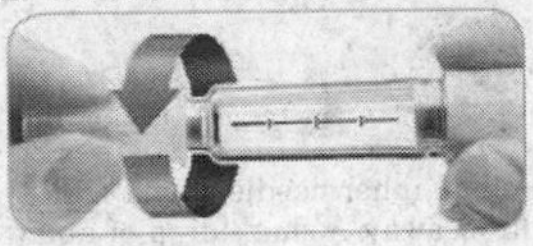

- Remove paper tab from outer needle shield.
- **Push** outer needle shield containing the needle **straight** onto the pen, then **screw** needle on until secure.

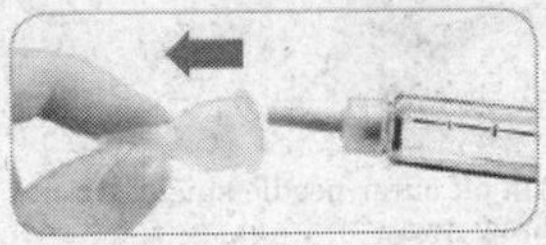

- Pull off outer needle shield. **Do not** throw away.

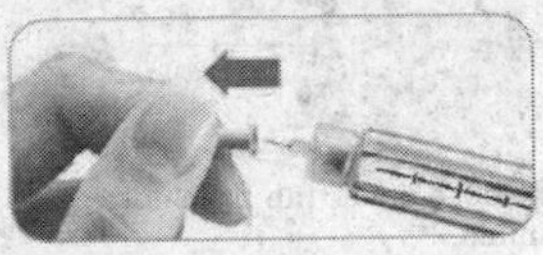

- Pull off inner needle shield and throw away. A small drop of liquid may appear. This is normal.

STEP C Dial the Dose

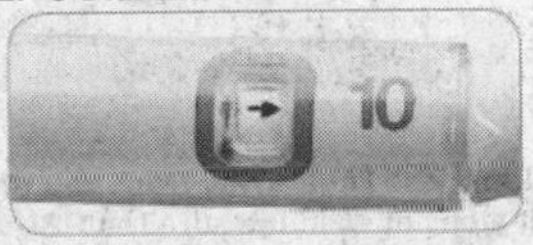

- Check that the ⊖ is in the dose window. If not, turn dose knob away from you (clockwise) **until it stops** and the ⊖ is in the dose window.

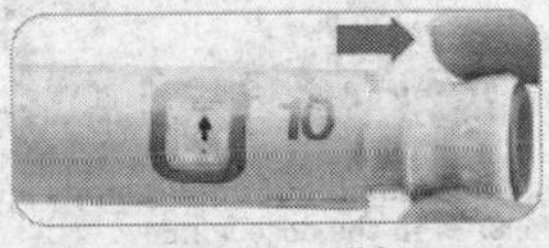

- **Pull dose knob out until it stops** and the ⊕ is in the dose window.

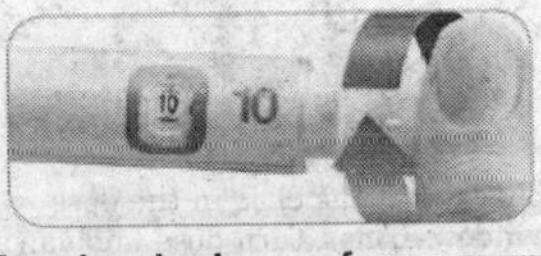

- **Turn dose knob away from you until it stops** at ⊞. Make sure that the 10 with the line under it is in the center of the dose window.

Note: If you cannot turn the dose knob away from you to the ⊞, see **Commonly Asked Questions,** number 7, in Section 4 of this user manual.

STEP D Prepare the Pen

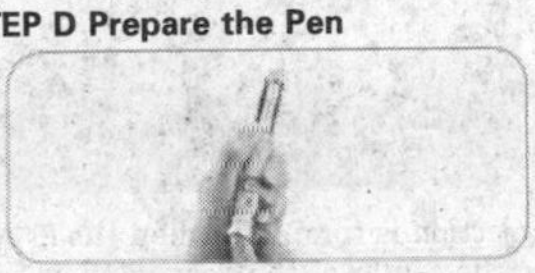

- Point the needle of the pen up and away from you.

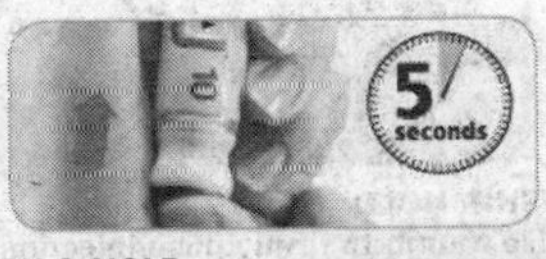

PUSH & HOLD
- **Use thumb to firmly push injection button in until it stops,** then continue holding the injection button in while **slowly counting to 5.**
- **If you do not see a stream or several drops come from the needle tip, repeat Steps C & D.**

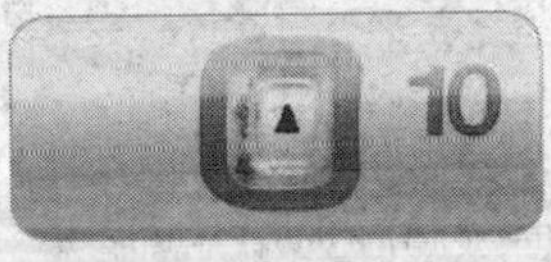

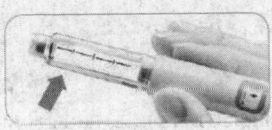

- Pen preparation is complete when the ⊡ is in the center of the dose window AND you have seen a stream or several drops come from the needle tip.

Note: If you do not see liquid after 4 times, see **Commonly Asked Questions,** number 3, in Section 4 of this user manual.

STEP E Complete New Pen Setup

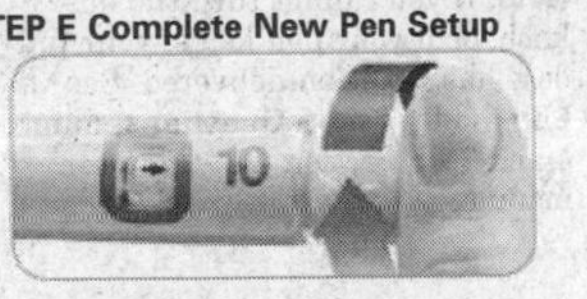

- **Turn dose knob away from you until it stops** and the ⊖ is in the dose window.
- **For routine use,** do not repeat this one-time-only new pen setup. If you do, you will run out of BYETTA before 30 days of use.
- You are now ready for your first dose of BYETTA.
- **Go to Section 3, Step 3, for instructions on how to inject your first routine dose.**

Note: If you cannot turn the dose knob, see **Commonly Asked Questions,** number 7, in Section 4 of user manual.

If you hear a click sound from your BYETTA Pen, ignore it. You must follow all the steps listed above to make sure your injection is complete.

6. Where should I inject BYETTA?

Inject BYETTA (exenatide) into your abdomen, thigh, or upper arm using the injection method explained to you by your healthcare provider.

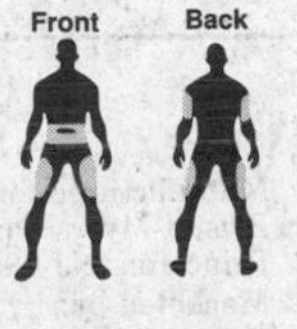

7. What if I cannot pull, turn, or push the dose knob?

Check the symbol in the dose window. Follow the steps next to the matching symbol.

If ⊖ is in the dose window:
- Pull the dose knob out until ⊕ appears.

If ⊕ is in the dose window and the dose knob will not turn:
- The cartridge in your BYETTA Pen may not have enough medicine to deliver a full dose. A small amount of BYETTA will always stay in the cartridge. If the cartridge contains a small amount and the dose knob will not turn, your pen does not have enough BYETTA (exenatide) and will not deliver any more doses. Obtain a new BYETTA Pen.

If ⊕ and part of ⊞ are in the dose window and the dose knob cannot be pushed in:
- The dose knob was not turned all the way. Continue turning the dose knob away from you until ⊞ is in the center of the dose window.

If part of ⊞ and part of ⊡ are in the dose window and the dose knob cannot be pushed in:
- The needle may be clogged, bent, or incorrectly attached.
- Attach a new needle. Make sure needle is on straight and screwed on all the way.
- Firmly push the injection button in all the way. BYETTA should come from needle tip.

If ⊡ is in the dose window and the dose knob will not turn:
- The injection button was not pushed in all the way and a complete dose was not delivered. **Talk with your healthcare provider about what to do about a partial dose.**
- Follow these steps to reset your pen for your next injection:

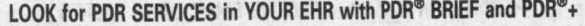

ROUTINE USE

STEP 1 Check the Pen

- Wash hands prior to use.
- Check pen label to make sure it is your 10 mcg pen.
- Pull off the blue pen cap.

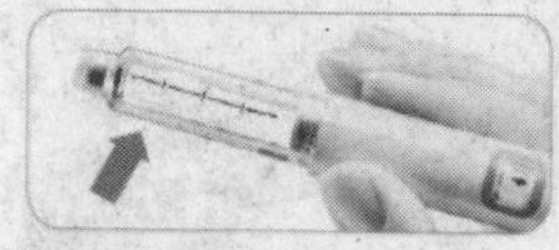

- Check BYETTA in the cartridge.
- The liquid should be clear, colorless, and free of particles. If it is not, do not use.

Note: A small air bubble will not harm you or affect your dose.

STEP 2 Attach the Needle

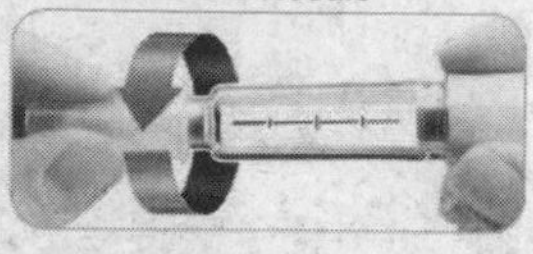

- Remove paper tab from outer needle shield.
- **Push** outer needle shield containing the needle **straight** onto pen, then **screw** needle on until secure.

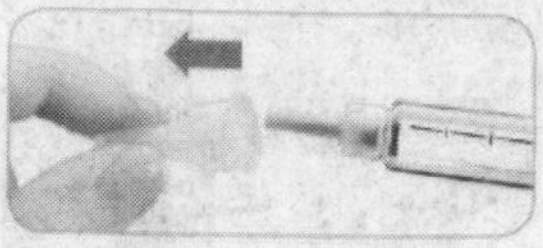

- Pull off outer needle shield. **Do not** throw away.

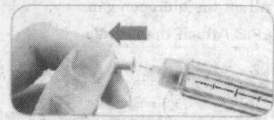

- Pull off inner needle shield and throw away. A small drop of liquid may appear. This is normal.

STEP 3 Dial the Dose

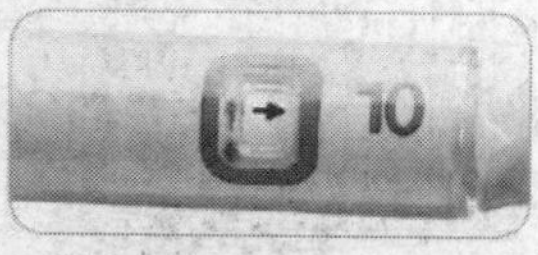

- Check that the ⊖ is in the dose window. If not, turn dose knob away from you (clockwise) **until it stops** and the ⊖ is in the dose window.

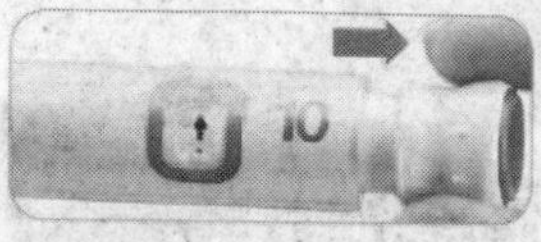

- **Pull dose knob out until it stops** and the ⊕ is in the dose window.

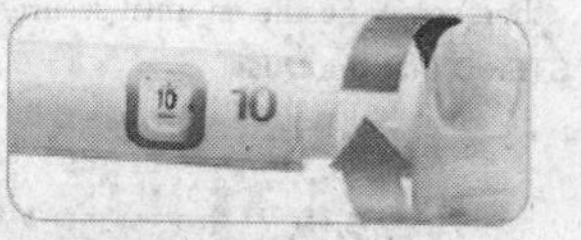

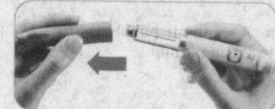

- **Turn dose knob away from you until it stops** at ⊞. Make sure that the 10 with the line under it is in the center of the dose window.

Note: If you cannot turn the dose knob away from you to the ⊞, see **Commonly Asked Questions,** number 7, in Section 4 of this user manual.

STEP 4 Inject the Dose

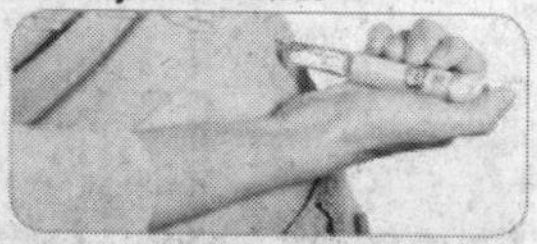

- Grip pen firmly.
- Insert needle into skin using the under-the-skin (subcutaneous) injection method explained by your healthcare provider.

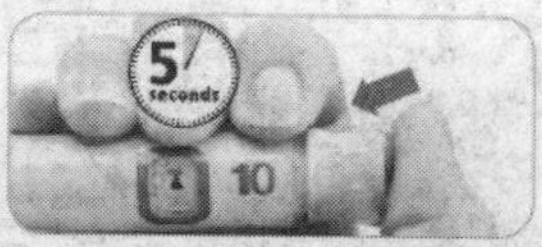

PUSH & HOLD

- **Use thumb to firmly push injection button in until it stops.** Continue holding in the injection button while **slowly counting to 5** to get a full dose.
- Remove needle from skin.

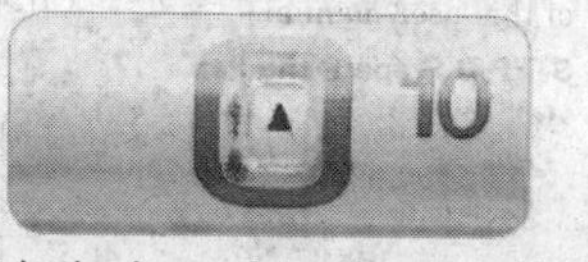

- Injection is complete when the ⊕ is in the center of the dose window.
- The pen is now ready to reset.

Note: If you see several drops of BYETTA leaking from the needle after the injection, you may not have received a complete dose. See **Commonly Asked Questions,** number 4, in Section 4 of this user manual.

STEP 5 Reset the Pen

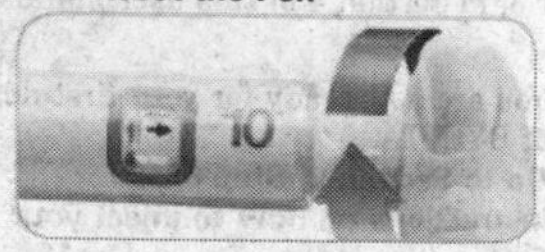

- **Turn dose knob away from you until it stops** and the ⊖ is in the dose window.

Note: If you cannot turn the dose knob, or if your pen leaks, your full dose has not been delivered. See **Commonly Asked Questions,** numbers 4 and 7, in Section 4 of this user manual.

STEP 6 Remove and Dispose of the Needle

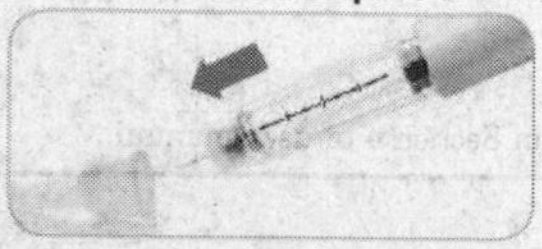

- Carefully put the outer needle shield back over the needle.
- **Remove the needle after each injection.**

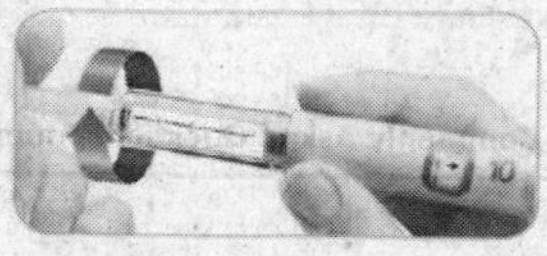

- Unscrew the needle.

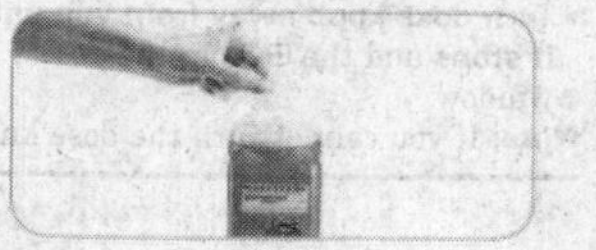

- Throw away needles in a puncture-resistant container or as recommended by your healthcare provider.

- Firmly push the injection button in all the way **until it stops.** Keep holding the injection button in and **slowly count to 5.** Then release the injection button and turn the dose knob away from you until ⊖ appears in the dose window.
- If you cannot turn the dose knob, the needle may be clogged. Replace the needle and repeat the step above.
- For your next dose, be sure to **firmly push and hold** the injection button in and **slowly count to 5** before removing needle from skin.

See the complete BYETTA *Medication Guide* that comes with BYETTA. For more information, call toll free 800-868-1190 or visit www.BYETTA.com

Manufactured for:
Bristol-Myers Squibb Company
Princeton, NJ 08543 USA
Marketed by:
Bristol-Myers Squibb Company
Princeton, NJ 08543
and
AstraZeneca Pharmaceuticals LP
Wilmington, DE 19850
BYETTA is a registered trademark of Amylin Pharmaceuticals, LLC.
925006-BB
Rev February 2013

Shown in Product Identification Guide, page 305

COUMADIN ℞

[COU-ma-din]
(warfarin sodium)
tablets, for oral use

COUMADIN

(warfarin sodium)
for injection, for intravenous use

HIGHLIGHTS OF PRESCRIBING INFORMATION
These highlights do not include all the information needed to use COUMADIN safely and effectively. See full prescribing information for COUMADIN.
COUMADIN (warfarin sodium) tablets, for oral use
COUMADIN (warfarin sodium) for injection, for intravenous use
Initial U.S. Approval: 1954

> **WARNING: BLEEDING RISK**
> ***See full prescribing information for complete boxed warning.***
> - **COUMADIN can cause major or fatal bleeding. (5.1)**
> - **Perform regular monitoring of INR in all treated patients. (2.1)**
> - **Drugs, dietary changes, and other factors affect INR levels achieved with COUMADIN therapy. (7)**
> - **Instruct patients about prevention measures to minimize risk of bleeding and to report signs and symptoms of bleeding. (17)**

RECENT MAJOR CHANGES

Contraindications (4)	10/2011
Warnings and Precautions, Use in Pregnant Women with Mechanical Heart Valves (5.5)	10/2011

INDICATIONS AND USAGE

COUMADIN is a vitamin K antagonist indicated for:
- Prophylaxis and treatment of venous thrombosis and its extension, pulmonary embolism (1)
- Prophylaxis and treatment of thromboembolic complications associated with atrial fibrillation and/or cardiac valve replacement (1)
- Reduction in the risk of death, recurrent myocardial infarction, and thromboembolic events such as stroke or systemic embolization after myocardial infarction (1)

Limitation of Use
COUMADIN has no direct effect on an established thrombus, nor does it reverse ischemic tissue damage. (1)

DOSAGE AND ADMINISTRATION

- Individualize dosing regimen for each patient, and adjust based on INR response. (2.1, 2.2)
- Knowledge of genotype can inform initial dose selection. (2.3)
- Monitoring: Obtain daily INR determinations upon initiation until stable in the therapeutic range. Obtain subsequent INR determinations every 1 to 4 weeks. (2.4)
- Review conversion instructions from other anticoagulants. (2.8)

DOSAGE FORMS AND STRENGTHS

- Scored tablets: 1, 2, 2-1/2, 3, 4, 5, 6, 7-1/2, or 10 mg (3)
- For injection: Vial containing 5 mg lyophilized powder (3)

CONTRAINDICATIONS

- Pregnancy, except in women with mechanical heart valves (4)
- Hemorrhagic tendencies or blood dyscrasias (4)
- Recent or contemplated surgery of the central nervous system (CNS) or eye, or traumatic surgery resulting in large open surfaces (4, 5.7)
- Bleeding tendencies associated with certain conditions (4)
- Threatened abortion, eclampsia, and preeclampsia (4)
- Unsupervised patients with potential high levels of non-compliance (4)
- Spinal puncture and other diagnostic or therapeutic procedures with potential for uncontrollable bleeding (4)
- Hypersensitivity to warfarin or any component of the product (4)
- Major regional or lumbar block anesthesia (4)
- Malignant hypertension (4)

WARNINGS AND PRECAUTIONS

- Tissue necrosis: Necrosis or gangrene of skin or other tissues can occur, with severe cases requiring debridement or amputation. Discontinue COUMADIN and consider alternative anticoagulants if necessary. (5.2)
- Systemic atheroemboli and cholesterol microemboli: Some cases have progressed to necrosis or death. Discontinue COUMADIN if such emboli occur. (5.3)
- Heparin-induced thrombocytopenia (HIT): Initial therapy with COUMADIN in HIT has resulted in cases of amputation and death. COUMADIN may be considered after platelet count has normalized. (5.4)
- Pregnant women with mechanical heart valves: COUMADIN may cause fetal harm; however, the benefits may outweigh the risks. (5.5)

ADVERSE REACTIONS

Most common adverse reactions to COUMADIN are fatal and nonfatal hemorrhage from any tissue or organ. (6)

To report SUSPECTED ADVERSE REACTIONS, contact Bristol-Myers Squibb at 1-800-721-5072 or FDA at 1-800-FDA-1088 or *www.fda.gov/medwatch*.

DRUG INTERACTIONS

- Consult labeling of all concurrently used drugs for complete information about interactions with COUMADIN (warfarin sodium) or increased risks for bleeding. (7)
- Inhibitors and inducers of CYP2C9, 1A2, or 3A4: May alter warfarin exposure. Monitor INR closely when any such drug is used with COUMADIN. (7.1)
- Drugs that increase bleeding risk: Closely monitor patients receiving any such drug (e.g., other anticoagulants, antiplatelet agents, nonsteroidal anti-inflammatory drugs, serotonin reuptake inhibitors). (7.2)
- Antibiotics and antifungals: Closely monitor INR when initiating or stopping an antibiotic or antifungal course of therapy. (7.3)
- Botanical (herbal) products: Some may influence patient response to COUMADIN necessitating close INR monitoring. (7.4)

USE IN SPECIFIC POPULATIONS

- Nursing mothers: Use with caution in a nursing woman. Monitor breast-feeding infants for bruising or bleeding. (8.3)

See 17 for PATIENT COUNSELING INFORMATION and Medication Guide

Revised: 10/2011

FULL PRESCRIBING INFORMATION: CONTENTS*

* Sections or subsections omitted from the full prescribing information are not listed

FULL PRESCRIBING INFORMATION

WARNING: BLEEDING RISK

- COUMADIN can cause major or fatal bleeding [see *Warnings and Precautions (5.1)*].
- Perform regular monitoring of INR in all treated patients [see *Dosage and Administration (2.1)*].
- Drugs, dietary changes, and other factors affect INR levels achieved with COUMADIN therapy [see *Drug Interactions (7)*].
- Instruct patients about prevention measures to minimize risk of bleeding and to report signs and symptoms of bleeding [see *Patient Counseling Information (17)*].

1 INDICATIONS AND USAGE

COUMADIN® (warfarin sodium) is indicated for:

- Prophylaxis and treatment of venous thrombosis and its extension, pulmonary embolism (PE).
- Prophylaxis and treatment of thromboembolic complications associated with atrial fibrillation (AF) and/or cardiac valve replacement.
- Reduction in the risk of death, recurrent myocardial infarction (MI), and thromboembolic events such as stroke or systemic embolization after myocardial infarction.

Limitations of Use

COUMADIN has no direct effect on an established thrombus, nor does it reverse ischemic tissue damage. Once a thrombus has occurred, however, the goals of anticoagulant treatment are to prevent further extension of the formed clot and to prevent secondary thromboembolic complications that may result in serious and possibly fatal sequelae.

2 DOSAGE AND ADMINISTRATION

2.1 Individualized Dosing

The dosage and administration of COUMADIN must be individualized for each patient according to the patient's INR response to the drug. Adjust the dose based on the patient's INR and the condition being treated. Consult the latest evidence-based clinical practice guidelines from the American College of Chest Physicians (ACCP) to assist in the determination of the duration and intensity of anticoagulation with COUMADIN [see *References (15)*].

2.2 Recommended Target INR Ranges and Durations for Individual Indications

An INR of greater than 4.0 appears to provide no additional therapeutic benefit in most patients and is associated with a higher risk of bleeding.

Venous Thromboembolism (including deep venous thrombosis [DVT] and PE)

Adjust the warfarin dose to maintain a target INR of 2.5 (INR range, 2.0-3.0) for all treatment durations. The duration of treatment is based on the indication as follows:

- For patients with a DVT or PE secondary to a transient (reversible) risk factor, treatment with warfarin for 3 months is recommended.
- For patients with an unprovoked DVT or PE, treatment with warfarin is recommended for at least 3 months. After 3 months of therapy, evaluate the risk-benefit ratio of long-term treatment for the individual patient.
- For patients with two episodes of unprovoked DVT or PE, long-term treatment with warfarin is recommended. For a patient receiving long-term anticoagulant treatment, periodically reassess the risk-benefit ratio of continuing such treatment in the individual patient.

Atrial Fibrillation

In patients with non-valvular AF, anticoagulate with warfarin to target INR of 2.5 (range, 2.0-3.0).

- In patients with non-valvular AF that is persistent or paroxysmal and at high risk of stroke (i.e., having any of the following features: prior ischemic stroke, transient ischemic attack, or systemic embolism, or 2 of the following risk factors: age greater than 75 years, moderately or severely impaired left ventricular systolic function and/or heart failure, history of hypertension, or diabetes mellitus), long-term anticoagulation with warfarin is recommended.
- In patients with non-valvular AF that is persistent or paroxysmal and at an intermediate risk of ischemic stroke (i.e., having 1 of the following risk factors: age greater than 75 years, moderately or severely impaired left ventricular systolic function and/or heart failure, history of hypertension, or diabetes mellitus), long-term anticoagulation with warfarin is recommended.
- For patients with AF and mitral stenosis, long-term anticoagulation with warfarin is recommended.
- For patients with AF and prosthetic heart valves, long-term anticoagulation with warfarin is recommended; the target INR may be increased and aspirin added depending on valve type and position, and on patient factors.

Mechanical and Bioprosthetic Heart Valves

- For patients with a bileaflet mechanical valve or a Medtronic Hall (Minneapolis, MN) tilting disk valve in the aortic position who are in sinus rhythm and without left atrial enlargement, therapy with warfarin to a target INR of 2.5 (range, 2.0-3.0) is recommended.
- For patients with tilting disk valves and bileaflet mechanical valves in the mitral position, therapy with warfarin to a target INR of 3.0 (range, 2.5-3.5) is recommended.
- For patients with caged ball or caged disk valves, therapy with warfarin to a target INR of 3.0 (range, 2.5-3.5) is recommended.
- For patients with a bioprosthetic valve in the mitral position, therapy with warfarin to a target INR of 2.5 (range, 2.0-3.0) for the first 3 months after valve insertion is recommended. If additional risk factors for thromboembolism are present (AF, previous thromboembolism, left ventricular dysfunction), a target INR of 2.5 (range, 2.0-3.0) is recommended.

Post-Myocardial Infarction

- For high-risk patients with MI (e.g., those with a large anterior MI, those with significant heart failure, those with intracardiac thrombus visible on transthoracic echocardiography, those with AF, and those with a history of a thromboembolic event), therapy with combined moderate-intensity (INR, 2.0-3.0) warfarin plus low-dose aspirin (≤100 mg/day) for at least 3 months after the MI is recommended.

Recurrent Systemic Embolism and Other Indications

Oral anticoagulation therapy with warfarin has not been fully evaluated by clinical trials in patients with valvular disease associated with AF, patients with mitral stenosis, and patients with recurrent systemic embolism of unknown etiology. However, a moderate dose regimen (INR 2.0-3.0) may be used for these patients.

2.3 Initial and Maintenance Dosing

The appropriate initial dosing of COUMADIN (warfarin sodium) varies widely for different patients. Not all factors responsible for warfarin dose variability are known, and the initial dose is influenced by:

- Clinical factors including age, race, body weight, sex, concomitant medications, and comorbidities
- Genetic factors (CYP2C9 and VKORC1 genotypes) [see *Clinical Pharmacology (12.5)*]

Select the initial dose based on the expected maintenance dose, taking into account the above factors. Modify this dose based on consideration of patient-specific clinical factors. Consider lower initial and maintenance doses for elderly and/or debilitated patients and in Asian patients [see *Use in Specific Populations (8.5)* and *Clinical Pharmacology (12.3)*]. Routine use of loading doses is not recommended as this practice may increase hemorrhagic and other complications and does not offer more rapid protection against clot formation.

Individualize the duration of therapy for each patient. In general, anticoagulant therapy should be continued until the danger of thrombosis and embolism has passed [see *Dosage and Administration (2.2)*].

Dosing Recommendations without Consideration of Genotype

If the patient's CYP2C9 and VKORC1 genotypes are not known, the initial dose of COUMADIN is usually 2 to 5 mg once daily. Determine each patient's dosing needs by close monitoring of the INR response and consideration of the indication being treated. Typical maintenance doses are 2 to 10 mg once daily.

Dosing Recommendations with Consideration of Genotype

Table 1 displays three ranges of expected maintenance COUMADIN doses observed in subgroups of patients having different combinations of CYP2C9 and VKORC1 gene variants [see *Clinical Pharmacology (12.5)*]. If the patient's CYP2C9 and/or VKORC1 genotype are known, consider these ranges in choosing the initial dose. Patients with CYP2C9 *1/*3, *2/*2, *2/*3, and *3/*3 may require more prolonged time (>2 to 4 weeks) to achieve maximum INR effect for a given dosage regimen than patients without these CYP variants.

[See table 1 at top of next page]

2.4 Monitoring to Achieve Optimal Anticoagulation

COUMADIN is a narrow therapeutic range (index) drug, and its action may be affected by factors such as other drugs and dietary vitamin K. Therefore, anticoagulation must be carefully monitored during COUMADIN therapy. Determine the INR daily after the administration of the initial dose until INR results stabilize in the therapeutic range. After stabilization, maintain dosing within the therapeutic range by performing periodic INRs. The frequency of performing INR should be based on the clinical situation but generally acceptable intervals for INR determinations are 1 to 4 weeks. Perform additional INR tests when other warfarin products are interchanged with COUMADIN, as well as whenever other medications are initiated, discontinued, or taken irregularly. Heparin, a common concomitant drug, increases the INR [see *Dosage and Administration (2.8)* and *Drug Interactions (7)*].

Table 1: Three Ranges of Expected Maintenance COUMADIN Daily Doses Based on CYP2C9 and VKORC1 Genotypes†

VKORC1	CYP2C9					
	*1/*1	*1/*2	*1/*3	*2/*2	*2/*3	*3/*3
GG	5-7 mg	5-7 mg	3-4 mg	3-4 mg	3-4 mg	0.5-2 mg
AG	5-7 mg	3-4 mg	3-4 mg	3-4 mg	0.5-2 mg	0.5-2 mg
AA	3-4 mg	3-4 mg	0.5-2 mg	0.5-2 mg	0.5-2 mg	0.5-2 mg

†Ranges are derived from multiple published clinical studies. VKORC1 –1639G>A (rs9923231) variant is used in this table. Other co-inherited VKORC1 variants may also be important determinants of warfarin dose.

Determinations of whole blood clotting and bleeding times are not effective measures for monitoring of COUMADIN (warfarin sodium) therapy.

2.5 Missed Dose

The anticoagulant effect of COUMADIN persists beyond 24 hours. If a patient misses a dose of COUMADIN at the intended time of day, the patient should take the dose as soon as possible on the same day. The patient should not double the dose the next day to make up for a missed dose.

2.6 Intravenous Route of Administration

The intravenous dose of COUMADIN is the same as the oral dose. After reconstitution, COUMADIN for injection should be administered as a slow bolus injection into a peripheral vein over 1 to 2 minutes. COUMADIN for injection is not recommended for intramuscular administration.

Reconstitute the vial with 2.7 mL of Sterile Water for Injection. The resulting yield is 2.5 mL of a 2 mg per mL solution (5 mg total). Parenteral drug products should be inspected visually for particulate matter and discoloration prior to administration. Do not use if particulate matter or discoloration is noted.

After reconstitution, COUMADIN for injection is stable for 4 hours at room temperature. It does not contain any antimicrobial preservative and, thus, care must be taken to assure the sterility of the prepared solution. The vial is for single use only, and any unused solution should be discarded.

2.7 Treatment During Dentistry and Surgery

Some dental or surgical procedures may necessitate the interruption or change in the dose of COUMADIN therapy. Consider the benefits and risks when discontinuing COUMADIN even for a short period of time. Determine the INR immediately prior to any dental or surgical procedure. In patients undergoing minimally invasive procedures who must be anticoagulated prior to, during, or immediately following these procedures, adjusting the dosage of COUMADIN to maintain the INR at the low end of the therapeutic range may safely allow for continued anticoagulation.

2.8 Conversion From Other Anticoagulants

Heparin

Since the full anticoagulant effect of COUMADIN is not achieved for several days, heparin is preferred for initial rapid anticoagulation. During initial therapy with COUMADIN, the interference with heparin anticoagulation is of minimal clinical significance. Conversion to COUMADIN may begin concomitantly with heparin therapy or may be delayed 3 to 6 days. To ensure therapeutic anticoagulation, continue full dose heparin therapy and overlap COUMADIN therapy with heparin for 4 to 5 days and until COUMADIN has produced the desired therapeutic response as determined by INR, at which point heparin may be discontinued.

As heparin may affect the INR, patients receiving both heparin and COUMADIN should have INR monitoring at least:

- 5 hours after the last intravenous bolus dose of heparin, or
- 4 hours after cessation of a continuous intravenous infusion of heparin, or
- 24 hours after the last subcutaneous heparin injection.

COUMADIN may increase the activated partial thromboplastin time (aPTT) test, even in the absence of heparin. A severe elevation (>50 seconds) in aPTT with an INR in the desired range has been identified as an indication of increased risk of postoperative hemorrhage.

Other Anticoagulants

Consult the labeling of other anticoagulants for instructions on conversion to COUMADIN.

3 DOSAGE FORMS AND STRENGTHS

COUMADIN tablets are single scored with one face imprinted numerically with 1, 2, 2-1/2, 3, 4, 5, 6, 7-1/2, or 10 superimposed and inscribed with "COUMADIN" and with the opposite face plain.

COUMADIN tablets are supplied in the following strengths:

COUMADIN Tablets

Strength	Color
1 mg	pink
2 mg	lavender
2-1/2 mg	green
3 mg	tan
4 mg	blue
5 mg	peach
6 mg	teal
7-1/2 mg	yellow
10 mg	white (dye-free)

COUMADIN for injection is available in a vial containing 5 mg of lyophilized powder.

4 CONTRAINDICATIONS

- Pregnancy

COUMADIN (warfarin sodium) is contraindicated in women who are pregnant except in pregnant women with mechanical heart valves, who are at high risk of thromboembolism [see *Warnings and Precautions (5.5)* and *Use in Specific Populations (8.1)*]. COUMADIN can cause fetal harm when administered to a pregnant woman. COUMADIN exposure during pregnancy causes a recognized pattern of major congenital malformations (warfarin embryopathy and fetotoxicity), fatal fetal hemorrhage, and an increased risk of spontaneous abortion and fetal mortality. If COUMADIN is used during pregnancy or if the patient becomes pregnant while taking this drug, the patient should be apprised of the potential hazard to a fetus [see *Warnings and Precautions (5.6)* and *Use in Specific Populations (8.1)*].

- Hemorrhagic tendencies or blood dyscrasias
- Recent or contemplated surgery of the central nervous system or eye, or traumatic surgery resulting in large open surfaces [see *Warnings and Precautions (5.7)*]
- Bleeding tendencies associated with:
  - Active ulceration or overt bleeding of the gastrointestinal, genitourinary, or respiratory tract
  - Central nervous system hemorrhage
  - Cerebral aneurysms, dissecting aorta
  - Pericarditis and pericardial effusions
  - Bacterial endocarditis
- Threatened abortion, eclampsia, and preeclampsia
- Unsupervised patients with conditions associated with potential high level of non-compliance
- Spinal puncture and other diagnostic or therapeutic procedures with potential for uncontrollable bleeding
- Hypersensitivity to warfarin or to any other components of this product (e.g., anaphylaxis) [see *Adverse Reactions (6)*]
- Major regional or lumbar block anesthesia
- Malignant hypertension

5 WARNINGS AND PRECAUTIONS

5.1 Hemorrhage

COUMADIN can cause major or fatal bleeding. Bleeding is more likely to occur within the first month. Risk factors for bleeding include high intensity of anticoagulation (INR >4.0), age greater than or equal to 65, history of highly variable INRs, history of gastrointestinal bleeding, hypertension, cerebrovascular disease, anemia, malignancy, trauma, renal impairment, certain genetic factors [see *Clinical Pharmacology (12.5)*], certain concomitant drugs [see *Drug Interactions (7)*], and long duration of warfarin therapy.

Perform regular monitoring of INR in all treated patients. Those at high risk of bleeding may benefit from more frequent INR monitoring, careful dose adjustment to desired INR, and a shortest duration of therapy appropriate for the clinical condition. However, maintenance of INR in the therapeutic range does not eliminate the risk of bleeding.

Drugs, dietary changes, and other factors affect INR levels achieved with COUMADIN therapy. Perform more frequent INR monitoring when starting or stopping other drugs, including botanicals, or when changing dosages of other drugs [see *Drug Interactions (7)*].

Instruct patients about prevention measures to minimize risk of bleeding and to report signs and symptoms of bleeding [see *Patient Counseling Information (17)*].

5.2 Tissue Necrosis

Necrosis and/or gangrene of skin and other tissues is an uncommon but serious risk (<0.1%). Necrosis may be associated with local thrombosis and usually appears within a few days of the start of COUMADIN (warfarin sodium) therapy. In severe cases of necrosis, treatment through debridement or amputation of the affected tissue, limb, breast, or penis has been reported.

Careful clinical evaluation is required to determine whether necrosis is caused by an underlying disease. Although various treatments have been attempted, no treatment for necrosis has been considered uniformly effective. Discontinue COUMADIN therapy if necrosis occurs. Consider alternative drugs if continued anticoagulation therapy is necessary.

5.3 Systemic Atheroemboli and Cholesterol Microemboli

Anticoagulation therapy with COUMADIN may enhance the release of atheromatous plaque emboli. Systemic atheroemboli and cholesterol microemboli can present with a variety of signs and symptoms depending on the site of embolization. The most commonly involved visceral organs are the kidneys followed by the pancreas, spleen, and liver. Some cases have progressed to necrosis or death. A distinct syndrome resulting from microemboli to the feet is known as "purple toes syndrome." Discontinue COUMADIN therapy if such phenomena are observed. Consider alternative drugs if continued anticoagulation therapy is necessary.

5.4 Heparin-Induced Thrombocytopenia

Do not use COUMADIN as initial therapy in patients with heparin-induced thrombocytopenia (HIT) and with heparin-induced thrombocytopenia with thrombosis syndrome (HITTS). Cases of limb ischemia, necrosis, and gangrene have occurred in patients with HIT and HITTS when heparin treatment was discontinued and warfarin therapy was started or continued. In some patients, sequelae have included amputation of the involved area and/or death. Treatment with COUMADIN may be considered after the platelet count has normalized.

5.5 Use in Pregnant Women with Mechanical Heart Valves

COUMADIN can cause fetal harm when administered to a pregnant woman. While COUMADIN is contraindicated during pregnancy, the potential benefits of using COUMADIN may outweigh the risks for pregnant women with mechanical heart valves at high risk of thromboembolism. In those individual situations, the decision to initiate or continue COUMADIN should be reviewed with the patient, taking into consideration the specific risks and benefits pertaining to the individual patient's medical situation, as well as the most current medical guidelines. COUMADIN exposure during pregnancy causes a recognized pattern of major congenital malformations (warfarin embryopathy and fetotoxicity), fatal fetal hemorrhage, and an increased risk of spontaneous abortion and fetal mortality. If this drug is used during pregnancy, or if the patient becomes pregnant while taking this drug, the patient should be apprised of the potential hazard to a fetus [see *Use in Specific Populations (8.1)*].

5.6 Females of Reproductive Potential

COUMADIN exposure during pregnancy can cause pregnancy loss, birth defects, or fetal death. Discuss pregnancy planning with females of reproductive potential who are on COUMADIN therapy [see *Contraindications (4)* and *Use in Specific Populations (8.8)*].

5.7 Other Clinical Settings with Increased Risks

In the following clinical settings, the risks of COUMADIN therapy may be increased:

- Moderate to severe hepatic impairment
- Infectious diseases or disturbances of intestinal flora (e.g., sprue, antibiotic therapy)
- Use of an indwelling catheter
- Severe to moderate hypertension
- Deficiency in protein C-mediated anticoagulant response: COUMADIN reduces the synthesis of the naturally occurring anticoagulants, protein C and protein S. Hereditary or acquired deficiencies of protein C or its cofactor, protein S, have been associated with tissue necrosis following warfarin administration. Concomitant anticoagulation therapy with heparin for 5 to 7 days during initiation of therapy with COUMADIN may minimize the incidence of tissue necrosis in these patients.
- Eye surgery: In cataract surgery, COUMADIN use was associated with a significant increase in minor complications of sharp needle and local anesthesia block but not associated with potentially sight-threatening operative hemorrhagic complications. As COUMADIN cessation or reduction may lead to serious thromboembolic complications, the decision to discontinue COUMADIN before a relatively less invasive and complex eye surgery, such as lens surgery, should be based upon the risks of anticoagulant therapy weighed against the benefits.
- Polycythemia vera
- Vasculitis
- Diabetes mellitus

5.8 Endogenous Factors Affecting INR

The following factors may be responsible for **increased** INR response: diarrhea, hepatic disorders, poor nutritional state, steatorrhea, or vitamin K deficiency.

The following factors may be responsible for **decreased** INR response: increased vitamin K intake or hereditary warfarin resistance.

6 ADVERSE REACTIONS

The following serious adverse reactions to COUMADIN (warfarin sodium) are discussed in greater detail in other sections of the labeling:

- Hemorrhage [see *Boxed Warning*, *Warnings and Precautions (5.1)*, and *Overdosage (10)*]
- Necrosis of skin and other tissues [see *Warnings and Precautions (5.2)*]
- Systemic atheroemboli and cholesterol microemboli [see *Warnings and Precautions (5.3)*]

Other adverse reactions to COUMADIN include:

- Immune system disorders: hypersensitivity/allergic reactions (including urticaria and anaphylactic reactions)
- Vascular disorders: vasculitis
- Hepatobiliary disorders: hepatitis, elevated liver enzymes. Cholestatic hepatitis has been associated with concomitant administration of COUMADIN and ticlopidine.
- Gastrointestinal disorders: nausea, vomiting, diarrhea, taste perversion, abdominal pain, flatulence, bloating
- Skin disorders: rash, dermatitis (including bullous eruptions), pruritus, alopecia
- Respiratory disorders: tracheal or tracheobronchial calcification
- General disorders: chills

7 DRUG INTERACTIONS

Drugs may interact with COUMADIN through pharmacodynamic or pharmacokinetic mechanisms. Pharmacodynamic mechanisms for drug interactions with COUMADIN are synergism (impaired hemostasis, reduced clotting factor synthesis), competitive antagonism (vitamin K), and alteration of the physiologic control loop for vitamin K metabolism (hereditary resistance). Pharmacokinetic mechanisms for drug interactions with COUMADIN are mainly enzyme induction, enzyme inhibition, and reduced plasma protein binding. It is important to note that some drugs may interact by more than one mechanism.

More frequent INR monitoring should be performed when starting or stopping other drugs, including botanicals, or when changing dosages of other drugs, including drugs intended for short-term use (e.g., antibiotics, antifungals, corticosteroids) [see *Boxed Warning*].

Consult the labeling of all concurrently used drugs to obtain further information about interactions with COUMADIN or adverse reactions pertaining to bleeding.

7.1 CYP450 Interactions

CYP450 isozymes involved in the metabolism of warfarin include CYP2C9, 2C19, 2C8, 2C18, 1A2, and 3A4. The more potent warfarin *S*-enantiomer is metabolized by CYP2C9 while the *R*-enantiomer is metabolized by CYP1A2 and 3A4.

- Inhibitors of CYP2C9, 1A2, and/or 3A4 have the potential to increase the effect (increase INR) of warfarin by increasing the exposure of warfarin.
- Inducers of CYP2C9, 1A2, and/or 3A4 have the potential to decrease the effect (decrease INR) of warfarin by decreasing the exposure of warfarin.

Examples of inhibitors and inducers of CYP2C9, 1A2, and 3A4 are below in Table 2; however, this list should not be considered all-inclusive. Consult the labeling of all concurrently used drugs to obtain further information about CYP450 interaction potential. The CYP450 inhibition and induction potential should be considered when starting, stopping, or changing dose of concomitant mediations. Closely monitor INR if a concomitant drug is a CYP2C9, 1A2, and/or 3A4 inhibitor or inducer.

Table 2: Examples of CYP450 Interactions with Warfarin

Enzyme	Inhibitors	Inducers
CYP2C9	amiodarone, capecitabine, cotrimoxazole, etravirine, fluconazole, fluvastatin, fluvoxamine, metronidazole, miconazole, oxandrolone, sulfinpyrazone, tigecycline, voriconazole, zafirlukast	aprepitant, bosentan, carbamazepine, phenobarbital, rifampin
CYP1A2	acyclovir, allopurinol, caffeine, cimetidine, ciprofloxacin, disulfiram, enoxacin, famotidine, fluvoxamine, methoxsalen, mexiletine, norfloxacin, oral contraceptives, phenylpropanolamine, propafenone, propranolol, terbinafine, thiabendazole, ticlopidine, verapamil, zileuton	montelukast, moricizine, omeprazole, phenobarbital, phenytoin, cigarette smoking
CYP3A4	alprazolam, amiodarone, amlodipine, amprenavir, aprepitant, atorvastatin, atazanavir, bicalutamide, cilostazol, cimetidine, ciprofloxacin, clarithromycin, conivaptan, cyclosporine, darunavir/ritonavir, diltiazem, erythromycin, fluconazole, fluoxetine, fluvoxamine, fosamprenavir, imatinib, indinavir, isoniazid, itraconazole, ketoconazole, lopinavir/ritonavir, nefazodone, nelfinavir, nilotinib, oral contraceptives, posaconazole, ranitidine, ranolazine, ritonavir, saquinavir, telithromycin, tipranavir, voriconazole, zileuton	armodafinil, amprenavir, aprepitant, bosentan, carbamazepine, efavirenz, etravirine, modafinil, nafcillin, phenytoin, pioglitazone, prednisone, rifampin, rufinamide

7.2 Drugs that Increase Bleeding Risk

Examples of drugs known to increase the risk of bleeding are presented in Table 3. Because bleeding risk is increased when these drugs are used concomitantly with warfarin, closely monitor patients receiving any such drug with warfarin.

Table 3: Drugs that Can Increase the Risk of Bleeding

Drug Class	Specific Drugs
Anticoagulants	argatroban, dabigatran, bivalirudin, desirudin, heparin, lepirudin
Antiplatelet Agents	aspirin, cilostazol, clopidogrel, dipyridamole, prasugrel, ticlopidine
Nonsteroidal Anti-Inflammatory Agents	celecoxib, diclofenac, diflunisal, fenoprofen, ibuprofen, indomethacin, ketoprofen, ketorolac, mefenamic acid, naproxen, oxaprozin, piroxicam, sulindac
Serotonin Reuptake Inhibitors	citalopram, desvenlafaxine, duloxetine, escitalopram, fluoxetine, fluvoxamine, milnacipran, paroxetine, sertraline, venlafaxine, vilazodone

7.3 Antibiotics and Antifungals

There have been reports of changes in INR in patients taking warfarin and antibiotics or antifungals, but clinical pharmacokinetic studies have not shown consistent effects of these agents on plasma concentrations of warfarin.

Closely monitor INR when starting or stopping any antibiotic or antifungal in patients taking warfarin.

7.4 Botanical (Herbal) Products and Foods

Exercise caution when botanical (herbal) products are taken concomitantly with COUMADIN (warfarin sodium). Few adequate, well-controlled studies evaluating the potential for metabolic and/or pharmacologic interactions between botanicals and COUMADIN exist. Due to a lack of manufacturing standardization with botanical medicinal preparations, the amount of active ingredients may vary. This could further confound the ability to assess potential interactions and effects on anticoagulation.

Some botanicals may cause bleeding events when taken alone (e.g., garlic and Ginkgo biloba) and may have anticoagulant, antiplatelet, and/or fibrinolytic properties. These effects would be expected to be additive to the anticoagulant effects of COUMADIN. Conversely, some botanicals may decrease the effects of COUMADIN (e.g., co-enzyme Q_{10}, St. John's wort, ginseng). Some botanicals and foods can interact with COUMADIN through CYP450 interactions (e.g., echinacea, grapefruit juice, ginkgo, goldenseal, St. John's wort).

Monitor the patient's response with additional INR determinations when initiating or discontinuing any botanicals.

8 USE IN SPECIFIC POPULATIONS

8.1 Pregnancy

Pregnancy Category D for women with mechanical heart valves [see *Warnings and Precautions (5.5)*] and **Pregnancy Category X** for other pregnant populations [see *Contraindications (4)*].

COUMADIN is contraindicated in women who are pregnant except in pregnant women with mechanical heart valves, who are at high risk of thromboembolism, and for whom the benefits of COUMADIN may outweigh the risks. COUMADIN (warfarin sodium) can cause fetal harm when administered to a pregnant woman. COUMADIN exposure during pregnancy causes a recognized pattern of major congenital malformations (warfarin embryopathy), fetal hemorrhage, and an increased risk of spontaneous abortion and fetal mortality. The reproductive and developmental effects of COUMADIN have not been evaluated in animals. If this drug is used during pregnancy or if the patient becomes pregnant while taking this drug, the patient should be apprised of the potential hazard to the fetus.

In humans, warfarin crosses the placenta, and concentrations in fetal plasma approach the maternal values. Exposure to warfarin during the first trimester of pregnancy caused a pattern of congenital malformations in about 5% of exposed offspring. Warfarin embryopathy is characterized by nasal hypoplasia with or without stippled epiphyses (chondrodysplasia punctata) and growth retardation (including low birth weight). Central nervous system and eye abnormalities have also been reported, including dorsal midline dysplasia characterized by agenesis of the corpus callosum, Dandy-Walker malformation, midline cerebellar atrophy, and ventral midline dysplasia characterized by optic atrophy. Mental retardation, blindness, schizencephaly, microcephaly, hydrocephalus, and other adverse pregnancy outcomes have been reported following warfarin exposure during the second and third trimesters of pregnancy [see *Contraindications (4)* and *Warnings and Precautions (5.6)*].

8.3 Nursing Mothers

Based on published data in 15 nursing mothers, warfarin was not detected in human milk. Among the 15 full-term newborns, 6 nursing infants had documented prothrombin times within the expected range. Prothrombin times were not obtained for the other 9 nursing infants. Monitor breast-feeding infants for bruising or bleeding. Effects in premature infants have not been evaluated. Caution should be exercised when COUMADIN is administered to a nursing woman.

8.4 Pediatric Use

Adequate and well-controlled studies with COUMADIN have not been conducted in any pediatric population, and the optimum dosing, safety, and efficacy in pediatric patients is unknown. Pediatric use of COUMADIN is based on adult data and recommendations, and available limited pediatric data from observational studies and patient registries. Pediatric patients administered COUMADIN should avoid any activity or sport that may result in traumatic injury.

The developing hemostatic system in infants and children results in a changing physiology of thrombosis and response to anticoagulants. Dosing of warfarin in the pediatric population varies by patient age, with infants generally having the highest, and adolescents having the lowest milligram per kilogram dose requirements to maintain target INRs. Because of changing warfarin requirements due to age, concomitant medications, diet, and existing medical condition, target INR ranges may be difficult to achieve and maintain in pediatric patients, and more frequent INR determinations are recommended. Bleeding rates varied by patient population and clinical care center in pediatric observational studies and patient registries.

Infants and children receiving vitamin K-supplemented nutrition, including infant formulas, may be resistant to warfarin therapy, while human milk-fed infants may be sensitive to warfarin therapy.

8.5 Geriatric Use

Of the total number of patients receiving warfarin sodium in controlled clinical trials for which data were available for analysis, 1885 patients (24.4%) were 65 years and older, while 185 patients (2.4%) were 75 years and older. No overall differences in effectiveness or safety were observed between these patients and younger patients, but greater sensitivity of some older individuals cannot be ruled out.

Patients 60 years or older appear to exhibit greater than expected INR response to the anticoagulant effects of warfarin [see *Clinical Pharmacology (12.3)*]. COUMADIN is contraindicated in any unsupervised patient with senility. Observe caution with administration of COUMADIN to elderly patients in any situation or with any physical condition where added risk of hemorrhage is present. Consider lower initiation and maintenance doses of COUMADIN in elderly patients [see *Dosage and Administration (2.2, 2.3)*].

8.6 Renal Impairment

Renal clearance is considered to be a minor determinant of anticoagulant response to warfarin. No dosage adjustment is necessary for patients with renal impairment.

8.7 Hepatic Impairment

Hepatic impairment can potentiate the response to warfarin through impaired synthesis of clotting factors and decreased metabolism of warfarin. Use caution when using COUMADIN in these patients.

8.8 Females of Reproductive Potential

COUMADIN exposure during pregnancy can cause spontaneous abortion, birth defects, or fetal death. Females of reproductive potential who are candidates for COUMADIN

Table 4: Clinical Studies of Warfarin in Non-Rheumatic AF Patients*

	N				Thromboembolism		% Major Bleeding	
Study	Warfarin-Treated Patients	Control Patients	PT Ratio	INR	% Risk Reduction	*p*-value	Warfarin-Treated Patients	Control Patients
AFASAK	335	336	1.5-2.0	2.8-4.2	60	0.027	0.6	0.0
SPAF	210	211	1.3-1.8	2.0-4.5	67	0.01	1.9	1.9
BAATAF	212	208	1.2-1.5	1.5-2.7	86	<0.05	0.9	0.5
CAFA	187	191	1.3-1.6	2.0-3.0	45	0.25	2.7	0.5
SPINAF	260	265	1.2-1.5	1.4-2.8	79	0.001	2.3	1.5

*All study results of warfarin vs. control are based on intention-to-treat analysis and include ischemic stroke and systemic thromboembolism, excluding hemorrhagic stroke and transient ischemic attacks.

therapy should be counseled regarding the benefits of therapy and potential reproductive risks. Discuss pregnancy planning with females of reproductive potential who are on COUMADIN (warfarin sodium) therapy. If the patient becomes pregnant while taking COUMADIN, she should be apprised of the potential risks to the fetus.

10 OVERDOSAGE

10.1 Signs and Symptoms

Bleeding (e.g., appearance of blood in stools or urine, hematuria, excessive menstrual bleeding, melena, petechiae, excessive bruising or persistent oozing from superficial injuries, unexplained fall in hemoglobin) is a manifestation of excessive anticoagulation.

10.2 Treatment

The treatment of excessive anticoagulation is based on the level of the INR, the presence or absence of bleeding, and clinical circumstances. Reversal of COUMADIN anticoagulation may be obtained by discontinuing COUMADIN therapy and, if necessary, by administration of oral or parenteral vitamin K_1.

The use of vitamin K_1 reduces response to subsequent COUMADIN therapy and patients may return to a pretreatment thrombotic status following the rapid reversal of a prolonged INR. Resumption of COUMADIN administration reverses the effect of vitamin K, and a therapeutic INR can again be obtained by careful dosage adjustment. If rapid re-anticoagulation is indicated, heparin may be preferable for initial therapy.

Prothrombin complex concentrate (PCC), fresh frozen plasma, or activated Factor VII treatment may be considered if the requirement to reverse the effects of COUMADIN is urgent. A risk of hepatitis and other viral diseases is associated with the use of blood products; PCC and activated Factor VII are also associated with an increased risk of thrombosis. Therefore, these preparations should be used only in exceptional or life-threatening bleeding episodes secondary to COUMADIN overdosage.

11 DESCRIPTION

COUMADIN (warfarin sodium) is an anticoagulant that acts by inhibiting vitamin K-dependent coagulation factors. Chemically, it is 3-(α-acetonylbenzyl)-4-hydroxycoumarin and is a racemic mixture of the *R*- and *S*-enantiomers. Crystalline warfarin sodium is an isopropanol clathrate. Its empirical formula is $C_{19}H_{15}NaO_4$, and its structural formula is represented by the following:

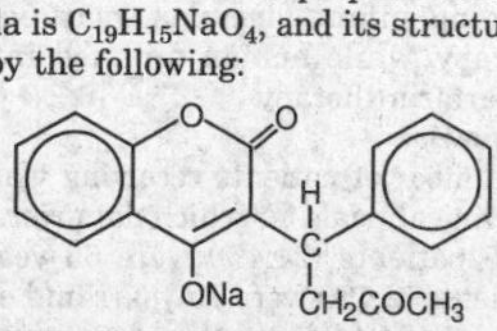

Crystalline warfarin sodium occurs as a white, odorless, crystalline powder that is discolored by light. It is very soluble in water, freely soluble in alcohol, and very slightly soluble in chloroform and ether.

COUMADIN tablets for oral use also contain:

All strengths:	Lactose, starch, and magnesium stearate
1 mg:	D&C Red No. 6 Barium Lake
2 mg:	FD&C Blue No. 2 Aluminum Lake and FD&C Red No. 40 Aluminum Lake
2-1/2 mg:	D&C Yellow No. 10 Aluminum Lake and FD&C Blue No. 1 Aluminum Lake
3 mg:	FD&C Yellow No. 6 Aluminum Lake, FD&C Blue No. 2 Aluminum Lake, and FD&C Red No. 40 Aluminum Lake
4 mg:	FD&C Blue No. 1 Aluminum Lake
5 mg:	FD&C Yellow No. 6 Aluminum Lake
6 mg:	FD&C Yellow No. 6 Aluminum Lake and FD&C Blue No. 1 Aluminum Lake
7-1/2 mg:	D&C Yellow No. 10 Aluminum Lake and FD&C Yellow No. 6 Aluminum Lake
10 mg:	Dye-free

COUMADIN for injection for intravenous use is supplied as a sterile, lyophilized powder, which, after reconstitution with 2.7 mL Sterile Water for Injection, contains:

Warfarin sodium	2 mg per mL
Sodium phosphate, dibasic, heptahydrate	4.98 mg per mL
Sodium phosphate, monobasic, monohydrate	0.194 mg per mL
Sodium chloride	0.1 mg per mL
Mannitol	38.0 mg per mL
Sodium hydroxide, as needed for pH adjustment to 8.1 to 8.3	

12 CLINICAL PHARMACOLOGY

12.1 Mechanism of Action

Warfarin acts by inhibiting the synthesis of vitamin K-dependent clotting factors, which include Factors II, VII, IX, and X, and the anticoagulant proteins C and S. Vitamin K is an essential cofactor for the post ribosomal synthesis of the vitamin K-dependent clotting factors. Vitamin K promotes the biosynthesis of γ-carboxyglutamic acid residues in the proteins that are essential for biological activity. Warfarin is thought to interfere with clotting factor synthesis by inhibition of the C1 subunit of vitamin K epoxide reductase (VKORC1) enzyme complex, thereby reducing the regeneration of vitamin K_1 epoxide [see *Clinical Pharmacology (12.5)*].

12.2 Pharmacodynamics

An anticoagulation effect generally occurs within 24 hours after warfarin administration. However, peak anticoagulant effect may be delayed 72 to 96 hours. The duration of action of a single dose of racemic warfarin is 2 to 5 days. The effects of COUMADIN (warfarin sodium) may become more pronounced as effects of daily maintenance doses overlap. This is consistent with the half-lives of the affected vitamin K-dependent clotting factors and anticoagulation proteins: Factor II - 60 hours, VII - 4 to 6 hours, IX - 24 hours, X - 48 to 72 hours, and proteins C and S are approximately 8 hours and 30 hours, respectively.

12.3 Pharmacokinetics

COUMADIN is a racemic mixture of the *R*- and *S*-enantiomers of warfarin. The *S*-enantiomer exhibits 2 to 5 times more anticoagulant activity than the *R*-enantiomer in humans, but generally has a more rapid clearance.

Absorption

Warfarin is essentially completely absorbed after oral administration, with peak concentration generally attained within the first 4 hours.

Distribution

Warfarin distributes into a relatively small apparent volume of distribution of about 0.14 L/kg. A distribution phase lasting 6 to 12 hours is distinguishable after rapid intravenous or oral administration of an aqueous solution. Approximately 99% of the drug is bound to plasma proteins.

Metabolism

The elimination of warfarin is almost entirely by metabolism. Warfarin is stereoselectively metabolized by hepatic cytochrome P-450 (CYP450) microsomal enzymes to inactive hydroxylated metabolites (predominant route) and by reductases to reduced metabolites (warfarin alcohols) with minimal anticoagulant activity. Identified metabolites of warfarin include dehydrowarfarin, two diastereoisomer alcohols, and 4′-, 6-, 7-, 8-, and 10-hydroxywarfarin. The CYP450 isozymes involved in the metabolism of warfarin include CYP2C9, 2C19, 2C8, 2C18, 1A2, and 3A4. CYP2C9, a polymorphic enzyme, is likely to be the principal form of human liver CYP450 that modulates the *in vivo* anticoagulant activity of warfarin. Patients with one or more variant CYP2C9 alleles have decreased S-warfarin clearance [see *Clinical Pharmacology (12.5)*].

Excretion

The terminal half-life of warfarin after a single dose is approximately 1 week; however, the effective half-life ranges from 20 to 60 hours, with a mean of about 40 hours. The clearance of R-warfarin is generally half that of S-warfarin, thus as the volumes of distribution are similar, the half-life of R-warfarin is longer than that of S-warfarin. The half-life of R-warfarin ranges from 37 to 89 hours, while that of S-warfarin ranges from 21 to 43 hours. Studies with radiolabeled drug have demonstrated that up to 92% of the orally administered dose is recovered in urine. Very little warfarin is excreted unchanged in urine. Urinary excretion is in the form of metabolites.

Geriatric Patients

Patients 60 years or older appear to exhibit greater than expected INR response to the anticoagulant effects of warfarin. The cause of the increased sensitivity to the anticoagulant effects of warfarin in this age group is unknown but may be due to a combination of pharmacokinetic and pharmacodynamic factors. Limited information suggests there is no difference in the clearance of S-warfarin; however, there may be a slight decrease in the clearance of R-warfarin in the elderly as compared to the young. Therefore, as patient age increases, a lower dose of warfarin is usually required to produce a therapeutic level of anticoagulation [see *Dosage and Administration (2.3, 2.4)*].

Asian Patients

Asian patients may require lower initiation and maintenance doses of warfarin. A non-controlled study of 151 Chinese outpatients stabilized on warfarin for various indications reported a mean daily warfarin requirement of 3.3 ± 1.4 mg to achieve an INR of 2 to 2.5. Patient age was the most important determinant of warfarin requirement in these patients, with a progressively lower warfarin requirement with increasing age.

12.5 Pharmacogenomics

CYP2C9 and VKORC1 Polymorphisms

The *S*-enantiomer of warfarin is mainly metabolized to 7-hydroxywarfarin by CYP2C9, a polymorphic enzyme. The variant alleles, CYP2C9*2 and CYP2C9*3, result in decreased *in vitro* CYP2C9 enzymatic 7-hydroxylation of S-warfarin. The frequencies of these alleles in Caucasians are approximately 11% and 7% for CYP2C9*2 and CYP2C9*3, respectively.

Other CYP2C9 alleles associated with reduced enzymatic activity occur at lower frequencies, including *5, *6, and *11 alleles in populations of African ancestry and *5, *9, and *11 alleles in Caucasians.

Warfarin reduces the regeneration of vitamin K from vitamin K epoxide in the vitamin K cycle through inhibition of VKOR, a multiprotein enzyme complex. Certain single nucleotide polymorphisms in the VKORC1 gene (e.g., –1639G>A) have been associated with variable warfarin dose requirements. VKORC1 and CYP2C9 gene variants generally explain the largest proportion of known variability in warfarin dose requirements.

CYP2C9 and VKORC1 genotype information, when available, can assist in selection of the initial dose of warfarin [see *Dosage and Administration (2.3)*].

13 NONCLINICAL TOXICOLOGY

13.1 Carcinogenesis, Mutagenesis, Impairment of Fertility

Carcinogenicity, mutagenicity, or fertility studies have not been performed with warfarin.

14 CLINICAL STUDIES

14.1 Atrial Fibrillation

In five prospective, randomized, controlled clinical trials involving 3711 patients with non-rheumatic AF, warfarin significantly reduced the risk of systemic thromboembolism including stroke (see Table 4). The risk reduction ranged from 60% to 86% in all except one trial (CAFA: 45%), which was stopped early due to published positive results from two of these trials. The incidence of major bleeding in these trials ranged from 0.6% to 2.7% (see Table 4).

[See table 4 above]

Trials in patients with both AF and mitral stenosis suggest a benefit from anticoagulation with COUMADIN (warfarin sodium) [see *Dosage and Administration (2.2)*].

14.2 Mechanical and Bioprosthetic Heart Valves

In a prospective, randomized, open-label, positive-controlled study in 254 patients with mechanical prosthetic heart valves, the thromboembolic-free interval was found to be significantly greater in patients treated with warfarin alone compared with dipyridamole/aspirin-treated patients (p<0.005) and pentoxifylline/aspirin-treated patients (p<0.05). The results of this study are presented in Table 5.

[See table 5 at top of next page]

In a prospective, open-label, clinical study comparing moderate (INR 2.65) vs. high intensity (INR 9.0) warfarin therapies in 258 patients with mechanical prosthetic heart valves, thromboembolism occurred with similar frequency in the two groups (4.0 and 3.7 events per 100 patient years, respectively). Major bleeding was more common in the high intensity group. The results of this study are presented in Table 6.

[See table 6 at top of next page]

In a randomized trial in 210 patients comparing two intensities of warfarin therapy (INR 2.0-2.25 vs. INR 2.5-4.0) for a three-month period following tissue heart valve replacement, thromboembolism occurred with similar frequency in the two groups (major embolic events 2.0% vs. 1.9%, respectively, and minor embolic events 10.8% vs. 10.2%, respectively). Major hemorrhages occurred in 4.6% of patients in the higher intensity INR group compared to zero in the lower intensity INR group.

14.3 Myocardial Infarction

WARIS (The Warfarin Re-Infarction Study) was a double-blind, randomized study of 1214 patients 2 to 4 weeks post-infarction treated with warfarin to a target INR of 2.8 to 4.8. The primary endpoint was a composite of total mortality and recurrent infarction. A secondary endpoint of cerebrovascular events was assessed. Mean follow-up of the patients was 37 months. The results for each endpoint separately, including an analysis of vascular death, are provided in Table 7.

[See table 7 below]

WARIS II (The Warfarin, Aspirin, Re-Infarction Study) was an open-label, randomized study of 3630 patients hospitalized for acute myocardial infarction treated with warfarin to a target INR 2.8 to 4.2, aspirin 160 mg per day, or warfarin to a target INR 2.0 to 2.5 plus aspirin 75 mg per day prior to hospital discharge. The primary endpoint was a composite of death, nonfatal reinfarction, or thromboembolic stroke. The mean duration of observation was approximately 4 years. The results for WARIS II are provided in Table 8.

[See table 8 below]

There were approximately four times as many major bleeding episodes in the two groups receiving warfarin than in the group receiving aspirin alone. Major bleeding episodes were not more frequent among patients receiving aspirin plus warfarin than among those receiving warfarin alone, but the incidence of minor bleeding episodes was higher in the combined therapy group.

Table 5: Prospective, Randomized, Open-Label, Positive-Controlled Clinical Study of Warfarin in Patients with Mechanical Prosthetic Heart Valves

Event	Patients Treated With		
	Warfarin	Dipyridamole/Aspirin	Pentoxifylline/Aspirin
Thromboembolism	2.2/100 py	8.6/100 py	7.9/100 py
Major Bleeding	2.5/100 py	0.0/100 py	0.9/100 py

py=patient years

Table 6: Prospective, Open-Label Clinical Study of Warfarin in Patients with Mechanical Prosthetic Heart Valves

Event	Moderate Warfarin Therapy INR 2.65	High Intensity Warfarin Therapy INR 9.0
Thromboembolism	4.0/100 py	3.7/100 py
Major Bleeding	0.95/100 py	2.1/100 py

py=patient years

Table 7: WARIS – Endpoint Analysis of Separate Events

Event	Warfarin (N=607)	Placebo (N=607)	RR (95% CI)	% Risk Reduction (*p*-value)
Total Patient Years of Follow-up	2018	1944		
Total Mortality	94 (4.7/100 py)	123 (6.3/100 py)	0.76 (0.60, 0.97)	24 (p=0.030)
Vascular Death	82 (4.1/100 py)	105 (5.4/100 py)	0.78 (0.60, 1.02)	22 (p=0.068)
Recurrent MI	82 (4.1/100 py)	124 (6.4/100 py)	0.66 (0.51, 0.85)	34 (p=0.001)
Cerebrovascular Event	20 (1.0/100 py)	44 (2.3/100 py)	0.46 (0.28, 0.75)	54 (p=0.002)

RR=Relative risk; Risk reduction=(1 - RR); CI=Confidence interval; MI=Myocardial infarction; py=patient years

Table 8: WARIS II - Distribution of Events According to Treatment Group

Event	Aspirin (N=1206)	Warfarin (N=1216)	Aspirin plus Warfarin (N=1208)	Rate Ratio (95% CI)	*p*-value
	No. of Events				
Major Bleeding[a]	8	33	28	3.35[b] (ND)	ND
				4.00[c] (ND)	ND
Minor Bleeding[d]	39	103	133	3.21[b] (ND)	ND
				2.55[c] (ND)	ND
Composite Endpoints[e]	241	203	181	0.81 (0.69-0.95)[b]	0.03
				0.71 (0.60-0.83)[c]	0.001
Reinfarction	117	90	69	0.56 (0.41-0.78)[b]	<0.001
				0.74 (0.55-0.98)[c]	0.03
Thromboembolic Stroke	32	17	17	0.52 (0.28-0.98)[b]	0.03
				0.52 (0.28-0.97)[c]	0.03
Death	92	96	95		0.82

[a] Major bleeding episodes were defined as nonfatal cerebral hemorrhage or bleeding necessitating surgical intervention or blood transfusion.
[b] The rate ratio is for aspirin plus warfarin as compared with aspirin.
[c] The rate ratio is for warfarin as compared with aspirin.
[d] Minor bleeding episodes were defined as non-cerebral hemorrhage not necessitating surgical intervention or blood transfusion.
[e] Includes death, nonfatal reinfarction, and thromboembolic cerebral stroke.
CI=confidence interval
ND=not determined

15 REFERENCES

- Ansell J, Hirsh J, Hylek E, Jacobson A, Crowther M, Palareti G. Pharmacology and management of the vitamin K antagonists. American College of Chest Physicians Evidence-Based Clinical Practice Guidelines. 8th Ed. *Chest*. 2008;133:160S-198S.
- Kearon C, Kahn SR, Agnelli G, Goldhaber S, Raskob GE, Comerota AJ. Antithrombotic therapy for venous thromboembolic disease. American College of Chest Physicians Evidence-Based Clinical Practice Guidelines. 8th Ed. *Chest*. 2008;133:454S-545S.
- Singer DE, Albers GW, Dalen JE, et al. Antithrombotic therapy in atrial fibrillation. American College of Chest Physicians Evidence-Based Clinical Practice Guidelines. 8th Ed. *Chest*. 2008;133:546S-592S.
- Becker RC, Meade TW, Berger PB, et al. The primary and secondary prevention of coronary artery disease. American College of Chest Physicians Evidence-Based Clinical Practice Guidelines. 8th Ed. *Chest*. 2008;133:776S-814S.
- Salem DN, O'Gara PT, Madias C, Pauker SG. Valvular and structural heart disease. American College of Chest Physicians Evidence-Based Clinical Practice Guidelines. 8th Ed. *Chest*. 2008;133:593S-629S.
- Monagle P, Chalmers E, Chan A, et al. Antithrombotic therapy in neonates and children. American College of Chest Physicians Evidence-Based Clinical Practice Guidelines. 8th Ed. *Chest*. 2008;133:887S-968S.

16 HOW SUPPLIED/STORAGE AND HANDLING

Tablets

COUMADIN (warfarin sodium) tablets are single-scored, with one face imprinted numerically with 1, 2, 2-1/2, 3, 4, 5, 6, 7-1/2, or 10 superimposed and inscribed with "COUMADIN" and with the opposite face plain. COUMADIN is available in bottles and hospital unit-dose blister packages with potencies and colors as follows:

[See table at top of next page]

Protect from light and moisture. Store at controlled room temperature (59°-86°F, 15°-30°C). Dispense in a tight, light-resistant container as defined in the USP.

Store the hospital unit-dose blister packages in the carton until contents have been used.

Injection

COUMADIN for injection vials yield 5 mg of warfarin after reconstitution with 2.7 mL of Sterile Water for Injection (maximum yield is 2.5 mL of a 2 mg/mL solution). Net content of vial is 5.4 mg lyophilized powder.

5-mg vial (box of 6) NDC 0590-0324-35

Protect from light. Keep vial in box until used. Store at controlled room temperature (59°-86°F, 15°-30°C).

After reconstitution, store at controlled room temperature (59°-86°F, 15°-30°C) and use within 4 hours. Do not refrigerate. Discard any unused solution.

17 PATIENT COUNSELING INFORMATION

See FDA-approved patient labeling (Medication Guide).

Advise patients to:

- Tell their physician if they fall often as this may increase their risk for complications.
- Strictly adhere to the prescribed dosage schedule. Do not take or discontinue any other drug, including salicylates (e.g., aspirin and topical analgesics), other over-the-counter drugs, and botanical (herbal) products except on advice of your physician.
- Notify their physician immediately if any unusual bleeding or symptoms occur. Signs and symptoms of bleeding include: pain, swelling or discomfort, prolonged bleeding from cuts, increased menstrual flow or vaginal bleeding, nosebleeds, bleeding of gums from brushing, unusual bleeding or bruising, red or dark brown urine, red or tar black stools, headache, dizziness, or weakness.
- Contact their doctor
  - immediately if they think they are pregnant
  - to discuss pregnancy planning
  - if they are considering breast-feeding
- Avoid any activity or sport that may result in traumatic injury.
- Obtain prothrombin time tests and make regular visits to their physician or clinic to monitor therapy.
- Carry identification stating that they are taking COUMADIN (warfarin sodium).
- If the prescribed dose of COUMADIN is missed, take the dose as soon as possible on the same day but do not take a double dose of COUMADIN the next day to make up for missed doses.
- Eat a normal, balanced diet to maintain a consistent intake of vitamin K. Avoid drastic changes in dietary habits, such as eating large amounts of leafy, green vegetables.
- Contact their physician to report any serious illness, such as severe diarrhea, infection, or fever.
- Be aware that if therapy with COUMADIN is discontinued, the anticoagulant effects of COUMADIN may persist for about 2 to 5 days.

	Bottles of 100	Bottles of 1000	Hospital Unit-Dose Blister Package of 100
1 mg pink	NDC 0056-0169-70	NDC 0056-0169-90	NDC 0056-0169-75
2 mg lavender	NDC 0056-0170-70	NDC 0056-0170-90	NDC 0056-0170-75
2-1/2 mg green	NDC 0056-0176-70	NDC 0056-0176-90	NDC 0056-0176-75
3 mg tan	NDC 0056-0188-70	NDC 0056-0188-90	NDC 0056-0188-75
4 mg blue	NDC 0056-0168-70	NDC 0056-0168-90	NDC 0056-0168-75
5 mg peach	NDC 0056-0172-70	NDC 0056-0172-90	NDC 0056-0172-75
6 mg teal	NDC 0056-0189-70	NDC 0056-0189-90	NDC 0056-0189-75
7-1/2 mg yellow	NDC 0056-0173-70		NDC 0056-0173-75
10 mg white (dye-free)	NDC 0056-0174-70		NDC 0056-0174-75

Distributed by:
Bristol-Myers Squibb Company
Princeton, New Jersey 08543 USA

Printed in USA
1274054A0 / 1274029A0 / 1274055A0 / 1274053A0
Rev October 2011

MEDICATION GUIDE
COUMADIN® (COU-ma-din)
(warfarin sodium)

Read this Medication Guide before you start taking COUMADIN (warfarin sodium) and each time you get a refill. There may be new information. This Medication Guide does not take the place of talking to your healthcare provider about your medical condition or treatment. You and your healthcare provider should talk about COUMADIN when you start taking it and at regular checkups.

What is the most important information I should know about COUMADIN?

COUMADIN can cause bleeding which can be serious and sometimes lead to death. This is because COUMADIN is a blood thinner medicine that lowers the chance of blood clots forming in your body.

- You may have a higher risk of bleeding if you take COUMADIN and:
  - are 65 years of age or older
  - have a history of stomach or intestinal bleeding
  - have high blood pressure (hypertension)
  - have a history of stroke, or "mini-stroke" (transient ischemic attack or TIA)
  - have serious heart disease
  - have a low blood count or cancer
  - have had trauma, such as an accident or surgery
  - have kidney problems
  - take other medicines that increase your risk of bleeding, including:
    - a medicine that contains heparin
    - other medicines to prevent or treat blood clots
    - nonsteroidal anti-inflammatory drugs (NSAIDs)
  - take warfarin sodium for a long time. Warfarin sodium is the active ingredient in COUMADIN.

Tell your healthcare provider if you take any of these medicines. Ask your healthcare provider if you are not sure if your medicine is one listed above.

Many other medicines can interact with COUMADIN and affect the dose you need or increase COUMADIN side effects. Do not change or stop any of your medicines or start any new medicines before you talk to your healthcare provider.

Do not take other medicines that contain warfarin sodium while taking COUMADIN.

- **Get your regular blood test to check for your response to COUMADIN.** This blood test is called an INR test. The INR test checks to see how fast your blood clots. Your healthcare provider will decide what INR numbers are best for you. Your dose of COUMADIN will be adjusted to keep your INR in a target range for you.
- **Call your healthcare provider right away if you get any of the following signs or symptoms of bleeding problems:**
  - pain, swelling, or discomfort
  - headaches, dizziness, or weakness
  - unusual bruising (bruises that develop without known cause or grow in size)
  - nosebleeds
  - bleeding gums
  - bleeding from cuts takes a long time to stop
  - menstrual bleeding or vaginal bleeding that is heavier than normal
  - pink or brown urine
  - red or black stools
  - coughing up blood
  - vomiting blood or material that looks like coffee grounds
- **Some foods and beverages can interact with COUMADIN and affect your treatment and dose.**
  - Eat a normal, balanced diet. Talk to your healthcare provider before you make any diet changes. Do not eat large amounts of leafy, green vegetables. Leafy, green vegetables contain vitamin K. Certain vegetable oils also contain large amounts of vitamin K. Too much vitamin K can lower the effect of COUMADIN (warfarin sodium).
- Always tell all of your healthcare providers that you take COUMADIN.
- Wear or carry information that you take COUMADIN.

See "What are the possible side effects of COUMADIN?" for more information about side effects.

What is COUMADIN?

COUMADIN is prescription medicine used to treat blood clots and to lower the chance of blood clots forming in your body. Blood clots can cause a stroke, heart attack, or other serious conditions if they form in the legs or lungs.

It is not known if COUMADIN is safe and effective in children.

Who should not take COUMADIN?

Do not take COUMADIN if:

- **your chance of having bleeding problems is higher than the possible benefit of treatment.** Your healthcare provider will decide if COUMADIN is right for you. Talk to your healthcare provider about all of your health conditions.
- **you are pregnant unless you have a mechanical heart valve.** COUMADIN may cause birth defects, miscarriage, or death of your unborn baby.
- **you are allergic to warfarin or any of the other ingredients in COUMADIN. See the end of this leaflet for a complete list of ingredients in COUMADIN.**

What should I tell my healthcare provider before taking COUMADIN?

Before you take COUMADIN, tell your healthcare provider if you:

- have bleeding problems
- fall often
- have liver or kidney problems
- have high blood pressure
- have a heart problem called congestive heart failure
- have diabetes
- plan to have any surgery or a dental procedure
- have any other medical conditions
- are pregnant or plan to become pregnant. See **"Who should not take COUMADIN?"**
- are breast-feeding. You and your healthcare provider should decide if you will take COUMADIN and breast-feed.

Tell all of your healthcare providers and dentists that you are taking COUMADIN. They should talk to the healthcare provider who prescribed COUMADIN for you before you have **any** surgery or dental procedure. Your COUMADIN may need to be stopped for a short time or you may need your dose adjusted.

Tell your healthcare provider about all the medicines you take, including prescription and non-prescription medicines, vitamins, and herbal supplements. Some of your other medicines may affect the way COUMADIN works. Certain medicines may increase your risk of bleeding. See **"What is the most important information I should know about COUMADIN?"**

Know the medicines you take. Keep a list of them to show your healthcare provider and pharmacist when you get a new medicine.

How should I take COUMADIN?

- **Take COUMADIN exactly as prescribed.** Your healthcare provider will adjust your dose from time to time depending on your response to COUMADIN.
- **You must have regular blood tests and visits with your healthcare provider to monitor your condition.**
- **If you miss a dose of COUMADIN, call your healthcare provider.** Take the dose as soon as possible on the same day. **Do not** take a double dose of COUMADIN (warfarin sodium) the next day to make up for a missed dose.
- Call your healthcare provider right away if you:
  - take too much COUMADIN
  - are sick with diarrhea, an infection, or have a fever
  - fall or injure yourself, especially if you hit your head. Your healthcare provider may need to check you

What should I avoid while taking COUMADIN?

- Do not do any activity or sport that may cause a serious injury.

What are the possible side effects of COUMADIN?

COUMADIN may cause serious side effects including:

- See **"What is the most important information I should know about COUMADIN?"**
  - **Death of skin tissue (skin necrosis or gangrene).** This can happen soon after starting COUMADIN. It happens because blood clots form and block blood flow to an area of your body. Call your healthcare provider right away if you have pain, color, or temperature change to any area of your body. You may need medical care right away to prevent death or loss (amputation) of your affected body part.
  - **"Purple toes syndrome."** Call your healthcare provider right away if you have pain in your toes and they look purple in color or dark in color.

Tell your healthcare provider if you have any side effect that bothers you or does not go away.

These are not all of the side effects of COUMADIN. For more information, ask your healthcare provider or pharmacist.

Call your doctor for medical advice about side effects. You may report side effects to FDA at 1-800-FDA-1088.

How should I store COUMADIN?

- Store COUMADIN at 59°F to 86°F (15°C to 30°C).
- Keep COUMADIN in a tightly closed container, and keep COUMADIN out of the light.

Keep COUMADIN and all medicines out of the reach of children.

General Information about COUMADIN.

Medicines are sometimes prescribed for purposes other than those listed in a Medication Guide. Do not use COUMADIN for a condition for which it was not prescribed. Do not give COUMADIN to other people, even if they have the same symptoms that you have. It may harm them.

This Medication Guide summarizes the most important information about COUMADIN. If you would like more information, talk with your healthcare provider. You can ask your healthcare provider or pharmacist for information about COUMADIN that is written for healthcare professionals.

If you would like more information, go to www.coumadin.com or call 1-800-321-1335.

What are the ingredients in COUMADIN?

Active ingredient: Warfarin Sodium

Inactive ingredients: Lactose, starch, and magnesium stearate. The following tablets contain:

1 mg:	D&C Red No. 6 Barium Lake
2 mg:	FD&C Blue No. 2 Aluminum Lake and FD&C Red No. 40 Aluminum Lake
2-1/2 mg:	D&C Yellow No. 10 Aluminum Lake and FD&C Blue No. 1 Aluminum Lake
3 mg:	FD&C Yellow No. 6 Aluminum Lake, FD&C Blue No. 2 Aluminum Lake, and FD&C Red No. 40 Aluminum Lake
4 mg:	FD&C Blue No. 1 Aluminum Lake
5 mg:	FD&C Yellow No. 6 Aluminum Lake
6 mg:	FD&C Yellow No. 6 Aluminum Lake and FD&C Blue No. 1 Aluminum Lake
7-1/2 mg:	D&C Yellow No. 10 Aluminum Lake and FD&C Yellow No. 6 Aluminum Lake

This Medication Guide has been approved by the U.S. Food and Drug Administration.

COUMADIN is distributed by:
Bristol-Myers Squibb Company
Princeton, New Jersey 08543 USA

1258498A3 / 1215385A4 / 1205734A4 / 1205736A4
Rev October 2011

Shown in Product Identification Guide, page 305

ELIQUIS ℞

[ELL eh kwiss]
(apixaban)
tablets for oral use

HIGHLIGHTS OF PRESCRIBING INFORMATION
These highlights do not include all the information needed to use ELIQUIS safely and effectively. See full prescribing information for ELIQUIS.

ELIQUIS (apixaban) tablets for oral use
Initial U.S. Approval: 2012

WARNING: DISCONTINUING ELIQUIS IN PATIENTS WITHOUT ADEQUATE CONTINUOUS ANTICOAGULATION INCREASES RISK OF STROKE
See full prescribing information for complete boxed warning.
Discontinuing ELIQUIS places patients at an increased risk of thrombotic events. An increased rate of stroke was observed following discontinuation of ELIQUIS in clinical trials in patients with nonvalvular atrial fibrillation. If anticoagulation with ELIQUIS must be discontinued for a reason other than pathological bleeding, coverage with another anticoagulant should be strongly considered. (2.4, 5.1)

INDICATIONS AND USAGE

ELIQUIS is a factor Xa inhibitor anticoagulant indicated to reduce the risk of stroke and systemic embolism in patients with nonvalvular atrial fibrillation. (1)

DOSAGE AND ADMINISTRATION

- The recommended dose is 5 mg orally twice daily. (2.1)
- In patients with at least 2 of the following characteristics: age ≥80 years, body weight ≤60 kg, or serum creatinine ≥1.5 mg/dL, the recommended dose is 2.5 mg orally twice daily. (2.2)

DOSAGE FORMS AND STRENGTHS

- Tablets: 2.5 mg and 5 mg (3)

CONTRAINDICATIONS

- Active pathological bleeding (4)
- Severe hypersensitivity to ELIQUIS (4)

WARNINGS AND PRECAUTIONS

- ELIQUIS can cause serious, potentially fatal bleeding. Promptly evaluate signs and symptoms of blood loss. (5.2)
- Prosthetic heart valves: ELIQUIS use not recommended. (5.3)

ADVERSE REACTIONS

Most common adverse reactions (>1%) are related to bleeding. (6.1)

To report SUSPECTED ADVERSE REACTIONS, contact Bristol-Myers Squibb at 1-800-721-5072 or FDA at 1-800-FDA-1088 or *www.fda.gov/medwatch*

DRUG INTERACTIONS

- Strong dual inhibitors of CYP3A4 and P-gp increase blood levels of apixaban: Reduce ELIQUIS dose to 2.5 mg or avoid concomitant use. (2.2, 7.1, 12.3)
- Simultaneous use of strong inducers of CYP3A4 and P-gp reduces blood levels of apixaban: Avoid concomitant use. (7.2, 12.3)

USE IN SPECIFIC POPULATIONS

- *Nursing Mothers:* Discontinue drug or discontinue nursing. (8.3)
- *Pregnancy:* Not recommended. (8.1)
- *Severe Hepatic Impairment:* Not recommended. (12.2)

See 17 for PATIENT COUNSELING INFORMATION and Medication Guide

Revised: 12/2012

FULL PRESCRIBING INFORMATION: CONTENTS*

*** Sections or subsections omitted from the full prescribing information are not listed**

FULL PRESCRIBING INFORMATION

WARNING: DISCONTINUING ELIQUIS IN PATIENTS WITHOUT ADEQUATE CONTINUOUS ANTICOAGULATION INCREASES RISK OF STROKE

Discontinuing ELIQUIS places patients at an increased risk of thrombotic events. An increased rate of stroke was observed following discontinuation of ELIQUIS in clinical trials in patients with nonvalvular atrial fibrillation. If anticoagulation with ELIQUIS must be discontinued for a reason other than pathological bleeding, coverage with another anticoagulant should be strongly considered *[see Dosage and Administration (2.4) and Warnings and Precautions (5.1)]*.

1 INDICATIONS AND USAGE

ELIQUIS® (apixaban) is indicated to reduce the risk of stroke and systemic embolism in patients with nonvalvular atrial fibrillation.

2 DOSAGE AND ADMINISTRATION

2.1 Recommended Dose

The recommended dose of ELIQUIS for most patients is 5 mg taken orally twice daily.

2.2 Dosage Adjustments

The recommended dose of ELIQUIS is 2.5 mg twice daily in patients with any 2 of the following characteristics:

- age ≥80 years
- body weight ≤60 kg
- serum creatinine ≥1.5 mg/dL

CYP3A4 and P-gp inhibitors: When ELIQUIS is coadministered with drugs that are strong dual inhibitors of cytochrome P450 3A4 (CYP3A4) and P-glycoprotein (P-gp) (e.g., ketoconazole, itraconazole, ritonavir, clarithromycin), the recommended dose is 2.5 mg twice daily *[see Clinical Pharmacology (12.3)]*.

In patients already taking 2.5 mg twice daily, coadministration of ELIQUIS with strong dual inhibitors of CYP3A4 and P-gp should be avoided.

2.3 Missed Dose

If a dose of ELIQUIS is not taken at the scheduled time, the dose should be taken as soon as possible on the same day and twice daily administration should be resumed. The dose should not be doubled to make up for a missed dose.

2.4 Discontinuation for Surgery and Other Interventions

ELIQUIS should be discontinued at least 48 hours prior to elective surgery or invasive procedures with a moderate or high risk of unacceptable or clinically significant bleeding. ELIQUIS should be discontinued at least 24 hours prior to elective surgery or invasive procedures with a low risk of bleeding or where the bleeding would be non-critical in location and easily controlled.

2.5 Converting from or to ELIQUIS

Switching from warfarin to ELIQUIS: Warfarin should be discontinued and ELIQUIS started when the international normalized ratio (INR) is below 2.0.

Switching from ELIQUIS to warfarin: ELIQUIS affects INR, so that INR measurements during coadministration with warfarin may not be useful for determining the appropriate dose of warfarin. If continuous anticoagulation is necessary, discontinue ELIQUIS and begin both a parenteral anticoagulant and warfarin at the time the next dose of ELIQUIS would have been taken, discontinuing the parenteral anticoagulant when INR reaches an acceptable range.

Switching between ELIQUIS and anticoagulants other than warfarin: Discontinue one being taken and begin the other at the next scheduled dose.

2.6 Hepatic Impairment

No dose adjustment is required in patients with mild hepatic impairment.

Because patients with moderate hepatic impairment may have intrinsic coagulation abnormalities and there is limited clinical experience with ELIQUIS (apixaban) in these patients, dosing recommendations cannot be provided *[see Clinical Pharmacology (12.2)]*.

ELIQUIS is not recommended in patients with severe hepatic impairment *[see Clinical Pharmacology (12.3)]*.

2.7 Renal Impairment

The dosing adjustment for moderate renal impairment is described above *[see Dosage and Administration (2.2)]*. No data inform use in patients with creatinine clearance <15 mL/min or on dialysis.

3 DOSAGE FORMS AND STRENGTHS

- 2.5 mg, yellow, round, biconvex, film-coated tablets with "893" debossed on one side and "2½" on the other side.
- 5 mg, pink, oval-shaped, biconvex, film-coated tablets with "894" debossed on one side and "5" on the other side.

4 CONTRAINDICATIONS

ELIQUIS is contraindicated in patients with the following conditions:

- Active pathological bleeding *[see Warnings and Precautions (5.2) and Adverse Reactions (6.1)]*
- Severe hypersensitivity reaction to ELIQUIS (i.e., anaphylactic reactions) *[see Adverse Reactions (6.1)]*

5 WARNINGS AND PRECAUTIONS

5.1 Increased Risk of Stroke with Discontinuation of ELIQUIS

Discontinuing ELIQUIS in the absence of adequate alternative anticoagulation increases the risk of thrombotic events. An increased rate of stroke was observed during the transition from ELIQUIS to warfarin in clinical trials in patients with nonvalvular atrial fibrillation. If ELIQUIS must be discontinued for a reason other than pathological bleeding, consider coverage with another anticoagulant *[see Dosage and Administration (2.3)]*.

5.2 Bleeding

ELIQUIS increases the risk of bleeding and can cause serious, potentially fatal, bleeding *[see Dosage and Administration (2.2) and Adverse Reactions (6.1)]*.

Concomitant use of drugs affecting hemostasis increases the risk of bleeding. These include aspirin and other antiplatelet agents, other anticoagulants, heparin, thrombolytic agents, selective serotonin reuptake inhibitors, serotonin norepinephrine reuptake inhibitor, and nonsteroidal anti-inflammatory drugs (NSAIDs) *[see Drug Interactions (7.3)]*.

Patients should be made aware of signs and symptoms of blood loss and instructed to report them immediately or go to an emergency room. ELIQUIS should be discontinued in patients with active pathological hemorrhage.

There is no established way to reverse the anticoagulant effect of apixaban, which can be expected to persist for about 24 hours after the last dose, i.e., for about two half-lives. A specific antidote for ELIQUIS is not available. Because of high plasma protein binding, apixaban is not expected to be dialyzable *[see Clinical Pharmacology (12.3)]*. Protamine sulfate and vitamin K would not be expected to affect the anticoagulant activity of apixaban. There is no experience with antifibrinolytic agents (tranexamic acid, aminocaproic acid) in individuals receiving apixaban. There is neither scientific rationale for reversal nor experience with systemic hemostatics (desmopressin and aprotinin) in individuals receiving apixaban. Use of procoagulant reversal agents such as prothrombin complex concentrate, activated prothrombin complex concentrate, or recombinant factor VIIa may be considered but has not been evaluated in clinical studies. Activated oral charcoal reduces absorption of apixaban, thereby lowering apixaban plasma concentration *[see Overdosage (10)]*.

5.3 Patients with Prosthetic Heart Valves

The safety and efficacy of ELIQUIS has not been studied in patients with prosthetic heart valves. Therefore, use of ELIQUIS is not recommended in these patients.

6 ADVERSE REACTIONS

The most serious adverse reactions reported with ELIQUIS were related to bleeding *[see Warnings and Precautions (5.2)]*.

6.1 Clinical Trials Experience

Because clinical trials are conducted under widely varying conditions, adverse reaction rates observed in the clinical trials of a drug cannot be directly compared to rates in the clinical trials of another drug and may not reflect the rates observed in practice.

The safety of ELIQUIS was evaluated in the ARISTOTLE and AVERROES studies *[see Clinical Studies (14)]*, including 11,284 patients exposed to ELIQUIS 5 mg twice daily and 602 patients exposed to ELIQUIS 2.5 mg twice daily. The duration of ELIQUIS exposure was ≥12 months for 9375 patients and ≥24 months for 3369 patients in the two

Table 1: Bleeding Events in Patients with Nonvalvular Atrial Fibrillation in ARISTOTLE

	ELIQUIS N=9088 n (%/year)	Warfarin N=9052 n (%/year)	Hazard Ratio (95% CI*)	P-value
Major†	327 (2.13)	462 (3.09)	0.69 (0.60, 0.80)	<0.0001
Gastrointestinal (GI)‡	128 (0.83)	141 (0.93)	0.89 (0.70, 1.14)	-
Intracranial	52 (0.33)	125 (0.82)	0.41 (0.30, 0.57)	-
Intraocular§	32 (0.21)	22 (0.14)	1.42 (0.83, 2.45)	-
Fatal¶	10 (0.06)	37 (0.24)	0.27 (0.13, 0.53)	-
CRNM**	318 (2.08)	444 (3.00)	0.70 (0.60, 0.80)	<0.0001

* Confidence interval.
† International Society on Thrombosis and Hemostasis (ISTH) major bleed assessed by sequential testing strategy for superiority designed to control the overall type I error in the trial.
‡ GI bleed includes upper GI, lower GI, and rectal bleeding.
§ Intraocular bleed is within the corpus of the eye (a conjunctival bleed is not an intraocular bleed).
¶ Fatal bleed is an adjudicated death because of bleeding during the treatment period and includes both fatal extracranial bleeds and fatal hemorrhagic stroke.
** CRNM = clinically relevant nonmajor bleeding.
Events associated with each endpoint were counted once per subject, but subjects may have contributed events to multiple endpoints.

Table 2: Bleeding Events in Patients with Nonvalvular Atrial Fibrillation in AVERROES

	ELIQUIS N=2978 n (%/year)	Aspirin N=2780 n (%/year)	Hazard Ratio (95% CI)	P-value
Major	45 (1.41)	29 (0.92)	1.54 (0.96, 2.45)	0.07
Fatal	5 (0.16)	5 (0.16)	0.99 (0.23, 4.29)	-
Intracranial	11 (0.34)	11 (0.35)	0.99 (0.39, 2.51)	-

Events associated with each endpoint were counted once per subject, but subjects may have contributed events to multiple endpoints.

studies. In ARISTOTLE, the mean duration of exposure was 89 weeks (>15,000 patient-years). In AVERROES, the mean duration of exposure was approximately 59 weeks (>3000 patients-years).

The most common reason for treatment discontinuation in both studies was for bleeding-related adverse reactions; in ARISTOTLE this occurred in 1.7% and 2.5% of patients treated with ELIQUIS (apixaban) and warfarin, respectively, and in AVERROES, in 1.5% and 1.3% on ELIQUIS and aspirin, respectively.

Bleeding in Patients with Nonvalvular Atrial Fibrillation in ARISTOTLE and AVERROES

Tables 1 and 2 show the number of patients experiencing major bleeding during the treatment period and the bleeding rate (percentage of subjects with at least one bleeding event per year) in ARISTOTLE and AVERROES.

Major bleeding was defined as clinically overt bleeding that was accompanied by one or more of the following: a decrease in hemoglobin of 2 g/dL or more; a transfusion of 2 or more units of packed red blood cells; bleeding that occurred in at least one of the following critical sites: intracranial, intraspinal, intraocular, pericardial, intra-articular, intramuscular with compartment syndrome, retroperitoneal; or bleeding that was fatal. Intracranial hemorrhage included intracerebral (hemorrhagic stroke), subarachnoid, and subdural bleeds.

[See table 1 above]

In ARISTOTLE, the results for major bleeding were generally consistent across most major subgroups including age, weight, $CHADS_2$ score (a scale from 0 to 6 used to estimate risk of stroke, with higher scores predicting greater risk), prior warfarin use, geographic region, ELIQUIS dose, type of AF, and aspirin use at randomization (Figure 1). Subjects treated with apixaban with diabetes bled more (3.0%/year) than did subjects without diabetes (1.9%/year).

[See figure 1 at top of next column]

[See table 2 above]

Other Adverse Reactions

Hypersensitivity reactions (including drug hypersensitivity, such as skin rash, and anaphylactic reactions, such as allergic edema) and syncope were reported in <1% of patients receiving ELIQUIS.

7 DRUG INTERACTIONS

Apixaban is a substrate of both CYP3A4 and P-gp. Inhibitors of CYP3A4 and P-gp increase exposure to apixaban and increase the risk of bleeding. Inducers of CYP3A4 and P-gp decrease exposure to apixaban and increase the risk of stroke.

7.1 Strong Dual Inhibitors of CYP3A4 and P-gp

The dose of ELIQUIS should be decreased to 2.5 mg twice daily when it is coadministered with drugs that are strong dual inhibitors of CYP3A4 and P-gp, (e.g., ketoconazole, itraconazole, ritonavir, or clarithromycin) *[see Dosage and Administration (2.2) and Clinical Pharmacology (12.3)]*.

Figure 1: Major Bleeding Hazard Ratios by Baseline Characteristics – ARISTOTLE Study

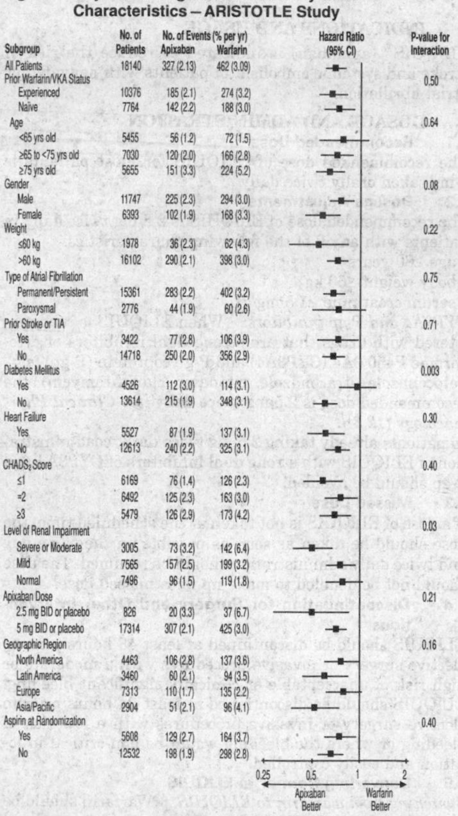

In patients already taking ELIQUIS (apixaban) at a dose of 2.5 mg twice daily, avoid coadministration with strong dual inhibitors of both CYP3A4 and P-gp *[see Dosage and Administration (2.2) and Clinical Pharmacology (12.3)]*.

7.2 Strong Dual Inducers of CYP3A4 and P-gp

Avoid concomitant use of ELIQUIS with strong dual inducers of CYP3A4 and P-gp (e.g., rifampin, carbamazepine, phenytoin, St. John's wort) because such drugs will decrease exposure to apixaban *[see Clinical Pharmacology (12.3)]*.

7.3 Anticoagulants and Antiplatelet Agents

Coadministration of antiplatelet agents, fibrinolytics, heparin, aspirin, and chronic NSAID use increases the risk of bleeding.

APPRAISE-2, a placebo-controlled clinical trial of apixaban in high-risk post-acute coronary syndrome patients treated with aspirin or the combination of aspirin and clopidogrel, was terminated early due to a higher rate of bleeding with apixaban compared to placebo. The rate of ISTH major bleeding was 2.77%/year with apixaban versus 0.62%/year with placebo in patients receiving single antiplatelet therapy and was 5.91%/year with apixaban versus 2.50%/year with placebo in those receiving dual antiplatelet therapy.

In ARISTOTLE, concomitant use of aspirin increased the bleeding risk on ELIQUIS (apixaban) from 1.8% per year to 3.4% per year and the bleeding risk on warfarin from 2.7% per year to 4.6% per year. In this clinical trial, there was limited (2.3%) use of dual antiplatelet therapy with ELIQUIS.

8 USE IN SPECIFIC POPULATIONS

8.1 Pregnancy

Pregnancy Category B

There are no adequate and well-controlled studies of ELIQUIS in pregnant women. Treatment is likely to increase the risk of hemorrhage during pregnancy and delivery. ELIQUIS should be used during pregnancy only if the potential benefit outweighs the potential risk to the mother and fetus.

Treatment of pregnant rats, rabbits, and mice after implantation until the end of gestation resulted in fetal exposure to apixaban, but was not associated with increased risk for fetal malformations or toxicity. No maternal or fetal deaths were attributed to bleeding. Increased incidence of maternal bleeding was observed in mice, rats, and rabbits at maternal exposures that were 19, 4, and 1 times, respectively, the human exposure of unbound drug, based on area under plasma-concentration time curve (AUC) comparisons at the maximum recommended human dose (MRHD) of 10 mg (5 mg twice daily).

8.2 Labor and Delivery

Safety and effectiveness of ELIQUIS during labor and delivery have not been studied in clinical trials. Consider the risks of bleeding and of stroke in using ELIQUIS in this setting *[see Warnings and Precautions (5.2)]*.

Treatment of pregnant rats from implantation (gestation Day 7) to weaning (lactation Day 21) with apixaban at a dose of 1000 mg/kg (about 5 times the human exposure based on unbound apixaban) did not result in death of offspring or death of mother rats during labor in association with uterine bleeding. However, increased incidence of maternal bleeding, primarily during gestation, occurred at apixaban doses of ≥25 mg/kg, a dose corresponding to ≥1.3 times the human exposure.

8.3 Nursing Mothers

It is unknown whether apixaban or its metabolites are excreted in human milk. Rats excrete apixaban in milk (12% of the maternal dose).

Women should be instructed either to discontinue breastfeeding or to discontinue ELIQUIS therapy, taking into account the importance of the drug to the mother.

8.4 Pediatric Use

Safety and effectiveness in pediatric patients have not been established.

8.5 Geriatric Use

Of the total subjects in clinical studies of apixaban, >69% were 65 and older, and >31% were 75 and older. The effects of ELIQUIS on the risk of stroke and major bleeding compared to warfarin were maintained in geriatric subjects.

10 OVERDOSAGE

There is no antidote to ELIQUIS. Overdose of ELIQUIS increases the risk of bleeding *[see Warnings and Precautions (5.2)]*.

In controlled clinical trials, orally administered apixaban in healthy subjects at doses up to 50 mg daily for 3 to 7 days (25 mg twice-daily for 7 days or 50 mg once-daily for 3 days) had no clinically relevant adverse effects.

In healthy subjects, administration of activated charcoal 2 and 6 hours after ingestion of a 20-mg dose of apixaban reduced mean apixaban AUC by 50% and 27%, respectively. Mean apparent half-life of apixaban decreased from 13.4 hours when apixaban was administered alone to 5.3 hours and 4.9 hours, respectively, when activated charcoal was administered 2 and 6 hours after apixaban, indicating that charcoal blocked the continued absorption of apixaban from the gut *[see Clinical Pharmacology (12.3)]*. Thus, administration of activated charcoal may be useful in the management of apixaban overdose or accidental ingestion by leading to a more rapid fall in apixaban blood levels.

11 DESCRIPTION

ELIQUIS (apixaban), a factor Xa (FXa) inhibitor, is chemically described as 1-(4-methoxyphenyl)-7-oxo-6-[4-(2-oxopiperidin-1-yl)phenyl]-4,5,6,7-tetrahydro-1*H*-pyrazolo-

[3,4-*c*]pyridine-3-carboxamide. Its molecular formula is $C_{25}H_{25}N_5O_4$, which corresponds to a molecular weight of 459.5. Apixaban has the following structural formula:

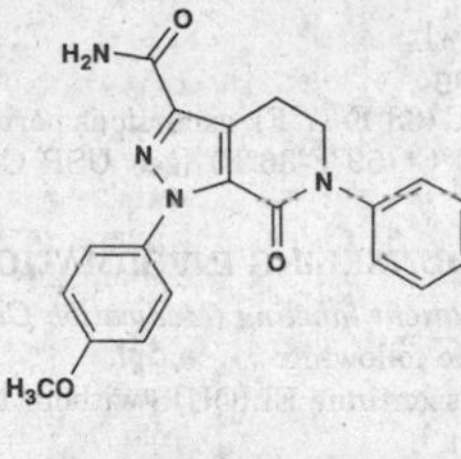

Apixaban is a white to pale-yellow powder. At physiological pH (1.2-6.8), apixaban does not ionize; its aqueous solubility across the physiological pH range is ~0.04 mg/mL.

ELIQUIS (apixaban) tablets are available for oral administration in strengths of 2.5 mg and 5 mg of apixaban with the following inactive ingredients: anhydrous lactose, microcrystalline cellulose, croscarmellose sodium, sodium lauryl sulfate, and magnesium stearate. The film coating contains lactose monohydrate, hypromellose, titanium dioxide, triacetin, and yellow iron oxide (2.5 mg tablets) or red iron oxide (5 mg tablets).

12 CLINICAL PHARMACOLOGY

12.1 Mechanism of Action

Apixaban is an oral, reversible, and selective active site inhibitor of FXa. It does not require antithrombin III for antithrombotic activity. Apixaban inhibits free and clot-bound FXa, and prothrombinase activity. Apixaban has no direct effect on platelet aggregation, but indirectly inhibits platelet aggregation induced by thrombin. By inhibiting FXa, apixaban decreases thrombin generation and thrombus development.

12.2 Pharmacodynamics

As a result of FXa inhibition, apixaban prolongs clotting tests such as prothrombin time (PT), INR, and activated partial thromboplastin time (aPTT). Changes observed in these clotting tests at the expected therapeutic dose, however, are small, subject to a high degree of variability, and not useful in monitoring the anticoagulation effect of apixaban.

The Rotachrom® Heparin chromogenic assay was used to measure the effect of apixaban on FXa activity in humans during the apixaban development program. A concentration-dependent increase in anti-FXa activity was observed in the dose range tested and was similar in healthy subjects and patients with AF.

This test is not recommended for assessing the anticoagulant effect of apixaban.

Pharmacodynamic Drug Interaction Studies

Pharmacodynamic drug interaction studies with aspirin, clopidogrel, aspirin and clopidogrel, enoxaparin, and naproxen were conducted. No pharmacodynamic interactions were observed with aspirin or clopidogrel, but a 50% to 60% increase in anti-FXa activity was observed when apixaban was coadministered with enoxaparin or naproxen.

Specific Populations

Renal impairment: Anti-FXa activity adjusted for exposure to apixaban was similar across renal function categories.

Hepatic impairment: Changes in anti-FXa activity were similar in patients with mild to moderate hepatic impairment and healthy subjects. However, in patients with moderate hepatic impairment, there is no clear understanding of the impact of this degree of hepatic function impairment on the coagulation cascade and its relationship to efficacy and bleeding. Patients with severe hepatic impairment were not studied.

Cardiac Electrophysiology

Apixaban has no effect on the QTc interval in humans at doses up to 50 mg.

12.3 Pharmacokinetics

Apixaban displays prolonged absorption. Thus, despite a short clearance half-life of about 6 hours, the apparent half-life during repeat dosing is about 12 hours, which allows twice-daily dosing to provide effective anticoagulation, but it also means that when the drug is stopped for surgery, anticoagulation persists for at least a day.

Absorption

The absolute bioavailability of apixaban is approximately 50% for doses up to 10 mg of ELIQUIS. Food does not affect the bioavailability of apixaban. Maximum concentrations (C_{max}) of apixaban appear 3 to 4 hours after oral administration of ELIQUIS. Apixaban is absorbed throughout the gastrointestinal tract with the distal small bowel and ascending colon contributing about 55% of apixaban absorption. Apixaban demonstrates linear pharmacokinetics with dose-proportional increases in exposure for oral doses up to 10 mg. At doses ≥25 mg, apixaban displays dissolution-limited absorption with decreased bioavailability.

Distribution

Plasma protein binding in humans is approximately 87%. The volume of distribution (Vss) is approximately 21 liters.

Metabolism

Approximately 25% of an orally administered apixaban dose is recovered in urine and feces as metabolites. Apixaban is metabolized mainly via CYP3A4 with minor contributions from CYP1A2, 2C8, 2C9, 2C19, and 2J2. O-demethylation and hydroxylation at the 3-oxopiperidinyl moiety are the major sites of biotransformation.

Unchanged apixaban is the major drug-related component in human plasma; there are no active circulating metabolites.

Elimination

Apixaban is eliminated in both urine and feces. Renal excretion accounts for about 27% of total clearance. Biliary and direct intestinal excretion contributes to elimination of apixaban in the feces.

Following intravenous administration, apixaban is eliminated with a dominant half-life of ~5 hours. Following oral administration, the apparent half-life is ~12 hours because of prolonged absorption.

Apixaban is a substrate of transport proteins: P-gp and breast cancer resistance protein.

Drug Interaction Studies

In vitro apixaban studies at concentrations significantly greater than therapeutic exposures, no inhibitory effect on the activity of CYP1A2, CYP2A6, CYP2B6, CYP2C8, CYP2C9, CYP2D6, CYP3A4/5 or CYP2C19, nor induction effect on the activity of CYP1A2, CYP2B6 or CYP3A4/5 were observed. Therefore, apixaban is not expected to alter the metabolic clearance of coadministered drugs that are metabolized by these enzymes. Apixaban is not a significant inhibitor of P-gp.

The effects of coadministered drugs on the pharmacokinetics of apixaban and associated dose recommendations are summarized in Figure 2 *[see also Warnings and Precautions (5.2) and Drug Interactions (7)]*.

Figure 2: Effect of Coadministered Drugs on the Pharmacokinetics of Apixaban

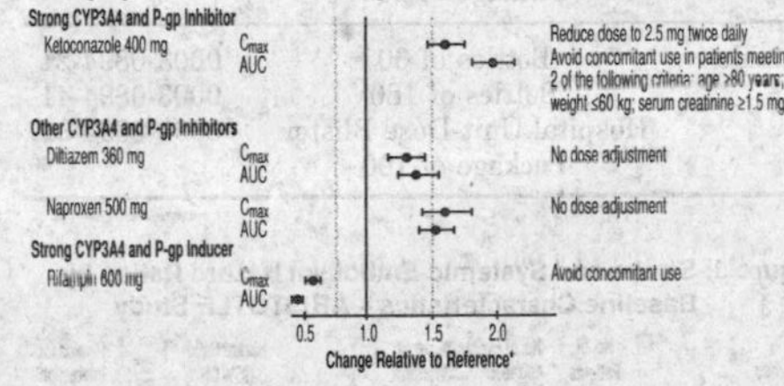

* Dashed vertical lines illustrate pharmacokinetic changes that were used to inform dosing recommendations. Dosing recommendations were also informed by clinical considerations *[see Warnings and Precautions (5.2) and Drug Interactions (7)]*.

In dedicated studies conducted in healthy subjects, famotidine, atenolol, and enoxaparin did not meaningfully alter the pharmacokinetics of apixaban.

In studies conducted in healthy subjects, apixaban did not meaningfully alter the pharmacokinetics of digoxin, naproxen, atenolol, or acetylsalicylic acid.

Specific Populations

The effects of level of renal impairment, age, body weight, level of hepatic impairment, gender, and ethnic origin on the pharmacokinetics of apixaban are summarized in Figure 3.

Figure 3: Effect of Specific Populations on the Pharmacokinetics of Apixaban

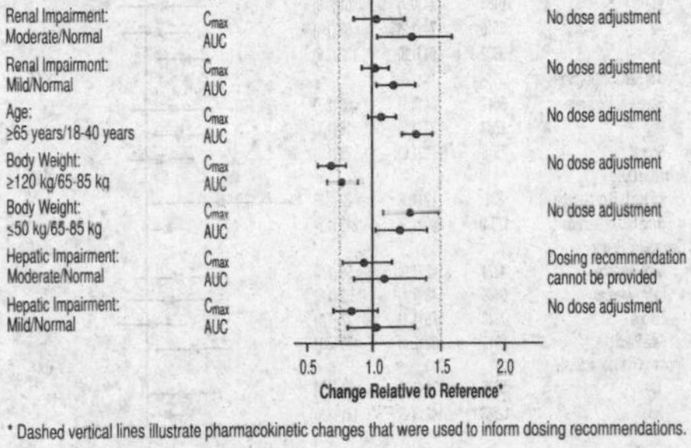

* Dashed vertical lines illustrate pharmacokinetic changes that were used to inform dosing recommendations.

A study in healthy subjects comparing the pharmacokinetics in males and females showed no meaningful difference. The results across pharmacokinetic studies in normal subjects showed no differences in apixaban pharmacokinetics among White/Caucasian, Asian, and Black/African American subjects. No dose adjustment is required based on race/ethnicity.

13 NONCLINICAL TOXICOLOGY

13.1 Carcinogenesis, Mutagenesis, Impairment of Fertility

Carcinogenesis: Apixaban was not carcinogenic when administered to mice and rats for up to 2 years. The systemic exposures (AUCs) of unbound apixaban in male and female mice at the highest doses tested (1500 and 3000 mg/kg/day) were 9 and 20 times, respectively, the human exposure of unbound drug at the MRHD of 10 mg/day. Systemic exposures of unbound apixaban in male and female rats at the highest dose tested (600 mg/kg/day) were 2 and 4 times, respectively, the human exposure.

Mutagenesis: Apixaban was neither mutagenic in the bacterial reverse mutation (Ames) assay, nor clastogenic in Chinese hamster ovary cells *in vitro*, in a 1-month *in vivo/in vitro* cytogenetics study in rat peripheral blood lymphocytes, or in a rat micronucleus study *in vivo*.

Impairment of Fertility: Apixaban had no effect on fertility in male or female rats when given at doses up to 600 mg/kg/day, a dose resulting in exposure levels that are 3 and 4 times, respectively, the human exposure.

Apixaban administered to female rats at doses up to 1000 mg/kg/day from implantation through the end of lactation produced no adverse findings in male offspring (F_1 generation) at doses up to 1000 mg/kg/day, a dose resulting in exposure that is 5 times the human exposure. Adverse effects in the F_1-generation female offspring were limited to decreased mating and fertility indices at 1000 mg/kg/day.

14 CLINICAL STUDIES

14.1 ARISTOTLE

Evidence for the efficacy and safety of ELIQUIS (apixaban) was derived from ARISTOTLE, a multinational, double-blind study in patients with nonvalvular atrial fibrillation (AF) comparing the effects of ELIQUIS and warfarin on the risk of stroke and non-central nervous system (CNS) systemic embolism. In ARISTOTLE, patients were randomized to ELIQUIS 5 mg orally twice daily (or 2.5 mg twice daily in subjects with at least 2 of the following characteristics: age ≥80 years, body weight ≤60 kg, or serum creatinine ≥1.5 mg/dL) or to warfarin (targeted to an INR range of 2.0-3.0). Patients had to have one or more of the following additional risk factors for stroke:

- prior stroke or transient ischemic attack (TIA)
- prior systemic embolism
- age ≥75 years
- arterial hypertension requiring treatment
- diabetes mellitus
- heart failure ≥New York Heart Association Class 2
- left ventricular ejection fraction ≤40%

The primary objective of ARISTOTLE was to determine whether ELIQUIS 5 mg twice daily (or 2.5 mg twice daily) was effective (noninferior to warfarin) in reducing the risk of stroke (ischemic or hemorrhagic) and systemic embolism. Superiority of ELIQUIS to warfarin was also examined for the primary endpoint (rate of stroke and systemic embolism), major bleeding, and death from any cause.

A total of 18,201 patients were randomized and followed on study treatment for a median of 89 weeks. Forty-three percent of patients were vitamin K antagonist (VKA) "naive," defined as having received ≤30 consecutive days of treatment with warfarin or another VKA before entering the study. The mean age was 69 years and the mean $CHADS_2$ score (a scale from 0 to 6 used to estimate risk of stroke, with higher scores predicting greater risk) was 2.1. The population was 65% male, 83% Caucasian, 14% Asian, and 1% Black. There was a history of stroke, TIA, or non-CNS systemic embolism in 19% of patients. Concomitant diseases of patients in this study included hypertension 88%, diabetes 25%, congestive heart failure (or left ventricular ejection fraction ≤40%) 35%, and prior myocardial infarction 14%. Patients treated with warfarin in ARISTOTLE had a mean percentage of time in therapeutic range (INR 2.0-3.0) of 62%.

ELIQUIS was superior to warfarin for the primary endpoint of reducing the risk of stroke and systemic embolism (Table 3 and Figure 4). Superiority to warfarin was primarily attributable to a reduction in hemorrhagic stroke and ischemic strokes with hemorrhagic conversion compared to warfarin. Purely ischemic strokes occurred with similar rates on both drugs.

ELIQUIS also showed significantly fewer major bleeds than warfarin *[see Adverse Reactions (6.1)]*.

[See table 3 at top of next page]

[See figure 4 at top of next column]

All-cause death was assessed using a sequential testing strategy that allowed testing for superiority if effects on earlier endpoints (stroke plus systemic embolus and major bleeding) were demonstrated. ELIQUIS treatment resulted

Table 3: Key Efficacy Outcomes in Patients with Nonvalvular Atrial Fibrillation in ARISTOTLE (Intent-to-Treat Analysis)

	ELIQUIS N=9120 n (%/year)	Warfarin N=9081 n (%/year)	Hazard Ratio (95% CI)	P-value
Stroke or systemic embolism	212 (1.27)	265 (1.60)	0.79 (0.66, 0.95)	0.01
Stroke	199 (1.19)	250 (1.51)	0.79 (0.65, 0.95)	
Ischemic without hemorrhage	140 (0.83)	136 (0.82)	1.02 (0.81, 1.29)	
Ischemic with hemorrhagic conversion	12 (0.07)	20 (0.12)	0.60 (0.29, 1.23)	
Hemorrhagic	40 (0.24)	78 (0.47)	0.51 (0.35, 0.75)	
Unknown	14 (0.08)	21 (0.13)	0.65 (0.33, 1.29)	
Systemic embolism	15 (0.09)	17 (0.10)	0.87 (0.44, 1.75)	

The primary endpoint was based on the time to first event (one per subject). Component counts are for subjects with any event, not necessarily the first.

Table 4: Key Efficacy Outcomes in Patients with Nonvalvular Atrial Fibrillation in AVERROES

	ELIQUIS N=2807 n (%/year)	Aspirin N=2791 n (%/year)	Hazard Ratio (95% CI)	P-value
Stroke or systemic embolism	51 (1.62)	113 (3.63)	0.45 (0.32, 0.62)	<0.0001
Stroke				
Ischemic or undetermined	43 (1.37)	97 (3.11)	0.44 (0.31, 0.63)	-
Hemorrhagic	6 (0.19)	9 (0.28)	0.67 (0.24, 1.88)	-
Systemic embolism	2 (0.06)	13 (0.41)	0.15 (0.03, 0.68)	-
MI	24 (0.76)	28 (0.89)	0.86 (0.50, 1.48)	-
All-cause death	111 (3.51)	140 (4.42)	0.79 (0.62, 1.02)	0.068
Vascular death	84 (2.65)	96 (3.03)	0.87 (0.65, 1.17)	-

Tablet Strength	Tablet Color/Shape	Tablet Markings	Package Size	NDC Code
2.5 mg	Yellow, round, biconvex	Debossed with "893" on one side and "2½" on the other side	Bottles of 60	0003-0893-21
			Bottles of 180	0003-0893-41
			Hospital Unit-Dose Blister Package of 100	0003-0893-31
5 mg	Pink, oval, biconvex	Debossed with "894" on one side and "5" on the other side	Bottles of 60	0003-0894-21
			Bottles of 180	0003-0894-41
			Hospital Unit-Dose Blister Package of 100	0003-0894-31

Figure 4: Kaplan-Meier Estimate of Time to First Stroke or Systemic Embolism in ARISTOTLE (Intent-to-Treat Population)

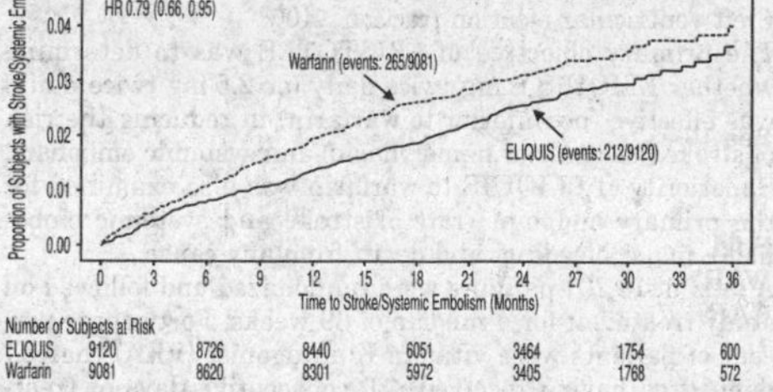

in a significantly lower rate of all-cause death (p = 0.046) than did treatment with warfarin, primarily because of a reduction in cardiovascular death, particularly stroke deaths. Non-vascular death rates were similar in the treatment arms.

In ARISTOTLE, the results for the primary efficacy endpoint were generally consistent across most major subgroups including weight, $CHADS_2$ score (a scale from 0 to 6 used to predict risk of stroke in patients with AF, with higher scores predicting greater risk), prior warfarin use, level of renal impairment, geographic region, ELIQUIS (apixaban) dose, type of AF, and aspirin use at randomization (Figure 5).

[See figure 5 at top of next column]

14.2 AVERROES

In AVERROES, patients with nonvalvular atrial fibrillation thought not to be candidates for warfarin therapy were randomized to treatment with ELIQUIS 5 mg orally twice daily (or 2.5 mg twice daily in selected patients) or aspirin 81 to 324 mg once daily. The primary objective of the study was to determine if ELIQUIS was superior to aspirin for preventing the composite outcome of stroke or systemic embolism. AVERROES was stopped early on the basis of a prespecified interim analysis showing a significant reduction in stroke and systemic embolism for ELIQUIS compared to aspirin

Figure 5: Stroke and Systemic Embolism Hazard Ratios by Baseline Characteristics – ARISTOTLE Study

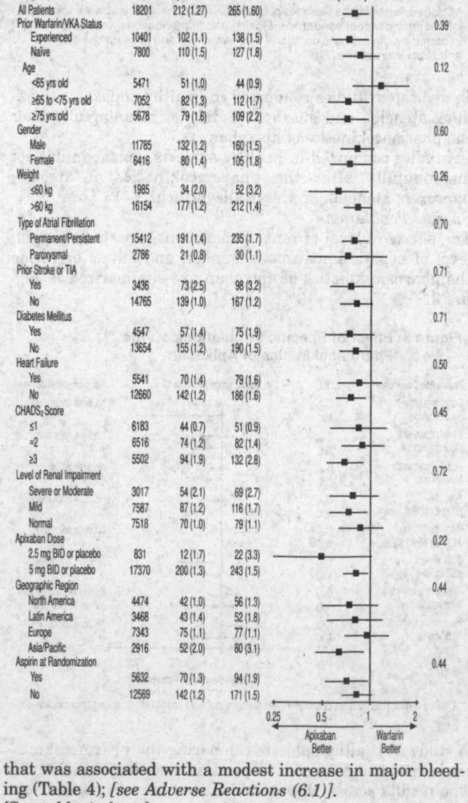
Subgroup | No. of Patients | No. of Events (% per yr) Apixaban | Warfarin | Hazard Ratio (95% CI) | P-value for Interaction
All Patients 18201 212 (1.27) 265 (1.60)
Prior Warfarin/VKA Status 0.39
Experienced 10401 102 (1.1) 138 (1.5)
Naïve 7800 110 (1.5) 127 (1.8)
Age 0.12
<65 yrs old 5471 51 (1.0) 44 (0.9)
≥65 to <75 yrs old 7052 82 (1.3) 112 (1.7)
≥75 yrs old 5678 79 (1.6) 109 (2.2)
Gender 0.60
Male 11785 132 (1.2) 160 (1.5)
Female 6416 80 (1.4) 105 (1.8)
Weight 0.26
≤60 kg 1985 34 (2.0) 52 (3.2)
>60 kg 16154 177 (1.2) 212 (1.4)
Type of Atrial Fibrillation 0.70
Permanent/Persistent 15412 191 (1.4) 235 (1.7)
Paroxysmal 2786 21 (0.8) 30 (1.1)
Prior Stroke or TIA 0.71
Yes 3436 73 (2.5) 98 (3.2)
No 14765 139 (1.0) 167 (1.2)
Diabetes Mellitus 0.71
Yes 4547 57 (1.4) 75 (1.9)
No 13654 155 (1.2) 190 (1.5)
Heart Failure 0.50
Yes 5541 70 (1.4) 79 (1.6)
No 12660 142 (1.2) 186 (1.6)
CHADS2 Score 0.45
≤1 6183 44 (0.7) 51 (0.9)
=2 6516 74 (1.2) 82 (1.4)
≥3 5502 94 (1.9) 132 (2.8)
Level of Renal Impairment 0.72
Severe or Moderate 3017 54 (2.1) 69 (2.7)
Mild 7587 87 (1.2) 116 (1.7)
Normal 7518 70 (1.0) 79 (1.1)
Apixaban Dose 0.22
2.5 mg BID or placebo 831 12 (1.7) 22 (3.3)
5 mg BID or placebo 17370 200 (1.3) 243 (1.5)
Geographic Region 0.44
North America 4474 42 (1.0) 56 (1.3)
Latin America 3468 43 (1.4) 52 (1.8)
Europe 7343 75 (1.1) 77 (1.1)
Asia/Pacific 2916 52 (2.0) 80 (3.1)
Aspirin at Randomization 0.44
Yes 5632 70 (1.3) 94 (1.9)
No 12569 142 (1.2) 171 (1.5)
0.25 0.5 1 2
Apixaban Better
Warfarin Better

that was associated with a modest increase in major bleeding (Table 4); *[see Adverse Reactions (6.1)]*.

[See table 4 above]

16 HOW SUPPLIED/STORAGE AND HANDLING

How Supplied

ELIQUIS (apixaban) tablets are available as listed in the table below.

[See third table below]

Storage and Handling

Store at 20°C to 25°C (68°F-77°F); excursions permitted between 15°C and 30°C (59°F-86°F) [see USP Controlled Room Temperature].

17 PATIENT COUNSELING INFORMATION

See FDA-approved patient labeling (Medication Guide).

Advise patients of the following:

- They should not discontinue ELIQUIS without talking to their physician first.
- They should be informed that it might take longer than usual for bleeding to stop, and they may bruise or bleed more easily when treated with ELIQUIS. Advise patients about how to recognize bleeding or symptoms of hypovolemia and of the urgent need to report any unusual bleeding to their physician.
- They should tell their physicians and dentists they are taking ELIQUIS, and/or any other product known to affect bleeding (including nonprescription products, such as aspirin or NSAIDs), before any surgery or medical or dental procedure is scheduled and before any new drug is taken.
- They should tell their physicians if they are pregnant or plan to become pregnant or are breastfeeding or intends to breastfeed during treatment with ELIQUIS *[see Use in Specific Populations (8.1, 8.3)]*.
- If a dose is missed, the dose should be taken as soon as possible on the same day and twice daily administration should be resumed. The dose should not be doubled to make up for a missed dose.

Manufactured by:
Bristol-Myers Squibb Company
Princeton, New Jersey 08543 USA
Marketed by:
Bristol-Myers Squibb Company
Princeton, New Jersey 08543 USA
and
Pfizer Inc
New York, New York 10017 USA

Rotachrom® is a registered trademark of Diagnostica Stago.
1289808 / 1298500 / 1289807
Issued December 2012

MEDICATION GUIDE
ELIQUIS® (ELL eh kwiss)
(apixaban)
tablets

What is the most important information I should know about ELIQUIS?

- People with atrial fibrillation (a type of irregular heartbeat) are at an increased risk of forming a blood clot in the heart, which can travel to the brain, causing a stroke, or to other parts of the body. ELIQUIS lowers your chance of having a stroke by helping to prevent clots from forming. If you stop taking ELIQUIS, you may have increased risk of forming a clot in your blood.

Do not stop taking ELIQUIS without talking to the doctor who prescribes it for you. Stopping ELIQUIS increases your risk of having a stroke.

ELIQUIS may need to be stopped, if possible, prior to surgery or a medical or dental procedure. Ask the doctor who prescribed ELIQUIS for you when you should stop taking it. Your doctor will tell you when you may start taking ELIQUIS again after your surgery or procedure. If you have to stop taking ELIQUIS, your doctor may prescribe another medicine to help prevent a blood clot from forming.

- **ELIQUIS can cause bleeding** which can be serious and rarely may lead to death. This is because ELIQUIS is a blood thinner medicine that reduces blood clotting.

You may have a higher risk of bleeding if you take ELIQUIS and take other medicines that increase your risk of bleeding, including:

- aspirin or aspirin-containing products
- long-term (chronic) use of nonsteroidal anti-inflammatory drugs (NSAIDs)
- warfarin sodium (COUMADIN®, JANTOVEN®)
- any medicine that contains heparin
- selective serotonin reuptake inhibitors (SSRIs) or serotonin norepinephrine reuptake inhibitors (SNRIs)
- other medicines to help prevent or treat blood clots

Tell your doctor if you take any of these medicines. Ask your doctor or pharmacist if you are not sure if your medicine is one listed above.

While taking ELIQUIS:

- you may bruise more easily
- it may take longer than usual for any bleeding to stop

Call your doctor or get medical help right away if you have any of these signs or symptoms of bleeding when taking ELIQUIS:

- unexpected bleeding, or bleeding that lasts a long time, such as:
  - unusual bleeding from the gums
  - nosebleeds that happen often
  - menstrual bleeding or vaginal bleeding that is heavier than normal
- bleeding that is severe or you cannot control
- red, pink, or brown urine
- red or black stools (looks like tar)
- cough up blood or blood clots
- vomit blood or your vomit looks like coffee grounds
- unexpected pain, swelling, or joint pain
- headaches, feeling dizzy or weak
- **ELIQUIS is not for patients with artificial heart valves.**

What is ELIQUIS?

ELIQUIS (apixaban) is a prescription medicine used to reduce the risk of stroke and blood clots in people who have atrial fibrillation.

It is not known if ELIQUIS is safe and effective in children.

Who should not take ELIQUIS?

Do not take ELIQUIS if you:

- currently have certain types of abnormal bleeding.
- have had a serious allergic reaction to ELIQUIS. Ask your doctor if you are not sure.

What should I tell my doctor before taking ELIQUIS?

Before you take ELIQUIS, tell your doctor if you:

- have kidney or liver problems
- have any other medical condition
- have ever had bleeding problems
- are pregnant or plan to become pregnant. It is not known if ELIQUIS will harm your unborn baby.
- are breastfeeding or plan to breastfeed. It is not known if ELIQUIS passes into your breast milk. You and your doctor should decide if you will take ELIQUIS or breastfeed. You should not do both.

Tell all of your doctors and dentists that you are taking ELIQUIS. They should talk to the doctor who prescribed ELIQUIS for you, before you have **any** surgery, medical or dental procedure.

Tell your doctor about all the medicines you take, including prescription and over-the-counter medicines, vitamins, and herbal supplements. Some of your other medicines may affect the way ELIQUIS works. Certain medicines may increase your risk of bleeding or stroke when taken with ELIQUIS. See **"What is the most important information I should know about ELIQUIS?"**

Know the medicines you take. Keep a list of them to show your doctor and pharmacist when you get a new medicine.

How should I take ELIQUIS?

- **Take ELIQUIS exactly as prescribed by your doctor.**
- Take ELIQUIS twice every day with or without food.
- Do not change your dose or stop taking ELIQUIS unless your doctor tells you to.
- If you miss a dose of ELIQUIS, take it as soon as you remember. Do not take more than one dose of ELIQUIS at the same time to make up for a missed dose.
- Your doctor will decide how long you should take ELIQUIS. **Do not stop taking it without first talking with your doctor. Stopping ELIQUIS may increase your risk of having a stroke.**
- **Do not run out of ELIQUIS. Refill your prescription before you run out.**
- If you take too much ELIQUIS, call your doctor or go to the nearest hospital emergency room right away.
- Call your doctor or healthcare provider right away if you fall or injure yourself, especially if you hit your head. Your doctor or healthcare provider may need to check you.

What are the possible side effects of ELIQUIS?

- See **"What is the most important information I should know about ELIQUIS?"**
- ELIQUIS can cause a skin rash or severe allergic reaction. Call your doctor or get medical help right away if you have any of the following symptoms:
  - chest pain or tightness
  - swelling of your face or tongue
  - trouble breathing or wheezing
  - feeling dizzy or faint

Tell your doctor if you have any side effect that bothers you or that does not go away.

These are not all of the possible side effects of ELIQUIS. For more information, ask your doctor or pharmacist.

Call your doctor for medical advice about side effects. You may report side effects to FDA at 1-800-FDA-1088.

How should I store ELIQUIS?

Store ELIQUIS at room temperature between 68°F to 77°F (20°C to 25°C).

Keep ELIQUIS and all medicines out of the reach of children.

General Information about ELIQUIS

Medicines are sometimes prescribed for purposes other than those listed in a Medication Guide. Do not use ELIQUIS for a condition for which it was not prescribed. Do not give ELIQUIS to other people, even if they have the same symptoms that you have. It may harm them.

If you would like more information, talk with your doctor. You can ask your pharmacist or doctor for information about ELIQUIS that is written for health professionals.

For more information, call 1-855-354-7847 (1-855-ELIQUIS) or go to www.ELIQUIS.com.

What are the ingredients in ELIQUIS?

Active ingredient: apixaban.

Inactive ingredients: anhydrous lactose, microcrystalline cellulose, croscarmellose sodium, sodium lauryl sulfate, and magnesium stearate. The film coating contains lactose monohydrate, hypromellose, titanium dioxide, triacetin, and yellow iron oxide (2.5 mg tablets) or red iron oxide (5 mg tablets).

This Medication Guide has been approved by the U.S. Food and Drug Administration.

Manufactured by:
Bristol-Myers Squibb Company
Princeton, New Jersey 08543 USA
Marketed by:
Bristol-Myers Squibb Company
Princeton, New Jersey 08543 USA
and
Pfizer Inc
New York, New York 10017 USA

COUMADIN® is a registered trademark of Bristol-Myers Squibb Pharma Company. All other trademarks are property of their respective companies.

1289808 / 1298500 / 1289807
1295958
Issued December 2012

Shown in Product Identification Guide, page 305

ERBITUX® ℞

[*ER-be-tux*]
(cetuximab)
injection, for intravenous infusion

HIGHLIGHTS OF PRESCRIBING INFORMATION
These highlights do not include all the information needed to use ERBITUX safely and effectively. See full prescribing information for ERBITUX.
ERBITUX® (cetuximab)
injection, for intravenous infusion
Initial U.S. Approval: 2004

> **WARNING: SERIOUS INFUSION REACTIONS and CARDIOPULMONARY ARREST**
>
> ***See full prescribing information for complete boxed warning.***
>
> - **Serious infusion reactions, some fatal, occurred in approximately 3% of patients. (5.1)**
> - **Cardiopulmonary arrest and/or sudden death occurred in 2% of patients with squamous cell carcinoma of the head and neck treated with Erbitux and radiation therapy and in 3% of patients with squamous cell carcinoma of the head and neck treated with cetuximab in combination with platinum-based therapy with 5-fluorouracil (5-FU). Closely monitor serum electrolytes, including serum magnesium, potassium, and calcium, during and after Erbitux administration. (5.2, 5.6)**

RECENT MAJOR CHANGES

Warnings and Precautions
Use of Erbitux in Combination With Radiation and Cisplatin (5.5) 03/2013

INDICATIONS AND USAGE

Erbitux® is an epidermal growth factor receptor (EGFR) antagonist indicated for treatment of:

Head and Neck Cancer

- Locally or regionally advanced squamous cell carcinoma of the head and neck in combination with radiation therapy. (1.1, 14.1)
- Recurrent locoregional disease or metastatic squamous cell carcinoma of the head and neck in combination with platinum-based therapy with 5-FU. (1.1, 14.1)
- Recurrent or metastatic squamous cell carcinoma of the head and neck progressing after platinum-based therapy. (1.1, 14.1)

Colorectal Cancer

K-Ras mutation-negative (wild-type), EGFR-expressing, metastatic colorectal cancer as determined by FDA-approved tests

- in combination with FOLFIRI for first-line treatment,
- in combination with irinotecan in patients who are refractory to irinotecan-based chemotherapy,
- as a single agent in patients who have failed oxaliplatin- and irinotecan-based chemotherapy or who are intolerant to irinotecan. (1.2, 5.7, 12.1, 14.2)

Limitation of Use: Erbitux is not indicated for treatment of *K-Ras* mutation-positive colorectal cancer. (5.7, 14.2)

DOSAGE AND ADMINISTRATION

- Premedicate with an H_1 antagonist. (2.3)
- Administer 400 mg/m^2 initial dose as a 120-minute intravenous infusion followed by 250 mg/m^2 weekly infused over 60 minutes. (2.1, 2.2)
- Initiate Erbitux one week prior to initiation of radiation therapy. Complete Erbitux administration 1 hour prior to platinum-based therapy with 5-FU (2.1) and FOLFIRI (2.2).
- Reduce the infusion rate by 50% for NCI CTC Grade 1 or 2 infusion reactions and non-serious NCI CTC Grade 3 infusion reaction. (2.4)
- Permanently discontinue for serious infusion reactions. (2.4)
- Withhold infusion for severe, persistent acneiform rash. Reduce dose for recurrent, severe rash. (2.4)

DOSAGE FORMS AND STRENGTHS

- 100 mg/50 mL, single-use vial (3)
- 200 mg/100 mL, single-use vial (3)

CONTRAINDICATIONS

None. (4)

WARNINGS AND PRECAUTIONS

- **Infusion Reactions:** Immediately stop and permanently discontinue Erbitux for serious infusion reactions. Monitor patients following infusion. (5.1)
- **Cardiopulmonary Arrest:** Closely monitor serum electrolytes during and after Erbitux. (5.2, 5.6)
- **Pulmonary Toxicity:** Interrupt therapy for acute onset or worsening of pulmonary symptoms. (5.3)
- **Dermatologic Toxicity:** Limit sun exposure. Monitor for inflammatory or infectious sequelae. (2.4, 5.4)
- **Hypomagnesemia:** Periodically monitor during and for at least 8 weeks following the completion of Erbitux. Replete electrolytes as necessary. (5.6)

ADVERSE REACTIONS

The most common adverse reactions (incidence ≥25%) are: cutaneous adverse reactions (including rash, pruritus, and nail changes), headache, diarrhea, and infection. (6)

To report SUSPECTED ADVERSE REACTIONS, contact Bristol-Myers Squibb at 1-800-721-5072 **or FDA at 1-800-FDA-1088 or www.fda.gov/medwatch.**

USE IN SPECIFIC POPULATIONS

- **Pregnancy:** Administer Erbitux to a pregnant woman only if the potential benefit justifies the potential risk to the fetus. (8.1)
- **Nursing Mothers:** Discontinue nursing during and for 60 days following treatment with Erbitux. (8.3)

See 17 for PATIENT COUNSELING INFORMATION

Revised: 08/2013

FULL PRESCRIBING INFORMATION: CONTENTS*

*** Sections or subsections omitted from the full prescribing information are not listed**

FULL PRESCRIBING INFORMATION

WARNING: SERIOUS INFUSION REACTIONS and CARDIOPULMONARY ARREST

Infusion Reactions: Serious infusion reactions occurred with the administration of Erbitux in approximately 3% of patients in clinical trials, with fatal outcome reported in less than 1 in 1000. [See *Warnings and Precautions (5.1), Adverse Reactions (6)*.] Immediately interrupt and permanently discontinue Erbitux infusion for serious infusion reactions. [See *Dosage and Administration (2.4), Warnings and Precautions (5.1)*.]

Cardiopulmonary Arrest: Cardiopulmonary arrest and/or sudden death occurred in 2% of patients with squamous cell carcinoma of the head and neck treated with Erbitux and radiation therapy in Study 1 and in 3% of patients with squamous cell carcinoma of the head and neck treated with European Union (EU)-approved cetuximab in combination with platinum-based therapy with 5-fluorouracil (5-FU) in Study 2. Closely monitor serum electrolytes, including serum magnesium, potassium, and calcium, during and after Erbitux administration. [See *Warnings and Precautions (5.2, 5.6), Clinical Studies (14.1)*.]

1 INDICATIONS AND USAGE

1.1 Squamous Cell Carcinoma of the Head and Neck (SCCHN)

Erbitux® (cetuximab) is indicated in combination with radiation therapy for the initial treatment of locally or regionally advanced squamous cell carcinoma of the head and neck. [See *Clinical Studies (14.1)*.]

Erbitux is indicated in combination with platinum-based therapy with 5-FU for the first-line treatment of patients with recurrent locoregional disease or metastatic squamous cell carcinoma of the head and neck. [See *Clinical Studies (14.1)*.]

Erbitux, as a single agent, is indicated for the treatment of patients with recurrent or metastatic squamous cell carcinoma of the head and neck for whom prior platinum-based therapy has failed. [See *Clinical Studies (14.1)*.]

1.2 *K-Ras* Mutation-negative, EGFR-expressing Colorectal Cancer

Erbitux is indicated for the treatment of *K-Ras* mutation-negative (wild-type), epidermal growth factor receptor (EGFR)-expressing, metastatic colorectal cancer (mCRC) as determined by FDA-approved tests for this use [see *Dosage and Administration (2.2), Warnings and Precautions (5.7), Clinical Studies (14.2)*]

- in combination with FOLFIRI (irinotecan, 5-fluorouracil, leucovorin) for first-line treatment,
- in combination with irinotecan in patients who are refractory to irinotecan-based chemotherapy,
- as a single agent in patients who have failed oxaliplatin- and irinotecan-based chemotherapy or who are intolerant to irinotecan. [See *Warnings and Precautions (5.7), Clinical Pharmacology (12.1), Clinical Studies (14.2)*.]

Limitation of Use: Erbitux is not indicated for treatment of *K-Ras* mutation-positive colorectal cancer [see *Warnings and Precautions (5.7), Clinical Studies (14.2)*].

2 DOSAGE AND ADMINISTRATION

2.1 Squamous Cell Carcinoma of the Head and Neck

Erbitux in combination with radiation therapy or in combination with platinum-based therapy with 5-FU:

- The recommended initial dose is 400 mg/m² administered one week prior to initiation of a course of radiation therapy or on the day of initiation of platinum-based therapy with 5-FU as a 120-minute intravenous infusion (maximum infusion rate 10 mg/min). Complete Erbitux administration 1 hour prior to platinum-based therapy with 5-FU.
- The recommended subsequent weekly dose (all other infusions) is 250 mg/m² infused over 60 minutes (maximum infusion rate 10 mg/min) for the duration of radiation therapy (6–7 weeks) or until disease progression or unacceptable toxicity when administered in combination with platinum-based therapy with 5-FU. Complete Erbitux administration 1 hour prior to radiation therapy or platinum-based therapy with 5-FU.

Erbitux (cetuximab) monotherapy:

- The recommended initial dose is 400 mg/m² administered as a 120-minute intravenous infusion (maximum infusion rate 10 mg/min).
- The recommended subsequent weekly dose (all other infusions) is 250 mg/m² infused over 60 minutes (maximum infusion rate 10 mg/min) until disease progression or unacceptable toxicity.

2.2 Colorectal Cancer

- Determine *K-Ras* mutation and EGFR-expression status using FDA-approved tests prior to initiating treatment. Only patients whose tumors are *K-Ras* mutation-negative (wild-type) should receive Erbitux.
- The recommended initial dose, either as monotherapy or in combination with irinotecan or FOLFIRI (irinotecan, 5-fluorouracil, leucovorin), is 400 mg/m² administered as a 120-minute intravenous infusion (maximum infusion rate 10 mg/min). Complete Erbitux (cetuximab) administration 1 hour prior to FOLFIRI.
- The recommended subsequent weekly dose, either as monotherapy or in combination with irinotecan or FOLFIRI, is 250 mg/m² infused over 60 minutes (maximum infusion rate 10 mg/min) until disease progression or unacceptable toxicity. Complete Erbitux administration 1 hour prior to FOLFIRI.

2.3 Recommended Premedication

Premedicate with an H_1 antagonist (eg, 50 mg of diphenhydramine) intravenously 30–60 minutes prior to the first dose; premedication should be administered for subsequent Erbitux doses based upon clinical judgment and presence/severity of prior infusion reactions.

2.4 Dose Modifications

Infusion Reactions

Reduce the infusion rate by 50% for NCI CTC Grade 1 or 2 and non-serious NCI CTC Grade 3 infusion reaction.

Immediately and permanently discontinue Erbitux for serious infusion reactions, requiring medical intervention and/or hospitalization. [See *Warnings and Precautions (5.1)*.]

Dermatologic Toxicity

Recommended dose modifications for severe (NCI CTC Grade 3 or 4) acneiform rash are specified in Table 1. [See *Warnings and Precautions (5.4)*.]

[See table 1 above]

Table 1: Erbitux Dose Modification Guidelines for Rash

Severe Acneiform Rash	Erbitux	Outcome	Erbitux Dose Modification
1st occurrence	Delay infusion 1 to 2 weeks	Improvement No Improvement	Continue at 250 mg/m² Discontinue Erbitux
2nd occurrence	Delay infusion 1 to 2 weeks	Improvement No Improvement	Reduce dose to 200 mg/m² Discontinue Erbitux
3rd occurrence	Delay infusion 1 to 2 weeks	Improvement No Improvement	Reduce dose to 150 mg/m² Discontinue Erbitux
4th occurrence	Discontinue Erbitux		

Table 2: Incidence of Selected Adverse Reactions (≥10%) in Patients with Locoregionally Advanced SCCHN

Body System Preferred Term	Erbitux plus Radiation (n=208)		Radiation Therapy Alone (n=212)	
	Grades 1–4	Grades 3 and 4	Grades 1–4	Grades 3 and 4
	% of Patients			
Body as a Whole				
Asthenia	56	4	49	5
Fever[a]	29	1	13	1
Headache	19	<1	8	<1
Infusion Reaction[b]	15	3	2	0
Infection	13	1	9	1
Chills[a]	16	0	5	0
Digestive				
Nausea	49	2	37	2
Emesis	29	2	23	4
Diarrhea	19	2	13	1
Dyspepsia	14	0	9	1
Metabolic/Nutritional				
Weight Loss	84	11	72	7
Dehydration	25	6	19	8
Alanine Transaminase, high[c]	43	2	21	1
Aspartate Transaminase, high[c]	38	1	24	1
Alkaline Phosphatase, high[c]	33	<1	24	0
Respiratory				
Pharyngitis	26	3	19	4
Skin/Appendages				
Acneiform Rash[d]	87	17	10	1
Radiation Dermatitis	86	23	90	18
Application Site Reaction	18	0	12	1
Pruritus	16	0	4	0

[a] Includes cases also reported as infusion reaction.

[b] Infusion reaction is defined as any event described at any time during the clinical study as "allergic reaction" or "anaphylactoid reaction", or any event occurring on the first day of dosing described as "allergic reaction", "anaphylactoid reaction", "fever", "chills", "chills and fever", or "dyspnea".

[c] Based on laboratory measurements, not on reported adverse reactions, the number of subjects with tested samples varied from 205–206 for Erbitux plus Radiation arm; 209–210 for Radiation alone.

[d] Acneiform rash is defined as any event described as "acne", "rash", "maculopapular rash", "pustular rash", "dry skin", or "exfoliative dermatitis".

2.5 Preparation for Administration

Do not administer Erbitux as an intravenous push or bolus.

Administer via infusion pump or syringe pump. Do not exceed an infusion rate of 10 mg/min.

Administer through a low protein binding 0.22-micrometer in-line filter.

Parenteral drug products should be inspected visually for particulate matter and discoloration prior to administration, whenever solution and container permit.

The solution should be clear and colorless and may contain a small amount of easily visible, white, amorphous, cetuximab particulates. **Do not shake or dilute.**

3 DOSAGE FORMS AND STRENGTHS

100 mg/50 mL, single-use vial

200 mg/100 mL, single-use vial

4 CONTRAINDICATIONS

None.

5 WARNINGS AND PRECAUTIONS

5.1 Infusion Reactions

Serious infusion reactions, requiring medical intervention and immediate, permanent discontinuation of Erbitux included rapid onset of airway obstruction (bronchospasm, stridor, hoarseness), hypotension, shock, loss of consciousness, myocardial infarction, and/or cardiac arrest. Severe (NCI CTC Grades 3 and 4) infusion reactions occurred in 2–5% of 1373 patients in Studies 1, 3, 5, and 6 receiving Erbitux, with fatal outcome in 1 patient. [See *Clinical Studies (14.1, 14.2).*]

Approximately 90% of severe infusion reactions occurred with the first infusion despite premedication with antihistamines.

Monitor patients for 1 hour following Erbitux infusions in a setting with resuscitation equipment and other agents necessary to treat anaphylaxis (eg, epinephrine, corticosteroids, intravenous antihistamines, bronchodilators, and oxygen). Monitor longer to confirm resolution of the event in patients requiring treatment for infusion reactions.

Immediately and permanently discontinue Erbitux in patients with serious infusion reactions. [See *Boxed Warning, Dosage and Administration (2.4).*]

5.2 Cardiopulmonary Arrest

Cardiopulmonary arrest and/or sudden death occurred in 4 (2%) of 208 patients treated with radiation therapy and Erbitux as compared to none of 212 patients treated with radiation therapy alone in Study 1. Three patients with prior history of coronary artery disease died at home, with myocardial infarction as the presumed cause of death. One of these patients had arrhythmia and one had congestive heart failure. Death occurred 27, 32, and 43 days after the last dose of Erbitux (cetuximab). One patient with no prior history of coronary artery disease died one day after the last dose of Erbitux. In Study 2, fatal cardiac disorders and/or sudden death occurred in 7 (3%) of 219 patients treated with EU-approved cetuximab and platinum-based therapy with 5-FU as compared to 4 (2%) of 215 patients treated with chemotherapy alone. Five of these 7 patients in the chemotherapy plus cetuximab arm received concomitant cisplatin and 2 patients received concomitant carboplatin. All 4 patients in the chemotherapy-alone arm received cisplatin. Carefully consider use of Erbitux in combination with radiation therapy or platinum-based therapy with 5-FU in head and neck cancer patients with a history of coronary artery disease, congestive heart failure, or arrhythmias in light of these risks. Closely monitor serum electrolytes, including serum magnesium, potassium, and calcium, during and after Erbitux. [See *Boxed Warning, Warnings and Precautions (5.6).*]

5.3 Pulmonary Toxicity

Interstitial lung disease (ILD), including 1 fatality, occurred in 4 of 1570 (<0.5%) patients receiving Erbitux in Studies 1, 3, and 6, as well as other studies, in colorectal cancer and head and neck cancer. Interrupt Erbitux for acute onset or worsening of pulmonary symptoms. Permanently discontinue Erbitux for confirmed ILD.

5.4 Dermatologic Toxicity

Dermatologic toxicities, including acneiform rash, skin drying and fissuring, paronychial inflammation, infectious sequelae (for example, *S. aureus* sepsis, abscess formation, cellulitis, blepharitis, conjunctivitis, keratitis/ulcerative keratitis with decreased visual acuity, cheilitis), and hypertrichosis occurred in patients receiving Erbitux therapy. Acneiform rash occurred in 76–88% of 1373 patients receiving Erbitux in Studies 1, 3, 5, and 6. Severe acneiform rash occurred in 1–17% of patients.

Acneiform rash usually developed within the first two weeks of therapy and resolved in a majority of the patients after cessation of treatment, although in nearly half, the event continued beyond 28 days. Monitor patients receiving Erbitux for dermatologic toxicities and infectious sequelae. Instruct patients to limit sun exposure during Erbitux therapy. [See *Dosage and Administration (2.4).*]

Table 3: Incidence of Selected Adverse Reactions (≥10%) in Patients with Recurrent Locoregional Disease or Metastatic SCCHN

System Organ Class Preferred Term	EU-Approved Cetuximab plus Platinum-based Therapy with 5-FU (n=219) Grades 1–4	EU-Approved Cetuximab plus Platinum-based Therapy with 5-FU (n=219) Grades 3 and 4	Platinum-based Therapy with 5-FU Alone (n=215) Grades 1–4	Platinum-based Therapy with 5-FU Alone (n=215) Grades 3 and 4
	% of Patients			
Eye Disorders				
Conjunctivitis	10	0	0	0
Gastrointestinal Disorders				
Nausea	54	4	47	4
Diarrhea	26	5	16	1
General Disorders and Administration Site Conditions				
Pyrexia	22	0	13	1
Infusion Reaction[a]	10	2	<1	0
Infections and Infestations				
Infection[b]	44	11	27	8
Metabolism and Nutrition Disorders				
Anorexia	25	5	14	1
Hypocalcemia	12	4	5	1
Hypokalemia	12	7	7	5
Hypomagnesemia	11	5	5	1
Skin and Subcutaneous Tissue Disorders				
Acneiform Rash[c]	70	9	2	0
Rash	28	5	2	0
Acne	22	2	0	0
Dermatitis Acneiform	15	2	0	0
Dry Skin	14	0	<1	0
Alopecia	12	0	7	0

[a] Infusion reaction defined as any event of "anaphylactic reaction", "hypersensitivity", "fever and/or chills", "dyspnea", or "pyrexia" on the first day of dosing.

[b] Infection – this term excludes sepsis-related events which are presented separately.

[c] Acneiform rash defined as any event described as "acne", "dermatitis acneiform", "dry skin", "exfoliative rash", "rash", "rash erythematous", "rash macular", "rash papular", or "rash pustular".

Chemotherapy = cisplatin + 5-fluorouracil or carboplatin + 5-fluorouracil

5.5 Use of Erbitux in Combination With Radiation and Cisplatin

In a controlled study, 940 patients with locally advanced SCCHN were randomized 1:1 to receive either Erbitux (cetuximab) in combination with radiation therapy and cisplatin or radiation therapy and cisplatin alone. The addition of Erbitux resulted in an increase in the incidence of Grade 3–4 mucositis, radiation recall syndrome, acneiform rash, cardiac events, and electrolyte disturbances compared to radiation and cisplatin alone. Adverse reactions with fatal outcome were reported in 20 patients (4.4%) in the Erbitux combination arm and 14 patients (3.0%) in the control arm. Nine patients in the Erbitux arm (2.0%) experienced myocardial ischemia compared to 4 patients (0.9%) in the control arm. The main efficacy outcome of the study was progression-free survival (PFS). The addition of Erbitux to radiation and cisplatin did not improve PFS.

5.6 Hypomagnesemia and Electrolyte Abnormalities

In patients evaluated during clinical trials, hypomagnesemia occurred in 55% of 365 patients receiving Erbitux in Study 5 and two other clinical trials in colorectal cancer and head and neck cancer, respectively, and was severe (NCI CTC Grades 3 and 4) in 6–17%.

In Study 2, where EU-approved cetuximab was administered in combination with platinum-based therapy, the addition of cetuximab to cisplatin and 5-FU resulted in an increased incidence of hypomagnesemia (14% vs. 6%) and of Grade 3–4 hypomagnesemia (7% vs. 2%) compared to cisplatin and 5-FU alone. In contrast, the incidences of hypomagnesemia were similar for those who received cetuximab, carboplatin, and 5-FU compared to carboplatin and 5-FU (4% vs. 4%). No patient experienced Grade 3–4 hypomagnesemia in either arm in the carboplatin subgroup.

The onset of hypomagnesemia and accompanying electrolyte abnormalities occurred days to months after initiation of Erbitux. Periodically monitor patients for hypomagnesemia, hypocalcemia, and hypokalemia, during and for at least 8 weeks following the completion of Erbitux. Replete electrolytes as necessary.

5.7 *K-Ras* Testing in Metastatic or Advanced Colorectal Cancer Patients

Determination of *K-Ras* mutational status in colorectal tumors using an FDA-approved test indicated for this use is necessary for selection of patients for treatment with Erbitux. Erbitux is indicated only for patients with EGFR-expressing *K-Ras* mutation-negative (wild-type) mCRC. Erbitux is not an effective treatment for patients with colorectal cancer that harbor somatic mutations in codons 12 and 13 (exon 2). Studies 4 and 5, conducted in patients with colorectal cancer, demonstrated a benefit with Erbitux (cetuximab) treatment only in the subset of patients whose tumors were *K-Ras* mutation-negative (wild-type). Erbitux is not effective for the treatment of *K-Ras* mutation-positive colorectal cancer as determined by an FDA-approved test for this use. [See *Indications and Usage (1.2), Clinical Pharmacology (12.1), Clinical Studies (14.2).*]

Perform the assesment for *K-Ras* mutation status in colorectal cancer in laboratories with demonstrated proficiency in the specific technology being utilized. Improper assay performance can lead to unreliable test results.

Refer to an FDA-approved test's package insert for instructions on the identification of patients eligible for the treatment of Erbitux.

5.8 Epidermal Growth Factor Receptor (EGFR) Expression and Response

Because expression of EGFR has been detected in nearly all SCCHN tumor specimens, patients enrolled in the head and neck cancer clinical studies were not required to have immunohistochemical evidence of EGFR tumor expression prior to study entry.

Patients enrolled in the colorectal cancer clinical studies were required to have immunohistochemical evidence of EGFR tumor expression. Primary tumor or tumor from a metastatic site was tested with the DakoCytomation EGFR pharmDx™ test kit. Specimens were scored based on the percentage of cells expressing EGFR and intensity (barely/faint, weak-to-moderate, and strong). Response rate did not correlate with either the percentage of positive cells or the intensity of EGFR expression.

6 ADVERSE REACTIONS

The following adverse reactions are discussed in greater detail in other sections of the label:

- Infusion reactions [See *Boxed Warning, Warnings and Precautions (5.1).*]
- Cardiopulmonary arrest [See *Boxed Warning, Warnings and Precautions (5.2).*]
- Pulmonary toxicity [See *Warnings and Precautions (5.3).*]
- Dermatologic toxicity [See *Warnings and Precautions (5.4).*]
- Hypomagnesemia and Electrolyte Abnormalities [See *Warnings and Precautions (5.6).*]

The most common adverse reactions in Erbitux clinical trials (incidence ≥25%) include cutaneous adverse reactions (including rash, pruritus, and nail changes), headache, diarrhea, and infection.

The most serious adverse reactions with Erbitux are infusion reactions, cardiopulmonary arrest, dermatologic toxicity and radiation dermatitis, sepsis, renal failure, interstitial lung disease, and pulmonary embolus.

Table 4: Incidence of Selected Adverse Reactions Occurring in ≥10% of Patients with *K-Ras* Mutation-negative (Wild-type) and EGFR-expressing, Metastatic Colorectal Cancer[a]

Body System Preferred Term	EU-Approved Cetuximab plus FOLFIRI (n=317)		FOLFIRI Alone (n=350)	
	Grades 1–4[b]	Grades 3 and 4	Grades 1–4	Grades 3 and 4
	% of Patients			
Blood and Lymphatic System Disorders				
Neutropenia	49	31	42	24
Eye Disorders				
Conjunctivitis	18	<1	3	0
Gastrointestinal Disorders				
Diarrhea	66	16	60	10
Stomatitis	31	3	19	1
Dyspepsia	16	0	9	0
General Disorders and Administration Site Conditions				
Infusion-related Reaction[c]	14	2	<1	0
Pyrexia	26	1	14	1
Infections and Infestations				
Paronychia	20	4	<1	0
Investigations				
Weight Decreased	15	1	9	1
Metabolism and Nutrition Disorders				
Anorexia	30	3	23	2
Skin and Subcutaneous Tissue Disorders				
Acne-like Rash[d]	86	18	13	<1
Rash	44	9	4	0
Dermatitis Acneiform	26	5	<1	0
Dry Skin	22	0	4	0
Acne	14	2	0	0
Pruritus	14	0	3	0
Palmar-plantar Erythrodysesthesia Syndrome	19	4	4	<1
Skin Fissures	19	2	1	0

[a] Adverse reactions occurring in at least 10% of Erbitux combination arm with a frequency at least 5% greater than that seen in the FOLFIRI arm.

[b] Adverse reactions were graded using the NCI CTC, V 2.0.

[c] Infusion related reaction is defined as any event meeting the medical concepts of allergy/anaphylaxis at any time during the clinical study or any event occurring on the first day of dosing and meeting the medical concepts of dyspnea and fever or by the following events using MedDRA preferred terms: "acute myocardial infarction", "angina pectoris", "angioedema", "autonomic seizure", "blood pressure abnormal", "blood pressure decreased", "blood pressure increased", "cardiac failure", "cardiopulmonary failure", "cardiovascular insufficiency", "clonus", "convulsion", "coronary no-reflow phenomenon", "epilepsy", "hypertension", "hypertensive crisis", "hypertensive emergency", "hypotension", "infusion related reaction", "loss of consciousness", "myocardial infarction", "myocardial ischaemia", "prinzmetal angina", "shock", "sudden death", "syncope", or "systolic hypertension".

[d] Acne-like rash is defined by the events using MedDRA preferred terms and included "acne", "acne pustular", "butterfly rash", "dermatitis acneiform", "drug rash with eosinophilia and systemic symptoms", "dry skin", "erythema", "exfoliative rash", "folliculitis", "genital rash", "mucocutaneous rash", "pruritus", "rash", "rash erythematous", "rash follicular", "rash generalized", "rash macular", "rash maculopapular", "rash maculovesicular", "rash morbilliform", "rash papular", "rash papulosquamous", "rash pruritic", "rash pustular", "rash rubelliform", "rash scarlatiniform", "rash vesicular", "skin exfoliation", "skin hyperpigmentation", "skin plaque", "telangiectasia", or "xerosis".

Across Studies 1, 3, 5, and 6, Erbitux (cetuximab) was discontinued in 3–10% of patients because of adverse reactions.

6.1 Clinical Trials Experience

Because clinical trials are conducted under widely varying conditions, adverse reaction rates observed in the clinical trials of a drug cannot be directly compared to rates in the clinical trials of another drug and may not reflect the rates observed in practice.

The data below reflect exposure to Erbitux in 1373 patients with SCCHN or colorectal cancer in randomized Phase 3 (Studies 1 and 5) or Phase 2 (Studies 3 and 6) trials treated at the recommended dose and schedule for medians of 7 to 14 weeks. [See *Clinical Studies (14)*.]

Infusion reactions: Infusion reactions, which included pyrexia, chills, rigors, dyspnea, bronchospasm, angioedema, urticaria, hypertension, and hypotension occurred in 15–21% of patients across studies. Grades 3 and 4 infusion reactions occurred in 2–5% of patients; infusion reactions were fatal in 1 patient.

Infections: The incidence of infection was variable across studies, ranging from 13–35%. Sepsis occurred in 1–4% of patients.

Renal: Renal failure occurred in 1% of patients with colorectal cancer.

Squamous Cell Carcinoma of the Head and Neck

Erbitux in Combination with Radiation Therapy

Table 2 contains selected adverse reactions in 420 patients receiving radiation therapy either alone or with Erbitux for locally or regionally advanced SCCHN in Study 1. Erbitux was administered at the recommended dose and schedule (400 mg/m^2 initial dose, followed by 250 mg/m^2 weekly). Patients received a median of 8 infusions (range 1–11).

[See table 2 at top of page 724]

The incidence and severity of mucositis, stomatitis, and xerostomia were similar in both arms of the study.

Late Radiation Toxicity

The overall incidence of late radiation toxicities (any grade) was higher in Erbitux (cetuximab) in combination with radiation therapy compared with radiation therapy alone. The following sites were affected: salivary glands (65% versus 56%), larynx (52% versus 36%), subcutaneous tissue (49% versus 45%), mucous membrane (48% versus 39%), esophagus (44% versus 35%), skin (42% versus 33%). The incidence of Grade 3 or 4 late radiation toxicities was similar between the radiation therapy alone and the Erbitux plus radiation treatment groups.

Study 2: EU-Approved Cetuximab in Combination with Platinum-based Therapy with 5-Fluorouracil

Study 2 used EU-approved cetuximab. Since U.S.-licensed Erbitux provides approximately 22% higher exposure relative to the EU-approved cetuximab, the data provided below may underestimate the incidence and severity of adverse reactions anticipated with Erbitux for this indication. However, the tolerability of the recommended dose is supported by safety data from additional studies of Erbitux [see *Clinical Pharmacology (12.3)*].

Table 3 contains selected adverse reactions in 434 patients with recurrent locoregional disease or metastatic SCCHN receiving EU-approved cetuximab in combination with platinum-based therapy with 5-FU or platinum-based therapy with 5-FU alone in Study 2. Cetuximab was administered at 400 mg/m^2 for the initial dose, followed by 250 mg/m^2 weekly. Patients received a median of 17 infusions (range 1–89).

[See table 3 at top of previous page]

For cardiac disorders, approximately 9% of subjects in both the EU-approved cetuximab plus chemotherapy and chemotherapy-only treatment arms in Study 2 experienced a cardiac event. The majority of these events occurred in patients who received cisplatin/5-FU, with or without cetuximab as follows: 11% and 12% in patients who received cisplatin/5-FU with or without cetuximab, respectively, and 6% or 4% in patients who received carboplatin/5-FU with or without cetuximab, respectively. In both arms, the incidence of cardiovascular events was higher in the cisplatin with 5-FU containing subgroup. Death attributed to cardiovascular event or sudden death was reported in 3% of the patients in the cetuximab plus platinum-based therapy with 5-FU arm and 2% in the platinum-based chemotherapy with 5-FU alone arm.

Colorectal Cancer

Study 4: EU-Approved Cetuximab in Combination with FOLFIRI

Study 4 used EU-approved cetuximab. U.S.-licensed Erbitux (cetuximab) provides approximately 22% higher exposure to cetuximab relative to the EU-approved cetuximab. The data provided below for Study 4 is consistent in incidence and severity of adverse reactions with those seen for Erbitux in this indication. The tolerability of the recommended dose is supported by safety data from additional studies of Erbitux [see *Clinical Pharmacology (12.3)*].

Table 4 contains selected adverse reactions in 667 patients with *K-Ras* mutation-negative (wild-type), EGFR-expressing, metastatic colorectal cancer receiving EU-approved cetuximab plus FOLFIRI or FOLFIRI alone in Study 4 [see *Warnings and Precautions (5.8)*]. Cetuximab was administered at the recommended dose and schedule (400 mg/m^2 initial dose, followed by 250 mg/m^2 weekly). Patients received a median of 26 infusions (range 1–224).

[See table 4 above]

Erbitux Monotherapy

Table 5 contains selected adverse reactions in 242 patients with *K-Ras* mutation-negative (wild-type), EGFR-expressing, metastatic colorectal cancer who received best supportive care (BSC) alone or with Erbitux in Study 5 [see *Warnings and Precautions (5.8)*]. Erbitux was administered at the recommended dose and schedule (400 mg/m^2 initial dose, followed by 250 mg/m^2 weekly). Patients received a median of 17 infusions (range 1–51).

[See table 5 at top of next page]

Erbitux in Combination with Irinotecan

The most frequently reported adverse reactions in 354 patients treated with Erbitux plus irinotecan in clinical trials were acneiform rash (88%), asthenia/malaise (73%), diarrhea (72%), and nausea (55%). The most common Grades 3–4 adverse reactions included diarrhea (22%), leukopenia (17%), asthenia/malaise (16%), and acneiform rash (14%).

6.2 Immunogenicity

As with all therapeutic proteins, there is potential for immunogenicity. Immunogenic responses to cetuximab were assessed using either a double antigen radiometric assay or an ELISA assay. Due to limitations in assay performance and sampling timing, the incidence of antibody development in patients receiving Erbitux has not been adequately determined. Non-neutralizing anti-cetuximab antibodies were detected in 5% (49 of 1001) of evaluable patients without apparent effect on the safety or antitumor activity of Erbitux.

The incidence of antibody formation is highly dependent on the sensitivity and specificity of the assay. Additionally, the observed incidence of antibody (including neutralizing antibody) positivity in an assay may be influenced by several factors including assay methodology, sample handling, timing of sample collection, concomitant medications, and underlying disease. For these reasons, comparison of the incidence of antibodies to Erbitux with the incidence of antibodies to other products may be misleading.

6.3 Postmarketing Experience

The following adverse reactions have been identified during post-approval use of Erbitux. Because these reactions are reported from a population of uncertain size, it is not always possible to reliably estimate their frequency or establish a causal relationship to drug exposure.

- Aseptic meningitis
- Mucosal inflammation

7 DRUG INTERACTIONS

A drug interaction study was performed in which Erbitux was administered in combination with irinotecan. There was no evidence of any pharmacokinetic interactions between Erbitux and irinotecan.

8 USE IN SPECIFIC POPULATIONS

8.1 Pregnancy

Pregnancy Category C

There are no adequate and well-controlled studies of Erbitux in pregnant women. Based on animal models, EGFR has been implicated in the control of prenatal development and may be essential for normal organogenesis, proliferation, and differentiation in the developing embryo. Human IgG is known to cross the placental barrier; therefore, Erbitux may be transmitted from the mother to the developing fetus, and has the potential to cause fetal harm when administered to pregnant women. Erbitux (cetuximab) should be used during pregnancy only if the potential benefit justifies the potential risk to the fetus.

Pregnant cynomolgus monkeys were treated weekly with 0.4 to 4 times the recommended human dose of cetuximab (based on body surface area) during the period of organogenesis (gestation day [GD] 20–48). Cetuximab was detected in the amniotic fluid and in the serum of embryos from treated dams at GD 49. No fetal malformations or other teratogenic effects occurred in offspring. However, significant increases in embryolethality and abortions occurred at doses of approximately 1.6 to 4 times the recommended human dose of cetuximab (based on total body surface area).

8.3 Nursing Mothers

It is not known whether Erbitux is secreted in human milk. IgG antibodies, such as Erbitux, can be excreted in human milk. Because many drugs are excreted in human milk and because of the potential for serious adverse reactions in nursing infants from Erbitux, a decision should be made whether to discontinue nursing or to discontinue the drug, taking into account the importance of the drug to the mother. If nursing is interrupted, based on the mean half-life of cetuximab [see *Clinical Pharmacology (12.3)*], nursing should not be resumed earlier than 60 days following the last dose of Erbitux.

8.4 Pediatric Use

The safety and effectiveness of Erbitux in pediatric patients have not been established. The pharmacokinetics of cetuximab, in combination with irinotecan, were evaluated in pediatric patients with refractory solid tumors in an open-label, single-arm, dose-finding study. Erbitux was administered once-weekly, at doses up to 250 mg/m^2, to 27 patients ranging from 1 to 12 years old; and in 19 patients ranging from 13 to 18 years old. No new safety signals were identified in pediatric patients. The pharmacokinetic profiles of cetuximab between the two age groups were similar at the 75 and 150 mg/m^2 single dose levels. The volume of the distribution appeared to be independent of dose and approximated the vascular space of 2–3 L/m^2. Following a single dose of 250 mg/m^2, the geometric mean $AUC_{0\text{-}inf}$ (CV%) value was 17.7 mg•h/mL (34%) in the younger age group (1–12 years, n=9) and 13.4 mg•h/mL (38%) in the adolescent group (13–18 years, n=6). The mean half-life of cetuximab was 110 hours (range 69 to 188 hours) for the younger age group, and 82 hours (range 55 to 117 hours) for the adolescent age group.

8.5 Geriatric Use

Of the 1662 patients who received Erbitux with irinotecan, FOLFIRI or Erbitux monotherapy in six studies of advanced colorectal cancer, 588 patients were 65 years of age or older. No overall differences in safety or efficacy were observed between these patients and younger patients.

Clinical studies of Erbitux conducted in patients with head and neck cancer did not include sufficient number of subjects aged 65 and over to determine whether they respond differently from younger subjects.

10 OVERDOSAGE

The maximum single dose of Erbitux administered is 1000 mg/m^2 in one patient. No adverse events were reported for this patient.

11 DESCRIPTION

Erbitux® (cetuximab) is a recombinant, human/mouse chimeric monoclonal antibody that binds specifically to the extracellular domain of the human epidermal growth factor receptor (EGFR). Cetuximab is composed of the Fv regions of a murine anti-EGFR antibody with human IgG1 heavy and kappa light chain constant regions and has an approximate molecular weight of 152 kDa. Cetuximab is produced in mammalian (murine myeloma) cell culture.

Erbitux is a sterile, clear, colorless liquid of pH 7.0 to 7.4, which may contain a small amount of easily visible, white, amorphous cetuximab particulates. Erbitux is supplied at a concentration of 2 mg/mL in either 100 mg (50 mL) or 200 mg (100 mL), single-use vials. Cetuximab is formulated in a solution with no preservatives, which contains 8.48 mg/mL sodium chloride, 1.88 mg/mL sodium phosphate dibasic heptahydrate, 0.41 mg/mL sodium phosphate monobasic monohydrate, and Water for Injection, USP.

12 CLINICAL PHARMACOLOGY

12.1 Mechanism of Action

The epidermal growth factor receptor (EGFR, HER1, c-ErbB-1) is a transmembrane glycoprotein that is a member of a subfamily of type I receptor tyrosine kinases including EGFR, HER2, HER3, and HER4. The EGFR is constitutively expressed in many normal epithelial tissues, including the skin and hair follicle. Expression of EGFR is also detected in many human cancers including those of the head and neck, colon, and rectum.

Cetuximab binds specifically to the EGFR on both normal and tumor cells, and competitively inhibits the binding of epidermal growth factor (EGF) and other ligands, such as transforming growth factor-alpha. *In vitro* assays and *in vivo* animal studies have shown that binding of cetuximab to the EGFR blocks phosphorylation and activation of receptor-associated kinases, resulting in inhibition of cell growth, induction of apoptosis, and decreased matrix metalloproteinase and vascular endothelial growth factor production. Signal transduction through the EGFR results in activation of wild-type *K-Ras* protein. However, in cells with activating *K-Ras* somatic mutations, the mutant *K-Ras* protein is continuously active and appears independent of EGFR regulation.

In vitro, cetuximab can mediate antibody-dependent cellular cytotoxicity (ADCC) against certain human tumor types. *In vitro* assays and *in vivo* animal studies have shown that cetuximab inhibits the growth and survival of tumor cells that express the EGFR. No anti-tumor effects of cetuximab were observed in human tumor xenografts lacking EGFR expression. The addition of cetuximab to radiation therapy or irinotecan in human tumor xenograft models in mice resulted in an increase in anti-tumor effects compared to radiation therapy or chemotherapy alone.

12.2 Pharmacodynamics

Effects on Electrocardiogram (ECG)

The effect of cetuximab on QT interval was evaluated in an open-label, single-arm, monotherapy trial in 37 subjects with advanced malignancies who received an initial dose of 400 mg/m^2, followed by weekly infusions of 250 mg/m^2 for a total of 5 weeks. No large changes in the mean QT interval of >20 ms from baseline were detected in the trial based on the Fridericia correction method. A small increase in the mean QTc interval of <10 ms cannot be excluded because of the limitations in the trial design.

12.3 Pharmacokinetics

Erbitux (cetuximab) administered as monotherapy or in combination with concomitant chemotherapy or radiation therapy exhibits nonlinear pharmacokinetics. The area under the concentration time curve (AUC) increased in a greater than dose proportional manner while clearance of cetuximab decreased from 0.08 to 0.02 L/h/m^2 as the dose increased from 20 to 200 mg/m^2, and at doses >200 mg/m^2, it appeared to plateau. The volume of the distribution for cetuximab appeared to be independent of dose and approximated the vascular space of 2–3 L/m^2.

Following the recommended dose regimen (400 mg/m^2 initial dose; 250 mg/m^2 weekly dose), concentrations of cetuximab reached steady-state levels by the third weekly infusion with mean peak and trough concentrations across studies ranging from 168 to 235 and 41 to 85 µg/mL, respectively. The mean half-life of cetuximab was approximately 112 hours (range 63–230 hours). The pharmacokinetics of cetuximab were similar in patients with SCCHN and those with colorectal cancer.

Erbitux (cetuximab) had an approximately 22% (90% confidence interval; 6%, 38%) higher systemic exposure relative to the EU-approved cetuximab used in Studies 2 and 4 based on a population pharmacokinetic analysis. [See *Clinical Studies (14.1)*.]

13 NONCLINICAL TOXICOLOGY

13.1 Carcinogenesis, Mutagenesis, Impairment of Fertility

Long-term animal studies have not been performed to test cetuximab for carcinogenic potential, and no mutagenic or clastogenic potential of cetuximab was observed in the *Salmonella-Escherichia coli* (Ames) assay or in the *in vivo* rat micronucleus test. Menstrual cyclicity was impaired in female cynomolgus monkeys receiving weekly doses of 0.4 to 4 times the human dose of cetuximab (based on total body surface area). Cetuximab-treated animals exhibited increased incidences of irregular or absent cycles, as compared to control animals. These effects were initially noted beginning week 25 of cetuximab treatment and continued through the 6-week recovery period. In this same study, there were no effects of cetuximab treatment on measured

Table 5: Incidence of Selected Adverse Reactions Occurring in ≥10% of Patients with *K-Ras* Mutation-negative (Wild-type), EGFR-expressing, Metastatic Colorectal Cancer Treated with Erbitux Monotherapy[a]

	Erbitux plus BSC (n=118)		BSC alone (n=124)	
Body System Preferred Term	**Grades 1–4[b]**	**Grades 3 and 4**	**Grades 1–4**	**Grades 3 and 4**
	% of Patients			
Dermatology/Skin				
Rash/Desquamation	95	16	21	1
Dry Skin	57	0	15	0
Pruritus	47	2	11	0
Other-Dermatology	35	0	7	2
Nail Changes	31	0	4	0
Constitutional Symptoms				
Fatigue	91	31	79	29
Fever	25	3	16	0
Infusion Reactions[c]	18	3	0	0
Rigors, Chills	16	1	3	0
Pain				
Pain-Other	59	18	37	10
Headache	38	2	11	0
Bone Pain	15	4	8	2
Pulmonary				
Dyspnea	49	16	44	13
Cough	30	2	19	2
Gastrointestinal				
Nausea	64	6	50	6
Constipation	53	3	38	3
Diarrhea	42	2	23	2
Vomiting	40	5	26	5
Stomatitis	32	1	10	0
Other-Gastrointestinal	22	12	16	5
Dehydration	13	5	3	0
Mouth Dryness	12	0	6	0
Taste Disturbance	10	0	5	0
Infection				
Infection without neutropenia	38	11	19	5
Musculoskeletal				
Arthralgia	14	3	6	0
Neurology				
Neuropathy-sensory	45	1	38	2
Insomnia	27	0	13	0
Confusion	18	6	10	2
Anxiety	14	1	5	1
Depression	14	0	5	0

[a] Adverse reactions occurring in at least 10% of Erbitux plus BSC arm with a frequency at least 5% greater than that seen in the BSC alone arm.

[b] Adverse reactions were graded using the NCI CTC, V 2.0.

[c] Infusion reaction is defined as any event (chills, rigors, dyspnea, tachycardia, bronchospasm, chest tightness, swelling, urticaria, hypotension, flushing, rash, hypertension, nausea, angioedema, pain, sweating, tremors, shaking, drug fever, or other hypersensitivity reaction) recorded by the investigator as infusion-related.

Table 6: Study 1: Clinical Efficacy in Locoregionally Advanced SCCHN

	Erbitux + Radiation (n=211)	Radiation Alone (n=213)	Hazard Ratio (95% CI[a])	Stratified Log-rank p-value
Locoregional Control				
Median duration (months)	24.4	14.9	0.68 (0.52–0.89)	0.005
Overall Survival				
Median duration (months)	49.0	29.3	0.74 (0.57–0.97)	0.03

[a] CI = confidence interval

Table 7: Study 2: Clinical Efficacy in Recurrent Locoregional Disease or Metastatic SCCHN

	EU-Approved Cetuximab + Platinum-based Therapy + 5-FU (n=222)	Platinum-based Therapy + 5-FU (n=220)	Hazard Ratio (95% CI[a])	Stratified Log-rank p-value
Overall Survival				
Median duration (months)	10.1	7.4	0.80 (0.64, 0.98)	0.034
Progression-free Survival				
Median duration (months)	5.5	3.3	0.57 (0.46, 0.72)	<0.0001
	EU-Approved Cetuximab + Platinum-based Therapy + 5-FU (n=222)	**Platinum-based Therapy + 5-FU (n=220)**	**Odds Ratio (95% CI[a])**	**CMH[b] test p-value**
Objective Response Rate	35.6%	19.5%	2.33 (1.50, 3.60)	0.0001

[a] CI = confidence interval
[b] CMH = Cochran-Mantel-Haenszel

male fertility parameters (ie, serum testosterone levels and analysis of sperm counts, viability, and motility) as compared to control male monkeys. It is not known if cetuximab can impair fertility in humans.

13.2 Animal Pharmacology and/or Toxicology

In cynomolgus monkeys, cetuximab, when administered at doses of approximately 0.4 to 4 times the weekly human exposure (based on total body surface area), resulted in dermatologic findings, including inflammation at the injection site and desquamation of the external integument. At the highest dose level, the epithelial mucosa of the nasal passage, esophagus, and tongue were similarly affected, and degenerative changes in the renal tubular epithelium occurred. Deaths due to sepsis were observed in 50% (5/10) of the animals at the highest dose level beginning after approximately 13 weeks of treatment.

14 CLINICAL STUDIES

Studies 2 and 4 were conducted outside the U.S. using an EU-approved cetuximab as the clinical trial material. Erbitux provides approximately 22% higher exposure relative to the EU-approved cetuximab used in Studies 2 and 4; these pharmacokinetic data, together with the results of Studies 2, 4, and other clinical trial data establish the efficacy of Erbitux (cetuximab) at the recommended dose in SCCHN and mCRC [see *Clinical Pharmacology (12.3)*].

14.1 Squamous Cell Carcinoma of the Head and Neck (SCCHN)

Study 1 was a randomized, multicenter, controlled trial of 424 patients with locally or regionally advanced SCCHN. Patients with Stage III/IV SCCHN of the oropharynx, hypopharynx, or larynx with no prior therapy were randomized (1:1) to receive either Erbitux plus radiation therapy or radiation therapy alone. Stratification factors were Karnofsky performance status (60–80 versus 90–100), nodal stage (N0 versus N+), tumor stage (T1–3 versus T4 using American Joint Committee on Cancer 1998 staging criteria), and radiation therapy fractionation (concomitant boost versus once-daily versus twice-daily). Radiation therapy was administered for 6–7 weeks as once-daily, twice-daily, or concomitant boost. Erbitux was administered as a 400 mg/m^2 initial dose beginning one week prior to initiation of radiation therapy, followed by 250 mg/m^2 weekly administered 1 hour prior to radiation therapy for the duration of radiation therapy (6–7 weeks).

Of the 424 randomized patients, the median age was 57 years, 80% were male, 83% were Caucasian, and 90% had baseline Karnofsky performance status ≥80. There were 258 patients enrolled in U.S. sites (61%). Sixty percent of patients had oropharyngeal, 25% laryngeal, and 15% hypopharyngeal primary tumors; 28% had AJCC T4 tumor stage. Fifty-six percent of the patients received radiation therapy with concomitant boost, 26% received once-daily regimen, and 18% twice-daily regimen.

The main outcome measure of this trial was duration of locoregional control. Overall survival was also assessed. Results are presented in Table 6.

[See table 6 above]

Study 2 was an open-label, randomized, multicenter, controlled trial of 442 patients with recurrent locoregional disease or metastatic SCCHN.

Patients with no prior therapy for recurrent locoregional disease or metastatic SCCHN were randomized (1:1) to receive EU-approved cetuximab plus cisplatin or carboplatin and 5-FU, or cisplatin or carboplatin and 5-FU alone. Choice of cisplatin or carboplatin was at the discretion of the treating physician. Stratification factors were Karnofsky performance status (<80 versus ≥80) and previous chemotherapy. Cisplatin (100 mg/m^2, Day 1) or carboplatin (AUC 5, Day 1) plus intravenous 5-FU (1000 mg/m^2/day, Days 1–4) were administered every 3 weeks (1 cycle) for a maximum of 6 cycles in the absence of disease progression or unacceptable toxicity. Cetuximab was administered at a 400 mg/m^2 initial dose, followed by a 250 mg/m^2 weekly dose in combination with chemotherapy. Patients demonstrating at least stable disease on cetuximab in combination with chemotherapy were to continue cetuximab monotherapy at 250 mg/m^2 weekly, in the absence of disease progression or unacceptable toxicity after completion of 6 planned courses of platinum-based therapy. For patients where treatment was delayed because of the toxic effects of chemotherapy, weekly cetuximab was continued. If chemotherapy was discontinued for toxicity, cetuximab could be continued as monotherapy until disease progression or unacceptable toxicity.

Of the 442 randomized patients, the median age was 57 years, 90% were male, 98% were Caucasian, and 88% had baseline Karnofsky performance status ≥80. Thirty-four percent of patients had oropharyngeal, 25% laryngeal, 20% oral cavity, and 14% hypopharyngeal primary tumors. Fifty-three percent of patients had recurrent locoregional disease only and 47% had metastatic disease. Fifty-eight percent had AJCC Stage IV disease and 21% had Stage III disease. Sixty-four percent of patients received cisplatin therapy and 34% received carboplatin as initial therapy. Approximately fifteen percent of the patients in the cisplatin alone arm switched to carboplatin during the treatment period.

The main outcome measure of this trial was overall survival. Results are presented in Table 7 and Figure 1.

[See table 7 above]

[See figure 1 at top of next column]

In exploratory subgroup analyses of Study 2 by initial platinum therapy (cisplatin or carboplatin), for patients (N=284) receiving cetuximab plus cisplatin with 5-FU compared to cisplatin with 5-FU alone, the difference in median overall survival was 3.3 months (10.6 versus 7.3 months, respectively; HR 0.71; 95% CI 0.54, 0.93). The difference in

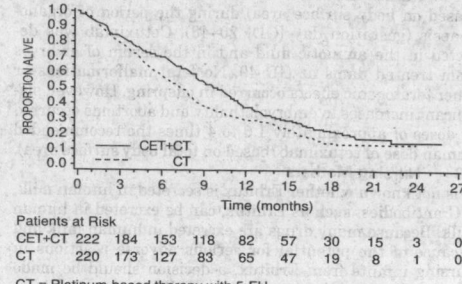

Figure 1: Kaplan-Meier Curve for Overall Survival in Patients with Recurrent Locoregional Disease or Metastatic Squamous Cell Carcinoma of the Head and Neck

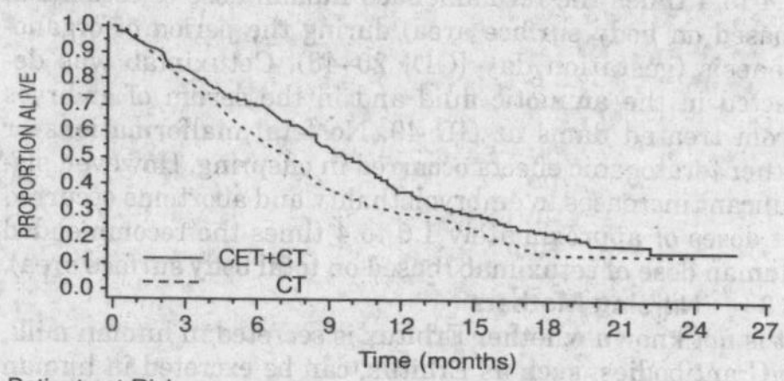

Patients at Risk

CET+CT	222	184	153	118	82	57	30	15	3	0
CT	220	173	127	83	65	47	19	8	1	0

CT = Platinum-based therapy with 5-FU
CET = EU-approved cetuximab

median progression-free survival was 2.1 months (5.6 versus 3.5 months, respectively; HR 0.55; 95% CI 0.41, 0.73). The objective response rate was 39% and 23%, respectively (OR 2.18; 95% CI 1.29, 3.69). For patients (N=149) receiving cetuximab plus carboplatin with 5-FU compared to carboplatin with 5-FU alone, the difference in median overall survival was 1.4 months (9.7 versus 8.3 months; HR 0.99; 95% CI 0.69, 1.43). The difference in median progression-free survival was 1.7 months (4.8 versus 3.1 months, respectively; HR 0.61; 95% CI 0.42, 0.89). The objective response rate was 30% and 15%, respectively (OR 2.45; 95% CI 1.10, 5.46).

Study 3 was a single-arm, multicenter clinical trial in 103 patients with recurrent or metastatic SCCHN. All patients had documented disease progression within 30 days of a platinum-based chemotherapy regimen. Patients received a 20-mg test dose of Erbitux on Day 1, followed by a 400 mg/m^2 initial dose, and 250 mg/m^2 weekly until disease progression or unacceptable toxicity.

The median age was 57 years, 82% were male, 100% Caucasian, and 62% had a Karnofsky performance status of ≥80.

The objective response rate was 13% (95% confidence interval 7%–21%). Median duration of response was 5.8 months (range 1.2–5.8 months).

14.2 Colorectal Cancer

Erbitux Clinical Trials in *K-Ras* Mutation-negative (Wild-type), EGFR-expressing, Metastatic Colorectal Cancer

Study 4 was a randomized, open-label, multicenter, study of 1217 patients with EGFR-expressing, metastatic colorectal cancer. Patients were randomized (1:1) to receive either EU-approved cetuximab in combination with FOLFIRI or FOLFIRI alone as first-line treatment. Stratification factors were Eastern Cooperative Oncology Group (ECOG) performance status (0 and 1 versus 2) and region (sites in Western Europe versus Eastern Europe versus other).

FOLFIRI regimen included 14-day cycles of irinotecan (180 mg/m^2 administered intravenously on Day 1), folinic acid (400 mg/m^2 [racemic] or 200 mg/m^2 [L-form] administered intravenously on Day 1), and 5-FU (400 mg/m^2 bolus on Day 1 followed by 2400 mg/m^2 as a 46-hour continuous infusion). Cetuximab was administered as a 400 mg/m^2 initial dose on Day 1, Week 1, followed by 250 mg/m^2 weekly administered 1 hour prior to chemotherapy. Study treatment continued until disease progression or unacceptable toxicity occurred.

Of the 1217 randomized patients, the median age was 61 years, 60% were male, 86% were Caucasian, and 96% had a baseline ECOG performance status 0–1, 60% had primary tumor localized in colon, 84% had 1–2 metastatic sites and 20% had received prior adjuvant and/or neoadjuvant chemotherapy. Demographics and baseline characteristics were similar between study arms.

K-Ras mutation status was available for 1079/1217 (89%) of the patients: 676 (63%) patients had *K-Ras* mutation-negative (wild-type) tumors and 403 (37%) patients had *K-Ras* mutation-positive tumors where testing assessed for the following somatic mutations in codons 12 and 13 (exon 2): G12A, G12D, G12R, G12C, G12S, G12V, G13D [see *Warnings and Precautions (5.7)*].

Baseline characteristics and demographics in the *K-Ras* mutation-negative (wild-type) subset were similar to that seen in the overall population [see *Warnings and Precautions (5.7)*].

The main outcome measure of this trial was progression-free survival assessed by an independent review committee (IRC). Overall survival and response rate were also assessed. A statistically significant improvement in PFS was observed for the cetuximab plus FOLFIRI arm compared with the FOLFIRI arm (median PFS 8.9 vs 8.1 months, HR 0.85 [95% CI 0.74, 0.99], p-value=0.036). Overall survival was not significantly different at the planned, final analysis based on 838 events [HR=0.93, 95% CI (0.8, 1.1), p-value 0.327].

Results of the planned PFS and ORR analysis in all randomized patients and post-hoc PFS and ORR analysis in subgroups of patients defined by *K-Ras* mutation status, and post-hoc analysis of updated OS based on additional follow-up (1000 events) in all randomized patients and in subgroups of patients defined by *K-Ras* mutation status are presented in Table 8 and Figure 2. The treatment effect in the all-randomized population for PFS was driven by treatment effects limited to patients who have *K-Ras* mutation-negative (wild-type) tumors. There is no evidence of effectiveness in the subgroup of patients with *K-Ras* mutation-positive tumors.

[See table above]

Table 8: Clinical Efficacy in First-line EGFR-expressing, Metastatic Colorectal Cancer (All Randomized and *K-Ras* Status)

	All Randomized		*K-Ras* Mutation-negative (Wild-type)		*K-Ras* Mutation-positive	
	EU-Approved Cetuximab plus FOLFIRI (n=608)	FOLFIRI (n=609)	EU-Approved Cetuximab plus FOLFIRI (n=320)	FOLFIRI (n=356)	EU-Approved Cetuximab plus FOLFIRI (n=216)	FOLFIRI (n=187)
Progression-Free Survival						
Number of Events (%)	343 (56)	371 (61)	165 (52)	214 (60)	138 (64)	112 (60)
Median (months)	8.9	8.1	9.5	8.1	7.5	8.2
(95% CI)	(8.0, 9.4)	(7.6, 8.8)	(8.9, 11.1)	(7.4, 9.2)	(6.7, 8.7)	(7.4, 9.2)
HR (95% CI)	0.85 (0.74, 0.99)		0.70 (0.57, 0.86)		1.13 (0.88, 1.46)	
p-value[a]	0.0358					
Overall Survival[b]						
Number of Events (%)	491 (81)	509 (84)	244 (76)	292 (82)	189 (88)	159 (85)
Median (months)	19.6	18.5	23.5	19.5	16.0	16.7
(95% CI)	(18, 21)	(17, 20)	(21, 26)	(17, 21)	(15, 18)	(15, 19)
HR (95% CI)	0.88 (0.78, 1.0)		0.80 (0.67, 0.94)		1.04 (0.84, 1.29)	
Objective Response Rate						
ORR (95% CI)	46% (42, 50)	38% (34, 42)	57% (51, 62)	39% (34, 44)	31% (25, 38)	35% (28, 43)

[a] Based on the Stratified Log-rank test.
[b] Post-hoc updated OS analysis, results based on an additional 162 events.

Figure 2: Kaplan-Meier Curve for Overall Survival in the *K-Ras* Mutation-negative (Wild-type) Population in Study 4

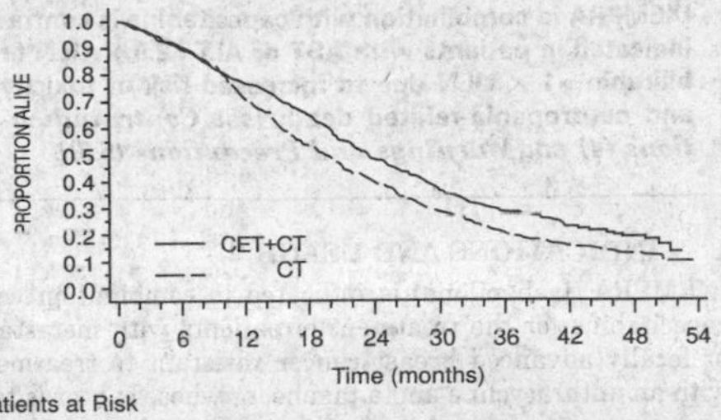

Patients at Risk										
CET+CT	320	282	237	198	144	108	82	65	21	4
CT	356	313	247	179	132	92	64	48	18	2

Study 5 was a multicenter, open-label, randomized, clinical trial conducted in 572 patients with EGFR-expressing, previously treated, recurrent mCRC. Patients were randomized (1:1) to receive either Erbitux plus best supportive care (BSC) or BSC alone. Erbitux was administered as a 400 mg/m^2 initial dose, followed by 250 mg/m^2 weekly until disease progression or unacceptable toxicity.

Of the 572 randomized patients, the median age was 63 years, 64% were male, 89% were Caucasian, and 77% had baseline ECOG performance status of 0–1. Demographics and baseline characteristics were similar between study arms. All patients were to have received and progressed on prior therapy including an irinotecan-containing regimen and an oxaliplatin-containing regimen.

K-Ras status was available for 453/572 (79%) of the patients: 245 (54%) patients had *K-Ras* mutation-negative (wild-type) tumors and 208 (46%) patients had *K-Ras* mutation-positive tumors where testing assessed for the following somatic mutations in codons 12 and 13 (exon 2): G12A, G12D, G12R, G12C, G12S, G12V, G13D [see *Warnings and Precautions (5.7)*].

The main outcome measure of the study was overall survival. Results are presented in Table 9 and Figure 3.

[See table above]

Table 9: Overall Survival in Previously Treated EGFR-expressing, Metastatic Colorectal Cancer (All Randomized and *K-Ras* Status)

	All Randomized		*K-Ras* Mutation-negative (Wild-type)		*K-Ras* Mutation-positive	
	Erbitux plus BSC (N=287)	BSC (N=285)	Erbitux plus BSC (N=117)	BSC (N=128)	Erbitux plus BSC (N=108)	BSC (N=100)
Median (months)	6.1	4.6	8.6	5.0	4.8	4.6
(95% CI)	(5.4, 6.7)	(4.2, 4.9)	(7.0, 10.3)	(4.3, 5.7)	(3.9, 5.6)	(3.6, 4.9)
HR	0.77		0.63		0.91	
(95% CI)	(0.64, 0.92)		(0.47, 0.84)		(0.67, 1.24)	
p-value[a]	0.0046					

[a] Based on the Stratified Log-rank test.

Figure 3: Kaplan-Meier Curve for Overall Survival in Patients with *K-Ras* Mutation-negative (Wild-type) Metastatic Colorectal Cancer in Study 5

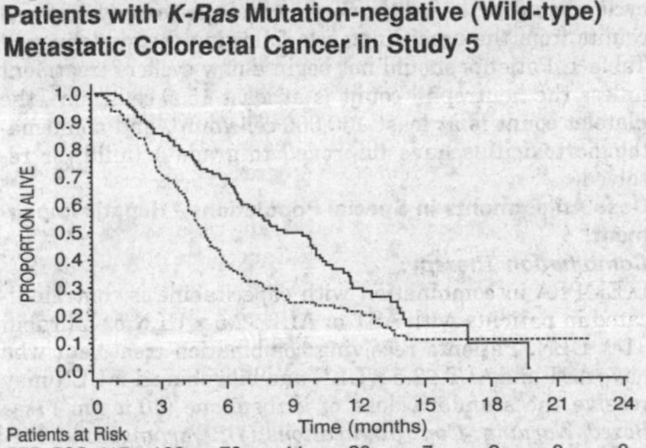

Patients at Risk									
ERB+BSC	117	100	76	44	20	7	2	0	0
BSC	128	89	45	24	15	7	5	1	0

—— ERB + BSC ---- BSC

Study 6 was a multicenter, clinical trial conducted in 329 patients with EGFR-expressing recurrent mCRC. Tumor specimens were not available for testing for *K-Ras* mutation status. Patients were randomized (2:1) to receive either Erbitux plus irinotecan (218 patients) or Erbitux monotherapy (111 patients). Erbitux (cetuximab) was administered as a 400 mg/m^2 initial dose, followed by 250 mg/m^2 weekly until disease progression or unacceptable toxicity. In the Erbitux plus irinotecan arm, irinotecan was added to Erbitux using the same dose and schedule for irinotecan as the patient had previously failed. Acceptable irinotecan schedules were 350 mg/m^2 every 3 weeks, 180 mg/m^2 every 2 weeks, or 125 mg/m^2 weekly times four doses every 6 weeks. Of the 329 patients, the median age was 59 years, 63% were male, 98% were Caucasian, and 88% had baseline Karnofsky performance status ≥80. Approximately two-thirds had previously failed oxaliplatin treatment.

The efficacy of Erbitux (cetuximab) plus irinotecan or Erbitux monotherapy, based on durable objective responses, was evaluated in all randomized patients and in two pre-specified subpopulations: irinotecan refractory patients, and irinotecan and oxaliplatin failures. In patients receiving Erbitux plus irinotecan, the objective response rate was 23% (95% confidence interval 18%–29%), median duration of response was 5.7 months, and median time to progression was 4.1 months. In patients receiving Erbitux monotherapy, the objective response rate was 11% (95% confidence interval 6%–18%), median duration of response was 4.2 months, and median time to progression was 1.5 months. Similar response rates were observed in the pre-defined subsets in both the combination arm and monotherapy arm of the study.

16 HOW SUPPLIED/STORAGE AND HANDLING

Erbitux® (cetuximab) is supplied at a concentration of 2 mg/mL as a 100 mg/50 mL, single-use vial or as a 200 mg/100 mL, single-use vial as a sterile, injectable liquid containing no preservatives.

NDC 66733-948-23	100 mg/50 mL, single-use vial, individually packaged in a carton
NDC 66733-958-23	200 mg/100 mL, single-use vial, individually packaged in a carton

Store vials under refrigeration at 2° C to 8° C (36° F to 46° F). **Do not freeze.** Increased particulate formation may occur at temperatures at or below 0° C. This product contains no preservatives. Preparations of Erbitux in infusion containers are chemically and physically stable for up to 12 hours at 2° C to 8° C (36° F to 46° F) and up to 8 hours at controlled room temperature (20° C to 25° C; 68° F to 77° F). Discard any remaining solution in the infusion container after 8 hours at controlled room temperature or after 12 hours at 2° C to 8° C. Discard any unused portion of the vial.

17 PATIENT COUNSELING INFORMATION

Advise patients:

- To report signs and symptoms of infusion reactions such as fever, chills, or breathing problems.
- Of the potential risks of using Erbitux during pregnancy or nursing and of the need to use adequate contraception in both males and females during and for 6 months following the last dose of Erbitux therapy.
- That nursing is not recommended during, and for 2 months following the last dose of Erbitux therapy.
- To limit sun exposure (use sunscreen, wear hats) while receiving and for 2 months following the last dose of Erbitux.

Erbitux® is a registered trademark of ImClone LLC a wholly-owned subsidiary of Eli Lilly and Company.

Manufactured by ImClone LLC a wholly-owned subsidiary of Eli Lilly and Company, Branchburg, NJ 08876 USA

Distributed and marketed by Bristol-Myers Squibb Company, Princeton, NJ 08543 USA

Co-marketed by Eli Lilly and Company, Indianapolis, IN 46285 USA

1236886B3

Rev August 2013

Shown in Product Identification Guide, page 305

IXEMPRA® *Kit* ℞

[*ĭk-sĕm-pră*]

(ixabepilone)

for Injection, for intravenous infusion only

HIGHLIGHTS OF PRESCRIBING INFORMATION

These highlights do not include all the information needed to use IXEMPRA® safely and effectively. See full prescribing information for IXEMPRA®.

IXEMPRA® *Kit* (ixabepilone) for Injection, for intravenous infusion only

Initial U.S. Approval: 2007

WARNING: TOXICITY IN HEPATIC IMPAIRMENT

See full prescribing information for complete boxed warning.

IXEMPRA® in combination with capecitabine must not be given to patients with AST or ALT >2.5 × ULN or bilirubin >1 × ULN due to increased risk of toxicity and neutropenia-related death. (4, 5.3)

INDICATIONS AND USAGE

- IXEMPRA, a microtubule inhibitor, in combination with capecitabine is indicated for the treatment of metastatic or locally advanced breast cancer in patients after failure of an anthracycline and a taxane (1).
- IXEMPRA as monotherapy is indicated for the treatment of metastatic or locally advanced breast cancer in patients after failure of an anthracycline, a taxane, and capecitabine (1).

DOSAGE AND ADMINISTRATION

- The recommended dose of IXEMPRA is 40 mg/m^2 infused intravenously over 3 hours every 3 weeks (2.1).
- Dose reduction is required in certain patients with elevated AST, ALT, or bilirubin (2.2, 8.6).

IXEMPRA (ixabepilone) for injection must be constituted with supplied DILUENT. The ixabepilone concentration in constituted solution is 2 mg/mL.

Constituted solution must be diluted with one of the specified fluids, to a final ixabepilone concentration of 0.2 mg/mL to 0.6 mg/mL. The final solution must be used within 6 hours of preparation (2.4).

DOSAGE FORMS AND STRENGTHS

- IXEMPRA for injection, 15 mg supplied with DILUENT for IXEMPRA, 8 mL (3)
- IXEMPRA for injection, 45 mg supplied with DILUENT for IXEMPRA, 23.5 mL (3)

CONTRAINDICATIONS

- Hypersensitivity to drugs formulated with Cremophor® EL (4).
- Baseline neutrophil count <1500 cells/mm^3 or a platelet count <100,000 cells/mm^3 (4).
- Patients with AST or ALT >2.5 × ULN or bilirubin >1 × ULN must not be treated with IXEMPRA in combination with capecitabine (4).

WARNINGS AND PRECAUTIONS

- Peripheral Neuropathy: Monitor for symptoms of neuropathy, primarily sensory. Neuropathy is cumulative, generally reversible, and should be managed by dose adjustment and delays (2.2, 5.1).
- Myelosuppression: Primarily neutropenia. Monitor with peripheral blood cell counts and adjust dose as appropriate (2.2, 5.2).
- Hypersensitivity reaction: Must premedicate all patients with an H_1 antagonist and an H_2 antagonist before treatment (2.3, 5.4).
- Fetal harm can occur when administered to a pregnant woman. Women should be advised not to become pregnant when taking IXEMPRA (5.5, 8.1).

ADVERSE REACTIONS

- The most common adverse reactions (≥20%) are peripheral sensory neuropathy, fatigue/asthenia, myalgia/arthralgia, alopecia, nausea, vomiting, stomatitis/mucositis, diarrhea, and musculoskeletal pain. Additional reactions occurred in ≥20% in combination treatment: palmar-plantar erythrodysesthesia syndrome, anorexia, abdominal pain, nail disorder, and constipation (6).
- Drug-associated hematologic abnormalities (>40%) include neutropenia, leukopenia, anemia, and thrombocytopenia (6).

To report SUSPECTED ADVERSE REACTIONS, contact Bristol-Myers Squibb at 1-800-721-5072 or FDA at 1-800-FDA-1088 or www.fda.gov/medwatch

DRUG INTERACTIONS

- Inhibitors of CYP3A4 may increase plasma concentrations of ixabepilone; dose of IXEMPRA must be reduced with strong CYP3A4 inhibitors (7.1).
- Inducers of CYP3A4 may decrease plasma concentrations of ixabepilone; alternative therapeutic agents with low enzyme induction potential should be considered (7.1).

See 17 for PATIENT COUNSELING INFORMATION and FDA-Approved Patient Labeling

Revised: 10/2011

FULL PRESCRIBING INFORMATION: CONTENTS*

*** Sections or subsections omitted from the full prescribing information are not listed**

FULL PRESCRIBING INFORMATION

WARNING: TOXICITY IN HEPATIC IMPAIRMENT

IXEMPRA in combination with capecitabine is contraindicated in patients with AST or ALT >2.5 × ULN or bilirubin >1 × ULN due to increased risk of toxicity and neutropenia-related death *[see Contraindications (4) and Warnings and Precautions (5.3)].*

1 INDICATIONS AND USAGE

IXEMPRA (ixabepilone) is indicated in combination with capecitabine for the treatment of patients with metastatic or locally advanced breast cancer resistant to treatment with an anthracycline and a taxane, or whose cancer is taxane resistant and for whom further anthracycline therapy is contraindicated. Anthracycline resistance is defined as progression while on therapy or within 6 months in the adjuvant setting or 3 months in the metastatic setting. Taxane resistance is defined as progression while on therapy or within 12 months in the adjuvant setting or 4 months in the metastatic setting.

IXEMPRA is indicated as monotherapy for the treatment of metastatic or locally advanced breast cancer in patients whose tumors are resistant or refractory to anthracyclines, taxanes, and capecitabine.

2 DOSAGE AND ADMINISTRATION

2.1 General Dosing Information

The recommended dosage of IXEMPRA is 40 mg/m^2 administered intravenously over 3 hours every 3 weeks. Doses for patients with body surface area (BSA) greater than 2.2 m^2 should be calculated based on 2.2 m^2.

2.2 Dose Modification

Dose Adjustments During Treatment

Patients should be evaluated during treatment by periodic clinical observation and laboratory tests including complete blood cell counts. If toxicities are present, treatment should be delayed to allow recovery. Dosing adjustment guidelines for monotherapy and combination therapy are shown in Table 1. If toxicities recur, an additional 20% dose reduction should be made.

[See table 1 below]

Re-treatment Criteria: Dose adjustments at the start of a cycle should be based on nonhematologic toxicity or blood counts from the preceding cycle following the guidelines in Table 1. Patients should not begin a new cycle of treatment unless the neutrophil count is at least 1500 cells/mm^3, the platelet count is at least 100,000 cells/mm^3, and nonhematologic toxicities have improved to grade 1 (mild) or resolved.

Dose Adjustments in Special Populations - Hepatic Impairment

Combination Therapy:

IXEMPRA in combination with capecitabine is contraindicated in patients with AST or ALT >2.5 × ULN or bilirubin >1 × ULN. Patients receiving combination treatment who have AST and ALT ≤2.5 × ULN and bilirubin ≤1 × ULN may receive the standard dose of ixabepilone (40 mg/m^2) *[see Boxed Warning, Contraindications (4), Warnings and Precautions (5.3), and Use in Specific Populations (8.6)].*

Monotherapy:

Patients with hepatic impairment should be dosed with IXEMPRA based on the guidelines in Table 2. Patients with moderate hepatic impairment should be started at 20 mg/m^2, the dosage in subsequent cycles may be escalated up to, but not exceeding, 30 mg/m^2 if tolerated. Use in patients with AST or ALT >10 × ULN or bilirubin >3 × ULN is not recommended. Limited data are available for patients with baseline AST or ALT >5 × ULN. Caution should be used when treating these patients *[see Warnings and Precautions (5.3) and Use in Specific Populations (8.6)].*

[See table 2 at top of next page]

Strong CYP3A4 Inhibitors

The use of concomitant strong CYP3A4 inhibitors should be avoided (eg, ketoconazole, itraconazole, clarithromycin, atazanavir, nefazodone, saquinavir, telithromycin, ritonavir, amprenavir, indinavir, nelfinavir, delavirdine, or voriconazole). Grapefruit juice may also increase plasma concentrations of IXEMPRA and should be avoided. Based on phar-

Table 1: Dose Adjustment Guidelines[a]

IXEMPRA (Monotherapy or Combination Therapy)	IXEMPRA Dose Modification
Nonhematologic:	
Grade 2 neuropathy (moderate) lasting ≥7 days	Decrease the dose by 20%
Grade 3 neuropathy (severe) lasting <7 days	Decrease the dose by 20%
Grade 3 neuropathy (severe) lasting ≥7 days or disabling neuropathy	Discontinue treatment
Any grade 3 toxicity (severe) other than neuropathy	Decrease the dose by 20%
Transient grade 3 arthralgia/myalgia or fatigue	No change in dose of IXEMPRA
Grade 3 hand-foot syndrome (palmar-plantar erythrodysesthesia)	
Any grade 4 toxicity (disabling)	Discontinue treatment
Hematologic:	
Neutrophil <500 cells/mm^3 for ≥7 days	Decrease the dose by 20%
Febrile neutropenia	Decrease the dose by 20%
Platelets <25,000/mm^3 or platelets <50,000/mm^3 with bleeding	Decrease the dose by 20%
Capecitabine (when used in combination with IXEMPRA)	**Capecitabine Dose Modification**
Nonhematologic:	Follow Capecitabine Label
Hematologic:	
Platelets <25,000/mm^{3}or <50,000/mm^3 with bleeding	Hold for concurrent diarrhea or stomatitis until platelet count >50,000/mm^3, then continue at same dose.
Neutrophils <500 cells/mm^3 for ≥7 days or febrile neutropenia	Hold for concurrent diarrhea or stomatitis until neutrophil count >1,000 cells/mm^3, then continue at same dose.

[a] Toxicities graded in accordance with National Cancer Institute (NCI) Common Terminology Criteria for Adverse Events (CTCAE v3.0).

macokinetic studies, if a strong CYP3A4 inhibitor must be coadministered, a dose reduction to 20 mg/m^2 is predicted to adjust the ixabepilone AUC to the range observed without inhibitors and should be considered. If the strong inhibitor is discontinued, a washout period of approximately 1 week should be allowed before the IXEMPRA (ixabepilone) dose is adjusted upward to the indicated dose *[see Drug Interactions (7.1)]*.

Strong CYP3A4 Inducers

The use of concomitant strong CYP3A4 inducers should be avoided (eg, phenytoin, carbamazepine, rifampin, rifabutin, dexamethasone, and phenobarbital). Selection of an alternative concomitant medication with no or minimal enzyme induction potential should be considered. Based on extrapolation from a drug interaction study with rifampin, the following guidance may be considered for dosing in patients requiring coadministration of a strong CYP3A4 inducer, if no alternatives are feasible. Once patients have been maintained on a strong CYP3A4 inducer, the dose of IXEMPRA may be gradually increased from 40 mg/m^2 to 60 mg/m^2 depending on tolerance. If the dose is increased, IXEMPRA should be given as a 4-hour intravenous infusion. This 60 mg/m^2 dose given intravenously over 4 hours is predicted to adjust the AUC to the range observed without inducers. However, there are no clinical data with this dose adjustment in patients receiving strong CYP3A4 inducers. Patients whose dose is increased above 40 mg/m^2 should be monitored carefully for toxicities associated with IXEMPRA. If the strong inducer is discontinued, the IXEMPRA dose should be returned to the dose used prior to initiation of the strong CYP3A4 inducer *[see Drug Interactions (7.1)]*.

2.3 Premedication

To minimize the chance of occurrence of a hypersensitivity reaction, all patients must be premedicated approximately 1 hour before the infusion of IXEMPRA with:

- An H_1 antagonist (eg, diphenhydramine 50 mg orally or equivalent) and
- An H_2 antagonist (eg, ranitidine 150 - 300 mg orally or equivalent).

Patients who experienced a hypersensitivity reaction to IXEMPRA require premedication with corticosteroids (eg, dexamethasone 20 mg intravenously, 30 minutes before infusion or orally, 60 minutes before infusion) in addition to pretreatment with H_1 and H_2 antagonists.

2.4 Instructions for Preparation and IV Administration

IXEMPRA *Kit* contains two vials, a vial labeled IXEMPRA (ixabepilone) for injection which contains ixabepilone powder and a vial containing DILUENT for IXEMPRA. Only supplied DILUENT must be used for constituting IXEMPRA (ixabepilone) for injection. IXEMPRA *Kit* must be stored in a refrigerator at 2° C - 8° C (36° F - 46° F) in the original package to protect from light. Prior to constituting IXEMPRA for injection, the *Kit* should be removed from the refrigerator and allowed to stand at room temperature for approximately 30 minutes. When the vials are first removed from the refrigerator, a white precipitate may be observed in the DILUENT vial. This precipitate will dissolve to form a clear solution once the DILUENT warms to room temperature. To allow for withdrawal losses, the vial labeled as 15 mg IXEMPRA for injection contains 16 mg of ixabepilone and the vial labeled as 45 mg IXEMPRA for injection contains 47 mg of ixabepilone. The 15-mg IXEMPRA *Kit* is supplied with a vial providing 8 mL of the DILUENT and the 45-mg IXEMPRA *Kit* is supplied with a vial providing 23.5 mL of the DILUENT. After constituting with the DILUENT, the concentration of ixabepilone is 2 mg/mL.

Please refer to Preparation and Handling Precautions [see Dosage and Administration (2.5)] before preparation.

A. To constitute:

1. With a suitable syringe, aseptically withdraw the DILUENT and slowly inject it into the IXEMPRA for injection vial. The 15-mg IXEMPRA is constituted with 8 mL of DILUENT and the 45-mg IXEMPRA is constituted with 23.5 mL of DILUENT.
2. Gently swirl and invert the vial until the powder in IXEMPRA is completely dissolved.

B. To dilute:

Before administration, the constituted solution must be further diluted with one of the specified infusion fluids listed below. The IXEMPRA infusion must be prepared in a DEHP [di-(2-ethylhexyl) phthalate] free bag.

The following infusion fluids have been qualified for use in the dilution of IXEMPRA:

- Lactated Ringer's Injection, USP
- 0.9% Sodium Chloride Injection, USP (pH adjusted with Sodium Bicarbonate Injection, USP)
  - When using a 250 mL or a 500 mL bag of 0.9% Sodium Chloride Injection to prepare the infusion, the pH must be adjusted to a pH between 6.0 and 9.0 by adding 2 mEq (ie, 2 mL of an 8.4% w/v solution or 4 mL of a 4.2% w/v solution) of Sodium Bicarbonate Injection, prior to the addition of the constituted IXEMPRA solution.
- PLASMA-LYTE A Injection pH 7.4®

Table 2: Dose Adjustments for IXEMPRA as Monotherapy in Patients with Hepatic Impairment

	Transaminase Levels		Bilirubin Levels[a]	IXEMPRA[b] (mg/m^2)
Mild	AST and ALT ≤2.5 × ULN	and	≤1 × ULN	40
	AST and ALT ≤10 × ULN	and	≤1.5 × ULN	32
Moderate	AST and ALT ≤10 × ULN	and	>1.5 × ULN - ≤3 × ULN	20 - 30

[a] Excluding patients whose total bilirubin is elevated due to Gilbert's disease.
[b] Dosage recommendations are for first course of therapy; further decreases in subsequent courses should be based on individual tolerance.

For most doses, a 250 mL bag of infusion fluid is sufficient. However, it is necessary to check the final IXEMPRA (ixabepilone) infusion concentration of each dose based on the volume of infusion fluid to be used.

The final concentration for infusion must be between 0.2 mg/mL and 0.6 mg/mL. To calculate the final infusion concentration, use the following formulas:

Total Infusion Volume = mL of Constituted Solution + mL of infusion fluid

Final Infusion Concentration = Dose of IXEMPRA (mg)/ Total Infusion Volume (mL)

1. Aseptically, withdraw the appropriate volume of constituted solution containing 2 mg of ixabepilone per mL.
2. Aseptically, transfer to an intravenous (IV) bag containing an appropriate volume of infusion fluid to achieve the final desired concentration of IXEMPRA.
3. Thoroughly mix the infusion bag by manual rotation.

The infusion solution must be administered through an appropriate in-line filter with a microporous membrane of 0.2 to 1.2 microns. DEHP-free infusion containers and administration sets must be used. Any remaining solution should be discarded according to institutional procedures for antineoplastics.

Stability

After constituting IXEMPRA, the constituted solution should be further diluted with infusion fluid as soon as possible, but may be stored in the vial (not the syringe) for a maximum of 1 hour at room temperature and room light. Once diluted with infusion fluid, the solution is stable at room temperature and room light for a maximum of 6 hours. Administration of diluted IXEMPRA must be completed within this 6-hour period. The infusion fluids previously mentioned are specified because their pH is in the range of 6.0 to 9.0, which is required to maintain IXEMPRA stability. Other infusion fluids should not be used with IXEMPRA.

2.5 Preparation and Handling Precautions

Procedures for proper handling and disposal of antineoplastic drugs *[see References (15)]* should be followed. To minimize the risk of dermal exposure, impervious gloves should be worn when handling vials containing IXEMPRA, regardless of the setting, including unpacking and inspection, transport within a facility, and dose preparation and administration.

3 DOSAGE FORMS AND STRENGTHS

IXEMPRA for injection, 15 mg supplied with DILUENT for IXEMPRA, 8 mL.

IXEMPRA for injection, 45 mg supplied with DILUENT for IXEMPRA, 23.5 mL.

4 CONTRAINDICATIONS

IXEMPRA is contraindicated in patients with a history of a severe (CTC grade 3/4) hypersensitivity reaction to agents containing Cremophor® EL or its derivatives (eg, polyoxyethylated castor oil) *[see Warnings and Precautions (5.4)]*.

IXEMPRA is contraindicated in patients who have a neutrophil count <1500 cells/mm^3 or a platelet count <100,000 cells/mm^3 *[see Warnings and Precautions (5.2)]*.

IXEMPRA in combination with capecitabine is contraindicated in patients with AST or ALT >2.5 × ULN or bilirubin >1 × ULN *[see Boxed Warning and Warnings and Precautions (5.3)]*.

5 WARNINGS AND PRECAUTIONS

5.1 Peripheral Neuropathy

Peripheral neuropathy was common (see Table 3). Patients treated with IXEMPRA should be monitored for symptoms of neuropathy, such as burning sensation, hyperesthesia, hypoesthesia, paresthesia, discomfort, or neuropathic pain. Neuropathy occurred early during treatment; ~75% of new onset or worsening neuropathy occurred during the first 3 cycles. Patients experiencing new or worsening symptoms may require a reduction or delay in the dose of IXEMPRA *[see Dosage and Administration (2.2)]*. In clinical studies, peripheral neuropathy was managed through dose reductions, dose delays, and treatment discontinuation. Neuropathy was the most frequent cause of treatment discontinuation due to drug toxicity. In Studies 046 and 081, 80% and 87%, respectively, of patients with peripheral neuropathy who received IXEMPRA had improvement or no worsening of their neuropathy following dose reduction. For patients with grade 3/4 neuropathy in Studies 046 and 081, 76% and 79%, respectively, had documented improvement to baseline or grade 1, twelve weeks after onset.

Table 3: Treatment-related Peripheral Neuropathy

	IXEMPRA with capecitabine Study 046	IXEMPRA as monotherapy Study 081
Peripheral neuropathy (all grades)[a,b]	67%	63%
Peripheral neuropathy (grade 3/4)[a,b]	23%	14%
Discontinuation due to neuropathy	21%	6%
Median number of cycles to onset of grade 3/4 neuropathy	4	4
Median time to improvement of grade 3/4 neuropathy to baseline or to grade 1	6.0 weeks	4.6 weeks

[a] Sensory and motor neuropathy combined.
[b] 24% and 27% of patients in 046 and 081, respectively, had preexisting neuropathy (grade 1).

A pooled analysis of 1540 cancer patients treated with IXEMPRA (ixabepilone) indicated that patients with diabetes mellitus or preexisting peripheral neuropathy may be at increased risk of severe neuropathy. Prior therapy with neurotoxic chemotherapy agents did not predict the development of neuropathy. Patients with moderate to severe neuropathy (grade 2 or greater) were excluded from studies with IXEMPRA. Caution should be used when treating patients with diabetes mellitus or preexisting peripheral neuropathy.

5.2 Myelosuppression

Myelosuppression is dose-dependent and primarily manifested as neutropenia. In clinical studies, grade 4 neutropenia (<500 cells/mm^3) occurred in 36% of patients treated with IXEMPRA in combination with capecitabine and 23% of patients treated with IXEMPRA monotherapy. Febrile neutropenia and infection with neutropenia were reported in 5% and 6% of patients treated with IXEMPRA in combination with capecitabine, respectively, and 3% and 5% of patients treated with IXEMPRA as monotherapy, respectively. Neutropenia-related death occurred in 1.9% of 414 patients with normal hepatic function or mild hepatic impairment treated with IXEMPRA in combination with capecitabine. The rate of neutropenia-related deaths was higher (29%, 5 out of 17) in patients with AST or ALT >2.5 × ULN or bilirubin >1.5 × ULN *[see Boxed Warning, Contraindications (4), and Warnings and Precautions (5.3)]*. Neutropenia-related death occurred in 0.4% of 240 patients treated with IXEMPRA as monotherapy. No neutropenia-related deaths were reported in 24 patients with AST or ALT >2.5 × ULN or bilirubin >1.5 × ULN treated with IXEMPRA monotherapy. IXEMPRA must not be administered to patients with a neutrophil count <1500 cells/mm^3. To monitor for myelosuppression, frequent peripheral blood cell counts are recommended for all patients receiving IXEMPRA. Patients who experience severe neutropenia or thrombocytopenia should have their dose reduced *[see Dosage and Administration (2.2)]*.

5.3 Hepatic Impairment

Patients with baseline AST or ALT >2.5 × ULN or bilirubin >1.5 × ULN experienced greater toxicity than patients with baseline AST or ALT ≤2.5 × ULN or bilirubin ≤1.5 × ULN when treated with IXEMPRA at 40 mg/m^2 in combination with capecitabine or as monotherapy in breast cancer studies. In combination with capecitabine, the overall frequency of grade 3/4 adverse reactions, febrile neutropenia, serious adverse reactions, and toxicity-related deaths was greater *[see Warnings and Precautions (5.2)]*. With monotherapy, grade 4 neutropenia, febrile neutropenia, and serious adverse reactions were more frequent. The safety and pharmacokinetics of IXEMPRA as monotherapy were evaluated in a dose escalation study in 56 patients with varying degrees of hepatic impairment. Exposure was increased in patients with elevated AST or bilirubin *[see Use in Specific Populations (8.6)]*.

IXEMPRA (ixabepilone) in combination with capecitabine is contraindicated in patients with AST or ALT >2.5 × ULN or bilirubin >1 × ULN due to increased risk of toxicity- and neutropenia-related death *[see Boxed Warning, Contraindications (4), and Warnings and Precautions (5.2)]*. Patients who are treated with IXEMPRA as monotherapy should receive a reduced dose depending on the degree of hepatic impairment *[see Dosage and Administration (2.2)]*. Use in patients with AST or ALT >10 × ULN or bilirubin >3 × ULN is not recommended. Limited data are available for patients with AST or ALT >5 × ULN. Caution should be used when treating these patients *[see Dosage and Administration (2.2)]*.

5.4 Hypersensitivity Reactions

Patients with a history of a severe hypersensitivity reaction to agents containing Cremophor® EL or its derivatives (eg, polyoxyethylated castor oil) should not be treated with IXEMPRA. All patients should be premedicated with an H_1 and an H_2 antagonist approximately 1 hour before IXEMPRA infusion and be observed for hypersensitivity reactions (eg, flushing, rash, dyspnea, and bronchospasm). In case of severe hypersensitivity reactions, infusion of IXEMPRA should be stopped and aggressive supportive treatment (eg, epinephrine, corticosteroids) started. Of the 1323 patients treated with IXEMPRA in clinical studies, 9 patients (1%) had experienced severe hypersensitivity reactions (including anaphylaxis). Three of the 9 patients were able to be retreated. Patients who experience a hypersensitivity reaction in one cycle of IXEMPRA must be premedicated in subsequent cycles with a corticosteroid in addition to the H_1 and H_2 antagonists, and extension of the infusion time should be considered *[see Dosage and Administration (2.3) and Contraindications (4)]*.

5.5 Pregnancy

Pregnancy Category D.

IXEMPRA may cause fetal harm when administered to pregnant women. There are no adequate and well-controlled studies with IXEMPRA in pregnant women. Women should be advised not to become pregnant when taking IXEMPRA. If this drug is used during pregnancy, or if the patient becomes pregnant while taking this drug, the patient should be apprised of the potential hazard to the fetus.

Ixabepilone was studied for effects on embryo-fetal development in pregnant rats and rabbits given IV doses of 0.02, 0.08, and 0.3 mg/kg/day and 0.01, 0.03, 0.11, and 0.3 mg/kg/day, respectively. There were no teratogenic effects. In rats, an increase in resorptions and post-implantation loss and a decrease in the number of live fetuses and fetal weight was observed at the maternally toxic dose of 0.3 mg/kg/day (approximately one-tenth the human clinical exposure based on AUC). Abnormalities included a reduced ossification of caudal vertebrae, sternebrae, and metacarpals. In rabbits, ixabepilone caused maternal toxicity (death) and embryo-fetal toxicity (resorptions) at 0.3 mg/kg/day (approximately one-tenth the human clinical dose based on body surface area). No fetuses were available at this dose for evaluation.

5.6 Cardiac Adverse Reactions

The frequency of cardiac adverse reactions (myocardial ischemia and ventricular dysfunction) was higher in the IXEMPRA in combination with capecitabine (1.9%) than in the capecitabine alone (0.3%) treatment group. Supraventricular arrhythmias were observed in the combination arm (0.5%) and not in the capecitabine alone arm. Caution should be exercised in patients with a history of cardiac disease. Discontinuation of IXEMPRA should be considered in patients who develop cardiac ischemia or impaired cardiac function.

5.7 Potential for Cognitive Impairment from Excipients

Since IXEMPRA contains dehydrated alcohol USP, consideration should be given to the possibility of central nervous system and other effects of alcohol *[see Description (11)]*.

6 ADVERSE REACTIONS

The following adverse reactions are discussed in greater detail in other sections.

- Peripheral neuropathy *[see Warnings and Precautions (5.1)]*
- Myelosuppression *[see Warnings and Precautions (5.2)]*
- Hypersensitivity reactions *[see Warnings and Precautions (5.4)]*

6.1 Clinical Trials Experience

Because clinical trials are conducted under widely varying conditions, the adverse reaction rates observed in the clinical trials of a drug cannot be directly compared to rates in other clinical trials and may not reflect the rates observed in clinical practice.

Unless otherwise specified, assessment of adverse reactions is based on one randomized study (Study 046) and one single-arm study (Study 081). In Study 046, 369 patients with metastatic breast cancer were treated with IXEMPRA (ixabepilone) 40 mg/m² administered intravenously over 3 hours every 21 days, combined with capecitabine 1000 mg/m² twice daily for 2 weeks followed by a 1-week rest period. Patients treated with capecitabine as monotherapy (n=368) in this study received 1250 mg/m² twice daily for 2 weeks every 21 days. In Study 081, 126 patients with metastatic or locally advanced breast cancer were treated with IXEMPRA (ixabepilone) 40 mg/m² administered intravenously over 3 hours every 3 weeks.

The most common adverse reactions (≥20%) reported by patients receiving IXEMPRA were peripheral sensory neuropathy, fatigue/asthenia, myalgia/arthralgia, alopecia, nausea, vomiting, stomatitis/mucositis, diarrhea, and musculoskeletal pain. The following additional reactions

Table 4: Nonhematologic Drug-related Adverse Reactions Occurring in at Least 5% of Patients with Metastatic or Locally Advanced Breast Cancer Treated with IXEMPRA

	Study 046				Study 081	
	IXEMPRA with capecitabine n=369		Capecitabine n=368		IXEMPRA monotherapy n=126	
System Organ Class[a]/ Preferred Term	Total (%)	Grade 3/4 (%)	Total (%)	Grade 3/4 (%)	Total (%)	Grade 3/4 (%)
Infections and Infestations						
Upper respiratory tract infection[b]	4	0	3	0	6	0
Blood and Lymphatic System Disorders						
Febrile neutropenia	5	4[c]	1	1[d]	3	3[d]
Immune System Disorders						
Hypersensitivity[b]	2	1[d]	0	0	5	1[d]
Metabolism and Nutrition Disorders						
Anorexia[b]	34	3[d]	15	1[d]	19	2[d]
Dehydration[b]	5	2	2	<1[d]	2	1[d]
Psychiatric Disorders						
Insomnia[b]	9	<1[d]	2	0	5	0
Nervous System Disorders						
Peripheral neuropathy						
Sensory neuropathy[b,e]	65	21	16	0	62	14
Motor neuropathy[b]	16	5[d]	<1	0	10	1[d]
Headache	8	<1[d]	3	0	11	0
Taste disorder[b]	12	0	4	0	6	0
Dizziness	8	1[d]	5	1[d]	7	0
Eye Disorders						
Lacrimation increased	5	0	4	<1[d]	4	0
Vascular Disorders						
Hot flush[b]	5	0	2	0	6	0
Respiratory, Thoracic, and Mediastinal Disorders						
Dyspnea[b]	7	1	4	1	9	1[d]
Cough[b]	6	0	2	0	2	0
Gastrointestinal Disorders						
Nausea	53	3[d]	40	2[d]	42	2[d]
Vomiting[b]	39	4[d]	24	2	29	1[d]
Stomatitis/mucositis[b]	31	4	20	3[d]	29	6
Diarrhea[b]	44	6[d]	39	9	22	1[d]
Constipation	22	0	6	<1[d]	16	2[d]
Abdominal pain[b]	24	2[d]	14	1[d]	13	2[d]
Gastroesophageal reflux disease[b]	7	1[d]	8	0	6	0
Skin and Subcutaneous Tissue Disorders						
Alopecia[b]	31	0	3	0	48	0
Skin rash[b]	17	1[d]	7	0	9	2[d]
Nail disorder[b]	24	2[d]	10	<1[d]	9	0
Palmar-plantar erythrodysesthesia syndrome[b,f]	64	18[d]	63	17[d]	8	2[d]
Pruritus	5	0	2	0	6	1[d]
Skin exfoliation[b]	5	<1[d]	3	0	2	0
Skin hyperpigmentation[b]	11	0	14	0	2	0
Musculoskeletal, Connective Tissue, and Bone Disorders						
Myalgia/arthralgia[b]	39	8[d]	5	<1[d]	49	8[d]
Musculoskeletal pain[b]	23	2[d]	5	0	20	3[d]
General Disorders and Administration Site Conditions						
Fatigue/asthenia[b]	60	16	29	4	56	13
Edema[b]	8	0	5	<1[d]	9	1[d]
Pyrexia	10	1[d]	4	0	8	1[d]
Pain[b]	9	1[d]	2	0	8	3[d]
Chest pain[b]	4	1[d]	<1	0	5	1[d]
Investigations						
Weight decreased	11	0	3	0	6	0

[a] System organ class presented as outlined in Guidelines for Preparing Core Clinical Safety Information on Drugs by the Council for International Organizations of Medical Sciences (CIOMS).

[b] A composite of multiple MedDRA Preferred Terms.

[c] NCI CTC grading for febrile neutropenia ranges from Grade 3 to 5. Three patients (1%) experienced Grade 5 (fatal) febrile neutropenia. Other neutropenia-related deaths (9) occurred in the absence of reported febrile neutropenia *[see Warnings and Precautions (5.2)]*.

[d] No grade 4 reports.

[e] Peripheral sensory neuropathy (graded with the NCI CTC scale) was defined as the occurrence of any of the following: areflexia, burning sensation, dysesthesia, hyperesthesia, hypoesthesia, hyporeflexia, neuralgia, neuritis, neuropathy, neuropathy peripheral, neurotoxicity, painful response to normal stimuli, paresthesia, pallanesthesia, peripheral sensory neuropathy, polyneuropathy, polyneuropathy toxic and sensorimotor disorder.
Peripheral motor neuropathy was defined as the occurrence of any of the following: multifocal motor neuropathy, neuromuscular toxicity, peripheral motor neuropathy, and peripheral sensorimotor neuropathy.

[f] Palmar-plantar erythrodysesthesia (hand-foot syndrome) was graded on a 1-3 severity scale in Study 046.

occurred in ≥20% in combination treatment: palmar-plantar erythrodysesthesia (hand-foot) syndrome, anorexia, abdominal pain, nail disorder, and constipation. The most common hematologic abnormalities (>40%) include neutropenia, leukopenia, anemia, and thrombocytopenia.

Table 4 presents nonhematologic adverse reactions reported in 5% or more of patients. Hematologic abnormalities are presented separately in Table 5.

[See table 4 at top of previous page]

[See table 5 above]

The following serious adverse reactions were also reported in 1323 patients treated with IXEMPRA (ixabepilone) as monotherapy or in combination with other therapies in Phase 2 and 3 studies.

Infections and Infestations: sepsis, pneumonia, infection, neutropenic infection, urinary tract infection, bacterial infection, enterocolitis, laryngitis, lower respiratory tract infection

Blood and Lymphatic System Disorders: coagulopathy, lymphopenia

Metabolism and Nutrition Disorders: hyponatremia, metabolic acidosis, hypokalemia, hypovolemia

Nervous System Disorders: cognitive disorder, syncope, cerebral hemorrhage, abnormal coordination, lethargy

Cardiac Disorders: myocardial infarction, supraventricular arrhythmia, left ventricular dysfunction, angina pectoris, atrial flutter, cardiomyopathy, myocardial ischemia

Vascular Disorders: hypotension, thrombosis, embolism, hemorrhage, hypovolemic shock, vasculitis

Respiratory, Thoracic, and Mediastinal Disorders: pneumonitis, hypoxia, respiratory failure, acute pulmonary edema, dysphonia, pharyngolaryngeal pain

Gastrointestinal Disorders: ileus, colitis, impaired gastric emptying, esophagitis, dysphagia, gastritis, gastrointestinal hemorrhage

Hepatobiliary Disorders: acute hepatic failure, jaundice

Skin and Subcutaneous Tissue Disorders: erythema multiforme

Musculoskeletal, Connective Tissue, and Bone Disorders: muscular weakness, muscle spasms, trismus

Renal and Urinary Disorders: nephrolithiasis, renal failure

General Disorders and Administration Site Conditions: chills

Investigations: increased transaminases, increased blood alkaline phosphatase, increased gamma-glutamyltransferase

6.2 Postmarketing Experience

Radiation recall has been reported during postmarketing use of IXEMPRA. Because this reaction was reported voluntarily from a population of uncertain size, it is not always possible to reliably estimate the frequency or establish a causal relationship to drug exposure.

7 DRUG INTERACTIONS

7.1 Effect of Other Drugs on Ixabepilone

Drugs That May Increase Ixabepilone Plasma Concentrations

CYP3A4 Inhibitors: Coadministration of ixabepilone with ketoconazole, a potent CYP3A4 inhibitor, increased ixabepilone AUC by 79% compared to ixabepilone treatment alone. If alternative treatment cannot be administered, a dose adjustment should be considered. The effect of mild or moderate inhibitors (eg, erythromycin, fluconazole, or verapamil) on exposure to ixabepilone has not been studied. Therefore, caution should be used when administering mild or moderate CYP3A4 inhibitors during treatment with IXEMPRA, and alternative therapeutic agents that do not inhibit CYP3A4 should be considered. Patients receiving CYP3A4 inhibitors during treatment with IXEMPRA should be monitored closely for acute toxicities (eg, frequent monitoring of peripheral blood counts between cycles of IXEMPRA) *[see Dosage and Administration (2.2)]*.

Drugs That May Decrease Ixabepilone Plasma Concentrations

CYP3A4 Inducers: IXEMPRA is a CYP3A4 substrate. Coadministration of IXEMPRA with rifampin, a potent CYP3A4 inducer, decreased ixabepilone AUC by 43% compared to IXEMPRA treatment alone. Other strong CYP3A4 inducers (eg, dexamethasone, phenytoin, carbamazepine, rifabutin, and phenobarbital) may also decrease ixabepilone concentrations leading to subtherapeutic levels. Therefore, therapeutic agents with low enzyme induction potential should be considered for coadministration with IXEMPRA. St. John's Wort may decrease ixabepilone plasma concentrations unpredictably and should be avoided. If patients must be coadministered a strong CYP3A4 inducer, a gradual dose adjustment may be considered *[see Dosage and Administration (2.2)]*.

7.2 Effect of Ixabepilone on Other Drugs

Ixabepilone does not inhibit CYP enzymes at relevant clinical concentrations and is not expected to alter the plasma concentrations of other drugs *[see Clinical Pharmacology (12.3)]*.

7.3 Capecitabine

In patients with cancer who received ixabepilone (40 mg/m^2) in combination with capecitabine (1000 mg/m^2), ixabepilone Cmax decreased by 19%, capecitabine Cmax decreased by 27%, and 5-fluorouracil AUC increased by 14%, as compared to ixabepilone or capecitabine administered separately. The interaction is not clinically significant given that the combination treatment is supported by efficacy data.

Table 5: Hematologic Abnormalities in Patients with Metastatic or Locally Advanced Breast Cancer Treated with IXEMPRA

	Study 046				Study 081	
	IXEMPRA with capecitabine n=369		Capecitabine n=368		IXEMPRA monotherapy n=126	
Hematology Parameter	Grade 3 (%)	Grade 4 (%)	Grade 3 (%)	Grade 4 (%)	Grade 3 (%)	Grade 4 (%)
Neutropenia[a]	32	36	9	2	31	23
Leukopenia (WBC)	41	16	5	1	36	13
Anemia (Hgb)	8	2	4	1	6	2
Thrombocytopenia	5	3	2	2	5	2

[a] G-CSF (granulocyte colony stimulating factor) or GM-CSF (granulocyte macrophage colony stimulating factor) was used in 20% and 17% of patients who received IXEMPRA in Study 046 and Study 081, respectively.

8 USE IN SPECIFIC POPULATIONS

8.1 Pregnancy

Pregnancy Category D *[see Warnings and Precautions (5.5)]*.

8.3 Nursing Mothers

It is not known whether ixabepilone is excreted into human milk. Following intravenous administration of radiolabeled ixabepilone to rats on days 7 to 9 postpartum, concentrations of radioactivity in milk were comparable with those in plasma and declined in parallel with the plasma concentrations. Because many drugs are excreted in human milk and because of the potential for serious adverse reactions in nursing infants from ixabepilone, a decision must be made whether to discontinue nursing or to discontinue IXEMPRA (ixabepilone) taking into account the importance of the drug to the mother.

8.4 Pediatric Use

The effectiveness of IXEMPRA in pediatric patients has not been established. IXEMPRA was evaluated in one Phase 1 and one Phase 2 trial. The pediatric patients had a safety profile consistent with that seen in adults, and no new safety signals were identified.

In the Phase 1 open-label, dose-finding trial, the safety of IXEMPRA was evaluated in 19 pediatric patients with advanced or refractory solid tumors and 2 with acute leukemias. IXEMPRA was administered as a one-hour IV infusion daily for the first five days of a 21-day cycle at one of 5 dose levels, ranging from 3 to 10 mg/m^2. Among the 21 patients, 12 ranged in age from 2 to 12 years and 9 ranged from 13 to 18 years. The maximum tolerated dose was 8 mg/m^2 IV daily for 5 days every 21 days. No significant activity was observed. The pharmacokinetics of ixabepilone were characterized by population pharmacokinetic analysis of data for 16 patients from this trial, who were aged 2 to 18 years (median 12 years). The pharmacokinetic parameters of ixabepilone in these pediatric patients were compared to the corresponding parameters of 130 adult patients enrolled in clinical trials using the same dosing schedule. The median BSA normalized clearance of ixabepilone in pediatric patients (17 L/h/m^2) was similar to that in adult patients (20 L/h/m^2).

In the Phase 2 trial of 59 patients with advanced or refractory solid tumors, 28 ranged in age from 3 to 12 years and 19 ranged in age from 13 to 18 years. Twelve additional patients over the age of 18 were treated in this trial. IXEMPRA was administered at a dose of 8 mg/m^2 IV daily for 5 days every 21 days. This trial was terminated early due to lack of efficacy.

8.5 Geriatric Use

Clinical studies of IXEMPRA did not include sufficient numbers of subjects aged sixty-five and over to determine whether they respond differently from younger subjects.

Forty-five of 431 patients treated with IXEMPRA in combination with capecitabine were ≥65 years of age and 3 patients were ≥75. Overall, the incidence of grade 3/4 adverse reactions was higher in patients ≥65 years of age versus those <65 years of age (82% versus 68%) including grade 3/4 stomatitis (9% versus 1%), diarrhea (9% versus 6%), palmar-plantar erythrodysesthesia syndrome (27% versus 20%), peripheral neuropathy (24% versus 22%), febrile neutropenia (9% versus 3%), fatigue (16% versus 12%), and asthenia (11% versus 6%). Toxicity-related deaths occurred in 2 (4.7%) of 43 patients ≥65 years with normal baseline hepatic function or mild impairment.

Thirty-two of 240 breast cancer patients treated with IXEMPRA as monotherapy were ≥65 years of age and 6 patients were ≥75. No overall differences in safety were observed in these patients compared to those <65 years of age.

8.6 Hepatic Impairment

IXEMPRA was evaluated in 56 patients with mild to severe hepatic impairment defined by bilirubin levels and AST levels. Compared to patients with normal hepatic function (n=17), the area under the curve ($AUC_{0\text{-infinity}}$) of ixabepilone increased by:

- 22% in patients with a) bilirubin >1 – 1.5 × ULN **or** b) AST >ULN but bilirubin <1.5 × ULN;
- 30% in patients with bilirubin >1.5 – 3 × ULN and any AST level; and
- 81% in patients with bilirubin >3 × ULN and any AST level.

Doses of 10 and 20 mg/m^2 as monotherapy were tolerated in 17 patients with severe hepatic impairment (bilirubin >3 × ULN).

IXEMPRA (ixabepilone) in combination with capecitabine must not be given to patients with AST or ALT >2.5 × ULN or bilirubin >1 × ULN *[see Boxed Warning, Contraindications (4), and Warnings and Precautions (5.3)]*. Dose reduction is recommended when administering IXEMPRA as monotherapy to patients with hepatic impairment *[see Dosage and Administration (2.3)]*. Because there is a need for dosage adjustment based upon hepatic function, assessment of hepatic function is recommended before initiation of IXEMPRA and periodically thereafter.

8.7 Renal Impairment

Ixabepilone is minimally excreted via the kidney. No controlled pharmacokinetic studies were conducted with IXEMPRA in patients with renal impairment. IXEMPRA in combination with capecitabine has not been evaluated in patients with calculated creatinine clearance of <50 mL/min. IXEMPRA as monotherapy has not been evaluated in patients with creatinine >1.5 times ULN. In a population pharmacokinetic analysis of IXEMPRA as monotherapy, there was no meaningful effect of mild and moderate renal insufficiency (CrCL >30 mL/min) on the pharmacokinetics of ixabepilone.

10 OVERDOSAGE

Experience with overdose of IXEMPRA is limited to isolated cases. The adverse reactions reported in these cases included peripheral neuropathy, fatigue, musculoskeletal pain/myalgia, and gastrointestinal symptoms (nausea, anorexia, diarrhea, abdominal pain, stomatitis). The highest dose mistakenly received was 100 mg/m^2 (total dose 185 mg).

There is no known antidote for overdosage of IXEMPRA. In case of overdosage, the patient should be closely monitored and supportive treatment should be administered. Management of overdose should include supportive medical interventions to treat the presenting clinical manifestations.

11 DESCRIPTION

IXEMPRA (ixabepilone) is a microtubule inhibitor belonging to a class of antineoplastic agents, the epothilones and their analogs. The epothilones are isolated from the myxobacterium *Sorangium cellulosum*. Ixabepilone is a semisynthetic analog of epothilone B, a 16-membered polyketide macrolide, with a chemically modified lactam substitution for the naturally existing lactone.

The chemical name for ixabepilone is (1*S*,3*S*,7*S*,10*R*,11*S*,12*S*,16*R*)-7,11-dihydroxy-8,8,10,12,16-pentamethyl-3-[(1*E*)-1-methyl-2-(2-methyl-4-thiazolyl)ethenyl]-17-oxa-4-azabicyclo[14.1.0] heptadecane-5,9-dione, and it has a molecular weight of 506.7. Ixabepilone has the following structural formula:

[See chemical structure at top of next column]

IXEMPRA (ixabepilone) for injection is intended for intravenous infusion only after constitution with the supplied DILUENT and after further dilution with a specified infusion fluid *[see Instructions for Preparation and IV Administration (2.4)]*. IXEMPRA (ixabepilone) for injection is supplied as a sterile, non-pyrogenic, single-use vial providing 15 mg or 45 mg ixabepilone as a lyophilized white powder. The DILUENT for IXEMPRA is a sterile, non-pyrogenic so-

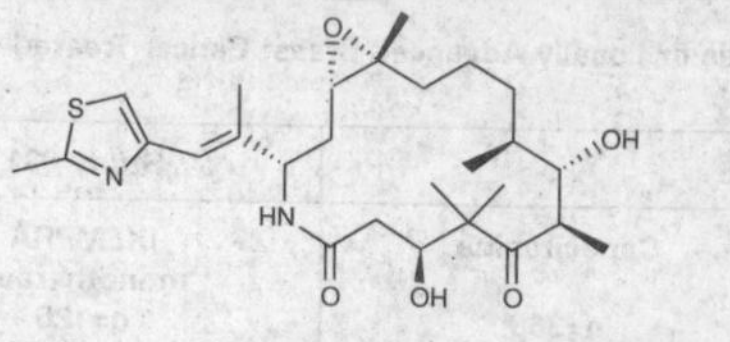

lution of 52.8% (w/v) purified polyoxyethylated castor oil and 39.8% (w/v) dehydrated alcohol, USP. The IXEMPRA (ixabepilone) for injection and the DILUENT for IXEMPRA are copackaged and supplied as IXEMPRA *Kit*.

12 CLINICAL PHARMACOLOGY

12.1 Mechanism of Action

Ixabepilone is a semi-synthetic analog of epothilone B. Ixabepilone binds directly to β-tubulin subunits on microtubules, leading to suppression of microtubule dynamics. Ixabepilone suppresses the dynamic instability of αβ-II and αβ-III microtubules. Ixabepilone possesses low *in vitro* susceptibility to multiple tumor resistance mechanisms including efflux transporters, such as MRP-1 and P-glycoprotein (P-gp). Ixabepilone blocks cells in the mitotic phase of the cell division cycle, leading to cell death.

12.2 Pharmacodynamics

In cancer patients, ixabepilone has a plasma concentration-dependent effect on tubulin dynamics in peripheral blood mononuclear cells that is observed as the formation of microtubule bundles. Ixabepilone has antitumor activity *in vivo* against multiple human tumor xenografts, including drug-resistant types that overexpress P-gp, MRP-1, and βIII tubulin isoforms, or harbor tubulin mutations. Ixabepilone is active in xenografts that are resistant to multiple agents including taxanes, anthracyclines, and vinca alkaloids. Ixabepilone demonstrated synergistic antitumor activity in combination with capecitabine *in vivo*. In addition to direct antitumor activity, ixabepilone has antiangiogenic activity.

12.3 Pharmacokinetics

Absorption

Following administration of a single 40 mg/m^2 dose of IXEMPRA in patients with cancer, the mean Cmax was 252 ng/mL (coefficient of variation, CV 56%) and the mean AUC was 2143 ng•hr/mL (CV 48%). Typically Cmax occurred at the end of the 3-hour infusion. In cancer patients, the pharmacokinetics of ixabepilone were linear at doses of 15 to 57 mg/m^2.

Distribution

The mean volume of distribution of 40 mg/m^2 ixabepilone at steady-state was in excess of 1000 L. *In vitro*, the binding of ixabepilone to human serum proteins ranged from 67 to 77%, and the blood-to-plasma concentration ratios in human blood ranged from 0.65 to 0.85 over a concentration range of 50 to 5000 ng/mL.

Metabolism

Ixabepilone is extensively metabolized in the liver. *In vitro* studies indicated that the main route of oxidative metabolism of ixabepilone is via CYP3A4. More than 30 metabolites of ixabepilone are excreted into human urine and feces. No single metabolite accounted for more than 6% of the administered dose. The biotransformation products generated from ixabepilone by human liver microsomes were not active when tested for *in vitro* cytotoxicity against a human tumor cell line.

In vitro studies using human liver microsomes indicate that clinically relevant concentrations of ixabepilone do not inhibit CYP3A4, CYP1A2, CYP2A6, CYP2B6, CYP2C8, CYP2C9, CYP2C19, or CYP2D6. Ixabepilone does not induce the activity or the corresponding mRNA levels of CYP1A2, CYP2B6, CYP2C9, or CYP3A4 in cultured human hepatocytes at clinically relevant concentrations. Therefore, it is unlikely that ixabepilone will affect the plasma levels of drugs that are substrates of CYP enzymes.

Elimination

Ixabepilone is eliminated primarily as metabolized drug. After an intravenous ^{14}[C]-ixabepilone dose to patients, approximately 86% of the dose was eliminated within 7 days in feces (65% of the dose) and in urine (21% of the dose). Unchanged ixabepilone accounted for approximately 1.6% and 5.6% of the dose in feces and urine, respectively. Ixabepilone has a terminal elimination half-life of approximately 52 hours. No accumulation in plasma is expected for ixabepilone administered every 3 weeks.

Drug Transport Systems

Ixabepilone is a substrate and a weak inhibitor for the drug efflux transporter P-glycoprotein (P-gp) *in vitro*.

Ixabepilone is not a substrate for the breast cancer resistance protein (BCRP) *in vitro*.

Effects of Age, Gender, and Race

Based upon a population pharmacokinetic analysis in 676 cancer patients, gender, race, and age do not have meaningful effects on the pharmacokinetics of ixabepilone.

12.4 Effect of Ixabepilone on QT/QTc Interval

The QT prolongation potential of ixabepilone was assessed as part of an uncontrolled, open-label, single-dose study in advanced cancer patients. Fourteen patients received a single dose of IXEMPRA (ixabepilone) 40 mg/m^2 intravenously over 3 hours and serial ECGs were collected over 24 hours. The maximum mean ΔQTcF was observed 1 hour after the end of infusion and was 8 ms (upper 95% CI: 12 ms). No patients had a QTcF interval >450 ms or ΔQTcF >30 ms after IXEMPRA administration. However, small increases in QTc interval with the use of ixabepilone cannot be excluded due to study design limitations.

13 NONCLINICAL TOXICOLOGY

13.1 Carcinogenesis, Mutagenesis, Impairment of Fertility

Carcinogenicity studies with ixabepilone have not been conducted. Ixabepilone did not induce mutations in the microbial mutagenesis (Ames) assay and was not clastogenic in an *in vitro* cytogenetic assay using primary human lymphocytes. Ixabepilone was clastogenic (induction of micronuclei) in the *in vivo* rat micronucleus assay at doses ≥0.625 mg/kg/day.

There were no effects on male or female rat mating or fertility at doses up to 0.2 mg/kg/day in both males and females (approximately one-fifteenth the expected human clinical exposure based on AUC). The effect of ixabepilone on human fertility is unknown. However, when rats were given an IV infusion of ixabepilone during breeding and through the first 7 days of gestation, a significant increase in resorptions and pre- and post-implantation loss and a decrease in the number of corpora lutea was observed at 0.2 mg/kg/day. Testicular atrophy or degeneration was observed in 6-month rat and 9-month dog studies when ixabepilone was given every 21 days at intravenous doses of 6.7 mg/kg (40 mg/m^2) in rats (approximately 2.1 times the expected clinical exposure based on AUC) and 0.5 and 0.75 mg/kg (10 and 15 mg/m^2) in dogs (approximately 0.2 and 0.4 times the expected clinical exposure based on AUC).

13.2 Animal Toxicology

Overdose

In rats, single intravenous doses of ixabepilone from 60 to 180 mg/m^2 (mean AUC values ≥8156 ng·h/mL) were associated with mortality occurring between 5 and 14 days after dosing, and toxicity was principally manifested in the gastrointestinal, hematopoietic (bone-marrow), lymphatic, peripheral-nervous, and male-reproductive systems. In dogs, a single intravenous dose of 100 mg/m^2 (mean AUC value of 6925 ng·h/mL) was markedly toxic, inducing severe gastrointestinal toxicity and death 3 days after dosing.

14 CLINICAL STUDIES

Combination Therapy

In an open-label, multicenter, multinational, randomized trial of 752 patients with metastatic or locally advanced breast cancer, the efficacy and safety of IXEMPRA (40 mg/m^2 every 3 weeks) in combination with capecitabine (at 1000 mg/m^2 twice daily for 2 weeks followed by 1 week rest) were assessed in comparison with capecitabine as monotherapy (at 1250 mg/m^2 twice daily for 2 weeks followed by 1 week rest). Patients were previously treated with anthracyclines and taxanes. Patients were required to have demonstrated tumor progression or resistance to taxanes and anthracyclines as follows:

- tumor progression within 3 months of the last anthracycline dose in the metastatic setting or recurrence within 6 months in the adjuvant or neoadjuvant setting, and
- tumor progression within 4 months of the last taxane dose in the metastatic setting or recurrence within 12 months in the adjuvant or neoadjuvant setting.

For anthracyclines, patients who received a minimum cumulative dose of 240 mg/m^2 of doxorubicin or 360 mg/m^2 of epirubicin were also eligible.

Sixty-seven percent of patients were White, 23% were Asian, and 3% were Black. Both arms were evenly matched with regards to race, age (median 53 years), baseline performance status (Karnofsky 70-100%), and receipt of prior adjuvant or neo-adjuvant chemotherapy (75%). Tumors were ER-positive in 47% of patients, ER-negative in 43%, HER2-positive in 15%, HER2-negative in 61%, and ER-negative, PR-negative, HER2-negative in 25%. The baseline disease characteristics and previous therapies for all patients (n=752) are shown in Table 6.

Table 6: Baseline Disease Characteristics and Previous Therapies

	IXEMPRA with capecitabine n=375	Capecitabine n=377
Site of disease		
Visceral disease (liver or lung)	316 (84%)	315 (84%)
Liver	245 (65%)	228 (61%)
Lung	180 (48%)	174 (46%)
Lymph node	250 (67%)	249 (66%)
Bone	168 (45%)	162 (43%)
Skin/soft tissue	60 (16%)	62 (16%)
Number of prior chemotherapy regimens in metastatic setting[a]		
0	27 (7%)	33 (9%)
1	179 (48%)	184 (49%)
2	152 (41%)	138 (37%)
≥3	17 (5%)	22 (6%)
Anthracycline resistance[b]	164 (44%)	165 (44%)
Taxane Resistance[c]		
Neoadjuvant/adjuvant setting	40 (11%)	44 (12%)
Metastatic setting	327 (87%)	319 (85%)

[a] For IXEMPRA (ixabepilone) plus capecitabine versus capecitabine only, prior treatment in the metastatic setting included cyclophosphamide (25% vs. 23%), fluorouracil (22% vs. 16%), vinorelbine (11% vs. 12%), gemcitabine (9% each arm), carboplatin (9% vs. 7%), liposomal doxorubicin (3% each arm), and cisplatin (2% vs. 3%).

[b] Tumor progression within 3 months in the metastatic setting or recurrence within 6 months in the adjuvant or neoadjuvant setting.

[c] 24% and 21% of patients had received 2 or more taxane-containing regimens in the combination and single agent treatment groups, respectively.

The patients in the combination treatment group received a median of 5 cycles of treatment and patients in the capecitabine monotherapy treatment group received a median of 4 cycles of treatment.

The primary endpoint of the study was progression-free survival (PFS) defined as time from randomization to radiologic progression as determined by Independent Radiologic Review (IRR), clinical progression of measurable skin lesions or death from any cause. Other study endpoints included objective tumor response based on Response Evaluation Criteria in Solid Tumors (RECIST), time to response, response duration, and overall survival.

IXEMPRA in combination with capecitabine resulted in a statistically significant improvement in PFS compared to capecitabine. The results of the study are presented in Table 7 and Figure 1.

Table 7: Efficacy of IXEMPRA in Combination with Capecitabine vs Capecitabine Alone – Intent-to-Treat Analysis

Efficacy Parameter	IXEMPRA with capecitabine n=375	Capecitabine n=377
PFS		
Number of events[a]	242	256
Median	5.7 months	4.1 months
(95% CI)	(4.8 - 6.7)	(3.1 - 4.3)
Hazard Ratio[b] (95% CI)	0.69 (0.58 - 0.83)	
p-value[c] (Log rank)	<0.0001	
Objective Tumor Response Rate	34.7%	14.3%
(95% CI)	(29.9 - 39.7)	(10.9 - 18.3)
p-value[c] (CMH)[d]	<0.0001	
Duration of Response, Median	6.4 months	5.6 months
(95% CI)	(5.6 - 7.1)	(4.2 - 7.5)

[a] Patients were censored for PFS at the last date of tumor assessment prior to the start of subsequent therapy. In patients where independent review was not available PFS was censored at the randomization date.

[b] For the hazard ratio, a value less than 1.00 favors combination treatment.

[c] Stratified by visceral metastasis in liver/lung, prior chemotherapy in metastatic setting, and anthracycline resistance.

[d] Cochran-Mantel-Haenszel test

[See figure 1 at top of next column]

There was no statistically significant difference in overall survival between treatment arms in this study, as well as in a second similar study. In the study described above, the median overall survivals were 12.9 months (95% CI: 11.5, 14.2) in the combination therapy arm and 11.1 months (95% CI: 10.0, 12.5) in the capecitabine alone arm [Hazard Ratio 0.90 (95% CI: 0.77, 1.05), p-value=0.19].

In the second trial, comparing IXEMPRA in combination with capecitabine versus capecitabine alone, conducted in

Figure 1: Progression-free Survival Kaplan Meier Curves

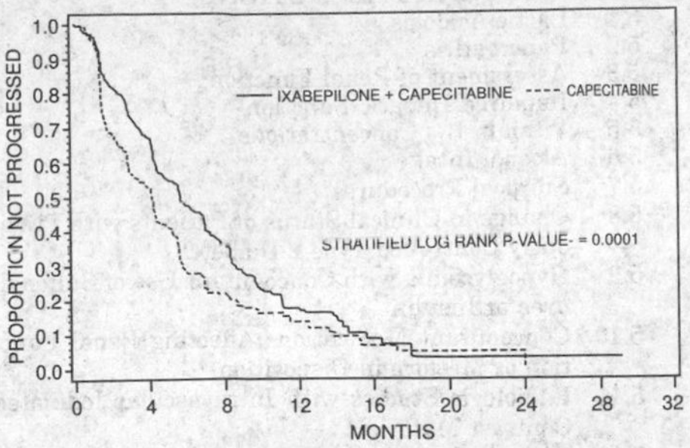

1221 patients pretreated with an anthracycline and a taxane, the median overall survivals were 16.4 months (95% CI: 15.0, 17.9) in the combination therapy arm and 15.6 months (95% CI: 13.9, 17.0), in the capecitabine alone arm [Hazard Ratio 0.90 (95% CI: 0.78, 1.03), p-value=0.12].

Monotherapy

IXEMPRA (ixabepilone) was evaluated as a single agent in a multicenter single-arm study in 126 women with metastatic or locally advanced breast cancer. The study enrolled patients whose tumors had recurred or had progressed following two or more chemotherapy regimens including an anthracycline, a taxane, and capecitabine. Patients who had received a minimum cumulative dose of 240 mg/m^2 of doxorubicin or 360 mg/m^2 of epirubicin were also eligible. Tumor progression or recurrence were prospectively defined as follows:

- Disease progression while on therapy in the metastatic setting (defined as progression while on treatment or within 8 weeks of last dose),
- Recurrence within 6 months of the last dose in the adjuvant or neoadjuvant setting (only for anthracycline and taxane),
- HER2-positive patients must also have progressed during or after discontinuation of trastuzumab.

In this study, the median age was 51 years (range, 30-78), and 79% were White, 5% Black, and 2% Asian, Karnofsky performance status was 70-100%, 88% had received two or more prior chemotherapy regimens for metastatic disease, and 86% had liver and/or lung metastases. Tumors were ER-positive in 48% of patients, ER-negative in 44%, HER2-positive in 7%, HER2-negative in 72%, and ER-negative, PR-negative, HER2-negative in 33%.

IXEMPRA was administered at a dose of 40 mg/m^2 intravenously over 3 hours every 3 weeks. Patients received a median of 4 cycles (range 1 to 18) of IXEMPRA therapy.

Objective tumor response was determined by independent radiologic and investigator review using RECIST. Efficacy results are presented in Table 8.

Table 8: Efficacy of IXEMPRA in Metastatic and Locally Advanced Breast Cancer

Endpoint	Result
Objective tumor response rate (95% CI)	
IRR Assessment[a] (n=113)	12.4% (6.9 - 19.9)
Investigator Assessment (n=126)	18.3% (11.9 - 26.1)
Time to response[b] (n=14)	
Median, weeks (min - max)	6.1 (5 - 54.4)
Duration of response[b] (n=14)	
Median, months (95% CI)	6.0 (5.0 - 7.6)

[a] All responses were partial.
[b] As assessed by IRR.

15 REFERENCES

1. Preventing Occupational Exposures to Antineoplastic and Other Hazardous Drugs in Health Care Settings. NIOSH Alert 2004-165.
2. OSHA Technical Manual, TED 1-0.15A, Section VI: Chapter 2. Controlling Occupational Exposure to Hazardous Drugs. OSHA, 1999. http://www.osha.gov/dts/osta/otm/otm_vi/otm_vi_2.html
3. American Society of Health-System Pharmacists. ASHP guidelines on handling hazardous drugs. *Am J Health-Syst Pharm.* 2006;63:1172-1193.
4. Polovich, M., White, J.M., & Kelleher, L.O. (eds.) 2005. Chemotherapy and biotherapy guidelines and recommendations for practice (2nd. ed.) Pittsburgh, PA: Oncology Nursing Society.

16 HOW SUPPLIED/STORAGE AND HANDLING

IXEMPRA is supplied as a *Kit* containing one vial of IXEMPRA® (ixabepilone) for injection and one vial of DILUENT for IXEMPRA.

NDC 0015-1910-12	IXEMPRA®*Kit* containing one vial of IXEMPRA® (ixabepilone) for injection, 15 mg and one vial of DILUENT for IXEMPRA, 8 mL
NDC 0015-1911-13	IXEMPRA®*Kit* containing one vial of IXEMPRA® (ixabepilone) for injection, 45 mg and one vial of DILUENT for IXEMPRA, 23.5 mL

IXEMPRA (ixabepilone) *Kit* must be stored in a refrigerator at 2° C to 8° C (36° F to 46° F). Retain in original package until time of use to protect from light.

Procedures for proper handling and disposal of antineoplastic drugs *[see References (15)]* should be followed. To minimize the risk of dermal exposure, impervious gloves should be worn when handling vials containing IXEMPRA, regardless of the setting, including unpacking and inspection, transport within a facility, and dose preparation and administration.

17 PATIENT COUNSELING INFORMATION

[see FDA-Approved Patient Labeling]

17.1 Peripheral Neuropathy

Patients should be advised to report to their physician any numbness and tingling of the hands or feet *[see Warnings and Precautions (5.1)]*.

17.2 Fever/Neutropenia

Patients should be instructed to call their physician if a fever of 100.5° F or greater or other evidence of potential infection such as chills, cough, or burning or pain on urination develops *[see Warnings and Precautions (5.2)]*.

17.3 Hypersensitivity Reactions

Patients should be advised to call their physician if they experience urticaria, pruritus, rash, flushing, swelling, dyspnea, chest tightness, or other hypersensitivity-related symptoms following an infusion of IXEMPRA *[see Warnings and Precautions (5.4)]*.

17.4 Pregnancy

Patients should be advised to use effective contraceptive measures to prevent pregnancy and to avoid nursing during treatment with IXEMPRA *[see Warnings and Precautions (5.5) and Use in Specific Populations (8.1, 8.3)]*.

17.5 Cardiac Adverse Reactions

Patients should be advised to report to their physician chest pain, difficulty breathing, palpitations, or unusual weight gain *[see Warnings and Precautions (5.6)]*.

FDA-Approved Patient Labeling
Patient Information
IXEMPRA®*Kit* (pronounced as ĭk-'sĕm-pră)
(ixabepilone)
for Injection, for intravenous infusion only

Read the Patient Information that comes with IXEMPRA before you start receiving it and before each injection. There may be new information. This leaflet does not take the place of talking with your healthcare provider about your medical condition or your treatment.

What is the most important information I should know about IXEMPRA?

Your healthcare provider should do blood tests to check your liver function:

- before you begin receiving IXEMPRA
- as needed while you are receiving IXEMPRA

If blood tests show that you have liver problems, do not receive injections of IXEMPRA along with the medicine capecitabine. Taking these two medicines together if you have liver problems increases your chance of serious problems. These include: serious infection and death due to a very low white blood cell count (neutropenia).

What is IXEMPRA?

IXEMPRA is a cancer medicine. IXEMPRA is used alone or with another cancer medicine called capecitabine. IXEMPRA is used to treat breast cancer, when certain other medicines have not worked or no longer work.

Who should not receive IXEMPRA?

Do not receive injections of IXEMPRA if you:

- are allergic to a medicine, such as TAXOL®, that contains Cremophor® EL or polyoxyethylated castor oil.
- have low white blood cell or platelet counts. Your healthcare provider will check your blood counts.
- are also taking a cancer medicine called capecitabine and you have liver problems. **See "What is the most important information I should know about IXEMPRA?"**

What should I tell my healthcare provider before receiving IXEMPRA?

IXEMPRA may not be right for you. Before you receive IXEMPRA, tell your healthcare provider about all of your medical conditions, including if you:

- have liver problems
- have heart problems or a history of heart problems
- have had an allergic reaction to IXEMPRA (ixabepilone). You will receive medicines before each injection of IXEMPRA to decrease the chance of an allergic reaction. **See "How will I receive IXEMPRA?"**
- are pregnant or plan to become pregnant. You should not receive IXEMPRA during pregnancy because it may harm your unborn baby. Talk with your healthcare provider about how to prevent pregnancy while receiving IXEMPRA. Tell your healthcare provider right away if you become pregnant or think you are pregnant while receiving IXEMPRA.
- are breast-feeding. It is not known if IXEMPRA passes into breast milk. You and your healthcare provider should decide if you will receive IXEMPRA or breast-feed. You should not do both.

Tell your healthcare provider about all the medicines you take, including prescription and non-prescription medicines, vitamins, and herbal supplements.

IXEMPRA and certain other medicines may affect each other causing side effects. IXEMPRA may affect the way other medicines work, and other medicines may affect how IXEMPRA works. Know the medicines you take. Keep a list of your medicines with you to show your healthcare provider.

How will I receive IXEMPRA?

IXEMPRA is given by an injection directly into your vein (intravenous infusion). IXEMPRA is usually given once every three weeks. Each treatment with IXEMPRA will take about 3 hours.

Your healthcare provider will decide how much IXEMPRA you will receive and how often you will receive it.

To lower the chance of allergic reaction, you will receive other medicines about 1 hour before each treatment with IXEMPRA. **See "What are the possible side effects of IXEMPRA?"**

If you have an allergic reaction to IXEMPRA, you will receive a steroid medicine before future doses of IXEMPRA. You may also need to receive your doses of IXEMPRA more slowly.

What should I avoid while receiving IXEMPRA?

IXEMPRA contains alcohol. If you are dizzy or drowsy, avoid activities that may be dangerous, such as driving or operating machinery.

Do not drink grapefruit juice while receiving IXEMPRA. Drinking grapefruit juice may cause you to have too much IXEMPRA in your blood and lead to side effects.

What are the possible side effects of IXEMPRA?

IXEMPRA may cause serious side effects including:

- **Numbness, tingling, or burning in the hands or feet can occur while receiving IXEMPRA (neuropathy).** These symptoms may be new or get worse while you are receiving IXEMPRA. These symptoms often occur early during treatment with IXEMPRA. Tell your healthcare provider if you have any of these symptoms. Your dose of IXEMPRA may need to be decreased, stopped until your symptoms get better, or totally stopped.
- **Low white blood cell count (neutropenia).** White blood cells help protect the body from infections caused by bacteria. If you get a fever or infection when your white blood cells are very low, you can become seriously ill and die. You may need treatment in the hospital with antibiotic medicines. Your healthcare provider will monitor your white blood cell count often with blood tests. Tell your healthcare provider right away or go to the nearest hospital emergency room if you have a fever (temperature above 100.5° F) or other sign of infection, such as chills, cough, burning or pain when you urinate, any time between treatments with IXEMPRA.
- **Allergic Reactions.** Severe allergic reactions can occur with IXEMPRA and may cause death in rare cases. Allergic reactions are most likely to occur while IXEMPRA is being injected into your vein. Tell your healthcare provider right away if you get any of the following signs and symptoms of an allergic reaction:
  - itching, hives (raised itchy welts), rash
  - flushed face
  - sudden swelling of face, throat or tongue
  - chest tightness, trouble breathing
  - feel dizzy or faint
  - feel your heart beating (palpitations)
  - **Harm to an unborn child. See "What should I tell my healthcare provider before receiving IXEMPRA?"**
  - **Heart problems.** IXEMPRA might cause decreased blood flow to the heart, problems with heart function, and abnormal heart beat. This is seen more often in patients who also take capecitabine. **Tell your healthcare provider right away if you have any of the following symptoms:**
  - chest pain,
  - difficulty breathing,
  - feel your heart beating (palpitations), or
  - unusual weight gain.

The most common side effects with IXEMPRA used alone or with capecitabine may include:

- tiredness
- loss of appetite
- disorders of toenails and fingernails
- hair loss

- fever
- decreased red blood cells (anemia)
- joint and muscle pain
- headache
- decreased platelets (thrombocytopenia)
- nausea, vomiting, diarrhea, constipation, and abdominal pain
- sores on the lip, in the mouth and esophagus
- tender, red palms and soles of feet (hand-foot syndrome) that looks like a sunburn; the skin may become dry and peel. There may also be numbness and tingling.

Tell your healthcare provider about any side effect that bothers you or that does not go away.

These are not all the side effects of IXEMPRA (ixabepilone). Ask your healthcare provider or pharmacist for more information if you have questions or concerns.

General information about IXEMPRA

This patient information leaflet summarizes the most important information about IXEMPRA. Medicines are sometimes prescribed for purposes other than those listed in a Patient Information Leaflet. If you would like more information about IXEMPRA, talk with your healthcare provider. You can ask your healthcare provider or pharmacist for information about IXEMPRA that is written for health professionals. For more information about IXEMPRA, call 1–888–IXEMPRA.

IXEMPRA® (ixabepilone) for injection Manufactured by: Baxter Oncology GmbH, 33790 Halle/Westfalen, Germany
DILUENT for IXEMPRA Manufactured by: Baxter Oncology GmbH, 33790 Halle/Westfalen, Germany
Distributed by Bristol-Myers Squibb Company, Princeton, NJ 08543 USA
1236925A7
5645-0006
Rev October 2011

Shown in Product Identification Guide, page 305

KOMBIGLYZE XR

[kom-be-glyze X-R] ℞

(saxagliptin and metformin hydrochloride extended-release) tablets, for oral use

HIGHLIGHTS OF PRESCRIBING INFORMATION

These highlights do not include all the information needed to use KOMBIGLYZE XR safely and effectively. See full prescribing information for KOMBIGLYZE XR.

KOMBIGLYZE XR (saxagliptin and metformin hydrochloride extended-release) tablets, for oral use

Initial U.S. Approval: 2010

WARNING: LACTIC ACIDOSIS

See full prescribing information for complete boxed warning.

- **Lactic acidosis can occur due to metformin accumulation. The risk increases with conditions such as sepsis, dehydration, excess alcohol intake, hepatic impairment, renal impairment, and acute congestive heart failure. (5.1)**
- **Symptoms include malaise, myalgias, respiratory distress, increasing somnolence, and nonspecific abdominal distress. Laboratory abnormalities include low pH, increased anion gap, and elevated blood lactate. (5.1)**
- **If acidosis is suspected, discontinue KOMBIGLYZE XR and hospitalize the patient immediately. (5.1)**

INDICATIONS AND USAGE

KOMBIGLYZE XR is a combination of saxagliptin, a dipeptidyl peptidase-4 (DPP4) inhibitor, and metformin, a biguanide, indicated as an adjunct to diet and exercise to improve glycemic control in adults with type 2 diabetes mellitus when treatment with both saxagliptin and metformin is appropriate. (1, 14)

Limitations of Use:
- Not for treatment of type 1 diabetes or diabetic ketoacidosis. (1.1)
- Has not been studied in patients with a history of pancreatitis. (1.1, 5.2)

DOSAGE AND ADMINISTRATION

- Administer once daily with the evening meal. (2.1)
- Individualize the starting dose based on the patient's current regimen then adjust the dosage based on effectiveness and tolerability. (2.1)
- Do not exceed a daily dosage of 5 mg saxagliptin/2000 mg metformin HCl extended-release. (2.1)
- Swallow whole. Never crush, cut, or chew. (2.1)
- Limit the saxagliptin dosage to 2.5 mg daily for patients also taking strong cytochrome P450 3A4/5 inhibitors (e.g., ketoconazole). (2.2, 7.1)

DOSAGE FORMS AND STRENGTHS

Tablets:
- 5 mg saxagliptin/500 mg metformin HCl extended-release (3)
- 5 mg saxagliptin/1000 mg metformin HCl extended-release (3)
- 2.5 mg saxagliptin/1000 mg metformin HCl extended-release (3)

CONTRAINDICATIONS

- Renal impairment. (4)
- Hypersensitivity to metformin hydrochloride. (4)
- Metabolic acidosis, including diabetic ketoacidosis. (4, 5.1)
- History of a serious hypersensitivity reaction (e.g., anaphylaxis, angioedema, exfoliative skin conditions) to KOMBIGLYZE XR or saxagliptin. (4)

WARNINGS AND PRECAUTIONS

- *Lactic Acidosis:* Warn patients against excessive alcohol intake. KOMBIGLYZE XR not recommended in hepatic impairment and contraindicated in renal impairment. Ensure normal renal function before initiating and at least annually thereafter. Temporarily discontinue KOMBIGLYZE XR in patients undergoing radiologic studies with intravascular administration of iodinated contrast materials or any surgical procedures necessitating restricted intake of food and fluids. (4, 5.1, 5.3, 5.4, 5.7, 5.10, 5.11)
- *Acute Pancreatitis (postmarketing reports):* If pancreatitis is suspected, promptly discontinue KOMBIGLYZE XR. (5.2, 6.2)
- *Vitamin B_{12} Deficiency:* Metformin may lower vitamin B_{12} levels. Measure hematological parameters annually. (5.5, 6.1)
- *Hypoglycemia:* In the saxagliptin add-on to sulfonylurea, add-on to insulin, and add-on to metformin plus sulfonylurea trials, confirmed hypoglycemia was reported more commonly in patients treated with saxagliptin compared to placebo. When used with an insulin secretagogue (e.g., sulfonylurea) or insulin, a lower dose of the insulin secretagogue or insulin may be required to minimize the risk of hypoglycemia. (5.9, 6.1)
- *Hypersensitivity-Related Events (e.g., urticaria, facial edema):* More common in patients treated with saxagliptin than in patients treated with placebo; and postmarketing reports of serious hypersensitivity reactions, such as anaphylaxis, angioedema, and exfoliative skin conditions in patients treated with saxagliptin. Promptly discontinue KOMBIGLYZE XR, assess for other potential causes, institute appropriate monitoring and treatment, and initiate alternative treatment for diabetes. (5.13, 6.1, 6.2)
- *Macrovascular Outcomes:* No conclusive evidence of macrovascular risk reduction with KOMBIGLYZE XR or any other antidiabetic drug. (5.14)

ADVERSE REACTIONS

- Adverse reactions reported in >5% of patients treated with metformin extended-release and more commonly than in patients treated with placebo are: diarrhea and nausea/vomiting. (6.1)
- Adverse reactions reported in ≥5% of patients treated with saxagliptin and more commonly than in patients treated with placebo are: upper respiratory tract infection, urinary tract infection, and headache. (6.1)
- Adverse reactions reported in ≥5% of treatment-naive patients treated with coadministered saxagliptin and metformin and more commonly than in patients treated with metformin alone are: headache and nasopharyngitis. (6.1)

To report SUSPECTED ADVERSE REACTIONS, contact Bristol-Myers Squibb at 1-800-721-5072 or FDA at 1-800-FDA-1088 or *www.fda.gov/medwatch*

DRUG INTERACTIONS

- Coadministration with strong CYP3A4/5 inhibitors (e.g., ketoconazole) significantly increases saxagliptin concentrations. Limit KOMBIGLYZE XR dose to 2.5 mg/1000 mg once daily. (2.2, 7.1)
- Cationic drugs eliminated by renal tubular secretion may reduce metformin elimination: use with caution. (5.10, 7.2)

USE IN SPECIFIC POPULATIONS

- No adequate and well-controlled studies in pregnant women. (8.1)

See 17 for PATIENT COUNSELING INFORMATION and Medication Guide

Revised: 05/2013

FULL PRESCRIBING INFORMATION: CONTENTS*

* Sections or subsections omitted from the full prescribing information are not listed

FULL PRESCRIBING INFORMATION

WARNING: LACTIC ACIDOSIS

Lactic acidosis is a rare, but serious, complication that can occur due to metformin accumulation. The risk increases with conditions such as sepsis, dehydration, excess alcohol intake, hepatic impairment, renal impairment, and acute congestive heart failure.
The onset of lactic acidosis is often subtle, accompanied only by nonspecific symptoms such as malaise, myalgias, respiratory distress, increasing somnolence, and nonspecific abdominal distress.
Laboratory abnormalities include low pH, increased anion gap, and elevated blood lactate.
If acidosis is suspected, KOMBIGLYZE XR should be discontinued and the patient hospitalized immediately. [See *Warnings and Precautions (5.1)*.]

1 INDICATIONS AND USAGE

KOMBIGLYZE XR (saxagliptin and metformin hydrochloride extended-release) is indicated as an adjunct to diet and exercise to improve glycemic control in adults with type 2 diabetes mellitus when treatment with both saxagliptin and metformin is appropriate. [See *Clinical Studies (14)*.]

1.1 Limitations of Use

KOMBIGLYZE XR should not be used for the treatment of type 1 diabetes mellitus or diabetic ketoacidosis.

KOMBIGLYZE XR has not been studied in patients with a history of pancreatitis. It is unknown whether patients with a history of pancreatitis are at an increased risk for the development of pancreatitis while using KOMBIGLYZE XR. [See *Warnings and Precautions (5.2)*.]

2 DOSAGE AND ADMINISTRATION

2.1 Recommended Dosage

The dosage of KOMBIGLYZE XR should be individualized on the basis of the patient's current regimen, effectiveness, and tolerability. KOMBIGLYZE XR should generally be administered once daily with the evening meal, with gradual dose titration to reduce the gastrointestinal side effects associated with metformin. The following dosage forms are available:

- KOMBIGLYZE XR (saxagliptin and metformin HCl extended-release) tablets 5 mg/500 mg
- KOMBIGLYZE XR (saxagliptin and metformin HCl extended-release) tablets 5 mg/1000 mg
- KOMBIGLYZE XR (saxagliptin and metformin HCl extended-release) tablets 2.5 mg/1000 mg

The recommended starting dose of KOMBIGLYZE XR in patients who need 5 mg of saxagliptin and who are not currently treated with metformin is 5 mg saxagliptin/500 mg metformin extended-release once daily with gradual dose escalation to reduce the gastrointestinal side effects due to metformin.

In patients treated with metformin, the dosage of KOMBIGLYZE XR should provide metformin at the dose already being taken, or the nearest therapeutically appropriate dose. Following a switch from metformin immediate-release to metformin extended-release, glycemic control should be closely monitored and dosage adjustments made accordingly.

Patients who need 2.5 mg saxagliptin in combination with metformin extended-release may be treated with KOMBIGLYZE XR 2.5 mg/1000 mg. Patients who need 2.5 mg saxagliptin who are either metformin naive or who require a dose of metformin higher than 1000 mg should use the individual components.

The maximum daily recommended dosage is 5 mg for saxagliptin and 2000 mg for metformin extended-release.

No studies have been performed specifically examining the safety and efficacy of KOMBIGLYZE XR in patients previously treated with other antihyperglycemic medications and switched to KOMBIGLYZE XR. Any change in therapy of type 2 diabetes should be undertaken with care and appropriate monitoring as changes in glycemic control can occur.

Inform patients that KOMBIGLYZE XR tablets must be swallowed whole and never crushed, cut, or chewed. Occasionally, the inactive ingredients of KOMBIGLYZE XR will be eliminated in the feces as a soft, hydrated mass that may resemble the original tablet.

2.2 Dosage Adjustments with Concomitant Use of Strong CYP3A4/5 Inhibitors

The maximum recommended dosage of saxagliptin is 2.5 mg once daily when coadministered with strong cytochrome P450 3A4/5 (CYP3A4/5) inhibitors (e.g., ketoconazole, atazanavir, clarithromycin, indinavir, itraconazole, nefazodone, nelfinavir, ritonavir, saquinavir, and telithromycin). For these patients, limit the KOMBIGLYZE XR dosage to 2.5 mg/1000 mg once daily. [See *Dosage and Administration (2.1), Drug Interactions (7.1),* and *Clinical Pharmacology (12.3).*]

2.3 Concomitant Use with an Insulin Secretagogue (e.g., Sulfonylurea) or with Insulin

When KOMBIGLYZE XR is used in combination with an insulin secretagogue (e.g., sulfonylurea) or with insulin, a lower dosage of the insulin secretagogue or insulin may be required to minimize the risk of hypoglycemia. [See *Warnings and Precautions (5.9).*]

3 DOSAGE FORMS AND STRENGTHS

- KOMBIGLYZE XR (saxagliptin and metformin HCl extended-release) 5 mg/500 mg tablets are light brown to brown, biconvex, capsule-shaped, film-coated tablets with "5/500" printed on one side and "4221" printed on the reverse side, in blue ink.
- KOMBIGLYZE XR (saxagliptin and metformin HCl extended-release) 5 mg/1000 mg tablets are pink, biconvex, capsule-shaped, film-coated tablets with "5/1000" printed on one side and "4223" printed on the reverse side, in blue ink.
- KOMBIGLYZE XR (saxagliptin and metformin HCl extended-release) 2.5 mg/1000 mg tablets are pale yellow to light yellow, biconvex, capsule shaped, film-coated tablets with "2.5/1000" printed on one side and "4222" printed on the reverse side, in blue ink.

4 CONTRAINDICATIONS

KOMBIGLYZE XR is contraindicated in patients with:

- Renal impairment (e.g., serum creatinine levels ≥1.5 mg/dL for men, ≥1.4 mg/dL for women, or abnormal creatinine clearance) which may also result from conditions such as cardiovascular collapse (shock), acute myocardial infarction, and septicemia.
- Hypersensitivity to metformin hydrochloride.
- Acute or chronic metabolic acidosis, including diabetic ketoacidosis. Diabetic ketoacidosis should be treated with insulin.
- History of a serious hypersensitivity reaction to KOMBIGLYZE XR (saxagliptin and metformin hydrochloride extended-release) or saxagliptin, such as anaphylaxis, angioedema, or exfoliative skin conditions. [See *Warnings and Precautions (5.13)* and *Adverse Reactions (6.2).*]

5 WARNINGS AND PRECAUTIONS

5.1 Lactic Acidosis

Lactic acidosis is a rare, but serious, metabolic complication that can occur due to metformin accumulation during treatment with KOMBIGLYZE XR; when it occurs, it is fatal in approximately 50% of cases. Lactic acidosis may also occur in association with a number of pathophysiologic conditions, including diabetes mellitus, and whenever there is significant tissue hypoperfusion and hypoxemia. Lactic acidosis is characterized by elevated blood lactate levels (>5 mmol/L), decreased blood pH, electrolyte disturbances with an increased anion gap, and an increased lactate/pyruvate ratio. When metformin is implicated as the cause of lactic acidosis, metformin plasma levels >5 μg/mL are generally found. The reported incidence of lactic acidosis in patients receiving metformin hydrochloride is very low (approximately 0.03 cases/1000 patient-years, with approximately 0.015 fatal cases/1000 patient-years). In more than 20,000 patient-years exposure to metformin in clinical trials, there were no reports of lactic acidosis. Reported cases have occurred primarily in diabetic patients with significant renal insufficiency, including both intrinsic renal disease and renal hypoperfusion, often in the setting of multiple concomitant medical/surgical problems and multiple concomitant medications. Patients with congestive heart failure requiring pharmacologic management, in particular those with unstable or acute congestive heart failure who are at risk of hypoperfusion and hypoxemia, are at increased risk of lactic acidosis. The risk of lactic acidosis increases with the degree of renal dysfunction and the patient's age. The risk of lactic acidosis may, therefore, be significantly decreased by regular monitoring of renal function in patients taking metformin and by use of the minimum effective dose of metformin. In particular, treatment of the elderly should be accompanied by careful monitoring of renal function. Metformin treatment should not be initiated in patients ≥80 years of age unless measurement of creatinine clearance demonstrates that renal function is not reduced, as these patients are more susceptible to developing lactic acidosis. In addition, metformin should be promptly withheld in the presence of any condition associated with hypoxemia, dehydration, or sepsis. Because impaired hepatic function may significantly limit the ability to clear lactate, metformin should generally be avoided in patients with clinical or laboratory evidence of hepatic disease. Patients should be cautioned against excessive alcohol intake when taking metformin since alcohol potentiates the effects of metformin hydrochloride on lactate metabolism. In addition, metformin should be temporarily discontinued prior to any intravascular radiocontrast study and for any surgical procedure [see *Warnings and Precautions (5.3, 5.6, 5.7, 5.11)*].

The onset of lactic acidosis often is subtle and accompanied only by nonspecific symptoms such as malaise, myalgias, respiratory distress, increasing somnolence, and nonspecific abdominal distress. There may be associated hypothermia, hypotension, and resistant bradyarrhythmias with more marked acidosis. The patient and the patient's physician must be aware of the possible importance of such symptoms and the patient should be instructed to notify the physician immediately if they occur [see *Warnings and Precautions (5.12)*]. Metformin should be withdrawn until the situation is clarified. Serum electrolytes, ketones, blood glucose, and if indicated, blood pH, lactate levels, and even blood metformin levels may be useful. Once a patient is stabilized on any dose level of metformin, gastrointestinal symptoms, which are common during initiation of therapy, are unlikely to be drug related. Later occurrence of gastrointestinal symptoms could be due to lactic acidosis or other serious disease.

Levels of fasting venous plasma lactate above the upper limit of normal, but less than 5 mmol/L, in patients taking metformin do not necessarily indicate impending lactic acidosis and may be explainable by other mechanisms, such as poorly controlled diabetes or obesity, vigorous physical activity, or technical problems in sample handling. [See *Warnings and Precautions (5.8).*]

Lactic acidosis should be suspected in any diabetic patient with metabolic acidosis lacking evidence of ketoacidosis (ketonuria and ketonemia).

Lactic acidosis is a medical emergency that must be treated in a hospital setting. In a patient with lactic acidosis who is taking metformin, the drug should be discontinued immediately and general supportive measures promptly instituted. Because metformin hydrochloride is dialyzable (with a clearance of up to 170 mL/min under good hemodynamic conditions), prompt hemodialysis is recommended to correct the acidosis and remove the accumulated metformin. Such management often results in prompt reversal of symptoms and recovery [see *Contraindications (4)* and *Warnings and Precautions (5.6, 5.7, 5.10, 5.11, 5.12)*].

5.2 Pancreatitis

There have been postmarketing reports of acute pancreatitis in patients taking saxagliptin. After initiation of KOMBIGLYZE XR (saxagliptin and metformin hydrochloride extended-release), patients should be observed carefully for signs and symptoms of pancreatitis. If pancreatitis is suspected, KOMBIGLYZE XR should promptly be discontinued and appropriate management should be initiated. It is unknown whether patients with a history of pancreatitis are at increased risk for the development of pancreatitis while using KOMBIGLYZE XR.

5.3 Assessment of Renal Function

Metformin is substantially excreted by the kidney, and the risk of metformin accumulation and lactic acidosis increases with the degree of impairment of renal function. Therefore, KOMBIGLYZE XR is contraindicated in patients with renal impairment [see *Contraindications (4)*].

Before initiation of KOMBIGLYZE XR, and at least annually thereafter, renal function should be assessed and verified as normal. In patients in whom development of renal impairment is anticipated (e.g., elderly), renal function should be assessed more frequently and KOMBIGLYZE XR discontinued if evidence of renal impairment is present.

5.4 Impaired Hepatic Function

Metformin use in patients with impaired hepatic function has been associated with some cases of lactic acidosis. Therefore, KOMBIGLYZE XR is not recommended in patients with hepatic impairment.

5.5 Vitamin B_{12} Concentrations

In controlled clinical trials of metformin of 29-week duration, a decrease to subnormal levels of previously normal serum vitamin B_{12} levels, without clinical manifestations, was observed in approximately 7% of patients. Such decrease, possibly due to interference with B_{12} absorption from the B_{12}-intrinsic factor complex, is, however, very rarely associated with anemia and appears to be rapidly reversible with discontinuation of metformin or vitamin B_{12} supplementation. Measurement of hematologic parameters on an annual basis is advised in patients on KOMBIGLYZE XR and any apparent abnormalities should be appropriately investigated and managed [see *Adverse Reactions (6.1)*].

Certain individuals (those with inadequate vitamin B_{12} or calcium intake or absorption) appear to be predisposed to developing subnormal vitamin B_{12} levels. In these patients, routine serum vitamin B_{12} measurements at 2- to 3-year intervals may be useful.

5.6 Alcohol Intake

Alcohol potentiates the effect of metformin on lactate metabolism. Patients should be warned against excessive alcohol intake while receiving KOMBIGLYZE XR.

5.7 Surgical Procedures

Use of KOMBIGLYZE XR should be temporarily suspended for any surgical procedure (except minor procedures not associated with restricted intake of food and fluids) and should not be restarted until the patient's oral intake has resumed and renal function has been evaluated as normal.

5.8 Change in Clinical Status of Patients with Previously Controlled Type 2 Diabetes

A patient with type 2 diabetes previously well controlled on KOMBIGLYZE XR who develops laboratory abnormalities or clinical illness (especially vague and poorly defined illness) should be evaluated promptly for evidence of ketoacidosis or lactic acidosis. Evaluation should include serum electrolytes and ketones, blood glucose and, if indicated, blood pH, lactate, pyruvate, and metformin levels. If acidosis of either form occurs, KOMBIGLYZE XR must be stopped immediately and other appropriate corrective measures initiated.

5.9 Hypoglycemia with Concomitant Use of Sulfonylurea or Insulin

Saxagliptin

When saxagliptin was used in combination with a sulfonylurea or with insulin, medications known to cause hypoglycemia, the incidence of confirmed hypoglycemia was increased over that of placebo used in combination with a sulfonylurea or with insulin. [See *Adverse Reactions (6.1).*] Therefore, a lower dose of the insulin secretagogue or insulin may be required to minimize the risk of hypoglycemia when used in combination with KOMBIGLYZE XR. [See *Dosage and Administration (2.3).*]

Metformin hydrochloride

Hypoglycemia does not occur in patients receiving metformin alone under usual circumstances of use, but could occur when caloric intake is deficient, when strenuous exercise is not compensated by caloric supplementation, or during concomitant use with other glucose-lowering agents (such as sulfonylureas and insulin) or ethanol. Elderly, debilitated, or malnourished patients and those with adrenal or pituitary insufficiency or alcohol intoxication are particularly susceptible to hypoglycemic effects. Hypoglycemia may be difficult to recognize in the elderly and in people who are taking beta-adrenergic blocking drugs.

5.10 Concomitant Medications Affecting Renal Function or Metformin Disposition

Concomitant medication(s) that may affect renal function or result in significant hemodynamic change or may interfere with the disposition of metformin, such as cationic drugs that are eliminated by renal tubular secretion [see *Drug Interactions (7.2)*], should be used with caution.

5.11 Radiologic Studies with Intravascular Iodinated Contrast Materials

Intravascular contrast studies with iodinated materials can lead to acute alteration of renal function and have been associated with lactic acidosis in patients receiving metformin. Therefore, in patients in whom any such study is planned, KOMBIGLYZE XR (saxagliptin and metformin hydrochloride extended-release) should be temporarily discontinued at the time of or prior to the procedure, and withheld for 48 hours subsequent to the procedure and reinstituted only after renal function has been re-evaluated and found to be normal.

5.12 Hypoxic States

Cardiovascular collapse (shock), acute congestive heart failure, acute myocardial infarction, and other conditions characterized by hypoxemia have been associated with lactic acidosis and may also cause prerenal azotemia. When such events occur in patients on KOMBIGLYZE XR therapy, the drug should be promptly discontinued.

5.13 Hypersensitivity Reactions

There have been postmarketing reports of serious hypersensitivity reactions in patients treated with saxagliptin. These reactions include anaphylaxis, angioedema, and exfoliative skin conditions. Onset of these reactions occurred within the first 3 months after initiation of treatment with saxagliptin, with some reports occurring after the first dose. If a serious hypersensitivity reaction is suspected, discontinue KOMBIGLYZE XR, assess for other potential causes for the event, and institute alternative treatment for diabetes. [See *Adverse Reactions (6.2).*]

Use caution in a patient with a history of angioedema to another dipeptidyl peptidase-4 (DPP4) inhibitor because it is unknown whether such patients will be predisposed to angioedema with KOMBIGLYZE XR.

5.14 Macrovascular Outcomes

There have been no clinical studies establishing conclusive evidence of macrovascular risk reduction with KOMBIGLYZE XR or any other antidiabetic drug.

6 ADVERSE REACTIONS

6.1 Clinical Trials Experience

Because clinical trials are conducted under widely varying conditions, adverse reaction rates observed in the clinical trials of a drug cannot be directly compared to rates in the clinical trials of another drug and may not reflect the rates observed in practice.

Adverse Reactions with Monotherapy and with Add-On Combination Therapy

Metformin hydrochloride

In placebo-controlled monotherapy trials of metformin extended-release, diarrhea and nausea/vomiting were reported in >5% of metformin-treated patients and more commonly than in placebo-treated patients (9.6% versus 2.6% for diarrhea and 6.5% versus 1.5% for nausea/vomiting). Diarrhea led to discontinuation of study medication in 0.6% of the patients treated with metformin extended-release.

Saxagliptin

In two placebo-controlled monotherapy trials of 24-week duration, patients were treated with saxagliptin 2.5 mg daily, saxagliptin 5 mg daily, and placebo. Three 24-week, placebo-controlled, add-on combination therapy trials were also conducted: one with metformin immediate-release, one with a thiazolidinedione (pioglitazone or rosiglitazone), and one with glyburide. In these three trials, patients were randomized to add-on therapy with saxagliptin 2.5 mg daily, saxagliptin 5 mg daily, or placebo. A saxagliptin 10 mg treatment arm was included in one of the monotherapy trials and in the add-on combination trial with metformin immediate-release. The 10 mg saxagliptin dosage is not an approved dosage.

In a prespecified pooled analysis of the 24-week data (regardless of glycemic rescue) from the two monotherapy trials, the add-on to metformin immediate-release trial, the add-on to thiazolidinedione (TZD) trial, and the add-on to glyburide trial, the overall incidence of adverse events in patients treated with saxagliptin 2.5 mg and saxagliptin 5 mg was similar to placebo (72% and 72.2% versus 70.6%, respectively). Discontinuation of therapy due to adverse events occurred in 2.2%, 3.3%, and 1.8% of patients receiving saxagliptin 2.5 mg, saxagliptin 5 mg, and placebo, respectively. The most common adverse events (reported in at least 2 patients treated with saxagliptin 2.5 mg or at least 2 patients treated with saxagliptin 5 mg) associated with premature discontinuation of therapy included lymphopenia (0.1% and 0.5% versus 0%, respectively), rash (0.2% and 0.3% versus 0.3%), blood creatinine increased (0.3% and 0% versus 0%), and blood creatine phosphokinase increased (0.1% and 0.2% versus 0%). The adverse reactions in this pooled analysis reported (regardless of investigator assessment of causality) in ≥5% of patients treated with saxagliptin 5 mg, and more commonly than in patients treated with placebo are shown in Table 1.

Table 1: Adverse Reactions in Placebo-Controlled Trials* Reported in ≥5% of Patients Treated with Saxagliptin 5 mg and More Commonly than in Patients Treated with Placebo

	Number (%) of Patients	
	Saxagliptin 5 mg N=882	Placebo N=799
Upper respiratory tract infection	68 (7.7)	61 (7.6)
Urinary tract infection	60 (6.8)	49 (6.1)
Headache	57 (6.5)	47 (5.9)

* The 5 placebo-controlled trials include two monotherapy trials and one add-on combination therapy trial with each of the following: metformin, thiazolidinedione, or glyburide. Table shows 24-week data regardless of glycemic rescue.

In patients treated with saxagliptin 2.5 mg, headache (6.5%) was the only adverse reaction reported at a rate ≥5% and more commonly than in patients treated with placebo. In this pooled analysis, adverse reactions that were reported in ≥2% of patients treated with saxagliptin 2.5 mg or saxagliptin 5 mg and ≥1% more frequently compared to placebo included: sinusitis (2.9% and 2.6% versus 1.6%, respectively), abdominal pain (2.4% and 1.7% versus 0.5%), gastroenteritis (1.9% and 2.3% versus 0.9%), and vomiting (2.2% and 2.3% versus 1.3%).

The incidence rate of fractures was 1.0 and 0.6 per 100 patient-years, respectively, for saxagliptin (pooled analysis of 2.5 mg, 5 mg, and 10 mg) and placebo. The 10 mg saxagliptin dosage is not an approved dosage. The incidence rate of fracture events in patients who received saxagliptin did not increase over time. Causality has not been established and nonclinical studies have not demonstrated adverse effects of saxagliptin on bone.

An event of thrombocytopenia, consistent with a diagnosis of idiopathic thrombocytopenic purpura, was observed in the clinical program. The relationship of this event to saxagliptin is not known.

Adverse Reactions with Concomitant Use with Insulin

In the add-on to insulin trial [see *Clinical Studies (14.4)*], the incidence of adverse events, including serious adverse events and discontinuations due to adverse events, was similar between saxagliptin and placebo, except for confirmed hypoglycemia [see *Adverse Reactions (6.1)*].

Adverse Reactions Associated with Saxagliptin Coadministered with Metformin Immediate-Release in Treatment-Naive Patients with Type 2 Diabetes

Table 2 shows the adverse reactions reported (regardless of investigator assessment of causality) in ≥5% of patients participating in an additional 24-week, active-controlled trial of coadministered saxagliptin and metformin in treatment-naive patients.

Table 2: Coadministration of Saxagliptin and Metformin Immediate-Release in Treatment-Naive Patients: Adverse Reactions Reported in ≥5% of Patients Treated with Combination Therapy of Saxagliptin 5 mg Plus Metformin Immediate-Release (and More Commonly than in Patients Treated with Metformin Immediate-Release Alone)

	Number (%) of Patients	
	Saxagliptin 5 mg + Metformin* N=320	Placebo + Metformin* N=328
Headache	24 (7.5)	17 (5.2)
Nasopharyngitis	22 (6.9)	13 (4.0)

* Metformin immediate-release was initiated at a starting dose of 500 mg daily and titrated up to a maximum of 2000 mg daily.

In patients treated with the combination of saxagliptin and metformin immediate-release, either as saxagliptin add-on to metformin immediate-release therapy or as coadministration in treatment-naive patients, diarrhea was the only gastrointestinal-related event that occurred with an incidence ≥5% in any treatment group in both studies. In the saxagliptin add-on to metformin immediate-release trial, the incidence of diarrhea was 9.9%, 5.8%, and 11.2% in the saxagliptin 2.5 mg, 5 mg, and placebo groups, respectively. When saxagliptin and metformin immediate-release were coadministered in treatment-naive patients, the incidence of diarrhea was 6.9% in the saxagliptin 5 mg + metformin immediate-release group and 7.3% in the placebo + metformin immediate-release group.

Hypoglycemia

In the saxagliptin clinical trials, adverse reactions of hypoglycemia were based on all reports of hypoglycemia. A concurrent glucose measurement was not required or was normal in some patients. Therefore, it is not possible to conclusively determine that all these reports reflect true hypoglycemia.

The incidence of reported hypoglycemia for saxagliptin 2.5 mg and saxagliptin 5 mg versus placebo given as monotherapy was 4% and 5.6% versus 4.1%, respectively. In the add-on to metformin immediate-release trial, the incidence of reported hypoglycemia was 7.8% with saxagliptin 2.5 mg, 5.8% with saxagliptin 5 mg, and 5% with placebo. When saxagliptin and metformin immediate-release were coadministered in treatment-naive patients, the incidence of reported hypoglycemia was 3.4% in patients given saxagliptin 5 mg + metformin immediate-release and 4% in patients given placebo + metformin immediate-release.

In the active-controlled trial comparing add-on therapy with saxagliptin 5 mg to glipizide in patients inadequately controlled on metformin alone, the incidence of reported hypoglycemia was 3% (19 events in 13 patients) with saxagliptin 5 mg versus 36.3% (750 events in 156 patients) with glipizide. Confirmed symptomatic hypoglycemia (accompanying fingerstick blood glucose ≤50 mg/dL) was reported in none of the saxagliptin-treated patients and in 35 glipizide-treated patients (8.1%) (p<0.0001).

In the saxagliptin add-on to insulin trial, the overall incidence of reported hypoglycemia was 18.4% for saxagliptin 5 mg and 19.9% for placebo. However, the incidence of confirmed symptomatic hypoglycemia (accompanying fingerstick blood glucose ≤50 mg/dL) was higher with saxagliptin 5 mg (5.3%) versus placebo (3.3%). Among the patients using insulin in combination with metformin, the incidence of confirmed symptomatic hypoglycemia was 4.8% with saxagliptin versus 1.9% with placebo.

In the saxagliptin add-on to metformin plus sulfonylurea trial, the overall incidence of reported hypoglycemia was 10.1% for saxagliptin 5 mg and 6.3% for placebo. Confirmed hypoglycemia was reported in 1.6% of the saxagliptin-treated patients and in none of the placebo-treated patients [see *Warnings and Precautions (5.9)*].

Hypersensitivity Reactions

Saxagliptin

Hypersensitivity-related events, such as urticaria and facial edema in the 5-study pooled analysis up to Week 24 were reported in 1.5%, 1.5%, and 0.4% of patients who received saxagliptin 2.5 mg, saxagliptin 5 mg, and placebo, respectively. None of these events in patients who received saxagliptin required hospitalization or were reported as life-threatening by the investigators. One saxagliptin-treated patient in this pooled analysis discontinued due to generalized urticaria and facial edema.

Infections

Saxagliptin

In the unblinded, controlled, clinical trial database for saxagliptin to date, there have been 6 (0.12%) reports of tuberculosis among the 4959 saxagliptin-treated patients (1.1 per 1000 patient-years) compared to no reports of tuberculosis among the 2868 comparator-treated patients. Two of these six cases were confirmed with laboratory testing. The remaining cases had limited information or had presumptive diagnoses of tuberculosis. None of the six cases occurred in the United States or in Western Europe. One case occurred in Canada in a patient originally from Indonesia who had recently visited Indonesia. The duration of treatment with saxagliptin until report of tuberculosis ranged from 144 to 929 days. Post-treatment lymphocyte counts were consistently within the reference range for four cases. One patient had lymphopenia prior to initiation of saxagliptin that remained stable throughout saxagliptin treatment. The final patient had an isolated lymphocyte count below normal approximately four months prior to the report of tuberculosis. There have been no spontaneous reports of tuberculosis associated with saxagliptin use. Causality has not been established and there are too few cases to date to determine whether tuberculosis is related to saxagliptin use.

There has been one case of a potential opportunistic infection in the unblinded, controlled clinical trial database to date in a saxagliptin-treated patient who developed suspected foodborne fatal salmonella sepsis after approximately 600 days of saxagliptin therapy. There have been no spontaneous reports of opportunistic infections associated with saxagliptin use.

Vital Signs

Saxagliptin

No clinically meaningful changes in vital signs have been observed in patients treated with saxagliptin alone or in combination with metformin.

Laboratory Tests

Absolute Lymphocyte Counts

Saxagliptin

There was a dose-related mean decrease in absolute lymphocyte count observed with saxagliptin. From a baseline mean absolute lymphocyte count of approximately 2200 cells/microL, mean decreases of approximately 100 and 120 cells/microL with saxagliptin 5 mg and 10 mg, respectively, relative to placebo were observed at 24 weeks in a pooled analysis of five placebo-controlled clinical studies. Similar effects were observed when saxagliptin 5 mg and metformin were coadministered in treatment-naive patients compared to placebo and metformin. There was no difference observed for saxagliptin 2.5 mg relative to placebo. The proportion of patients who were reported to have a lymphocyte count ≤750 cells/microL was 0.5%, 1.5%, 1.4%, and 0.4% in the saxagliptin 2.5 mg, 5 mg, 10 mg, and placebo groups, respectively. In most patients, recurrence was not observed with repeated exposure to saxagliptin although some patients had recurrent decreases upon rechallenge that led to discontinuation of saxagliptin. The decreases in lymphocyte count were not associated with clinically relevant adverse reactions. The 10 mg saxagliptin dosage is not an approved dosage.

The clinical significance of this decrease in lymphocyte count relative to placebo is not known. When clinically indicated, such as in settings of unusual or prolonged infection, lymphocyte count should be measured. The effect of saxagliptin on lymphocyte counts in patients with lymphocyte abnormalities (e.g., human immunodeficiency virus) is unknown.

Vitamin B_{12} Concentrations

Metformin hydrochloride

Metformin may lower serum vitamin B_{12} concentrations. Measurement of hematologic parameters on an annual basis is advised in patients on KOMBIGLYZE XR (saxagliptin and metformin hydrochloride extended-release) and any apparent abnormalities should be appropriately investigated and managed. [See *Warnings and Precautions (5.5)*.]

6.2 Postmarketing Experience

Additional adverse reactions have been identified during postapproval use of saxagliptin. Because these reactions are reported voluntarily from a population of uncertain size, it is generally not possible to reliably estimate their frequency or establish a causal relationship to drug exposure.

- Hypersensitivity reactions including anaphylaxis, angioedema, and exfoliative skin conditions. [See *Contraindications (4)* and *Warnings and Precautions (5.13)*.]
- Acute pancreatitis. [See *Indications and Usage (1.1)* and *Warnings and Precautions (5.2)*.]

7 DRUG INTERACTIONS

7.1 Strong Inhibitors of CYP3A4/5 Enzymes

Saxagliptin

Ketoconazole significantly increased saxagliptin exposure. Similar significant increases in plasma concentrations of saxagliptin are anticipated with other strong CYP3A4/5 inhibitors (e.g., atazanavir, clarithromycin, indinavir, itraconazole, nefazodone, nelfinavir, ritonavir, saquinavir, and telithromycin). The dose of saxagliptin should be limited to 2.5 mg when coadministered with a strong CYP3A4/5 inhibitor. [See *Dosage and Administration (2.2)* and *Clinical Pharmacology (12.3)*.]

7.2 Cationic Drugs

Metformin hydrochloride

Cationic drugs (e.g., amiloride, digoxin, morphine, procainamide, quinidine, quinine, ranitidine, triamterene, trimethoprim, or vancomycin) that are eliminated by renal tubular secretion theoretically have the potential for interaction with metformin by competing for common renal tubular transport systems. Such interaction between metformin and oral cimetidine has been observed in healthy volunteers. Although such interactions remain theoretical (except for cimetidine), careful patient monitoring and dose adjustment of KOMBIGLYZE XR and/or the interfering drug is recommended in patients who are taking cationic medications that are excreted via the proximal renal tubular secretory system.

7.3 Use with Other Drugs

Metformin hydrochloride

Some medications can predispose to hyperglycemia and may lead to loss of glycemic control. These medications include the thiazides and other diuretics, corticosteroids, phenothiazines, thyroid products, estrogens, oral contraceptives, phenytoin, nicotinic acid, sympathomimetics, calcium channel blockers, and isoniazid. When such drugs are administered to a patient receiving KOMBIGLYZE XR, the patient should be closely observed for loss of glycemic control. When such drugs are withdrawn from a patient receiving KOMBIGLYZE XR, the patient should be observed closely for hypoglycemia.

8 USE IN SPECIFIC POPULATIONS

8.1 Pregnancy

Pregnancy Category B

There are no adequate and well-controlled studies in pregnant women with KOMBIGLYZE XR (saxagliptin and metformin hydrochloride extended-release) or its individual components. Because animal reproduction studies are not always predictive of human response, KOMBIGLYZE XR, like other antidiabetic medications, should be used during pregnancy only if clearly needed.

Coadministration of saxagliptin and metformin, to pregnant rats and rabbits during the period of organogenesis, was neither embryolethal nor teratogenic in either species when tested at doses yielding systemic exposures (AUC) up to 100 and 10 times the maximum recommended human doses (MRHD; saxagliptin 5 mg and metformin 2000 mg), respectively, in rats; and 249 and 1.1 times the MRHDs in rabbits. In rats, minor developmental toxicity was limited to an increased incidence of wavy ribs; associated maternal toxicity was limited to weight decrements of 11% to 17% over the course of the study, and related reductions in maternal food consumption. In rabbits, coadministration was poorly tolerated in a subset of mothers (12 of 30), resulting in death, moribundity, or abortion. However, among surviving mothers with evaluable litters, maternal toxicity was limited to marginal reductions in body weight over the course of gestation days 21 to 29; and associated developmental toxicity in these litters was limited to fetal body weight decrements of 7%, and a low incidence of delayed ossification of the fetal hyoid.

Saxagliptin

Saxagliptin was not teratogenic at any dose tested when administered to pregnant rats and rabbits during periods of organogenesis. Incomplete ossification of the pelvis, a form of developmental delay, occurred in rats at a dose of 240 mg/kg, or approximately 1503 and 66 times human exposure to saxagliptin and the active metabolite, respectively, at the MRHD of 5 mg. Maternal toxicity and reduced fetal body weights were observed at 7986 and 328 times the human exposure at the MRHD for saxagliptin and the active metabolite, respectively. Minor skeletal variations in rabbits occurred at a maternally toxic dose of 200 mg/kg, or approximately 1432 and 992 times the MRHD.

Saxagliptin administered to female rats from gestation day 6 to lactation day 20 resulted in decreased body weights in male and female offspring only at maternally toxic doses (exposures ≥1629 and 53 times saxagliptin and its active metabolite at the MRHD). No functional or behavioral toxicity was observed in offspring of rats administered saxagliptin at any dose.

Saxagliptin crosses the placenta into the fetus following dosing in pregnant rats.

Metformin hydrochloride

Metformin was not teratogenic in rats and rabbits at doses up to 600 mg/kg/day. This represents an exposure of about 2 and 6 times the maximum recommended human daily dose of 2000 mg based on body surface area comparisons for rats and rabbits, respectively. Determination of fetal concentrations demonstrated a partial placental barrier to metformin.

8.3 Nursing Mothers

No studies in lactating animals have been conducted with the combined components of KOMBIGLYZE XR. In studies performed with the individual components, both saxagliptin and metformin are secreted in the milk of lactating rats. It is not known whether saxagliptin or metformin are secreted in human milk. Because many drugs are secreted in human milk, caution should be exercised when KOMBIGLYZE XR is administered to a nursing woman.

8.4 Pediatric Use

Safety and effectiveness of KOMBIGLYZE XR in pediatric patients under 18 years of age have not been established. Additionally, studies characterizing the pharmacokinetics of KOMBIGLYZE XR in pediatric patients have not been performed.

8.5 Geriatric Use

KOMBIGLYZE XR

Elderly patients are more likely to have decreased renal function. Because metformin is contraindicated in patients with renal impairment, carefully monitor renal function in the elderly and use KOMBIGLYZE XR with caution as age increases. [See *Warnings and Precautions (5.1, 5.3)* and *Clinical Pharmacology (12.3)*.]

Saxagliptin

In the six, double-blind, controlled clinical safety and efficacy trials of saxagliptin, 634 (15.3%) of the 4148 randomized patients were 65 years and over, and 59 (1.4%) patients were 75 years and over. No overall differences in safety or effectiveness were observed between patients ≥65 years old and the younger patients. While this clinical experience has not identified differences in responses between the elderly and younger patients, greater sensitivity of some older individuals cannot be ruled out.

Metformin hydrochloride

Controlled clinical studies of metformin did not include sufficient numbers of elderly patients to determine whether they respond differently from younger patients, although other reported clinical experience has not identified differences in responses between the elderly and young patients. Metformin is known to be substantially excreted by the kidney. Because the risk of lactic acidosis with metformin is greater in patients with impaired renal function, KOMBIGLYZE XR (saxagliptin and metformin hydrochloride extended-release) should only be used in patients with normal renal function. The initial and maintenance dosing of metformin should be conservative in patients with advanced age due to the potential for decreased renal function in this population. Any dose adjustment should be based on a careful assessment of renal function. [See *Contraindications (4)*, *Warnings and Precautions (5.3)*, and *Clinical Pharmacology (12.3)*.]

10 OVERDOSAGE

Saxagliptin

In a controlled clinical trial, once-daily, orally administered saxagliptin in healthy subjects at doses up to 400 mg daily for 2 weeks (80 times the MRHD) had no dose-related clinical adverse reactions and no clinically meaningful effect on QTc interval or heart rate.

In the event of an overdose, appropriate supportive treatment should be initiated as dictated by the patient's clinical status. Saxagliptin and its active metabolite are removed by hemodialysis (23% of dose over 4 hours).

Metformin hydrochloride

Overdose of metformin hydrochloride has occurred, including ingestion of amounts greater than 50 grams. Hypoglycemia was reported in approximately 10% of cases, but no causal association with metformin hydrochloride has been established. Lactic acidosis has been reported in approximately 32% of metformin overdose cases [see *Warnings and Precautions (5.1)*]. Metformin is dialyzable with a clearance of up to 170 mL/min under good hemodynamic conditions. Therefore, hemodialysis may be useful for removal of accumulated drug from patients in whom metformin overdosage is suspected.

11 DESCRIPTION

KOMBIGLYZE XR (saxagliptin and metformin HCl extended-release) tablets contain two oral antihyperglycemic medications used in the management of type 2 diabetes: saxagliptin and metformin hydrochloride.

Saxagliptin

Saxagliptin is an orally active inhibitor of the dipeptidyl-peptidase-4 (DPP4) enzyme.

Saxagliptin monohydrate is described chemically as (1*S*,3*S*,5*S*)-2-[(2*S*)-2-Amino-2-(3-hydroxytricyclo[3.3.1.1^{3,7}]dec-1-yl)-acetyl]-2-azabicyclo[3.1.0]hexane-3-carbonitrile, monohydrate or (1*S*,3*S*,5*S*)-2-[(2*S*)-2-Amino-2-(3-hydroxyadamantan-1-yl)acetyl]-2-azabicyclo[3.1.0]hexane-3-carbonitrile hydrate. The empirical formula is $C_{18}H_{25}N_3O_2 \cdot H_2O$ and the molecular weight is 333.43. The structural formula is:

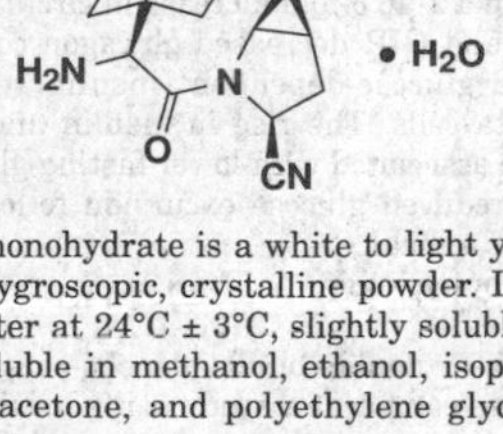

Saxagliptin monohydrate is a white to light yellow or light brown, non-hygroscopic, crystalline powder. It is sparingly soluble in water at 24°C ± 3°C, slightly soluble in ethyl acetate, and soluble in methanol, ethanol, isopropyl alcohol, acetonitrile, acetone, and polyethylene glycol 400 (PEG 400).

Metformin hydrochloride

Metformin hydrochloride (*N,N*-dimethylimidodicarbonimidic diamide hydrochloride) is a white to off-white crystalline compound with a molecular formula of $C_4H_{11}N_5 \cdot HCl$ and a molecular weight of 165.63. Metformin hydrochloride is freely soluble in water, slightly soluble in alcohol, and is practically insoluble in acetone, ether, and chloroform. The pK_a of metformin is 12.4. The pH of a 1% aqueous solution of metformin hydrochloride is 6.68. The structural formula is:

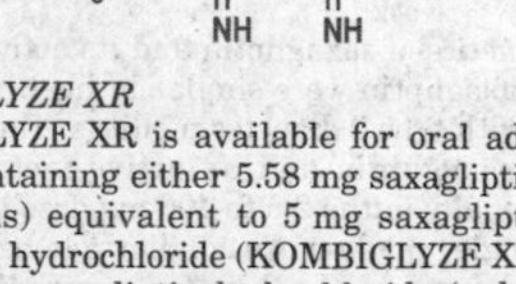

KOMBIGLYZE XR

KOMBIGLYZE XR is available for oral administration as tablets containing either 5.58 mg saxagliptin hydrochloride (anhydrous) equivalent to 5 mg saxagliptin and 500 mg metformin hydrochloride (KOMBIGLYZE XR 5 mg/500 mg), or 5.58 mg saxagliptin hydrochloride (anhydrous) equivalent to 5 mg saxagliptin and 1000 mg metformin hydrochloride (KOMBIGLYZE XR 5 mg/1000 mg), or 2.79 mg saxagliptin hydrochloride (anhydrous) equivalent to 2.5 mg saxagliptin and 1000 mg metformin hydrochloride (KOMBIGLYZE XR 2.5 mg/1000 mg). Each film-coated tablet of KOMBIGLYZE XR (saxagliptin and metformin hydrochloride extended-release) contains the following inactive ingredients: carboxymethylcellulose sodium, hypromellose 2208, and magnesium stearate. The 5 mg/500 mg strength tablet of KOMBIGLYZE XR also contains microcrystalline cellulose and hypromellose 2910. In addition, the film coatings contain the following inactive ingredients: polyvinyl alcohol, polyethylene glycol 3350, titanium dioxide, talc, and iron oxides.

The biologically inert components of the tablet may occasionally remain intact during gastrointestinal transit and will be eliminated in the feces as a soft, hydrated mass.

12 CLINICAL PHARMACOLOGY

12.1 Mechanism of Action

KOMBIGLYZE XR

KOMBIGLYZE XR combines two antihyperglycemic medications with complementary mechanisms of action to improve glycemic control in adults with type 2 diabetes: saxagliptin, a dipeptidyl-peptidase-4 (DPP4) inhibitor, and metformin hydrochloride, a biguanide.

Saxagliptin

Increased concentrations of the incretin hormones such as glucagon-like peptide-1 (GLP-1) and glucose-dependent insulinotropic polypeptide (GIP) are released into the bloodstream from the small intestine in response to meals. These hormones cause insulin release from the pancreatic beta cells in a glucose-dependent manner but are inactivated by the DPP4 enzyme within minutes. GLP-1 also lowers glucagon secretion from pancreatic alpha cells, reducing hepatic glucose production. In patients with type 2 diabetes, concentrations of GLP-1 are reduced but the insulin response to GLP-1 is preserved. Saxagliptin is a competitive DPP4 inhibitor that slows the inactivation of the incretin hormones, thereby increasing their bloodstream concentrations and reducing fasting and postprandial glucose concentrations in a glucose-dependent manner in patients with type 2 diabetes mellitus.

Metformin hydrochloride

Metformin improves glucose tolerance in patients with type 2 diabetes, lowering both basal and postprandial plasma glucose. Metformin decreases hepatic glucose production, decreases intestinal absorption of glucose, and improves insulin sensitivity by increasing peripheral glucose uptake and utilization. Unlike sulfonylureas, metformin does not produce hypoglycemia in patients with type 2 diabetes or in healthy subjects except in unusual circumstances [see *Warnings and Precautions (5.9)*] and does not cause hyperinsulinemia. With metformin therapy, insulin secretion remains unchanged while fasting insulin levels and day-long plasma insulin response may actually decrease.

12.2 Pharmacodynamics

Saxagliptin

In patients with type 2 diabetes mellitus, administration of saxagliptin inhibits DPP4 enzyme activity for a 24-hour period. After an oral glucose load or a meal, this DPP4 inhibition resulted in a 2- to 3-fold increase in circulating levels of active GLP-1 and GIP, decreased glucagon concentrations, and increased glucose-dependent insulin secretion from pancreatic beta cells. The rise in insulin and decrease in glucagon were associated with lower fasting glucose concentrations and reduced glucose excursion following an oral glucose load or a meal.

Cardiac Electrophysiology

Saxagliptin

In a randomized, double-blind, placebo-controlled, 4-way crossover, active comparator study using moxifloxacin in 40 healthy subjects, saxagliptin was not associated with clinically meaningful prolongation of the QTc interval or heart rate at daily doses up to 40 mg (8 times the MRHD).

12.3 Pharmacokinetics

KOMBIGLYZE XR

Bioequivalence and food effect of KOMBIGLYZE XR was characterized under low calorie diet. The low calorie diet consisted of 324 kcal with meal composition that contained 11.1% protein, 10.5% fat, and 78.4% carbohydrate. The results of bioequivalence studies in healthy subjects demonstrated that KOMBIGLYZE XR combination tablets are bioequivalent to coadministration of corresponding doses of saxagliptin (ONGLYZA®) and metformin hydrochloride extended-release (GLUCOPHAGE® XR) as individual tablets under fed conditions.

Saxagliptin

The pharmacokinetics of saxagliptin and its active metabolite, 5-hydroxy saxagliptin were similar in healthy subjects and in patients with type 2 diabetes mellitus. The C_{max} and AUC values of saxagliptin and its active metabolite increased proportionally in the 2.5 to 400 mg dose range. Following a 5 mg single oral dose of saxagliptin to healthy subjects, the mean plasma AUC values for saxagliptin and its active metabolite were 78 ng•h/mL and 214 ng•h/mL, respectively. The corresponding plasma C_{max} values were 24 ng/mL and 47 ng/mL, respectively. The average variability (%CV) for AUC and C_{max} for both saxagliptin and its active metabolite was less than 25%.

No appreciable accumulation of either saxagliptin or its active metabolite was observed with repeated once-daily dosing at any dose level. No dose- and time-dependence were observed in the clearance of saxagliptin and its active metabolite over 14 days of once-daily dosing with saxagliptin at doses ranging from 2.5 to 400 mg.

Metformin hydrochloride

Metformin extended-release C_{max} is achieved with a median value of 7 hours and a range of 4 to 8 hours. At steady state, the AUC and C_{max} are less than dose proportional for metformin extended-release within the range of 500 to 2000 mg. After repeated administration of metformin extended-release, metformin did not accumulate in plasma. Metformin is excreted unchanged in the urine and does not undergo hepatic metabolism. Peak plasma levels of metformin extended-release tablets are approximately 20% lower compared to the same dose of metformin immediate-release tablets, however, the extent of absorption (as measured by AUC) is similar between extended-release tablets and immediate-release tablets.

Absorption

Saxagliptin

The median time to maximum concentration (T_{max}) following the 5 mg once daily dose was 2 hours for saxagliptin and 4 hours for its active metabolite. Administration with a high-fat meal resulted in an increase in T_{max} of saxagliptin by approximately 20 minutes as compared to fasted conditions. There was a 27% increase in the AUC of saxagliptin when given with a meal as compared to fasted conditions. Saxagliptin may be administered with or without food. Food has no significant effect on the pharmacokinetics of saxagliptin when administered as KOMBIGLYZE XR (saxagliptin and metformin hydrochloride extended-release) combination tablets.

Metformin hydrochloride

Following a single oral dose of metformin extended-release, C_{max} is achieved with a median value of 7 hours and a range of 4 to 8 hours. Although the extent of metformin absorption (as measured by AUC) from the metformin extended-release tablet increased by approximately 50% when given with food, there was no effect of food on C_{max} and T_{max} of metformin. Both high and low fat meals had the same effect on the pharmacokinetics of metformin extended-release. Food has no significant effect on the pharmacokinetics of metformin when administered as KOMBIGLYZE XR combination tablets.

Distribution

Saxagliptin

The *in vitro* protein binding of saxagliptin and its active metabolite in human serum is negligible. Therefore, changes in blood protein levels in various disease states (e.g., renal or hepatic impairment) are not expected to alter the disposition of saxagliptin.

Metformin hydrochloride

Distribution studies with extended-release metformin have not been conducted; however, the apparent volume of distribution (V/F) of metformin following single oral doses of immediate-release metformin 850 mg averaged 654 ± 358 L. Metformin is negligibly bound to plasma proteins, in contrast to sulfonylureas, which are more than 90% protein bound. Metformin partitions into erythrocytes, most likely as a function of time. Metformin is negligibly bound to plasma proteins and is, therefore, less likely to interact with highly protein-bound drugs such as salicylates, sulfonamides, chloramphenicol, and probenecid, as compared to the sulfonylureas, which are extensively bound to serum proteins.

Metabolism

Saxagliptin

The metabolism of saxagliptin is primarily mediated by cytochrome P450 3A4/5 (CYP3A4/5). The major metabolite of saxagliptin is also a DPP4 inhibitor, which is one-half as potent as saxagliptin. Therefore, strong CYP3A4/5 inhibitors and inducers will alter the pharmacokinetics of saxagliptin and its active metabolite. [See *Drug Interactions (7.1)*.]

Metformin hydrochloride

Intravenous single-dose studies in healthy subjects demonstrate that metformin is excreted unchanged in the urine and does not undergo hepatic metabolism (no metabolites have been identified in humans) or biliary excretion.

Metabolism studies with extended-release metformin tablets have not been conducted.

Excretion

Saxagliptin

Saxagliptin is eliminated by both renal and hepatic pathways. Following a single 50 mg dose of ^{14}C-saxagliptin, 24%, 36%, and 75% of the dose was excreted in the urine as saxagliptin, its active metabolite, and total radioactivity, respectively. The average renal clearance of saxagliptin (~230 mL/min) was greater than the average estimated glomerular filtration rate (~120 mL/min), suggesting some active renal excretion. A total of 22% of the administered radioactivity was recovered in feces representing the fraction of the saxagliptin dose excreted in bile and/or unabsorbed drug from the gastrointestinal tract. Following a single oral dose of saxagliptin 5 mg to healthy subjects, the mean plasma terminal half-life ($t_{1/2}$) for saxagliptin and its active metabolite was 2.5 and 3.1 hours, respectively.

Metformin hydrochloride

Renal clearance is approximately 3.5 times greater than creatinine clearance, which indicates that tubular secretion is the major route of metformin elimination. Following oral administration, approximately 90% of the absorbed drug is eliminated via the renal route within the first 24 hours, with a plasma elimination half-life of approximately 6.2 hours. In blood, the elimination half-life is approximately 17.6 hours, suggesting that the erythrocyte mass may be a compartment of distribution.

Specific Populations

Renal Impairment

KOMBIGLYZE XR

In patients with decreased renal function (based on measured creatinine clearance), the plasma and blood half-life of metformin is prolonged and the renal clearance is decreased in proportion to the decrease in creatinine clearance. Use of metformin in patients with renal impairment increases the risk for lactic acidosis. Because KOMBIGLYZE XR (saxagliptin and metformin hydrochloride extended-release) contains metformin, KOMBIGLYZE XR is contraindicated in patients with renal impairment [see *Contraindications (4)* and *Warnings and Precautions (5.3)*].

Hepatic Impairment

No pharmacokinetic studies of metformin have been conducted in patients with hepatic impairment. Use of metformin in patients with hepatic impairment has been associated with some cases of lactic acidosis. Because KOMBIGLYZE XR contains metformin, KOMBIGLYZE XR is not recommended in patients with hepatic impairment [see *Warnings and Precautions (5.4)*].

Body Mass Index

Saxagliptin

No dosage adjustment is recommended based on body mass index (BMI) which was not identified as a significant covariate on the apparent clearance of saxagliptin or its active metabolite in the population pharmacokinetic analysis.

Gender

Saxagliptin

No dosage adjustment is recommended based on gender. There were no differences observed in saxagliptin pharmacokinetics between males and females. Compared to males, females had approximately 25% higher exposure values for the active metabolite than males, but this difference is unlikely to be of clinical relevance. Gender was not identified as a significant covariate on the apparent clearance of saxagliptin and its active metabolite in the population pharmacokinetic analysis.

Metformin hydrochloride

Metformin pharmacokinetic parameters did not differ significantly between healthy subjects and patients with type 2 diabetes when analyzed according to gender (males=19, females=16). Similarly, in controlled clinical studies in patients with type 2 diabetes, the antihyperglycemic effect of metformin was comparable in males and females.

Geriatric

Saxagliptin

No dosage adjustment is recommended based on age alone. Elderly subjects (65-80 years of age) had 23% and 59% higher geometric mean C_{max} and geometric mean AUC values, respectively, for saxagliptin than young subjects (18-40 years of age). Differences in active metabolite pharmacokinetics between elderly and young subjects generally reflected the differences observed in saxagliptin pharmacokinetics. The difference between the pharmacokinetics of saxagliptin and the active metabolite in young and elderly subjects is likely due to multiple factors including declining renal function and metabolic capacity with increasing age. Age was not identified as a significant covariate on the apparent clearance of saxagliptin and its active metabolite in the population pharmacokinetic analysis.

Metformin hydrochloride

Limited data from controlled pharmacokinetic studies of metformin in healthy elderly subjects suggest that total plasma clearance of metformin is decreased, the half-life is prolonged, and C_{max} is increased, compared to healthy young subjects. From these data, it appears that the change in metformin pharmacokinetics with aging is primarily accounted for by a change in renal function.

KOMBIGLYZE XR should not be initiated in patients of any age unless measurement of creatinine clearance demonstrates that renal function is normal [see *Warnings and Precautions (5.1, 5.3)*].

Race and Ethnicity

Saxagliptin

No dosage adjustment is recommended based on race. The population pharmacokinetic analysis compared the pharmacokinetics of saxagliptin and its active metabolite in 309

Caucasian subjects with 105 non-Caucasian subjects (consisting of six racial groups). No significant difference in the pharmacokinetics of saxagliptin and its active metabolite were detected between these two populations.

Metformin hydrochloride

No studies of metformin pharmacokinetic parameters according to race have been performed. In controlled clinical studies of metformin in patients with type 2 diabetes, the antihyperglycemic effect was comparable in whites (n=249), blacks (n=51), and Hispanics (n=24).

Drug Interaction Studies

Specific pharmacokinetic drug interaction studies with KOMBIGLYZE XR (saxagliptin and metformin hydrochloride extended-release) have not been performed, although such studies have been conducted with the individual saxagliptin and metformin components.

In Vitro Assessment of Drug Interactions

In *in vitro* studies, saxagliptin and its active metabolite did not inhibit CYP1A2, 2A6, 2B6, 2C9, 2C19, 2D6, 2E1, or 3A4, or induce CYP1A2, 2B6, 2C9, or 3A4. Therefore, saxagliptin is not expected to alter the metabolic clearance of coadministered drugs that are metabolized by these enzymes. Saxagliptin is a P-glycoprotein (P-gp) substrate, but is not a significant inhibitor or inducer of P-gp.

In Vivo Assessment of Drug Interactions

[See table 3 above]
[See table 4 at top of next page]
[See table 5 at top of next page]
[See table 6 at top of page 743]

Table 3: Effect of Coadministered Drug on Saxagliptin and 5-hydroxy Saxagliptin Systemic Exposures

Coadministered Drug	Dosage of Coadministered Drug*	Dosage of Saxagliptin*	Geometric Mean Ratio (ratio with/without coadministered drug) No Effect = 1.00	AUC[†]	C_{max}
No dosing adjustments required for the following:					
Metformin	1000 mg	100 mg	saxagliptin 5-hydroxy saxagliptin	0.98 0.99	0.79 0.88
Glyburide	5 mg	10 mg	saxagliptin 5-hydroxy saxagliptin	0.98 ND	1.08 ND
Pioglitazone[‡]	45 mg QD for 10 days	10 mg QD for 5 days	saxagliptin 5-hydroxy saxagliptin	1.11 ND	1.11 ND
Digoxin	0.25 mg q6h first day followed by q12h second day followed by QD for 5 days	10 mg QD for 7 days	saxagliptin 5-hydroxy saxagliptin	1.05 1.06	0.99 1.02
Simvastatin	40 mg QD for 8 days	10 mg QD for 4 days	saxagliptin 5-hydroxy saxagliptin	1.12 1.02	1.21 1.08
Diltiazem	360 mg LA QD for 9 days	10 mg	saxagliptin 5-hydroxy saxagliptin	2.09 0.66	1.63 0.57
Rifampin[§]	600 mg QD for 6 days	5 mg	saxagliptin 5-hydroxy saxagliptin	0.24 1.03	0.47 1.39
Omeprazole	40 mg QD for 5 days	10 mg	saxagliptin 5-hydroxy saxagliptin	1.13 ND	0.98 ND
Aluminum hydroxide + magnesium hydroxide + simethicone	aluminum hydroxide: 2400 mg magnesium hydroxide: 2400 mg simethicone: 240 mg	10 mg	saxagliptin 5-hydroxy saxagliptin	0.97 ND	0.74 ND
Famotidine	40 mg	10 mg	saxagliptin 5-hydroxy saxagliptin	1.03 ND	1.14 ND
Limit KOMBIGLYZE XR dose to 2.5 mg/1000 mg once daily when coadministered with strong CYP3A4/5 inhibitors [see *Drug Interactions (7.1)* and *Dosage and Administration (2.2)*]					
Ketoconazole	200 mg BID for 9 days	100 mg	saxagliptin 5-hydroxy saxagliptin	2.45 0.12	1.62 0.05
Ketoconazole	200 mg BID for 7 days	20 mg	saxagliptin 5-hydroxy saxagliptin	3.67 ND	2.44 ND

* Single dose unless otherwise noted.
† AUC = AUC(INF) for drugs given as single dose and AUC = AUC(TAU) for drugs given in multiple doses
‡ Results exclude one subject.
§ The plasma dipeptidyl peptidase-4 (DPP4) activity inhibition over a 24-hour dose interval was not affected by rifampin.
ND=not determined; QD=once daily; q6h=every 6 hours; q12h=every 12 hours; BID=twice daily; LA=long acting

13 NONCLINICAL TOXICOLOGY

13.1 Carcinogenesis, Mutagenesis, Impairment of Fertility

Carcinogenesis

KOMBIGLYZE XR

No animal studies have been conducted with KOMBIGLYZE XR to evaluate carcinogenesis, mutagenesis, or impairment of fertility. The following data are based on the findings in the studies with saxagliptin and metformin individually.

Saxagliptin

Saxagliptin did not induce tumors in either mice (50, 250, and 600 mg/kg) or rats (25, 75, 150, and 300 mg/kg) at the highest doses evaluated. The highest doses evaluated in mice were equivalent to approximately 870 (males) and 1165 (females) times the human exposure at the MRHD of 5 mg/day. In rats, exposures were approximately 355 (males) and 2217 (females) times the MRHD.

Metformin hydrochloride

Long-term carcinogenicity studies have been performed in rats (dosing duration of 104 weeks) and mice (dosing duration of 91 weeks) at doses up to and including 900 mg/kg/day and 1500 mg/kg/day, respectively. These doses are both approximately 4 times the maximum recommended human daily dose of 2000 mg based on body surface area comparisons. No evidence of carcinogenicity with metformin was found in either male or female mice. Similarly, there was no tumorigenic potential observed with metformin in male rats. There was, however, an increased incidence of benign stromal uterine polyps in female rats treated with 900 mg/kg/day.

Mutagenesis

Saxagliptin

Saxagliptin was not mutagenic or clastogenic with or without metabolic activation in an *in vitro* Ames bacterial assay, an *in vitro* cytogenetics assay in primary human lymphocytes, an *in vivo* oral micronucleus assay in rats, an *in vivo* oral DNA repair study in rats, and an oral *in vivo/in vitro* cytogenetics study in rat peripheral blood lymphocytes. The active metabolite was not mutagenic in an *in vitro* Ames bacterial assay.

Metformin hydrochloride

There was no evidence of a mutagenic potential of metformin in the following *in vitro* tests: Ames test (*S. typhimurium*), gene mutation test (mouse lymphoma cells), or chromosomal aberrations test (human lymphocytes). Results in the *in vivo* mouse micronucleus test were also negative.

Impairment of Fertility

Saxagliptin

In a rat fertility study, males were treated with oral gavage doses for 2 weeks prior to mating, during mating, and up to scheduled termination (approximately 4 weeks total) and females were treated with oral gavage doses for 2 weeks prior to mating through gestation day 7. No adverse effects on fertility were observed at exposures of approximately 603 (males) and 776 (females) times the MRHD. Higher doses that elicited maternal toxicity also increased fetal resorptions (approximately 2069 and 6138 times the MRHD). Additional effects on estrous cycling, fertility, ovulation, and implantation were observed at approximately 6138 times the MRHD.

Metformin hydrochloride

Fertility of male or female rats was unaffected by metformin when administered at doses as high as 600 mg/kg/day, which is approximately 3 times the maximum recommended human daily dose based on body surface area comparisons.

13.2 Animal Toxicology and/or Pharmacology

Saxagliptin

Saxagliptin produced adverse skin changes in the extremities of cynomolgus monkeys (scabs and/or ulceration of tail, digits, scrotum, and/or nose). Skin lesions were reversible at ≥20 times the MRHD but in some cases were irreversible and necrotizing at higher exposures. Adverse skin changes were not observed at exposures similar to (1-3 times) the MRHD of 5 mg. Clinical correlates to skin lesions in monkeys have not been observed in human clinical trials of saxagliptin.

14 CLINICAL STUDIES

There have been no clinical efficacy or safety studies conducted with KOMBIGLYZE XR (saxagliptin and metformin hydrochloride extended-release) to characterize its effect on hemoglobin A1c (A1C) reduction. Bioequivalence of KOMBIGLYZE XR with coadministered saxagliptin and metformin hydrochloride extended-release tablets has been demonstrated; however, relative bioavailability studies between KOMBIGLYZE XR and coadministered saxagliptin and metformin hydrochloride immediate-release tablets have not been conducted. The metformin hydrochloride extended-release tablets and metformin hydrochloride immediate-release tablets have a similar extent of absorption (as measured by AUC) while peak plasma levels of extended-release tablets are approximately 20% lower than those of immediate-release tablets at the same dose.

The coadministration of saxagliptin and metformin immediate-release tablets has been studied in adults with type 2 diabetes inadequately controlled on metformin alone and in treatment-naive patients inadequately controlled on diet and exercise alone. In these two trials, treatment with saxagliptin dosed in the morning plus metformin immediate-release tablets at all doses produced clinically relevant and statistically significant improvements in hemoglobin A1c (A1C), fasting plasma glucose (FPG), and 2-hour postprandial glucose (PPG) following a standard oral glucose tolerance test (OGTT), compared to control. Reductions in A1C were seen across subgroups including gender, age, race, and baseline BMI.

In these two trials, decrease in body weight in the treatment groups given saxagliptin in combination with metformin immediate-release was similar to that in the groups given metformin immediate-release alone. Saxagliptin plus metformin immediate-release was not associated with significant changes from baseline in fasting serum lipids compared to metformin alone.

The coadministration of saxagliptin and metformin immediate-release tablets has also been evaluated in an active-controlled trial comparing add-on therapy with saxagliptin to glipizide in 858 patients inadequately controlled on metformin alone, in a placebo-controlled trial where a subgroup of 314 patients inadequately controlled on insulin plus metformin received add-on therapy with saxagliptin or placebo, and a trial comparing saxagliptin to placebo in 257 patients inadequately controlled on metformin plus a sulfonylurea.

In a 24-week, double-blind, randomized trial, patients treated with metformin immediate-release 500 mg twice daily for at least 8 weeks were randomized to continued treatment with metformin immediate-release 500 mg twice daily or to metformin extended-release either 1000 mg once daily or 1500 mg once daily. The mean change in A1C from baseline to Week 24 was 0.1% (95% confidence interval 0%, 0.3%) for the metformin immediate-release treatment arm,

Table 4: Effect of Saxagliptin on Coadministered Drug Systemic Exposures

Coadministered Drug	Dosage of Coadministered Drug*	Dosage of Saxagliptin*	Geometric Mean Ratio (ratio with/without saxagliptin) No Effect = 1.00		
				AUC†	C_{max}
No dosing adjustments required for the following:					
Metformin	1000 mg	100 mg	metformin	1.20	1.09
Glyburide	5 mg	10 mg	glyburide	1.06	1.16
Pioglitazone‡	45 mg QD for 10 days	10 mg QD for 5 days	pioglitazone hydroxy-pioglitazone	1.08 ND	1.14 ND
Digoxin	0.25 mg q6h first day followed by q12h second day followed by QD for 5 days	10 mg QD for 7 days	digoxin	1.06	1.09
Simvastatin	40 mg QD for 8 days	10 mg QD for 4 days	simvastatin simvastatin acid	1.04 1.16	0.88 1.00
Diltiazem	360 mg LA QD for 9 days	10 mg	diltiazem	1.10	1.16
Ketoconazole	200 mg BID for 9 days	100 mg	ketoconazole	0.87	0.84
Ethinyl estradiol and Norgestimate	ethinyl estradiol 0.035 mg and norgestimate 0.250 mg for 21 days	5 mg QD for 21 days	ethinyl estradiol norelgestromin norgestrel	1.07 1.10 1.13	0.98 1.09 1.17

* Single dose unless otherwise noted.
† AUC = AUC(INF) for drugs given as single dose and AUC = AUC(TAU) for drugs given in multiple doses
‡ Results include all subjects.
ND=not determined; QD=once daily; q6h=every 6 hours; q12h=every 12 hours; BID=twice daily; LA=long acting

Table 5: Effect of Coadministered Drug on Plasma Metformin Systemic Exposure

Coadministered Drug	Dose of Coadministered Drug*	Dose of Metformin*	Geometric Mean Ratio (ratio with/without coadministered drug) No Effect = 1.00		
				AUC†	C_{max}
No dosing adjustments required for the following:					
Glyburide	5 mg	850 mg	metformin	0.91‡	0.93‡
Furosemide	40 mg	850 mg	metformin	1.09‡	1.22‡
Nifedipine	10 mg	850 mg	metformin	1.16	1.21
Propranolol	40 mg	850 mg	metformin	0.90	0.94
Ibuprofen	400 mg	850 mg	metformin	1.05‡	1.07‡
Cationic drugs eliminated by renal tubular secretion may reduce metformin elimination: use with caution. [See *Warnings and Precautions (5.10)* and *Drug Interactions (7.2)*.]					
Cimetidine	400 mg	850 mg	metformin	1.40	1.61

* All metformin and coadministered drugs were given as single doses.
† AUC = AUC(INF)
‡ Ratio of arithmetic means

0.3% (95% confidence interval 0.1%, 0.4%) for the 1000 mg metformin extended-release treatment arm, and 0.1% (95% confidence interval 0%, 0.3%) for the 1500 mg metformin extended-release treatment arm. Results of this trial suggest that patients receiving metformin immediate-release treatment may be safely switched to metformin extended-release once daily at the same total daily dose, up to 2000 mg once daily. Following a switch from metformin immediate-release to metformin extended-release, glycemic control should be closely monitored and dosage adjustments made accordingly.

Saxagliptin Morning and Evening Dosing

A 24-week monotherapy trial was conducted to assess a range of dosing regimens for saxagliptin. Treatment-naive patients with inadequately controlled diabetes (A1C ≥7% to ≤10%) underwent a 2-week, single-blind diet, exercise, and placebo lead-in period. A total of 365 patients were randomized to 2.5 mg every morning, 5 mg every morning, 2.5 mg with possible titration to 5 mg every morning, or 5 mg every evening of saxagliptin, or placebo. Patients who failed to meet specific glycemic goals during the study were treated with metformin rescue therapy added on to placebo or saxagliptin; the number of patients randomized per treatment group ranged from 71 to 74.

Treatment with either saxagliptin 5 mg every morning or 5 mg every evening provided significant improvements in A1C versus placebo (mean placebo-corrected reductions of −0.4% and −0.3%, respectively).

14.1 Coadministration of Saxagliptin with Metformin Immediate-Release in Treatment-Naive Patients

A total of 1306 treatment-naive patients with type 2 diabetes mellitus participated in this 24-week, randomized, double-blind, active-controlled trial to evaluate the efficacy and safety of saxagliptin coadministered with metformin immediate-release in patients with inadequate glycemic control (A1C ≥8% to ≤12%) on diet and exercise alone. Patients were required to be treatment-naive to be enrolled in this study.

Patients who met eligibility criteria were enrolled in a single-blind, 1-week, dietary and exercise placebo lead-in period. Patients were randomized to one of four treatment arms: saxagliptin 5 mg + metformin immediate-release 500 mg, saxagliptin 10 mg + metformin immediate-release 500 mg, saxagliptin 10 mg + placebo, or metformin immediate-release 500 mg + placebo (the maximum recommended approved saxagliptin dose is 5 mg daily; the 10 mg daily dose of saxagliptin does not provide greater efficacy than the 5 mg daily dose and the 10 mg dosage is not an approved dosage). Saxagliptin was dosed once daily. In the 3 treatment groups using metformin immediate-release, the metformin dose was up-titrated weekly in 500 mg per day increments, as tolerated, to a maximum of 2000 mg per day based on FPG. Patients who failed to meet specific glycemic goals during this study were treated with pioglitazone rescue as add-on therapy.

Coadministration of saxagliptin 5 mg plus metformin immediate-release provided significant improvements in A1C, FPG, and PPG compared with placebo plus metformin immediate-release (Table 7).

[See table 7 at top of next page]

14.2 Addition of Saxagliptin to Metformin Immediate-Release

A total of 743 patients with type 2 diabetes participated in this 24-week, randomized, double-blind, placebo-controlled trial to evaluate the efficacy and safety of saxagliptin in combination with metformin immediate-release in patients with inadequate glycemic control (A1C ≥7% and ≤10%) on metformin alone. To qualify for enrollment, patients were required to be on a stable dose of metformin (1500-2550 mg daily) for at least 8 weeks.

Patients who met eligibility criteria were enrolled in a single-blind, 2-week, dietary and exercise placebo lead-in period during which patients received metformin immediate-release at their pre-study dose, up to 2500 mg daily, for the duration of the study. Following the lead-in period, eligible patients were randomized to 2.5 mg, 5 mg, or 10 mg of saxagliptin or placebo in addition to their current dose of open-label metformin immediate-release (the maximum recommended approved saxagliptin dose is 5 mg daily; the 10 mg daily dose of saxagliptin does not provide greater efficacy than the 5 mg daily dose and the 10 mg dosage is not an approved dosage). Patients who failed to meet specific glycemic goals during the study were treated with pioglitazone rescue therapy, added on to existing study medications. Dose titrations of saxagliptin and metformin immediate-release were not permitted.

Saxagliptin 2.5 mg and 5 mg add-on to metformin immediate-release provided significant improvements in A1C, FPG, and PPG compared with placebo add-on to metformin immediate-release (Table 8). Mean changes from baseline for A1C over time and at endpoint are shown in Figure 1. The proportion of patients who discontinued for lack of glycemic control or who were rescued for meeting prespecified glycemic criteria was 15% in the saxagliptin 2.5 mg add-on to metformin immediate-release group, 13% in the saxagliptin 5 mg add-on to metformin immediate-release group, and 27% in the placebo add-on to metformin immediate-release group.

[See table 8 at bottom of next page]

Figure 1: Mean Change from Baseline in A1C in a Placebo-Controlled Trial of Saxagliptin as Add-On Combination Therapy with Metformin Immediate-Release*

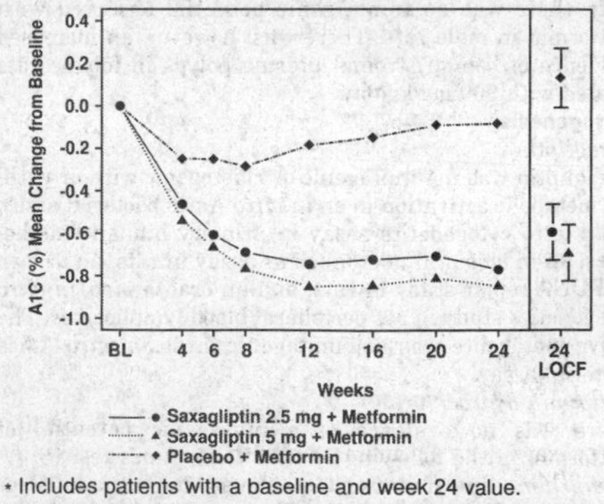

* Includes patients with a baseline and week 24 value.

Week 24 (LOCF) includes intent-to-treat population using last observation on study prior to pioglitazone rescue therapy for patients needing rescue. Mean change from baseline is adjusted for baseline value.

14.3 Saxagliptin Add-On Combination Therapy with Metformin Immediate-Release versus Glipizide Add-On Combination Therapy with Metformin Immediate-Release

In this 52-week, active-controlled trial, a total of 858 patients with type 2 diabetes and inadequate glycemic control (A1C >6.5% and ≤10%) on metformin immediate-release alone were randomized to double-blind add-on therapy with saxagliptin or glipizide. Patients were required to be on a stable dose of metformin immediate-release (at least 1500 mg daily) for at least 8 weeks prior to enrollment.

Patients who met eligibility criteria were enrolled in a single-blind, 2-week, dietary and exercise placebo lead-in period during which patients received metformin immediate-release (1500-3000 mg based on their prestudy dose). Following the lead-in period, eligible patients were randomized to 5 mg of saxagliptin or 5 mg of glipizide in addition to their current dose of open-label metformin immediate-release. Patients in the glipizide plus metformin immediate-release group underwent blinded titration of the glipizide dose during the first 18 weeks of the trial up to a maximum glipizide dose of 20 mg per day. Titration was based on a goal FPG ≤110 mg/dL or the highest tolerable glipizide dose. Fifty percent (50%) of the glipizide-treated patients were titrated to the 20-mg daily dose; 21% of the glipizide-treated patients had a final daily glipizide dose of 5 mg or less. The mean final daily dose of glipizide was 15 mg.

After 52 weeks of treatment, saxagliptin and glipizide resulted in similar mean reductions from baseline in A1C when added to metformin immediate-release therapy (Table 9). This conclusion may be limited to patients with baseline A1C comparable to those in the trial (91% of patients had baseline A1C <9%).

From a baseline mean body weight of 89 kg, there was a statistically significant mean reduction of 1.1 kg in patients treated with saxagliptin compared to a mean weight gain of 1.1 kg in patients treated with glipizide (p<0.0001).

[See table 9 at top of next page]

14.4 Saxagliptin Add-On Combination Therapy with Insulin (with or without Metformin Immediate-Release)

A total of 455 patients with type 2 diabetes participated in this 24-week, randomized, double-blind, placebo-controlled trial to evaluate the efficacy and safety of saxagliptin in combination with insulin in patients with inadequate glycemic control (A1C ≥7.5% and ≤11%) on insulin alone (N=141) or on insulin in combination with a stable dose of metformin immediate-release (N=314). Patients were required to be on a stable dose of insulin (≥30 units to ≤150 units daily) with ≤20% variation in total daily dose for ≥8 weeks prior to screening. Patients entered the trial on intermediate- or long-acting (basal) insulin or premixed insulin. Patients using short-acting insulins were excluded unless the short-acting insulin was administered as part of a premixed insulin.

Patients who met eligibility criteria were enrolled in a single-blind, four-week, dietary and exercise placebo lead-in period during which patients received insulin (and metformin immediate-release if applicable) at their pretrial dose(s). Following the lead-in period, eligible patients were randomized to add-on therapy with either saxagliptin 5 mg or placebo. Doses of the antidiabetic therapies were to remain stable but patients were rescued and allowed to adjust the insulin regimen if specific glycemic goals were not met or if the investigator learned that the patient had self-increased the insulin dose by >20%. Data after rescue were excluded from the primary efficacy analyses.

Add-on therapy with saxagliptin 5 mg provided significant improvements from baseline to Week 24 in A1C and PPG compared with add-on placebo (Table 10). Similar mean reductions in A1C versus placebo were observed for patients using saxagliptin 5 mg add-on to insulin alone and saxagliptin 5 mg add-on to insulin in combination with metformin immediate-release (−0.4% and −0.4%, respectively). The percentage of patients who discontinued for lack of glycemic control or who were rescued was 23% in the saxagliptin group and 32% in the placebo group.

The mean daily insulin dose at baseline was 53 units in patients treated with saxagliptin 5 mg and 55 units in patients treated with placebo. The mean change from baseline in daily dose of insulin was 2 units for the saxagliptin 5 mg group and 5 units for the placebo group.

[See table 10 at top of next page]

The change in fasting plasma glucose from baseline to Week 24 was also tested, but was not statistically significant. The percent of patients achieving an A1C <7% was 17% (52/300) with saxagliptin in combination with insulin compared to 7% (10/149) with placebo. Significance was not tested.

14.5 Saxagliptin Add-On Combination Therapy with Metformin plus Sulfonylurea

A total of 257 subjects with type 2 diabetes participated in this 24-week, randomized, double-blind, placebo-controlled trial to evaluate the efficacy and safety of saxagliptin in combination with metformin plus a sulfonylurea in patients with inadequate glycemic control (A1C ≥7% and ≤10%). Patients were to be on a stable combined dose of metformin extended-release or immediate-release (at maximum tolerated dose, with minimum dose for enrollment being 1500 mg) and a sulfonylurea (at maximum tolerated dose, with minimum dose for enrollment being ≥50% of the maximum recommended dose) for ≥8 weeks prior to enrollment. Patients who met eligibility criteria were entered in a 2-week enrollment period to allow assessment of inclusion/exclusion criteria. Following the 2-week enrollment period, eligible patients were randomized to either double-blind saxagliptin (5 mg once daily) or double-blind matching placebo for 24 weeks. During the 24-week double-blind treatment period, patients were to receive metformin and a sul-

Table 6: Effect of Metformin on Coadministered Drug Systemic Exposure

Coadministered Drug	Dose of Coadministered Drug*	Dose of Metformin*	Geometric Mean Ratio (ratio with/without metformin) No Effect = 1.00		
				AUC†	C_{max}
No dosing adjustments required for the following:					
Glyburide	5 mg	850 mg	glyburide	0.78‡	0.63‡
Furosemide	40 mg	850 mg	furosemide	0.87‡	0.69‡
Nifedipine	10 mg	850 mg	nifedipine	1.10§	1.08
Propranolol	40 mg	850 mg	propranolol	1.01§	1.02
Ibuprofen	400 mg	850 mg	ibuprofen	0.97¶	1.01¶
Cimetidine	400 mg	850 mg	cimetidine	0.95§	1.01

* All metformin and coadministered drugs were given as single doses.
† AUC = AUC(INF) unless otherwise noted
‡ Ratio of arithmetic means, p-value of difference <0.05
§ AUC(0-24 hr) reported
¶ Ratio of arithmetic means

Table 7: Glycemic Parameters at Week 24 in a Placebo-Controlled Trial of Saxagliptin Coadministration with Metformin Immediate-Release in Treatment-Naive Patients*

Efficacy Parameter	Saxagliptin 5 mg + Metformin N=320	Placebo + Metformin N=328
Hemoglobin A1C (%)	**N=306**	**N=313**
Baseline (mean)	9.4	9.4
Change from baseline (adjusted mean†)	−2.5	−2.0
Difference from placebo + metformin (adjusted mean†)	−0.5‡	
95% Confidence Interval	(−0.7, −0.4)	
Percent of patients achieving A1C <7%	60%§ (185/307)	41% (129/314)
Fasting Plasma Glucose (mg/dL)	**N=315**	**N=320**
Baseline (mean)	199	199
Change from baseline (adjusted mean†)	−60	−47
Difference from placebo + metformin (adjusted mean†)	−13‡	
95% Confidence Interval	(−19, −6)	
2-hour Postprandial Glucose (mg/dL)	**N=146**	**N=141**
Baseline (mean)	340	355
Change from baseline (adjusted mean†)	−138	−97
Difference from placebo + metformin (adjusted mean†)	−41‡	
95% Confidence Interval	(−57, −25)	

* Intent-to-treat population using last observation on study or last observation prior to pioglitazone rescue therapy for patients needing rescue.
† Least squares mean adjusted for baseline value.
‡ p-value <0.0001 compared to placebo + metformin
§ p-value <0.05 compared to placebo + metformin

Table 8: Glycemic Parameters at Week 24 in a Placebo-Controlled Study of Saxagliptin as Add-On Combination Therapy with Metformin Immediate-Release*

Efficacy Parameter	Saxagliptin 2.5 mg + Metformin N=192	Saxagliptin 5 mg + Metformin N=191	Placebo + Metformin N=179
Hemoglobin A1C (%)	**N=186**	**N=186**	**N=175**
Baseline (mean)	8.1	8.1	8.1
Change from baseline (adjusted mean†)	−0.6	−0.7	+0.1
Difference from placebo (adjusted mean†)	−0.7‡	−0.8‡	
95% Confidence Interval	(−0.9, −0.5)	(−1.0, −0.6)	
Percent of patients achieving A1C <7%	37%§ (69/186)	44%§ (81/186)	17% (29/175)
Fasting Plasma Glucose (mg/dL)	**N=188**	**N=187**	**N=176**
Baseline (mean)	174	179	175
Change from baseline (adjusted mean†)	−14	−22	+1
Difference from placebo (adjusted mean†)	−16§	−23§	
95% Confidence Interval	(−23, −9)	(−30, −16)	
2-hour Postprandial Glucose (mg/dL)	**N=155**	**N=155**	**N=135**
Baseline (mean)	294	296	295
Change from baseline (adjusted mean†)	−62	−58	−18
Difference from placebo (adjusted mean†)	−44§	−40§	
95% Confidence Interval	(−60, −27)	(−56, −24)	

* Intent-to-treat population using last observation on study or last observation prior to pioglitazone rescue therapy for patients needing rescue.
† Least squares mean adjusted for baseline value.
‡ p-value <0.0001 compared to placebo + metformin
§ p-value <0.05 compared to placebo + metformin

Table 9: Glycemic Parameters at Week 52 in an Active-Controlled Trial of Saxagliptin versus Glipizide in Combination with Metformin Immediate-Release*

Efficacy Parameter	Saxagliptin 5 mg + Metformin N=428	Titrated Glipizide + Metformin N=430
Hemoglobin A1C (%)	N=423	N=423
Baseline (mean)	7.7	7.6
Change from baseline (adjusted mean†)	−0.6	−0.7
Difference from glipizide + metformin (adjusted mean†)	0.1	
95% Confidence Interval	(−0.02, 0.2)‡	
Fasting Plasma Glucose (mg/dL)	N=420	N=420
Baseline (mean)	162	161
Change from baseline (adjusted mean†)	−9	−16
Difference from glipizide + metformin (adjusted mean†)	6	
95% Confidence Interval	(2, 11)§	

* Intent-to-treat population using last observation on study.
† Least squares mean adjusted for baseline value.
‡ Saxagliptin + metformin is considered non-inferior to glipizide + metformin because the upper limit of this confidence interval is less than the prespecified non-inferiority margin of 0.35%.
§ Significance not tested.

Table 10: Glycemic Parameters at Week 24 in a Placebo-Controlled Trial of Saxagliptin as Add-On Combination Therapy with Insulin*

Efficacy Parameter	Saxagliptin 5 mg + Insulin (+/− Metformin) N=304	Placebo + Insulin (+/− Metformin) N=151
Hemoglobin A1C (%)	N=300	N=149
Baseline (mean)	8.7	8.7
Change from baseline (adjusted mean†)	−0.7	−0.3
Difference from placebo (adjusted mean†)	−0.4‡	
95% Confidence Interval	(−0.6, −0.2)	
2-hour Postprandial Glucose (mg/dL)	N=262	N=129
Baseline (mean)	251	255
Change from baseline (adjusted mean†)	−27	−4
Difference from placebo (adjusted mean†)	−23§	
95% Confidence Interval	(−37, −9)	

* Intent-to-treat population using last observation on study or last observation prior to insulin rescue therapy for patients needing rescue.
† Least squares mean adjusted for baseline value and metformin use at baseline.
‡ p-value <0.0001 compared to placebo + insulin
§ p-value <0.05 compared to placebo + insulin

Table 11: Glycemic Parameters at Week 24 in a Placebo-Controlled Trial of Saxagliptin as Add-On Combination Therapy with Metformin plus Sulfonylurea*

Efficacy Parameter	Saxagliptin 5 mg + Metformin plus Sulfonylurea N=129	Placebo + Metformin plus Sulfonylurea N=128
Hemoglobin A1C (%)	N=127	N=127
Baseline (mean)	8.4	8.2
Change from baseline (adjusted mean†)	−0.7	−0.1
Difference from placebo (adjusted mean†)	−0.7‡	
95% Confidence Interval	(−0.9, −0.5)	
2-hour Postprandial Glucose (mg/dL)	N=115	N=113
Baseline (mean)	268	262
Change from baseline (adjusted mean†)	−12	5
Difference from placebo (adjusted mean†)	−17§	
95% Confidence Interval	(−32, −2)	

* Intent-to-treat population using last observation prior to discontinuation.
† Least squares mean adjusted for baseline value.
‡ p-value <0.0001 compared to placebo + metformin plus sulfonylurea
§ p-value <0.05 compared to placebo + metformin plus sulfonylurea

fonylurea at the same constant dose ascertained during enrollment. Sulfonylurea dose could be down titrated once in the case of a major hypoglycemic event or recurring minor hypoglycemic events. In the absence of hypoglycemia, titration (up or down) of study medication during the treatment period was prohibited.

Saxagliptin in combination with metformin plus a sulfonylurea provided significant improvements in A1C and PPG compared with placebo in combination with metformin plus a sulfonylurea (Table 11). The percentage of patients who discontinued for lack of glycemic control was 6% in the saxagliptin group and 5% in the placebo group.

[See table 1 above]

The change in fasting plasma glucose from baseline to Week 24 was also tested, but was not statistically significant. The percent of patients achieving an A1C <7% was 31% (39/127) with saxagliptin in combination with metformin plus a sulfonylurea compared to 9% (12/127) with placebo. Significance was not tested.

16 HOW SUPPLIED/STORAGE AND HANDLING

How Supplied

KOMBIGLYZE™ XR (saxagliptin and metformin HCl extended-release) tablets have markings on both sides and are available in the strengths and packages listed in Table 12.

[See table 12 at top of next page]

Storage and Handling

Store at 20°C to 25°C (68°F to 77°F); excursions permitted between 15°C and 30°C (59°F and 86°F) [see USP Controlled Room Temperature].

17 PATIENT COUNSELING INFORMATION

See FDA-approved patient labeling (Medication Guide).

Medication Guide

Healthcare providers should instruct their patients to read the Medication Guide before starting KOMBIGLYZE XR therapy and to reread it each time the prescription is renewed. Patients should be instructed to inform their healthcare provider if they develop any unusual symptom or if any existing symptom persists or worsens.

Patients should be informed of the potential risks and benefits of KOMBIGLYZE XR and of alternative modes of therapy. Patients should also be informed about the importance of adherence to dietary instructions, regular physical activity, periodic blood glucose monitoring and A1C testing, recognition and management of hypoglycemia and hyperglycemia, and assessment of diabetes complications. During periods of stress such as fever, trauma, infection, or surgery, medication requirements may change and patients should be advised to seek medical advice promptly.

Lactic Acidosis

The risks of lactic acidosis due to the metformin component, its symptoms and conditions that predispose to its development, as noted in Warnings and Precautions (5.1), should be explained to patients. Patients should be advised to discontinue KOMBIGLYZE XR immediately and to promptly notify their healthcare provider if unexplained hyperventilation, myalgia, malaise, unusual somnolence, dizziness, slow or irregular heart beat, sensation of feeling cold (especially in the extremities), or other nonspecific symptoms occur. Gastrointestinal symptoms are common during initiation of metformin treatment and may occur during initiation of KOMBIGLYZE XR therapy; however, patients should consult their physician if they develop unexplained symptoms. Although gastrointestinal symptoms that occur after stabilization are unlikely to be drug related, such an occurrence of symptoms should be evaluated to determine if it may be due to lactic acidosis or other serious disease.

Patients should be counseled against excessive alcohol intake while receiving KOMBIGLYZE XR.

Patients should be informed about the importance of regular testing of renal function and hematological parameters when receiving treatment with KOMBIGLYZE XR.

Pancreatitis

Patients should be informed that acute pancreatitis has been reported during postmarketing use of saxagliptin. Before initiating KOMBIGLYZE XR, patients should be questioned about other risk factors for pancreatitis, such as a history of pancreatitis, alcoholism, gallstones, or hypertriglyceridemia. Patients should also be informed that persistent severe abdominal pain, sometimes radiating to the back, which may or may not be accompanied by vomiting, is the hallmark symptom of acute pancreatitis. Patients should be instructed to promptly discontinue KOMBIGLYZE XR and contact their physician if persistent severe abdominal pain occurs [see *Warnings and Precautions (5.2)*].

Hypoglycemia

Patients should be informed that the incidence of hypoglycemia may be increased when KOMBIGLYZE XR is added to an insulin secretagogue (e.g., sulfonylurea) or insulin.

Hypersensitivity Reactions

Patients should be informed that serious allergic (hypersensitivity) reactions, such as angioedema, anaphylaxis, and exfoliative skin conditions, have been reported during postmarketing use of saxagliptin. If symptoms of these allergic reactions (such as rash, skin flaking or peeling, urticaria, swelling of the skin, or swelling of the face, lips, tongue, and throat that may cause difficulty in breathing or swallowing) occur, patients must stop taking KOMBIGLYZE XR and seek medical advice promptly.

Administration Instructions

Patients should be informed that KOMBIGLYZE XR must be swallowed whole and not crushed or chewed, and that the inactive ingredients may occasionally be eliminated in the feces as a soft mass that may resemble the original tablet.

Missed Dose

Patients should be informed that if they miss a dose of KOMBIGLYZE XR, they should take the next dose as prescribed, unless otherwise instructed by their healthcare provider. Patients should be instructed not to take an extra dose the next day.

GLUCOPHAGE® is a registered trademark of Merck Santé S.A.S., a subsidiary of Merck KGaA of Darmstadt, Germany, licensed to Bristol-Myers Squibb Company.

ONGLYZA® is a trademark of Bristol-Myers Squibb Company.

Manufactured by:
Bristol-Myers Squibb Company
Princeton, NJ 08543 USA
Marketed by:
Bristol-Myers Squibb Company
Princeton, NJ 08543
and
AstraZeneca Pharmaceuticals LP
Wilmington, DE 19850
1281913A2

MEDICATION GUIDE
KOMBIGLYZE XR (kom-be-glyze X-R)
(saxagliptin and metformin HCl extended-release)
tablets

Read this Medication Guide carefully before you start taking KOMBIGLYZE XR and each time you get a refill. There may be new information. This information does not take the place of talking with your healthcare provider about your medical condition or treatment. If you have any questions about KOMBIGLYZE XR, ask your healthcare provider.

What is the most important information I should know about KOMBIGLYZE XR?

Serious side effects can happen in people taking KOMBIGLYZE XR, including:

1. **Lactic Acidosis.** Metformin hydrochloride, one of the medicines in KOMBIGLYZE XR, can cause a rare, but serious, side effect called lactic acidosis (a build-up of lactic acid in the blood) that can cause death. Lactic acidosis is a medical emergency and must be treated in a hospital.
   Stop taking KOMBIGLYZE XR and call your healthcare provider right away if you get any of the following symptoms of lactic acidosis:
   - feel very weak and tired
   - have unusual (not normal) muscle pain
   - have trouble breathing
   - have unusual sleepiness or sleep longer than usual
   - have unexplained stomach or intestinal problems with nausea and vomiting, or diarrhea
   - feel cold, especially in your arms and legs
   - feel dizzy or lightheaded
   - have a slow or irregular heartbeat

   You have a higher chance of getting lactic acidosis if you:
   - have kidney problems. People whose kidneys are not working properly should not take KOMBIGLYZE XR.
   - have liver problems.
   - have congestive heart failure that requires treatment with medicines.
   - drink a lot of alcohol (very often or short-term "binge" drinking).
   - get dehydrated (lose a large amount of body fluids). This can happen if you are sick with a fever, vomiting, or diarrhea. Dehydration can also happen when you sweat a lot with activity or exercise and do not drink enough fluids.
   - have certain x-ray tests with injectable dyes or contrast agents.
   - have surgery.
   - have a heart attack, severe infection, or stroke.
   - are 80 years of age or older and have not had your kidney function tested.
2. **Inflammation of the pancreas (pancreatitis)** which may be severe and lead to death.
   Certain medical problems make you more likely to get pancreatitis.
   Before you start taking KOMBIGLYZE XR:
   Tell your healthcare provider if you have ever had
   - inflammation of your pancreas (pancreatitis)
   - stones in your gallbladder (gallstones)
   - a history of alcoholism
   - high blood triglyceride levels

   It is not known if having these medical problems will make you more likely to get pancreatitis with KOMBIGLYZE XR.
   Stop taking KOMBIGLYZE XR and contact your healthcare provider right away if you have pain in your stomach area (abdomen) that is severe and will not go away. The pain may be felt going from your abdomen through to your back. The pain may happen with or without vomiting. These may be symptoms of pancreatitis.

What is KOMBIGLYZE XR?
- KOMBIGLYZE XR is a prescription medicine that contains saxagliptin and metformin hydrochloride. KOMBIGLYZE XR is used with diet and exercise to help control high blood sugar (hyperglycemia) in adults with type 2 diabetes.
- KOMBIGLYZE XR is not for people with type 1 diabetes.
- KOMBIGLYZE XR is not for people with diabetic ketoacidosis (increased ketones in your blood or urine).
- If you have had inflammation of the pancreas (pancreatitis) in the past, it is not known if you have a higher chance of getting pancreatitis while you take KOMBIGLYZE XR.

It is not known if KOMBIGLYZE XR is safe and effective in children younger than 18 years old.

Table 12: KOMBIGLYZE XR Tablet Presentations

Tablet Strength (saxagliptin and metformin HCl extended-release)	Film-Coated Tablet Color/Shape	Tablet Markings	Package Size	NDC Code
5 mg/500 mg	light brown to brown, biconvex, capsule-shaped	"5/500" on one side and "4221" on the reverse, in blue ink	Bottles of 30	0003-4221-11
5 mg/1000 mg	pink, biconvex, capsule-shaped	"5/1000" on one side and "4223" on the reverse, in blue ink	Bottles of 30 Bottles of 90 Bottles of 500	0003-4223-11 0003-4223-21 0003-4223-31
2.5 mg/1000 mg	pale yellow to light yellow, biconvex, capsule-shaped	"2.5/1000" on one side and "4222" on the reverse, in blue ink	Bottles of 60 Bottles of 500	0003-4222-16 0003-4222-31

Who should not take KOMBIGLYZE XR?
Do not take KOMBIGLYZE XR if you:
- have kidney problems.
- are allergic to metformin hydrochloride, saxagliptin, or any of the ingredients in KOMBIGLYZE XR (saxagliptin and metformin hydrochloride extended-release). See the end of this Medication Guide for a complete list of ingredients in KOMBIGLYZE XR.
  Symptoms of a serious allergic reaction to KOMBIGLYZE XR may include:
  - swelling of your face, lips, throat, and other areas on your skin
  - difficulty with swallowing or breathing
  - raised, red areas on your skin (hives)
  - skin rash, itching, flaking, or peeling

  If you have these symptoms, stop taking KOMBIGLYZE XR and contact your healthcare provider right away.
- have a condition called metabolic acidosis or diabetic ketoacidosis (increased ketones in your blood or urine).

What should I tell my healthcare provider before taking KOMBIGLYZE XR?
Before you take KOMBIGLYZE XR, tell your healthcare provider if you:
- have type 1 diabetes. KOMBIGLYZE XR should not be used to treat type 1 diabetes.
- have a history or risk for diabetic ketoacidosis (high levels of certain acids, known as ketones, in the blood or urine). KOMBIGLYZE XR should not be used for the treatment of diabetic ketoacidosis.
- have kidney problems.
- have liver problems.
- have heart problems, including congestive heart failure.
- are older than 80 years. If you are over 80 years old you should not take KOMBIGLYZE XR unless your kidneys have been checked and they are normal.
- drink alcohol very often, or drink a lot of alcohol in short-term "binge" drinking.
- are going to get an injection of dye or contrast agents for an x-ray procedure or if you are going to have surgery and will not be able to eat or drink much. In these situations, KOMBIGLYZE XR will need to be stopped for a short time. Talk to your healthcare provider about when you should stop KOMBIGLYZE XR and when you should start KOMBIGLYZE XR again. See **"What is the most important information I should know about KOMBIGLYZE XR?"**
- have any other medical conditions.
- are pregnant or plan to become pregnant. It is not known if KOMBIGLYZE XR will harm your unborn baby. If you are pregnant, talk with your healthcare provider about the best way to control your blood sugar while you are pregnant.
- are breast-feeding or plan to breast-feed. It is not known if KOMBIGLYZE XR passes into your breast milk. Talk with your healthcare provider about the best way to feed your baby while you take KOMBIGLYZE XR.

Tell your healthcare provider about all the medicines you take, including prescription and nonprescription medicines, vitamins, and herbal supplements. Know the medicines you take. Keep a list of them to show your healthcare provider and pharmacist when you get a new medicine.

KOMBIGLYZE XR may affect the way other medicines work, and other medicines may affect how KOMBIGLYZE XR works.

Tell your healthcare provider if you will be starting or stopping certain other types of medicines, such as antibiotics, or medicines that treat fungus or HIV/AIDS, because your dose of KOMBIGLYZE XR might need to be changed.

How should I take KOMBIGLYZE XR?
- Take KOMBIGLYZE XR exactly as your healthcare provider tells you.
- KOMBIGLYZE XR should be taken with meals to help lessen an upset stomach side effect.
- Swallow KOMBIGLYZE XR whole. Do not crush, cut, or chew KOMBIGLYZE XR.
- You may sometimes pass a soft mass in your stools (bowel movement) that looks like KOMBIGLYZE XR (saxagliptin and metformin hydrochloride extended-release) tablets.
- When your body is under some types of stress, such as fever, trauma (such as a car accident), infection, or surgery, the amount of diabetes medicine that you need may change. Tell your healthcare provider right away if you have any of these problems.
- Your healthcare provider should do blood tests to check how well your kidneys are working before and during your treatment with KOMBIGLYZE XR.
- Your healthcare provider will check your diabetes with regular blood tests, including your blood sugar levels and your hemoglobin A1C.
- Follow your healthcare provider's instructions for treating blood sugar that is too low (hypoglycemia). Talk to your healthcare provider if low blood sugar is a problem for you. See **"What are the possible side effects of KOMBIGLYZE XR?"**
- Check your blood sugar as your healthcare provider tells you to.
- Stay on your prescribed diet and exercise program while taking KOMBIGLYZE XR.
- If you miss a dose of KOMBIGLYZE XR, take your next dose as prescribed unless your healthcare provider tells you differently. Do not take an extra dose the next day.
- If you take too much KOMBIGLYZE XR, call your healthcare provider, local Poison Control Center, or go to the nearest hospital emergency room right away.

What are the possible side effects of KOMBIGLYZE XR?
KOMBIGLYZE XR can cause serious side effects, including:
- See **"What is the most important information I should know about KOMBIGLYZE XR?"**
- **Allergic (hypersensitivity) reactions,** such as:
  - swelling of your face, lips, throat, and other areas on your skin
  - difficulty with swallowing or breathing
  - raised, red areas on your skin (hives)
  - skin rash, itching, flaking, or peeling

  If you have these symptoms, stop taking KOMBIGLYZE XR and contact your healthcare provider right away.

Low blood sugar (hypoglycemia) may become worse in people who also take another medication to treat diabetes, such as sulfonylureas or insulin. Tell your healthcare provider if you take other diabetes medicines. If you have symptoms of low blood sugar, you should check your blood sugar and treat if low, then call your healthcare provider. Symptoms of low blood sugar include:
- shaking
- sweating
- rapid heartbeat
- change in vision
- hunger
- headache
- change in mood

Common side effects of KOMBIGLYZE XR include:
- upper respiratory tract infection
- stuffy or runny nose and sore throat
- urinary tract infection
- headache
- diarrhea
- nausea and vomiting

Taking KOMBIGLYZE XR with meals can help lessen the common stomach side effects of metformin. If you have unexplained stomach problems, tell your healthcare provider. Stomach problems that start later during treatment may be a sign of something more serious.

Tell your healthcare provider if you have any side effects that bother you or that do not go away.

These are not all of the possible side effects of KOMBIGLYZE XR. For more information, ask your healthcare provider or pharmacist.

Call your doctor for medical advice about side effects. You may report side effects to the FDA at 1-800-FDA-1088.

How should I store KOMBIGLYZE XR?
Store KOMBIGLYZE XR (saxagliptin and metformin hydrochloride extended-release) between 68°F and 77°F (20°C and 25°C).

Keep KOMBIGLYZE XR and all medicines out of the reach of children.

General information about the use of KOMBIGLYZE XR
Medicines are sometimes prescribed for purposes other than those listed in a Medication Guide. Do not use KOMBIGLYZE XR for a condition for which it was not prescribed. Do not give KOMBIGLYZE XR to other people, even if they have the same symptoms you have. It may harm them.
This Medication Guide summarizes the most important information about KOMBIGLYZE XR. If you would like more information, talk with your healthcare provider. You can ask your pharmacist or healthcare provider for information about KOMBIGLYZE XR that is written for healthcare professionals.
For more information, go to www.kombiglyzexr.com or call 1-800-664-5992.

What are the ingredients of KOMBIGLYZE XR?
Active ingredients: saxagliptin and metformin hydrochloride.
Inactive ingredients in each tablet: carboxymethylcellulose sodium, hypromellose 2208, and magnesium stearate. The 5 mg/500 mg tablet also contains: microcrystalline cellulose and hypromellose 2910.
Tablet film coat contains: polyvinyl alcohol, polyethylene glycol 3350, titanium dioxide, talc, and iron oxides.

What is type 2 diabetes?
Type 2 diabetes is a condition in which your body does not make enough insulin, and the insulin that your body produces does not work as well as it should. Your body can also make too much sugar. When this happens, sugar (glucose) builds up in the blood. This can lead to serious medical problems.
The main goal of treating diabetes is to lower your blood sugar so that it is as close to normal as possible. High blood sugar can be lowered by diet and exercise, and by certain medicines when necessary.
Talk to your healthcare provider about how to prevent, recognize, and take care of low blood sugar (hypoglycemia), high blood sugar (hyperglycemia), and problems you have because of your diabetes.
This Medication Guide has been approved by the U.S. Food and Drug Administration.

KOMBIGLYZE XR (saxagliptin and metformin HCl extended-release) tablets
Manufactured by:
Bristol-Myers Squibb Company
Princeton, NJ 08543 USA
Marketed by:
Bristol-Myers Squibb Company
Princeton, NJ 08543
and
AstraZeneca Pharmaceuticals LP
Wilmington, DE 19850
1281913A2
Rev May 2013

Shown in Product Identification Guide, page 306

NULOJIX ℞
[*noo-LOJ-jiks*]
(belatacept)
For injection, for intravenous use

HIGHLIGHTS OF PRESCRIBING INFORMATION
These highlights do not include all the information needed to use NULOJIX safely and effectively. See full prescribing information for NULOJIX.
NULOJIX (belatacept)
For injection, for intravenous use
Initial U.S. Approval: 2011

WARNING: POST-TRANSPLANT LYMPHOPROLIFERATIVE DISORDER, OTHER MALIGNANCIES, AND SERIOUS INFECTIONS
See full prescribing information for complete boxed warning.
- **Increased risk for developing post-transplant lymphoproliferative disorder (PTLD), predominantly involving the central nervous system (CNS). Recipients without immunity to Epstein-Barr virus (EBV) are at a particularly increased risk; therefore, use in EBV seropositive patients only. Do not use NULOJIX in transplant recipients who are EBV seronegative or with unknown serostatus. (4, 5.1)**
- **Only physicians experienced in immunosuppressive therapy and management of kidney transplant patients should prescribe NULOJIX. (5.2)**
- **Increased susceptibility to infection and the possible development of malignancies may result from immunosuppression. (5.1, 5.3, 5.4, 5.5)**
- **Use in liver transplant patients is not recommended due to an increased risk of graft loss and death. (5.6)**

RECENT MAJOR CHANGES
Dosage and Administration, Dosage in Adult Kidney Transplant Recipients (2.1) 04/2013
Warnings and Precautions, Acute Rejection and Graft Loss with Corticosteroid Minimization (5.7) 04/2013

INDICATIONS AND USAGE
- NULOJIX is a selective T-cell costimulation blocker indicated for prophylaxis of organ rejection in adult patients receiving a kidney transplant. (1.1)
- Use in combination with basiliximab induction, mycophenolate mofetil, and corticosteroids. (1.1)

Limitations of Use:
- Use only in patients who are EBV seropositive. (1.2, 4, 5.1)
- Use has not been established for the prophylaxis of organ rejection in transplanted organs other than the kidney. (1.2, 5.6)

DOSAGE AND ADMINISTRATION
- Use of higher than recommended or more frequent dosing is not recommended due to increased risk of serious infections and malignancy. (5.1, 5.4, 6.1)
- For complete dosing instructions, see full prescribing information. (2.1)

Dosing of NULOJIX for Kidney Transplant Recipients (2.1)

Dosing for Initial Phase	**Dose**
Day 1 (day of transplantation, prior to implantation) and Day 5 (approximately 96 hours after Day 1 dose)	10 mg per kg
End of Week 2 and Week 4 after transplantation	10 mg per kg
End of Week 8 and Week 12 after transplantation	10 mg per kg
Dosing for Maintenance Phase	**Dose**
End of Week 16 after transplantation and every 4 weeks (plus or minus 3 days) thereafter	5 mg per kg

- For intravenous infusion only; administer over 30 minutes. (2.1, 2.2)
- Only use the enclosed *silicone-free disposable syringe* to prepare for administration. (2.2)

DOSAGE FORMS AND STRENGTHS
- Lyophilized powder for injection: 250 mg per vial (3)

CONTRAINDICATIONS
- Patients who are EBV seronegative or with unknown EBV serostatus. (4)

WARNINGS AND PRECAUTIONS
- Post-Transplant Lymphoproliferative Disorder (PTLD): increased risk, predominantly involving the CNS; monitor for new or worsening neurological, cognitive, or behavioral signs and symptoms. (Boxed Warning, 4, 5.1, 5.6)
- Other malignancies: increased risk with all immunosuppressants; appears related to intensity and duration of use. Avoid prolonged exposure to UV light and sunlight. (5.3)
- Progressive Multifocal Leukoencephalopathy (PML): increased risk; consider in the diagnosis of patients reporting new or worsening neurological, cognitive, or behavioral signs and symptoms. Recommended doses of immunosuppressants should not be exceeded. (5.4)
- Other serious infections: increased risk of bacterial, viral, fungal, and protozoal infections, including opportunistic infections and tuberculosis. Some infections were fatal. Polyoma virus-associated nephropathy can lead to kidney graft loss; consider reduction in immunosuppression. Evaluate for tuberculosis and initiate treatment for latent infection prior to NULOJIX use. Cytomegalovirus and pneumocystis prophylaxis are recommended after transplantation. (5.1, 5.4, 5.5)
- Liver transplant: use is not recommended. (5.6)
- Acute Rejection and Graft Loss with Corticosteroid Minimization: corticosteroid utilization should be consistent with the NULOJIX clinical trial experience. (2.1, 5.7, 14.1)
- Immunizations: avoid use of live vaccines during treatment. (5.8)

ADVERSE REACTIONS
Most common adverse reactions (≥20% on NULOJIX treatment) are anemia, diarrhea, urinary tract infection, peripheral edema, constipation, hypertension, pyrexia, graft dysfunction, cough, nausea, vomiting, headache, hypokalemia, hyperkalemia, and leukopenia. (6.1)

To report SUSPECTED ADVERSE REACTIONS, contact Bristol-Myers Squibb at 1-800-721-5072 or FDA at 1-800-FDA-1088 or *www.fda.gov/medwatch*

USE IN SPECIFIC POPULATIONS
- Pregnancy: Based on animal data, may cause fetal harm; pregnancy registry available. (8.1)
- Nursing Mothers: Discontinue drug or nursing, taking into consideration importance of drug to mother. (8.3)

See 17 for PATIENT COUNSELING INFORMATION and Medication Guide

Revised: 04/2013

FULL PRESCRIBING INFORMATION: CONTENTS*

*** Sections or subsections omitted from the full prescribing information are not listed**

FULL PRESCRIBING INFORMATION

WARNING: POST-TRANSPLANT LYMPHOPROLIFERATIVE DISORDER, OTHER MALIGNANCIES, AND SERIOUS INFECTIONS
Increased risk for developing post-transplant lymphoproliferative disorder (PTLD), predominantly involving the central nervous system (CNS). Recipients without immunity to Epstein-Barr virus (EBV) are at a particularly increased risk; therefore, use in EBV seropositive patients only. Do not use NULOJIX in transplant recipients who are EBV seronegative or with unknown EBV serostatus [see *Contraindications (4)* and *Warnings and Precautions (5.1)*].

Only physicians experienced in immunosuppressive therapy and management of kidney transplant patients should prescribe NULOJIX. Patients receiving the drug should be managed in facilities equipped and staffed with adequate laboratory and supportive medical resources. The physician responsible for maintenance therapy should have complete information requisite for the follow-up of the patient [see *Warnings and Precautions (5.2)*].

Increased susceptibility to infection and the possible development of malignancies may result from immunosuppression [see *Warnings and Precautions (5.1, 5.3, 5.4, 5.5)*].

Use in liver transplant patients is not recommended due to an increased risk of graft loss and death [see *Warnings and Precautions (5.6)*].

1 INDICATIONS AND USAGE

1.1 Adult Kidney Transplant Recipients

NULOJIX® (belatacept) is indicated for prophylaxis of organ rejection in adult patients receiving a kidney transplant. NULOJIX is to be used in combination with basiliximab induction, mycophenolate mofetil, and corticosteroids.

1.2 Limitations of Use

Use NULOJIX only in patients who are EBV seropositive [see *Contraindications (4)* and *Warnings and Precautions (5.1)*].

Use of NULOJIX for the prophylaxis of organ rejection in transplanted organs other than kidney has not been established [see *Warnings and Precautions (5.6)*].

2 DOSAGE AND ADMINISTRATION

2.1 Dosage in Adult Kidney Transplant Recipients

NULOJIX should be administered in combination with basiliximab induction, mycophenolate mofetil (MMF), and corticosteroids. In clinical trials the median (25th-75th percentile) corticosteroid doses were tapered to approximately 15 mg (10-20 mg) per day by the first 6 weeks and remained at approximately 10 mg (5-10 mg) per day for the first 6 months post-transplant. Corticosteroid utilization should be consistent with the NULOJIX clinical trial experience [see *Warnings and Precautions (5.7)* and *Clinical Studies (14.1)*].

Due to an increased risk of post-transplant lymphoproliferative disorder (PTLD) predominantly involving the central nervous system (CNS), progressive multifocal leukoencephalopathy (PML), and serious CNS infections, administration of higher than the recommended doses or more frequent dosing of NULOJIX is not recommended [see *Warnings and Precautions (5.1, 5.4, 5.5)* and *Adverse Reactions (6.1)*].

NULOJIX is for intravenous infusion only. Patients do not require premedication prior to administration of NULOJIX. Dosing instructions are provided in Table 1.

- The total infusion dose of NULOJIX should be based on the actual body weight of the patient at the time of transplantation, and should not be modified during the course of therapy, unless there is a change in body weight of greater than 10%.
- The prescribed dose of NULOJIX must be evenly divisible by 12.5 mg in order for the dose to be prepared accurately using the reconstituted solution and the *silicone-free disposable syringe* provided. Evenly divisible increments are 0, 12.5, 25, 37.5, 50, 62.5, 75, 87.5, and 100. For example:
  - *A patient weighs 64 kg. The dose is 10 mg per kg.*
  - *Calculated Dose: 64 kg × 10 mg per kg = 640 mg*
  - *The closest doses evenly divisible by 12.5 mg below and above 640 mg are 637.5 mg and 650 mg.*
  - *The nearest dose to 640 mg is 637.5 mg.*
  - *Therefore, the actual prescribed dose for the patient should be 637.5 mg.*

Table 1: Dosing*,† of NULOJIX for Kidney Transplant Recipients

Dosing for Initial Phase	Dose
Day 1 (day of transplantation, prior to implantation) and Day 5 (approximately 96 hours after Day 1 dose)	10 mg per kg
End of Week 2 and Week 4 after transplantation	10 mg per kg
End of Week 8 and Week 12 after transplantation	10 mg per kg
Dosing for Maintenance Phase	**Dose**
End of Week 16 after transplantation and every 4 weeks (plus or minus 3 days) thereafter	5 mg per kg

* [See *Clinical Studies (14.1)*.]

† The dose prescribed for the patient must be evenly divisible by 12.5 mg (see instructions above; e.g., evenly divisible increments are 0, 12.5, 25, 37.5, 50, 62.5, 75, 87.5, and 100).

2.2 Preparation and Administration Instructions

NULOJIX (belatacept) is for intravenous infusion only.

Caution: NULOJIX must be reconstituted/prepared using only the *silicone-free disposable syringe* provided with each vial.

If the *silicone-free disposable syringe* is dropped or becomes contaminated, use a new *silicone-free disposable syringe* from inventory. For information on obtaining additional *silicone-free disposable syringes*, contact Bristol-Myers Squibb at 1-888-NULOJIX.

Preparation for Administration

1. Calculate the number of NULOJIX vials required to provide the total infusion dose. Each vial contains 250 mg of belatacept lyophilized powder.
2. Reconstitute the contents of each vial of NULOJIX with 10.5 mL of a suitable diluent using the *silicone-free disposable syringe* provided with each vial and an 18- to 21-gauge needle. Suitable diluents include: sterile water for injection (SWFI), 0.9% sodium chloride (NS), or 5% dextrose in water (D5W).
   Note: If the NULOJIX powder is accidentally reconstituted using a different syringe than the one provided, the solution may develop a few translucent particles. Discard any solutions prepared using siliconized syringes.
3. To reconstitute the NULOJIX powder, remove the flip-top from the vial and wipe the top with an alcohol swab. Insert the syringe needle into the vial through the center of the rubber stopper and direct the stream of diluent (10.5 mL of SWFI, NS, or D5W) to the glass wall of the vial.
4. To minimize foam formation, rotate the vial and invert with gentle swirling until the contents are completely dissolved. Avoid prolonged or vigorous agitation. Do not shake.
5. The reconstituted solution contains a belatacept concentration of 25 mg/mL and should be clear to slightly opalescent and colorless to pale yellow. Do not use if opaque particles, discoloration, or other foreign particles are present.
6. Calculate the total volume of the reconstituted 25 mg/mL NULOJIX solution required to provide the total infusion dose.
   Volume of 25 mg/mL NULOJIX solution (in mL) = Prescribed Dose (in mg) ÷ 25 mg/mL
7. Prior to intravenous infusion, the required volume of the reconstituted NULOJIX solution must be further diluted with a suitable infusion fluid (NS or D5W). NULOJIX should be reconstituted with:
   - SWFI should be further diluted with either NS or D5W
   - NS should be further diluted with NS
   - D5W should be further diluted with D5W
8. From the appropriate size infusion container, withdraw a volume of infusion fluid that is equal to the volume of the reconstituted NULOJIX solution required to provide the prescribed dose. With the same *silicone-free disposable syringe* used for reconstitution, withdraw the required amount of belatacept solution from the vial, inject it into the infusion container, and gently rotate the infusion container to ensure mixing.
   The final belatacept concentration in the infusion container should range from 2 mg/mL to 10 mg/mL. Typically, an infusion volume of 100 mL will be appropriate for most patients and doses, but total infusion volumes ranging from 50 mL to 250 mL may be used. Any unused solution remaining in the vials must be discarded.
9. Prior to administration, the NULOJIX infusion should be inspected visually for particulate matter and discoloration. Discard the infusion if any particulate matter or discoloration is observed.
10. The entire NULOJIX infusion should be administered over a period of 30 minutes and must be administered with an infusion set and a sterile, non-pyrogenic, low-protein-binding filter (with a pore size of 0.2-1.2 μm).
    - The reconstituted solution should be transferred from the vial to the infusion bag or bottle immediately. The NULOJIX infusion must be completed within 24 hours of reconstitution of the NULOJIX lyophilized powder. If not used immediately, the infusion solution may be stored under refrigeration conditions: 2°-8°C (36°-46°F) and protected from light for up to 24 hours (a maximum of 4 hours of the total 24 hours can be at room temperature: 20°-25°C [68°-77°F] and room light).
    - Infuse NULOJIX in a separate line from other concomitantly infused agents. NULOJIX should not be infused concomitantly in the same intravenous line with other agents. No physical or biochemical compatibility studies have been conducted to evaluate the coadministration of NULOJIX with other agents.

3 DOSAGE FORMS AND STRENGTHS

Lyophilized powder for injection: 250 mg per vial.

4 CONTRAINDICATIONS

NULOJIX (belatacept) is contraindicated in transplant recipients who are Epstein-Barr virus (EBV) seronegative or with unknown EBV serostatus due to the risk of post-transplant lymphoproliferative disorder (PTLD), predominantly involving the central nervous system (CNS) [see *Boxed Warning* and *Warnings and Precautions (5.1)*].

5 WARNINGS AND PRECAUTIONS

5.1 Post-Transplant Lymphoproliferative Disorder

NULOJIX-treated patients have an increased risk for developing post-transplant lymphoproliferative disorder (PTLD), predominantly involving the CNS, compared to patients on a cyclosporine-based regimen [see *Adverse Reactions (6.1)* and *Table 2*]. As the total burden of immunosuppression is a risk factor for PTLD, higher than the recommended doses or more frequent dosing of NULOJIX and higher than recommended doses of concomitant immunosuppressive agents are not recommended [see *Dosage and Administration (2.1)* and *Warnings and Precautions (5.6)*]. Physicians should consider PTLD in patients reporting new or worsening neurological, cognitive, or behavioral signs or symptoms.

EBV Serostatus

The risk of PTLD was higher in EBV seronegative patients compared to EBV seropositive patients. EBV seropositive patients are defined as having evidence of acquired immunity shown by the presence of IgG antibodies to viral capsid antigen (VCA) and EBV nuclear antigen (EBNA).

Epstein-Barr virus serology should be ascertained before starting administration of NULOJIX, and only patients who are EBV seropositive should receive NULOJIX. Transplant recipients who are EBV seronegative, or with unknown serostatus, should not receive NULOJIX [see *Boxed Warning* and *Contraindications (4)*].

Other Risk Factors

Other known risk factors for PTLD include cytomegalovirus (CMV) infection and T-cell-depleting therapy. T-cell-depleting therapies to treat acute rejection should be used cautiously. CMV prophylaxis is recommended for at least 3 months after transplantation [see *Warnings and Precautions (5.5)*].

Patients who are EBV seropositive and CMV seronegative may be at increased risk for PTLD compared to patients who are EBV seropositive and CMV seropositive [see *Adverse Reactions (6.1)*]. Since CMV seronegative patients are at increased risk for CMV disease (a known risk factor for PTLD), the clinical significance of CMV serology for PTLD remains to be determined; however, these findings should be considered when prescribing NULOJIX.

5.2 Management of Immunosuppression

Only physicians experienced in management of systemic immunosuppressant therapy in transplantation should prescribe NULOJIX. Patients receiving the drug should be managed in facilities equipped and staffed with adequate laboratory and supportive medical resources. The physician responsible for the maintenance therapy should have complete information requisite for the follow-up of the patient [see *Boxed Warning*].

5.3 Other Malignancies

Patients receiving immunosuppressants, including NULOJIX, are at increased risk of developing malignancies, in addition to PTLD, including the skin [see *Boxed Warning* and *Warnings and Precautions (5.1)*]. Exposure to sunlight and ultraviolet (UV) light should be limited by wearing protective clothing and using a sunscreen with a high protection factor.

5.4 Progressive Multifocal Leukoencephalopathy

Progressive multifocal leukoencephalopathy (PML) is an often rapidly progressive and fatal opportunistic infection of the CNS that is caused by the JC virus, a human polyoma virus. In clinical trials with NULOJIX, two cases of PML were reported in patients receiving NULOJIX at higher cumulative doses and more frequently than the recommended regimen, along with mycophenolate mofetil (MMF) and corticosteroids; one case occurred in a kidney transplant recipient and the second case occurred in a liver transplant recipient [see *Warnings and Precautions (5.6)*]. As PML has been associated with high levels of overall immunosuppression, the recommended doses and frequency of NULOJIX and concomitant immunosuppressives, including MMF, should not be exceeded.

Physicians should consider PML in the differential diagnosis in patients with new or worsening neurological, cognitive, or behavioral signs or symptoms. PML is usually diagnosed by brain imaging, cerebrospinal fluid (CSF) testing for JC viral DNA by polymerase chain reaction (PCR), and/or brain biopsy. Consultation with a specialist (e.g., neurologist and/or infectious disease) should be considered for any suspected or confirmed cases of PML.

If PML is diagnosed, consideration should be given to reduction or withdrawal of immunosuppression taking into account the risk to the allograft.

5.5 Other Serious Infections

Patients receiving immunosuppressants, including NULOJIX, are at increased risk of developing bacterial, viral (cytomegalovirus [CMV] and herpes), fungal, and protozoal infections, including opportunistic infections. These in-

Table 2: Summary of PTLD Reported in Studies 1, 2, and 3 Through Three Years of Treatment

Trial	NULOJIX Non-Recommended Regimen* (N=477)			NULOJIX Recommended Regimen† (N=472)			Cyclosporine (N=476)		
	EBV Positive (n=406)	EBV Negative (n=43)	EBV Unknown (n=28)	EBV Positive (n=404)	EBV Negative (n=48)	EBV Unknown (n=20)	EBV Positive (n=399)	EBV Negative (n=57)	EBV Unknown (n=20)
Study 1									
CNS PTLD	1	1							
Non-CNS PTLD		1		2				1	
Study 2									
CNS PTLD	1	1		1	1				
Non-CNS PTLD					1				
Study 3									
CNS PTLD		2							
Non-CNS PTLD			1						
Total (%)	**2 (0.5)**	**5 (11.6)**	**1 (3.6)**	**3 (0.7)**	**2 (4.1)**	**0**	**0**	**1 (1.8)**	**0**

* Regimen with higher cumulative dose and more frequent dosing than the recommended NULOJIX regimen.
† In Studies 1 and 2 the NULOJIX regimen is identical to the recommended regimen, but is slightly different in Study 3.

fections may lead to serious, including fatal, outcomes [see *Boxed Warning* and *Adverse Reactions (6.1)*].
Prophylaxis for cytomegalovirus is recommended for at least 3 months after transplantation. Prophylaxis for *Pneumocystis jiroveci* is recommended after transplantation.

Tuberculosis
Tuberculosis was more frequently observed in patients receiving NULOJIX (belatacept) than cyclosporine in clinical trials [see *Adverse Reactions (6.1)*]. Patients should be evaluated for tuberculosis and tested for latent infection prior to initiating NULOJIX. Treatment of latent tuberculosis infection should be initiated prior to NULOJIX use.

Polyoma Virus Nephropathy
In addition to cases of JC virus-associated PML [see *Warnings and Precautions (5.4)*], cases of polyoma virus-associated nephropathy (PVAN), mostly due to BK virus infection, have been reported. PVAN is associated with serious outcomes; including deteriorating renal function and kidney graft loss [see *Adverse Reactions (6.1)*]. Patient monitoring may help detect patients at risk for PVAN. Reductions in immunosuppression should be considered for patients who develop evidence of PVAN. Physicians should also consider the risk that reduced immunosuppression represents to the functioning allograft.

5.6 Liver Transplant
Use of NULOJIX in liver transplant patients is not recommended [see *Boxed Warning*]. In a clinical trial of liver transplant patients, use of NULOJIX regimens with more frequent administration of belatacept than any of those studied in kidney transplant, along with mycophenolate mofetil (MMF) and corticosteroids, was associated with a higher rate of graft loss and death compared to the tacrolimus control arms. In addition, two cases of PTLD involving the liver allograft (one fatal) and one fatal case of PML were observed among the 147 patients randomized to NULOJIX. The two cases of PTLD were reported among the 140 EBV seropositive patients (1.4%). The fatal case of PML was reported in a patient receiving higher than recommended doses of NULOJIX and MMF [see *Warnings and Precautions (5.4)*].

5.7 Acute Rejection and Graft Loss with Corticosteroid Minimization
In postmarketing experience, use of NULOJIX in conjunction with basiliximab induction, MMF, and corticosteroid minimization to 5 mg per day between Day 3 and Week 6 post-transplant was associated with an increased rate and grade of acute rejection, particularly Grade III rejection. These Grade III rejections occurred in patients with 4 to 6 HLA mismatches. Graft loss was a consequence of Grade III rejection in some patients.
Corticosteroid utilization should be consistent with the NULOJIX clinical trial experience [see *Dosage and Administration (2.1)* and *Clinical Studies (14.1)*].

5.8 Immunizations
The use of live vaccines should be avoided during treatment with NULOJIX, including but not limited to the following: intranasal influenza, measles, mumps, rubella, oral polio, BCG, yellow fever, varicella, and TY21a typhoid vaccines.

6 ADVERSE REACTIONS
The most serious adverse reactions reported with NULOJIX (belatacept) are:
- PTLD, predominantly CNS PTLD, and other malignancies [see *Boxed Warning* and *Warnings and Precautions (5.1, 5.3)*]
- Serious infections, including JC virus-associated PML and polyoma virus nephropathy [see *Warnings and Precautions (5.4, 5.5, 5.6)*]

6.1 Clinical Studies Experience
The data described below primarily derive from two randomized, active-controlled three-year trials of NULOJIX in *de novo* kidney transplant patients. In Study 1 and Study 2, NULOJIX was studied at the recommended dose and frequency [see *Dosage and Administration (2.1)*] in a total of 401 patients compared to a cyclosporine control regimen in a total of 405 patients. These two trials also included a total of 403 patients treated with a NULOJIX regimen of higher cumulative dose and more frequent dosing than recommended [see *Clinical Studies (14.1)*]. All patients also received basiliximab induction, mycophenolate mofetil, and corticosteroids. Patients were treated and followed for 3 years.
CNS PTLD, PML, and other CNS infections were more frequently observed in association with a NULOJIX regimen of higher cumulative dose and more frequent dosing compared to the recommended regimen; therefore, administration of higher than the recommended doses and/or more frequent dosing of NULOJIX is not recommended [see *Dosage and Administration (2.1)*].
The average age of patients in Studies 1 and 2 in the NULOJIX recommended dose and cyclosporine control regimens was 49 years, ranging from 18 to 79 years. Approximately 70% of patients were male; 67% were white, 11% were black, and 22% other races. About 25% of patients were from the United States and 75% from other countries.
Because clinical trials are conducted under widely varying conditions, the adverse reaction rates observed cannot be directly compared to rates in other trials and may not reflect the rates observed in clinical practice.
The most commonly reported adverse reactions occurring in ≥20% of patients treated with the recommended dose and frequency of NULOJIX were anemia, diarrhea, urinary tract infection, peripheral edema, constipation, hypertension, pyrexia, graft dysfunction, cough, nausea, vomiting, headache, hypokalemia, hyperkalemia, and leukopenia.
The proportion of patients who discontinued treatment due to adverse reactions was 13% for the recommended NULOJIX regimen and 19% for the cyclosporine control arm through three years of treatment. The most common adverse reactions leading to discontinuation in NULOJIX-treated patients were cytomegalovirus infection (1.5%) and complications of transplanted kidney (1.5%).
Information on selected significant adverse reactions observed during clinical trials is summarized below.

Post-Transplant Lymphoproliferative Disorder
Reported cases of post-transplant lymphoproliferative disorder (PTLD) up to 36 months post transplant were obtained for NULOJIX (belatacept) by pooling both dosage regimens of NULOJIX in Studies 1 and 2 (804 patients) with data from a third study in kidney transplantation (Study 3, 145 patients) which evaluated two NULOJIX dosage regimens similar, but slightly different, from those of Studies 1 and 2 (see Table 2). The total number of NULOJIX patients from these three studies (949) was compared to the pooled cyclosporine control groups from all three studies (476 patients). Among 401 patients in Studies 1 and 2 treated with the recommended regimen of NULOJIX and the 71 patients in Study 3 treated with a very similar (but non-identical) NULOJIX regimen, there were 5 cases of PTLD: 3 in EBV seropositive patients and 2 in EBV seronegative patients. Two of the 5 cases presented with CNS involvement.
Among the 477 patients in Studies 1, 2, and 3 treated with the NULOJIX regimen of higher cumulative dose and more frequent dosing than recommended, there were 8 cases of PTLD: 2 in EBV seropositive patients and 6 in EBV seronegative or serostatus unknown patients. Six of the 8 cases presented with CNS involvement. Therefore, administration of higher than the recommended doses or more frequent dosing of NULOJIX is not recommended. [See *Dosage and Administration (2.1)* and *Warnings and Precautions (5.1)*.]
One of the 476 patients treated with cyclosporine developed PTLD, without CNS involvement.
All cases of PTLD reported up to 36 months post transplant in NULOJIX- or cyclosporine-treated patients presented within 18 months of transplantation.
Overall, the rate of PTLD in 949 patients treated with any of the NULOJIX regimens was 9-fold higher in those who were EBV seronegative or EBV serostatus unknown (8/139) compared to those who were EBV seropositive (5/810 patients). Therefore NULOJIX is recommended for use only in patients who are EBV seropositive [see *Boxed Warning* and *Contraindications (4)*].
[See table 2 above]

EBV Seropositive Subpopulation
Among the 806 EBV seropositive patients with known CMV serostatus treated with either NULOJIX regimen in Studies 1, 2, and 3, two percent (2%; 4/210) of CMV seronegative patients developed PTLD compared to 0.2% (1/596) of CMV seropositive patients. Among the 404 EBV seropositive recipients treated with the recommended dosage regimen of NULOJIX, three PTLD cases were detected among 99 CMV seronegative patients (3%) and there was no case detected among 303 CMV seropositive patients. The clinical significance of CMV serology as a risk factor for PTLD remains to be determined; however, these findings should be considered when prescribing NULOJIX [see *Warnings and Precautions (5.1)*].

Other Malignancies
Malignancies, excluding non-melanoma skin cancer and PTLD, were reported in Study 1 and Study 2 in 3.5% (14/401) of patients treated with the recommended NULOJIX regimen and 3.7% (15/405) of patients treated with the cyclosporine control regimen. Non-melanoma skin cancer was reported in 1.5% (6/401) of patients treated with the recommended NULOJIX regimen and in 3.7% (15/405) of patients treated with cyclosporine [see *Warnings and Precautions (5.3)*].

Progressive Multifocal Leukoencephalopathy
Two fatal cases of progressive multifocal leukoencephalopathy (PML) have been reported among 1096 patients treated with a NULOJIX-containing regimen: one patient in clinical trials of kidney transplant (Studies 1, 2, and 3 described above) and one patient in a trial of liver transplant (trial of 250 patients). No cases of PML were reported in patients treated with the recommended NULOJIX regimen or the control regimen in these trials.
The kidney transplant recipient was treated with the NULOJIX regimen of higher cumulative dose and more frequent dosing than recommended, mycophenolate mofetil (MMF), and corticosteroids for 2 years. The liver transplant recipient was treated with 6 months of a NULOJIX dosage regimen that was more intensive than that studied in kidney transplant recipients, MMF at doses higher than the recommended dose, and corticosteroids [see *Warnings and Precautions (5.4)*].

Bacterial, Mycobacterial, Viral, and Fungal Infections
Adverse reactions of infectious etiology were reported based on clinical assessment by physicians. The causative organisms for these reactions are identified when provided by the physician. The overall number of infections, serious infections, and select infections with identified etiology reported in patients treated with the NULOJIX recommended regimen or the cyclosporine control in Studies 1 and 2 are shown in Table 3. Fungal infections were reported in 18% of patients receiving NULOJIX compared to 22% receiving cyclosporine, primarily due to skin and mucocutaneous fungal infections. Tuberculosis and herpes infections were reported more frequently in patients receiving NULOJIX than cyclosporine. Of the patients who developed tuberculosis through 3 years, all but one NULOJIX patient lived in countries

with a high prevalence of tuberculosis [see *Warnings and Precautions (5.5)*].

[See table 3 above]

Infections Reported in the CNS

Following three years of treatment in Studies 1 and 2, cryptococcal meningitis was reported in one patient out of 401 patients treated with the NULOJIX (belatacept) recommended regimen (0.2%) and one patient out of the 405 treated with the cyclosporine control (0.2%).

Six patients out of the 403 who were treated with the NULOJIX regimen of higher cumulative dose and more frequent dosing than recommended in Studies 1 and 2 (1.5%) were reported to have developed CNS infections, including 2 cases of cryptococcal meningitis, one case of Chagas encephalitis with cryptococcal meningitis, one case of cerebral aspergillosis, one case of West Nile encephalitis, and one case of PML (discussed above).

Infusion Reactions

There were no reports of anaphylaxis or drug hypersensitivity in patients treated with NULOJIX in Studies 1 and 2 through three years.

Infusion-related reactions within one hour of infusion were reported in 5% of patients treated with the recommended dose of NULOJIX, similar to the placebo rate. No serious events were reported through Year 3. The most frequent reactions were hypotension and hypertension.

Proteinuria

At Month 1 after transplantation in Studies 1 and 2, the frequency of 2+ proteinuria on urine dipstick in patients treated with the NULOJIX recommended regimen was 33% (130/390) and 28% (107/384) in patients treated with the cyclosporine control regimen. The frequency of 2+ proteinuria was similar between the two treatment groups between one and three years after transplantation (<10% in both studies). There were no differences in the occurrence of 3+ proteinuria (<4% in both studies) at any time point, and no patients experienced 4+ proteinuria. The clinical significance of this increase in early proteinuria is unknown.

Immunogenicity

Antibodies directed against the belatacept molecule were assessed in 398 patients treated with the NULOJIX recommended regimen in Studies 1 and 2 (212 of these patients were treated for at least 2 years). Of the 372 patients with immunogenicity assessment at baseline (prior to receiving belatacept treatment), 29 patients tested positive for anti-belatacept antibodies; 13 of these patients had antibodies to the modified cytotoxic T-lymphocyte-associated antigen 4 (CTLA-4). Anti-belatacept antibody titers did not increase during treatment in these 29 patients.

Eight (2%) patients developed antibodies during treatment with the NULOJIX recommended regimen. In the patients who developed antibodies during treatment, the median titer (by dilution method) was 8, with a range of 5 to 80. Of 56 patients who tested negative for antibodies during treatment and reassessed approximately 7 half-lives after discontinuation of NULOJIX, 1 tested antibody positive. Anti-belatacept antibody development was not associated with altered clearance of belatacept.

Samples from 6 patients with confirmed binding activity to the modified cytotoxic T-lymphocyte-associated antigen 4 (CTLA-4) region of the belatacept molecule were assessed by an *in vitro* bioassay for the presence of neutralizing antibodies. Three of these 6 patients tested positive for neutralizing antibodies. However, the development of neutralizing antibodies may be underreported due to lack of assay sensitivity.

The clinical impact of anti-belatacept antibodies (including neutralizing anti-belatacept antibodies) could not be determined in the studies.

The data reflect the percentage of patients whose test results were positive for antibodies to belatacept in specific assays. The observed incidence of antibody (including neutralizing antibody) positivity in an assay may be influenced by several factors including assay sensitivity and specificity, assay methodology, sample handling, timing of sample collection, concomitant medications, and underlying disease. For these reasons, comparison of the incidence of antibodies to belatacept with the incidence of antibodies to other products may be misleading.

New-Onset Diabetes After Transplantation

The incidence of new-onset diabetes after transplantation (NODAT) was defined in Studies 1 and 2 as use of an anti-diabetic agent for ≥30 days or ≥2 fasting plasma glucose values ≥126 mg/dL (7.0 mmol/L) post-transplantation. Of the patients treated with the NULOJIX recommended regimen, 5% (14/304) developed NODAT by the end of one year compared to 10% (27/280) of patients on the cyclosporine control regimen. However, by the end of the third year, the cumulative incidence of NODAT was 8% (24/304) in patients treated with the NULOJIX recommended regimen and 10% (29/280) in patients treated with the cyclosporine regimen.

Table 3: Overall Infections and Select Infections with Identified Etiology by Treatment Group following One and Three Years of Treatment in Studies 1 and 2*

	Up to Year 1		Up to Year 3†	
	NULOJIX Recommended Regimen N=401 n (%)	Cyclosporine N=405 n (%)	NULOJIX Recommended Regimen N=401 n (%)	Cyclosporine N=405 n (%)
All infections‡	287 (72)	299 (74)	329 (82)	327 (81)
Serious infections§	98 (24)	113 (28)	144 (36)	157 (39)
CMV	44 (11)	52 (13)	53 (13)	56 (14)
Polyoma virus¶	10 (3)	23 (6)	17 (4)	27 (7)
Herpes#	27 (7)	26 (6)	55 (14)	46 (11)
Tuberculosis	2 (1)	1 (<1)	6 (2)	1 (<1)

* Studies 1 and 2 were not designed to support comparative claims for NULOJIX for the adverse reactions reported in this table.

† Median exposure in days for pooled studies: 1203 for NULOJIX recommended regimen and 1163 for cyclosporine in Studies 1 and 2.

‡ All infections include bacterial, viral, fungal, and other organisms. For infectious adverse reactions, the causative organism is reported if specified by the physician in the clinical trials.

§ A medically important event that may be life-threatening or result in death or hospitalization or prolongation of existing hospitalization. Infections not meeting these criteria are considered non-serious.

¶ BK virus-associated nephropathy was reported in 6 NULOJIX patients (4 of which resulted in graft loss) and 6 cyclosporine patients (none of which resulted in graft loss) by Year 3.

\# Most herpes infections were non-serious and 1 led to treatment discontinuation.

Hypertension

Blood pressure and use of antihypertensive medications were reported in Studies 1 and 2. By Year 3, one or more antihypertensive medications were used in 85% of NULOJIX-treated patients and 92% of cyclosporine-treated patients. At one year after transplantation, systolic blood pressures were 8 mmHg lower and diastolic blood pressures were 3 mmHg lower in patients treated with the NULOJIX (belatacept) recommended regimen compared to the cyclosporine control regimen. At three years after transplantation, systolic blood pressures were 6 mmHg lower and diastolic blood pressures were 3 mmHg lower in NULOJIX-treated patients compared to cyclosporine-treated patients. Hypertension was reported as an adverse reaction in 32% of NULOJIX-treated patients and 37% of cyclosporine-treated patients (see Table 4).

Dyslipidemia

Mean values of total cholesterol, HDL, LDL, and triglycerides were reported in Studies 1 and 2. At one year after transplantation these values were 183 mg/dL, 50 mg/dL, 102 mg/dL, and 151 mg/dL, respectively, in 401 patients treated with the NULOJIX recommended regimen and 196 mg/dL, 48 mg/dL, 108 mg/dL, and 195 mg/dL, respectively, in 405 patients treated with the cyclosporine control regimen. At three years after transplantation, the total cholesterol, HDL, LDL, and triglycerides were 176 mg/dL, 49 mg/dL, 100 mg/dL, and 141 mg/dL, respectively, in NULOJIX-treated patients compared to 193 mg/dL, 48 mg/dL, 106 mg/dL, and 180 mg/dL in cyclosporine-treated patients.

The clinical significance of the lower mean triglyceride values in NULOJIX-treated patients at one and three years is unknown.

Other Adverse Reactions

Adverse reactions that occurred at a frequency of ≥10% in patients treated with the NULOJIX recommended regimen or cyclosporine control regimen in Studies 1 and 2 through three years are summarized by preferred term in decreasing order of frequency within Table 4.

Table 4: Adverse Reactions Reported by ≥10% of Patients Treated with Either the NULOJIX Recommended Regimen or Control in Studies 1 and 2 Through Three Years*,†

Adverse Reaction	NULOJIX Recommended Regimen N=401 %	Cyclosporine N=405 %
Infections and Infestations		
Urinary tract infection	37	36
Upper respiratory infection	15	16
Nasopharyngitis	13	16
Cytomegalovirus infection	12	12
Influenza	11	8
Bronchitis	10	7
Gastrointestinal Disorders		
Diarrhea	39	36
Constipation	33	35
Nausea	24	27
Vomiting	22	20
Abdominal pain	19	16
Abdominal pain upper	9	10
Metabolism and Nutrition Disorders		
Hyperkalemia	20	20
Hypokalemia	21	14
Hypophosphatemia	19	13
Dyslipidemia	19	24
Hyperglycemia	16	17
Hypocalcemia	13	11
Hypercholesterolemia	11	11
Hypomagnesemia	7	10
Hyperuricemia	5	12
Procedural Complications		
Graft dysfunction	25	34
General Disorders		
Peripheral edema	34	42
Pyrexia	28	26
Blood and Lymphatic System Disorders		
Anemia	45	44

Leukopenia	20	23
Renal and Urinary Disorders		
Hematuria	16	18
Proteinuria	16	12
Dysuria	11	11
Renal tubular necrosis	9	13
Vascular Disorders		
Hypertension	32	37
Hypotension	18	12
Respiratory, Thoracic, and Mediastinal Disorders		
Cough	24	18
Dyspnea	12	15
Investigations		
Blood creatinine increased	15	20
Musculoskeletal and Connective Tissue Disorders		
Arthralgia	17	13
Back pain	13	13
Nervous System Disorders		
Headache	21	18
Dizziness	9	10
Tremor	8	17
Skin and Subcutaneous Tissue Disorders		
Acne	8	11
Psychiatric Disorders		
Insomnia	15	18
Anxiety	10	11

* All randomized and transplanted patients in Studies 1 and 2.

† Studies 1 and 2 were not designed to support comparative claims for NULOJIX for the adverse reactions reported in this table.

Selected adverse reactions occurring in <10% from NULOJIX-treated patients in either regimen through three years in Studies 1 and 2 are listed below:

Immune System Disorders: Guillain-Barré syndrome

Infections and Infestations: see Table 3

Gastrointestinal Disorders: stomatitis, including aphthous stomatitis

Injury, Poisoning, and Procedural Complications: chronic allograft nephropathy, complications of transplanted kidney, including wound dehiscence, arteriovenous fistula thrombosis

Blood and Lymphatic System Disorders: neutropenia

Renal and Urinary Disorders: renal impairment, including acute renal failure, renal artery stenosis, urinary incontinence, hydronephrosis

Vascular Disorders: hematoma, lymphocele

Musculoskeletal and Connective Tissue Disorders: musculoskeletal pain

Skin and Subcutaneous Tissue Disorders: alopecia, hyperhidrosis

Cardiac Disorders: atrial fibrillation

7 DRUG INTERACTIONS

7.1 Cytochrome P450 Substrates

No formal drug interaction studies have been conducted with NULOJIX (belatacept). Other biologic therapies that are cytokines or cytokine modulators have been shown to affect the expression and/or functional activities of cytochrome P450 (CYP450) enzymes *in vitro* and/or *in vivo*. *In vitro* studies have shown that NULOJIX (belatacept) inhibits the production of certain cytokines during an alloimmune response. No studies in kidney transplant patients have been conducted to assess if NULOJIX inhibits cytokine production *in vivo*. The potential for NULOJIX to alter the systemic concentrations of drugs that are CYP450 substrates has not been studied; however, in the event that kidney transplant patients receiving NULOJIX exhibit signs and symptoms of altered efficacy or adverse events associated with coadministered drugs which are known to be metabolized by CYP450, the clinician should be aware of potentially altered CYP450 metabolism of these drugs.

7.2 Use with Mycophenolate Mofetil

In a pharmacokinetic substudy of Studies 1 and 2, the plasma concentrations of mycophenolic acid (MPA) were measured in 41 patients who received fixed mycophenolate mofetil (MMF) doses of 500 mg to 1500 mg twice daily with either 5 mg per kg of NULOJIX or cyclosporine. The mean dose-normalized MPA C_{max} and AUC_{0-12} were approximately 20% and 40% higher, respectively, with NULOJIX coadministration than with cyclosporine coadministration. Clinicians should be aware that there is also a potential change of MPA exposure after crossover from cyclosporine to NULOJIX or from NULOJIX to cyclosporine in patients concomitantly receiving MMF.

8 USE IN SPECIFIC POPULATIONS

8.1 Pregnancy

Pregnancy Category C

NULOJIX should not be used in pregnancy unless the potential benefit to the mother outweighs the potential risk to the fetus. There are no studies of NULOJIX treatment in pregnant women. Belatacept is known to cross the placenta of animals. Belatacept was not teratogenic in pregnant rats and rabbits at doses approximately 16 and 19 times greater than the exposure associated with the maximum recommended human dose (MRHD) of 10 mg per kg administered over the first month of treatment, based on area under the concentration-time curve (AUC).

Belatacept administered to female rats daily during gestation and throughout the lactation period was associated with maternal toxicity (infections) in a small percentage of dams at doses of ≥20 mg per kg (≥3 times the MRHD exposure based on AUC) resulting in increased pup mortality (up to 100% pup mortality in some dams). In pups that survived, there were no abnormalities or malformations at doses up to 200 mg per kg (19 times the MRHD exposure).

In vitro data indicate that belatacept has lower binding affinity to CD80/CD86 and lower potency in rodents than in humans. Although the rat toxicity studies with belatacept were done at pharmacologically saturating doses, the *in vivo* difference in potency between rats and humans is unknown. Therefore, the relevance of the rat toxicities to humans and the significance of the magnitude of the relative exposures (rats: humans) are unknown.

Abatacept, a fusion protein that differs from belatacept by 2 amino acids, binds to the same ligands (CD80/CD86) and blocks T-cell costimulation like belatacept, but is more active than belatacept in rodents. Therefore, toxicities identified with abatacept in rodents, including infections and autoimmunity, may be predictive of adverse effects in humans treated with belatacept [see *Nonclinical Toxicology (13.2)*].

Autoimmunity was observed in one rat offspring exposed to abatacept *in utero* and/or during lactation and in juvenile rats after treatment with abatacept. However, the clinical relevance of autoimmunity in rats to patients or a fetus exposed *in utero* is unknown [see *Nonclinical Toxicology (13.2)*].

Pregnancy Registry: To monitor maternal-fetal outcomes of pregnant women who have received NULOJIX or whose partners have received NULOJIX, healthcare providers are strongly encouraged to register pregnant patients in the National Transplant Pregnancy Registry (NTPR) by calling 1-877-955-6877.

8.3 Nursing Mothers

It is not known whether belatacept is excreted in human milk or absorbed systemically after ingestion by a nursing infant. However, belatacept is excreted in rat milk. Because many drugs are excreted in human milk and because of the potential for serious adverse reactions from NULOJIX in nursing infants, a decision should be made whether to discontinue nursing or to discontinue the drug, taking into account the importance of the drug to the mother.

8.4 Pediatric Use

The safety and efficacy of NULOJIX in patients under 18 years of age have not been established. Because T cell development continues into the teenage years, the potential concern for autoimmunity in neonates applies to pediatric use as well [see *Use in Specific Populations (8.1)*].

8.5 Geriatric Use

Of 401 patients treated with the recommended dosage regimen of NULOJIX, 15% were 65 years of age and older, while 3% were 75 and older. No overall differences in safety or effectiveness were observed between these subjects and younger subjects, but greater sensitivity or less efficacy in older individuals cannot be ruled out.

10 OVERDOSAGE

Single doses up to 20 mg per kg of NULOJIX (belatacept) have been administered to healthy subjects without apparent toxic effect. The administration of NULOJIX of higher cumulative dose and more frequent dosing than recommended in kidney transplant patients resulted in a higher frequency of CNS-related adverse reactions [see *Adverse Reactions (6.1)*]. In case of overdosage, it is recommended that the patient be monitored for any signs or symptoms of adverse reactions and appropriate symptomatic treatment instituted.

11 DESCRIPTION

NULOJIX® (belatacept), a selective T-cell costimulation blocker, is a soluble fusion protein consisting of the modified extracellular domain of CTLA-4 fused to a portion (hinge-CH2-CH3 domains) of the Fc domain of a human immunoglobulin G1 antibody. Belatacept is produced by recombinant DNA technology in a mammalian cell expression system. Two amino acid substitutions (L104 to E; A29 to Y) were made in the ligand binding region of CTLA-4. As a result of these modifications, belatacept binds CD80 and CD86 more avidly than abatacept, the parent CTLA4-Immunoglobulin (CTLA4-Ig) molecule from which it is derived. The molecular weight of belatacept is approximately 90 kilodaltons.

NULOJIX is supplied as a sterile, white or off-white lyophilized powder for intravenous administration. Prior to use, the lyophile is reconstituted with a suitable fluid to obtain a clear to slightly opalescent, colorless to pale yellow solution, with a pH in the range of 7.2 to 7.8. Suitable fluids for constitution of the lyophile include SWFI, 0.9% NS, or D5W [see *Dosage and Administration (2.2)*]. Each 250 mg single-use vial of NULOJIX also contains: monobasic sodium phosphate (34.5 mg), sodium chloride (5.8 mg), and sucrose (500 mg).

12 CLINICAL PHARMACOLOGY

12.1 Mechanism of Action

Belatacept, a selective T-cell (lymphocyte) costimulation blocker, binds to CD80 and CD86 on antigen-presenting cells thereby blocking CD28 mediated costimulation of T lymphocytes. *In vitro*, belatacept inhibits T lymphocyte proliferation and the production of the cytokines interleukin-2, interferon-γ, interleukin-4, and TNF-α. Activated T lymphocytes are the predominant mediators of immunologic rejection.

In non-human primate models of renal transplantation, belatacept monotherapy prolonged graft survival and decreased the production of anti-donor antibodies, compared to vehicle.

12.2 Pharmacodynamics

Belatacept-mediated costimulation blockade results in the inhibition of cytokine production by T cells required for antigen-specific antibody production by B cells. In clinical trials, greater reductions in mean immunoglobulin (IgG, IgM, and IgA) concentrations were observed from baseline to Month 6 and Month 12 post-transplant in belatacept-treated patients compared to cyclosporine-treated patients. In an exploratory subset analysis, a trend of decreasing IgG concentrations with increasing belatacept trough concentrations was observed at Month 6. Also in this exploratory subset analysis, belatacept-treated patients with CNS PTLD, CNS infections including PML, other serious infections, and malignancies were observed to have a higher incidence of IgG concentrations below the lower limit of the normal range (<694 mg/dL) at Month 6 than those patients who did not experience these adverse events. This observation was more pronounced with the higher than recommended dose of belatacept. A similar trend was also observed for cyclosporine-treated patients with serious infections and malignancies.

However, it is unclear whether any causal relationship between an IgG concentration below the lower level of normal and these adverse events exists, as the analysis may have been confounded by other factors (e.g., age greater than 60 years, receipt of an extended criteria donor kidney, exposure to lymphocyte depleting agents) which were also associated with IgG below the lower level of normal at Month 6 in these trials.

12.3 Pharmacokinetics

Table 5 summarizes the pharmacokinetic parameters of belatacept in healthy adult subjects after a single 10 mg per kg intravenous infusion; and in kidney transplant patients after the 10 mg per kg intravenous infusion at Week 12, and after 5 mg per kg intravenous infusion every 4 weeks at Month 12 post-transplant or later.

[See table 5 at top of next page]

In healthy subjects, the pharmacokinetics of belatacept was linear and the exposure to belatacept increased proportionally after a single intravenous infusion dose of 1 to 20 mg per kg. The pharmacokinetics of belatacept in *de novo* kidney transplant patients and healthy subjects are comparable. Following the recommended regimen, the mean belatacept serum concentration reached steady-state by Week 8 in the initial phase following transplantation and by Month 6 during the maintenance phase. Following once monthly intravenous infusion of 10 mg per kg and 5 mg per kg, there was about 20% and 10% systemic accumulation of belatacept in kidney transplant patients, respectively.

Based on population pharmacokinetic analysis of 924 kidney transplant patients up to 1 year post-transplant, the pharmacokinetics of belatacept were similar at different time periods post-transplant. In clinical trials, trough concentrations of belatacept were consistently maintained from Month 6 up to 3 years post-transplant. Population pharmacokinetic analyses in kidney transplant patients revealed that there was a trend toward higher clearance of belatacept with increasing body weight. Age, gender, race, renal function (measured by calculated glomerular filtration rate [GFR]), hepatic function (measured by albumin), diabetes, and concomitant dialysis did not affect the clearance of belatacept.

13 NONCLINICAL TOXICOLOGY

13.1 Carcinogenesis, Mutagenesis, Impairment of Fertility

A carcinogenicity study was not conducted with belatacept. However, a murine carcinogenicity study was conducted with abatacept (a more active analog in rodents) to determine the carcinogenic potential of CD28 blockade. Weekly subcutaneous injections of 20, 65, or 200 mg per kg of abatacept were associated with increases in the incidence of malignant lymphomas (all doses) and mammary gland tumors (intermediate- and high-dose in females) at clinically relevant exposures. The mice in this study were infected with endogenous murine leukemia and mouse mammary tumor viruses which are associated with an increased incidence of lymphomas and mammary gland tumors, respectively, in immunosuppressed mice. Although the precise relevance of these findings to the clinical use of NULOJIX (belatacept) is unknown, cases of PTLD (a premalignant or malignant proliferation of B lymphocytes) were reported in clinical trials.

Genotoxicity testing is not required for protein therapeutics; therefore, no genotoxicity studies were conducted with belatacept.

Belatacept had no adverse effects on male or female fertility in rats at doses up to 200 mg per kg daily (25 times the MRHD exposure).

13.2 Animal Toxicology and/or Pharmacology

Abatacept, a fusion protein that differs from belatacept by 2 amino acids, binds to the same ligands (CD80/CD86) and blocks T-cell costimulation like belatacept, but is more active than belatacept in rodents. Therefore, toxicities identified with abatacept in rodents may be predictive of adverse effects in humans treated with belatacept.

Studies in rats exposed to abatacept have shown immune system abnormalities including a low incidence of infections leading to death (observed in juvenile rats and pregnant rats) as well as autoimmunity of the thyroid and pancreas (observed in rats exposed *in utero*, as juveniles or as adults). Studies of abatacept in adult mice and monkeys, as well as belatacept in adult monkeys, have not demonstrated similar findings.

The increased susceptibility to opportunistic infections observed in juvenile rats is likely associated with the exposure to abatacept before the complete development of memory immune responses. In pregnant rats, the increased susceptibility to opportunistic infections may be due to the inherent lapses in immunity that occur in rats during late pregnancy/lactation. Infections related to NULOJIX have been observed in human clinical trials [see *Warnings and Precautions (5.5)*].

Administration of abatacept to rats was associated with a significant decrease in T-regulatory cells (up to 90%). Deficiency of T-regulatory cells in humans has been associated with autoimmunity. The occurrence of autoimmune events across the core clinical trials was infrequent. However, the possibility that patients administered NULOJIX could develop autoimmunity (or that fetuses exposed to NULOJIX *in utero* could develop autoimmunity) cannot be excluded.

In a 6-month toxicity study with belatacept in cynomolgus monkeys administered weekly doses up to 50 mg per kg (6 times the MRHD exposure) and in a 1-year toxicity study with abatacept in adult cynomolgus monkeys administered weekly doses up to 50 mg per kg, no significant drug-related toxicities were observed. Reversible pharmacological effects consisted of minimal transient decreases in serum IgG and minimal to severe lymphoid depletion of germinal centers in the spleen and/or lymph nodes.

Following 5 doses (10 mg per kg or 50 mg per kg, once a week for 5 weeks) of systemic administration, belatacept was not detected in brain tissue of normal healthy cynomolgus monkeys. The number of cells expressing major histocompatibility complex (MHC) class-II antigens (potential marker of immune cell activation) in the brain were increased in monkeys administered belatacept compared to vehicle control. However, distribution of some other cells expressing CD68, CD20, CD80, and CD86, typically expressed on MHC class II-positive cells, was not altered and there were no other histological changes in the brain. The clinical relevance of the findings is unknown.

Table 5: Pharmacokinetic Parameters (Mean±SD [Range]) of Belatacept in Healthy Subjects and Kidney Transplant Patients After 5 and 10 mg per kg Intravenous Infusions Administered Over 30 Minutes

Pharmacokinetic Parameter	Healthy Subjects (After 10 mg per kg Single Dose) N=15	Kidney Transplant Patients (After 10 mg per kg Multiple Doses) N=10	Kidney Transplant Patients (After 5 mg per kg Multiple Doses) N=14
Peak concentration (C_{max}) [μg/mL]	300±77 (190-492)	247±68 (161-340)	139±28 (80-176)
AUC* [μg•h/mL]	26398±5175 (18964-40684)	22252±7868 (13575-42144)	14090±3860 (7906-20510)
Terminal half-life ($t_{1/2}$) [days]	9.8±2.8 (6.4-15.6)	9.8±3.2 (6.1-15.1)	8.2±2.4 (3.1-11.9)
Systemic clearance (CL) [mL/h/kg]	0.39±0.07 (0.25-0.53)	0.49±0.13 (0.23-0.70)	0.51±0.14 (0.33-0.75)
Volume of distribution (Vss) [L/kg]	0.09±0.02 (0.07-0.15)	0.11±0.03 (0.067-0.17)	0.12±0.03 (0.09-0.17)

* AUC=AUC (INF) after single dose and AUC (TAU) after multiple dose, where TAU=4 weeks

14 CLINICAL STUDIES

14.1 Prevention of Organ Rejection in Kidney Transplant Recipients

The efficacy and safety of NULOJIX (belatacept) in *de novo* kidney transplantation were assessed in two open-label, randomized, multicenter, active-controlled trials (Study 1 and Study 2). These trials evaluated two dose regimens of NULOJIX, the recommended dosage regimen [see *Dosage and Administration (2.1)*] and a regimen with higher cumulative doses and more frequent dosing than the recommended dosage regimen, compared to a cyclosporine control regimen. All treatment groups also received basiliximab induction, mycophenolate mofetil (MMF), and corticosteroids.

Treatment Regimen

The NULOJIX recommended regimen consisted of a 10 mg per kg dose administered on Day 1 (the day of transplantation, prior to implantation), Day 5 (approximately 96 hours after the Day 1 dose), end of Weeks 2 and 4; then every 4 weeks through Week 12 after transplantation. Starting at Week 16 after transplantation, NULOJIX was administered at the maintenance dose of 5 mg per kg every 4 weeks (plus or minus 3 days). NULOJIX was administered as an intravenous infusion over 30 minutes [see *Dosage and Administration (2.1)*].

Basiliximab 20 mg was administered intravenously on the day of transplantation and 4 days later.

The initial dose of MMF was 1 gram twice daily and was adjusted, as needed based on clinical signs of adverse events or efficacy failure.

The protocol-specified dosing of corticosteroids in Studies 1 and 2 at Day 1 was methylprednisolone (as sodium succinate) 500 mg IV on arrival in the operating room, Day 2, methylprednisolone 250 mg IV, and Day 3, prednisone 100 mg orally. Actual median corticosteroid doses used with the NULOJIX recommended regimen from Week 1 through Month 6 are summarized in the table below (Table 6).

Table 6: Actual Corticosteroid* Dosing in Studies 1 and 2

Day of Dosing	Median (Q1–Q3) Daily Dose[†,‡]	
	Study 1	Study 2
Week 1	31.7 mg (26.7-50 mg)	30 mg (26.7-50 mg)
Week 2	25 mg (20-30 mg)	25 mg (20-30 mg)
Week 4	20 mg (15-20 mg)	20 mg (15-22.5 mg)
Week 6	15 mg (10-20 mg)	16.7 mg (12.5-20 mg)
Month 6	10 mg (5-10 mg)	10 mg (5-12.5 mg)

* Corticosteroid = prednisone or prednisolone.

† The protocols allowed for flexibility in determining corticosteroid dose and rapidity of taper after Day 15. It is not possible to distinguish corticosteroid doses used to treat acute rejection versus doses used in a maintenance regimen.

‡ Q1 and Q3 are the 25th and 75th percentiles of daily corticosteroid doses, respectively.

Study 1 enrolled recipients of living donor and standard criteria deceased donor organs and Study 2 enrolled recipients of extended criteria donor organs. Standard criteria donor organs were defined as organs from a deceased donor with anticipated cold ischemia time of <24 hours and not meeting the definition of extended criteria donor organs. Extended criteria donors were defined as deceased donors with at least one of the following: (1) donor age ≥60 years; (2) donor age ≥50 years and other donor comorbidities (≥2 of the following: stroke, hypertension, serum creatinine >1.5 mg/dL); (3) donation of organ after cardiac death; or (4) anticipated cold ischemia time of the organ of ≥24 hours. Study 1 excluded recipients undergoing a first transplant whose current Panel Reactive Antibodies (PRA) were ≥50% and recipients undergoing a retransplantation whose current PRA were ≥30%; Study 2 excluded recipients with a current PRA ≥30%. Both studies excluded recipients with HIV, hepatitis C, or evidence of current hepatitis B infection; recipients with active tuberculosis; and recipients in whom intravenous access was difficult to obtain.

Efficacy data are presented for the NULOJIX recommended regimen and cyclosporine regimen in Studies 1 and 2.

The NULOJIX (belatacept) regimen with higher cumulative doses and more frequent dosing of belatacept was associated with more efficacy failures. Higher doses and/or more frequent dosing of NULOJIX are not recommended [see *Dosage and Administration (2.1)*, *Warnings and Precautions (5.1)*, and *Adverse Reactions (6.1)*].

Study 1: Recipients of Living Donor and Standard Criteria Deceased Donor Kidneys

In Study 1, 666 patients were enrolled, randomized, and transplanted: 226 to the NULOJIX recommended regimen, 219 to the NULOJIX regimen with higher cumulative doses and more frequent dosing than recommended, and 221 to cyclosporine control regimen. The median age was 45 years; 58% of organs were from living donors; 3% were retransplanted; 69% of the study population was male; 61% of patients were white, 8% were black/African-American, 31% were categorized as of other races; 16% had PRA ≥10%; 41% had 4 to 6 HLA mismatches; and 27% had diabetes prior to transplant. The incidence of delayed graft function was similar in all treatment arms (14% to 18%).

Premature discontinuation from treatment at the end of the first year occurred in 19% of patients receiving the NULOJIX recommended regimen and 19% of patients on the cyclosporine regimen. Among the patients who received the NULOJIX recommended regimen, 10% discontinued due to lack of efficacy, 5% due to adverse events, and 4% for other reasons. Among the patients who received the cyclosporine regimen, 9% discontinued due to adverse events, 5% due to lack of efficacy, and 5% for other reasons.

At the end of three years, 25% of patients receiving the NULOJIX recommended regimen and 34% of patients receiving the cyclosporine regimen had discontinued from treatment. Among the patients who received the NULOJIX recommended regimen, 12% discontinued due to lack of efficacy, 7% due to adverse events, and 6% for other reasons. Among the patients who received the cyclosporine regimen, 15% discontinued due to adverse events, 8% due to lack of efficacy, and 11% for other reasons.

Assessment of Efficacy

Table 7 summarizes the results of Study 1 following one and three years of treatment with the NULOJIX recommended dosage regimen and the cyclosporine control regimen. Efficacy failure at one year was defined as the occurrence of bi-

Table 7: Efficacy Outcomes by Years 1 and 3 for Study 1: Recipients of Living and Standard Criteria Deceased Donor Kidneys

Parameter	NULOJIX Recommended Regimen N=226 n (%)	Cyclosporine CSA N=221 n (%)	NULOJIX-CSA (97.3% CI)
Efficacy Failure by Year 1	49 (21.7)	37 (16.7)	4.9 (−3.3, 13.2)
Components of Efficacy Failure*			
Biopsy Proven Acute Rejection	45 (19.9)	23 (10.4)	
Graft Loss	5 (2.2)	8 (3.6)	
Death	4 (1.8)	7 (3.2)	
Lost to follow-up	0	1 (0.5)	
Efficacy Failure by Year 3	58 (25.7)	57 (25.8)	−0.1 (−9.3, 9)
Components of Efficacy Failure*			
Biopsy Proven Acute Rejection	50 (22.1)	31 (14)	
Graft Loss	9 (4)	10 (4.5)	
Death	10 (4.4)	15 (6.8)	
Lost to follow-up	2 (0.9)	5 (2.3)	
Patient and graft survival†			
Year 1	218 (96.5)	206 (93.2)	3.2 (−1.5, 8.4)
Year 3	206 (91.2)	192 (86.9)	4.3 (−2.2, 10.8)

* Patients may have experienced more than one event.
† Patients known to be alive with a functioning graft.

Table 8: Measured and Calculated GFR for Study 1: Recipients of Living and Standard Criteria Deceased Donor Kidneys

Parameter	NULOJIX Recommended Regimen N=226	Cyclosporine (CSA) N=221	NULOJIX-CSA (97.3% CI)
Measured GFR* mL/min/1.73 m² mean (SD)			
Year 1	63.4 (27.7) (n=206)	50.4 (18.7) (n=199)	13.0 (7.3, 18.7)
Year 2†	67.9 (29.9) (n=199)	50.5 (20.5) (n=185)	17.4 (11.5, 23.4)
Calculated GFR‡ mL/min/1.73 m² mean (SD)			
Year 1	65.4 (22.9) (n=200)	50.1 (21.1) (n=199)	15.3 (10.3, 20.3)
Year 2	65.4 (25.2) (n=201)	47.9 (23) (n=182)	17.5 (12, 23.1)
Year 3	65.8 (27) (n=190)	44.4 (23.6) (n=171)	21.4 (15.4, 27.4)

* GFR was measured using the cold-iothalamate method.
† Measured GFR was not assessed at Year 3.
‡ GFR was calculated using the MDRD formula.

opsy proven acute rejection (BPAR), graft loss, death, or lost to follow-up. BPAR was defined as histologically confirmed acute rejection by a central pathologist on a biopsy done for any reason, whether or not accompanied by clinical signs of rejection. Patient and graft survival was also assessed separately.

[See table 7 above]

In Study 1, the rate of BPAR at one year and three years was higher in patients treated with the NULOJIX (belatacept) recommended regimen than the cyclosporine regimen. Of the patients who experienced BPAR with NULOJIX, 70% experienced BPAR by Month 3, and 84% experienced BPAR by Month 6. By three years, recurrent BPAR occurred with similar frequency across treatment groups (<3%). The component of BPAR determined by biopsy only (subclinical protocol-defined acute rejection) was 5% in both treatment groups.

Patients treated with the NULOJIX recommended regimen experienced episodes of BPAR classified as Banff grade IIb or higher (6% [14/226] at one year and 7% [15/226] at three years) more frequently compared to patients treated with the cyclosporine regimen (2% [4/221] at one year and 2% [5/221] at three years). Also, T-cell depleting therapy was used more frequently to treat episodes of BPAR in NULOJIX-treated patients (10%; 23/226) compared to cyclosporine-treated patients (2%; 5/221). At Month 12, the difference in mean calculated glomerular filtration rate (GFR) between patients with and without history of BPAR was 19 mL/min/1.73 m² among NULOJIX-treated patients compared to 7 mL/min/1.73 m² among cyclosporine-treated patients. By three years, 22% (11/50) of NULOJIX-treated patients with a history of BPAR experienced graft loss and/or death compared to 10% (3/31) of cyclosporine-treated patients with a history of BPAR; at that time point, 10% (5/50) of NULOJIX-treated patients experienced graft loss and 12% (6/50) of NULOJIX-treated patients had died following an episode of BPAR, whereas 7% (2/31) of cyclosporine-treated patients experienced graft loss and 7% (2/31) of cyclosporine-treated patients had died following an episode of BPAR. The overall prevalence of donor-specific antibodies was 5% and 11% for the NULOJIX (belatacept) recommended regimen and cyclosporine, respectively, up to 36 months post-transplant.

While the difference in GFR in patients with BPAR versus those without BPAR was greater in patients treated with NULOJIX than cyclosporine, the mean GFR following BPAR was similar in NULOJIX (49 mL/min/1.73 m²) and cyclosporine treated patients (43 mL/min/1.73 m²) at one year. The relationship between BPAR, GFR, and patient and graft survival is unclear due to the limited number of patients who experienced BPAR, differences in renal hemodynamics (and, consequently, GFR) across maintenance immunosuppression regimens, and the high rate of switching treatment regimens after BPAR.

Assessment of Efficacy in the EBV Seropositive Subpopulation

NULOJIX is recommended for use only in EBV seropositive patients [see *Indications and Usage (1.2)*].

In Study 1, approximately 87% of patients were EBV seropositive prior to transplant. Efficacy results in the EBV seropositive subpopulation were consistent with those in the total population studied.

By one year, the efficacy failure rate in the EBV seropositive population was 21% (42/202) in patients treated with the NULOJIX recommended regimen and 17% (31/184) in patients treated with cyclosporine (difference=4%, 97.3% CI [−4.8, 12.8]). Patient and graft survival was 98% (198/202) in NULOJIX-treated patients and 92% (170/184) in cyclosporine-treated patients (difference=5.6%, 97.3% CI [0.8, 10.4]).

By three years, efficacy failure was 25% in both treatment groups and patient and graft survival was 94% (187/202) in NULOJIX-treated patients compared with 88% (162/184) in cyclosporine-treated patients (difference=4.6%, 97.3% CI [−2.1, 11.3]).

Assessment of Glomerular Filtration Rate (GFR)

Glomerular Filtration Rate (GFR) was measured at one and two years and was calculated using the Modification of Diet in Renal Disease (MDRD) formula at one, two, and three years after transplantation. As shown in Table 8, both measured and calculated GFR was higher in patients treated with the NULOJIX (belatacept) recommended regimen compared to patients treated with the cyclosporine control regimen at all time points. As shown in Figure 1, the differences in GFR were apparent in the first month after transplant and were maintained up to three years (36 months). An analysis of change of calculated mean GFR between three and 36 months demonstrated an increase of 0.8 mL/min/year (95% CI [−0.2, 1.8]) for NULOJIX-treated patients and a decrease of 2.2 mL/min/year (95% CI [−3.2, −1.2]) for cyclosporine-treated patients.

[See table 8 below]

Figure 1: Calculated (MDRD) GFR through Month 36; Study 1: Recipients of Living and Standard Criteria Deceased Donor Kidneys

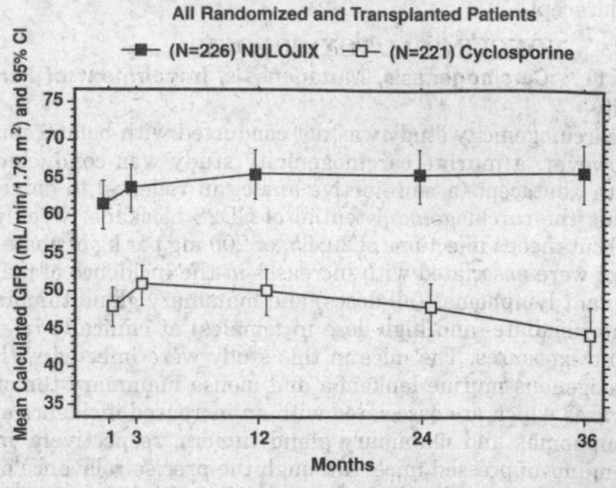

Assessment of Chronic Allograft Nephropathy (CAN)

The prevalence of chronic allograft nephropathy (CAN) at one year, as defined by the Banff '97 classification system, was 24% (54/226) in patients treated with the NULOJIX recommended regimen and in 32% (71/219) of patients treated with the cyclosporine control regimen. CAN was not evaluated after the first year following transplantation. The clinical significance of this finding is unknown.

Study 2: Recipients of Extended Criteria Donor Kidneys

In Study 2, 543 patients were enrolled, randomized, and transplanted: 175 to the NULOJIX recommended regimen, 184 to the NULOJIX regimen with higher cumulative doses and more frequent dosing than recommended, and 184 to the cyclosporine control regimen. The median age was 58 years; 67% of the study population was male; 75% of patients were white, 13% were black/African-American, 12% were categorized as of other races; 3% had PRA ≥10%; 53% had 4 to 6 HLA mismatches; and 29% had diabetes prior to transplantation. The incidence of delayed graft function was similar in all treatment arms (47% to 49%).

Premature discontinuation from treatment at the end of the first year occurred in 25% of patients receiving the NULOJIX recommended regimen and 30% of patients receiving the cyclosporine control regimen. Among the patients who received the NULOJIX recommended regimen, 14% discontinued due to adverse events, 9% due to lack of efficacy, and 2% for other reasons. Among the patients who received the cyclosporine regimen, 17% discontinued due to adverse events, 7% due to lack of efficacy, and 6% for other reasons.

At the end of three years, 35% of patients receiving the NULOJIX recommended regimen and 44% of patients receiving the cyclosporine regimen had discontinued from treatment. Among the patients who received the NULOJIX recommended regimen, 20% discontinued due to adverse events, 9% due to lack of efficacy, and 6% for other reasons. Among the patients who received the cyclosporine regimen, 25% discontinued due to adverse events, 10% due to lack of efficacy, and 10% for other reasons.

Assessment of Efficacy

Table 9 summarizes the results of Study 2 following one and three years of treatment with the NULOJIX recommended dosage regimen and the cyclosporine control regimen. Efficacy failure at one year was defined as the occurrence of biopsy proven acute rejection (BPAR), graft loss, death, or lost to follow-up. BPAR was defined as histologically confirmed acute rejection by a central pathologist on a biopsy done for any reason, whether or not accompanied by clinical signs of rejection. Patient and graft survival was also assessed.

[See table 9 at top of next page]

In Study 2, the rate of BPAR at one year and three years was similar in patients treated with NULOJIX and cyclosporine. Of the patients who experienced BPAR with NULOJIX, 62% experienced BPAR by Month 3, and 76% experienced BPAR by Month 6. By three years, recurrent BPAR occurred with similar frequency across treatment groups (<3%). The component of BPAR determined by biopsy only (subclinical protocol-defined acute rejection) was 5% in both treatment groups.

A similar proportion of patients in the NULOJIX (belatacept) recommended regimen group experienced BPAR classified as Banff grade IIb or higher (5% [9/175] at one year and 6% [10/175] at three years) compared to patients treated with the cyclosporine regimen (4% [7/184] at one year and 5% [9/184] at three years). Also, T-cell depleting therapy was used with similar frequency to treat any episode of BPAR in NULOJIX-treated patients (5% or 9/175) compared to cyclosporine-treated patients (4% or 7/184). At Month 12, the difference in mean calculated GFR between patients with and without a history of BPAR was 10 mL/min/1.73 m^2 among NULOJIX-treated patients compared to 14 mL/min/1.73 m^2 among cyclosporine-treated patients. By three years, 24% (10/42) of NULOJIX-treated patients with a history of BPAR experienced graft loss and/or death compared to 31% (13/42) of cyclosporine-treated patients with a history of BPAR; at that time point, 17% (7/42) of NULOJIX-treated patients experienced graft loss and 14% (6/42) of NULOJIX-treated patients had died following an episode of BPAR, whereas 19% (8/42) of cyclosporine-treated patients experienced graft loss and 19% (8/42) of cyclosporine-treated patients had died following an episode of BPAR. The overall prevalence of donor-specific antibodies was 6% and 15% for the NULOJIX recommended regimen and cyclosporine, respectively, up to 36 months post-transplant.

The mean GFR following BPAR was 36 mL/min/1.73 m^2 in NULOJIX patients and 24 mL/min/1.73 m^2 in cyclosporine-treated patients at one year. The relationship between BPAR, GFR, and patient and graft survival is unclear due to the limited number of patients who experienced BPAR, differences in renal hemodynamics (and, consequently, GFR) across maintenance immunosuppression regimens, and the high rate of switching treatment regimens after BPAR.

Assessment of Efficacy in the EBV Seropositive Subpopulation

NULOJIX is recommended for use only in EBV seropositive patients [see *Indications and Usage (1.2)*].

In Study 2, approximately 91% of the patients were EBV seropositive prior to transplant. Efficacy results in the EBV seropositive subpopulation were consistent with those in the total population studied.

By one year, the efficacy failure rate in the EBV seropositive population was 29% (45/156) in patients treated with the NULOJIX recommended regimen and 28% (47/168) in patients treated with cyclosporine (difference=0.8%, 97.3% CI [–10.3, 11.9]). Patient and graft survival rate in the EBV seropositive population was 89% (139/156) in the NULOJIX-treated patients and 86% (144/168) in cyclosporine-treated patients (difference=3.4%, 97.3% CI [–4.7, 11.5]).

By three years, efficacy failure was 35% (54/156) in NULOJIX-treated patients and 36% (61/168) in cyclosporine-treated patients. Patient and graft survival was 83% (130/156) in NULOJIX-treated patients compared with 77% (130/168) in cyclosporine-treated patients (difference=5.9%, 97.3% CI [–3.8, 15.6]).

Assessment of Glomerular Filtration Rate (GFR)

Glomerular Filtration Rate (GFR) was measured at one and two years and was calculated using the Modification of Diet in Renal Disease (MDRD) formula at one, two, and three years after transplantation. As shown in Table 10, both measured and calculated GFR was higher in patients treated with the NULOJIX recommended regimen compared to patients treated with the cyclosporine control regimen at all time points. As shown in Figure 2, the differences in GFR were apparent in the first month after transplant and were maintained up to three years (36 months). An analysis of change of calculated mean GFR between Month 3 and Month 36 demonstrated a decrease of 0.8 mL/min/year (95% CI [–1.9, 0.3]) for NULOJIX-treated patients and a decrease of 2.0 mL/min/year (95% CI [–3.1, –0.8]) for cyclosporine-treated patients.

[See table 10 above]

[See figure 2 at top of next column]

Assessment of Chronic Allograft Nephropathy (CAN)

The prevalence of chronic allograft nephropathy (CAN) at one year, as defined by the Banff '97 classification system, was 46% (80/174) in patients treated with the NULOJIX recommended regimen and 52% (95/184) of patients treated with the cyclosporine control regimen. CAN was not evaluated after the first year following transplantation. The clinical significance of this finding is unknown.

16 HOW SUPPLIED/STORAGE AND HANDLING

NULOJIX® (belatacept) lyophilized powder for intravenous infusion is supplied as a single-use vial with a *silicone-free disposable syringe* in the following packaging configuration:

Description		NDC Number
One 250-mg vial	One 12 mL Syringe	0003-0371-13

16.1 Storage

NULOJIX (belatacept) lyophilized powder is stored refrigerated at 2°-8°C (36°-46°F). Protect NULOJIX from light by storing in the original package until time of use.

The reconstituted solution should be transferred from the vial to the infusion bag or bottle immediately. The NULOJIX infusion must be completed within 24 hours of constitution of the NULOJIX lyophilized powder. If not used immediately, the infusion solution may be stored under refrigeration conditions: 2°-8°C (36°-46°F) for up to 24 hours (a maximum of 4 hours of the total 24 hours can be at room temperature: 20°-25°C [68°-77°F] and room light) [see *Dosage and Administration (2.2)*].

Table 9: Efficacy Outcomes by Years 1 and 3 for Study 2: Recipients of Extended Criteria Donor Kidneys

Parameter	NULOJIX Recommended Regimen N=175 n (%)	Cyclosporine (CSA) N=184 n (%)	NULOJIX-CSA (97.3% CI)
Efficacy Failure by Year 1	51 (29.1)	52 (28.3)	0.9 (–9.7, 11.5)
Components of Efficacy Failure*			
Biopsy Proven Acute Rejection	37 (21.1)	34 (18.5)	
Graft Loss	16 (9.1)	20 (10.9)	
Death	5 (2.9)	8 (4.3)	
Lost to follow-up	0	2 (1.1)	
Efficacy Failure by Year 3	63 (36)	68 (37)	–1.0 (–12.1, 10.3)
Components of Efficacy Failure*			
Biopsy Proven Acute Rejection	42 (24)	42 (22.8)	
Graft Loss	21 (12)	23 (12.5)	
Death	15 (8.6)	17 (9.2)	
Lost to follow-up	1 (0.6)	5 (2.7)	
Patient and graft survival†			
Year 1	155 (88.6)	157 (85.3)	3.2 (–4.8, 11.3)
Year 3	143 (81.7)	143 (77.7)	4.0 (–5.4, 13.4)

* Patients may have experienced more than one event.
† Patients known to be alive with a functioning graft.

Table 10: Measured and Calculated GFR for Study 2: Recipients of Extended Criteria Donor Kidneys

Parameter	NULOJIX Recommended Regimen N=175	Cyclosporine (CSA) N=184	NULOJIX-CSA (97.3% CI)
Measured GFR* mL/min/1.73 m^2 mean (SD)			
Year 1	49.6 (25.8) (n=151)	45.2 (21.1) (n=154)	4.3 (–1.5, 10.2)
Year 2†	49.7 (23.7) (n=139)	45.0 (27.2) (n=136)	4.7 (–1.8, 11.3)
Calculated GFR‡ mL/min/1.73 m^2 mean (SD)			
Year 1	44.5 (21.8) (n=158)	36.5 (21.1) (n=159)	8.0 (2.5, 13.4)
Year 2	42.8 (24.1) (n=158)	34.9 (21.6) (n=154)	8.0 (1.9, 14)
Year 3	42.2 (25.2) (n=154)	31.5 (22.1) (n=143)	10.7 (4.3, 17.2)

* GFR was measured using the cold-iothalamate method.
† Measured GFR was not assessed at Year 3.
‡ GFR was calculated using the MDRD formula.

Figure 2: Calculated (MDRD) GFR through Month 36; Study 2: Recipients of Extended Criteria Donor Kidneys

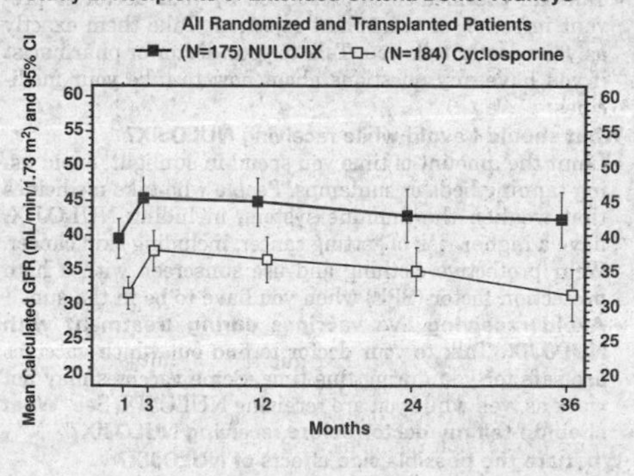

17 PATIENT COUNSELING INFORMATION

See FDA-approved patient labeling (Medication Guide).

17.1 Post-Transplant Lymphoproliferative Disorder

The overall risk of PTLD, especially CNS PTLD, was elevated in NULOJIX-treated patients. Instruct patients to immediately report any of the following neurological, cognitive, or behavioral signs and symptoms during and after therapy with NULOJIX (belatacept) [see *Boxed Warning* and *Warnings and Precautions (5.1)*]:

- changes in mood or usual behavior
- confusion, problems thinking, loss of memory
- changes in walking or talking
- decreased strength or weakness on one side of the body
- changes in vision

17.2 Other Malignancies

Inform patients about the increased risk of malignancies, in addition to PTLD, while taking immunosuppressive therapy, especially skin cancer. Instruct patients to limit exposure to sunlight and UV light by wearing protective clothing and using a sunscreen with a high protection factor. Instruct patients to look for any signs and symptoms of skin cancer, such as suspicious moles or lesions [see *Warnings and Precautions (5.3)*].

17.3 Progressive Multifocal Leukoencephalopathy

Cases of PML have been reported in NULOJIX-treated patients. Instruct patients to immediately report any of the following neurological, cognitive, or behavioral signs and symptoms during and after therapy with NULOJIX [see *Warnings and Precautions (5.4)*]:

- changes in mood or usual behavior
- confusion, problems thinking, loss of memory
- changes in walking or talking
- decreased strength or weakness on one side of the body
- changes in vision

17.4 Other Serious Infections

Inform patients about the increased risk of infection while taking immunosuppressive therapy. Instruct patients to adhere to antimicrobial prophylaxis regimens as prescribed. Tell patients to immediately report any signs and symptoms of infection during therapy with NULOJIX [see *Warnings and Precautions (5.5)*].

17.5 Immunizations

Inform patients that vaccinations may be less effective while they are being treated with NULOJIX (belatacept). Advise patients that live vaccines should be avoided [see *Warnings and Precautions (5.8)*].

17.6 Pregnant Women and Nursing Mothers

Inform patients that NULOJIX has not been studied in pregnant women or nursing mothers so the effects of NULOJIX on pregnant women or nursing infants are not known. Instruct patients to tell their healthcare provider if they are pregnant, become pregnant, or are thinking about becoming pregnant [see *Use in Specific Populations (8.1)*]. Instruct patients to tell their healthcare provider if they plan to breast-feed their infant [see *Use in Specific Populations (8.3)*].

Bristol-Myers Squibb Company
Princeton, New Jersey 08543
1274492A0
Rev April 2013

MEDICATION GUIDE
NULOJIX® (noo-LOJ-jiks)
(belatacept)
For Injection, For Intravenous Use

Read this Medication Guide before you start receiving NULOJIX and before each treatment. There may be new information. This Medication Guide does not take the place of talking with your doctor about your medical condition or your treatment.

What is the most important information I should know about NULOJIX?

NULOJIX increases your risk of serious side effects, including:

- **Post-transplant lymphoproliferative disorder (PTLD).** PTLD is a condition that can happen if certain white blood cells grow out of control after an organ transplant because your immune system is weak. PTLD can get worse and become a type of cancer. PTLD can lead to death.
  People treated with NULOJIX have a higher risk of getting PTLD. If you get PTLD with NULOJIX you are at especially high risk of getting it in your brain. Your risk for PTLD is also higher if you:
  - have never been exposed to the Epstein-Barr virus (EBV). Your doctor should test you for EBV. Do not receive NULOJIX unless you are EBV positive (you have been exposed to EBV).
  - get an infection with a virus called cytomegalovirus (CMV).
  - receive treatment for transplant rejection that lowers certain white blood cells called T lymphocytes.
- **Increased risk of getting cancers other than PTLD.** People who take medicines that weaken the immune system, including NULOJIX, have a higher risk of getting other cancers, including skin cancer. Talk to your doctor about your risk for cancer. See **"What should I avoid while receiving NULOJIX?"**
- **Progressive multifocal leukoencephalopathy (PML).** PML is a rare, serious brain infection caused by JC virus. People with weakened immune systems are at risk for getting PML. PML can result in death or severe disability. There is no known prevention, treatment, or cure for PML.
- **Increased risk of getting other serious infections, including tuberculosis (TB) and other infections caused by bacteria, viruses, or fungi.** These serious infections may lead to death. Also, a virus called BK virus can affect how your kidney works and cause your transplanted kidney to fail.

Tell your doctor right away if you get any of the following symptoms during treatment with NULOJIX:

- change in mood or your usual behavior
- confusion or problems thinking or with memory
- change in the way you walk or talk
- decreased strength or weakness on one side of your body
- change in vision
- fever, night sweats, or tiredness that does not go away
- weight loss
- swollen glands
- flu, cold symptoms, or cough
- stomach-area pain
- vomiting or diarrhea
- tenderness over your transplanted kidney
- change in the amount of urine that you make, blood in your urine, pain or burning on urination
- a new skin lesion or bump, or change in size or color of a mole

See **"What are the possible side effects of NULOJIX?"** for more information about side effects.

Liver transplant patients should not receive NULOJIX because of an increased risk of losing the transplanted liver (graft loss) and death. Talk to your doctor if you would like more information about this risk.

What is NULOJIX?

NULOJIX is a prescription medicine used in adults to prevent transplant rejection in people who have received a kidney transplant. Transplant rejection happens when the body's immune system senses that the new transplanted kidney is different or foreign, and attacks it. NULOJIX is used with corticosteroids and certain other medicines to help prevent rejection of your new kidney.

It is not known if NULOJIX (belatacept) is safe and effective in children under 18 years of age.

NULOJIX is only used in people who have been exposed to the EBV virus.

It is not known if NULOJIX is safe and effective in people who receive an organ transplant other than a kidney transplant.

Who should not receive NULOJIX?

Do not receive treatment with NULOJIX if you are EBV negative. Your doctor will do a test to see if you were exposed to EBV in the past.

What should I tell my doctor before receiving NULOJIX?

Before receiving NULOJIX, tell your doctor if you:

- plan to receive any vaccines. Talk to your doctor about which vaccines are safe for you to receive during your treatment with NULOJIX. See **"What should I avoid while receiving NULOJIX?"**
- have any other medical conditions
- are pregnant or plan to become pregnant. It is not known if NULOJIX will harm your unborn baby. If you become pregnant while taking NULOJIX:
  - **Tell your doctor right away.** You and your doctor should decide if you will keep receiving NULOJIX while you are pregnant.
  - Talk with your doctor about enrolling in the National Transplant Pregnancy Registry (NTPR). This Registry collects information about pregnancies in women who have received NULOJIX or if their partner has received NULOJIX, and had a transplant. You can also enroll by calling 1-877-955-6877.
- are breast-feeding or plan to breast-feed. It is not known if NULOJIX passes into your breast milk. You and your doctor should decide if you will receive NULOJIX or breastfeed. You should not do both.

Tell your doctor about all of the medicines you take, including prescription and non-prescription medicines, vitamins, and herbal supplements.

Know the medicines you take. Keep a list of them to show your doctor and pharmacist when you get a new medicine. Do not take any new medicine without talking with your transplant doctor first.

How will I receive NULOJIX?

- To help prevent rejection of your new kidney, you will receive NULOJIX regularly as prescribed by your doctor. It is important for you to keep all your appointments for NULOJIX treatment and follow up.
- You will receive NULOJIX as an intravenous (IV) infusion in your arm. Each IV infusion takes about 30 minutes.
- During treatment with NULOJIX, your doctor will test your blood and urine to check how your kidney is working.
- Take all the medicines prescribed by your doctor to prevent infection or transplant rejection. Take them exactly as your doctor tells you. Talk to your doctor or pharmacist if you have any questions about how to take your medicines.

What should I avoid while receiving NULOJIX?

- Limit the amount of time you spend in sunlight. Avoid using tanning beds or sunlamps. People who take medicines that weaken the immune system, including NULOJIX, have a higher risk of getting cancer, including skin cancer. Wear protective clothing and use sunscreen with a high protection factor (SPF) when you have to be in the sun.
- **Avoid receiving live vaccines during treatment with NULOJIX.** Talk to your doctor to find out which vaccines are safe for you during this time. Some vaccines may not work as well while you are receiving NULOJIX. See **"What should I tell my doctor before receiving NULOJIX?"**

What are the possible side effects of NULOJIX?

NULOJIX increases your risk of serious side effects that can cause death. See **"What is the most important information I should know about NULOJIX?"**

Common side effects of NULOJIX include:

- low red blood count (anemia)
- diarrhea
- kidney or bladder infection
- swollen legs, feet, or ankles
- constipation
- high blood pressure
- fever
- new kidney not working well
- cough
- nausea or vomiting
- headache
- low potassium or high potassium in your blood
- low white blood cell count

Tell your doctor about any side effect that bothers you or that does not go away. These are not all the possible side effects of NULOJIX. For more information, ask your doctor or pharmacist.

Call your doctor for medical advice about side effects. You may report side effects to FDA at 1-800-FDA-1088.

You may also report side effects to BMS at 1-800-321-1335.

General information about NULOJIX

Medicines are sometimes prescribed for purposes other than those listed in a Medication Guide. This Medication Guide summarizes the most important information about NULOJIX (belatacept). If you would like more information about NULOJIX, talk with your doctor. You can ask your pharmacist or doctor for information about NULOJIX that is written for healthcare professionals.

For more information, go to www.NULOJIX.com or call 1-800-321-1335.

What are the ingredients in NULOJIX?

Active ingredient: belatacept

Inactive ingredients: monobasic sodium phosphate, sodium chloride, and sucrose

This Medication Guide has been approved by the U.S. Food and Drug Administration.

Bristol-Myers Squibb Company
Princeton, New Jersey 08543
1274492A0
Rev April 2013

Shown in Product Identification Guide, page 306

ONGLYZA ℞
[*on-GLY-zah*]
(saxagliptin)
tablets, for oral use

HIGHLIGHTS OF PRESCRIBING INFORMATION

These highlights do not include all the information needed to use ONGLYZA safely and effectively. See full prescribing information for ONGLYZA.

ONGLYZA (saxagliptin) tablets, for oral use
Initial U.S. Approval: 2009

INDICATIONS AND USAGE

ONGLYZA is a dipeptidyl peptidase-4 (DPP4) inhibitor indicated as an adjunct to diet and exercise to improve glycemic control in adults with type 2 diabetes mellitus in multiple clinical settings. (1.1, 14)

Limitations of Use:

- Should not be used for the treatment of type 1 diabetes mellitus or diabetic ketoacidosis. (1.2)
- Has not been studied in patients with a history of pancreatitis. (1.2, 5.1)

DOSAGE AND ADMINISTRATION

- Recommended dosage is 2.5 mg or 5 mg once daily taken regardless of meals. (2.1)
- Patients with moderate or severe renal impairment, or end-stage renal disease (CrCl ≤ 50 mL/min): Recommended dosage is 2.5 mg once daily regardless of meals. (2.2)
- Assess renal function before starting ONGLYZA and periodically thereafter. (2.2)
- 2.5 mg daily is recommended for patients also taking strong cytochrome P450 3A4/5 (CYP3A4/5) inhibitors (e.g., ketoconazole). (2.3, 7.1)

DOSAGE FORMS AND STRENGTHS

- Tablets: 5 mg and 2.5 mg (3)

CONTRAINDICATIONS

- History of a serious hypersensitivity reaction (e.g., anaphylaxis, angioedema, exfoliative skin conditions) to ONGLYZA. (4)

WARNINGS AND PRECAUTIONS

- *Acute Pancreatitis (postmarketing reports):* If pancreatitis is suspected, promptly discontinue ONGLYZA. (5.1)
- *Hypoglycemia:* In add-on to sulfonylurea, add-on to insulin, and add-on to metformin plus sulfonylurea trials, confirmed hypoglycemia was more common in patients treated with ONGLYZA compared to placebo. When used with an insulin secretagogue (e.g., sulfonylurea) or insulin, a lower dose of the insulin secretagogue or insulin may be required to minimize the risk of hypoglycemia. (5.2, 6.1)
- *Hypersensitivity-Related Events (e.g., urticaria, facial edema):* More common in patients treated with ONGLYZA than in patients treated with placebo; and postmarketing reports of serioius hypersensitivity reactions such as anaphylaxis, angioedema, and exfoliative skin conditions. Promptly discontinue ONGLYZA, assess for other potential causes, institute appropriate monitoring and treatment, and initiate alternative treatment for diabetes. (5.3,6.1, 6.2)
- There have been no clinical studies establishing conclusive evidence of macrovascular risk reduction with ONGLYZA or any other antidiabetic drug. (5.4)

ADVERSE REACTIONS

- Adverse reactions reported in ≥5% of patients treated with ONGLYZA and more commonly than in patients treated with placebo are upper respiratory tract infection, urinary tract infection, and headache. (6.1)
- Peripheral edema was reported more commonly in patients treated with the combination of ONGLYZA and a thiazolidinedione (TZD) than in patients treated with the combination of placebo and TZD. (6.1)

To report SUSPECTED ADVERSE REACTIONS, contact Bristol-Myers Squibb at 1-800-721-5072 or FDA at 1-800-FDA-1088 or *www.fda.gov/medwatch*

DRUG INTERACTIONS

- *Strong CYP3A4/5 inhibitors (e.g., ketoconazole):* Coadministration with ONGLYZA significantly increases saxagliptin concentrations. Recommend limiting ONGLYZA dosage to 2.5 mg once daily. (2.3, 7.1)

USE IN SPECIFIC POPULATIONS

- No adequate and well-controlled studies in pregnant women. (8.1)

See 17 for PATIENT COUNSELING INFORMATION and Medication Guide

Revised: 05/2013

FULL PRESCRIBING INFORMATION: CONTENTS*

*** Sections or subsections omitted from the full prescribing information are not listed**

FULL PRESCRIBING INFORMATION

1 INDICATIONS AND USAGE

1.1 Monotherapy and Combination Therapy

ONGLYZA (saxagliptin) is indicated as an adjunct to diet and exercise to improve glycemic control in adults with type 2 diabetes mellitus in multiple clinical settings. [See *Clinical Studies (14)*.]

1.2 Limitations of Use

ONGLYZA should not be used for the treatment of type 1 diabetes mellitus or diabetic ketoacidosis, as it would not be effective in these settings.

ONGLYZA has not been studied in patients with a history of pancreatitis. It is unknown whether patients with a history of pancreatitis are at an increased risk for the development of pancreatitis while using ONGLYZA. [See *Warnings and Precautions (5.1)*.]

2 DOSAGE AND ADMINISTRATION

2.1 Recommended Dosage

The recommended dosage of ONGLYZA is 2.5 mg or 5 mg once daily taken regardless of meals.

ONGLYZA tablets must not be split or cut.

2.2 Dosage in Patients with Renal Impairment

No dosage adjustment for ONGLYZA is recommended for patients with mild renal impairment (creatinine clearance [CrCl] >50 mL/min).

The dosage of ONGLYZA (saxagliptin) is 2.5 mg once daily (regardless of meals) for patients with moderate or severe renal impairment, or with end-stage renal disease (ESRD) requiring hemodialysis (creatinine clearance [CrCl] ≤50 mL/min) [see *Clinical Pharmacology (12.3)* and *Clinical Studies (14.3)*]. ONGLYZA should be administered following hemodialysis. ONGLYZA has not been studied in patients undergoing peritoneal dialysis.

Because the dosage of ONGLYZA should be limited to 2.5 mg based upon renal function, assessment of renal function is recommended prior to initiation of ONGLYZA and periodically thereafter. Renal function can be estimated from serum creatinine using the Cockcroft-Gault formula or Modification of Diet in Renal Disease formula. [See *Clinical Pharmacology (12.3)*.]

2.3 Dosage Adjustment with Concomitant Use of Strong CYP3A4/5 Inhibitors

The dosage of ONGLYZA is 2.5 mg once daily when coadministered with strong cytochrome P450 3A4/5 (CYP3A4/5) inhibitors (e.g., ketoconazole, atazanavir, clarithromycin, indinavir, itraconazole, nefazodone, nelfinavir, ritonavir, saquinavir, and telithromycin). [See *Drug Interactions (7.1)* and *Clinical Pharmacology (12.3)*.]

2.4 Concomitant Use with an Insulin Secretagogue (e.g., Sulfonylurea) or with Insulin

When ONGLYZA is used in combination with an insulin secretagogue (e.g., sulfonylurea) or with insulin, a lower dose of the insulin secretagogue or insulin may be required to minimize the risk of hypoglycemia. [See *Warnings and Precautions (5.2)*.]

3 DOSAGE FORMS AND STRENGTHS

- ONGLYZA (saxagliptin) 5 mg tablets are pink, biconvex, round, film-coated tablets with "5" printed on one side and "4215" printed on the reverse side, in blue ink.
- ONGLYZA (saxagliptin) 2.5 mg tablets are pale yellow to light yellow, biconvex, round, film-coated tablets with "2.5" printed on one side and "4214" printed on the reverse side, in blue ink.

4 CONTRAINDICATIONS

ONGLYZA is contraindicated in patients with a history of a serious hypersensitivity reaction to ONGLYZA, such as anaphylaxis, angioedema, or exfoliative skin conditions. [See *Warnings and Precautions (5.3) and Adverse Reactions (6.2)*.]

5 WARNINGS AND PRECAUTIONS

5.1 Pancreatitis

There have been postmarketing reports of acute pancreatitis in patients taking ONGLYZA. After initiation of ONGLYZA, patients should be observed carefully for signs and symptoms of pancreatitis. If pancreatitis is suspected, ONGLYZA should promptly be discontinued and appropriate management should be initiated. It is unknown whether patients with a history of pancreatitis are at increased risk for the development of pancreatitis while using ONGLYZA.

5.2 Hypoglycemia with Cocomitant Use of Sulfonylurea or Insulin

When ONGLYZA was used in combination with a sulfonylurea or with insulin, medications known to cause hypoglycemia, the incidence of confirmed hypoglycemia was increased over that of placebo used in combination with a sulfonylurea or with insulin. [See *Adverse Reactions (6.1)*.] Therefore, a lower dose of the insulin secretagogue or insulin may be required to minimize the risk of hypoglycemia when used in combination with ONGLYZA. [See *Dosage and Administration (2.4)*.]

5.3 Hypersensitivity Reactions

There have been postmarketing reports of serious hypersensitivity reactions in patients treated with ONGLYZA. These reactions include anaphylaxis, angioedema, and exfoliative skin conditions. Onset of these reactions occurred within the first 3 months after initiation of treatment with ONGLYZA, with some reports occurring after the first dose. If a serious hypersensitivity reaction is suspected, discontinue ONGLYZA, assess for other potential causes for the event, and institute alternative treatment for diabetes. [See *Adverse Reactions (6.2)*.]

Use caution in a patient with a history of angioedema to another dipeptidyl peptidase-4 (DPP4) inhibitor because it is unknown whether such patients will be predisposed to angioedema with ONGLYZA.

5.4 Macrovascular Outcomes

There have been no clinical studies establishing conclusive evidence of macrovascular risk reduction with ONGLYZA or any other antidiabetic drug.

6 ADVERSE REACTIONS

6.1 Clinical Trials Experience

Because clinical trials are conducted under widely varying conditions, adverse reaction rates observed in the clinical trials of a drug cannot be directly compared to rates in the clinical trials of another drug and may not reflect the rates observed in practice.

Adverse Reactions with Monotherapy and with Add-On Combination Therapy

In two placebo-controlled monotherapy trials of 24-weeks duration, patients were treated with ONGLYZA 2.5 mg daily, ONGLYZA (saxagliptin) 5 mg daily, and placebo. Three 24-week, placebo-controlled, add-on combination therapy trials were also conducted: one with metformin, one with a thiazolidinedione (pioglitazone or rosiglitazone), and one with glyburide. In these three trials, patients were randomized to add-on therapy with ONGLYZA 2.5 mg daily, ONGLYZA 5 mg daily, or placebo. A saxagliptin 10 mg treatment arm was included in one of the monotherapy trials and in the add-on combination trial with metformin. The 10 mg dosage is not an approved dosage.

In a prespecified pooled analysis of the 24-week data (regardless of glycemic rescue) from the two monotherapy trials, the add-on to metformin trial, the add-on to thiazolidinedione (TZD) trial, and the add-on to glyburide trial, the overall incidence of adverse events in patients treated with ONGLYZA 2.5 mg and ONGLYZA 5 mg was similar to placebo (72% and 72.2% versus 70.6%, respectively). Discontinuation of therapy due to adverse events occurred in 2.2%, 3.3%, and 1.8% of patients receiving ONGLYZA 2.5 mg, ONGLYZA 5 mg, and placebo, respectively. The most common adverse events (reported in at least 2 patients treated with ONGLYZA 2.5 mg or at least 2 patients treated with ONGLYZA 5 mg) associated with premature discontinuation of therapy included lymphopenia (0.1% and 0.5% versus 0%, respectively), rash (0.2% and 0.3% versus 0.3%), blood creatinine increased (0.3% and 0% versus 0%), and blood creatine phosphokinase increased (0.1% and 0.2% versus 0%). The adverse reactions in this pooled analysis reported (regardless of investigator assessment of causality) in ≥5% of patients treated with ONGLYZA 5 mg, and more commonly than in patients treated with placebo are shown in Table 1.

Table 1: Adverse Reactions in Placebo-Controlled Trials* Reported in ≥5% of Patients Treated with ONGLYZA 5 mg and More Commonly than in Patients Treated with Placebo

	Number (%) of Patients	
	ONGLYZA 5 mg N=882	Placebo N=799
Upper respiratory tract infection	68 (7.7)	61 (7.6)
Urinary tract infection	60 (6.8)	49 (6.1)
Headache	57 (6.5)	47 (5.9)

* The 5 placebo-controlled trials include two monotherapy trials and one add-on combination therapy trial with each of the following: metformin, thiazolidinedione, or glyburide. Table shows 24-week data regardless of glycemic rescue.

In patients treated with ONGLYZA 2.5 mg, headache (6.5%) was the only adverse reaction reported at a rate ≥5% and more commonly than in patients treated with placebo.

In this pooled analysis, adverse reactions that were reported in ≥2% of patients treated with ONGLYZA 2.5 mg or ONGLYZA 5 mg and ≥1% more frequently compared to placebo included: sinusitis (2.9% and 2.6% versus 1.6%, respectively), abdominal pain (2.4% and 1.7% versus 0.5%), gastroenteritis (1.9% and 2.3% versus 0.9%), and vomiting (2.2% and 2.3% versus 1.3%).

In the add-on to TZD trial, the incidence of peripheral edema was higher for ONGLYZA 5 mg versus placebo (8.1% and 4.3%, respectively). The incidence of peripheral edema for ONGLYZA 2.5 mg was 3.1%. None of the reported adverse reactions of peripheral edema resulted in study drug discontinuation. Rates of peripheral edema for ONGLYZA 2.5 mg and ONGLYZA 5 mg versus placebo were 3.6% and 2% versus 3% given as monotherapy, 2.1% and 2.1% versus 2.2% given as add-on therapy to metformin, and 2.4% and 1.2% versus 2.2% given as add-on therapy to glyburide.

The incidence rate of fractures was 1.0 and 0.6 per 100 patient-years, respectively, for ONGLYZA (pooled analysis of 2.5 mg, 5 mg, and 10 mg) and placebo. The 10 mg dosage is not an approved dosage. The incidence rate of fracture events in patients who received ONGLYZA did not increase over time. Causality has not been established and nonclinical studies have not demonstrated adverse effects of ONGLYZA on bone.

An event of thrombocytopenia, consistent with a diagnosis of idiopathic thrombocytopenic purpura, was observed in the clinical program. The relationship of this event to ONGLYZA is not known.

Adverse Reactions in Patients with Renal Impairment

ONGLYZA (saxagliptin) 2.5 mg was compared to placebo in a 12-week trial in 170 patients with type 2 diabetes and moderate or severe renal impairment or end-stage renal disease (ESRD). The incidence of adverse events, including serious adverse events and discontinuations due to adverse events, was similar between ONGLYZA and placebo.

Adverse Reactions with Concomitant Use with Insulin

In the add-on to insulin trial [see *Clinical Studies (14.2)*], the incidence of adverse events, including serious adverse events and discontinuations due to adverse events, was similar between ONGLYZA and placebo, except for confirmed hypoglycemia [See *Adverse Reactions (6.1)*].

Adverse Reactions with Concomitant Use with Metformin in Treatment-Naive Patients with Type 2 Diabetes

Table 2 shows the adverse reactions reported (regardless of investigator assessment of causality) in ≥5% of patients participating in an additional 24-week, active-controlled trial of coadministered ONGLYZA and metformin in treatment-naive patients.

Table 2: Initial Therapy with Combination of ONGLYZA and Metformin in Treatment-Naive Patients: Adverse Reactions Reported in ≥5% of Patients Treated with Combination Therapy of ONGLYZA 5 mg Plus Metformin (and More Commonly than in Patients Treated with Metformin Alone)

	Number (%) of Patients	
	ONGLYZA 5 mg + Metformin* N=320	Metformin* N=328
Headache	24 (7.5)	17 (5.2)
Nasopharyngitis	22 (6.9)	13 (4.0)

* Metformin was initiated at a starting dose of 500 mg daily and titrated up to a maximum of 2000 mg daily.

Hypoglycemia

Adverse reactions of hypoglycemia were based on all reports of hypoglycemia. A concurrent glucose measurement was not required or was normal in some patients. Therefore, it is not possible to conclusively determine that all these reports reflect true hypoglycemia.

In the add-on to glyburide study, the overall incidence of reported hypoglycemia was higher for ONGLYZA 2.5 mg and ONGLYZA 5 mg (13.3% and 14.6%) versus placebo (10.1%). The incidence of confirmed hypoglycemia in this study, defined as symptoms of hypoglycemia accompanied by a fingerstick glucose value of ≤50 mg/dL, was 2.4% and 0.8% for ONGLYZA 2.5 mg and ONGLYZA 5 mg and 0.7% for placebo [see *Warnings and Precautions (5.2)*]. The incidence of reported hypoglycemia for ONGLYZA 2.5 mg and ONGLYZA 5 mg versus placebo given as monotherapy was 4% and 5.6% versus 4.1%, respectively, 7.8% and 5.8% versus 5% given as add-on therapy to metformin, and 4.1% and 2.7% versus 3.8% given as add-on therapy to TZD. The incidence of reported hypoglycemia was 3.4% in treatment-naive patients given ONGLYZA 5 mg plus metformin and 4% in patients given metformin alone.

In the active-controlled trial comparing add-on therapy with ONGLYZA 5 mg to glipizide in patients inadequately controlled on metformin alone, the incidence of reported hypoglycemia was 3% (19 events in 13 patients) with ONGLYZA 5 mg versus 36.3% (750 events in 156 patients) with glipizide. Confirmed symptomatic hypoglycemia (accompanying fingerstick blood glucose ≤50 mg/dL) was reported in none of the ONGLYZA-treated patients and in 35 glipizide-treated patients (8.1%) (p<0.0001).

During 12 weeks of treatment in patients with moderate or severe renal impairment or ESRD, the overall incidence of reported hypoglycemia was 20% among patients treated with ONGLYZA 2.5 mg and 22% among patients treated with placebo. Four ONGLYZA-treated patients (4.7%) and three placebo-treated patients (3.5%) reported at least one episode of confirmed symptomatic hypoglycemia (accompanying fingerstick glucose ≤50 mg/dL).

In the add-on to insulin trial, the overall incidence of reported hypoglycemia was 18.4% for ONGLYZA 5 mg and 19.9% for placebo. However, the incidence of confirmed symptomatic hypoglycemia (accompanying fingerstick blood glucose ≤50 mg/dL) was higher with ONGLYZA 5 mg (5.3%) versus placebo (3.3%).

In the add-on to metformin plus sulfonylurea trial, the overall incidence of reported hypoglycemia was 10.1% for ONGLYZA 5 mg and 6.3% for placebo. Confirmed hypoglycemia was reported in 1.6% of the ONGLYZA-treated patients and in none of the placebo-treated patients [see *Warnings and Precautions (5.2)*].

Hypersensitivity Reactions

Hypersensitivity-related events, such as urticaria and facial edema in the 5-study pooled analysis up to Week 24 were reported in 1.5%, 1.5%, and 0.4% of patients who received ONGLYZA 2.5 mg, ONGLYZA (saxagliptin) 5 mg, and placebo, respectively. None of these events in patients who received ONGLYZA required hospitalization or were reported as life-threatening by the investigators. One ONGLYZA-treated patient in this pooled analysis discontinued due to generalized urticaria and facial edema.

Infections

In the unblinded, controlled, clinical trial database for ONGLYZA to date, there have been 6 (0.12%) reports of tuberculosis among the 4959 ONGLYZA-treated patients (1.1 per 1000 patient-years) compared to no reports of tuberculosis among the 2868 comparator-treated patients. Two of these six cases were confirmed with laboratory testing. The remaining cases had limited information or had presumptive diagnoses of tuberculosis. None of the six cases occurred in the United States or in Western Europe. One case occurred in Canada in a patient originally from Indonesia who had recently visited Indonesia. The duration of treatment with ONGLYZA until report of tuberculosis ranged from 144 to 929 days. Post-treatment lymphocyte counts were consistently within the reference range for four cases. One patient had lymphopenia prior to initiation of ONGLYZA that remained stable throughout ONGLYZA treatment. The final patient had an isolated lymphocyte count below normal approximately four months prior to the report of tuberculosis. There have been no spontaneous reports of tuberculosis associated with ONGLYZA use. Causality has not been estimated and there are too few cases to date to determine whether tuberculosis is related to ONGLYZA use.

There has been one case of a potential opportunistic infection in the unblinded, controlled clinical trial database to date in an ONGLYZA-treated patient who developed suspected foodborne fatal salmonella sepsis after approximately 600 days of ONGLYZA therapy. There have been no spontaneous reports of opportunistic infections associated with ONGLYZA use.

Vital Signs

No clinically meaningful changes in vital signs have been observed in patients treated with ONGLYZA.

Laboratory Tests

Absolute Lymphocyte Counts

There was a dose-related mean decrease in absolute lymphocyte count observed with ONGLYZA. From a baseline mean absolute lymphocyte count of approximately 2200 cells/microL, mean decreases of approximately 100 and 120 cells/microL with ONGLYZA 5 mg and 10 mg, respectively, relative to placebo were observed at 24 weeks in a pooled analysis of five placebo-controlled clinical studies. Similar effects were observed when ONGLYZA 5 mg was given in initial combination with metformin compared to metformin alone. There was no difference observed for ONGLYZA 2.5 mg relative to placebo. The proportion of patients who were reported to have a lymphocyte count ≤750 cells/microL was 0.5%, 1.5%, 1.4%, and 0.4% in the ONGLYZA 2.5 mg, 5 mg, 10 mg, and placebo groups, respectively. In most patients, recurrence was not observed with repeated exposure to ONGLYZA although some patients had recurrent decreases upon rechallenge that led to discontinuation of ONGLYZA. The decreases in lymphocyte count were not associated with clinically relevant adverse reactions. The 10 mg dosage is not an approved dosage.

The clinical significance of this decrease in lymphocyte count relative to placebo is not known. When clinically indicated, such as in settings of unusual or prolonged infection, lymphocyte count should be measured. The effect of ONGLYZA on lymphocyte counts in patients with lymphocyte abnormalities (e.g., human immunodeficiency virus) is unknown.

6.2 Postmarketing Experience

Additional adverse reactions have been identified during postapproval use of ONGLYZA. Because these reactions are reported voluntarily from a population of uncertain size, it is generally not possible to reliably estimate their frequency or establish a causal relationship to drug exposure.

- Hypersensitivity reactions including anaphylaxis, angioedema, and exfoliative skin conditions. [See *Contraindications (4)* and *Warnings and Precautions (5.3)*.]
- Acute pancreatitis. [See *Indications and Usage (1.2)* and *Warnings and Precautions (5.1)*.]

7 DRUG INTERACTIONS

7.1 Strong Inhibitors of CYP3A4/5 Enzymes

Ketoconazole significantly increased saxagliptin exposure. Similar significant increases in plasma concentrations of saxagliptin are anticipated with other strong CYP3A4/5 inhibitors (e.g., atazanavir, clarithromycin, indinavir, itraconazole, nefazodone, nelfinavir, ritonavir, saquinavir, and telithromycin). The dose of ONGLYZA should be limited to 2.5 mg when coadministered with a strong CYP3A4/5 inhibitor. [See *Dosage and Administration (2.3)* and *Clinical Pharmacology (12.3)*.]

8 USE IN SPECIFIC POPULATIONS

8.1 Pregnancy

Pregnancy Category B

There are no adequate and well-controlled studies in pregnant women. Because animal reproduction studies are not always predictive of human response, ONGLYZA (saxagliptin), like other antidiabetic medications, should be used during pregnancy only if clearly needed.

Saxagliptin was not teratogenic at any dose tested when administered to pregnant rats and rabbits during periods of organogenesis. Incomplete ossification of the pelvis, a form of developmental delay, occurred in rats at a dose of 240 mg/kg, or approximately 1503 and 66 times human exposure to saxagliptin and the active metabolite, respectively, at the maximum recommended human dose (MRHD) of 5 mg. Maternal toxicity and reduced fetal body weights were observed at 7986 and 328 times the human exposure at the MRHD for saxagliptin and the active metabolite, respectively. Minor skeletal variations in rabbits occurred at a maternally toxic dose of 200 mg/kg, or approximately 1432 and 992 times the MRHD.

Coadministration of saxagliptin and metformin, to pregnant rats and rabbits during the period of organogenesis, was neither embryolethal nor teratogenic in either species when tested at doses yielding systemic exposures (AUC) up to 100 and 10 times the MRHD (saxagliptin 5 mg and metformin 2000 mg), respectively, in rats; and 249 and 1.1 times the MRHDs in rabbits. In rats, minor developmental toxicity was limited to an increased incidence of wavy ribs; associated maternal toxicity was limited to weight decrements of 11% to 17% over the course of the study, and related reductions in maternal food consumption. In rabbits, coadministration was poorly tolerated in a subset of mothers (12 of 30), resulting in death, moribundity, or abortion. However, among surviving mothers with evaluable litters, maternal toxicity was limited to marginal reductions in body weight over the course of gestation days 21 to 29; and associated developmental toxicity in these litters was limited to fetal body weight decrements of 7%, and a low incidence of delayed ossification of the fetal hyoid.

Saxagliptin administered to female rats from gestation day 6 to lactation day 20 resulted in decreased body weights in male and female offspring only at maternally toxic doses (exposures ≥1629 and 53 times saxagliptin and its active metabolite at the MRHD). No functional or behavioral toxicity was observed in offspring of rats administered saxagliptin at any dose.

Saxagliptin crosses the placenta into the fetus following dosing in pregnant rats.

8.3 Nursing Mothers

Saxagliptin is secreted in the milk of lactating rats at approximately a 1:1 ratio with plasma drug concentrations. It is not known whether saxagliptin is secreted in human milk. Because many drugs are secreted in human milk, caution should be exercised when ONGLYZA is administered to a nursing woman.

8.4 Pediatric Use

Safety and effectiveness of ONGLYZA in pediatric patients under 18 years of age have not been established. Additionally, studies characterizing the pharmacokinetics of ONGLYZA in pediatric patients have not been performed.

8.5 Geriatric Use

In the six, double-blind, controlled clinical safety and efficacy trials of ONGLYZA, 634 (15.3%) of the 4148 randomized patients were 65 years and over, and 59 (1.4%) patients were 75 years and over. No overall differences in safety or effectiveness were observed between patients ≥65 years old and the younger patients. While this clinical experience has not identified differences in responses between the elderly and younger patients, greater sensitivity of some older individuals cannot be ruled out.

Saxagliptin and its active metabolite are eliminated in part by the kidney. Because elderly patients are more likely to have decreased renal function, care should be taken in dose selection in the elderly based on renal function. [See *Dosage and Administration (2.2)* and *Clinical Pharmacology (12.3)*.]

10 OVERDOSAGE

In a controlled clinical trial, once-daily, orally-administered ONGLYZA in healthy subjects at doses up to 400 mg daily for 2 weeks (80 times the MRHD) had no dose-related clinical adverse reactions and no clinically meaningful effect on QTc interval or heart rate.

In the event of an overdose, appropriate supportive treatment should be initiated as dictated by the patient's clinical status. Saxagliptin and its active metabolite are removed by hemodialysis (23% of dose over 4 hours).

11 DESCRIPTION

Saxagliptin is an orally-active inhibitor of the DPP4 enzyme.

Saxagliptin monohydrate is described chemically as (1*S*,3*S*,5*S*)-2-[(2*S*)-2-Amino-2-(3-hydroxytricyclo[3.3.1.1^{3,7}]dec-1-yl)acetyl]-2-azabicyclo[3.1.0]hexane-3-carbonitrile, monohydrate or (1*S*,3*S*,5*S*)-2-[(2*S*)-2-Amino-2-(3-hydroxy-adamantan-1-yl)acetyl]-2-azabicyclo[3.1.0]hexane-3-carbonitrile hydrate. The empirical formula is $C_{18}H_{25}N_3O_2 \bullet H_2O$ and the molecular weight is 333.43. The structural formula is:

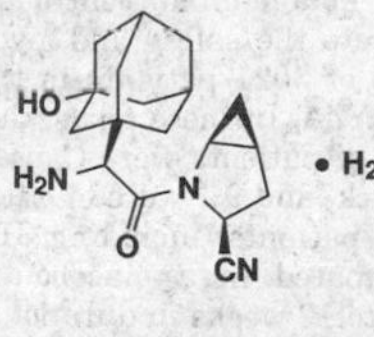

Saxagliptin monohydrate is a white to light yellow or light brown, non-hygroscopic, crystalline powder. It is sparingly soluble in water at 24°C ± 3°C, slightly soluble in ethyl acetate, and soluble in methanol, ethanol, isopropyl alcohol, acetonitrile, acetone, and polyethylene glycol 400 (PEG 400).

Each film-coated tablet of ONGLYZA (saxagliptin) for oral use contains either 2.79 mg saxagliptin hydrochloride (anhydrous) equivalent to 2.5 mg saxagliptin or 5.58 mg saxagliptin hydrochloride (anhydrous) equivalent to 5 mg saxagliptin and the following inactive ingredients: lactose monohydrate, microcrystalline cellulose, croscarmellose sodium, and magnesium stearate. In addition, the film coating contains the following inactive ingredients: polyvinyl alcohol, polyethylene glycol, titanium dioxide, talc, and iron oxides.

12 CLINICAL PHARMACOLOGY

12.1 Mechanism of Action

Increased concentrations of the incretin hormones such as glucagon-like peptide-1 (GLP-1) and glucose-dependent insulinotropic polypeptide (GIP) are released into the bloodstream from the small intestine in response to meals. These hormones cause insulin release from the pancreatic beta cells in a glucose-dependent manner but are inactivated by the DPP4 enzyme within minutes. GLP-1 also lowers glucagon secretion from pancreatic alpha cells, reducing hepatic glucose production. In patients with type 2 diabetes, concentrations of GLP-1 are reduced but the insulin response to GLP-1 is preserved. Saxagliptin is a competitive DPP4 inhibitor that slows the inactivation of the incretin hormones, thereby increasing their bloodstream concentrations and reducing fasting and postprandial glucose concentrations in a glucose-dependent manner in patients with type 2 diabetes mellitus.

12.2 Pharmacodynamics

In patients with type 2 diabetes mellitus, administration of ONGLYZA inhibits DPP4 enzyme activity for a 24-hour period. After an oral glucose load or a meal, this DPP4 inhibition resulted in a 2- to 3-fold increase in circulating levels of active GLP-1 and GIP, decreased glucagon concentrations, and increased glucose-dependent insulin secretion from pancreatic beta cells. The rise in insulin and decrease in glucagon were associated with lower fasting glucose concentrations and reduced glucose excursion following an oral glucose load or a meal.

Cardiac Electrophysiology

In a randomized, double-blind, placebo-controlled, 4-way crossover, active comparator study using moxifloxacin in 40 healthy subjects, ONGLYZA was not associated with clinically meaningful prolongation of the QTc interval or heart rate at daily doses up to 40 mg (8 times the MRHD).

12.3 Pharmacokinetics

The pharmacokinetics of saxagliptin and its active metabolite, 5-hydroxy saxagliptin were similar in healthy subjects and in patients with type 2 diabetes mellitus. The C_{max} and AUC values of saxagliptin and its active metabolite increased proportionally in the 2.5 to 400 mg dose range. Following a 5 mg single oral dose of saxagliptin to healthy subjects, the mean plasma AUC values for saxagliptin and its active metabolite were 78 ng•h/mL and 214 ng•h/mL, respectively. The corresponding plasma C_{max} values were 24 ng/mL and 47 ng/mL, respectively. The average variability (%CV) for AUC and C_{max} for both saxagliptin and its active metabolite was less than 25%.

No appreciable accumulation of either saxagliptin or its active metabolite was observed with repeated once-daily dosing at any dose level. No dose- and time-dependence were observed in the clearance of saxagliptin and its active metabolite over 14 days of once-daily dosing with saxagliptin at doses ranging from 2.5 to 400 mg.

Absorption

The median time to maximum concentration (T_{max}) following the 5 mg once daily dose was 2 hours for saxagliptin and 4 hours for its active metabolite. Administration with a high-fat meal resulted in an increase in T_{max} of saxagliptin by approximately 20 minutes as compared to fasted conditions. There was a 27% increase in the AUC of saxagliptin when given with a meal as compared to fasted conditions. ONGLYZA may be administered with or without food.

Table 3: Effect of Coadministered Drugs on Systemic Exposures of Saxagliptin and its Active Metabolite, 5-hydroxy Saxagliptin

Coadministered Drug	Dosage of Coadministered Drug*	Dosage of Saxagliptin*	Geometric Mean Ratio (ratio with/without coadministered drug) No Effect = 1.00		
				AUC†	C_{max}
No dosing adjustments required for the following:					
Metformin	1000 mg	100 mg	saxagliptin 5-hydroxy saxagliptin	0.98 0.99	0.79 0.88
Glyburide	5 mg	10 mg	saxagliptin 5-hydroxy saxagliptin	0.98 ND	1.08 ND
Pioglitazone‡	45 mg QD for 10 days	10 mg QD for 5 days	saxagliptin 5-hydroxy saxagliptin	1.11 ND	1.11 ND
Digoxin	0.25 mg q6h first day followed by q12h second day followed by QD for 5 days	10 mg QD for 7 days	saxagliptin 5-hydroxy saxagliptin	1.05 1.06	0.99 1.02
Simvastatin	40 mg QD for 8 days	10 mg QD for 4 days	saxagliptin 5-hydroxy saxagliptin	1.12 1.02	1.21 1.08
Diltiazem	360 mg LA QD for 9 days	10 mg	saxagliptin 5-hydroxy saxagliptin	2.09 0.66	1.63 0.57
Rifampin§	600 mg QD for 6 days	5 mg	saxagliptin 5-hydroxy saxagliptin	0.24 1.03	0.47 1.39
Omeprazole	40 mg QD for 5 days	10 mg	saxagliptin 5-hydroxy saxagliptin	1.13 ND	0.98 ND
Aluminum hydroxide + magnesium hydroxide + simethicone	aluminum hydroxide: 2400 mg magnesium hydroxide: 2400 mg simethicone: 240 mg	10 mg	saxagliptin 5-hydroxy saxagliptin	0.97 ND	0.74 ND
Famotidine	40 mg	10 mg	saxagliptin 5-hydroxy saxagliptin	1.03 ND	1.14 ND
Limit ONGLYZA dose to 2.5 mg once daily when coadministered with strong CYP3A4/5 inhibitors [see *Drug Interactions (7.1)* and *Dosage and Administration (2.3)*]:					
Ketoconazole	200 mg BID for 9 days	100 mg	saxagliptin 5-hydroxy saxagliptin	2.45 0.12	1.62 0.05
Ketoconazole	200 mg BID for 7 days	20 mg	saxagliptin 5-hydroxy saxagliptin	3.67 ND	2.44 ND

* Single dose unless otherwise noted

† AUC = AUC(INF) for drugs given as single dose and AUC = AUC(TAU) for drugs given in multiple doses

‡ Results exclude one subject

§ The plasma dipeptidyl peptidase-4 (DPP4) activity inhibition over a 24-hour dose interval was not affected by rifampin.

ND=not determined; QD=once daily; q6h=every 6 hours; q12h=every 12 hours; BID=twice daily; LA=long acting

Distribution

The *in vitro* protein binding of saxagliptin and its active metabolite in human serum is negligible. Therefore, changes in blood protein levels in various disease states (e.g., renal or hepatic impairment) are not expected to alter the disposition of saxagliptin.

Metabolism

The metabolism of saxagliptin is primarily mediated by cytochrome P450 3A4/5 (CYP3A4/5). The major metabolite of saxagliptin is also a DPP4 inhibitor, which is one-half as potent as saxagliptin. Therefore, strong CYP3A4/5 inhibitors and inducers will alter the pharmacokinetics of saxagliptin and its active metabolite. [See *Drug Interactions (7.1)*.]

Excretion

Saxagliptin is eliminated by both renal and hepatic pathways. Following a single 50 mg dose of ^{14}C-saxagliptin, 24%, 36%, and 75% of the dose was excreted in the urine as saxagliptin, its active metabolite, and total radioactivity, respectively. The average renal clearance of saxagliptin (~230 mL/min) was greater than the average estimated glomerular filtration rate (~120 mL/min), suggesting some active renal excretion. A total of 22% of the administered radioactivity was recovered in feces representing the fraction of the saxagliptin dose excreted in bile and/or unabsorbed drug from the gastrointestinal tract. Following a single oral dose of ONGLYZA (saxagliptin) 5 mg to healthy subjects, the mean plasma terminal half-life ($t_{1/2}$) for saxagliptin and its active metabolite was 2.5 and 3.1 hours, respectively.

Specific Populations

Renal Impairment

A single-dose, open-label study was conducted to evaluate the pharmacokinetics of saxagliptin (10 mg dose) in subjects with varying degrees of chronic renal impairment (N=8 per group) compared to subjects with normal renal function. The 10 mg dosage is not an approved dosage. The study included patients with renal impairment classified on the basis of creatinine clearance as mild (>50 to ≤80 mL/min), moderate (30 to ≤50 mL/min), and severe (<30 mL/min), as well as patients with end-stage renal disease on hemodialysis. Creatinine clearance was estimated from serum creatinine based on the Cockcroft-Gault formula:

$$CrCl = \frac{[140 - \text{age (years)}] \times \text{weight (kg)}}{[72 \times \text{serum creatinine (mg/dL)}]} \quad \{\times 0.85 \text{ for female patients}\}$$

The degree of renal impairment did not affect the C_{max} of saxagliptin or its active metabolite. In subjects with mild renal impairment, the AUC values of saxagliptin and its active metabolite were 20% and 70% higher, respectively, than AUC values in subjects with normal renal function. Because increases of this magnitude are not considered to be clinically relevant, dosage adjustment in patients with mild renal impairment is not recommended. In subjects with moderate or severe renal impairment, the AUC values of saxagliptin and its active metabolite were up to 2.1- and 4.5-fold higher, respectively, than AUC values in subjects with normal renal function. To achieve plasma exposures of saxagliptin and its active metabolite similar to those in patients with normal renal function, the recommended dose is 2.5 mg once daily in patients with moderate and severe renal impairment, as well as in patients with end-stage renal disease requiring hemodialysis. Saxagliptin is removed by hemodialysis.

Table 4: Effect of Saxagliptin on Systemic Exposures of Coadministered Drugs

Coadministered Drug	Dosage of Coadministered Drug*	Dosage of Saxagliptin*	Geometric Mean Ratio (ratio with/without saxagliptin) No Effect = 1.00		
				AUC†	C_{max}
No dosing adjustments required for the following:					
Metformin	1000 mg	100 mg	metformin	1.20	1.09
Glyburide	5 mg	10 mg	glyburide	1.06	1.16
Pioglitazone‡	45 mg QD for 10 days	10 mg QD for 5 days	pioglitazone hydroxy-pioglitazone	1.08 ND	1.14 ND
Digoxin	0.25 mg q6h first day followed by q12h second day followed by QD for 5 days	10 mg QD for 7 days	digoxin	1.06	1.09
Simvastatin	40 mg QD for 8 days	10 mg QD for 4 days	simvastatin simvastatin acid	1.04 1.16	0.88 1.00
Diltiazem	360 mg LA QD for 9 days	10 mg	diltiazem	1.10	1.16
Ketoconazole	200 mg BID for 9 days	100 mg	ketoconazole	0.87	0.84
Ethinyl estradiol and Norgestimate	ethinyl estradiol 0.035 mg and norgestimate 0.250 mg for 21 days	5 mg QD for 21 days	ethinyl estradiol norelgestromin norgestrel	1.07 1.10 1.13	0.98 1.09 1.17

* Single dose unless otherwise noted
† AUC = AUC(INF) for drugs given as single dose and AUC = AUC(TAU) for drugs given in multiple doses
‡ Results include all subjects
ND=not determined; QD=once daily; q6h=every 6 hours; q12h=every 12 hours; BID=twice daily; LA=long acting

Hepatic Impairment

In subjects with hepatic impairment (Child-Pugh classes A, B, and C), mean C_{max} and AUC of saxagliptin were up to 8% and 77% higher, respectively, compared to healthy matched controls following administration of a single 10 mg dose of saxagliptin. The 10 mg dosage is not an approved dosage. The corresponding C_{max} and AUC of the active metabolite were up to 59% and 33% lower, respectively, compared to healthy matched controls. These differences are not considered to be clinically meaningful. No dosage adjustment is recommended for patients with hepatic impairment.

Body Mass Index

No dosage adjustment is recommended based on body mass index (BMI) which was not identified as a significant covariate on the apparent clearance of saxagliptin or its active metabolite in the population pharmacokinetic analysis.

Gender

No dosage adjustment is recommended based on gender. There were no differences observed in saxagliptin pharmacokinetics between males and females. Compared to males, females had approximately 25% higher exposure values for the active metabolite than males, but this difference is unlikely to be of clinical relevance. Gender was not identified as a significant covariate on the apparent clearance of saxagliptin and its active metabolite in the population pharmacokinetic analysis.

Geriatric

No dosage adjustment is recommended based on age alone. Elderly subjects (65-80 years) had 23% and 59% higher geometric mean C_{max} and geometric mean AUC values, respectively, for saxagliptin than young subjects (18-40 years). Differences in active metabolite pharmacokinetics between elderly and young subjects generally reflected the differences observed in saxagliptin pharmacokinetics. The difference between the pharmacokinetics of saxagliptin and the active metabolite in young and elderly subjects is likely due to multiple factors including declining renal function and metabolic capacity with increasing age. Age was not identified as a significant covariate on the apparent clearance of saxagliptin and its active metabolite in the population pharmacokinetic analysis.

Race and Ethnicity

No dosage adjustment is recommended based on race. The population pharmacokinetic analysis compared the pharmacokinetics of saxagliptin and its active metabolite in 309 Caucasian subjects with 105 non-Caucasian subjects (consisting of six racial groups). No significant difference in the pharmacokinetics of saxagliptin and its active metabolite were detected between these two populations.

Drug Interaction Studies

In Vitro Assessment of Drug Interactions

The metabolism of saxagliptin is primarily mediated by CYP3A4/5.

In *in vitro* studies, saxagliptin and its active metabolite did not inhibit CYP1A2, 2A6, 2B6, 2C9, 2C19, 2D6, 2E1, or 3A4, or induce CYP1A2, 2B6, 2C9, or 3A4. Therefore, saxagliptin is not expected to alter the metabolic clearance of coadministered drugs that are metabolized by these enzymes. Saxagliptin is a P-glycoprotein (P-gp) substrate but is not a significant inhibitor or inducer of P-gp.

In Vivo Assessment of Drug Interactions

[See table 3 at top of previous page]
[See table 4 above]

13 NONCLINICAL TOXICOLOGY

13.1 Carcinogenesis, Mutagenesis, Impairment of Fertility

Carcinogenesis

Saxagliptin did not induce tumors in either mice (50, 250, and 600 mg/kg) or rats (25, 75, 150, and 300 mg/kg) at the highest doses evaluated. The highest doses evaluated in mice were equivalent to approximately 870 (males) and 1165 (females) times the human exposure at the MRHD of 5 mg/day. In rats, exposures were approximately 355 (males) and 2217 (females) times the MRHD.

Mutagenesis

Saxagliptin was not mutagenic or clastogenic with or without metabolic activation in an *in vitro* Ames bacterial assay, an *in vitro* cytogenetics assay in primary human lymphocytes, an *in vivo* oral micronucleus assay in rats, an *in vivo* oral DNA repair study in rats, and an oral *in vivo/in vitro* cytogenetics study in rat peripheral blood lymphocytes. The active metabolite was not mutagenic in an *in vitro* Ames bacterial assay.

Impairment of Fertility

In a rat fertility study, males were treated with oral gavage doses for 2 weeks prior to mating, during mating, and up to scheduled termination (approximately 4 weeks total) and females were treated with oral gavage doses for 2 weeks prior to mating through gestation day 7. No adverse effects on fertility were observed at exposures of approximately 603 (males) and 776 (females) times the MRHD. Higher doses that elicited maternal toxicity also increased fetal resorptions (approximately 2069 and 6138 times the MRHD). Additional effects on estrous cycling, fertility, ovulation, and implantation were observed at approximately 6138 times the MRHD.

13.2 Animal Toxicology and/or Pharmacology

Saxagliptin produced adverse skin changes in the extremities of cynomolgus monkeys (scabs and/or ulceration of tail, digits, scrotum, and/or nose). Skin lesions were reversible at ≥20 times the MRHD but in some cases were irreversible and necrotizing at higher exposures. Adverse skin changes were not observed at exposures similar to (1 to 3 times) the MRHD of 5 mg. Clinical correlates to skin lesions in monkeys have not been observed in human clinical trials of saxagliptin.

14 CLINICAL STUDIES

ONGLYZA (saxagliptin) has been studied as monotherapy and in combination with metformin, glyburide, and thiazolidinedione (pioglitazone and rosiglitazone) therapy.

A total of 4148 patients with type 2 diabetes mellitus were randomized in six, double-blind, controlled clinical trials conducted to evaluate the safety and glycemic efficacy of ONGLYZA. A total of 3021 patients in these trials were treated with ONGLYZA. In these trials, the mean age was 54 years, and 71% of patients were Caucasian, 16% were Asian, 4% were black, and 9% were of other racial groups. An additional 423 patients, including 315 who received ONGLYZA, participated in a placebo-controlled, dose-ranging study of 6 to 12 weeks in duration.

In these six, double-blind trials, ONGLYZA was evaluated at doses of 2.5 mg and 5 mg once daily. Three of these trials also evaluated a saxagliptin dose of 10 mg daily. The 10 mg daily dose of saxagliptin did not provide greater efficacy than the 5 mg daily dose. The 10 mg dosage is not an approved dosage. Treatment with ONGLYZA 5 mg and 2.5 mg doses produced clinically relevant and statistically significant improvements in hemoglobin A1c (A1C), fasting plasma glucose (FPG), and 2-hour postprandial glucose (PPG) following a standard oral glucose tolerance test (OGTT), compared to control. Reductions in A1C were seen across subgroups including gender, age, race, and baseline BMI.

ONGLYZA was not associated with significant changes from baseline in body weight or fasting serum lipids compared to placebo.

ONGLYZA has also been evaluated in four additional trials in patients with type 2 diabetes: an active-controlled trial comparing add-on therapy with ONGLYZA to glipizide in 858 patients inadequately controlled on metformin alone, a trial comparing ONGLYZA to placebo in 455 patients inadequately controlled on insulin alone or on insulin in combination with metformin, a trial comparing ONGLYZA to placebo in 257 patients inadequately controlled on metformin plus a sulfonylurea, and a trial comparing ONGLYZA to placebo in 170 patients with type 2 diabetes and moderate or severe renal impairment or ESRD.

14.1 Monotherapy

A total of 766 patients with type 2 diabetes inadequately controlled on diet and exercise (A1C ≥7% to ≤10%) participated in two 24-week, double-blind, placebo-controlled trials evaluating the efficacy and safety of ONGLYZA monotherapy.

In the first trial, following a 2-week single-blind diet, exercise, and placebo lead-in period, 401 patients were randomized to 2.5 mg, 5 mg, or 10 mg of ONGLYZA or placebo. The 10 mg dosage is not an approved dosage. Patients who failed to meet specific glycemic goals during the study were treated with metformin rescue therapy, added on to placebo or ONGLYZA. Efficacy was evaluated at the last measurement prior to rescue therapy for patients needing rescue. Dose titration of ONGLYZA was not permitted.

Treatment with ONGLYZA 2.5 mg and 5 mg daily provided significant improvements in A1C, FPG, and PPG compared to placebo (Table 5). The percentage of patients who discontinued for lack of glycemic control or who were rescued for meeting prespecified glycemic criteria was 16% in the ONGLYZA 2.5 mg treatment group, 20% in the ONGLYZA 5 mg treatment group, and 26% in the placebo group.

[See table 5 at top of next page]

A second 24-week monotherapy trial was conducted to assess a range of dosing regimens for ONGLYZA. Treatment-naive patients with inadequately controlled diabetes (A1C ≥7% to ≤10%) underwent a 2-week, single-blind diet, exercise, and placebo lead-in period. A total of 365 patients were randomized to 2.5 mg every morning, 5 mg every morning, 2.5 mg with possible titration to 5 mg every morning, or 5 mg every evening of ONGLYZA, or placebo. Patients who failed to meet specific glycemic goals during the study were treated with metformin rescue therapy added on to placebo or ONGLYZA; the number of patients randomized per treatment group ranged from 71 to 74.

Treatment with either ONGLYZA 5 mg every morning or 5 mg every evening provided significant improvements in A1C versus placebo (mean placebo-corrected reductions of −0.4% and −0.3%, respectively). Treatment with ONGLYZA 2.5 mg every morning also provided significant improvement in A1C versus placebo (mean placebo-corrected reduction of −0.4%).

14.2 Combination Therapy

Add-On Combination Therapy with Metformin

A total of 743 patients with type 2 diabetes participated in this 24-week, randomized, double-blind, placebo-controlled trial to evaluate the efficacy and safety of ONGLYZA in combination with metformin in patients with inadequate glycemic control (A1C ≥7% and ≤10%) on metformin alone. To qualify for enrollment, patients were required to be on a stable dose of metformin (1500-2550 mg daily) for at least 8 weeks.

Patients who met eligibility criteria were enrolled in a single-blind, 2-week, dietary and exercise placebo lead-in period during which patients received metformin at their pre-study dose, up to 2500 mg daily. Following the lead-in period, eligible patients were randomized to 2.5 mg, 5 mg, or 10 mg of ONGLYZA (saxagliptin) or placebo in addition to their current dose of open-label metformin. The 10 mg dosage is not an approved dosage. Patients who failed to meet specific glycemic goals during the study were treated with pioglitazone rescue therapy, added on to existing study medications. Dose titrations of ONGLYZA and metformin were not permitted.

ONGLYZA 2.5 mg and 5 mg add-on to metformin provided significant improvements in A1C, FPG, and PPG compared with placebo add-on to metformin (Table 6). Mean changes from baseline for A1C over time and at endpoint are shown in Figure 1. The proportion of patients who discontinued for lack of glycemic control or who were rescued for meeting prespecified glycemic criteria was 15% in the ONGLYZA 2.5 mg add-on to metformin group, 13% in the ONGLYZA 5 mg add-on to metformin group, and 27% in the placebo add-on to metformin group.

[See table 6 below]

Figure 1: Mean Change from Baseline in A1C in a Placebo-Controlled Trial of ONGLYZA as Add-On Combination Therapy with Metformin*

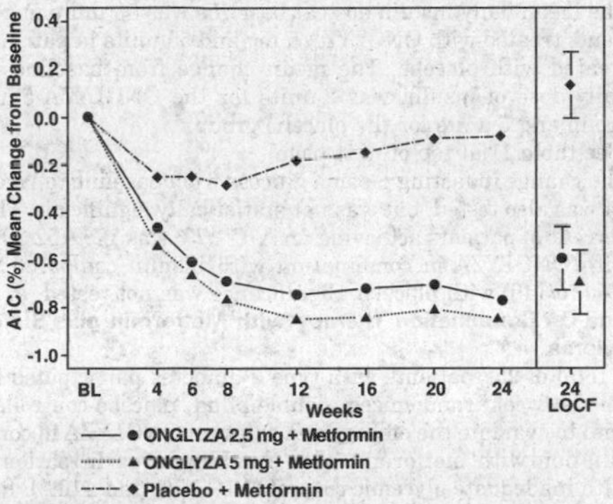

* Includes patients with a baseline and week 24 value. Week 24 (LOCF) includes intent-to-treat population using last observation on study prior to pioglitazone rescue therapy for patients needing rescue. Mean change from baseline is adjusted for baseline value.

Add-On Combination Therapy with a Thiazolidinedione

A total of 565 patients with type 2 diabetes participated in this 24-week, randomized, double-blind, placebo-controlled trial to evaluate the efficacy and safety of ONGLYZA in combination with a thiazolidinedione (TZD) in patients with inadequate glycemic control (A1C ≥7% to ≤10.5%) on TZD alone. To qualify for enrollment, patients were required to be on a stable dose of pioglitazone (30-45 mg once daily) or rosiglitazone (4 mg once daily or 8 mg either once daily or in two divided doses of 4 mg) for at least 12 weeks.

Patients who met eligibility criteria were enrolled in a single-blind, 2-week, dietary and exercise placebo lead-in period during which patients received TZD at their pre-study dose. Following the lead-in period, eligible patients were randomized to 2.5 mg or 5 mg of ONGLYZA or placebo in addition to their current dose of TZD. Patients who failed to meet specific glycemic goals during the study were treated with metformin rescue, added on to existing study medications. Dose titration of ONGLYZA or TZD was not permitted during the study. A change in TZD regimen from rosiglitazone to pioglitazone at specified, equivalent therapeutic doses was permitted at the investigator's discretion if believed to be medically appropriate.

ONGLYZA 2.5 mg and 5 mg add-on to TZD provided significant improvements in A1C, FPG, and PPG compared with placebo add-on to TZD (Table 7). The proportion of patients who discontinued for lack of glycemic control or who were rescued for meeting prespecified glycemic criteria was 10% in the ONGLYZA 2.5 mg add-on to TZD group, 6% for the ONGLYZA 5 mg add-on to TZD group, and 10% in the placebo add-on to TZD group.

[See table 7 at top of next page]

Add-On Combination Therapy with Glyburide

A total of 768 patients with type 2 diabetes participated in this 24-week, randomized, double-blind, placebo-controlled trial to evaluate the efficacy and safety of ONGLYZA in combination with a sulfonylurea (SU) in patients with inadequate glycemic control at enrollment (A1C ≥7.5% to ≤10%) on a submaximal dose of SU alone. To qualify for enrollment, patients were required to be on a submaximal dose of SU for 2 months or greater. In this study, ONGLYZA in combination with a fixed, intermediate dose of SU was compared to titration to a higher dose of SU.

Table 5: Glycemic Parameters at Week 24 in a Placebo-Controlled Study of ONGLYZA Monotherapy in Patients with Type 2 Diabetes*

Efficacy Parameter	ONGLYZA 2.5 mg N=102	ONGLYZA 5 mg N=106	Placebo N=95
Hemoglobin A1C (%)	N=100	N=103	N=92
Baseline (mean)	7.9	8.0	7.9
Change from baseline (adjusted mean†)	−0.4	−0.5	+0.2
Difference from placebo (adjusted mean†)	−0.6‡	−0.6‡	
95% Confidence Interval	(−0.9, −0.3)	(−0.9, −0.4)	
Percent of patients achieving A1C <7%	35% (35/100)	38%§ (39/103)	24% (22/92)
Fasting Plasma Glucose (mg/dL)	N=101	N=105	N=92
Baseline (mean)	178	171	172
Change from baseline (adjusted mean†)	−15	−9	+6
Difference from placebo (adjusted mean†)	−21§	−15§	
95% Confidence Interval	(−31, −10)	(−25, −4)	
2-hour Postprandial Glucose (mg/dL)	N=78	N=84	N=71
Baseline (mean)	279	278	283
Change from baseline (adjusted mean†)	−45	−43	−6
Difference from placebo (adjusted mean†)	−39¶	−37§	
95% Confidence Interval	(−61, −16)	(−59, −15)	

* Intent-to-treat population using last observation on study or last observation prior to metformin rescue therapy for patients needing rescue.
† Least squares mean adjusted for baseline value.
‡ p-value <0.0001 compared to placebo
§ p-value <0.05 compared to placebo
¶ Significance was not tested for the 2-hour PPG for the 2.5 mg dose of ONGLYZA.

Table 6: Glycemic Parameters at Week 24 in a Placebo-Controlled Study of ONGLYZA as Add-On Combination Therapy with Metformin*

Efficacy Parameter	ONGLYZA 2.5 mg + Metformin N=192	ONGLYZA 5 mg + Metformin N=191	Placebo + Metformin N=179
Hemoglobin A1C (%)	N=186	N=186	N=175
Baseline (mean)	8.1	8.1	8.1
Change from baseline (adjusted mean†)	−0.6	−0.7	+0.1
Difference from placebo (adjusted mean†)	−0.7‡	−0.8‡	
95% Confidence Interval	(−0.9, −0.5)	(−1.0, −0.6)	
Percent of patients achieving A1C <7%	37%§ (69/186)	44%§ (81/186)	17% (29/175)
Fasting Plasma Glucose (mg/dL)	N=188	N=187	N=176
Baseline (mean)	174	179	175
Change from baseline (adjusted mean†)	−14	−22	+1
Difference from placebo (adjusted mean†)	−16§	−23§	
95% Confidence Interval	(−23, −9)	(−30, −16)	
2-hour Postprandial Glucose (mg/dL)	N=155	N=155	N=135
Baseline (mean)	294	296	295
Change from baseline (adjusted mean†)	−62	−58	−18
Difference from placebo (adjusted mean†)	−44§	−40§	
95% Confidence Interval	(−60, −27)	(−56, −24)	

* Intent-to-treat population using last observation on study or last observation prior to pioglitazone rescue therapy for patients needing rescue.
† Least squares mean adjusted for baseline value.
‡ p-value <0.0001 compared to placebo + metformin
§ p-value <0.05 compared to placebo + metformin

Patients who met eligibility criteria were enrolled in a single-blind, 4-week, dietary and exercise lead-in period, and placed on glyburide 7.5 mg once daily. Following the lead-in period, eligible patients with A1C ≥7% to ≤10% were randomized to either 2.5 mg or 5 mg of ONGLYZA (saxagliptin) add-on to 7.5 mg glyburide or to placebo plus a 10 mg total daily dose of glyburide. Patients who received placebo were eligible to have glyburide up-titrated to a total daily dose of 15 mg. Up-titration of glyburide was not permitted in patients who received ONGLYZA 2.5 mg or 5 mg. Glyburide could be down-titrated in any treatment group once during the 24-week study period due to hypoglycemia as deemed necessary by the investigator. Approximately 92% of patients in the placebo plus glyburide group were up-titrated to a final total daily dose of 15 mg during the first 4 weeks of the study period. Patients who failed to meet specific glycemic goals during the study were treated with metformin rescue, added on to existing study medication. Dose titration of ONGLYZA was not permitted during the study.

In combination with glyburide, ONGLYZA 2.5 mg and 5 mg provided significant improvements in A1C, FPG, and PPG compared with the placebo plus up-titrated glyburide group (Table 8). The proportion of patients who discontinued for lack of glycemic control or who were rescued for meeting prespecified glycemic criteria was 18% in the ONGLYZA 2.5 mg add-on to glyburide group, 17% in the ONGLYZA (saxagliptin) 5 mg add-on to glyburide group, and 30% in the placebo plus up-titrated glyburide group.

[See table 8 at top of next page]

Coadministration with Metformin in Treatment-Naive Patients

A total of 1306 treatment-naive patients with type 2 diabetes mellitus participated in this 24-week, randomized, double-blind, active-controlled trial to evaluate the efficacy and safety of ONGLYZA coadministered with metformin in patients with inadequate glycemic control (A1C ≥8% to ≤12%) on diet and exercise alone. Patients were required to be treatment-naive to be enrolled in this study.

Patients who met eligibility criteria were enrolled in a single-blind, 1-week, dietary and exercise placebo lead-in period. Patients were randomized to one of four treatment arms: ONGLYZA 5 mg + metformin 500 mg, saxagliptin 10 mg + metformin 500 mg, saxagliptin 10 mg + placebo, or metformin 500 mg + placebo. The 10 mg dosage is not an approved dosage. ONGLYZA was dosed once daily. In the 3 treatment groups using metformin, the metformin dose was up-titrated weekly in 500 mg per day increments, as tolerated, to a maximum of 2000 mg per day based on FPG. Patients who failed to meet specific glycemic goals during the studies were treated with pioglitazone rescue as add-on therapy.

Table 7: Glycemic Parameters at Week 24 in a Placebo-Controlled Study of ONGLYZA as Add-On Combination Therapy with a Thiazolidinedione*

Efficacy Parameter	ONGLYZA 2.5 mg + TZD N=195	ONGLYZA 5 mg + TZD N=186	Placebo + TZD N=184
Hemoglobin A1C (%)	**N=192**	**N=183**	**N=180**
Baseline (mean)	8.3	8.4	8.2
Change from baseline (adjusted mean†)	−0.7	−0.9	−0.3
Difference from placebo (adjusted mean†)	−0.4§	−0.6‡	
95% Confidence Interval	(−0.6, −0.2)	(−0.8, −0.4)	
Percent of patients achieving A1C <7%	42%§ (81/192)	42%§ (77/184)	26% (46/180)
Fasting Plasma Glucose (mg/dL)	**N=193**	**N=185**	**N=181**
Baseline (mean)	163	160	162
Change from baseline (adjusted mean†)	−14	−17	−3
Difference from placebo (adjusted mean†)	−12§	−15§	
95% Confidence Interval	(−20, −3)	(−23, −6)	
2-hour Postprandial Glucose (mg/dL)	**N=156**	**N=134**	**N=127**
Baseline (mean)	296	303	291
Change from baseline (adjusted mean†)	−55	−65	−15
Difference from placebo (adjusted mean†)	−40§	−50§	
95% Confidence Interval	(−56, −24)	(−66, −34)	

* Intent-to-treat population using last observation on study or last observation prior to metformin rescue therapy for patients needing rescue.
† Least squares mean adjusted for baseline value.
‡ p-value <0.0001 compared to placebo + TZD
§ p-value <0.05 compared to placebo + TZD

Table 8: Glycemic Parameters at Week 24 in a Placebo-Controlled Study of ONGLYZA as Add-On Combination Therapy with Glyburide*

Efficacy Parameter	ONGLYZA 2.5 mg + Glyburide 7.5 mg N=248	ONGLYZA 5 mg + Glyburide 7.5 mg N=253	Placebo + Up-Titrated Glyburide N=267
Hemoglobin A1C (%)	**N=246**	**N=250**	**N=264**
Baseline (mean)	8.4	8.5	8.4
Change from baseline (adjusted mean†)	−0.5	−0.6	+0.1
Difference from up-titrated glyburide (adjusted mean†)	−0.6‡	−0.7‡	
95% Confidence Interval	(−0.8, −0.5)	(−0.9, −0.6)	
Percent of patients achieving A1C <7%	22%§ (55/246)	23%§ (57/250)	9% (24/264)
Fasting Plasma Glucose (mg/dL)	**N=247**	**N=252**	**N=265**
Baseline (mean)	170	175	174
Change from baseline (adjusted mean†)	−7	−10	+1
Difference from up-titrated glyburide (adjusted mean†)	−8§	−10§	
95% Confidence Interval	(−14, −1)	(−17, −4)	
2-hour Postprandial Glucose (mg/dL)	**N=195**	**N=202**	**N=206**
Baseline (mean)	309	315	323
Change from baseline (adjusted mean†)	−31	−34	+8
Difference from up-titrated glyburide (adjusted mean†)	−38§	−42§	
95% Confidence Interval	(−50, −27)	(−53, −31)	

* Intent-to-treat population using last observation on study or last observation prior to metformin rescue therapy for patients needing rescue.
† Least squares mean adjusted for baseline value.
‡ p-value <0.0001 compared to placebo + up-titrated glyburide
§ p-value <0.05 compared to placebo + up-titrated glyburide

Coadministration of ONGLYZA (saxagliptin) 5 mg plus metformin provided significant improvements in A1C, FPG, and PPG compared with placebo plus metformin (Table 9).
[See table 9 at top of next page]

Add-On Combination Therapy with Metformin versus Glipizide Add-On Combination Therapy with Metformin

In this 52-week, active-controlled trial, a total of 858 patients with type 2 diabetes and inadequate glycemic control (A1C >6.5% and ≤10%) on metformin alone were randomized to double-blind add-on therapy with ONGLYZA or glipizide. Patients were required to be on a stable dose of metformin (at least 1500 mg daily) for at least 8 weeks prior to enrollment.

Patients who met eligibility criteria were enrolled in a single-blind, 2-week, dietary and exercise placebo lead-in period during which patients received metformin (1500-3000 mg based on their pre-study dose). Following the lead-in period, eligible patients were randomized to 5 mg of ONGLYZA or 5 mg of glipizide in addition to their current dose of open-label metformin. Patients in the glipizide plus metformin group underwent blinded titration of the glipizide dose during the first 18 weeks of the trial up to a maximum glipizide dose of 20 mg per day. Titration was based on a goal FPG ≤110 mg/dL or the highest tolerable glipizide dose. Fifty percent (50%) of the glipizide-treated patients were titrated to the 20-mg daily dose; 21% of the glipizide-treated patients had a final daily glipizide dose of 5 mg or less. The mean final daily dose of glipizide was 15 mg.

After 52 weeks of treatment, ONGLYZA (saxagliptin) and glipizide resulted in similar mean reductions from baseline in A1C when added to metformin therapy (Table 10). This conclusion may be limited to patients with baseline A1C comparable to those in the trial (91% of patients had baseline A1C <9%).

From a baseline mean body weight of 89 kg, there was a statistically significant mean reduction of 1.1 kg in patients treated with ONGLYZA compared to a mean weight gain of 1.1 kg in patients treated with glipizide (p<0.0001).
[See table 10 at top of next page]

Add-On Combination Therapy with Insulin (with or without metformin)

A total of 455 patients with type 2 diabetes participated in this 24-week, randomized, double-blind, placebo-controlled trial to evaluate the efficacy and safety of ONGLYZA in combination with insulin in patients with inadequate glycemic control (A1C ≥7.5% and ≤11%) on insulin alone (N=141) or on insulin in combination with a stable dose of metformin (N=314). Patients were required to be on a stable dose of insulin (≥30 units to ≤150 units daily) with ≤20% variation in total daily dose for ≥8 weeks prior to screening. Patients entered the trial on intermediate- or long-acting (basal) insulin or premixed insulin. Patients using short-acting insulins were excluded unless the short-acting insulin was administered as part of a premixed insulin.

Patients who met eligibility criteria were enrolled in a single-blind, four-week, dietary and exercise placebo lead-in period during which patients received insulin (and metformin if applicable) at their pretrial dose(s). Following the lead-in period, eligible patients were randomized to add-on therapy with either ONGLYZA (saxagliptin) 5 mg or placebo. Doses of the antidiabetic therapies were to remain stable but patients were rescued and allowed to adjust the insulin regimen if specific glycemic goals were not met or if the investigator learned that the patient had self-increased the insulin dose by >20%. Data after rescue were excluded from the primary efficacy analyses.

Add-on therapy with ONGLYZA 5 mg provided significant improvements from baseline to Week 24 in A1C and PPG compared with add-on placebo (Table 11). Similar mean reductions in A1C versus placebo were observed for patients using ONGLYZA 5 mg add-on to insulin alone and ONGLYZA 5 mg add-on to insulin in combination with metformin (−0.4% and −0.4%, respectively). The percentage of patients who discontinued for lack of glycemic control or who were rescued was 23% in the ONGLYZA group and 32% in the placebo group.

The mean daily insulin dose at baseline was 53 units in patients treated with ONGLYZA 5 mg and 55 units in patients treated with placebo. The mean change from baseline in daily dose of insulin was 2 units for the ONGLYZA 5 mg group and 5 units for the placebo group.
[See table 11 at top of next page]

The change in fasting plasma glucose from baseline to Week 24 was also tested, but was not statistically significant. The percent of patients achieving an A1C <7% was 17% (52/300) with ONGLYZA in combination with insulin compared to 7% (10/149) with placebo. Significance was not tested.

Add-On Combination Therapy with Metformin plus Sulfonylurea

A total of 257 patients with type 2 diabetes participated in this 24-week, randomized, double-blind, placebo-controlled trial to evaluate the efficacy and safety of ONGLYZA in combination with metformin plus a sulfonylurea in patients with inadequate glycemic control (A1C ≥7% and ≤10%). Patients were to be on a stable combined dose of metformin extended-release or immediate-release (at maximum tolerated dose, with minimum dose for enrollment being 1500 mg) and a sulfonylurea (at maximum tolerated dose, with minimum dose for enrollment being ≥50% of the maximum recommended dose) for ≥8 weeks prior to enrollment. Patients who met eligibility criteria were entered in a 2-week enrollment period to allow assessment of inclusion/exclusion criteria. Following the 2-week enrollment period, eligible patients were randomized to either double-blind ONGLYZA (5 mg once daily) or double-blind matching placebo for 24 weeks. During the 24-week double-blind treatment period, patients were to receive metformin and a sulfonylurea at the same constant dose ascertained during enrollment. Sulfonylurea dose could be down titrated once in the case of a major hypoglycemic event or recurring minor hypoglycemic events. In the absence of hypoglycemia, titration (up or down) of study medication during the treatment period was prohibited.

ONGLYZA in combination with metformin plus a sulfonylurea provided significant improvements in A1C and PPG compared with placebo in combination with metformin plus a sulfonylurea (Table 12). The percentage of patients who discontinued for a lack of glycemic control was 6% in the ONGLYZA group and 5% in the placebo group.
[See table 12 at top of page 762]

The change in fasting plasma glucose from baseline to Week 24 was also tested, but was not statistically significant. The percent of patients achieving an A1C <7% was 31% (39/127) with ONGLYZA in combination with metformin plus a sulfonylurea compared to 9% (12/127) with placebo. Significance was not tested.

14.3 Renal Impairment

A total of 170 patients participated in a 12-week, randomized, double-blind, placebo-controlled trial conducted to evaluate the efficacy and safety of ONGLYZA 2.5 mg once daily compared with placebo in patients with type 2 diabetes and moderate (n=90) or severe (n=41) renal impairment or ESRD (n=39). In this trial, 98% of the patients were using background antidiabetic medications (75% were using insulin and 31% were using oral antidiabetic medications, mostly sulfonylureas).

After 12 weeks of treatment, ONGLYZA 2.5 mg provided significant improvement in A1C compared to placebo (Table 13). In the subgroup of patients with ESRD, ONGLYZA and placebo resulted in comparable reductions in A1C from baseline to Week 12. This finding is inconclusive because the trial was not adequately powered to show efficacy within specific subgroups of renal impairment.

Table 9: Glycemic Parameters at Week 24 in a Placebo-Controlled Trial of ONGLYZA Coadministration with Metformin in Treatment-Naive Patients*

Efficacy Parameter	ONGLYZA 5 mg + Metformin N=320	Placebo + Metformin N=328
Hemoglobin A1C (%)	N=306	N=313
Baseline (mean)	9.4	9.4
Change from baseline (adjusted mean†)	−2.5	−2.0
Difference from placebo + metformin (adjusted mean†)	−0.5‡	
95% Confidence Interval	(−0.7, −0.4)	
Percent of patients achieving A1C <7%	60%§ (185/307)	41% (129/314)
Fasting Plasma Glucose (mg/dL)	N=315	N=320
Baseline (mean)	199	199
Change from baseline (adjusted mean†)	−60	−47
Difference from placebo + metformin (adjusted mean†)	−13§	
95% Confidence Interval	(−19, −6)	
2-hour Postprandial Glucose (mg/dL)	N=146	N=141
Baseline (mean)	340	355
Change from baseline (adjusted mean†)	−138	−97
Difference from placebo + metformin (adjusted mean†)	−41§	
95% Confidence Interval	(−57, −25)	

* Intent-to-treat population using last observation on study or last observation prior to pioglitazone rescue therapy for patients needing rescue.
† Least squares mean adjusted for baseline value.
‡ p-value <0.0001 compared to placebo + metformin
§ p-value <0.05 compared to placebo + metformin

Table 10: Glycemic Parameters at Week 52 in an Active-Controlled Trial of ONGLYZA versus Glipizide in Combination with Metformin*

Efficacy Parameter	ONGLYZA 5 mg + Metformin N=428	Titrated Glipizide + Metformin N=430
Hemoglobin A1C (%)	N=423	N=423
Baseline (mean)	7.7	7.6
Change from baseline (adjusted mean†)	−0.6	−0.7
Difference from glipizide + metformin (adjusted mean†)	0.1	
95% Confidence Interval	(−0.02, 0.2)‡	
Fasting Plasma Glucose (mg/dL)	N=420	N=420
Baseline (mean)	162	161
Change from baseline (adjusted mean†)	−9	−16
Difference from glipizide + metformin (adjusted mean†)	6	
95% Confidence Interval	(2, 11)§	

* Intent-to-treat population using last observation on study.
† Least squares mean adjusted for baseline value.
‡ ONGLYZA + metformin is considered non-inferior to glipizide + metformin because the upper limit of this confidence interval is less than the prespecified non-inferiority margin of 0.35%.
§ Significance not tested.

Table 11: Glycemic Parameters at Week 24 in a Placebo-Controlled Trial of ONGLYZA as Add-On Combination Therapy with Insulin*

Efficacy Parameter	ONGLYZA 5 mg + Insulin (+/− Metformin) N=304	Placebo + Insulin (+/− Metformin) N=151
Hemoglobin A1C (%)	N=300	N=149
Baseline (mean)	8.7	8.7
Change from baseline (adjusted mean†)	−0.7	−0.3
Difference from placebo (adjusted mean†)	−0.4‡	
95% Confidence Interval	(−0.6, −0.2)	
2-hour Postprandial Glucose (mg/dL)	N=262	N=129
Baseline (mean)	251	255
Change from baseline (adjusted mean†)	−27	−4
Difference from placebo (adjusted mean†)	−23§	
95% Confidence Interval	(−37, −9)	

* Intent-to-treat population using last observation on study or last observation prior to insulin rescue therapy for patients needing rescue.
† Least squares mean adjusted for baseline value and metformin use at baseline.
‡ p-value <0.0001 compared to placebo + insulin
§ p-value <0.05 compared to placebo + insulin

After 12 weeks of treatment, the mean change in FPG was −12 mg/dL with ONGLYZA 2.5 mg and −13 mg/dL with placebo. Compared to placebo, the mean change in FPG with ONGLYZA was −12 mg/dL in the subgroup of patients with moderate renal impairment, −4 mg/dL in the subgroup of patients with severe renal impairment, and +44 mg/dL in the subgroup of patients with ESRD. These findings are inconclusive because the trial was not adequately powered to show efficacy within specific subgroups of renal impairment. [See table 13 at top of next page]

16 HOW SUPPLIED/STORAGE AND HANDLING

How Supplied

ONGLYZA® (saxagliptin) tablets have markings on both sides and are available in the strengths and packages listed in Table 14.

[See table 14 at top of next page]

Storage and Handling

Store at 20°-25°C (68°-77°F); excursions permitted to 15°-30°C (59°-86°F) [see USP Controlled Room Temperature].

17 PATIENT COUNSELING INFORMATION

See FDA-approved Patient Labeling (Medication Guide).

Medication Guide

Healthcare providers should instruct their patients to read the Medication Guide before starting ONGLYZA therapy and to reread it each time the prescription is renewed. Patients should be instructed to inform their healthcare provider if they develop any unusual symptom or if any existing symptom persists or worsens.

Patients should be informed of the potential risks and benefits of ONGLYZA and of alternative modes of therapy. Patients should also be informed about the importance of adherence to dietary instructions, regular physical activity, periodic blood glucose monitoring and A1C testing, recognition and management of hypoglycemia and hyperglycemia, and assessment of diabetes complications. During periods of stress such as fever, trauma, infection, or surgery, medication requirements may change and patients should be advised to seek medical advice promptly.

Pancreatitis

Patients should be informed that acute pancreatitis has been reported during postmarketing use of ONGLYZA. Before initiating ONGLYZA, patients should be questioned about other risk factors for pancreatitis, such as a history of pancreatitis, alcoholism, gallstones, or hypertriglyceridemia. Patients should also be informed that persistent severe abdominal pain, sometimes radiating to the back, which may or may not be accompanied by vomiting, is the hallmark symptom of acute pancreatitis. Patients should be instructed to promptly discontinue ONGLYZA and contact their healthcare provider if persistent severe abdominal pain occurs [see *Warnings and Precautions (5.1)*].

Hypersensitivity Reactions

Patients should be informed that serious allergic (hypersensitivity) reactions, such as angioedema, anaphylaxis, and exfoliative skin conditions, have been reported during postmarketing use of ONGLYZA. If symptoms of these allergic reactions (such as rash, skin flaking or peeling, urticaria, swelling of the skin, or swelling of the face, lips, tongue, and throat that may cause difficulty in breathing or swallowing) occur, patients must stop taking ONGLYZA and seek medical advice promptly.

Missed Dose

Patients should be informed that if they miss a dose of ONGLYZA they should take the next dose as prescribed, unless otherwise instructed by their healthcare provider. Patients should be instructed not to take an extra dose the next day.

Administration Instructions

Patients should be informed that ONGLYZA tablets must not be split or cut.

Laboratory Tests

Patients should be informed that response to all diabetic therapies should be monitored by periodic measurements of blood glucose and A1C, with a goal of decreasing these levels toward the normal range. A1C is especially useful for evaluating long-term glycemic control. Patients should be informed of the potential need to adjust their dose based on changes in renal function tests over time.

Manufactured by:
Bristol-Myers Squibb Company
Princeton, NJ 08543 USA
Marketed by:
Bristol-Myers Squibb Company
Princeton, NJ 08543
and
AstraZeneca Pharmaceuticals LP
Wilmington, DE 19850
1297954A0/1256314A4

MEDICATION GUIDE
ONGLYZA (on-GLY-zah)
(saxagliptin)
tablets

Read this Medication Guide carefully before you start taking ONGLYZA and each time you get a refill. There may be new information. This information does not take the place of talking with your healthcare provider about your medical condition or treatment. If you have any questions about ONGLYZA, ask your healthcare provider.

Table 12: Glycemic Parameters at Week 24 in a Placebo-Controlled Trial of ONGLYZA as Add-On Combination Therapy with Metformin plus Sulfonylurea*

Efficacy Parameter	ONGLYZA 5 mg + Metformin plus Sulfonylurea N=129	Placebo + Metformin plus Sulfonylurea N=128
Hemoglobin A1C (%)	N=127	N=127
Baseline (mean)	8.4	8.2
Change from baseline (adjusted mean†)	−0.7	−0.1
Difference from placebo (adjusted mean†)	−0.7‡	
95% Confidence Interval	(−0.9, −0.5)	
2-hour Postprandial Glucose (mg/dL)	N=115	N=113
Baseline (mean)	268	262
Change from baseline (adjusted mean†)	−12	5
Difference from placebo (adjusted mean†)	−17§	
95% Confidence Interval	(−32, −2)	

* Intent-to-treat population using last observation prior to discontinuation.
† Least squares mean adjusted for baseline value.
‡ p-value <0.0001 compared to placebo + metformin plus sulfonylurea
§ p-value <0.05 compared to placebo + metformin plus sulfonylurea

Table 13: A1C at Week 12 in a Placebo-Controlled Trial of ONGLYZA in Patients with Renal Impairment*

Efficacy Parameter	ONGLYZA 2.5 mg N=85	Placebo N=85
Hemoglobin A1C (%)	N=81	N=83
Baseline (mean)	8.4	8.1
Change from baseline (adjusted mean†)	−0.9	−0.4
Difference from placebo (adjusted mean†)	−0.4‡	
95% Confidence Interval	(−0.7, −0.1)	

* Intent-to-treat population using last observation on study.
† Least squares mean adjusted for baseline value.
‡ p-value <0.01 compared to placebo

Table 14: ONGLYZA Tablet Presentations

Tablet Strength	Film-Coated Tablet Color/Shape	Tablet Markings	Package Size	NDC Code
5 mg	pink biconvex, round	"5" on one side and "4215" on the reverse, in blue ink	Bottles of 30 Bottles of 90 Bottles of 500 Blister of 100	0003-4215-11 0003-4215-21 0003-4215-31 0003-4215-41
2.5 mg	pale yellow to light yellow biconvex, round	"2.5" on one side and "4214" on the reverse, in blue ink	Bottles of 30 Bottles of 90	0003-4214-11 0003-4214-21

What is the most important information I should know about ONGLYZA?

Serious side effects can happen to people taking ONGLYZA, including inflammation of the pancreas (pancreatitis) which may be severe and lead to death.

Certain medical problems make you more likely to get pancreatitis.

Before you start taking ONGLYZA:

Tell your healthcare provider if you have ever had
- inflammation of your pancreas (pancreatitis)
- stones in your gallbladder (gallstones)
- a history of alcoholism
- high blood triglyceride levels

It is not known if having these medical problems will make you more likely to get pancreatitis with ONGLYZA (saxagliptin).

Stop taking ONGLYZA and contact your healthcare provider right away if you have pain in your stomach area (abdomen) that is severe and will not go away. The pain may be felt going from your abdomen through to your back. The pain may happen with or without vomiting. These may be symptoms of pancreatitis.

What is ONGLYZA?
- ONGLYZA is a prescription medicine used with diet and exercise to control high blood sugar (hyperglycemia) in adults with type 2 diabetes.
- ONGLYZA lowers blood sugar by helping the body increase the level of insulin after meals.
- ONGLYZA is unlikely by itself to cause your blood sugar to be lowered to a dangerous level (hypoglycemia) because it does not work well when your blood sugar is low. However, hypoglycemia may still occur with ONGLYZA. Your risk for getting hypoglycemia is higher if you take ONGLYZA with some other diabetes medicines, such as a sulfonylurea or insulin.
- ONGLYZA is not for people with type 1 diabetes.
- ONGLYZA (saxagliptin) is not for people with diabetic ketoacidosis (increased ketones in your blood or urine).
- If you have had pancreatitis in the past, it is not known if you have a higher chance of getting pancreatitis while you take ONGLYZA.

It is not known if ONGLYZA is safe and effective in children younger than 18 years old.

Who should not take ONGLYZA?

Do not take ONGLYZA if you:
- are allergic to any ingredients in ONGLYZA. See the end of this Medication Guide for a complete list of ingredients in ONGLYZA.

  Symptoms of a serious allergic reaction to ONGLYZA may include:
  - swelling of your face, lips, throat, and other areas on your skin
  - difficulty with swallowing or breathing
  - raised, red areas on your skin (hives)
  - skin rash, itching, flaking, or peeling

  If you have these symptoms, stop taking ONGLYZA and contact your healthcare provider right away.

What should I tell my healthcare provider before taking ONGLYZA?

Before you take ONGLYZA, tell your healthcare provider if you:
- have kidney problems.
- are pregnant or plan to become pregnant. It is not known if ONGLYZA will harm your unborn baby. If you are pregnant, talk with your healthcare provider about the best way to control your blood sugar while you are pregnant.
- are breast-feeding or plan to breast-feed. ONGLYZA may be passed in your milk to your baby. Talk with your healthcare provider about the best way to feed your baby while you take ONGLYZA.

Tell your healthcare provider about all the medicines you take, including prescription and nonprescription medicines, vitamins, and herbal supplements.

Know the medicines you take. Keep a list of your medicines and show it to your healthcare provider and pharmacist when you get a new medicine.

ONGLYZA (saxagliptin) may affect the way other medicines work, and other medicines may affect how ONGLYZA works. Contact your healthcare provider if you will be starting or stopping certain other types of medications, such as antibiotics, or medicines that treat fungus or HIV/AIDS, because your dose of ONGLYZA might need to be changed.

How should I take ONGLYZA?
- Take ONGLYZA by mouth one time each day exactly as directed by your healthcare provider. Do not change your dose without talking to your healthcare provider.
- ONGLYZA can be taken with or without food.
- Do not split or cut ONGLYZA tablets.
- During periods of stress on the body, such as:
  - fever
  - trauma
  - infection
  - surgery

  Contact your healthcare provider right away as your medication needs may change.
- Your healthcare provider should test your blood to measure how well your kidneys are working before and during your treatment with ONGLYZA. You may need a lower dose of ONGLYZA if your kidneys are not working well.
- Follow your healthcare provider's instructions for treating blood sugar that is too low (hypoglycemia). Talk to your healthcare provider if low blood sugar is a problem for you.
- If you miss a dose of ONGLYZA, take it as soon as you remember. If it is almost time for your next dose, skip the missed dose. Just take the next dose at your regular time. Do not take two doses at the same time unless your healthcare provider tells you to do so. Talk to your healthcare provider if you have questions about a missed dose.
- If you take too much ONGLYZA, call your healthcare provider or Poison Control Center at 1-800-222-1222, or go to the nearest hospital emergency room right away.

What are the possible side effects of ONGLYZA?

ONGLYZA can cause serious side effects, including:
- See **"What is the most important information I should know about ONGLYZA?"**
- **Allergic (hypersensitivity) reactions**, such as:
  - swelling of your face, lips, throat, and other areas on your skin
  - difficulty with swallowing or breathing
  - raised, red areas on your skin (hives)
  - skin rash, itching, flaking, or peeling

  If you have these symptoms, stop taking ONGLYZA and contact your healthcare provider right away.

Common side effects of ONGLYZA include:
- upper respiratory tract infection
- urinary tract infection
- headache

Low blood sugar (hypoglycemia) may become worse in people who also take another medication to treat diabetes, such as sulfonylureas or insulin. Tell your healthcare provider if you take other diabetes medicines. If you have symptoms of low blood sugar, you should check your blood sugar and treat if low, then call your healthcare provider. Symptoms of low blood sugar include:
- shaking
- sweating
- rapid heartbeat
- change in vision
- hunger
- headache
- change in mood

Swelling or fluid retention in your hands, feet, or ankles (peripheral edema) may become worse in people who also take a thiazolidinedione to treat diabetes. If you do not know whether you are already on this type of medication, ask your healthcare provider.

These are not all of the possible side effects of ONGLYZA. Tell your healthcare provider if you have any side effects that bother you or that do not go away. For more information, ask your healthcare provider.

Call your healthcare provider for medical advice about side effects. You may report side effects to the FDA at 1-800-FDA-1088.

How should I store ONGLYZA?

Store ONGLYZA between 68°F and 77°F (20°C and 25°C).

Keep ONGLYZA and all medicines out of the reach of children.

General information about the use of ONGLYZA

Medicines are sometimes prescribed for conditions that are not mentioned in Medication Guides. Do not use ONGLYZA for a condition for which it was not prescribed. Do not give ONGLYZA to other people, even if they have the same symptoms you have. It may harm them.

This Medication Guide summarizes the most important information about ONGLYZA. If you would like to know more information about ONGLYZA, talk with your healthcare provider. You can ask your healthcare provider for additional information about ONGLYZA (saxagliptin) that is written for healthcare professionals. For more information, go to www.ONGLYZA.com or call 1-800-ONGLYZA.

What are the ingredients of ONGLYZA?

Active ingredient: saxagliptin

Inactive ingredients: lactose monohydrate, microcrystalline cellulose, croscarmellose sodium, and magnesium stearate. In addition, the film coating contains the following inactive ingredients: polyvinyl alcohol, polyethylene glycol, titanium dioxide, talc, and iron oxides.

What is type 2 diabetes?

Type 2 diabetes is a condition in which your body does not make enough insulin, and the insulin that your body produces does not work as well as it should. Your body can also make too much sugar. When this happens, sugar (glucose) builds up in the blood. This can lead to serious medical problems.

The main goal of treating diabetes is to lower your blood sugar so that it is as close to normal as possible.

High blood sugar can be lowered by diet and exercise, and by certain medicines when necessary.

This Medication Guide has been approved by the U.S. Food and Drug Administration.

ONGLYZA (saxagliptin) tablets

Manufactured by:
Bristol-Myers Squibb Company
Princeton, NJ 08543 USA
Marketed by:
Bristol-Myers Squibb Company
Princeton, NJ 08543
and
AstraZeneca Pharmaceuticals LP
Wilmington, DE 19850
1297954A0/1256314A4/1296566A1
Rev May 2013

Shown in Product Identification Guide, page 306

ORENCIA ℞

[oh-REN-see-ah]
(abatacept)
for injection for intravenous use
injection, for subcutaneous use

HIGHLIGHTS OF PRESCRIBING INFORMATION
These highlights do not include all the information needed to use ORENCIA safely and effectively. See full prescribing information for ORENCIA.
ORENCIA (abatacept)
for injection for intravenous use
injection, for subcutaneous use
Initial U.S. Approval: 2005

INDICATIONS AND USAGE

ORENCIA is a selective T cell costimulation modulator indicated for:

Adult Rheumatoid Arthritis (RA) (1.1)
- moderately to severely active RA in adults. ORENCIA may be used as monotherapy or concomitantly with DMARDs other than TNF antagonists (1.1).

Juvenile Idiopathic Arthritis (1.2)
- moderately to severely active polyarticular juvenile idiopathic arthritis in pediatric patients 6 years of age and older. ORENCIA may be used as monotherapy or concomitantly with methotrexate (1.2).

Important Limitations of Use (1.3)
- should not be given concomitantly with TNF antagonists (1.3, 5.1).

DOSAGE AND ADMINISTRATION

Intravenous Administration for Adult RA (2.1)

Body Weight of Patient	Dose	Number of Vials
Less than 60 kg	500 mg	2
60 to 100 kg	750 mg	3
More than 100 kg	1000 mg	4

Subcutaneous Administration for Adult RA (2.1)
- After a single intravenous infusion as a loading dose (as per body weight categories above), 125 mg administered by a subcutaneous injection should be given within a day, followed by 125 mg subcutaneously once a week.
- Patients who are unable to receive an infusion may initiate weekly injections of subcutaneous ORENCIA without an intravenous loading dose.
- Patients transitioning from ORENCIA intravenous therapy to subcutaneous administration should administer the first subcutaneous dose instead of the next scheduled intravenous dose.

Juvenile Idiopathic Arthritis (2.2)
- Pediatric patients weighing less than 75 kg receive 10 mg/kg intravenously based on the patient's body weight. Pediatric patients weighing 75 kg or more should be administered ORENCIA following the adult intravenous dosing regimen, not to exceed a maximum dose of 1000 mg (2.2).

General Dosing Information for Intravenous Administration (2.1)
- Administer as a 30-minute intravenous infusion (2.1)
- Following initial dose, give at 2 and 4 weeks, then every 4 weeks (2.1)
- Prepare ORENCIA using only the silicone-free disposable syringe (2.3)
- Use only sterile water to reconstitute the powder (2.3)
- The reconstituted product must be administered using a filter (2.3)

DOSAGE FORMS AND STRENGTHS

- 250 mg lyophilized powder in a single-use vial for intravenous infusion (3)
- 125 mg/mL solution in a single-dose prefilled syringe (3)

CONTRAINDICATIONS

- None (4)

WARNINGS AND PRECAUTIONS

- Concomitant use with a TNF antagonist can increase the risk of infections and serious infections (5.1)
- Hypersensitivity, anaphylaxis, and anaphylactoid reactions (5.2)
- Patients with a history of recurrent infections or underlying conditions predisposing to infections may experience more infections (5.3, 8.5)
- Discontinue if a serious infection develops (5.3)
- Screen for latent TB infection prior to initiating therapy. Patients testing positive should be treated prior to initiating ORENCIA (5.3)
- Live vaccines should not be given concurrently or within 3 months of discontinuation (5.4)
- Patients with juvenile idiopathic arthritis should be brought up to date with all immunizations prior to ORENCIA therapy (5.4)
- Based on its mechanism of action, ORENCIA may blunt the effectiveness of some immunizations (5.4)
- COPD patients may develop more frequent respiratory adverse events (5.5)

ADVERSE REACTIONS

Most common adverse events (≥10%) are headache, upper respiratory tract infection, nasopharyngitis, and nausea (6.1).

To report SUSPECTED ADVERSE REACTIONS, contact Bristol-Myers Squibb at 1-800-721-5072 or FDA at 1-800-FDA-1088 or *www.fda.gov/medwatch.*

USE IN SPECIFIC POPULATIONS

- Pregnancy: Registry available. Based on animal data, may cause fetal harm (8.1).

See 17 for PATIENT COUNSELING INFORMATION and FDA-approved patient labeling

Revised: 07/2013

FULL PRESCRIBING INFORMATION: CONTENTS*

*** Sections or subsections omitted from the full prescribing information are not listed**

FULL PRESCRIBING INFORMATION

1 INDICATIONS AND USAGE

1.1 Adult Rheumatoid Arthritis (RA)

ORENCIA® (abatacept) is indicated for reducing signs and symptoms, inducing major clinical response, inhibiting the progression of structural damage, and improving physical function in adult patients with moderately to severely active rheumatoid arthritis. ORENCIA may be used as monotherapy or concomitantly with disease-modifying antirheumatic drugs (DMARDs) other than tumor necrosis factor (TNF) antagonists.

1.2 Juvenile Idiopathic Arthritis

ORENCIA is indicated for reducing signs and symptoms in pediatric patients 6 years of age and older with moderately to severely active polyarticular juvenile idiopathic arthritis. ORENCIA may be used as monotherapy or concomitantly with methotrexate (MTX).

1.3 Important Limitations of Use

ORENCIA should not be administered concomitantly with TNF antagonists. ORENCIA is not recommended for use concomitantly with other biologic rheumatoid arthritis (RA) therapy, such as anakinra.

2 DOSAGE AND ADMINISTRATION

2.1 Adult Rheumatoid Arthritis

For adult patients with RA, ORENCIA may be administered as an intravenous infusion or a subcutaneous injection.

ORENCIA may be used as monotherapy or concomitantly with DMARDs other than TNF antagonists.

For pediatric juvenile idiopathic arthritis, a dose calculated based on each patient's body weight is used [see *Dosage and Administration (2.2)*].

Intravenous Dosing Regimen

ORENCIA intravenous should be administered as a 30-minute intravenous infusion utilizing the weight range-based dosing specified in Table 1. Following the initial intravenous administration, an intravenous infusion should be given at 2 and 4 weeks after the first infusion and every 4 weeks thereafter.

Table 1: Dose of ORENCIA for Intravenous Infusion in Adult RA Patients

Body Weight of Patient	Dose	Number of Vials[a]
Less than 60 kg	500 mg	2
60 to 100 kg	750 mg	3
More than 100 kg	1000 mg	4

[a] Each vial provides 250 mg of abatacept for administration.

Subcutaneous Dosing Regimen

Following a single intravenous loading dose (as per body weight categories listed in Table 1), the first 125 mg subcutaneous injection of ORENCIA should be given within a day, followed by 125 mg subcutaneous injections once weekly.

Patients who are unable to receive an infusion may initiate weekly injections of subcutaneous ORENCIA without an intravenous loading dose.

Patients transitioning from ORENCIA intravenous therapy to subcutaneous administration should administer the first subcutaneous dose instead of the next scheduled intravenous dose.

2.2 Juvenile Idiopathic Arthritis

The recommended dose of ORENCIA (abatacept) for patients 6 to 17 years of age with juvenile idiopathic arthritis who weigh less than 75 kg is 10 mg/kg intravenously calculated based on the patient's body weight at each administration. Pediatric patients weighing 75 kg or more should be administered ORENCIA following the adult intravenous dosing regimen, not to exceed a maximum dose of 1000 mg. ORENCIA should be administered as a 30-minute intravenous infusion. Following the initial administration, ORENCIA should be given at 2 and 4 weeks after the first infusion and every 4 weeks thereafter. Any unused portions in the vials must be immediately discarded.

The safety and efficacy of subcutaneous ORENCIA injection has not been studied in patients under 18 years of age.

2.3 Preparation and Administration Instructions for Intravenous Infusion

Use aseptic technique.

ORENCIA is provided as a lyophilized powder in preservative-free, single-use vials. Each ORENCIA vial provides 250 mg of abatacept for administration. The ORENCIA powder in each vial must be reconstituted with 10 mL of Sterile Water for Injection, USP, using *only the silicone-free disposable syringe provided with each vial* and an 18- to 21-gauge needle. After reconstitution, the concentration of abatacept in the vial will be 25 mg/mL. If the ORENCIA powder is accidentally reconstituted using a siliconized syringe, the solution may develop a few translucent particles. Discard any solutions prepared using siliconized syringes.

If the *silicone-free disposable syringe* is dropped or becomes contaminated, use a new *silicone-free disposable syringe* from inventory. For information on obtaining additional *silicone-free disposable syringes*, contact Bristol-Myers Squibb 1-800-ORENCIA.

1) Use 10 mL of Sterile Water for Injection, USP to reconstitute the ORENCIA powder. To reconstitute the ORENCIA powder, remove the flip-top from the vial and wipe the top with an alcohol swab. Insert the syringe needle into the vial through the center of the rubber stopper and direct the stream of Sterile Water for Injection, USP, to the glass wall of the vial. Do not use the vial if the vacuum is not present. Rotate the vial with gentle swirling to minimize foam formation, until the contents are completely dissolved. Do not shake. Avoid prolonged or vigorous agitation.
2) Upon complete dissolution of the lyophilized powder, the vial should be vented with a needle to dissipate any foam that may be present. After reconstitution, each milliliter will contain 25 mg (250 mg/10 mL). The solution should be clear and colorless to pale yellow. Do not use if opaque particles, discoloration, or other foreign particles are present.
3) The reconstituted ORENCIA solution must be further diluted to 100 mL as follows. From a 100 mL infusion bag or bottle, withdraw a volume of 0.9% Sodium Chloride Injection, USP, equal to the volume of the reconstituted ORENCIA solution required for the patient's dose. Slowly add the reconstituted ORENCIA solution into the infusion bag or bottle using the same *silicone-free disposable syringe provided with each vial*. Gently mix. *Do not shake the bag or bottle*. The final concentration of abatacept in the bag or bottle will depend upon the amount of drug added, but will be no more than 10 mg/mL. Any unused portions in the vials must be immediately discarded.
4) Prior to administration, the ORENCIA solution should be inspected visually for particulate matter and discoloration. Discard the solution if any particulate matter or discoloration is observed.
5) The entire, fully diluted ORENCIA solution should be administered over a period of 30 minutes and must be administered with an infusion set and a *sterile, non-pyrogenic, low-protein-binding filter* (pore size of 0.2 µm to 1.2 µm).
6) The infusion of the fully diluted ORENCIA solution must be completed within 24 hours of reconstitution of the ORENCIA vials. The fully diluted ORENCIA solution may be stored at room temperature or refrigerated at 2°C to 8°C (36°F to 46°F) before use. Discard the fully diluted solution if not administered within 24 hours.
7) ORENCIA should not be infused concomitantly in the same intravenous line with other agents. No physical or biochemical compatibility studies have been conducted to evaluate the coadministration of ORENCIA with other agents.

2.4 General Considerations for Subcutaneous Administration

ORENCIA Injection, 125 mg/syringe is not intended for intravenous infusion.

ORENCIA Injection is intended for use under the guidance of a physician or healthcare practitioner. After proper training in subcutaneous injection technique, a patient may self-inject with ORENCIA if a physician/healthcare practitioner determines that it is appropriate. Patients should be instructed to follow the directions provided in the Instructions for Use for additional details on medication administration. Parenteral drug products should be inspected visually for particulate matter and discoloration prior to administration, whenever solution and container permit. Do not use ORENCIA (abatacept) prefilled syringes exhibiting particulate matter or discoloration. ORENCIA should be clear and colorless to pale yellow.

Patients using ORENCIA for subcutaneous administration should be instructed to inject the full amount in the syringe (1 mL), which provides 125 mg of ORENCIA, according to the directions provided in the Instructions for Use.

Injection sites should be rotated and injections should never be given into areas where the skin is tender, bruised, red, or hard.

3 DOSAGE FORMS AND STRENGTHS

- **Lyophilized Powder for Intravenous Infusion**
  250 mg single-use vial
- **Solution for Subcutaneous Injection**
  125 mg/mL single-dose prefilled glass syringe

4 CONTRAINDICATIONS

None.

5 WARNINGS AND PRECAUTIONS

5.1 Concomitant Use with TNF Antagonists

In controlled clinical trials in patients with adult RA, patients receiving concomitant intravenous ORENCIA and TNF antagonist therapy experienced more infections (63%) and serious infections (4.4%) compared to patients treated with only TNF antagonists (43% and 0.8%, respectively) [see *Adverse Reactions (6.1)*]. These trials failed to demonstrate an important enhancement of efficacy with concomitant administration of ORENCIA with TNF antagonist; therefore, concurrent therapy with ORENCIA and a TNF antagonist is not recommended. While transitioning from TNF antagonist therapy to ORENCIA therapy, patients should be monitored for signs of infection.

5.2 Hypersensitivity

In controlled, double-blind and open-label clinical trials, the occurrence of anaphylaxis and anaphylactoid reactions was rare (<0.1%) and was only observed in patients dosed with intravenous ORENCIA. Other reactions potentially associated with drug hypersensitivity, such as hypotension, urticaria, and dyspnea that occurred within 24 hours of ORENCIA infusion, were uncommon (<1%). Of the 190 patients with juvenile idiopathic arthritis treated with ORENCIA in clinical trials, there was one case of a hypersensitivity reaction (0.5%). Appropriate medical support measures for the treatment of hypersensitivity reactions should be available for immediate use in the event of a reaction [see *Adverse Reactions (6.1, 6.3)*]. Anaphylaxis or anaphylactoid reactions can occur after the first infusion and can be life threatening. In postmarketing experience, a case of fatal anaphylaxis following the first infusion of ORENCIA has been reported. If an anaphylactic or other serious allergic reaction occurs, administration of ORENCIA should be stopped immediately with appropriate therapy instituted, and the use of ORENCIA should be permanently discontinued.

5.3 Infections

Serious infections, including sepsis and pneumonia, have been reported in patients receiving ORENCIA. Some of these infections have been fatal. Many of the serious infections have occurred in patients on concomitant immunosuppressive therapy which in addition to their underlying disease, could further predispose them to infection. Physicians should exercise caution when considering the use of ORENCIA in patients with a history of recurrent infections, underlying conditions which may predispose them to infections, or chronic, latent, or localized infections. Patients who develop a new infection while undergoing treatment with ORENCIA should be monitored closely. Administration of ORENCIA should be discontinued if a patient develops a serious infection [see *Adverse Reactions (6.1)*]. A higher rate of serious infections has been observed in adult RA patients treated with concurrent TNF antagonists and ORENCIA [see *Warnings and Precautions (5.1)*].

Prior to initiating immunomodulatory therapies, including ORENCIA, patients should be screened for latent tuberculosis infection with a tuberculin skin test. ORENCIA has not been studied in patients with a positive tuberculosis screen, and the safety of ORENCIA in individuals with latent tuberculosis infection is unknown. Patients testing positive in tuberculosis screening should be treated by standard medical practice prior to therapy with ORENCIA.

Antirheumatic therapies have been associated with hepatitis B reactivation. Therefore, screening for viral hepatitis should be performed in accordance with published guidelines before starting therapy with ORENCIA. In clinical studies with ORENCIA, patients who screened positive for hepatitis were excluded from study.

5.4 Immunizations

Live vaccines should not be given concurrently with ORENCIA or within 3 months of its discontinuation. No data are available on the secondary transmission of infection from persons receiving live vaccines to patients receiving ORENCIA (abatacept). The efficacy of vaccination in patients receiving ORENCIA is not known. Based on its mechanism of action, ORENCIA may blunt the effectiveness of some immunizations.

It is recommended that patients with juvenile idiopathic arthritis be brought up to date with all immunizations in agreement with current immunization guidelines prior to initiating ORENCIA therapy.

5.5 Use in Patients with Chronic Obstructive Pulmonary Disease (COPD)

Adult COPD patients treated with ORENCIA developed adverse events more frequently than those treated with placebo, including COPD exacerbations, cough, rhonchi, and dyspnea. Use of ORENCIA in patients with RA and COPD should be undertaken with caution and such patients should be monitored for worsening of their respiratory status [see *Adverse Reactions (6.1)*].

5.6 Immunosuppression

The possibility exists for drugs inhibiting T cell activation, including ORENCIA, to affect host defenses against infections and malignancies since T cells mediate cellular immune responses. The impact of treatment with ORENCIA on the development and course of malignancies is not fully understood [see *Adverse Reactions (6.1)*]. In clinical trials in patients with adult RA, a higher rate of infections was seen in ORENCIA-treated patients compared to placebo [see *Adverse Reactions (6.1)*].

6 ADVERSE REACTIONS

6.1 Clinical Studies Experience in Adult RA Patients Treated with Intravenous ORENCIA

Because clinical trials are conducted under widely varying and controlled conditions, adverse reaction rates observed in clinical trials of a drug cannot be directly compared to rates in the clinical trials of another drug and may not predict the rates observed in a broader patient population in clinical practice.

The data described herein reflect exposure to ORENCIA administered intravenously in patients with active RA in placebo-controlled studies (1955 patients with ORENCIA, 989 with placebo). The studies had either a double-blind, placebo-controlled period of 6 months (258 patients with ORENCIA, 133 with placebo) or 1 year (1697 patients with ORENCIA, 856 with placebo). A subset of these patients received concomitant biologic DMARD therapy, such as a TNF blocking agent (204 patients with ORENCIA, 134 with placebo).

The majority of patients in RA clinical studies received one or more of the following concomitant medications with ORENCIA: methotrexate, nonsteroidal anti-inflammatory drugs (NSAIDs), corticosteroids, TNF blocking agents, azathioprine, chloroquine, gold, hydroxychloroquine, leflunomide, sulfasalazine, and anakinra.

The most serious adverse reactions were serious infections and malignancies.

The most commonly reported adverse events (occurring in ≥10% of patients treated with ORENCIA) were headache, upper respiratory tract infection, nasopharyngitis, and nausea.

The adverse events most frequently resulting in clinical intervention (interruption or discontinuation of ORENCIA) were due to infection. The most frequently reported infections resulting in dose interruption were upper respiratory tract infection (1.0%), bronchitis (0.7%), and herpes zoster (0.7%). The most frequent infections resulting in discontinuation were pneumonia (0.2%), localized infection (0.2%), and bronchitis (0.1%).

Infections

In the placebo-controlled trials, infections were reported in 54% of ORENCIA-treated patients and 48% of placebo-treated patients. The most commonly reported infections (reported in 5%-13% of patients) were upper respiratory tract infection, nasopharyngitis, sinusitis, urinary tract infection, influenza, and bronchitis. Other infections reported in fewer than 5% of patients at a higher frequency (>0.5%) with ORENCIA compared to placebo, were rhinitis, herpes simplex, and pneumonia [see *Warnings and Precautions (5.3)*].

Serious infections were reported in 3.0% of patients treated with ORENCIA and 1.9% of patients treated with placebo. The most common (0.2%-0.5%) serious infections reported with ORENCIA were pneumonia, cellulitis, urinary tract infection, bronchitis, diverticulitis, and acute pyelonephritis [see *Warnings and Precautions (5.3)*].

Malignancies

In the placebo-controlled portions of the clinical trials (1955 patients treated with ORENCIA for a median of 12 months), the overall frequencies of malignancies were similar in the ORENCIA- and placebo-treated patients (1.3% and 1.1%, respectively). However, more cases of lung cancer were observed in ORENCIA-treated patients (4, 0.2%) than placebo-treated patients (0). In the cumulative ORENCIA clinical trials (placebo-controlled and uncontrolled, open-label) a total of 8 cases of lung cancer (0.21 cases per 100 patient-years) and 4 lymphomas (0.10 cases per 100 patient-years) were observed in 2688 patients (3827 patient-years). The rate observed for lymphoma is approximately 3.5-fold higher than expected in an age- and gender-matched general population based on the National Cancer Institute's Surveillance, Epidemiology, and End Results Database. Patients with RA, particularly those with highly active disease, are at a higher risk for the development of lymphoma. Other malignancies included skin, breast, bile duct, bladder, cervical, endometrial, lymphoma, melanoma, myelodysplastic syndrome, ovarian, prostate, renal, thyroid, and uterine cancers [see *Warnings and Precautions (5.6)*]. The potential role of ORENCIA in the development of malignancies in humans is unknown.

Infusion-Related Reactions and Hypersensitivity Reactions

Acute infusion-related events (adverse reactions occurring within 1 hour of the start of the infusion) in Studies III, IV, and V [see *Clinical Studies (14.1)*] were more common in the ORENCIA-treated patients than the placebo patients (9% for ORENCIA (abatacept), 6% for placebo). The most frequently reported events (1%-2%) were dizziness, headache, and hypertension.

Acute infusion-related events that were reported in >0.1% and ≤1% of patients treated with ORENCIA included cardiopulmonary symptoms, such as hypotension, increased blood pressure, and dyspnea; other symptoms included nausea, flushing, urticaria, cough, hypersensitivity, pruritus, rash, and wheezing. Most of these reactions were mild (68%) to moderate (28%). Fewer than 1% of ORENCIA-treated patients discontinued due to an acute infusion-related event. In controlled trials, 6 ORENCIA-treated patients compared to 2 placebo-treated patients discontinued study treatment due to acute infusion-related events.

Anaphylaxis was observed in patients dosed with ORENCIA administered intravenously in controlled and open-label clinical trials, and the occurrence was rare (<0.1%). Other reactions potentially associated with drug hypersensitivity, such as hypotension, urticaria, and dyspnea that occurred within 24 hours of ORENCIA infusion, were uncommon (<1%). Appropriate medical support measures for the treatment of hypersensitivity reactions should be available for immediate use in the event of a reaction [see *Warnings and Precautions (5.2)*].

Adverse Reactions in Patients with COPD

In Study V [see *Clinical Studies (14.1)*], there were 37 patients with chronic obstructive pulmonary disease (COPD) who were treated with ORENCIA and 17 COPD patients who were treated with placebo. The COPD patients treated with ORENCIA developed adverse events more frequently than those treated with placebo (97% vs 88%, respectively). Respiratory disorders occurred more frequently in ORENCIA-treated patients compared to placebo-treated patients (43% vs 24%, respectively) including COPD exacerbation, cough, rhonchi, and dyspnea. A greater percentage of ORENCIA-treated patients developed a serious adverse event compared to placebo-treated patients (27% vs 6%), including COPD exacerbation (3 of 37 patients [8%]) and pneumonia (1 of 37 patients [3%]) [see *Warnings and Precautions (5.5)*].

Other Adverse Reactions

Adverse events occurring in 3% or more of patients and at least 1% more frequently in ORENCIA-treated patients during placebo-controlled RA studies are summarized in Table 2.

Table 2: Adverse Events Occurring in 3% or More of Patients and at Least 1% More Frequently in ORENCIA-Treated Patients During Placebo-Controlled RA Studies

Adverse Event (Preferred Term)	ORENCIA (n=1955)[a] Percentage	Placebo (n=989)[b] Percentage
Headache	18	13
Nasopharyngitis	12	9
Dizziness	9	7
Cough	8	7
Back pain	7	6
Hypertension	7	4
Dyspepsia	6	4
Urinary tract infection	6	5
Rash	4	3
Pain in extremity	3	2

[a] Includes 204 patients on concomitant biologic DMARDs (adalimumab, anakinra, etanercept, or infliximab).

[b] Includes 134 patients on concomitant biologic DMARDs (adalimumab, anakinra, etanercept, or infliximab).

Immunogenicity

Antibodies directed against the entire abatacept molecule or to the CTLA-4 portion of abatacept were assessed by ELISA assays in RA patients for up to 2 years following repeated treatment with ORENCIA (abatacept). Thirty-four of 1993 (1.7%) patients developed binding antibodies to the entire abatacept molecule or to the CTLA-4 portion of abatacept. Because trough levels of abatacept can interfere with assay results, a subset analysis was performed. In this analysis it was observed that 9 of 154 (5.8%) patients that had discontinued treatment with ORENCIA for over 56 days developed antibodies.

Samples with confirmed binding activity to CTLA-4 were assessed for the presence of neutralizing antibodies in a cell-based luciferase reporter assay. Six of 9 (67%) evaluable patients were shown to possess neutralizing antibodies. However, the development of neutralizing antibodies may be underreported due to lack of assay sensitivity.

No correlation of antibody development to clinical response or adverse events was observed.

The data reflect the percentage of patients whose test results were positive for antibodies to abatacept in specific assays. The observed incidence of antibody (including neutralizing antibody) positivity in an assay is highly dependent on several factors, including assay sensitivity and specificity, assay methodology, sample handling, timing of sample collection, concomitant medication, and underlying disease. For these reasons, comparison of the incidence of antibodies to abatacept with the incidence of antibodies to other products may be misleading.

Clinical Experience in Methotrexate-Naive Patients

Study VI was an active-controlled clinical trial in methotrexate-naive patients [see *Clinical Studies (14.1)*]. The safety experience in these patients was consistent with Studies I-V.

6.2 Clinical Experience in Adult RA Patients Treated with Subcutaneous ORENCIA

Because clinical trials are conducted under widely varying and controlled conditions, adverse reaction rates observed in clinical trials of a drug cannot be directly compared to rates in the clinical trials of another drug and may not predict the rates observed in a broader patient population in clinical practice.

Study SC-I was a randomized, double-blind, double-dummy, non-inferiority study that compared the efficacy and safety of abatacept administered subcutaneously (SC) and intravenously (IV) in 1457 subjects with rheumatoid arthritis, receiving background methotrexate, and experiencing an inadequate response to methotrexate (MTX-IR) [see *Clinical Studies (14.1)*]. The safety experience and immunogenicity for ORENCIA administered subcutaneously was consistent with intravenous Studies I-VI. Due to the route of administration, injection site reactions and immunogenicity were evaluated in Study SC-I and two other smaller studies discussed in the sections below.

Injection Site Reactions in Adult RA Patients Treated with Subcutaneous ORENCIA

Study SC-I compared the safety of abatacept including injection site reactions following subcutaneous or intravenous administration. The overall frequency of injection site reactions was 2.6% (19/736) and 2.5% (18/721) for the subcutaneous abatacept group and the intravenous abatacept group (subcutaneous placebo), respectively. All these injection site reactions (including hematoma, pruritus, and erythema) were mild (83%) to moderate (17%) in severity, and none necessitated drug discontinuation.

Immunogenicity in Adult RA Patients Treated with Subcutaneous ORENCIA

Study SC-I compared the immunogenicity to abatacept following subcutaneous or intravenous administration. The overall immunogenicity frequency to abatacept was 1.1% (8/725) and 2.3% (16/710) for the subcutaneous and intravenous groups, respectively. The rate is consistent with previous experience, and there was no correlation of immunogenicity with effects on pharmacokinetics, safety, or efficacy.

Immunogenicity and Safety of Subcutaneous ORENCIA Administration as Monotherapy without an Intravenous Loading Dose

Study SC-II was conducted to determine the effect of monotherapy use of ORENCIA on immunogenicity following subcutaneous administration without an intravenous load in 100 RA patients, who had not previously received abatacept or other CTLA4Ig, who received either subcutaneous ORENCIA plus methotrexate (n=51) or subcutaneous ORENCIA monotherapy (n=49). No patients in either group developed anti-product antibodies after 4 months of treatment. The safety observed in this study was consistent with that observed in the other subcutaneous studies.

Immunogenicity and Safety of Subcutaneous ORENCIA upon Withdrawal (Three Months) and Restart of Treatment

Study SC-III in the subcutaneous program was conducted to investigate the effect of withdrawal (three months) and restart of ORENCIA subcutaneous treatment on immunogenicity in RA patients treated concomitantly with methotrexate. One hundred sixty-seven patients were enrolled in the first 3-month treatment period and responders (n=120) were randomized to either subcutaneous ORENCIA (abatacept) or placebo for the second 3-month period (withdrawal period). Patients from this period then received open-label ORENCIA treatment in the final 3-month period of the study (period 3). At the end of the withdrawal period, 0/38 patients who continued to receive subcutaneous ORENCIA developed anti-product antibodies compared to 7/73 (9.6%) of patients who had subcutaneous ORENCIA withdrawn during this period. Half of the patients receiving subcutaneous placebo during the withdrawal period received a single intravenous infusion of ORENCIA at the start of period 3 and half received intravenous placebo. At the end of period 3, when all patients again received subcutaneous ORENCIA, the immunogenicity rates were 1/38 (2.6%) in the group receiving subcutaneous ORENCIA throughout, and 2/73 (2.7%) in the group that had received placebo during the withdrawal period. Upon reinitiating therapy, there were no injection reactions and no differences in response to therapy in patients who were withdrawn from subcutaneous therapy for up to 3 months relative to those who remained on subcutaneous therapy, whether therapy was reintroduced with or without an intravenous loading dose. The safety observed in this study was consistent with that observed in the other studies.

6.3 Clinical Studies Experience in Juvenile Idiopathic Arthritis

In general, the adverse events in pediatric patients were similar in frequency and type to those seen in adult patients [see *Warnings and Precautions (5), Adverse Reactions (6)*]. ORENCIA has been studied in 190 pediatric patients, 6 to 17 years of age, with polyarticular juvenile idiopathic arthritis. Overall frequency of adverse events in the 4-month, lead-in, open-label period of the study was 70%; infections occurred at a frequency of 36% [see *Clinical Studies (14.2)*]. The most common infections were upper respiratory tract infection and nasopharyngitis. The infections resolved without sequelae, and the types of infections were consistent with those commonly seen in outpatient pediatric populations. Other events that occurred at a prevalence of at least 5% were headache, nausea, diarrhea, cough, pyrexia, and abdominal pain.

A total of 6 serious adverse events (acute lymphocytic leukemia, ovarian cyst, varicella infection, disease flare [2], and joint wear) were reported during the initial 4 months of treatment with ORENCIA.

Of the 190 patients with juvenile idiopathic arthritis treated with ORENCIA in clinical trials, there was one case of a hypersensitivity reaction (0.5%). During Periods A, B, and C, acute infusion-related reactions occurred at a frequency of 4%, 2%, and 3%, respectively, and were consistent with the types of events reported in adults.

Upon continued treatment in the open-label extension period, the types of adverse events were similar in frequency and type to those seen in adult patients, except for a single patient diagnosed with multiple sclerosis while on open-label treatment.

Immunogenicity

Antibodies directed against the entire abatacept molecule or to the CTLA-4 portion of abatacept were assessed by ELISA assays in patients with juvenile idiopathic arthritis following repeated treatment with ORENCIA throughout the open-label period. For patients who were withdrawn from therapy for up to 6 months during the double-blind period, the rate of antibody formation to the CTLA-4 portion of the molecule was 41% (22/54), while for those who remained on therapy the rate was 13% (7/54). Twenty of these patients had samples that could be tested for antibodies with neutralizing activity; of these, 8 (40%) patients were shown to possess neutralizing antibodies.

The presence of antibodies was generally transient and titers were low. The presence of antibodies was not associated with adverse events, changes in efficacy, or an effect on serum concentrations of abatacept. For patients who were withdrawn from ORENCIA during the double-blind period for up to 6 months, no serious acute infusion-related events were observed upon re-initiation of ORENCIA therapy.

6.4 Postmarketing Experience

Adverse reactions have been reported during the postapproval use of ORENCIA. Because these reactions are reported voluntarily from a population of uncertain size, it is not always possible to reliably estimate their frequency or establish a causal relationship to ORENCIA. Based on the postmarketing experience in adult RA patients, the following adverse reaction has been identified during postapproval use with ORENCIA.

- Vasculitis (including cutaneous vasculitis and leukocytoclastic vasculitis)

7 DRUG INTERACTIONS

7.1 TNF Antagonists

Concurrent administration of a TNF antagonist with ORENCIA has been associated with an increased risk of serious infections and no significant additional efficacy over use of the TNF antagonists alone. Concurrent therapy with ORENCIA and TNF antagonists is not recommended [see *Warnings and Precautions (5.1)*].

7.2 Other Biologic RA Therapy

There is insufficient experience to assess the safety and efficacy of ORENCIA (abatacept) administered concurrently with other biologic RA therapy, such as anakinra, and therefore such use is not recommended.

7.3 Blood Glucose Testing

Parenteral drug products containing maltose can interfere with the readings of blood glucose monitors that use test strips with glucose dehydrogenase pyrroloquinolinequinone (GDH-PQQ). The GDH-PQQ based glucose monitoring systems may react with the maltose present in ORENCIA for intravenous administration, resulting in falsely elevated blood glucose readings on the day of infusion. When receiving ORENCIA through intravenous administration, patients that require blood glucose monitoring should be advised to consider methods that do not react with maltose, such as those based on glucose dehydrogenase nicotine adenine dinucleotide (GDH-NAD), glucose oxidase, or glucose hexokinase test methods.

ORENCIA for subcutaneous administration does not contain maltose; therefore, patients do not need to alter their glucose monitoring.

8 USE IN SPECIFIC POPULATIONS

8.1 Pregnancy

Pregnancy Category C

There are no adequate and well-controlled studies of ORENCIA use in pregnant women. Abatacept has been shown to cross the placenta in animals, and in animal reproduction studies alterations in immune function occurred. ORENCIA should be used during pregnancy only if the potential benefit to the mother justifies the potential risk to the fetus.

Abatacept was not teratogenic when administered to pregnant mice at doses up to 300 mg/kg and in pregnant rats and rabbits at doses up to 200 mg/kg daily representing approximately 29 times the exposure associated with the maximum recommended human dose (MRHD) of 10 mg/kg based on AUC (area under the time-concentration curve).

Abatacept administered to female rats every three days during early gestation and throughout the lactation period, produced no adverse effects in offspring at doses up to 45 mg/kg, representing 3 times the exposure associated with the MRHD of 10 mg/kg based on AUC. However, at 200 mg/kg, 11 times the MRHD exposure, alterations in immune function were observed consisting of a 9-fold increase in T-cell dependent antibody response in female pups and thyroid inflammation in one female pup. It is not known whether these findings indicate a risk for development of autoimmune diseases in humans exposed *in utero* to abatacept. However, exposure to abatacept in the juvenile rat, which may be more representative of the fetal immune system state in the human, resulted in immune system abnormalities including inflammation of the thyroid and pancreas [see *Nonclinical Toxicology (13.2)*].

Pregnancy Registry: To monitor maternal-fetal outcomes of pregnant women exposed to ORENCIA, a pregnancy registry has been established. Healthcare professionals are encouraged to register patients and pregnant women are encouraged to enroll themselves by calling 1-877-311-8972.

8.3 Nursing Mothers

It is not known whether ORENCIA is excreted into human milk or absorbed systemically after ingestion by a nursing infant. However, abatacept was excreted in rat milk. Because many drugs are excreted in human milk, and because of the potential for serious adverse reactions in nursing infants from ORENCIA, a decision should be made whether to discontinue nursing or to discontinue the drug, taking into account the importance of the drug to the mother.

8.4 Pediatric Use

Intravenous ORENCIA is indicated for reducing signs and symptoms in pediatric patients with moderately to severely active polyarticular juvenile idiopathic arthritis ages 6 years and older. ORENCIA may be used as monotherapy or concomitantly with methotrexate.

Studies in juvenile rats exposed to ORENCIA prior to immune system maturity have shown immune system abnormalities including an increase in the incidence of infections leading to death as well as inflammation of the thyroid and pancreas [see *Nonclinical Toxicology (13.2)*]. Studies in adult mice and monkeys have not demonstrated similar findings. As the immune system of the rat is undeveloped in the first few weeks after birth, the relevance of these results to humans greater than 6 years of age (where the immune system is largely developed) is unknown.

ORENCIA is not recommended for use in patients below the age of 6 years.

The safety and effectiveness of ORENCIA in pediatric patients below 6 years of age have not been established. The safety and efficacy of ORENCIA in pediatric patients for uses other than juvenile idiopathic arthritis have not been established.

The safety and efficacy of subcutaneous ORENCIA has not been studied in patients under 18 years of age.

8.5 Geriatric Use

A total of 323 patients 65 years of age and older, including 53 patients 75 years and older, received ORENCIA (abatacept) in clinical studies. No overall differences in safety or effectiveness were observed between these patients and younger patients, but these numbers are too low to rule out differences. The frequency of serious infection and malignancy among ORENCIA-treated patients over age 65 was higher than for those under age 65. Because there is a higher incidence of infections and malignancies in the elderly population in general, caution should be used when treating the elderly.

10 OVERDOSAGE

Doses up to 50 mg/kg have been administered intravenously without apparent toxic effect. In case of overdosage, it is recommended that the patient be monitored for any signs or symptoms of adverse reactions and appropriate symptomatic treatment instituted.

11 DESCRIPTION

ORENCIA® (abatacept) is a soluble fusion protein that consists of the extracellular domain of human cytotoxic T-lymphocyte-associated antigen 4 (CTLA-4) linked to the modified Fc (hinge, CH2, and CH3 domains) portion of human immunoglobulin G1 (IgG1). Abatacept is produced by recombinant DNA technology in a mammalian cell expression system. The apparent molecular weight of abatacept is 92 kilodaltons.

ORENCIA lyophilized powder for intravenous infusion is supplied as a sterile, white, preservative-free, lyophilized powder for intravenous administration. Following reconstitution of the lyophilized powder with 10 mL of Sterile Water for Injection, USP, the solution of ORENCIA is clear, colorless to pale yellow, with a pH range of 7.2 to 7.8. Each single-use vial of ORENCIA provides 250 mg abatacept, maltose (500 mg), monobasic sodium phosphate (17.2 mg), and sodium chloride (14.6 mg) for administration.

ORENCIA solution for subcutaneous administration is supplied as a sterile, preservative-free, clear, colorless to pale-yellow solution with a pH of 6.8 to 7.4. Each single dose of subcutaneous injection provides 125 mg abatacept, dibasic sodium phosphate anhydrous (0.838 mg), monobasic sodium phosphate monohydrate (0.286 mg), poloxamer 188 (8 mg), sucrose (170 mg), and quantity sufficient to 1 mL with water for injection. Unlike the intravenous formulation, ORENCIA solution for subcutaneous administration contains no maltose.

12 CLINICAL PHARMACOLOGY

12.1 Mechanism of Action

Abatacept, a selective costimulation modulator, inhibits T cell (T lymphocyte) activation by binding to CD80 and CD86, thereby blocking interaction with CD28. This interaction provides a costimulatory signal necessary for full activation of T lymphocytes. Activated T lymphocytes are implicated in the pathogenesis of RA and are found in the synovium of patients with RA.

In vitro, abatacept decreases T cell proliferation and inhibits the production of the cytokines TNF alpha (TNFα), interferon-γ, and interleukin-2. In a rat collagen-induced arthritis model, abatacept suppresses inflammation, decreases anti-collagen antibody production, and reduces antigen specific production of interferon-γ. The relationship of these biological response markers to the mechanisms by which ORENCIA exerts its effects in RA is unknown.

12.2 Pharmacodynamics

In clinical trials with ORENCIA at doses approximating 10 mg/kg, decreases were observed in serum levels of soluble interleukin-2 receptor (sIL-2R), interleukin-6 (IL-6), rheumatoid factor (RF), C-reactive protein (CRP), matrix metalloproteinase-3 (MMP3), and TNFα. The relationship of these biological response markers to the mechanisms by which ORENCIA exerts its effects in RA is unknown.

12.3 Pharmacokinetics

Healthy Adults and Adult RA - Intravenous Administration

The pharmacokinetics of abatacept were studied in healthy adult subjects after a single 10 mg/kg intravenous infusion and in RA patients after multiple 10 mg/kg intravenous infusions (see Table 3).

Table 3: Pharmacokinetic Parameters (Mean, Range) in Healthy Subjects and RA Patients After 10 mg/kg Intravenous Infusion(s)

PK Parameter	Healthy Subjects (After 10 mg/kg Single Dose) n=13	RA Patients (After 10 mg/kg Multiple Doses[a]) n=14
Peak Concentration (C_{max}) [mcg/mL]	292 (175-427)	295 (171-398)
Terminal half-life ($t_{1/2}$) [days]	16.7 (12-23)	13.1 (8-25)
Systemic clearance (CL) [mL/h/kg]	0.23 (0.16-0.30)	0.22 (0.13-0.47)
Volume of distribution (Vss) [L/kg]	0.09 (0.06-0.13)	0.07 (0.02-0.13)

[a] Multiple intravenous infusions were administered at days 1, 15, 30, and monthly thereafter.

The pharmacokinetics of abatacept in RA patients and healthy subjects appeared to be comparable. In RA patients, after multiple intravenous infusions, the pharmacokinetics of abatacept showed proportional increases of C_{max} and AUC over the dose range of 2 mg/kg to 10 mg/kg. At 10 mg/kg, serum concentration appeared to reach a steady-state by day 60 with a mean (range) trough concentration of 24 mcg/mL (1 to 66 mcg/mL). No systemic accumulation of abatacept occurred upon continued repeated treatment with 10 mg/kg at monthly intervals in RA patients.

Population pharmacokinetic analyses in RA patients revealed that there was a trend toward higher clearance of abatacept with increasing body weight. Age and gender (when corrected for body weight) did not affect clearance. Concomitant methotrexate, NSAIDs, corticosteroids, and TNF blocking agents did not influence abatacept clearance.

No formal studies were conducted to examine the effects of either renal or hepatic impairment on the pharmacokinetics of abatacept.

Juvenile Idiopathic Arthritis

In patients 6 to 17 years of age, the mean (range) steady-state serum peak and trough concentrations of abatacept were 217 mcg/mL (57 to 700 mcg/mL) and 11.9 mcg/mL (0.15 to 44.6 mcg/mL). Population pharmacokinetic analyses of the serum concentration data showed that clearance of abatacept increased with baseline body weight. The estimated mean (range) clearance of abatacept in the juvenile idiopathic arthritis patients was 0.4 mL/h/kg (0.20 to 1.12 mL/h/kg). After accounting for the effect of body weight, the clearance of abatacept was not related to age and gender. Concomitant methotrexate, corticosteroids, and NSAIDs were also shown not to influence abatacept clearance.

Adult RA - Subcutaneous Administration

Abatacept exhibited linear pharmacokinetics following subcutaneous administration. The mean (range) for C_{min} and C_{max} at steady state observed after 85 days of treatment was 32.5 mcg/mL (6.6 to 113.8 mcg/mL) and 48.1 mcg/mL (9.8 to 132.4 mcg/mL), respectively. The bioavailability of abatacept following subcutaneous administration relative to intravenous administration is 78.6%. Mean estimates for systemic clearance (0.28 mL/h/kg), volume of distribution (0.11 L/kg), and terminal half-life (14.3 days) were comparable between subcutaneous and intravenous administration.

Study SC-II was conducted to determine the effect of monotherapy use of ORENCIA (abatacept) on immunogenicity following subcutaneous administration without an intravenous load. When the intravenous loading dose was not administered, a mean trough concentration of 12.6 mcg/mL was achieved after 2 weeks of dosing.

Consistent with the intravenous data, population pharmacokinetic analyses for subcutaneous abatacept in RA patients revealed that there was a trend toward higher clearance of abatacept with increasing body weight. Age and gender (when corrected for body weight) did not affect apparent clearance. Concomitant medication, such as methotrexate, corticosteroids, and NSAIDs, did not influence abatacept apparent clearance.

13 NONCLINICAL TOXICOLOGY

13.1 Carcinogenesis, Mutagenesis, Impairment of Fertility

In a mouse carcinogenicity study, weekly subcutaneous injections of 20, 65, or 200 mg/kg of abatacept administered for up to 84 weeks in males and 88 weeks in females were associated with increases in the incidence of malignant lymphomas (all doses) and mammary gland tumors (intermediate- and high-dose in females). The mice from this study were infected with murine leukemia virus and mouse mammary tumor virus. These viruses are associated with an increased incidence of lymphomas and mammary gland tumors, respectively, in immunosuppressed mice. The doses used in these studies produced exposures 0.8, 2.0, and 3.0 times higher, respectively, than the exposure associated with the maximum recommended human dose (MRHD) of 10 mg/kg based on AUC (area under the time-concentration curve). The relevance of these findings to the clinical use of ORENCIA is unknown.

In a one-year toxicity study in cynomolgus monkeys, abatacept was administered intravenously once weekly at doses up to 50 mg/kg (producing 9 times the MRHD exposure based on AUC). Abatacept was not associated with any significant drug-related toxicity. Reversible pharmacological effects consisted of minimal transient decreases in serum IgG and minimal to severe lymphoid depletion of germinal centers in the spleen and/or lymph nodes. No evidence of lymphomas or preneoplastic morphologic changes was observed, despite the presence of a virus (lymphocryptovirus) known to cause these lesions in immunosuppressed monkeys within the time frame of this study. The relevance of these findings to the clinical use of ORENCIA (abatacept) is unknown.

No mutagenic potential of abatacept was observed in the *in vitro* bacterial reverse mutation (Ames) or Chinese hamster ovary/hypoxanthine guanine phosphoribosyl-transferase (CHO/HGPRT) forward point mutation assays with or without metabolic activation, and no chromosomal aberrations were observed in human lymphocytes treated with abatacept with or without metabolic activation.

Abatacept had no adverse effects on male or female fertility in rats at doses up to 200 mg/kg every three days (11 times the MRHD exposure based on AUC).

13.2 Animal Toxicology and/or Pharmacology

A juvenile animal study was conducted in rats dosed with abatacept from 4 to 94 days of age in which an increase in the incidence of infections leading to death occurred at all doses compared with controls. Altered T-cell subsets including increased T-helper cells and reduced T-regulatory cells were observed. In addition, inhibition of T-cell-dependent antibody responses (TDAR) was observed. Upon following these animals into adulthood, lymphocytic inflammation of the thyroid and pancreatic islets was observed.

In studies of adult mice and monkeys, inhibition of TDAR was apparent. However, infection and mortality, altered T-helper cells, and inflammation of thyroid and pancreas were not observed.

14 CLINICAL STUDIES

14.1 Adult Rheumatoid Arthritis

The efficacy and safety of ORENCIA for intravenous administration were assessed in six randomized, double-blind, controlled studies (five placebo-controlled and one active-controlled) in patients ≥18 years of age with active RA diagnosed according to American College of Rheumatology (ACR) criteria. Studies I, II, III, IV, and VI required patients to have at least 12 tender and 10 swollen joints at randomization. Study V did not require any specific number of tender or swollen joints. ORENCIA or placebo treatment was given intravenously at weeks 0, 2, and 4 and then every 4 weeks thereafter in intravenous Studies I, II, III, IV, and VI. The safety and efficacy of ORENCIA for subcutaneous administration were assessed in Study SC-I, which was a randomized, double-blind, double-dummy, non-inferiority study that compared abatacept administered subcutaneously and intravenously in 1457 subjects with rheumatoid arthritis (RA), receiving background methotrexate (MTX), and experiencing an inadequate response to methotrexate (MTX-IR).

Study I evaluated ORENCIA as monotherapy in 122 patients with active RA who had failed at least one non-biologic DMARD or etanercept. In Study II and Study III, the efficacy and safety of ORENCIA were assessed in patients with an inadequate response to methotrexate and who were continued on their stable dose of methotrexate. In Study IV, the efficacy and safety of ORENCIA were assessed in patients with an inadequate response to a TNF blocking agent, with the TNF blocking agent discontinued prior to randomization; other DMARDs were permitted. Study V primarily assessed safety in patients with active RA requiring additional intervention in spite of current therapy with DMARDs; all DMARDs used at enrollment were continued. Patients in Study V were not excluded for comorbid medical conditions. In Study VI, the efficacy and safety of ORENCIA were assessed in methotrexate-naive patients with RA of less than 2 years disease duration. In Study VI, patients previously naive to methotrexate were randomized to receive ORENCIA plus methotrexate or methotrexate plus placebo. In Study SC-I, the goal was to demonstrate the efficacy and safety of ORENCIA subcutaneous relative to ORENCIA intravenous administration in subjects with moderate to severely active RA and experiencing inadequate response to methotrexate, using a non-inferiority study design.

Study I patients were randomized to receive one of three doses of ORENCIA (0.5, 2, or 10 mg/kg) or placebo ending at week 8. Study II patients were randomized to receive ORENCIA 2 or 10 mg/kg or placebo for 12 months. Study III, IV, V, and VI patients were randomized to receive a dose of ORENCIA based on weight range or placebo for 12 months (Studies III, V, and VI) or 6 months (Study IV). The dose of ORENCIA was 500 mg for patients weighing less than 60 kg, 750 mg for patients weighing 60 to 100 kg, and 1000 mg for patients weighing greater than 100 kg. In Study SC-I, patients were randomized with stratification by body weight (<60 kg, 60 to 100 kg, >100 kg) to receive ORENCIA 125 mg subcutaneous injections weekly, after a single intravenous loading dose of ORENCIA based on body weight or ORENCIA intravenously on Days 1, 15, 29, and every four weeks thereafter. Subjects continued taking their current dose of methotrexate from the day of randomization.

Table 4: Clinical Responses in Controlled Trials

	Percent of Patients									
	Intravenous Administration								Subcutaneous Administration	
	Inadequate Response to DMARDs		Inadequate Response to Methotrexate (MTX)		Inadequate Response to TNF Blocking Agent		MTX-Naive		Inadequate Response to MTX	
	Study I		Study III		Study IV		Study VI		Study SC-I	
Response Rate	ORN[a] n=32	PBO n=32	ORN[b] +MTX n=424	PBO +MTX n=214	ORN[b] + DMARDs n=256	PBO + DMARDs n=133	ORN[b] +MTX n=256	PBO +MTX n=253	ORN[e] SC +MTX n=693	ORN[e] IV +MTX n=678
ACR 20										
Month 3	53%	31%	62%‡	37%	46%‡	18%	64%*	53%	68%	69%
Month 6	NA	NA	68%‡	40%	50%‡	20%	75%†	62%	76%§	76%
Month 12	NA	NA	73%‡	40%	NA	NA	76%‡	62%	NA	NA
ACR 50										
Month 3	16%	6%	32%†	8%	18%†	6%	40%‡	23%	33%	39%
Month 6	NA	NA	40%‡	17%	20%‡	4%	53%‡	38%	52%	50%
Month 12	NA	NA	48%‡	18%	NA	NA	57%‡	42%	NA	NA
ACR 70										
Month 3	6%	0	13%‡	3%	6%*	1%	19%†	10%	13%	16%
Month 6	NA	NA	20%‡	7%	10%†	2%	32%†	20%	26%	25%
Month 12	NA	NA	29%‡	6%	NA	NA	43%‡	27%	NA	NA
Major Clinical Response[c]	NA	NA	14%‡	2%	NA	NA	27%‡	12%	NA	NA
DAS28-CRP <2.6[d]										
Month 12	NA	NA	NA	NA	NA	NA	41%‡	23%	NA	NA

* $p<0.05$, ORENCIA (ORN) vs placebo (PBO) or MTX.
† $p<0.01$, ORENCIA vs placebo or MTX.
‡ $p<0.001$, ORENCIA vs placebo or MTX.
§ 95% CI: −4.2, 4.8 (based on prespecified margin for non-inferiority of −7.5%).
a 10 mg/kg.
b Dosing based on weight range [see *Dosage and Administration (2.1)*].
c Major clinical response is defined as achieving an ACR 70 response for a continuous 6-month period.
d Refer to text for additional description of remaining joint activity.
e Per protocol data is presented in table. For ITT; n=736, 721 for SC and IV ORENCIA, respectively.

Clinical Response

The percent of ORENCIA-treated patients achieving ACR 20, 50, and 70 responses and major clinical response in Studies I, III, IV, and VI are shown in Table 4. ORENCIA-treated patients had higher ACR 20, 50, and 70 response rates at 6 months compared to placebo-treated patients. Month 6 ACR response rates in Study II for the 10 mg/kg group were similar to the ORENCIA (abatacept) group in Study III.

In Studies III and IV, improvement in the ACR 20 response rate versus placebo was observed within 15 days in some patients and within 29 days versus methotrexate in Study VI. In Studies II, III, and VI, ACR response rates were maintained to 12 months in ORENCIA-treated patients. ACR responses were maintained up to three years in the open-label extension of Study II. In Study III, ORENCIA-treated patients experienced greater improvement than placebo-treated patients in morning stiffness.

In Study VI, a greater proportion of patients treated with ORENCIA plus methotrexate achieved a low level of disease activity as measured by a DAS28-CRP less than 2.6 at 12 months compared to those treated with methotrexate plus placebo (Table 4). Of patients treated with ORENCIA plus methotrexate who achieved DAS28-CRP less than 2.6, 54% had no active joints, 17% had one active joint, 7% had two active joints, and 22% had three or more active joints, where an active joint was a joint that was rated as tender or swollen or both.

In Study SC-I, the main outcome measure was ACR 20 at 6 months. The pre-specified non-inferiority margin was a treatment difference of −7.5%. As shown in Table 4, the study demonstrated non-inferiority of ORENCIA administered subcutaneously to intravenous infusions of ORENCIA with respect to ACR 20 responses up to 6 months of treatment. ACR 50 and 70 responses are also shown in Table 4. No major differences in ACR responses were observed between intravenous and subcutaneous treatment groups in subgroups based on weight categories (less than 60 kg, 60 to 100 kg, and more than 100 kg; data not shown).

[See table 4 above]

The results of the components of the ACR response criteria for Studies III, IV, and SC-I are shown in Table 5 (results at Baseline [BL] and 6 months [6 M]). In ORENCIA-treated patients, greater improvement was seen in all ACR response criteria components through 6 and 12 months than in placebo-treated patients.

[See table 5 at top of next page]

The percent of patients achieving the ACR 50 response for Study III by visit is shown in Figure 1. The time course for the ORENCIA (abatacept) group in Study VI was similar to that in Study III.

Figure 1: Percent of Patients Achieving ACR 50 Response by Visit* (Study III)

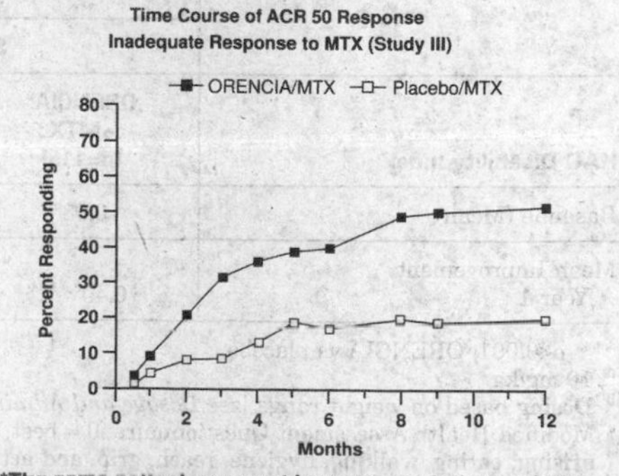

*The same patients may not have responded at each time point.

The percent of patients achieving the ACR 50 response for Study SC-I in the ORENCIA subcutaneous (SC) and intravenous (IV) treatment arms at each treatment visit was as follows: Day 15—SC 3%, IV 5%; Day 29—SC 11%, IV 14%; Day 57—SC 24%, IV 30%; Day 85—SC 33%, IV 38%; Day 113—SC 39%, IV 41%; Day 141—SC 46%, IV 47%; Day 169—SC 51%, IV 50%.

Radiographic Response

In Study III and Study VI, structural joint damage was assessed radiographically and expressed as change from baseline in the Genant-modified Total Sharp Score (TSS) and its components, the Erosion Score (ES) and Joint Space Nar-

Table 5: Components of ACR Responses at 6 Months

	Intravenous Administration								Subcutaneous Administration			
	Inadequate Response to Methotrexate (MTX)				Inadequate Response to TNF Blocking Agent				Inadequate Response to MTX			
	Study III				Study IV				Study SC-I[c]			
	ORN +MTX n=424		PBO +MTX n=214		ORN +DMARDs n=256		PBO +DMARDs n=133		ORN SC +MTX n=693		ORN IV +MTX n=678	
Component (median)	BL	6 M	BL	6 M	BL	6 M	BL	6 M	BL	6 M	BL	6 M
Number of tender joints (0-68)	28	7[‡]	31	14	30	13[‡]	31	24	27	5	27	6
Number of swollen joints (0-66)	19	5[‡]	20	11	21	10[‡]	20	14	18	4	18	3
Pain[a]	67	27[‡]	70	50	73	43[†]	74	64	71	25	70	28
Patient global assessment[a]	66	29[‡]	64	48	71	44[‡]	73	63	70	26	68	27
Disability index[b]	1.75	1.13[‡]	1.75	1.38	1.88	1.38[‡]	2.00	1.75	1.88	1.00	1.75	1.00
Physician global assessment[a]	69	21[‡]	68	40	71	32[‡]	69	54	65	16	65	15
CRP (mg/dL)	2.2	0.9[‡]	2.1	1.8	3.4	1.3[‡]	2.8	2.3	1.6	0.7	1.8	0.7

[†] p<0.01, ORENCIA (ORN) vs placebo (PBO), based on mean percent change from baseline.
[‡] p<0.001, ORENCIA vs placebo, based on mean percent change from baseline.
[a] Visual analog scale: 0 = best, 100 = worst.
[b] Health Assessment Questionnaire: 0 = best, 3 = worst; 20 questions; 8 categories: dressing and grooming, arising, eating, walking, hygiene, reach, grip, and activities.
[c] SC-I is a non-inferiority study. Per protocol data is presented in table.

Table 6: Mean Radiographic Changes in Study III[a] and Study VI[b]

Parameter	ORENCIA/MTX	Placebo/MTX	Differences	P-value[d]
Study III				
First Year				
TSS	1.07	2.43	1.36	<0.01
ES	0.61	1.47	0.86	<0.01
JSN score	0.46	0.97	0.51	<0.01
Second Year				
TSS	0.48	0.74[c]	-	-
ES	0.23	0.22[c]	-	-
JSN score	0.25	0.51[c]	-	-
Study VI				
First Year				
TSS	0.6	1.1	0.5	0.04

[a] Patients with an inadequate response to MTX.
[b] MTX-naive patients.
[c] Patients received 1 year of placebo/MTX followed by 1 year of ORENCIA/MTX.
[d] Based on a nonparametric ANCOVA model.

Table 7: Mean Improvement from Baseline in Health Assessment Questionnaire Disability Index (HAQ-DI)

	Inadequate Response to Methotrexate			
	Study II		Study III	
HAQ Disability Index	ORENCIA[a] +MTX (n=115)	Placebo +MTX (n=119)	ORENCIA[b] +MTX (n=422)	Placebo +MTX (n=212)
Baseline (Mean)	0.98[c]	0.97[c]	1.69[d]	1.69[d]
Mean Improvement Year 1	0.40[c,***]	0.15[c]	0.66[d,***]	0.37[d]

*** p<0.001, ORENCIA vs placebo.
[a] 10 mg/kg.
[b] Dosing based on weight range [see *Dosage and Administration (2.1)*].
[c] Modified Health Assessment Questionnaire: 0 = best, 3 = worst; 8 questions; 8 categories: dressing and grooming, arising, eating, walking, hygiene, reach, grip, and activities.
[d] Health Assessment Questionnaire: 0 = best, 3 = worst; 20 questions; 8 categories: dressing and grooming, arising, eating, walking, hygiene, reach, grip, and activities.

rowing (JSN) score. ORENCIA/methotrexate slowed the progression of structural damage compared to placebo/methotrexate after 12 months of treatment as shown in Table 6.

[See table 6 above]

In the open-label extension of Study III, 75% of patients initially randomized to ORENCIA/methotrexate and 65% of patients initially randomized to placebo/methotrexate were evaluated radiographically at Year 2. As shown in Table 6, progression of structural damage in ORENCIA/methotrexate-treated patients was further reduced in the second year of treatment.

Following 2 years of treatment with ORENCIA/methotrexate, 51% of patients had no progression of structural damage as defined by a change in the TSS of zero or less compared with baseline. Fifty-six percent (56%) of ORENCIA/methotrexate-treated patients had no progression during the first year compared to 45% of placebo/methotrexate-treated patients. In their second year of treatment with ORENCIA/methotrexate, more patients had no progression than in the first year (65% vs 56%).

Physical Function Response and Health-Related Outcomes

Improvement in physical function was measured by the Health Assessment Questionnaire Disability Index (HAQ-DI). In the HAQ-DI, ORENCIA (abatacept) demonstrated greater improvement from baseline versus placebo in Studies II-V and versus methotrexate in Study VI. In Study SC-I, improvement from baseline as measured by HAQ-DI at 6 months and over time was similar between subcutaneous and intravenous administration. The results from Studies II and III are shown in Table 7. Similar results were observed in Study V compared to placebo and in Study VI compared to methotrexate. During the open-label period of Study II, the improvement in physical function has been maintained for up to 3 years.

[See table 7 below]

Health-related quality of life was assessed by the SF-36 questionnaire at 6 months in Studies II, III, and IV and at 12 months in Studies II and III. In these studies, improvement was observed in the ORENCIA group as compared with the placebo group in all 8 domains of the SF-36 as well as the Physical Component Summary (PCS) and the Mental Component Summary (MCS).

14.2 Juvenile Idiopathic Arthritis

The safety and efficacy of ORENCIA were assessed in a three-part study including an open-label extension in children with polyarticular juvenile idiopathic arthritis (JIA). Patients 6 to 17 years of age (n=190) with moderately to severely active polyarticular JIA who had an inadequate response to one or more DMARDs, such as methotrexate or TNF antagonists, were treated. Patients had a disease duration of approximately 4 years with moderately to severely active disease at study entry, as determined by baseline counts of active joints (mean, 16) and joints with loss of motion (mean, 16); patients had elevated C-reactive protein (CRP) levels (mean, 3.2 mg/dL) and ESR (mean, 32 mm/h). The patients enrolled had subtypes of JIA that at disease onset included Oligoarticular (16%), Polyarticular (64%; 20% were rheumatoid factor positive), and Systemic (20%). At study entry, 74% of patients were receiving methotrexate (mean dose, 13.2 mg/m^2 per week) and remained on a stable dose of methotrexate (those not receiving methotrexate did not initiate methotrexate treatment during the study).

In Period A (open-label, lead-in), patients received 10 mg/kg (maximum 1000 mg per dose) intravenously on days 1, 15, 29, and monthly thereafter. Response was assessed utilizing the ACR Pediatric 30 definition of improvement, defined as ≥30% improvement in at least 3 of the 6 JIA core set variables and ≥30% worsening in not more than 1 of the 6 JIA core set variables. Patients demonstrating an ACR Pedi 30 response at the end of Period A were randomized into the double-blind phase (Period B) and received either ORENCIA or placebo for 6 months or until disease flare. Disease flare was defined as a ≥30% worsening in at least 3 of the 6 JIA core set variables with ≥30% improvement in not more than 1 of the 6 JIA core set variables; ≥2 cm of worsening of the Physician or Parent Global Assessment was necessary if used as 1 of the 3 JIA core set variables used to define flare, and worsening in ≥2 joints was necessary if the number of active joints or joints with limitation of motion was used as 1 of the 3 JIA core set variables used to define flare.

At the conclusion of Period A, pediatric ACR 30/50/70 responses were 65%, 50%, and 28%, respectively. Pediatric ACR 30 responses were similar in all subtypes of JIA studied.

During the double-blind randomized withdrawal phase (Period B), ORENCIA-treated patients experienced significantly fewer disease flares compared to placebo-treated patients (20% vs 53%); 95% CI of the difference (15%, 52%). The risk of disease flare among patients continuing on ORENCIA was less than one-third than that for patients withdrawn from ORENCIA treatment (hazard ratio=0.31, 95% CI [0.16, 0.59]). Among patients who received ORENCIA throughout the study (Period A, Period B, and the open-label extension Period C), the proportion of pediatric ACR 30/50/70 responders has remained consistent for 1 year.

16 HOW SUPPLIED/STORAGE AND HANDLING

For Intravenous Infusion

ORENCIA® (abatacept) lyophilized powder for intravenous infusion is supplied as an individually packaged, single-use vial with a silicone-free disposable syringe, providing 250 mg of abatacept in a 15-mL vial: NDC 0003-2187-10.

For Subcutaneous Injection

ORENCIA® (abatacept) injection solution for subcutaneous administration is supplied either as a single-dose disposable prefilled glass syringe with UltraSafe Passive® needle guard with flange extenders or as a single-dose disposable prefilled glass syringe with flange extender. The Type I glass syringe has a coated stopper and fixed stainless steel needle (5 bevel, 29-gauge thin wall, ½-inch needle) covered with a rigid needle shield. The prefilled syringe provides 125 mg of abatacept in 1 mL and is provided in the following packages:

NDC 0003-2188-11: pack of 4 syringes with a passive needle safety guard

NDC 0003-2188-31: pack of 4 syringes without a passive needle safety guard

Storage

ORENCIA (abatacept) lyophilized powder supplied in a vial should be refrigerated at 2°C to 8°C (36°F to 46°F). Do not use beyond the expiration date on the vial. Protect the vials from light by storing in the original package until time of use.

ORENCIA solution supplied in a prefilled syringe should be refrigerated at 2°C to 8°C (36°F to 46°F). Do not use beyond the expiration date on the prefilled syringe. Protect from light by storing in the original package until time of use. Do not allow the prefilled syringe to freeze.

17 PATIENT COUNSELING INFORMATION

See FDA-Approved Patient Labeling (Patient Information and Instructions for Use)

17.1 Concomitant Use With Biologic Medications for RA

Patients should be informed that they should not receive ORENCIA treatment concomitantly with a TNF antagonist, such as adalimumab, etanercept, and infliximab because such combination therapy may increase their risk for infections [see *Indications and Usage (1.3), Warnings and Precautions (5.1)*, and *Drug Interactions (7.1)*], and that they should not receive ORENCIA concomitantly with other biologic RA therapy, such as anakinra because there is not enough information to assess the safety and efficacy of such combination therapy [see *Indications and Usage (1.3), Drug Interactions (7.2)*].

17.2 Hypersensitivity

Patients should be instructed to immediately tell their healthcare professional if they experience symptoms of an allergic reaction during or for the first day after the administration of ORENCIA [see *Warnings and Precautions (5.2)*].

17.3 Infections

Patients should be asked if they have a history of recurrent infections, have underlying conditions which may predispose them to infections, or have chronic, latent, or localized infections. Patients should be asked if they have had tuberculosis (TB), a positive skin test for TB, or recently have been in close contact with someone who has had TB. Patients should be instructed that they may be tested for TB before they receive ORENCIA. Patients should be informed to tell their healthcare professional if they develop an infection during therapy with ORENCIA [see *Warnings and Precautions (5.3)*].

17.4 Immunizations

Patients should be informed that live vaccines should not be given concurrently with ORENCIA or within 3 months of its discontinuation. Caregivers of patients with juvenile idiopathic arthritis should be informed that the patient should be brought up to date with all immunizations in agreement with current immunization guidelines prior to initiating ORENCIA therapy and to discuss with their healthcare provider how best to handle future immunizations once ORENCIA therapy has been initiated [see *Warnings and Precautions (5.4)*].

17.5 Pregnancy and Nursing Mothers

Patients should be informed that ORENCIA has not been studied in pregnant women or nursing mothers so the effects of ORENCIA on pregnant women or nursing infants are not known. Patients should be instructed to tell their healthcare professional if they are pregnant, become pregnant, or are thinking about becoming pregnant [see *Use in Specific Populations (8.1)*]. Patients should be instructed to tell their healthcare professional if they plan to breastfeed their infant [see *Use in Specific Populations (8.3)*].

17.6 Blood Glucose Testing

Intravenous Administration

Patients should be asked if they have diabetes. Maltose is contained in ORENCIA for intravenous administration and can give falsely elevated blood glucose readings with certain blood glucose monitors on the day of ORENCIA infusion. If a patient is using such a monitor, the patient should be advised to discuss with their healthcare professional methods that do not react with maltose [see *Drug Interactions (7.3)*].

Subcutaneous Administration

ORENCIA for subcutaneous administration does not contain maltose; therefore, patients do not need to alter their glucose monitoring.

Bristol-Myers Squibb Company
Princeton, New Jersey 08543 USA
1292618A2 / 1294018A1
Rev July 2013

PATIENT INFORMATION
ORENCIA® (oh-REN-see-ah)
(abatacept)
Lyophilized Powder for Intravenous Infusion
ORENCIA®(oh-REN-see-ah)
(abatacept)
Injection, Solution for Subcutaneous Administration

Read this Patient Information before you start using ORENCIA and each time you get a refill. There may be new information. This information does not take the place of talking with your healthcare provider about your medical condition or your treatment.

What is ORENCIA?

ORENCIA is a prescription medicine that reduces signs and symptoms in:

- adults with moderate to severe rheumatoid arthritis (RA), including those who have not been helped enough by other medicines for RA. ORENCIA may prevent further damage to your bones and joints and may help your ability to perform daily activities. In adults, ORENCIA may be used alone or with other RA treatments other than tumor necrosis factor (TNF) antagonists.
- children and adolescents 6 years of age and older with moderate to severe polyarticular juvenile idiopathic arthritis (JIA). ORENCIA may be used alone or with methotrexate.

It is not known if ORENCIA is safe and effective in children under 6 years of age.

It is not known if ORENCIA is safe and effective in children for uses other than juvenile idiopathic arthritis.

ORENCIA for subcutaneous injection has not been studied in children under 18 years of age; therefore, it is not known if ORENCIA for subcutaneous injection is safe and effective in children under 18 years of age.

What should I tell my healthcare provider before using ORENCIA?

Before you use ORENCIA, tell your healthcare provider if you:

- have any kind of infection even if it is small (such as an open cut or sore), or an infection that is in your whole body (such as the flu). If you have an infection when taking ORENCIA, you may have a higher chance for getting serious side effects.
- have an infection that will not go away or an infection that keeps coming back
- are allergic to abatacept or any of the ingredients in ORENCIA. See the end of this leaflet for a list of the ingredients in ORENCIA.
- have or have had inflammation of your liver due to an infection (viral hepatitis). Before you use ORENCIA, your healthcare provider may examine you for hepatitis.
- have had a lung infection called tuberculosis (TB), a positive skin test for TB, or you recently have been in close contact with someone who has had TB. Before you use ORENCIA, your healthcare provider may examine you for TB or perform a skin test. Symptoms of TB may include:
  - a cough that does not go away
  - weight loss
  - fever
  - night sweats
- are scheduled to have surgery.
- recently received a vaccination or are scheduled for a vaccination. If you are receiving ORENCIA, and for 3 months after you stop receiving ORENCIA, you should not receive live vaccines.
- have a history of a breathing problem called chronic obstructive pulmonary disease (COPD).
- have diabetes and use a blood glucose monitor to check your blood sugar (blood glucose) levels. ORENCIA for intravenous infusion (given through a needle placed in a vein) contains maltose, a type of sugar that can give false high blood sugar readings with certain types of blood glucose monitors, on the day of ORENCIA infusion. Your doctor may tell you to use a different way to monitor your blood sugar levels.
- ORENCIA for subcutaneous injection (injected under the skin) does not contain maltose. You do not need to change your blood sugar monitoring if you are taking ORENCIA subcutaneously.
- have any other medical conditions.
- are pregnant or planning to become pregnant. It is not known if ORENCIA can harm your unborn baby.
  Bristol-Myers Squibb Company has a registry for pregnant women exposed to ORENCIA. The purpose of this registry is to check the health of the pregnant mother and her child. Women are encouraged to call the registry themselves or ask their doctors to contact the registry for them by calling 1-877-311-8972.
- are breastfeeding or plan to breastfeed. It is not known if ORENCIA passes into your breast milk. You and your healthcare provider should decide if you will use ORENCIA or breastfeed. You should not do both.

Tell your healthcare provider about all the medicines you take, including prescription and non-prescription medicines, vitamins, and herbal supplements.

ORENCIA may affect the way other medicines work, and other medicines may affect the way ORENCIA works causing serious side effects.

Especially tell your healthcare provider if you take other biologic medicines to treat RA or JIA that may affect your immune system, such as:

- Enbrel® (etanercept)
- Humira® (adalimumab)
- Remicade® (infliximab)
- Kineret® (anakinra)
- Rituxan® (rituximab)
- Simponi® (golimumab)
- Cimzia® (certolizumab pegol)
- Actemra® (tocilizumab)

You may have a higher chance of getting a serious infection if you take ORENCIA (abatacept) with other biologic medicines for your RA or JIA.

Know the medicines you take. Keep a list of your medicines and show it to your healthcare provider and pharmacist when you get a new prescription.

How should I use ORENCIA?

- You may receive ORENCIA given by a healthcare provider through a vein in your arm (IV or intravenous infusion). It takes about 30 minutes to give you the full dose of medicine. You will then receive ORENCIA 2 weeks and 4 weeks after the first dose and then every 4 weeks.
- You may also receive ORENCIA as an injection under your skin (subcutaneous). If your healthcare provider decides that you or a caregiver can give your injections of ORENCIA at home, you or your caregiver should receive training on the right way to prepare and inject ORENCIA. Do not try to inject ORENCIA until you have been shown the right way to give the injections by your healthcare provider.
- Your healthcare provider will tell you how much ORENCIA to use and when to use it.
- **See the Instructions for Use at the end of this Patient Information leaflet for instructions about the right way to prepare and give your ORENCIA injections at home.**

What are the possible side effects of ORENCIA?

ORENCIA can cause serious side effects including:

- **infections.** ORENCIA can make you more likely to get infections or make the infection that you have get worse. Some patients have died from these infections. Call your healthcare provider right away if you have any symptoms of an infection. Symptoms of an infection may include:
  - fever
  - feel very tired
  - have a cough
  - have flu-like symptoms
  - warm, red, or painful skin
- **allergic reactions.** Allergic reactions can happen to people who use ORENCIA. Call your healthcare provider or go to the emergency room right away if you have any symptoms of an allergic reaction. Symptoms of an allergic reaction may include:
  - hives
  - swollen face, eyelids, lips, or tongue
  - trouble breathing
- **hepatitis B infection** in people who carry the virus in their blood. If you are a carrier of the hepatitis B virus (a virus that affects the liver), the virus can become active while you use ORENCIA. Your healthcare provider may do a blood test before you start treatment with ORENCIA while you use ORENCIA.
- **vaccinations.** You should not receive ORENCIA with certain types of vaccines (live vaccines). ORENCIA may also cause some vaccinations to be less effective. Talk with your healthcare provider about your vaccination plans.
- **breathing problems in patients with Chronic Obstructive Pulmonary Disease (COPD).** Some people may get certain respiratory problems more often if you receive ORENCIA and have COPD. Symptoms of respiratory problems include:
  - COPD that becomes worse
  - cough
  - trouble breathing
- **cancer (malignancies).** Certain kinds of cancer have been reported in people using ORENCIA. It is not known if ORENCIA increases your chance of getting certain kinds of cancer.

Common side effects of ORENCIA include:

- headache
- upper respiratory tract infection
- sore throat
- nausea

In children and adolescents, other side effects may include:

- diarrhea
- cough
- fever
- abdominal pain

Tell your healthcare provider if you have any side effect that bothers you or that does not go away.

These are not all the possible side effects of ORENCIA (abatacept). For more information, ask your healthcare provider or pharmacist.

Call your doctor for medical advice about side effects. You may report side effects to FDA at 1-800-FDA-1088.

How should I store ORENCIA?

- Store ORENCIA in the refrigerator at 36°F to 46°F (2°C to 8°C).
- Keep ORENCIA in the original package and out of the light.
- Do not freeze ORENCIA.
- Safely throw away medicine that is out of date or no longer needed.

Keep ORENCIA and all medicines out of the reach of children.

General information about the safe and effective use of ORENCIA

Medicines are sometimes prescribed for purposes other than those listed in this Patient Information leaflet. Do not use ORENCIA for a condition for which it was not prescribed. Do not give ORENCIA to other people, even if they have the same symptoms that you have. It may harm them.

This Patient Information leaflet summarizes the most important information about ORENCIA. If you would like more information, talk to your healthcare provider.

You can ask your pharmacist or healthcare provider for information about ORENCIA that is written for health professionals.

For more information, go to www.ORENCIA.com or call 1-800-ORENCIA.

What are the ingredients in ORENCIA?

Active ingredient: abatacept

Intravenous inactive ingredients: maltose, monobasic sodium phosphate, sodium chloride for administration

Subcutaneous inactive ingredients: sucrose, poloxamer 188, monobasic sodium phosphate monohydrate, dibasic sodium phosphate anhydrous, water for injection

This Patient Information has been approved by the U.S. Food and Drug Administration.

Bristol-Myers Squibb Company
Princeton, NJ 08543 USA

All other trademarks are property of their respective companies.

1292618A2 / 1294018A1
Rev July 2013

INSTRUCTIONS FOR USE
ORENCIA® (oh-REN-see-ah)
(abatacept)
Prefilled Syringe

Read and follow these Instructions for Use that come with your ORENCIA prefilled syringe before you start using it and each time you get a refill. Before you use ORENCIA prefilled syringe for the first time, make sure your healthcare provider shows you the right way to use it.

Do not remove the needle cover (the cap) until you are ready to inject ORENCIA. Do not put the needle cover back on the needle once removed.

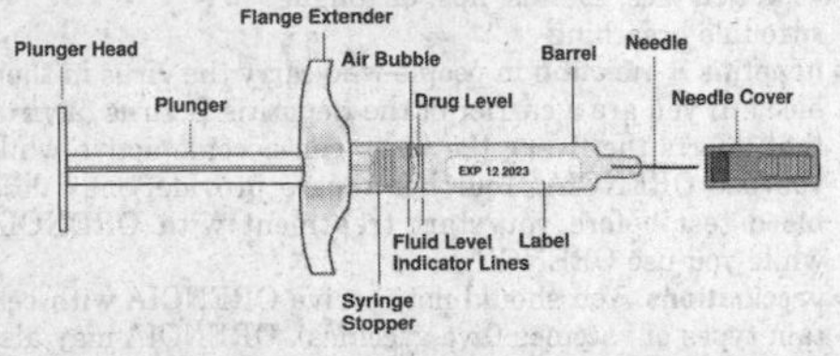

Figure A

- The ORENCIA prefilled syringe has a flange extender that makes it easier to hold the syringe and inject (**see Figure A**).

Supplies needed for your ORENCIA Prefilled Syringe Injection (see Figure B):

- a new ORENCIA prefilled syringe
- alcohol swab
- cotton ball or gauze
- adhesive bandage
- puncture resistant container (sharps container)

[See figure B at top of next column]

STEP 1: Preparing for an ORENCIA Injection

Find a comfortable space with a clean, flat, working surface.

- Check the expiration date on the ORENCIA prefilled syringe (**see Figure A**). **Do not** use it if the expiration date has passed. Throw it away and get a new one.
- Remove 1 single-use ORENCIA prefilled syringe from the refrigerator and let it warm up for 30 to 60 minutes to allow it to reach room temperature.
  - **Do not** speed up the warming process in any way, such as using the microwave or placing the syringe in warm water.

Do not remove the needle cover while allowing ORENCIA prefilled syringe to reach room temperature.

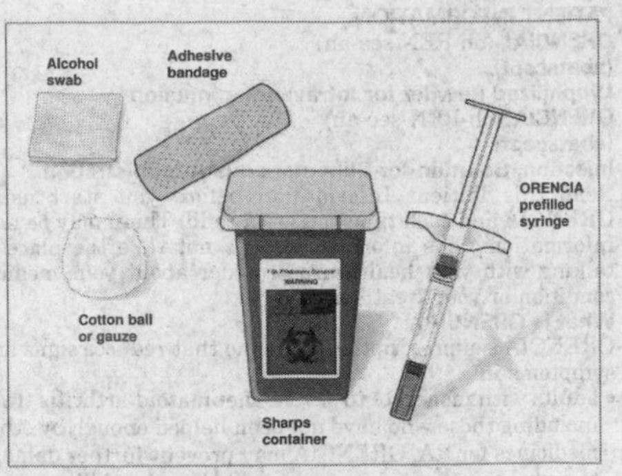

Figure B

- Keep your unused syringes in their original carton and keep in the refrigerator at 36°F to 46°F (2°C to 8°C). **Do not** freeze.
- Hold your ORENCIA (abatacept) prefilled syringe by the barrel with the covered needle pointing down (**see Figure C**).

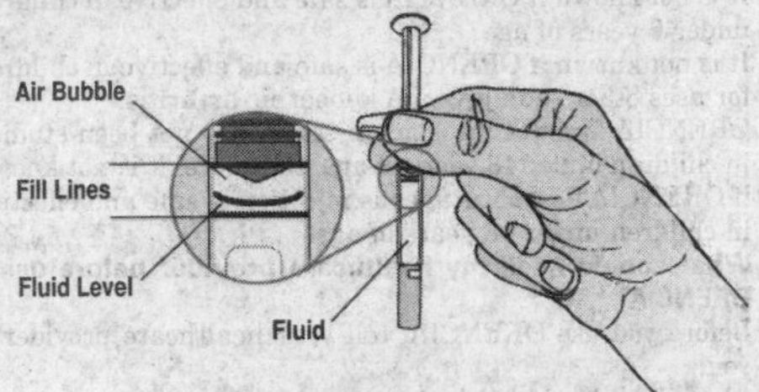

Figure C

- Check the liquid in the ORENCIA prefilled syringe. It should be clear and colorless to pale yellow. **Do not** inject ORENCIA if the liquid is cloudy, discolored, or has lumps or particles in it. Throw the syringe away and get a new one.
- Check that the amount of liquid in your ORENCIA prefilled syringe is the correct amount. The liquid should be between the two lines on the syringe barrel (**see Figure C**).
- **Do not** inject ORENCIA if it does not have the correct amount of liquid. Throw the ORENCIA prefilled syringe away and get a new one. It is normal to see an air bubble. There is no reason to remove it.
- Wash your hands well with soap and water.

STEP 2: Choose and Prepare an Injection Site

Choose an Injection Site

- The front of your thigh is a recommended injection area. You may use your abdomen except for the 2-inch area around your navel (**see Figure D**).
- The outer area of the upper arms may also be used only if the injection is being given by a caregiver. Do not attempt to use the upper arm area by yourself (**see Figure E**).

Rotate Injection Site

- Choose a different injection site for each new injection. You may use the same thigh for weekly injections, as long as each injection is at least 1 inch away from the last area you injected.
- Do not inject into areas where your skin is tender, bruised, red, scaly, or hard. Avoid any areas with scars or stretch marks.

Areas for self-injection and caregiver injection

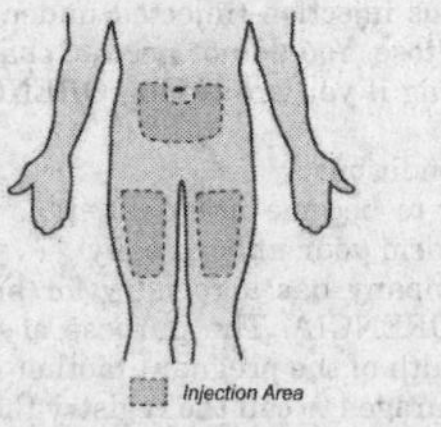

Figure D

Additional injection area for caregivers only

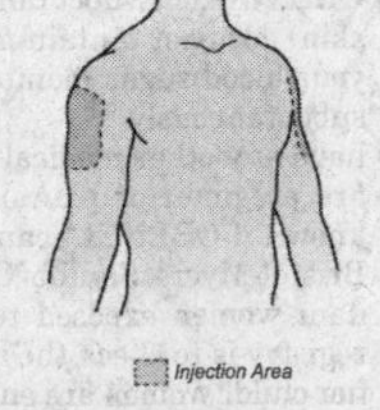

Figure E

Prepare the Injection Site

- Wipe the injection site with an alcohol swab in a circular motion and let it air dry. **Do not** touch the injection site again before giving the injection.
- **Do not** fan or blow on the clean area.

STEP 3: Inject ORENCIA

- Remove the needle cover only when you are ready to administer the injection.Hold the barrel of the ORENCIA (abatacept) prefilled syringe with one hand and pull the needle cover straight off with your other hand (**see Figure F**). **Do not** touch the plunger while you remove the needle cover.

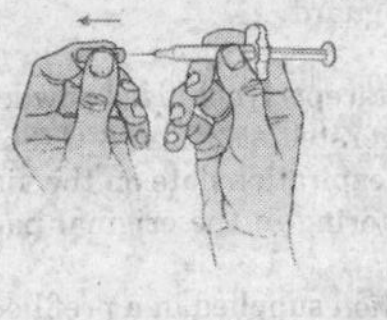

Figure F

- **Do not** put the needle cover back on the needle once removed. Throw away the needle cover in your household trash.
- **Do not** use the syringe if there are visible signs of needle damage or bending.
- There may be a small air bubble in the ORENCIA prefilled syringe barrel. You do not need to remove it.
- You may notice a drop of fluid leaving the needle. This is normal and will not affect your dose.
- **Do not** touch the needle or let it touch any surfaces.
- **Do not** use the prefilled syringe if it is dropped without the needle cover in place.
- Hold the barrel of your ORENCIA prefilled syringe in one hand between the thumb and index finger (**see Figure G**).

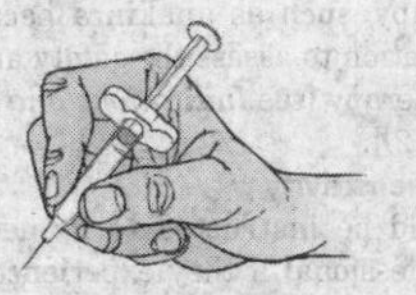

Figure G

- **Do not** pull back on the plunger of the syringe.
- Use your other hand and gently pinch the area of skin you cleaned. Hold firmly.
- Insert the needle with a quick motion into the pinched skin at a 45° angle (**see Figure H**).

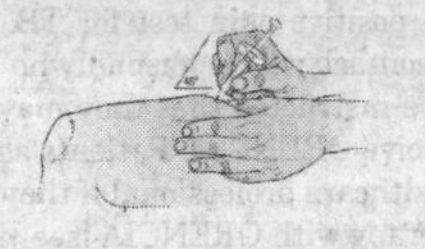

Figure H

- To inject all of the medicine, use your thumb to push down on the plunger head until the plunger head is pushed in as far as it will go (**see Figure I**).

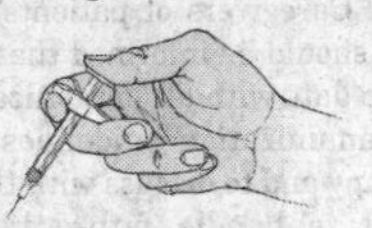

Figure I

- Remove the needle from the skin and let go of the surrounding skin.

After the Injection

- There may be a little bleeding at the injection site. You can press a cotton ball or gauze over the injection site.
- **Do not** rub the injection site.
- If needed, you may cover the injection site with a small bandage.

STEP 4: Disposal and Recordkeeping

- The ORENCIA prefilled syringe should not be reused.
- Put the used syringe into your puncture resistant container (see "**How do I throw away used syringes?**").
- **Do not** put the needle cover back on the needle.
- **If your injection is given by another person, this person must also be careful when removing the syringe and disposing of the syringe to prevent accidental needle stick injury and passing infection.**

How do I throw away used syringes?

Check with your healthcare provider or pharmacist for instructions about the right way to throw away used syringes. There may be special local or state laws about how to throw away used syringes.

- **Do not** throw away used syringes in the household trash and do not recycle them.
- Put used and empty ORENCIA prefilled syringes in a biohazard container made specifically for disposing of used syringes (called a "sharps" container) or in a hard plastic container with a screw-on cap (such as an empty detergent

bottle) or in a metal container with a plastic lid (such as a coffee can). Sharps containers can be purchased at your local pharmacy or many retail outlets.
- When the container is full, tape around the cap or lid to make sure the cap or lid does not come off.
- **Keep ORENCIA prefilled syringes and the disposal container out of the reach of children.**

Record your Injection
- Write the date, time, and specific part of your body where you injected yourself. It may also be helpful to write any questions or concerns about the injection so you can ask your healthcare provider.

If you have questions or concerns about your ORENCIA prefilled syringe, please contact a healthcare provider familiar with ORENCIA or call our toll-free help line at 1-800-ORENCIA (1-800-673-6242).

Frequently Asked Questions

Injecting with the ORENCIA prefilled syringe

I feel a little bit of burning or pain during injection. Is this normal?
- When giving yourself an injection, you may feel a prick from the needle. Sometimes, the medicine can cause slight irritation near the injection site. This may happen and the discomfort should be mild to moderate. If you have any side effects, including pain, swelling, or discoloration near the injection site, contact your healthcare provider.

Traveling with ORENCIA prefilled syringes

How should I keep my prefilled syringes cool while traveling?
- If you need to take your prefilled syringes with you, store them in a cool carrier between 36°F to 46°F (2°C to 8°C) until you are ready to use.
- **Do not** freeze ORENCIA (abatacept).
- Keep ORENCIA in the original carton and protected from light. Your healthcare provider may know about special carrying cases for injectable medicines.

Can I take my prefilled syringes on an airplane?
- Generally you are allowed to carry ORENCIA prefilled syringes with you on an airplane. **Be sure to carry the prefilled syringes with you on board the plane, and do not put them in your "checked" luggage.** You should carry ORENCIA prefilled syringes with you in your travel cooler at a temperature of 36°F to 46°F (2°C to 8°C) until you are ready to use.
- Keep ORENCIA in the original carton, with its original preprinted labels and protected from light.

What if my syringe does not stay cool for an extended period of time? Is it dangerous to use?
- Contact 1-800-ORENCIA (1-800-673-6242) for details.

If you have questions or concerns about your ORENCIA prefilled syringe, please contact a healthcare provider familiar with ORENCIA or call our toll-free help line at 1-800-ORENCIA (1-800-673-6242).

Bristol-Myers Squibb Company
Princeton, NJ 08543 USA

This Instructions for Use has been approved by the U.S. Food and Drug Administration.

All other trademarks are property of their respective companies.

1292618A2 / 1294018A1
Rev July 2013

INSTRUCTIONS FOR USE
ORENCIA® (oh-REN-see-ah)
(abatacept)
Prefilled Syringe with UltraSafe Passive® Needle Guard

Read and follow these Instructions for Use that come with your ORENCIA prefilled syringe before you start using it and each time you get a refill. Before you use ORENCIA prefilled syringe for the first time, make sure your healthcare provider shows you the right way to use it.

Do not remove the needle cover (the cap) until you are ready to inject ORENCIA. Do not put the needle cover back on the needle once removed.

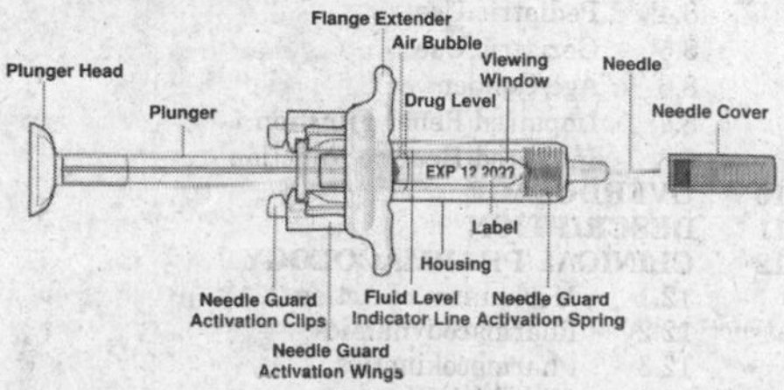

Figure A

- The ORENCIA prefilled syringe has a flange extender that makes it easier to hold the syringe and inject, and a needle guard that automatically extends over the needle after the injection is complete (**see Figure A**).

Supplies needed for your ORENCIA Prefilled Syringe Injection (see Figure B):
- a new ORENCIA (abatacept) prefilled syringe
- alcohol swab
- cotton ball or gauze
- adhesive bandage
- puncture resistant container (sharps container)

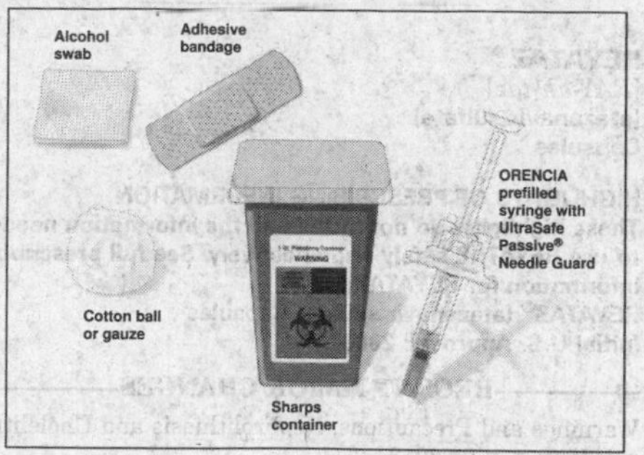

Figure B

STEP 1: Preparing for an ORENCIA Injection

Find a comfortable space with a clean, flat, working surface.
- Check the expiration date on the ORENCIA prefilled syringe (**see Figure A**). **Do not** use it if the expiration date has passed. Throw it away and get a new one.
- Remove 1 single-use ORENCIA prefilled syringe from the refrigerator and let it warm up for 30 to 60 minutes to allow it to reach room temperature.
  - **Do not** speed up the warming process in any way, such as using the microwave or placing the syringe in warm water.

Do not remove the needle cover while allowing ORENCIA prefilled syringe to reach room temperature.
- Keep your unused syringes in their original carton and keep in the refrigerator at 36°F to 46°F (2°C to 8°C). **Do not** freeze.
- Hold your ORENCIA prefilled syringe by the housing with the covered needle pointing down (**see Figure C**).

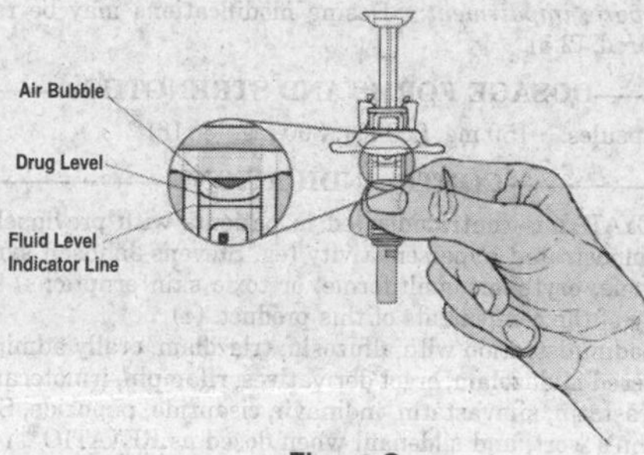

Figure C

- Check the liquid in the ORENCIA prefilled syringe. It should be clear and colorless to pale yellow. **Do not** inject ORENCIA if the liquid is cloudy, discolored, or has lumps or particles in it. Throw the syringe away and get a new one.
- Check that the amount of liquid in your ORENCIA prefilled syringe is the correct amount. Confirm the drug level is above the fluid level indicator line (**see Figure C**).
- **Do not** inject ORENCIA if it does not have the correct amount of liquid. Throw the ORENCIA prefilled syringe away and get a new one. It is normal to see an air bubble. There is no reason to remove it.
- Wash your hands well with soap and water.

STEP 2: Choose and Prepare an Injection Site

Choose an Injection Site
- The front of your thigh is a recommended injection area. You may use your abdomen except for the 2-inch area around your navel (**see Figure D**).
- The outer area of the upper arms may also be used only if the injection is being given by a caregiver. Do not attempt to use the upper arm area by yourself (**see Figure E**).

Rotate Injection Site
- Choose a different injection site for each new injection. You may use the same thigh for weekly injections, as long as each injection is at least 1 inch away from the last area you injected.
- Do not inject into areas where your skin is tender, bruised, red, scaly, or hard. Avoid any areas with scars or stretch marks.

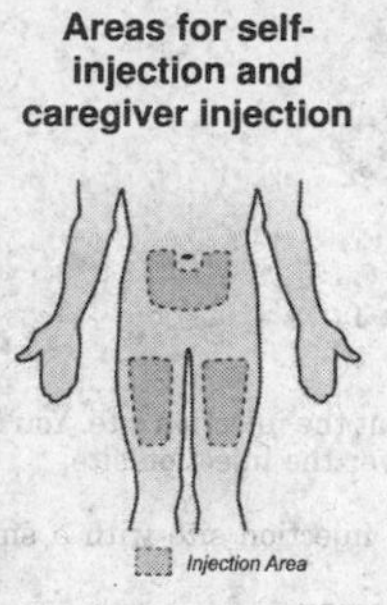

Figure D

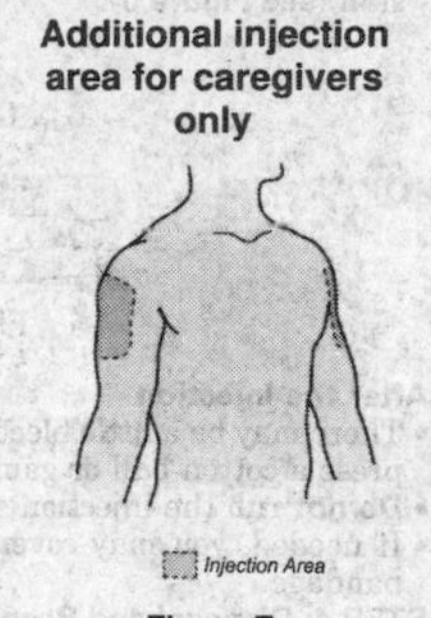

Figure E

Prepare the Injection Site
- Wipe the injection site with an alcohol swab in a circular motion and let it air dry. **Do not** touch the injection site again before giving the injection.
- **Do not** fan or blow on the clean area.

STEP 3: Inject ORENCIA
- Remove the needle cover only when you are ready to administer the injection. Hold the housing of the ORENCIA (abatacept) prefilled syringe with one hand and pull the needle cover straight off with your other hand (**see Figure F**). **Do not** touch the plunger while you remove the needle cover.

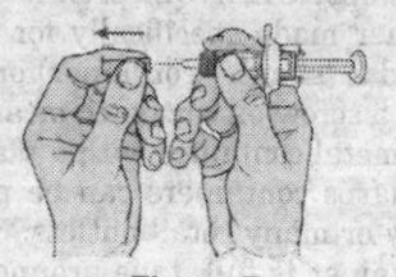

Figure F

- **Do not** put the needle cover back on the needle once removed. Throw away the needle cover in your household trash.
- **Do not** use the syringe if there are visible signs of needle damage or bending.
- There may be a small air bubble in the ORENCIA prefilled syringe housing. You do not need to remove it.
- You may notice a drop of fluid leaving the needle. This is normal and will not affect your dose.
- **Do not** touch the needle or let it touch any surfaces.
- **Do not** use the prefilled syringe if it is dropped without the needle cover in place.
- Hold the housing of your ORENCIA prefilled syringe in one hand between the thumb and index finger (**see Figure G**).

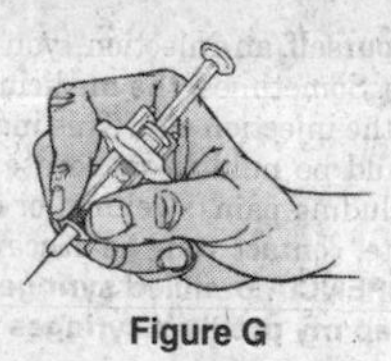

Figure G

- **Do not** pull back on the plunger of the syringe.
- Use your other hand and gently pinch the area of skin you cleaned. Hold firmly.
- Insert the needle with a quick motion into the pinched skin at a 45° angle (**see Figure H**).

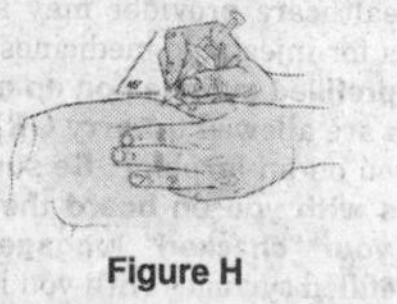

Figure H

- To inject all of the medicine, use your thumb to push the plunger until the plunger head is pushed in as far as it will go.
- Slowly lift your thumb from the plunger head. This allows the needle to be completely covered by the needle guard as it is removed from the skin (**see Figure I**).

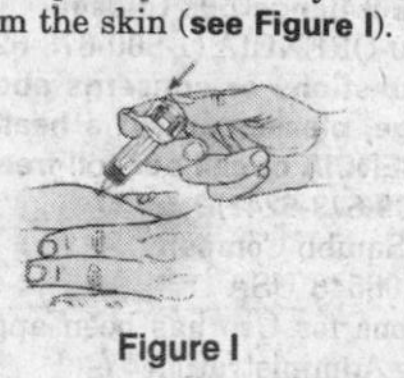

Figure I

- Remove the prefilled syringe and let go of the surrounding skin (**see Figure J**).

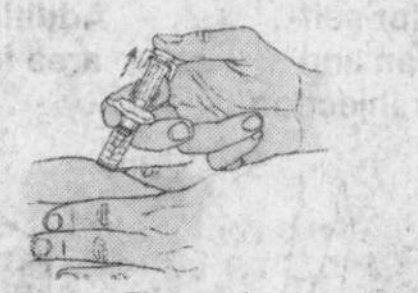

Figure J

After the Injection

- There may be a little bleeding at the injection site. You can press a cotton ball or gauze over the injection site.
- **Do not** rub the injection site.
- If needed, you may cover the injection site with a small bandage.

STEP 4: Disposal and Recordkeeping

- The ORENCIA (abatacept) prefilled syringe should not be reused.
- Put the used syringe into your puncture resistant container (see **"How do I throw away used syringes?"**).
- **Do not** put the needle cover back on the needle.
- **If your injection is given by another person, this person must also be careful when removing the syringe and disposing of the syringe to prevent accidental needle stick injury and passing infection.**

How do I throw away used syringes?

Check with your healthcare provider or pharmacist for instructions about the right way to throw away used syringes. There may be special local or state laws about how to throw away used syringes.

- **Do not** throw away used syringes in the household trash and do not recycle them.
- Put used and empty ORENCIA prefilled syringes in a biohazard container made specifically for disposing of used syringes (called a "sharps" container) or in a hard plastic container with a screw-on cap (such as an empty detergent bottle) or in a metal container with a plastic lid (such as a coffee can). Sharps containers can be purchased at your local pharmacy or many retail outlets.
- When the container is full, tape around the cap or lid to make sure the cap or lid does not come off.
- **Keep ORENCIA prefilled syringes and the disposal container out of the reach of children.**

Record your Injection

- Write the date, time, and specific part of your body where you injected yourself. It may also be helpful to write any questions or concerns about the injection so you can ask your healthcare provider.

If you have questions or concerns about your ORENCIA prefilled syringe, please contact a healthcare provider familiar with ORENCIA or call our toll-free help line at 1-800-ORENCIA (1-800-673-6242).

Frequently Asked Questions

<u>Injecting with the ORENCIA prefilled syringe</u>

I feel a little bit of burning or pain during injection. Is this normal?

- When giving yourself an injection, you may feel a prick from the needle. Sometimes, the medicine can cause slight irritation near the injection site. This may happen and the discomfort should be mild to moderate. If you have any side effects, including pain, swelling, or discoloration near the injection site, contact your healthcare provider.

<u>Traveling with ORENCIA prefilled syringes</u>

How should I keep my prefilled syringes cool while traveling?

- If you need to take your prefilled syringes with you, store them in a cool carrier between 36°F to 46°F (2°C to 8°C) until you are ready to use.
- **Do not** freeze ORENCIA.
- Keep ORENCIA in the original carton and protected from light. Your healthcare provider may know about special carrying cases for injectable medicines.

Can I take my prefilled syringes on an airplane?

- Generally you are allowed to carry ORENCIA prefilled syringes with you on an airplane. **Be sure to carry the prefilled syringes with you on board the plane, and do not put them in your "checked" luggage.** You should carry ORENCIA prefilled syringes with you in your travel cooler at a temperature of 36°F to 46°F (2°C to 8°C) until you are ready to use.
- Keep ORENCIA in the original carton, with its original preprinted labels and protected from light.

What if my syringe does not stay cool for an extended period of time? Is it dangerous to use?

- Contact 1-800-ORENCIA (1-800-673-6242) for details.

If you have questions or concerns about your ORENCIA prefilled syringe, please contact a healthcare provider familiar with ORENCIA or call our toll-free help line at 1-800-ORENCIA (1-800-673-6242).

Bristol-Myers Squibb Company
Princeton, NJ 08543 USA

This Instructions for Use has been approved by the U.S. Food and Drug Administration.

UltraSafe Passive® is a registered trademark of Safety Syringes, Inc.
All other trademarks are property of their respective companies.
1292618A2 / 1294018A1
Iss July 2013

Shown in Product Identification Guide, page 306

REYATAZ® ℞

[*RAY-ah-taz*]
(atazanavir sulfate)
Capsules

HIGHLIGHTS OF PRESCRIBING INFORMATION
These highlights do not include all the information needed to use REYATAZ safely and effectively. See full prescribing information for REYATAZ.
REYATAZ® (atazanavir sulfate) Capsules
Initial U.S. Approval: 2003

RECENT MAJOR CHANGES

Warnings and Precautions, Nephrolithiasis and Cholelithiasis (5.6) 01/2013

INDICATIONS AND USAGE

REYATAZ is a protease inhibitor indicated for use in combination with other antiretroviral agents for the treatment of HIV-1 infection. (1)

DOSAGE AND ADMINISTRATION

- *Treatment-naive patients:* REYATAZ 300 mg with ritonavir 100 mg once daily with food or REYATAZ 400 mg once daily with food. When coadministered with tenofovir, the recommended dose is REYATAZ 300 mg with ritonavir 100 mg. (2.1)
- *Treatment-experienced patients:* REYATAZ 300 mg with ritonavir 100 mg once daily with food. (2.1)
- *Pediatric patients (6 to less than 18 years of age):* Dosage is based on body weight not to exceed the adult dose. (2.2)
- *Pregnancy:* REYATAZ 300 mg with ritonavir 100 mg once daily with food, with dosing modifications for some concomitant medications. (2.3)
- *Concomitant therapy:* Dosing modifications may be required. (2.1, 7)
- *Renal impairment:* Dosing modifications may be required. (2.4)
- *Hepatic impairment:* Dosing modifications may be required. (2.5)

DOSAGE FORMS AND STRENGTHS

- Capsules: 150 mg, 200 mg, 300 mg. (3, 16)

CONTRAINDICATIONS

- REYATAZ is contraindicated in patients with previously demonstrated hypersensitivity (eg, Stevens-Johnson syndrome, erythema multiforme, or toxic skin eruptions) to any of the components of this product. (4)
- Coadministration with alfuzosin, triazolam, orally administered midazolam, ergot derivatives, rifampin, irinotecan, lovastatin, simvastatin, indinavir, cisapride, pimozide, St. John's wort, and sildenafil when dosed as REVATIO®. (4)

WARNINGS AND PRECAUTIONS

- *Cardiac conduction abnormalities:* PR interval prolongation may occur in some patients. Use with caution in patients with preexisting conduction system disease or when administered with other drugs that may prolong the PR interval. (5.2, 6.4, 7.3, 12.2, 17.3)
- *Rash:* Discontinue if severe rash develops. (5.3, 6.4, 17.4)
- *Hyperbilirubinemia:* Most patients experience asymptomatic increases in indirect bilirubin, which is reversible upon discontinuation. Do not dose reduce. If a concomitant transaminase increase occurs, evaluate for alternative etiologies. (5.4, 6.2)
- *Hepatotoxicity:* REYATAZ should be used with caution in patients with hepatic impairment (5.5). Patients with hepatitis B or C infection are at risk of increased transaminases or hepatic decompensation. Monitor hepatic laboratory tests prior to therapy and during treatment. (2.5, 5.5, 6.3, 6.4, 8.8)
- *Nephrolithiasis and cholelithiasis* have been reported. Consider temporary interruption or discontinuation. (5.6, 6.4)
- Patients receiving REYATAZ may develop new onset or exacerbations of diabetes mellitus/hyperglycemia (5.7, 6.4), immune reconstitution syndrome (5.8), and redistribution/accumulation of body fat (5.9).
- *Hemophilia:* Spontaneous bleeding may occur and additional factor VIII may be required. (5.10)

ADVERSE REACTIONS

Most common adverse reactions (≥2%) are nausea, jaundice/scleral icterus, rash, headache, abdominal pain, vomiting, insomnia, peripheral neurologic symptoms, dizziness, myalgia, diarrhea, depression, and fever. (6.1, 6.2)

To report SUSPECTED ADVERSE REACTIONS, contact Bristol-Myers Squibb at 1-800-721-5072 or FDA at 1-800-FDA-1088 or www.fda.gov/medwatch

DRUG INTERACTIONS

Coadministration of REYATAZ can alter the concentration of other drugs and other drugs may alter the concentration of atazanavir. The potential drug-drug interactions must be considered prior to and during therapy. (4, 5.1, 7, 12.3)

USE IN SPECIFIC POPULATIONS

- *Pregnancy:* Use only if the potential benefit justifies the potential risk. (8.1)
- *Nursing mothers* should be instructed not to breastfeed due to the potential for postnatal HIV transmission. (8.3)
- *Hepatitis B or C co-infection:* Monitor liver enzymes. (5.5, 6.3)
- *Renal impairment:* Do not use in treatment-experienced patients with end stage renal disease managed with hemodialysis. (2.4, 8.7)
- *Hepatic impairment:* REYATAZ should be used with caution in patients with mild to moderate hepatic impairment. Do not use REYATAZ in patients with severe hepatic impairment. REYATAZ/ritonavir is not recommended. (2.5, 8.8)

See 17 for PATIENT COUNSELING INFORMATION and FDA-approved patient labeling

Revised: 08/2013

FULL PRESCRIBING INFORMATION: CONTENTS*

*** Sections or subsections omitted from the full prescribing information are not listed**

FULL PRESCRIBING INFORMATION

1 INDICATIONS AND USAGE

REYATAZ® (atazanavir sulfate) is indicated in combination with other antiretroviral agents for the treatment of HIV-1 infection. This indication is based on analyses of plasma HIV-1 RNA levels and CD4+ cell counts from controlled studies of 96 weeks duration in antiretroviral-naive and 48 weeks duration in antiretroviral-treatment-experienced adult and pediatric patients at least 6 years of age.

The following points should be considered when initiating therapy with REYATAZ:

- In Study AI424-045, REYATAZ/ritonavir and lopinavir/ritonavir were similar for the primary efficacy outcome measure of time-averaged difference in change from baseline in HIV RNA level. This study was not large enough to reach a definitive conclusion that REYATAZ/ritonavir and lopinavir/ritonavir are equivalent on the secondary efficacy outcome measure of proportions below the HIV RNA lower limit of detection [see *Clinical Studies (14.2)*].
- The number of baseline primary protease inhibitor mutations affects the virologic response to REYATAZ/ritonavir [see *Clinical Pharmacology (12.4)*].

2 DOSAGE AND ADMINISTRATION

General Dosing Recommendations:

- REYATAZ Capsules must be taken with food.
- Do not open the capsules.
- The recommended oral dosage of REYATAZ depends on the treatment history of the patient and the use of other coadministered drugs. When coadministered with H_2-receptor antagonists or proton-pump inhibitors, dose separation may be required [see *Dosage and Administration (2.1)*].
- When coadministered with didanosine buffered or enteric-coated formulations, REYATAZ should be given (with food) 2 hours before or 1 hour after didanosine.
- REYATAZ without ritonavir is not recommended for treatment-experienced adult or pediatric patients with prior virologic failure [see *Clinical Studies (14)*].
- Efficacy and safety of REYATAZ with ritonavir in doses greater than 100 mg once daily have not been established. The use of higher ritonavir doses might alter the safety profile of atazanavir (cardiac effects, hyperbilirubinemia) and, therefore, is not recommended. Prescribers should consult the complete prescribing information for NORVIR® (ritonavir) when using this agent.

2.1 Recommended Adult Dosage

Table 1 summarizes the recommended REYATAZ dosing regimen in adults. All REYATAZ dosing regimens are to be administered as a single dose with food.

Table 1: REYATAZ Dosing Regimens

Treatment-Naive Patients	**REYATAZ 300 mg with ritonavir 100 mg once daily**
If unable to tolerate ritonavir	**REYATAZ 400 mg once daily**
When combined with any of the following: Tenofovir, H_2-receptor antagonist, Proton-pump inhibitor	**REYATAZ 300 mg with ritonavir 100 mg once daily**

- The H_2-receptor antagonist dose should not exceed a dose comparable to famotidine 40 mg twice daily. Administer REYATAZ and ritonavir simultaneously with, and/or at least 10 hours after the H_2-receptor antagonist.
- If unable to tolerate ritonavir, administer REYATAZ 400 mg once daily at least 2 hours before and at least 10 hours after the H_2-receptor antagonist. No single dose of the H_2-receptor antagonist should exceed a dose comparable to famotidine 20 mg and the total daily dose should not exceed a dose comparable to famotidine 40 mg.
- The proton-pump inhibitor dose should not exceed a dose comparable to omeprazole 20 mg daily and must be taken approximately 12 hours prior to REYATAZ and ritonavir.

When combined with efavirenz	**REYATAZ 400 mg with ritonavir 100 mg once daily**

- Efavirenz should be administered on an empty stomach, preferably at bedtime.

Treatment-Experienced Patients	**REYATAZ 300 mg with ritonavir 100 mg once daily**

Do not coadminister with proton-pump inhibitors or efavirenz in treatment-experienced patients.

When given with an H_2-receptor antagonist	**REYATAZ 300 mg with ritonavir 100 mg once daily**

- The H_2-receptor antagonist dose should not exceed a dose comparable to famotidine 20 mg twice daily. Administer REYATAZ and ritonavir simultaneously with, and/or at least 10 hours after the H_2-receptor antagonist.

When given with both tenofovir *and* an H_2-receptor antagonist	**REYATAZ 400 mg with ritonavir 100 mg once daily**

- The H_2-receptor antagonist dose should not exceed a dose comparable to famotidine 20 mg twice daily. Administer REYATAZ and ritonavir simultaneously with, and/or at least 10 hours after the H_2-receptor antagonist.

[For these drugs and other antiretroviral agents for which dosing modification may be appropriate, see *Drug Interactions (7)*.]

2.2 Recommended Pediatric Dosage

The recommended daily dosage of REYATAZ for pediatric patients (6 to less than 18 years of age) is based on body weight and should not exceed the recommended adult dosage. REYATAZ (atazanavir sulfate) Capsules must be taken with food. The data are insufficient to recommend dosing of REYATAZ for any of the following: (1) patients less than 6 years of age, (2) without ritonavir in any pediatric patient less than 13 years of age, and (3) patients less than 40 kg receiving concomitant tenofovir, H_2-receptor antagonists, or proton-pump inhibitors.

The recommended dosage of REYATAZ with ritonavir in pediatric patients at least 6 years of age is shown in Table 2.

Table 2: Dosage for Pediatric Patients (6 to less than 18 years of age) for REYATAZ Capsules with ritonavir[a]

Body Weight	REYATAZ dose	ritonavir dose
15 kg to less than 20 kg	150 mg	100 mg
20 kg to less than 40 kg	200 mg	100 mg
at least 40 kg	300 mg	100 mg

[a] The REYATAZ and ritonavir dose should be taken together once daily with food.

For treatment-naive patients at least 13 years of age and at least 40 kg, who are unable to tolerate ritonavir, the recommended dose is REYATAZ (atazanavir sulfate) 400 mg (without ritonavir) once daily with food. For patients at least 13 years of age and at least 40 kg receiving concomitant tenofovir, H_2-receptor antagonists, or proton-pump inhibitors, REYATAZ should not be administered without ritonavir.

2.3 Pregnancy

Dosing During Pregnancy and the Postpartum Period:

- REYATAZ should not be administered without ritonavir.
- REYATAZ should only be administered to pregnant women with HIV-1 strains susceptible to atazanavir.
- For pregnant patients, no dose adjustment is required for REYATAZ with the following exceptions:
  - For treatment-experienced pregnant women during the second or third trimester, when REYATAZ is coadministered with either an H_2-receptor antagonist or tenofovir, REYATAZ 400 mg with ritonavir 100 mg once daily is recommended. There are insufficient data to recommend a REYATAZ dose for use with both an H_2-receptor antagonist *and* tenofovir in treatment-experienced pregnant women.
- No dose adjustment is required for postpartum patients. However, patients should be closely monitored for adverse events because atazanavir exposures could be higher during the first 2 months after delivery. [See *Use in Specific Populations (8.1)* and *Clinical Pharmacology (12.3)*.]

2.4 Renal Impairment

For patients with renal impairment, including those with severe renal impairment who are not managed with hemo-

Table 3: Drugs That Are Contraindicated with REYATAZ (atazanavir) (Information in the table applies to REYATAZ with or without ritonavir, unless otherwise indicated)

Drug Class	Drugs within class that are contraindicated with REYATAZ	Clinical Comment
Alpha 1-Adrenoreceptor Antagonist	Alfuzosin	Potential for increased alfuzosin concentrations, which can result in hypotension.
Antimycobacterials	Rifampin	Rifampin substantially decreases plasma concentrations of atazanavir, which may result in loss of therapeutic effect and development of resistance.
Antineoplastics	Irinotecan	Atazanavir inhibits UGT1A1 and may interfere with the metabolism of irinotecan, resulting in increased irinotecan toxicities.
Benzodiazepines	Triazolam, orally administered midazolam[a]	Triazolam and orally administered midazolam are extensively metabolized by CYP3A4. Coadministration of triazolam or orally administered midazolam with REYATAZ may cause large increases in the concentration of these benzodiazepines. Potential for serious and/or life-threatening events such as prolonged or increased sedation or respiratory depression.
Ergot Derivatives	Dihydroergotamine, ergotamine, ergonovine, methylergonovine	Potential for serious and/or life-threatening events such as acute ergot toxicity characterized by peripheral vasospasm and ischemia of the extremities and other tissues.
GI Motility Agent	Cisapride	Potential for serious and/or life-threatening reactions such as cardiac arrhythmias.
Herbal Products	St. John's wort (*Hypericum perforatum*)	Patients taking REYATAZ should not use products containing St. John's wort because coadministration may be expected to reduce plasma concentrations of atazanavir. This may result in loss of therapeutic effect and development of resistance.
HMG-CoA Reductase Inhibitors	Lovastatin, simvastatin	Potential for serious reactions such as myopathy including rhabdomyolysis.
Neuroleptic	Pimozide	Potential for serious and/or life-threatening reactions such as cardiac arrhythmias.
PDE5 Inhibitor	Sildenafil[b] when dosed as REVATIO® for the treatment of pulmonary arterial hypertension	A safe and effective dose in combination with REYATAZ has not been established for sildenafil (REVATIO®) when used for the treatment of pulmonary hypertension. There is increased potential for sildenafil-associated adverse events (which include visual disturbances, hypotension, priapism, and syncope).
Protease Inhibitors	Indinavir	Both REYATAZ and indinavir are associated with indirect (unconjugated) hyperbilirubinemia.

[a] See *Drug Interactions, Table 13 (7)* for parenterally administered midazolam.
[b] See *Drug Interactions, Table 13 (7)* for sildenafil when dosed as VIAGRA® for erectile dysfunction.

Table 4: Selected Treatment-Emergent Adverse Reactions[a] of Moderate or Severe Intensity Reported in ≥2% of Adult Treatment-Naive Patients,[b] Study AI424-138

	96 weeks[c] REYATAZ 300 mg with ritonavir 100 mg (once daily) and tenofovir with emtricitabine[d] (n=441)	96 weeks[c] lopinavir 400 mg with ritonavir 100 mg (twice daily) and tenofovir with emtricitabine[d] (n=437)
Digestive System		
Nausea	4%	8%
Jaundice/scleral icterus	5%	*
Diarrhea	2%	12%
Skin and Appendages		
Rash	3%	2%

* None reported in this treatment arm.
[a] Includes events of possible, probable, certain, or unknown relationship to treatment regimen.
[b] Based on the regimen containing REYATAZ.
[c] Median time on therapy.
[d] As a fixed-dose combination: 300 mg tenofovir, 200 mg emtricitabine once daily.

Table 5: Selected Treatment-Emergent Adverse Reactions[a] of Moderate or Severe Intensity Reported in ≥2% of Adult Treatment-Naive Patients,[b] Studies AI424-034, AI424-007, and AI424-008

	Study AI424-034		Studies AI424-007, -008	
	64 weeks[c] REYATAZ 400 mg once daily + lamivudine + zidovudine[e] (n=404)	64 weeks[c] efavirenz 600 mg once daily + lamivudine + zidovudine[e] (n=401)	120 weeks[c,d] REYATAZ 400 mg once daily + stavudine + lamivudine or didanosine (n=279)	73 weeks[c,d] nelfinavir 750 mg TID or 1250 mg BID + stavudine + lamivudine or didanosine (n=191)
Body as a Whole				
Headache	6%	6%	1%	2%
Digestive System				
Nausea	14%	12%	6%	4%
Jaundice/scleral icterus	7%	*	7%	*
Vomiting	4%	7%	3%	3%
Abdominal pain	4%	4%	4%	2%
Diarrhea	1%	2%	3%	16%
Nervous System				
Insomnia	3%	3%	<1%	*
Dizziness	2%	7%	<1%	*
Peripheral neurologic symptoms	<1%	1%	4%	3%
Skin and Appendages				
Rash	7%	10%	5%	1%

* None reported in this treatment arm.
[a] Includes events of possible, probable, certain, or unknown relationship to treatment regimen.
[b] Based on regimens containing REYATAZ.
[c] Median time on therapy.
[d] Includes long-term follow-up.
[e] As a fixed-dose combination: 150 mg lamivudine, 300 mg zidovudine twice daily.

dialysis, no dose adjustment is required for REYATAZ. (atazanavir sulfate) Treatment-naive patients with end stage renal disease managed with hemodialysis should receive REYATAZ 300 mg with ritonavir 100 mg. REYATAZ should not be administered to HIV-treatment-experienced patients with end stage renal disease managed with hemodialysis. [See *Use in Specific Populations (8.7)*.]

2.5 Hepatic Impairment

REYATAZ should be used with caution in patients with mild-to-moderate hepatic impairment. For patients with moderate hepatic impairment (Child-Pugh Class B) who have not experienced prior virologic failure, a dose reduction to 300 mg once daily should be considered. REYATAZ should not be used in patients with severe hepatic impairment (Child-Pugh Class C). REYATAZ/ritonavir has not been studied in subjects with hepatic impairment and is not recommended. [See *Warnings and Precautions (5.5)* and *Use in Specific Populations (8.8)*.]

3 DOSAGE FORMS AND STRENGTHS

- 150 mg capsule with blue cap and powder blue body, printed with white ink "BMS 150 mg" on the cap and with blue ink "3624" on the body.
- 200 mg capsule with blue cap and blue body, printed with white ink "BMS 200 mg" on the cap and with white ink "3631" on the body.
- 300 mg capsule with red cap and blue body, printed with white ink "BMS 300 mg" on the cap and with white ink "3622" on the body.

4 CONTRAINDICATIONS

REYATAZ (atazanavir sulfate) is contraindicated:

- in patients with previously demonstrated clinically significant hypersensitivity (eg, Stevens-Johnson syndrome, erythema multiforme, or toxic skin eruptions) to any of the components of this product.
- when coadministered with drugs that are highly dependent on CYP3A or UGT1A1 for clearance, and for which elevated plasma concentrations are associated with serious and/or life-threatening events. These and other contraindicated drugs are listed in Table 3.

[See table 3 at top of previous page]

5 WARNINGS AND PRECAUTIONS

5.1 Drug Interactions

See Table 3 for a listing of drugs that are contraindicated for use with REYATAZ (atazanavir sulfate) due to potentially life-threatening adverse events, significant drug interactions, or loss of virologic activity. [See *Contraindications (4)*.] Please refer to Table 13 for established and other potentially significant drug interactions [see *Drug Interactions (7.3)*].

5.2 Cardiac Conduction Abnormalities

Atazanavir has been shown to prolong the PR interval of the electrocardiogram in some patients. In healthy volunteers and in patients, abnormalities in atrioventricular (AV) conduction were asymptomatic and generally limited to first-degree AV block. There have been reports of second-degree AV block and other conduction abnormalities [see *Adverse Reactions (6.4)* and *Overdosage (10)*]. In clinical trials that included electrocardiograms, asymptomatic first-degree AV block was observed in 5.9% of atazanavir-treated patients (n=920), 5.2% of lopinavir/ritonavir-treated patients (n=252), 10.4% of nelfinavir-treated patients (n=48), and 3.0% of efavirenz-treated patients (n=329). In Study AI424-045, asymptomatic first-degree AV block was observed in 5% (6/118) of atazanavir/ritonavir-treated patients and 5% (6/116) of lopinavir/ritonavir-treated patients who had on-study electrocardiogram measurements. Because of limited clinical experience in patients with preexisting conduction system disease (eg, marked first-degree AV block or second- or third-degree AV block), atazanavir should be used with caution in these patients. [See *Clinical Pharmacology (12.2)*.]

Atazanavir in combination with diltiazem increased diltiazem plasma concentration by 2-fold with an additive effect on the PR interval. When used in combination with atazanavir, a dose reduction of diltiazem by one-half should be considered and ECG monitoring is recommended. In a pharmacokinetic study between atazanavir 400 mg once daily and atenolol 50 mg once daily, no clinically significant additive effect of atazanavir and atenolol on the PR interval was observed. Dose adjustment of atenolol is not required when used in combination with atazanavir. [See *Drug Interactions (7)* and *Clinical Pharmacology (12.2)*.] Pharmacokinetic studies between atazanavir and other drugs that prolong the PR interval including beta blockers [other than atenolol, see *Drug Interactions (7)*], verapamil, and digoxin have not been performed. An additive effect of atazanavir and these drugs cannot be excluded; therefore, caution should be exercised when atazanavir is given concurrently with these drugs, especially those that are metabolized by CYP3A (eg, verapamil).

5.3 Rash

In controlled clinical trials, rash (all grades, regardless of causality) occurred in approximately 20% of patients treated with REYATAZ (atazanavir sulfate). The median time to onset of rash in clinical studies was 7.3 weeks and the median duration of rash was 1.4 weeks. Rashes were generally mild-to-moderate maculopapular skin eruptions. Treatment-emergent adverse reactions of moderate or severe rash (occurring at a rate of ≥2%) are presented for the individual clinical studies [see *Adverse Reactions (6.1)*]. Dosing with REYATAZ (atazanavir sulfate) was often continued without interruption in patients who developed rash. The discontinuation rate for rash in clinical trials was <1%. REYATAZ should be discontinued if severe rash develops. Cases of Stevens-Johnson syndrome, erythema multiforme, and toxic skin eruptions, including drug rash, eosinophilia and systemic symptoms (DRESS) syndrome, have been reported in patients receiving REYATAZ. [See *Contraindications (4)*.]

5.4 Hyperbilirubinemia

Most patients taking REYATAZ experience asymptomatic elevations in indirect (unconjugated) bilirubin related to inhibition of UDP-glucuronosyl transferase (UGT). This hyperbilirubinemia is reversible upon discontinuation of REYATAZ. Hepatic transaminase elevations that occur with hyperbilirubinemia should be evaluated for alternative etiologies. No long-term safety data are available for patients experiencing persistent elevations in total bilirubin >5 times ULN. Alternative antiretroviral therapy to REYATAZ may be considered if jaundice or scleral icterus associated with bilirubin elevations presents cosmetic concerns for patients. Dose reduction of atazanavir is not recommended since long-term efficacy of reduced doses has not been established. [See *Adverse Reactions (6.1, 6.2)*.]

5.5 Hepatotoxicity

Caution should be exercised when administering REYATAZ to patients with hepatic impairment because atazanavir concentrations may be increased. [See *Dosage and Administration (2.5)*.] Patients with underlying hepatitis B or C viral infections or marked elevations in transaminases before treatment may be at increased risk for developing further transaminase elevations or hepatic decompensation. In these patients, hepatic laboratory testing should be conducted prior to initiating therapy with REYATAZ and during treatment. [See *Adverse Reactions (6.3)* and *Use in Specific Populations (8.8)*.]

5.6 Nephrolithiasis and Cholelithiasis

Cases of nephrolithiasis and/or cholelithiasis have been reported during postmarketing surveillance in HIV-infected patients receiving REYATAZ therapy. Some patients required hospitalization for additional management and some had complications. Because these events were reported voluntarily during clinical practice, estimates of frequency cannot be made. If signs or symptoms of nephrolithiasis and/or cholelithiasis occur, temporary interruption or discontinuation of therapy may be considered. [See *Adverse Reactions (6.4)*.]

5.7 Diabetes Mellitus/Hyperglycemia

New-onset diabetes mellitus, exacerbation of preexisting diabetes mellitus, and hyperglycemia have been reported during postmarketing surveillance in HIV-infected patients receiving protease inhibitor therapy. Some patients required either initiation or dose adjustments of insulin or oral hypoglycemic agents for treatment of these events. In some cases, diabetic ketoacidosis has occurred. In those patients who discontinued protease inhibitor therapy, hyperglycemia persisted in some cases. Because these events have been reported voluntarily during clinical practice, estimates of frequency cannot be made and a causal relationship between protease inhibitor therapy and these events has not been established. [See *Adverse Reactions (6.4)*.]

5.8 Immune Reconstitution Syndrome

Immune reconstitution syndrome has been reported in patients treated with combination antiretroviral therapy, including REYATAZ (atazanavir sulfate). During the initial phase of combination antiretroviral treatment, patients whose immune system responds may develop an inflammatory response to indolent or residual opportunistic infections (such as *Mycobacterium avium* infection, cytomegalovirus, *Pneumocystis jiroveci* pneumonia, or tuberculosis), which may necessitate further evaluation and treatment. Autoimmune disorders (such as Graves' disease, polymyositis, and Guillain-Barré syndrome) have also been reported to occur in the setting of immune reconstitution; however, the time to onset is more variable, and can occur many months after initiation of treatment.

5.9 Fat Redistribution

Redistribution/accumulation of body fat including central obesity, dorsocervical fat enlargement (buffalo hump), peripheral wasting, facial wasting, breast enlargement, and "cushingoid appearance" have been observed in patients receiving antiretroviral therapy. The mechanism and long-term consequences of these events are currently unknown. A causal relationship has not been established.

5.10 Hemophilia

There have been reports of increased bleeding, including spontaneous skin hematomas and hemarthrosis, in patients with hemophilia type A and B treated with protease inhibitors. In some patients additional factor VIII was given. In more than half of the reported cases, treatment with protease inhibitors was continued or reintroduced. A causal relationship between protease inhibitor therapy and these events has not been established.

5.11 Resistance/Cross-Resistance

Various degrees of cross-resistance among protease inhibitors have been observed. Resistance to atazanavir may not preclude the subsequent use of other protease inhibitors. [See *Clinical Pharmacology (12.4)*.]

6 ADVERSE REACTIONS

The following adverse reactions are discussed in greater detail in other sections of the labeling:

- cardiac conduction abnormalities [see *Warnings and Precautions (5.2)*]
- rash [see *Warnings and Precautions (5.3)*]
- hyperbilirubinemia [see *Warnings and Precautions (5.4)*]
- nephrolithiasis and cholelithiasis [see *Warnings and Precautions (5.6)*]

Because clinical trials are conducted under widely varying conditions, adverse reaction rates observed in the clinical trials of a drug cannot be directly compared to rates in the clinical trials of another drug and may not reflect the rates observed in practice.

6.1 Clinical Trial Experience in Adults

Treatment-Emergent Adverse Reactions in Treatment-Naive Patients

The safety profile of REYATAZ in treatment-naive adults is based on 1625 HIV-1 infected patients in clinical trials. 536 patients received REYATAZ 300 mg with ritonavir 100 mg and 1089 patients received REYATAZ 400 mg or higher (without ritonavir).

The most common adverse reactions are nausea, jaundice/scleral icterus, and rash.

Selected clinical adverse reactions of moderate or severe intensity reported in ≥2% of treatment-naive patients receiving combination therapy including REYATAZ 300 mg with ritonavir 100 mg and REYATAZ 400 mg (without ritonavir) are presented in Tables 4 and 5, respectively.

[See table 4 at top of previous page]
[See table 5 at top of previous page]

Treatment-Emergent Adverse Reactions in Treatment-Experienced Patients

The safety profile of REYATAZ in treatment-experienced adults is based on 119 HIV-1 infected patients in clinical trials.

The most common adverse reactions are jaundice/scleral icterus and myalgia.

Selected clinical adverse reactions of moderate or severe intensity reported in ≥2% of treatment-experienced patients receiving REYATAZ/ritonavir are presented in Table 6.

[See table 6 above]

Laboratory Abnormalities in Treatment-Naive Patients

The percentages of adult treatment-naive patients treated with combination therapy including REYATAZ (atazanavir sulfate) 300 mg with ritonavir 100 mg and REYATAZ 400 mg (without ritonavir) with Grade 3–4 laboratory abnormalities are presented in Tables 7 and 8, respectively.

[See table 7 above]
[See table 8 above]

Table 6: Selected Treatment-Emergent Adverse Reactions[a] of Moderate or Severe Intensity Reported in ≥2% of Adult Treatment-Experienced Patients,[b] Study AI424-045

	48 weeks[c] REYATAZ/ritonavir 300/100 mg once daily + tenofovir + NRTI (n=119)	48 weeks[c] lopinavir/ritonavir 400/100 mg twice daily[d] + tenofovir + NRTI (n=118)
Body as a Whole		
Fever	2%	*
Digestive System		
Jaundice/scleral icterus	9%	*
Diarrhea	3%	11%
Nausea	3%	2%
Nervous System		
Depression	2%	<1%
Musculoskeletal System		
Myalgia	4%	*

* None reported in this treatment arm.
[a] Includes events of possible, probable, certain, or unknown relationship to treatment regimen.
[b] Based on the regimen containing REYATAZ.
[c] Median time on therapy.
[d] As a fixed-dose combination.

Table 7: Grade 3–4 Laboratory Abnormalities Reported in ≥2% of Adult Treatment-Naive Patients,[a] Study AI424-138

Variable	Limit[c]	96 weeks[b] REYATAZ 300 mg with ritonavir 100 mg (once daily) and tenofovir with emtricitabine[d] (n=441)	96 weeks[b] lopinavir 400 mg with ritonavir 100 mg (twice daily) and tenofovir with emtricitabine[d] (n=437)
Chemistry	High		
SGOT/AST	≥5.1 × ULN	3%	1%
SGPT/ALT	≥5.1 × ULN	3%	2%
Total Bilirubin	≥2.6 × ULN	44%	<1%
Lipase	≥2.1 × ULN	2%	2%
Creatine Kinase	≥5.1 × ULN	8%	7%
Total Cholesterol	≥240 mg/dL	11%	25%
Hematology	Low		
Neutrophils	<750 cells/mm³	5%	2%

[a] Based on the regimen containing REYATAZ.
[b] Median time on therapy.
[c] ULN = upper limit of normal.
[d] As a fixed-dose combination. 300 mg tenofovir, 200 mg emtricitabine once daily.

Table 8: Grade 3–4 Laboratory Abnormalities Reported in ≥2% of Adult Treatment-Naive Patients,[a] Studies AI424-034, AI424-007, and AI424-008

		Study AI424-034		Studies AI424-007, -008	
Variable	Limit[d]	64 weeks[b] REYATAZ 400 mg once daily + lamivudine + zidovudine[e] (n=404)	64 weeks[b] efavirenz 600 mg once daily + lamivudine + zidovudine[e] (n=401)	120 weeks[b,c] REYATAZ 400 mg once daily + stavudine + lamivudine or + stavudine + didanosine (n=279)	73 weeks[b,c] nelfinavir 750 mg TID or 1250 mg BID + stavudine + lamivudine or + stavudine + didanosine (n=191)
Chemistry	High				
SGOT/AST	≥5.1 × ULN	2%	2%	7%	5%
SGPT/ALT	≥5.1 × ULN	4%	3%	9%	7%
Total Bilirubin	≥2.6 × ULN	35%	<1%	47%	3%
Amylase	≥2.1 × ULN	*	*	14%	10%
Lipase	≥2.1 × ULN	<1%	1%	4%	5%
Creatine Kinase	≥5.1 × ULN	6%	6%	11%	9%
Total Cholesterol	≥240 mg/dL	6%	24%	19%	48%
Triglycerides	≥751 mg/dL	<1%	3%	4%	2%
Hematology	Low				
Hemoglobin	<8.0 g/dL	5%	3%	<1%	4%
Neutrophils	<750 cells/mm³	7%	9%	3%	7%

* None reported in this treatment arm.
[a] Based on regimen(s) containing REYATAZ.
[b] Median time on therapy.
[c] Includes long-term follow-up.
[d] ULN = upper limit of normal.
[e] As a fixed-dose combination: 150 mg lamivudine, 300 mg zidovudine twice daily.

Laboratory Abnormalities in Treatment-Experienced Patients

The percentages of adult treatment-experienced patients treated with combination therapy including REYATAZ/ritonavir with Grade 3–4 laboratory abnormalities are presented in Table 9.

[See table 9 at top of next page]

Lipids, Change from Baseline in Treatment-Naive Patients

For Study AI424-138 and Study AI424-034, changes from baseline in LDL-cholesterol, HDL-cholesterol, total cholesterol, and triglycerides are shown in Tables 10 and 11, respectively.

[See table 10 at top of next page]
[See table 11 at top of next page]

Table 9: Grade 3–4 Laboratory Abnormalities Reported in ≥2% of Adult Treatment-Experienced Patients, Study AI424-045[a]

Variable	Limit[c]	48 weeks[b] REYATAZ/ritonavir 300/100 mg once daily + tenofovir + NRTI (n=119)	48 weeks[b] lopinavir/ritonavir 400/100 mg twice daily[d] + tenofovir + NRTI (n=118)
Chemistry	High		
SGOT/AST	≥5.1 × ULN	3%	3%
SGPT/ALT	≥5.1 × ULN	4%	3%
Total Bilirubin	≥2.6 × ULN	49%	<1%
Lipase	≥2.1 × ULN	5%	6%
Creatine Kinase	≥5.1 × ULN	8%	8%
Total Cholesterol	≥240 mg/dL	25%	26%
Triglycerides	≥751 mg/dL	8%	12%
Glucose	≥251 mg/dL	5%	<1%
Hematology	Low		
Platelets	<50,000 cells/mm^3	2%	3%
Neutrophils	<750 cells/mm^3	7%	8%

[a] Based on regimen(s) containing REYATAZ.
[b] Median time on therapy.
[c] ULN = upper limit of normal.
[d] As a fixed-dose combination.

Table 10: Lipid Values, Mean Change from Baseline, Study AI424-138

	REYATAZ/ritonavir[a,b] Baseline mg/dL (n=428[e])	Week 48 mg/dL (n=372[e])	Week 48 Change[d] (n=372[e])	Week 96 mg/dL (n=342[e])	Week 96 Change[d] (n=342[e])	lopinavir/ritonavir[b,c] Baseline mg/dL (n=424[e])	Week 48 mg/dL (n=335[e])	Week 48 Change[d] (n=335[e])	Week 96 mg/dL (n=291[e])	Week 96 Change[d] (n=291[e])
LDL-Cholesterol[f]	92	105	+14%	105	+14%	93	111	+19%	110	+17%
HDL-Cholesterol[f]	37	46	+29%	44	+21%	36	48	+37%	46	+29%
Total Cholesterol[f]	149	169	+13%	169	+13%	150	187	+25%	186	+25%
Triglycerides[f]	126	145	+15%	140	+13%	129	194	+52%	184	+50%

[a] REYATAZ 300 mg with ritonavir 100 mg once daily with the fixed-dose combination: 300 mg tenofovir, 200 mg emtricitabine once daily.
[b] Values obtained after initiation of serum lipid-reducing agents were not included in these analyses. At baseline, serum lipid-reducing agents were used in 1% in the lopinavir/ritonavir treatment arm and 1% in the REYATAZ/ritonavir arm. Through Week 48, serum lipid-reducing agents were used in 8% in the lopinavir/ritonavir treatment arm and 2% in the REYATAZ/ritonavir arm. Through Week 96, serum lipid-reducing agents were used in 10% in the lopinavir/ritonavir treatment arm and 3% in the REYATAZ/ritonavir arm.
[c] Lopinavir 400 mg with ritonavir 100 mg twice daily with the fixed-dose combination 300 mg tenofovir, 200 mg emtricitabine once daily.
[d] The change from baseline is the mean of within-patient changes from baseline for patients with both baseline and Week 48 or Week 96 values and is not a simple difference of the baseline and Week 48 or Week 96 mean values, respectively.
[e] Number of patients with LDL-cholesterol measured.
[f] Fasting.

Table 11: Lipid Values, Mean Change from Baseline, Study AI424-034

	REYATAZ[a,b] Baseline mg/dL (n=383[e])	Week 48 mg/dL (n=283[e])	Week 48 Change[d] (n=272[e])	efavirenz[b,c] Baseline mg/dL (n=378[e])	Week 48 mg/dL (n=264[e])	Week 48 Change[d] (n=253[e])
LDL-Cholesterol[f]	98	98	+1%	98	114	+18%
HDL-Cholesterol	39	43	+13%	38	46	+24%
Total Cholesterol	164	168	+2%	162	195	+21%
Triglycerides[f]	138	124	-9%	129	168	+23%

[a] REYATAZ 400 mg once daily with the fixed-dose combination: 150 mg lamivudine, 300 mg zidovudine twice daily.
[b] Values obtained after initiation of serum lipid-reducing agents were not included in these analyses. At baseline, serum lipid-reducing agents were used in 0% in the efavirenz treatment arm and <1% in the REYATAZ arm. Through Week 48, serum lipid-reducing agents were used in 3% in the efavirenz treatment arm and 1% in the REYATAZ arm.
[c] Efavirenz 600 mg once daily with the fixed-dose combination: 150 mg lamivudine, 300 mg zidovudine twice daily.
[d] The change from baseline is the mean of within-patient changes from baseline for patients with both baseline and Week 48 values and is not a simple difference of the baseline and Week 48 mean values.
[e] Number of patients with LDL-cholesterol measured.
[f] Fasting.

Lipids, Change from Baseline in Treatment-Experienced Patients

For Study AI424-045, changes from baseline in LDL-cholesterol, HDL-cholesterol, total cholesterol, and triglycerides are shown in Table 12. The observed magnitude of dyslipidemia was less with REYATAZ/ritonavir than with lopinavir/ritonavir. However, the clinical impact of such findings has not been demonstrated.

[See table 12 at top of next page]

6.2 Clinical Trial Experience in Pediatric Patients

The safety and tolerability of REYATAZ (atazanavir sulfate) Capsules with and without ritonavir have been established in pediatric patients at least 6 years of age from the open-label, multicenter clinical trial PACTG 1020A. Use of REYATAZ (atazanavir sulfate) in pediatric patients less than 6 years of age is under investigation.

The safety profile of REYATAZ in pediatric patients (6 to less than 18 years of age) was generally similar to that observed in clinical studies of REYATAZ in adults. The most common Grade 2–4 adverse events (≥5%, regardless of causality) reported in pediatric patients were cough (21%), fever (18%), jaundice/scleral icterus (15%), rash (14%), vomiting (12%), diarrhea (9%), headache (8%), peripheral edema (7%), extremity pain (6%), nasal congestion (6%), oropharyngeal pain (6%), wheezing (6%), and rhinorrhea (6%). Asymptomatic second-degree atrioventricular block was reported in <2% of patients. The most common Grade 3–4 laboratory abnormalities occurring in pediatric patients were elevation of total bilirubin (≥3.2 mg/dL, 58%), neutropenia (9%), and hypoglycemia (4%). All other Grade 3–4 laboratory abnormalities occurred with a frequency of less than 3%.

6.3 Patients Co-infected With Hepatitis B and/or Hepatitis C Virus

Liver function tests should be monitored in patients with a history of hepatitis B or C.

In study AI424-138, 60 patients treated with REYATAZ/ritonavir 300 mg/100 mg once daily, and 51 patients treated with lopinavir/ritonavir 400 mg/100 mg twice daily, each with fixed dose tenofovir-emtricitabine, were seropositive for hepatitis B and/or C at study entry. ALT levels >5 times ULN developed in 10% (6/60) of the REYATAZ/ritonavir-treated patients and 8% (4/50) of the lopinavir/ritonavir-treated patients. AST levels >5 times ULN developed in 10% (6/60) of the REYATAZ/ritonavir-treated patients and none (0/50) of the lopinavir/ritonavir-treated patients.

In study AI424-045, 20 patients treated with REYATAZ/ritonavir 300 mg/100 mg once daily, and 18 patients treated with lopinavir/ritonavir 400 mg/100 mg twice daily, were seropositive for hepatitis B and/or C at study entry. ALT levels >5 times ULN developed in 25% (5/20) of the REYATAZ/ritonavir-treated patients and 6% (1/18) of the lopinavir/ritonavir-treated patients. AST levels >5 times ULN developed in 10% (2/20) of the REYATAZ/ritonavir-treated patients and 6% (1/18) of the lopinavir/ritonavir-treated patients.

In studies AI424-008 and AI424-034, 74 patients treated with 400 mg of REYATAZ (atazanavir sulfate) once daily, 58 who received efavirenz, and 12 who received nelfinavir were seropositive for hepatitis B and/or C at study entry. ALT levels >5 times the upper limit of normal (ULN) developed in 15% of the REYATAZ-treated patients, 14% of the efavirenz-treated patients, and 17% of the nelfinavir-treated patients. AST levels >5 times ULN developed in 9% of the REYATAZ-treated patients, 5% of the efavirenz-treated patients, and 17% of the nelfinavir-treated patients. Within atazanavir and control regimens, no difference in frequency of bilirubin elevations was noted between seropositive and seronegative patients. [See *Warnings and Precautions (5.5)*.]

6.4 Postmarketing Experience

The following events have been identified during postmarketing use of REYATAZ. Because these reactions are reported voluntarily from a population of unknown size, it is not always possible to reliably estimate their frequency or establish a causal relationship to drug exposure.

Body as a Whole: edema

Cardiovascular System: second-degree AV block, third-degree AV block, left bundle branch block, QTc prolongation [see *Warnings and Precautions (5.2)*]

Gastrointestinal System: pancreatitis

Hepatic System: hepatic function abnormalities

Hepatobiliary Disorders: cholelithiasis [see *Warnings and Precautions (5.6)*], cholecystitis, cholestasis

Metabolic System and Nutrition Disorders: diabetes mellitus, hyperglycemia [see *Warnings and Precautions (5.7)*]

Musculoskeletal System: arthralgia

Renal System: nephrolithiasis [see *Warnings and Precautions (5.6)*], interstitial nephritis

Skin and Appendages: alopecia, maculopapular rash [see *Contraindications (4)* and *Warnings and Precautions (5.3)*], pruritus, angioedema

7 DRUG INTERACTIONS

See also *Contraindications (4)* and *Clinical Pharmacology (12.3)*.

7.1 Potential for REYATAZ to Affect Other Drugs

Atazanavir is an inhibitor of CYP3A and UGT1A1. Coadministration of REYATAZ and drugs primarily metabolized by CYP3A or UGT1A1 may result in increased plasma concentrations of the other drug that could increase or prolong its therapeutic and adverse effects.

Atazanavir is a weak inhibitor of CYP2C8. Caution should be used when REYATAZ without ritonavir is coadministered with drugs highly dependent on CYP2C8 with narrow therapeutic indices (eg, paclitaxel, repaglinide). When REYATAZ with ritonavir is coadministered with substrates of CYP2C8, clinically significant interactions are not expected. [See *Clinical Pharmacology, Table 14 (12.3)*.]

The magnitude of CYP3A-mediated drug interactions on coadministered drug may change when REYATAZ is coadministered with ritonavir. See the complete prescribing information for NORVIR® (ritonavir) for information on drug interactions with ritonavir.

7.2 Potential for Other Drugs to Affect Atazanavir

Atazanavir is a CYP3A4 substrate; therefore, drugs that induce CYP3A4 may decrease atazanavir plasma concentrations and reduce REYATAZ's therapeutic effect.

Atazanavir solubility decreases as pH increases. Reduced plasma concentrations of atazanavir are expected if proton-pump inhibitors, antacids, buffered medications, or H_2-receptor antagonists are administered with atazanavir.

7.3 Established and Other Potentially Significant Drug Interactions

Table 13 provides dosing recommendations as a result of drug interactions with REYATAZ (atazanavir sulfate). These recommendations are based on either drug interaction studies or predicted interactions due to the expected magnitude of interaction and potential for serious events or loss of efficacy.

[See table 13 below and on pages 778 through 781]

7.4 Drugs with No Observed or Predicted Interactions with REYATAZ

Clinically significant interactions are not expected between atazanavir and substrates of CYP2C19, CYP2C9, CYP2D6, CYP2B6, CYP2A6, CYP1A2, or CYP2E1. Clinically significant interactions are not expected between atazanavir when administered with ritonavir and substrates of CYP2C8. See the complete prescribing information for NORVIR® for information on other potential drug interactions with ritonavir.

Based on known metabolic profiles, clinically significant drug interactions are not expected between REYATAZ (atazanavir sulfate) and dapsone, trimethoprim/sulfamethoxazole, azithromycin, or erythromycin. REYATAZ does not interact with substrates of CYP2D6 (eg, nortriptyline, desipramine, metoprolol). Additionally, no clinically significant drug interactions were observed when REYATAZ was coadministered with methadone, fluconazole, acetaminophen, or atenolol. [See *Clinical Pharmacology, Tables 17* and *18 (12.3)*.]

8 USE IN SPECIFIC POPULATIONS

8.1 Pregnancy

Pregnancy Category B

Antiretroviral Pregnancy Registry: To monitor maternal-fetal outcomes of pregnant women exposed to REYATAZ, an Antiretroviral Pregnancy Registry has been established. Physicians are encouraged to register patients by calling 1-800-258-4263.

Risk Summary

Atazanavir has been evaluated in a limited number of women during pregnancy and postpartum. Available human and animal data suggest that atazanavir does not increase the risk of major birth defects overall compared to the background rate. However, because the studies in humans cannot rule out the possibility of harm, REYATAZ should be used during pregnancy only if clearly needed.

Cases of lactic acidosis syndrome, sometimes fatal, and symptomatic hyperlactatemia have occurred in pregnant women using REYATAZ in combination with nucleoside analogues. Nucleoside analogues are associated with an increased risk of lactic acidosis syndrome.

Hyperbilirubinemia occurs frequently in patients who take REYATAZ, including pregnant women. All infants, including neonates exposed to REYATAZ *in-utero*, should be monitored for the development of severe hyperbilirubinemia during the first few days of life.

Clinical Considerations

Dosing During Pregnancy and the Postpartum Period:

- REYATAZ should not be administered without ritonavir.
- REYATAZ should only be administered to pregnant women with HIV-1 strains susceptible to atazanavir.
- For pregnant patients, no dose adjustment is required for REYATAZ with the following exceptions:
  - For treatment-experienced pregnant women during the second or third trimester, when REYATAZ is coadministered with either an H_2-receptor antagonist **or** tenofovir, REYATAZ 400 mg with ritonavir 100 mg once daily is recommended. There are insufficient data to recommend a REYATAZ dose for use with both an H_2-receptor antagonist *and* tenofovir in treatment-experienced pregnant women.
- No dose adjustment is required for postpartum patients. However, patients should be closely monitored for adverse events because atazanavir exposures could be higher during the first 2 months after delivery. [See *Dosage and Administration (2, 2.3)* and *Clinical Pharmacology (12.3)*.]

Human Data

Clinical Trials: In clinical trial AI424-182, REYATAZ/ritonavir (300/100 mg or 400/100 mg) in combination with zidovudine/lamivudine was administered to 41 HIV-infected pregnant women during the second or third trimester. Among the 39 women who completed the study, 38 women achieved an HIV RNA <50 copies/mL at time of delivery. Six of 20 (30%) women on REYATAZ/ritonavir 300/100 mg and 13 of 21 (62%) women on REYATAZ/ritonavir 400/100 mg experienced hyperbilirubinemia (total bilirubin greater than or equal to 2.6 times the upper limit of normal). There were no cases of lactic acidosis observed in clinical trial AI424-182.

Atazanavir drug concentrations in fetal umbilical cord blood were approximately 12–19% of maternal concentrations. Among the 40 infants born to 40 HIV-infected pregnant women, all had test results that were negative for HIV-1 DNA at the time of delivery and/or during the first 6 months postpartum. All 40 infants received antiretroviral prophylactic treatment containing zidovudine. No evidence of severe hyperbilirubinemia (total bilirubin levels greater than 20 mg/dL) or acute or chronic bilirubin encephalopathy was observed among neonates in this study. However, 10/36 (28%) infants (6 greater than or equal to 38 weeks gestation and 4 less than 38 weeks gestation) had bilirubin levels of 4 mg/dL or greater within the first day of life.

Table 12: Lipid Values, Mean Change from Baseline, Study AI424-045

	REYATAZ/ritonavir[a,b]			lopinavir/ritonavir[b,c]		
	Baseline mg/dL (n=111[e])	Week 48 mg/dL (n=75[e])	Week 48 Change[d] (n=74[e])	Baseline mg/dL (n=108[e])	Week 48 mg/dL (n=76[e])	Week 48 Change[d] (n=73[e])
LDL Cholesterol[f]	108	98	-10%	104	103	+1%
HDL-Cholesterol	40	39	-7%	39	41	+2%
Total Cholesterol	188	170	-8%	181	187	+6%
Triglycerides[f]	215	161	-4%	196	224	+30%

[a] REYATAZ 300 mg once daily + ritonavir + tenofovir + 1 NRTI.

[b] Values obtained after initiation of serum lipid-reducing agents were not included in these analyses. At baseline, serum lipid-reducing agents were used in 4% in the lopinavir/ritonavir treatment arm and 4% in the REYATAZ/ritonavir arm. Through Week 48, serum lipid-reducing agents were used in 19% in the lopinavir/ritonavir treatment arm and 8% in the REYATAZ/ritonavir arm.

[c] Lopinavir/ritonavir (400/100 mg) BID + tenofovir + 1 NRTI.

[d] The change from baseline is the mean of within-patient changes from baseline for patients with both baseline and Week 48 values and is not a simple difference of the baseline and Week 48 mean values.

[e] Number of patients with LDL-cholesterol measured.

[f] Fasting.

Table 13: Established and Other Potentially Significant Drug Interactions: Alteration in Dose or Regimen May Be Recommended Based on Drug Interaction Studies[a] or Predicted Interactions (Information in the table applies to REYATAZ with or without ritonavir, unless otherwise indicated)

Concomitant Drug Class: Specific Drugs	Effect on Concentration of Atazanavir or Concomitant Drug	Clinical Comment
HIV Antiviral Agents		
Nucleoside Reverse Transcriptase Inhibitors (NRTIs): didanosine buffered formulations enteric-coated (EC) capsules	↓ atazanavir ↓ didanosine	Coadministration of REYATAZ with didanosine buffered tablets resulted in a marked decrease in atazanavir exposure. It is recommended that REYATAZ be given (with food) 2 h before or 1 h after didanosine buffered formulations. Simultaneous administration of didanosine EC and REYATAZ with food results in a decrease in didanosine exposure. Thus, REYATAZ and didanosine EC should be administered at different times.
Nucleotide Reverse Transcriptase Inhibitors: tenofovir disoproxil fumarate	↓ atazanavir ↑ tenofovir	Tenofovir may decrease the AUC and C_{min} of atazanavir. When coadministered with tenofovir, it is recommended that REYATAZ 300 mg be given with ritonavir 100 mg and tenofovir 300 mg (all as a single daily dose with food). **REYATAZ without ritonavir should not be coadministered with tenofovir.** REYATAZ increases tenofovir concentrations. The mechanism of this interaction is unknown. Higher tenofovir concentrations could potentiate tenofovir-associated adverse events, including renal disorders. Patients receiving REYATAZ and tenofovir should be monitored for tenofovir-associated adverse events. For pregnant women taking REYATAZ with ritonavir *and* tenofovir, see *Dosage and Administration (2.3)*.
Non-nucleoside Reverse Transcriptase Inhibitors (NNRTIs): efavirenz	↓ atazanavir	Efavirenz decreases atazanavir exposure. ***In treatment-naive patients:*** If REYATAZ is combined with efavirenz, REYATAZ 400 mg (two 200-mg capsules) with ritonavir 100 mg should be administered once daily all as a single dose with food, and efavirenz 600 mg should be administered once daily on an empty stomach, preferably at bedtime. ***In treatment-experienced patients:*** Do not coadminister REYATAZ with efavirenz in treatment-experienced patients due to decreased atazanavir exposure.
nevirapine	↓ atazanavir ↑ nevirapine	Do not coadminister REYATAZ with nevirapine because: • Nevirapine substantially decreases atazanavir exposure. • Potential risk for nevirapine associated toxicity due to increased nevirapine exposures.
Protease Inhibitors: saquinavir (soft gelatin capsules)	↑ saquinavir	Appropriate dosing recommendations for this combination, with or without ritonavir, with respect to efficacy and safety have not been established. In a clinical study, saquinavir 1200 mg coadministered with REYATAZ 400 mg and tenofovir 300 mg (all given once daily) plus nucleoside analogue reverse transcriptase inhibitors did not provide adequate efficacy [see *Clinical Studies (14.2)*].
ritonavir	↑ atazanavir	If REYATAZ is coadministered with ritonavir, it is recommended that REYATAZ 300 mg once daily be given with ritonavir 100 mg once daily with food. See the complete prescribing information for NORVIR® (ritonavir) for information on drug interactions with ritonavir.
others	↑ other protease inhibitor	***REYATAZ/ritonavir:*** Although not studied, the coadministration of REYATAZ/ritonavir and other protease inhibitors would be expected to increase exposure to the other protease inhibitor. Such coadministration is not recommended.

(Table continued on next page)

Table 13 *(cont.)*: Established and Other Potentially Significant Drug Interactions: Alteration in Dose or Regimen May Be Recommended Based on Drug Interaction Studies[a] or Predicted Interactions (Information in the table applies to REYATAZ with or without ritonavir, unless otherwise indicated)

Concomitant Drug Class: Specific Drugs	Effect on Concentration of Atazanavir or Concomitant Drug	Clinical Comment
HCV Antiviral Agents		
Protease Inhibitors: boceprevir	↓ atazanavir ↓ ritonavir	Concomitant administration of boceprevir and atazanavir/ritonavir resulted in reduced steady-state exposures to atazanavir and ritonavir. Coadministration of REYATAZ/ritonavir and boceprevir is not recommended.
telaprevir	↓ telaprevir ↑ atazanavir	Concomitant administration of telaprevir and atazanavir/ritonavir resulted in reduced steady-state telaprevir exposure, while steady-state atazanavir exposure was increased.
Other Agents		
Antacids and buffered medications	↓ atazanavir	Reduced plasma concentrations of atazanavir are expected if antacids, including buffered medications, are administered with REYATAZ. REYATAZ should be administered 2 hours before or 1 hour after these medications.
Antiarrhythmics: amiodarone, bepridil, lidocaine (systemic), quinidine	↑ amiodarone, bepridil, lidocaine (systemic), quinidine	Coadministration with REYATAZ has the potential to produce serious and/or life-threatening adverse events and has not been studied. Caution is warranted and therapeutic concentration monitoring of these drugs is recommended if they are used concomitantly with REYATAZ (atazanavir sulfate).
Anticoagulants: warfarin	↑ warfarin	Coadministration with REYATAZ has the potential to produce serious and/or life-threatening bleeding and has not been studied. It is recommended that INR (International Normalized Ratio) be monitored.
Antidepressants: tricyclic antidepressants	↑ tricyclic antidepressants	Coadministration with REYATAZ has the potential to produce serious and/or life-threatening adverse events and has not been studied. Concentration monitoring of these drugs is recommended if they are used concomitantly with REYATAZ.
trazodone	↑ trazodone	Concomitant use of trazodone and REYATAZ with or without ritonavir may increase plasma concentrations of trazodone. Adverse events of nausea, dizziness, hypotension, and syncope have been observed following coadministration of trazodone and ritonavir. If trazodone is used with a CYP3A4 inhibitor such as REYATAZ, the combination should be used with caution and a lower dose of trazodone should be considered.
Antiepileptics: carbamazepine	↓ atazanavir ↑ carbamazepine	Plasma concentrations of atazanavir may be decreased when carbamazepine is administered with REYATAZ without ritonavir. Coadministration of carbamazepine and REYATAZ without ritonavir is not recommended. Ritonavir may increase plasma levels of carbamazepine. If patients beginning treatment with REYATAZ/ritonavir have been titrated to a stable dose of carbamazepine, a dose reduction for carbamazepine may be necessary.
phenytoin, phenobarbital	↓ atazanavir ↓ phenytoin ↓ phenobarbital	Plasma concentrations of atazanavir may be decreased when phenytoin or phenobarbital is administered with REYATAZ without ritonavir. Coadministration of phenytoin or phenobarbital and REYATAZ without ritonavir is not recommended. Ritonavir may decrease plasma levels of phenytoin and phenobarbital. When REYATAZ with ritonavir is coadministered with either phenytoin or phenobarbital, a dose adjustment of phenytoin or phenobarbital may be required.
lamotrigine	↓ lamotrigine	Coadministration of lamotrigine and REYATAZ ***with*** ritonavir may decrease lamotrigine plasma concentrations. Dose adjustment of lamotrigine may be required when coadministered with REYATAZ and ritonavir. Coadministration of lamotrigine and REYATAZ ***without*** ritonavir is not expected to decrease lamotrigine plasma concentrations. No dose adjustment of lamotrigine is required when coadministered with REYATAZ without ritonavir.
Antifungals: ketoconazole, itraconazole	***REYATAZ/ritonavir:*** ↑ ketoconazole ↑ itraconazole	Coadministration of ketoconazole has only been studied with REYATAZ without ritonavir (negligible increase in atazanavir AUC and C_{max}). Due to the effect of ritonavir on ketoconazole, high doses of ketoconazole and itraconazole (>200 mg/day) should be used cautiously with REYATAZ/ritonavir.
voriconazole	***REYATAZ/ritonavir in subjects with a functional CYP2C19 allele:*** ↓ voriconazole ↓ atazanavir	Voriconazole should not be administered to patients receiving REYATAZ/ritonavir, unless an assessment of the benefit/risk to the patient justifies the use of voriconazole. Patients should be carefully monitored for voriconazole-associated adverse events and loss of either voriconazole or atazanavir efficacy during the coadministration of voriconazole and REYATAZ/ritonavir.
	REYATAZ/ritonavir in subjects without a functional CYP2C19 allele: ↑ voriconazole ↓ atazanavir	Coadministration of voriconazole with REYATAZ (without ritonavir) may affect atazanavir concentrations; however, no data are available.

(Table continued on next page)

Lack of ethnic diversity was a study limitation. In the study population, 33/40 (83%) infants were Black/African American, who have a lower incidence of neonatal hyperbilirubinemia than Caucasians and Asians. In addition, women with Rh incompatibility were excluded, as well as women who had a previous infant who developed hemolytic disease and/or had neonatal pathologic jaundice (requiring phototherapy).

Additionally, of the 38 infants who had glucose samples collected in the first day of life, 3 had adequately collected serum glucose samples with values of <40 mg/dL that could not be attributed to maternal glucose intolerance, difficult delivery, or sepsis.

Antiretroviral Pregnancy Registry Data: As of January 2010, the Antiretroviral Pregnancy Registry (APR) has received prospective reports of 635 exposures to atazanavir-containing regimens (425 exposed in the first trimester and 160 and 50 exposed in second and third trimester, respectively). Birth defects occurred in 9 of 393 (2.3%) live births (first trimester exposure) and 5 of 212 (2.4%) live births (second/third trimester exposure). Among pregnant women in the U.S. reference population, the background rate of birth defects is 2.7%. There was no association between atazanavir and overall birth defects observed in the APR.

Pharmacokinetics of Atazanavir in Pregnancy

[See *Clinical Pharmacology (12.3).*]

Animal Data

In animal reproduction studies, there was no evidence of teratogenicity in offspring born to animals at systemic drug exposure levels (AUC) 0.7 (in rabbits) to 1.2 (in rats) times those observed at the human clinical dose (300 mg/day atazanavir boosted with 100 mg/day ritonavir). In pre- and post-natal development studies in the rat, atazanavir caused body weight loss or weight gain suppression in the animal offspring with maternal drug exposure (AUC) 1.3 times the human exposure at this clinical dose. However, maternal toxicity also occurred at this exposure level.

8.3 Nursing Mothers

The Centers for Disease Control and Prevention recommend that HIV-infected mothers not breastfeed their infants to avoid risking postnatal transmission of HIV. It is not known whether atazanavir is present in human milk. Because of both the potential for HIV transmission and the potential for serious adverse reactions in nursing infants, **mothers should be instructed not to breastfeed if they are taking REYATAZ.**

8.4 Pediatric Use

REYATAZ (atazanavir sulfate) should not be administered to pediatric patients below the age of 3 months due to the risk of kernicterus.

The safety, activity, and pharmacokinetic profiles of REYATAZ in pediatric patients ages 3 months to less than 6 years have not been established.

The safety, pharmacokinetic profile, and virologic response of REYATAZ were evaluated in pediatric patients in an open-label, multicenter clinical trial PACTG 1020A [see *Clinical Pharmacology (12.3)* and *Clinical Studies (14.3)*]. The safety profile in pediatric patients was generally similar to that observed in adults [see *Adverse Reactions (6.2)*]. Please see *Dosage and Administration (2.2)* for dosing recommendations for pediatric patients 6 years of age and older.

8.5 Geriatric Use

Clinical studies of REYATAZ did not include sufficient numbers of patients aged 65 and over to determine whether they respond differently from younger patients. Based on a comparison of mean single-dose pharmacokinetic values for C_{max} and AUC, a dose adjustment based upon age is not recommended. In general, appropriate caution should be exercised in the administration and monitoring of REYATAZ in elderly patients reflecting the greater frequency of decreased hepatic, renal, or cardiac function, and of concomitant disease or other drug therapy.

8.6 Age/Gender

A study of the pharmacokinetics of atazanavir was performed in young (n=29; 18–40 years) and elderly (n=30; ≥65 years) healthy subjects. There were no clinically important pharmacokinetic differences observed due to age or gender.

8.7 Impaired Renal Function

In healthy subjects, the renal elimination of unchanged atazanavir was approximately 7% of the administered dose. REYATAZ has been studied in adult subjects with severe renal impairment (n=20), including those on hemodialysis, at multiple doses of 400 mg once daily. The mean atazanavir C_{max} was 9% lower, AUC was 19% higher, and C_{min} was 96% higher in subjects with severe renal impairment not undergoing hemodialysis (n=10), than in age, weight, and gender matched subjects with normal renal function. Atazanavir was not appreciably cleared during hemodialysis. In a 4-hour dialysis session, 2.1% of the administered dose was removed. When atazanavir was administered either prior to, or following hemodialysis (n=10), the geometric means for C_{max}, AUC, and C_{min} were approximately 25 to 43% lower compared to subjects with normal renal function. The mechanism of this decrease is unknown. REYATAZ should not be administered to HIV-treatment-experienced patients with end stage renal disease managed with hemodialysis. [See *Dosage and Administration (2.4).*]

8.8 Impaired Hepatic Function

Atazanavir is metabolized and eliminated primarily by the liver. REYATAZ (atazanavir sulfate) has been studied in adult subjects with moderate to severe hepatic impairment (14 Child-Pugh B and 2 Child-Pugh C subjects) after a single 400-mg dose. The mean $AUC_{(0-\infty)}$ was 42% greater in subjects with impaired hepatic function than in healthy vol-

Table 13 *(cont.)*: Established and Other Potentially Significant Drug Interactions: Alteration in Dose or Regimen May Be Recommended Based on Drug Interaction Studies[a] or Predicted Interactions (Information in the table applies to REYATAZ with or without ritonavir, unless otherwise indicated)

Concomitant Drug Class: Specific Drugs	Effect on Concentration of Atazanavir or Concomitant Drug	Clinical Comment
Antigout: colchicine	↑ colchicine	REYATAZ should not be coadministered with colchicine to patients with renal or hepatic impairment. ***Recommended dosage of colchicine when administered with REYATAZ:*** ***Treatment of gout flares:*** 0.6 mg (1 tablet) for 1 dose, followed by 0.3 mg (half tablet) 1 hour later. Not to be repeated before 3 days. ***Prophylaxis of gout flares:*** If the original regimen was 0.6 mg *twice* a day, the regimen should be adjusted to 0.3 mg *once a day*. If the original regimen was 0.6 mg *once* a day, the regimen should be adjusted to 0.3 mg *once every other day*. ***Treatment of familial Mediterranean fever (FMF):*** Maximum daily dose of 0.6 mg (may be given as 0.3 mg twice a day).
Antimycobacterials: rifabutin	↑ rifabutin	A rifabutin dose reduction of up to 75% (eg, 150 mg every other day or 3 times per week) is recommended. Increased monitoring for rifabutin-associated adverse reactions including neutropenia is warranted.
Benzodiazepines: parenterally administered midazolam[b]	↑ midazolam	Concomitant use of parenteral midazolam with REYATAZ may increase plasma concentrations of midazolam. Coadministration should be done in a setting which ensures close clinical monitoring and appropriate medical management in case of respiratory depression and/or prolonged sedation. Dosage reduction for midazolam should be considered, especially if more than a single dose of midazolam is administered. Coadministration of oral midazolam with REYATAZ is CONTRAINDICATED.
Calcium channel blockers: diltiazem	↑ diltiazem and desacetyl-diltiazem	Caution is warranted. A dose reduction of diltiazem by 50% should be considered. ECG monitoring is recommended. Coadministration of REYATAZ/ritonavir with diltiazem has not been studied.
felodipine, nifedipine, nicardipine, and verapamil	↑ calcium channel blocker	Caution is warranted. Dose titration of the calcium channel blocker should be considered. ECG monitoring is recommended.
Endothelin receptor antagonists: bosentan	↓ atazanavir ↑ bosentan	Plasma concentrations of atazanavir may be decreased when bosentan is administered with REYATAZ without ritonavir. Coadministration of bosentan and REYATAZ without ritonavir is not recommended. ***Coadministration of bosentan in patients on REYATAZ/ritonavir:*** For patients who have been receiving REYATAZ/ritonavir for at least 10 days, start bosentan at 62.5 mg once daily or every other day based on individual tolerability. ***Coadministration of REYATAZ/ritonavir in patients on bosentan:*** Discontinue bosentan at least 36 hours before starting REYATAZ/ritonavir. At least 10 days after starting REYATAZ/ritonavir, resume bosentan at 62.5 mg once daily or every other day based on individual tolerability.
HMG-CoA reductase inhibitors: atorvastatin, rosuvastatin	↑ atorvastatin ↑ rosuvastatin	Titrate atorvastatin dose carefully and use the lowest necessary dose. Rosuvastatin dose should not exceed 10 mg/day. The risk of myopathy, including rhabdomyolysis, may be increased when HIV protease inhibitors, including REYATAZ, are used in combination with these drugs.
H_2-Receptor antagonists	↓ atazanavir	Plasma concentrations of atazanavir were substantially decreased when REYATAZ 400 mg once daily was administered simultaneously with famotidine 40 mg twice daily, which may result in loss of therapeutic effect and development of resistance. ***In treatment-naive patients:*** REYATAZ 300 mg with ritonavir 100 mg once daily with food should be administered simultaneously with, and/or at least 10 hours after, a dose of the H_2-receptor antagonist. An H_2-receptor antagonist dose comparable to famotidine 20 mg once daily up to a dose comparable to famotidine 40 mg twice daily can be used with REYATAZ 300 mg with ritonavir 100 mg in treatment-naive patients. OR For patients unable to tolerate ritonavir, REYATAZ 400 mg once daily with food should be administered at least 2 hours before and at least 10 hours after a dose of the H_2-receptor antagonist. No single dose of the H_2-receptor antagonist should exceed a dose comparable to famotidine 20 mg, and the total daily dose should not exceed a dose comparable to famotidine 40 mg. However, REYATAZ should not be used without ritonavir in pregnant women.

(Table continued on next page)

unteers. The mean half-life of atazanavir in hepatically impaired subjects was 12.1 hours compared to 6.4 hours in healthy volunteers. Increased concentrations of atazanavir are expected in patients with moderately or severely impaired hepatic function. The pharmacokinetics of REYATAZ (atazanavir sulfate) in combination with ritonavir have not been studied in subjects with hepatic impairment. REYATAZ should not be administered to patients with severe hepatic impairment. REYATAZ/ritonavir is not recommended for use in patients with hepatic impairment. [See *Dosage and Administration (2.5)* and *Warnings and Precautions (5.5)*.]

10 OVERDOSAGE

Human experience of acute overdose with REYATAZ (atazanavir sulfate) is limited. Single doses up to 1200 mg have been taken by healthy volunteers without symptomatic untoward effects. A single self-administered overdose of 29.2 g of REYATAZ (atazanavir sulfate) in an HIV-infected patient (73 times the 400-mg recommended dose) was associated with asymptomatic bifascicular block and PR interval prolongation. These events resolved spontaneously. At high doses that lead to high drug exposures, jaundice due to indirect (unconjugated) hyperbilirubinemia (without associated liver function test changes) or PR interval prolongation may be observed. [See *Warnings and Precautions (5.2, 5.4)* and *Clinical Pharmacology (12.2)*.]

Treatment of overdosage with REYATAZ should consist of general supportive measures, including monitoring of vital signs and ECG, and observations of the patient's clinical status. If indicated, elimination of unabsorbed atazanavir should be achieved by emesis or gastric lavage. Administration of activated charcoal may also be used to aid removal of unabsorbed drug. There is no specific antidote for overdose with REYATAZ. Since atazanavir is extensively metabolized by the liver and is highly protein bound, dialysis is unlikely to be beneficial in significant removal of this medicine.

11 DESCRIPTION

REYATAZ® (atazanavir sulfate) is an azapeptide inhibitor of HIV-1 protease.

The chemical name for atazanavir sulfate is (3*S*,8*S*,9*S*,12*S*)-3,12-Bis(1,1-dimethylethyl)-8-hydroxy-4,11-dioxo-9-(phenylmethyl)-6-[[4-(2-pyridinyl)phenyl]methyl]-2,5,6,10,13-pentaazatetradecanedioic acid dimethyl ester, sulfate (1:1). Its molecular formula is $C_{38}H_{52}N_6O_7 \cdot H_2SO_4$, which corresponds to a molecular weight of 802.9 (sulfuric acid salt). The free base molecular weight is 704.9. Atazanavir sulfate has the following structural formula:

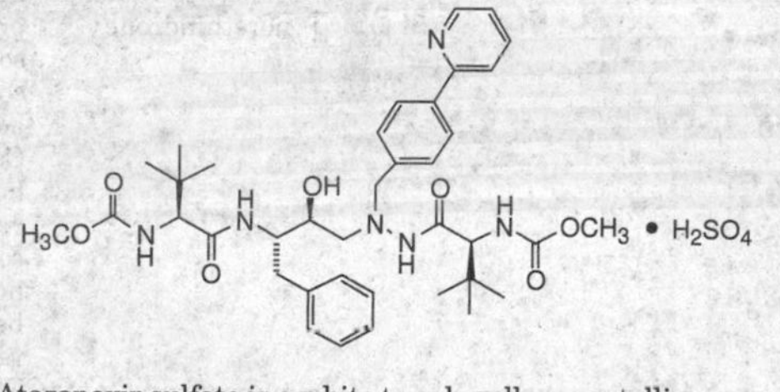

Atazanavir sulfate is a white to pale yellow crystalline powder. It is slightly soluble in water (4–5 mg/mL, free base equivalent) with the pH of a saturated solution in water being about 1.9 at 24 ± 3° C.

REYATAZ Capsules are available for oral administration in strengths containing the equivalent of 150 mg, 200 mg, or 300 mg of atazanavir as atazanavir sulfate and the following inactive ingredients: crospovidone, lactose monohydrate, and magnesium stearate. The capsule shells contain the following inactive ingredients: gelatin, FD&C Blue No. 2, titanium dioxide, black iron oxide, red iron oxide, and yellow iron oxide. The capsules are printed with ink containing shellac, titanium dioxide, FD&C Blue No. 2, isopropyl alcohol, ammonium hydroxide, propylene glycol, n-butyl alcohol, simethicone, and dehydrated alcohol.

12 CLINICAL PHARMACOLOGY

12.1 Mechanism of Action

Atazanavir is an antiviral drug [see *Clinical Pharmacology (12.4)*].

12.2 Pharmacodynamics

Effects on Electrocardiogram

Concentration- and dose-dependent prolongation of the PR interval in the electrocardiogram has been observed in healthy volunteers receiving atazanavir. In a placebo-controlled study (AI424-076), the mean (±SD) maximum change in PR interval from the predose value was 24 (±15) msec following oral dosing with 400 mg of atazanavir (n=65) compared to 13 (±11) msec following dosing with placebo (n=67). The PR interval prolongations in this study were asymptomatic. There is limited information on the potential for a pharmacodynamic interaction in humans between atazanavir and other drugs that prolong the PR interval of the electrocardiogram. [See *Warnings and Precautions (5.2)*.]

Electrocardiographic effects of atazanavir were determined in a clinical pharmacology study of 72 healthy subjects. Oral doses of 400 mg and 800 mg were compared with placebo; there was no concentration-dependent effect of atazanavir on the QTc interval (using Fridericia's correction). In 1793 HIV-infected patients receiving antiretroviral regimens, QTc prolongation was comparable in the atazanavir and comparator regimens. No atazanavir-treated healthy subject or HIV-infected patient in clinical trials had a QTc interval >500 msec. [See *Warnings and Precautions (5.2)*.]

In a pharmacokinetic study between atazanavir 400 mg once daily and diltiazem 180 mg once daily, a CYP3A substrate, there was a 2-fold increase in the diltiazem plasma concentration and an additive effect on the PR interval. In a pharmacokinetic study between atazanavir 400 mg once

Table 13 *(cont.)*: Established and Other Potentially Significant Drug Interactions: Alteration in Dose or Regimen May Be Recommended Based on Drug Interaction Studies[a] or Predicted Interactions (Information in the table applies to REYATAZ with or without ritonavir, unless otherwise indicated)

Concomitant Drug Class: Specific Drugs	Effect on Concentration of Atazanavir or Concomitant Drug	Clinical Comment
		In treatment-experienced patients: Whenever an H_2-receptor antagonist is given to a patient receiving REYATAZ with ritonavir, the H_2-receptor antagonist dose should not exceed a dose comparable to famotidine 20 mg twice daily, and the REYATAZ and ritonavir doses should be administered simultaneously with, and/or at least 10 hours after, the dose of the H_2-receptor antagonist. • REYATAZ 300 mg with ritonavir 100 mg once daily (all as a single dose with food) if taken with an H_2-receptor antagonist. For pregnant women taking REYATAZ with ritonavir and an H_2-receptor antagonist, see *Dosage and Administration (2.3)*. • REYATAZ 400 mg with ritonavir 100 mg once daily (all as a single dose with food) if taken with both tenofovir and an H_2-receptor antagonist. For pregnant women taking REYATAZ with ritonavir and both tenofovir and an H_2-receptor antagonist, see *Dosage and Administration (2.3)*.
Hormonal contraceptives: ethinyl estradiol and norgestimate or norethindrone	↓ ethinyl estradiol ↑ norgestimate[c]	Use with caution if coadministration of REYATAZ or REYATAZ/ritonavir with oral contraceptives is considered. If an oral contraceptive is administered with REYATAZ plus ritonavir, it is recommended that the oral contraceptive contain at least 35 mcg of ethinyl estradiol. If REYATAZ is administered without ritonavir, the oral contraceptive should contain no more than 30 mcg of ethinyl estradiol.
	↑ ethinyl estradiol ↑ norethindrone[d]	Potential safety risks include substantial increases in progesterone exposure. The long-term effects of increases in concentration of the progestational agent are unknown and could increase the risk of insulin resistance, dyslipidemia, and acne. Coadministration of REYATAZ or REYATAZ/ritonavir with other hormonal contraceptives (eg, contraceptive patch, contraceptive vaginal ring, or injectable contraceptives) or oral contraceptives containing progestogens other than norethindrone or norgestimate, or less than 25 mcg of ethinyl estradiol, has not been studied; therefore, alternative methods of contraception are recommended.
Immunosuppressants: cyclosporin, sirolimus, tacrolimus	↑ immunosuppressants	Therapeutic concentration monitoring is recommended for immunosuppressant agents when coadministered with REYATAZ (atazanavir sulfate).
Inhaled beta agonist: salmeterol	↑ salmeterol	Coadministration of salmeterol with REYATAZ is not recommended. Concomitant use of salmeterol and REYATAZ may result in increased risk of cardiovascular adverse events associated with salmeterol, including QT prolongation, palpitations, and sinus tachycardia.
Inhaled/nasal steroid: fluticasone	***REYATAZ*** ↑ fluticasone	Concomitant use of fluticasone propionate and REYATAZ (without ritonavir) may increase plasma concentrations of fluticasone propionate. Use with caution. Consider alternatives to fluticasone propionate, particularly for long-term use.
	REYATAZ/ritonavir ↑ fluticasone	Concomitant use of fluticasone propionate and REYATAZ/ritonavir may increase plasma concentrations of fluticasone propionate, resulting in significantly reduced serum cortisol concentrations. Systemic corticosteroid effects, including Cushing's syndrome and adrenal suppression, have been reported during postmarketing use in patients receiving ritonavir and inhaled or intranasally administered fluticasone propionate. Coadministration of fluticasone propionate and REYATAZ/ritonavir is not recommended unless the potential benefit to the patient outweighs the risk of systemic corticosteroid side effects [see *Warnings and Precautions (5.1)*].
Macrolide antibiotics: clarithromycin	↑ clarithromycin ↓ 14-OH clarithromycin ↑ atazanavir	Increased concentrations of clarithromycin may cause QTc prolongations; therefore, a dose reduction of clarithromycin by 50% should be considered when it is coadministered with REYATAZ. In addition, concentrations of the active metabolite 14-OH clarithromycin are significantly reduced; consider alternative therapy for indications other than infections due to *Mycobacterium avium* complex. Coadministration of REYATAZ/ritonavir with clarithromycin has not been studied.
Opioids: Buprenorphine	↑ buprenorphine ↑ norbuprenorphine	Coadministration of buprenorphine and REYATAZ with or without ritonavir increases the plasma concentration of buprenorphine and norbuprenorphine. Coadministration of REYATAZ plus ritonavir with buprenorphine warrants clinical monitoring for sedation and cognitive effects. A dose reduction of buprenorphine may be considered. Coadministration of buprenorphine and REYATAZ with ritonavir is not expected to decrease atazanavir plasma concentrations. Coadministration of buprenorphine and REYATAZ without ritonavir may decrease atazanavir plasma concentrations. REYATAZ without ritonavir should not be coadministered with buprenorphine.

(Table continued on next page)

daily and atenolol 50 mg once daily, there was no substantial additive effect of atazanavir and atenolol on the PR interval. [See *Warnings and Precautions (5.2)*.]

12.3 Pharmacokinetics

The pharmacokinetics of atazanavir were evaluated in healthy adult volunteers and in HIV-infected patients after administration of REYATAZ 400 mg once daily and after administration of REYATAZ 300 mg with ritonavir 100 mg once daily (see Table 14).

[See table 14 at bottom of next page]

Figure 1 displays the mean plasma concentrations of atazanavir at steady state after REYATAZ 400 mg once daily (as two 200-mg capsules) with a light meal and after REYATAZ 300 mg (as two 150-mg capsules) with ritonavir 100 mg once daily with a light meal in HIV-infected adult patients.

Figure 1: Mean (SD) Steady-State Plasma Concentrations of Atazanavir 400 mg (n=13) and 300 mg with Ritonavir (n=10) for HIV-Infected Adult Patients

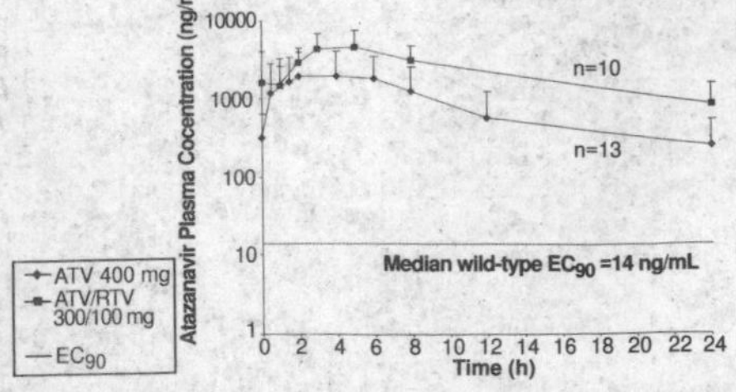

Absorption

Atazanavir is rapidly absorbed with a T_{max} of approximately 2.5 hours. Atazanavir demonstrates nonlinear pharmacokinetics with greater than dose-proportional increases in AUC and C_{max} values over the dose range of 200–800 mg once daily. Steady state is achieved between Days 4 and 8, with an accumulation of approximately 2.3-fold.

Food Effect

Administration of REYATAZ (atazanavir sulfate) with food enhances bioavailability and reduces pharmacokinetic variability. Administration of a single 400-mg dose of REYATAZ with a light meal (357 kcal, 8.2 g fat, 10.6 g protein) resulted in a 70% increase in AUC and 57% increase in C_{max} relative to the fasting state. Administration of a single 400-mg dose of REYATAZ with a high-fat meal (721 kcal, 37.3 g fat, 29.4 g protein) resulted in a mean increase in AUC of 35% with no change in C_{max} relative to the fasting state. Administration of REYATAZ (atazanavir sulfate) with either a light meal or high-fat meal decreased the coefficient of variation of AUC and C_{max} by approximately one-half compared to the fasting state.

Coadministration of a single 300-mg dose of REYATAZ and a 100-mg dose of ritonavir with a light meal (336 kcal, 5.1 g fat, 9.3 g protein) resulted in a 33% increase in the AUC and a 40% increase in both the C_{max} and the 24-hour concentration of atazanavir relative to the fasting state. Coadministration with a high-fat meal (951 kcal, 54.7 g fat, 35.9 g protein) did not affect the AUC of atazanavir relative to fasting conditions and the C_{max} was within 11% of fasting values. The 24-hour concentration following a high-fat meal was increased by approximately 33% due to delayed absorption; the median T_{max} increased from 2.0 to 5.0 hours. Coadministration of REYATAZ with ritonavir with either a light or a high-fat meal decreased the coefficient of variation of AUC and C_{max} by approximately 25% compared to the fasting state.

Distribution

Atazanavir is 86% bound to human serum proteins and protein binding is independent of concentration. Atazanavir binds to both alpha-1-acid glycoprotein (AAG) and albumin to a similar extent (89% and 86%, respectively). In a multiple-dose study in HIV-infected patients dosed with REYATAZ 400 mg once daily with a light meal for 12 weeks, atazanavir was detected in the cerebrospinal fluid and semen. The cerebrospinal fluid/plasma ratio for atazanavir (n=4) ranged between 0.0021 and 0.0226 and seminal fluid/plasma ratio (n=5) ranged between 0.11 and 4.42.

Metabolism

Atazanavir is extensively metabolized in humans. The major biotransformation pathways of atazanavir in humans consisted of monooxygenation and dioxygenation. Other minor biotransformation pathways for atazanavir or its metabolites consisted of glucuronidation, N-dealkylation, hydrolysis, and oxygenation with dehydrogenation. Two minor metabolites of atazanavir in plasma have been characterized. Neither metabolite demonstrated *in vitro* antiviral activity. *In vitro* studies using human liver microsomes suggested that atazanavir is metabolized by CYP3A.

Elimination

Following a single 400-mg dose of ^{14}C-atazanavir, 79% and 13% of the total radioactivity was recovered in the feces and urine, respectively. Unchanged drug accounted for approximately 20% and 7% of the administered dose in the feces and urine, respectively. The mean elimination half-life of atazanavir in healthy volunteers (n=214) and HIV-infected adult patients (n=13) was approximately 7 hours at steady state following a dose of 400 mg daily with a light meal.

Special Populations

Pediatrics

The pharmacokinetic parameters for atazanavir at steady state in pediatric patients were predicted by a population pharmacokinetic model and are summarized in Table 15 by weight ranges that correspond to the recommended doses. [See *Dosage and Administration (2.2)*.]

[See table 15 at top of next page]

Pregnancy

The pharmacokinetic data from HIV-infected pregnant women receiving REYATAZ (atazanavir sulfate) Capsules with ritonavir are presented in Table 16.

[See table 16 at top of next page]

Drug Interaction Data

Atazanavir is a metabolism-dependent CYP3A inhibitor, with a K_{inact} value of 0.05 to 0.06 min^{-1} and K_i value of 0.84 to 1.0 μM. Atazanavir is also a direct inhibitor for UGT1A1 (K_i=1.9 μM) and CYP2C8 (K_i=2.1 μM).

Atazanavir has been shown *in vivo* not to induce its own metabolism, nor to increase the biotransformation of some drugs metabolized by CYP3A. In a multiple-dose study, REYATAZ decreased the urinary ratio of endogenous 6β-OH cortisol to cortisol versus baseline, indicating that CYP3A production was not induced.

Drug interaction studies were performed with REYATAZ and other drugs likely to be coadministered and some drugs commonly used as probes for pharmacokinetic interactions. The effects of coadministration of REYATAZ on the AUC, C_{max}, and C_{min} are summarized in Tables 17 and 18 . For information regarding clinical recommendations, see *Drug Interactions (7)*.

[See table 17 on pages 782 through 784]

[See table 18 on pages 785 and 786]

12.4 Microbiology

Mechanism of Action

Atazanavir (ATV) is an azapeptide HIV-1 protease inhibitor (PI). The compound selectively inhibits the virus-specific processing of viral Gag and Gag-Pol polyproteins in HIV-1 infected cells, thus preventing formation of mature virions.

Antiviral Activity in Cell Culture

Atazanavir exhibits anti-HIV-1 activity with a mean 50% effective concentration (EC_{50}) in the absence of human serum of 2 to 5 nM against a variety of laboratory and clinical HIV-1 isolates grown in peripheral blood mononuclear cells, macrophages, CEM-SS cells, and MT-2 cells. ATV has activity against HIV-1 Group M subtype viruses A, B, C, D, AE, AG, F, G, and J isolates in cell culture. ATV has variable activity against HIV-2 isolates (1.9 to 32 nM), with EC_{50} values above the EC_{50} values of failure isolates. Two-drug combination antiviral activity studies with ATV showed no antagonism in cell culture with NNRTIs (delavirdine, efavirenz, and nevirapine), PIs (amprenavir, indinavir, lopinavir, nelfinavir, ritonavir, and saquinavir), NRTIs (abacavir, didanosine, emtricitabine, lamivudine, stavudine, tenofovir, zalcitabine, and zidovudine), the HIV-1 fusion inhibitor enfuvirtide, and two compounds used in the treatment of viral hepatitis, adefovir and ribavirin, without enhanced cytotoxicity.

Resistance

In Cell Culture: HIV-1 isolates with a decreased susceptibility to ATV have been selected in cell culture and obtained from patients treated with ATV or atazanavir/ritonavir (ATV/RTV). HIV-1 isolates with 93- to 183-fold reduced susceptibility to ATV from three different viral strains were selected in cell culture by 5 months. The substitutions in these HIV-1 viruses that contributed to ATV resistance include I50L, N88S, I84V, A71V, and M46I. Changes were also observed at the protease cleavage sites following drug selection. Recombinant viruses containing the I50L substitution without other major PI substitutions were growth impaired and displayed increased susceptibility in cell culture to other PIs (amprenavir, indinavir, lopinavir, nelfinavir, ritonavir, and saquinavir). The I50L and I50V substitutions yielded selective resistance to ATV and amprenavir, respectively, and did not appear to be cross-resistant.

Clinical Studies of Treatment-Naive Patients: Comparison of Ritonavir-Boosted REYATAZ vs. Unboosted REYATAZ: Study AI424-089 compared REYATAZ 300 mg once daily with ritonavir 100 mg vs. REYATAZ 400 mg once daily when administered with lamivudine and extended-release stavudine in HIV-infected treatment-naive patients. A summary of the number of virologic failures and virologic failure isolates with ATV resistance in each arm is shown in Table 19.

[See table 19 at top of page 787]

Clinical Studies of Treatment-Naive Patients Receiving REYATAZ 300 mg With Ritonavir 100 mg: In Phase III study AI424-138, an as-treated genotypic and phenotypic analysis was conducted on samples from patients who experienced virologic failure (HIV-1 RNA ≥400 copies/mL) or discontinued before achieving suppression on ATV/RTV (n=39; 9%) and LPV/RTV (n=39; 9%) through 96 weeks of treatment. In the ATV/RTV arm, one of the virologic failure isolates had a 56-fold decrease in ATV susceptibility emerge on therapy with the development of PI resistance-associated substitutions L10F, V32I, K43T, M46I, A71I, G73S, I85I/V, and L90M. The NRTI resistance-associated substitution M184V also emerged on treatment in this isolate conferring

Table 13 *(cont.)*: Established and Other Potentially Significant Drug Interactions: Alteration in Dose or Regimen May Be Recommended Based on Drug Interaction Studies[a] or Predicted Interactions (Information in the table applies to REYATAZ with or without ritonavir, unless otherwise indicated)

Concomitant Drug Class: Specific Drugs	Effect on Concentration of Atazanavir or Concomitant Drug	Clinical Comment
PDE5 inhibitors: sildenafil, tadalafil, vardenafil	↑ sildenafil ↑ tadalafil ↑ vardenafil	Coadministration with REYATAZ has not been studied but may result in an increase in PDE5 inhibitor-associated adverse events, including hypotension, syncope, visual disturbances, and priapism. ***Use of PDE5 inhibitors for pulmonary arterial hypertension (PAH):*** Use of REVATIO® (sildenafil) for the treatment of pulmonary hypertension (PAH) is contraindicated with REYATAZ [see *Contraindications (4)*]. The following dose adjustments are recommended for the use of ADCIRCA® (tadalafil) with REYATAZ: Coadministration of ADCIRCA® in patients on REYATAZ (with or without ritonavir): • For patients receiving REYATAZ (with or without ritonavir) for at least one week, start ADCIRCA® at 20 mg once daily. Increase to 40 mg once daily based on individual tolerability. Coadministration of REYATAZ (with or without ritonavir) in patients on ADCIRCA®: • Avoid the use of ADCIRCA® when starting REYATAZ (with or without ritonavir). Stop ADCIRCA® at least 24 hours before starting REYATAZ (with or without ritonavir). At least one week after starting REYATAZ (with or without ritonavir), resume ADCIRCA® at 20 mg once daily. Increase to 40 mg once daily based on individual tolerability. ***Use of PDE5 inhibitors for erectile dysfunction:*** Use VIAGRA® (sildenafil) with caution at reduced doses of 25 mg every 48 hours with increased monitoring for adverse events. Use CIALIS® (tadalafil) with caution at reduced doses of 10 mg every 72 hours with increased monitoring for adverse events. ***REYATAZ/ritonavir:*** Use LEVITRA® (vardenafil) with caution at reduced doses of no more than 2.5 mg every 72 hours with increased monitoring for adverse events. ***REYATAZ:*** Use LEVITRA® (vardenafil) with caution at reduced doses of no more than 2.5 mg every 24 hours with increased monitoring for adverse events.
Proton-pump inhibitors: omeprazole	↓ atazanavir	Plasma concentrations of atazanavir were substantially decreased when REYATAZ 400 mg or REYATAZ 300 mg/ritonavir 100 mg once daily was administered with omeprazole 40 mg once daily, which may result in loss of therapeutic effect and development of resistance. ***In treatment-naive patients:*** The proton-pump inhibitor dose should not exceed a dose comparable to omeprazole 20 mg and must be taken approximately 12 hours prior to the REYATAZ 300 mg with ritonavir 100 mg dose. ***In treatment-experienced patients:*** Proton-pump inhibitors should not be used in treatment-experienced patients receiving REYATAZ.

[a] For magnitude of interactions see *Clinical Pharmacology, Tables 17* and *18 (12.3)*.
[b] See *Contraindications (4), Table 3* for orally administered midazolam.
[c] In combination with atazanavir 300 mg and ritonavir 100 mg once daily.
[d] In combination with atazanavir 400 mg once daily.

Table 14: Steady-State Pharmacokinetics of Atazanavir in Healthy Subjects or HIV-Infected Patients in the Fed State

	400 mg once daily		300 mg with ritonavir 100 mg once daily	
Parameter	**Healthy Subjects (n=14)**	**HIV-Infected Patients (n=13)**	**Healthy Subjects (n=28)**	**HIV-Infected Patients (n=10)**
C_{max} (ng/mL)				
Geometric mean (CV%)	5199 (26)	2298 (71)	6129 (31)	4422 (58)
Mean (SD)	5358 (1371)	3152 (2231)	6450 (2031)	5233 (3033)
T_{max} (h)				
Median	2.5	2.0	2.7	3.0
AUC (ng•h/mL)				
Geometric mean (CV%)	28132 (28)	14874 (91)	57039 (37)	46073 (66)
Mean (SD)	29303 (8263)	22262 (20159)	61435 (22911)	53761 (35294)
T-half (h)				
Mean (SD)	7.9 (2.9)	6.5 (2.6)	18.1 (6.2)[a]	8.6 (2.3)
C_{min} (ng/mL)				
Geometric mean (CV%)	159 (88)	120 (109)	1227 (53)	636 (97)
Mean (SD)	218 (191)	273 (298)[b]	1441 (757)	862 (838)

[a] n=26.
[b] n=12.

Table 15: Predicted Steady-State Pharmacokinetics of Atazanavir (capsule formulation) with ritonavir in HIV-Infected Pediatric Patients

Body Weight (range in kg)	atazanavir/ritonavir Dose (mg)	C_{max} ng/mL Geometric Mean (CV%)	AUC ng·h/mL Geometric Mean (CV%)	C_{min} ng/mL Geometric Mean (CV%)
15 – <20	150/100	5213 (78.7%)	42902 (77.0%)	504 (99.5%)
20 – <40	200/100	4954 (81.7%)	42999 (78.5%)	562 (98.9%)
≥40	300/100	5040 (84.6%)	46777 (80.6%)	691 (98.5%)

Table 16: Steady-State Pharmacokinetics of Atazanavir with ritonavir in HIV-Infected Pregnant Women in the Fed State

Pharmacokinetic Parameter	Atazanavir 300 mg with ritonavir 100 mg 2nd Trimester (n=5[a])	3rd Trimester (n=20)	Postpartum[b] (n=34)
C_{max} ng/mL Geometric mean (CV%)	3078.85 (50)	3291.46 (48)	5721.21 (31)
AUC ng•h/mL Geometric mean (CV%)	27657.1 (43)	34251.5 (43)	61990.4 (32)
C_{min} ng/mL[c] Geometric mean (CV%)	538.70 (46)	668.48 (50)	1462.59 (45)

[a] Available data during the 2nd trimester are limited.
[b] Atazanavir peak concentrations and AUCs were found to be approximately 28–43% higher during the postpartum period (4–12 weeks) than those observed historically in HIV-infected, non-pregnant patients. Atazanavir plasma trough concentrations were approximately 2.2-fold higher during the postpartum period when compared to those observed historically in HIV-infected, non-pregnant patients.
[c] C_{min} is concentration 24 hours post-dose.

Table 17: Drug Interactions: Pharmacokinetic Parameters for Atazanavir in the Presence of Coadministered Drugs[a]

Coadministered Drug	Coadministered Drug Dose/Schedule	REYATAZ Dose/Schedule	Ratio (90% Confidence Interval) of Atazanavir Pharmacokinetic Parameters with/without Coadministered Drug; No Effect = 1.00 C_{max}	AUC	C_{min}
atenolol	50 mg QD, d 7–11 (n=19) and d 19–23	400 mg QD, d 1–11 (n=19)	1.00 (0.89, 1.12)	0.93 (0.85, 1.01)	0.74 (0.65, 0.86)
boceprevir	800 mg TID, d 1–6, 25–31	300 mg QD/ritonavir 100 mg QD, d 10–31	atazanavir: 0.75 (0.64–0.88) ritonavir: 0.73 (0.64–0.83)	atazanavir: 0.65 (0.55–0.78) ritonavir: 0.64 (0.58–0.72)	atazanavir: 0.51 (0.44–0.61) ritonavir: 0.55 (0.45–0.67)
clarithromycin	500 mg BID, d 7–10 (n=29) and d 18–21	400 mg QD, d 1–10 (n=29)	1.06 (0.93, 1.20)	1.28 (1.16, 1.43)	1.91 (1.66, 2.21)
didanosine (ddI) (buffered tablets) plus stavudine (d4T)[b]	ddI: 200 mg × 1 dose, d4T: 40 mg × 1 dose (n=31)	400 mg × 1 dose simultaneously with ddI and d4T (n=31)	0.11 (0.06, 0.18)	0.13 (0.08, 0.21)	0.16 (0.10, 0.27)
	ddI: 200 mg × 1 dose, d4T: 40 mg × 1 dose (n=32)	400 mg × 1 dose 1 h after ddI + d4T (n=32)	1.12 (0.67, 1.18)	1.03 (0.64, 1.67)	1.03 (0.61, 1.73)
ddI (enteric-coated [EC] capsules)[c]	400 mg d 8 (fed) (n=34)	400 mg QD, d 2–8 (n=34)	1.03 (0.93, 1.14)	0.99 (0.91, 1.08)	0.98 (0.89, 1.08)
	400 mg d 19 (fed) (n=31)	300 mg/ritonavir 100 mg QD, d 9–19 (n=31)	1.04 (1.01, 1.07)	1.00 (0.96, 1.03)	0.87 (0.82, 0.92)
diltiazem	180 mg QD, d 7–11 (n=30) and d 19–23	400 mg QD, d 1–11 (n=30)	1.04 (0.96, 1.11)	1.00 (0.95, 1.05)	0.98 (0.90, 1.07)
efavirenz	600 mg QD, d 7–20 (n=27)	400 mg QD, d 1–20 (n=27)	0.41 (0.33, 0.51)	0.26 (0.22, 0.32)	0.07 (0.05, 0.10)
	600 mg QD, d 7–20 (n=13)	400 mg QD, d 1–6 (n=23) then 300 mg/ ritonavir 100 mg QD, 2 h before efavirenz, d 7–20 (n=13)	1.14 (0.83, 1.58)	1.39 (1.02, 1.88)	1.48 (1.24, 1.76)
	600 mg QD, d 11–24 (pm) (n=14)	300 mg QD/ritonavir 100 mg QD, d 1–10 (pm) (n=22), then 400 mg QD/ritonavir 100 mg QD, d 11–24 (pm), (simultaneous with efavirenz) (n=14)	1.17 (1.08, 1.27)	1.00 (0.91, 1.10)	0.58 (0.49, 0.69)
famotidine	40 mg BID, d 7–12 (n=15)	400 mg QD, d 1–6 (n=45), d 7–12 (simultaneous administration) (n=15)	0.53 (0.34, 0.82)	0.59 (0.40, 0.87)	0.58 (0.37, 0.89)

(Table continued on next page)

emtricitabine resistance. Two ATV/RTV-virologic failure isolates had baseline phenotypic ATV resistance and IAS-defined major PI resistance-associated substitutions at baseline. The I50L substitution emerged on study in one of these failure isolates and was associated with a 17-fold decrease in ATV susceptibility from baseline and the other failure isolate with baseline ATV resistance and PI substitutions (M46M/I and I84I/V) had additional IAS-defined major PI substitutions (V32I, M46I, and I84V) emerge on ATV treatment associated with a 3-fold decrease in ATV susceptibility from baseline. Five of the treatment failure isolates in the ATV/RTV arm developed phenotypic emtricitabine resistance with the emergence of either the M184I (n=1) or the M184V (n=4) substitution on therapy and none developed phenotypic tenofovir disoproxil resistance. In the LPV/RTV arm, one of the virologic failure patient isolates had a 69-fold decrease in LPV susceptibility emerge on therapy with the development of PI substitutions L10V, V11I, I54V, G73S, and V82A in addition to baseline PI substitutions L10L/I, V32I, I54I/V, A71I, G73G/S, V82V/A, L89V, and L90M. Six LPV/RTV virologic failure isolates developed the M184V substitution and phenotypic emtricitabine resistance and two developed phenotypic tenofovir disoproxil resistance.

Clinical Studies of Treatment-Naive Patients Receiving REYATAZ 400 mg Without Ritonavir: ATV-resistant clinical isolates from treatment-naive patients who experienced virologic failure on REYATAZ (atazanavir sulfate) 400 mg treatment without ritonavir often developed an I50L substitution (after an average of 50 weeks of ATV therapy), often in combination with an A71V substitution, but also developed one or more other PI substitutions (eg, V32I, L33F, G73S, V82A, I85V, or N88S) with or without the I50L substitution. In treatment-naive patients, viral isolates that developed the I50L substitution, without other major PI substitutions, showed phenotypic resistance to ATV but retained in cell culture susceptibility to other PIs (amprenavir, indinavir, lopinavir, nelfinavir, ritonavir, and saquinavir); however, there are no clinical data available to demonstrate the effect of the I50L substitution on the efficacy of subsequently administered PIs.

Clinical Studies of Treatment-Experienced Patients: In studies of treatment-experienced patients treated with ATV or ATV/RTV, most ATV-resistant isolates from patients who experienced virologic failure developed substitutions that were associated with resistance to multiple PIs and displayed decreased susceptibility to multiple PIs. The most common protease substitutions to develop in the viral isolates of patients who failed treatment with ATV 300 mg once daily and RTV 100 mg once daily (together with tenofovir and an NRTI) included V32I, L33F/V/I, E35D/G, M46I/L, I50L, F53L/V, I54V, A71V/T/I, G73S/T/C, V82A/T/L, I85V, and L89V/Q/M/T. Other substitutions that developed on ATV/RTV treatment including E34K/A/Q, G48V, I84V, N88S/D/T, and L90M occurred in less than 10% of patient isolates. Generally, if multiple PI resistance substitutions were present in the HIV-1 virus of the patient at baseline, ATV resistance developed through substitutions associated with resistance to other PIs and could include the development of the I50L substitution. The I50L substitution has been detected in treatment-experienced patients experiencing virologic failure after long-term treatment. Protease cleavage site changes also emerged on ATV treatment but their presence did not correlate with the level of ATV resistance.

Cross-Resistance

Cross-resistance among PIs has been observed. Baseline phenotypic and genotypic analyses of clinical isolates from ATV clinical trials of PI-experienced patients showed that isolates cross-resistant to multiple PIs were cross-resistant to ATV. Greater than 90% of the isolates with substitutions that included I84V or G48V were resistant to ATV. Greater than 60% of isolates containing L90M, G73S/T/C, A71V/T, I54V, M46I/L, or a change at V82 were resistant to ATV, and 38% of isolates containing a D30N substitution in addition to other changes were resistant to ATV. Isolates resistant to ATV were also cross-resistant to other PIs with >90% of the isolates resistant to indinavir, lopinavir, nelfinavir, ritonavir, and saquinavir, and 80% resistant to amprenavir. In treatment-experienced patients, PI-resistant viral isolates that developed the I50L substitution in addition to other PI resistance-associated substitution were also cross-resistant to other PIs.

Baseline Genotype/Phenotype and Virologic Outcome Analyses

Genotypic and/or phenotypic analysis of baseline virus may aid in determining ATV susceptibility before initiation of ATV/RTV therapy. An association between virologic response at 48 weeks and the number and type of primary PI resistance-associated substitutions detected in baseline HIV-1 isolates from antiretroviral-experienced patients receiving ATV/RTV once daily or lopinavir (LPV)/RTV twice daily in Study AI424-045 is shown in Table 20.

Overall, both the number and type of baseline PI substitutions affected response rates in treatment-experienced patients. In the ATV/RTV group, patients had lower response

Table 17 *(cont.)*: Drug Interactions: Pharmacokinetic Parameters for Atazanavir in the Presence of Coadministered Drugs[a]

Coadministered Drug	Coadministered Drug Dose/Schedule	REYATAZ Dose/Schedule	Ratio (90% Confidence Interval) of Atazanavir Pharmacokinetic Parameters with/without Coadministered Drug; No Effect = 1.00		
			C_{max}	AUC	C_{min}
	40 mg BID, d 7–12 (n=14)	400 mg QD (pm), d 1–6 (n=14), d 7–12 (10 h after, 2 h before famotidine) (n=14)	1.08 (0.82, 1.41)	0.95 (0.74, 1.21)	0.79 (0.60, 1.04)
	40 mg BID, d 11–20 (n=14)[d]	300 mg QD/ritonavir 100 mg QD, d 1–10 (n=46), d 11–20[d] (simultaneous administration) (n=14)	0.86 (0.79, 0.94)	0.82 (0.75, 0.89)	0.72 (0.64, 0.81)
	20 mg BID, d 11–17 (n=18)	300 mg QD/ritonavir 100 mg QD/tenofovir 300 mg QD, d 1–10 (am) (n=39), d 11–17 (am) (simultaneous administration with am famotidine) (n=18)[e,f]	0.91 (0.84, 0.99)	0.90 (0.82, 0.98)	0.81 (0.69, 0.94)
	40 mg QD (pm), d 18–24 (n=20)	300 mg QD/ritonavir 100 mg QD/tenofovir 300 mg QD, d 1–10 (am) (n=39), d 18–24 (am) (12 h after pm famotidine) (n=20)[f]	0.89 (0.81, 0.97)	0.88 (0.80, 0.96)	0.77 (0.63, 0.93)
	40 mg BID, d 18–24 (n=18)	300 mg QD/ritonavir 100 mg QD/tenofovir 300 mg QD, d 1–10 (am) (n=39), d 18–24 (am) (10 h after pm famotidine and 2 h before am famotidine) (n=18)[f]	0.74 (0.66, 0.84)	0.79 (0.70, 0.88)	0.72 (0.63, 0.83)
	40 mg BID, d 11–20 (n=15)	300 mg QD/ritonavir 100 mg QD, d 1–10 (am) (n=46), then 400 mg QD/ritonavir 100 mg QD, d 11–20 (am) (n=15)	1.02 (0.87, 1.18)	1.03 (0.86, 1.22)	0.86 (0.68, 1.08)
fluconazole	200 mg QD, d 11–20 (n=29)	300 mg QD/ritonavir 100 mg QD, d 1–10 (n=19), d 11–20 (n=29)	1.03 (0.95, 1.11)	1.04 (0.95, 1.13)	0.98 (0.85, 1.13)
ketoconazole	200 mg QD, d 7–13 (n=14)	400 mg QD, d 1–13 (n=14)	0.99 (0.77, 1.28)	1.10 (0.89, 1.37)	1.03 (0.53, 2.01)
nevirapine[g,h]	200 mg BID, d 1–23 (n=23)	300 mg QD/ritonavir 100 mg QD, d 4–13, then 400 mg QD/ritonavir 100 mg QD, d 14–23 (n=23)[i]	0.72 (0.60, 0.86) 1.02 (0.85, 1.24)	0.58 (0.48, 0.71) 0.81 (0.65, 1.02)	0.28 (0.20, 0.40) 0.41 (0.27, 0.60)
omeprazole	40 mg QD, d 7–12 (n=16)[j]	400 mg QD, d 1–6 (n=48), d 7–12 (n=16)	0.04 (0.04, 0.05)	0.06 (0.05, 0.07)	0.05 (0.03, 0.07)
	40 mg QD, d 11–20 (n=15)[j]	300 mg QD/ritonavir 100 mg QD, d 1–20 (n=15)	0.28 (0.24, 0.32)	0.24 (0.21, 0.27)	0.22 (0.19, 0.26)
	20 mg QD, d 17–23 (am) (n=13)	300 mg QD/ritonavir 100 mg QD, d 7–16 (pm) (n=27), d 17–23 (pm) (n=13)[k,l]	0.61 (0.46, 0.81)	0.58 (0.44, 0.75)	0.54 (0.41, 0.71)
	20 mg QD, d 17–23 (am) (n=14)	300 mg QD/ritonavir 100 mg QD, d 7–16 (am) (n=27), then 400 mg QD/ritonavir 100 mg QD, d 17–23 (am) (n=14)[m,n]	0.69 (0.58, 0.83)	0.70 (0.57, 0.86)	0.69 (0.54, 0.88)
pitavastatin	4 mg QD for 5 days	300 mg QD for 5 days	1.13 (0.96, 1.32)	1.06 (0.90, 1.26)	NA
rifabutin	150 mg QD, d 15–28 (n=7)	400 mg QD, d 1–28 (n=7)	1.34 (1.14, 1.59)	1.15 (0.98, 1.34)	1.13 (0.68, 1.87)
rifampin	600 mg QD, d 17–26 (n=16)	300 mg QD/ritonavir 100 mg QD, d 7–16 (n=48), d 17–26 (n=16)	0.47 (0.41, 0.53)	0.28 (0.25, 0.32)	0.02 (0.02, 0.03)
ritonavir[o]	100 mg QD, d 11–20 (n=28)	300 mg QD, d 1–20 (n=28)	1.86 (1.69, 2.05)	3.38 (3.13, 3.63)	11.89 (10.23, 13.82)
telaprevir	750 mg q8h for 10 days (n=7)	300 mg QD/ritonavir 100 mg QD for 20 days (n=7)	0.85 (0.73, 0.98)	1.17 (0.97, 1.43)	1.85 (1.40, 2.44)

(Table continued on next page)

rates when 3 or more baseline PI substitutions, including a substitution at position 36, 71, 77, 82, or 90, were present compared to patients with 1–2 PI substitutions, including one of these substitutions.

[See table 20 at top of page 787]

The response rates of antiretroviral-experienced patients in Study AI424-045 were analyzed by baseline phenotype (shift in susceptibility in cell culture relative to reference, Table 21). The analyses are based on a select patient population with 62% of patients receiving an NNRTI-based regimen before study entry compared to 35% receiving a PI-based regimen. Additional data are needed to determine clinically relevant break points for REYATAZ (atazanavir sulfate).

Table 21: Baseline Phenotype by Outcome, Antiretroviral-Experienced Patients in Study AI424-045, As-Treated Analysis

Baseline Phenotype[a]	Virologic Response = HIV RNA <400 copies/mL[b]	
	ATV/RTV (n=111)	LPV/RTV (n=111)
0–2	71% (55/78)	70% (56/80)
>2–5	53% (8/15)	44% (4/9)
>5–10	13% (1/8)	33% (3/9)
>10	10% (1/10)	23% (3/13)

[a] Fold change susceptibility in cell culture relative to the wild-type reference.

[b] Results should be interpreted with caution because the subgroups were small.

13 NONCLINICAL TOXICOLOGY

13.1 Carcinogenesis, Mutagenesis, Impairment of Fertility

Carcinogenesis

Long-term carcinogenicity studies in mice and rats were carried out with atazanavir for two years. In the mouse study, drug-related increases in hepatocellular adenomas were found in females at 360 mg/kg/day. The systemic drug exposure (AUC) at the NOAEL (no observable adverse effect level) in females, (120 mg/kg/day) was 2.8 times and in males (80 mg/kg/day) was 2.9 times higher than those in humans at the clinical dose (300 mg/day atazanavir boosted with 100 mg/day ritonavir, non-pregnant patients). In the rat study, no drug-related increases in tumor incidence were observed at doses up to 1200 mg/kg/day, for which AUCs were 1.1 (males) or 3.9 (females) times those measured in humans at the clinical dose.

Mutagenesis

Atazanavir tested positive in an *in vitro* clastogenicity test using primary human lymphocytes, in the absence and presence of metabolic activation. Atazanavir tested negative in the *in vitro* Ames reverse-mutation assay, *in vivo* micronucleus and DNA repair tests in rats, and *in vivo* DNA damage test in rat duodenum (comet assay).

Impairment of Fertility

At the systemic drug exposure levels (AUC) 0.9 (in male rats) or 2.3 (in female rats) times that of the human clinical dose, (300 mg/day atazanavir boosted with 100 mg/day ritonavir) significant effects on mating, fertility, or early embryonic development were not observed.

14 CLINICAL STUDIES

14.1 Adult Patients Without Prior Antiretroviral Therapy

Study AI424-138: a 96-week study comparing the antiviral efficacy and safety of atazanavir/ritonavir with lopinavir/ritonavir, each in combination with fixed-dose tenofovir-emtricitabine in HIV-1 infected treatment-naive subjects. Study AI424-138 was a 96-week, open-label, randomized, multicenter study, comparing REYATAZ (300 mg once daily) with ritonavir (100 mg once daily) to lopinavir with ritonavir (400/100 mg twice daily), each in combination with fixed-dose tenofovir with emtricitabine (300/200 mg once daily), in 878 antiretroviral treatment-naive treated patients. Patients had a mean age of 36 years (range: 19–72), 49% were Caucasian, 18% Black, 9% Asian, 23% Hispanic/Mestizo/mixed race, and 68% were male. The median baseline plasma CD4+ cell count was 204 cells/mm^3 (range: 2 to 810 cells/mm^3) and the mean baseline plasma HIV-1 RNA level was 4.94 $\log_{10}$ copies/mL (range: 2.60 to 5.88 $\log_{10}$ copies/mL). Treatment response and outcomes through Week 96 are presented in Table 22.

[See table 22 at top of page 787]

Through 96 weeks of therapy, the proportion of responders among patients with high viral loads (ie, baseline HIV RNA ≥100,000 copies/mL) was comparable for the REYATAZ/ritonavir (165 of 223 patients, 74%) and lopinavir/ritonavir (148 of 222 patients, 67%) arms. At 96 weeks, the median increase from baseline in CD4+ cell count was 261 cells/mm^3 for the REYATAZ/ritonavir arm and 273 cells/mm^3 for the lopinavir/ritonavir arm.

Table 17 *(cont.)*: Drug Interactions: Pharmacokinetic Parameters for Atazanavir in the Presence of Coadministered Drugs[a]

Coadministered Drug	Coadministered Drug Dose/Schedule	REYATAZ Dose/Schedule	Ratio (90% Confidence Interval) of Atazanavir Pharmacokinetic Parameters with/without Coadministered Drug; No Effect = 1.00		
			C_{max}	AUC	C_{min}
tenofovir[p]	300 mg QD, d 9–16 (n=34)	400 mg QD, d 2–16 (n=34)	0.79 (0.73, 0.86)	0.75 (0.70, 0.81)	0.60 (0.52, 0.68)
	300 mg QD, d 15–42 (n=10)	300 mg/ritonavir 100 mg QD, d 1–42 (n=10)	0.72[q] (0.50, 1.05)	0.75[q] (0.58, 0.97)	0.77[q] (0.54, 1.10)
voriconazole (Subjects with at least one functional CYP2C19 allele)	200 mg BID, d 2–3, 22–30; 400 mg BID, d 1, 21 (n=20)	300 mg/ritonavir 100 mg QD, d 11–30 (n=20)	0.87 (0.80, 0.96)	0.88 (0.82, 0.95)	0.80 (0.72, 0.90)
voriconazole (Subjects without a functional CYP2C19 allele)	50 mg BID, d 2–3, 22–30; 100 mg BID, d 1, 21 (n=8)	300 mg/ritonavir 100 mg QD, d 11–30 (n=8)	0.81 (0.66, 1.00)	0.80 (0.65, 0.97)	0.69 (0.54, 0.87)

[a] Data provided are under fed conditions unless otherwise noted.
[b] All drugs were given under fasted conditions.
[c] 400 mg ddI EC and REYATAZ were administered together with food on Days 8 and 19.
[d] REYATAZ 300 mg plus ritonavir 100 mg once daily coadministered with famotidine 40 mg twice daily resulted in atazanavir geometric mean C_{max} that was similar and AUC and C_{min} values that were 1.79- and 4.46-fold higher relative to REYATAZ 400 mg once daily alone.
[e] Similar results were noted when famotidine 20 mg BID was administered 2 hours after and 10 hours before atazanavir 300 mg and ritonavir 100 mg plus tenofovir 300 mg.
[f] Atazanavir/ritonavir/tenofovir was administered after a light meal.
[g] Study was conducted in HIV-infected individuals.
[h] Compared with atazanavir 400 mg historical data without nevirapine (n=13), the ratio of geometric means (90% confidence intervals) for C_{max}, AUC, and C_{min} were 1.42 (0.98, 2.05), 1.64 (1.11, 2.42), and 1.25 (0.66, 2.36), respectively, for atazanavir/ritonavir 300/100 mg; and 2.02 (1.42, 2.87), 2.28 (1.54, 3.38), and 1.80 (0.94, 3.45), respectively, for atazanavir/ritonavir 400/100 mg.
[i] Parallel group design; n=23 for atazanavir/ritonavir plus nevirapine, n=22 for atazanavir 300 mg/ritonavir 100 mg without nevirapine. Subjects were treated with nevirapine prior to study entry.
[j] Omeprazole 40 mg was administered on an empty stomach 2 hours before REYATAZ.
[k] Omeprazole 20 mg was administered 30 minutes prior to a light meal in the morning and REYATAZ 300 mg plus ritonavir 100 mg in the evening after a light meal, separated by 12 hours from omeprazole.
[l] REYATAZ 300 mg plus ritonavir 100 mg once daily separated by 12 hours from omeprazole 20 mg daily resulted in increases in atazanavir geometric mean AUC (10%) and C_{min} (2.4-fold), with a decrease in C_{max} (29%) relative to REYATAZ 400 mg once daily in the absence of omeprazole (study days 1–6).
[m] Omeprazole 20 mg was given 30 minutes prior to a light meal in the morning and REYATAZ 400 mg plus ritonavir 100 mg once daily after a light meal, 1 hour after omeprazole. Effects on atazanavir concentrations were similar when REYATAZ 400 mg plus ritonavir 100 mg was separated from omeprazole 20 mg by 12 hours.
[n] REYATAZ 400 mg plus ritonavir 100 mg once daily administered with omeprazole 20 mg once daily resulted in increases in atazanavir geometric mean AUC (32%) and C_{min} (3.3-fold), with a decrease in C_{max} (26%) relative to REYATAZ 400 mg once daily in the absence of omeprazole (study days 1–6).
[o] Compared with atazanavir 400 mg QD historical data, administration of atazanavir/ritonavir 300/100 mg QD increased the atazanavir geometric mean values of C_{max}, AUC, and C_{min} by 18%, 103%, and 671%, respectively.
[p] Note that similar results were observed in studies where administration of tenofovir and REYATAZ was separated by 12 hours.
[q] Ratio of atazanavir plus ritonavir plus tenofovir to atazanavir plus ritonavir. Atazanavir 300 mg plus ritonavir 100 mg results in higher atazanavir exposure than atazanavir 400 mg (see footnote [o]). The geometric mean values of atazanavir pharmacokinetic parameters when coadministered with ritonavir and tenofovir were: C_{max} = 3190 ng/mL, AUC = 34459 ng•h/mL, and C_{min} = 491 ng/mL. Study was conducted in HIV-infected individuals.
NA = not available.

Study AI424-034: REYATAZ once daily compared to efavirenz once daily, each in combination with fixed-dose lamivudine + zidovudine twice daily. Study AI424-034 was a randomized, double-blind, multicenter trial comparing REYATAZ (atazanavir sulfate) (400 mg once daily) to efavirenz (600 mg once daily), each in combination with a fixed-dose combination of lamivudine (3TC) (150 mg) and zidovudine (ZDV) (300 mg) given twice daily, in 810 antiretroviral treatment-naive patients. Patients had a mean age of 34 years (range: 18 to 73), 36% were Hispanic, 33% were Caucasian, and 65% were male. The mean baseline CD4+ cell count was 321 cells/mm^3 (range: 64 to 1424 cells/mm^3) and the mean baseline plasma HIV-1 RNA level was 4.8 log_{10} copies/mL (range: 2.2 to 5.9 log_{10} copies/mL). Treatment response and outcomes through Week 48 are presented in Table 23.

[See table 23 at top of page 788]

Through 48 weeks of therapy, the proportion of responders among patients with high viral loads (ie, baseline HIV RNA ≥100,000 copies/mL) was comparable for the REYATAZ and efavirenz arms. The mean increase from baseline in CD4+ cell count was 176 cells/mm^3 for the REYATAZ arm and 160 cells/mm^3 for the efavirenz arm.

Study AI424-008: REYATAZ 400 mg once daily compared to REYATAZ 600 mg once daily, and compared to nelfinavir 1250 mg twice daily, each in combination with stavudine and lamivudine twice daily. Study AI424-008 was a 48-week, randomized, multicenter trial, blinded to dose of REYATAZ, comparing REYATAZ at two dose levels (400 mg and 600 mg once daily) to nelfinavir (1250 mg twice daily), each in combination with stavudine (40 mg) and lamivudine (150 mg) given twice daily, in 467 antiretroviral treatment-naive patients. Patients had a mean age of 35 years (range: 18 to 69), 55% were Caucasian, and 63% were male. The mean baseline CD4+ cell count was 295 cells/mm^3 (range: 4 to 1003 cells/mm^3) and the mean baseline plasma HIV-1 RNA level was 4.7 log_{10} copies/mL (range: 1.8 to 5.9 log_{10} copies/mL). Treatment response and outcomes through Week 48 are presented in Table 24.

[See table 24 at top of page 788]

Through 48 weeks of therapy, the mean increase from baseline in CD4+ cell count was 234 cells/mm^3 for the REYATAZ 400-mg arm and 211 cells/mm^3 for the nelfinavir arm.

14.2 Adult Patients With Prior Antiretroviral Therapy

Study AI424-045: REYATAZ once daily + ritonavir once daily compared to REYATAZ once daily + saquinavir (soft gelatin capsules) once daily, and compared to lopinavir + ritonavir twice daily, each in combination with tenofovir + one NRTI. Study AI424-045 was a randomized, multicenter trial comparing REYATAZ (atazanavir sulfate) (300 mg once daily) with ritonavir (100 mg once daily) to REYATAZ (400 mg once daily) with saquinavir soft gelatin capsules (1200 mg once daily), and to lopinavir + ritonavir (400/100 mg twice daily), each in combination with tenofovir and one NRTI, in 347 (of 358 randomized) patients who experienced virologic failure on HAART regimens containing PIs, NRTIs, and NNRTIs. The mean time of prior exposure to antiretrovirals was 139 weeks for PIs, 283 weeks for NRTIs, and 85 weeks for NNRTIs. The mean age was 41 years (range: 24 to 74); 60% were Caucasian, and 78% were male. The mean baseline CD4+ cell count was 338 cells/mm^3 (range: 14 to 1543 cells/mm^3) and the mean baseline plasma HIV-1 RNA level was 4.4 log_{10} copies/mL (range: 2.6 to 5.88 log_{10} copies/mL).

Treatment outcomes through Week 48 for the REYATAZ/ritonavir and lopinavir/ritonavir treatment arms are presented in Table 25. REYATAZ/ritonavir and lopinavir/ritonavir were similar for the primary efficacy outcome measure of time-averaged difference in change from baseline in HIV RNA level. Study AI424-045 was not large enough to reach a definitive conclusion that REYATAZ/ritonavir and lopinavir/ritonavir are equivalent on the secondary efficacy outcome measure of proportions below the HIV RNA lower limit of detection. [See *Clinical Pharmacology, Tables 20* and *21 (12.4)*.]

[See table 25 at top of page 788]

No patients in the REYATAZ/ritonavir treatment arm and three patients in the lopinavir/ritonavir treatment arm experienced a new-onset CDC Category C event during the study.

In Study AI424-045, the mean change from baseline in plasma HIV-1 RNA for REYATAZ (atazanavir sulfate) 400 mg with saquinavir (n=115) was −1.55 log_{10} copies/mL, and the time-averaged difference in change in HIV-1 RNA levels versus lopinavir/ritonavir was 0.33. The corresponding mean increase in CD4+ cell count was 72 cells/mm^3. Through 48 weeks of treatment, the proportion of patients in this treatment arm with plasma HIV-1 RNA <400 (<50) copies/mL was 38% (26%). In this study, coadministration of REYATAZ and saquinavir did not provide adequate efficacy [see *Drug Interactions (7)*].

Study AI424-045 also compared changes from baseline in lipid values. [See *Adverse Reactions (6.1)*.]

Study AI424-043: Study AI424-043 was a randomized, open-label, multicenter trial comparing REYATAZ (400 mg once daily) to lopinavir/ritonavir (400/100 mg twice daily), each in combination with two NRTIs, in 300 patients who experienced virologic failure to only one prior PI-containing regimen. Through 48 weeks, the proportion of patients with plasma HIV-1 RNA <400 (<50) copies/mL was 49% (35%) for patients randomized to REYATAZ (n=144) and 69% (53%) for patients randomized to lopinavir/ritonavir (n=146). The mean change from baseline was −1.59 log_{10} copies/mL in the REYATAZ treatment arm and −2.02 log_{10} copies/mL in the lopinavir/ritonavir arm. Based on the results of this study, REYATAZ without ritonavir is inferior to lopinavir/ritonavir in PI-experienced patients with prior virologic failure and is not recommended for such patients.

14.3 Pediatric Patients

Assessment of the pharmacokinetics, safety, tolerability, and efficacy of REYATAZ is based on data from the open-label, multicenter clinical trial PACTG 1020A conducted in patients from 3 months to 21 years of age. In this study, 193 patients (86 antiretroviral-naive and 107 antiretroviral-experienced) received once daily REYATAZ, with or without ritonavir, in combination with two NRTIs.

One-hundred five patients (6 to less than 18 years of age) treated with the REYATAZ capsule formulation, with or without ritonavir, were evaluated. Using an ITT analysis, the overall proportions of antiretroviral-naive and -experienced patients with HIV RNA <400 copies/mL at Week 96 were 51% (22/43) and 34% (21/62), respectively. The overall proportions of antiretroviral-naive and -experienced patients with HIV RNA <50 copies/mL at Week 96 were 47% (20/43) and 24% (15/62), respectively. The median increase from baseline in absolute CD4 count at 96 weeks of therapy was 335 cells/mm^3 in antiretroviral-naive patients and 220 cells/mm^3 in antiretroviral-experienced patients.

16 HOW SUPPLIED/STORAGE AND HANDLING

REYATAZ® (atazanavir sulfate) Capsules are available in the following strengths and configurations of plastic bottles with child-resistant closures.

[See fourth table at top of page 788]

REYATAZ (atazanavir sulfate) Capsules should be stored at 25° C (77° F); excursions permitted to 15–30° C (59–86° F) [see USP Controlled Room Temperature].

17 PATIENT COUNSELING INFORMATION

See *FDA-approved patient labeling (Patient Information)*.

A statement to patients and healthcare providers is included on the product's bottle label: **ALERT: Find out about medicines that should NOT be taken with REYATAZ.**

REYATAZ is not a cure for HIV-1 infection and patients may continue to experience illnesses associated with HIV-1 infection, including opportunistic infections. Patients should remain under the care of a physician when using REYATAZ.

Patients should be advised to avoid doing things that can spread HIV-1 infection to others.

- **Do not share needles or other injection equipment.**
- **Do not share personal items that can have blood or body fluids on them, like toothbrushes and razor blades.**
- **Do not have any kind of sex without protection.** Always practice safe sex by using a latex or polyurethane condom to lower the chance of sexual contact with semen, vaginal secretions, or blood.
- **Do not breastfeed.** It is not known if REYATAZ can be passed to your baby in your breast milk and whether it could harm your baby. Also, mothers with HIV-1 should not breastfeed because HIV-1 can be passed to the baby in breast milk.

17.1 Dosing Instructions

Patients should be told that sustained decreases in plasma HIV RNA have been associated with a reduced risk of progression to AIDS and death. Patients should remain under the care of a physician while using REYATAZ (atazanavir sulfate). Patients should be advised to take REYATAZ with food every day and take other concomitant antiretroviral therapy as prescribed. REYATAZ must always be used in combination with other antiretroviral drugs. Patients should not alter the dose or discontinue therapy without consulting with their doctor. If a dose of REYATAZ is missed, patients should take the dose as soon as possible and then return to their normal schedule. However, if a dose is skipped the patient should not double the next dose.

17.2 Drug Interactions

REYATAZ may interact with some drugs; therefore, patients should be advised to report to their doctor the use of any other prescription, nonprescription medication, or herbal products, particularly St. John's wort.

Patients receiving a PDE5 inhibitor and atazanavir should be advised that they may be at an increased risk of PDE5 inhibitor-associated adverse events including hypotension, syncope, visual disturbances, and priapism, and should promptly report any symptoms to their doctor.

Patients should be informed that REVATIO® (used to treat pulmonary arterial hypertension) is contraindicated with REYATAZ and that dose adjustments are necessary when REYATAZ is used with CIALIS®, LEVITRA®, or VIAGRA® (used to treat erectile dysfunction), or ADCIRCA® (used to treat pulmonary arterial hypertension).

17.3 Cardiac Conduction Abnormalities

Patients should be informed that atazanavir may produce changes in the electrocardiogram (eg, PR prolongation). Patients should consult their physician if they are experiencing symptoms such as dizziness or lightheadedness.

17.4 Rash

Patients should be informed that mild rashes without other symptoms have been reported with REYATAZ use. These rashes go away within two weeks with no change in treatment. However, there have been a few reports of severe skin reactions (eg, Stevens-Johnson syndrome, erythema multiforme, and toxic skin eruptions) with REYATAZ use. Patients developing signs or symptoms of severe skin reactions or hypersensitivity reactions (including, but not limited to, severe rash or rash accompanied by one or more of the following: fever, general malaise, muscle or joint aches, blisters, oral lesions, conjunctivitis, facial edema, hepatitis, eosinophilia, granulocytopenia, lymphadenopathy, and renal dysfunction) must discontinue REYATAZ and seek medical evaluation immediately.

17.5 Hyperbilirubinemia

Patients should be informed that asymptomatic elevations in indirect bilirubin have occurred in patients receiving REYATAZ. This may be accompanied by yellowing of the skin or whites of the eyes and alternative antiretroviral therapy may be considered if the patient has cosmetic concerns.

17.6 Fat Redistribution

Patients should be informed that redistribution or accumulation of body fat may occur in patients receiving antiretroviral therapy including protease inhibitors and that the cause and long-term health effects of these conditions are not known at this time. It is unknown whether long-term use of REYATAZ will result in a lower incidence of lipodystrophy than with other protease inhibitors.

17.7 Nephrolithiasis and Cholelithiasis

Patients should be informed that kidney stones and/or gallstones have been reported with REYATAZ use. Some patients with kidney stones and/or gallstones required hospitalization for additional management and some had complications. Discontinuation of REYATAZ may be necessary as part of the medical management of these adverse events.

Patient Information

REYATAZ® (RAY-ah-taz)

(generic name = **atazanavir sulfate**)

Capsules

ALERT: Find out about medicines that should NOT be taken with REYATAZ. Read the section "What important information should I know about taking REYATAZ (atazanavir sulfate) with other medicines?"

Read the Patient Information that comes with REYATAZ before you start using it and each time you get a refill. There may be new information. This leaflet provides a summary about REYATAZ and does not include everything there is to know about your medicine. This information does not take the place of talking with your healthcare provider about your medical condition or treatment.

What is REYATAZ?

REYATAZ (atazanavir sulfate) is a prescription medicine used with other anti-HIV medicines to treat people 6 years of age and older who are infected with the human immunodeficiency virus (HIV). HIV is the virus that causes acquired

Table 18: Drug Interactions: Pharmacokinetic Parameters for Coadministered Drugs in the Presence of REYATAZ[a]

Coadministered Drug	Coadministered Drug Dose/Schedule	REYATAZ Dose/Schedule	Ratio (90% Confidence Interval) of Coadministered Drug Pharmacokinetic Parameters with/without REYATAZ; No Effect = 1.00		
			C_{max}	AUC	C_{min}
acetaminophen	1 gm BID, d 1–20 (n=10)	300 mg QD/ritonavir 100 mg QD, d 11–20 (n=10)	0.87 (0.77, 0.99)	0.97 (0.91, 1.03)	1.26 (1.08, 1.46)
atenolol	50 mg QD, d 7–11 (n=19) and d 19–23	400 mg QD, d 1–11 (n=19)	1.34 (1.26, 1.42)	1.25 (1.16, 1.34)	1.02 (0.88, 1.19)
boceprevir	800 mg TID, d 1–6, 25–31	300 mg QD/ritonavir 100 mg QD, d 10–31	0.93 (0.80, 1.08)	0.95 (0.87, 1.05)	0.82 (0.68, 0.98)
clarithromycin	500 mg BID, d 7–10 (n=21) and d 18–21	400 mg QD, d 1–10 (n=21)	1.50 (1.32, 1.71) OH-clarithromycin: 0.28 (0.24, 0.33)	1.94 (1.75, 2.16) OH-clarithromycin: 0.30 (0.26, 0.34)	2.60 (2.35, 2.88) OH-clarithromycin: 0.38 (0.34, 0.42)
didanosine (ddI) (buffered tablets) plus stavudine (d4T)[b]	ddI: 200 mg × 1 dose, d4T: 40 mg × 1 dose (n=31)	400 mg × 1 dose simultaneous with ddI and d4T (n=31)	ddI: 0.92 (0.84, 1.02) d4T: 1.08 (0.96, 1.22)	ddI: 0.98 (0.92, 1.05) d4T: 1.00 (0.97, 1.03)	NA d4T: 1.04 (0.94, 1.16)
ddI (enteric-coated [EC] capsules)[c]	400 mg d 1 (fasted), d 8 (fed) (n=34)	400 mg QD, d 2–8 (n=34)	0.64 (0.55, 0.74)	0.66 (0.60, 0.74)	1.13 (0.91, 1.41)
	400 mg d 1 (fasted), d 19 (fed) (n=31)	300 mg QD/ritonavir 100 mg QD, d 9–19 (n=31)	0.62 (0.52, 0.74)	0.66 (0.59, 0.73)	1.25 (0.92, 1.69)
diltiazem	180 mg QD, d 7–11 (n=28) and d 19–23	400 mg QD, d 1–11 (n=28)	1.98 (1.78, 2.19) desacetyl-diltiazem: 2.72 (2.44, 3.03)	2.25 (2.09, 2.16) desacetyl-diltiazem: 2.65 (2.45, 2.87)	2.42 (2.14, 2.73) desacetyl-diltiazem: 2.21 (2.02, 2.42)
ethinyl estradiol & norethindrone[d]	Ortho-Novum® 7/7/7 QD, d 1–29 (n=19)	400 mg QD, d 16–29 (n=19)	ethinyl estradiol: 1.15 (0.99, 1.32) norethindrone: 1.67 (1.42, 1.96)	ethinyl estradiol: 1.48 (1.31, 1.68) norethindrone: 2.10 (1.68, 2.62)	ethinyl estradiol: 1.91 (1.57, 2.33) norethindrone: 3.62 (2.57, 5.09)
ethinyl estradiol & norgestimate[e]	Ortho Tri-Cyclen® QD, d 1–28 (n=18), then Ortho Tri-Cyclen® LO QD, d 29–42[f] (n=14)	300 mg QD/ritonavir 100 mg QD, d 29–42 (n=14)	ethinyl estradiol: 0.84 (0.74, 0.95) 17-deacetyl norgestimate:[g] 1.68 (1.51, 1.88)	ethinyl estradiol: 0.81 (0.75, 0.87) 17-deacetyl norgestimate:[g] 1.85 (1.67, 2.05)	ethinyl estradiol: 0.63 (0.55, 0.71) 17-deacetyl norgestimate:[g] 2.02 (1.77, 2.31)
fluconazole	200 mg QD, d 1–10 (n=11) and 200 mg QD, d 11–20 (n=29)	300 mg QD/ritonavir 100 mg QD, d 11–20 (n=29)	1.05 (0.99, 1.10)	1.08 (1.02, 1.15)	1.07 (1.00, 1.15)
methadone	Stable maintenance dose, d 1–15 (n=16)	400 mg QD, d 2–15 (n=16)	(R)-methadone[h] 0.91 (0.84, 1.0) total: 0.85 (0.78, 0.93)	(R)-methadone[h] 1.03 (0.95, 1.10) total: 0.94 (0.87, 1.02)	(R)-methadone[h] 1.11 (1.02, 1.20) total: 1.02 (0.93, 1.12)
nevirapine[i,j]	200 mg BID, d 1–23 (n=23)	300 mg QD/ritonavir 100 mg QD, d 4–13, then 400 mg QD/ritonavir 100 mg QD, d 14–23 (n=23)	1.17 (1.09, 1.25) 1.21 (1.11, 1.32)	1.25 (1.17, 1.34) 1.26 (1.17, 1.36)	1.32 (1.22, 1.43) 1.35 (1.25, 1.47)
omeprazole[k]	40 mg single dose, d 7 and d 20 (n=16)	400 mg QD, d 1–12 (n=16)	1.24 (1.04, 1.47)	1.45 (1.20, 1.76)	NA
rifabutin	300 mg QD, d 1–10 then 150 mg QD, d 11–20 (n=3)	600 mg QD,[l] d 11–20 (n=3)	1.18 (0.94, 1.48) 25-O-desacetyl-rifabutin: 8.20 (5.90, 11.40)	2.10 (1.57, 2.79) 25-O-desacetyl-rifabutin: 22.01 (15.97, 30.34)	3.43 (1.98, 5.96) 25-O-desacetyl-rifabutin: 75.6 (30.1, 190.0)
	150 mg twice weekly, d 1–15 (n=7)	300 mg QD/ritonavir 100 mg QD, d 1–17 (n=7)	2.49[m] (2.03, 3.06) 25-O-desacetyl-rifabutin: 7.77 (6.13, 9.83)	1.48[m] (1.19, 1.84) 25-O-desacetyl-rifabutin: 10.90 (8.14, 14.61)	1.40[m] (1.05, 1.87) 25-O-desacetyl-rifabutin: 11.45 (8.15, 16.10)

(Table continued on next page)

immune deficiency syndrome (AIDS). REYATAZ (atazanavir sulfate) is a type of anti-HIV medicine called a protease inhibitor. HIV infection destroys CD4+ (T) cells, which are important to the immune system. The immune system helps fight infection. After a large number of (T) cells are destroyed, AIDS develops. REYATAZ helps to block HIV protease, an enzyme that is needed for the HIV virus to multiply. REYATAZ may lower the amount of HIV in your blood, help your body keep its supply of CD4+ (T) cells, and reduce the risk of death and illness associated with HIV.

Does REYATAZ cure HIV or AIDS?

REYATAZ does not cure HIV infection or AIDS and you may continue to experience illnesses associated with HIV-1 infection, including opportunistic infections. You should remain under the care of a doctor when using REYATAZ.

Avoid doing things that can spread HIV-1 infection.

- **Do not share needles or other injection equipment.**
- **Do not share personal items that can have blood or body fluids on them, like toothbrushes and razor blades.**
- **Do not have any kind of sex without protection.** Always practice safe sex by using a latex or polyurethane condom to lower the chance of sexual contact with semen, vaginal secretions, or blood.

Who should not take REYATAZ?

Do not take REYATAZ if you:

- **are taking certain medicines.** (See "What important information should I know about taking REYATAZ with other medicines?") Serious life-threatening side effects or death may happen. Before you take REYATAZ, tell your healthcare provider about all medicines you are taking or planning to take. These include other prescription and nonprescription medicines, vitamins, and herbal supplements.
- **are allergic to REYATAZ or to any of its ingredients.** The active ingredient is atazanavir sulfate. See the end of this leaflet for a complete list of ingredients in REYATAZ. Tell your healthcare provider if you think you have had an allergic reaction to any of these ingredients.

What should I tell my healthcare provider before I take REYATAZ?

Tell your healthcare provider:

- **If you are pregnant or plan to become pregnant.** REYATAZ use during pregnancy has not been associated with an increase in birth defects. Pregnant women have experienced serious side effects when taking REYATAZ with other HIV medicines called nucleoside analogues. You and your healthcare provider will need to decide if REYATAZ is right for you. If you use REYATAZ while you are pregnant, talk to your healthcare provider about the Antiretroviral Pregnancy Registry.
  - **After your baby is born**, tell your healthcare provider if your baby's skin or the white part of his/her eyes turns yellow.
- **If you are breastfeeding. Do not breastfeed.** It is not known if REYATAZ can be passed to your baby in your breast milk and whether it could harm your baby. Also, mothers with HIV-1 should not breastfeed because HIV-1 can be passed to the baby in the breast milk.
- **If you have liver problems or are infected with the hepatitis B or C virus.** See "What are the possible side effects of REYATAZ?"
- **If you have end stage kidney disease** managed with hemodialysis.
- **If you have diabetes.** See "What are the possible side effects of REYATAZ?"
- **If you have hemophilia.** See "What are the possible side effects of REYATAZ?"
- **About all the medicines you take** including prescription and nonprescription medicines, vitamins, and herbal supplements. Keep a list of your medicines with you to show your healthcare provider. For more information, see "What important information should I know about taking REYATAZ with other medicines?" and "Who should not take REYATAZ?" Some medicines can cause serious side effects if taken with REYATAZ.

How should I take REYATAZ?

- **Take REYATAZ once every day exactly as instructed by your healthcare provider.** Your healthcare provider will prescribe the amount of REYATAZ that is right for you.
- **Always take REYATAZ with food** (a meal or snack) to help it work better. Swallow the capsules whole. **Do not open the capsules.** Take REYATAZ at the same time each day.
- **If you are taking antacids or didanosine (VIDEX® or VIDEX® EC)**, take REYATAZ 2 hours before or 1 hour after these medicines.
- **If you are taking medicines for indigestion, heartburn, or ulcers such as AXID® (nizatidine), PEPCID AC® (famotidine), TAGAMET® (cimetidine), ZANTAC® (ranitidine), AcipHex® (rabeprazole), NEXIUM® (esomeprazole), PREVACID® (lansoprazole), PRILOSEC® (omeprazole), or PROTONIX® (pantoprazole)**, talk to your healthcare provider.
- **Do not change your dose or stop taking REYATAZ without first talking with your healthcare provider.** It is important to stay under a healthcare provider's care while taking REYATAZ (atazanavir sulfate).
- **When your supply of REYATAZ starts to run low**, get more from your healthcare provider or pharmacy. It is important not to run out of REYATAZ. The amount of HIV in your blood may increase if the medicine is stopped for even a short time.
- **If you miss a dose of REYATAZ**, take it as soon as possible and then take your next scheduled dose at its regular time. If, however, it is within 6 hours of your next dose, do not take the missed dose. Wait and take the next dose at the regular time. Do not double the next dose. **It is important that you do not miss any doses of REYATAZ or your other anti-HIV medicines.**
- **If you take more than the prescribed dose of REYATAZ,** call your healthcare provider or poison control center right away.

What are the possible side effects of REYATAZ?

The following list of side effects is **not** complete. Report any new or continuing symptoms to your healthcare provider. If you have questions about side effects, ask your healthcare provider. Your healthcare provider may be able to help you manage these side effects.

Table 18 *(cont.)*: Drug Interactions: Pharmacokinetic Parameters for Coadministered Drugs in the Presence of REYATAZ[a]

Coadministered Drug	Coadministered Drug Dose/Schedule	REYATAZ Dose/Schedule	Ratio (90% Confidence Interval) of Coadministered Drug Pharmacokinetic Parameters with/without REYATAZ; No Effect = 1.00		
			C_{max}	AUC	C_{min}
pitavastatin	4 mg QD for 5 days	300 mg QD for 5 days	1.60 (1.39, 1.85)	1.31 (1.23, 1.39)	NA
rosiglitazone[n]	4 mg single dose, d 1, 7, 17 (n=14)	400 mg QD, d 2–7, then 300 mg QD/ ritonavir 100 mg QD, d 8–17 (n=14)	1.08 (1.03, 1.13) 0.97 (0.91, 1.04)	1.35 (1.26, 1.44) 0.83 (0.77, 0.89)	NA NA
rosuvastatin	10 mg single dose	300 mg QD/ ritonavir 100 mg QD for 7 days	↑ 7-fold[o]	↑ 3-fold[o]	NA
saquinavir[p] (soft gelatin capsules)	1200 mg QD, d 1–13 (n=7)	400 mg QD, d 7–13 (n=7)	4.39 (3.24, 5.95)	5.49 (4.04, 7.47)	6.86 (5.29, 8.91)
telaprevir	750 mg q8h for 10 days (n=14)	300 mg QD/ ritonavir 100 mg QD for 20 days (n=14)	0.79 (0.74, 0.84)	0.80 (0.76, 0.85)	0.85 (0.75, 0.98)
tenofovir[q]	300 mg QD, d 9–16 (n=33) and d 24–30 (n=33)	400 mg QD, d 2–16 (n=33)	1.14 (1.08, 1.20)	1.24 (1.21, 1.28)	1.22 (1.15, 1.30)
	300 mg QD, d 1–7 (pm) (n=14) d 25–34 (pm) (n=12)	300 mg QD/ritonavir 100 mg QD, d 25–34 (am) (n=12)[r]	1.34 (1.20, 1.51)	1.37 (1.30, 1.45)	1.29 (1.21, 1.36)
voriconazole (Subjects with at least one functional CYP2C19 allele)	200 mg BID, d 2–3, 22–30; 400 mg BID, d 1, 21 (n=20)	300 mg/ritonavir 100 mg QD, d 11–30 (n=20)	0.90 (0.78, 1.04)	0.67 (0.58, 0.78)	0.61 (0.51, 0.72)
voriconazole (Subjects without a functional CYP2C19 allele)	50 mg BID, d 2–3, 22–30; 100 mg BID, d 1, 21 (n=8)	300 mg/ritonavir 100 mg QD, d 11–30 (n=8)	4.38 (3.55, 5.39)	5.61 (4.51, 6.99)	7.65 (5.71, 10.2)
lamivudine + zidovudine	150 mg lamivudine + 300 mg zidovudine BID, d 1–12 (n=19)	400 mg QD, d 7–12 (n=19)	lamivudine: 1.04 (0.92, 1.16) zidovudine: 1.05 (0.88, 1.24) zidovudine glucuronide: 0.95 (0.88, 1.02)	lamivudine: 1.03 (0.98, 1.08) zidovudine: 1.05 (0.96, 1.14) zidovudine glucuronide: 1.00 (0.97, 1.03)	lamivudine: 1.12 (1.04, 1.21) zidovudine: 0.69 (0.57, 0.84) zidovudine glucuronide: 0.82 (0.62, 1.08)

[a] Data provided are under fed conditions unless otherwise noted.
[b] All drugs were given under fasted conditions.
[c] 400 mg ddI EC and REYATAZ were administered together with food on Days 8 and 19.
[d] Upon further dose normalization of ethinyl estradiol 25 mcg with atazanavir relative to ethinyl estradiol 35 mcg without atazanavir, the ratio of geometric means (90% confidence intervals) for C_{max}, AUC, and C_{min} were 0.82 (0.73, 0.92), 1.06 (0.95, 1.17), and 1.35 (1.11, 1.63), respectively.
[e] Upon further dose normalization of ethinyl estradiol 35 mcg with atazanavir/ritonavir relative to ethinyl estradiol 25 mcg without atazanavir/ritonavir, the ratio of geometric means (90% confidence intervals) for C_{max}, AUC, and C_{min} were 1.17 (1.03, 1.34), 1.13 (1.05, 1.22), and 0.88 (0.77, 1.00), respectively.
[f] All subjects were on a 28 day lead-in period; one full cycle of Ortho Tri-Cyclen®. Ortho Tri-Cyclen® contains 35 mcg of ethinyl estradiol. Ortho Tri-Cyclen® LO contains 25 mcg of ethinyl estradiol. Results were dose normalized to an ethinyl estradiol dose of 35 mcg.
[g] 17-deacetyl norgestimate is the active component of norgestimate.
[h] (R)-methadone is the active isomer of methadone.
[i] Study was conducted in HIV-infected individuals.
[j] Subjects were treated with nevirapine prior to study entry.
[k] Omeprazole was used as a metabolic probe for CYP2C19. Omeprazole was given 2 hours after REYATAZ on Day 7; and was given alone 2 hours after a light meal on Day 20.
[l] Not the recommended therapeutic dose of atazanavir.
[m] When compared to rifabutin 150 mg QD alone d1–10 (n=14). Total of Rifabutin + 25-O-desacetyl-rifabutin: AUC 2.19 (1.78, 2.69).
[n] Rosiglitazone used as a probe substrate for CYP2C8.
[o] Mean ratio (with/without coadministered drug). ↑ indicates an increase in rosuvastatin exposure.
[p] The combination of atazanavir and saquinavir 1200 mg QD produced daily saquinavir exposures similar to the values produced by the standard therapeutic dosing of saquinavir at 1200 mg TID. However, the C_{max} is about 79% higher than that for the standard dosing of saquinavir (soft gelatin capsules) alone at 1200 mg TID.
[q] Note that similar results were observed in a study where administration of tenofovir and REYATAZ was separated by 12 hours.
[r] Administration of tenofovir and REYATAZ was temporally separated by 12 hours.
NA = not available.

The following side effects have been reported with REYATAZ:

- **mild rash** (redness and itching) without other symptoms sometimes occurs in patients taking REYATAZ (atazanavir sulfate), most often in the first few weeks after the medicine is started. Rashes usually go away within 2 weeks with no change in treatment. Tell your healthcare provider if rash occurs.
- **severe rash:** Rash may develop in association with other symptoms which could be serious and potentially cause death.

  If you develop a rash with any of the following symptoms stop using REYATAZ and call your healthcare provider right away:
  - shortness of breath
  - general ill feeling or "flu-like" symptoms
  - fever
  - muscle or joint aches
  - conjunctivitis (red or inflamed eyes, like "pink eye")
  - blisters
  - mouth sores
  - swelling of your face
- **yellowing of the skin or eyes.** These effects may be due to increases in bilirubin levels in the blood (bilirubin is made by the liver). Although these effects may not be damaging to your liver, skin, or eyes, call your healthcare provider promptly if your skin or the white part of your eyes turn yellow.
- **a change in the way your heart beats (heart rhythm change).** Call your healthcare provider right away if you get dizzy or lightheaded. These could be symptoms of a heart problem.
- **diabetes and high blood sugar (hyperglycemia)** sometimes happen in patients taking protease inhibitor medicines like REYATAZ. Some patients had diabetes before taking protease inhibitors while others did not. Some patients may need changes in their diabetes medicine.
- **if you have liver disease** including hepatitis B or C, your liver disease may get worse when you take anti-HIV medicines like REYATAZ.
- **kidney stones** have been reported in patients taking REYATAZ. If you develop signs or symptoms of kidney stones (pain in your side, blood in your urine, pain when you urinate) tell your healthcare provider promptly.
- **gallbladder disorders** (which may include gallstones and gallbladder inflammation) have been reported in patients taking REYATAZ. If you develop signs or symptoms of gallstones (pain in the right or middle upper stomach, fever, nausea and vomiting, or yellowing of skin and whites of the eyes), tell your healthcare provider promptly.
- **some patients with hemophilia** have increased bleeding problems with protease inhibitors like REYATAZ.
- **changes in body fat.** These changes may include an increased amount of fat in the upper back and neck ("buffalo hump"), breast, and around the trunk. Loss of fat from the legs, arms, and face may also happen. The cause and long-term health effects of these conditions are not known at this time.
- **immune reconstitution syndrome.** In some patients with advanced HIV infection (AIDS) and a history of opportunistic infection, signs and symptoms of inflammation from previous infections may occur soon after anti-HIV treatment, including REYATAZ, is started.

Other common side effects of REYATAZ taken with other anti-HIV medicines include nausea; headache; stomach pain; vomiting; diarrhea; depression; fever; dizziness; trouble sleeping; numbness, tingling, or burning of hands or feet; and muscle pain.

What important information should I know about taking REYATAZ with other medicines?

Do not take REYATAZ if you take the following medicines (not all brands may be listed; tell your healthcare provider about all the medicines you take). REYATAZ may cause serious, life-threatening side effects or death when used with these medicines.

- Ergot medicines: dihydroergotamine, ergonovine, ergotamine, and methylergonovine such as CAFERGOT®, MIGRANAL®, D.H.E. 45®, ergotrate maleate, METHERGINE®, and others (used for migraine headaches).
- ORAP® (pimozide, used for Tourette's disorder).
- PROPULSID® (cisapride, used for certain stomach problems).
- Triazolam, also known as HALCION® (used for insomnia).
- Midazolam, also known as VERSED® (used for sedation), when taken by mouth.

Do not take the following medicines with REYATAZ because of possible serious side effects:

- CAMPTOSAR® (irinotecan, used for cancer).
- CRIXIVAN® (indinavir, used for HIV infection). Both REYATAZ and CRIXIVAN sometimes cause increased levels of bilirubin in the blood.
- Cholesterol-lowering medicines MEVACOR® (lovastatin) or ZOCOR® (simvastatin).

Table 19: Summary of Virologic Failures[a] at Week 96 in Study AI424-089: Comparison of Ritonavir Boosted REYATAZ vs. Unboosted REYATAZ: Randomized Patients

	REYATAZ 300 mg + ritonavir 100 mg (n=95)	REYATAZ 400 mg (n=105)
Virologic Failure (≥50 copies/mL) at Week 96	15 (16%)	34 (32%)
Virologic Failure with Genotypes and Phenotypes Data	5	17
Virologic Failure Isolates with ATV-resistance at Week 96	0/5 (0%)[b]	4/17 (24%)[b]
Virologic Failure Isolates with I50L Emergence at Week 96[c]	0/5 (0%)[b]	2/17 (12%)[b]
Virologic Failure Isolates with Lamivudine Resistance at Week 96	2/5 (40%)[b]	11/17 (65%)[b]

[a] Virologic failure includes patients who were never suppressed through Week 96 and on study at Week 96, had virologic rebound or discontinued due to insufficient viral load response.
[b] Percentage of Virologic Failure Isolates with genotypic and phenotypic data.
[c] Mixture of I50I/L emerged in 2 other ATV 400 mg-treated patients. Neither isolate was phenotypically resistant to ATV.

Table 20: HIV RNA Response by Number and Type of Baseline PI Substitution, Antiretroviral-Experienced Patients in Study AI424-045, As-Treated Analysis

Number and Type of Baseline PI Substitutions[a]	Virologic Response = HIV RNA <400 copies/mL[b] ATV/RTV (n=110)	LPV/RTV (n=113)
3 or more primary PI substitutions including:[c]		
D30N	75% (6/8)	50% (3/6)
M36I/V	19% (3/16)	33% (6/18)
M46I/L/T	24% (4/17)	23% (5/22)
I54V/L/T/M/A	31% (5/16)	31% (5/16)
A71V/T/I/G	34% (10/29)	39% (12/31)
G73S/A/C/T	14% (1/7)	38% (3/8)
V77I	47% (7/15)	44% (7/16)
V82A/F/T/S/I	29% (6/21)	27% (7/26)
I84V/A	11% (1/9)	33% (2/6)
N88D	63% (5/8)	67% (4/6)
L90M	10% (2/21)	44% (11/25)
Number of baseline primary PI substitutions[a]		
All patients, as-treated	58% (64/110)	59% (67/113)
0–2 PI substitutions	75% (50/67)	75% (50/67)
3–4 PI substitutions	41% (14/34)	43% (12/28)
5 or more PI substitutions	0% (0/9)	28% (5/18)

[a] Primary substitutions include any change at D30, V32, M36, M46, I47, G48, I50, I54, A71, G73, V77, V82, I84, N88, and L90.
[b] Results should be interpreted with caution because the subgroups were small.
[c] There were insufficient data (n<3) for PI substitutions V32I, I47V, G48V, I50V, and F53L.

Table 22: Outcomes of Treatment Through Week 96 (Study AI424-138)

Outcome	REYATAZ 300 mg + ritonavir 100 mg (once daily) with tenofovir/emtricitabine (once daily)[a] (n=441) 96 Weeks	lopinavir 400 mg + ritonavir 100 mg (twice daily) with tenofovir/emtricitabine (once daily)[a] (n=437) 96 Weeks
Responder[b,c,d]	75%	68%
Virologic failure[e]	17%	19%
Rebound	8%	10%
Never suppressed through Week 96	9%	9%
Death	1%	1%
Discontinued due to adverse event	3%	5%
Discontinued for other reasons[f]	4%	7%

[a] As a fixed-dose combination: 300 mg tenofovir, 200 mg emtricitabine once daily.
[b] Patients achieved HIV RNA <50 copies/mL at Week 96. Roche Amplicor®, v1.5 ultra-sensitive assay.
[c] Pre-specified ITT analysis at Week 48 using as-randomized cohort: ATV/RTV 78% and LPV/RTV 76% [difference estimate: 1.7% (95% confidence interval: −3.8%, 7.1%)].
[d] Pre-specified ITT analysis at Week 96 using as-randomized cohort: ATV/RTV 74% and LPV/RTV 68% [difference estimate: 6.1% (95% confidence interval: 0.3%, 12.0%)].
[e] Includes viral rebound and failure to achieve confirmed HIV RNA <50 copies/mL through Week 96.
[f] Includes lost to follow-up, patient's withdrawal, noncompliance, protocol violation, and other reasons.

- UROXATRAL® (alfuzosin, used to treat benign enlargement of the prostate).
- REVATIO® (sildenafil, used to treat pulmonary arterial hypertension).

Do not take the following medicines with REYATAZ because they may lower the amount of REYATAZ in your blood. This may lead to an increased HIV viral load. Resistance to REYATAZ (atazanavir sulfate) or cross-resistance to other HIV medicines may develop:

- Rifampin (also known as RIMACTANE®, RIFADIN®, RIFATER®, or RIFAMATE®, used for tuberculosis).
- St. John's wort (*Hypericum perforatum*), an herbal product sold as a dietary supplement, or products containing St. John's wort.
- VIRAMUNE® (nevirapine, used for HIV infection).

The following medicines are not recommended with REYATAZ:

- SEREVENT DISKUS® (salmeterol) and ADVAIR® (salmeterol with fluticasone), used to treat asthma, emphysema/chronic obstructive pulmonary disease also known as COPD.
- VICTRELIS® (boceprevir), used to treat chronic hepatitis C infection in adults.
- VFEND® (voriconazole), used to treat fungal infections.

The following medicines may require your healthcare provider to monitor your therapy more closely (for some medicines a change in the dose or dose schedule may be needed):

- CIALIS® (tadalafil), LEVITRA® (vardenafil), or VIAGRA® (sildenafil), used to treat erectile dysfunction. REYATAZ (atazanavir sulfate) may increase the chances of serious side effects that can happen with CIALIS, LEVITRA, or VIAGRA. Do not use CIALIS, LEVITRA, or VIAGRA while you are taking REYATAZ unless your healthcare provider tells you it is okay.
- ADCIRCA® (tadalafil) or TRACLEER® (bosentan), used to treat pulmonary arterial hypertension.
- LIPITOR® (atorvastatin) or CRESTOR® (rosuvastatin). There is an increased chance of serious side effects if you take REYATAZ with this cholesterol-lowering medicine.
- Medicines for abnormal heart rhythm: CORDARONE® (amiodarone), lidocaine, quinidine (also known as CARDIOQUIN®, QUINIDEX®, and others).
- MYCOBUTIN® (rifabutin, an antibiotic used to treat tuberculosis).
- BUPRENEX®, SUBUTEX®, SUBOXONE® (buprenorphine or buprenorphine/naloxone, used to treat pain and addiction to narcotic painkillers).
- VASCOR® (bepridil, used for chest pain).
- COUMADIN® (warfarin).
- Tricyclic antidepressants such as ELAVIL® (amitriptyline), NORPRAMIN® (desipramine), SINEQUAN® (doxepin), SURMONTIL® (trimipramine), TOFRANIL® (imipramine), or VIVACTIL® (protriptyline).
- Medicines to prevent organ transplant rejection: SANDIMMUNE® or NEORAL® (cyclosporin), RAPAMUNE® (sirolimus), or PROGRAF® (tacrolimus).
- The antidepressant trazodone (DESYREL® and others).
- Fluticasone propionate (FLONASE®, FLOVENT®), given by nose or inhaled to treat allergic symptoms or asthma. Your doctor may choose not to keep you on fluticasone, especially if you are also taking NORVIR®.
- Colchicine (COLCRYS®), used to prevent or treat gout or treat familial Mediterranean fever.

The following medicines may require a change in the dose or dose schedule of either REYATAZ or the other medicine:

- INVIRASE® (saquinavir).
- NORVIR® (ritonavir).
- SUSTIVA® (efavirenz).
- Antacids or buffered medicines.
- VIDEX® (didanosine).
- VIREAD® (tenofovir disoproxil fumarate).
- MYCOBUTIN® (rifabutin).
- Calcium channel blockers such as CARDIZEM® or TIAZAC® (diltiazem), COVERA-HS® or ISOPTIN SR® (verapamil) and others.
- BIAXIN® (clarithromycin).
- Medicines for indigestion, heartburn, or ulcers such as AXID® (nizatidine), PEPCID AC® (famotidine), TAGAMET® (cimetidine), or ZANTAC® (ranitidine).
- Antiepileptic medicines such as CARBATROL® or EPITOL®(carbamazepine), DILANTIN® (phenytoin), or phenobarbital, or LAMICTAL® (lamotrigine).

Talk to your healthcare provider about choosing an effective method of contraception. REYATAZ may affect the safety and effectiveness of hormonal contraceptives such as birth control pills or the contraceptive patch. Hormonal contraceptives do not prevent the spread of HIV to others.

Remember:

1. **Know all the medicines you take.**
2. **Tell your healthcare provider about all the medicines you take.**
3. **Do not start a new medicine without talking to your healthcare provider.**

How should I store REYATAZ?

- Store REYATAZ Capsules at room temperature, 59° to 86° F (15° to 30° C). Do **not** store this medicine in a damp place such as a bathroom medicine cabinet or near the kitchen sink.
- Keep your medicine in a tightly closed container.
- Keep all medicines out of the reach of children and pets at all times. Do not keep medicine that is out of date or that you no longer need. Dispose of unused medicines through community take-back disposal programs when available or place REYATAZ in an unrecognizable, closed container in the household trash.

General information about REYATAZ

This medicine was prescribed for your particular condition. Do not use REYATAZ for another condition. Do not give REYATAZ to other people, even if they have the same symptoms you have. It may harm them. **Keep REYATAZ and all medicines out of the reach of children and pets.**

This summary does not include everything there is to know about REYATAZ. Medicines are sometimes prescribed for conditions that are not mentioned in patient information leaflets. Remember no written summary can replace careful discussion with your healthcare provider. If you would like more information, talk with your healthcare provider or you can call 1-800-321-1335.

What are the ingredients in REYATAZ?

Active Ingredient: atazanavir sulfate

Table 23: Outcomes of Randomized Treatment Through Week 48 (Study AI424-034)

Outcome	REYATAZ 400 mg once daily + lamivudine + zidovudine[d] (n=405)	efavirenz 600 mg once daily + lamivudine + zidovudine[d] (n=405)
Responder[a]	67% (32%)	62% (37%)
Virologic failure[b]	20%	21%
Rebound	17%	16%
Never suppressed through Week 48	3%	5%
Death	–	<1%
Discontinued due to adverse event	5%	7%
Discontinued for other reasons[c]	8%	10%

[a] Patients achieved and maintained confirmed HIV RNA <400 copies/mL (<50 copies/mL) through Week 48. Roche Amplicor® HIV-1 Monitor™ Assay, test version 1.0 or 1.5 as geographically appropriate.
[b] Includes viral rebound and failure to achieve confirmed HIV RNA <400 copies/mL through Week 48.
[c] Includes lost to follow-up, patient's withdrawal, noncompliance, protocol violation, and other reasons.
[d] As a fixed-dose combination: 150 mg lamivudine, 300 mg zidovudine twice daily.

Table 24: Outcomes of Randomized Treatment Through Week 48 (Study AI424-008)

Outcome	REYATAZ 400 mg once daily + lamivudine + stavudine (n=181)	nelfinavir 1250 mg twice daily + lamivudine + stavudine (n=91)
Responder[a]	67% (33%)	59% (38%)
Virologic failure[b]	24%	27%
Rebound	14%	14%
Never suppressed through Week 48	10%	13%
Death	<1%	–
Discontinued due to adverse event	1%	3%
Discontinued for other reasons[c]	7%	10%

[a] Patients achieved and maintained confirmed HIV RNA <400 copies/mL (<50 copies/mL) through Week 48. Roche Amplicor® HIV-1 Monitor™ Assay, test version 1.0 or 1.5 as geographically appropriate.
[b] Includes viral rebound and failure to achieve confirmed HIV RNA <400 copies/mL through Week 48.
[c] Includes lost to follow-up, patient's withdrawal, noncompliance, protocol violation, and other reasons.

Table 25: Outcomes of Treatment Through Week 48 in Study AI424-045 (Patients with Prior Antiretroviral Experience)

Outcome	REYATAZ 300 mg + ritonavir 100 mg once daily + tenofovir + 1 NRTI (n=119)	lopinavir/ritonavir (400/100 mg) twice daily + tenofovir + 1 NRTI (n=118)	Difference[a] (REYATAZ-lopinavir/ritonavir) (CI)
HIV RNA Change from Baseline (log_{10} copies/mL)[b]	−1.58	−1.70	+0.12[c] (−0.17, 0.41)
CD4+ Change from Baseline (cells/mm^3)[d]	116	123	−7 (−67, 52)
Percent of Patients Responding[e]			
HIV RNA <400 copies/mL[b]	55%	57%	-2.2% (−14.8%, 10.5%)
HIV RNA <50 copies/mL[b]	38%	45%	−7.1% (−19.6%, 5.4%)

[a] Time-averaged difference through Week 48 for HIV RNA; Week 48 difference in HIV RNA percentages and CD4+ mean changes, REYATAZ/ritonavir vs lopinavir/ritonavir; CI = 97.5% confidence interval for change in HIV RNA; 95% confidence interval otherwise.
[b] Roche Amplicor® HIV-1 Monitor™ Assay, test version 1.5.
[c] Protocol-defined primary efficacy outcome measure.
[d] Based on patients with baseline and Week 48 CD4+ cell count measurements (REYATAZ/ritonavir, n=85; lopinavir/ritonavir, n=93).
[e] Patients achieved and maintained confirmed HIV-1 RNA <400 copies/mL (<50 copies/mL) through Week 48.

Product Strength*	Capsule Shell Color (cap/body)	Markings on Capsule (ink color) cap	body	Capsules per Bottle	NDC Number
150 mg	blue/powder blue	BMS 150 mg (white)	3624 (blue)	60	0003-3624-12
200 mg	blue/blue	BMS 200 mg (white)	3631 (white)	60	0003-3631-12
300 mg	red/blue	BMS 300 mg (white)	3622 (white)	30	0003-3622-12

* atazanavir equivalent as atazanavir sulfate.

Inactive Ingredients: Crospovidone, lactose monohydrate (milk sugar), magnesium stearate, gelatin, FD&C Blue No. 2, and titanium dioxide.

VIDEX® and REYATAZ® are registered trademarks of Bristol-Myers Squibb Company. COUMADIN® and SUSTIVA® are registered trademarks of Bristol-Myers

Squibb Pharma Company. DESYREL® is a registered trademark of Mead Johnson and Company. Other brands listed are the trademarks of their respective owners and are not trademarks of Bristol-Myers Squibb Company.
Bristol-Myers Squibb Company
Princeton, NJ 08543 USA
1246226B5
Rev August 2013

Shown in Product Identification Guide, page 306

SPRYCEL® ℞
[*Spry-sell*]
(dasatinib)
Tablet for Oral Use

HIGHLIGHTS OF PRESCRIBING INFORMATION
These highlights do not include all the information needed to use SPRYCEL safely and effectively. See full prescribing information for SPRYCEL.
SPRYCEL® (dasatinib) Tablet for Oral Use
Initial U.S. Approval: 2006

INDICATIONS AND USAGE

SPRYCEL is a kinase inhibitor indicated for the treatment of

- newly diagnosed adults with Philadelphia chromosome-positive (Ph+) chronic myeloid leukemia (CML) in chronic phase. The trial is ongoing and further data will be required to determine long-term outcome. (1, 14)
- adults with chronic, accelerated, or myeloid or lymphoid blast phase Ph+ CML with resistance or intolerance to prior therapy including imatinib. (1, 14)
- adults with Philadelphia chromosome-positive acute lymphoblastic leukemia (Ph+ ALL) with resistance or intolerance to prior therapy. (1, 14)

DOSAGE AND ADMINISTRATION

- Chronic phase CML: 100 mg once daily. (2)
- Accelerated phase CML, myeloid or lymphoid blast phase CML, or Ph+ ALL: 140 mg once daily. (2)

Administer orally, with or without a meal. Do not crush or cut. (2)

DOSAGE FORMS AND STRENGTHS

Tablets: 20 mg, 50 mg, 70 mg, 80 mg, 100 mg, and 140 mg. (3, 16)

CONTRAINDICATIONS

None. (4)

WARNINGS AND PRECAUTIONS

- *Myelosuppression and Bleeding Events:* Severe thrombocytopenia, neutropenia, and anemia may occur. Use caution if used concomitantly with medications that inhibit platelet function or anticoagulants. Monitor complete blood counts regularly. Transfuse and interrupt SPRYCEL when indicated. (2.3, 5.1, 5.2, 6.1)
- *Fluid Retention:* Fluid retention, sometimes severe, including ascites, edema, and pleural and pericardial effusions. Manage with appropriate supportive care measures. (5.3, 6.1)
- *QT Prolongation:* Use SPRYCEL with caution in patients who have or may develop prolongation of the QT interval. (5.4)
- *Cardiac Dysfunction:* Monitor patients for signs or symptoms and treat appropriately. (5.5, 6.1)
- *Pulmonary Arterial Hypertension (PAH):* SPRYCEL may increase the risk of developing PAH which may be reversible on discontinuation. Consider baseline risk and evaluate patients for signs and symptoms of PAH during treatment. Stop SPRYCEL if PAH is confirmed. (5.6)
- *Use in Pregnancy:* Fetal harm may occur when administered to a pregnant woman. Women should be advised of the potential hazard to the fetus and to avoid becoming pregnant. (5.7, 8.1)

ADVERSE REACTIONS

Most common adverse reactions (≥15%) in patients with newly diagnosed chronic phase CML included myelosuppression, fluid retention, and diarrhea. Most common adverse reactions (≥20%) in patients with resistance or intolerance to prior imatinib therapy included myelosuppression, fluid retention events, headache, diarrhea, fatigue, dyspnea, and musculoskeletal pain. (6.1)

To report SUSPECTED ADVERSE REACTIONS, contact Bristol-Myers Squibb at 1-800-721-5072 or FDA at 1-800-FDA-1088 or www.fda.gov/medwatch.

DRUG INTERACTIONS

- *CYP3A4 Inhibitors:* May increase dasatinib drug levels and should be avoided. If coadministration cannot be avoided, monitor closely and consider reducing SPRYCEL dose. (2.1, 7.1)
- *CYP3A4 Inducers:* May decrease dasatinib drug levels. If coadministration cannot be avoided, consider increasing SPRYCEL dose. (2.1, 7.2)
- *Antacids:* May decrease dasatinib drug levels. Avoid simultaneous administration. If needed, administer the antacid at least 2 hours prior to or 2 hours after the dose of SPRYCEL. (7.2)
- *H_2 Antagonists/Proton Pump Inhibitors:* May decrease dasatinib drug levels. Consider antacids in place of H_2 antagonists or proton pump inhibitors. (7.2)

USE IN SPECIFIC POPULATIONS

- *Hepatic Impairment:* Use SPRYCEL with caution in patients with hepatic impairment. (8.6)

See 17 for PATIENT COUNSELING INFORMATION and FDA-approved patient labeling

Revised: 06/2013

FULL PRESCRIBING INFORMATION: CONTENTS*

*** Sections or subsections omitted from the full prescribing information are not listed**

FULL PRESCRIBING INFORMATION

1 INDICATIONS AND USAGE

SPRYCEL® (dasatinib) is indicated for the treatment of adults with

- newly diagnosed Philadelphia chromosome-positive (Ph+) chronic myeloid leukemia (CML) in chronic phase. The effectiveness of SPRYCEL is based on cytogenetic response and major molecular response rates *[see Clinical Studies (14.1)]*. The trial is ongoing and further data will be required to determine long-term outcome.
- chronic, accelerated, or myeloid or lymphoid blast phase Ph+ CML with resistance or intolerance to prior therapy including imatinib.
- Philadelphia chromosome-positive acute lymphoblastic leukemia (Ph+ ALL) with resistance or intolerance to prior therapy.

2 DOSAGE AND ADMINISTRATION

The recommended starting dosage of SPRYCEL (dasatinib) for chronic phase CML is 100 mg administered orally once daily. The recommended starting dosage of SPRYCEL for accelerated phase CML, myeloid or lymphoid blast phase CML, or Ph+ ALL is 140 mg administered orally once daily. Tablets should not be crushed or cut; they should be swallowed whole. SPRYCEL can be taken with or without a meal, either in the morning or in the evening.

In clinical studies, treatment with SPRYCEL was continued until disease progression or until no longer tolerated by the patient. The effect of stopping treatment after the achievement of a complete cytogenetic response (CCyR) has not been investigated.

2.1 Dose Modification

Concomitant Strong CYP3A4 inducers: The use of concomitant strong CYP3A4 inducers may decrease dasatinib plasma concentrations and should be avoided (eg, dexamethasone, phenytoin, carbamazepine, rifampin, rifabutin, phenobarbital). St. John's Wort may decrease dasatinib plasma concentrations unpredictably and should be avoided. If patients must be coadministered a strong CYP3A4 inducer, based on pharmacokinetic studies, a SPRYCEL dose increase should be considered. If the dose of SPRYCEL is increased, the patient should be monitored carefully for toxicity *[see Drug Interactions (7.2)]*.

Concomitant Strong CYP3A4 inhibitors: CYP3A4 inhibitors (eg, ketoconazole, itraconazole, clarithromycin, atazanavir, indinavir, nefazodone, nelfinavir, ritonavir, saquinavir, telithromycin, and voriconazole) may increase dasatinib plasma concentrations. Grapefruit juice may also increase plasma concentrations of dasatinib and should be avoided. Selection of an alternate concomitant medication with no or minimal enzyme inhibition potential, if possible, is recommended. If SPRYCEL must be administered with a strong CYP3A4 inhibitor, a dose decrease should be considered. Based on pharmacokinetic studies, a dose decrease to 20 mg daily should be considered for patients taking SPRYCEL 100 mg daily. For patients taking SPRYCEL 140 mg daily, a dose decrease to 40 mg daily should be considered. These reduced doses of SPRYCEL are predicted to adjust the area under the curve (AUC) to the range observed without CYP3A4 inhibitors. However, there are no clinical data with these dose adjustments in patients receiving strong CYP3A4 inhibitors. If SPRYCEL is not tolerated after dose reduction, either the strong CYP3A4 inhibitor must be discontinued, or SPRYCEL should be stopped until treatment with the inhibitor has ceased. When the strong inhibitor is discontinued, a washout period of approximately 1 week should be allowed before the SPRYCEL dose is increased. *[See Drug Interactions (7.1).]*

2.2 Dose Escalation

In clinical studies of adult CML and Ph+ ALL patients, dose escalation to 140 mg once daily (chronic phase CML) or 180 mg once daily (advanced phase CML and Ph+ ALL) was allowed in patients who did not achieve a hematologic or cytogenetic response at the recommended starting dosage.

2.3 Dose Adjustment for Adverse Reactions

Myelosuppression

In clinical studies, myelosuppression was managed by dose interruption, dose reduction, or discontinuation of study therapy. Hematopoietic growth factor has been used in patients with resistant myelosuppression. Guidelines for dose modifications are summarized in Table 1.

[See table 1 at top of next page]

Non-hematological adverse reactions

If a severe non-hematological adverse reaction develops with SPRYCEL use, treatment must be withheld until the event has resolved or improved. Thereafter, treatment can be resumed as appropriate at a reduced dose depending on the initial severity of the event.

3 DOSAGE FORMS AND STRENGTHS

SPRYCEL (dasatinib) Tablets are available as 20-mg, 50-mg, 70-mg, 80-mg, 100-mg, and 140-mg white to off-white, biconvex, film-coated tablets. *[See How Supplied (16.1).]*

4 CONTRAINDICATIONS

None.

5 WARNINGS AND PRECAUTIONS

5.1 Myelosuppression

Treatment with SPRYCEL is associated with severe (NCI CTC Grade 3 or 4) thrombocytopenia, neutropenia, and anemia. Their occurrence is more frequent in patients with advanced phase CML or Ph+ ALL than in chronic phase CML. In a dose-optimization trial in patients with resistance or intolerance to prior imatinib therapy and chronic phase CML, Grade 3 or 4 myelosuppression was reported less frequently in patients treated with 100 mg once daily than in patients treated with other dosing regimens.

Table 1: Dose Adjustments for Neutropenia and Thrombocytopenia

Chronic Phase CML (starting dose 100 mg once daily)	ANC* <0.5 × 10^9/L or Platelets <50 × 10^9/L	1. Stop SPRYCEL until ANC ≥1.0 × 10^9/L and platelets ≥50 × 10^9/L. 2. Resume treatment with SPRYCEL at the original starting dose if recovery occurs in ≤7 days. 3. If platelets <25 × 10^9/L or recurrence of ANC <0.5 × 10^9/L for >7 days, repeat Step 1 and resume SPRYCEL at a reduced dose of 80 mg once daily for second episode. For third episode, further reduce dose to 50 mg once daily (for newly diagnosed patients) or discontinue SPRYCEL (for patients resistant or intolerant to prior therapy including imatinib).
Accelerated Phase CML, Blast Phase CML and Ph+ ALL (starting dose 140 mg once daily)	ANC* <0.5 × 10^9/L or Platelets <10 × 10^9/L	1. Check if cytopenia is related to leukemia (marrow aspirate or biopsy). 2. If cytopenia is unrelated to leukemia, stop SPRYCEL until ANC ≥1.0 × 10^9/L and platelets ≥20 × 10^9/L and resume at the original starting dose. 3. If recurrence of cytopenia, repeat Step 1 and resume SPRYCEL at a reduced dose of 100 mg once daily (second episode) or 80 mg once daily (third episode). 4. If cytopenia is related to leukemia, consider dose escalation to 180 mg once daily.

* ANC: absolute neutrophil count

Table 2: Adverse Reactions Reported in ≥10% of Patients with Newly Diagnosed Chronic Phase CML (minimum of 36 months follow up)

	All Grades		Grade 3/4	
	SPRYCEL (n=258)	Imatinib (n=258)	SPRYCEL (n=258)	Imatinib (n=258)
Preferred Term	Percent (%) of Patients			
Fluid retention	31	44	3	1
Pleural effusion	19	<1	2	0
Superficial localized edema	13	37	0	<1
Generalized edema	3	7	0	0
Congestive heart failure/ cardiac dysfunction[a]	2	1	<1	<1
Pericardial effusion	3	1	1	0
Pulmonary hypertension	2	0	<1	0
Pulmonary edema	1	0	0	0
Diarrhea	21	22	1	1
Headache	13	11	0	0
Musculoskeletal pain	13	17	0	<1
Rash[b]	13	18	0	2
Nausea	10	24	0	0
Fatigue	9	11	<1	0
Myalgia	6	12	0	0
Hemorrhage[c]	7	7	1	1
Gastrointestinal bleeding	2	1	1	0
Other bleeding[d]	6	5	0	1
CNS bleeding	0	<1	0	<1
Vomiting	5	11	0	0
Muscle spasms	5	21	0	<1

[a] Includes cardiac failure acute, cardiac failure congestive, cardiomyopathy, diastolic dysfunction, ejection fraction decreased, and left ventricular dysfunction.
[b] Includes erythema, erythema multiforme, rash, rash generalized, rash macular, rash papular, rash pustular, skin exfoliation, and rash vesicular.
[c] Adverse reaction of special interest with <10% frequency.
[d] Includes conjunctival hemorrhage, ear hemorrhage, ecchymosis, epistaxis, eye hemorrhage, gingival bleeding, hematoma, hematuria, hemoptysis, intra-abdominal hematoma, petechiae, scleral hemorrhage, uterine hemorrhage, and vaginal hemorrhage.

Perform complete blood counts weekly for the first 2 months and then monthly thereafter, or as clinically indicated. Myelosuppression was generally reversible and usually managed by withholding SPRYCEL (dasatinib) temporarily or dose reduction *[see Dosage and Administration (2.3)* and *Adverse Reactions (6.1)]*.

5.2 Bleeding Related Events

In addition to causing thrombocytopenia in human subjects, dasatinib caused platelet dysfunction *in vitro*. In all clinical studies, severe central nervous system (CNS) hemorrhages, including fatalities, occurred in 1% of patients receiving SPRYCEL. Severe gastrointestinal hemorrhage, including fatalities, occurred in 4% of patients and generally required treatment interruptions and transfusions. Other cases of severe hemorrhage occurred in 2% of patients. Most bleeding events were associated with severe thrombocytopenia.

Patients were excluded from participation in initial SPRYCEL clinical studies if they took medications that inhibit platelet function or anticoagulants. In subsequent trials, the use of anticoagulants, aspirin, and non-steroidal anti-inflammatory drugs (NSAIDs) was allowed concurrently with SPRYCEL if the platelet count was >50,000–75,000 per microliter. Exercise caution if patients are required to take medications that inhibit platelet function or anticoagulants.

5.3 Fluid Retention

SPRYCEL (dasatinib) is associated with fluid retention. In clinical trials, severe fluid retention was reported in up to 10% of patients. Severe ascites, pulmonary edema, and generalized edema were each reported in ≤1% of patients. Patients who develop symptoms suggestive of pleural effusion, such as dyspnea or dry cough, should be evaluated by chest X-ray. Severe pleural effusion may require thoracentesis and oxygen therapy. Fluid retention events were typically managed by supportive care measures that include diuretics or short courses of steroids. In dose-optimization studies, fluid retention events were reported less frequently with once daily dosing than with other dosing regimens.

5.4 QT Prolongation

In vitro data suggest that dasatinib has the potential to prolong cardiac ventricular repolarization (QT interval). Of the 2440 patients treated with SPRYCEL in clinical studies, 16 patients (1%) had QTc prolongation reported as an adverse reaction. Twenty-two patients (1%) experienced a QTcF >500 ms. In 865 patients with leukemia treated with SPRYCEL (dasatinib) in five Phase 2 single-arm studies, the maximum mean changes in QTcF (90% upper bound CI) from baseline ranged from 7.0 ms to 13.4 ms.

Administer SPRYCEL with caution to patients who have or may develop prolongation of QTc. These include patients with hypokalemia or hypomagnesemia, patients with congenital long QT syndrome, patients taking anti-arrhythmic medicines or other medicinal products that lead to QT prolongation, and cumulative high-dose anthracycline therapy. Correct hypokalemia or hypomagnesemia prior to SPRYCEL administration.

5.5 Congestive Heart Failure, Left Ventricular Dysfunction, and Myocardial Infarction

Cardiac adverse reactions were reported in 7% of 258 patients taking SPRYCEL, including, 1.6% of patients with cardiomyopathy, heart failure congestive, diastolic dysfunction, fatal myocardial infarction, and left ventricular dysfunction. Monitor patients for signs or symptoms consistent with cardiac dysfunction and treat appropriately.

5.6 Pulmonary Arterial Hypertension

SPRYCEL may increase the risk of developing pulmonary arterial hypertension (PAH) which may occur any time after initiation, including after more than one year of treatment. Manifestations include dyspnea, fatigue, hypoxia, and fluid retention. PAH may be reversible on discontinuation of SPRYCEL. Evaluate patients for signs and symptoms of underlying cardiopulmonary disease prior to initiating SPRYCEL and during treatment. If PAH is confirmed, SPRYCEL should be permanently discontinued.

5.7 Use in Pregnancy

SPRYCEL may cause fetal harm when administered to a pregnant woman. In nonclinical studies, at plasma concentrations below those observed in humans receiving therapeutic doses of dasatinib, embryo-fetal toxicities, including skeletal malformations, were observed in rats and rabbits. There are no adequate and well-controlled studies of SPRYCEL in pregnant women. Women of childbearing potential should be advised to avoid becoming pregnant while receiving treatment with SPRYCEL *[see Use in Specific Populations (8.1)]*.

6 ADVERSE REACTIONS

The following adverse reactions are discussed in greater detail in other sections of the labeling:

- Myelosuppression *[see Dosage and Administration (2.3)* and *Warnings and Precautions (5.1)]*.
- Bleeding related events *[see Warnings and Precautions (5.2)]*.
- Fluid retention *[see Warnings and Precautions (5.3)]*.
- QT prolongation *[see Warnings and Precautions (5.4)]*.
- Congestive heart failure, left ventricular dysfunction, and myocardial infarction *[see Warnings and Precautions (5.5)]*.
- Pulmonary Arterial Hypertension *[see Warnings and Precautions (5.6)]*.

Because clinical trials are conducted under widely varying conditions, adverse reaction rates observed in the clinical trials of a drug cannot be directly compared to rates in the clinical trials of another drug and may not reflect the rates observed in practice.

The data described below reflect exposure to SPRYCEL in clinical studies including 258 patients with newly diagnosed chronic phase CML and in 2182 patients with imatinib resistant or intolerant CML or Ph+ ALL.

In the newly diagnosed chronic phase CML trial with a minimum of 36 months follow up and median duration of therapy of 37 months, the median average daily dose was 99 mg. In the imatinib resistant or intolerant CML or Ph+ ALL clinical trials, 1520 patients had a minimum of 2 years follow up and 662 patients with chronic phase CML had a minimum of 60 months follow up (starting dosage 100 mg once daily, 140 mg once daily, 50 mg twice daily, or 70 mg twice daily). Among patients with chronic phase CML and resistance or intolerance to prior imatinib therapy, the median duration of treatment with SPRYCEL 100 mg once daily was 37 months (range 1–65 months). The median duration of treatment with SPRYCEL 140 mg once daily was 15 months (range 0.03–36 months) for accelerated phase CML, 3 months (range 0.03–29 months) for myeloid blast phase CML, and 3 months (range 0.1–10 months) for lymphoid blast CML.

The majority of SPRYCEL-treated patients experienced adverse reactions at some time. In the newly diagnosed chronic phase CML trial, drug was discontinued for adverse reactions in 6% of SPRYCEL-treated patients with a minimum of 12 months follow up. After a minimum of 36 month follow up, the cumulative discontinuation rate was 9%. Among patients with resistance or intolerance to prior imatinib therapy, the rates of discontinuation for adverse reactions at 2 years were 15% in chronic phase CML for all dosages, 16% in accelerated phase CML, 15% in myeloid blast phase CML, 8% in lymphoid blast phase CML, and 8% in Ph+ ALL. In a dose-optimization trial in patients with resistance or intolerance to prior imatinib therapy and chronic phase CML with a minimum of 60 months follow up, the rate of discontinuation for adverse reactions was 18% in patients treated with 100 mg once daily.

The most frequently reported adverse reactions reported in ≥10% of patients in newly diagnosed chronic phase CML included myelosuppression, fluid retention events (pleural effusion, superficial localized edema, generalized edema), diarrhea, headache, musculoskeletal pain, rash, and nausea. Pleural effusions were reported in 50 patients (see Table 2).

The most frequently reported adverse reactions reported in ≥20% of patients with resistance or intolerance to prior imatinib therapy included myelosuppression, fluid retention events, diarrhea, headache, dyspnea, skin rash, fatigue, nausea, and hemorrhage.

The most frequently reported serious adverse reactions in patients with newly diagnosed chronic phase CML included pleural effusion (4%), hemorrhage (2%), congestive heart failure (1%), pulmonary hypertension (1%), and pyrexia (1%). The most frequently reported serious adverse reactions in patients with resistance or intolerance to prior imatinib therapy included pleural effusion (11%), gastrointestinal bleeding (4%), febrile neutropenia (4%), dyspnea (3%), pneumonia (3%), pyrexia (3%), diarrhea (3%), infection (2%), congestive heart failure/cardiac dysfunction (2%), pericardial effusion (1%), and CNS hemorrhage (1%).

6.1 Chronic Myeloid Leukemia (CML)

Adverse reactions (excluding laboratory abnormalities) that were reported in at least 10% of patients are shown in Table 2 for newly diagnosed patients with chronic phase CML and Tables 3 and 4 for CML patients with resistance or intolerance to prior imatinib therapy.

[See table 2 at top of previous page]

The cumulative rates of the majority of adverse reactions (all grades) in newly diagnosed patients with chronic phase CML were similar after 12 and 36 months minimum follow up including congestive heart failure/cardiac dysfunction (2% vs 2%), pericardial effusion (2% vs 3%), pulmonary edema (<1% vs 1%), gastrointestinal bleeding (2% vs 2%), diarrhea (18% vs 21%), and generalized edema (3% vs 3%). Cumulative adverse reaction rates (all grades) that increased between 12 months and 36 months minimum follow up included overall fluid retention (23% vs 31%), pleural effusion (12% vs 19%), and superficial edema (10% vs 13%). A total of 9 patients (3.5%) discontinued due to pleural effusion in the trial.

At 36 months, there were 17 deaths in the dasatinib-treated patients (6.6%) and 20 deaths in the imatinib-treated patients (7.7%); 1 in each group was judged by the investigator as related to study therapy.

Table 3: Adverse Reactions Reported in ≥10% of Patients with Chronic Phase CML Resistant or Intolerant to Prior Imatinib Therapy (minimum of 60 months follow up)

	100 mg Once Daily	
	Chronic (n=165)	
	All Grades	Grade 3/4
Preferred Term	Percent (%) of Patients	
Fluid retention	42	5
Superficial localized edema	21	0
Pleural effusion	24	4
Generalized edema	4	0
Pericardial effusion	2	1
Congestive heart failure/ cardiac dysfunction[a]	0	0
Pulmonary edema	0	0
Headache	33	1
Diarrhea	28	2
Fatigue	26	4
Dyspnea	24	2
Musculoskeletal pain	22	2
Nausea	18	1
Skin rash[b]	18	2
Myalgia	13	0
Arthralgia	12	1
Infection (including bacterial, viral, fungal, and non-specified)	13	1
Abdominal pain	12	1
Hemorrhage	11	1
Gastrointestinal bleeding	2	1
CNS bleeding	0	0
Pruritus	10	1
Pain	10	1

[a] Includes ventricular dysfunction, cardiac failure, cardiac failure congestive, cardiomyopathy, congestive cardiomyopathy, diastolic dysfunction, ejection fraction decreased, and ventricular failure.

[b] Includes drug eruption, erythema, erythema multiforme, erythrosis, exfoliative rash, generalized erythema, genital rash, heat rash, milia, rash, rash erythematous, rash follicular, rash generalized, rash macular, rash maculopapular, rash papular, rash pruritic, rash pustular, skin exfoliation, skin irritation, urticaria vesiculosa, and rash vesicular.

Table 4: Adverse Reactions Reported in ≥10% of Patients with Advanced Phase CML Resistant or Intolerant to Prior Imatinib Therapy

	140 mg Once Daily					
	Accelerated (n=157)		Myeloid Blast (n=74)		Lymphoid Blast (n=33)	
	All Grades	Grade 3/4	All Grades	Grade 3/4	All Grades	Grade 3/4
Preferred Term	Percent (%) of Patients					
Fluid retention	35	8	34	7	21	6
Superficial localized edema	18	1	14	0	3	0
Pleural effusion	21	7	20	7	21	6
Generalized edema	1	0	3	0	0	0
Pericardial effusion	3	1	0	0	0	0
Congestive heart failure/cardiac dysfunction[a]	0	0	4	0	0	0
Pulmonary edema	1	0	4	3	0	0
Headache	27	1	18	1	15	3
Diarrhea	31	3	20	5	18	0
Fatigue	19	2	20	1	9	3
Dyspnea	20	3	15	3	3	3
Musculoskeletal pain	11	0	8	1	0	0
Nausea	19	1	23	1	21	3
Skin rash[b]	15	0	16	1	21	0
Arthralgia	10	0	5	1	0	0
Infection (including bacterial, viral, fungal, and non-specified)	10	6	14	7	9	0
Hemorrhage	26	8	19	9	24	9
Gastrointestinal bleeding	8	6	9	7	9	3
CNS bleeding	1	1	0	0	3	3
Vomiting	11	1	12	0	15	0
Pyrexia	11	2	18	3	6	0
Febrile neutropenia	4	4	12	12	12	12

[a] Includes ventricular dysfunction, cardiac failure, cardiac failure congestive, cardiomyopathy, congestive cardiomyopathy, diastolic dysfunction, ejection fraction decreased, and ventricular failure.

[b] Includes drug eruption, erythema, erythema multiforme, erythrosis, exfoliative rash, generalized erythema, genital rash, heat rash, milia, rash, rash erythematous, rash follicular, rash generalized, rash macular, rash maculopapular, rash papular, rash pruritic, rash pustular, skin exfoliation, skin irritation, urticaria vesiculosa, and rash vesicular.

With a minimum follow up of 60 months (see Table 3), the cumulative rates of the majority of adverse reactions (all grades) in patients with chronic phase CML treated with a starting dose of 100 mg once daily were identical with a minimum follow up of 24 and 60 months including congestive heart failure/cardiac dysfunction, pericardial effusion, pulmonary edema, and gastrointestinal bleeding or similar for diarrhea (27% vs 28%), and generalized edema (3% vs 4%). Cumulative adverse reaction rates (all grades) that increased between 24 months and 60 months minimum follow up included: overall fluid retention (34% vs 42%), pleural effusion (18% vs 24%), and superficial edema (18% vs 21%). The cumulative rate of Grade 3 or 4 pleural effusion was 2% vs 4%, respectively.

[See table 4 above]

Laboratory Abnormalities

Myelosuppression was commonly reported in all patient populations. The frequency of Grade 3 or 4 neutropenia, thrombocytopenia, and anemia was higher in patients with advanced phase CML than in chronic phase CML (Tables 5 and 6). Myelosuppression was reported in patients with normal baseline laboratory values as well as in patients with pre-existing laboratory abnormalities.

In patients who experienced severe myelosuppression, recovery generally occurred following dose interruption or reduction; permanent discontinuation of treatment occurred in 2% of patients with newly diagnosed chronic phase CML and 5% of patients with resistance or intolerance to prior imatinib therapy *[see Warnings and Precautions (5.1)]*.

Grade 3 or 4 elevations of transaminase or bilirubin and Grade 3 or 4 hypocalcemia, hypokalemia, and hypophosphatemia were reported in patients with all phases of CML but were reported with an increased frequency in patients with myeloid or lymphoid blast phase CML. Elevations in transaminase or bilirubin were usually managed with dose reduction or interruption. Patients developing Grade 3 or 4 hypocalcemia during the course of SPRYCEL therapy often had recovery with oral calcium supplementation.

Laboratory abnormalities reported in patients with newly diagnosed chronic phase CML are shown in Table 5. There were no discontinuations of SPRYCEL therapy in this patient population due to biochemical laboratory parameters.

Table 5: CTC Grade 3/4 Laboratory Abnormalities in Patients with Newly Diagnosed Chronic Phase CML (minimum of 36 months follow up)

	SPRYCEL (n=258)	Imatinib (n=258)
	Percent (%) of Patients	
Hematology Parameters		
Neutropenia	24	21
Thrombocytopenia	19	11
Anemia	12	9
Biochemistry Parameters		
Hypophosphatemia	7	28
Hypokalemia	0	2
Hypocalcemia	3	2
Elevated SGPT (ALT)	<1	2
Elevated SGOT (AST)	<1	1
Elevated Bilirubin	1	0
Elevated Creatinine	1	1

CTC grades: neutropenia (Grade 3 ≥0.5–<1.0 × 10^9/L, Grade 4 <0.5 × 10^9/L); thrombocytopenia (Grade 3 ≥25–<50 × 10^9/L, Grade 4 <25 × 10^9/L); anemia (hemoglobin Grade 3 ≥65–<80 g/L, Grade 4 <65 g/L); elevated creatinine (Grade 3 >3–6 × upper limit of normal range (ULN), Grade 4 >6 × ULN); elevated bilirubin (Grade 3 >3–10 × ULN, Grade 4 >10 × ULN); elevated SGOT or SGPT (Grade 3 >5–20 × ULN, Grade 4 >20 × ULN); hypocalcemia (Grade 3 <7.0–6.0 mg/dL, Grade 4 <6.0 mg/dL); hypophosphatemia (Grade 3 <2.0–1.0 mg/dL, Grade 4 <1.0 mg/dL); hypokalemia (Grade 3 <3.0–2.5 mmol/L, Grade 4 <2.5 mmol/L).

Laboratory abnormalities reported in patients with CML resistant or intolerant to imatinib who received the recommended starting doses of SPRYCEL are shown by disease phase in Table 6.

[See table 6 at top of next page]

Among chronic phase CML patients with resistance or intolerance to prior imatinib therapy, cumulative Grade 3 or 4 cytopenias were similar at 2 and 5 years including: neutropenia (36% vs 36%), thrombocytopenia (23% vs 24%) and anemia (13% vs 13%).

Table 6: CTC Grade 3/4 Laboratory Abnormalities in Clinical Studies of CML: Resistance or Intolerance to Prior Imatinib Therapy

	Chronic Phase CML	Advanced Phase CML 140 mg Once Daily		
	100 mg Once Daily (n=165)	Accelerated Phase (n=157)	Myeloid Blast Phase (n=74)	Lymphoid Blast Phase (n=33)
	Percent (%) of Patients			
Hematology Parameters*				
Neutropenia	36	58	77	79
Thrombocytopenia	24	63	78	85
Anemia	13	47	74	52
Biochemistry Parameters				
Hypophosphatemia	10	13	12	18
Hypokalemia	2	7	11	15
Hypocalcemia	<1	4	9	12
Elevated SGPT (ALT)	0	2	5	3
Elevated SGOT (AST)	<1	0	4	3
Elevated Bilirubin	<1	1	3	6
Elevated Creatinine	0	2	8	0

CTC grades: neutropenia (Grade 3 ≥0.5–<1.0 × 10^9/L, Grade 4 <0.5 × 10^9/L); thrombocytopenia (Grade 3 ≥25–<50 × 10^9/L, Grade 4 <25 × 10^9/L); anemia (hemoglobin Grade 3 ≥65–<80 g/L, Grade 4 <65 g/L); elevated creatinine (Grade 3 >3–6 × upper limit of normal range (ULN), Grade 4 >6 × ULN); elevated bilirubin (Grade 3 >3–10 × ULN, Grade 4 >10 × ULN); elevated SGOT or SGPT (Grade 3 >5–20 × ULN, Grade 4 >20 × ULN); hypocalcemia (Grade 3 <7.0–6.0 mg/dL, Grade 4 <6.0 mg/dL); hypophosphatemia (Grade 3 <2.0–1.0 mg/dL, Grade 4 <1.0 mg/dL); hypokalemia (Grade 3 <3.0–2.5 mmol/L, Grade 4 <2.5 mmol/L).

* Hematology parameters for 100 mg once-daily dosing in chronic phase CML reflects 60 month minimum follow up.

6.2 Philadelphia Chromosome-Positive Acute Lymphoblastic Leukemia (Ph+ ALL)

A total of 135 patients with Ph+ ALL were treated with SPRYCEL (dasatinib) in clinical studies. The median duration of treatment was 3 months (range 0.03–31 months). The safety profile of patients with Ph+ ALL was similar to those with lymphoid blast phase CML. The most frequently reported adverse reactions included fluid retention events, such as pleural effusion (24%) and superficial edema (19%), and gastrointestinal disorders, such as diarrhea (31%), nausea (24%), and vomiting (16%). Hemorrhage (19%), pyrexia (17%), rash (16%), and dyspnea (16%) were also frequently reported. The most frequently reported serious adverse reactions included pleural effusion (11%), gastrointestinal bleeding (7%), febrile neutropenia (6%), infection (5%), pyrexia (4%), pneumonia (3%), diarrhea (3%), nausea (2%), vomiting (2%), and colitis (2%).

6.3 Additional Data From Clinical Trials

The following adverse reactions were reported in patients in the SPRYCEL clinical studies at a frequency of ≥10%, 1%–<10%, 0.1%–<1%, or <0.1%. These events are included on the basis of clinical relevance.

Gastrointestinal Disorders: *1%–<10%* – mucosal inflammation (including mucositis/stomatitis), dyspepsia, abdominal distension, constipation, gastritis, colitis (including neutropenic colitis), oral soft tissue disorder; *0.1%–<1%* – ascites, dysphagia, anal fissure, upper gastrointestinal ulcer, esophagitis, pancreatitis; *<0.1%* – protein losing gastroenteropathy, ileus.

General Disorders and Administration Site Conditions: *1%–<10%* – asthenia, pain, chest pain, chills; *0.1%–<1%* – malaise, temperature intolerance.

Skin and Subcutaneous Tissue Disorders: *1%–<10%* – pruritus, alopecia, acne, dry skin, hyperhidrosis, urticaria, dermatitis (including eczema); *0.1%–<1%* – pigmentation disorder, skin ulcer, bullous conditions, photosensitivity, nail disorder, acute febrile neutrophilic dermatosis, panniculitis, palmar-plantar erythrodysesthesia syndrome.

Respiratory, Thoracic, and Mediastinal Disorders: *≥10%* - cough; *1%–<10%* – lung infiltration, pneumonitis, pulmonary hypertension; *0.1%–<1%* – asthma, bronchospasm; *<0.1%* – acute respiratory distress syndrome.

Nervous System Disorders: *1%–<10%* – neuropathy (including peripheral neuropathy), dizziness, dysgeusia, somnolence; *0.1%–<1%* – amnesia, tremor, syncope; *<0.1%* – convulsion, cerebrovascular accident, transient ischemic attack, optic neuritis, VIIth nerve paralysis.

Blood and Lymphatic System Disorders: *1%–<10%* – pancytopenia; *<0.1%* – aplasia pure red cell.

Musculoskeletal and Connective Tissue Disorders: *1%–<10%* – muscular weakness, musculoskeletal stiffness, muscle spasm; *0.1%–<1%* – rhabdomyolysis, tendonitis, muscle inflammation.

Investigations: *1%–<10%* – weight increased, weight decreased; *0.1%–<1%* – blood creatine phosphokinase increased.

Infections and Infestations: *1%–<10%* – pneumonia (including bacterial, viral, and fungal), upper respiratory tract infection/inflammation, herpes virus infection, enterocolitis infection, sepsis (including fatal outcomes (0.2%)).

Metabolism and Nutrition Disorders: *1%–<10%* – anorexia, appetite disturbances, hyperuricemia; *0.1%–<1%* – hypoalbuminemia.

Cardiac Disorders: *1%–<10%* – arrhythmia (including tachycardia), palpitations; *0.1%–<1%* – angina pectoris, cardiomegaly, pericarditis, ventricular arrhythmia (including ventricular tachycardia); *<0.1%* – cor pulmonale, myocarditis, acute coronary syndrome.

Eye Disorders: *1%–<10%* – visual disorder (including visual disturbance, vision blurred, and visual acuity reduced), dry eye; *0.1% –<1%* – conjunctivitis; *<0.1%* – visual impairment.

Vascular Disorders: *1%–<10%* – flushing, hypertension; *0.1%–<1%* – hypotension, thrombophlebitis; *<0.1%* – livedo reticularis.

Psychiatric Disorders: *1%–<10%* – insomnia, depression; *0.1%–<1%* – anxiety, affect lability, confusional state, libido decreased.

Reproductive System and Breast Disorders: *0.1%–<1%* – gynecomastia, menstruation irregular.

Injury, Poisoning, and Procedural Complications: *1%–<10%* – contusion.

Ear and Labyrinth Disorders: *1%–<10%* – tinnitus; *0.1%–<1%* – vertigo.

Hepatobiliary Disorders: *0.1%–<1%* – cholestasis, cholecystitis, hepatitis.

Renal and Urinary Disorders: *0.1%–<1%* – urinary frequency, renal failure, proteinuria.

Neoplasms Benign, Malignant, and Unspecified: *0.1%–<1%* – tumor lysis syndrome.

Immune System Disorders: *0.1%–<1%* – hypersensitivity (including erythema nodosum).

6.4 Postmarketing Experience

The following additional adverse reactions have been identified during post approval use of SPRYCEL. Because these reactions are reported voluntarily from a population of uncertain size, it is not always possible to reliably estimate their frequency or establish a causal relationship to drug exposure.

Cardiac disorders: atrial fibrillation/atrial flutter

Vascular disorders: thrombosis/embolism (including pulmonary embolism, deep vein thrombosis)

Respiratory, thoracic, and mediastinal disorders: interstitial lung disease, pulmonary arterial hypertension

7 DRUG INTERACTIONS

7.1 Drugs That May Increase Dasatinib Plasma Concentrations

CYP3A4 Inhibitors: Dasatinib is a CYP3A4 substrate. In a trial of 18 patients with solid tumors, 20-mg SPRYCEL (dasatinib) once daily coadministered with 200 mg of ketoconazole twice daily increased the dasatinib C_{max} and AUC by four- and five-fold, respectively. Concomitant use of SPRYCEL and drugs that inhibit CYP3A4 may increase exposure to dasatinib and should be avoided. In patients receiving treatment with SPRYCEL, close monitoring for toxicity and a SPRYCEL dose reduction should be considered if systemic administration of a potent CYP3A4 inhibitor cannot be avoided *[see Dosage and Administration (2.1)]*.

7.2 Drugs That May Decrease Dasatinib Plasma Concentrations

CYP3A4 Inducers: When a single morning dose of SPRYCEL (dasatinib) was administered following 8 days of continuous evening administration of 600 mg of rifampin, a potent CYP3A4 inducer, the mean C_{max} and AUC of dasatinib were decreased by 81% and 82%, respectively. Alternative agents with less enzyme induction potential should be considered. If SPRYCEL must be administered with a CYP3A4 inducer, a dose increase in SPRYCEL should be considered *[see Dosage and Administration (2.1)]*.

Antacids: Nonclinical data demonstrate that the solubility of dasatinib is pH dependent. In a trial of 24 healthy subjects, administration of 30 mL of aluminum hydroxide/magnesium hydroxide 2 hours prior to a single 50-mg dose of SPRYCEL was associated with no relevant change in dasatinib AUC; however, the dasatinib C_{max} increased 26%. When 30 mL of aluminum hydroxide/magnesium hydroxide was administered to the same subjects concomitantly with a 50-mg dose of SPRYCEL, a 55% reduction in dasatinib AUC and a 58% reduction in C_{max} were observed. Simultaneous administration of SPRYCEL with antacids should be avoided. If antacid therapy is needed, the antacid dose should be administered at least 2 hours prior to or 2 hours after the dose of SPRYCEL.

H_2 Antagonists/Proton Pump Inhibitors: Long-term suppression of gastric acid secretion by H_2 antagonists or proton pump inhibitors (eg, famotidine and omeprazole) is likely to reduce dasatinib exposure. In a trial of 24 healthy subjects, administration of a single 50-mg dose of SPRYCEL 10 hours following famotidine reduced the AUC and C_{max} of dasatinib by 61% and 63%, respectively. In a trial of 14 healthy subjects, administration of a single 100-mg dose of SPRYCEL 22 hours following a 40-mg omeprazole dose at steady state reduced the AUC and C_{max} of dasatinib by 43% and 42%, respectively. The concomitant use of H_2 antagonists or proton pump inhibitors with SPRYCEL is not recommended. The use of antacids (at least 2 hours prior to or 2 hours after the dose of SPRYCEL) should be considered in place of H_2 antagonists or proton pump inhibitors in patients receiving SPRYCEL therapy.

7.3 Drugs That May Have Their Plasma Concentration Altered By Dasatinib

CYP3A4 Substrates: Single-dose data from a trial of 54 healthy subjects indicate that the mean C_{max} and AUC of simvastatin, a CYP3A4 substrate, were increased by 37% and 20%, respectively, when simvastatin was administered in combination with a single 100-mg dose of SPRYCEL. Therefore, CYP3A4 substrates known to have a narrow therapeutic index such as alfentanil, astemizole, terfenadine, cisapride, cyclosporine, fentanyl, pimozide, quinidine, sirolimus, tacrolimus, or ergot alkaloids (ergotamine, dihydroergotamine) should be administered with caution in patients receiving SPRYCEL.

8 USE IN SPECIFIC POPULATIONS

8.1 Pregnancy

Pregnancy Category D

SPRYCEL may cause fetal harm when administered to a pregnant woman. There are no adequate and well-controlled studies of SPRYCEL in pregnant women. Women of childbearing potential should be advised of the potential hazard to the fetus and to avoid becoming pregnant. If SPRYCEL is used during pregnancy, or if the patient becomes pregnant while taking SPRYCEL, the patient should be apprised of the potential hazard to the fetus.

In nonclinical studies, at plasma concentrations below those observed in humans receiving therapeutic doses of dasatinib, embryo-fetal toxicities were observed in rats and rabbits. Fetal death was observed in rats. In both rats and rabbits, the lowest doses of dasatinib tested (rat: 2.5 mg/kg/day [15 mg/m^2/day] and rabbit: 0.5 mg/kg/day [6 mg/m^2/day]) resulted in embryo-fetal toxicities. These doses produced maternal AUCs of 105 ng•hr/mL (0.3-fold the human AUC in females at a dose of 70 mg twice daily) and 44 ng•hr/mL (0.1-fold the human AUC) in rats and rabbits, respectively. Embryo-fetal toxicities included skeletal malformations at multiple sites (scapula, humerus, femur, radius, ribs, and clavicle), reduced ossification (sternum; thoracic, lumbar, and sacral vertebrae; forepaw phalanges; pelvis; and hyoid body), edema, and microhepatia.

8.3 Nursing Mothers

It is unknown whether SPRYCEL is excreted in human milk. Because many drugs are excreted in human milk and because of the potential for serious adverse reactions in nursing infants from SPRYCEL, a decision should be made whether to discontinue nursing or to discontinue the drug, taking into account the importance of the drug to the mother.

8.4 Pediatric Use

The safety and efficacy of SPRYCEL in patients less than 18 years of age have not been established.

8.5 Geriatric Use

In the newly diagnosed chronic phase CML trial, 25 patients (10%) were 65 years of age and over and 7 patients

(3%) were 75 years of age and over. Of the 2182 patients in clinical studies of SPRYCEL (dasatinib) with resistance or intolerance to imatinib therapy, 547 (25%) were 65 years of age and over and 105 (5%) were 75 years of age and over. No differences in efficacy were observed between older and younger patients. Compared to patients under age 65 years, patients aged 65 years and older are more likely to experience toxicity.

8.6 Hepatic Impairment

The effect of hepatic impairment on the pharmacokinetics of dasatinib was evaluated in healthy volunteers with normal liver function and patients with moderate (Child-Pugh class B) and severe (Child-Pugh class C) hepatic impairment. Compared to the healthy volunteers with normal hepatic function, the dose normalized pharmacokinetic parameters were decreased in the patients with hepatic impairment.

No dosage adjustment is necessary in patients with hepatic impairment *[see Clinical Pharmacology (12.3)]*. Caution is recommended when administering SPRYCEL to patients with hepatic impairment.

8.7 Renal Impairment

There are currently no clinical studies with SPRYCEL in patients with impaired renal function. Less than 4% of dasatinib and its metabolites are excreted via the kidney.

10 OVERDOSAGE

Experience with overdose of SPRYCEL in clinical studies is limited to isolated cases. The highest overdosage of 280 mg per day for 1 week was reported in two patients and both developed severe myelosuppression and bleeding. Since SPRYCEL is associated with severe myelosuppression, *[see Warnings and Precautions (5.1)* and *Adverse Reactions (6.1)]*, patients who ingested more than the recommended dosage should be closely monitored for myelosuppression and given appropriate supportive treatment.

Acute overdose in animals was associated with cardiotoxicity. Evidence of cardiotoxicity included ventricular necrosis and valvular/ventricular/atrial hemorrhage at single doses ≥100 mg/kg (600 mg/m^2) in rodents. There was a tendency for increased systolic and diastolic blood pressure in monkeys at single doses ≥10 mg/kg (120 mg/m^2).

11 DESCRIPTION

SPRYCEL (dasatinib) is a kinase inhibitor. The chemical name for dasatinib is N-(2-chloro-6-methylphenyl)-2-[[6-[4-(2-hydroxyethyl)-1-piperazinyl]-2-methyl-4-pyrimidinyl]-amino]-5-thiazolecarboxamide, monohydrate. The molecular formula is $C_{22}H_{26}ClN_7O_2S \bullet H_2O$, which corresponds to a formula weight of 506.02 (monohydrate). The anhydrous free base has a molecular weight of 488.01. Dasatinib has the following chemical structure:

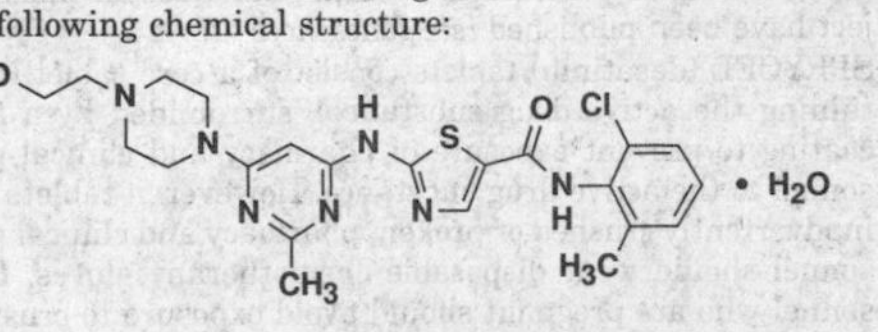

Dasatinib is a white to off-white powder. The drug substance is insoluble in water and slightly soluble in ethanol and methanol. SPRYCEL tablets are white to off-white, biconvex, film-coated tablets containing dasatinib, with the following inactive ingredients: lactose monohydrate, microcrystalline cellulose, croscarmellose sodium, hydroxypropyl cellulose, and magnesium stearate. The tablet coating consists of hypromellose, titanium dioxide, and polyethylene glycol.

12 CLINICAL PHARMACOLOGY

12.1 Mechanism of Action

Dasatinib, at nanomolar concentrations, inhibits the following kinases: BCR-ABL, SRC family (SRC, LCK, YES, FYN), c-KIT, EPHA2, and PDGFRβ. Based on modeling studies, dasatinib is predicted to bind to multiple conformations of the ABL kinase.

In vitro, dasatinib was active in leukemic cell lines representing variants of imatinib mesylate sensitive and resistant disease. Dasatinib inhibited the growth of chronic myeloid leukemia (CML) and acute lymphoblastic leukemia (ALL) cell lines overexpressing BCR-ABL. Under the conditions of the assays, dasatinib was able to overcome imatinib resistance resulting from BCR-ABL kinase domain mutations, activation of alternate signaling pathways involving the SRC family kinases (LYN, HCK), and multi-drug resistance gene overexpression.

12.3 Pharmacokinetics

Absorption

Maximum plasma concentrations (C_{max}) of dasatinib are observed between 0.5 and 6 hours (T_{max}) following oral administration. Dasatinib exhibits dose proportional increases in AUC and linear elimination characteristics over the dose range of 15 mg to 240 mg/day. The overall mean terminal half-life of dasatinib is 3–5 hours.

Data from a trial of 54 healthy subjects administered a single, 100-mg dose of dasatinib 30 minutes following consumption of a high-fat meal resulted in a 14% increase in the mean AUC of dasatinib. The observed food effects were not clinically relevant.

Distribution

In patients, dasatinib has an apparent volume of distribution of 2505 L, suggesting that the drug is extensively distributed in the extravascular space. Binding of dasatinib and its active metabolite to human plasma proteins *in vitro* was approximately 96% and 93%, respectively, with no concentration dependence over the range of 100–500 ng/mL.

Metabolism

Dasatinib is extensively metabolized in humans, primarily by the cytochrome P450 enzyme 3A4. CYP3A4 was the primary enzyme responsible for the formation of the active metabolite. Flavin-containing monooxygenase 3 (FMO-3) and uridine diphosphate-glucuronosyltransferase (UGT) enzymes are also involved in the formation of dasatinib metabolites.

The exposure of the active metabolite, which is equipotent to dasatinib, represents approximately 5% of the dasatinib AUC. This indicates that the active metabolite of dasatinib is unlikely to play a major role in the observed pharmacology of the drug. Dasatinib also had several other inactive oxidative metabolites.

Dasatinib is a weak time-dependent inhibitor of CYP3A4. At clinically relevant concentrations, dasatinib does not inhibit CYP1A2, 2A6, 2B6, 2C8, 2C9, 2C19, 2D6, or 2E1. Dasatinib is not an inducer of human CYP enzymes.

Elimination

Elimination is primarily via the feces. Following a single oral dose of [^{14}C]-labeled dasatinib, approximately 4% and 85% of the administered radioactivity was recovered in the urine and feces, respectively, within 10 days. Unchanged dasatinib accounted for 0.1% and 19% of the administered dose in urine and feces, respectively, with the remainder of the dose being metabolites.

Effects of Age and Gender

Pharmacokinetic analyses of demographic data indicate that there are no clinically relevant effects of age and gender on the pharmacokinetics of dasatinib.

Hepatic Impairment

Dasatinib doses of 50 mg and 20 mg were evaluated in eight patients with moderate (Child-Pugh class B) and seven patients with severe (Child-Pugh class C) hepatic impairment, respectively. Matched controls with normal hepatic function (n=15) were also evaluated and received a dasatinib dose of 70 mg. Compared to subjects with normal liver function, patients with moderate hepatic impairment had decreases in dose normalized C_{max} and AUC by 47% and 8%, respectively. Patients with severe hepatic impairment had dose normalized C_{max} decreased by 43% and AUC decreased by 28% compared to the normal controls.

These differences in C_{max} and AUC are not clinically relevant. Dose adjustment is not necessary in patients with hepatic impairment.

13 NONCLINICAL TOXICOLOGY

13.1 Carcinogenesis, Mutagenesis, Impairment of Fertility

In a two-year carcinogenicity study, rats were administered oral doses of dasatinib at 0.3, 1, and 3 mg/kg/day. The highest dose resulted in a plasma drug exposure (AUC) level equivalent to human exposure at 70 mg twice daily. Dasatinib induced a statistically significant increase in the combined incidence of squamous cell carcinomas and papillomas in the uterus and cervix of high-dose females and prostate adenoma in low-dose males.

Dasatinib was clastogenic when tested *in vitro* in Chinese hamster ovary cells, with and without metabolic activation. Dasatinib was not mutagenic when tested in an *in vitro* bacterial cell assay (Ames test) and was not genotoxic in an *in vivo* rat micronucleus study.

The effects of dasatinib on male and female fertility have not been studied. However, results of repeat-dose toxicity studies in multiple species indicate the potential for dasatinib to impair reproductive function and fertility. Effects evident in male animals included reduced size and secretion of seminal vesicles, and immature prostate, seminal vesicle, and testis. The administration of dasatinib resulted in uterine inflammation and mineralization in monkeys, and cystic ovaries and ovarian hypertrophy in rodents.

14 CLINICAL STUDIES

14.1 Newly Diagnosed Chronic Phase CML

An open-label, multicenter, international, randomized trial was conducted in adult patients with newly diagnosed chronic phase CML. A total of 519 patients were randomized to receive either SPRYCEL 100 mg once daily or imatinib 400 mg once daily. Patients with a history of cardiac disease were included in this trial except those which had a myocardial infarction within 6 months, congestive heart failure within 3 months, significant arrhythmias, or QTc prolongation. The primary endpoint was the rate of confirmed complete cytogenetic response (CCyR) within 12 months. Confirmed CCyR was defined as a CCyR noted on two consecutive occasions (at least 28 days apart).

Median age was 46 years in the SPRYCEL (dasatinib) group and 49 years in the imatinib groups, with 10% and 11% of patients ≥65 years of age. There were slightly more male than female patients in both groups (59% vs 41%). Fifty-three percent of all patients were Caucasian, and 39% were Asian. At baseline, the distribution of Hasford Scores was similar in the SPRYCEL and imatinib treatment groups (low risk: 33% and 34%; intermediate risk: 48% and 47%; high risk: 19% and 19%, respectively). With a minimum of 12 months follow up, 85% of patients randomized to SPRYCEL and 81% of patients randomized to imatinib were still on study.

With a minimum of 24 months follow up, 77% of patients randomized to SPRYCEL and 75% of patients randomized to imatinib were still on study and with a minimum of 36 months follow up, 71% and 69% of patients, respectively, were still on study.

Efficacy results are summarized in Table 7.

[See table 7 above]

Table 7: Efficacy Results in Newly Diagnosed Patients with Chronic Phase CML

	SPRYCEL (n=259)	Imatinib (n=260)	p-value
	Response rate (95% CI)		
Confirmed CCyR[a]			
within 12 months	76.8% (71.2–81.8)	66.2% (60.1–71.9)	p=0.007*
within 24 months	80.3%	74.2%	–**
within 36 months	82.6%	77.3%	–**
Major Molecular Response[b]			
12 months	52.1% (45.9–58.3)	33.8% (28.1–39.9)	p=<0.0001*
24 months	64.5% (58.3–70.3)	50% (43.8–56.2)	–**
36 months	69.1% (63.1–74.7)	56.2% (49.9–62.3)	–**

[a] Confirmed CCyR is defined as a CCyR noted on two consecutive occasions at least 28 days apart.

[b] Major molecular response (at any time) was defined as BCR-ABL ratios ≤0.1% by RQ-PCR in peripheral blood samples standardized on the International scale. These are cumulative rates representing minimum follow up for the time frame specified.

* Adjusted for Hasford Score and indicated statistical significance at a pre-defined nominal level of significance.

** Formal statistical comparison of cCCyR and MMR rates was only performed at the time of the primary endpoint (cCCyR within 12 months).

CI = confidence interval.

After 36 months follow up, median time to confirmed CCyR was 3.1 months in 214 SPRYCEL responders and 5.8 months in 201 imatinib responders. Median time to MMR after 36 months follow up was 8.9 months in 179 SPRYCEL responders and 13.4 months in 146 imatinib responders.

At 36 months, 8 patients (3%) on the dasatinib arm progressed to either accelerated phase or blast crisis while 13 patients (5%) on the imatinib arm progressed to either accelerated phase or blast crisis.

The rate of MMR at any time in each risk group determined by Hasford score was higher in the SPRYCEL group compared with the imatinib group (low risk: 81% and 64%; intermediate risk: 64% and 56%; high risk: 61% and 42%, respectively).

BCR-ABL sequencing was performed on blood samples from patients in the newly diagnosed trial who discontinued dasatinib or imatinib therapy. Among dasatinib-treated patients the mutations detected were T315I, F317I/L, and V299L.

Table 9: Efficacy of SPRYCEL in Imatinib Resistant or Intolerant Advanced Phase CML and Ph+ ALL

	140 mg Once Daily			
	Accelerated (n=158)	**Myeloid Blast (n=75)**	**Lymphoid Blast (n=33)**	**Ph+ ALL (n=40)**
MaHR[a]	66%	28%	42%	38%
(95% CI)	(59–74)	(18–40)	(26–61)	(23–54)
CHR[a]	47%	17%	21%	33%
(95% CI)	(40–56)	(10–28)	(9–39)	(19–49)
NEL[a]	19%	11%	21%	5%
(95% CI)	(13–26)	(5–20)	(9–39)	(1–17)
MCyR[b]	39%	28%	52%	70%
(95% CI)	(31–47)	(18–40)	(34–69)	(54–83)
CCyR	32%	17%	39%	50%
(95% CI)	(25–40)	(10–28)	(23–58)	(34–66)

[a] Hematologic response criteria (all responses confirmed after 4 weeks): Major hematologic response: (MaHR) = complete hematologic response (CHR) + no evidence of leukemia (NEL).
CHR: WBC ≤ institutional ULN, ANC ≥1000/mm^3, platelets ≥100,000/mm^3, no blasts or promyelocytes in peripheral blood, bone marrow blasts ≤5%, <5% myelocytes plus metamyelocytes in peripheral blood, basophils in peripheral blood <20%, and no extramedullary involvement.
NEL: same criteria as for CHR but ANC ≥500/mm^3 and <1000/mm^3, or platelets ≥20,000/mm^3 and ≤100,000/mm^3.
[b] MCyR combines both complete (0% Ph+ metaphases) and partial (>0%–35%) responses.
CI = confidence interval ULN = upper limit of normal range.

Dasatinib does not appear to be active against the T315I mutation, based on *in vitro* data.

14.2 Imatinib Resistant or Intolerant CML or Ph+ ALL

The efficacy and safety of SPRYCEL (dasatinib) were investigated in adult patients with CML or Ph+ ALL whose disease was resistant to or who were intolerant to imatinib: 1158 patients had chronic phase CML, 858 patients had accelerated phase, myeloid blast phase, or lymphoid blast phase CML, and 130 patients had Ph+ ALL. In a clinical trial in chronic phase CML, resistance to imatinib was defined as failure to achieve a complete hematologic response (CHR; after 3 months), major cytogenetic response (MCyR; after 6 months), or complete cytogenetic response (CCyR; after 12 months); or loss of a previous molecular response (with concurrent ≥10% increase in Ph+ metaphases), cytogenetic response, or hematologic response. Imatinib intolerance was defined as inability to tolerate 400 mg or more of imatinib per day or discontinuation of imatinib because of toxicity.

Results described below are based on a minimum of 2 years follow up after the start of SPRYCEL therapy in patients with a median time from initial diagnosis of approximately 5 years. Across all studies, 48% of patients were women, 81% were white, 15% were black or Asian, 25% were 65 years of age or older, and 5% were 75 years of age or older. Most patients had long disease histories with extensive prior treatment, including imatinib, cytotoxic chemotherapy, interferon, and stem cell transplant. Overall, 80% of patients had imatinib-resistant disease and 20% of patients were intolerant to imatinib. The maximum imatinib dose had been 400–600 mg/day in about 60% of the patients and >600 mg/day in 40% of the patients.

The primary efficacy endpoint in chronic phase CML was MCyR, defined as elimination (CCyR) or substantial diminution (by at least 65%, partial cytogenetic response) of Ph+ hematopoietic cells. The primary efficacy endpoint in accelerated phase, myeloid blast phase, lymphoid blast phase CML, and Ph+ ALL was major hematologic response (MaHR), defined as either a CHR or no evidence of leukemia (NEL).

Chronic Phase CML

Dose-Optimization Trial: A randomized, open-label trial was conducted in patients with chronic phase CML to evaluate the efficacy and safety of SPRYCEL administered once daily compared with SPRYCEL administered twice daily. Patients with significant cardiac diseases, including myocardial infarction within 6 months, congestive heart failure within 3 months, significant arrhythmias, or QTc prolongation were excluded from the trial. The primary efficacy endpoint was MCyR in patients with imatinib-resistant CML. A total of 670 patients, of whom 497 had imatinib-resistant disease, were randomized to the SPRYCEL 100 mg once daily, 140 mg once daily, 50 mg twice daily, or 70 mg twice daily group. Median duration of treatment was 22 months. Efficacy was achieved across all SPRYCEL treatment groups with the once daily schedule demonstrating comparable efficacy (non-inferiority) to the twice daily schedule on the primary efficacy endpoint (difference in MCyR 1.9%; 95% CI [-6.8%–10.6%]).

Efficacy results are presented in Table 8 for patients with chronic phase CML who received the recommended starting dose of 100 mg once daily. Additional efficacy results in this patient population are described after the table. Results for all patients with chronic phase CML, regardless of dosage (a starting dosage of 100 mg once daily, 140 mg once daily, 50 mg twice daily, or 70 mg twice daily), were consistent with those for patients treated with 100 mg once daily.

Table 8: Efficacy of SPRYCEL in Imatinib Resistant or Intolerant Chronic Phase CML (minimum of 24 months follow up)

	100 mg Once Daily (n=167)
CHR[a]% (95% CI)	92% (86–95)
MCyR[b]% (95% CI)	63% (56–71)
CCyR% (95% CI)	50% (42–58)

[a] CHR (response confirmed after 4 weeks): WBC ≤ institutional ULN, platelets <450,000/mm^3, no blasts or promyelocytes in peripheral blood, <5% myelocytes plus metamyelocytes in peripheral blood, basophils in peripheral blood <20%, and no extramedullary involvement.
[b] MCyR combines both complete (0% Ph+ metaphases) and partial (>0%–35%) responses.

In the SPRYCEL 100 mg once daily group, median time to MCyR was 2.9 months (95% CI: [2.8–3.0]) with a minimum of 24 months follow up. Based on the Kaplan-Meier estimates, 93% (95% CI: [88%–98%]) of patients who had achieved an MCyR maintained that response for 18 months. In the 100 mg once daily group, MMR in all patients assessed for MMR was achieved in 43% within 5 years. The estimated rate of progression-free survival and overall survival at 2 years in all patients treated with 100 mg once daily was 80% (95% CI: [73%–87%]) and 91% (95% CI: [86%–96%]), respectively. Based on data six years after the last patient was enrolled in the trial, 64% were known to be alive at 5 years, 22% were known to have died prior to 5 years and 14% had an unknown 5-year survival status.

By 5 years, transformation to either accelerated or blast phase occurred in eight patients on treatment.

Advanced Phase CML and Ph+ ALL

Dose-Optimization Trial: One randomized open-label trial was conducted in patients with advanced phase CML (accelerated phase CML, myeloid blast phase CML, or lymphoid blast phase CML) to evaluate the efficacy and safety of SPRYCEL (dasatinib) administered once daily compared with SPRYCEL administered twice daily. The primary efficacy endpoint was MaHR. A total of 611 patients were randomized to either the SPRYCEL 140 mg once daily or 70 mg twice daily group. Median duration of treatment was approximately 6 months for both treatment groups. The once daily schedule demonstrated comparable efficacy (non-inferiority) to the twice daily schedule on the primary efficacy endpoint.

The efficacy and safety of SPRYCEL were also investigated in patients with Ph+ ALL in one randomized trial (starting dosage 140 mg once daily or 70 mg twice daily) and one single-arm trial (starting dosage 70 mg twice daily). The primary efficacy endpoint was MaHR. A total of 130 patients were enrolled in these studies. The median duration of therapy was 3 months.

Response rates are presented in Table 9.

[See table 9 above]

In the SPRYCEL (dasatinib) 140 mg once daily group, the median time to MaHR was 1.9 months for patients with accelerated phase CML, 1.9 months for patients with myeloid blast phase CML, and 1.8 months for patients with lymphoid blast phase CML.

In patients with myeloid blast phase CML, the median duration of MaHR was 8 months and 9 months for the 140 mg once daily group and the 70 mg twice daily group, respectively. In patients with lymphoid blast phase CML, the median duration of MaHR was 5 months and 8 months for the 140 mg once daily group and the 70 mg twice daily group, respectively. In patients with Ph+ ALL who were treated with SPRYCEL 140 mg once daily, the median duration of MaHR was 4.6 months. The medians of progression-free survival for patients with Ph+ ALL treated with SPRYCEL 140 mg once daily and 70 mg twice daily were 4.0 months and 3.5 months, respectively.

15 REFERENCES

1. NIOSH Alert: Preventing occupational exposures to antineoplastic and other hazardous drugs in healthcare settings. 2004. U.S. Department of Health and Human Services, Public Health Service, Centers for Disease Control and Prevention, National Institute for Occupational Safety and Health, DHHS (NIOSH) Publication No. 2004–165.
2. OSHA Technical Manual, TED 1-0.15A, Section VI: Chapter 2. Controlling Occupational Exposure to Hazardous Drugs. OSHA, 1999, http://www.osha.gov/dts/osta/otm/otm_vi/otm_vi_2.html.
3. American Society of Health-System Pharmacists. ASHP guidelines on handling hazardous drugs. *Am J Health-Syst Pharm.* (2006) 63:1172–1193.
4. Polovich M, White JM, Kelleher LO (eds). 2005. Chemotherapy and biotherapy guidelines and recommendations for practice (2nd ed). Pittsburgh, PA: Oncology Nursing Society.

16 HOW SUPPLIED/STORAGE AND HANDLING

16.1 How Supplied

SPRYCEL® (dasatinib) tablets are available as described in Table 10.

[See table 10 at top of next page]

16.2 Storage

SPRYCEL® tablets should be stored at 20° to 25°C (68° to 77°F); excursions permitted between 15°–30°C (59°–86°F) [see USP Controlled Room Temperature].

16.3 Handling and Disposal

Procedures for proper handling and disposal of anticancer drugs should be considered. Several guidelines on this subject have been published *[see References (15)]*.

SPRYCEL (dasatinib) tablets consist of a core tablet (containing the active drug substance), surrounded by a film coating to prevent exposure of pharmacy and clinical personnel to the active drug substance. However, if tablets are inadvertently crushed or broken, pharmacy and clinical personnel should wear disposable chemotherapy gloves. Personnel who are pregnant should avoid exposure to crushed or broken tablets.

17 PATIENT COUNSELING INFORMATION

See FDA-Approved Patient Labeling.

17.1 Bleeding

Patients should be informed of the possibility of serious bleeding and to report immediately any signs or symptoms suggestive of hemorrhage (unusual bleeding or easy bruising).

17.2 Myelosuppression

Patients should be informed of the possibility of developing low blood cell counts; they should be instructed to report immediately should fever develop, particularly in association with any suggestion of infection.

17.3 Fluid Retention

Patients should be informed of the possibility of developing fluid retention (swelling, weight gain, or shortness of breath) and to seek medical attention if those symptoms arise.

17.4 Pregnancy

Patients should be informed that dasatinib may cause fetal harm when administered to a pregnant woman. Women should be advised of the potential hazard to the fetus and to avoid becoming pregnant. If SPRYCEL is used during pregnancy, or if the patient becomes pregnant while taking SPRYCEL, the patient should be apprised of the potential hazard to the fetus *[see Warnings and Precautions (5.7)]*.

17.5 Gastrointestinal Complaints

Patients should be informed that they may experience nausea, vomiting, or diarrhea with SPRYCEL. If these symptoms are significant, they should seek medical attention.

17.6 Pain

Patients should be informed that they may experience headache or musculoskeletal pain with SPRYCEL. If these symptoms are significant, they should seek medical attention.

17.7 Fatigue
Patients should be informed that they may experience fatigue with SPRYCEL (dasatinib). If this symptom is significant, they should seek medical attention.
17.8 Rash
Patients should be informed that they may experience skin rash with SPRYCEL. If this symptom is significant, they should seek medical attention.
17.9 Lactose
Patients should be informed that SPRYCEL contains 135 mg of lactose monohydrate in a 100-mg daily dose and 189 mg of lactose monohydrate in a 140-mg daily dose.
17.10 Missed Dose
If the patient misses a dose of SPRYCEL, the patient should take the next scheduled dose at its regular time. The patient should not take two doses at the same time.

FDA-Approved Patient Labeling
PATIENT INFORMATION
SPRYCEL®
(Spry-sell)
(dasatinib)
Tablets

Read the Patient Information that comes with SPRYCEL before you start taking it and each time you get a refill. There may be new information. This leaflet does not take the place of talking with your healthcare provider about your medical condition or treatment.

What is SPRYCEL?
SPRYCEL® is a prescription medicine used to treat adults who have:
- newly diagnosed Philadelphia chromosome-positive (Ph+) chronic myeloid leukemia (CML) in chronic phase.
- Ph+ CML who no longer benefit from, or did not tolerate, other treatment, including Gleevec® (imatinib mesylate).
- Philadelphia chromosome-positive acute lymphoblastic leukemia (Ph+ ALL) who no longer benefit from, or did not tolerate, other treatment.

It is not known if SPRYCEL is safe and effective in children younger than 18 years old.

What should I tell my healthcare provider before taking SPRYCEL?
Before you take SPRYCEL, tell your healthcare provider if you:
- have problems with your immune system
- have liver problems
- have heart problems
- are lactose intolerant
- have any other medical conditions
- are pregnant or planning to become pregnant. SPRYCEL may harm your unborn baby. Women should not become pregnant while taking SPRYCEL. Talk to your healthcare provider right away if you are pregnant or plan to become pregnant.
- are breastfeeding or plan to breastfeed. It is not known if SPRYCEL passes into your breast milk or if it can harm your baby. You and your healthcare provider should decide if you will take SPRYCEL or breastfeed. You should not do both.

Tell your healthcare provider about all the medicines you take, including prescription and non-prescription medicines, vitamins, antacids, and herbal supplements.
Especially tell your healthcare provider if you take:
- **medicines that increase the amount of SPRYCEL in your bloodstream, such as:**
  Nizoral® (ketoconazole), Sporanox® (itraconazole), Norvir® (ritonavir), Reyataz® (atazanavir sulfate), Crixivan® (indinavir), Viracept® (nelfinavir), Nefazodone (serzone, nefadar), Invirase® (saquinavir), Ketek® (telithromycin), E-mycin® (erythromycin), Biaxin® (clarithromycin).
- **medicines that decrease the amount of SPRYCEL in your bloodstream, such as:**
  Decadron® (dexamethasone), Dilantin® (phenytoin), Tegretol® (carbamazepine), Rimactane® (rifampin), Luminal® (phenobarbital).
- **medicines whose blood levels might change by taking SPRYCEL, such as:**
  Sandimmune® (cyclosporine), Alfenta® (alfentanil), Fentanyl® (fentanyl), Orap® (pimozide), Rapamune® (sirolimus), Prograf® (tacrolimus), Ergomar® (ergotamine).

SPRYCEL is best absorbed from your stomach into your bloodstream in the presence of stomach acid. You should avoid taking medicines that reduce stomach acid, such as:
Tagamet® (cimetidine), Pepcid® (famotidine), Zantac® (ranitidine), Prilosec® (omeprazole), Protonix® (pantoprazole sodium), Nexium® (esomeprazole), AcipHex® (rabeprazole), Prevacid® (lansoprazole).

Table 10: SPRYCEL Trade Presentations

NDC Number	Strength	Description	Tablets per Bottle
0003-0527-11	20 mg	white to off-white, biconvex, round, film-coated tablet with "BMS" debossed on one side and "527" on the other side	60
0003-0528-11	50 mg	white to off-white, biconvex, oval, film-coated tablet with "BMS" debossed on one side and "528" on the other side	60
0003-0524-11	70 mg	white to off-white, biconvex, round, film-coated tablet with "BMS" debossed on one side and "524" on the other side	60
0003-0855-22	80 mg	white to off-white, biconvex, triangle, film-coated tablet with "BMS" and "80" (BMS over 80) debossed on one side and "855" on the other side	30
0003-0852-22	100 mg	white to off-white, biconvex, oval, film-coated tablet with "BMS 100" debossed on one side and "852" on the other side	30
0003-0857-22	140 mg	white to off-white, biconvex, round, film-coated tablet with "BMS" and "140" (BMS over 140) debossed on one side and "857" on the other side	30

Medicines that neutralize stomach acid, such as Maalox® (aluminum hydroxide/magnesium hydroxide), Tums® (calcium carbonate), or Rolaids® (calcium carbonate and magnesia), may be taken up to 2 hours before or 2 hours after SPRYCEL (dasatinib).

Since SPRYCEL therapy may cause bleeding, tell your healthcare provider if you are using blood thinner medicine, such as Coumadin® (warfarin sodium) or aspirin.

Know the medicines you take. Keep a list of your medicines and show it to your healthcare provider and pharmacist when you get a new medicine.

How should I take SPRYCEL?
Take SPRYCEL exactly as prescribed by your healthcare provider.
- Take SPRYCEL with or without food. Try to take SPRYCEL at the same time each day.
- Swallow SPRYCEL tablets whole. Do not break, cut, or crush the tablets.
- You should not drink grapefruit juice while taking SPRYCEL.
- **Your healthcare provider may:**
  - **change your dose of SPRYCEL or**
  - **tell you to temporarily stop taking SPRYCEL.**
- **Do not change your dose or stop taking SPRYCEL without first talking with your healthcare provider.**
- **If you miss a dose of SPRYCEL,** take your next scheduled dose at its regular time. Do not take two doses at the same time. Call your healthcare provider or pharmacist if you are not sure what to do.
- **If you take too much SPRYCEL,** call your healthcare provider or go to the nearest hospital emergency room right away.

What are the possible side effects of SPRYCEL?
SPRYCEL may cause serious side effects, including:
- **Low Blood Cell Counts:** SPRYCEL may cause low red blood cell counts (anemia), low white blood cell counts (neutropenia), and low platelet counts (thrombocytopenia). Your healthcare provider will do blood tests to check your blood cell counts regularly during your treatment with SPRYCEL. Call your healthcare provider right away if you have a fever or any signs of an infection while taking SPRYCEL.
- **Bleeding:** SPRYCEL may cause severe bleeding that can lead to death. Call your healthcare provider right away if you have:
  - unusual bleeding or bruising of your skin
  - bright red or dark tar-like stools
  - a decrease in your level of consciousness, headache, or change in speech.
- **Your body may hold too much fluid (fluid retention):** In severe cases, fluid may build up in the lining of your lungs, the sac around your heart, or your stomach cavity. Call your healthcare provider right away if you get any of these symptoms during treatment with SPRYCEL:
  - swelling all over your body
  - weight gain
  - shortness of breath and cough.
- **Heart problems.** SPRYCEL may cause an abnormal heart rate, heart problems or a heart attack. Your healthcare provider will monitor the potassium and magnesium levels in your blood, and your heart function.
- **Pulmonary Arterial Hypertension (PAH).** SPRYCEL may cause high blood pressure in the vessels of your lungs. PAH may happen at any time during your treatment with SPRYCEL. Your healthcare provider should check your heart and lungs before and during your treatment with SPRYCEL. Call your healthcare provider right away if you have shortness of breath, tiredness, or swelling all over your body (fluid retention).

Other common side effects of SPRYCEL therapy include:
- diarrhea
- headache
- cough
- skin rash
- fever
- nausea
- tiredness
- vomiting
- muscle pain
- weakness
- infections

Tell your healthcare provider if you have any side effect that bothers you or that does not go away.

These are not all of the possible side effects of SPRYCEL. For more information, ask your healthcare provider or pharmacist.

Call your doctor for medical advice about side effects. You may report side effects to FDA at 1-800-FDA-1088.

How should I store SPRYCEL?
- Store SPRYCEL (dasatinib) at room temperature, between 68°F to 77°F (20°C to 25°C).
- Ask your healthcare provider or pharmacist about the right way to throw away outdated or unused SPRYCEL.
- Women who are pregnant should not handle crushed or broken SPRYCEL tablets.
- **Keep SPRYCEL and all medicines out of the reach of children and pets.**

General information about SPRYCEL
Medicines are sometimes prescribed for purposes other than those listed in the Patient Information leaflet. Do not use SPRYCEL for a condition for which it is not prescribed. Do not give SPRYCEL to other people even if they have the same symptoms you have. It may harm them.

This Patient Information leaflet summarizes the most important information about SPRYCEL. If you would like more information, talk with your healthcare provider. You can ask your healthcare provider or pharmacist for information about SPRYCEL that is written for healthcare professionals.

For more information, go to www.sprycel.com or call 1-800-332-2056.

What are the ingredients in SPRYCEL?
Active ingredient: dasatinib
Inactive ingredients: lactose monohydrate, microcrystalline cellulose, croscarmellose sodium, hydroxypropyl cellulose, and magnesium stearate. The tablet coating consists of hypromellose, titanium dioxide, and polyethylene glycol.

This Patient Package Insert has been approved by the U.S. Food and Drug Administration.

Manufactured by:
Bristol-Myers Squibb Company
Princeton, NJ 08543 USA
1284903A2
Rev June 2010

Shown in Product Identification Guide, page 306

SUSTIVA® ℞
[sus-TEE-vah]
(efavirenz)
capsules for oral use
SUSTIVA®
(efavirenz)
tablets for oral use

HIGHLIGHTS OF PRESCRIBING INFORMATION
These highlights do not include all the information needed to use SUSTIVA safely and effectively. See full prescribing information for SUSTIVA.

SUSTIVA® (efavirenz) capsules for oral use
SUSTIVA® (efavirenz) tablets for oral use
Initial U.S. Approval: 1998

RECENT MAJOR CHANGES

Indications and Usage (1)	05/2013
Dosage and Administration	
Adults (2.1)	05/2013
Pediatric Patients (2.2)	05/2013
Capsule Sprinkle Method of Administration (2.3)	05/2013
Warnings and Precautions	
Coadministration with Related Products (5.3)	08/2012
Rash (5.7)	08/2012
Immune Reconstitution Syndrome (5.11)	08/2012

INDICATIONS AND USAGE

SUSTIVA is a non-nucleoside reverse transcriptase inhibitor indicated in combination with other antiretroviral agents for the treatment of human immunodeficiency virus type 1 infection in adults and in pediatric patients at least 3 months old and weighing at least 3.5 kg. (1)

DOSAGE AND ADMINISTRATION

- SUSTIVA should be taken orally once daily on an empty stomach, preferably at bedtime. (2)
- Recommended adult dose: 600 mg. (2.1)
- With voriconazole, increase voriconazole maintenance dose to 400 mg every 12 hours and decrease SUSTIVA dose to 300 mg once daily using the capsule formulation. (2.1)
- With rifampin, increase SUSTIVA dose to 800 mg once daily for patients weighing 50 kg or more. (2.1)
- Pediatric dosing is based on weight. (2.2)

DOSAGE FORMS AND STRENGTHS

- Capsules: 200 mg and 50 mg (3)
- Tablets: 600 mg (3)

CONTRAINDICATIONS

- SUSTIVA is contraindicated in patients with previously demonstrated hypersensitivity (eg, Stevens-Johnson syndrome, erythema multiforme, or toxic skin eruptions) to any of the components of this product. (4.1)
- For some drugs, competition for CYP3A by efavirenz could result in inhibition of their metabolism and create the potential for serious and/or life-threatening adverse reactions (eg, cardiac arrhythmias, prolonged sedation, or respiratory depression). (4.2)

WARNINGS AND PRECAUTIONS

- *Do not use as a single agent* or add on as a sole agent to a failing regimen. Consider potential for cross resistance when choosing other agents. (5.2)
- Not recommended with ATRIPLA, which contains efavirenz, emtricitabine, and tenofovir disoproxil fumarate, unless needed for dose adjustment when coadministered with rifampin. (5.3)
- *Serious psychiatric symptoms:* Immediate medical evaluation is recommended for serious psychiatric symptoms such as severe depression or suicidal ideation. (5.4, 17.5)
- *Nervous system symptoms (NSS):* NSS are frequent, usually begin 1-2 days after initiating therapy and resolve in 2-4 weeks. Dosing at bedtime may improve tolerability. NSS are not predictive of onset of psychiatric symptoms. (5.5, 6.1, 17.4)
- *Pregnancy:* Fetal harm can occur when administered to a pregnant woman during the first trimester. Women should be apprised of the potential harm to the fetus. (5.6, 17.7) Pregnancy registry is available. (8.1)
- *Hepatotoxicity:* Monitor liver function tests before and during treatment in patients with underlying hepatic disease, including hepatitis B or C coinfection, marked transaminase elevations, or who are taking medications associated with liver toxicity. Among reported cases of hepatic failure, a few occurred in patients with no pre-existing hepatic disease. (5.8, 6.1, 8.6)
- *Rash:* Rash usually begins within 1-2 weeks after initiating therapy and resolves within 4 weeks. Discontinue if severe rash develops. (5.7, 6.1, 17.6)
- *Convulsions:* Use caution in patients with a history of seizures. (5.9)
- *Lipids:* Total cholesterol and triglyceride elevations. Monitor before therapy and periodically thereafter. (5.10)
- *Immune reconstitution syndrome:* May necessitate further evaluation and treatment. (5.11)
- *Redistribution/accumulation of body fat:* Observed in patients receiving antiretroviral therapy. (5.12, 17.8)

ADVERSE REACTIONS

Most common adverse reactions (>5%, moderate-severe) are rash, dizziness, nausea, headache, fatigue, insomnia, and vomiting. (6)

To report SUSPECTED ADVERSE REACTIONS, contact Bristol-Myers Squibb at 1-800-721-5072 or FDA at 1-800-FDA-1088 or www.fda.gov/medwatch.

DRUG INTERACTIONS

Coadministration of efavirenz can alter the concentrations of other drugs and other drugs may alter the concentrations of efavirenz. The potential for drug-drug interactions must be considered before and during therapy. (4.2, 7.1, 12.3)

USE IN SPECIFIC POPULATIONS

- *Pregnancy:* Women should avoid pregnancy during SUSTIVA therapy and for 12 weeks after discontinuation. (5.6)
- *Nursing mothers:* Women infected with HIV should be instructed not to breast-feed. (8.3)
- *Hepatic impairment:* SUSTIVA is not recommended for patients with moderate or severe hepatic impairment. Use caution in patients with mild hepatic impairment. (8.6)
- *Pediatric patients:* The incidence of rash was higher than in adults. (5.7, 6.2, 8.4)

See 17 for PATIENT COUNSELING INFORMATION and FDA-approved patient labeling

Revised: 05/2013

FULL PRESCRIBING INFORMATION: CONTENTS*

*** Sections or subsections omitted from the full prescribing information are not listed**

FULL PRESCRIBING INFORMATION

1 INDICATIONS AND USAGE

SUSTIVA® (efavirenz) in combination with other antiretroviral agents is indicated for the treatment of human immunodeficiency virus type 1 (HIV-1) infection in adults and in pediatric patients at least 3 months old and weighing at least 3.5 kg.

2 DOSAGE AND ADMINISTRATION

2.1 Adults

The recommended dosage of SUSTIVA (efavirenz) is 600 mg orally, once daily, in combination with a protease inhibitor and/or nucleoside analogue reverse transcriptase inhibitors (NRTIs). It is recommended that SUSTIVA be taken on an empty stomach, preferably at bedtime. The increased efavirenz concentrations observed following administration of SUSTIVA with food may lead to an increase in frequency of adverse reactions [see *Clinical Pharmacology (12.3)*]. Dosing at bedtime may improve the tolerability of nervous system symptoms [see *Warnings and Precautions (5.5), Adverse Reactions (6.1),* and *Patient Counseling Information (17.4)*]. SUSTIVA capsules or tablets should be swallowed intact with liquid. For patients who cannot swallow capsules or tablets, the capsule sprinkle method of administration is recommended [see *Dosage and Administration (2.3)*].

Concomitant Antiretroviral Therapy

SUSTIVA must be given in combination with other antiretroviral medications [see *Indications and Usage (1), Warnings and Precautions (5.2), Drug Interactions (7.1),* and *Clinical Pharmacology (12.3)*].

Dosage Adjustment

If SUSTIVA is coadministered with voriconazole, the voriconazole maintenance dose should be increased to 400 mg every 12 hours and the SUSTIVA dose should be decreased to 300 mg once daily using the capsule formulation (one 200 mg and two 50 mg capsules or six 50 mg capsules). SUSTIVA tablets should not be broken. See *Drug Interactions (7.1, Table 6)* and *Clinical Pharmacology (12.3, Tables 8 and 9)*.

If SUSTIVA is coadministered with rifampin to patients weighing 50 kg or more, an increase in the dose of SUSTIVA to 800 mg once daily is recommended [see *Drug Interactions (7.1, Table 6)* and *Clinical Pharmacology (12.3, Table 9)*].

2.2 Pediatric Patients

It is recommended that SUSTIVA be taken on an empty stomach, preferably at bedtime. Table 1 describes the recommended dose of SUSTIVA for pediatric patients 3 months of age or older and weighing between 3.5 kg and 40 kg [see *Clinical Pharmacology (12.3)*]. The recommended dosage of SUSTIVA for pediatric patients weighing 40 kg or greater is 600 mg once daily. For pediatric patients who cannot swallow capsules, the capsule contents can be administered with a small amount of food or infant formula using the capsule sprinkle method of administration [see *Dosage and Administration (2.3)*].

[See table 1 below]

2.3 Capsule Sprinkle Method of Administration

For pediatric patients at least 3 months old and weighing at least 3.5 kg and adults who cannot swallow capsules or tablets, the capsule contents may be administered with a small amount (1 to 2 teaspoons) of food. Use of infant formula for mixing should only be considered for those young infants who cannot reliably consume solid foods. Patients and caregivers must be instructed to open the capsule carefully to avoid spillage or dispersion of the capsule contents into the air. The capsule should be held horizontally over a small container and carefully twisted to open. For patients able to tolerate solid foods, the entire capsule contents should be gently mixed with an age-appropriate soft food, such as applesauce, grape jelly, or yogurt, in the small container.

Table 1: SUSTIVA Dosing in Pediatric Patients

Patient Body Weight	SUSTIVA Daily Dose	Number of Capsules[a] or Tablets[b] and Strength to Administer
3.5 kg to less than 5 kg	100 mg	two 50 mg capsules
5 kg to less than 7.5 kg	150 mg	three 50 mg capsules
7.5 kg to less than 15 kg	200 mg	one 200 mg capsule
15 kg to less than 20 kg	250 mg	one 200 mg + one 50 mg capsule
20 kg to less than 25 kg	300 mg	one 200 mg + two 50 mg capsules
25 kg to less than 32.5 kg	350 mg	one 200 mg + three 50 mg capsules
32.5 kg to less than 40 kg	400 mg	two 200 mg capsules
at least 40 kg	600 mg	one 600 mg tablet OR three 200 mg capsules

[a] Capsules can be administered intact or as sprinkles [see *Dosage and Administration (2.3)*].
[b] Tablets must not be crushed.

For young infants receiving the capsule sprinkle-infant formula mixture, the entire capsule contents should be gently mixed into 2 teaspoons (10 mL) of reconstituted room temperature infant formula in a medicine cup by carefully stirring with a small spoon, and then drawing up the mixture into a 10 mL oral dosing syringe for administration. After administration of the SUSTIVA-food or -formula mixture, an additional small amount (approximately 2 teaspoons) of food or formula must be added to the empty mixing container, stirred to disperse any remaining SUSTIVA (efavirenz) residue, and administered to the patient. The SUSTIVA-food or -formula mixture should be administered within 30 of mixing. No additional food should be consumed for 2 hours after administration of SUSTIVA.

Further patient instructions on the capsule sprinkle method of administration are provided in the FDA-approved patient labeling (see Patient Information and Instructions for Use).

3 DOSAGE FORMS AND STRENGTHS

- *Capsules*

  200 mg capsules are gold color, reverse printed with "SUSTIVA" on the body and imprinted "200 mg" on the cap.

  50 mg capsules are gold color and white, printed with "SUSTIVA" on the gold color cap and reverse printed "50 mg" on the white body.

- *Tablets*

  600 mg tablets are yellow, capsular-shaped, film-coated tablets, with "SUSTIVA" printed on both sides.

4 CONTRAINDICATIONS

4.1 Hypersensitivity

SUSTIVA is contraindicated in patients with previously demonstrated clinically significant hypersensitivity (eg, Stevens-Johnson syndrome, erythema multiforme, or toxic skin eruptions) to any of the components of this product.

4.2 Contraindicated Drugs

For some drugs, competition for CYP3A by efavirenz could result in inhibition of their metabolism and create the potential for serious and/or life-threatening adverse reactions (eg, cardiac arrhythmias, prolonged sedation, or respiratory depression). Drugs that are contraindicated with SUSTIVA are listed in Table 2.

[See table 2 above]

Table 2: Drugs That Are Contraindicated or Not Recommended for Use With SUSTIVA

Drug Class: Drug Name	Clinical Comment
Antimigraine: ergot derivatives (dihydroergotamine, ergonovine, ergotamine, methylergonovine)	Potential for serious and/or life-threatening reactions such as acute ergot toxicity characterized by peripheral vasospasm and ischemia of the extremities and other tissues.
Benzodiazepines: midazolam, triazolam	Potential for serious and/or life-threatening reactions such as prolonged or increased sedation or respiratory depression.
Calcium channel blocker: bepridil	Potential for serious and/or life-threatening reactions such as cardiac arrhythmias.
GI motility agent: cisapride	Potential for serious and/or life-threatening reactions such as cardiac arrhythmias.
Neuroleptic: pimozide	Potential for serious and/or life-threatening reactions such as cardiac arrhythmias.
St. John's wort *(Hypericum perforatum)*	May lead to loss of virologic response and possible resistance to efavirenz or to the class of non-nucleoside reverse transcriptase inhibitors (NNRTIs).

5 WARNINGS AND PRECAUTIONS

5.1 Drug Interactions

Efavirenz plasma concentrations may be altered by substrates, inhibitors, or inducers of CYP3A. Likewise, efavirenz may alter plasma concentrations of drugs metabolized by CYP3A or CYP2B6 [see *Contraindications (4.2)* and *Drug Interactions (7.1)*].

5.2 Resistance

SUSTIVA must not be used as a single agent to treat HIV-1 infection or added on as a sole agent to a failing regimen. Resistant virus emerges rapidly when efavirenz is administered as monotherapy. The choice of new antiretroviral agents to be used in combination with efavirenz should take into consideration the potential for viral cross-resistance.

5.3 Coadministration with Related Products

Coadministration of SUSTIVA with ATRIPLA (efavirenz 600 mg/emtricitabine 200 mg/tenofovir disoproxil fumarate 300 mg) is not recommended unless needed for dose adjustment (eg, with rifampin), since efavirenz is one of its active ingredients.

5.4 Psychiatric Symptoms

Serious psychiatric adverse experiences have been reported in patients treated with SUSTIVA. In controlled trials of 1008 patients treated with regimens containing SUSTIVA for a mean of 2.1 years and 635 patients treated with control regimens for a mean of 1.5 years, the frequency (regardless of causality) of specific serious psychiatric events among patients who received SUSTIVA or control regimens, respectively, were severe depression (2.4%, 0.9%), suicidal ideation (0.7%, 0.3%), nonfatal suicide attempts (0.5%, 0), aggressive behavior (0.4%, 0.5%), paranoid reactions (0.4%, 0.3%), and manic reactions (0.2%, 0.3%). When psychiatric symptoms similar to those noted above were combined and evaluated as a group in a multifactorial analysis of data from Study 006, treatment with efavirenz was associated with an increase in the occurrence of these selected psychiatric symptoms. Other factors associated with an increase in the occurrence of these psychiatric symptoms were history of injection drug use, psychiatric history, and receipt of psychiatric medication at study entry; similar associations were observed in both the SUSTIVA and control treatment groups. In Study 006, onset of new serious psychiatric symptoms occurred throughout the study for both SUSTIVA-treated and control-treated patients. One percent of SUSTIVA-treated patients discontinued or interrupted treatment because of one or more of these selected psychiatric symptoms. There have also been occasional postmarketing reports of death by suicide, delusions, and psychosis-like behavior, although a causal relationship to the use of SUSTIVA cannot be determined from these reports. Patients with serious psychiatric adverse experiences should seek immediate medical evaluation to assess the possibility that the symptoms may be related to the use of SUSTIVA (efavirenz), and if so, to determine whether the risks of continued therapy outweigh the benefits. See *Adverse Reactions (6.1)*.

5.5 Nervous System Symptoms

Fifty-three percent (531/1008) of patients receiving SUSTIVA in controlled trials reported central nervous system symptoms (any grade, regardless of causality) compared to 25% (156/635) of patients receiving control regimens [see *Adverse Reactions (6.1, Table 4)*]. These symptoms included, but were not limited to, dizziness (28.1% of the 1008 patients), insomnia (16.3%), impaired concentration (8.3%), somnolence (7.0%), abnormal dreams (6.2%), and hallucinations (1.2%). These symptoms were severe in 2.0% of patients, and 2.1% of patients discontinued therapy as a result. These symptoms usually begin during the first or second day of therapy and generally resolve after the first 2-4 weeks of therapy. After 4 weeks of therapy, the prevalence of nervous system symptoms of at least moderate severity ranged from 5% to 9% in patients treated with regimens containing SUSTIVA and from 3% to 5% in patients treated with a control regimen. Patients should be informed that these common symptoms were likely to improve with continued therapy and were not predictive of subsequent onset of the less frequent psychiatric symptoms [see *Warnings and Precautions (5.4)*]. Dosing at bedtime may improve the tolerability of these nervous system symptoms [see *Dosage and Administration (2)*].

Analysis of long-term data from Study 006 (median follow-up 180 weeks, 102 weeks, and 76 weeks for patients treated with SUSTIVA + zidovudine + lamivudine, SUSTIVA + indinavir, and indinavir + zidovudine + lamivudine, respectively) showed that, beyond 24 weeks of therapy, the incidences of new-onset nervous system symptoms among SUSTIVA-treated patients were generally similar to those in the indinavir-containing control arm.

Patients receiving SUSTIVA should be alerted to the potential for additive central nervous system effects when SUSTIVA is used concomitantly with alcohol or psychoactive drugs.

Patients who experience central nervous system symptoms such as dizziness, impaired concentration, and/or drowsiness should avoid potentially hazardous tasks such as driving or operating machinery.

5.6 Reproductive Risk Potential

Pregnancy Category D. Efavirenz may cause fetal harm when administered during the first trimester to a pregnant woman. Pregnancy should be avoided in women receiving SUSTIVA. Barrier contraception must always be used in combination with other methods of contraception (eg, oral or other hormonal contraceptives). Because of the long half-life of efavirenz, use of adequate contraceptive measures for 12 weeks after discontinuation of SUSTIVA is recommended. Women of childbearing potential should undergo pregnancy testing before initiation of SUSTIVA. If this drug is used during the first trimester of pregnancy, or if the patient becomes pregnant while taking this drug, the patient should be apprised of the potential harm to the fetus.

There are no adequate and well-controlled studies in pregnant women. SUSTIVA should be used during pregnancy only if the potential benefit justifies the potential risk to the fetus, such as in pregnant women without other therapeutic options. [See *Use in Specific Populations (8.1)*.]

5.7 Rash

In controlled clinical trials, 26% (266/1008) of adult patients treated with 600 mg SUSTIVA experienced new-onset skin rash compared with 17% (111/635) of those treated in control groups [see *Adverse Reactions (6.1)*]. Rash associated with blistering, moist desquamation, or ulceration occurred in 0.9% (9/1008) of patients treated with SUSTIVA. The incidence of Grade 4 rash (eg, erythema multiforme, Stevens-Johnson syndrome) in adult patients treated with SUSTIVA in all studies and expanded access was 0.1%. Rashes are usually mild-to-moderate maculopapular skin eruptions that occur within the first 2 weeks of initiating therapy with efavirenz (median time to onset of rash in adults was 11 days) and, in most patients continuing therapy with efavirenz, rash resolves within 1 month (median duration, 16 days). The discontinuation rate for rash in adult clinical trials was 1.7% (17/1008).

Rash was reported in 59 of 182 pediatric patients (32%) treated with SUSTIVA [see *Adverse Reactions (6.2)*]. Two pediatric patients experienced Grade 3 rash (confluent rash with fever, generalized rash), and four patients had Grade 4 rash (erythema multiforme). The median time to onset of rash in pediatric patients was 28 days (range 3-1642 days). Prophylaxis with appropriate antihistamines before initiating therapy with SUSTIVA in pediatric patients should be considered.

SUSTIVA (efavirenz) can be reinitiated in patients interrupting therapy because of rash. SUSTIVA should be discontinued in patients developing severe rash associated with blistering, desquamation, mucosal involvement, or fever. Appropriate antihistamines and/or corticosteroids may improve the tolerability and hasten the resolution of rash. For patients who have had a life-threatening cutaneous reaction (eg, Stevens-Johnson syndrome), alternative therapy should be considered [see also *Contraindications (4.1)*].

5.8 Hepatotoxicity

Monitoring of liver enzymes before and during treatment is recommended for patients with underlying hepatic disease, including hepatitis B or C infection; patients with marked transaminase elevations; and patients treated with other medications associated with liver toxicity [see *Adverse Reactions (6.1)* and *Use in Specific Populations (8.6)*]. A few of the postmarketing reports of hepatic failure occurred in patients with no pre-existing hepatic disease or other identifiable risk factors [see *Adverse Reactions (6.3)*]. Liver enzyme monitoring should also be considered for patients without pre-existing hepatic dysfunction or other risk factors. In patients with persistent elevations of serum transaminases to greater than five times the upper limit of the normal range, the benefit of continued therapy with SUSTIVA needs to be weighed against the unknown risks of significant liver toxicity.

5.9 Convulsions

Convulsions have been observed in adult and pediatric patients receiving efavirenz, generally in the presence of known medical history of seizures [see *Nonclinical Toxicology (13.2)*]. Caution must be taken in any patient with a history of seizures. Patients who are receiving concomitant anticonvulsant medications primarily metabolized by the liver, such as phenytoin and phenobarbital, may require periodic monitoring of plasma levels [see *Drug Interactions (7.1)*].

5.10 Lipid Elevations

Treatment with SUSTIVA has resulted in increases in the concentration of total cholesterol and triglycerides [see *Adverse Reactions (6.1)*]. Cholesterol and triglyceride testing should be performed before initiating SUSTIVA therapy and at periodic intervals during therapy.

5.11 Immune Reconstitution Syndrome

Immune reconstitution syndrome has been reported in patients treated with combination antiretroviral therapy, including SUSTIVA. During the initial phase of combination antiretroviral treatment, patients whose immune system responds may develop an inflammatory response to indolent or residual opportunistic infections [such as *Mycobacterium avium* infection, cytomegalovirus, *Pneumocystis jiroveci* pneumonia (PCP), or tuberculosis], which may necessitate further evaluation and treatment.

Autoimmune disorders (such as Graves' disease, polymyositis, and Guillain-Barré syndrome) have also been reported to occur in the setting of immune reconstitution; however, the time to onset is more variable, and can occur many months after initiation of treatment.

5.12 Fat Redistribution

Redistribution/accumulation of body fat including central obesity, dorsocervical fat enlargement (buffalo hump), pe-

Table 3: Selected Treatment-Emergent[a] Adverse Reactions of Moderate or Severe Intensity Reported in ≥2% of SUSTIVA-Treated Patients in Studies 006 and ACTG 364

	Study 006 LAM-, NNRTI-, and Protease Inhibitor-Naive Patients			Study ACTG 364 NRTI-experienced, NNRTI-, and Protease Inhibitor-Naive Patients		
Adverse Reactions	SUSTIVA[b] + ZDV/LAM (n=412) 180 weeks[c]	SUSTIVA[b] + Indinavir (n=415) 102 weeks[c]	Indinavir + ZDV/LAM (n=401) 76 weeks[c]	SUSTIVA[b] + Nelfinavir + NRTIs (n=64) 71.1 weeks[c]	SUSTIVA[b] + NRTIs (n=65) 70.9 weeks[c]	Nelfinavir + NRTIs (n=66) 62.7 weeks[c]
Body as a Whole						
Fatigue	8%	5%	9%	0	2%	3%
Pain	1%	2%	8%	13%	6%	17%
Central and Peripheral Nervous System						
Dizziness	9%	9%	2%	2%	6%	6%
Headache	8%	5%	3%	5%	2%	3%
Insomnia	7%	7%	2%	0	0	2%
Concentration impaired	5%	3%	<1%	0	0	0
Abnormal dreams	3%	1%	0	—	—	—
Somnolence	2%	2%	<1%	0	0	0
Anorexia	1%	<1%	<1%	0	2%	2%
Gastrointestinal						
Nausea	10%	6%	24%	3%	2%	2%
Vomiting	6%	3%	14%	—	—	—
Diarrhea	3%	5%	6%	14%	3%	9%
Dyspepsia	4%	4%	6%	0	0	2%
Abdominal pain	2%	2%	5%	3%	3%	3%
Psychiatric						
Anxiety	2%	4%	<1%	—	—	—
Depression	5%	4%	<1%	3%	0	5%
Nervousness	2%	2%	0	2%	0	2%
Skin & Appendages						
Rash[d]	11%	16%	5%	9%	5%	9%
Pruritus	<1%	1%	1%	9%	5%	9%

[a] Includes adverse events at least possibly related to study drug or of unknown relationship for Study 006. Includes all adverse events regardless of relationship to study drug for Study ACTG 364.
[b] SUSTIVA provided as 600 mg once daily.
[c] Median duration of treatment.
[d] Includes erythema multiforme, rash, rash erythematous, rash follicular, rash maculopapular, rash petechial, rash pustular, and urticaria for Study 006 and macules, papules, rash, erythema, redness, inflammation, allergic rash, urticaria, welts, hives, itchy, and pruritus for ACTG 364.
— = Not Specified.
ZDV = zidovudine, LAM = lamivudine.

Table 4: Percent of Patients with One or More Selected Nervous System Symptoms[a,b]

Percent of Patients with:	SUSTIVA 600 mg Once Daily (n=1008) %	Control Groups (n=635) %
Symptoms of any severity	52.7	24.6
Mild symptoms[c]	33.3	15.6
Moderate symptoms[d]	17.4	7.7
Severe symptoms[e]	2.0	1.3
Treatment discontinuation as a result of symptoms	2.1	1.1

[a] Includes events reported regardless of causality.
[b] Data from Study 006 and three Phase 2/3 studies.
[c] "Mild" = Symptoms which do not interfere with patient's daily activities.
[d] "Moderate" = Symptoms which may interfere with daily activities.
[e] "Severe" = Events which interrupt patient's usual daily activities.

ripheral wasting, facial wasting, breast enlargement, and "cushingoid appearance" have been observed in patients receiving antiretroviral therapy. The mechanism and long-term consequences of these events are currently unknown. A causal relationship has not been established.

6 ADVERSE REACTIONS

The most significant adverse reactions observed in patients treated with SUSTIVA (efavirenz) are:

- psychiatric symptoms [see *Warnings and Precautions (5.4)*],
- nervous system symptoms [see *Warnings and Precautions (5.5)*],
- rash [see *Warnings and Precautions (5.7)*].

The most common (>5% in either efavirenz treatment group) adverse reactions of at least moderate severity among patients in Study 006 treated with SUSTIVA in combination with zidovudine/lamivudine or indinavir were rash, dizziness, nausea, headache, fatigue, insomnia, and vomiting.

6.1 Clinical Trials Experience in Adults

Because clinical studies are conducted under widely varying conditions, the adverse reaction rates reported cannot be directly compared to rates in other clinical studies and may not reflect the rates observed in clinical practice.

Selected clinical adverse reactions of moderate or severe intensity observed in ≥2% of SUSTIVA-treated patients in two controlled clinical trials are presented in Table 3.

[See table 3 above]

Pancreatitis has been reported, although a causal relationship with efavirenz has not been established. Asymptomatic increases in serum amylase levels were observed in a significantly higher number of patients treated with efavirenz 600 mg than in control patients (see *Laboratory Abnormalities*).

Nervous System Symptoms

For 1008 patients treated with regimens containing SUSTIVA (efavirenz) and 635 patients treated with a control regimen in controlled trials, Table 4 lists the frequency of symptoms of different degrees of severity and gives the discontinuation rates for one or more of the following nervous system symptoms: dizziness, insomnia, impaired concentration, somnolence, abnormal dreaming, euphoria, confusion, agitation, amnesia, hallucinations, stupor, abnormal thinking, and depersonalization [see *Warnings and Precautions (5.5)*]. The frequencies of specific central and peripheral nervous system symptoms are provided in Table 3.

[See table 4 above]

Psychiatric Symptoms

Serious psychiatric adverse experiences have been reported in patients treated with SUSTIVA (efavirenz). In controlled trials, psychiatric symptoms observed at a frequency greater than 2% among patients treated with SUSTIVA or control regimens, respectively, were depression (19%, 16%), anxiety (13%, 9%), and nervousness (7%, 2%).

Rash

In controlled clinical trials, the frequency of rash (all grades, regardless of causality) was 26% for 1008 adults treated with regimens containing SUSTIVA and 17% for 635 adults treated with a control regimen. Most reports of rash were mild or moderate in severity. The frequency of Grade 3 rash was 0.8% for SUSTIVA-treated patients and 0.3% for control groups, and the frequency of Grade 4 rash was 0.1% for SUSTIVA and 0 for control groups. The discontinuation rates as a result of rash were 1.7% for SUSTIVA-treated patients and 0.3% for control groups [see *Warnings and Precautions (5.7)*].

Experience with SUSTIVA in patients who discontinued other antiretroviral agents of the NNRTI class is limited. Nineteen patients who discontinued nevirapine because of rash have been treated with SUSTIVA. Nine of these patients developed mild-to-moderate rash while receiving therapy with SUSTIVA, and two of these patients discontinued because of rash.

Laboratory Abnormalities

Selected Grade 3-4 laboratory abnormalities reported in ≥2% of SUSTIVA-treated patients in two clinical trials are presented in Table 5.

[See table 5 at top of next page]

Patients Coinfected with Hepatitis B or C

Liver function tests should be monitored in patients with a history of hepatitis B and/or C. In the long-term data set from Study 006, 137 patients treated with SUSTIVA-containing regimens (median duration of therapy, 68 weeks) and 84 treated with a control regimen (median duration, 56 weeks) were seropositive at screening for hepatitis B (surface antigen positive) and/or C (hepatitis C antibody positive). Among these coinfected patients, elevations in AST to greater than five times ULN developed in 13% of patients in the SUSTIVA arms and 7% of those in the control arm, and elevations in ALT to greater than five times ULN developed in 20% of patients in the SUSTIVA arms and 7% of patients in the control arm. Among coinfected patients, 3% of those treated with SUSTIVA-containing regimens and 2% in the control arm discontinued from the study because of liver or biliary system disorders [see *Warnings and Precautions (5.8)*].

Lipids

Increases from baseline in total cholesterol of 10-20% have been observed in some uninfected volunteers receiving SUSTIVA. In patients treated with SUSTIVA + zidovudine + lamivudine, increases from baseline in nonfasting total cholesterol and HDL of approximately 20% and 25%, respectively, were observed. In patients treated with SUSTIVA + indinavir, increases from baseline in nonfasting cholesterol and HDL of approximately 40% and 35%, respectively, were observed. Nonfasting total cholesterol levels ≥240 mg/dL and ≥300 mg/dL were reported in 34% and 9%, respectively, of patients treated with SUSTIVA + zidovudine + lamivudine; 54% and 20%, respectively, of patients treated with SUSTIVA + indinavir; and 28% and 4%, respectively, of patients treated with indinavir + zidovudine + lamivudine. The effects of SUSTIVA on triglycerides and LDL in this study were not well characterized since samples were taken from nonfasting patients. The clinical significance of these findings is unknown [see *Warnings and Precautions (5.10)*].

6.2 Clinical Trial Experience in Pediatric Patients

Assessment of adverse reactions is based on three clinical trials in 182 HIV-1 infected pediatric patients (3 months to 21 years of age) who received SUSTIVA in combination with other antiretroviral agents for a median of 123 weeks. The adverse reactions observed in the three trials were similar to those observed in clinical trials in adults except that rash was more common in pediatric patients (32% for all grades regardless of causality) and more often of higher grade (ie, more severe). Two (1.1%) pediatric patients experienced Grade 3 rash (confluent rash with fever, generalized rash), and four (2.2%) pediatric patients had Grade 4 rash (all erythema multiforme). Five pediatric patients (2.7%) discontinued from the study because of rash [see *Warnings and Precautions (5.7)*].

6.3 Postmarketing Experience

The following adverse reactions have been identified during postapproval use of SUSTIVA. Because these reactions are reported voluntarily from a population of unknown size, it is not always possible to reliably estimate their frequency or establish a causal relationship to drug exposure.

Body as a Whole: allergic reactions, asthenia, redistribution/accumulation of body fat [see *Warnings and Precautions (5.12)*]

Central and Peripheral Nervous System: abnormal coordination, ataxia, cerebellar coordination and balance disturbances, convulsions, hypoesthesia, paresthesia, neuropathy, tremor, vertigo

Endocrine: gynecomastia
Gastrointestinal: constipation, malabsorption
Cardiovascular: flushing, palpitations
Liver and Biliary System: hepatic enzyme increase, hepatic failure, hepatitis. A few of the postmarketing reports of hepatic failure, including cases in patients with no preexisting hepatic disease or other identifiable risk factors, were characterized by a fulminant course, progressing in some cases to transplantation or death.
Metabolic and Nutritional: hypercholesterolemia, hypertriglyceridemia
Musculoskeletal: arthralgia, myalgia, myopathy
Psychiatric: aggressive reactions, agitation, delusions, emotional lability, mania, neurosis, paranoia, psychosis, suicide
Respiratory: dyspnea
Skin and Appendages: erythema multiforme, photoallergic dermatitis, Stevens-Johnson syndrome
Special Senses: abnormal vision, tinnitus

7 DRUG INTERACTIONS

7.1 Drug-Drug Interactions

Efavirenz has been shown *in vivo* to induce CYP3A and CYP2B6. Other compounds that are substrates of CYP3A or CYP2B6 may have decreased plasma concentrations when coadministered with SUSTIVA (efavirenz). *In vitro* studies have demonstrated that efavirenz inhibits CYP2C9, 2C19, and 3A4 isozymes in the range of observed efavirenz plasma concentrations. Coadministration of efavirenz with drugs primarily metabolized by these isozymes may result in altered plasma concentrations of the coadministered drug. Therefore, appropriate dose adjustments may be necessary for these drugs.

Drugs that induce CYP3A activity (eg, phenobarbital, rifampin, rifabutin) would be expected to increase the clearance of efavirenz resulting in lowered plasma concentrations.

Drug interactions with SUSTIVA are summarized in Tables 2 and 6 [for pharmacokinetics data see *Clinical Pharmacology (12.3, Tables 8* and *9)*]. The tables include potentially significant interactions, but are not all inclusive.

[See table 6 on pages 800 through 802]

Other Drugs

Based on the results of drug interaction studies [see *Clinical Pharmacology (12.3, Tables 8* and *9)*], no dosage adjustment is recommended when SUSTIVA (efavirenz) is given with the following: aluminum/magnesium hydroxide antacids, azithromycin, cetirizine, famotidine, fluconazole, lamivudine, lorazepam, nelfinavir, paroxetine, tenofovir disoproxil fumarate, and zidovudine.

Specific drug interaction studies have not been performed with SUSTIVA and NRTIs other than lamivudine and zidovudine. Clinically significant interactions would not be expected since the NRTIs are metabolized via a different route than efavirenz and would be unlikely to compete for the same metabolic enzymes and elimination pathways.

7.2 Cannabinoid Test Interaction

Efavirenz does not bind to cannabinoid receptors. False-positive urine cannabinoid test results have been observed in non-HIV-infected volunteers receiving SUSTIVA when the Microgenics CEDIA DAU Multi-Level THC assay was used for screening. Negative results were obtained when more specific confirmatory testing was performed with gas chromatography/mass spectrometry.

Of the three assays analyzed (Microgenics CEDIA DAU Multi-Level THC assay, Cannabinoid Enzyme Immunoassay [Diagnostic Reagents, Inc], and AxSYM Cannabinoid Assay), only the Microgenics CEDIA DAU Multi-Level THC assay showed false-positive results. The other two assays provided true-negative results. The effects of SUSTIVA on cannabinoid screening tests other than these three are unknown. The manufacturers of cannabinoid assays should be contacted for additional information regarding the use of their assays with patients receiving efavirenz.

8 USE IN SPECIFIC POPULATIONS

8.1 Pregnancy

Pregnancy Category D: See *Warnings and Precautions (5.6)*.

Antiretroviral Pregnancy Registry: To monitor fetal outcomes of pregnant women exposed to SUSTIVA, an Antiretroviral Pregnancy Registry has been established. Physicians are encouraged to register patients by calling 1-800-258-4263.

As of July 2010, the Antiretroviral Pregnancy Registry has received prospective reports of 792 pregnancies exposed to efavirenz-containing regimens, nearly all of which were first-trimester exposures (718 pregnancies). Birth defects occurred in 17 of 604 live births (first-trimester exposure) and 2 of 69 live births (second/third-trimester exposure). One of these prospectively reported defects with first-trimester exposure was a neural tube defect. A single case of anophthalmia with first-trimester exposure to efavirenz has also been prospectively reported; however, this case included severe oblique facial clefts and amniotic banding, a known association with anophthalmia. There have been six retrospective reports of findings consistent with neural tube defects, including meningomyelocele. All mothers were exposed to efavirenz-containing regimens in the first trimester. Although a causal relationship of these events to the use of SUSTIVA has not been established, similar defects have been observed in preclinical studies of efavirenz.

Table 5: Selected Grade 3-4 Laboratory Abnormalities Reported in ≥2% of SUSTIVA-Treated Patients in Studies 006 and ACTG 364

		Study 006 LAM-, NNRTI-, and Protease Inhibitor-Naive Patients			Study ACTG 364 NRTI-experienced, NNRTI-, and Protease Inhibitor-Naive Patients		
Variable	Limit	SUSTIVA[a] + ZDV/LAM (n=412) 180 weeks[b]	SUSTIVA[a] + Indinavir (n=415) 102 weeks[b]	Indinavir + ZDV/LAM (n=401) 76 weeks[b]	SUSTIVA[a] + Nelfinavir + NRTIs (n=64) 71.1 weeks[b]	SUSTIVA[a] + NRTIs (n=65) 70.9 weeks[b]	Nelfinavir + NRTIs (n=66) 62.7 weeks[b]
Chemistry							
ALT	>5 × ULN	5%	8%	5%	2%	6%	3%
AST	>5 × ULN	5%	6%	5%	6%	8%	8%
GGT[c]	>5 × ULN	8%	7%	3%	5%	0	5%
Amylase	>2 × ULN	4%	4%	1%	0	6%	2%
Glucose	>250 mg/dL	3%	3%	3%	5%	2%	3%
Triglycerides[d]	≥751 mg/dL	9%	6%	6%	11%	8%	17%
Hematology							
Neutrophils	<750/mm^3	10%	3%	5%	2%	3%	2%

[a] SUSTIVA provided as 600 mg once daily.
[b] Median duration of treatment.
[c] Isolated elevations of GGT in patients receiving SUSTIVA may reflect enzyme induction not associated with liver toxicity.
[d] Nonfasting.
ZDV = zidovudine, LAM = lamivudine, ULN = Upper limit of normal, ALT = alanine aminotransferase, AST = aspartate aminotransferase, GGT = gamma-glutamyltransferase.

Animal Data

Effects of efavirenz on embryo-fetal development have been studied in three nonclinical species (cynomolgus monkeys, rats, and rabbits). In monkeys, efavirenz 60 mg/kg/day was administered to pregnant females throughout pregnancy (gestation days 20 through 150). The maternal systemic drug exposures (AUC) were 1.3 times the exposure in humans at the recommended clinical dose (600 mg/day), with fetal umbilical venous drug concentrations approximately 0.7 times the maternal values. Three fetuses of 20 fetuses/infants had one or more malformations; there were no malformed fetuses or infants from placebo-treated mothers. The malformations that occurred in these three monkey fetuses included anencephaly and unilateral anophthalmia in one fetus, microophthalmia in a second, and cleft palate in the third. There was no NOAEL (no observable adverse effect level) established for this study because only one dosage was evaluated. In rats, efavirenz was administered either during organogenesis (gestation days 7 to 18) or from gestation day 7 through lactation day 21 at 50, 100, or 200 mg/kg/day. Administration of 200 mg/kg/day in rats was associated with increase in the incidence of early resorptions; and doses 100 mg/kg/day and greater were associated with early neonatal mortality. The AUC at the NOAEL (50 mg/kg/day) in this rat study was 0.1 times that in humans at the recommended clinical dose. Drug concentrations in the milk on lactation day 10 were approximately 8 times higher than those in maternal plasma. In pregnant rabbits, efavirenz was neither embryo lethal nor teratogenic when administered at doses of 25, 50, and 75 mg/kg/day over the period of organogenesis (gestation days 6 through 18). The AUC at the NOAEL (75 mg/kg/day) in rabbits was 0.4 times that in humans at the recommended clinical dose.

8.3 Nursing Mothers

The Centers for Disease Control and Prevention recommend that HIV-infected mothers not breast-feed their infants to avoid risking postnatal transmission of HIV. Although it is not known if efavirenz is secreted in human milk, efavirenz is secreted into the milk of lactating rats. Because of the potential for HIV transmission and the potential for serious adverse effects in nursing infants, mothers should be instructed not to breast-feed if they are receiving SUSTIVA (efavirenz).

8.4 Pediatric Use

The safety, pharmacokinetic profile, and virologic and immunologic responses of SUSTIVA were evaluated in antiretroviral-naive and -experienced HIV-1 infected pediatric patients 3 months to 21 years of age in three open-label clinical trials [see *Adverse Reactions (6.2)*, *Clinical Pharmacology (12.3)*, and *Clinical Studies (14.2)*]. The type and frequency of adverse reactions in these trials were generally similar to those of adult patients with the exception of a higher frequency of rash, including a higher frequency of Grade 3 or 4 rash, in pediatric patients compared to adults [see *Warnings and Precautions (5.7)* and *Adverse Reactions (6.2)*].

Use of SUSTIVA in patients younger than 3 months of age OR less than 3.5 kg body weight is not recommended because the safety, pharmacokinetics, and antiviral activity of SUSTIVA (efavirenz) have not been evaluated in this age group and there is a risk of developing HIV resistance if SUSTIVA is underdosed. See *Dosage and Administration (2.2)* for dosing recommendations for pediatric patients.

8.5 Geriatric Use

Clinical studies of SUSTIVA did not include sufficient numbers of subjects aged 65 years and over to determine whether they respond differently from younger subjects. In general, dose selection for an elderly patient should be cautious, reflecting the greater frequency of decreased hepatic, renal, or cardiac function and of concomitant disease or other therapy.

8.6 Hepatic Impairment

SUSTIVA is not recommended for patients with moderate or severe hepatic impairment because there are insufficient data to determine whether dose adjustment is necessary. Patients with mild hepatic impairment may be treated with efavirenz without any adjustment in dose. Because of the extensive cytochrome P450-mediated metabolism of efavirenz and limited clinical experience in patients with hepatic impairment, caution should be exercised in administering SUSTIVA to these patients [see *Warnings and Precautions (5.8)* and *Clinical Pharmacology (12.3)*].

10 OVERDOSAGE

Some patients accidentally taking 600 mg twice daily have reported increased nervous system symptoms. One patient experienced involuntary muscle contractions.

Treatment of overdose with SUSTIVA should consist of general supportive measures, including monitoring of vital signs and observation of the patient's clinical status. Administration of activated charcoal may be used to aid removal of unabsorbed drug. There is no specific antidote for overdose with SUSTIVA. Since efavirenz is highly protein bound, dialysis is unlikely to significantly remove the drug from blood.

11 DESCRIPTION

SUSTIVA® (efavirenz) is an HIV-1 specific, non-nucleoside, reverse transcriptase inhibitor (NNRTI). Efavirenz is chemically described as (S)-6-chloro-4-(cyclopropylethynyl)-1,4-dihydro-4-(trifluoromethyl)-2H-3,1-benzoxazin-2-one. Its empirical formula is $C_{14}H_9ClF_3NO_2$ and its structural formula is:

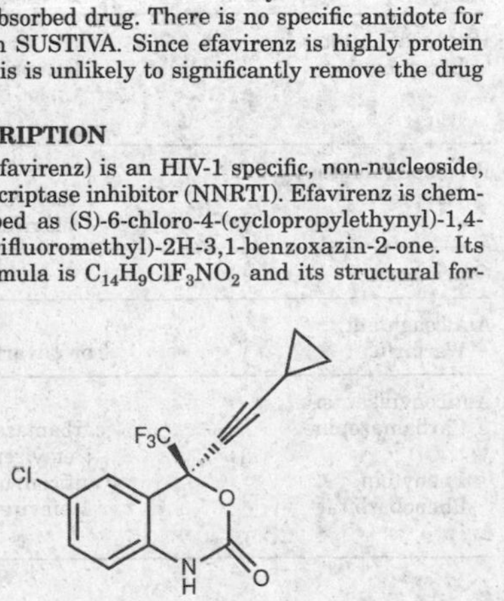

Efavirenz is a white to slightly pink crystalline powder with a molecular mass of 315.68. It is practically insoluble in water (<10 microgram/mL).

Table 6: Established and Other Potentially Significant Drug Interactions: Alteration in Dose or Regimen May Be Recommended Based on Drug Interaction Studies or Predicted Interaction

Concomitant Drug Class: Drug Name	Effect	Clinical Comment
HIV antiviral agents		
Protease inhibitor: Fosamprenavir calcium	↓ amprenavir	Fosamprenavir (unboosted): Appropriate doses of the combinations with respect to safety and efficacy have not been established. Fosamprenavir/ritonavir: An additional 100 mg/day (300 mg total) of ritonavir is recommended when SUSTIVA is administered with fosamprenavir/ritonavir once daily. No change in the ritonavir dose is required when SUSTIVA is administered with fosamprenavir plus ritonavir twice daily.
Protease inhibitor: Atazanavir sulfate	↓ atazanavir*	*Treatment-naive patients:* When coadministered with SUSTIVA, the recommended dose of atazanavir is 400 mg with ritonavir 100 mg (together once daily with food) and SUSTIVA 600 mg (once daily on an empty stomach, preferably at bedtime). *Treatment-experienced patients:* Coadministration of SUSTIVA and atazanavir is not recommended.
Protease inhibitor: Indinavir	↓ indinavir*	The optimal dose of indinavir, when given in combination with SUSTIVA, is not known. Increasing the indinavir dose to 1000 mg every 8 hours does not compensate for the increased indinavir metabolism due to SUSTIVA. When indinavir at an increased dose (1000 mg every 8 hours) was given with SUSTIVA (600 mg once daily), the indinavir AUC and C_{min} were decreased on average by 33-46% and 39-57%, respectively, compared to when indinavir (800 mg every 8 hours) was given alone.
Protease inhibitor: Lopinavir/ritonavir	↓ lopinavir*	Lopinavir/ritonavir tablets should not be administered once daily in combination with SUSTIVA. In antiretroviral-naive patients, lopinavir/ritonavir tablets can be used twice daily in combination with SUSTIVA with no dose adjustment. A dose increase of lopinavir/ritonavir tablets to 600/150 mg (3 tablets) twice daily may be considered when used in combination with SUSTIVA in treatment-experienced patients where decreased susceptibility to lopinavir is clinically suspected (by treatment history or laboratory evidence). A dose increase of lopinavir/ritonavir oral solution to 533/133 mg (6.5 mL) twice daily taken with food is recommended when used in combination with SUSTIVA.
Protease inhibitor: Ritonavir	↑ ritonavir* ↑ efavirenz*	When ritonavir 500 mg q12h was coadministered with SUSTIVA 600 mg once daily, the combination was associated with a higher frequency of adverse clinical experiences (eg, dizziness, nausea, paresthesia) and laboratory abnormalities (elevated liver enzymes). Monitoring of liver enzymes is recommended when SUSTIVA is used in combination with ritonavir.
Protease inhibitor: Saquinavir	↓ saquinavir*	Should not be used as sole protease inhibitor in combination with SUSTIVA.
NNRTI: Other NNRTIs	↑ or ↓ efavirenz and/or NNRTI	Combining two NNRTIs has not been shown to be beneficial. SUSTIVA should not be coadministered with other NNRTIs.
CCR5 co-receptor antagonist: Maraviroc	↓ maraviroc*	Refer to the full prescribing information for maraviroc for guidance on coadministration with efavirenz.
Integrase strand transfer inhibitor: Raltegravir	↓ raltegravir*	SUSTIVA reduces plasma concentrations of raltegravir. The clinical significance of this interaction has not been directly assessed.
Hepatitis C antiviral agents		
Protease inhibitor: Boceprevir	↓ boceprevir*	Plasma trough concentrations of boceprevir were decreased when boceprevir was coadministered with SUSTIVA, which may result in loss of therapeutic effect. The combination should be avoided.
Protease inhibitor: Telaprevir	↓ telaprevir* ↓ efavirenz*	Concomitant administration of telaprevir and SUSTIVA resulted in reduced steady-state exposures to telaprevir and efavirenz.
Other agents		
Anticoagulant: Warfarin	↑ or ↓ warfarin	Plasma concentrations and effects potentially increased or decreased by SUSTIVA.
Anticonvulsants: Carbamazepine	↓ carbamazepine* ↓ efavirenz*	There are insufficient data to make a dose recommendation for efavirenz. Alternative anticonvulsant treatment should be used.
Phenytoin Phenobarbital	↓ anticonvulsant ↓ efavirenz	Potential for reduction in anticonvulsant and/or efavirenz plasma levels; periodic monitoring of anticonvulsant plasma levels should be conducted.

(Table continued on next page)

Capsules: SUSTIVA is available as capsules for oral administration containing either 50 mg or 200 mg of efavirenz and the following inactive ingredients: lactose monohydrate, magnesium stearate, sodium lauryl sulfate, and sodium starch glycolate. The capsule shell contains the following inactive ingredients and dyes: gelatin, sodium lauryl sulfate, titanium dioxide, and/or yellow iron oxide. The capsule shells may also contain silicon dioxide. The capsules are printed with ink containing carmine 40 blue, FD&C Blue No. 2, and titanium dioxide.

Tablets: SUSTIVA (efavirenz) is available as film-coated tablets for oral administration containing 600 mg of efavirenz and the following inactive ingredients: croscarmellose sodium, hydroxypropyl cellulose, lactose monohydrate, magnesium stearate, microcrystalline cellulose, and sodium lauryl sulfate. The film coating contains Opadry Yellow and Opadry Clear. The tablets are polished with carnauba wax and printed with purple ink, Opacode WB.

12 CLINICAL PHARMACOLOGY

12.1 Mechanism of Action

Efavirenz is an antiviral drug [see *Microbiology (12.4)*].

12.3 Pharmacokinetics

Absorption

Peak efavirenz plasma concentrations of 1.6-9.1 μM were attained by 5 hours following single oral doses of 100 mg to 1600 mg administered to uninfected volunteers. Dose-related increases in C_{max} and AUC were seen for doses up to 1600 mg; the increases were less than proportional suggesting diminished absorption at higher doses.

In HIV-1-infected patients at steady state, mean C_{max}, mean C_{min}, and mean AUC were dose proportional following 200 mg, 400 mg, and 600 mg daily doses. Time-to-peak plasma concentrations were approximately 3-5 hours and steady-state plasma concentrations were reached in 6-10 days. In 35 patients receiving SUSTIVA 600 mg once daily, steady-state C_{max} was 12.9 ± 3.7 μM (mean ± SD), steady-state C_{min} was 5.6 ± 3.2 μM, and AUC was 184 ± 73 μM•h.

Effect of Food on Oral Absorption:

Capsules: Administration of a single 600 mg dose of efavirenz capsules with a high-fat/high-caloric meal (894 kcal, 54 g fat, 54% calories from fat) or a reduced-fat/normal-caloric meal (440 kcal, 2 g fat, 4% calories from fat) was associated with a mean increase of 22% and 17% in efavirenz AUC_{∞} and a mean increase of 39% and 51% in efavirenz C_{max}, respectively, relative to the exposures achieved when given under fasted conditions. See *Dosage and Administration (2)* and *Patient Counseling Information (17.3)*.

Tablets: Administration of a single 600 mg efavirenz tablet with a high-fat/high-caloric meal (approximately 1000 kcal, 500-600 kcal from fat) was associated with a 28% increase in mean AUC_{∞} of efavirenz and a 79% increase in mean C_{max} of efavirenz relative to the exposures achieved under fasted conditions. See *Dosage and Administration (2)* and *Patient Counseling Information (17.3)*.

Bioavailability of capsule contents mixed with food vehicles: In healthy adult subjects, the efavirenz AUC when administered as the contents of three 200 mg capsules mixed with 2 teaspoons of certain food vehicles (applesauce, grape jelly or yogurt, or infant formula) met bioequivalency criteria for the AUC of the intact capsule formulation administered under fasted conditions.

Distribution

Efavirenz is highly bound (approximately 99.5-99.75%) to human plasma proteins, predominantly albumin. In HIV-1 infected patients (n=9) who received SUSTIVA 200 to 600 mg once daily for at least one month, cerebrospinal fluid concentrations ranged from 0.26 to 1.19% (mean 0.69%) of the corresponding plasma concentration. This proportion is approximately 3-fold higher than the non-protein-bound (free) fraction of efavirenz in plasma.

Metabolism

Studies in humans and *in vitro* studies using human liver microsomes have demonstrated that efavirenz is principally metabolized by the cytochrome P450 system to hydroxylated metabolites with subsequent glucuronidation of these hydroxylated metabolites. These metabolites are essentially inactive against HIV-1. The *in vitro* studies suggest that CYP3A and CYP2B6 are the major isozymes responsible for efavirenz metabolism.

Efavirenz has been shown to induce CYP enzymes, resulting in the induction of its own metabolism. Multiple doses of 200-400 mg per day for 10 days resulted in a lower than predicted extent of accumulation (22-42% lower) and a shorter terminal half-life of 40-55 hours (single dose half-life 52-76 hours).

Elimination

Efavirenz has a terminal half-life of 52-76 hours after single doses and 40-55 hours after multiple doses. A one-month mass balance/excretion study was conducted using 400 mg per day with a ^{14}C-labeled dose administered on Day 8. Approximately 14-34% of the radiolabel was recovered in the urine and 16-61% was recovered in the feces. Nearly all of the urinary excretion of the radiolabeled drug was in the form of metabolites. Efavirenz accounted for the majority of the total radioactivity measured in feces.

Special Populations

Pediatric: The pharmacokinetic parameters for efavirenz at steady state in pediatric patients were predicted by a population pharmacokinetic model and are summarized in Table 7 by weight ranges that correspond to the recommended doses.

[See table 7 at top of next page]

Gender and race: The pharmacokinetics of efavirenz in patients appear to be similar between men and women and among the racial groups studied.

Renal impairment: The pharmacokinetics of efavirenz have not been studied in patients with renal insufficiency; however, less than 1% of efavirenz is excreted unchanged in the urine, so the impact of renal impairment on efavirenz elimination should be minimal.

Hepatic impairment: A multiple-dose study showed no significant effect on efavirenz pharmacokinetics in patients with mild hepatic impairment (Child-Pugh Class A) compared with controls. There were insufficient data to determine whether moderate or severe hepatic impairment (Child-Pugh Class B or C) affects efavirenz pharmacokinetics.

Drug Interaction Studies

Efavirenz has been shown *in vivo* to cause hepatic enzyme induction, thus increasing the biotransformation of some drugs metabolized by CYP3A and CYP2B6. *In vitro* studies have shown that efavirenz inhibited CYP isozymes 2C9, 2C19, and 3A4 with K_i values (8.5-17 μM) in the range of observed efavirenz plasma concentrations. In *in vitro* studies, efavirenz did not inhibit CYP2E1 and inhibited CYP2D6 and CYP1A2 (K_i values 82-160 μM) only at concentrations well above those achieved clinically. The inhibitory effect on CYP3A is expected to be similar between 200 mg, 400 mg, and 600 mg doses of efavirenz. Coadministration of efavirenz with drugs primarily metabolized by CYP2C9, CYP2C19, CYP3A, or CYP2B6 isozymes may result in altered plasma concentrations of the coadministered drug. Drugs which induce CYP3A and CYP2B6 activity would be expected to increase the clearance of efavirenz resulting in lowered plasma concentrations.

Drug interaction studies were performed with efavirenz and other drugs likely to be coadministered or drugs commonly used as probes for pharmacokinetic interaction. The effects of coadministration of efavirenz on the C_{max}, AUC, and C_{min} are summarized in Table 8 (effect of efavirenz on other drugs) and Table 9 (effect of other drugs on efavirenz). For information regarding clinical recommendations see *Contraindications (4.2)* and *Drug Interactions (7.1)*.

[See table 8 on pages 803 and 804]

[See table 9 on pages 805 and 806]

12.4 Microbiology

Mechanism of Action

Efavirenz is an NNRTI of HIV-1. Efavirenz activity is mediated predominantly by noncompetitive inhibition of HIV-1 reverse transcriptase. HIV-2 reverse transcriptase and human cellular DNA polymerases α, β, γ, and δ are not inhibited by efavirenz.

Antiviral Activity in Cell Culture

The concentration of efavirenz inhibiting replication of wild-type laboratory adapted strains and clinical isolates in cell culture by 90-95% (EC_{90-95}) ranged from 1.7 to 25 nM in lymphoblastoid cell lines, peripheral blood mononuclear cells (PBMCs), and macrophage/monocyte cultures. Efavirenz demonstrated antiviral activity against clade B and most non-clade B isolates (subtypes A, AE, AG, C, D, F, G, J, N), but had reduced antiviral activity against group O viruses. Efavirenz demonstrated additive antiviral activity without cytotoxicity against HIV-1 in cell culture when combined with the NNRTIs delavirdine and nevirapine, NRTIs (abacavir, didanosine, emtricitabine, lamivudine, stavudine, tenofovir, zalcitabine, zidovudine), PIs (amprenavir, indinavir, lopinavir, nelfinavir, ritonavir, saquinavir), and the fusion inhibitor enfuvirtide. Efavirenz demonstrated additive to antagonistic antiviral activity in cell culture with atazanavir. Efavirenz was not antagonistic with adefovir, used for the treatment of hepatitis B virus infection, or ribavirin, used in combination with interferon for the treatment of hepatitis C virus infection.

Resistance

In cell culture

In cell culture, HIV-1 isolates with reduced susceptibility to efavirenz (>380-fold increase in EC_{90} value) emerged rapidly in the presence of drug. Genotypic characterization of these viruses identified single amino acid substitutions L100I or V179D, double substitutions L100I/V108I, and triple substitutions L100I/V179D/Y181C in reverse transcriptase.

Clinical studies

Clinical isolates with reduced susceptibility in cell culture to efavirenz have been obtained. One or more substitutions at amino acid positions 98, 100, 101, 103, 106, 108, 188, 190, 225, and 227 in reverse transcriptase were observed in patients failing treatment with efavirenz in combination with indinavir, or with zidovudine plus lamivudine. The K103N substitution was the most frequently observed. Long-term resistance surveillance (average 52 weeks, range 4-106 weeks) analyzed 28 matching baseline and virologic failure isolates. Sixty-one percent (17/28) of these failure isolates had decreased efavirenz susceptibility in cell culture with a median 88-fold change in efavirenz susceptibility (EC_{50} value) from reference. The most frequent NNRTI substitution to develop in these patient isolates was K103N (54%). Other NNRTI substitutions that developed included L100I (7%), K101E/Q/R (14%), V108I (11%), G190S/T/A (7%), P225H (18%), and M230I/L (11%).

Cross-Resistance

Cross-resistance among NNRTIs has been observed. Clinical isolates previously characterized as efavirenz-resistant were also phenotypically resistant in cell culture to delavirdine and nevirapine compared to baseline. Delavirdine-

Table 6 *(cont.)*: Established and Other Potentially Significant Drug Interactions: Alteration in Dose or Regimen May Be Recommended Based on Drug Interaction Studies or Predicted Interaction

Concomitant Drug Class: Drug Name	Effect	Clinical Comment
Antidepressants:		
Bupropion	↓ bupropion*	The effect of efavirenz on bupropion exposure is thought to be due to the induction of bupropion metabolism. Increases in bupropion dosage should be guided by clinical response, but the maximum recommended dose of bupropion should not be exceeded.
Sertraline	↓ sertraline*	Increases in sertraline dosage should be guided by clinical response.
Antifungals:		
Voriconazole	↓ voriconazole* ↑ efavirenz*	SUSTIVA and voriconazole must not be coadministered at standard doses. Efavirenz significantly decreases voriconazole plasma concentrations, and coadministration may decrease the therapeutic effectiveness of voriconazole. Also, voriconazole significantly increases efavirenz plasma concentrations, which may increase the risk of SUSTIVA-associated side effects. When voriconazole is coadministered with SUSTIVA, voriconazole maintenance dose should be increased to 400 mg every 12 hours and SUSTIVA dose should be decreased to 300 mg once daily using the capsule formulation. SUSTIVA tablets should not be broken. [See *Dosage and Administration (2.1)* and *Clinical Pharmacology (12.3, Tables 8* and *9)*.]
Itraconazole	↓ itraconazole* ↓ hydroxyitraconazole*	Since no dose recommendation for itraconazole can be made, alternative antifungal treatment should be considered.
Ketoconazole	↓ ketoconazole	Drug interaction studies with SUSTIVA and ketoconazole have not been conducted. SUSTIVA has the potential to decrease plasma concentrations of ketoconazole.
Posaconazole	↓ posaconazole*	Avoid concomitant use unless the benefit outweighs the risks.
Anti-infective:		
Clarithromycin	↓ clarithromycin* ↑ 14-OH metabolite*	Plasma concentrations decreased by SUSTIVA; clinical significance unknown. In uninfected volunteers, 46% developed rash while receiving SUSTIVA and clarithromycin. No dose adjustment of SUSTIVA is recommended when given with clarithromycin. Alternatives to clarithromycin, such as azithromycin, should be considered (see *Other Drugs*, following table). Other macrolide antibiotics, such as erythromycin, have not been studied in combination with SUSTIVA.
Antimycobacterials:		
Rifabutin	↓ rifabutin*	Increase daily dose of rifabutin by 50%. Consider doubling the rifabutin dose in regimens where rifabutin is given 2 or 3 times a week.
Rifampin	↓ efavirenz*	If SUSTIVA is coadministered with rifampin to patients weighing 50 kg or more, an increase in the dose of SUSTIVA to 800 mg once daily is recommended.
Calcium channel blockers:		
Diltiazem	↓ diltiazem* ↓ desacetyl diltiazem* ↓ N-monodesmethyl diltiazem*	Diltiazem dose adjustments should be guided by clinical response (refer to the full prescribing information for diltiazem). No dose adjustment of efavirenz is necessary when administered with diltiazem.
Others (eg, felodipine, nicardipine, nifedipine, verapamil)	↓ calcium channel blocker	No data are available on the potential interactions of efavirenz with other calcium channel blockers that are substrates of CYP3A. The potential exists for reduction in plasma concentrations of the calcium channel blocker. Dose adjustments should be guided by clinical response (refer to the full prescribing information for the calcium channel blocker).
HMG-CoA reductase inhibitors: Atorvastatin Pravastatin Simvastatin	↓ atorvastatin* ↓ pravastatin* ↓ simvastatin*	Plasma concentrations of atorvastatin, pravastatin, and simvastatin decreased. Consult the full prescribing information for the HMG-CoA reductase inhibitor for guidance on individualizing the dose.
Hormonal contraceptives:		
Oral		
Ethinyl estradiol/ Norgestimate	↓ active metabolites of norgestimate*	A reliable method of barrier contraception must be used in addition to hormonal contraceptives. Efavirenz had no effect on ethinyl estradiol concentrations, but progestin levels (norelgestromin and levonorgestrel) were markedly decreased. No effect of ethinyl estradiol/norgestimate on efavirenz plasma concentrations was observed.
Implant		
Etonogestrel	↓ etonogestrel	A reliable method of barrier contraception must be used in addition to hormonal contraceptives. The interaction between etonogestrel and efavirenz has not been studied. Decreased exposure of etonogestrel may be expected. There have been postmarketing reports of contraceptive failure with etonogestrel in efavirenz-exposed patients.

(Table continued on next page)

Table 6 *(cont.)*: Established and Other Potentially Significant Drug Interactions: Alteration in Dose or Regimen May Be Recommended Based on Drug Interaction Studies or Predicted Interaction

Concomitant Drug Class: Drug Name	Effect	Clinical Comment
Immunosuppressants: Cyclosporine, tacrolimus, sirolimus, and others metabolized by CYP3A	↓ immunosuppressant	Decreased exposure of the immunosuppressant may be expected due to CYP3A induction. These immunosuppressants are not anticipated to affect exposure of efavirenz. Dose adjustments of the immunosuppressant may be required. Close monitoring of immunosuppressant concentrations for at least 2 weeks (until stable concentrations are reached) is recommended when starting or stopping treatment with efavirenz.
Narcotic analgesic: Methadone	↓ methadone*	Coadministration in HIV-infected individuals with a history of injection drug use resulted in decreased plasma levels of methadone and signs of opiate withdrawal. Methadone dose was increased by a mean of 22% to alleviate withdrawal symptoms. Patients should be monitored for signs of withdrawal and their methadone dose increased as required to alleviate withdrawal symptoms.

* The interaction between SUSTIVA and the drug was evaluated in a clinical study. All other drug interactions shown are predicted.

This table is not all-inclusive.

Table 7: Predicted Steady-State Pharmacokinetics of Recommended Doses of Efavirenz (Capsules/Capsule Sprinkles) in HIV-Infected Pediatric Patients

Body Weight	Dose	Mean AUC $_{(0-24)}$ μM•h	Mean C_{max} μg/mL	Mean C_{min} μg/mL
3.5-5 kg	100 mg	220.52	5.81	2.43
5-7.5 kg	150 mg	262.62	7.07	2.71
7.5-10 kg	200 mg	284.28	7.75	2.87
10-15 kg	200 mg	238.14	6.54	2.32
15-20 kg	250 mg	233.98	6.47	2.3
20-25 kg	300 mg	257.56	7.04	2.55
25-32.5 kg	350 mg	262.37	7.12	2.68
32.5-40 kg	400 mg	259.79	6.96	2.69
>40 kg	600 mg	254.78	6.57	2.82

and/or nevirapine-resistant clinical viral isolates with NNRTI resistance-associated substitutions (A98G, L100I, K101E/P, K103N/S, V106A, Y181X, Y188X, G190X, P225H, F227L, or M230L) showed reduced susceptibility to efavirenz in cell culture. Greater than 90% of NRTI-resistant clinical isolates tested in cell culture retained susceptibility to efavirenz.

13 NONCLINICAL TOXICOLOGY

13.1 Carcinogenesis, Mutagenesis, Impairment of Fertility

Carcinogenesis

Long-term carcinogenicity studies in mice and rats were carried out with efavirenz. Mice were dosed with 0, 25, 75, 150, or 300 mg/kg/day for 2 years. Incidences of hepatocellular adenomas and carcinomas and pulmonary alveolar/bronchiolar adenomas were increased above background in females. No increases in tumor incidence above background were seen in males. There was no NOAEL in females established for this study because tumor findings occurred at all doses. AUC at the NOAEL (150 mg/kg) in the males was approximately 0.9 times that in humans at the recommended clinical dose. In the rat study, no increases in tumor incidence were observed at doses up to 100 mg/kg/day, for which AUCs were 0.1 (males) or 0.2 (females) times those in humans at the recommended clinical dose.

Mutagenesis

Efavirenz tested negative in a battery of *in vitro* and *in vivo* genotoxicity assays. These included bacterial mutation assays in *S. typhimurium* and *E. coli*, mammalian mutation assays in Chinese hamster ovary cells, chromosome aberration assays in human peripheral blood lymphocytes or Chinese hamster ovary cells, and an *in vivo* mouse bone marrow micronucleus assay.

Impairment of Fertility

Efavirenz did not impair mating or fertility of male or female rats, and did not affect sperm of treated male rats. The reproductive performance of offspring born to female rats given efavirenz was not affected. The AUCs at the NOAEL values in male (200 mg/kg) and female (100 mg/kg) rats were approximately ≤0.15 times that in humans at the recommended clinical dose.

13.2 Animal Toxicology

Nonsustained convulsions were observed in 6 of 20 monkeys receiving efavirenz at doses yielding plasma AUC values 4- to 13-fold greater than those in humans given the recommended dose [see *Warnings and Precautions (5.9)*].

14 CLINICAL STUDIES

14.1 Adults

Study 006, a randomized, open-label trial, compared SUSTIVA (efavirenz) (600 mg once daily) + zidovudine (ZDV, 300 mg q12h) + lamivudine (LAM, 150 mg q12h) or SUSTIVA (600 mg once daily) + indinavir (IDV, 1000 mg q8h) with indinavir (800 mg q8h) + zidovudine (300 mg q12h) + lamivudine (150 mg q12h). Twelve hundred sixty-six patients (mean age 36.5 years [range 18-81], 60% Caucasian, 83% male) were enrolled. All patients were efavirenz-, lamivudine-, NNRTI-, and PI-naive at study entry. The median baseline CD4+ cell count was 320 cells/mm^3 and the median baseline HIV-1 RNA level was 4.8 $\log_{10}$ copies/mL. Treatment outcomes with standard assay (assay limit
400 copies/mL) through 48 and 168 weeks are shown in Table 10. Plasma HIV RNA levels were quantified with standard (assay limit 400 copies/mL) and ultrasensitive (assay limit 50 copies/mL) versions of the AMPLICOR HIV-1 MONITOR assay. During the study, version 1.5 of the assay was introduced in Europe to enhance detection of non-clade B virus.

[See table 10 at top of page 806]

For patients treated with SUSTIVA + zidovudine + lamivudine, SUSTIVA + indinavir, or indinavir + zidovudine + lamivudine, the percentage of responders with HIV-1 RNA <50 copies/mL was 65%, 50%, and 45%, respectively, through 48 weeks, and 43%, 31%, and 23%, respectively, through 168 weeks. A Kaplan-Meier analysis of time to loss of virologic response (HIV RNA <400 copies/mL) suggests that both the trends of virologic response and differences in response continue through 4 years.

ACTG 364 is a randomized, double-blind, placebo-controlled, 48-week study in NRTI-experienced patients who had completed two prior ACTG studies. One-hundred ninety-six patients (mean age 41 years [range 18-76], 74% Caucasian, 88% male) received NRTIs in combination with SUSTIVA (efavirenz) (600 mg once daily), or nelfinavir (NFV, 750 mg three times daily), or SUSTIVA (600 mg once daily) + nelfinavir in a randomized, double-blinded manner. The mean baseline CD4+ cell count was 389 cells/mm^3 and mean baseline HIV-1 RNA level was 8130 copies/mL. Upon entry into the study, all patients were assigned a new open-label NRTI regimen, which was dependent on their previous NRTI treatment experience. There was no significant difference in the mean CD4+ cell count among treatment groups; the overall mean increase was approximately 100 cells at 48 weeks among patients who continued on study regimens. Treatment outcomes are shown in Table 11. Plasma HIV RNA levels were quantified with the AMPLICOR HIV-1 MONITOR assay using a lower limit of quantification of 500 copies/mL.

[See table 11 at bottom of page 806]

A Kaplan-Meier analysis of time to treatment failure through 72 weeks demonstrates a longer duration of virologic suppression (HIV RNA <500 copies/mL) in the SUSTIVA-containing treatment arms.

14.2 Pediatric Patients

Study AI266922 is an open-label study to evaluate the pharmacokinetics, safety, tolerability, and antiviral activity of SUSTIVA (efavirenz) in combination with didanosine and emtricitabine in antiretroviral-naive and -experienced pediatric patients. Thirty-seven patients 3 months to 6 years of age (median 0.7 years) were treated with SUSTIVA. At baseline, median plasma HIV-1 RNA was 5.88 $\log_{10}$ copies/mL, median CD4+ cell count was 1144 cells/mm^3, and median CD4+ percentage was 25%. The median time on study therapy was 60 weeks; 27% of patients discontinued before Week 48. Using an ITT analysis, the overall proportions of patients with HIV RNA <400 copies/mL and <50 copies/mL at Week 48 were 57% (21/37) and 46% (17/37), respectively. The median increase from baseline in CD4+ count at 48 weeks was 196 cells/mm^3 and the median increase in CD4+ percentage was 6%.

Study PACTG 1021 was an open-label study to evaluate the pharmacokinetics, safety, tolerability, and antiviral activity of SUSTIVA in combination with didanosine and emtricitabine in pediatric patients who were antiretroviral therapy naive. Forty-three patients 3 months to 21 years of age (median 9.6 years) were dosed with SUSTIVA. At baseline, median plasma HIV-1 RNA was 4.8 $\log_{10}$ copies/mL, median CD4+ cell count was 367 cells/mm^3, and median CD4+ percentage was 18%. The median time on study therapy was 181 weeks; 16% of patients discontinued before Week 48. Using an ITT analysis, the overall proportions of patients with HIV RNA <400 copies/mL and <50 copies/mL at Week 48 were 77% (33/43) and 70% (30/43), respectively. The median increase from baseline in CD4+ count at 48 weeks of therapy was 238 cells/mm^3 and the median increase in CD4+ percentage was 13%.

Study PACTG 382 was an open-label study to evaluate the pharmacokinetics, safety, tolerability, and antiviral activity of SUSTIVA in combination with nelfinavir and an NRTI in antiretroviral-naive and NRTI-experienced pediatric patients. One hundred two patients 3 months to 16 years of age (median 5.7 years) were treated with SUSTIVA. Eighty-seven percent of patients had received prior antiretroviral therapy. At baseline, median plasma HIV-1 RNA was 4.57 $\log_{10}$ copies/mL, median CD4+ cell count was 755 cells/mm^3, and median CD4+ percentage was 30%. The median time on study therapy was 118 weeks; 25% of patients discontinued before Week 48. Using an ITT analysis, the overall proportion of patients with HIV RNA <400 copies/mL and <50 copies/mL at Week 48 were 57% (58/102) and 43% (44/102), respectively. The median increase from baseline in CD4+ count at 48 weeks of therapy was 128 cells/mm^3 and the median increase in CD4+ percentage was 5%.

16 HOW SUPPLIED/STORAGE AND HANDLING

16.1 Capsules

SUSTIVA® (efavirenz) capsules are available as follows:

Capsules 200 mg are gold color, reverse printed with "SUSTIVA" on the body and imprinted "200 mg" on the cap.

Bottles of 90 NDC 0056-0474-92

Capsules 50 mg are gold color and white, printed with "SUSTIVA" on the gold color cap and reverse printed "50 mg" on the white body.

Bottles of 30 NDC 0056-0470-30

16.2 Tablets

SUSTIVA® (efavirenz) tablets are available as follows:

Tablets 600 mg are yellow, capsular-shaped, film-coated tablets, with "SUSTIVA" printed on both sides.

Bottles of 30 NDC 0056-0510-30

16.3 Storage

SUSTIVA capsules and SUSTIVA tablets should be stored at 25° C (77° F); excursions permitted to 15°–30° C (59°–86° F) [see USP Controlled Room Temperature].

17 PATIENT COUNSELING INFORMATION

See *FDA-approved patient labeling (Patient Information and Instructions for Use)*.

17.1 Drug Interactions

A statement to patients and healthcare providers is included on the product's bottle labels:

ALERT: Find out about medicines that should NOT be taken with SUSTIVA.

SUSTIVA may interact with some drugs; therefore, patients should be advised to report to their doctor the use of any other prescription, nonprescription medication, or herbal products, particularly St. John's wort.

17.2 General Information for Patients

Patients should be informed that SUSTIVA is not a cure for HIV-1 infection and patients may continue to experience illnesses associated with HIV-1 infection, including opportunistic infections. Patients should remain under the care of a physician while taking SUSTIVA.

Patients should be advised to avoid doing things that can spread HIV-1 infection to others.

- **Do not share needles or other injection equipment.**
- **Do not share personal items that can have blood or body fluids on them, like toothbrushes and razor blades.**
- **Do not have any kind of sex without protection.** Always practice safe sex by using a latex or polyurethane condom to lower the chance of sexual contact with semen, vaginal secretions, or blood.
- **Do not breast-feed.** It is not known if SUSTIVA (efavirenz) can be passed to your baby in your breast milk and whether it could harm your baby. Also, mothers with HIV-1 should not breast-feed because HIV-1 can be passed to the baby in breast milk.

17.3 Dosing Instructions

Patients should be advised to take SUSTIVA every day as prescribed. SUSTIVA must always be used in combination with other antiretroviral drugs. Patients should be advised to take SUSTIVA on an empty stomach, preferably at bedtime. Taking SUSTIVA with food increases efavirenz concentrations and may increase the frequency of adverse reactions. Dosing at bedtime may improve the tolerability of nervous system symptoms [see *Dosage and Administration (2)* and *Adverse Reactions (6.1)*]. Healthcare providers should assist parents or caregivers in determining the best SUSTIVA dosing schedule for infants and young children.

For adult and pediatric patients who cannot swallow capsules or tablets, patients or their caregivers should be advised to read and carefully follow the instructions for administering the capsule contents in a small amount of food or infant formula [see *Dosage and Administration (2.3)* and *FDA-approved patient labeling (Patient Information and Instructions for Use)*]. Patients should call their healthcare provider or pharmacist if they have any questions.

17.4 Nervous System Symptoms

Patients should be informed that central nervous system symptoms (NSS) including dizziness, insomnia, impaired concentration, drowsiness, and abnormal dreams are commonly reported during the first weeks of therapy with SUSTIVA [see *Warnings and Precautions (5.5)*]. Dosing at bedtime may improve the tolerability of these symptoms, which are likely to improve with continued therapy. Patients should be alerted to the potential for additive effects when SUSTIVA is used concomitantly with alcohol or psychoactive drugs. Patients should be instructed that if they experience NSS they should avoid potentially hazardous tasks such as driving or operating machinery.

17.5 Psychiatric Symptoms

Patients should be informed that serious psychiatric symptoms including severe depression, suicide attempts, aggressive behavior, delusions, paranoia, and psychosis-like symptoms have been reported in patients receiving SUSTIVA [see *Warnings and Precautions (5.4)*]. If they experience severe psychiatric adverse experiences they should seek immediate medical evaluation. Patients should be advised to inform their physician of any history of mental illness or substance abuse.

17.6 Rash

Patients should be informed that a common side effect is rash [see *Warnings and Precautions (5.7)*]. Rashes usually go away without any change in treatment. However, since rash may be serious, patients should be advised to contact their physician promptly if rash occurs.

17.7 Reproductive Risk Potential

Women receiving SUSTIVA should be instructed to avoid pregnancy [see *Warnings and Precautions (5.6)*]. A reliable form of barrier contraception must always be used in combination with other methods of contraception, including oral or other hormonal contraception. Because of the long half-life of efavirenz, use of adequate contraceptive measures for 12 weeks after discontinuation of SUSTIVA is recommended. Women should be advised to notify their physician if they become pregnant or plan to become pregnant while taking SUSTIVA. If this drug is used during the first trimester of pregnancy, or if the patient becomes pregnant while taking this drug, she should be apprised of the potential harm to the fetus.

17.8 Fat Redistribution

Patients should be informed that redistribution or accumulation of body fat may occur in patients receiving antiretroviral therapy and that the cause and long-term health effects of these conditions are not known [see *Warnings and Precautions (5.12)*].

SUSTIVA is a registered trademark of Bristol-Myers Squibb Pharma Company, ATRIPLA is a trademark of Bristol-Myers Squibb & Gilead Sciences, LLC, PRAVACHOL is a registered trademark of ER Squibb & Sons, LLC, and REYATAZ is a registered trademark of Bristol-Myers Squibb Company. Other brands listed are the trademarks of their respective owners.

Distributed by:
Bristol-Myers Squibb Company
Princeton, NJ 08543 USA
SUSTIVA® (efavirenz) capsules made in India.

Rev May 2013

Table 8: Effect of Efavirenz on Coadministered Drug Plasma C_{max}, AUC, and C_{min}

Coadministered Drug	Dose	Efavirenz Dose	Number of Subjects	Coadministered Drug (mean % change)		
				C_{max} (90% CI)	AUC (90% CI)	C_{min} (90% CI)
Atazanavir	400 mg qd with a light meal d 1-20	600 mg qd with a light meal d 7-20	27	↓ 59% (49-67%)	↓ 74% (68-78%)	↓ 93% (90-95%)
	400 mg qd d 1-6, then 300 mg qd d 7-20 with ritonavir 100 mg qd and a light meal	600 mg qd 2 h after atazanavir and ritonavir d 7-20	13	↑ 14%[a] (↓ 17-↑ 58%)	↑ 39%[a] (2-88%)	↑ 48%[a] (24-76%)
	300 mg qd/ritonavir 100 mg qd d 1-10 (pm), then 400 mg qd/ritonavir 100 mg qd d 11-24 (pm) (simultaneous with efavirenz)	600 mg qd with a light snack d 11-24 (pm)	14	↑ 17% (8-27%)	↔	↓ 42% (31-51%)
Indinavir	1000 mg q8h × 10 days	600 mg qd × 10 days	20			
	After morning dose			↔[b]	↓ 33%[b] (26-39%)	↓ 39%[b] (24-51%)
	After afternoon dose			↔[b]	↓ 37%[b] (26-46%)	↓ 52%[b] (47-57%)
	After evening dose			↓ 29%[b] (11-43%)	↓ 46%[b] (37-54%)	↓ 57%[b] (50-63%)
Lopinavir/ ritonavir	400/100 mg capsule q12h × 9 days	600 mg qd × 9 days	11,7[c]	↔[d]	↓ 19%[d] (↓ 36-↑ 3%)	↓ 39%[d] (3-62%)
	600/150 mg tablet q12h × 10 days with efavirenz compared to 400/100 mg q12h alone	600 mg qd × 9 days	23	↑ 36%[d] (28-44%)	↑ 36%[d] (28-44%)	↑ 32%[d] (21-44%)
Nelfinavir	750 mg q8h × 7 days	600 mg qd × 7 days	10	↑ 21% (10-33%)	↑ 20% (8-34%)	↔
Metabolite AG-1402				↓ 40% (30-48%)	↓ 37% (25-48%)	↓ 43% (21-59%)
Ritonavir	500 mg q12h × 8 days	600 mg qd × 10 days	11			
	After AM dose			↑ 24% (12-38%)	↑ 18% (6-33%)	↑ 42% (9-86%)[e]
	After PM dose			↔	↔	↑ 24% (3-50%)[e]
Saquinavir SGC[f]	1200 mg q8h × 10 days	600 mg qd × 10 days	12	↓ 50% (28-66%)	↓ 62% (45-74%)	↓ 56% (16-77%)[e]
Lamivudine	150 mg q12h × 14 days	600 mg qd × 14 days	9	↔	↔	↑ 265% (37-873%)
Tenofovir[g]	300 mg qd	600 mg qd × 14 days	29	↔	↔	↔
Zidovudine	300 mg q12h × 14 days	600 mg qd × 14 days	9	↔	↔	↑ 225% (43-640%)
Maraviroc	100 mg bid	600 mg qd	12	↓ 51% (37-62%)	↓ 45% (38-51%)	↓ 45% (28-57%)
Raltegravir	400 mg single dose	600 mg qd	9	↓ 36% (2-59%)	↓ 36% (20-48%)	↓ 21% (↓ 51-↑ 28%)
Boceprevir	800 mg tid × 6 days	600 mg qd × 16 days	NA	↓ 8% (↓ 22-↑ 8%)	↓ 19% (11-25%)	↓ 44% (26-58%)
Telaprevir	750 mg q8h × 10 days	600 mg qd × 20 days	21	↓ 9% (↓ 18-↑ 2%)	↓ 26% (16-35%)	↓ 47% (35-56%)
Azithromycin	600 mg single dose	400 mg qd × 7 days	14	↑ 22% (4-42%)	↔	NA
Clarithromycin	500 mg q12h × 7 days	400 mg qd × 7 days	11	↓ 26% (15-35%)	↓ 39% (30-46%)	↓ 53% (42-63%)
14-OH metabolite				↑ 49% (32-69%)	↑ 34% (18-53%)	↑ 26% (9-45%)
Fluconazole	200 mg × 7 days	400 mg qd × 7 days	10	↔	↔	↔
Itraconazole	200 mg q12h × 28 days	600 mg qd × 14 days	18	↓ 37% (20-51%)	↓ 39% (21-53%)	↓ 44% (27-58%)
Hydroxy-itraconazole				↓ 35% (12-52%)	↓ 37% (14-55%)	↓ 43% (18-60%)
Posaconazole	400 mg (oral suspension) bid × 10 and 20 days	400 mg qd × 10 and 20 days	11	↓ 45% (34-53%)	↓ 50% (40-57%)	NA
Rifabutin	300 mg qd × 14 days	600 mg qd × 14 days	9	↓ 32% (15-46%)	↓ 38% (28-47%)	↓ 45% (31-56%)

(Table continued on next page)

Patient Information
SUSTIVA® (sus-TEE-vah)
[efavirenz (eh-FAH-vih-rehnz)**]**
capsules and tablets

ALERT: Find out about medicines that should NOT be taken with SUSTIVA.

Please also read the section **"MEDICINES YOU SHOULD NOT TAKE WITH SUSTIVA."**

Read this information before you start taking SUSTIVA. Read it again each time you refill your prescription, in case there is any new information. This leaflet provides a summary about SUSTIVA and does not include everything there is to know about your medicine. This information is not meant to take the place of talking with your doctor.

What is SUSTIVA?

SUSTIVA is a medicine used with other antiretroviral medicines to help treat infection with Human Immunodeficiency Virus type 1 (HIV-1) in adults and children 3 months or older and who weigh 7 pounds 12 ounces (3.5 kg) or more. HIV-1 is the virus that causes AIDS (acquired immune deficiency syndrome). SUSTIVA is a type of anti-HIV drug called a "non-nucleoside reverse transcriptase inhibitor" (NNRTI). NNRTIs are not used in the treatment of Human Immunodeficiency Virus type 2 (HIV-2) infection.

SUSTIVA works by lowering the amount of HIV-1 in the blood (viral load). SUSTIVA must be taken with other anti-HIV medicines. When taken with other anti-HIV medicines, SUSTIVA has been shown to reduce viral load and increase the number of CD4+ cells, a type of immune cell in blood. SUSTIVA may not have these effects in every patient.

SUSTIVA does not cure HIV or AIDS and you may continue to experience illnesses associated with HIV-1 infection, including opportunistic infections. You should remain under the care of a doctor when using SUSTIVA.

Avoid doing things that can spread HIV-1 infection.

- **Do not share needles or other injection equipment.**
- **Do not share personal items that can have blood or body fluids on them, like toothbrushes and razor blades.**
- **Do not have any kind of sex without protection.** Always practice safe sex by using a latex or polyurethane condom to lower the chance of sexual contact with semen, vaginal secretions, or blood.

What are the possible side effects of SUSTIVA?

Serious psychiatric problems. A small number of patients experience severe depression, strange thoughts, or angry behavior while taking SUSTIVA. Some patients have thoughts of suicide and a few have actually committed suicide. These problems tend to occur more often in patients who have had mental illness. Contact your doctor right away if you think you are having these psychiatric symptoms, so your doctor can decide if you should continue to take SUSTIVA (efavirenz).

Common side effects. Many patients have dizziness, trouble sleeping, drowsiness, trouble concentrating, and/or unusual dreams during treatment with SUSTIVA. These side effects may be reduced if you take SUSTIVA at bedtime on an empty stomach. They also tend to go away after you have taken the medicine for a few weeks. If you have these common side effects, such as dizziness, it does not mean that you will also have serious psychiatric problems, such as severe depression, strange thoughts, or angry behavior. Tell your doctor right away if any of these side effects continue or if they bother you. It is possible that these symptoms may be more severe if SUSTIVA is used with alcohol or mood altering (street) drugs.

If you are dizzy, have trouble concentrating, or are drowsy, avoid activities that may be dangerous, such as driving or operating machinery.

Rash is common. Rashes usually go away without any change in treatment. In a small number of patients, rash may be serious. If you develop a rash, call your doctor right away. **Rash may be a serious problem in some children.** Tell your child's doctor right away if you notice rash or any other side effects while your child is taking SUSTIVA.

Other common side effects include tiredness, upset stomach, vomiting, and diarrhea. Some patients taking SUSTIVA have experienced increased levels of lipids (cholesterol and triglycerides) in the blood.

Changes in body fat. Changes in body fat develop in some patients taking anti-HIV medicine. These changes may include an increased amount of fat in the upper back and neck ("buffalo hump"), in the breasts, and around the trunk. Loss of fat from the legs, arms, and face may also happen. The cause and long-term health effects of these fat changes are not known.

Liver problems. Some patients taking SUSTIVA have experienced serious liver problems including liver failure resulting in transplantation or death. Most of these serious side effects occurred in patients with a chronic liver disease such as hepatitis infection, but there have also been a few reports in patients without any existing liver disease.

Table 8 *(cont.)*: Effect of Efavirenz on Coadministered Drug Plasma C_{max}, AUC, and C_{min}

Coadministered Drug	Dose	Efavirenz Dose	Number of Subjects	Coadministered Drug (mean % change) C_{max} (90% CI)	AUC (90% CI)	C_{min} (90% CI)
Voriconazole	400 mg po q12h × 1 day, then 200 mg po q12h × 8 days	400 mg qd × 9 days	NA	↓ 61%[h]	↓ 77%[h]	NA
	300 mg po q12h days 2-7	300 mg qd × 7 days	NA	↓ 36%[i] (21-49%)	↓ 55%[i] (45-62%)	NA
	400 mg po q12h days 2-7	300 mg qd × 7 days	NA	↑ 23%[i] (↓ 1-↑ 53%)	↓ 7%[i] (↓ 23-↑ 13%)	NA
Atorvastatin	10 mg qd × 4 days	600 mg qd × 15 days	14	↓ 14% (1-26%)	↓ 43% (34-50%)	↓ 69% (49-81%)
Total active (including metabolites)				↓ 15% (2-26%)	↓ 32% (21-41%)	↓ 48% (23-64%)
Pravastatin	40 mg qd × 4 days	600 mg qd × 15 days	13	↓ 32% (↓ 59-↑ 12%)	↓ 44% (26-57%)	↓ 19% (0-35%)
Simvastatin	40 mg qd × 4 days	600 mg qd × 15 days	14	↓ 72% (63-79%)	↓ 68% (62-73%)	↓ 45% (20-62%)
Total active (including metabolites)				↓ 68% (55-78%)	↓ 60% (52-68%)	NA[j]
Carbamazepine	200 mg qd × 3 days, 200 mg bid × 3 days, then 400 mg qd × 29 days	600 mg qd × 14 days	12	↓ 20% (15-24%)	↓ 27% (20-33%)	↓ 35% (24-44%)
Epoxide metabolite				↔	↔	↓ 13% (↓ 30-↑ 7%)
Cetirizine	10 mg single dose	600 mg qd × 10 days	11	↓ 24% (18-30%)	↔	NA
Diltiazem	240 mg × 21 days	600 mg qd × 14 days	13	↓ 60% (50-68%)	↓ 69% (55-79%)	↓ 63% (44-75%)
Desacetyl diltiazem				↓ 64% (57-69%)	↓ 75% (59-84%)	↓ 62% (44-75%)
N-monodesmethyl diltiazem				↓ 28% (7-44%)	↓ 37% (17-52%)	↓ 37% (17-52%)
Ethinyl estradiol/ Norgestimate	0.035 mg/ 0.25 mg × 14 days	600 mg qd × 14 days				
Ethinyl estradiol			21	↔	↔	↔
Norelgestromin			21	↓ 46% (39-52%)	↓ 64% (62-67%)	↓ 82% (79-85%)
Levonorgestrel			6	↓ 80% (77-83%)	↓ 83% (79-87%)	↓ 86% (80-90%)
Lorazepam	2 mg single dose	600 mg qd × 10 days	12	↑ 16% (2-32%)	↔	NA
Methadone	Stable maintenance 35-100 mg daily	600 mg qd × 14-21 days	11	↓ 45% (25-59%)	↓ 52% (33-66%)	NA
Bupropion	150 mg single dose (sustained-release)	600 mg qd × 14 days	13	↓ 34% (21-47%)	↓ 55% (48-62%)	NA
Hydroxy-bupropion				↑ 50% (20-80%)	↔	NA
Paroxetine	20 mg qd × 14 days	600 mg qd × 14 days	16	↔	↔	↔
Sertraline	50 mg qd × 14 days	600 mg qd × 14 days	13	↓ 29% (15-40%)	↓ 39% (27-50%)	↓ 46% (31-58%)

↑ Indicates increase ↓ Indicates decrease ↔ Indicates no change or a mean increase or decrease of <10%.
[a] Compared with atazanavir 400 mg qd alone.
[b] Comparator dose of indinavir was 800 mg q8h × 10 days.
[c] Parallel-group design; n for efavirenz + lopinavir/ritonavir, n for lopinavir/ritonavir alone.
[d] Values are for lopinavir; the pharmacokinetics of ritonavir in this study were unaffected by concurrent efavirenz.
[e] 95% CI.
[f] Soft Gelatin Capsule.
[g] Tenofovir disoproxil fumarate.
[h] 90% CI not available.
[i] Relative to steady-state administration of voriconazole (400 mg for 1 day, then 200 mg po q12h for 2 days).
[j] Not available because of insufficient data.
NA = not available.

Tell your doctor or healthcare provider if you notice any side effects while taking SUSTIVA (efavirenz).

Contact your doctor before stopping SUSTIVA because of side effects or for any other reason.

This is not a complete list of side effects possible with SUSTIVA (efavirenz). Ask your doctor or pharmacist for a more complete list of side effects of SUSTIVA and all the medicines you will take.

How should I take SUSTIVA?

- Take SUSTIVA (efavirenz) exactly as your doctor tells you to. Do not stop taking SUSTIVA unless your doctor tells you to.
- SUSTIVA must be used with other anti-HIV medicines.
- You should take SUSTIVA on an empty stomach at bedtime. Some side effects may bother you less if you take SUSTIVA at bedtime.
- SUSTIVA comes as tablets or capsules.
- The usual dose of SUSTIVA for adults is 600 mg (one tablet or three 200 mg capsules) taken 1 time each day
- SUSTIVA tablets should not be broken.
- Swallow SUSTIVA tablets or capsules whole with liquid.
- If you have difficulty swallowing tablets or capsules, tell your doctor. If your doctor recommends opening the SUSTIVA capsule and mixing the contents with food or infant formula, see the detailed "Instructions for Use" at the end of this Patient Information leaflet for information about the right way to take a dose of SUSTIVA using the capsule sprinkle method.
- Ask your doctor or pharmacist if you have any questions about how to take a dose of SUSTIVA using the capsule sprinkle method.
- The dose of SUSTIVA for children may be lower than the dose for adults. Capsules containing lower amounts of SUSTIVA are available. Your child's doctor will prescribe the right dose based on your child's weight.
- Taking SUSTIVA with food increases the amount of medicine in your body. This may cause side effects to happen more often.
- Adults and children who take SUSTIVA using the capsule sprinkle method should not eat for 2 hours after taking a dose of SUSTIVA.
- Babies should not be given infant formula for 2 hours after taking a dose of SUSTIVA using the capsule sprinkle method.
- Talk with your doctor to help decide the best schedule for giving your baby SUSTIVA mixed with infant formula using the capsule sprinkle method.
- Do not miss a dose of SUSTIVA. If you forget to take SUSTIVA, take the missed dose right away, unless it is almost time for your next dose. Do not take 2 doses at one time. Just take your next dose at your regularly scheduled time. If you need help in planning the best times to take your medicine, ask your doctor or pharmacist.
- If you believe you took more than the prescribed amount of SUSTIVA, contact your local Poison Control Center or emergency room right away.
- Tell your doctor if you start any new medicine or change how you take any of your current medicines. Your doses may need to be changed.
- When your SUSTIVA supply starts to run low, get more from your doctor or pharmacy. This is very important because the amount of virus in your blood may increase if the medicine is stopped for even a short time. The virus may develop resistance to SUSTIVA and become harder to treat.
- Your doctor may want to do blood tests to check for certain side effects while you take SUSTIVA (efavirenz).

Who should not take SUSTIVA?

Do not take SUSTIVA if you are allergic to efavirenz or any of the ingredients in SUSTIVA. You can ask your doctor or pharmacist for a list of the ingredients in SUSTIVA.

What should I avoid while taking SUSTIVA?

- **Women should not become pregnant while taking SUSTIVA and for 12 weeks after stopping it.** Serious birth defects have been seen in the offspring of animals and women treated with SUSTIVA during pregnancy. It is not known whether SUSTIVA caused these defects. **Tell your doctor right away if you are pregnant.** Also talk with your doctor if you want to become pregnant.
- Women should not rely only on hormone-based birth control, such as pills, injections, or implants, because SUSTIVA may make these contraceptives ineffective. Women must use a reliable form of barrier contraception, such as a condom or diaphragm, even if they also use other methods of birth control. SUSTIVA may remain in your blood for a time after therapy is stopped. Therefore, you should continue to use contraceptive measures for 12 weeks after you stop taking SUSTIVA.
- **Do not breast-feed if you are taking SUSTIVA.** It is not known if SUSTIVA can be passed to your baby in your breast milk and whether it could harm your baby. Also, mothers with HIV-1 should not breast-feed because HIV-1 can be passed to the baby in the breast milk. Talk with your doctor if you are breast-feeding. You may need to stop breast-feeding or use a different medicine.
- Taking SUSTIVA with alcohol or other medicines causing similar side effects as SUSTIVA, such as drowsiness, may increase those side effects.
- Do not take any other medicines without checking with your doctor. These medicines include prescription and nonprescription medicines and herbal products, especially St. John's wort *(Hypericum perforatum)*.

Before using SUSTIVA, tell your doctor if you

- **have problems with your liver or have hepatitis.** Your doctor may want to do tests to check your liver while you take SUSTIVA or may switch you to another medicine.
- **have ever had mental illness or are using drugs or alcohol.**
- **have ever had seizures or are taking medicine for seizures** [for example, Dilantin (phenytoin), Tegretol (carbamazepine), or phenobarbital]. Your doctor may want to switch you to another medicine or check drug levels in your blood from time to time.

What important information should I know about taking other medicines with SUSTIVA?

SUSTIVA may change the effect of other medicines, including ones for HIV, and cause serious side effects. Your doctor may change your other medicines or change their doses. Other medicines, including herbal products, may affect SUSTIVA (efavirenz). For this reason, **it is very important to:**

- let all your doctors and pharmacists know that you take SUSTIVA (efavirenz).
- tell your doctors and pharmacists about all medicines you take. This includes those you buy over-the-counter and herbal or natural remedies.

Bring all your prescription and nonprescription medicines as well as any herbal remedies that you are taking when you see a doctor, or make a list of their names, how much you take, and how often you take them. This will give your doctor a complete picture of the medicines you use. Then he or she can decide the best approach for your situation.

Do not take SUSTIVA with St. John's wort *(Hypericum perforatum)*, an herbal product sold as a dietary supplement, or products containing St. John's wort. Taking St. John's wort

Table 9: Effect of Coadministered Drug on Efavirenz Plasma C_{max}, AUC, and C_{min}

Coadministered Drug	Dose	Efavirenz Dose	Number of Subjects	Efavirenz (mean % change) C_{max} (90% CI)	AUC (90% CI)	C_{min} (90% CI)
Indinavir	800 mg q8h × 14 days	200 mg qd × 14 days	11	↔	↔	↔
Lopinavir/ ritonavir	400/100 mg q12h × 9 days	600 mg qd × 9 days	11,12[a]	↔	↓ 16% (↓ 38-↑ 15%)	↓ 16% (↓ 42-↑ 20%)
Nelfinavir	750 mg q8h × 7 days	600 mg qd × 7 days	10	↓ 12% (↓ 32-↑ 13%)[b]	↓ 12% (↓ 35-↑ 18%)[b]	↓ 21% (↓ 53-↑ 33%)
Ritonavir	500 mg q12h × 8 days	600 mg qd × 10 days	9	↑ 14% (4-26%)	↑ 21% (10-34%)	↑ 25% (7-46%)[b]
Saquinavir SGC[c]	1200 mg q8h × 10 days	600 mg qd × 10 days	13	↓ 13% (5-20%)	↓ 12% (4-19%)	↓ 14% (2-24%)[b]
Tenofovir[d]	300 mg qd	600 mg qd × 14 days	30	↔	↔	↔
Boceprevir	800 mg tid × 6 days	600 mg qd × 16 days	NA	↑ 11% (2-20%)	↑ 20% (15-26%)	NA
Telaprevir	750 mg q8h × 10 days	600 mg qd × 20 days	21	↓ 16% (7-24%)	↓ 7% (2-13%)	↓ 2% (↓ 6-↑ 2%)
Telaprevir, coadministered with tenofovir disoproxil fumarate (TDF)	1125 mg q8h × 7 days	600 mg efavirenz/300 mg TDF qd × 7 days	15	↓ 24% (15-32%)	↓ 18% (10-26%)	↓ 10% (↓ 19-↑ 1%)
	1500 mg q12h × 7 days	600 mg efavirenz/300 mg TDF qd × 7 days	16	↓ 20% (14-26%)	↓ 15% (9-21%)	↓ 11% (4-18%)
Azithromycin	600 mg single dose	400 mg qd × 7 days	14	↔	↔	↔
Clarithromycin	500 mg q12h × 7 days	400 mg qd × 7 days	12	↑ 11% (3-19%)	↔	↔
Fluconazole	200 mg × 7 days	400 mg qd × 7 days	10	↔	↑ 16% (6-26%)	↑ 22% (5-41%)
Itraconazole	200 mg q12h × 14 days	600 mg qd × 28 days	16	↔	↔	↔
Rifabutin	300 mg qd × 14 days	600 mg qd × 14 days	11	↔	↔	↓ 12% (↓ 24-↑ 1%)
Rifampin	600 mg × 7 days	600 mg qd × 7 days	12	↓ 20% (11-28%)	↓ 26% (15-36%)	↓ 32% (15-46%)
Voriconazole	400 mg po q12h × 1 day, then 200 mg po q12h × 8 days	400 mg qd × 9 days	NA	↑ 38%[e]	↑ 44%[e]	NA
	300 mg po q12h days 2-7	300 mg qd × 7 days	NA	↓ 14%[f] (7-21%)	↔[f]	NA
	400 mg po q12h days 2-7	300 mg qd × 7 days	NA	↔[f]	↑ 17%[f] (6-29%)	NA
Atorvastatin	10 mg qd × 4 days	600 mg qd × 15 days	14	↔	↔	↔
Pravastatin	40 mg qd × 4 days	600 mg qd × 15 days	11	↔	↔	↔
Simvastatin	40 mg qd × 4 days	600 mg qd × 15 days	14	↓ 12% (↓ 28-↑ 8%)	↔	↓ 12% (↓ 25-↑ 3%)

(Table continued on next page)

Table 9 *(cont.)*: Effect of Coadministered Drug on Efavirenz Plasma C_{max}, AUC, and C_{min}

Coadministered Drug	Dose	Efavirenz Dose	Number of Subjects	Efavirenz (mean % change) C_{max} (90% CI)	AUC (90% CI)	C_{min} (90% CI)
Aluminum hydroxide 400 mg, magnesium hydroxide 400 mg, plus simethicone 40 mg	30 mL single dose	400 mg single dose	17	↔	↔	NA
Carbamazepine	200 mg qd × 3 days, 200 mg bid × 3 days, then 400 mg qd × 15 days	600 mg qd × 35 days	14	↓ 21% (15-26%)	↓ 36% (32-40%)	↓ 47% (41-53%)
Cetirizine	10 mg single dose	600 mg qd × 10 days	11	↔	↔	↔
Diltiazem	240 mg × 14 days	600 mg qd × 28 days	12	↑ 16% (6-26%)	↑ 11% (5-18%)	↑ 13% (1-26%)
Famotidine	40 mg single dose	400 mg single dose	17	↔	↔	NA
Paroxetine	20 mg qd × 14 days	600 mg qd × 14 days	12	↔	↔	↔
Sertraline	50 mg qd × 14 days	600 mg qd × 14 days	13	↑ 11% (6-16%)	↔	↔

↑ Indicates increase ↓ Indicates decrease ↔ Indicates no change or a mean increase or decrease of <10%.
[a] Parallel-group design; n for efavirenz + lopinavir/ritonavir, n for efavirenz alone.
[b] 95% CI.
[c] Soft Gelatin Capsule.
[d] Tenofovir disoproxil fumarate.
[e] 90% CI not available.
[f] Relative to steady-state administration of efavirenz (600 mg once daily for 9 days).
NA = not available.

Table 10: Outcomes of Randomized Treatment Through 48 and 168 Weeks, Study 006

Outcome	SUSTIVA + ZDV + LAM (n=422) Week 48	Week 168	SUSTIVA + IDV (n=429) Week 48	Week 168	IDV + ZDV + LAM (n=415) Week 48	Week 168
Responder[a]	69%	48%	57%	40%	50%	29%
Virologic failure[b]	6%	12%	15%	20%	13%	19%
Discontinued for adverse events	7%	8%	6%	8%	16%	20%
Discontinued for other reasons[c]	17%	31%	22%	32%	21%	32%
CD4+ cell count (cells/mm^3)						
Observed subjects (n)	(279)	(205)	(256)	(158)	(228)	(129)
Mean change from baseline	190	329	191	319	180	329

[a] Patients achieved and maintained confirmed HIV-1 RNA <400 copies/mL through Week 48 or Week 168.
[b] Includes patients who rebounded, patients who were on study at Week 48 and failed to achieve confirmed HIV-1 RNA <400 copies/mL at time of discontinuation, and patients who discontinued due to lack of efficacy.
[c] Includes consent withdrawn, lost to follow-up, noncompliance, never treated, missing data, protocol violation, death, and other reasons. Patients with HIV-1 RNA levels <400 copies/mL who chose not to continue in the voluntary extension phases of the study were censored at date of last dose of study medication.

Table 11: Outcomes of Randomized Treatment Through 48 Weeks, Study ACTG 364*

Outcome	SUSTIVA + NFV + NRTIs (n=65)	SUSTIVA + NRTIs (n=65)	NFV + NRTIs (n=66)
HIV-1 RNA <500 copies/mL[a]	71%	63%	41%
HIV-1 RNA ≥500 copies/mL[b]	17%	34%	54%
CDC Category C Event	2%	0%	0%
Discontinuations for adverse events[c]	3%	3%	5%
Discontinuations for other reasons[d]	8%	0%	0%

* For some patients, Week 56 data were used to confirm the status at Week 48.
[a] Subjects achieved virologic response (two consecutive viral loads <500 copies/mL) and maintained it through Week 48.
[b] Includes viral rebound and failure to achieve confirmed <500 copies/mL by Week 48.
[c] See *Adverse Reactions (6.1)* for a safety profile of these regimens.
[d] Includes loss to follow-up, consent withdrawn, noncompliance.

may decrease SUSTIVA (efavirenz) levels and lead to increased viral load and possible resistance to SUSTIVA or cross-resistance to other anti-HIV drugs.

MEDICINES YOU SHOULD NOT TAKE WITH SUSTIVA

- The following medicines may cause serious and life-threatening side effects when taken with SUSTIVA. You should not take any of these medicines while taking SUSTIVA:
  - Vascor (bepridil)
  - Propulsid (cisapride)
  - Versed (midazolam)
  - Orap (pimozide)
  - Halcion (triazolam)
  - Ergot medications (for example, Wigraine and Cafergot)

You should not take SUSTIVA with ATRIPLA (efavirenz, emtricitabine, tenofovir disoproxil fumarate) unless your doctor tells you to.

The following medicines may need to be replaced with another medicine when taken with SUSTIVA:

- Fortovase, Invirase (saquinavir)
- Biaxin (clarithromycin)
- Carbatrol, Tegretol (carbamazepine)
- Noxafil (posaconazole)
- Sporanox (itraconazole)
- REYATAZ (atazanavir sulfate), if this is not the first time you are receiving treatment for your HIV infection
- Victrelis (boceprevir)

The following medicines may require a change in the dose of either SUSTIVA or the other medicine:

- Calcium channel blockers such as Cardizem or Tiazac (diltiazem), Covera HS or Isoptin SR (verapamil), and others.
- The cholesterol-lowering medicines Lipitor (atorvastatin), PRAVACHOL (pravastatin sodium), and Zocor (simvastatin).
- Crixivan (indinavir)
- Kaletra (lopinavir/ritonavir)
- Methadone
- Mycobutin (rifabutin)
- REYATAZ (atazanavir sulfate). If you are taking SUSTIVA and REYATAZ, you should also be taking Norvir (ritonavir).
- Rifadin (rifampin) or the rifampin-containing medicines Rifamate and Rifater.
- Selzentry (maraviroc)
- Vfend (voriconazole) and SUSTIVA must not be taken together at standard doses. Some doses of voriconazole can be taken at the same time as a lower dose of SUSTIVA, but you must check with your doctor first.
- Zoloft (sertraline)
- Wellbutrin, Wellbutrin SR, Wellbutrin XL, or Zyban (bupropion)
- The immunosuppressant medicines cyclosporine (Gengraf, Neoral, Sandimmune, and others), Prograf (tacrolimus), or Rapamune (sirolimus).

These are not all the medicines that may cause problems if you take SUSTIVA. Be sure to tell your doctor about all medicines that you take.

General advice about SUSTIVA:

Medicines are sometimes prescribed for conditions that are not mentioned in patient information leaflets. Do not use SUSTIVA for a condition for which it was not prescribed. Do not give SUSTIVA to other people, even if they have the same symptoms you have. It may harm them.

Keep SUSTIVA at room temperature between 68°F to 77°F (20°C to 25°C).

Keep SUSTIVA out of the reach of children.

This leaflet summarizes the most important information about SUSTIVA. If you would like more information, talk with your doctor. You can ask your pharmacist or doctor for the full prescribing information about SUSTIVA, or you can visit the SUSTIVA website at *www.sustiva.com* or call 1-800-321-1335.

SUSTIVA is a registered trademark of Bristol-Myers Squibb Pharma Company, ATRIPLA is a trademark of Bristol-Myers Squibb & Gilead Sciences, LLC, PRAVACHOL is a registered trademark of ER Squibb & Sons, LLC, and REYATAZ is a registered trademark of Bristol-Myers Squibb Company. Other brands listed are the trademarks of their respective owners.

Distributed by:
Bristol-Myers Squibb Company
Princeton, NJ 08543 USA
SUSTIVA® (efavirenz) capsules made in India.

Rev May 2013

Instructions for Use
SUSTIVA (sus-TEE-vah)
efavirenz
capsules

Preparing a dose of SUSTIVA using the capsule sprinkle method

Read this Instructions for Use before you prepare your first dose of SUSTIVA mixed with food or infant formula using the capsule sprinkle method, each time you get a refill, and as needed. There may be new information. This information does not take the place of talking to your doctor about your medical condition or treatment. Ask your doctor or pharmacist if you have any questions about how to mix or give a dose of SUSTIVA (efavirenz) using the capsule sprinkle method.

Important Information:

- For more information about SUSTIVA capsules, see the Patient Information leaflet.
- The capsule sprinkle method for mixing the contents of SUSTIVA capsules with soft food or infant formula may be used for adults or children who cannot swallow capsules or tablets.
- You should take SUSTIVA on an empty stomach at bedtime.
- You should not eat for 2 hours after taking SUSTIVA mixed with food.
- Babies who are old enough to swallow food should be given SUSTIVA using the capsule sprinkle method mixed with food instead of with infant formula.
- Talk with your doctor to help decide the best schedule for giving your baby SUSTIVA mixed with infant formula using the capsule sprinkle method.

Preparing a dose of SUSTIVA mixed with food using the capsule sprinkle method.

Before you prepare a dose of SUSTIVA mixed with food using the capsule sprinkle method, gather the following supplies:

- paper towels
- small spoon
- **small** clean container (such as a **small** cup or bowl)
- soft food such as applesauce, grape jelly, or yogurt

Step 1. Choose a clean, flat work surface. Place a clean paper towel on the work surface. Then place the other supplies on the paper towel.

Step 2. Wash and dry your hands well.

Step 3. Place 1 to 2 teaspoons of soft food such as applesauce, grape jelly, or yogurt in the small container (see Figure A). The color and thickness of the food may change when mixed with the medicine.

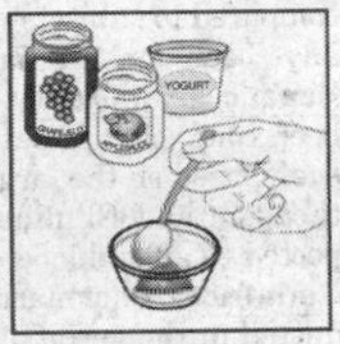

Figure A

Step 4. There are 2 parts of the SUSTIVA capsule. Look at the SUSTIVA capsule to see which part of the capsule overlaps the other part (see Figure B).

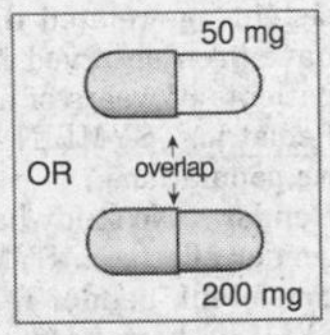

Figure B

Step 5. Turn the SUSTIVA capsule so that you are holding it in a sideways (horizontal) position directly over the container of food. Hold each end of the SUSTIVA capsule between your thumbs and index (pointer) fingers (see Figure C).

Figure C

Step 6. Use your thumb and index finger to pinch near the end of the overlapping part of the SUSTIVA capsule (see Figure D).

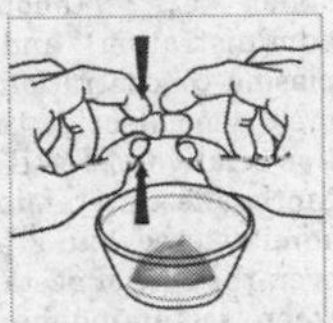

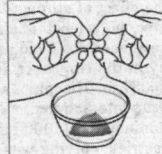

Figure D

Then, carefully twist both ends of the SUSTIVA capsule in opposite directions to open it (see Figure E). Be careful not to spill the capsule contents or spread it in the air.

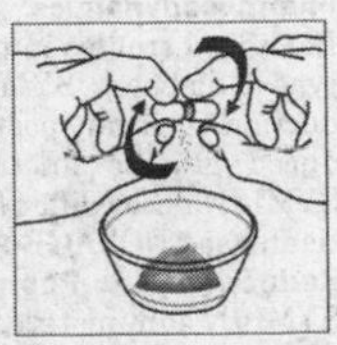

Figure E

Step 7. Sprinkle the contents of the SUSTIVA capsule onto the food (see Figure F). Throw away the empty capsule shells.

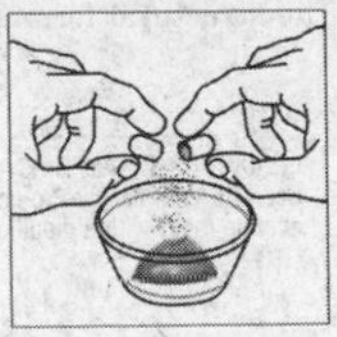

Figure F

If the total prescribed dose is more than 1 capsule, follow Steps 4 through 7 for each capsule. Do not add more food.

Steps 8 through 11 must be completed **within 30 minutes** of mixing the medicine.

Step 8. Use a spoon to gently mix the capsule contents and food together (see Figure G).

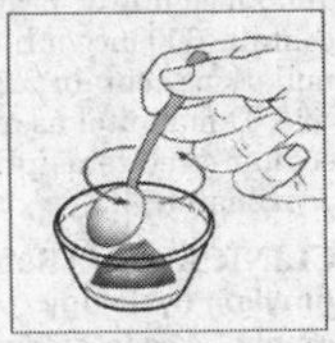

Figure G

Step 9. Use the spoon to take the food and capsule contents mixture or feed it to your child. Swallow all of the mixture. If you are giving the mixture to your child, look in your child's mouth to make sure that all of the mixture is swallowed.

Step 10. Add about 2 teaspoons more of the food to the empty container and gently stir to mix with any capsule contents that may still be in the container.

Step 11. Use the spoon to take the mixture or feed it to your child. Swallow all of the mixture. If you are giving the mixture to your child, look in your child's mouth to make sure that all of the mixture is swallowed.

Step 12. Wash the container and spoon. Throw away the paper towel and clean the work surface.

Step 13. Wash your hands.

Preparing a dose of SUSTIVA mixed with infant formula using the capsule sprinkle method

Before you prepare a dose of SUSTIVA mixed with infant formula using the capsule sprinkle method, gather the following supplies:

- paper towels
- small spoon
- 30 milliliter (mL) medicine cup (ask your pharmacist for this). See Figure H.
- 10 mL oral dosing syringe (ask your pharmacist for this). See Figure H.
- infant formula at room temperature. If you are using powdered formula, you should prepare the formula according to the formula directions before mixing with SUSTIVA capsule contents.

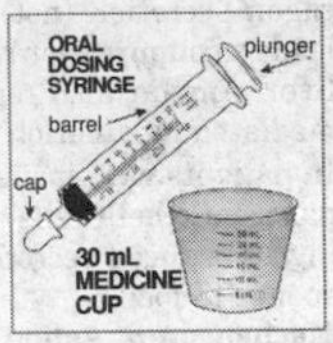

Figure H

Step 1. Choose a clean, flat work surface. Place a clean paper towel on the work surface. Place the supplies you will need on the paper towel.

Step 2. Wash and dry your hands well.

Step 3. Pour 10 mL of room temperature infant formula into the 30 mL medicine cup (see Figure I).

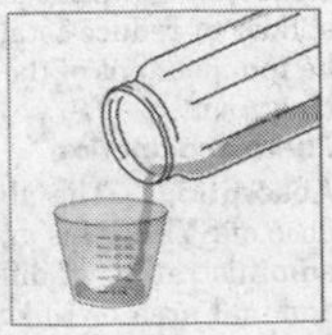

Figure I

Step 4. There are 2 parts of the SUSTIVA capsule. Look at the SUSTIVA capsule to see which part of the capsule overlaps the other part (see Figure J).

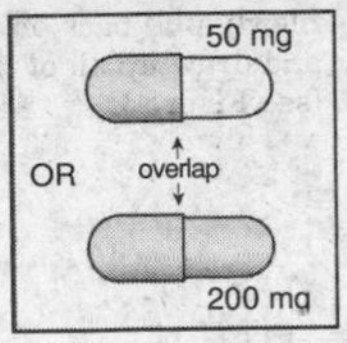

Figure J

Step 5. Turn the SUSTIVA capsule so that you are holding it in a sideways (horizontal) position directly over the medicine cup that contains the infant formula. Hold each end of the SUSTIVA capsule between your thumbs and index (pointer) fingers (see Figure K).

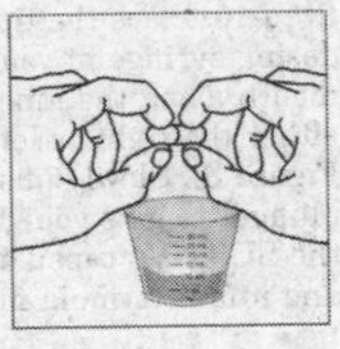

Figure K

Step 6. Use your thumb and index finger to pinch near the end of the overlapping part of the SUSTIVA capsule (see Figure L).

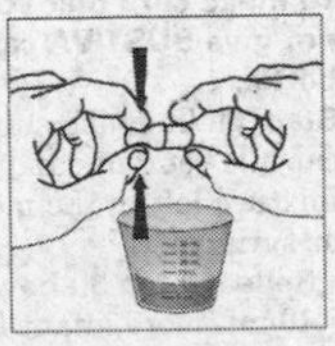

Figure L

Then, carefully twist both ends of the SUSTIVA capsule in opposite directions to open it (see Figure M). Be careful not to spill the capsule contents or spread it in the air.

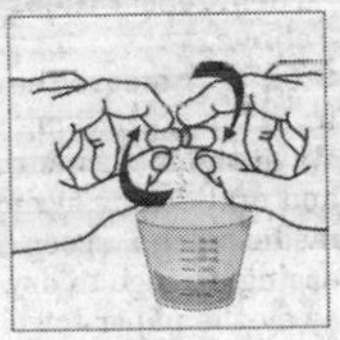

Figure M

Step 7. Sprinkle the contents of the SUSTIVA capsule onto the infant formula (see Figure N). Throw away the empty capsule shells.

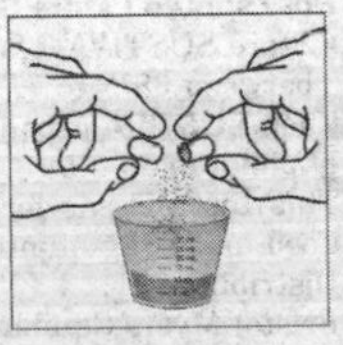

Figure N

If the total prescribed dose is more than 1 capsule, follow Steps 4 through 7 for each capsule. Do not add more infant formula.

Steps 8 through 11 must be completed **within 30 minutes** of mixing the medicine.

Step 8. Hold the medicine cup with one hand. With your other hand, use the small spoon to gently mix the capsule contents and the infant formula (see Figure O).

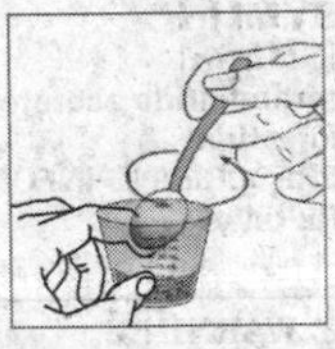

Figure O

Step 9. Draw up the capsule contents and infant formula mixture into the 10 mL oral dosing syringe as follows:

- Check that the plunger is completely pushed into barrel of the syringe (see Figure P).

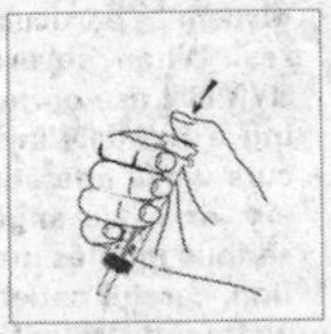

Figure P

- Place the tip of the syringe into the capsule contents and infant formula mixture in the medicine cup (see Figure Q).

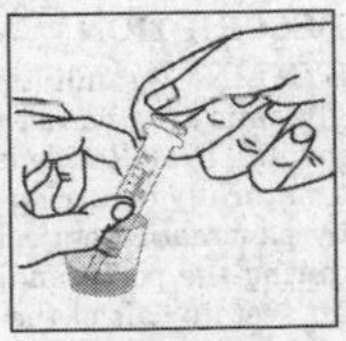

Figure Q

- Slowly pull back on the plunger and draw up all of the mixture (see Figure R).

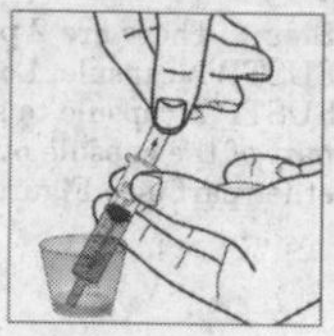

Figure R

Step 10. Place the tip of the oral dosing syringe in your baby's mouth along the inner cheek on either the right or left side (see Figure S). Slowly push on the plunger to give your baby all of the SUSTIVA capsule contents and infant formula mixture.

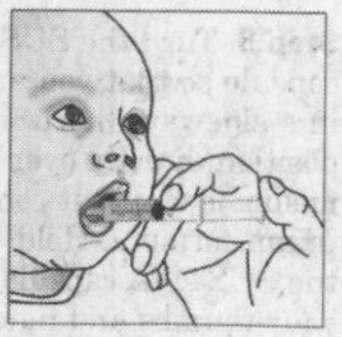

Figure S

To make sure that your baby gets all of the medicine, do not give SUSTIVA capsule contents to your baby in a bottle.

Step 11. To make sure there is no capsule contents and formula mixture left in the medicine cup or syringe:

- **Repeat Step 3 above** to add 10 mL more infant formula into the medicine cup.
- Stir with a small spoon.
- Then, repeat **Steps 9 and 10 above.**

Step 12. Remove the plunger from the oral dosing syringe. Wash the medicine cup, spoon, and oral dosing syringe. Allow the medicine cup, spoon, and oral dosing syringe to dry. Throw away the paper towel and clean the work surface.

Step 13. Wash your hands.

How should I store SUSTIVA capsules?

- Store SUSTIVA (efavirenz) capsules at room temperature between 68°F to 77°F (20°C to 25°C).

Keep SUSTIVA capsules and all medicines out of the reach of children.

This Instructions for Use has been approved by the U.S. Food and Drug Administration.

Distributed by:
Bristol-Myers Squibb Company
Princeton, NJ 08543 USA
SUSTIVA® (efavirenz) capsules made in India.
Issued: May 2013

Shown in Product Identification Guide, page 306

SYMLIN® ℞

[SĬM-lĭn]
(pramlintide acetate)
injection
PRESCRIBING INFORMATION
Rx only

WARNING

SYMLIN is used with insulin and has been associated with an increased risk of insulin-induced severe hypoglycemia, particularly in patients with type 1 diabetes. When severe hypoglycemia associated with SYMLIN use occurs, it is seen within 3 hours following a SYMLIN injection. If severe hypoglycemia occurs while operating a motor vehicle, heavy machinery, or while engaging in other high-risk activities, serious injuries may occur. Appropriate patient selection, careful patient instruction, and insulin dose adjustments are critical elements for reducing this risk.

DESCRIPTION

SYMLIN® (pramlintide acetate) injection is an antihyperglycemic drug for use in patients with diabetes treated with insulin. Pramlintide is a synthetic analog of human amylin, a naturally occurring neuroendocrine hormone synthesized by pancreatic beta cells that contributes to glucose control during the postprandial period. Pramlintide is provided as an acetate salt of the synthetic 37-amino acid polypeptide, which differs in amino acid sequence from human amylin by replacement with proline at positions 25 (alanine), 28 (serine), and 29 (serine).

The structural formula of pramlintide acetate is as shown:

Lys-Cys-Asn-Thr-Ala-Thr-Cys-Ala-Thr-Gln-Arg-Leu-Ala-Asn-Phe-Leu-Val-His-Ser-Ser-Asn-Asn-Phe-Gly-Pro-Ile-Leu-Pro-Pro-Thr-Asn-Val-Gly-Ser-Asn-Thr-Tyr-NH_2 acetate (salt) with a disulfide bridge between the two Cys residues.

Pramlintide acetate is a white powder that has a molecular formula of $C_{171}H_{267}N_{51}O_{53}S2 \bullet \times C_2H_4O_2$ ($3 \leq \times \leq 8$); the molecular weight is 3949.4. Pramlintide acetate is soluble in water.

SYMLIN (pramlintide acetate) is formulated as a clear, isotonic, sterile solution for subcutaneous (SC) administration. The disposable multidose SymlinPen® pen-injector contains 1000 mcg/mL of pramlintide (as acetate); SYMLIN vials contain 600 mcg/mL of pramlintide (as acetate). Both formulations contain 2.25 mg/mL of metacresol as a preservative, D-mannitol as a tonicity modifier, and acetic acid and sodium acetate as pH modifiers. SYMLIN has a pH of approximately 4.0.

CLINICAL PHARMACOLOGY

Amylin Physiology

Amylin is co-located with insulin in secretory granules and co-secreted with insulin by pancreatic beta cells in response to food intake. Amylin and insulin show similar fasting and postprandial patterns in healthy individuals **(Figure 1)**.

Figure 1: Secretion Profile of Amylin and Insulin in Healthy Adults

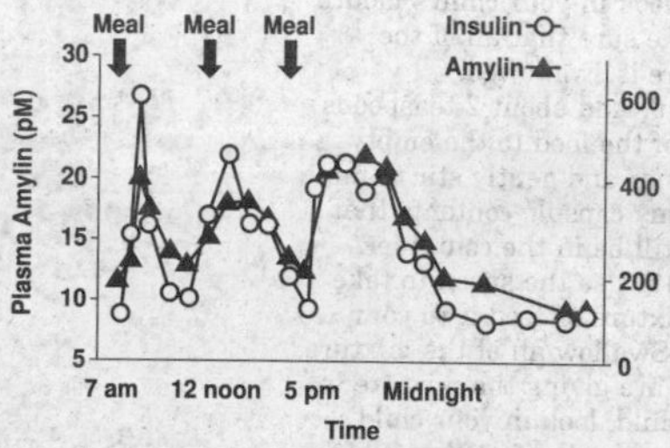

Amylin affects the rate of postprandial glucose appearance through a variety of mechanisms. Amylin slows gastric emptying (i.e., the rate at which food is released from the stomach to the small intestine) without altering the overall absorption of nutrients. In addition, amylin suppresses glucagon secretion (not normalized by insulin alone), which leads to suppression of endogenous glucose output from the liver. Amylin also regulates food intake due to centrally-mediated modulation of appetite.

In patients with insulin-using type 2 or type 1 diabetes, the pancreatic beta cells are dysfunctional or damaged, resulting in reduced secretion of both insulin and amylin in response to food.

Mechanism of Action

SYMLIN, by acting as an amylinomimetic agent, has the following effects: 1) modulation of gastric emptying; 2) prevention of the postprandial rise in plasma glucagon; and 3) satiety leading to decreased caloric intake and potential weight loss.

Gastric Emptying. The gastric-emptying rate is an important determinant of the postprandial rise in plasma glucose. SYMLIN slows the rate at which food is released from the stomach to the small intestine following a meal and, thus, it reduces the initial postprandial increase in plasma glucose. This effect lasts for approximately 3 hours following SYMLIN administration. SYMLIN does not alter the net absorption of ingested carbohydrate or other nutrients.

Postprandial Glucagon Secretion. In patients with diabetes, glucagon concentrations are abnormally elevated during the postprandial period, contributing to hyperglycemia. SYMLIN has been shown to decrease postprandial glucagon concentrations in insulin-using patients with diabetes.

Satiety. SYMLIN administered prior to a meal has been shown to reduce total caloric intake. This effect appears to be independent of the nausea that can accompany SYMLIN treatment.

Pharmacokinetics

Absorption. The absolute bioavailability of a single SC dose of SYMLIN is approximately 30 to 40%. Subcutaneous administration of different doses of SYMLIN into the abdominal area or thigh of healthy subjects resulted in dose-proportionate maximum plasma concentrations (C_{max}) and overall exposure (expressed as area under the plasma concentration curve or (AUC)) **(Table 1)**.

Table 1: Mean Pharmacokinetic Parameters Following Administration of Single SC Doses of SYMLIN

SC Dose (mcg)	$AUC_{(0-\infty)}$ (pmol*min/L)	C_{max} (pmol/L)	T_{max} (min)	Elimination $t_{1/2}$ (min)
30	3750	39	21	55
60	6778	79	20	49
90	8507	102	19	51
120	11970	147	21	48

Injection of SYMLIN (pramlintide acetate) into the arm showed higher exposure with greater variability, compared with exposure after injection of SYMLIN into the abdominal area or thigh.

There was no strong correlation between the degree of adiposity as assessed by BMI or skin fold thickness measurements and relative bioavailability. Injections administered with 6.0-mm and 12.7-mm needles yielded similar bioavailability.

Distribution. SYMLIN does not extensively bind to blood cells or albumin (approximately 40% of the drug is unbound in plasma), and thus SYMLIN's pharmacokinetics should be insensitive to changes in binding sites.

Metabolism and Elimination. In healthy subjects, the half-life of SYMLIN is approximately 48 minutes. SYMLIN is metabolized primarily by the kidneys. Des-lys[1] pramlintide (2–37 pramlintide), the primary metabolite, has a similar half-life and is biologically active both *in vitro* and *in vivo* in rats. AUC values are relatively constant with repeat dosing, indicating no bioaccumulation.

Special Populations.

Renal Insufficiency: Patients with moderate or severe renal impairment (Cl_{Cr} >20 to ≤50 mL/min) did not show increased SYMLIN exposure or reduced SYMLIN clearance, compared to subjects with normal renal function. No studies have been done in dialysis patients.

Hepatic Insufficiency: Pharmacokinetic studies have not been conducted in patients with hepatic insufficiency. However, based on the large degree of renal metabolism (see Metabolism and Elimination), hepatic dysfunction is not expected to affect blood concentrations of SYMLIN.

Geriatric: Pharmacokinetic studies have not been conducted in the geriatric population. SYMLIN should only be used in patients known to fully understand and adhere to proper insulin adjustments and glucose monitoring. No consistent age-related differences in the activity of SYMLIN have been observed in the geriatric population (n=539 for patients 65 years of age or older in the clinical trials).

Pediatric: SYMLIN has not been evaluated in the pediatric population.

Gender: No study has been conducted to evaluate possible gender effects on SYMLIN pharmacokinetics. However, no consistent gender-related differences in the activity of SYMLIN have been observed in the clinical trials (n=2799 for male and n=2085 for female).

Race/Ethnicity: No study has been conducted to evaluate the effect of ethnicity on SYMLIN pharmacokinetics. However, no consistent differences in the activity of SYMLIN have been observed among patients of differing race/ethnicity in the clinical trials (n=4257 for white, n=229 for black, n=337 for Hispanic, and n=61 for other ethnic origins).

Drug Interactions: The effect of SYMLIN (120 mcg) on acetaminophen (1000 mg) pharmacokinetics as a marker of gastric-emptying was evaluated in patients with type 2 diabetes (n=24). SYMLIN did not significantly alter the AUC of acetaminophen. However, SYMLIN decreased acetaminophen C_{max} (about 29% with simultaneous co-administration) and increased the time to maximum plasma concentration or t_{max} (ranging from 48 to 72 minutes) dependent on the time of acetaminophen administration relative to SYMLIN injection. SYMLIN did not significantly affect acetaminophen t_{max} when acetaminophen was administered 1 to 2 hours before SYMLIN injection. However, the t_{max} of acetaminophen was significantly increased when acetaminophen was administered simultaneously with or up to 2 hours following SYMLIN injection (see PRECAUTIONS, Drug Interactions).

Pharmacodynamics

In clinical studies in patients with insulin-using type 2 and type 1 diabetes, SYMLIN administration resulted in a reduction in mean postprandial glucose concentrations, reduced glucose fluctuations, and reduced food intake. SYMLIN doses differ for insulin-using type 2 and type 1 patients (see DOSAGE AND ADMINISTRATION).

Reduction in Postprandial Glucose Concentrations. SYMLIN administered subcutaneously immediately prior to a meal reduced plasma glucose concentrations following the meal when used with regular insulin or rapid-acting insulin analogs **(Figure 2). This reduction in postprandial glucose**

decreased the amount of short-acting insulin required and limited glucose fluctuations based upon 24-hour glucose monitoring. When rapid-acting analog insulins were used, plasma glucose concentrations tended to rise during the interval between 150 minutes following SYMLIN (pramlintide acetate) injection and the next meal (see DOSAGE and ADMINISTRATION).

Figure 2: Postprandial Plasma Glucose Profiles in Patients With Type 2 and Type 1 Diabetes Receiving SYMLIN and/or Insulin

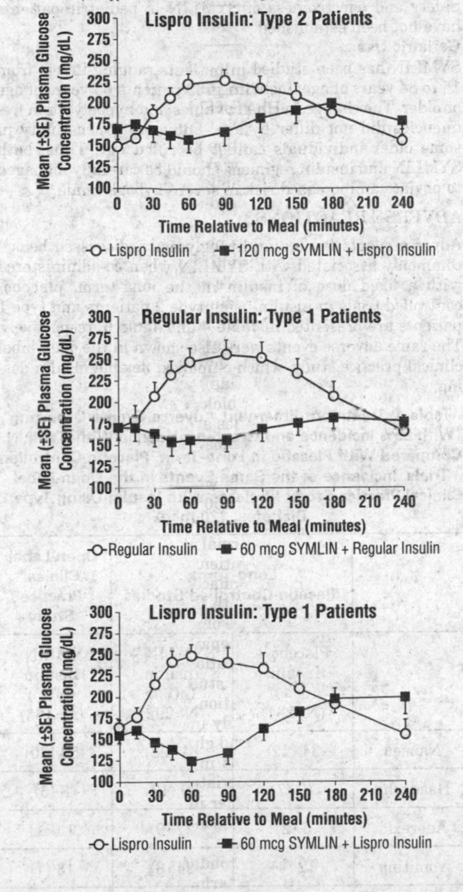

Reduced Food Intake. A single, subcutaneous dose of SYMLIN 120 mcg (type 2) or 30 mcg (type 1) administered 1 hour prior to an unlimited buffet meal was associated with reductions in total caloric intake (placebo-subtracted mean changes of ~23% and 21%, respectively), which occurred without decreases in meal duration.

CLINICAL STUDIES

A total of 5325 patients and healthy volunteers received SYMLIN in clinical studies. This includes 1688 with type 2 diabetes and 2375 with type 1 diabetes in short- and long-term controlled clinical trials, long-term uncontrolled clinical trials, and an open-label study in the clinical practice setting.

Clinical Studies in Type 2 Diabetes

The efficacy of a range of SYMLIN doses was evaluated in several placebo-controlled and open-label clinical trials in insulin-using patients with type 2 diabetes. Based on results obtained in these studies, the recommended dose of SYMLIN for patients with insulin-using type 2 diabetes is 120 mcg administered immediately prior to major meals.

Two, long-term (26 to 52 week), randomized, double-blind, placebo-controlled studies of SYMLIN were conducted in patients with type 2 diabetes using fixed dose insulin to isolate the SYMLIN effect. Demographic and baseline characteristics for the 871 SYMLIN-treated patients are as follows: mean baseline HbA1c ranged from 9.0 to 9.4%, mean age was 56.4 to 59.1 years, mean duration of diabetes ranged from 11.5 to 14.4 years, and mean BMI ranged from 30.1 to 34.4 kg/m^2. In both of these studies, SYMLIN or placebo was added to the participants' existing diabetes therapies, which included insulin with or without a sulfonylurea agent and/or metformin.

Table 2 summarizes the composite results across both studies for patients assigned to the 120-mcg dose after 6 months of treatment.

Table 2: Mean (SE) Change in HbA1c, Weight, and Insulin at 6 Months in the Double-Blind, Placebo-Controlled Studies in Patients With Insulin-Using Type 2 Diabetes

Variable	Placebo	SYMLIN (120 mcg)
Baseline HbA1c (%)	9.3 (0.08)	9.1 (0.06)
Change in HbA1c at 6 Months Relative to Baseline (%)	-0.17 (0.07)	-0.57 (0.06)*
Placebo-Subtracted HbA1c Change at 6 Months (%)	NA	-0.40 (0.09)*
Baseline Weight (kg)	91.3 (1.2)	92.5 (1.2)
Change in Weight at 6 Months Relative to Baseline (kg)	+0.2 (0.2)	-1.5 (0.2)*
Placebo-Subtracted Weight Change at 6 Months (kg)	NA	-1.7 (0.3)*
Percent Change in Insulin Doses at 6 Months: Rapid/Short-Acting	+6.5 (2.7)	-3.0 (1.6)*
Percent Change in Insulin Doses at 6 Months: Long-Acting	+5.2 (1.4)	-0.2 (1.3)*

* Statistically significant reduction compared with placebo (p-value < 0.05).

In a cohort of 145 patients who completed two years of SYMLIN (pramlintide acetate) treatment the baseline-subtracted HbA1c and weight reductions were: -0.40% and -0.36 kg, respectively.

Open-Label Study in the Clinical Practice Setting. An open-label study of SYMLIN was conducted at the recommended dose of 120 mcg in 166 patients with insulin-using type 2 diabetes who were unable to achieve glycemic targets using insulin alone. A flexible-dose insulin regimen was employed in these patients (see DOSAGE and ADMINISTRATION). In this study, patients adjusted their insulin regimen based on pre- and post-meal glucose monitoring. At baseline, mean HbA1c was 8.3%, mean age was 54.4 years, mean duration of diabetes was 13.3 years, and mean BMI was 38.6 kg/m^2. SYMLIN was administered with major meals. SYMLIN plus insulin treatment for 6 months resulted in a baseline-subtracted mean HbA1c reduction of -0.56 ± 0.15% and a baseline-subtracted mean weight reduction of −2.76 ± 0.34 kg. These changes were accomplished with reductions in doses of total, short-acting, and long-acting insulin (-6.4 ± 2.66, -10.3 ± 4.84, and -4.20 ± 2.42%, respectively).

Clinical Studies in Type 1 Diabetes

The efficacy of a range of SYMLIN doses was evaluated in several placebo-controlled and open-label clinical trials conducted in patients with type 1 diabetes. Based on results obtained in these studies, the recommended dose of SYMLIN for patients with type 1 diabetes is 30 mcg or 60 mcg administered immediately prior to major meals.

Three, long-term (26 to 52 week), randomized, double-blind, placebo-controlled studies of SYMLIN were conducted in patients with type 1 diabetes (N=1717). Two of these studies allowed only minimal insulin adjustments in order to isolate the SYMLIN effect; in the third study, insulin adjustments were made according to standard medical practice. Demographic and baseline characteristics for the 1179 SYMLIN-treated patients were as follows: mean baseline HbA1c range was 8.7 to 9.0%, mean age range was 37.3 to 41.9 years, mean duration of diabetes range was 15.5 to 19.2 years, and mean BMI range was 25.0 to 26.8 kg/m^2. SYMLIN or placebo was added to existing insulin therapies. **Table 3** summarizes the composite results across these studies for patients assigned to the 30 or 60 mcg dose after 6 months of treatment.

Table 3: Mean (SE) Change in HbA1c, Weight, and Insulin at 6 Months in the Double-Blind, Placebo-Controlled Studies in Patients With Type 1 Diabetes

Variable	Placebo	SYMLIN (30 or 60 mcg)
Baseline HbA1c (%)	9.0 (0.06)	8.9 (0.04)
Change in HbA1c at 6 Months Relative to Baseline (%)	-0.10 (0.05)	-0.43 (0.04)*
Placebo-Subtracted HbA1c Change at 6 Months (%)	NA	-0.33 (0.06)*
Baseline Weight (kg)	75.1 (0.6)	76.1 (0.5)
Change in Weight at 6 Months Relative to Baseline (kg)	+0.6 (0.1)	1.1 (0.1)*
Placebo-Subtracted Weight Change at 6 Months (kg)	NA	-1.7 (0.1)*
Percent Change in Insulin Doses at 6 Months: Rapid/Short-Acting	+1.7 (3.3)	-3.6 (2.9)
Percent Change in Insulin Doses at 6 Months: Long-Acting	+2.5 (1.9)	+1.9 (1.3)

* Statistically significant reduction compared with placebo (p-value < 0.05).

In a cohort of 73 patients who completed two years of SYMLIN (pramlintide acetate) treatment the baseline-subtracted HbA1c and weight changes were: -0.35% and 0.60 kg, respectively.

SYMLIN Dose-Titration Trial. A dose-titration study of SYMLIN was conducted in patients with type 1 diabetes. Patients with relatively good baseline glycemic control (mean HbA1c = 8.1%) were randomized to receive either insulin plus placebo or insulin plus SYMLIN. Other baseline and demographics characteristics were: mean age of 41 years, mean duration of diabetes of 20 years, mean BMI of 28 kg/m^2. SYMLIN was initiated at a dose of 15 mcg and titrated upward at weekly intervals by 15-mcg increments to doses of 30 mcg or 60 mcg, based on whether patients experienced nausea. Once a tolerated dose of either 30 mcg or 60 mcg was reached, the SYMLIN dose was maintained for the remainder of the study (SYMLIN was administered before major meals). During SYMLIN titration, the insulin dose (mostly the short/rapid-acting insulin) was reduced by 30–50% in order to reduce the occurrence of hypoglycemia. Once a tolerated SYMLIN dose was reached, insulin dose adjustments were made according to standard clinical practice, based on pre- and post-meal blood glucose monitoring. By 6 months of treatment, patients treated with SYMLIN and insulin and patients treated with insulin and placebo had equivalent reductions in mean HbA1c (−0.47 ± 0.07% vs. −0.49 ± 0.07%, respectively); patients on SYMLIN lost weight (−1.33 ± 0.31 kg relative to baseline and −2.6 kg relative to placebo plus insulin-treated patients). SYMLIN-treated patients used less total insulin (−11.7% relative to baseline) and less short/rapid-acting insulin (−22.8%) relative to baseline.

Open-Label Study in the Clinical Practice Setting. An open-label study of SYMLIN was conducted in patients with type 1 diabetes who were unable to achieve glycemic targets using insulin alone. A flexible-dose insulin regimen was employed in these patients after SYMLIN titration was completed (see DOSAGE and ADMINISTRATION). In this study, patients adjusted their insulin regimen based on pre- and post-meal glucose monitoring. At baseline, mean HbA1c was 8.0%, mean age was 42.7 years, mean duration of diabetes was 21.2 years, and mean BMI was 28.6 kg/m^2. SYMLIN daily dosage was 30 mcg or 60 mcg with major meals.

SYMLIN plus insulin reduced HbA1c and body weight from baseline at 6 months by a mean of 0.18% and 3.0 kg, respectively. These changes in glycemic control and body weight were achieved with reductions in doses of total, short-acting, and long-acting insulin (-12.0 ± 1.36, -21.7 ± 2.81, and -0.4 ± 1.59%, respectively).

INDICATIONS AND USAGE

SYMLIN is given at mealtimes and is indicated for:

- Type 1 diabetes, as an adjunct treatment in patients who use mealtime insulin therapy and who have failed to achieve desired glucose control despite optimal insulin therapy.
- Type 2 diabetes, as an adjunct treatment in patients who use mealtime insulin therapy and who have failed to achieve desired glucose control despite optimal insulin therapy, with or without a concurrent sulfonylurea agent and/or metformin.

CONTRAINDICATIONS

SYMLIN is contraindicated in patients with any of the following:

- a known hypersensitivity to SYMLIN or any of its components, including metacresol;
- a confirmed diagnosis of gastroparesis;
- hypoglycemia unawareness.

WARNINGS

Patient Selection

Proper patient selection is critical to safe and effective use of SYMLIN. Before initiation of therapy, the patient's HbA1c, recent blood glucose monitoring data, history of insulin-induced hypoglycemia, current insulin regimen, and body weight should be reviewed. SYMLIN (pramlintide acetate) therapy should only be considered in patients with insulin-using type 2 or type 1 diabetes who fulfill the following criteria:

- have failed to achieve adequate glycemic control despite individualized insulin management;
- are receiving ongoing care under the guidance of a healthcare professional skilled in the use of insulin and supported by the services of diabetes educator(s).

Patients meeting any of the following criteria should NOT be considered for SYMLIN therapy:

- poor compliance with current insulin regimen;
- poor compliance with prescribed self-blood glucose monitoring;
- have an HbA1c >9%;
- recurrent severe hypoglycemia requiring assistance during the past 6 months;
- presence of hypoglycemia unawareness;
- confirmed diagnosis of gastroparesis;
- require the use of drugs that stimulate gastrointestinal motility;
- pediatric patients.

Hypoglycemia. SYMLIN alone does not cause hypoglycemia. However, SYMLIN is indicated to be co-administered with insulin therapy and in this setting SYMLIN increases the risk of insulin-induced severe hypoglycemia, particularly in patients with type 1 diabetes. Severe hypoglycemia associated with SYMLIN occurs within the first 3 hours following a SYMLIN injection. If severe hypoglycemia occurs while operating a motor vehicle, heavy machinery, or while engaging in other high-risk activities, serious injuries may occur. Therefore, when introducing SYMLIN therapy, appropriate precautions need to be taken to avoid increasing the risk for insulin-induced severe hypoglycemia. These precautions include **frequent pre- and post-meal glucose monitoring combined with an initial 50% reduction in pre-meal doses of short-acting insulin (see DOSAGE and ADMINISTRATION).**

Symptoms of hypoglycemia may include hunger, headache, sweating, tremor, irritability, or difficulty concentrating. Rapid reductions in blood glucose concentrations may induce such symptoms regardless of glucose values. More severe symptoms of hypoglycemia include loss of consciousness, coma, or seizure.

Early warning symptoms of hypoglycemia may be different or less pronounced under certain conditions, such as long duration of diabetes; diabetic nerve disease; use of medications such as beta-blockers, clonidine, guanethidine, or reserpine; or intensified diabetes control.

The addition of any antihyperglycemic agent such as SYMLIN to an existing regimen of one or more antihyperglycemic agents (e.g., insulin, sulfonylurea), or other agents that can increase the risk of hypoglycemia may necessitate further insulin dose adjustments and particularly close monitoring of blood glucose.

The following are examples of substances that may increase the blood glucose-lowering effect and susceptibility to hypoglycemia: oral anti-diabetic products, ACE inhibitors, disopyramide, fibrates, fluoxetine, MAO inhibitors, pentoxifylline, propoxyphene, salicylates, and sulfonamide antibiotics.

Clinical studies employing a controlled hypoglycemic challenge have demonstrated that SYMLIN does not alter the counter-regulatory hormonal response to insulin-induced hypoglycemia. Likewise, in SYMLIN-treated patients, the perception of hypoglycemic symptoms was not altered with plasma glucose concentrations as low as 45 mg/dL.

PRECAUTIONS

General

Hypoglycemia (See WARNINGS).

SYMLIN should be prescribed with caution to persons with visual or dexterity impairment.

Information for Patients: Healthcare providers should inform patients of the potential risks and advantages of SYMLIN therapy. Healthcare providers should also inform patients about self-management practices including glucose monitoring, proper injection technique, timing of dosing, and proper storage of SYMLIN. In addition, reinforce the importance of adherence to meal planning, physical activity, recognition and management of hypoglycemia and hyperglycemia, and assessment of diabetes complications. Refer patients to the SYMLIN Medication Guide and Patient Instructions for Use for additional information.

Instruct patients on handling of special situations such as intercurrent conditions (illness or stress), an inadequate or omitted insulin dose, inadvertent administration of increased insulin or SYMLIN dose, inadequate food intake or missed meals.

SYMLIN and insulin should always be administered as separate injections and never be mixed.

Women with diabetes should be advised to inform their healthcare professional if they are pregnant or contemplating pregnancy.

Renal Impairment: The dosing requirements for SYMLIN (pramlintide acetate) are not altered in patients with moderate or severe renal impairment (Cl_{Cr} >20 to ≤50 mL/min). No studies have been done in dialysis patients (see CLINICAL PHARMACOLOGY; Special Populations).

Hepatic Impairment: Studies have not been performed in patients with hepatic impairment. However, hepatic dysfunction is not expected to affect blood concentrations of SYMLIN (see CLINICAL PHARMACOLOGY; Special Populations).

Allergy:

Local allergy. Patients may experience redness, swelling, or itching at the site of injection. These minor reactions usually resolve in a few days to a few weeks. In some instances, these reactions may be related to factors other than SYMLIN, such as irritants in a skin cleansing agent or improper injection technique.

Systemic Allergy. In controlled clinical trials up to 12 months, potential systemic allergic reactions were reported in 65 (5%) of type 2 patients and 59 (5%) of type 1 SYMLIN-treated patients. Similar reactions were reported by 18 (4%) and 28 (5%) of placebo-treated type 2 and type 1 patients, respectively. No patient receiving SYMLIN was withdrawn from a trial due to a potential systemic allergic reaction.

Drug Interactions

Due to its effects on gastric emptying, SYMLIN therapy should not be considered for patients taking drugs that alter gastrointestinal motility (e.g., anticholinergic agents such as atropine) and agents that slow the intestinal absorption of nutrients (e.g., α-glucosidase inhibitors). Patients using these drugs have not been studied in clinical trials.

SYMLIN has the potential to delay the absorption of concomitantly administered oral medications.When the rapid onset of a concomitant orally administered agent is a critical determinant of effectiveness (such as analgesics), the agent should be administered at least 1 hour prior to or 2 hours after SYMLIN injection.

In clinical trials, the concomitant use of sulfonylureas or biguanides did not alter the adverse event profile of SYMLIN. No formal interaction studies have been performed to assess the effect of SYMLIN on the kinetics of oral antidiabetic agents.

Mixing SYMLIN and Insulin

The pharmacokinetic parameters of SYMLIN were altered when mixed with regular, NPH, and 70/30 premixed formulations of recombinant human insulin immediately prior to injection. **Thus, SYMLIN and insulin should not be mixed and must be administered separately.**

Carcinogenesis, Mutagenesis, Impairment of Fertility

Carcinogenesis. A two-year carcinogenicity study was conducted in CD-1 mice with doses of 0.2, 0.5, and 1.2 mg/kg/day of SYMLIN (32, 67, and 159 times the exposure resulting from the maximum recommended human dose based on area under the plasma concentration curve or AUC, respectively). No drug-induced tumors were observed. A two-year carcinogenicity study was conducted in Sprague-Dawley rats with doses of 0.04, 0.2, and 0.5 mg/kg/day of SYMLIN (3, 9, and 25 times the exposure resulting from the maximum recommended human dose based on AUC, respectively). No drug-induced tumors were observed in any organ.

Mutagenesis. SYMLIN was not mutagenic in the Ames test and did not increase chromosomal aberration in the human lymphocytes assay. SYMLIN was not clastogenic in the *in vivo* mouse micronucleus test or in the chromosomal aberration assay utilizing Chinese hamster ovary cells.

Impairment of Fertility. Administration of 0.3, 1, or 3 mg/kg/day of SYMLIN (8, 17, and 82 times the exposure resulting from the maximum recommended human dose based on body surface area) had no significant effects on fertility in male or female rats. The highest dose of 3 mg/kg/day resulted in dystocia in 8/12 female rats secondary to significant decreases in serum calcium levels.

Pregnancy

Teratogenic Effects: Pregnancy Category C. No adequate and well-controlled studies have been conducted in pregnant women. Studies in perfused human placenta indicate that SYMLIN has low potential to cross the maternal/fetal placental barrier. Embryofetal toxicity studies with SYMLIN have been performed in rats and rabbits. Increases in congenital abnormalities (neural tube defect, cleft palate, exencephaly) were observed in fetuses of rats treated during organogenesis with 0.3 and 1.0 mg/kg/day (10 and 47 times the exposure resulting from the maximum recommended human dose based on AUC, respectively). Administration of doses up to 0.3 mg/kg/day SYMLIN (9 times maximum recommended dose based on AUC) to pregnant rabbits had no adverse effects in embryofetal development; however, animal reproduction studies are not always predictive of human response. SYMLIN (pramlintide acetate) should be used during pregnancy only if it is determined by the healthcare professional that the potential benefit justifies the potential risk to the fetus.

Nursing Mothers

It is unknown whether SYMLIN is excreted in human milk. Many drugs, including peptide drugs, are excreted in human milk. Therefore, SYMLIN should be administered to nursing women only if it is determined by the healthcare professional that the potential benefit outweighs the potential risk to the infant.

Pediatric Use

Safety and effectiveness of SYMLIN in pediatric patients have not been established.

Geriatric Use

SYMLIN has been studied in patients ranging in age from 15 to 84 years of age, including 539 patients 65 years of age or older. The change in HbA1c values and hypoglycemia frequencies did not differ by age, but greater sensitivity in some older individuals cannot be ruled out. Thus, both SYMLIN and insulin regimens should be carefully managed to obviate an increased risk of severe hypoglycemia.

ADVERSE REACTIONS

Adverse events (excluding hypoglycemia, discussed below) commonly associated with SYMLIN when co-administered with a fixed dose of insulin in the long-term, placebo-controlled trials in insulin-using type 2 patients and type 1 patients are presented in **Table 4** and **Table 5**, respectively. The same adverse events were also shown in the open-label clinical practice study, which employed flexible insulin dosing.

Table 4: Treatment-Emergent Adverse Events Occurring With ≥5% Incidence and Greater Incidence With SYMLIN Compared With Placebo in Long-Term, Placebo-Controlled Trials. Incidence of the Same Events in the Open-Label Clinical Practice Study (Patients With Insulin-Using Type 2 Diabetes, 120 mcg)

	Long-Term, Placebo-Controlled Studies		Open-Label, Clinical Practice Study
	Placebo + Insulin (n(%)) (N=284)	SYMLIN + Insulin (n(%)) (N=292)	SYMLIN + Insulin (n(%)) (N=166)
Nausea	34 (12)	81 (28)	53 (30)
Headache	19 (7)	39 (13)	8 (5)
Anorexia	5 (2)	27 (9)	1 (<1)
Vomiting	12 (4)	24 (8)	13 (7)
Abdominal Pain	19 (7)	23 (8)	3 (2)
Fatigue	11 (4)	20 (7)	5 (3)
Dizziness	11 (4)	17 (6)	3 (2)
Coughing	12 (4)	18 (6)	4 (2)
Pharyngitis	7 (2)	15 (5)	6 (3)

Table 5: Treatment-Emergent Adverse Events Occurring With ≥5% Incidence and Greater Incidence With SYMLIN Compared to Placebo in Long-Term, Placebo-Controlled Studies. Incidence of the Same Events in the Open-Label Clinical Practice Study (Patients With Type 1 Diabetes, 30 or 60 mcg)

	Long-Term, Placebo-Controlled Studies		Open-Label, Clinical Practice Study
	Placebo + Insulin (n(%)) (N=538)	SYMLIN + Insulin (n(%)) (N=716)	SYMLIN + Insulin (n(%)) (N=265)
Nausea	92 (17)	342 (48)	98 (37)
Anorexia	12 (2)	122 (17)	0 (0)
Inflicted Injury	55 (10)	97 (14)	20 (8)
Vomiting	36 (7)	82 (11)	18 (7)

Arthralgia	27 (5)	51 (7)	6 (2)
Fatigue	22 (4)	51 (7)	12 (4.5)
Allergic Reaction	28 (5)	41 (6)	1 (< 1)
Dizziness	21 (4)	34 (5)	5 (2)

Most adverse events were gastrointestinal in nature. In patients with type 2 or type 1 diabetes, the incidence of nausea was higher at the beginning of SYMLIN (pramlintide acetate) treatment and decreased with time in most patients. The incidence and severity of nausea are reduced when SYMLIN is gradually titrated to the recommended doses (see DOSAGE and ADMINISTRATION).

Severe Hypoglycemia

SYMLIN alone (without the concomitant administration of insulin) does not cause hypoglycemia. However, SYMLIN is indicated as an adjunct treatment in patients who use mealtime insulin therapy and co-administration of SYMLIN with insulin can increase the risk of insulin-induced hypoglycemia, particularly in patients with type 1 diabetes (see Boxed Warning). The incidence of severe hypoglycemia during the SYMLIN clinical development program is summarized in **Table 6** and **Table 7**.

[See table 6 above]
[See table 7 below]

Table 6: Incidence and Event Rate of Severe Hypoglycemia in Long-Term, Placebo-Controlled and Open-Label, Clinical Practice Studies in Patients With Insulin-Using Type 2 Diabetes

	Long-Term, Placebo-Controlled Studies (No Insulin Dose-Reduction During Initiation)				Open-Label, Clinical Practice Study (Insulin Dose-Reduction During Initiation)	
	Placebo + Insulin		SYMLIN + Insulin		SYMLIN + Insulin	
Severe Hypoglycemia	0–3 Months (n=284)	>3–6 Months (n=251)	0–3 Months (n=292)	>3–6 Months (n=255)	0–3 Months (n=166)	>3–6 Months (n=150)
Patient-Ascertained*						
Event Rate (event rate/patient year)	0.24	0.13	0.45	0.39	0.05	0.03
Incidence (%)	2.1	2.4	8.2	4.7	0.6	0.7
Medically Assisted**						
Event Rate (event rate/patient year)	0.06	0.07	0.09	0.02	0.05	0.03
Incidence (%)	0.7	1.2	1.7	0.4	0.6	0.7

* Patient-ascertained severe hypoglycemia: Requiring the assistance of another individual (including aid in ingestion of oral carbohydrate); and/or requiring the administration of glucagon injection, intravenous glucose, or other medical intervention.

** Medically assisted severe hypoglycemia: Requiring glucagon, IV glucose, hospitalization, paramedic assistance, emergency room visit, and/or assessed as an SAE by the investigator.

Table 7: Incidence and Event Rate of Severe Hypoglycemia in Long-Term, Placebo-Controlled and Open-Label, Clinical Practice Studies in Patients With Type 1 Diabetes

	Long-Term, Placebo-Controlled Studies (No Insulin Dose-Reduction During Initiation)				Open-Label, Clinical Practice Study (Insulin Dose-Reduction During Initiation)	
	Placebo + Insulin		SYMLIN + Insulin		SYMLIN + Insulin	
Severe Hypoglycemia	0–3 Months (n=538)	>3–6 Months (n=470)	0–3 Months (n=716)	>3–6 Months (n=576)	0–3 Months (n=265)	>3–6 Months (n=213)
Patient-Ascertained*						
Event Rate (event rate/patient year)	1.33	1.06	1.55	0.82	0.29	0.16
Incidence (%)	10.8	8.7	16.8	11.1	5.7	3.8
Medically Assisted**						
Event Rate (event rate/patient year)	0.19	0.24	0.50	0.27	0.10	0.04
Incidence (%)	3.3	4.3	7.3	5.2	2.3	0.9

* Patient-ascertained severe hypoglycemia: Requiring the assistance of another individual (including aid in ingestion of oral carbohydrate); and/or requiring the administration of glucagon injection, intravenous glucose, or other medical intervention.

** Medically assisted severe hypoglycemia: Requiring glucagon, IV glucose, hospitalization, paramedic assistance, emergency room visit, and/or assessed as an SAE by the investigator.

Post Marketing Experience

Since market introduction of SYMLIN, the following adverse reactions have been reported. Because these events are reported voluntarily from a population of uncertain size, it is not always possible to reliably estimate their frequency or establish a causal relationship to drug exposure.

General: Injection site reactions.

OVERDOSAGE

Single 10 mg doses of SYMLIN (83 times the maximum dose of 120 mcg) were administered to three healthy volunteers. Severe nausea was reported in all three individuals and was associated with vomiting, diarrhea, vasodilatation, and dizziness. No hypoglycemia was reported. SYMLIN has a short half-life and in the case of overdose, supportive measures are indicated.

DOSAGE AND ADMINISTRATION

SYMLIN dosage differs depending on whether the patient has type 2 or type 1 diabetes (see below). When initiating therapy with SYMLIN, initial insulin dose reduction is required in all patients (both type 2 and type 1) to reduce the risk of insulin-induced hypoglycemia. As this reduction in insulin can lead to glucose elevations, patients should be monitored at regular intervals to assess SYMLIN tolerability and the effect on blood glucose, so that **individualized** insulin adjustments can be initiated. If SYMLIN therapy is discontinued for any reason (e.g., surgery or illnesses), the same initiation protocol should be followed when SYMLIN therapy is re-instituted (see below).

Initiation of SYMLIN therapy

Patients With Insulin-Using Type 2 Diabetes

In patients with insulin-using type 2 diabetes, SYMLIN should be initiated at a dose of 60 mcg and increased to a dose of 120 mcg as tolerated.

Patients should be instructed to:

- Initiate SYMLIN at 60 mcg subcutaneously, immediately prior to major meals;
- Reduce preprandial, rapid-acting or short-acting insulin dosages, including fixed-mix insulins (70/30) by **50%**;
- Monitor blood glucose frequently, including pre- and post-meals and at bedtime;
- Increase the SYMLIN dose to 120 mcg when no clinically significant nausea has occurred for 3–7 days. **SYMLIN dose adjustments should be made only as directed by the healthcare professional.** If significant nausea persists at the 120 mcg dose, the SYMLIN dose should be decreased to 60 mcg;
- Adjust insulin doses to optimize glycemic control once the target dose of SYMLIN is achieved and nausea (if experienced) has subsided. **Insulin dose adjustments should be made only as directed by the healthcare professional;**
- Contact a healthcare professional skilled in the use of insulin to review SYMLIN and insulin dose adjustments at least once a week until a target dose of SYMLIN is achieved, SYMLIN is well-tolerated, and blood glucose concentrations are stable.

Patients With Type 1 Diabetes

In patients with type 1 diabetes, SYMLIN should be initiated at a dose of 15 mcg and titrated at 15-mcg increments to a maintenance dose of 30 mcg or 60 mcg as tolerated.

Patients should be instructed to:

- Initiate SYMLIN at a starting dose of 15 mcg subcutaneously, immediately prior to major meals;
- Reduce preprandial, rapid-acting or short-acting insulin dosages, including fixed-mix insulins (e.g., 70/30) by **50%**;
- Monitor blood glucose frequently, including pre- and post-meals and at bedtime;
- Increase the SYMLIN (pramlintide acetate) dose to the next increment (30 mcg, 45 mcg, or 60 mcg) when no clinically significant nausea has occurred for at least 3 days. **SYMLIN dose adjustments should be made only as directed by the healthcare professional.** If significant nausea persists at the 45 or 60 mcg dose level, the SYMLIN dose should be decreased to 30 mcg. If the 30 mcg dose is not tolerated, discontinuation of SYMLIN therapy should be considered;
- Adjust insulin doses to optimize glycemic control once the target dose of SYMLIN is achieved and nausea (if experienced) has subsided. **Insulin dose adjustments should be made only as directed by the healthcare professional;**
- Contact a healthcare professional skilled in the use of insulin to review SYMLIN and insulin dose adjustments at least once a week until a target dose of SYMLIN is achieved, SYMLIN is well-tolerated, and blood glucose concentrations are stable.

Once Target Dose of SYMLIN is Achieved in Type 2 or Type 1 Patients

After a maintenance dose of SYMLIN is achieved, both insulin-using patients with type 2 diabetes and patients with type 1 diabetes should be instructed to:

- Adjust insulin doses to optimize glycemic control once the target dose of SYMLIN is achieved and nausea (if experienced) has subsided. **Insulin dose adjustments should be made only as directed by a healthcare professional;**
- Contact a healthcare professional in the event of recurrent nausea or hypoglycemia. An increased frequency of mild to moderate hypoglycemia should be viewed as a warning sign of increased risk for severe hypoglycemia.

Administration

SYMLIN (pramlintide acetate) should be administered subcutaneously immediately prior to each major meal (≥250 kcal or containing ≥30 g of carbohydrate).

SYMLIN should be at room temperature before injecting to reduce potential injection site reactions. Each SYMLIN dose should be administered subcutaneously into the abdomen or thigh (administration into the arm is not recommended because of variable absorption). Injection sites should be rotated so that the same site is not used repeatedly. The injection site selected should also be distinct from the site chosen for any concomitant insulin injection.

- **SYMLIN and insulin should always be administered as separate injections.**
- **SYMLIN should not be mixed with any type of insulin.**
- **If a SYMLIN dose is missed, wait until the next scheduled dose and administer the usual amount.**

SymlinPen® pen-injector

The SymlinPen® pen-injector is available in two presentations:

- SymlinPen® 60 pen-injector for doses of 15 mcg, 30 mcg, 45 mcg and 60 mcg.
- SymlinPen® 120 pen-injector for doses of 60 mcg and 120 mcg.

See the accompanying Patient Instructions for Use for instructions for using the SymlinPen® pen-injector.

The patient should be advised:

- to confirm they are using the correct pen-injector that will deliver their prescribed dose;
- on proper use of the pen-injector, emphasizing how and when to set up a new pen-injector;
- **not to transfer SYMLIN from the pen-injector to a syringe. Doing so could result in a higher dose than intended, because SYMLIN in the pen-injector is a higher concentration than SYMLIN in the SYMLIN vial;**
- not to share the pen-injector and needles with others;
- that needles are not included with the pen-injector and must be purchased separately;
- which needle length and gauge should be used;
- to use a new needle for each injection.

SYMLIN vials

To administer SYMLIN (pramlintide acetate) from vials, use a U-100 insulin syringe (preferably a 0.3 mL [0.3 cc] size) for optimal accuracy. If using a syringe calibrated for use with U-100 insulin, use the chart below **(Table 8)** to measure the microgram dosage in unit increments.

Table 8: Conversion of SYMLIN Dose to Insulin Unit Equivalents

Dosage Prescribed (mcg)	Increment Using a U-100 Syringe (Units)	Volume (cc or mL)
15	2½	0.025
30	5	0.05
45	7½	0.075
60	10	0.1
120	20	0.2

Always use separate, new syringes and needles to give SYMLIN and insulin injections.

Discontinuation of Therapy

SYMLIN therapy should be discontinued if any of the following occur:

- Recurrent unexplained hypoglycemia that requires medical assistance;
- Persistent clinically significant nausea;
- Noncompliance with self-monitoring of blood glucose concentrations;
- Noncompliance with insulin dose adjustments;
- Noncompliance with scheduled healthcare professional contacts or recommended clinic visits.

Preparation and Handling

SYMLIN should be inspected visually for particulate matter or discoloration prior to administration whenever the solution and the container permit.

HOW SUPPLIED

SYMLIN is supplied as a sterile injection in the following dosage forms:

- 1.5 mL disposable multidose SymlinPen® 60 pen-injector containing 1000 mcg/mL pramlintide (as acetate).
- 2.7 mL disposable multidose SymlinPen® 120 pen-injector containing 1000 mcg/mL pramlintide (as acetate).
- 5 mL vial, containing 600 mcg/mL pramlintide (as acetate), for use with an insulin syringe.

To administer SYMLIN from vials, use a U-100 insulin syringe (preferably a 0.3 mL [0.3 cc] size). If using a syringe calibrated for use with U-100 insulin, use the chart **(Table 8)** in the DOSAGE AND ADMINISTRATION section to measure the microgram dosage in unit increments.

Do not mix SYMLIN with insulin.

SYMLIN Injection is available in the following package sizes:

- SymlinPen® 60 pen-injector, containing 1000 mcg/mL pramlintide (as acetate) 2×1.5 mL disposable multidose pen-injector (NDC 66780-115-02)
- SymlinPen® 120 pen-injector, containing 1000 mcg/mL pramlintide (as acetate) 2×2.7 mL disposable multidose pen-injector (NDC 66780-121-02)
- 5 mL vial, containing 600 mcg/mL pramlintide (as acetate), for use with an insulin syringe (NDC 66780-110-01)

STORAGE

SYMLIN pen-injectors and vials not in use: Refrigerate (36°F to 46°F; 2°C to 8°C), and protect from light. Do not freeze. Do not use if product has been frozen. Unused SYMLIN (pramlintide acetate) (opened or unopened) should not be used after the expiration (EXP) date printed on the carton and the label.

SYMLIN pen-injectors and vials in use: After first use, refrigerate or keep at a temperature not greater than 86°F (30°C) for 30 days. Use within 30 days, whether or not refrigerated.

Storage conditions are summarized in **Table 9.**

[See table 9 below]

Table 9: Storage Conditions

Dosage Form	Unopened (not in use) Refrigerated	Open (in use) Refrigerated or Temperature Up To 86°F (30°C)
1.5 mL pen-injector 2.7 mL pen-injector 5 mL vial	Until Expiration Date	Use Within 30 Days

The SymlinPen® pen-injectors and SYMLIN vials are manufactured for:

Amylin Pharmaceuticals, Inc.
San Diego, CA 92121 USA
1-800-349 8919
http://www.SYMLIN.com

Rx only

The SYMLIN mark, SYMLIN design mark, and SymlinPen are registered trademarks of Amylin Pharmaceuticals, Inc.

Literature Revised July 2008 812003-CC

Medication Guide

SYMLIN® (SĬM-lĭn)

(pramlintide acetate) injection

Read the Medication Guide and the "Patient Instructions for Use" that come with your SYMLIN product before you start using it and each time you get a refill. There may be new information. This Medication Guide does not take the place of talking to your doctor about your medical condition or treatment.

What is the most important information I should know about SYMLIN?

- **SYMLIN is used with insulin to lower blood sugar, especially high blood sugar that happens after meals.**
- **SYMLIN is given at mealtimes. The use of SYMLIN does not replace your daily insulin but may lower the amount of insulin you need, especially before meals.**
- **Even when SYMLIN is carefully added to your mealtime insulin therapy, your blood sugar may drop too low, especially if you have type 1 diabetes. If this low blood sugar (severe hypoglycemia) happens, it is seen within 3 hours after a SYMLIN injection. Severe low blood sugar makes it hard to think clearly, drive a car, use heavy machinery or do other risky activities where you could hurt yourself or others.**
- **SYMLIN should only be used by people with type 2 and type 1 diabetes who:**
  - already use their insulin as prescribed, but still need better blood sugar control.
  - will follow their doctor's instructions exactly.
  - will follow up with their doctor often.
  - will test their blood sugar levels before and after every meal, and at bedtime.
  - understand how to adjust SYMLIN and insulin doses.

What is SYMLIN?

SYMLIN is an injectable medicine for adults with type 2 and type 1 diabetes to control blood sugar. SYMLIN slows down the movement of food through your stomach. This affects how fast sugar enters your blood after eating. SYMLIN is always used with insulin to help lower blood sugar during the 3 hours after meals.

Who should not use SYMLIN?

Do not use SYMLIN if you:

- cannot tell when your blood sugar is low (hypoglycemia unawareness).
- have a stomach problem called gastroparesis. This is when your stomach does not empty as fast as it should.
- are allergic to SYMLIN or any ingredients in SYMLIN. See the end of this Medication Guide for a complete list of ingredients.

SYMLIN has not been studied in children.

What should I tell my doctor before starting SYMLIN?

Tell your doctor about all of your medical conditions including if you:

- **are pregnant or planning to become pregnant.** It is not known if SYMLIN (pramlintide acetate) can harm your unborn baby. You and your doctor will decide how to best control your blood sugar levels during pregnancy.
- **are breastfeeding.** It is not known if SYMLIN passes into your milk and if it can harm your baby. You and your doctor will decide the best way to feed your baby if you are using SYMLIN.

Keep a list of all the medicines you take. Tell your doctor about all the medicines you take including prescription and non-prescription medicines, vitamins, and herbal supplements. SYMLIN can slow down how other medicines pass through your stomach and may affect how much of them get into your body. You may have to change the times you take certain medicines.

How should I use SYMLIN?

- **You must use SYMLIN exactly as prescribed. The amount of SYMLIN you use will depend on whether you have type 2 or type 1 diabetes.** You and your doctor will decide if you can use SYMLIN.
- It is important for you to carefully read, understand and follow the "Patient Instructions for Use" that comes along with this Medication Guide and your SYMLIN.
- **SYMLIN is available in vials and two SymlinPen® pen-injectors. Your doctor will prescribe the type of SYMLIN that is right for you.**
  - If you have been using the SYMLIN vial with an insulin syringe and you are changing to the SymlinPen® pen-injector: **Your doctor will prescribe the SymlinPen® pen-injector that is right for you, tell you how much SYMLIN to inject and when to inject it.**
  - **It is important that you understand how to inject the right SYMLIN dose. Read the "Patient Instructions for Use" carefully BEFORE giving your first dose with the SymlinPen® pen-injector. The SYMLIN in the pen-injector is a different strength than the SYMLIN in the vial.**
- The way you inject SYMLIN is similar to the way you inject insulin. **Inject SYMLIN under the skin (subcutaneously) of your stomach area (abdomen) or upper leg (thigh).** Inject SYMLIN at a site that is more than 2 inches away from your insulin injection. Do not inject SYMLIN and insulin in the same site.
- To help reduce the chances of getting a reaction at the injection site, allow SYMLIN to come to room temperature before injecting.
- Use a new needle for each SYMLIN injection.
- **Never mix SYMLIN and insulin.** Insulin can affect SYMLIN when the two are mixed together.
- Do not use SYMLIN if the liquid looks cloudy.
- If you take more than your prescribed dose of SYMLIN, you may get nauseous or vomit, and you may not be able to eat the amount of food you usually eat. If you take more SYMLIN than your prescribed dose, pay careful attention to the amount of insulin you use because you may be at more risk for low blood sugar. Contact your doctor for guidance.
- If you miss or forget a dose of SYMLIN, wait until the next meal and take your usual dose of SYMLIN at that meal. Do not take more than your usual dose of SYMLIN.

Using SYMLIN and insulin with Type 2 Diabetes

1. Start SYMLIN at 60 mcg injected under your skin, just before major meals. A major meal must have at least 250 calories or 30 grams of carbohydrate.
2. Reduce your rapid-acting or short-acting insulin, including fixed-mix insulin such as 70/30, used before meals by **50 percent**. This means half of the dose you usually use.
3. You must check your blood sugar before and after every meal and at bedtime.
4. Increase your dose of SYMLIN to 120 mcg on your doctor's instructions if you have not had any nausea for 3 days or more.
5. Tell your doctor right away if you have nausea with the 120 mcg dose. Your doctor will tell you how to adjust your dose of SYMLIN.
6. Your doctor may make changes to your insulin doses to better control your blood sugar once you are using the 120 mcg dose of SYMLIN. All insulin changes should be directed by your doctor.

Using SYMLIN and insulin with Type 1 Diabetes

1. Start SYMLIN at 15 mcg injected under your skin, just before major meals. A major meal must have at least 250 calories or 30 grams of carbohydrate.
2. When starting SYMLIN, reduce your rapid-acting or short-acting insulin, including fixed-mix insulin such as 70/30, used before meals by **50 percent**. This means half of the dose you usually use. All insulin changes should be directed by your doctor.
3. You must check your blood sugar before and after every meal and at bedtime.
4. Increase your dose of SYMLIN to 30 mcg on your doctor's instructions if you have not had any nausea for 3 days or more. If you have nausea with SYMLIN at 30 mcg, call your doctor right away. Your doctor may decide that you should stop SYMLIN.

5. Increase your dose of SYMLIN (pramlintide acetate) to 45 mcg on your doctor's instructions if you have not had any nausea for 3 days or more while using the 30 mcg dose.
6. Increase your dose of SYMLIN to 60 mcg on your doctor's instructions if you have not had any nausea for 3 days or more while using the 45 mcg dose.
7. Call your doctor right away if you are bothered with nausea on the 45 mcg or 60 mcg dose. Your doctor may decide that you should reduce SYMLIN to the 30 mcg dose.
8. Your doctor may make changes to your insulin doses to better control your blood sugar once you are on a dose of SYMLIN that is right for you. All insulin changes should be directed by your doctor.

Staying on SYMLIN

- Once you reach your recommended dose of SYMLIN, talk to your doctor about changing your insulin doses to better control your blood sugar. You may have to increase your long-acting insulin to prevent high blood sugar (hyperglycemia) between meals. **Insulin changes should always be directed by your doctor based on blood sugar testing.**
- Call your doctor if nausea or low blood sugar continues while on your recommended dose of SYMLIN. Low blood sugar that happens often is a warning sign of possible severe low blood sugar, especially if you have type 1 diabetes.
- **If you stop taking SYMLIN for any reason, such as surgery or illness, talk to your doctor about how to re-start SYMLIN.**

When should I not use SYMLIN?

Do not use SYMLIN if:

- your blood sugar is too low.
- you do not plan to eat. Do not inject SYMLIN if you skip a meal.
- you plan to eat a meal with less than 250 calories or 30 grams of carbohydrate.
- you are sick and can't eat your usual meal.
- you are having surgery or a medical test where you cannot eat.
- you are pregnant or breastfeeding and have not talked to your doctor.

Talk to your doctor if you have any of these conditions.

What should I avoid while taking SYMLIN?

- Do not drive or operate dangerous machinery until you know how SYMLIN affects your blood sugar. Low blood sugar makes it hard to think clearly, drive a car, use heavy machinery or do other risky activities where you could hurt yourself or others. Discuss with your doctor what activities you should avoid.
- Alcohol may increase the risk of low blood sugar.
- **Your doctor will tell you which medicines you can take while using SYMLIN. Do not take other medicines that slow stomach emptying.**

What are the possible side effects of SYMLIN?

Low blood sugar (hypoglycemia)

- **SYMLIN is used with insulin to lower your blood sugar, but your blood sugar may drop too low, especially if you have type 1 diabetes.** See "What is the most important information I should know about SYMLIN?"
- When starting SYMLIN, reduce your doses of insulin before meals as recommended by your doctor to reduce the chance of low blood sugar. You and your doctor should talk about a plan to treat low blood sugar. You should have fast-acting sugar (such as hard candy, glucose tablets, juice) or glucagon with you at all times. Call your doctor if you have low blood sugar more often than normal or severe low blood sugar.

Your chance for low blood sugar is higher if you:

- do not reduce your insulin dose before meals at the beginning of SYMLIN treatment, as directed by your doctor.
- use more SYMLIN or insulin than prescribed by your doctor.
- change your insulin dose without checking your blood sugar.
- eat less food than your usual meal.
- are sick and cannot eat.
- are more active than usual.
- have a low blood sugar level before eating.
- drink alcohol.

Always have fast acting sugar (such as hard candy, glucose tablets, juice) or glucagon available to treat low blood sugar.

Nausea: Nausea is the most common side effect with SYMLIN. Mild nausea is more likely during the first weeks after starting SYMLIN and usually does not last long. It is very important to start SYMLIN at a low dose and increase it as directed by your doctor. See "How should I use SYMLIN?" If nausea continues or bothers you, call your doctor right away.

Other Side Effects: SYMLIN also may cause the following side effects: decreased appetite, vomiting, stomach pain, tiredness, dizziness, or indigestion.

SYMLIN also can cause reactions at the injection site including redness, minor bruising, or pain. See the detailed "Patient Instructions for Use." Follow the directions under "How should I use SYMLIN?" to reduce the chance of an injection site reaction.

Tell your doctor if you have any side effects that bother you or that do not go away.

These are not all the side effects with SYMLIN (pramlintide acetate). Ask your doctor or pharmacist for more information.

How should I store SYMLIN?

- Store SYMLIN that has not been opened in the refrigerator, between 36°F to 46°F (2°C to 8°C), until you are ready to use it. Protect SYMLIN from light.
- After a vial or pen-injector has been used for the first time, it can be refrigerated or kept at a temperature up to 86°F (30°C) for 30 days. Do not leave **above** 86°F (30°C). Any vial or pen-injector in use should be thrown away after 30 days, even if it still has medicine in it.
- Unused SYMLIN (opened or unopened) should not be used after the expiration (EXP) date printed on the carton and the label.
- **Do not freeze SYMLIN. Do not use SYMLIN if it has been frozen.**

Keep SYMLIN and all medicines out of the reach of children.

General information about the safe and effective use of SYMLIN

Medicines are sometimes prescribed for purposes other than those listed in a Medication Guide. Do not use SYMLIN for a condition for which it was not prescribed. Do not give SYMLIN to other people, even if they have the same symptoms that you have. It may harm them.

This Medication Guide summarizes the most important information about SYMLIN. Also see the "Patient Instructions for Use" on using the SymlinPen® pen-injector or vial. You can ask your doctor for more about SYMLIN, including information that is written for doctors.

More information on SYMLIN can be found at http://www.SYMLIN.com.

SYMLIN Customer Service is available 24 hours a day at 1-800-349-8919.

Call your doctor for medical advice about side effects. You may report side effects to FDA at 1-800-FDA-1088.

What are the ingredients in SYMLIN?

Active ingredient: pramlintide acetate

Inactive ingredients: metacresol, D-mannitol, acetic acid, and sodium acetate.

This Medication Guide has been approved by the U.S. Food and Drug Administration.

Literature Revised July 2008

Manufactured for Amylin Pharmaceuticals, Inc.
San Diego CA 92121, USA
1-800-349-8919
http://www.SYMLIN.com

813006-FF

Symlin®
(pramlintide acetate)
injection
600 mcg/mL
5 mL vial

Patient Instructions for Use

Read the Medication Guide on the reverse side first.

These instructions do not take the place of talking with your doctor about your diabetes treatment. Ask your doctor about your dose and preferred injection technique. If you have questions or concerns about SYMLIN, please visit www.SYMLIN.com or call **Amylin Customer Support** toll free at **1-800-349-8919.**

Prepare and Inject Your Dose

1. Inspect your SYMLIN vial. The liquid in the vial should be clear and colorless.
2. Check the expiration date (EXP) on the label to be sure your SYMLIN is not expired (see Figure A).
3. Clean the top of the SYMLIN vial with an alcohol swab.

Figure A

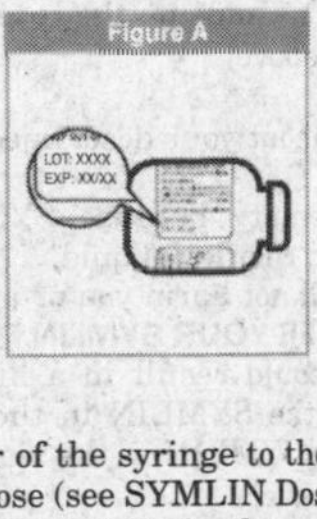

4. Pull the plunger of the syringe to the line that matches your SYMLIN dose (see SYMLIN Dosing Chart and Figure B). The amount of air in the syringe should equal the amount of SYMLIN you plan to take.

Figure B

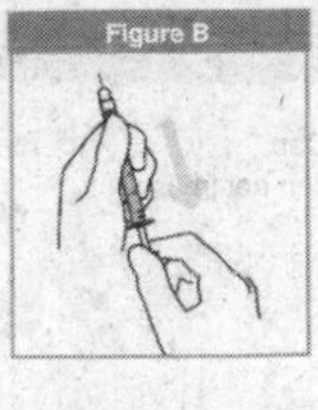

5. Push the needle through the center of the rubber top of the SYMLIN vial (see Figure C).
6. Push the plunger to inject the air into the vial.

Figure C

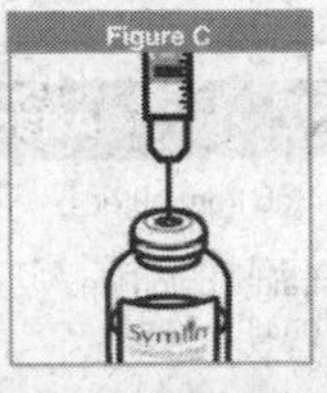

7. Turn the vial and syringe upside down.
8. Slowly pull the plunger down to draw the SYMLIN into the syringe until you have your correct dose (see Figure D).
9. BEFORE removing the syringe from the vial, look for air bubbles inside the syringe. If you see bubbles, push the SYMLIN back into the vial. Then slowly pull the plunger down to draw the SYMLIN into the syringe until you have your correct dose.

Figure D

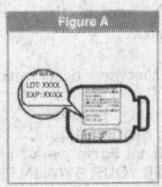

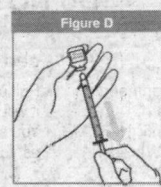

10. Check to be sure your dose is **correct**, then remove the syringe from the vial.
11. Give your injection as directed by your healthcare provider.
12. Dispose of the used syringe as directed by your healthcare provider.

Care and Storage

- Store SYMLIN that has not been opened in the refrigerator, between 36°F to 46°F (2°C to 8°C), until you are ready to use it. Protect SYMLIN from light.
- After a vial has been used for the first time, it can be refrigerated or kept at a temperature up to 86°F (30°C) for 30 days. Do not leave above 86°F (30°C).
- Any vial in use should be thrown away after 30 days, even if it still has medicine in it.
- Unused SYMLIN (opened or unopened) should not be used after the expiration (EXP) date printed on the carton and the label.
- **Do not freeze SYMLIN.** Do not use SYMLIN if it has been frozen.
- **Keep SYMLIN and all medicines out of the reach of children.**

About SYMLIN

- The way you inject SYMLIN (pramlintide acetate) is similar to the way you inject insulin. **Inject SYMLIN under the skin (subcutaneously) of your stomach area (abdomen) or upper leg (thigh).** Inject SYMLIN at a site that is more than 2 inches away from your insulin injection. To help reduce the chances of getting a reaction at the injection site, allow SYMLIN to come to room temperature before injecting. Also, use a new needle for each SYMLIN injection.
- If you take more than your prescribed dose of SYMLIN, you may get nauseous or vomit, and you may not be able to eat the amount of food you usually eat. Pay careful attention to the amount of insulin you use at this time as you may be at more risk for low blood sugar. Contact your doctor for guidance.
- If you miss or forget a dose of SYMLIN, wait until the next meal and take your usual dose of SYMLIN at that meal. Do not take more than your usual dose of SYMLIN.
- **Never mix SYMLIN and insulin. Use different syringes for SYMLIN and insulin.** Insulin can affect SYMLIN when the two are mixed together.
- Your prescription may be written in micrograms, and your insulin syringe is labeled in units. Use the chart below to convert micrograms to units

Pen Parts

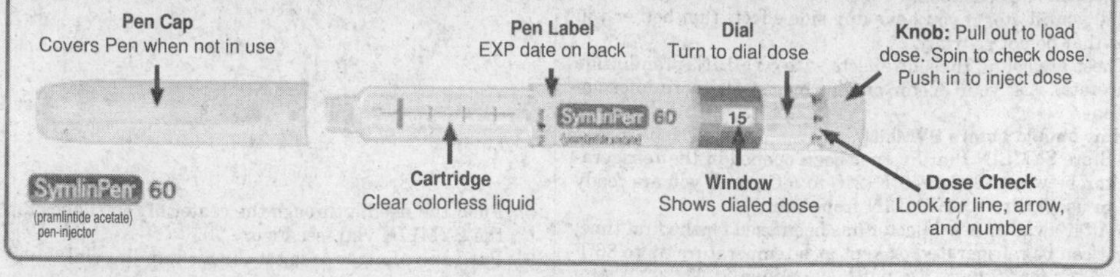

Attach Pen Needle (needles not included)

- Remove paper tab from outer needle cover.
- Push needle straight onto Pen.
- Screw needle on until tight.

- Remove outer needle cover and save for needle removal.
- Remove inner needle cover and throw away.

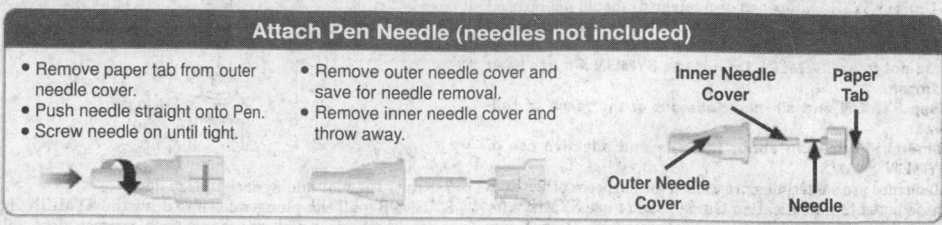

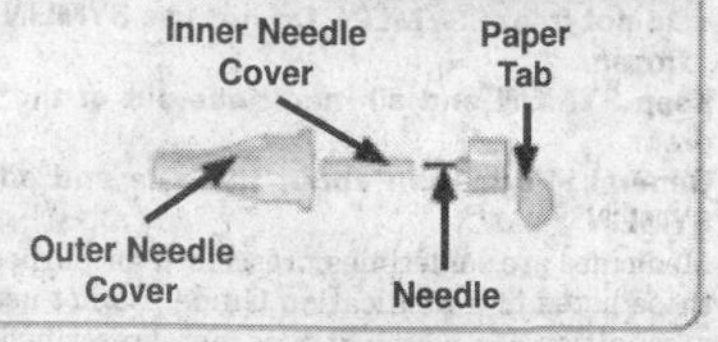

START HERE

New Pen Setup (REQUIRED before the first dose with each new Pen).

Do NOT repeat setup before each dose.

Dial

- Attach a new pen needle (see above).
- Turn the **Dial** until 15 appears in the **Window**.

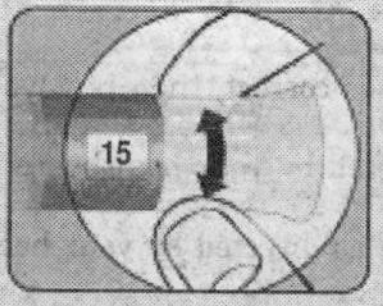

Load

- Pull out the **Knob** as far as it will go.
- You should hear "clicking" as you pull the **Knob**.

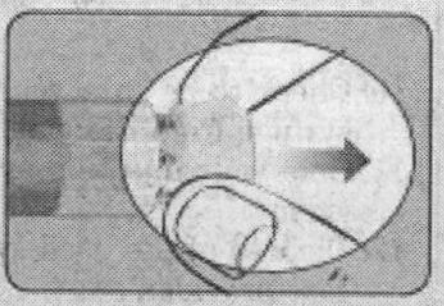

Watch For Stream

- Before you give your first injection, you need to see a stream of liquid from the needle.
- With the needle pointing up, use your thumb to firmly push in the **Knob** all the way until it stops.
- You should hear "clicking" as you push the **Knob**.
- If no stream, pull out and push in **Knob** (up to 6 times) until you see a stream.
- After Setup, go to **Routine Use**.

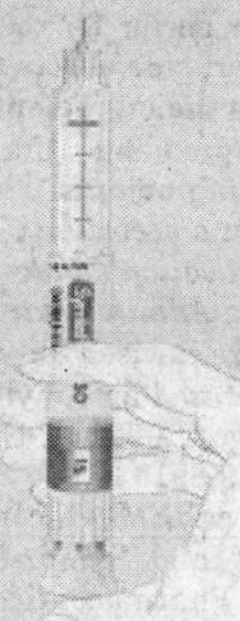

NOTE: If you drop your Pen, repeat Pen Setup to make sure the Pen works.

Routine Use (For Every Dose)

1. Dial
- Attach a new pen needle (see above).
- Turn the **Dial** until your dose appears in the **Window**.

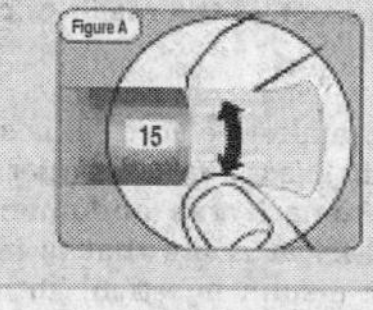

2. Load
- Pull out the **Knob** as far as it will go.
- You should hear "clicking" as you pull the **Knob**.

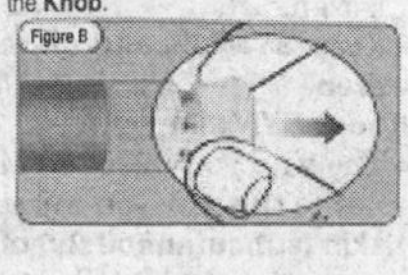

3. Check
- Use line on **Dose Check** (K15) to confirm you have loaded your full dose.

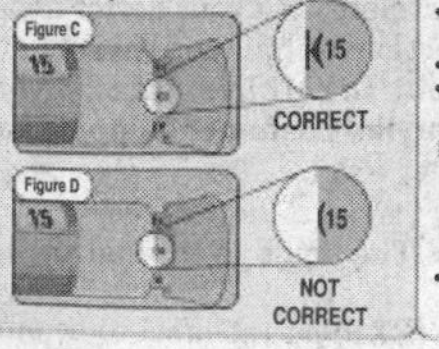

4. Inject
- Insert needle into thigh or abdomen at least 2 inches from your insulin injection site.
- Use thumb to push in the **Knob** all the way until it stops.
- You should hear "clicking" as you push the **Knob**.
- Push and hold the **Knob** for 10 seconds to give your full dose.

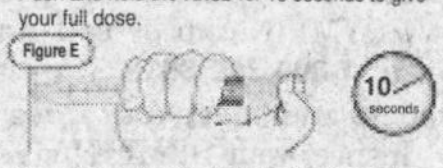

- Remove needle with outer needle cover and throw away.

SYMLIN Dosing Chart

Find Your Dose in Micrograms (mcg)	Draw Up This Amount in U-100 Insulin Syringe (Units)
15 mcg	2½ units
30 mcg	5 units
45 mcg	7½ units
60 mcg	10 units
120 mcg	20 units

Literature Issued September 2007
815004-BB

[See first figure above]

SymlinPen® 60 Pen-Injector Patient Instructions for Use

Read the Medication Guide on the reverse side first

[See second figure above]

Important Notes

- Ask your doctor about your dose, injection technique, and needle size.
- Pen may look empty because SYMLIN (pramlintide acetate) is a clear, colorless liquid.
- Small bubbles will not harm you or affect your dose.
- **DO NOT TRANSFER YOUR SYMLIN FROM THE PEN TO A SYRINGE.** This could result in a higher dose than intended, because the SYMLIN in the Pen is a different strength than the SYMLIN in the vial.

[See third figure above]

[See fourth figure above]

Literature Revised July 2008

SymlinPen® pen-injector (Pen)

Read these instructions carefully before using your Pen. Failure to follow these instructions may cause an incorrect dose, a broken Pen, or an infection.

- Check Pen label before each use to make sure you have the 15•30•45•60 mcg Pen.
- Check the expiration date (EXP) on the Pen label (see Pen Parts), and make sure the Pen is not expired.
- If you drop your Pen, go to **New Pen Setup** to confirm Pen works.
- If any part of your Pen appears broken or damaged, do not use.
- This Pen is not recommended for use by blind or visually impaired persons without the assistance of a person trained in the proper use of this Pen.
- If SYMLIN (pramlintide acetate) in the Cartridge (see Pen Parts) is not clear, colorless, and free of particles, do not use Pen.

Needles

- Use a new needle for each injection. Remove the needle from the Pen after completing each injection. This will help prevent leakage of SYMLIN, keep out air bubbles, reduce needle clogs, and reduce risk of infection.
- Pen needles are not included with the Pen. Use 29, 30, or 31 gauge disposable needles with the Pen. Ask your healthcare provider which needle gauge and length is best for you.
- Do not share your Pen or needles with anyone.
- Be sure the needle is completely attached to the Pen before use (see Attach Pen Needle). Do not push the Knob unless a needle is attached to Pen.
- Throw away used needles in a puncture-resistant container or as directed by your healthcare provider. Do not throw away the Pen with a needle attached.
- Follow local or institutional policies regarding needle handling and disposal.

Care and Storage

- Pen that has never been used:
  - Refrigerate (36°F to 46°F, 2°C to 8°C).
  - Protect from light.
  - **Do not freeze.** Do not use a Pen that has been frozen.
- Pen in use:
  - After the Pen is used for the first time (first use), refrigerate or keep at a temperature up to 86°F (30°C) for 30 days. Throw away Pen 30 days after first use, even if it still has SYMLIN in it.
- Pen should not be used after the expiration (EXP) date printed on the label.
- Do not store Pen with needle attached, or with Knob pulled out.
- If needed, wipe only the outside of Pen with a clean, damp cloth (water only).
- White particles may appear where the needle attaches during normal use. You may remove the particles with an alcohol wipe or alcohol swab.
- Keep Pen and needles out of the reach of children.

About SYMLIN

- The way you inject SYMLIN is similar to the way you inject insulin. **Inject SYMLIN under the skin (subcutaneously) of your stomach area (abdomen) or upper leg (thigh).** Inject SYMLIN at a site that is more than 2 inches away from your insulin injection. To help reduce the chances of getting a reaction at the injection site, allow SYMLIN to come to room temperature before injecting. Also, use a new needle for each SYMLIN injection.
- If you take more than your prescribed dose of SYMLIN, you may get nauseous or vomit, and you may not be able to eat the amount of food you usually eat. Pay careful attention to the amount of insulin you use at this time as you may be at more risk for low blood sugar. Contact your doctor for guidance.
- If you miss or forget a dose of SYMLIN, wait until the next meal and take your usual dose of SYMLIN at that meal. **Do not take more than your usual dose of SYMLIN.**

Questions and Answers (Q&A)

Why does my new Pen look empty?

- Because SYMLIN is clear and colorless, the Cartridge (see Pen Parts) may look empty, even though there is medicine in it.
- To be sure there is SYMLIN in the Cartridge, perform Pen setup (see New Pen Setup).

What should I do if I see air bubbles?

- The Cartridge may contain small air bubbles. Small air bubbles are normal and will not harm you or affect your dose.
- Perform **New Pen Setup** before the first dose with each new Pen (see New Pen Setup).
- To prevent more air bubbles, do NOT store Pen with needle attached.

Why can't I turn the Dial?

- If the Knob has been pulled out, the Dial will not move and you cannot reset your dose. Push in the Knob to discard the dose and repeat the instructions (see Routine Use).
- If the Knob is pushed in all the way, and you cannot rotate the Dial, call Amylin Customer Support.

What should I do if I do not see a stream of liquid when I perform the setup?
- Watch for a stream when you start to push the Knob.
- The liquid is clear and colorless, so it may be difficult to see.
- Pull out the Knob all the way - you will hear clicking.
- Firmly push in the Knob all the way - you will hear clicking.
- If there is no stream of liquid after 6 attempts, replace the needle and repeat setup.
- If still no stream, call Amylin Customer Support.

What should I do if I load an incorrect dose?
- **Do not inject an incorrect dose.** Point the needle away from you and discard the dose by pushing in the Knob all the way. Dial your correct dose.

How do I make sure I am getting my correct dose of SYMLIN?
- Before pulling out Knob, be sure the number in Window matches your prescribed SYMLIN (pramlintide acetate) dose (see Figure A).
- Pull out the Knob all the way - you will hear clicking (see Figure B).
- Be sure that number on the Dose Check matches your dose in Window. You must see **line, arrow, and number**

on Dose Check (see Figure C).
- Firmly push in the Knob all the way - you will hear clicking.
- Hold Knob for 10 seconds before removing needle from skin (see Figure E).

Why do I see SYMLIN leaking from my needle after I inject?
- You may see one or two drops - this is normal.
- If you see more than 2 drops:
  - You may not have received your full dose.
  - **Do not inject another dose.**
  - Talk to your healthcare provider.
- To prevent dripping or leaking, be sure to firmly push and hold Knob with your thumb for 10 seconds before removing needle from skin.

How do I know when my pen is empty?
- **Check Your Dose** after pulling out the Knob (see Figure C).
- The lines on the Cartridge show approximately how much SYMLIN is left in the Pen. When the Plunger is at the thickest line on the Cartridge, your Pen is almost empty (see Figure F).

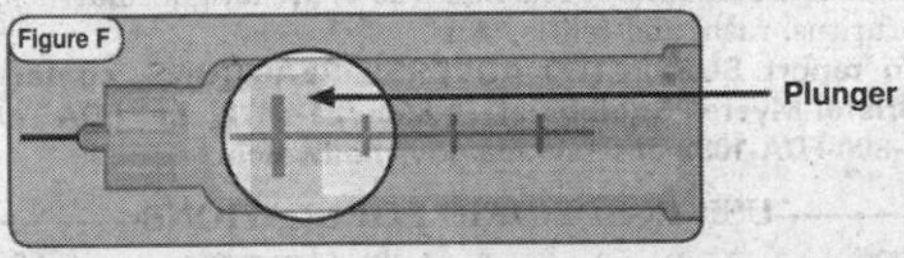
Figure F
Plunger

- If you cannot see the **line, arrow, and number**

that match your prescribed dose, you do not have enough SYMLIN to give your full dose (see Figure H). Throw away this Pen, and use a new Pen to give your dose.

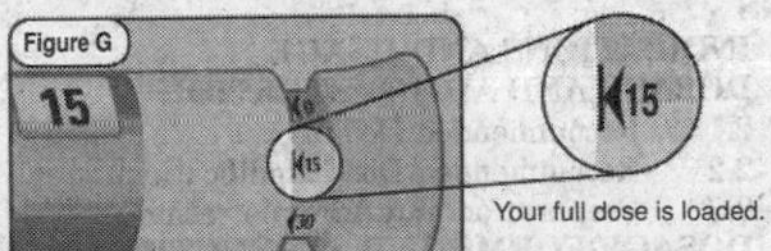

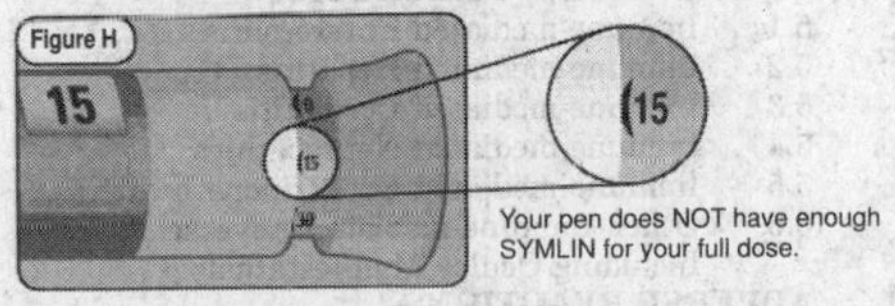
Figure H
15
15
Your pen does NOT have enough SYMLIN for your full dose.

The Patient Instructions for Use do not take the place of talking with your doctor about your diabetes treatment. Ask your doctor about your dose and preferred injection technique. If you are having problems using your Pen, please visit **www.SYMLIN.com** or call **Amylin Customer Support** toll free at **1-800-349-8919.**

815002-FF

[See first figure above]

SymlinPen® 120 Pen-Injector Patient Instructions for Use

Read the Medication Guide on the reverse side first

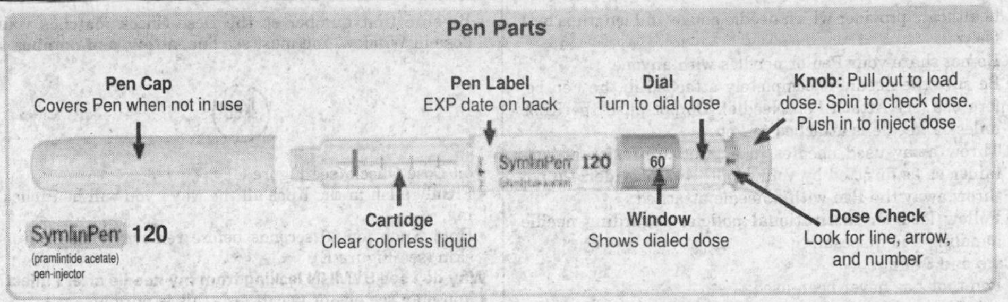
Pen Parts
Pen Cap
Covers Pen when not in use
Pen Label
EXP date on back
Dial
Turn to dial dose
Knob: Pull out to load dose. Spin to check dose. Push in to inject dose
SymlinPen 120
60
SymlinPen 120
(pramlintide acetate) pen-injector
Cartidge
Clear colorless liquid
Window
Shows dialed dose
Dose Check
Look for line, arrow, and number

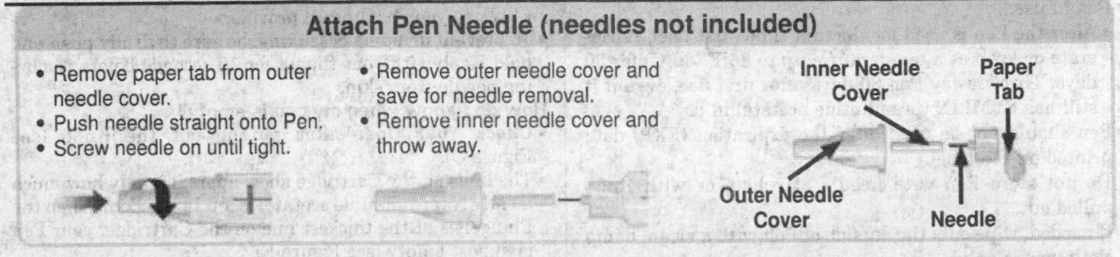
Attach Pen Needle (needles not included)
• Remove paper tab from outer needle cover.
• Push needle straight onto Pen.
• Screw needle on until tight.
• Remove outer needle cover and save for needle removal.
• Remove inner needle cover and throw away.
Inner Needle Cover
Paper Tab
Outer Needle Cover
Needle

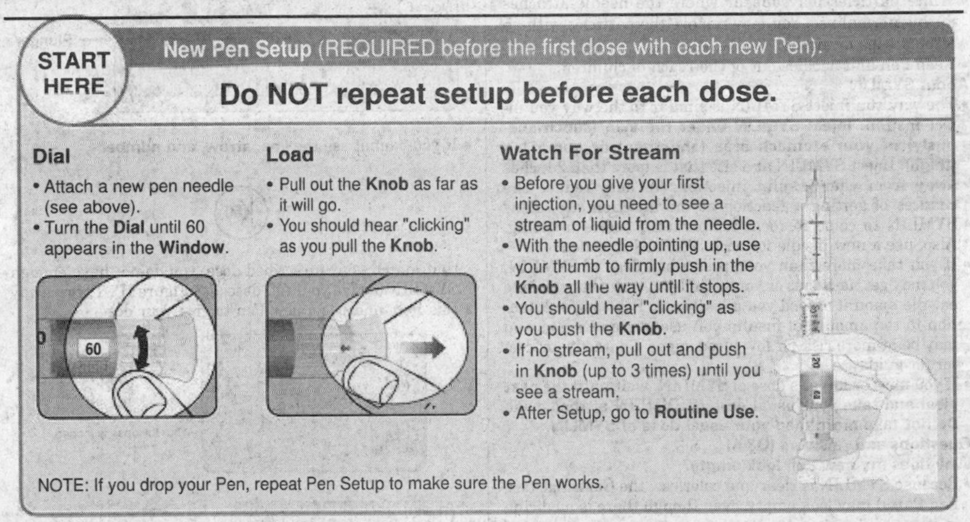
START HERE
New Pen Setup (REQUIRED before the first dose with each new Pen).
Do NOT repeat setup before each dose.
Dial
• Attach a new pen needle (see above).
• Turn the Dial until 60 appears in the Window.
60
Load
• Pull out the Knob as far as it will go.
• You should hear "clicking" as you pull the Knob.
Watch For Stream
• Before you give your first injection, you need to see a stream of liquid from the needle.
• With the needle pointing up, use your thumb to firmly push in the Knob all the way until it stops.
• You should hear "clicking" as you push the Knob.
• If no stream, pull out and push in Knob (up to 3 times) until you see a stream.
• After Setup, go to Routine Use.
NOTE: If you drop your Pen, repeat Pen Setup to make sure the Pen works.

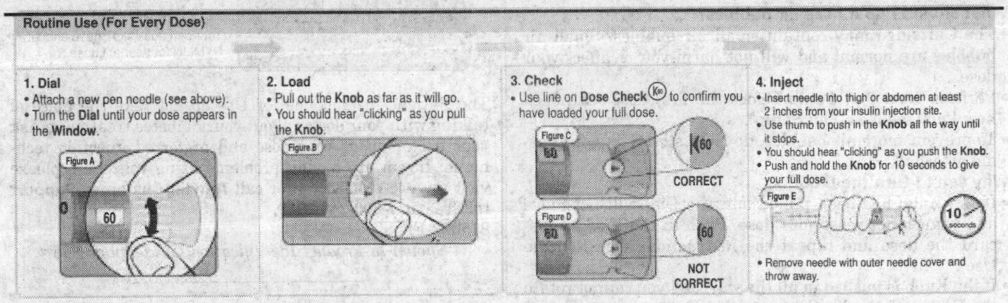
Routine Use (For Every Dose)
1. Dial
• Attach a new pen needle (see above).
• Turn the Dial until your dose appears in the Window.
Figure A
60
2. Load
• Pull out the Knob as far as it will go.
• You should hear "clicking" as you pull the Knob.
Figure B
3. Check
• Use line on Dose Check to confirm you have loaded your full dose.
Figure C
60
CORRECT
Figure D
60
NOT CORRECT
4. Inject
• Insert needle into thigh or abdomen at least 2 inches from your insulin injection site.
• Use thumb to push in the Knob all the way until it stops.
• You should hear "clicking" as you push the Knob.
• Push and hold the Knob for 10 seconds to give your full dose.
Figure E
10 seconds
• Remove needle with outer needle cover and throw away.

[See second figure above]

Important Notes
- Ask your doctor about your dose, injection technique, and needle size.
- Pen may look empty because SYMLIN (pramlintide acetate) is a clear, colorless liquid.
- Small bubbles will not harm you or affect your dose.
- **DO NOT TRANSFER YOUR SYMLIN FROM THE PEN TO A SYRINGE.** This could result in a higher dose than intended, because the SYMLIN in the Pen is a different strength than the SYMLIN in the vial.

[See third figure above]

[See fourth figure above]

Literature Revised July 2008

SymlinPen® pen-injector (Pen)

Read these instructions carefully before using your Pen. Failure to follow these instructions may cause an incorrect dose, a broken Pen, or an infection.
- Check Pen label before each use to make sure you have the 60•120 mcg Pen.
- Check the expiration date (EXP) on the Pen label (see Pen Parts), and make sure the Pen is not expired.
- If you drop your Pen, go to **New Pen Setup** to confirm Pen works.
- If any part of your Pen appears broken or damaged, do not use.
- This Pen is not recommended for use by blind or visually impaired persons without the assistance of a person trained in the proper use of this Pen.
- If SYMLIN (pramlintide acetate) in the Cartridge (see Pen Parts) is not clear, colorless, and free of particles, do not use Pen.

Needles
- Use a new needle for each injection. Remove the needle from the Pen after completing each injection. This will help prevent leakage of SYMLIN, keep out air bubbles, reduce needle clogs, and reduce risk of infection.
- Pen needles are not included with the Pen. Use 29, 30, or 31 gauge disposable needles with the Pen. Ask your

healthcare provider which needle gauge and length is best for you.
- Do not share your Pen or needles with anyone.
- Be sure the needle is completely attached to the Pen before use (see Attach Pen Needle). Do not push the Knob unless a needle is attached to Pen.
- Throw away used needles in a puncture-resistant container or as directed by your healthcare provider. Do not throw away the Pen with a needle attached.
- Follow local or institutional policies regarding needle handling and disposal.

Care and Storage
- Pen that has never been used:
  - Refrigerate (36°F to 46°F, 2°C to 8°C).
  - Protect from light.
  - **Do not freeze**. Do not use a Pen that has been frozen.
- Pen in use:
  - After the Pen is used for the first time (first use), refrigerate or keep at a temperature up to 86°F (30°C) for 30 days. Throw away Pen 30 days after first use, even if it still has SYMLIN (pramlintide acetate) in it.
- Pen should not be used after the expiration (EXP) date printed on the label.
- Do not store Pen with needle attached, or with Knob pulled out.
- If needed, wipe only the outside of Pen with a clean, damp cloth (water only).
- White particles may appear where the needle attaches during normal use. You may remove the particles with an alcohol wipe or alcohol swab.
- Keep Pen and needles out of the reach of children.

About SYMLIN
- The way you inject SYMLIN is similar to the way you inject insulin. **Inject SYMLIN under the skin (subcutaneously) of your stomach area (abdomen) or upper leg (thigh).** Inject SYMLIN at a site that is more than 2 inches away from your insulin injection. To help reduce the chances of getting a reaction at the injection site, allow SYMLIN to come to room temperature before injecting. Also, use a new needle for each SYMLIN injection.
- If you take more than your prescribed dose of SYMLIN, you may get nauseous or vomit, and you may not be able to eat the amount of food you usually eat. Pay careful attention to the amount of insulin you use at this time as you may be at more risk for low blood sugar. Contact your doctor for guidance.
- If you miss or forget a dose of SYMLIN, wait until the next meal and take your usual dose of SYMLIN at that meal. **Do not take more than your usual dose of SYMLIN.**

Questions and Answers (Q&A)

Why does my new Pen look empty?
- Because SYMLIN is clear and colorless, the Cartridge (see Pen Parts) may look empty, even though there is medicine in it.
- To be sure there is SYMLIN in the Cartridge, perform Pen setup (see New Pen Setup).

What should I do if I see air bubbles?
- The Cartridge may contain small air bubbles. Small air bubbles are normal and will not harm you or affect your dose.
- Perform **New Pen Setup** before the first dose with each new Pen (see New Pen Setup).
- To prevent more air bubbles, do NOT store Pen with needle attached.

Why can't I turn the Dial?
- If the Knob has been pulled out, the Dial will not move and you cannot reset your dose. Push in the Knob to discard the dose and repeat the instructions (see Routine Use).
- If the Knob is pushed in all the way, and you cannot rotate the Dial, call Amylin Customer Support.

What should I do if I do not see a stream of liquid when I perform the setup?
- Watch for a stream when you start to push the Knob.
- The liquid is clear and colorless, so it may be difficult to see.
- Pull out the Knob all the way - you will hear clicking.
- Firmly push in the Knob all the way - you will hear clicking.
- If there is no stream of liquid after 3 attempts, replace the needle and repeat setup.
- If still no stream, call Amylin Customer Support.

What should I do if I load an incorrect dose?
- **Do not inject an incorrect dose.** Point the needle away from you and discard the dose by pushing in the Knob all the way. Dial your correct dose.

How do I make sure I am getting my correct dose of SYMLIN?
- Before pulling out Knob, be sure the number in Window matches your prescribed SYMLIN dose (see Figure A).
- Pull out the Knob all the way - you will hear clicking (see Figure B).
- Be sure that number on the Dose Check matches your dose in Window. You must see **line, arrow, and number**

on Dose Check (see Figure C).
- Firmly push in the Knob all the way - you will hear clicking.
- Hold Knob for 10 seconds before removing needle from skin (see Figure E).

Why do I see SYMLIN leaking from my needle after I inject?
- You may see one or two drops - this is normal.
- If you see more than 2 drops:
  - You may not have received your full dose.
  - **Do not inject another dose.**
  - Talk to your healthcare provider.
- To prevent dripping or leaking, be sure to firmly push and hold Knob with your thumb for 10 seconds before removing needle from skin.

How do I know when my pen is empty?
- **Check Your Dose** after pulling out the Knob (see Figure C).
- The lines on the Cartridge show approximately how much SYMLIN (pramlintide acetate) is left in the Pen. When the Plunger is at the thickest line on the Cartridge, your Pen is almost empty (see Figure F).

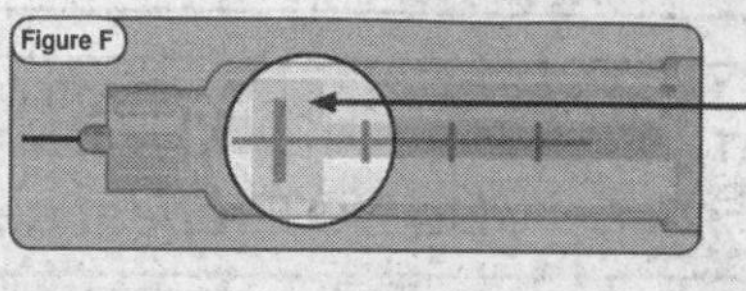
Figure F
Plunger

- If you cannot see the **line, arrow, and number**

that match your prescribed dose, you do not have enough SYMLIN to give your full dose (see Figure H). Throw away this Pen, and use a new Pen to give your dose.

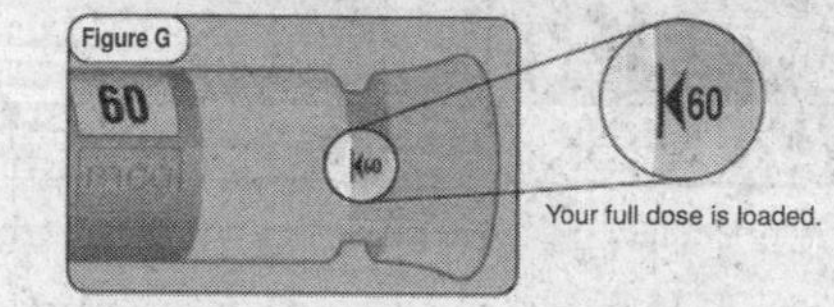
Figure G
60
Your full dose is loaded.

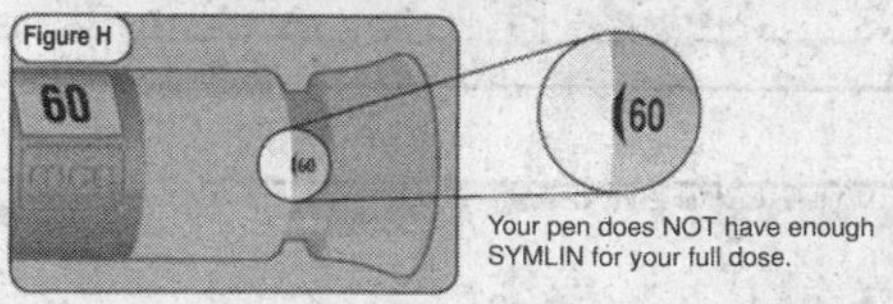
Figure H
60
Your pen does NOT have enough SYMLIN for your full dose.

The Patient Instructions for Use do not take the place of talking with your doctor about your diabetes treatment. Ask your doctor about your dose and preferred injection technique. If you are having problems using your Pen, please visit **www.SYMLIN.com** or call **Amylin Customer Support** toll free at **1-800-349-8919.**
815003-FF

Shown in Product Identification Guide, page 306

YERVOY® ℞
[yur-voi]
(ipilimumab)
Injection, for intravenous infusion

HIGHLIGHTS OF PRESCRIBING INFORMATION
These highlights do not include all the information needed to use YERVOY safely and effectively. See full prescribing information for YERVOY.
YERVOY® (ipilimumab)
Injection, for intravenous infusion
Initial U.S. Approval: 2011

WARNING: IMMUNE-MEDIATED ADVERSE REACTIONS
See full prescribing information for complete boxed warning.
YERVOY can result in severe and fatal immune-mediated adverse reactions due to T-cell activation and proliferation. These immune-mediated reactions may involve any organ system; however, the most common severe immune-mediated adverse reactions are enterocolitis, hepatitis, dermatitis (including toxic epidermal necrolysis), neuropathy, and endocrinopathy. The majority of these immune-mediated reactions initially manifested during treatment; however, a minority occurred weeks to months after discontinuation of YERVOY.
Permanently discontinue YERVOY and initiate systemic high-dose corticosteroid therapy for severe immune-mediated reactions. (2.2)
Assess patients for signs and symptoms of enterocolitis, dermatitis, neuropathy, and endocrinopathy and evaluate clinical chemistries including liver function tests and thyroid function tests at baseline and before each dose. (5.1, 5.2, 5.3, 5.4, 5.5)

INDICATIONS AND USAGE

YERVOY is a human cytotoxic T-lymphocyte antigen 4 (CTLA-4)-blocking antibody indicated for the treatment of unresectable or metastatic melanoma. (1)

DOSAGE AND ADMINISTRATION

- YERVOY 3 mg/kg administered intravenously over 90 minutes every 3 weeks for a total of four doses. (2.1)
- Permanently discontinue for severe adverse reactions. (2.2)

DOSAGE FORMS AND STRENGTHS

- 50 mg/10 mL (5 mg/mL) (3)
- 200 mg/40 mL (5 mg/mL) (3)

CONTRAINDICATIONS

None. (4)

WARNINGS AND PRECAUTIONS

Immune-mediated adverse reactions: Permanently discontinue for severe reactions. Withhold dose for moderate immune-mediated adverse reactions until return to baseline, improvement to mild severity, or complete resolution, and patient is receiving less than 7.5 mg prednisone or equivalent per day. Administer systemic high-dose corticosteroids for severe, persistent, or recurring immune-mediated reactions. (5.1, 5.2, 5.3, 5.4, 5.5)
- Immune-mediated hepatitis: Evaluate liver function tests before each dose of YERVOY. (5.2)
- Immune-mediated endocrinopathies: Monitor thyroid function tests and clinical chemistries prior to each dose. Evaluate at each visit for signs and symptoms of endocrinopathy. Institute hormone replacement therapy as needed. (5.5)

ADVERSE REACTIONS

Most common adverse reactions (≥5%) are fatigue, diarrhea, pruritus, rash, and colitis. (6.1)
To report SUSPECTED ADVERSE REACTIONS, contact Bristol-Myers Squibb at 1-800-721-5072 or FDA at 1-800-FDA-1088 or www.fda.gov/medwatch.

USE IN SPECIFIC POPULATIONS

- Pregnancy: Based on animal data, YERVOY may cause fetal harm. (8.1)
- Nursing mothers: Discontinue nursing or discontinue YERVOY. (8.3)

See 17 for PATIENT COUNSELING INFORMATION and Medication Guide

Revised: 05/2013

FULL PRESCRIBING INFORMATION: CONTENTS*

*** Sections or subsections omitted from the full prescribing information are not listed**

FULL PRESCRIBING INFORMATION

WARNING: IMMUNE-MEDIATED ADVERSE REACTIONS

YERVOY can result in severe and fatal immune-mediated adverse reactions due to T-cell activation and proliferation. These immune-mediated reactions may involve any organ system; however, the most common severe immune-mediated adverse reactions are enterocolitis, hepatitis, dermatitis (including toxic epidermal necrolysis), neuropathy, and endocrinopathy. The majority of these immune-mediated reactions initially manifested during treatment; however, a minority occurred weeks to months after discontinuation of YERVOY.

Permanently discontinue YERVOY and initiate systemic high-dose corticosteroid therapy for severe immune-mediated reactions. *[See Dosage and Administration (2.2).]*

Assess patients for signs and symptoms of enterocolitis, dermatitis, neuropathy, and endocrinopathy and evaluate clinical chemistries including liver function tests and thyroid function tests at baseline and before each dose. *[See Warnings and Precautions (5.1, 5.2, 5.3, 5.4, 5.5).]*

1 INDICATIONS AND USAGE

YERVOY (ipilimumab) is indicated for the treatment of unresectable or metastatic melanoma.

2 DOSAGE AND ADMINISTRATION

2.1 Recommended Dosing

The recommended dose of YERVOY is 3 mg/kg administered intravenously over 90 minutes every 3 weeks for a total of 4 doses.

2.2 Recommended Dose Modifications

- Withhold scheduled dose of YERVOY for any moderate immune-mediated adverse reactions or for symptomatic endocrinopathy. For patients with complete or partial resolution of adverse reactions (Grade 0–1), and who are receiving less than 7.5 mg prednisone or equivalent per day, resume YERVOY at a dose of 3 mg/kg every 3 weeks until administration of all 4 planned doses or 16 weeks from first dose, whichever occurs earlier.
- Permanently discontinue YERVOY for any of the following:
  - Persistent moderate adverse reactions or inability to reduce corticosteroid dose to 7.5 mg prednisone or equivalent per day.
  - Failure to complete full treatment course within 16 weeks from administration of first dose.
  - Severe or life-threatening adverse reactions, including any of the following:
    - Colitis with abdominal pain, fever, ileus, or peritoneal signs; increase in stool frequency (7 or more over baseline), stool incontinence, need for intravenous hydration for more than 24 hours, gastrointestinal hemorrhage, and gastrointestinal perforation
    - Aspartate aminotransferase (AST) or alanine aminotransferase (ALT) >5 times the upper limit of normal or total bilirubin >3 times the upper limit of normal
    - Stevens-Johnson syndrome, toxic epidermal necrolysis, or rash complicated by full thickness dermal ulceration, or necrotic, bullous, or hemorrhagic manifestations
    - Severe motor or sensory neuropathy, Guillain-Barré syndrome, or myasthenia gravis
    - Severe immune-mediated reactions involving any organ system (eg, nephritis, pneumonitis, pancreatitis, non-infectious myocarditis)
    - Immune-mediated ocular disease that is unresponsive to topical immunosuppressive therapy

2.3 Preparation and Administration

- Do not shake product.
- Inspect parenteral drug products visually for particulate matter and discoloration prior to administration. Discard vial if solution is cloudy, there is pronounced discoloration (solution may have pale-yellow color), or there is foreign particulate matter other than translucent-to-white, amorphous particles.

Preparation of Solution

- Allow the vials to stand at room temperature for approximately 5 minutes prior to preparation of infusion.
- Withdraw the required volume of YERVOY (ipilimumab) and transfer into an intravenous bag.
- Dilute with 0.9% Sodium Chloride Injection, USP or 5% Dextrose Injection, USP to prepare a diluted solution with a final concentration ranging from 1 mg/mL to 2 mg/mL. Mix diluted solution by gentle inversion.
- Store the diluted solution for no more than 24 hours under refrigeration (2°C to 8°C, 36°F to 46°F) or at room temperature (20°C to 25°C, 68°F to 77°F).
- Discard partially used vials or empty vials of YERVOY.

Administration Instructions

- Do not mix YERVOY with, or administer as an infusion with, other medicinal products.
- Flush the intravenous line with 0.9% Sodium Chloride Injection, USP or 5% Dextrose Injection, USP after each dose.
- Administer diluted solution over 90 minutes through an intravenous line containing a sterile, non-pyrogenic, low-protein-binding in-line filter.

3 DOSAGE FORMS AND STRENGTHS

50 mg/10 mL (5 mg/mL)
200 mg/40 mL (5 mg/mL)

4 CONTRAINDICATIONS

None.

5 WARNINGS AND PRECAUTIONS

YERVOY can result in severe and fatal immune-mediated reactions due to T-cell activation and proliferation. *[See Boxed Warning.]*

5.1 Immune-mediated Enterocolitis

In Study 1, severe, life-threatening, or fatal (diarrhea of 7 or more stools above baseline, fever, ileus, peritoneal signs; Grade 3–5) immune-mediated enterocolitis occurred in 34 (7%) YERVOY-treated patients, and moderate (diarrhea with up to 6 stools above baseline, abdominal pain, mucus or blood in stool; Grade 2) enterocolitis occurred in 28 (5%) YERVOY-treated patients. Across all YERVOY-treated patients (n=511), 5 (1%) patients developed intestinal perforation, 4 (0.8%) patients died as a result of complications, and 26 (5%) patients were hospitalized for severe enterocolitis.

The median time to onset was 7.4 weeks (range: 1.6–13.4) and 6.3 weeks (range: 0.3–18.9) after the initiation of YERVOY for patients with Grade 3–5 enterocolitis and with Grade 2 enterocolitis, respectively.

Twenty-nine patients (85%) with Grade 3–5 enterocolitis were treated with high-dose (≥40 mg prednisone equivalent per day) corticosteroids, with a median dose of 80 mg/day of prednisone or equivalent; the median duration of treatment was 2.3 weeks (ranging up to 13.9 weeks) followed by corticosteroid taper. Of the 28 patients with moderate enterocolitis, 46% were not treated with systemic corticosteroids, 29% were treated with <40 mg prednisone or equivalent per day for a median duration of 5.1 weeks, and 25% were treated with high-dose corticosteroids for a median duration of 10 days prior to corticosteroid taper. Infliximab was administered to 5 of the 62 patients (8%) with moderate, severe, or life-threatening immune-mediated enterocolitis following inadequate response to corticosteroids.

Of the 34 patients with Grade 3–5 enterocolitis, 74% experienced complete resolution, 3% experienced improvement to Grade 2 severity, and 24% did not improve. Among the 28 patients with Grade 2 enterocolitis, 79% experienced complete resolution, 11% improved, and 11% did not improve.

Monitor patients for signs and symptoms of enterocolitis (such as diarrhea, abdominal pain, mucus or blood in stool, with or without fever) and of bowel perforation (such as peritoneal signs and ileus). In symptomatic patients, rule out infectious etiologies and consider endoscopic evaluation for persistent or severe symptoms.

Permanently discontinue YERVOY in patients with severe enterocolitis and initiate systemic corticosteroids at a dose of 1 to 2 mg/kg/day of prednisone or equivalent. Upon improvement to Grade 1 or less, initiate corticosteroid taper and continue to taper over at least 1 month. In clinical trials, rapid corticosteroid tapering resulted in recurrence or worsening symptoms of enterocolitis in some patients.

Withhold YERVOY dosing for moderate enterocolitis; administer anti-diarrheal treatment and, if persistent for more than 1 week, initiate systemic corticosteroids at a dose of 0.5 mg/kg/day prednisone or equivalent. *[See Dosage and Administration (2.2).]*

5.2 Immune-mediated Hepatitis

In Study 1, severe, life-threatening, or fatal hepatotoxicity (AST or ALT elevations of more than 5 times the upper limit of normal or total bilirubin elevations more than 3 times the upper limit of normal; Grade 3–5) occurred in 8 (2%) YERVOY-treated patients, with fatal hepatic failure in 0.2% and hospitalization in 0.4% of YERVOY-treated patients. An additional 13 (2.5%) patients experienced moderate hepatotoxicity manifested by liver function test abnormalities (AST or ALT elevations of more than 2.5 times but not more than 5 times the upper limit of normal or total bilirubin elevation of more than 1.5 times but not more than 3 times the upper limit of normal; Grade 2). The underlying pathology was not ascertained in all patients but in some instances included immune-mediated hepatitis. There were insufficient numbers of patients with biopsy-proven hepatitis to characterize the clinical course of this event.

Monitor liver function tests (hepatic transaminase and bilirubin levels) and assess patients for signs and symptoms of hepatotoxicity before each dose of YERVOY (ipilimumab). In patients with hepatotoxicity, rule out infectious or malignant causes and increase frequency of liver function test monitoring until resolution.

Permanently discontinue YERVOY in patients with Grade 3–5 hepatotoxicity and administer systemic corticosteroids at a dose of 1 to 2 mg/kg/day of prednisone or equivalent. When liver function tests show sustained improvement or return to baseline, initiate corticosteroid tapering and continue to taper over 1 month. Across the clinical development program for YERVOY, mycophenolate treatment has been administered in patients who have persistent severe hepatitis despite high-dose corticosteroids. Withhold YERVOY in patients with Grade 2 hepatotoxicity. *[See Dosage and Administration (2.2).]*

5.3 Immune-mediated Dermatitis

In Study 1, severe, life-threatening, or fatal immune-mediated dermatitis (eg, Stevens-Johnson syndrome, toxic epidermal necrolysis, or rash complicated by full thickness dermal ulceration, or necrotic, bullous, or hemorrhagic manifestations; Grade 3–5) occurred in 13 (2.5%) YERVOY-treated patients. One (0.2%) patient died as a result of toxic epidermal necrolysis and one additional patient required hospitalization for severe dermatitis. There were 63 (12%) patients with moderate (Grade 2) dermatitis.

The median time to onset of moderate, severe, or life-threatening immune-mediated dermatitis was 3.1 weeks and ranged up to 17.3 weeks from the initiation of YERVOY. Seven (54%) YERVOY-treated patients with severe dermatitis received high-dose corticosteroids (median dose 60 mg prednisone/day or equivalent) for up to 14.9 weeks followed by corticosteroid taper. Of these 7 patients, 6 had complete resolution; time to resolution ranged up to 15.6 weeks.

Of the 63 patients with moderate dermatitis, 25 (40%) were treated with systemic corticosteroids (median of 60 mg/day of prednisone or equivalent) for a median of 2.1 weeks, 7 (11%) were treated with only topical corticosteroids, and 31 (49%) did not receive systemic or topical corticosteroids. Forty-four (70%) patients with moderate dermatitis were reported to have complete resolution, 7 (11%) improved to mild (Grade 1) severity, and 12 (19%) had no reported improvement.

Monitor patients for signs and symptoms of dermatitis such as rash and pruritus. Unless an alternate etiology has been identified, signs or symptoms of dermatitis should be considered immune-mediated.

Permanently discontinue YERVOY in patients with Stevens-Johnson syndrome, toxic epidermal necrolysis, or rash complicated by full thickness dermal ulceration, or necrotic, bullous, or hemorrhagic manifestations. Administer systemic corticosteroids at a dose of 1 to 2 mg/kg/day of prednisone or equivalent. When dermatitis is controlled, corticosteroid tapering should occur over a period of at least 1 month. Withhold YERVOY dosing in patients with moderate to severe signs and symptoms. *[See Dosage and Administration (2.2).]*

For mild to moderate dermatitis, such as localized rash and pruritus, treat symptomatically. Administer topical or systemic corticosteroids if there is no improvement of symptoms within 1 week.

5.4 Immune-mediated Neuropathies

In Study 1, 1 case of fatal Guillain-Barré syndrome and 1 case of severe (Grade 3) peripheral motor neuropathy were reported. Across the clinical development program of YERVOY, myasthenia gravis and additional cases of Guillain-Barré syndrome have been reported.

Monitor for symptoms of motor or sensory neuropathy such as unilateral or bilateral weakness, sensory alterations, or paresthesia. Permanently discontinue YERVOY in patients with severe neuropathy (interfering with daily activities) such as Guillain-Barré-like syndromes. Institute medical intervention as appropriate for management of severe neuropathy. Consider initiation of systemic corticosteroids at a dose of 1 to 2 mg/kg/day prednisone or equivalent for severe neuropathies. Withhold YERVOY dosing in patients with moderate neuropathy (not interfering with daily activities). *[See Dosage and Administration (2.2).]*

5.5 Immune-mediated Endocrinopathies

In Study 1, severe to life-threatening immune-mediated endocrinopathies (requiring hospitalization, urgent medical intervention, or interfering with activities of daily living;

Table 1: Selected Adverse Reactions in Study 1

System Organ Class/ Preferred Term	Percentage (%) of Patients[a]					
	YERVOY 3 mg/kg n=131		YERVOY 3 mg/kg+gp100 n=380		gp100 n=132	
	Any Grade	Grade 3–5	Any Grade	Grade 3–5	Any Grade	Grade 3–5
Gastrointestinal Disorders						
Diarrhea	32	5	37	4	20	1
Colitis	8	5	5	3	2	0
Skin and Subcutaneous Tissue Disorders						
Pruritus	31	0	21	<1	11	0
Rash	29	2	25	2	8	0
General Disorders and Administration Site Conditions						
Fatigue	41	7	34	5	31	3

[a] Incidences presented in this table are based on reports of adverse events regardless of causality.

Grade 3–4) occurred in 9 (1.8%) YERVOY-treated patients. All 9 patients had hypopituitarism and some had additional concomitant endocrinopathies such as adrenal insufficiency, hypogonadism, and hypothyroidism. Six of the 9 patients were hospitalized for severe endocrinopathies. Moderate endocrinopathy (requiring hormone replacement or medical intervention; Grade 2) occurred in 12 (2.3%) patients and consisted of hypothyroidism, adrenal insufficiency, hypopituitarism, and 1 case each of hyperthyroidism and Cushing's syndrome. The median time to onset of moderate to severe immune-mediated endocrinopathy was 11 weeks and ranged up to 19.3 weeks after the initiation of YERVOY (ipilimumab).

Of the 21 patients with moderate to life-threatening endocrinopathy, 17 patients required long-term hormone replacement therapy including, most commonly, adrenal hormones (n=10) and thyroid hormones (n=13).

Monitor patients for clinical signs and symptoms of hypophysitis, adrenal insufficiency (including adrenal crisis), and hyper- or hypothyroidism. Patients may present with fatigue, headache, mental status changes, abdominal pain, unusual bowel habits, and hypotension, or nonspecific symptoms which may resemble other causes such as brain metastasis or underlying disease. Unless an alternate etiology has been identified, signs or symptoms of endocrinopathies should be considered immune-mediated.

Monitor thyroid function tests and clinical chemistries at the start of treatment, before each dose, and as clinically indicated based on symptoms. In a limited number of patients, hypophysitis was diagnosed by imaging studies through enlargement of the pituitary gland.

Withhold YERVOY dosing in symptomatic patients. Initiate systemic corticosteroids at a dose of 1 to 2 mg/kg/day of prednisone or equivalent, and initiate appropriate hormone replacement therapy. *[See Dosage and Administration (2.2).]*

5.6 Other Immune-mediated Adverse Reactions, Including Ocular Manifestations

The following clinically significant immune-mediated adverse reactions were seen in less than 1% of YERVOY-treated patients in Study 1: nephritis, pneumonitis, meningitis, pericarditis, uveitis, iritis, and hemolytic anemia.

Across the clinical development program for YERVOY, the following likely immune-mediated adverse reactions were also reported with less than 1% incidence: myocarditis, angiopathy, temporal arteritis, vasculitis, polymyalgia rheumatica, conjunctivitis, blepharitis, episcleritis, scleritis, leukocytoclastic vasculitis, erythema multiforme, psoriasis, pancreatitis, arthritis, autoimmune thyroiditis, sarcoidosis, neurosensory hypoacusis, autoimmune central neuropathy (encephalitis), myositis, polymyositis, and ocular myositis.

Permanently discontinue YERVOY for clinically significant or severe immune-mediated adverse reactions. Initiate systemic corticosteroids at a dose of 1 to 2 mg/kg/day prednisone or equivalent for severe immune-mediated adverse reactions.

Administer corticosteroid eye drops to patients who develop uveitis, iritis, or episcleritis. Permanently discontinue YERVOY for immune-mediated ocular disease that is unresponsive to local immunosuppressive therapy. *[See Dosage and Administration (2.2).]*

6 ADVERSE REACTIONS

The following adverse reactions are discussed in greater detail in other sections of the labeling.

- Immune-mediated enterocolitis *[see Warnings and Precautions (5.1)].*
- Immune-mediated hepatitis *[see Warnings and Precautions (5.2)].*
- Immune-mediated dermatitis *[see Warnings and Precautions (5.3)].*
- Immune-mediated neuropathies *[see Warnings and Precautions (5.4)].*
- Immune-mediated endocrinopathies *[see Warnings and Precautions (5.5)].*
- Other immune-mediated adverse reactions, including ocular manifestations *[see Warnings and Precautions (5.6)].*

6.1 Clinical Trials Experience

Because clinical trials are conducted under widely varying conditions, the adverse reaction rates observed cannot be directly compared with rates in other clinical trials or experience with therapeutics in the same class and may not reflect the rates observed in clinical practice.

The clinical development program excluded patients with active autoimmune disease or those receiving systemic immunosuppression for organ transplantation. Exposure to YERVOY 3 mg/kg for 4 doses given by intravenous infusion in previously treated patients with unresectable or metastatic melanoma was assessed in a randomized, double-blind clinical study (Study 1). *[See Clinical Studies (14).]* One hundred thirty-one patients (median age 57 years, 60% male) received YERVOY (ipilimumab) as a single agent, 380 patients (median age 56 years, 61% male) received YERVOY with an investigational gp100 peptide vaccine (gp100), and 132 patients (median age 57 years, 54% male) received gp100 peptide vaccine alone. Patients in the study received a median of 4 doses (range: 1–4 doses). YERVOY was discontinued for adverse reactions in 10% of patients.

The most common adverse reactions (≥5%) in patients who received YERVOY at 3 mg/kg were fatigue, diarrhea, pruritus, rash, and colitis.

Table 1 presents selected adverse reactions from Study 1, which occurred in at least 5% of patients in the YERVOY-containing arms and with at least 5% increased incidence over the control gp100 arm for all-grade events and at least 1% incidence over the control group for Grade 3–5 events. [See table 1 above]

Table 2 presents the per-patient incidence of severe, life-threatening, or fatal immune-mediated adverse reactions from Study 1.

Table 2: Severe to Fatal Immune-mediated Adverse Reactions in Study 1

	Percentage (%) of Patients	
	YERVOY 3 mg/kg n=131	YERVOY 3 mg/kg+gp100 n=380
Any Immune-mediated Adverse Reaction	15	12
Enterocolitis[a,b]	7	7
Hepatotoxicity[a]	1	2
Dermatitis[a]	2	3
Neuropathy[a]	1	<1
Endocrinopathy	4	1
Hypopituitarism	4	1
Adrenal insufficiency	0	1
Other		
Pneumonitis	0	<1
Meningitis	0	<1
Nephritis	1	0
Eosinophilia[c]	1	0
Pericarditis[a,c]	0	<1

[a] Including fatal outcome.
[b] Including intestinal perforation.
[c] Underlying etiology not established.

Across clinical studies that utilized YERVOY doses ranging from 0.3 to 10 mg/kg, the following adverse reactions were also reported (incidence less than 1% unless otherwise noted): urticaria (2%), large intestinal ulcer, esophagitis, acute respiratory distress syndrome, renal failure, and infusion reaction.

Based on the experience in the entire clinical program for melanoma, the incidence and severity of enterocolitis and hepatitis appear to be dose dependent.

6.2 Immunogenicity

In clinical studies, 1.1% of 1024 evaluable patients tested positive for binding antibodies against ipilimumab in an electrochemiluminescent (ECL) based assay. This assay has substantial limitations in detecting anti-ipilimumab antibodies in the presence of ipilimumab. Infusion-related or peri-infusional reactions consistent with hypersensitivity or anaphylaxis were not reported in these 11 patients nor were neutralizing antibodies against ipilimumab detected.

Because trough levels of ipilimumab interfere with the ECL assay results, a subset analysis was performed in the dose cohort with the lowest trough levels. In this analysis, 6.9% of 58 evaluable patients, who were treated with 0.3 mg/kg dose, tested positive for binding antibodies against ipilimumab.

Immunogenicity assay results are highly dependent on several factors including assay sensitivity and specificity, assay methodology, sample handling, timing of sample collection, concomitant medications, and underlying disease. For these reasons, comparison of incidence of antibodies to YERVOY (ipilimumab) with the incidences of antibodies to other products may be misleading.

7 DRUG INTERACTIONS

No formal pharmacokinetic drug interaction studies have been conducted with YERVOY.

8 USE IN SPECIFIC POPULATIONS

8.1 Pregnancy

Pregnancy Category C

There are no adequate and well-controlled studies of YERVOY in pregnant women. Use YERVOY during pregnancy only if the potential benefit justifies the potential risk to the fetus.

In a combined study of embryo-fetal and peri-postnatal development, pregnant cynomolgus monkeys received ipilimumab every 3 weeks from the onset of organogenesis in the first trimester through parturition, at exposure levels either 2.6 or 7.2 times higher by AUC than the exposures at the clinical dose of 3 mg/kg of ipilimumab. No treatment-related adverse effects on reproduction were detected during the first two trimesters of pregnancy. Beginning in the third trimester, the ipilimumab treated groups experienced higher incidences of severe toxicities including abortion, stillbirth, premature delivery (with corresponding lower birth weight), and higher incidences of infant mortality in a dose-related manner compared to controls. *[See Nonclinical Toxicology (13.2).]*

Human IgG1 is known to cross the placental barrier and ipilimumab is an IgG1; therefore, ipilimumab has the potential to be transmitted from the mother to the developing fetus.

8.3 Nursing Mothers

It is not known whether ipilimumab is secreted in human milk. In monkeys treated at dose levels resulting in exposures 2.6 and 7.2 times higher than those in humans at the recommended dose, ipilimumab was present in milk at concentrations of 0.1 and 0.4 mcg/mL, representing a ratio of up to 0.3% of the serum concentration of the drug. Because many drugs are secreted in human milk and because of the potential for serious adverse reactions in nursing infants from YERVOY, a decision should be made whether to discontinue nursing or to discontinue YERVOY, taking into account the importance of YERVOY to the mother.

8.4 Pediatric Use

Safety and effectiveness of YERVOY have not been established in pediatric patients.

8.5 Geriatric Use

Of the 511 patients treated with YERVOY at 3 mg/kg, 28% were 65 years and over. No overall differences in safety or efficacy were reported between the elderly patients (65 years and over) and younger patients (less than 65 years).

8.6 Renal Impairment

No dose adjustment is needed for patients with renal impairment. *[See Clinical Pharmacology (12.3).]*

8.7 Hepatic Impairment

No dose adjustment is needed for patients with mild hepatic impairment (total bilirubin [TB] >1.0 × to 1.5 × the upper limit of normal [ULN] or AST >ULN). YERVOY has not been studied in patients with moderate (TB >1.5 × to 3.0 × ULN and any AST) or severe (TB >3 × ULN and any AST) hepatic impairment. *[See Clinical Pharmacology (12.3).]*

10 OVERDOSAGE

There is no information on overdosage with YERVOY.

11 DESCRIPTION

YERVOY (ipilimumab) is a recombinant, human monoclonal antibody that binds to the cytotoxic T-lymphocyte-associated antigen 4 (CTLA-4). Ipilimumab is an IgG1 kappa immunoglobulin with an approximate molecular weight of 148 kDa. Ipilimumab is produced in mammalian (Chinese hamster ovary) cell culture.

YERVOY (ipilimumab) is a sterile, preservative-free, clear to slightly opalescent, colorless to pale-yellow solution for intravenous infusion, which may contain a small amount of visible translucent-to white, amorphous ipilimumab particulates. It is supplied in single-use vials of 50 mg/10 mL and 200 mg/40 mL. Each milliliter contains 5 mg of ipilimumab and the following inactive ingredients: diethylene triamine pentaacetic acid (DTPA) (0.04 mg), mannitol (10 mg), polysorbate 80 (vegetable origin) (0.1 mg), sodium chloride (5.85 mg), tris hydrochloride (3.15 mg), and Water for Injection, USP at a pH of 7.

12 CLINICAL PHARMACOLOGY

12.1 Mechanism of Action

CTLA-4 is a negative regulator of T-cell activation. Ipilimumab binds to CTLA-4 and blocks the interaction of CTLA-4 with its ligands, CD80/CD86. Blockade of CTLA-4 has been shown to augment T-cell activation and proliferation. The mechanism of action of ipilimumab's effect in patients with melanoma is indirect, possibly through T-cell mediated anti-tumor immune responses.

12.3 Pharmacokinetics

The pharmacokinetics of ipilimumab were studied in 785 patients with unresectable or metastatic melanoma who received doses of 0.3, 3, or 10 mg/kg once every 3 weeks for 4 doses. Peak concentration (C_{max}), trough concentration (C_{min}), and area under the plasma concentration versus time curve (AUC) of ipilimumab increased dose proportionally within the dose range examined. Upon repeated dosing every 3 weeks, the clearance (CL) of ipilimumab was found to be time-invariant, and systemic accumulation was 1.5-fold or less. Steady-state concentrations of ipilimumab were reached by the third dose; the mean C_{min} at steady-state was 19.4 mcg/mL following repeated doses of 3 mg/kg. The mean value (% coefficient of variation) generated through population pharmacokinetic analysis for the terminal half-life ($t_{1/2}$) was 15.4 days (34%) and for CL was 16.8 mL/h (38%).

Specific Populations: The effects of various covariates on the pharmacokinetics of ipilimumab were assessed in population pharmacokinetic analyses. The CL of ipilimumab increased with increasing body weight; however, no dose adjustment is recommended for body weight after administration on a mg/kg basis. The following factors had no clinically important effect on the CL of ipilimumab: age (range: 23–88 years), gender, performance status, renal impairment, mild hepatic impairment, previous cancer therapy, and baseline lactate dehydrogenase (LDH) levels. The effect of race was not examined due to limited data available in non-Caucasian ethnic groups.

Renal Impairment: The effect of renal impairment on the CL of ipilimumab was evaluated in patients with mild (GFR <90 and ≥60 mL/min/1.73 m^2; n=349), moderate (GFR <60 and ≥30 mL/min/1.73 m^2; n=82), or severe (GFR <30 and ≥15 mL/min/1.73 m^2; n=4) renal impairment compared to patients with normal renal function (GFR ≥90 mL/min/1.73 m^2; n=350) in population pharmacokinetic analyses. No clinically important differences in the CL of ipilimumab were found between patients with renal impairment and patients with normal renal function. *[See Use in Specific Populations (8.6).]*

Hepatic Impairment: The effect of hepatic impairment on the CL of ipilimumab was evaluated in patients with mild hepatic impairment (TB 1.0 × to 1.5 × ULN or AST >ULN as defined using the National Cancer Institute criteria of hepatic dysfunction; n=76) compared to patients with normal hepatic function (TB and AST ≤ULN; n=708) in the population pharmacokinetic analyses. No clinically important differences in the CL of ipilimumab were found between patients with mild hepatic impairment and normal hepatic function. YERVOY has not been studied in patients with moderate (TB >1.5 × to 3 × ULN and any AST) or severe hepatic impairment (TB >3 × ULN and any AST). *[See Use in Specific Populations (8.7).]*

13 NONCLINICAL TOXICOLOGY

13.1 Carcinogenesis, Mutagenesis, Impairment of Fertility

Carcinogenesis

The carcinogenic potential of ipilimumab has not been evaluated in long-term animal studies.

Mutagenesis

The genotoxic potential of ipilimumab has not been evaluated.

Impairment of Fertility

Fertility studies have not been performed with ipilimumab.

13.2 Animal Toxicology and/or Pharmacology

In addition to the severe findings of abortion, stillbirths, and postnatal deaths observed in pregnant cynomolgus monkeys that received ipilimumab every 3 weeks from the onset of organogenesis in the first trimester through parturition *[see Use in Specific Populations (8.1)]*, developmental abnormalities were identified in the urogenital system of 2 infant monkeys exposed *in utero* to 30 mg/kg of ipilimumab (7.2 times the AUC in humans at the clinically recommended dose). One female infant monkey had unilateral renal agenesis of the left kidney and ureter, and 1 male infant monkey had an imperforate urethra with associated urinary obstruction and subcutaneous scrotal edema.

Genetically engineered mice heterozygous for CTLA-4 (CTLA-4+/–), the target for ipilimumab, appeared healthy and gave birth to healthy CTLA-4+/– heterozygous offspring. Mated CTLA-4+/– heterozygous mice also produced offspring deficient in CTLA-4 (homozygous negative, CTLA-4–/–). The CTLA-4–/– homozygous negative offspring appeared healthy at birth, exhibited signs of multiorgan lymphoproliferative disease by 2 weeks of age, and all died by 3–4 weeks of age with massive lymphoproliferation and multiorgan tissue destruction.

14 CLINICAL STUDIES

The safety and efficacy of YERVOY (ipilimumab) were investigated in a randomized (3:1:1), double-blind, double-dummy study (Study 1) that included 676 randomized patients with unresectable or metastatic melanoma previously treated with one or more of the following: aldesleukin, dacarbazine, temozolomide, fotemustine, or carboplatin. Of these 676 patients, 403 were randomized to receive YERVOY at 3 mg/kg in combination with an investigational peptide vaccine with incomplete Freund's adjuvant (gp100), 137 were randomized to receive YERVOY at 3 mg/kg, and 136 were randomized to receive gp100 alone. The study enrolled only patients with HLA-A2*0201 genotype; this HLA genotype facilitates the immune presentation of the investigational peptide vaccine. The study excluded patients with active autoimmune disease or those receiving systemic immunosuppression for organ transplantation. YERVOY/placebo was administered at 3 mg/kg as an intravenous infusion every 3 weeks for 4 doses. Gp100/placebo was administered at a dose of 2 mg peptide by deep subcutaneous injection every 3 weeks for 4 doses. Assessment of tumor response was conducted at weeks 12 and 24, and every 3 months thereafter. Patients with evidence of objective tumor response at 12 or 24 weeks had assessment for confirmation of durability of response at 16 or 28 weeks, respectively.

The major efficacy outcome measure was overall survival (OS) in the YERVOY+gp100 arm compared to that in the gp100 arm. Secondary efficacy outcome measures were OS in the YERVOY+gp100 arm compared to the YERVOY arm, OS in the YERVOY (ipilimumab) arm compared to the gp100 arm, best overall response rate (BORR) at week 24 between each of the study arms, and duration of response.

Of the randomized patients, 61%, 59%, and 54% in the YERVOY+gp100, YERVOY, and gp100 arms, respectively, were men. Twenty-nine percent were ≥65 years of age, the median age was 57 years, 71% had M1c stage, 12% had a history of previously treated brain metastasis, 98% had ECOG performance status of 0 and 1, 23% had received aldesleukin, and 38% had elevated LDH level. Sixty-one percent of patients randomized to either YERVOY-containing arm received all 4 planned doses. The median duration of follow-up was 8.9 months.

The OS results are shown in Table 3 and Figure 1.

[See table 3 above]

[See figure 1 above]

Table 3: Overall Survival Results

	YERVOY n=137	YERVOY+gp100 n=403	gp100 n=136
Hazard Ratio (vs. gp100)	0.66	0.68	
(95% CI)	(0.51, 0.87)	(0.55, 0.85)	
p-value	p=0.0026[a]	p=0.0004	
Hazard Ratio (vs. YERVOY)		1.04	
(95% CI)		(0.83, 1.30)	
Median (months)	10	10	6
(95% CI)	(8.0, 13.8)	(8.5, 11.5)	(5.5, 8.7)

[a] Not adjusted for multiple comparisons.

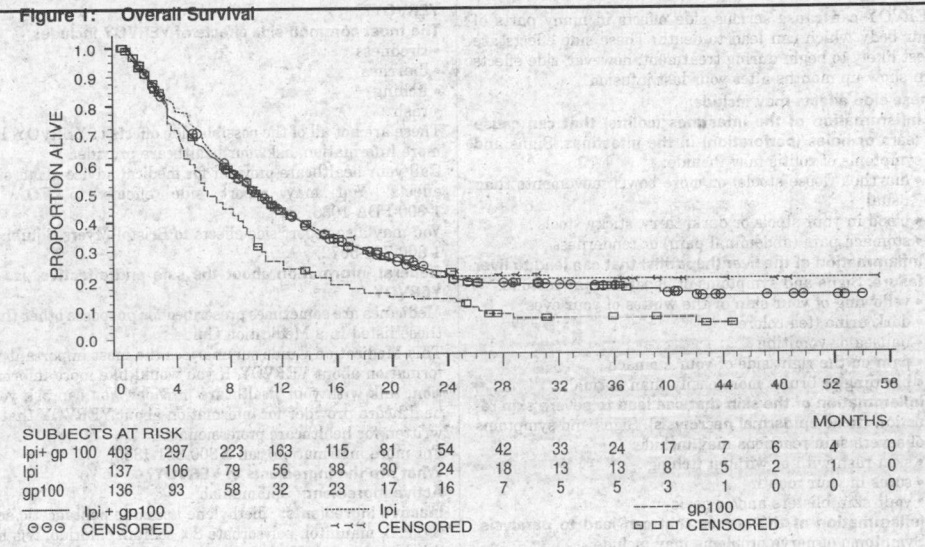

Figure 1: Overall Survival

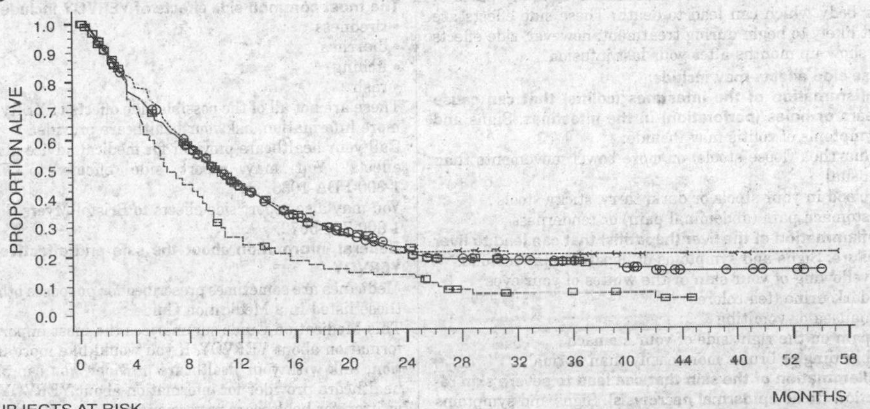

SUBJECTS AT RISK														
Ipi+ gp 100	403	297	223	163	115	81	54	42	33	24	17	7	6	4	0
Ipi	137	106	79	56	38	30	24	18	13	13	8	5	2	1	0
gp100	136	93	58	32	23	17	16	7	5	5	3	1	0	0	0

——— Ipi + gp100 ⊖⊖⊖ CENSORED
------- Ipi ⊣⊣⊣ CENSORED
- - - - gp100 □□□ CENSORED

The best overall response rate (BORR) as assessed by the investigator was 5.7% (95% CI: 3.7%, 8.4%) in the YERVOY+gp100 arm, 10.9% (95% CI: 6.3%, 17.4%) in the YERVOY arm, and 1.5% (95% CI: 0.2%, 5.2%) in the gp100 arm. The median duration of response was 11.5 months in the YERVOY+gp100 arm and has not been reached in the YERVOY or gp100 arm.

16 HOW SUPPLIED/STORAGE AND HANDLING

YERVOY is available as follows:

Carton Contents	NDC
One 50 mg vial (5 mg/mL), single-use vial	NDC 0003-2327-11
One 200 mg vial (5 mg/mL), single-use vial	NDC 0003-2328-22

Store YERVOY under refrigeration at 2°C to 8°C (36°F to 46°F). Do not freeze. Protect vials from light.

17 PATIENT COUNSELING INFORMATION

See MEDICATION GUIDE.

- Inform patients of the potential risk of immune-mediated adverse reactions.
- Advise patients to read the YERVOY Medication Guide before each YERVOY infusion.
- Advise women that YERVOY may cause fetal harm.
- Advise nursing mothers not to breastfeed while taking YERVOY.

Manufactured by:
Bristol-Myers Squibb Company
Princeton, NJ 08543 USA
U.S. License No. 1713
1281558A4
Rev May 2013

MEDICATION GUIDE

YERVOY® (yur-voi)

(ipilimumab)

Read this Medication Guide before you start receiving YERVOY (ipilimumab) and before each infusion. There may be new information. This Medication Guide does not take the place of talking with your healthcare provider about your medical condition or your treatment.

What is the most important information I should know about YERVOY?

YERVOY can cause serious side effects in many parts of your body which can lead to death. These side effects are most likely to begin during treatment; however, side effects can show up months after your last infusion.

These side effects may include:

1. **Inflammation of the intestines (colitis) that can cause tears or holes (perforation) in the intestines.** Signs and symptoms of colitis may include:
   - diarrhea (loose stools) or more bowel movements than usual
   - blood in your stools or dark, tarry, sticky stools
   - stomach pain (abdominal pain) or tenderness
2. **Inflammation of the liver (hepatitis) that can lead to liver failure.** Signs and symptoms of hepatitis may include:
   - yellowing of your skin or the whites of your eyes
   - dark urine (tea colored)
   - nausea or vomiting
   - pain on the right side of your stomach
   - bleeding or bruise more easily than normal
3. **Inflammation of the skin that can lead to severe skin reaction (toxic epidermal necrolysis).** Signs and symptoms of severe skin reactions may include:
   - skin rash with or without itching
   - sores in your mouth
   - your skin blisters and/or peels
4. **Inflammation of the nerves that can lead to paralysis.** Symptoms of nerve problems may include:
   - unusual weakness of legs, arms, or face
   - numbness or tingling in hands or feet
5. **Inflammation of hormone glands (especially the pituitary, adrenal, and thyroid glands) that may affect how these glands work.** Signs and symptoms that your glands are not working properly may include:
   - persistent or unusual headaches
   - unusual sluggishness, feeling cold all the time, or weight gain
   - changes in mood or behavior such as decreased sex drive, irritability, or forgetfulness
   - dizziness or fainting
6. **Inflammation of the eyes.** Symptoms may include:
   - blurry vision, double vision, or other vision problems
   - eye pain or redness

Call your healthcare provider if you have any of these signs or symptoms or they get worse. Do not try to treat symptoms yourself.

Getting medical treatment right away may keep the problem from becoming more serious. Your oncologist may decide to delay or stop YERVOY.

What is YERVOY?

YERVOY is a prescription medicine used in adults to treat melanoma (a kind of skin cancer) that has spread or cannot be removed by surgery.

It is not known if YERVOY is safe and effective in children less than 18 years of age.

What should I tell my healthcare provider before getting YERVOY?

Before you are given YERVOY, tell your healthcare provider about all your health problems if you:

- have an active condition where your immune system attacks your body (autoimmune disease), such as ulcerative colitis, Crohn's disease, lupus, or sarcoidosis
- had an organ transplant, such as a kidney transplant
- have liver damage from diseases or drugs
- have any other medical conditions
- are pregnant or plan to become pregnant. YERVOY may cause stillbirth, premature delivery, and/or death of your unborn baby
- are breastfeeding

Tell your healthcare provider about all the medicines you take, including all prescription and non-prescription medicines, steroids or other medicines that lower your immune response, vitamins, and herbal supplements.

Know the medicines you take. Keep a list to show your doctors and pharmacists each time you get a new medicine.

You should not start a new medicine before you talk with the healthcare provider who prescribes you YERVOY.

How will I receive YERVOY?

You will get YERVOY (ipilimumab) through an intravenous line in your vein (infusion). It takes about 90 minutes to get a full dose.

- YERVOY is usually given every 3 weeks for up to 4 doses. Your healthcare provider may change how often you receive YERVOY or how long the infusion may take.
- Your healthcare provider should perform blood tests before starting and during treatment with YERVOY.

It is important for you to keep all appointments with your healthcare provider. Call your healthcare provider if you miss an appointment. There may be special instructions for you.

What are the possible side effects of YERVOY?

YERVOY can cause serious side effects. See **"What is the most important information I should know about YERVOY?"**

The most common side effects of YERVOY include:

- tiredness
- diarrhea
- itching
- rash

These are not all of the possible side effects of YERVOY. For more information, ask your healthcare provider.

Call your healthcare provider for medical advice about side effects. You may report side effects to FDA at 1-800-FDA-1088.

You may also report side effects to Bristol-Myers Squibb at 1-800-721-5072.

General information about the safe and effective use of YERVOY.

Medicines are sometimes prescribed for purposes other than those listed in a Medication Guide.

This Medication Guide summarizes the most important information about YERVOY. If you would like more information, talk with your healthcare provider. You can ask your healthcare provider for information about YERVOY that is written for healthcare professionals.

For more information, call 1-800-321-1335.

What are the ingredients of YERVOY?

Active ingredient: ipilimumab

Inactive ingredients: diethylene triamine pentaacetic acid (DTPA), mannitol, polysorbate 80, sodium chloride, tris hydrochloride, and Water for Injection, USP

This Medication Guide has been approved by the U.S. Food and Drug Administration.

Manufactured by:
Bristol-Myers Squibb Company
Princeton, NJ 08543 USA
U.S. License No. 1713
1281558A4
1281915A3
Rev May 2013

Shown in Product Identification Guide, page 306

Bristol-Myers Squibb & Gilead Sciences, LLC

333 LAKESIDE DRIVE
FOSTER CITY, CA 94404

For Medical Information:
1-888-547-4267
medicalinformation@bms-gilead.com
To Report Adverse Events:
1-800-445-3235, press option 3
For Business Operations:
1-800-445-3235, press option 8

ATRIPLA® ℞

[uh TRIP luh]

(efavirenz/emtricitabine/tenofovir disoproxil fumarate) tablets, for oral use

HIGHLIGHTS OF PRESCRIBING INFORMATION

These highlights do not include all the information needed to use ATRIPLA safely and effectively. See full prescribing information for ATRIPLA.

ATRIPLA® (efavirenz/emtricitabine/tenofovir disoproxil fumarate) tablets, for oral use

Initial U.S. Approval: 2006

WARNING: LACTIC ACIDOSIS/SEVERE HEPATOMEGALY WITH STEATOSIS and POST TREATMENT EXACERBATION OF HEPATITIS B

See full prescribing information for complete boxed warning.

- **Lactic acidosis and severe hepatomegaly with steatosis, including fatal cases, have been reported with the use of nucleoside analogs, including tenofovir disoproxil fumarate, a component of ATRIPLA. (5.1)**
- **ATRIPLA is not approved for the treatment of chronic hepatitis B virus (HBV) infection. Severe acute exacerbations of hepatitis B have been reported in patients coinfected with HBV and HIV-1 who have discontinued EMTRIVA or VIREAD, two of the components of ATRIPLA. Hepatic function should be monitored closely in these patients. If appropriate, initiation of anti-hepatitis B therapy may be warranted. (5.2)**

RECENT MAJOR CHANGES

Indications and Usage (1)	06/2012
Dosage and Administration (2)	06/2012
Warnings and Precautions	
Drug Interactions (5.3)	06/2012
Coadministration with Related Products (5.4)	04/2013
Rash (5.9)	04/2013
Decreases in Bone Mineral Density (5.11)	06/2012
Immune Reconstitution Syndrome (5.13)	06/2012

INDICATIONS AND USAGE

ATRIPLA, a combination of 2 nucleoside analog HIV-1 reverse transcriptase inhibitors and 1 non-nucleoside HIV-1 reverse transcriptase inhibitor, is indicated for use alone as a complete regimen or in combination with other antiretroviral agents for the treatment of HIV-1 infection in adults and pediatric patients 12 years of age and older. (1)

DOSAGE AND ADMINISTRATION

- Recommended dose in adults and pediatric patients (12 years of age and older and weighing at least 40 kg): One tablet once daily taken orally on an empty stomach, preferably at bedtime. (2)
- Dose in renal impairment: Should not be administered in patients with creatinine clearance below 50 mL/min. (2)
- With rifampin coadministration, an additional 200 mg/day of efavirenz is recommended for patients weighing 50 kg or more. (2)

DOSAGE FORMS AND STRENGTHS

Tablet containing 600 mg of efavirenz, 200 mg of emtricitabine and 300 mg of tenofovir disoproxil fumarate. (3)

CONTRAINDICATIONS

- Previously demonstrated hypersensitivity (e.g., Stevens-Johnson syndrome, erythema multiforme, or toxic skin eruptions) to efavirenz, a component of ATRIPLA. (4.1)
- For some drugs, competition for CYP3A by efavirenz could result in inhibition of their metabolism and create the potential for serious and/or life-threatening adverse reactions (e.g., cardiac arrhythmias, prolonged sedation, or respiratory depression). (4.2)

WARNINGS AND PRECAUTIONS

- Serious psychiatric symptoms: Immediate medical evaluation is recommended. (5.5, 6.1)
- Nervous system symptoms (NSS): NSS are frequent, usually begin 1–2 days after initiating therapy and resolve in 2–4 weeks. Dosing at bedtime may improve tolerability. NSS are not predictive of onset of psychiatric symptoms. (2, 5.6)
- New onset or worsening renal impairment: Can include acute renal failure and Fanconi syndrome. Assess creatinine clearance (CrCl) before initiating treatment with ATRIPLA. Monitor CrCl and serum phosphorus in patients at risk. Avoid administering ATRIPLA with concurrent or recent use of nephrotoxic drugs. (5.7)
- Pregnancy: Fetal harm can occur when administered to a pregnant woman during the first trimester. Women should be apprised of the potential harm to the fetus. A pregnancy registry is available. (5.8, 8.1)
- Rash: Discontinue if severe rash develops. (5.9, 6.1)
- Hepatotoxicity: Monitor liver function tests before and during treatment in patients with underlying hepatic disease, including hepatitis B or C coinfection, marked transaminase elevations, or who are taking medications associated with liver toxicity. Among reported cases of hepatic failure, a few occurred in patients with no pre-existing hepatic disease. (5.10, 6.3, 8.6)
- Decreases in bone mineral density (BMD): Consider assessment of BMD in patients with a history of pathological fracture or other risk factors for osteoporosis or bone loss. (5.11)
- Convulsions: Use caution in patients with a history of seizures. (5.12)
- Immune reconstitution syndrome: May necessitate further evaluation and treatment. (5.13)
- Redistribution/accumulation of body fat: Observed in patients receiving antiretroviral therapy. (5.14)
- Coadministration with other products: Do not use with drugs containing emtricitabine or tenofovir disoproxil

fumarate including COMPLERA, EMTRIVA, STRIBILD, TRUVADA, or VIREAD; or with drugs containing lamivudine. SUSTIVA (efavirenz) should not be coadministered with ATRIPLA unless required for dose-adjustment when coadministered with rifampin. (5.4) Do not administer in combination with HEPSERA. (5.2)

ADVERSE REACTIONS

Most common adverse reactions (incidence greater than or equal to 10%) observed in an active-controlled clinical trial of efavirenz, emtricitabine, and tenofovir DF are diarrhea, nausea, fatigue, headache, dizziness, depression, insomnia, abnormal dreams, and rash. (6)

To report SUSPECTED ADVERSE REACTIONS, contact Gilead Sciences, Inc. at 1-800-GILEAD-5 or FDA at 1-800-FDA-1088 or www.fda.gov/medwatch

DRUG INTERACTIONS

- Efavirenz: Coadministration of efavirenz can alter the concentrations of other drugs and other drugs may alter the concentrations of efavirenz. The potential for drug-drug interactions must be considered before and during therapy. (4.2, 7.1, 12.3)
- Didanosine: Tenofovir disoproxil fumarate increases didanosine concentrations. Use with caution and monitor for evidence of didanosine toxicity (e.g., pancreatitis, neuropathy) when coadministered. Consider dose reductions or discontinuations of didanosine if warranted. (7.2)
- Atazanavir: Coadministration of ATRIPLA and atazanavir or atazanavir/ritonavir is not recommended. (7.3)
- Lopinavir/ritonavir: Coadministration increases tenofovir concentrations. Monitor for evidence of tenofovir toxicity. (7.3)

USE IN SPECIFIC POPULATIONS

- Pregnancy: Women should avoid pregnancy while receiving ATRIPLA and for 12 weeks after discontinuation. (5.8)
- Nursing mothers: Women infected with HIV should be instructed not to breastfeed. (8.3)
- Hepatic impairment: ATRIPLA is not recommended for patients with moderate or severe hepatic impairment. Use caution in patients with mild hepatic impairment. (5.10, 8.6)
- Pediatrics: The incidence of rash was higher than in adults. (5.9, 6.1)

See 17 for PATIENT COUNSELING INFORMATION and FDA-approved patient labeling

Revised: 06/2013

FULL PRESCRIBING INFORMATION: CONTENTS*

*** Sections or subsections omitted from the full prescribing information are not listed**

Table 1 Drugs That Are Contraindicated or Not Recommended for Use With ATRIPLA

Drug Class: Drug Name	Clinical Comment
Antifungal: voriconazole	Efavirenz significantly decreases voriconazole plasma concentrations, and coadministration may decrease the therapeutic effectiveness of voriconazole. Also, voriconazole significantly increases efavirenz plasma concentrations, which may increase the risk of efavirenz-associated side effects. Because ATRIPLA is a fixed-dose combination product, the dose of efavirenz cannot be altered. *[See Clinical Pharmacology (12.3) Tables 5 and 6]*
Ergot derivatives (dihydroergotamine, ergonovine, ergotamine, methylergonovine)	Potential for serious and/or life-threatening reactions such as acute ergot toxicity characterized by peripheral vasospasm and ischemia of the extremities and other tissues.
Benzodiazepines: midazolam, triazolam	Potential for serious and/or life-threatening reactions such as prolonged or increased sedation or respiratory depression.
Calcium channel blocker: bepridil	Potential for serious and/or life-threatening reactions such as cardiac arrhythmias.
GI motility agent: cisapride	Potential for serious and/or life-threatening reactions such as cardiac arrhythmias.
Neuroleptic: pimozide	Potential for serious and/or life-threatening reactions such as cardiac arrhythmias.
St. John's wort (*Hypericum perforatum*)	May lead to loss of virologic response and possible resistance to efavirenz or to the class of non-nucleoside reverse transcriptase inhibitors (NNRTIs).

FULL PRESCRIBING INFORMATION

WARNING: LACTIC ACIDOSIS/SEVERE HEPATOMEGALY WITH STEATOSIS and POST TREATMENT EXACERBATION OF HEPATITIS B

Lactic acidosis and severe hepatomegaly with steatosis, including fatal cases, have been reported with the use of nucleoside analogs, including tenofovir disoproxil fumarate, a component of ATRIPLA, in combination with other antiretrovirals *[See Warnings and Precautions (5.1)]*.

ATRIPLA is not approved for the treatment of chronic hepatitis B virus (HBV) infection and the safety and efficacy of ATRIPLA have not been established in patients coinfected with HBV and HIV-1. Severe acute exacerbations of hepatitis B have been reported in patients who have discontinued EMTRIVA or VIREAD, which are components of ATRIPLA. Hepatic function should be monitored closely with both clinical and laboratory follow-up for at least several months in patients who are coinfected with HIV-1 and HBV and discontinue ATRIPLA. If appropriate, initiation of anti-hepatitis B therapy may be warranted *[See Warnings and Precautions (5.2)]*.

1 INDICATIONS AND USAGE

ATRIPLA® is indicated for use alone as a complete regimen or in combination with other antiretroviral agents for the treatment of HIV-1 infection in adults and pediatric patients 12 years of age and older.

2 DOSAGE AND ADMINISTRATION

Adults and pediatric patients 12 years of age and older with body weight at least 40 kg (at least 88 lbs): The dose of ATRIPLA is one tablet once daily taken orally on an empty stomach. Dosing at bedtime may improve the tolerability of nervous system symptoms.

Renal Impairment: Because ATRIPLA is a fixed-dose combination, it should not be prescribed for patients requiring dosage adjustment such as those with moderate or severe renal impairment (creatinine clearance below 50 mL/min).

Rifampin Coadministration: When ATRIPLA is administered with rifampin to patients weighing 50 kg or more, an additional 200 mg/day of efavirenz is recommended *[See Drug Interactions (7.3), Table 4, and Clinical Pharmacology (12.3), Table 5]*.

3 DOSAGE FORMS AND STRENGTHS

ATRIPLA is available as tablets. Each tablet contains 600 mg of efavirenz, 200 mg of emtricitabine and 300 mg of tenofovir disoproxil fumarate (tenofovir DF, which is equivalent to 245 mg of tenofovir disoproxil). The tablets are pink, capsule-shaped, film-coated, debossed with "123" on one side and plain-faced on the other side.

4 CONTRAINDICATIONS

4.1 Hypersensitivity

ATRIPLA is contraindicated in patients with previously demonstrated clinically significant hypersensitivity (e.g., Stevens-Johnson syndrome, erythema multiforme, or toxic skin eruptions) to efavirenz, a component of ATRIPLA.

4.2 Contraindicated Drugs

For some drugs, competition for CYP3A by efavirenz could result in inhibition of their metabolism and create the potential for serious and/or life-threatening adverse reactions (e.g., cardiac arrhythmias, prolonged sedation, or respiratory depression). Drugs that are contraindicated with ATRIPLA are listed in Table 1.

[See table 1 above]

5 WARNINGS AND PRECAUTIONS

5.1 Lactic Acidosis/Severe Hepatomegaly with Steatosis

Lactic acidosis and severe hepatomegaly with steatosis, including fatal cases, have been reported with the use of nucleoside analogs including tenofovir DF, a component of ATRIPLA, in combination with other antiretrovirals. A majority of these cases have been in women. Obesity and prolonged nucleoside exposure may be risk factors. Particular caution should be exercised when administering nucleoside analogs to any patient with known risk factors for liver disease; however, cases have also been reported in patients with no known risk factors. Treatment with ATRIPLA should be suspended in any patient who develops clinical or laboratory findings suggestive of lactic acidosis or pronounced hepatotoxicity (which may include hepatomegaly and steatosis even in the absence of marked transaminase elevations).

5.2 Patients Coinfected with HIV-1 and HBV

It is recommended that all patients with HIV-1 be tested for the presence of chronic HBV before initiating antiretroviral therapy. ATRIPLA is not approved for the treatment of chronic HBV infection, and the safety and efficacy of

ATRIPLA have not been established in patients coinfected with HBV and HIV-1. Severe acute exacerbations of hepatitis B have been reported in patients who are coinfected with HBV and HIV-1 and have discontinued emtricitabine or tenofovir DF, two of the components of ATRIPLA. In some patients infected with HBV and treated with emtricitabine, the exacerbations of hepatitis B were associated with liver decompensation and liver failure. Patients who are coinfected with HIV-1 and HBV should be closely monitored with both clinical and laboratory follow-up for at least several months after stopping treatment with ATRIPLA. If appropriate, initiation of anti-hepatitis B therapy may be warranted.

ATRIPLA should not be administered with HEPSERA® (adefovir dipivoxil) *[See Drug Interactions (7.2)]*.

5.3 Drug Interactions

Efavirenz plasma concentrations may be altered by substrates, inhibitors, or inducers of CYP3A. Likewise, efavirenz may alter plasma concentrations of drugs metabolized by CYP3A or CYP2B6 *[See Contraindications (4.2), Drug Interactions (7.1)]*.

5.4 Coadministration with Related Products

Related drugs not for coadministration with ATRIPLA include COMPLERA® (emtricitabine/rilpivirine/tenofovir DF), EMTRIVA® (emtricitabine), STRIBILD® (elvitegravir/cobicistat/emtricitabine/tenofovir DF), TRUVADA® (emtricitabine/tenofovir DF), and VIREAD® (tenofovir DF), which contain the same active components as ATRIPLA. SUSTIVA® (efavirenz) should not be coadministered with ATRIPLA unless needed for dose-adjustment (e.g., with rifampin) *[See Dosage and Administration (2), Drug Interactions (7.1)]*. Due to similarities between emtricitabine and lamivudine, ATRIPLA should not be coadministered with drugs containing lamivudine, including Combivir (lamivudine/zidovudine), Epivir, or Epivir-HBV (lamivudine), Epzicom (abacavir sulfate/lamivudine), or Trizivir (abacavir sulfate/lamivudine/zidovudine).

5.5 Psychiatric Symptoms

Serious psychiatric adverse experiences have been reported in patients treated with efavirenz. In controlled trials of 1008 subjects treated with regimens containing efavirenz for a mean of 2.1 years and 635 subjects treated with control regimens for a mean of 1.5 years, the frequency (regardless of causality) of specific serious psychiatric events among subjects who received efavirenz or control regimens, respectively, were: severe depression (2.4%, 0.9%), suicidal ideation (0.7%, 0.3%), nonfatal suicide attempts (0.5%, 0%), aggressive behavior (0.4%, 0.5%), paranoid reactions (0.4%, 0.3%), and manic reactions (0.2%, 0.3%). When psychiatric symptoms similar to those noted above were combined and evaluated as a group in a multifactorial analysis of data from Study AI266006 (006), treatment with efavirenz was associated with an increase in the occurrence of these selected psychiatric symptoms. Other factors associated with an increase in the occurrence of these psychiatric symptoms were history of injection drug use, psychiatric history, and receipt of psychiatric medication at trial entry; similar associations were observed in both the efavirenz and control treatment groups. In Study 006, onset of new serious psychiatric symptoms occurred throughout the trial for both efavirenz-treated and control-treated subjects. One percent of efavirenz-treated subjects discontinued or interrupted treatment because of one or more of these selected psychiatric symptoms. There have also been occasional postmarketing reports of death by suicide, delusions, and psychosis-like behavior, although a causal relationship to the use of efavirenz cannot be determined from these reports. Patients with serious psychiatric adverse experiences should seek immediate medical evaluation to assess the possibility that the symptoms may be related to the use of efavirenz, and if so, to determine whether the risks of continued therapy outweigh the benefits *[See Adverse Reactions (6)]*.

5.6 Nervous System Symptoms

Fifty-three percent (531/1008) of subjects receiving efavirenz in controlled trials reported central nervous system symptoms (any grade, regardless of causality) compared to 25% (156/635) of subjects receiving control regimens. These symptoms included dizziness (28.1% of the 1008 subjects), insomnia (16.3%), impaired concentration (8.3%), somnolence (7.0%), abnormal dreams (6.2%), and hallucinations (1.2%). Other reported symptoms were euphoria, confusion, agitation, amnesia, stupor, abnormal thinking, and depersonalization. The majority of these symptoms were mild-to-moderate (50.7%); symptoms were severe in 2.0% of subjects. Overall, 2.1% of subjects discontinued therapy as a result. These symptoms usually begin during the first or second day of therapy and generally resolve after the first 2–4 weeks of therapy. After 4 weeks of therapy, the prevalence of nervous system symptoms of at least moderate severity ranged from 5% to 9% in subjects treated with regimens containing efavirenz and from 3% to 5% in subjects treated with a control regimen. Patients should be informed that these common symptoms were likely to improve with continued therapy and were not predictive of subsequent onset of the less frequent psychiatric symptoms *[See Warnings and Precautions (5.5)]*. Dosing at bedtime may improve the tolerability of these nervous system symptoms *[See Dosage and Administration (2)]*.

Analysis of long-term data from Study 006 (median follow-up 180 weeks, 102 weeks, and 76 weeks for subjects treated with efavirenz + zidovudine + lamivudine, efavirenz + indinavir, and indinavir + zidovudine + lamivudine, respectively) showed that, beyond 24 weeks of therapy, the incidences of new-onset nervous system symptoms among efavirenz-treated subjects were generally similar to those in the indinavir-containing control arm.

Patients receiving ATRIPLA should be alerted to the potential for additive central nervous system effects when ATRIPLA is used concomitantly with alcohol or psychoactive drugs.

Patients who experience central nervous system symptoms such as dizziness, impaired concentration, and/or drowsiness should avoid potentially hazardous tasks such as driving or operating machinery.

5.7 New Onset or Worsening Renal Impairment

Emtricitabine and tenofovir are principally eliminated by the kidney; however, efavirenz is not. Since ATRIPLA is a combination product and the dose of the individual components cannot be altered, patients with creatinine clearance below 50 mL/min should not receive ATRIPLA.

Renal impairment, including cases of acute renal failure and Fanconi syndrome (renal tubular injury with severe hypophosphatemia), has been reported with the use of tenofovir DF *[See Adverse Reactions (6.3)]*.

It is recommended that creatinine clearance be calculated in all patients prior to initiating therapy and as clinically appropriate during therapy with ATRIPLA. Routine monitoring of calculated creatinine clearance and serum phosphorus should be performed in patients at risk for renal impairment, including patients who have previously experienced renal events while receiving HEPSERA.

ATRIPLA should be avoided with concurrent or recent use of a nephrotoxic agent.

5.8 Reproductive Risk Potential

Pregnancy Category D: Efavirenz may cause fetal harm when administered during the first trimester to a pregnant woman. Pregnancy should be avoided in women receiving ATRIPLA. Barrier contraception must always be used in combination with other methods of contraception (e.g., oral or other hormonal contraceptives). Because of the long half-life of efavirenz, use of adequate contraceptive measures for 12 weeks after discontinuation of ATRIPLA is recommended. Women of childbearing potential should undergo pregnancy testing before initiation of ATRIPLA. If this drug is used during the first trimester of pregnancy, or if the patient becomes pregnant while taking this drug, the patient should be apprised of the potential harm to the fetus.

There are no adequate and well-controlled trials of ATRIPLA in pregnant women. ATRIPLA should be used during pregnancy only if the potential benefit justifies the potential risk to the fetus, such as in pregnant women without other therapeutic options *[See Use in Specific Populations (8.1)]*.

5.9 Rash

In controlled clinical trials, 26% (266/1008) of subjects treated with 600 mg efavirenz experienced new-onset skin rash compared with 17% (111/635) of subjects treated in control groups. Rash associated with blistering, moist desquamation, or ulceration occurred in 0.9% (9/1008) of subjects treated with efavirenz. The incidence of Grade 4 rash (e.g., erythema multiforme, Stevens-Johnson syndrome) in subjects treated with efavirenz in all trials and expanded access was 0.1%. Rashes are usually mild-to-moderate maculopapular skin eruptions that occur within the first 2 weeks of initiating therapy with efavirenz (median time to onset of rash in adults was 11 days) and, in most subjects continuing therapy with efavirenz, rash resolves within 1 month (median duration, 16 days). The discontinuation rate for rash in clinical trials was 1.7% (17/1008). ATRIPLA can be reinitiated in patients interrupting therapy because of rash. ATRIPLA should be discontinued in patients developing severe rash associated with blistering, desquamation, mucosal involvement, or fever. Appropriate antihistamines and/or corticosteroids may improve the tolerability and hasten the resolution of rash. For patients who have had a life-threatening cutaneous reaction (e.g., Stevens-Johnson syndrome), alternative therapy should be considered *[See also Contraindications (4.1)]*.

Experience with efavirenz in subjects who discontinued other antiretroviral agents of the NNRTI class is limited. Nineteen subjects who discontinued nevirapine because of rash have been treated with efavirenz. Nine of these subjects developed mild-to-moderate rash while receiving therapy with efavirenz, and two of these subjects discontinued because of rash.

Rash was reported in 26 of 57 pediatric subjects (46%) treated with efavirenz *[See Adverse Reactions (6.1)]*. One pediatric subject experienced Grade 3 rash (confluent rash with fever), and two subjects had Grade 4 rash (erythema multiforme). The median time to onset of rash in pediatric subjects was 8 days. Prophylaxis with appropriate antihistamines before initiating therapy with ATRIPLA in pediatric patients should be considered.

5.10 Hepatotoxicity

Monitoring of liver enzymes before and during treatment is recommended for patients with underlying hepatic disease, including hepatitis B or C infection; patients with marked transaminase elevations; and patients treated with other medications associated with liver toxicity *[See also Warnings and Precautions (5.2)]*. A few of the postmarketing reports of hepatic failure occurred in patients with no pre-existing hepatic disease or other identifiable risk factors *[See Adverse Reactions (6.3)]*. Liver enzyme monitoring should also be considered for patients without pre-existing hepatic dysfunction or other risk factors. In patients with persistent elevations of serum transaminases to greater than five times the upper limit of the normal range, the benefit of continued therapy with ATRIPLA needs to be weighed against the unknown risks of significant liver toxicity *[See Adverse Reactions (6.2)]*.

5.11 Decreases in Bone Mineral Density

Assessment of bone mineral density (BMD) should be considered for patients who have a history of pathologic bone fracture or other risk factors for osteoporosis or bone loss. Although the effect of supplementation with calcium and vitamin D was not studied, such supplementation may be beneficial for all patients. If bone abnormalities are suspected then appropriate consultation should be obtained.

In a 144-week trial of treatment-naive adult subjects receiving tenofovir DF, decreases in BMD were seen at the lumbar spine and hip in both arms of the trial. At Week 144, there was a significantly greater mean percentage decrease from baseline in BMD at the lumbar spine in subjects receiving tenofovir DF + lamivudine + efavirenz compared with subjects receiving stavudine + lamivudine + efavirenz. Changes in BMD at the hip were similar between the two treatment groups. In both groups, the majority of the reduction in BMD occurred in the first 24–48 weeks of the trial and this reduction was sustained through 144 weeks. Twenty-eight percent of tenofovir DF-treated subjects vs. 21% of the comparator subjects lost at least 5% of BMD at the spine or 7% of BMD at the hip. Clinically relevant fractures (excluding fingers and toes) were reported in 4 subjects in the tenofovir DF group and 6 subjects in the comparator group. Tenofovir DF was associated with significant increases in biochemical markers of bone metabolism (serum bone-specific alkaline phosphatase, serum osteocalcin, serum C-telopeptide, and urinary N-telopeptide), suggesting increased bone turnover. Serum parathyroid hormone levels and 1,25 Vitamin D levels were also higher in subjects receiving tenofovir DF.

In a clinical trial of HIV-1 infected pediatric subjects 12 years of age and older (Study 321), bone effects were similar to adult subjects. Under normal circumstances BMD increases rapidly in this age group. In this trial, the mean rate of bone gain was less in the tenofovir DF-treated group compared to the placebo group. Six tenofovir DF-treated subjects and one placebo-treated subject had significant (greater than 4%) lumbar spine BMD loss at 48 weeks. Among 28 subjects receiving 96 weeks of tenofovir DF, Z-scores declined by -0.341 for lumbar spine and -0.458 for total body. Skeletal growth (height) appeared to be unaffected. Markers of bone turnover in tenofovir DF-treated pediatric subjects 12 years of age and older suggest increased bone turnover, consistent with the effects observed in adults.

The effects of tenofovir DF-associated changes in BMD and biochemical markers on long-term bone health and future fracture risk are unknown. For additional information, consult the VIREAD prescribing information.

Cases of osteomalacia (associated with proximal renal tubulopathy and which may contribute to fractures) have been reported in association with the use of tenofovir DF *[See Adverse Reactions (6.3)]*.

5.12 Convulsions

Convulsions have been observed in patients receiving efavirenz, generally in the presence of known medical history of seizures. Caution must be taken in any patient with a history of seizures.

Patients who are receiving concomitant anticonvulsant medications primarily metabolized by the liver, such as phenytoin and phenobarbital, may require periodic monitoring of plasma levels *[See Drug Interactions (7.3)]*.

5.13 Immune Reconstitution Syndrome

Immune reconstitution syndrome has been reported in patients treated with combination antiretroviral therapy, including the components of ATRIPLA. During the initial phase of combination antiretroviral treatment, patients whose immune system responds may develop an inflammatory response to indolent or residual opportunistic infections [such as *Mycobacterium avium* infection, cytomegalovirus, *Pneumocystis jirovecii* pneumonia (PCP), or tuberculosis], which may necessitate further evaluation and treatment.

Autoimmune disorders (such as Graves' disease, polymyositis, and Guillain-Barré syndrome) have also been reported to occur in the setting of immune reconstitution, however, the time to onset is more variable, and can occur many months after initiation of treatment.

5.14 Fat Redistribution

Redistribution/accumulation of body fat including central obesity, dorsocervical fat enlargement (buffalo hump), peripheral wasting, facial wasting, breast enlargement, and "cushingoid appearance" have been observed in patients receiving antiretroviral therapy. The mechanism and long-term consequences of these events are currently unknown. A causal relationship has not been established.

6 ADVERSE REACTIONS

Efavirenz, Emtricitabine and Tenofovir Disoproxil Fumarate: The following adverse reactions are discussed in other sections of the labeling:

- Lactic Acidosis/Severe Hepatomegaly with Steatosis *[See Boxed Warning, Warnings and Precautions (5.1)].*
- Severe Acute Exacerbations of Hepatitis B *[See Boxed Warning, Warnings and Precautions (5.2)].*
- Psychiatric Symptoms *[See Warnings and Precautions (5.5)].*
- Nervous System Symptoms *[See Warnings and Precautions (5.6)].*
- New Onset or Worsening Renal Impairment *[See Warnings and Precautions (5.7)].*
- Rash *[See Warnings and Precautions (5.9)].*
- Hepatotoxicity *[See Warnings and Precautions (5.10)].*
- Decreases in Bone Mineral Density *[See Warnings and Precautions (5.11)].*
- Immune Reconstitution Syndrome *[See Warnings and Precautions (5.13)].*
- Drug Interactions *[See Contraindications (4.2), Warnings and Precautions (5.3) and Drug Interactions (7)].*

For additional safety information about SUSTIVA (efavirenz), EMTRIVA (emtricitabine), or VIREAD (tenofovir DF) in combination with other antiretroviral agents, consult the prescribing information for these products.

6.1 Adverse Reactions from Clinical Trials Experience

Because clinical trials are conducted under widely varying conditions, adverse reaction rates observed in the clinical trials of a drug cannot be directly compared to rates in the clinical trials of another drug and may not reflect the rates observed in practice.

Clinical Trials in Adult Subjects

Study 934

Study 934 was an open-label active-controlled trial in which 511 antiretroviral-naive subjects received either emtricitabine + tenofovir DF administered in combination with efavirenz (N=257) or zidovudine/lamivudine administered in combination with efavirenz (N=254).

The most common adverse reactions (incidence greater than or equal to 10%, any severity) occurring in Study 934 include diarrhea, nausea, fatigue, headache, dizziness, depression, insomnia, abnormal dreams, and rash. Adverse reactions observed in Study 934 were generally consistent with those seen in previous trials of the individual components (Table 2).

Table 2 Selected Treatment-Emergent Adverse Reactions* (Grades 2–4) Reported in ≥5% in Either Treatment Group in Study 934 (0–144 Weeks)

	FTC + TDF + EFV†	AZT/3TC + EFV
	N=257	N=254
Gastrointestinal Disorder		
Diarrhea	9%	5%
Nausea	9%	7%
Vomiting	2%	5%
General Disorders and Administration Site Condition		
Fatigue	9%	8%
Infections and Infestations		
Sinusitis	8%	4%
Upper respiratory tract infections	8%	5%
Nasopharyngitis	5%	3%
Nervous System Disorders		
Headache	6%	5%
Dizziness	8%	7%
Psychiatric Disorders		
Anxiety	5%	4%
Depression	9%	7%
Insomnia	5%	7%
Skin and Subcutaneous Tissue Disorders		
Rash Event‡	7%	9%

* Frequencies of adverse reactions are based on all treatment-emergent adverse events, regardless of relationship to study drug.

† From Weeks 96 to 144 of the trial, subjects received emtricitabine/tenofovir DF administered in combination with efavirenz in place of emtricitabine + tenofovir DF with efavirenz.

‡ Rash event includes rash, exfoliative rash, rash generalized, rash macular, rash maculo-papular, rash pruritic, and rash vesicular.

Study 073

In Study 073, subjects with stable, virologic suppression on antiretroviral therapy and no history of virologic failure were randomized to receive ATRIPLA or to stay on their baseline regimen. The adverse reactions observed in Study 073 were generally consistent with those seen in Study 934 and those seen with the individual components of ATRIPLA when each was administered in combination with other antiretroviral agents.

Efavirenz, Emtricitabine, or Tenofovir Disoproxil Fumarate

In addition to the adverse reactions in Study 934 and Study 073, the following adverse reactions were observed in clinical trials of efavirenz, emtricitabine, or tenofovir DF in combination with other antiretroviral agents.

Efavirenz: The most significant adverse reactions observed in subjects treated with efavirenz are nervous system symptoms *[See Warnings and Precautions (5.6)]*, psychiatric symptoms *[See Warnings and Precautions (5.5)]*, and rash *[See Warnings and Precautions (5.9)]*.

Selected adverse reactions of moderate-to-severe intensity observed in greater than or equal to 2% of efavirenz-treated subjects in two controlled clinical trials included pain, impaired concentration, abnormal dreams, somnolence, anorexia, dyspepsia, abdominal pain, nervousness, and pruritus.

Pancreatitis has also been reported, although a causal relationship with efavirenz has not been established. Asymptomatic increases in serum amylase levels were observed in a significantly higher number of subjects treated with efavirenz 600 mg than in control subjects.

Emtricitabine and Tenofovir Disoproxil Fumarate: Adverse reactions that occurred in at least 5% of treatment-experienced or treatment-naive subjects receiving emtricitabine or tenofovir DF with other antiretroviral agents in clinical trials include arthralgia, increased cough, dyspepsia, fever, myalgia, pain, abdominal pain, back pain, paresthesia, peripheral neuropathy (including peripheral neuritis and neuropathy), pneumonia, rhinitis and rash event (including rash, pruritus, maculopapular rash, urticaria, vesiculobullous rash, pustular rash, and allergic reaction).

Skin discoloration has been reported with higher frequency among emtricitabine-treated subjects; it was manifested by hyperpigmentation on the palms and/or soles and was generally mild and asymptomatic. The mechanism and clinical significance are unknown.

Clinical Trials in Pediatric Subjects

Efavirenz: In a pediatric clinical trial in 57 NRTI-experienced subjects aged 3 to 16 years, the type and frequency of adverse experiences was generally similar to that of adult subjects with the exception of a higher incidence of rash, which was reported in 46% (26/57) of pediatric subjects compared to 26% of adults, and a higher frequency of Grade 3 or 4 rash reported in 5% (3/57) of pediatric subjects compared to 0.9% of adults *[See Warnings and Precautions (5.9)]*. For additional information, please consult the SUSTIVA prescribing information.

Emtricitabine: In addition to the adverse reactions reported in adults, anemia and hyperpigmentation were observed in 7% and 32%, respectively, of pediatric subjects (3 months to less than 18 years of age) who received treatment with emtricitabine in the larger of two open-label, uncontrolled pediatric trials (N=116). For additional information, please consult the EMTRIVA prescribing information.

Tenofovir Disoproxil Fumarate: In a pediatric clinical trial conducted in subjects 12 to less than 18 years of age, the adverse reactions observed in pediatric subjects who received treatment with tenofovir DF were consistent with those observed in clinical trials of tenofovir DF in adults *[See Warnings and Precautions (5.11)]*.

6.2 Laboratory Abnormalities

Efavirenz, Emtricitabine and Tenofovir Disoproxil Fumarate: Laboratory abnormalities observed in Study 934 were generally consistent with those seen in previous trials (Table 3).

Table 3 Significant Laboratory Abnormalities Reported in ≥1% of Subjects in Either Treatment Group in Study 934 (0–144 Weeks)

	FTC + TDF + EFV*	AZT/3TC + EFV
	N=257	N=254
Any ≥ Grade 3 Laboratory Abnormality	30%	26%
Fasting Cholesterol (>240 mg/dL)	22%	24%
Creatine Kinase (M: >990 U/L) (F: >845 U/L)	9%	7%
Serum Amylase (>175 U/L)	8%	4%
Alkaline Phosphatase (>550 U/L)	1%	0%
AST (M: >180 U/L) (F: >170 U/L)	3%	3%
ALT (M: >215 U/L) (F: >170 U/L)	2%	3%
Hemoglobin (<8.0 mg/dL)	0%	4%
Hyperglycemia (>250 mg/dL)	2%	1%
Hematuria (>75 RBC/HPF)	3%	2%
Glycosuria (≥3+)	<1%	1%
Neutrophils (<750/mm^3)	3%	5%
Fasting Triglycerides (>750 mg/dL)	4%	2%

* From Weeks 96 to 144 of the trial, subjects received emtricitabine/tenofovir DF administered in combination with efavirenz in place of emtricitabine + tenofovir DF with efavirenz.

Laboratory abnormalities observed in Study 073 were generally consistent with those in Study 934.

In addition to the laboratory abnormalities described for Study 934 (Table 3), Grade 3/4 laboratory abnormalities of increased bilirubin (greater than 2.5 × upper limit of normal (ULN)), increased pancreatic amylase (greater than 2.0 × ULN), increased or decreased serum glucose (less than 40 or greater than 250 mg/dL), and increased serum lipase (greater than 2.0 × ULN) occurred in up to 3% of subjects treated with emtricitabine or tenofovir DF with other antiretroviral agents in clinical trials.

Hepatic Events: In Study 934, 19 subjects treated with efavirenz, emtricitabine, and tenofovir DF and 20 subjects treated with efavirenz and fixed-dose zidovudine/lamivudine were hepatitis B surface antigen or hepatitis C antibody positive. Among these coinfected subjects, one subject (1/19) in the efavirenz, emtricitabine and tenofovir DF arm had elevations in transaminases to greater than five times ULN through 144 weeks. In the fixed-dose zidovudine/lamivudine arm, two subjects (2/20) had elevations in transaminases to greater than five times ULN through 144 weeks. No HBV and/or HCV coinfected subject discontinued from the trial due to hepatobiliary disorders *[See Warnings and Precautions (5.10)]*.

6.3 Postmarketing Experience

The following adverse reactions have been identified during postapproval use of efavirenz, emtricitabine, or tenofovir DF. Because postmarketing reactions are reported voluntarily from a population of uncertain size, it is not always possible to reliably estimate their frequency or establish a causal relationship to drug exposure.

Efavirenz:

Cardiac Disorders

Palpitations

Ear and Labyrinth Disorders

Tinnitus, vertigo

Endocrine Disorders

Gynecomastia

Eye Disorders

Abnormal vision

Gastrointestinal Disorders

Constipation, malabsorption

General Disorders and Administration Site Conditions

Asthenia

Hepatobiliary Disorders
Hepatic enzyme increase, hepatic failure, hepatitis. A few of the postmarketing reports of hepatic failure, including cases in patients with no pre-existing hepatic disease or other identifiable risk factors, were characterized by a fulminant course, progressing in some cases to transplantation or death.
Immune System Disorders
Allergic reactions
Metabolism and Nutrition Disorders
Redistribution/accumulation of body fat *[See Warnings and Precautions (5.14)]*, hypercholesterolemia, hypertriglyceridemia
Musculoskeletal and Connective Tissue Disorders
Arthralgia, myalgia, myopathy
Nervous System Disorders
Abnormal coordination, ataxia, cerebellar coordination and balance disturbances, convulsions, hypoesthesia, paresthesia, neuropathy, tremor
Psychiatric Disorders
Aggressive reactions, agitation, delusions, emotional lability, mania, neurosis, paranoia, psychosis, suicide
Respiratory, Thoracic and Mediastinal Disorders
Dyspnea
Skin and Subcutaneous Tissue Disorders
Flushing, erythema multiforme, photoallergic dermatitis, Stevens-Johnson syndrome
Emtricitabine: No postmarketing adverse reactions have been identified for inclusion in this section.
Tenofovir Disoproxil Fumarate:
Immune System Disorders
Allergic reaction, including angioedema
Metabolism and Nutrition Disorders
Lactic acidosis, hypokalemia, hypophosphatemia
Respiratory, Thoracic, and Mediastinal Disorders
Dyspnea
Gastrointestinal Disorders
Pancreatitis, increased amylase, abdominal pain
Hepatobiliary Disorders
Hepatic steatosis, hepatitis, increased liver enzymes (most commonly AST, ALT, gamma GT)
Skin and Subcutaneous Tissue Disorders
Rash
Musculoskeletal and Connective Tissue Disorders
Rhabdomyolysis, osteomalacia (manifested as bone pain and which may contribute to fractures), muscular weakness, myopathy
Renal and Urinary Disorders
Acute renal failure, renal failure, acute tubular necrosis, Fanconi syndrome, proximal renal tubulopathy, interstitial nephritis (including acute cases), nephrogenic diabetes insipidus, renal insufficiency, increased creatinine, proteinuria, polyuria
General Disorders and Administration Site Conditions
Asthenia
The following adverse reactions, listed under the body system headings above, may occur as a consequence of proximal renal tubulopathy: rhabdomyolysis, osteomalacia, hypokalemia, muscular weakness, myopathy, hypophosphatemia.

7 DRUG INTERACTIONS

This section describes clinically relevant drug interactions with ATRIPLA. Drug interaction trials are described elsewhere in the labeling *[See Clinical Pharmacology (12.3)]*.

7.1 Efavirenz

Efavirenz has been shown in vivo to induce CYP3A and CYP2B6. Other compounds that are substrates of CYP3A or CYP2B6 may have decreased plasma concentrations when coadministered with efavirenz. In vitro studies have demonstrated that efavirenz inhibits CYP2C9, 2C19, and 3A4 isozymes in the range of observed efavirenz plasma concentrations. Coadministration of efavirenz with drugs primarily metabolized by these isozymes may result in altered plasma concentrations of the coadministered drug. Therefore, appropriate dose adjustments may be necessary for these drugs.

Drugs that induce CYP3A activity (e.g., phenobarbital, rifampin, rifabutin) would be expected to increase the clearance of efavirenz, resulting in lowered plasma concentrations *[See Dosage and Administration (2)]*.

7.2 Emtricitabine and Tenofovir Disoproxil Fumarate

Since emtricitabine and tenofovir are primarily eliminated by the kidneys, coadministration of ATRIPLA with drugs that reduce renal function or compete for active tubular secretion may increase serum concentrations of emtricitabine, tenofovir, and/or other renally eliminated drugs. Some examples include, but are not limited to, acyclovir, adefovir dipivoxil, cidofovir, ganciclovir, valacyclovir, and valganciclovir.

Coadministration of tenofovir DF and didanosine should be undertaken with caution and patients receiving this combination should be monitored closely for didanosine-associated adverse reactions. Didanosine should be discontinued in patients who develop didanosine-associated adverse reactions [for didanosine dosing adjustment recommendations, see *Table 4]*. Suppression of CD4+ cell counts has been observed in patients receiving tenofovir DF with didanosine 400 mg daily.

Lopinavir/ritonavir has been shown to increase tenofovir concentrations. The mechanism of this interaction is unknown. Patients receiving lopinavir/ritonavir with ATRIPLA should be monitored for tenofovir-associated adverse reactions. ATRIPLA should be discontinued in patients who develop tenofovir-associated adverse reactions *[See Table 4]*.

Coadministration of atazanavir with ATRIPLA is not recommended since coadministration of atazanavir with either efavirenz or tenofovir DF has been shown to decrease plasma concentrations of atazanavir. Also, atazanavir has

Table 4 Established and Other Potentially Significant* Drug Interactions: Alteration in Dose or Regimen May Be Recommended Based on Drug Interaction Trials or Predicted Interaction

Concomitant Drug Class: Drug Name	Effect	Clinical Comment
HIV antiviral agents		
Protease inhibitor: atazanavir	↓atazanavir ↑ tenofovir	Coadministration of atazanavir with ATRIPLA is not recommended. Coadministration of atazanavir with either efavirenz or tenofovir DF decreases plasma concentrations of atazanavir. The combined effect of efavirenz plus tenofovir DF on atazanavir plasma concentrations is not known. Also, atazanavir has been shown to increase tenofovir concentrations. There are insufficient data to support dosing recommendations for atazanavir or atazanavir/ritonavir in combination with ATRIPLA.
Protease inhibitor: fosamprenavir calcium	↓ amprenavir	Fosamprenavir (unboosted): Appropriate doses of fosamprenavir and ATRIPLA with respect to safety and efficacy have not been established. Fosamprenavir/ritonavir: An additional 100 mg/day (300 mg total) of ritonavir is recommended when ATRIPLA is administered with fosamprenavir/ritonavir once daily. No change in the ritonavir dose is required when ATRIPLA is administered with fosamprenavir plus ritonavir twice daily.
Protease inhibitor: indinavir	↓ indinavir	The optimal dose of indinavir, when given in combination with efavirenz, is not known. Increasing the indinavir dose to 1000 mg every 8 hours does not compensate for the increased indinavir metabolism due to efavirenz.
Protease inhibitor: lopinavir/ritonavir	↓ lopinavir ↑ tenofovir	Do not use once daily administration of lopinavir/ritonavir. Dose adjustment of lopinavir/ritonavir is recommended when coadministered with efavirenz. Refer to the full prescribing information for lopinavir/ritonavir for guidance on coadministration with efavirenz- or tenofovir-containing regimens, such as ATRIPLA. Patients should be monitored for tenofovir-associated adverse reactions.
Protease inhibitor: ritonavir	↑ ritonavir ↑ efavirenz	When ritonavir 500 mg every 12 hours was coadministered with efavirenz 600 mg once daily, the combination was associated with a higher frequency of adverse clinical experiences (e.g., dizziness, nausea, paresthesia) and laboratory abnormalities (elevated liver enzymes). Monitoring of liver enzymes is recommended when ATRIPLA is used in combination with ritonavir.
Protease inhibitor: saquinavir	↓ saquinavir	Appropriate doses of the combination of efavirenz and saquinavir/ritonavir with respect to safety and efficacy have not been established.
CCR5 co-receptor antagonist: maraviroc	↓ maraviroc	Efavirenz decreases plasma concentrations of maraviroc. Refer to the full prescribing information for maraviroc for guidance on coadministration with ATRIPLA.
NRTI: didanosine	↑ didanosine	Coadministration of ATRIPLA and didanosine should be undertaken with caution and patients receiving this combination should be monitored closely for didanosine-associated adverse reactions including pancreatitis, lactic acidosis, and neuropathy. A dose reduction of didanosine is recommended when coadministered with tenofovir DF. For additional information on coadministration with tenofovir DF-containing products, please refer to the didanosine prescribing information.
NNRTI: Other NNRTIs	↑ or ↓ efavirenz and/or NNRTI	Combining two NNRTIs has not been shown to be beneficial. ATRIPLA contains efavirenz and should not be coadministered with other NNRTIs.
Integrase strand transfer inhibitor: raltegravir	↓ raltegravir	Efavirenz reduces plasma concentrations of raltegravir. The clinical significance of this interaction has not been directly assessed.
Hepatitis C antiviral agents		
Protease inhibitor: boceprevir	↓ boceprevir	Plasma trough concentrations of boceprevir were decreased when boceprevir was coadministered with efavirenz, which may result in loss of therapeutic effect. The combination should be avoided.
Protease inhibitor: telaprevir	↓ telaprevir ↓ efavirenz	Concomitant administration of telaprevir and efavirenz resulted in reduced steady-state exposures to telaprevir and efavirenz.

(Table continued on next page)

been shown to increase tenofovir concentrations. There are insufficient data to support dosing recommendations for atazanavir or atazanavir/ritonavir in combination with ATRIPLA *[See Table 4]*.

7.3 Efavirenz, Emtricitabine and Tenofovir Disoproxil Fumarate

Other important drug interaction information for ATRIPLA is summarized in Table 1 and Table 4. The drug interactions described are based on trials conducted with efavirenz, emtricitabine or tenofovir DF as individual agents or are potential drug interactions; no drug interaction trials have been conducted using ATRIPLA [for pharmacokinetics data see *Clinical Pharmacology (12.3)*, Tables 5–8]. The tables include potentially significant interactions, but are not all inclusive.

[See table 4 on pages 824 through 826]

7.4 Efavirenz Assay Interference

Cannabinoid Test Interaction: Efavirenz does not bind to cannabinoid receptors. False-positive urine cannabinoid test results have been observed in non-HIV-infected volunteers receiving efavirenz when the Microgenics Cedia DAU Multi-Level THC assay was used for screening. Negative results were obtained when more specific confirmatory testing was performed with gas chromatography/mass spectrometry. For more information, please consult the SUSTIVA prescribing information.

8 USE IN SPECIFIC POPULATIONS

8.1 Pregnancy

Pregnancy Category D *[See Warnings and Precautions (5.8)]*

Antiretroviral Pregnancy Registry: To monitor fetal outcomes of pregnant women, an Antiretroviral Pregnancy Registry has been established. Physicians are encouraged to register patients who become pregnant by calling (800) 258-4263.

Efavirenz: As of July 2010, the Antiretroviral Pregnancy Registry has received prospective reports of 792 pregnancies exposed to efavirenz-containing regimens, nearly all of which were first-trimester exposures (718 pregnancies). Birth defects occurred in 17 of 604 live births (first-trimester exposure) and 2 of 69 live births (second/third-trimester exposure). One of these prospectively reported defects with first-trimester exposure was a neural tube defect. A single case of anophthalmia with first-trimester exposure to efavirenz has also been prospectively reported, however, this case included severe oblique facial clefts and amniotic banding, a known association with anophthalmia. There have been six retrospective reports of findings consistent with neural tube defects, including meningomyelocele. All mothers were exposed to efavirenz-containing regimens in the first trimester. Although a causal relationship of these events to the use of efavirenz has not been established, similar defects have been observed in preclinical studies of efavirenz.

Animal Data

Effects of efavirenz on embryo-fetal development have been studied in three nonclinical species (cynomolgus monkeys, rats, and rabbits). In monkeys, efavirenz 60 mg/kg/day was administered to pregnant females throughout pregnancy (gestation Days 20 through 150). The maternal systemic drug exposures (AUC) were 1.3 times the exposure in humans at the recommended clinical dose (600 mg/day), with fetal umbilical venous drug concentrations approximately 0.7 times the maternal values. Three fetuses of 20 fetuses/infants had one or more malformations; there were no malformed fetuses or infants from placebo-treated mothers. The malformations that occurred in these three monkey fetuses included anencephaly and unilateral anophthalmia in one fetus, microophthalmia in a second, and cleft palate in the third. There was no NOAEL (no observable adverse effect level) established for this study because only one dosage was evaluated. In rats, efavirenz was administered either during organogenesis (gestation Days 7 to 18) or from gestation Day 7 through lactation Day 21 at 50, 100, or 200 mg/kg/day. Administration of 200 mg/kg/day in rats was associated with an increase in the incidence of early resorptions, and doses 100 mg/kg/day and greater were associated with early neonatal mortality. The AUC at the NOAEL (50 mg/kg/day) in this rat study was 0.1 times that in humans at the recommended clinical dose. Drug concentrations in the milk on lactation Day 10 were approximately 8 times higher than those in maternal plasma. In pregnant rabbits, efavirenz was neither embryo lethal nor teratogenic when administered at doses of 25, 50, and 75 mg/kg/day over the period of organogenesis (gestation Days 6 through 18). The AUC at the NOAEL (75 mg/kg/day) in rabbits was 0.4 times that in humans at the recommended clinical dose.

8.3 Nursing Mothers

The Centers for Disease Control and Prevention recommend that HIV-1 infected mothers not breastfeed their infants to avoid risking postnatal transmission of HIV-1. Studies in rats have demonstrated that efavirenz is secreted in milk. Studies in humans have shown that both tenofovir and emtricitabine are excreted in human milk. Because the risks of low level exposure to emtricitabine and tenofovir to infants are unknown, and because of the potential for HIV-1 transmission, **mothers should be instructed not to breastfeed if they are receiving ATRIPLA**.

Emtricitabine

Samples of breast milk obtained from five HIV-1 infected mothers show that emtricitabine is secreted in human milk. Breastfeeding infants whose mothers are being treated with emtricitabine may be at risk for developing viral resistance to emtricitabine. Other emtricitabine-associated risks in infants breastfed by mothers being treated with emtricitabine are unknown.

Tenofovir Disoproxil Fumarate

Samples of breast milk obtained from five HIV-1 infected mothers show that tenofovir is secreted in human milk. Tenofovir-associated risks, including the risk of viral resistance to tenofovir, in infants breastfed by mothers being treated with tenofovir disoproxil fumarate are unknown.

8.4 Pediatric Use

ATRIPLA should only be administered to pediatric patients 12 years of age and older with a body weight greater than or equal to 40 kg (greater than or equal to 88 lbs). Because ATRIPLA is a fixed-dose combination tablet, the dose adjustments recommended for pediatric patients younger than

Table 4 *(cont.)* Established and Other Potentially Significant* Drug Interactions: Alteration in Dose or Regimen May Be Recommended Based on Drug Interaction Trials or Predicted Interaction

Concomitant Drug Class: Drug Name	Effect	Clinical Comment
Other agents		
Anticoagulant: warfarin	↑ or ↓ warfarin	Plasma concentrations and effects potentially increased or decreased by efavirenz.
Anticonvulsants: carbamazepine phenytoin phenobarbital	↓ carbamazepine ↓ efavirenz ↓ anticonvulsant ↓ efavirenz	There are insufficient data to make a dose recommendation for ATRIPLA. Alternative anticonvulsant treatment should be used. Potential for reduction in anticonvulsant and/or efavirenz plasma levels; periodic monitoring of anticonvulsant plasma levels should be conducted.
Antidepressants: bupropion	↓ buproprion	The effect of efavirenz on bupropion exposure is thought to be due to the induction of bupropion metabolism. Increases in bupropion dosage should be guided by clinical response, but the maximum recommended dose of bupropion should not be exceeded.
sertraline	↓ sertraline	Increases in sertraline dose should be guided by clinical response.
Antifungals: itraconazole ketoconazole	↓ itraconazole ↓ hydroxy-itraconazole ↓ ketoconazole	Since no dose recommendation for itraconazole can be made, alternative antifungal treatment should be considered. Drug interaction trials with ATRIPLA and ketoconazole have not been conducted. Efavirenz has the potential to decrease plasma concentrations of ketoconazole.
posaconazole	↓ posaconazole	Avoid concomitant use unless the benefit outweighs the risks.
Anti-infective: clarithromycin	↓ clarithromycin ↑ 14-OH metabolite	Clinical significance unknown. In uninfected volunteers, 46% developed rash while receiving efavirenz and clarithromycin. No dose adjustment of ATRIPLA is recommended when given with clarithromycin. Alternatives to clarithromycin, such as azithromycin, should be considered. Other macrolide antibiotics, such as erythromycin, have not been studied in combination with ATRIPLA.
Antimycobacterial: rifabutin	↓ rifabutin	Increase daily dose of rifabutin by 50%. Consider doubling the rifabutin dose in regimens where rifabutin is given 2 or 3 times a week.
rifampin	↓ efavirenz	If ATRIPLA is coadministered with rifampin to patients weighing 50 kg or more, an additional 200 mg/day of efavirenz is recommended.
Calcium channel blockers: diltiazem	↓ diltiazem ↓ desacetyl diltiazem ↓ N-monodes-methyl diltiazem	Diltiazem dose adjustments should be guided by clinical response (refer to the full prescribing information for diltiazem). No dose adjustment of ATRIPLA is necessary when administered with diltiazem.
Others (e.g., felodipine, nicardipine, nifedipine, verapamil)	↓ calcium channel blocker	No data are available on the potential interactions of efavirenz with other calcium channel blockers that are substrates of CYP3A. The potential exists for reduction in plasma concentrations of the calcium channel blocker. Dose adjustments should be guided by clinical response (refer to the full prescribing information for the calcium channel blocker).
HMG-CoA reductase inhibitors: atorvastatin pravastatin simvastatin	↓ atorvastatin ↓ pravastatin ↓ simvastatin	Plasma concentrations of atorvastatin, pravastatin, and simvastatin decreased with efavirenz. Consult the full prescribing information for the HMG-CoA reductase inhibitor for guidance on individualizing the dose.
Hormonal contraceptives: Oral: ethinyl estradiol/norgestimate	↓ active metabolites of norgestimate	A reliable method of barrier contraception must be used in addition to hormonal contraceptives. Efavirenz had no effect on ethinyl estradiol concentrations, but progestin levels (norelgestromin and levonorgestrel) were markedly decreased. No effect of ethinyl estradiol/norgestimate on efavirenz plasma concentrations was observed.
Implant: etonogestrel	↓ etonogestrel	A reliable method of barrier contraception must be used in addition to hormonal contraceptives. The interaction between etonogestrel and efavirenz has not been studied. Decreased exposure of etonogestrel may be expected. There have been postmarketing reports of contraceptive failure with etonogestrel in efavirenz-exposed patients.

(Table continued on next page)

Table 4 *(cont.)* Established and Other Potentially Significant* Drug Interactions: Alteration in Dose or Regimen May Be Recommended Based on Drug Interaction Trials or Predicted Interaction

Concomitant Drug Class: Drug Name	Effect	Clinical Comment
Immunosuppressants: cyclosporine, tacrolimus, sirolimus, and others metabolized by CYP3A	↓ immuno-suppressant	Decreased exposure of the immunosuppressant may be expected due to CYP3A induction by efavirenz. These immunosuppressants are not anticipated to affect exposure of efavirenz. Dose adjustments of the immunosuppressant may be required. Close monitoring of immunosuppressant concentrations for at least 2 weeks (until stable concentrations are reached) is recommended when starting or stopping treatment with ATRIPLA.
Narcotic analgesic: methadone	↓ methadone	Coadministration of efavirenz in HIV-1 infected individuals with a history of injection drug use resulted in decreased plasma levels of methadone and signs of opiate withdrawal. Methadone dose was increased by a mean of 22% to alleviate withdrawal symptoms. Patients should be monitored for signs of withdrawal and their methadone dose increased as required to alleviate withdrawal symptoms.

* This table is not all inclusive.

12 years of age for each individual component cannot be made with ATRIPLA *[See Warnings and Precautions (5.9, 5.11), Adverse Reactions (6.1) and Clinical Pharmacology (12.3)]*.

8.5 Geriatric Use

Clinical trials of efavirenz, emtricitabine, or tenofovir DF did not include sufficient numbers of subjects aged 65 and over to determine whether they respond differently from younger subjects. In general, dose selection for elderly patients should be cautious, keeping in mind the greater frequency of decreased hepatic, renal, or cardiac function, and of concomitant disease or other drug therapy.

8.6 Hepatic Impairment

ATRIPLA is not recommended for patients with moderate or severe hepatic impairment because there are insufficient data to determine an appropriate dose. Patients with mild hepatic impairment may be treated with ATRIPLA at the approved dose. Because of the extensive cytochrome P450-mediated metabolism of efavirenz and limited clinical experience in patients with hepatic impairment, caution should be exercised in administering ATRIPLA to these patients *[See Warnings and Precautions (5.10) and Clinical Pharmacology (12.3)]*.

8.7 Renal Impairment

Because ATRIPLA is a fixed-dose combination, it should not be prescribed for patients requiring dosage adjustment such as those with moderate or severe renal impairment (creatinine clearance below 50 mL/min) *[See Warnings and Precautions (5.7)]*.

10 OVERDOSAGE

If overdose occurs, the patient should be monitored for evidence of toxicity, including monitoring of vital signs and observation of the patient's clinical status; standard supportive treatment should then be applied as necessary. Administration of activated charcoal may be used to aid removal of unabsorbed efavirenz. Hemodialysis can remove both emtricitabine and tenofovir DF (refer to detailed information below), but is unlikely to significantly remove efavirenz from the blood.

Efavirenz: Some patients accidentally taking 600 mg twice daily have reported increased nervous system symptoms. One patient experienced involuntary muscle contractions.

Emtricitabine: Limited clinical experience is available at doses higher than the therapeutic dose of emtricitabine. In one clinical pharmacology trial single doses of emtricitabine 1200 mg were administered to 11 subjects. No severe adverse reactions were reported.

Hemodialysis treatment removes approximately 30% of the emtricitabine dose over a 3-hour dialysis period starting within 1.5 hours of emtricitabine dosing (blood flow rate of 400 mL/min and a dialysate flow rate of 600 mL/min). It is not known whether emtricitabine can be removed by peritoneal dialysis.

Tenofovir Disoproxil Fumarate: Limited clinical experience at doses higher than the therapeutic dose of tenofovir DF 300 mg is available. In one trial, 600 mg tenofovir DF was administered to 8 subjects orally for 28 days, and no severe adverse reactions were reported. The effects of higher doses are not known.

Tenofovir is efficiently removed by hemodialysis with an extraction coefficient of approximately 54%. Following a single 300 mg dose of tenofovir DF, a 4-hour hemodialysis session removed approximately 10% of the administered tenofovir dose.

11 DESCRIPTION

ATRIPLA is a fixed-dose combination tablet containing efavirenz, emtricitabine, and tenofovir disoproxil fumarate (tenofovir DF). SUSTIVA is the brand name for efavirenz, a non-nucleoside reverse transcriptase inhibitor. EMTRIVA is the brand name for emtricitabine, a synthetic nucleoside analog of cytidine. VIREAD is the brand name for tenofovir DF, which is converted in vivo to tenofovir, an acyclic nucleoside phosphonate (nucleotide) analog of adenosine 5′-monophosphate. VIREAD and EMTRIVA are the components of TRUVADA.

ATRIPLA tablets are for oral administration. Each tablet contains 600 mg of efavirenz, 200 mg of emtricitabine, and 300 mg of tenofovir DF (which is equivalent to 245 mg of tenofovir disoproxil) as active ingredients. The tablets include the following inactive ingredients: croscarmellose sodium, hydroxypropyl cellulose, magnesium stearate, microcrystalline cellulose, and sodium lauryl sulfate. The tablets are film-coated with a coating material containing black iron oxide, polyethylene glycol, polyvinyl alcohol, red iron oxide, talc, and titanium dioxide.

Efavirenz: Efavirenz is chemically described as (*S*)-6-chloro-4-(cyclopropylethynyl)-1,4-dihydro-4-(trifluoromethyl)-2*H*-3,1-benzoxazin-2-one. Its molecular formula is $C_{14}H_9ClF_3NO_2$ and its structural formula is:

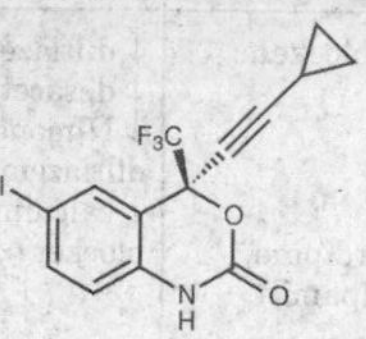

Efavirenz is a white to slightly pink crystalline powder with a molecular mass of 315.68. It is practically insoluble in water (less than 10 µg/mL).

Emtricitabine: The chemical name of emtricitabine is 5-fluoro-1-(2*R*,5*S*)-[2-(hydroxymethyl)-1,3-oxathiolan-5-yl]cytosine. Emtricitabine is the (-) enantiomer of a thio analog of cytidine, which differs from other cytidine analogs in that it has a fluorine in the 5-position.

It has a molecular formula of $C_8H_{10}FN_3O_3S$ and a molecular weight of 247.24. It has the following structural formula:

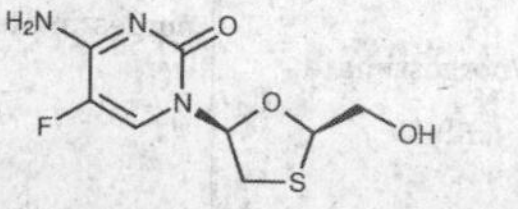

Emtricitabine is a white to off-white crystalline powder with a solubility of approximately 112 mg/mL in water at 25 °C.

Tenofovir Disoproxil Fumarate: Tenofovir DF is a fumaric acid salt of the *bis*-isopropoxycarbonyloxymethyl ester derivative of tenofovir. The chemical name of tenofovir disoproxil fumarate is 9-[(*R*)-2[[bis[[(isopropoxycarbonyl)oxy]- methoxy]phosphinyl]methoxy]propyl]adenine fumarate (1:1). It has a molecular formula of $C_{19}H_{30}N_5O_{10}P \cdot C_4H_4O_4$ and a molecular weight of 635.52. It has the following structural formula:

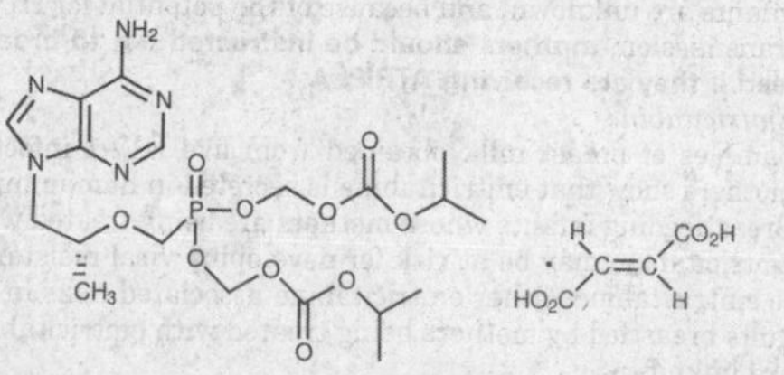

Tenofovir DF is a white to off-white crystalline powder with a solubility of 13.4 mg/mL in water at 25 °C.

12 CLINICAL PHARMACOLOGY

For additional information on Mechanism of Action, Antiviral Activity, Resistance and Cross Resistance, please consult the SUSTIVA, EMTRIVA and VIREAD prescribing information.

12.1 Mechanism of Action

ATRIPLA is a fixed-dose combination of antiviral drugs efavirenz, emtricitabine and tenofovir disoproxil fumarate *[See Clinical Pharmacology (12.4)]*.

12.3 Pharmacokinetics

ATRIPLA: One ATRIPLA tablet is bioequivalent to one SUSTIVA tablet (600 mg) plus one EMTRIVA capsule (200 mg) plus one VIREAD tablet (300 mg) following single-dose administration to fasting healthy subjects (N=45).

Efavirenz: In HIV-1 infected subjects time-to-peak plasma concentrations were approximately 3–5 hours and steady-state plasma concentrations were reached in 6–10 days. In 35 HIV-1 infected subjects receiving efavirenz 600 mg once daily, steady-state C_{max} was 12.9 ± 3.7 µM (mean ± SD), C_{min} was 5.6 ± 3.2 µM, and AUC was 184 ± 73 µM•hr. Efavirenz is highly bound (approximately 99.5–99.75%) to human plasma proteins, predominantly albumin. Following administration of ^{14}C-labeled efavirenz, 14–34% of the dose was recovered in the urine (mostly as metabolites) and 16–61% was recovered in feces (mostly as parent drug). In vitro studies suggest CYP3A and CYP2B6 are the major isozymes responsible for efavirenz metabolism. Efavirenz has been shown to induce CYP enzymes, resulting in induction of its own metabolism. Efavirenz has a terminal half-life of 52–76 hours after single doses and 40–55 hours after multiple doses.

Emtricitabine: Following oral administration, emtricitabine is rapidly absorbed, with peak plasma concentrations occurring at 1–2 hours post-dose. Following multiple dose oral administration of emtricitabine to 20 HIV-1 infected subjects, the steady-state plasma emtricitabine C_{max} was 1.8 ± 0.7 µg/mL (mean ± SD) and the AUC over a 24-hour dosing interval was 10.0 ± 3.1 µg•hr/mL. The mean steady-state plasma trough concentration at 24 hours post-dose was 0.09 µg/mL. The mean absolute bioavailability of emtricitabine was 93%. Less than 4% of emtricitabine binds to human plasma proteins *in vitro* and the binding is independent of concentration over the range of 0.02–200 µg/mL. Following administration of radiolabelled emtricitabine, approximately 86% is recovered in the urine and 13% is recovered as metabolites. The metabolites of emtricitabine include 3′-sulfoxide diastereomers and their glucuronic acid conjugate. Emtricitabine is eliminated by a combination of glomerular filtration and active tubular secretion with a renal clearance in adults with normal renal function of 213 ± 89 mL/min (mean ± SD). Following a single oral dose, the plasma emtricitabine half-life is approximately 10 hours.

Tenofovir Disoproxil Fumarate: Following oral administration of a single 300 mg dose of tenofovir DF to HIV-1 infected subjects in the fasted state, maximum serum concentrations (C_{max}) were achieved in 1.0 ± 0.4 hrs (mean ± SD) and C_{max} and AUC values were 296 ± 90 ng/mL and 2287 ± 685 ng•hr/mL, respectively. The oral bioavailability of tenofovir from tenofovir DF in fasted subjects is approximately 25%. Less than 0.7% of tenofovir binds to human plasma proteins *in vitro* and the binding is independent of concentration over the range of 0.01–25 µg/mL. Approximately 70–80% of the intravenous dose of tenofovir is recovered as unchanged drug in the urine. Tenofovir is eliminated by a combination of glomerular filtration and active tubular secretion with a renal clearance in adults with normal renal function of 243 ± 33 mL/min (mean ± SD). Following a single oral dose, the terminal elimination half-life of tenofovir is approximately 17 hours.

Effects of Food on Oral Absorption

ATRIPLA has not been evaluated in the presence of food. Administration of efavirenz tablets with a high fat meal increased the mean AUC and C_{max} of efavirenz by 28% and 79%, respectively, compared to administration in the fasted state. Compared to fasted administration, dosing of tenofovir DF and emtricitabine in combination with either a high fat meal or a light meal increased the mean AUC and C_{max} of tenofovir by 35% and 15%, respectively, without affecting emtricitabine exposures *[See Dosage and Administration (2) and Patient Counseling Information (17.7)]*.

Special Populations

Race

Efavirenz: The pharmacokinetics of efavirenz in HIV-1 infected subjects appear to be similar among the racial groups studied.

Emtricitabine: No pharmacokinetic differences due to race have been identified following the administration of emtricitabine.

Tenofovir Disoproxil Fumarate: There were insufficient numbers from racial and ethnic groups other than Caucasian to adequately determine potential pharmacokinetic differences among these populations following the administration of tenofovir DF.

Gender

Efavirenz, Emtricitabine, and Tenofovir Disoproxil Fumarate: Efavirenz, emtricitabine, and tenofovir pharmacokinetics are similar in male and female subjects.

Pediatric Patients

ATRIPLA should only be administered to pediatric patients 12 years of age and weighing greater than or equal to 40 kg (greater than or equal to 88 lb).

Efavirenz: In an open-label trial in NRTI-experienced pediatric subjects (mean age 8 years, range 3–16), the pharmacokinetics of efavirenz in pediatric subjects were similar to the pharmacokinetics in adults who received a 600 mg daily dose of efavirenz. In 48 pediatric subjects, receiving the equivalent of a 600 mg dose of efavirenz, mean (± SD) steady-state C_{max} was 14.2 ± 5.8 μM, steady-state C_{min} was 5.6 ± 4.1 μM, and AUC was 218 ± 104 μM•hr.

Emtricitabine: The pharmacokinetics of emtricitabine at steady state were determined in 27 HIV-1-infected pediatric subjects 13 to 17 years of age receiving a daily dose of 6 mg/kg up to a maximum dose of 240 mg oral solution or a 200 mg capsule; 26 of 27 subjects in this age group received the 200 mg EMTRIVA capsule. Mean (± SD) C_{max} and AUC were 2.7 ± 0.9 μg/mL and 12.6 ± 5.4 μg•hr/mL, respectively. Exposures achieved in pediatric subjects 12 to less than 18 years of age were similar to those achieved in adults receiving a once daily dose of 200 mg.

Tenofovir Disoproxil Fumarate: Steady-state pharmacokinetics of tenofovir were evaluated in 8 HIV-1 infected pediatric subjects (12 to less than 18 years). Mean (± SD) C_{max} and AUC_{tau} are 0.38 ± 0.13 μg/mL and 3.39 ± 1.22 μg•hr/mL, respectively. Tenofovir exposure achieved in these pediatric subjects receiving oral daily doses of VIREAD 300 mg was similar to exposures achieved in adults receiving once-daily doses of VIREAD 300 mg.

Geriatric Patients

Pharmacokinetics of efavirenz, emtricitabine and tenofovir have not been fully evaluated in the elderly (65 years of age and older) *[See Use in Specific Populations (8.5)].*

Patients with Impaired Renal Function

Efavirenz: The pharmacokinetics of efavirenz have not been studied in subjects with renal insufficiency; however, less than 1% of efavirenz is excreted unchanged in the urine, so the impact of renal impairment on efavirenz elimination should be minimal.

Emtricitabine and Tenofovir Disoproxil Fumarate: The pharmacokinetics of emtricitabine and tenofovir DF are altered in subjects with renal impairment. In subjects with creatinine clearance below 50 mL/min, C_{max} and $AUC_{0-\infty}$ of emtricitabine and tenofovir were increased *[See Warnings and Precautions (5.7)].*

Patients with Hepatic Impairment

Efavirenz: A multiple-dose trial showed no significant effect on efavirenz pharmacokinetics in subjects with mild hepatic impairment (Child-Pugh Class A) compared with controls. There were insufficient data to determine whether moderate or severe hepatic impairment (Child-Pugh Class B or C) affects efavirenz pharmacokinetics *[See Warnings and Precautions (5.10) and Use in Specific Populations (8.6)].*

Emtricitabine: The pharmacokinetics of emtricitabine have not been studied in subjects with hepatic impairment; however, emtricitabine is not significantly metabolized by liver enzymes, so the impact of liver impairment should be limited.

Tenofovir Disoproxil Fumarate: The pharmacokinetics of tenofovir following a 300 mg dose of tenofovir DF have been studied in non-HIV infected subjects with moderate to severe hepatic impairment. There were no substantial alterations in tenofovir pharmacokinetics in subjects with hepatic impairment compared with unimpaired subjects.

Assessment of Drug Interactions

The drug interaction trials described were conducted with efavirenz, emtricitabine, or tenofovir DF as individual agents; no drug interaction trials have been conducted using ATRIPLA.

Efavirenz: The steady-state pharmacokinetics of efavirenz and tenofovir were unaffected when efavirenz and tenofovir DF were administered together versus each agent dosed alone. Specific drug interaction trials have not been performed with efavirenz and NRTIs other than tenofovir, lamivudine, and zidovudine. Clinically significant interactions would not be expected based on NRTIs elimination pathways.

Efavirenz has been shown *in vivo* to cause hepatic enzyme induction, thus increasing the biotransformation of some drugs metabolized by CYP3A and CYP2B6. In vitro studies have shown that efavirenz inhibited CYP isozymes 2C9, 2C19, and 3A4 with K_i values (8.5–17 μM) in the range of observed efavirenz plasma concentrations. In in vitro studies, efavirenz did not inhibit CYP2E1 and inhibited CYP2D6 and CYP1A2 (K_i values 82–160 μM) only at concentrations well above those achieved clinically. Coadministration of efavirenz with drugs primarily metabolized by 2C9, 2C19, and 3A4 isozymes may result in altered plasma concentrations of the coadministered drug. Drugs which induce CYP3A activity would be expected to increase the clearance of efavirenz resulting in lowered plasma concentrations.

Drug interaction trials were performed with efavirenz and other drugs likely to be coadministered or drugs commonly used as probes for pharmacokinetic interaction. There was no clinically significant interaction observed between efavirenz and zidovudine, lamivudine, azithromycin, fluconazole, lorazepam, cetirizine, or paroxetine. Single doses of famotidine or an aluminum and magnesium antacid with simethicone had no effects on efavirenz exposures. The effects of coadministration of efavirenz on C_{max}, AUC, and C_{min} are summarized in Table 5 (effect of other drugs on efavirenz) and Table 6 (effect of efavirenz on other drugs). For information regarding clinical recommendations see *Drug Interactions (7).*

Table 5 Drug Interactions: Changes in Pharmacokinetic Parameters for Efavirenz in the Presence of the Coadministered Drug

Coadministered Drug	Dose of Coadministered Drug (mg)	Efavirenz Dose (mg)	N	Mean % Change of Efavirenz Pharmacokinetic Parameters* (90% CI) C_{max}	AUC	C_{min}
Indinavir	800 mg q8h × 14 days	200 mg qd × 14 days	11	↔	↔	↔
Lopinavir/ ritonavir	400/100 mg q12h × 9 days	600 mg qd × 9 days	11, 12[†]	↔	↓ 16 (↓ 38 to ↑ 15)	↓ 16 (↓ 42 to ↑ 20)
Nelfinavir	750 mg q8h × 7 days	600 mg qd × 7 days	10	↓ 12 (↓ 32 to ↑ 13)[‡]	↓ 12 (↓ 35 to ↑ 18)[‡]	↓ 21 (↓ 53 to ↑ 33)
Ritonavir	500 mg q12h × 8 days	600 mg qd × 10 days	9	↑ 14 (↑ 4 to ↑ 26)	↑ 21 (↑ 10 to ↑ 34)	↑ 25 (↑ 7 to ↑ 46)[‡]
Saquinavir SGC[§]	1200 mg q8h × 10 days	600 mg qd × 10 days	13	↓ 13 (↓ 5 to ↓ 20)	↓ 12 (↓ 4 to ↓ 19)	↓ 14 (↓ 2 to ↓ 24)[‡]
Boceprevir	800 mg tid × 6 days	600 mg qd × 16 days	NA	↑ 11 (↑ 2 to ↑ 20)	↑ 20 (↑ 15 to ↑ 26)	NA
Telaprevir	750 mg q8h × 10 days	600 mg qd × 20 days	21	↓ 16 (↓ 7 to ↓ 24)	↓ 7 (↓ 2 to ↓ 13)	↓ 2 (↓ 6 to ↑ 2)
Telaprevir, coadministered with tenofovir disoproxil fumarate (TDF)	1125 mg q8h × 7 days	600 mg efavirenz/ 300 mg TDF qd × 7 days	15	↓ 24 (↓ 15 to ↓ 32)	↓ 18 (↓ 10 to ↓ 26)	↓ 10 (↓ 19 to ↑ 1)
	1500 mg q12h × 7 days	600 mg efavirenz/ 300 mg TDF qd × 7 days	16	↓ 20 (↓ 14 to ↓ 26)	↓ 15 (↓ 9 to ↓ 21)	↓ 11 (↓ 4 to ↓ 18)
Clarithromycin	500 mg q12h × 7 days	400 mg qd × 7 days	12	↑ 11 (↑ 3 to ↑ 19)	↔	↔
Itraconazole	200 mg q12h × 14 days	600 mg qd × 28 days	16	↔	↔	↔
Rifabutin	300 mg qd × 14 days	600 mg qd × 14 days	11	↔	↔	↓ 12 (↓ 24 to ↑ 1)
Rifampin	600 mg × 7 days	600 mg qd × 7 days	12	↓ 20 (↓ 11 to ↓ 28)	↓ 26 (↓ 15 to ↓ 36)	↓ 32 (↓ 15 to ↓ 46)
Atorvastatin	10 mg qd × 4 days	600 mg qd × 15 days	14	↔	↔	↔
Pravastatin	40 mg qd × 4 days	600 mg qd × 15 days	11	↔	↔	↔
Simvastatin	40 mg qd × 4 days	600 mg qd × 15 days	14	↓ 12 (↓ 28 to ↑ 8)	↔	↓ 12 (↓ 25 to ↑ 3)
Carbamazepine	200 mg qd × 3 days, 200 mg bid × 3 days, then 400 mg qd × 15 days	600 mg qd × 35 days	14	↓ 21 (↓ 15 to ↓ 26)	↓ 36 (↓ 32 to ↓ 40)	↓ 47 (↓ 41 to ↓ 53)
Diltiazem	240 mg × 14 days	600 mg qd × 28 days	12	↑ 16 (↑ 6 to ↑ 26)	↑ 11 (↑ 5 to ↑ 18)	↑ 13 (↑ 1 to ↑ 26)

(Table continued on next page)

[See table 5 above and on next page]

[See table 6 on pages 829 through 831]

Emtricitabine and Tenofovir Disoproxil Fumarate: The steady-state pharmacokinetics of emtricitabine and tenofovir were unaffected when emtricitabine and tenofovir DF were administered together versus each agent dosed alone.

Table 5 *(cont.)* Drug Interactions: Changes in Pharmacokinetic Parameters for Efavirenz in the Presence of the Coadministered Drug

Coadministered Drug	Dose of Coadministered Drug (mg)	Efavirenz Dose (mg)	N	Mean % Change of Efavirenz Pharmacokinetic Parameters* (90% CI) C_{max}	AUC	C_{min}
Sertraline	50 mg qd × 14 days	600 mg qd × 14 days	13	↑ 11 (↑ 6 to ↑ 16)	↔	↔
Voriconazole	400 mg po q12h × 1 day then 200 mg po q12h × 8 days	400 mg qd × 9 days	NA	↑ 38¶	↑ 44¶	NA
	300 mg po q12h days 2–7	300 mg qd × 7 days	NA	↓ 14# (↓ 7 to ↓ 21)	↔#	NA
	400 mg po q12h days 2–7	300 mg qd × 7 days	NA	↔#	↑ 17# (↑ 6 to ↑ 29)	NA

NA = not available
* Increase = ↑; Decrease = ↓; No Effect = ↔
† Parallel-group design; N for efavirenz + lopinavir/ritonavir, N for efavirenz alone.
‡ 95% CI
§ Soft Gelatin Capsule
¶ 90% CI not available
\# Relative to steady-state administration of efavirenz (600 mg once daily for 9 days).

In vitro and clinical pharmacokinetic drug-drug interaction studies have shown that the potential for CYP mediated interactions involving emtricitabine and tenofovir with other medicinal products is low.

Emtricitabine and tenofovir are primarily excreted by the kidneys by a combination of glomerular filtration and active tubular secretion. No drug-drug interactions due to competition for renal excretion have been observed; however, coadministration of emtricitabine and tenofovir DF with drugs that are eliminated by active tubular secretion may increase concentrations of emtricitabine, tenofovir, and/or the coadministered drug.

Drugs that decrease renal function may increase concentrations of emtricitabine and/or tenofovir.

No clinically significant drug interactions have been observed between emtricitabine and famciclovir, indinavir, stavudine, tenofovir DF and zidovudine. Similarly, no clinically significant drug interactions have been observed between tenofovir DF and abacavir, efavirenz, emtricitabine, entecavir, indinavir, lamivudine, lopinavir/ritonavir, methadone, nelfinavir, oral contraceptives, ribavirin, saquinavir/ritonavir or tacrolimus in trials conducted in healthy volunteers.

Following multiple dosing to HIV-negative subjects receiving either chronic methadone maintenance therapy, oral contraceptives, or single doses of ribavirin, steady-state tenofovir pharmacokinetics were similar to those observed in previous trials, indicating a lack of clinically significant drug interactions between these agents and tenofovir DF.

The effects of coadministered drugs on the C_{max}, AUC, and C_{min} of tenofovir are shown in Table 7. The effects of coadministration of tenofovir DF on C_{max}, AUC, and C_{min} of coadministered drugs are shown in Table 8.

[See table 7 at top of page 831]

[See table 8 at top of page 832]

Coadministration of tenofovir DF with didanosine results in changes in the pharmacokinetics of didanosine that may be of clinical significance. Concomitant dosing of tenofovir DF with didanosine enteric-coated capsules significantly increases the C_{max} and AUC of didanosine. When didanosine 250 mg enteric-coated capsules were administered with tenofovir DF, systemic exposures of didanosine were similar to those seen with the 400 mg enteric-coated capsules alone under fasted conditions. The mechanism of this interaction is unknown [for didanosine dosing adjustment recommendations see *Drug Interactions (7.3)*, Table 4].

12.4 Microbiology

Mechanism of Action

Efavirenz: Efavirenz is a non-nucleoside reverse transcriptase (RT) inhibitor of HIV-1. Efavirenz activity is mediated predominantly by noncompetitive inhibition of HIV-1 reverse transcriptase (RT). HIV-2 RT and human cellular DNA polymerases α, β, γ, and σ are not inhibited by efavirenz.

Emtricitabine: Emtricitabine, a synthetic nucleoside analog of cytidine, is phosphorylated by cellular enzymes to form emtricitabine 5′-triphosphate. Emtricitabine 5′-triphosphate inhibits the activity of the HIV-1 RT by competing with the natural substrate deoxycytidine 5′-triphosphate and by being incorporated into nascent viral DNA which results in chain termination. Emtricitabine 5′-triphosphate is a weak inhibitor of mammalian DNA polymerase α, β, ϵ, and mitochondrial DNA polymerase γ.

Tenofovir Disoproxil Fumarate: Tenofovir DF is an acyclic nucleoside phosphonate diester analog of adenosine monophosphate. Tenofovir DF requires initial diester hydrolysis for conversion to tenofovir and subsequent phosphorylations by cellular enzymes to form tenofovir diphosphate. Tenofovir diphosphate inhibits the activity of HIV-1 RT by competing with the natural substrate deoxyadenosine 5′-triphosphate and, after incorporation into DNA, by DNA chain termination. Tenofovir diphosphate is a weak inhibitor of mammalian DNA polymerases α, β, and mitochondrial DNA polymerase γ.

Antiviral Activity

Efavirenz, Emtricitabine, and Tenofovir Disoproxil Fumarate: In combination studies evaluating the antiviral activity in cell culture of emtricitabine and efavirenz together, efavirenz and tenofovir together, and emtricitabine and tenofovir together, additive to synergistic antiviral effects were observed.

Efavirenz: The concentration of efavirenz inhibiting replication of wild-type laboratory adapted strains and clinical isolates in cell culture by 90–95% (EC_{90-95}) ranged from 1.7–25 nM in lymphoblastoid cell lines, peripheral blood mononuclear cells, and macrophage/monocyte cultures. Efavirenz demonstrated additive antiviral activity against HIV-1 in cell culture when combined with non-nucleoside reverse transcriptase inhibitors (NNRTIs) (delavirdine and nevirapine), nucleoside reverse transcriptase inhibitors (NRTIs) (abacavir, didanosine, lamivudine, stavudine, zalcitabine, and zidovudine), protease inhibitors (PIs) (amprenavir, indinavir, lopinavir, nelfinavir, ritonavir, and saquinavir), and the fusion inhibitor enfuvirtide. Efavirenz demonstrated additive to antagonistic antiviral activity in cell culture with atazanavir. Efavirenz demonstrated antiviral activity against clade B and most non-clade B isolates (subtypes A, AE, AG, C, D, F, G, J, and N), but had reduced antiviral activity against group O viruses. Efavirenz is not active against HIV-2.

Emtricitabine: The antiviral activity in cell culture of emtricitabine against laboratory and clinical isolates of HIV-1 was assessed in lymphoblastoid cell lines, the MAGI-CCR5 cell line, and peripheral blood mononuclear cells. The 50% effective concentration (EC_{50}) values for emtricitabine were in the range of 0.0013–0.64 µM (0.0003–0.158 µg/mL). In drug combination studies of emtricitabine with NRTIs (abacavir, lamivudine, stavudine, zalcitabine, and zidovudine), NNRTIs (delavirdine, efavirenz, and nevirapine), and PIs (amprenavir, nelfinavir, ritonavir, and saquinavir), additive to synergistic effects were observed. Emtricitabine displayed antiviral activity in cell culture against HIV-1 clades A, B, C, D, E, F, and G (EC_{50} values ranged from 0.007–0.075 µM) and showed strain specific activity against HIV-2 (EC_{50} values ranged from 0.007–1.5 µM).

Tenofovir Disoproxil Fumarate: The antiviral activity in cell culture of tenofovir against laboratory and clinical isolates of HIV-1 was assessed in lymphoblastoid cell lines, primary monocyte/macrophage cells and peripheral blood lymphocytes. The EC_{50} values for tenofovir were in the range of 0.04–8.5 µM. In drug combination studies of tenofovir with NRTIs (abacavir, didanosine, lamivudine, stavudine, zalcitabine, and zidovudine), NNRTIs (delavirdine, efavirenz, and nevirapine), and PIs (amprenavir, indinavir, nelfinavir, ritonavir, and saquinavir), additive to synergistic effects were observed. Tenofovir displayed antiviral activity in cell culture against HIV-1 clades A, B, C, D, E, F, G and O (EC_{50} values ranged from 0.5–2.2 µM) and showed strain specific activity against HIV-2 (EC_{50} values ranged from 1.6 µM–5.5 µM).

Resistance

Efavirenz, Emtricitabine, and Tenofovir Disoproxil Fumarate: HIV-1 isolates with reduced susceptibility to the combination of emtricitabine and tenofovir have been selected in cell culture and in clinical trials. Genotypic analysis of these isolates identified the M184V/I and/or K65R amino acid substitutions in the viral RT.

In a clinical trial of treatment-naive subjects *[Study 934, see Clinical Studies (14)]* resistance analysis was performed on HIV-1 isolates from all confirmed virologic failure subjects with greater than 400 copies/mL of HIV-1 RNA at Week 144 or early discontinuations. Genotypic resistance to efavirenz, predominantly the K103N substitution, was the most common form of resistance that developed. Resistance to efavirenz occurred in 13/19 analyzed subjects in the emtricitabine + tenofovir DF group and in 21/29 analyzed subjects in the zidovudine/lamivudine fixed-dose combination group. The M184V amino acid substitution, associated with resistance to emtricitabine and lamivudine, was observed in 2/19 analyzed subject isolates in the emtricitabine + tenofovir DF group and in 10/29 analyzed subject isolates in the zidovudine/lamivudine group. Through 144 weeks of Study 934, no subjects developed a detectable K65R substitution in their HIV-1 as analyzed through standard genotypic analysis.

In a clinical trial of treatment-naive subjects, isolates from 8/47 (17%) analyzed subjects receiving tenofovir DF developed the K65R substitution through 144 weeks of therapy; 7 of these occurred in the first 48 weeks of treatment and one at Week 96. In treatment experienced subjects, 14/304 (5%) of tenofovir DF treated subjects with virologic failure through Week 96 showed greater than 1.4-fold (median 2.7) reduced susceptibility to tenofovir. Genotypic analysis of the resistant isolates showed a substitution in the HIV-1 RT gene resulting in the K65R amino acid substitution.

Efavirenz: Clinical isolates with reduced susceptibility in cell culture to efavirenz have been obtained. The most frequently observed amino acid substitution in clinical trials with efavirenz is K103N (54%). One or more RT substitutions at amino acid positions 98, 100, 101, 103, 106, 108, 188, 190, 225, 227, and 230 were observed in subjects failing treatment with efavirenz in combination with other antiretrovirals. Other resistance substitutions observed to emerge commonly included L100I (7%), K101E/Q/R (14%), V108I (11%), G190S/T/A (7%), P225H (18%), and M230I/L (11%).

HIV-1 isolates with reduced susceptibility to efavirenz (greater than 380-fold increase in EC_{90} value) emerged rapidly under selection in cell culture. Genotypic characterization of these viruses identified substitutions resulting in single amino acid substitutions L100I or V179D, double substitutions L100I/V108I, and triple substitutions L100I/V179D/Y181C in RT.

Emtricitabine: Emtricitabine-resistant isolates of HIV-1 have been selected in cell culture and in clinical trials. Genotypic analysis of these isolates showed that the reduced susceptibility to emtricitabine was associated with a substitution in the HIV-1 RT gene at codon 184 which resulted in an amino acid substitution of methionine by valine or isoleucine (M184V/I).

Tenofovir Disoproxil Fumarate: HIV-1 isolates with reduced susceptibility to tenofovir have been selected in cell culture. These viruses expressed a K65R substitution in RT and showed a 2- to 4-fold reduction in susceptibility to tenofovir.

Cross Resistance

Efavirenz, Emtricitabine, and Tenofovir Disoproxil Fumarate: Cross-resistance has been recognized among NNRTIs. Cross resistance has also been recognized among certain NRTIs. The M184V/I and/or K65R substitutions selected in cell culture by the combination of emtricitabine and tenofovir are also observed in some HIV-1 isolates from subjects failing treatment with tenofovir in combination with either lamivudine or emtricitabine, and either abacavir or didanosine. Therefore, cross-resistance among these drugs may occur in patients whose virus harbors either or both of these amino acid substitutions.

Efavirenz: Clinical isolates previously characterized as efavirenz-resistant were also phenotypically resistant in cell culture to delavirdine and nevirapine compared to baseline. Delavirdine- and/or nevirapine-resistant clinical viral isolates with NNRTI resistance-associated substitutions (A98G, L100I, K101E/P, K103N/S, V106A, Y181X, Y188X, G190X, P225H, F227L, or M230L) showed reduced susceptibility to efavirenz in cell culture. Greater than 90% of NRTI-resistant isolates tested in cell culture retained susceptibility to efavirenz.

Emtricitabine: Emtricitabine-resistant isolates (M184V/I) were cross-resistant to lamivudine and zalcitabine but retained susceptibility in cell culture to didanosine, stavudine, tenofovir, zidovudine, and NNRTIs (delavirdine, efavirenz, and nevirapine). HIV-1 isolates containing the K65R substitution, selected in vivo by abacavir, didanosine, tenofovir, and zalcitabine, demonstrated reduced susceptibility to inhibition by emtricitabine. Viruses harboring substitutions conferring reduced susceptibility to stavudine and zidovudine (M41L, D67N, K70R, L210W, T215Y/F, and K219Q/E) or didanosine (L74V) remained sensitive to emtricitabine.

Tenofovir Disoproxil Fumarate: The K65R substitution selected by tenofovir is also selected in some HIV-1 infected patients treated with abacavir, didanosine, or zalcitabine. HIV-1 isolates with the K65R substitution also showed reduced susceptibility to emtricitabine and lamivudine. Therefore, cross-resistance among these drugs may occur in patients whose virus harbors the K65R substitution. HIV-1 isolates from subjects (N=20) whose HIV-1 expressed a mean of 3 zidovudine-associated RT amino acid substitutions (M41L, D67N, K70R, L210W, T215Y/F, or K219Q/E/N) showed a 3.1-fold decrease in the susceptibility to tenofovir. Subjects whose virus expressed an L74V substitution without zidovudine resistance associated substitutions (N=8) had reduced response to VIREAD. Limited data are available for patients whose virus expressed a Y115F substitution (N=3), Q151M substitution (N=2), or T69 insertion (N=4), all of whom had a reduced response.

13 NONCLINICAL TOXICOLOGY

13.1 Carcinogenesis, Mutagenesis, Impairment of Fertility

Efavirenz: Long-term carcinogenicity studies in mice and rats were carried out with efavirenz. Mice were dosed with 0, 25, 75, 150, or 300 mg/kg/day for 2 years. Incidences of hepatocellular adenomas and carcinomas and pulmonary alveolar/bronchiolar adenomas were increased above background in females. No increases in tumor incidence above background were seen in males. In studies in which rats were administered efavirenz at doses of 0, 25, 50, or 100 mg/kg/day for 2 years, no increases in tumor incidence above background were observed. The systemic exposure (based on AUCs) in mice was approximately 1.7-fold that in humans receiving the 600-mg/day dose. The exposure in rats was lower than that in humans. The mechanism of the carcinogenic potential is unknown. However, in genetic toxicology assays, efavirenz showed no evidence of mutagenic or clastogenic activity in a battery of in vitro and in vivo studies. These included bacterial mutation assays in *S. typhimurium* and *E. coli*, mammalian mutation assays in Chinese hamster ovary cells, chromosome aberration assays in human peripheral blood lymphocytes or Chinese hamster ovary cells, and an in vivo mouse bone marrow micronucleus assay. Given the lack of genotoxic activity of efavirenz, the relevance to humans of neoplasms in efavirenz-treated mice is not known.

Efavirenz did not impair mating or fertility of male or female rats, and did not affect sperm of treated male rats. The reproductive performance of offspring born to female rats given efavirenz was not affected. As a result of the rapid clearance of efavirenz in rats, systemic drug exposures achieved in these studies were equivalent to or below those achieved in humans given therapeutic doses of efavirenz.

Emtricitabine: In long-term carcinogenicity studies of emtricitabine, no drug-related increases in tumor incidence were found in mice at doses up to 750 mg/kg/day (26 times the human systemic exposure at the therapeutic dose of 200 mg/day) or in rats at doses up to 600 mg/day (31 times the human systemic exposure at the therapeutic dose).

Emtricitabine was not genotoxic in the reverse mutation bacterial test (Ames test), mouse lymphoma or mouse micronucleus assays.

Emtricitabine did not affect fertility in male rats at approximately 140-fold or in male and female mice at approximately 60-fold higher exposures (AUC) than in humans given the recommended 200 mg daily dose. Fertility was normal in the offspring of mice exposed daily from before birth (in utero) through sexual maturity at daily exposures (AUC) of approximately 60-fold higher than human exposures at the recommended 200 mg daily dose.

Tenofovir Disoproxil Fumarate: Long-term oral carcinogenicity studies of tenofovir DF in mice and rats were carried out at exposures up to approximately 16 times (mice) and 5 times (rats) those observed in humans at the therapeutic dose for HIV-1 infection. At the high dose in female mice, liver adenomas were increased at exposures 16 times that in humans. In rats, the study was negative for carcinogenic findings at exposures up to 5 times that observed in humans at the therapeutic dose.

Table 6 Drug Interactions: Changes in Pharmacokinetic Parameters for Coadministered Drug in the Presence of Efavirenz

Coadministered Drug	Dose of Coadministered Drug (mg)	Efavirenz Dose (mg)	N	Mean % Change of Coadministered Drug Pharmacokinetic Parameters* (90% CI): C_{max}	AUC	C_{min}
Atazanavir	400 mg qd with a light meal d 1–20	600 mg qd with a light meal d 7–20	27	↓ 59 (↓ 49 to ↓ 67)	↓ 74 (↓ 68 to ↓ 78)	↓ 93 (↓ 90 to ↓ 95)
	400 mg qd d 1–6, then 300 mg qd d 7–20 with ritonavir 100 mg qd and a light meal	600 mg qd 2 h after atazanavir and ritonavir d 7–20	13	↑ 14[†] (↓ 17 to ↑ 58)	↑ 39[†] (↑ 2 to ↑ 88)	↑ 48[†] (↑ 24 to ↑ 76)
	300 mg qd/ritonavir 100 mg qd d 1–10 (pm), then 400 mg qd/ritonavir 100 mg qd d 11–24 (pm) (simultaneous with efavirenz)	600 mg qd with a light snack d 11–24 (pm)	14	↑ 17 (↑ 8 to ↑ 27)	↔	↓ 42 (↓ 31 to ↓ 51)
Indinavir	1000 mg q8h × 10 days	600 mg qd × 10 days	20			
	After morning dose			↔[‡]	↓ 33[‡] (↓ 26 to ↓ 39)	↓ 39[‡] (↓ 24 to ↓ 51)
	After afternoon dose			↔[‡]	↓ 37[‡] (↓ 26 to ↓ 46)	↓ 52[†] (↓ 47 to ↓ 57)
	After evening dose			↓ 29[‡] (↓ 11 to ↓ 43)	↓ 46[‡] (↓ 37 to ↓ 54)	↓ 57[‡] (↓ 50 to ↓ 63)
Lopinavir/ ritonavir	400/100 mg q12h × 9 days	600 mg qd × 9 days	11, 7[§]	↔[¶]	↓ 19[¶] (↓ 36 to ↑ 3)	↓ 39[¶] (↓ 3 to ↓ 62)
Nelfinavir	750 mg q8h × 7 days	600 mg qd × 7 days	10	↑ 21 (↑ 10 to ↑ 33)	↑ 20 (↑ 8 to ↑ 34)	↔
Metabolite AG-1402				↓ 40 (↓ 30 to ↓ 48)	↓ 37 (↓ 25 to ↓ 48)	↓ 43 (↓ 21 to ↓ 59)
Ritonavir	500 mg q12h × 8 days	600 mg qd × 10 days	11			
	After AM dose			↑ 24 (↑ 12 to ↑ 38)	↑ 18 (↑ 6 to ↑ 33)	↑ 42 (↑ 9 to ↑ 86)[#]
	After PM dose			↔	↔	↑ 24 (↑ 3 to ↑ 50)[#]
Saquinavir SGC[b]	1200 mg q8h × 10 days	600 mg qd × 10 days	12	↓ 50 (↓ 28 to ↓ 66)	↓ 62 (↓ 45 to ↓ 74)	↓ 56 (↓ 16 to ↓ 77)[#]
Maraviroc	100 mg bid	600 mg qd	12	↓ 51 (↓ 37 to ↓ 62)	↓ 45 (↓ 38 to ↓ 51)	↓ 45 (↓ 28 to ↓ 57)
Raltegravir	400 mg single dose	600 mg qd	9	↓ 36 (↓ 2 to ↓ 59)	↓ 36 (↓ 20 to ↓ 48)	↓ 21 (↓ 51 to ↑ 28)
Boceprevir	800 mg tid × 6 days	600 mg qd × 16 days	NA	↓ 8 (↓ 22 to ↑ 8)	↓ 19 (↓ 11 to ↓ 25)	↓ 44 (↓ 26 to ↓ 58)
Telaprevir	750 mg q8h × 10 days	600 mg qd × 20 days	21	↓ 9 (↓18 to ↑ 2)	↓ 26 (↓16 to ↓ 35)	↓ 47 (↓ 35 to ↓ 56)

(Table continued on next page)

Tenofovir DF was mutagenic in the in vitro mouse lymphoma assay and negative in an in vitro bacterial mutagenicity test (Ames test). In an in vivo mouse micronucleus assay, tenofovir DF was negative when administered to male mice.

There were no effects on fertility, mating performance or early embryonic development when tenofovir DF was administered to male rats at a dose equivalent to 10 times the human dose based on body surface area comparisons for 28 days prior to mating and to female rats for 15 days prior to mating through Day seven of gestation. There was, however, an alteration of the estrous cycle in female rats.

13.2 Animal Toxicology and/or Pharmacology

Efavirenz: Nonsustained convulsions were observed in 6 of 20 monkeys receiving efavirenz at doses yielding plasma AUC values 4- to 13-fold greater than those in humans given the recommended dose.

Table 6 *(cont.)* Drug Interactions: Changes in Pharmacokinetic Parameters for Coadministered Drug in the Presence of Efavirenz

Coadministered Drug	Dose of Coadministered Drug (mg)	Efavirenz Dose (mg)	N	Mean % Change of Coadministered Drug Pharmacokinetic Parameters* (90% CI) C_{max}	AUC	C_{min}
Clarithromycin	500 mg q12h × 7 days	400 mg qd × 7 days	11	↓ 26 (↓ 15 to ↓ 35)	↓ 39 (↓ 30 to ↓ 46)	↓ 53 (↓ 42 to ↓ 63)
14-OH metabolite				↑ 49 (↑ 32 to ↑ 69)	↑ 34 (↑ 18 to ↑ 53)	↑ 26 (↑ 9 to ↑ 45)
Itraconazole	200 mg q12h × 28 days	600 mg qd × 14 days	18	↓ 37 (↓ 20 to ↓ 51)	↓ 39 (↓ 21 to ↓ 53)	↓ 44 (↓ 27 to ↓ 58)
Hydroxy-itraconazole				↓ 35 (↓ 12 to ↓ 52)	↓ 37 (↓ 14 to ↓ 55)	↓ 43 (↓ 18 to ↓ 60)
Posaconazole	400 mg (oral suspension) bid × 10 and 20 days	400 mg qd × 10 and 20 days	11	↓ 45 (↓ 34 to ↓ 53)	↓ 50 (↓ 40 to ↓ 57)	NA
Rifabutin	300 mg qd × 14 days	600 mg qd × 14 days	9	↓ 32 (↓ 15 to ↓ 46)	↓ 38 (↓ 28 to ↓ 47)	↓ 45 (↓ 31 to ↓ 56)
Atorvastatin	10 mg qd × 4 days	600 mg qd × 15 days	14	↓ 14 (↓ 1 to ↓ 26)	↓ 43 (↓ 34 to ↓ 50)	↓ 69 (↓ 49 to ↓ 81)
Total active (including metabolites)				↓ 15 (↓ 2 to ↓ 26)	↓ 32 (↓ 21 to ↓ 41)	↓ 48 (↓ 23 to ↓ 64)
Pravastatin	40 mg qd × 4 days	600 mg qd × 15 days	13	↓ 32 (↓ 59 to ↑ 12)	↓ 44 (↓ 26 to ↓ 57)	↓ 19 (↓ 0 to ↓ 35)
Simvastatin	40 mg qd × 4 days	600 mg qd × 15 days	14	↓ 72 (↓ 63 to ↓ 79)	↓ 68 (↓ 62 to ↓ 73)	↓ 45 (↓ 20 to ↓ 62)
Total active (including metabolites)				↓ 68 (↓ 55 to ↓ 78)	↓ 60 (↓ 52 to ↓ 68)	NA[β]
Carbamazepine	200 mg qd × 3 days, 200 mg bid × 3 days, then 400 mg qd × 29 days	600 mg qd × 14 days	12	↓ 20 (↓ 15 to ↓ 24)	↓ 27 (↓ 20 to ↓ 33)	↓ 35 (↓ 24 to ↓ 44)
Epoxide metabolite				↔	↔	↓ 13 (↓ 30 to ↑ 7)
Diltiazem	240 mg × 21 days	600 mg qd × 14 days	13	↓ 60 (↓ 50 to ↓ 68)	↓ 69 (↓ 55 to ↓ 79)	↓ 63 (↓ 44 to ↓ 75)
Desacetyl diltiazem				↓ 64 (↓ 57 to ↓ 69)	↓ 75 (↓ 59 to ↓ 84)	↓ 62 (↓ 44 to ↓ 75)
N-monodesmethyl diltiazem				↓ 28 (↓ 7 to ↓ 44)	↓ 37 (↓ 17 to ↓ 52)	↓ 37 (↓ 17 to ↓ 52)
Ethinyl estradiol/ Norgestimate	0.035 mg/0.25 mg × 14 days	600 mg qd × 14 days				
Ethinyl estradiol			21	↔	↔	↔
Norelgestromin			21	↓ 46 (↓39 to ↓ 52)	↓ 64 (↓ 62 to ↓ 67)	↓ 82 (↓ 79 to ↓ 85)
Levonorgestrel			6	↓ 80 (↓77 to ↓ 83)	↓ 83 (↓79 to ↓ 87)	↓ 86 (↓80 to ↓ 90)
Methadone	Stable maintenance 35–100 mg daily	600 mg qd × 14–21 days	11	↓ 45 (↓ 25 to ↓ 59)	↓ 52 (↓ 33 to ↓ 66)	NA

(Table continued on next page)

Tenofovir Disoproxil Fumarate: Tenofovir and tenofovir DF administered in toxicology studies to rats, dogs and monkeys at exposures (based on AUCs) greater than or equal to 6-fold those observed in humans caused bone toxicity. In monkeys the bone toxicity was diagnosed as osteomalacia. Osteomalacia observed in monkeys appeared to be reversible upon dose reduction or discontinuation of tenofovir. In rats and dogs, the bone toxicity manifested as reduced bone mineral density. The mechanism(s) underlying bone toxicity is unknown.

Evidence of renal toxicity was noted in 4 animal species administered tenofovir and tenofovir DF. Increases in serum creatinine, BUN, glycosuria, proteinuria, phosphaturia and/or calciuria and decreases in serum phosphate were observed to varying degrees in these animals. These toxicities were noted at exposures (based on AUCs) 2- to 20-times higher than those observed in humans. The relationship of the renal abnormalities, particularly the phosphaturia, to the bone toxicity is not known.

14 CLINICAL STUDIES

Clinical Study 934 supports the use of ATRIPLA tablets in antiretroviral treatment-naive HIV-1 infected patients. Additional data in support of the use of ATRIPLA in treatment- naive patients can be found in the prescribing information for VIREAD.

Clinical Study 073 provides clinical experience in subjects with stable, virologic suppression and no history of virologic failure who switched from their current regimen to ATRIPLA.

In antiretroviral treatment-experienced patients, the use of ATRIPLA tablets may be considered for patients with HIV-1 strains that are expected to be susceptible to the components of ATRIPLA as assessed by treatment history or by genotypic or phenotypic testing *[See Clinical Pharmacology (12.4)]*.

Study 934: Data through 144 weeks are reported for Study 934, a randomized, open-label, active-controlled multicenter trial comparing emtricitabine + tenofovir DF administered in combination with efavirenz versus zidovudine/lamivudine fixed-dose combination administered in combination with efavirenz in 511 antiretroviral-naive subjects. From Weeks 96 to 144 of the trial, subjects received emtricitabine/tenofovir DF fixed-dose combination with efavirenz in place of emtricitabine + tenofovir DF with efavirenz. Subjects had a mean age of 38 years (range 18–80), 86% were male, 59% were Caucasian and 23% were Black. The mean baseline $CD4^+$ cell count was 245 cells/mm^3 (range 2–1191) and median baseline plasma HIV-1 RNA was 5.01 log_{10} copies/mL (range 3.56–6.54). Subjects were stratified by baseline $CD4^+$ cell count (< or ≥200 cells/mm^3) and 41% had $CD4^+$ cell counts <200 cells/mm^3. Fifty-one percent (51%) of subjects had baseline viral loads >100,000 copies/mL. Treatment outcomes through 48 and 144 weeks for those subjects who did not have efavirenz resistance at baseline (N=487) are presented in Table 9.

[See table 9 at top of page 832]

Through Week 48, 84% and 73% of subjects in the emtricitabine + tenofovir DF group and the zidovudine/lamivudine group, respectively, achieved and maintained HIV-1 RNA <400 copies/mL (71% and 58% through Week 144). The difference in the proportion of subjects who achieved and maintained HIV-1 RNA <400 copies/mL through 48 weeks largely results from the higher number of discontinuations due to adverse events and other reasons in the zidovudine/lamivudine group in this open-label trial. In addition, 80% and 70% of subjects in the emtricitabine + tenofovir DF group and the zidovudine/lamivudine group, respectively, achieved and maintained HIV-1 RNA <50 copies/mL through Week 48 (64% and 56% through Week 144). The mean increase from baseline in $CD4^+$ cell count was 190 cells/mm^3 in the emtricitabine + tenofovir DF group and 158 cells/mm^3 in the zidovudine/lamivudine group at Week 48 (312 and 271 cells/mm^3 at Week 144).

Through 48 weeks, 7 subjects in the emtricitabine + tenofovir DF group and 5 subjects in the zidovudine/lamivudine group experienced a new CDC Class C event (10 and 6 subjects through 144 weeks).

Study 073: Study 073 was a 48-week open-label, randomized clinical trial in subjects with stable virologic suppression on combination antiretroviral therapy consisting of at least two nucleoside reverse transcriptase inhibitors (NRTIs) administered in combination with a protease inhibitor (with or without ritonavir) or a non-nucleoside reverse transcriptase inhibitor (NNRTI).

To be enrolled, subjects were to have HIV-1 RNA <200 copies/mL for at least 12 weeks on their current regimen prior to trial entry with no known HIV-1 substitutions conferring resistance to the components of ATRIPLA and no history of virologic failure.

The trial compared the efficacy of switching to ATRIPLA or staying on the baseline antiretroviral regimen (SBR). Subjects were randomized in a 2:1 ratio to switch to ATRIPLA (N=203) or stay on SBR (N=97). Subjects had a mean age of 43 years (range 22–73 years), 88% were male, 68% were white, 29% were Black or African-American, and 3% were of other races. At baseline, median $CD4^+$ cell count was 516 cells/mm^3 and 96% had HIV-1 RNA <50 copies/mL. The median time since onset of antiretroviral therapy was 3 years and 88% of subjects were receiving their first antiretroviral regimen at trial enrollment.

At Week 48, 89% and 87% of subjects who switched to ATRIPLA maintained HIV RNA <200 copies/mL and <50 copies/mL, respectively, compared to 88% and 85% who remained on SBR; this difference was not statistically significant. No changes in $CD4^+$ cell counts from baseline to Week 48 were observed in either treatment arm.

Table 6 *(cont.)* Drug Interactions: Changes in Pharmacokinetic Parameters for Coadministered Drug in the Presence of Efavirenz

Coadministered Drug	Dose of Coadministered Drug (mg)	Efavirenz Dose (mg)	N	Mean % Change of Coadministered Drug Pharmacokinetic Parameters* (90% CI)		
				C_{max}	AUC	C_{min}
Bupropion	150 mg single dose (sustained-release)	600 mg qd × 14 days	13	↓ 34 (↓21 to ↓47)	↓ 55 (↓48 to ↓62)	NA
Hydroxybupropion				↑ 50 (↑ 20 to ↑ 80)	↔	NA
Sertraline	50 mg qd × 14 days	600 mg qd × 14 days	13	↓ 29 (↓ 15 to ↓ 40)	↓ 39 (↓ 27 to ↓ 50)	↓ 46 (↓ 31 to ↓ 58)
Voriconazole	400 mg po q12h × 1 day then 200 mg po q12h × 8 days	400 mg qd × 9 days	NA	↓ 61[à]	↓ 77[à]	NA
	300 mg po q12h days 2–7	300 mg qd × 7 days	NA	↓ 36[è] (↓ 21 to ↓ 49)	↓ 55[è] (↓ 45 to ↓ 62)	NA
	400 mg po q12h days 2–7	300 mg qd × 7 days	NA	↑ 23[è] (↓ 1 to ↑ 53)	↓ 7[è] (↓ 23 to ↑ 13)	NA

NA = not available
* Increase = ↑; Decrease = ↓; No Effect = ↔
† Compared with atazanavir 400 mg qd alone.
‡ Comparator dose of indinavir was 800 mg q8h × 10 days.
§ Parallel-group design; N for efavirenz + lopinavir/ritonavir, N for lopinavir/ritonavir alone.
¶ Values are for lopinavir. The pharmacokinetics of ritonavir 100 mg q12h are unaffected by concurrent efavirenz.
\# 95% CI
Þ Soft Gelatin Capsule
ß Not available because of insufficient data.
à 90% CI not available
è Relative to steady-state administration of voriconazole (400 mg for 1 day, then 200 mg po q12h for 2 days).

Table 7 Drug Interactions: Changes in Pharmacokinetic Parameters for Tenofovir in the Presence of the Coadministered Drug*,†

Coadministered Drug	Dose of Coadministered Drug (mg)	N	Mean % Change of Tenofovir Pharmacokinetic Parameters‡ (90% CI)		
			C_{max}	AUC	C_{min}
Atazanavir§	400 once daily × 14 days	33	↑ 14 (↑ 8 to ↑ 20)	↑ 24 (↑ 21 to ↑ 28)	↑ 22 (↑ 15 to ↑ 30)
Didanosine¶	250 or 400 once daily × 7 days	14	↔	↔	↔
Lopinavir/ ritonavir	400/100 twice daily × 14 days	24	↔	↑ 32 (↑ 25 to ↑ 38)	↑ 51 (↑ 37 to ↑ 66)

* All interaction trials conducted in healthy volunteers.
† Subjects received tenofovir DF 300 mg once daily.
‡ Increase = ↑; Decrease = ↓; No Effect = ↔
§ Reyataz Prescribing Information
¶ Subjects received didanosine buffered tablets.

16 HOW SUPPLIED/STORAGE AND HANDLING

ATRIPLA tablets are pink, capsule-shaped, film-coated, debossed with "123" on one side and plain-faced on the other side. Each bottle contains 30 tablets (NDC 15584-0101-1) and silica gel desiccant, and is closed with a child-resistant closure.

Store at 25 °C (77 °F); excursions permitted to 15–30 °C (59–86 °F) *[See USP Controlled Room Temperature]*.
- Keep container tightly closed.
- Dispense only in original container.
- Do not use if seal over bottle opening is broken or missing.

17 PATIENT COUNSELING INFORMATION

See FDA-approved patient labeling (Patient Information)

17.1 Drug Interactions

A statement to patients and healthcare providers is included on the product's bottle labels: *ALERT: Find out about medicines that should NOT be taken with ATRIPLA.* ATRIPLA may interact with some drugs; therefore, patients should be advised to report to their doctor the use of any other prescription, nonprescription medication, or herbal products, particularly St. John's wort.

17.2 General Information for Patients

Patients should be advised that:
- ATRIPLA is not a cure for HIV-1 infection and patients may continue to experience illnesses associated with HIV-1 infection, including opportunistic infections. Patients should remain under the care of a physician when using ATRIPLA.
- Patients should avoid doing things that can spread HIV-1 to others.
  - **Do not share needles or other injection equipment.**
  - **Do not share personal items that can have blood or body fluids on them, like toothbrushes and razor blades.**
  - **Do not have any kind of sex without protection.** Always practice safe sex by using a latex or polyurethane condom to lower the chance of sexual contact with semen, vaginal secretions, or blood.
  - **Do not breastfeed.** Some of the medicines in ATRIPLA can be passed to your baby in your breast milk. We do not know whether it could harm your baby. Also, mothers with HIV-1 should not breastfeed because HIV-1 can be passed to the baby in the breast milk.
- The long-term effects of ATRIPLA are unknown.
- Redistribution or accumulation of body fat may occur in patients receiving antiretroviral therapy and that the cause and long-term health effects of these conditions are not known.
- ATRIPLA should not be coadministered with COMPLERA, EMTRIVA, STRIBILD, TRUVADA, or VIREAD; or drugs containing lamivudine, including Combivir, Epivir, Epivir-HBV, Epzicom, or Trizivir. SUSTIVA should not be coadministered with ATRIPLA unless needed for dose adjustment *[See Warnings and Precautions (5.4)]*.
- ATRIPLA should not be administered with HEPSERA *[See Warnings and Precautions (5.2)]*.

17.3 Lactic Acidosis/Severe Hepatomegaly with Steatosis

Patients should be informed that lactic acidosis and severe hepatomegaly with steatosis, including fatal cases, have been reported. Treatment will be suspended in any patients who develop clinical symptoms suggestive of lactic acidosis or pronounced hepatotoxicity (including nausea, vomiting, unusual or unexpected stomach discomfort, and weakness) *[See Warnings and Precautions (5.1)]*.

17.4 Patients Coinfected with HIV-1 and HBV

Patients with HIV-1 should be tested for hepatitis B virus (HBV) before initiating antiretroviral therapy.

Patients should be advised that severe acute exacerbations of hepatitis B have been reported in patients who are coinfected with HBV and HIV-1 and have discontinued EMTRIVA (emtricitabine) or VIREAD (tenofovir DF), which are components of ATRIPLA.

17.5 New Onset or Worsening Renal Impairment

Renal impairment, including cases of acute renal failure and Fanconi syndrome, has been reported. ATRIPLA should be avoided with concurrent or recent use of a nephrotoxic agent *[See Warnings and Precautions (5.7)]*.

17.6 Decreases in Bone Mineral Density

Patients should be informed that decreases in bone mineral density have been observed with the use of tenofovir DF. Bone mineral density monitoring may be performed in patients who have a history of pathologic bone fracture or other risk factors for osteoporosis or bone loss *[See Warnings and Precautions (5.11)]*.

17.7 Dosing Instructions

Patients should be advised to take ATRIPLA orally on an empty stomach and that it is important to take ATRIPLA on a regular dosing schedule to avoid missing doses.

17.8 Nervous System Symptoms

Patients should be informed that central nervous system symptoms (NSS) including dizziness, insomnia, impaired concentration, drowsiness, and abnormal dreams are commonly reported during the first weeks of therapy with efavirenz. Dosing at bedtime may improve the tolerability of these symptoms, which are likely to improve with continued therapy. Patients should be alerted to the potential for additive effects when ATRIPLA is used concomitantly with alcohol or psychoactive drugs. Patients should be instructed that if they experience NSS they should avoid potentially hazardous tasks such as driving or operating machinery *[See Warnings and Precautions (5.6) and Dosage and Administration (2)]*.

17.9 Psychiatric Symptoms

Patients should be informed that serious psychiatric symptoms including severe depression, suicide attempts, aggressive behavior, delusions, paranoia, and psychosis-like symptoms have been reported in patients receiving efavirenz. If they experience severe psychiatric adverse experiences they should seek immediate medical evaluation. Patients should be advised to inform their physician of any history of mental illness or substance abuse *[See Warnings and Precautions (5.5)]*.

17.10 Rash

Patients should be informed that a common side effect is rash. Rashes usually go away without any change in treatment. However, since rash may be serious, patients should be advised to contact their physician promptly if rash occurs.

17.11 Reproductive Risk Potential

Women receiving ATRIPLA should be instructed to avoid pregnancy *[See Warnings and Precautions (5.8)]*. A reliable form of barrier contraception must always be used in combination with other methods of contraception, including oral or other hormonal contraception. Because of the long half-life of efavirenz, use of adequate contraceptive measures for 12 weeks after discontinuation of ATRIPLA is recommended. Women should be advised to notify their physician if they become pregnant or plan to become pregnant while taking ATRIPLA. If this drug is used during the first trimester of pregnancy, or if the patient becomes pregnant while taking this drug, she should be apprised of the potential harm to the fetus.

Patient Information

ATRIPLA® (uh TRIP luh) Tablets

ALERT: Find out about medicines that should NOT be taken with ATRIPLA.

Please also read the section **"MEDICINES YOU SHOULD NOT TAKE WITH ATRIPLA."**

Table 8 Drug Interactions: Changes in Pharmacokinetic Parameters for Coadministered Drug in the Presence of Tenofovir Disoproxil Fumarate*,†

Coadministered Drug	Dose of Coadministered Drug (mg)	N	Mean % Change of Coadministered Drug Pharmacokinetic Parameters‡ (90% CI)		
			C_{max}	AUC	C_{min}
Atazanavir[§]	400 once daily × 14 days	34	$\downarrow$ 21 ($\downarrow$ 27 to $\downarrow$ 14)	$\downarrow$ 25 ($\downarrow$ 30 to $\downarrow$ 19)	$\downarrow$ 40 ($\downarrow$ 48 to $\downarrow$ 32)
	Atazanavir/ritonavir 300/100 once daily × 42 days	10	$\downarrow$ 28 ($\downarrow$ 50 to $\uparrow$ 5)	$\downarrow$ 25[¶] ($\downarrow$ 42 to $\downarrow$ 3)	$\downarrow$ 23[¶] ($\downarrow$ 46 to $\uparrow$ 10)
Didanosine[#]	250 once, simultaneously with tenofovir DF and a light meal[Þ]	33	$\downarrow$ 20 ($\downarrow$ 32 to $\downarrow$ 7)[ß]	$\leftrightarrow$[ß]	NA
Lopinavir	Lopinavir/ritonavir 400/100 twice daily × 14 days	24	$\leftrightarrow$	$\leftrightarrow$	$\leftrightarrow$
Ritonavir	Lopinavir/ritonavir 400/100 twice daily × 14 days	24	$\leftrightarrow$	$\leftrightarrow$	$\leftrightarrow$

* All interaction trials conducted in healthy volunteers.
† Subjects received tenofovir DF 300 mg once daily.
‡ Increase = $\uparrow$; Decrease = $\downarrow$; No Effect = $\leftrightarrow$
§ Reyataz Prescribing Information.
¶ In HIV-infected patients, addition of tenofovir DF to atazanavir 300 mg plus ritonavir 100 mg, resulted in AUC and C_{min} values of atazanavir that were 2.3- and 4-fold higher than the respective values observed for atazanavir 400 mg when given alone.
\# Videx EC Prescribing Information. Subjects received didanosine enteric-coated capsules.
Þ 373 kcal, 8.2 g fat.
ß Compared with didanosine (enteric-coated) 400 mg administered alone under fasting conditions.

Table 9 Outcomes of Randomized Treatment at Weeks 48 and 144 (Study 934)

Outcomes	At Week 48		At Week 144	
	FTC + TDF + EFV (N=244)	AZT/3TC + EFV (N=243)	FTC + TDF + EFV (N=227)*	AZT/3TC + EFV (N=229)*
Responder[†]	84%	73%	71%	58%
Virologic failure[‡]	2%	4%	3%	6%
Rebound	1%	3%	2%	5%
Never suppressed	0%	0%	0%	0%
Change in antiretroviral regimen	1%	1%	1%	1%
Death	<1%	1%	1%	1%
Discontinued due to adverse event	4%	9%	5%	12%
Discontinued for other reasons[§]	10%	14%	20%	22%

* Subjects who were responders at Week 48 or Week 96 (HIV-1 RNA <400 copies/mL) but did not consent to continue trial after Week 48 or Week 96 were excluded from analysis.
† Subjects achieved and maintained confirmed HIV-1 RNA <400 copies/mL through Weeks 48 and 144.
‡ Includes confirmed viral rebound and failure to achieve confirmed HIV-1 RNA <400 copies/mL through Weeks 48 and 144.
§ Includes lost to follow-up, patient withdrawal, noncompliance, protocol violation and other reasons.

Generic name: efavirenz, emtricitabine and tenofovir disoproxil fumarate (eh FAH vih renz, em tri SIT uh bean and te NOE' fo veer dye soe PROX il FYOU mar ate)

Read the Patient Information that comes with ATRIPLA before you start taking it and each time you get a refill since there may be new information. This information does not take the place of talking to your healthcare provider about your medical condition or treatment. You should stay under a healthcare provider's care when taking ATRIPLA. **Do not change or stop your medicine without first talking with your healthcare provider.** Talk to your healthcare provider or pharmacist if you have any questions about ATRIPLA.

What is the most important information I should know about ATRIPLA?

- **Some people who have taken medicine like ATRIPLA (which contains nucleoside analogs) have developed a serious condition called lactic acidosis** (build up of an acid in the blood). Lactic acidosis can be a medical emergency and may need to be treated in the hospital. **Call your healthcare provider right away if you get the following signs or symptoms of lactic acidosis:**
  - You feel very weak or tired.
  - You have unusual (not normal) muscle pain.
  - You have trouble breathing.
  - You have stomach pain with nausea and vomiting.
  - You feel cold, especially in your arms and legs.
  - You feel dizzy or lightheaded.
  - You have a fast or irregular heartbeat.
- **Some people who have taken medicines like ATRIPLA have developed serious liver problems called hepatotoxicity**, with liver enlargement (hepatomegaly) and fat in the liver (steatosis). **Call your healthcare provider right away if you get the following signs or symptoms of liver problems:**
  - Your skin or the white part of your eyes turns yellow (jaundice).
  - Your urine turns dark.
  - Your bowel movements (stools) turn light in color.
  - You don't feel like eating food for several days or longer.
  - You feel sick to your stomach (nausea).
  - You have lower stomach area (abdominal) pain.
- **You may be more likely to get lactic acidosis or liver problems** if you are female, very overweight (obese), or have been taking nucleoside analog-containing medicines, like ATRIPLA, for a long time.
- **If you also have hepatitis B virus (HBV) infection and you stop taking ATRIPLA, you may get a "flare-up" of your hepatitis. A "flare-up" is when the disease suddenly returns in a worse way than before.** Patients with HBV who stop taking ATRIPLA need close medical follow-up for several months, including medical exams and blood tests to check for hepatitis that could be getting worse. ATRIPLA is not approved for the treatment of HBV, so you must discuss your HBV therapy with your healthcare provider.

What is ATRIPLA?

ATRIPLA contains 3 medicines, SUSTIVA® (efavirenz), EMTRIVA® (emtricitabine) and VIREAD® (tenofovir disoproxil fumarate also called tenofovir DF) combined in one pill. EMTRIVA and VIREAD are HIV-1 (human immunodeficiency virus) nucleoside analog reverse transcriptase inhibitors (NRTIs) and SUSTIVA is an HIV-1 non-nucleoside analog reverse transcriptase inhibitor (NNRTI). VIREAD and EMTRIVA are the components of TRUVADA®. ATRIPLA can be used alone as a complete regimen, or in combination with other anti-HIV-1 medicines to treat people with HIV-1 infection. ATRIPLA is for adults and children 12 years of age and older who weigh at least 40 kg (at least 88 lbs). ATRIPLA is not recommended for children younger than 12 years of age. ATRIPLA has not been studied in adults over 65 years of age.

HIV infection destroys CD4⁺ T cells, which are important to the immune system. The immune system helps fight infection. After a large number of T cells are destroyed, acquired immune deficiency syndrome (AIDS) develops.

ATRIPLA helps block HIV-1 reverse transcriptase, a viral chemical in your body (enzyme) that is needed for HIV-1 to multiply. ATRIPLA lowers the amount of HIV-1 in the blood (viral load). ATRIPLA may also help to increase the number of T cells (CD4⁺ cells), allowing your immune system to improve. Lowering the amount of HIV-1 in the blood lowers the chance of death or infections that happen when your immune system is weak (opportunistic infections).

Does ATRIPLA cure HIV-1 or AIDS?

ATRIPLA does not cure HIV-1 infection or AIDS and you may continue to experience illnesses associated with HIV-1 infection, including opportunistic infections. You should remain under the care of a doctor when using ATRIPLA.

Who should not take ATRIPLA?

Together with your healthcare provider, you need to decide whether ATRIPLA is right for you.

Do not take ATRIPLA if you are allergic to ATRIPLA or any of its ingredients. The active ingredients of ATRIPLA are efavirenz, emtricitabine, and tenofovir DF. See the end of this leaflet for a complete list of ingredients.

What should I tell my healthcare provider before taking ATRIPLA?

Tell your healthcare provider if you:

- **Are pregnant or planning to become pregnant** (see "What should I avoid while taking ATRIPLA?").
- **Are breastfeeding** (see "What should I avoid while taking ATRIPLA?").
- **Have kidney problems or are undergoing kidney dialysis treatment.**
- **Have bone problems.**
- **Have liver problems, including hepatitis B virus infection.** Your healthcare provider may want to do tests to check your liver while you take ATRIPLA or may switch you to another medicine.
- **Have ever had mental illness or are using drugs or alcohol.**
- **Have ever had seizures or are taking medicine for seizures.**

What important information should I know about taking other medicines with ATRIPLA?

ATRIPLA may change the effect of other medicines, including the ones for HIV-1, and may cause serious side effects. Your healthcare provider may change your other medicines or change their doses. Other medicines, including herbal products, may affect ATRIPLA. For this reason, **it is very important to** let all your healthcare providers and pharmacists know what medications, herbal supplements, or vitamins you are taking.

MEDICINES YOU SHOULD NOT TAKE WITH ATRIPLA

- The following medicines may cause serious and life-threatening side effects when taken with ATRIPLA. You should not take any of these medicines while taking ATRIPLA: Vascor (bepridil), Propulsid (cisapride), Versed (midazolam), Orap (pimozide), Halcion (triazolam), ergot medications (for example, Wigraine and Cafergot).
- ATRIPLA also should not be used with Combivir (lamivudine/zidovudine), COMPLERA®, EMTRIVA, Epivir, Epivir-HBV (lamivudine), Epzicom (abacavir sulfate/lamivudine), STRIBILD®, Trizivir (abacavir sulfate/lamivudine/zidovudine), TRUVADA, or VIREAD. ATRIPLA also should not be used with SUSTIVA unless recommended by your healthcare provider.

- Vfend (voriconazole) should not be taken with ATRIPLA since it may lose its effect or may increase the chance of having side effects from ATRIPLA.
- **Do not take St. John's wort (*Hypericum perforatum*), or products containing St. John's wort with ATRIPLA.** St. John's wort is an herbal product sold as a dietary supplement. Talk with your healthcare provider if you are taking or are planning to take St. John's wort. Taking St. John's wort may decrease ATRIPLA levels and lead to increased viral load and possible resistance to ATRIPLA or cross-resistance to other anti-HIV-1 drugs.
- ATRIPLA should not be used with HEPSERA® (adefovir dipivoxil).

It is also important to tell your healthcare provider if you are taking any of the following:

- Fortovase, Invirase (saquinavir), Biaxin (clarithromycin), Noxafil (posaconazole), Sporanox (itraconazole), or Victrelis (boceprevir); **these medicines may need to be replaced with another medicine when taken with ATRIPLA.**
- Calcium channel blockers such as Cardizem or Tiazac (diltiazem), Covera HS or Isoptin (verapamil) and others; Crixivan (indinavir), Selzentry (maraviroc); the immunosuppressant medicines cyclosporine (Gengraf, Neoral, Sandimmune, and others), Prograf (tacrolimus), or Rapamune (sirolimus); Methadone; Mycobutin (rifabutin); Rifampin; cholesterol-lowering medicines such as Lipitor (atorvastatin), Pravachol (pravastatin sodium), and Zocor (simvastatin); or the anti-depressant medications bupropion (Wellbutrin, Wellbutrin SR, Wellbutrin XL, and Zyban) or Zoloft (sertraline); **dose changes may be needed when these drugs are taken with ATRIPLA.**
- Videx, Videx EC (didanosine); tenofovir DF (a component of ATRIPLA) may increase the amount of didanosine in your blood, which could result in more side effects. **You may need to be monitored more carefully** if you are taking ATRIPLA and didanosine together. Also, the dose of didanosine may need to be changed.
- Reyataz (atazanavir sulfate) or Kaletra (lopinavir/ritonavir); these medicines may increase the amount of tenofovir DF (a component of ATRIPLA) in your blood, which could result in more side effects. Reyataz is not recommended with ATRIPLA. **You may need to be monitored more carefully** if you are taking ATRIPLA and Kaletra together. Also, the dose of Kaletra may need to be changed.
- Medicine for seizures [for example, Dilantin (phenytoin), Tegretol (carbamazepine), or phenobarbital]; your healthcare provider may want to switch you to another medicine or check drug levels in your blood from time to time.

These are not all the medicines that may cause problems if you take ATRIPLA. Be sure to tell your healthcare provider about all medicines that you take.

Keep a complete list of all the prescription and nonprescription medicines as well as any herbal remedies that you are taking, how much you take, and how often you take them. Make a new list when medicines or herbal remedies are added or stopped, or if the dose changes. Give copies of this list to all of your healthcare providers and pharmacists **every** time you visit your healthcare provider or fill a prescription. This will give your healthcare provider a complete picture of the medicines you use. Then he or she can decide the best approach for your situation.

How should I take ATRIPLA?

- Take the exact amount of ATRIPLA your healthcare provider prescribes. Never change the dose on your own. Do not stop this medicine unless your healthcare provider tells you to stop.
- You should take ATRIPLA on an empty stomach.
- Swallow ATRIPLA with water.
- Taking ATRIPLA at bedtime may make some side effects less bothersome.
- Do not miss a dose of ATRIPLA. If you forget to take ATRIPLA, take the missed dose right away, unless it is almost time for your next dose. Do not double the next dose. Carry on with your regular dosing schedule. If you need help in planning the best times to take your medicine, ask your healthcare provider or pharmacist.
- If you believe you took more than the prescribed amount of ATRIPLA, contact your local poison control center or emergency room right away.
- Tell your healthcare provider if you start any new medicine or change how you take old ones. Your doses may need adjustment.
- When your ATRIPLA supply starts to run low, get more from your healthcare provider or pharmacy. This is very important because the amount of virus in your blood may increase if the medicine is stopped for even a short time. The virus may develop resistance to ATRIPLA and become harder to treat.
- Your healthcare provider may want to do blood tests to check for certain side effects while you take ATRIPLA.

What should I avoid while taking ATRIPLA?

- **Women should not become pregnant while taking ATRIPLA and for 12 weeks after stopping it.** Serious birth defects have been seen in the babies of animals and women treated with efavirenz (a component of ATRIPLA) during pregnancy. It is not known whether efavirenz caused these defects. **Tell your healthcare provider right away if you are pregnant.** Also talk with your healthcare provider if you want to become pregnant.
- Women should not rely only on hormone-based birth control, such as pills, injections, or implants, because ATRIPLA may make these contraceptives ineffective. Women must use a reliable form of barrier contraception, such as a condom or diaphragm, even if they also use other methods of birth control. Efavirenz, a component of ATRIPLA, may remain in your blood for a time after therapy is stopped. Therefore, you should continue to use contraceptive measures for 12 weeks after you stop taking ATRIPLA.
- **Do not breastfeed if you are taking ATRIPLA.** Some of the medicines in ATRIPLA can be passed to your baby in your breast milk. We do not know whether it could harm your baby. Also, mothers with HIV-1 should not breastfeed because HIV-1 can be passed to the baby in the breast milk. Talk with your healthcare provider if you are breastfeeding. You should stop breastfeeding or may need to use a different medicine.
- Taking ATRIPLA with alcohol or other medicines causing similar side effects as ATRIPLA, such as drowsiness, may increase those side effects.
- Do not take any other medicines, including prescription and nonprescription medicines and herbal products, without checking with your healthcare provider.
- Avoid doing things that can spread HIV-1 to others.
  - **Do not share needles or other injection equipment.**
  - **Do not share personal items that can have blood or body fluids on them, like toothbrushes and razor blades.**
  - **Do not have any kind of sex without protection.** Always practice safe sex by using a latex or polyurethane condom to lower the chance of sexual contact with semen, vaginal secretions, or blood.

What are the possible side effects of ATRIPLA?

ATRIPLA may cause the following serious side effects:

- **Lactic acidosis** (buildup of an acid in the blood). Lactic acidosis can be a medical emergency and may need to be treated in the hospital. **Call your healthcare provider right away if you get signs of lactic acidosis.** (See "What is the most important information I should know about ATRIPLA?")
- **Serious liver problems (hepatotoxicity)**, with liver enlargement (hepatomegaly) and fat in the liver (steatosis). Call your healthcare provider right away if you get any signs of liver problems. (See "What is the most important information I should know about ATRIPLA?")
- **"Flare-ups" of hepatitis B virus (HBV) infection**, in which the disease suddenly returns in a worse way than before, can occur if you have HBV and you stop taking ATRIPLA. Your healthcare provider will monitor your condition for several months after stopping ATRIPLA if you have both HIV-1 and HBV infection and may recommend treatment for your HBV. ATRIPLA is not approved for the treatment of hepatitis B virus infection. If you have advanced liver disease and stop treatment with ATRIPLA, the "flare-up" of hepatitis B may cause your liver function to decline.
- **Serious psychiatric problems.** A small number of patients may experience severe depression, strange thoughts, or angry behavior while taking ATRIPLA. Some patients have thoughts of suicide and a few have actually committed suicide. These problems may occur more often in patients who have had mental illness. Contact your healthcare provider right away if you think you are having these psychiatric symptoms, so your healthcare provider can decide if you should continue to take ATRIPLA.
- **Kidney problems** (including decline or failure of kidney function). If you have had kidney problems in the past or take other medicines that can cause kidney problems, your healthcare provider should do regular blood tests to check your kidneys. Symptoms that may be related to kidney problems include a high volume of urine, thirst, muscle pain, and muscle weakness.
- **Other serious liver problems.** Some patients have experienced serious liver problems including liver failure resulting in transplantation or death. Most of these serious side effects occurred in patients with a chronic liver disease such as hepatitis infection, but there have also been a few reports in patients without any existing liver disease.
- **Changes in bone mineral density (thinning bones).** Laboratory tests show changes in the bones of patients treated with tenofovir DF, a component of ATRIPLA. Some HIV patients treated with tenofovir DF developed thinning of the bones (osteopenia) which could lead to fractures. If you have had bone problems in the past, your healthcare provider may need to do tests to check your bone mineral density or may prescribe medicines to help your bone mineral density. Additionally, bone pain and softening of the bone (which may contribute to fractures) may occur as a consequence of kidney problems.

Common side effects:

Patients may have dizziness, headache, trouble sleeping, drowsiness, trouble concentrating, and/or unusual dreams during treatment with ATRIPLA. These side effects may be reduced if you take ATRIPLA at bedtime on an empty stomach. They also tend to go away after you have taken the medicine for a few weeks. If you have these common side effects, such as dizziness, it does not mean that you will also have serious psychiatric problems, such as severe depression, strange thoughts, or angry behavior. Tell your healthcare provider right away if any of these side effects continue or if they bother you. It is possible that these symptoms may be more severe if ATRIPLA is used with alcohol or mood altering (street) drugs.

If you are dizzy, have trouble concentrating, or are drowsy, avoid activities that may be dangerous, such as driving or operating machinery.

Rash may be common. Rashes usually go away without any change in treatment. In a small number of patients, rash may be serious. If you develop a rash, call your healthcare provider right away. **Rash may be a serious problem in some children.** Tell your child's healthcare provider right away if you notice rash or any other side effects while your child is taking ATRIPLA.

Other common side effects include tiredness, upset stomach, vomiting, gas, and diarrhea.

Other possible side effects with ATRIPLA:

- Changes in body fat. Changes in body fat develop in some patients taking anti HIV-1 medicine. These changes may include an increased amount of fat in the upper back and neck ("buffalo hump"), in the breasts, and around the trunk. Loss of fat from the legs, arms, and face may also happen. The cause and long-term health effects of these fat changes are not known.
- Skin discoloration (small spots or freckles) may also happen with ATRIPLA.
- In some patients with advanced HIV infection (AIDS), signs and symptoms of inflammation from previous infections may occur soon after anti-HIV treatment is started. It is believed that these symptoms are due to an improvement in the body's immune response, enabling the body to fight infections that may have been present with no obvious symptoms. If you notice any symptoms of infection, please inform your doctor immediately.
- Additional side effects are inflammation of the pancreas, allergic reaction (including swelling of the face, lips, tongue, or throat), shortness of breath, pain, stomach pain, weakness and indigestion.

Tell your healthcare provider or pharmacist if you notice any side effects while taking ATRIPLA.

Contact your healthcare provider before stopping ATRIPLA because of side effects or for any other reason.

This is not a complete list of side effects possible with ATRIPLA. Ask your healthcare provider or pharmacist for a more complete list of side effects of ATRIPLA and all the medicines you will take.

How do I store ATRIPLA?

- **Keep ATRIPLA and all other medicines out of reach of children.**
- Store ATRIPLA at room temperature 77 °F (25 °C).
- Keep ATRIPLA in its original container and keep the container tightly closed.
- Do not keep medicine that is out of date or that you no longer need. If you throw any medicines away make sure that children will not find them.

General information about ATRIPLA:

Medicines are sometimes prescribed for conditions that are not mentioned in patient information leaflets. Do not use ATRIPLA for a condition for which it was not prescribed. Do not give ATRIPLA to other people, even if they have the same symptoms you have. It may harm them.

This leaflet summarizes the most important information about ATRIPLA. If you would like more information, talk with your healthcare provider. You can ask your healthcare provider or pharmacist for information about ATRIPLA that is written for health professionals.

Do not use ATRIPLA if the seal over bottle opening is broken or missing.

What are the ingredients of ATRIPLA?

Active Ingredients: efavirenz, emtricitabine, and tenofovir disoproxil fumarate

Inactive Ingredients: croscarmellose sodium, hydroxypropyl cellulose, microcrystalline cellulose, magnesium stearate, sodium lauryl sulfate. The film coating contains black iron oxide, polyethylene glycol, polyvinyl alcohol, red iron oxide, talc, and titanium dioxide.

June 2013

ATRIPLA is a trademark of Bristol-Myers Squibb & Gilead Sciences, LLC. COMPLERA, EMTRIVA, HEPSERA, STRIBILD, TRUVADA, and VIREAD are trademarks of Gilead Sciences, Inc., or its related companies. SUSTIVA is a trademark of Bristol-Myers Squibb Pharma Company. Reyataz and Videx are trademarks of Bristol-Myers Squibb

Company. Pravachol is a trademark of ER Squibb & Sons, LLC. Other brands listed are the trademarks of their respective owners.
21-937-GS-012

Ferring Pharmaceuticals Inc.
4 GATEHALL DRIVE
3RD FLOOR
PARSIPPANY, NJ 07054

Phone: (973)796-1600
Fax: (973)796-1616

PREPOPIK ℞
(sodium picosulfate, magnesium oxide, and anhydrous citric acid)
for oral solution

HIGHLIGHTS OF PRESCRIBING INFORMATION
These highlights do not include all the information needed to use PREPOPIK safely and effectively. See full prescribing information for PREPOPIK.
PREPOPIK (sodium picosulfate, magnesium oxide, and anhydrous citric acid) for oral solution
Initial U.S. Approval: 2012

INDICATIONS AND USAGE

PREPOPIK is a combination of sodium picosulfate, a stimulant laxative, and magnesium oxide and anhydrous citric acid which form magnesium citrate, an osmotic laxative, indicated for cleansing of the colon as a preparation for colonoscopy in adults (1)

DOSAGE AND ADMINISTRATION

- PREPOPIK, supplied as a powder, must be reconstituted with cold water right before its use (2.1, 2.2).
- Two dosing regimens, each requires two separate dosing times (2.1)
- "Split Dose" method is preferred method (2.3)
  - First dose: during evening before the colonoscopy
  - Second dose: next day, during the morning prior to the colonoscopy
- "Day Before" method is alternative method if "Split Dose" is not appropriate (2.4)
  - First dose: during afternoon or early evening before the colonoscopy
  - Second dose: 6 hours later during evening before colonoscopy
- Additional clear liquids (no solid food or milk) must be consumed after every dose in both dosing regimens (2.3, 2.4).

DOSAGE FORMS AND STRENGTHS

For oral solution: each of 2 packets contains 16.1 g of powder: 10 mg sodium picosulfate, 3.5 g magnesium oxide, and 12 g anhydrous citric acid (3)

CONTRAINDICATIONS

- Patients with severely reduced renal function (creatinine clearance less than 30 mL/minute (4)
- Gastrointestinal (GI) obstruction or ileus (4)
- Bowel perforation (4)
- Toxic colitis or toxic megacolon (4)
- Gastric retention (4)

WARNINGS AND PRECAUTIONS

- *Risk of fluid and electrolyte abnormalities, arrhythmia, seizures, and renal impairment:* Encourage adequate hydration, assess concurrent medications, and consider laboratory assessments prior to and after use (5.1, 5.2, 5.3, 5.4)
- *Risks in patients with renal insufficiency or patients taking concomitant medications that affect renal function:* Use caution, ensure adequate hydration and consider testing (5.3)
- *Mucosal ulcerations:* Consider potential for mucosal ulcerations when interpreting colonoscopy findings in patients with known or suspected inflammatory bowel disease (5.5)
- *Suspected GI obstruction or perforation:* Rule out diagnosis before administration (4, 5.6)
- *Patients at risk for aspiration:* Observe during administration (5.7)
- *Not for direct ingestion:* Dissolve and take with additional water (5.8)

ADVERSE REACTIONS

Most common adverse reactions (>1%) are nausea, headache and vomiting (abdominal bloating, distension, pain/cramping, and watery diarrhea not requiring an intervention were not collected) (6.1)

To report SUSPECTED ADVERSE REACTIONS, contact Ferring at (1-888-FERRING (1-888-337-7464) or FDA at 1-800-FDA-1088 or *www.fda.gov/medwatch*.

DRUG INTERACTIONS

- Drugs that increase risks due to fluid and electrolyte change (7.1)
- *Oral medication taken within 1 hour of start of each dosing:* Might not be properly absorbed (7.2)
- *Antibiotics:* Prior or concomitant use of antibiotics may reduce efficacy of PREPOPIK (7.3)

USE IN SPECIFIC POPULATIONS

Pregnancy: PREPOPIK should be used during pregnancy only if clearly needed (8.1)

See 17 for PATIENT COUNSELING INFORMATION and Medication Guide

Revised: 07/2012

FULL PRESCRIBING INFORMATION: CONTENTS*

*** Sections or subsections omitted from the full prescribing information are not listed**

FULL PRESCRIBING INFORMATION

1 INDICATIONS AND USAGE

PREPOPIK™ (sodium picosulfate, magnesium oxide and anhydrous citric acid) for oral solution is indicated for cleansing of the colon as a preparation for colonoscopy in adults.

2 DOSAGE AND ADMINISTRATION

2.1 Dosing Overview

PREPOPIK, supplied as a powder, must be reconstituted with cold water right before its use *[see Dosage and Administration (2.2)]*. There are two dosing regimens, each requires two separate dosing times:

- The preferred method is the "Split Dose" method and consists of two separate doses: the first dose during the evening before the colonoscopy and the second dose the next day, during the morning prior to the colonoscopy *[see Dosage and Administration (2.3)]*
- The alternative method is the "Day Before" method and consists of two separate doses: the first dose during the afternoon or early evening before the colonoscopy and the second dose 6 hours later during the evening before the colonoscopy) *[see Dosage and Administration (2.4)]*.

Additional fluids must be consumed after every dose in both dosing regimens *[see Dosage and Administration (2.3, 2.4)]*. Instruct patients to consume only clear liquids (no solid food or milk) on the day before the colonoscopy up until 2 hours before the time of the colonoscopy. Instruct patients that if they experience severe bloating, distention, or abdominal pain following the first dose, delay the second dose until their symptoms resolve.

2.2 Reconstitution of the PREPOPIK Powder

(a) Reconstitute the PREPOPIK powder right before each administration. Do not prepare the solution in advance.
(b) Fill the supplied dosing cup with cold water up to the lower (5-ounce) line on the cup and pour in the contents of one packet of PREPOPIK powder.
(c) Stir for 2 to 3 minutes. The reconstituted PREPOPIK solution may become slightly warm as the powder dissolves.

2.3 Split-Dose Dosing Regimen (Preferred Method)

The Split-Dose regimen is the preferred dosing method. Instruct patients to take two separate doses in conjunction with fluids, as follows:

- Take the first dose during the evening before the colonoscopy (e.g., 5:00 to 9:00 PM) followed by five 8-ounce drinks (upper line on the dosing cup) of clear liquids before bed. Consume clear liquids within 5 hours.
- Take second dose, the next day approximately 5 hours before the colonoscopy followed by at least three 8-ounce drinks of clear liquids before the colonoscopy. Consume clear liquids within 5 hours up until 2 hour before the time of the colonoscopy.

2.4 Day-Before Dosing Regimen (Alternative Method)

The Day-Before regimen is the alternative dosing method for patients for whom the Split-Dosing is inappropriate. Instruct patients to take two separate doses in conjunction with fluids, as follows:

- Take the first dose in the afternoon or early evening (e.g., 4:00 to 6:00 PM) before the colonoscopy followed by five 8-ounce drinks (upper line on the dosing cup) of clear liquids before the next dose. Consume clear liquids within 5 hours.
- Take the second dose approximately 6 hours later in the late evening (e.g., 10:00 PM to 12:00 AM), the night before the colonoscopy followed by three 8-ounce drinks of clear liquids before bed. Consume clear liquids within 5 hours.

3 DOSAGE FORMS AND STRENGTHS

For oral solution: each of the two packets contains 10 mg of sodium picosulfate, 3.5 grams of magnesium oxide, and 12.0 grams of anhydrous citric acid in 16.1 grams of powder

4 CONTRAINDICATIONS

PREPOPIK is contraindicated in the following conditions:

- Patients with severely reduced renal function (creatinine clearance less than 30 mL/minute) which may result in accumulation of magnesium *[see Warnings and Precautions (5.3)]*
- Gastrointestinal obstruction or ileus *[see Warnings and Precautions (5.6)]*
- Bowel perforation
- Toxic colitis or toxic megacolon
- Gastric retention
- An allergy to any of the ingredients in PREPOPIK

5 WARNINGS AND PRECAUTIONS

5.1 Serious Fluid and Serum Chemistry Abnormalities

Advise patients to hydrate adequately before, during, and after the use of PREPOPIK. Use caution in patients with congestive heart failure when replacing fluids. If a patient develops significant vomiting or signs of dehydration including signs of orthostatic hypotension after taking PREPOPIK, consider performing post-colonoscopy lab tests (electrolytes, creatinine, and BUN) and treat accordingly. Approximately 20% of patients in both arms (PREPOPIK, 2L of PEG + E plus two × 5-mg bisacodyl tablets) of clinical trials of PREPOPIK had orthostatic changes (changes in blood pressure and/or heart rate) on the day of colonoscopy. In clinical trials orthostatic changes were documented out to seven days post colonoscopy. *[see Adverse Reactions (6.1, 6.2)]*

Fluid and electrolyte disturbances can lead to serious adverse events including cardiac arrhythmias or seizures and renal impairment. Fluid and electrolyte abnormalities should be corrected before treatment with PREPOPIK. In addition, use caution when prescribing Prepopik for patients who have conditions or who are using medications that increase the risk for fluid and electrolyte disturbances or that may increase the risk of adverse events of seizure, arrhythmia, and renal impairment.

5.2 Seizures

There have been reports of generalized tonic-clonic seizures with the use of bowel preparation products in patients with no prior history of seizures. The seizure cases were associated with electrolyte abnormalities (e.g., hyponatremia, hypokalemia, hypocalcemia, and hypomagnesemia) and low serum osmolality. The neurologic abnormalities resolved with correction of fluid and electrolyte abnormalities.

Use caution when prescribing PREPOPIK for patients with a history of seizures and in patients at risk of seizure, such as patients taking medications that lower the seizure threshold (e.g., tricyclic antidepressants), patients withdrawing from alcohol or benzodiazepines, patients with known or suspected hyponatremia. *[see Adverse Reactions (6.2)]*

5.3 Use in Patients with Renal Impairment

As in other magnesium containing bowel preparations, use caution when prescribing PREPOPIK for patients with impaired renal function or patients taking concomitant medications that may affect renal function (such as diuretics, angiotensin converting enzyme inhibitors, angiotensin receptor blockers, or non-steroidal anti-inflammatory drugs). These patients may be at increased risk for renal injury. Advise these patients of the importance of adequate hydration before during and after the use of PREPOPIK. Consider performing baseline and post-colonoscopy laboratory tests (electrolytes, creatinine, and BUN) in these patients. In patients with severely reduced renal function (creatinine clearance < 30 mL/min), accumulation of magnesium in plasma may occur.

5.4 Cardiac Arrhythmias

There have been rare reports of serious arrhythmias associated with the use of ionic osmotic laxative products for bowel preparation. Use caution when prescribing PREPOPIK for patients at increased risk of arrhythmias (e.g., patients with a history of prolonged QT, uncontrolled arrhythmias, recent myocardial infarction, unstable angina, congestive heart failure, or cardiomyopathy). Pre-dose and post-colonoscopy ECGs should be considered in patients at increased risk of serious cardiac arrhythmias.

5.5 Colonic Mucosal Ulceration, Ischemic Colitis and Ulcerative Colitis

Osmotic laxatives may produce colonic mucosal aphthous ulcerations and there have been reports of more serious cases of ischemic colitis requiring hospitalization. Concurrent use of additional stimulant laxatives with PREPOPIK may increase this risk. The potential for mucosal ulcerations should be considered when interpreting colonoscopy findings in patients with known or suspected inflammatory bowel disease. *[see Adverse Reactions (6.2)]*

5.6 Use in Patients with Significant Gastrointestinal Disease

If gastrointestinal obstruction or perforation is suspected, perform appropriate diagnostic studies to rule out these conditions before administering PREPOPIK. Use with caution in patients with severe active ulcerative colitis.

5.7 Aspiration

Patients with impaired gag reflex and patients prone to regurgitation or aspiration should be observed during the administration of PREPOPIK. Use with caution in these patients.

5.8 Not for Direct Ingestion

Each packet must be dissolved in 5 ounces of cold water and administered at separate times according to the dosing regimen. Ingestion of additional water is important to patient tolerance. Direct ingestion of the undissolved powder may increase the risk of nausea, vomiting, dehydration, and electrolyte disturbances.

6 ADVERSE REACTIONS

6.1 Clinical Trials Experience

Because clinical trials are conducted under widely varying conditions, adverse reaction rates observed in the clinical trials of a drug cannot be directly compared to rates in clinical trials of another drug and may not reflect the rates observed in practice.

In randomized, multicenter, controlled clinical trials, nausea, headache, and vomiting were the most common adverse reactions (>1%) following PREPOPIK administration. The patients were not blinded to the study drug. Since abdominal bloating, distension, pain/cramping, and watery diarrhea are known to occur in response to colon cleansing preparations, these effects were documented as adverse events in the clinical trials only if they required medical intervention (such as a change in study drug or led to study discontinuation, therapeutic or diagnostic procedures, met the criteria for a serious adverse event), or showed clinically significant worsening during the study that was not in the frame of the usual clinical course, as determined by the investigator.

PREPOPIK was compared for colon cleansing effectiveness with a preparation containing two liters (2L) of polyethylene glycol plus electrolytes solution (PEG + E) and two 5-mg bisacodyl tablets, all administered the day before the procedure. Table 1 displays the most common adverse reactions in Study 1 and Study 2 for the PREPOPIK Split-Dose and Day-Before dosing regimens, respectively, each as compared to the comparator preparation.

[See table 1 above]

Table 1: Treatment-Emergent Adverse Reactions observed in at Least (>1%) of Patients using the Split-Dose Regimen and Day –Before Regimen *

Adverse Reaction	Study 1: Split-Dose Regimen		Study 2: Day-Before Regimen	
	PREPOPIK (N=305) n (% = n/N)	2L PEG+E† with 2 × 5-mg bisacodyl tablets (N=298) n (% = n/N)	PREPOPIK (N=296) n (% = n/N)	2L PEG+E† with 2 × 5-mg bisacodyl tablets (N=302) n (% = n/N)
Nausea	8 (2.6)	11 (3.7)	9 (3.0)	13 (4.3)
Headache	5 (1.6)	5 (1.7)	8 (2.7)	5 (1.7)
Vomiting	3 (1.0)	10 (3.4)	4 (1.4)	6 (2.0)

* abdominal bloating, distension, pain/cramping, and watery diarrhea not requiring an intervention were not collected

† 2L PEG + E = two liters polyethylene glycol plus electrolytes solution.

Electrolyte Abnormalities

In general, PREPOPIK was associated with numerically higher rates of abnormal electrolyte shifts on the day of colonoscopy compared to the preparation containing 2L of PEG + E plus two × 5-mg bisacodyl tablets (Table 2). These shifts were transient in nature and numerically similar between treatment arms at the Day 30 visit.

[See table 2 at top of next page]

6.2 Postmarketing Experience

The following foreign spontaneous reports have been identified during use of formulations similar to PREPOPIK. Because these events are reported voluntarily from a population of uncertain size, it is not always possible to reliably estimate their frequency or establish a causal relationship to drug exposure.

Allergic reactions

Cases of hypersensitivity reactions including rash, urticaria, and purpura have been reported.

Electrolyte abnormalities

There have been reports of hypokalemia, hyponatremia and hypermagnesemia with the use of PREPOPIK for colon preparation prior to colonoscopy

Gastrointestinal:

Abdominal pain, diarrhea, fecal incontinence, and proctalgia have been reported with the use of PREPOPIK for colon preparation prior to colonoscopy. There have been isolated reports of reversible aphthoid ileal ulcers. Ischemic colitis has been reported with the use of PREPOPIK for colon preparation prior to colonoscopy. However, a causal relationship between these ischemic colitis cases and the use of PREPOPIK has not been established.

Neurologic,

There have been reports of generalized tonic-clonic seizures associated with and without hyponatremia in epileptic patients.

7 DRUG INTERACTIONS

7.1 Drugs That May Increase Risks of Fluid and Electrolyte Abnormalities

Use caution when prescribing PREPOPIK for patients with conditions or who are using medications that increase the risk for fluid and electrolyte disturbances or may increase the risk of seizure, arrhythmias, and prolonged QT in the setting of fluid and electrolyte abnormalities. This includes patients receiving drugs which may be associated with hypokalemia (such as diuretics or corticosteroids, or drugs where hypokalemia is a particular risk, such as cardiac glycosides) or hyponatremia. Use caution when PREPOPIK is used in patients on nonsteroidal anti-inflammatory drugs (NSAIDS) or drugs known to induce Antidiuretic Hormone Secretion (SIADH), such as tricyclic antidepressants, selective serotonin re-uptake inhibitors, antipsychotic drugs and carbamazepine, as these drugs may increase the risk of water retention and/or electrolyte imbalance. Consider additional patient evaluations as appropriate. *[see Adverse Reactions (6.1, 6.2)]*

7.2 Potential for Altered Drug Absorption

Oral medication administered within one hour of the start of administration of PREPOPIK solution may be flushed from the GI tract and the medication may not be absorbed. Tetracycline and fluoroquinolone antibiotics, iron, digoxin, chlorpromazine and penicillamine, should be taken at least 2 hours before and not less than 6 hours after administration of PREPOPIK to avoid chelation with magnesium.

7.3 Antibiotics

Prior or concomitant use of antibiotics with PREPOPIK may reduce efficacy of PREPOPIK as conversion of sodium picosulfate to its active metabolite BHPM is mediated by colonic bacteria.

8 USE IN SPECIFIC POPULATIONS

8.1 Pregnancy

Pregnancy Category B

Reproduction studies with PREPOPIK have been performed in pregnant rats at oral doses up to 2000 mg/kg/day (about 1.2 times the recommended human dose based on the body surface area), and did not reveal any evidence of impaired fertility or harm to the fetus due to PREPOPIK. The reproduction study in rabbits was not adequate, as treatment-related mortalities were observed at all doses. A pre and postnatal development study in rats showed no evidence of any adverse effect on pre and postnatal development at oral doses up to 2000 mg/kg twice daily (about 1.2 times the recommended human dose based on the body surface area). There are, however, no adequate and well-controlled studies in pregnant women. Because animal reproduction studies are not always predictive of human response, PREPOPIK should be used during pregnancy only if clearly needed.

8.3 Nursing Mothers

It is not known whether this drug is excreted in human milk. Because many drugs are excreted in human milk, caution should be exercised when PREPOPIK is administered to a nursing woman.

8.4 Pediatric Use

The safety and effectiveness of PREPOPIK in pediatric patients has not been established.

8.5 Geriatric Use

In controlled clinical trials of PREPOPIK, 215 of 1201 (18%) patients were 65 years of age or older. The overall incidence of treatment-emergent adverse events was similar among patients ≥65 years of age (73%) and patients <65 years of age (71%). Among all patients ≥65 years of age, the proportion of patients with successful colon cleansing was greater in the PREPOPIK group (81.1%) than in the comparator group (70.9%).

8.6 Renal Insufficiency

Patients with impaired renal function or patients taking concomitant medications that may affect renal function (such as diuretics, angiotensin converting enzyme inhibitors, angiotensin receptor blockers, or non-steroidal anti-inflammatory drugs) may be at increased risk for further renal injury. Advise these patients of the importance of adequate hydration before during and after the use of PREPOPIK. Consider performing baseline and post-colonoscopy laboratory tests (electrolytes, creatinine, and BUN) in these patients. In patients with severely reduced renal function (creatinine clearance < 30 mL/min), accumulation of magnesium in plasma may occur. The signs and symptoms of hypermagnesemia may include, but are not limited to, diminished or absent deep tendon reflexes, somnolence, hypocalcemia, hypotension, bradycardia, muscle, respiratory paralysis, complete heart block, and cardiac arrest.

10 OVERDOSAGE

The patient who has taken an overdose should be monitored carefully, and treated symptomatically for complications.

11 DESCRIPTION

PREPOPIK (sodium picosulfate, magnesium oxide and anhydrous citric acid) for oral solution is provided in two packets, the contents of each to be dissolved in 5 ounces of cold water and consumed.

Each packet contains 10 mg sodium picosulfate, 3.5 g magnesium oxide and 12 g anhydrous citric acid. The product also contains the following inactive ingredients, potassium hydrogen carbonate, saccharine sodium, and spray dried orange flavor which contains acacia gum, lactose, ascorbic acid and butylated hydroxyanisole. The following is a description of the three active ingredients:

Sodium picosulfate is a stimulant laxative.

Sodium picosulfate

- Chemical name: 4,4′-(2-pyridylmethylene) diphenyl bis-(hydrogen sulfate) disodium salt, monohydrate

Table 2: Shifts from Normal Baseline to Outside the Normal Range at Day 7 and Day 30

Laboratory Parameter (direction of change)	Visit	Study 1: Split-Dose Regimen		Study 2: Day-Before Regimen	
		PREPOPIK	2L PEG+E with 2× 5 mg bisacodyl tablets	PREPOPIK	2L PEG+E with 2× 5 mg bisacodyl tablets
		n/N (%)		n/N (%)	
Potassium (low)	Day of Colonoscopy	19/260 (7.3)	11/268 (4.1)	13/274 (4.7)	13/271 (4.8)
	24-48 hours	3/302 (1.0)	2/294 (0.7)	3/287 (1.0)	5/292 (1.7)
	Day 7	11/285 (3.9)	8/279 (2.9)	6/276 (2.2)	14/278 (5.0)
	Day 30	11/284 (3.9)	8/278 (2.9)	7/275 (2.5)	8/284 (2.8)
Sodium (low)	Day of Colonoscopy	11/298 (3.7)	3/295 (1.0)	3/286 (1.0)	3/295 (1.0)
	24-48 hours	1/303 (0.3)	1/295 (0.3)	1/288 (0.3)	1/293 (0.3)
	Day 7	2/300 (0.7)	1/292 (0.3)	1/285 (0.4)	1/291 (0.3)
	Day 30	2/299(0.7)	3/291 (1.0)	1/284(0.4)	1/296 (0.3)
Chloride (low)	Day of Colonoscopy	11/301 (3.7)	1/298 (0.3)	3/287 (1.0)	0/297 (0.0)
	24-48 hours	1/303 (0.3)	0/295 (0.0)	2/288 (0.7)	0/293 (0.0)
	Day 7	1/303 (0.3)	3/295 (1.0)	0/285 (0.0)	0/293 (0.0)
	Day 30	2/302 (0.7)	3/294 (1.0)	0/285 (0.0)	0/298 (0.0)
Magnesium (high)	Day of Colonoscopy	34/294 (11.6)	0/294 (0.0)	25/288 (8.7)	1/289 (0.3)
	24-48 hours	0/303 (0.0)	0/295 (0.0)	0/288 (0.0)	0/293 (0.0)
	Day 7	0/297 (0.0)	1/291 (0.3)	1/286 (0.3)	1/285 (0.4)
	Day 30	1/296 (0.3)	2/290 (0.7)	0/286 (0.0)	0/290 (0.0)
Calcium (low)	Day of Colonoscopy	2/292 (0.7)	1/286 (0.3)	0/276 (0.0)	2/282 (0.7)
	24-48 hours	0/303 (0.0)	0/295 (0.0)	0/288 (0.0)	0/293 (0.0)
	Day 7	0/293 (0.0)	1/283 (0.4)	0/274 (0.0)	0/278 (0.0)
	Day 30	0/292 (0.0)	1/282 (0.4)	0/274 (0.0)	1 /283(0.4)
Creatinine (high)	Day of Colonoscopy	5/260 (1.9)	13/268 (4.9)	12/266 (4.5)	16/270 (5.9)
	24-48 hours	1/303 (0.3)	0/295 (0.0)	0/288 (0.0)	0/293 (0.0)
	Day 7	10/264 (0.4)	13/267 (4.8)	10/264 (3.8)	10/265 (3.8)
	Day 30	11/264 (4.2)	14/265(5.3)	18/264 (6.8)	10/272 (3.7)
eGFR (low)	Day of Colonoscopy	22/221 (10.0)	17/214 (7.9)	26/199 (13.1)	25/224 (11.2)
	24-48 hours	76/303 (25.1)	72/295 (24.4)	82/288 (28.5)	62/293 (21.2)
	Day 7	22/223 (10.0)	17/213 (8.0)	11/198 (5.6)	28/219 (12.8)
	Day 30	24/223(10.8)	21/211 (10.0)	21/199 (10.6)	24/224 (10.7)

• Chemical formula: $C_{18}H_{13}NNa_2O_8S_2.H_2O$
• Molecular weight: 499.4
• Structural formula:

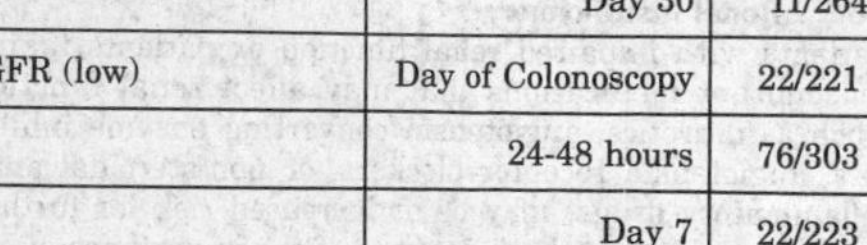

• Sodium picosulfate

Magnesium citrate, which is formed in solution by the combination of magnesium oxide and anhydrous citric acid, is an osmotic laxative.

Magnesium oxide
• Chemical name: Magnesium oxide
• Chemical formula: Mg O
• Molecular weight: 40.3
• Structural formula: Mg O

Anhydrous citric acid
• Chemical name: 2-hydroxypropane-1,2,3-tricarboxylic acid
• Chemical formula: $C_6H_8O_7$
• Molecular weight: 192.1
• Structural formula:

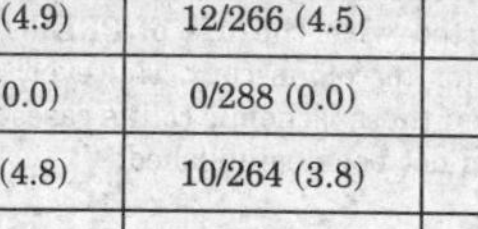

Anhydrous citric acid

12 CLINICAL PHARMACOLOGY

12.1 Mechanism of Action

Sodium picosulfate is hydrolyzed by colonic bacteria to form an active metabolite: bis-(p-hydroxy-phenyl)-pyridyl-2-methane, BHPM, which acts directly on the colonic mucosa to stimulate colonic peristalsis.

Magnesium oxide and citric acid react to create magnesium citrate in solution, which is an osmotic agent that causes water to be retained within the gastrointestinal tract.

12.2 Pharmacodynamics

The stimulant laxative activity of sodium picosulfate together with the osmotic laxative activity of magnesium citrate produces a purgative effect which, when ingested with additional fluids, produces watery diarrhea.

12.3 Pharmacokinetics

Sodium picosulfate, which is a prodrug, is converted to its active metabolite, BHPM, by colonic bacteria. After administration of 2 packets of PREPOPIK separated by 6 hours, in 16 healthy volunteers, sodium picosulfate reached a mean C_{max} of 3.2 ng/mL at approximately 7 hours (T_{max}). After the first packet the corresponding values were 2.3 ng/mL at 2 hours. The terminal half-life of sodium picosulfate was 7.4 hours. The fraction of the absorbed sodium picosulfate dose excreted unchanged in urine was 0.19%. Plasma levels of the free BHPM were low, with 13 out of 16 subjects studied having plasma BHPM concentrations below the lower limit of quantification (0.1 ng/mL). Urinary samples show that the majority of excreted BHPM was in the glucuronide-conjugated form. Magnesium oxide and citric acid react in water to create magnesium citrate. Baseline uncorrected magnesium concentration reached a maximum (C_{max}) of approximately 1.9 mEq/L, which occurred at 10 hours post initial packet administration (T_{max}). This represent an approximately 20% increase from the baseline.

Drug Interaction Studies

In an *in vitro* study using human liver microsomes, sodium picosulfate did not inhibit the major CYP enzymes (CYP 1A2, 2B6, 2C8, 2C9, 2C19, 2D6 and 3A4/5) evaluated. Based on an *in vitro* study using freshly isolated hepatocyte culture, sodium picosulfate is not an inducer of CYP1A2, CYP2B6 or CYP3A4/5.

13 NONCLINICAL TOXICOLOGY

13.1 Carcinogenesis, Mutagenesis, Impairment of Fertility

Long-term studies in animals to evaluate carcinogenic potential or studies to evaluate mutagenic potential have not been performed with PREPOPIK. However, sodium picosulfate was not mutagenic in the Ames test, the mouse lymphoma assay and the mouse bone marrow micronucleus test.

In an oral fertility study in rats, PREPOPIK did not cause any significant adverse effect on male or female fertility parameters up to a maximum dose of 2000 mg/kg twice daily (about 1.2 times the recommended human dose based on the body surface area).

14 CLINICAL STUDIES

The colon cleansing efficacy of PREPOPIK was evaluated for non-inferiority against a comparator in two randomized, investigator-blinded, active-controlled, multicenter US trials in patients scheduled to have an elective colonoscopy. In all, 1195 adult patients were included in the primary efficacy analysis: 601 from Study 1, and 594 from Study 2. Patients ranged in age from 18 to 80 years (mean age 56 years); 61% were female and 39% male. Self-identified race was distributed as follows: 90% White, 10% Black, and less than 1% other. Of these, 3% self-identified their ethnicity as Hispanic or Latino.

Patients randomized to Prepopik in the two studies were treated with one of two dosing regimens:

• In Study 1, PREPOPIK was given by "Split-Dose" (evening before and day of) dosing, where the first packet was taken the evening before the colonoscopy (between 5:00 and 9:00 PM), followed by five (5) 8-ounce glasses of clear liquid, and the second packet was taken the morning of the colonoscopy (at least 5 hours prior to but no more than 9 hours prior to colonoscopy), followed by three (3) 8-ounce glasses of clear liquid.
• In Study 2, PREPOPIK was given by "Day-Before" (afternoon/evening before only) dosing, where both packets were taken separately on the day before the colonoscopy, with the first packet taken in the afternoon (between 4:00 and 6:00 PM), followed by five (5) 8-ounce glasses of clear liquid, and the second packet taken in the late evening (approximately 6 hours later, between 10:00 PM and 12:00 AM), followed by three (3) 8-ounce glasses of clear liquid.

The comparator was a preparation containing two liters of polyethylene glycol plus electrolytes solution (PEG + E) and two 5-mg bisacodyl tablets, administered the day before the procedure. All patients in both the Prepopik and comparator groups were limited to a clear liquid diet on the day before the procedure (24 hours before).

The primary efficacy endpoint was the proportion of patients with successful colon cleansing, as assessed by blinded colonoscopists using the Aronchick Scale. The Aronchick scale is a tool used to assess overall colon cleansing. Successful colon cleansing was defined as bowel preparations with >90% of the mucosa seen and mostly liquid stool that were graded excellent (minimal suctioning needed for adequate visualization) or good (significant suctioning needed for adequate visualization) by the colonoscopist.

In both studies, PREPOPIK was non-inferior to the comparator. In addition, PREPOPIK provided by Split-Dose dosing met the pre-specified criteria for superiority to the comparator for colon cleansing in Study 1. The comparator in that study was administered entirely on the day prior to colonoscopy. See Tables 3 and 4 below.

[See table 3 at top of next page]
[See table 4 at top of next page]

16 HOW SUPPLIED/STORAGE AND HANDLING

How Supplied

PREPOPIK is supplied in a carton containing 2 packets, each holding 16.1 grams of powder for oral solution, along with a pre-marked dosing cup. Each packet contains 10 mg sodium picosulfate, 3.5 g magnesium oxide and 12 g anhydrous citric acid. The excipients include potassium hydrogen carbonate, sodium saccharin, spray dried orange flavor which contains acacia gum, lactose, ascorbic acid, and butylated hydroxyanisole.

Storage

Store at 25°C (77°F). Excursions permitted at 15°C to 30°C (59°F to 86°F) [See USP Controlled Room Temperature].

NDC# 55566-9300-2 Kit, 2 packets and cup

17 PATIENT COUNSELING INFORMATION

See FDA-approved patient labeling (Medication Guide).

- Ask patients to let you know if they have trouble swallowing or are prone to regurgitation or aspiration.
- Tell patients not to take other laxatives while they are taking PREPOPIK.
- Tell patients that if they experience severe bloating, distention or abdominal pain following the first packet of PREPOPIK, delay the second administration until the symptoms resolve.
- Instruct patients to contact their healthcare provider if they develop signs and symptoms of dehydration.
- Not for Direct Ingestion: Each packet must be dissolved in 5 ounces of cold water and administered at separate times according to the dosing regimen. Ingestion of additional water is important to patient tolerance. Direct ingestion of the undissolved powder may increase the risk of nausea, vomiting, dehydration, and electrolyte disturbances. Inform patients that oral medication administered within one hour of the start of administration of PREPOPIK solution may not be absorbed completely.

Manufactured by:
Ferring Pharmaceuticals (China) Co., Ltd.
No. 6 HuiLing Lu (Ferring Road)
National Health Technology Park
Zhongshan City, Guangdong Province, CHINA

Manufactured for:
Ferring Pharmaceuticals Inc.
Parsippany, N.J. 07054

Medication Guide

PREPOPIK (prep-ō-pik)

(sodium picosulfate, magnesium oxide and anhydrous citric acid) for oral solution

Read this Medication Guide instructions before you start taking PREPOPIK and each time you get a refill. There may be new information. This information does not take the place of talking with your healthcare provider about your medical condition or your treatment.

What is the most important information I should know about PREPOPIK?

PREPOPIK and other bowel preparations can cause serious side effects, including:

Serious loss of body fluid (dehydration) and changes in blood salts (electrolytes) in your blood. These changes can cause:

- abnormal heartbeats that can cause death
- seizures. This can happen even if you have never had a seizure.
- kidney problems

Your chance of having fluid loss and changes in blood salts with PREPOPIK is higher if you:

- have heart problems
- have kidney problems
- take water pills or non-steroidal anti-inflammatory drugs (NSAIDS)

Tell your healthcare provider right away if you have any of these symptoms of a loss of too much body fluid (dehydration) while taking PREPOPIK:

- vomiting that prevents you from keeping down the additional prescribed amounts of clear liquids that you must drink after taking your PREPOPIK
- dizziness
- urinating less often than normal
- headache

See "What are the possible side effects of PREPOPIK?" for more information about side effects.

What is PREPOPIK?

PREPOPIK is a prescription medicine used by adults to clean the colon before a colonoscopy. Prepopik cleans your colon by causing you to have diarrhea. Cleaning your colon helps your healthcare provider see the inside of your colon more clearly during your colonoscopy.

It is not known if PREPOPIK is safe and effective in children.

Who should not take PREPOPIK?

Do not take PREPOPIK if your healthcare provider has told you that you have:

- serious kidney problems
- a blockage in your intestine (bowel obstruction)

Table 3: Proportion of Patients with Successful Colon Cleansing in Study 1 Split –Dose Regimen

PREPOPIK Split-Dose Regimen	2L PEG+E* with 2 × 5-mg bisacodyl tablets	Difference between treatment groups	
% (n/N)	% (n/N)	Difference	95% CI
84.2% (256/304)	74.4% (221/297)	9.8%	(3.4%, 16.2%)†

* 2L PEG + E = two liters polyethylene glycol plus electrolytes solution.
† Non-inferior and superior 2L PEG+E with 2 × 5-mg bisacodyl tablets

Table 4: Proportion of Patients with Successful Colon Cleansing in Study 2 Day-Before Regimen

PREPOPIK Day-Before Regimen	2L PEG+E* with 2 × 5-mg bisacodyl tablets	Difference between treatment groups	
% (n/N)	% (n/N)	Difference	95% CI
83.0% (244/294)	79.7% (239/300)	3.3%	(-2.9%, 9.6%)†

* 2L PEG + E = two liters polyethylene glycol plus electrolytes solution.
† . Non-inferior

- an opening in the wall of your stomach or intestines (bowel perforation)
- a very dilated intestine (toxic megacolon)
- problems with the emptying of food and fluid from your stomach (gastric retention)
- an allergy to any of the ingredients in PREPOPIK. See the end of this leaflet for a complete list of ingredients in PREPOPIK.

What should I tell my healthcare provider before taking PREPOPIK?

Before you take PREPOPIK, tell your healthcare provider if you:

- have heart problems
- have stomach or bowel problems
- have ulcerative colitis
- have problems with swallowing or gastric reflux
- are withdrawing from drinking alcohol and benzodiazepines
- have kidney problems
- have low blood salt (sodium) level
- any other medical conditions
- are pregnant. It is not known if Prepopik will harm your unborn baby. Talk to your provider if you are pregnant or plan to become pregnant.
- are breastfeeding or plan to breastfeed. It is not known if Prepopik passes into your breast milk. You and your healthcare provider should decide if you will take Prepopik while breastfeeding.

Tell your healthcare provider about all the medicines you take, including prescription and non-prescription medicines, vitamins, and herbal supplements.

Prepopik may affect how other medicines work. Medicines taken by mouth may not be absorbed properly when taken within 1 hour before the start of PREPOPIK.

Especially tell your healthcare provider if you take:

- medicines for blood pressure or heart problems
- medicines for kidney problems
- medicines for seizures
- water pills (diuretics)
- nonsteroidal anti-inflammatory medicines (pain medicines)
- medicines for depression or mental health problems
- laxatives
- the following medicines should be taken at least 2 hours before starting PREPOPIK and not less than 6 hours after taking PREPOPIK:
  - tetracycline
  - fluoroquinolone antibiotics
  - iron
  - digoxin (Lanoxin)
  - chlorpromazine
  - penicillamine (Cuprimine, Depen)

Ask your healthcare provider or pharmacist for a list of these medicines if you are not sure if you are taking the medicines listed above.

Know the medicines you take. Keep a list of them to show your healthcare provider and pharmacist when you get a new medicine.

How should I take PREPOPIK?

See the Instructions for Use on the outer product carton for dosing. You must read, understand, and follow these instructions to take PREPOPIK the right way.

- **Take PREPOPIK exactly as your healthcare provider tells you to take it**. Your healthcare provider will prescribe the Split-Dosing option or the Day Before Dosing option, depending on colonoscopy scheduling, distance traveled, and other personal circumstances.
- A complete preparation requires 2 packets of PREPOPIK for oral solution taken separately, each followed by additional fluids.
- It is important for you to drink the additional prescribed amount of clear liquids after taking PREPOPIK to prevent fluid loss (dehydration).
- Examples of clear liquids include water, clear broth, apple juice, white cranberry juice, white grape juice, and ginger ale, plain jello (not red or purple) and frozen juice bars(not purple or red).
- Do not eat solid foods or drink milk while taking PREPOPIK
- Drink clear liquids until your colonoscopy.
- Do not take other laxatives while taking PREPOPIK.
- Stop drinking PREPOPIK temporarily or allow for longer time between each dose if you have bloating, distension, or stomach (abdominal) pain until your symptoms improve.
- Stop taking PREPOPIK and, and call your healthcare provider right away if you develop hives or rash after you take your first packet of PREPOPIK. These may be signs of an allergic reaction.

See the Instructions for Use on the outer product carton for dosing. You must read, understand, and follow these instructions to take PREPOPIK the right way.

1) Split-Dose (evening-before and day of the procedure) Dosing

Take your first packet of PREPOPIK the night before your colonoscopy, and take your second dose the next day, in the morning before your colonoscopy.

On the day before your colonoscopy procedure – 1 packet:

- Dissolve 1 packet of powder in 5 ounces of cold water in the evening, followed by five 8-ounce drinks (upper line on the dosing cup) of clear liquids before bed.

On the day of the colonoscopy procedure – 1 packet:

- Dissolve 1 packet of powder in 5 ounces of cold water in the morning (5 hours before the colonoscopy), followed by at least three 8-ounce drinks of clear liquids before the colonoscopy.

You may continue to drink clear liquids until 2 hours before the time of the colonoscopy.

2) Day-Before (afternoon and evening-before the procedure) Dosing

Take your first PREPOPIK packet in the afternoon or early evening and take your second packet 6 hours later, the night before the colonoscopy.

On the day before the colonoscopy procedure – 2 packets:

- Dissolve 1 packet of powder in 5 ounces of cold water in the afternoon or early evening, followed by five 8-ounce drinks (upper line on the dosing cup) of clear liquids before the next dose.
- Dissolve 1 packet of powder in 5 ounces of cold water in the late evening (followed by three 8-ounce drinks (upper line on the dosing cup) of clear liquids before bed.

You may continue to drink clear liquids until 2 hours before the time of the colonoscopy.

What are the possible side effects of PREPOPIK?

PREPOPIK can cause serious side effects, including:

See **"What Is the most important information I should know about PREPOPIK"?**

- **changes in certain blood tests.** Your healthcare provider may do blood tests after you take PREPOPIK to check your blood for changes. Tell your healthcare provider if you have any symptoms of too much fluid loss, including:
  - Vomiting
  - Nausea
  - Bloating

- Dizziness
- Stomach(abdominal)cramping
- Urinate less than usual
- Trouble drinking clear liquids
- Troubles swallowing
- Seizures
- Heart problems (arrhythmia). PREPOPIK may cause irregular heartbeats
- Ulcers of the bowel or bowel problems (ischemic colitis). Tell your healthcare provider right away if you have severe stomach (abdominal) pain or rectal bleeding. These may be symptoms of decreased blood flow to the intestine.

The most common side effects of PREPOPIK include:

- nausea
- headache
- vomiting

Tell your healthcare provider if you have any side effect that bothers you or that does not go away.

These are not all the possible side effects of PREPOPIK. For more information, ask your healthcare provider or pharmacist.

Call your doctor for medical advice about side effects. You may report side effects to FDA at 1-800-FDA-1088.

How should I store PREPOPIK?

- Store PREPOPIK at room temperature, between 68 to 77°F (20 to 25°C).

Keep PREPOPIK and all medicines out of the reach of children.

General information about the safe and effective use of PREPOPIK.

Medicines are sometimes prescribed for purposes other than those listed in a Medication Guide. Do not use PREPOPIK for a condition for which it was not prescribed. Do not give PREPOPIK to other people, even if they are going to have the same procedure you are. It may harm them.

This Medication Guide summarizes the most important information about PREPOPIK. If you would like more information, talk with your healthcare provider. You can also ask your pharmacist or healthcare provider for information that is written for healthcare professionals.

For more information, go to www.ferring.com or call 1-888-337-7464.

What are the ingredients in PREPOPIK?

Active ingredients: sodium picosulfate, magnesium oxide and anhydrous citric acid

Inactive ingredients: potassium hydrogen carbonate, saccharin sodium, spray dried orange flavor which contains acacia gum, lactose, ascorbic acid and butylated hydroxyanisole

This Medication Guide has been approved by the U.S. Food and Drug Administration.

Ferring Pharmaceuticals Inc.
Parsippany, NJ 07054, USA
Issued July/2012

Shown in Product Identification Guide, page 306

Fleet Laboratories Division of C. B. Fleet Company, Incorporated

LYNCHBURG, VA 24502

Direct Inquiries to:
Sherrie McNamara, RN, MSN, MBA
Director, Global Medical Affairs and Pharmacovigilance
1-888-999-9711
www.fleetlabs.com

BOUDREAUX'S BUTT PASTE® OTC
ORIGINAL FORMULA OINTMENT
ALL NATURAL FORMULA OINTMENT
MAXIMUM STRENGTH FORMULA OINTMENT
DIAPER RASH SKIN PROTECTANT

COMPOSITION

Original: 16% Zinc Oxide
All-Natural: 16% Zinc Oxide
Maximum Strength: 40% Zinc Oxide

ACTIONS AND USES

Zinc oxide is a skin protectant used to help treat and prevent diaper rash. It protects chafed skin due to diaper rash and helps seal out wetness. Zinc oxide is effective as a skin protectant due to its absorbent and lubricant properties. It has a low range of sensitization, and has cooling, slightly astringent, antiseptic, antibacterial and protective actions.

GENERAL SKIN PROTECTANT WARNINGS

For external use only. When using this product avoid contact with the eyes. Stop use and ask a doctor if condition worsens or does not improve after seven (7) days.

Keep this and all drugs out of the reach of children to prevent accidental ingestion. In case of accidental ingestion, get medical help or contact a Poison Control Center right away.

DIRECTIONS FOR USE

Change wet and soiled diaper immediately. Cleanse the diaper area and allow to dry. Remove foil seal from the tube's tip. Apply ointment liberally and as often as necessary, with each diaper change and especially when exposed to wet diapers for a prolonged period of time, such as bedtime.

INACTIVE INGREDIENTS

Original formula: castor oil, mineral oil, paraffin, Peruvian balsam, white petrolatum.

All Natural formula: Aloe Vera, beeswax, carnauba wax, castor oil, citric acid, hydrogenated castor oil, Peruvian balsam oil.

Maximum Strength formula: castor oil, mineral oil, paraffin, Peruvian balsam, white petrolatum.

HOW SUPPLIED

Original formula is available in 2 oz (NDC 0132033322), 4 oz (NDC 0132033344) and 16 oz (NDC 0132033316) containers. **All Natural formula** is available in 2 oz (NDC 0132033422) and 4 oz (NDC 0132033444) containers. **Maximum Strength formula** is available in 2 oz (NDC 0132032322) and 4 oz (NDC 0132032344) containers.

IS THIS PRODUCT OTC?
Yes.

QUESTIONS? Call 1-855-785-2888 or visit www.buttpaste.com

FLEET® GLYCERIN LAXATIVES: OTC
FLEET® GLYCERIN SUPPOSITORIES,
FLEET® PEDIA-LAX® GLYCERIN SUPPOSITORIES,
FLEET® BABYLAX® AND
FLEET® PEDIA-LAX® LIQUID GLYCERIN SUPPOSITORIES AND
FLEET® LIQUID GLYCERIN SUPPOSITORIES
A HYPEROSMOTIC LAXATIVE

COMPOSITION

FLEET® Pedia-Lax® and Babylax® Liquid Glycerin Suppositories for Children 2 to under 6 years—Each rectal applicator delivers 2.8 g of glycerin.

FLEET® Liquid Glycerin Suppositories for Adults and Children 6 years of age and over—Each rectal applicator delivers 5.4 g of glycerin.

FLEET® Glycerin Suppositories for Adults—Each suppository contains 2 g of glycerin.

FLEET® Pedia-Lax® Glycerin Suppositories for Children 2 to under 6 years—Each suppository contains 1 g of glycerin.

ACTIONS AND USES

Glycerin is a hyperosmotic laxative, given rectally, which usually produces a bowel movement within 15 minutes to 1 hour. Hyperosmotic laxatives encourage bowel movements by drawing water into the bowel from surrounding tissues. This produces a softer stool mass and increased bowel action. These products are used for fast, predictable relief of occasional constipation. However, rectal irritation may occur with its use.

INFORMATION FOR PATIENT

WARNINGS

This product may cause rectal discomfort or a burning sensation.

GENERAL LAXATIVE WARNINGS

Do not use a laxative product when nausea, vomiting or abdominal pain is present unless directed by a physician. If you notice a sudden change in bowel habits that persists over a period of 2 weeks, consult a physician before using a laxative. Rectal bleeding or failure to have a bowel movement after 1 hour of using this laxative product may indicate a serious condition. Discontinue use and consult a physician. Laxative products should not be used longer than 1 week unless directed by a physician. If constipation continues after one week of use, contact your doctor.

Keep this and all drugs out of the reach of children to prevent accidental ingestion. In case of accidental overdose or ingestion, seek professional assistance or contact a Poison Control Center right away.

DOSAGE AND ADMINISTRATION

FLEET® Pedia-Lax® and Babylax® Liquid Glycerin Suppositories—Children 2 to under 6 years: only 1 suppository per 24 hours or as directed by a physician. Children under 2 years: Consult a physician.

Positions for using the liquid suppository:

- **Left-side position:** Place child on left side with knees bent, and arms resting comfortably.
- **Knee-chest position:** Have child kneel, then lower head and chest forward until left side of face is resting on surface with left arm folded comfortably.

REMOVE ORANGE PROTECTIVE SHIELD FROM TIP BEFORE INSERTING. Hold the unit upright, grasping the bulb with fingers. Grasp the orange protective shield with the other hand; pull gently to remove.

- With steady pressure, gently insert tip into rectum with a slight side-to-side movement, with tip pointing toward navel. Insertion may be easier if child receiving the liquid suppository bears down, as if having a bowel movement. This helps relax the muscles around the anus.
- **DISCONTINUE USE IF RESISTANCE IS ENCOUNTERED. FORCING THE TIP INTO RECTUM CAN CAUSE INJURY.**
- Squeeze bulb until nearly all liquid is gone. It is not necessary to empty the bulb completely, as it contains more liquid than needed. A small amount of liquid will remain in the bulb after squeezing.
- Remove tip from rectum and discard the bulb. The liquid suppository will usually cause a bowel movement after 15 minutes but may take up to 1 hour. Do not allow child to retain liquid suppository for more than 1 hour.
- Stop using this product and consult a doctor if your child doesn't have a bowel movement within 1 hour of using this product.

FLEET® Liquid Glycerin Suppositories for Adults and Children 6 years of age and older: only 1 suppository per 24 hours or as directed by a physician. Children 2 to under 6 years use Fleet® Pedia-Lax® or Fleet® Babylax® Liquid Glycerin Suppositories. Children under 2 years, consult a physician.

Positions for using the liquid suppository:

- **Left-side position:** Lie on left side with knee bent, and arms resting comfortably.
- **Knee-chest position:** Kneel, then lower head and chest forward until left side of face is resting on surface with left arm folded comfortably.

REMOVE ORANGE PROTECTIVE SHIELD FROM TIP BEFORE INSERTING. Hold the unit upright, grasping the bulb with fingers. Grasp the orange protective shield with the other hand; pull gently to remove.

- With steady pressure, gently insert tip into rectum with a slight side-to-side movement, with tip pointing toward navel. Insertion may be easier if person receiving the liquid suppository bears down, as if having a bowel movement. This helps relax the muscles around the anus.
- **DISCONTINUE USE IF RESISTANCE IS ENCOUNTERED. FORCING THE TIP INTO RECTUM CAN CAUSE INJURY.**
- Squeeze bulb until nearly all liquid is gone. It is not necessary to empty the bulb completely, as it contains more liquid than needed. A small amount of liquid will remain in the bulb after squeezing.
- Remove tip from rectum and discard the bulb. The liquid suppository will usually cause a bowel movement after 15 minutes but may take up to 1 hour. Do not retain liquid suppository for more than 1 hour.
- Stop using this product and consult a doctor if you don't have a bowel movement within 1 hour of using this product.

FLEET® Glycerin Suppositories—Adults and Children 6 years of age and older: only 1 suppository per 24 hours or as directed by a physician.

Positions for using the suppository:

- **Left-side position:** Lie on left side with knee bent, and arms resting comfortably.
- **Knee-chest position:** Kneel, then lower head and chest forward until left side of face is resting on surface with left arm folded comfortably.
- Insert one suppository fully into the rectum. The suppository need not melt completely to produce laxative action. The suppository is designed to partially dissolve which may or may not be noticeable.
- The suppository will usually cause a bowel movement after 15 minutes but may take up to 1 hour.
- Do not retain suppository for more than 1 hour.
- Stop using this product and consult a doctor if you don't have a bowel movement within 1 hour of using this product.

Store the container tightly closed and keep away from excessive heat.

FLEET® Pedia-Lax® Glycerin Suppositories—Children 2 to under 6 years: only 1 suppository per 24 hours or as directed by a physician.

Children under 2 years: Consult a physician.

Positions for using the suppository:
- **Left-side position:** Place child on left side with knees bent, and arms resting comfortably.
- **Knee-chest position:** Have child kneel, then lower head and chest forward until left side of face is resting on surface with left arm folded comfortably.
- Insert one suppository fully into the rectum. The suppository need not melt completely to produce laxative action. The suppository is designed to partially dissolve which may or may not be noticeable.
- The suppository will usually cause a bowel movement after 15 minutes but may take up to 1 hour. Do not allow child to retain suppository for more than 1 hour.
- Stop using this product and consult a doctor if your child doesn't have a bowel movement within 1 hour of using this product.

Store the container tightly closed and keep away from excessive heat.

HOW SUPPLIED

FLEET® Pedia-Lax® and Babylax® Liquid Glycerin Suppositories for children 2 to under 6 years—Each box contains 6 child rectal applicators (4 mL each). NDC code: 0132019012 or 0132019024 (8×3 bundle)

FLEET® Liquid Glycerin Suppositories for Adults and Children 6 years of age and over—Each box contains 4 adult rectal applicators (7.5 mL each). NDC code: 0132018582

FLEET® Glycerin Suppositories—Available in jars of 12, 24, 50 and 100 adult suppositories. NDC code: 0132007912 (12 count); NDC code: 0132007924 (24 count); NDC code: 0132007950 (50 count) or 0132007953 (2×6 bundle); NDC code: 0132007900 (100 count)

FLEET® Pedia-Lax® Glycerin Suppositories—Available in jars of 12. NDC code: 0132008112.

IS THIS PRODUCT OTC? Yes.

QUESTIONS? Call 1-866-255-6960 or visit www.fleetlabs.com or www.pedia-lax.com.

FLEET® BISACODYL LAXATIVES: ENEMA AND TABLETS OTC
A STIMULANT LAXATIVE

COMPOSITION

FLEET® Bisacodyl Enema - 10 mg bisacodyl enema solution in a 37-mL ready-to-use squeeze bottle which is **not made with natural rubber latex**, with a 2-inch, prelubricated Comfortip®. It is disposable after a single use.

FLEET® Stimulant Laxative Tablets - Enteric-coated 5 mg bisacodyl each tablet.

ACTION AND USES

Bisacodyl is a stimulant laxative given either orally or rectally, acting directly on the colonic mucosa where it stimulates sensory nerve endings to produce parasympathetic reflexes resulting in increased peristaltic contractions of the colon. The contact action of the drug is restricted to the colon, and motility in the small intestine is not appreciably influenced. FLEET® Stimulant Laxative Tablets usually work within 6-12 hours, and the FLEET® Bisacodyl Enema produces a bowel movement within 5–20 minutes. Bisacodyl is useful as a laxative for relief of occasional constipation and in bowel cleansing in preparation for x-ray or endoscopic examination. Bisacodyl may be used as a laxative in postoperative, antepartum, or postpartum care or in preparation for delivery under guidance of a healthcare professional.

Store at controlled room temperature 68-77°F (20-25°C).

WARNINGS: Do not administer Fleet® Bisacodyl Enema to children under 12 years of age.

GENERAL LAXATIVE WARNINGS
INFORMATION FOR PATIENT

Do not use a laxative product when nausea, vomiting or abdominal pain is present unless directed by a physician. If you notice a sudden change in bowel habits that persists over a period of 2 weeks, consult a physician before using a laxative. Rectal bleeding or failure to have a bowel movement after use of a laxative may indicate a serious condition. Discontinue use and consult a physician. Laxative products should not be used longer than 1 week unless directed by a physician. If constipation continues after one week of use, contact your doctor. As with any drug, if you are pregnant or nursing a baby, seek the advice of a healthcare professional before using this product. All bisacodyl products may cause abdominal discomfort, faintness and mild cramps. Rectal products may also cause rectal burning.

Keep this and all drugs out of the reach of children to prevent accidental ingestion. In case of accidental overdose or ingestion, seek professional assistance or contact a Poison Control Center right away.

DOSAGE AND ADMINISTRATION
Enema

SHAKE BEFORE USING.

Dosage:

Adults and children 12 years of age and over: Use one 1.25 fl. oz. bottle (30-mL delivered dose) as a single daily dose (per 24 hours).

Children under 12 years of age: DO NOT USE.

Positions for using this enema:
- **Left-side position:** Lie on left side with knee bent, and arms resting comfortably.
- **Knee-chest position:** Kneel, then lower head and chest forward until left side of face is resting on surface with left arm folded comfortably.

Fleet® Bisacodyl Enema should be used at room temperature.

How to use this enema:
- Shake bottle well before removing protective shield
- **REMOVE ORANGE PROTECTIVE SHIELD FROM ENEMA COMFORTIP® BEFORE INSERTING.**
- With steady pressure, gently insert enema tip into rectum with a slight side-to-side movement, with tip pointing toward navel. Insertion may be easier if person receiving enema bears down, as if having a bowel movement. This helps relax the muscles around the anus.
- **DO NOT FORCE THE ENEMA TIP INTO RECTUM AS THIS CAN CAUSE INJURY.**
- Squeeze bottle until nearly all liquid is gone. It is not necessary to empty the bottle completely, as it contains more liquid than needed. A small amount of liquid will remain in the bottle after squeezing.
- Remove Comfortip® from rectum and discard bottle.
- Maintain position until urge to evacuate is strong (usually 5 to 20 minutes). Do not retain enema solution for more than 20 minutes.
- Stop using this product and consult a doctor if you don't have a bowel movement within 20 minutes of using this product.

The diaphragm at the base of the tube prevents reflux and assures controlled flow of the enema solution.

IMPORTANT: FLEET® Bisacodyl Enema IS NOT INTENDED FOR ORAL CONSUMPTION in any dosage size.

PROFESSIONAL ADMINISTRATION

FLEET® Bisacodyl Enema should not be used in children under 12 years of age. Careful consideration of the use of enemas in children in general is recommended. Proper and safe use of FLEET® enemas also requires that the products be administered according to the directions. Healthcare professionals should remember when administering the product to gently insert the enema into the rectum with the tip pointing toward the navel. Insertion may be made easier by having the patient bear down as if having a bowel movement. Care during insertion is necessary due to lack of sensory innervation of the rectum and due to the possibility of bowel perforation. Once inserted, squeeze the bottle until nearly all the liquid is expelled. If resistance is encountered on insertion of the nozzle or in administering the solution, the procedure should be discontinued. **Forcing the enema can result in perforation and/or abrasion of the rectum.**

Tablets

Adults and children 12 years of age and over: Take 1 to 3 tablets (usually 2) in a single dose once daily (per 24 hours).

Children 6 to under 12 years of age: Take 1 tablet once daily (per 24 hours).

Children under 6 years of age: Consult a physician.

Expect results in 6–12 hours if taken at bedtime or within 6 hours if taken before breakfast. Swallow tablets whole. Do not chew or crush tablets. Do not administer tablets within 1 hour after taking an antacid, milk, or milk products.

HOW SUPPLIED
Enema

FLEET® Bisacodyl Enema is supplied in a 1.25 fl. oz. (37-mL) ready-to-use squeeze bottle.

NDC code: 0132070336.

Tablets

FLEET® Stimulant Laxative Tablets are supplied in cartons of 25 tablets (5 mg bisacodyl in each tablet) wrapped in a foil seal.

NDC code: 0132070402

IS THIS PRODUCT OTC? Yes.

QUESTIONS? Call 1-866-255-6960 or visit www.fleetlabs.com

FLEET® ENEMA, A SALINE LAXATIVE OTC FLEET® ENEMA EXTRA®, A SALINE LAXATIVE FLEET® PEDIA-LAX® ENEMA, A SALINE LAXATIVE, FLEET® ENEMA FOR CHILDREN, A SALINE LAXATIVE

FLEET® enemas are designed for quick, convenient administration by nurse, patient or caregiver according to instructions. Each is disposable after a single use.

COMPOSITION

FLEET® ENEMA: Each FLEET® Enema unit, with a 2-inch, pre-lubricated Comfortip®, contains 4.5 fl. oz. (133 mL) of enema solution in a ready-to-use squeeze bottle which is **not made with natural rubber latex.** Each enema unit delivers a dose of 118 mL, which contains 19 g monobasic sodium phosphate monohydrate and 7 g dibasic sodium phosphate heptahydrate. Each Fleet® Enema 118 mL delivered dose contains 4.4 grams sodium.

FLEET® ENEMA EXTRA®: Each FLEET® Enema EXTRA® unit, with a 2-inch, pre-lubricated Comfortip®, contains 7.8 fl. oz. (230 mL) of enema solution in a ready-to-use squeeze bottle which is **not made with natural rubber latex.** Each enema unit delivers a dose of 197 mL, which contains 19 g monobasic sodium phosphate monohydrate and 7 g dibasic sodium phosphate heptahydrate. Each Fleet® Enema EXTRA® 197 mL delivered dose contains 4.4 grams sodium.

FLEET® PEDIA-LAX® ENEMA and FLEET® ENEMA FOR CHILDREN: Each Fleet® Pedia-Lax® Enema and FLEET® Enema for Children unit, with a 2-inch, pre-lubricated Comfortip®, contains 2.25 fl. oz. (66 mL) of enema solution in a ready-to-use squeeze bottle which is **not made with natural rubber latex.** Each enema unit delivers a dose of 59 mL, which contains 9.5 g monobasic sodium phosphate monohydrate and 3.5 g dibasic sodium phosphate heptahydrate. Each Fleet® Enema for Children and Fleet® Pedia-Lax® Enema 59 mL delivered dose contains 2.2 grams sodium.

ELEMENTAL AND ELECTROLYTIC CONTENT (Fleet® Enema, Fleet® Pedia-Lax® Enema and Fleet® Enema for Children)	
mEq Phosphate (PO_4) per mL	4.15
mEq Sodium (Na) per mL	1.61
mg Sodium (Na) per mL	37
mmole Phosphorus (P) per mL	1.38

ELEMENTAL AND ELECTROLYTIC CONTENT (Fleet® Enema EXTRA®)	
mEq Phosphate (PO_4) per mL	2.484
mEq Sodium (Na) per mL	0.961
mg Sodium (Na) per mL	22.1
mmole Phosphorus (P) per mL	0.828

ACTION AND USES

FLEET® Enema, FLEET® Enema EXTRA®, Fleet® Pedia-Lax® Enema and FLEET® Enema for Children are useful as laxatives in the relief of occasional constipation and as part of a bowel cleansing regimen in preparing the colon for surgery, x-ray or endoscopic examination.

When used as directed, FLEET® Enema, FLEET® Enema EXTRA®, Fleet® Pedia-Lax® Enema and FLEET® Enema for Children provide thorough yet safe cleansing action and induce complete emptying of the left colon, usually within 1 to 5 minutes, without pain or spasm.

INFORMATION FOR PATIENT

WARNINGS

Using more than one enema in 24 hours can be harmful.

AFTER THE ENEMA SOLUTION IS ADMINISTERED, THE RETENTION TIME SHOULD NOT EXCEED 10 MINUTES. IF THE RETENTION TIME EXCEEDS 10 MINUTES OR THERE IS NO RETURN OF ENEMA SOLUTION, CONTACT A PHYSICIAN IMMEDIATELY, AS ELECTROLYTE DISTURBANCES AND CONSEQUENT SERIOUS SIDE EFFECTS COULD OCCUR.

DO NOT USE ANY FLEET® ENEMA IN CHILDREN UNDER 2 YEARS OF AGE.

DO NOT ADMINISTER THE 4.5 FL. OZ. (133 mL) ADULT SIZE OR THE 7.8 FL.OZ. (230 mL) EXTRA® SIZE TO CHILDREN UNDER 12 YEARS OF AGE.

DO NOT ADMINISTER A FULL 2.25 FL. OZ. (66 mL) CHILDREN'S SIZE TO CHILDREN UNDER 5 YEARS OF AGE.

FOR CHILDREN 2 TO UNDER 5 YEARS, USE ONE-HALF BOTTLE OF 2.25 FL. OZ. (66 mL) CHILDREN'S SIZE. (SEE **DOSAGE AND ADMINISTRATION**).

IMPORTANT: FLEET® Enema (Adult size), FLEET® Enema EXTRA®, Fleet® Pedia-Lax® Enema and Fleet® Enema for Children ARE NOT INTENDED FOR ORAL CONSUMPTION in any dosage size.

When using any of these Fleet® enemas, patient may experience anal discomfort.

GENERAL LAXATIVE WARNINGS

Do not use laxative products when nausea, vomiting or abdominal pain is present unless directed by a physician. If you notice a sudden change in bowel habits that persists over a period of 2 weeks, consult a physician. Fleet® enemas should be administered according to the instructions for use and handling. Stop use if resistance is encountered as forced administration of the enema may cause injury. Stop using this product and consult a doctor if you have rectal bleeding following the use of this product as this may indicate a serious condition. Failure to have bowel movement within 30 minutes of using this product may also indicate a serious condition. Discontinue use and consult a physician. Stop use and ask a doctor if you have any symptoms that your body is losing more fluids than you are drinking. This is called dehydration. Early symptoms of dehydration include feeling thirsty, dizziness, urinating less often than normal and vomiting. Laxative products should not be used longer than 1 week unless directed by a physician. If constipation continues after one week of use, contact your doctor. As with any drug, if you are pregnant or nursing a baby, seek the advice of a healthcare professional before using this product. As sodium phosphate may pass into the breast milk, it is advised that breast milk is expressed and discarded for at least 24 hours after receiving the Fleet® enema.

Keep this and all drugs out of the reach of children to prevent accidental ingestion. In case of accidental overdose or ingestion, seek professional assistance or contact a Poison Control Center right away.

PROFESSIONAL USE INFORMATION
CONTRAINDICATIONS

Do not use in patients with
- Congestive heart failure
- Clinically significant impairment of renal function
- Known or suspected gastrointestinal obstruction
- Megacolon (congenital or acquired)
- Paralytic ileus
- Perforation
- Active inflammatory bowel disease
- Imperforate anus
- Dehydration
- Generally in all cases where absorption capacity is increased or elimination capacity is decreased
- Children under 2 years of age
- Hypersensitivity to active ingredients or to any of the excipients of the product

PRECAUTIONS

Use with caution in patients
- With impaired renal function
- Taking medications known to affect renal perfusion or function, or hydration status
- With pre-existing electrolyte disturbances or who are taking diuretics or other medications which may affect electrolyte levels
- Who are taking medications known to prolong the QT interval
- Ascites
- With a colostomy
- In children 2-11 years of age
- 65 or older and under a doctor's care for any medical condition
- Who are pregnant or nursing a baby

Patients with conditions that may predispose to dehydration or those taking medications which may decrease glomerular filtration rate, such as diuretics, angiotensin converting enzyme inhibitors (ACE-Is), angiotensin receptor blockers (ARBs), or non-steroidal anti-inflammatory drugs (NSAIDs), should be assessed for hydration status prior to use and managed appropriately.

Fleet® Pedia-Lax® Enema and Fleet® Enema for Children should be used with caution in children of any age. Careful consideration of the use of enemas in children in general is recommended.

Careful consideration of the use of sodium phosphates enemas in the elderly with co-morbidities is also recommended. See PROFESSIONAL USE WARNINGS. In those cases where complications have been reported, elderly patients with co-morbidities are often involved.

Since FLEET® enemas contain sodium phosphates, in all patients there is a risk of elevated serum levels of sodium and phosphate and decreased levels of calcium and potassium, and consequently hypernatremia, hyperphosphatemia, hypocalcemia and hypokalemia may occur which could result in metabolic acidosis, tetany, renal failure, QT prolongation and/or, in more severe cases, multi-organ failure, cardiac arrhythmia/arrest and death. This is of particular concern in children with megacolon or any other condition where there is retention of enema solution, and in patients with co-morbidities, particularly gastrointestinal, renal and neurological disorders. If any patient develops vomiting and/or signs of dehydration, measure post-administration labs (phosphate, calcium, potassium, sodium, creatinine, GFR and BUN).

SINCE FLEET® BRAND ENEMAS ARE AVAILABLE IN ADULT, ADULT EXTRA, AND CHILDREN'S SIZES, PRESCRIBE CAREFULLY.

DRUG INTERACTIONS

NO OTHER SODIUM PHOSPHATES PREPARATIONS INCLUDING SODIUM PHOSPHATES ORAL SOLUTION OR TABLETS SHOULD BE GIVEN CONCOMITANTLY.

Electrolyte disturbances and hypovolemia from purgation may be exacerbated by inadequate oral fluid intake, nausea, vomiting, loss of appetite, or use of diuretics, angiotensin converting enzyme inhibitors (ACE-Is), angiotensin receptor blockers (ARBs), non-steroidal anti-inflammatory drugs (NSAIDs), and lithium or other medications that may affect electrolyte levels, and may result in metabolic acidosis, tetany, renal failure, QT prolongation and, in more severe cases, multi-organ failure, cardiac arrhythmia/arrest and death.

As hypernatremia is associated with lower lithium levels, concomitant use of Fleet® enemas and lithium therapy could lead to a fall in serum lithium levels with a lessening of effectiveness.

POSSIBLE SIDE EFFECTS

Hypersensitivity
Pruritis
Dehydration
Hyperphosphatemia
Hypocalcemia
Hypokalemia
Hypernatremia
Metabolic Acidosis
Nausea
Vomiting
Abdominal Pain
Abdominal Distension
Diarrhea
Gastrointestinal Pain
Chills
Blistering
Stinging
Anal Discomfort
Proctalgia

HYDRATION

Additional liquids by mouth are recommended.

Encourage patients to drink large amounts of clear liquids to prevent dehydration. Inadequate fluid intake when using any effective purgative may lead to excessive fluid loss, possibly producing dehydration and hypovolemia.

OVERDOSAGE OR RETENTION

Overdosage (more than one enema in a 24-hour period), no return of enema solution, retention time greater than 10 minutes or failure to have a bowel movement within 30 minutes of enema use may lead to severe electrolyte disturbances, including hypernatremia, hyperphosphatemia, hypocalcemia, and hypokalemia, as well as dehydration and hypovolemia, with attendant signs and symptoms of these disturbances (such as metabolic acidosis, renal failure, and tetany), QT prolongation and/or, in more severe cases, multi-organ failure, cardiac arrhythmia/arrest and death. The patient who has taken an overdose or who has retained the product for more than 10 minutes should be monitored carefully. If any patient develops vomiting and/or signs of dehydration, measure post-procedure labs (phosphate, calcium, potassium, sodium, creatinine, GFR and BUN). **Treatment of electrolyte imbalance may require immediate medical intervention with appropriate electrolyte and fluid replacement therapy.**

DOSAGE AND ADMINISTRATION

Dosage: FLEET® Enema (Adult size) and FLEET® Enema EXTRA®:

Use only 1 enema per 24 hours.

Do not use more unless directed by a doctor. See Warnings. Do not use if taking another sodium phosphates product.

Age	Daily Dose (per 24 hours)
adults and children 12 years and older	one bottle
children 2 to 11 years	use Fleet® Pedia-Lax® Enema or FLEET® Enema for Children (See below)
children under 2 years	**DO NOT USE**

How to use this enema:
- **REMOVE ORANGE PROTECTIVE SHIELD FROM ENEMA COMFORTIP® BEFORE INSERTING.**
- With steady pressure, gently insert enema tip into rectum with a slight side-to-side movement, with tip pointing toward navel. Insertion may be easier if person receiving enema bears down, as if having a bowel movement. This helps relax the muscles around the anus.
- **DO NOT FORCE THE ENEMA TIP INTO RECTUM AS THIS CAN CAUSE INJURY.**
- Squeeze bottle until nearly all liquid is gone. It is not necessary to empty the bottle completely, as it contains more liquid than needed.
- Remove Comfortip® from rectum and maintain position until urge to evacuate is strong (usually 1 to 5 minutes). Do not retain enema solution for more than 10 minutes. Contact a doctor if there is no bowel movement within 30 minutes of enema use.

Positions for using this enema:
- **Left-side position:** Lie on left side with knee bent, and arms resting comfortably.
- **Knee-chest position:** Kneel, then lower head and chest forward until left side of face is resting on surface with left arm folded comfortably.

The diaphragm at base of tube prevents reflux and assures controlled flow of the enema solution. Fleet® Enema should be used at room temperature.

Dosage: Fleet® Pedia-Lax® Enema and FLEET® Enema for Children:

Use only 1 enema per 24 hours.

Do not use more unless directed by a doctor. See Warnings. **Do not use if child is taking another sodium phosphates product.**

Age	Daily Dose (per 24 hours)
children 5 to 11 years	one bottle or as directed by a doctor
children 2 to under 5 years	one-half bottle (see below) or as directed by a doctor
children under 2 years	**DO NOT USE**

One-half bottle preparation: Unscrew cap and remove 2 Tablespoons of liquid with a measuring spoon. Replace cap and follow DIRECTIONS on back of carton.

How to use this enema:
- **REMOVE ORANGE PROTECTIVE SHIELD FROM ENEMA COMFORTIP® BEFORE INSERTING.**
- With steady pressure, gently insert enema tip into rectum with a slight side-to-side movement, with tip pointing toward navel. Insertion may be easier if child receiving enema bears down, as if having a bowel movement. This helps relax the muscles around the anus.
- **DO NOT FORCE THE ENEMA TIP INTO RECTUM AS THIS CAN CAUSE INJURY.**
- Squeeze bottle until nearly all liquid is gone. It is not necessary to empty the bottle completely, as it contains more liquid than needed.
- Remove Comfortip® from rectum and keep child in position until urge to evacuate is strong (usually 1 to 5 minutes). Do not allow child to retain enema solution for more than 10 minutes. Contact a doctor if the child doesn't have a bowel movement within 30 minutes of enema use.

Positions for using this enema:
- **Left-side position:** Place child on left side with knees bent, and arms resting comfortably.
- **Knee-chest position:** Have child kneel, then lower head and chest forward until left side of face is resting on surface with left arm folded comfortably.

The diaphragm at base of tube prevents reflux and assures controlled flow of the enema solution. Fleet® Pedia-Lax® Enema and FLEET® Enema for Children should be used at room temperature.

PROFESSIONAL DOSAGE AND ADMINISTRATION

Administration of more than one enema in 24 hours can be harmful. In those cases where complications have been reported, overdoses are often involved.

NO OTHER SODIUM PHOSPHATES PREPARATIONS INCLUDING SODIUM PHOSPHATES ORAL SOLUTION OR TABLETS SHOULD BE GIVEN CONCOMITANTLY.

FLEET® Enema (Adult size) and FLEET® Enema EXTRA® should not be used in children under 12 years of age. In those cases where complications have been reported, infants and young children are often involved. Fleet® Pedia-Lax® Enema and FLEET® Enema for Children should be used with caution in children of any age. Careful consideration of the use of enemas in children in general is recommended.

Careful consideration of the use of sodium phosphates enemas in the elderly with co-morbidities is also recommended. See PROFESSIONAL USE WARNINGS. In those cases where complications have been reported, elderly patients with co-morbidities are often involved.

See **DOSAGE AND ADMINISTRATION** for dosing detail. Proper and safe use of FLEET® Enemas also requires that the products be administered according to the Directions. Healthcare professionals should remember when administering the product to gently insert the enema into the rectum with the tip pointing toward the navel. Insertion may be made easier by having the patient bear down as if having a bowel movement. Care during insertion is necessary due to lack of sensory innervation of the rectum and due to possibility of bowel perforation. Once inserted, squeeze the bottle until nearly all the liquid is expelled. If resistance is encountered on insertion of the nozzle or in administering the solution, the procedure should be discontinued. **Forcing the enema can result in perforation and/or abrasion of the rectum.**

If an enema containing phosphate or sodium is not advised, consider using FLEET® Bisacodyl Enema.

HOW SUPPLIED

FLEET® Enema is supplied in a 4.5 fl. oz. (133-mL) ready-to-use squeeze bottle. NDC code: 0132020140 (single), 0132020142 (twin), 0132020145 (4-pack), 0132011946 (6-pack), Fleet® Enema EXTRA® is supplied in a 7.8 fl. oz. (230-mL) ready-to-use squeeze bottle. NDC code: 0132020110 Fleet® Pedia-Lax® Enema and Fleet® Enema for Children are supplied in a 2.25 fl. oz. (66 mL) ready-to-use squeeze bottle. NDC code: 0132020220
IS THIS PRODUCT OTC? Yes.
QUESTIONS? Call 1-866-255-6960 or visit www.fleetlabs.com

FLEET® MINERAL OIL ENEMA — OTC
A LUBRICANT LAXATIVE

COMPOSITION

FLEET® Mineral Oil Enema unit, with a 2-inch, pre-lubricated Comfortip®, delivers 118 mL of mineral oil, 100%, in a ready-to-use squeeze bottle **not made with natural rubber latex.** FLEET® Mineral Oil Enema is sodium-free. The unit is disposable after a single use.

ACTION AND USES

FLEET® Mineral Oil Enema serves to soften and lubricate hard stools, easing their passage without irritating the mucosa. Results approximate a normal bowel movement in that only the rectum, sigmoid, and part or all of the descending colon are evacuated. FLEET® Mineral Oil Enema is indicated for relief of fecal impaction; is valuable in relief of occasional constipation when straining must be avoided (in hypertension, coronary occlusion, proctologic procedures, or postoperative care); is indicated for removal of barium sulfate residues from the colon after barium administration and is indicated for obtaining the laxative benefits of mineral oil while avoiding possible untoward effects of oral administration such as (1) interference with intestinal absorption of fat-soluble vitamins A, D, E and K and other nutrients, (2) danger of systemic absorption, or (3) possible risk of lipid pneumonia due to aspiration. It is generally effective in 2 to 15 minutes.

WARNINGS

DO NOT ADMINISTER TO CHILDREN UNDER 2 YEARS OF AGE.

GENERAL LAXATIVE WARNINGS
INFORMATION FOR PATIENT

Do not use laxative products when nausea, vomiting or abdominal pain is present unless directed by a physician. If you notice a sudden change in bowel habits that persists over a period of 2 weeks, consult a physician before using a laxative. Rectal bleeding or failure to have a bowel movement after use of a laxative may indicate a serious condition. Discontinue use and consult a physician. Laxative products should not be used longer than 1 week unless directed by a physician. If constipation continues after one week of use, contact your doctor. As with any drug, if you are pregnant or nursing a baby, seek the advice of a healthcare professional before using this product.
Keep this and all drugs out of the reach of children to prevent accidental ingestion. In case of accidental overdose or ingestion, seek professional assistance or contact a Poison Control Center right away.

DOSAGE AND ADMINISTRATION

Use only 1 enema per 24 hours.

Adults & children 12 years of age and over	1 bottle
Children 2 to 11 years of age	One-half bottle
Children under 2 years of age	DO NOT USE

Positions for using this enema:
- **Left-side position:** Lie on left side with knee bent, and arms resting comfortably.
- **Knee-chest position:** Kneel, then lower head and chest forward until left side of face is resting on surface with left arm folded comfortably.

REMOVE ORANGE PROTECTIVE SHIELD FROM ENEMA COMFORTIP® BEFORE INSERTING.
- With steady pressure, gently insert enema tip into rectum with a slight side-to-side movement, with tip pointing toward navel. Insertion may be easier if person receiving enema bears down, as if having a bowel movement. This helps relax the muscles around the anus.
- **DISCONTINUE USE IF RESISTANCE IS ENCOUNTERED. FORCING THE TIP INTO RECTUM CAN CAUSE INJURY**
- Squeeze bottle until nearly all liquid is gone. It is not necessary to empty the bottle completely, as it contains more liquid than needed. A small amount of liquid will remain in the bottle after squeezing.
- Remove tip from rectum and discard bottle. The enema will usually cause a bowel movement within 2 to 15 minutes. Do not retain liquid for more than 15 minutes.
- Stop using this product and consult a doctor if you don't have a bowel movement within 15 minutes of using this product.

The diaphragm at base of tube prevents reflux and assures controlled flow of the enema solution. The enema should be used at room temperature.

PROFESSIONAL DOSAGE AND ADMINISTRATION

FLEET® Mineral Oil Enema should not be used in children under 2 years of age and should be used with caution in children of any age. In general, careful consideration of the use of enemas in children is recommended.
Proper and safe use of FLEET® Mineral Oil Enema also requires that the product be administered according to the Directions. Healthcare professionals should remember when administering the product to gently insert the enema into the rectum with the tip pointing toward the navel. Insertion may be made easier by having the patient bear down as if having a bowel movement. Care during insertion is necessary due to lack of sensory innervation of the rectum and due to the possibility of bowel perforation. Once inserted, squeeze the bottle until nearly all the liquid is expelled. If resistance is encountered on insertion of the nozzle or in administering the solution, the procedure should be discontinued. **Forcing the enema can result in perforation and/or abrasion of the rectum.**

HOW SUPPLIED

FLEET® Mineral Oil Enema is supplied in 4.5 fl. oz. (133-mL) ready-to-use squeeze bottle.
NDC code: 0132030140.
IS THIS PRODUCT OTC? Yes.
QUESTIONS? Call 1-866-255-6960 or visit www.fleetlabs.com

FLEET® PEDIA-LAX® DOCUSATE SODIUM LIQUID STOOL SOFTENER — OTC
Stool softener laxative

COMPOSITION

Active ingredient (in each tablespoon – 15 mL)	**Purpose**
Docusate sodium 50 mg	Stool softener

Each tablespoon (15 mL) contains 13 mg sodium.

USES
- to help prevent dry, hard stools
- to relieve occasional constipation

DESCRIPTION

Docusate sodium is a stool softener laxative, given orally, which usually produces a bowel movement within 12 to 72 hours. Stool softener laxatives penetrate and soften the stool, thereby promoting bowel movement.

INFORMATION FOR PATIENT

DRUG INTERACTION PRECAUTION: Do not give this product to child if child is presently taking mineral oil, unless directed by a doctor.

WARNINGS

Ask a doctor before using any laxative if your child has
- abdominal pain, nausea or vomiting
- a sudden change in bowel habits lasting more than 2 weeks
- already used a laxative for more than 1 week

Stop using this product and consult a doctor if your child has
- rectal bleeding
- no bowel movement within 72 hours of using this product
- if constipation continues after one week of use, contact your child's doctor.

These symptoms may be signs of a serious condition.
Keep this and all drugs out of the reach of children to prevent accidental ingestion. In case of overdose, get medical help or contact a Poison Control Center right away.

DIRECTIONS

Doses may be taken as a single daily dose or in divided doses in a 24-hour period.
Doses must be given in a 6-8 ounce glass of milk or juice, to prevent throat irritation.

Dosing Chart

Age	Starting Dose	Maximum Dose per Day (24 hours)
Children 2 to 11 years	1–3 tablespoons	3 tablespoons
Children under 2	Ask a doctor	Ask a doctor

Inactive ingredients: citric acid, edetate disodium, FD&C Red #3, flavor, methylparaben, polyethylene glycol, povidone, propylene glycol, propylparaben, sodium citrate, sorbitol, sucralose, water, xanthan gum, xylitol.

HOW SUPPLIED

4 fl.oz. (118 mL) bottles with child-resistant cap, and sealed for your protection. Fruit punch flavor.
NDC code: 0132010624
IS THIS PRODUCT OTC? Yes.
QUESTIONS? Call 1-866-255-6960 or visit www.Pedia-Lax.com

FLEET® PEDIA-LAX® MAGNESIUM HYDROXIDE CHEWABLE TABLETS — OTC
Saline laxative

COMPOSITION

Active ingredient (in each tablet):	**Purpose**
Magnesium hydroxide 400 mg	Saline laxative

Each tablet contains 170 mg magnesium.

USE
- to relieve occasional constipation

DESCRIPTION

Magnesium hydroxide is a saline laxative, given orally, which usually produces a bowel movement within 30 minutes to 6 hours. Saline laxatives increase water in the intestine thereby promoting bowel movement.

INFORMATION FOR PATIENT
WARNINGS

Ask a physician before using this product if child has a magnesium-restricted diet or kidney disease.
Ask a doctor before using any laxative if your child has
- abdominal pain, nausea or vomiting
- a sudden change in bowel habits lasting more than 2 weeks
- already used a laxative for more than 1 week

Stop using this product and consult a doctor if your child has
- rectal bleeding
- no bowel movement within 6 hours of taking this product
- if constipation continues after one week of use, contact your child's doctor.

These symptoms may be signs of a serious condition.
Keep this and all drugs out of the reach of children to prevent accidental ingestion. In case of overdose, get medical help or contact a Poison Control Center right away.

DIRECTIONS

Doses may be taken as a single daily dose or in divided doses in a 24-hour period. **Have child drink a full glass (8 fluid ounces) of liquid with each dose.**

Dosing Chart

Age	Starting Dose	Maximum Dose per Day (24 hours)
Children 6 to 11 years	3–6 tablets	6 tablets
Children 2 to 5 years	1–3 tablets	3 tablets
Children under 2	Ask a doctor	Ask a doctor

Inactive ingredients: colloidal silicon dioxide, FD&C Red #40 aluminum lake, flavor, magnesium stearate, maltodextrin, mannitol, sorbitol, stearic acid, sucralose

HOW SUPPLIED

30 Pedia-Lax Chewable Tablets per bottle with child-resistant cap, sealed for your protection. Watermelon flavor.
NDC code: 0132065501
IS THIS PRODUCT OTC? Yes
QUESTIONS?
Call 1-866-255-6960 or visit www.Pedia-Lax.com

PHAZYME® ULTRA STRENGTH **OTC**
SIMETHICONE SOFTGEL
ANTIGAS

COMPOSITION

Each softgel contains 180mg of Simethicone

ACTIONS AND USES

Simethicone is used to relieve bloating, pressure or fullness commonly referred to as gas. Simethicone reduces the surface tension of gas bubbles in the stomach, allowing them to break up or create a larger gas mass which is more easily expelled from the gastrointestinal tract.

INFORMATION FOR PATIENT

GENERAL WARNINGS

Stop use and ask a doctor if condition persists.
Keep out of the reach of children.

Due to the low potential for acute toxicity resulting from accidental ingestion, the labeling for antiflatulent drug products containing simethicone is exempt from the requirement that the labeling bear the general warning statement "In case of accidental overdose, seek professional assistance or contact a poison control center immediately."

DOSAGE AND ADMINISTRATION

The maximum daily dose for Simethicone is 500 mg.
Swallow one or two softgels after a meal. Do not exceed two softgels per day except under the advice and supervision of a physician.

PROFESSIONAL DOSAGE AND ADMINISTRATION

There is no dosage limitation at this time for professional labeling.
Phazyme® Ultra Strength may be used to relieve postoperative gas pain or for use in endoscopic examination.

INACTIVE INGREDIENTS

FD&C yellow no. 6, gelatin, glycerin, purified water, white edible ink.

HOW SUPPLIED

Phazyme® Ultra Strength is available in 12 (NDC 0132020612) count blister packs and 60 (NDC 0132020860) count bottles.
IS THIS PRODUCT OTC?
Yes.

QUESTIONS?

Call 1-855-727-4277 or visit www.phazyme.com

Forest Pharmaceuticals, Inc.
(Subsidiary of Forest Laboratories, Inc.)
13600 SHORELINE DRIVE
ST. LOUIS, MO 63045

Direct Inquiries to:
Medical Information and Communications
Forest Pharmaceuticals, Inc.
13600 Shoreline Drive
St. Louis, MO 63045
(800) 678-1605

LINZESS ℞
(linaclotide)
capsules, for oral use

HIGHLIGHTS OF PRESCRIBING INFORMATION
These highlights do not include all the information needed to use LINZESS safely and effectively. See full prescribing information for LINZESS.
LINZESS (linaclotide) capsules, for oral use
Initial U.S. Approval: 2012

> **WARNING: PEDIATRIC RISK**
> ***See full prescribing information for complete boxed warning.***
> **LINZESS is contraindicated in pediatric patients up to 6 years of age. Avoid use of LINZESS in pediatric patients 6 through 17 years of age. Linaclotide caused deaths in young juvenile mice (4, 5.1, 8.4, 13.2).**

INDICATIONS AND USAGE

LINZESS is a guanylate cyclase-C agonist indicated in adults for treatment of:
- Irritable bowel syndrome with constipation (IBS-C) (1.1)
- Chronic idiopathic constipation (CIC) (1.2)

DOSAGE AND ADMINISTRATION

- IBS-C: Take 290 mcg orally once daily (2.1)
- CIC: Take 145 mcg orally once daily (2.2)
- Take on empty stomach at least 30 minutes prior to first meal of the day (2.1, 2.2)

DOSAGE FORMS AND STRENGTHS

Capsules: 145 mcg and 290 mcg (3)

CONTRAINDICATIONS

- Pediatric patients up to 6 years of age (4)
- Patients with known or suspected mechanical gastrointestinal obstruction (4)

WARNINGS AND PRECAUTIONS

- *Diarrhea:* Patients may experience severe diarrhea. Hold or stop LINZESS (5.2)

ADVERSE REACTIONS

Most common adverse reactions (incidence of at least 2%) reported in IBS-C or CIC patients are diarrhea, abdominal pain, flatulence and abdominal distension. (6.1)
To report SUSPECTED ADVERSE REACTIONS, contact Forest Pharmaceuticals, Inc., at 1- 800- 678-1605 or FDA at 1-800-FDA-1088 or www.fda.gov/medwatch.
See 17 for PATIENT COUNSELING INFORMATION and Medication Guide

Revised: 08/2013

FULL PRESCRIBING INFORMATION: CONTENTS*

*** Sections or subsections omitted from the full prescribing information are not listed**

FULL PRESCRIBING INFORMATION

> **WARNING: PEDIATRIC RISK**
> **LINZESS is contraindicated in pediatric patients up to 6 years of age. Avoid use in pediatric patients 6 through 17 years of age. In nonclinical studies, administration of a single, clinically relevant adult oral dose of linaclotide caused deaths in young juvenile mice *[see Contraindications (4), Warnings and Precautions (5.1), Use in Specific Populations (8.4) and Nonclinical Toxicology (13.2)].***

1 INDICATIONS AND USAGE

1.1 Irritable Bowel Syndrome with Constipation (IBS-C)

LINZESS (linaclotide) is indicated in adults for the treatment of irritable bowel syndrome with constipation (IBS-C).

1.2 Chronic Idiopathic Constipation (CIC)

LINZESS is indicated in adults for the treatment of chronic idiopathic constipation (CIC).

2 DOSAGE AND ADMINISTRATION

2.1 Irritable Bowel Syndrome with Constipation (IBS-C)

The recommended dose of LINZESS is 290 mcg taken orally once daily on an empty stomach, at least 30 minutes prior to the first meal of the day.

2.2 Chronic Idiopathic Constipation (CIC)

The recommended dose of LINZESS is 145 mcg taken orally once daily on an empty stomach, at least 30 minutes prior to the first meal of the day.

2.3 Important Administration Instructions

Swallow capsules whole; do not break apart or chew.

3 DOSAGE FORMS AND STRENGTHS

- 145 mcg capsules are white to off-white opaque with gray imprint "FL 145"
- 290 mcg capsules are white to off-white opaque with gray imprint "FL 290"

4 CONTRAINDICATIONS

LINZESS is contraindicated in:
- Pediatric patients up to 6 years of age *[see Warnings and Precautions (5.1), Use in Specific Populations (8.4) and Nonclinical Toxicology (13.2)]*
- Patients with known or suspected mechanical gastrointestinal obstruction

5 WARNINGS AND PRECAUTIONS

5.1 Pediatric Risk

LINZESS is contraindicated in pediatric patients up to 6 years of age. In nonclinical studies, deaths occurred within 24 hours in young juvenile mice (1 to 3 week-old mice; approximately equivalent to human pediatric patients less than 2 years of age) following administration of one or two daily oral doses of linaclotide *[see Contraindications (4), Use in Specific Populations (8.4) and Nonclinical Toxicology (13.2)]*.
Avoid the use of LINZESS in pediatric patients 6 through 17 years of age. Linaclotide did not cause deaths in older juvenile mice (approximately equivalent to humans ages 12 to 17 years). Although there were no deaths in older juvenile mice, given the deaths in young juvenile mice and the lack of clinical safety and efficacy data in pediatric patients, avoid the use of LINZESS in pediatric patients 6 through 17 years of age *[see Use in Specific Populations (8.4) and Nonclinical Toxicology (13.2)]*.

5.2 Diarrhea

Diarrhea was the most common adverse reaction of LINZESS-treated patients in the pooled IBS-C and CIC double-blind placebo-controlled trials. Severe diarrhea was reported in 2% of the LINZESS-treated patients. The incidence of diarrhea was similar between the IBS-C and CIC populations *[see Adverse Reactions (6.1)]*.
Instruct patients to stop LINZESS if severe diarrhea occurs and to contact their healthcare provider, who should consider dose suspension *[see Patient Counseling Information (17)]*.

6 ADVERSE REACTIONS

6.1 Clinical Trials Experience

Because clinical trials are conducted under widely varying conditions, adverse reaction rates observed in the clinical trials of a drug cannot be directly compared with rates in the clinical trials of another drug and may not reflect the rates observed in practice.
During clinical development, approximately 2570, 2040, and 1220 patients with either IBS-C or CIC were treated with LINZESS for 6 months or longer, 1 year or longer, and 18 months or longer, respectively (not mutually exclusive).

Irritable Bowel Syndrome with Constipation (IBS-C)

Most Common Adverse Reactions

The data described below reflect exposure to LINZESS in the two placebo-controlled clinical trials involving 1605 adult patients with IBS-C (Trials 1 and 2). Patients were randomized to receive placebo or 290 mcg LINZESS once daily on an empty stomach for up to 26 weeks. Demographic characteristics were comparable between treatment groups *[see Clinical Studies (14.1)]*. **Table 1** provides the incidence of adverse reactions reported in at least 2% of IBS-C patients in the LINZESS treatment group and at an incidence that was greater than in the placebo group.

Table 1: Adverse Reactions Reported in at least 2% of LINZESS-treated Patients and at an Incidence Greater than in Placebo Group Patients in the Two Phase 3 Placebo-controlled Trials (1 and 2) in IBS-C

Adverse Reactions	LINZESS 290 mcg [N=807] %	Placebo [N=798] %
Gastrointestinal		
Diarrhea	20	3
Abdominal pain[a]	7	5
Flatulence	4	2
Abdominal distension	2	1

Infections and Infestations		
Viral Gastroenteritis	3	1
Nervous System Disorders		
Headache	4	3

a: "Abdominal pain" term includes abdominal pain, upper abdominal pain, and lower abdominal pain.

Diarrhea

Diarrhea was the most commonly reported adverse reaction of the LINZESS-treated patients in the pooled IBS-C pivotal placebo-controlled trials. In these trials, 20% of LINZESS-treated patients reported diarrhea compared to 3% of placebo-treated patients. Severe diarrhea was reported in 2% of the LINZESS-treated patients versus less than 1% of the placebo-treated patients, and 5% of LINZESS-treated patients discontinued due to diarrhea vs less than 1% of placebo-treated patients. The majority of reported cases of diarrhea started within the first 2 weeks of LINZESS treatment. Fecal incontinence and dehydration were each reported in less than or equal to 1% of patients in the LINZESS treatment group *[see Warnings and Precautions (5.2)]*.

Adverse Reactions Leading to Discontinuation

In placebo-controlled trials in patients with IBS-C, 9% of patients treated with LINZESS and 3% of patients treated with placebo discontinued prematurely due to adverse reactions. In the LINZESS treatment group, the most common reasons for discontinuation due to adverse reactions were diarrhea (5%) and abdominal pain (1%). In comparison, less than 1% of patients in the placebo group withdrew due to diarrhea or abdominal pain.

Adverse Reactions Leading to Dose Reductions

In the open-label, long-term trials, 2147 patients with IBS-C received 290 mcg of LINZESS daily for up to 18 months. In these trials, 29% of patients had their dose reduced or suspended secondary to adverse reactions, the majority of which were diarrhea or other GI adverse reactions.

Other Adverse Reactions

Adverse reactions that were reported in at least 1% and less than 2% of IBS-C patients in the LINZESS treatment group and at an incidence greater than in the placebo treatment group are listed below by body system:

Gastrointestinal Disorders: gastroesophageal reflux disease, vomiting

General Disorders and Administration Site Conditions: fatigue

Other Adverse Events

In placebo-controlled trials in patients with IBS-C, less than 1% LINZESS-treated patients and no placebo-treated patients reported hematochezia; no patient in either treatment group reported melena. Less than 1% of LINZESS-treated and placebo-treated patients reported allergic reactions, urticaria, or hives as adverse events.

Chronic Idiopathic Constipation (CIC)

Most Common Adverse Reactions

The data described below reflect exposure to LINZESS in the two double-blind placebo-controlled clinical trials of 1275 adult patients with CIC (Trials 3 and 4). Patients were randomized to receive placebo or 145 mcg LINZESS or 290 mcg LINZESS once daily on an empty stomach, for at least 12 weeks. Demographic characteristics were comparable between both LINZESS treatment groups and placebo *[see Clinical Studies (14.2)]*. Only data for the recommended LINZESS 145 mcg dose and placebo are presented. **Table 2** provides the incidence of adverse reactions reported in at least 2% of CIC patients in the 145 mcg LINZESS treatment group and at an incidence that was greater than in the placebo treatment group.

Table 2: Adverse Reactions Reported in at least 2% of 145 mcg LINZESS-treated Patients and at an Incidence Greater than in Placebo Group Patients in the Two Phase 3 Placebo-controlled Trials (3 and 4) in CIC

Adverse Reactions	LINZESS 145 mcg [N=430] %	Placebo [N=423] %
Gastrointestinal		
Diarrhea	16	5
Abdominal pain[a]	7	6
Flatulence	6	5
Abdominal distension	3	2
Infections and Infestations		
Upper respiratory tract infection	5	4
Sinusitis	3	2

a: "Abdominal pain" term includes abdominal pain, upper abdominal pain, and lower abdominal pain.

Diarrhea

Diarrhea was the most commonly reported adverse reaction of the LINZESS-treated patients in the pooled CIC placebo-controlled trials. In these trials, 16% of LINZESS-treated patients reported diarrhea compared to 5% of placebo-treated patients. Severe diarrhea was reported in 2% of the 145 mcg LINZESS-treated patients versus less than 1% of the placebo-treated patients, and 5% of LINZESS-treated patients discontinued due to diarrhea vs less than 1% of placebo-treated patients. The majority of reported cases of diarrhea started within the first 2 weeks of LINZESS treatment. Fecal incontinence was reported in 1% of patients in the LINZESS treatment group, compared with less than 1% in the placebo group. Dehydration was reported in less than 1% of patients in the LINZESS treatment group *[see Warnings and Precautions (5.2)]*.

Adverse Reactions Leading to Discontinuation

In placebo-controlled trials in patients with CIC, 8% of patients treated with LINZESS and 4% of patients treated with placebo discontinued prematurely due to adverse reactions. In the 145 mcg LINZESS treatment group, the most common reasons for discontinuation due to adverse reactions were diarrhea (5%) and abdominal pain (1%). In comparison, less than 1% of patients in the placebo group withdrew due to diarrhea or abdominal pain.

Adverse Reactions Leading to Dose Reductions

In the open-label, long-term trials, 1129 patients with CIC received 290 mcg of LINZESS daily for up to 18 months. In these trials, 27% of patients had their dose reduced or suspended secondary to adverse reactions, the majority of which were diarrhea or other GI adverse reactions.

Other Adverse Reactions

Adverse reactions that were reported in at least 1% of and less than 2% of CIC patients in the 145 mcg LINZESS treatment group and at an incidence greater than in the placebo treatment group are listed below by body system:

Gastrointestinal Disorders: dyspepsia, fecal incontinence

Infections and Infestations: viral gastroenteritis

Other Adverse Events

In placebo-controlled trials in patients with CIC, less than 1% of both LINZESS-treated and placebo-treated patients reported rectal hemorrhage, hematochezia or melena. Less than 1% of LINZESS-treated and placebo-treated patients reported allergic reactions, urticaria, or hives as adverse events.

7 DRUG INTERACTIONS

No drug-drug interaction studies have been conducted with LINZESS. Linaclotide and its active metabolite are not measurable in plasma following administration of the recommended clinical doses; hence, no systemic drug-drug interactions or drug interactions mediated by plasma protein binding of linaclotide or its metabolite are anticipated *[see Clinical Pharmacology (12.3)]*.

Linaclotide does not interact with the cytochrome P450 enzyme system based on the results of *in vitro* studies. In addition, linaclotide is neither a substrate nor an inhibitor of the efflux transporter P-glycoprotein (P-gp).

8 USE IN SPECIFIC POPULATIONS

8.1 Pregnancy

Pregnancy Category C

Risk Summary

There are no adequate and well-controlled studies with LINZESS in pregnant women. In animal developmental studies, adverse fetal effects were observed only with maternal toxicity and at doses of linaclotide much higher than the maximum recommended human dose. LINZESS should be used during pregnancy only if the potential benefit justifies the potential risk to the fetus.

Animal Data

The potential for linaclotide to cause teratogenic effects was studied in rats, rabbits and mice. Oral administration of up to 100,000 mcg/kg/day in rats and 40,000 mcg/kg/day in rabbits produced no maternal toxicity and no effects on embryo-fetal development. In mice, oral dose levels of at least 40,000 mcg/kg/day produced severe maternal toxicity including death, reduction of gravid uterine and fetal weights, and effects on fetal morphology. Oral doses of 5000 mcg/kg/day did not produce maternal toxicity or any adverse effects on embryo-fetal development in mice.

The maximum recommended human dose is approximately 5 mcg/kg/day, based on a 60-kg body weight. Limited systemic exposure to linaclotide was achieved at the tested dose levels in animals (AUC = 40, 640, and 25 ng•hr/mL in rats, rabbits, and mice, respectively, at the highest dose levels), whereas no detectable exposure occurred in humans. Therefore, animal and human doses should not be compared directly for evaluating relative exposure.

8.3 Nursing Mothers

It is not known whether linaclotide is excreted in human milk; however, linaclotide and its active metabolite are not measurable in plasma following administration of the recommended clinical doses *[see Clinical Pharmacology (12.3)]*. Caution should be exercised when LINZESS is administered to nursing women *[see Contraindications (4), Warnings and Precautions (5.1) and Use in Specific Populations (8.4)]*.

8.4 Pediatric Use

Safety and effectiveness in pediatric patients have not been established.

LINZESS is contraindicated in pediatric patients up to 6 years of age. In nonclinical studies, deaths occurred within 24 hours in young juvenile mice (1 to 3 week-old-mice; approximately equivalent to human pediatric patients less than 2 years of age) following administration of one or two daily oral doses of linaclotide *[see Contraindications (4), Warnings and Precautions (5.1) and Nonclinical Toxicology (13.2)]*.

Avoid the use of LINZESS in pediatric patients 6 through 17 years of age. Linaclotide did not cause deaths in older juvenile mice (approximately equivalent to humans age 12 to 17 years). Although there were no deaths in older juvenile mice, given the deaths in young juvenile mice and the lack of clinical safety and efficacy data in pediatric patients, avoid the use of LINZESS in pediatric patients 6 through 17 years of age *[see Warnings and Precautions (5.1) and Nonclinical Toxicology (13.2)]*.

8.5 Geriatric Use

Irritable Bowel Syndrome with Constipation (IBS-C)

Of 1605 IBS-C patients in the placebo-controlled clinical studies of LINZESS, 85 (5%) were at least 65 years of age, while 20 (1%) were at least 75 years old. Clinical studies of LINZESS did not include sufficient numbers of subjects aged 65 and over to determine whether they respond differently from younger subjects.

Chronic Idiopathic Constipation (CIC)

Of 1275 CIC patients in the placebo-controlled clinical studies of LINZESS, 155 (12%) were at least 65 years of age, while 30 (2%) were at least 75 years old. Clinical trials of LINZESS did not include sufficient numbers of subjects aged 65 and over to determine whether they respond differently from younger subjects.

8.6 Hepatic or Renal Impairment

No dose adjustment is necessary based on hepatic or renal function *[see Clinical Pharmacology (12.3)]*.

10 OVERDOSAGE

There is limited experience with overdose of LINZESS. During the clinical development program of LINZESS, single doses of 2897 mcg were administered to 22 healthy volunteers; the safety profile in these subjects was consistent with that in the overall LINZESS-treated population, with diarrhea being the most commonly reported adverse reaction.

11 DESCRIPTION

LINZESS (linaclotide) is a guanylate cyclase-C agonist. Linaclotide is a 14-amino acid peptide with the following chemical name: L-cysteinyl-L-cysteinyl-L-glutamyl-L-tyrosyl-L-cysteinyl-L-cysteinyl-L-asparaginyl-L-prolyl-L-alanyl-L-cysteinyl-L-threonyl-glycyl-L-cysteinyl-L-tyrosine, cyclic (1-6), (2-10), (5-13)-tris (disulfide).

The molecular formula of linaclotide is $C_{59}H_{79}N_{15}O_{21}S_6$ and its molecular weight is 1526.8. The amino acid sequence for linaclotide is shown below:

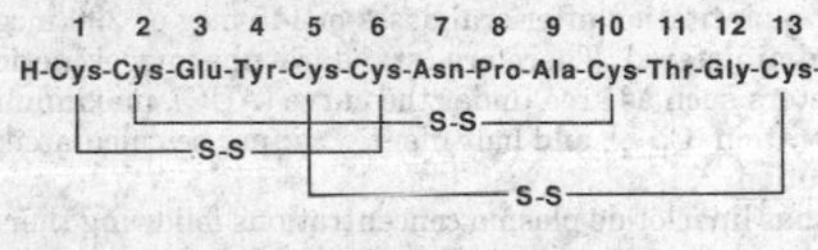

Linaclotide is an amorphous, white to off-white powder. It is slightly soluble in water and aqueous sodium chloride (0.9%). LINZESS contains linaclotide-coated beads in hard gelatin capsules. LINZESS is available as 145 mcg and 290 mcg capsules for oral administration.

The inactive ingredients of LINZESS capsules include: calcium chloride dihydrate, L-leucine, hypromellose, microcrystalline cellulose, gelatin, and titanium dioxide.

12 CLINICAL PHARMACOLOGY

12.1 Mechanism of Action

Linaclotide is a guanylate cyclase-C (GC-C) agonist. Both linaclotide and its active metabolite bind to GC-C and act locally on the luminal surface of the intestinal epithelium. Activation of GC-C results in an increase in both intracellular and extracellular concentrations of cyclic guanosine monophosphate (cGMP). Elevation in intracellular cGMP stimulates secretion of chloride and bicarbonate into the intestinal lumen, mainly through activation of the cystic fibrosis transmembrane conductance regulator (CFTR) ion channel, resulting in increased intestinal fluid and accelerated transit. In animal models, linaclotide has been shown to both accelerate GI transit and reduce intestinal pain. The linaclotide-induced reduction in visceral pain in animals is

Table 3: Efficacy Responder Rates in the Two Placebo-controlled IBS-C Trials: at Least 9 Out of 12 Weeks

	Trial 1			Trial 2		
	LINZESS 290 mcg (N=405)	Placebo (N=395)	Treatment Difference [95% CI]	LINZESS 290 mcg (N=401)	Placebo (N=403)	Treatment Difference [95% CI]
Combined Responder* (Abdominal Pain and CSBM Responder)	12.1%	5.1%	7.0% [3.2%, 10.9%]	12.7%	3.0%	9.7% [6.1%, 13.4%]
Abdominal Pain Responder* (≥ 30% Abdominal Pain Reduction)	34.3%	27.1%	7.2% [0.9%, 13.6%]	38.9%	19.6%	19.3% [13.2%, 25.4%]
CSBM Responder* (≥ 3 CSBMs and Increase ≥1 CSBM from Baseline)	19.5%	6.3%	13.2% [8.6%, 17.7%]	18.0%	5.0%	13.0% [8.7%, 17.3%]

* Primary Endpoints
Note: Analyses based on first 12 weeks of treatment for both Trials 1 and 2
CI =Confidence Interval

Table 4: Efficacy Responder Rates in the Two Placebo-controlled IBS-C Trials: at Least 6 Out of 12 Weeks

	Trial 1			Trial 2		
	LINZESS 290 mcg (N=405)	Placebo (N=395)	Treatment Difference [95% CI]	LINZESS 290 mcg (N=401)	Placebo (N=403)	Treatment Difference [95% CI]
Combined Responder* (Abdominal Pain and CSBM Responder)	33.6%	21.0%	12.6% [6.5%, 18.7%]	33.7%	13.9%	19.8% [14.0%, 25.5%]
Abdominal Pain Responder** (≥ 30% Abdominal Pain Reduction)	50.1%	37.5%	12.7% [5.8%, 19.5%]	48.9%	34.5%	14.4% [7.6%, 21.1%]
CSBM Responder** (Increase ≥ 1 CSBM from Baseline)	48.6%	29.6%	19.0% [12.4%, 25.7%]	47.6%	22.6%	25.1% [18.7%, 31.4%]

* Primary Endpoint, ** Secondary Endpoints
Note: Analyses based on first 12 weeks of treatment for both Trials 1 and 2
CI =Confidence Interval

thought to be mediated by increased extracellular cGMP, which was shown to decrease the activity of pain-sensing nerves.

12.2 Pharmacodynamics

Although the pharmacologic effects of LINZESS in humans have not been fully evaluated, in clinical studies, LINZESS has been shown to change stool consistency as measured by the Bristol Stool Form Scale (BSFS) and increase stool frequency.

12.3 Pharmacokinetics

Absorption

LINZESS is minimally absorbed with low systemic availability following oral administration. Concentrations of linaclotide and its active metabolite in plasma are below the limit of quantitation after oral doses of 145 mcg or 290 mcg were administered. Therefore, standard pharmacokinetic parameters such as area under the curve (AUC), maximum concentration (C_{max}), and half-life ($t_{1/2}$) cannot be calculated.

Distribution

Given that linaclotide plasma concentrations following therapeutic oral doses are not measurable, linaclotide is expected to be minimally distributed to tissues.

Metabolism

Linaclotide is metabolized within the gastrointestinal tract to its principal, active metabolite by loss of the terminal tyrosine moiety. Both linaclotide and the metabolite are proteolytically degraded within the intestinal lumen to smaller peptides and naturally occurring amino acids.

Elimination

Active peptide recovery in the stool samples of fed and fasted subjects following the daily administration of 290 mcg of LINZESS for seven days averaged about 5% (fasted) and about 3% (fed) and virtually all as the active metabolite.

Food Effect

In a cross-over study, 18 healthy subjects were given LINZESS 290 mcg for 7 days both in the non-fed and fed state. Neither linaclotide nor its active metabolite was detected in the plasma. Taking LINZESS immediately after the high fat breakfast resulted in looser stools and a higher stool frequency compared with taking it in the fasted state *[see Dosage and Administration (2.1, 2.2)]*. In clinical trials, LINZESS was administered on an empty stomach, at least 30 minutes before breakfast.

Specific Populations

Age and Gender

Clinical studies to determine the impact of age and gender on the pharmacokinetics of LINZESS have not been conducted. See *Use in Specific Populations (8.5)* for information regarding patients aged 65 years and older.

Hepatic Impairment

LINZESS has not been specifically studied in patients who have hepatic impairment. Hepatic impairment is not expected to affect the metabolism or clearance of the parent drug or its metabolite because linaclotide is metabolized within the gastrointestinal tract *[see Use in Specific Populations (8.6)]*.

Renal Impairment

LINZESS has not been specifically studied in patients who have renal impairment. Renal impairment is not expected to affect clearance of the parent drug or its metabolite because linaclotide has low systemic availability following oral administration and is metabolized within the gastrointestinal tract *[see Use in Specific Populations (8.6)]*.

13 NONCLINICAL TOXICOLOGY

13.1 Carcinogenesis, Mutagenesis, Impairment of Fertility

Carcinogenesis

In 2-year carcinogenicity studies, linaclotide was not tumorigenic in rats at doses up to 3500 mcg/kg/day or in mice at doses up to 6000 mcg/kg/day. The maximum recommended human dose is approximately 5 mcg/kg/day based on a 60-kg bodyweight. Limited systemic exposure to linaclotide was achieved at the tested dose levels in animals, whereas no detectable exposure occurred in humans. Therefore, animal and human doses should not be compared directly for evaluating relative exposure.

Mutagenesis

Linaclotide was not genotoxic in an *in vitro* bacterial reverse mutation (Ames) assay or in the *in vitro* chromosomal aberration assay in cultured human peripheral blood lymphocytes.

Impairment of Fertility

Linaclotide had no effect on fertility or reproductive function in male and female rats at oral doses of up to 100,000 mcg/kg/day.

13.2 Animal Toxicology and/or Pharmacology

Linaclotide caused deaths in two separate toxicology studies in juvenile mice. The mechanism for these deaths is unknown *[see Contraindications (4) and Warnings and Precautions (5.1)]*.

Linaclotide caused deaths at 10 mcg/kg/day in neonatal mice after oral administration of 1 or 2 daily doses, starting on post partum day 7. Deaths were also observed in juvenile mice after a single oral administration on post partum day 14 (100 mcg/kg) and post partum day 21 (600 mcg/kg). The deaths were identified in mice with ages approximately equivalent to human infants and children less than 2 years of age. There were no deaths in the control groups. There are currently no data for mice between ages of 21 days and 6 weeks. Linaclotide did not cause death in a study in older juvenile mice age 6 weeks (approximately equivalent to humans age 12 to 17 years) at a dose of 20,000 mcg/kg/day for 28 days. Linaclotide did not cause death in adult mice, rats, rabbits and monkeys at dose levels up to 5,000 mcg/kg/day. The maximum recommended dose in adults is approximately 5 mcg/kg/day, based on a 60-kg body weight. Animal and human doses of linaclotide should not be compared directly for evaluating relative exposure *[see Nonclinical Toxicology (13.1)]*.

14 CLINICAL STUDIES

14.1 Irritable Bowel Syndrome with Constipation (IBS-C)

The efficacy of LINZESS for the management of symptoms of IBS-C was established in two double-blind, placebo-controlled, randomized, multicenter trials in adult patients (Trials 1 and 2). A total of 800 patients in Trial 1 and 804 patients in Trial 2 [overall mean age of 44 years (range 18 - 87 years with 5% at least 65 years of age), 90% female, 77% white, 19% black, and 12% Hispanic] received treatment with LINZESS 290 mcg or placebo once daily and were evaluated for efficacy. All patients met Rome II criteria for IBS and were required, during the 2-week baseline period, to meet the following criteria:

- a mean abdominal pain score of at least 3 on a 0-to-10-point numeric rating scale
- less than 3 complete spontaneous bowel movements (CSBMs) per week [a CSBM is a spontaneous bowel movement (SBM) that is associated with a sense of complete evacuation; a SBM is a bowel movement occurring in the absence of laxative use], and
- less than or equal to 5 SBMs per week.

The trial designs were identical through the first 12 weeks, and thereafter differed only in that Trial 1 included a 4-week randomized withdrawal (RW) period, and Trial 2 continued for 14 additional weeks (total of 26 weeks) of double-blind treatment. During the trials, patients were allowed to continue stable doses of bulk laxatives or stool softeners but were not allowed to take laxatives, bismuth, prokinetic agents, or other drugs to treat IBS-C or chronic constipation.

Efficacy of LINZESS was assessed using overall responder analyses and change-from-baseline endpoints. Results for endpoints were based on information provided daily by patients in diaries.

The 4 primary efficacy responder endpoints were based on a patient being a weekly responder for either at least 9 out of the first 12 weeks of treatment or at least 6 out of the first 12 weeks of treatment. For the 9 out of 12 weeks combined primary responder endpoint, a patient had to have at least a 30% reduction from baseline in mean abdominal pain, at least 3 CSBMs and an increase of at least 1 CSBM from baseline, all in the same week, for at least 9 out of the first 12 weeks of treatment. Each of the 2 components of the 9 out of 12 weeks combined responder endpoint, abdominal pain and CSBMs, was also a primary endpoint.

For the 6 out of 12 weeks combined primary responder endpoint, a patient had to have at least a 30% reduction from baseline in mean abdominal pain and an increase of at least 1 CSBM from baseline, all in the same week, for at least 6 out of the first 12 weeks of treatment. To be considered a responder for this analysis, patients did not have to have at least 3 CSBMs per week.

The efficacy results for the 9 out of 12 weeks and the 6 out of 12 weeks responder endpoints are shown in **Tables 3 and 4**, respectively. In both trials, the proportion of patients who were responders to LINZESS 290 mcg was statistically significantly higher than with placebo.

[See table 3 above]
[See table 4 above]

In each trial, improvement from baseline in abdominal pain and CSBM frequency was seen over the first 12-weeks of the treatment periods. For change from baseline in the 11-point abdominal pain scale, LINZESS 290 mcg began to separate from placebo in the first week. Maximum effects were seen at weeks 6 - 9 and were maintained until the end of the study. The mean treatment difference from placebo at week 12 was a decrease in pain score of approximately 1.0 point in both trials (using an 11-point scale). Maximum effect on

CSBM frequency occurred within the first week, and for change from baseline in CSBM frequency at week 12, the difference between placebo and LINZESS was approximately 1.5 CSBMs per week in both trials.

During the 4-week randomized withdrawal period in Trial 1, patients who received LINZESS during the 12-week treatment period were re-randomized to receive placebo or continue treatment on LINZESS 290 mcg. In LINZESS-treated patients re-randomized to placebo, CSBM frequency and abdominal-pain severity returned toward baseline within 1 week and did not result in worsening compared to baseline. Patients who continued on LINZESS maintained their response to therapy over the additional 4 weeks. Patients on placebo who were allocated to LINZESS had an increase in CSBM frequency and a decrease in abdominal pain levels that were similar to the levels observed in patients taking LINZESS during the treatment period.

14.2 Chronic Idiopathic Constipation (CIC)

The efficacy of LINZESS for the management of symptoms of CIC was established in two double-blind, placebo-controlled, randomized, multicenter clinical trials in adult patients (Trials 3 and 4). A total of 642 patients in Trial 3 and 630 patients in Trial 4 [overall mean age of 48 years (range 18 - 85 years with 12% at least 65 years of age), 89% female, 76% white, 22% black, 10% Hispanic] received treatment with LINZESS 145 mcg, 290 mcg, or placebo once daily and were evaluated for efficacy. All patients met modified Rome II criteria for functional constipation. Modified Rome II criteria were less than 3 Spontaneous Bowel Movements (SBMs) per week and 1 of the following symptoms for at least 12 weeks, which need not be consecutive, in the preceding 12 months:

- Straining during greater than 25% of bowel movements
- Lumpy or hard stools during greater than 25% of bowel movements
- Sensation of incomplete evacuation during greater than 25% of bowel movements

Patients were also required to have less than 3 CSBMs per week and less than or equal to 6 SBMs per week during a 2-week baseline period. Patients were excluded if they met criteria for IBS-C or had fecal impaction that required emergency room treatment.

The trial designs were identical through the first 12 weeks. Trial 3 also included an additional 4-week randomized withdrawal (RW) period. During the trials, patients were allowed to continue stable doses of bulk laxatives or stool softeners but were not allowed to take laxatives, bismuth, prokinetic agents, or other drugs to treat chronic constipation.

Efficacy of LINZESS was assessed using overall responder analysis and change-from-baseline endpoints. Results for endpoints were based on information provided daily by patients in diaries.

A CSBM overall responder in the CIC trials was defined as a patient who had at least 3 CSBMs and an increase of at least 1 CSBM from baseline in a given week for at least 9 weeks out of the 12-week treatment period. The CSBM responder rates are shown in **Table 5**. During the individual double-blind placebo-controlled trials, LINZESS 290 mcg did not consistently offer additional clinically meaningful treatment benefit over placebo than that observed with the LINZESS 145 mcg dose. Therefore, the 145 mcg dose is the recommended dose. Only the data for the approved 145 mcg dose of LINZESS are presented in **Table 5**.

In Trials 3 and 4, the proportion of patients who were CSBM responders was statistically significantly greater with the LINZESS 145 mcg dose than with placebo.

[See table 5 above]

Table 5: Efficacy Responder Rates in the Two Placebo-controlled CIC Trials: at Least 9 Out of 12 Weeks

	Trial 3			Trial 4		
	LINZESS 145 mcg (N=217)	**Placebo (N=209)**	**Treatment Difference [95% CI]**	**LINZESS 145 mcg (N=213)**	**Placebo (N=215)**	**Treatment Difference [95% CI]**
CSBM Overall Responder* (≥ 3 CSBMs and Increase ≥ 1 CSBM from Baseline)	20.3%	3.3%	16.9% [11.0%, 22.8%]	15.5%	5.6%	9.9% [4.2%, 15.7%]

*Primary Endpoint
CI=Confidence Interval

CSBM frequency reached maximum level during week 1 and was also demonstrated over the remainder of the 12-week treatment period in Trial 3 and Trial 4. For the mean change from baseline in CSBM frequency at week 12, the difference between placebo and LINZESS was approximately 1.5 CSBMs.

On average, patients who received LINZESS across the 2 trials had significantly greater improvements compared with patients receiving placebo in stool frequency (CSBMs/week and SBMs/week), and stool consistency (as measured by the BSFS).

During the 4-week randomized withdrawal period in Trial 3, patients who received LINZESS during the 12-week treatment period were re-randomized to receive placebo or continue treatment on the same dose of LINZESS taken during the treatment period. In LINZESS-treated patients re-randomized to placebo, CSBM and SBM frequency returned toward baseline within 1 week and did not result in worsening compared to baseline. Patients who continued on LINZESS maintained their response to therapy over the additional 4 weeks. Patients on placebo who were allocated to LINZESS had an increase in CSBM and SBM frequency similar to the levels observed in patients taking LINZESS during the treatment period.

16 HOW SUPPLIED/STORAGE AND HANDLING

How Supplied

- **145 mcg Capsules**: White to off-white opaque hard gelatin capsules with grey imprint "FL 145"
  Bottle of 30: NDC 0456-1201-30
- **290 mcg Capsules**: White to off-white opaque hard gelatin capsules with grey imprint "FL 290"
  Bottle of 30: NDC 0456-1202-30

Storage

Store at 25°C (77°F); excursions permitted between 15°C and 30°C (59°F and 86°F) [see USP Controlled Room Temperature].

Keep LINZESS in the original container. Do not subdivide or repackage. Protect from moisture. Do not remove desiccant from the container. Keep bottles tightly closed in a dry place.

17 PATIENT COUNSELING INFORMATION

See FDA-approved patient labeling (Medication Guide).

Patients should be instructed as follows:

- **Do not give LINZESS to children who are under 6 years of age. You should not give LINZESS to children 6 to 17 years of age. It may harm them** *[see Contraindications (4), Warnings and Precautions (5.1), Use in Specific Populations (8.4) and Nonclinical Toxicology (13.2)]*.
- Keep LINZESS in the original container. Do not subdivide or repackage. Protect from moisture. Do not remove desiccant from the container. Keep bottles closed tightly in a dry place *[see How Supplied/Storage and Handling (16)]*.
- Take LINZESS once daily on an empty stomach as prescribed. Swallow the capsule whole and do not break apart or chew *[see Dosage and Administration (2.1 and 2.2)]*.
- If you miss a dose, skip the missed dose. Just take the next dose at your regular time. Do not take 2 doses at the same time.
- Stop LINZESS and contact your physician if you experience severe diarrhea *[see Warnings and Precautions (5.2)]*.
- Seek immediate medical attention if you develop unusual or severe abdominal pain, and /or severe diarrhea, especially if in combination with hematochezia or melena *[see Adverse Reactions (6.1)]*.

LINZESS® is a registered trademark of Ironwood Pharmaceuticals, Inc.

Distributed by:
Forest Pharmaceuticals, Inc.
Subsidiary of Forest Laboratories, Inc.
St. Louis, Missouri, 63045

Marketed by:
Forest Pharmaceuticals, Inc.
Subsidiary of Forest Laboratories, Inc.
St. Louis, Missouri, 63045
Ironwood Pharmaceuticals, Inc.
Cambridge, MA, 02142

MEDICATION GUIDE
LINZESS® (lin-ZESS)
(linaclotide)
capsules

Read this Medication Guide before you start taking LINZESS and each time you get a refill. There may be new information. This information does not take the place of talking to your doctor about your medical condition or your treatment.

What is the most important information I should know about LINZESS?

- **Do not give LINZESS to children who are under 6 years of age. It may harm them.**
- **You should not give LINZESS to children 6 to 17 years of age. It may harm them.**

See the section **"What are the possible side effects of LINZESS?"** for more information about side effects.

What is LINZESS?

LINZESS is a prescription medication used in adults to treat

- irritable bowel syndrome with constipation (IBS-C)
- a type of constipation called chronic idiopathic constipation (CIC). "Idiopathic" means the cause of the constipation is unknown.

It is not known if LINZESS is safe and effective in children.

Who should not take LINZESS?

- **Do not give LINZESS to children who are under 6 years of age.**
- Do not take LINZESS if a doctor has told you that you have a bowel blockage (intestinal obstruction).

What should I tell my doctor before taking LINZESS?

Before you take LINZESS, tell your doctor if you:

- have any other medical conditions
- are pregnant or plan to become pregnant. It is not known if LINZESS will harm your unborn baby.
- are breastfeeding or plan to breastfeed. It is not known if LINZESS passes into your breast milk. Talk with your doctor about the best way to feed your baby, if you take LINZESS.

Tell your doctor about all the medicines you take, including prescription and non-prescription medicines, vitamins and herbal supplements.

How should I take LINZESS?

- Take LINZESS exactly as your doctor tells you to take it.
- Take LINZESS one time each day on an empty stomach, at least 30 minutes before your first meal of the day.
- Swallow LINZESS capsules whole. Do not break or chew the capsules.
- If you miss a dose, skip the missed dose. Just take the next dose at your regular time. Do not take 2 doses at the same time.

What are the possible side effects of LINZESS?

LINZESS can cause serious side effects, including:

- **See "What is the most important information I should know about LINZESS?"**
- **Diarrhea is the most common side effect of LINZESS, and it can sometimes be severe.**
  - Diarrhea often begins within the first 2 weeks of LINZESS treatment.
  - **Stop taking LINZESS and call your doctor right away if you get severe diarrhea during treatment with LINZESS.**

Other common side effects of LINZESS include:

- gas
- stomach-area (abdomen) pain
- swelling, or a feeling of fullness or pressure in your abdomen (distention)

Tell your doctor if you have any side effect that bothers you or that does not go away.

These are not all the possible side effects of LINZESS. For more information, ask your doctor or pharmacist.

In addition, call your doctor or go to the nearest hospital emergency room right away, if you develop unusual or severe stomach-area (abdomen) pain, especially if you also have bright red, bloody stools or black stools that look like tar.

Call your doctor for medical advice about side effects. You may report side effects to FDA at 1-800-FDA-1088.

How should I store LINZESS?

- Store LINZESS at room temperature between 68°F to 77°F (20°C to 25°C).
- Keep LINZESS in the bottle that it comes in.
- The LINZESS bottle contains a desiccant packet to help keep your medicine dry (protect it from moisture). Do not remove the desiccant packet from the bottle.
- Keep the container of LINZESS tightly closed and in a dry place.

Keep LINZESS and all medicines out of the reach of children.

General information about LINZESS

Medicines are sometimes prescribed for purposes other than those listed in a Medication Guide. Do not use LINZESS for a condition for which it was not prescribed. Do not give LINZESS to other people, even if they have the same symptoms that you have. It may harm them.

This Medication Guide summarizes the most important information about LINZESS. If you would like more information, talk with your doctor. You can ask your doctor or pharmacist for information about LINZESS that is written for health professionals. For more information, go to www.LINZESS.com or call 1-800-678-1605.

What are the ingredients in LINZESS?
Active ingredient: linaclotide
Inactive ingredients: calcium chloride dihydrate, L-leucine, hypromellose, microcrystalline cellulose, gelatin, and titanium dioxide.
This Medication Guide has been approved by the U.S. Food and Drug Administration.
Revised: August 2013
LINZESS® is a registered trademark of Ironwood Pharmaceuticals, Inc.
Distributed by:
Forest Pharmaceuticals, Inc.
Subsidiary of Forest Laboratories, Inc.
St. Louis, Missouri, 63045
Marketed by:
Forest Pharmaceuticals, Inc.
Subsidiary of Forest Laboratories, Inc.
St. Louis, Missouri, 63045
Ironwood Pharmaceuticals, Inc.
Cambridge, MA, 02142

Shown in Product Identification Guide, page 306

NAMENDA XR ℞
(memantine hydrochloride)
extended release capsules

HIGHLIGHTS OF PRESCRIBING INFORMATION
These highlights do not include all the information needed to use NAMENDA XR capsules safely and effectively. See full prescribing information for NAMENDA XR capsules.
NAMENDA XR (memantine hydrochloride) extended release capsules
Initial U.S. Approval: 2003

INDICATIONS AND USAGE
NAMENDA XR contains memantine HCl, an NMDA receptor antagonist indicated for the treatment of moderate to severe dementia of the Alzheimer's type. (1)

DOSAGE AND ADMINISTRATION
Initial Dose 7 mg NAMENDA XR once daily (2.1)
Maintenance Dose 28 mg NAMENDA XR once daily (2.1)
A minimum of 1 week of treatment with the previous dose should be observed before increasing the dose. (2.1)
A target dose of 14 mg once daily is recommended in patients with severe renal impairment. (2.1)

DOSAGE FORMS AND STRENGTHS
NAMENDA XR is available as an extended-release capsule (3.1) in the following strengths: 7 mg, 14 mg, 21 mg, 28 mg (3.1, 3.2)

CONTRAINDICATIONS
NAMENDA XR is contraindicated in patients with known hypersensitivity to memantine hydrochloride or to any excipients used in the formulation. (4.1)

WARNINGS AND PRECAUTIONS
Conditions that raise urine pH may decrease the urinary elimination of memantine resulting in increased plasma levels of memantine. (5.1)

ADVERSE REACTIONS
The most commonly observed adverse reactions occurring at a frequency of at least 5% and greater than placebo with administration of NAMENDA XR 28 mg/day were headache, diarrhea and dizziness. Other less common and sometimes serious adverse events have been reported. (6)
To report SUSPECTED ADVERSE REACTIONS, Contact Forest Laboratories, Inc. at 1-800-678-1605 or FDA at 1-800-FDA-1088 or www.fda.gov/medwatch.

DRUG INTERACTIONS
Use with other NMDA antagonists (amantadine, ketamine, and dextromethorphan) has not been systematically evaluated and such use should be approached with caution. (7.1)

USE IN SPECIFIC POPULATIONS
Pediatric Use: The safety and effectiveness of NAMENDA XR in pediatric patients have not been established. (8.4)
See 17 for PATIENT COUNSELING INFORMATION and FDA-approved patient labeling
Revised: 04/2013

FULL PRESCRIBING INFORMATION: CONTENTS*

*** Sections or subsections omitted from the full prescribing information are not listed**

FULL PRESCRIBING INFORMATION

1 INDICATIONS AND USAGE
NAMENDA XR (memantine hydrochloride) extended-release capsules are indicated for the treatment of moderate to severe dementia of the Alzheimer's type.

2 DOSAGE AND ADMINISTRATION
2.1 Recommended Dosing
The dosage of NAMENDA XR shown to be effective in a controlled clinical trial is 28 mg once daily.
The recommended starting dose of NAMENDA XR is 7 mg once daily. The recommended target dose is 28 mg once daily. The dose should be increased in 7 mg increments to 28 mg once daily. The minimum recommended interval between dose increases is one week, and only if the previous dose has been well tolerated. The maximum recommended dose is 28 mg once daily.
NAMENDA XR can be taken with or without food. NAMENDA XR capsules can be taken intact or may be opened, sprinkled on applesauce, and thereby swallowed. The entire contents of each NAMENDA XR capsule should be consumed; the dose should not be divided.
Except when opened and sprinkled on applesauce, as described above, NAMENDA XR should be swallowed whole. NAMENDA XR capsules should not be divided, chewed, or crushed.
Switching from NAMENDA Tablets to NAMENDA XR Capsules:
Patients treated with NAMENDA tablets may be switched to NAMENDA XR capsules as follows:
It is recommended that a patient who is on a regimen of 10 mg twice daily of NAMENDA tablets be switched to NAMENDA XR 28 mg once daily capsules the day following the last dose of a 10 mg NAMENDA tablet. There is no study addressing the comparative efficacy of these 2 regimens.
In a patient with severe renal impairment, it is recommended that a patient who is on a regimen of 5 mg twice daily of NAMENDA tablets be switched to NAMENDA XR 14 mg once daily capsules the day following the last dose of a 5 mg NAMENDA tablet.
Special Populations:
Hepatic Impairment
No dosage adjustment is recommended in patients with mild or moderate hepatic impairment. NAMENDA XR should be administered with caution to patients with severe hepatic impairment.
Renal Impairment
No dosage adjustment is recommended in patients with mild or moderate renal impairment.
A target dose of 14 mg/day is recommended in patients with severe renal impairment (creatinine clearance of 5 – 29 mL/min, based on the Cockroft-Gault equation).

3 DOSAGE FORMS AND STRENGTHS
3.1 Dosage Form
Capsule:
Each capsule contains 7 mg, 14 mg, 21 mg or 28 mg of memantine HCl.
The 7 mg capsules are a yellow opaque #4 size capsule, with "FLI 7 mg" black imprint.
The 14 mg capsules are a yellow cap and dark green opaque body #4 size capsule, with "FLI 14 mg" black imprint on the yellow cap.
The 21 mg capsules are a white to off-white cap and dark green opaque body #4 size capsule, with "FLI 21 mg" black imprint on the white to off-white cap.
The 28 mg capsules are a dark green opaque #3 size capsule, with "FLI 28 mg" white imprint.
3.2 Dosage Strengths
- Each 7 mg capsule contains 7 mg memantine HCl.
- Each 14 mg capsule contains 14 mg memantine HCl.
- Each 21 mg capsule contains 21 mg memantine HCl.
- Each 28 mg capsule contains 28 mg memantine HCl.

For a full list of excipients, see *Description (11)*.

4 CONTRAINDICATIONS
4.1 Hypersensitivity
NAMENDA XR is contraindicated in patients with known hypersensitivity to memantine hydrochloride or to any excipients used in the formulation *[See Description (11)]*.

5 WARNINGS AND PRECAUTIONS
5.1 Genitourinary Conditions
Conditions that raise urine pH may decrease the urinary elimination of memantine resulting in increased plasma levels of memantine.
5.2 Seizures
NAMENDA XR has not been systematically evaluated in patients with a seizure disorder. In clinical trials of memantine, seizures occurred in 0.3% of patients treated with memantine and 0.6% of patients treated with placebo.

6 ADVERSE REACTIONS
6.1 Clinical Trial Data Sources
NAMENDA XR was evaluated in a double-blind placebo-controlled trial treating a total of 676 patients with moderate to severe dementia of the Alzheimer's type (341 patients treated with NAMENDA XR 28 mg/day dose and 335 patients treated with placebo) for a treatment period up to 24 weeks.
Because clinical trials are conducted under widely varying conditions, adverse reaction rates observed in the clinical trials of a drug cannot be directly compared to rates in the clinical trials of another drug and may not reflect the rates observed in practice.
6.2 Adverse Reactions Leading to Discontinuation
In the placebo-controlled clinical trial of NAMENDA XR [See *Clinical Studies (14)*], which treated a total of 676 patients, the proportion of patients in the NAMENDA XR 28 mg/day dose and placebo groups who discontinued treatment due to adverse events were 10.0% and 6.3%, respectively. The most common adverse reaction in the NAMENDA XR treated group that led to treatment discontinuation in this study was dizziness at a rate of 1.5%.
6.3 Most Common Adverse Reactions
The most commonly observed adverse reactions seen in patients administered NAMENDA XR in the controlled clinical trial, defined as those occurring at a frequency of at least 5% in the NAMENDA XR group and at a higher frequency than placebo were headache, diarrhea and dizziness.
Table 1 lists treatment-emergent adverse reactions that were observed at an incidence of ≥ 2% in the NAMENDA XR treated group and occurred at a rate greater than placebo.

Table 1: Adverse reactions observed with a frequency of ≥ 2% and occurring with a rate greater than placebo

Adverse reaction	*Placebo (n = 335) %*	*NAMENDA XR 28mg (n = 341) %*
Gastrointestinal Disorders		
Diarrhea	4	5
Constipation	1	3
Abdominal pain	1	2

Vomiting	1	2
Infections and infestations		
Influenza	3	4
Investigations		
Weight, increased	1	3
Musculoskeletal and connective tissue disorders		
Back pain	1	3
Nervous system disorders		
Headache	5	6
Dizziness	1	5
Somnolence	1	3
Psychiatric disorders		
Anxiety	3	4
Depression	1	3
Aggression	1	2
Renal and urinary disorders		
Urinary incontinence	1	2
Vascular disorders		
Hypertension	2	4
Hypotension	1	2

6.4 Vital Sign Changes

NAMENDA XR and placebo groups were compared with respect to (1) mean change from baseline in vital signs (pulse, systolic blood pressure, diastolic blood pressure, and weight) and (2) the incidence of patients meeting criteria for potentially clinically significant changes from baseline in these variables. There were no clinically important changes in vital signs in patients treated with NAMENDA XR. A comparison of supine and standing vital sign measures for NAMENDA XR and placebo in Alzheimer's patients indicated that NAMENDA XR treatment is not associated with orthostatic changes.

6.5 Laboratory Changes

NAMENDA XR and placebo groups were compared with respect to (1) mean change from baseline in various serum chemistry, hematology, and urinalysis variables and (2) the incidence of patients meeting criteria for potentially clinically significant changes from baseline in these variables. These analyses revealed no clinically important changes in laboratory test parameters associated with NAMENDA XR treatment.

6.6 ECG Changes

NAMENDA XR and placebo groups were compared with respect to (1) mean change from baseline in various ECG parameters and (2) the incidence of patients meeting criteria for potentially clinically significant changes from baseline in these variables. These analyses revealed no clinically important changes in ECG parameters associated with NAMENDA XR treatment.

6.7 Other Adverse Reactions Observed During Clinical Trials of NAMENDA XR

Following is a list of treatment-emergent adverse reactions reported from 750 patients treated with NAMENDA XR for periods up to 52 weeks in double-blind or open-label clinical trials. The listing does not include those events already listed in Table 1, those events for which a drug cause was remote, those events for which descriptive terms were so lacking in specificity as to be uninformative, and those events reported only once which did not have a substantial probability of being immediately life threatening. Events are categorized by body system.

Blood and Lymphatic System Disorders: anemia.

Cardiac Disorders: bradycardia, myocardial infarction.

Gastrointestinal Disorders: fecal incontinence, nausea.

General Disorders: asthenia, fatigue, gait disturbance, irritability, peripheral edema, pyrexia.

Infections and Infestations: bronchitis, nasopharyngitis, pneumonia, upper respiratory tract infection, urinary tract infection.

Injury, Poisoning and Procedural Complications: fall.

Investigations: weight decreased.

Metabolism and Nutrition Disorders: anorexia, dehydration, decreased appetite, hyperglycemia.

Musculoskeletal and Connective Tissue Disorders: arthralgia, pain in extremity.

Nervous System Disorders: convulsion, dementia Alzheimer's type, syncope, tremor.

Psychiatric Disorders: agitation, confusional state, delirium, delusion, disorientation, hallucination, insomnia, restlessness.

Respiratory, Thoracic and Mediastinal Disorders: cough, dyspnea.

6.8 Memantine Immediate Release Clinical Trial and Post Marketing Spontaneous Reports

The following additional adverse reactions have been identified from previous worldwide experience with memantine (immediate release) use. These adverse reactions have been chosen for inclusion because of a combination of seriousness, frequency of reporting, or potential causal connection to memantine and have not been listed elsewhere in labeling. However, because some of these adverse reactions were reported voluntarily from a population of uncertain size, it is not always possible to reliably estimate their frequency or establish a causal relationship between their occurrence and the administration of memantine. These events include:

Blood and Lymphatic System Disorders: agranulocytosis, leukopenia (including neutropenia), pancytopenia, thrombocytopenia. thrombotic thrombocytopenic purpura.

Cardiac Disorders: atrial fibrillation, atrioventricular block (including 2nd and 3rd degree block), cardiac failure, orthostatic hypotension, and torsades de pointes.

Endocrine Disorders: inappropriate antidiuretic hormone secretion.

Gastrointestinal disorders: colitis, pancreatitis.

General disorders and administration site conditions: malaise, sudden death.

Hepatobiliary Disorders: hepatitis (including abnormal hepatic function test, cytolytic and cholestatic hepatitis), hepatic failure.

Infections and infestations: sepsis.

Investigations: electrocardiogram QT prolonged, international normalized ratio increased.

Metabolism and Nutrition Disorders: hypoglycaemia, hyponatraemia.

Nervous System Disorders: convulsions (including grand mal), cerebrovascular accident, dyskinesia, extrapyramidal disorder, hypertonia, loss of consciousness, neuroleptic malignant syndrome, Parkinsonism, tardive dyskinesia, transient ischemic attack.

Psychiatric Disorders: hallucinations (both visual and auditory), restlessness, suicidal ideation.

Renal and Urinary Disorders: acute renal failure (including abnormal renal function test), urinary retention.

Skin Disorders: rash, Stevens Johnson syndrome.

Vascular Disorders: pulmonary embolism, thrombophlebitis, deep venous thrombosis.

The following adverse events have been reported to be temporally associated with memantine treatment and are not described elsewhere in the product labeling: aspiration pneumonia, bone fracture, carpal tunnel syndrome, cerebral infarction, chest pain, cholelithiasis, claudication, depressed level of consciousness (including rare reports of coma), dysphagia, encephalopathy, gastritis, gastroesophageal reflux, intracranial hemorrhage, hyperglycemia, hyperlipidemia, ileus, impotence, lethargy, myoclonus, supraventricular tachycardia, and tachycardia. However, there is again no evidence that any of these additional adverse events are caused by memantine.

7 DRUG INTERACTIONS

No drug-drug interaction studies have been conducted with NAMENDA XR, specifically.

7.1 Use with other N-methyl-D-aspartate (NMDA) Antagonists

The combined use of NAMENDA XR with other NMDA antagonists (amantadine, ketamine, and dextromethorphan) has not been systematically evaluated and such use should be approached with caution.

7.2 Effect of Memantine on the Metabolism of Other Drugs

In vitro studies conducted with marker substrates of CYP450 enzymes (CYP1A2, -2A6, -2C9, -2D6, -2E1, -3A4) showed minimal inhibition of these enzymes by memantine. In addition, *in vitro* studies indicate that at concentrations exceeding those associated with efficacy, memantine does not induce the cytochrome P450 isozymes CYP1A2, -2C9, -2E1 and -3A4/5. No pharmacokinetic interactions with drugs metabolized by these enzymes are expected.

Pharmacokinetic studies evaluated the potential of memantine for interaction with donepezil (See *Section 7.7 Use with Cholinesterase Inhibitors*) and bupropion. Coadministration of memantine with the AChE inhibitor donepezil HCl does not affect the pharmacokinetics of either compound. Memantine did not affect the pharmacokinetics of the CYP2B6 substrate bupropion or its metabolite hydroxybupropion.

7.3 Effect of Other Drugs on Memantine

Memantine is predominantly renally eliminated, and drugs that are substrates and/or inhibitors of the CYP450 system are not expected to alter the pharmacokinetics of memantine. A clinical drug-drug interaction study indicated that bupropion did not affect the pharmacokinetics of memantine.

7.4 Drugs Eliminated via Renal Mechanisms

Because memantine is eliminated in part by tubular secretion, coadministration of drugs that use the same renal cationic system, including hydrochlorothiazide (HCTZ), triamterene (TA), metformin, cimetidine, ranitidine, quinidine, and nicotine, could potentially result in altered plasma levels of both agents. However, coadministration of memantine and HCTZ/TA did not affect the bioavailability of either memantine or TA, and the bioavailability of HCTZ decreased by 20%. In addition, coadministration of memantine with the antihyperglycemic drug Glucovance® (glyburide and metformin HCl) did not affect the pharmacokinetics of memantine, metformin and glyburide. Furthermore, memantine did not modify the serum glucose lowering effect of Glucovance®, indicating the absence of a pharmacodynamic interaction.

7.5 Drugs That Make the Urine Alkaline

The clearance of memantine was reduced by about 80% under alkaline urine conditions at pH 8. Therefore, alterations of urine pH towards the alkaline condition may lead to an accumulation of the drug with a possible increase in adverse effects. Urine pH is altered by diet, drugs (e.g. carbonic anhydrase inhibitors, sodium bicarbonate) and clinical state of the patient (e.g. renal tubular acidosis or severe infections of the urinary tract). Hence, memantine should be used with caution under these conditions.

7.6 Drugs Highly Bound to Plasma Proteins

Because the plasma protein binding of memantine is low (45%), an interaction with drugs that are highly bound to plasma proteins, such as warfarin and digoxin, is unlikely *[see Section 7.]*

7.7 Use with Cholinesterase Inhibitors

Coadministration of memantine with the AChE inhibitor donepezil HCl did not affect the pharmacokinetics of either compound. In a 24-week controlled clinical study in patients with moderate to severe Alzheimer's disease, the adverse event profile observed with a combination of memantine immediate-release and donepezil was similar to that of donepezil alone.

8. USE IN SPECIFIC POPULATIONS

8.1 Pregnancy

Pregnancy Category B: There are no adequate and well-controlled studies of NAMENDA XR in pregnant women. NAMENDA XR should be used during pregnancy only if the potential benefit justifies the potential risk to the fetus.

Memantine given orally to pregnant rats and pregnant rabbits during the period of organogenesis was not teratogenic up to the highest doses tested (18 mg/kg/day in rats and 30 mg/kg/day in rabbits, which are 6 and 21 times, respectively, the maximum recommended human dose [MRHD] on a mg/m^2 basis).

Slight maternal toxicity, decreased pup weights and an increased incidence of non-ossified cervical vertebrae were seen at an oral dose of 18 mg/kg/day in a study in which rats were given oral memantine beginning pre-mating and continuing through the postpartum period. Slight maternal toxicity and decreased pup weights were also seen at this dose in a study in which rats were treated from day 15 of gestation through the post-partum period. The no-effect dose for these effects was 6 mg/kg, which is 2 times the MRHD on a mg/m^2 basis.

8.3 Nursing Mothers

It is not known whether memantine is excreted in human milk. Because many drugs are excreted in human milk, caution should be exercised when memantine is administered to a nursing mother.

8.4 Pediatric Use

The safety and effectiveness of memantine in pediatric patients have not been established.

9 DRUG ABUSE AND DEPENDENCE

Memantine is not a controlled substance. Memantine is a low to moderate affinity uncompetitive NMDA antagonist that did not produce any evidence of drug-seeking behavior or withdrawal symptoms upon discontinuation in 3,254 patients who participated in clinical trials at therapeutic doses. Post marketing data, outside the U.S., retrospectively collected, has provided no evidence of drug abuse or dependence.

10 OVERDOSAGE

Signs and symptoms most often accompanying overdosage with other formulations of memantine in clinical trials and from worldwide marketing experience, alone or in combination with other drugs and/or alcohol, include agitation, asthenia, bradycardia, confusion, coma, dizziness, ECG changes, increased blood pressure, lethargy, loss of consciousness, psychosis, restlessness, slowed movement, somnolence, stupor, unsteady gait, visual hallucinations, vertigo, vomiting, and weakness. The largest known ingestion of memantine worldwide was 2 grams in an individual who took memantine in conjunction with unspecified antidiabetic medications. This person experienced coma, diplopia, and agitation, but subsequently recovered.

One patient participating in a NAMENDA XR clinical trial unintentionally took 112 mg of NAMENDA XR daily for 31 days and experienced an elevated serum uric acid, elevated serum alkaline phosphatase, and low platelet count.

No fatalities have been noted with overdoses of memantine alone. A fatal outcome has very rarely been reported when memantine has been ingested as part of overdosing with multiple drugs; in those instances, the relationship between memantine and a fatal outcome has been unclear.

Because strategies for the management of overdose are continually evolving, it is advisable to contact a poison control center to determine the latest recommendations for the management of an overdose of any drug. As in any cases of overdose, general supportive measures should be utilized, and treatment should be symptomatic. Elimination of memantine can be enhanced by acidification of urine.

11 DESCRIPTION

NAMENDA XR is an orally active NMDA receptor antagonist. The chemical name for memantine hydrochloride is 1-amino-3,5-dimethyladamantane hydrochloride with the following structural formula:

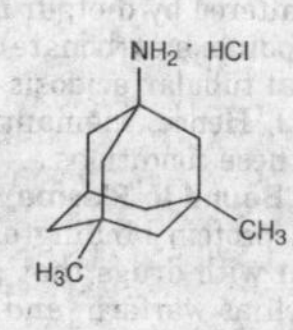

The molecular formula is $C_{12}H_{21}N \bullet HCl$ and the molecular weight is 215.76. Memantine HCl occurs as a fine white to off-white powder and is soluble in water.

NAMENDA XR capsules are supplied for oral administration as 7, 14, 21 and 28 mg capsules (see *How Supplied* Section 16). Each capsule contains extended release beads with the labeled amount of memantine HCl and the following inactive ingredients: sugar spheres, polyvinylpyrrolidone, hypromellose, talc, polyethylene glycol, ethylcellulose, ammonium hydroxide, oleic acid, and medium chain triglycerides in hard gelatin capsules.

12 CLINICAL PHARMACOLOGY

12.1 Mechanism of Action

Persistent activation of central nervous system N-methyl-D-aspartate (NMDA) receptors by the excitatory amino acid glutamate has been hypothesized to contribute to the symptomatology of Alzheimer's disease. Memantine is postulated to exert its therapeutic effect through its action as a low to moderate affinity uncompetitive (open-channel) NMDA receptor antagonist which binds preferentially to the NMDA receptor-operated cation channels. There is no evidence that memantine prevents or slows neurodegeneration in patients with Alzheimer's disease.

12.2 Pharmacodynamics

Memantine showed low to negligible affinity for GABA, benzodiazepine, dopamine, adrenergic, histamine and glycine receptors and for voltage-dependent Ca^{2+}, Na^{+} or K^{+} channels. Memantine also showed antagonistic effects at the $5HT_3$ receptor with a potency similar to that for the NMDA receptor and blocked nicotinic acetylcholine receptors with one-sixth to one-tenth the potency.

In vitro studies have shown that memantine does not affect the reversible inhibition of acetylcholinesterase by donepezil, galantamine, or tacrine.

12.3 Pharmacokinetics

Memantine is well absorbed after oral administration and has linear pharmacokinetics over the therapeutic dose range. It is excreted predominantly unchanged in urine and has a terminal elimination half life of about 60-80 hours. In a study comparing 28 mg once daily NAMENDA XR to 10 mg twice daily NAMENDA C_{max} and $AUC_{0\text{-}24}$ values were 48% and 33% higher for the XR dosage regimen, respectively.

Absorption

After multiple dose administration of NAMENDA XR, memantine peak concentrations occur around 9-12 hours postdose. There is no difference in the absorption of NAMENDA XR when the capsule is taken intact or when the contents are sprinkled on applesauce.

There is no difference in memantine exposure, based on C_{max} or AUC, for NAMENDA XR whether that drug product is administered with food or on an empty stomach. However, peak plasma concentrations are achieved about 18 hours after administration with food versus approximately 25 hours after administration on an empty stomach.

Distribution

The mean volume of distribution of memantine is 9-11 L/kg and the plasma protein binding is low (45%).

Metabolism

Memantine undergoes partial hepatic metabolism. The hepatic microsomal CYP450 enzyme system does not play a significant role in the metabolism of memantine.

Elimination

Memantine is excreted predominantly in the urine, unchanged, and has a terminal elimination half life of about 60-80 hours. About 48% of administered drug is excreted unchanged in urine; the remainder is converted primarily to three polar metabolites which possess minimal NMDA receptor antagonistic activity: the N-glucuronide conjugate, 6-hydroxy memantine, and 1-nitroso-deaminated memantine. A total of 74% of the administered dose is excreted as the sum of the parent drug and the N-glucuronide conjugate. Renal clearance involves active tubular secretion moderated by pH dependent tubular reabsorption.

12.4 Pharmacokinetics in Special Populations

Hepatic Impairment

Memantine pharmacokinetics were evaluated following the administration of single oral doses of 20 mg in 8 subjects with moderate hepatic impairment (Child-Pugh Class B,score 7-9) and 8 subjects who were age-, gender-, and weight-matched to the hepatically-impaired subjects. There was no change in memantine exposure (based on Cmax and AUC) in subjects with moderate hepatic impairment as compared with healthy subjects. However, terminal elimination half-life increased by about 16% in subjects with moderate hepatic impairment as compared with healthy subjects. No dose adjustment is recommended for patients with mild and moderate hepatic impairment. NAMENDA XR should be administered with caution to patients with severe hepatic impairment as the pharmacokinetics of memantine have not been evaluated in that population.

Renal Impairment

Memantine pharmacokinetics were evaluated following single oral administration of 20 mg memantine HCl in 8 subjects with mild renal impairment (creatinine clearance, CLcr, > 50 – 80 mL/min), 8 subjects with moderate renal impairment (CLcr 30 – 49 mL/min), 7 subjects with severe renal impairment (CLcr 5 – 29 mL/min) and 8 healthy subjects (CLcr > 80 mL/min) matched as closely as possible by age, weight and gender to the subjects with renal impairment. Mean $AUC_{0-\infty}$ increased by 4%, 60%, and 115% in subjects with mild, moderate, and severe renal impairment, respectively, compared to healthy subjects. The terminal elimination half-life increased by 18%, 41%, and 95% in subjects with mild, moderate, and severe renal impairment, respectively, compared to healthy subjects.

No dosage adjustment is recommended for patients with mild and moderate renal impairment. Dosage should be reduced in patients with severe renal impairment [See *Dosage and Administration (2)*].

Gender

Following multiple dose administration of memantine HCl 20 mg daily, females had about 45% higher exposure than males, but there was no difference in exposure when body weight was taken into account.

Elderly

The pharmacokinetics of memantine in young and elderly subjects are similar.

13 NONCLINICAL TOXICOLOGY

13.1 Carcinogenesis, Mutagenesis, Impairment of Fertility

There was no evidence of carcinogenicity in a 113-week oral study in mice at doses up to 40 mg/kg/day (7 times the maximum recommended human dose [MRHD] on a mg/m^2 basis). There was also no evidence of carcinogenicity in rats orally dosed at up to 40 mg/kg/day for 71 weeks followed by 20 mg/kg/day (14 and 7 times the MRHD on a mg/m^2 basis, respectively) through 128 weeks.

Memantine produced no evidence of genotoxic potential when evaluated in the *in vitro S. typhimurium* or *E. coli* reverse mutation assay, an *in vitro* chromosomal aberration test in human lymphocytes, an *in vivo* cytogenetics assay for chromosome damage in rats, and the *in vivo* mouse micronucleus assay. The results were equivocal in an *in vitro* gene mutation assay using Chinese hamster V79 cells.

No impairment of fertility or reproductive performance was seen in rats administered up to 18 mg/kg/day (6 times the MRHD on a mg/m^2 basis) orally from 14 days prior to mating through gestation and lactation in females, or for 60 days prior to mating in males.

13.2 Animal Toxicology

Memantine induced neuronal lesions (vacuolation and necrosis) in the multipolar and pyramidal cells in cortical layers III and IV of the posterior cingulate and retrosplenial neocortices in rats, similar to those which are known to occur in rodents administered other NMDA receptor antagonists. Lesions were seen after a single dose of memantine. In a study in which rats were given daily oral doses of memantine for 14 days, the no-effect dose for neuronal necrosis was 4 times the maximum recommended human dose (MRHD of 28 mg/day) on a mg/m^2 basis.

In a neurotoxicity study, female rats were given oral doses of memantine (3, 10, 30, 60 mg/kg/day) alone or in combination with donepezil (3, 10 mg/kg/day) for 28 days. When administered alone, memantine induced neurodegeneration only at 60 mg/kg/day; however, when administered in combination with 10 mg/kg/day donepezil, memantine induced neurodegeneration at doses of 30 and 60 mg/kg/day. When 60 mg/kg/day memantine and 10 mg/kg/day donepezil were administered in combination, the incidence and severity of neurodegeneration was increased compared to that with 60 mg/kg/day memantine alone or with 30 mg/kg/day memantine in combination with 10 mg/kg/day donepezil. In addition, the combination of 60 mg/kg/day memantine and 10 mg/kg/day donepezil was associated with widespread neurodegeneration in cortical areas (perirhinal, temporal, entorhinal, frontal, insular, piriform) and in olfactory nucleus and subiculum, whereas in the other affected groups, there was limited cortical (entorhinal, retrosplenial) involvement. At the no-effect level of the combination (10 mg/kg/day memantine + 10 mg/kg/day donepezil), plasma exposures of memantine were similar to (AUC) or two times (Cmax) those expected in humans at the MRHD; plasma exposures of donepezil were 3 (AUC) or 6 (Cmax) times those in humans at the MRHD of donepezil (10 mg/day). In a published study, similar donepezil-mediated exacerbation of memantine-induced neurodegeneration was observed in female rats given single doses of memantine in combination with donepezil, both administered by intraperitoneal injection.

The potential for induction of central neurodegenerative lesions by NMDA receptor antagonists in humans is unknown.

14 CLINICAL STUDIES

The effectiveness of NAMENDA XR as a treatment for patients with moderate to severe Alzheimer's disease was based on the results of a double-blind, placebo-controlled trial.

24-week Study of NAMENDA XR Capsules

This was a randomized double-blind clinical investigation in outpatients with moderate to severe Alzheimer's disease (diagnosed by DSM-IV criteria and NINCDS-ADRDA criteria for AD with a Mini Mental State Examination (MMSE) score ≥ 3 and ≤ 14 at Screening and Baseline) receiving acetylcholinesterase inhibitor (AChEI) therapy at a stable dose for 3 months prior to screening. The mean age of patients participating in this trial was 76.5 years with a range of 49-97 years. Approximately 72% of patients were female and 94% were Caucasian.

Study Outcome Measures

The effectiveness of NAMENDA XR was evaluated in this study using the co-primary efficacy parameters of Severe Impairment Battery (SIB) and the Clinician's Interview-Based Impression of Change (CIBIC-Plus).

The ability of NAMENDA XR to improve cognitive performance was assessed with the Severe Impairment Battery (SIB), a multi-item instrument that has been validated for the evaluation of cognitive function in patients with moderate to severe dementia. The SIB examines selected aspects of cognitive performance, including elements of attention, orientation, language, memory, visuospatial ability, construction, praxis, and social interaction. The SIB scoring range is from 0 to 100, with lower scores indicating greater cognitive impairment.

The ability of NAMENDA XR to produce an overall clinical effect was assessed using a Clinician's Interview Based Impression of Change that required the use of caregiver information, the CIBIC-Plus. The CIBIC-Plus is not a single instrument and is not a standardized instrument like the ADCS-ADL or SIB. Clinical trials for investigational drugs have used a variety of CIBIC formats, each different in terms of depth and structure. As such, results from a CIBIC-Plus reflect clinical experience from the trial or trials in which it was used and cannot be compared directly with the results of CIBIC-Plus evaluations from other clinical trials. The CIBIC-Plus used in this trial was a structured instrument based on a comprehensive evaluation at baseline and subsequent time-points of four domains: general (overall clinical status), functional (including activities of daily living), cognitive, and behavioral. It represents the assessment of a skilled clinician using validated scales based on his/her observation during an interview with the patient, in combination with information supplied by a caregiver familiar with the behavior of the patient over the interval rated. The CIBIC-Plus is scored as a seven point categorical rating, ranging from a score of 1, indicating "marked improvement" to a score of 4, indicating "no change" to a score of 7, indicating "marked worsening." The CIBIC-Plus has not been systematically compared directly to assessments not using information from caregivers (CIBIC) or other global methods.

Study Results

In this study, 677 patients were randomized to one of the following 2 treatments: NAMENDA XR 28 mg/day or placebo while still receiving an AChEI (either donepezil, galantamine, or rivastigmine).

Effects on Severe Impairment Battery (SIB)

Figure 1 shows the time course for the change from baseline in SIB score for the two treatment groups completing the 24 weeks of the study. At 24 weeks of treatment, the mean difference in the SIB change scores for the NAMENDA XR 28 mg/AChEI-treated (combination therapy) patients compared to the patients on placebo/AChEI (monotherapy) was 2.6 units. Using an LOCF analysis, NAMENDA XR 28 mg/AChEI treatment was statistically significantly superior to placebo/AChEI.

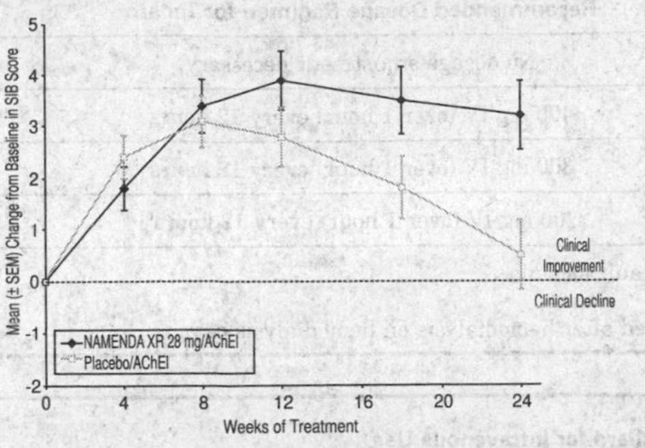

Figure 1: Time course of the change from baseline in SIB score for patients completing 24 weeks of treatment.

Figure 2 shows the cumulative percentages of patients from each treatment group who had attained at least the measure of improvement in SIB score shown on the X axis. The curves show that both patients assigned to NAMENDA XR 28 mg/AChEI and placebo/AChEI have a wide range of responses, but that the NAMENDA XR 28 mg/AChEI group is more likely to show an improvement or a smaller decline.

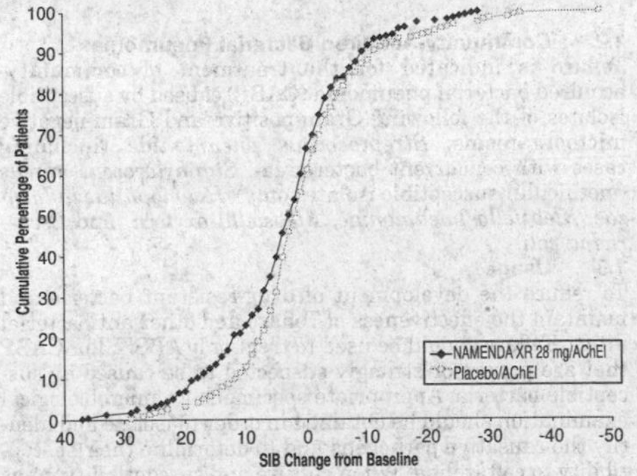

Figure 2: Cumulative percentage of patients completing 24 weeks of double-blind treatment with specified changes from baseline in SIB scores.

Figure 3 shows the time course for the CIBIC-Plus score for patients in the two treatment groups completing the 24 weeks of the study. At 24 weeks of treatment, the mean difference in the CIBIC-Plus scores for the NAMENDA XR 28 mg/AChEI-treated patients compared to the patients on placebo/AChEI was 0.3 units. Using an LOCF analysis, NAMENDA XR 28 mg/AChEI treatment was statistically significantly superior to placebo/AChEI.

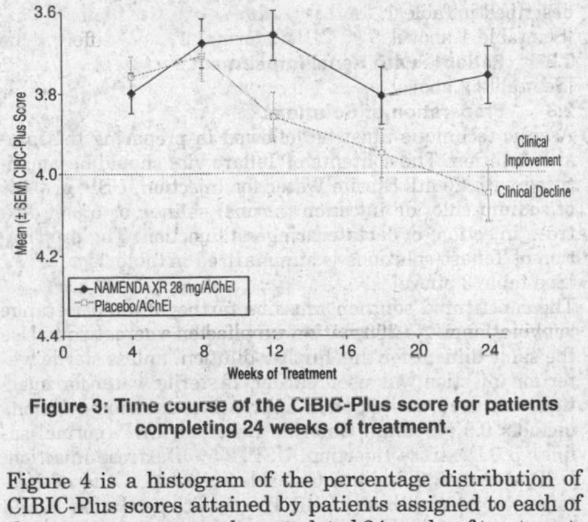

Figure 3: Time course of the CIBIC-Plus score for patients completing 24 weeks of treatment.

Figure 4 is a histogram of the percentage distribution of CIBIC-Plus scores attained by patients assigned to each of the treatment groups who completed 24 weeks of treatment.

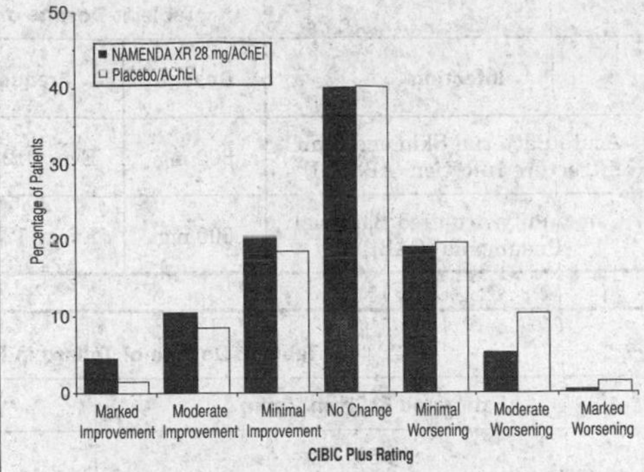

Figure 4: Distribution of CIBIC-Plus ratings at week 24

16 HOW SUPPLIED/STORAGE AND HANDLING

7 mg Capsule:

Yellow opaque capsule, with "FLI 7 mg" black imprint.
Bottle of 30: NDC# 0456-3407-33

14 mg Capsule:

Yellow cap and dark green opaque capsule with "FLI 14 mg" black imprint on the yellow cap.
Bottle of 30: NDC# 0456-3414-33
Bottle of 90: NDC# 0456-3414-90
10 × 10 Unit Dose: NDC# 0456-3414-63

21 mg Capsule:

White to off-white cap and dark green opaque capsule, with "FLI 21 mg" black imprint on the white to off-white cap.
Bottle of 30: NDC# 0456-3421-33

28 mg Capsule:

Dark green opaque capsule, with "FLI 28 mg" white imprint.
Bottle of 30: NDC# 0456-3428-33
Bottle of 90: NDC# 0456-3428-90
10 × 10 Unit Dose: NDC# 0456-3428-63

Titration Pack: NDC# 0456-3400-29

Contains 28 capsules (7 × 7 mg, 7 × 14 mg, 7 × 21 mg, 7 × 28 mg)

Storage

Store at 25°C (77°F); excursions permitted to 15-30°C (59-86°F) [see USP Controlled Room Temperature].

17 PATIENT COUNSELING INFORMATION

See FDA-approved patient labeling.

To assure safe and effective use of NAMENDA XR, the information and instructions provided in the patient information section should be discussed with patients and caregivers.

Patients and caregivers should be instructed to take NAMENDA XR only once per day, as prescribed.

Patients and caregivers should be instructed that NAMENDA XR capsules be swallowed whole. Alternatively, NAMENDA XR capsules may be opened and sprinkled on applesauce and the entire contents should be consumed. The capsules should not be divided, chewed or crushed.

Patients and caregivers should be advised that the product may cause headache, diarrhea and dizziness.

Manufactured for:Forest Pharmaceuticals, Inc.
Subsidiary of Forest Laboratories, Inc.
St. Louis, MO 63045
Manufactured by:
Forest Laboratories Ireland Ltd
Licensed from Merz Pharmaceuticals GmbH

PATIENT INFORMATION

NAMENDA XR [Nuh-MEN-dah Eks-Are]

(memantine hydrochloride) Extended Release Capsules

What is NAMENDA XR and what is it used for?

NAMENDA XR belongs to a class of substances called NMDA antagonists. It is used for the treatment of patients with Alzheimer's disease.

Do not take NAMENDA XR in the following cases:

If you know that you are allergic (hyper-sensitive) to memantine (the active substance in NAMENDA XR) or to any of the other ingredients of NAMENDA XR [see *Description (11)*].

Take special care with NAMENDA XR if:

- You have, or ever had seizures.
- You have, or ever had difficulty passing urine.

If any of these apply to you, your doctor may need to monitor you more closely while you are on this medicine.

NAMENDA XR with food and drink:

NAMENDA XR may be taken with or without food. NAMENDA XR capsules may be opened and sprinkled on applesauce before swallowing, but the contents of the entire capsule should be taken and the dose should not be divided. Except when opened and sprinkled on applesauce, NAMENDA XR capsules must be swallowed whole and never crushed, divided or chewed [see *Dosage and Administration (2)*].

NAMENDA XR and older people:

NAMENDA XR can be used by patients over the age of 65, as well as by patients with Alzheimer's Disease who are aged 65 years or younger.

NAMENDA XR and children:

The use of NAMENDA XR in children is not recommended.

Pregnant women:

Tell your doctor if you are pregnant or planning to become pregnant. In the event of pregnancy, the benefits of NAMENDA XR must be assessed against the possible effects on your unborn child. Ask your doctor or pharmacist for advice before taking any medicine during pregnancy.

Breast-feeding mothers:

You should not breast-feed during treatment with NAMENDA XR. Ask your doctor or pharmacist for advice before taking any medicine while you are breast-feeding.

Taking other medicines:

Tell your doctor or pharmacist about any other medicines you are taking or have recently taken, including any you have taken without a prescription.

How to use NAMENDA XR:

Follow all instructions given to you by your doctor carefully, even if they differ from the ones given in this leaflet.

How to start treatment:

Treatment begins at a low dose (7 mg, once a day) and is gradually increased until the target dose (28 mg, once a day) is reached. To be effective, NAMENDA XR must be taken correctly, according to the following schedule:

Week 1: Start on Day 1
Take one 7 mg capsule each day.
Week 2: Start on Day 8
Take one 14 mg capsule each day.
Week 3: Start on Day 15
Take one 21 mg capsule each day.
Week 4: Start on Day 22
Take one 28 mg capsule each day.

Once the target dose (28 mg, once a day) has been reached, you can continue with that daily schedule unless told otherwise by your healthcare professional. (For patients with severe renal impairment, 14 mg once a day is the recommended dose.)

During the course of treatment, your healthcare professional may change the dose to suit your individual needs.

If you are currently taking another formulation of memantine, talk to your healthcare professional about how to switch to NAMENDA XR.

What to do if you take more NAMENDA XR capsules than you should:

If you accidentally take more NAMENDA XR capsules than you should, inform your healthcare professional that you have accidentally taken more NAMENDA XR than you should have. You may require medical attention. Some people who have accidentally taken too much memantine have experienced dizziness, unsteadiness, weakness, tiredness, confusion, as well as other symptoms.

If you forget to take NAMENDA XR:

If you forget to take one dose of NAMENDA XR, do not double-up on your next dose. Take only your next dose as scheduled.

If you have forgotten to take NAMENDA XR for several days, do not take the next dose until you have talked to your healthcare professional.

Possible side effects:

Like all medicines, NAMENDA XR can cause side effects, although not everyone gets them.

Do not be alarmed by this list of possible side effects. You may not experience any of them.

The most common side effects in patients taking NAMENDA XR were headache, diarrhea and dizziness.

How to store NAMENDA XR:

Do not use NAMENDA XR after the expiration date shown on the carton and bottle.

Store at 25°C (77°F).

Do not use any capsules of NAMENDA XR that are damaged or show signs of tampering.

Keep NAMENDA XR out of the reach and sight of children and pets.

Manufactured for:Forest Pharmaceuticals, Inc.
Subsidiary of Forest Laboratories, Inc.
St. Louis, MO 63045
Manufactured by:
Forest Laboratories Ireland Ltd
Licensed from Merz Pharmaceuticals GmbH

Shown in Product Identification Guide, page 306

TEFLARO® ℞
(ceftaroline fosamil)
injection for intravenous (IV) use

HIGHLIGHTS OF PRESCRIBING INFORMATION

These highlights do not include all the information needed to use TEFLARO safely and effectively. See full prescribing information for TEFLARO.

TEFLARO® (ceftaroline fosamil) injection for intravenous (IV) use
Initial U.S. Approval: 2010

To reduce the development of drug-resistant bacteria and maintain the effectiveness of TEFLARO and other antibacterial drugs, Teflaro should be used only to treat infections that are proven or strongly suspected to be caused by bacteria.

RECENT MAJOR CHANGES

Dosage and Administration (2.3) 10/2012

INDICATIONS AND USAGE

Teflaro® is a cephalosporin antibacterial indicated for the treatment of the following infections caused by designated susceptible bacteria:

- Acute bacterial skin and skin structure infections (ABSSSI) (1.1)
- Community-acquired bacterial pneumonia (CABP) (1.2)

DOSAGE AND ADMINISTRATION

- 600 mg every 12 hours by IV infusion administered over 1 hour in adults ≥ 18 years of age (2.1)
- Dosage adjustment in patients with renal impairment (2.2)

Estimated Creatinine Clearance[#] (mL/min)	Teflaro Dosage Regimen
>50	No dosage adjustment necessary
>30 to ≤ 50	400 mg IV (over 1 hour) every 12 hours
≥ 15 to ≤ 30	300 mg IV (over 1 hour) every 12 hours
End-stage renal disease (ESRD), including hemodialysis	200 mg IV (over 1 hour) every 12 hours

[#]As calculated using the Cockcroft-Gault formula

DOSAGE FORMS AND STRENGTHS

600 mg or 400 mg of sterile Teflaro powder in single-use 20 mL vials. (3)

CONTRAINDICATIONS

- Known serious hypersensitivity to ceftaroline or other members of the cephalosporin class. (4)

WARNINGS AND PRECAUTIONS

- Serious hypersensitivity (anaphylactic) reactions have been reported with beta-lactam antibiotics, including ceftaroline. Exercise caution in patients with known hypersensitivity to beta-lactam antibiotics. (5.1)
- *Clostridium difficile*-associated diarrhea (CDAD) has been reported with nearly all systemic antibacterial agents, including Teflaro. Evaluate if diarrhea occurs. (5.2)
- Direct Coombs' test seroconversion has been reported with Teflaro. If anemia develops during or after therapy, a diagnostic workup for drug-induced hemolytic anemia should be performed and consideration given to discontinuation of Teflaro. (5.3)

ADVERSE REACTIONS

The most common adverse reactions occurring in >2 % of patients are diarrhea, nausea, and rash. (6.3)

To report SUSPECTED ADVERSE REACTIONS, contact Forest Pharmaceuticals, Inc., at 1-800-678-1605 or FDA at 1-800-FDA-1088 orwww.fda.gov/medwatch.

USE IN SPECIFIC POPULATIONS

Dosage adjustment is required in patients with moderate or severe renal impairment and in ESRD patients, including patients on hemodialysis. (2.2,12.3)

See 17 for PATIENT COUNSELING INFORMATION

Revised: 07/2013

FULL PRESCRIBING INFORMATION: CONTENTS*

*** Sections or subsections omitted from the full prescribing information are not listed**

FULL PRESCRIBING INFORMATION

1. INDICATIONS AND USAGE

Teflaro® (ceftaroline fosamil) is indicated for the treatment of patients with the following infections caused by susceptible isolates of the designated microorganisms.

1.1 Acute Bacterial Skin and Skin Structure Infections

Teflaro is indicated for the treatment of acute bacterial skin and skin structure infections (ABSSSI) caused by susceptible isolates of the following Gram-positive and Gram-negative microorganisms: *Staphylococcus aureus* (including methicillin-susceptible and -resistant isolates), *Streptococcus pyogenes, Streptococcus agalactiae, Escherichia coli, Klebsiella pneumoniae, and Klebsiella oxytoca.*

1.2 Community-Acquired Bacterial Pneumonia

Teflaro is indicated for the treatment of community-acquired bacterial pneumonia (CABP) caused by susceptible isolates of the following Gram-positive and Gram-negative microorganisms: *Streptococcus pneumoniae* (including cases with concurrent bacteremia), *Staphylococcus aureus* (methicillin-susceptible isolates only), *Haemophilus influenzae, Klebsiella pneumoniae, Klebsiella oxytoca,* and *Escherichia coli.*

1.3 Usage

To reduce the development of drug-resistant bacteria and maintain the effectiveness of Teflaro and other antibacterial drugs, Teflaro should be used to treat only ABSSSI or CABP that are proven or strongly suspected to be caused by susceptible bacteria. Appropriate specimens for microbiological examination should be obtained in order to isolate and identify the causative pathogens and to determine their susceptibility to ceftaroline. When culture and susceptibility information are available, they should be considered in selecting or modifying antibacterial therapy. In the absence of such data, local epidemiology and susceptibility patterns may contribute to the empiric selection of therapy.

2. DOSAGE AND ADMINISTRATION

2.1 Recommended Dosage

The recommended dosage of Teflaro is 600 mg administered every 12 hours by intravenous (IV) infusion over 1 hour in patients ≥ 18 years of age. The duration of therapy should be guided by the severity and site of infection and the patient's clinical and bacteriological progress.

The recommended dosage and administration by infection is described inTable 1.

[See table 1 above]

Table 1: Dosage of Teflaro by Infection

Infection	Dosage	Frequency	Infusion Time (hours)	Recommended Duration of Total Antimicrobial Treatment
Acute Bacterial Skin and Skin Structure Infection (ABSSSI)	600 mg	Every 12 hours	1	5-14 days
Community-Acquired Bacterial Pneumonia (CABP)	600 mg	Every 12 hours	1	5-7 days

2.2 Patients with Renal Impairment

[See table 2 above]

Table 2: Dosage of Teflaro in Patients with Renal Impairment

Estimated CrCl[a](mL/min)	Recommended Dosage Regimen for Teflaro
>50	No dosage adjustment necessary
>30 to ≤ 50	400 mg IV (over 1 hour) every 12 hours
≥ 15 to ≤ 30	300 mg IV (over 1 hour) every 12 hours
End-stage renal disease, including hemodialysis[b]	200 mg IV (over 1 hour) every 12 hours[c]

[a]Creatinine clearance (CrCl) estimated using the Cockcroft-Gault formula.
[b]End-stage renal disease is defined as CrCl < 15 mL/min.
[c]Teflaro is hemodialyzable; thus Teflaro should be administered after hemodialysis on hemodialysis days.

2.3 Preparation of Solutions

Aseptic technique must be followed in preparing the infusion solution. The contents of Teflaro vial should be constituted with 20 mL Sterile Water for Injection, USP; or 0.9% of sodium chloride injection (normal saline); or 5% of dextrose injection; or lactated ringer's injection. The preparation of Teflaro solutions is summarized inTable 3.

[See table 3 above]

Table 3: Preparation of Teflaro for Intravenous Use

Dosage Strength (mg)	Volume of Diluent To Be Added (mL)	Approximate Ceftaroline fosamil Concentration (mg/mL)	Amount to Be Withdrawn
400	20	20	Total Volume
600	20	30	Total Volume

The constituted solution must be further diluted in range between 50 mL to 250 mL before infusion into patients. Use the same diluent for this further dilution, unless sterile water for injection was used earlier. If sterile water for injection was used earlier, then appropriate infusion solutions include: 0.9% Sodium Chloride Injection, USP (normal saline); 5% Dextrose Injection, USP; 2.5% Dextrose Injection, USP, and 0.45% Sodium Chloride Injection, USP; or Lactated Ringer's Injection, USP. The resulting solution should be administered over approximately 1 hour.

Constitution time is less than 2 minutes. Mix gently to constitute and check to see that the contents have dissolved completely. Parenteral drug products should be inspected visually for particulate matter prior to administration.
The color of Teflaro infusion solutions ranges from clear, light to dark yellow depending on the concentration and storage conditions. When stored as recommended, the product potency is not affected.
Studies have shown that the constituted solution in the infusion bag should be used within 6 hours when stored at room temperature or within 24 hours when stored under refrigeration at 2 to 8° C (36 to 46° F).
The compatibility of Teflaro with other drugs has not been established. Teflaro should not be mixed with or physically added to solutions containing other drugs.

Only for the 50 mL infusion bags dilution, see the instructions listed in 2.3.1 and 2.3.2.

2.3.1 Preparation of 600 mg of Teflaro dose in 50 mL
Withdraw 20 mL of diluent from the infusion bag. Proceed to inject entire content of the Teflaro vial into the bag to provide a total volume of 50 mL. The resultant concentration is approximately 12 mg/mL.

2.3.2 Preparation of 400 mg of Teflaro dose in 50 mL
Withdraw 20 mL of diluent from the infusion bag. Proceed to inject entire content of the Teflaro vial into the bag to provide a total volume of 50 mL. The resultant concentration is approximately 8 mg/mL.

3. DOSAGE FORMS AND STRENGTHS

Teflaro is supplied in single-use, clear glass vials containing either 600 mg or 400 mg of sterile ceftaroline fosamil powder.

4. CONTRAINDICATIONS

Teflaro is contraindicated in patients with known serious hypersensitivity to ceftaroline or other members of the cephalosporin class. Anaphylaxis and anaphylactoid reactions have been reported with ceftaroline.

5. WARNINGS AND PRECAUTIONS

5.1 Hypersensitivity Reactions

Serious and occasionally fatal hypersensitivity (anaphylactic) reactions and serious skin reactions have been reported in patients receiving beta-lactam antibacterials. Before therapy with Teflaro is instituted, careful inquiry about previous hypersensitivity reactions to other cephalosporins, penicillins, or carbapenems should be made. If this product is to be given to a penicillin- or other beta-lactam-allergic patient, caution should be exercised because cross sensitivity among beta-lactam antibacterial agents has been clearly established.
If an allergic reaction to Teflaro occurs, the drug should be discontinued. Serious acute hypersensitivity (anaphylactic) reactions require emergency treatment with epinephrine and other emergency measures, that may include airway management, oxygen, intravenous fluids, antihistamines, corticosteroids, and vasopressors as clinically indicated.

5.2 *Clostridium difficile*-associated Diarrhea

Clostridium difficile-associated diarrhea (CDAD) has been reported for nearly all systemic antibacterial agents, including Teflaro, and may range in severity from mild diarrhea to fatal colitis.
Treatment with antibacterial agents alters the normal flora of the colon and may permit overgrowth of *C. difficile*.
C. difficile produces toxins A and B which contribute to the development of CDAD. Hypertoxin-producing strains of *C. difficile* cause increased morbidity and mortality, as these infections can be refractory to antimicrobial therapy and may require colectomy. CDAD must be considered in all patients who present with diarrhea following antibiotic use. Careful medical history is necessary because CDAD has been reported to occur more than 2 months after the administration of antibacterial agents.
If CDAD is suspected or confirmed, antibacterials not directed against *C. difficile* should be discontinued, if possible. Appropriate fluid and electrolyte management, protein supplementation, antibiotic treatment of *C. difficile*, and surgical evaluation should be instituted as clinically indicated *[see Adverse Reactions (6.3)]*.

5.3 Direct Coombs' Test Seroconversion

Seroconversion from a negative to a positive direct Coombs' test result occurred in 120/1114 (10.8%) of patients receiving Teflaro and 49/1116 (4.4%) of patients receiving comparator drugs in the four pooled Phase 3 trials.
In the pooled Phase 3 CABP trials, 51/520 (9.8%) of Teflaro-treated patients compared to 24/534 (4.5%) of ceftriaxone-treated patients seroconverted from a negative to a positive direct Coombs' test result. No adverse reactions representing hemolytic anemia were reported in any treatment group.
If anemia develops during or after treatment with Teflaro, drug-induced hemolytic anemia should be considered. Diagnostic studies including a direct Coombs' test, should be performed. If drug-induced hemolytic anemia is suspected, discontinuation of Teflaro should be considered and supportive care should be administered to the patient (i.e. transfusion) if clinically indicated.

5.4 Development of Drug-Resistant Bacteria

Prescribing Teflaro in the absence of a proven or strongly suspected bacterial infection is unlikely to provide benefit to the patient and increases the risk of the development of drug-resistant bacteria.

6. ADVERSE REACTIONS

The following serious events are described in greater detail in the Warnings and Precautions section
- Hypersensitivity reactions *[see Warnings and Precautions (5.1)]*
- *Clostridium difficile*-associated diarrhea *[see Warnings and Precautions (5.2)]*
- Direct Coombs' test seroconversion *[see Warnings and Precautions (5.3)]*

6.1 Adverse Reactions from Clinical Trials

Because clinical trials are conducted under widely varying conditions, adverse reaction rates observed in clinical trials of a drug cannot be compared directly to rates from clinical trials of another drug and may not reflect rates observed in practice.
Teflaro was evaluated in four controlled comparative Phase 3 clinical trials (two in ABSSSI and two in CABP) which included 1300 adult patients treated with Teflaro (600 mg administered by IV over 1 hour every 12h) and 1297 patients treated with comparator (vancomycin plus aztreonam or ceftriaxone) for a treatment period up to 21 days. The median age of patients treated with Teflaro was 54 years, ranging between 18 and 99 years old. Patients treated with Teflaro were predominantly male (63%) and Caucasian (82%).

6.2 Serious Adverse Events and Adverse Events Leading to Discontinuation

In the four pooled Phase 3 clinical trials, serious adverse events occurred in 98/1300 (7.5%) of patients receiving Teflaro and 100/1297 (7.7%) of patients receiving comparator drugs. The most common SAEs in both the Teflaro and comparator treatment groups were in the respiratory and infection system organ classes (SOC). Treatment discontinuation due to adverse events occurred in 35/1300 (2.7%) of patients receiving Teflaro and 48/1297 (3.7%) of patients receiving comparator drugs with the most common adverse events leading to discontinuation being hypersensitivity for both treatment groups at a rate of 0.3% in the Teflaro group and 0.5% in comparator group.

6.3 Most Common Adverse Reactions

No adverse reactions occurred in greater than 5% of patients receiving Teflaro. The most common adverse reactions occurring in > 2% of patients receiving Teflaro in the pooled phase 3 clinical trials were diarrhea, nausea, and rash.
Table 4 lists adverse reactions occurring in ≥ 2% of patients receiving Teflaro in the pooled Phase 3 clinical trials.

Table 4: Adverse Reactions Occurring in ≥ 2% of Patients Receiving Teflaro in the Pooled Phase 3 Clinical Trials

System Organ Class/ Preferred Term	Pooled Phase 3 Clinical Trials (four trials, two in ABSSSI and two in CABP)	
	Teflaro (N=1300)	Pooled Comparators[a] (N=1297)
Gastrointestinal disorders		
Diarrhea	5 %	3 %
Nausea	4 %	4 %
Constipation	2 %	2 %
Vomiting	2 %	2 %
Investigations		
Increased transaminases	2%	3 %
Metabolism and nutrition disorders		
Hypokalemia	2 %	3 %
Skin and subcutaneous tissue disorders		
Rash	3%	2%
Vascular disorders		
Phlebitis	2%	1%

[a]Comparators included vancomycin 1 gram IV every 12h plus aztreonam 1 gram IV every 12h in the Phase 3 ABSSSI trials, and ceftriaxone 1 gram IV every 24h in the Phase 3 CABP trials.

6.4 Other Adverse Reactions Observed During Clinical Trials of Teflaro

Following is a list of additional adverse reactions reported by the 1740 patients who received Teflaro in any clinical trial with incidences less than 2%. Events are categorized by System Organ Class.
Blood and lymphatic system disorders- Anemia, Eosinophilia, Neutropenia, Thrombocytopenia
Cardiac disorders- Bradycardia, Palpitations
Gastrointestinal disorders- Abdominal pain
General disorders and administration site conditions- Pyrexia
Hepatobiliary disorders -Hepatitis
Immune system disorders- Hypersensitivity, Anaphylaxis
Infections and infestations- *Clostridium difficile* colitis
Metabolism and nutrition disorders- Hyperglycemia, Hyperkalemia
Nervous system disorders- Dizziness, Convulsion
Renal and urinary disorders- Renal failure
Skin and subcutaneous tissue disorders- Urticaria

7. DRUG INTERACTIONS

No clinical drug-drug interaction studies have been conducted with Teflaro. There is minimal potential for drug-drug interactions between Teflaro and CYP450 substrates, inhibitors, or inducers; drugs known to undergo active renal secretion; and drugs that may alter renal blood flow *[see Clinical Pharmacology (12.3)]*.

8. USE IN SPECIFIC POPULATIONS

8.1 Pregnancy

Category B.
Developmental toxicity studies performed with ceftaroline fosamil in rats at IV doses up to 300 mg/kg demonstrated no maternal toxicity and no effects on the fetus. A separate toxicokinetic study showed that ceftaroline exposure in rats (based on AUC) at this dose level was approximately 8 times the exposure in humans given 600 mg every 12 hours. There were no drug-induced malformations in the offspring of rabbits given IV doses of 25, 50, and 100 mg/kg, despite maternal toxicity. Signs of maternal toxicity appeared secondary to the sensitivity of the rabbit gastrointestinal system to broad-spectrum antibacterials and included changes in fecal output in all groups and dose-related reductions in body weight gain and food consumption at ≥ 50 mg/kg; these were associated with an increase in spontaneous abortion at 50 and 100 mg/kg. The highest dose was also associated with maternal moribundity and mortality. An increased incidence of a common rabbit skeletal variation, angulated hyoid alae, was also observed at the maternally toxic doses of 50 and 100 mg/kg. A separate toxicokinetic study showed that ceftaroline exposure in rabbits (based on AUC) was approximately 0.8 times the exposure in humans given 600 mg every 12 hours at 25 mg/kg and 1.5 times the human exposure at 50 mg/kg.
Ceftaroline fosamil did not affect the postnatal development or reproductive performance of the offspring of rats given IV doses up to 450 mg/kg/day. Results from a toxicokinetic study conducted in pregnant rats with doses up to 300 mg/kg suggest that exposure was ≥ 8 times the exposure in humans given 600 mg every 12 hours.
There are no adequate and well-controlled trials in pregnant women. Teflaro should be used during pregnancy only if the potential benefit justifies the potential risk to the fetus.

8.3 Nursing Mothers

It is not known whether ceftaroline is excreted in human milk. Because many drugs are excreted in human milk, caution should be exercised when Teflaro is administered to a nursing woman.

8.4 Pediatric Use

Safety and effectiveness in pediatric patients have not been established.

8.5 Geriatric Use

Of the 1300 patients treated with Teflaro in the Phase 3 ABSSSI and CABP trials, 397 (30.5%) were ≥ 65 years of age. The clinical cure rates in the Teflaro group (Clinically Evaluable [CE] Population) were similar in patients ≥ 65 years of age compared with patients < 65 years of age in both the ABSSSI and CABP trials.
The adverse event profiles in patients ≥ 65 years of age and in patients < 65 years of age were similar. The percentage of patients in the Teflaro group who had at least one adverse event was 52.4% in patients ≥ 65 years of age and 42.8% in patients < 65 years of age for the two indications combined. Ceftaroline is excreted primarily by the kidney, and the risk of adverse reactions may be greater in patients with impaired renal function. Because elderly patients are more likely to have decreased renal function, care should be

taken in dose selection in this age group and it may be useful to monitor renal function. Elderly subjects had greater ceftaroline exposure relative to non-elderly subjects when administered the same single dose of Teflaro. However, higher exposure in elderly subjects was mainly attributed to age-related changes in renal function. Dosage adjustment for elderly patients should be based on renal function *[see Dosage and Administration (2.2) and Clinical Pharmacology (12.3)]*.

8.6 Patients with Renal Impairment

Dosage adjustment is required in patients with moderate (CrCl > 30 to ≤ 50 mL/min) or severe (CrCl ≥ 15 to ≤ 30 mL/min) renal impairment and in patients with end-stage renal disease (ESRD – defined as CrCl < 15 mL/min), including patients on hemodialysis (HD) *[see Dosage and Administration (2.2) and Clinical Pharmacology (12.3)]*.

10. OVERDOSAGE

In the event of overdose, Teflaro should be discontinued and general supportive treatment given.

Ceftaroline can be removed by hemodialysis. In subjects with ESRD administered 400 mg of Teflaro, the mean total recovery of ceftaroline in the dialysate following a 4-hour hemodialysis session started 4 hours after dosing was 76.5 mg (21.6% of the dose). However, no information is available on the use of hemodialysis to treat overdosage *[see Clinical Pharmacology (12.3)]*.

11. DESCRIPTION

Teflaro is a sterile, semi-synthetic, broad-spectrum, prodrug antibacterial of cephalosporin class of beta-lactams (β-lactams). Chemically, the prodrug, ceftaroline fosamil monoacetate monohydrate is (6*R*,7*R*)-7-{(2*Z*)-2-(ethoxyimino)-2-[5-(phosphonoamino)-1,2,4-thiadiazol-3-yl]acetamido}-3-{[4-(1-methylpyridin-1-ium-4-yl)-1,3-thiazol-2-yl]sulfanyl}-8-oxo-5-thia-1-azabicyclo[4.2.0]oct-2-ene-2-carboxylate monoacetate monohydrate. Its molecular weight is 762.75. The empirical formula is $C_{22}H_{21}N_8O_8PS_4.C_2H_4O_2.H_2O$.

Figure 1: Chemical structure of ceftaroline fosamil

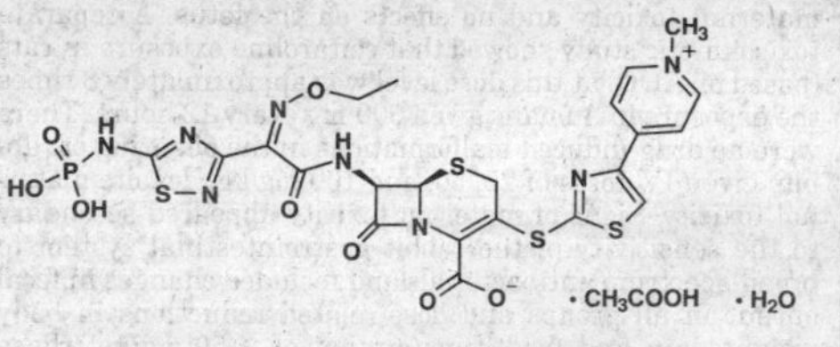

Teflaro vials contain either 600 mg or 400 mg of anhydrous ceftaroline fosamil. The powder for injection is formulated from ceftaroline fosamil monoacetate monohydrate, a pale yellowish-white to light yellow sterile powder. All references to ceftaroline activity are expressed in terms of the prodrug, ceftaroline fosamil. The powder is constituted for IV injection *[see Dosage and Administration (2.3)]*.

Each vial of Teflaro contains ceftaroline fosamil and L-arginine, which results in a constituted solution at pH 4.8 to 6.5.

12. CLINICAL PHARMACOLOGY

Ceftaroline fosamil is the water-soluble prodrug of the bioactive ceftaroline *[see Clinical Pharmacology (12.3)]*.

12.1 Mechanism of Action

Ceftaroline is an antibacterial drug *[see Clinical Pharmacology (12.4)]*.

12.2 Pharmacodynamics

As with other beta-lactam antimicrobial agents, the time that unbound plasma concentration of ceftaroline exceeds the minimum inhibitory concentration (MIC) of the infecting organism has been shown to best correlate with efficacy in a neutropenic murine thigh infection model with *S. aureus* and *S. pneumoniae*.

Exposure-response analysis of Phase 2/3 ABSSSI trials supports the recommended dosage regimen of Teflaro 600 mg every 12 hours by IV infusion over 1 hour. For Phase 3 CABP trials, an exposure-response relationship could not be identified due to the limited range of ceftaroline exposures in the majority of patients.

Cardiac Electrophysiology

In a randomized, positive- and placebo-controlled crossover thorough QTc study, 54 healthy subjects were each administered a single dose of Teflaro 1500 mg, placebo, and a positive control by IV infusion over 1 hour. At the 1500 mg dose of Teflaro, no significant effect on QTc interval was detected at peak plasma concentration or at any other time.

12.3 Pharmacokinetics

The mean pharmacokinetic parameters of ceftaroline in healthy adults (n=6) with normal renal function after single and multiple 1-hour IV infusions of 600 mg ceftaroline fosamil administered every 12 hours are summarized in Table 5. Pharmacokinetic parameters were similar for single and multiple dose administration.

Table 5: Mean (Standard Deviation) Pharmacokinetic Parameters of Ceftaroline IV in Healthy Adults

Parameter	Single 600 mg Dose Administered as a 1-Hour Infusion(n=6)	Multiple 600 mg Doses Administered Every 12 Hours as 1-Hour Infusions for 14 Days(n=6)
C_{max}(mcg/mL)	19.0 (0.71)	21.3 (4.10)
T_{max}(h)[a]	1.00 (0.92-1.25)	0.92 (0.92-1.08)
AUC (mcg·h/mL)[b]	56.8 (9.31)	56.3 (8.90)
$T_{1/2}$(h)	1.60 (0.38)	2.66 (0.40)
CL (L/h)	9.58 (1.85)	9.60 (1.40)

[a]Reported as median (range)

[b]$AUC_{0-\infty}$ for single-dose administration, AUC_{0-tau} for multiple-dose administration, C_{max}, maximum observed concentration; T_{max}, time of C_{max}; $AUC_{0-\infty}$, area under concentration-time curve from time 0 to infinity; AUC_{0-tau}, area under concentration-time curve over dosing interval (0-12 hours); $T_{1/2}$, terminal elimination half-life; CL, plasma clearance

The C_{max} and AUC of ceftaroline increase approximately in proportion to dose within the single dose range of 50 to 1000 mg. No appreciable accumulation of ceftaroline is observed following multiple IV infusions of 600 mg administered every 12 hours for up to 14 days in healthy adults with normal renal function.

Distribution

The average binding of ceftaroline to human plasma proteins is approximately 20% and decreases slightly with increasing concentrations over 1-50 mcg/mL (14.5-28.0%). The median (range) steady-state volume of distribution of ceftaroline in healthy adult males (n=6) following a single 600 mg IV dose of radiolabeled ceftaroline fosamil was 20.3 L (18.3-21.6 L), similar to extracellular fluid volume.

Metabolism

Ceftaroline fosamil is converted into bioactive ceftaroline in plasma by a phosphatase enzyme and concentrations of the prodrug are measurable in plasma primarily during IV infusion. Hydrolysis of the beta-lactam ring of ceftaroline occurs to form the microbiologically inactive, open-ring metabolite ceftaroline M-1. The mean (SD) plasma ceftaroline M-1 to ceftaroline $AUC_{0-\infty}$ ratio following a single 600 mg IV infusion of ceftaroline fosamil in healthy adults (n=6) with normal renal function is 28% (3.1%).

When incubated with pooled human liver microsomes, ceftaroline was metabolically stable (< 12% metabolic turnover), indicating that ceftaroline is not a substrate for hepatic CYP450 enzymes.

Excretion

Ceftaroline and its metabolites are primarily eliminated by the kidneys. Following administration of a single 600 mg IV dose of radiolabeled ceftaroline fosamil to healthy male adults (n=6), approximately 88% of radioactivity was recovered in urine and 6% in feces within 48 hours. Of the radioactivity recovered in urine approximately 64% was excreted as ceftaroline and approximately 2% as ceftaroline M-1. The mean (SD) renal clearance of ceftaroline was 5.56 (0.20) L/h, suggesting that ceftaroline is predominantly eliminated by glomerular filtration.

Specific Populations

Renal Impairment

Following administration of a single 600 mg IV dose of Teflaro, the geometric mean $AUC_{0-\infty}$ of ceftaroline in subjects with mild (CrCl > 50 to ≤ 80 mL/min, n=6) or moderate (CrCl > 30 to ≤ 50 mL/min, n=6) renal impairment was 19% and 52% higher, respectively, compared to healthy subjects with normal renal function (CrCl > 80 mL/min, n=6). Following administration of a single 400 mg IV dose of Teflaro, the geometric mean $AUC_{0-\infty}$ of ceftaroline in subjects with severe (CrCl ≥ 15 to ≤30 mL/min, n=6) renal impairment was 115% higher compared to healthy subjects with normal renal function (CrCl > 80 mL/min, n=6). Dosage adjustment is recommended in patients with moderate and severe renal impairment *[see Dosage and Administration (2.2)]*.

A single 400 mg dose of Teflaro was administered to subjects with ESRD (n=6) either 4 hours prior to or 1 hour after hemodialysis (HD). The geometric mean ceftaroline $AUC_{0-\infty}$ following the post-HD infusion was 167% higher compared to healthy subjects with normal renal function (CrCL > 80 mL/min, n=6). The mean recovery of ceftaroline in the dialysate following a 4-hour HD session was 76.5 mg, or 21.6% of the administered dose. Dosage adjustment is recommended in patients with ESRD (defined as CrCL < 15 mL/min), including patients on HD *[see Dosage and Administration (2.2)]*.

Hepatic Impairment

The pharmacokinetics of ceftaroline in patients with hepatic impairment have not been established. As ceftaroline does not appear to undergo significant hepatic metabolism, the systemic clearance of ceftaroline is not expected to be significantly affected by hepatic impairment.

Geriatric Patients

Following administration of a single 600 mg IV dose of Teflaro to healthy elderly subjects (≥ 65 years of age, n=16), the geometric mean $AUC_{0-\infty}$ of ceftaroline was ~33% higher compared to healthy young adult subjects (18-45 years of age, n=16). The difference in $AUC_{0-\infty}$ was mainly attributable to age-related changes in renal function. Dosage adjustment for Teflaro in elderly patients should be based on renal function *[see Dosage and Administration (2.2)]*.

Pediatric Patients

The pharmacokinetics of ceftaroline were evaluated in adolescent patients (ages 12 to 17, n=7) with normal renal function following administration of a single 8 mg/kg IV dose of Teflaro (or 600 mg for subjects weighing > 75 kg). The mean plasma clearance and terminal phase volume of distribution for ceftaroline in adolescent subjects were similar to healthy adults (n=6) in a separate study following administration of a single 600 mg IV dose. However, the mean C_{max} and $AUC_{0-\infty}$ for ceftaroline in adolescent subjects who received a single 8 mg/kg dose were 10% and 23% less than in healthy adult subjects who received a single 600 mg IV dose.

Gender

Following administration of a single 600 mg IV dose of Teflaro to healthy elderly males (n=10) and females (n=6) and healthy young adult males (n=6) and females (n=10), the mean C_{max} and $AUC_{0-\infty}$ for ceftaroline were similar between males and females, although there was a trend for higher C_{max} (17%) and $AUC_{0-\infty}$ (6-15%) in female subjects. Population pharmacokinetic analysis did not identify any significant differences in ceftaroline AUC_{0-tau} based on gender in Phase 2/3 patients with ABSSSI or CABP. No dose adjustment is recommended based on gender.

Race

A population pharmacokinetic analysis was performed to evaluate the impact of race on the pharmacokinetics of ceftaroline using data from Phase 2/3 ABSSSI and CABP trials. No significant differences in ceftaroline AUC_{0-tau} was observed across White (n=35), Hispanic (n=34), and Black (n=17) race groups for ABSSSI patients. Patients enrolled in CABP trials were predominantly categorized as White (n=115); thus there were too few patients of other races to draw any conclusions. No dosage adjustment is recommended based on race.

Drug Interactions

In vitro studies in human liver microsomes indicate that ceftaroline does not inhibit the major cytochrome P450 isoenzymes CYP1A1, CYP1A2, CYP2A6, CYP2B6, CYP2C8, CYP2C9, CYP2C19, CYP2D6, CYP2E1 and CYP3A4. *In vitro* studies in human hepatocytes also demonstrate that ceftaroline and its inactive open-ring metabolite are not inducers of CYP1A2, CYP2B6, CYP2C8, CYP2C9, CYP2C19, or CYP3A4/5. Therefore Teflaro is not expected to inhibit or induce the clearance of drugs that are metabolized by these metabolic pathways in a clinically relevant manner.

Population pharmacokinetic analysis did not identify any clinically relevant differences in ceftaroline exposure (C_{max}, and AUC_{0-tau}) in Phase 2/3 patients with ABSSSI or CABP who were taking concomitant medications that are known inhibitors, inducers, or substrates of the cytochrome P450 system; anionic or cationic drugs known to undergo active renal secretion; and vasodilator or vasoconstrictor drugs that may alter renal blood flow.

12.4 Microbiology

Mode of Action

Ceftaroline is a cephalosporin with *in vitro* activity against Gram-positive and -negative bacteria. The bactericidal action of ceftaroline is mediated through binding to essential penicillin-binding proteins (PBPs). Ceftaroline is bactericidal against *S. aureus* due to its affinity for PBP2a and against *Streptococcus pneumoniae* due to its affinity for PBP2x.

Mechanisms of Resistance

Ceftaroline is not active against Gram-negative bacteria producing extended spectrum beta-lactamases (ESBLs) from the TEM, SHV or CTX-M families, serine carbapenemases (such as KPC), class B metallo-beta-lactamases, or class C (AmpC cephalosporinases).

Cross-Resistance

Although cross-resistance may occur, some isolates resistant to other cephalosporins may be susceptible to ceftaroline.

Interaction with Other Antimicrobials

In vitro studies have not demonstrated any antagonism between ceftaroline or other commonly used antibacterial agents (e.g., vancomycin, linezolid, daptomycin, levofloxacin, azithromycin, amikacin, aztreonam, tigecycline, and meropenem).

Ceftaroline has been shown to be active against most of the following bacteria, both *in vitro* and in clinical infections *[see Indications and Usage (1)]*.

Skin Infections

Gram-positive bacteria
Staphylococcus aureus (including methicillin-susceptible and -resistant isolates)
Streptococcus pyogenes
Streptococcus agalactiae
Gram-negative bacteria
Escherichia coli
Klebsiella pneumoniae
Klebsiella oxytoca

Community-Acquired Bacterial Pneumonia (CABP)

Gram-positive bacteria
Streptococcus pneumoniae
Staphylococcus aureus (methicillin-susceptible isolates only)
Gram-negative bacteria
Haemophilus influenzae
Klebsiella pneumoniae
Klebsiella oxytoca
Escherichia coli

The following *in vitro* data are available, but their clinical significance is unknown. Ceftaroline exhibits *in vitro* MICs of 1 mcg/mL or less against most (≥ 90%) isolates of the following bacteria; however, the safety and effectiveness of Teflaro in treating clinical infections due to these bacteria have not been established in adequate and well-controlled clinical trials.

Gram-positive bacteria
Streptococcus dysgalactiae
Gram-negative bacteria
Citrobacter koseri
Citrobacter freundii
Enterobacter cloacae
Enterobacter aerogenes
Moraxella catarrhalis
Morganella morganii
Proteus mirabilis
Haemophilus parainfluenzae

Susceptibility Test Methods

When available, the clinical microbiology laboratory should provide the results of *in vitro* susceptibility test results for antimicrobial drugs used in local hospitals and practice areas to the physician as periodic reports that describe the susceptibility profile of nosocomial and community-acquired pathogens. These reports should aid the physician in selecting an antibacterial drug product for treatment.

Dilution Techniques

Quantitative methods are used to determine antimicrobial minimum inhibitory concentrations (MICs). These MICs provide estimates of the susceptibility of bacteria to antimicrobial compounds. The MICs should be determined using a standardized test method[1,3], (broth, and/or agar). Broth dilution MICs need to be read within 18 hours due to degradation of ceftaroline activity by 24 hours. The MIC values should be interpreted according to the criteria in Table 6.

Diffusion Techniques

Quantitative methods that require measurement of zone diameters can also provide reproducible estimates of the susceptibility of bacteria to antimicrobial compounds. The zone size provides an estimate of the susceptibility of bacteria to antimicrobial compounds. The zone size should be determined using a standardized method. This procedure uses paper disks impregnated with 30 mcg of ceftaroline to test the susceptibility of bacteria to ceftaroline. The disk diffusion interpretive criteria are provided in Table 6.

[See table 6 above]

A report of "Susceptible" indicates that the antimicrobial is likely to inhibit growth of the pathogen if the antimicrobial compound reaches the concentration at the infection site necessary to inhibit growth of the pathogen. A report of "Intermediate" indicates that the result should be considered equivocal, and if the microorganism is not fully susceptible to alternative clinically feasible drugs, the test should be repeated. This category implies possible clinical applicability in body sites where the drug is physiologically concentrated. This category also provides a buffer zone that prevents small uncontrolled technical factors from causing major discrepancies in interpretation. A report of "Resistant" indicates that the antimicrobial is not likely to inhibit growth of the pathogen if the antimicrobial compound reaches the concentrations usually achievable at the infection site; other therapy should be selected.

Quality Control

Standardized susceptibility test procedures require the use of laboratory controls to monitor and ensure the accuracy and precision of supplies and reagents used in the assay, and the techniques of the individuals performing the test.[1, 2, 3] Standard ceftaroline powder should provide the following range of MIC values provided in Table 7. For the diffusion technique using the 30-mcg ceftaroline disk the criteria provided in Table 7 should be achieved.

[See table 7 above]

Table 6: Susceptibility Interpretive Criteria for Ceftaroline

Pathogen and Isolate Source	Minimum Inhibitory Concentrations (mcg/mL)			Disk Diffusion Zone Diameter (mm)		
	S	I	R	S	I	R
Staphylococcus aureus (includes methicillin-resistant isolates - skin isolates only) -See **NOTE** below	≤ 1	2	≥ 4	≥ 24	21-23	≤ 20
Streptococcus agalactiae[a] (skin isolates only)	≤ 0.5	—	—	≥ 26	—	—
Streptococcus pyogenes[a] (skin isolates only)	≤ 0.5	—	—	≥ 26	—	—
Streptococcus pneumoniae[a] (CABP isolates only)	≤ 0.5	—	—	≥ 26	—	—
Haemophilus influenzae[a] (CABP isolates only)	≤ 0. 5	—	—	≥ 30	—	—
Enterobacteriaceae [b] (CABP and skin isolates)	≤ 0.5	1	≥ 2	≥ 23	20-22	≤ 19

S = susceptible, I = intermediate, R = resistant

NOTE: Clinical efficacy of Teflaro to treat lower respiratory infections such as community-acquired bacterial pneumonia due to MRSA has not been studied in adequate and well controlled trials (See "Clinical Trials" section 14)

[a] The current absence of resistant isolates precludes defining any results other than "Susceptible." Isolates yielding MIC results other than "Susceptible" should be submitted to a reference laboratory for further testing.

[b] Clinical efficacy was shown for the following *Enterobacteriaceae: Escherichia coli, Klebsiella pneumoniae, and Klebsiella oxytoca.*

Table 7: Acceptable Quality Control Ranges for Susceptibility Testing

Quality Control Organism	Minimum Inhibitory Concentrations (mcg/mL)	Disk Diffusion (zone diameters in mm)
Staphylococcus aureus ATCC 25923	Not Applicable	26-35
Staphylococcus aureus ATCC 29213	0.12-0.5	Not Applicable
Escherichia coli ATCC 25922	0.03-0.12	26-34
Haemophilus influenzae ATCC 49247	0.03-0.12	29-39
Streptococcus pneumoniae ATCC 49619	0.008-0.03	31-41

ATCC = American Type Culture Collection

Table 8: Clinical Responders at Study Day 3 from Two Phase 3 ABSSSI Trials

	Teflaro n/N (%)	Vancomycin/ Aztreonam n/N (%)	Treatment Difference (2-sided 95% CI)
ABSSSI Trial 1	148/200 (74.0)	135/209 (64.6)	9.4 (0.4, 18.2)
ABSSSI Trial 2	148/200 (74.0)	128/188 (68.1)	5.9 (-3.1, 14.9)

13. NONCLINICAL TOXICOLOGY

13.1 Carcinogenesis, Mutagenesis, Impairment of Fertility

Long-term carcinogenicity studies have not been conducted with ceftaroline.

Ceftaroline fosamil did not show evidence of mutagenic activity in *in vitro* tests that included a bacterial reverse mutation assay and the mouse lymphoma assay. Ceftaroline was not mutagenic in an *in vitro* mammalian cell assay. *In vivo*, ceftaroline fosamil did not induce unscheduled DNA synthesis in rat hepatocytes and did not induce the formation of micronucleated erythrocytes in mouse or rat bone marrow. Both ceftaroline fosamil and ceftaroline were clastogenic in the absence of metabolic activation in an *in vitro* chromosomal aberration assays, but not in the presence of metabolic activation.

IV injection of ceftaroline fosamil had no adverse effects on fertility of male and female rats given up to 450 mg/kg. This is approximately 4-fold higher than the maximum recommended human dose based on body surface area.

14. CLINICAL TRIALS

14.1 Acute Bacterial Skin and Skin Structure Infections (ABSSSI)

A total of 1396 adults with clinically documented complicated skin and skin structure infection were enrolled in two identical randomized, multi-center, multinational, double-blind, non-inferiority trials (Trials 1 and 2) comparing Teflaro (600 mg administered IV over 1 hour every 12 hours) to vancomycin plus aztreonam (1 g vancomycin administered IV over 1 hour followed by 1 g aztreonam administered IV over 1 hour every 12 hours). Treatment duration was 5 to 14 days. A switch to oral therapy was not allowed. The Modified Intent-to-Treat (MITT) population included all patients who received any amount of study drug according to their randomized treatment group. The CE population included patients in the MITT population who demonstrated sufficient adherence to the protocol.

To evaluate the treatment effect of ceftaroline, an analysis was conducted in 797 patients with ABSSSI (such as deep/extensive cellulitis or a wound infection [surgical or traumatic]) for whom the treatment effect of antibacterials may be supported by historical evidence. This analysis evaluated responder rates based on achieving both cessation of lesion spread and absence of fever on Trial Day 3 in the following subgroup of patients:

Patients with lesion size ≥ 75 cm^2 and having one of the following infection types:

- Major abscess with ≥ 5 cm of surrounding erythema
- Wound infection
- Deep/extensive cellulitis

The results of this analysis are shown in Table 8.

Table 9: Clinical Cure Rates at TOC from Two Phase 3 ABSSSI Trials

	Teflaro n/N (%)	Vancomycin/ Aztreonam n/N (%)	Treatment Difference (2-sided 95% CI)
Trial 1			
CE	288/316 (91.1)	280/300 (93.3)	-2.2 (-6.6, 2.1)
MITT	304/351 (86.6)	297/347 (85.6)	1.0 (-4.2, 6.2)
Trial 2			
CE	271/294 (92.2)	269/292 (92.1)	0.1 (-4.4., 4.5)
MITT	291/342 (85.1)	289/338 (85.5)	-0.4 (-5.8, 5.0)

Table 10: Clinical Cure Rates at TOC by Pathogen from Two Integrated Phase 3 ABSSSI Trials

	Teflaro n/N (%)	Vancomycin/Aztreonam n/N (%)
Gram-positive:		
MSSA (methicillin-susceptible)	212/228 (93.0%)	225/238 (94.5%)
MRSA (methicillin-resistant)	142/152 (93.4%)	115/122 (94.3%)
Streptococcus pyogenes	56/56 (100%)	56/58 (96.6%)
Streptococcus agalactiae	21/22 (95.5%)	18/18 (100%)
Gram-negative:		
Escherichia coli	20/21 (95.2%)	19/21 (90.5%)
Klebsiella pneumoniae	17/18 (94.4%)	13/14 (92.9%)
Klebsiella oxytoca	10/12 (83.3%)	6/6 (100%)

Table 11: Response Rates at Study Day 4 (72-96 hours) from Two Phase 3 CABP Trials

	Teflaro n/N (%)	Ceftriaxone n/N (%)	Treatment Difference (2-sided 95% CI)
CABP Trial 1	48/69 (69.6%)	42/72 (58.3%)	11.2 (-4.6,26.5)
CABP Trial 2	58/84 (69.0%)	51/83 (61.4%)	7.6 (-6.8,21.8)

Table 12: Clinical Cure Rates at TOC from Two Phase 3 CABP Trials

	Teflaro n/N (%)	Ceftriaxone n/N (%)	Treatment Difference (2-sided 95% CI)
CABP Trial 1			
CE	194/224 (86.6%)	183/234 (78.2%)	8.4 (1.4, 15.4)
MITTE	244/291 (83.8%)	233/300 (77.7%)	6.2 (-0.2, 12.6)
CABP Trial 2			
CE	191/232 (82.3%)	165/214 (77.1%)	5.2 (-2.2, 12.8)
MITTE	231/284 (81.3%)	203/269 (75.5%)	5.9 (-1.0, 12.8)

[See table 8 at top of previous page]

The protocol-specified analyses included clinical cure rates at the Test of Cure (TOC) (visit 8 to 15 days after the end of therapy) in the co-primary CE and MITT populations (Table 9) and clinical cure rates at TOC by pathogen in the Microbiologically Evaluable (ME) population (Table 10). However, there are insufficient historical data to establish the magnitude of drug effect for antibacterial drugs compared with placebo at a TOC time point. Therefore, comparisons of Teflaro to vancomycin plus aztreonam based on clinical response rates at TOC can not be utilized to establish non-inferiority.

[See table 9 above]
[See table 10 above]

14.2 Community-Acquired Bacterial Pneumonia (CABP)

A total of 1231 adults with a diagnosis of CABP were enrolled in two randomized, multi-center, multinational, double-blind, non-inferiority trials (Trials 1 and 2) comparing Teflaro (600 mg administered IV over 1 hour every 12 hours) with ceftriaxone (1 g ceftriaxone administered IV over 30 minutes every 24 hours). In both treatment groups of CABP Trial 1, two doses of oral clarithromycin (500 mg every 12 hours), were administered as adjunctive therapy starting on Study Day 1. No adjunctive macrolide therapy was used in CABP Trial 2. Patients with known or suspected MRSA were excluded from both trials. Patients with new or progressive pulmonary infiltrate(s) on chest radiography and signs and symptoms consistent with CABP with the need for hospitalization and IV therapy were enrolled in the trials. Treatment duration was 5 to 7 days. A switch to oral therapy was not allowed. Among all subjects who received any amount of study drug in the two CABP trials, the 30-day all-cause mortality rates were 11/609 (1.8%) for the Teflaro group vs. 12/610 (2.0%) for the ceftriaxone group, and the difference in mortality rates was not statistically significant.

To evaluate the treatment effect of ceftaroline, an analysis was conducted in CABP patients for whom the treatment effect of antibacterials may be supported by historical evidence. The analysis endpoint required subjects to meet sign and symptom criteria at Day 4 of therapy: a responder had to both (a) be in stable condition according to consensus treatment guidelines of the Infectious Diseases Society of America and American Thoracic Society, based on temperature, heart rate, respiratory rate, blood pressure, oxygen saturation, and mental status;[4] (b) show improvement from baseline on at least one symptom of cough, dyspnea, pleuritic chest pain, or sputum production, while not worsening on any of these four symptoms. The analysis used a microbiological intent-to-treat population (mITT population) containing only subjects with a confirmed bacterial pathogen at baseline. Results for this analysis are presented in Table 11.

[See table 11 above]

The protocol-specified analyses included clinical cure rates at the TOC (8 to 15 days after the end of therapy) in the co-primary Modified Intent-to-Treat Efficacy (MITTE) and CE populations (Table 12) and clinical cure rates at TOC by pathogen in the Microbiologically Evaluable (ME) population (Table 13). However, there are insufficient historical data to establish the magnitude of drug effect for antibacterials drugs compared with placebo at a TOC time point. Therefore, comparisons of Teflaro to ceftriaxone based on clinical response rates at TOC cannot be utilized to establish non-inferiority. Neither trial established that Teflaro was statistically superior to ceftriaxone in terms of clinical response rates. The MITTE population included all patients who received any amount of study drug according to their randomized treatment group and were in PORT (Pneumonia Outcomes Research Team) Risk Class III or IV. The CE population included patients in the MITTE population who demonstrated sufficient adherence to the protocol.

[See table 12 above]
[See table 13 at top of next page]

15. REFERENCES

1. Clinical and Laboratory Standards Institute (CLSI). *Methods for Dilution Antimicrobial Susceptibility Tests for Bacteria that Grow Aerobically; Approved Standard - Ninth Edition*. CLSI document M07-A9, Clinical and Laboratory Standards Institute, 950 West Valley Road, Suite 2500, Wayne, Pennsylvania 19087, USA, 2012.
2. Clinical and Laboratory Standards Institute (CLSI). *Performance Standards for Antimicrobial Disk Diffusion Susceptibility Tests; Approved Standard – Eleventh Edition* CLSI document M02-A11, Clinical and Laboratory Standards Institute, 950 West Valley Road, Suite 2500, Wayne, Pennsylvania 19087, USA, 2012.
3. Clinical and Laboratory Standards Institute (CLSI). *Performance Standards for Antimicrobial Susceptibility Testing; Twenty-third Informational Supplement*, CLSI document M100-S23. CLSI document M100-S23, Clinical and Laboratory Standards Institute, 950 West Valley Road, Suite 2500, Wayne, Pennsylvania 19087, USA, 2013.
4. Mandell, L.A., Wunderink, R.G., Anzueto, A., Bartlett, J.G., Campbell, G.D., Dean, N.C., Dowell, S.F., File, T.M., Musher, D.M., Niederman, M.S., Torres, A., Whitney, C.G. Infectious Diseases Society of America/American Thoracic Society consensus guidelines on the management of community-acquired pneumonia in adults. Clinical Infectious Disease. 2007; 44:S27-72.

16. HOW SUPPLIED/STORAGE AND HANDLING

Teflaro (ceftaroline fosamil) for injection is supplied in single-use, clear glass vials containing:

- 600 mg - individual vial (NDC 0456-0600-01) and carton containing 10 vials (NDC 0456-0600-10)
- 400 mg - individual vial (NDC 0456-0400-01) and carton containing 10 vials (NDC 0456-0400-10)

Unreconstituted Teflaro vials should be stored at 25°C (77°F); excursions permitted to 15-30°C (59-86°F) [see USP Controlled Room Temperature].

17. PATIENT COUNSELING INFORMATION

- Patients should be advised that allergic reactions, including serious allergic reactions, could occur and that serious reactions require immediate treatment. They should inform their healthcare provider about any previous hypersensitivity reactions to Teflaro, other beta-lactams (including cephalosporins) or other allergens.
- Patients should be counseled that antibacterial drugs including Teflaro should be used to treat only bacterial infections. They do not treat viral infections (e.g., the common cold). When Teflaro is prescribed to treat a bacterial infection, patients should be told that although it is common to feel better early in the course of therapy, the medication should be taken exactly as directed. Skipping doses or not completing the full course of therapy may (1) decrease the effectiveness of the immediate treatment and (2) increase the likelihood that bacteria will develop resistance and will not be treatable by Teflaro or other antibacterial drugs in the future.
- Patients should be advised that diarrhea is a common problem caused by antibacterial drugs and usually resolves when the drug is discontinued. Sometimes, frequent watery or bloody diarrhea may occur and may be a sign of a more serious intestinal infection. If severe watery or bloody diarrhea develops, patients should contact their healthcare provider.
- Keep out of reach of children

Table 13: Clinical Cure Rates at TOC by Pathogen from Two Integrated Phase 3 CABP Trials

	Teflaro n/N (%)	Ceftriaxone n/N (%)
Gram-positive: *Streptococcus pneumoniae*	54/63 (85.7%)	41/59 (69.5%)
Staphylococcus aureus (methicillin-susceptible isolates only)	18/25 (72.0%)	14/25 (56.0%)
Gram-negative: *Haemophilus influenzae*	15/18 (83.3%)	17/20 (85.0%)
Klebsiella pneumoniae	12/12 (100%)	10/12 (83.3%)
Klebsiella oxytoca	5/6 (83.3%)	7/8 (87.5%)
Escherichia coli	10/12 (83.3%)	9/12 (75.0%)

Teflaro® (ceftaroline fosamil) for injection

Distributed by:
Forest Pharmaceuticals, Inc.
Subsidiary of Forest Laboratories, Inc.
St. Louis, MO 63045, USA

Manufactured by:
Facta Farmaceutici S.p.A.
Nucleo Industriale S. Atto–S. Nicolò a Tordino
64020 Teramo, Italy

Teflaro® is a registered trademark of Forest Laboratories, Inc.

IF95USCFR08

Shown in Product Identification Guide, page 306

TUDORZA™ PRESSAIR™ ℞

(aclidinium bromide inhalation powder)
FOR ORAL INHALATION ONLY

HIGHLIGHTS OF PRESCRIBING INFORMATION

These highlights do not include all the information needed to use TUDORZA PRESSAIR safely and effectively. See full prescribing information for TUDORZA PRESSAIR.
TUDORZA™ PRESSAIR™ (aclidinium bromide inhalation powder)
FOR ORAL INHALATION ONLY
Initial U.S. Approval: 2012

INDICATIONS AND USAGE

TUDORZA PRESSAIR is an anticholinergic indicated for the long-term maintenance treatment of bronchospasm associated with chronic obstructive pulmonary disease (COPD), including chronic bronchitis and emphysema. (1)

DOSAGE AND ADMINISTRATION

For oral inhalation only
- One inhalation of TUDORZA PRESSAIR 400 mcg twice daily. (2)

DOSAGE FORMS AND STRENGTHS

- Inhalation powder; The multi-dose device is a dry powder inhaler metering 400 mcg of aclidinium bromide per actuation. (3)

CONTRAINDICATIONS

None. (4)

WARNINGS AND PRECAUTIONS

- Not for acute use: Not for use as a rescue medication. (5.1)
- Paradoxical bronchospasm: Discontinue TUDORZA PRESSAIR and consider other treatments if paradoxical bronchospasm occurs. (5.2)
- Worsening of narrow-angle glaucoma may occur. Use with caution in patients with narrow-angle glaucoma and instruct patients to consult a physician immediately if this occurs. (5.3)
- Worsening of urinary retention may occur. Use with caution in patients with prostatic hyperplasia or bladder-neck obstruction and instruct patients to consult a physician immediately if this occurs. (5.4)
- Immediate hypersensitivity reactions: Use with caution in patients with severe hypersensitivity to milk proteins. (5.5)

ADVERSE REACTIONS

Most common adverse reactions (≥3% incidence and greater than placebo) are headache, nasopharyngitis and cough. (6.1)

To report SUSPECTED ADVERSE REACTIONS, Contact Forest Laboratories, Inc. at 1-800-678-1605 or FDA at 1-800-FDA-1088 orwww.fda.gov/medwatch.

DRUG INTERACTIONS

Anticholinergics: May interact additively with concomitantly used anticholinergic medications. Avoid administrations of TUDORZA PRESSAIR with other anticholinergic-containing drugs. (7.2)

See 17 for PATIENT COUNSELING INFORMATION and FDA-approved patient labeling

Revised: 07/2012

FULL PRESCRIBING INFORMATION: CONTENTS*

*** Sections or subsections omitted from the full prescribing information are not listed**

FULL PRESCRIBING INFORMATION

1 INDICATIONS AND USAGE

TUDORZA™ PRESSAIR™ (aclidinium bromide inhalation powder) is indicated for the long-term, maintenance treatment of bronchospasm associated with chronic obstructive pulmonary disease (COPD), including chronic bronchitis and emphysema.

2 DOSAGE AND ADMINISTRATION

The recommended dose of TUDORZA PRESSAIR is one oral inhalation of 400 mcg, twice daily.

3 DOSAGE FORMS AND STRENGTHS

Inhalation Powder. TUDORZA PRESSAIR is a breath-actuated multi-dose dry powder inhaler metering 400 mcg of aclidinium bromide per actuation. Each actuation delivers 375 mcg of aclidinium bromide from the mouthpiece.

4 CONTRAINDICATIONS

None.

5 WARNINGS AND PRECAUTIONS

5.1 Not for Acute Use

TUDORZA PRESSAIR is intended as a twice-daily maintenance treatment for COPD and is not indicated for the initial treatment of acute episodes of bronchospasm (i.e., rescue therapy).

5.2 Paradoxical Bronchospasm

Inhaled medicines, including TUDORZA PRESSAIR, may cause paradoxical bronchospasm. If this occurs, treatment with TUDORZA PRESSAIR should be stopped and other treatments considered.

5.3 Worsening of Narrow-Angle Glaucoma

TUDORZA PRESSAIR should be used with caution in patients with narrow-angle glaucoma. Prescribers and patients should be alert for signs and symptoms of acute narrow-angle glaucoma (e.g., eye pain or discomfort, blurred vision, visual halos or colored images in association with red eyes from conjunctival congestion and corneal edema). Instruct patients to consult a physician immediately should any of these signs or symptoms develop.

5.4 Worsening of Urinary Retention

TUDORZA PRESSAIR should be used with caution in patients with urinary retention. Prescribers and patients should be alert for signs and symptoms of prostatic hyperplasia or bladder-neck obstruction (e.g., difficulty passing urine, painful urination). Instruct patients to consult a physician immediately should any of these signs or symptoms develop.

5.5 Immediate Hypersensitivity Reactions

Immediate hypersensitivity reactions may occur after administration of TUDORZA PRESSAIR. If such a reaction occurs, therapy with TUDORZA PRESSAIR should be stopped at once and alternative treatments should be considered. Given the similar structural formula of atropine to aclidinium, patients with a history of hypersensitivity reactions to atropine should be closely monitored for similar hypersensitivity reactions to TUDORZA PRESSAIR. In addition, TUDORZA PRESSAIR should be used with caution in patients with severe hypersensitivity to milk proteins.

6 ADVERSE REACTIONS

The following adverse reactions are described in greater detail in other sections:
- Paradoxical bronchospasm *[see Warnings and Precautions (5.2)]*
- Worsening of narrow-angle glaucoma *[see Warnings and Precautions (5.3)]*
- Worsening of urinary retention *[see Warnings and Precautions (5.4)]*

6.1 Clinical Trials Experience

Because clinical trials are conducted under widely varying conditions, adverse reaction rates observed in the clinical trials of a drug cannot be directly compared to rates in the clinical trials of another drug and may not reflect the rates observed in practice.

3-Month and 6-Month Trials

TUDORZA PRESSAIR was studied in two 3-month (Trials B and C) and one 6-month (Trial D) placebo-controlled trials in patients with COPD. In these trials, 636 patients were treated with TUDORZA PRESSAIR at the recommended dose of 400 mcg twice daily.

The population had a mean age of 64 years (ranging from 40 to 89 years), with 58% males, 94% Caucasian, and had COPD with a mean pre-bronchodilator forced expiratory volume in one second (FEV_1) percent predicted of 48%. Patients with unstable cardiac disease, narrow-angle glaucoma, or symptomatic prostatic hypertrophy or bladder outlet obstruction were excluded from these trials.

Table 1shows all adverse reactions that occurred with a frequency of greater than or equal to 1% in the TUDORZA PRESSAIR group in the two 3-month and one 6-month placebo-controlled trials where the rates in the TUDORZA PRESSAIR group exceeded placebo.

Table 1: Adverse Reactions (% Patients) in Placebo-Controlled Clinical Trials

Adverse Reactions	Treatment	
	TUDORZA PRESSAIR	Placebo
Preferred Term	(N=636)	(N=640)
	n (%)	n (%)
Headache	42 (6.6)	32 (5.0)
Nasopharyngitis	35 (5.5)	25 (3.9)

Cough	19 (3.0)	14 (2.2)
Diarrhea	17 (2.7)	9 (1.4)
Sinusitis	11 (1.7)	5 (0.8)
Rhinitis	10 (1.6)	8 (1.2)
Toothache	7 (1.1)	5 (0.8)
Fall	7 (1.1)	3 (0.5)
Vomiting	7 (1.1)	3 (0.5)

In addition, among the adverse reactions observed in the clinical trials with an incidence of less than 1% were diabetes mellitus, dry mouth, 1st degree AV block, osteoarthritis, cardiac failure, and cardio-respiratory arrest.

Long-term Safety Trials

TUDORZA PRESSAIR was studied in three long term safety trials, two double blind and one open label, ranging from 40 to 52 weeks in patients with moderate to severe COPD. Two of these trials were extensions of the 3-month trials, and one was a dedicated long term safety trial. In these trials, 891 patients were treated with TUDORZA PRESSAIR at the recommended dose of 400 mcg twice daily. The demographic and baseline characteristics of the long term safety trials were similar to those of the placebo-controlled trials. The adverse events reported in the long term safety trials were similar to those occurring in the placebo-controlled trials of 3 to 6 months. No new safety findings were reported compared to the placebo controlled trials.

7 DRUG INTERACTIONS

In vitro studies suggest limited potential for CYP450-related metabolic drug interactions, thus no formal drug interaction studies have been performed with TUDORZA PRESSAIR *[see Clinical Pharmacology (12.3)]*.

7.1 Sympathomimetics, Methylxanthines, Steroids

In clinical studies, concurrent administration of aclidinium bromide and other drugs commonly used in the treatment of COPD including sympathomimetics (short-acting beta$_2$ agonists), methylxanthines, and oral and inhaled steroids showed no increases in adverse drug reactions.

7.2 Anticholinergics

There is a potential for an additive interaction with concomitantly used anticholinergic medications. Therefore, avoid coadministration of TUDORZA PRESSAIR with other anticholinergic-containing drugs as this may lead to an increase in anticholinergic effects.

8 USE IN SPECIFIC POPULATIONS

8.1 Pregnancy

Teratogenic effects: Pregnancy Category C: There are no adequate and well controlled studies in pregnant women. Adverse development effects were observed in rats and rabbits exposed to aclidinium bromide. TUDORZA PRESSAIR should be used during pregnancy only if the potential benefit justifies the potential risk to the fetus.

Effects of aclidinium bromide on embryo-fetal development were examined in rats and rabbits. No evidence of structural alterations was observed in rats exposed during the period of organogenesis at approximately 15 times the recommended human daily dose (RHDD) [based on summed AUCs of aclidinium bromide and its metabolites at inhaled doses less than or equal to 5.0 mg/kg/day]. However, decreased pup weights were observed from dams exposed during the lactation period at approximately 5 times the RHDD [based on summed AUCs of aclidinium bromide and its metabolites at inhaled doses greater than or equal to 0.2 mg/kg/day]. Maternal toxicity was also observed at inhaled doses greater than or equal to 0.2 mg/kg/day.

No evidence of structural alterations was observed in Himalayan rabbits exposed during the period of organogenesis at approximately 20 times the RHDD [based on summed AUCs of aclidinium bromide and its metabolites at inhaled doses less than or equal to 3.6 mg/kg/day]. However, increased incidences of additional liver lobes (3-5%), as compared to 0% in the control group, were observed at approximately 1,400 times the RHDD [based on summed AUCs of aclidinium bromide and its metabolites at oral doses greater than or equal to 150 mg/kg/day], and decreased fetal body weights were observed at approximately 2,300 times the RHDD [based on summed AUCs of aclidinium bromide and its metabolites at oral doses greater than or equal to 300 mg/kg/day]. These fetal findings were observed in the presence of maternal toxicity.

8.2 Labor and Delivery

The effect of TUDORZA PRESSAIR on labor and delivery is unknown. TUDORZA PRESSAIR should be used during labor and delivery only if the potential benefit to the patient justifies the potential risk to the fetus.

8.3 Nursing Mothers

Aclidinium bromide is excreted into the milk of lactating female rats, and decreased pup weights were observed. Excretion of aclidinium into human milk is probable. There are no human studies that have investigated the effects of TUDORZA PRESSAIR on breast-fed infants. Caution should be exercised when TUDORZA PRESSAIR is administered to nursing women.

8.4 Pediatric Use

TUDORZA PRESSAIR is approved for use in the maintenance treatment of bronchospasm associated with COPD. COPD does not normally occur in children. The safety and effectiveness of TUDORZA PRESSAIR in pediatric patients have not been established.

8.5 Geriatric Use

Of the 636 COPD patients exposed to TUDORZA PRESSAIR 400 mcg twice daily for up to 24 weeks in three placebo-controlled clinical trials, 197 were less than 60 years, 272 were greater than or equal to 60 to less than 70 years, and 167 were greater than or equal to 70 years of age. No overall differences in safety or effectiveness were observed between these subjects and younger subjects. Other reported clinical experience has not identified differences in responses between the elderly and younger patients, but greater sensitivity of some older individuals cannot be ruled out. Based on available data for TUDORZA PRESSAIR, no adjustment of dosage in geriatric patients is warranted *[see Clinical Pharmacology (12.3)]*.

8.6 Renal Impairment

The pharmacokinetics of TUDORZA PRESSAIR were investigated in subjects with normal renal function and in subjects with mild, moderate and severe renal impairment *[see Clinical Pharmacology (12.3)]*. No clinically significant differences in aclidinium pharmacokinetics were noted between these populations. Based on available data for TUDORZA PRESSAIR, no adjustment of dosage in renally impaired subjects is warranted.

8.7 Hepatic Impairment

The effects of hepatic impairment on the pharmacokinetics of TUDORZA PRESSAIR were not studied *[see Clinical Pharmacology (12.3)]*.

10 OVERDOSAGE

10.1 Human Experience

No case of overdose has been reported in clinical studies with TUDORZA PRESSAIR. There were no systemic anticholinergic or other adverse effects following a single inhaled dose of up to 6,000 mcg aclidinium bromide (7.5 times the RHDD) in 16 healthy volunteers.

11 DESCRIPTION

TUDORZA PRESSAIR consists of a dry powder formulation of aclidinium bromide for oral inhalation only.

Aclidinium bromide, the active component of TUDORZA PRESSAIR is an anticholinergic with specificity for muscarinic receptors. Aclidinium bromide is a synthetic, quaternary ammonium compound, chemically described as 1-Azoniabicyclo[2.2.2]octane, 3-[(hydroxydi-2-thienylacetyl)-oxy]-1-(3-phenoxypropyl)-, bromide, (3*R*)-. The structural formula is:

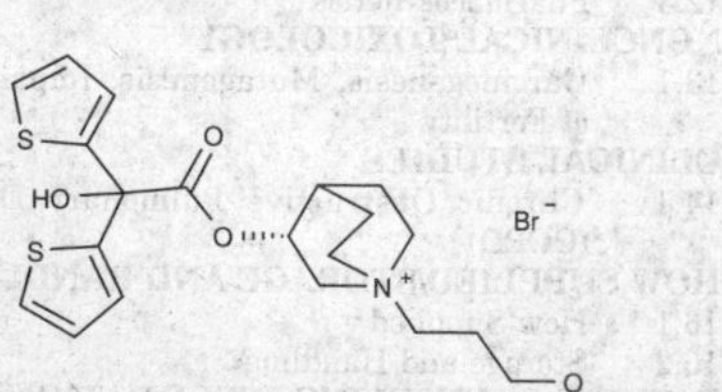

Aclidinium bromide is a white powder with a molecular formula of $C_{26}H_{30}NO_4S_2Br$ and a molecular mass of 564.56. It is very slightly soluble in water and ethanol and sparingly soluble in methanol.

TUDORZA PRESSAIR is a breath-actuated multi-dose dry powder inhaler. Each actuation of TUDORZA PRESSAIR provides a metered dose of 13 mg of the formulation which contains lactose monohydrate (which may contain milk proteins) as the carrier and 400 mcg of aclidinium bromide. This results in delivery of 375 mcg aclidinium bromide from the mouthpiece, based on *in vitro* testing at an average flow rate of 63 L/min with constant volume of 2 L. The amount of drug delivered to the lungs will vary depending on patient factors such as inspiratory flow rate and inspiratory time. The PRESSAIR inhaler delivers the target dose at flow rates as low as 35 L/min. Based on a study in adult patients with moderate (N=24) and severe (N=24) COPD the mean peak inspiratory flow (PIF) was 95.3 L/min (range: 54.6 to 129.4 L/min) and 88.7 L/min (range: 72.0 to 106.4 L/min) respectively.

12 CLINICAL PHARMACOLOGY

12.1 Mechanism of Action

Aclidinium bromide is a long-acting antimuscarinic agent, which is often referred to as an anticholinergic. It has similar affinity to the subtypes of muscarinic receptors M_1 to M_5. In the airways, it exhibits pharmacological effects through inhibition of M_3 receptor at the smooth muscle leading to bronchodilation. The competitive and reversible nature of antagonism was shown with human and animal origin receptors and isolated organ preparations. In preclinical *in vitro* as well as *in vivo* studies, prevention of acetylcholine-induced bronchoconstriction effects was dose-dependent and lasted longer than 24 hours. The clinical relevance of these findings is unknown. The bronchodilation following inhalation of aclidinium bromide is predominantly a site-specific effect.

12.2 Pharmacodynamics

Cardiovascular Effects

In a thorough QT Study, 200 mcg and 800 mcg TUDORZA PRESSAIR was administered to healthy volunteers once daily for 3 days; no effects on prolongation of QT interval were observed using QTcF heart-rate correction methods.

Additionally, the effect of TUDORZA PRESSAIR on cardiac rhythm was assessed in 336 COPD patients, 164 patients received aclidinium bromide 400 mcg twice daily and 172 patients received placebo, using 24-hr Holter monitoring. No clinically significant effects on cardiac rhythm were observed.

12.3 Pharmacokinetics

Absorption

The absolute bioavailability of aclidinium bromide is approximately 6% in healthy volunteers. Following twice-daily oral inhalation administration of 400 mcg aclidinium bromide in healthy subjects, peak steady state plasma levels were observed within 10 minutes after inhalation.

Distribution

Aclidinium bromide shows a volume of distribution of approximately 300 L following intravenous administration of 400 mcg in humans.

Metabolism

Clinical pharmacokinetics studies, including a mass balance study, indicate that the major route of metabolism of aclidinium bromide is hydrolysis, which occurs both chemically and enzymatically by esterases. Aclidinium bromide is rapidly and extensively hydrolyzed to its alcohol and dithienylglycolic acid derivatives, neither of which binds to muscarinic receptors and are devoid of pharmacologic activity.

Therefore, due to the low plasma levels achieved at the clinically relevant doses, aclidinium bromide and its metabolites are not expected to alter the disposition of drugs metabolized by the human CYP450 enzymes.

Elimination

Total clearance was approximately 170 L/h after an intravenous dose of aclidinium bromide in young healthy volunteers with an inter-individual variability of 36%. Intravenously administered radiolabelled aclidinium bromide was administered to healthy volunteers and was extensively metabolized with 1% excreted as unchanged aclidinium. Approximately 54% to 65% of the radioactivity was excreted in urine and 20% to 33% of the dose was excreted in feces. The combined results indicated that almost the entire aclidinium bromide dose was eliminated by hydrolysis. After dry powder inhalation, urinary excretion of aclidinium is about 0.09% of the dose and the estimated effective half-life is 5 to 8 hours.

Drug Interactions

Formal drug interaction studies were not performed. *In vitro* studies using human liver microsomes indicated that aclidinium bromide and its major metabolites do not inhibit CYP450, 1A2, 2A6, 2B6, 2C8, 2C9, 2C19, 2D6, 2E1, 3A4/5 or 4A9/11 at concentrations up to 1,000-fold higher than the maximum plasma concentration that would be expected to be achieved at the therapeutic dose. Therefore, it is unlikely that aclidinium bromide causes CYP450 related drug interactions *[see Drug Interactions (7)]*.

Specific Populations

Elderly Patients

The pharmacokinetic profile of aclidinium bromide and its main metabolites was assessed in 12 elderly COPD patients (aged 70 years or older) compared to a younger cohort of 12 COPD patients (40-59 years) that were administered 400 mcg aclidinium bromide once daily for 3 days via inhalation. No clinically significant differences in systemic exposure (AUC and C_{max}) were observed when the two groups were compared. No dosage adjustment is necessary in elderly patients *[Use in Specific Populations (8.5)]*.

Renal Impairment

The impact of renal disease upon the pharmacokinetics of aclidinium bromide was studied in 18 subjects with mild, moderate, or severe renal impairment. Systemic exposure (AUC and C_{max}) to aclidinium bromide and its main metabolites following single doses of 400 mcg aclidinium bromide was similar in renally impaired patients compared with 6 matched healthy control subjects. No dose adjustment is necessary in renally impaired patients *[see Use in Specific Populations (8.6)]*.

Hepatic Impairment

The effects of hepatic impairment on the pharmacokinetics of aclidinium bromide were not studied. However, hepatic insufficiency is not expected to have relevant influence on aclidinium bromide pharmacokinetics, since it is predominantly metabolized by chemical and enzymatic hydrolysis to products that do not bind to muscarinic receptors *[see Use in Specific Populations (8.7)]*.

13 NONCLINICAL TOXICOLOGY

13.1 Carcinogenesis, Mutagenesis, Impairment of Fertility

Two-year inhalation studies were conducted in mice and rats to assess the carcinogenic potential of aclidinium bromide. No evidence of tumorigenicity was observed in rats and mice at aclidinium doses up to 0.20 and 2.4 mg/kg/day, respectively [approximately 10 and 80 times the Recommended Human Daily Dose (RHDD), respectively, based on summed AUCs of aclidinium bromide and its metabolites].

Aclidinium bromide was positive in the *in vitro* bacterial gene mutation assay and the *in vitro* thymidine locus mouse lymphoma assay. However, aclidinium bromide was negative in the *in vivo* mouse micronucleus assay and the *in vivo/in vitro* unscheduled DNA synthesis assay with rat liver.

Aclidinium bromide impaired several fertility and reproductive performance indices (increased number of days to mate, decreased conception rate, decreased number of corpora lutea, increased pre-implantation loss with consequent decreased number of implantations and live embryos) in both male and female rats administered inhaled doses greater than or equal to 0.8 mg/kg/day [approximately 15 times the RHDD based on summed AUCs of aclidinium bromide and its metabolites]. These adverse fertility effects were observed in the presence of paternal toxicity as evidenced by mortality and decreased body weight gain. However, there were no effects on mating index and sperm number and morphology. In the separate fertility assessments (treated males mated with untreated females; treated females mated with untreated males), no effect was observed in male and female rats at inhaled doses of 1.9 and 0.8 mg/kg/day, respectively [approximately 30 and 15 times the RHDD, respectively, based on summed AUCs of aclidinium bromide and its metabolites].

14 CLINICAL STUDIES

14.1 Chronic Obstructive Pulmonary Disease (COPD)

The TUDORZA PRESSAIR clinical development program included a dose-ranging trial (Trial A) for nominal dose selection and three confirmatory trials (Trials B, C, and D).

Dose-ranging trial

Trial A was a randomized, double-blind, placebo-controlled, active-controlled, crossover trial with 7-day treatment periods separated by 5-day washout periods. Trial A enrolled 79 patients who had a clinical diagnosis of COPD, were 40 years of age or older, had a history of smoking at least 10 pack-years, had a forced expiratory volume in one second (FEV_1) of at least 30% and less than 80% of predicted normal value, and a ratio of FEV_1 over forced vital capacity (FEV_1/FVC) of less than 0.7. Trial A included TUDORZA PRESSAIR doses of 400 mcg, 200 mcg and 100 mcg twice daily, formoterol active control, and placebo. Trial A demonstrated that the effect on trough FEV_1 and serial FEV_1 in patients treated with the TUDORZA PRESSAIR 100 mcg twice daily and 200 mcg twice daily doses was lower compared to patients treated with the TUDORZA PRESSAIR 400 mcg twice daily dose (Figure 1).

Figure 1. Change from baseline in FEV_1 Over Time (prior to and after administration of study drug) at Week 1 in Trial A

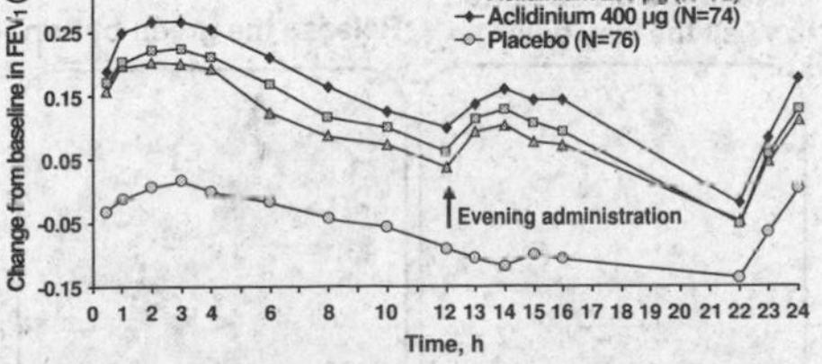

Confirmatory trials

Trials B, C, and D were three randomized, double-blind, placebo-controlled trials in patients with COPD. Trials B and C were 3 months in duration, and Trial D was 6 months in duration. These trials enrolled 1,276 patients who had a clinical diagnosis of COPD, were 40 years of age or older, had a history of smoking at least 10 pack-years, had an FEV_1 of at least 30% and less than 80% of predicted normal value, and a ratio of FEV_1/FVC of less than 0.7; 59% were male, and 93% were Caucasian.

These clinical trials evaluated TUDORZA PRESSAIR 400 mcg twice daily (636 patients) and placebo (640 patients). TUDORZA PRESSAIR 400 mcg resulted in statistically significantly greater bronchodilation as measured by change from baseline in morning pre-dose FEV_1 at 12 weeks (the primary efficacy endpoint) compared to placebo in all three trials (Table 2).

Table 2: Change from Baseline in Trough FEV_1(L) at Week 12

Treatment Arm	Baseline	Change from Baseline LS Mean (SE)	Treatment Difference LS Mean (95% CI)
Trial B (N=375)			
Aclidinium 400 mcg	1.33	0.10 (0.01)	0.12 (0.08, 0.16)
Placebo	1.38	-0.02 (0.02)	
Trial C (N=359)			
Aclidinium 400 mcg	1.25	0.06 (0.02)	0.07 (0.03, 0.12)
Placebo	1.46	-0.01 (0.02)	
Trial D* (N=542)			
Aclidinium 400 mcg	1.51	0.06 (0.02)	0.11 (0.07, 0.14)
Placebo	1.50	-0.05 (0.02)	

SE=standard error, and LS mean=least square mean. LS mean, and 95% confidence interval were obtained from an ANCOVA model with change from baseline in trough FEV_1 as response, with treatment group and sex as factors and baseline trough FEV_1 and age as covariates.

*In the 6-month Trial D, placebo adjusted change from baseline in Trough FEV_1 at 24 weeks was 0.13 (0.09, 0.17).

[See table 2 above]

Serial spirometric evaluations were performed throughout daytime hours in a subset of patients in the three trials. The serial FEV_1 values over 12 hours for one of the 3-month trials (Trial B) are displayed in Figure 2. Results for the other two placebo-controlled trials were similar to the results for Trial B. Improvement of lung function was maintained for 12 hours after a single dose and was consistent over the 3- or 6-month treatment period.

Figure 2. Mean FEV_1 Over Time (prior to and after administration of study drug) on Day 1 and Week 12 in Subset of Patients Participating in the 12 hours Serial Spirometry Substudy for Trial B (a 3-month Placebo-Controlled Study)

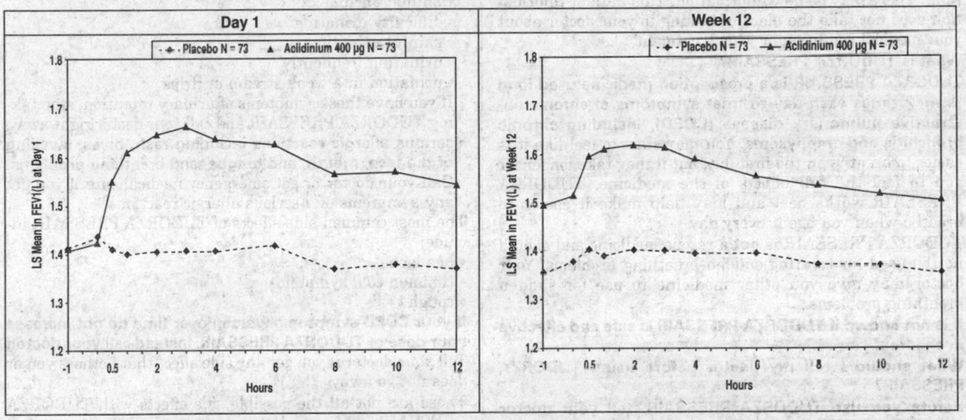

[See figure 2 above]

Mean peak improvements in FEV_1, for TUDORZA PRESSAIR relative to baseline were assessed in all patients in trials B, C and D after the first dose on day 1 and were similar at week 12. In Trials B and D but not in Trial C, patients treated with TUDORZA PRESSAIR used less daily rescue albuterol during the trial compared to patients treated with placebo.

16 HOW SUPPLIED/STORAGE AND HANDLING

16.1 How Supplied

TUDORZA™ PRESSAIR™ (aclidinium bromide inhalation powder) 400 mcg is supplied in a sealed labeled aluminum pouch and is available in 60 metered doses (NDC 0456-0800-60) and 30 metered doses (NDC 0456-0800-31).

The active ingredient is administered using a multi-dose dry powder inhaler, PRESSAIR™, which delivers 60 doses or 30 doses of aclidinium bromide powder for oral inhalation. The PRESSAIR inhaler is a white and green colored device and is comprised of an assembled plastic dosing mechanism with a dose indicator, a drug-product storage unit containing the drug-product formulation, and a mouthpiece covered by a green protective cap. The inhaler should be discarded when the marking "0" with a red background shows in the middle of the dose indicator or when the device locks out, whichever comes first.

16.2 Storage and Handling

Store TUDORZA PRESSAIR in a dry place at 25 C (77 F); excursions permitted to 15-30 C (59-86 F) *[see USP Controlled Room Temperature]*.

The PRESSAIR inhaler should be stored inside the sealed pouch and only be opened immediately before use.

Discard the PRESSAIR inhaler 45 days after opening the pouch, after the marking "0" with a red background shows in the middle of the dose indicator, or when the device locks out, whichever comes first.

Keep out of reach of children.

17 PATIENT COUNSELING INFORMATION

See FDA-approved Patient Labeling (Patient Information and Instructions for Use)

17.1 Instructions for Administering TUDORZA PRESSAIR

It is important for patients to understand how to correctly use TUDORZA PRESSAIR.

Inform patients that if they miss a dose, they should take their next dose at the usual time; they should not take 2 doses at one time.

17.2 Acute Bronchospasm

Instruct patients that TUDORZA PRESSAIR is a twice daily maintenance bronchodilator and should not be used for immediate relief of breathing problems (i.e., as a rescue medication) *[see Warnings and Precautions (5.1)]*.

17.3 Paradoxical Bronchospasm

Inform patients that TUDORZA PRESSAIR can cause paradoxical bronchospasm. Advise patients that if paradoxical bronchospasm occurs, patients should discontinue TUDORZA PRESSAIR *[see Warnings and Precautions (5.2)]*.

17.4 Visual Effects

Eye pain or discomfort, blurred vision, visual halos or colored images in association with red eyes from conjunctival congestion and corneal edema may be signs of acute narrow-angle glaucoma. Inform patients to consult a physician immediately should any of these signs and symptoms develop.

Advise patients that miotic eyedrops alone are not considered to be effective treatment *[see Warnings and Precautions (5.3)]*.

Inform patients that care must be taken not to allow the powder to enter into the eyes as this may cause blurring of vision and pupil dilation.

17.5 Urinary Retention

Difficulty passing urine and dysuria may be symptoms of new or worsening prostatic hyperplasia or bladder outlet obstruction. Patients should be instructed to consult a physician immediately should any of these signs or symptoms develop *[see Warnings and Precautions (5.4)]*.

Distributed by:
Forest Pharmaceuticals, Inc.
Subsidiary of Forest Laboratories, Inc.
St. Louis, MO 63045

FOREST PHARMACEUTICALS, INC.
Subsidiary of Forest Laboratories, Inc.
St. Louis, Missouri 63045
Under license of ALMIRALL, S.A.
Almirall

TUDORZA™ and **PRESSAIR™** are trademarks of ALMIRALL, S.A.

Patient Information

TUDORZA™ PRESSAIR™ (TU-door-za PRESS-air)
(aclidinium bromide inhalation powder)

FOR ORAL INHALATION ONLY

Read the Patient Information that comes with TUDORZA PRESSAIR before you start using it and each time you get a refill. There may be new information. This Patient Information does not take the place of talking to your doctor about your medical condition or your treatment.

What is TUDORZA PRESSAIR?

TUDORZA PRESSAIR is a prescription medicine used long term, 2 times each day to treat symptoms of chronic obstructive pulmonary disease (COPD), including chronic bronchitis and emphysema. You may start to feel like it is easier to breathe on the first day, but it may take longer for you to feel the full effects of the medicine. TUDORZA PRESSAIR works best and may help make it easier to breathe when you use it every day.

TUDORZA PRESSAIR is **not** a rescue medicine and should not be used for treating sudden breathing problems. Your doctor may give you other medicine to use for sudden breathing problems.

It is not known if TUDORZA PRESSAIR is safe and effective in children.

What should I tell my doctor before using TUDORZA PRESSAIR?

Before you use TUDORZA PRESSAIR, tell your doctor about all your medical conditions, including if you:

- have eye problems, especially glaucoma. TUDORZA PRESSAIR may make your glaucoma worse.
- have prostate or bladder problems, or problems passing urine. TUDORZA PRESSAIR may make these problems worse.
- have a severe allergy to milk proteins. Ask your doctor if you are not sure.
- are pregnant or plan to become pregnant. It is not known if TUDORZA PRESSAIR can harm your unborn baby.
- are breast-feeding or plan to breast-feed. TUDORZA PRESSAIR may pass into your breast milk. You and your doctor should decide if you will take TUDORZA PRESSAIR.

Tell your doctor about all the medicines you take, including prescription and non-prescription medicines and eyedrops, vitamins, and herbal supplements.

TUDORZA PRESSAIR and certain other medicines may interact with each other. This may cause serious side effects. Especially tell your doctor if you take:

- anticholinergics (including Tiotropium, Ipratropium)
- atropine

Ask your doctor or pharmacist for a list of these medicines if you are not sure.

Know the medicines you take. Keep a list of them to show your doctor and pharmacist each time you get a new medicine.

How should I use TUDORZA PRESSAIR?

See the step-by-step instructions for using TUDORZA PRESSAIR at the end of this Patient Information.

- Use TUDORZA PRESSAIR exactly as prescribed.
- The usual dose of TUDORZA PRESSAIR is one oral inhalation 2 times a day. Each dose should be about 12 hours apart.
- If you miss a dose, just skip the dose. Take your next dose at your usual time. Do not take 2 doses at one time.

TUDORZA PRESSAIR does not relieve sudden symptoms of COPD. Always have a rescue inhaler medicine with you to treat sudden symptoms. If you do not have a rescue inhaler medicine, call your doctor to have one prescribed for you.

Do not use TUDORZA PRESSAIR more often than prescribed or take more medicine than prescribed for you.

- **Call your doctor or get emergency medical care right away if:**
  - your breathing problems worsen with TUDORZA PRESSAIR
  - you need to use your rescue inhaler medicine more often than usual
  - your rescue inhaler medicine does not work as well for you at relieving symptoms

What are the possible side effects of TUDORZA PRESSAIR?

TUDORZA PRESSAIR can cause serious side effects including:

- **sudden shortness of breath immediately after use of TUDORZA PRESSAIR.** If you have this symptom, stop taking TUDORZA PRESSAIR and call your doctor right away or go to the nearest hospital emergency room.
- **new or worsened increased pressure in your eyes (acute narrow-angle glaucoma).** Acute narrow-angle glaucoma can lead to permanent loss of vision if not treated. Symptoms of acute narrow-angle glaucoma may include:
  - eye pain or discomfort
  - nausea or vomiting
  - blurred vision
  - seeing halos or bright colors around lights
  - red eyes

  Using only eyedrops to treat these symptoms may not work. If you have these symptoms, stop taking TUDORZA PRESSAIR and call your doctor right away.
- **new or worsened urinary retention.** Urinary retention can be caused by blockage in your bladder or, if you are a male, a larger than normal prostate. Symptoms of urinary retention may include:
  - difficulty urinating
  - painful urination
  - urinating frequently
  - urination in a weak stream or drips

  If you have these symptoms of urinary retention, stop taking TUDORZA PRESSAIR and call your doctor right away.
- **serious allergic reactions including rash, hives, swelling of the face, mouth, and tongue, and breathing problems.** Call your doctor or get emergency medical care if you get any symptoms of a serious allergic reaction.

The most common side effects of TUDORZA PRESSAIR include:

- headache
- common cold symptoms
- cough

If your COPD symptoms worsen over time do not increase your dose of TUDORZA PRESSAIR, instead call your doctor.

Tell your doctor if you get any side effect that bothers you or does not go away.

These are not all the possible side effects with TUDORZA PRESSAIR. Ask your doctor or pharmacist for more information.

Call your doctor for medical advice about side effects. You may report side effects to FDA at 1-800-FDA-1088.

How should I store TUDORZA PRESSAIR?

Store TUDORZA PRESSAIR at room temperature between 68 F to 77 F (20 to 25 C) in the protective pouch. **Do not open the sealed pouch until you are ready to use a dose of TUDORZA PRESSAIR. Once a sealed pouch is opened, start using your TUDORZA PRESSAIR.** Discard the PRESSAIR inhaler 45 days after opening the pouch, after the marking "0" with a red background shows in the middle of the dose indicator, or when the device locks out, whichever comes first.

- Keep TUDORZA PRESSAIR in a dry place.
- Do not store the inhaler on a vibrating surface.

Keep TUDORZA PRESSAIR and all medicines out of the reach of children.

General information about the safe and effective use of TUDORZA PRESSAIR

Medicines are sometimes prescribed for purposes other than those listed in Patient Information leaflets. Do not use TUDORZA PRESSAIR for a condition for which it was not prescribed. Do not give TUDORZA PRESSAIR to other people even if they have the same symptoms that you have. It may harm them.

This patient leaflet summarizes the most important information about TUDORZA PRESSAIR. If you would like more information, talk with your doctor. You can ask your pharmacist or doctor for information about TUDORZA PRESSAIR that is written for health professionals.

For more information, go to www.tudorza.com, or call 1-800-678-1605.

What are the ingredients in TUDORZA PRESSAIR?

Active ingredient: aclidinium bromide
Inactive ingredient: lactose monohydrate

Instructions for Use

TUDORZA™ PRESSAIR™ (TU-door-za PRESS-air)
(aclidinium bromide inhalation powder)

FOR ORAL INHALATION ONLY

Read this Instructions for Use before you start using TUDORZA PRESSAIR and each time you get a refill. There may be new information. This information does not take the place of talking to your doctor about your medical condition or your treatment.

Your TUDORZA PRESSAIR INHALER:

When you are ready to use TUDORZA PRESSAIR for the first time, remove the TUDORZA PRESSAIR inhaler from the pouch. To remove the inhaler from the pouch, tear along the "notch." The pouch may then be discarded.

Look at the parts of the inhaler so you become familiar with them. **(See Figure A)**

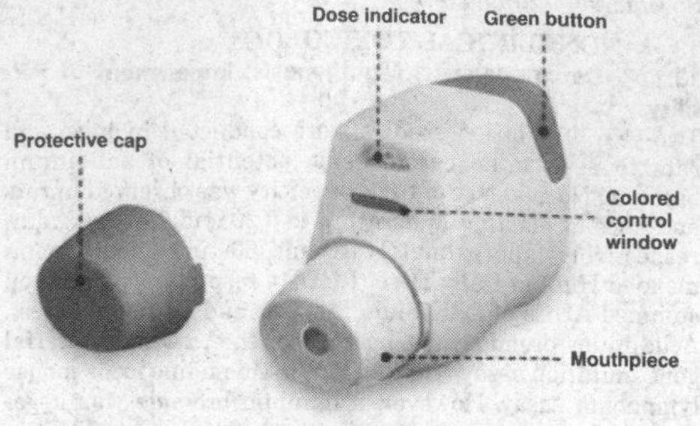

Figure A

Taking a dose from the TUDORZA PRESSAIR Inhaler requires you to press, release, and inhale. See the step-by-step instructions for using TUDORZA PRESSAIR below.

How to prepare and use your TUDORZA PRESSAIR Inhaler

Step 1. Remove the protective cap by **lightly squeezing the arrows** marked on each side of the cap and pulling outwards. **(See Figure B)**

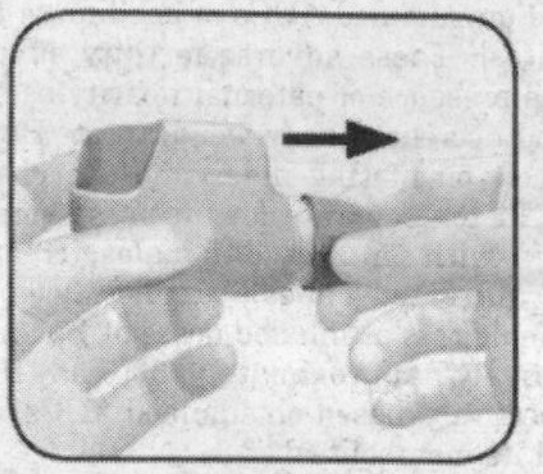

Figure B

- Look to see that nothing is blocking the mouthpiece.

Step 2. Hold the TUDORZA PRESSAIR inhaler with the mouthpiece facing you, but not inside your mouth. The green button should be facing straight up. **(See Figure C)**

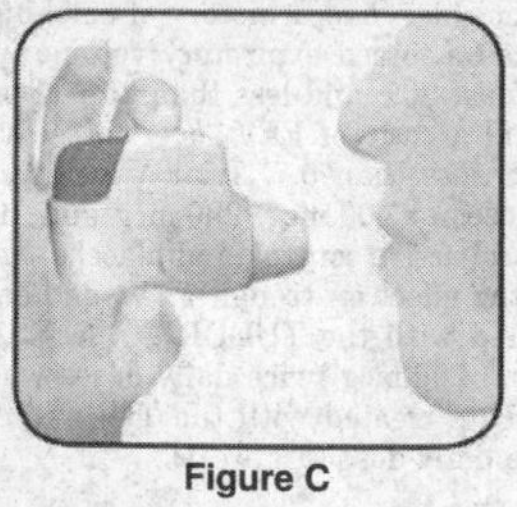

Hold with the green button facing straight up. Do not tilt.

Figure C

Step 3. Before you put the inhaler into your mouth, **press** the green button all the way down. **(See Figure D)**

- Then **release** the green button. **(See Figure E)**
- **Do not continue to hold the green button down.**

Press the green button all the way down

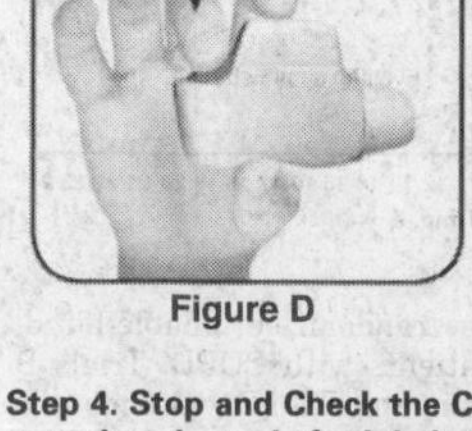

Figure D

Release the green button

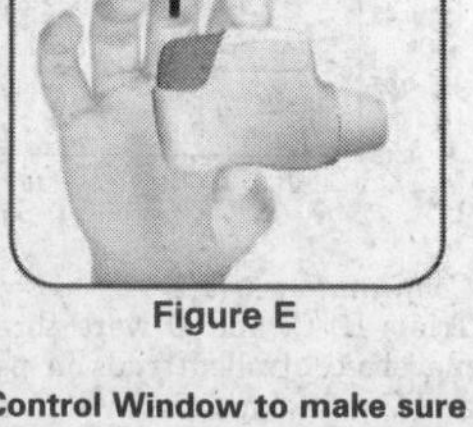

Figure E

Step 4. Stop and Check the Control Window to make sure your dose is ready for inhalation. Look to see if the colored control window has changed from **red (See Figure F)**, to **green (See Figure G)**

- The green control window tells you that your medicine is ready for inhalation. **(See Figure G)**

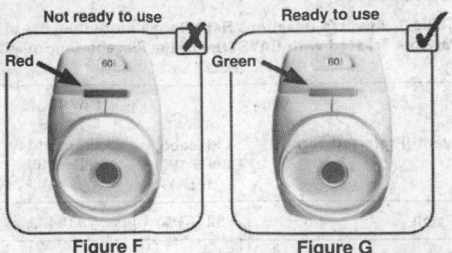

Figure F

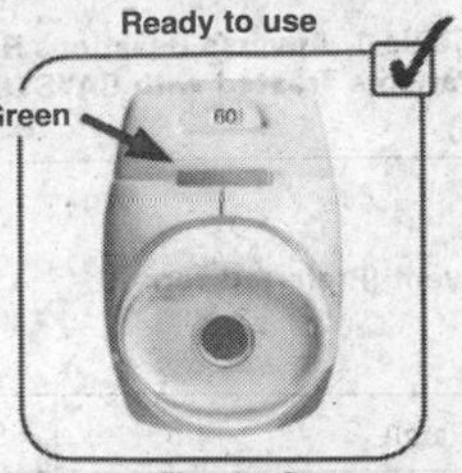

Figure G

- **If the control window stays red (See Figure F), repeat the Press and Release actions in Step 3 until the control window is green.**

Now the dose is ready to be inhaled.

Step 5. Before you put the inhaler into your mouth, breathe out completely. Do not breathe out into the inhaler.

- Put your lips tightly around the mouthpiece of the TUDORZA PRESSAIR inhaler. Breathe in **quickly** and **deeply** through your mouth. **(See Figure H)**. This quick, deep breath makes sure that you get enough of the medication from the inhaler into your lungs.
- Breathe in until you hear a **"click"** sound. Keep breathing in, even after you have heard the inhaler **"click"** to be sure you get the full dose.

Attention: Do not hold the green button down while you are inhaling

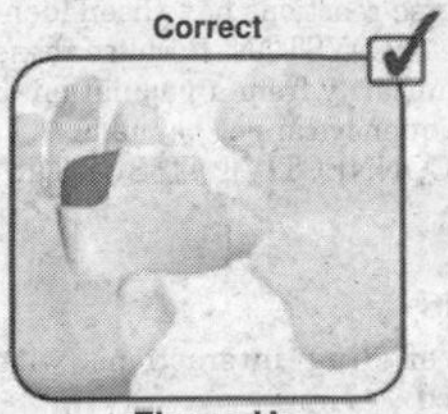

Figure H

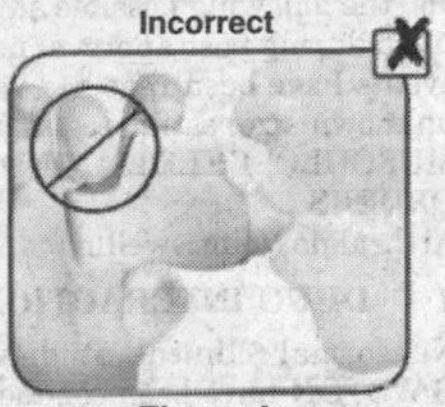

Figure I

- **Do not hold down the green button while you are breathing in. (See Figure I)**

Step 6. Remove the TUDORZA PRESSAIR inhaler from your mouth and hold your breath for as long as is comfortable **(See Figure J)**, then breathe out slowly through your nose.

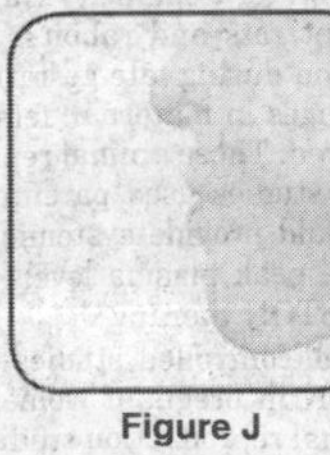

Figure J

Some people may taste the medicine during their inhalation. Do not take an extra dose even if you do not taste anything after inhaling.

Step 7. Stop and Check the Control Window. Make sure you have used your TUDORZA PRESSAIR inhaler correctly.

- Look at the control window to see if it has turned to **red- (See Figure K)** from **green (See Figure L)**. If the window is **red** you have inhaled your full dose of medicine correctly.

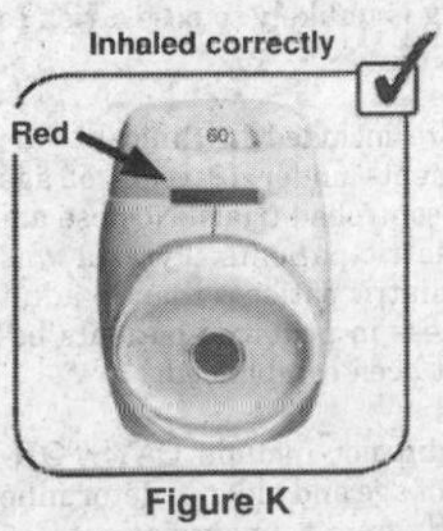

Figure K

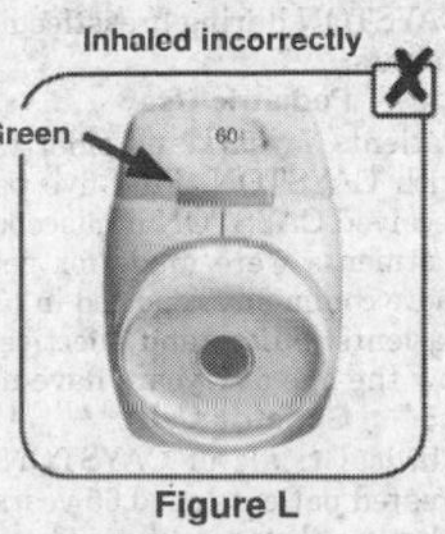

Figure L

If the colored control window is still green, repeat **Step 5**.

- If the window still does not change to **red**, you may have forgotten to release the **green** button before inhaling or may not have inhaled correctly. If that happens repeat **Step 5** again.
- Make sure you have released the green button and take a **quick** and **deep** breath in through the mouthpiece.
- If you are unable to inhale correctly after several attempts, call your doctor.

Step 8. Once the window has turned **red**, place the protective cap back onto the inhaler by pressing it back onto the mouthpiece. **(See Figure M)**

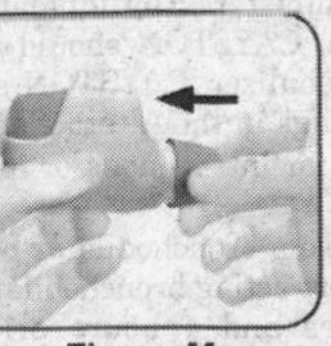

Figure M

Additional information about the safe and effective use of TUDORZA PRESSAIR inhaler

The "click" sound and colored control window:

- The **"click"** that you hear while inhaling tells you that you are using the TUDORZA PRESSAIR inhaler correctly.
- When you use the inhaler correctly the colored control window changes from **green** to **red**.
- Each time you are ready to use the TUDORZA PRESSAIR inhaler again, you will need to make sure the inhaler is ready by pressing and releasing the green button as seen in **Step 3**. When you press and release the green button the colored control window will change from **red** to **green**.

When should you get a new TUDORZA PRESSAIR inhaler?

- The TUDORZA PRESSAIR inhaler has a dose indicator to show you how many doses are left in your inhaler. Each TUDORZA PRESSAIR inhaler has 60 doses of medicine.
  - When you start using the inhaler for the first time you will see the number **60** in the dose indicator.
  - You will see the number of doses count down in the dose indicator as you use the inhaler. The dose indicator moves down slowly, displaying intervals of 10 (60, 50, 40, 30, 20, 10, 0).
  - When a red band begins to appear in the dose indicator **(See Figure N)**, this means you are nearing your last dose and should obtain a new PRESSAIR inhaler.

Dose indicator goes down by intervals of 10: 60, 50, 40, 30, 20, 10, 0.

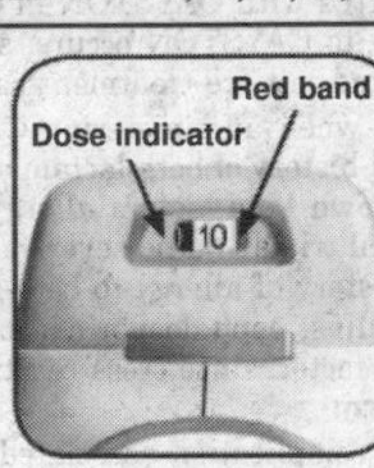

Figure N

  - You should discard the inhaler and start a new one when
    - the marking "0" with the red background shows in the middle of the dose indicator **(See Figure O)**, or
    - the device locks out **(See Figure P)**, or
    - 45 days after you took the inhaler out of the sealed pouch, whichever comes first.

[See figures O and P at top of next column]

- If your TUDORZA PRESSAIR inhaler appears to be damaged or if you lose the cap, your inhaler should be replaced.
- You **do not need** to clean your TUDORZA PRESSAIR inhaler. If you wish to clean it, wipe the outside of the mouthpiece with a dry tissue or paper towel. **Do not** use water to clean your TUDORZA PRESSAIR inhaler, as this may damage your medicine.

This Patient Information and Instructions for Use have been approved by the U.S. Food and Drug Administration.

Distributed by:
Forest Pharmaceuticals, Inc.
Subsidiary of Forest Laboratories, Inc.
St. Louis, MO 63045

FOREST PHARMACEUTICALS, INC.
Subsidiary of Forest Laboratories, Inc.
St. Louis, Missouri 63045

Under license of ALMIRALL, S.A.
Almirall

TUDORZA™ and **PRESSAIR™** are trademarks of ALMIRALL, S.A.

Approved July 2012
Revised September 2012

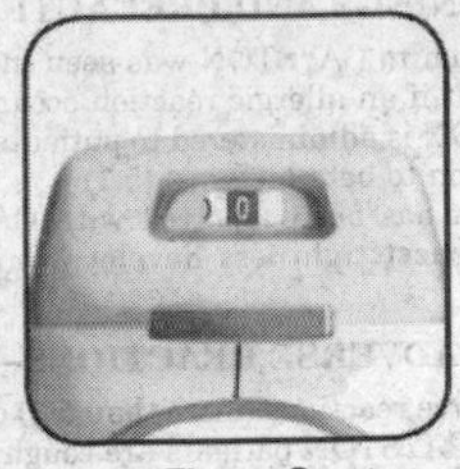

Figure O

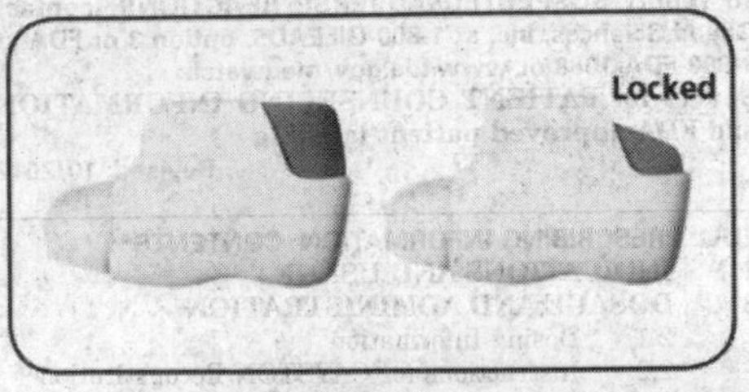

Figure P

Gilead Sciences, Inc.

333 LAKESIDE DRIVE
FOSTER CITY, CA 94404
www.gilead.com

For Medical Information:
1-800-445-3235, press option 2
medicalinformation@gilead.com
To Report Adverse Events:
1-800-445-3235, press option 3
For Business Operations:
1-800-445-3235, press option 8

ATRIPLA®

ATRIPLA® is co-marketed by Bristol-Myers Squibb and Gilead Sciences. Please see Bristol-Myers Squibb & Gilead Sciences, LLC for full prescribing information.

Shown in Product Identification Guide, page 306

CAYSTON® ℞

[kay-stun]
(aztreonam for inhalation solution)

HIGHLIGHTS OF PRESCRIBING INFORMATION

These highlights do not include all the information needed to use CAYSTON safely and effectively. See full prescribing information for CAYSTON.

CAYSTON® (aztreonam for inhalation solution)
Initial U.S. Approval: 1986

To reduce the development of drug-resistant bacteria and maintain the effectiveness of CAYSTON and other antibacterial drugs, CAYSTON should be used only to treat patients with cystic fibrosis (CF) known to have *Pseudomonas aeruginosa* in the lungs.

INDICATIONS AND USAGE

CAYSTON is a monobactam antibacterial indicated to improve respiratory symptoms in cystic fibrosis (CF) patients with *Pseudomonas aeruginosa*. Safety and effectiveness have not been established in pediatric patients below the age of 7 years, patients with FEV_1 <25% or >75% predicted, or patients colonized with *Burkholderia cepacia*. (1)

DOSAGE AND ADMINISTRATION

- Administer one dose (one single use vial and one ampule of diluent) 3 times a day for 28 days. (2.1)
- Use dose immediately after reconstitution. (2.2)
- Administer only with the Altera® Nebulizer System. Do not administer with any other type of nebulizer. (2.3)

DOSAGE FORMS AND STRENGTHS

- Lyophilized aztreonam (75 mg/vial) (3)
- Diluent (0.17% sodium chloride): 1 mL/ampule (3)

CONTRAINDICATIONS

- Do not administer to patients with a known allergy to aztreonam. (4)

WARNINGS AND PRECAUTIONS

- Allergic reaction to CAYSTON was seen in clinical trials. Stop treatment if an allergic reaction occurs. Use caution when CAYSTON is administered to patients with a known allergic reaction to beta-lactams. (5.1)
- Bronchospasm has been reported with CAYSTON. Stop treatment if chest tightness develops during nebulizer use. (5.2)

ADVERSE REACTIONS

- Common adverse reactions (more than 5%) occurring more frequently in CAYSTON patients are cough, nasal congestion, wheezing, pharyngolaryngeal pain, pyrexia, chest discomfort, abdominal pain and vomiting. (6.1)

To report SUSPECTED ADVERSE REACTIONS, contact Gilead Sciences, Inc. at 1-800-GILEAD5, option 3 or FDA at 1-800-FDA-1088 or www.fda.gov/medwatch.

See 17 for PATIENT COUNSELING INFORMATION and FDA-approved patient labeling

Revised: 10/2012

FULL PRESCRIBING INFORMATION: CONTENTS*

*** Sections or subsections omitted from the full prescribing information are not listed**

FULL PRESCRIBING INFORMATION

1 INDICATIONS AND USAGE

CAYSTON® is indicated to improve respiratory symptoms in cystic fibrosis (CF) patients with *Pseudomonas aeruginosa*. Safety and effectiveness have not been established in pediatric patients below the age of 7 years, patients with FEV_1 <25% or >75% predicted, or patients colonized with *Burkholderia cepacia* [*see Clinical Studies (14)*].

To reduce the development of drug-resistant bacteria and maintain the effectiveness of CAYSTON and other antibacterial drugs, CAYSTON should be used only to treat patients with CF known to have *Pseudomonas aeruginosa* in the lungs.

2 DOSAGE AND ADMINISTRATION

2.1 Dosing Information

The recommended dose of CAYSTON for both adults and pediatric patients 7 years of age and older is one single-use vial (75 mg of aztreonam) reconstituted with 1 mL of sterile diluent administered 3 times a day for a 28-day course (followed by 28 days off CAYSTON therapy). Dosage is not based on weight or adjusted for age. Doses should be taken at least 4 hours apart.

CAYSTON is administered by inhalation using an Altera® Nebulizer System. Patients should use a bronchodilator before administration of CAYSTON.

2.2 Instructions for CAYSTON Reconstitution

CAYSTON should be administered immediately after reconstitution. Do not reconstitute CAYSTON until ready to administer a dose.

Take one amber glass vial containing CAYSTON and one diluent ampule from the carton. To open the glass vial, carefully remove the metal ring by pulling the tab and remove the gray rubber stopper. Twist the tip off the diluent ampule and squeeze the liquid into the glass vial. Replace the rubber stopper, then gently swirl the vial until contents have completely dissolved.

The empty vial, stopper, and diluent ampule should be disposed of properly upon completion of dosing.

2.3 Instructions for CAYSTON Administration

CAYSTON is administered by inhalation using an Altera Nebulizer System. CAYSTON should not be administered with any other nebulizer. CAYSTON should not be mixed with any other drugs in the Altera Nebulizer Handset.

CAYSTON is not for intravenous or intramuscular administration.

Patients should use a bronchodilator before administration of CAYSTON. Short-acting bronchodilators can be taken between 15 minutes and 4 hours prior to each dose of CAYSTON. Alternatively, long-acting bronchodilators can be taken between 30 minutes and 12 hours prior to administration of CAYSTON. For patients taking multiple inhaled therapies, the recommended order of administration is as follows: bronchodilator, mucolytics, and lastly, CAYSTON.

To administer CAYSTON, pour the reconstituted solution into the handset of the nebulizer system. Turn the unit on. Place the mouthpiece of the handset in your mouth and breathe normally only through your mouth. Administration typically takes between 2 and 3 minutes. Further patient instructions on how to administer CAYSTON are provided in the FDA-approved patient labeling. Instructions on testing nebulizer functionality and cleaning the handset are provided in the Instructions for Use included with the nebulizer system.

3 DOSAGE FORMS AND STRENGTHS

A dose of CAYSTON consists of a single-use vial of sterile, lyophilized aztreonam (75 mg) reconstituted with a 1 mL ampule of sterile diluent (0.17% sodium chloride). Reconstituted CAYSTON is administered by inhalation.

4 CONTRAINDICATIONS

CAYSTON is contraindicated in patients with a known allergy to aztreonam.

5 WARNINGS AND PRECAUTIONS

5.1 Allergic Reactions

Severe allergic reactions have been reported following administration of aztreonam for injection to patients with no known history of exposure to aztreonam. In addition, allergic reaction with facial rash, facial swelling, and throat tightness was reported with CAYSTON in clinical trials. If an allergic reaction to CAYSTON occurs, stop administration of CAYSTON and initiate treatment as appropriate.

Caution is advised when administering CAYSTON to patients if they have a history of beta-lactam allergy, although patients with a known beta-lactam allergy have received CAYSTON in clinical trials and no severe allergic reactions were reported. A history of allergy to beta-lactam antibiotics, such as penicillins, cephalosporins, and/or carbapenems, may be a risk factor, since cross-reactivity may occur.

5.2 Bronchospasm

Bronchospasm is a complication associated with nebulized therapies, including CAYSTON. Reduction of 15% or more in forced expiratory volume in 1 second (FEV_1) immediately following administration of study medication after pretreatment with a bronchodilator was observed in 3% of patients treated with CAYSTON.

5.3 Decreases in FEV_1 After 28-Day Treatment Cycle

In clinical trials, patients with increases in FEV_1 during a 28-day course of CAYSTON were sometimes treated for pulmonary exacerbations when FEV_1 declined after the treatment period. Healthcare providers should consider a patient's baseline FEV_1 measured prior to CAYSTON therapy and the presence of other symptoms when evaluating whether post-treatment changes in FEV_1 are caused by a pulmonary exacerbation.

5.4 Development of Drug-Resistant Bacteria

Prescribing CAYSTON in the absence of known *Pseudomonas aeruginosa* infection in patients with CF is unlikely to provide benefit and increases the risk of development of drug-resistant bacteria.

6 ADVERSE REACTIONS

6.1 Clinical Trials Experience

Because clinical trials are conducted under widely varying conditions, adverse reaction rates observed in the clinical trials of drugs cannot be directly compared to rates in the clinical trials of another drug and may not reflect the rates observed in practice.

The safety of CAYSTON was evaluated in 344 patients from two placebo-controlled trials and one open-label follow-on trial. In controlled trials, 146 patients with CF received 75 mg CAYSTON 3 times a day for 28 days.

Table 1 displays adverse reactions reported in more than 5% of patients treated with CAYSTON 3 times a day in placebo-controlled trials. The listed adverse reactions occurred more frequently in CAYSTON-treated patients than in placebo-treated patients.

Table 1. Adverse Reactions Reported in more than 5% of Patients Treated with CAYSTON in the Placebo-Controlled Trials

Event (Preferred Term)	Placebo (N = 160) n (%)	CAYSTON 75 mg 3 times a day (N = 146) n (%)
Cough	82 (51%)	79 (54%)
Nasal congestion	19 (12%)	23 (16%)
Wheezing	16 (10%)	23 (16%)
Pharyngolaryngeal pain	17 (11%)	18 (12%)
Pyrexia	9 (6%)	19 (13%)
Chest discomfort	10 (6%)	11 (8%)
Abdominal Pain	8 (5%)	10 (7%)
Vomiting	7 (4%)	9 (6%)

Adverse reactions that occurred in less than 5% of patients treated with CAYSTON were bronchospasm (3%) [*see Warnings and Precautions (5.2)*] and rash (2%).

6.2 Postmarketing Experience

In addition to adverse reactions reported from clinical trials, the following possible adverse reactions have been identified during post-approval use of CAYSTON. Because these events have been reported voluntarily from a population of unknown size, estimates of frequency cannot be made.

MUSCULOSKELETAL AND CONNECTIVE TISSUE DISORDERS

Arthralgia, joint swelling

7 DRUG INTERACTIONS

No formal clinical studies of drug interactions with CAYSTON have been conducted.

8 USE IN SPECIFIC POPULATIONS

8.1 Pregnancy

Pregnancy Category B

No reproductive toxicology studies have been conducted with CAYSTON. However, studies were conducted with aztreonam for injection. Aztreonam has been shown to cross the placenta and enter fetal circulation. No evidence of embryo or fetotoxicity or teratogenicity has been shown in studies with pregnant rats and rabbits. In rats receiving aztreonam for injection during late gestation and lactation, no drug induced changes in maternal, fetal or neonatal parameters were observed. These animal reproduction and developmental toxicity studies used parenteral routes of administration that would provide systemic exposures far in excess of the average peak plasma levels measured in humans following CAYSTON therapy.

No adequate and well-controlled studies of aztreonam for injection or CAYSTON in pregnant women have been conducted. Because animal reproduction studies are not always predictive of human response, CAYSTON should be used during pregnancy only if clearly needed.

8.3 Nursing Mothers

Following administration of aztreonam for injection, aztreonam is excreted in human milk at concentrations that are less than one percent of those determined in simultaneously obtained maternal serum. Peak plasma concentrations of aztreonam following administration of CAYSTON (75 mg) are approximately 1% of peak concentrations observed following IV aztreonam (500 mg). Therefore, use of CAYSTON during breastfeeding is unlikely to pose a risk to infants.

8.4 Pediatric Use

Patients 7 years and older were included in clinical trials with CAYSTON. Fifty-five patients under 18 years of age received CAYSTON in placebo-controlled trials. No dose adjustments were made for pediatric patients. Pyrexia was more commonly reported in pediatric patients than in adult patients. Safety and effectiveness in pediatric patients below the age of 7 years have not been established.

8.5 Geriatric Use

Clinical trials of CAYSTON did not include CAYSTON-treated patients aged 65 years of age and older to determine whether they respond differently from younger patients.

8.6 Use in Patients with Renal Impairment

Aztreonam is known to be excreted by the kidney. Placebo-controlled clinical trials with CAYSTON excluded patients with abnormal baseline renal function (defined as serum creatinine greater than 2 times the upper limit of normal range). Given the low systemic exposure of aztreonam following administration of CAYSTON, clinically relevant accumulation of aztreonam is unlikely to occur in patients with renal impairment. Therefore, CAYSTON may be administered to patients with mild, moderate and severe renal impairment with no dosage adjustment.

10 OVERDOSAGE

No overdoses have been reported with CAYSTON in clinical trials to date. In clinical trials, 225 mg doses of CAYSTON via inhalation were associated with higher rates of drug-related respiratory adverse reactions, particularly cough. Since the peak plasma concentration of aztreonam following administration of CAYSTON (75 mg) is approximately 0.6 mcg/mL, compared to a serum concentration of 54 mcg/mL following administration of aztreonam for injection (500 mg), no systemic safety issues associated with CAYSTON overdose are anticipated.

11 DESCRIPTION

A dose of CAYSTON consists of a 2 mL amber glass vial containing lyophilized aztreonam (75 mg) and lysine (46.7 mg), and a low-density polyethylene ampule containing 1 mL sterile diluent (0.17% sodium chloride). The reconstituted solution is for inhalation. The formulation contains no preservatives or arginine.

The active ingredient in CAYSTON is aztreonam, a monobactam antibacterial. The monobactams are structurally different from beta-lactam antibiotics (e.g., penicillins, cephalosporins, carbapenems) due to a monocyclic nucleus. This nucleus contains several side chains; sulfonic acid in the 1-position activates the nucleus, an aminothiazolyl oxime side chain in the 3-position confers specificity for aerobic Gram negative bacteria including *Pseudomonas spp.*, and a methyl group in the 4-position enhances beta-lactamase stability.

Aztreonam is designated chemically as (*Z*)-2-[[[(2-amino-4-thiazolyl)[[(2*S*,3*S*)-2-methyl-4-oxo-1-sulfo-3-azetidinyl]carbamoyl]methylene]amino]oxy]-2-methylpropionic acid. The structural formula is presented below:

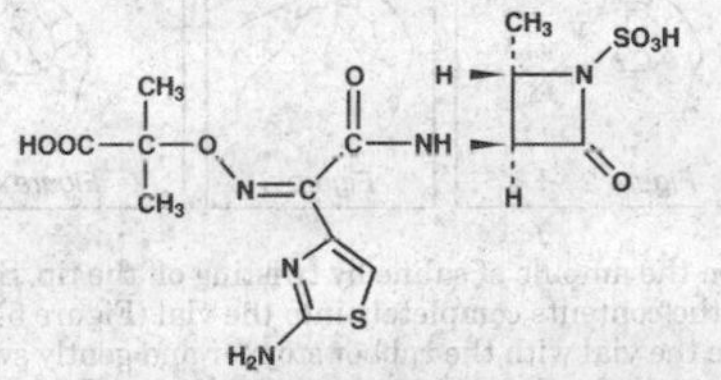

CAYSTON is a white to off-white powder. CAYSTON is sterile, hygroscopic, and light sensitive. Once reconstituted with the supplied diluent, the pH range is 4.5 to 6.0.

12 CLINICAL PHARMACOLOGY

12.1 Mechanism of Action

Aztreonam is an antibacterial drug [*see Clinical Pharmacology (12.4)*].

12.3 Pharmacokinetics

Sputum Concentrations

Sputum aztreonam concentrations exhibited considerable variability between patients receiving CAYSTON (75 mg) in clinical trials. The mean sputum concentration 10 minutes following the first dose of CAYSTON (n = 195 patients with CF) was 726 mcg/g. Mean sputum concentrations of aztreonam in patients receiving CAYSTON 3 times a day for 28 days were 984 mcg/g, 793 mcg/g, and 715 mcg/g 10 minutes after dose administration on Days 0, 14, and 28, respectively, indicating no accumulation of aztreonam in sputum.

Plasma Concentrations

Plasma aztreonam concentrations exhibited considerable variability between patients receiving CAYSTON (75 mg) in the clinical trials. The mean plasma concentration one hour following the first dose of CAYSTON (at approximately the peak plasma concentration) was 0.59 mcg/mL. Mean peak plasma concentrations in patients receiving CAYSTON 3 times a day for 28 days were 0.55 mcg/mL, 0.67 mcg/mL, and 0.65 mcg/mL on Days 0, 14, and 28, respectively, indicating no systemic accumulation of aztreonam. In contrast, the serum concentration of aztreonam following administration of aztreonam for injection (500 mg) is approximately 54 mcg/mL.

Absorption

Evaluation of plasma and urine aztreonam concentrations following administration of CAYSTON indicates low systemic absorption of aztreonam. Approximately 10% of the total CAYSTON dose is excreted in the urine as unchanged drug, as compared to 60–65% following intravenous administration of aztreonam for injection.

Distribution

The protein binding of aztreonam in serum is approximately 56% and is independent of dose.

Metabolism

Following intramuscular administration of aztreonam for injection 500 mg every 8 hours for 7 days, approximately 6% of the dose was excreted as a microbiologically inactive open β-lactam ring hydrolysis product in an 8-hour urine collection on the last day of multiple dosing.

Excretion

The elimination half-life of aztreonam from plasma is approximately 2.1 hours following administration of CAYSTON to adult patients with CF, similar to what has been reported for aztreonam for injection. Approximately 10% of the total CAYSTON dose is excreted in the urine as unchanged drug. Systemically absorbed aztreonam is eliminated about equally by active tubular secretion and glomerular filtration. Following administration of a single intravenous dose of radiolabeled aztreonam for injection, about 12% of the dose was recovered in the feces.

12.4 Microbiology

Mechanism of Action

Aztreonam exhibits activity *in vitro* against Gram-negative aerobic pathogens including *P. aeruginosa*. Aztreonam binds to penicillin-binding proteins of susceptible bacteria, which leads to inhibition of bacterial cell wall synthesis and death of the cell. Aztreonam activity is not decreased in the presence of CF lung secretions.

Susceptibility Testing

A single sputum sample from a patient with CF may contain multiple morphotypes of *P. aeruginosa* and each morphotype may have a different level of *in vitro* susceptibility to aztreonam. There are no *in vitro* susceptibility test interpretive criteria for isolates of *P. aeruginosa* obtained from the sputum of CF patients.[1]

Development of Resistance

No changes in the susceptibility of *P. aeruginosa* to aztreonam were observed following a 28-day course of CAYSTON in the placebo-controlled trials.

Cross-Resistance

No cross-resistance to other classes of antibiotics, including aminoglycosides, quinolones, and beta-lactams, was observed following a 28-day course of CAYSTON in the Phase 3 placebo-controlled trials or in an open-label follow-on trial of up to nine 28-day courses of 75 mg CAYSTON 3 times a day.

Other

No trends in the treatment-emergent isolation of other bacterial respiratory pathogens (*Burkholderia cepacia*, *Stenotrophomonas maltophilia*, *Achromobacter xylosoxidans*, and *Staphylococcus aureus*) were observed in clinical trials. There was a slight increase in the isolation of *Candida spp.* following up to nine 28-day courses of CAYSTON therapy.

13 NONCLINICAL TOXICOLOGY

13.1 Carcinogenesis, Mutagenesis, Impairment of Fertility

A 104-week rat inhalation toxicology study to assess the carcinogenic potential of aztreonam demonstrated no drug-related increase in the incidence of tumors. Rats were exposed to aztreonam for up to 4 hours per day. Peak plasma levels of aztreonam averaging approximately 6.8 mcg/mL were measured in rats at the highest dose level. This is approximately 12-fold higher than the average peak plasma level measured in humans following CAYSTON therapy.

Genetic toxicology studies performed *in vitro* demonstrated that aztreonam did not induce structural chromosome aberrations in CHO cells and did not induce mutations at the TK locus in mouse lymphoma L5178Y $TK^{+/-}$ cells. Likewise, genetic toxicology studies performed *in vivo* did not reveal evidence of mutagenic potential.

Aztreonam did not impair the fertility of rats when administered at doses that would provide systemic exposures far in excess of peak plasma levels measured in humans following CAYSTON therapy.

14 CLINICAL STUDIES

CAYSTON was evaluated over a period of 28 days of treatment in a randomized, double-blind, placebo-controlled, multicenter trial that enrolled patients with CF and *P. aeruginosa*. This trial was designed to evaluate improvement in respiratory symptoms. Patients 7 years of age and older and with FEV_1 of 25% to 75% predicted were enrolled. All patients received CAYSTON or placebo on an outpatient basis administered with the Altera Nebulizer System. All patients were required to take a dose of an inhaled bronchodilator (beta-agonist) prior to taking a dose of CAYSTON or placebo. Patients were receiving standard care for CF, including drugs for obstructive airway diseases.

The trial enrolled 164 patients with CF and *P. aeruginosa*. The mean age was 30 years, and the mean baseline FEV_1 % predicted was 55%; 43% were females and 96% were Caucasian. These patients were randomized in a 1:1 ratio to receive either CAYSTON (75 mg) or volume-matched placebo administered by inhalation 3 times a day for 28 days. Patients were required to have been off antibiotics for at least 28 days before treatment with study drug. The primary efficacy endpoint was improvement in respiratory symptoms on the last day of treatment with CAYSTON or placebo. Respiratory symptoms were also assessed two weeks after the completion of treatment with CAYSTON or placebo. Changes in respiratory symptoms were assessed using a questionnaire that asks patients to report on symptoms like cough, wheezing, and sputum production.

Improvement in respiratory symptoms was noted for CAYSTON-treated patients relative to placebo-treated patients on the last day of drug treatment. Statistically significant improvements were seen in both adult and pediatric patients, but were substantially smaller in adult patients. Two weeks after completion of treatment, a difference in respiratory symptoms between treatment groups was still present, though the difference was smaller.

Pulmonary function, as measured by FEV_1 (L), increased from baseline in patients treated with CAYSTON (see Figure 1). The treatment difference at Day 28 between CAYSTON-treated and placebo-treated patients for percent change in FEV_1 (L) was statistically significant at 10% (95% CI: 6%, 14%). Improvements in FEV_1 were comparable between adult and pediatric patients. Two weeks after completion of drug treatment, the difference in FEV_1 between CAYSTON and placebo groups had decreased to 6% (95% CI: 2%, 9%).

Figure 1. Adjusted Mean Percent Change in FEV_1 from Baseline to Study End (Days 0–42).

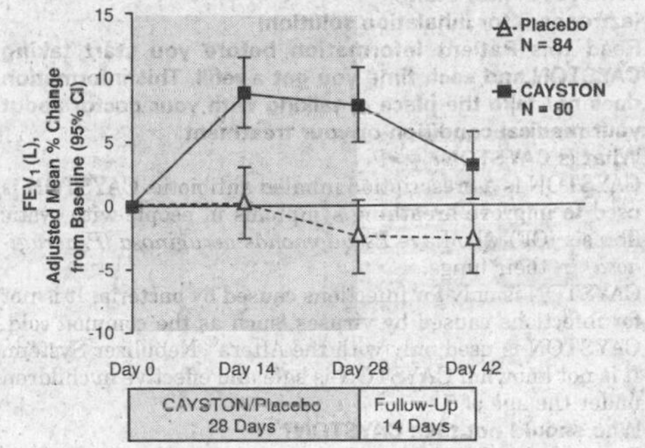

15 REFERENCES

1. Clinical and Laboratory Standards Institute (CLSI). Methods for Dilution Antimicrobial Susceptibility Tests for Bacteria that Grow Aerobically—Eighth Edition; Approved Standard. CLSI Document M7-A8. CLSI, Wayne, PA 19087. January, 2009.

16 HOW SUPPLIED/STORAGE AND HANDLING

Each kit for a 28-day course of CAYSTON contains 84 sterile vials of CAYSTON and 88 ampules of sterile diluent packed in 2 cartons, each carton containing a 14-day supply. The four additional diluent ampules are provided in case of spillage.

Package Configuration	Dosage Strength	NDC No.
28-Day Kit	75 mg	61958-0901-1

CAYSTON vials and diluent ampules should be stored in the refrigerator at 2 °C to 8 °C (36 °F to 46 °F) until needed. Once removed from the refrigerator, CAYSTON and diluent may be stored at room temperature (up to 25 °C/77 °F) for up to 28 days. Do not separate the CAYSTON vials from the diluent ampules. CAYSTON should be protected from light. Do not use CAYSTON if it has been stored at room temperature for more than 28 days. Do not use CAYSTON beyond the expiration date stamped on the vial. Do not use diluent beyond the expiration date embossed on the ampule.

CAYSTON should be used immediately upon reconstitution. Do not reconstitute more than one dose at a time.

Do not use diluent or reconstituted CAYSTON if it is cloudy or if there are particles in the solution.

17 PATIENT COUNSELING INFORMATION

See FDA-Approved Patient Labeling

Patients should be advised that CAYSTON is for inhalation use only and that CAYSTON should only be administered using the Altera Nebulizer System. Patients should be instructed only to reconstitute CAYSTON with the provided diluent and not mix other drugs with CAYSTON in the Altera Nebulizer System.

Patients should be advised to complete the full 28-day course of CAYSTON even if they are feeling better. Inform the patient that if they miss a dose, they should take all 3 daily doses as long as the doses are at least 4 hours apart.

Patients should be advised to use a bronchodilator prior to administration of CAYSTON. Patients taking several inhaled medications should be advised to use the medications in the following order of administration: bronchodilator, mucolytics, and lastly, CAYSTON.

Patients should be advised to tell their doctor if they have new or worsening symptoms. Patients who believe they are experiencing an allergic reaction to CAYSTON should be advised to contact their doctor immediately.

Patients should be counseled that antibacterial drugs including CAYSTON should only be used to treat bacterial infections. They do not treat viral infection (e.g., the common cold). When CAYSTON is prescribed to treat a bacterial infection, patients should be told that although it is common to feel better early in the course of therapy, the medication should be taken as directed. Skipping doses or not completing the full course of therapy may (1) decrease the effectiveness of the immediate treatment and (2) increase the likelihood that bacteria will develop resistance and will not be treatable by CAYSTON or other antibacterial drugs in the future.

Manufactured by: Gilead Sciences, Inc., Foster City, CA 94404

CAYSTON is a trademark of Gilead Sciences, Inc. All other trademarks referenced herein are the property of their respective owners.

50-814-GS-001

FDA-Approved Patient Labeling

Patient Information

CAYSTON® (kay-stun)

(aztreonam for inhalation solution)

Read this Patient Information before you start taking CAYSTON and each time you get a refill. This information does not take the place of talking with your doctor about your medical condition or your treatment.

What is CAYSTON?

CAYSTON is a prescription inhaled antibiotic. CAYSTON is used to improve breathing symptoms in people with cystic fibrosis (CF) who have *Pseudomonas aeruginosa (P. aeruginosa)* in their lungs.

CAYSTON is only for infections caused by bacteria. It is not for infections caused by viruses, such as the common cold.

CAYSTON is used only with the Altera® Nebulizer System.

It is not known if CAYSTON is safe and effective in children under the age of 7.

Who should not take CAYSTON?

Do not take CAYSTON if you are allergic to aztreonam (AZACTAM®).

What should I tell my doctor before taking CAYSTON?

Before taking CAYSTON, tell your doctor if you:
- are allergic to any antibiotics.
- are pregnant or plan to become pregnant.
- are breast-feeding or plan to breast feed. Talk to your doctor about the best way to breast feed your baby if you take CAYSTON.

Tell your doctor about all the medicine you take, including prescription and non-prescription medicines, vitamins and herbal supplements.

Know the medicines you take. Keep a list of them to show your doctor and pharmacist when you get a new medicine.

How should I take CAYSTON?
- Take CAYSTON exactly as prescribed by your doctor.
- The dose of CAYSTON for both adults and children 7 years of age and older is one vial of CAYSTON, mixed with one ampule of saline (diluent) 3 times a day.
- Doses of CAYSTON should be taken at least 4 hours apart (for example: morning, after school, and before bed).
- CAYSTON should be taken for 28 days.
- CAYSTON is taken as a breathing treatment (inhalation) with the Altera Nebulizer System. Do not use any other nebulizer for your CAYSTON treatment.
- You should use an inhaled bronchodilator (a type of medicine used to relax and open your airways) before taking a dose of CAYSTON. If you do not have an inhaled bronchodilator, ask your doctor to prescribe one for you.
- If you are taking several medicines or treatments to treat your cystic fibrosis, you should take your medicines or other treatments in this order:
  1) bronchodilator
  2) mucolytics (medicines to help clear mucus from your lungs)
  3) CAYSTON
- You should take CAYSTON as prescribed, in courses of 28 days on CAYSTON, followed by at least 28 days off CAYSTON, as directed by your doctor.
- Do not mix CAYSTON with any other medicines in your Altera Nebulizer System.
- Do not mix CAYSTON with the saline until right before you are ready to use it. Do not mix more than one dose of CAYSTON at a time.
- Each treatment should take about 2 to 3 minutes.
- If you miss a dose of CAYSTON, you can still take all 3 daily doses as long as they are at least 4 hours apart.
- It is important for you to finish taking the full 28-day course of CAYSTON even if you are feeling better. If you skip doses or do not finish the full 28-day course of CAYSTON, your infection may not be fully treated and CAYSTON may not work as well as a treatment for infections in the future.
- See the end of this Patient Information leaflet for the Patient Instructions for Use on how to take CAYSTON the right way.

What are the possible side effects of CAYSTON?

CAYSTON can cause serious side effects, including:
- **Severe allergic reactions. Stop your treatment with CAYSTON and call your doctor right away if you have any symptoms of an allergic reaction, including:**
  - Rash or swelling of your face
  - Throat tightness
- **Trouble breathing right after treatment with CAYSTON (bronchospasm).** To decrease the chance of this happening, be sure to use your inhaled bronchodilator medicine before each treatment with CAYSTON. See "How should I take CAYSTON?"

Common side effects of CAYSTON include:
- Cough
- Nasal congestion
- Wheezing
- Sore throat
- Fever. Fever may be more common in children than in adults.
- Chest discomfort
- Stomach area (abdominal) pain
- Vomiting

Other possible side effects of CAYSTON include:
- Swelling or pain of joints

Tell your doctor if you have any new or worsening symptoms while taking CAYSTON. Tell your doctor about any side effect that bothers you or that does not go away.

These are not all the possible side effects of CAYSTON. For more information, ask your doctor or pharmacist.

Call your doctor for medical advice about side effects. You may report side effects to FDA at 1-800-FDA-1088.

How should I store CAYSTON?
- Each CAYSTON kit contains enough vials of CAYSTON and ampules of saline for 28 days of treatment. There are 4 extra saline ampules in case some saline spills.
- Always keep your CAYSTON and saline together.
- Store CAYSTON and saline in the refrigerator at 36 °F to 46 °F (2 °C to 8 °C) until needed.
- When you remove CAYSTON and saline from the refrigerator, they may be stored at room temperature (less than 77 °F) for up to 28 days. Do not use any CAYSTON that has been stored at room temperature for more than 28 days.
- Keep CAYSTON away from light.
- Do not use CAYSTON after the expiration date on the vial. Do not use the saline after the expiration date on the ampule.

Keep CAYSTON and all medicines out of the reach of children.

General information about CAYSTON

Medicines are sometimes prescribed for purposes other than those listed in a Patient Information leaflet. Do not use CAYSTON for a condition for which it was not prescribed. Do not give CAYSTON to other people, even if they have the same symptoms that you have. It may harm them.

This Patient Information leaflet summarizes the most important information about CAYSTON. If you would like more information, talk with your doctor. You can ask your pharmacist or doctor for information about CAYSTON that is written for health professionals.

For more information, call 1-877-7CAYSTON (1-877-722-9786).

What are the ingredients in CAYSTON?

Active ingredient: aztreonam

Inactive ingredient: lysine, sodium chloride (diluent)

Patient Instructions for Use

CAYSTON®

(aztreonam for inhalation solution)

Be sure that you read, understand and follow the Patient Instructions for Use below for the right way to take CAYSTON. If you have any questions, ask your doctor or pharmacist.

You will need the following supplies (Figure 1):
- 1 amber colored CAYSTON vial
- 1 ampule of saline (diluent)
- Altera Nebulizer System

[See figure 1 at top of next column]

Check to make sure that your Altera Nebulizer System works properly before starting your treatment with CAYSTON. See the manufacturer's instructions for use that comes with your Altera Nebulizer System. This should have complete information about how to put together (assemble), prepare, use, and care for your Altera Nebulizer System.

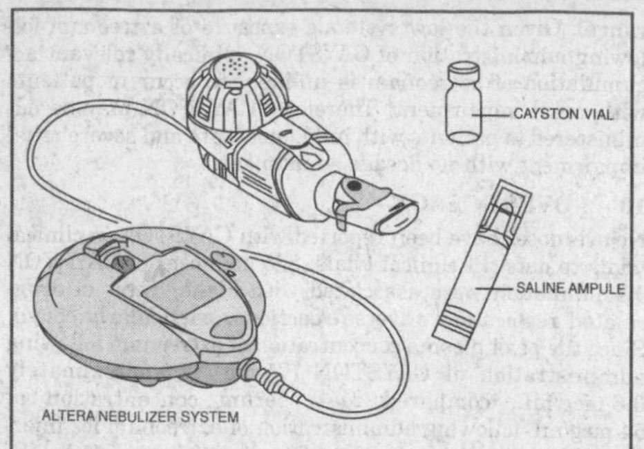

Figure 1

Step 1 Preparing your CAYSTON for inhalation
1. Mix (reconstitute) CAYSTON with the saline only when ready to take a dose. Take one amber vial of CAYSTON and one ampule of saline from the carton. Separate the saline ampules by gently pulling apart.
2. Look at the ampule of saline. If it looks cloudy do not use it. Throw away this ampule and get another ampule of saline.
3. Gently tap the vial so that the powder settles to the bottom of the vial. This helps you get the proper dose of medicine. Open the amber drug vial by lifting up the metal flap on the top (Figure 2) and pulling down (Figure 3) to carefully remove the entire metal ring from the vial (Figure 4). Safely dispose of the ring in household garbage. Carefully remove the rubber stopper.

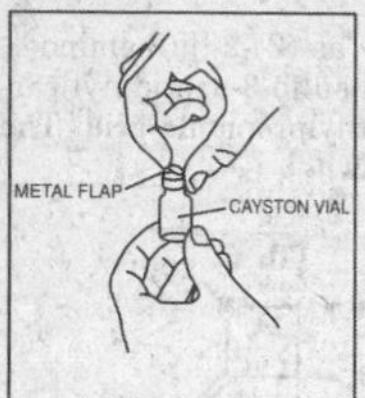

Figure 2

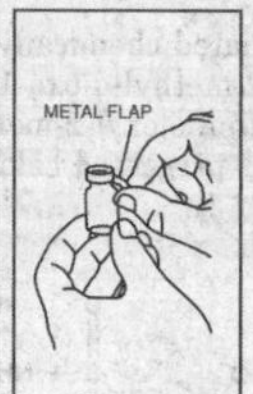

Figure 3

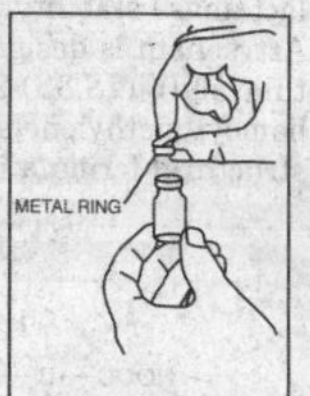

Figure 4

4. Open the ampule of saline by twisting off the tip. Squeeze out the contents completely into the vial (Figure 5). Next, close the vial with the rubber stopper and gently swirl the vial until the powder has completely dissolved and the liquid is clear.

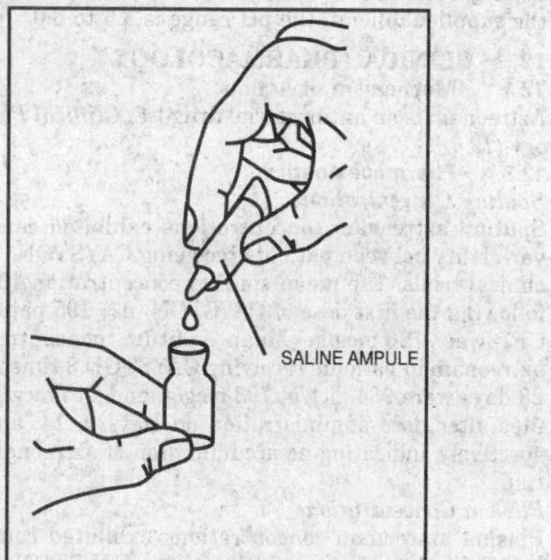

Figure 5

5. After mixing CAYSTON with the saline, check to make sure the diluted medicine is clear. If it is cloudy or has particles in it, do not use this medicine. Throw away this dose of medicine and start over again with a new vial of CAYSTON and a new ampule of saline.
6. Use CAYSTON right away after you mix with the saline.

Step 2 Taking your CAYSTON treatment

See the manufacturer's instructions for use that comes with your Altera Nebulizer System for complete instructions on taking a treatment, and how to clean and disinfect your Altera Nebulizer Handset.

7. Make sure the handset is on a flat, stable surface.
8. Remove the rubber stopper from the vial, then pour all of the mixed CAYSTON and saline into the Medication Reservoir of the handset (Figure 6). Be sure to completely empty the vial, gently tapping the vial against the side of the Medication Reservoir if necessary. Close the Medication Reservoir (Figure 7).

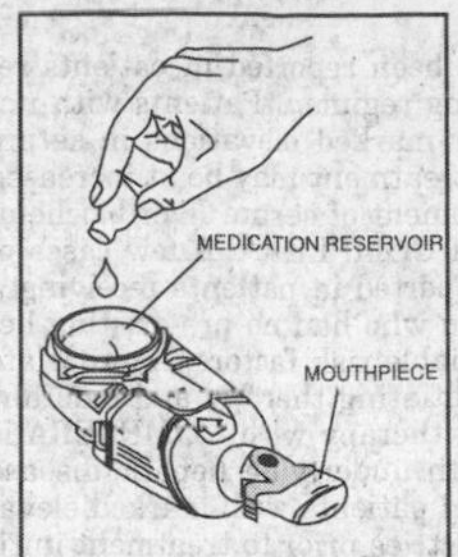

Figure 6

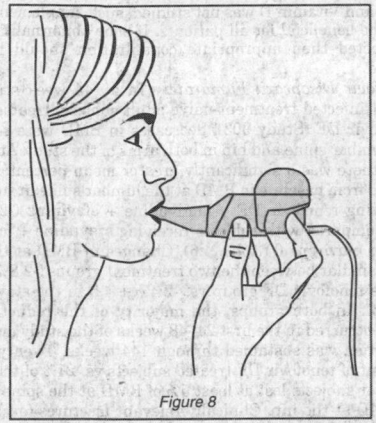

Figure 7

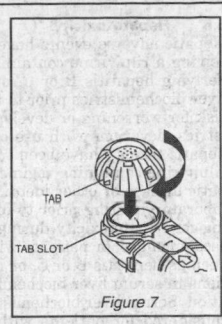

9. Begin your treatment by sitting in a relaxed, upright position. Hold the handset level, and place the Mouthpiece in your mouth. Close your lips around the Mouthpiece (Figure 8).

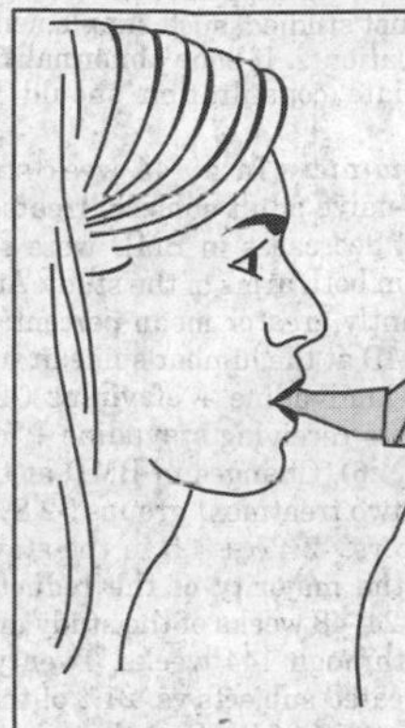
Figure 8

10. Breathe in and out normally (inhale and exhale) through the Mouthpiece. **Avoid breathing through your nose**. Continue to inhale and exhale comfortably until the treatment is finished.
11. The empty vial, stopper and saline ampule should be disposed of in household garbage upon completion of dosing.

Manufactured by: Gilead Sciences, Inc., Foster City, CA 94404

CAYSTON is a trademark of Gilead Sciences, Inc. All other trademarks referenced herein are the property of their respective owners.

50-814-GS-001

Shown in Product Identification Guide, page 306

COMPLERA® ℞

[*kom-PLEH-rah*]

(emtricitabine/rilpivirine/tenofovir disoproxil fumarate) tablets, for oral use

HIGHLIGHTS OF PRESCRIBING INFORMATION

These highlights do not include all the information needed to use COMPLERA safely and effectively. See full prescribing information for COMPLERA.

COMPLERA®(emtricitabine/rilpivirine/tenofovir disoproxil fumarate) tablets, for oral use

Initial U.S. Approval: 2011

WARNING: LACTIC ACIDOSIS/SEVERE HEPATOMEGALY WITH STEATOSIS and POST TREATMENT ACUTE EXACERBATION OF HEPATITIS B

See full prescribing information for complete boxed warning.

- **Lactic acidosis and severe hepatomegaly with steatosis, including fatal cases, have been reported with the use of nucleoside analogs, including tenofovir disoproxil fumarate, a component of COMPLERA. (5.1)**
- **COMPLERA is not approved for the treatment of chronic hepatitis B virus (HBV) infection. Severe acute exacerbations of hepatitis B have been reported in patients coinfected with HIV-1 and HBV who have discontinued EMTRIVA or VIREAD, two of the components of COMPLERA. Hepatic function should be monitored closely in these patients. If appropriate, initiation of anti-hepatitis B therapy may be warranted. (5.2)**

RECENT MAJOR CHANGES

Indications and Usage (1)	01/2013
Dosage and Administration (2)	06/2013
Contraindications (4)	01/2013
Warnings and Precautions	
Depressive Disorders (5.5)	01/2013
Hepatotoxicity (5.6)	01/2013
Coadministration with Other Products (5.8)	01/2013
Immune Reconstitution Syndrome (5.10)	08/2012

INDICATIONS AND USAGE

COMPLERA, a combination of 2 nucleoside analog HIV-1 reverse transcriptase inhibitors (emtricitabine and tenofovir disoproxil fumarate) and 1 non-nucleoside reverse transcriptase inhibitor (rilpivirine), is indicated for use as a complete regimen for the treatment of HIV-1 infection in treatment-naive adult patients with HIV-1 RNA less than or equal to 100,000 copies/mL. (1)

This indication is based on safety and efficacy analyses through 96 weeks from 2 randomized, double-blind, active controlled, Phase 3 trials in treatment-naïve subjects. (14)

The following points should be considered when initiating therapy with COMPLERA:

- More rilpivirine-treated subjects with HIV-1 RNA greater than 100,000 copies/mL at the start of therapy experienced virologic failure (HIV-1 RNA ≥50 copies/mL) compared to rilpivirine-treated subjects with HIV-1 RNA less than or equal to 100,000 copies/mL.
- Regardless of HIV-1 RNA level at the start of therapy, more rilpivirine-treated subjects with CD4+ cell count less than 200 cells/mm^3 at the start of therapy experienced virologic failure compared to subjects with CD4+ cell count greater than or equal to 200 cells/mm^3.
- The observed virologic failure rate in rilpivirine-treated subjects conferred a higher rate of overall treatment resistance and cross-resistance to the NNRTI class compared to efavirenz.
- More subjects treated with rilpivirine developed tenofovir and lamivudine/emtricitabine associated resistance compared to efavirenz. (1, 12.4, 14)
- COMPLERA is not recommended for patients less than 18 years of age. (8.4)

DOSAGE AND ADMINISTRATION

- Recommended dose: One tablet (containing 200 mg of emtricitabine, 25 mg of rilpivirine, and 300 mg of tenofovir disoproxil fumarate) taken once daily with food. (2)
- Dose in renal impairment: Should not be administered in patients with creatinine clearance below 50 mL per minute. (2)

DOSAGE FORMS AND STRENGTHS

Tablets: 200 mg of emtricitabine, 25 mg of rilpivirine, and 300 mg of tenofovir disoproxil fumarate. (3)

CONTRAINDICATIONS

Coadministration of COMPLERA is contraindicated with drugs where significant decreases in rilpivirine plasma concentrations may occur, which may result in loss of virologic response and possible resistance and cross-resistance. (4)

WARNINGS AND PRECAUTIONS

- New onset or worsening renal impairment: Can include acute renal failure and Fanconi syndrome. Assess creatinine clearance (CrCl) before initiating treatment with COMPLERA. Monitor CrCl and serum phosphorus in patients at risk. Avoid administering COMPLERA with concurrent or recent use of nephrotoxic drugs. (5.3)
- Caution should be given to prescribing COMPLERA with drugs that may reduce the exposure of rilpivirine. (5.4)
- Caution should be given to prescribing COMPLERA with drugs with a known risk of Torsade de Pointes. (5.4)
- Depressive disorders: Severe depressive disorders have been reported. Immediate medical evaluation is recommended for severe depressive disorders. (5.5)
- Hepatotoxicity: Hepatic adverse events have been reported in patients receiving a rilpivirine-containing regimen. Monitor serum liver biochemistries before and during treatment with COMPLERA in patients with underlying hepatic disease or marked elevations in serum liver biochemistries. Also consider monitoring serum liver biochemistries in patients without risk factors. (5.6)
- Decreases in bone mineral density (BMD): Consider monitoring BMD in patients with a history of pathologic fracture or other risk factors of osteoporosis or bone loss. (5.7)
- Coadministration with other products: Do not use with drugs containing emtricitabine, rilpivirine or tenofovir disoproxil fumarate including ATRIPLA, EDURANT, EMTRIVA, STRIBILD, TRUVADA, VIREAD, or with drugs containing lamivudine. Do not administer in combination with HEPSERA. (5.8)
- Redistribution/accumulation of body fat: Observed in patients receiving antiretroviral therapy. (5.9)
- Immune reconstitution syndrome: May necessitate further evaluation and treatment. (5.10)

ADVERSE REACTIONS

Most common adverse drug reactions to rilpivirine (incidence greater than or equal to 2%, Grades 2–4) are depressive disorders, insomnia, and headache. (6.1)

Most common adverse drug reactions to emtricitabine and tenofovir disoproxil fumarate (incidence ≥10%) are diarrhea, nausea, fatigue, headache, dizziness, depression, insomnia, abnormal dreams, and rash. (6.1)

To report SUSPECTED ADVERSE REACTIONS, contact Gilead Sciences, Inc. at 1-800-GILEAD-5 or FDA at 1-800-FDA-1088 or www.fda.gov/medwatch

DRUG INTERACTIONS

- COMPLERA is a complete regimen for the treatment of HIV-1 infection; therefore, COMPLERA should not be administered with other antiretroviral medications for treatment of HIV-1 infection.
- CYP3A4 inducers or inhibitors: Drugs that induce or inhibit CYP3A4 may affect the plasma concentrations of rilpivirine. (7.1)
- Drugs that increase gastric pH: Drugs that increase gastric pH may decrease plasma concentrations of rilpivirine. (7.2)

USE IN SPECIFIC POPULATIONS

- Pregnancy: Use during pregnancy only if the potential benefit justifies the potential risk. (8.1)
- Nursing mothers: Women infected with HIV should be instructed not to breastfeed due to the potential for HIV transmission. (8.3)
- Pediatrics: Not recommended for patients less than 18 years of age. (8.4)

See 17 for PATIENT COUNSELING INFORMATION and FDA-approved patient labeling

Revised: 06/2013

FULL PRESCRIBING INFORMATION: CONTENTS*

*** Sections or subsections omitted from the full prescribing information are not listed**

FULL PRESCRIBING INFORMATION

WARNING: LACTIC ACIDOSIS/SEVERE HEPATOMEGALY WITH STEATOSIS and POST TREATMENT ACUTE EXACERBATION OF HEPATITIS B

Lactic acidosis and severe hepatomegaly with steatosis, including fatal cases, have been reported with the use of nucleoside analogs, including tenofovir disoproxil fumarate, a component of COMPLERA, in combination with other antiretrovirals *[See Warnings and Precautions (5.1)]*.

COMPLERA is not approved for the treatment of chronic hepatitis B virus (HBV) infection and the safety and efficacy of COMPLERA have not been established in patients coinfected with HBV and HIV-1. Severe acute exacerbations of hepatitis B have been reported in patients who are coinfected with HBV and HIV-1 and have discontinued EMTRIVA or VIREAD, which are components of COMPLERA. Hepatic function should be monitored closely with both clinical and laboratory follow-up for at least several months in patients who are coinfected with HIV-1 and HBV and discontinue COMPLERA. If appropriate, initiation of anti-hepatitis B therapy may be warranted *[See Warnings and Precautions (5.2)]*.

1 INDICATIONS AND USAGE

COMPLERA® (emtricitabine/rilpivirine/tenofovir disoproxil fumarate) is indicated for use as a complete regimen for the treatment of HIV-1 infection in antiretroviral treatment-naive adult patients with HIV-1 RNA less than or equal to 100,000 copies/mL at the start of therapy.

This indication is based on safety and efficacy analyses through 96 weeks from 2 randomized, double-blind, active controlled, Phase 3 trials in treatment-naive subjects comparing rilpivirine to efavirenz *[See Clinical Studies (14)]*.

The following points should be considered when initiating therapy with COMPLERA:

- More rilpivirine-treated subjects with HIV-1 RNA greater than 100,000 copies/mL at the start of therapy experienced virologic failure (HIV-1 RNA ≥50 copies/mL) compared to rilpivirine-treated subjects with HIV-1 RNA less than or equal to 100,000 copies/mL *[See Clinical Studies (14)]*.
- Regardless of HIV-1 RNA level at the start of therapy, more rilpivirine-treated subjects with CD4+ cell count less than 200 cells/mm^3 experienced virologic failure compared to rilpivirine-treated subjects with CD4+ cell count greater than or equal to 200 cells/mm^3 *[See Clinical Studies (14)]*.
- The observed virologic failure rate in rilpivirine-treated subjects conferred a higher rate of overall treatment resistance and cross-resistance to the NNRTI class compared to efavirenz *[See Microbiology (12.4)]*.
- More subjects treated with rilpivirine developed tenofovir and lamivudine/emtricitabine associated resistance compared to efavirenz *[See Microbiology (12.4)]*.

COMPLERA is not recommended for patients less than 18 years of age *[See Use in Specific Populations (8.4)]*.

2 DOSAGE AND ADMINISTRATION

Adults: The recommended dose of COMPLERA is one tablet taken orally once daily with food *[See Clinical Pharmacology (12.3)]*.

Renal Impairment: Because COMPLERA is a fixed-dose combination, it should not be prescribed for patients requiring dose adjustment such as those with moderate or severe renal impairment (creatinine clearance below 50 mL per minute).

3 DOSAGE FORMS AND STRENGTHS

COMPLERA is available as tablets. Each tablet contains 200 mg of emtricitabine (FTC), 27.5 mg of rilpivirine hydrochloride (equivalent to 25 mg of rilpivirine) and 300 mg of tenofovir disoproxil fumarate (tenofovir DF or TDF, equivalent to 245 mg of tenofovir disoproxil).

The tablets are purplish-pink, capsule-shaped, film-coated, debossed with "GSI" on one side and plain-faced on the other side.

4 CONTRAINDICATIONS

COMPLERA should not be coadministered with the following drugs, as significant decreases in rilpivirine plasma concentrations may occur due to CYP3A enzyme induction or gastric pH increase, which may result in loss of virologic response and possible resistance to COMPLERA or to the class of NNRTIs *[See Drug Interactions (7) and Clinical Pharmacology (12.3)]*:

- the anticonvulsants carbamazepine, oxcarbazepine, phenobarbital, phenytoin
- the antimycobacterials rifabutin, rifampin, rifapentine
- proton pump inhibitors, such as dexlansoprazole, esomeprazole, lansoprazole, omeprazole, pantoprazole, rabeprazole
- the glucocorticoid systemic dexamethasone (more than a single dose)
- St. John's wort (*Hypericum perforatum*)

5 WARNINGS AND PRECAUTIONS

5.1 Lactic Acidosis/Severe Hepatomegaly with Steatosis

Lactic acidosis and severe hepatomegaly with steatosis, including fatal cases, have been reported with the use of nucleoside analogs, including tenofovir DF, a component of COMPLERA, in combination with other antiretrovirals. A majority of these cases have been in women. Obesity and prolonged nucleoside exposure may be risk factors. Particular caution should be exercised when administering nucleoside analogs to any patient with known risk factors for liver disease; however, cases have also been reported in patients with no known risk factors. Treatment with COMPLERA should be suspended in any patient who develops clinical or laboratory findings suggestive of lactic acidosis or pronounced hepatotoxicity (which may include hepatomegaly and steatosis even in the absence of marked transaminase elevations).

5.2 Patients Coinfected with HIV-1 and HBV

It is recommended that all patients with HIV-1 be tested for the presence of chronic hepatitis B virus before initiating antiretroviral therapy. COMPLERA is not approved for the treatment of chronic HBV infection and the safety and efficacy of COMPLERA have not been established in patients coinfected with HBV and HIV-1. Severe acute exacerbations of hepatitis B have been reported in patients who are coinfected with HBV and HIV-1 and have discontinued emtricitabine or tenofovir DF, two of the components of COMPLERA. In some patients infected with HBV and treated with EMTRIVA®, the exacerbations of hepatitis B were associated with liver decompensation and liver failure. Patients who are coinfected with HIV-1 and HBV should be closely monitored with both clinical and laboratory follow-up for at least several months after stopping treatment with COMPLERA. If appropriate, initiation of anti-hepatitis B therapy may be warranted.

5.3 New Onset or Worsening Renal Impairment

Renal impairment, including cases of acute renal failure and Fanconi syndrome (renal tubular injury with severe hypophosphatemia), has been reported with the use of tenofovir DF *[See Adverse Reactions (6.2)]*.

It is recommended that creatinine clearance be calculated in all patients prior to initiating therapy and as clinically appropriate during therapy with COMPLERA. Routine monitoring of calculated creatinine clearance and serum phosphorus should be performed in patients at risk for renal impairment, including patients who have previously experienced renal events while receiving HEPSERA®.

COMPLERA should be avoided with concurrent or recent use of a nephrotoxic agent.

Emtricitabine and tenofovir are principally eliminated by the kidney; however, rilpivirine is not. Since COMPLERA is a combination product and the dose of the individual components cannot be altered, patients with creatinine clearance below 50 mL per minute should not receive COMPLERA.

5.4 Drug Interactions

Caution should be given to prescribing COMPLERA with drugs that may reduce the exposure of rilpivirine *[See Contraindications (4), Drug Interactions (7), and Clinical Pharmacology (12.3)]*.

In healthy subjects, supratherapeutic doses of rilpivirine (75 mg once daily and 300 mg once daily) have been shown to prolong the QTc interval of the electrocardiogram *[See Drug Interactions (7) and Clinical Pharmacology (12.2)]*. COMPLERA should be used with caution when coadministered with a drug with a known risk of Torsade de Pointes.

5.5 Depressive Disorders

The adverse reaction depressive disorders (depressed mood, depression, dysphoria, major depression, mood altered, negative thoughts, suicide attempt, suicidal ideation) has been reported with rilpivirine. During the Phase 3 trials (N=1368) through 96 weeks, the incidence of depressive disorders (regardless of causality, severity) reported among rilpivirine (N=686) or efavirenz (N=682) was 9% and 8%, respectively. Most events were mild or moderate in severity. The incidence of Grades 3 and 4 depressive disorders (regardless of causality) was 1% for both rilpivirine and efavirenz. The incidence of discontinuation due to depressive disorders among rilpivirine or efavirenz was 1% in each arm. Suicidal ideation was reported in 4 subjects in each arm while suicide attempt was reported in 2 subjects in the rilpivirine arm. Patients with severe depressive symptoms should seek immediate medical evaluation to assess the possibility that the symptoms are related to COMPLERA, and if so, to determine whether the risks of continued therapy outweigh the benefits.

5.6 Hepatotoxicity

Hepatic adverse events have been reported in patients receiving a rilpivirine containing regimen. Patients with underlying hepatitis B or C, or marked elevations in serum liver biochemistries prior to treatment may be at increased risk for worsening or development of serum liver biochemistries elevations with use of COMPLERA. A few cases of hepatic toxicity have been reported in patients receiving a rilpivirine containing regimen who had no pre-existing hepatic disease or other identifiable risk factors. Appropriate laboratory testing prior to initiating therapy and monitoring for hepatotoxicity during therapy with COMPLERA is recommended in patients with underlying hepatic disease such as hepatitis B or C, or in patients with marked elevations in serum liver biochemistries prior to treatment initiation. Serum liver biochemistries monitoring should also be considered for patients without pre-existing hepatic dysfunction or other risk factors.

5.7 Decreases in Bone Mineral Density

Bone mineral density (BMD) monitoring should be considered for HIV-1 infected patients who have a history of pathologic bone fracture or other risk factors for osteoporosis or bone loss. Although the effect of supplementation with calcium and Vitamin D was not studied, such supplementation may be beneficial for all patients. If bone abnormalities are suspected then appropriate consultation should be obtained.

Tenofovir Disoproxil Fumarate: In a 144 week study of HIV-1 infected treatment-naive adult subjects treated with tenofovir DF (Study 903), decreases in BMD were seen at the lumbar spine and hip in both arms of the study. At Week 144, there was a significantly greater mean percentage decrease from baseline in BMD at the lumbar spine in subjects receiving tenofovir DF + lamivudine + efavirenz (-2.2% ± 3.9) compared with subjects receiving stavudine + lamivudine + efavirenz (-1.0% ± 4.6). Changes in BMD at the hip were similar between the two treatment groups (-2.8% ± 3.5 in the tenofovir DF group vs. -2.4% ± 4.5 in the stavudine group). In both groups, the majority of the reduction in BMD occurred in the first 24–48 weeks of the study and this reduction was sustained through 144 weeks. Twenty-eight percent of tenofovir DF-treated subjects vs. 21% of the comparator subjects lost at least 5% of BMD at the spine or 7% of BMD at the hip. Clinically relevant fractures (excluding fingers and toes) were reported in 4 subjects in the tenofovir DF group and 6 subjects in the comparator group. Tenofovir DF was associated with significant increases in biochemical markers of bone metabolism (serum bone-specific alkaline phosphatase, serum osteocalcin, serum C telopeptide, and urinary N telopeptide), suggesting increased bone turnover. Serum parathyroid hormone levels and 1,25 Vitamin D levels were also higher in subjects receiving tenofovir DF.

The effects of tenofovir DF-associated changes in BMD and biochemical markers on long-term bone health and future fracture risk are unknown. For additional information, please consult the VIREAD® prescribing information.

Cases of osteomalacia (associated with proximal renal tubulopathy and which may contribute to fractures) have been reported in association with the use of VIREAD *[See Adverse Reactions (6.2)]*.

5.8 Coadministration with Other Products

COMPLERA should not be administered concurrently with other medicinal products containing any of the same active components, emtricitabine, rilpivirine, or tenofovir DF (ATRIPLA®, Edurant®, EMTRIVA, STRIBILD®, TRUVADA®, VIREAD), with medicinal products containing lamivudine (Epivir®, Epivir-HBV®, Epzicom®, Combivir®, Trizivir®), or with adefovir dipivoxil (HEPSERA).

5.9 Fat Redistribution

Redistribution/accumulation of body fat including central obesity, dorsocervical fat enlargement (buffalo hump), peripheral wasting, facial wasting, breast enlargement, and "cushingoid appearance" have been observed in patients receiving antiretroviral therapy. The mechanism and long-term consequences of these events are unknown. A causal relationship has not been established.

5.10 Immune Reconstitution Syndrome

Immune reconstitution syndrome has been reported in patients treated with combination antiretroviral therapy, including the components of COMPLERA. During the initial phase of combination antiretroviral treatment, patients whose immune system responds may develop an inflammatory response to indolent or residual opportunistic infections [such as *Mycobacterium avium* infection, cytomegalovirus, *Pneumocystis jirovecii* pneumonia (PCP), or tuberculosis], which may necessitate further evaluation and treatment.

Autoimmune disorders (such as Graves' disease, polymyositis, and Guillain-Barré syndrome) have also been reported to occur in the setting of immune reconstitution, however, the time to onset is more variable, and can occur many months after initiation of treatment.

6 ADVERSE REACTIONS

The following adverse drug reactions are discussed in other sections of the labeling:

- Lactic Acidosis/Severe Hepatomegaly with Steatosis *[See Boxed Warning, Warnings and Precautions (5.1)]*.
- Severe Acute Exacerbations of Hepatitis B *[See Boxed Warning, Warnings and Precautions (5.2)]*.
- New Onset or Worsening Renal Impairment *[See Warnings and Precautions (5.3)]*.
- Depressive Disorders *[See Warnings and Precautions (5.5)]*.
- Hepatotoxicity *[See Warnings and Precautions (5.6)]*.
- Decreases in Bone Mineral Density *[See Warnings and Precautions (5.7)]*.
- Immune Reconstitution Syndrome *[See Warnings and Precautions (5.10)]*.

6.1 Adverse Reactions from Clinical Trials Experience

Because clinical trials are conducted under widely varying conditions, adverse reaction rates observed in the clinical trials of a drug cannot be directly compared to rates in the clinical trials of another drug and may not reflect the rates observed in practice.

Studies C209 and C215 – Treatment-Emergent Adverse Drug Reactions: The safety assessment of rilpivirine, used in combination with other antiretroviral drugs, is based on the Week 96 pooled data from 1368 subjects in the Phase 3 trials TMC278-C209 (ECHO) and TMC278-C215 (THRIVE) in antiretroviral treatment-naive HIV-1 infected adult subjects. A total of 686 subjects received rilpivirine in combination with other antiretroviral drugs as background regimen; most (N=550) received emtricitabine/tenofovir DF as background regimen. The number of subjects randomized to the control arm efavirenz was 682, of which 546 received emtricitabine/tenofovir DF as background regimen *[See Clinical Studies (14)]*. The median duration of exposure for subjects in either treatment arm was 104 weeks.

Adverse drug reactions (ADR) observed at Week 96 in subjects who received rilpivirine or efavirenz plus emtricitabine/tenofovir DF as background regimen are shown in Table 1. No new types of adverse reactions were identified between Week 48 and Week 96. The adverse drug reactions observed in this subset of subjects were generally consistent with those seen for the overall patient population participating in these studies (refer to the prescribing information for EDURANT).

The proportion of subjects who discontinued treatment with rilpivirine or efavirenz + emtricitabine/tenofovir DF due to ADR, regardless of severity, was 2% and 5%, respectively. The most common ADRs leading to discontinuation were psychiatric disorders: 9 (1.6%) subjects in the rilpivirine + emtricitabine/tenofovir DF arm and 12 (2.2%) subjects in the efavirenz + emtricitabine/tenofovir DF arm. Rash led to discontinuation in 1 (0.2%) subjects in the rilpivirine + emtricitabine/tenofovir DF arm and 10 (1.8%) subjects in the efavirenz + emtricitabine/tenofovir DF arm.

Common Adverse Drug Reactions

Clinical ADRs to rilpivirine or efavirenz of at least moderate intensity (≥ Grade 2) reported in at least 2% of adult subjects are shown in Table 1.

Table 1 Selected Treatment-Emergent Adverse Drug Reactions* (Grades 2–4) Reported in ≥2% of Subjects Receiving Rilpivirine or Efavirenz in Combination with Emtricitabine/Tenofovir DF in Studies C209 and C215 (Week 96 analysis)

	Rilpivirine + FTC/TDF	Efavirenz + FTC/TDF
	N=550	N=546
Gastrointestinal Disorder		
Nausea	1%	2%
Nervous System Disorders		
Headache	2%	2%
Dizziness	1%	7%
Psychiatric Disorders		
Depressive disorders†	2%	2%
Insomnia	2%	2%
Abnormal dreams	1%	3%
Skin and Subcutaneous Tissue Disorders		
Rash	1%	5%

* Frequencies of adverse reactions are based on all Grades 2–4) treatment-emergent adverse events assessed to be related to study drug.

† Includes adverse drug reactions reported as depressed mood, depression, dysphoria, major depression, mood altered, negative thoughts, suicide attempt, suicide ideation.

Rilpivirine: Treatment-emergent adverse drug reactions of at least moderate intensity (≥ Grade 2) that occurred in less than 2% of subjects treated with rilpivirine plus any of the allowed background regimens (N=686) in clinical studies C209 and C215 include (grouped by Body System): vomiting, diarrhea, abdominal discomfort, abdominal pain, fatigue, cholecystitis, cholelithiasis, decreased appetite, somnolence, sleep disorders, anxiety, glomerulonephritis membranous, glomerulonephritis mesangioproliferative, and nephrolithiasis.

Emtricitabine and Tenofovir Disoproxil Fumarate: The following adverse reactions were observed in clinical trials of emtricitabine or tenofovir DF in combination with other antiretroviral agents:

The most common adverse drug reactions occurred in at least 10% of treatment-naive subjects in a phase 3 clinical trial of emtricitabine and tenofovir DF in combination with another antiretroviral agent are diarrhea, nausea, fatigue, headache, dizziness, depression, insomnia, abnormal dreams, and rash. In addition, adverse drug reactions that occurred in at least 5% of treatment-experienced or treatment-naive subjects receiving emtricitabine or tenofovir DF with other antiretroviral agents in clinical trials include abdominal pain, dyspepsia, vomiting, fever, pain, nasopharyngitis, pneumonia, sinusitis, upper respiratory tract infection, arthralgia, back pain, myalgia, paresthesia, peripheral neuropathy (including peripheral neuritis and neuropathy), anxiety, increased cough, and rhinitis.

Skin discoloration has been reported with higher frequency among emtricitabine-treated subjects; it was manifested by hyperpigmentation on the palms and/or soles and was generally mild and asymptomatic. The mechanism and clinical significance are unknown.

Laboratory Abnormalities: The percentage of subjects treated with rilpivirine + emtricitabine/tenofovir DF or efavirenz + emtricitabine/tenofovir DF in studies C209 and C215 with selected treatment-emergent laboratory abnormalities (Grades 1 to 4), representing worst grade toxicity are presented in Table 2.

[See table 2 above]

Table 2 Selected Laboratory Abnormalities (Grades 1–4) Reported in Subjects Who Received Rilpivirine or Efavirenz in Combination with Emtricitabine/Tenofovir DF in Studies C209 and C215 (Week 96 Analysis)

Laboratory Parameter Abnormality, (%)	DAIDS Toxicity Range	Rilpivirine + FTC/TDF N=550	Efavirenz + FTC/TDF N=546
BIOCHEMISTRY			
Increased Creatinine			
Grade 1	1.1–1.3 × ULN*	6%	1%
Grade 2	>1.3–1.8 × ULN	1%	1%
Grade 3	>1.8–3.4 × ULN	<1%	0
Grade 4	>3.4 × ULN	0	<1%
Increased AST			
Grade 1	1.25–2.5 × ULN	16%	19%
Grade 2	>2.5–5.0 × ULN	4%	7%
Grade 3	>5.0–10.0 × ULN	2%	3%
Grade 4	>10.0 × ULN	1%	1%
Increased ALT			
Grade 1	1.25–2.5 × ULN	19%	22%
Grade 2	>2.5–5.0 × ULN	5%	7%
Grade 3	>5.0–10.0 × ULN	1%	2%
Grade 4	>10.0 × ULN	1%	1%
Increased Total Bilirubin			
Grade 1	1.1–1.5 × ULN	6%	<1%
Grade 2	>1.5–2.5 × ULN	3%	1%
Grade 3	>2.5–5.0 × ULN	1%	<1%
Increased Total Cholesterol (fasted)			
Grade 1	200–239 mg/dL	14%	31%
Grade 2	240–300 mg/dL	6%	18%
Grade 3	>300 mg/dL	<1%	2%
Increased LDL Cholesterol (fasted)			
Grade 1	130–159 mg/dL	13%	28%
Grade 2	160–190 mg/dL	5%	13%
Grade 3	>190 mg/dL	1%	4%
Increased Triglycerides (fasted)			
Grade 2	500–750 mg/dL	1%	2%
Grade 3	751–1,200 mg/dL	1%	2%
Grade 4	>1,200 mg/dL	0	1%

N = number of subjects per treatment group

Note: Percentages were calculated versus the number of subjects in ITT population with emtricitabine + tenofovir DF as background regimen.

* ULN = Upper limit of normal value.

Table 3 Lipid Values Reported in Subjects Receiving Rilpivirine or Efavirenz in Combination with Emtricitabine/Tenofovir DF in Studies C209 and C215*

	Pooled Data from the Week 96 Analysis of C209 and C215 Trials							
	Rilpivirine + FTC/TDF N=550				Efavirenz + FTC/TDF N=546			
	N	Baseline	Week 96		N	Baseline	Week 96	
Mean		Mean (mg/dL)	Mean (mg/dL)	Mean Change† (mg/dL)		Mean (mg/dL)	Mean (mg/dL)	Mean Change† (mg/dL)
Total Cholesterol (fasted)	430	162	164	2	401	160	186	26
HDL-cholesterol (fasted)	429	42	45	4	399	40	50	11
LDL-cholesterol (fasted)	427	97	97	-1	397	96	110	14
Triglycerides (fasted)	430	123	109	-14	401	127	133	6

N = number of subjects per treatment group
* Excludes subjects who received lipid lowering agents during the treatment period.
† The change from baseline is the mean of within-patient changes from baseline for patients with both baseline and Week 96 values.

Emtricitabine or Tenofovir Disoproxil Fumarate: The following laboratory abnormalities have been previously reported in subjects treated with emtricitabine or tenofovir DF with other antiretroviral agents in other clinical trials: Grade 3 or 4 laboratory abnormalities of increased pancreatic amylase (>2.0 × ULN), increased serum amylase (>175 U/L), increased lipase (>3.0 × ULN), increased alkaline phosphatase (>550 U/L), increased or decreased serum glucose (<40 or >250 mg/dL), increased glycosuria (≥3+), increased creatine kinase (M: >990 U/L; F: >845 U/L), decreased neutrophils (<750/mm^3) and increased hematuria (>75 RBC/HPF) occurred.

Adrenal Function

In the pooled Phase 3 trials of C209 and C215, in subjects treated with rilpivirine plus any of the allowed background regimen (N=686), at Week 96, there was an overall mean change from baseline in basal cortisol of -19.1 (95% CI: -30.9; -7.4) nmol/L in the rilpivirine group, and of +0.1 (95% CI: -12.6; 12.8) nmol/L in the efavirenz group. At Week 96, the mean change from baseline in ACTH-stimulated cortisol levels was lower in the rilpivirine group (+18.4± 8.36 nmol/L) than in the efavirenz group (+54.1± 7.24 nmol/L). Mean values for both basal and ACTH-stimulated cortisol values at Week 96 were within the normal range. Overall, there were no serious adverse events, deaths, or treatment discontinuations that could clearly be attributed to adrenal insufficiency. Effects on adrenal function were comparable by background N(t)RTIs.

Serum Creatinine

In the pooled Phase 3 trials of C209 and C215 trials in subjects treated with rilpivirine plus any of the allowed background regimen (N=686), there was a small increase in serum creatinine over 96 weeks of treatment with rilpivirine. Most of this increase occurred within the first four weeks of treatment with a mean change of 0.1 mg/dL (range: -0.3 mg/dL to 0.6 mg/dL) observed through Week 96. In subjects who entered the trial with mild or moderate renal impairment, the serum creatinine increase observed was similar to that seen in subjects with normal renal function. These changes are not considered to be clinically relevant and no subject discontinued treatment due to increases in serum creatinine. Creatinine increases were comparable by background N(t)RTIs.

Serum Lipids

Changes from baseline in total cholesterol, LDL-cholesterol and triglycerides are presented in Table 3.

[See table 3 above]

Subjects Coinfected with Hepatitis B and/or Hepatitis C Virus

In patients coinfected with hepatitis B or C virus receiving rilpivirine in studies C209 and C215, the incidence of hepatic enzyme elevation was higher than in subjects receiving rilpivirine who were not coinfected. The same increase was also observed in the efavirenz arm. The pharmacokinetic exposure of rilpivirine in coinfected subjects was comparable to that in subjects without coinfection.

6.2 Postmarketing Experience

The following adverse reactions have been identified during postapproval use of emtricitabine or tenofovir DF. Because postmarketing reactions are reported voluntarily from a population of uncertain size, it is not always possible to reliably estimate their frequency or establish a causal relationship to drug exposure.

Rilpivirine:

Renal and Urinary Disorders

nephrotic syndrome

Emtricitabine:

No postmarketing adverse reactions have been identified for inclusion in this section.

Tenofovir Disoproxil Fumarate:

Immune System Disorders

allergic reaction, including angioedema

Metabolism and Nutrition Disorders

lactic acidosis, hypokalemia, hypophosphatemia

Respiratory, Thoracic, and Mediastinal Disorders

dyspnea

Gastrointestinal Disorders

pancreatitis, increased amylase, abdominal pain

Hepatobiliary Disorders

hepatic steatosis, hepatitis, increased liver enzymes (most commonly AST, ALT gamma GT)

Skin and Subcutaneous Tissue Disorders

rash

Musculoskeletal and Connective Tissue Disorders

rhabdomyolysis, osteomalacia (manifested as bone pain and which may contribute to fractures), muscular weakness, myopathy

Renal and Urinary Disorders

acute renal failure, renal failure, acute tubular necrosis, Fanconi syndrome, proximal renal tubulopathy, interstitial nephritis (including acute cases), nephrogenic diabetes insipidus, renal insufficiency, increased creatinine, proteinuria, polyuria

General Disorders and Administration Site Conditions

asthenia

The following adverse reactions, listed under the body system headings above, may occur as a consequence of proximal renal tubulopathy: rhabdomyolysis, osteomalacia, hypokalemia, muscular weakness, myopathy, hypophosphatemia.

7 DRUG INTERACTIONS

COMPLERA is a complete regimen for the treatment of HIV-1 infection; therefore, COMPLERA should not be administered with other antiretroviral medications. Information regarding potential drug-drug interactions with other antiretroviral medications is not provided. Please refer to the EDURANT, VIREAD and EMTRIVA prescribing information as needed.

There were no drug-drug interaction trials conducted with the fixed-dose combination tablet. Drug interaction studies were conducted with emtricitabine, rilpivirine, or tenofovir DF, the components of COMPLERA. This section describes clinically relevant drug interactions with COMPLERA *[See Contraindications (4) and Clinical Pharmacology (12.3)].*

7.1 Drugs Inducing or Inhibiting CYP3A Enzymes

Rilpivirine is primarily metabolized by cytochrome P450 (CYP) 3A, and drugs that induce or inhibit CYP3A may thus affect the clearance of rilpivirine *[See Clinical Pharmacology (12.3), Contraindications (4)].* Coadministration of rilpivirine and drugs that induce CYP3A may result in decreased plasma concentrations of rilpivirine and loss of virologic response and possible resistance to rilpivirine or to the class of NNRTIs. Coadministration of rilpivirine and drugs that inhibit CYP3A may result in increased plasma concentrations of rilpivirine.

Rilpivirine at a dose of 25 mg once daily is not likely to have a clinically relevant effect on the exposure of drugs metabolized by CYP enzymes.

7.2 Drugs Increasing Gastric pH

Coadministration of rilpivirine with drugs that increase gastric pH may decrease plasma concentrations of rilpivirine and loss of virologic response and possible resistance to rilpivirine or to the class of NNRTIs *[See Table 4].*

7.3 Drugs Affecting Renal Function

Because emtricitabine and tenofovir are primarily eliminated by the kidneys through a combination of glomerular filtration and active tubular secretion, coadministration of COMPLERA with drugs that reduce renal function or compete for active tubular secretion may increase serum concentrations of emtricitabine, tenofovir, and/or other renally eliminated drugs. Some examples of drugs that are eliminated by active tubular secretion include, but are not limited to, acyclovir, adefovir dipivoxil, cidofovir, ganciclovir, valacyclovir, and valganciclovir.

7.4 QT Prolonging Drugs

There is limited information available on the potential for a pharmacodynamic interaction between rilpivirine and drugs that prolong the QTc interval of the electrocardiogram. In a study of healthy subjects, supratherapeutic doses of rilpivirine (75 mg once daily and 300 mg once daily) have been shown to prolong the QTc interval of the electrocardiogram *[See Clinical Pharmacology (12.2)].* COMPLERA should be used with caution when coadministered with a drug with a known risk of Torsade de Pointes.

7.5 Established and Other Potentially Significant Drug Interactions

Important drug interaction information for COMPLERA is summarized in Table 4. The drug interactions described are based on studies conducted with emtricitabine, rilpivirine, or tenofovir DF as individual medications that may occur with COMPLERA or are potential drug interactions; no drug interaction studies have been conducted using COMPLERA [for pharmacokinetic data see *Clinical Pharmacology (12.3)*, Tables 6–7]. The tables include potentially significant interactions, but are not all inclusive.

[See table 4 at top of next page]

7.6 Drugs with No Observed or Predicted Interactions with COMPLERA

No clinically significant drug interactions have been observed between emtricitabine and the following medications: famciclovir or tenofovir DF. Similarly, no clinically significant drug interactions have been observed between tenofovir DF and the following medications: entecavir, methadone, oral contraceptives, ribavirin, or tacrolimus in studies conducted in healthy subjects.

No clinically significant drug interactions have been observed between rilpivirine and the following medications: acetaminophen, atorvastatin, chlorzoxazone, digoxin, ethinyl estradiol, norethindrone, sildenafil, telaprevir, or tenofovir DF. No clinically relevant drug-drug interaction is expected when rilpivirine is coadministered with ribavirin.

8 USE IN SPECIFIC POPULATIONS

8.1 Pregnancy

Pregnancy Category B

Emtricitabine: The incidence of fetal variations and malformations was not increased in embryofetal toxicity studies performed with emtricitabine in mice at exposures (AUC) approximately 60 times higher and in rabbits at approximately 120-times higher than human exposures at the recommended daily dose.

Rilpivirine: Studies in animals have shown no evidence of embryonic or fetal toxicity or an effect on reproductive function. In offspring from rat and rabbit dams treated with rilpivirine during pregnancy and lactation, there were no toxicologically significant effects on developmental endpoints. The exposures at the embryo-fetal No Observed Adverse Effects Levels in rats and rabbits were respectively 15 and 70 times higher than the exposure in humans at the recommended dose of 25 mg once daily.

Tenofovir Disoproxil Fumarate: Reproduction studies have been performed in rats and rabbits at doses up to 14 and 19 times the human dose based on body surface area comparisons and revealed no evidence of impaired fertility or harm to the fetus due to tenofovir.

There are, however, no adequate and well-controlled studies in pregnant women. Because animal reproduction studies are not always predictive of human response, COMPLERA should be used during pregnancy only if the potential benefit justifies the potential risk to the fetus.

Antiretroviral Pregnancy Registry: To monitor fetal outcomes of pregnant women exposed to COMPLERA, an Antiretroviral Pregnancy Registry has been established. Healthcare providers are encouraged to register patients by calling 1-800-258-4263.

8.3 Nursing Mothers

The Centers for Disease Control and Prevention recommend that HIV infected mothers not breastfeed their infants to avoid risking postnatal transmission of HIV.

Emtricitabine: Samples of breast milk obtained from five HIV-1 infected mothers show that emtricitabine is secreted in human milk. Breastfeeding infants whose mothers are being treated with emtricitabine may be at risk for developing viral resistance to emtricitabine. Other emtricitabine-associated risks in infants breastfed by mothers being treated with emtricitabine are unknown.

Rilpivirine: Studies in lactating rats and their offspring indicate that rilpivirine was present in rat milk. It is not known whether rilpivirine is secreted in human milk.

Tenofovir Disoproxil Fumarate: Samples of breast milk obtained from five HIV-1 infected mothers in the first postpartum week show that tenofovir is excreted in human milk. The impact of this exposure in breastfed infants is unknown.

Because of both the potential for HIV transmission and the potential for serious adverse reactions in nursing infants, **mothers should be instructed not to breastfeed if they are receiving COMPLERA.**

8.4 Pediatric Use

COMPLERA is not recommended for patients less than 18 years of age because not all the individual components of the COMPLERA have safety, efficacy and dosing recommendations available for all pediatric age groups *[See Clinical Pharmacology (12.3)]*.

8.5 Geriatric Use

Clinical studies of emtricitabine, rilpivirine, or tenofovir DF did not include sufficient numbers of subjects aged 65 and over to determine whether they respond differently from younger subjects. In general, dose selection for the elderly patients should be cautious, keeping in mind the greater frequency of decreased hepatic, renal, or cardiac function, and of concomitant disease or other drug therapy *[See Clinical Pharmacology (12.3)]*.

8.6 Renal Impairment

Because COMPLERA is a fixed-dose combination, it should not be prescribed for patients requiring dosage adjustment such as those with moderate, severe or end stage renal impairment (creatinine clearance below 50 mL per minute) or that require dialysis *[See Warnings and Precautions (5.3), Clinical Pharmacology (12.3)]*.

8.7 Hepatic Impairment

No dose adjustment of COMPLERA is required in patients with mild (Child-Pugh Class A) or moderate (Child-Pugh Class B) hepatic impairment. COMPLERA has not been studied in patients with severe hepatic impairment (Child-Pugh Class C) *[See Clinical Pharmacology (12.3)]*.

10 OVERDOSAGE

If overdose occurs the patient must be monitored for evidence of toxicity. Treatment of overdose with COMPLERA consists of general supportive measures including monitoring of vital signs and ECG (QT interval) as well as observation of the clinical status of the patient.

Emtricitabine: Limited clinical experience is available at doses higher than the therapeutic dose of EMTRIVA. In one clinical pharmacology study, single doses of emtricitabine 1200 mg were administered to 11 subjects. No severe adverse reactions were reported. The effects of higher doses are not known.

Hemodialysis treatment removes approximately 30% of the emtricitabine dose over a 3-hour dialysis period starting within 1.5 hours of emtricitabine dosing (blood flow rate of 400 mL per minute and a dialysate flow rate of 600 mL per minute). It is not known whether emtricitabine can be removed by peritoneal dialysis.

Rilpivirine: There is no specific antidote for overdose with rilpivirine. Human experience of overdose with rilpivirine is limited. Since rilpivirine is highly bound to plasma protein, dialysis is unlikely to result in significant removal of rilpivirine.

If indicated, elimination of unabsorbed active substance may be achieved by gastric lavage. Administration of activated charcoal may also be used to aid in removal of unabsorbed active substance.

Tenofovir Disoproxil Fumarate: Limited clinical experience at doses higher than the therapeutic dose of VIREAD 300 mg is available. In one study, 600 mg tenofovir DF was administered to 8 subjects orally for 28 days, and no severe adverse reactions were reported. The effects of higher doses are not known.

Tenofovir is efficiently removed by hemodialysis with an extraction coefficient of approximately 54%. Following a single 300 mg dose of VIREAD, a four-hour hemodialysis session removed approximately 10% of the administered tenofovir dose.

11 DESCRIPTION

COMPLERA is a fixed-dose combination tablet containing emtricitabine, rilpivirine hydrochloride, and tenofovir DF. EMTRIVA is the brand name for emtricitabine, a synthetic nucleoside analog of cytidine. EDURANT is the brand name for rilpivirine, a non-nucleoside reverse transcriptase inhibitor. VIREAD is the brand name for tenofovir DF, which is converted *in vivo* to tenofovir, an acyclic nucleoside phosphonate (nucleotide) analog of adenosine 5′-monophosphate. VIREAD and EMTRIVA are the components of TRUVADA.

Table 4 Established and Other Potentially Significant* Drug Interactions: Alteration in Dose or Regimen May Be Recommended Based on Drug Interaction Studies or Predicted Interaction

Concomitant Drug Class: Drug Name	Effect on Concentration†	Clinical Comment
Antacids: antacids (e.g., aluminium, magnesium hydroxide, or calcium carbonate)	↔ rilpivirine (antacids taken at least 2 hours before or at least 4 hours after rilpivirine) ↓ rilpivirine (concomitant intake)	The combination of COMPLERA and antacids should be used with caution as coadministration may cause significant decreases in rilpivirine plasma concentrations (increase in gastric pH). Antacids should only be administered either at least 2 hours before or at least 4 hours after COMPLERA.
Azole Antifungal Agents: fluconazole itraconazole ketoconazole posaconazole voriconazole	↑ rilpivirine‡,§ ↓ ketoconazole‡,§	Concomitant use of COMPLERA with azole antifungal agents may cause an increase in the plasma concentrations of rilpivirine (inhibition of CYP3A enzymes). No dose adjustment is required when COMPLERA is coadministered with azole antifungal agents. Clinically monitor for breakthrough fungal infections when azole antifungals are coadministered with COMPLERA.
H_2-Receptor Antagonists: cimetidine famotidine nizatidine ranitidine	↔ rilpivirine‡,§ (famotidine taken 12 hours before rilpivirine or 4 hours after rilpivirine) ↓ rilpivirine‡,§ (famotidine taken 2 hours before rilpivirine)	The combination of COMPLERA and H_2-receptor antagonists should be used with caution as coadministration may cause significant decreases in rilpivirine plasma concentrations (increase in gastric pH). H_2-receptor antagonists should only be administered at least 12 hours before or at least 4 hours after COMPLERA.
Macrolide or Ketolide Antibiotics: clarithromycin erythromycin troleandomycin	↑ rilpivirine ↔ clarithromycin ↔ erythromycin ↔ troleandomycin	Concomitant use of COMPLERA with clarithromycin, erythromycin or telithromycin may cause an increase in the plasma concentrations of rilpivirine (inhibition of CYP3A enzymes). Where possible, alternatives such as azithromycin should be considered.
Narcotic Analgesics: methadone	↓ R(−) methadone‡ ↓ S(+) methadone‡ ↔ rilpivirine‡ ↔ methadone‡(when used with tenofovir)	No dose adjustments are required when initiating coadministration of methadone with COMPLERA. However, clinical monitoring is recommended as methadone maintenance therapy may need to be adjusted in some patients.

* This table is not all inclusive.
† Increase = ↑; Decrease = ↓; No Effect = ↔
‡ The interaction was evaluated in a clinical study. All other drug-drug interactions shown are predicted.
§ This interaction study has been performed with a dose higher than the recommended dose for rilpivirine. The dosing recommendation is applicable to the recommended dose of rilpivirine 25 mg once daily.

COMPLERA tablets are for oral administration. Each tablet contains 200 mg of emtricitabine, 27.5 mg of rilpivirine hydrochloride (equivalent to 25 mg of rilpivirine), and 300 mg of tenofovir DF (equivalent to 245 mg of tenofovir disoproxil) as active ingredients. The tablets include the following inactive ingredients: pregelatinized starch, lactose monohydrate, microcrystalline cellulose, croscarmellose sodium, magnesium stearate, povidone, polysorbate 20. The tablets are film-coated with a coating material containing polyethylene glycol, hypromellose, lactose monohydrate, triacetin, titanium dioxide, iron oxide red, FD&C Blue #2 aluminum lake, FD&C Yellow #6 aluminum lake.

Emtricitabine: The chemical name of emtricitabine is 5-fluoro-1-[(2*R*,5*S*)-2-(hydroxymethyl)-1,3-oxathiolan-5-yl] cytosine. Emtricitabine is the (−) enantiomer of a thio analog of cytidine, which differs from other cytidine analogs in that it has a fluorine in the 5-position.

It has a molecular formula of $C_8H_{10}FN_3O_3S$ and a molecular weight of 247.24. It has the following structural formula:

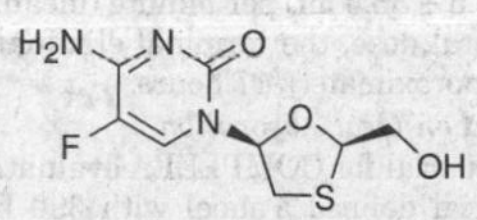

Emtricitabine is a white to off-white crystalline powder with a solubility of approximately 112 mg per mL in water at 25 °C.

Rilpivirine: Rilpivirine is available as the hydrochloride salt. The chemical name for rilpivirine hydrochloride is 4-[[4-[[4-[(E)-2-cyanoethenyl]-2,6-dimethylphenyl]amino]-2-pyrimidinyl]amino]benzonitrile monohydrochloride. Its molecular formula is $C_{22}H_{18}N_6 \cdot HCl$ and its molecular weight is 402.88. Rilpivirine hydrochloride has the following structural formula:

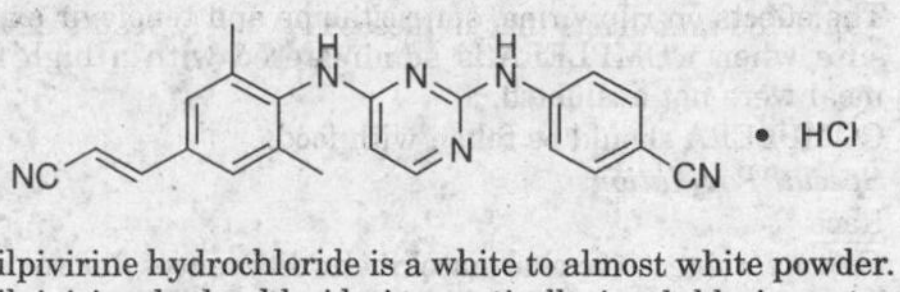

Rilpivirine hydrochloride is a white to almost white powder. Rilpivirine hydrochloride is practically insoluble in water over a wide pH range.

Tenofovir Disoproxil Fumarate: Tenofovir DF is a fumaric acid salt of the bis-isopropoxycarbonyloxymethyl ester derivative of tenofovir. The chemical name of tenofovir DF is 9-[(*R*)-2 [[bis[[(isopropoxycarbonyl)oxy]- methoxy]phosphinyl]methoxy]propyl]adenine fumarate (1:1). It has a molecular formula of $C_{19}H_{30}N_5O_{10}P \cdot C_4H_4O_4$ and a molecular weight of 635.52. It has the following structural formula:

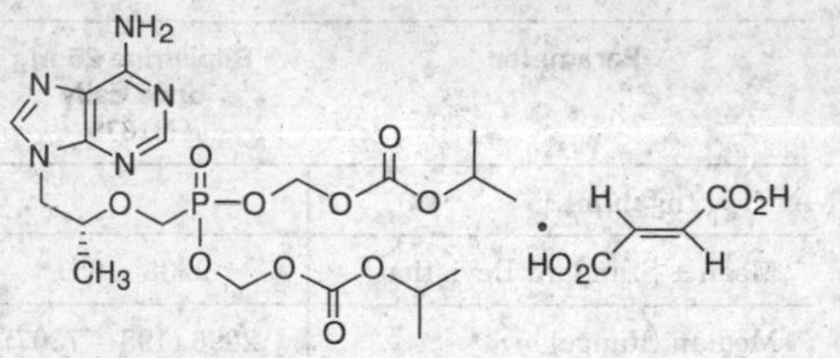

Tenofovir DF is a white to off-white crystalline powder with a solubility of 13.4 mg per mL in water at 25 °C. All dosages are expressed in terms of tenofovir DF except where otherwise noted.

12 CLINICAL PHARMACOLOGY

12.1 Mechanism of Action

COMPLERA is a fixed-dose combination of the antiretroviral drugs emtricitabine, rilpivirine and tenofovir disoproxil fumarate *[See Microbiology (12.4)]*.

12.2 Pharmacodynamics

Effects on Electrocardiogram

The effect of rilpivirine at the recommended dose of 25 mg once daily on the QTcF interval was evaluated in a randomized, placebo and active (moxifloxacin 400 mg once daily) controlled crossover study in 60 healthy adults, with 13 measurements over 24 hours at steady state. The maximum mean time-matched (95% upper confidence bound) differences in QTcF interval from placebo after baseline-correction was 2.0 (5.0) milliseconds (i.e., below the threshold of clinical concern).

When supratherapeutic doses of 75 mg once daily and 300 mg once daily of rilpivirine were studied in healthy adults, the maximum mean time-matched (95% upper confidence bound) differences in QTcF interval from placebo after baseline-correction were 10.7 (15.3) and 23.3 (28.4) milliseconds, respectively. Steady-state administration of rilpivirine 75 mg once daily and 300 mg once daily resulted in a mean steady-state C_{max} approximately 2.6-fold and 6.7-fold, respectively, higher than the mean C_{max} observed with the recommended 25 mg once daily dose of rilpivirine *[See Warnings and Precautions (5.4)]*.

12.3 Pharmacokinetics

COMPLERA: Under fed conditions (total calorie content of the meal was approximately 400 kcal with approximately 13 grams of fat), rilpivirine, emtricitabine and tenofovir exposures were bioequivalent when comparing COMPLERA to EMTRIVA capsules (200 mg) plus EDURANT tablets (25 mg) plus VIREAD tablets (300 mg) following single-dose administration to healthy subjects (N=34).

Single-dose administration of COMPLERA tablet to healthy subjects under fasted conditions provided approximately 25% higher exposure of rilpivirine compared to administration of EMTRIVA capsules (200 mg) plus EDURANT tablets (25 mg) plus VIREAD tablets (300 mg), while exposures of emtricitabine and tenofovir were comparable (N=15).

Emtricitabine: Following oral administration, emtricitabine is absorbed with peak plasma concentrations occurring at 1–2 hours post-dose. Following multiple dose oral administration of EMTRIVA to 20 HIV-1 infected subjects, the mean steady-state plasma emtricitabine C_{max} was 1.8 ± 0.7 µg per mL and the AUC over a 24-hour dosing interval was 10.0 ± 3.1 µg•hr per mL. The mean steady state plasma trough concentration at 24 hours post-dose was 0.09 µg per mL. The mean absolute bioavailability of EMTRIVA capsules was 93%. Less than 4% of emtricitabine binds to human plasma proteins *in vitro* over the range of 0.02 to 200 µg per mL. Following administration of radiolabelled emtricitabine, approximately 86% is recovered in the urine, approximately 14% in the feces and 13% is recovered as metabolites in the urine. The metabolites of emtricitabine include 3′-sulfoxide diastereomers (approximately 9% of the dose) and the glucuronic acid conjugate (approximately 4% of the dose). Emtricitabine is eliminated by a combination of glomerular filtration and active tubular secretion with a renal clearance in adults with creatinine clearance >80 mL per minute of 213 ± 89 mL per minute (mean ± SD). The plasma emtricitabine half-life is approximately 10 hours.

Rilpivirine: The pharmacokinetic properties of rilpivirine have been evaluated in adult healthy subjects and in adult antiretroviral treatment-naive HIV-1 infected subjects. Exposure to rilpivirine was generally lower in HIV-1 infected subjects than in healthy subjects. After oral administration, the C_{max} of rilpivirine is achieved within 4–5 hours. The absolute bioavailability of rilpivirine is unknown.

Table 5 Population Pharmacokinetic Estimates of Rilpivirine 25 mg Once Daily in Antiretroviral Treatment-Naive HIV-1-infected Subjects (Pooled Data from Phase 3 Trials through Week 96)

Parameter	Rilpivirine 25 mg once daily N=679
AUC_{24h} (ng•h/mL)	
Mean ± Standard Deviation	2235 ± 851
Median (Range)	2096 (198 – 7307)
C_{0h} (ng/mL)	
Mean ± Standard Deviation	79 ± 35
Median (Range)	73 (2 – 288)

Rilpivirine is approximately 99.7% bound to plasma proteins *in vitro*, primarily to albumin. *In vitro* experiments indicate that rilpivirine primarily undergoes oxidative metabolism by the cytochrome CYP3A system. The terminal elimination half-life of rilpivirine is approximately 50 hours. After single dose oral administration of ^{14}C-rilpivirine, on average 85% and 6.1% of the radioactivity could be retrieved in feces and urine, respectively. In feces, unchanged rilpivirine accounted for on average 25% of the administered dose. Only trace amounts of unchanged rilpivirine (less than 1% of dose) were detected in urine.

Tenofovir Disoproxil Fumarate: Following oral administration of a single 300 mg dose of VIREAD to HIV-1 infected subjects in the fasted state, C_{max} was achieved in one hour. C_{max} and AUC values were 0.30 ± 0.09 µg per mL and 2.29 ± 0.69 µg•hr per mL, respectively. The oral bioavailability of tenofovir from VIREAD in fasted subjects is approximately 25%. Less than 0.7% of tenofovir binds to human plasma proteins *in vitro* over the range of 0.01 to 25 µg per mL. Approximately 70–80% of the intravenous dose of tenofovir is recovered as unchanged drug in the urine within 72 hours of dosing. Tenofovir is eliminated by a combination of glomerular filtration and active tubular secretion with a renal clearance in adults with creatinine clearance >80 mL per minute of 243.5 ± 33.3 mL per minute (mean ± SD). Following a single oral dose, the terminal elimination half-life of tenofovir is approximately 17 hours.

Table 6 Drug Interactions: Changes in Pharmacokinetic Parameters for Rilpivirine in the Presence of the Coadministered Drugs

Coadministered Drug	Dose of Coadministered Drug (mg)	Dose of Rilpivirine	N*	Mean % Change of Rilpivirine Pharmacokinetic Parameters† (90% CI)		
				C_{max}	AUC	C_{min}
Acetaminophen	500 mg single dose	150 mg once daily‡	16	↑ 9 (↑ 1 to ↑ 18)	↑ 16 (↑ 10 to ↑ 22)	↑ 26 (↑ 16 to ↑ 38)
Atorvastatin	40 mg once daily	150 mg once daily‡	16	↓ 9 (↓ 21 to↑ 6)	↓ 10 (↓ 19 to ↓ 1)	↓ 10 (↓ 16 to ↓ 4)
Chlorzoxazone	500 mg single dose	150 mg once daily‡	16	↑ 17 (↑ 8 to ↑ 27)	↑ 25 (↑ 16 to ↑ 35)	↑ 18 (↑ 9 to ↑ 28)
Ethinyl estradiol/ Norethindrone	0.035 mg once daily/1 mg once daily	25 mg once daily	16	↔§	↔§	↔§
Famotidine	40 mg single dose taken 12 hours before rilpivirine	150 mg single dose‡	24	↓ 1 (↓ 16 to↑ 16)	↓ 9 (↓ 22 to↑ 7)	NA
	40 mg single dose taken 2 hours before rilpivirine	150 mg single dose‡	23	↓ 85 (↓ 88 to ↓ 81)	↓ 76 (↓ 80 to ↓ 72)	NA
	40 mg single dose taken 4 hours after rilpivirine	150 mg single dose‡	24	↑ 21 (↑ 6 to↑ 39)	↑ 13 (↑ 1 to↑ 27)	NA
Ketoconazole	400 mg once daily	150 mg once daily‡	15	↑ 30 (↑ 13 to ↑ 48)	↑ 49 (↑ 31 to ↑ 70)	↑ 76 (↑ 57 to ↑ 97)
Methadone	60 –100 mg once daily individualized dose	25 mg once daily	12	↔§	↔§	↔§
Omeprazole	20 mg once daily	150 mg once daily‡	16	↓ 40 (↓ 52 to ↓ 27)	↓ 40 (↓ 49 to ↓ 29)	↓ 33 (↓ 42 to ↓ 22)
Rifabutin	300 mg once daily	150 mg once daily‡	16	↓ 35 (↓ 42 to ↓ 26)	↓ 46 (↓ 50 to ↓ 42)	↓ 49 (↓ 52 to ↓ 46)
Rifampin	600 mg once daily	150 mg once daily‡	16	↓ 69 (↓ 73 to ↓ 64)	↓ 80 (↓ 82 to ↓ 77)	↓ 89 (↓ 90 to ↓ 87)
Sildenafil	50 mg single dose	75 mg once daily	16	↓ 8 (↓ 15 to ↓ 1)	↓ 2 (↓ 8 to ↑ 5)	↑ 4 (↓ 2 to ↑ 9)
Telaprevir	750 mg every 8 hours	25 mg once daily	16	↑ 49 (↑ 20 to ↑ 84)	↑ 78 (↑ 44 to ↑ 120)	↑ 93 (↑ 55 to ↑ 141)

NA = not available

* N=maximum number of subjects for C_{max}, AUC, or C_{min}

† Increase = ↑; Decrease = ↓; No Effect = ↔

‡ The Interaction study has been performed with a dose higher than the recommended dose for rilpivirine (25 mg once daily) assessing the maximal effect on the coadministered drug.

§ Comparison based on historic controls.

Effects of Food on Oral Absorption

The food effect trial for COMPLERA evaluated two types of meals. The trial defined a meal with 390 kcal containing 12 g fat as a light meal, and a meal with 540 kcal containing 21 g fat as a standard meal. Relative to fasting conditions, the administration of COMPLERA to healthy adult subjects with both types of meals resulted in increased exposures of rilpivirine and tenofovir. The C_{max} and AUC of rilpivirine increased 34% and 9% with a light meal, while increasing 26% and 16% with a standard meal, respectively. The C_{max} and AUC of tenofovir increased 12% and 28% with a light meal, while increasing 32% and 38% with a standard meal, respectively. Emtricitabine exposures were not affected by food.

The effects on rilpivirine, emtricitabine and tenofovir exposure when COMPLERA is administered with a high fat meal were not evaluated.

COMPLERA should be taken with food.

Special Populations

Race

Emtricitabine: No pharmacokinetic differences due to race have been identified following the administration of EMTRIVA.

Rilpivirine: Population pharmacokinetic analysis of rilpivirine in HIV-1 infected subjects indicated that race had no clinically relevant effect on the exposure to rilpivirine.

Tenofovir Disoproxil Fumarate: There were insufficient numbers from racial and ethnic groups other than Caucasian to adequately determine potential pharmacokinetic differences among these populations following the administration of VIREAD.

Gender

No clinically relevant pharmacokinetic differences have been observed between men and women for emtricitabine, rilpivirine, and tenofovir DF.

Pediatric Patients

Emtricitabine has been studied in pediatric subjects from 3 months to 17 years of age. Tenofovir DF has been studied in adolescent subjects (12 to less than 18 years of age). The pharmacokinetics of rilpivirine in pediatric subjects have not been established.

Geriatric Patients

Pharmacokinetics of emtricitabine, rilpivirine and tenofovir have not been fully evaluated in the elderly (65 years of age and older) *[See Use in Specific Populations (8.5)]*.

Patients with Renal Impairment

Emtricitabine and Tenofovir Disoproxil Fumarate: The pharmacokinetics of emtricitabine and tenofovir DF are altered in subjects with renal impairment. In subjects with creatinine clearance below 50 mL per minute or with end stage renal disease requiring dialysis, C_{max}, and AUC of emtricitabine and tenofovir were increased *[See Warnings and Precautions (5.3) and Use in Specific Populations (8.6)]*.

Rilpivirine: Population pharmacokinetic analysis indicated that rilpivirine exposure was similar in HIV-1 infected subjects with mild renal impairment relative to HIV-1 infected subjects with normal renal function. There is limited or no information regarding the pharmacokinetics of rilpivirine in patients with moderate or severe renal impairment or in patients with end-stage renal disease, and rilpivirine concentrations may be increased due to alteration of drug absorption, distribution, and metabolism secondary to renal dysfunction *[See Use in Specific Populations (8.6)].*

Patients with Hepatic Impairment

Emtricitabine: The pharmacokinetics of emtricitabine have not been studied in subjects with hepatic impairment; however, emtricitabine is not significantly metabolized by liver enzymes, so the impact of liver impairment should be limited.

Rilpivirine: Rilpivirine is primarily metabolized and eliminated by the liver. In a study comparing 8 subjects with mild hepatic impairment (Child-Pugh score A) to 8 matched controls and 8 subjects with moderate hepatic impairment (Child-Pugh score B) to 8 matched controls, the multiple dose exposure of rilpivirine was 47% higher in subjects with mild hepatic impairment and 5% higher in subjects with moderate hepatic impairment *[See Use in Specific Populations (8.7)].*

Tenofovir Disoproxil Fumarate: The pharmacokinetics of tenofovir following a 300 mg dose of VIREAD have been studied in non-HIV infected subjects with moderate to severe hepatic impairment. There were no substantial alterations in tenofovir pharmacokinetics in subjects with hepatic impairment compared with unimpaired subjects.

Hepatitis B and/or Hepatitis C Virus Coinfection

Pharmacokinetics of emtricitabine and tenofovir DF have not been fully evaluated in hepatitis B and/or C virus-coinfected patients. Population pharmacokinetic analysis indicated that hepatitis B and/or C virus coinfection had no clinically relevant effect on the exposure to rilpivirine.

Assessment of Drug Interactions

COMPLERA is a complete regimen for the treatment of HIV-1 infection; therefore, COMPLERA should not be administered with other HIV antiretroviral medications. Information regarding potential drug-drug interactions with other antiretroviral medications is not provided. Please refer to the EDURANT, VIREAD and EMTRIVA prescribing information as needed.

The drug interaction studies described were conducted with emtricitabine, rilpivirine, or tenofovir DF as individual agents; no drug interaction studies have been conducted using COMPLERA.

Emtricitabine and Tenofovir Disoproxil Fumarate: In vitro and clinical pharmacokinetic drug-drug interaction studies have shown that the potential for CYP mediated interactions involving emtricitabine and tenofovir with other medicinal products is low.

Emtricitabine and tenofovir are primarily excreted by the kidneys by a combination of glomerular filtration and active tubular secretion. No drug-drug interactions due to competition for renal excretion have been observed; however, coadministration of emtricitabine and tenofovir DF with drugs that are eliminated by active tubular secretion may increase concentrations of emtricitabine, tenofovir, and/or the coadministered drug *[See Drug Interactions (7.6)].*

Drugs that decrease renal function may increase concentrations of emtricitabine and/or tenofovir.

Drug interaction studies were performed for emtricitabine and the following medications: tenofovir DF and famciclovir. Tenofovir increased the C_{min} of emtricitabine by 20% (90% confidence interval [CI]: [↑12 to ↑29]) and had no effect on emtricitabine C_{max} and AUC. Emtricitabine had no effect on the C_{max}, AUC and C_{min} of tenofovir. Coadministration of emtricitabine and famciclovir had no effect on the C_{max} or AUC of either medication.

Drug interaction studies were performed for tenofovir DF and the following medications: entecavir, methadone, oral contraceptives (ethinyl estradiol/norgestimate), ribavirin, and tacrolimus. Tacrolimus increased the C_{max} of tenofovir by 13% (90% CI: [↑1 to ↑27]) and had no effect on the tenofovir AUC and C_{min}. Tenofovir had no effect on the C_{max}, AUC and C_{min} of tacrolimus.

The C_{max}, AUC and C_{min} of tenofovir were not affected in the presence of entecavir. Tenofovir increased the AUC of entecavir by 13% (90% CI: [↑11 to ↑15]) and had no effect on the entecavir C_{max} and C_{min}.

Tenofovir had no effect on the C_{max}, AUC and C_{min} of methadone or ethinyl estradiol/norgestimate or the C_{max} and AUC of ribavirin.

Rilpivirine: Rilpivirine is primarily metabolized by cytochrome CYP3A, and drugs that induce or inhibit CYP3A may thus affect the clearance of rilpivirine. Coadministration of COMPLERA and drugs that induce CYP3A may result in decreased plasma concentrations of rilpivirine and loss of virologic response and possible resistance. Coadministration of COMPLERA and drugs that inhibit CYP3A may result in increased plasma concentrations of rilpivirine. Coadministration of COMPLERA with drugs that increase gastric pH may result in decreased plasma concentrations of rilpivirine and loss of virologic response and possible resistance to rilpivirine and to the class of NNRTIs.

Rilpivirine at a dose of 25 mg once daily is not likely to have a clinically relevant effect on the exposure of medicinal products metabolized by CYP enzymes.

The effects of coadministration of other drugs on the AUC, C_{max} and C_{min} values of rilpivirine are summarized in Table 6. The effect of coadministration of rilpivirine on the AUC, C_{max} and C_{min} values of other drugs are summarized in Table 7. For information regarding clinical recommendations, see *Drug Interactions (7).*

[See table 6 at top of previous page]

[See table 7 above]

Table 7 Drug Interactions: Changes in Pharmacokinetic Parameters for Coadministered Drug in the Presence of Rilpivirine

Coadministered Drug	Dose of Coadministered Drug (mg)	Dose of Rilpivirine	N*	Mean % Change of Coadministered Drug Pharmacokinetic Parameters† (90% CI)		
				C_{max}	AUC	C_{min}
Acetaminophen	500 mg single dose	150 mg once daily‡	16	↓ 3 (↓ 14 to ↑ 10)	↓ 9 (↓ 14 to ↓ 3)	NA
Atorvastatin	40 mg once daily	150 mg once daily‡	16	↑ 35 (↑ 8 to ↑ 68)	↑ 4 (↓ 3 to ↑ 12)	↓ 15 (↓ 31 to ↑ 3)
2-hydroxy-atorvastatin			16	↑ 58 (↑ 33 to ↑ 87)	↑ 39 (↑ 29 to ↑ 50)	↑ 32 (↑ 10 to ↑ 58)
4-hydroxy-atorvastatin			16	↑ 28 (↑ 15 to ↑ 43)	↑ 23 (↑ 13 to ↑ 33)	NA
Chlorzoxazone	500 mg single dose taken 2 hours after rilpivirine	150 mg once daily‡	16	↓ 2 (↓ 15 to ↑ 13)	↑ 3 (↓ 5 to ↑ 13)	NA
Digoxin	0.5 mg single dose	25 mg once daily	22	↑ 6 (↓ 3 to ↑ 17)	↓ 2 (↓ 7 to ↑ 4)§	NA
Ethinyl estradiol	0.035 mg once daily	25 mg once daily	17	↑ 17 (↑ 6 to ↑ 30)	↑ 14 (↑ 10 to ↑ 19)	↑ 9 (↑ 3 to ↑ 16)
Norethindrone	1 mg once daily		17	↓ 6 (↓ 17 to ↑ 6)	↓ 11 (↓ 16 to ↓ 6)	↓ 1 (↓ 10 to ↑ 8)
Ketoconazole	400 mg once daily	150 mg once daily‡	14	↓ 15 (↓ 20 to ↓ 10)	↓ 24 (↓ 30 to ↓ 18)	↓ 66 (↓ 75 to ↓ 54)
R(–) methadone	60–100 mg once daily individualized dose	25 mg once daily	13	↓ 14 (↓ 22 to ↓ 5)	↓ 16 (↓ 26 to ↓ 5)	↓ 22 (↓ 33 to ↓ 9)
S(+) methadone			13	↓ 13 (↓ 22 to ↓ 3)	↓ 16 (↓ 26 to ↓ 4)	↓ 21 (↓ 33 to ↓ 8)
Omeprazole	20 mg once daily	150 mg once daily‡	15	↓ 14 (↓ 32 to ↑ 9)	↓ 14 (↓ 24 to ↓ 3)	NA
Rifampin	600 mg once daily	150 mg once daily‡	16	↑ 2 (↓ 7 to ↑ 12)	↓ 1 (↓ 8 to ↑ 7)	NA
25-desacetylrifampin			16	↔ (↓ 13 to ↑ 15)	↓ 9 (↓ 23 to ↑ 7)	NA
Sildenafil	50 mg single dose	75 mg once daily‡	16	↓ 7 (↓ 20 to ↑ 8)	↓ 3 (↓ 13 to ↑ 8)	NA
N-desmethyl-sildenafil			16	↓ 10 (↓ 20 to ↑ 2)	↓ 8 (↓ 15 to ↓ 1)§	NA
Telaprevir	750 mg every 8 hours	25 mg once daily	13	↓ 3 (↓ 21 to ↑ 21)	↓ 5 (↓ 24 to ↑ 18)	↓ 11 (↓ 33 to ↑ 18)

NA = not available

* N=maximum number of subjects for C_{max}, AUC, or C_{min}

† Increase = ↑; Decrease = ↓; No Effect = ↔

‡ The Interaction study has been performed with a dose higher than the recommended dose for rilpivirine (25 mg once daily).

§ $AUC_{(0\text{-last})}$

12.4 Microbiology

Mechanism of Action

Emtricitabine: Emtricitabine, a synthetic nucleoside analog of cytidine, is phosphorylated by cellular enzymes to form emtricitabine 5′-triphosphate. Emtricitabine 5′-triphosphate inhibits the activity of the HIV-1 RT by competing with the natural substrate deoxycytidine 5′-triphosphate and by being incorporated into nascent viral DNA which results in chain termination. Emtricitabine 5′-triphosphate is a weak inhibitor of mammalian DNA polymerase α, β, ε, and mitochondrial DNA polymerase γ.

Rilpivirine: Rilpivirine is a diarylpyrimidine non-nucleoside reverse transcriptase inhibitor of HIV-1 and inhibits HIV-1 replication by non-competitive inhibition of HIV-1 RT. Rilpivirine does not inhibit the human cellular DNA polymerases α, β, and mitochondrial DNA polymerase γ.

Tenofovir Disoproxil Fumarate: Tenofovir DF is an acyclic nucleoside phosphonate diester analog of adenosine monophosphate. Tenofovir DF requires initial diester hydrolysis for conversion to tenofovir and subsequent phosphorylations by cellular enzymes to form tenofovir diphosphate. Tenofovir diphosphate inhibits the activity of HIV-1 RT by competing with the natural substrate deoxyadenosine 5′-triphosphate and, after incorporation into DNA, by DNA chain termination. Tenofovir diphosphate is a weak inhibitor of mammalian DNA polymerases α, β, and mitochondrial DNA polymerase γ.

Antiviral Activity

Emtricitabine, Rilpivirine, and Tenofovir Disoproxil Fumarate: The triple combination of emtricitabine, rilpivirine, and tenofovir was not antagonistic in cell culture.

Emtricitabine: The antiviral activity of emtricitabine against laboratory and clinical isolates of HIV-1 was assessed in lymphoblastoid cell lines, the MAGI-CCR5 cell line, and peripheral blood mononuclear cells. The 50% effective concentration (EC_{50}) values for emtricitabine were in the range of 0.0013–0.64 µM. Emtricitabine displayed antiviral activity in cell culture against HIV-1 clades A, B, C, D, E, F, and G (EC_{50} values ranged from 0.007–0.075 µM) and showed strain specific activity against HIV-2 (EC_{50} values ranged from 0.007–1.5 µM). In drug combination studies of emtricitabine with nucleoside reverse transcriptase inhibitors (abacavir, lamivudine, stavudine, tenofovir, zidovudine), non-nucleoside reverse transcriptase inhibitors (delavirdine, efavirenz, nevirapine, and rilpivirine), and protease inhibitors (amprenavir, nelfinavir, ritonavir, saquinavir), no antagonistic effects were observed.

Rilpivirine: Rilpivirine exhibited activity against laboratory strains of wild-type HIV-1 in an acutely infected T-cell line with a median EC_{50} value for HIV-1_{IIIB} of 0.73 nM. Rilpivirine demonstrated limited activity in cell culture against HIV-2 with a median EC_{50} value of 5220 nM (range 2510 to 10830 nM). Rilpivirine demonstrated antiviral activity against a broad panel of HIV-1 group M (subtype A, B, C, D, F, G, H) primary isolates with EC_{50} values ranging from 0.07 to 1.01 nM and was less active against group O primary isolates with EC_{50} values ranging from 2.88 to 8.45 nM. The antiviral activity of rilpivirine was not antagonistic when combined with the NNRTIs efavirenz, etravirine or nevirapine; N(t)RTIs abacavir, didanosine, emtricitabine, lamivudine, stavudine, tenofovir or zidovudine; the PIs amprenavir, atazanavir, darunavir, indinavir, lopinavir, nelfinavir, ritonavir, saquinavir or tipranavir; the fusion inhibitor enfuvirtide; the CCR5 co-receptor antagonist maraviroc or the integrase strand transfer inhibitor raltegravir.

Tenofovir Disoproxil Fumarate: The antiviral activity of tenofovir against laboratory and clinical isolates of HIV-1 was assessed in lymphoblastoid cell lines, primary monocyte/macrophage cells and peripheral blood lymphocytes. The EC_{50} values for tenofovir were in the range of 0.04–8.5 µM. Tenofovir displayed antiviral activity in cell culture against HIV-1 clades A, B, C, D, E, F, G, and O (EC_{50} values ranged from 0.5–2.2 µM) and showed strain specific activity against HIV-2 (EC_{50} values ranged from 1.6 µM–5.5 µM). In drug combination studies of tenofovir with NRTIs (abacavir, didanosine, emtricitabine, lamivudine, stavudine, and zidovudine), NNRTIs (delavirdine, efavirenz, nevirapine, and rilpivirine), and PIs (amprenavir, indinavir, nelfinavir, ritonavir, saquinavir), no antagonistic effects were observed.

Resistance

In Cell Culture

Emtricitabine and Tenofovir Disoproxil Fumarate: HIV-1 isolates with reduced susceptibility to emtricitabine or tenofovir have been selected in cell culture. Reduced susceptibility to emtricitabine was associated with M184V/I substitutions in HIV-1 RT. HIV-1 isolates selected by tenofovir expressed a K65R substitution in HIV-1 RT and showed a 2–4 fold reduction in susceptibility to tenofovir.

Rilpivirine: Rilpivirine-resistant strains were selected in cell culture starting from wild-type HIV-1 of different origins and subtypes as well as NNRTI resistant HIV-1. The frequently observed amino acid substitutions that emerged and conferred decreased phenotypic susceptibility to rilpivirine included: L100I, K101E, V106I and A, V108I, E138K and G, Q, R, V179F and I, Y181C and I, V189I, G190E, H221Y, F227C and M230I and L.

In Treatment-Naive HIV-1-infected Subjects

In the Week 96 pooled resistance analysis for subjects receiving rilpivirine or efavirenz in combination with emtricitabine/tenofovir DF in the Phase 3 clinical trials C209 and C215, the emergence of resistance was greater among subjects' viruses in the rilpivirine plus emtricitabine/tenofovir DF arm compared to the efavirenz plus emtricitabine/tenofovir DF arm and was dependent on baseline viral load. In the pooled resistance analysis, 61% (47/77) of the subjects who qualified for resistance analysis (resistance analysis subjects) in the rilpivirine plus emtricitabine/tenofovir DF arm had virus with genotypic and/or phenotypic resistance to rilpivirine compared to 42% (18/43) of the resistance analysis subjects in the efavirenz plus emtricitabine/tenofovir DF arm who had genotypic and/or phenotypic resistance to efavirenz. Moreover, genotypic and/or phenotypic resistance to emtricitabine or tenofovir emerged in viruses from 57% (44/77) of the resistance analysis subjects in the rilpivirine arm compared to 26% (11/43) in the efavirenz arm.

Emerging NNRTI substitutions in the rilpivirine resistance analysis of subjects' viruses included V90I, K101E/P/T, E138K/A/Q/G, V179I/L, Y181C/I, V189I, H221Y, F227C/L and M230L, which were associated with a rilpivirine phenotypic fold change range of 2.6–621. The E138K substitution emerged most frequently during rilpivirine treatment commonly in combination with the M184I substitution. The emtricitabine and lamivudine resistance-associated substitutions M184I or V and NRTI resistance-associated substitutions (K65R/N, A62V, D67N/G, K70E, Y115F, K219E/R) emerged more frequently in the rilpivirine resistance analysis subjects than in efavirenz resistance analysis subjects (See Table 8).

NNRTI- and NRTI-resistance substitutions emerged less frequently in the resistance analysis of viruses from subjects with baseline viral loads of ≤100,000 copies/mL compared to viruses from subjects with baseline viral loads of >100,000 copies/mL: 23% (10/44) compared to 77% (34/44) of NNRTI-resistance substitutions and 20% (9/44) compared to 80% (35/44) of NRTI-resistance substitutions. This difference was also observed for the individual emtricitabine/lamivudine and tenofovir resistance substitutions: 22% (9/41) compared to 78% (32/41) for M184I/V and 0% (0/8) compared to 100% (8/8) for K65R/N. Additionally, NNRTI and/or NRTI-resistance substitutions emerged less frequently in the resistance analysis of the viruses from subjects with baseline CD4+ cell counts ≥200 cells/mm³ compared to the viruses from subjects with baseline CD4+ cell counts <200 cells/mm³: 32% (14/44) compared to 68% (30/44) of NNRTI-resistance substitutions and 27% (12/44) compared to 73% (32/44) of NRTI-resistance substitutions.

Table 8 Proportion of Frequently Emerging Reverse Transcriptase Substitutions in the HIV-1 Virus of Resistance Analysis Subjects* Who Received Rilpivirine or Efavirenz in Combination with Emtricitabine/Tenofovir DF from Pooled Phase 3 TMC278-C209 and TMC278-C215 Trials in the Week 96 Analysis

	C209 and C215 N=1096	
	Rilpivirine + FTC/TDF	**Efavirenz + FTC/TDF**
	N=550	**N=546**
Subjects who Qualified for Resistance Analysis	14% (77/550)	8% (43/546)
Subjects with Evaluable Post-Baseline Resistance Data	70	31
Emergent NNRTI Substitutions†		
Any	63% (44/70)	55% (17/31)
V90I	14% (10/70)	0
K101E/P/T/Q	19% (13/70)	10% (3/31)
K103N	1% (1/70)	39% (12/31)
E138K/A/Q/G	40% (28/70)	0
E138K+M184I‡	30% (21/70)	0
V179I/D	6% (4/70)	10% (3/31)
Y181C/I/S	13% (9/70)	3% (1/31)
V189I	9% (6/70)	0
H221Y	10% (7/70)	0
Emergent NRTI Substitutions§		
Any	63% (44/70)	32% (10/31)
M184I/V	59% (41/70)	26% (8/31)
K65R/N	11% (8/70)	6% (2/31)
A62V, D67N/G, K70E, Y115F, or K219E/R¶	20% (14/70)	3% (1/31)

* Subjects who qualified for resistance analysis

† V90, L100, K101, K103, V106, V108, E138, V179, Y181, Y188, V189, G190, H221, P225, F227, and M230

‡ This combination of NRTI and NNRTI substitutions is a subset of those with the E138K.

§ A62V, K65R/N, D67N/G, K70E, L74I, Y115F, M184V/I, L210F, K219E/R

¶ These substitutions emerged in addition to the primary substitutions M184V/I or K65R; A62V (n=2), D67N/G (n=3), K70E (n=4), Y115F (n=2), K219E/R (n=8) in rilpivirine resistance analysis subjects.

Cross Resistance

Emtricitabine, Rilpivirine, and Tenofovir Disoproxil Fumarate:

In Cell Culture

No significant cross-resistance has been demonstrated between rilpivirine-resistant HIV-1 variants and emtricitabine or tenofovir, or between emtricitabine- or tenofovir-resistant variants and rilpivirine.

Rilpivirine:

Site-Directed NNRTI Mutant Virus

Cross-resistance has been observed among NNRTIs. The single NNRTI substitutions K101P, Y181I and Y181V conferred 52-fold, 15-fold and 12-fold decreased susceptibility to rilpivirine, respectively. The combination of E138K and M184I showed 6.7-fold reduced susceptibility to rilpivirine compared to 2.8-fold for E138K alone. The K103N substitution did not show reduced susceptibility to rilpivirine by itself. However, the combination of K103N and L100I resulted in a 7-fold reduced susceptibility to rilpivirine. In another study, the Y188L substitution resulted in a reduced susceptibility to rilpivirine of 9-fold for clinical isolates and 6-fold for site-directed mutants. Combinations of 2 or 3 NNRTI resistance-associated substitutions gave decreased susceptibility to rilpivirine (fold change range of 3.7–554) in 38% and 66% of mutants, respectively.

In Treatment-Naive HIV-1-infected Subjects

Considering all of the available cell culture and clinical data, any of the following amino acid substitutions, when present at baseline, are likely to decrease the antiviral activity of rilpivirine: K101E, K101P, E138A, E138G, E138K, E138R, E138Q, V179L, Y181C, Y181I, Y181V, Y188L, H221Y, F227C, M230I or M230L.

Cross-resistance to efavirenz, etravirine and/or nevirapine is likely after virologic failure and development of rilpivirine resistance. In a pooled 96-Week analysis for subjects receiving rilpivirine in combination with emtricitabine/tenofovir DF in the Phase 3 clinical trials TMC278-C209 and TMC278-C215, 43 of the 70 (61%) rilpivirine resistance analysis subjects with post-baseline resistance data had virus with decreased susceptibility to rilpivirine (≥2.5-fold). Of these, 84% (n=36/43) were resistant to efavirenz (≥3.3 fold change), 88% (n=38/43) were resistant to etravirine (≥3.2 fold change) and 60% (n=26/43) were resistant to nevirapine (≥6 fold change). In the efavirenz arm, 3 of the 15 (20%) efavirenz resistance analysis subjects had viruses with resistance to etravirine and rilpivirine, and 93% (14/15) had resistance to nevirapine. Virus from subjects experiencing virologic failure on rilpivirine in combination with emtricitabine/tenofovir DF developed more NNRTI resistance-associated substitutions conferring more cross-resistance to the NNRTI class and had a higher likelihood of cross-resistance to all NNRTIs in the class than subjects who failed on efavirenz.

Emtricitabine: Emtricitabine-resistant isolates (M184V/I) were cross-resistant to lamivudine but retained susceptibility in cell culture to didanosine, stavudine, tenofovir, zidovudine, and NNRTIs (delavirdine, efavirenz, nevirapine, and rilpivirine). HIV-1 isolates containing the K65R substitution, selected *in vivo* by abacavir, didanosine, and tenofovir, demonstrated reduced susceptibility to inhibition by emtricitabine. Viruses harboring substitutions conferring reduced susceptibility to stavudine and zidovudine (M41L, D67N, K70R, L210W, T215Y/F, K219Q/E), or didanosine (L74V) remained sensitive to emtricitabine. HIV-1 containing the substitutions associated with NNRTI resistance K103N or rilpivirine-associated substitutions were susceptible to emtricitabine.

Tenofovir Disoproxil Fumarate: The K65R substitution selected by tenofovir is also selected in some HIV-1 infected patients treated with abacavir or didanosine. HIV-1 isolates with the K65R substitution also showed reduced susceptibility to emtricitabine and lamivudine. Therefore, cross-resistance among these NRTIs may occur in patients whose virus harbors the K65R substitution. HIV-1 isolates from patients (N=20) whose HIV-1 expressed a mean of 3 zidovudine-associated RT amino acid substitutions (M41L, D67N, K70R, L210W, T215Y/F, or K219Q/E/N) showed a 3.1-fold decrease in the susceptibility to tenofovir.

Subjects whose virus expressed an L74V substitution without zidovudine resistance associated substitutions (N=8) had reduced response to VIREAD. Limited data are available for patients whose virus expressed a Y115F substitution (N=3), Q151M substitution (N=2), or T69 insertion (N=4), all of whom had a reduced response.

HIV-1 containing the substitutions associated with NNRTI resistance K103N and Y181C, or rilpivirine-associated substitutions were susceptible to tenofovir.

13 NONCLINICAL TOXICOLOGY

13.1 Carcinogenesis, Mutagenesis, Impairment of Fertility

Emtricitabine: In long-term carcinogenicity studies of emtricitabine, no drug-related increases in tumor incidence were found in mice at doses up to 750 mg per kg per day (26 times the human systemic exposure at the therapeutic dose of 200 mg per day) or in rats at doses up to 600 mg per kg per day (31 times the human systemic exposure at the therapeutic dose).

Emtricitabine was not genotoxic in the reverse mutation bacterial test (Ames test), mouse lymphoma or mouse micronucleus assays.

Emtricitabine did not affect fertility in male rats at approximately 140-fold or in male and female mice at approximately 60-fold higher exposures (AUC) than in humans given the recommended 200 mg daily dose. Fertility was normal in the offspring of mice exposed daily from before birth (in utero) through sexual maturity at daily exposures (AUC) of approximately 60-fold higher than human exposures at the recommended 200 mg daily dose.

Rilpivirine: Rilpivirine was evaluated for carcinogenic potential by oral gavage administration to mice and rats up to 104 weeks. Daily doses of 20, 60 and 160 mg per kg per day were administered to mice and doses of 40, 200, 500 and 1500 mg per kg per day were administered to rats. In rats, there were no drug related neoplasms. In mice, rilpivirine was positive for hepatocellular neoplasms in both males and females. The observed hepatocellular findings in mice may be rodent-specific. At the lowest tested doses in the carcinogenicity studies, the systemic exposures (based on AUC) to rilpivirine were 21 fold (mice) and 3 fold (rats), relative to those observed in humans at the recommended dose (25 mg once daily).

Rilpivirine has tested negative in the absence and presence of a metabolic activation system, in the *in vitro* Ames reverse mutation assay and *in vitro* clastogenicity mouse lymphoma assay. Rilpivirine did not induce chromosomal damage in the *in vivo* micronucleus test in mice.

In a study conducted in rats, there were no effects on mating or fertility with rilpivirine up to 400 mg per kg per day, a dose of rilpivirine that showed maternal toxicity. This dose is associated with an exposure that is approximately 40 times higher than the exposure in humans at the recommended dose of 25 mg once daily.

Tenofovir Disoproxil Fumarate: Long-term oral carcinogenicity studies of tenofovir DF in mice and rats were carried out at exposures up to approximately 16 times (mice) and 5 times (rats) those observed in humans at the therapeutic dose for HIV-1 infection. At the high dose in female mice, liver adenomas were increased at exposures 16 times that in humans. In rats, the study was negative for carcinogenic findings at exposures up to 5 times that observed in humans at the therapeutic dose.

Tenofovir DF was mutagenic in the *in vitro* mouse lymphoma assay and negative in an *in vitro* bacterial mutagenicity test (Ames test). In an *in vivo* mouse micronucleus assay, tenofovir DF was negative when administered to male mice.

There were no effects on fertility, mating performance or early embryonic development when tenofovir DF was administered to male rats at a dose equivalent to 10 times the human dose based on body surface area comparisons for 28 days prior to mating and to female rats for 15 days prior to mating through day seven of gestation. There was, however, an alteration of the estrous cycle in female rats.

13.2 Animal Toxicology and/or Pharmacology

Tenofovir Disoproxil Fumarate: Tenofovir and tenofovir DF administered in toxicology studies to rats, dogs and monkeys at exposures (based on AUCs) greater than or equal to 6-fold those observed in humans caused bone toxicity. In monkeys the bone toxicity was diagnosed as osteomalacia. Osteomalacia observed in monkeys appeared to be reversible upon dose reduction or discontinuation of tenofovir. In rats and dogs, the bone toxicity manifested as reduced bone mineral density. The mechanism(s) underlying bone toxicity is unknown.

Evidence of renal toxicity was noted in 4 animal species. Increases in serum creatinine, BUN, glycosuria, proteinuria, phosphaturia, and/or calciuria and decreases in serum phosphate were observed to varying degrees in these animals. These toxicities were noted at exposures (based on AUCs) 2–20 times higher than those observed in humans. The relationship of the renal abnormalities, particularly the phosphaturia, to the bone toxicity is not known.

14 CLINICAL STUDIES

The efficacy of COMPLERA is based on the analyses of 48- and 96-week data from two randomized, double-blind, controlled studies C209 (ECHO) and C215 (THRIVE) in treatment-naive, HIV-1 infected subjects (N=1368). The studies are identical in design with the exception of the background regimen (BR). Subjects were randomized in a 1:1 ratio to receive either rilpivirine 25 mg (N=686) once daily or efavirenz 600 mg (N=682) once daily in addition to a BR. In Study C209 (N=690), the BR was emtricitabine/tenofovir DF. In Study C215 (N=678), the BR consisted of 2 NRTIs: emtricitabine/tenofovir DF (60%, N=406) or lamivudine/zidovudine (30%, N=204) or abacavir plus lamivudine (10%, N=68).

For subjects who received emtricitabine/tenofovir DF (N=1096) in C209 and C215, the mean age was 37 years (range 18–78), 78% were male, 62% were White, 24% were Black, and 11% were Asian. The mean baseline CD4+ cell count was 265 cells/mm^3 (range 1–888) and 31% had CD4+ cell counts <200 cells/mm^3. The median baseline plasma HIV-1 RNA was 5 $\log_{10}$ copies/mL (range 2–7). Subjects were stratified by baseline HIV-1 RNA. Fifty percent of subjects had baseline viral loads ≤100,000 copies/mL, 39% of subjects had baseline viral load between 100,000 copies/mL to 500,000 copies/mL and 11% of subject had baseline viral load >500,000 copies/mL.

Treatment outcomes through 96 weeks for the subset of subjects receiving emtricitabine/tenofovir DF in studies C209 and C215 (Table 9) are generally consistent with treatment outcomes for all participating subjects (presented in the prescribing information for EDURANT). The incidence of virologic failure was higher in the rilpivirine arm than the efavirenz arm at Week 96. Virologic failures and discontinuations due to adverse events mostly occurred in the first 48 weeks of treatment.

Table 9 Virologic Outcome of Randomized Treatment of Studies C209 and C215 (Pooled Data for Subjects Receiving Rilpivirine or Efavirenz in Combination with Emtricitabine/Tenofovir DF) at Week 96*

	Rilpivirine + FTC/TDF	Efavirenz + FTC/TDF
	N=550	N=546
HIV-1 RNA <50 copies/mL†	77%	77%
HIV-1 RNA ≥50 copies/mL‡	14%	8%
No virologic data at Week 96 window Reasons		
Discontinued study due to adverse event or death§	4%	9%
Discontinued study for other reasons¶ and the last available HIV-1 RNA <50 copies/mL (or missing)	4%	6%
Missing data during window but on study	<1%	<1%
HIV-1 RNA <50 copies/mL by Baseline HIV-1 RNA (copies/mL)		
≤100,000	83%	80%
>100,000	71%	74%
HIV-1 RNA ≥50 copies/mL‡ by Baseline HIV-1 RNA (copies/mL)		
≤100,000	7%	5%
>100,000	22%	12%
HIV-1 RNA <50 copies/mL by Baseline CD4+ Cell Count (cells/mm^3)		
<200	68%	72%
≥200	82%	79%
HIV-1 RNA ≥50 copies/mL‡ by Baseline CD4+ Cell Count (cells/mm^3)		
<200	27%	12%
≥200	8%	7%

* Analyses were based on the last observed viral load data within the Week 96 window (Week 90–103).

† Predicted difference (95% CI) of response rate is 0.5% (-4.5% to 5.5%) at Week 96.

‡ Includes subjects who had ≥50 copies/mL in the Week 96 window, subjects who discontinued early due to lack or loss of efficacy, subjects who discontinued for reasons other than an adverse event, death or lack or loss of efficacy and at the time of discontinuation had a viral value of ≥50 copies/mL, and subjects who had a switch in background regimen that was not permitted by the protocol.

§ Includes subjects who discontinued due to an adverse event or death if this resulted in no on-treatment virologic data in the Week 96 window.

¶ Includes subjects who discontinued for reasons other than an adverse event, death or lack or loss of efficacy, e.g., withdrew consent, loss to follow-up, etc.

Based on the pooled data from studies C209 and C215, the mean CD4+ cell count increase from baseline at Week 96 was 226 cells/mm^3 for rilpivirine plus emtricitabine/tenofovir DF-treated subjects and 223 cells/mm^3 for efavirenz plus emtricitabine/tenofovir DF-treated subjects.

16 HOW SUPPLIED/STORAGE AND HANDLING

COMPLERA tablets are purplish-pink, capsule-shaped, film-coated, debossed with "GSI" on one side and plain-faced on the other side. Each bottle contains 30 tablets (NDC 61958-1101-1), a silica gel desiccant, polyester fiber coil, and is closed with a child-resistant closure.

Store at 25 °C (77 °F), excursions permitted to 15 °C–30 °C (59 °F–86 °F) (see USP Controlled Room Temperature).

- Keep container tightly closed
- Dispense only in original container
- Do not use if seal over bottle opening is broken or missing.

17 PATIENT COUNSELING INFORMATION

See FDA-Approved Patient Labeling (Patient Information)

A statement to patients and healthcare providers is included on the product's bottle label: **ALERT: Find out about medicines that should NOT be taken with COMPLERA.** A Patient Package Insert for COMPLERA is available for patient information.

Information for Patients

Patients should be advised that:

- Patients should remain under the care of a healthcare provider when using COMPLERA.
- Patients should be informed that COMPLERA is not a cure for HIV infection. Patients should stay on continuous HIV therapy to control HIV infection and decrease HIV-related illnesses. Patients should be told that sustained decreases in plasma HIV RNA have been associated with a reduced risk of progression to AIDS and death.
- Patients should be advised to continue to practice safer sex and to use latex or polyurethane condoms to lower the chance of sexual contact with any body fluids such as semen, vaginal secretions or blood. Patients should be advised never to re-use or share needles.
- Patients should be advised not to breastfeed because at least two of the drugs contained in COMPLERA can be passed to the baby in breast milk. It is not known whether this could harm the baby. Also, mothers with HIV-1 should not breastfeed because HIV-1 can be passed to the baby in breast milk.
- It is important to take COMPLERA on a regular dosing schedule with food and to avoid missing doses. A protein drink is not a substitute for food. If the healthcare provider decides to stop COMPLERA and the patient is switched to new medicines to treat HIV that includes rilpivirine tablets, the rilpivirine tablets should be taken only with a meal.
- If the patient misses a dose of COMPLERA within 12 hours of the time it is usually taken, the patient should take COMPLERA with food as soon as possible and then take the next dose of COMPLERA at the regularly scheduled time. If a patient misses a dose of COMPLERA by more than 12 hours, the patient should not take the missed dose, but resume the usual dosing schedule. Inform the patient that he or she should not take more or less than the prescribed dose of COMPLERA at any one time.
- Lactic acidosis and severe hepatomegaly with steatosis, including fatal cases, have been reported. Treatment with COMPLERA should be suspended in any patients who develop clinical symptoms suggestive of lactic acidosis or pronounced hepatotoxicity (including nausea, vomiting, unusual or unexpected stomach discomfort, and weakness) *[See Warnings and Precautions (5.1)]*.
- Patients with HIV-1 should be tested for hepatitis B virus (HBV) before initiating antiretroviral therapy. Severe acute exacerbations of hepatitis B have been reported in patients who are coinfected with HBV and HIV-1 and have discontinued EMTRIVA or VIREAD *[See Warnings and Precautions (5.2)]*. COMPLERA should not be discontinued without first informing their healthcare provider.
- Renal impairment, including cases of acute renal failure and Fanconi syndrome, has been reported in association with the use of VIREAD. COMPLERA should be avoided with concurrent or recent use of a nephrotoxic agent *[See Warnings and Precautions (5.3)]*.
- COMPLERA may interact with many drugs; therefore, patients should be advised to report to their healthcare provider the use of any other prescription or nonprescription medication or herbal products, including St. John's wort *[See Warnings and Precautions (5.4)]*.
- COMPLERA should not be coadministered with the following drugs, as significant decreases in rilpivirine plasma concentrations may occur due to CYP3A enzyme

induction or gastric pH increase, which may result in loss of virologic response and possible resistance to COMPLERA or to the class of NNRTIs: the anticonvulsants carbamazepine, oxcarbazepine, phenobarbital, phenytoin; the antimycobacterials rifabutin, rifampin, rifapentine; proton pump inhibitors, such as esomeprazole, lansoprazole, omeprazole, pantoprazole, rabeprazole; the glucocorticoid systemic dexamethasone (more than a single dose); or St. John's wort (*Hypericum perforatum*) *[See Contraindications (4)]*.

- Patients should be informed that depressive disorders (depressed mood, depression, dysphoria, major depression, mood altered, negative thoughts, suicide attempt, suicidal ideation) have been reported with COMPLERA. If they experience depressive symptoms, they should seek immediate medical evaluation *[See Warnings and Precautions (5.5)]*.
- Patients should be informed that hepatotoxicity has been reported with COMPLERA *[See Warnings and Precautions (5.6)]*.
- Decreases in bone mineral density have been observed with the use of VIREAD. Bone mineral density (BMD) monitoring should be considered in patients who have a history of pathologic bone fracture or other risk factors for osteoporosis or bone loss *[See Warnings and Precautions (5.7)]*.
- COMPLERA should not be coadministered with ATRIPLA, Edurant, EMTRIVA, STRIBILD, TRUVADA, or VIREAD; or with drugs containing lamivudine, including Combivir, Epivir or Epivir-HBV, Epzicom, or Trizivir; or with HEPSERA *[See Warnings and Precautions (5.8)]*.
- Redistribution or accumulation of body fat may occur in patients receiving antiretroviral therapy and that the cause and long-term health effects of these conditions are not known *[See Warnings and Precautions (5.9)]*.
- In some patients with advanced HIV infection (AIDS), signs and symptoms of inflammation from previous infections may occur soon after anti-HIV treatment is started. It is believed that these symptoms are due to an improvement in the body's immune response, enabling the body to fight infections that may have been present with no obvious symptoms. Patients should be advised to inform their healthcare provider immediately of any symptoms of infection *[See Warnings and Precautions (5.10)]*.

Manufactured and distributed by:
Gilead Sciences, Inc.
Foster City, CA 94404

Patient Information
COMPLERA® (kom-PLEH-rah)
(emtricitabine, rilpivirine, tenofovir disoproxil fumarate)
Tablets

Important: Ask your healthcare provider or pharmacist about medicines that should not be taken with COMPLERA. For more information, see the section "What should I tell my healthcare provider before taking COMPLERA?"

Read this Patient Information before you start taking COMPLERA and each time you get a refill. There may be new information. This information does not take the place of talking to your healthcare provider about your medical condition or treatment.

What is the most important information I should know about COMPLERA?

COMPLERA can cause serious side effects, including:

1. **Build-up of an acid in your blood (lactic acidosis).** Lactic acidosis can happen in some people who take COMPLERA or similar (nucleoside analogs) medicines. **Lactic acidosis** is a serious medical emergency that can lead to death.
   Lactic acidosis can be hard to identify early, because the symptoms could seem like symptoms of other health problems. **Call your healthcare provider right away if you get any of the following symptoms which could be signs of lactic acidosis:**
   - feeling very weak or tired
   - have unusual (not normal) muscle pain
   - have trouble breathing
   - have stomach pain with
     - nausea (feel sick to your stomach)
     - vomiting
   - feel cold, especially in your arms and legs
   - feel dizzy or lightheaded
   - have a fast or irregular heartbeat
2. **Severe liver problems.** Severe liver problems can happen in people who take COMPLERA or similar medicines. In some cases these liver problems can lead to death. Your liver may become large (hepatomegaly) and you may develop fat in your liver (steatosis) when you take COMPLERA.
   Call your healthcare provider right away if you have any of the following symptoms of liver problems:
   - your skin or the white part of your eyes turns yellow (jaundice)
   - dark "tea-colored" urine
   - light-colored bowel movements (stools)
   - loss of appetite for several days or longer
   - nausea
   - stomach pain

You may be more likely to get lactic acidosis or severe liver problems if you are female, very overweight (obese), or have been taking COMPLERA or a similar medicine containing nucleoside analogs for a long time.

3. **Worsening of Hepatitis B infection.** If you also have hepatitis B virus (HBV) infection and you stop taking COMPLERA, your HBV infection may become worse (flare-up). A "flare-up" is when your HBV infection suddenly returns in a worse way than before. COMPLERA is not approved for the treatment of HBV, so you must discuss your HBV therapy with your healthcare provider.
   - Do not let your COMPLERA run out. Refill your prescription or talk to your healthcare provider before your COMPLERA is all gone.
   - Do not stop taking COMPLERA without first talking to your healthcare provider.
   - If you stop taking COMPLERA, your healthcare provider will need to check your health often and do blood tests regularly to check your HBV infection. Tell your healthcare provider about any new or unusual symptoms you may have after you stop taking COMPLERA.

What is COMPLERA?

COMPLERA is a prescription HIV (Human Immunodeficiency Virus) medicine that:
- is used to treat HIV-1 in adults who have **never** taken HIV medicines before, **and**
- who have an amount of HIV in their blood (this is called 'viral load') that is no more than 100,000 copies/mL. Your healthcare provider will measure your viral load.

HIV is the virus that causes AIDS (Acquired Immunodeficiency Syndrome).

COMPLERA contains 3 medicines, (rilpivirine, emtricitabine, tenofovir disoproxil fumarate) combined in one tablet. Emtricitabine (EMTRIVA®) and tenofovir disoproxil fumarate (VIREAD®) are HIV-1 (human immunodeficiency virus) nucleoside analog reverse transcriptase inhibitors (NRTIs). Rilpivirine (Edurant®) is an HIV-1 non-nucleoside analog reverse transcriptase inhibitor (NNRTI). It is not known if COMPLERA is safe and effective in children under the age of 18 years.

COMPLERA may help:
- Reduce the amount of HIV in your blood.
- Increase the number of white blood cells called CD4+ (T) cells in your blood that help fight off other infections.

Reducing the amount of HIV and increasing the CD4+ (T) cells in your blood may help improve your immune system. This may reduce your risk of death or getting infections that can happen when your immune system is weak (opportunistic infections).

COMPLERA does not cure HIV infections or AIDS.

You must stay on continuous HIV therapy to control HIV infection and decrease HIV-related illnesses.

Avoid doing things that can spread HIV-1 infection to others.
- Do not share or re-use needles or other injection equipment.
- Do not share personal items that can have blood or body fluids on them, like toothbrushes and razor blades.
- Do not have any kind of sex without protection. Always practice safer sex by using a latex or polyurethane condom to lower the chance of sexual contact with any body fluids such as semen, vaginal secretions, or blood.

Ask your healthcare provider if you have any questions about how to prevent passing HIV to other people.

Who should not take COMPLERA?

Do not take COMPLERA if:
- your HIV infection has been previously treated with HIV medicines.
- you are taking any of the following medicines:
  - anti-seizure medicines:
    - carbamazepine (Carbatrol®, Equetro®, Tegretol®, Tegretol- XR®, Teril®, Epitol®)
    - oxcarbazepine (Trileptal®)
    - phenobarbital (Luminal®)
    - phenytoin (Dilantin®, Dilantin-125®, Phenytek®)
  - anti-tuberculosis (anti-TB) medicines:
    - rifabutin (Mycobutin®)
    - rifampin (Rifater®,Rifamate®, Rimactane®, Rifadin®)
    - rifapentine (Priftin®)
  - proton pump inhibitor (PPI) medicine for certain stomach or intestinal problems:
    - dexlansoprazole (Dexilant®)
    - esomeprazole (Nexium®, Vimovo®)
    - lansoprazole (Prevacid®)
    - omeprazole (Prilosec®, Zegerid®)
    - pantoprazole sodium (Protonix®)
    - rabeprazole (Aciphex®)
  - more than 1 dose of the steroid medicine dexamethasone or dexamethasone sodium phosphate
  - St. John's wort (Hypericum perforatum)

What should I tell my healthcare provider before taking COMPLERA?

Before you take COMPLERA, tell your healthcare provider if you:
- have liver problems, including hepatitis B or C virus infection
- have kidney problems
- have ever had a mental health problem
- have bone problems
- are pregnant or plan to become pregnant. It is not known if COMPLERA can harm your unborn child.
  Pregnancy Registry. There is a pregnancy registry for women who take antiretroviral medicines during pregnancy. The purpose of this registry is to collect information about the health of you and your baby. Talk to your healthcare provider about how you can take part in this registry.
- are breast-feeding or plan to breast-feed. You should not breastfeed if you have HIV because of the risk of passing HIV to your baby. Do not breastfeed if you are taking COMPLERA. At least two of the medicines contained in COMPLERA can be passed to your baby in your breast milk. We do not know whether this could harm your baby. Talk to your healthcare provider about the best way to feed your baby.

Tell your healthcare provider about all the medicines you take, including prescription and nonprescription medicines, vitamins, and herbal supplements.

COMPLERA may affect the way other medicines work, and other medicines may affect how COMPLERA works, and may cause serious side effects. If you take certain medicines with COMPLERA, the amount of COMPLERA in your body may be too low and it may not work to help control your HIV infection. The HIV virus in your body may become resistant to COMPLERA or other HIV medicines that are like it.

COMPLERA provides a complete treatment for HIV infection. Do not take other HIV medicines with COMPLERA.

If you take COMPLERA, you should not take:
- other medicines that contain tenofovir (VIREAD, TRUVADA®, STRIBILD®, ATRIPLA®)
- other medicines that contain emtricitabine or lamivudine (EMTRIVA, Combivir®, Epivir® or Epivir-HBV®, Epzicom®, Trizivir®, ATRIPLA, TRUVADA, STRIBILD)
- rilpivirine (Edurant)
- adefovir (HEPSERA®)

Especially tell your healthcare provider if you take:
- an antacid medicine that contains aluminum, magnesium hydroxide, or calcium carbonate. If you take an antacid during treatment with COMPLERA, take the antacid **at least 2 hours before or at least 4 hours after** you take COMPLERA.
- a medicine to block the acid in your stomach, including cimetidine (Tagamet®), famotidine (Pepcid®), nizatidine (Axid®), or ranitidine hydrochloride (Zantac®). If you take one of these medicines during treatment with COMPLERA, take the acid blocker **at least 12 hours before or at least 4 hours after** you take COMPLERA.
- any of these medicines (if taken by mouth or injection):
  - clarithromycin (Biaxin®)
  - erythromycin (E-Mycin®, Eryc®, Ery-Tab®, PCE®, Pediazole®, Iloson®)
  - fluconazole (Diflucan®)
  - itraconazole (Sporanox®)
  - ketoconazole (Nizoral®)
  - methadone (Dolophine®)
  - posaconazole (Noxafil®)
  - telithromycin (Ketek®)
  - voriconazole (Vfend®)
- medicines that are eliminated by the kidney, including acyclovir (Zovirax®), cidofovir (VISTIDE®), ganciclovir (Cytovene IV®, Vitrasert®), valacyclovir (Valtrex®), and valganciclovir (Valcyte®)

Ask your healthcare provider or pharmacist if you are not sure if your medicine is one that is listed above.

Know the medicines you take. Keep a list of your medicines and show it to your healthcare provider and pharmacist when you get a new medicine. Your healthcare provider and your pharmacist can tell you if you can take these medicines with COMPLERA. Do not start any new medicines while you are taking COMPLERA without first talking with your healthcare provider or pharmacist. You can ask your healthcare provider or pharmacist for a list of medicines that can interact with COMPLERA.

How should I take COMPLERA?
- **Stay under the care of your healthcare provider during treatment with COMPLERA.**
- **Take COMPLERA exactly as your healthcare provider tells you to take it.**
- **Always take COMPLERA with food.** Taking COMPLERA with food is important to help get the right amount of medicine in your body. A protein drink does not replace food. If your healthcare provider decides to stop

COMPLERA and you are switched to new medicines to treat HIV that includes rilpivirine tablets, the rilpivirine tablets should be taken only with a meal.
- Do not change your dose or stop taking COMPLERA without first talking with your healthcare provider. See your healthcare provider regularly while taking COMPLERA.
- If you miss a dose of COMPLERA within 12 hours of the time you usually take it, take your dose of COMPLERA **with food** as soon as possible. Then, take your next dose of COMPLERA at the regularly scheduled time. If you miss a dose of COMPLERA by more than 12 hours of the time you usually take it, wait and then take the next dose of COMPLERA at the regularly scheduled time.
- Do not take more than your prescribed dose to make up for a missed dose.
- When your COMPLERA supply starts to run low, get more from your healthcare provider or pharmacy. It is very important not to run out of COMPLERA. The amount of virus in your blood may increase if the medicine is stopped for even a short time.
- If you take too much COMPLERA, contact your local poison control center or go to the nearest hospital emergency room right away.

What are the possible side effects of COMPLERA?

COMPLERA can cause serious side effects, including:
- **See "What is the most important information I should know about COMPLERA?"**
- **New or worse kidney problems, including kidney failure,** can happen in some people who take COMPLERA. Your healthcare provider should do blood tests to check your kidneys before starting treatment with COMPLERA. If you have had kidney problems in the past or need to take another medicine that can cause kidney problems, your healthcare provider may need to do blood tests to check your kidneys during your treatment with COMPLERA.
- **Depression or mood changes. Tell your healthcare provider right away if you have any of the following symptoms:**
  - feeling sad or hopeless
  - feeling anxious or restless
  - have thoughts of hurting yourself (suicide) or have tried to hurt yourself
- **Change in liver enzymes.** People with a history of hepatitis B or C virus infection or who have certain liver enzyme changes may have an increased risk of developing new or worsening liver problems during treatment with COMPLERA. Liver problems can also happen during treatment with COMPLERA in people without a history of liver disease. Your healthcare provider may need to do tests to check your liver enzymes before and during treatment with COMPLERA.
- **Bone problems** can happen in some people who take COMPLERA. Bone problems include bone pain, softening or thinning (which may lead to fractures). Your healthcare provider may need to do additional tests to check your bones.
- **Changes in body fat** can happen in people taking HIV medicine. These changes may include increased amount of fat in the upper back and neck ("buffalo hump"), breast, and around the main part of your body (trunk). Loss of fat from the legs, arms and face may also happen. The cause and long term health effect of these conditions are not known.
- **Changes in your immune system (Immune Reconstitution Syndrome)** can happen when you start taking HIV medicines. Your immune system may get stronger and begin to fight infections that have been hidden in your body for a long time. Tell your healthcare provider if you start having new symptoms after starting your HIV medicine.

The most common side effects of COMPLERA include:
- trouble sleeping (insomnia)
- abnormal dreams
- headache
- dizziness
- diarrhea
- nausea
- rash
- tiredness
- depression

Additional common side effects include:
- vomiting
- stomach pain or discomfort
- skin discoloration (small spots or freckles)
- pain

Tell your healthcare provider if you have any side effect that bothers you or that does not go away.

These are not all the possible side effects of COMPLERA. For more information, ask your healthcare provider or pharmacist.

Call your doctor for medical advice about side effects. You may report side effects to FDA at 1-800-FDA-1088 (1-800-332-1088).

How do I store COMPLERA?
- Store COMPLERA at room temperature between 68 °F to 77 °F (20 °C to 25 °C).
- Keep COMPLERA in its original container and keep the container tightly closed.
- Do not use COMPLERA if the seal over the bottle opening is broken or missing.

Keep COMPLERA and all other medicines out of reach of children.

General information about COMPLERA:

Medicines are sometimes prescribed for purposes other than those listed in a Patient Information leaflet. Do not use COMPLERA for a condition for which it was not prescribed. Do not give COMPLERA to other people, even if they have the same symptoms you have. It may harm them.

This leaflet summarizes the most important information about COMPLERA. If you would like more information, talk with your healthcare provider. You can ask your healthcare provider or pharmacist for information about COMPLERA that is written for health professionals. For more information, call 1-800-445-3235 or go to www.COMPLERA.com.

What are the ingredients of COMPLERA?

Active ingredients: emtricitabine, rilpivirine hydrochloride, and tenofovir disoproxil fumarate.

Inactive ingredients: pregelatinized starch, lactose monohydrate, microcrystalline cellulose, croscarmellose sodium, magnesium stearate, povidone, polysorbate 20. The tablet film coating contains polyethylene glycol, hypromellose, lactose monohydrate, triacetin, titanium dioxide, iron oxide red, FD&C Blue #2 aluminum lake, FD&C Yellow #6 aluminum lake.

This Patient Information has been approved by the U.S. Food and Drug Administration

Manufactured and distributed by:
Gilead Sciences, Inc.
Foster City, CA 94404
Revised: June 2013

COMPLERA, EMTRIVA, HEPSERA, TRUVADA, VIREAD, and VISTIDE are trademarks of Gilead Sciences, Inc., or its related companies. Edurant is a trademark of Janssen Pharmaceuticals, Inc. ATRIPLA is a trademark of Bristol-Myers Squibb & Gilead Sciences, LLC. All other trademarks referenced herein are the property of their respective owners.

202123-GS-003

Shown in Product Identification Guide, page 306

LETAIRIS® ℞

[le-TAIR-is]
(ambrisentan)
tablets, for oral use

HIGHLIGHTS OF PRESCRIBING INFORMATION

These highlights do not include all the information needed to use Letairis® safely and effectively. See full prescribing information for Letairis.

Letairis (ambrisentan) tablets, for oral use
Initial U.S. Approval: 2007

> **WARNING: EMBRYO-FETAL TOXICITY**
>
> ***See full prescribing information for complete boxed warning.***
> - **Do not administer Letairis to a pregnant female because it may cause fetal harm (4.1, 5.1, 8.1).**
> - **Females of reproductive potential: Exclude pregnancy before the start of treatment, monthly during treatment, and 1 month after stopping treatment. Prevent pregnancy during treatment and for one month after stopping treatment by using acceptable methods of contraception (2.2, 8.6).**
> - **For all female patients, Letairis is available only through a restricted program called the Letairis Risk Evaluation and Mitigation Strategy (REMS). (5.2)**

RECENT MAJOR CHANGES

• Boxed Warning	08/2013
• Dosage and Administration (2.2)	08/2013
• Contraindications, Idiopathic Pulmonary Fibrosis (4.2)	10/2012
• Warnings and Precautions, Embryo-fetal Toxicity (5.1)	08/2013
• Warnings and Precautions, Letairis REMS Program (5.2)	08/2013

INDICATIONS AND USAGE

Letairis is an endothelin receptor antagonist indicated for the treatment of pulmonary arterial hypertension (PAH) (WHO Group 1) to improve exercise ability and delay clinical worsening. Studies establishing effectiveness included predominantly patients with WHO Functional Class II–III symptoms and etiologies of idiopathic or heritable PAH (64%) or PAH associated with connective tissue diseases (32%) (1).

DOSAGE AND ADMINISTRATION

- Initiate treatment at 5 mg once daily with or without food, and consider increasing the dose to 10 mg once daily if 5 mg is tolerated (2.1).
- Tablets should not be split, crushed, or chewed (2.1).

DOSAGE FORMS AND STRENGTHS

Tablet: 5 mg and 10 mg (3)

CONTRAINDICATIONS

Pregnancy (4.1)
Idiopathic Pulmonary Fibrosis (4.2)

WARNINGS AND PRECAUTIONS

- Fluid retention may require intervention (5.3).
- If patients develop acute pulmonary edema during initiation of therapy with Letairis, consider underlying pulmonary veno-occlusive disease and discontinue treatment if necessary (5.4).
- Decreases in sperm count have been observed in patients taking endothelin receptor antagonists (5.5).
- Decreases in hemoglobin have been observed within the first few weeks; measure hemoglobin at initiation, at 1 month, and periodically thereafter (5.6).

ADVERSE REACTIONS

Most common adverse reactions (>3% compared to placebo) are peripheral edema, nasal congestion, sinusitis, and flushing (6.1).

To report SUSPECTED ADVERSE REACTIONS, contact Gilead Sciences, Inc. at (1-800-445-3235, Option 3) or FDA at 1-800-FDA-1088 or www.fda.gov/medwatch.

DRUG INTERACTIONS

Multiple dose co-administration of ambrisentan and cyclosporine resulted in an about 2-fold increase in ambrisentan exposure in healthy volunteers. When co-administered with cyclosporine, limit the dose to 5 mg once daily (7).

USE IN SPECIFIC POPULATIONS

- Breastfeeding: Choose Letairis or breastfeeding (8.3).
- Not recommended in patients with moderate or severe hepatic impairment (8.8).

See 17 for PATIENT COUNSELING INFORMATION and Medication Guide

Revised: 08/2013

FULL PRESCRIBING INFORMATION: CONTENTS*

*** Sections or subsections omitted from the full prescribing information are not listed**

FULL PRESCRIBING INFORMATION

WARNING: EMBRYO-FETAL TOXICITY

Do not administer Letairis to a pregnant female because it may cause fetal harm. Letairis is very likely to produce serious birth defects if used by pregnant females, as this effect has been seen consistently when it is administered to animals *[see Contraindications (4.1), Use in Specific Populations (8.1)]*.

Exclude pregnancy before the initiation of treatment with Letairis. Females of reproductive potential must use acceptable methods of contraception during treatment with Letairis and for one month after treatment. Obtain monthly pregnancy tests during treatment and 1 month after discontinuation of treatment *[see Use in Specific Populations (8.6)]*.

Because of the risk of embryo-fetal toxicity, females can only receive Letairis through a restricted program called the Letairis REMS program *[see Warnings and Precautions (5.2)]*.

1 INDICATIONS AND USAGE

Letairis is indicated for the treatment of pulmonary arterial hypertension (PAH) (WHO Group 1) to improve exercise ability and delay clinical worsening. Studies establishing effectiveness included predominantly patients with WHO Functional Class II–III symptoms and etiologies of idiopathic or heritable PAH (64%) or PAH associated with connective tissue diseases (32%).

2 DOSAGE AND ADMINISTRATION

2.1 Adult Dosage

Initiate treatment at 5 mg once daily, and consider increasing the dose to 10 mg once daily if 5 mg is tolerated.

Tablets may be administered with or without food. Tablets should not be split, crushed, or chewed. Doses higher than 10 mg once daily have not been studied in patients with pulmonary arterial hypertension (PAH).

2.2 Pregnancy Testing in Females of Reproductive Potential

Initiate treatment with Letairis in females of reproductive potential only after a negative pregnancy test. Obtain monthly pregnancy tests during treatment *[see Use in Specific Populations (8.6)]*.

3 DOSAGE FORMS AND STRENGTHS

5 mg and 10 mg film-coated tablets for oral administration

- Each 5 mg tablet is square convex, pale pink, with "5" on one side and "GSI" on the other side.
- Each 10 mg tablet is oval convex, deep pink, with "10" on one side and "GSI" on the other side.

4 CONTRAINDICATIONS

4.1 Pregnancy

Letairis may cause fetal harm when administered to a pregnant female. Letairis is contraindicated in females who are pregnant. Letairis was consistently shown to have teratogenic effects when administered to animals. If this drug is used during pregnancy, or if the patient becomes pregnant while taking this drug, the patient should be apprised of the potential hazard to a fetus *[see Warnings and Precautions (5.1, 5.2) and Use in Specific Populations (8.1)]*.

4.2 Idiopathic Pulmonary Fibrosis

Letairis is contraindicated in patients with Idiopathic Pulmonary Fibrosis (IPF) including IPF patients with pulmonary hypertension (WHO Group 3) *[see Clinical Studies (14.3)]*.

5 WARNINGS AND PRECAUTIONS

5.1 Embryo-fetal Toxicity

Letairis may cause fetal harm when administered during pregnancy and is contraindicated for use in females who are pregnant. In females of reproductive potential, exclude pregnancy prior to initiation of therapy, ensure use of acceptable contraceptive methods and obtain monthly pregnancy tests *[see Dosage and Administration (2.2), and Use in Specific Populations (8.1, 8.6)]*.

Letairis is only available for females through a restricted program under a REMS *[see Warnings and Precautions (5.2)]*.

5.2 Letairis REMS Program

For all females, Letairis is available only through a restricted program called the Letairis REMS, because of the risk of embryo-fetal toxicity *[see Contraindications (4.1), Warnings and Precautions (5.1), and Use in Specific Populations (8.1, 8.6)]*.

Notable requirements of the Letairis REMS program include the following:

- Prescribers must be certified with the program by enrolling and completing training.
- All females, regardless of reproductive potential, must enroll in the Letairis REMS program prior to initiating Letairis. Male patients are not enrolled in the REMS.
  - Females of reproductive potential must comply with the pregnancy testing and contraception requirements *[see Use in Specific Populations (8.6)]*.
- Pharmacies that dispense Letairis must be certified with the program and must dispense to female patients who are authorized to receive Letairis.

Further information is available at www.letairisrems.com or 1-866-664-5327.

5.3 Fluid Retention

Peripheral edema is a known class effect of endothelin receptor antagonists, and is also a clinical consequence of PAH and worsening PAH. In the placebo-controlled studies, there was an increased incidence of peripheral edema in patients treated with doses of 5 or 10 mg Letairis compared to placebo *[see Adverse Reactions (6.1)]*. Most edema was mild to moderate in severity, and it occurred with greater frequency and severity in elderly patients.

In addition, there have been post-marketing reports of fluid retention in patients with pulmonary hypertension, occurring within weeks after starting Letairis. Patients required intervention with a diuretic, fluid management, or, in some cases, hospitalization for decompensating heart failure.

If clinically significant fluid retention develops, with or without associated weight gain, further evaluation should be undertaken to determine the cause, such as Letairis or underlying heart failure, and the possible need for specific treatment or discontinuation of Letairis therapy.

5.4 Pulmonary Edema with Pulmonary Veno-occlusive Disease (PVOD)

If patients develop acute pulmonary edema during initiation of therapy with vasodilating agents such as Letairis, the possibility of PVOD should be considered, and if confirmed Letairis should be discontinued.

5.5 Decreased Sperm Counts

Decreased sperm counts have been observed in human and animal studies with another endothelin receptor antagonist and in animal fertility studies with ambrisentan. Letairis may have an adverse effect on spermatogenesis. Counsel patients about potential effects on fertility *[see Special Populations (8.6) and Nonclinical Toxicology (13.1)]*.

5.6 Hematological Changes

Decreases in hemoglobin concentration and hematocrit have followed administration of other endothelin receptor antagonists and were observed in clinical studies with Letairis. These decreases were observed within the first few weeks of treatment with Letairis, and stabilized thereafter. The mean decrease in hemoglobin from baseline to end of treatment for those patients receiving Letairis in the 12-week placebo-controlled studies was 0.8 g/dL.

Marked decreases in hemoglobin (>15% decrease from baseline resulting in a value below the lower limit of normal) were observed in 7% of all patients receiving Letairis (and 10% of patients receiving 10 mg) compared to 4% of patients receiving placebo. The cause of the decrease in hemoglobin is unknown, but it does not appear to result from hemorrhage or hemolysis.

In the long-term open-label extension of the two pivotal clinical studies, mean decreases from baseline (ranging from 0.9 to 1.2 g/dL) in hemoglobin concentrations persisted for up to 4 years of treatment.

There have been postmarketing reports of decreases in hemoglobin concentration and hematocrit that have resulted in anemia requiring transfusion.

Measure hemoglobin prior to initiation of Letairis, at one month, and periodically thereafter. Initiation of Letairis therapy is not recommended for patients with clinically significant anemia. If a clinically significant decrease in hemoglobin is observed and other causes have been excluded, consider discontinuing Letairis.

6 ADVERSE REACTIONS

Clinically significant adverse reactions that appear in other sections of the labeling include:

- Embryo-fetal toxicity *[see Warnings and Precautions (5.1), Use in Specific Populations (8.1)]*
- Fluid Retention *[see Warnings and Precautions (5.3)]*
- Pulmonary Edema with PVOD *[see Warnings and Precautions (5.4)]*
- Decreased Sperm Count *[see Warnings and Precautions (5.5)]*
- Hematologic changes *[see Warnings and Precautions (5.6)]*

6.1 Clinical Trials Experience

Because clinical trials are conducted under widely varying conditions, adverse reaction rates observed in the clinical trials of a drug cannot be directly compared to rates in the clinical trials of another drug and may not reflect the rates observed in practice.

Safety data for Letairis were obtained from two 12-week, placebo-controlled studies in patients with pulmonary arterial hypertension (PAH) (ARIES-1 and ARIES-2) and four nonplacebo-controlled studies in 483 patients with PAH who were treated with doses of 1, 2.5, 5, or 10 mg once daily. The exposure to Letairis in these studies ranged from 1 day to 4 years (N=418 for at least 6 months and N=343 for at least 1 year).

In ARIES-1 and ARIES-2, a total of 261 patients received Letairis at doses of 2.5, 5, or 10 mg once daily and 132 patients received placebo. The adverse reactions that occurred in >3% more patients receiving Letairis than receiving placebo are shown in Table 1.

Table 1 Adverse Reactions with Placebo-Adjusted Rates >3%

	Placebo (N=132)	Letairis (N=261)	
Adverse reaction	n (%)	n (%)	Placebo-adjusted (%)
Peripheral edema	14 (11)	45 (17)	6
Nasal congestion	2 (2)	15 (6)	4
Sinusitis	0 (0)	8 (3)	3
Flushing	1 (1)	10 (4)	3

Most adverse drug reactions were mild to moderate and only nasal congestion was dose-dependent.

Few notable differences in the incidence of adverse reactions were observed for patients by age or sex. Peripheral edema was similar in younger patients (<65 years) receiving Letairis (14%; 29/205) or placebo (13%; 13/104), and was greater in elderly patients (≥65 years) receiving Letairis (29%; 16/56) compared to placebo (4%; 1/28). The results of such subgroup analyses must be interpreted cautiously.

The incidence of treatment discontinuations due to adverse events other than those related to PAH during the clinical trials in patients with PAH was similar for Letairis (2%; 5/261 patients) and placebo (2%; 3/132 patients). The incidence of patients with serious adverse events other than those related to PAH during the clinical trials in patients with PAH was similar for placebo (7%; 9/132 patients) and for Letairis (5%; 13/261 patients).

During 12-week controlled clinical trials, the incidence of aminotransferase elevations >3 × upper limit of normal (ULN) were 0% on Letairis and 2.3% on placebo. In practice, cases of hepatic injury should be carefully evaluated for cause.

<u>*Use in Patients with Prior Endothelin Receptor Antagonist (ERA) Related Serum Liver Enzyme Abnormalities*</u>

In an uncontrolled, open-label study, 36 patients who had previously discontinued endothelin receptor antagonists (ERAs: bosentan, an investigational drug, or both) due to aminotransferase elevations >3 × ULN were treated with Letairis. Prior elevations were predominantly moderate, with 64% of the ALT elevations <5 × ULN, but 9 patients had elevations >8 × ULN. Eight patients had been re-challenged with bosentan and/or the investigational ERA and all eight had a recurrence of aminotransferase abnormalities that required discontinuation of ERA therapy. All patients had to have normal aminotransferase levels on entry to this study. Twenty-five of the 36 patients were also receiving prostanoid and/or phosphodiesterase type 5 (PDE5) inhibitor therapy. Two patients discontinued early (including one of the patients with a prior 8 × ULN elevation). Of the remaining 34 patients, one patient experienced a mild aminotransferase elevation at 12 weeks on Letairis 5 mg that resolved with decreasing the dosage to 2.5 mg, and that did not recur with later escalations to 10 mg. With a median follow-up of 13 months and with 50% of patients increasing the dose of Letairis to 10 mg, no patients were discontinued for aminotransferase elevations. While the uncontrolled study design does not provide information about what would have occurred with re-administration of previously used ERAs or show that Letairis led to fewer aminotransferase elevations than would have been seen with those drugs, the study indicates that Letairis may be tried in patients who have experienced asymptomatic aminotransferase elevations on other ERAs after aminotransferase levels have returned to normal.

6.2 Postmarketing Experience

The following adverse reactions were identified during postapproval use of Letairis. Because these reactions were reported voluntarily from a population of uncertain size, it is not possible to estimate reliably the frequency or to establish a causal relationship to drug exposure: anemia *[see Warnings and Precautions (5.6)]*, asthenia, dizziness, fatigue, fluid retention *[see Warnings and Precautions (5.3)]*, heart failure (associated with fluid retention), hypersensitivity (e.g., angioedema, rash), nausea, and vomiting.

Elevations of liver aminotransferases (ALT, AST) have been reported with Letairis use; in most cases alternative causes of the liver injury could be identified (heart failure, hepatic congestion, hepatitis, alcohol use, hepatotoxic medications). Other endothelin receptor antagonists have been associated with elevations of aminotransferases, hepatotoxicity, and cases of liver failure *[see Adverse Reactions (6.1)]*.

7 DRUG INTERACTIONS

Multiple dose co-administration of ambrisentan and cyclosporine resulted in an approximately 2-fold increase in ambrisentan exposure in healthy volunteers; therefore, limit the dose of ambrisentan to 5 mg once daily when co-administered with cyclosporine *[see Clinical Pharmacology (12.3)]*.

8 USE IN SPECIFIC POPULATIONS

8.1 Pregnancy

Pregnancy Category X

Risk Summary

Letairis may cause fetal harm when administered to a pregnant woman and is contraindicated during pregnancy. Letairis was teratogenic in rats and rabbits at doses which resulted in exposures of 3.5 and 1.7 times respectively the human dose of 10 mg per day. If this drug is used during pregnancy, or if the patient becomes pregnant while taking this drug, advise the patient of the potential hazard to a fetus *[see Contraindications (4.1), Warnings and Precautions (5.1)]*.

Animal Data

Letairis was teratogenic at oral doses of ≥ 15 mg/kg/day (AUC 51.7 h•μg/mL) in rats and ≥ 7 mg/kg/day (24.7 h•μg/mL) in rabbits; it was not studied at lower doses. These doses are of 3.5 and 1.7 times respectively the human dose of 10 mg per day (14.8 h•μg/mL) based on AUC. In both species, there were abnormalities of the lower jaw and hard and soft palate, malformation of the heart and great vessels, and failure of formation of the thymus and thyroid.

A preclinical study in rats has shown decreased survival of newborn pups (mid and high doses) and effects on testicle size and fertility of pups (high dose) following maternal treatment with ambrisentan from late gestation through weaning. Doses tested were 17×, 51×, and 170× (on a mg/kg:mg/m^2 basis) the maximum oral human dose of 10 mg and an average adult body weight of 70 kg.

8.3 Nursing Mothers

It is not known whether ambrisentan is present in human milk. Because many drugs are present in human milk and because of the potential for serious adverse reactions in nursing infants from Letairis, a decision should be made whether to discontinue nursing or discontinue Letairis, taking into account the importance of the drug to the mother.

8.4 Pediatric Use

Safety and effectiveness of Letairis in pediatric patients have not been established.

8.5 Geriatric Use

In the two placebo-controlled clinical studies of Letairis, 21% of patients were ≥65 years old and 5% were ≥75 years old. The elderly (age ≥65 years) showed less improvement in walk distances with Letairis than younger patients did, but the results of such subgroup analyses must be interpreted cautiously. Peripheral edema was more common in the elderly than in younger patients.

8.6 Females and Males of Reproductive Potential

Pregnancy Testing

Female patients of reproductive potential must have a negative pregnancy test prior to initiation of treatment, monthly pregnancy test during treatment, and 1 month after stopping treatment with Letairis. Advise patients to contact their health care provider if they become pregnant or suspect they may be pregnant. Perform a pregnancy test if pregnancy is suspected for any reason. For positive pregnancy tests, counsel patient on the potential risk to the fetus and patient options *[see Boxed Warning and Dosage and Administration (2.2)]*.

Contraception

Female patients of reproductive potential must use acceptable methods of contraception during treatment with Letairis and for 1 month after stopping treatment with Letairis. Patients may choose one highly effective form of contraception (intrauterine devices (IUD), contraceptive implants, or tubal sterilization) or a combination of methods (hormone method with a barrier method or two barrier methods). If a partner's vasectomy is the chosen method of contraception, a hormone or barrier method must be used along with this method. Counsel patients on pregnancy planning and prevention, including emergency contraception, or designate counseling by another healthcare provider trained in contraceptive counseling *[see Boxed Warning]*.

Infertility

Males

In a 6-month study of another endothelin receptor antagonist, bosentan, 25 male patients with WHO functional class III and IV PAH and normal baseline sperm count were evaluated for effects on testicular function. There was a decline in sperm count of at least 50% in 25% of the patients after 3 or 6 months of treatment with bosentan. One patient developed marked oligospermia at 3 months and the sperm count remained low with 2 follow-up measurements over the subsequent 6 weeks. Bosentan was discontinued and after 2 months the sperm count had returned to baseline levels. In 22 patients who completed 6 months of treatment, sperm count remained within the normal range and no changes in sperm morphology, sperm motility, or hormone levels were observed. Based on these findings and preclinical data *[see Nonclinical Toxicology (13.1)]* from endothelin receptor antagonists, it cannot be excluded that endothelin receptor antagonists such as Letairis have an adverse effect on spermatogenesis. Counsel patients about the potential effects on fertility *[see Warnings and Precautions (5.5)]*.

8.7 Renal Impairment

The impact of renal impairment on the pharmacokinetics of ambrisentan has been examined using a population pharmacokinetic approach in PAH patients with creatinine clearances ranging between 20 and 150 mL/min. There was no significant impact of mild or moderate renal impairment on exposure to ambrisentan *[see Clinical Pharmacology (12.3)]*. Dose adjustment of Letairis in patients with mild or moderate renal impairment is therefore not required. There is no information on the exposure to ambrisentan in patients with severe renal impairment.

The impact of hemodialysis on the disposition of ambrisentan has not been investigated.

8.8 Hepatic Impairment

Pre-existing hepatic impairment

The influence of pre-existing hepatic impairment on the pharmacokinetics of ambrisentan has not been evaluated. Because there is *in vitro* and *in vivo* evidence of significant metabolic and biliary contribution to the elimination of ambrisentan, hepatic impairment would be expected to have significant effects on the pharmacokinetics of ambrisentan *[see Clinical Pharmacology (12.3)]*. Letairis is not recommended in patients with moderate or severe hepatic impairment. There is no information on the use of Letairis in patients with mild pre-existing impaired liver function; however, exposure to ambrisentan may be increased in these patients.

Elevation of Liver Transaminases

Other endothelin receptor antagonists (ERAs) have been associated with aminotransferase (AST, ALT) elevations, hepatotoxicity, and cases of liver failure *[see Adverse Reactions (6.1, 6.2)]*. In patients who develop hepatic impairment after Letairis initiation, the cause of liver injury should be fully investigated. Discontinue Letairis if elevations of liver aminotransferases are >5× ULN or if elevations are accompanied by bilirubin >2× ULN, or by signs or symptoms of liver dysfunction and other causes are excluded.

10 OVERDOSAGE

There is no experience with overdosage of Letairis. The highest single dose of Letairis administered to healthy volunteers was 100 mg and the highest daily dose administered to patients with PAH was 10 mg once daily. In healthy volunteers, single doses of 50 mg and 100 mg (5 to 10 times the maximum recommended dose) were associated with headache, flushing, dizziness, nausea, and nasal congestion. Massive overdosage could potentially result in hypotension that may require intervention.

11 DESCRIPTION

Letairis is the brand name for ambrisentan, an endothelin receptor antagonist that is selective for the endothelin type-A (ET_A) receptor. The chemical name of ambrisentan is (+)-(2*S*)-2-[(4,6-dimethylpyrimidin-2-yl)oxy]-3-methoxy-3,3-diphenylpropanoic acid. It has a molecular formula of $C_{22}H_{22}N_2O_4$ and a molecular weight of 378.42. It contains a single chiral center determined to be the (*S*) configuration and has the following structural formula:

Figure 1 Ambrisentan Structural Formula

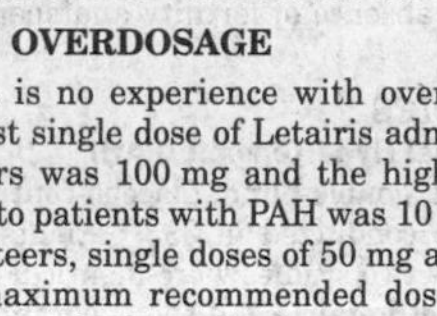

Ambrisentan is a white to off-white, crystalline solid. It is a carboxylic acid with a pKa of 4.0. Ambrisentan is practically insoluble in water and in aqueous solutions at low pH. Solubility increases in aqueous solutions at higher pH. In the solid state ambrisentan is very stable, is not hygroscopic, and is not light sensitive.

Letairis is available as 5 mg and 10 mg film-coated tablets for once daily oral administration. The tablets include the following inactive ingredients: croscarmellose sodium, lactose monohydrate, magnesium stearate and microcrystalline cellulose. The tablets are film-coated with a coating material containing FD&C Red #40 aluminum lake, lecithin, polyethylene glycol, polyvinyl alcohol, talc, and titanium dioxide. Each square, pale pink Letairis tablet contains 5 mg of ambrisentan. Each oval, deep pink Letairis tablet contains 10 mg of ambrisentan. Letairis tablets are unscored.

12 CLINICAL PHARMACOLOGY

12.1 Mechanism of Action

Endothelin-1 (ET-1) is a potent autocrine and paracrine peptide. Two receptor subtypes, ET_A and ET_B, mediate the effects of ET-1 in the vascular smooth muscle and endothelium. The primary actions of ET_A are vasoconstriction and cell proliferation, while the predominant actions of ET_B are vasodilation, antiproliferation, and ET-1 clearance.

In patients with PAH, plasma ET-1 concentrations are increased as much as 10-fold and correlate with increased mean right atrial pressure and disease severity. ET-1 and ET-1 mRNA concentrations are increased as much as 9-fold in the lung tissue of patients with PAH, primarily in the endothelium of pulmonary arteries. These findings suggest that ET-1 may play a critical role in the pathogenesis and progression of PAH.

Ambrisentan is a high affinity (K_i=0.011 nM) ET_A receptor antagonist with a high selectivity for the ET_A versus ET_B receptor (>4000-fold). The clinical impact of high selectivity for ET_A is not known.

12.2 Pharmacodynamics

Cardiac Electrophysiology

In a randomized, positive- and placebo-controlled, parallel-group study, healthy subjects received either Letairis 10 mg daily followed by a single dose of 40 mg, placebo followed by a single dose of moxifloxacin 400 mg, or placebo alone. Letairis 10 mg daily had no significant effect on the QTc interval. The 40 mg dose of Letairis increased mean QTc at t_{max} by 5 ms with an upper 95% confidence limit of 9 ms. For patients receiving Letairis 5–10 mg daily and not taking metabolic inhibitors, no significant QT prolongation is expected.

12.3 Pharmacokinetics

The pharmacokinetics of ambrisentan (S-ambrisentan) in healthy subjects are dose proportional. The absolute bioavailability of ambrisentan is not known. Ambrisentan is absorbed with peak concentrations occurring approximately 2 hours after oral administration in healthy subjects and PAH patients. Food does not affect its bioavailability. *In vitro* studies indicate that ambrisentan is a substrate of P-gp. Ambrisentan is highly bound to plasma proteins (99%). The elimination of ambrisentan is predominantly by non-renal pathways, but the relative contributions of metabolism and biliary elimination have not been well characterized. In plasma, the AUC of 4-hydroxymethyl ambrisentan accounts for approximately 4% relative to parent ambrisentan AUC. The *in vivo* inversion of S-ambrisentan to R-ambrisentan is negligible. The mean oral clearance of ambrisentan is 38 mL/min and 19 mL/min in healthy subjects and in PAH patients, respectively. Although ambrisentan has a 15-hour terminal half-life, the mean trough concentration of ambrisentan at steady-state is about 15% of the mean peak concentration and the accumulation factor is about 1.2 after long-term daily dosing, indicating that the effective half-life of ambrisentan is about 9 hours.

Drug Interactions

In vitro studies

Studies with human liver tissue indicate that ambrisentan is metabolized by CYP3A, CYP2C19, and uridine 5′-diphosphate glucuronosyltransferases (UGTs) 1A9S, 2B7S, and 1A3S. *In vitro* studies suggest that ambrisentan is a substrate of the Organic Anion Transporting Polypeptides OATP1B1 and OATP1B3, and a substrate but not an inhibitor of P-glycoprotein (P-gp). Drug interactions might be expected because of these factors; however, a clinically relevant interaction has been demonstrated only with cyclosporine *[see Drug Interactions (7)]*. Ambrisentan does not inhibit or induce drug metabolizing enzymes at clinically relevant concentrations.

In vivo studies

The effects of other drugs on ambrisentan pharmacokinetics and the effects of ambrisentan on the exposure to other drugs are shown in Figure 2 and Figure 3, respectively.

[See figure 2 at top of next column]

[See figure 3 at top of next column]

13 NONCLINICAL TOXICOLOGY

13.1 Carcinogenesis, Mutagenesis, Impairment of Fertility

Oral carcinogenicity studies of up to two years duration were conducted at starting doses of 10, 30, and 60 mg/kg/day in rats [8 to 48 times the maximum recommended human dose (MRHD) on a mg/m^2 basis] and at 50, 150 and 250 mg/kg/day in mice (28 to 140 times the MRHD). In the rat study, the high and mid-dose male and female groups had their doses lowered to 40 and 20 mg/kg/day, respectively, in week 51 because of effects on survival. The high dose males and females were taken off drug completely in weeks 69 and 93, respectively. The only evidence of

Figure 2 Effects of Other Drugs on Ambrisentan Pharmacokinetics

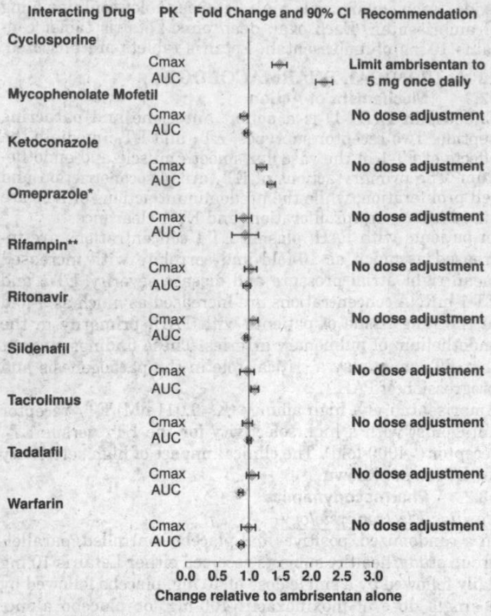

* Omeprazole: based on population pharmacokinetic analysis in PAH patients

** Rifampin: AUC and C_{max} were measured at steady-state. On Day 3 of co-administration a transient 2-fold increase in AUC was noted that was no longer evident by Day 7. Day 7 results are presented.

Figure 3 Effects of Ambrisentan on Other Drugs

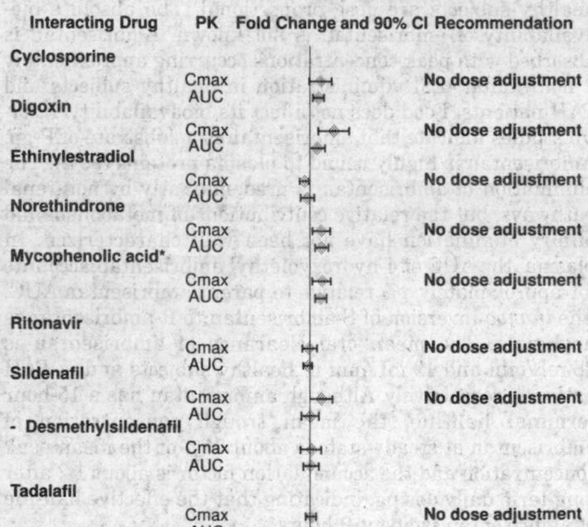

* Active metabolite of mycophenolate mofetil

** GMR (95% CI) for INR

ambrisentan-related carcinogenicity was a positive trend in male rats, for the combined incidence of benign basal cell tumor and basal cell carcinoma of skin/subcutis in the mid-dose group (high-dose group excluded from analysis), and the occurrence of mammary fibroadenomas in males in the high-dose group. In the mouse study, high dose male and female groups had their doses lowered to 150 mg/kg/day in week 39 and were taken off drug completely in week 96 (males) or week 76 (females). In mice, ambrisentan was not associated with excess tumors in any dosed group.

Positive findings of clastogenicity were detected, at drug concentrations producing moderate to high toxicity, in the chromosome aberration assay in cultured human lymphocytes. There was no evidence for genetic toxicity of ambrisentan when tested *in vitro* in bacteria (Ames test) or *in vivo* in rats (micronucleus assay, unscheduled DNA synthesis assay).

The development of testicular tubular atrophy and impaired fertility has been linked to the chronic administration of endothelin receptor antagonists in rodents. Testicular tubular degeneration was observed in rats treated with

Table 2 Changes from Baseline in 6-Minute Walk Distance (meters)

	ARIES-1			ARIES-2		
	Placebo (N=67)	**5 mg (N=67)**	**10 mg (N=67)**	**Placebo (N=65)**	**2.5 mg (N=64)**	**5 mg (N=63)**
Baseline	342 ± 73	340 ± 77	342 ± 78	343 ± 86	347 ± 84	355 ± 84
Mean change from baseline	-8 ± 79	23 ± 83	44 ± 63	-10 ± 94	22 ± 83	49 ± 75
Placebo-adjusted mean change from baseline	–	31	51	–	32	59
Placebo-adjusted median change from baseline	–	27	39	–	30	45
p-value*	–	0.008	<0.001	–	0.022	<0.001

Mean ± standard deviation

* p-values are Wilcoxon rank sum test comparisons of Letairis to placebo at Week 12 stratified by idiopathic or heritable PAH and non-idiopathic, non-heritable PAH patients

Table 3 Time to Clinical Worsening

	ARIES-1		ARIES-2	
	Placebo (N=67)	**Letairis (N=134)**	**Placebo (N=65)**	**Letairis (N=127)**
Clinical worsening, no. (%)	7 (10%)	4 (3%)	13 (22%)	8 (6%)
Hazard ratio	–	0.28	–	0.30
p-value, Fisher exact test	–	0.044	–	0.006
p-value, Log-rank test	–	0.030	–	0.005

Intention-to-treat population

Note: Patients may have had more than one reason for clinical worsening.

Nominal p-values

ambrisentan for two years at doses ≥10 mg/kg/day (8-fold MRHD). Increased incidences of testicular findings were also observed in mice treated for two years at doses ≥50 mg/kg/day (28-fold MRHD). Effects on sperm count, sperm morphology, mating performance and fertility were observed in fertility studies in which male rats were treated with ambrisentan at oral doses of 300 mg/kg/day (236-fold MRHD). At doses of ≥10 mg/kg/day, observations of testicular histopathology in the absence of fertility and sperm effects were also present.

14 CLINICAL STUDIES

14.1 Pulmonary Arterial Hypertension (PAH)

Two 12-week, randomized, double-blind, placebo-controlled, multicenter studies were conducted in 393 patients with PAH (WHO Group 1). The two studies were identical in design except for the doses of Letairis and the geographic region of the investigational sites. ARIES-1 compared once-daily doses of 5 mg and 10 mg Letairis to placebo, while ARIES-2 compared once-daily doses of 2.5 mg and 5 mg Letairis to placebo. In both studies, Letairis or placebo was added to current therapy, which could have included a combination of anticoagulants, diuretics, calcium channel blockers, or digoxin, but not epoprostenol, treprostinil, iloprost, bosentan, or sildenafil. The primary study endpoint was 6-minute walk distance. In addition, clinical worsening, WHO functional class, dyspnea, and SF-36® Health Survey were assessed.

Patients had idiopathic or heritable PAH (64%) or PAH associated with connective tissue diseases (32%), HIV infection (3%), or anorexigen use (1%). There were no patients with PAH associated with congenital heart disease.

Patients had WHO functional class I (2%), II (38%), III (55%), or IV (5%) symptoms at baseline. The mean age of patients was 50 years, 79% of patients were female, and 77% were Caucasian.

Submaximal Exercise Ability

Results of the 6-minute walk distance at 12 weeks for the ARIES-1 and ARIES-2 studies are shown in Table 2 and Figure 4.

[See table 2 above]

[See figure 4 at top of next column]

In both studies, treatment with Letairis resulted in a significant improvement in 6-minute walk distance for each dose of Letairis and the improvements increased with dose. An increase in 6-minute walk distance was observed after 4 weeks of treatment with Letairis, with a dose-response observed after 12 weeks of treatment. Improvements in walk distance with Letairis were smaller for elderly patients (age ≥65) than younger patients and for patients with secondary

Figure 4 Mean Change in 6-Minute Walk Distance

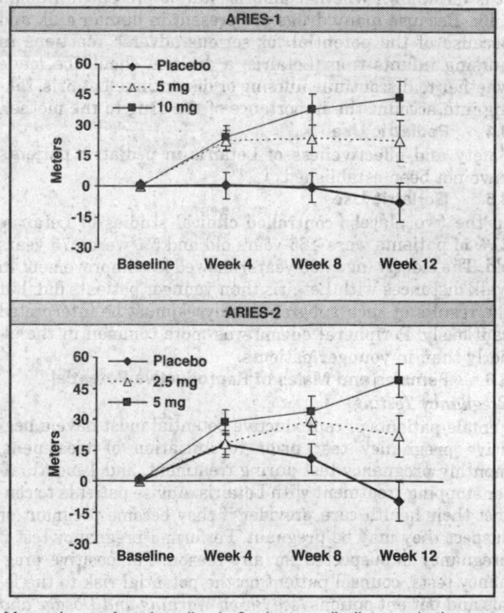

Mean change from baseline in 6-minute walk distance in the placebo and Letairis groups

Values are expressed as mean ± standard error of the mean.

PAH than for patients with idiopathic or heritable PAH. The results of such subgroup analyses must be interpreted cautiously.

The effects of Letairis on walk distances at trough drug levels are not known. Because only once daily dosing was studied in the clinical trials, the efficacy and safety of more frequent dosing regimens for Letairis are not known. If exercise ability is not sustained throughout the day in a patient, consider other PAH treatments that have been studied with more frequent dosing regimens.

Clinical Worsening

Time to clinical worsening of PAH was defined as the first occurrence of death, lung transplantation, hospitalization for PAH, atrial septostomy, study withdrawal due to the addition of other PAH therapeutic agents or study withdrawal due to early escape. Early escape was defined as meeting two or more of the following criteria: a 20% decrease in the

6-minute walk distance; an increase in WHO functional class; worsening right ventricular failure; rapidly progressing cardiogenic, hepatic, or renal failure; or refractory systolic hypotension. The clinical worsening events during the 12-week treatment period of the Letairis clinical trials are shown in Table 3 and Figure 5.

[See table 3 at top of previous page]

There was a significant delay in the time to clinical worsening for patients receiving Letairis compared to placebo. Results in subgroups such as the elderly were also favorable.

Figure 5 Time to Clinical Worsening

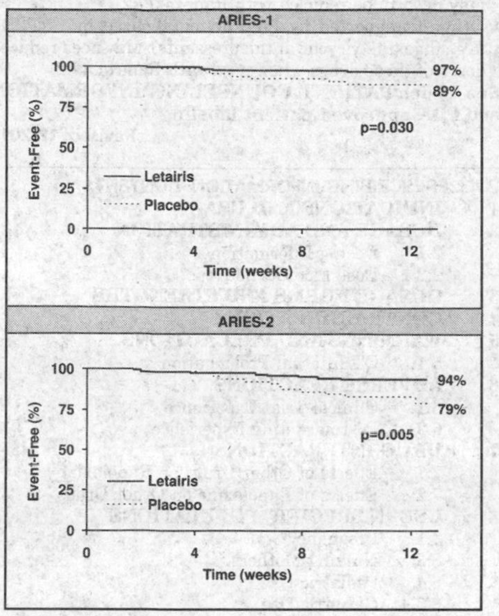

Time from randomization to clinical worsening with Kaplan-Meier estimates of the proportions of failures in ARIES-1 and ARIES-2. p-values shown are the log-rank comparisons of Letairis to placebo stratified by idiopathic or heritable PAH and non-idiopathic, non-heritable PAH patients

14.2 Long-term Treatment of PAH

In long-term follow-up of patients who were treated with Letairis (2.5 mg, 5 mg, or 10 mg once daily) in the two pivotal studies and their open-label extension (N=383), Kaplan-Meier estimates of survival at 1, 2, and 3 years were 93%, 85%, and 79%, respectively. Of the patients who remained on Letairis for up to 3 years, the majority received no other treatment for PAH. These uncontrolled observations do not allow comparison with a group not given Letairis and cannot be used to determine the long-term effect of Letairis on mortality.

14.3 Adverse Effects in Idiopathic Pulmonary Fibrosis (IPF)

A randomized controlled study in patients with IPF, with or without pulmonary hypertension (WHO Group 3), compared Letairis (n=329) to placebo (n=163). The study was terminated after 34 weeks for lack of efficacy, and was found to demonstrate a greater risk of disease progression or death on Letairis. More patients taking Letairis died (8% vs. 4%), had a respiratory hospitalization (13% vs. 6%), and had a decrease in FVC/DLCO (17% vs. 12%) *[see Contraindications (4.2)]*.

16 HOW SUPPLIED/STORAGE AND HANDLING

Letairis film-coated, tablets are supplied as follows:

Tablet Strength	Package Configuration	NDC No.	Description of Tablet; Debossed on Tablet; Size
5 mg	30 count blister	61958-0801-2	Square convex; pale pink; "5" on side 1 and "GSI" on side 2; 6.6 mm Square
	30 count bottle	61958-0801-1	
	10 count blister	61958-0801-3	
	10 count bottle	61958-0801-5	
10 mg	30 count blister	61958-0802-2	Oval convex; deep pink; "10" on side 1 and "GSI" on side 2; 9.8 mm × 4.9 mm Oval
	30 count bottle	61958-0802-1	
	10 count blister	61958-0802-3	
	10 count bottle	61958-0802-5	

Acceptable Birth Control Options

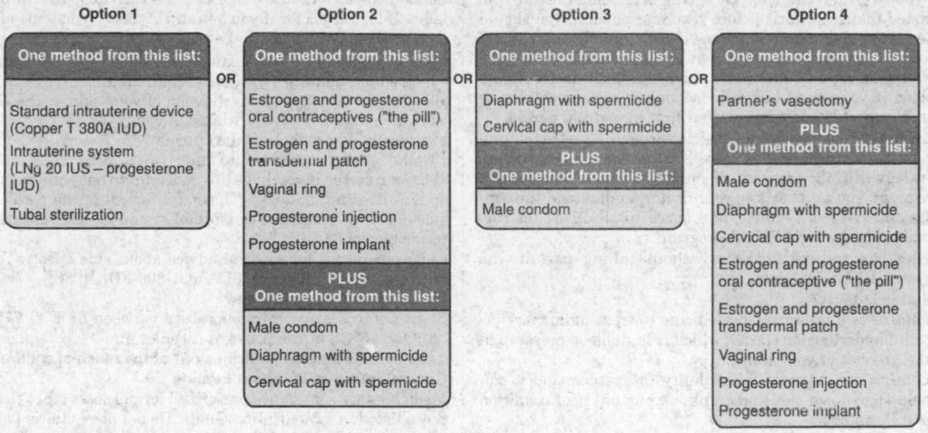

Store at 25°C (77°F); excursions permitted to 15–30°C (59–86°F) *[see USP controlled room temperature]*. Store Letairis in its original packaging.

17 PATIENT COUNSELING INFORMATION

See FDA-approved patient labeling (Medication Guide).

17.1 Embryo-fetal toxicity

Instruct patients on the risk of fetal harm when Letairis is used in pregnancy *[see Warnings and Precautions (5.1) and Use in Special Populations (8)]*. Female patients must enroll in the Letairis REMS program. Instruct females of reproductive potential to immediately contact their physician if they suspect they may be pregnant.

17.2 Letairis REMS Program

For female patients, Letairis is only available through a restricted program called the Letairis REMS *[see Contraindications (4.1), Warnings and Precautions (5.2)]*. Male patients are not enrolled in the Letairis REMS.

Inform female patients (and their guardians, if applicable) of the following notable requirements:

- All female patients must sign an enrollment form.
- Advise female patients of reproductive potential that they must comply with the pregnancy testing and contraception requirements *[see Use in Specific Populations (8.6)]*.
- Educate and counsel females of reproductive potential on the use of emergency contraception in the event of unprotected sex or known or suspected contraceptive failure.
- Advise pre-pubertal females to report any changes in their reproductive status immediately to their prescriber.

Review the Letairis Medication Guide and REMS educational material with female patients.

A limited number of pharmacies are certified to dispense Letairis. Therefore, provide patients with the telephone number and website for information on how to obtain the product.

17.3 Hepatic Effects

Some members of this pharmacological class are hepatotoxic. Patients should be educated on the symptoms of potential liver injury (such as anorexia, nausea, vomiting, fever, malaise, fatigue, right upper quadrant abdominal discomfort, jaundice, dark urine or itching) and instructed to report any of these symptoms to their physician.

17.4 Hematological Change

Patients should be advised of the importance of hemoglobin testing.

17.5 Other Risks Associated with Letairis

Instruct patients that the risks associated with Letairis also include the following:

- Decreases in hemoglobin and hematocrit
- Decreases in sperm count
- Fluid overload

17.6 Administration

Patients should be advised not to split, crush, or chew tablets.

Gilead Sciences, Inc., Foster City, CA 94404

Letairis is a registered trademark of Gilead Sciences, Inc. Gilead and the Gilead logo are trademarks of Gilead Sciences, Inc. Other brands noted herein are the property of their respective owners.

GS22-081-012

Medication Guide

Letairis® (le-TAIR-is)
(ambrisentan)
Tablets

Read this Medication Guide before you start taking Letairis and each time you get a refill. There may be new information. This Medication Guide does not take the place of talking with your doctor about your medical condition or your treatment.

What is the most important information I should know about Letairis?

- **Serious birth defects.**

  Letairis can cause serious birth defects if taken during pregnancy.

  - **Females must not be pregnant when they start taking Letairis or become pregnant during treatment with Letairis.**
  - Females who are able to get pregnant must have a negative pregnancy test before beginning treatment with Letairis and each month during treatment with Letairis. Talk to your doctor about your menstrual cycle. Your doctor will decide when to do the tests, and order the tests for you depending on your menstrual cycle.
    - Females who are able to get pregnant are females who:
      - Have entered puberty, even if they have not started their period, **and**
      - Have a uterus, **and**
      - Have not gone through menopause (have not had a period for at least 12 months for natural reasons, or who have had their ovaries removed)
    - Females who are not able to get pregnant are females who:
      - Have not yet entered puberty, **or**
      - Do not have a uterus, **or**
      - Have gone through menopause (have not had a period for at least 12 months for natural reasons, or who have had their ovaries removed)

  Females who are able to get pregnant must use two acceptable forms of birth control, during treatment with Letairis, and for one month after stopping Letairis because the medicine may still be in the body.

  - If you have had a tubal sterilization or have an IUD (intrauterine device), these methods can be used alone and no other form of birth control is needed.
  - Talk with your doctor or gynecologist (a doctor who specializes in female reproduction) to find out about options for acceptable forms of birth control that you may use to prevent pregnancy during treatment with Letairis.
  - If you decide that you want to change the form of birth control that you use, talk with your doctor or gynecologist to be sure that you choose another acceptable form of birth control.

  See the chart below for Acceptable Birth Control Options during treatment with Letairis.

[See figure above]

  - **Do not have unprotected sex. Talk to your doctor or pharmacist right away if you have unprotected sex or if you think your birth control has failed. Your doctor may tell you to use emergency birth control.**
  - **Tell your doctor right away if you miss a menstrual period or think you may be pregnant for any reason.**

If you are the parent or caregiver of a female child who started taking Letairis before reaching puberty, you should check your child regularly to see if she is developing signs of puberty. Tell your doctor right away if you notice that she is developing breast buds or any pubic hair. Your doctor should decide if your child has reached puberty. **Your child may reach puberty before having her first menstrual period.**

Females can only receive Letairis through a restricted program called the Letairis Risk Evaluation and Mitigation Strategy (REMS) program. If you are a female who can get pregnant, you must talk to your doctor, understand the benefits and risks of Letairis, and agree to all of the instructions in the Letairis REMS program.

Males can receive Letairis without taking part in the Letairis REMS program.

What is Letairis?

- Letairis is a prescription medicine to treat pulmonary arterial hypertension (PAH), which is high blood pressure in the arteries of your lungs.
- Letairis can improve your ability to exercise and it can help slow down the worsening of your physical condition and symptoms.
- It is not known if Letairis is safe and effective in children.

Who should not take Letairis?

Do not take Letairis if:

- **you are pregnant, plan to become pregnant, or become pregnant during treatment with Letairis. Letairis can cause serious birth defects.** (See the Medication Guide section above called "What is the most important information I should know about Letairis?") Serious birth defects from Letairis happen early in pregnancy.
- you have a condition called Idiopathic Pulmonary Fibrosis (IPF).

Tell your doctor about all your medical conditions and all the medicines you take including prescription and nonprescription medicines. Letairis and other medicines may affect each other causing side effects. Do not start any new medicines until you check with your doctor.

Especially tell your doctor if you take the medicine cyclosporine (Gengraf, Neoral, Sandimmune). Your doctor may need to change your dose of Letairis. You should not take more than 5 mg of Letairis each day if you also take cyclosporine.

How should I take Letairis?

Letairis will be mailed to you by a certified pharmacy. Your doctor will give you complete details.

- Take Letairis exactly as your doctor tells you. Do not stop taking Letairis unless your doctor tells you.
- You can take Letairis with or without food.
- Do not split, crush or chew Letairis tablets.
- It will be easier to remember to take Letairis if you take it at the same time each day.
- If you take more than your regular dose of Letairis, call your doctor right away.
- If you miss a dose, take it as soon as you remember that day. Take your next dose at the regular time. Do not take two doses at the same time to make up for a missed dose.

What should I avoid while taking Letairis?

- **Do not get pregnant** while taking Letairis. (See the serious birth defects section of the Medication Guide above called "What is the most important information I should know about Letairis?") If you miss a menstrual period, or think you might be pregnant, call your doctor right away.

It is not known if Letairis passes into your breast milk. You should not breastfeed if you are taking Letairis. Talk to your doctor about the best way to feed your baby if you take Letairis.

What are the possible side effects of Letairis?

Letairis can cause serious side effects including:

- **Serious birth defects.** (See "What is the most important information I should know about Letairis?")
- **Swelling all over the body** (fluid retention) can happen within weeks after starting Letairis. Tell your doctor right away if you have any unusual weight gain, tiredness, or trouble breathing while taking Letairis. These may be symptoms of a serious health problem. You may need to be treated with medicine or need to go to the hospital.
- **Sperm count reduction.** Reduced sperm counts have been observed in some men taking a drug similar to Letairis, an effect which might impair their ability to father a child. Tell your doctor if remaining fertile is important to you.
- **Low red blood cell levels** (anemia) can happen during the first weeks after starting Letairis. If this happens, you may need a blood transfusion. Your doctor will do blood tests to check your red blood cells before starting Letairis. Your doctor may also do these tests during treatment with Letairis.

The most common side effects of Letairis are:

- Swelling of hands, legs, ankles and feet (peripheral edema)
- Stuffy nose (nasal congestion)
- Inflamed nasal passages (sinusitis)
- Hot flashes or getting red in the face (flushing)

Some medicines that are like Letairis can cause liver problems. Tell your doctor if you get any of these symptoms of a liver problem while taking Letairis:

- loss of appetite
- nausea or vomiting
- fever
- achiness
- generally do not feel well
- pain in the upper right stomach (abdominal) area
- yellowing of your skin or the whites of your eyes
- dark urine
- itching

Tell your doctor if you have any side effect that bothers you or that does not go away. These are not all of the possible side effects of Letairis. For more information, ask your doctor or pharmacist.

Call your doctor for medical advice about side effects. You may report side effects to FDA at 1-800-FDA-1088.

How should I store Letairis?

Store Letairis at room temperature between 68°F to 77°F (20°C to 25°C), in the package it comes in.

Keep Letairis and all medicines out of the reach of children.

General information about Letairis

Medicines are sometimes prescribed for purposes other than those listed in a Medication Guide. Do not use Letairis for a condition for which it was not prescribed. Do not give Letairis to other people, even if they have the same symptoms that you have. It may harm them.

This Medication Guide summarizes the most important information about Letairis. If you would like more information, ask your doctor. You can ask your doctor or pharmacist for information about Letairis that is written for health professionals.

For more information, call 1-866-664- 5327 or visit www.letairis.com or www.gilead.com.

What are the ingredients in Letairis?

Active ingredient: ambrisentan.

Inactive Ingredients: croscarmellose sodium, lactose monohydrate, magnesium stearate and microcrystalline cellulose. The tablets are film-coated with a coating material containing FD&C Red #40 aluminum lake, lecithin, polyethylene glycol, polyvinyl alcohol, talc, and titanium dioxide.

This Medication Guide has been approved by the U.S. Food and Drug Administration.

Gilead Sciences, Inc., Foster City, CA 94404

Revised August 2013

Letairis is a registered trademark of Gilead Sciences, Inc. Gilead and the Gilead logo are trademarks of Gilead Sciences, Inc. Other brands noted herein are the property of their respective owners.

GS22-081-012

Shown in Product Identification Guide, page 306

RANEXA® ℞

[rAn-ex-a]

(ranolazine)

extended-release tablets

HIGHLIGHTS OF PRESCRIBING INFORMATION

These highlights do not include all the information needed to use Ranexa safely and effectively. See full prescribing information for Ranexa.

Ranexa® (ranolazine) extended-release tablets

Initial U.S. Approval: 2006

INDICATIONS AND USAGE

Ranexa is indicated for the treatment of chronic angina. (1)

DOSAGE AND ADMINISTRATION

- 500 mg twice daily and increase to 1000 mg twice daily, based on clinical symptoms (2.1)

DOSAGE FORMS AND STRENGTHS

Extended-release tablets: 500 mg, 1000 mg (3)

CONTRAINDICATIONS

- Strong CYP3A inhibitors (e.g., ketoconazole, clarithromycin, nelfinavir) (4, 7.1)
- CYP3A inducers (e.g., rifampin, phenobarbital, St. John's wort) (4, 7.1)
- Liver cirrhosis (4, 8.6)

WARNINGS AND PRECAUTIONS

- QT interval prolongation: Can occur with ranolazine. Little data available on high doses, long exposure, use with QT interval-prolonging drugs, potassium channel variants causing prolonged QT interval, in patients with a family history of (or congenital) long QT syndrome, or in patients with known acquired QT interval prolongation. (5.1)

ADVERSE REACTIONS

Most common adverse reactions (> 4% and more common than with placebo) are dizziness, headache, constipation, nausea. (6.1)

To report SUSPECTED ADVERSE REACTIONS, contact Gilead Sciences, Inc., at 1-800-GILEAD-5 or FDA at 1-800-FDA-1088 or *www.fda.gov/medwatch.*

DRUG INTERACTIONS

- Moderate CYP3A inhibitors (e.g., diltiazem, verapamil, erythromycin): Limit Ranexa to 500 mg twice daily. (7.1)
- P-gp inhibitors (e.g., cyclosporine): Ranolazine exposure increased. Titrate Ranexa based on clinical response. (7.1)
- CYP3A substrates: Limit simvastatin to 20 mg when used with Ranexa. Doses of other sensitive CYP3A substrates (e.g., lovastatin) and CYP3A substrates with narrow therapeutic range (e.g., cyclosporine, tacrolimus, sirolimus) may need to be reduced with Ranexa. (7.2)
- Drugs transported by P-gp or metabolized by CYP2D6 (e.g., digoxin, tricyclic antidepressants): May need reduced doses of these drugs when used with Ranexa. (7.2)

See 17 for PATIENT COUNSELING INFORMATION and FDA-approved patient labeling

Revised: 12/2011

FULL PRESCRIBING INFORMATION: CONTENTS*

*** Sections or subsections omitted from the full prescribing information are not listed**

FULL PRESCRIBING INFORMATION

1 INDICATIONS AND USAGE

Ranexa is indicated for the treatment of chronic angina.

Ranexa may be used with beta-blockers, nitrates, calcium channel blockers, anti-platelet therapy, lipid-lowering therapy, ACE inhibitors, and angiotensin receptor blockers.

2 DOSAGE AND ADMINISTRATION

2.1 Dosing Information

Initiate Ranexa dosing at 500 mg twice daily and increase to 1000 mg twice daily, as needed, based on clinical symptoms. Take Ranexa with or without meals. Swallow Ranexa tablets whole; do not crush, break, or chew.

The maximum recommended daily dose of Ranexa is 1000 mg twice daily.

If a dose of Ranexa is missed, take the prescribed dose at the next scheduled time; do not double the next dose.

2.2 Dose Modification

Dose adjustments may be needed when Ranexa is taken in combination with certain other drugs *[see Drug Interactions (7.1)]*. Limit the maximum dose of Ranexa to 500 mg twice daily in patients on moderate CYP3A inhibitors such as diltiazem, verapamil, and erythromycin. Use of Ranexa with strong CYP3A inhibitors is contraindicated *[see Contraindications (4), Drug Interactions (7.1)]*.

Use of P-gp inhibitors, such as cyclosporine, may increase exposure to Ranexa. Titrate Ranexa based on clinical response *[see Drug Interactions (7.1)]*.

3 DOSAGE FORMS AND STRENGTHS

Ranexa is supplied as film-coated, oblong-shaped, extended-release tablets in the following strengths:
- 500 mg tablets are light orange, with GSI500 on one side
- 1000 mg tablets are pale yellow, with GSI1000 on one side

4 CONTRAINDICATIONS

Ranexa is contraindicated in patients:
- Taking strong inhibitors of CYP3A *[see Drug Interactions (7.1)]*
- Taking inducers of CYP3A *[see Drug Interactions (7.1)]*
- With liver cirrhosis *[see Use in Specific Populations (8.6)]*

5 WARNINGS AND PRECAUTIONS

5.1 QT Interval Prolongation

Ranolazine blocks I_{Kr} and prolongs the QTc interval in a dose-related manner.

Clinical experience in an acute coronary syndrome population did not show an increased risk of proarrhythmia or sudden death *[see Clinical Studies (14.2)]*. However, there is little experience with high doses (> 1000 mg twice daily) or exposure, other QT-prolonging drugs, potassium channel variants resulting in a long QT interval, in patients with a family history of (or congenital) long QT syndrome, or in patients with known acquired QT interval prolongation.

6 ADVERSE REACTIONS

6.1 Clinical Trial Experience

Because clinical trials are conducted under widely varying conditions, adverse reaction rates observed in the clinical trials of a drug cannot be directly compared to rates in the clinical trials of another drug and may not reflect the rates observed in practice.

A total of 2,018 patients with chronic angina were treated with ranolazine in controlled clinical trials. Of the patients treated with Ranexa, 1,026 were enrolled in three double-blind, placebo-controlled, randomized studies (CARISA, ERICA, MARISA) of up to 12 weeks duration. In addition, upon study completion, 1,251 patients received treatment with Ranexa in open-label, long-term studies; 1,227 patients were exposed to Ranexa for more than 1 year, 613 patients for more than 2 years, 531 patients for more than 3 years, and 326 patients for more than 4 years.

At recommended doses, about 6% of patients discontinued treatment with Ranexa because of an adverse event in controlled studies in angina patients compared to about 3% on placebo. The most common adverse events that led to discontinuation more frequently on Ranexa than placebo were dizziness (1.3% versus 0.1%), nausea (1% versus 0%), asthenia, constipation, and headache (each about 0.5% versus 0%). Doses above 1000 mg twice daily are poorly tolerated.

In controlled clinical trials of angina patients, the most frequently reported treatment-emergent adverse reactions (> 4% and more common on Ranexa than on placebo) were dizziness (6.2%), headache (5.5%), constipation (4.5%), and nausea (4.4%). Dizziness may be dose-related. In open-label, long-term treatment studies, a similar adverse reaction profile was observed.

The following additional adverse reactions occurred at an incidence of 0.5 to 4.0% in patients treated with Ranexa and were more frequent than the incidence observed in placebo-treated patients:

Cardiac Disorders – bradycardia, palpitations
Ear and Labyrinth Disorders – tinnitus, vertigo
Eye Disorders – blurred vision
Gastrointestinal Disorders – abdominal pain, dry mouth, vomiting, dyspepsia
General Disorders and Administrative Site Adverse Events – asthenia, peripheral edema
Metabolism and Nutrition Disorders – anorexia
Nervous System Disorders – syncope (vasovagal)
Psychiatric Disorders – confusional state
Renal and Urinary Disorders – hematuria
Respiratory, Thoracic, and Mediastinal Disorders – dyspnea
Skin and Subcutaneous Tissue Disorders – hyperhidrosis
Vascular Disorders – hypotension, orthostatic hypotension

Other (< 0.5%) but potentially medically important adverse reactions observed more frequently with Ranexa than placebo treatment in all controlled studies included: angioedema, renal failure, eosinophilia, chromaturia, blood urea increased, hypoesthesia, paresthesia, tremor, pulmonary fibrosis, thrombocytopenia, leukopenia, and pancytopenia.

A large clinical trial in acute coronary syndrome patients was unsuccessful in demonstrating a benefit for Ranexa, but there was no apparent proarrhythmic effect in these high-risk patients *[see Clinical Trials (14.2)]*.

Laboratory Abnormalities

Ranexa produces small reductions in hemoglobin A1c. Ranexa is not a treatment for diabetes.

Ranexa produces elevations of serum creatinine by 0.1 mg/dL, regardless of previous renal function. The elevation has a rapid onset, shows no signs of progression during long-term therapy, is reversible after discontinuation of Ranexa, and is not accompanied by changes in BUN. In healthy volunteers, Ranexa 1000 mg twice daily had no effect upon the glomerular filtration rate. The elevated creatinine levels are likely due to a blockage of creatinine's tubular secretion by ranolazine or one of its metabolites.

6.2 Postmarketing Experience

The following adverse reactions have been identified during postapproval use of Ranexa. Because these reactions are reported voluntarily from a population of uncertain size, it is not always possible to reliably estimate their frequency or establish a causal relationship to drug exposure:

Nervous System Disorders – tremor, paresthesia, hypoesthesia
Psychiatric Disorders – hallucination
Skin and Subcutaneous Tissue Disorders – angioedema, rash, pruritus

7 DRUG INTERACTIONS

7.1 Effects of Other Drugs on Ranolazine

Strong CYP3A Inhibitors

Do not use Ranexa with strong CYP3A inhibitors, including ketoconazole, itraconazole, clarithromycin, nefazodone, nelfinavir, ritonavir, indinavir, and saquinavir *[see Contraindications (4), Clinical Pharmacology (12.3)]*.

Moderate CYP3A Inhibitors

Limit the dose of Ranexa to 500 mg twice daily in patients on moderate CYP3A inhibitors, including diltiazem, verapamil, erythromycin, fluconazole, and grapefruit juice or grapefruit-containing products *[see Dosage and Administration (2.2), Clinical Pharmacology (12.3)]*.

P-gp Inhibitors

Concomitant use of Ranexa and P-gp inhibitors, such as cyclosporine, may result in increases in ranolazine concentrations. Titrate Ranexa based on clinical response in patients concomitantly treated with predominant P-gp inhibitors such as cyclosporine *[see Dosage and Administration (2.2)]*.

CYP3A Inducers

Do not use Ranexa with CYP3A inducers such as rifampin, rifabutin, rifapentin, phenobarbital, phenytoin, carbamazepine, and St. John's wort *[see Contraindications (4), Clinical Pharmacology (12.3)]*.

7.2 Effects of Ranolazine on Other Drugs

Drugs Metabolized by CYP3A

Limit the dose of simvastatin in patients on any dose of Ranexa to 20 mg once daily, when ranolazine is co-administered. Dose adjustment of other sensitive CYP3A substrates (e.g., lovastatin) and CYP3A substrates with a narrow therapeutic range (e.g., cyclosporine, tacrolimus, sirolimus) may be required as Ranexa may increase plasma concentrations of these drugs *[see Clinical Pharmacology (12.3)]*.

Drugs Transported by P-gp

Concomitant use of ranolazine and digoxin results in increased exposure to digoxin. The dose of digoxin may have to be adjusted *[see Clinical Pharmacology (12.3)]*.

Drugs Metabolized by CYP2D6

The exposure to CYP2D6 substrates, such as tricyclic antidepressants and antipsychotics, may be increased during co-administration with Ranexa, and lower doses of these drugs may be required.

8 USE IN SPECIFIC POPULATIONS

8.1 Pregnancy

Pregnancy Category C

In animal studies, ranolazine at exposures 1.5 (rabbit) to 2 (rat) times the usual human exposure caused maternal toxicity and misshapen sternebrae and reduced ossification in offspring. These doses in rats and rabbits were associated with an increased maternal mortality rate *[see Reproductive Toxicology Studies (13.3)]*. There are no adequate well-controlled studies in pregnant women. Ranexa should be used during pregnancy only when the potential benefit to the patient justifies the potential risk to the fetus.

8.3 Nursing Mothers

It is not known whether ranolazine is excreted in human milk. Because many drugs are excreted in human milk and because of the potential for serious adverse reactions from ranolazine in nursing infants, decide whether to discontinue nursing or to discontinue Ranexa, taking into account the importance of the drug to the mother.

8.4 Pediatric Use

Safety and effectiveness have not been established in pediatric patients.

8.5 Geriatric Use

Of the chronic angina patients treated with Ranexa in controlled studies, 496 (48%) were ≥ 65 years of age, and 114 (11%) were ≥ 75 years of age. No overall differences in efficacy were observed between older and younger patients. There were no differences in safety for patients ≥ 65 years compared to younger patients, but patients ≥ 75 years of age on Ranexa, compared to placebo, had a higher incidence of adverse events, serious adverse events, and drug discontinuations due to adverse events. In general, dose selection for an elderly patient should usually start at the low end of the dosing range, reflecting the greater frequency of decreased hepatic, renal, or cardiac function, and of concomitant disease, or other drug therapy.

8.6 Use in Patients with Hepatic Impairment

Ranexa is contraindicated in patients with liver cirrhosis. In a study of cirrhotic patients, the C_{max} of ranolazine was increased 30% in cirrhotic patients with mild (Child-Pugh Class A) hepatic impairment, but increased 80% in cirrhotic patients with moderate (Child-Pugh Class B) hepatic impairment compared to patients without hepatic impairment. This increase was not enough to account for the 3-fold increase in QT prolongation seen in cirrhotic patients with mild to moderate hepatic impairment *[see Clinical Pharmacology (12.2)]*.

8.7 Use in Patients with Renal Impairment

Compared to patients with no renal impairment, C_{max} was increased between 40% and 50% in patients with mild, moderate or severe renal impairment suggesting a similar increase in exposure in patients with renal failure independent of the degree of impairment. The pharmacokinetics of ranolazine has not been assessed in patients on dialysis.

8.8 Use in Patients with Heart Failure

Heart failure (NYHA Class I to IV) had no significant effect on ranolazine pharmacokinetics. Ranexa had minimal effects on heart rate and blood pressure in patients with angina and heart failure NYHA Class I to IV. No dose adjustment of Ranexa is required in patients with heart failure.

8.9 Use in Patients with Diabetes Mellitus

A population pharmacokinetic evaluation of data from angina patients and healthy subjects showed no effect of diabetes on ranolazine pharmacokinetics. No dose adjustment is required in patients with diabetes.

Ranexa produces small reductions in HbA1c in patients with diabetes, the clinical significance of which is unknown. Ranexa should not be considered a treatment for diabetes.

10 OVERDOSAGE

High oral doses of ranolazine produce dose-related increases in dizziness, nausea, and vomiting. High intravenous exposure also produces diplopia, paresthesia, confusion, and syncope. In addition to general supportive measures, continuous ECG monitoring may be warranted in the event of overdose.

Since ranolazine is about 62% bound to plasma proteins, hemodialysis is unlikely to be effective in clearing ranolazine.

11 DESCRIPTION

Ranexa (ranolazine) is available as a film-coated, non-scored, extended-release tablet for oral administration.

Ranolazine is a racemic mixture, chemically described as 1-piperazineacetamide, *N*-(2,6-dimethylphenyl)-4-[2-hydroxy-3-(2-methoxyphenoxy)propyl]-, (±)-. It has an empirical formula of $C_{24}H_{33}N_3O_4$, a molecular weight of 427.54 g/mole, and the following structural formula:

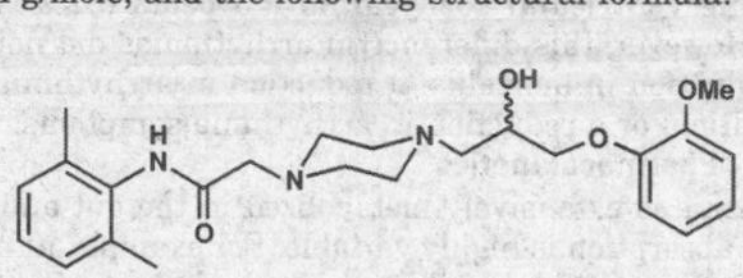

Ranolazine is a white to off-white solid. Ranolazine is soluble in dichloromethane and methanol; sparingly soluble in tetrahydrofuran, ethanol, acetonitrile, and acetone; slightly soluble in ethyl acetate, isopropanol, toluene, and ethyl ether; and very slightly soluble in water.

Ranexa tablets contain 500 mg or 1000 mg of ranolazine and the following inactive ingredients: carnauba wax, hypromellose, magnesium stearate, methacrylic acid copolymer (Type C), microcrystalline cellulose, polyethylene glycol, sodium hydroxide, and titanium dioxide. Additional inactive ingredients for the 500 mg tablet include polyvinyl alcohol, talc, Iron Oxide Yellow, and Iron Oxide Red; additional inactive ingredients for the 1000 mg tablet include lactose monohydrate, triacetin, and Iron Oxide Yellow.

12 CLINICAL PHARMACOLOGY

12.1 Mechanism of Action

The mechanism of action of ranolazine's antianginal effects has not been determined. Ranolazine has anti-ischemic and antianginal effects that do not depend upon reductions in heart rate or blood pressure. It does not affect the rate-pressure product, a measure of myocardial work, at maximal exercise. Ranolazine at therapeutic levels can inhibit the cardiac late sodium current (I_{Na}). However, the relationship of this inhibition to angina symptoms is uncertain.

The QT prolongation effect of ranolazine on the surface electrocardiogram is the result of inhibition of I_{Kr}, which prolongs the ventricular action potential.

12.2 Pharmacodynamics

Hemodynamic Effects

Patients with chronic angina treated with Ranexa in controlled clinical studies had minimal changes in mean heart rate (< 2 bpm) and systolic blood pressure (< 3 mm Hg). Similar results were observed in subgroups of patients with CHF NYHA Class I or II, diabetes, or reactive airway disease, and in elderly patients.

Table 2 Angina Frequency and Nitroglycerin Use (CARISA)

		Placebo	Ranexa 750 mg*	Ranexa 1000 mg*
Angina Frequency (attacks/week)	N	258	272	261
	Mean	3.3	2.5	2.1
	p-value vs placebo	—	*0.006*	*< 0.001*
Nitroglycerin Use (doses/week)	N	252	262	244
	Mean	3.1	2.1	1.8
	p-value vs placebo	—	*0.016*	*< 0.001*

* Twice daily

Electrocardiographic Effects

Dose and plasma concentration-related increases in the QTc interval *[see Warnings and Precautions (5.1)]*, reductions in T wave amplitude, and, in some cases, notched T waves, have been observed in patients treated with Ranexa. These effects are believed to be caused by ranolazine and not by its metabolites. The relationship between the change in QTc and ranolazine plasma concentrations is linear, with a slope of about 2.6 msec/1000 ng/mL, through exposures corresponding to doses several-fold higher than the maximum recommended dose of 1000 mg twice daily. The variable blood levels attained after a given dose of ranolazine give a wide range of effects on QTc. At T_{max} following repeat dosing at 1000 mg twice daily, the mean change in QTc is about 6 msec, but in the 5% of the population with the highest plasma concentrations, the prolongation of QTc is at least 15 msec. In cirrhotic subjects with mild or moderate hepatic impairment, the relationship between plasma level of ranolazine and QTc is much steeper *[see Contraindications (4)]*.

Age, weight, gender, race, heart rate, congestive heart failure, diabetes, and renal impairment did not alter the slope of the QTc-concentration relationship of ranolazine.

No proarrhythmic effects were observed on 7-day Holter recordings in 3,162 acute coronary syndrome patients treated with Ranexa. There was a significantly lower incidence of arrhythmias (ventricular tachycardia, bradycardia, supraventricular tachycardia, and new atrial fibrillation) in patients treated with Ranexa (80%) versus placebo (87%), including ventricular tachycardia ≥ 3 beats (52% versus 61%). However, this difference in arrhythmias did not lead to a reduction in mortality, a reduction in arrhythmia hospitalization, or a reduction in arrhythmia symptoms.

12.3 Pharmacokinetics

Ranolazine is extensively metabolized in the gut and liver and its absorption is highly variable. For example, at a dose of 1000 mg twice daily, the mean steady-state C_{max} was 2600 ng/mL with 95% confidence limits of 400 and 6100 ng/mL. The pharmacokinetics of the (+) R- and (-) S-enantiomers of ranolazine are similar in healthy volunteers. The apparent terminal half-life of ranolazine is 7 hours. Steady state is generally achieved within 3 days of twice-daily dosing with Ranexa. At steady state over the dose range of 500 to 1000 mg twice daily, C_{max} and $AUC_{0-\tau}$ increase slightly more than proportionally to dose, 2.2- and 2.4-fold, respectively. With twice-daily dosing, the trough:peak ratio of the ranolazine plasma concentration is 0.3 to 0.6. The pharmacokinetics of ranolazine is unaffected by age, gender, or food.

Absorption and Distribution

After oral administration of Ranexa, peak plasma concentrations of ranolazine are reached between 2 and 5 hours. After oral administration of ^{14}C-ranolazine as a solution, 73% of the dose is systemically available as ranolazine or metabolites. The bioavailability of ranolazine from Ranexa tablets relative to that from a solution of ranolazine is 76%. Because ranolazine is a substrate of P-gp, inhibitors of P-gp may increase the absorption of ranolazine.

Food (high-fat breakfast) has no important effect on the C_{max} and AUC of ranolazine. Therefore, Ranexa may be taken without regard to meals. Over the concentration range of 0.25 to 10 µg/mL, ranolazine is approximately 62% bound to human plasma proteins.

Metabolism and Excretion

Ranolazine is metabolized mainly by CYP3A and, to a lesser extent, by CYP2D6. Following a single oral dose of ranolazine solution, approximately 75% of the dose is excreted in urine and 25% in feces. Ranolazine is metabolized rapidly and extensively in the liver and intestine; less than 5% is excreted unchanged in urine and feces. The pharmacologic activity of the metabolites has not been well characterized. After dosing to steady state with 500 mg to 1500 mg twice daily, the four most abundant metabolites in plasma have AUC values ranging from about 5 to 33% that of ranolazine, and display apparent half-lives ranging from 6 to 22 hours.

Drug Interactions

Effect of other drugs on ranolazine

In vitro data indicate that ranolazine is a substrate of CYP3A and, to a lesser degree, of CYP2D6. Ranolazine is also a substrate of P-glycoprotein.

Strong CYP3A Inhibitors

Plasma levels of ranolazine with Ranexa 1000 mg twice daily are 3.2-fold higher if coadministered with ketoconazole 200 mg twice daily *[see Contraindications (4)]*.

Moderate CYP3A Inhibitors

Plasma levels of ranolazine with Ranexa 1000 mg twice daily are increased about 50 to 130% by diltiazem 180 to 360 mg, respectively. Plasma levels of ranolazine with Ranexa 750 mg twice daily are increased about 100% by verapamil 120 mg three times daily *[see Drug Interactions 7.1]*.

Weak CYP3A Inhibitors

The weak CYP3A inhibitors simvastatin (20 mg once daily) and cimetidine (400 mg three times daily) do not increase the exposure to ranolazine in healthy volunteers.

CYP3A Inducers

Rifampin 600 mg once daily decreases the plasma concentrations of ranolazine (1000 mg twice daily) by approximately 95% *[see Contraindications (4)]*.

CYP2D6 Inhibitors

Paroxetine 20 mg once daily increased ranolazine concentrations 20% in healthy volunteers receiving Ranexa 1000 mg twice daily. No dose adjustment of Ranexa is required in patients treated with CYP2D6 inhibitors.

Digoxin

Plasma concentrations of ranolazine are not significantly altered by concomitant digoxin at 0.125 mg once daily.

Effect of ranolazine on other drugs

In vitro ranolazine and its O-demethylated metabolite are weak inhibitors of CYP3A and moderate inhibitors of CYP2D6 and P-gp. *In vitro* ranolazine is an inhibitor of OCT2.

CYP3A Substrates

The plasma levels of simvastatin, a CYP3A substrate, and its active metabolite are each doubled in healthy subjects receiving 80 mg once daily and Ranexa 1000 mg twice daily *[see Drug Interactions (7.2)]*.

Diltiazem

The pharmacokinetics of diltiazem is not affected by ranolazine in healthy volunteers receiving diltiazem 60 mg three times daily and Ranexa 1000 mg twice daily.

P-gp Substrates

Ranolazine increases digoxin concentrations 50% in healthy volunteers receiving Ranexa 1000 mg twice daily and digoxin 0.125 mg once daily *[see Drug Interactions (7.2)]*.

CYP2D6 Substrates

Ranexa 750 mg twice daily increases the plasma concentrations of a single dose of immediate release metoprolol (100 mg), a CYP2D6 substrate, by 80% in extensive CYP2D6 metabolizers with no need for dose adjustment of metoprolol. In extensive metabolizers of dextromethorphan, a substrate of CYP2D6, ranolazine inhibits partially the formation of the main metabolite dextrorphan.

13 NONCLINICAL TOXICOLOGY

13.1 Carcinogenesis, Mutagenesis, Impairment of Fertility

Ranolazine tested negative for genotoxic potential in the following assays: Ames bacterial mutation assay, Saccharomyces assay for mitotic gene conversion, chromosomal aberrations assay in Chinese hamster ovary (CHO) cells, mammalian CHO/HGPRT gene mutation assay, and mouse and rat bone marrow micronucleus assays.

There was no evidence of carcinogenic potential in mice or rats. The highest oral doses used in the carcinogenicity studies were 150 mg/kg/day for 21 months in rats (900 mg/m²/day) and 50 mg/kg/day for 24 months in mice (150 mg/m²/day). These maximally tolerated doses are 0.8 and 0.1 times, respectively, the maximum recommended human dose (MRHD) of 2 grams on a surface area basis. A published study reported that ranolazine promoted tumor formation and progression to malignancy when given to transgenic APC (min/+) mice at a dose of 30 mg/kg twice daily *[see References (15)]*. The clinical significance of this finding is unclear.

13.3 Reproductive Toxicology Studies

Animal reproduction studies with ranolazine were conducted in rats and rabbits.

There was an increased incidence of misshapen sternebrae and reduced ossification of pelvic and cranial bones in fetuses of pregnant rats dosed at 400 mg/kg/day (2 times the MRHD on a surface area basis). Reduced ossification of sternebrae was observed in fetuses of pregnant rabbits dosed at 150 mg/kg/day (1.5 times the MRHD on a surface area basis). These doses in rats and rabbits were associated with an increased maternal mortality rate.

14 CLINICAL STUDIES

14.1 Chronic Stable Angina

CARISA (Combination Assessment of Ranolazine In Stable Angina) was a study in 823 chronic angina patients randomized to receive 12 weeks of treatment with twice-daily Ranexa 750 mg, 1000 mg, or placebo, who also continued on daily doses of atenolol 50 mg, amlodipine 5 mg, or diltiazem CD 180 mg. Sublingual nitrates were used in this study as needed.

In this trial, statistically significant ($p < 0.05$) increases in modified Bruce treadmill exercise duration and time to angina were observed for each Ranexa dose versus placebo, at both trough (12 hours after dosing) and peak (4 hours after dosing) plasma levels, with minimal effects on blood pressure and heart rate. The changes versus placebo in exercise parameters are presented in Table 1. Exercise treadmill results showed no increase in effect on exercise at the 1000 mg dose compared to the 750 mg dose.

Table 1 Exercise Treadmill Results (CARISA)

	Mean Difference from Placebo (sec)	
Study	**CARISA (N = 791)**	
Ranexa Twice-daily Dose	**750 mg**	**1000 mg**
Exercise Duration		
Trough	24*	24*
Peak	34†	26*
Time to Angina		
Trough	30*	26*
Peak	38†	38†
Time to 1 mm ST-Segment Depression		
Trough	20	21
Peak	41†	35†

* p-value ≤ 0.05
† p-value ≤ 0.005

The effects of Ranexa on angina frequency and nitroglycerin use are shown in Table 2.

[See table 2 above]

Tolerance to Ranexa did not develop after 12 weeks of therapy. Rebound increases in angina, as measured by exercise duration, have not been observed following abrupt discontinuation of Ranexa.

Ranexa has been evaluated in patients with chronic angina who remained symptomatic despite treatment with the maximum dose of an antianginal agent. In the ERICA (Efficacy of Ranolazine In Chronic Angina) trial, 565 patients were randomized to receive an initial dose of Ranexa 500 mg twice daily or placebo for 1 week, followed by 6 weeks of treatment with Ranexa 1000 mg twice daily or placebo, in addition to concomitant treatment with amlodipine 10 mg once daily. In addition, 45% of the study population also received long-acting nitrates. Sublingual nitrates were used as needed to treat angina episodes. Results are shown in Table 3. Statistically significant decreases in angina attack frequency ($p = 0.028$) and nitroglycerin use ($p = 0.014$) were observed with Ranexa compared to placebo. These treatment effects appeared consistent across age and use of long-acting nitrates.

Table 3 Angina Frequency and Nitroglycerin Use (ERICA)

		Placebo	Ranexa*
Angina Frequency (attacks/week)	N	281	277
	Mean	4.3	3.3
	Median	2.4	2.2

Nitroglycerin Use (doses/week)	N	281	277
	Mean	3.6	2.7
	Median	1.7	1.3

* 1000 mg twice daily

Gender

Effects on angina frequency and exercise tolerance were considerably smaller in women than in men. In CARISA, the improvement in Exercise Tolerance Test (ETT) in females was about 33% of that in males at the 1000 mg twice-daily dose level. In ERICA, where the primary endpoint was angina attack frequency, the mean reduction in weekly angina attacks was 0.3 for females and 1.3 for males.

Race

There were insufficient numbers of non-Caucasian patients to allow for analyses of efficacy or safety by racial subgroup.

14.2 Lack of Benefit in Acute Coronary Syndrome

In a large (n = 6,560) placebo-controlled trial (MERLIN-TIMI 36) in patients with acute coronary syndrome, there was no benefit shown on outcome measures. However, the study is somewhat reassuring regarding proarrhythmic risks, as ventricular arrhythmias were less common on ranolazine *[see Clinical Pharmacology (12.2)]*, and there was no difference between Ranexa and placebo in the risk of all-cause mortality (relative risk ranolazine:placebo 0.99 with an upper 95% confidence limit of 1.22).

15 REFERENCES

M.A. Suckow et al. The anti-ischemia agent ranolazine promotes the development of intestinal tumors in APC (min/+) mice. Cancer Letters 209(2004):165–9.

16 HOW SUPPLIED/STORAGE AND HANDLING

Ranexa is supplied as film-coated, oblong-shaped, extended-release tablets in the following strengths:

- 500 mg tablets are light orange, with GSI500 on one side
- 1000 mg tablets are pale yellow, with GSI1000 on one side

Ranexa (ranolazine) extended-release tablets are available in:

	Strength	NDC
Unit-of-Use Bottle (60 Tablets)	500 mg	61958-1003-1
Unit-of-Use Bottle (60 Tablets)	1000 mg	61958-1004-1

Store Ranexa tablets at 25 °C (77 °F) with excursions permitted to 15 ° to 30 °C (59 ° to 86 °F).

17 PATIENT COUNSELING INFORMATION

To ensure safe and effective use of Ranexa, the following information and instructions should be communicated to the patient when appropriate.

Patients should be advised:

- that Ranexa will not abate an acute angina episode
- to inform their physician of any other medications when taken concurrently with Ranexa, including over-the-counter medications
- that Ranexa may produce changes in the electrocardiogram (QTc interval prolongation)
- to inform their physician of any personal or family history of QTc prolongation, congenital long QT syndrome, or if they are receiving drugs that prolong the QTc interval such as Class Ia (e.g., quinidine) or Class III (e.g., dofetilide, sotalol, amiodarone) antiarrhythmic agents, erythromycin, and certain antipsychotics (e.g., thioridazine, ziprasidone)
- that Ranexa should not be used in patients who are receiving drugs that are strong CYP3A inhibitors (e.g., ketoconazole, clarithromycin, nefazodone, ritonavir)
- that initiation of treatment with Ranexa should be avoided during administration of inducers of CYP3A (e.g., rifampin, rifabutin, rifapentin, barbiturates, carbamazepine, phenytoin, St. John's wort)
- to inform their physician if they are receiving drugs that are moderate CYP3A inhibitors (e.g., diltiazem, verapamil, erythromycin)
- to inform their physician if they are receiving P-gp inhibitors (e.g., cyclosporine)
- that grapefruit juice or grapefruit products should be limited when taking Ranexa
- that Ranexa should not be used in patients with liver cirrhosis
- that doses of Ranexa higher than 1000 mg twice daily should not be used
- that if a dose is missed, the usual dose should be taken at the next scheduled time. The next dose should not be doubled
- that Ranexa may be taken with or without meals
- that Ranexa tablets should be swallowed whole and not crushed, broken, or chewed
- to contact their physician if they experience fainting spells while taking Ranexa
- that Ranexa may cause dizziness and lightheadedness; therefore, patients should know how they react to this drug before they operate an automobile, or machinery, or engage in activities requiring mental alertness or coordination

Manufactured for:
Gilead Sciences, Inc.
Foster City, CA 94404

Ranexa is a registered trademark of Gilead Sciences, Inc.

21-526-GS-011

PATIENT INFORMATION

Ranexa® (rah **NEX** ah)
(ranolazine)
extended-release tablets

Dosing Strengths:
500 mg tablets
1000 mg tablets

Read this Patient Information before you start taking Ranexa and each time you get a refill. There may be new information. This information does not take the place of talking with your doctor about your medical condition or treatment.

What is Ranexa?

Ranexa is a prescription medicine used to treat angina that keeps coming back (chronic angina).

Ranexa may be used with other medicines that are used for heart problems and blood pressure control.

It is not known if Ranexa is safe and effective in children.

Who should not take Ranexa?

Do not take Ranexa if:

- you take any of the following medicines:
  - for fungus infection: ketoconazole (Nizoral®), itraconazole (Sporanox®, Onmel)
  - for infection: clarithromycin (Biaxin®)
  - for depression: nefazodone
  - for HIV: nelfinavir (Viracept®), ritonavir (Norvir®), lopinavir and ritonavir (Kaletra®) indinavir (Crixivan®), saquinavir (Invirase®)
  - for tuberculosis (TB): rifampin (Rifadin®), rifabutin (Mycobutin®), rifapentin (Priftin®)
  - for seizures: phenobarbital, phenytoin (Phenytek®, Dilantin® Dilantin-125®), carbamazepine (Tegretol®)
  - St. John's wort (Hypericum perforatum)
- you have scarring (cirrhosis) of your liver

What should I tell my doctor before taking Ranexa?

Before you take Ranexa, tell your doctor if you:

- have or have a family history of a heart problem, called 'QT prolongation' or 'long QT syndrome'.
- have liver problems.
- are pregnant or plan to become pregnant. It is not known if Ranexa will harm your unborn baby.
- are breast-feeding or plan to breast-feed. It is not known if Ranexa passes into your breast milk. You and your doctor should decide if you will take Ranexa or breast-feed. You should not do both.

Tell your doctor about all the medicines you take, including all prescription and non-prescription medicines, vitamins and herbal supplements. Ranexa may affect the way other medicines work and other medicines may affect how Ranexa works.

Tell your doctor if you take medicines:

- for your heart
- for cholesterol
- for infection
- for fungus
- for transplant
- for nausea and vomiting because of cancer treatments
- for mental problems

Know the medicines you take. Keep a list of them to show your doctor or pharmacist when you get a new medicine.

How should I take Ranexa?

- Take Ranexa exactly as your doctor tells you.
- Your doctor will tell you how much Ranexa to take and when to take it.
  - Do not change your dose unless your doctor tells you to.
- Tell your doctor if you still have symptoms of angina after starting Ranexa.
- Take Ranexa by mouth, with or without food.
- Swallow the Ranexa tablets whole. Do not crush, break, or chew Ranexa tablets before swallowing.
- If you miss a dose of Ranexa, wait to take the next dose of Ranexa at your regular time. Do not make up for the missed dose. Do not take more than 1 dose at a time.
- If you take too much Ranexa, call your doctor, or go to the nearest emergency room right away.

What should I avoid while taking Ranexa?

- Grapefruit and grapefruit juice. Limit products that have grapefruit in them. They can cause your blood levels of Ranexa to increase.
- Ranexa can cause dizziness, lightheadness, or fainting. If you have these symptoms, do not drive a car, use machinery, or do anything that needs you to be alert.

What are the possible side effects of Ranexa?

Ranexa may cause serious side effects, including:

- changes in the electrical activity of your heart called QT prolongation. Your doctor may check the electrical activity of your heart with an ECG. Tell your doctor right away if you feel faint, lightheaded, or feel your heart beating irregularly or fast while taking Ranexa. These may be symptoms related to QT prolongation.

The most common side effects of Ranexa include:

- dizziness
- headache
- constipation
- nausea

Tell your doctor if you have any side effect that bothers you or does not go away.

These are not all the possible side effects of Ranexa. For more information, ask your doctor or pharmacist.

Call your doctor for medical advice about side effects. You may report side effects to FDA at 1-800-FDA-1088.

How should I store Ranexa?

Store Ranexa tablets at room temperature between 59° to 86°F (15° to 30°C)

Keep Ranexa and all medicines out of the reach of children.

General information about Ranexa

Medicines are sometimes prescribed for purposes other than those listed in Patient Information. Do not use Ranexa for a condition for which it was not prescribed. Do not give Ranexa to other people, even if they have the same condition you have. It may harm them.

The Patient Information summarizes the most important information about Ranexa. If you would like more information, talk with your doctor. You can ask your pharmacist or doctor for information about Ranexa that is written for health professionals.

For more information, go to www.ranexa.com or call Gilead Sciences, Inc. at 1-800-445-3235.

What is chronic angina?

Chronic angina means pain or discomfort in the chest, jaw, shoulder, back, or arm that keeps coming back. There are other possible signs and symptoms of angina including shortness of breath. Angina usually comes on when you are active or under stress. Chronic angina is a symptom of a heart problem called coronary heart disease (CHD), also known as coronary artery disease (CAD). When you have CHD, the blood vessels in your heart become stiff and narrow. Oxygen-rich blood cannot reach your heart muscle easily. Angina comes on when too little oxygen reaches your heart muscle.

What are the ingredients in Ranexa?

Active ingredient: ranolazine

Inactive ingredients:

500 mg tablet: carnauba wax, hypromellose, magnesium stearate, methacrylic acid copolymer (Type C), microcrystalline cellulose, polyethylene glycol, sodium hydroxide, titanium dioxide, polyvinyl alcohol, talc, Iron Oxide Yellow, and Iron Oxide Red.

1000 mg tablet: carnauba wax, hypromellose, magnesium stearate, methacrylic acid copolymer (Type C), microcrystalline cellulose, polyethylene glycol, sodium hydroxide, titanium dioxide, lactose monohydrate, triacetin, and Iron Oxide Yellow.

This Patient Information has been approved by the U.S. Food and Drug Administration.

Manufactured for:
Gilead Sciences, Inc.
Foster City, CA 94404

Issued December 2011

Ranexa is a registered trademark of Gilead Sciences, Inc.

D-21-526-GS-011

Shown in Product Identification Guide, page 306

STRIBILD™ ℞

(elvitegravir, cobicistat, emtricitabine, tenofovir disoproxil fumarate)
Tablets, for oral use

HIGHLIGHTS OF PRESCRIBING INFORMATION

These highlights do not include all the information needed to use STRIBILD safely and effectively. See full prescribing information for STRIBILD.

STRIBILD™ (elvitegravir, cobicistat, emtricitabine, tenofovir disoproxil fumarate) Tablets, for oral use

Initial U.S. Approval: 2012

WARNING: LACTIC ACIDOSIS/SEVERE HEPATOMEGALY WITH STEATOSIS and POST TREATMENT ACUTE EXACERBATION OF HEPATITIS B

See full prescribing information for complete boxed warning.

- **Lactic acidosis and severe hepatomegaly with steatosis, including fatal cases, have been reported with the use of nucleoside analogs, including tenofovir disoproxil fumarate, a component of STRIBILD. (5.1)**
- **STRIBILD is not approved for the treatment of chronic hepatitis B virus (HBV) infection. Severe acute exacerbations of hepatitis B have been reported in patients coinfected with HIV-1 and HBV who have discontinued EMTRIVA or VIREAD, two of the components of STRIBILD. Hepatic function should be monitored closely in these patients. If appropriate, initiation of anti-hepatitis B therapy may be warranted. (5.2)**

INDICATIONS AND USAGE

STRIBILD, a combination of 1 integrase strand transfer inhibitor, 1 pharmacokinetic enhancer, and 2 nucleos(t)ide analog HIV-1 reverse transcriptase inhibitors, is indicated as a complete regimen for the treatment of HIV-1 infection in adults who are antiretroviral treatment-naïve. (1)

DOSAGE AND ADMINISTRATION

- Recommended dose: One tablet taken once daily with food. (2)
- Dosing in renal impairment: STRIBILD should not be initiated in patients with estimated creatinine clearance below 70 mL per minute. Discontinue in patients with estimated creatinine clearance below 50 mL per minute. (2)

DOSAGE FORMS AND STRENGTHS

Tablets: 150 mg of elvitegravir, 150 mg of cobicistat, 200 mg of emtricitabine, and 300 mg of tenofovir disoproxil fumarate. (3)

CONTRAINDICATIONS

- Coadministration of STRIBILD with drugs that:
  - are highly dependent on CYP3A for clearance and for which elevated plasma concentrations are associated with serious and/or life-threatening adverse events. (4)
  - strongly induce CYP3A which may lead to lower exposure of one or more components and loss of efficacy of STRIBILD which may result in loss of virologic response and possible resistance. (4)

WARNINGS AND PRECAUTIONS

- New onset or worsening renal impairment: Can include acute renal failure and Fanconi syndrome. Assess creatinine clearance (CLcr), urine glucose and urine protein before initiating treatment with STRIBILD. Monitor CLcr, urine glucose, and urine protein in all patients. Monitor serum phosphorus in patients at risk for renal impairment. Avoid administering STRIBILD with concurrent or recent use of nephrotoxic drugs. (5.3)
- Coadministration with other products: Do not use with drugs containing emtricitabine or tenofovir disoproxil fumarate including ATRIPLA, COMPLERA, EMTRIVA, TRUVADA, or VIREAD; with drugs containing lamivudine; or with drugs or regimens containing ritonavir. Do not administer in combination with HEPSERA. (5.4)
- Decreases in bone mineral density (BMD): Consider monitoring BMD in patients with a history of pathologic fracture or other risk factors of osteoporosis or bone loss. (5.5)
- Redistribution/accumulation of body fat: Observed in patients receiving antiretroviral therapy. (5.6)
- Immune reconstitution syndrome: May necessitate further evaluation and treatment. (5.7)

ADVERSE REACTIONS

Most common adverse drug reactions to STRIBILD (incidence greater than or equal to 10%, all grades) are nausea and diarrhea. (6.1)

To report SUSPECTED ADVERSE REACTIONS, contact Gilead Sciences, Inc. at 1-800-GILEAD-5 or FDA at 1-800-FDA-1088 or www.fda.gov/medwatch.

DRUG INTERACTIONS

- STRIBILD is a complete regimen for the treatment of HIV-1 infection; therefore, STRIBILD should not be administered with other antiretroviral medications for treatment of HIV-1 infection. (5.4, 7)
- STRIBILD can alter the concentration of drugs metabolized by CYP3A or CYP2D6. Drugs that induce CYP3A can alter the concentrations of one or more components of STRIBILD. Consult the full prescribing information prior to and during treatment for potential drug-drug interactions. (4, 7, 12.3)

USE IN SPECIFIC POPULATIONS

- Pregnancy: Use during pregnancy only if the potential benefit justifies the potential risk. (8.1)
- Nursing mothers: Women infected with HIV should be instructed not to breastfeed due to the potential for HIV transmission. (8.3)

See 17 for PATIENT COUNSELING INFORMATION and FDA-approved patient labeling

Revised: 08/2012

FULL PRESCRIBING INFORMATION: CONTENTS*

*** Sections or subsections omitted from the full prescribing information are not listed**

FULL PRESCRIBING INFORMATION

WARNING: LACTIC ACIDOSIS/SEVERE HEPATOMEGALY WITH STEATOSIS and POST TREATMENT ACUTE EXACERBATION OF HEPATITIS B

Lactic acidosis and severe hepatomegaly with steatosis, including fatal cases, have been reported with the use of nucleoside analogs, including tenofovir disoproxil fumarate, a component of STRIBILD, in combination with other antiretrovirals *[See Warnings and Precautions (5.1)]*.

STRIBILD is not approved for the treatment of chronic hepatitis B virus (HBV) infection and the safety and efficacy of STRIBILD have not been established in patients coinfected with HBV and HIV-1. Severe acute exacerbations of hepatitis B have been reported in patients who are coinfected with HBV and human immunodeficiency virus-1 (HIV-1) and have discontinued EMTRIVA or VIREAD, which are components of STRIBILD. Hepatic function should be monitored closely with both clinical and laboratory follow-up for at least several months in patients who are coinfected with HIV-1 and HBV and discontinue STRIBILD. If appropriate, initiation of anti-hepatitis B therapy may be warranted *[See Warnings and Precautions (5.2)]*.

1 INDICATION AND USAGE

STRIBILD™ is indicated as a complete regimen for the treatment of HIV-1 infection in adults who are antiretroviral treatment-naïve.

2 DOSAGE AND ADMINISTRATION

The recommended dose of STRIBILD is one tablet taken orally once daily with food *[See Clinical Pharmacology (12.3)]*.

Renal Impairment: STRIBILD should not be initiated in patients with estimated creatinine clearance below 70 mL per min. Because STRIBILD is a fixed-dose combination tablet, STRIBILD should be discontinued if estimated creatinine clearance declines below 50 mL per min during treatment with STRIBILD as dose interval adjustment required for emtricitabine and tenofovir disoproxil fumarate (tenofovir DF) cannot be achieved *[See Warnings and Precautions (5.3), Adverse Reactions (6.1), Use in Specific Populations (8.6), Clinical Pharmacology (12.3), and Clinical Studies (14)]*.

Hepatic Impairment: No dose adjustment of STRIBILD is required in patients with mild (Child-Pugh Class A) or moderate (Child-Pugh Class B) hepatic impairment. No pharmacokinetic or safety data are available regarding the use of STRIBILD in patients with severe hepatic impairment (Child-Pugh Class C). Therefore, STRIBILD is not recommended for use in patients with severe hepatic impairment *[See Use in Specific Populations (8.7) and Clinical Pharmacology (12.3)]*.

3 DOSAGE FORMS AND STRENGTHS

STRIBILD is available as tablets. Each tablet contains 150 mg of elvitegravir, 150 mg of cobicistat, 200 mg of emtricitabine, and 300 mg of tenofovir disoproxil fumarate (tenofovir DF, equivalent to 245 mg of tenofovir disoproxil). The tablets are green, capsule-shaped, film-coated, debossed with "GSI" on one side and the number "1" surrounded by a square box (1) on the other side of the tablet.

4 CONTRAINDICATIONS

Coadministration of STRIBILD is contraindicated with drugs that are highly dependent on CYP3A for clearance and for which elevated plasma concentrations are associated with serious and/or life-threatening events. These drugs and other contraindicated drugs (which may lead to reduced efficacy of STRIBILD and possible resistance) are listed in Table 1 *[See Drug Interactions (7.4), Clinical Pharmacology (12.3)]*.

[See table 1 at top of next page]

5 WARNINGS AND PRECAUTIONS

5.1 Lactic Acidosis/Severe Hepatomegaly with Steatosis

Lactic acidosis and severe hepatomegaly with steatosis, including fatal cases, have been reported with the use of nucleoside analogs, including tenofovir DF, a component of STRIBILD, in combination with other antiretrovirals. A majority of these cases have been in women. Obesity and prolonged nucleoside exposure may be risk factors. Particular caution should be exercised when administering nucleoside analogs to any patient with known risk factors for liver disease; however, cases have also been reported in patients with no known risk factors. Treatment with STRIBILD should be suspended in any patient who develops clinical or laboratory findings suggestive of lactic acidosis or pronounced hepatotoxicity (which may include hepatomegaly and steatosis even in the absence of marked transaminase elevations).

5.2 Patients Coinfected with HIV-1 and HBV

It is recommended that all patients with HIV-1 be tested for the presence of chronic hepatitis B virus (HBV) before initiating antiretroviral therapy. STRIBILD is not approved for the treatment of chronic HBV infection and the safety and efficacy of STRIBILD have not been established in patients coinfected with HBV and HIV-1. Severe acute exacerbations of hepatitis B have been reported in patients who are coinfected with HBV and HIV-1 and have discontinued emtricitabine or tenofovir DF, two of the components of STRIBILD. In some patients infected with HBV and treated with EMTRIVA, the exacerbations of hepatitis B were associated with liver decompensation and liver failure. Patients who are coinfected with HIV-1 and HBV should be closely monitored with both clinical and laboratory follow-up for at least several months after stopping treatment with STRIBILD. If appropriate, initiation of anti-hepatitis B therapy may be warranted.

5.3 New Onset or Worsening Renal Impairment

Renal impairment, including cases of acute renal failure and Fanconi syndrome (renal tubular injury with severe hypophosphatemia), has been reported with the use of tenofovir DF and with the use of STRIBILD *[See Adverse Reactions (6.2)]*.

In the clinical trials of STRIBILD over 48 weeks (N=701), 8 (1.1%) subjects in the STRIBILD group and 1 (0.1%) subject in the combined comparator groups discontinued study drug due to a renal adverse event. Four (0.6%) of the subjects who received STRIBILD developed laboratory findings consistent with proximal renal tubular dysfunction leading to discontinuation of STRIBILD compared to none in the comparator groups. Two of these four subjects had renal impairment (i.e. estimated creatinine clearance less than 70 mL per min) at baseline. The laboratory findings in these 4 subjects with evidence of proximal tubulopathy improved but did not completely resolve in all subjects upon discontinuation of STRIBILD. Renal replacement therapy was not required for these subjects.

Estimated creatinine clearance, urine glucose and urine protein should be documented in all patients prior to initiating therapy. STRIBILD should not be initiated in patients with estimated creatinine clearance below 70 mL per min. Routine monitoring of estimated creatinine clearance, urine glucose, and urine protein should be performed during STRIBILD therapy in all patients. Additionally, serum phosphorus should be measured in patients at risk for renal impairment.

Although cobicistat may cause modest increases in serum creatinine and modest declines in estimated creatinine clearance without affecting renal glomerular function *[See Adverse Reactions (6.1)]*, patients who experience a confirmed increase in serum creatinine of greater than 0.4 mg per dL from baseline should be closely monitored for renal safety.

STRIBILD should be avoided with concurrent or recent use of a nephrotoxic agent.

The emtricitabine and tenofovir DF components of STRIBILD are primarily excreted by the kidney. STRIBILD should be discontinued if estimated creatinine clearance declines below 50 mL per min as dose interval adjustment required for emtricitabine and tenofovir DF cannot be achieved with the fixed-dose combination tablet.

5.4 Use with Other Antiretroviral Products

STRIBILD is indicated for use as a complete regimen for the treatment of HIV-1 infection and should not be coadministered with other antiretroviral products.

STRIBILD should not be coadministered with products containing any of the same active components, emtricitabine or tenofovir DF (ATRIPLA, COMPLERA, EMTRIVA, TRUVADA, VIREAD); or with products containing lamivudine (COMBIVIR, EPIVIR, EPIVIR-HBV, EPZICOM, TRIZIVIR). STRIBILD should not be administered with adefovir dipivoxil (HEPSERA).

5.5 Decreases in Bone Mineral Density

In previous clinical trials, tenofovir DF has been associated with decreases in bone mineral density (BMD) and increases in biochemical markers of bone metabolism (serum bone-specific alkaline phosphatase, serum osteocalcin, serum C telopeptide, and urinary N telopeptide), suggesting increased bone turnover. Serum parathyroid hormone levels and 1.25 Vitamin D levels were also higher in subjects receiving VIREAD. The effects of tenofovir DF-associated changes in BMD on future fracture risk are unknown. For additional information, please consult the VIREAD prescribing information.

Cases of osteomalacia (associated with proximal renal tubulopathy and which may contribute to fractures) have been reported in association with the use of tenofovir DF *[See Adverse Reactions (6.2)]*.

In Study 103, BMD was assessed by DEXA in a non-random subset of 120 subjects. Mean percentage decreases in BMD from baseline to Week 48 in the STRIBILD group (N = 54) were comparable to the atazanavir + ritonavir +TRUVADA group (N = 66) at the lumbar spine (-2.6% versus -3.3%, respectively) and at the hip (-3.1% versus -3.9%, respectively). In Studies 102 and 103, bone fractures occurred in 9 subjects (1.3%) in the STRIBILD group, 6 subjects (1.7%) in the ATRIPLA group, and 6 subjects (1.7%) in the atazanavir + ritonavir + TRUVADA group. These findings were consistent with data from an earlier 144-week trial of treatment-naïve subjects receiving tenofovir DF + lamivudine + efavirenz.

Assessment of BMD should be considered for HIV-1 infected patients who have a history of pathologic bone fracture or other risk factors for osteoporosis or bone loss. Although the effect of supplementation with calcium and vitamin D was not studied, such supplementation may be beneficial in all patients. If bone abnormalities are suspected, then appropriate consultation should be obtained.

5.6 Fat Redistribution

Redistribution/accumulation of body fat including central obesity, dorsocervical fat enlargement (buffalo hump), peripheral wasting, facial wasting, breast enlargement, and "cushingoid appearance" have been observed in patients receiving antiretroviral therapy. The mechanism and long-term consequences of these events are currently unknown. A causal relationship has not been established.

5.7 Immune Reconstitution Syndrome

Immune reconstitution syndrome has been reported in patients treated with combination antiretroviral therapy, including STRIBILD. During the initial phase of combination antiretroviral treatment, patients whose immune system responds may develop an inflammatory response to indolent or residual opportunistic infections [such as *Mycobacterium avium* infection, cytomegalovirus, *Pneumocystis jirovecii* pneumonia (PCP), or tuberculosis], which may necessitate further evaluation and treatment.

Table 1 Drugs that are Contraindicated with STRIBILD

Drug Class	Drugs within class that are contraindicated with STRIBILD	Clinical Comment
Alpha 1-Adrenoreceptor Antagonist	Alfuzosin	Potential for increased alfuzosin concentrations, which can result in hypotension.
Antimycobacterial	Rifampin	Rifampin is a potent inducer of CYP450 metabolism. STRIBILD should not be used in combination with rifampin, as this may cause significant decrease in the plasma concentration of elvitegravir and cobicistat. This may result in loss of therapeutic effect to STRIBILD.
Ergot Derivatives	Dihydroergotamine Ergotamine Methylergonovine	Potential for serious and/or life-threatening events such as acute ergot toxicity characterized by peripheral vasospasm and ischemia of the extremities and other tissues.
GI Motility Agent	Cisapride	Potential for serious and/or life-threatening events such as cardiac arrhythmias.
Herbal Products	St. John's wort (*Hypericum perforatum*)	Patients taking STRIBILD should not use products containing St. John's wort because coadministration may result in reduced plasma concentrations of elvitegravir and cobicistat. This may result in loss of therapeutic effect and development of resistance.
HMG-CoA Reductase Inhibitors	Lovastatin Simvastatin	Potential for serious reactions such as myopathy, including rhabdomyolysis.
Neuroleptic	Pimozide	Potential for serious and/or life-threatening events such as cardiac arrhythmias.
Phosphodiesterase-5 (PDE5) Inhibitor	Sildenafil* when dosed as REVATIO for the treatment of pulmonary arterial hypertension	A safe and effective dose in combination with STRIBILD has not been established for sildenafil (REVATIO) when used for the treatment of pulmonary hypertension. There is increased potential for sildenafil-associated adverse events (which include visual disturbances, hypotension, priapism, and syncope).
Sedative/hypnotics	Triazolam Orally administered midazolam†	Triazolam and orally administered midazolam are extensively metabolized by CYP3A4. Coadministration of triazolam or orally administered midazolam with STRIBILD may cause large increases in the concentration of these benzodiazepines. The potential exists for serious and/or life threatening events such as prolonged or increased sedation or respiratory depression.

* See Drug Interactions (7), Table 5 for sildenafil when dosed as VIAGRA for erectile dysfunction.
† See Drug Interactions (7), Table 5 for parenterally administered midazolam.

Autoimmune disorders (such as Graves' disease, polymyositis, and Guillain-Barré syndrome) have also been reported to occur in the setting of immune reconstitution, however, the time to onset is more variable, and can occur many months after initiation of treatment.

6 ADVERSE REACTIONS

The following adverse drug reactions are discussed in other sections of the labeling:

- Lactic Acidosis/Severe Hepatomegaly with Steatosis *[See Boxed Warning, Warnings and Precautions (5.1)]*.
- Severe Acute Exacerbations of Hepatitis B *[See Boxed Warning, Warnings and Precautions (5.2)]*.
- New Onset or Worsening Renal Impairment *[See Warnings and Precautions (5.3)]*.
- Decreases in Bone Mineral Density *[See Warnings and Precautions (5.5)]*.
- Immune Reconstitution Syndrome *[See Warnings and Precautions (5.7)]*.

6.1 Adverse Reactions from Clinical Trials Experience

Because clinical trials are conducted under widely varying conditions, adverse reaction rates observed in the clinical trials of a drug cannot be directly compared to rates in the clinical trials of another drug and may not reflect the rates observed in practice.

The safety assessment of STRIBILD is based on pooled data from 1408 subjects in two comparative clinical trials, Study 102 and Study 103, in antiretroviral treatment-naive HIV-1 infected adult subjects. A total of 701 subjects received STRIBILD once daily for at least 48 weeks.

The proportion of subjects who discontinued treatment with STRIBILD, ATRIPLA (efavirenz 600 mg/emtricitabine 200 mg/tenofovir DF 300 mg) or atazanavir + ritonavir + TRUVADA (emtricitabine 200 mg/tenofovir DF 300 mg) due to adverse events, regardless of severity, was 3.7%, 5.1% and 5.1%, respectively. Table 2 displays the frequency of adverse drug reactions greater than or equal to 5%.

Table 2 Treatment-Emergent Adverse Drug Reactions* (all grades) Reported in ≥ 5% of Subjects in Any Treatment Arm in Studies 102 and 103 (Week 48 analysis)

	STRIBILD N=701	ATRIPLA N=352	Atazanavir + ritonavir + TRUVADA N=355
EYE DISORDERS			
Ocular icterus	<1%	0%	13%
GASTRO-INTESTINAL DISORDERS			
Diarrhea	12%	11%	16%
Flatulence	2%	<1%	7%
Nausea	16%	9%	13%
GENERAL DISORDERS AND ADMINISTRATION SITE CONDITIONS			
Fatigue	5%	7%	6%
HEPATOBILIARY DISORDERS			
Jaundice	0%	<1%	8%
NERVOUS SYSTEM DISORDERS			
Somnolence	1%	7%	1%
Headache	7%	4%	6%
Dizziness	3%	20%	4%

PSYCHIATRIC DISORDERS			
Insomnia	3%	8%	1%
Abnormal dreams	9%	26%	3%
SKIN AND SUBCUTANEOUS TISSUE DISORDERS			
Rash†	3%	15%	6%

* Frequencies of adverse reactions are based on all treatment-emergent adverse events, attributed to study drugs.
† Rash event includes dermatitis, drug eruption, eczema, pruritus, pruritus generalized, rash, rash erythematous, rash generalized, rash macular, rash maculo-papular, rash morbilliform, rash popular, rash pruritic, and urticaria.

See *Warnings and Precautions (5.3)*, for a discussion of renal adverse events from clinical trials experience with STRIBILD.

Emtricitabine and Tenofovir Disoproxil Fumarate; In addition to the adverse drug reactions observed with STRIBILD, the following adverse drug reactions occurred in at least 5% of treatment-experienced or treatment-naive subjects receiving emtricitabine or tenofovir DF with other antiretroviral agents in other clinical trials: depression, abdominal pain, dyspepsia, vomiting, fever, pain, nasopharyngitis, pneumonia, sinusitis, upper respiratory tract infection, arthralgia, back pain, myalgia, paresthesia, peripheral neuropathy (including peripheral neuritis and neuropathy), anxiety, increased cough, and rhinitis.

Skin discoloration has been reported with higher frequency among emtricitabine-treated subjects; it was manifested by hyperpigmentation on the palms and/or soles and was generally mild and asymptomatic. The mechanism and clinical significance are unknown.

Laboratory Abnormalities: The frequency of treatment-emergent laboratory abnormalities (Grades 3–4) occurring in at least 2% of subjects receiving STRIBILD in Studies 102 and 103 are presented in Table 3.

Table 3 Laboratory Abnormalities (Grades 3–4) Reported in ≥ 2% of Subjects Receiving STRIBILD in Studies 102 and 103 (Week 48 analysis)

	STRIBILD	ATRIPLA	Atazanavir + ritonavir + TRUVADA
Laboratory Parameter Abnormality	N=701	N=352	N=355
AST (>5.0 × ULN)	2%	3%	4%
Amylase* (>2.0 × ULN)	2%	2%	4%
Creatine Kinase (≥ 10.0 × ULN)	5%	11%	7%
Urine RBC (Hematuria) (> 75 RBC/HPF)	3%	1%	2%

* For subjects with serum amylase > 1.5 × upper limit of normal, lipase test was also performed. The frequency of increased lipase (Grades 3–4) occurring in STRIBILD (N=58), ATRIPLA (N=33), and atazanavir + ritonavir + TRUVADA (N=33) was 12%, 15%, and 21%, respectively.

Proteinuria (all grades) occurred in 39% of subjects receiving STRIBILD, 29% of subjects receiving ATRIPLA, and 24% of subjects receiving atazanavir + ritonavir + TRUVADA.

The cobicistat component of STRIBILD has been shown to increase serum creatinine and decrease estimated creatinine clearance due to inhibition of tubular secretion of creatinine without affecting renal glomerular function. In Studies 102 and 103, increases in serum creatinine and decreases in estimated creatinine clearance occurred early in treatment with STRIBILD, after which they stabilized. The mean ± SD change in serum creatinine after 48 weeks of treatment was 0.14 mg per dL ± 0.13 mg per dL for STRIBILD, 0.01 mg per dL ± 0.12 mg per dL for ATRIPLA, and 0.09 mg per dL ± 0.13 mg per dL for atazanavir + ritonavir + TRUVADA. The mean ± SD change in estimated glomerular filtration rate (eGFR) by Cockcroft-Gault method after 48 weeks of treatment was -13.9 ± 14.9 mL per min for STRIBILD, -1.6 ± 16.5 mL per min for ATRIPLA, and -9.3 ± 15.8 mL per min for atazanavir + ritonavir + TRUVADA. Elevation in serum creatinine (all grades) occurred in 7% of subjects receiving STRIBILD, 1% of subjects receiving ATRIPLA, and 4% of subjects receiving atazanavir + ritonavir + TRUVADA.

Emtricitabine or Tenofovir Disoproxil Fumarate: In addition to the laboratory abnormalities observed with STRIBILD, the following laboratory abnormalities have been previously reported in subjects treated with emtricitabine or tenofovir DF with other antiretroviral agents in other clinical trials: Grades 3 or 4 laboratory abnormalities of ALT (M: greater than 215 U per L; F: greater than 170 U per L), alkaline phosphatase (greater than 550 U per L), bilirubin (greater than 2.5 × ULN), serum glucose (less than 40 or greater than 250 mg per dL), glycosuria (greater than or equal to 3+), neutrophils (less than 750 per mm^3), fasting cholesterol (greater than 240 mg per dL), and fasting triglycerides (greater than 750 mg per dL).

Serum Lipids: In the clinical trials of STRIBILD, a similar percentage of subjects receiving STRIBILD, ATRIPLA, and atazanavir + ritonavir + TRUVADA were on lipid lowering agents at baseline (11%, 11%, and 12%, respectively). While receiving study drug through Week 48, an additional 4% of STRIBILD subjects were started on lipid lowering agents, compared to 5% of ATRIPLA and 7% of atazanavir + ritonavir + TRUVADA subjects. During the first 48 weeks of study drug exposure, 1% or fewer subjects in any treatment arm experienced Grades 3 or 4 elevations in fasting cholesterol (greater than 300 mg per dL) or fasting triglycerides (greater than 750 mg per dL).

Changes from baseline in total cholesterol, HDL-cholesterol, LDL-cholesterol, and triglycerides are presented in Table 4.

[See table 4 above]

Table 4 Lipid Values, Mean Change from Baseline, Reported in Subjects Receiving STRIBILD or Comparator in Studies 102 and 103

	STRIBILD N=701		ATRIPLA N=352		Atazanavir + ritonavir + TRUVADA N=355	
	Baseline mg/dL	Week 48 Change*	Baseline mg/dL	Week 48 Change*	Baseline mg/dL	Week 48 Change*
Total Cholesterol (fasted)	166 [N=675]	+11 [N=606]	161 [N=343]	+19 [N=298]	168 [N=337]	+9 [N=287]
HDL-cholesterol (fasted)	43 [N=675]	+6 [N=605]	43 [N=343]	+8 [N=298]	42 [N=335]	+5 [N=284]
LDL-cholesterol (fasted)	100 [N=675]	+10 [N=606]	97 [N=343]	+17 [N=298]	101 [N=337]	+11 [N=288]
Triglycerides (fasted)	122 [N=675]	+13 [N=606]	121 [N=343]	+13 [N=298]	132 [N=337]	+29 [N=287]

* The change from baseline is the mean of within-patient changes from baseline for patients with both baseline and Week 48 values.

6.2 Postmarketing Experience

Because postmarketing reactions are reported voluntarily from a population of uncertain size, it is not always possible to reliably estimate their frequency or establish a causal relationship to drug exposure. The following adverse reactions have been identified during post approval use of tenofovir DF. No additional postmarketing adverse reactions specific for emtricitabine have been identified.

Immune System Disorders
allergic reaction, including angioedema
Metabolism and Nutrition Disorders
lactic acidosis, hypokalemia, hypophosphatemia
Respiratory, Thoracic, and Mediastinal Disorders
dyspnea
Gastrointestinal Disorders
pancreatitis, increased amylase, abdominal pain
Hepatobiliary Disorders
hepatic steatosis, hepatitis, increased liver enzymes (most commonly AST, ALT gamma GT)
Skin and Subcutaneous Tissue Disorders
rash
Musculoskeletal and Connective Tissue Disorders
rhabdomyolysis, osteomalacia (manifested as bone pain and which may contribute to fractures), muscular weakness, myopathy
Renal and Urinary Disorders
acute renal failure, renal failure, acute tubular necrosis, Fanconi syndrome, proximal renal tubulopathy, interstitial nephritis (including acute cases), nephrogenic diabetes insipidus, renal insufficiency, increased creatinine, proteinuria, polyuria
General Disorders and Administration Site Conditions
asthenia

The following adverse reactions, listed under the body system headings above, may occur as a consequence of proximal renal tubulopathy: rhabdomyolysis, osteomalacia, hypokalemia, muscular weakness, myopathy, hypophosphatemia.

7 DRUG INTERACTIONS

See also *Contraindications (4)* and *Clinical Pharmacology (12.3)*.

STRIBILD is a complete regimen for the treatment of HIV-1 infection; therefore, STRIBILD should not be administered with other antiretroviral medications for treatment of HIV-1 infection. Complete information regarding potential drug-drug interactions with other antiretroviral medications is not provided.

STRIBILD should not be used in conjunction with protease inhibitors or non-nucleoside reverse transcriptase inhibitors due to potential drug-drug interactions including altered and/or suboptimal pharmacokinetics of cobicistat, elvitegravir, and/or the coadministered antiretroviral products. STRIBILD should not be administered concurrently with products containing ritonavir or regimens containing ritonavir due to similar effects of cobicistat and ritonavir on CYP3A.

7.1 Potential for STRIBILD to Affect Other Drugs

Cobicistat, a component of STRIBILD, is an inhibitor of CYP3A and CYP2D6. The transporters that cobicistat inhibits include p-glycoprotein (P-gp), BCRP, OATP1B1 and OATP1B3. Thus, coadministration of STRIBILD with drugs that are primarily metabolized by CYP3A or CYP2D6, or are substrates of P-gp, BCRP, OATP1B1 or OATP1B3 may result in increased plasma concentrations of such drugs. Elvitegravir is a modest inducer of CYP2C9 and may decrease the plasma concentrations of CYP2C9 substrates.

7.2 Potential for Other Drugs to Affect One or More Components of STRIBILD

Elvitegravir and cobicistat, components of STRIBILD, are metabolized by CYP3A. Cobicistat is also metabolized, to a minor extent, by CYP2D6.

Drugs that induce CYP3A activity are expected to increase the clearance of elvitegravir and cobicistat, resulting in decreased plasma concentration of cobicistat and elvitegravir, which may lead to loss of therapeutic effect of STRIBILD and development of resistance (see Table 5).

Coadministration of STRIBILD with other drugs that inhibit CYP3A may decrease the clearance and increase the plasma concentration of cobicistat (see Table 5).

7.3 Drugs Affecting Renal Function

Because emtricitabine and tenofovir, components of STRIBILD are primarily excreted by the kidneys by a combination of glomerular filtration and active tubular secretion, coadministration of STRIBILD with drugs that reduce renal function or compete for active tubular secretion may increase concentrations of emtricitabine, tenofovir, and other renally eliminated drugs. Some examples of drugs that are eliminated by active tubular secretion include, but are not limited to acyclovir, cidofovir, ganciclovir, valacyclovir, and valganciclovir.

7.4 Established and Other Potentially Significant Interactions

Table 5 provides a listing of established or potentially clinically significant drug-drug interactions. The drug interactions described are based on studies conducted with either STRIBILD, the components of STRIBILD, (elvitegravir, cobicistat, emtricitabine, and tenofovir DF) as individual agents and/or in combination, or are predicted drug interactions that may occur with STRIBILD [for magnitude of in-

Table 5 Established and Other Potentially Significant* Drug Interactions: Alteration in Dose or Regimen May Be Recommended Based on Drug Interaction Studies or Predicted Interaction

Concomitant Drug Class: Drug Name	Effect on Concentration†	Clinical Comment
Acid Reducing Agents: Antacids‡ (for example aluminum and magnesium hydroxide) **Proton Pump Inhibitors** H_2 Receptor Antagonists	↓ elvitegravir ⇔ elvitegravir	Elvitegravir plasma concentrations are lower when STRIBILD is administered simultaneously with antacids. It is recommended to separate STRIBILD and antacid administration by at least 2 hours. No dose adjustment is needed when STRIBILD is combined with either H_2 receptor antagonists or proton pump inhibitors.
Antiarrhythmics: e.g. amiodarone bepridil digoxin‡ disopyramide flecainide systemic lidocaine mexiletine propafenone quinidine	↑ antiarrhythmics ↑ digoxin	Concentrations of these antiarrhythmic drugs may be increased when coadministered with STRIBILD. Caution is warranted and therapeutic concentration monitoring, if available, is recommended for antiarrhythmics when coadministered with STRIBILD.
Antibacterials: clarithromycin telithromycin	↑ clarithromycin ↑ telithromycin ↑ cobicistat	Concentrations of clarithromycin and/or cobicistat may be altered when clarithromycin is coadministered with STRIBILD. <u>Patients with CLcr greater than or equal to 60 mL/min:</u> No dose adjustment of clarithromycin is required. <u>Patients with CLcr between 50 mL/min and 60 mL/min:</u> The dose of clarithromycin should be reduced by 50%. Concentrations of telithromycin and/or cobicistat may be increased when telithromycin is coadministered with STRIBILD.
Anticoagulants: warfarin	Effect on warfarin unknown	Concentrations of warfarin may be affected upon coadministration with STRIBILD. It is recommended that the international normalized ratio (INR) be monitored upon coadministration with STRIBILD.
Anticonvulsants: carbamazepine oxcarbazepine phenobarbital phenytoin	↑ carbamazepine ↓ elvitegravir ↓ cobicistat	Coadministration of carbamazepine, oxcarbazepine, phenobarbital, or phenytoin with STRIBILD may significantly decrease cobicistat and elvitegravir plasma concentrations, which may result in loss of therapeutic effect and development of resistance. Alternative anticonvulsants should be considered.
clonazepam ethosuximide	↑ clonazepam ↑ ethosuximide	Concentrations of clonazepam and ethosuximide may be increased when coadministered with STRIBILD. Clinical monitoring is recommended upon coadministration with STRIBILD.
Antidepressants: Selective Serotonin Reuptake Inhibitors (SSRIs) e.g. paroxetine Tricyclic Antidepressants (TCAs) e.g. amitriptyline desipramine imipramine nortriptyline buproprion trazodone	↑ SSRIs ↑ TCAs ↑ trazodone	Concentrations of these antidepressant agents may be increased when coadministered with STRIBILD. Careful dose titration of the antidepressant and monitoring for antidepressant response is recommended.
Antifungals: itraconazole ketoconazole‡ voriconazole	↑ elvitegravir ↑ cobicistat ↑ itraconazole ↑ ketoconazole ↑voriconazole	Concentrations of ketoconazole, itraconazole and voriconazole may increase upon coadministration with STRIBILD. When administering with STRIBILD, the maximum daily dose of ketoconazole or itraconazole should not exceed 200 mg per day. An assessment of benefit/risk ratio is recommended to justify use of voriconazole with STRIBILD.

(Table continued on next page)

teraction, see *Clinical Pharmacology (12.3)*]. The table includes potentially significant interactions but is not all inclusive.

[See table 5 above and on pages 886 and 887]

7.5 Drugs without Clinically Significant Interactions with STRIBILD

Based on drug interaction studies conducted with the components of STRIBILD, no clinically significant drug interactions have been either observed or are expected when STRIBILD is combined with the following drugs: entecavir, famciclovir, and ribavirin.

8 USE IN SPECIFIC POPULATIONS

8.1 Pregnancy

Pregnancy Category B

There are no adequate and well-controlled studies in pregnant women. Because animal reproduction studies are not always predictive of human response, STRIBILD should be used during pregnancy only if the potential benefit justifies the potential risk to the fetus.

Antiretroviral Pregnancy Registry: To monitor fetal outcomes of pregnant women exposed to STRIBILD, an Antiretroviral Pregnancy Registry has been established. Healthcare providers are encouraged to register patients by calling 1-800-258-4263.

<u>Animal Data</u>

Elvitegravir: Studies in animals have shown no evidence of teratogenicity or an effect on reproductive function. In offspring from rat and rabbit dams treated with elvitegravir during pregnancy, there were no toxicologically significant effects on developmental endpoints. The exposures (AUC) at the embryo-fetal No Observed Adverse Effects Levels (NOAELs) in rats and rabbits were respectively 23 and 0.2 times higher than the exposure in humans at the recommended daily dose of 150 mg.

Cobicistat: Studies in animals have shown no evidence of teratogenicity or an effect on reproductive function. In offspring from rat and rabbit dams treated with cobicistat during pregnancy, there were no toxicologically significant effects on developmental endpoints. The exposures (AUC) at the embryo-fetal NOAELs in rats and rabbits were respectively 1.8 and 4.3 times higher than the exposure in humans at the recommended daily dose of 150 mg.

Emtricitabine: The incidence of fetal variations and malformations was not increased in embryofetal toxicity studies performed with emtricitabine in mice at exposures (AUC) approximately 60 times higher and in rabbits at approximately 120 times higher than human exposures at the recommended daily dose.

Tenofovir Disoproxil Fumarate: Reproduction studies have been performed in rats and rabbits at doses up to 14 and 19 times the human dose based on body surface area comparisons and revealed no evidence of impaired fertility or harm to the fetus due to tenofovir.

8.3 Nursing Mothers

The Centers for Disease Control and Prevention recommend that HIV infected mothers not breastfeed their infants to avoid risking postnatal transmission of HIV. Studies in rats have demonstrated that elvitegravir, cobicistat, and tenofovir are secreted in milk. It is not known whether elvitegravir or cobicistat is excreted in human milk.

In humans, samples of breast milk obtained from five HIV-1 infected mothers show that emtricitabine is secreted in human milk. Breastfeeding infants whose mothers are being treated with emtricitabine may be at risk for developing viral resistance to emtricitabine. Other emtricitabine-associated risks in infants breastfed by mothers being treated with emtricitabine are unknown.

Samples of breast milk obtained from five HIV-1 infected mothers show that tenofovir is secreted in human milk. Tenofovir-associated risks, including the risk of viral resistance to tenofovir, in infants breastfed by mothers being treated with tenofovir disoproxil fumarate are unknown.

Because of both the potential for HIV transmission and the potential for serious adverse reactions in nursing infants, **mothers should be instructed not to breastfeed if they are receiving STRIBILD.**

8.4 Pediatric Use

Safety and effectiveness of STRIBILD in pediatric patients less than 18 years of age have not been established *[See Clinical Pharmacology (12.3)]*.

8.5 Geriatric Use

Clinical studies of STRIBILD did not include sufficient numbers of subjects aged 65 and over to determine whether they respond differently from younger subjects. In general, dose selection for the elderly patients should be cautious, keeping in mind the greater frequency of decreased hepatic, renal, or cardiac function, and of concomitant disease or other drug therapy *[See Clinical Pharmacology (12.3)]*.

8.6 Renal Impairment

STRIBILD should not be initiated in patients with estimated creatinine clearance below 70 mL per min. Because STRIBILD is a fixed-dose combination tablet, STRIBILD should be discontinued if estimated creatinine clearance declines below 50 mL per min during treatment with STRIBILD as dose interval adjustment required for emtricitabine and tenofovir DF cannot be achieved *[See Warnings and Precautions (5.3), Adverse Reactions (6.1), Clinical Pharmacology (12.3), and Clinical Studies (14)]*.

8.7 Hepatic Impairment

No dose adjustment of STRIBILD is required in patients with mild (Child-Pugh Class A) or moderate (Child-Pugh Class B) hepatic impairment. No pharmacokinetic or safety data are available regarding the use of STRIBILD in patients with severe hepatic impairment (Child-Pugh Class C). Therefore, STRIBILD is not recommended for use in patients with severe hepatic impairment *[See Dosage and Administration (2) and Clinical Pharmacology (12.3)]*.

10 OVERDOSAGE

If overdose occurs the patient must be monitored for evidence of toxicity. Treatment of overdose with STRIBILD consists of general supportive measures including monitoring of vital signs as well as observation of the clinical status of the patient.

Elvitegravir: Limited clinical experience is available at doses higher than the therapeutic dose of elvitegravir. In one study, boosted elvitegravir equivalent to 2 times the therapeutic dose of 150 mg once daily for 10 days was administered to 42 healthy subjects. No severe adverse reactions were reported. The effects of higher doses are not known. As elvitegravir is highly bound to plasma proteins, it is unlikely that it will be significantly removed by hemodialysis or peritoneal dialysis.

Table 5 *(cont.)* Established and Other Potentially Significant* Drug Interactions: Alteration in Dose or Regimen May Be Recommended Based on Drug Interaction Studies or Predicted Interaction

Concomitant Drug Class: Drug Name	Effect on Concentration†	Clinical Comment
Anti-gout: colchicine	↑ colchicine	STRIBILD should not be coadministered with colchicine to patients with renal or hepatic impairment. Treatment of gout-flares – coadministration of colchicine in patients receiving STRIBILD: 0.6 mg (1 tablet) × 1 dose, followed by 0.3 mg (half tablet) 1 hour later. Treatment course to be repeated no earlier than 3 days. Prophylaxis of gout-flares – coadministration of colchicine in patients receiving STRIBILD: If the original regimen was 0.6 mg twice a day, the regimen should be adjusted to 0.3 mg once a day. If the original regimen was 0.6 mg once a day, the regimen should be adjusted to 0.3 mg once every other day. Treatment of familial Mediterranean fever – coadministration of colchicine in patients receiving STRIBILD: Maximum daily dose of 0.6 mg (may be given as 0.3 mg twice a day).
Antimycobacterial: rifabutin‡ rifapentine	↓ elvitegravir ↓ cobicistat	Coadministration of rifabutin and rifapentine with STRIBILD may significantly decrease elvitegravir and cobicistat plasma concentrations, which may result in loss of therapeutic effect and development of resistance. Coadministration of STRIBILD with rifabutin or rifapentine is not recommended.
Beta-Blockers: e.g. metoprolol timolol	↑ beta-blockers	Concentrations of beta-blockers may be increased when coadministered with STRIBILD. Clinical monitoring is recommended and a dose decrease of the beta blocker may be necessary when these agents are coadministered with STRIBILD.
Calcium Channel Blockers: e.g. amlodipine diltiazem felodipine nicardipine nifedipine verapamil	↑ calcium channel blockers	Concentrations of calcium channel blockers may be increased when coadministered with STRIBILD. Caution is warranted and clinical monitoring is recommended upon coadministration with STRIBILD.
Corticosteroid: Systemic: dexamethasone	↓ elvitegravir ↓ cobicistat	Systemic dexamethasone, a CYP3A inducer, may significantly decrease elvitegravir and cobicistat plasma concentrations, which may result in loss of therapeutic effect and development of resistance.
Corticosteroid: Inhaled/Nasal: fluticasone	↑ fluticasone	Concomitant use of inhaled or nasal fluticasone and STRIBILD may increase plasma concentrations of fluticasone, resulting in reduced serum cortisol concentrations. Alternative corticosteroids should be considered, particularly for long term use.
Endothelin Receptor Antagonists: bosentan	↑ bosentan	Coadministration of bosentan in patients on STRIBILD: In patients who have been receiving STRIBILD for at least 10 days, start bosentan at 62.5 mg once daily or every other day based upon individual tolerability. Coadministration of STRIBILD in patients on bosentan: Discontinue use of bosentan at least 36 hours prior to initiation of STRIBILD. After at least 10 days following the initiation of STRIBILD, resume bosentan at 62.5 mg once daily or every other day based upon individual tolerability.
HMG-CoA Reductase Inhibitors: atorvastatin	↑ atorvastatin	Initiate with the lowest starting dose of atorvastatin and titrate carefully while monitoring for safety.

(Table continued on next page)

Cobicistat: Limited clinical experience is available at doses higher than the therapeutic dose of cobicistat. In two studies, a single dose of cobicistat 400 mg was administered to a total of 60 healthy subjects. No severe adverse reactions were reported. The effects of higher doses are not known. As cobicistat is highly bound to plasma proteins, it is unlikely that it will be significantly removed by hemodialysis or peritoneal dialysis.

Emtricitabine: Limited clinical experience is available at doses higher than the therapeutic dose of EMTRIVA. In one clinical pharmacology study, single doses of emtricitabine 1200 mg were administered to 11 subjects. No severe adverse reactions were reported. The effects of higher doses are not known.

Hemodialysis treatment removes approximately 30% of the emtricitabine dose over a 3 hour dialysis period starting within 1.5 hours of emtricitabine dosing (blood flow rate of 400 mL per minute and a dialysate flow rate of 600 mL per minute). It is not known whether emtricitabine can be removed by peritoneal dialysis.

Tenofovir Disoproxil Fumarate: Limited clinical experience at doses higher than the therapeutic dose of VIREAD 300 mg is available. In one study, 600 mg tenofovir DF was administered to 8 subjects orally for 28 days, and no severe adverse reactions were reported. The effects of higher doses are not known. Tenofovir is efficiently removed by hemodialysis with an extraction coefficient of approximately 54%. Following a single 300 mg dose of VIREAD, a 4-hour hemodialysis session removed approximately 10% of the administered tenofovir dose.

11 DESCRIPTION

STRIBILD is a fixed-dose combination tablet containing elvitegravir, cobicistat, emtricitabine, and tenofovir DF. Elvitegravir is a HIV-1 integrase strand transfer inhibitor. Cobicistat is a mechanism-based inhibitor of cytochrome P450 (CYP) enzymes of the CYP3A family. Tenofovir DF is converted *in vivo* to tenofovir, an acyclic nucleoside phosphonate (nucleotide) analog of adenosine 5′-monophosphate. VIREAD is the brand name for tenofovir DF. Emtricitabine is a synthetic nucleoside analog of cytidine. EMTRIVA is the brand name for emtricitabine.

STRIBILD tablets are for oral administration. Each tablet contains 150 mg of elvitegravir, 150 mg of cobicistat, 200 mg of emtricitabine, and 300 mg of tenofovir DF (equivalent to 245 mg of tenofovir disoproxil). The tablets include the following inactive ingredients: lactose monohydrate, microcrystalline cellulose, silicon dioxide, croscarmellose sodium, hydroxypropyl cellulose, sodium lauryl sulfate, and magnesium stearate. The tablets are film-coated with a coating material containing indigo carmine (FD&C Blue #2) aluminum lake, polyethylene glycol, polyvinyl alcohol, talc, titanium dioxide, and yellow iron oxide.

Elvitegravir: The chemical name of elvitegravir is 6-(3-Chloro-2-fluorobenzyl)-1-[(2*S*)-1-hydroxy-3-methylbutan-2-yl]-7-methoxy-4-oxo-1,4-dihydroquinoline-3-carboxylic acid. It has a molecular formula of $C_{23}H_{23}ClFNO_5$ and a molecular weight of 447.9. It has the following structural formula:

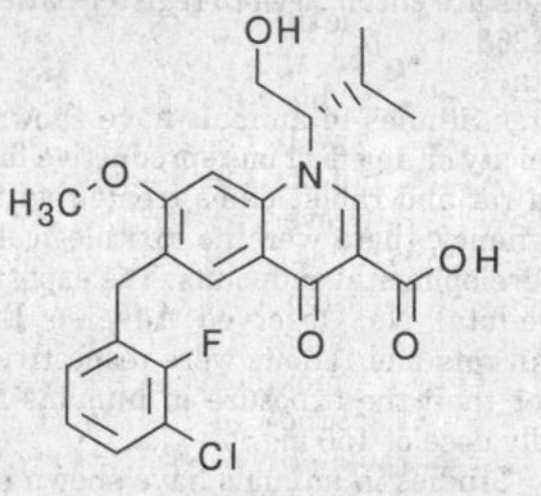

Elvitegravir is a white to pale yellow powder with a solubility of less than 0.3 micrograms per mL in water at 20 °C.

Cobicistat: The chemical name for cobicistat is 1,3-thiazol-5-ylmethyl [(2*R*,5*R*)-5-{[(2*S*)-2-[(methyl{[2-(propan-2-yl)-1,3-thiazol-4-yl]methyl}carbamoyl)amino]-4-(morpholin-4-yl)-butanoyl]amino}-1,6-diphenylhexan-2-yl]carbamate.

It has a molecular formula of $C_{40}H_{53}N_7O_5S_2$ and a molecular weight of 776.0. It has the following structural formula:

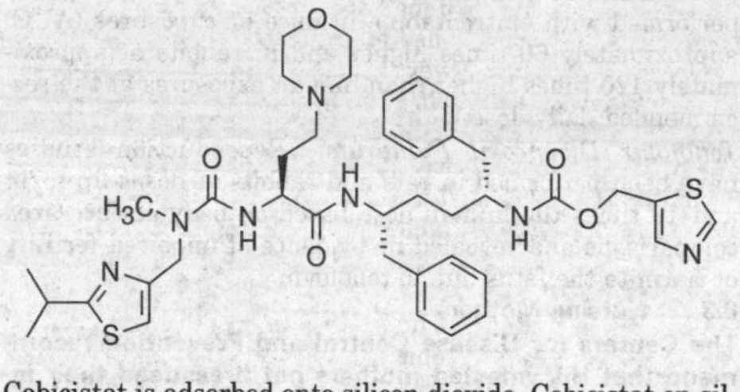

Cobicistat is adsorbed onto silicon dioxide. Cobicistat on silicon dioxide is a white to pale yellow solid with a solubility of 0.1 mg per mL in water at 20 °C.

Emtricitabine: The chemical name of emtricitabine is 5-fluoro-1-[(2*R*,5*S*)-2-(hydroxymethyl)-1,3-oxathiolan-5-yl]-cytosine. Emtricitabine is the (-)enantiomer of a thio analog of cytidine, which differs from other cytidine analogs in that it has a fluorine in the 5-position.

It has a molecular formula of $C_8H_{10}FN_3O_3S$ and a molecular weight of 247.25. It has the following structural formula:

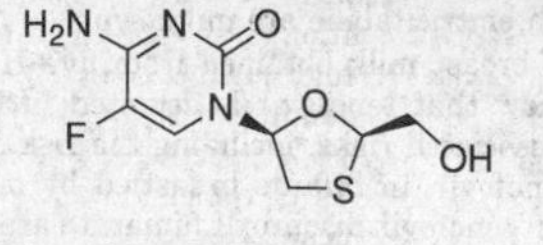

Emtricitabine is a white to off-white crystalline powder with a solubility of approximately 112 mg per mL in water at 25 °C.

Tenofovir Disoproxil Fumarate: Tenofovir DF is a fumaric acid salt of the bis-isopropoxycarbonyloxymethyl ester derivative of tenofovir. The chemical name of tenofovir DF is 9-[(*R*)-2-[[bis[[(isopropoxycarbonyl)oxy]-methoxy]phosphinyl]methoxy]propyl]adenine fumarate (1:1). It has a molecular formula of $C_{19}H_{30}N_5O_{10}P \bullet C_4H_4O_4$ and a molecular weight of 635.51. It has the following structural formula:

[See chemical structure at top of next column]

Tenofovir DF is a white to off-white crystalline powder with a solubility of 13.4 mg per mL in water at 25 °C. All dosages are expressed in terms of tenofovir DF except where otherwise noted.

12 CLINICAL PHARMACOLOGY

12.1 Mechanism of Action

STRIBILD is a fixed-dose combination of antiviral drugs elvitegravir boosted by the pharmacokinetic enhancer cobicistat, emtricitabine, and tenofovir DF *[See Microbiology (12.4)]*.

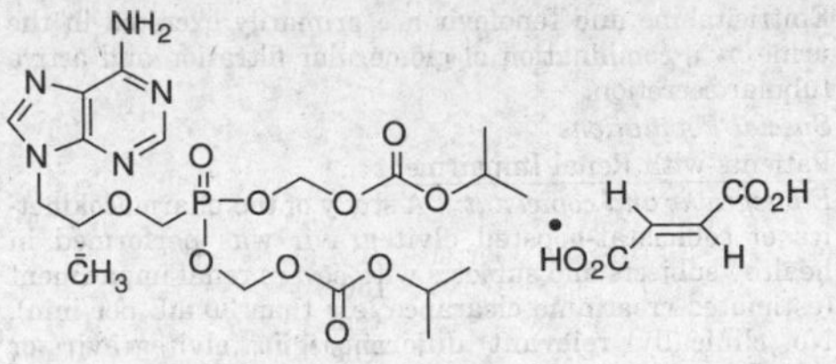

12.2 Pharmacodynamics

Effects on Electrocardiogram

Thorough QT studies have been conducted for elvitegravir and cobicistat. The effect of the other two components, tenofovir and emtricitabine, or the combination regimen STRIBILD on the QT interval is not known.

The effect of multiple doses of elvitegravir 125 and 250 mg (coadministered with 100 mg ritonavir) on QTc interval was evaluated in a randomized, placebo- and active-controlled (moxifloxacin 400 mg) parallel group thorough QT study in 126 healthy subjects. In a study with demonstrated ability to detect small effects, the upper bound of the one-sided 95% confidence interval for the largest placebo adjusted, baseline-corrected QTc based on Fridericia's correction method (QTcF) was below 10 ms, the threshold for regulatory concern. The dose of 250 mg elvitegravir (with 100 mg ritonavir) is expected to cover the high exposure clinical scenario.

The effect of a single dose of cobicistat 250 mg and 400 mg on QTc interval was evaluated in a randomized, placebo- and active-controlled (moxifloxacin 400 mg) four-period crossover thorough QT study in 48 healthy subjects. In a study with demonstrated ability to detect small effects, the upper bound of the one-sided 95% confidence interval for the largest placebo adjusted, baseline-corrected QTc based on individual correction method (QTc) was below 10 ms, the threshold for regulatory concern. The dose of 400 mg cobicistat is expected to cover the high exposure clinical scenario. Prolongation of the PR interval was noted in subjects receiving cobicistat in the same study. The maximum mean (95% upper confidence bound) difference in PR from placebo after baseline-correction was 9.5 (12.1) ms for 250 mg dose and 20.2 (22.8) for 400 mg dose cobicistat. Because the 150 mg cobicistat dose used in the STRIBILD fixed-dose combination tablet is lower than the lowest dose studied in the thorough QT study, it is unlikely that treatment with STRIBILD will result in clinically relevant PR prolongation.

12.3 Pharmacokinetics

Pharmacokinetics in Adults

Absorption and Bioavailability

STRIBILD: Following oral administration of STRIBILD with food in HIV-1 infected subjects, peak plasma concentrations were observed 4 hours post-dose for elvitegravir, 3 hours post-dose for cobicistat, 3 hours post-dose for emtricitabine, and 2 hours for tenofovir following the rapid conversion of tenofovir DF (see Table 6 for additional pharmacokinetic parameters).

[See table 6 at top of next page]

Effect of Food on Oral Absorption

Relative to fasting conditions, the administration of single dose STRIBILD with a light meal (~373 kcal, 20% fat) increased the mean systemic exposure of elvitegravir and tenofovir by 34% and 24%, respectively. The alterations in mean systemic exposures of cobicistat and emtricitabine were not clinically significant.

Relative to fasting conditions, the administration of single dose STRIBILD with a high fat meal (~ 800 kcal, 50% fat) increased the mean systemic exposure of elvitegravir and tenofovir by 87% and 23%, respectively. The alterations in mean systemic exposures of cobicistat and emtricitabine were not clinically significant.

STRIBILD should be taken with food.

Distribution

Elvitegravir: Elvitegravir is 98–99% bound to human plasma proteins and binding is independent of drug concentration over the range of 1 ng per mL to 1.6 micrograms per mL. The mean blood-to-plasma ratio was 0.73.

Cobicistat: Cobicistat is 97–98% bound to human plasma proteins and the mean blood-to-plasma ratio was approximately 0.5.

Emtricitabine: *In vitro* binding of emtricitabine to human plasma proteins is less than 4% and is independent of drug concentration over the range of 0.02–200 micrograms per mL.

Tenofovir Disoproxil Fumarate: *In vitro* binding of tenofovir to human plasma proteins is less than 0.7% and is independent of concentration over the range of 0.01–25 micrograms per mL.

Metabolism

Elvitegravir: The majority of elvitegravir metabolism is mediated by CYP3A enzymes. Elvitegravir also undergoes glucuronidation via UGT1A1/3 enzymes.

Table 5 *(cont.)* Established and Other Potentially Significant* Drug Interactions: Alteration in Dose or Regimen May Be Recommended Based on Drug Interaction Studies or Predicted Interaction

Concomitant Drug Class: Drug Name	Effect on Concentration†	Clinical Comment
Hormonal Contraceptives: norgestimate/ethinyl estradiol‡	↑ norgestimate ↓ ethinyl estradiol	The effects of increases in the concentration of the progestational component norgestimate are not fully known and can include increased risk of insulin resistance, dyslipidemia, acne, and venous thrombosis. The potential risks and benefits associated with coadministration of norgestimate/ethinyl estradiol with STRIBILD should be considered, particularly in women who have risk factors for these events. Coadministration of STRIBILD with other hormonal contraceptives (e.g., contraceptive patch, contraceptive vaginal ring, or injectable contraceptives) or oral contraceptives containing progestogens other than norgestimate has not been studied; therefore, alternative (non hormonal) methods of contraception can be considered.
Immuno-suppressants: e.g. cyclosporine sirolimus tacrolimus	↑ immuno-suppressants	Concentrations of these immunosuppressant agents may be increased when coadministered with STRIBILD. Therapeutic monitoring of the immunosuppressive agents is recommended upon coadministration with STRIBILD.
Inhaled Beta Agonist: salmeterol	↑ salmeterol	Coadministration of salmeterol and STRIBILD is not recommended. Coadministration of salmeterol with STRIBILD may result in increased risk of cardiovascular adverse events associated with salmeterol, including QT prolongation, palpitations, and sinus tachycardia.
Neuroleptics: e.g. perphenazine risperidone thioridazine	↑ neuroleptics	A decrease in dose of the neuroleptic may be needed when coadministered with STRIBILD.
Phosphodiesterase-5 (PDE5) Inhibitors: sildenafil tadalafil vardenafil	↑ PDE5 inhibitors	Coadministration with STRIBILD may result in an increase in PDE-5 inhibitor associated adverse events, including hypotension, syncope, visual disturbances, and priapism. Use of PDE-5 inhibitors for pulmonary arterial hypertension (PAH): • Use of sildenafil is contraindicated when used for the treatment of pulmonary arterial hypertension (PAH). • The following dose adjustments are recommended for the use of tadalafil with STRIBILD: *Coadministration of tadalafil in patients on STRIBILD:* In patients receiving STRIBILD for at least 1 week, start tadalafil at 20 mg once daily. Increase tadalafil dose to 40 mg once daily based upon individual tolerability. *Coadministration of STRIBILD in patients on tadalafil:* Avoid use of tadalafil during the initiation of STRIBILD. Stop tadalafil at least 24 hours prior to starting STRIBILD. After at least one week following initiation of STRIBILD, resume tadalafil at 20 mg once daily. Increase tadalafil dose to 40 mg once daily based upon individual tolerability. Use of PDE-5 inhibitors for erectile dysfunction: Sildenafil at a single dose not exceeding 25 mg in 48 hours, vardenafil at a single dose not exceeding 2.5 mg in 72 hours, or tadalafil at a single dose not exceeding 10 mg in 72 hours can be used with increased monitoring for PDE-5 inhibitor associated with adverse events.
Sedative/hypnotics: Benzodiazepines: e.g. Parenterally administered midazolam clorazepate diazepam estazolam flurazepam buspirone zolpidem	↑ sedatives/hypnotics	Concomitant use of parenteral midazolam with STRIBILD may increase plasma concentrations of midazolam. Coadministration should be done in a setting that ensures close clinical monitoring and appropriate medical management in case of respiratory depression and/or prolonged sedation. Dosage reduction for midazolam should be considered, especially if more than a single dose of midazolam is administered. Coadministration of oral midazolam with STRIBILD is contraindicated. With other sedative/hypnotics, dose reduction may be necessary and clinical monitoring is recommended.

* This table is not all inclusive.
† ↑ = Increase, ↓ = Decrease, ⇔ = No Effect
‡ Indicates that a drug-drug interaction trial was conducted.

Cobicistat: Cobicistat is metabolized by CYP3A and to a minor extent by CYP2D6 enzymes and does not undergo glucuronidation.

Emtricitabine and tenofovir are not significantly metabolized.

Elimination

Elvitegravir: The median terminal plasma half-life of elvitegravir following administration of STRIBILD is approximately 12.9 hours. After single dose administration of [^{14}C] elvitegravir (coadministered with 100 mg ritonavir),

Table 6 Pharmacokinetic Parameters of Elvitegravir, Cobicistat, Emtricitabine, and Tenofovir Exposure Following Oral Administration of STRIBILD in HIV-Infected Subjects

Parameter Mean ± SD [range: min:max]	Elvitegravir*	Cobicistat†	Emtricitabine†	Tenofovir†
C_{max} (microgram per mL)	1.7 ± 0. 4 [0.4:3.7]	1.1 ± 0.4 [0.1:2.1]	1.9 ± 0.5 [0.6:3.6]	0.45 ± 0.2 [0.2:1.2]
AUC_{tau} (microgram•hour per mL)	23.0 ± 7.5 [4.4:69.8]	8.3 ± 3.8 [0.5:18.3]	12.7 ± 4.5 [5.2:34.1]	4.4 ± 2.2 [2.1:18.2]
C_{trough} (microgram per mL)	0.45 ± 0.26 [0.05:2.34]	0.05 ± 0.13 [0.01:0.92]	0.14 ± 0.25 [0.04:1.94]	0.10 ± 0.08 [0.04:0.58]

SD = Standard Deviation
* From Population Pharmacokinetic analysis, N=419.
† From Intensive Pharmacokinetic analysis, N=61–62, except cobicistat C_{trough} N=53.

Table 7 Drug Interactions: Changes in Pharmacokinetic Parameters for Elvitegravir in the Presence of the Coadministered Drug*

Coadministered Drug	Dose of Coadministered Drug (mg)	Elvitegravir Dose (mg)	Cobicistat or Ritonavir Booster Dose (mg)	N	Mean Ratio of Elvitegravir Pharmacokinetic Parameters (90% CI); No effect = 1.00		
					C_{max}	AUC	C_{min}
Antacids	20 mL single dose given 4 hours before elvitegravir	50 single dose	Ritonavir 100 single dose	8	0.95 (0.84,1.07)	0.96 (0.88,1.04)	1.04 (0.93,1.17)
	20 mL single dose given 4 hours after elvitegravir			10	0.98 (0.88,1.10)	0.98 (0.91,1.06)	1.00 (0.90,1.11)
	20 mL single dose given 2 hours before elvitegravir			11	0.82 (0.74,0.91)	0.85 (0.79,0.91)	0.90 (0.82,0.99)
	20 mL single dose given 2 hours after elvitegravir			10	0.79 (0.71,0.88)	0.80 (0.75,0.86)	0.80 (0.73,0.89)
Famotidine	40 once daily given 12 hours after elvitegravir	150 once daily	Cobicistat 150 once daily	10	1.02 (0.89,1.17)	1.03 (0.95,1.13)	1.18 (1.05,1.32)
	40 once daily given simultaneously with elvitegravir			16	1.00 (0.92,1.10)	1.03 (0.98,1.08)	1.07 (0.98,1.17)
Ketoconazole	200 twice daily	150 once daily	Ritonavir 100 once daily	18	1.17 (1.04,1.33)	1.48 (1.36,1.62)	1.67 (1.48,1.88)
	40 once daily given 2 hours before elvitegravir	50 once daily	Ritonavir 100 once daily	9	0.93 (0.83,1.04)	0.99 (0.91,1.07)	0.94 (0.85,1.04)
Omeprazole	20 once daily given 2 hours before elvitegravir	150 once daily	Cobicistat 150 once daily	11	1.16 (1.04,1.30)	1.10 (1.02,1.19)	1.13 (0.96,1.34)
	20 once daily given 12 hours after elvitegravir			11	1.03 (0.92,1.15)	1.05 (0.93,1.18)	1.10 (0.92,1.32)
Rifabutin	150 once every other day	150 once daily	Cobicistat 150 once daily	12	0.91 (0.84,0.99)	0.79 (0.74,0.85)	0.33 (0.27,0.40)
Rosuvastatin	10 single dose	150 once daily	Cobicistat 150 once daily	10	0.94 (0.83,1.07)	1.02 (0.91,1.14)	0.98 (0.83,1.16)

* All interaction studies conducted in healthy volunteers.

94.8 % and 6.7 % of the administered dose was excreted in feces and urine, respectively.

Cobicistat: The median terminal plasma half-life of cobicistat following administration of STRIBILD is approximately 3.5 hours. With single dose administration of [^{14}C] cobicistat after multiple dosing of cobicistat for six days, 86.2 % and 8.2 % of the administered dose was excreted in feces and urine, respectively.

Emtricitabine and tenofovir are primarily excreted in the urine by a combination of glomerular filtration and active tubular secretion.

Special Populations

Patients with Renal Impairment

Elvitegravir and cobicistat: A study of the pharmacokinetics of cobicistat-boosted elvitegravir was performed in healthy subjects and subjects with severe renal impairment (estimated creatinine clearance less than 30 mL per min). No clinically relevant differences in elvitegravir or cobicistat pharmacokinetics were observed between healthy subjects and subjects with severe renal impairment.

Emtricitabine and Tenofovir Disoproxil Fumarate: The pharmacokinetics of emtricitabine and tenofovir are altered in subjects with estimated creatinine clearance below 50 mL per min or with end stage renal disease requiring dialysis, *[See Warnings and Precautions (5.3) and Use in Specific Populations (8.6)]*.

Patients with Hepatic Impairment

Elvitegravir and cobicistat: A study of the pharmacokinetics of cobicistat-boosted elvitegravir was performed in healthy subjects and subjects with moderate hepatic impairment. No clinically relevant differences in elvitegravir or cobicistat pharmacokinetics were observed between subjects with moderate hepatic impairment (Child-Pugh Class B) and healthy subjects. No dosage adjustment of elvitegravir or cobicistat is necessary for patients with mild to moderate hepatic impairment. The effect of severe hepatic impairment (Child-Pugh Class C) on the pharmacokinetics of elvitegravir or cobicistat has not been studied *[See Use in Specific Populations (8.7)]*.

Emtricitabine: The pharmacokinetics of emtricitabine has not been studied in subjects with hepatic impairment; however, emtricitabine is not significantly metabolized by liver enzymes, so the impact of liver impairment should be limited.

Tenofovir Disoproxil Fumarate: The pharmacokinetics of tenofovir following a 300 mg dose of VIREAD has been studied in healthy subjects with moderate to severe hepatic impairment. No clinically relevant differences in tenofovir pharmacokinetics were observed between subjects with hepatic impairment and healthy subjects.

Hepatitis B and/or Hepatitis C Virus Co-infection

Elvitegravir: Limited data from population pharmacokinetic analysis (N=24) indicated that hepatitis B and/or C virus infection had no clinically relevant effect on the exposure of cobicistat boosted elvitegravir.

Cobicistat: There were insufficient pharmacokinetic data in the clinical trials to determine the effect of hepatitis B and/or C virus infection on the pharmacokinetics of cobicistat.

Emtricitabine and Tenofovir: Pharmacokinetics of emtricitabine and tenofovir DF have not been fully evaluated in subjects coinfected with hepatitis B and/or C virus.

Race

Elvitegravir: Population pharmacokinetic analysis of elvitegravir in HIV-1 infected subjects indicated that race had no clinically relevant effect on the exposure of cobicistat-boosted elvitegravir.

Cobicistat: There were insufficient pharmacokinetic data in the clinical trials to determine the effect of race on the pharmacokinetics of cobicistat.

Emtricitabine: No pharmacokinetic differences due to race have been identified following the administration of EMTRIVA.

Tenofovir Disoproxil Fumarate: There were insufficient numbers from racial and ethnic groups other than Caucasian to adequately determine potential pharmacokinetic differences among these populations following the administration of VIREAD.

Gender

No clinically relevant pharmacokinetic differences have been observed between men and women for cobicistat-boosted elvitegravir, emtricitabine and tenofovir DF. There was insufficient pharmacokinetic data in clinical trials to determine the effect of gender on the pharmacokinetics of cobicistat.

Pediatric Patients

Emtricitabine has been studied in pediatric subjects from 3 months to 17 years of age. Tenofovir DF has been studied in pediatric subjects from 2 years to less than 18 years of age. The pharmacokinetics of elvitegravir or cobicistat in pediatric subjects have not been established *[See Use in Specific Populations (8.4)]*.

Geriatric Patients

Pharmacokinetics of elvitegravir, cobicistat, emtricitabine and tenofovir have not been fully evaluated in elderly (65 years of age and older) patients *[See Use in Specific Populations (8.5)]*.

Assessment of Drug Interactions

[See also *Contraindications (4)* and *Drug Interactions (7)*]

The drug-drug interaction studies described in Tables 7 and 8 were conducted with STRIBILD, elvitegravir (coadministered with cobicistat or ritonavir), or cobicistat administered alone.

As STRIBILD is indicated for use as a complete regimen for the treatment of HIV-1 infection and should not be administered with other antiretroviral medications, information regarding drug-drug interactions with other antiretrovirals agents is not provided *[See Warnings and Precautions (5.4)].*

The effects of coadministered drugs on the exposure of elvitegravir are shown in Table 7. The effects of elvitegravir or cobicistat on the exposure of coadministered drugs are shown in Table 8. For information regarding clinical recommendations, see *Drug Interactions (7).*

[See table 7 at top of previous page]
[See table 8 above]

12.4 Microbiology

Mechanism of Action

Elvitegravir: Elvitegravir inhibits the strand transfer activity of HIV-1 integrase (integrase strand transfer inhibitor; INSTI), an HIV-1 encoded enzyme that is required for viral replication. Inhibition of integrase prevents the integration of HIV-1 DNA into host genomic DNA, blocking the formation of the HIV-1 provirus and propagation of the viral infection. Elvitegravir does not inhibit human topoisomerases I or II.

Cobicistat: Cobicistat is a selective, mechanism-based inhibitor of cytochromes P450 of the CYP3A subfamily. Inhibition of CYP3A-mediated metabolism by cobicistat enhances the systemic exposure of CYP3A substrates, such as elvitegravir, where bioavailability is limited and half-life is shortened by CYP3A-dependent metabolism.

Emtricitabine: Emtricitabine, a synthetic nucleoside analog of cytidine, is phosphorylated by cellular enzymes to form emtricitabine 5′-triphosphate. Emtricitabine 5′-triphosphate inhibits the activity of the HIV-1 RT by competing with the natural substrate deoxycytidine 5′-triphosphate and by being incorporated into nascent viral DNA which results in chain termination. Emtricitabine 5′-triphosphate is a weak inhibitor of mammalian DNA polymerases α, β, ϵ, and mitochondrial DNA polymerase γ.

Tenofovir Disoproxil Fumarate: Tenofovir DF is an acyclic nucleoside phosphonate diester analog of adenosine monophosphate. Tenofovir DF requires initial diester hydrolysis for conversion to tenofovir and subsequent phosphorylations by cellular enzymes to form tenofovir diphosphate. Tenofovir diphosphate inhibits the activity of HIV-1 RT by competing with the natural substrate deoxyadenosine 5′-triphosphate and, after incorporation into DNA, by DNA chain termination. Tenofovir diphosphate is a weak inhibitor of mammalian DNA polymerases α, β, and mitochondrial DNA polymerase γ.

Antiviral Activity in Cell Culture

Elvitegravir, Cobicistat, Emtricitabine, and Tenofovir Disoproxil Fumarate: The triple combination of elvitegravir, emtricitabine, and tenofovir was not antagonistic in cell culture combination antiviral activity assays and was not affected by the addition of cobicistat.

Elvitegravir: The antiviral activity of elvitegravir against laboratory and clinical isolates of HIV-1 was assessed in T lymphoblastoid cell lines, monocyte/macrophage cells, and primary peripheral blood lymphocytes. The 50% effective concentrations (EC_{50}) ranged from 0.02 to 1.7 nM. Elvitegravir displayed antiviral activity in cell culture against HIV-1 clades A, B, C, D, E, F, G, and O (EC_{50} values ranged from 0.1 to 1.3 nM) and activity against HIV-2 (EC_{50} value of 0.53 nM). The antiviral activity of elvitegravir with antiretroviral drugs in two-drug combination studies was not antagonistic when combined with the INSTI raltegravir, NNRTIs (efavirenz, etravirine, or nevirapine), NRTIs (abacavir, didanosine, emtricitabine, lamivudine, stavudine, tenofovir, or zidovudine), PIs (amprenavir, atazanavir, darunavir, indinavir, lopinavir, nelfinavir, ritonavir, saquinavir, or tipranavir), the fusion inhibitor enfuvirtide, or the CCR5 co-receptor antagonist maraviroc. Elvitegravir did not show inhibition of replication of HBV or HCV in cell culture.

Cobicistat: Cobicistat has no detectable antiviral activity in cell culture against HIV-1, HBV, or HCV and does not antagonize the antiviral activity of elvitegravir, emtricitabine, or tenofovir.

Emtricitabine: The antiviral activity of emtricitabine against laboratory and clinical isolates of HIV-1 was assessed in T lymphoblastoid cell lines, the MAGI-CCR5 cell line, and primary peripheral blood mononuclear cells. The EC_{50} values for emtricitabine were in the range of 0.0013–0.64 micromolar. Emtricitabine displayed antiviral activity in cell culture against HIV-1 clades A, B, C, D, E, F, and G (EC_{50} values ranged from 0.007–0.075 micromolar) and showed strain specific activity against HIV-2 (EC_{50} values ranged from 0.007–1.5 micromolar). No antagonistic effects were observed in two-drug combination studies of emtricitabine with NRTIs (abacavir, lamivudine, stavudine, tenofovir, or zidovudine), NNRTIs (delavirdine, efavirenz, nevirapine, or rilpivirine), PIs (amprenavir, nelfinavir, ritonavir, or saquinavir), or the INSTI elvitegravir.

Table 8 Drug Interactions: Changes in Pharmacokinetic Parameters for Coadministered Drug in the Presence of Elvitegravir, Elvitegravir plus Cobicistat, Cobicistat, or STRIBILD*

Coadministered Drug	Dose of Coadministered Drug (mg)	Elvitegravir Dose[†] (mg)	Cobicistat or Ritonavir Booster Dose (mg)	N	Mean Ratio of Coadministered Drug Pharmacokinetic Parameters[‡] (90% CI); No effect = 1.00		
					C_{max}	AUC	C_{min}
Desipramine	50 single dose	N/A	Cobicistat 150 once daily	8	1.24 (1.08,1.44)	1.65 (1.36,2.02)	NC
Digoxin	0.5 single dose	N/A	Cobicistat 150 once daily	22	1.41 (1.29,1.55)	1.08 (1.00, 1.17)	NC
Norgestimate/ ethinyl estradiol	0.180/0.215/ 0.250 norgestimate once daily	150 once daily[§]	Cobicistat 150 once daily[§]	13	2.08 (2.00,2.17)	2.26 (2.15,2.37)	2.67 (2.43,2.92)
	0.025 ethinyl estradiol once daily				0.94 (0.86,1.04)	0.75 (0.69,0.81)	0.56 (0.52,0.61)
Rifabutin	150 once every other day	150 once daily	Cobicistat 150 once daily	12	1.09 (0.98,1.20)[¶]	0.92 (0.83,1.03)[¶]	0.94 (0.85,1.04)[¶]
25-O-desacetyl-rifabutin				12	4.84 (4.09,5.74)[¶]	6.25 (5.08,7.69)[¶]	4.94 (4.04,6.04)[¶]
Rosuvastatin	10 single dose	150 single dose	Cobicistat 150 single dose	10	1.89 (1.48,2.42)	1.38 (1.14,1.67)	NC

* All interaction studies conducted in healthy volunteers.
† N/A = Not Applicable
‡ NC = Not Calculated
§ Study conducted with STRIBILD.
¶ Comparison based on rifabutin 300 mg once daily.

Tenofovir Disoproxil Fumarate: The antiviral activity of tenofovir against laboratory and clinical isolates of HIV-1 was assessed in T lymphoblastoid cell lines, primary monocyte/macrophage cells and peripheral blood lymphocytes. The EC_{50} values for tenofovir were in the range of 0.04–8.5 micromolar. Tenofovir displayed antiviral activity in cell culture against HIV-1 clades A, B, C, D, E, F, G, and O (EC_{50} values ranged from 0.5–2.2 micromolar) and showed strain specific activity against HIV-2 (EC_{50} values ranged from 1.6–5.5 micromolar). No antagonistic effects were observed in two-drug combination studies of tenofovir with NRTIs (abacavir, didanosine, emtricitabine, lamivudine, stavudine, or zidovudine), NNRTIs (delavirdine, efavirenz, nevirapine, or rilpivirine), PIs (amprenavir, indinavir, nelfinavir, ritonavir, or saquinavir), or the INSTI elvitegravir.

Resistance

In Cell Culture:

Elvitegravir: HIV-1 isolates with reduced susceptibility to elvitegravir have been selected in cell culture. Reduced susceptibility to elvitegravir was associated with the primary integrase substitutions T66A/I, E92G/Q, S147G, and Q148R. Additional integrase substitutions observed in cell culture selection included D10E, S17N, H51Y, F121Y, S153F/Y, E157Q, D232N, R263K, and V281M.

Emtricitabine and Tenofovir Disoproxil Fumarate: HIV-1 isolates with reduced susceptibility to emtricitabine or tenofovir have been selected in cell culture. Reduced susceptibility to emtricitabine was associated with M184V/I substitutions in HIV-1 RT. HIV-1 isolates selected by tenofovir expressed a K65R substitution in HIV-1 RT and showed a 2–4 fold reduction in susceptibility to tenofovir.

In Treatment-Naïve HIV-1-Infected Subjects:

Virus samples from STRIBILD-treatment failure subjects in Studies 102 and 103 who were viremic with HIV-1 RNA greater than 400 copies per mL at virologic failure, at Week 48, or at the time of early study drug discontinuation were evaluated for STRIBILD resistance (genotypic and phenotypic data available for 23 subjects [3%, 23/669]). The development of one or more primary substitutions associated with resistance to elvitegravir, emtricitabine, and/or tenofovir was observed in 57% (13/23) of the viremic subjects with evaluable genotypic data. The most common substitutions that emerged were M184V/I (N=12) in HIV-1 RT and the primary elvitegravir resistance-associated substitutions T66I (N=2), E92Q (N=8), Q148R (N=3), and N155H (N=3) in integrase; K65R in RT was also detected (N=4). In isolates with primary elvitegravir resistance substitutions, additional substitutions in integrase associated with resistance to elvitegravir were H51Y, L68I/V, G140C, S153A, E157Q, V165I, and H183P. Failure isolates expressing primary elvitegravir resistance-associated substitutions (N=11) had median decreases in susceptibility to elvitegravir of 44-fold (range: 6- to greater than 198-fold) and 33-fold (range: 4- to greater than 122-fold) compared to wild-type reference HIV-1 and to the respective baseline isolates, respectively. Most subjects (N=10) who developed integrase substitutions associated with elvitegravir resistance also developed the M184I/V RT substitutions, conferring reduced susceptibility to both elvitegravir and emtricitabine. In phenotypic analyses, 50% (11/22) of the viremic subjects with evaluable data had HIV-1 isolates with reduced susceptibility to elvitegravir, 57% (12/21) had reduced susceptibility to emtricitabine, and 10% (2/21) had reduced susceptibility to tenofovir.

Cross Resistance

STRIBILD-treatment failure subject isolates exhibited varying degrees of cross resistance within the INSTI and NRTI drug classes depending on the specific substitutions observed. These isolates remained susceptible to all NNRTIs and protease inhibitors.

Elvitegravir: Cross-resistance has been observed among INSTIs. Elvitegravir-resistant viruses showed varying degrees of cross-resistance in cell culture to raltegravir depending on the type and number of substitutions in HIV-1 integrase. Among the four primary elvitegravir resistance-associated substitutions detected in the STRIBILD-treatment virologic failure isolates, E92Q, Q148R, and N155H individually conferred reduced susceptibility both to elvitegravir (greater than 32-fold) and raltegravir (greater than 5-fold) when introduced into a wild-type virus by site-directed mutagenesis. The T66I substitution conferred greater than 14-fold reduced susceptibility to elvitegravir but less than 3-fold to raltegravir. Among the three primary raltegravir resistance-associated substitutions (Y143H/R, Q148H/K/R, and N155H), all but one (Y143H) conferred significant reductions in susceptibility to elvitegravir (greater than 5-fold).

Emtricitabine: Cross-resistance has been observed among NRTIs. Emtricitabine-resistant isolates harboring an M184V/I substitution in HIV-1 RT were cross-resistant to lamivudine. HIV-1 isolates containing the K65R RT substitution, selected *in vivo* by abacavir, didanosine, and tenofovir, demonstrated reduced susceptibility to inhibition by emtricitabine.

Tenofovir Disoproxil Fumarate: Cross-resistance has been observed among NRTIs. The K65R substitution in HIV-1 RT selected by tenofovir is also selected in some HIV-1-infected patients treated with abacavir or didanosine. HIV-1 isolates with the K65R substitution also showed reduced susceptibility to emtricitabine and lamivudine. Therefore, cross-resistance among these NRTIs may occur in patients whose virus harbors the K65R substitution. HIV-1 isolates from

Table 9 Virologic Outcome of Randomized Treatment of Study 102 and Study 103 at Week 48*

	Study 102		Study 103	
	STRIBILD (N=348)	**ATRIPLA (N=352)**	**STRIBILD (N=353)**	**ATV + RTV + TRUVADA (N=355)**
Virologic Success HIV-1 RNA < 50 copies/mL	88%	84%	90%	87%
Treatment Difference	3.6% (95% CI = -1.6%, 8.8%)		3.0% (95% CI = -1.9%, 7.8%)	
Virologic Failure†	7%	7%	5%	5%
No Virologic Data at Week 48 Window				
Discontinued Study Drug Due to AE or Death‡	3%	5 %	3%	5%
Discontinued Study Drug Due to Other Reasons and Last Available HIV-1 RNA < 50 copies/mL§	2%	3%	2%	3%
Missing Data During Window but on Study Drug	0%	<1 %	0%	<1 %

* Week 48 window is between Day 309 and 378 (inclusive).
† Includes subjects who had ≥50 copies/mL in the Week 48 window, subjects who discontinued early due to lack or loss of efficacy, subjects who discontinued for reasons other than an adverse event, death or lack or loss of efficacy and at the time of discontinuation had a viral value of ≥50 copies/mL.
‡ Includes patients who discontinued due to adverse event or death at any time point from Day 1 through the time window if this resulted in no virologic data on treatment during the specified window.
§ Includes subjects who discontinued for reasons other than an adverse event, death or lack or loss of efficacy, e.g., withdrew consent, loss to follow-up, etc.

patients (N=20) whose HIV-1 expressed a mean of 3 zidovudine-associated RT amino acid substitutions (M41L, D67N, K70R, L210W, T215Y/F, or K219Q/E/N) showed a 3.1-fold decrease in the susceptibility to tenofovir. Subjects whose virus expressed an L74V RT substitution without zidovudine resistance-associated substitutions (N=8) had reduced response to VIREAD. Limited data are available for patients whose virus expressed a Y115F substitution (N=3), Q151M substitution (N=2), or T69 insertion (N=4) in HIV-1 RT, all of whom had a reduced response in clinical trials.

13 NONCLINICAL TOXICOLOGY

13.1 Carcinogenesis, Mutagenesis, Impairment of Fertility

Elvitegravir: Long-term carcinogenicity studies of elvitegravir were carried out in mice (104 weeks) and in rats for up to 88 weeks (males) and 90 weeks (females). No drug-related increases in tumor incidence were found in mice at doses up to 2000 mg per kg per day alone or in combination with 25 mg per kg per day ritonavir at exposures 3- and 14-fold, respectively, the human systemic exposure at the recommended daily dose of 150 mg. No drug-related increases in tumor incidence were found in rats at doses up to 2000 mg per kg per day at exposures 12- to 27-fold, respectively in male and female, the human systemic exposure.
Elvitegravir was not genotoxic in the reverse mutation bacterial test (Ames test) and the rat micronucleus assay. In an *in vitro* chromosomal aberration test, elvitegravir was negative with metabolic activation; however, an equivocal response was observed without activation.
Elvitegravir did not affect fertility in male and female rats at approximately 16- and 30-fold higher exposures (AUC), respectively, than in humans at the therapeutic 150 mg daily dose.
Fertility was normal in the offspring of rats exposed daily from before birth (*in utero*) through sexual maturity at daily exposures (AUC) of approximately 18-fold higher than human exposures at the recommended 150 mg daily dose.
Cobicistat: The assessment of the carcinogenicity studies of cobicistat is ongoing.
Cobicistat was not genotoxic in the reverse mutation bacterial test (Ames test), mouse lymphoma or rat micronucleus assays.
Cobicistat did not affect fertility in male or female rats at daily exposures (AUC) approximately 4-fold higher than human exposures at the recommended 150 mg daily dose.
Fertility was normal in the offspring of rats exposed daily from before birth (*in utero*) through sexual maturity at daily exposures (AUC) of approximately 1.2-fold higher than human exposures at the recommended 150 mg daily dose.
Emtricitabine: In long-term carcinogenicity studies of emtricitabine, no drug-related increases in tumor incidence were found in mice at doses up to 750 mg per kg per day (23 times the human systemic exposure at the therapeutic dose of 200 mg per day) or in rats at doses up to 600 mg per kg per day (28 times the human systemic exposure at the therapeutic dose).
Emtricitabine was not genotoxic in the reverse mutation bacterial test (Ames test), mouse lymphoma or mouse micronucleus assays.
Emtricitabine did not affect fertility in male rats at approximately 140-fold or in male and female mice at approximately 60-fold higher exposures (AUC) than in humans given the recommended 200 mg daily dose. Fertility was normal in the offspring of mice exposed daily from before birth (*in utero*) through sexual maturity at daily exposures (AUC) of approximately 60-fold higher than human exposures at the recommended 200 mg daily dose.
Tenofovir Disoproxil Fumarate: Long-term oral carcinogenicity studies of tenofovir DF in mice and rats were carried out at exposures up to approximately 10 times (mice) and 4 times (rats) those observed in humans at the therapeutic dose for HIV 1 infection. At the high dose in female mice, liver adenomas were increased at exposures 10 times of that in humans. In rats, the study was negative for carcinogenic findings at exposures up to 4 times that observed in humans at the therapeutic dose.
Tenofovir DF was mutagenic in the *in vitro* mouse lymphoma assay and negative in an *in vitro* bacterial mutagenicity test (Ames test). In an *in vivo* mouse micronucleus assay, tenofovir DF was negative when administered to male mice.
There were no effects on fertility, mating performance or early embryonic development when tenofovir DF was administered to male rats at a dose equivalent to 10 times the human dose based on body surface area comparisons for 28 days prior to mating and to female rats for 15 days prior to mating through day seven of gestation. There was, however, an alteration of the estrous cycle in female rats.

14 CLINICAL STUDIES

The efficacy of STRIBILD is based on the analyses of 48-week data from two randomized, double-blind, active-controlled trials, Study 102 and Study 103, in treatment-naive, HIV-1 infected subjects (N=1408, randomized and dosed) with baseline estimated creatinine clearance above 70 mL per min.
In Study 102, subjects were randomized in a 1:1 ratio to receive either STRIBILD (N=348) once daily or ATRIPLA (efavirenz 600 mg/emtricitabine 200 mg/tenofovir DF 300 mg; N=352) once daily. The mean age was 38 years (range 18–67), 89% were male, 63% were White, 28% were Black, and 2% were Asian. Twenty-four percent of subjects identified as Hispanic/Latino. The mean baseline plasma HIV-1 RNA was 4.8 $\log_{10}$ copies per mL (range 2.6–6.5). The mean baseline CD4+ cell count was 386 cells per mm^3 (range 3–1348) and 13% had CD4+ cell counts less than 200 cells per mm^3. Thirty-three percent of subjects had baseline viral loads greater than 100,000 copies per mL.
In Study 103, subjects were randomized in a 1:1 ratio to receive either STRIBILD (N=353) once daily or atazanavir 300 mg + ritonavir 100 mg (ATV+RTV) + TRUVADA (emtricitabine 200 mg/tenofovir DF 300 mg) (N=355) once daily. The mean age was 38 years (range 19–72), 90% were male, 74% were White, 17% were Black, and 5% were Asian. Sixteen percent of subjects identified as Hispanic/Latino. The mean baseline plasma HIV-1 RNA was 4.8 $\log_{10}$ copies per mL (range 1.7–6.6). The mean baseline CD4+ cell count was 370 cells per mm^3 (range 5–1132) and 13% had CD4+ cell count less than 200 cells per mm^3. Forty-one percent of subjects had baseline viral loads greater than 100,000 copies per mL.
In both studies, subjects were stratified by baseline HIV-1 RNA (less than or equal to 100,000 copies per mL or greater than 100,000 copies per mL).
Treatment outcomes of Study 102 and Study 103 through 48 weeks are presented in Table 9.
[See table 9 above]
In Study 102, the mean increase from baseline in CD4+ cell count at Week 48 was 230 cells per mm^3 in the STRIBILD-treated subjects and 193 cells per mm^3 in the ATRIPLA-treated subjects. In Study 103, the mean increase from baseline in CD4+ cell count at Week 48 was 202 cells per mm^3 in the STRIBILD-treated subjects and 201 cells per mm^3 in the atazanavir + ritonavir + TRUVADA-treated subjects.

16 HOW SUPPLIED/STORAGE AND HANDLING

STRIBILD tablets are green, capsule-shaped, film-coated, debossed with "GSI" on one side and the number "1" surrounded by a square box (1) on the other side. Each bottle contains 30 tablets (NDC 61958-1201-1), a silica gel desiccant and closed with a child-resistant closure.
Store at 25 °C (77 °F), excursions permitted to 15–30 °C (59–86 °F) (see USP Controlled Room Temperature).
- Keep container tightly closed.
- Dispense only in original container.
- Do not use if seal over bottle opening is broken or missing.

17 PATIENT COUNSELING INFORMATION

- *See FDA-Approved Patient Labeling (Patient Information)*

A statement to patients and healthcare providers is included on the product's bottle label: **ALERT: Find out about medicines that should NOT be taken with STRIBILD.** A Patient Package Insert for STRIBILD is available for patient information.

Information for Patients

Patients should be advised that:
- STRIBILD may interact with many drugs; therefore, patients should be advised to report to their healthcare provider the use of any other prescription or non-prescription medication or herbal products including St. John's wort.
- Patients should remain under the care of a healthcare provider when using STRIBILD.
- Patients should be informed that STRIBILD is not a cure for HIV-1 infection. Patients should stay on continuous HIV therapy to control HIV-1 infection and decrease HIV-related illnesses. Patients should be told that sustained decreases in plasma HIV RNA have been associated with a reduced risk of progression to AIDS and death.
- Patients should avoid doing things that can spread HIV-1 infection to others.
  - **Do not share needles or other injection equipment.**
  - **Do not share personal items that can have blood or body fluids on them, like toothbrushes and razor blades.**
  - **Do not have any kind of sex without protection.** Always practice safer sex by using a latex or polyurethane condom to lower the chance of sexual contact with semen, vaginal secretions, or blood.
  - **Do not breastfeed.** At least two of the drugs contained in STRIBILD can be passed to the baby in breast milk. It is not known whether this could harm the baby. Also, mothers with HIV-1 should not breastfeed because HIV-1 can be passed to the baby in breast milk.
  - It is important to take STRIBILD on a regular dosing schedule with food and to avoid missing doses.
  - Do not miss a dose of STRIBILD. If a patient misses a dose of STRIBILD, the patient should take the missed dose as soon as they remember. If it is almost time for the next dose of STRIBILD, the patient should not take the missed dose, but resume the usual dosing schedule. Inform the patient that he or she should not take more or less than the prescribed dose of STRIBILD at any one time.
- Lactic acidosis and severe hepatomegaly with steatosis, including fatal cases, have been reported. Treatment with STRIBILD should be suspended in any patients who develop clinical symptoms suggestive of lactic acidosis or pronounced hepatotoxicity (including nausea, vomiting, unusual or unexpected stomach discomfort, and weakness) *[See Warnings and Precautions (5.1)]*.
- Patients with HIV-1 should be tested for hepatitis B virus (HBV) before initiating antiretroviral therapy. Severe acute exacerbations of hepatitis B have been reported in patients who are coinfected with HBV and HIV-1 and have discontinued EMTRIVA or VIREAD *[See Warnings and Precautions (5.2)]*. STRIBILD should not be discontinued without first informing their healthcare provider.
- Renal impairment, including cases of acute renal failure and Fanconi syndrome, has been reported in association with the use of STRIBILD. STRIBILD should be avoided with concurrent or recent use of a nephrotoxic agent *[See Warnings and Precautions (5.3)]*.
- STRIBILD should not be coadministered with other antiretroviral products because it provides a complete treatment regimen and because of potential drug interactions *[See Warnings and Precautions (5.4) and Drug Interactions (7)]*.

- STRIBILD should not be administered in combination with ATRIPLA, COMPLERA, EMTRIVA, TRUVADA, or VIREAD; with drugs containing lamivudine, including COMBIVIR, EPIVIR or EPIVIR-HBV, EPZICOM, or TRIZIVIR; with drugs containing ritonavir or regimens containing ritonavir; or with HEPSERA *[See Warnings and Precautions (5.4)]*.
- Decreases in bone mineral density have been observed with the use of STRIBILD. Assessment of bone mineral density (BMD) should be considered in patients who have a history of pathologic bone fracture or other risk factors for osteoporosis or bone loss *[See Warnings and Precautions (5.5)]*.
- Redistribution or accumulation of body fat may occur in patients receiving antiretroviral therapy and that the cause and long-term health effects of these conditions are not known *[See Warnings and Precautions (5.6)]*.
- In some patients with advanced HIV infection (AIDS), signs and symptoms of inflammation from previous infections may occur soon after anti-HIV treatment is started. It is believed that these symptoms are due to an improvement in the body's immune response, enabling the body to fight infections that may have been present with no obvious symptoms. Patients should be advised to inform their healthcare provider immediately of any symptoms of infection *[See Warnings and Precautions (5.7)]*.

Patient Information
STRIBILD™ (STRY-bild)
(elvitegravir, cobicistat, emtricitabine, and tenofovir disoproxil fumarate)
Tablets

Important: Ask your healthcare provider or pharmacist about medicines that should not be taken with STRIBILD. For more information, see the section "What should I tell my healthcare provider before taking STRIBILD?"

Read this Patient Information before you start taking STRIBILD and each time you get a refill. There may be new information. This information does not take the place of talking with your healthcare provider about your medical condition or treatment.

What is the most important information I should know about STRIBILD?

STRIBILD can cause serious side effects, including:

1. **Build-up of lactic acid in your blood (lactic acidosis).** Lactic acidosis can happen in some people who take STRIBILD or similar (nucleoside analogs) medicines. Lactic acidosis is a serious medical emergency that can lead to death.
   Lactic acidosis can be hard to identify early, because the symptoms could seem like symptoms of other health problems. **Call your healthcare provider right away if you get any of the following symptoms which could be signs of lactic acidosis:**
   - feel very weak or tired
   - have unusual (not normal) muscle pain
   - have trouble breathing
   - have stomach pain with
     - nausea
     - vomiting
   - feel cold, especially in your arms and legs
   - feel dizzy or lightheaded
   - have a fast or irregular heartbeat
2. **Severe liver problems.** Severe liver problems can happen in people who take STRIBILD. In some cases, these liver problems can lead to death. Your liver may become large (hepatomegaly) and you may develop fat in your liver (steatosis).
   Call your healthcare provider right away if you get any of the following symptoms of liver problems:
   - your skin or the white part of your eyes turns yellow (jaundice)
   - dark "tea-colored" urine
   - light-colored bowel movements (stools)
   - loss of appetite for several days or longer
   - nausea
   - stomach pain

   You may be more likely to get lactic acidosis or severe liver problems if you are female, very overweight (obese), or have been taking STRIBILD for a long time.
3. **Worsening of Hepatitis B infection. If you have hepatitis B virus (HBV) infection and take STRIBILD, your HBV may get worse (flare-up) if you stop taking STRIBILD. A "flare-up" is when your HBV infection suddenly returns in a worse way than before.**
   - Do not run out of STRIBILD. Refill your prescription or talk to your healthcare provider before your STRIBILD is all gone.
   - Do not stop taking STRIBILD without first talking to your healthcare provider.
   - If you stop taking STRIBILD, your healthcare provider will need to check your health often and do blood tests regularly for several months to check your HBV infection. Tell your healthcare provider about any new or unusual symptoms you may have after you stop taking STRIBILD.

For more information about side effects, see the section **"What are the possible side effects of STRIBILD?"**

What is STRIBILD?

STRIBILD is a prescription medicine that is used without other antiretroviral medicines to treat Human Immunodeficiency Virus-1 (HIV-1) in adults who have never taken HIV-1 medicines before. HIV-1 is the virus that causes AIDS (Acquired Immune Deficiency Syndrome).

STRIBILD contains the prescription medicines elvitegravir, cobicistat, emtricitabine (EMTRIVA®) and tenofovir disoproxil fumarate (VIREAD®).

It is not known if STRIBILD is safe and effective in children under 18 years of age.

When used to treat HIV-1 infection, STRIBILD may:

- Reduce the amount of HIV-1 in your blood. This is called "viral load".
- Increase the number of CD4+ (T) cells in your blood that help fight off other infections.
- Reduce the amount of HIV-1 and increasing the CD4+ (T) cells in your blood may help improve your immune system. This may reduce your risk of death or getting infections that can happen when your immune system is weak (opportunistic infections).

STRIBILD does not cure HIV-1 infections or AIDS. You must stay on continuous HIV-1 therapy to control HIV-1 infection and decrease HIV-related illnesses.

Avoid doing things that can spread HIV-1 infection to others.

- Do not share or re-use needles or other injection equipment.
- Do not share personal items that can have blood or body fluids on them, like toothbrushes and razor blades.
- Do not have any kind of sex without protection. Always practice safer sex by using a latex or polyurethane condom to lower the chance of sexual contact with semen, vaginal secretions, or blood.

Ask your healthcare provider if you have any questions about how to prevent passing HIV-1 to other people.

Who should not take STRIBILD?

Do not take STRIBILD if you also take a medicine that contains:

- alfuzosin hydrochloride (UROXATRAL®)
- cisapride (PROPULSID®, PROPULSID QUICKSOLV®)
- ergot-containing medicines, including:
  - dihydroergotamine mesylate (D.H.E. 45®, MIGRANAL®)
  - ergotamine tartrate (CAFERGOT®, MIGERGOT®, ERGOSTAT®, MEDIHALER ERGOTAMINE®, WIGRAINE®, WIGRETTES®)
  - methylergonovine maleate (ERGOTRATE®, METHERGINE®)
- lovastatin (ADVICOR®, ALTOPREV®, MEVACOR®)
- oral midazolam
- pimozide (ORAP®)
- rifampin (RIFADIN®, RIFAMATE®, RIFATER®, RIMACTANE®)
- sildenafil (REVATIO®), when used for treating the lung problem, pulmonary arterial hypertension (PAH)
- simvastatin (SIMCOR®, VYTORIN®, ZOCOR®)
- triazolam (HALCION®)
- St. John's wort (*Hypericum perforatum*) or a product that contains St. John's wort

What should I tell my healthcare provider before taking STRIBILD?

Before taking STRIBILD, tell your healthcare provider if you:

- have liver problems including hepatitis B infection
- have kidney problems
- have bone problems
- have any other medical conditions
- are pregnant or plan to become pregnant. It is not known if STRIBILD can harm your unborn baby. Tell your healthcare provider if you become pregnant while taking STRIBILD.
  Pregnancy Registry. There is a pregnancy registry for women who take antiviral medicines during pregnancy. The purpose of this registry is to collect information about the health of you and your baby. Talk with your healthcare provider about how you can take part in this registry.
- are breastfeeding or plan to breastfeed. Do not breastfeed if you take STRIBILD.
  - You should not breastfeed if you have HIV-1 because of the risk of passing HIV-1 to your baby.
  - Two of the medicines in STRIBILD can pass to your baby in your breast milk. It is not known if the other medicines in STRIBILD can pass into your breast milk.

Talk with your healthcare provider about the best way to feed your baby.

Tell your healthcare provider about all the medicines you take, including prescription and nonprescription medicines, vitamins, and herbal supplements. STRIBILD may affect the way other medicines work, and other medicines may affect how STRIBILD works.

You should not take STRIBILD if you also take:

- any other medicines to treat HIV-1 infection
- other medicines that contain tenofovir (ATRIPLA®, COMPLERA®, VIREAD®, TRUVADA®)
- other medicines that contain emtricitabine or lamivudine (COMBIVIR®, EMTRIVA®, EPIVIR® or EPIVIR-HBV®, EPZICOM®, TRIZIVIR®)
- adefovir (HEPSERA®)

Especially tell your healthcare provider if you take:

- hormone-based contraceptives (birth control pills and patches)
- an antacid medicine that contains aluminum, magnesium hydroxide, or calcium carbonate. Take antacids at least 2 hours before or after you take STRIBILD.
- medicines to treat depression
- medicines to prevent organ transplant rejection
- medicines to treat high blood pressure
- any of the following medicines:
  - amiodarone (CORDARONE®, PACERONE®)
  - atorvastatin (LIPITOR®, CADUET®)
  - bepridil hydrochloric (VASCOR®, BEPADIN®)
  - bosentan (TRACLEER®)
  - buspirone
  - carbamazepine (CARBATROL®, EPITOL®, EQUETRO®, TEGRETO®)
  - clarithromycin (BIAXIN®, PREVPAC®)
  - clonazepam (KLONOPIN®)
  - clorazepate (GEN-XENE®, TRANXENE®)
  - colchicine (Colcrys®)
  - medicines that contain dexamethasone
  - diazepam (VALIUM®)
  - digoxin (LANOXIN®)
  - disopyramide (NORPACE®)
  - estazolam
  - ethosuximide (ZARONTIN®)
  - flecainide (TAMBOCOR®)
  - flurazepam
  - fluticasone (FLOVENT®, FLONASE®, FLOVENT® DISKUS, FLOVENT® HFA, VERAMYST®)
  - itraconazole (SPORANOX®)
  - ketoconazole (NIZORAL®)
  - lidocaine (XYLOCAINE®)
  - mexiletine
  - oxcarbazepine (TRILEPTAL®)
  - perphenazine
  - phenobarbital (LUMINAL®)
  - phenytoin (DILANTIN®, PHENYTEK®)
  - propafenone (RYTHMOL®)
  - quinidine (NEUDEXTA®)
  - rifabutin (MYCOBUTIN®)
  - rifapentine (PRIFTIN®)
  - risperidone (RISPERDAL®, RISPERDAL CONSTA®)
  - salmeterol (SEREVENT®) or salmeterol when taken in combination with fluticasone (ADVAIR DISKUS®, ADVAIR HFA®)
  - sildenafil (VIAGRA®), tadalafil (CIALIS®) or vardenafil (LEVITRA®, STAXYN®), for the treatment of erectile dysfunction (ED). If you get dizzy or faint (low blood pressure), have vision changes or have an erection that last longer than 4 hours, call your healthcare provider or get medical help right away.
  - tadalafil (ADCIRCA®), for the treatment of pulmonary arterial hypertension
  - telithromycin (KETEK®)
  - thioridazine
  - voriconazole (VFEND®)
  - warfarin (COUMADIN®, JANTOVEN®)
  - zolpidem (AMBIEN®, EDLULAR®, INTERMEZZO®, ZOLPIMIST®)

Ask your healthcare provider or pharmacist if you are not sure if your medicine is one that is listed above. Do not start any new medicines while you are taking STRIBILD without first talking with your healthcare provider or pharmacist. Know the medicines you take. Keep a list of your medicines and show it to your healthcare provider and pharmacist when you get a new medicine.

How should I take STRIBILD?

- Take STRIBILD exactly as your healthcare provider tells you to take it. **STRIBILD is taken by itself (not with other antiretroviral medicines) to treat HIV-1 infection.**
- STRIBILD is usually taken 1 time each day.
- Take STRIBILD with food.
- Do not change your dose or stop taking STRIBILD without first talking with your healthcare provider. Stay under a healthcare provider's care when taking STRIBILD.
- Do not miss a dose of STRIBILD. If you miss a dose of STRIBILD, take the missed dose as soon as you remember. If it is almost time for your next dose of STRIBILD, do not take the missed dose. Take the next dose of STRIBILD at your regular time. Do not take 2 doses at the same time to make up for a missed dose.
- If you take too much STRIBILD, call your healthcare provider or go to the nearest hospital emergency room right away.

• When your STRIBILD supply starts to run low, get more from your healthcare provider or pharmacy. This is very important because the amount of virus in your blood may increase if the medicine is stopped for even a short time. The virus may develop resistance to STRIBILD and become harder to treat.

What are the possible side effects of STRIBILD?

STRIBILD may cause the following serious side effects, including:

• **See "What is the most important information I should know about STRIBILD?"**

• **New or worse kidney problems, including kidney failure.** Your healthcare provider should do blood and urine tests to check your kidneys before you start and while you are taking STRIBILD. Your healthcare provider may tell you to stop taking STRIBILD if you develop new or worse kidney problems.

• **Bone problems** can happen in some people who take STRIBILD. Bone problems include bone pain, softening or thinning (which may lead to fractures). Your healthcare provider may need to do tests to check your bones.

• **Changes in body fat can happen in people who take HIV-1 medicine.** These changes may include increased amount of fat in the upper back and neck ("buffalo hump"), breast, and around the middle of your body (trunk). Loss of fat from the legs, arms and face may also happen. The exact cause and long-term health effects of these conditions are not known.

• **Changes in your immune system (Immune Reconstitution Syndrome)** can happen when you start taking HIV-1 medicines. Your immune system may get stronger and begin to fight infections that have been hidden in your body for a long time. Tell your healthcare provider right away if you start having any new symptoms after starting your HIV-1 medicine.

The most common side effects of STRIBILD include:

• nausea

• diarrhea

Tell your healthcare provider if you have any side effect that bothers you or that does not go away.

These are not all the possible side effects of STRIBILD. For more information, ask your healthcare provider or pharmacist.

Call your healthcare provider for medical advice about side effects. You may report side effects to FDA at 1-800-FDA-1088.

How should I store STRIBILD?

• Store STRIBILD at room temperature between 68°F to 77°F (20°C to 25°C).

• Keep STRIBILD in its original container.

• Keep the container tightly closed.

• Do not use STRIBILD if the seal over the bottle opening is broken or missing.

Keep STRIBILD and all medicines out of reach of children.

General information about STRIBILD.

Medicines are sometimes prescribed for purposes other than those listed in a Patient Information leaflet. Do not use STRIBILD for a condition for which it was not prescribed. Do not give STRIBILD to other people, even if they have the same symptoms you have. It may harm them.

This leaflet summarizes the most important information about STRIBILD. If you would like more information, talk with your healthcare provider. You can ask your healthcare provider or pharmacist for information about STRIBILD that is written for health professionals.

For more information, call 1-800-445-3235 or go to www.STRIBILD.com.

What are the ingredients in STRIBILD?

Active ingredients: elvitegravir, cobicistat, emtricitabine, and tenofovir disoproxil fumarate

Inactive ingredients: lactose monohydrate, microcrystalline cellulose, silicon dioxide, croscarmellose sodium, hydroxypropyl cellulose, sodium lauryl sulfate, and magnesium stearate. The tablets are film-coated with a coating material containing indigo carmine (FD&C blue #2) aluminum lake, polyethylene glycol, polyvinyl alcohol, talc, titanium dioxide, and yellow iron oxide.

This Patient Information has been approved by the U.S. Food and Drug Administration.

Manufactured and distributed by:
Gilead Sciences, Inc.
Foster City, CA 94404
Issued: August 2012

COMPLERA, EMTRIVA, HEPSERA, STRIBILD, TRUVADA, and VIREAD are trademarks of Gilead Sciences, Inc., or its related companies. ATRIPLA is a trademark of Bristol-Myers Squibb & Gilead Sciences, LLC. All other trademarks referenced herein are the property of their respective owners.

203100-GS-000

Shown in Product Identification Guide, page 306

TRUVADA® ℞

[tru-VAH-dah]

(emtricitabine/tenofovir disoproxil fumarate) tablets, for oral use

HIGHLIGHTS OF PRESCRIBING INFORMATION

These highlights do not include all the information needed to use TRUVADA safely and effectively. See full prescribing information for TRUVADA.

TRUVADA® (emtricitabine/tenofovir disoproxil fumarate) tablets, for oral use

Initial U.S. Approval: 2004

WARNING: LACTIC ACIDOSIS/SEVERE HEPATOMEGALY WITH STEATOSIS, POST-TREATMENT ACUTE EXACERBATION OF HEPATITIS B, and RISK OF DRUG RESISTANCE WITH USE OF TRUVADA FOR PrEP IN UNDIAGNOSED HIV-1 INFECTION

See full prescribing information for complete boxed warning.

• **Lactic acidosis and severe hepatomegaly with steatosis, including fatal cases, have been reported with the use of nucleoside analogs, including VIREAD, a component of TRUVADA. (5.1)**

• **TRUVADA is not approved for the treatment of chronic hepatitis B virus (HBV) infection. Severe acute exacerbations of hepatitis B have been reported in patients coinfected with HIV-1 and HBV who have discontinued TRUVADA. Therefore, hepatic function should be monitored closely in HBV-infected patients who discontinue TRUVADA. If appropriate, initiation of anti-hepatitis B therapy may be warranted. (5.2)**

• **TRUVADA used for a PrEP indication must only be prescribed to individuals confirmed to be HIV-negative immediately prior to initial use and periodically during use. Drug-resistant HIV-1 variants have been identified with the use of TRUVADA for a PrEP indication following undetected acute HIV-1 infection. Do not initiate TRUVADA for a PrEP indication if signs or symptoms of acute HIV infection are present unless negative infection status is confirmed. (5.9)**

RECENT MAJOR CHANGES

Boxed Warning	07/2012
Indications and Usage	
Treatment of HIV-1 infection (1.1)	06/2013
Pre-exposure Prophylaxis (1.2)	07/2012
Dosage and Administration (2)	07/2012
Contraindications (4)	07/2012
Warnings and Precautions	
New Onset or Worsening Renal Impairment (5.3)	07/2012
Coadministration with Other Products (5.4)	06/2013
Decreases in Bone Mineral Density (5.5)	07/2012
Immune Reconstitution Syndrome (5.7)	07/2012
Comprehensive Management to Reduce the Risk of Acquiring HIV-1 (5.9)	07/2012

INDICATIONS AND USAGE

TRUVADA is a combination of EMTRIVA and VIREAD, both nucleoside analog HIV-1 reverse transcriptase inhibitors.

TRUVADA is indicated in combination with other antiretroviral agents for the treatment of HIV-1 infection in adults and pediatric patients 12 years of age and older. (1)

TRUVADA is indicated in combination with safer sex practices for pre-exposure prophylaxis (PrEP) to reduce the risk of sexually acquired HIV-1 in adults at high risk. (1)

DOSAGE AND ADMINISTRATION

Treatment of HIV-1 Infection (2.1)

• Recommended dose in adults and pediatric patients (12 years of age and older and weighing greater than or equal to 35 kg): One tablet once daily taken orally with or without food. (2.1)

• Recommended dose in renally impaired HIV-1 infected adult patients: Creatinine clearance 30–49 mL/min: 1 tablet every 48 hours. (2.3) CrCl below 30 mL/min or hemodialysis: Do not use TRUVADA. (2.3)

Pre-exposure Prophylaxis (2.2)

• Recommended dose in HIV-1 uninfected adults: One tablet once daily taken orally with or without food. (2.2)

• Recommended dose in renally impaired HIV-uninfected individuals: Do not use TRUVADA in HIV-uninfected individuals if CrCl is below 60 mL/min. If a decrease in CrCl is observed in uninfected individuals while using TRUVADA for PrEP, evaluate potential causes and reassess potential risks and benefits of continued use. (2.3)

DOSAGE FORMS AND STRENGTHS

Tablets: 200 mg of emtricitabine and 300 mg of tenofovir disoproxil fumarate. (3)

CONTRAINDICATIONS

Do not use TRUVADA for pre-exposure prophylaxis in individuals with unknown or positive HIV-1 status. TRUVADA should be used in HIV-infected patients only in combination with other antiretroviral agents. (4)

WARNINGS AND PRECAUTIONS

• New onset or worsening renal impairment: Can include acute renal failure and Fanconi syndrome. Assess creatinine clearance (CrCl) before initiating treatment with TRUVADA. Monitor CrCl and serum phosphorus in patients at risk. Avoid administering Truvada with concurrent or recent use of nephrotoxic drugs. (5.3)

• Coadministration with Other Products: Do not use with drugs containing emtricitabine or tenofovir disoproxil fumarate including ATRIPLA, COMPLERA, EMTRIVA, STRIBILD, VIREAD; or with drugs containing lamivudine. Do not administer in combination with HEPSERA. (5.4)

• Decreases in bone mineral density (BMD): Consider assessment of BMD in patients with a history of pathologic fracture or other risk factors for osteoporosis or bone loss. (5.5)

• Redistribution/accumulation of body fat: Observed in patients receiving antiretroviral therapy. (5.6)

• Immune reconstitution syndrome: May necessitate further evaluation and treatment. (5.7)

• Triple nucleoside-only regimens: Early virologic failure has been reported in HIV-infected patients. Monitor carefully and consider treatment modification. (5.8)

• Comprehensive management to reduce the risk of acquiring HIV-1: Use as part of a comprehensive prevention strategy including other prevention measures; strictly adhere to dosing schedule. (5.9)

• Management to reduce the risk of acquiring HIV-1 drug resistance:

Prior to initiating TRUVADA for PrEP - if clinical symptoms consistent with acute viral infection are present and recent (<1 month) exposures are suspected, delay starting PrEP for at least one month and reconfirm negative HIV-1 status or use a test approved by the FDA as an aid in the diagnosis of HIV-1 infection, including acute or primary HIV-1 infection.

While using TRUVADA for PrEP - HIV-1 screening tests should be repeated at least every 3 months. (5.9)

ADVERSE REACTIONS

In HIV1 infected patients, the most common adverse reactions (incidence greater than or equal to 10%) are diarrhea, nausea, fatigue, headache, dizziness, depression, insomnia, abnormal dreams, and rash. (6.1)

In HIV-1 uninfected individuals in PrEP trials, adverse reactions that were reported by more than 2% of TRUVADA subjects and more frequently than by placebo subjects were headache, abdominal pain and weight decreased. (6.2)

To report SUSPECTED ADVERSE REACTIONS, contact Gilead Sciences, Inc. at 1-800-445-3235 or FDA at 1-800-FDA-1088 or www.fda.gov/medwatch

DRUG INTERACTIONS

• Didanosine: Tenofovir disoproxil fumarate increases didanosine concentrations. Use with caution and monitor for evidence of didanosine toxicity (e.g., pancreatitis, neuropathy) when coadministered. Consider dose reductions or discontinuations of didanosine if warranted. (7.1)

• Atazanavir: Coadministration decreases atazanavir concentrations and increases tenofovir concentrations. Use atazanavir with TRUVADA only with ritonavir; monitor for evidence of tenofovir toxicity. (7.2)

• Lopinavir/ritonavir: Coadministration increases tenofovir concentrations. Monitor for evidence of tenofovir toxicity. (7.3)

USE IN SPECIFIC POPULATIONS

• Nursing mothers: Women infected with HIV-1 should be instructed not to breast feed. (8.3)

See 17 for PATIENT COUNSELING INFORMATION and Medication Guide

Revised: 06/2013

FULL PRESCRIBING INFORMATION: CONTENTS*

*** Sections or subsections omitted from the full prescribing information are not listed**

FULL PRESCRIBING INFORMATION

WARNING: LACTIC ACIDOSIS/SEVERE HEPATOMEGALY WITH STEATOSIS, POST TREATMENT ACUTE EXACERBATION OF HEPATITIS B, and RISK OF DRUG RESISTANCE WITH USE OF TRUVADA FOR PRE-EXPOSURE PROPHYLAXIS (PrEP) IN UNDIAGNOSED EARLY HIV-1 INFECTION

Lactic acidosis and severe hepatomegaly with steatosis, including fatal cases, have been reported with the use of nucleoside analogs, including VIREAD, a component of TRUVADA, in combination with other antiretrovirals *[See Warnings and Precautions (5.1)]*.

TRUVADA is not approved for the treatment of chronic hepatitis B virus (HBV) infection and the safety and efficacy of TRUVADA have not been established in patients coinfected with HBV and HIV-1. Severe acute exacerbations of hepatitis B have been reported in patients who are coinfected with HBV and HIV-1 and have discontinued TRUVADA. Therefore, hepatic function should be monitored closely with both clinical and laboratory follow-up for at least several months in patients who are infected with HBV and discontinue TRUVADA. If appropriate, initiation of anti-hepatitis B therapy may be warranted *[See Warnings and Precautions (5.2)]*.

TRUVADA used for a PrEP indication must only be prescribed to individuals confirmed to be HIV-negative immediately prior to initiating and periodically (at least every 3 months) during use. Drug-resistant HIV-1 variants have been identified with use of TRUVADA for a PrEP indication following undetected acute HIV-1 infection. Do not initiate TRUVADA for a PrEP indication if signs or symptoms of acute HIV-1 infection are present unless negative infection status is confirmed *[See Warnings and Precautions (5.9)]*.

1 INDICATIONS AND USAGE

1.1 Treatment of HIV-1 Infection

TRUVADA®, a combination of EMTRIVA® and VIREAD®, is indicated in combination with other antiretroviral agents (such as non-nucleoside reverse transcriptase inhibitors or protease inhibitors) for the treatment of HIV-1 infection in adults and pediatric patients 12 years of age and older.

The following points should be considered when initiating therapy with TRUVADA for the treatment of HIV-1 infection:

- It is not recommended that TRUVADA be used as a component of a triple nucleoside regimen.
- TRUVADA should not be coadministered with ATRIPLA®, COMPLERA®, EMTRIVA, STRIBILD®, VIREAD or lamivudine-containing products *[See Warnings and Precautions (5.4)]*.
- In treatment experienced patients, the use of TRUVADA should be guided by laboratory testing and treatment history *[See Clinical Pharmacology (12.4)]*.

1.2 Pre-Exposure Prophylaxis

TRUVADA is indicated in combination with safer sex practices for pre-exposure prophylaxis (PrEP) to reduce the risk of sexually acquired HIV-1 in adults at high risk. This indication is based on clinical trials in men who have sex with men (MSM) at high risk for HIV-1 infection and in heterosexual serodiscordant couples *[See Clinical Studies (14.2, 14.3)]*.

When considering TRUVADA for pre-exposure prophylaxis the following factors may help to identify individuals at high risk:

- has partner(s) known to be HIV-1 infected, or
- engages in sexual activity within a high prevalence area or social network and one or more of the following:
  - inconsistent or no condom use
  - diagnosis of sexually transmitted infections
  - exchange of sex for commodities (such as money, food, shelter, or drugs)
  - use of illicit drugs or alcohol dependence
  - incarceration
  - partner(s) of unknown HIV-1 status with any of the factors listed above

When prescribing TRUVADA for pre-exposure prophylaxis, healthcare providers must:

- prescribe TRUVADA as part of a comprehensive prevention strategy because TRUVADA is not always effective in preventing the acquisition of HIV-1 infection *[See Warnings and Precautions (5.9)]*;
- counsel all uninfected individuals to strictly adhere to the recommended TRUVADA dosing schedule because the effectiveness of TRUVADA in reducing the risk of acquiring HIV-1 was strongly correlated with adherence as demonstrated by measurable drug levels in clinical trials *[See Warnings and Precautions (5.9)]*;
- confirm a negative HIV-1 test immediately prior to initiating TRUVADA for a PrEP indication. If clinical symptoms consistent with acute viral infection are present and recent (<1 month) exposures are suspected, delay starting PrEP for at least one month and reconfirm HIV-1 status or use a test approved by the FDA as an aid in the diagnosis of HIV-1 infection, including acute or primary HIV-1 infection. *[See Warnings and Precautions (5.9)]*; and
- screen for HIV-1 infection at least once every 3 months while taking TRUVADA for PrEP.

2 DOSAGE AND ADMINISTRATION

2.1 Recommended Dose for Treatment of HIV-1 Infection

The recommended dose of TRUVADA in adults and in pediatric patients 12 years of age and older with body weight greater than or equal to 35 kg (greater than or equal to 77 lb) is one tablet (containing 200 mg of emtricitabine and 300 mg of tenofovir disoproxil fumarate) once daily taken orally with or without food.

2.2 Recommended Dose for Pre-exposure Prophylaxis

The dose of TRUVADA in HIV-1 uninfected adults is one tablet (containing 200 mg of emtricitabine and 300 mg of tenofovir disoproxil fumarate) once daily taken orally with or without food.

2.3 Dose Adjustment for Renal Impairment

Treatment of HIV-1 Infection

Significantly increased drug exposures occurred when EMTRIVA or VIREAD were administered to subjects with moderate to severe renal impairment *[See EMTRIVA or VIREAD Package Insert]*. Therefore, adjust the dosing interval of TRUVADA in HIV-1 infected adult patients with baseline creatinine clearance 30–49 mL/min using the recommendations in Table 1. These dosing interval recommendations are based on modeling of single-dose pharmacokinetic data in non-HIV infected subjects. The safety and effectiveness of these dosing interval adjustment recommendations have not been clinically evaluated in patients with moderate renal impairment, therefore clinical response to treatment and renal function should be closely monitored in these patients *[See Warnings and Precautions (5.3)]*.

No dose adjustment is necessary for HIV-1 infected patients with mild renal impairment (creatinine clearance 50–80 mL/min). No data are available to make dose recommendations in pediatric patients with renal impairment.

Table 1 Dosage Adjustment for HIV-1 Infected Adult Patients with Altered Creatinine Clearance

	Creatinine Clearance (mL/min)*		
	≥50	30–49	<30 (Including Patients Requiring Hemodialysis)
Recommended Dosing Interval	Every 24 hours	Every 48 hours	TRUVADA should not be administered.

* Calculated using ideal (lean) body weight

Routine monitoring of calculated creatinine clearance and serum phosphorus should be performed in all individuals with mild renal impairment *[See Warnings and Precautions (5.3)]*.

Pre-exposure Prophylaxis

Do not use TRUVADA for a PrEP indication in HIV-1 uninfected individuals with creatinine clearance below 60 mL/min *[See Warnings and Precautions (5.3)]*.

Routine monitoring of calculated creatinine clearance and serum phosphorus should be performed in all individuals with mild renal impairment. If a decrease in creatinine clearance is observed in uninfected individuals while using TRUVADA for PrEP, evaluate potential causes and re-assess potential risks and benefits of continued use *[See Warnings and Precautions (5.3)]*.

3 DOSAGE FORMS AND STRENGTHS

TRUVADA is available as tablets. Each tablet contains 200 mg of emtricitabine and 300 mg of tenofovir disoproxil fumarate (which is equivalent to 245 mg of tenofovir disoproxil). The tablets are blue, capsule-shaped, film-coated, debossed with "GILEAD" on one side and with "701" on the other side.

4 CONTRAINDICATIONS

Do not use TRUVADA for pre-exposure prophylaxis in individuals with unknown or positive HIV-1 status. TRUVADA should be used in HIV-infected patients only in combination with other antiretroviral agents.

5 WARNINGS AND PRECAUTIONS

5.1 Lactic Acidosis/Severe Hepatomegaly with Steatosis

Lactic acidosis and severe hepatomegaly with steatosis, including fatal cases, have been reported with the use of nucleoside analogs, including VIREAD, a component of TRUVADA, in combination with other antiretrovirals. A majority of these cases have been in women. Obesity and prolonged nucleoside exposure may be risk factors. Particular caution should be exercised when administering nucleoside analogs to any patient or uninfected individual with known risk factors for liver disease; however, cases have also been reported in HIV-1 infected patients with no known risk factors. Treatment with TRUVADA should be suspended in any patient or uninfected individual who develops clinical or laboratory findings suggestive of lactic acidosis or pronounced hepatotoxicity (which may include hepatomegaly and steatosis even in the absence of marked transaminase elevations).

5.2 HBV Infection

It is recommended that all individuals be tested for the presence of chronic hepatitis B virus (HBV) before initiating TRUVADA. TRUVADA is not approved for the treatment of chronic HBV infection and the safety and efficacy of TRUVADA have not been established in patients infected with HBV. Severe acute exacerbations of hepatitis B have been reported in patients who are coinfected with HBV and HIV-1 and have discontinued TRUVADA. In some patients infected with HBV and treated with EMTRIVA, the exacerbations of hepatitis B were associated with liver decompensation and liver failure. Patients who are infected with HBV should be closely monitored with both clinical and laboratory follow-up for at least several months after stopping treatment with TRUVADA. If appropriate, initiation of anti-hepatitis B therapy may be warranted. HBV -uninfected individuals should be offered vaccination.

5.3 New Onset or Worsening Renal Impairment

Emtricitabine and tenofovir are principally eliminated by the kidney. Renal impairment, including cases of acute renal failure and Fanconi syndrome (renal tubular injury with severe hypophosphatemia), has been reported with the use of VIREAD *[See Adverse Reactions (6.2)]*.

It is recommended that creatinine clearance be calculated in all individuals prior to initiating therapy and as clinically appropriate during therapy with TRUVADA.

Routine monitoring of calculated creatinine clearance and serum phosphorus should be performed in all individuals at risk for renal impairment, including individuals who have previously experienced renal events while receiving HEPSERA®.

TRUVADA should be avoided with concurrent or recent use of a nephrotoxic agent.

Treatment of HIV-1 Infection

Dosing interval adjustment of TRUVADA and close monitoring of renal function are recommended in all patients with creatinine clearance 30–49 mL/min, *[See Dosage and Administration (2.3)]*. No safety or efficacy data are available in patients with renal impairment who received TRUVADA using these dosing guidelines, so the potential benefit of TRUVADA therapy should be assessed against the potential risk of renal toxicity. TRUVADA should not be administered to patients with creatinine clearance below 30 mL/min or patients requiring hemodialysis.

Pre-exposure Prophylaxis

TRUVADA for a PrEP indication should not be used if creatinine clearance is less than 60 mL/min. If a decrease in creatinine clearance is observed in uninfected individuals while using TRUVADA for PrEP, evaluate potential causes and re-assess potential risks and benefits of continued use *[See Dosage and Administration (2.3)]*.

5.4 Coadministration with Other Products

TRUVADA is a fixed-dose combination of emtricitabine and tenofovir disoproxil fumarate. Do not coadminister TRUVADA with ATRIPLA, COMPLERA, EMTRIVA, STRIBILD, or VIREAD. Due to similarities between emtricitabine and lamivudine, do not coadminister TRUVADA with other drugs containing lamivudine, including Combivir (lamivudine/zidovudine), Epivir or Epivir-HBV (lamivudine), Epzicom (abacavir sulfate/lamivudine), or Trizivir (abacavir sulfate/lamivudine/zidovudine).

Do not coadminister TRUVADA with HEPSERA (adefovir dipivoxil).

5.5 Decreases in Bone Mineral Density

Assessment of bone mineral density (BMD) should be considered for adults and in pediatric patients 12 years of age and older who have a history of pathologic bone fracture or other risk factors for osteoporosis or bone loss. Although the effect of supplementation with calcium and vitamin D was not studied, such supplementation may be beneficial. If bone abnormalities are suspected then appropriate consultation should be obtained.

Tenofovir Disoproxil Fumarate: In a 144-week trial of treatment-naive HIV-1 infected adult subjects, decreases in BMD were seen at the lumbar spine and hip in both arms of the trial. At Week 144, there was a significantly greater mean percentage decrease from baseline in BMD at the lumbar spine in subjects receiving VIREAD + lamivudine + efavirenz compared with subjects receiving stavudine + lamivudine + efavirenz. Changes in BMD at the hip were similar between the two treatment groups. In both groups, the majority of the reduction in BMD occurred in the first 24–48 weeks of the trial and this reduction was sustained through 144 weeks. Twenty-eight percent of VIREAD-treated subjects vs. 21% of the comparator subjects lost at least 5% of BMD at the spine or 7% of BMD at the hip. Clinically relevant fractures (excluding fingers and toes) were reported in 4 subjects in the VIREAD group and 6 subjects in the comparator group. Tenofovir disoproxil fumarate was associated with significant increases in biochemical markers of bone metabolism (serum bone-specific alkaline phosphatase, serum osteocalcin, serum C-telopeptide, and urinary N-telopeptide), suggesting increased bone turnover. Serum parathyroid hormone levels and 1,25 Vitamin D levels were also higher in subjects receiving VIREAD.

In a clinical trial of HIV-1 infected pediatric subjects 12 years of age and older (Study 321), bone effects were similar to adult subjects. Under normal circumstances, BMD increases rapidly in this age group. In this trial, the mean rate of bone gain was less in the VIREAD-treated group compared to the placebo group. Six VIREAD treated subjects and one placebo treated subject had significant (greater than 4%) lumbar spine BMD loss in 48 weeks. Among 28 subjects receiving 96 weeks of VIREAD, Z-scores declined by -0.341 for lumbar spine and -0.458 for total body. Skeletal growth (height) appeared to be unaffected. Markers of bone turnover in VIREAD-treated pediatric subjects 12 years of age and older suggest increased bone turnover, consistent with the effects observed in adults.

In clinical trials of HIV-1 uninfected individuals, decreases in BMD were observed. In the iPrEx trial, a substudy of 503 subjects found mean changes from baseline in BMD ranging from -0.4% to -1.0% across total hip, spine, femoral neck, and trochanter in the TRUVADA group compared with the placebo group, which returned toward baseline after discontinuation of treatment. Thirteen percent of subjects receiving TRUVADA vs. 6% of subjects receiving placebo lost at least 5% of BMD at the spine during treatment. Bone fractures were reported in 1.7% of the TRUVADA group compared with 1.4% in the placebo group. No correlation between BMD and fractures was noted *[See Clinical Studies (14.2)]*. The Partners PrEP trial found similar fracture rates between treatment and placebo groups (0.8% and 0.6%, respectively). No BMD evaluations were conducted during this trial *[See Clinical Studies (14.3)]*.

The effects of VIREAD-associated changes in BMD and biochemical markers on long-term bone health and future fracture risk are unknown. For additional information, please consult the VIREAD prescribing information.

Cases of osteomalacia (associated with proximal renal tubulopathy and which may contribute to fractures) have been reported in association with the use of VIREAD *[See Adverse Reactions (6.2)]*.

5.6 Fat Redistribution

Redistribution/accumulation of body fat including central obesity, dorsocervical fat enlargement (buffalo hump), peripheral wasting, facial wasting, breast enlargement, and "cushingoid appearance" have been observed in HIV-1 infected patients receiving antiretroviral therapy. The mechanism and long-term consequences of these events are currently unknown. A causal relationship has not been established.

5.7 Immune Reconstitution Syndrome

Immune reconstitution syndrome has been reported in HIV-1 infected patients treated with combination antiretroviral therapy, including TRUVADA. During the initial phase of combination antiretroviral treatment, HIV-1 infected patients whose immune system responds may develop an inflammatory response to indolent or residual opportunistic infections [such as *Mycobacterium avium* infection, cytomegalovirus, *Pneumocystis jirovecii* pneumonia (PCP), or tuberculosis], which may necessitate further evaluation and treatment.

Autoimmune disorders (such as Graves' disease, polymyositis, and Guillain-Barré syndrome) have also been reported to occur in the setting of immune reconstitution, however, the time to onset is more variable, and can occur many months after initiation of treatment.

5.8 Early Virologic Failure

Clinical trials in HIV-1 infected subjects have demonstrated that certain regimens that only contain three nucleoside reverse transcriptase inhibitors (NRTI) are generally less effective than triple drug regimens containing two NRTIs in combination with either a non-nucleoside reverse transcriptase inhibitor or a HIV-1 protease inhibitor. In particular, early virological failure and high rates of resistance substitutions have been reported. Triple nucleoside regimens should therefore be used with caution. Patients on a therapy utilizing a triple nucleoside-only regimen should be carefully monitored and considered for treatment modification.

5.9 Comprehensive Management to Reduce the Risk of Acquiring HIV-1

Use TRUVADA for pre-exposure prophylaxis only as part of a comprehensive prevention strategy that includes other prevention measures, such as safer sex practices, because TRUVADA is not always effective in preventing the acquisition of HIV-1 *[See Clinical Studies (14.2 and 14.3)]*.

- Counsel uninfected individuals about safer sex practices that include consistent and correct use of condoms, knowledge of their HIV-1 status and that of their partner(s), and regular testing for other sexually transmitted infections that can facilitate HIV-1 transmission (such as syphilis and gonorrhea).
- Inform uninfected individuals about and support their efforts in reducing sexual risk behavior.

Use TRUVADA to reduce the risk of acquiring HIV-1 only in individuals confirmed to be HIV-negative. HIV-1 resistance substitutions may emerge in individuals with undetected HIV-1 infection who are taking only TRUVADA, because TRUVADA alone does not constitute a complete treatment regimen for HIV-1 treatment *[See Microbiology: Resistance (12.4)]*; therefore, care should be taken to minimize drug exposure in HIV-infected individuals.

- Many HIV-1 tests, such as rapid tests, detect anti-HIV antibodies and may not identify HIV-1 during the acute stage of infection. Prior to initiating TRUVADA for a PrEP indication, evaluate seronegative individuals for current or recent signs or symptoms consistent with acute viral infections (e.g., fever, fatigue, myalgia, skin rash, etc.) and ask about potential exposure events (e.g., unprotected, or condom broke during sex with an HIV-1 infected partner) that may have occurred within the last month.
  - If clinical symptoms consistent with acute viral infection are present and recent (<1 month) exposures are suspected, delay starting PrEP for at least one month and reconfirm HIV-1 status or use a test approved by the FDA as an aid in the diagnosis of HIV-1 infection, including acute or primary HIV-1 infection.
- While using TRUVADA for a PrEP indication, HIV-1 screening tests should be repeated at least every 3 months. If symptoms consistent with acute HIV-1 infection develop following a potential exposure event, PrEP should be discontinued until negative infection status is confirmed using a test approved by the FDA as an aid in the diagnosis of HIV-1, including acute or primary HIV-1 infection.

Counsel uninfected individuals to strictly adhere to the recommended TRUVADA dosing schedule. The effectiveness of TRUVADA in reducing the risk of acquiring HIV-1 is strongly correlated with adherence as demonstrated by measurable drug levels in clinical trials *[See Clinical Studies (14.2 and 14.3)]*.

6 ADVERSE REACTIONS

The following adverse reactions are discussed in other sections of the labeling:

- Lactic Acidosis/Severe Hepatomegaly with Steatosis *[See Boxed Warning, Warnings and Precautions (5.1)]*.
- Severe Acute Exacerbations of hepatitis B *[See Boxed Warning, Warnings and Precautions (5.2)]*.
- New Onset or Worsening Renal Impairment *[See Warnings and Precautions (5.3)]*.
- Decreases in Bone Mineral Density *[See Warnings and Precautions (5.5)]*.
- Immune Reconstitution Syndrome *[See Warnings and Precautions (5.7)]*.

6.1 Adverse Reactions from Clinical Trials Experience in HIV-1 Infected Subjects

Because clinical trials are conducted under widely varying conditions, adverse reaction rates observed in the clinical trials of a drug cannot be directly compared to rates in the clinical trials of another drug and may not reflect the rates observed in practice.

Clinical Trials in Adult Subjects

The most common adverse reactions (incidence greater than or equal to 10%, any severity) occurring in Study 934, an active-controlled clinical trial of efavirenz, emtricitabine, and tenofovir disoproxil fumarate, include diarrhea, nausea, fatigue, headache, dizziness, depression, insomnia, abnormal dreams, and rash. See also Table 2 for the frequency of treatment-emergent adverse reactions (Grades 2–4) occurring in greater than or equal to 5% of subjects treated in any treatment group in this trial.

Skin discoloration, manifested by hyperpigmentation on the palms and/or soles, was generally mild and asymptomatic. The mechanism and clinical significance are unknown.

Study 934 - Treatment Emergent Adverse Reactions: In Study 934, 511 antiretroviral-naive subjects received either VIREAD + EMTRIVA administered in combination with efavirenz (N=257) or zidovudine/lamivudine administered in combination with efavirenz (N=254) for 144 weeks. Subjects had a mean age of 40 years (range 20 to 73 years) and were predominantly male (88%). Overall, 65% were White, 17% were Black, and 13% were Hispanic. Adverse reactions observed in this trial were generally consistent with those seen in other trials in treatment-experienced or treatment-naive subjects receiving VIREAD and/or EMTRIVA (Table 2).

Table 2 Selected Treatment-Emergent Adverse Reactions* (Grades 2–4) Reported in ≥5% in Any Treatment Group in Study 934 (0–144 Weeks)

	FTC + TDF + EFV† N=257	AZT/3TC + EFV N=254
Gastrointestinal Disorder		
Diarrhea	9%	5%
Nausea	9%	7%
Vomiting	2%	5%
General Disorders and Administration Site Condition		
Fatigue	9%	8%
Infections and Infestations		
Sinusitis	8%	4%
Upper respiratory tract infections	8%	5%
Nasopharyngitis	5%	3%
Nervous System Disorders		
Headache	6%	5%
Dizziness	8%	7%
Psychiatric Disorders		
Depression	9%	7%
Insomnia	5%	7%
Skin and Subcutaneous Tissue Disorders		
Rash event‡	7%	9%

* Frequencies of adverse reactions are based on all treatment-emergent adverse events, regardless of relationship to study drug.

† From Weeks 96 to 144 of the trial, subjects received TRUVADA with efavirenz in place of VIREAD + EMTRIVA with efavirenz.

‡ Rash event includes rash, exfoliative rash, rash generalized, rash macular, rash maculo-papular, rash pruritic, and rash vesicular.

Laboratory Abnormalities: Laboratory abnormalities observed in this trial were generally consistent with those seen in other trials of VIREAD and/or EMTRIVA (Table 3).

Table 3 Significant Laboratory Abnormalities Reported in ≥1% of Subjects in Any Treatment Group in Study 934 (0–144 Weeks)

	FTC + TDF + EFV*	AZT/3TC + EFV
	N=257	N=254
Any ≥ Grade 3 Laboratory Abnormality	30%	26%
Fasting Cholesterol (>240 mg/dL)	22%	24%
Creatine Kinase (M: >990 U/L) (F: >845 U/L)	9%	7%
Serum Amylase (>175 U/L)	8%	4%
Alkaline Phosphatase (>550 U/L)	1%	0%
AST (M: >180 U/L) (F: >170 U/L)	3%	3%
ALT (M: >215 U/L) (F: >170 U/L)	2%	3%
Hemoglobin (<8.0 mg/dL)	0%	4%
Hyperglycemia (>250 mg/dL)	2%	1%
Hematuria (>75 RBC/HPF)	3%	2%
Glycosuria (≥3+)	<1%	1%
Neutrophils (<750/mm^3)	3%	5%
Fasting Triglycerides (>750 mg/dL)	4%	2%

* From Weeks 96 to 144 of the trial, subjects received TRUVADA with efavirenz in place of VIREAD + EMTRIVA with efavirenz.

In addition to the events described above for Study 934, other adverse reactions that occurred in at least 5% of subjects receiving EMTRIVA or VIREAD with other antiretroviral agents in clinical trials include anxiety, arthralgia, increased cough, dyspepsia, fever, myalgia, pain, abdominal pain, back pain, paresthesia, peripheral neuropathy (including peripheral neuritis and neuropathy), pneumonia, and rhinitis.

In addition to the laboratory abnormalities described above for Study 934, Grades 3–4 laboratory abnormalities of increased bilirubin (>2.5 × ULN), increased pancreatic amylase (>2.0 × ULN), increased or decreased serum glucose (<40 or >250 mg/dL), and increased serum lipase (>2.0 × ULN) occurred in up to 3% of subjects treated with EMTRIVA or VIREAD with other antiretroviral agents in clinical trials.

Clinical Trials in Pediatric Subjects 12 Years of Age and Older

Emtricitabine: In addition to the adverse reactions reported in adults, anemia and hyperpigmentation were observed in 7% and 32%, respectively, of pediatric subjects (3 months to less than 18 years of age) who received treatment with EMTRIVA in the larger of two open-label, uncontrolled pediatric trials (N=116). For additional information, please consult the EMTRIVA prescribing information.

Tenofovir Disoproxil Fumarate: In a pediatric clinical trial conducted in subjects 12 to less than 18 years of age, the adverse reactions observed in pediatric subjects who received treatment with VIREAD were consistent with those observed in clinical trials of VIREAD in adults *[See Warnings and Precautions (5.5)]*.

6.2 Adverse Reactions from Clinical Trial Experience in HIV-1 Uninfected Adult Subjects

No new adverse reactions to TRUVADA were identified from two randomized placebo-controlled clinical trials (iPrEx, Partners PrEP) in which 2830 HIV-1 uninfected adults received TRUVADA once daily for pre-exposure prophylaxis. Subjects were followed for a median of 71 weeks and 87 weeks, respectively. These trials enrolled HIV-negative individuals ranging in age from 18 to 67 years. The iPrEx trial enrolled only males or transgender females of Hispanic/Latino (72%), White (18%), Black (9%) and Asian (5%) race. The Partners PrEP trial enrolled both males (61–64% across treatment groups) and females in Kenya and Uganda. Table 4 provides a list of all adverse events that occurred ≥2% of subjects in any treatment group in the iPrEx and Partners PrEP trials.

Table 4 Selected Adverse Events (All Grades) Reported in ≥2% in Any Treatment Group in the iPrEx Trial and Partners PrEP Trial

	iPrEx Trial		Partners PrEP Trial	
	FTC/TDF (N=1251)	Placebo (N=1248)	FTC/TDF (N-1579)	Placebo (N= 1584)
Gastrointestinal Disorders				
Diarrhea	7%	8%	2%	3%
Abdominal pain	4%	2%	-*	-
Infections and Infestations				
Pharyngitis	13%	16%	-	-
Urethritis	5%	7%	-	-
Urinary tract infection	2%	2%	5%	7%
Syphilis	6%	5%	-	-
Secondary syphilis	6%	4%	-	-
Anogenital warts	2%	3%	-	-
Musculoskeletal and Connective Tissue Disorders				
Back pain	5%	5%	-	-
Nervous System Disorders				
Headache	7%	6%	-	-
Psychiatric Disorders				
Depression	6%	7%	-	-
Anxiety	3%	3%	-	-
Reproductive System and Breast Disorders				
Genital ulceration	2%	2%	2%	2%
Investigations				
Weight decreased	3%	2%	-	-

* Not reported or reported below 2%.

Laboratory Abnormalities: Table 5 provides a list of laboratory abnormalities observed in both trials. Six subjects in the TDF-containing arms of the Partners PrEP trial discontinued participation in the study due to an increase in blood creatinine compared with no discontinuations in the placebo group. One subject in the TRUVADA arm of the iPrEx trial discontinued from the study due to an increase in blood creatinine and another due to low phosphorous.

In addition to the laboratory abnormalities described above, Grade 1 proteinuria (1+) occurred in 6% of subjects receiving TRUVADA in the iPrEx trial. Grades 2–3 proteinuria (2–4+) and glycosuria (3+) occurred in less than 1% of subjects treated with TRUVADA in the iPrEx trial and Partners PrEP trial.

[See table 4 above]

[See table 5 at top of next page]

6.3 Postmarketing Experience

The following adverse reactions have been identified during postapproval use of VIREAD. No additional adverse reactions have been identified during postapproval use of EMTRIVA. Because postmarketing reactions are reported voluntarily from a population of uncertain size, it is not always possible to reliably estimate their frequency or establish a causal relationship to drug exposure.

Immune System Disorders

allergic reaction, including angioedema

Metabolism and Nutrition Disorders

lactic acidosis, hypokalemia, hypophosphatemia

Respiratory, Thoracic, and Mediastinal Disorders

dyspnea

Gastrointestinal Disorders

pancreatitis, increased amylase, abdominal pain

Hepatobiliary Disorders

hepatic steatosis, hepatitis, increased liver enzymes (most commonly AST, ALT gamma GT)

Skin and Subcutaneous Tissue Disorders

rash

Musculoskeletal and Connective Tissue Disorders

rhabdomyolysis, osteomalacia (manifested as bone pain and which may contribute to fractures), muscular weakness, myopathy

Renal and Urinary Disorders

acute renal failure, renal failure, acute tubular necrosis, Fanconi syndrome, proximal renal tubulopathy, interstitial nephritis (including acute cases), nephrogenic diabetes insipidus, renal insufficiency, increased creatinine, proteinuria, polyuria

General Disorders and Administration Site Conditions

asthenia

The following adverse reactions, listed under the body system headings above, may occur as a consequence of proximal renal tubulopathy: rhabdomyolysis, osteomalacia, hypokalemia, muscular weakness, myopathy, hypophosphatemia.

7 DRUG INTERACTIONS

No drug interaction trials have been conducted using TRUVADA tablets. Drug interaction trials have been conducted with emtricitabine and tenofovir disoproxil fumarate, the components of TRUVADA. This section describes clinically relevant drug interactions observed with emtricitabine and tenofovir disoproxil fumarate *[See Clinical Pharmacology (12.3)]*.

7.1 Didanosine

Coadministration of TRUVADA and didanosine should be undertaken with caution and patients receiving this combination should be monitored closely for didanosine-associated adverse reactions. Didanosine should be discontinued in patients who develop didanosine-associated adverse reactions.

When tenofovir disoproxil fumarate was administered with didanosine the C_{max} and AUC of didanosine increased significantly *[See Clinical Pharmacology (12.3)]*. The mechanism of this interaction is unknown. Higher didanosine concentrations could potentiate didanosine-associated adverse reactions, including pancreatitis, and neuropathy. Suppression of CD4$^+$ cell counts has been observed in patients receiving tenofovir DF with didanosine 400 mg daily.

In patients weighing greater than 60 kg, the didanosine dose should be reduced to 250 mg when it is coadministered with TRUVADA. Data are not available to recommend a dose adjustment of didanosine for adult or pediatric patients weighing less than 60 kg. When coadministered, TRUVADA and Videx EC may be taken under fasted conditions or with a light meal (less than 400 kcal, 20% fat).

7.2 Atazanavir

Atazanavir has been shown to increase tenofovir concentrations *[See Clinical Pharmacology (12.3)]*. The mechanism of this interaction is unknown. Patients receiving atazanavir and TRUVADA should be monitored for TRUVADA-associated adverse reactions. TRUVADA should be discontinued in patients who develop TRUVADA-associated adverse reactions.

Tenofovir decreases the AUC and C_{min} of atazanavir *[See Clinical Pharmacology (12.3)]*. When coadministered with

Table 5 Laboratory Abnormalities (Highest Toxicity Grade) Reported for Each Subject in the iPrEx Trial and Partners PrEP Trial

Grade*			iPrEx Trial FTC/TDF N= 1251	iPrEx Trial Placebo N= 1248	Partners PrEP Trial FTC/TDF N=1579	Partners PrEP Trial Placebo N=1584
Creatinine	1	(1.1–1.3 × ULN)	27 (2%)	21 (2%)	18 (1%)	12 (<1%)
	2–4	(> 1.4 × ULN)	5 (<1%)	3 (<1%)	2 (<1%)	1 (<1%)
Phosphorus	1	(2.5 – <LLN mg/dL)	81 (7%)	110 (9%)	NR †	NR †
	2–4	(<2.0 mg/dL)	123 (10%)	101 (8%)	140 (9%)	136 (9%)
AST	1	(1.25–<2.5 × ULN)	175 (14%)	175 (14%)	20 (1%)	25 (2%)
	2–4	(> 2.6 × ULN)	57 (5%)	61 (5%)	10 (<1%)	4 (<1%)
ALT	1	(1.25–<2.5 × ULN)	178 (14%)	194 (16%)	21 (1%)	13 (<1%)
	2–4	(> 2.6 × ULN)	84 (7%)	82 (7%)	4 (<1%)	6 (<1%)
Hemoglobin	1	(8.5 – 10 mg/dL)	49 (4%)	62 (5%)	56 (4%)	39 (2%)
	2–4	(<9.4 mg/dL)	13 (1%)	19 (2%)	28 (2%)	39 (2%)
Neutrophils	1	(1000–1300/mm^3)	23 (2%)	25 (2%)	208 (13%)	163 (10%)
	2–4	(<750/mm^3)	7 (<1%)	7 (<1%)	73 (5%)	56 (3%)

* Grading is per DAIDS criteria.
† Grade 1 phosphorus was not reported for the Partners PrEP trial.

TRUVADA, it is recommended that atazanavir 300 mg is given with ritonavir 100 mg. Atazanavir without ritonavir should not be coadministered with TRUVADA.

7.3 Lopinavir/Ritonavir

Lopinavir/ritonavir has been shown to increase tenofovir concentrations *[See Clinical Pharmacology (12.3)]*. The mechanism of this interaction is unknown. Patients receiving lopinavir/ritonavir and TRUVADA should be monitored for TRUVADA-associated adverse reactions. TRUVADA should be discontinued in patients who develop TRUVADA-associated adverse reactions.

7.4 Drugs Affecting Renal Function

Emtricitabine and tenofovir are primarily excreted by the kidneys by a combination of glomerular filtration and active tubular secretion *[See Clinical Pharmacology (12.3)]*. No drug-drug interactions due to competition for renal excretion have been observed; however, coadministration of TRUVADA with drugs that are eliminated by active tubular secretion may increase concentrations of emtricitabine, tenofovir, and/or the coadministered drug. Some examples include, but are not limited to acyclovir, adefovir dipivoxil, cidofovir, ganciclovir, valacyclovir, and valganciclovir. Drugs that decrease renal function may increase concentrations of emtricitabine and/or tenofovir.

8 USE IN SPECIFIC POPULATIONS

8.1 Pregnancy

Pregnancy Category B

Antiretroviral Pregnancy Registry: To monitor fetal outcomes of pregnant women exposed to TRUVADA, an Antiretroviral Pregnancy Registry (APR) has been established. Healthcare providers are encouraged to register patients by calling 1-800-258-4263.

Risk Summary

TRUVADA has been evaluated in a limited number of women during pregnancy and postpartum. Available human and animal data suggest that TRUVADA does not increase the risk of major birth defects overall compared to the background rate. There are, however, no adequate and well-controlled trials in pregnant women. Because the studies in humans cannot rule out the possibility of harm, TRUVADA should be used during pregnancy only if clearly needed. If an uninfected individual becomes pregnant while taking TRUVADA for a PrEP indication, careful consideration should be given to whether use of TRUVADA should be continued, taking into account the potential increased risk of HIV-1 infection during pregnancy.

Clinical Considerations

As of July 2011, the APR has received prospective reports of 764 and 1219 exposures to emtricitabine- and tenofovir-containing regimens, respectively in the first trimester, 321 and 455 exposures, respectively, in second trimester, and 140 and 257 exposures, respectively, in the third trimester. Birth defects occurred in 18 of 764 (2.4%) live births for emtricitabine-containing regimens and 27 of 1219 (2.2%) live births for tenofovir-containing regimens (first trimester exposure) and 10 of 461 (2.2%) live births for emtricitabine-containing regimens and 15 of 714 (2.1%) live births for tenofovir-containing regimens (second/third trimester exposure). Among pregnant women in the U.S. reference population, the background rate of birth defects is 2.7%. There was no association between emtricitabine or tenofovir and overall birth defects observed in the APR.

Animal Data

Emtricitabine:

The incidence of fetal variations and malformations was not increased in embryofetal toxicity studies performed with emtricitabine in mice at exposures (AUC) approximately 60-fold higher and in rabbits at approximately 120-fold higher than human exposures at the recommended daily dose.

Tenofovir Disoproxil Fumarate:

Reproduction studies have been performed in rats and rabbits at doses up to 14 and 19 times the human dose based on body surface area comparisons and revealed no evidence of impaired fertility or harm to the fetus due to tenofovir.

8.3 Nursing Mothers

Nursing Mothers: The Centers for Disease Control and Prevention recommend that HIV-1 infected mothers not breast-feed their infants to avoid risking postnatal transmission of HIV-1.

Studies in humans have shown that both tenofovir and emtricitabine are excreted in human milk. Because the risks of low level exposure to emtricitabine and tenofovir to infants are unknown, **mothers should be instructed not to breast-feed if they are receiving TRUVADA,** whether they are taking TRUVADA for treatment or to reduce the risk of acquiring HIV-1.

Emtricitabine

Samples of breast milk obtained from five HIV-1 infected mothers show that emtricitabine is secreted in human milk. Breastfeeding infants whose mothers are being treated with emtricitabine may be at risk for developing viral resistance to emtricitabine. Other emtricitabine-associated risks in infants breastfed by mothers being treated with emtricitabine are unknown.

Tenofovir Disoproxil Fumarate

Samples of breast milk obtained from five HIV-1 infected mothers show that tenofovir is secreted in human milk. Tenofovir-associated risks, including the risk of viral resistance to tenofovir, in infants breastfed by mothers being treated with tenofovir disoproxil fumarate are unknown.

8.4 Pediatric Use

TRUVADA should only be administered to HIV-1 infected pediatric patients 12 years of age and older with body weight greater than or equal to 35 kg. Because it is a fixed-dose combination tablet, TRUVADA cannot be adjusted for patients of lower age and weight. Safety and efficacy have not been established in pediatric patients less than 12 years of age or weighing less than 35 kg *[See Warnings and Precautions (5.5), Adverse Reactions (6.1) and Clinical Pharmacology (12.3)]*.

8.5 Geriatric Use

Clinical trials of EMTRIVA or VIREAD did not include sufficient numbers of subjects aged 65 and over to determine whether they respond differently from younger subjects. In general, dose selection for the elderly patients should be cautious, keeping in mind the greater frequency of decreased hepatic, renal, or cardiac function, and of concomitant disease or other drug therapy.

8.6 Patients with Impaired Renal Function

Treatment of HIV-1 Infection

The dosing interval for TRUVADA should be modified in HIV-infected adult patients with creatinine clearance of 30–49 mL/min. TRUVADA should not be used in patients with creatinine clearance below 30 mL/min and in patients with end-stage renal disease requiring dialysis. *[See Dosage and Administration (2.3)].*

Pre-exposure Prophylaxis

TRUVADA for a PrEP indication should not be used in HIV-1 uninfected individuals with creatinine clearance below 60 mL/min. If a decrease in creatinine clearance is observed in uninfected individuals while using TRUVADA for PrEP, evaluate potential causes and re-assess potential risks and benefits of continued use *[See Dosage and Administration (2.3)].*

10 OVERDOSAGE

If overdose occurs, the patient must be monitored for evidence of toxicity, and standard supportive treatment applied as necessary.

Emtricitabine: Limited clinical experience is available at doses higher than the therapeutic dose of EMTRIVA. In one clinical pharmacology trial, single doses of emtricitabine 1200 mg were administered to 11 subjects. No severe adverse reactions were reported.

Hemodialysis treatment removes approximately 30% of the emtricitabine dose over a 3-hour dialysis period starting within 1.5 hours of emtricitabine dosing (blood flow rate of 400 mL/min and a dialysate flow rate of 600 mL/min). It is not known whether emtricitabine can be removed by peritoneal dialysis.

Tenofovir Disoproxil Fumarate: Limited clinical experience at doses higher than the therapeutic dose of VIREAD 300 mg is available. In one trial, 600 mg tenofovir disoproxil fumarate was administered to 8 subjects orally for 28 days, and no severe adverse reactions were reported. The effects of higher doses are not known.

Tenofovir is efficiently removed by hemodialysis with an extraction coefficient of approximately 54%. Following a single 300 mg dose of VIREAD, a four-hour hemodialysis session removed approximately 10% of the administered tenofovir dose.

11 DESCRIPTION

TRUVADA tablets are fixed dose combination tablets containing emtricitabine and tenofovir disoproxil fumarate. EMTRIVA is the brand name for emtricitabine, a synthetic nucleoside analog of cytidine. Tenofovir disoproxil fumarate (tenofovir DF) is converted in vivo to tenofovir, an acyclic nucleoside phosphonate (nucleotide) analog of adenosine 5'-monophosphate. Both emtricitabine and tenofovir exhibit inhibitory activity against HIV-1 reverse transcriptase.

Emtricitabine: The chemical name of emtricitabine is 5-fluoro-1-(2*R*,5*S*)-[2-(hydroxymethyl)-1,3-oxathiolan-5-yl]cytosine. Emtricitabine is the (-) enantiomer of a thio analog of cytidine, which differs from other cytidine analogs in that it has a fluorine in the 5-position.

It has a molecular formula of $C_8H_{10}FN_3O_3S$ and a molecular weight of 247.24. It has the following structural formula:

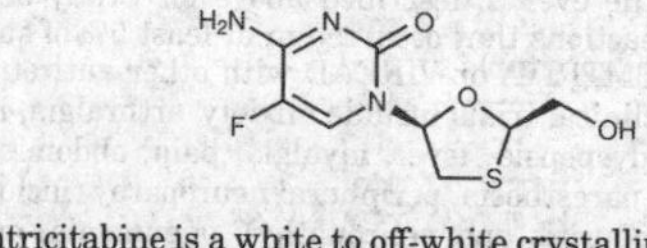

Emtricitabine is a white to off-white crystalline powder with a solubility of approximately 112 mg/mL in water at 25 °C. The partition coefficient (log p) for emtricitabine is -0.43 and the pKa is 2.65.

Tenofovir Disoproxil Fumarate: Tenofovir disoproxil fumarate is a fumaric acid salt of the bis-isopropoxycarbonyloxymethyl ester derivative of tenofovir. The chemical name of tenofovir disoproxil fumarate is 9-[(*R*)-2 [[bis[[(isopropoxycarbonyl)oxy]- methoxy]phosphinyl]methoxy]propyl]adenine fumarate (1:1). It has a molecular formula of $C_{19}H_{30}N_5O_{10}P \cdot C_4H_4O_4$ and a molecular weight of 635.52. It has the following structural formula:

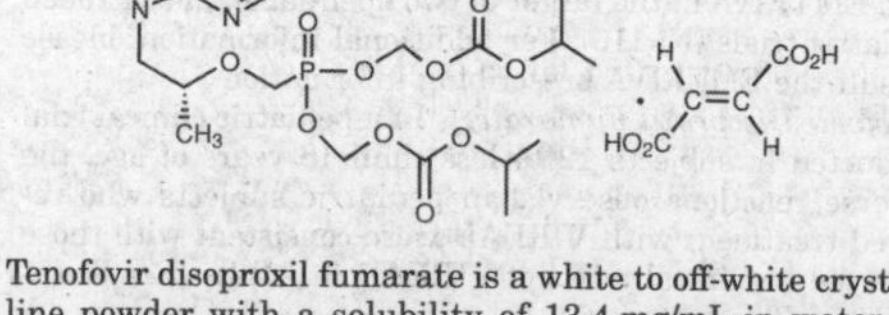

Tenofovir disoproxil fumarate is a white to off-white crystalline powder with a solubility of 13.4 mg/mL in water at 25 °C. The partition coefficient (log p) for tenofovir disoproxil is 1.25 and the pKa is 3.75. All dosages are expressed in terms of tenofovir disoproxil fumarate except where otherwise noted.

TRUVADA tablets are for oral administration. Each film-coated tablet contains 200 mg of emtricitabine and 300 mg of tenofovir disoproxil fumarate, (which is equivalent to 245 mg of tenofovir disoproxil), as active ingredients. The tablets also include the following inactive ingredients: croscarmellose sodium, lactose monohydrate, magnesium stearate, microcrystalline cellulose, and pregelatinized starch (gluten free). The tablets are coated with Opadry II Blue Y-30-10701, which contains FD&C Blue #2 aluminum lake, hydroxypropyl methylcellulose 2910, lactose monohydrate, titanium dioxide, and triacetin.

12 CLINICAL PHARMACOLOGY

For additional information on Mechanism of Action, Antiviral Activity, Resistance and Cross Resistance, please consult the EMTRIVA and VIREAD prescribing information.

12.1 Mechanism of Action

TRUVADA is a fixed-dose combination of antiviral drugs emtricitabine and tenofovir disoproxil fumarate *[See Clinical Pharmacology (12.4)]*.

12.3 Pharmacokinetics

TRUVADA: One TRUVADA tablet was bioequivalent to one EMTRIVA capsule (200 mg) plus one VIREAD tablet (300 mg) following single-dose administration to fasting healthy subjects (N=39).

Emtricitabine: The pharmacokinetic properties of emtricitabine are summarized in Table 6. Following oral administration of EMTRIVA, emtricitabine is rapidly absorbed with peak plasma concentrations occurring at 1–2 hours post-dose. Less than 4% of emtricitabine binds to human plasma proteins in vitro and the binding is independent of concentration over the range of 0.02–200 µg/mL. Following administration of radiolabelled emtricitabine, approximately 86% is recovered in the urine and 13% is recovered as metabolites. The metabolites of emtricitabine include 3'-sulfoxide diastereomers and their glucuronic acid conjugate. Emtricitabine is eliminated by a combination of glomerular filtration and active tubular secretion. Following a single oral dose of EMTRIVA, the plasma emtricitabine half-life is approximately 10 hours.

Tenofovir Disoproxil Fumarate: The pharmacokinetic properties of tenofovir disoproxil fumarate are summarized in Table 6. Following oral administration of VIREAD, maximum tenofovir serum concentrations are achieved in 1.0 ± 0.4 hour. Less than 0.7% of tenofovir binds to human plasma proteins in vitro and the binding is independent of concentration over the range of 0.01–25 µg/mL. Approximately 70–80% of the intravenous dose of tenofovir is recovered as unchanged drug in the urine. Tenofovir is eliminated by a combination of glomerular filtration and active tubular secretion. Following a single oral dose of VIREAD, the terminal elimination half-life of tenofovir is approximately 17 hours.

Table 6 Single Dose Pharmacokinetic Parameters for Emtricitabine and Tenofovir in Adults*

	Emtricitabine	Tenofovir
Fasted Oral Bioavailability† (%)	92 (83.1–106.4)	25 (NC–45.0)
Plasma Terminal Elimination Half-Life† (hr)	10 (7.4–18.0)	17 (12.0–25.7)
C_{max}‡ (µg/mL)	1.8 ± 0.72§	0.30 ± 0.09
AUC‡ (µg•hr/mL)	10.0 ± 3.12§	2.29 ± 0.69
CL/F‡ (mL/min)	302 ± 94	1043 ± 115
CL_{renal}‡ (mL/min)	213 ± 89	243 ± 33

* NC = Not calculated
† Median (range)
‡ Mean (± SD)
§ Data presented as steady state values

Effects of Food on Oral Absorption

TRUVADA may be administered with or without food. Administration of TRUVADA following a high fat meal (784 kcal; 49 grams of fat) or a light meal (373 kcal; 8 grams of fat) delayed the time of tenofovir C_{max} by approximately 0.75 hour. The mean increases in tenofovir AUC and C_{max} were approximately 35% and 15%, respectively, when administered with a high fat or light meal, compared to administration in the fasted state. In previous safety and efficacy trials, VIREAD (tenofovir) was taken under fed conditions. Emtricitabine systemic exposures (AUC and C_{max}) were unaffected when TRUVADA was administered with either a high fat or a light meal.

Special Populations

Race

Emtricitabine: No pharmacokinetic differences due to race have been identified following the administration of EMTRIVA.

Table 7 Drug Interactions: Changes in Pharmacokinetic Parameters for Emtricitabine in the Presence of the Coadministered Drug*

Coadministered Drug	Dose of Coadministered Drug (mg)	Emtricitabine Dose (mg)	N	% Change of Emtricitabine Pharmacokinetic Parameters† (90% CI)		
				C_{max}	AUC	C_{min}
Tenofovir DF	300 once daily × 7 days	200 once daily × 7 days	17	⇔	⇔	↑ 20 (↑ 12 to ↑ 29)
Zidovudine	300 twice daily × 7 days	200 once daily × 7 days	27	⇔	⇔	⇔
Indinavir	800 × 1	200 × 1	12	⇔	⇔	NA
Famciclovir	500 × 1	200 × 1	12	⇔	⇔	NA
Stavudine	40 × 1	200 × 1	6	⇔	⇔	NA

* All interaction trials conducted in healthy volunteers
† ↑ = Increase; ↓ = Decrease; ⇔ = No Effect; NA = Not Applicable

Table 8 Drug Interactions: Changes in Pharmacokinetic Parameters for Coadministered Drug in the Presence of Emtricitabine*

Coadministered Drug	Dose of Coadministered Drug (mg)	Emtricitabine Dose (mg)	N	% Change of Coadministered Drug Pharmacokinetic Parameters† (90% CI)		
				C_{max}	AUC	C_{min}
Tenofovir DF	300 once daily × 7 days	200 once daily × 7 days	17	⇔	⇔	⇔
Zidovudine	300 twice daily × 7 days	200 once daily × 7 days	27	↑ 17 (↑ 0 to ↑ 38)	↑ 13 (↑ 5 to ↑ 20)	⇔
Indinavir	800 × 1	200 × 1	12	⇔	⇔	NA
Famciclovir	500 × 1	200 × 1	12	⇔	⇔	NA
Stavudine	40 × 1	200 × 1	6	⇔	⇔	NA

* All interaction trials conducted in healthy volunteers
† ↑ = Increase; ↓ = Decrease; ⇔ = No Effect; NA = Not Applicable

Tenofovir Disoproxil Fumarate: There were insufficient numbers from racial and ethnic groups other than Caucasian to adequately determine potential pharmacokinetic differences among these populations following the administration of VIREAD.

Gender

Emtricitabine and Tenofovir Disoproxil Fumarate: Emtricitabine and tenofovir pharmacokinetics are similar in male and female subjects.

Pediatric Patients

TRUVADA should not be administered to HIV-1 infected pediatric patients less than 12 years of age or weighing less than 35 kg (less than 77 lb).

Emtricitabine: The pharmacokinetics of emtricitabine at steady state were determined in 27 HIV-1-infected pediatric subjects 13 to 17 years of age receiving a daily dose of 6 mg/kg up to a maximum dose of 240 mg oral solution or a 200 mg capsule; 26 of 27 subjects in this age group received the 200 mg EMTRIVA capsule. Mean (± SD) C_{max} and AUC were 2.7 ± 0.9 µg/mL and 12.6 ± 5.4 µg•hr/mL, respectively. Exposures achieved in pediatric subjects 12 to less than 18 years of age were similar to those achieved in adults receiving a once daily dose of 200 mg.

Tenofovir Disoproxil Fumarate: Steady-state pharmacokinetics of tenofovir were evaluated in 8 HIV-1 infected pediatric subjects (12 to less than 18 years). Mean (± SD) C_{max} and AUC_{tau} are 0.38 ± 0.13 µg/mL and 3.39 ± 1.22 µg•hr/mL, respectively. Tenofovir exposure achieved in these pediatric subjects receiving oral daily doses of VIREAD 300 mg was similar to exposures achieved in adults receiving once-daily doses of VIREAD 300 mg.

Geriatric Patients

Pharmacokinetics of emtricitabine and tenofovir have not been fully evaluated in the elderly (65 years of age and older).

Patients with Impaired Renal Function

The pharmacokinetics of emtricitabine and tenofovir are altered in subjects with renal impairment *[See Warnings and Precautions (5.3)]*. In adult subjects with creatinine clearance below 50 mL/min, C_{max}, and $AUC_{0-\infty}$ of emtricitabine and tenofovir were increased. It is recommended that the dosing interval for TRUVADA be modified in HIV-infected adult patients with creatinine clearance 30–49 mL/min. No data are available to make dose recommendations in pediatric patients with renal impairment. TRUVADA should not be used in patients with creatinine clearance below 30 mL/min and in patients with end-stage renal disease requiring dialysis *[See Dosage and Administration (2.3)]*.

TRUVADA for a PrEP indication should not be used in HIV-1 uninfected individuals with creatinine clearance below 60 mL/min. If a decrease in creatinine clearance is observed in uninfected individuals while using TRUVADA for PrEP, evaluate potential causes and re-assess potential risks and benefits of continued use *[See Dosage and Administration (2.3)]*.

Patients with Hepatic Impairment

The pharmacokinetics of tenofovir following a 300 mg dose of VIREAD have been studied in non-HIV infected subjects with moderate to severe hepatic impairment. There were no substantial alterations in tenofovir pharmacokinetics in subjects with hepatic impairment compared with unimpaired subjects. The pharmacokinetics of TRUVADA or emtricitabine have not been studied in subjects with hepatic impairment; however, emtricitabine is not significantly metabolized by liver enzymes, so the impact of liver impairment should be limited.

Assessment of Drug Interactions

The steady state pharmacokinetics of emtricitabine and tenofovir were unaffected when emtricitabine and tenofovir disoproxil fumarate were administered together versus each agent dosed alone.

In vitro studies and clinical pharmacokinetic drug-drug interaction trials have shown that the potential for CYP mediated interactions involving emtricitabine and tenofovir with other medicinal products is low.

No clinically significant drug interactions have been observed between emtricitabine and famciclovir, indinavir, stavudine, tenofovir disoproxil fumarate, and zidovudine (see Tables 7 and 8). Similarly, no clinically significant drug interactions have been observed between tenofovir disoproxil fumarate and efavirenz, methadone, nelfinavir, oral contraceptives, or ribavirin in trials conducted in healthy volunteers (see Tables 9 and 10).

[See table 7 above]
[See table 8 above]
[See table 9 at top of next page]
[See table 10 at top of page 899]

Coadministration of tenofovir disoproxil fumarate with didanosine results in changes in the pharmacokinetics of didanosine that may be of clinical significance. Concomitant

Table 9 Drug Interactions: Changes in Pharmacokinetic Parameters for Tenofovir* in the Presence of the Coadministered Drug

Coadministered Drug	Dose of Coadministered Drug (mg)	N	% Change of Tenofovir Pharmacokinetic Parameters† (90% CI)		
			C_{max}	AUC	C_{min}
Abacavir	300 once	8	⇔	⇔	NC
Atazanavir‡	400 once daily × 14 days	33	↑ 14 (↑ 8 to ↑ 20)	↑ 24 (↑ 21 to ↑ 28)	↑ 22 (↑ 15 to ↑ 30)
Didanosine§	250 or 400 once daily × 7 days	14	⇔	⇔	⇔
Emtricitabine	200 once daily × 7 days	17	⇔	⇔	⇔
Entecavir	1 mg once daily × 10 days	28	⇔	⇔	⇔
Indinavir	800 three times daily × 7 days	13	↑ 14 (↓ 3 to ↑ 33)	⇔	⇔
Lamivudine	150 twice daily × 7 days	15	⇔	⇔	⇔
Lopinavir/ Ritonavir	400/100 twice daily × 14 days	24	⇔	↑ 32 (↑ 25 to ↑ 38)	↑ 51 (↑ 37 to ↑ 66)
Saquinavir/ Ritonavir	1000/100 twice daily × 14 days	35	⇔	⇔	↑ 23 (↑ 16 to ↑ 30)
Tacrolimus	0.05 mg/kg twice daily × 7 days	21	↑ 13 (↑ 1 to ↑ 27)	⇔	⇔

* Subjects received VIREAD 300 mg once daily
† Increase = ↑; Decrease = ↓; No Effect = ⇔; NC = Not Calculated
‡ Reyataz Prescribing Information
§ Subjects received didanosine buffered tablets.

dosing of tenofovir disoproxil fumarate with didanosine enteric-coated capsules significantly increases the C_{max} and AUC of didanosine. When didanosine 250 mg enteric-coated capsules were administered with tenofovir disoproxil fumarate, systemic exposures of didanosine were similar to those seen with the 400 mg enteric-coated capsules alone under fasted conditions. The mechanism of this interaction is unknown. See *Drug Interactions (7.1)* regarding use of didanosine with VIREAD.

12.4 Microbiology

Mechanism of Action

Emtricitabine: Emtricitabine, a synthetic nucleoside analog of cytidine, is phosphorylated by cellular enzymes to form emtricitabine 5′-triphosphate. Emtricitabine 5′-triphosphate inhibits the activity of the HIV-1 reverse transcriptase (RT) by competing with the natural substrate deoxycytidine 5′-triphosphate and by being incorporated into nascent viral DNA which results in chain termination.Emtricitabine 5′-triphosphate is a weak inhibitor of mammalian DNA polymerase α, β, ϵ and mitochondrial DNA polymerase γ.

Tenofovir Disoproxil Fumarate: Tenofovir disoproxil fumarate is an acyclic nucleoside phosphonate diester analog of adenosine monophosphate. Tenofovir disoproxil fumarate requires initial diester hydrolysis for conversion to tenofovir and subsequent phosphorylations by cellular enzymes to form tenofovir diphosphate. Tenofovir diphosphate inhibits the activity of HIV-1 RT by competing with the natural substrate deoxyadenosine 5′-triphosphate and, after incorporation into DNA, by DNA chain termination. Tenofovir diphosphate is a weak inhibitor of mammalian DNA polymerases α, β, and mitochondrial DNA polymerase γ.

Antiviral Activity

Emtricitabine and Tenofovir Disoproxil Fumarate: In combination studies evaluating the cell culture antiviral activity of emtricitabine and tenofovir together, synergistic antiviral effects were observed.

Emtricitabine: The antiviral activity of emtricitabine against laboratory and clinical isolates of HIV-1 was assessed in lymphoblastoid cell lines, the MAGI-CCR5 cell line, and peripheral blood mononuclear cells. The 50% effective concentration (EC_{50}) values for emtricitabine were in the range of 0.0013–0.64 μM (0.0003–0.158 μg/mL). In drug combination studies of emtricitabine with nucleoside reverse transcriptase inhibitors (abacavir, lamivudine, stavudine, zalcitabine, zidovudine), non-nucleoside reverse transcriptase inhibitors (delavirdine, efavirenz, nevirapine), and protease inhibitors (amprenavir, nelfinavir, ritonavir, saquinavir), additive to synergistic effects were observed. Emtricitabine displayed antiviral activity in cell culture against HIV-1 clades A, B, C, D, E, F, and G (EC_{50} values ranged from 0.007–0.075 μM) and showed strain specific activity against HIV-2 (EC_{50} values ranged from 0.007–1.5 μM).

Tenofovir Disoproxil Fumarate: The antiviral activity of tenofovir against laboratory and clinical isolates of HIV-1 was assessed in lymphoblastoid cell lines, primary monocyte/macrophage cells and peripheral blood lymphocytes. The EC_{50} values for tenofovir were in the range of 0.04–8.5 μM. In drug combination studies of tenofovir with nucleoside reverse transcriptase inhibitors (abacavir, didanosine, lamivudine, stavudine, zalcitabine, zidovudine), non-nucleoside reverse transcriptase inhibitors (delavirdine, efavirenz, nevirapine), and protease inhibitors (amprenavir, indinavir, nelfinavir, ritonavir, saquinavir), additive to synergistic effects were observed. Tenofovir displayed antiviral activity in cell culture against HIV-1 clades A, B, C, D, E, F, G and O (EC_{50} values ranged from 0.5–2.2 μM) and showed strain specific activity against HIV-2 (EC_{50} values ranged from 1.6 μM to 5.5 μM).

Prophylactic Activity in a Nonhuman Primate Model of HIV Transmission

Emtricitabine and Tenofovir Disoproxil Fumarate: The prophylactic activity of the combination of daily oral emtricitabine (FTC) and tenofovir disoproxil fumarate (TDF) was evaluated in a controlled study of macaques inoculated once weekly for 14 weeks with SIV/HIV-1 chimeric virus (SHIV) applied to the rectal surface. Of the 18 control animals, 17 became infected after a median of 2 weeks. In contrast, 4 of the 6 animals treated daily with oral FTC and TDF remained uninfected and the two infections that did occur were significantly delayed until 9 and 12 weeks and exhibited reduced viremia. An M184I-expressing FTC-resistant variant emerged in 1 of the 2 macaques after 3 weeks of continued drug exposure.

Resistance

Emtricitabine and Tenofovir Disoproxil Fumarate: HIV-1 isolates with reduced susceptibility to the combination of emtricitabine and tenofovir have been selected in cell culture. Genotypic analysis of these isolates identified the M184V/I and/or K65R amino acid substitutions in the viral RT.

In a clinical trial of treatment-naive subjects *[Study 934, see Clinical Studies (14.1)]*, resistance analysis was performed on HIV-1 isolates from all confirmed virologic failure subjects with greater than 400 copies/mL of HIV-1 RNA at Week 144 or early discontinuation. Development of efavirenz resistance-associated substitutions occurred most frequently and was similar between the treatment arms. The M184V amino acid substitution, associated with resistance to EMTRIVA and lamivudine, was observed in 2/19 analyzed subject isolates in the EMTRIVA + VIREAD group and in 10/29 analyzed subject isolates in the zidovudine/lamivudine group. Through 144 weeks of Study 934, no subjects have developed a detectable K65R substitution in their HIV-1 as analyzed through standard genotypic analysis.

Emtricitabine: Emtricitabine-resistant isolates of HIV-1 have been selected in cell culture and in vivo. Genotypic analysis of these isolates showed that the reduced susceptibility to emtricitabine was associated with a substitution in the HIV-1 RT gene at codon 184 which resulted in an amino acid substitution of methionine by valine or isoleucine (M184V/I).

Tenofovir Disoproxil Fumarate: HIV-1 isolates with reduced susceptibility to tenofovir have been selected in cell culture. These viruses expressed a K65R substitution in RT and showed a 2–4 fold reduction in susceptibility to tenofovir.

In treatment-naive subjects, isolates from 8/47 (17%) analyzed subjects developed the K65R substitution in the VIREAD arm through 144 weeks; 7 occurred in the first 48 weeks of treatment and 1 at Week 96. In treatment-experienced subjects, 14/304 (5%) isolates from subjects failing VIREAD through Week 96 showed greater than 1.4 fold (median 2.7) reduced susceptibility to tenofovir. Genotypic analysis of the resistant isolates showed a substitution in the HIV-1 RT gene resulting in the K65R amino acid substitution.

iPrEx Trial: In a clinical study of HIV-1 seronegative subjects *[iPrEx Trial, see Clinical Studies (14.2)]*, no amino acid substitutions associated with resistance to emtricitabine or tenofovir were detected at the time of seroconversion among 48 subjects in the TRUVADA group and 83 subjects in the placebo group who became infected with HIV-1 during the trial. Ten subjects were observed to be HIV-1 infected at time of enrollment. The M184V/I substitutions associated with resistance to emtricitabine were observed in 3 of the 10 subjects (2 of 2 in the TRUVADA group and 1 of 8 in the placebo group). One of the two subjects in the TRUVADA group harbored wild type virus at enrollment and developed the M184V substitution 4 weeks after enrollment. The other subject had indeterminate resistance at enrollment but was found to have the M184I substitution 4 weeks after enrollment.

Partners PrEP Trial: In a clinical study of HIV-1 seronegative subjects *[Partners PrEP Trial, see Clinical Studies (14.3)]*, no variants expressing amino acid substitutions associated with resistance to emtricitabine or tenofovir were detected at the time of seroconversion among 12 subjects in the TRUVADA group, 15 subjects in the VIREAD group, and 51 subjects in the placebo group. Fourteen subjects were observed to be HIV-1 infected at the time of enrollment (3 in the TRUVADA group, 5 in the VIREAD group, and 6 in the placebo group). One of the three subjects in the TRUVADA group who was infected with wild type virus at enrollment selected an M184V expressing virus by week 12. Two of the five subjects in the VIREAD group had tenofovir-resistant viruses at the time of seroconversion; one subject infected with wild type virus at enrollment developed a K65R substitution by week 16, while the second subject had virus expressing the combination of D67N and K70R substitutions upon seroconversion at week 60, although baseline virus was not genotyped and it is unclear if the resistance emerged or was transmitted. Following enrollment, 4 subjects (2 in the VIREAD group, 1 in the TRUVADA group, and 1 in the placebo group) had virus expressing K103N or V106A substitutions, which confer high-level resistance to NNRTIs but have not been associated with tenofovir or emtricitabine and may have been present in the infecting virus.

Cross Resistance

Emtricitabine and Tenofovir Disoproxil Fumarate: Cross-resistance among certain nucleoside reverse transcriptase inhibitors (NRTIs) has been recognized. The M184V/I and/or K65R substitutions selected in cell culture by the combination of emtricitabine and tenofovir are also observed in some HIV-1 isolates from subjects failing treatment with tenofovir in combination with either lamivudine or emtricitabine, and either abacavir or didanosine. Therefore, cross-resistance among these drugs may occur in patients whose virus harbors either or both of these amino acid substitutions.

Emtricitabine: Emtricitabine-resistant isolates (M184V/I) were cross-resistant to lamivudine and zalcitabine but retained susceptibility in cell culture to didanosine, stavudine, tenofovir, zidovudine, and NNRTIs (delavirdine, efavirenz, and nevirapine). HIV-1 isolates containing the K65R substitution, selected in vivo by abacavir, didanosine, tenofovir, and zalcitabine, demonstrated reduced susceptibility to inhibition by emtricitabine. Viruses harboring substitutions conferring reduced susceptibility to stavudine and zidovudine (M41L, D67N, K70R, L210W, T215Y/F, K219Q/E), or didanosine (L74V) remained sensitive to emtricitabine. HIV-1 containing the K103N substitution associated with resistance to NNRTIs was susceptible to emtricitabine.

Tenofovir Disoproxil Fumarate: HIV-1 isolates from subjects (N=20) whose HIV-1 expressed a mean of 3 zidovudine-associated RT amino acid substitutions (M41L, D67N, K70R, L210W, T215Y/F, or K219Q/E/N) showed a 3.1-fold decrease in the susceptibility to tenofovir. Subjects whose virus expressed an L74V substitution without zidovudine resistance associated substitutions (N=8) had reduced response to VIREAD. Limited data are available for patients whose virus expressed a Y115F substitution (N=3), Q151M substitution (N=2), or T69 insertion (N=4), all of whom had a reduced response.

13 NONCLINICAL TOXICOLOGY

13.1 Carcinogenesis, Mutagenesis, Impairment of Fertility

Emtricitabine: In long-term oral carcinogenicity studies of emtricitabine, no drug-related increases in tumor incidence were found in mice at doses up to 750 mg/kg/day (26 times the human systemic exposure at the therapeutic dose of 200 mg/day) or in rats at doses up to 600 mg/kg/day (31 times the human systemic exposure at the therapeutic dose).

Emtricitabine was not genotoxic in the reverse mutation bacterial test (Ames test), mouse lymphoma or mouse micronucleus assays.

Emtricitabine did not affect fertility in male rats at approximately 140-fold or in male and female mice at approximately 60-fold higher exposures (AUC) than in humans given the recommended 200 mg daily dose. Fertility was normal in the offspring of mice exposed daily from before birth (in utero) through sexual maturity at daily exposures (AUC) of approximately 60-fold higher than human exposures at the recommended 200 mg daily dose.

Tenofovir Disoproxil Fumarate: Long-term oral carcinogenicity studies of tenofovir disoproxil fumarate in mice and rats were carried out at exposures up to approximately 16 times (mice) and 5 times (rats) those observed in humans at the therapeutic dose for HIV-1 infection. At the high dose in female mice, liver adenomas were increased at exposures 16 times that in humans. In rats, the study was negative for carcinogenic findings at exposures up to 5 times that observed in humans at the therapeutic dose.

Tenofovir disoproxil fumarate was mutagenic in the in vitro mouse lymphoma assay and negative in an in vitro bacterial mutagenicity test (Ames test). In an in vivo mouse micronucleus assay, tenofovir disoproxil fumarate was negative when administered to male mice.

There were no effects on fertility, mating performance or early embryonic development when tenofovir disoproxil fumarate was administered to male rats at a dose equivalent to 10 times the human dose based on body surface area comparisons for 28 days prior to mating and to female rats for 15 days prior to mating through day seven of gestation. There was, however, an alteration of the estrous cycle in female rats.

13.2 Animal Toxicology and/or Pharmacology

Tenofovir and tenofovir disoproxil fumarate administered in toxicology studies to rats, dogs and monkeys at exposures (based on AUCs) greater than or equal to 6-fold those observed in humans caused bone toxicity. In monkeys the bone toxicity was diagnosed as osteomalacia. Osteomalacia observed in monkeys appeared to be reversible upon dose reduction or discontinuation of tenofovir. In rats and dogs, the bone toxicity manifested as reduced bone mineral density. The mechanism(s) underlying bone toxicity is unknown.

Evidence of renal toxicity was noted in 4 animal species. Increases in serum creatinine, BUN, glycosuria, proteinuria, phosphaturia, and/or calciuria and decreases in serum phosphate were observed to varying degrees in these animals. These toxicities were noted at exposures (based on AUCs) 2–20 times higher than those observed in humans. The relationship of the renal abnormalities, particularly the phosphaturia, to the bone toxicity is not known.

14 CLINICAL STUDIES

Clinical Study 934 supports the use of TRUVADA tablets for the treatment of HIV-1 infection. Additional data in support of the use of TRUVADA are derived from clinical Study 903, in which lamivudine and tenofovir disoproxil fumarate (tenofovir DF) were used in combination in treatment-naive adults, and clinical Study 303 in which emtricitabine and lamivudine demonstrated comparable efficacy, safety and resistance patterns as part of multidrug regimens. For additional information about these trials, please consult the prescribing information for tenofovir DF and emtricitabine. The iPrEx study and Partners PrEP study support the use of TRUVADA to help reduce the risk of acquiring HIV-1.

14.1 Study 934

Data through 144 weeks are reported for Study 934, a randomized, open-label, active-controlled multicenter trial comparing emtricitabine + tenofovir DF administered in combination with efavirenz versus zidovudine/lamivudine fixed-dose combination administered in combination with efavirenz in 511 antiretroviral-naive subjects. From Weeks 96 to 144 of the trial, subjects received TRUVADA with efavirenz in place of emtricitabine + tenofovir DF with efavirenz. Subjects had a mean age of 38 years (range 18–80), 86% were male, 59% were Caucasian and 23% were Black. The mean baseline $CD4^+$ cell count was 245 cells/mm^3 (range 2–1191) and median baseline plasma HIV-1 RNA was 5.01 $\log_{10}$ copies/mL (range 3.56–6.54). Subjects were stratified by baseline $CD4^+$ cell count (< or ≥200 cells/mm^3); 41% had $CD4^+$ cell counts <200 cells/mm^3 and 51% of subjects had baseline viral loads >100,000 copies/mL. Treatment outcomes through 48 and 144 weeks for those subjects who did not have efavirenz resistance at baseline are presented in Table 11.

[See table 11 at top of next page]

Through Week 48, 84% and 73% of subjects in the emtricitabine + tenofovir DF group and the zidovudine/lamivudine group, respectively, achieved and maintained HIV-1 RNA <400 copies/mL (71% and 58% through Week 144). The difference in the proportion of subjects who achieved and maintained HIV-1 RNA <400 copies/mL through 48 weeks largely results from the higher number of discontinuations due to adverse events and other reasons in the zidovudine/lamivudine group in this open-label trial. In addition, 80% and 70% of subjects in the emtricitabine + tenofovir DF group and the zidovudine/lamivudine group, respectively, achieved and maintained HIV-1 RNA <50 copies/mL through Week 48 (64% and 56% through Week 144). The mean increase from baseline in $CD4^+$ cell count was 190 cells/mm^3 in the emtricitabine + tenofovir DF group and 158 cells/mm^3 in the zidovudine/lamivudine group at Week 48 (312 and 271 cells/mm^3 at Week 144).

Through 48 weeks, 7 subjects in the emtricitabine + tenofovir DF group and 5 subjects in the zidovudine/lamivudine group experienced a new CDC Class C event (10 and 6 subjects through 144 weeks).

14.2 iPrEx Trial

The iPrEx trial was a randomized double-blind placebo-controlled multinational study evaluating TRUVADA in 2499 HIV-seronegative men or transgender women who have sex with men and with evidence of high risk behavior for HIV-1 infection. Evidence of high risk behavior included any one of the following reported to have occurred up to six months prior to study screening: no condom use during anal intercourse with an HIV-1 positive partner or a partner of unknown HIV status; anal intercourse with more than 3 sex partners; exchange of money, gifts, shelter or drugs for anal sex; sex with male partner and diagnosis of sexually transmitted infection; no consistent use of condoms with sex partner known to be HIV-1 positive.

All subjects received monthly HIV-1 testing, risk-reduction counseling, condoms and management of sexually transmitted infections. Of the 2499 enrolled, 1251 received TRUVADA and 1248 received placebo. The mean age of subjects was 27 years, 5% were Asian, 9% Black, 18% White, and 72% Hispanic/Latino.

Subjects were followed for 4237 person-years. The primary outcome measure for the study was the incidence of documented HIV seroconversion. At the end of treatment, emergent HIV-1 seroconversion was observed in 131 subjects, of which 48 occurred in the TRUVADA group and 83 occurred in the placebo group, indicating a 42% (95% CI: 18% to 60%) reduction in risk. Risk reduction was found to be higher (53%; 95% CI: 34% to 72%) among subjects who reported previous unprotected anal intercourse (URAI) at screening (732 and 753 subjects reported URAI within the last 12 weeks at screening in the TRUVADA and placebo groups, respectively). In a post-hoc case control study of plasma and intracellular drug levels in about 10% of study subjects, risk reduction appeared to be the greatest in subjects with detectable intracellular tenofovir. Efficacy was therefore strongly correlated with adherence.

Table 10 Drug Interactions: Changes in Pharmacokinetic Parameters for Coadministered Drug in the Presence of Tenofovir

Coadministered Drug	Dose of Coadministered Drug (mg)	N	% Change of Coadministered Drug Pharmacokinetic Parameters* (90% CI)		
			C_{max}	AUC	C_{min}
Abacavir	300 once	8	↑ 12 (↓ 1 to ↑ 26)	⇔	NA
Atazanavir†	400 once daily × 14 days	34	↓ 21 (↓ 27 to ↓ 14)	↓ 25 (↓ 30 to ↓ 19)	↓ 40 (↓ 48 to ↓ 32)
Atazanavir†	Atazanavir/Ritonavir 300/100 once daily × 42 days	10	↓ 28 (↓ 50 to ↑ 5)	↓ 25‡ (↓ 42 to ↓ 3)	↓ 23‡ (↓ 46 to ↑ 10)
Didanosine§	250 once, simultaneously with tenofovir DF and a light meal¶	33	↓ 20# (↓ 32 to ↓ 7)	⇔#	NA
Emtricitabine	200 once daily × 7 days	17	⇔	⇔	↑ 20 (↑ 12 to ↑ 29)
Indinavir	800 three times daily × 7 days	12	↓ 11 (↓ 30 to ↑ 12)	⇔	⇔
Entecavir	1 mg once daily × 10 days	28	⇔	↑ 13 (↑ 11 to ↑ 15)	⇔
Lamivudine	150 twice daily × 7 days	15	↓ 24 (↓ 34 to ↓ 12)	⇔	⇔
Lopinavir Ritonavir	Lopinavir/Ritonavir 400/100 twice daily × 14 days	24	⇔ ⇔	⇔ ⇔	⇔ ⇔
Saquinavir	Saquinavir/Ritonavir 1000/100 twice daily × 14 days	32	↑ 22 (↑ 6 to ↑ 41)	↑ 29Þ (↑ 12 to ↑ 48)	↑ 47Þ (↑ 23 to ↑ 76)
Ritonavir			⇔	⇔	↑ 23 (↑ 3 to ↑ 46)
Tacrolimus	0.05 mg/kg twice daily × 7 days	21	⇔	⇔	⇔

* Increase = ↑; Decrease = ↓; No Effect = ⇔; NA = Not Applicable

† Reyataz Prescribing Information

‡ In HIV-infected subjects, addition of tenofovir DF to atazanavir 300 mg plus ritonavir 100 mg, resulted in AUC and C_{min} values of atazanavir that were 2.3 and 4-fold higher than the respective values observed for atazanavir 400 mg when given alone.

§ Videx EC Prescribing Information. Subjects received didanosine enteric-coated capsules.

¶ 373 kcal, 8.2 g fat

#Compared with didanosine (enteric-coated) 400 mg administered alone under fasting conditions.

Þ Increases in AUC and C_{min} are not expected to be clinically relevant; hence no dose adjustments are required when tenofovir DF and ritonavir-boosted saquinavir are coadministered.

Table 11 Outcomes of Randomized Treatment at Week 48 and 144 (Study 934)

Outcomes	At Week 48		At Week 144	
	FTC + TDF + EFV (N=244)	AZT/3TC + EFV (N=243)	FTC + TDF + EFV (N=227)*	AZT/3TC + EFV (N=229)*
Responder†	84%	73%	71%	58%
Virologic failure‡	2%	4%	3%	6%
Rebound	1%	3%	2%	5%
Never suppressed	0%	0%	0%	0%
Change in antiretroviral regimen	1%	1%	1%	1%
Death	<1%	1%	1%	1%
Discontinued due to adverse event	4%	9%	5%	12%
Discontinued for other reasons§	10%	14%	20%	22%

* Subjects who were responders at Week 48 or Week 96 (HIV-1 RNA <400 copies/mL) but did not consent to continue trial after Week 48 or Week 96 were excluded from analysis.
† Subjects achieved and maintained confirmed HIV-1 RNA <400 copies/mL through Weeks 48 and 144.
‡ Includes confirmed viral rebound and failure to achieve confirmed <400 copies/mL through Weeks 48 and 144.
§ Includes lost to follow-up, subject withdrawal, noncompliance, protocol violation and other reasons.

14.3 Partners PrEP Trial

The Partners PrEP trial was a randomized, double-blind, placebo-controlled 3 arm trial conducted in 4758 serodiscordant heterosexual couples in Kenya and Uganda to evaluate the efficacy and safety of TDF (N=1589) and FTC/TDF (N=1583) versus (parallel comparison) placebo (N=1586), in preventing HIV-1 acquisition by the uninfected partner.

All subjects received monthly HIV-1 testing, evaluation of adherence, assessment of sexual behavior, and safety evaluations. Women were also tested monthly for pregnancy. Women who became pregnant during the trial had study drug interrupted for the duration of the pregnancy and while breastfeeding. The uninfected partner subjects were predominantly male (61–64% across study drug groups), and had a mean age of 33–34 years.

Following 7827 person-years of follow up, 82 emergent HIV-1 seroconversions were reported, with an overall observed seroincidence rate of 1.05 per 100 person-years. Of the 82 seroconversions, 13 and 52 occurred in partner subjects randomized to TRUVADA and placebo, respectively. Two of the 13 seroconversions in the TRUVADA arm and 3 of the 52 seroconversions in the placebo arm occurred in women during treatment interruptions for pregnancy. The risk reduction for TRUVADA relative to placebo was 75% (95% CI: 55% to 87%). In a post-hoc case control study of plasma drug levels in about 10% of study subjects, risk reduction appeared to be the greatest in subjects with detectable plasma tenofovir. Efficacy was therefore strongly correlated with adherence.

16 HOW SUPPLIED/STORAGE AND HANDLING

The blue, capsule-shaped, film-coated, tablets contain 200 mg of emtricitabine and 300 mg of tenofovir disoproxil fumarate (which is equivalent to 245 mg of tenofovir disoproxil), are debossed with "GILEAD" on one side and with "701" on the other side, and are available in unit of use bottles [containing a dessicant (silica gel canister or sachet) and closed with a child-resistant closure] of:

- 30 tablets (NDC 61958-0701-1)

Store at 25 °C (77 °F), excursions permitted to 15 °C –30 °C (59 °F –86 °F) (see USP Controlled Room Temperature).

- Keep container tightly closed
- Dispense only in original container
- Do not use if seal over bottle opening is broken or missing

17 PATIENT COUNSELING INFORMATION

As a part of patient counseling, healthcare providers must review the TRUVADA Medication Guide with every uninfected individual taking TRUVADA to reduce the risk of acquiring HIV.

See FDA-approved patient labeling (Medication Guide)

17.1 Important Information for All Patients and Uninfected Individuals

Advise patients and uninfected individuals that:

- The long term effects of TRUVADA are unknown.
- TRUVADA tablets are for oral ingestion only.
- Patients and uninfected individuals should not discontinue TRUVADA without first informing their physicians.
- Patients and uninfected individuals should remain under the care of a physician when using TRUVADA.
- It is important to take TRUVADA on a regular dosing schedule to avoid missing doses.
- Lactic acidosis and severe hepatomegaly with steatosis, including fatal cases, have been reported. Treatment with TRUVADA should be suspended in patients or uninfected individuals who develop clinical symptoms suggestive of lactic acidosis or pronounced hepatotoxicity (including nausea, vomiting, unusual or unexpected stomach discomfort, and weakness) *[See Warnings and Precautions (5.1)]*.
- Severe acute exacerbations of hepatitis B have been reported in patients who are coinfected with hepatitis B virus (HBV) and HIV-1 and have discontinued TRUVADA. Before initiating TRUVADA, test all patients and uninfected individuals for HBV. All patients who are infected with HBV need close medical follow-up for several months after stopping TRUVADA to monitor for exacerbations of hepatitis *[See Warnings and Precautions (5.2)]*.
- Renal impairment, including cases of acute renal failure and Fanconi syndrome, has been reported in association with the use of VIREAD. TRUVADA should be avoided with concurrent or recent use of a nephrotoxic agent *[See Warnings and Precautions (5.3)]*. Dosing interval of TRUVADA may need adjustment in HIV-1 infected patients with renal impairment. TRUVADA for a PrEP indication should not be used in HIV-1 uninfected individuals if creatinine clearance is less than 60 mL/min. If a decrease in creatinine clearance is observed in uninfected individuals while using TRUVADA for PrEP, evaluate potential causes and re-assess potential risks and benefits of continued use *[See Dosage and Administration (2.3)]*.
- Do not administer TRUVADA with ATRIPLA, COMPLERA, EMTRIVA, STRIBILD, or VIREAD; or with drugs containing lamivudine, including Combivir (lamivudine/zidovudine), Epivir or Epivir-HBV (lamivudine), Epzicom (abacavir sulfate/lamivudine), or Trizivir (abacavir sulfate/lamivudine/zidovudine) *[See Warnings and Precautions (5.4)]*.
- Do not administer TRUVADA with HEPSERA *[See Warnings and Precautions (5.4)]*.
- Decreases in bone mineral density have been observed with the use of VIREAD or TRUVADA. Consider bone monitoring in patients and uninfected individuals who have a history of pathologic bone fracture or at risk for osteopenia *[See Warnings and Precautions (5.5)]*.
- Patients and uninfected individuals should avoid doing things that can spread HIV-1 or HBV infection.
  - Do not share needles or other injection equipment.
  - Do not share personal items that can have blood or body fluids on them, like toothbrushes and razor blades.
  - Do not have any kind of sex without protection. Always practice safer sex by using a latex or polyurethane condom to lower the chance of sexual contact with semen, vaginal secretions, or blood.
  - Patients and uninfected individuals should not breastfeed because the drugs in TRUVADA can be passed to the baby in breast milk, and it is not known whether they can harm the baby. HIV-positive women should also not breastfeed because of the risk of passing the HIV-1 virus to the baby.

17.2 Treatment of HIV-1 Infection

When TRUVADA is used in the treatment of HIV-infection, advise patients that:

- TRUVADA is not a cure for HIV-1 infection and patients may continue to experience illnesses associated with HIV-1 infection, including opportunistic infections.
- It is important to take TRUVADA in a regular dosing schedule with combination therapy to avoid missing doses.
- All patients with HIV-1 should be tested for hepatitis B virus (HBV) before initiating and monitored after discontinuing taking TRUVADA.

17.3 Pre-Exposure Prophylaxis

When TRUVADA is used to reduce the risk of acquiring HIV-1, advise uninfected individuals about the importance of the following:

- Confirming that they are HIV-negative before starting to take TRUVADA to reduce the risk of acquiring HIV-1.
- TRUVADA should only be used as part of a complete prevention strategy including other prevention measures. In clinical trials, TRUVADA only protected some subjects from acquiring HIV-1.
- Using condoms consistently and correctly to lower the chance of sexual contact with any body fluids such as semen, vaginal secretions, or blood.
- Knowing their HIV status and the status of their partner(s).
- Getting tested regularly (at least every 3 months) for HIV-1 and ask their partner(s) to get tested as well.
- HIV-1 resistance substitutions may emerge in individuals with undetected HIV-1 infection who are taking TRUVADA, because TRUVADA alone does not constitute a complete regimen for HIV-1 treatment *[See Warnings and Precautions (5.9)]*
- Reporting any symptoms of acute HIV-1 infection (flu-like symptoms) to their healthcare provider immediately.
  - Signs and symptoms of acute infection include: fever, headache, fatigue, arthralgia, vomiting, myalgia, diarrhea, pharyngitis, rash, night sweats, and adenopathy (cervical and inguinal).
- Getting tested for other sexually transmitted infections such as syphilis and gonorrhea that may facilitate HIV-1 transmission.
- Learning about sexual risk behavior and getting support to help reduce sexual risk behavior.
- Taking TRUVADA on a regular dosing schedule and strictly adhere to the recommended dosing schedule to reduce the risk of acquiring HIV-1. Uninfected individuals who miss doses are at greater risk of acquiring HIV-1 than those who do not miss doses. *[See Warnings and Precautions (5.9)]*.
- Women who are pregnant should learn about the risks and benefits of TRUVADA to reduce the risk of acquiring HIV-1 during their pregnancy.
- Encourage use of the Agreement Form for Initiating TRUVADA for PrEP of Sexually Acquired HIV-1 Infection.

COMPLERA, EMTRIVA, HEPSERA, STRIBILD, TRUVADA, and VIREAD are trademarks of Gilead Sciences, Inc., or its related companies. ATRIPLA is a trademark of Bristol-Myers Squibb & Gilead Sciences, LLC. All other trademarks referenced herein are the property of their respective owners.

Manufactured for and distributed by:
Gilead Sciences, Inc.
Foster City, CA 94404
21-752-GS-026

Medication Guide
TRUVADA ® (tru-VAH-dah)
(emtricitabine and tenofovir disoproxil fumarate)
Tablets

Read this Medication Guide before you start taking TRUVADA and each time you get a refill. There may be new information. This information does not take the place of talking to your healthcare provider about your medical condition or your treatment.

What is the most important information I should know about TRUVADA?

TRUVADA can cause serious side effects, including:

1. Build-up of an acid in your blood (lactic acidosis). Lactic acidosis is a serious medical emergency that can lead to death.

Lactic acidosis can be hard to identify early, because the symptoms could seem like symptoms of other health problems. **Call your healthcare provider right away if you get the following symptoms which could be signs of lactic acidosis:**

- feeling very weak or tired
- unusual muscle pain
- trouble breathing
- stomach pain with
  - nausea
  - vomiting
- feel cold, especially in your arms and legs
- feel dizzy or lightheaded
- have a fast or irregular heartbeat

2. Severe liver problems. Severe liver problems can happen in people who take TRUVADA. In some cases these liver problems can lead to death. Your liver may become large (hepatomegaly) and you may develop fat in your liver (steatosis) when you take TRUVADA. **Call your healthcare provider right away if you get the following symptoms:**

- your skin or the white part of your eyes turns yellow (jaundice)

- dark "tea colored" urine
- light-colored bowel movements (stools)
- loss of appetite for several days or longer
- nausea
- stomach pain

You may be more likely to get lactic acidosis or severe liver problems if you are female, very overweight (obese), or have been taking TRUVADA for a long time.

3. Worsening of your hepatitis B infection. If you have hepatitis B virus (HBV) infection it may become worse (flare-up) if you take TRUVADA and then stop it. A "flare-up" is when your HBV infection suddenly returns in a worse way than before.

- Do not run out of TRUVADA. Refill your prescription or talk to your healthcare provider before your TRUVADA is all gone.
- Do not stop taking TRUVADA without first talking to your healthcare provider.
- If you stop taking TRUVADA, your healthcare provider will need to check your health often and do blood tests regularly for several months to check your HBV infection. Tell your healthcare provider about any new or unusual symptoms you may have after you stop taking TRUVADA.

For more information about side effects, see the section **"What are the possible side effects of TRUVADA?".**

Before taking TRUVADA to help prevent you from getting HIV:

- **You must get tested to be sure you are HIV-negative.** It is important that you also get tested at least every 3 months as recommended by your healthcare provider while taking TRUVADA. **Do not take TRUVADA to reduce the risk of getting HIV unless you are confirmed to be HIV-negative.**
- Tell your healthcare provider if you have any of the following symptoms within the last month before you start taking TRUVADA or at any time while taking TRUVADA:
  - tiredness
  - fever
  - sweating a lot (especially at night)
  - rash
  - vomiting
  - diarrhea
  - joint or muscle aches
  - headache
  - sore throat
  - enlarged lymph nodes in the neck or groin

  These may be signs of HIV infection and you may need to have a different kind of test to diagnose HIV. Also, tell your healthcare provider if you think you were exposed to the HIV virus. If you are already taking TRUVADA to prevent HIV-1 infection, your healthcare provider may tell you to stop taking TRUVADA until an HIV test confirms that you do not have HIV-1 infection.
- **TRUVADA by itself is not a complete treatment for HIV.** If you already have HIV or get HIV and take TRUVADA by itself without other medicines, you may develop resistance to TRUVADA. This means that the HIV virus may become harder to treat.
- **Just taking TRUVADA may not keep you from getting HIV. TRUVADA does not always prevent HIV.**
- **You must still practice safer sex at all times. Do not have any kind of sex without protection.** Always practice safer sex by using a latex or polyurethane condom to lower the chance of sexual contact with semen, vaginal secretions, or blood.
- **You must also use other prevention methods to keep from getting HIV.**
  - Know your HIV status and the HIV status of your partners. While taking TRUVADA, get tested at least every 3 months for HIV, as recommended by your healthcare provider. Ask your partners to get tested.
  - Get tested for other sexually transmitted infections such as syphilis and gonorrhea. These infections make it easier for HIV to infect you.
  - Get information and support to help reduce risky sexual behavior.
  - Have fewer sex partners.
- **Do not miss any doses of TRUVADA. Missing doses increases your risk of getting HIV.**
- **See the section "What is TRUVADA?" and talk to your healthcare provider for more information about how to prevent HIV infection.**

What is TRUVADA?

TRUVADA contains the prescription medicines emtricitabine (EMTRIVA®) and tenofovir disoproxil fumarate (VIREAD®). TRUVADA is used:

- with other antiviral medicines to treat Human Immunodeficiency Virus-1 (HIV-1) in adults and children age 12 years and older. HIV is the virus that causes AIDS (Acquired Immune Deficiency Syndrome).
- **with safer sex practices at all times,** to reduce the risk of getting HIV-1 in men who have sex with men who are at high risk of getting infected with HIV-1 through sex, and heterosexual couples where one partner has HIV-1 and the other does not. This is called Pre-Exposure Prophylaxis or PrEP.

It is not known if TRUVADA is safe and effective in children with HIV-1 infection who are under 12 years of age or who weigh less than 77 pounds.

When used with other HIV medicines to treat HIV-1 infection, TRUVADA may help:

- Reduce the amount of HIV in your blood. This is called "viral load."
- Increase the number of CD4+ (T) cells in your blood that help fight off other infections.
- Reducing the amount of HIV and increasing the CD4+ (T) cells in your blood may help improve your immune system. This may reduce your risk of death or infections that can happen when your immune system is weak (opportunistic infections).

TRUVADA does not cure HIV infection or AIDS. If you have HIV infection, you must stay on continuous HIV therapy to control HIV infection and decrease HIV-related illnesses.

Avoid doing things that can increase your risk of getting HIV infection or spreading HIV infection to other people:

- Do not share or re-use needles or other injection equipment.
- Do not share personal items that can have blood or body fluids on them, like toothbrushes and razor blades.
- Do not have any kind of sex without protection. Always practice safer sex by using a latex or polyurethane condom to lower the chance of sexual contact with semen, vaginal secretions, or blood.

Ask your healthcare provider if you have any questions on how to prevent getting HIV infection or spreading HIV infection to other people.

Who should not take TRUVADA?

Do not take TRUVADA to prevent HIV infection if you are HIV positive or if your HIV status is not known.

What should I tell my healthcare provider before taking TRUVADA?

See "What is the most important information I should know about TRUVADA?".

Before taking TRUVADA, tell your healthcare provider if you:

- have liver problems including hepatitis B virus infection
- have kidney problems or receive kidney dialysis treatment
- have bone problems
- have any other medical conditions
- are pregnant or plan to become pregnant. It is not known if TRUVADA can harm your unborn baby.

  If you are a female who is taking TRUVADA to prevent HIV infection and you become pregnant while taking TRUVADA, talk to your healthcare provider about whether you will continue taking TRUVADA.

  Pregnancy Registry. There is a pregnancy registry for women who take antiviral medicines during pregnancy. The purpose of this registry is to collect information about the health of you and your baby. Talk to your healthcare provider about how you can take part in this registry.
- are breastfeeding or plan to breastfeed. Do not breastfeed if you take TRUVADA.
  - You should not breastfeed if you have HIV because of the risk of passing HIV to your baby.
  - TRUVADA can pass to your baby in your breast milk.

  Talk with your healthcare provider about the best way to feed your baby.

Tell your healthcare provider about all the medicines you take, including prescription and non-prescription medicines, vitamins, and herbal supplements. TRUVADA may affect the way other medicines work, and other medicines may affect how TRUVADA works.

Do not take TRUVADA if you also take:

- other medicines that contain tenofovir or emtricitabine (ATRIPLA®, COMPLERA®, EMTRIVA, STRIBILD®, VIREAD)
- medicines that contain lamivudine (Combivir, Epivir, Epivir-HBV, Epzicom, Trizivir)
- adefovir (HEPSERA®)

Especially tell your healthcare provider if you take:

- didanosine (VIDEX EC)
- atazanavir (REYATAZ)
- lopinavir with ritonavir (KALETRA)

Know the medicines you take. Keep a list of them to show your healthcare provider or pharmacist when you get a new medicine.

How should I take TRUVADA?

- Take TRUVADA exactly as prescribed.
- **Do not change your dose or stop taking TRUVADA without first talking with your healthcare provider.** Stay under a healthcare provider's care when taking TRUVADA.
- TRUVADA is usually taken 1 time each day. If you have kidney problems, your healthcare provider may tell you to take TRUVADA less often.
- **When used to treat HIV-1 infection, TRUVADA is always used with other HIV-1 medicines.**
- **If you take TRUVADA to reduce the risk of getting HIV-1, you must also use other methods to reduce your risk of getting HIV. See "What is the most important information I should know about TRUVADA?".**
- Take TRUVADA by mouth, with or without food.
- Take TRUVADA at the same time each day.
- If you miss a dose of TRUVADA, take it as soon as you remember that day. Do not take more than 1 dose of TRUVADA in a day. Do not take 2 doses at the same time to make up for a missed dose. Call your healthcare provider or pharmacist if you are not sure what to do.
- It is important that you do not miss any doses of TRUVADA or your other HIV-1 medicines.
- When your TRUVADA supply starts to run low, get more from your healthcare provider or pharmacy. This is very important because the amount of virus in your blood may increase if the medicine is stopped for even a short time. The virus may develop resistance to TRUVADA and become harder to treat.
- If you take too much TRUVADA, call your healthcare provider or go to the nearest hospital emergency room right away.

What are the possible side effects of TRUVADA?

TRUVADA may cause the following serious side effects, including:

- **See "What is the most important information I should know about TRUVADA?".**
- **New or worse kidney problems,** including kidney failure. If you have had kidney problems in the past or need to take another medicine that can cause kidney problems, your healthcare provider may need to do blood tests to check your kidneys before you start and while you are taking TRUVADA. Your healthcare provider may tell you to take TRUVADA less often, or to stop taking TRUVADA if you have kidney problems.
- **Bone problems** can happen in some people who take TRUVADA. Bone problems include bone pain, softening or thinning (which may lead to fractures). Your healthcare provider may need to do tests to check your bones.
- **Changes in body fat can happen in people who take HIV medicines.** These changes may include increased amount of fat in the upper back and neck ("buffalo hump"), breast, and around the middle of your body (trunk). Loss of fat from the legs, arms, and face may also happen. The exact cause and long-term health effects of these problems are not known.
- **Changes in your immune system (Immune Reconstitution Syndrome)** can happen when an HIV-infected person starts taking HIV medicines. Your immune system may get stronger and begin to fight infections that have been hidden in your body for a long time. Tell your healthcare provider right away if you start having any new symptoms after starting your HIV medicine.

The most common side effects of TRUVADA in people with HIV-1 infection include:

- diarrhea
- nausea
- tiredness
- headache
- dizziness
- depression
- problems sleeping
- abnormal dreams
- rash

Common side effects in people who take TRUVADA to prevent HIV-1 infection include:

- stomach-area (abdomen) pain
- headache
- decreased weight

Tell your healthcare provider if you have any side effect that bothers you or that does not go away.

These are not all the possible side effects of TRUVADA. For more information, ask your healthcare provider or pharmacist.

Call your doctor for medical advice about side effects. You may report side effects to FDA at 1-800-FDA-1088.

How should I store TRUVADA?

- Store TRUVADA at room temperature between 68°F to 77°F (20°C to 25°C).
- Keep TRUVADA in its original container and keep the container tightly closed.
- Do not use TRUVADA if seal over bottle opening is broken or missing.

Keep TRUVADA and all other medicines out of reach of children.

General information about TRUVADA.

Medicines are sometimes prescribed for purposes other than those listed in a Medication Guide. Do not use TRUVADA for a condition for which it was not prescribed. Do not give TRUVADA to other people, even if they have the same symptoms you have. It may harm them.

This Medication Guide summarizes the most important information about TRUVADA. If you would like more information, talk with your healthcare provider. You can ask your healthcare provider or pharmacist for information about TRUVADA that is written for health professionals. For more information, call 1-800-445-3235 or go to www.TRUVADA.com.

What are the ingredients in TRUVADA?

Active ingredients: emtricitabine and tenofovir disoproxil fumarate.

Inactive ingredients: Croscarmellose sodium, lactose monohydrate, magnesium stearate, microcrystalline cellulose, and pregelatinized starch (gluten free). The tablets are coated with Opadry II Blue Y-30-10701 which contains FD&C Blue #2 aluminum lake, hydroxypropyl methylcellulose 2910, lactose monohydrate, titanium dioxide, and triacetin.

This Medication Guide has been approved by the U.S. Food and Drug Administration.

Manufactured for and distributed by:
Gilead Sciences, Inc.
Foster City, CA 94404
Issued June 2013
21-752-GS-026

Shown in Product Identification Guide, page 306

VIREAD® ℞
[VEER-ee-ad]
(tenofovir disoproxil fumarate)
tablets, for oral use

VIREAD®
(tenofovir disoproxil fumarate)
powder, for oral use

HIGHLIGHTS OF PRESCRIBING INFORMATION

These highlights do not include all the information needed to use VIREAD safely and effectively. See full prescribing information for VIREAD.

VIREAD® (tenofovir disoproxil fumarate) tablets, for oral use
VIREAD® (tenofovir disoproxil fumarate) powder, for oral use
Initial U.S. Approval: 2001

WARNING: LACTIC ACIDOSIS/SEVERE HEPATOMEGALY WITH STEATOSIS and POST TREATMENT EXACERBATION OF HEPATITIS

See full prescribing information for complete boxed warning.

- **Lactic acidosis and severe hepatomegaly with steatosis, including fatal cases, have been reported with the use of nucleoside analogs, including VIREAD. (5.1)**
- **Severe acute exacerbations of hepatitis have been reported in HBV-infected patients who have discontinued anti-hepatitis B therapy, including VIREAD. Hepatic function should be monitored closely in these patients. If appropriate, resumption of anti-hepatitis B therapy may be warranted. (5.2)**

RECENT MAJOR CHANGES

Indications and Usage (1.1)	11/2012
Indications and Usage (1.2)	07/2013
Dosage and Administration (2.1, 2.2)	08/2012
Warnings and Precautions	
Coadministration with Other Products (5.4)	11/2012
Decreases in Bone Mineral Density (5.6)	08/2012

INDICATIONS AND USAGE

VIREAD is a nucleotide analog HIV-1 reverse transcriptase inhibitor and an HBV reverse transcriptase inhibitor.

VIREAD is indicated in combination with other antiretroviral agents for the treatment of HIV-1 infection in adults and pediatric patients 2 years of age and older. (1)

VIREAD is indicated for the treatment of chronic hepatitis B in adults and pediatric patients 12 years of age and older. (1)

DOSAGE AND ADMINISTRATION

- Recommended dose for the treatment of HIV-1 or chronic hepatitis B in adults and pediatric patients 12 years of age and older (35 kg or more): 300 mg once daily taken orally without regard to food. (2.1)
- Recommended dose for the treatment of HIV-1 in pediatric patients (2 to less than 12 years of age):
  Tablets: for pediatric patients weighing greater than or equal to 17 kg who can swallow an intact tablet, one VIREAD tablet (150, 200, 250 or 300 mg based on body weight) once daily taken orally without regard to food. (2.2)
  Oral powder: 8 mg/kg VIREAD oral powder (up to a maximum of 300 mg) once daily with food. (2.2)
- Dose recommended in renal impairment in adults:
  Creatinine clearance 30–49 mL/min: 300 mg every 48 hours. (2.3)
  Creatinine clearance 10–29 mL/min: 300 mg every 72 to 96 hours. (2.3)
  Hemodialysis: 300 mg every 7 days or after approximately 12 hours of dialysis. (2.3)

DOSAGE FORMS AND STRENGTHS

Tablets: 150, 200, 250 and 300 mg (3)
Oral Powder: 40 mg per 1 g of oral powder (3)

CONTRAINDICATIONS

None. (4)

WARNINGS AND PRECAUTIONS

- New onset or worsening renal impairment: Can include acute renal failure and Fanconi syndrome. Assess creatinine clearance (CrCl) before initiating treatment with VIREAD. Monitor CrCl and serum phosphorus in patients at risk. Avoid administering VIREAD with concurrent or recent use of nephrotoxic drugs. (5.3)
- Coadministration with Other Products: Do not use with other tenofovir-containing products (e.g., ATRIPLA, COMPLERA, STRIBILD and TRUVADA). Do not administer in combination with HEPSERA. (5.4)
- HIV testing: HIV antibody testing should be offered to all HBV-infected patients before initiating therapy with VIREAD. VIREAD should only be used as part of an appropriate antiretroviral combination regimen in HIV-infected patients with or without HBV coinfection. (5.5)
- Decreases in bone mineral density (BMD): Consider assessment of BMD in patients with a history of pathologic fracture or other risk factors for osteoporosis or bone loss. (5.6)
- Redistribution/accumulation of body fat: Observed in HIV-infected patients receiving antiretroviral combination therapy. (5.7)
- Immune reconstitution syndrome: Observed in HIV-infected patients. May necessitate further evaluation and treatment. (5.8)
- Triple nucleoside-only regimens: Early virologic failure has been reported in HIV-infected patients. Monitor carefully and consider treatment modification. (5.9)

ADVERSE REACTIONS

In HIV-infected adult subjects: Most common adverse reactions (incidence greater than or equal to 10%, Grades 2–4) are rash, diarrhea, headache, pain, depression, asthenia, and nausea. (6.1)

In HBV-infected subjects with compensated liver disease: most common adverse reaction (all grades) was nausea (9%). (6.1)

In pediatric subjects: Adverse reactions in pediatric subjects were consistent with those observed in adults. (6.1)

In HBV-infected subjects with decompensated liver disease: most common adverse reactions (incidence greater than or equal to 10%, all grades) were abdominal pain, nausea, insomnia, pruritus, vomiting, dizziness, and pyrexia. (6.1)

To report SUSPECTED ADVERSE REACTIONS, contact Gilead Sciences, Inc. at 1-800-GILEAD-5 or FDA at 1-800-FDA-1088 or www.fda.gov/medwatch

DRUG INTERACTIONS

- Didanosine: Coadministration increases didanosine concentrations. Use with caution and monitor for evidence of didanosine toxicity (e.g., pancreatitis, neuropathy). Consider dose reductions or discontinuations of didanosine if warranted. (7.1)
- Atazanavir: Coadministration decreases atazanavir concentrations and increases tenofovir concentrations. Use atazanavir with VIREAD only with additional ritonavir; monitor for evidence of tenofovir toxicity. (7.2)
- Lopinavir/ritonavir: Coadministration increases tenofovir concentrations. Monitor for evidence of tenofovir toxicity. (7.3)

USE IN SPECIFIC POPULATIONS

- Nursing mothers: Women infected with HIV should be instructed not to breast feed. (8.3)

See 17 for PATIENT COUNSELING INFORMATION and FDA-approved patient labeling

Revised: 08/2013

FULL PRESCRIBING INFORMATION: CONTENTS*

*** Sections or subsections omitted from the full prescribing information are not listed**

FULL PRESCRIBING INFORMATION

WARNING: LACTIC ACIDOSIS/SEVERE HEPATOMEGALY WITH STEATOSIS and POST TREATMENT EXACERBATION OF HEPATITIS

Lactic acidosis and severe hepatomegaly with steatosis, including fatal cases, have been reported with the use of nucleoside analogs, including VIREAD, in combination with other antiretrovirals *[See Warnings and Precautions (5.1)]*.

Severe acute exacerbations of hepatitis have been reported in HBV-infected patients who have discontinued anti-hepatitis B therapy, including VIREAD. Hepatic function should be monitored closely with both clinical and laboratory follow-up for at least several months in patients who discontinue anti-hepatitis B therapy, including VIREAD. If appropriate, resumption of anti-hepatitis B therapy may be warranted *[See Warnings and Precautions (5.2)]*.

1 INDICATIONS AND USAGE

1.1 HIV-1 Infection

VIREAD® is indicated in combination with other antiretroviral agents for the treatment of HIV-1 infection in adults and pediatric patients 2 years of age and older.

The following points should be considered when initiating therapy with VIREAD for the treatment of HIV-1 infection:

- VIREAD should not be used in combination with ATRIPLA®, COMPLERA®, STRIBILD®, or TRUVADA® *[See Warnings and Precautions (5.4)]*.

1.2 Chronic Hepatitis B

VIREAD is indicated for the treatment of chronic hepatitis B in adults and pediatric patients 12 years of age and older.

The following points should be considered when initiating therapy with VIREAD for the treatment of HBV infection:

- The indication in adults is based on safety and efficacy data from treatment of subjects who were nucleoside-treatment-naïve and subjects who were treatment-experienced with documented resistance to lamivudine. Subjects were adults with HBeAg-positive and HBeAg-negative chronic hepatitis B with compensated liver disease *[See Clinical Studies (14.2)]*.
- VIREAD was evaluated in a limited number of subjects with chronic hepatitis B and decompensated liver disease *[See Adverse Reactions (6.1), Clinical Studies (14.2)]*.
- The numbers of subjects in clinical trials who had adefovir resistance-associated substitutions at baseline were too small to reach conclusions of efficacy *[See Microbiology (12.4), Clinical Studies (14.2)]*.

2 DOSAGE AND ADMINISTRATION

2.1 Recommended Dose in Adults and Pediatric Patients 12 Years of Age and Older (35 kg or more)

For the treatment of HIV-1 or chronic hepatitis B: The dose is one 300 mg VIREAD tablet once daily taken orally, without regard to food.

For patients unable to swallow VIREAD tablets, the oral powder formulation (7.5 scoops) may be used.

In the treatment of chronic hepatitis B, the optimal duration of treatment is unknown. Safety and efficacy in pediatric patients with chronic hepatitis B weighing less than 35 kg have not been established.

2.2 Recommended Dose in Pediatric Patients 2 Years to Less Than 12 Years of Age

HIV-1 Infection

For the treatment of HIV-1 in pediatric patients 2 years of age and older, the recommended oral dose of VIREAD is 8 mg of tenofovir disoproxil fumarate per kilogram of body weight (up to a maximum of 300 mg) once daily administered as oral powder or tablets.

VIREAD oral powder should be measured only with the supplied dosing scoop. One level scoop delivers 1 g of powder which contains 40 mg of tenofovir disoproxil fumarate. VIREAD oral powder should be mixed in a container with 2 to 4 ounces of soft food not requiring chewing (e.g., applesauce, baby food, yogurt). The entire mixture should be ingested immediately to avoid a bitter taste. Do not administer VIREAD oral powder in a liquid as the powder may float on top of the liquid even after stirring. Further patient instructions on how to administer VIREAD oral powder with the supplied dosing scoop are provided in the FDA-approved patient labeling (Patient Information).

VIREAD is also available as tablets in 150, 200, 250 and 300 mg strengths for pediatric patients who weigh greater than or equal to 17 kg and who are able to reliably swallow intact tablets. The dose is one tablet once daily taken orally, without regard to food.

Tables 1 and 2 contain dosing recommendations for VIREAD oral powder and tablets based on body weight. Weight should be monitored periodically and the VIREAD dose adjusted accordingly.

Table 1 Dosing Recommendations for Pediatric Patients ≥2 Years of Age Using VIREAD Oral Powder

Body Weight Kilogram (kg)	Oral Powder Once Daily Scoops of Powder
10 to <12	2
12 to <14	2.5
14 to <17	3
17 to <19	3.5
19 to <22	4
22 to <24	4.5
24 to <27	5
27 to <29	5.5
29 to <32	6
32 to <34	6.5
34 to <35	7
≥35	7.5

Table 2 Dosing Recommendations for Pediatric Patients ≥2 Years of Age and Weighing ≥17 kg Using VIREAD Tablets

Body Weight Kilogram (kg)	Tablets Once Daily
17 to <22	150 mg
22 to <28	200 mg
28 to <35	250 mg
≥35	300 mg

Chronic Hepatitis B

Safety and efficacy of VIREAD in patients younger than 12 years of age have not been established.

2.3 Dose Adjustment for Renal Impairment in Adults

Significantly increased drug exposures occurred when VIREAD was administered to subjects with moderate to severe renal impairment *[See Clinical Pharmacology (12.3)]*.

Table 3 Dosage Adjustment for Patients with Altered Creatinine Clearance

	Creatinine Clearance (mL/min)*			
	≥50	30–49	10–29	Hemodialysis Patients
Recommended 300 mg Dosing Interval	Every 24 hours	Every 48 hours	Every 72 to 96 hours	Every 7 days or after a total of approximately 12 hours of dialysis†

* Calculated using ideal (lean) body weight.

† Generally once weekly assuming three hemodialysis sessions a week of approximately 4 hours duration. VIREAD should be administered following completion of dialysis.

Therefore, the dosing interval of VIREAD tablets 300 mg should be adjusted in patients with baseline creatinine clearance below 50 mL/min using the recommendations in Table 3. These dosing interval recommendations are based on modeling of single-dose pharmacokinetic data in non-HIV and non-HBV infected subjects with varying degrees of renal impairment, including end-stage renal disease requiring hemodialysis. The safety and effectiveness of these dosing interval adjustment recommendations have not been clinically evaluated in patients with moderate or severe renal impairment, therefore clinical response to treatment and renal function should be closely monitored in these patients *[See Warnings and Precautions (5.3)]*. There are no data to recommend use of VIREAD tablets 150, 200 or 250 mg or VIREAD oral powder in patients with renal impairment.

No dose adjustment of VIREAD tablets 300 mg is necessary for patients with mild renal impairment (creatinine clearance 50–80 mL/min). Routine monitoring of calculated creatinine clearance and serum phosphorus should be performed in patients with mild renal impairment *[See Warnings and Precautions (5.3)]*.

[See table 3 above]

The pharmacokinetics of tenofovir have not been evaluated in non-hemodialysis patients with creatinine clearance below 10 mL/min; therefore, no dosing recommendation is available for these patients.

No data are available to make dose recommendations in pediatric patients with renal impairment.

3 DOSAGE FORMS AND STRENGTHS

VIREAD is available as tablets or as an oral powder.

VIREAD tablets 150 mg contain 150 mg of tenofovir disoproxil fumarate, which is equivalent to 123 mg of tenofovir disoproxil. The tablets are triangle-shaped, white, film-coated, and debossed with "GSI" on one side and "150" on the other side.

VIREAD tablets 200 mg contain 200 mg of tenofovir disoproxil fumarate, which is equivalent to 163 mg of tenofovir disoproxil. The tablets are round-shaped, white, film-coated, and debossed with "GSI" on one side and "200" on the other side.

VIREAD tablets 250 mg contain 250 mg of tenofovir disoproxil fumarate, which is equivalent to 204 mg of tenofovir disoproxil. The tablets are capsule-shaped, white, film-coated, and debossed with "GSI" on one side and "250" on the other side.

VIREAD tablets 300 mg contain 300 mg of tenofovir disoproxil fumarate, which is equivalent to 245 mg of tenofovir disoproxil. The tablets are almond-shaped, light blue, film-coated, and debossed with "GILEAD" and "4331" on one side and with "300" on the other side.

The oral powder consists of white, taste-masked, coated granules containing 40 mg of tenofovir disoproxil fumarate, which is equivalent to 33 mg of tenofovir disoproxil, per level scoop. Each level scoop contains 1 gram of oral powder.

4 CONTRAINDICATIONS

None.

5 WARNINGS AND PRECAUTIONS

5.1 Lactic Acidosis/Severe Hepatomegaly with Steatosis

Lactic acidosis and severe hepatomegaly with steatosis, including fatal cases, have been reported with the use of nucleoside analogs, including VIREAD, in combination with other antiretrovirals. A majority of these cases have been in women. Obesity and prolonged nucleoside exposure may be risk factors. Particular caution should be exercised when administering nucleoside analogs to any patient with known risk factors for liver disease; however, cases have also been reported in patients with no known risk factors. Treatment with VIREAD should be suspended in any patient who develops clinical or laboratory findings suggestive of lactic acidosis or pronounced hepatotoxicity (which may include hepatomegaly and steatosis even in the absence of marked transaminase elevations).

5.2 Exacerbation of Hepatitis after Discontinuation of Treatment

Discontinuation of anti-HBV therapy, including VIREAD, may be associated with severe acute exacerbations of hepatitis. Patients infected with HBV who discontinue VIREAD should be closely monitored with both clinical and laboratory follow-up for at least several months after stopping treatment. If appropriate, resumption of anti-hepatitis B therapy may be warranted.

5.3 New Onset or Worsening Renal Impairment

Tenofovir is principally eliminated by the kidney. Renal impairment, including cases of acute renal failure and Fanconi syndrome (renal tubular injury with severe hypophosphatemia), has been reported with the use of VIREAD *[See Adverse Reactions (6.2)]*.

It is recommended that creatinine clearance be calculated in all patients prior to initiating therapy and as clinically appropriate during therapy with VIREAD. Routine monitoring of calculated creatinine clearance and serum phosphorus should be performed in patients at risk for renal impairment, including patients who have previously experienced renal events while receiving HEPSERA®.

Dosing interval adjustment of VIREAD and close monitoring of renal function are recommended in all patients with creatinine clearance below 50 mL/min *[See Dosage and Administration (2.3)]*. No safety or efficacy data are available in patients with renal impairment who received VIREAD using these dosing guidelines, so the potential benefit of VIREAD therapy should be assessed against the potential risk of renal toxicity.

VIREAD should be avoided with concurrent or recent use of a nephrotoxic agent.

5.4 Coadministration with Other Products

VIREAD should not be used in combination with the fixed-dose combination products ATRIPLA, COMPLERA, STRIBILD, or TRUVADA since tenofovir disoproxil fumarate is a component of these products.

VIREAD should not be administered in combination with HEPSERA (adefovir dipivoxil) *[See Drug Interactions (7.4)]*.

5.5 Patients Coinfected with HIV-1 and HBV

Due to the risk of development of HIV-1 resistance, VIREAD should only be used in HIV-1 and HBV coinfected patients as part of an appropriate antiretroviral combination regimen.

HIV-1 antibody testing should be offered to all HBV-infected patients before initiating therapy with VIREAD. It is also recommended that all patients with HIV-1 be tested for the presence of chronic hepatitis B before initiating treatment with VIREAD.

5.6 Decreases in Bone Mineral Density

Assessment of bone mineral density (BMD) should be considered for adults and pediatric patients who have a history of pathologic bone fracture or other risk factors for osteoporosis or bone loss. Although the effect of supplementation with calcium and vitamin D was not studied, such supplementation may be beneficial for all patients. If bone abnormalities are suspected then appropriate consultation should be obtained.

Adult Patients

In HIV-1 infected adult subjects treated with VIREAD in Study 903 through 144 weeks, decreases from baseline in BMD were seen at the lumbar spine and hip in both arms of the trial. At Week 144, there was a significantly greater mean percentage decrease from baseline in BMD at the lumbar spine in subjects receiving VIREAD + lamivudine + efavirenz (-2.2% ± 3.9) compared with subjects receiving stavudine + lamivudine + efavirenz (-1.0% ± 4.6). Changes in BMD at the hip were similar between the two treatment groups (-2.8% ± 3.5 in the VIREAD group vs. -2.4% ± 4.5 in the stavudine group). In both groups, the majority of the reduction in BMD occurred in the first 24–48 weeks of the trial and this reduction was sustained through Week 144. Twenty-eight percent of VIREAD-treated subjects vs. 21%

of the stavudine-treated subjects lost at least 5% of BMD at the spine or 7% of BMD at the hip. Clinically relevant fractures (excluding fingers and toes) were reported in 4 subjects in the VIREAD group and 6 subjects in the stavudine group. In addition, there were significant increases in biochemical markers of bone metabolism (serum bone-specific alkaline phosphatase, serum osteocalcin, serum C-telopeptide, and urinary N-telopeptide) in the VIREAD group relative to the stavudine group, suggesting increased bone turnover. Serum parathyroid hormone levels and 1,25 Vitamin D levels were also higher in the VIREAD group. Except for bone specific alkaline phosphatase, these changes resulted in values that remained within the normal range.

Pediatric Patients

In clinical trials evaluating VIREAD in HIV-1 infected pediatric subjects 2 to less than 18 years of age, bone effects were similar to those observed in adult subjects. Under normal circumstances BMD increases rapidly in pediatric patients. In Study 352 (2 to less than 12 years), the mean rate of BMD gain in lumbar spine at Week 48 was similar between the VIREAD and the d4T or AZT treatment groups. Total body BMD gain was less in the VIREAD compared to the d4T or AZT treatment group. One VIREAD-treated subject and none of the d4T or AZT-treated subjects experienced significant (greater than 4%) lumbar spine BMD loss at Week 48. Changes from baseline in BMD Z-scores were -0.012 for lumbar spine and -0.338 for total body in the 64 subjects who were treated with VIREAD for 96 weeks. In Study 321 (12 to less than 18 years), the mean rate of BMD gain at Week 48 was less in the VIREAD compared to the placebo treatment group. Six VIREAD treated subjects and one placebo treated subject had significant (greater than 4%) lumbar spine BMD loss at Week 48. Changes from baseline BMD Z-scores were -0.341 for lumbar spine and -0.458 for total body in the 28 subjects who were treated with VIREAD for 96 weeks. In both trials, skeletal growth (height) appeared to be unaffected. Markers of bone turnover in VIREAD-treated pediatric subjects suggest increased bone turnover, consistent with the effects observed in adults.

In a clinical trial (Study 115) conducted in pediatric subjects 12 to less than 18 years of age with chronic hepatitis B infection, both the VIREAD and placebo treatment arms experienced an overall increase in mean lumbar spine BMD over 72 weeks, as expected for an adolescent population. The BMD gains from baseline to Week 72 in lumbar spine and total body BMD in VIREAD-treated subjects (+5% and +3%, respectively) were less than the BMD gains observed in placebo-treated subjects (+8% and +5%, respectively). Three subjects in the VIREAD group and two subjects in the placebo group had significant (greater than 4%) lumbar spine BMD loss at Week 72. At baseline, mean BMD Z-scores in subjects randomized to VIREAD were −0.43 for lumbar spine and −0.20 for total body, and mean BMD Z-scores in subjects randomized to placebo were −0.28 for lumbar spine and −0.26 for total body. In subjects receiving VIREAD for 72 weeks, the mean change in BMD Z-score was −0.05 for lumbar spine and −0.15 for total body compared to +0.07 and +0.06, respectively, in subjects receiving placebo. As observed in pediatric studies of HIV-infected patients, skeletal growth (height) appeared to be unaffected.

The effects of VIREAD-associated changes in BMD and biochemical markers on long-term bone health and future fracture risk are unknown.

Cases of osteomalacia (associated with proximal renal tubulopathy and which may contribute to fractures) have been reported in association with the use of VIREAD *[See Adverse Reactions (6.2)]*.

5.7 Fat Redistribution

In HIV-infected patients redistribution/accumulation of body fat including central obesity, dorsocervical fat enlargement (buffalo hump), peripheral wasting, facial wasting, breast enlargement, and "cushingoid appearance" have been observed in patients receiving combination antiretroviral therapy. The mechanism and long-term consequences of these events are currently unknown. A causal relationship has not been established.

5.8 Immune Reconstitution Syndrome

Immune reconstitution syndrome has been reported in HIV-infected patients treated with combination antiretroviral therapy, including VIREAD. During the initial phase of combination antiretroviral treatment, patients whose immune system responds may develop an inflammatory response to indolent or residual opportunistic infections [such as *Mycobacterium avium* infection, cytomegalovirus, *Pneumocystis jirovecii* pneumonia (PCP), or tuberculosis], which may necessitate further evaluation and treatment.

Autoimmune disorders (such as Graves' disease, polymyositis, and Guillain-Barré syndrome) have also been reported to occur in the setting of immune reconstitution, however, the time to onset is more variable, and can occur many months after initiation of treatment.

5.9 Early Virologic Failure

Clinical trials in HIV-infected subjects have demonstrated that certain regimens that only contain three nucleoside reverse transcriptase inhibitors (NRTI) are generally less effective than triple drug regimens containing two NRTIs in combination with either a non-nucleoside reverse transcriptase inhibitor or a HIV-1 protease inhibitor. In particular, early virological failure and high rates of resistance substitutions have been reported. Triple nucleoside regimens should therefore be used with caution. Patients on a therapy utilizing a triple nucleoside-only regimen should be carefully monitored and considered for treatment modification.

6 ADVERSE REACTIONS

The following adverse reactions are discussed in other sections of the labeling:

- Lactic Acidosis/Severe Hepatomegaly with Steatosis *[See Boxed Warning, Warnings and Precautions (5.1)]*.
- Severe Acute Exacerbation of Hepatitis *[See Boxed Warning, Warnings and Precautions (5.2)]*.
- New Onset or Worsening Renal Impairment *[See Warnings and Precautions (5.3)]*.
- Decreases in Bone Mineral Density *[See Warnings and Precautions (5.6)]*.
- Immune Reconstitution Syndrome *[See Warnings and Precautions (5.8)]*.

6.1 Adverse Reactions from Clinical Trials Experience

Because clinical trials are conducted under widely varying conditions, adverse reaction rates observed in the clinical trials of a drug cannot be directly compared to rates in the clinical trials of another drug and may not reflect the rates observed in practice.

Clinical Trials in Adult Patients with HIV-1 Infection

More than 12,000 subjects have been treated with VIREAD alone or in combination with other antiretroviral medicinal products for periods of 28 days to 215 weeks in clinical trials and expanded access programs. A total of 1,544 subjects have received VIREAD 300 mg once daily in clinical trials; over 11,000 subjects have received VIREAD in expanded access programs.

The most common adverse reactions (incidence greater than or equal to 10%, Grades 2–4) identified from any of the 3 large controlled clinical trials include rash, diarrhea, headache, pain, depression, asthenia, and nausea.

Treatment-Naïve Patients

Study 903 - Treatment-Emergent Adverse Reactions: The most common adverse reactions seen in a double-blind comparative controlled trial in which 600 treatment-naïve subjects received VIREAD (N=299) or stavudine (N=301) in combination with lamivudine and efavirenz for 144 weeks (Study 903) were mild to moderate gastrointestinal events and dizziness.

Mild adverse reactions (Grade 1) were common with a similar incidence in both arms, and included dizziness, diarrhea, and nausea. Selected treatment-emergent moderate to severe adverse reactions are summarized in Table 4.

Table 4 Selected Treatment-Emergent Adverse Reactions* (Grades 2–4) Reported in ≥5% in Any Treatment Group in Study 903 (0–144 Weeks)

	VIREAD + 3TC + EFV	d4T + 3TC + EFV
	N=299	N=301
Body as a Whole		
Headache	14%	17%
Pain	13%	12%
Fever	8%	7%
Abdominal pain	7%	12%
Back pain	9%	8%
Asthenia	6%	7%
Digestive System		
Diarrhea	11%	13%
Nausea	8%	9%
Dyspepsia	4%	5%
Vomiting	5%	9%
Metabolic Disorders		
Lipodystrophy†	1%	8%
Musculoskeletal		
Arthralgia	5%	7%
Myalgia	3%	5%
Nervous System		
Depression	11%	10%
Insomnia	5%	8%
Dizziness	3%	6%
Peripheral neuropathy‡	1%	5%
Anxiety	6%	6%
Respiratory		
Pneumonia	5%	5%
Skin and Appendages		
Rash event§	18%	12%

* Frequencies of adverse reactions are based on all treatment-emergent adverse events, regardless of relationship to study drug.

† Lipodystrophy represents a variety of investigator-described adverse events not a protocol-defined syndrome.

‡ Peripheral neuropathy includes peripheral neuritis and neuropathy.

§ Rash event includes rash, pruritus, maculopapular rash, urticaria, vesiculobullous rash, and pustular rash.

Laboratory Abnormalities: With the exception of fasting cholesterol and fasting triglyceride elevations that were more common in the stavudine group (40% and 9%) compared with VIREAD (19% and 1%) respectively, laboratory abnormalities observed in this trial occurred with similar frequency in the VIREAD and stavudine treatment arms. A summary of Grades 3–4 laboratory abnormalities is provided in Table 5.

Table 5 Grades 3–4 Laboratory Abnormalities Reported in ≥1% of VIREAD-Treated Subjects in Study 903 (0–144 Weeks)

	VIREAD + 3TC + EFV	d4T + 3TC + EFV
	N=299	N=301
Any ≥ Grade 3 Laboratory Abnormality	36%	42%
Fasting Cholesterol (>240 mg/dL)	19%	40%
Creatine Kinase (M: >990 U/L; F: >845 U/L)	12%	12%
Serum Amylase (>175 U/L)	9%	8%
AST (M: >180 U/L; F: >170 U/L)	5%	7%
ALT (M: >215 U/L; F: >170 U/L)	4%	5%
Hematuria (>100 RBC/HPF)	7%	7%
Neutrophils (<750/mm^3)	3%	1%
Fasting Triglycerides (>750 mg/dL)	1%	9%

Study 934 - Treatment Emergent Adverse Reactions: In Study 934, 511 antiretroviral-naïve subjects received either VIREAD + EMTRIVA® administered in combination with efavirenz (N=257) or zidovudine/lamivudine administered in combination with efavirenz (N=254). Adverse reactions observed in this trial were generally consistent with those seen in previous studies in treatment-experienced or treatment-naïve subjects (Table 6).

Table 6 Selected Treatment-Emergent Adverse Reactions* (Grades 2–4) Reported in ≥5% in Any Treatment Group in Study 934 (0–144 Weeks)

	VIREAD† + FTC + EFV	AZT/3TC + EFV
	N=257	N=254
Gastrointestinal Disorder		
Diarrhea	9%	5%
Nausea	9%	7%
Vomiting	2%	5%
General Disorders and Administration Site Condition		
Fatigue	9%	8%
Infections and Infestations		
Sinusitis	8%	4%
Upper respiratory tract infections	8%	5%
Nasopharyngitis	5%	3%
Nervous System Disorders		
Headache	6%	5%
Dizziness	8%	7%

Psychiatric Disorders		
Depression	9%	7%
Insomnia	5%	7%
Skin and Subcutaneous Tissue Disorders		
Rash event‡	7%	9%

* Frequencies of adverse reactions are based on all treatment-emergent adverse events, regardless of relationship to study drug.
† From Weeks 96 to 144 of the trial, subjects received TRUVADA with efavirenz in place of VIREAD + EMTRIVA with efavirenz.
‡ Rash event includes rash, exfoliative rash, rash generalized, rash macular, rash maculopapular, rash pruritic, and rash vesicular.

Laboratory Abnormalities: Laboratory abnormalities observed in this trial were generally consistent with those seen in previous trials (Table 7).

Table 7 Significant Laboratory Abnormalities Reported in ≥1% of Subjects in Any Treatment Group in Study 934 (0–144 Weeks)

	VIREAD* + FTC + EFV	AZT/3TC + EFV
	N=257	N=254
Any ≥ Grade 3 Laboratory Abnormality	30%	26%
Fasting Cholesterol (>240 mg/dL)	22%	24%
Creatine Kinase (M: >990 U/L; F: >845 U/L)	9%	7%
Serum Amylase (>175 U/L)	8%	4%
Alkaline Phosphatase (>550 U/L)	1%	0%
AST (M: >180 U/L; F: >170 U/L)	3%	3%
ALT (M: >215 U/L; F: >170 U/L)	2%	3%
Hemoglobin (<8.0 mg/dL)	0%	4%
Hyperglycemia (>250 mg/dL)	2%	1%
Hematuria (>75 RBC/HPF)	3%	2%
Glycosuria (≥3+)	<1%	1%
Neutrophils (<750/mm³)	3%	5%
Fasting Triglycerides (>750 mg/dL)	4%	2%

* From Weeks 96 to 144 of the trial, subjects received TRUVADA with efavirenz in place of VIREAD + EMTRIVA with efavirenz.

Treatment-Experienced Patients

Treatment-Emergent Adverse Reactions: The adverse reactions seen in treatment experienced subjects were generally consistent with those seen in treatment naïve subjects including mild to moderate gastrointestinal events, such as nausea, diarrhea, vomiting, and flatulence. Less than 1% of subjects discontinued participation in the clinical trials due to gastrointestinal adverse reactions (Study 907).

A summary of moderate to severe, treatment-emergent adverse reactions that occurred during the first 48 weeks of Study 907 is provided in Table 8.

[See table 8 above]

Laboratory Abnormalities: Laboratory abnormalities observed in this trial occurred with similar frequency in the VIREAD and placebo-treated groups. A summary of Grades 3–4 laboratory abnormalities is provided in Table 9.

[See table 9 above]

Clinical Trials in Pediatric Subjects 2 Years of Age and Older with HIV-1 Infection

Assessment of adverse reactions is based on two randomized trials (Studies 352 and 321) in 184 HIV-1 infected pediatric subjects (2 to less than 18 years of age) who received treatment with VIREAD (N=93) or placebo/active comparator (N=91) in combination with other antiretroviral agents for 48 weeks. The adverse reactions observed in subjects who received treatment with VIREAD were consistent with those observed in clinical trials in adults.

Table 8 Selected Treatment-Emergent Adverse Reactions* (Grades 2–4) Reported in ≥3% in Any Treatment Group in Study 907 (0–48 Weeks)

	VIREAD (N=368) (Week 0–24)	Placebo (N=182) (Week 0–24)	VIREAD (N=368) (Week 0–48)	Placebo Crossover to VIREAD (N=170) (Week 24–48)
Body as a Whole				
Asthenia	7%	6%	11%	1%
Pain	7%	7%	12%	4%
Headache	5%	5%	8%	2%
Abdominal pain	4%	3%	7%	6%
Back pain	3%	3%	4%	2%
Chest pain	3%	1%	3%	2%
Fever	2%	2%	4%	2%
Digestive System				
Diarrhea	11%	10%	16%	11%
Nausea	8%	5%	11%	7%
Vomiting	4%	1%	7%	5%
Anorexia	3%	2%	4%	1%
Dyspepsia	3%	2%	4%	2%
Flatulence	3%	1%	4%	1%
Respiratory				
Pneumonia	2%	0%	3%	2%
Nervous System				
Depression	4%	3%	8%	4%
Insomnia	3%	2%	4%	4%
Peripheral neuropathy†	3%	3%	5%	2%
Dizziness	1%	3%	3%	1%
Skin and Appendage				
Rash event‡	5%	4%	7%	1%
Sweating	3%	2%	3%	1%
Musculoskeletal				
Myalgia	3%	3%	4%	1%
Metabolic				
Weight loss	2%	1%	4%	2%

* Frequencies of adverse reactions are based on all treatment-emergent adverse events, regardless of relationship to study drug.
† Peripheral neuropathy includes peripheral neuritis and neuropathy.
‡ Rash event includes rash, pruritus, maculopapular rash, urticaria, vesiculobullous rash, and pustular rash.

Table 9 Grades 3–4 Laboratory Abnormalities Reported in ≥1% of VIREAD-Treated Subjects in Study 907 (0–48 Weeks)

	VIREAD (N=368) (Week 0–24)	Placebo (N=182) (Week 0–24)	VIREAD (N=368) (Week 0–48)	Placebo Crossover to VIREAD (N=170) (Week 24–48)
Any ≥ Grade 3 Laboratory Abnormality	25%	38%	35%	34%
Triglycerides (>750 mg/dL)	8%	13%	11%	9%
Creatine Kinase (M: >990 U/L; F: >845 U/L)	7%	14%	12%	12%
Serum Amylase (>175 U/L)	6%	7%	7%	6%
Glycosuria (≥3+)	3%	3%	3%	2%
AST (M: >180 U/L; F: >170 U/L)	3%	3%	4%	5%
ALT (M: >215 U/L; F: >170 U/L)	2%	2%	4%	5%
Serum Glucose (>250 U/L)	2%	4%	3%	3%
Neutrophils (<750/mm³)	1%	1%	2%	1%

Bone effects observed in pediatric subjects 2 years of age and older were consistent with those observed in adult clinical trials *[See Warnings and Precautions (5.6)]*.

Eighty-nine pediatric subjects received VIREAD in Study 352 (48 who were initially randomized to VIREAD and 41 who were initially randomized to continue stavudine or zidovudine and then received VIREAD in the extension phase) for a median exposure of 104 weeks. Of these, 4 subjects discontinued from the trial due to adverse reactions consistent with proximal renal tubulopathy. Three of these 4 subjects presented with hypophosphatemia and also had decreases in total body or spine BMD Z score *[See Warnings and Precautions (5.6)]*.

Clinical Trials in Adult Subjects with Chronic Hepatitis B and Compensated Liver Disease

Treatment-Emergent Adverse Reactions: In controlled clinical trials in 641 subjects with chronic hepatitis B (0102 and 0103), more subjects treated with VIREAD during the 48-week double-blind period experienced nausea: 9% with VIREAD versus 2% with HEPSERA. Other treatment-emergent adverse reactions reported in more than 5% of subjects treated with VIREAD included: abdominal pain, diarrhea, headache, dizziness, fatigue, nasopharyngitis, back pain and skin rash.

During the open-label phase of treatment with VIREAD (weeks 48–240) in Studies 0102 and 0103, less than 1% of subjects (5/585) experienced a confirmed increase in serum creatinine of 0.5 mg/dL from baseline. No significant change in the tolerability profile was observed with continued treatment for up to 240 weeks.

Laboratory Abnormalities: A summary of Grades 3–4 laboratory abnormalities through Week 48 is provided in Table 10. Grades 3–4 laboratory abnormalities were similar in subjects continuing VIREAD treatment for up to 240 weeks in these trials.

Table 10 Grades 3–4 Laboratory Abnormalities Reported in ≥1% of VIREAD-Treated Subjects in Studies 0102 and 0103 (0–48 Weeks)

	VIREAD (N=426)	HEPSERA (N=215)
Any ≥ Grade 3 Laboratory Abnormality	19%	13%
Creatine Kinase (M: >990 U/L; F: >845 U/L)	2%	3%
Serum Amylase (>175 U/L)	4%	1%
Glycosuria (≥3+)	3%	<1%
AST (M: >180 U/L; F: >170 U/L)	4%	4%
ALT (M: >215 U/L; F: >170 U/L)	10%	6%

The overall incidence of on-treatment ALT flares (defined as serum ALT greater than 2 × baseline and greater than 10 × ULN, with or without associated symptoms) was similar between VIREAD (2.6%) and HEPSERA (2%). ALT flares generally occurred within the first 4–8 weeks of treatment and were accompanied by decreases in HBV DNA levels. No subject had evidence of decompensation. ALT flares typically resolved within 4 to 8 weeks without changes in study medication.

The adverse reactions observed in subjects with chronic hepatitis B and lamivudine resistance who received treatment with VIREAD were consistent with those observed in other hepatitis B clinical trials in adults.

Clinical Trials in Adult Subjects with Chronic Hepatitis B and Decompensated Liver Disease

In a small randomized, double-blind, active-controlled trial (0108), subjects with CHB and decompensated liver disease received treatment with VIREAD or other antiviral drugs for up to 48 weeks *[See Clinical Studies (14.2)]*. Among the 45 subjects receiving VIREAD, the most frequently reported treatment-emergent adverse reactions of any severity were abdominal pain (22%), nausea (20%), insomnia (18%), pruritus (16%), vomiting (13%), dizziness (13%), and pyrexia (11%). Two of 45 (4%) subjects died through Week 48 of the trial due to progression of liver disease. Three of 45 (7%) subjects discontinued treatment due to an adverse event. Four of 45 (9%) subjects experienced a confirmed increase in serum creatinine of 0.5 mg/dL (1 subject also had a confirmed serum phosphorus less than 2 mg/dL through Week 48). Three of these subjects (each of whom had a Child-Pugh score greater than or equal to 10 and MELD score greater than or equal to 14 at entry) developed renal failure. Because both VIREAD and decompensated liver disease may have an impact on renal function, the contribution of VIREAD to renal impairment in this population is difficult to ascertain.

One of 45 subjects experienced an on-treatment hepatic flare during the 48 Week trial.

Clinical Trials in Pediatric Subjects 12 Years of Age and Older with Chronic Hepatitis B

Assessment of adverse reactions is based on one randomized study (Study GS-US-174-0115) in 106 pediatric subjects (12 to less than 18 years of age) infected with chronic hepatitis B receiving treatment with VIREAD (N = 52) or placebo (N = 54) for 72 weeks. The adverse reactions observed in pediatric subjects who received treatment with VIREAD were consistent with those observed in clinical trials of VIREAD in adults.

The mean rate of bone mineral density gain was less in VIREAD-treated subjects compared to placebo *[See Warnings and Precautions (5.6)]*.

6.2 Postmarketing Experience

The following adverse reactions have been identified during postapproval use of VIREAD. Because postmarketing reactions are reported voluntarily from a population of uncertain size, it is not always possible to reliably estimate their frequency or establish a causal relationship to drug exposure.

Immune System Disorders
allergic reaction, including angioedema
Metabolism and Nutrition Disorders
lactic acidosis, hypokalemia, hypophosphatemia
Respiratory, Thoracic, and Mediastinal Disorders
dyspnea
Gastrointestinal Disorders
pancreatitis, increased amylase, abdominal pain
Hepatobiliary Disorders
hepatic steatosis, hepatitis, increased liver enzymes (most commonly AST, ALT gamma GT)
Skin and Subcutaneous Tissue Disorders
rash
Musculoskeletal and Connective Tissue Disorders
rhabdomyolysis, osteomalacia (manifested as bone pain and which may contribute to fractures), muscular weakness, myopathy
Renal and Urinary Disorders
acute renal failure, renal failure, acute tubular necrosis, Fanconi syndrome, proximal renal tubulopathy, interstitial nephritis (including acute cases), nephrogenic diabetes insipidus, renal insufficiency, increased creatinine, proteinuria, polyuria
General Disorders and Administration Site Conditions
asthenia

The following adverse reactions, listed under the body system headings above, may occur as a consequence of proximal renal tubulopathy: rhabdomyolysis, osteomalacia, hypokalemia, muscular weakness, myopathy, hypophosphatemia.

7 DRUG INTERACTIONS

This section describes clinically relevant drug interactions with VIREAD. Drug interactions trials are described elsewhere in the labeling *[See Clinical Pharmacology (12.3)]*.

7.1 Didanosine

Coadministration of VIREAD and didanosine should be undertaken with caution and patients receiving this combination should be monitored closely for didanosine-associated adverse reactions. Didanosine should be discontinued in patients who develop didanosine-associated adverse reactions. When administered with VIREAD, C_{max} and AUC of didanosine increased significantly *[See Clinical Pharmacology (12.3)]*. The mechanism of this interaction is unknown. Higher didanosine concentrations could potentiate didanosine-associated adverse reactions, including pancreatitis and neuropathy. Suppression of $CD4^+$ cell counts has been observed in patients receiving VIREAD with didanosine 400 mg daily.

In patients weighing greater than 60 kg, the didanosine dose should be reduced to 250 mg once daily when it is coadministered with VIREAD. In patients weighing less than 60 kg, the didanosine dose should be reduced to 200 mg once daily when it is coadministered with VIREAD. When coadministered, VIREAD and didanosine EC may be taken under fasted conditions or with a light meal (less than 400 kcal, 20% fat). For additional information on coadministration of VIREAD and didanosine, please refer to the full prescribing information for didanosine.

7.2 Atazanavir

Atazanavir has been shown to increase tenofovir concentrations *[See Clinical Pharmacology (12.3)]*. The mechanism of this interaction is unknown. Patients receiving atazanavir and VIREAD should be monitored for VIREAD-associated adverse reactions. VIREAD should be discontinued in patients who develop VIREAD-associated adverse reactions.

VIREAD decreases the AUC and C_{min} of atazanavir *[See Clinical Pharmacology (12.3)]*. When coadministered with VIREAD, it is recommended that atazanavir 300 mg is given with ritonavir 100 mg. Atazanavir without ritonavir should not be coadministered with VIREAD.

7.3 Lopinavir/Ritonavir

Lopinavir/ritonavir has been shown to increase tenofovir concentrations *[See Clinical Pharmacology (12.3)]*. The mechanism of this interaction is unknown. Patients receiving lopinavir/ritonavir and VIREAD should be monitored for VIREAD-associated adverse reactions. VIREAD should be discontinued in patients who develop VIREAD-associated adverse reactions.

7.4 Drugs Affecting Renal Function

Since tenofovir is primarily eliminated by the kidneys *[See Clinical Pharmacology (12.3)]*, coadministration of VIREAD with drugs that reduce renal function or compete for active tubular secretion may increase serum concentrations of tenofovir and/or increase the concentrations of other renally eliminated drugs. Some examples include, but are not limited to cidofovir, acyclovir, valacyclovir, ganciclovir, and valganciclovir. Drugs that decrease renal function may also increase serum concentrations of tenofovir.

In the treatment of chronic hepatitis B, VIREAD should not be administered in combination with HEPSERA (adefovir dipivoxil).

8 USE IN SPECIFIC POPULATIONS

8.1 Pregnancy

Pregnancy Category B

There are no adequate and well-controlled studies in pregnant women. Because animal reproduction studies are not always predictive of human response, VIREAD should be used during pregnancy only if clearly needed.

Antiretroviral Pregnancy Registry: To monitor fetal outcomes of pregnant women exposed to VIREAD, an Antiretroviral Pregnancy Registry has been established. Healthcare providers are encouraged to register patients by calling 1-800-258-4263.

Animal Data

Reproduction studies have been performed in rats and rabbits at doses up to 14 and 19 times the human dose based on body surface area comparisons and revealed no evidence of impaired fertility or harm to the fetus due to tenofovir.

8.3 Nursing Mothers

Nursing Mothers: The Centers for Disease Control and Prevention recommend that HIV-1-infected mothers not breast-feed their infants to avoid risking postnatal transmission of HIV-1. Samples of breast milk obtained from five HIV-1 infected mothers in the first post-partum week show that tenofovir is secreted in human milk. The impact of this exposure in breastfed infants is unknown. Because of both the potential for HIV-1 transmission and the potential for serious adverse reactions in nursing infants, **mothers should be instructed not to breast-feed if they are receiving VIREAD.**

8.4 Pediatric Use

Pediatric Patients 2 Years of Age and Older with HIV-1 infection

The safety of VIREAD in pediatric patients aged 2 to less than 18 years is supported by data from two randomized trials in which VIREAD was administered to HIV-1 infected treatment-experienced subjects. In addition, the pharmacokinetic profile of tenofovir in patients 2 to less than 18 years of age at the recommended doses was similar to that found to be safe and effective in adult clinical trials *[See Clinical Pharmacology (12.3)]*.

In Study 352, 92 treatment-experienced subjects 2 to less than 12 years of age with stable, virologic suppression on stavudine- or zidovudine-containing regimen were randomized to either replace stavudine or zidovudine with VIREAD (N = 44) or continue their original regimen (N = 48) for 48 weeks. Five additional subjects over the age of 12 were enrolled and randomized (VIREAD N=4, original regimen N=1) but are not included in the efficacy analysis. After 48 weeks, all eligible subjects were allowed to continue in the study receiving open-label VIREAD. At Week 48, 89% of subjects in the VIREAD treatment group and 90% of subjects in the stavudine or zidovudine treatment group had HIV-1 RNA concentrations less than 400 copies/mL. During the 48 week randomized phase of the study, 1 subject in the VIREAD group discontinued the study prematurely because of virologic failure/lack of efficacy and 3 subjects (2 subjects in the VIREAD group and 1 subject in the stavudine or zidovudine group) discontinued for other reasons.

In Study 321, 87 treatment-experienced subjects 12 to less than 18 years of age were treated with VIREAD (N=45) or placebo (N=42) in combination with an optimized background regimen (OBR) for 48 weeks. The mean baseline CD4 cell count was 374 cells/mm^3 and the mean baseline plasma HIV-1 RNA was 4.6 log_{10} copies/mL. At baseline, 90% of subjects harbored NRTI resistance-associated substitutions in their HIV-1 isolates. Overall, the trial failed to show a difference in virologic response between the VIREAD and placebo treatment groups. Subgroup analyses suggest the lack of difference in virologic response may be attributable to imbalances between treatment arms in baseline viral susceptibility to VIREAD and OBR.

Although changes in HIV-1 RNA in these highly treatment-experienced subjects were less than anticipated, the comparability of the pharmacokinetic and safety data to that observed in adults supports the use of VIREAD in pediatric patients 12 years of age and older who weigh greater than or equal to 35 kg and whose HIV-1 isolate is expected to be sensitive to VIREAD. *[See Warnings and Precautions (5.6), Adverse Reactions (6.1), and Clinical Pharmacology (12.3)]*.

Safety and effectiveness of VIREAD in pediatric patients younger than 2 years of age with HIV-1 infection have not been established.

Pediatric Patients 12 Years of Age and Older with Chronic Hepatitis B

In Study 115, 106 HBeAg negative (9%) and positive (91%) subjects aged 12 to less than 18 years with chronic HBV infection were randomized to receive blinded treatment with VIREAD 300 mg (N = 52) or placebo (N = 54) for 72 weeks. At study entry, the mean HBV DNA was 8.1 log_{10} copies/mL and mean ALT was 101 U/L. Of 52 subjects treated with VIREAD, 20 subjects were nucleos(t)ide-naïve and 32 subjects were nucleos(t)ide-experienced. Thirty-one of the 32 nucleos(t)ide-experienced subjects had prior lamivudine experience. At Week 72, 88% (46/52) of subjects in the VIREAD group and 0% (0/54) of subjects in the placebo group had HBV DNA <400 copies/mL. Among subjects with abnormal ALT at baseline, 74% (26/35) of subjects receiving VIREAD had normalized ALT at Week 72 compared to 31% (13/42) in the placebo group. One VIREAD-treated subject experienced sustained HBsAg-loss and seroconversion to anti-HBs during the first 72 weeks of study participation.

Safety and effectiveness of VIREAD in pediatric patients younger than 12 years of age or less than 35 kg with chronic hepatitis B have not been established.

8.5 Geriatric Use

Clinical trials of VIREAD did not include sufficient numbers of subjects aged 65 and over to determine whether they respond differently from younger subjects. In general, dose selection for the elderly patient should be cautious, keeping in mind the greater frequency of decreased hepatic, renal, or cardiac function, and of concomitant disease or other drug therapy.

8.6 Patients with Impaired Renal Function

It is recommended that the dosing interval for VIREAD be modified in patients with creatinine clearance below 50 mL/min or in patients with ESRD who require dialysis *[See Dosage and Administration (2.3), Clinical Pharmacology (12.3)].*

10 OVERDOSAGE

Limited clinical experience at doses higher than the therapeutic dose of VIREAD 300 mg is available. In Study 901, 600 mg tenofovir disoproxil fumarate was administered to 8 subjects orally for 28 days. No severe adverse reactions were reported. The effects of higher doses are not known.

If overdose occurs the patient must be monitored for evidence of toxicity, and standard supportive treatment applied as necessary.

Tenofovir is efficiently removed by hemodialysis with an extraction coefficient of approximately 54%. Following a single 300 mg dose of VIREAD, a four-hour hemodialysis session removed approximately 10% of the administered tenofovir dose.

11 DESCRIPTION

VIREAD is the brand name for tenofovir disoproxil fumarate (a prodrug of tenofovir) which is a fumaric acid salt of bis-isopropoxycarbonyloxymethyl ester derivative of tenofovir. *In vivo* tenofovir disoproxil fumarate is converted to tenofovir, an acyclic nucleoside phosphonate (nucleotide) analog of adenosine 5′-monophosphate. Tenofovir exhibits activity against HIV-1 reverse transcriptase.

The chemical name of tenofovir disoproxil fumarate is 9-[(*R*)-2-[[bis[[(isopropoxycarbonyl)oxy]methoxy]phosphinyl]methoxy]propyl]adenine fumarate (1:1). It has a molecular formula of $C_{19}H_{30}N_5O_{10}P \bullet C_4H_4O_4$ and a molecular weight of 635.52. It has the following structural formula:

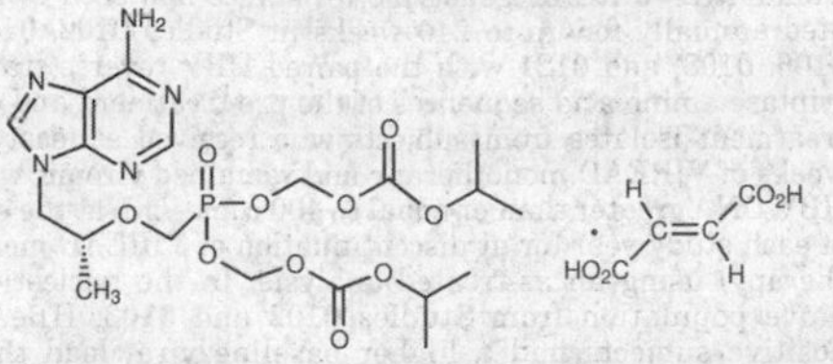

Tenofovir disoproxil fumarate is a white to off-white crystalline powder with a solubility of 13.4 mg/mL in distilled water at 25 °C. It has an octanol/phosphate buffer (pH 6.5) partition coefficient (log p) of 1.25 at 25 °C.

VIREAD is available as tablets or as an oral powder.

VIREAD tablets are for oral administration in strengths of 150, 200, 250, and 300 mg of tenofovir disoproxil fumarate, which are equivalent to 123, 163, 204 and 245 mg of tenofovir disoproxil, respectively. Each tablet contains the following inactive ingredients: croscarmellose sodium, lactose monohydrate, magnesium stearate, microcrystalline cellulose, and pregelatinized starch. The 300 mg tablets are coated with Opadry II Y-30-10671-A, which contains FD&C blue #2 aluminum lake, hypromellose 2910, lactose monohydrate, titanium dioxide, and triacetin. The 150, 200, and 250 mg tablets are coated with Opadry II 32K-18425, which contains hypromellose 2910, lactose monohydrate, titanium dioxide, and triacetin.

VIREAD oral powder is available for oral administration as white, taste-masked, coated granules containing 40 mg of tenofovir disoproxil fumarate per gram of oral powder, which is equivalent to 33 mg of tenofovir disoproxil. The oral powder contains the following inactive ingredients: mannitol, hydroxypropyl cellulose, ethylcellulose, and silicon dioxide.

In this insert, all dosages are expressed in terms of tenofovir disoproxil fumarate except where otherwise noted.

12 CLINICAL PHARMACOLOGY

12.1 Mechanism of Action

Tenofovir disoproxil fumarate is an antiviral drug *[See Microbiology (12.4)].*

12.3 Pharmacokinetics

The pharmacokinetics of tenofovir disoproxil fumarate have been evaluated in healthy volunteers and HIV-1 infected individuals. Tenofovir pharmacokinetics are similar between these populations.

Absorption

VIREAD is a water soluble diester prodrug of the active ingredient tenofovir. The oral bioavailability of tenofovir from VIREAD in fasted subjects is approximately 25%. Following oral administration of a single dose of VIREAD 300 mg to HIV-1 infected subjects in the fasted state, maximum serum concentrations (C_{max}) are achieved in 1.0 ± 0.4 hrs. C_{max} and AUC values are 0.30 ± 0.09 µg/mL and 2.29 ± 0.69 µg•hr/mL, respectively.

The pharmacokinetics of tenofovir are dose proportional over a VIREAD dose range of 75 to 600 mg and are not affected by repeated dosing.

Table 12 Pharmacokinetic Parameters (Mean ± SD) of Tenofovir* in Subjects with Varying Degrees of Renal Function

Baseline Creatinine Clearance (mL/min)	>80 (N=3)	50–80 (N=10)	30–49 (N=8)	12–29 (N=11)
C_{max} (µg/mL)	0.34 ± 0.03	0.33 ± 0.06	0.37 ± 0.16	0.60 ± 0.19
$AUC_{0-\infty}$ (µg•hr/mL)	2.18 ± 0.26	3.06 ± 0.93	6.01 ± 2.50	15.98 ± 7.22
CL/F (mL/min)	1043.7 ± 115.4	807.7 ± 279.2	444.4 ± 209.8	177.0 ± 97.1
CL_{renal} (mL/min)	243.5 ± 33.3	168.6 ± 27.5	100.6 ± 27.5	43.0 ± 31.2

* 300 mg, single dose of VIREAD

In a single-dose bioequivalence study conducted under non-fasted conditions (dose administered with 4 oz. applesauce) in healthy adult volunteers, the mean C_{max} of tenofovir was 26% lower for the oral powder relative to the tablet formulation. Mean AUC of tenofovir was similar between the oral powder and tablet formulations.

Distribution

In vitro binding of tenofovir to human plasma or serum proteins is less than 0.7 and 7.2%, respectively, over the tenofovir concentration range 0.01 to 25 µg/mL. The volume of distribution at steady-state is 1.3 ± 0.6 L/kg and 1.2 ± 0.4 L/kg, following intravenous administration of tenofovir 1.0 mg/kg and 3.0 mg/kg.

Metabolism and Elimination

In vitro studies indicate that neither tenofovir disoproxil nor tenofovir are substrates of CYP enzymes.

Following IV administration of tenofovir, approximately 70–80% of the dose is recovered in the urine as unchanged tenofovir within 72 hours of dosing. Following single dose, oral administration of VIREAD, the terminal elimination half-life of tenofovir is approximately 17 hours. After multiple oral doses of VIREAD 300 mg once daily (under fed conditions), 32 ± 10% of the administered dose is recovered in urine over 24 hours.

Tenofovir is eliminated by a combination of glomerular filtration and active tubular secretion. There may be competition for elimination with other compounds that are also renally eliminated.

Effects of Food on Oral Absorption

Administration of VIREAD 300 mg tablets following a high-fat meal (~700 to 1000 kcal containing 40 to 50% fat) increases the oral bioavailability, with an increase in tenofovir $AUC_{0-\infty}$ of approximately 40% and an increase in C_{max} of approximately 14%. However, administration of VIREAD with a light meal did not have a significant effect on the pharmacokinetics of tenofovir when compared to fasted administration of the drug. Food delays the time to tenofovir C_{max} by approximately 1 hour. C_{max} and AUC of tenofovir are 0.33 ± 0.12 µg/mL and 3.32 ± 1.37 µg•hr/mL following multiple doses of VIREAD 300 mg once daily in the fed state, when meal content was not controlled.

Special Populations

Race: There were insufficient numbers from racial and ethnic groups other than Caucasian to adequately determine potential pharmacokinetic differences among these populations.

Gender: Tenofovir pharmacokinetics are similar in male and female subjects.

Pediatric Patients 2 Years of Age and Older: Steady-state pharmacokinetics of tenofovir were evaluated in 31 HIV-1 infected pediatric subjects 2 to less than 18 years (Table 11). Tenofovir exposure achieved in these pediatric subjects receiving oral once daily doses of VIREAD 300 mg (tablet) or 8 mg/kg of body weight (powder) up to a maximum dose of 300 mg was similar to exposures achieved in adults receiving once-daily doses of VIREAD 300 mg.

Table 11 Mean (± SD) Tenofovir Pharmacokinetic Parameters by Age Groups for HIV-1-infected Pediatric Patients

Dose and Formulation	300 mg Tablet	8 mg/kg Oral Powder
	12 to <18 Year (N=8)	2 to <12 Years (N=23)
C_{max} (µg/mL)	0.38 ± 0.13	0.24 ± 0.13
AUC_{tau} (µg•hr/mL)	3.39 ± 1.22	2.59 ± 1.06

Tenofovir exposures in 52 HBV-infected pediatric subjects (12 to less than 18 years of age) receiving oral once-daily doses of VIREAD 300 mg tablet were comparable to exposures achieved in HIV-1-infected adults and adolescents receiving once-daily doses of 300 mg.

Geriatric Patients: Pharmacokinetic trials have not been performed in the elderly (65 years and older).

Patients with Impaired Renal Function: The pharmacokinetics of tenofovir are altered in subjects with renal impairment *[See Warnings and Precautions (5.3)].* In subjects with creatinine clearance below 50 mL/min or with end-stage renal disease (ESRD) requiring dialysis, C_{max}, and $AUC_{0-\infty}$ of tenofovir were increased (Table 12). It is recommended that the dosing interval for VIREAD be modified in patients with creatinine clearance below 50 mL/min or in patients with ESRD who require dialysis *[See Dosage and Administration (2.3)].*

[See table 12 above]

Tenofovir is efficiently removed by hemodialysis with an extraction coefficient of approximately 54%. Following a single 300 mg dose of VIREAD, a four-hour hemodialysis session removed approximately 10% of the administered tenofovir dose.

Patients with Hepatic Impairment: The pharmacokinetics of tenofovir following a 300 mg single dose of VIREAD have been studied in non-HIV infected subjects with moderate to severe hepatic impairment. There were no substantial alterations in tenofovir pharmacokinetics in subjects with hepatic impairment compared with unimpaired subjects. No change in VIREAD dosing is required in patients with hepatic impairment.

Assessment of Drug Interactions

At concentrations substantially higher (~300-fold) than those observed *in vivo*, tenofovir did not inhibit *in vitro* drug metabolism mediated by any of the following human CYP isoforms: CYP3A4, CYP2D6, CYP2C9, or CYP2E1. However, a small (6%) but statistically significant reduction in metabolism of CYP1A substrate was observed. Based on the results of *in vitro* experiments and the known elimination pathway of tenofovir, the potential for CYP mediated interactions involving tenofovir with other medicinal products is low.

VIREAD has been evaluated in healthy volunteers in combination with other antiretroviral and potential concomitant drugs. Tables 13 and 14 summarize pharmacokinetic effects of coadministered drug on tenofovir pharmacokinetics and effects of VIREAD on the pharmacokinetics of coadministered drug. Coadministration of VIREAD with didanosine results in changes in the pharmacokinetics of didanosine that may be of clinical significance. Concomitant dosing of VIREAD with didanosine significantly increases the Cmax and AUC of didanosine. When didanosine 250 mg enteric-coated capsules were administered with VIREAD, systemic exposures of didanosine were similar to those seen with the 400 mg enteric-coated capsules alone under fasted conditions (Table 14). The mechanism of this interaction is unknown.

No clinically significant drug interactions have been observed between VIREAD and efavirenz, methadone, nelfinavir, oral contraceptives, or ribavirin.

[See table 13 at top of next page]

[See table 14 at top of page 909]

12.4 Microbiology

Mechanism of Action

Tenofovir disoproxil fumarate is an acyclic nucleoside phosphonate diester analog of adenosine monophosphate. Tenofovir disoproxil fumarate requires initial diester hydrolysis for conversion to tenofovir and subsequent phosphorylations by cellular enzymes to form tenofovir diphosphate, an obligate chain terminator. Tenofovir diphosphate inhibits the activity of HIV-1 reverse transcriptase and HBV reverse transcriptase by competing with the natural substrate deoxyadenosine 5′-triphosphate and, after incorporation into DNA, by DNA chain termination. Tenofovir diphosphate is a weak inhibitor of mammalian DNA polymerases α, β, and mitochondrial DNA polymerase γ.

Activity against HIV

Antiviral Activity

The antiviral activity of tenofovir against laboratory and clinical isolates of HIV-1 was assessed in lymphoblastoid cell lines, primary monocyte/macrophage cells and peripheral blood lymphocytes. The EC_{50} (50% effective concentration) values for tenofovir were in the range of 0.04 µM to 8.5 µM. In drug combination studies, tenofovir was not an-

Table 13 Drug Interactions: Changes in Pharmacokinetic Parameters for Tenofovir* in the Presence of the Coadministered Drug

Coadministered Drug	Dose of Coadministered Drug (mg)	N	% Change of Tenofovir Pharmacokinetic Parameters† (90% CI)		
			C_{max}	AUC	C_{min}
Abacavir	300 once	8	⇔	⇔	NC
Atazanavir‡	400 once daily × 14 days	33	↑ 14 (↑ 8 to ↑ 20)	↑ 24 (↑ 21 to ↑ 28)	↑ 22 (↑ 15 to ↑ 30)
Didanosine§	250 or 400 once daily × 7 days	14	⇔	⇔	⇔
Emtricitabine	200 once daily × 7 days	17	⇔	⇔	⇔
Entecavir	1 mg once daily × 10 days	28	⇔	⇔	⇔
Indinavir	800 three times daily × 7 days	13	↑ 14 (↓ 3 to ↑ 33)	⇔	⇔
Lamivudine	150 twice daily × 7 days	15	⇔	⇔	⇔
Lopinavir/Ritonavir	400/100 twice daily × 14 days	24	⇔	↑ 32 (↑ 25 to ↑ 38)	↑ 51 (↑ 37 to ↑ 66)
Saquinavir/Ritonavir	1000/100 twice daily × 14 days	35	⇔	⇔	↑ 23 (↑ 16 to ↑ 30)
Tacrolimus	0.05 mg/kg twice daily × 7 days	21	↑ 13 (↑ 1 to ↑ 27)	⇔	⇔

* Subjects received VIREAD 300 mg once daily.
† Increase = ↑; Decrease = ↓; No Effect = ⇔; NC = Not Calculated
‡ Reyataz Prescribing Information
§ Subjects received didanosine buffered tablets.

tagonistic with nucleoside reverse transcriptase inhibitors (abacavir, didanosine, lamivudine, stavudine, zalcitabine, zidovudine), non-nucleoside reverse transcriptase inhibitors (delavirdine, efavirenz, nevirapine), and protease inhibitors (amprenavir, indinavir, nelfinavir, ritonavir, saquinavir). Tenofovir displayed antiviral activity in cell culture against HIV-1 clades A, B, C, D, E, F, G, and O (EC_{50} values ranged from 0.5 µM to 2.2 µM) and strain specific activity against HIV-2 (EC_{50} values ranged from 1.6 µM to 5.5 µM).

Resistance

HIV-1 isolates with reduced susceptibility to tenofovir have been selected in cell culture. These viruses expressed a K65R substitution in reverse transcriptase and showed a 2–4 fold reduction in susceptibility to tenofovir.

In Study 903 of treatment-naïve subjects (VIREAD + lamivudine + efavirenz versus stavudine + lamivudine + efavirenz) *[See Clinical Studies (14.1)]*, genotypic analyses of isolates from subjects with virologic failure through Week 144 showed development of efavirenz and lamivudine resistance-associated substitutions to occur most frequently and with no difference between the treatment arms. The K65R substitution occurred in 8/47 (17%) analyzed patient isolates on the VIREAD arm and in 2/49 (4%) analyzed patient isolates on the stavudine arm. Of the 8 subjects whose virus developed K65R in the VIREAD arm through 144 weeks, 7 of these occurred in the first 48 weeks of treatment and one at Week 96. Other substitutions resulting in resistance to VIREAD were not identified in this trial.

In Study 934 of treatment-naïve subjects (VIREAD + EMTRIVA + efavirenz versus zidovudine (AZT)/lamivudine (3TC) + efavirenz) *[See Clinical Studies (14.1)]*, genotypic analysis performed on HIV-1 isolates from all confirmed virologic failure subjects with greater than 400 copies/mL of HIV-1 RNA at Week 144 or early discontinuation showed development of efavirenz resistance-associated substitutions occurred most frequently and was similar between the two treatment arms. The M184V substitution, associated with resistance to EMTRIVA and lamivudine, was observed in 2/19 analyzed subject isolates in the VIREAD + EMTRIVA group and in 10/29 analyzed subject isolates in the zidovudine/lamivudine group. Through 144 weeks of Study 934, no subjects have developed a detectable K65R substitution in their HIV-1 as analyzed through standard genotypic analysis.

Cross-Resistance

Cross-resistance among certain reverse transcriptase inhibitors has been recognized. The K65R substitution selected by tenofovir is also selected in some HIV-1 infected subjects treated with abacavir, didanosine, or zalcitabine. HIV-1 isolates with this substitution also show reduced susceptibility to emtricitabine and lamivudine. Therefore, cross-resistance among these drugs may occur in patients whose virus harbors the K65R substitution. HIV-1 isolates from subjects (N=20) whose HIV-1 expressed a mean of 3 zidovudine-associated reverse transcriptase substitutions (M41L, D67N, K70R, L210W, T215Y/F, or K219Q/E/N), showed a 3.1-fold decrease in the susceptibility to tenofovir.

In Studies 902 and 907 conducted in treatment-experienced subjects (VIREAD + Standard Background Therapy (SBT) compared to Placebo + SBT) *[See Clinical Studies (14.1)]*, 14/304 (5%) of the VIREAD-treated subjects with virologic failure through Week 96 had greater than 1.4-fold (median 2.7-fold) reduced susceptibility to tenofovir. Genotypic analysis of the baseline and failure isolates showed the development of the K65R substitution in the HIV-1 reverse transcriptase gene.

The virologic response to VIREAD therapy has been evaluated with respect to baseline viral genotype (N=222) in treatment-experienced subjects participating in Studies 902 and 907. In these clinical trials, 94% of the participants evaluated had baseline HIV-1 isolates expressing at least one NRTI substitution. Virologic responses for subjects in the genotype substudy were similar to the overall trial results.

Several exploratory analyses were conducted to evaluate the effect of specific substitutions and substitutional patterns on virologic outcome. Because of the large number of potential comparisons, statistical testing was not conducted. Varying degrees of cross-resistance of VIREAD to pre-existing zidovudine resistance-associated substitutions (M41L, D67N, K70R, L210W, T215Y/F, or K219Q/E/N) were observed and appeared to depend on the type and number of specific substitutions. VIREAD-treated subjects whose HIV-1 expressed 3 or more zidovudine resistance-associated substitutions that included either the M41L or L210W reverse transcriptase substitution showed reduced responses to VIREAD therapy; however, these responses were still improved compared with placebo. The presence of the D67N, K70R, T215Y/F, or K219Q/E/N substitution did not appear to affect responses to VIREAD therapy. Subjects whose virus expressed an L74V substitution without zidovudine resistance associated substitutions (N=8) had reduced response to VIREAD. Limited data are available for subjects whose virus expressed a Y115F substitution (N=3), Q151M substitution (N=2), or T69 insertion (N=4), all of whom had a reduced response.

In the protocol defined analyses, virologic response to VIREAD was not reduced in subjects with HIV-1 that expressed the abacavir/emtricitabine/lamivudine resistance-associated M184V substitution. HIV-1 RNA responses among these subjects were durable through Week 48.

Studies 902 and 907 Phenotypic Analyses

Phenotypic analysis of baseline HIV-1 from treatment-experienced subjects (N=100) demonstrated a correlation between baseline susceptibility to VIREAD and response to VIREAD therapy. Table 15 summarizes the HIV-1 RNA response by baseline VIREAD susceptibility.

Table 15 HIV-1 RNA Response at Week 24 by Baseline VIREAD Susceptibility (Intent-To-Treat)*

Baseline VIREAD Susceptibility†	Change in HIV-1 RNA‡ (N)
<1	-0.74 (35)
>1 and ≤3	-0.56 (49)
>3 and ≤4	-0.3 (7)
>4	-0.12 (9)

* Tenofovir susceptibility was determined by recombinant phenotypic Antivirogram assay (Virco).
† Fold change in susceptibility from wild-type.
‡ Average HIV-1 RNA change from baseline through Week 24 ($DAVG_{24}$) in log_{10} copies/mL.

Activity against HBV

Antiviral Activity

The antiviral activity of tenofovir against HBV was assessed in the HepG2 2.2.15 cell line. The EC_{50} values for tenofovir ranged from 0.14 to 1.5 µM, with CC_{50} (50% cytotoxicity concentration) values greater than 100 µM. In cell culture combination antiviral activity studies of tenofovir with the nucleoside HBV reverse transcriptase inhibitors entecavir, lamivudine, and telbivudine, and with the nucleoside HIV-1 reverse transcriptase inhibitor emtricitabine, no antagonistic activity was observed.

Resistance

Cumulative VIREAD genotypic resistance has been evaluated annually for up to 240 weeks in Studies 0102, 0103, 0106, 0108, and 0121 with the paired HBV reverse transcriptase amino acid sequences of the pre-treatment and on-treatment isolates from subjects who received at least 24 weeks of VIREAD monotherapy and remained viremic with HBV DNA greater than or equal to 400 copies/mL at the end of each study year (or at discontinuation of VIREAD monotherapy) using an as-treated analysis. In the nucleotide-naïve population from Studies 0102 and 0103, HBeAg-positive subjects had a higher baseline viral load than HBeAg-negative subjects and a significantly higher proportion of the subjects remained viremic at their last time point on VIREAD monotherapy (15% versus 4%, respectively). HBV isolates from these subjects who remained viremic showed treatment-emergent substitutions (Table 16); however, no specific substitutions occurred at a sufficient frequency to be associated with resistance to VIREAD (genotypic and phenotypic analyses).

[See table 16 at bottom of next page]

Cross-Resistance

Cross-resistance has been observed between HBV nucleoside/nucleotide analogue reverse transcriptase inhibitors.

In cell based assays, HBV strains expressing the rtV173L, rtL180M, and rtM204I/V substitutions associated with resistance to lamivudine and telbivudine showed a susceptibility to tenofovir ranging from 0.7- to 3.4-fold that of wild type virus. The rtL180M and rtM204I/V double substitutions conferred 3.4-fold reduced susceptibility to tenofovir.

HBV strains expressing the rtL180M, rtT184G, rtS202G/I, rtM204V, and rtM250V substitutions associated with resistance to entecavir showed a susceptibility to tenofovir ranging from 0.6- to 6.9-fold that of wild type virus.

HBV strains expressing the adefovir resistance-associated substitutions rtA181V and/or rtN236T showed reductions in susceptibility to tenofovir ranging from 2.9- to 10-fold that of wild type virus. Strains containing the rtA181T substitution showed changes in susceptibility to tenofovir ranging from 0.9- to 1.5-fold that of wild type virus.

One hundred fifty-two subjects initiating VIREAD therapy in Studies 0102, 0103, 0106, 0108, and 0121 harbored HBV with known resistance substitutions to HBV nucleos(t)ide analogue reverse transcriptase inhibitors: 14 with adefovir resistance-associated substitutions (rtA181S/T/V and/or rtN236T), 135 with lamivudine resistance-associated substitutions (rtM204I/V), and 3 with both adefovir and lamivudine resistance-associated substitutions. Following up to 240 weeks of VIREAD treatment, 11 of the 14 subjects with adefovir-resistant HBV, 124 of the 135 subjects with lamivudine-resistant HBV, and 2 of the 3 subjects with both adefovir- and lamivudine-resistant HBV achieved and maintained virologic suppression (HBV DNA less than 400 copies/mL). Three of the 5 subjects whose virus harbored both the rtA181T/V and rtN236T substitutions remained viremic.

13 NONCLINICAL TOXICOLOGY

13.1 Carcinogenesis, Mutagenesis, Impairment of Fertility

Carcinogenesis

Long-term oral carcinogenicity studies of tenofovir disoproxil fumarate in mice and rats were carried out at ex-

Table 14 Drug Interactions: Changes in Pharmacokinetic Parameters for Coadministered Drug in the Presence of VIREAD

Coadministered Drug	Dose of Coadministered Drug (mg)	N	% Change of Coadministered Drug Pharmacokinetic Parameters* (90% CI)		
			C_{max}	AUC	C_{min}
Abacavir	300 once	8	↑ 12 (↓ 1 to ↑ 26)	⇔	NA
Atazanavir†	400 once daily × 14 days	34	↓ 21 (↓ 27 to ↓ 14)	↓ 25 (↓ 30 to ↓ 19)	↓ 40 (↓ 48 to ↓ 32)
Atazanavir†	Atazanavir/ Ritonavir 300/100 once daily × 42 days	10	↓ 28 (↓ 50 to ↑ 5)	↓ 25‡ (↓ 42 to ↓ 3)	↓ 23‡ (↓ 46 to ↑ 10)
Didanosine§	250 once, simultaneously with VIREAD and a light meal¶	33	↓ 20# (↓ 32 to ↓ 7)	⇔#	NA
Emtricitabine	200 once daily × 7 days	17	⇔	⇔	↑ 20 (↑ 12 to ↑ 29)
Entecavir	1 mg once daily × 10 days	28	⇔	↑ 13 (↑ 11 to ↑ 15)	⇔
Indinavir	800 three times daily × 7 days	12	↓ 11 (↓ 30 to ↑ 12)	⇔	⇔
Lamivudine	150 twice daily × 7 days	15	↓ 24 (↓ 34 to ↓ 12)	⇔	⇔
Lopinavir	Lopinavir/Ritonavir 400/100 twice daily × 14 days	24	⇔	⇔	⇔
Ritonavir			⇔	⇔	⇔
Saquinavir	Saquinavir/Ritonavir 1000/100 twice daily × 14 days	32	↑ 22 (↑ 6 to ↑ 41)	↑ 29Þ (↑ 12 to ↑ 48)	↑ 47Þ (↑ 23 to ↑ 76)
Ritonavir			⇔	⇔	↑ 23 (↑ 3 to ↑ 46)
Tacrolimus	0.05 mg/kg twice daily × 7 days	21	⇔	⇔	⇔

* Increase = ↑; Decrease = ↓; No Effect = ⇔; NA = Not Applicable
† Reyataz Prescribing Information
‡ In HIV-infected subjects, addition of tenofovir DF to atazanavir 300 mg plus ritonavir 100 mg, resulted in AUC and C_{min} values of atazanavir that were 2.3- and 4-fold higher than the respective values observed for atazanavir 400 mg when given alone.
§ Videx EC Prescribing Information. Subjects received didanosine enteric-coated capsules.
¶ 373 kcal, 8.2 g fat
\# Compared with didanosine (enteric-coated) 400 mg administered alone under fasting conditions.
Þ Increases in AUC and C_{min} are not expected to be clinically relevant; hence no dose adjustments are required when tenofovir DF and ritonavir-boosted saquinavir are coadministered.

Table 16 Amino Acid Substitutions in Viremic Subjects across HBV Trials of VIREAD

	Compensated Liver Disease			Decompensated Liver Disease (N=39)*
	Nucleotide-Naïve (N=417)†	HEPSERA-Experienced (N=247)‡	Lamivudine-Resistant (N=136)§	
Viremic at Last Time Point on VIREAD	35/417 (8%)	34/247 (14%)	9/136 (7%)	7/39 (18%)
Treatment-Emergent Amino Acid Substitutions¶	19#/33 (58%)	10Þ/27 (37%)	6ß/8 (75%)	3/5 (60%)

* Subjects with decompensated liver disease from Study 0108 (N=39) receiving up to 48 weeks of treatment with VIREAD.
† Nucleotide-naïve subjects from Studies 0102 (N=246) and 0103 (N=171) receiving up to 240 weeks of treatment with VIREAD.
‡ HEPSERA-experienced subjects from Studies 0102/0103 (N=195) and 0106 (N=52) receiving up to 192 weeks of treatment with VIREAD after switching to VIREAD from HEPSERA. Study 0106, a randomized, double-blind, 168-week Phase 2 trial, has been completed.
§ Lamivudine-resistant subjects from Study 0121 (N=136) receiving up to 96 weeks of treatment with VIREAD after switching to VIREAD from lamivudine.
¶ Denominator includes those subjects who were viremic at last time point on VIREAD monotherapy and had evaluable paired genotypic data.
\# Of the 19 subjects with treatment-emergent amino acid substitutions during Studies 0102 and 0103, 5 subjects had substitutions at conserved sites and 14 subjects had substitutions only at polymorphic sites, and 8 subjects had only transient substitutions that were not detected at the last time point on VIREAD.
Þ Of the 10 HEPSERA-experienced subjects with treatment-emergent amino acid substitutions, 2 subjects had substitutions at conserved sites and 8 had substitutions only at polymorphic sites.
ß Of the 6 lamivudine-resistant subjects with treatment-emergent substitutions during Study 0121, 3 subjects had substitutions at conserved sites and 3 had substitutions only at polymorphic sites.

posures up to approximately 16 times (mice) and 5 times (rats) those observed in humans at the therapeutic dose for HIV-1 infection. At the high dose in female mice, liver adenomas were increased at exposures 16 times that in humans. In rats, the study was negative for carcinogenic findings at exposures up to 5 times that observed in humans at the therapeutic dose.

Mutagenesis

Tenofovir disoproxil fumarate was mutagenic in the *in vitro* mouse lymphoma assay and negative in an *in vitro* bacterial mutagenicity test (Ames test). In an *in vivo* mouse micronucleus assay, tenofovir disoproxil fumarate was negative when administered to male mice.

Impairment of Fertility

There were no effects on fertility, mating performance or early embryonic development when tenofovir disoproxil fumarate was administered to male rats at a dose equivalent to 10 times the human dose based on body surface area comparisons for 28 days prior to mating and to female rats for 15 days prior to mating through day seven of gestation. There was, however, an alteration of the estrous cycle in female rats.

13.2 Animal Toxicology and/or Pharmacology

Tenofovir and tenofovir disoproxil fumarate administered in toxicology studies to rats, dogs, and monkeys at exposures (based on AUCs) greater than or equal to 6 fold those observed in humans caused bone toxicity. In monkeys the bone toxicity was diagnosed as osteomalacia. Osteomalacia observed in monkeys appeared to be reversible upon dose reduction or discontinuation of tenofovir. In rats and dogs, the bone toxicity manifested as reduced bone mineral density. The mechanism(s) underlying bone toxicity is unknown.

Evidence of renal toxicity was noted in 4 animal species. Increases in serum creatinine, BUN, glycosuria, proteinuria, phosphaturia, and/or calciuria and decreases in serum phosphate were observed to varying degrees in these animals. These toxicities were noted at exposures (based on AUCs) 2–20 times higher than those observed in humans. The relationship of the renal abnormalities, particularly the phosphaturia, to the bone toxicity is not known.

14 CLINICAL STUDIES

14.1 Clinical Efficacy in Adults with HIV-1 Infection

Treatment-Naïve Adult Patients

Study 903

Data through 144 weeks are reported for Study 903, a double-blind, active-controlled multicenter trial comparing VIREAD (300 mg once daily) administered in combination with lamivudine and efavirenz versus stavudine (d4T), lamivudine, and efavirenz in 600 antiretroviral-naïve subjects. Subjects had a mean age of 36 years (range 18–64), 74% were male, 64% were Caucasian and 20% were Black. The mean baseline CD4+ cell count was 279 cells/mm³ (range 3–956) and median baseline plasma HIV-1 RNA was 77,600 copies/mL (range 417–5,130,000). Subjects were stratified by baseline HIV-1 RNA and CD4+ cell count. Forty-three percent of subjects had baseline viral loads >100,000 copies/mL and 39% had CD4+ cell counts <200 cells/mm³. Treatment outcomes through 48 and 144 weeks are presented in Table 17.

[See table 17 at top of next page]

Achievement of plasma HIV-1 RNA concentrations of less than 400 copies/mL at Week 144 was similar between the two treatment groups for the population stratified at baseline on the basis of HIV-1 RNA concentration (> or ≤100,000 copies/mL) and CD4+ cell count (< or ≥200 cells/mm³). Through 144 weeks of therapy, 62% and 58% of subjects in the VIREAD and stavudine arms, respectively achieved and maintained confirmed HIV-1 RNA <50 copies/mL. The mean increase from baseline in CD4+ cell count was 263 cells/mm³ for the VIREAD arm and 283 cells/mm³ for the stavudine arm.

Through 144 weeks, 11 subjects in the VIREAD group and 9 subjects in the stavudine group experienced a new CDC Class C event.

Study 934

Data through 144 weeks are reported for Study 934, a randomized, open-label, active-controlled multicenter trial comparing emtricitabine + VIREAD administered in combination with efavirenz versus zidovudine/lamivudine fixed-dose combination administered in combination with efavirenz in 511 antiretroviral-naïve subjects. From Weeks 96 to 144 of the trial, subjects received a fixed-dose combination of emtricitabine and tenofovir DF with efavirenz in place of emtricitabine + VIREAD with efavirenz. Subjects had a mean age of 38 years (range 18–80), 86% were male, 59% were Caucasian and 23% were Black. The mean baseline CD4+ cell count was 245 cells/mm³ (range 2–1191) and median baseline plasma HIV-1 RNA was 5.01 $\log_{10}$ copies/mL (range 3.56–6.54). Subjects were stratified by baseline CD4+ cell count (< or ≥200 cells/mm³); 41% had CD4+ cell counts <200 cells/mm³ and 51% of subjects had baseline viral loads >100,000 copies/mL. Treatment outcomes through 48 and 144 weeks for those subjects who did not have efavirenz resistance at baseline are presented in Table 18.

[See table 18 at top of next page]

Through Week 48, 84% and 73% of subjects in the emtricitabine + VIREAD group and the zidovudine/lamivudine group, respectively, achieved and maintained HIV-1 RNA

Table 17 Outcomes of Randomized Treatment at Week 48 and 144 (Study 903)

Outcomes	At Week 48		At Week 144	
	VIREAD+3TC +EFV (N=299)	d4T+3TC +EFV (N=301)	VIREAD+3TC +EFV (N=299)	d4T+3TC +EFV (N=301)
Responder*	79%	82%	68%	62%
Virologic failure†	6%	4%	10%	8%
Rebound	5%	3%	8%	7%
Never suppressed	0%	1%	0%	0%
Added an antiretroviral agent	1%	1%	2%	1%
Death	<1%	1%	<1%	2%
Discontinued due to adverse event	6%	6%	8%	13%
Discontinued for other reasons‡	8%	7%	14%	15%

* Subjects achieved and maintained confirmed HIV-1 RNA <400 copies/mL through Week 48 and 144.
† Includes confirmed viral rebound and failure to achieve confirmed <400 copies/mL through Week 48 and 144.
‡ Includes lost to follow-up, subject's withdrawal, noncompliance, protocol violation and other reasons.

Table 18 Outcomes of Randomized Treatment at Week 48 and 144 (Study 934)

Outcomes	At Week 48		At Week 144	
	FTC +VIREAD +EFV (N=244)	AZT/3TC +EFV (N=243)	FTC +VIREAD +EFV (N=227)*	AZT/3TC +EFV (N=229)*
Responder†	84%	73%	71%	58%
Virologic failure‡	2%	4%	3%	6%
Rebound	1%	3%	2%	5%
Never suppressed	0%	0%	0%	0%
Change in antiretroviral regimen	1%	1%	1%	1%
Death	<1%	1%	1%	1%
Discontinued due to adverse event	4%	9%	5%	12%
Discontinued for other reasons§	10%	14%	20%	22%

* Subjects who were responders at Week 48 or Week 96 (HIV-1 RNA <400 copies/mL) but did not consent to continue the trial after Week 48 or Week 96 were excluded from analysis.
† Subjects achieved and maintained confirmed HIV-1 RNA <400 copies/mL through Weeks 48 and 144.
‡ Includes confirmed viral rebound and failure to achieve confirmed <400 copies/mL through Weeks 48 and 144.
§ Includes lost to follow-up, subject withdrawal, noncompliance, protocol violation and other reasons.

<400 copies/mL (71% and 58% through Week 144). The difference in the proportion of subjects who achieved and maintained HIV-1 RNA <400 copies/mL through 48 weeks largely results from the higher number of discontinuations due to adverse events and other reasons in the zidovudine/lamivudine group in this open-label trial. In addition, 80% and 70% of subjects in the emtricitabine + VIREAD group and the zidovudine/lamivudine group, respectively, achieved and maintained HIV-1 RNA <50 copies/mL through Week 48 (64% and 56% through Week 144). The mean increase from baseline in $CD4^+$ cell count was 190 cells/mm^3 in the EMTRIVA + VIREAD group and 158 cells/mm^3 in the zidovudine/lamivudine group at Week 48 (312 and 271 cells/mm^3 at Week 144).

Through 48 weeks, 7 subjects in the emtricitabine + VIREAD group and 5 subjects in the zidovudine/lamivudine group experienced a new CDC Class C event (10 and 6 subjects through 144 weeks).

Treatment-Experienced Adult Patients

Study 907

Study 907 was a 24-week, double-blind placebo-controlled multicenter trial of VIREAD added to a stable background regimen of antiretroviral agents in 550 treatment-experienced subjects. After 24 weeks of blinded trial treatment, all subjects continuing on trial were offered open-label VIREAD for an additional 24 weeks. Subjects had a mean baseline $CD4^+$ cell count of 427 cells/mm^3 (range 23–1385), median baseline plasma HIV-1 RNA of 2340 (range 50–75,000) copies/mL, and mean duration of prior HIV-1 treatment was 5.4 years. Mean age of the subjects was 42 years, 85% were male and 69% were Caucasian, 17% Black and 12% Hispanic.

The percent of subjects with HIV-1 RNA <400 copies/mL and outcomes of subjects through 48 weeks are summarized in Table 19.

[See table 19 at top of next page]

At 24 weeks of therapy, there was a higher proportion of subjects in the VIREAD arm compared to the placebo arm with HIV-1 RNA <50 copies/mL (19% and 1%, respectively). Mean change in absolute $CD4^+$ cell counts by Week 24 was +11 cells/mm^3 for the VIREAD group and -5 cells/mm^3 for the placebo group. Mean change in absolute $CD4^+$ cell counts by Week 48 was +4 cells/mm^3 for the VIREAD group. Through Week 24, one subject in the VIREAD group and no subjects in the placebo arm experienced a new CDC Class C event.

14.2 Clinical Efficacy in Adults with Chronic Hepatitis B

HBeAg-Negative Chronic Hepatitis B

Study 0102 was a Phase 3, randomized, double-blind, active-controlled trial of VIREAD 300 mg compared to HEPSERA 10 mg in 375 HBeAg- (anti-HBe+) subjects with compensated liver function, the majority of whom were nucleoside-naïve. The mean age of subjects was 44 years, 77% were male, 25% were Asian, 65% were Caucasian, 17% had previously received alpha-interferon therapy and 18% were nucleoside-experienced (16% had prior lamivudine experience). At baseline, subjects had a mean Knodell necroinflammatory score of 7.8; mean plasma HBV DNA was 6.9 $\log_{10}$ copies/mL; and mean serum ALT was 140 U/L.

HBeAg-Positive Chronic Hepatitis B

Study 0103 was a Phase 3, randomized, double-blind, active-controlled trial of VIREAD 300 mg compared to HEPSERA 10 mg in 266 HBeAg+ nucleoside-naïve subjects with compensated liver function. The mean age of subjects was 34 years, 69% were male, 36% were Asian, 52% were Caucasian, 16% had previously received alpha-interferon therapy, and <5% were nucleoside experienced. At baseline, subjects had a mean Knodell necroinflammatory score of 8.4; mean plasma HBV DNA was 8.7 $\log_{10}$ copies /mL; and mean serum ALT was 147 U/L.

The primary data analysis was conducted after all subjects reached 48 weeks of treatment and results are summarized below.

The primary efficacy endpoint in both trials was complete response to treatment defined as HBV DNA <400 copies/mL and Knodell necroinflammatory score improvement of at least 2 points, without worsening in Knodell fibrosis at Week 48 (Table 20).

[See table 20 at top of next page]

Treatment Beyond 48 Weeks

In Studies 0102 (HBeAg-negative) and 0103 (HBeAg-positive), subjects who completed double-blind treatment (389 and 196 subjects who were originally randomized to VIREAD and HEPSERA, respectively) were eligible to roll over to open-label VIREAD with no interruption in treatment.

In Study 0102, 304 of 375 subjects (81%) continued in the study through Week 240. Among subjects randomized to VIREAD followed by open-label treatment with VIREAD, 82% had HBV DNA < 400 copies/mL, and 69% had ALT normalization at Week 240. Among subjects randomized to HEPSERA followed by open-label treatment with VIREAD, 88% had HBV DNA < 400 copies/mL and 76% had ALT normalization through Week 240. No subject in either treatment group experienced HBsAg loss/seroconversion through Week 240.

In Study 0103, 185 of 266 subjects (69%) continued in the study through Week 240. Among subjects randomized to VIREAD, 63% had HBV DNA < 400 copies/mL, 44% had ALT normalization, and 34% had HBeAg loss (26% seroconversion to anti-HBe antibody) through Week 240. Among subjects randomized to HEPSERA followed by up to 192 weeks of open-label treatment with VIREAD, 64% had HBV DNA < 400 copies/mL, 54% had ALT normalization, and 34% had HBeAg loss (29% seroconversion to anti-HBe antibody) through Week 240. At Week 240, HBsAg loss was 9% in both treatment groups, and seroconversion to anti-HBs was 7% for the subjects initially randomized to VIREAD and 9% for subjects initially randomized to HEPSERA.

Of the originally randomized and treated 641 subjects in the two studies, liver biopsy data from 328 subjects who received continuing open-label treatment with VIREAD monotherapy were available for analysis at baseline, Week 48 and Week 240. There were no apparent differences between the subset of subjects who had liver biopsy data at Week 240 and those subjects remaining on open-label VIREAD without biopsy data that would be expected to affect histological outcomes at Week 240. Among the 328 subjects evaluated, the observed histological response rates were 80% and 88% at Week 48 and Week 240, respectively. In the subjects without cirrhosis at baseline (Ishak fibrosis score 0–4), 92% (216/235) and 95% (223/235) had either improvement or no change in Ishak fibrosis score at Week 48 and Week 240, respectively. In subjects with cirrhosis at baseline (Ishak fibrosis score 5–6), 97% (90/93) and 99% (92/93) had either improvement or no change in Ishak fibrosis score at Week 48 and Week 240, respectively. Twenty-nine percent (27/93) and 72% (67/93) of subjects with cirrhosis at baseline experienced regression of cirrhosis by Week 48 and Week 240, respectively, with a reduction in Ishak fibrosis score of at least 2 points. No definitive conclusions can be established about the remaining study population who were not part of this subset analysis.

Patients with Lamivudine-Resistant Chronic Hepatitis B

Study 121 was a randomized, double-blind, active-controlled trial evaluating the safety and efficacy of VIREAD compared to an unapproved antiviral regimen in subjects with chronic hepatitis B, persistent viremia (HBV DNA ≥ 1,000 IU/mL), and genotypic evidence of lamivudine resistance (rtM204I/V +/- rtL180M). One hundred forty-one adult subjects were randomized to the VIREAD treatment arm. The mean age of subjects randomized to VIREAD was 47 years (range 18–73), 74% were male, 59% were Caucasian, and 37% were Asian. At baseline, 54% of subjects were HBeAg-negative, 46% were HBeAg-positive, and 56% had abnormal ALT. Subjects had a mean HBV DNA of 6.4 $\log_{10}$ copies/mL and mean serum ALT of 71 U/L at baseline.

After 96 weeks of treatment, 126 of 141 subjects (89%) randomized to VIREAD had HBV DNA < 400 copies/mL, and 49 of 79 subjects (62%) with abnormal ALT at baseline had ALT normalization. Among the HBeAg-positive subjects randomized to VIREAD, 10 of 65 subjects (15%) experienced HBeAg loss, and 7 of 65 subjects (11%) experienced anti-HBe seroconversion through Week 96. The proportion of subjects with HBV DNA concentrations below 400 copies/mL at Week 96 was similar between the VIREAD monotherapy and the comparator arms.

Across the combined chronic hepatitis B treatment trials, the number of subjects with adefovir-resistance associated substitutions at baseline was too small to establish efficacy in this subgroup.

Patients with Chronic Hepatitis B and Decompensated Liver Disease

VIREAD was studied in a small randomized, double-blind, active-controlled trial evaluating the safety of VIREAD compared to other antiviral drugs in subjects with chronic

hepatitis B and decompensated liver disease through 48 weeks (Study 0108).
Forty-five adult subjects (37 males and 8 females) were randomized to the VIREAD treatment arm. At baseline, 69% subjects were HBeAg-negative, and 31% were HBeAg-positive. Subjects had a mean Child-Pugh score of 7, a mean MELD score of 12, mean HBV DNA of 5.8 $\log_{10}$ copies/mL and mean serum ALT of 61 U/L at baseline. Trial endpoints were discontinuation due to an adverse event and confirmed increase in serum creatinine ≥ 0.5 mg/dL or confirmed serum phosphorus of < 2 mg/dL *[See Adverse Reactions (6.1)]*.
At 48 weeks, 31/44 (70%) and 12/26 (46%) Viread-treated subjects achieved an HBV DNA < 400 copies/mL, and normalized ALT, respectively. The trial was not designed to evaluate treatment impact on clinical endpoints such as progression of liver disease, need for liver transplantation, or death.

16 HOW SUPPLIED/STORAGE AND HANDLING

Tablets

VIREAD tablets, 150 mg, are triangle-shaped, white, film-coated tablets containing 150 mg of tenofovir disoproxil fumarate, which is equivalent to 123 mg of tenofovir disoproxil, are debossed with "GSI" on one side and with "150" on the other side. Each bottle contains 30 tablets, a desiccant (silica gel canister or sachet), and closed with a child-resistant closure. (NDC 61958-0404-1)
VIREAD tablets, 200 mg, are round-shaped, white, film-coated tablets containing 200 mg of tenofovir disoproxil fumarate, which is equivalent to 163 mg of tenofovir disoproxil, are debossed with "GSI" on one side and with "200" on the other side. Each bottle contains 30 tablets, a desiccant (silica gel canister or sachet), and closed with a child-resistant closure. (NDC 61958-0405-1)
VIREAD tablets, 250 mg, are capsule-shaped, white, film-coated tablets containing 250 mg of tenofovir disoproxil fumarate, which is equivalent to 204 mg of tenofovir disoproxil, are debossed with "GSI" on one side and with "250" on the other side. Each bottle contains 30 tablets, a desiccant (silica gel canister or sachet), and closed with a child-resistant closure. (NDC 61958-0406-1)
VIREAD tablets, 300 mg, are almond-shaped, light blue, film-coated tablets containing 300 mg of tenofovir disoproxil fumarate, which is equivalent to 245 mg of tenofovir disoproxil, are debossed with "GILEAD" and "4331" on one side and with "300" on the other side. Each bottle contains 30 tablets, a desiccant (silica gel canister or sachet), and closed with a child-resistant closure. (NDC 61958-0401-1)

Oral Powder

VIREAD oral powder consists of white, coated granules containing 40 mg of tenofovir disoproxil fumarate, which is equivalent to 33 mg of tenofovir disoproxil, per gram of powder and is available in multi-use bottles containing 60 grams of oral powder, closed with a child-resistant closure, and co-packaged with a dosing scoop. (NDC 61958-0403-1)
Store VIREAD tablets and oral powder at 25 °C (77 °F), excursions permitted to 15–30 °C (59–86 °F) (see USP Controlled Room Temperature).
Keep the bottle tightly closed. Dispense only in original container. Do not use if seal over bottle opening is broken or missing.

17 PATIENT COUNSELING INFORMATION

See FDA-approved patient labeling (Patient Information and Instructions for Use).

Information for Patients

Patients should be advised that:
- VIREAD is not a cure for HIV-1 infection and patients may continue to experience illnesses associated with HIV-1 infection, including opportunistic infections. Patients should remain under the care of a physician when using VIREAD.
- Patients should avoid doing things that can spread HIV or HBV to others.
  - **Do not share needles or other injection equipment.**
  - **Do not share personal items that can have blood or body fluids on them, like toothbrushes and razor blades.**
  - **Do not have any kind of sex without protection.** Always practice safer sex by using a latex or polyurethane condom to lower the chance of sexual contact with semen, vaginal secretions, or blood.
  - **Do not breastfeed.** Tenofovir is excreted in breast milk and it is not known whether it can harm the baby. Mothers with HIV-1 should not breastfeed because HIV-1 can be passed to the baby in the breast milk.
- The long term effects of VIREAD are unknown.
- VIREAD tablets and oral powder are for oral ingestion only.
- VIREAD should not be discontinued without first informing their physician.
- If you have HIV-1 infection, with or without HBV coinfection, it is important to take VIREAD with combination therapy.
- It is important to take VIREAD on a regular dosing schedule and to avoid missing doses.

Table 19 Outcomes of Randomized Treatment (Study 907)

Outcomes	0–24 weeks VIREAD (N=368)	0–24 weeks Placebo (N=182)	0–48 weeks VIREAD (N=368)	24–48 weeks Placebo Crossover to VIREAD (N=170)
HIV-1 RNA <400 copies/mL*	40%	11%	28%	30%
Virologic failure†	53%	84%	61%	64%
Discontinued due to adverse event	3%	3%	5%	5%
Discontinued for other reasons‡	3%	3%	5%	1%

* Subjects with HIV-1 RNA <400 copies/mL and no prior study drug discontinuation at Week 24 and 48 respectively.
† Subjects with HIV-1 RNA ≥400 copies/mL efficacy failure or missing HIV-1 RNA at Week 24 and 48 respectively.
‡ Includes lost to follow-up, subject withdrawal, noncompliance, protocol violation and other reasons.

Table 20 Histological, Virological, Biochemical, and Serological Response at Week 48

	0102 (HBeAg-) VIREAD (N=250)	0102 (HBeAg-) HEPSERA (N=125)	0103 (HBeAg+) VIREAD (N=176)	0103 (HBeAg+) HEPSERA (N=90)
Complete Response	71%	49%	67%	12%
Histology Histological Response*	72%	69%	74%	68%
HBV DNA <400 copies/mL (<69 IU/mL)	93%	63%	76%	13%
ALT Normalized ALT†	76%	77%	68%	54%
Serology HBeAg Loss/Seroconversion	NA‡	NA‡	20%/19%	16%/16%
HBsAg Loss/Seroconversion	0/0	0/0	3%/1%	0/0

* Knodell necroinflammatory score improvement of at least 2 points without worsening in Knodell fibrosis.
† The population used for analysis of ALT normalization included only subjects with ALT above ULN at baseline.
‡ NA = Not Applicable

- Lactic acidosis and severe hepatomegaly with steatosis, including fatal cases, have been reported. Treatment with VIREAD should be suspended in any patient who develops clinical symptoms suggestive of lactic acidosis or pronounced hepatotoxicity (including nausea, vomiting, unusual or unexpected stomach discomfort, and weakness) *[See Warnings and Precautions (5.1)]*.
- Severe acute exacerbations of hepatitis have been reported in patients who are infected with HBV or coinfected with HBV and HIV-1 and have discontinued VIREAD *[See Warnings and Precautions (5.2)]*.
- Renal impairment, including cases of acute renal failure and Fanconi syndrome, has been reported. VIREAD should be avoided with concurrent or recent use of a nephrotoxic agent *[See Warnings and Precautions (5.3)]*. Dosing interval of VIREAD may need adjustment in patients with renal impairment *[See Dosage and Administration (2.3)]*.
- VIREAD should not be coadministered with the fixed-dose combination products ATRIPLA, COMPLERA, STRIBILD, and TRUVADA since it is a component of these products *[See Warnings and Precautions (5.4)]*.
- VIREAD should not be administered in combination with HEPSERA *[See Warnings and Precautions (5.4)]*.
- Patients with HIV-1 should be tested for Hepatitis B virus (HBV) before initiating antiretroviral therapy *[See Warnings and Precautions (5.5)]*.
- In patients with chronic hepatitis B, it is important to obtain HIV antibody testing prior to initiating VIREAD *[See Warnings and Precautions (5.5)]*.
- Decreases in bone mineral density have been observed with the use of VIREAD. Bone mineral density monitoring should be considered in patients who have a history of pathologic bone fracture or at risk for osteopenia *[See Warnings and Precautions (5.6)]*.
- In the treatment of chronic hepatitis B, the optimal duration of treatment is unknown. The relationship between response and long-term prevention of outcomes such as hepatocellular carcinoma is not known.

PATIENT INFORMATION

VIREAD® (VEER-ee-ad)
(tenofovir disoproxil fumarate)
tablets and oral powder

Read this Patient Information before you start taking VIREAD and each time you get a refill. There may be new information. This information does not take the place of talking with your healthcare provider about your medical condition or your treatment.

What is the most important information I should know about VIREAD?

VIREAD can cause serious side effects, including:

1. **Build-up of an acid in your blood (lactic acidosis).** Lactic acidosis can happen in some people who take VIREAD. **Lactic acidosis** is a serious medical emergency that can lead to death.
   Lactic acidosis can be hard to identify early, because the symptoms could seem like symptoms of other health problems. **Call your healthcare provider right away if you get the following symptoms which could be signs of lactic acidosis:**
   - feeling very weak or tired
   - have unusual (not normal) muscle pain
   - have trouble breathing
   - have stomach pain with
     - nausea (feel sick to your stomach)
     - vomiting
   - feel cold, especially in your arms and legs
   - feel dizzy or lightheaded
   - have a fast or irregular heartbeat
2. **Severe liver problems.** Severe liver problems can happen in people who take VIREAD or similar medicines. In some cases these liver problems can lead to death. Your liver may become large (hepatomegaly) and you may develop fat in your liver (steatosis) when you take VIREAD. **Call your healthcare provider right away if you have any of the following symptoms of liver problems:**
   - Your skin or the white part of your eyes turns yellow (jaundice).
   - dark "tea-colored" urine
   - light-colored bowel movements (stools)
   - loss of appetite for several days or longer
   - nausea
   - stomach pain

You may be more likely to get lactic acidosis or severe liver problems if you are female, very overweight (obese), or have been taking VIREAD for a long time.

3. **Worsening of your Hepatitis B infection.** Your hepatitis B Virus (HBV) infection may become worse (flare-up) if you

take VIREAD and then stop it. A "flare-up" is when your HBV infection suddenly returns in a worse way than before.

- Do not let your VIREAD run out. Refill your prescription or talk to your healthcare provider before your VIREAD is all gone.
- Do not stop taking VIREAD without first talking to your healthcare provider.
- If you stop taking VIREAD, your healthcare provider will need to check your health often and do blood tests regularly to check your HBV infection. Tell your healthcare provider about any new or unusual symptoms you may have after you stop taking VIREAD.

4. Talk to your doctor about taking an HIV test before starting treatment with VIREAD for chronic hepatitis B. You should also get a test for HBV if you are taking VIREAD for treatment of HIV.

What is VIREAD?

VIREAD is a prescription medicine used:

1. with other antiviral medicines to treat Human Immunodeficiency Virus-1 (HIV-1) in people 2 years of age and older. HIV is the virus that causes AIDS (Acquired Immune Deficiency Syndrome).

- When used with other HIV medicines, VIREAD may reduce the amount of HIV in your blood (called "viral load"). VIREAD may also help to increase the number of CD4 (T) cells in your blood which help fight off other infections. Reducing the amount of HIV and increasing the CD4 (T) cell count may improve your immune system. This may reduce your risk of death or infections that can happen when your immune system is weak (opportunistic infections).
- **VIREAD does not cure HIV infection or AIDS.** People taking VIREAD may still develop infections or other conditions associated with HIV infection.
- You must stay on continuous HIV therapy to control infection and decrease HIV-related illnesses.
- It is very important that you stay under the care of your healthcare provider.
- It is not known if VIREAD is safe and effective for the treatment of HIV-1 infection in children under the age of 2 years.

2. to treat chronic (long-lasting) hepatitis B virus (HBV) in people 12 years of age and older.

- VIREAD will not cure HBV.
- VIREAD may lower the amount of HBV in your body.
- VIREAD may improve the condition of your liver.
- The long-term effects of taking VIREAD for treatment of chronic hepatitis B infection are not known.
- It is not known if VIREAD is safe and effective for treatment of chronic hepatitis B in children under the age of 12 years.

What should I tell my healthcare provider before taking VIREAD?

Before you take VIREAD, tell your healthcare provider if you:

- have liver problems, including hepatitis B (HBV) infection.
- have kidney problems.
- have bone problems.
- have any other medical conditions, including HIV infection.
- are pregnant or plan to become pregnant. It is not known if VIREAD will harm your unborn baby.
  Pregnancy Registry. There is a pregnancy registry for women who take antiviral medicines during pregnancy. Its purpose is to collect information about the health of you and your baby. Talk to your healthcare provider about how you can take part in this registry.
- are breastfeeding or plan to breastfeed. **Do not breastfeed if you are taking VIREAD.** Tenofovir passes into your breast milk. You should not breastfeed because of the risk of passing HIV to your baby. Talk to your healthcare provider about the best way to feed your baby.

Tell your healthcare provider about all the medicines you take, including prescription and non-prescription medicines, vitamins and herbal supplements.

VIREAD may affect the way other medicines work, and other medicines may affect how VIREAD works.

Do not take VIREAD if you also take:

- other medicines that contain tenofovir (ATRIPLA®, COMPLERA®, STRIBILD®, TRUVADA®)
- adefovir (HEPSERA®)

Especially tell your healthcare provider if you take the following medications. The dose of these other medications may need to be changed.

- didanosine (VIDEX, VIDEX EC)
- atazanavir (REYATAZ)
- lopinavir with ritonavir (KALETRA)

Know the medicines you take. Keep a list of them to show your healthcare provider or pharmacist when you get a new medicine.

How should I take VIREAD?

- See "What is the most important information I should know about VIREAD?"
- Take VIREAD exactly as your healthcare provider tells you to take it.
- Take VIREAD at the same time every day.
- For adults and children 12 years of age and older, the usual dose of VIREAD is one 300 mg tablet each day.
- If you are an adult with kidney problems, your healthcare provider may tell you to take VIREAD less often.
- Adults and children 12 years of age and older who are unable to swallow VIREAD tablets whole may take 7½ scoops of VIREAD oral powder.
- For children 2 to 12 years of age, your healthcare provider will prescribe the right dose of VIREAD oral powder or tablets based on your child's body weight.
- Tell your healthcare provider if your child has problems with swallowing tablets.
- See the "Instructions for Use" section at the end of this Patient Information leaflet for information about the right way to measure and take VIREAD oral powder.
- Take VIREAD tablets by mouth, with or without food.
- Do not miss a dose of VIREAD. If you miss a dose of VIREAD, take the missed dose as soon as you remember. If it is almost time for your next dose of VIREAD, do not take the missed dose. Take the next dose of VIREAD at your regular time.
- If you take too much VIREAD, call your local poison control center or go right away to the nearest hospital emergency room.

What are the possible side effects of VIREAD?

VIREAD may cause serious side effects, including:

- **See "What is the most important information I should know about VIREAD?"**
- **New or worse kidney problems, including kidney failure,** can happen in some people who take VIREAD. Your healthcare provider should do blood tests to check your kidneys before you start treatment with VIREAD. If you have had kidney problems in the past or need to take another medicine that can cause kidney problems, your healthcare provider may need to do blood tests to check your kidneys during your treatment with VIREAD.
- **Bone problems** can happen in some people who take VIREAD. Bone problems include bone pain, softening or thinning (which may lead to fractures). Your healthcare provider may need to do additional tests to check your bones.
- **Changes in body fat** can happen in some people who take antiviral medicines. These changes may include increased amount of fat in the upper back and neck ("buffalo hump"), breast, and around the main part of your body (trunk). Loss of fat from the legs, arms, and face may also happen. The cause and long-term health effects of these conditions are not known.
- **Changes in your immune system (Immune Reconstitution Syndrome)** can happen when you start taking HIV medicines. Your immune system may get stronger and begin to fight infections that have been hidden in your body for a long time. Tell your healthcare provider if you start having new symptoms after starting your HIV medicine.

The most common side effects in all people who take VIREAD are:

- nausea
- rash
- diarrhea
- headache
- pain
- depression
- weakness

In some people with advanced HBV-infection, other common side effects may include:

- sleeping problems
- itching
- vomiting
- dizziness
- fever

Tell your healthcare provider if you have any side effect that bothers you or that does not go away.

These are not all the possible side effects of VIREAD. For more information, ask your healthcare provider or pharmacist.

Call your doctor for medical advice about side effects. You may report side effects to FDA at 1-800-FDA-1088.

How should I store VIREAD?

- Store VIREAD tablets or oral powder at room temperature between 68 °F to 77 °F (20 °C to 25 °C).
- Keep VIREAD in the original container.
- Do not use VIREAD if the seal over the bottle opening is broken or missing.
- Keep the bottle tightly closed.

Keep VIREAD and all medicines out of the reach of children.

General information about VIREAD:

Medicines are sometimes prescribed for purposes other than those listed in a Patient Information leaflet. Do not use VIREAD for a condition for which it was not prescribed. Do not give VIREAD to other people, even if they have the same condition you have. It may harm them.

Avoid doing things that can spread HIV-1 or HBV infection to others.

- **Do not share or re-use needles or other injection equipment.**
- **Do not share personal items that can have blood or body fluids on them, like toothbrushes and razor blades.**
- **Do not have any kind of sex without protection.** Always practice safe sex by using a latex or polyurethane condom to lower the chance of sexual contact with semen, vaginal secretions, or blood.

A vaccine is available to protect people at risk for becoming infected with HBV. You can ask your healthcare provider for information about this vaccine.

This leaflet summarizes the most important information about VIREAD. If you would like more information, talk with your healthcare provider. You can ask your pharmacist or healthcare provider for information about VIREAD that is written for health professionals.

For more information, go to www.viread.com or call Gilead Sciences, Inc. at 1-800-GILEAD-5 (1-800-445-3235).

What are the ingredients in VIREAD?

Active Ingredient: tenofovir disoproxil fumarate

Inactive Ingredients:

VIREAD tablets: croscarmellose sodium, lactose monohydrate, magnesium stearate, microcrystalline cellulose, and pregelatinized starch.

VIREAD Oral Powder: mannitol, hydroxypropyl cellulose, ethylcellulose, and silicon dioxide.

Tablet Coating:

VIREAD tablets 300 mg: Opadry II Y–30–10671–A, which contains FD&C blue #2 aluminum lake, hypromellose 2910, lactose monohydrate, titanium dioxide, and triacetin.

VIREAD tablets 150, 200 and 250 mg: Opadry II 32K-18425, which contains hypromellose 2910, lactose monohydrate, titanium dioxide, and triacetin.

Instructions for Use of VIREAD oral powder

Read the Instructions for Use below before you give VIREAD oral powder. Be sure you can understand and follow them. If you have any questions, ask your healthcare provider or pharmacist.

Important information

- VIREAD oral powder comes in a box that has a bottle of VIREAD and a dosing scoop (see Figure A).

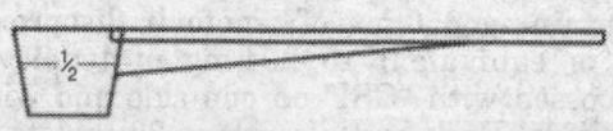

Figure A

- **Only use the dosing scoop to measure VIREAD oral powder.**
- **Only mix VIREAD oral powder with soft foods** that can be swallowed without chewing. Examples of soft foods you can use are: applesauce, baby food, or yogurt.
- **Do not mix VIREAD oral powder with liquid.** The powder may float to the top even after stirring.
- **Give the entire dose right away after mixing** to avoid a bad taste.

How do I prepare and give VIREAD oral powder?

1. Wash and dry your hands.
2. Measure ¼ to ½ cup of soft food into a cup or bowl.
3. To open a new bottle of powder, press down on the bottle lid and turn to remove (see picture on the top of the bottle cap). Peel off the foil.
4. Measure the number of scoops prescribed by your healthcare provider.
   - For each full scoop prescribed:
     - Fill the dosing scoop to the top.
     - Use the flat edge of clean knife to make the powder even with the top of the scoop (see Figure B).

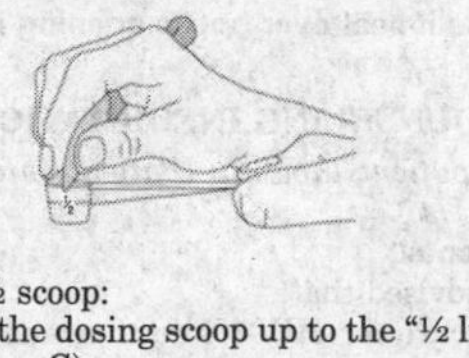

Figure B

   - For ½ scoop:
     - Fill the dosing scoop up to the "½ line" on the side (see Figure C).

½ line

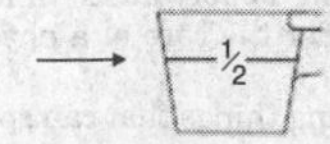

Figure C

5. Sprinkle the VIREAD oral powder on the soft food. Stir with a spoon until well mixed. **Give the entire dose right away after mixing** to avoid a bad taste.
6. Close the bottle of VIREAD tightly.
7. Wash and dry the dosing scoop. Do not store the dosing scoop in the bottle.

See the section "How should I store VIREAD?" for information about how to store VIREAD oral powder.

This Patient Information has been approved by the U.S. Food and Drug Administration.

Manufactured for and distributed by:
Gilead Sciences, Inc.
Foster City, CA 94404

Revised July 2013

COMPLERA, EMTRIVA, GSI, HEPSERA, STRIBILD, TRUVADA, and VIREAD are trademarks or registered trademarks of Gilead Sciences, Inc., or its related companies. ATRIPLA is a registered trademark of Bristol-Myers Squibb & Gilead Sciences, LLC. All other trademarks herein are the property of their respective owners.

21-356-GS-034

Shown in Product Identification Guide, page 307

GlaxoSmithKline
FIVE MOORE DRIVE
RESEARCH TRIANGLE PARK, NC 27709

For all inquiries, including adverse event and quality assurance reporting, contact the GSK Response Center at 1-888-825-5249.
For updates to the product information listed below, also consult www.gsk.com.

ADVAIR DISKUS 100/50 ℞
[ad' vair disk' us]
(fluticasone propionate 100 mcg and salmeterol 50 mcg inhalation powder)
ADVAIR DISKUS 250/50
(fluticasone propionate 250 mcg and salmeterol 50 mcg inhalation powder)
ADVAIR DISKUS 500/50
(fluticasone propionate 500 mcg and salmeterol 50 mcg inhalation powder)
FOR ORAL INHALATION

HIGHLIGHTS OF PRESCRIBING INFORMATION
These highlights do not include all the information needed to use ADVAIR DISKUS safely and effectively. See full prescribing information for ADVAIR DISKUS.
ADVAIR DISKUS 100/50
(fluticasone propionate 100 mcg and salmeterol 50 mcg inhalation powder)
ADVAIR DISKUS 250/50
(fluticasone propionate 250 mcg and salmeterol 50 mcg inhalation powder)
ADVAIR DISKUS 500/50
(fluticasone propionate 500 mcg and salmeterol 50 mcg inhalation powder)
FOR ORAL INHALATION
Initial U.S. Approval: 2000

> WARNING: ASTHMA-RELATED DEATH
> ***See full prescribing information for complete boxed warning***
> - **Long-acting beta$_2$-adrenergic agonists (LABAs), such as salmeterol, one of the active ingredients in ADVAIR DISKUS, increase the risk of asthma-related death. A US study showed an increase in asthma-related deaths in patients receiving salmeterol (13 deaths out of 13,176 patients treated for 28 weeks on salmeterol versus 3 out of 13,179 patients on placebo). Currently available data are inadequate to determine whether concurrent use of inhaled corticosteroids or other long-term asthma control drugs mitigates the increased risk of asthma-related death from LABAs. Available data from controlled clinical trials suggest that LABAs increase the risk of asthma-related hospitalization in pediatric and adolescent patients. (5.1)**
> - **When treating patients with asthma, only prescribe ADVAIR DISKUS for patients not adequately controlled on a long-term asthma control medication, such as an inhaled corticosteroid, or whose disease severity clearly warrants initiation of treatment with both an inhaled corticosteroid and a LABA. Once asthma control is achieved and maintained, assess the patient at regular intervals and step down therapy (e.g., discontinue ADVAIR DISKUS) if possible without loss of asthma control and maintain the patient on a long-term asthma control medication, such as an inhaled corticosteroid. Do not use ADVAIR DISKUS for patients whose asthma is adequately controlled on low- or medium-dose inhaled corticosteroids. (1.1, 5.1)**

INDICATIONS AND USAGE

ADVAIR DISKUS is a combination product containing a corticosteroid and a LABA indicated for:
- Treatment of asthma in patients aged 4 years and older. (1.1)
- Maintenance treatment of airflow obstruction and reducing exacerbations in patients with chronic obstructive pulmonary disease (COPD). (1.2)

Important limitation:
- Not indicated for the relief of acute bronchospasm. (1.1, 1.2)

DOSAGE AND ADMINISTRATION

For oral inhalation only.
- Treatment of asthma in patients ≥12 years: 1 inhalation of ADVAIR DISKUS 100/50, 250/50, or 500/50 twice daily. Starting dosage is based on asthma severity. (2.1)
- Treatment of asthma in patients aged 4 to 11 years: 1 inhalation of ADVAIR DISKUS 100/50 twice daily. (2.1)
- Maintenance treatment of COPD: 1 inhalation of ADVAIR DISKUS 250/50 twice daily. (2.2)

DOSAGE FORMS AND STRENGTHS

DISKUS device containing a combination of fluticasone propionate (100, 250, or 500 mcg) and salmeterol (50 mcg) as an oral inhalation powder. (3)

CONTRAINDICATIONS

- Primary treatment of status asthmaticus or acute episodes of asthma or COPD requiring intensive measures. (4)
- Severe hypersensitivity to milk proteins. (4)

WARNINGS AND PRECAUTIONS

- Asthma-related death: LABAs increase the risk. Prescribe only for recommended patient populations. (5.1)
- Deterioration of disease and acute episodes: Do not initiate in acutely deteriorating asthma or to treat acute symptoms. (5.2)
- Use with additional LABA: Do not use in combination because of risk of overdose. (5.3)
- Localized infections: *Candida albicans* infection of the mouth and throat may occur. Monitor patients periodically for signs of adverse effects on the oral cavity. Advise patients to rinse the mouth following inhalation. (5.4)
- Pneumonia: Increased risk in patients with COPD. Monitor patients for signs and symptoms of pneumonia. (5.5)
- Immunosuppression: Potential worsening of infections (e.g., existing tuberculosis, fungal, bacterial, viral, or parasitic infection; ocular herpes simplex). Use with caution in patients with these infections. More serious or even fatal course of chickenpox or measles can occur in susceptible patients. (5.6)
- Transferring patients from systemic corticosteroids: Risk of impaired adrenal function when transferring from oral steroids. Taper patients slowly from systemic corticosteroids if transferring to ADVAIR DISKUS. (5.7)
- Hypercorticism and adrenal suppression: May occur with very high dosages or at the regular dosage in susceptible individuals. If such changes occur, discontinue ADVAIR DISKUS slowly. (5.8)
- Strong cytochrome P450 3A4 inhibitors (e.g., ritonavir): Risk of increased systemic corticosteroid and cardiovascular effects. Use not recommended with ADVAIR DISKUS. (5.9)
- Paradoxical bronchospasm: Discontinue ADVAIR DISKUS and institute alternative therapy if paradoxical bronchospasm occurs. (5.10)
- Patients with cardiovascular or central nervous system disorders: Use with caution because of beta-adrenergic stimulation. (5.12)
- Decreases in bone mineral density: Assess bone mineral density initially and periodically thereafter. (5.13)
- Effects on growth: Monitor growth of pediatric patients. (5.14)
- Glaucoma and cataracts: Close monitoring is warranted. (5.15)
- Metabolic effects: Be alert to eosinophilic conditions, hypokalemia, and hyperglycemia. (5.16, 5.18)
- Coexisting conditions: Use with caution in patients with convulsive disorders, thyrotoxicosis, diabetes mellitus, and ketoacidosis. (5.17)

ADVERSE REACTIONS

Most common adverse reactions (incidence ≥3%) are:
- Asthma: upper respiratory tract infection or inflammation, pharyngitis, dysphonia, oral candidiasis, bronchitis, cough, headaches, nausea and vomiting. (6.1)
- COPD: pneumonia, oral candidiasis, throat irritation, dysphonia, viral respiratory infections, headaches, musculoskeletal pain. (6.2)

To report SUSPECTED ADVERSE REACTIONS, contact GlaxoSmithKline at 1-888-825-5249 or FDA at 1-800-FDA-1088 or www.fda.gov/medwatch.

DRUG INTERACTIONS

- Strong cytochrome P450 3A4 inhibitors (e.g., ritonavir): Use not recommended. May cause systemic corticosteroid and cardiovascular effects. (7.1)
- Monoamine oxidase inhibitors and tricyclic antidepressants: Use with extreme caution. May potentiate effect of salmeterol on vascular system. (7.2)
- Beta-blockers: Use with caution. May block bronchodilatory effects of beta-agonists and produce severe bronchospasm. (7.3)
- Diuretics: Use with caution. Electrocardiographic changes and/or hypokalemia associated with nonpotassium-sparing diuretics may worsen with concomitant beta-agonists. (7.4)

USE IN SPECIFIC POPULATIONS

Hepatic impairment: Monitor patients for signs of increased drug exposure. (8.6)

See 17 for PATIENT COUNSELING INFORMATION and Medication Guide
Revised: 09/2011

FULL PRESCRIBING INFORMATION: CONTENTS*

*** Sections or subsections omitted from the full prescribing information are not listed**

FULL PRESCRIBING INFORMATION

> WARNING: ASTHMA-RELATED DEATH
> **Long-acting beta$_2$-adrenergic agonists (LABAs), such as salmeterol, one of the active ingredients in ADVAIR DISKUS®, increase the risk of asthma-related death. Data from a large placebo-controlled US study that compared the safety of salmeterol**

(SEREVENT®showed an increase in asthma-related deaths in patients receiving salmeterol (13 deaths out of 13,176 patients treated for 28 weeks on salmeterol versus 3 o Inhalation Aerosol) or placebo added to usual asthma therapy ut of 13,179 patients on placebo). Currently available data are inadequate to determine whether concurrent use of inhaled corticosteroids or other long-term asthma control drugs mitigates the increased risk of asthma-related death from LABAs. Available data from controlled clinical trials suggest that LABAs increase the risk of asthma-related hospitalization in pediatric and adolescent patients.

Therefore, when treating patients with asthma, physicians should only prescribe ADVAIR DISKUS for patients not adequately controlled on a long-term asthma control medication, such as an inhaled corticosteroid, or whose disease severity clearly warrants initiation of treatment with both an inhaled corticosteroid and a LABA. Once asthma control is achieved and maintained, assess the patient at regular intervals and step down therapy (e.g., discontinue ADVAIR DISKUS) if possible without loss of asthma control and maintain the patient on a long-term asthma control medication, such as an inhaled corticosteroid. Do not use ADVAIR DISKUS for patients whose asthma is adequately controlled on low- or medium-dose inhaled corticosteroids *[see Warnings and Precautions (5.1)]*.

Table 1. Asthma-Related Deaths in the 28-Week Salmeterol Multi-center Asthma Research Trial (SMART)

	Salmeterol n (%[a])	Placebo n (%[a])	Relative Risk[b] (95% Confidence Interval)	Excess Deaths Expressed per 10,000 Patients[c] (95% Confidence Interval)
Total Population[d]				
Salmeterol: N = 13,176	13 (0.10%)		4.37 (1.25, 15.34)	8 (3, 13)
Placebo: N = 13,179		3 (0.02%)		
Caucasian				
Salmeterol: N = 9,281	6 (0.07%)		5.82 (0.70, 48.37)	6 (1, 10)
Placebo: N = 9,361		1 (0.01%)		
African American				
Salmeterol: N = 2,366	7 (0.31%)		7.26 (0.89, 58.94)	27 (8, 46)
Placebo: N = 2,319		1 (0.04%)		

[a]Life-table 28-week estimate, adjusted according to the patients' actual lengths of exposure to study treatment to account for early withdrawal of patients from the study.
[b]Relative risk is the ratio of the rate of asthma-related death in the salmeterol group and the rate in the placebo group. The relative risk indicates how many more times likely an asthma-related death occurred in the salmeterol group than in the placebo group in a 28-week treatment period.
[c]Estimate of the number of additional asthma-related deaths in patients treated with salmeterol in SMART, assuming 10,000 patients received salmeterol for a 28-week treatment period. Estimate calculated as the difference between the salmeterol and placebo groups in the rates of asthma-related death multiplied by 10,000.
[d]The Total Population includes the following ethnic origins listed on the case report form: Caucasian, African American, Hispanic, Asian, and "Other." In addition, the Total Population includes those patients whose ethnic origin was not reported. The results for Caucasian and African American subpopulations are shown above. No asthma-related deaths occurred in the Hispanic (salmeterol n = 996, placebo n = 999), Asian (salmeterol n = 173, placebo n = 149), or "Other" (salmeterol n = 230, placebo n = 224) subpopulations. One asthma-related death occurred in the placebo group in the subpopulation whose ethnic origin was not reported (salmeterol n = 130, placebo n = 127).

1 INDICATIONS AND USAGE

1.1 Treatment of Asthma

ADVAIR DISKUS is indicated for the treatment of asthma in patients aged 4 years and older.

Long-acting beta$_2$-adrenergic agonists (LABAs), such as salmeterol, one of the active ingredients in ADVAIR DISKUS, increase the risk of asthma-related death. Available data from controlled clinical trials suggest that LABAs increase the risk of asthma-related hospitalization in pediatric and adolescent patients *[see Warnings and Precautions (5.1)]*. Therefore, when treating patients with asthma, physicians should only prescribe ADVAIR DISKUS for patients not adequately controlled on a long-term asthma control medication, such as an inhaled corticosteroid, or whose disease severity clearly warrants initiation of treatment with both an inhaled corticosteroid and a LABA. Once asthma control is achieved and maintained, assess the patient at regular intervals and step down therapy (e.g., discontinue ADVAIR DISKUS) if possible without loss of asthma control and maintain the patient on a long-term asthma control medication, such as an inhaled corticosteroid. Do not use ADVAIR DISKUS for patients whose asthma is adequately controlled on low- or medium-dose inhaled corticosteroids.

Important Limitation of Use: ADVAIR DISKUS is NOT indicated for the relief of acute bronchospasm.

1.2 Maintenance Treatment of Chronic Obstructive Pulmonary Disease

ADVAIR DISKUS 250/50 is indicated for the twice-daily maintenance treatment of airflow obstruction in patients with chronic obstructive pulmonary disease (COPD), including chronic bronchitis and/or emphysema. ADVAIR DISKUS 250/50 is also indicated to reduce exacerbations of COPD in patients with a history of exacerbations. ADVAIR DISKUS 250/50 twice daily is the only approved dosage for the treatment of COPD because an efficacy advantage of the higher strength ADVAIR DISKUS 500/50 over ADVAIR DISKUS 250/50 has not been demonstrated.

Important Limitation of Use: ADVAIR DISKUS is NOT indicated for the relief of acute bronchospasm.

2 DOSAGE AND ADMINISTRATION

ADVAIR DISKUS should be administered twice daily every day by the orally inhaled route only. After inhalation, the patient should rinse the mouth with water without swallowing *[see Patient Counseling Information (17.4)]*.

More frequent administration or a higher number of inhalations (more than 1 inhalation twice daily) of the prescribed strength of ADVAIR DISKUS is not recommended as some patients are more likely to experience adverse effects with higher doses of salmeterol. Patients using ADVAIR DISKUS should not use additional LABAs for any reason. *[See Warnings and Precautions (5.3, 5.12).]*

2.1 Asthma

If asthma symptoms arise in the period between doses, an inhaled, short-acting beta$_2$-agonist should be taken for immediate relief.

Adult and Adolescent Patients Aged 12 Years and Older: For patients aged 12 years and older, the dosage is 1 inhalation twice daily (morning and evening, approximately 12 hours apart).

The recommended starting dosages for ADVAIR DISKUS for patients aged 12 years and older are based upon patients' asthma severity.

The maximum recommended dosage is ADVAIR DISKUS 500/50 twice daily.

Improvement in asthma control following inhaled administration of ADVAIR DISKUS can occur within 30 minutes of beginning treatment, although maximum benefit may not be achieved for 1 week or longer after starting treatment. Individual patients will experience a variable time to onset and degree of symptom relief.

For patients who do not respond adequately to the starting dosage after 2 weeks of therapy, replacing the current strength of ADVAIR DISKUS with a higher strength may provide additional improvement in asthma control.

If a previously effective dosage regimen of ADVAIR DISKUS fails to provide adequate improvement in asthma control, the therapeutic regimen should be reevaluated and additional therapeutic options (e.g., replacing the current strength of ADVAIR DISKUS with a higher strength, adding additional inhaled corticosteroid, initiating oral corticosteroids) should be considered.

Pediatric Patients Aged 4 to 11 Years: For patients with asthma aged 4 to 11 years who are not controlled on an inhaled corticosteroid, the dosage is 1 inhalation of ADVAIR DISKUS 100/50 twice daily (morning and evening, approximately 12 hours apart).

2.2 Chronic Obstructive Pulmonary Disease

The recommended dosage for patients with COPD is 1 inhalation of ADVAIR DISKUS 250/50 twice daily (morning and evening, approximately 12 hours apart).

If shortness of breath occurs in the period between doses, an inhaled, short-acting beta$_2$-agonist should be taken for immediate relief.

3 DOSAGE FORMS AND STRENGTHS

Disposable purple device with 60 blisters containing a combination of fluticasone propionate (100, 250, or 500 mcg) and salmeterol (50 mcg) as an oral inhalation powder formulation. An institutional pack containing 14 blisters is also available.

4 CONTRAINDICATIONS

The use of ADVAIR DISKUS is contraindicated in the following conditions:

- Primary treatment of status asthmaticus or other acute episodes of asthma or COPD where intensive measures are required
- Severe hypersensitivity to milk proteins *[see Warnings and Precautions (5.11), Description (11)]*

5 WARNINGS AND PRECAUTIONS

5.1 Asthma-Related Death

LABAs, such as salmeterol, one of the active ingredients in ADVAIR DISKUS, increase the risk of asthma-related death. Currently available data are inadequate to determine whether concurrent use of inhaled corticosteroids or other long-term asthma control drugs mitigates the increased risk of asthma-related death from LABAs. Available data from controlled clinical trials suggest that LABAs increase the risk of asthma-related hospitalization in pediatric and adolescent patients. Therefore, when treating patients with asthma, physicians should only prescribe ADVAIR DISKUS for patients not adequately controlled on a long-term asthma control medication, such as an inhaled corticosteroid, or whose disease severity clearly warrants initiation of treatment with both an inhaled corticosteroid and a LABA. Once asthma control is achieved and maintained, assess the patient at regular intervals and step down therapy (e.g., discontinue ADVAIR DISKUS) if possible without loss of asthma control and maintain the patient on a long-term asthma control medication, such as an inhaled corticosteroid. Do not use ADVAIR DISKUS for patients whose asthma is adequately controlled on low- or medium-dose inhaled corticosteroids.

A large placebo-controlled US study that compared the safety of salmeterol with placebo, each added to usual asthma therapy, showed an increase in asthma-related deaths in patients receiving salmeterol. The Salmeterol Multi-center Asthma Research Trial (SMART) was a randomized double-blind study that enrolled LABA-naive patients with asthma to assess the safety of salmeterol (SEREVENT® Inhalation Aerosol) 42 mcg twice daily over 28 weeks compared with placebo when added to usual asthma therapy. A planned interim analysis was conducted when approximately half of the intended number of patients had been enrolled (N = 26,355), which led to premature termination of the study. The results of the interim analysis showed that patients receiving salmeterol were at increased risk for fatal asthma events (see Table 1 and Figure 1). In the total population, a higher rate of asthma-related death occurred in patients treated with salmeterol than those treated with placebo (0.10% versus 0.02%, relative risk: 4.37 [95% CI: 1.25, 15.34]).

Post-hoc subpopulation analyses were performed. In Caucasians, asthma-related death occurred at a higher rate in patients treated with salmeterol than in patients treated with placebo (0.07% versus 0.01%, relative risk: 5.82 [95% CI: 0.70, 48.37]). In African Americans also, asthma-related death occurred at a higher rate in patients treated with salmeterol than those treated with placebo (0.31% versus 0.04%, relative risk: 7.26 [95% CI: 0.89, 58.94]). Although the relative risks of asthma-related death were similar in Caucasians and African Americans, the estimate of excess deaths in patients treated with salmeterol was greater in African Americans because there was a higher overall rate of asthma-related death in African American patients (see Table 1). Given the similar basic mechanisms of action of beta$_2$-agonists, the findings seen in the SMART study are considered a class effect.

Post-hoc analyses in pediatric patients aged 12 to 18 years were also performed. Pediatric patients accounted for approximately 12% of patients in each treatment arm. Respiratory-related death or life-threatening experience occurred at a similar rate in the salmeterol group (0.12% [2/1,653]) and the placebo group (0.12% [2/1,622]; relative risk: 1.0 [95% CI: 0.1, 7.2]). All-cause hospitalization, however, was increased in the salmeterol group (2% [35/1,653]) versus the placebo group (<1% [16/1,622]; relative risk: 2.1 [95% CI: 1.1, 3.7]).

The data from the SMART study are not adequate to determine whether concurrent use of inhaled corticosteroids, such as fluticasone propionate, the other active ingredient in ADVAIR DISKUS, or other long-term asthma control therapy mitigates the risk of asthma-related death.
[See table 1 at top of previous page]

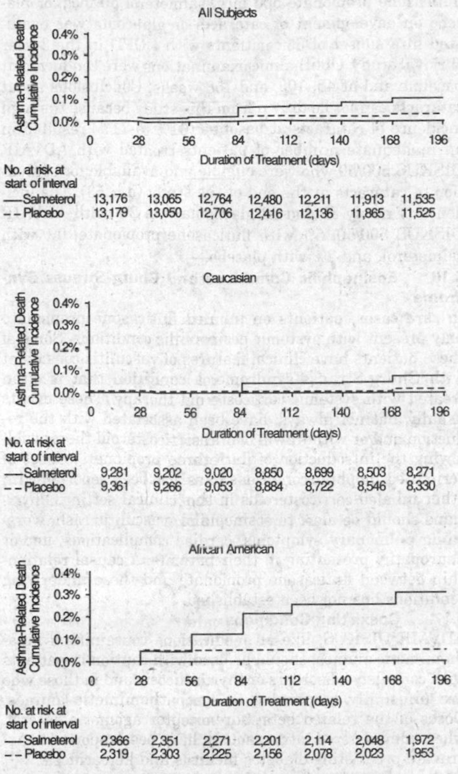

Figure 1. Cumulative Incidence of Asthma-Related Deaths in the 28-Week Salmeterol Multi-center Asthma Research Trial (SMART), by Duration of Treatment

A 16-week clinical study performed in the United Kingdom, the Salmeterol Nationwide Surveillance (SNS) study, showed results similar to the SMART study. In the SNS study, the rate of asthma-related death was numerically, though not statistically significantly, greater in patients with asthma treated with salmeterol (42 mcg twice daily) than those treated with albuterol (180 mcg 4 times daily) added to usual asthma therapy.

The SNS and SMART studies enrolled patients with asthma. No studies have been conducted that were primarily designed to determine whether the rate of death in patients with COPD is increased by LABAs.

5.2 Deterioration of Disease and Acute Episodes

ADVAIR DISKUS should not be initiated in patients during rapidly deteriorating or potentially life-threatening episodes of asthma or COPD. ADVAIR DISKUS has not been studied in patients with acutely deteriorating asthma or COPD. The initiation of ADVAIR DISKUS in this setting is not appropriate.

Serious acute respiratory events, including fatalities, have been reported when salmeterol, a component of ADVAIR DISKUS, has been initiated in patients with significantly worsening or acutely deteriorating asthma. In most cases, these have occurred in patients with severe asthma (e.g., patients with a history of corticosteroid dependence, low pulmonary function, intubation, mechanical ventilation, frequent hospitalizations, previous life-threatening acute asthma exacerbations) and in some patients with acutely deteriorating asthma (e.g., patients with significantly increasing symptoms; increasing need for inhaled, short-acting beta$_2$-agonists; decreasing response to usual medications; increasing need for systemic corticosteroids; recent emergency room visits; deteriorating lung function). However, these events have occurred in a few patients with less severe asthma as well. It was not possible from these reports to determine whether salmeterol contributed to these events.

Increasing use of inhaled, short-acting beta$_2$-agonists is a marker of deteriorating asthma. In this situation, the patient requires immediate reevaluation with reassessment of the treatment regimen, giving special consideration to the possible need for replacing the current strength of ADVAIR DISKUS with a higher strength, adding additional inhaled corticosteroid, or initiating systemic corticosteroids. Patients should not use more than 1 inhalation twice daily (morning and evening) of ADVAIR DISKUS.

ADVAIR DISKUS should not be used for the relief of acute symptoms, i.e., as rescue therapy for the treatment of acute episodes of bronchospasm. An inhaled, short-acting beta$_2$-agonist, not ADVAIR DISKUS, should be used to relieve acute symptoms such as shortness of breath. When prescribing ADVAIR DISKUS, the physician must also provide the patient with an inhaled, short-acting beta$_2$-agonist (e.g., albuterol) for treatment of acute symptoms, despite regular twice-daily (morning and evening) use of ADVAIR DISKUS.

When beginning treatment with ADVAIR DISKUS, patients who have been taking oral or inhaled, short-acting beta$_2$-agonists on a regular basis (e.g., 4 times a day) should be instructed to discontinue the regular use of these drugs.

5.3 Excessive Use of ADVAIR DISKUS and Use With Other Long-Acting Beta$_2$-Agonists

As with other inhaled drugs containing beta$_2$-adrenergic agents, ADVAIR DISKUS should not be used more often than recommended, at higher doses than recommended, or in conjunction with other medications containing LABAs, as an overdose may result. Clinically significant cardiovascular effects and fatalities have been reported in association with excessive use of inhaled sympathomimetic drugs. Patients using ADVAIR DISKUS should not use an additional LABA (e.g., salmeterol, formoterol fumarate, arformoterol tartrate) for any reason, including prevention of exercise-induced bronchospasm (EIB) or the treatment of asthma or COPD.

5.4 Local Effects

In clinical studies, the development of localized infections of the mouth and pharynx with *Candida albicans* has occurred in patients treated with ADVAIR DISKUS. When such an infection develops, it should be treated with appropriate local or systemic (i.e., oral antifungal) therapy while treatment with ADVAIR DISKUS continues, but at times therapy with ADVAIR DISKUS may need to be interrupted. Patients should rinse the mouth after inhalation of ADVAIR DISKUS.

5.5 Pneumonia

Physicians should remain vigilant for the possible development of pneumonia in patients with COPD as the clinical features of pneumonia and exacerbations frequently overlap.

Lower respiratory tract infections, including pneumonia, have been reported in patients with COPD following the inhaled administration of corticosteroids, including fluticasone propionate and ADVAIR DISKUS. In 2 replicate 12-month studies of 1,579 patients with COPD, there was a higher incidence of pneumonia reported in patients receiving ADVAIR DISKUS 250/50 (7%) than in those receiving salmeterol 50 mcg (3%). The incidence of pneumonia in the patients treated with ADVAIR DISKUS was higher in patients over 65 years of age (9%) compared with the incidence in patients less than 65 years of age (4%). *[See Adverse Reactions (6.2), Use in Specific Populations (8.5).]*

In a 3-year study of 6,184 patients with COPD, there was a higher incidence of pneumonia reported in patients receiving ADVAIR DISKUS 500/50 compared with placebo (16% with ADVAIR DISKUS 500/50, 14% with fluticasone propionate 500 mcg, 11% with salmeterol 50 mcg, and 9% with placebo). Similar to what was seen in the 1-year studies with ADVAIR DISKUS 250/50, the incidence of pneumonia was higher in patients over 65 years of age (18% with ADVAIR DISKUS 500/50 versus 10% with placebo) compared with patients less than 65 years of age (14% with ADVAIR DISKUS 500/50 versus 8% with placebo). *[See Adverse Reactions (6.2), Use in Specific Populations (8.5).]*

5.6 Immunosuppression

Persons who are using drugs that suppress the immune system are more susceptible to infections than healthy individuals. Chickenpox and measles, for example, can have a more serious or even fatal course in susceptible children or adults using corticosteroids. In such children or adults who have not had these diseases or been properly immunized, particular care should be taken to avoid exposure. How the dose, route, and duration of corticosteroid administration affect the risk of developing a disseminated infection is not known. The contribution of the underlying disease and/or prior corticosteroid treatment to the risk is also not known. If a patient is exposed to chickenpox, prophylaxis with varicella zoster immune globulin (VZIG) may be indicated. If a patient is exposed to measles, prophylaxis with pooled intramuscular immunoglobulin (IG) may be indicated. (See the respective package inserts for complete VZIG and IG prescribing information.) If chickenpox develops, treatment with antiviral agents may be considered.

Inhaled corticosteroids should be used with caution, if at all, in patients with active or quiescent tuberculosis infections of the respiratory tract; untreated systemic fungal, bacterial, viral, or parasitic infections; or ocular herpes simplex.

5.7 Transferring Patients From Systemic Corticosteroid Therapy

Particular care is needed for patients who have been transferred from systemically active corticosteroids to inhaled corticosteroids because deaths due to adrenal insufficiency have occurred in patients with asthma during and after transfer from systemic corticosteroids to less systemically available inhaled corticosteroids. After withdrawal from systemic corticosteroids, a number of months are required for recovery of hypothalamic-pituitary-adrenal (HPA) function.

Patients who have been previously maintained on 20 mg or more per day of prednisone (or its equivalent) may be most susceptible, particularly when their systemic corticosteroids have been almost completely withdrawn. During this period of HPA suppression, patients may exhibit signs and symptoms of adrenal insufficiency when exposed to trauma, surgery, or infection (particularly gastroenteritis) or other conditions associated with severe electrolyte loss. Although ADVAIR DISKUS may provide control of asthma symptoms during these episodes, in recommended doses it supplies less than normal physiological amounts of glucocorticoid systemically and does NOT provide the mineralocorticoid activity that is necessary for coping with these emergencies.

During periods of stress or a severe asthma attack, patients who have been withdrawn from systemic corticosteroids should be instructed to resume oral corticosteroids (in large doses) immediately and to contact their physicians for further instruction. These patients should also be instructed to carry a warning card indicating that they may need supplementary systemic corticosteroids during periods of stress or a severe asthma attack.

Patients requiring oral corticosteroids should be weaned slowly from systemic corticosteroid use after transferring to ADVAIR DISKUS. Prednisone reduction can be accomplished by reducing the daily prednisone dose by 2.5 mg on a weekly basis during therapy with ADVAIR DISKUS. Lung function (mean forced expiratory volume in 1 second [FEV$_1$] or morning peak expiratory flow [PEF]), beta-agonist use, and asthma symptoms should be carefully monitored during withdrawal of oral corticosteroids. In addition to monitoring asthma signs and symptoms, patients should be observed for signs and symptoms of adrenal insufficiency, such as fatigue, lassitude, weakness, nausea and vomiting, and hypotension.

Transfer of patients from systemic corticosteroid therapy to inhaled corticosteroids or ADVAIR DISKUS may unmask conditions previously suppressed by the systemic corticosteroid therapy (e.g., rhinitis, conjunctivitis, eczema, arthritis, eosinophilic conditions). Some patients may experience symptoms of systemically active corticosteroid withdrawal (e.g., joint and/or muscular pain, lassitude, depression) despite maintenance or even improvement of respiratory function.

5.8 Hypercorticism and Adrenal Suppression

Fluticasone propionate, a component of ADVAIR DISKUS, will often help control asthma symptoms with less suppression of HPA function than therapeutically equivalent oral doses of prednisone. Since fluticasone propionate is absorbed into the circulation and can be systemically active at higher doses, the beneficial effects of ADVAIR DISKUS in minimizing HPA dysfunction may be expected only when recommended dosages are not exceeded and individual patients are titrated to the lowest effective dose. A relationship between plasma levels of fluticasone propionate and inhibitory effects on stimulated cortisol production has been shown after 4 weeks of treatment with fluticasone propionate inhalation aerosol. Since individual sensitivity to effects on cortisol production exists, physicians should consider this information when prescribing ADVAIR DISKUS.

Because of the possibility of systemic absorption of inhaled corticosteroids, patients treated with ADVAIR DISKUS should be observed carefully for any evidence of systemic corticosteroid effects. Particular care should be taken in observing patients postoperatively or during periods of stress for evidence of inadequate adrenal response.

It is possible that systemic corticosteroid effects such as hypercorticism and adrenal suppression (including adrenal crisis) may appear in a small number of patients, particularly when fluticasone propionate is administered at higher than recommended doses over prolonged periods of time. If such effects occur, the dosage of ADVAIR DISKUS should be reduced slowly, consistent with accepted procedures for reducing systemic corticosteroids and for management of asthma symptoms.

5.9 Drug Interactions With Strong Cytochrome P450 3A4 Inhibitors

The use of strong cytochrome P450 3A4 (CYP3A4) inhibitors (e.g., ritonavir, atazanavir, clarithromycin, indinavir, itraconazole, nefazodone, nelfinavir, saquinavir, ketoconazole, telithromycin) with ADVAIR DISKUS is not recommended because increased systemic corticosteroid and increased cardiovascular adverse effects may occur *[see Drug interactions (7.1), Clinical Pharmacology (12.3)]*.

5.10 Paradoxical Bronchospasm and Upper Airway Symptoms

As with other inhaled medications, ADVAIR DISKUS can produce paradoxical bronchospasm, which may be life

Table 2. Adverse Reactions With ≥3% Incidence With ADVAIR DISKUS in Adult and Adolescent Patients With Asthma

Adverse Event	ADVAIR DISKUS 100/50 (N = 92) %	ADVAIR DISKUS 250/50 (N = 84) %	Fluticasone Propionate 100 mcg (N = 90) %	Fluticasone Propionate 250 mcg (N = 84) %	Salmeterol 50 mcg (N = 180) %	Placebo (N = 175) %
Ear, nose, & throat						
Upper respiratory tract infection	27	21	29	25	19	14
Pharyngitis	13	10	7	12	8	6
Upper respiratory inflammation	7	6	7	8	8	5
Sinusitis	4	5	6	1	3	4
Hoarseness/dysphonia	5	2	2	4	<1	<1
Oral candidiasis	1	4	2	2	0	0
Lower respiratory						
Viral respiratory infections	4	4	4	10	6	3
Bronchitis	2	8	1	2	2	2
Cough	3	6	0	0	3	2
Neurology						
Headaches	12	13	14	8	10	7
Gastrointestinal						
Nausea & vomiting	4	6	3	4	1	1
Gastrointestinal discomfort & pain	4	1	0	2	1	1
Diarrhea	4	2	2	2	1	1
Viral gastrointestinal infections	3	0	3	1	2	2
Non-site specific						
Candidiasis unspecified site	3	0	1	4	0	1
Musculoskeletal						
Musculoskeletal pain	4	2	1	5	3	3

threatening. If paradoxical bronchospasm occurs following dosing with ADVAIR DISKUS, it should be treated immediately with an inhaled, short-acting bronchodilator; ADVAIR DISKUS should be discontinued immediately; and alternative therapy should be instituted. Upper airway symptoms of laryngeal spasm, irritation, or swelling, such as stridor and choking, have been reported in patients receiving fluticasone propionate and salmeterol.

5.11 Immediate Hypersensitivity Reactions

Immediate hypersensitivity reactions may occur after administration of ADVAIR DISKUS, as demonstrated by cases of urticaria, angioedema, rash, and bronchospasm. There have been reports of anaphylactic reactions in patients with severe milk protein allergy; therefore, patients with severe milk protein allergy should not take ADVAIR DISKUS *[see Contraindications (4)]*.

5.12 Cardiovascular and Central Nervous System Effects

Excessive beta-adrenergic stimulation has been associated with seizures, angina, hypertension or hypotension, tachycardia with rates up to 200 beats/min, arrhythmias, nervousness, headache, tremor, palpitation, nausea, dizziness, fatigue, malaise, and insomnia *[see Overdosage (10)]*. Therefore, ADVAIR DISKUS, like all products containing sympathomimetic amines, should be used with caution in patients with cardiovascular disorders, especially coronary insufficiency, cardiac arrhythmias, and hypertension.

Salmeterol, a component of ADVAIR DISKUS, can produce a clinically significant cardiovascular effect in some patients as measured by pulse rate, blood pressure, and/or symptoms. Although such effects are uncommon after administration of salmeterol at recommended doses, if they occur, the drug may need to be discontinued. In addition, beta-agonists have been reported to produce electrocardiogram (ECG) changes, such as flattening of the T wave, prolongation of the QTc interval, and ST segment depression. The clinical significance of these findings is unknown. Large doses of inhaled or oral salmeterol (12 to 20 times the recommended dose) have been associated with clinically significant prolongation of the QTc interval, which has the potential for producing ventricular arrhythmias. Fatalities have been reported in association with excessive use of inhaled sympathomimetic drugs.

5.13 Reduction in Bone Mineral Density

Decreases in bone mineral density (BMD) have been observed with long-term administration of products containing inhaled corticosteroids. The clinical significance of small changes in BMD with regard to long-term consequences such as fracture is unknown. Patients with major risk factors for decreased bone mineral content, such as prolonged immobilization, family history of osteoporosis, postmenopausal status, tobacco use, advanced age, poor nutrition, or chronic use of drugs that can reduce bone mass (e.g., anticonvulsants, oral corticosteroids) should be monitored and treated with established standards of care. Since patients with COPD often have multiple risk factors for reduced BMD, assessment of BMD is recommended prior to initiating ADVAIR DISKUS and periodically thereafter. If significant reductions in BMD are seen and ADVAIR DISKUS is still considered medically important for that patient's COPD therapy, use of medication to treat or prevent osteoporosis should be strongly considered.

2-Year Fluticasone Propionate Study: A 2-year study of 160 patients (females aged 18 to 40 years, males 18 to 50) with asthma receiving CFC-propelled fluticasone propionate inhalation aerosol 88 or 440 mcg twice daily demonstrated no statistically significant changes in BMD at any time point (24, 52, 76, and 104 weeks of double-blind treatment) as assessed by dual-energy x-ray absorptiometry at lumbar regions L1 through L4.

3-Year Bone Mineral Density Study: Effects of treatment with ADVAIR DISKUS 250/50 or salmeterol 50 mcg on BMD at the L_1-L_4 lumbar spine and total hip were evaluated in 186 patients with COPD (aged 43 to 87 years) in a 3-year double-blind study. Of those enrolled, 108 patients (72 males and 36 females) were followed for the entire 3 years. BMD evaluations were conducted at baseline and at 6-month intervals. Conclusions cannot be drawn from this study regarding BMD decline in patients treated with ADVAIR DISKUS versus salmeterol due to the inconsistency of treatment differences across gender and between lumbar spine and total hip.

In this study there were 7 non-traumatic fractures reported in 5 patients treated with ADVAIR DISKUS and 1 non-traumatic fracture in 1 patient treated with salmeterol. None of the non-traumatic fractures occurred in the vertebrae, hip, or long bones.

3-Year Survival Study: Effects of treatment with ADVAIR DISKUS 500/50, fluticasone propionate 500 mcg, salmeterol 50 mcg, or placebo on BMD was evaluated in a subset of 658 patients (females and males aged 40 to 80 years) with COPD in the 3-year survival study. BMD evaluations were conducted at baseline and at 48, 108, and 158 weeks. Conclusions cannot be drawn from this study because of the large number of drop outs (>50%) before the end of the follow-up and the maldistribution of covariates among the treatment groups that can affect BMD.

Fracture risk was estimated for the entire population of patients with COPD in the survival study (N = 6,184). The probability of a fracture over 3 years was 6.3% for ADVAIR DISKUS, 5.4% for fluticasone propionate, 5.1% for salmeterol, and 5.1% for placebo.

5.14 Effect on Growth

Orally inhaled corticosteroids may cause a reduction in growth velocity when administered to pediatric patients. Monitor the growth of pediatric patients receiving ADVAIR DISKUS routinely (e.g., via stadiometry). To minimize the systemic effects of orally inhaled corticosteroids, including ADVAIR DISKUS, titrate each patient's dose to the lowest dosage that effectively controls his/her symptoms. *[See Dosage and Administration (2.1), Use in Specific Populations (8.4).]*

5.15 Glaucoma and Cataracts

Glaucoma, increased intraocular pressure, and cataracts have been reported in patients with asthma and COPD following the long-term administration of inhaled corticosteroids, including fluticasone propionate, a component of ADVAIR DISKUS. Therefore, close monitoring is warranted in patients with a change in vision or with a history of increased intraocular pressure, glaucoma, and/or cataracts.

Effects of treatment with ADVAIR DISKUS 500/50, fluticasone propionate 500 mcg, salmeterol 50 mcg, or placebo on development of cataracts or glaucoma was evaluated in a subset of 658 patients with COPD in the 3-year survival study. Ophthalmic examinations were conducted at baseline and at 48, 108, and 158 weeks. Conclusions about cataracts cannot be drawn from this study because the high incidence of cataracts at baseline (61% to 71%) resulted in an inadequate number of patients treated with ADVAIR DISKUS 500/50 who were eligible and available for evaluation of cataracts at the end of the study (n = 53). The incidence of newly diagnosed glaucoma was 2% with ADVAIR DISKUS 500/50, 5% with fluticasone propionate, 0% with salmeterol, and 2% with placebo.

5.16 Eosinophilic Conditions and Churg-Strauss Syndrome

In rare cases, patients on inhaled fluticasone propionate may present with systemic eosinophilic conditions. Some of these patients have clinical features of vasculitis consistent with Churg-Strauss syndrome, a condition that is often treated with systemic corticosteroid therapy. These events usually, but not always, have been associated with the reduction and/or withdrawal of oral corticosteroid therapy following the introduction of fluticasone propionate. Cases of serious eosinophilic conditions have also been reported with other inhaled corticosteroids in this clinical setting. Physicians should be alert to eosinophilia, vasculitic rash, worsening pulmonary symptoms, cardiac complications, and/or neuropathy presenting in their patients. A causal relationship between fluticasone propionate and these underlying conditions has not been established.

5.17 Coexisting Conditions

ADVAIR DISKUS, like all medications containing sympathomimetic amines, should be used with caution in patients with convulsive disorders or thyrotoxicosis and in those who are unusually responsive to sympathomimetic amines. Doses of the related beta$_2$-adrenoceptor agonist albuterol, when administered intravenously, have been reported to aggravate preexisting diabetes mellitus and ketoacidosis.

5.18 Hypokalemia and Hyperglycemia

Beta-adrenergic agonist medications may produce significant hypokalemia in some patients, possibly through intracellular shunting, which has the potential to produce adverse cardiovascular effects *[see Clinical Pharmacology (12.2)]*. The decrease in serum potassium is usually transient, not requiring supplementation. Clinically significant changes in blood glucose and/or serum potassium were seen infrequently during clinical studies with ADVAIR DISKUS at recommended doses.

6 ADVERSE REACTIONS

LABAs, such as salmeterol, one of the active ingredients in ADVAIR DISKUS, increase the risk of asthma-related death. Data from a large placebo-controlled US study that compared the safety of salmeterol (SEREVENT Inhalation Aerosol) or placebo added to usual asthma therapy showed an increase in asthma-related deaths in patients receiving salmeterol *[see Warnings and Precautions (5.1)]*. Currently available data are inadequate to determine whether concurrent use of inhaled corticosteroids or other long-term asthma control drugs mitigates the increased risk of asthma-related death from LABA. Available data from controlled clinical trials suggest that LABA increase the risk of asthma-related hospitalization in pediatric and adolescent patients.

Systemic and local corticosteroid use may result in the following:

- *Candida albicans* infection *[see Warnings and Precautions (5.4)]*
- Pneumonia in patients with COPD *[see Warnings and Precautions (5.5)]*
- Immunosuppression *[see Warnings and Precautions (5.6)]*
- Hypercorticism and adrenal suppression *[see Warnings and Precautions (5.8)]*
- Growth effects *[see Warnings and Precautions (5.14)]*
- Glaucoma and cataracts *[see Warnings and Precautions (5.15)]*

Because clinical trials are conducted under widely varying conditions, adverse reaction rates observed in the clinical trials of a drug cannot be directly compared with rates in the clinical trials of another drug and may not reflect the rates observed in practice.

6.1 Clinical Trials Experience in Asthma

Adult and Adolescent Patients Aged 12 Years and Older: The incidence of adverse reactions associated with ADVAIR DISKUS in Table 2 is based upon 2 placebo-controlled, 12-week, US clinical studies (Studies 1 and 2). A total of 705 adult and adolescent patients (349 females and 356 males) previously treated with salmeterol or inhaled corticosteroids were treated twice daily with ADVAIR DISKUS (100/50- or 250/50-mcg doses), fluticasone propionate inhalation powder (100- or 250-mcg doses), salmeterol inhalation powder 50 mcg, or placebo. The average duration of exposure was 60 to 79 days in the active treatment groups compared with 42 days in the placebo group.

[See table 2 at top of previous page]

The types of adverse reactions and events reported in Study 3, a 28-week, non-US clinical study of 503 patients previously treated with inhaled corticosteroids who were treated twice daily with ADVAIR DISKUS 500/50, fluticasone propionate inhalation powder 500 mcg and salmeterol inhalation powder 50 mcg used concurrently, or fluticasone propionate inhalation powder 500 mcg, were similar to those reported in Table 2.

Additional Adverse Reactions: Other adverse reactions not previously listed, whether considered drug-related or not by the investigators, that were reported more frequently by patients with asthma treated with ADVAIR DISKUS compared with patients treated with placebo include the following: lymphatic signs and symptoms; muscle injuries; fractures; wounds and lacerations; contusions and hematomas; ear signs and symptoms; nasal signs and symptoms; nasal sinus disorders; keratitis and conjunctivitis; dental discomfort and pain; gastrointestinal signs and symptoms; oral ulcerations; oral discomfort and pain; lower respiratory signs and symptoms; pneumonia; muscle stiffness, tightness, and rigidity; bone and cartilage disorders; sleep disorders; compressed nerve syndromes; viral infections; pain; chest symptoms; fluid retention; bacterial infections; unusual taste; viral skin infections; skin flakiness and acquired ichthyosis; disorders of sweat and sebum.

Pediatric Patients Aged 4 to 11 Years: The safety data for pediatric patients aged 4 to 11 years is based upon 1 US trial of 12 weeks' treatment duration. A total of 203 patients (74 females and 129 males) who were receiving inhaled corticosteroids at study entry were randomized to either ADVAIR DISKUS 100/50 or fluticasone propionate inhalation powder 100 mcg twice daily. Common adverse reactions (≥3% and greater than placebo) seen in the pediatric patients but not reported in the adult and adolescent clinical trials include: throat irritation and ear, nose, and throat infections.

Laboratory Test Abnormalities: Elevation of hepatic enzymes was reported in ≥1% of patients in clinical trials. The elevations were transient and did not lead to discontinuation from the studies. In addition, there were no clinically relevant changes noted in glucose or potassium.

6.2 Clinical Trials Experience in Chronic Obstructive Pulmonary Disease

Short-Term (6 Months to 1 Year) Trials: The short-term safety data are based on exposure to ADVAIR DISKUS 250/50 twice daily in one 6-month and two 1-year clinical trials. In the 6-month trial, a total of 723 adult patients (266 females and 457 males) were treated twice daily with ADVAIR DISKUS 250/50, fluticasone propionate inhalation powder 250 mcg, salmeterol inhalation powder, or placebo. The mean age of the patients was 64, and the majority (93%) was Caucasian. In this trial, 70% of the patients treated with ADVAIR DISKUS reported an adverse reaction compared with 64% on placebo. The average duration of exposure to ADVAIR DISKUS 250/50 was 141.3 days compared with 131.6 days for placebo. The incidence of adverse reactions in the 6-month study is shown in Table 3.

[See table 3 above]

Table 3. Overall Adverse Reactions With ≥3% Incidence With ADVAIR DISKUS 250/50 in Patients With Chronic Obstructive Pulmonary Disease Associated With Chronic Bronchitis

Adverse Event	ADVAIR DISKUS 250/50 (N = 178) %	Fluticasone Propionate 250 mcg (N = 183) %	Salmeterol 50 mcg (N = 177) %	Placebo (N = 185) %
Ear, nose, & throat				
Candidiasis mouth/throat	10	6	3	1
Throat irritation	8	5	4	7
Hoarseness/dysphonia	5	3	<1	0
Sinusitis	3	8	5	3
Lower respiratory				
Viral respiratory infections	6	4	3	3
Neurology				
Headaches	16	11	10	12
Dizziness	4	<1	3	2
Non-site specific				
Fever	4	3	0	3
Malaise & fatigue	3	2	2	3
Musculoskeletal				
Musculoskeletal pain	9	8	12	9
Muscle cramps & spasms	3	3	1	1

In the two 1-year studies, ADVAIR DISKUS 250/50 was compared with salmeterol in 1,579 patients (863 males and 716 females). The mean age of the patients was 65, and the majority (94%) was Caucasian. To be enrolled, all of the patients had to have had a COPD exacerbation in the previous 12 months. In this trial, 88% of the patients treated with ADVAIR DISKUS and 86% of the patients treated with salmeterol reported an adverse event. The most common events that occurred with a frequency of >5% and more frequently in the patients treated with ADVAIR DISKUS were nasopharyngitis, upper respiratory tract infection, nasal congestion, back pain, sinusitis, dizziness, nausea, pneumonia, candidiasis, and dysphonia. Overall, 55 (7%) of the patients treated with ADVAIR DISKUS and 25 (3%) of the patients treated with salmeterol developed pneumonia.

The incidence of pneumonia was higher in patients over 65 years of age, 9% in the patients treated with ADVAIR DISKUS compared with 4% in the patients treated with ADVAIR DISKUS less than 65 years of age. In the patients treated with salmeterol, the incidence of pneumonia was the same (3%) in both age-groups. *[See Warnings and Precautions (5.5), Use in Specific Populations (8.5).]*

Long-Term (3-Year) Trial: The safety of ADVAIR DISKUS 500/50 was evaluated in a randomized, double-blind, placebo-controlled, multicenter, international, 3-year study in 6,184 adult patients with COPD (4,684 males and 1,500 females). The mean age of the patients was 65, and the majority (82%) was Caucasian. The distribution of adverse events was similar to that seen in the 1-year trials with ADVAIR DISKUS 250/50. In addition, pneumonia was reported in a significantly increased number of patients treated with ADVAIR DISKUS 500/50 and fluticasone propionate 500 mcg (16% and 14%, respectively) compared with patients treated with salmeterol 50 mcg or placebo (11% and 9%, respectively). When adjusted for time on treatment, the rates of pneumonia were 84 and 88 events per 1,000 treatment-years in the groups treated with fluticasone propionate 500 mcg and with ADVAIR DISKUS 500/50, respectively, compared with 52 events per 1,000 treatment-years in the salmeterol and placebo groups. Similar to what was seen in the 1-year studies with ADVAIR DISKUS 250/50, the incidence of pneumonia was higher in patients over 65 years of age (18% with ADVAIR DISKUS 500/50 versus 10% with placebo) compared with patients less than 65 years of age (14% with ADVAIR DISKUS 500/50 versus 8% with placebo). *[See Warnings and Precautions (5.5), Use in Specific Populations (8.5).]*

Additional Adverse Reactions: Other adverse reactions not previously listed, whether considered drug-related or not by the investigators, that were reported more frequently by patients with COPD treated with ADVAIR DISKUS compared with patients treated with placebo include the following: syncope; ear, nose, and throat infections; ear signs and symptoms; laryngitis; nasal congestion/blockage; nasal sinus disorders; pharyngitis/throat infection; hypothyroidism; dry eyes; eye infections; gastrointestinal signs and symptoms; oral lesions; abnormal liver function tests; bacterial infections; edema and swelling; viral infections.

Laboratory Abnormalities: There were no clinically relevant changes in these trials. Specifically, no increased reporting of neutrophilia or changes in glucose or potassium was noted.

6.3 Postmarketing Experience

In addition to adverse events reported from clinical trials, the following events have been identified during worldwide use of any formulation of ADVAIR, fluticasone propionate, and/or salmeterol regardless of indication. Because they are reported voluntarily from a population of unknown size, estimates of frequency cannot be made. These events have been chosen for inclusion due to either their seriousness, frequency of reporting, or causal connection to ADVAIR DISKUS, fluticasone propionate, and/or salmeterol or a combination of these factors.

Cardiac Disorders: Arrhythmias (including atrial fibrillation, extrasystoles, supraventricular tachycardia), ventricular tachycardia.

Endocrine Disorders: Cushing's syndrome, Cushingoid features, growth velocity reduction in children/adolescents, hypercorticism.

Eye Disorders: Glaucoma.

Gastrointestinal Disorders: Abdominal pain, dyspepsia, xerostomia.

Immune System Disorders: Immediate and delayed hypersensitivity reaction (including very rare anaphylactic reaction). Very rare anaphylactic reaction in patients with severe milk protein allergy.

Metabolic and Nutrition Disorders: Hyperglycemia, weight gain.

Musculoskeletal, Connective Tissue, and Bone Disorders: Arthralgia, cramps, myositis, osteoporosis.

Nervous System Disorders: Paresthesia, restlessness.

Psychiatric Disorders: Agitation, aggression, depression. Behavioral changes, including hyperactivity and irritability, have been reported very rarely and primarily in children.

Reproductive System and Breast Disorders: Dysmenorrhea.

Respiratory, Thoracic, and Mediastinal Disorders: Chest congestion; chest tightness; dyspnea; facial and oropharyngeal edema, immediate bronchospasm; paradoxical bronchospasm; tracheitis; wheezing; reports of upper respiratory symptoms of laryngeal spasm, irritation, or swelling such as stridor or choking.

Skin and Subcutaneous Tissue Disorders: Ecchymoses, photodermatitis.

Vascular Disorders: Pallor.

7 DRUG INTERACTIONS

ADVAIR DISKUS has been used concomitantly with other drugs, including short-acting beta$_2$-agonists, methylxanthines, and intranasal corticosteroids, commonly used in patients with asthma or COPD, without adverse drug reactions. No formal drug interaction studies have been performed with ADVAIR DISKUS.

7.1 Inhibitors of Cytochrome P450 3A4

Fluticasone propionate and salmeterol, the individual components of ADVAIR DISKUS, are substrates of CYP3A4. The use of strong CYP3A4 inhibitors (e.g., ritonavir, atazanavir, clarithromycin, indinavir, itraconazole, nefazodone, nelfinavir, saquinavir, ketoconazole, telithromycin) with ADVAIR DISKUS is not recommended because increased systemic corticosteroid and increased cardiovascular adverse effects may occur.

Ritonavir: *Fluticasone Propionate:* A drug interaction study with fluticasone propionate aqueous nasal spray in healthy subjects has shown that ritonavir (a strong CYP3A4 inhibitor) can significantly increase plasma fluticasone propionate exposure, resulting in significantly reduced serum cortisol concentrations *[see Clinical Pharmacology (12.3)]*. During postmarketing use, there have been reports of clinically significant drug interactions in patients receiving fluticasone propionate and ritonavir, resulting in systemic corticosteroid effects including Cushing's syndrome and adrenal suppression.

Ketoconazole: *Fluticasone Propionate:* Coadministration of orally inhaled fluticasone propionate (1,000 mcg) and ketoconazole (200 mg once daily) resulted in increased plasma fluticasone propionate exposure and reduced plasma cortisol area under the curve (AUC), but had no effect on urinary excretion of cortisol.

Salmeterol: In a drug interaction study in 20 healthy subjects, coadministration of inhaled salmeterol (50 mcg twice daily) and oral ketoconazole (400 mg once daily) for 7 days resulted in greater systemic exposure to salmeterol (AUC increased 16-fold and C_{max} increased 1.4-fold). Three (3) subjects were withdrawn due to beta$_2$-agonist side effects (2 with prolonged QTc and 1 with palpitations and sinus tachycardia). Although there was no statistical effect on the mean QTc, coadministration of salmeterol and ketoconazole was associated with more frequent increases in QTc duration compared with salmeterol and placebo administration.

7.2 Monoamine Oxidase Inhibitors and Tricyclic Antidepressants

ADVAIR DISKUS should be administered with extreme caution to patients being treated with monoamine oxidase inhibitors or tricyclic antidepressants, or within 2 weeks of discontinuation of such agents, because the action of salmeterol, a component of ADVAIR DISKUS, on the vascular system may be potentiated by these agents.

7.3 Beta-Adrenergic Receptor Blocking Agents

Beta-blockers not only block the pulmonary effect of beta-agonists, such as salmeterol, a component of ADVAIR DISKUS, but may also produce severe bronchospasm in patients with reversible obstructive airways disease. Therefore, patients with asthma or COPD should not normally be treated with beta-blockers. However, under certain circumstances, there may be no acceptable alternatives to the use of beta-adrenergic blocking agents for these patients; cardioselective beta-blockers could be considered, although they should be administered with caution.

7.4 Diuretics

The ECG changes and/or hypokalemia that may result from the administration of nonpotassium-sparing diuretics (such as loop or thiazide diuretics) can be acutely worsened by beta-agonists, especially when the recommended dose of the beta-agonist is exceeded. Although the clinical relevance of these effects is not known, caution is advised in the coadministration of beta-agonists with nonpotassium-sparing diuretics.

8 USE IN SPECIFIC POPULATIONS

8.1 Pregnancy

Teratogenic Effects: Pregnancy Category C. There are no adequate and well-controlled studies with ADVAIR DISKUS in pregnant women. ADVAIR DISKUS was teratogenic in mice and not in rats, although it lowered fetal weight in rats. Fluticasone propionate alone was teratogenic in mice, rats, and rabbits, and salmeterol alone was teratogenic in rabbits and not in rats. From the reproduction toxicity studies in mice and rats, no evidence of enhanced toxicity was seen using combinations of fluticasone propionate and salmeterol when compared with toxicity data from the components administered separately.

ADVAIR DISKUS should be used during pregnancy only if the potential benefit justifies the potential risk to the fetus.

ADVAIR DISKUS: In the mouse reproduction assay, fluticasone propionate by the subcutaneous route at a dose approximately 3/5 the maximum recommended human daily inhalation dose (MRHD) on an mg/m^2 basis combined with oral salmeterol at a dose approximately 410 times the MRHD on an mg/m^2 basis produced cleft palate, fetal death, increased implantation loss, and delayed ossification. These observations are characteristic of glucocorticoids. No developmental toxicity was observed at combination doses of fluticasone propionate subcutaneously up to approximately 1/6 the MRHD on an mg/m^2 basis and oral doses of salmeterol up to approximately 55 times the MRHD on an mg/m^2 basis. In rats, combining fluticasone propionate subcutaneously at a dose equivalent to the MRHD on an mg/m^2 basis and an oral dose of salmeterol at approximately 810 times the MRHD on an mg/m^2 basis produced decreased fetal weight, umbilical hernia, delayed ossification, and changes in the occipital bone. No such effects were seen when combining fluticasone propionate subcutaneously at a dose less than the MRHD on an mg/m^2 basis and an oral dose of salmeterol at approximately 80 times the MRHD on an mg/m^2 basis.

Fluticasone Propionate: Subcutaneous studies in mice at a dose less than the MRHD on an mg/m^2 basis and in rats at a dose equivalent to the MRHD on an mg/m^2 basis revealed fetal toxicity characteristic of potent corticosteroid compounds, including embryonic growth retardation, omphalocele, cleft palate, and retarded cranial ossification.

In rabbits, fetal weight reduction and cleft palate were observed at a subcutaneous dose less than the MRHD on an mg/m^2 basis. However, no teratogenic effects were reported at oral doses up to approximately 5 times the MRHD on an mg/m^2 basis. No fluticasone propionate was detected in the plasma in this study, consistent with the established low bioavailability following oral administration *[see Clinical Pharmacology (12.3)]*.

Experience with oral corticosteroids since their introduction in pharmacologic, as opposed to physiologic, doses suggests that rodents are more prone to teratogenic effects from corticosteroids than humans. In addition, because there is a natural increase in corticosteroid production during pregnancy, most women will require a lower exogenous corticosteroid dose and many will not need corticosteroid treatment during pregnancy.

Salmeterol: No teratogenic effects occurred in rats at oral doses approximately 160 times the MRHD on an mg/m^2 basis. In pregnant Dutch rabbits administered oral doses approximately 50 times the MRHD based on comparison of the AUCs, salmeterol exhibited fetal toxic effects characteristically resulting from beta-adrenoceptor stimulation. These included precocious eyelid openings, cleft palate, sternebral fusion, limb and paw flexures, and delayed ossification of the frontal cranial bones. No such effects occurred at an oral dose approximately 20 times the MRHD based on comparison of the AUCs.

New Zealand White rabbits were less sensitive since only delayed ossification of the frontal cranial bones was seen at an oral dose approximately 1,600 times the MRHD on an mg/m^2 basis. Extensive use of other beta-agonists has provided no evidence that these class effects in animals are relevant to their use in humans.

8.2 Labor and Delivery

There are no well-controlled human studies that have investigated effects of ADVAIR DISKUS on preterm labor or labor at term. Because of the potential for beta-agonist interference with uterine contractility, use of ADVAIR DISKUS during labor should be restricted to those patients in whom the benefits clearly outweigh the risks.

8.3 Nursing Mothers

Plasma levels of salmeterol, a component of ADVAIR DISKUS, after inhaled therapeutic doses are very low. In rats, salmeterol xinafoate is excreted in the milk. There are no data from controlled trials on the use of salmeterol by nursing mothers. It is not known whether fluticasone propionate, a component of ADVAIR DISKUS, is excreted in human breast milk. However, other corticosteroids have been detected in human milk. Subcutaneous administration to lactating rats of tritiated fluticasone propionate resulted in measurable radioactivity in milk.

Since there are no data from controlled trials on the use of ADVAIR DISKUS by nursing mothers, a decision should be made whether to discontinue nursing or to discontinue ADVAIR DISKUS, taking into account the importance of ADVAIR DISKUS to the mother.

Caution should be exercised when ADVAIR DISKUS is administered to a nursing woman.

8.4 Pediatric Use

Use of ADVAIR DISKUS 100/50 in patients aged 4 to 11 years is supported by extrapolation of efficacy data from older patients and by safety and efficacy data from a study of ADVAIR DISKUS 100/50 in children with asthma aged 4 to 11 years *[see Adverse Reactions (6.1), Clinical Studies (14.1)]*. The safety and effectiveness of ADVAIR DISKUS in children with asthma less than 4 years of age have not been established.

Inhaled corticosteroids, including fluticasone propionate, a component of ADVAIR DISKUS, may cause a reduction in growth velocity in children and adolescents *[see Warnings and Precautions (5.14)]*. The growth of pediatric patients receiving orally inhaled corticosteroids, including ADVAIR DISKUS, should be monitored.

A 52-week placebo-controlled study to assess the potential growth effects of fluticasone propionate inhalation powder (FLOVENT® ROTADISK®) at 50 and 100 mcg twice daily was conducted in the US in 325 prepubescent children (244 males and 81 females) aged 4 to 11 years. The mean growth velocities at 52 weeks observed in the intent-to-treat population were 6.32 cm/year in the placebo group (N = 76), 6.07 cm/year in the 50-mcg group (N = 98), and 5.66 cm/year in the 100-mcg group (N = 89). An imbalance in the proportion of children entering puberty between groups and a higher dropout rate in the placebo group due to poorly controlled asthma may be confounding factors in interpreting these data. A separate subset analysis of children who remained prepubertal during the study revealed growth rates at 52 weeks of 6.10 cm/year in the placebo group (n = 57), 5.91 cm/year in the 50-mcg group (n = 74), and 5.67 cm/year in the 100-mcg group (n = 79). In children aged 8.5 years, the mean age of children in this study, the range for expected growth velocity is: boys – 3rd percentile = 3.8 cm/year, 50th percentile = 5.4 cm/year, and 97th percentile = 7.0 cm/year; girls – 3rd percentile = 4.2 cm/year, 50th percentile = 5.7 cm/year, and 97th percentile = 7.3 cm/year. The clinical relevance of these growth data is not certain.

If a child or adolescent on any corticosteroid appears to have growth suppression, the possibility that he/she is particularly sensitive to this effect of corticosteroids should be considered. The potential growth effects of prolonged treatment should be weighed against the clinical benefits obtained. To minimize the systemic effects of orally inhaled corticosteroids, including ADVAIR DISKUS, each patient should be titrated to the lowest strength that effectively controls his/her asthma *[see Dosage and Administration (2.1)]*.

8.5 Geriatric Use

Clinical studies of ADVAIR DISKUS for asthma did not include sufficient numbers of patients aged 65 years and older to determine whether older patients with asthma respond differently than younger patients.

Of the total number of patients in clinical studies receiving ADVAIR DISKUS for COPD, 1,621 were aged 65 years or older and 379 were aged 75 years or older. Patients with COPD aged 65 years and older had a higher incidence of serious adverse events compared with patients less than 65 years of age. Although the distribution of adverse events was similar in the 2 age-groups, patients over 65 years of age experienced more severe events. In two 1-year studies, the excess risk of pneumonia that was seen in patients treated with ADVAIR DISKUS compared with those treated with salmeterol was greater in patients over 65 years of age than in patients less than 65 years of age *[see Adverse Reactions (6.2)]*. As with other products containing beta$_2$-agonists, special caution should be observed when using ADVAIR DISKUS in geriatric patients who have concomitant cardiovascular disease that could be adversely affected by beta$_2$-agonists. Based on available data for ADVAIR DISKUS or its active components, no adjustment of dosage of ADVAIR DISKUS in geriatric patients is warranted.

No relationship between fluticasone propionate systemic exposure and age was observed in 57 patients with COPD (aged 40 to 82 years) given 250 or 500 mcg twice daily.

8.6 Hepatic Impairment

Formal pharmacokinetic studies using ADVAIR DISKUS have not been conducted in patients with hepatic impairment. However, since both fluticasone propionate and salmeterol are predominantly cleared by hepatic metabolism, impairment of liver function may lead to accumulation of fluticasone propionate and salmeterol in plasma. Therefore, patients with hepatic disease should be closely monitored.

8.7 Renal Impairment

Formal pharmacokinetic studies using ADVAIR DISKUS have not been conducted in patients with renal impairment.

10 OVERDOSAGE

No human overdosage data has been reported for ADVAIR DISKUS.

No deaths occurred in rats given an inhaled single-dose combination of salmeterol 3.6 mg/kg (approximately 290 and 140 times the MRHD for adults and children, respectively, on an mg/m^2 basis) and 1.9 mg/kg of fluticasone propionate (approximately 15 and 35 times the MRHD for adults and children, respectively, on an mg/m^2 basis).

Fluticasone Propionate: Chronic overdosage with fluticasone propionate may result in signs/symptoms of hypercorticism *[see Warnings and Precautions (5.7)]*. Inhalation by healthy volunteers of a single dose of 4,000 mcg of fluticasone propionate inhalation powder or single doses of 1,760 or 3,520 mcg of fluticasone propionate CFC inhalation aerosol was well tolerated. Fluticasone propionate given by inhalation aerosol at dosages of 1,320 mcg twice daily for 7 to 15 days to healthy human volunteers was also well tolerated. Repeat oral doses up to 80 mg daily for 10 days in healthy volunteers and repeat oral doses up to 20 mg daily for 42 days in patients were well tolerated. Adverse reactions were of mild or moderate severity, and incidences were similar in active and placebo treatment groups.

No deaths were seen in mice given an oral dose of 1,000 mg/kg (4,100 and 9,600 times the MRHD dose for adults and children, respectively, on an mg/m^2 basis). No deaths were seen in rats given an oral dose of 1,000 mg/kg (8,100 and 19,200 times the MRHD for adults and children, respectively, on an mg/m^2 basis).

Salmeterol: The expected signs and symptoms with overdosage of salmeterol are those of excessive beta-adrenergic stimulation and/or occurrence or exaggeration of any of the following: seizures, angina, hypertension or hypotension, tachycardia with rates up to 200 beats/min, arrhythmias, nervousness, headache, tremor, muscle cramps, dry mouth, palpitation, nausea, dizziness, fatigue, malaise, and insomnia. Overdosage with salmeterol can lead to clinically significant prolongation of the QTc interval, which can produce ventricular arrhythmias. Other signs of overdosage may include hypokalemia and hyperglycemia.

As with all sympathomimetic medications, cardiac arrest and even death may be associated with abuse of salmeterol. Treatment consists of discontinuation of salmeterol together with appropriate symptomatic therapy. The judicious use of a cardioselective beta-receptor blocker may be considered, bearing in mind that such medication can produce bronchospasm. There is insufficient evidence to determine if dialysis is beneficial for overdosage of salmeterol. Cardiac monitoring is recommended in cases of overdosage.

No deaths were seen in rats given salmeterol at an inhalation dose of 2.9 mg/kg (approximately 240 and 110 times the MRHD for adults and children, respectively, on an mg/m^2 basis) and in dogs at an inhalation dose of 0.7 mg/kg (approximately 190 and 90 times the MRHD for adults and children, respectively, on an mg/m^2 basis). By the oral route, no deaths occurred in mice at 150 mg/kg (approximately 6,100 and 2,900 times the MRHD for adults and children, respectively, on an mg/m^2 basis) and in rats at 1,000 mg/kg (approximately 81,000 and 38,000 times the MRHD for adults and children, respectively, on an mg/m^2 basis).

11 DESCRIPTION

ADVAIR DISKUS 100/50, ADVAIR DISKUS 250/50, and ADVAIR DISKUS 500/50 are combinations of fluticasone propionate and salmeterol xinafoate.

One active component of ADVAIR DISKUS is fluticasone propionate, a corticosteroid having the chemical name *S*-(fluoromethyl) 6α,9-difluoro-11β,17-dihydroxy-16α-methyl-3-oxoandrosta-1,4-diene-17β-carbothioate, 17-propionate and the following chemical structure:

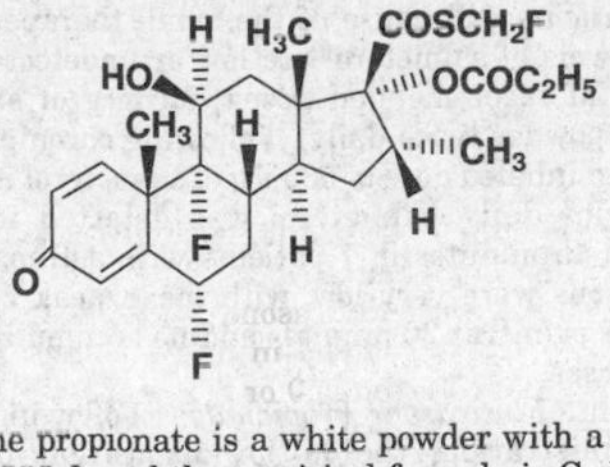

Fluticasone propionate is a white powder with a molecular weight of 500.6, and the empirical formula is $C_{25}H_{31}F_3O_5S$. It is practically insoluble in water, freely soluble in dimethyl sulfoxide and dimethylformamide, and slightly soluble in methanol and 95% ethanol.

The other active component of ADVAIR DISKUS is salmeterol xinafoate, a $beta_2$-adrenergic bronchodilator. Salmeterol xinafoate is the racemic form of the 1-hydroxy-2-naphthoic acid salt of salmeterol. The chemical name of salmeterol xinafoate is 4-hydroxy-α^1-[[[6-(4-phenylbutoxy) hexyl]amino]methyl]-1,3-benzenedimethanol, 1-hydroxy-2-naphthalenecarboxylate, and it has the following chemical structure:

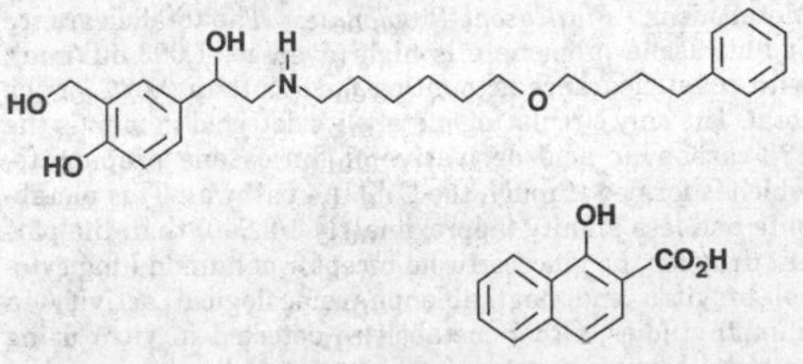

Salmeterol xinafoate is a white powder with a molecular weight of 603.8, and the empirical formula is $C_{25}H_{37}NO_4 \bullet C_{11}H_8O_3$. It is freely soluble in methanol; slightly soluble in ethanol, chloroform, and isopropanol; and sparingly soluble in water.

ADVAIR DISKUS 100/50, ADVAIR DISKUS 250/50, and ADVAIR DISKUS 500/50 are specially designed plastic devices containing a double-foil blister strip of a powder formulation of fluticasone propionate and salmeterol xinafoate intended for oral inhalation only. Each blister on the double-foil strip within the device contains 100, 250, or 500 mcg of microfine fluticasone propionate and 72.5 mcg of microfine salmeterol xinafoate salt, equivalent to 50 mcg of salmeterol base, in 12.5 mg of formulation containing lactose (which contains milk proteins). Each blister contains 1 complete dose of both medications. After a blister containing medication is opened by activating the device, the medication is dispersed into the airstream created by the patient inhaling through the mouthpiece.

Under standardized in vitro test conditions, ADVAIR DISKUS delivers 93, 233, and 465 mcg of fluticasone propionate and 45 mcg of salmeterol base per blister from ADVAIR DISKUS 100/50, 250/50, and 500/50, respectively, when tested at a flow rate of 60 L/min for 2 seconds. In adult patients with obstructive lung disease and severely compromised lung function (mean FEV_1 20% to 30% of predicted), mean peak inspiratory flow (PIF) through a DISKUS® inhalation device was 82.4 L/min (range: 46.1 to 115.3 L/min).

Inhalation profiles for adolescent (N = 13, aged 12 to 17 years) and adult (N = 17, aged 18 to 50 years) patients with asthma inhaling maximally through the DISKUS device show mean PIF of 122.2 L/min (range: 81.6 to 152.1 L/min). Inhalation profiles for pediatric patients with asthma inhaling maximally through the DISKUS device show a mean PIF of 75.5 L/min (range: 49.0 to 104.8 L/min) for the 4-year-old patient set (N = 20) and 107.3 L/min (range: 82.8 to 125.6 L/min) for the 8-year-old patient set (N = 20).

The actual amount of drug delivered to the lung will depend on patient factors, such as inspiratory flow profile.

12 CLINICAL PHARMACOLOGY

12.1 Mechanism of Action

ADVAIR DISKUS: Since ADVAIR DISKUS contains both fluticasone propionate and salmeterol, the mechanisms of action described below for the individual components apply to ADVAIR DISKUS. These drugs represent 2 classes of medications (a synthetic corticosteroid and a selective LABA) that have different effects on clinical and physiological indices.

Fluticasone Propionate: Fluticasone propionate is a synthetic trifluorinated corticosteroid with potent anti-inflammatory activity. In vitro assays using human lung cytosol preparations have established fluticasone propionate as a human glucocorticoid receptor agonist with an affinity 18 times greater than dexamethasone, almost twice that of beclomethasone-17-monopropionate (BMP), the active metabolite of beclomethasone dipropionate, and over 3 times that of budesonide. Data from the McKenzie vasoconstrictor assay in man are consistent with these results.

Inflammation is an important component in the pathogenesis of asthma. Corticosteroids have been shown to inhibit multiple cell types (e.g., mast cells, eosinophils, basophils, lymphocytes, macrophages, neutrophils) and mediator production or secretion (e.g., histamine, eicosanoids, leukotrienes, cytokines) involved in the asthmatic response. These anti-inflammatory actions of corticosteroids contribute to their efficacy in asthma.

Inflammation is also a component in the pathogenesis of COPD. In contrast to asthma, however, the predominant inflammatory cells in COPD include neutrophils, CD8+ T-lymphocytes, and macrophages. The effects of corticosteroids in the treatment of COPD are not well defined and inhaled corticosteroids and fluticasone propionate when used apart from ADVAIR DISKUS are not indicated for the treatment of COPD.

Salmeterol Xinafoate: Salmeterol is a selective LABA. In vitro studies show salmeterol to be at least 50 times more selective for $beta_2$-adrenoceptors than albuterol. Although $beta_2$-adrenoceptors are the predominant adrenergic receptors in bronchial smooth muscle and $beta_1$-adrenoceptors are the predominant receptors in the heart, there are also $beta_2$-adrenoceptors in the human heart comprising 10% to 50% of the total beta-adrenoceptors. The precise function of these receptors has not been established, but their presence raises the possibility that even highly selective $beta_2$-agonists may have cardiac effects.

The pharmacologic effects of $beta_2$-adrenoceptor agonist drugs, including salmeterol, are at least in part attributable to stimulation of intracellular adenyl cyclase, the enzyme that catalyzes the conversion of adenosine triphosphate (ATP) to cyclic-3′,5′-adenosine monophosphate (cyclic AMP). Increased cyclic AMP levels cause relaxation of bronchial smooth muscle and inhibition of release of mediators of immediate hypersensitivity from cells, especially from mast cells.

In vitro tests show that salmeterol is a potent and long-lasting inhibitor of the release of mast cell mediators, such as histamine, leukotrienes, and prostaglandin D_2, from human lung. Salmeterol inhibits histamine-induced plasma protein extravasation and inhibits platelet-activating factor-induced eosinophil accumulation in the lungs of guinea pigs when administered by the inhaled route. In humans, single doses of salmeterol administered via inhalation aerosol attenuate allergen-induced bronchial hyper-responsiveness.

12.2 Pharmacodynamics

ADVAIR DISKUS: *Healthy Subjects: Cardiovascular Effects:* Since systemic pharmacodynamic effects of salmeterol are not normally seen at the therapeutic dose, higher doses were used to produce measurable effects. Four (4) studies were conducted in healthy adult subjects: (1) a single-dose crossover study using 2 inhalations of ADVAIR DISKUS 500/50, fluticasone propionate powder 500 mcg and salmeterol powder 50 mcg given concurrently, or fluticasone propionate powder 500 mcg given alone, (2) a cumulative dose study using 50 to 400 mcg of salmeterol powder given alone or as ADVAIR DISKUS 500/50, (3) a repeat-dose study for 11 days using 2 inhalations twice daily of ADVAIR DISKUS 250/50, fluticasone propionate powder 250 mcg, or salmeterol powder 50 mcg, and (4) a single-dose study using 5 inhalations of ADVAIR DISKUS 100/50, fluticasone propionate powder 100 mcg alone, or placebo. In these studies no significant differences were observed in the pharmacodynamic effects of salmeterol (pulse rate, blood pressure, QTc interval, potassium, and glucose) whether the salmeterol was given as ADVAIR DISKUS, concurrently with fluticasone propionate from separate inhalers, or as salmeterol alone. The systemic pharmacodynamic effects of salmeterol were not altered by the presence of fluticasone propionate in ADVAIR DISKUS. The potential effect of salmeterol on the effects of fluticasone propionate on the HPA axis was also evaluated in these studies.

HPA Axis Effects: No significant differences across treatments were observed in 24-hour urinary cortisol excretion and, where measured, 24-hour plasma cortisol AUC. The systemic pharmacodynamic effects of fluticasone propionate were not altered by the presence of salmeterol in ADVAIR DISKUS in healthy subjects.

Asthma: Adult and Adolescent Patients: Cardiovascular Effects: In clinical studies with ADVAIR DISKUS in adult and adolescent patients aged 12 years and older with asthma, no significant differences were observed in the systemic pharmacodynamic effects of salmeterol (pulse rate, blood pressure, QTc interval, potassium, and glucose) whether the salmeterol was given alone or as ADVAIR DISKUS. In 72 adult and adolescent patients with asthma given either ADVAIR DISKUS 100/50 or ADVAIR DISKUS 250/50, continuous 24-hour electrocardiographic monitoring was performed after the first dose and after 12 weeks of therapy, and no clinically significant dysrhythmias were noted.

HPA Axis Effects: In a 28-week study in adult and adolescent patients with asthma, ADVAIR DISKUS 500/50 twice daily was compared with the concurrent use of salmeterol powder 50 mcg plus fluticasone propionate powder 500 mcg from separate inhalers or fluticasone propionate powder 500 mcg alone. No significant differences across treatments were observed in serum cortisol AUC after 12 weeks of dosing or in 24-hour urinary cortisol excretion after 12 and 28 weeks.

In a 12-week study in adult and adolescent patients with asthma, ADVAIR DISKUS 250/50 twice daily was compared with fluticasone propionate powder 250 mcg alone, salmeterol powder 50 mcg alone, and placebo. For most patients, the ability to increase cortisol production in response to stress, as assessed by 30-minute cosyntropin stimulation, remained intact with ADVAIR DISKUS. One patient (3%) who received ADVAIR DISKUS 250/50 had an abnormal response (peak serum cortisol <18 mcg/dL) after dosing, compared with 2 patients (6%) who received placebo, 2 patients (6%) who received fluticasone propionate 250 mcg, and no patients who received salmeterol.

In a repeat-dose, 3-way crossover study, 1 inhalation twice daily of ADVAIR DISKUS 100/50, FLOVENT® DISKUS® 100 mcg (fluticasone propionate inhalation powder, 100 mcg), or placebo was administered to 20 adult and adolescent patients with asthma. After 28 days of treatment, geometric mean serum cortisol AUC over 12 hours showed no significant difference between ADVAIR DISKUS and FLOVENT DISKUS or between either active treatment and placebo.

Pediatric Patients: HPA Axis Effects: In a 12-week study in patients with asthma aged 4 to 11 years who were receiving inhaled corticosteroids at study entry, ADVAIR DISKUS 100/50 twice daily was compared with fluticasone propionate inhalation powder 100 mcg administered twice daily via the DISKUS. The values for 24-hour urinary cortisol excretion at study entry and after 12 weeks of treatment were similar within each treatment group. After 12 weeks, 24-hour urinary cortisol excretion was also similar between the 2 groups.

Chronic Obstructive Pulmonary Disease: Cardiovascular Effects: In clinical studies with ADVAIR DISKUS in patients with COPD, no significant differences were seen in pulse rate, blood pressure, potassium, and glucose between ADVAIR DISKUS, the individual components of ADVAIR DISKUS, and placebo. In a study of ADVAIR DISKUS 250/50, 8 patients (2 [1.1%] in the group given ADVAIR DISKUS 250/50, 1 [0.5%] in the fluticasone propionate 250-mcg group, 3 [1.7%] in the salmeterol group, and 2 [1.1%] in the placebo group) had QTc intervals >470 msec at least 1 time during the treatment period. Five (5) of these 8 patients had a prolonged QTc interval at baseline.

In a 24-week study, 130 patients with COPD received continuous 24-hour electrocardiographic monitoring prior to the first dose and after 4 weeks of twice-daily treatment with either ADVAIR DISKUS 500/50, fluticasone propionate powder 500 mcg, salmeterol powder 50 mcg, or placebo. No significant differences in ventricular or supraventricular arrhythmias and heart rate were observed among the groups treated with ADVAIR DISKUS 500/50, the individual components, or placebo. One (1) subject in the fluticasone propionate group experienced atrial flutter/atrial fibrillation, and 1 subject in the group given ADVAIR DISKUS 500/50 experienced heart block. There were 3 cases of non-sustained ventricular tachycardia (1 each in the placebo, salmeterol, and fluticasone propionate 500-mcg treatment groups).

In 24-week clinical studies in patients with COPD, the incidence of clinically significant ECG abnormalities (myocardial ischemia, ventricular hypertrophy, clinically significant conduction abnormalities, clinically significant arrhythmias) was lower for patients who received salmeterol (1%, 9 of 688 patients who received either salmeterol 50 mcg or ADVAIR DISKUS) compared with placebo (3%, 10 of 370 patients).

No significant differences with salmeterol 50 mcg alone or in combination with fluticasone propionate as ADVAIR DISKUS 500/50 were observed on pulse rate and systolic and diastolic blood pressure in a subset of patients with COPD who underwent 12-hour serial vital sign measurements after the first dose (N = 183) and after 12 weeks of therapy (N = 149). Median changes from baseline in pulse rate and systolic and diastolic blood pressure were similar to those seen with placebo.

HPA Axis Effects: Short-cosyntropin stimulation testing was performed both at Day 1 and Endpoint in 101 patients with COPD receiving twice-daily ADVAIR DISKUS 250/50, fluticasone propionate powder 250 mcg, salmeterol powder 50 mcg, or placebo. For most patients, the ability to increase cortisol production in response to stress, as assessed by short cosyntropin stimulation, remained intact with ADVAIR DISKUS 250/50. One (1) patient (3%) who received ADVAIR DISKUS 250/50 had an abnormal stimulated cortisol response (peak cortisol <14.5 mcg/dL assessed by high-performance liquid chromatography) after dosing, compared with 2 patients (9%) who received fluticasone propionate

250 mcg, 2 patients (7%) who received salmeterol 50 mcg, and 1 patient (4%) who received placebo following 24 weeks of treatment or early discontinuation from study.

After 36 weeks of dosing, serum cortisol concentrations in a subset of patients with COPD (n = 83) were 22% lower in patients receiving ADVAIR DISKUS 500/50 and 21% lower in patients receiving fluticasone propionate 500 mcg than in patients receiving placebo.

Other Fluticasone Propionate Products: *Asthma: HPA Axis Effects:* In clinical trials with fluticasone propionate inhalation powder using doses up to and including 250 mcg twice daily, occasional abnormal short cosyntropin tests (peak serum cortisol <18 mcg/dL assessed by radioimmunoassay) were noted both in patients receiving fluticasone propionate and in patients receiving placebo. The incidence of abnormal tests at 500 mcg twice daily was greater than placebo. In a 2-year study carried out with the DISKHALER® inhalation device in 64 patients with mild, persistent asthma (mean FEV_1 91% of predicted) randomized to fluticasone propionate 500 mcg twice daily or placebo, no patient receiving fluticasone propionate had an abnormal response to 6-hour cosyntropin infusion (peak serum cortisol <18 mcg/dL). With a peak cortisol threshold of <35 mcg/dL, 1 patient receiving fluticasone propionate (4%) had an abnormal response at 1 year; repeat testing at 18 months and 2 years was normal. Another patient receiving fluticasone propionate (5%) had an abnormal response at 2 years. No patient on placebo had an abnormal response at 1 or 2 years.

Chronic Obstructive Pulmonary Disease: HPA Axis Effects: After 4 weeks of dosing, the steady-state fluticasone propionate pharmacokinetics and serum cortisol levels were described in a subset of patients with COPD (n = 86) randomized to twice-daily fluticasone propionate inhalation powder via the DISKUS 500 mcg, fluticasone propionate inhalation powder 250 mcg, or placebo. Serial serum cortisol concentrations were measured across a 12-hour dosing interval. Serum cortisol concentrations following 250- and 500-mcg twice-daily dosing were 10% and 21% lower than placebo, respectively, indicating a dose-dependent increase in systemic exposure to fluticasone propionate.

Other Salmeterol Xinafoate Products: *Asthma: Cardiovascular Effects:* Inhaled salmeterol, like other beta-adrenergic agonist drugs, can produce dose-related cardiovascular effects and effects on blood glucose and/or serum potassium *[see Warnings and Precautions (5.12, 5.18)]*. The cardiovascular effects (heart rate, blood pressure) associated with salmeterol occur with similar frequency, and are of similar type and severity, as those noted following albuterol administration.

The effects of rising doses of inhaled salmeterol and standard inhaled doses of albuterol were studied in volunteers and in patients with asthma. Salmeterol doses up to 84 mcg administered as inhalation aerosol resulted in heart rate increases of 3 to 16 beats/min, about the same as albuterol dosed at 180 mcg by inhalation aerosol (4 to 10 beats/min). Adolescent and adult patients receiving 50-mcg doses of salmeterol inhalation powder (N = 60) underwent continuous electrocardiographic monitoring during two 12-hour periods after the first dose and after 1 month of therapy, and no clinically significant dysrhythmias were noted.

Concomitant Use of ADVAIR DISKUS With Other Respiratory Medications: *Short-Acting $Beta_2$-Agonists:* In clinical trials with patients with asthma, the mean daily need for albuterol by 166 adult and adolescent patients aged 12 years and older using ADVAIR DISKUS was approximately 1.3 inhalations/day and ranged from 0 to 9 inhalations/day. Five percent (5%) of patients using ADVAIR DISKUS in these trials averaged 6 or more inhalations per day over the course of the 12-week trials. No increase in frequency of cardiovascular adverse reactions was observed among patients who averaged 6 or more inhalations per day.

In a COPD clinical trial, the mean daily need for albuterol for patients using ADVAIR DISKUS 250/50 was 4.1 inhalations/day. Twenty-six percent (26%) of patients using ADVAIR DISKUS 250/50 averaged 6 or more inhalations per day over the course of the 24-week trial. No increase in frequency of cardiovascular adverse reactions was observed among patients who averaged 6 or more inhalations of albuterol per day.

Methylxanthines: The concurrent use of intravenously or orally administered methylxanthines (e.g., aminophylline, theophylline) by adult and adolescent patients aged 12 years and older receiving ADVAIR DISKUS has not been completely evaluated. In clinical trials with patients with asthma, 39 patients receiving ADVAIR DISKUS 100/50, 250/50, or 500/50 twice daily concurrently with a theophylline product had adverse event rates similar to those in 304 patients receiving ADVAIR DISKUS without theophylline. Similar results were observed in patients receiving salmeterol 50 mcg plus fluticasone propionate 500 mcg twice daily concurrently with a theophylline product (n = 39) or without theophylline (n = 132).

In a COPD clinical trial, 17 patients receiving ADVAIR DISKUS 250/50 twice daily concurrently with a theophylline product had adverse event rates similar to those in 161 patients receiving ADVAIR DISKUS without theophylline. Based on the available data, the concomitant administration of methylxanthines with ADVAIR DISKUS did not alter the observed adverse event profile.

Fluticasone Propionate Nasal Spray: In adult and adolescent patients aged 12 years and older taking ADVAIR DISKUS in clinical trials, no difference in the profile of adverse events or HPA axis effects was noted between patients who were taking FLONASE® (fluticasone propionate) Nasal Spray, 50 mcg concurrently (n = 46) and those who were not (n = 130).

12.3 Pharmacokinetics

Absorption: *Fluticasone Propionate: Healthy Subjects:* Fluticasone propionate acts locally in the lung; therefore, plasma levels do not predict therapeutic effect. Studies using oral dosing of labeled and unlabeled drug have demonstrated that the oral systemic bioavailability of fluticasone propionate is negligible (<1%), primarily due to incomplete absorption and presystemic metabolism in the gut and liver. In contrast, the majority of the fluticasone propionate delivered to the lung is systemically absorbed.

Following administration of ADVAIR DISKUS to healthy adult subjects, peak plasma concentrations of fluticasone propionate were achieved in 1 to 2 hours. In a single-dose crossover study, a higher-than-recommended dose of ADVAIR DISKUS was administered to 14 healthy adult subjects. Two (2) inhalations of the following treatments were administered: ADVAIR DISKUS 500/50, fluticasone propionate powder 500 mcg and salmeterol powder 50 mcg given concurrently, and fluticasone propionate powder 500 mcg alone. Mean peak plasma concentrations of fluticasone propionate averaged 107, 94, and 120 pg/mL, respectively, indicating no significant changes in systemic exposures of fluticasone propionate.

In 15 healthy subjects, systemic exposure to fluticasone propionate from 4 inhalations of ADVAIR® HFA 230/21 (fluticasone propionate 230 mcg and salmeterol 21 mcg) Inhalation Aerosol (920/84 mcg) and 2 inhalations of ADVAIR DISKUS 500/50 (1,000/100 mcg) were similar between the 2 inhalers (i.e., 799 versus 832 pg•hr/mL, respectively), but approximately half the systemic exposure from 4 inhalations of fluticasone propionate CFC inhalation aerosol 220 mcg (880 mcg, AUC = 1,543 pg•hr/mL). Similar results were observed for peak fluticasone propionate plasma concentrations (186 and 182 pg/mL from ADVAIR HFA and ADVAIR DISKUS, respectively, and 307 pg/mL from the fluticasone propionate CFC inhalation aerosol). Absolute bioavailability of fluticasone propionate was 5.3% and 5.5% following administration of ADVAIR HFA and ADVAIR DISKUS, respectively.

Asthma and COPD Patients: Peak steady-state fluticasone propionate plasma concentrations in adult patients with asthma (N = 11) ranged from undetectable to 266 pg/mL after a 500-mcg twice-daily dose of fluticasone propionate inhalation powder using the DISKUS device. The mean fluticasone propionate plasma concentration was 110 pg/mL.

Full pharmacokinetic profiles were obtained from 9 female and 16 male patients with asthma given fluticasone propionate inhalation powder 500 mcg twice daily using the DISKUS device and from 14 female and 43 male patients with COPD given 250 or 500 mcg twice daily. No overall differences in fluticasone propionate pharmacokinetics were observed.

Peak steady-state fluticasone propionate plasma concentrations in patients with COPD averaged 53 pg/mL (range: 19.3 to 159.3 pg/mL) after treatment with 250 mcg twice daily (N = 30) and 84 pg/mL (range: 24.3 to 197.1 pg/mL) after treatment with 500 mcg twice daily (N = 27) via the fluticasone propionate DISKUS device. In another study in patients with COPD, peak steady-state fluticasone propionate plasma concentrations averaged 115 pg/mL (range: 52.6 to 366.0 pg/mL) after treatment with 500 mcg twice daily via the fluticasone propionate DISKUS device (N = 15) and 105 pg/mL (range: 22.5 to 299.0 pg/mL) via ADVAIR DISKUS (N = 24).

Salmeterol Xinafoate: Healthy Subjects: Salmeterol xinafoate, an ionic salt, dissociates in solution so that the salmeterol and 1-hydroxy-2-naphthoic acid (xinafoate) moieties are absorbed, distributed, metabolized, and eliminated independently. Salmeterol acts locally in the lung; therefore, plasma levels do not predict therapeutic effect.

Following administration of ADVAIR DISKUS to healthy adult subjects, peak plasma concentrations of salmeterol were achieved in about 5 minutes.

In 15 healthy subjects receiving ADVAIR HFA 230/21 Inhalation Aerosol (920/84 mcg) and ADVAIR DISKUS 500/50 (1,000/100 mcg), systemic exposure to salmeterol was higher (317 versus 169 pg•hr/mL) and peak salmeterol concentrations were lower (196 versus 223 pg/mL) following ADVAIR HFA compared with ADVAIR DISKUS, although pharmacodynamic results were comparable.

Asthma Patients: Because of the small therapeutic dose, systemic levels of salmeterol are low or undetectable after inhalation of recommended doses (50 mcg of salmeterol inhalation powder twice daily). Following chronic administration of an inhaled dose of 50 mcg of salmeterol inhalation powder twice daily, salmeterol was detected in plasma within 5 to 45 minutes in 7 patients with asthma; plasma concentrations were very low, with mean peak concentrations of 167 pg/mL at 20 minutes and no accumulation with repeated doses.

Distribution: *Fluticasone Propionate:* Following intravenous administration, the initial disposition phase for fluticasone propionate was rapid and consistent with its high lipid solubility and tissue binding. The volume of distribution averaged 4.2 L/kg.

The percentage of fluticasone propionate bound to human plasma proteins averages 91%. Fluticasone propionate is weakly and reversibly bound to erythrocytes and is not significantly bound to human transcortin.

Salmeterol: The percentage of salmeterol bound to human plasma proteins averages 96% in vitro over the concentration range of 8 to 7,722 ng of salmeterol base per milliliter, much higher concentrations than those achieved following therapeutic doses of salmeterol.

Metabolism: *Fluticasone Propionate:* The total clearance of fluticasone propionate is high (average, 1,093 mL/min), with renal clearance accounting for less than 0.02% of the total. The only circulating metabolite detected in man is the 17β-carboxylic acid derivative of fluticasone propionate, which is formed through the CYP3A4 pathway. This metabolite had less affinity (approximately 1/2,000) than the parent drug for the glucocorticoid receptor of human lung cytosol in vitro and negligible pharmacological activity in animal studies. Other metabolites detected in vitro using cultured human hepatoma cells have not been detected in man.

Salmeterol: Salmeterol base is extensively metabolized by hydroxylation, with subsequent elimination predominantly in the feces. No significant amount of unchanged salmeterol base was detected in either urine or feces.

An in vitro study using human liver microsomes showed that salmeterol is extensively metabolized to α-hydroxysalmeterol (aliphatic oxidation) by CYP3A4. Ketoconazole, a strong inhibitor of CYP3A4, essentially completely inhibited the formation of α-hydroxysalmeterol in vitro.

Elimination: *Fluticasone Propionate:* Following intravenous dosing, fluticasone propionate showed polyexponential kinetics and had a terminal elimination half-life of approximately 7.8 hours. Less than 5% of a radiolabeled oral dose was excreted in the urine as metabolites, with the remainder excreted in the feces as parent drug and metabolites. Terminal half-life estimates of fluticasone propionate for ADVAIR HFA, ADVAIR DISKUS, and fluticasone propionate CFC inhalation aerosol were similar and averaged 5.6 hours.

Salmeterol: In 2 healthy adult subjects who received 1 mg of radiolabeled salmeterol (as salmeterol xinafoate) orally, approximately 25% and 60% of the radiolabeled salmeterol was eliminated in urine and feces, respectively, over a period of 7 days. The terminal elimination half-life was about 5.5 hours (1 volunteer only).

The xinafoate moiety has no apparent pharmacologic activity. The xinafoate moiety is highly protein bound (>99%) and has a long elimination half-life of 11 days. No terminal half-life estimates were calculated for salmeterol following administration of ADVAIR DISKUS.

Special Populations: A population pharmacokinetic analysis was performed for fluticasone propionate and salmeterol utilizing data from 9 controlled clinical trials that included 350 patients with asthma aged 4 to 77 years who received treatment with ADVAIR DISKUS, the combination of HFA-propelled fluticasone propionate and salmeterol inhalation aerosol (ADVAIR HFA), fluticasone propionate inhalation powder (FLOVENT DISKUS), HFA-propelled fluticasone propionate inhalation aerosol (FLOVENT® HFA), or CFC-propelled fluticasone propionate inhalation aerosol. The population pharmacokinetic analyses for fluticasone propionate and salmeterol showed no clinically relevant effects of age, gender, race, body weight, body mass index, or percent of predicted FEV_1 on apparent clearance and apparent volume of distribution.

Age: When the population pharmacokinetic analysis for fluticasone propionate was divided into subgroups based on fluticasone propionate strength, formulation, and age (adolescents/adults and children), there were some differences in fluticasone propionate exposure. Higher fluticasone propionate exposure from ADVAIR DISKUS 100/50 compared with FLOVENT DISKUS 100 mcg was observed in adolescents and adults (ratio 1.52 [90% CI: 1.08, 2.13]). However, in clinical studies of up to 12 weeks' duration comparing ADVAIR DISKUS 100/50 and FLOVENT DISKUS 100 mcg in adolescents and adults, no differences in systemic effects of corticosteroid treatment (e.g., HPA axis effects) were observed. Similar fluticasone propionate exposure was observed from ADVAIR DISKUS 500/50 and FLOVENT DISKUS 500 mcg (ratio 0.83 [90% CI: 0.65, 1.07]) in adolescents and adults.

Steady-state systemic exposure to salmeterol when delivered as ADVAIR DISKUS 100/50, ADVAIR DISKUS 250/50, or ADVAIR HFA 115/21 (fluticasone propionate 115 mcg and salmeterol 21 mcg) Inhalation Aerosol was evaluated in 127 patients aged 4 to 57 years. The geometric mean AUC was 325 pg•hr/mL (90% CI: 309, 341) in adolescents and adults.

The population pharmacokinetic analysis included 160 patients with asthma aged 4 to 11 years who received ADVAIR DISKUS 100/50 or FLOVENT DISKUS 100 mcg. Higher fluticasone propionate exposure (AUC) was observed in children from ADVAIR DISKUS 100/50 compared with FLOVENT DISKUS 100 mcg (ratio 1.20 [90% CI: 1.06, 1.37]). Higher fluticasone propionate exposure (AUC) from ADVAIR DISKUS 100/50 was observed in children compared with adolescents and adults (ratio 1.63 [90% CI: 1.35, 1.96]). However, in clinical studies of up to 12 weeks' duration comparing ADVAIR DISKUS 100/50 and FLOVENT DISKUS 100 mcg in both adolescents and adults and in children, no differences in systemic effects of corticosteroid treatment (e.g., HPA axis effects) were observed.

Exposure to salmeterol was higher in children compared with adolescents and adults who received ADVAIR DISKUS 100/50 (ratio 1.23 [90% CI: 1.10, 1.38]). However, in clinical studies of up to 12 weeks' duration with ADVAIR DISKUS 100/50 in both adolescents and adults and in children, no differences in systemic effects of beta$_2$-agonist treatment (e.g., cardiovascular effects, tremor) were observed.

Gender: The population pharmacokinetic analysis involved 202 males and 148 females with asthma who received fluticasone propionate alone or in combination with salmeterol and showed no gender differences for fluticasone propionate pharmacokinetics.

The population pharmacokinetic analysis involved 76 males and 51 females with asthma who received salmeterol in combination with fluticasone propionate and showed no gender differences for salmeterol pharmacokinetics.

Hepatic and Renal Impairment: Formal pharmacokinetic studies using ADVAIR DISKUS have not been conducted in patients with hepatic or renal impairment. However, since both fluticasone propionate and salmeterol are predominantly cleared by hepatic metabolism, impairment of liver function may lead to accumulation of fluticasone propionate and salmeterol in plasma. Therefore, patients with hepatic disease should be closely monitored.

Drug Interactions: In the repeat- and single-dose studies, there was no evidence of significant drug interaction in systemic exposure between fluticasone propionate and salmeterol when given as ADVAIR DISKUS. The population pharmacokinetic analysis from 9 controlled clinical trials in 350 patients with asthma showed no significant effects on fluticasone propionate or salmeterol pharmacokinetics following co-administration with beta$_2$-agonists, corticosteroids, antihistamines, or theophyllines.

Inhibitors of Cytochrome P450 3A4: Ritonavir: Fluticasone Propionate: Fluticasone propionate is a substrate of CYP3A4. Coadministration of fluticasone propionate and the strong CYP3A4 inhibitor ritonavir is not recommended based upon a multiple-dose, crossover drug interaction study in 18 healthy subjects. Fluticasone propionate aqueous nasal spray (200 mcg once daily) was coadministered for 7 days with ritonavir (100 mg twice daily). Plasma fluticasone propionate concentrations following fluticasone propionate aqueous nasal spray alone were undetectable (<10 pg/mL) in most subjects, and when concentrations were detectable peak levels (C_{max}) averaged 11.9 pg/mL (range: 10.8 to 14.1 pg/mL) and $AUC_{(0-\tau)}$ averaged 8.43 pg•hr/mL (range: 4.2 to 18.8 pg•hr/mL). Fluticasone propionate C_{max} and $AUC_{(0-\tau)}$ increased to 318 pg/mL (range: 110 to 648 pg/mL) and 3,102.6 pg•hr/mL (range: 1,207.1 to 5,662.0 pg•hr/mL), respectively, after coadministration of ritonavir with fluticasone propionate aqueous nasal spray. This significant increase in plasma fluticasone propionate exposure resulted in a significant decrease (86%) in serum cortisol AUC.

Ketoconazole: Fluticasone Propionate: In a placebo-controlled, crossover study in 8 healthy adult volunteers, coadministration of a single dose of orally inhaled fluticasone propionate (1,000 mcg) with multiple doses of ketoconazole (200 mg) to steady state resulted in increased plasma fluticasone propionate exposure, a reduction in plasma cortisol AUC, and no effect on urinary excretion of cortisol.

Salmeterol: In a placebo-controlled, crossover drug interaction study in 20 healthy male and female subjects, coadministration of salmeterol (50 mcg twice daily) and the strong CYP3A4 inhibitor ketoconazole (400 mg once daily) for 7 days resulted in a significant increase in plasma salmeterol exposure as determined by a 16-fold increase in AUC (ratio with and without ketoconazole 15.76 [90% CI: 10.66, 23.31]) mainly due to increased bioavailability of the swallowed portion of the dose. Peak plasma salmeterol concentrations were increased by 1.4-fold (90% CI: 1.23, 1.68). Three (3) out of 20 subjects (15%) were withdrawn from salmeterol and ketoconazole coadministration due to beta-agonist–mediated systemic effects (2 with QTc prolongation and 1 with palpitations and sinus tachycardia). Coadministration of salmeterol and ketoconazole did not result in a clinically significant effect on mean heart rate, mean blood potassium, or mean blood glucose. Although there was no statistical effect on the mean QTc, coadministration of salmeterol and ketoconazole was associated with more frequent increases in QTc duration compared with salmeterol and placebo administration.

Erythromycin: Fluticasone Propionate: In a multiple-dose drug interaction study, coadministration of orally inhaled fluticasone propionate (500 mcg twice daily) and erythromycin (333 mg 3 times daily) did not affect fluticasone propionate pharmacokinetics.

Salmeterol: In a repeat-dose study in 13 healthy subjects, concomitant administration of erythromycin (a moderate CYP3A4 inhibitor) and salmeterol inhalation aerosol resulted in a 40% increase in salmeterol C_{max} at steady state (ratio with and without erythromycin 1.4 [90% CI: 0.96, 2.03], p = 0.12), a 3.6-beat/min increase in heart rate ([95% CI: 0.19, 7.03], p<0.04), a 5.8-msec increase in QTc interval ([95% CI: -6.14, 17.77], p = 0.34), and no change in plasma potassium.

13 NONCLINICAL TOXICOLOGY

13.1 Carcinogenesis, Mutagenesis, Impairment of Fertility

Fluticasone Propionate: Fluticasone propionate demonstrated no tumorigenic potential in mice at oral doses up to 1,000 mcg/kg (approximately 4 and 10 times the MRHD for adults and children, respectively, on an mg/m^2 basis) for 78 weeks or in rats at inhalation doses up to 57 mcg/kg (less than and approximately equivalent to the MRHD for adults and children, respectively, on an mg/m^2 basis) for 104 weeks.

Fluticasone propionate did not induce gene mutation in prokaryotic or eukaryotic cells in vitro. No significant clastogenic effect was seen in cultured human peripheral lymphocytes in vitro or in the in vivo mouse micronucleus test.

No evidence of impairment of fertility was observed in reproductive studies conducted in rats at subcutaneous doses up to 50 mcg/kg (less than the MRHD on an mg/m^2 basis). Prostate weight was significantly reduced.

Salmeterol: In an 18-month carcinogenicity study in CD-mice, salmeterol at oral doses of 1.4 mg/kg and above (approximately 20 times the MRHD for adults and children based on comparison of the plasma AUCs) caused a dose-related increase in the incidence of smooth muscle hyperplasia, cystic glandular hyperplasia, leiomyomas of the uterus, and ovarian cysts. No tumors were seen at 0.2 mg/kg (approximately 3 times the MRHD for adults and children based on comparison of the AUCs).

In a 24-month oral and inhalation carcinogenicity study in Sprague Dawley rats, salmeterol caused a dose-related increase in the incidence of mesovarian leiomyomas and ovarian cysts at doses of 0.68 mg/kg and above (approximately 55 and 25 times the MRHD for adults and children, respectively, on an mg/m^2 basis). No tumors were seen at 0.21 mg/kg (approximately 15 and 8 times the MRHD for adults and children, respectively, on an mg/m^2 basis). These findings in rodents are similar to those reported previously for other beta-adrenergic agonist drugs. The relevance of these findings to human use is unknown.

Salmeterol produced no detectable or reproducible increases in microbial and mammalian gene mutation in vitro. No clastogenic activity occurred in vitro in human lymphocytes or in vivo in a rat micronucleus test. No effects on fertility were identified in rats treated with salmeterol at oral doses up to 2 mg/kg (approximately 160 times the MRHD for adults on an mg/m^2 basis).

13.2 Animal Toxicology and/or Pharmacology

Preclinical: Studies in laboratory animals (minipigs, rodents, and dogs) have demonstrated the occurrence of cardiac arrhythmias and sudden death (with histologic evidence of myocardial necrosis) when beta-agonists and methylxanthines are administered concurrently. The clinical relevance of these findings is unknown.

Reproductive Toxicology Studies: *ADVAIR DISKUS:* In mice, combining 150 mcg/kg subcutaneously of fluticasone propionate (less than the MRHD on an mg/m^2 basis) with 10 mg/kg orally of salmeterol (approximately 410 times the MRHD on an mg/m^2 basis) produced cleft palate, fetal death, increased implantation loss, and delayed ossification. No such effects were observed at combination subcutaneous doses up to 40 mcg/kg subcutaneously of fluticasone propionate (less than the MRHD on an mg/m^2 basis) and up to 1.4 mg/kg orally doses of salmeterol (approximately 55 times the MRHD on an mg/m^2 basis).

In rats, combining 100 mcg/kg subcutaneously of fluticasone propionate (equivalent to the MRHD on an mg/m^2 basis) and 10 mg/kg orally of salmeterol (approximately 810 times the MRHD on an mg/m^2 basis) produced decreased fetal weight, umbilical hernia, delayed ossification, and changes in the occipital bone. No such effects were observed at combination doses up to 30 mcg/kg subcutaneously of fluticasone propionate (less than the MRHD on an mg/m^2 basis) and up to 1 mg/kg orally of salmeterol (approximately 80 times the MRHD on an mg/m^2 basis).

Fluticasone Propionate: Subcutaneous studies in the mouse and rat at 45 and 100 mcg/kg (less than and equivalent to the MRHD on an mg/m^2 basis), respectively, revealed fetal toxicity characteristic of potent corticosteroid compounds, including embryonic growth retardation, omphalocele, cleft palate, and retarded cranial ossification.

In the rabbit, fetal weight reduction and cleft palate were observed at a subcutaneous dose of 4 mcg/kg (less than the MRHD on an mg/m^2 basis). However, no teratogenic effects were reported at oral doses up to 300 mcg/kg (approximately 5 times the MRHD on an mg/m^2 basis) of fluticasone propionate. No fluticasone propionate was detected in the plasma in this study, consistent with the established low bioavailability following oral administration *[see Clinical Pharmacology (12.3)]*.

Fluticasone propionate crossed the placenta following subcutaneous administration to mice and rats and oral administration to rabbits.

Salmeterol: No teratogenic effects occurred in rats at oral doses up to 2 mg/kg (approximately 160 times the MRHD on an mg/m^2 basis).

In Dutch rabbits administered oral doses of 1 mg/kg and above (approximately 50 times and above the MRHD based on comparison of the AUCs), salmeterol exhibited fetal toxic effects characteristically resulting from beta-adrenoceptor stimulation. These included precocious eyelid openings, cleft palate, sternebral fusion, limb and paw flexures, and delayed ossification of the frontal cranial bones. No such effects occurred at an oral dose of 0.6 mg/kg (approximately 20 times the MRHD based on comparison of the AUCs). New Zealand White rabbits were less sensitive since only delayed ossification of the frontal bones was seen at an oral dose of 10 mg/kg (approximately 1,600 times the MRHD on an mg/m^2 basis).

Salmeterol crossed the placenta following oral administration to mice and rats.

14 CLINICAL STUDIES

14.1 Asthma

Adult and Adolescent Patients Aged 12 Years and Older: In clinical trials comparing ADVAIR DISKUS with its individual components, improvements in most efficacy endpoints were greater with ADVAIR DISKUS than with the use of either fluticasone propionate or salmeterol alone. In addition, clinical trials showed similar results between ADVAIR DISKUS and the concurrent use of fluticasone propionate plus salmeterol at corresponding doses from separate inhalers.

Studies Comparing ADVAIR DISKUS to Fluticasone Propionate Alone or Salmeterol Alone: Three (3) double-blind, parallel-group clinical trials were conducted with ADVAIR DISKUS in 1,208 adolescent and adult patients (≥12 years, baseline FEV$_1$ 63% to 72% of predicted normal) with asthma that was not optimally controlled on their current therapy. All treatments were inhalation powders given as 1 inhalation from the DISKUS device twice daily, and other maintenance therapies were discontinued.

Study 1: Clinical Trial With ADVAIR DISKUS 100/50: This placebo-controlled, 12-week, US study compared ADVAIR DISKUS 100/50 with its individual components, fluticasone propionate 100 mcg and salmeterol 50 mcg. The study was stratified according to baseline asthma maintenance therapy; patients were using either inhaled corticosteroids (N = 250) (daily doses of beclomethasone dipropionate 252 to 420 mcg; flunisolide 1,000 mcg; fluticasone propionate inhalation aerosol 176 mcg; or triamcinolone acetonide 600 to 1,000 mcg) or salmeterol (N = 106). Baseline FEV$_1$ measurements were similar across treatments: ADVAIR DISKUS 100/50, 2.17 L; fluticasone propionate 100 mcg, 2.11 L; salmeterol, 2.13 L; and placebo, 2.15 L.

Predefined withdrawal criteria for lack of efficacy, an indicator of worsening asthma, were utilized for this placebo-controlled study. Worsening asthma was defined as a clinically important decrease in FEV$_1$ or PEF, increase in use of VENTOLIN® (albuterol, USP) Inhalation Aerosol, increase in night awakenings due to asthma, emergency intervention or hospitalization due to asthma, or requirement for asthma medication not allowed by the protocol. As shown in Table 4, statistically significantly fewer patients receiving ADVAIR DISKUS 100/50 were withdrawn due to worsening asthma compared with fluticasone propionate, salmeterol, and placebo.

Table 4. Percent of Patients Withdrawn Due to Worsening Asthma in Patients Previously Treated With Either Inhaled Corticosteroids or Salmeterol (Study 1)

ADVAIR DISKUS 100/50 (N = 87)	Fluticasone Propionate 100 mcg (N = 85)	Salmeterol 50 mcg (N = 86)	Placebo (N = 77)
3%	11%	35%	49%

The FEV_1 results are displayed in Figure 2. Because this trial used predetermined criteria for worsening asthma, which caused more patients in the placebo group to be withdrawn, FEV_1 results at Endpoint (last available FEV_1 result) are also provided. Patients receiving ADVAIR DISKUS 100/50 had significantly greater improvements in FEV_1 (0.51 L, 25%) compared with fluticasone propionate 100 mcg (0.28 L, 15%), salmeterol (0.11 L, 5%), and placebo (0.01 L, 1%). These improvements in FEV_1 with ADVAIR DISKUS were achieved regardless of baseline asthma maintenance therapy (inhaled corticosteroids or salmeterol).

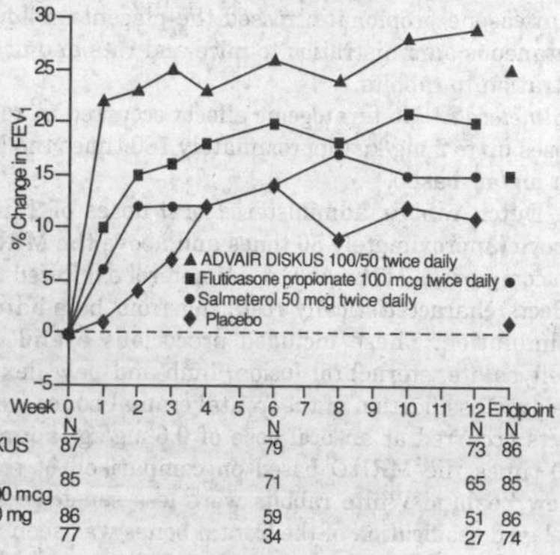

Figure 2. Mean Percent Change From Baseline in FEV_1 in Patients With Asthma Previously Treated With Either Inhaled Corticosteroids or Salmeterol (Study 1)

The effect of ADVAIR DISKUS 100/50 on morning and evening PEF endpoints is shown in Table 5.

[See table 5 below]

The subjective impact of asthma on patients' perception of health was evaluated through use of an instrument called the Asthma Quality of Life Questionnaire (AQLQ) (based on a 7-point scale where 1 = maximum impairment and 7 = none). Patients receiving ADVAIR DISKUS 100/50 had clinically meaningful improvements in overall asthma-specific quality of life as defined by a difference between groups of ≥0.5 points in change from baseline AQLQ scores (difference in AQLQ score of 1.25 compared with placebo).

Study 2: Clinical Trial With ADVAIR DISKUS 250/50: This placebo-controlled, 12-week, US study compared ADVAIR DISKUS 250/50 with its individual components, fluticasone propionate 250 mcg and salmeterol 50 mcg, in 349 patients with asthma using inhaled corticosteroids (daily doses of beclomethasone dipropionate 462 to 672 mcg; flunisolide 1,250 to 2,000 mcg; fluticasone propionate inhalation aerosol 440 mcg; or triamcinolone acetonide 1,100 to 1,600 mcg). Baseline FEV_1 measurements were similar across treatments: ADVAIR DISKUS 250/50, 2.23 L; fluticasone propionate 250 mcg, 2.12 L; salmeterol, 2.20 L; and placebo, 2.19 L.

Efficacy results in this study were similar to those observed in Study 1. Patients receiving ADVAIR DISKUS 250/50 had significantly greater improvements in FEV_1 (0.48 L, 23%) compared with fluticasone propionate 250 mcg (0.25 L, 13%), salmeterol (0.05 L, 4%), and placebo (decrease of 0.11 L, decrease of 5%). Statistically significantly fewer patients receiving ADVAIR DISKUS 250/50 were withdrawn from this study for worsening asthma (4%) compared with fluticasone propionate (22%), salmeterol (38%), and placebo (62%). In addition, ADVAIR DISKUS 250/50 was superior to fluticasone propionate, salmeterol, and placebo for improvements in morning and evening PEF. Patients receiving ADVAIR DISKUS 250/50 also had clinically meaningful improvements in overall asthma-specific quality of life as described in Study 1 (difference in AQLQ score of 1.29 compared with placebo).

Study 3: Clinical Trial With ADVAIR DISKUS 500/50: This 28-week, non-US study compared ADVAIR DISKUS 500/50 with fluticasone propionate 500 mcg alone and concurrent therapy (salmeterol 50 mcg plus fluticasone propionate 500 mcg administered from separate inhalers) twice daily in 503 patients with asthma using inhaled corticosteroids (daily doses of beclomethasone dipropionate 1,260 to 1,680 mcg; budesonide 1,500 to 2,000 mcg; flunisolide 1,500 to 2,000 mcg; or fluticasone propionate inhalation aerosol 660 to 880 mcg [750 to 1,000 mcg inhalation powder]). The primary efficacy parameter, morning PEF, was collected daily for the first 12 weeks of the study. The primary purpose of weeks 13 to 28 was to collect safety data. Baseline PEF measurements were similar across treatments: ADVAIR DISKUS 500/50, 359 L/min; fluticasone propionate 500 mcg, 351 L/min; and concurrent therapy, 345 L/min. Morning PEF improved significantly with ADVAIR DISKUS 500/50 compared with fluticasone propionate 500 mcg over the 12-week treatment period. Improvements in morning PEF observed with ADVAIR DISKUS 500/50 were similar to improvements observed with concurrent therapy.

Onset of Action and Progression of Improvement in Asthma Control: The onset of action and progression of improvement in asthma control were evaluated in the 2 placebo-controlled US trials. Following the first dose, the median time to onset of clinically significant bronchodilatation (≥15% improvement in FEV_1) in most patients was seen within 30 to 60 minutes. Maximum improvement in FEV_1 generally occurred within 3 hours, and clinically significant improvement was maintained for 12 hours (see Figure 3). Following the initial dose, predose FEV_1 relative to Day 1 baseline improved markedly over the first week of treatment and continued to improve over the 12 weeks of treatment in both studies. No diminution in the 12-hour bronchodilator effect was observed with either ADVAIR DISKUS 100/50 (Figures 3 and 4) or ADVAIR DISKUS 250/50 as assessed by FEV_1 following 12 weeks of therapy.

[See figure 3 at top of next column]

[See figure 4 at top of next column]

Reduction in asthma symptoms, use of rescue VENTOLIN Inhalation Aerosol, and improvement in morning and evening PEF also occurred within the first day of treatment with ADVAIR DISKUS, and continued to improve over the 12 weeks of therapy in both studies.

Pediatric Patients: In a 12-week US study, ADVAIR DISKUS 100/50 twice daily was compared with fluticasone propionate inhalation powder 100 mcg twice daily in 203 children with asthma aged 4 to 11 years. At study entry, the children were symptomatic on low doses of inhaled corticosteroids (beclomethasone dipropionate 252 to 336 mcg/day; budesonide 200 to 400 mcg/day; flunisolide 1,000 mcg/day; triamcinolone acetonide 600 to 1,000 mcg/day; or fluticasone propionate 88 to 250 mcg/day). The primary objective of this study was to determine the safety of ADVAIR DISKUS 100/50 compared with fluticasone propionate inhalation powder 100 mcg in this age-group; however, the study also included secondary efficacy measures of pulmonary function. Morning predose FEV_1 was obtained at baseline and Endpoint (last available FEV_1 result) in children aged 6 to 11 years. In patients receiving ADVAIR DISKUS 100/50, FEV_1 increased from 1.70 L at baseline (N = 79) to 1.88 L at Endpoint (N = 69) compared with an increase from 1.65 L at baseline (N = 83) to 1.77 L at Endpoint (N = 75) in patients receiving fluticasone propionate 100 mcg.

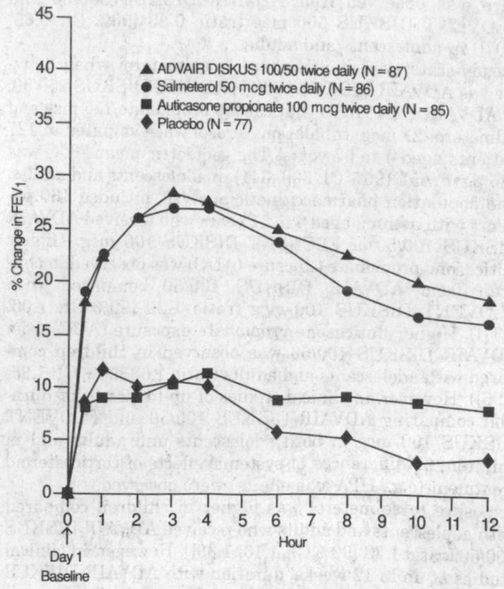

Figure 3. Percent Change in Serial 12-hour FEV_1 in Patients With Asthma Previously Using Either Inhaled Corticosteroids or Salmeterol (Study 1)

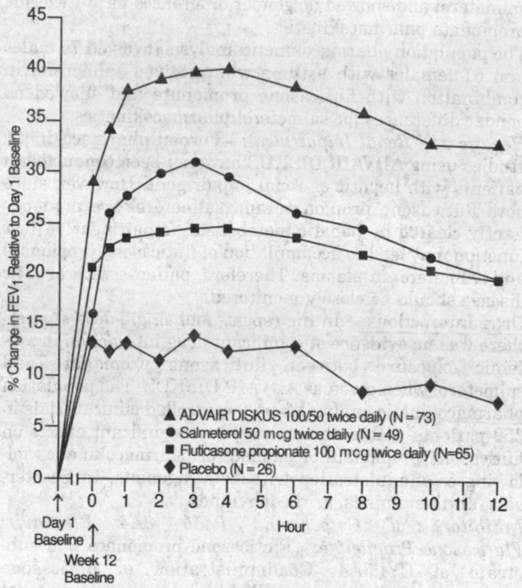

Figure 4. Percent Change in Serial 12-hour FEV_1 in Patients With Asthma Previously Using Either Inhaled Corticosteroids or Salmeterol (Study 1)

The findings of this study, along with extrapolation of efficacy data from patients aged 12 years and older, support the overall conclusion that ADVAIR DISKUS 100/50 is efficacious in the treatment of asthma in patients aged 4 to 11 years.

14.2 Chronic Obstructive Pulmonary Disease

The efficacy of ADVAIR DISKUS 250/50 and ADVAIR DISKUS 500/50 in the treatment of patients with COPD was evaluated in 6 randomized, double-blind, parallel-group clinical trials in adult patients aged 40 years and older. These trials were primarily designed to evaluate the efficacy of ADVAIR DISKUS on lung function (3 trials), exacerbations (2 trials), and survival (1 trial).

Lung Function: Two of the 3 clinical trials primarily designed to evaluate the efficacy of ADVAIR DISKUS on lung function were conducted in 1,414 patients with COPD associated with chronic bronchitis. In these 2 trials, all the patients had a history of cough productive of sputum that was not attributable to another disease process on most days for at least 3 months of the year for at least 2 years. The trials were randomized, double-blind, parallel-group, 24-week treatment duration. One trial evaluated the efficacy of ADVAIR DISKUS 250/50 compared with its components fluticasone propionate 250 mcg and salmeterol 50 mcg and with placebo, and the other trial evaluated the efficacy of ADVAIR DISKUS 500/50 compared with its components fluticasone propionate 500 mcg and salmeterol 50 mcg and with placebo. Study treatments were inhalation powders given as 1 inhalation from the DISKUS device twice daily.

Table 5. Peak Expiratory Flow Results for Patients With Asthma Previously Treated With Either Inhaled Corticosteroids or Salmeterol (Study 1)

Efficacy Variable[a]	ADVAIR DISKUS 100/50 (N = 87)	Fluticasone Propionate 100 mcg (N = 85)	Salmeterol 50 mcg (N = 86)	Placebo (N = 77)
AM PEF (L/min)				
Baseline	393	374	369	382
Change from baseline	53	17	-2	-24
PM PEF (L/min)				
Baseline	418	390	396	398
Change from baseline	35	18	-7	-13

[a]Change from baseline = change from baseline at Endpoint (last available data).

Maintenance COPD therapies were discontinued, with the exception of theophylline. The patients had a mean pre-bronchodilator FEV_1 of 41% and 20% reversibility at study entry. Percent reversibility was calculated as 100 times (FEV_1 post-albuterol minus FEV_1 pre-albuterol)/FEV_1 pre-albuterol.

Improvements in lung function (as defined by predose and postdose FEV_1) were significantly greater with ADVAIR DISKUS than with fluticasone propionate, salmeterol, or placebo. The improvement in lung function with ADVAIR DISKUS 500/50 was similar to the improvement seen with ADVAIR DISKUS 250/50.

Figures 5 and 6 display predose and 2-hour postdose, respectively, FEV_1 results for the study with ADVAIR DISKUS 250/50. To account for patient withdrawals during the study, FEV_1 at Endpoint (last evaluable FEV_1) was evaluated. Patients receiving ADVAIR DISKUS 250/50 had significantly greater improvements in predose FEV_1 at Endpoint (165 mL, 17%) compared with salmeterol 50 mcg (91 mL, 9%) and placebo (1 mL, 1%), demonstrating the contribution of fluticasone propionate to the improvement in lung function with ADVAIR DISKUS (Figure 5). Patients receiving ADVAIR DISKUS 250/50 had significantly greater improvements in postdose FEV_1 at Endpoint (281 mL, 27%) compared with fluticasone propionate 250 mcg (147 mL, 14%) and placebo (58 mL, 6%), demonstrating the contribution of salmeterol to the improvement in lung function with ADVAIR DISKUS (Figure 6).

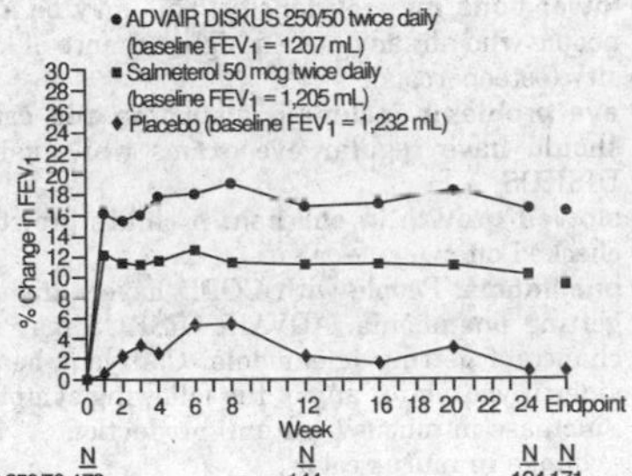

	N	N	N	N
ADVAIR DISKUS 250/50	178	144	124	171
Salmeterol 50 mcg	177	135	119	168
Placebo	185	139	125	172

Figure 5. Predose FEV_1: Mean Percent Change From Baseline in Patients With Chronic Obstructive Pulmonary Disease

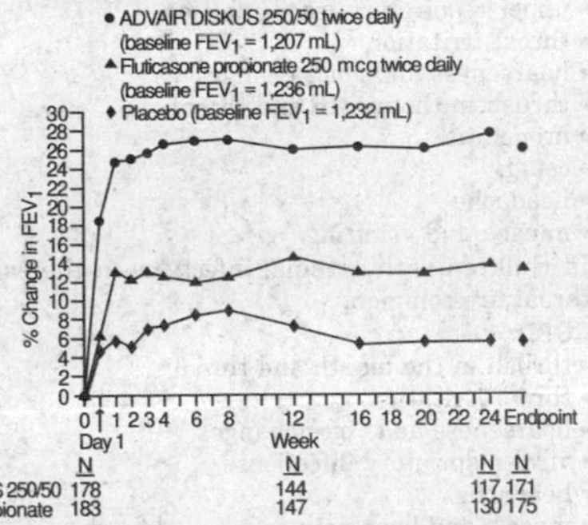

	N	N	N	N
ADVAIR DISKUS 250/50	178	144	117	171
Fluticasone propionate 250 mcg	183	147	130	175
Placebo	185	139	119	172

Figure 6. Two-Hour Postdose FEV_1: Mean Percent Changes From Baseline Over Time in Patients With Chronic Obstructive Pulmonary Disease

The third trial was a 1-year study that evaluated ADVAIR DISKUS 500/50, fluticasone propionate 500 mcg, salmeterol 50 mcg, and placebo in 1,465 patients. The patients had an established history of COPD and exacerbations, a pre-bronchodilator FEV_1 <70% of predicted at study entry, and 8.3% reversibility. The primary endpoint was the comparison of pre-bronchodilator FEV_1 in the groups receiving ADVAIR DISKUS 500/50 or placebo. Patients treated with ADVAIR DISKUS 500/50 had greater improvements in FEV_1 (113 mL, 10%) compared with fluticasone propionate 500 mcg (7 mL, 2%), salmeterol (15 mL, 2%), and placebo (-60 mL, -3%).

Exacerbations: Two studies were primarily designed to evaluate the effect of ADVAIR DISKUS 250/50 on exacerbations. In these 2 studies, exacerbations were defined as worsening of 2 or more major symptoms (dyspnea, sputum volume, and sputum purulence) or worsening of any 1 major symptom together with any 1 of the following minor symptoms: sore throat, colds (nasal discharge and/or nasal congestion), fever without other cause, and increased cough or wheeze for at least 2 consecutive days. COPD exacerbations were considered of moderate severity if treatment with systemic corticosteroids and/or antibiotics was required and were considered severe if hospitalization was required.

Exacerbations were also evaluated as a secondary outcome in the 1- and 3-year trials with ADVAIR DISKUS 500/50. There was not a symptomatic definition of exacerbation in these 2 trials. Exacerbations were defined in terms of severity requiring treatment with antibiotics and/or systemic corticosteroids (moderately severe) or requiring hospitalization (severe).

The 2 exacerbation trials with ADVAIR DISKUS 250/50 were identical studies designed to evaluate the effect of ADVAIR DISKUS 250/50 and salmeterol 50 mcg, each given twice daily, on exacerbations of COPD over a 12-month period. A total of 1,579 patients had an established history of COPD (but no other significant respiratory disorders). Patients had a pre-bronchodilator FEV_1 of 33% of predicted, a mean reversibility of 23% at baseline, and a history of ≥1 COPD exacerbation in the previous year that was moderate or severe. All patients were treated with ADVAIR DISKUS 250/50 twice daily during a 4-week run-in period prior to being assigned study treatment with twice-daily ADVAIR DISKUS 250/50 or salmeterol 50 mcg. In both studies, treatment with ADVAIR DISKUS 250/50 resulted in a significantly lower annual rate of moderate/severe COPD exacerbations compared with salmeterol (30.5% reduction [95% CI: 17.0, 41.8], p<0.001) in the first study and (30.4% reduction [95% CI: 16.9, 41.7], p<0.001) in the second study. Patients treated with ADVAIR DISKUS 250/50 also had a significantly lower annual rate of exacerbations requiring treatment with oral corticosteroids compared with patients treated with salmeterol (39.7% reduction [95% CI: 22.8, 52.9], p <0.001) in the first study and (34.3% reduction [95% CI: 18.6, 47.0], p<0.001) in the second study. Secondary endpoints including pulmonary function and symptom scores improved more in patients treated with ADVAIR DISKUS 250/50 than with salmeterol 50 mcg in both studies

Exacerbations were evaluated in the 1- and the 3-year trials with ADVAIR DISKUS 500/50 as 1 of the secondary efficacy endpoints. In the 1-year trial, the group receiving ADVAIR DISKUS 500/50 had a significantly lower rate of moderate and severe exacerbations compared with placebo (25.4% reduction compared with placebo [95% CI: 13.5, 35.7]) but not when compared with its components (7.5% reduction compared with fluticasone propionate [95% CI: -7.3, 20.3] and 7% reduction compared with salmeterol [95% CI: -8.0, 19.9]). In the 3-year trial, the group receiving ADVAIR DISKUS 500/50 had a significantly lower rate of moderate and severe exacerbations compared with each of the other treatment groups (25.1% reduction compared with placebo [95% CI: 18.6, 31.1], 9.0% reduction compared with fluticasone propionate [95% CI: 1.2, 16.2], and 12.2% reduction compared with salmeterol [95% CI: 4.6, 19.2]).

There were no studies conducted to directly compare the efficacy of ADVAIR DISKUS 250/50 with ADVAIR DISKUS 500/50 on exacerbations. Across studies, the reduction in exacerbations seen with ADVAIR DISKUS 500/50 was not greater than the reduction in exacerbations seen with ADVAIR DISKUS 250/50.

Survival: A 3-year multicenter, international study evaluated the efficacy of ADVAIR DISKUS 500/50 compared with fluticasone propionate 500 mcg, salmeterol 50 mcg, and placebo on survival in 6,112 patients with COPD. During the study patients were permitted usual COPD therapy with the exception of other inhaled corticosteroids and long-acting bronchodilators. The patients were aged 40 to 80 years with an established history of COPD, a pre-bronchodilator FEV_1 <60% of predicted at study entry, and <10% of predicted reversibility. Each patient who withdrew from double-blind treatment for any reason was followed for the full 3-year study period to determine survival status. The primary efficacy endpoint was all-cause mortality. Survival with ADVAIR DISKUS 500/50 was not significantly improved compared with placebo or the individual components (all-cause mortality rate 12.6% ADVAIR DISKUS versus 15.2% placebo). The rates for all-cause mortality were 13.5% and 16.0% in the groups treated with salmeterol 50 mcg and fluticasone propionate 500 mcg, respectively. Secondary outcomes, including pulmonary function (post-bronchodilator FEV_1), improved with ADVAIR DISKUS 500/50, salmeterol, and fluticasone propionate 500/50 compared with placebo.

16 HOW SUPPLIED/STORAGE AND HANDLING

ADVAIR DISKUS 100/50 is supplied as a disposable purple device containing 60 blisters. The DISKUS inhalation device is packaged within a plastic-coated, moisture-protective foil pouch (NDC 0173-0695-00). ADVAIR DISKUS 100/50 is also supplied in an institutional pack of 1 disposable purple device containing 14 blisters. The DISKUS inhalation device is packaged within a plastic-coated, moisture-protective foil pouch (NDC 0173-0695-04).

ADVAIR DISKUS 250/50 is supplied as a disposable purple device containing 60 blisters. The DISKUS inhalation device is packaged within a plastic-coated, moisture-protective foil pouch (NDC 0173-0696-00). ADVAIR DISKUS 250/50 is also supplied in an institutional pack of 1 disposable purple device containing 14 blisters. The DISKUS inhalation device is packaged within a plastic-coated, moisture-protective foil pouch (NDC 0173-0696-04).

ADVAIR DISKUS 500/50 is supplied as a disposable purple device containing 60 blisters. The DISKUS inhalation device is packaged within a plastic-coated, moisture-protective foil pouch (NDC 0173-0697-00). ADVAIR DISKUS 500/50 is also supplied in an institutional pack of 1 disposable purple device containing 14 blisters. The DISKUS inhalation device is packaged within a plastic-coated, moisture-protective foil pouch (NDC 0173-0697-04).

Store at controlled room temperature (see USP), 20° to 25°C (68° to 77°F), in a dry place away from direct heat or sunlight. Keep out of reach of children. The DISKUS inhalation device is not reusable. The device should be discarded 1 month after removal from the moisture-protective foil overwrap pouch or after all blisters have been used (when the dose indicator reads "0"), whichever comes first. Do not attempt to take the device apart.

17 PATIENT COUNSELING INFORMATION

See FDA-approved Medication Guide.

17.1 Asthma-Related Death

Patients with asthma should be informed that salmeterol, one of the active ingredients in ADVAIR DISKUS, increases the risk of asthma-related death and may increase the risk of asthma-related hospitalization in pediatric and adolescent patients. They should also be informed that currently available data are inadequate to determine whether concurrent use of inhaled corticosteroids or other long-term asthma control drugs mitigates the increased risk of asthma-related death from LABAs.

17.2 Not for Acute Symptoms

ADVAIR DISKUS is not meant to relieve acute asthma symptoms or exacerbations of COPD and extra doses should not be used for that purpose. Acute symptoms should be treated with an inhaled, short-acting $beta_2$-agonist such as albuterol. The physician should provide the patient with such medication and instruct the patient in how it should be used.

Patients should be instructed to notify their physician immediately if they experience any of the following:

- Decreasing effectiveness of inhaled, short-acting $beta_2$-agonists
- Need for more inhalations than usual of inhaled, short-acting $beta_2$-agonists
- Significant decrease in lung function as outlined by the physician

Patients should not stop therapy with ADVAIR DISKUS without physician/provider guidance since symptoms may recur after discontinuation.

17.3 Do Not Use Additional Long-Acting $Beta_2$-Agonists

When patients are prescribed ADVAIR DISKUS, other LABAs for asthma and COPD should not be used.

17.4 Risks Associated With Corticosteroid Therapy

Local Effects: Patients should be advised that localized infections with *Candida albicans* occurred in the mouth and pharynx in some patients. If oropharyngeal candidiasis develops, it should be treated with appropriate local or systemic (i.e., oral) antifungal therapy while still continuing therapy with ADVAIR DISKUS, but at times therapy with ADVAIR DISKUS may need to be temporarily interrupted under close medical supervision. Rinsing the mouth after inhalation is advised.

Pneumonia: Patients with COPD have a higher risk of pneumonia and should be instructed to contact their healthcare provider if they develop symptoms of pneumonia.

Immunosuppression: Patients who are on immunosuppressant doses of corticosteroids should be warned to avoid exposure to chickenpox or measles and, if exposed, to consult their physician without delay. Patients should be informed of potential worsening of existing tuberculosis, fungal, bacterial, viral, or parasitic infections, or ocular herpes simplex.

Hypercorticism and Adrenal Suppression: Patients should be advised that ADVAIR DISKUS may cause systemic corticosteroid effects of hypercorticism and adrenal suppression. Additionally, patients should be instructed that deaths due to adrenal insufficiency have occurred during and after transfer from systemic corticosteroids. Patients should taper slowly from systemic corticosteroids if transferring to ADVAIR DISKUS.

Reduction in Bone Mineral Density: Patients who are at an increased risk for decreased BMD should be advised that the use of corticosteroids may pose an additional risk.

Reduced Growth Velocity: Patients should be informed that orally inhaled corticosteroids, including fluticasone propionate, a component of ADVAIR DISKUS, may cause a reduction in growth velocity when administered to pediatric patients. Physicians should closely follow the growth of children and adolescents taking corticosteroids by any route.

Ocular Effects: Long-term use of inhaled corticosteroids may increase the risk of some eye problems (cataracts or glaucoma); regular eye examinations should be considered.

17.5 Risks Associated With Beta-Agonist Therapy

Patients should be informed of adverse effects associated with beta$_2$-agonists, such as palpitations, chest pain, rapid heart rate, tremor, or nervousness.

ADVAIR, ADVAIR DISKUS, DISKHALER, DISKUS, FLONASE, FLOVENT, ROTADISK, SEREVENT, and VENTOLIN are registered trademarks of GlaxoSmithKline.

GlaxoSmithKline
Research Triangle Park, NC 27709

September 2011
ADD: 9PI

MEDICATION GUIDE

ADVAIR [*ad' vair*] DISKUS® 100/50
(fluticasone propionate 100 mcg and salmeterol 50 mcg inhalation powder)
ADVAIR DISKUS® 250/50
(fluticasone propionate 250 mcg and salmeterol 50 mcg inhalation powder)
ADVAIR DISKUS® 500/50
(fluticasone propionate 500 mcg and salmeterol 50 mcg inhalation powder)

Read the Medication Guide that comes with ADVAIR DISKUS before you start using it and each time you get a refill. There may be new information. This Medication Guide does not take the place of talking to your healthcare provider about your medical condition or treatment.

What is the most important information I should know about ADVAIR DISKUS?

ADVAIR DISKUS can cause serious side effects, including:

1. **People with asthma who take long-acting beta$_2$-adrenergic agonist (LABA) medicines, such as salmeterol (one of the medicines in ADVAIR DISKUS), have an increased risk of death from asthma problems.** It is not known whether fluticasone propionate, the other medicine in ADVAIR DISKUS, reduces the risk of death from asthma problems seen with salmeterol.
   - **Call your healthcare provider if breathing problems worsen over time while using ADVAIR DISKUS. You may need different treatment.**
   - **Get emergency medical care if:**
     - breathing problems worsen quickly and
     - you use your rescue inhaler medicine, but it does not relieve your breathing problems.
2. ADVAIR DISKUS should be used only if your healthcare provider decides that your asthma is not well controlled with a long-term asthma control medicine, such as inhaled corticosteroids.
3. When your asthma is well controlled, your healthcare provider may tell you to stop taking ADVAIR DISKUS. Your healthcare provider will decide if you can stop ADVAIR DISKUS without loss of asthma control. Your healthcare provider may prescribe a different asthma control medicine for you, such as an inhaled corticosteroid.
4. Children and adolescents who take LABA medicines may have an increased risk of being hospitalized for asthma problems.

What is ADVAIR DISKUS?

- ADVAIR DISKUS combines an inhaled corticosteroid medicine, fluticasone propionate (the same medicine found in FLOVENT®), and a LABA medicine, salmeterol (the same medicine found in SEREVENT®).
  - Inhaled corticosteroids help to decrease inflammation in the lungs. Inflammation in the lungs can lead to asthma symptoms.
  - LABA medicines are used in people with asthma and chronic obstructive pulmonary disease (COPD). LABA medicines help the muscles around the airways in your lungs stay relaxed to prevent symptoms, such as wheezing and shortness of breath. These symptoms can happen when the muscles around the airways tighten. This makes it hard to breathe. In severe cases, wheezing can stop your breathing and cause death if not treated right away.
- ADVAIR DISKUS is used for asthma and COPD as follows:

Asthma:

ADVAIR DISKUS is used to control symptoms of asthma and to prevent symptoms such as wheezing in adults and children aged 4 years and older.

ADVAIR DISKUS contains salmeterol (the same medicine found in SEREVENT). LABA medicines, such as salmeterol, increase the risk of death from asthma problems.

ADVAIR DISKUS is not for adults and children with asthma who are well controlled with an asthma control medicine, such as a low to medium dose of an inhaled corticosteroid medicine.

COPD:

COPD is a chronic lung disease that includes chronic bronchitis, emphysema, or both. ADVAIR DISKUS 250/50 is used long term, 2 times each day to help improve lung function for better breathing in adults with COPD. ADVAIR DISKUS 250/50 has been shown to decrease the number of flare-ups and worsening of COPD symptoms (exacerbations).

Who should not use ADVAIR DISKUS?

Do not use ADVAIR DISKUS:
- to treat sudden, severe symptoms of asthma or COPD and
- if you have a severe allergy to milk proteins. Ask your doctor if you are not sure.

What should I tell my healthcare provider before using ADVAIR DISKUS?

Tell your healthcare provider about all of your health conditions, including if you:
- **have heart problems**
- **have high blood pressure**
- **have seizures**
- **have thyroid problems**
- **have diabetes**
- **have liver problems**
- **have osteoporosis**
- **have an immune system problem**
- **are pregnant or planning to become pregnant.** It is not known if ADVAIR DISKUS may harm your unborn baby.
- **are breastfeeding.** It is not known if ADVAIR DISKUS passes into your milk and if it can harm your baby.
- **are allergic to any of the ingredients in ADVAIR DISKUS, any other medicines, or food products.** See the end of this Medication Guide for a complete list of the ingredients in ADVAIR DISKUS.
- **are exposed to chickenpox or measles**

Tell your healthcare provider about all the medicines you take including prescription and non-prescription medicines, vitamins, and herbal supplements. ADVAIR DISKUS and certain other medicines may interact with each other. This may cause serious side effects. Especially, tell your healthcare provider if you take ritonavir. The anti-HIV medicines NORVIR® (ritonavir capsules) Soft Gelatin, NORVIR (ritonavir oral solution), and KALETRA® (lopinavir/ritonavir) Tablets contain ritonavir.

Know the medicines you take. Keep a list and show it to your healthcare provider and pharmacist each time you get a new medicine.

How do I use ADVAIR DISKUS?

See the step-by-step instructions for using ADVAIR DISKUS at the end of this Medication Guide. Do not use ADVAIR DISKUS unless your healthcare provider has taught you and you understand everything. Ask your healthcare provider or pharmacist if you have any questions.

- Children should use ADVAIR DISKUS with an adult's help, as instructed by the child's healthcare provider.
- Use ADVAIR DISKUS exactly as prescribed. **Do not use ADVAIR DISKUS more often than prescribed.** ADVAIR DISKUS comes in 3 strengths. Your healthcare provider has prescribed the one that is best for your condition.
- The usual dosage of ADVAIR DISKUS is 1 inhalation 2 times each day (morning and evening). The 2 doses should be about 12 hours apart. Rinse your mouth with water after using ADVAIR DISKUS.
- If you take more ADVAIR DISKUS than your doctor has prescribed, get medical help right away if you have any unusual symptoms, such as worsening shortness of breath, chest pain, increased heart rate, or shakiness.
- If you miss a dose of ADVAIR DISKUS, just skip that dose. Take your next dose at your usual time. Do not take 2 doses at one time.
- Do not use a spacer device with ADVAIR DISKUS.
- Do not breathe into ADVAIR DISKUS.
- **While you are using ADVAIR DISKUS 2 times each day, do not use other medicines that contain a LABA for any reason.** Ask your healthcare provider or pharmacist if any of your other medicines are LABA medicines.
- Do not stop using ADVAIR DISKUS or other asthma medicines unless told to do so by your healthcare provider because your symptoms might get worse. Your healthcare provider will change your medicines as needed.
- ADVAIR DISKUS does not relieve sudden symptoms. Always have a rescue inhaler medicine with you to treat sudden symptoms. If you do not have an inhaled, short-acting bronchodilator, call your healthcare provider to have one prescribed for you.
- Call your healthcare provider or get medical care right away if:
  - your breathing problems worsen with ADVAIR DISKUS
  - you need to use your rescue inhaler medicine more often than usual
  - your rescue inhaler medicine does not work as well for you at relieving symptoms
  - you need to use 4 or more inhalations of your rescue inhaler medicine for 2 or more days in a row
  - you use 1 whole canister of your rescue inhaler medicine in 8 weeks' time
  - your peak flow meter results decrease. Your healthcare provider will tell you the numbers that are right for you.
  - you have asthma and your symptoms do not improve after using ADVAIR DISKUS regularly for 1 week

What are the possible side effects with ADVAIR DISKUS?

ADVAIR DISKUS can cause serious side effects, including:
- **See "What is the most important information I should know about ADVAIR DISKUS?"**
- **serious allergic reactions.** Call your healthcare provider or get emergency medical care if you get any of the following symptoms of a serious allergic reaction:
  - rash
  - hives
  - swelling of the face, mouth, and tongue
  - breathing problems
- **sudden breathing problems immediately after inhaling your medicine**
- **effects on heart**
  - increased blood pressure
  - a fast and irregular heartbeat
  - chest pain
- **effects on nervous system**
  - tremor
  - nervousness
- **reduced adrenal function (may result in loss of energy)**
- **changes in blood (sugar, potassium, certain types of white blood cells)**
- **weakened immune system and a higher chance of infections**
- **lower bone mineral density.** This may be a problem for people who already have a higher chance of low bone density (osteoporosis).
- **eye problems including glaucoma and cataracts.** You should have regular eye exams while using ADVAIR DISKUS.
- **slowed growth in children.** A child's growth should be checked often.
- **pneumonia.** People with COPD have a higher chance of getting pneumonia. ADVAIR DISKUS may increase the chance of getting pneumonia. Call your healthcare provider if you notice any of the following symptoms:
  - increase in mucus (sputum) production
  - change in mucus color
  - fever
  - chills
  - increased cough
  - increased breathing problems

Common side effects of ADVAIR DISKUS include:

Asthma:
- upper respiratory tract infection
- throat irritation
- hoarseness and voice changes
- thrush in the mouth and throat
- bronchitis
- cough
- headache
- nausea and vomiting

In children with asthma, infections in the ear, nose, and throat are common.

COPD:
- thrush in the mouth and throat
- throat irritation
- hoarseness and voice changes
- viral respiratory infections
- headache
- muscle and bone pain

Tell your healthcare provider about any side effect that bothers you or that does not go away.

These are not all the side effects with ADVAIR DISKUS. Ask your healthcare provider or pharmacist for more information.

Call your doctor for medical advice about side effects. You may report side effects to FDA at 1-800-FDA-1088.

How do I store ADVAIR DISKUS?
- Store ADVAIR DISKUS at room temperature between 68°F to 77°F (20°C to 25°C). Keep in a dry place away from heat and sunlight.
- Safely discard ADVAIR DISKUS 1 month after you remove it from the foil pouch, or after the dose indicator reads "0", whichever comes first.
- Keep ADVAIR DISKUS and all medicines out of the reach of children.

General Information about ADVAIR DISKUS

Medicines are sometimes prescribed for purposes not mentioned in a Medication Guide. Do not use ADVAIR DISKUS for a condition for which it was not prescribed. Do not give your ADVAIR DISKUS to other people, even if they have the same condition that you have. It may harm them.

This Medication Guide summarizes the most important information about ADVAIR DISKUS. If you would like more information, talk with your healthcare provider or pharmacist. You can ask your healthcare provider or pharmacist for information about ADVAIR DISKUS that was written for healthcare professionals. You can also contact the company that makes ADVAIR DISKUS (toll free) at 1-888-825-5249 or at www.advair.com.

What are the ingredients in ADVAIR DISKUS?

Active ingredients: fluticasone propionate, salmeterol xinafoate

Inactive ingredient: lactose (contains milk proteins)

Instructions for Using ADVAIR DISKUS

Follow the instructions below for using your ADVAIR DISKUS. **You will breathe in (inhale) the medicine from the DISKUS®.** If you have any questions, ask your healthcare provider or pharmacist.

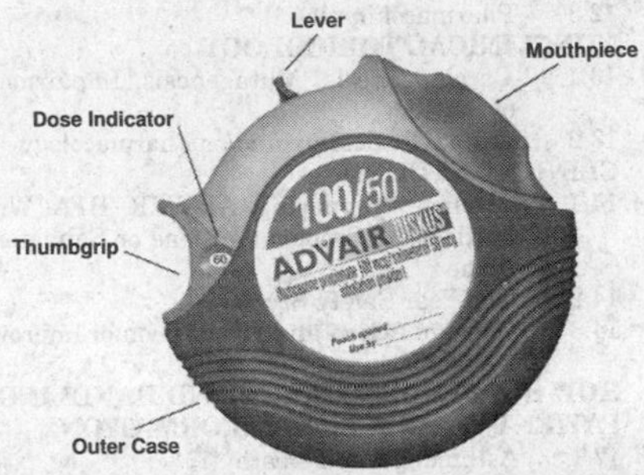

Take ADVAIR DISKUS out of the box and foil pouch. Write the **"Pouch opened"** and **"Use by"** dates on the label on top of the DISKUS. **The "Use by" date is 1 month from date of opening the pouch.**

- The DISKUS will be in the closed position when the pouch is opened.
- The **dose indicator** on the top of the DISKUS tells you how many doses are left. The dose indicator number will decrease each time you use the DISKUS. After you have used 55 doses from the DISKUS, the numbers 5 to 0 will appear in **red** to warn you that there are only a few doses left *(see Figure 1)*. If you are using a "sample" DISKUS, the numbers 5 to 0 will appear in red after 9 doses.

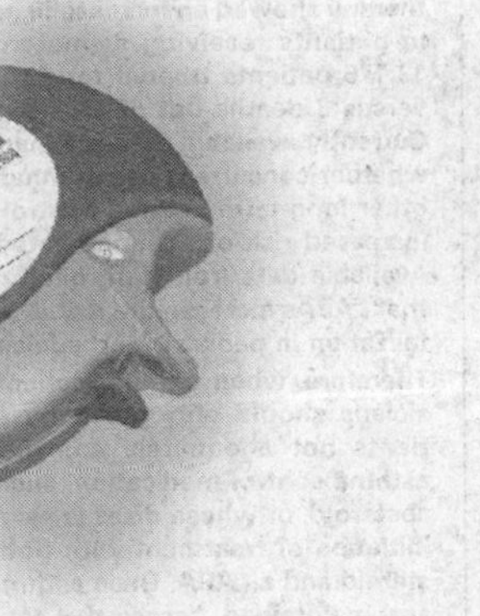

Figure 1

Taking a dose from the DISKUS requires the following 3 simple steps: Open, Click, Inhale.

1. OPEN

Hold the DISKUS in one hand and put the thumb of your other hand on the **thumbgrip**. Push your thumb away from you as far as it will go until the mouthpiece appears and snaps into position *(see Figure 2)*.

[See figure 2 at top of next column]

2. CLICK

Hold the DISKUS in a level, flat position with the mouthpiece towards you. Slide the **lever** away from you as far as it will go until it **clicks***(see Figure 3)*. The DISKUS is now ready to use.

[See figure 3 at top of next column]

Every time the **lever** is pushed back, a dose is ready to be inhaled. This is shown by a decrease in numbers on the dose counter. **To avoid releasing or wasting doses once the DISKUS is ready:**

- **Do not close the DISKUS.**
- **Do not tilt the DISKUS.**
- **Do not play with the lever.**
- **Do not move the lever more than once.**

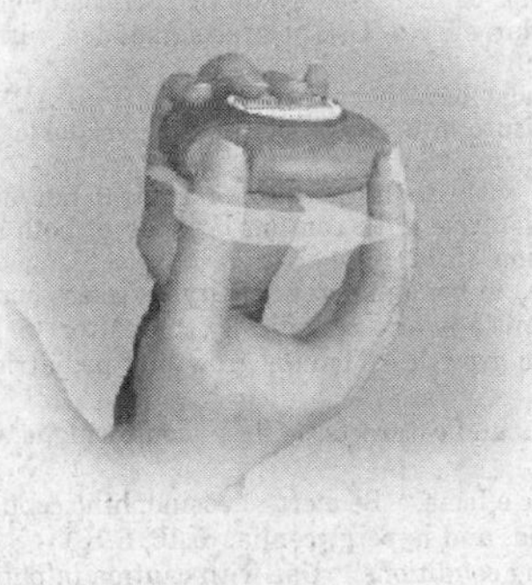

Figure 2

Figure 3

3. INHALE

Before inhaling your dose from the DISKUS, breathe out (exhale) fully while holding the DISKUS level and away from your mouth *(see Figure 4)*. **Remember, never breathe out into the DISKUS mouthpiece.**

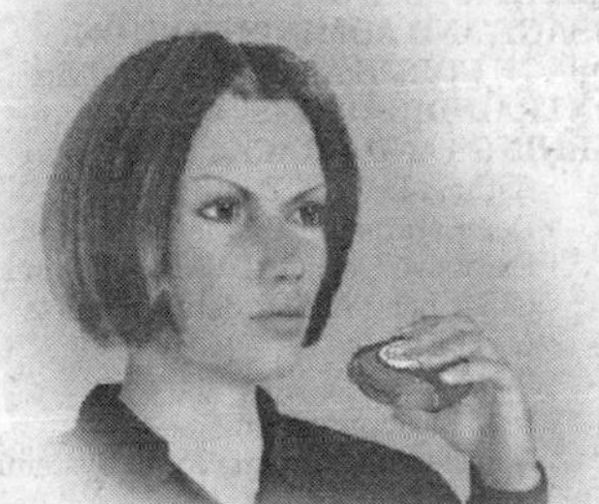

Figure 4

Put the mouthpiece to your lips *(see Figure 5)*. Breathe in quickly and deeply through the DISKUS. Do not breathe in through your nose.

[See figure 5 at top of next column]

Remove the DISKUS from your mouth. Hold your breath for about 10 seconds, or for as long as is comfortable. Breathe out slowly.

The DISKUS delivers your dose of medicine as a very fine powder. Patients may or may not taste or feel the powder. Do not use an extra dose from the DISKUS if you do not feel or taste the medicine.

Rinse your mouth with water after breathing-in the medicine. Spit the water out. Do not swallow.

4. Close the DISKUS when you are finished taking a dose so that the DISKUS will be ready for you to take your next dose. Put your thumb on the thumbgrip and slide the thumbgrip back towards you as far as it will go *(see Figure*

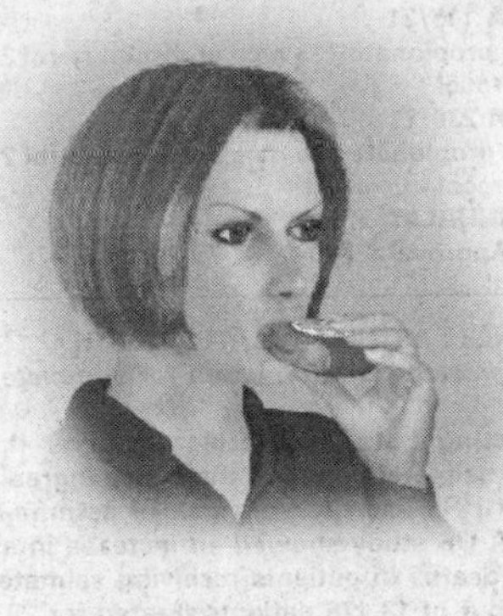

Figure 5

6). The DISKUS will click shut. The lever will automatically return to its original position. The DISKUS is now ready for you to take your next scheduled dose, due in about 12 hours. (Repeat steps 1 to 4.)

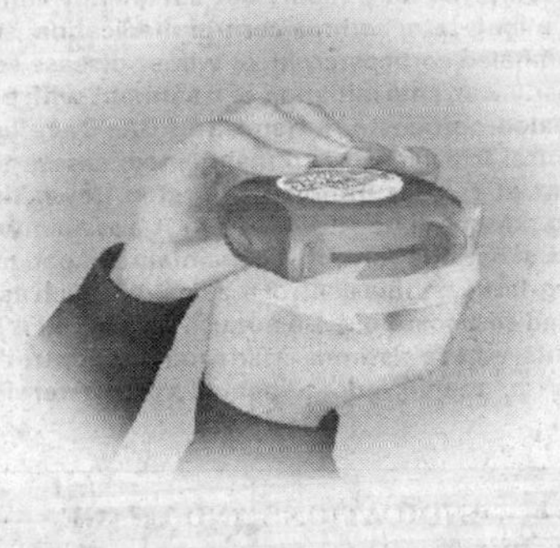

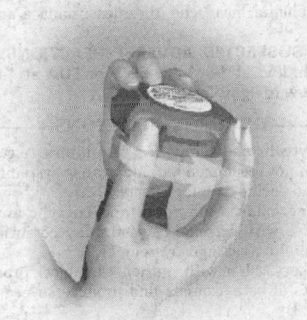

Figure 6

Remember:

- Never breathe into the DISKUS.
- Never take the DISKUS apart.
- Always ready and use the DISKUS in a level, flat position.
- Do not use the DISKUS with a spacer device.
- After each dose, rinse your mouth with water and spit the water out. Do not swallow.
- Never wash the mouthpiece or any part of the DISKUS. **Keep it dry.**
- Always keep the DISKUS in a dry place.
- Never take an extra dose, even if you did not taste or feel the medicine.

This Medication Guide has been approved by the U.S. Food and Drug Administration.

GlaxoSmithKline
Research Triangle Park, NC 27709

January 2011
ADD:7MG

ADVAIR HFA 45/21 ℞

[ad' vair]

(fluticasone propionate 45 mcg and salmeterol 21 mcg)
Inhalation Aerosol

ADVAIR HFA 115/21

(fluticasone propionate 115 mcg and salmeterol 21 mcg)
Inhalation Aerosol

ADVAIR HFA 230/21

(fluticasone propionate 230 mcg and salmeterol 21 mcg)
Inhalation Aerosol
FOR ORAL INHALATION

HIGHLIGHTS OF PRESCRIBING INFORMATION

These highlights do not include all the information needed to use ADVAIR HFA safely and effectively. See full prescribing information for ADVAIR HFA.

ADVAIR HFA 45/21
(fluticasone propionate 45 mcg and salmeterol 21 mcg) Inhalation Aerosol
ADVAIR HFA 115/21
(fluticasone propionate 115 mcg and salmeterol 21 mcg) Inhalation Aerosol
ADVAIR HFA 230/21
(fluticasone propionate 230 mcg and salmeterol 21 mcg) Inhalation Aerosol
FOR ORAL INHALATION
Initial U.S. Approval: 2000

WARNING: ASTHMA-RELATED DEATH
See full prescribing information for complete boxed warning

- **Long-acting $beta_2$-adrenergic agonists (LABAs), such as salmeterol, one of the active ingredients in ADVAIR HFA, increase the risk of asthma-related death. A US study showed an increase in asthma-related deaths in patients receiving salmeterol (13 deaths out of 13,176 patients treated for 28 weeks on salmeterol versus 3 out of 13,179 patients on placebo). Currently available data are inadequate to determine whether concurrent use of inhaled corticosteroids or other long-term asthma control drugs mitigates the increased risk of asthma-related death from LABAs. Available data from controlled clinical trials suggest that LABAs increase the risk of asthma-related hospitalization in pediatric and adolescent patients. (5.1)**
- **When treating patients with asthma, only prescribe ADVAIR HFA for patients not adequately controlled on a long-term asthma control medication, such as an inhaled corticosteroid, or whose disease severity clearly warrants initiation of treatment with both an inhaled corticosteroid and a LABA. Once asthma control is achieved and maintained, assess the patient at regular intervals and step down therapy (e.g., discontinue ADVAIR HFA) if possible without loss of asthma control and maintain the patient on a long-term asthma control medication, such as an inhaled corticosteroid. Do not use ADVAIR HFA for patients whose asthma is adequately controlled on low- or medium-dose inhaled corticosteroids. (1, 5.1)**

INDICATIONS AND USAGE

ADVAIR HFA is a combination product containing a corticosteroid and a LABA indicated for treatment of asthma in patients aged 12 years and older. (1)
Important limitation: (1)
- Not indicated for the relief of acute bronchospasm. (1)

DOSAGE AND ADMINISTRATION

For oral inhalation only. (2)
Treatment of asthma in patients ≥12 years: 2 inhalations of ADVAIR HFA 45/21, 115/21, or 230/21 twice daily. Starting dosage is based on asthma severity. (2)

DOSAGE FORMS AND STRENGTHS

Inhalation aerosol: delivers a combination of fluticasone propionate (45, 115, or 230 mcg) and salmeterol (21 mcg) from mouthpiece per actuation. (3)

CONTRAINDICATIONS

- Primary treatment of status asthmaticus or acute episodes of asthma requiring intensive measures. (4)
- Hypersensitivity to any ingredient. (4)

WARNINGS AND PRECAUTIONS

- Asthma-related death: LABAs increase the risk. Prescribe only for recommended patient populations. (5.1)
- Deterioration of disease and acute episodes: Do not initiate in acutely deteriorating asthma or to treat acute symptoms. (5.2)
- Use with additional LABA: Do not use in combination because of risk of overdose. (5.3)
- Localized infections: *Candida albicans* infection of the mouth and throat may occur. Monitor patients periodically for signs of adverse effects on the oral cavity. Advise patients to rinse the mouth following inhalation. (5.4)
- Pneumonia: Increased risk in patients with COPD. Monitor patients for signs and symptoms of pneumonia. (5.5)
- Immunosuppression: Potential worsening of infections (e.g., existing tuberculosis, fungal, bacterial, viral, or parasitic infection; ocular herpes simplex). Use with caution in patients with these infections. More serious or even fatal course of chickenpox or measles can occur in susceptible patients. (5.6)
- Transferring patients from systemic corticosteroids: Risk of impaired adrenal function when transferring from oral steroids. Taper patients slowly from systemic corticosteroids if transferring to ADVAIR HFA. (5.7)
- Hypercorticism and adrenal suppression: May occur with very high dosages or at the regular dosage in susceptible individuals. If such changes occur, discontinue ADVAIR HFA slowly. (5.8)
- Strong cytochrome P450 3A4 inhibitors (e.g., ritonavir): Risk of increased systemic corticosteroid and cardiovascular effects. Use not recommended with ADVAIR HFA. (5.9)
- Paradoxical bronchospasm: Discontinue ADVAIR HFA and institute alternative therapy if paradoxical bronchospasm occurs. (5.10)
- Patients with cardiovascular or central nervous system disorders: Use with caution because of beta-adrenergic stimulation. (5.12)
- Decreases in bone mineral density: Assess bone mineral density initially and periodically thereafter. (5.13)
- Effects on growth: Monitor growth of pediatric patients. (5.14)
- Glaucoma and cataracts: Close monitoring is warranted. (5.15)
- Metabolic effects: Be alert to eosinophilic conditions, hypokalemia, and hyperglycemia. (5.16, 5.18)
- Coexisting conditions: Use with caution in patients with convulsive disorders, thyrotoxicosis, diabetes mellitus, and ketoacidosis. (5.17)

ADVERSE REACTIONS

Most common adverse reactions (incidence ≥3%) are: upper respiratory tract infection or inflammation, throat irritation, dysphonia, headache, dizziness, nausea and vomiting. (6.1)
To report SUSPECTED ADVERSE REACTIONS, contact GlaxoSmithKline at 1-888-825-5249 or FDA at 1-800-FDA-1088 or www.fda.gov/medwatch.

DRUG INTERACTIONS

- Strong cytochrome P450 3A4 inhibitors (e.g., ritonavir): Use not recommended. May cause systemic corticosteroid and cardiovascular effects. (7.1)
- Monoamine oxidase inhibitors and tricyclic antidepressants: Use with extreme caution. May potentiate effect of salmeterol on vascular system. (7.2)
- Beta-blockers: Use with caution. May block bronchodilatory effects of beta-agonists and produce severe bronchospasm. (7.3)
- Diuretics: Use with caution. Electrocardiographic changes and/or hypokalemia associated with nonpotassium-sparing diuretics may worsen with concomitant beta-agonists. (7.4)

USE IN SPECIFIC POPULATIONS

Hepatic impairment: Monitor patients for signs of increased drug exposure. (8.6)
See 17 for PATIENT COUNSELING INFORMATION and Medication Guide

Revised: 03/2013

FULL PRESCRIBING INFORMATION: CONTENTS*

*** Sections or subsections omitted from the full prescribing information are not listed**

FULL PRESCRIBING INFORMATION

WARNING: ASTHMA-RELATED DEATH

Long-acting $beta_2$-adrenergic agonists (LABAs), such as salmeterol, one of the active ingredients in ADVAIR® HFA, increase the risk of asthma-related death. Data from a large placebo-controlled US study that compared the safety of salmeterol (SEREVENT® Inhalation Aerosol) or placebo added to usual asthma therapy showed an increase in asthma-related deaths in patients receiving salmeterol (13 deaths out of 13,176 patients treated for 28 weeks on salmeterol versus 3 deaths out of 13,179 patients on placebo). Currently available data are inadequate to determine whether concurrent use of inhaled corticosteroids or other long-term asthma control drugs mitigates the increased risk of asthma-related death from LABAs. Available data from controlled clinical trials suggest that LABAs increase the risk of asthma-related hospitalization in pediatric and adolescent patients.

Therefore, when treating patients with asthma, physicians should only prescribe ADVAIR HFA for patients not adequately controlled on a long-term asthma control medication, such as an inhaled corticosteroid, or whose disease severity clearly warrants initiation of treatment with both an inhaled corticosteroid and a LABA. Once asthma control is achieved and maintained, assess the patient at regular intervals and step down therapy (e.g., discontinue ADVAIR HFA) if possible without loss of asthma control and maintain the patient on a long-term asthma control medication, such as an inhaled corticosteroid. Do not use ADVAIR HFA for patients whose asthma is adequately controlled on low- or medium-dose inhaled corticosteroids *[see Warnings and Precautions (5.1)]*.

1 INDICATIONS AND USAGE

ADVAIR HFA is indicated for the treatment of asthma in patients aged 12 years and older.
Long-acting $beta_2$-adrenergic agonists (LABAs), such as salmeterol, one of the active ingredients in ADVAIR HFA, increase the risk of asthma-related death. Available data from controlled clinical trials suggest that LABAs increase the risk of asthma-related hospitalization in pediatric and adolescent patients *[see Warnings and Precautions (5.1)]*. Therefore, when treating patients with asthma, physicians should only prescribe ADVAIR HFA for patients not adequately controlled on a long-term asthma control medication, such as an inhaled corticosteroid, or whose disease severity clearly warrants initiation of treatment with both an inhaled corticosteroid and a LABA. Once asthma control is

Table 1. Asthma-Related Deaths in the 28-Week Salmeterol Multi-center Asthma Research Trial (SMART)

	Salmeterol n (%[a])	Placebo n (%[a])	Relative Risk[b] (95% Confidence Interval)	Excess Deaths Expressed per 10,000 Patients[c] (95% Confidence Interval)
Total Population[d]				
Salmeterol: n = 13,176	13 (0.10%)		4.37 (1.25, 15.34)	8 (3, 13)
Placebo: n = 13,179		3 (0.02%)		
Caucasian				
Salmeterol: n = 9,281	6 (0.07%)		5.82 (0.70, 48.37)	6 (1, 10)
Placebo: n = 9,361		1 (0.01%)		
African American				
Salmeterol: n = 2,366	7 (0.31%)		7.26 (0.89, 58.94)	27 (8, 46)
Placebo: n = 2,319		1 (0.04%)		

[a]Life-table 28-week estimate, adjusted according to the patients' actual lengths of exposure to study treatment to account for early withdrawal of patients from the study.
[b]Relative risk is the ratio of the rate of asthma-related death in the salmeterol group and the rate in the placebo group. The relative risk indicates how many more times likely an asthma-related death occurred in the salmeterol group than in the placebo group in a 28-week treatment period.
[c]Estimate of the number of additional asthma-related deaths in patients treated with salmeterol in SMART, assuming 10,000 patients received salmeterol for a 28-week treatment period. Estimate calculated as the difference between the salmeterol and placebo groups in the rates of asthma-related death multiplied by 10,000.
[d]The Total Population includes the following ethnic origins listed on the case report form: Caucasian, African American, Hispanic, Asian, and "Other." In addition, the Total Population includes those patients whose ethnic origin was not reported. The results for Caucasian and African American subpopulations are shown above. No asthma-related deaths occurred in the Hispanic (salmeterol n = 996, placebo n = 999), Asian (salmeterol n = 173, placebo n = 149), or "Other" (salmeterol n = 230, placebo n = 224) subpopulations. One asthma-related death occurred in the placebo group in the subpopulation whose ethnic origin was not reported (salmeterol n = 130, placebo n = 127).

achieved and maintained, assess the patient at regular intervals and step down therapy (e.g., discontinue ADVAIR HFA) if possible without loss of asthma control and maintain the patient on a long-term asthma control medication, such as an inhaled corticosteroid. Do not use ADVAIR HFA for patients whose asthma is adequately controlled on low- or medium-dose inhaled corticosteroids.

Important Limitation of Use: ADVAIR HFA is NOT indicated for the relief of acute bronchospasm.

2 DOSAGE AND ADMINISTRATION

ADVAIR HFA should be administered twice daily every day by the orally inhaled route only. After inhalation, the patient should rinse the mouth with water without swallowing *[see Patient Counseling Information (17.4)]*.

More frequent administration or a higher number of inhalations (more than 2 inhalations twice daily) of the prescribed strength of ADVAIR HFA is not recommended as some patients are more likely to experience adverse effects with higher doses of salmeterol. Patients using ADVAIR HFA should not use additional LABAs for any reason. *[See Warnings and Precautions (5.3, 5.12).]*

If asthma symptoms arise in the period between doses, an inhaled, short-acting beta$_2$–agonist should be taken for immediate relief.

For patients aged 12 years and older, the dosage is 2 inhalations twice daily (morning and evening, approximately 12 hours apart).

The recommended starting dosages for ADVAIR HFA for patients aged 12 years and older are based upon patients' asthma severity.

The maximum recommended dosage is 2 inhalations of ADVAIR HFA 230/21 twice daily.

Improvement in asthma control following inhaled administration of ADVAIR HFA can occur within 30 minutes of beginning treatment, although maximum benefit may not be achieved for 1 week or longer after starting treatment. Individual patients will experience a variable time to onset and degree of symptom relief.

For patients who do not respond adequately to the starting dosage after 2 weeks of therapy, replacing the current strength of ADVAIR HFA with a higher strength may provide additional improvement in asthma control.

If a previously effective dosage regimen of ADVAIR HFA fails to provide adequate improvement in asthma control, the therapeutic regimen should be reevaluated and additional therapeutic options (e.g., replacing the current strength of ADVAIR HFA with a higher strength, adding additional inhaled corticosteroid, initiating oral corticosteroids) should be considered.

ADVAIR HFA should be primed before using for the first time by releasing 4 test sprays into the air away from the face, shaking well for 5 seconds before each spray. In cases where the inhaler has not been used for more than 4 weeks or when it has been dropped, prime the inhaler again by releasing 2 test sprays into the air away from the face, shaking well for 5 seconds before each spray.

3 DOSAGE FORMS AND STRENGTHS

ADVAIR HFA is an inhalation aerosol. Each actuation delivers a combination of fluticasone propionate (45, 115, or 230 mcg) and salmeterol (21 mcg) from the actuator. ADVAIR HFA is supplied in 8- and 12-g pressurized aluminum canisters containing 60 and 120 metered inhalations, respectively. Each canister is fitted with a counter and a purple actuator with a light purple strapcap.

4 CONTRAINDICATIONS

The use of ADVAIR HFA is contraindicated in the following conditions:

- Primary treatment of status asthmaticus or other acute episodes of asthma where intensive measures are required.
- Hypersensitivity to any of the ingredients of these preparations contraindicates their use *[see Description (11)]*.

5 WARNINGS AND PRECAUTIONS

5.1 Asthma-Related Death

LABAs, such as salmeterol, one of the active ingredients in ADVAIR HFA, increase the risk of asthma-related death. Currently available data are inadequate to determine whether concurrent use of inhaled corticosteroids or other long-term asthma control drugs mitigates the increased risk of asthma-related death from LABAs. Available data from controlled clinical trials suggest that LABAs increase the risk of asthma-related hospitalization in pediatric and adolescent patients. Therefore, when treating patients with asthma, physicians should only prescribe ADVAIR HFA for patients not adequately controlled on a long-term asthma control medication such as an inhaled corticosteroid, or whose disease severity clearly warrants initiation of treatment with both an inhaled corticosteroid and a LABA. Once asthma control is achieved and maintained, assess the patient at regular intervals and step down therapy (e.g., discontinue ADVAIR HFA) if possible without loss of asthma control and maintain the patient on a long-term asthma control medication, such as an inhaled corticosteroid. Do not use ADVAIR HFA for patients whose asthma is adequately controlled on low- or medium-dose inhaled corticosteroids.

A large placebo-controlled US study that compared the safety of salmeterol with placebo, each added to usual asthma therapy, showed an increase in asthma-related deaths in patients receiving salmeterol. The Salmeterol Multi-center Asthma Research Trial (SMART) was a randomized double-blind study that enrolled LABA-naive patients with asthma to assess the safety of salmeterol (SEREVENT Inhalation Aerosol) 42 mcg twice daily over 28 weeks compared with placebo when added to usual asthma therapy. A planned interim analysis was conducted when approximately half of the intended number of patients had been enrolled (N = 26,355), which led to premature termination of the study. The results of the interim analysis showed that patients receiving salmeterol were at increased risk for fatal asthma events (see Table 3 and Figure 5). In the total population, a higher rate of asthma-related death occurred in patients treated with salmeterol than those treated with placebo (0.10% versus 0.02%; relative risk: 4.37 [95% CI: 1.25, 15.34]).

Post-hoc subpopulation analyses were performed. In Caucasians, asthma-related death occurred at a higher rate in patients treated with salmeterol than in patients treated with placebo (0.07% versus 0.01%; relative risk: 5.82 [95% CI: 0.70, 48.37]). In African Americans also, asthma-related death occurred at a higher rate in patients treated with salmeterol than those treated with placebo (0.31% versus 0.04%; relative risk: 7.26 [95% CI: 0.89, 58.94]). Although the relative risks of asthma-related death were similar in Caucasians and African Americans, the estimate of excess deaths in patients treated with salmeterol was greater in African Americans because there was a higher overall rate of asthma-related death in African American patients (see Table 3). Given the similar basic mechanisms of action of beta$_2$-agonists, the findings seen in the SMART study are considered a class effect.

Post-hoc analyses in pediatric patients aged 12 to 18 years were also performed. Pediatric patients accounted for approximately 12% of patients in each treatment arm. Respiratory-related death or life-threatening experience occurred at a similar rate in the salmeterol group (0.12% [2/1,653]) and the placebo group (0.12% [2/1,622]; relative risk: 1.0 [95% CI: 0.1, 7.2]). All–cause hospitalization, however, was increased in the salmeterol group (2% [35/1,653]) versus the placebo group (<1% [16/1,622]; relative risk: 2.1 [95% CI: 1.1, 3.7]).

The data from the SMART study are not adequate to determine whether concurrent use of inhaled corticosteroids, such as fluticasone propionate, the other active ingredient in ADVAIR HFA, or other long-term asthma control therapy mitigates the risk of asthma-related death.

[See table 1 above]

Figure 1. Cumulative Incidence of Asthma-Related Deaths in the 28-Week Salmeterol Multi-center Asthma Research Trial (SMART), by Duration of Treatment

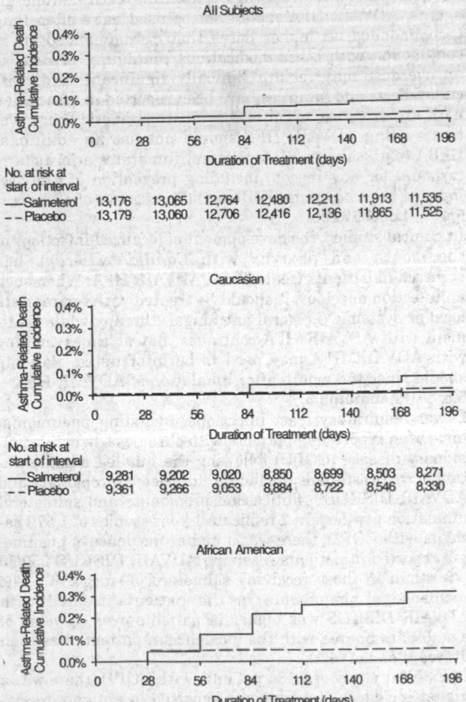

A 16-week clinical study performed in the United Kingdom, the Salmeterol Nationwide Surveillance (SNS) study, showed results similar to the SMART study. In the SNS study, the rate of asthma-related death was numerically, though not statistically significantly, greater in patients with asthma treated with salmeterol (42 mcg twice daily) than those treated with albuterol (180 mcg 4 times daily) added to usual asthma therapy.

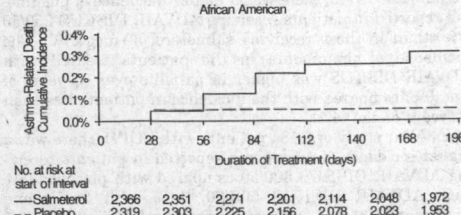

5.2 Deterioration of Disease and Acute Episodes
ADVAIR HFA should not be initiated in patients during rapidly deteriorating or potentially life-threatening episodes of asthma. ADVAIR HFA has not been studied in patients with acutely deteriorating asthma. The initiation of ADVAIR HFA in this setting is not appropriate.
Serious acute respiratory events, including fatalities, have been reported when salmeterol, a component of ADVAIR HFA, has been initiated in patients with significantly worsening or acutely deteriorating asthma. In most cases, these have occurred in patients with severe asthma (e.g., patients with a history of corticosteroid dependence, low pulmonary function, intubation, mechanical ventilation, frequent hospitalizations, previous life-threatening acute asthma exacerbations) and in some patients with acutely deteriorating asthma (e.g., patients with significantly increasing symptoms; increasing need for inhaled, short-acting beta$_2$-agonists; decreasing response to usual medications; increasing need for systemic corticosteroids; recent emergency room visits; deteriorating lung function). However, these events have occurred in a few patients with less severe asthma as well. It was not possible from these reports to determine whether salmeterol contributed to these events.
Increasing use of inhaled, short-acting beta$_2$-agonists is a marker of deteriorating asthma. In this situation, the patient requires immediate reevaluation with reassessment of the treatment regimen, giving special consideration to the possible need for replacing the current strength of ADVAIR HFA with a higher strength, adding additional inhaled corticosteroid, or initiating systemic corticosteroids. Patients should not use more than 2 inhalations twice daily (morning and evening) of ADVAIR HFA.
ADVAIR HFA should not be used for the relief of acute symptoms, i.e., as rescue therapy for the treatment of acute episodes of bronchospasm. An inhaled, short-acting beta$_2$–agonist, not ADVAIR HFA, should be used to relieve acute symptoms such as shortness of breath. When prescribing ADVAIR HFA, the physician must also provide the patient with an inhaled, short-acting beta$_2$-agonist (e.g., albuterol) for treatment of acute symptoms, despite regular twice-daily (morning and evening) use of ADVAIR HFA.
When beginning treatment with ADVAIR HFA, patients who have been taking oral or inhaled, short-acting beta$_2$-agonists on a regular basis (e.g., 4 times a day) should be instructed to discontinue the regular use of these drugs.

5.3 Excessive Use of ADVAIR HFA and Use With Other Long-Acting Beta$_2$-Agonists
As with other inhaled drugs containing beta$_2$-adrenergic agents, ADVAIR HFA should not be used more often than recommended, at higher doses than recommended, or in conjunction with other medications containing LABAs, as an overdose may result. Clinically significant cardiovascular effects and fatalities have been reported in association with excessive use of inhaled sympathomimetic drugs. Patients using ADVAIR HFA should not use an additional LABA (e.g., salmeterol, formoterol fumarate, arformoterol tartrate) for any reason, including prevention of exercise-induced bronchospasm (EIB) or the treatment of asthma.

5.4 Local Effects
In clinical studies, the development of localized infections of the mouth and pharynx with *Candida albicans* has occurred in patients treated with ADVAIR HFA. When such an infection develops, it should be treated with appropriate local or systemic (i.e., oral antifungal) therapy while treatment with ADVAIR HFA continues, but at times therapy with ADVAIR HFA may need to be interrupted. Patients should rinse the mouth after inhalation of ADVAIR HFA.

5.5 Pneumonia
Lower respiratory tract infections, including pneumonia, have been reported in patients with chronic obstructive pulmonary disease (COPD) following the inhaled administration of corticosteroids, including fluticasone propionate and ADVAIR DISKUS® (fluticasone propionate and salmeterol inhalation powder). In 2 replicate 1-year studies of 1,579 patients with COPD, there was a higher incidence of pneumonia reported in patients receiving ADVAIR DISKUS 250/50 (7%) than in those receiving salmeterol 50 mcg (3%). The incidence of pneumonia in the patients treated with ADVAIR DISKUS was higher in patients over 65 years of age (9%) compared with the incidence in patients less than 65 years of age (4%).
In a 3-year study of 6,184 patients with COPD, there was a higher incidence of pneumonia reported in patients receiving ADVAIR DISKUS 500/50 compared with placebo (16% with ADVAIR DISKUS 500/50, 14% with fluticasone propionate 500 mcg, 11% with salmeterol 50 mcg, and 9% with placebo). Similar to what was seen in the 1-year studies with ADVAIR DISKUS 250/50, the incidence of pneumonia was higher in patients over 65 years of age (18% with ADVAIR DISKUS 500/50 versus 10% with placebo) compared with patients less than 65 years of age (14% with ADVAIR DISKUS 500/50 versus 8% with placebo).

5.6 Immunosuppression
Persons who are using drugs that suppress the immune system are more susceptible to infections than healthy individuals. Chickenpox and measles, for example, can have a more serious or even fatal course in susceptible children or adults using corticosteroids. In such children or adults who have not had these diseases or been properly immunized, particular care should be taken to avoid exposure. How the dose, route, and duration of corticosteroid administration affect the risk of developing a disseminated infection is not known. The contribution of the underlying disease and/or prior corticosteroid treatment to the risk is also not known. If a patient is exposed to chickenpox, prophylaxis with varicella zoster immune globulin (VZIG) may be indicated. If a patient is exposed to measles, prophylaxis with pooled intramuscular immunoglobulin (IG) may be indicated. (See the respective package inserts for complete VZIG and IG prescribing information.) If chickenpox develops, treatment with antiviral agents may be considered.
Inhaled corticosteroids should be used with caution, if at all, in patients with active or quiescent tuberculosis infections of the respiratory tract; untreated systemic fungal, bacterial, viral, or parasitic infections; or ocular herpes simplex.

5.7 Transferring Patients From Systemic Corticosteroid Therapy
Particular care is needed for patients who have been transferred from systemically active corticosteroids to inhaled corticosteroids because deaths due to adrenal insufficiency have occurred in patients with asthma during and after transfer from systemic corticosteroids to less systemically available inhaled corticosteroids. After withdrawal from systemic corticosteroids, a number of months are required for recovery of hypothalamic-pituitary-adrenal (HPA) function.
Patients who have been previously maintained on 20 mg or more per day of prednisone (or its equivalent) may be most susceptible, particularly when their systemic corticosteroids have been almost completely withdrawn. During this period of HPA suppression, patients may exhibit signs and symptoms of adrenal insufficiency when exposed to trauma, surgery, or infection (particularly gastroenteritis) or other conditions associated with severe electrolyte loss. Although ADVAIR HFA may provide control of asthma symptoms during these episodes, in recommended doses it supplies less than normal physiologic amounts of glucocorticoid systemically and does NOT provide the mineralocorticoid activity that is necessary for coping with these emergencies.
During periods of stress or a severe asthma attack, patients who have been withdrawn from systemic corticosteroids should be instructed to resume oral corticosteroids (in large doses) immediately and to contact their physicians for further instruction. These patients should also be instructed to carry a warning card indicating that they may need supplementary systemic corticosteroids during periods of stress or a severe asthma attack.
Patients requiring oral corticosteroids should be weaned slowly from systemic corticosteroid use after transferring to ADVAIR HFA. Prednisone reduction can be accomplished by reducing the daily prednisone dose by 2.5 mg on a weekly basis during therapy with ADVAIR HFA. Lung function (mean forced expiratory volume in 1 second [FEV$_1$] or morning peak expiratory flow [PEF]), beta-agonist use, and asthma symptoms should be carefully monitored during withdrawal of oral corticosteroids. In addition to monitoring asthma signs and symptoms, patients should be observed for signs and symptoms of adrenal insufficiency, such as fatigue, lassitude, weakness, nausea and vomiting, and hypotension.
Transfer of patients from systemic corticosteroid therapy to inhaled corticosteroids or ADVAIR HFA may unmask conditions previously suppressed by the systemic corticosteroid therapy (e.g., rhinitis, conjunctivitis, eczema, arthritis, eosinophilic conditions). Some patients may experience symptoms of systemically active corticosteroid withdrawal (e.g., joint and/or muscular pain, lassitude, depression) despite maintenance or even improvement of respiratory function.

5.8 Hypercorticism and Adrenal Suppression
Fluticasone propionate, a component of ADVAIR HFA, will often help control asthma symptoms with less suppression of HPA function than therapeutically equivalent oral doses of prednisone. Since fluticasone propionate is absorbed into the circulation and can be systemically active at higher doses, the beneficial effects of ADVAIR HFA in minimizing HPA dysfunction may be expected only when recommended dosages are not exceeded and individual patients are titrated to the lowest effective dose. A relationship between plasma levels of fluticasone propionate and inhibitory effects on stimulated cortisol production has been shown after 4 weeks of treatment with fluticasone propionate inhalation aerosol. Since individual sensitivity to effects on cortisol production exists, physicians should consider this information when prescribing ADVAIR HFA.
Because of the possibility of systemic absorption of inhaled corticosteroids, patients treated with ADVAIR HFA should be observed carefully for any evidence of systemic corticosteroid effects. Particular care should be taken in observing patients postoperatively or during periods of stress for evidence of inadequate adrenal response.
It is possible that systemic corticosteroid effects such as hypercorticism and adrenal suppression (including adrenal crisis) may appear in a small number of patients, particularly when fluticasone propionate is administered at higher than recommended doses over prolonged periods of time. If such effects occur, the dosage of ADVAIR HFA should be reduced slowly, consistent with accepted procedures for reducing systemic corticosteroids and for management of asthma symptoms.

5.9 Drug Interactions With Strong Cytochrome P450 3A4 Inhibitors
The use of strong cytochrome P450 3A4 (CYP3A4) inhibitors (e.g., ritonavir, atazanavir, clarithromycin, indinavir, itraconazole, nefazodone, nelfinavir, saquinavir, ketoconazole, telithromycin) with ADVAIR HFA is not recommended because increased systemic corticosteroid and increased cardiovascular adverse effects may occur *[see Drug Interactions (7.1), Clinical Pharmacology (12.3)]*.

5.10 Paradoxical Bronchospasm and Upper Airway Symptoms
As with other inhaled medications, ADVAIR HFA can produce paradoxical bronchospasm, which may be life threatening. If paradoxical bronchospasm occurs following dosing with ADVAIR HFA, it should be treated immediately with an inhaled, short-acting bronchodilator; ADVAIR HFA should be discontinued immediately; and alternative therapy should be instituted. Upper airway symptoms of laryngeal spasm, irritation, or swelling, such as stridor and choking, have been reported in patients receiving fluticasone propionate and salmeterol.

5.11 Immediate Hypersensitivity Reactions
Immediate hypersensitivity reactions may occur after administration of ADVAIR HFA, as demonstrated by cases of urticaria, angioedema, rash, and bronchospasm *[see Adverse Reactions (6.2)]*.

5.12 Cardiovascular and Central Nervous System Effects
Excessive beta-adrenergic stimulation has been associated with seizures, angina, hypertension or hypotension, tachycardia with rates up to 200 beats/min, arrhythmias, nervousness, headache, tremor, palpitation, nausea, dizziness, fatigue, malaise, and insomnia *[see Overdosage (10)]*. Therefore, ADVAIR HFA, like all products containing sympathomimetic amines, should be used with caution in patients with cardiovascular disorders, especially coronary insufficiency, cardiac arrhythmias, and hypertension.
Salmeterol, a component of ADVAIR HFA, can produce a clinically significant cardiovascular effect in some patients as measured by pulse rate, blood pressure, and/or symptoms. Although such effects are uncommon after administration of salmeterol at recommended doses, if they occur, the drug may need to be discontinued. In addition, beta-agonists have been reported to produce electrocardiogram (ECG) changes, such as flattening of the T wave, prolongation of the QTc interval, and ST segment depression. The clinical significance of these findings is unknown. Large doses of inhaled or oral salmeterol (12 to 20 times the recommended dose) have been associated with clinically significant prolongation of the QTc interval, which has the potential for producing ventricular arrhythmias. Fatalities have been reported in association with excessive use of inhaled sympathomimetic drugs.

5.13 Reduction in Bone Mineral Density
Decreases in bone mineral density (BMD) have been observed with long-term administration of products containing inhaled corticosteroids. The clinical significance of small changes in BMD with regard to long-term consequences such as fracture is unknown. Patients with major risk factors for decreased bone mineral content, such as prolonged immobilization, family history of osteoporosis, postmenopausal status, tobacco use, advanced age, poor nutrition, or chronic use of drugs that can reduce bone mass (e.g., anticonvulsants, oral corticosteroids) should be monitored and treated with established standards of care.
2-Year Fluticasone Propionate Study: A 2-year study of 160 patients (females aged 18 to 40 years, males 18 to 50) with asthma receiving CFC-propelled fluticasone propionate inhalation aerosol 88 or 440 mcg twice daily demonstrated no statistically significant changes in BMD at any time point (24, 52, 76, and 104 weeks of double-blind treatment) as assessed by dual-energy x-ray absorptiometry at lumbar regions L1 through L4.

5.14 Effect on Growth
Orally inhaled corticosteroids may cause a reduction in growth velocity when administered to pediatric patients. Monitor the growth of pediatric patients receiving ADVAIR HFA routinely (e.g., via stadiometry). To minimize the systemic effects of orally inhaled corticosteroids, including ADVAIR HFA, titrate each patient's dose to the lowest dosage that effectively controls his/her symptoms *[see Use in Specific Populations (8.4)]*.

5.15 Glaucoma and Cataracts
Glaucoma, increased intraocular pressure, and cataracts have been reported in patients with asthma following the

long-term administration of inhaled corticosteroids, including fluticasone propionate, a component of ADVAIR HFA. Therefore, close monitoring is warranted in patients with a change in vision or with a history of increased intraocular pressure, glaucoma, and/or cataracts.

5.16 Eosinophilic Conditions and Churg-Strauss Syndrome

In rare cases, patients on inhaled fluticasone propionate, a component of ADVAIR HFA, may present with systemic eosinophilic conditions. Some of these patients have clinical features of vasculitis consistent with Churg-Strauss syndrome, a condition that is often treated with systemic corticosteroid therapy. These events usually, but not always, have been associated with the reduction and/or withdrawal of oral corticosteroid therapy following the introduction of fluticasone propionate. Cases of serious eosinophilic conditions have also been reported with other inhaled corticosteroids in this clinical setting. Physicians should be alert to eosinophilia, vasculitic rash, worsening pulmonary symptoms, cardiac complications, and/or neuropathy presenting in their patients. A causal relationship between fluticasone propionate and these underlying conditions has not been established.

5.17 Coexisting Conditions

ADVAIR HFA, like all medications containing sympathomimetic amines, should be used with caution in patients with convulsive disorders or thyrotoxicosis and in those who are unusually responsive to sympathomimetic amines. Doses of the related beta$_2$-adrenoceptor agonist albuterol, when administered intravenously, have been reported to aggravate preexisting diabetes mellitus and ketoacidosis.

5.18 Hypokalemia and Hyperglycemia

Beta-adrenergic agonist medications may produce significant hypokalemia in some patients, possibly through intracellular shunting, which has the potential to produce adverse cardiovascular effects *[see Clinical Pharmacology (12.2)]*. The decrease in serum potassium is usually transient, not requiring supplementation. Clinically significant changes in blood glucose and/or serum potassium were seen infrequently during clinical studies with ADVAIR HFA at recommended doses.

6 ADVERSE REACTIONS

LABAs, such as salmeterol, one of the active ingredients in ADVAIR HFA, increase the risk of asthma-related death. Data from a large placebo-controlled US study that compared the safety of salmeterol (SEREVENT Inhalation Aerosol) or placebo added to usual asthma therapy showed an increase in asthma-related deaths in patients receiving salmeterol *[see Warnings and Precautions (5.1)]*. Currently available data are inadequate to determine whether concurrent use of inhaled corticosteroids or other long-term asthma control drugs mitigates the increased risk of asthma-related death from LABAs. Available data from controlled clinical trials suggest that LABAs increase the risk of asthma-related hospitalization in pediatric and adolescent patients.

Systemic and local corticosteroid use may result in the following:

- *Candida albicans* infection *[see Warnings and Precautions (5.4)]*
- Pneumonia in patients with COPD *[see Warnings and Precautions (5.5)]*
- Immunosuppression *[see Warnings and Precautions (5.6)]*
- Hypercorticism and adrenal suppression *[see Warnings and Precautions (5.8)]*
- Growth effects *[see Warnings and Precautions (5.14)]*
- Glaucoma and cataracts *[see Warnings and Precautions (5.15)]*

6.1 Clinical Trials Experience

Because clinical trials are conducted under widely varying conditions, adverse reaction rates observed in the clinical trials of a drug cannot be directly compared with rates in the clinical trials of another drug and may not reflect the rates observed in practice.

Adult and Adolescent Patients Aged 12 Years and Older: The incidence of adverse reactions associated with ADVAIR HFA in Table 2 is based upon 2 placebo-controlled 12-week US clinical studies (Studies 1 and 3) and 1 active-controlled 12-week US clinical study (Study 2). A total of 1,008 adult and adolescent patients with asthma (556 females and 452 males) previously treated with albuterol alone, salmeterol, or inhaled corticosteroids were treated twice daily with 2 inhalations of ADVAIR HFA 45/21 or ADVAIR HFA 115/21, fluticasone propionate chlorofluorocarbon (CFC) inhalation aerosol (44- or 110-mcg doses), salmeterol CFC inhalation aerosol 21 mcg, or placebo HFA inhalation aerosol. The average duration of exposure was 71 to 81 days in the active treatment groups compared with 51 days in the placebo group.

[See table 2 above]

The incidence of common adverse reactions reported in Study 4, a 12-week non-US clinical study of 509 patients previously treated with inhaled corticosteroids who were

Table 2. Adverse Reactions With ≥3% Incidence With ADVAIR HFA Inhalation Aerosol in Adult and Adolescent Patients With Asthma

Adverse Event	ADVAIR HFA Inhalation Aerosol		Fluticasone Propionate CFC Inhalation Aerosol		Salmeterol CFC Inhalation Aerosol	Placebo HFA Inhalation Aerosol
	45/21 (n = 187) %	115/21 (n = 94) %	44 mcg (n = 186) %	110 mcg (n = 91) %	21 mcg (n = 274) %	(n = 176) %
Ear, nose, & throat						
Upper respiratory tract infection	16	24	13	15	17	13
Throat irritation	9	7	12	13	9	7
Upper respiratory inflammation	4	4	3	7	5	3
Hoarseness/dysphonia	3	1	2	0	1	0
Lower respiratory						
Viral respiratory infection	3	5	4	5	3	4
Neurology						
Headache	21	15	24	16	20	11
Dizziness	4	1	1	0	<1	0
Gastrointestinal						
Nausea & vomiting	5	3	4	2	2	3
Viral gastrointestinal infection	4	2	2	0	1	2
Gastrointestinal signs & symptoms	3	2	2	1	1	1
Musculoskeletal						
Musculoskeletal pain	5	7	8	2	4	4
Muscle pain	4	1	1	1	3	<1

treated twice daily with 2 inhalations of ADVAIR HFA 230/21, fluticasone propionate CFC inhalation aerosol 220 mcg, or 1 inhalation of ADVAIR DISKUS 500/50 was similar to the incidences reported in Table 2.

Additional Adverse Reactions: Other adverse reactions not previously listed, whether considered drug-related or not by the investigators, that occurred in the groups receiving ADVAIR HFA with an incidence of 1% to 3% and that occurred at a greater incidence than with placebo include the following: tachycardia, arrhythmias, myocardial infarction, postoperative complications, wounds and lacerations, soft tissue injuries, ear signs and symptoms, rhinorrhea/postnasal drip, epistaxis, nasal congestion/blockage, laryngitis, unspecified oropharyngeal plaques, dryness of nose, weight gain, allergic eye disorders, eye edema and swelling, gastrointestinal discomfort and pain, dental discomfort and pain, candidiasis mouth/throat, hyposalivation, gastrointestinal infections, disorders of hard tissue of teeth, abdominal discomfort and pain, oral abnormalities, arthralgia and articular rheumatism, muscle cramps and spasms, musculoskeletal inflammation, bone and skeletal pain, muscle injuries, sleep disorders, migraines, allergies and allergic reactions, viral infections, bacterial infections, candidiasis unspecified site, congestion, inflammation, bacterial reproductive infections, lower respiratory signs and symptoms, lower respiratory infections, lower respiratory hemorrhage, eczema, dermatitis and dermatosis, urinary infections.

Laboratory Test Abnormalities: In Study 3, there were more reports of hyperglycemia among adults and adolescents receiving ADVAIR HFA, but this was not seen in Studies 1 and 2.

6.2 Postmarketing Experience

In addition to adverse reactions reported from clinical trials, the following adverse reactions have been identified during postmarketing use of any formulation of ADVAIR, fluticasone propionate, and/or salmeterol regardless of indication. Because these reactions are reported voluntarily from a population of uncertain size, it is not always possible to reliably estimate their frequency or establish a causal relationship to drug exposure. These events have been chosen for inclusion due to either their seriousness, frequency of reporting, or causal connection to ADVAIR, fluticasone propionate, and/or salmeterol or a combination of these factors.

Cardiovascular: Arrhythmias (including atrial fibrillation, extrasystoles, supraventricular tachycardia), hypertension, ventricular tachycardia.

Ear, Nose, and Throat: Aphonia, earache, facial and oropharyngeal edema, paranasal sinus pain, rhinitis, throat soreness, tonsillitis.

Endocrine and Metabolic: Cushing's syndrome, Cushingoid features, growth velocity reduction in children/adolescents, hypercorticism, osteoporosis.

Eye: Cataracts, glaucoma.

Gastrointestinal: Dyspepsia, xerostomia.

Hepatobiliary Tract and Pancreas: Abnormal liver function tests.

Immune System: Immediate and delayed hypersensitivity reactions, including rash and rare events of angioedema, bronchospasm, and anaphylaxis.

Musculoskeletal: Back pain, myositis.

Neurology: Paresthesia, restlessness.

Non-Site Specific: Fever, pallor.

Psychiatry: Agitation, aggression, anxiety, depression. Behavioral changes, including hyperactivity and irritability, have been reported very rarely and primarily in children.

Respiratory: Asthma; asthma exacerbation; chest congestion; chest tightness; cough; dyspnea; immediate bronchospasm; influenza; paradoxical bronchospasm; tracheitis; wheezing; pneumonia; reports of upper respiratory symptoms of laryngeal spasm, irritation, or swelling such as stridor or choking.

Skin: Contact dermatitis, contusions, ecchymoses, photodermatitis, pruritus.

Urogenital: Dysmenorrhea, irregular menstrual cycle, pelvic inflammatory disease, vaginal candidiasis, vaginitis, vulvovaginitis.

7 DRUG INTERACTIONS

ADVAIR HFA has been used concomitantly with other drugs, including short-acting beta$_2$-agonists, methylxanthines, and intranasal corticosteroids, commonly used in patients with asthma, without adverse drug reactions *[see Clinical Pharmacology (12.2)]*. No formal drug interaction studies have been performed with ADVAIR HFA.

7.1 Inhibitors of Cytochrome P450 3A4

Fluticasone propionate and salmeterol, the individual components of ADVAIR HFA, are substrates of CYP3A4. The use of strong CYP3A4 inhibitors (e.g., ritonavir, atazanavir, clarithromycin, indinavir, itraconazole, nefazodone, nelfinavir, saquinavir, ketoconazole, telithromycin) with ADVAIR HFA is not recommended because increased systemic corticosteroid and increased cardiovascular adverse effects may occur.

Ritonavir: *Fluticasone Propionate:* A drug interaction study with fluticasone propionate aqueous nasal spray in healthy subjects has shown that ritonavir (a strong CYP3A4 inhibitor) can significantly increase plasma fluticasone propionate exposure, resulting in significantly reduced serum cortisol concentrations *[see Clinical Pharmacology (12.3)]*. During postmarketing use, there have been reports of clinically significant drug interactions in patients receiving fluticasone propionate and ritonavir, resulting in systemic corticosteroid effects including Cushing's syndrome and adrenal suppression.

Ketoconazole: *Fluticasone Propionate:* Coadministration of orally inhaled fluticasone propionate (1,000 mcg) and ketoconazole (200 mg once daily) resulted in increased plasma fluticasone propionate exposure and reduced plasma cortisol area under the curve (AUC), but had no effect on urinary excretion of cortisol.

Salmeterol: In a drug interaction study in 20 healthy subjects, coadministration of inhaled salmeterol (50 mcg twice daily) and oral ketoconazole (400 mg once daily) for 7 days resulted in greater systemic exposure to salmeterol (AUC increased 16-fold and C_{max} increased 1.4-fold). Three (3) subjects were withdrawn due to beta$_2$-agonist side effects (2 with prolonged QTc and 1 with palpitations and sinus tachycardia). Although there was no statistical effect on the mean QTc, coadministration of salmeterol and ketoconazole was associated with more frequent increases in QTc duration compared with salmeterol and placebo administration.

7.2 Monoamine Oxidase Inhibitors and Tricyclic Antidepressants

ADVAIR HFA should be administered with extreme caution to patients being treated with monoamine oxidase inhibitors or tricyclic antidepressants, or within 2 weeks of discontinuation of such agents, because the action of salmeterol, a component of ADVAIR HFA, on the vascular system may be potentiated by these agents.

7.3 Beta-Adrenergic Receptor Blocking Agents

Beta-blockers not only block the pulmonary effect of beta-agonists, such as salmeterol, a component of ADVAIR HFA, but may produce severe bronchospasm in patients with reversible obstructive airways disease. Therefore, patients with asthma should not normally be treated with beta-blockers. However, under certain circumstances, there may be no acceptable alternatives to the use of beta-adrenergic blocking agents for these patients; cardioselective beta-blockers could be considered, although they should be administered with caution.

7.4 Diuretics

The ECG changes and/or hypokalemia that may result from the administration of nonpotassium-sparing diuretics (such as loop or thiazide diuretics) can be acutely worsened by beta-agonists such as salmeterol, a component of ADVAIR HFA, especially when the recommended dose of the beta-agonist is exceeded. Although the clinical relevance of these effects is not known, caution is advised in the coadministration of ADVAIR HFA with nonpotassium-sparing diuretics.

8 USE IN SPECIFIC POPULATIONS

8.1 Pregnancy

Teratogenic Effects: Pregnancy Category C. There are no adequate and well-controlled studies with ADVAIR HFA in pregnant women. The combination of fluticasone propionate and salmeterol was teratogenic in mice and rats. Fluticasone propionate alone was teratogenic in mice, rats, and rabbits, and salmeterol alone was teratogenic in rabbits and not in rats. From the reproduction toxicity studies in mice and rats, no evidence of enhanced toxicity was seen using combinations of fluticasone propionate and salmeterol when compared with toxicity data from the components administered separately.

ADVAIR HFA should be used during pregnancy only if the potential benefit justifies the potential risk to the fetus.

Combination of Fluticasone Propionate and Salmeterol: In the mouse reproduction assay, fluticasone propionate by the subcutaneous route at a dose approximately equivalent to the maximum recommended human daily inhalation dose (MRHD) (on a mcg/m^2 basis at a maternal dose of 150 mcg/kg) combined with oral salmeterol at a dose approximately 580 times the MRHD (on a mg/m^2 basis at a maternal dose of 10 mg/kg) produced cleft palate, fetal death, increased implantation loss, and delayed ossification. These observations are characteristic of glucocorticoids. No developmental toxicity was observed at combination doses of fluticasone propionate subcutaneously up to approximately 1/5 the MRHD (on a mcg/m^2 basis at a maternal dose of 40 mcg/kg) and oral doses of salmeterol up to approximately 80 times the MRHD (on a mg/m^2 basis at a maternal dose of 1.4 mg/kg). In rats, combining fluticasone propionate subcutaneously at a dose equivalent to the MRHD (on a mcg/m^2 basis at a maternal dose of 100 mcg/kg) and an oral dose of salmeterol at approximately 1,200 times the MRHD (on a mg/m^2 basis at a maternal dose of 10 mg/kg) produced decreased fetal weight, umbilical hernia, delayed ossification, and changes in the occipital bone. No such effects were seen when combining fluticasone propionate subcutaneously at a dose less than the MRHD (on a mcg/m^2 basis at a maternal dose of 30 mcg/kg) and an oral dose of salmeterol at approximately 120 times the MRHD (on a mg/m^2 basis at a maternal dose of 1 mg/kg).

Fluticasone Propionate: Subcutaneous studies in mice at a dose less than the MRHD (on a mcg/m^2 basis at a maternal dose of 45 mcg/kg) and in rats at a dose equivalent to the MRHD (on a mcg/m^2 basis at a maternal dose of 100 mcg/kg) revealed fetal toxicity characteristic of potent corticosteroid compounds, including embryonic growth retardation, omphalocele, cleft palate, and retarded cranial ossification. No teratogenicity was seen in rats at inhalation doses approximately equivalent to the MRHD (on a mcg/m^2 basis at maternal doses up to 68.7 mcg/kg).

In rabbits, fetal weight reduction and cleft palate were observed at a subcutaneous dose less than the MRHD (on a mcg/m^2 basis at a maternal dose of 4 mcg/kg). However, no teratogenic effects were reported at oral doses up to approximately 6 times the MRHD (on a mcg/m^2 basis at maternal doses up to 300 mcg/kg). No fluticasone propionate was detected in the plasma in this study, consistent with the established low bioavailability following oral administration *[see Clinical Pharmacology (12.3)]*.

Fluticasone propionate crossed the placenta following subcutaneous administration to mice and rats and oral administration to rabbits.

Experience with oral corticosteroids since their introduction in pharmacologic, as opposed to physiologic, doses suggests that rodents are more prone to teratogenic effects from corticosteroids than humans. In addition, because there is a natural increase in corticosteroid production during pregnancy, most women will require a lower exogenous corticosteroid dose and many will not need corticosteroid treatment during pregnancy.

Salmeterol: No teratogenic effects occurred in rats at oral doses approximately 230 times the MRHD (on a mg/m^2 basis at maternal doses up to 2 mg/kg). In Dutch rabbits administered oral doses approximately 25 times the MRHD (on an AUC basis at maternal doses of 1 mg/kg and higher), salmeterol exhibited fetal toxic effects characteristically resulting from beta-adrenoceptor stimulation. These included precocious eyelid openings, cleft palate, sternebral fusion, limb and paw flexures, and delayed ossification of the frontal cranial bones. No such effects occurred at an oral dose approximately 10 times the MRHD (on an AUC basis at a maternal dose of 0.6 mg/kg).

New Zealand White rabbits were less sensitive since only delayed ossification of the frontal cranial bones was seen at an oral dose approximately 2,300 times the MRHD (on a mg/m^2 basis at a maternal dose of 10 mg/kg). Extensive use of other beta-agonists has provided no evidence that these class effects in animals are relevant to their use in humans.

Salmeterol xinafoate crossed the placenta following oral administration to mice and rats.

8.2 Labor and Delivery

There are no well-controlled human studies that have investigated effects of ADVAIR HFA on preterm labor or labor at term. Because of the potential for beta-agonist interference with uterine contractility, use of ADVAIR HFA during labor should be restricted to those patients in whom the benefits clearly outweigh the risks.

8.3 Nursing Mothers

Plasma levels of salmeterol, a component of ADVAIR HFA, after inhaled therapeutic doses are very low. In rats, salmeterol xinafoate is excreted in the milk. There are no data from controlled trials on the use of salmeterol by nursing mothers. It is not known whether fluticasone propionate is excreted in human breast milk. However, other corticosteroids have been detected in human milk. Subcutaneous administration to lactating rats of tritiated fluticasone propionate resulted in measurable radioactivity in milk.

Since there are no data from controlled trials on the use of ADVAIR HFA by nursing mothers, caution should be exercised when ADVAIR HFA is administered to a nursing woman.

8.4 Pediatric Use

Thirty-eight (38) patients aged 12 to 17 years were treated with ADVAIR HFA in US pivotal clinical trials. Patients in this age-group demonstrated efficacy results similar to those observed in patients aged 18 years and older. There were no obvious differences in the type or frequency of adverse events reported in this age-group compared with patients aged 18 years and older.

In a 12-week study, the safety of ADVAIR HFA 45/21 given as 2 inhalations twice daily was compared with that of fluticasone propionate 44 mcg HFA (FLOVENT® HFA) 2 inhalations twice daily in 350 subjects aged 4 to 11 years with persistent asthma currently being treated with inhaled corticosteroids. No new safety concerns were observed in children aged 4 to 11 years treated for 12 weeks with ADVAIR HFA 45/21 compared with adults and adolescents aged 12 years and older. Common adverse reactions (≥3%) seen in children aged 4 to 11 years treated with ADVAIR HFA 45/21 but not reported in the adult and adolescent clinical trials of ADVAIR HFA include: pyrexia, cough, pharyngolaryngeal pain, rhinitis, and sinusitis *[see Adverse Reactions (6.1)]*.This study was not designed to assess the effect of salmeterol, a component of ADVAIR HFA, on asthma hospitalizations and death in patients aged 4 to 11 years.

The pharmacokinetics and pharmacodynamic effect on serum cortisol of 21 days of treatment with ADVAIR HFA 45/21 (2 inhalations twice daily with or without a spacer) or ADVAIR DISKUS 100/50 (1 inhalation twice daily) was evaluated in a study of 31 children aged 4 to 11 years with mild asthma. Systemic exposure to salmeterol xinafoate was similar for ADVAIR HFA, ADVAIR HFA delivered with a spacer, and ADVAIR DISKUS while the systemic exposure to fluticasone propionate was lower with ADVAIR HFA compared with that of ADVAIR HFA delivered with a spacer or ADVAIR DISKUS. There were reductions in serum cortisol from baseline in all treatment groups (14%, 22%, and 13% for ADVAIR HFA, ADVAIR HFA delivered with a spacer, and ADVAIR DISKUS, respectively) *[see Clinical Pharmacology (12.2, 12.3)]*.

The safety and effectiveness of ADVAIR HFA in children less than 12 years have not been established.

Effects on Growth: Inhaled corticosteroids, including fluticasone propionate, a component of ADVAIR HFA, may cause a reduction in growth velocity in children and adolescents *[see Warnings and Precautions (5.14)]*. The growth of pediatric patients receiving orally inhaled corticosteroids, including ADVAIR HFA, should be monitored.

A 52-week placebo-controlled study to assess the potential growth effects of fluticasone propionate inhalation powder (FLOVENT® ROTADISK®) at 50 and 100 mcg twice daily was conducted in the US in 325 prepubescent children (244 males and 81 females) aged 4 to 11 years. The mean growth velocities at 52 weeks observed in the intent-to-treat population were 6.32 cm/year in the placebo group (n = 76), 6.07 cm/year in the 50-mcg group (n = 98), and 5.66 cm/year in the 100-mcg group (n = 89). An imbalance in the proportion of children entering puberty between groups and a higher dropout rate in the placebo group due to poorly controlled asthma may be confounding factors in interpreting these data. A separate subset analysis of children who remained prepubertal during the study revealed growth rates at 52 weeks of 6.10 cm/year in the placebo group (n = 57), 5.91 cm/year in the 50-mcg group (n = 74), and 5.67 cm/year in the 100-mcg group (n = 79). In children aged 8.5 years, the mean age of children in this study, the range for expected growth velocity is: boys – 3rd percentile = 3.8 cm/year, 50th percentile = 5.4 cm/year, and 97th percentile = 7.0 cm/year; girls – 3rd percentile = 4.2 cm/year, 50th percentile = 5.7 cm/year, and 97th percentile = 7.3 cm/year. The clinical relevance of these growth data is not certain.

If a child or adolescent on any corticosteroid appears to have growth suppression, the possibility that he/she is particularly sensitive to this effect of corticosteroids should be considered. The potential growth effects of prolonged treatment should be weighed against the clinical benefits obtained. To minimize the systemic effects of orally inhaled corticosteroids, including ADVAIR HFA, each patient should be titrated to the lowest strength that effectively controls his/her asthma.

8.5 Geriatric Use

Clinical studies of ADVAIR HFA did not include sufficient numbers of patients aged 65 years and older to determine whether older patients respond differently than younger patients. In general, dose selection for an elderly patient should be cautious, usually starting at the low end of the dosing range, reflecting the greater frequency of decreased hepatic, renal, or cardiac function, and of concomitant disease or other drug therapy. In addition, as with other products containing beta$_2$-agonists, special caution should be observed when using ADVAIR HFA in geriatric patients who have concomitant cardiovascular disease that could be adversely affected by beta$_2$–agonists.

8.6 Hepatic Impairment

Formal pharmacokinetic studies using ADVAIR HFA have not been conducted in patients with hepatic impairment. However, since both fluticasone propionate and salmeterol are predominantly cleared by hepatic metabolism, impairment of liver function may lead to accumulation of fluticasone propionate and salmeterol in plasma. Therefore, patients with hepatic disease should be closely monitored.

8.7 Renal Impairment

Formal pharmacokinetic studies using ADVAIR HFA have not been conducted in patients with renal impairment.

10 OVERDOSAGE

Fluticasone Propionate: Chronic overdosage with fluticasone propionate may result in signs/symptoms of hypercorticism *[see Warnings and Precautions (5.7)]*. Inhalation by healthy volunteers of a single dose of 4,000 mcg of fluticasone propionate inhalation powder or single doses of 1,760 or 3,520 mcg of fluticasone propionate CFC inhalation aerosol was well tolerated. Fluticasone propionate given by inhalation aerosol at dosages of 1,320 mcg twice daily for 7 to 15 days to healthy human volunteers was also well tolerated. Repeat oral doses up to 80 mg daily for 10 days in healthy volunteers and repeat oral doses up to 20 mg daily for 42 days in patients were well tolerated. Adverse reactions were of mild or moderate severity, and incidences were similar in active and placebo treatment groups.

Salmeterol: The expected signs and symptoms with overdosage of salmeterol are those of excessive beta-adrenergic stimulation and/or occurrence or exaggeration of any of the following: seizures, angina, hypertension or hypotension, tachycardia with rates up to 200 beats/min, arrhythmias, nervousness, headache, tremor, muscle cramps, dry mouth, palpitation, nausea, dizziness, fatigue, malaise, and insomnia. Overdosage with salmeterol can lead to clinically significant prolongation of the QTc interval, which can produce ventricular arrhythmias. Other signs of overdosage may include hypokalemia and hyperglycemia.

As with all sympathomimetic medications, cardiac arrest and even death may be associated with abuse of salmeterol. Treatment consists of discontinuation of salmeterol together with appropriate symptomatic therapy. The judicious use of a cardioselective beta-receptor blocker may be considered, bearing in mind that such medication can produce bronchospasm. There is insufficient evidence to determine if dialysis is beneficial for overdosage of salmeterol. Cardiac monitoring is recommended in cases of overdosage.

11 DESCRIPTION

ADVAIR HFA 45/21 Inhalation Aerosol, ADVAIR HFA 115/21 Inhalation Aerosol, and ADVAIR HFA 230/21 Inhalation Aerosol are combinations of fluticasone propionate and salmeterol xinafoate.

One active component of ADVAIR HFA is fluticasone propionate, a corticosteroid having the chemical name S-(fluoromethyl) 6α,9-difluoro-11β,17-dihydroxy-16α-methyl-3-oxoandrosta-1,4-diene-17β carbothioate, 17-propionate and the following chemical structure:

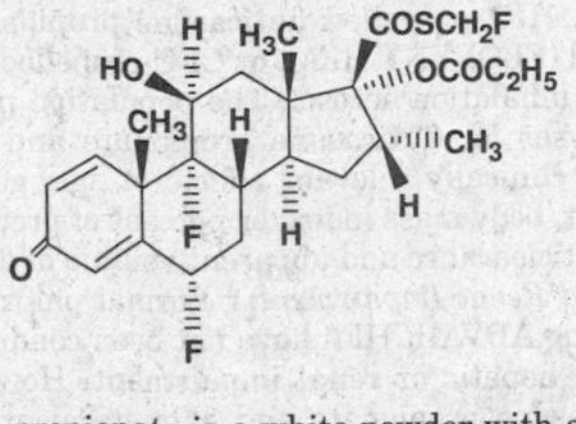

Fluticasone propionate is a white powder with a molecular weight of 500.6, and the empirical formula is $C_{25}H_{31}F_3O_5S$. It is practically insoluble in water, freely soluble in dimethyl sulfoxide and dimethylformamide, and slightly soluble in methanol and 95% ethanol.

The other active component of ADVAIR HFA is salmeterol xinafoate, a beta$_2$-adrenergic bronchodilator. Salmeterol xinafoate is the racemic form of the 1-hydroxy-2-naphthoic acid salt of salmeterol. The chemical name of salmeterol xinafoate is 4-hydroxy-α^1-[[[6-(4-phenylbutoxy)hexyl] amino]methyl]-1,3-benzenedimethanol, 1-hydroxy-2-naphthalenecarboxylate, and it has the following chemical structure:

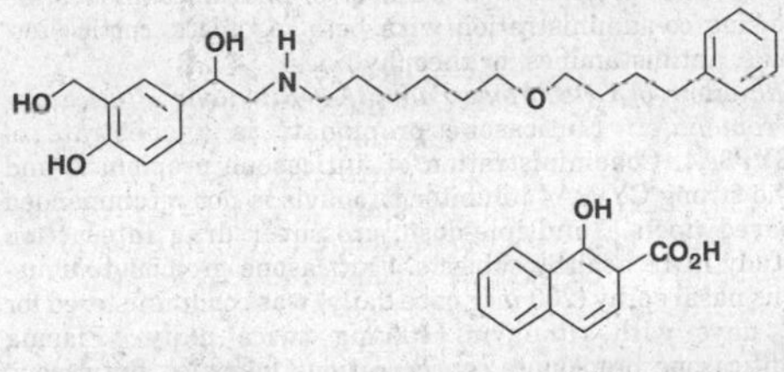

Salmeterol xinafoate is a white powder with a molecular weight of 603.8, and the empirical formula is $C_{25}H_{37}NO_4 \bullet C_{11}H_8O_3$. It is freely soluble in methanol; slightly soluble in ethanol, chloroform, and isopropanol; and sparingly soluble in water.

ADVAIR HFA 45/21 Inhalation Aerosol, ADVAIR HFA 115/21 Inhalation Aerosol, and ADVAIR HFA 230/21 Inhalation Aerosol are pressurized metered-dose aerosol units fitted with a counter. ADVAIR HFA is intended for oral inhalation only. Each unit contains a microcrystalline suspension of fluticasone propionate (micronized) and salmeterol xinafoate (micronized) in propellant HFA-134a (1,1,1,2-tetrafluoroethane). It contains no other excipients.

After priming, each actuation of the inhaler delivers 50, 125, or 250 mcg of fluticasone propionate and 25 mcg of salmeterol in 75 mg of suspension from the valve. Each actuation delivers 45, 115, or 230 mcg of fluticasone propionate and 21 mcg of salmeterol from the actuator. Twenty-one micrograms (21 mcg) of salmeterol base is equivalent to 30.45 mcg of salmeterol xinafoate. The actual amount of drug delivered to the lung may depend on patient factors, such as the coordination between the actuation of the device and inspiration through the delivery system.

Each 8-g canister contains 60 inhalations. Each 12-g canister provides 120 inhalations.

ADVAIR HFA should be primed before using for the first time by releasing 4 test sprays into the air away from the face, shaking well for 5 seconds before each spray. In cases where the inhaler has not been used for more than 4 weeks or when it has been dropped, prime the inhaler again by releasing 2 test sprays into the air away from the face, shaking well for 5 seconds before each spray.

12 CLINICAL PHARMACOLOGY

12.1 Mechanism of Action

ADVAIR HFA: Since ADVAIR HFA contains both fluticasone propionate and salmeterol, the mechanisms of action described below for the individual components apply to ADVAIR HFA. These drugs represent 2 classes of medications (a synthetic corticosteroid and a selective LABA) that have different effects on clinical, physiologic, and inflammatory indices of asthma.

Fluticasone Propionate: Fluticasone propionate is a synthetic trifluorinated corticosteroid with potent anti-inflammatory activity. In vitro assays using human lung cytosol preparations have established fluticasone propionate as a human glucocorticoid receptor agonist with an affinity 18 times greater than dexamethasone, almost twice that of beclomethasone-17-monopropionate (BMP), the active metabolite of beclomethasone dipropionate, and over 3 times that of budesonide. Data from the McKenzie vasoconstrictor assay in man are consistent with these results.

Inflammation is an important component in the pathogenesis of asthma. Corticosteroids have been shown to inhibit multiple cell types (e.g., mast cells, eosinophils, basophils, lymphocytes, macrophages, neutrophils) and mediator production or secretion (e.g., histamine, eicosanoids, leukotrienes, cytokines) involved in the asthmatic response. These anti-inflammatory actions of corticosteroids contribute to their efficacy in asthma.

Salmeterol Xinafoate: Salmeterol is a selective LABA. In vitro studies show salmeterol to be at least 50 times more selective for beta$_2$-adrenoceptors than albuterol. Although beta$_2$-adrenoceptors are the predominant adrenergic receptors in bronchial smooth muscle and beta$_1$-adrenoceptors are the predominant receptors in the heart, there are also beta$_2$-adrenoceptors in the human heart comprising 10% to 50% of the total beta-adrenoceptors. The precise function of these receptors has not been established, but their presence raises the possibility that even selective beta$_2$-agonists may have cardiac effects.

The pharmacologic effects of beta$_2$-adrenoceptor agonist drugs, including salmeterol, are at least in part attributable to stimulation of intracellular adenyl cyclase, the enzyme that catalyzes the conversion of adenosine triphosphate (ATP) to cyclic-3′,5′-adenosine monophosphate (cyclic AMP). Increased cyclic AMP levels cause relaxation of bronchial smooth muscle and inhibition of release of mediators of immediate hypersensitivity from cells, especially from mast cells.

In vitro tests show that salmeterol is a potent and long-lasting inhibitor of the release of mast cell mediators, such as histamine, leukotrienes, and prostaglandin D_2, from human lung. Salmeterol inhibits histamine-induced plasma protein extravasation and inhibits platelet activating factor-induced eosinophil accumulation in the lungs of guinea pigs when administered by the inhaled route. In humans, single doses of salmeterol administered via inhalation aerosol attenuate allergen-induced bronchial hyperresponsiveness.

12.2 Pharmacodynamics

ADVAIR HFA: *Healthy Subjects: Cardiovascular Effects:* Since systemic pharmacodynamic effects of salmeterol are not normally seen at the therapeutic dose, higher doses were used to produce measurable effects. Four (4) placebo-controlled crossover studies were conducted in healthy subjects: (1) a cumulative-dose study using 42 to 336 mcg of salmeterol CFC inhalation aerosol given alone or as ADVAIR HFA 115/21, (2) a single-dose study using 4 inhalations of ADVAIR HFA 230/21, salmeterol CFC inhalation aerosol 21 mcg, or fluticasone propionate CFC inhalation aerosol 220 mcg, (3) a single-dose study using 8 inhalations of ADVAIR HFA 45/21, ADVAIR HFA 115/21, or ADVAIR HFA 230/21, and (4) a single-dose study using 4 inhalations of ADVAIR HFA 230/21; 2 inhalations of ADVAIR DISKUS 500/50; 4 inhalations of fluticasone propionate CFC inhalation aerosol 220 mcg; or 1,010 mcg of fluticasone propionate given intravenously. In these studies pulse rate, blood pressure, QTc interval, glucose, and/or potassium were measured. Comparable or lower effects were observed for ADVAIR HFA compared with ADVAIR DISKUS or salmeterol alone. The effect of salmeterol on pulse rate and potassium was not altered by the presence of different amounts of fluticasone propionate in ADVAIR HFA.

Hypothalamic-Pituitary-Adrenal Axis Effects: The potential effect of salmeterol on the effects of fluticasone propionate on the HPA axis was also evaluated in 3 of these studies. Compared with fluticasone propionate CFC inhalation aerosol, ADVAIR HFA had less effect on 24-hour urinary cortisol excretion and less or comparable effect on 24-hour serum cortisol. In these crossover studies in healthy subjects, ADVAIR HFA and ADVAIR DISKUS had similar effects on urinary and serum cortisol.

Patients With Asthma: Cardiovascular Effects: In clinical studies with ADVAIR HFA in adult and adolescent patients aged 12 years and older with asthma, systemic pharmacodynamic effects of salmeterol (pulse rate, blood pressure, QTc interval, potassium, and glucose) were similar to or slightly lower in patients treated with ADVAIR HFA compared with patients treated with salmeterol CFC inhalation aerosol 21 mcg. In 61 adult and adolescent patients with asthma given ADVAIR HFA (45/21 or 115/21 mcg), continuous 24-hour electrocardiographic monitoring was performed after the first dose and after 12 weeks of twice-daily therapy, and no clinically significant dysrhythmias were noted.

The effect of 21 days of treatment with ADVAIR HFA 45/21 (2 inhalations twice daily with or without a spacer) or ADVAIR DISKUS 100/50 (1 inhalation twice daily) was evaluated in 31 children aged 4 to 11 years with mild asthma. There were no notable changes from baseline for QTc, heart rate, or systolic and diastolic blood pressure.

Hypothalamic-Pituitary-Adrenal Axis Effects: A 4-way crossover study in 13 patients with asthma compared pharmacodynamics at steady state following 4 weeks of twice-daily treatment with 2 inhalations of ADVAIR HFA 115/21, 1 inhalation of ADVAIR DISKUS 250/50 mcg, 2 inhalations of fluticasone propionate HFA inhalation aerosol 110 mcg, and placebo. No significant differences in serum cortisol AUC were observed between active treatments and placebo. Mean 12-hour serum cortisol AUC ratios comparing active treatment with placebo ranged from 0.9 to 1.2. No statistically or clinically significant increases in heart rate or QTc interval were observed for any active treatment compared with placebo.

In a 12-week study in adult and adolescent patients with asthma, ADVAIR HFA 115/21 was compared with the individual components, fluticasone propionate CFC inhalation aerosol 110 mcg and salmeterol CFC inhalation aerosol 21 mcg, and placebo *[see Clinical Studies (14.1)]*. All treatments were administered as 2 inhalations twice daily. After 12 weeks of treatment with these therapeutic doses, the geometric mean ratio of urinary cortisol excretion compared with baseline was 0.9 for ADVAIR HFA and fluticasone propionate and 1.0 for placebo and salmeterol. In addition, the ability to increase cortisol production in response to stress, as assessed by 30-minute cosyntropin stimulation in 23 to 32 patients per treatment group, remained intact for the majority of patients and was similar across treatments. Three patients who received ADVAIR HFA 115/21 had an abnormal response (peak serum cortisol <18 mcg/dL) after dosing, compared with 1 patient who received placebo, 2 patients who received fluticasone propionate 110 mcg, and 1 patient who received salmeterol.

In another 12-week study in adult and adolescent patients with asthma, ADVAIR HFA 230/21 (2 inhalations twice daily) was compared with ADVAIR DISKUS 500/50 (1 inhalation twice daily) and fluticasone propionate CFC inhalation aerosol 220 mcg (2 inhalations twice daily) *[see Clinical Studies (14.1)]*. The geometric mean ratio of 24-hour urinary cortisol excretion at week 12 compared with baseline was 0.9 for all 3 treatment groups.

The effect of 21 days of treatment with ADVAIR HFA 45/21 (2 inhalations twice daily with or without a spacer) or ADVAIR DISKUS 100/50 (1 inhalation twice daily) on serum cortisol was evaluated in 31 children aged 4 to 11 years with mild asthma. There were reductions in serum cortisol from baseline in all treatment groups (14%, 22%, and 13% for ADVAIR HFA, ADVAIR HFA with spacer, and ADVAIR DISKUS, respectively).

Other Fluticasone Propionate Products: *Patients With Asthma: Hypothalamic-Pituitary-Adrenal Axis Effects:* In clinical trials with fluticasone propionate inhalation powder using dosages up to and including 250 mcg twice daily, occasional abnormal short cosyntropin tests (peak serum cortisol <18 mcg/dL assessed by radioimmunoassay) were noted both in patients receiving fluticasone propionate and in patients receiving placebo. The incidence of abnormal tests at 500 mcg twice daily was greater than placebo. In a 2-year study carried out with the DISKHALER® inhalation device in 64 patients with mild, persistent asthma (mean FEV_1 91% of predicted) randomized to fluticasone propionate 500 mcg twice daily or placebo, no patient receiving fluticasone propionate had an abnormal response to 6-hour cosyntropin infusion (peak serum cortisol <18 mcg/dL). With a peak cortisol threshold of <35 mcg/dL, 1 patient receiving fluticasone propionate (4%) had an abnormal response at 1 year; repeat testing at 18 months and 2 years was normal. Another patient receiving fluticasone propionate (5%) had an abnormal response at 2 years. No patient on placebo had an abnormal response at 1 or 2 years.

Other Salmeterol Xinafoate Products: *Patients With Asthma: Cardiovascular Effects:* Inhaled salmeterol, like other beta-adrenergic agonist drugs, can produce dose-related cardiovascular effects and effects on blood glucose and/or serum potassium *[see Warnings and Precautions (5.12, 5.18)]*. The cardiovascular effects (heart rate, blood pressure) associated with salmeterol occur with similar frequency, and are of similar type and severity, as those noted following albuterol administration.

The effects of rising inhaled doses of salmeterol and standard inhaled doses of albuterol were studied in volunteers and in patients with asthma. Salmeterol doses up to 84 mcg administered as inhalation aerosol resulted in heart rate increases of 3 to 16 beats/min, about the same as albuterol dosed at 180 mcg by inhalation aerosol (4 to 10 beats/min). In 2 double-blind asthma studies, patients receiving either 42 mcg of salmeterol inhalation aerosol twice daily (n = 81) or 180 mcg of albuterol inhalation aerosol 4 times daily (n = 80) underwent continuous electrocardiographic monitoring during four 24-hour periods; no clinically significant dysrhythmias were noted.

Concomitant Use of ADVAIR HFA With Other Respiratory Medications: *Short-Acting Beta$_2$-Agonists:* In three 12-week US clinical trials, the mean daily need for additional

$beta_2$-agonist use in 277 patients receiving ADVAIR HFA was approximately 1.2 inhalations/day and ranged from 0 to 9 inhalations/day. Two percent (2%) of patients receiving ADVAIR HFA in these trials averaged 6 or more inhalations per day over the course of the 12-week trials. No increase in frequency of cardiovascular adverse reactions was observed among patients who averaged 6 or more inhalations per day.

Methylxanthines: The concurrent use of intravenously or orally administered methylxanthines (e.g., aminophylline, theophylline) by patients receiving ADVAIR HFA has not been completely evaluated. In five 12-week clinical trials (3 US and 2 non-US), 45 patients receiving ADVAIR HFA 45/21, 115/21, or 230/21 twice daily concurrently with a theophylline product had adverse event rates similar to those in 577 patients receiving ADVAIR HFA without theophylline.

Fluticasone Propionate Nasal Spray: In patients receiving ADVAIR HFA in three 12-week US clinical trials, no difference in the profile of adverse events or HPA axis effects was noted between patients receiving FLONASE® (fluticasone propionate) Nasal Spray, 50 mcg concurrently (n = 89) and those who were not (n = 192).

12.3 Pharmacokinetics

Absorption: *Fluticasone Propionate: Healthy Subjects:* Fluticasone propionate acts locally in the lung; therefore, plasma levels do not predict therapeutic effect. Studies using oral dosing of labeled and unlabeled drug have demonstrated that the oral systemic bioavailability of fluticasone propionate is negligible (<1%), primarily due to incomplete absorption and presystemic metabolism in the gut and liver. In contrast, the majority of the fluticasone propionate delivered to the lung is systemically absorbed.

Three single-dose placebo-controlled crossover studies were conducted in healthy subjects: (1) a study using 4 inhalations of ADVAIR HFA 230/21, salmeterol CFC inhalation aerosol 21 mcg, or fluticasone propionate CFC inhalation aerosol 220 mcg, (2) a study using 8 inhalations of ADVAIR HFA 45/21, ADVAIR HFA 115/21, or ADVAIR HFA 230/21, and (3) a study using 4 inhalations of ADVAIR HFA 230/21; 2 inhalations of ADVAIR DISKUS 500/50; 4 inhalations of fluticasone propionate CFC inhalation aerosol 220 mcg; or 1,010 mcg of fluticasone propionate given intravenously. Peak plasma concentrations of fluticasone propionate were achieved in 0.33 to 1.5 hours and those of salmeterol were achieved in 5 to 10 minutes.

Peak plasma concentrations of fluticasone propionate (N = 20 subjects) following 8 inhalations of ADVAIR HFA 45/21, ADVAIR HFA 115/21, and ADVAIR HFA 230/21 averaged 41, 108, and 173 pg/mL, respectively.

Systemic exposure (N = 20 subjects) from 4 inhalations of ADVAIR HFA 230/21 was 53% of the value from the individual inhaler for fluticasone propionate CFC inhalation aerosol and 42% of the value from the individual inhaler for salmeterol CFC inhalation aerosol. Peak plasma concentrations from ADVAIR HFA for fluticasone propionate (86 versus 120 pg/mL) and salmeterol (170 versus 510 pg/mL) were significantly lower compared with individual inhalers.

In 15 healthy subjects, systemic exposure (AUC) to fluticasone propionate from 4 inhalations of ADVAIR HFA 230/21 (920/84 mcg) and 2 inhalations of ADVAIR DISKUS 500/50 (1,000/100 mcg) were similar between the 2 inhalers (i.e., 799 versus 832 pg•hr/mL, respectively) but approximately half the systemic exposure from 4 inhalations of fluticasone propionate CFC inhalation aerosol 220 mcg (880 mcg, AUC = 1,543 pg•hr/mL). Similar results were observed for peak fluticasone propionate plasma concentrations (186 and 182 pg/mL from ADVAIR HFA and ADVAIR DISKUS, respectively, and 307 pg/mL from the fluticasone propionate CFC inhalation aerosol). Absolute bioavailability of fluticasone propionate was 5.3% and 5.5% following administration of ADVAIR HFA and ADVAIR DISKUS, respectively.

Patients With Asthma: A double-blind crossover study was conducted in 13 adult patients with asthma to evaluate the steady-state pharmacokinetics of fluticasone propionate and salmeterol following administration of 2 inhalations of ADVAIR HFA 115/21 twice daily or 1 inhalation of ADVAIR DISKUS 250/50 twice daily for 4 weeks. Systemic exposure (AUC) to fluticasone propionate was similar for ADVAIR HFA (274 pg•hr/mL [95% CI: 150, 502]) and ADVAIR DISKUS (338 pg•hr/mL [95% CI: 197, 581]).

The effect of 21 days of treatment with ADVAIR HFA 45/21 (2 inhalations twice daily with or without a spacer) or ADVAIR DISKUS 100/50 (1 inhalation twice daily) was evaluated in a study of 31 children aged 4 to 11 years with mild asthma. Systemic exposure to fluticasone propionate was similar with ADVAIR DISKUS and ADVAIR HFA with a spacer (138 pg•hr/mL [95% CI: 69, 273] and 107 pg•hr/mL [95% CI: 46, 252], respectively) and lower with ADVAIR HFA without a spacer (24 pg•hr/mL [95% CI: 10, 60]).

Salmeterol: Healthy Subjects: Salmeterol xinafoate, an ionic salt, dissociates in solution so that the salmeterol and 1-hydroxy-2-naphthoic acid (xinafoate) moieties are absorbed, distributed, metabolized, and eliminated independently. Salmeterol acts locally in the lung; therefore, plasma levels do not predict therapeutic effect.

Peak plasma concentrations of salmeterol (N = 20 subjects) following 8 inhalations of ADVAIR HFA 45/21, ADVAIR HFA 115/21, and ADVAIR HFA 230/21 ranged from 220 to 470 pg/mL.

In 15 healthy subjects receiving ADVAIR HFA 230/21 (920/84 mcg) and ADVAIR DISKUS 500/50 (1,000/100 mcg), systemic exposure to salmeterol was higher (317 versus 169 pg•hr/mL) and peak salmeterol concentrations were lower (196 versus 223 pg/mL) following ADVAIR HFA compared with ADVAIR DISKUS, although pharmacodynamic results were comparable.

Patients With Asthma: Because of the small therapeutic dose, systemic levels of salmeterol are low or undetectable after inhalation of recommended dosages (42 mcg of salmeterol inhalation aerosol twice daily). Following chronic administration of an inhaled dosage of 42 mcg of salmeterol inhalation aerosol twice daily, salmeterol was detected in plasma within 5 to 10 minutes in 6 patients with asthma; plasma concentrations were very low, with mean peak concentrations of 150 pg/mL at 20 minutes and no accumulation with repeated doses.

A double-blind crossover study was conducted in 13 adult patients with asthma to evaluate the steady-state pharmacokinetics of fluticasone propionate and salmeterol following administration of 2 inhalations of ADVAIR HFA 115/21 twice daily or 1 inhalation of ADVAIR DISKUS 250/50 twice daily for 4 weeks. Systemic exposure to salmeterol was similar for ADVAIR HFA (53 pg•hr/mL [95% CI: 17, 164]) and ADVAIR DISKUS (70 pg•hr/mL [95% CI: 19, 254]).

The effect of 21 days of treatment with ADVAIR HFA 45/21 (2 inhalations twice daily with or without a spacer) or ADVAIR DISKUS 100/50 (1 inhalation twice daily) was evaluated in 31 children aged 4 to 11 years with mild asthma. Systemic exposure to salmeterol was similar for ADVAIR HFA, ADVAIR HFA with spacer, and ADVAIR DISKUS (126 pg•hr/mL [95% CI: 70, 225], 103 pg•hr/mL [95% CI: 54, 200], and 110 pg•hr/mL [95% CI: 55, 219], respectively).

Distribution: *Fluticasone Propionate:* Following intravenous administration, the initial disposition phase for fluticasone propionate was rapid and consistent with its high lipid solubility and tissue binding. The volume of distribution averaged 4.2 L/kg.

The percentage of fluticasone propionate bound to human plasma proteins averages 99%. Fluticasone propionate is weakly and reversibly bound to erythrocytes and is not significantly bound to human transcortin.

Salmeterol: The percentage of salmeterol bound to human plasma proteins averages 96% in vitro over the concentration range of 8 to 7,722 ng of salmeterol base per milliliter, much higher concentrations than those achieved following therapeutic doses of salmeterol.

Metabolism: *Fluticasone Propionate:* The total clearance of fluticasone propionate is high (average, 1,093 mL/min), with renal clearance accounting for less than 0.02% of the total. The only circulating metabolite detected in man is the 17β-carboxylic acid derivative of fluticasone propionate, which is formed through the CYP3A4 pathway. This metabolite had less affinity (approximately 1/2,000) than the parent drug for the glucocorticoid receptor of human lung cytosol in vitro and negligible pharmacological activity in animal studies. Other metabolites detected in vitro using cultured human hepatoma cells have not been detected in man.

Salmeterol: Salmeterol base is extensively metabolized by hydroxylation, with subsequent elimination predominantly in the feces. No significant amount of unchanged salmeterol base was detected in either urine or feces.

An in vitro study using human liver microsomes showed that salmeterol is extensively metabolized to α-hydroxysalmeterol (aliphatic oxidation) by CYP3A4. Ketoconazole, a strong inhibitor of CYP3A4, essentially completely inhibited the formation of α-hydroxysalmeterol in vitro.

Elimination: *Fluticasone Propionate:* Following intravenous dosing, fluticasone propionate showed polyexponential kinetics and had a terminal elimination half-life of approximately 7.8 hours. Less than 5% of a radiolabeled oral dose was excreted in the urine as metabolites, with the remainder excreted in the feces as parent drug and metabolites. Terminal half-life estimates of fluticasone propionate for ADVAIR HFA, ADVAIR DISKUS, and fluticasone propionate CFC inhalation aerosol were similar and averaged 5.6 hours.

Salmeterol: In 2 healthy adult subjects who received 1 mg of radiolabeled salmeterol (as salmeterol xinafoate) orally, approximately 25% and 60% of the radiolabeled salmeterol was eliminated in urine and feces, respectively, over a period of 7 days. The terminal elimination half-life was about 5.5 hours (1 volunteer only).

The xinafoate moiety has no apparent pharmacologic activity. The xinafoate moiety is highly protein bound (>99%) and has a long elimination half-life of 11 days. No terminal half-life estimates were calculated for salmeterol following administration of ADVAIR HFA.

Special Populations: A population pharmacokinetic analysis was performed for fluticasone propionate and salmeterol utilizing data from 9 controlled clinical trials that included 350 patients with asthma aged 4 to 77 years who received treatment with ADVAIR DISKUS, ADVAIR HFA, fluticasone propionate inhalation powder (FLOVENT® DISKUS®), HFA-propelled fluticasone propionate inhalation aerosol (FLOVENT HFA), or CFC-propelled fluticasone propionate inhalation aerosol. The population pharmacokinetic analyses for fluticasone propionate and salmeterol showed no clinically relevant effects of age, gender, race, body weight, body mass index, or percent of predicted FEV_1 on apparent clearance and apparent volume of distribution.

Hepatic and Renal Impairment: Formal pharmacokinetic studies using ADVAIR HFA have not been conducted in patients with hepatic or renal impairment. However, since both fluticasone propionate and salmeterol are predominantly cleared by hepatic metabolism, impairment of liver function may lead to accumulation of fluticasone propionate and salmeterol in plasma. Therefore, patients with hepatic disease should be closely monitored.

Drug Interactions: In the repeat- and single-dose studies, there was no evidence of significant drug interaction in systemic exposure between fluticasone propionate and salmeterol when given alone or in combination via the DISKUS. Similar definitive studies have not been performed with ADVAIR HFA. The population pharmacokinetic analysis from 9 controlled clinical trials in 350 patients with asthma showed no significant effects on fluticasone propionate or salmeterol pharmacokinetics following co-administration with $beta_2$-agonists, corticosteroids, antihistamines, or theophyllines.

Inhibitors of Cytochrome P450 3A4: Ritonavir: Fluticasone Propionate: Fluticasone propionate is a substrate of CYP3A4. Coadministration of fluticasone propionate and the strong CYP3A4 inhibitor ritonavir is not recommended based upon a multiple-dose, crossover drug interaction study in 18 healthy subjects. Fluticasone propionate aqueous nasal spray (200 mcg once daily) was coadministered for 7 days with ritonavir (100 mg twice daily). Plasma fluticasone propionate concentrations following fluticasone propionate aqueous nasal spray alone were undetectable (<10 pg/mL) in most subjects, and when concentrations were detectable peak levels (C_{max}) averaged 11.9 pg/mL (range: 10.8 to 14.1 pg/mL) and $AUC_{(0-\tau)}$ averaged 8.43 pg•hr/mL (range: 4.2 to 18.8 pg•hr/mL). Fluticasone propionate C_{max} and $AUC_{(0-\tau)}$ increased to 318 pg/mL (range: 110 to 648 pg/mL) and 3,102.6 pg•hr/mL (range: 1,207.1 to 5,662.0 pg•hr/mL), respectively, after coadministration of ritonavir with fluticasone propionate aqueous nasal spray. This significant increase in plasma fluticasone propionate exposure resulted in a significant decrease (86%) in serum cortisol AUC.

Ketoconazole: Fluticasone Propionate: In a placebo-controlled, crossover study in 8 healthy adult volunteers, coadministration of a single dose of orally inhaled fluticasone propionate (1,000 mcg) with multiple doses of ketoconazole (200 mg) to steady state resulted in increased plasma fluticasone propionate exposure, a reduction in plasma cortisol AUC, and no effect on urinary excretion of cortisol.

Salmeterol: In a placebo-controlled, crossover drug interaction study in 20 healthy male and female subjects, coadministration of salmeterol (50 mcg twice daily) and the strong CYP3A4 inhibitor ketoconazole (400 mg once daily) for 7 days resulted in a significant increase in plasma salmeterol exposure as determined by a 16-fold increase in AUC (ratio with and without ketoconazole 15.76 [90% CI: 10.66, 23.31]) mainly due to increased bioavailability of the swallowed portion of the dose. Peak plasma salmeterol concentrations were increased by 1.4-fold (90% CI: 1.23, 1.68). Three (3) out of 20 subjects (15%) were withdrawn from salmeterol and ketoconazole coadministration due to beta-agonist–mediated systemic effects (2 with QTc prolongation and 1 with palpitations and sinus tachycardia). Coadministration of salmeterol and ketoconazole did not result in a clinically significant effect on mean heart rate, mean blood potassium, or mean blood glucose. Although there was no statistical effect on the mean QTc, coadministration of salmeterol and ketoconazole was associated with more frequent increases in QTc duration compared with salmeterol and placebo administration.

Erythromycin: Fluticasone Propionate: In a multiple-dose drug interaction study, coadministration of orally inhaled fluticasone propionate (500 mcg twice daily) and erythromycin (333 mg 3 times daily) did not affect fluticasone propionate pharmacokinetics.

Salmeterol: In a repeat-dose study in 13 healthy subjects, concomitant administration of erythromycin (a moderate CYP3A4 inhibitor) and salmeterol inhalation aerosol resulted in a 40% increase in salmeterol C_{max} at steady state (ratio with and without erythromycin 1.4 [90% CI: 0.96, 2.03], p = 0.12), a 3.6-beat/min increase in heart rate ([95% CI: 0.19, 7.03], p<0.04), a 5.8-msec increase in QTc interval ([95% CI: -6.14, 17.77], p = 0.34), and no change in plasma potassium.

13 NONCLINICAL TOXICOLOGY

13.1 Carcinogenesis, Mutagenesis, Impairment of Fertility

Fluticasone Propionate: Fluticasone propionate demonstrated no tumorigenic potential in mice at oral doses up to 1,000 mcg/kg (approximately 5 times the MRHD on a mcg/m^2 basis) for 78 weeks or in rats at inhalation doses up to 57 mcg/kg (less than the MRHD on a mcg/m^2 basis) for 104 weeks.

Fluticasone propionate did not induce gene mutation in prokaryotic or eukaryotic cells in vitro. No significant clastogenic effect was seen in cultured human peripheral lymphocytes in vitro or in the in vivo mouse micronucleus test.

No evidence of impairment of fertility was observed in reproductive studies conducted in rats at subcutaneous doses up to 50 mcg/kg (less than the MRHD on a mcg/m^2 basis). Prostate weight was significantly reduced.

Salmeterol: In an 18-month carcinogenicity study in CD-mice, salmeterol at oral doses of 1.4 mg/kg and above (approximately 10 times the MRHD based on comparison of the plasma AUCs) caused a dose-related increase in the incidence of smooth muscle hyperplasia, cystic glandular hyperplasia, leiomyomas of the uterus, and ovarian cysts. No tumors were seen at 0.2 mg/kg (approximately 2 times the MRHD for adults based on comparison of the AUCs).

In a 24-month oral and inhalation carcinogenicity study in Sprague Dawley rats, salmeterol caused a dose-related increase in the incidence of mesovarian leiomyomas and ovarian cysts at doses of 0.68 mg/kg and above (approximately 80 times the MRHD on a mg/m^2 basis). No tumors were seen at 0.21 mg/kg (approximately 25 times the MRHD on a mg/m^2 basis). These findings in rodents are similar to those reported previously for other beta–adrenergic agonist drugs. The relevance of these findings to human use is unknown.

Salmeterol produced no detectable or reproducible increases in microbial and mammalian gene mutation in vitro. No clastogenic activity occurred in vitro in human lymphocytes or in vivo in a rat micronucleus test. No effects on fertility were identified in rats treated with salmeterol at oral doses up to 2 mg/kg (approximately 230 times the MRHD on a mg/m^2 basis).

13.2 Animal Toxicology and/or Pharmacology

Preclinical: Studies in laboratory animals (minipigs, rodents, and dogs) have demonstrated the occurrence of cardiac arrhythmias and sudden death (with histologic evidence of myocardial necrosis) when beta-agonists and methylxanthines are administered concurrently. The clinical relevance of these findings is unknown.

Propellant HFA 134a: In animals and humans, propellant HFA-134a was found to be rapidly absorbed and rapidly eliminated, with an elimination half-life of 3 to 27 minutes in animals and 5 to 7 minutes in humans. Time to maximum plasma concentration (T_{max}) and mean residence time are both extremely short, leading to a transient appearance of HFA-134a in the blood with no evidence of accumulation.

Propellant HFA-134a is devoid of pharmacological activity except at very high doses in animals (i.e., 380 to 1,300 times the maximum human exposure based on comparisons of area under the plasma concentration versus time curve [AUC] values), primarily producing ataxia, tremors, dyspnea, or salivation. These events are similar to effects produced by the structurally related CFCs, which have been used extensively in metered-dose inhalers. In drug interaction studies in male and female dogs, there was a slight increase in the salmeterol-related effect on heart rate (a known effect of beta$_2$-agonists) when given in combination with high doses of fluticasone propionate. This effect was not observed in clinical studies.

14 CLINICAL STUDIES

ADVAIR HFA has been studied in patients with asthma aged 12 years and older. ADVAIR HFA has not been studied in patients less than 12 years of age or in patients with COPD. In clinical trials comparing ADVAIR HFA Inhalation Aerosol with its individual components, improvements in most efficacy endpoints were greater with ADVAIR HFA than with the use of either fluticasone propionate or salmeterol alone. In addition, clinical trials showed comparable results between Advair HFA and Advair Diskus.

14.1 Studies Comparing ADVAIR HFA With Fluticasone Propionate Alone or Salmeterol Alone

Four (4) double-blind parallel-group clinical trials were conducted with ADVAIR HFA in 1,517 adult and adolescent patients (≥12 years, mean baseline FEV$_1$ 65% to 75% of predicted normal) with asthma that was not optimally controlled on their current therapy. All metered-dose inhaler treatments were inhalation aerosols given as 2 inhalations twice daily, and other maintenance therapies were discontinued.

Table 5. Secondary Efficacy Variable Results for Patients Previously Treated With Beta$_2$-Agonists (Albuterol or Salmeterol) or Inhaled Corticosteroids (Study 1)

Efficacy Variable[a]	ADVAIR HFA 45/21 Inhalation Aerosol (n = 92)	Fluticasone Propionate CFC Inhalation Aerosol 44 mcg (n = 89)	Salmeterol CFC Inhalation Aerosol 21 mcg (n = 92)	Placebo HFA Inhalation Aerosol (n = 87)
AM PEF (L/min)				
Baseline	377	369	381	382
Change from baseline	58	27	25	1
PM PEF (L/min)				
Baseline	397	387	402	407
Change from baseline	48	20	16	3
Use of VENTOLIN Inhalation Aerosol (inhalations/day)				
Baseline	3.1	2.4	2.7	2.7
Change from baseline	-2.1	-0.4	-0.8	0.2
Asthma symptom score/day				
Baseline	1.8	1.6	1.7	1.7
Change from baseline	-1.0	-0.3	-0.4	0

[a] Change from baseline = change from baseline at Endpoint (last available data).

Study 1: Clinical Trial With ADVAIR HFA 45/21 Inhalation Aerosol: This placebo-controlled 12-week US study compared ADVAIR HFA 45/21 with fluticasone propionate CFC inhalation aerosol 44 mcg or salmeterol CFC inhalation aerosol 21 mcg, each given as 2 inhalations twice daily. The primary efficacy endpoints were predose FEV$_1$ and withdrawals due to worsening asthma. This study was stratified according to baseline asthma therapy: patients using beta-agonists (albuterol alone [n = 142], salmeterol [n = 84], or inhaled corticosteroids [n = 134] [daily doses of beclomethasone dipropionate 252 to 336 mcg; budesonide 400 to 600 mcg; flunisolide 1,000 mcg; fluticasone propionate inhalation aerosol 176 mcg; fluticasone propionate inhalation powder 200 mcg; or triamcinolone acetonide 600 to 800 mcg]). Baseline FEV$_1$ measurements were similar across treatments: ADVAIR HFA 45/21, 2.29 L; fluticasone propionate 44 mcg, 2.20 L; salmeterol, 2.33 L; and placebo, 2.27 L.

Predefined withdrawal criteria for lack of efficacy, an indicator of worsening asthma, were utilized for this placebo-controlled study. Worsening asthma was defined as a clinically important decrease in FEV$_1$ or PEF, increase in use of VENTOLIN® (albuterol, USP) Inhalation Aerosol, increase in night awakenings due to asthma, emergency intervention or hospitalization due to asthma, or requirement for asthma medication not allowed by the protocol. As shown in Table 4, statistically significantly fewer patients receiving ADVAIR HFA 45/21 were withdrawn due to worsening asthma compared with salmeterol and placebo. Fewer patients receiving ADVAIR HFA 45/21 were withdrawn due to worsening asthma compared with fluticasone propionate 44 mcg; however, the difference was not statistically significant.

Table 4. Percent of Patients Withdrawn Due to Worsening Asthma in Patients Previously Treated With Beta$_2$-Agonists (Albuterol or Salmeterol) or Inhaled Corticosteroids (Study 1)

ADVAIR HFA 45/21 Inhalation Aerosol (n = 92)	Fluticasone Propionate CFC Inhalation Aerosol 44 mcg (n = 89)	Salmeterol CFC Inhalation Aerosol 21 mcg (n = 92)	Placebo HFA Inhalation Aerosol (n = 87)
2%	8%	25%	28%

The FEV$_1$ results are displayed in Figure 2. Because this trial used predetermined criteria for worsening asthma, which caused more patients in the placebo group to be withdrawn, FEV$_1$ results at Endpoint (last available FEV$_1$ result) are also provided. Patients receiving ADVAIR HFA 45/21 had significantly greater improvements in FEV$_1$ (0.58 L, 27%) compared with fluticasone propionate 44 mcg (0.36 L, 18%), salmeterol (0.25 L, 12%), and placebo (0.14 L, 5%). These improvements in FEV$_1$ with ADVAIR HFA 45/21 were achieved regardless of baseline asthma therapy (albuterol alone, salmeterol, or inhaled corticosteroids).

Figure 2. Mean Percent Change From Baseline in FEV$_1$ in Patients Previously Treated With Either Beta$_2$-Agonists (Albuterol or Salmeterol or Inhaled Corticosteroids (Study 1)

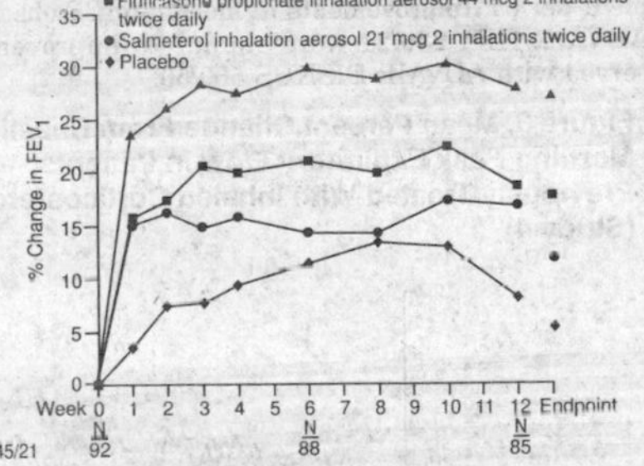

	N (Week 0)	N (Week 6)	N (Week 12)
ADVAIR HFA45/21	92	88	85
Fluticasone propionate inhalation aerosol 44 mcg	89	84	76
Salmeterol inhalation aerosol 21 mcg	92	72	65
Placebo	87	63	58

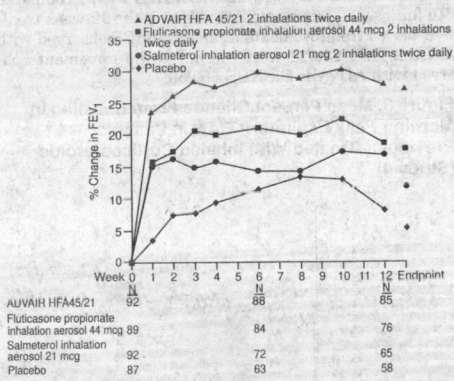

The effect of ADVAIR HFA 45/21 on the secondary efficacy parameters, including morning and evening PEF, usage of VENTOLIN Inhalation Aerosol, and asthma symptoms over 24 hours on a scale of 0 to 5 is shown in Table 5.

[See table 5 above]

The subjective impact of asthma on patients' perceptions of health was evaluated through use of an instrument called the Asthma Quality of Life Questionnaire (AQLQ) (based on a 7- point scale where 1 = maximum impairment and 7 = none). Patients receiving ADVAIR HFA 45/21 had clinically meaningful improvements in overall asthma-specific quality of life as defined by a difference between groups of ≥0.5 points in change from baseline AQLQ scores (difference in AQLQ score of 1.14 [95% CI: 0.85, 1.44] compared with placebo).

Study 2: Clinical Trial With ADVAIR HFA 45/21 Inhalation Aerosol: This active-controlled 12-week US study compared ADVAIR HFA 45/21 with fluticasone propionate CFC inhalation aerosol 44 mcg and salmeterol CFC inhalation aerosol 21 mcg, each given as 2 inhalations twice daily, in 283 patients using as-needed albuterol alone. The primary efficacy endpoint was predose FEV$_1$. Baseline FEV$_1$ measurements were similar across treatments: ADVAIR HFA 45/21, 2.37 L; fluticasone propionate 44 mcg, 2.31 L; and salmeterol, 2.34 L.

Efficacy results in this study were similar to those observed in Study 1. Patients receiving ADVAIR HFA 45/21 had significantly greater improvements in FEV$_1$ (0.69 L, 33%) compared with fluticasone propionate 44 mcg (0.51 L, 25%) and salmeterol (0.47 L, 22%).

Study 3: Clinical Trial With ADVAIR HFA 115/21 Inhalation Aerosol: This placebo-controlled 12-week US study compared ADVAIR HFA 115/21 with fluticasone propionate CFC inhalation aerosol 110 mcg or salmeterol CFC inhalation aerosol 21 mcg, each given as 2 inhalations twice daily, in 365 patients using inhaled corticosteroids (daily doses of beclomethasone dipropionate 378 to 840 mcg; budesonide 800 to 1,200 mcg; flunisolide 1,250 to 2,000 mcg; fluticasone propionate inhalation aerosol 440 to 660 mcg; fluticasone propionate inhalation powder 400 to 600 mcg; or triamcinolone acetonide 900 to 1,600 mcg). The primary efficacy endpoints were predose FEV_1 and withdrawals due to worsening asthma. Baseline FEV_1 measurements were similar across treatments: ADVAIR HFA 115/21, 2.23 L; fluticasone propionate 110 mcg, 2.18 L; salmeterol, 2.22 L; and placebo, 2.17 L.

Efficacy results in this study were similar to those observed in Studies 1 and 2. Patients receiving ADVAIR HFA 115/21 had significantly greater improvements in FEV_1 (0.41 L, 20%) compared with fluticasone propionate 110 mcg (0.19 L, 9%), salmeterol (0.15 L, 8%), and placebo (-0.12 L, -6%). Significantly fewer patients receiving ADVAIR HFA 115/21 were withdrawn from this study for worsening asthma (7%) compared with salmeterol (24%) and placebo (54%). Fewer patients receiving ADVAIR HFA 115/21 were withdrawn due to worsening asthma (7%) compared with fluticasone propionate 110 mcg (11%); however, the difference was not statistically significant.

Study 4: Clinical Trial With ADVAIR HFA 230/21 Inhalation Aerosol: This active-controlled 12-week non-US study compared ADVAIR HFA 230/21 with fluticasone propionate CFC inhalation aerosol 220 mcg, each given as 2 inhalations twice daily, and with ADVAIR DISKUS 500/50 given as 1 inhalation twice daily in 509 patients using inhaled corticosteroids (daily doses of beclomethasone dipropionate CFC inhalation aerosol 1,500 to 2,000 mcg; budesonide 1,500 to 2,000 mcg; flunisolide 1,500 to 2,000 mcg; fluticasone propionate inhalation aerosol 660 to 880 mcg; or fluticasone propionate inhalation powder 750 to 1,000 mcg). The primary efficacy endpoint was morning PEF.

Baseline morning PEF measurements were similar across treatments: ADVAIR HFA 230/21, 327 L/min; ADVAIR DISKUS 500/50, 341 L/min; and fluticasone propionate 220 mcg, 345 L/min. As shown in Figure 3, morning PEF improved significantly with ADVAIR HFA 230/21 compared with fluticasone propionate 220 mcg over the 12-week treatment period. Improvements in morning PEF observed with ADVAIR HFA 230/21 were similar to improvements observed with ADVAIR DISKUS 500/50.

Figure 3. Mean Percent Change From Baseline in Morning Peak Expiratory Flow in Patients Previously Treated With Inhaled Corticosteroids (Study 4)

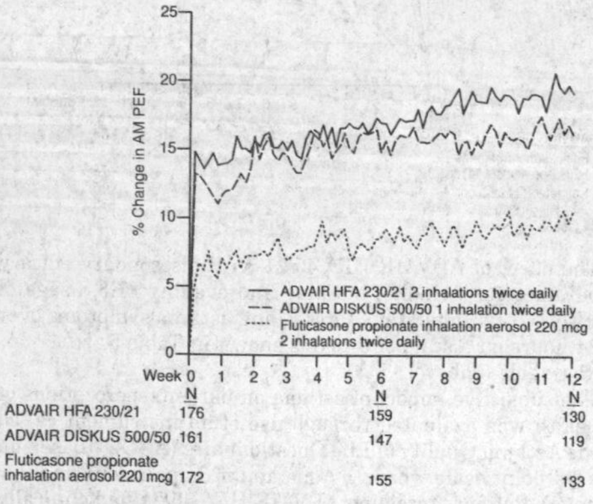

14.2 One-Year Safety Study

Clinical Trial With ADVAIR HFA 45/21, 115/21, and 230/21 Inhalation Aerosol: This 1-year open-label non-US study evaluated the safety of ADVAIR HFA 45/21, 115/21, and 230/21 given as 2 inhalations twice daily in 325 patients. This study was stratified into 3 groups according to baseline asthma therapy: patients using short-acting $beta_2$-agonists alone (n = 42), salmeterol (n = 91), or inhaled corticosteroids (n = 277). Patients treated with short-acting $beta_2$–agonists alone, salmeterol, or low doses of inhaled corticosteroids with or without concurrent salmeterol received ADVAIR HFA 45/21. Patients treated with moderate doses of inhaled corticosteroids with or without concurrent salmeterol received ADVAIR HFA 115/21. Patients treated with high doses of inhaled corticosteroids with or without concurrent salmeterol received ADVAIR HFA 230/21. Baseline FEV_1 measurements ranged from 2.3 to 2.6 L.

Improvements in FEV_1 (0.17 to 0.35 L at 4 weeks) were seen across all 3 treatments and were sustained throughout the 52–week treatment period. Few patients (3%) were withdrawn due to worsening asthma over 1 year.

14.3 Onset of Action and Progression of Improvement in Control

The onset of action and progression of improvement in asthma control were evaluated in 2 placebo-controlled US trials and 1 active-controlled US trial. Following the first dose, the median time to onset of clinically significant bronchodilatation (≥15% improvement in FEV_1) in most patients was seen within 30 to 60 minutes. Maximum improvement in FEV_1 occurred within 4 hours, and clinically significant improvement was maintained for 12 hours (see Figure 4).

Following the initial dose, predose FEV_1 relative to Day 1 baseline improved markedly over the first week of treatment and continued to improve over the 12 weeks of treatment in all 3 studies.

No diminution in the 12-hour bronchodilator effect was observed with either ADVAIR HFA 45/21 (Figures 4 and 5) or ADVAIR HFA 230/21 as assessed by FEV_1 following 12 weeks of therapy.

Figure 4. Percent Change in Serial 12-Hour FEV_1 in Patients Previously Using Either $Beta_2$-Agonists (Albuterol or Salmeterol) or Inhaled Corticosteroids (Study 1)

First Treatment Day

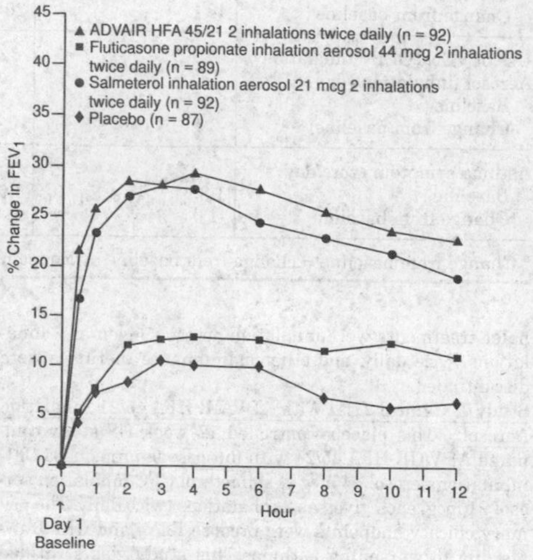

Figure 5. Percent Change in Serial 12-Hour FEV_1 in Patients Previously Using Either $Beta_2$-Agonists (Albuterol or Salmeterol) or Inhaled Corticosteroids (Study 1)

Last Treatment Day (Week 12)

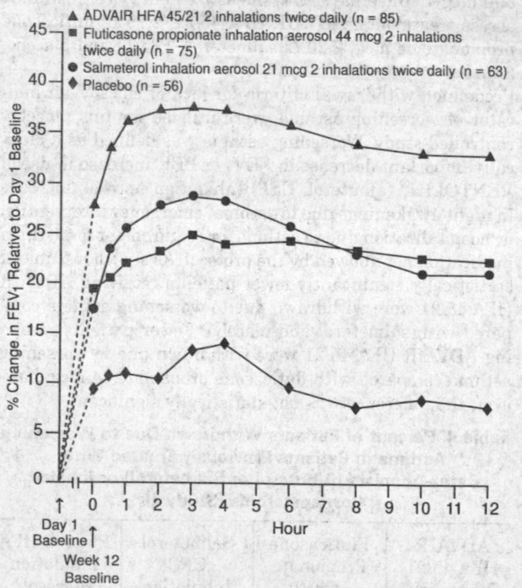

Reduction in asthma symptoms and use of rescue VENTOLIN Inhalation Aerosol and improvement in morning and evening PEF also occurred within the first day of treatment with ADVAIR HFA, and continued to improve over the 12 weeks of therapy in all 3 studies.

16 HOW SUPPLIED/STORAGE AND HANDLING

ADVAIR HFA 45/21 Inhalation Aerosol is supplied in 12-g pressurized aluminum canisters containing 120 metered actuations in boxes of 1 (NDC 0173-0715-20) and 8-g pressurized aluminum canisters containing 60 metered actuations in institutional pack boxes of 1 (NDC 0173-0715-22).

ADVAIR HFA 115/21 Inhalation Aerosol is supplied in 12-g pressurized aluminum canisters containing 120 metered actuations in boxes of 1 (NDC 0173-0716-20) and 8-g pressurized aluminum canisters containing 60 metered actuations in institutional pack boxes of 1 (NDC 0173-0716-22).

ADVAIR HFA 230/21 Inhalation Aerosol is supplied in 12-g pressurized aluminum canisters containing 120 metered actuations in boxes of 1 (NDC 0173-0717-20) and 8-g pressurized aluminum canisters containing 60 metered actuations in institutional pack boxes of 1 (NDC 0173-0717-22).

Each canister is fitted with a counter, supplied with a purple actuator with a light purple strapcap, and sealed in a plastic-coated, moisture-protective foil pouch with a desiccant that should be discarded when the pouch is opened. Each canister is packaged with a Medication Guide leaflet.

The purple actuator supplied with ADVAIR HFA Inhalation Aerosol should not be used with any other product canisters, and actuators from other products should not be used with an ADVAIR HFA Inhalation Aerosol canister.

The correct amount of medication in each actuation cannot be assured after the counter reads 000, even though the canister is not completely empty and will continue to operate. The inhaler should be discarded when the counter reads 000.

Keep out of reach of children. Avoid spraying in eyes.

Contents Under Pressure: Do not puncture. Do not use or store near heat or open flame. Exposure to temperatures above 120°F may cause bursting. Never throw container into fire or incinerator.

Store at 25°C (77°F); excursions permitted to 15°-30°C (59°-86°F). Store the inhaler with the mouthpiece down. For best results, the inhaler should be at room temperature before use. Shake well FOR 5 SECONDS before using.

17 PATIENT COUNSELING INFORMATION

See FDA-approved patient labeling (Medication Guide).

17.1 Asthma-Related Death

Patients should be informed that salmeterol, one of the active ingredients in ADVAIR HFA, increases the risk of asthma-related death and may increase the risk of asthma-related hospitalization in pediatric and adolescent patients. They should also be informed that currently available data are inadequate to determine whether concurrent use of inhaled corticosteroids or other long-term asthma control drugs mitigates the increased risk of asthma-related death from LABAs.

17.2 Not for Acute Symptoms

ADVAIR HFA is not meant to relieve acute asthma symptoms, and extra doses should not be used for that purpose. Acute symptoms should be treated with an inhaled, short-acting $beta_2$-agonist such as albuterol. The healthcare provider should provide the patient with such medication and instruct the patient in how it should be used.

Patients should be instructed to seek medical attention immediately if they experience any of the following:

- Decreasing effectiveness of inhaled, short-acting $beta_2$-agonists
- Need for more inhalations than usual of inhaled, short-acting $beta_2$-agonists
- Significant decrease in lung function as outlined by the physician

Patients should not stop therapy with ADVAIR HFA without physician/provider guidance since symptoms may recur after discontinuation.

17.3 Do Not Use Additional Long-Acting $Beta_2$-Agonists

When patients are prescribed ADVAIR HFA, other LABAs for asthma should not be used.

17.4 Risks Associated With Corticosteroid Therapy

Local Effects: Patients should be advised that localized infections with *Candida albicans* occurred in the mouth and pharynx in some patients. If oropharyngeal candidiasis develops, it should be treated with appropriate local or systemic (i.e., oral) antifungal therapy while still continuing therapy with ADVAIR HFA, but at times therapy with ADVAIR HFA may need to be temporarily interrupted under close medical supervision. Rinsing the mouth after inhalation is advised.

Pneumonia: Patients with COPD have a higher risk of pneumonia and should be instructed to contact their healthcare provider if they develop symptoms of pneumonia.

Immunosuppression: Patients who are on immunosuppressant doses of corticosteroids should be warned to avoid exposure to chickenpox or measles and if they are exposed to consult their physicians without delay. Patients should be informed of potential worsening of existing tuberculosis; fungal, bacterial, viral, or parasitic infections; or ocular herpes simplex.

Hypercorticism and Adrenal Suppression: Patients should be advised that ADVAIR HFA may cause systemic corticosteroid effects of hypercorticism and adrenal suppression. Additionally, patients should be instructed that deaths due to adrenal insufficiency have occurred during and after transfer from systemic corticosteroids. Patients should taper slowly from systemic corticosteroids if transferring to ADVAIR HFA.

Reduction in Bone Mineral Density: Patients who are at an increased risk for decreased BMD should be advised that the use of corticosteroids may pose an additional risk.

Reduced Growth Velocity: Patients should be informed that orally inhaled corticosteroids, including fluticasone propionate, may cause a reduction in growth velocity when administered to pediatric patients. Physicians should closely follow the growth of children and adolescents taking corticosteroids by any route.

Ocular Effects: Long-term use of inhaled corticosteroids may increase the risk of some eye problems (cataracts or glaucoma); regular eye examinations should be considered.

17.5 Risks Associated With Beta-Agonist Therapy

Patients should be informed of adverse effects associated with $beta_2$ agonists, such as palpitations, chest pain, rapid heart rate, tremor, or nervousness.

ADVAIR, ADVAIR DISKUS, DISKUS, FLOVENT, FLONASE, ROTADISK, SEREVENT, and VENTOLIN are registered trademarks of GlaxoSmithKline.

The other brands listed are trademarks of their respective owners and are not trademarks of GlaxoSmithKline. The makers of these brands are not affiliated with and do not endorse GlaxoSmithKline or its products.

GlaxoSmithKline
Research Triangle Park, NC 27709

March 2013
ADH:8PI

PHARMACIST—DETACH HERE AND GIVE MEDICATION GUIDE TO PATIENT

MEDICATION GUIDE

ADVAIR® HFA [*ad' vair*] 45/21 Inhalation Aerosol
(fluticasone propionate 45 mcg and salmeterol 21 mcg)
ADVAIR® HFA 115/21 Inhalation Aerosol
(fluticasone propionate 115 mcg and salmeterol 21 mcg)
ADVAIR® HFA 230/21 Inhalation Aerosol
(fluticasone propionate 230 mcg and salmeterol 21 mcg)

Read the Medication Guide that comes with ADVAIR HFA Inhalation Aerosol before you start using it and each time you get a refill. There may be new information. This Medication Guide does not take the place of talking to your healthcare provider about your medical condition or treatment.

What is the most important information I should know about ADVAIR HFA?

ADVAIR HFA can cause serious side effects, including:

1. **People with asthma who take long-acting $beta_2$-adrenergic agonist (LABA) medicines, such as salmeterol (one of the medicines in ADVAIR HFA), have an increased risk of death from asthma problems.** It is not known whether fluticasone propionate, the other medicine in ADVAIR HFA, reduces the risk of death from asthma problems seen with salmeterol.
   - **Call your healthcare provider if breathing problems worsen over time while using ADVAIR HFA.** You may need different treatment.
   - **Get emergency medical care if:**
     - breathing problems worsen quickly and
     - you use your rescue inhaler medicine, but it does not relieve your breathing problems.
2. ADVAIR HFA should be used only if your healthcare provider decides that your asthma is not well controlled with a long-term asthma control medicine, such as inhaled corticosteroids.
3. When your asthma is well controlled, your healthcare provider may tell you to stop taking ADVAIR HFA. Your healthcare provider will decide if you can stop ADVAIR HFA without loss of asthma control. Your healthcare provider may prescribe a different long-term asthma control medicine for you, such as an inhaled corticosteroid.
4. Children and adolescents who take LABA medicines may have an increased risk of being hospitalized for asthma problems.

What is ADVAIR HFA?

- ADVAIR HFA combines an inhaled corticosteroid medicine, fluticasone propionate (the same medicine found in FLOVENT®), and a LABA medicine, salmeterol (the same medicine found in SEREVENT®).
  - Inhaled corticosteroids help to decrease inflammation in the lungs. Inflammation in the lungs can lead to asthma symptoms.
  - LABA medicines are used in people with asthma and chronic obstructive pulmonary disease (COPD). LABA medicines help the muscles around the airways in your lungs stay relaxed to prevent symptoms, such as wheezing and shortness of breath. These symptoms can happen when the muscles around the airways tighten. This makes it hard to breathe. In severe cases, wheezing can stop your breathing and cause death if not treated right away.
- ADVAIR HFA is used to control symptoms of asthma and to prevent symptoms such as wheezing in adults and adolescents aged 12 years and older
- ADVAIR HFA should not be used as a rescue inhaler.
- ADVAIR HFA contains salmeterol (the same medicine found in SEREVENT). LABA medicines, such as salmeterol, increase the risk of death from asthma problems.

ADVAIR HFA is not for adults and adolescents with asthma who are well controlled with an asthma control medicine, such as a low to medium dose of an inhaled corticosteroid medicine.

Who should not use ADVAIR HFA?

Do not use ADVAIR HFA:
- to treat sudden, severe symptoms of asthma and
- if you are allergic to any of the ingredients in ADVAIR HFA. See the end of this Medication Guide for a list of ingredients in ADVAIR HFA.

What should I tell my healthcare provider before using ADVAIR HFA?

Tell your healthcare provider about all of your health conditions, including if you:
- **have heart problems**
- **have high blood pressure**
- **have seizures**
- **have thyroid problems**
- **have diabetes**
- **have liver problems**
- **have osteoporosis**
- **have an immune system problem**
- **have eye problems such as increased pressure in the eye (glaucoma) or cataracts**
- **are pregnant or planning to become pregnant.** It is not known if ADVAIR HFA may harm your unborn baby.
- **are breastfeeding.** It is not known if ADVAIR HFA passes into your milk and if it can harm your baby.
- **are allergic to ADVAIR HFA or any other medicines**
- **are exposed to chickenpox or measles**

Tell your healthcare provider about all the medicines you take including prescription and non-prescription medicines, vitamins, and herbal supplements. ADVAIR HFA and certain other medicines may interact with each other. This may cause serious side effects. Especially, tell your healthcare provider if you take ritonavir. The anti-HIV medicines NORVIR® (ritonavir capsules) Soft Gelatin, NORVIR (ritonavir oral solution), and KALETRA® (lopinavir/ritonavir) Tablets contain ritonavir.

Know the medicines you take. Keep a list and show it to your healthcare provider and pharmacist each time you get a new medicine.

How do I use ADVAIR HFA?

See the step-by-step instructions for using ADVAIR HFA at the end of this Medication Guide. Do not use ADVAIR HFA unless your healthcare provider has taught you and you understand everything. Ask your healthcare provider or pharmacist if you have any questions.
- Use ADVAIR HFA exactly as prescribed. **Do not use ADVAIR HFA more often than prescribed.** ADVAIR HFA comes in 3 strengths. Your healthcare provider has prescribed the one that is best for your condition.
- The usual dosage of ADVAIR HFA is 2 inhalations 2 times each day (morning and evening). The 2 doses should be about 12 hours apart. Rinse your mouth with water after using ADVAIR HFA.
- If you take more ADVAIR HFA than your doctor has prescribed, get medical help right away if you have any unusual symptom, such as worsening shortness of breath, chest pain, increased heart rate, or shakiness.
- If you miss a dose of ADVAIR HFA, just skip that dose. Take your next dose at your usual time. Do not take 2 doses at one time.
- **While you are using ADVAIR HFA 2 times each day, do not use other medicines that contain a LABA for any reason.** Ask your healthcare provider or pharmacist if any of your other medicines are LABA medicines.
- Do not stop using ADVAIR HFA or other asthma medicines unless told to do so by your healthcare provider because your symptoms might get worse. Your healthcare provider will change your medicines as needed.
- ADVAIR HFA does not relieve sudden symptoms. Always have a rescue inhaler medicine with you to treat sudden symptoms. If you do not have a short-acting bronchodilator rescue inhaler, call your healthcare provider to have one prescribed for you.
- Call your healthcare provider or get medical care right away if:
  - your breathing problems worsen with ADVAIR HFA
  - you need to use your rescue inhaler medicine more often than usual
  - your rescue inhaler medicine does not work as well for you at relieving symptoms
  - you need to use 4 or more inhalations of your rescue inhaler medicine for 2 or more days in a row
  - you use 1 whole canister of your rescue inhaler medicine in 8 weeks' time
  - your peak flow meter results decrease. Your healthcare provider will tell you the numbers that are right for you.
  - your asthma symptoms do not improve after using ADVAIR HFA regularly for 1 week

What are the possible side effects with ADVAIR HFA?

ADVAIR HFA can cause serious side effects, including:
- **See "What is the most important information I should know about ADVAIR HFA?"**
- **serious allergic reactions.** Call your healthcare provider or get emergency medical care if you get any of the following symptoms of a serious allergic reaction:
  - rash
  - hives
  - swelling of the face, mouth, and tongue
  - breathing problems
- **sudden breathing problems immediately after inhaling your medicine**
- **effects on heart**
  - increased blood pressure
  - a fast and irregular heartbeat
  - chest pain
- **effects on nervous system**
  - tremor
  - nervousness
- **reduced adrenal function (may result in loss of energy)**
- **changes in blood (sugar, potassium, certain types of white blood cells)**
- **weakened immune system and a higher chance of infections**
- **lower bone mineral density.** This may be a problem for people who already have a higher chance of low bone density (osteoporosis).
- **eye problems including glaucoma and cataracts.** You should have regular eye exams while using ADVAIR HFA.
- **slowed growth in children.** A child's growth should be checked often.
- **throat tightness**
- **pneumonia.** ADVAIR HFA contains the same medicine found in ADVAIR DISKUS®. ADVAIR DISKUS is used to treat people with asthma and people with chronic obstructive pulmonary disease (COPD). People with COPD have a higher chance of getting pneumonia. ADVAIR DISKUS may increase the chance of getting pneumonia. ADVAIR HFA has not been studied in people with COPD. Call your healthcare provider if you notice any of the following symptoms:
  - increase in mucus (sputum) production
  - change in mucus color
  - fever
  - chills
  - increased cough
  - increased breathing problems

Common side effects of ADVAIR HFA include:
- upper respiratory tract infection
- throat irritation
- hoarseness and voice changes
- headache
- dizziness
- nausea and vomiting

Tell your healthcare provider about any side effect that bothers you or that does not go away.

These are not all the side effects with ADVAIR HFA. Ask your healthcare provider or pharmacist for more information.

Call your doctor for medical advice about side effects. You may report side effects to FDA at 1-800-FDA-1088.

How do I store ADVAIR HFA?
- Store ADVAIR HFA at room temperature between 59°F to 86°F (15°C to 30°C), with the mouthpiece down.
- **Contents Under Pressure:** Do not puncture. Do not use or store near heat or open flame. Exposure to temperatures above 120°F may cause bursting.
- Do not throw into fire or an incinerator.
- Keep ADVAIR HFA and all medicines out of the reach of children.

General Information about ADVAIR HFA

Medicines are sometimes prescribed for purposes not mentioned in a Medication Guide. Do not use ADVAIR HFA for a condition for which it was not prescribed. Do not give your ADVAIR HFA to other people, even if they have the same condition that you have. It may harm them.

This Medication Guide summarizes the most important information about ADVAIR HFA. If you would like more information, talk with your healthcare provider or pharmacist. You can ask your healthcare provider or pharmacist for information about ADVAIR HFA that was written for healthcare professionals. You can also contact the company that makes ADVAIR HFA (toll free) at 1-888-825-5249 or at www.advair.com.

What are the ingredients in ADVAIR HFA?

Active ingredients: fluticasone propionate, salmeterol xinafoate

Inactive ingredient: propellant HFA-134a

Instructions for using your ADVAIR HFA

The parts of your ADVAIR HFA

There are 2 main parts to your ADVAIR HFA inhaler—the metal canister that holds the medicine and the purple plastic actuator that sprays the medicine from the canister (see Figure 1).

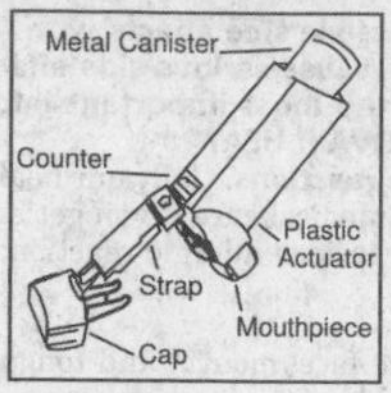

Figure 1

The canister has a counter to show how many sprays of medicine you have left. The number shows through a window in the back of the actuator. The counter starts at 124, or at 064 if you have a sample or institutional canister. The number will count down by 1 each time you spray the inhaler. The counter will stop counting at 000.

Never try to change the numbers or take the counter off the metal canister. The counter cannot be reset, and it is permanently attached to the canister.

The mouthpiece of the actuator is covered by a cap. The strap on the cap keeps it attached to the actuator.

Do not use the actuator with a canister of medicine from any other inhaler. Do not use an ADVAIR HFA canister with an actuator from any other inhaler.

Using your ADVAIR HFA

- The inhaler should be at room temperature before you use it.
- Take your ADVAIR HFA inhaler out of the moisture-protective pouch just before you use it for the first time. Safely throw away the foil pouch and the drying packet that comes inside the pouch.

Priming your ADVAIR HFA

Before you use ADVAIR HFA for the first time, you must prime the inhaler so that you will get the right amount of medicine when you use it. To prime the inhaler, take the cap off the mouthpiece and shake the inhaler well for 5 seconds. Then spray the inhaler 1 time into the air away from your face. **Avoid spraying in eyes.** Shake and spray the inhaler like this 3 more times to finish priming it. The counter should now read 120, or 060 if you have a sample or institutional canister.

You must prime your inhaler again if you have not used it in more than 4 weeks or if you drop it. Take the cap off the mouthpiece, shake the inhaler well for 5 seconds. Then spray it into the air away from your face. Shake and spray the inhaler like this 1 more time to finish priming it.

Read the following 7 steps before using ADVAIR HFA and follow them at each use. If you have any questions, ask your doctor or pharmacist.

1. **Take the cap off the mouthpiece of the actuator** (see Figure 2).
   Look inside the mouthpiece for foreign objects, and take out any you see.
   Make sure the canister fits firmly in the actuator.
   Shake the inhaler well for 5 seconds.

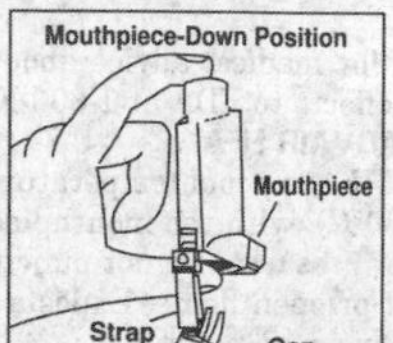

Figure 2

2. Hold the inhaler with the mouthpiece down (see Figure 2).
   Breathe out through your mouth and push as much air from your lungs as you can. Put the mouthpiece in your mouth and close your lips around it.
3. **Push the top of the canister all the way down while you breathe in deeply and slowly through your mouth** (see Figure 3).
   Right after the spray comes out, take your finger off the canister. After you have breathed in all the way, take the inhaler out of your mouth and close your mouth.

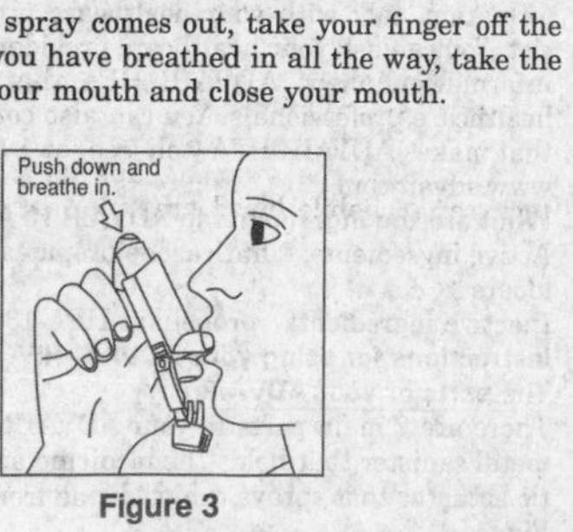

Figure 3

4. **Hold your breath as long as you can**, up to 10 seconds, then breathe normally.
5. **Wait about 30 seconds and shake the inhaler** well for 5 seconds. Repeat steps 2 through 4.
6. After you finish taking this medicine, rinse your mouth with water. Spit out the water. Do not swallow it.
7. Put the cap back on the mouthpiece after every time you use the inhaler. Make sure it snaps firmly into place.

Cleaning your ADVAIR HFA

Clean your inhaler at least 1 time each week after your evening dose. It is important to keep the canister and plastic actuator clean so the medicine will not build-up and block the spray.

1. Take the cap off the mouthpiece. The strap on the cap will stay attached to the actuator. Do not take the canister out of the plastic actuator.
2. Use a dry cotton swab to clean the small circular opening where the medicine sprays out of the canister. Carefully twist the swab in a circular motion to take off any medicine (see Figure 4).

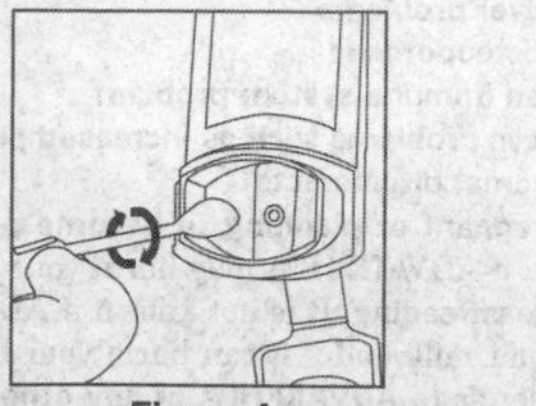

Figure 4

3. Wipe the inside of the mouthpiece with a clean tissue dampened with water. Let the actuator air-dry overnight.
4. Put the cap back on the mouthpiece after the actuator has dried.

Replacing your ADVAIR HFA

- **When the counter reads 020,** you should refill your prescription or ask your doctor if you need another prescription for ADVAIR HFA.
- **When the counter reads 000, throw the inhaler away.** You should not keep using the inhaler when the counter reads 000 because you will not receive the right amount of medicine.
- **Do not use the inhaler** after the expiration date, which is on the packaging it comes in.

This Medication Guide has been approved by the U.S. Food and Drug Administration.

ADVAIR, ADVAIR DISKUS, FLOVENT, and SEREVENT are registered trademarks of GlaxoSmithKline. The other brands listed are trademarks of their respective owners and are not trademarks of GlaxoSmithKline. The makers of these brands are not affiliated with and do not endorse GlaxoSmithKline or its products.

GlaxoSmithKline
Research Triangle Park, NC 27709

December 2012
ADH:8MG

AMERGE® ℞

[ə-merj']
(naratriptan hydrochloride)
Tablets

DESCRIPTION

AMERGE Tablets contain naratriptan as the hydrochloride, which is a selective 5-hydroxytryptamine$_1$ receptor subtype agonist. Naratriptan hydrochloride is chemically designated as N-methyl-3-(1-methyl-4-piperidinyl)-1H-indole-5-ethanesulfonamide monohydrochloride, and it has the following structure:

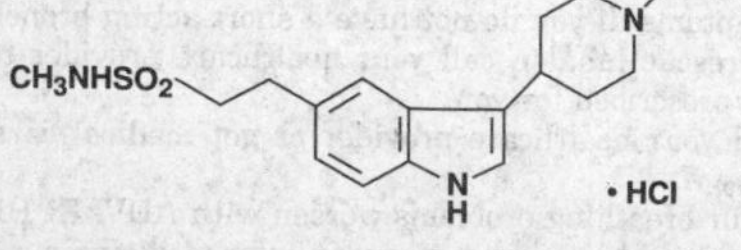

The empirical formula is $C_{17}H_{25}N_3O_2S \bullet HCl$, representing a molecular weight of 371.93. Naratriptan hydrochloride is a white to pale yellow powder that is readily soluble in water. Each AMERGE Tablet for oral administration contains 1.11 or 2.78 mg of naratriptan hydrochloride equivalent to 1 or 2.5 mg of naratriptan, respectively. Each tablet also contains the inactive ingredients croscarmellose sodium; hypromellose; lactose; magnesium stearate; microcrystalline cellulose; triacetin; and titanium dioxide, iron oxide yellow (2.5-mg tablet only), and indigo carmine aluminum lake (FD&C Blue No. 2) (2.5-mg tablet only) for coloring.

CLINICAL PHARMACOLOGY

Mechanism of Action

Naratriptan binds with high affinity to 5-HT_{1D} and 5-HT_{1B} receptors and has no significant affinity or pharmacological activity at 5-HT_{2-4} receptor subtypes or at adrenergic α_1, α_2, or β; dopaminergic D_1 or D_2; muscarinic; or benzodiazepine receptors.

The therapeutic activity of naratriptan in migraine is generally attributed to its agonist activity at 5-$HT_{1D/1B}$ receptors. Two current theories have been proposed to explain the efficacy of 5-$HT_{1D/1B}$ receptor agonists in migraine. One theory suggests that activation of 5-$HT_{1D/1B}$ receptors located on intracranial blood vessels, including those on the arteriovenous anastomoses, leads to vasoconstriction, which is correlated with the relief of migraine headache. The other hypothesis suggests that activation of 5-$HT_{1D/1B}$ receptors on sensory nerve endings in the trigeminal system results in the inhibition of pro-inflammatory neuropeptide release.

In the anesthetized dog, naratriptan has been shown to reduce the carotid arterial blood flow with little or no effect on arterial blood pressure or total peripheral resistance. While the effect on blood flow was selective for the carotid arterial bed, increases in vascular resistance of up to 30% were seen in the coronary arterial bed. Naratriptan has also been shown to inhibit trigeminal nerve activity in rat and cat. In 10 human subjects with suspected coronary artery disease (CAD) undergoing coronary artery catheterization, there was a 1% to 10% reduction in coronary artery diameter following subcutaneous injection of 1.5 mg of naratriptan.

Pharmacokinetics

Naratriptan tablets are well absorbed, with about 70% oral bioavailability. Following administration of a 2.5-mg tablet orally, the peak concentrations are obtained in 2 to 3 hours. After administration of 1- or 2.5-mg tablets, the C_{max} is somewhat (about 50%) higher in women (not corrected for milligram-per-kilogram dose) than in men. During a migraine attack, absorption was slower, with a T_{max} of 3 to 4 hours. Food does not affect the pharmacokinetics of naratriptan. Naratriptan displays linear kinetics over the therapeutic dose range.

The steady-state volume of distribution of naratriptan is 170 L. Plasma protein binding is 28% to 31% over the concentration range of 50 to 1,000 ng/mL.

Naratriptan is predominantly eliminated in urine, with 50% of the dose recovered unchanged and 30% as metabolites in urine. In vitro, naratriptan is metabolized by a wide range of cytochrome P450 isoenzymes into a number of inactive metabolites.

The mean elimination half-life of naratriptan is 6 hours. The systemic clearance of naratriptan is 6.6 mL/min/kg. The renal clearance (220 mL/min) exceeds glomerular filtration rate, indicating active tubular secretion. Repeat administration of naratriptan tablets does not result in drug accumulation.

Special Populations

Age: A small decrease in clearance (approximately 26%) was observed in healthy elderly subjects (65 to 77 years) compared to younger patients, resulting in slightly higher exposure (see PRECAUTIONS).

Race: The effect of race on the pharmacokinetics of naratriptan has not been examined.

Renal Impairment: Clearance of naratriptan was reduced by 50% in patients with moderate renal impairment (creatinine clearance: 18 to 39 mL/min) compared to the normal group. Decrease in clearances resulted in an increase of mean half-life from 6 hours (healthy) to 11 hours (range: 7 to 20 hours). The mean C_{max} increased by approximately 40%. The effects of severe renal impairment (creatinine clearance: ≤15 mL/min) on the pharmacokinetics of naratriptan has not been assessed (see CONTRAINDICATIONS and DOSAGE AND ADMINISTRATION).

Hepatic Impairment: Clearance of naratriptan was decreased by 30% in patients with moderate hepatic impairment (Child-Pugh grade A or B). This resulted in an approximately 40% increase in the half-life (range: 8 to 16 hours). The effects of severe hepatic impairment (Child-Pugh grade C) on the pharmacokinetics of naratriptan have not been assessed (see CONTRAINDICATIONS and DOSAGE AND ADMINISTRATION).

Drug Interactions

In normal volunteers, coadministration of single doses of naratriptan tablets and alcohol did not result in substantial modification of naratriptan pharmacokinetic parameters.

From population pharmacokinetic analyses, coadministration of naratriptan and fluoxetine, beta-blockers, or tricyclic antidepressants did not affect the clearance of naratriptan.

Naratriptan does not inhibit monoamine oxidase (MAO) enzymes and is a poor inhibitor of P450; metabolic interactions between naratriptan and drugs metabolized by P450 or MAO are therefore unlikely.

Oral Contraceptives: Oral contraceptives reduced clearance by 32% and volume of distribution by 22%, resulting in slightly higher concentrations of naratriptan. Hormone replacement therapy had no effect on pharmacokinetics in older female patients.

Smoking increased the clearance of naratriptan by 30%.

CLINICAL TRIALS

The efficacy of AMERGE Tablets in the acute treatment of migraine headaches was evaluated in 6 randomized, double-blind, placebo-controlled studies of which 4 used the recommended dosing regimen and were conducted as outpatient trials. Three of these studies enrolled adult patients who were predominantly female (86%) and Caucasian (96%) with a mean age of 41 (range: 18 to 65). One study enrolled adolescents with a mean age of 14 (range: 12 to 17). In the adolescent study, 54% of the patients were female and 89% were Caucasian. In all studies, patients were instructed to treat at least 1 moderate to severe headache. Headache response, defined as a reduction in headache severity from moderate or severe pain to mild or no pain, was assessed up to 4 hours after dosing. Associated symptoms such as nausea, vomiting, photophobia, and phonophobia were also assessed. Maintenance of response was assessed for up to 24 hours postdose. A second dose of AMERGE Tablets or other medication was allowed 4 to 24 hours after the initial treatment for recurrent headache. The frequency and time to use of these additional treatments were also determined.

In all 3 trials in adults utilizing the recommended dosage regimen and outpatient use, the percentage of patients achieving headache response 4 hours after treatment, the primary outcome measure, was significantly greater among patients receiving AMERGE compared to those who received placebo. In all studies, response to 2.5 mg was numerically greater than response to 1 mg and in the largest of the 3 studies, there was a statistically significant greater percentage of patients with headache response at 4 hours in the 2.5-mg group compared to the 1-mg group. The results are summarized in Table 1.

Table 1. Percentage of Adult Patients With Headache Response (Mild or No Headache) 4 Hours Following Treatment

	Placebo	AMERGE 1.0 mg	AMERGE 2.5 mg
Study 1	34% (n = 122)	50%[a] (n = 117)	60%[a] (n = 127)
Study 2	27% (n = 104)	52%[a] (n = 208)	66%[ab] (n = 199)
Study 3	32% (n = 169)	54%[a] (n = 166)	65%[a] (n = 167)

[a] $P<0.05$ in comparison with placebo.
[b] $P<0.05$ in comparison with 1 mg.

In the single study in adolescents, there were no statistically significant differences between any of the treatment groups. The headache response rates at 4 hours (n) were 65% (n = 74), 67% (n = 78), and 64% (n = 71) for placebo, 1-mg, and 2.5-mg groups, respectively.

Comparisons of drug performance based upon results obtained in different clinical trials are never reliable. Because studies are conducted at different times, with different samples of patients, by different investigators, employing different criteria and/or different interpretations of the same criteria, under different conditions (dose, dosing regimen, etc.), quantitative estimates of treatment response and the timing of response may be expected to vary considerably from study to study.

The estimated probability of achieving an initial headache response in adults over the 4 hours following treatment is depicted in Figure 1.

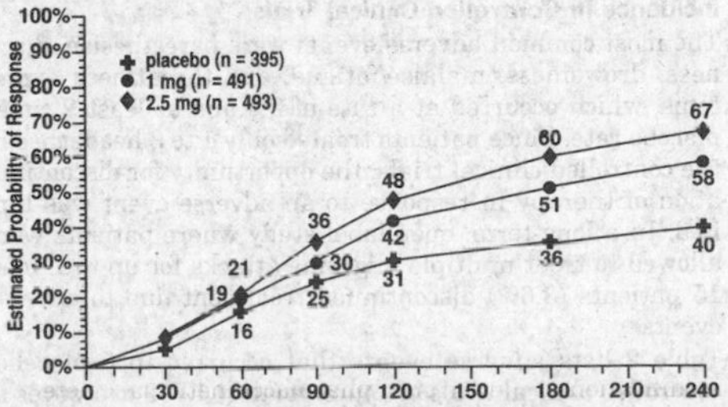

Figure 1. Estimated Probability of Achieving Initial Headache Response Within 4 Hours[a]

[a] The figure shows the probability over time of obtaining headache response (no or mild pain) following treatment with AMERGE Tablets. The averages displayed are based on pooled data from the 3 controlled clinical trials providing evidence of efficacy (Studies 1, 2, and 3). In this Kaplan-Meier plot, patients not achieving response within 240 minutes were censored at 240 minutes.

For patients with migraine-associated nausea, photophobia, and phonophobia at baseline, there was a lower incidence of these symptoms 4 hours following administration of 1- and 2.5-mg AMERGE Tablets compared to placebo.

Four to 24 hours following the initial dose of study treatment, patients were allowed to use additional treatment for pain relief in the form of a second dose of study treatment or other medication. The estimated probability of patients taking a second dose or other medication for migraine over the 24 hours following the initial dose of study treatment is summarized in Figure 2.

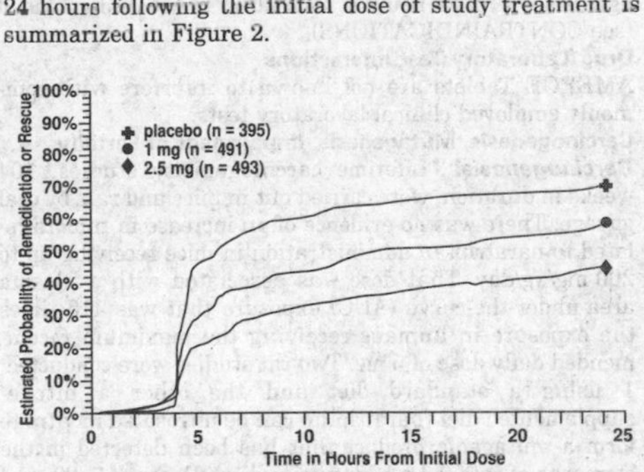

Figure 2. Estimated Probability of Patients Taking a Second Dose of AMERGE Tablets or Other Medication for Migraine Over the 24 Hours Following the Initial Dose of Study Treatment[a]

[a] Kaplan-Meier plot based on data obtained in the 3 controlled clinical trials (Studies 1, 2, and 3) providing evidence of efficacy with patients not using additional treatments censored at 24 hours. The plot also includes patients who had no response to the initial dose. Remedication was discouraged prior to 4 hours postdose.

There is no evidence that doses of 5 mg provide a greater effect than 2.5 mg. There was no evidence to suggest that treatment with AMERGE was associated with an increase in the severity or frequency of migraine attacks. The efficacy of AMERGE Tablets was unaffected by presence of aura; gender, age, or weight of the patient; oral contraceptive use; or concomitant use of common migraine prophylactic drugs (e.g., beta-blockers, calcium channel blockers, tricyclic antidepressants). There was insufficient data to assess the impact of race on efficacy.

INDICATIONS AND USAGE

AMERGE Tablets are indicated for the acute treatment of migraine attacks with or without aura in adults.

AMERGE Tablets are not intended for the prophylactic therapy of migraine or for use in the management of hemiplegic or basilar migraine (see CONTRAINDICATIONS). Safety and effectiveness of AMERGE Tablets have not been established for cluster headache, which is present in an older, predominantly male population.

CONTRAINDICATIONS

AMERGE Tablets should not be given to patients with history, symptoms, or signs of ischemic cardiac, cerebrovascular, or peripheral vascular syndromes. In addition, patients with other significant underlying cardiovascular diseases should not receive AMERGE Tablets. Ischemic cardiac syndromes include, but are not limited to, angina pectoris of any type (e.g., stable angina of effort, vasospastic forms of angina such as the Prinzmetal variant), all forms of myocardial infarction, and silent myocardial ischemia. Cerebrovascular syndromes include, but are not limited to, strokes of any type as well as transient ischemic attacks. Peripheral vascular disease includes, but is not limited to, ischemic bowel disease (see WARNINGS).

Because AMERGE Tablets may increase blood pressure, they should not be given to patients with uncontrolled hypertension (see WARNINGS).

AMERGE Tablets are contraindicated in patients with severe renal impairment (creatinine clearance, <15 mL/min) (see CLINICAL PHARMACOLOGY and DOSAGE and ADMINISTRATION).

AMERGE Tablets are contraindicated in patients with severe hepatic impairment (Child-Pugh grade C) (see CLINICAL PHARMACOLOGY and DOSAGE AND ADMINISTRATION).

AMERGE Tablets should not be administered to patients with hemiplegic or basilar migraine.

AMERGE Tablets should not be used within 24 hours of treatment with another 5-HT$_1$ agonist, an ergotamine-containing or ergot-type medication like dihydroergotamine or methysergide.

AMERGE Tablets are contraindicated in patients with hypersensitivity to naratriptan or any of the components.

WARNINGS

AMERGE Tablets should only be used where a clear diagnosis of migraine has been established.

Risk of Myocardial Ischemia and/or Infarction and Other Adverse Cardiac Events

Because of the potential of this class of compounds (5-HT$_{1B/1D}$ agonists) to cause coronary vasospasm, naratriptan should not be given to patients with documented ischemic or vasospastic coronary artery disease (CAD) (see CONTRAINDICATIONS). It is strongly recommended that 5-HT$_1$ agonists (including naratriptan) not be given to patients in whom unrecognized CAD is predicted by the presence of risk factors (e.g., hypertension, hypercholesterolemia, smoker, obesity, diabetes, strong family history of CAD, female with surgical or physiological menopause, male over 40 years of age) unless a cardiovascular evaluation provides satisfactory clinical evidence that the patient is reasonably free of coronary artery and ischemic myocardial disease or other significant underlying cardiovascular disease. The sensitivity of cardiac diagnostic procedures to detect cardiovascular disease or predisposition to coronary artery vasospasm is modest, at best. If, during the cardiovascular evaluation, the patient's medical history, electrocardiographic, or other investigations reveal findings indicative of, or consistent with, coronary artery vasospasm or myocardial ischemia, naratriptan should not be administered (see CONTRAINDICATIONS).

For patients with risk factors predictive of CAD, who are determined to have a satisfactory cardiovascular evaluation, it is strongly recommended that administration of the first dose of naratriptan take place in the setting of a physician's office or similar medically staffed and equipped facility. Because cardiac ischemia can occur in the absence of clinical symptoms, consideration should be given to obtaining on the first occasion of use an electrocardiogram (ECG) during the interval immediately following administration of AMERGE Tablets, in these patients with risk factors.

It is recommended that patients who are intermittent long-term users of 5-HT$_1$ agonists, including AMERGE Tablets, and who have or acquire risk factors predictive of CAD, as described above, undergo periodic cardiovascular evaluation as they continue to use AMERGE Tablets.

The systematic approach described above is intended to reduce the likelihood that patients with unrecognized cardiovascular disease will be inadvertently exposed to naratriptan.

Cardiac Events and Fatalities Associated With 5-HT$_1$ Agonists

Naratriptan can cause coronary artery vasospasm (see CLINICAL PHARMACOLOGY). Serious adverse cardiac events, including acute myocardial infarction, life-threatening disturbances of cardiac rhythm, and death have been reported within a few hours following the administration of 5-HT$_1$ agonists. Considering the extent of use of 5-HT$_1$ agonists in patients with migraine, the incidence of these events is extremely low.

Premarketing Experience With AMERGE Tablets: Among approximately 3,500 patients with migraine who participated in premarketing clinical trials of naratriptan tablets, 4 patients treated with single oral doses of naratriptan ranging from 1 to 10 mg experienced asymptomatic ischemic ECG changes with at least 1, who took 7.5 mg, likely due to coronary vasospasm.

Cerebrovascular Events and Fatalities With 5-HT$_1$ Agonists

Cerebral hemorrhage, subarachnoid hemorrhage, stroke, and other cerebrovascular events have been reported in patients treated with 5-HT$_1$ agonists, and some have resulted in fatalities. In a number of cases, it appears possible that the cerebrovascular events were primary, the agonist having been administered in the incorrect belief that the symptoms experienced were a consequence of migraine, when they were not. It should be noted that patients with migraine may be at increased risk of certain cerebrovascular events (e.g., stroke, hemorrhage, transient ischemic attack).

Other Vasospasm-Related Events

5-HT$_1$ agonists may cause vasospastic reactions other than coronary artery spasm. Both peripheral vascular ischemia and colonic ischemia with abdominal pain and bloody diarrhea have been reported with naratriptan.

Serotonin Syndrome

Serotonin syndrome may occur with triptans, including AMERGE, particularly during combined use with selective serotonin reuptake inhibitors (SSRIs) or serotonin norepinephrine reuptake inhibitors (SNRIs). Serotonin syndrome symptoms may include mental status changes (e.g., agitation, hallucinations, coma), autonomic instability (e.g., tachycardia, labile blood pressure, hyperthermia), neuromuscular aberrations (e.g., hyperreflexia, incoordination), and/or gastrointestinal symptoms (e.g., nausea, vomiting, diarrhea). The onset of symptoms can occur within minutes to hours of receiving a new or a greater dose of a serotonergic medication. Treatment with AMERGE should be discontinued if serotonin syndrome is suspected.

Increase in Blood Pressure

In healthy volunteers, dose-related increases in systemic blood pressure have been observed after administration of up to 20 mg of oral naratriptan. At the recommended doses, the elevations are generally small, although an increase of systolic pressure of 32 mmHg was seen in 1 patient following a single 2.5-mg dose. The effect may be more pronounced in the elderly and hypertensive patients. A patient who was mildly hypertensive (the baseline blood pressure was 150/98) experienced a significant increase in blood pressure to 204/144 mmHg 225 minutes after administration of a 10-mg oral dose. Significant elevation in blood pressure, including hypertensive crisis, has been reported on rare occasions in patients receiving 5-HT_1 agonists with and without a history of hypertension. Naratriptan is contraindicated in patients with uncontrolled hypertension (see CONTRAINDICATIONS).

An 18% increase in mean pulmonary artery pressure and an 8% increase in mean aortic pressure was seen following dosing with 1.5 mg of subcutaneous naratriptan in a study evaluating 10 subjects with suspected CAD undergoing cardiac catheterization.

Hypersensitivity

Hypersensitivity (anaphylaxis/anaphylactoid) reactions may occur in patients receiving naratriptan. Such reactions can be life threatening or fatal. In general, hypersensitivity reactions to drugs are more likely to occur in individuals with a history of sensitivity to multiple allergens (see CONTRAINDICATIONS).

PRECAUTIONS

General

Chest discomfort (including pain, pressure, heaviness, tightness) has been reported after administration of 5-HT_1 agonists, including AMERGE Tablets. These events have not been associated with arrhythmias or ischemic ECG changes in clinical trials with AMERGE Tablets. Because naratriptan may cause coronary artery vasospasm, patients who experience signs or symptoms suggestive of angina following naratriptan should be evaluated for the presence of CAD or a predisposition to Prinzmetal variant angina before receiving additional doses of naratriptan, and should be monitored electrocardiographically if dosing is resumed and similar symptoms recur. Similarly, patients who experience other symptoms or signs suggestive of decreased arterial flow, such as ischemic bowel syndrome or Raynaud syndrome following naratriptan administration should be evaluated for atherosclerosis or predisposition to vasospasm (see CONTRAINDICATIONS and WARNINGS).

AMERGE Tablets should also be administered with caution to patients with diseases that may alter the absorption, metabolism, or excretion of drugs, such as impaired renal or hepatic function (see CLINICAL PHARMACOLOGY, CONTRAINDICATIONS, and DOSAGE AND ADMINISTRATION).

Care should be taken to exclude other potentially serious neurological conditions before treating headache in patients not previously diagnosed with migraine or who experience a headache that is atypical for them. There have been rare reports where patients received 5-HT_1 agonists for severe headaches that were subsequently shown to have been secondary to an evolving neurologic lesion (see WARNINGS).

For a given attack, if a patient has no response to the first dose of AMERGE, the diagnosis of migraine should be reconsidered before administration of a second dose.

Overuse

Overuse of acute migraine drugs (e.g., ergotamine, triptans, opioids, or a combination of drugs for 10 or more days per month) may lead to exacerbation of headache (medication overuse headache). Medication overuse headache may present as migraine-like daily headaches, or as a marked increase in frequency of migraine attacks. Detoxification of patients, including withdrawal of the overused drugs, and treatment of withdrawal symptoms (which often includes a transient worsening of headache) may be necessary. Migraine patients should be informed about the risks of medication overuse and encouraged to record headache frequency and drug use.

Information for Patients

See PATIENT INFORMATION at the end of the full prescribing information for the text of the separate leaflet provided for patients.

Patients should be cautioned about the risk of serotonin syndrome with the use of naratriptan or other triptans, especially during combined use with SSRIs or SNRIs.

Laboratory Tests

No specific laboratory tests are recommended for monitoring patients prior to and/or after treatment with AMERGE Tablets.

Drug Interactions

Selective Serotonin Reuptake Inhibitors/Serotonin Norepinephrine Reuptake Inhibitors and Serotonin Syndrome: Cases of life-threatening serotonin syndrome have been reported during combined use of SSRIs or SNRIs and triptans (see WARNINGS).

Ergot-Containing Drugs: Ergot-containing drugs have been reported to cause prolonged vasospastic reactions. Because there is a theoretical basis that these effects may be additive, use of ergotamine-containing or ergot-type medications (like dihydroergotamine or methysergide) and naratriptan within 24 hours is contraindicated (see CONTRAINDICATIONS).

Other 5-HT_1 Agonists: The administration of naratriptan with other 5-HT_1 agonists has not been evaluated in migraine patients. Because their vasospastic effects may be additive, coadministration of naratriptan and other 5-HT_1 agonists within 24 hours of each other is not recommended (see CONTRAINDICATIONS).

Drug/Laboratory Test Interactions

AMERGE Tablets are not known to interfere with commonly employed clinical laboratory tests.

Carcinogenesis, Mutagenesis, Impairment of Fertility

Carcinogenesis: Lifetime carcinogenicity studies, 104 weeks in duration, were carried out in mice and rats by oral gavage. There was no evidence of an increase in tumors related to naratriptan administration in mice receiving up to 200 mg/kg/day. That dose was associated with a plasma area-under-the-curve (AUC) exposure that was 110 times the exposure in humans receiving the maximum recommended daily dose of 5 mg. Two rat studies were conducted, 1 using a standard diet and the other a nitrite-supplemented diet (naratriptan can be nitrosated in vitro to form a mutagenic product that has been detected in the stomachs of rats fed a high nitrite diet). Doses of 5, 20, and 90 mg/kg were associated with week 13 AUC exposures that in the standard diet study were 7, 40, and 236 times, respectively, and in the nitrite-supplemented diet study were 7, 29, and 180 times, respectively, the exposure attained in humans given the maximum recommended daily dose of 5 mg. In both studies, there was an increase in the incidence of thyroid follicular hyperplasia in high-dose males and females and in thyroid follicular adenomas in high-dose males. In the standard diet study only, there was also an increase in the incidence of benign c-cell adenomas in the thyroid of high-dose males and females. The exposures achieved at the no-effect dose for thyroid tumors were 40 (standard diet) and 29 (nitrite-supplemented diet) times the exposure achieved in humans receiving the maximum recommended daily dose of 5 mg. In the nitrite-supplemented diet study only, the incidence of benign lymphocytic thymoma was increased in all treated groups of females. It was not determined if the nitrosated product is systemically absorbed. However, no changes were seen in the stomachs of rats in that study.

Mutagenesis: Naratriptan was not mutagenic when tested in 2 gene mutation assays, the Ames test and the in vitro thymidine locus mouse lymphoma assay. It was not clastogenic in 2 cytogenetics assays, the in vitro human lymphocyte assay and the in vivo mouse micronucleus assay. Naratriptan can be nitrosated in vitro to form a mutagenic product (WHO nitrosation assay) that has been detected in the stomachs of rats fed a nitrite-supplemented diet.

Impairment of Fertility: In a reproductive toxicity study in which male and female rats were dosed prior to and throughout the mating period with 10, 60, 170, or 340 mg/kg/day (plasma exposures [AUC] approximately 11, 70, 230, and 470 times, respectively, the human exposure at the maximum recommended daily dose [MRDD] of 5 mg), there was a treatment-related decrease in the number of females exhibiting normal estrous cycles at doses of 170 mg/kg/day or greater and an increase in preimplantation loss at 60 mg/kg/day or greater. In high-dose group males, testicular/epididymal atrophy accompanied by spermatozoa depletion reduced mating success and may have contributed to the observed preimplantation loss. The exposures achieved at the no-effect doses for preimplantation loss, anestrus, and testicular effects were approximately 11, 70, and 230 times, respectively, the exposures in humans receiving the MRDD.

In a study in which rats were dosed orally with 10, 60, or 340 mg/kg/day for 6 months, changes in the female reproductive tract including atrophic or cystic ovaries and anestrus were seen at the high dose. The exposure at the no-effect dose of 60 mg/kg was approximately 85 times the exposure in humans receiving the MRDD.

Pregnancy

Pregnancy Category C. There are no adequate and well-controlled studies in pregnant women; therefore, naratriptan should be used during pregnancy only if the potential benefit justifies the potential risk to the fetus.

In reproductive toxicity studies in rats and rabbits, oral administration of naratriptan was associated with developmental toxicity (embryolethality, fetal abnormalities, pup mortality, offspring growth retardation) at doses producing maternal plasma drug exposures as low as 11 and 2.5 times, respectively, the exposure in humans receiving the MRDD of 5 mg.

When pregnant rats were administered naratriptan during the period of organogenesis at doses of 10, 60, or 340 mg/kg/day, there was a dose-related increase in embryonic death, with a statistically significant difference at the highest dose, and incidences of fetal structural variations (incomplete/irregular ossification of skull bones, sternebrae, ribs) were increased at all doses. The maternal plasma exposures (AUC) at these doses were approximately 11, 70, and 470 times the exposure in humans at the MRDD. The high dose was maternally toxic, as evidenced by decreased maternal body weight gain during gestation. A no-effect dose for developmental toxicity in rats exposed during organogenesis was not established.

When doses of 1, 5, or 30 mg/kg/day were given to pregnant Dutch rabbits throughout organogenesis, the incidence of a specific fetal skeletal malformation (fused sternebrae) was increased at the high dose, and increased incidences of embryonic death and fetal variations (major blood vessel variations, supernumerary ribs, incomplete skeletal ossification) were observed at all doses (4, 20, and 120 times, respectively, the MRDD on a body surface area basis). Maternal toxicity (decreased body weight gain) was evident at the high dose in this study. In a similar study in New Zealand White rabbits (1, 5, or 30 mg/kg/day throughout organogenesis), decreased fetal weights and increased incidences of fetal skeletal variations were observed at all doses (maternal exposures equivalent to 2.5, 19, and 140 times exposure in humans receiving the MRDD), while maternal body weight gain was reduced at 5 mg/kg or greater. A no-effect dose for developmental toxicity in rabbits exposed during organogenesis was not established.

When female rats were treated with 10, 60, or 340 mg/kg/day during late gestation and lactation, offspring behavioral impairment (tremors) and decreased offspring viability and growth were observed at doses of 60 mg/kg or greater, while maternal toxicity occurred only at the highest dose. Maternal exposures at the no-effect dose for developmental effects in this study were approximately 11 times the exposure in humans receiving the MRDD.

Nursing Mothers

Naratriptan-related material is excreted in the milk of rats. Therefore, caution should be exercised when considering the administration of AMERGE Tablets to a nursing woman.

Pediatric Use

Safety and effectiveness of AMERGE Tablets in pediatric patients (younger than 18 years) have not been established. One randomized, placebo-controlled clinical trial evaluating oral naratriptan (0.25 to 2.5 mg) in pediatric patients aged 12 to 17 years evaluated a total of 300 adolescent migraineurs. This study did not establish the efficacy of oral naratriptan compared to placebo in the treatment of migraine in adolescents (see CLINICAL TRIALS). Adverse events observed in this clinical trial were similar in nature to those reported in clinical trials in adults.

Geriatric Use

The use of AMERGE Tablets in elderly patients is not recommended.

Naratriptan is known to be substantially excreted by the kidney, and the risk of adverse reactions to this drug may be greater in elderly patients who have reduced renal function. In addition, elderly patients are more likely to have decreased hepatic function; they are at higher risk for CAD; and blood pressure increases may be more pronounced in the elderly. Clinical studies of AMERGE Tablets did not include patients over 65 years of age.

ADVERSE REACTIONS

Serious cardiac events, including some that have been fatal, have occurred following the use of 5-HT_1 agonists. These events are extremely rare and most have been reported in patients with risk factors predictive of CAD. Events reported have included coronary artery vasospasm, transient myocardial ischemia, myocardial infarction, ventricular tachycardia, and ventricular fibrillation (see CONTRAINDICATIONS, WARNINGS, and PRECAUTIONS).

Incidence in Controlled Clinical Trials

The most common adverse events were paresthesias, dizziness, drowsiness, malaise/fatigue, and throat/neck symptoms, which occurred at a rate of 2% and at least 2 times placebo rate. Since patients treated only 1 to 3 headaches in the controlled clinical trials, the opportunity for discontinuation of therapy in response to an adverse event was limited. In a long-term, open-label study where patients were allowed to treat multiple migraine attacks for up to 1 year, 15 patients (3.6%) discontinued treatment due to adverse events.

Table 2 lists adverse events that occurred in 5 placebo-controlled clinical trials of approximately 1,752 exposures to placebo and AMERGE Tablets in adult migraine patients. The events cited reflect experience gained under closely monitored conditions of clinical trials in a highly selected patient population. In actual clinical practice or in other clinical trials, these frequency estimates may not apply, as the conditions of use, reporting behavior, and the kinds of patients treated may differ. Only events that occurred at a frequency of 2% or more in the group treated with AMERGE Tablets 2.5 mg and were more frequent in that group than in the placebo group are included in Table 2. From this table, it appears that many of these adverse events are dose related.

[See table 2 above]

One event (vomiting) present in more than 1% of patients receiving AMERGE Tablets occurred more frequently on placebo than on naratriptan 2.5 mg.

AMERGE Tablets are generally well tolerated. Most adverse reactions were mild and transient.

The incidence of adverse events in placebo-controlled clinical trials was not affected by age or weight of the patients, duration of headache prior to treatment, presence of aura, use of prophylactic medications, or tobacco use. There was insufficient data to assess the impact of race on the incidence of adverse events.

Table 2. Treatment-Emergent Adverse Events Reported by at Least 2% of Patients in Placebo-Controlled Migraine Trials

Adverse Event Type	Placebo (n = 498)	AMERGE 1 mg (n = 627)	AMERGE 2.5 mg (n = 627)
Atypical sensation	1%	2%	4%
Paresthesias (all types)	<1%	1%	2%
Gastrointestinal	5%	6%	7%
Nausea	4%	4%	5%
Neurological	3%	4%	7%
Dizziness	1%	1%	2%
Drowsiness	<1%	1%	2%
Malaise/fatigue	1%	2%	2%
Pain and pressure sensation	2%	2%	4%
Throat/neck symptoms	1%	1%	2%

Other Events Observed in Association With the Administration of AMERGE Tablets

In the paragraphs that follow, the frequencies of less commonly reported adverse clinical events are presented. Because the reports include events observed in open and uncontrolled studies, the role of AMERGE Tablets in their causation cannot be reliably determined. Furthermore, variability associated with adverse event reporting, the terminology used to describe adverse events, etc., limit the value of the quantitative frequency estimates provided. Event frequencies are calculated as the number of patients reporting an event divided by the total number of patients (n = 3,557) exposed to oral naratriptan doses up to 10 mg. All reported events are included except those already listed in the previous table, those too general to be informative, and those not reasonably associated with the use of the drug. Events are further classified within body system categories and enumerated in order of decreasing frequency using the following definitions: frequent adverse events are those occurring in at least 1/100 patients, infrequent adverse events are those occurring in 1/100 to 1/1,000 patients, and rare adverse events are those occurring in fewer than 1/1,000 patients.

Atypical Sensations: Frequent were warm/cold temperature sensations. Infrequent were feeling strange and burning/stinging sensation.

Cardiovascular: Infrequent were palpitations, increased blood pressure, tachyarrhythmias, and abnormal ECG (PR prolongation, QT_c prolongation, ST/T wave abnormalities, premature ventricular contractions, atrial flutter, or atrial fibrillation), and syncope. Rare were bradycardia, varicosities, hypotension, and heart murmurs.

Ear, Nose, and Throat: Frequent were ear, nose, and throat infections. Infrequent were phonophobia, sinusitis, upper respiratory inflammation, and tinnitus. Rare were allergic rhinitis; labyrinthitis; ear, nose, and throat hemorrhage; and hearing difficulty.

Endocrine and Metabolic: Infrequent were thirst and polydipsia, dehydration, and fluid retention. Rare were hyperlipidemia, hypercholesterolemia, hypothyroidism, hyperglycemia, glycosuria and ketonuria, and parathyroid neoplasm.

Eye: Frequent was photophobia. Infrequent was blurred vision. Rare were eye pain and discomfort, sensation of eye pressure, eye hemorrhage, dry eyes, difficulty focusing, and scotoma.

Gastrointestinal: Frequent were hyposalivation and vomiting. Infrequent were dyspeptic symptoms, diarrhea, gastrointestinal discomfort and pain, gastroenteritis, and constipation. Rare were abnormal liver function tests, abnormal bilirubin levels, hemorrhoids, gastritis, esophagitis, salivary gland inflammation, oral itching and irritation, regurgitation and reflux, and gastric ulcers.

Hematological Disorders: Infrequent was increased white cells. Rare were thrombocytopenia, quantitative red cell or hemoglobin defects, anemia, and purpura.

Lower Respiratory Tract: Infrequent were bronchitis, cough, and pneumonia. Rare were tracheitis, asthma, pleuritis, and airway constriction and obstruction.

Musculoskeletal: Infrequent were muscle pain, arthralgia and articular rheumatism, muscle cramps and spasms, joint and muscle stiffness, tightness, and rigidity. Rare were bone and skeletal pain.

Neurological: Frequent was vertigo. Infrequent were tremors, cognitive function disorders, sleep disorders, and disorders of equilibrium. Rare were compressed nerve syndromes, confusion, sedation, hyperesthesia, coordination disorders, paralysis of cranial nerves, decreased consciousness, dreams, altered sense of taste, neuralgia, neuritis, aphasia, hypoesthesia, motor retardation, muscle twitching and fasciculation, psychomotor restlessness, and convulsions.

Non-Site Specific: Infrequent were chills and/or fever, descriptions of odor or taste, edema and swelling, allergies, and allergic reactions. Rare were spasms and mobility disorders.

Pain and Pressure Sensations: Frequent were pressure/tightness/heaviness sensations.

Psychiatry: Infrequent were anxiety, depressive disorders, and detachment. Rare were aggression and hostility, agitation, hallucinations, panic, and hyperactivity.

Reproduction: Rare were lumps of female reproductive tract, breast inflammation, inflammation of vagina, inflammation of fallopian tube, breast discharge, endometrium disorders, decreased libido, and lumps of breast.

Skin: Infrequent were sweating, skin rashes, pruritus, and urticaria. Rare were skin erythema, dermatitis and dermatosis, hair loss and alopecia, pruritic skin rashes, acne and folliculitis, allergic skin reactions, macular skin/rashes, skin photosensitivity, photodermatitis, skin flakiness, and dry skin.

Urology: Infrequent were bladder inflammation and polyuria and diuresis. Rare were urinary tract hemorrhage, urinary urgency, pyelitis, and urinary incontinence.

Observed During Clinical Practice

The following section enumerates potentially important adverse events that have occurred in clinical practice and that have been reported spontaneously to various surveillance systems. The events enumerated represent reports arising from both domestic and nondomestic use of naratriptan. These events do not include those already listed in the ADVERSE REACTIONS section above. Because the reports cite events reported spontaneously from worldwide postmarketing experience, frequency of events and the role of naratriptan in their causation cannot be reliably determined.

Cardiovascular: Angina, myocardial infarction (see WARNINGS).

Gastrointestinal: Colonic ischemia (see WARNINGS).

Lower Respiratory: Dyspnea.

Miscellaneous: Hypersensitivity, including anaphylaxis/anaphylactoid reactions, in some cases severe (e.g., circulatory collapse) (see WARNINGS).

Neurologic: Cerebral vascular accident, including transient ischemic attack, subarachnoid hemorrhage, and cerebral infarction (see WARNINGS); serotonin syndrome.

DRUG ABUSE AND DEPENDENCE

In one clinical study enrolling 12 subjects, all of whom had experience using oral opiates and other psychoactive drugs, AMERGE Tablets produced less intense subjective responses ordinarily associated with many drugs of abuse than did codeine (30 to 90 mg).

OVERDOSAGE

A patient who was mildly hypertensive experienced a significant increase in blood pressure after administration of a 10-mg dose starting at 30 minutes (baseline value of 150/98 to 204/144 mmHg 225 minutes). This event resolved after treatment with antihypertensive therapy. Oral administration of 25 mg of naratriptan in 1 healthy young male subject increased blood pressure from 120/67 mmHg pretreatment up to 191/113 mmHg at approximately 6 hours postdose and resulted in adverse events including lightheadedness, tension in the neck, tiredness, and loss of coordination. Blood pressure returned to near baseline by 8 hours after dosing without any pharmacological intervention.

Another subject experienced asymptomatic ischemic ECG changes likely due to coronary artery vasospasm approximately 2 hours following a 7.5-mg oral dose.

The elimination half-life of naratriptan is about 6 hours (see CLINICAL PHARMACOLOGY), and therefore monitoring of patients after overdose with AMERGE Tablets should continue for at least 24 hours or while symptoms or signs persist. There is no specific antidote to naratriptan. Standard supportive treatment should be applied as required. If the patient presents with chest pain or other symptoms consistent with angina pectoris, ECG monitoring should be performed for evidence of ischemia. It is unknown what effect hemodialysis or peritoneal dialysis has on the serum concentrations of naratriptan.

DOSAGE AND ADMINISTRATION

In controlled clinical trials, single doses of 1 and 2.5 mg of AMERGE Tablets taken with fluid were effective for the acute treatment of migraines in adults. A greater proportion of patients had headache response following a 2.5-mg dose than following a 1-mg dose (see CLINICAL TRIALS). Individuals may vary in response to doses of AMERGE Tablets. The choice of dose should therefore be made on an individual basis, weighing the possible benefit of the 2.5-mg dose with the potential for a greater risk of adverse events. If the headache returns or if the patient has only partial response, the dose may be repeated once after 4 hours, for a maximum dose of 5 mg in a 24-hour period. There is evidence that doses of 5 mg do not provide a greater effect than 2.5 mg. The safety of treating, on average, more than 4 headaches in a 30-day period has not been established.

Renal Impairment

The use of AMERGE is contraindicated in patients with severe renal impairment (creatinine clearance, <15 mL/min) because of decreased clearance of the drug (see CONTRAINDICATIONS and CLINICAL PHARMACOLOGY). In patients with mild to moderate renal impairment, the maximum daily dose should not exceed 2.5 mg over a 24-hour period and a lower starting dose should be considered.

Hepatic Impairment

The use of AMERGE is contraindicated in patients with severe hepatic impairment (Child-Pugh grade C) because of decreased clearance (see CONTRAINDICATIONS and CLINICAL PHARMACOLOGY). In patients with mild or moderate hepatic impairment, the maximum daily dose should not exceed 2.5 mg over a 24-hour period and a lower starting dose should be considered (see CLINICAL PHARMACOLOGY).

HOW SUPPLIED

AMERGE Tablets 1 and 2.5 mg of naratriptan (base) as the hydrochloride. AMERGE Tablets, 1 mg, are white, D-shaped, film-coated tablets debossed with "GX CE3" on one side in blister packs of 9 tablets (NDC 0173-0561-00). AMERGE Tablets, 2.5 mg, are green, D-shaped, film-coated tablets debossed with "GX CE5" on one side in blister packs of 9 tablets (NDC 0173-0562-00).

Store at controlled room temperature, 20° to 25°C (68° to 77°F) (see USP).

GlaxoSmithKline
Research Triangle Park, NC 27709

March 2012
AMG:3PI

PATIENT INFORMATION

The following wording is contained in a separate leaflet provided for patients.

Patient Information
AMERGE® (a-MERJ)
(naratriptan hydrochloride)
Tablets

Read this Patient Information before you start taking AMERGE and each time you get a refill. There may be new information. This information does not take the place of talking with your healthcare provider about your medical condition or treatment.

What is the most important information I should know about AMERGE?

AMERGE can cause serious side effects, including:

Heart attack and other heart problems. Heart problems may lead to death.

Stop taking AMERGE and get emergency medical help right away if you have any of the following symptoms of a heart attack:

- discomfort in the center of your chest that lasts for more than a few minutes, or that goes away and comes back.

- chest pain or chest discomfort that feels like heavy pressure, squeezing, or fullness
- pain or discomfort in your arms, back, neck, jaw, or stomach

shortness of breath with or without chest discomfort
- breaking out in a cold sweat
- nausea or vomiting
- feeling lightheaded

AMERGE is not for people with risk factors for heart disease unless a heart exam is done and shows no problem. You have a higher risk for heart disease if you:
- have high blood pressure
- have high cholesterol levels
- smoke
- are overweight
- have diabetes
- have a family history of heart disease
- are a female who has gone through menopause
- are a male over age 40

Serotonin syndrome. Serotonin syndrome is a serious and life-threatening problem that can happen in people taking AMERGE, especially if AMERGE is used with antidepressant medicines called selective serotonin reuptake inhibitors (SSRIs) or selective norepinephrine reuptake inhibitors (SNRIs).

Ask your healthcare provider or pharmacist for a list of these medicines if you are not sure.

Call your healthcare provider right away if you have any of the following symptoms of serotonin syndrome:
- mental changes such as seeing things that are not there (hallucinations), agitation, or coma
- fast heartbeat
- changes in blood pressure
- high body temperature
- tight muscles
- trouble walking
- nausea, vomiting, or diarrhea

What is AMERGE?

AMERGE is a prescription medicine used to treat acute migraine headaches with or without aura in adults.

AMERGE is not used to prevent or decrease the number of migraine headaches you have.

AMERGE is not used to treat other types of headaches such as hemiplegic migraines (that make you unable to move on one side of your body) or basilar migraines (rare form of migraine with aura).

It is not known if AMERGE is safe and effective to treat cluster headaches.

It is not known if AMERGE is safe and effective in children under 18 years of age.

Who should not take AMERGE?

Do not take AMERGE if you have:
- heart problems or a history of heart problems
- narrowing of blood vessels to your legs, arms, stomach, or kidney (peripheral vascular disease)
- uncontrolled high blood pressure
- severe kidney problems
- severe liver problems
- hemiplegic migraines or basilar migraines. If you are not sure if you have these types of migraines, ask your healthcare provider.
- had a stroke, transient ischemic attacks (TIAs), or problems with your blood circulation
- taken any of the following medicines in the last 24 hours:
  - almotriptan (AXERT®)
  - eletriptan (RELPAX®)
  - frovatriptan (FROVA®)
  - rizatriptan (MAXALT®, MAXALT-MLT®)
  - sumatriptan (IMITREX®, SUMAVEL® DosePro®)
  - sumatriptan and naproxen (TREXIMET®)
  - ergotamines (CAFERGOT®, ERGOMAR®, MIGERGOT®)
  - dihydroergotamine (D.H.E. 45®, MIGRANAL®)

Ask your doctor if you are not sure if your medicine is listed above.
- an allergy to naratriptan hydrochloride or any of the ingredients in AMERGE. See the end of this leaflet for a complete list of ingredients in AMERGE.

What should I tell my healthcare provider before taking AMERGE?

Before you take AMERGE, tell your healthcare provider about all of your medical conditions, including if you:
- have high blood pressure
- have high cholesterol
- have diabetes
- smoke
- are overweight
- are a female who has gone through menopause
- have heart disease or a family history of heart disease or stroke
- have kidney problems
- have liver problems
- have had epilepsy or seizures
- are not using effective birth control
- are pregnant or plan to become pregnant. It is not known if AMERGE will harm your unborn baby.
- become pregnant while taking AMERGE
- are breastfeeding or plan to breastfeed. AMERGE passes into your breast milk and may harm your baby. Talk with your healthcare provider about the best way to feed your baby if you take AMERGE.

Tell your healthcare provider about all the medicines you take, including prescription and nonprescription medicines, vitamins, and herbal supplements.

AMERGE and other medicines may affect each other, causing side effects.

Especially tell your healthcare provider if you take antidepressant medicines called:
- selective serotonin reuptake inhibitors (SSRIs)
- serotonin norepinephrine reuptake inhibitors (SNRIs)
- monoamine oxidase inhibitors (MAOIs)

Ask your healthcare provider or pharmacist for a list of these medicines if you are not sure.

Know the medicines you take. Keep a list of them to show your healthcare provider or pharmacist when you get a new medicine.

How should I take AMERGE?
- Certain people should take their first dose of AMERGE in their healthcare provider's office or in another medical setting. Ask your healthcare provider if you should take your first dose in a medical setting.
- Take AMERGE exactly as your healthcare provider tells you to take it.
- Your healthcare provider may change your dose. Do not change your dose without first talking with your healthcare provider.
- Take AMERGE with water or other liquids.
- If you do not get any relief after your first AMERGE tablet, do not take a second tablet without first talking with your healthcare provider.
- If your headache comes back or you only get some relief from your headache, you can take a second tablet 4 hours after the first tablet.
- Do not take more than a total of 5 mg of AMERGE in a 24-hour period.
- Some people who take too many AMERGE tablets may have worse headaches (medication overuse headache). If your headaches get worse, your healthcare provider may decide to stop your treatment with AMERGE.
- If you take too much AMERGE, call your healthcare provider or go to the nearest hospital emergency room right away.
- You should write down when you have headaches and when you take AMERGE so you can talk with your healthcare provider about how AMERGE is working for you.

What should I avoid while taking AMERGE?

AMERGE can cause dizziness, weakness, or drowsiness. If you have these symptoms, do not drive a car, use machinery, or do anything where you need to be alert.

What are the possible side effects of AMERGE?

AMERGE may cause serious side effects. See "What is the most important information I should know about AMERGE?"

These serious side effects include:
- changes in color or sensation in your fingers and toes (Raynaud's syndrome)
- stomach and intestinal problems (gastrointestinal and colonic ischemic events). Symptoms of gastrointestinal and colonic ischemic events include:
  - sudden or severe stomach pain
  - stomach pain after meals
  - weight loss
  - nausea or vomiting
  - constipation or diarrhea
  - bloody diarrhea
  - fever
- problems with blood circulation to your legs and feet (peripheral vascular ischemia). Symptoms of peripheral vascular ischemia include:
  - cramping and pain in your legs or hips
  - feeling of heaviness or tightness in your leg muscles
  - burning or aching pain in your feet or toes while resting
  - numbness, tingling, or weakness in your legs
  - cold feeling or color changes in 1 or both legs or feet
- shortness of breath or wheezing
- hives (itchy bumps); swelling of your tongue, mouth, or throat

The most common side effects of AMERGE include:
- dizziness
- warm, hot, burning feeling to your face (flushing)
- cold and hot temperature sensations
- sensitivity to light or vision problems
- ear, nose, and throat infections
- feeling weak, drowsy, or tired
- decrease in saliva

Tell your healthcare provider if you have any side effect that bothers you or that does not go away.

These are not all the possible side effects of AMERGE. For more information, ask your healthcare provider or pharmacist.

Call your doctor for medical advice about side effects. You may report side effects to FDA at 1-800-FDA-1088.

How should I store AMERGE?

Store AMERGE between 68°F to 77°F (20°C to 25°C).

Keep AMERGE and all medicines out of the reach of children.

General information about the safe and effective use of AMERGE.

Medicines are sometimes prescribed for purposes other than those listed in Patient Information leaflets. Do not use AMERGE for a condition for which it was not prescribed. Do not give AMERGE to other people, even if they have the same symptoms you have. It may harm them.

This Patient Information leaflet summarizes the most important information about AMERGE. If you would like more information, talk with your healthcare provider. You can ask your healthcare provider or pharmacist for information about AMERGE that is written for healthcare professionals. For more information, go to www.gsk.com or call 1-888-825-5249.

What are the ingredients in AMERGE?

Active ingredient: naratriptan hydrochloride

Inactive ingredients: croscarmellose sodium, hypromellose, lactose, magnesium stearate, microcrystalline cellulose, triacetin, titanium dioxide

2.5-mg tablets also contain iron oxide yellow and indigo carmine aluminum lake (FD&C Blue No. 2) for coloring.

AMERGE, IMITREX, and TREXIMET are registered trademarks of GlaxoSmithKline. The other brands listed are trademarks of their respective owners and are not trademarks of GlaxoSmithKline. The makers of these brands are not affiliated with and do not endorse GlaxoSmithKline or its products.

This Patient Information has been approved by the U.S. Food and Drug Administration.

GlaxoSmithKline
Research Triangle Park, NC 27709

March 2012
AMG:3PIL

ARGATROBAN ℞

[är-ga' trō-ban]
Injection

DESCRIPTION

Argatroban is a synthetic direct thrombin inhibitor derived from L-arginine. The chemical name for Argatroban is 1-[5-[(aminoiminomethyl)amino]-1-oxo-2-[[(1,2,3,4-tetrahydro-3-methyl-8-quinolinyl)sulfonyl]amino]pentyl]-4-methyl-2-piperidinecarboxylic acid, monohydrate. Argatroban has 4 asymmetric carbons. One of the asymmetric carbons has an *R* configuration (stereoisomer Type I) and an *S* configuration (stereoisomer Type II). Argatroban consists of a mixture of *R* and *S* stereoisomers at a ratio of approximately 65:35.

The molecular formula of Argatroban is $C_{23}H_{36}N_6O_5S \bullet H_2O$. Its molecular weight is 526.66. The structural formula is shown below:

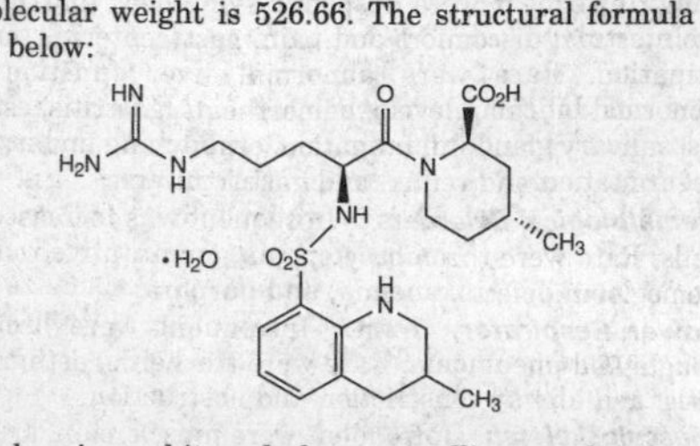

Argatroban is a white, odorless crystalline powder that is freely soluble in glacial acetic acid, slightly soluble in ethanol, and insoluble in acetone, ethyl acetate, and ether. Argatroban Injection is a sterile clear, colorless to pale yellow, slightly viscous solution. Argatroban is available in 250-mg (in 2.5-mL) single-use amber vials, with gray fliptop caps. Each mL of sterile, nonpyrogenic solution contains 100 mg Argatroban. Inert ingredients: 750 mg D-sorbitol, 1,000 mg dehydrated alcohol.

CLINICAL PHARMACOLOGY

Mechanism of Action

Argatroban is a direct thrombin inhibitor that reversibly binds to the thrombin active site. Argatroban does not require the co-factor antithrombin III for antithrombotic activity. Argatroban exerts its anticoagulant effects by inhibiting thrombin-catalyzed or -induced reactions, including fibrin formation; activation of coagulation factors V, VIII, and XIII; activation of protein C; and platelet aggregation.

Argatroban is highly selective for thrombin with an inhibitory constant (K_i) of 0.04 μM. At therapeutic concentrations, Argatroban has little or no effect on related serine proteases (trypsin, factor Xa, plasmin, and kallikrein).

Argatroban is capable of inhibiting the action of both free and clot-associated thrombin.

Argatroban does not interact with heparin-induced antibodies. Evaluation of sera in 12 healthy subjects and 8 patients who received multiple doses of Argatroban did not reveal antibody formation to Argatroban (see CLINICAL STUDIES).

Pharmacokinetics

Distribution: Argatroban distributes mainly in the extracellular fluid as evidenced by an apparent steady-state volume of distribution of 174 mL/kg (12.18 L in a 70-kg adult). Argatroban is 54% bound to human serum proteins, with binding to albumin and α_1-acid glycoprotein being 20% and 34%, respectively.

Metabolism: The main route of Argatroban metabolism is hydroxylation and aromatization of the 3-methyltetrahydroquinoline ring in the liver. The formation of each of the 4 known metabolites is catalyzed in vitro by the human liver microsomal cytochrome P450 enzymes CYP3A4/5. The primary metabolite (M1) exerts 3- to 5-fold weaker anticoagulant effects than Argatroban. Unchanged Argatroban is the major component in plasma. The plasma concentrations of M1 range between 0% and 20% of that of the parent drug. The other metabolites (M2 to M4) are found only in very low quantities in the urine and have not been detected in plasma or feces. These data, together with the lack of effect of erythromycin (a potent CYP3A4/5 inhibitor) on Argatroban pharmacokinetics, suggest that CYP3A4/5-mediated metabolism is not an important elimination pathway in vivo.

Total body clearance is approximately 5.1 mL/kg/min (0.31 L/kg/hr) for infusion doses up to 40 mcg/kg/min. The terminal elimination half-life of Argatroban ranges between 39 and 51 minutes.

There is no interconversion of the 21–(R):21–(S) diastereoisomers. The plasma ratio of these diastereoisomers is unchanged by metabolism or hepatic impairment, remaining constant at 65:35 (± 2%).

Excretion: Argatroban is excreted primarily in the feces, presumably through biliary secretion. In a study in which ^{14}C-Argatroban (5 mcg/kg/min) was infused for 4 hours into healthy subjects, approximately 65% of the radioactivity was recovered in the feces within 6 days of the start of infusion with little or no radioactivity subsequently detected. Approximately 22% of the radioactivity appeared in the urine within 12 hours of the start of infusion. Little or no additional urinary radioactivity was subsequently detected. Average percent recovery of unchanged drug, relative to total dose, was 16% in urine and at least 14% in feces.

Pharmacokinetic/Pharmacodynamic Relationship

When Argatroban is administered by continuous infusion, anticoagulant effects and plasma concentrations of Argatroban follow similar, predictable temporal response profiles, with low intersubject variability. Immediately upon initiation of Argatroban infusion, anticoagulant effects are produced as plasma Argatroban concentrations begin to rise. Steady-state levels of both drug and anticoagulant effect are typically attained within 1 to 3 hours and are maintained until the infusion is discontinued or the dosage adjusted. Steady-state plasma Argatroban concentrations increase proportionally with dose (for infusion doses up to 40 mcg/kg/min in healthy subjects) and are well correlated with steady-state anticoagulant effects. For infusion doses up to 40 mcg/kg/min, Argatroban increases in a dose-dependent fashion, the activated partial thromboplastin time (aPTT), the activated clotting time (ACT), the prothrombin time (PT), the International Normalized Ratio (INR), and the thrombin time (TT) in healthy volunteers and cardiac patients. Representative steady-state plasma Argatroban concentrations and anticoagulant effects are shown below for Argatroban infusion doses up to 10 mcg/kg/min (see Figure 1).

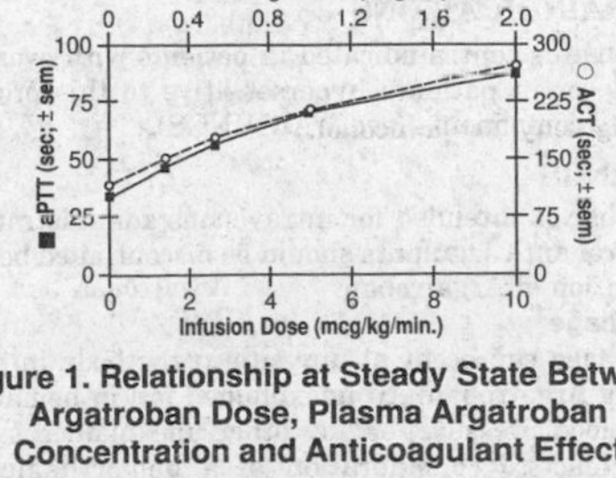

Figure 1. Relationship at Steady State Between Argatroban Dose, Plasma Argatroban Concentration and Anticoagulant Effect

Effect on International Normalized Ratio (INR)

Because Argatroban is a direct thrombin inhibitor, co-administration of Argatroban and warfarin produces a combined effect on the laboratory measurement of the INR. However, concurrent therapy, compared to warfarin monotherapy, exerts no additional effect on vitamin K–dependent factor Xa activity.

The relationship between INR on co-therapy and warfarin alone is dependent on both the dose of Argatroban and the thromboplastin reagent used. This relationship is influenced by the International Sensitivity Index (ISI) of the thromboplastin. Data for 2 commonly utilized thromboplastins with ISI values of 0.88 (Innovin, Dade) and 1.78 (Thromboplastin C Plus, Dade) are presented in Figure 2 for an Argatroban dose of 2 mcg/kg/min. Thromboplastins with higher ISI values than shown result in higher INRs on combined therapy of warfarin and Argatroban. These data are based on results obtained in normal individuals (see PRECAUTIONS, Drug Interactions and DOSAGE AND ADMINISTRATION, Conversion to Oral Anticoagulant Therapy).

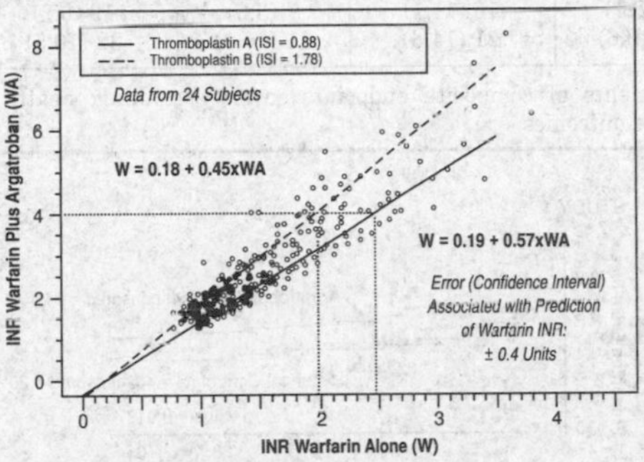

Figure 2. INR Relationship of Argatroban Plus Warfarin Versus Warfarin Alone

Figure 2 demonstrates the relationship between INR for warfarin alone and INR for warfarin co-administered with Argatroban at a dose of 2 mcg/kg/min. To calculate INR for warfarin alone (INR_W), based on INR for co-therapy of warfarin and Argatroban (INR_{WA}), when the Argatroban dose is 2 mcg/kg/min, use the equation next to the appropriate curve. Example: At a dose of 2 mcg/kg/min and an INR performed with Thromboplastin A, the equation 0.19 + 0.57 (INR_{WA}) = INR_W would allow a prediction of the INR on warfarin alone (INR_W). Thus, using an INR_{WA} value of 4.0 obtained on combined therapy: $INR_W = 0.19 + 0.57\ (4) = 2.47$ as the value for INR on warfarin alone. The error (confidence interval) associated with a prediction is ± 0.4 units. Similar linear relationships and prediction errors exist for Argatroban at a dose of 1 mcg/kg/min. Thus, for Argatroban doses of 1 or 2 mcg/kg/min, INR_W can be predicted from INR_{WA}. For Argatroban doses greater than 2 mcg/kg/min, the error associated with predicting INR_W from INR_{WA} is ± 1. Thus, INR_W cannot be reliably predicted from INR_{WA} at doses greater than 2 mcg/kg/min.

SPECIAL POPULATIONS

Renal Impairment

No dosage adjustment is necessary in patients with renal dysfunction. The effect of renal disease on the pharmacokinetics of Argatroban was studied in 6 subjects with normal renal function (mean Clcr = 95 ± 16 mL/min) and in 18 subjects with mild (mean Clcr = 64 ± 10 mL/min), moderate (mean Clcr = 41 ± 5.8 mL/min), and severe (mean Clcr = 5 ± 7 mL/min) renal impairment. The pharmacokinetics and pharmacodynamics of Argatroban at dosages up to 5 mcg/kg/min were not significantly affected by renal dysfunction. Use of Argatroban was evaluated in a study of 12 patients with stable end-stage renal disease undergoing chronic intermittent hemodialysis. Argatroban was administered at a rate of 2 to 3 mcg/kg/min (begun at least 4 hours prior to dialysis) or as a bolus dose of 250 mcg/kg at the start of dialysis followed by a continuous infusion of 2 mcg/kg/min. Although these regimens did not achieve the goal of maintaining ACT values at 1.8 times the baseline value throughout most of the hemodialysis period, the hemodialysis sessions were successfully completed with both of these regimens. The mean ACTs produced in this study ranged from 1.39 to 1.82 times baseline, and the mean aPTTs ranged from 1.96 to 3.4 times baseline. When Argatroban was administered as a continuous infusion of 2 mcg/kg/min prior to and during a 4-hour hemodialysis session, approximately 20% was cleared through dialysis.

Hepatic Impairment

The dosage of Argatroban should be decreased in patients with hepatic impairment (see PRECAUTIONS and DOSAGE AND ADMINISTRATION). Patients with hepatic impairment were not studied in percutaneous coronary intervention (PCI) trials. At a dose of 2.5 mcg/kg/min, hepatic impairment is associated with decreased clearance and increased elimination half-life of Argatroban (to 1.9 mL/kg/min and 181 minutes, respectively, for patients with a Child-Pugh score >6).

Gender

Gender has not been shown to significantly affect Argatroban pharmacokinetics or pharmacodynamics (e.g., aPTT).

Age

Adult: Age has not been shown to significantly affect Argatroban pharmacokinetics or pharmacodynamics (e.g., aPTT).

Pediatric: Argatroban clearance is decreased in seriously ill pediatric patients. Pharmacokinetic parameters of Argatroban were characterized in a population pharmacokinetic/pharmacodynamic analysis with sparse data from 15 seriously ill pediatric patients. Clearance in pediatric patients (0.16 L/hr/kg) was 50% lower compared to healthy adults (0.31 L/hr/kg). Four pediatric patients with elevated bilirubin (secondary to cardiac complications or hepatic impairment) had, on average, 80% lower clearance (0.03 L/hr/kg) when compared to pediatric patients with normal bilirubin levels. (See PRECAUTIONS, Pediatric Use.)

Drug-Drug Interactions

Digoxin: In 12 healthy volunteers, intravenous infusion of Argatroban (2 mcg/kg/min) over 5 days (study days 11 to 15) did not affect the steady-state pharmacokinetics of oral digoxin (0.375 mg daily for 15 days).

Erythromycin: In 10 healthy subjects, orally administered erythromycin (a potent inhibitor of CYP3A4/5) at 500 mg four times daily for 7 days had no effect on the pharmacokinetics of Argatroban at a dose of 1 mcg/kg/min for 5 hours. These data suggest oxidative metabolism by CYP3A4/5 is not an important elimination pathway in vivo for Argatroban.

CLINICAL STUDIES

Heparin-Induced Thrombocytopenia

Heparin-induced thrombocytopenia (HIT) is a potentially serious, immune-mediated complication of heparin therapy that is strongly associated with subsequent venous and arterial thrombosis. Whereas initial treatment of HIT is to discontinue administration of all heparin, patients may require anticoagulation for prevention and treatment of thromboembolic events.

The conclusion that Argatroban is an effective treatment for heparin-induced thrombocytopenia (HIT) and heparin-induced thrombocytopenia and thrombosis syndrome (HITTS) is based upon the data from an historically controlled efficacy and safety study (Study 1) and a follow-on efficacy and safety study (Study 2). These studies were comparable with regard to study design, study objectives, dosing regimens as well as study outline, conduct, and monitoring.

In these studies, 568 adult patients were treated with Argatroban and 193 adult patients made up the historical control group. Patients were required to have a clinical diagnosis of heparin-induced thrombocytopenia, either without thrombosis (HIT) or with thrombosis (HITTS) and be males or non-pregnant females between the age of 18 and 80 years old. HIT/HITTS was defined by a fall in platelet count to less than 100,000/μL or a 50% decrease in platelets after the initiation of heparin therapy with no apparent explanation other than HIT. Patients with HITTS also had presence of an arterial or venous thrombosis documented by appropriate imaging techniques or supported by clinical evidence such as acute myocardial infarction, stroke, pulmonary embolism, or other clinical indications of vascular occlusion. Patients who required anticoagulation with documented histories of positive HIT antibody test were also eligible in the absence of thrombocytopenia or heparin challenge (e.g., patients with latent disease).

Patients with documented unexplained aPTT >200% of control at baseline, documented coagulation disorder or bleeding diathesis unrelated to HITTS, a lumbar puncture within the past 7 days or a history of previous aneurysm, hemorrhagic stroke, or recent thrombotic stroke, within the past 6 months, unrelated to HITTS were excluded from these studies.

The initial dose of Argatroban was 2 mcg/kg/min, not to exceed 10 mcg/kg/min. Two hours after the start of the Argatroban infusion, an aPTT level was obtained and dose adjustments were made to achieve a steady-state aPTT value that was 1.5 to 3.0 times the baseline value, not to exceed 100 seconds. In Study 1, the mean aPTT level for HIT patients was 38 seconds prior to start of Argatroban infusion. At first assessment,* during the Argatroban infusion, mean aPTT level for HIT patients was 64 seconds. Overall the mean aPTT level during the Argatroban infusion for HIT patients was 62.5 seconds. In Study 1, the mean aPTT level for HITTS patients was 34 seconds prior to start of Argatroban infusion. At first assessment,* during the Argatroban infusion, mean aPTT level for HITTS patients was 70 seconds. Overall, the mean aPTT level during

Table 1. Efficacy Results of Study 1: Composite Endpoint*

Parameter, N (%)	HIT		HITTS		HIT/HITTS	
	Control n = 147	Argatroban n = 160	Control n = 46	Argatroban n = 144	Control n = 193	Argatroban n = 304
Composite Endpoint	57 (38.8)	41 (25.6)	26 (56.5)	63 (43.8)	83 (43.0)	104 (34.2)

* Death (all causes), amputation (all causes), or new thrombosis within 37-day study period.

Table 2. Efficacy Results of Study 1: Components of the Composite Endpoint, Ranked by Severity*

Parameter, N (%)	HIT		HITTS		HIT/HITTS	
	Control n = 147	Argatroban n = 160	Control n = 46	Argatroban n = 144	Control n = 193	Argatroban n = 304
Death	32 (21.8)	27 (16.9)	13 (28.3)	26 (18.1)	45 (23.3)	53 (17.4)
Amputation	3 (2.0)	3 (1.9)	4 (8.7)	16 (11.1)	7 (3.6)	19 (6.2)
New Thrombosis	22 (15.0)	11 (6.9)	9 (19.6)	21 (14.6)	31 (16.1)	32 (10.5)

* Reported as the most severe outcome among the components of composite endpoint (severity ranking: death > amputation > new thrombosis); patients may have had multiple outcomes.

the Argatroban infusion for HITTS patients was 64.5 seconds (see DOSAGE AND ADMINISTRATION). (*First assessment was defined as occurring at least 2 hours post-infusion start time.)

The primary efficacy analysis was based on a comparison of event rates for a composite endpoint that included death (all causes), amputation (all causes) or new thrombosis during the treatment and follow-up period (study days 0 to 37). Secondary analyses included evaluation of the event rates for the components of the composite endpoint as well as time-to-event analyses.

In Study 1, 304 patients were enrolled having active HIT (129/304, 42%), active HITTS (144/304, 47%), or latent disease (31/304, 10%). Among the 193 historical controls, 139 (72%) had active HIT, 46 (24%) had active HITTS, and 8 (4%) had latent disease. Within each group, those with active HIT and those with latent disease were analyzed together. Positive laboratory confirmation of HIT/HITTS by the heparin-induced platelet aggregation test or serotonin release assay was demonstrated in 174 of 304 (57%) Argatroban-treated patients (i.e., in 80 with HIT or latent disease and 94 with HITTS) and in 149 of 193 (77%) historical controls (i.e., in 119 with HIT or latent disease and 30 with HITTS). The test results for the remainder of the patients and controls were either negative or not determined.

A categorical analysis showed a significant improvement in the composite outcome in patients with HIT and HITTS treated with Argatroban versus those in the historical control group (see Table 1). The components of the composite endpoint are shown in Table 2.

[See table 1 above]
[See table 2 above]

Time-to-event analyses showed significant improvements in the time-to-first event in patients with HIT or HITTS treated with Argatroban versus those in the historical control group. The between-group differences in the proportion of patients who remained free of death, amputation, or new thrombosis were statistically significant in favor of Argatroban by these analyses (p = 0.007 in patients with HIT and p = 0.018 in patients with HITTS, according to log-rank test).

A time-to-event analysis for the composite endpoint is shown in Figure 3 for patients with HIT and Figure 4 for patients with HITTS.

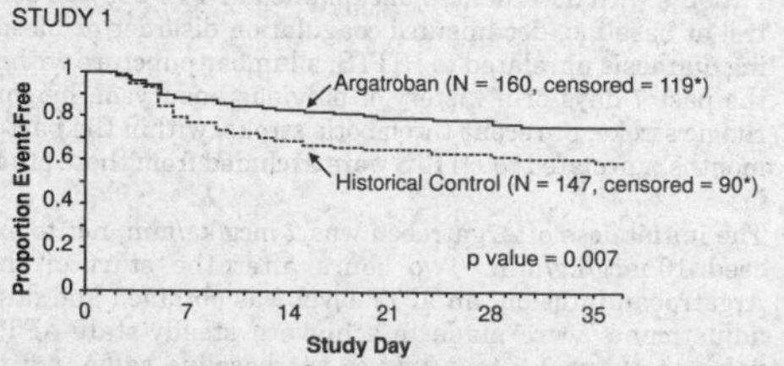

Figure 3. Time–to–First Event for the Composite Efficacy Endpoint: HIT Patients

* Censored indicates no clinical endpoint (defined as death, amputation, or new thrombosis) was observed during the follow-up period (maximum period of follow-up was 37 days).

[See figure 4 at top of next column]

In Study 2, 264 patients were enrolled, having either HIT (125/264, 47.3%) or HITTS (139/264, 52.7%), and then treated with Argatroban. Categorical analysis demon-

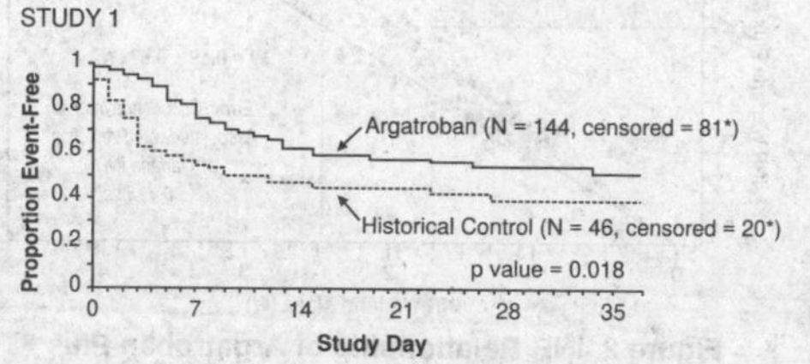

Figure 4. Time–to–First Event for the Composite Efficacy Endpoint: HITTS Patients

* Censored indicates no clinical endpoint (defined as death, amputation, or new thrombosis) was observed during the follow-up period (maximum period of follow-up was 37 days).

strated significant improvement in the composite efficacy outcome for Argatroban-treated patients, versus the same historical control group from Study 1, among patients having HIT (25.6% vs. 38.8%), patients having HITTS (41.0% vs. 56.5%), and patients having either HIT or HITTS (33.7% vs. 43.0%). Time-to-event analyses showed significant improvements in the time-to-first event in patients with HIT or HITTS treated with Argatroban versus those in the historical control group. The between-group differences in the proportion of patients who remained free of death, amputation, or new thrombosis were statistically significant in favor of Argatroban.

Anticoagulant Effect: In Study 1, the mean (± SE) dose of Argatroban administered was 2.0 ± 0.1 mcg/kg/min in the HIT arm and 1.9 ± 0.1 mcg/kg/min in the HITTS arm. Seventy-six percent of patients with HIT and 81% of patients with HITTS achieved a target aPTT at least 1.5-fold greater than the baseline aPTT at the first assessment occurring on average at 4.6 hours (HIT) and 3.9 hours (HITTS) following initiation of Argatroban therapy.

No enhancement of aPTT response was observed in subjects receiving repeated administration of Argatroban.

Platelet Count Recovery: In Study 1, the majority of patients, 53% of those with HIT and 58% of those with HITTS, had a recovery of platelet count by day 3. Platelet Count Recovery was defined as an increase in platelet count to >100,000/μL or to at least 1.5-fold greater than the baseline count (platelet count at study initiation) by day 3 of the study.

Percutaneous Coronary Intervention (PCI) in HIT/HITTS Patients

In 3 similarly designed trials, Argatroban was administered to 91 patients with current or previous clinical diagnosis of HIT/HITTS or heparin-dependent antibodies, who underwent a total of 112 percutaneous coronary interventions (PCIs) including percutaneous transluminal coronary angioplasty (PTCA), coronary stent placement, or atherectomy. Among the 91 patients undergoing their first PCI with Argatroban, notable ongoing or recent medical history included myocardial infarction (n = 35), unstable angina (n = 23), and chronic angina (n = 34). There were 33 females and 58 males. The average age was 67.6 years (median 70.7, range 44 to 86), and the average weight was 82.5 kg (median 81.0 kg, range 49 to 141).

Due to the history or presence of the heparin-dependent antibody or HIT/HITTS, these patients required alternative anticoagulation. Twenty-one of the 91 patients had a repeat PCI using Argatroban an average of 150 days after their initial PCI. Seven of 91 patients received glycoprotein IIb/IIIa inhibitors. Safety and efficacy were assessed against historical control populations.

Per protocol, all patients received oral aspirin (325 mg) 2 to 24 hours prior to the interventional procedure. After venous or arterial sheaths were in place, anticoagulation was initiated with a bolus of Argatroban of 350 mcg/kg via a large-bore IV line or through the venous sheath over 3 to 5 minutes. Simultaneously, a maintenance infusion of 25 mcg/kg/min was initiated to achieve a therapeutic activated clotting time (ACT) of 300 to 450 seconds. If necessary to achieve this therapeutic range, the maintenance infusion dose was titrated (15 to 40 mcg/kg/min) and/or an additional bolus dose of 150 mcg/kg could be given. Each patient's ACT was checked 5 to 10 minutes following the bolus dose. The ACT was checked as clinically indicated thereafter. Arterial and venous sheaths were removed no sooner than 2 hours after discontinuation of Argatroban and when the ACT was less than 160 seconds.

If a patient required anticoagulation after the procedure, Argatroban could be continued, but at a lower infusion dose between 2.5 and 5 mcg/kg/min. An aPTT was drawn 2 hours after this dose reduction and the dose of Argatroban then adjusted as clinically indicated (not to exceed 10 mcg/kg/min), to reach an aPTT between 1.5 and 3 times baseline value (not to exceed 100 seconds).

Ninety-one patients were treated with Argatroban on their first PCI, and 21 patients were reexposed to Argatroban on subsequent PCIs. In 92 of the 112 interventions (82%), the patient received the initial bolus of 350 mcg/kg and an initial infusion dose of 25 mcg/kg/min. The majority of patients did not require additional bolus dosing during the PCI procedure. The mean value for the initial ACT measurement after the start of dosing for all interventions was 379 sec (median 338 sec; 5th percentile-95th percentile 238 to 675 sec). The mean ACT value per intervention over all measurements taken during the procedure was 416 sec (median 390 sec; 5th percentile-95th percentile 261 to 698 sec). About 65% of patients had ACTs within the recommended range of 300 to 450 seconds throughout the procedure. The investigators did not achieve anticoagulation within the recommended range in about 23% of patients. However, in this small sample, patients with ACTs below 300 seconds did not have more coronary thrombotic events, and patients with ACTs over 450 seconds did not have higher bleeding rates.

Acute procedural success was defined as lack of death, emergent coronary artery bypass graft (CABG), or Q-wave myocardial infarction. Acute procedural success was reported in 98.2% of patients who underwent PCIs with Argatroban anticoagulation compared with 94.3% of historical control patients anticoagulated with heparin (p = NS).

Among the 112 interventions, 2 patients had emergency CABGs, 3 had repeat PTCAs, 4 had non-Q-wave myocardial infarctions, 3 had myocardial ischemia, 1 had an abrupt closure, and 1 had an impending closure (some patients may have experienced more than 1 event). No patients died. Two patients had protocol-defined major bleeding, 1 of which was retroperitoneal and the other gastrointestinal. Minor bleeding, defined as spontaneous and observed with hemoglobin decreasing >3g/dL or with no bleeding site and hemoglobin decreasing >4g/dL, occurred in 4.5% of interventions.

Additional Information

Cardiac Therapy: The safety and effectiveness of Argatroban for cardiac indications outside of percutaneous coronary intervention in patients with HIT have not been established.

Reexposure and Lack of Antibody Formation: Plasma from 12 healthy volunteers treated with Argatroban over 6 days showed no evidence of neutralizing antibodies. Repeated administration of Argatroban to more than 40 patients was tolerated with no loss of anticoagulant activity. No change in the dose is required.

INDICATIONS AND USAGE

Argatroban is indicated as an anticoagulant for prophylaxis or treatment of thrombosis in patients with heparin-induced thrombocytopenia.

Argatroban is indicated as an anticoagulant in patients with or at risk for heparin-induced thrombocytopenia undergoing percutaneous coronary intervention (PCI).

CONTRAINDICATIONS

Argatroban is contraindicated in patients with overt major bleeding, or in patients hypersensitive to this product or any of its components (see WARNINGS).

WARNINGS

Argatroban is intended for intravenous administration. All parenteral anticoagulants should be discontinued before administration of Argatroban.

Hemorrhage

Hemorrhage can occur at any site in the body in patients receiving Argatroban. An unexplained fall in hematocrit, a fall in blood pressure, or any other unexplained symptom should lead to consideration of a hemorrhagic event.

Argatroban should be used with extreme caution in disease states and other circumstances in which there is an increased danger of hemorrhage. These include severe hypertension; immediately following lumbar puncture; spinal anesthesia; major surgery, especially involving the brain, spinal cord, or eye; hematologic conditions associated with increased bleeding tendencies such as congenital or acquired bleeding disorders and gastrointestinal lesions such as ulcerations.

PRECAUTIONS

Hepatic Impairment

Caution should be exercised when administering Argatroban to patients with hepatic impairment by starting with a lower dose and carefully titrating until the desired level of anticoagulation is achieved. Achievement of steady state aPTT levels may take longer and require more Argatroban dose adjustments in patients with hepatic impairment compared to patients with normal hepatic function (see PRECAUTIONS, Pediatric Use). Also, upon cessation of Argatroban infusion in the hepatically impaired patient, full reversal of anticoagulant effects may require longer than 4 hours due to decreased clearance and increased elimination half-life of Argatroban (see DOSAGE AND ADMINISTRATION). Use of high doses of Argatroban in PCI patients with clinically significant hepatic disease or AST/ALT levels ≥3 times the upper limit of normal should be avoided. Such patients were not studied in PCI trials.

Laboratory Tests

Anticoagulation effects associated with Argatroban infusion at doses up to 40 mcg/kg/min correlate with increases of the activated partial thromboplastin time (aPTT).

Although other global clot-based tests including prothrombin time (PT), the International Normalized Ratio (INR), and thrombin time (TT) are affected by Argatroban, the therapeutic ranges for these tests have not been identified for Argatroban therapy. Plasma Argatroban concentrations also correlate well with anticoagulant effects (see CLINICAL PHARMACOLOGY).

In clinical trials in PCI, the activated clotting time (ACT) was used for monitoring Argatroban anticoagulant activity during the procedure.

The concomitant use of Argatroban and warfarin results in prolongation of the PT and INR beyond that produced by warfarin alone. Alternative approaches for monitoring concurrent Argatroban and warfarin therapy are described in a subsequent section (see DOSAGE AND ADMINISTRATION).

Drug Interactions

Heparin: Since heparin is contraindicated in patients with heparin-induced thrombocytopenia, the co-administration of Argatroban and heparin is unlikely for this indication. However, if Argatroban is to be initiated after cessation of heparin therapy, allow sufficient time for heparin's effect on the aPTT to decrease prior to initiation of Argatroban therapy.

Aspirin/Acetaminophen: Pharmacokinetic or pharmacodynamic drug-drug interactions have not been demonstrated between Argatroban and concomitantly administered aspirin (162.5 mg orally given 26 and 2 hours prior to initiation of Argatroban 1 mcg/kg/min over 4 hours) or acetaminophen (1,000 mg orally given 12, 6, and 0 hours prior to, and 6 and 12 hours subsequent to, initiation of Argatroban 1.5 mcg/kg/min over 18 hours).

Oral Anticoagulant Agents: Pharmacokinetic drug-drug interactions between Argatroban and warfarin (7.5 mg single oral dose) have not been demonstrated. However, the concomitant use of Argatroban and warfarin (5 to 7.5 mg initial oral dose, followed by 2.5 to 6 mg/day orally for 6 to 10 days) results in prolongation of the prothrombin time (PT) and International Normalized Ratio (INR) (see CLINICAL PHARMACOLOGY and DOSAGE AND ADMINISTRATION).

Thrombolytic Agents: The safety and effectiveness of Argatroban with thrombolytic agents have not been established (see ADVERSE REACTIONS, *Intracranial Bleeding*).

Glycoprotein IIb/IIIa Antagonists: The safety and effectiveness of Argatroban with glycoprotein IIb/IIIa antagonists have not been established.

Co-Administration: Concomitant use of Argatroban with antiplatelet agents, thrombolytics, and other anticoagulants may increase the risk of bleeding (see WARNINGS). Drug-drug interactions have not been observed between Argatroban and digoxin or erythromycin (see CLINICAL PHARMACOLOGY, Drug-Drug Interactions).

Carcinogenesis, Mutagenesis, Impairment of Fertility

No long-term studies in animals have been performed to evaluate the carcinogenic potential of Argatroban.

Argatroban was not genotoxic in the Ames test, the Chinese hamster ovary cell (CHO/HGPRT) forward mutation test, the Chinese hamster lung fibroblast chromosome aberration test, the rat hepatocyte, and WI-38 human fetal lung cell unscheduled DNA synthesis (UDS) tests, or the mouse micronucleus test.

Table 3. Major and Minor Hemorrhagic Adverse Events in HIT/HITTS Patients

Major Hemorrhagic Events*	Argatroban-treated Patients (Study 1 and Study 2) (n = 568) %	Historical Control (n = 193) %
Overall bleeding	5.3	6.7
Gastrointestinal	2.3	1.6
Genitourinary and hematuria	0.9	0.5
Decrease in hemoglobin and hematocrit	0.7	0
Multisystem hemorrhage and DIC	0.5	1
Limb and BKA stump	0.5	0
Intracranial hemorrhage	0[†]	0.5
Minor Hemorrhagic Events*	**Argatroban-treated Patients (Study 1 and Study 2) (n = 568) %**	**Historical Control (n = 193) %**
Gastrointestinal	14.4	18.1
Genitourinary and hematuria	11.6	0.8
Decrease in hemoglobin and hematocrit	10.4	0
Groin	5.4	3.1
Hemoptysis	2.9	0.8
Brachial	2.4	0.8

* Patients may have experienced more than 1 adverse event.

† One patient experienced intracranial hemorrhage 4 days after discontinuation of Argatroban and following therapy with urokinase and oral anticoagulation.

DIC = disseminated intravascular coagulation.

BKA = below-the-knee amputation.

Argatroban at intravenous doses up to 27 mg/kg/day (0.3 times the recommended maximum human dose based on body surface area) was found to have no effect on fertility and reproductive performance of male and female rats.

Pregnancy

Teratogenic Effects: Pregnancy Category B. Teratology studies have been performed in rats with intravenous doses up to 27 mg/kg/day (0.3 times the recommended maximum human dose based on body surface area) and rabbits at intravenous doses up to 10.8 mg/kg/day (0.2 times the recommended maximum human dose based on body surface area) and have revealed no evidence of impaired fertility or harm to the fetus due to Argatroban. There are, however, no adequate and well-controlled studies in pregnant women. Because animal reproduction studies are not always predictive of human response, this drug should be used during pregnancy only if clearly needed.

Nursing Mothers

Experiments in rats show that Argatroban is detected in milk. It is not known whether this drug is excreted in human milk. Because many drugs are excreted in human milk and because of the potential for serious adverse reactions in nursing infants from Argatroban, a decision should be made whether to discontinue nursing or to discontinue the drug, taking into account the importance of the drug to the mother.

Geriatric Use

In the clinical studies of adult patients with HIT or HITTS, the effectiveness of Argatroban was not affected by age.

Pediatric Use

The safety and effectiveness of Argatroban, including the appropriate anticoagulation goals and duration of therapy, have not been established among pediatric patients.

Argatroban was studied among 18 seriously ill pediatric patients who required an alternative to heparin anticoagulation. Most patients were diagnosed with HIT or suspected HIT. Age ranges of patients were <6 months, n = 8; six months to <8 years, n = 6; 8 to 16 years, n = 4. All patients had serious underlying conditions and were receiving multiple concomitant medications. Thirteen patients received Argatroban solely as a continuous infusion (no bolus dose). Dosing was initiated in the majority of these 13 patients at 1 mcg/kg/min. Dosing was titrated as needed to achieve and maintain an aPTT of 1.5 to 3 times the baseline value. Most patients required multiple dose adjustments to maintain anticoagulation parameters within the desired range. During the 30-day study period, thrombotic events occurred during Argatroban administration to two patients and following Argatroban discontinuation in three other patients. Major bleeding occurred among two patients; one patient experienced an intracranial hemorrhage after 4 days of Argatroban therapy in the setting of sepsis and thrombocytopenia. Another patient completed 14 days of Argatroban treatment in the study, but experienced an intracranial hemorrhage while receiving Argatroban following completion of the study treatment period.

When Argatroban is used among seriously ill pediatric patients with HIT/HITTS who require an alternative to heparin and who have normal hepatic function, initiate a continuous infusion of Argatroban at a dose of 0.75 mcg/kg/min. Initiate the infusion at a dose of 0.2 mcg/kg/min among seriously ill pediatric patients with impaired hepatic function (see CLINICAL PHARMACOLOGY, Pharmacokinetics). Check the aPTT two hours after the initiation of the Argatroban infusion and adjust the dose to achieve the target aPTT. These dose recommendations are based upon a goal of aPTT prolongation of 1.5 to 3 times the baseline value and avoidance of an aPTT >100 seconds. Increments of 0.1 to 0.25 mcg/kg/min for pediatric patients with normal hepatic function and increments of 0.05 mcg/kg/min or lower for pediatric patients with impaired hepatic function may be considered but dose selection must take into account multiple factors including the current Argatroban dose, the current aPTT, target aPTT, and the clinical status of the patient. These dose recommendations are based upon a goal of aPTT prolongation of 1.5 to 3 times the baseline value and avoidance of an aPTT >100 seconds.

ADVERSE REACTIONS

Adverse Events Reported in HIT/HITTS Patients

The following safety information is based on all 568 patients treated with Argatroban in Study 1 and Study 2. The safety profile of the patients from these studies is compared with that of 193 historical controls in which the adverse events were collected retrospectively. The adverse events reported in this section include all events regardless of relationship to treatment. Adverse events are separated into hemorrhagic and non-hemorrhagic events.

Major bleeding was defined as bleeding that was overt and associated with a hemoglobin decrease ≥2 g/dL, that led to a transfusion of ≥2 units, or that was intracranial, retroperitoneal, or into a major prosthetic joint. Minor bleeding was overt bleeding that did not meet the criteria for major bleeding.

Table 3 gives an overview of the most frequently observed hemorrhagic events, presented separately by major and minor bleeding, sorted by decreasing occurrence among Argatroban-treated HIT/HITTS patients.

[See table 3 at top of previous page]

Table 4 gives an overview of the most frequently observed non-hemorrhagic events sorted by decreasing frequency of occurrence (≥2%) among Argatroban-treated HIT/HITTS patients.

[See table 4 above]

Table 4. Non-hemorrhagic Adverse Events in HIT/HITTS Patients*

	Argatroban-treated Patients (Study 1 and Study 2) (n = 568) %	Historical Control (n = 193) %
Dyspnea	8.1	8.8
Hypotension	7.2	2.6
Fever	6.9	2.1
Diarrhea	6.2	1.6
Sepsis	6.0	12.4
Cardiac arrest	5.8	3.1
Nausea	4.8	0.5
Ventricular tachycardia	4.8	3.1
Pain	4.6	3.1
Urinary tract infection	4.6	5.2
Vomiting	4.2	0
Infection	3.7	3.6
Pneumonia	3.3	9.3
Atrial fibrillation	3.0	11.4
Coughing	2.8	1.6
Abnormal renal function	2.8	4.7
Abdominal pain	2.6	1.6
Cerebrovascular disorder	2.3	4.1

* Patients may have experienced more than 1 adverse event.

Adverse Events Reported in HIT/HITTS Patients Undergoing PCI

The following safety information is based on 91 patients initially treated with Argatroban and 21 patients subsequently re-exposed to Argatroban for a total of 112 PCIs with Argatroban anticoagulation. The adverse events reported in this section include all events regardless of relationship to treatment. Adverse events are separated into hemorrhagic (Table 5) and non-hemorrhagic (Table 6) events.

Major bleeding was defined as bleeding that was overt and associated with a hemoglobin decrease ≥5 g/dL, that led to a transfusion of ≥2 units, or that was intracranial, retroperitoneal, or into a major prosthetic joint.

The rate of major bleeding events and intracranial hemorrhage in the PCI trials was 1.8% and in the placebo arm of the EPILOG trial (placebo plus standard dose, weight-adjusted heparin) was 3.1%.

Table 5. Major and Minor Hemorrhagic Adverse Events in HIT/HITTS Patients Undergoing PCI

Major Hemorrhagic Events*

	Argatroban-treated Patients (n = 112)† %
Retroperitoneal	0.9
Gastrointestinal	0.9
Intracranial	0

Minor Hemorrhagic Events*

	Argatroban-treated Patients (n = 112)† %
Groin (bleeding or hematoma)	3.6
Gastrointestinal (includes hematemesis)	2.6
Genitourinary (includes hematuria)	1.8
Decrease in hemoglobin and/or hematocrit	1.8
CABG (coronary arteries)	1.8
Access site	0.9
Hemoptysis	0.9
Other	0.9

* Patients may have experienced more than 1 adverse event.

† 91 patients who underwent 112 interventions.

CABG = coronary artery bypass graft.

Table 6 gives an overview of the most frequently observed non-hemorrhagic events (>2%), sorted by decreasing frequency of occurrence among Argatroban-treated PCI patients.

Table 6. Non-hemorrhagic Adverse Events* in HIT/HITTS Patients Undergoing PCI

	Argatroban Procedures* (n = 112)† %	Controls (n = 2226)‡ %
Chest pain	15.2	9.3
Hypotension	10.7	10.3
Back pain	8.0	13.7
Nausea	7.1	11.5
Vomiting	6.3	6.8
Headache	5.4	5.5
Bradycardia	4.5	3.5
Abdominal pain	3.6	2.2
Fever	3.6	<0.5
Myocardial infarction	3.6	NR§

* Patients may have experienced more than 1 adverse event.

† 91 patients who underwent 112 interventions.

‡ Controls from EPIC (Evaluation of c7E3 Fab in the Prevention of Ischemic Complications), EPILOG (Evaluation in PTCA to Improve Long-Term Outcome with Abciximab GP IIb/IIIa Blockade Study) and CAPTURE (Chimeric 7E3 Antiplatelet Therapy in Unstable angina Refractory to standard treatment) trials. Source: ReoPro® Prescribing Information.

§ NR = not reported.

There were 22 serious adverse events in 17 PCI patients (19.6% in 112 interventions). The types of events, which are listed regardless of relationship to treatment, are shown in Table 7. Table 7 lists the serious adverse events occurring in Argatroban-treated HIT/HITTS patients undergoing PCI.

Table 7. Serious Adverse Events in HIT/HITTS Patients Undergoing PCI*

Coded Term	Argatroban Procedures† (n = 112)
Chest pain	1 (0.9%)
Fever	1 (0.9%)
Retroperitoneal hemorrhage	1 (0.9%)
Angina pectoris	2 (1.8%)
Aortic stenosis	1 (0.9%)
Coronary thrombosis	2 (1.8%)
Arterial thrombosis	1 (0.9%)
Myocardial infarction	4 (3.5%)
Myocardial ischemia	2 (1.8%)
Occlusion coronary	2 (1.8%)
Gastrointestinal hemorrhage	1 (0.9%)
Gastrointestinal disorder (GERD)	1 (0.9%)
Cerebrovascular disorder	1 (0.9%)
Lung edema	1 (0.9%)
Vascular disorder	1 (0.9%)

* Individual events may also have been reported elsewhere (see Table 5 and 6).

† 91 patients underwent 112 procedures. Some patients may have experienced more than 1 event.

Adverse Events Reported in Other Populations

Intracranial Bleeding: The overall frequency of intracranial bleeding among patients with acute myocardial infarction receiving both Argatroban and thrombolytic therapy (streptokinase or tissue plasminogen activator) was 1% (8 out of 810 patients). Intracranial bleeding was not observed in 317 subjects or patients who did not receive concomitant thrombolysis (see PRECAUTIONS, Drug Interactions).

Intracranial bleeding was also observed in a prospective, placebo-controlled study of Argatroban in patients who had onset of acute stroke within 12 hours of study entry. Symptomatic intracranial hemorrhage was reported in 5 of 117 patients (4.3%) who received Argatroban at 1.0 to 3.0 mcg/kg/min and in none of the 54 patients who received placebo. Asymptomatic intracranial hemorrhage occurred in 5 (4.3%) and 2 (3.7%) of the patients, respectively.

Allergic Reactions: 156 allergic reactions or suspected allergic reactions were observed in 1,127 individuals who were treated with Argatroban in clinical pharmacology studies or for various clinical indications. About 95% (148/156) of these reactions occurred in patients who concomitantly received thrombolytic therapy (e.g., streptokinase) for acute myocardial infarction and/or contrast media for coronary angiography.

Allergic reactions or suspected allergic reactions in populations other than HIT/HITTS patients include (in descending order of frequency[1]):

- Airway reactions (coughing, dyspnea): 10% or more
- Skin reactions (rash, bullous eruption): 1 to <10%
- General reactions (vasodilation): 1 to 10%

[1]The CIOMS (Council for International Organization of Medical Sciences) III standard categories are used for classification of frequencies.

OVERDOSAGE

Symptoms/Treatment

Excessive anticoagulation, with or without bleeding, may be controlled by discontinuing Argatroban or by decreasing the Argatroban infusion dosage (see WARNINGS). In clinical studies at therapeutic levels, anticoagulation parameters generally return to baseline within 2 to 4 hours after discontinuation of the drug. Reversal of anticoagulant effect may take longer in patients with hepatic impairment.

No specific antidote to Argatroban is available; if life-threatening bleeding occurs and excessive plasma levels of Argatroban are suspected, Argatroban should be discontinued immediately, aPTT and other coagulation tests should be determined. Symptomatic and supportive therapy should be provided to the patient (see WARNINGS). When Argatroban was administered as a continuous infusion (2 mcg/kg/min) prior to and during a 4-hour hemodialysis session, approximately 20% of Argatroban was cleared through dialysis.

Single intravenous doses of Argatroban at 200, 124, 150, and 200 mg/kg were lethal to mice, rats, rabbits, and dogs, respectively. The symptoms of acute toxicity were loss of righting reflex, tremors, clonic convulsions, paralysis of hind limbs, and coma.

DOSAGE AND ADMINISTRATION

Each 2.5-mL vial contains 250 mg of Argatroban; and, as supplied, is a concentrated drug (100 mg/mL), which must be diluted 100-fold prior to infusion. Argatroban should not be mixed with other drugs prior to dilution in a suitable intravenous fluid.

Preparation for Intravenous Administration

Argatroban should be diluted in 0.9% Sodium Chloride Injection, 5% Dextrose Injection, or Lactated Ringer's Injection to a final concentration of 1 mg/mL. The contents of each 2.5-mL vial should be diluted 100-fold by mixing with 250 mL of diluent. Use 250 mg (2.5 mL) per 250 mL of diluent or 500 mg (5 mL) per 500 mL of diluent.

The constituted solution must be mixed by repeated inversion of the diluent bag for 1 minute. Upon preparation, the solution may show slight but brief haziness due to the formation of microprecipitates that rapidly dissolve upon mixing. Use of diluent at room temperature is recommended. Colder temperatures can slow down the rate of dissolution of precipitates. The final solution must be clear before use. The pH of the intravenous solution prepared as recommended is 3.2 to 7.5.

Heparin-Induced Thrombocytopenia (HIT/HITTS)

Initial Dosage: Before administering Argatroban, discontinue heparin therapy and obtain a baseline aPTT. The recommended initial dose of Argatroban for adult patients without hepatic impairment is 2 mcg/kg/min, administered as a continuous infusion (see Table 8).

Table 8. Recommended Doses and Infusion Rates for 2 mcg/kg/min Dose of Argatroban for Patients With HIT/HITTS (Without Hepatic Impairment) (1 mg/mL Final Concentration)

Body Weight (kg)	Dose (mcg/min)	Infusion Rate (mL/hr)
50	100	6
60	120	7
70	140	8
80	160	10
90	180	11
100	200	12
110	220	13
120	240	14
130	260	16
140	280	17

Monitoring Therapy: In general, therapy with Argatroban is monitored using the aPTT. Tests of anticoagulant effects (including the aPTT) typically attain steady-state levels within one to three hours following initiation of Argatroban. Dose adjustment may be required to attain the target aPTT. Check the aPTT two hours after initiation of therapy and any dose change to confirm that the patient has attained the desired therapeutic range.

Dosage Adjustment: After the initial dose of Argatroban, the dose can be adjusted as clinically indicated (not to exceed 10 mcg/kg/min), until the steady-state aPTT is 1.5 to 3 times the initial baseline value (not to exceed 100 seconds) (see CLINICAL STUDIES for mean values of aPTT obtained after initial doses of Argatroban).

Table 9. Recommended Doses and Infusion Rates of Argatroban for Patients Undergoing PCI (Without Hepatic Impairment) (1 mg/mL Final Concentration)

Body Weight (kg)	For ACT 300-450 seconds Initial Dosage* 25 mcg/kg/min			If ACT <300 seconds Dosage Adjustment† 30 mcg/kg/min			If ACT >450 seconds Dosage Adjustment 15 mcg/kg/min	
	Bolus Dose (mcg)	Infusion Dose (mcg/min)	Infusion Rate (mL/hr)	Bolus Dose (mcg)	Infusion Dose (mcg/min)	Infusion Rate (mL/hr)	Infusion Dose (mcg/min)	Infusion Rate (mL/hr)
50	17500	1250	75	7500	1500	90	750	45
60	21000	1500	90	9000	1800	108	900	54
70	24500	1750	105	10500	2100	126	1050	63
80	28000	2000	120	12000	2400	144	1200	72
90	31500	2250	135	13500	2700	162	1350	81
100	35000	2500	150	15000	3000	180	1500	90
110	38500	2750	165	16500	3300	198	1650	99
120	42000	3000	180	18000	3600	216	1800	108
130	45500	3250	195	19500	3900	234	1950	117
140	49000	3500	210	21000	4200	252	2100	126

NOTE: 1 mg = 1000 mcg; 1 kg = 2.2 lbs

* Initial IV bolus dose of 350 mcg/kg should be administered.

† Additional IV bolus dose of 150 mcg/kg should be administered if ACT <300 seconds.

Percutaneous Coronary Interventions (PCI) in HIT/HITTS Patients

Initial Dosage: An infusion of Argatroban should be started at 25 mcg/kg/min and a bolus of 350 mcg/kg administered via a large bore intravenous (IV) line over 3 to 5 minutes (see Table 9). Activated clotting time (ACT) should be checked 5 to 10 minutes after the bolus dose is completed. The procedure may proceed if the ACT is greater than 300 seconds.

Dosage Adjustment: If the ACT is less than 300 seconds, an additional IV bolus dose of 150 mcg/kg should be administered, the infusion dose increased to 30 mcg/kg/min, and the ACT checked 5 to 10 minutes later (see Table 9). If the ACT is greater than 450 seconds, the infusion rate should be decreased to 15 mcg/kg/min, and the ACT checked 5 to 10 minutes later (see Table 9). Once a therapeutic ACT (between 300 and 450 seconds) has been achieved, this infusion dose should be continued for the duration of the procedure. [See table 9 above]

In case of dissection, impending abrupt closure, thrombus formation during the procedure, or inability to achieve or maintain an ACT over 300 seconds, additional bolus doses of 150 mcg/kg may be administered and the infusion dose increased to 40 mcg/kg/min. The ACT should be checked after each additional bolus or change in the rate of infusion.

Monitoring therapy: Therapy with Argatroban is monitored using ACT. ACTs should be obtained before dosing, 5 to 10 minutes after bolus dosing and after change in the infusion rate, and at the end of the PCI procedure. Additional ACTs should be drawn about every 20 to 30 minutes during a prolonged procedure.

Continued Anticoagulation after PCI: If a patient requires anticoagulation after the procedure, Argatroban may be continued, but at a lower infusion dose [see DOSAGE AND ADMINISTRATION, Heparin-Induced Thrombocytopenia (HIT/HITTS)].

Dosing in Special Populations

Hepatic Impairment: For adult patients with heparin-induced thrombocytopenia with hepatic impairment, the initial dose of Argatroban should be reduced. For adult patients with moderate hepatic impairment, an initial dose of 0.5 mcg/kg/min is recommended, based on the approximate 4-fold decrease in Argatroban clearance relative to those with normal hepatic function. The aPTT should be monitored closely, and the dosage should be adjusted as clinically indicated (see PRECAUTIONS).

Hepatic Impairment in HIT/HITTS Patients Undergoing PCI: Carefully titrate Argatroban until the desired level of anticoagulation is achieved (see PRECAUTIONS, Hepatic Impairment).

Renal Impairment: No dosage adjustment is necessary in patients with renal impairment (see SPECIAL POPULATIONS, Renal Impairment).

Pediatric HIT/HITTS Patients: Initial Argatroban infusion doses are lower for seriously ill pediatric patients compared to adults with normal hepatic function (see PRECAUTIONS, Pediatric Use).

Monitoring Therapy: In general, therapy with Argatroban is monitored using the aPTT. Tests of anticoagulant effects (including the aPTT) typically attain steady-state levels within one to three hours following initiation of Argatroban in patients without hepatic impairment (see PRECAUTIONS, Hepatic Impairment). Dose adjustment may be required to attain the target aPTT. Check the aPTT two hours after initiation of therapy and after any dose change to confirm that the patient has attained the desired therapeutic range.

Dosage Adjustment: See PRECAUTIONS, Pediatric Use.

CONVERSION TO ORAL ANTICOAGULANT THERAPY

Initiating Oral Anticoagulant Therapy

Once the decision is made to initiate oral anticoagulant therapy, recognize the potential for combined effects on INR with co-administration of Argatroban and warfarin. A loading dose of warfarin should not be used. Initiate therapy using the expected daily dose of warfarin. To avoid prothrombotic effects and to ensure continuous anticoagulation when initiating warfarin, it is suggested that Argatroban and warfarin therapy be overlapped. There are insufficient data available to recommend the duration of the overlap.

Co-Administration of Warfarin and Argatroban at Doses Up to 2 mcg/kg/min

Use of Argatroban with warfarin results in prolongation of INR beyond that produced by warfarin alone. To avoid prothrombotic effects and to ensure continuous anticoagulation when initiating warfarin, it is suggested that warfarin be co-administered before discontinuing Argatroban. There are insufficient data available to recommend the duration of the co-administration. The previously established relationship between INR and bleeding risk is altered. The combination of Argatroban and warfarin does not cause further reduction in the vitamin K–dependent factor Xa activity than that which is seen with warfarin alone. The relationship between INR obtained on combined therapy and INR obtained on warfarin alone is dependent on both the dose of Argatroban and the thromboplastin reagent used. The INR value on warfarin alone (INR_W) can be calculated from the INR value on combination Argatroban and warfarin therapy (see CLINICAL PHARMACOLOGY, Figure 2 explanation and PRECAUTIONS, Drug Interactions).

INR should be measured daily while Argatroban and warfarin are co-administered. In general, with doses of

Argatroban up to 2 mcg/kg/min, Argatroban can be discontinued when the INR is >4 on combined therapy. After Argatroban is discontinued, repeat the INR measurement in 4 to 6 hours. If the repeat INR is below the desired therapeutic range, resume the infusion of Argatroban and repeat the procedure daily until the desired therapeutic range on warfarin alone is reached.

Co-Administration of Warfarin and Argatroban at Doses Greater than 2 mcg/kg/min

For doses greater than 2 mcg/kg/min, the relationship of INR between warfarin alone to the INR on warfarin plus Argatroban is less predictable. In this case, in order to predict the INR on warfarin alone, temporarily reduce the dose of Argatroban to a dose of 2 mcg/kg/min. Repeat the INR on Argatroban and warfarin 4 to 6 hours after reduction of the Argatroban dose and follow the process outlined above for administering Argatroban at doses up to 2 mcg/kg/min.

STABILITY/COMPATIBILITY

Argatroban is a clear, colorless to pale yellow, slightly viscous solution. If the solution is cloudy, or if an insoluble precipitate is noted, the vial should be discarded.

Solutions prepared as recommended are stable at 25°C (77°F), with excursions permitted to 15° to 30°C (59° to 86°F) in ambient indoor light for 24 hours; therefore, light-resistant measures such as foil protection for intravenous lines are unnecessary. Solutions are physically and chemically stable for up to 96 hours when protected from light and stored at controlled room temperature, 20° to 25°C (68° to 77°F) (see USP), or at refrigerated conditions, 5° ± 3°C (41°± 5°F). Prepared solutions should not be exposed to direct sunlight. No significant potency losses have been noted following simulated delivery of the solution through intravenous tubing.

HOW SUPPLIED

Argatroban Injection is supplied in 2.5-mL solution in single-use vials at the concentration of 100 mg/mL. Each vial contains 250 mg of Argatroban.

NDC 0007-4407-01 (Package of 1)

Storage

Store the vials in original cartons at room temperature [25°C (77°F), with excursions permitted to 15° to 30°C (59° to 86°F)]. Do not freeze. Retain in the original carton to protect from light.

Manufactured, Distributed, and Marketed by **GlaxoSmithKline**

Research Triangle Park, NC 27709

April 2012 ARG:12PI

ARIXTRA ℞

[ə-rix' trə]

(fondaparinux sodium)

Solution for subcutaneous injection

HIGHLIGHTS OF PRESCRIBING INFORMATION

These highlights do not include all the information needed to use ARIXTRA safely and effectively. See full prescribing information for ARIXTRA.

ARIXTRA (fondaparinux sodium) Solution for subcutaneous injection

Initial U.S. Approval: 2001

WARNING: SPINAL/EPIDURAL HEMATOMAS

Epidural or spinal hematomas may occur in patients who are anticoagulated with low molecular weight heparins (LMWH), heparinoids, or fondaparinux sodium and are receiving neuraxial anesthesia or undergoing spinal puncture. These hematomas may result in long-term or permanent paralysis. Consider these risks when scheduling patients for spinal procedures. Factors that can increase the risk of developing epidural or spinal hematomas in these patients include:

- **use of indwelling epidural catheters**
- **concomitant use of other drugs that affect hemostasis, such as non-steroidal anti-inflammatory drugs (NSAIDs), platelet inhibitors, or other anticoagulants**
- **a history of traumatic or repeated epidural or spinal puncture**
- **a history of spinal deformity or spinal surgery**

Monitor patients frequently for signs and symptoms of neurologic impairment. If neurologic compromise is noted, urgent treatment is necessary.

Consider the benefit and risks before neuraxial intervention in patients anticoagulated or to be anticoagulated for thromboprophylaxis. *[See Warnings and Precautions (5.5) and Drug Interactions (7).]*

INDICATIONS AND USAGE

ARIXTRA is a Factor Xa inhibitor (anticoagulant) indicated for:

- Prophylaxis of deep vein thrombosis (DVT) in patients undergoing hip fracture surgery (including extended prophylaxis), hip replacement surgery, knee replacement surgery, or abdominal surgery. (1.1)
- Treatment of DVT or acute pulmonary embolism (PE) when administered in conjunction with warfarin. (1.2, 1.3)

DOSAGE AND ADMINISTRATION

- Prophylaxis of deep vein thrombosis: ARIXTRA 2.5 mg subcutaneously once daily after hemostasis has been established. The initial dose should be given no earlier than 6 to 8 hours after surgery and continued for 5 to 9 days. For patients undergoing hip fracture surgery, extended prophylaxis up to 24 additional days is recommended. (2.1, 2.2)
- Treatment of deep vein thrombosis and pulmonary embolism: ARIXTRA 5 mg (body weight <50 kg), 7.5 mg (50 to 100 kg), or 10 mg (>100 kg) subcutaneously once daily. Treatment should continue for at least 5 days until INR 2 to 3 achieved with warfarin sodium. (2.3)

Do not use as intramuscular injection. For subcutaneous use, do not mix with other injections or infusions.

DOSAGE FORMS AND STRENGTHS

Single-dose, prefilled syringes containing 2.5 mg, 5 mg, 7.5 mg, or 10 mg of fondaparinux. (3)

CONTRAINDICATIONS

ARIXTRA is contraindicated in the following conditions: (4)

- Severe renal impairment (creatinine clearance <30 mL/min) in prophylaxis or treatment of venous thromboembolism.
- Active major bleeding.
- Bacterial endocarditis.
- Thrombocytopenia associated with a positive *in vitro* test for anti-platelet antibody in the presence of fondaparinux sodium.
- Body weight <50 kg (venous thromboembolism prophylaxis only).

WARNINGS AND PRECAUTIONS

- Use with caution in patients who have conditions or are taking concomitant medications that increase risk of hemorrhage. (5.1)
- Bleeding risk is increased in renal impairment and in patients with low body weight <50 kg. (5.2, 5.3)
- Thrombocytopenia can occur with administration of ARIXTRA. (5.4)
- Periodic routine complete blood counts (including platelet counts), serum creatinine level, and stool occult blood tests are recommended (5.6)
- The packaging (needle guard) contains dry natural rubber and may cause allergic reactions in latex sensitive individuals (5.7)

ADVERSE REACTIONS

The most common adverse reactions associated with the use of ARIXTRA are bleeding complications. (6.1) Mild local irritation (injection site bleeding, rash, and pruritus) may occur following subcutaneous injection. (6.2)

Anemia, insomnia, increased wound drainage, hypokalemia, dizziness, hypotension, confusion, bullous eruption, hematoma, post-operative hemorrhage, and purpura may occur. (6.4)

To report SUSPECTED ADVERSE REACTIONS, contact GlaxoSmithKline at 1-888-825-5249 or FDA at 1-800-FDA-1088 or www.fda.gov/medwatch.

DRUG INTERACTIONS

Discontinue agents that may enhance the risk of hemorrhage prior to initiation of therapy with ARIXTRA unless essential. If co-administration is necessary, monitor patients closely for hemorrhage. (7)

USE IN SPECIFIC POPULATIONS

- Safety and effectiveness of ARIXTRA in pediatric patients have not been established. Because the risk for bleeding during treatment with ARIXTRA is increased in adults who weigh <50 kg, bleeding may be a particular safety concern for use of ARIXTRA in the pediatric population. (4, 5.3)
- Because elderly patients are more likely to have reduced renal function, ARIXTRA should be used with caution in these patients. (8.5)
- The risk of bleeding is increased with reduced renal or hepatic function. (8.6, 8.7)

See 17 for PATIENT COUNSELING INFORMATION and FDA-approved patient labeling

Revised: 01/2012

FULL PRESCRIBING INFORMATION: CONTENTS*

*** Sections or subsections omitted from the full prescribing information are not listed**

FULL PRESCRIBING INFORMATION

WARNING: SPINAL/EPIDURAL HEMATOMAS

Epidural or spinal hematomas may occur in patients who are anticoagulated with low molecular weight heparins (LMWH), heparinoids, or fondaparinux sodium and are receiving neuraxial anesthesia or undergoing spinal puncture. These hematomas may result in long-term or permanent paralysis. Consider these risks when scheduling patients for spinal procedures. Factors that can increase the risk of developing epidural or spinal hematomas in these patients include:

- use of indwelling epidural catheters
- concomitant use of other drugs that affect hemostasis, such as non-steroidal anti-inflammatory drugs (NSAIDs), platelet inhibitors, or other anticoagulants
- a history of traumatic or repeated epidural or spinal puncture
- a history of spinal deformity or spinal surgery

Monitor patients frequently for signs and symptoms of neurologic impairment. If neurologic compromise is noted, urgent treatment is necessary.

Consider the benefit and risks before neuraxial intervention in patients anticoagulated or to be anticoagulated for thromboprophylaxis. *[See Warnings and Precautions (5.5) and Drug Interactions (7).]*

1 INDICATIONS AND USAGE

1.1 Prophylaxis of Deep Vein Thrombosis

ARIXTRA® is indicated for the prophylaxis of deep vein thrombosis (DVT), which may lead to pulmonary embolism (PE):

- in patients undergoing hip fracture surgery, including extended prophylaxis;
- in patients undergoing hip replacement surgery;
- in patients undergoing knee replacement surgery;
- in patients undergoing abdominal surgery who are at risk for thromboembolic complications.

1.2 Treatment of Acute Deep Vein Thrombosis

ARIXTRA is indicated for the treatment of acute deep vein thrombosis when administered in conjunction with warfarin sodium.

1.3 Treatment of Acute Pulmonary Embolism

ARIXTRA is indicated for the treatment of acute pulmonary embolism when administered in conjunction with warfarin sodium when initial therapy is administered in the hospital.

2 DOSAGE AND ADMINISTRATION

Do not mix other medications or solutions with ARIXTRA. Administer ARIXTRA only subcutaneously.

2.1 Deep Vein Thrombosis Prophylaxis Following Hip Fracture, Hip Replacement, and Knee Replacement Surgery

In patients undergoing hip fracture, hip replacement, or knee replacement surgery, the recommended dose of ARIXTRA is 2.5 mg administered by subcutaneous injection once daily after hemostasis has been established. Administer the initial dose no earlier than 6 to 8 hours after surgery. Administration of ARIXTRA earlier than 6 hours after surgery increases the risk of major bleeding. The usual duration of therapy is 5 to 9 days; up to 11 days of therapy was administered in clinical trials.

In patients undergoing hip fracture surgery, an extended prophylaxis course of up to 24 additional days is recommended. In patients undergoing hip fracture surgery, a total of 32 days (peri-operative and extended prophylaxis) was administered in clinical trials. *[See Warnings and Precautions (5.6), Adverse Reactions (6), and Clinical Studies (14)].*

2.2 Deep Vein Thrombosis Prophylaxis Following Abdominal Surgery

In patients undergoing abdominal surgery, the recommended dose of ARIXTRA is 2.5 mg administered by subcutaneous injection once daily after hemostasis has been established. Administer the initial dose no earlier than 6 to 8 hours after surgery. Administration of ARIXTRA earlier than 6 hours after surgery increases the risk of major bleeding. The usual duration of administration is 5 to 9 days, and up to 10 days of ARIXTRA was administered in clinical trials.

2.3 Deep Vein Thrombosis and Pulmonary Embolism Treatment

In patients with acute symptomatic DVT and in patients with acute symptomatic PE, the recommended dose of ARIXTRA is 5 mg (body weight <50 kg), 7.5 mg (body weight 50 to 100 kg), or 10 mg (body weight >100 kg) by subcutaneous injection once daily (ARIXTRA treatment regimen). Initiate concomitant treatment with warfarin sodium as soon as possible, usually within 72 hours. Continue treatment with ARIXTRA for at least 5 days and until a therapeutic oral anticoagulant effect is established (INR 2 to 3). The usual duration of administration of ARIXTRA is 5 to 9 days; up to 26 days of ARIXTRA injection was administered in clinical trials. *[See Warnings and Precautions (5.6), Adverse Reactions (6), and Clinical Studies (14)].*

2.4 Hepatic Impairment

No dose adjustment is recommended in patients with mild to moderate hepatic impairment, based upon single-dose pharmacokinetic data. Pharmacokinetic data are not available for patients with severe hepatic impairment. Patients with hepatic impairment may be particularly vulnerable to bleeding during ARIXTRA therapy. Observe these patients closely for signs and symptoms of bleeding. *[See Clinical Pharmacology (12.4).]*

2.5 Instructions for Use

ARIXTRA Injection is provided in a single-dose, prefilled syringe affixed with an automatic needle protection system. ARIXTRA is administered by subcutaneous injection. It must not be administered by intramuscular injection. ARIXTRA is intended for use under a physician's guidance. Patients may self-inject only if their physician determines that it is appropriate and the patients are trained in subcutaneous injection techniques.

Prior to administration, visually inspect ARIXTRA to ensure the solution is clear and free of particulate matter.

To avoid the loss of drug when using the prefilled syringe, do not expel the air bubble from the syringe before the injection. Administration should be made in the fatty tissue, alternating injection sites (e.g., between the left and right anterolateral or the left and right posterolateral abdominal wall).

To administer ARIXTRA:

1. Wipe the surface of the injection site with an alcohol swab.
2. Hold the syringe with either hand and use your other hand to twist the rigid needle guard (covers the needle) counter-clockwise. Pull the rigid needle guard straight off the needle (Figure 1). Discard the needle guard.
3. Do not try to remove the air bubbles from the syringe before giving the injection.
4. Pinch a fold of skin at the injection site between your thumb and forefinger and hold it throughout the injection.
5. Hold the syringe with your thumb on the top pad of the plunger rod and your next 2 fingers on the finger grips on the syringe barrel. Pay attention to avoid sticking yourself with the exposed needle (Figure 2).

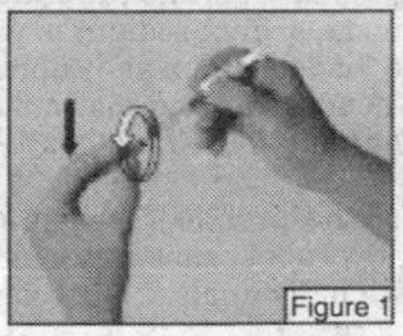
Figure 1

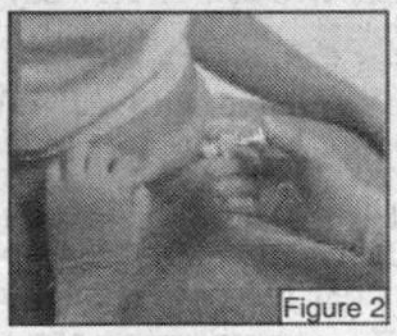
Figure 2

6. Insert the full length of the syringe needle perpendicularly into the skin fold held between the thumb and forefinger (Figure 3).
7. Push the plunger rod firmly with your thumb as far as it will go. This will ensure you have injected all the contents of the syringe (Figure 4).

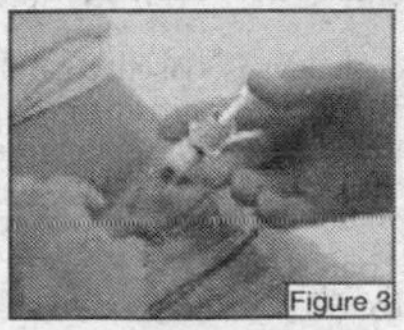
Figure 3

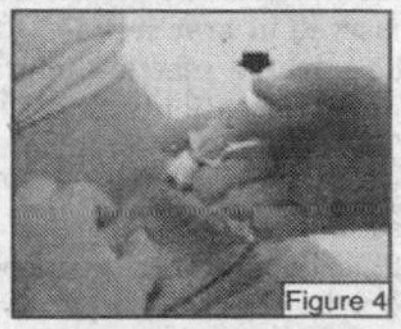
Figure 4

8. When you have injected all the contents of the syringe, the plunger should be released. The plunger will then rise automatically while the needle withdraws from the skin and retracts into the security sleeve. Discard the syringe into the sharps container.
9. You will know that the syringe has worked when:
- The needle is pulled back into the security sleeve and the white safety indicator appears above the upper body.
- You may also hear or feel a soft click when the plunger rod is released fully.

3 DOSAGE FORMS AND STRENGTHS

Single-dose, prefilled syringes containing either 2.5 mg, 5 mg, 7.5 mg, or 10 mg of fondaparinux.

4 CONTRAINDICATIONS

ARIXTRA is contraindicated in the following conditions:

- Severe renal impairment (creatinine clearance [CrCl] <30 mL/min). *[See Warnings and Precautions (5.2) and Use in Specific Populations (8.6).]*
- Active major bleeding.
- Bacterial endocarditis.
- Thrombocytopenia associated with a positive *in vitro* test for anti-platelet antibody in the presence of fondaparinux sodium.
- Body weight <50 kg (venous thromboembolism [VTE] prophylaxis only) *[see Warnings and Precautions (5.3)].*

5 WARNINGS AND PRECAUTIONS

5.1 Hemorrhage

Use ARIXTRA with extreme caution in conditions with increased risk of hemorrhage, such as congenital or acquired bleeding disorders, active ulcerative and angiodysplastic gastrointestinal disease, hemorrhagic stroke, uncontrolled arterial hypertension, diabetic retinopathy, or shortly after brain, spinal, or ophthalmological surgery. Isolated cases of elevated aPTT temporally associated with bleeding events have been reported following administration of ARIXTRA (with or without concomitant administration of other anticoagulants) *[See Adverse Reactions (6.5)].*

Do not administer agents that enhance the risk of hemorrhage with ARIXTRA unless essential for the management of the underlying condition, such as vitamin K antagonists for the treatment of VTE. If co-administration is essential, closely monitor patients for signs and symptoms of bleeding.

Do not administer the initial dose of ARIXTRA earlier than 6 to 8 hours after surgery. Administration earlier than 6 hours after surgery increases risk of major bleeding *[see Dosage and Administration (2) and Adverse Reactions (6.1)].*

5.2 Renal Impairment and Bleeding Risk

ARIXTRA increases the risk of bleeding in patients with impaired renal function due to reduced clearance *[see Clinical Pharmacology (12.4)].*

The incidence of major bleeding by renal function status reported in clinical trials of patients receiving ARIXTRA for VTE surgical prophylaxis is provided in Table 1. In these patient populations, the following is recommended:

- Do not use ARIXTRA for VTE prophylaxis and treatment in patients with CrCl <30 mL/min *[see Contraindications (4)].*
- Use ARIXTRA with caution in patients with CrCl 30 to 50 mL/min.

[See table 1 above]

Table 1. Incidence of Major Bleeding in Patients Treated With ARIXTRA by Renal Function Status for Surgical Prophylaxis and Treatment of Deep Vein Thrombosis (DVT) and Pulmonary Embolism (PE)

		Degree of Renal Impairment			
Population	**Timing of Dose**	**Normal % (n/N)**	**Mild % (n/N)**	**Moderate % (n/N)**	**Severe % (n/N)**
CrCl (mL/min)		**≥80**	**≥50 - <80**	**≥30 - <50**	**<30**
Orthopedic surgery[a]	Overall	1.6% (25/1,565)	2.4% (31/1,288)	3.8% (19/504)	4.8% (4/83)
	6-8 hours after surgery	1.8% (16/905)	2.2% (15/675)	2.3% (6/265)	0% (0/40)
Abdominal surgery	Overall	2.1% (13/606)	3.6% (22/613)	6.7% (12/179)	7.1% (1/14)
	6-8 hours after surgery	2.1% (10/467)	3.3% (16/481)	5.8% (8/137)	7.7% (1/13)
DVT and PE Treatment		0.4% (4/1,132)	1.6% (12/733)	2.2% (7/318)	7.3% (4/55)

CrCl = creatinine clearance.

[a] Hip fracture, hip replacement, and knee replacement surgery prophylaxis.

Assess renal function periodically in patients receiving ARIXTRA. Discontinue the drug immediately in patients who develop severe renal impairment while on therapy. After discontinuation of ARIXTRA, its anticoagulant effects may persist for 2 to 4 days in patients with normal renal function (i.e., at least 3 to 5 half-lives). The anticoagulant effects of ARIXTRA may persist even longer in patients with renal impairment *[see Clinical Pharmacology (12.4)].*

5.3 Body Weight <50 Kg and Bleeding Risk

ARIXTRA increases the risk for bleeding in patients who weigh less than 50 kg, compared to patients with higher weights.

In patients who weigh less than 50 kg:

- Do not administer ARIXTRA as prophylactic therapy for patients undergoing hip fracture, hip replacement, or knee replacement surgery and abdominal surgery *[see Contraindications (4)].*

Table 2. Bleeding Across Randomized, Controlled Hip Fracture, Hip Replacement, and Knee Replacement Surgery Studies

	Peri-Operative Prophylaxis (Day 1 to Day 7 ± 1 post-surgery)		Extended Prophylaxis (Day 8 to Day 28 ± 2 post-surgery)	
	ARIXTRA 2.5 mg SC once daily N = 3,616	Enoxaparin Sodium[a, b] N = 3,956	ARIXTRA 2.5 mg SC once daily N = 327	Placebo SC once daily N = 329
Major bleeding[c]	96 (2.7%)	75 (1.9%)	8 (2.4%)	2 (0.6%)
Hip fracture	18/831 (2.2%)	19/842 (2.3%)	8/327 (2.4%)	2/329 (0.6%)
Hip replacement	67/2,268 (3.0%)	55/2,597 (2.1%)	—	—
Knee replacement	11/517 (2.1%)	1/517 (0.2%)	—	—
Fatal bleeding	0 (0.0%)	1 (<0.1%)	0 (0.0%)	0 (0.0%)
Non-fatal bleeding at critical site	0 (0.0%)	1 (<0.1%)	0 (0.0%)	0 (0.0%)
Re-operation due to bleeding	12 (0.3%)	10 (0.3%)	2 (0.6%)	2 (0.6%)
BI ≥2[d]	84 (2.3%)	63 (1.6%)	6 (1.8%)	0 (0.0%)
Minor bleeding[e]	109 (3.0%)	116 (2.9%)	5 (1.5%)	2 (0.6%)

[a] Enoxaparin sodium dosing regimen: 30 mg every 12 hours or 40 mg once daily.
[b] Not approved for use in patients undergoing hip fracture surgery.
[c] Major bleeding was defined as clinically overt bleeding that was (1) fatal, (2) bleeding at critical site (e.g. intracranial, retroperitoneal, intraocular, pericardial, spinal, or into adrenal gland), (3) associated with re-operation at operative site, or (4) with a bleeding index (BI) ≥2.
[d] BI ≥2: Overt bleeding associated only with a bleeding index (BI) ≥2 calculated as [number of whole blood or packed red blood cell units transfused + [(pre-bleeding) – (post-bleeding)] hemoglobin (g/dL) values].
[e] Minor bleeding was defined as clinically overt bleeding that was not major.

• Use ARIXTRA with caution in the treatment of PE and DVT.

During the randomized clinical trials of VTE prophylaxis in the peri-operative period following hip fracture, hip replacement, or knee replacement surgery and abdominal surgery, major bleeding occurred at a higher rate among patients with a body weight <50 kg compared to those with a body weight >50 kg (5.4% versus 2.1% in patients undergoing hip fracture, hip replacement, or knee replacement surgery; 5.3% versus 3.3% in patients undergoing abdominal surgery).

5.4 Thrombocytopenia

Thrombocytopenia can occur with the administration of ARIXTRA. Thrombocytopenia of any degree should be monitored closely. Discontinue ARIXTRA if the platelet count falls below 100,000/mm^3. Moderate thrombocytopenia (platelet counts between 100,000/mm^3 and 50,000/mm^3) occurred at a rate of 3.0% in patients given ARIXTRA 2.5 mg in the peri-operative hip fracture, hip replacement, or knee replacement surgery and abdominal surgery clinical trials. Severe thrombocytopenia (platelet counts less than 50,000/mm^3) occurred at a rate of 0.2% in patients given ARIXTRA 2.5 mg in these clinical trials. During extended prophylaxis, no cases of moderate or severe thrombocytopenia were reported.

Moderate thrombocytopenia occurred at a rate of 0.5% in patients given the ARIXTRA treatment regimen in the DVT and PE treatment clinical trials. Severe thrombocytopenia occurred at a rate of 0.04% in patients given the ARIXTRA treatment regimen in the DVT and PE treatment clinical trials.

Isolated occurrences of thrombocytopenia with thrombosis that manifested similar to heparin-induced thrombocytopenia have been reported with the use of ARIXTRA in postmarketing experience. *[See Adverse Reactions (6.5).]*

5.5 Neuraxial Anesthesia and Post-operative Indwelling Epidural Catheter Use

Spinal or epidural hematomas, which may result in long-term or permanent paralysis, can occur with the use of anticoagulants and neuraxial (spinal/epidural) anesthesia or spinal puncture. The risk of these events may be higher with post-operative use of indwelling epidural catheters or concomitant use of other drugs affecting hemostasis such as NSAIDs *[see Boxed Warning]*. In the postmarketing experience, epidural or spinal hematoma has been reported in association with the use of ARIXTRA by subcutaneous (SC) injection. Monitor patients undergoing these procedures for signs and symptoms of neurologic impairment. Consider the potential risks and benefits before neuraxial intervention in patients anticoagulated or who may be anticoagulated for thromboprophylaxis.

5.6 Monitoring: Laboratory Tests

Routine coagulation tests such as Prothrombin Time (PT) and Activated Partial Thromboplastin Time (aPTT) are relatively insensitive measures of the activity of ARIXTRA and international standards of heparin or LMWH are not calibrators to measure anti-Factor Xa activity of ARIXTRA. If unexpected changes in coagulation parameters or major bleeding occur during therapy with ARIXTRA, discontinue ARIXTRA. In postmarketing experience, isolated occurrences of aPTT elevations have been reported following administration of ARIXTRA *[see Adverse Reactions (6.5)]*.

Periodic routine complete blood counts (including platelet count), serum creatinine level, and stool occult blood tests are recommended during the course of treatment with ARIXTRA.

The anti-Factor Xa activity of fondaparinux sodium can be measured by anti-Xa assay using the appropriate calibrator (fondaparinux). The activity of fondaparinux sodium is expressed in milligrams (mg) of the fondaparinux and cannot be compared with activities of heparin or low molecular weight heparins. *[See Clinical Pharmacology (12.2, 12.3).]*

5.7 Latex

The packaging (needle guard) of the prefilled syringe of ARIXTRA contains dry natural latex rubber that may cause allergic reactions in latex sensitive individuals.

6 ADVERSE REACTIONS

The most serious adverse reactions reported with ARIXTRA are bleeding complications and thrombocytopenia *[see Warnings and Precautions (5)]*.

Because clinical trials are conducted under widely varying conditions, adverse reaction rates observed in the clinical trials of a drug cannot be directly compared to rates in the clinical trials of another drug and may not reflect the rates observed in practice.

The adverse reaction information below is based on data from 8,877 patients exposed to ARIXTRA in controlled trials of hip fracture, hip replacement, major knee, or abdominal surgeries, and DVT and PE treatment. These trials consisted of the following:

- 2 peri-operative dose-response trials (n = 989)
- 4 active-controlled peri-operative VTE prophylaxis trials with enoxaparin sodium (n = 3,616), an extended VTE prophylaxis trial (n = 327), and an active-controlled trial with dalteparin sodium (n = 1,425)
- a dose-response trial (n = 111) and an active-controlled trial with enoxaparin sodium in DVT treatment (n = 1,091)
- an active-controlled trial with heparin in PE treatment (n = 1,092)

6.1 Hemorrhage

During administration of ARIXTRA, the most common adverse reactions were bleeding complications *[see Warnings and Precautions (5.1)]*.

Hip Fracture, Hip Replacement, and Knee Replacement Surgery: The rates of major bleeding events reported during the hip fracture, hip replacement, or knee replacement surgery clinical trials with ARIXTRA 2.5 mg are provided in Table 2.

[See table 2 above]

A separate analysis of major bleeding across all randomized, controlled, peri-operative, prophylaxis clinical studies of hip fracture, hip replacement, or knee replacement surgery according to the time of the first injection of ARIXTRA after surgical closure was performed in patients who received ARIXTRA only post-operatively. In this analysis, the incidences of major bleeding were as follows: <4 hours was 4.8% (5/104), 4 to 6 hours was 2.3% (28/1,196), 6 to 8 hours was 1.9% (38/1,965). In all studies, the majority (≥75%) of the major bleeding events occurred during the first 4 days after surgery.

Abdominal Surgery: In a randomized study of patients undergoing abdominal surgery, ARIXTRA 2.5 mg once daily (n = 1,433) was compared with dalteparin 5,000 IU once daily (n = 1,425). Bleeding rates are shown in Table 3.

Table 3. Bleeding in the Abdominal Surgery Study

	ARIXTRA 2.5 mg SC once daily N = 1,433	Dalteparin Sodium 5,000 IU SC once daily N = 1,425
Major bleeding[a]	49 (3.4%)	34 (2.4%)
Fatal bleeding	2 (0.1%)	2 (0.1%)
Non-fatal bleeding at critical site	0 (0.0%)	0 (0.0%)
Other non-fatal major bleeding		
Surgical site	38 (2.7%)	26 (1.8%)
Non-surgical site	9 (0.6%)	6 (0.4%)
Minor bleeding[b]	31 (2.2%)	23 (1.6%)

[a] Major bleeding was defined as bleeding that was (1) fatal, (2) bleeding at the surgical site leading to intervention, (3) non-surgical bleeding at a critical site (e.g. intracranial, retroperitoneal, intraocular, pericardial, spinal, or into adrenal gland), or leading to an intervention, and/or with a bleeding index (BI) ≥2.
[b] Minor bleeding was defined as clinically overt bleeding that was not major.

The rates of major bleeding according to the time interval following the first ARIXTRA injection were as follows: <6 hours was 3.4% (9/263) and 6 to 8 hours was 2.9% (32/1112).

Treatment of Deep Vein Thrombosis and Pulmonary Embolism: The rates of bleeding events reported during the DVT and PE clinical trials with the ARIXTRA injection treatment regimen are provided in Table 4.

[See table 4 at top of next page]

6.2 Local Reactions

Local irritation (injection site bleeding, rash, and pruritus) may occur following subcutaneous injection of ARIXTRA.

6.3 Elevations of Serum Aminotransferases

In the peri-operative prophylaxis randomized clinical trials of 7 ± 2 days, asymptomatic increases in aspartate (AST) and alanine (ALT) aminotransferase levels greater than 3 times the upper limit of normal were reported in 1.7% and 2.6% of patients, respectively, during treatment with ARIXTRA 2.5 mg once daily versus 3.2% and 3.9% of patients, respectively, during treatment with enoxaparin sodium 30 mg every 12 hours or 40 mg once daily enoxaparin sodium. These elevations are reversible and rarely associated with increases in bilirubin. In the extended prophylaxis clinical trial, no significant differences in AST and ALT levels between ARIXTRA 2.5 mg and placebo-treated patients were observed.

In the DVT and PE treatment clinical trials, asymptomatic increases in AST and ALT levels greater than 3 times the upper limit of normal of the laboratory reference range were reported in 0.7% and 1.3% of patients, respectively, during treatment with ARIXTRA. In comparison, these increases were reported in 4.8% and 12.3% of patients, respectively, in the DVT treatment trial during treatment with enoxaparin sodium 1 mg/kg every 12 hours and in 2.9% and 8.7% of patients, respectively, in the PE treatment trial during treatment with aPTT adjusted heparin.

Since aminotransferase determinations are important in the differential diagnosis of myocardial infarction, liver disease, and pulmonary emboli, elevations that might be caused by drugs like ARIXTRA should be interpreted with caution.

6.4 Other Adverse Reactions

Other adverse reactions that occurred during treatment with ARIXTRA in clinical trials with patients undergoing hip fracture, hip replacement, or knee replacement surgery are provided in Table 5.

[See table 5 above]

Adverse reactions in the abdominal surgery study and in the VTE treatment trials generally occurred at lower rates than in the hip and knee surgery trials described above. The most common adverse reaction in the abdominal surgery trial was post-operative wound infection (4.9%), and the most common adverse reaction in the VTE treatment trials was epistaxis (1.3%).

6.5 Postmarketing Experience

The following adverse reactions have been identified during post-approval use of ARIXTRA. Because these reactions are reported voluntarily from a population of uncertain size, it is not always possible to reliably estimate their frequency or establish a causal relationship to drug exposure.

Isolated occurrences of thrombocytopenia with thrombosis that manifested similar to heparin-induced thrombocytopenia have been reported in the postmarketing experience and isolated cases of elevated aPTT temporally associated with bleeding events have been reported following administration of ARIXTRA (with or without concomitant administration of other anticoagulants) *[see Warnings and Precautions (5.4)]*.

7 DRUG INTERACTIONS

In clinical studies performed with ARIXTRA, the concomitant use of oral anticoagulants (warfarin), platelet inhibitors (acetylsalicylic acid), NSAIDs (piroxicam), and digoxin did not significantly affect the pharmacokinetics/pharmacodynamics of fondaparinux sodium. In addition, ARIXTRA neither influenced the pharmacodynamics of warfarin, acetylsalicylic acid, piroxicam, and digoxin, nor the pharmacokinetics of digoxin at steady state.

Agents that may enhance the risk of hemorrhage should be discontinued prior to initiation of therapy with ARIXTRA unless these agents are essential. If co-administration is necessary, monitor patients closely for hemorrhage. *[See Warnings and Precautions (5.1).]*

In an *in vitro* study in human liver microsomes, inhibition of CYP2A6 hydroxylation of coumarin by fondaparinux (200 micromolar i.e., 350 mg/L) was 17 to 28%. Inhibition of the other isozymes evaluated (CYPs 1A2, 2C9, 2C19, 2D6, 3A4, and 3E1) was 0 to 16%. Since fondaparinux does not markedly inhibit CYP450s (CYP1A2, CYP2A6, CYP2C9, CYP2C19, CYP2D6, CYP2E1, or CYP3A4) *in vitro*, fondaparinux sodium is not expected to significantly interact with other drugs *in vivo* by inhibition of metabolism mediated by these isozymes.

Since fondaparinux sodium does not bind significantly to plasma proteins other than ATIII, no drug interactions by protein-binding displacement are expected.

8 USE IN SPECIFIC POPULATIONS

8.1 Pregnancy

Pregnancy Category B. Reproduction studies have been performed in pregnant rats at subcutaneous doses up to 10 mg/kg/day (about 32 times the recommended human dose based on body surface area) and pregnant rabbits at subcutaneous doses up to 10 mg/kg/day (about 65 times the recommended human dose based on body surface area) and have revealed no evidence of impaired fertility or harm to the fetus due to fondaparinux sodium. There are, however, no adequate and well-controlled studies in pregnant women. Because animal reproduction studies are not always predictive of human response, ARIXTRA should be used during pregnancy only if clearly needed.

8.3 Nursing Mothers

Fondaparinux sodium was found to be excreted in the milk of lactating rats. However, it is not known whether this drug is excreted in human milk. Because many drugs are excreted in human milk, caution should be exercised when ARIXTRA is administered to a nursing mother.

8.4 Pediatric Use

Safety and effectiveness of ARIXTRA in pediatric patients have not been established. Because risk for bleeding during treatment with ARIXTRA is increased in adults who weigh <50 kg, bleeding may be a particular safety concern for use of ARIXTRA in the pediatric population *[see Warnings and Precautions (5.3)]*.

8.5 Geriatric Use

In clinical trials the efficacy of ARIXTRA in the elderly (65 years or older) was similar to that seen in patients younger than 65 years; however, serious adverse events increased with age. Exercise caution when using ARIXTRA in elderly patients, paying particular attention to dosing directions and concomitant medications (especially anti-platelet medication). *[See Warnings and Precautions (5.1).]*

Fondaparinux sodium is substantially excreted by the kidney, and the risk of adverse reactions to ARIXTRA may be greater in patients with impaired renal function. Because elderly patients are more likely to have decreased renal function, assess renal function prior to ARIXTRA administration. *[See Contraindications (4), Warnings and Precautions (5.2), and Clinical Pharmacology (12.4).]*

In the peri-operative hip fracture, hip replacement, or knee replacement surgery clinical trials with patients receiving

Table 4. Bleeding[a] in Deep Vein Thrombosis and Pulmonary Embolism Treatment Studies

	ARIXTRA N = 2,294	Enoxaparin Sodium N = 1,101	Heparin aPTT adjusted IV N = 1,092
Major bleeding[b]	28 (1.2%)	13 (1.2%)	12 (1.1%)
Fatal bleeding	3 (0.1%)	0 (0.0%)	1 (0.1%)
Non-fatal bleeding at a critical site	3 (0.1%)	0 (0.0%)	2 (0.2%)
Intracranial bleeding	3 (0.1%)	0 (0.0%)	1 (0.1%)
Retro-peritoneal bleeding	0 (0.0%)	0 (0.0%)	1 (0.1%)
Other clinically overt bleeding[c]	22 (1.0%)	13 (1.2%)	10 (0.9%)
Minor bleeding[d]	70 (3.1%)	33 (3.0%)	57 (5.2%)

[a] Bleeding rates are during the study drug treatment period (approximately 7 days). Patients were also treated with vitamin K antagonists initiated within 72 hours after the first study drug administration.
[b] Major bleeding was defined as clinically overt: –and/or contributing to death – and/or in a critical organ including intracranial, retroperitoneal, intraocular, spinal, pericardial, or adrenal gland – and/or associated with a fall in hemoglobin level ≥2 g/dL – and/or leading to a transfusion ≥2 units of packed red blood cells or whole blood.
[c] Clinically overt bleeding with a 2 g/dL fall in hemoglobin and/or leading to transfusion of PRBC or whole blood ≥2 units.
[d] Minor bleeding was defined as clinically overt bleeding that was not major.

Table 5. Adverse Reactions Across Randomized, Controlled, Hip Fracture Surgery, Hip Replacement Surgery, and Knee Replacement Surgery Studies

	Peri-Operative Prophylaxis (Day 1 to Day 7 ± 1 post-surgery)		Extended Prophylaxis (Day 8 to Day 28 ± 2 post-surgery)	
Adverse Reactions	ARIXTRA 2.5 mg SC once daily	Enoxaparin Sodium[a, b]	ARIXTRA 2.5 mg SC once daily	Placebo SC once daily
	N = 3,616	N = 3,956	N = 327	N = 329
Anemia	707 (19.6%)	670 (16.9%)	5 (1.5%)	4 (1.2%)
Insomnia	179 (5.0%)	214 (5.4%)	3 (0.9%)	1 (0.3%)
Wound drainage increased	161 (4.5%)	184 (4.7%)	2 (0.6%)	0 (0.0%)
Hypokalemia	152 (4.2%)	164 (4.1%)	0 (0.0%)	0 (0.0%)
Dizziness	131 (3.6%)	165 (4.2%)	2 (0.6%)	0 (0.0%)
Purpura	128 (3.5%)	137 (3.5%)	0 (0.0%)	0 (0.0%)
Hypotension	126 (3.5%)	125 (3.2%)	1 (0.3%)	0 (0.0%)
Confusion	113 (3.1%)	132 (3.3%)	4 (1.2%)	1 (0.3%)
Bullous eruption[c]	112 (3.1%)	102 (2.6%)	0 (0.0%)	1 (0.3%)
Hematoma	103 (2.8%)	109 (2.8%)	7 (2.1%)	1 (0.3%)
Post-operative hemorrhage	85 (2.4%)	69 (1.7%)	2 (0.6%)	2 (0.6%)

[a] Enoxaparin sodium dosing regimen: 30 mg every 12 hours or 40 mg once daily.
[b] Not approved for use in patients undergoing hip fracture surgery.
[c] Localized blister coded as bullous eruption.

ARIXTRA 2.5 mg, serious adverse events increased with age for patients receiving ARIXTRA. The incidence of major bleeding in clinical trials of ARIXTRA by age is provided in Table 6.

[See table 6 at top of next page]

8.6 Renal Impairment

Patients with impaired renal function are at increased risk of bleeding due to reduced clearance of ARIXTRA *[see Contraindications (4) and Warnings and Precautions (5.2)]*. Assess renal function periodically in patients receiving ARIXTRA. Discontinue ARIXTRA immediately in patients who develop severe renal impairment while on therapy. After discontinuation of ARIXTRA, its anticoagulant effects may persist for 2 to 4 days in patients with normal renal function (i.e., at least 3 to 5 half-lives). The anticoagulant effects of ARIXTRA may persist even longer in patients with renal impairment *[see Clinical Pharmacology (12.4)]*.

8.7 Hepatic Impairment

Following a single, subcutaneous dose of 7.5 mg of ARIXTRA in patients with moderate hepatic impairment (Child-Pugh Category B) compared to subjects with normal liver function, changes from baseline in aPTT, PT/INR, and antithrombin III were similar in the two groups. However, a higher incidence of hemorrhage was observed in subjects with moderate hepatic impairment than in normal subjects, especially mild hematomas at the blood sampling or injection site. The pharmacokinetics of fondaparinux have not been studied in patients with severe hepatic impairment. *[See Dosage and Administration (2.4) and Clinical Pharmacology (12.4).]*

10 OVERDOSAGE

There is no known antidote for ARIXTRA. Overdose of ARIXTRA may lead to hemorrhagic complications. Discontinue treatment and initiate appropriate therapy if bleeding complications associated with overdosage occur.

Data obtained in patients undergoing chronic intermittent hemodialysis suggest that clearance of ARIXTRA can increase by 20% during hemodialysis.

11 DESCRIPTION

ARIXTRA (fondaparinux sodium) Injection is a sterile solution containing fondaparinux sodium. It is a synthetic and specific inhibitor of activated Factor X (Xa). Fondaparinux sodium is methyl O-2-deoxy-6-O-sulfo-2-(sulfoamino)-α-D-glucopyranosyl-(1→4)-O-β-D-glucopyra-nuronosyl-(1→4)-O-2-deoxy-3,6-di-O-sulfo-2-(sulfoamino)-α-D-glucopyranosyl-(1→4)-O-2-O-sulfo-α-L-idopyranuronosyl-(1→4)-2-deoxy-6-O-sulfo-2-(sulfoamino)-α-D-glucopyranoside, decasodium salt.

Table 6. Incidence of Major Bleeding in Patients Treated With ARIXTRA by Age

	Age		
	<65 years % (n/N)	65 to 74 years % (n/N)	≥75 years % (n/N)
Orthopedic surgery[a]	1.8% (23/1,253)	2.2% (24/1,111)	2.7% (33/1,277)
Extended prophylaxis	1.9% (1/52)	1.4% (1/71)	2.9% (6/204)
Abdominal surgery	3.0% (19/644)	3.2% (16/507)	5.0% (14/282)
DVT and PE treatment	0.6% (7/1,151)	1.6% (9/560)	2.1% (12/583)

[a] Includes hip fracture, hip replacement, and knee replacement surgery prophylaxis.

Table 7. Efficacy of ARIXTRA in the Peri-operative Prophylaxis of Thromboembolic Events Following Hip Fracture Surgery

Endpoint	Peri-operative Prophylaxis (Day 1 to Day 7 ± 2 post-surgery)			
	ARIXTRA 2.5 mg SC once daily		Enoxaparin Sodium 40 mg SC once daily	
	n/N[a]	% (95% CI)	n/N[a]	% (95% CI)
VTE	52/626	8.3%[b] (6.3, 10.8)	119/624	19.1% (16.1, 22.4)
All DVT	49/624	7.9%[b] (5.9, 10.2)	117/623	18.8% (15.8, 22.1)
Proximal DVT	6/650	0.9%[b] (0.3, 2.0)	28/646	4.3% (2.9, 6.2)
Symptomatic PE	3/831	0.4%[c] (0.1, 1.1)	3/840	0.4% (0.1, 1.0)

[a] N = all evaluable hip fracture surgery patients. Evaluable patients were those who were treated and underwent the appropriate surgery (i.e., hip fracture surgery of the upper third of the femur), with an adequate efficacy assessment up to Day 11.
[b] *P* value versus enoxaparin sodium <0.001.
[c] *P* value versus enoxaparin sodium: NS.

The molecular formula of fondaparinux sodium is $C_{31}H_{43}N_3Na_{10}O_{49}S_8$ and its molecular weight is 1728. The structural formula is provided below:

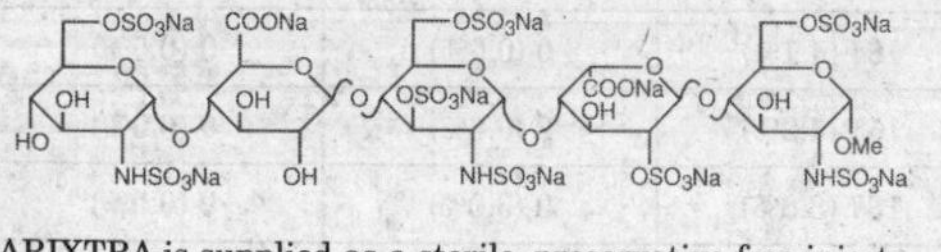

ARIXTRA is supplied as a sterile, preservative-free injectable solution for subcutaneous use.

Each single-dose, prefilled syringe of ARIXTRA, affixed with an automatic needle protection system, contains 2.5 mg of fondaparinux sodium in 0.5 mL, 5.0 mg of fondaparinux sodium in 0.4 mL, 7.5 mg of fondaparinux sodium in 0.6 mL, or 10.0 mg of fondaparinux sodium in 0.8 mL of an isotonic solution of sodium chloride and water for injection. The final drug product is a clear and colorless to slightly yellow liquid with a pH between 5.0 and 8.0.

12 CLINICAL PHARMACOLOGY

12.1 Mechanism of Action

The antithrombotic activity of fondaparinux sodium is the result of antithrombin III (ATIII)-mediated selective inhibition of Factor Xa. By selectively binding to ATIII, fondaparinux sodium potentiates (about 300 times) the innate neutralization of Factor Xa by ATIII. Neutralization of Factor Xa interrupts the blood coagulation cascade and thus inhibits thrombin formation and thrombus development.

Fondaparinux sodium does not inactivate thrombin (activated Factor II) and has no known effect on platelet function. At the recommended dose, fondaparinux sodium does not affect fibrinolytic activity or bleeding time.

12.2 Pharmacodynamics

Anti-Xa Activity: The pharmacodynamics/pharmacokinetics of fondaparinux sodium are derived from fondaparinux plasma concentrations quantified via anti-Factor Xa activity. Only fondaparinux can be used to calibrate the anti-Xa assay. (The international standards of heparin or LMWH are not appropriate for this use.) As a result, the activity of fondaparinux sodium is expressed as milligrams (mg) of the fondaparinux calibrator. The anti-Xa activity of the drug increases with increasing drug concentration, reaching maximum values in approximately three hours.

12.3 Pharmacokinetics

Absorption: Fondaparinux sodium administered by subcutaneous injection is rapidly and completely absorbed (absolute bioavailability is 100%). Following a single subcutaneous dose of fondaparinux sodium 2.5 mg in young male subjects, C_{max} of 0.34 mg/L is reached in approximately 2 hours. In patients undergoing treatment with fondaparinux sodium injection 2.5 mg, once daily, the peak steady-state plasma concentration is, on average, 0.39 to 0.50 mg/L and is reached approximately 3 hours post-dose. In these patients, the minimum steady-state plasma concentration is 0.14 to 0.19 mg/L. In patients with symptomatic deep vein thrombosis and pulmonary embolism undergoing treatment with fondaparinux sodium injection 5 mg (body weight <50 kg), 7.5 mg (body weight 50 to 100 kg), and 10 mg (body weight >100 kg) once daily, the body-weight-adjusted doses provide similar mean steady-state peaks and minimum plasma concentrations across all body weight categories. The mean peak steady-state plasma concentration is in the range of 1.20 to 1.26 mg/L. In these patients, the mean minimum steady-state plasma concentration is in the range of 0.46 to 0.62 mg/L.

Distribution: In healthy adults, intravenously or subcutaneously administered fondaparinux sodium distributes mainly in blood and only to a minor extent in extravascular fluid as evidenced by steady state and non-steady state apparent volume of distribution of 7 to 11 L. Similar fondaparinux distribution occurs in patients undergoing elective hip surgery or hip fracture surgery. *In vitro,* fondaparinux sodium is highly (at least 94%) and specifically bound to antithrombin III (ATIII) and does not bind significantly to other plasma proteins (including platelet Factor 4 [PF4]) or red blood cells.

Metabolism: *In vivo* metabolism of fondaparinux has not been investigated since the majority of the administered dose is eliminated unchanged in urine in individuals with normal kidney function.

Elimination: In individuals with normal kidney function, fondaparinux is eliminated in urine mainly as unchanged drug. In healthy individuals up to 75 years of age, up to 77% of a single subcutaneous or intravenous fondaparinux dose is eliminated in urine as unchanged drug in 72 hours. The elimination half-life is 17 to 21 hours.

12.4 Special Populations

Renal Impairment: Fondaparinux elimination is prolonged in patients with renal impairment since the major route of elimination is urinary excretion of unchanged drug. In patients undergoing prophylaxis following elective hip surgery or hip fracture surgery, the total clearance of fondaparinux is approximately 25% lower in patients with mild renal impairment (CrCl 50 to 80 mL/min), approximately 40% lower in patients with moderate renal impairment (CrCl 30 to 50 mL/min), and approximately 55% lower in patients with severe renal impairment (<30 mL/min) compared to patients with normal renal function. A similar relationship between fondaparinux clearance and extent of renal impairment was observed in DVT treatment patients. *[See Contraindications (4) and Warnings and Precautions (5.2).]*

Hepatic Impairment: Following a single, subcutaneous dose of 7.5 mg of ARIXTRA in patients with moderate hepatic impairment (Child-Pugh Category B), C_{max} and AUC were decreased by 22% and 39%, respectively, compared to subjects with normal liver function. The changes from baseline in pharmacodynamic parameters, such as aPTT, PT/INR, and antithrombin III, were similar in normal subjects and in patients with moderate hepatic impairment. Based on these data, no dosage adjustment is recommended in these patients. However, a higher incidence of hemorrhage was observed in subjects with moderate hepatic impairment than in normal subjects *[see Use in Specific Populations (8.7)]*. The pharmacokinetics of fondaparinux have not been studied in patients with severe hepatic impairment. *[See Dosage and Administration (2.4).]*

Pediatric: The pharmacokinetics of fondaparinux have not been investigated in pediatric patients. *[See Contraindications (4), Warnings and Precautions (5.3), and Pediatric Use (8.4).]*

Geriatric: Fondaparinux elimination is prolonged in patients older than 75 years. In studies evaluating fondaparinux sodium 2.5 mg prophylaxis in hip fracture surgery or elective hip surgery, the total clearance of fondaparinux was approximately 25% lower in patients older than 75 years as compared to patients younger than 65 years. A similar relationship between fondaparinux clearance and age was observed in DVT treatment patients. *[See Use in Specific Populations (8.5).]*

Patients Weighing Less Than 50 kg: Total clearance of fondaparinux sodium is decreased by approximately 30% in patients weighing less than 50 kg *[see Dosage and Administration (2.3) and Contraindications (4)]*.

Gender: The pharmacokinetic properties of fondaparinux sodium are not significantly affected by gender.

Race: Pharmacokinetic differences due to race have not been studied prospectively. However, studies performed in Asian (Japanese) healthy subjects did not reveal a different pharmacokinetic profile compared to Caucasian healthy subjects. Similarly, no plasma clearance differences were observed between black and Caucasian patients undergoing orthopedic surgery.

13 NONCLINICAL TOXICOLOGY

13.1 Carcinogenesis, Mutagenesis, Impairment of Fertility

No long-term studies in animals have been performed to evaluate the carcinogenic potential of fondaparinux sodium. Fondaparinux sodium was not genotoxic in the Ames test, the mouse lymphoma cell (L5178Y/TK$^{+/-}$) forward mutation test, the human lymphocyte chromosome aberration test, the rat hepatocyte unscheduled DNA synthesis (UDS) test, or the rat micronucleus test.

At subcutaneous doses up to 10 mg/kg/day (about 32 times the recommended human dose based on body surface area), fondaparinux sodium was found to have no effect on fertility and reproductive performance of male and female rats.

14 CLINICAL STUDIES

14.1 Prophylaxis of Thromboembolic Events Following Hip Fracture Surgery

In a randomized, double-blind, clinical trial in patients undergoing hip fracture surgery, ARIXTRA 2.5 mg SC once daily was compared to enoxaparin sodium 40 mg SC once daily, which is not approved for use in patients undergoing hip fracture surgery. A total of 1,711 patients were randomized and 1,673 were treated. Patients ranged in age from 17 to 101 years (mean age 77 years) with 25% men and 75% women. Patients were 99% Caucasian, 1% other races. Patients with multiple traumas affecting more than one organ system, serum creatinine level more than 2 mg/dL (180 micromol/L), or platelet count less than 100,000/mm^3 were excluded from the trial. ARIXTRA was initiated after surgery in 88% of patients (mean 6 hours) and enoxaparin sodium was initiated after surgery in 74% of patients (mean 18 hours). For both drugs, treatment was continued for 7 ± 2 days. The primary efficacy endpoint, venous thromboembolism (VTE), was a composite of documented deep vein thrombosis (DVT) and/or documented symptomatic pulmonary embolism (PE) reported up to Day 11. The efficacy data are provided in Table 7 and demonstrate that under the conditions of the trial ARIXTRA was associated with a VTE rate of 8.3% compared with a VTE rate of 19.1% for enoxaparin sodium for a relative risk reduction of 56% (95% CI: 39%, 70%; *P* <0.001). Major bleeding episodes occurred in 2.2% of patients receiving ARIXTRA and 2.3% of enoxaparin sodium patients *[see Adverse Reactions (6.1)]*.

[See table 7 above]

14.2 Extended Prophylaxis of Thromboembolic Events Following Hip Fracture Surgery

In a noncomparative, unblinded manner, 737 patients undergoing hip fracture surgery were initially treated during the peri-operative period with ARIXTRA 2.5 mg once daily for 7 ± 1 days. Eighty-one (81) of the 737 patients were not eligible for randomization into the 3-week double-blind period. Three hundred twenty-six (326) patients and 330 patients were randomized to receive ARIXTRA 2.5 mg once daily or placebo, respectively, in or out of the hospital for 21 ± 2 days. Patients ranged in age from 23 to 96 years (mean age 75 years) and were 29% men and 71% women. Patients were 99% Caucasian and 1% other races. Patients with multiple traumas affecting more than one organ system or serum creatinine level more than 2 mg/dL (180 micromol/L) were excluded from the trial. The primary efficacy endpoint, venous thromboembolism (VTE), was a composite of documented deep vein thrombosis (DVT) and/or documented symptomatic pulmonary embolism (PE) reported for up to 24 days following randomization. The efficacy data are provided in Table 8 and demonstrate that extended prophylaxis with ARIXTRA was associated with a VTE rate of 1.4% compared with a VTE rate of 35.0% for placebo for a relative risk reduction of 95.9% (95% CI = [98.7; 87.1], *P* <0.0001). Major bleeding rates during the 3-week extended prophylaxis period for ARIXTRA occurred in 2.4% of patients receiving ARIXTRA and 0.6% of placebo-treated patients *[see Adverse Reactions (6.1)]*.

[See table 8 above]

14.3 Prophylaxis of Thromboembolic Events Following Hip Replacement Surgery

In 2 randomized, double-blind, clinical trials in patients undergoing hip replacement surgery, ARIXTRA 2.5 mg SC once daily was compared to either enoxaparin sodium 30 mg SC every 12 hours (Study 1) or to enoxaparin sodium 40 mg SC once a day (Study 2). In Study 1, a total of 2,275 patients were randomized and 2,257 were treated. Patients ranged in age from 18 to 92 years (mean age 65 years) with 48% men and 52% women. Patients were 94% Caucasian, 4% black, <1% Asian, and 2% others. In Study 2, a total of 2,309 patients were randomized and 2,273 were treated. Patients ranged in age from 24 to 97 years (mean age 65 years) with 42% men and 58% women. Patients were 99% Caucasian, and 1% other races. Patients with serum creatinine level more than 2 mg/dL (180 micromol/L), or platelet count less than 100,000/mm^3 were excluded from both trials. In Study 1, ARIXTRA was initiated 6 ± 2 hours (mean 6.5 hours) after surgery in 92% of patients and enoxaparin sodium was initiated 12 to 24 hours (mean 20.25 hours) after surgery in 97% of patients. In Study 2, ARIXTRA was initiated 6 ± 2 hours (mean 6.25 hours) after surgery in 86% of patients and enoxaparin sodium was initiated 12 hours before surgery in 78% of patients. The first post-operative enoxaparin sodium dose was given within 12 hours after surgery in 60% of patients and 12 to 24 hours after surgery in 35% of patients with a mean of 13 hours. For both studies, both study treatments were continued for 7 ± 2 days. The efficacy data are provided in Table 9. Under the conditions of Study 1, ARIXTRA was associated with a VTE rate of 6.1% compared with a VTE rate of 8.3% for enoxaparin sodium for a relative risk reduction of 26% (95% CI: -11%, 53%; *P* = NS). Under the conditions of Study 2, fondaparinux sodium was associated with a VTE rate of 4.1% compared with a VTE rate of 9.2% for enoxaparin sodium for a relative risk reduction of 56% (95% CI: 33%, 73%; *P* <0.001). For the 2 studies combined, the major bleeding episodes occurred in 3.0% of patients receiving ARIXTRA and 2.1% of enoxaparin sodium patients *[see Adverse Reactions (6.1)]*.

[See table 9 above]

14.4 Prophylaxis of Thromboembolic Events Following Knee Replacement Surgery

In a randomized, double-blind, clinical trial in patients undergoing knee replacement surgery (i.e., surgery requiring resection of the distal end of the femur or proximal end of the tibia), ARIXTRA 2.5 mg SC once daily was compared to enoxaparin sodium 30 mg SC every 12 hours. A total of 1,049 patients were randomized and 1,034 were treated. Patients ranged in age from 19 to 94 years (mean age 68 years) with 41% men and 59% women. Patients were 88% Caucasian, 8% black, <1% Asian, and 3% others. Patients with serum creatinine level more than 2 mg/dL (180 micromol/L), or platelet count less than 100,000/mm^3 were excluded from the trial. ARIXTRA was initiated 6 ± 2 hours (mean 6.25 hours) after surgery in 94% of patients, and enoxaparin sodium was initiated 12 to 24 hours (mean 21 hours) after surgery in 96% of patients. For both drugs, treatment was continued for 7 ± 2 days. The efficacy data are provided in Table 10 and demonstrate that under the conditions of the trial, ARIXTRA was associated with a VTE rate of 12.5% compared with a VTE rate of 27.8% for enoxaparin sodium for a relative risk reduction of 55% (95% CI: 36%, 70%; *P* <0.001). Major bleeding episodes occurred in 2.1% of patients receiving ARIXTRA and 0.2% of enoxaparin sodium patients *[see Adverse Reactions (6.1)]*.

[See table 10 at top of next page]

14.5 Prophylaxis of Thromboembolic Events Following Abdominal Surgery in Patients at Risk for Thromboembolic Complications

Abdominal surgery patients at risk included the following: Those undergoing surgery under general anesthesia lasting longer than 45 minutes who are older than 60 years with or without additional risk factors; and those undergoing surgery under general anesthesia lasting longer than 45 minutes who are older than 40 years with additional risk factors. Risk factors included neoplastic disease, obesity, chronic obstructive pulmonary disease, inflammatory bowel disease, history of deep vein thrombosis (DVT) or pulmonary embolism (PE), or congestive heart failure.

In a randomized, double-blind, clinical trial in patients undergoing abdominal surgery, ARIXTRA 2.5 mg SC once daily started postoperatively was compared to dalteparin sodium 5,000 IU SC once daily, with one 2,500 IU SC preoperative injection and a 2,500 IU SC first postoperative injection. A total of 2,927 patients were randomized and 2,858 were treated. Patients ranged in age from 17 to 93 years (mean age 65 years) with 55% men and 45% women. Patients were 97% Caucasian, 1% black, 1% Asian, and 1% others. Patients with serum creatinine level more than 2 mg/dL (180 micromol/L), or platelet count less than 100,000/mm^3 were excluded from the trial. Sixty nine percent (69%) of study patients underwent cancer-related abdominal surgery. Study treatment was continued for 7 ± 2 days. The efficacy data are provided in Table 11 and demonstrate that prophylaxis with ARIXTRA was associated with a VTE rate of 4.6% compared with a VTE rate of 6.1% for dalteparin sodium (*P* = NS).

[See table 11 at top of next page]

14.6 Treatment of Deep Vein Thrombosis

In a randomized, double-blind, clinical trial in patients with a confirmed diagnosis of acute symptomatic DVT without PE, ARIXTRA 5 mg (body weight <50 kg), 7.5 mg (body weight 50 to 100 kg), or 10 mg (body weight >100 kg) SC once daily (ARIXTRA treatment regimen) was compared to enoxaparin sodium 1 mg/kg SC every 12 hours. Almost all patients started study treatment in hospital. Approximately 30% of patients in both groups were discharged home from the hospital while receiving study treatment. A total of 2,205 patients were randomized and 2,192 were treated. Patients ranged in age from 18 to 95 years (mean age 61 years) with 53% men and 47% women. Patients were 97% Caucasian, 2% black, and 1% other races. Patients with serum creatinine level more than 2 mg/dL (180 micromol/L), or platelet count less than 100,000/mm^3 were excluded from the trial. For both groups, treatment continued for at least 5 days with a treatment duration range of 7 ± 2 days, and both treatment groups received vitamin K antagonist therapy initiated within 72 hours after the first study drug administration and continued for 90 ± 7 days, with regular dose adjustments to achieve an INR of 2 to 3. The primary efficacy endpoint was confirmed, symptomatic, recurrent VTE reported up to Day 97. The efficacy data are provided in Table 12.

[See table 12 at top of next page]

During the initial treatment period, 18 (1.6%) of patients treated with fondaparinux sodium and 10 (0.9%) of patients treated with enoxaparin sodium had a VTE endpoint (95% CI for the treatment difference [fondaparinux sodium-enoxaparin sodium] for VTE rates: -0.2%; 1.7%).

14.7 Treatment of Pulmonary Embolism

In a randomized, open-label, clinical trial in patients with a confirmed diagnosis of acute symptomatic PE, with or without DVT, ARIXTRA 5 mg (body weight <50 kg), 7.5 mg (body weight 50 to 100 kg), or 10 mg (body weight >100 kg) SC once daily (ARIXTRA treatment regimen) was compared to heparin IV bolus (5,000 USP units) followed by a continuous IV infusion adjusted to maintain 1.5 to 2.5 times aPTT control value. Patients with a PE requiring thrombolysis or

Table 8. Efficacy of ARIXTRA Injection in the Extended Prophylaxis of Thromboembolic Events Following Hip Fracture Surgery

	Extended Prophylaxis (Day 8 to Day 28 ± 2 post-surgery)			
Endpoint	**ARIXTRA 2.5 mg SC once daily**		**Placebo SC once daily**	
	n/N[a]	**% (95% CI)**	**n/N[a]**	**% (95% CI)**
VTE	3/208	1.4%[b] (0.3, 4.2)	77/220	35.0% (28.7, 41.7)
All DVT	3/208	1.4%[b] (0.3, 4.2)	74/218	33.9% (27.7, 40.6)
Proximal DVT	2/221	0.9%[b] (0.1, 3.2)	35/222	15.8% (11.2, 21.2)
Symptomatic VTE (all)	1/326	0.3%[c] (0.0, 1.7)	9/330	2.7% (1.3, 5.1)
Symptomatic PE	0/326	0.0%[d] (0.0, 1.1)	3/330	0.9% (0.2, 2.6)

[a] N = all randomized evaluable hip fracture surgery patients. Evaluable patients were those who were treated in the post-randomization period, with an adequate efficacy assessment for up to 24 days following randomization.
[b] *P* value versus placebo <0.001
[c] *P* value versus placebo = 0.021.
[d] *P* value versus placebo = NS.

Table 9. Efficacy of ARIXTRA in the Prophylaxis of Thromboembolic Events Following Hip Replacement Surgery

	Study 1 n/N[a] % (95% CI)		Study 2 n/N[a] % (95% CI)	
Endpoint	**ARIXTRA 2.5 mg SC once daily**	**Enoxaparin Sodium 30 mg SC every 12 hr**	**ARIXTRA 2.5 mg SC once daily**	**Enoxaparin Sodium 40 mg SC once daily**
VTE[b]	48/787 6.1%[c] (4.5, 8.0)	66/797 8.3% (6.5, 10.4)	37/908 4.1%[e] (2.9, 5.6)	85/919 9.2% (7.5, 11.3)
All DVT	44/784 5.6%[d] (4.1, 7.5)	65/796 8.2% (6.4, 10.3)	36/908 4.0%[e] (2.8, 5.4)	83/918 9.0% (7.3, 11.1)
Proximal DVT	14/816 1.7%[c] (0.9, 2.9)	10/830 1.2% (0.6, 2.2)	6/922 0.7%[f] (0.2, 1.4)	23/927 2.5% (1.6, 3.7)
Symptomatic PE	5/1,126 0.4%[c] (0.1, 1.0)	1/1,128 0.1% (0.0, 0.5)	2/1,129 0.2%[c] (0.0, 0.6)	2/1,123 0.2% (0.0, 0.6)

[a] N = all evaluable hip replacement surgery patients. Evaluable patients were those who were treated and underwent the appropriate surgery (i.e., hip replacement surgery), with an adequate efficacy assessment up to Day 11.
[b] VTE was a composite of documented DVT and/or documented symptomatic PE reported up to Day 11.
[c] *P* value versus enoxaparin sodium: NS.
[d] *P* value versus enoxaparin sodium in study 1: <0.05.
[e] *P* value versus enoxaparin sodium in study 2: <0.001.
[f] *P* value versus enoxaparin sodium in study 2: <0.01.

Table 10. Efficacy of ARIXTRA in the Prophylaxis of Thromboembolic Events Following Knee Replacement Surgery

Endpoint	ARIXTRA 2.5 mg SC once daily		Enoxaparin Sodium 30 mg SC every 12 hours	
	n/N[a]	% (95% CI)	n/N[a]	% (95% CI)
VTE[b]	45/361	12.5%[c] (9.2, 16.3)	101/363	27.8% (23.3, 32.7)
All DVT	45/361	12.5%[c] (9.2, 16.3)	98/361	27.1% (22.6, 32.0)
Proximal DVT	9/368	2.4%[d] (1.1, 4.6)	20/372	5.4% (3.3, 8.2)
Symptomatic PE	1/517	0.2%[d] (0.0, 1.1)	4/517	0.8% (0.2, 2.0)

[a] N = all evaluable knee replacement surgery patients. Evaluable patients were those who were treated and underwent the appropriate surgery (i.e., knee replacement surgery), with an adequate efficacy assessment up to Day 11.
[b] VTE was a composite of documented DVT and/or documented symptomatic PE reported up to Day 11.
[c] *P* value versus enoxaparin sodium <0.001.
[d] *P* value versus enoxaparin sodium: NS.

Table 11. Efficacy of ARIXTRA In Prophylaxis of Thromboembolic Events Following Abdominal Surgery

Endpoint	ARIXTRA 2.5 mg SC once daily		Dalteparin Sodium 5,000 IU SC once daily	
	n/N[a]	% (95% CI)	n/N[a]	% (95% CI)
VTE[b]	47/1,027	4.6%[c] (3.4, 6.0)	62/1,021	6.1% (4.7, 7.7)
All DVT	43/1,024	4.2% (3.1, 5.6)	59/1,018	5.8% (4.4, 7.4)
Proximal DVT	5/1,076	0.5% (0.2, 1.1)	5/1,077	0.5% (0.2, 1.1)
Symptomatic VTE	6/1,465	0.4% (0.2, 0.9)	5/1,462	0.3% (0.1, 0.8)

[a] N = all evaluable abdominal surgery patients. Evaluable patients were those who were randomized and had an adequate efficacy assessment up to Day 10; non-treated patients and patients who did not undergo surgery did not get a VTE assessment.
[b] VTE was a composite of venogram positive DVT, symptomatic DVT, non-fatal PE and/or fatal PE reported up to Day 10.
[c] *P* value versus dalteparin sodium: NS.

Table 12. Efficacy of ARIXTRA in the Treatment of Deep Vein Thrombosis (All Randomized)

Endpoint	ARIXTRA 5, 7.5, or 10 mg SC once daily N = 1,098		Enoxaparin Sodium 1 mg/kg SC every 12 hours N = 1,107	
	n	% (95% CI)	n	% (95% CI)
Total VTE[a]	43	3.9% (2.8, 5.2)	45	4.1% (3.0, 5.4)
DVT only	18	1.6% (1.0, 2.6)	28	2.5% (1.7, 3.6)
Non-fatal PE	20	1.8% (1.1, 2.8)	12	1.1% (0.6, 1.9)
Fatal PE	5	0.5% (0.1, 1.1)	5	0.5% (0.1, 1.1)

[a] VTE was a composite of symptomatic recurrent non-fatal VTE or fatal PE reported up to Day 97. The 95% confidence interval for the treatment difference for total VTE was: (-1.8% to 1.5%).

Table 13. Efficacy of ARIXTRA in the Treatment of Pulmonary Embolism (All Randomized)

Endpoint	ARIXTRA 5, 7.5, or 10 mg SC once daily N = 1,103		Heparin aPTT adjusted IV N = 1,110	
	n	% (95% CI)	n	% (95% CI)
Total VTE[a]	42	3.8% (2.8, 5.1)	56	5.0% (3.8, 6.5)
DVT only	12	1.1% (0.6, 1.9)	17	1.5% (0.9, 2.4)
Non-fatal PE	14	1.3% (0.7, 2.1)	24	2.2% (1.4, 3.2)
Fatal PE	16	1.5% (0.8, 2.3)	15	1.4% (0.8, 2.2)

[a] VTE was a composite of symptomatic recurrent non-fatal VTE or fatal PE reported up to Day 97. The 95% confidence interval for the treatment difference for total VTE was: (-3.0% to 0.5%).

surgical thrombectomy were excluded from the trial. All patients started study treatment in hospital. Approximately 15% of patients were discharged home from the hospital while receiving ARIXTRA therapy. A total of 2,213 patients were randomized and 2,184 were treated. Patients ranged in age from 18 to 97 years (mean age 62 years) with 44% men and 56% women. Patients were 94% Caucasian, 5% black, and 1% other races. Patients with serum creatinine level more than 2 mg/dL (180 micromol/L), or platelet count less than 100,000/mm^3 were excluded from the trial. For both groups, treatment continued for at least 5 days with a treatment duration range 7 ± 2 days, and both treatment groups received vitamin K antagonist therapy initiated within 72 hours after the first study drug administration and continued for 90 ± 7 days, with regular dose adjustments to achieve an INR of 2 to 3. The primary efficacy endpoint was confirmed, symptomatic, recurrent VTE reported up to Day 97. The efficacy data are provided in Table 13. [See table 13 above]

During the initial treatment period, 12 (1.1%) of patients treated with fondaparinux sodium and 19 (1.7%) of patients treated with heparin had a VTE endpoint (95% CI for the treatment difference [fondaparinux sodium-heparin] for VTE rates: -1.6%; 0.4%).

16 HOW SUPPLIED/STORAGE AND HANDLING

ARIXTRA Injection is available in the following strengths and package sizes:

2.5 mg ARIXTRA in 0.5 mL single-dose prefilled syringe, affixed with a 27-gauge × ½-inch needle and an automatic needle protection system with white plunger rod.

NDC 0007-3230-02	2 Single Unit Syringes
NDC 0007-3230-11	10 Single Unit Syringes

5 mg ARIXTRA in 0.4 mL single-dose prefilled syringe, affixed with a 27-gauge × ½-inch needle and an automatic needle protection system with white plunger rod.

NDC 0007-3232-02	2 Single Unit Syringes
NDC 0007-3232-11	10 Single Unit Syringes

7.5 mg ARIXTRA in 0.6 mL single-dose prefilled syringe, affixed with a 27-gauge × ½-inch needle and an automatic needle protection system with white plunger rod.

NDC 0007-3234-02	2 Single Unit Syringes
NDC 0007-3234-11	10 Single Unit Syringes

10 mg ARIXTRA in 0.8 mL single-dose prefilled syringe, affixed with a 27-gauge × ½-inch needle and an automatic needle protection system with white plunger rod.

NDC 0007-3236-02	2 Single Unit Syringes
NDC 0007-3236-11	10 Single Unit Syringes

Store at 25°C (77°F); excursions permitted to 15–30°C (59–86°F).

17 PATIENT COUNSELING INFORMATION

See FDA-Approved Patient Labeling (17.2)

17.1 Patient Advice

If the patients have had neuraxial anesthesia or spinal puncture, and particularly, if they are taking concomitant NSAIDS, platelet inhibitors, or other anticoagulants, they should be informed to watch for signs and symptoms of spinal or epidural hematomas, such as tingling, numbness (especially in the lower limbs) and muscular weakness. If any of these symptoms occur, the patients should contact his or her physician immediately.

The use of aspirin and other NSAIDS may enhance the risk of hemorrhage. Their use should be discontinued prior to ARIXTRA therapy whenever possible; if co-administration is essential, the patient's clinical and laboratory status should be closely monitored. *[See Drug Interactions (7).]*

If patients must self-administer ARIXTRA (e.g., if ARIXTRA is used at home), they should be advised of the following:

- ARIXTRA should be given by subcutaneous injection. Patients must be instructed in the proper technique for administration.
- As with all anticoagulants, the most important risk with ARIXTRA administration is bleeding. Patients should be counseled on signs and symptoms of possible bleeding.
- It may take them longer than usual to stop bleeding.
- They may bruise and/or bleed more easily when they are treated with ARIXTRA.
- They should report any unusual bleeding, bruising, or signs of thrombocytopenia (such as a rash of dark red spots under the skin) to their physician *[see Warnings and Precautions (5.1, 5.4)]*.
- To tell their physicians and dentists they are taking ARIXTRA and/or any other product known to affect bleeding before any surgery is scheduled and before any new drug is taken *[see Warnings and Precautions (5.1)]*.
- To tell their physicians and dentists of all medications they are taking, including those obtained without a prescription, such as aspirin or other NSAIDs. *[See Drug Interactions (7)]*.

Keep out of the reach of children.

17.2 FDA-Approved Patient Labeling

Patient labeling is provided as a tear-off leaflet at the end of this full prescribing information.

ARIXTRA is a registered trademark of GlaxoSmithKline.

GlaxoSmithKline
Research Triangle Park, NC 27709

February 2011
ARX:9PI

PHARMACIST-DETACH HERE AND GIVE INSTRUCTIONS TO PATIENT

PATIENT INFORMATION

ARIXTRA® (Ah-RIX-trah)

fondaparinux sodium injection

Read the Patient Information that comes with ARIXTRA before you start taking it and each time you get a refill. There may be new information. This information does not take the place of talking with your doctor about your medical condition or your treatment. If you have any questions about ARIXTRA, ask your doctor or pharmacist.

What is the most important information I should know about ARIXTRA?

Certain medical procedures involving the spine, such as an epidural (pain medication given through the spine), spinal anesthesia, or spinal puncture, may be used during your hospital stay. If you need any of these procedures while receiving ARIXTRA, heparins, heparinoids, or low-molecular weight heparins (anticoagulants), you may be at risk for having a blood clot (hematoma) in or around your spine. This type of clot is very serious, as it can cause long-term and possibly permanent paralysis (loss of the ability to move).

If you receive ARIXTRA after an epidural or spinal anesthetic is used, as the anesthesia for your surgery, your doctor will watch you closely for problems with feeling (sensation) and being able to move. Tell your doctor right away if you have any of these signs and symptoms, especially in your legs and feet:

- tingling
- numbness
- muscle weakness

Because the risk of bleeding may be higher, tell your doctor before taking ARIXTRA if you:

- are also taking certain other medicines that affect blood clotting such as aspirin, an NSAID (for example, ibuprofen or naproxen), clopidogrel, or warfarin sodium.
- have bleeding problems.
- had problems in the past with pain medication given through the spine.
- have had surgery to your spine.
- have a spinal deformity.

What is ARIXTRA?

ARIXTRA is a prescription medicine that "thins your blood" (also known as an anticoagulant). ARIXTRA is used to:

- help prevent blood clots from forming in patients who have had certain surgeries of the hip, knee, or the stomach area (abdominal surgery)
- treat people who have blood clots in their legs or blood clots that travel to their lungs

It is not known if ARIXTRA is safe and effective for use in children younger than 18 years of age.

Who should not take ARIXTRA?

Do not take ARIXTRA if you have:

- certain kidney problems
- active bleeding problems
- an infection in your heart
- low platelet counts and if you test positive for a certain antibody while you are taking ARIXTRA.

People who weigh less than 110 pounds (50 kg) should not use ARIXTRA to prevent blood clots from forming after surgery.

What should I tell my doctor before taking ARIXTRA?

Tell your doctor about all of your medical conditions, including if you:

- have had any bleeding problems (such as stomach ulcers)
- have had a stroke
- have had recent surgeries, including eye surgery
- have diabetic eye disease
- have kidney problems
- have uncontrolled high blood pressure
- have a latex allergy. The packaging (needle guard) for ARIXTRA contains dry natural rubber.
- are pregnant. It is not known if ARIXTRA will harm your unborn baby. If you are pregnant, talk to your doctor about the best way for you to prevent or treat blood clots.
- are breast-feeding. It is not known if ARIXTRA passes into breast milk.

Tell your doctor about all the medicines you take including prescriptions and non-prescription medicines, vitamins, and herbal supplements. Some medicines can increase your risk of bleeding. Especially tell your doctor if you take:

- aspirin
- NSAIDS (such as ibuprofen or naproxen)
- other blood thinner medicines, such as clopidogrel or warfarin

See "What is the most important information I should know about ARIXTRA?" Do not start taking any new medicines without first talking to your doctor.

Know the medicines you take. Tell all your doctors and dentist that you take ARIXTRA, especially if you need to have any kind of surgery or a dental procedure. Keep a list of your medicines and show it to all your doctors and pharmacist before you start a new medicine.

How should I take ARIXTRA?

- Take ARIXTRA exactly as prescribed by your doctor.
- ARIXTRA is given by injection under the skin (subcutaneous injection). See "How should I give an injection of ARIXTRA?"
- If your doctor tells you that you may give yourself injections of ARIXTRA at home, you will be shown how to give the injections first before you do them on your own.
- Tell your doctor if you have any bleeding or bruising while taking ARIXTRA.
- If you miss a dose of ARIXTRA, take your dose as soon as you remember. Do not take 2 doses at the same time.
- If you take too much ARIXTRA, call your doctor right away.
- Do not use ARIXTRA if:
  - the solution appears discolored (the solution should normally appear clear),
  - you see any particles in the solution, or
  - the syringe is damaged.

What are possible side effects of ARIXTRA?

ARIXTRA can cause serious side effects. See "What is the most important information I should know about ARIXTRA?"

- Severe **bleeding**
  Certain conditions can increase your risk for severe bleeding, including:
  -some bleeding problems
  -some gastrointestinal problems including ulcers
  -some types of strokes
  -uncontrolled high blood pressure
  -diabetic eye disease
  -soon after brain, spine, or eye surgery
  - **Certain kidney problems can also increase your risk of bleeding with ARIXTRA**. Your doctor may check your kidney function while you are taking ARIXTRA.
  - **People undergoing surgery who weigh less than 110 pounds.** See "Who should not take ARIXTRA?"
  - **Low blood platelets**. Low blood platelets can happen when you take ARIXTRA. Platelets are blood cells that help your blood to clot normally. Your doctor may check your platelet counts while you take ARIXTRA.
  You may bruise or bleed more easily while taking ARIXTRA, and it may take longer than usual for bleeding to stop.
  Tell your doctor if you have any of these signs or symptoms of bleeding while taking ARIXTRA.
  -any bleeding
  -bruising
  -rash of dark red spots under the skin
- **Allergic reactions.** See "What should I tell my doctor before taking ARIXTRA?"

Other side effects include:

- **Injection site reactions**. Bleeding, rash, and itching can happen at the place where you inject ARIXTRA.
- **Low red blood cell counts (anemia)**.Your doctor may check your red blood cell counts while you are taking ARIXTRA.
- **Increased liver enzyme test results.** Your doctor may check your liver function while you are taking ARIXTRA.
- **Sleep problems (insomnia)**.

These are not all the possible side effects of ARIXTRA. Call your doctor if you have any side effects that bother you or don't go away.

Call your doctor for medical advice about side effects. You may report side effects to the FDA at 1-800-FDA-1088.

How should I store ARIXTRA?

Store ARIXTRA at room temperature 59°F to 86°F (15°C to 30°C). Do not freeze.

Safely, throw away ARIXTRA that is out of date or no longer needed.

Keep ARIXTRA and all medicines out of the reach of children.

General information about ARIXTRA

Medicines are sometimes prescribed for purposes other than those described in patient information leaflets. Do not use ARIXTRA for a condition for which it was not prescribed. Do not give ARIXTRA to other people. It may harm them.

This leaflet summarizes the most important information about ARIXTRA. If you would like more information, talk with your doctor. You can ask your doctor or pharmacist for information about ARIXTRA that is written for healthcare professionals. For more information about ARIXTRA, go to www.ARIXTRA.com or call 1-888-825-5249.

What are the ingredients in ARIXTRA?

Active Ingredient: fondaparinux sodium

Inactive Ingredients: sodium chloride and water for injection

How should I give an injection of ARIXTRA?

ARIXTRA is injected into a skin fold of the lower stomach area (abdomen). Do not inject ARIXTRA into muscle. Usually a doctor or nurse will give this injection to you. In some cases you may be taught how to do this yourself. Be sure that you read, understand, and follow the step-by-step instructions in this leaflet, on how to give yourself an injection of ARIXTRA.

Instructions for self-administration

The different parts of ARIXTRA safety syringe are:

1. Rigid needle guard
2. Plunger
3. Finger-grip
4. Security sleeve

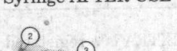

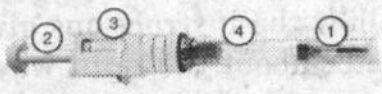

Syringe BEFORE USE

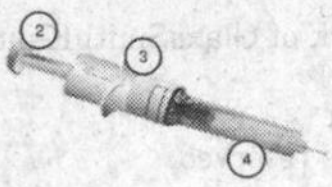

Syringe AFTER USE

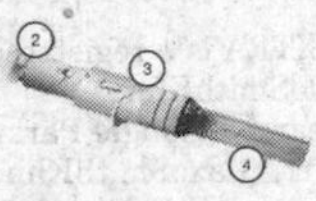

1. Wash your hands thoroughly with soap and water. Towel dry.

2. Sit or lie down in a comfortable position. Choose a spot on the lower stomach area (abdomen), at least 2 inches below your belly button (Figure A). Change (alternate) between using the left and right side of the lower abdomen for each injection. If you have any questions talk to your nurse or doctor.

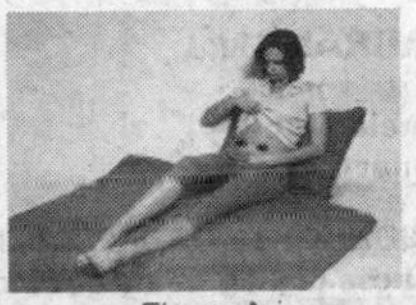

Figure A.

3. Clean the injection area with an alcohol swab.

4. Remove the needle guard, by first twisting it and then pulling it in a straight line away from the body of the syringe (Figure B). Discard the needle guard. **To prevent infection, do not touch the needle or let it come in contact with any surface before the injection.** A small air bubble in the syringe is normal. To be sure that you do not lose any medicine from the syringe, do not try to remove air bubbles from the syringe before giving the injection.

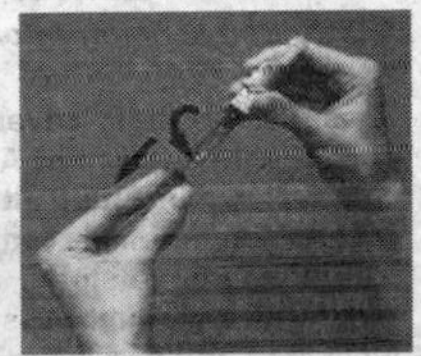

Figure B.

5. Gently pinch the skin that has been cleaned to make a fold. Hold the fold between the thumb and the forefinger of one hand during the entire injection (Figure C).

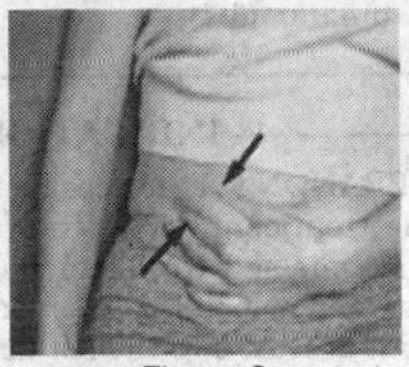

Figure C.

6. Hold the syringe firmly in your other hand using the finger grip. Insert the full length of the needle directly up and down (at an angle of 90°) into the skin fold (Figure D).

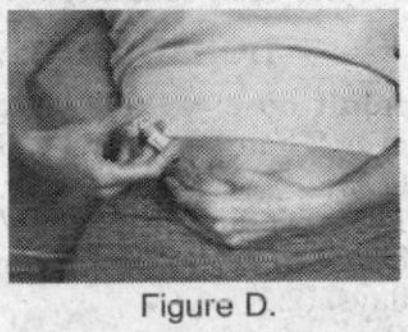

Figure D.

7. Inject all of the medicine in the syringe by pressing down on the plunger as far as it goes. This will activate the automatic needle protection system (Figure E).

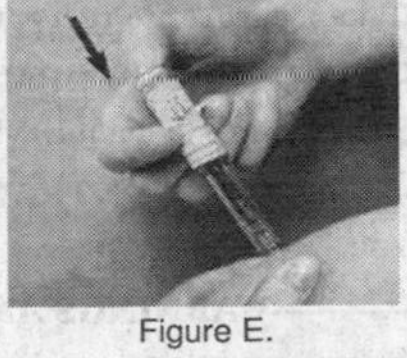

Figure E.

8. Release the plunger. The needle will withdraw automatically from the skin, and pull back (retract) into the security sleeve where it will be locked (Figure F).

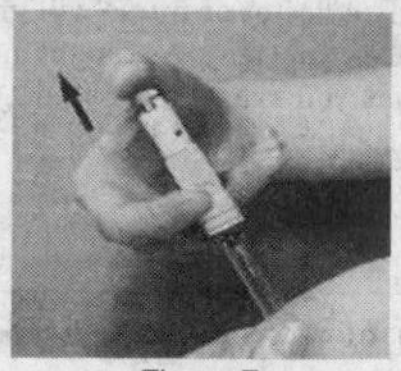

Figure F.

Follow the instructions given to you by your nurse or doctor about the right way to throw away used syringes and needles. There may be state laws about the right way to dispose of used syringes, needles, and disposal containers.

ARIXTRA is a registered trademark of GlaxoSmithKline.
GlaxoSmithKline
Research Triangle Park, NC 27709

Revised: February 2011
ARX:5PIL

ARRANON ℞

[air'ə-non]
(nelarabine)
Injection

HIGHLIGHTS OF PRESCRIBING INFORMATION
These highlights do not include all the information needed to use ARRANON safely and effectively. See full prescribing information for ARRANON.
ARRANON (nelarabine) Injection
Initial U.S. Approval: 2005

> **WARNING: NEUROLOGIC ADVERSE REACTIONS**
> ***See full prescribing information for complete boxed warning.***
> **Severe neurologic adverse reactions have been reported with the use of ARRANON. These adverse reactions have included altered mental states including severe somnolence, central nervous system effects including convulsions, and peripheral neuropathy ranging from numbness and paresthesias to motor weakness and paralysis. There have also been reports of adverse reactions associated with demyelination, and ascending peripheral neuropathies similar in appearance to Guillain-Barré syndrome. (5.1)**
> **Full recovery from these adverse reactions has not always occurred with cessation of therapy with ARRANON. Close monitoring for neurologic adverse reactions is strongly recommended, and ARRANON should be discontinued for neurologic adverse reactions of NCI Common Toxicity Criteria grade 2 or greater. (5.1)**

INDICATIONS AND USAGE

ARRANON is a nucleoside metabolic inhibitor indicated for the treatment of patients with T-cell acute lymphoblastic leukemia and T-cell lymphoblastic lymphoma whose disease has not responded to or has relapsed following treatment with at least two chemotherapy regimens. This use is based on the induction of complete responses. Randomized trials demonstrating increased survival or other clinical benefit have not been conducted. (1)

DOSAGE AND ADMINISTRATION

- Adult dose: 1,500 mg/m^2 administered intravenously over 2 hours on days 1, 3, and 5 repeated every 21 days. (2.1)
- Pediatric dose: 650 mg/m^2 administered intravenously over 1 hour daily for 5 consecutive days repeated every 21 days. (2.1)
- Discontinue treatment for ≥grade 2 neurologic reactions. (2.2)
- Dosage may be delayed for hematologic reactions (2.2)
- Take measures to prevent hyperuricemia. (2.4)

DOSAGE FORMS AND STRENGTHS

250 mg/50 mL (5 mg/mL) vial (3)

CONTRAINDICATIONS

None.

WARNINGS AND PRECAUTIONS

- Severe neurologic reactions have been reported. Monitor for signs and symptoms of neurologic toxicity. (5.1)
- Hematologic Reactions: Complete blood counts including platelets should be monitored regularly. (5.2)
- Fetal harm can occur if administered to a pregnant woman. Women should be advised not to become pregnant when taking ARRANON. (5.3)

ADVERSE REACTIONS

The most common (≥ 20%) adverse reactions were:
- Adult: anemia, thrombocytopenia, neutropenia, nausea, diarrhea, vomiting, constipation, fatigue, pyrexia, cough, and dyspnea (6.1)
- Pediatric: anemia, neutropenia, thrombocytopenia, and leukopenia (6.1)

The most common (>10%) neurological adverse reactions were:
- Adult: somnolence, dizziness, peripheral neurologic disorders, hypoesthesia, headache, and paresthesia (6.1)
- Pediatric: headache and peripheral neurologic disorders (6.1)

To report SUSPECTED ADVERSE REACTIONS, contact GlaxoSmithKline at 1-888-825-5249 or FDA at 1-800-FDA-1088 or www.fda.gov/medwatch.

DRUG INTERACTIONS

Administration in combination with adenosine deaminase inhibitors, such as pentostatin, is not recommended. (7, 12.3)

USE IN SPECIFIC POPULATIONS

- Renal Impairment: Closely monitor patients with moderate or severe renal impairment for toxicities. (8.6)
- Hepatic Impairment: Closely monitor patients with severe hepatic impairment for toxicities. (8.7)

See 17 for PATIENT COUNSELING INFORMATION and FDA-approved patient labeling

Revised: 12/2011

FULL PRESCRIBING INFORMATION: CONTENTS*

*** Sections or subsections omitted from the full prescribing information are not listed**

FULL PRESCRIBING INFORMATION

> **WARNING: NEUROLOGIC ADVERSE REACTIONS**
> Severe neurologic adverse reactions have been reported with the use of ARRANON. These adverse reactions have included altered mental states including severe somnolence, central nervous system effects including convulsions, and peripheral neuropathy ranging from numbness and paresthesias to motor weakness and paralysis. There have also been reports of adverse reactions associated with demyelination, and ascending peripheral neuropathies similar in appearance to Guillain-Barré syndrome *[see Warnings and Precautions (5.1)]*.
> Full recovery from these adverse reactions has not always occurred with cessation of therapy with ARRANON. Close monitoring for neurologic adverse reactions is strongly recommended, and ARRANON should be discontinued for neurologic adverse reactions of NCI Common Toxicity Criteria grade 2 or greater *[see Warnings and Precautions (5.1)]*.

1 INDICATIONS AND USAGE

ARRANON® is indicated for the treatment of patients with T-cell acute lymphoblastic leukemia and T-cell lymphoblastic lymphoma whose disease has not responded to or has relapsed following treatment with at least two chemotherapy regimens. This use is based on the induction of complete responses. Randomized trials demonstrating increased survival or other clinical benefit have not been conducted.

2 DOSAGE AND ADMINISTRATION

2.1 Recommended Dosage

This product is for intravenous use only.

The recommended duration of treatment for adult and pediatric patients has not been clearly established. In clinical trials, treatment was generally continued until there was evidence of disease progression, the patient experienced unacceptable toxicity, the patient became a candidate for bone marrow transplant, or the patient no longer continued to benefit from treatment.

Adult Dosage: The recommended adult dose of ARRANON is 1,500 mg/m^2 administered intravenously over 2 hours on days 1, 3, and 5 repeated every 21 days. ARRANON is administered undiluted.

Pediatric Dosage: The recommended pediatric dose of ARRANON is 650 mg/m^2 administered intravenously over 1 hour daily for 5 consecutive days repeated every 21 days. ARRANON is administered undiluted.

2.2 Dosage Modification

ARRANON administration should be discontinued for neurologic adverse reactions of NCI Common Toxicity Criteria grade 2 or greater. Dosage may be delayed for other toxicity including hematologic toxicity. *[See Boxed Warning and Warnings and Precautions (5.1, 5.2).]*

2.3 Adjustment of Dose in Special Populations

ARRANON has not been studied in patients with renal or hepatic dysfunction *[see Use in Specific Populations (8.6, 8.7)]*. No dose adjustment is recommended for patients with a creatinine clearance (CL_{cr}) ≥50 mL/min *[see Clinical Pharmacology (12.3)]*. There are insufficient data to support a dose recommendation for patients with a CL_{cr} <50 mL/min.

2.4 Prevention of Hyperuricemia

Appropriate measures (e.g., hydration, urine alkalinization, and prophylaxis with allopurinol) must be taken to prevent hyperuricemia *[see Warnings and Precautions (5.4)]*.

2.5 Instructions for Handling, Preparation, and Administration

Handling: ARRANON is a cytotoxic agent. Caution should be used during handling and preparation. Use of gloves and other protective clothing to prevent skin contact is recommended. Proper aseptic technique should be used. Guidelines for proper handling and disposal of anticancer drugs have been published.[1-4]

Preparation and Administration: Do not dilute ARRANON prior to administration. The appropriate dose of ARRANON is transferred into polyvinylchloride (PVC) infusion bags or glass containers and administered as a two-hour infusion in adult patients and as a one-hour infusion in pediatric patients.

Prior to administration, inspect the drug product visually for particulate matter and discoloration.

Stability: ARRANON Injection is stable in polyvinylchloride (PVC) infusion bags and glass containers for up to 8 hours at up to 30° C.

3 DOSAGE FORMS AND STRENGTHS

250 mg/50 mL (5 mg/mL) vial

4 CONTRAINDICATIONS

None.

5 WARNINGS AND PRECAUTIONS

5.1 Neurologic Adverse Reactions

Neurotoxicity is the dose-limiting toxicity of nelarabine. Patients undergoing therapy with ARRANON should be

Table 2. Neurologic Adverse Reactions (≥2%) Regardless of Causality in Adult Patients Treated with 1,500 mg/m² of ARRANON Administered Intravenously Over 2 Hours on Days 1, 3, and 5 Repeated Every 21 Days

Nervous System Disorders Preferred Term	Percentage of Patients (N =103) Grade 1 %	Grade 2 %	Grade 3 %	Grade 4 %	All Grades %
Somnolence	20	3	0	0	23
Dizziness	14	8	0	0	21
Peripheral neurologic disorders, any adverse reaction	8	12	2	0	21
Neuropathy	0	4	0	0	4
Peripheral neuropathy	2	2	1	0	5
Peripheral motor neuropathy	3	3	1	0	7
Peripheral sensory neuropathy	7	6	0	0	13
Hypoesthesia	5	10	2	0	17
Headache	11	3	1	0	15
Paresthesia	11	4	0	0	15
Ataxia	1	6	2	0	9
Depressed level of consciousness	4	1	0	1	6
Tremor	2	3	0	0	5
Amnesia	2	1	0	0	3
Dysgeusia	2	1	0	0	3
Balance disorder	1	1	0	0	2
Sensory loss	0	2	0	0	2

closely observed for signs and symptoms of neurologic toxicity *[see Boxed Warning and Dosage and Administration (2.2)]*. Common signs and symptoms of nelarabine-related neurotoxicity include somnolence, confusion, convulsions, ataxia, paresthesias, and hypoesthesia. Severe neurologic toxicity can manifest as coma, status epilepticus, craniospinal demyelination, or ascending neuropathy similar in presentation to Guillain-Barré syndrome.

Patients treated previously or concurrently with intrathecal chemotherapy or previously with craniospinal irradiation may be at increased risk for neurologic adverse events.

5.2 Hematologic Adverse Reactions

Leukopenia, thrombocytopenia, anemia, and neutropenia, including febrile neutropenia have been associated with nelarabine therapy. Complete blood counts including platelets should be monitored regularly *[see Dosage and Administration (2.2) and Adverse Reactions (6.1)]*.

5.3 Pregnancy

Pregnancy Category D

ARRANON can cause fetal harm when administered to a pregnant woman.

Nelarabine administered during the period of organogenesis caused increased incidences of fetal malformations, anomalies, and variations in rabbits *(see Use in Specific Populations (8.1))*.

There are no adequate and well-controlled studies of ARRANON in pregnant women. If this drug is used during pregnancy, or if the patient becomes pregnant while taking this drug, the patient should be apprised of the potential hazard to the fetus. Women of child-bearing potential should be advised to avoid becoming pregnant while receiving treatment with ARRANON.

5.4 Hyperuricemia

Patients receiving ARRANON should receive intravenous hydration according to standard medical practice for the management of hyperuricemia in patients at risk for tumor lysis syndrome. Consideration should be given to the use of allopurinol in patients at risk of hyperuricemia *[see Dosage and Administration (2.4)]*.

5.5 Vaccinations

Administration of live vaccines to immunocompromised patients should be avoided.

6 ADVERSE REACTIONS

The following serious adverse reactions are discussed in greater detail in other sections of the label:

- Neurologic *[see Boxed Warning and Warnings and Precautions (5.1)]*
- Hematologic *[see Warnings and Precautions (5.2)]*
- Hyperuricemia *[see Warnings and Precautions (5.4)]*

6.1 Clinical Trials Experience

Because clinical trials are conducted under widely varying conditions, adverse reaction rates observed in the clinical trials of a drug cannot be directly compared to rates in the clinical trials of another drug and may not reflect the rates observed in practice.

ARRANON was studied in 459 patients in Phase I and Phase II clinical trials.

Adults: The safety profile of ARRANON is based on data from 103 adult patients treated with the recommended dose and schedule in 2 studies: an adult T-cell acute lymphoblastic leukemia (T-ALL)/T-cell lymphoblastic lymphoma (T-LBL) study and an adult chronic lymphocytic leukemia study.

The most common adverse reactions in adults, regardless of causality, were fatigue; gastrointestinal (GI) disorders (nausea, diarrhea, vomiting, and constipation); hematologic disorders (anemia, neutropenia, and thrombocytopenia); respiratory disorders (cough and dyspnea); nervous system disorders (somnolence and dizziness); and pyrexia.

The most common adverse reactions in adults, by System Organ Class, regardless of causality, including severe or life threatening adverse reactions (NCI Common Toxicity Criteria grade 3 or grade 4) and fatal adverse reactions (grade 5) are shown in Table 1.

Table 1. Most Commonly Reported (≥5% Overall) Adverse Reactions Regardless of Causality in Adult Patients Treated with 1,500 mg/m² of ARRANON Administered Intravenously Over 2 Hours on Days 1, 3, and 5 Repeated Every 21 Days

System Organ Class Preferred Term	Percentage of Patients (N = 103) Toxicity Grade: Grade 3 %	Grade 4 and 5[a] %	All Grades %
Blood and Lymphatic System Disorders			
Anemia	20	14	99
Thrombocytopenia	37	22	86
Neutropenia	14	49	81
Febrile neutropenia	9	1	12
Cardiac Disorders			
Sinus tachycardia	1	0	8
Gastrointestinal Disorders			
Nausea	0	0	41
Diarrhea	1	0	22
Vomiting	1	0	22
Constipation	1	0	21
Abdominal pain	1	0	9
Stomatitis	1	0	8
Abdominal distension	0	0	6
General Disorders and Administration Site Conditions			
Fatigue	10	2	50
Pyrexia	5	0	23
Asthenia	0	1	17
Edema, peripheral	0	0	15
Edema	0	0	11
Pain	3	0	11
Rigors	0	0	8
Gait, abnormal	0	0	6
Chest pain	0	0	5
Non-cardiac chest pain	0	1	5
Infections			
Infection	2	1	9
Pneumonia	4	1	8
Sinusitis	1	0	7
Hepatobiliary Disorders			
AST increased	1	1	6
Metabolism and Nutrition Disorders			
Anorexia	0	0	9
Dehydration	3	1	7
Hyperglycemia	1	0	6
Musculoskeletal and Connective Tissue Disorders			
Myalgia	1	0	13
Arthralgia	1	0	9
Back pain	0	0	8
Muscular weakness	5	0	8
Pain in extremity	1	0	7
Nervous System Disorders (see Table 2)			
Psychiatric Disorders			
Confusional state	2	0	8
Insomnia	0	0	7
Depression	1	0	6
Respiratory, Thoracic, and Mediastinal Disorders			
Cough	0	0	25
Dyspnea	4	2	20
Pleural effusion	5	1	10
Epistaxis	0	0	8
Dyspnea, exertional	0	0	7

Table 4. Neurologic Adverse Reactions (≥2%) Regardless of Causality in Pediatric Patients Treated with 650 mg/m^2 of ARRANON Administered Intravenously Over 1 Hour Daily for 5 Consecutive Days Repeated Every 21 Days

Nervous System Disorders Preferred Term	Percentage of Patients (N = 84)				
	Grade 1 %	Grade 2 %	Grade 3 %	Grade 4 and 5[a] %	All Grades %
Headache	8	2	4	2	17
Peripheral neurologic disorders, any adverse reaction	1	4	7	0	12
Peripheral neuropathy	0	4	2	0	6
Peripheral motor neuropathy	1	0	2	0	4
Peripheral sensory neuropathy	0	0	6	0	6
Somnolence	1	4	1	1	7
Hypoesthesia	1	1	4	0	6
Seizures	0	0	0	6	6
Convulsions	0	0	0	3	4
Grand mal convulsions	0	0	0	1	1
Status epilepticus	0	0	0	1	1
Motor dysfunction	1	1	1	0	4
Nervous system disorder	1	2	0	0	4
Paresthesia	0	2	1	0	4
Tremor	1	2	0	0	4
Ataxia	1	0	1	0	2

[a] One (1) patient had a fatal neurologic adverse reaction, status epilepticus.

Wheezing	0	0	5
Vascular Disorders			
Petechiae	2	0	12
Hypotension	1	1	8

[a] Five patients had a fatal adverse reaction. Fatal adverse reactions included hypotension (n = 1), respiratory arrest (n = 1), pleural effusion/pneumothorax (n = 1), pneumonia (n = 1), and cerebral hemorrhage/coma/leukoencephalopathy (n = 1).

Other Adverse Events: Blurred vision was also reported in 4% of adult patients.

There was a single report of biopsy confirmed progressive multifocal leukoencephalopathy in the adult patient population.

Neurologic Adverse Reactions: Nervous system adverse reactions, regardless of drug relationship, were reported for 76% of adult patients across the Phase I and Phase II studies. The most common neurologic adverse reactions (≥2%) in adult patients, regardless of causality, including all grades (NCI Common Toxicity Criteria) are shown in Table 2.

[See table 2 at top of previous page]

One patient had a fatal neurologic adverse reaction, cerebral hemorrhage/coma/leukoencephalopathy.

Most nervous system adverse reactions in the adult patients were evaluated as grade 1 or 2. The additional grade 3 adverse reactions in adult patients, regardless of causality, were aphasia, convulsion, hemiparesis, and loss of consciousness, each reported in 1 patient (1%). The additional grade 4 adverse reactions, regardless of causality, were cerebral hemorrhage, coma, intracranial hemorrhage, leukoencephalopathy, and metabolic encephalopathy, each reported in one patient (1%).

The other neurologic adverse reactions, regardless of causality, reported as grade 1, 2, or unknown in adult patients were abnormal coordination, burning sensation, disturbance in attention, dysarthria, hyporeflexia, neuropathic pain, nystagmus, peroneal nerve palsy, sciatica, sensory disturbance, sinus headache, and speech disorder, each reported in one patient (1%).

Pediatrics: The safety profile for children is based on data from 84 pediatric patients treated with the recommended dose and schedule in a T-cell acute lymphoblastic leukemia (T-ALL)/T-cell lymphoblastic lymphoma (T-LBL) treatment study.

The most common adverse reactions in pediatric patients, regardless of causality, were hematologic disorders (anemia, leukopenia, neutropenia, and thrombocytopenia). Of the non-hematologic adverse reactions in pediatric patients, the most frequent adverse reactions reported were headache, increased transaminase levels, decreased blood potassium, decreased blood albumin, increased blood bilirubin, and vomiting.

The most common adverse reactions in pediatric patients, by System Organ Class, regardless of causality, including severe or life threatening adverse reactions (NCI Common Toxicity Criteria grade 3 or grade 4) and fatal adverse reactions (grade 5) are shown in Table 3.

Table 3. Most Commonly Reported (≥5% Overall) Adverse Reactions Regardless of Causality in Pediatric Patients Treated with 650 mg/m^2 of ARRANON Administered Intravenously Over 1 Hour Daily for 5 Consecutive Days Repeated Every 21 Days

System Organ Class Preferred Term	Percentage of Patients (N = 84) Toxicity Grade		
	Grade 3 %	Grade 4 and 5[a] %	All Grades %
Blood and Lymphatic System Disorders			
Anemia	45	10	95
Neutropenia	17	62	94
Thrombocytopenia	27	32	88
Leukopenia	14	7	38
Hepatobiliary Disorders			
Transaminases increased	4	0	12
Blood albumin decreased	5	1	10
Blood bilirubin increased	7	2	10
Metabolic/Laboratory			
Blood potassium decreased	4	2	11
Blood calcium decreased	1	1	8
Blood creatinine increased	0	0	6
Blood glucose decreased	4	0	6
Blood magnesium decreased	2	0	6
Nervous System Disorders (see Table 4)			
Gastrointestinal Disorders			
Vomiting	0	0	10
General Disorders & Administration Site Conditions			
Asthenia	1	0	6
Infections & Infestations			
Infection	2	1	5

[a] Three patients had a fatal adverse reaction. Fatal adverse reactions included neutropenia and pyrexia (n = 1), status epilepticus/seizure (n = 1), and fungal pneumonia (n = 1).

Neurologic Adverse Reactions: Nervous system adverse reactions, regardless of drug relationship, were reported for 42% of pediatric patients across the Phase I and Phase II studies. The most common neurologic adverse reactions (≥2%) in pediatric patients, regardless of causality, including all grades (NCI Common Toxicity Criteria) are shown in Table 4.

[See table 4 above]

The other grade 3 neurologic adverse reaction in pediatric patients, regardless of causality, was hypertonia reported in 1 patient (1%). The additional grade 4 neurologic adverse reactions, regardless of causality, were 3rd nerve paralysis, and 6th nerve paralysis, each reported in 1 patient (1%).

The other neurologic adverse reactions, regardless of causality, reported as grade 1, 2, or unknown in pediatric patients were dysarthria, encephalopathy, hydrocephalus, hyporeflexia, lethargy, mental impairment, paralysis, and sensory loss, each reported in 1 patient (1%).

6.2 Postmarketing Experience

The following adverse reactions have been identified during post-approval use of ARRANON. Because these reactions are reported voluntarily from a population of uncertain size, it is not always possible to reliably estimate their frequency or establish a causal relationship to drug exposure.

Infections and Infestations: Fatal opportunistic infections.

Metabolism and Nutrition Disorders: Tumor lysis syndrome.

Nervous System Disorders: Demyelination and ascending peripheral neuropathies similar in appearance to Guillain-Barré syndrome.

Musculoskeletal and Connective Disorders: Rhabdomyolysis, blood creatine phosphokinase increased.

7 DRUG INTERACTIONS

Administration of nelarabine in combination with adenosine deaminase inhibitors, such as pentostatin, is not recommended *[see Clinical Pharmacology (12.3)]*.

8 USE IN SPECIFIC POPULATIONS

8.1 Pregnancy

Pregnancy Category D *[see Warnings and Precautions (5.3)]*

ARRANON can cause fetal harm when administered to a pregnant woman. Nelarabine administered to rabbits during the period of organogenesis caused increased incidences of fetal malformations, anomalies, and variations at doses ≥360 mg/m^2/day (8-hour IV infusion; approximately ¼ the adult dose compared on a mg/m^2 basis), which was the lowest dose tested. Cleft palate was seen in rabbits given 3,600 mg/m^2/day (approximately 2-fold the adult dose), absent pollices (digits) in rabbits given ≥1,200 mg/m^2/day (approximately ¾ the adult dose), while absent gall bladder, absent accessory lung lobes, fused or extra sternebrae and delayed ossification was seen at all doses. Maternal body weight gain and fetal body weights were reduced in rabbits given 3,600 mg/m^2/day (approximately 2-fold the adult dose), but could not account for the increased incidence of malformations seen at this or lower administered doses.

There are no adequate and well-controlled studies of ARRANON in pregnant women. If this drug is used during pregnancy, or if the patient becomes pregnant while taking this drug, the patient should be apprised of the potential hazard to the fetus. Women of child-bearing potential should be advised to avoid becoming pregnant while receiving treatment with ARRANON.

8.3 Nursing Mothers

It is not known whether nelarabine or ara-G are excreted in human milk. Because many drugs are excreted in human milk and because of the potential for serious adverse reactions in nursing infants from ARRANON, a decision should be made whether to discontinue nursing or to discontinue the drug, taking into account the importance of the drug to the mother.

8.4 Pediatric Use

The safety and effectiveness of ARRANON has been established in pediatric patients *[see Dosage and Administration (2.1) and Clinical Studies (14.2]*.

8.5 Geriatric Use

Clinical studies of ARRANON did not include sufficient numbers of patients aged 65 and over to determine whether they respond differently from younger patients. In an exploratory analysis, increasing age, especially age 65 years and older, appeared to be associated with increased rates of neurologic adverse reactions. Because elderly patients are more likely to have decreased renal function, care should be taken in dose selection, and it may be useful to monitor renal function.

8.6 Renal Impairment

Ara-G clearance decreased as renal function decreased *[see Clinical Pharmacology (12.3)]*. Because the risk of adverse reactions to this drug may be greater in patients with moderate (CL_{cr} 30 to 50 mL/min) or severe (CL_{cr} <30 mL/min) renal impairment, these patients should be closely monitored for toxicities when treated with ARRANON *[see Dosage and Administration (2.3)]*.

8.7 Hepatic Impairment

The influence of hepatic impairment on the pharmacokinetics of nelarabine has not been evaluated. Because the risk of adverse reactions to this drug may be greater in patients with severe hepatic impairment (total bilirubin >3 times upper limit of normal), these patients should be closely monitored for toxicities when treated with ARRANON.

10 OVERDOSAGE

There is no known antidote for overdoses of ARRANON. It is anticipated that overdosage would result in severe neurotoxicity (possibly including paralysis, coma), myelosuppression, and potentially death. In the event of overdose, supportive care consistent with good clinical practice should be provided.

Nelarabine has been administered in clinical trials up to a dose of 2,900 mg/m² on days 1, 3, and 5 to 2 adult patients. At a dose of 2,200 mg/m² given on days 1, 3, and 5 every 21 days, 2 patients developed a significant grade 3 ascending sensory neuropathy. MRI evaluations of the 2 patients demonstrated findings consistent with a demyelinating process in the cervical spine.

11 DESCRIPTION

ARRANON (nelarabine) is a pro-drug of the cytotoxic deoxyguanosine analogue, 9-β-*D*-arabinofuranosylguanine (ara-G).

The chemical name for nelarabine is 2-amino-9-β-*D*-arabinofuranosyl-6-methoxy-9*H*-purine. It has the molecular formula $C_{11}H_{15}N_5O_5$ and a molecular weight of 297.27. Nelarabine has the following structural formula:

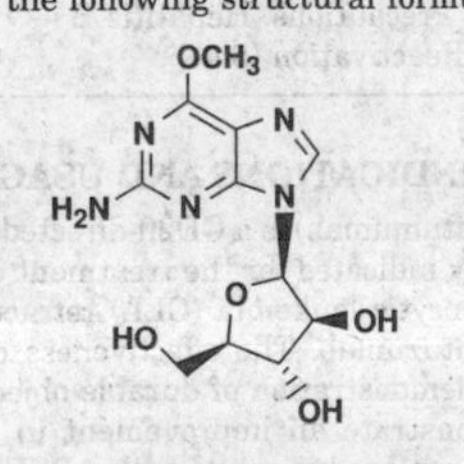

Nelarabine is slightly soluble to soluble in water and melts with decomposition between 209° and 217° C.

ARRANON Injection is supplied as a clear, colorless, sterile solution in glass vials. Each vial contains 250 mg of nelarabine (5 mg nelarabine per mL) and the inactive ingredient sodium chloride (4.5 mg per mL) in 50 mL Water for Injection, USP. ARRANON is intended for intravenous infusion.

Hydrochloric acid and sodium hydroxide may have been used to adjust the pH. The solution pH ranges from 5.0 to 7.0.

12 CLINICAL PHARMACOLOGY

12.1 Mechanism of Action

Nelarabine is a pro-drug of the deoxyguanosine analogue 9-β-*D*-arabinofuranosylguanine (ara-G), a nucleoside metabolic inhibitor. Nelarabine is demethylated by adenosine deaminase (ADA) to ara-G, mono-phosphorylated by deoxyguanosine kinase and deoxycytidine kinase, and subsequently converted to the active 5′-triphosphate, ara-GTP. Accumulation of ara-GTP in leukemic blasts allows for incorporation into deoxyribonucleic acid (DNA), leading to inhibition of DNA synthesis and cell death. Other mechanisms may contribute to the cytotoxic and systemic toxicity of nelarabine.

12.3 Pharmacokinetics

Absorption: Following intravenous administration of nelarabine to adult patients with refractory leukemia or lymphoma, plasma ara-G C_{max} values generally occurred at the end of the nelarabine infusion and were generally higher than nelarabine C_{max} values, suggesting rapid and extensive conversion of nelarabine to ara-G. Mean plasma nelarabine and ara-G C_{max} values were 5.0 ± 3.0 µg/mL and 31.4 ± 5.6 µg/mL, respectively, after a 1,500 mg/m² nelarabine dose infused over 2 hours in adult patients. The area under the concentration-time curve (AUC) of ara-G is 37 times higher than that for nelarabine on Day 1 after nelarabine IV infusion of 1,500 mg/m² dose (162 ± 49 µg.h/mL versus 4.4 ± 2.2 µg.h/mL, respectively). Comparable C_{max} and AUC values were obtained for nelarabine between Days 1 and 5 at the nelarabine adult dosage of 1,500 mg/m², indicating that nelarabine does not accumulate after multiple-dosing. There are not enough ara-G data to make a comparison between Day 1 and Day 5. After a nelarabine adult dose of 1,500 mg/m², intracellular C_{max} for ara-GTP appeared within 3 to 25 hours on Day 1. Exposure (AUC) to intracellular ara-GTP was 532 times higher than that for nelarabine and 14 times higher than that for ara-G (2,339 ± 2,628 µg.h/mL versus 4.4 ± 2.2 µg.h/mL and 162 ± 49 µg.h/mL, respectively). Because the intracellular levels of ara-GTP were so prolonged, its elimination half-life could not be accurately estimated.

Distribution: Nelarabine and ara-G are extensively distributed throughout the body. For nelarabine, V_{SS} values were 197 ± 216 L/m² in adult patients. For ara-G, V_{SS}/F values were 50 ± 24 L/m² in adult patients.

Nelarabine and ara-G are not substantially bound to human plasma proteins (<25%) in vitro, and binding is independent of nelarabine or ara-G concentrations up to 600 µM.

Metabolism: The principal route of metabolism for nelarabine is O-demethylation by adenosine deaminase to form ara-G, which undergoes hydrolysis to form guanine. In addition, some nelarabine is hydrolyzed to form methylguanine, which is O-demethylated to form guanine. Guanine is N-deaminated to form xanthine, which is further oxidized to yield uric acid.

Excretion: Nelarabine and ara-G are partially eliminated by the kidneys. Mean urinary excretion of nelarabine and ara-G was 6.6 ± 4.7% and 27 ± 15% of the administered dose, respectively, in 28 adult patients over the 24 hours after nelarabine infusion on Day 1. Renal clearance averaged 24 ± 23 L/h for nelarabine and 6.2 ± 5.0 L/h for ara-G in 21 adult patients. Combined Phase 1 pharmacokinetic data at nelarabine doses of 199 to 2,900 mg/m² (n = 66 adult patients) indicate that the mean clearance (CL) of nelarabine is 197 ± 189 L/h/m² on Day 1. The apparent clearance of ara-G (CL/F) is 10.5 ± 4.5 L/h/m² on Day 1. Nelarabine and ara-G are rapidly eliminated from plasma with a mean half-life of 18 minutes and 3.2 hours, respectively, in adult patients.

Pediatrics: No pharmacokinetic data are available in pediatric patients at the once daily 650 mg/m² nelarabine dosage. Combined Phase 1 pharmacokinetic data at nelarabine doses of 104 to 2,900 mg/m² indicate that the mean clearance (CL) of nelarabine is about 30% higher in pediatric patients than in adult patients (259 ± 409 L/h/m² versus 197 ± 189 L/h/m², respectively) (n = 66 adults, n = 22 pediatric patients) on Day 1. The apparent clearance of ara-G (CL/F) is comparable between the two groups (10.5 ± 4.5 L/h/m² in adult patients and 11.3 ± 4.2 L/h/m² in pediatric patients) on Day 1. Nelarabine and ara-G are extensively distributed throughout the body. For nelarabine, V_{SS} values were 213 ± 358 L/m² in pediatric patients. For ara-G, V_{SS}/F values were 33 ± 9.3 L/m² in pediatric patients. Nelarabine and ara-G are rapidly eliminated from plasma in pediatric patients, with a half-life of 13 minutes and 2 hours, respectively.

Effect of Age: Age has no effect on the pharmacokinetics of nelarabine or ara-G in adults. Decreased renal function, which is more common in the elderly, may reduce ara-G clearance *[see Use in Specific Populations (8.5)]*.

Effect of Gender: Gender has no effect on nelarabine or ara-G pharmacokinetics.

Effect of Race: In general, nelarabine mean clearance and volume of distribution values tend to be higher in Whites (n = 63) than in Blacks (by about 10%) (n = 15). The opposite is true for ara-G; mean apparent clearance and volume of distribution values tend to be lower in Whites than in Blacks (by about 15-20%). No differences in safety or effectiveness were observed between these groups.

Effect of Renal Impairment: The pharmacokinetics of nelarabine and ara-G have not been specifically studied in renally impaired or hemodialyzed patients. Nelarabine is excreted by the kidney to a small extent (5 to 10% of the administered dose). Ara-G is excreted by the kidney to a greater extent (20 to 30% of the administered nelarabine dose). In the combined Phase 1 studies, patients were categorized into 3 groups: normal with CL_{cr} >80 mL/min (n = 67), mild with CL_{cr} = 50-80 mL/min (n = 15), and moderate with CL_{cr} <50 mL/min (n = 3). The mean apparent clearance (CL/F) of ara-G was about 15% and 40% lower in patients with mild and moderate renal impairment, respectively, than in patients with normal renal function *[see Use in Specific Populations (8.6) and Dosage and Administration (2.3)]*. No differences in safety or effectiveness were observed.

Effect of Hepatic Impairment: The influence of hepatic impairment on the pharmacokinetics of nelarabine has not been evaluated *[see Use in Specific Populations (8.7)]*.

Drug Interactions: *Cytochrome P450:* Nelarabine and ara-G did not significantly inhibit the activities of the human hepatic cytochrome P450 isoenzymes 1A2, 2A6, 2B6, 2C8, 2C9, 2C19, 2D6, or 3A4 in vitro at concentrations of nelarabine and ara-G up to 100 µM.

Fludarabine: Administration of fludarabine 30 mg/m² as a 30-minute infusion 4 hours before a 1,200 mg/m² infusion of nelarabine did not affect the pharmacokinetics of nelarabine, ara-G, or ara-GTP in 12 patients with refractory leukemia.

Pentostatin: There is in vitro evidence that pentostatin is a strong inhibitor of adenosine deaminase. Inhibition of adenosine deaminase may result in a reduction in the conversion of the pro-drug nelarabine to its active moiety and consequently in a reduction in efficacy of nelarabine and/or change in adverse reaction profile of either drug *[see Drug Interactions (7)]*.

13 NONCLINICAL TOXICOLOGY

13.1 Carcinogenesis, Mutagenesis, Impairment of Fertility

Carcinogenicity testing of nelarabine has not been done. However, nelarabine was mutagenic when tested in vitro in L5178Y/TK mouse lymphoma cells with and without metabolic activation. No studies have been conducted in animals to assess genotoxic potential or effects on fertility. The effect on human fertility is unknown.

14 CLINICAL STUDIES

The safety and efficacy of ARRANON were evaluated in two open-label, single-arm, multicenter studies.

14.1 Adult Clinical Study

The safety and efficacy of ARRANON in adult patients were studied in a clinical trial which included 39 treated patients, 28 who had T-cell acute lymphoblastic leukemia (T-ALL) or T-cell lymphoblastic lymphoma (T-LBL) that had relapsed following or was refractory to at least two prior induction regimens. A 1,500 mg/m² dose of ARRANON was administered intravenously over 2 hours on days 1, 3, and 5 repeated every 21 days. Patients who experienced signs or symptoms of grade 2 or greater neurologic toxicity on therapy were to be discontinued from further therapy with ARRANON. Seventeen patients had a diagnosis of T-ALL and 11 had a diagnosis of T-LBL. For patients with ≥2 prior inductions, the age range was 16-65 years (mean 34 years) and most patients were male (82%) and Caucasian (61%). Patients with central nervous system (CNS) disease were not eligible.

Complete response (CR) in this study was defined as bone marrow blast counts ≤5%, no other evidence of disease, and full recovery of peripheral blood counts. Complete response without complete hematologic recovery (CR*) was also assessed. The results of the study for patients who had received ≥2 prior inductions are shown in Table 5.

Table 5. Efficacy Results in Adult Patients With ≥2 Prior Inductions Treated with 1,500 mg/m² of ARRANON Administered Intravenously Over 2 Hours on Days 1, 3, and 5 Repeated Every 21 Days

	N = 28
CR plus CR* % (n) [95% CI]	21% (6) [8%, 41%]
CR % (n) [95% CI]	18% (5) [6%, 37%]
CR* % (n) [95% CI]	4% (1) [0%, 18%]
Duration of CR plus CR* (range in weeks)[a]	4 to 195+
Median overall survival (weeks) [95% CI]	20.6 weeks [10.4, 36.4]

CR = Complete response

CR* = Complete response without hematologic recovery

[a] Does not include 1 patient who was transplanted (duration of response was 156+ weeks)

The mean number of days on therapy was 56 days (range of 10 to 136 days). Time to CR plus CR* ranged from 2.9 to 11.7 weeks.

14.2 Pediatric Clinical Study

The safety and efficacy of ARRANON in pediatric patients were studied in a clinical trial which included patients 21 years of age and younger, who had relapsed or refractory T-cell acute lymphoblastic leukemia (T-ALL) or T-cell lymphoblastic lymphoma (T-LBL). Eighty-four (84) patients, 39 of whom had received two or more prior induction regimens, were treated with 650 mg/m²/day of ARRANON administered intravenously over 1 hour daily for 5 consecutive days repeated every 21 days (see Table 6). Patients who experienced signs or symptoms of grade 2 or greater neurologic toxicity on therapy were to be discontinued from further therapy with ARRANON.

Table 6. Pediatric Clinical Study - Patient Allocation

Patient Population	N
Patients treated at 650 mg/m²/day × 5 days every 21 days.	84
Patients with T-ALL or T-LBL with two or more prior induction treated at 650 mg/m²/day × 5 days every 21 days.	39
Patients with T-ALL or T-LBL with one prior induction treated at 650 mg/m²/day × 5 days every 21 days.	31

The 84 patients ranged in age from 2.5-21.7 years (overall mean, 11.9 years), 52% were 3 to 12 years of age and most were male (74%) and Caucasian (62%). The majority (77%) of patients had a diagnosis of T-ALL.

Complete response (CR) in this study was defined as bone marrow blast counts ≤5%, no other evidence of disease, and full recovery of peripheral blood counts. Complete response without full hematologic recovery (CR*) was also assessed as a meaningful outcome in this heavily pretreated population. Duration of response is reported from date of response to date of relapse, and may include subsequent stem cell transplant. Efficacy results are presented in Table 7.

Table 7. Efficacy Results in Patients 21 Years of Age and Younger at Diagnosis With ≥2 Prior Inductions Treated with 650 mg/m² of ARRANON Administered Intravenously Over 1 Hour Daily for 5 Consecutive Days Repeated Every 21 Days

	N = 39
CR plus CR* % (n) [95% CI]	23% (9) [11%, 39%]
CR % (n) [95% CI]	13% (5) [4%, 27%]
CR* % (n) [95% CI]	10% (4) [3%, 24%]
Duration of CR plus CR* (range in weeks)[a]	3.3 to 9.3
Median overall survival (weeks) [95% CI]	13.1 [8.7, 17.4]

CR = Complete response
CR* = Complete response without hematologic recovery
[a] Does not include 5 patients who were transplanted or had subsequent systemic chemotherapy (duration of response in these 5 patients was 4.7 to 42.1 weeks).

The mean number of days on therapy was 46 days (range of 7 to 129 days). Median time to CR plus CR* was 3.4 weeks (95% CI: 3.0, 3.7).

15 REFERENCES

1. Preventing Occupational Exposures to Antineoplastic and Other Hazardous Drugs in Health Care Settings. NIOSH Alert 2004-165.
2. OSHA Technical Manual, TED 1-0.15A, Section VI: Chapter 2. Controlling Occupational Exposure to Hazardous Drugs. OSHA, 1999. http://www.osha.gov/dts/osta/otm/otm_vi/otm_vi_2.html
3. American Society of Health-System Pharmacists. ASHP Guidelines on Handling Hazardous Drugs. *Am J Health-Syst Pharm.* 2006;63:1172-1193.
4. Polovich M, White JM, Kelleher LO (eds.) 2005. Chemotherapy and Biotherapy Guidelines and Recommendations for Practice. (2nd ed) Pittsburgh, PA: Oncology Nursing Society.

16 HOW SUPPLIED/STORAGE AND HANDLING

ARRANON Injection is supplied as a clear, colorless, sterile solution in Type I, clear glass vials with a gray butyl rubber (latex-free) stopper and a red snap-off aluminum seal. Each vial contains 250 mg of nelarabine (5 mg nelarabine per mL) and the inactive ingredient sodium chloride (4.5 mg per mL) in 50 mL Water for Injection, USP. Vials are available in the following carton size:

NDC 0007-4401-06 (package of 6)

Store at 25° C (77° F); excursions permitted to 15° to 30° C (59° to 86° F) [see USP Controlled Room Temperature].

17 PATIENT COUNSELING INFORMATION

Patient labeling is provided as a tear-off leaflet at the end of this full prescribing information. However, inform the patients of the following:

- Since patients receiving nelarabine therapy may experience somnolence, they should be cautioned about operating hazardous machinery, including automobiles.
- Patients should be instructed to contact their physician if they experience new or worsening symptoms of peripheral neuropathy *(see Boxed Warning, Warnings and Precautions (5.1), and Dosage and Administration (2.3))*. These signs and symptoms include: tingling or numbness in fingers, hands, toes, or feet; difficulty with the fine motor coordination tasks such as buttoning clothing; unsteadiness while walking; weakness arising from a low chair; weakness in climbing stairs; increased tripping while walking over uneven surfaces.
- Patients should be instructed that seizures have been known to occur in patients who receive nelarabine. If a seizure occurs, the physician administering ARRANON should be promptly informed.
- Patients who develop fever or signs of infection while on therapy should notify their physician promptly.
- Patients should be advised to use effective contraceptive measures to prevent pregnancy and to avoid breastfeeding during treatment with ARRANON.

ARRANON is a registered trademark of GlaxoSmithKline.
GlaxoSmithKline
Research Triangle Park, NC 27709

December 2011
ARR:2PI

PHARMACIST-DETACH HERE AND GIVE INSTRUCTIONS TO PATIENT

PATIENT INFORMATION LEAFLET
ARRANON® (AIR-ra-non)
Nelarabine Injection

Read the Patient Information that comes with ARRANON before you or your child start treatment with ARRANON. Read the information you get each time before each treatment with ARRANON. There may be new information. This information does not take the place of talking with the doctor about your or your child's medical condition or treatment. Talk to your or your child's doctor, if you have any questions.

What is the most important information I should know about ARRANON?

ARRANON may cause serious nervous system problems including:
- extreme sleepiness
- seizures
- coma
- numbness and tingling in the hands, fingers, feet, or toes (peripheral neuropathy)
- weakness and paralysis

Call the doctor right away if you or your child has the following symptoms:
- seizures
- numbness and tingling in the hands, fingers, feet, or toes
- problems with fine motor skills such as buttoning clothes
- unsteadiness while walking
- increased tripping while walking
- weakness when getting out of a chair or walking up stairs

These symptoms may not go away even when treatment with ARRANON is stopped.

What is ARRANON?

ARRANON is an anti-cancer medicine used to treat adults and children who have:
- T-cell acute lymphoblastic leukemia
- T-cell lymphoblastic lymphoma

What should you tell the doctor before you or your child starts ARRANON?

Tell the doctor about all health conditions you or your child have, including if you or your child:
- have any nervous system problems.
- have kidney problems.
- are breast-feeding or plan to breast-feed. It is not known whether ARRANON passes through breast milk. You should not breast-feed during treatment with ARRANON.
- are pregnant or plan to become pregnant. ARRANON may harm an unborn baby. You should use effective birth control to avoid getting pregnant. Talk with your doctor about your choices.

Tell the doctor about all the medicines you or your child take, including prescription and nonprescription medicines, vitamins, and herbal supplements.

How is ARRANON given?

ARRANON is an intravenous medicine. This means it is given through a tube in your vein.

What should you or your child avoid during treatment with ARRANON?
- You or your child should not drive or operate dangerous machines. ARRANON may cause sleepiness.
- You or your child should not receive vaccines made with live germs during treatment with ARRANON.

What are the possible side effects of ARRANON?

ARRANON may cause serious nervous system problems. See "What is the most important information I should know about ARRANON?"

ARRANON may also cause:
- decreased blood counts such as low red blood cells, low white blood cells, and low platelets. Blood tests should be done regularly to check blood counts. Call the doctor right away if you or your child:
  - is more tired than usual, pale, or has trouble breathing
  - has a fever or other signs of an infection
  - bruises easy or has any unusual bleeding
- stomach area problems such as nausea, vomiting, diarrhea, and constipation
- headache
- sleepiness
- blurry eyesight

Call your doctor right away if you experience unexplained muscle pain, tenderness, or weakness while taking ARRANON. This is because on rare occasions, muscle problems can be serious.

These are not all the side effects associated with ARRANON. Ask your doctor or pharmacist for more information.

General Advice about ARRANON

This leaflet summarizes important information about ARRANON. If you have questions or problems, talk with your or your child's doctor. You can ask your doctor or pharmacist for information about ARRANON that is written for healthcare providers or it is available at www.GSK.com.

ARRANON is a registered trademark of GlaxoSmithKline.
GlaxoSmithKline
Research Triangle Park, NC 27709

December 2011
ARR:2PIL

ARZERRA® ℞

[ar-zer-ra]
(ofatumumab)
Injection, for intravenous infusion

HIGHLIGHTS OF PRESCRIBING INFORMATION
These highlights do not include all the information needed to use ARZERRA safely and effectively. See full prescribing information for ARZERRA.
ARZERRA (ofatumumab)
Injection, for intravenous infusion
Initial U.S. Approval: 2009

RECENT MAJOR CHANGES

Dosage and Administration, Preparation and Administration (2.5)	04/2011
Warnings and Precautions, Hepatitis B Infection and Reactivation (5.4)	09/2011

INDICATIONS AND USAGE

ARZERRA (ofatumumab) is a CD20-directed cytolytic monoclonal antibody indicated for the treatment of patients with chronic lymphocytic leukemia (CLL) refractory to fludarabine and alemtuzumab. The effectiveness of ARZERRA is based on the demonstration of durable objective responses. No data demonstrate an improvement in disease-related symptoms or increased survival with ARZERRA. (1, 14)

DOSAGE AND ADMINISTRATION

- Dilute and administer as an intravenous infusion. Do not administer as an intravenous push or bolus. (2.1)
- Recommended dosage and schedule is 12 doses administered as follows:
  - 300 mg initial dose, followed 1 week later by
  - 2,000 mg weekly for 7 doses, followed 4 weeks later by
  - 2,000 mg every 4 weeks for 4 doses. (2.1)
- Premedicate with oral acetaminophen, oral or intravenous antihistamine, and intravenous corticosteroid. (2.4)

DOSAGE FORMS AND STRENGTHS

- 100 mg/5 mL single-use vial. (3)
- 1,000 mg/50 mL single-use vial. (3)

CONTRAINDICATIONS

None. (4)

WARNINGS AND PRECAUTIONS

- Infusion Reactions: Premedicate with an intravenous corticosteroid (as appropriate), an oral analgesic, and an oral or intravenous antihistamine. Monitor patients closely during infusions. Interrupt infusion if infusion reactions occur. (2.3, 2.4, 5.1)
- Cytopenias: Monitor blood counts at regular intervals for neutropenia and thrombocytopenia. (5.2)
- Progressive Multifocal Leukoencephalopathy (PML): Monitor neurologic function and discontinue ARZERRA if PML is suspected. (5.3)

• Hepatitis B Infection and Reactivation: Screen high-risk patients. Discontinue ARZERRA in patients who develop viral hepatitis or reactivation of viral hepatitis. (5.4)

ADVERSE REACTIONS

Most common adverse reactions (≥10%) were neutropenia, pneumonia, pyrexia, cough, diarrhea, anemia, fatigue, dyspnea, rash, nausea, bronchitis, and upper respiratory tract infections. (6)

To report SUSPECTED ADVERSE REACTIONS, contact GlaxoSmithKline at 1-888-825-5249 or FDA at 1-800-FDA-1088 or www.fda.gov/medwatch.

USE IN SPECIFIC POPULATIONS

• Pregnancy: Based on animal data, may cause fetal harm. (8.1)
• Nursing mothers: Published data suggest that consumption of breast milk does not result in substantial absorption of maternal antibodies into circulation. (8.3)

See 17 for PATIENT COUNSELING INFORMATION

Revised: 09/2011

FULL PRESCRIBING INFORMATION: CONTENTS*

*** Sections or subsections omitted from the full prescribing information are not listed**

FULL PRESCRIBING INFORMATION

1 INDICATIONS AND USAGE

ARZERRA® (ofatumumab) is indicated for the treatment of patients with chronic lymphocytic leukemia (CLL) refractory to fludarabine and alemtuzumab.

The effectiveness of ARZERRA is based on the demonstration of durable objective responses *[see Clinical Studies (14)]*. No data demonstrate an improvement in disease-related symptoms or increased survival with ARZERRA.

2 DOSAGE AND ADMINISTRATION

2.1 Recommended Dosage Regimen

• Do not administer as an intravenous push or bolus.
• Premedicate before each infusion *[see Dosage and Administration (2.4)]*.
• Administer with an in-line filter set supplied with product.

The recommended dosage and schedule is 12 doses administered as follows:

• 300 mg initial dose (Dose 1), followed 1 week later by
• 2,000 mg weekly for 7 doses (Doses 2 through 8), followed 4 weeks later by
• 2,000 mg every 4 weeks for 4 doses (Doses 9 through 12)

2.2 Administration

Prepare all doses in 1,000 mL of 0.9% Sodium Chloride Injection, USP *[see Dosage and Administration (2.5)]*.

• Dose 1: Initiate infusion at a rate of 3.6 mg/hour (12 mL/hour).
• Dose 2: Initiate infusion at a rate of 24 mg/hour (12 mL/hour).
• Doses 3 through 12: Initiate infusion at a rate of 50 mg/hour (25 mL/hour).

In the absence of infusional toxicity, the rate of infusion may be increased every 30 minutes as described in Table 1. Do not exceed the infusion rates in Table 1.

Table 1. Infusion Rates for ARZERRA

Interval After Start of Infusion(min)	Dose 1[a] (mL/hour)	Dose 2[b] (mL/hour)	Doses 3-12[b] (mL/hour)
0-30	12	12	25
31-60	25	25	50
61-90	50	50	100
91-120	100	100	200
>120	200	200	400

[a] Dose 1 = 300 mg (0.3 mg/mL).

[b] Doses 2 and 3-12 = 2,000 mg (2 mg/mL).

2.3 Dose Modification

• Interrupt infusion for infusion reactions of any severity *[see Warnings and Precautions (5.1)]*.
• For Grade 4 infusion reactions, do not resume the infusion.
• For Grade 1, 2, or 3 infusion reaction, if the infusion reaction resolves or remains less than or equal to Grade 2, resume infusion with the following modifications according to the initial Grade of the infusion reaction.

Grade 1 or 2: Infuse at one-half of the previous infusion rate.

Grade 3: Infuse at a rate of 12 mL/hour.

• After resuming the infusion, the infusion rate may be increased according to Table 1 above, based on patient tolerance.

2.4 Premedication

• Premedicate 30 minutes to 2 hours prior to each dose with oral acetaminophen 1,000 mg (or equivalent), oral or intravenous antihistamine (cetirizine 10 mg or equivalent), and intravenous corticosteroid (prednisolone 100 mg or equivalent).
• Do not reduce corticosteroid dose for Doses 1, 2, and 9.
• Corticosteroid dose may be reduced as follows for Doses 3 through 8 and 10 through 12:
  ◦ Doses 3 through 8: Gradually reduce corticosteroid dose with successive infusions if a Grade 3 or greater infusion reaction did not occur with the preceding dose.
  ◦ Doses 10 through 12: Administer prednisolone 50 mg to 100 mg or equivalent if a Grade 3 or greater infusion reaction did not occur with Dose 9.

2.5 Preparation and Administration

• Do not shake product.
• Inspect parenteral drug products visually for particulate matter and discoloration prior to administration. ARZERRA should be a clear to opalescent, colorless solution and may contain a small amount of visible translucent-to-white, amorphous, ofatumumab particles. The solution should not be used if discolored or cloudy, or if foreign particulate matter is present.

Preparation of Solution:

• 300-mg dose: Withdraw and discard 15 mL from a 1,000-mL bag of 0.9% Sodium Chloride Injection, USP. Withdraw 5 mL from each of 3 single-use 100 mg vials of ARZERRA and add to the bag. Mix diluted solution by gentle inversion.
• 2,000-mg dose: Withdraw and discard 100 mL from a 1,000-mL bag of 0.9% Sodium Chloride Injection, USP. Withdraw 50 mL from each of 2 single-use 1,000 mg vials of ARZERRA and add to the bag. Mix diluted solution by gentle inversion.
• Store diluted solution between 2° to 8°C (36° to 46°F).
• No incompatibilities between ARZERRA and polyvinylchloride or polyolefin bags and administration sets have been observed.

Administration Instructions:

• Do not mix ARZERRA with, or administer as an infusion with, other medicinal products.
• Administer using an infusion pump with an administration set and the provided in-line filter set.
• Flush the intravenous line with 0.9% Sodium Chloride Injection, USP before and after each dose.
• Start infusion within 12 hours of preparation.
• Discard prepared solution after 24 hours.

3 DOSAGE FORMS AND STRENGTHS

• 100 mg/5 mL single-use vial.
• 1,000 mg/50 mL single-use vial.

4 CONTRAINDICATIONS

None.

5 WARNINGS AND PRECAUTIONS

5.1 Infusion Reactions

ARZERRA can cause serious infusion reactions manifesting as bronchospasm, dyspnea, laryngeal edema, pulmonary edema, flushing, hypertension, hypotension, syncope, cardiac ischemia/infarction, back pain, abdominal pain, pyrexia, rash, urticaria, and angioedema. Infusion reactions occur more frequently with the first 2 infusions *[see Adverse Reactions (6.1)]*.

Premedicate with acetaminophen, an antihistamine, and a corticosteroid *[see Dosage and Administration (2.1, 2.4)]*. Interrupt infusion for infusion reactions of any severity. Institute medical management for severe infusion reactions including angina or other signs and symptoms of myocardial ischemia *[see Dosage and Administration (2.3)]*.

In a study of patients with moderate to severe chronic obstructive pulmonary disease, an indication for which ARZERRA is not approved, 2 of 5 patients developed Grade 3 bronchospasm during infusion.

5.2 Cytopenias

Prolonged (≥1 week) severe neutropenia and thrombocytopenia can occur with ARZERRA. Monitor complete blood counts (CBC) and platelet counts at regular intervals during therapy, and increase the frequency of monitoring in patients who develop Grade 3 or 4 cytopenias.

5.3 Progressive Multifocal Leukoencephalopathy

Progressive multifocal leukoencephalopathy (PML), including fatal PML, can occur with ARZERRA. Consider PML in any patient with new onset of or changes in pre-existing neurological signs or symptoms. Discontinue ARZERRA if PML is suspected, and initiate evaluation for PML including consultation with a neurologist, brain MRI, and lumbar puncture.

5.4 Hepatitis B Infection and Reactivation

Fulminant and fatal hepatitis B virus (HBV) infection and reactivation can occur in patients following treatment with ARZERRA. Screen patients at high risk of HBV infection before initiation of ARZERRA. Closely monitor carriers of hepatitis B for clinical and laboratory signs of active HBV infection during treatment with ARZERRA and for 6 to 12 months following the last infusion of ARZERRA. Discontinue ARZERRA in patients who develop viral hepatitis or reactivation of viral hepatitis, and institute appropriate treatment. Insufficient data exist regarding the safety of administration of ARZERRA in patients with active hepatitis.

5.5 Intestinal Obstruction

Obstruction of the small intestine can occur in patients receiving ARZERRA. Perform a diagnostic evaluation if obstruction is suspected.

5.6 Immunizations

The safety of immunization with live viral vaccines during or following administration of ARZERRA has not been studied. Do not administer live viral vaccines to patients who have recently received ARZERRA. The ability to generate an immune response to any vaccine following administration of ARZERRA has not been studied.

6 ADVERSE REACTIONS

The following serious adverse reactions are discussed in greater detail in other sections of the labeling:

• Infusion Reactions *[see Warnings and Precautions (5.1)]*
• Cytopenias *[see Warnings and Precautions (5.2)]*
• Progressive Multifocal Leukoencephalopathy *[see Warnings and Precautions (5.3)]*
• Hepatitis B Reactivation *[see Warnings and Precautions (5.4)]*
• Intestinal Obstruction *[see Warnings and Precautions (5.5)]*

The most common adverse reactions (≥10%) in Study 1 were neutropenia, pneumonia, pyrexia, cough, diarrhea, anemia, fatigue, dyspnea, rash, nausea, bronchitis, and upper respiratory tract infections.

The most common serious adverse reactions in Study 1 were infections (including pneumonia and sepsis), neutropenia, and pyrexia. Infections were the most common adverse reactions leading to drug discontinuation in Study 1.

6.1 Clinical Trials Experience

Because clinical trials are conducted under widely varying conditions, adverse reaction rates observed in the clinical trials of a drug cannot be directly compared to rates in the clinical trials of another drug and may not reflect the rates observed in practice.

The safety of monotherapy with ARZERRA was evaluated in 181 patients with relapsed or refractory CLL in 2 open-label, non-randomized, single-arm studies. In these studies, ARZERRA was administered at 2,000 mg beginning with the second dose for 11 doses (Study 1 [n = 154]) or 3 doses (Study 2 [n = 27]).

The data described in Table 2 and other sections below are derived from 154 patients in Study 1. All patients received 2,000 mg weekly from the second dose onward. Ninety percent of patients received at least 8 infusions of ARZERRA and 55% received all 12 infusions. The median age was 63 years (range: 41 to 86 years), 72% were male, and 97% were White.

[See table 2 above]

Infusion Reactions: Infusion reactions occurred in 44% of patients on the day of the first infusion (300 mg), 29% on the day of the second infusion (2,000 mg), and less frequently during subsequent infusions.

Infections: A total of 108 patients (70%) experienced bacterial, viral, or fungal infections. A total of 45 patients (29%) experienced ≥Grade 3 infections, of which 19 (12%) were fatal. The proportion of fatal infections in the fludarabine- and alemtuzumab-refractory group was 17%.

Neutropenia: Of 108 patients with normal neutrophil counts at baseline, 45 (42%) developed ≥Grade 3 neutropenia. Nineteen (18%) developed Grade 4 neutropenia. Some patients experienced new onset Grade 4 neutropenia >2 weeks in duration.

6.2 Immunogenicity

There is a potential for immunogenicity with therapeutic proteins such as ofatumumab. Serum samples from patients with CLL in Study 1 were tested by enzyme-linked immunosorbent assay (ELISA) for anti-ofatumumab antibodies during and after the 24-week treatment period. Results were negative in 46 patients after the 8th infusion and in 33 patients after the 12th infusion.

Immunogenicity assay results are highly dependent on several factors including assay sensitivity and specificity, assay methodology, sample handling, timing of sample collection, concomitant medications, and underlying disease. For these reasons, comparison of incidence of antibodies to ARZERRA with the incidence of antibodies to other products may be misleading.

7 DRUG INTERACTIONS

No formal drug-drug interaction studies have been conducted with ARZERRA.

8 USE IN SPECIFIC POPULATIONS

8.1 Pregnancy

Pregnancy Category C: There are no adequate or well-controlled studies of ofatumumab in pregnant women. A reproductive study in pregnant cynomolgus monkeys that received ofatumumab at doses up to 3.5 times the recommended human dose of ofatumumab did not demonstrate maternal toxicity or teratogenicity. Ofatumumab crossed the placental barrier, and fetuses exhibited depletion of peripheral B cells and decreased spleen and placental weights. ARZERRA should be used during pregnancy only if the potential benefit to the mother justifies the potential risk to the fetus.

There are no human or animal data on the potential short- and long-term effects of perinatal B-cell depletion in offspring following in utero exposure to ofatumumab. Ofatumumab does not bind normal human tissues other than B lymphocytes. It is not known if binding occurs to unique embryonic or fetal tissue targets. In addition, the kinetics of B-lymphocyte recovery are unknown in offspring with B-cell depletion *[see Nonclinical Toxicology (13.3)]*.

8.3 Nursing Mothers

It is not known whether ofatumumab is secreted in human milk; however, human IgG is secreted in human milk. Published data suggest that neonatal and infant consumption of breast milk does not result in substantial absorption of these maternal antibodies into circulation. Because the effects of local gastrointestinal and limited systemic exposure to ofatumumab are unknown, caution should be exercised when ARZERRA is administered to a nursing woman.

8.4 Pediatric Use

Safety and effectiveness of ARZERRA have not been established in children.

8.5 Geriatric Use

Clinical studies of ARZERRA did not include sufficient numbers of subjects aged 65 and over to determine whether they respond differently from younger subjects *[see Clinical Pharmacology (12.3)]*.

8.6 Renal Impairment

No formal studies of ARZERRA in patients with renal impairment have been conducted *[see Clinical Pharmacology (12.3)]*.

8.7 Hepatic Impairment

No formal studies of ARZERRA in patients with hepatic impairment have been conducted.

10 OVERDOSAGE

No data are available regarding overdosage with ARZERRA.

11 DESCRIPTION

ARZERRA (ofatumumab) is an IgG1κ human monoclonal antibody with a molecular weight of approximately 149 kDa. The antibody was generated via transgenic mouse and hybridoma technology and is produced in a recombinant murine cell line (NS0) using standard mammalian cell cultivation and purification technologies.

ARZERRA is a sterile, clear to opalescent, colorless, preservative-free liquid concentrate for intravenous administration. ARZERRA is supplied at a concentration of 20 mg/mL in single-use vials. Each single-use vial contains either 100 mg ofatumumab in 5 mL of solution or 1,000 mg ofatumumab in 50 mL of solution.

Inactive ingredients include: 10 mg/mL arginine, diluted hydrochloric acid, 0.019 mg/mL edetate disodium,

Table 2. Incidence of All Adverse Reactions Occurring in ≥5% of Patients in Study 1 and in the Fludarabine- and Alemtuzumab-Refractory Subset of Study 1 (MedDRA 9.0)

Body System/Adverse Event	Total Population (n = 154) All Grades %	Total Population (n = 154) Grade ≥3 %	Fludarabine- and Alemtuzumab-Refractory (n = 59) All Grades %	Fludarabine- and Alemtuzumab-Refractory (n = 59) Grade ≥3 %
Infections and infestations				
Pneumonia[a]	23	14	25	15
Upper respiratory tract infection	11	0	3	0
Bronchitis	11	<1	19	2
Sepsis[b]	8	8	10	10
Nasopharyngitis	8	0	8	0
Herpes zoster	6	1	7	2
Sinusitis	5	2	3	2
Blood and lymphatic system disorders				
Anemia	16	5	17	8
Psychiatric disorders				
Insomnia	7	0	10	0
Nervous system disorders				
Headache	6	0	7	0
Cardiovascular disorders				
Hypertension	5	0	8	0
Hypotension	5	0	3	0
Tachycardia	5	<1	7	2
Respiratory, thoracic, and mediastinal disorders				
Cough	19	0	19	0
Dyspnea	14	2	19	5
Gastrointestinal disorders				
Diarrhea	18	0	19	0
Nausea	11	0	12	0
Skin and subcutaneous tissue disorders				
Rash[c]	14	<1	17	2
Urticaria	8	0	5	0
Hyperhidrosis	5	0	5	0
Musculoskeletal and connective tissue disorders				
Back pain	8	1	12	2
Muscle spasms	5	0	3	0
General disorders and administration site conditions				
Pyrexia	20	3	25	5
Fatigue	15	0	15	0
Edema peripheral	9	<1	8	2
Chills	8	0	10	0

[a] Pneumonia includes pneumonia, lung infection, lobar pneumonia, and bronchopneumonia.

[b] Sepsis includes sepsis, neutropenic sepsis, bacteremia, and septic shock.

[c] Rash includes rash, rash macular, and rash vesicular.

0.2 mg/mL polysorbate 80, 6.8 mg/mL sodium acetate, 2.98 mg/mL sodium chloride, and Water for Injection, USP. The pH is 5.5.

12 CLINICAL PHARMACOLOGY

12.1 Mechanism of Action

Ofatumumab binds specifically to both the small and large extracellular loops of the CD20 molecule. The CD20 molecule is expressed on normal B lymphocytes (pre-B- to mature B-lymphocyte) and on B-cell CLL. The CD20 molecule is not shed from the cell surface and is not internalized following antibody binding.

The Fab domain of ofatumumab binds to the CD20 molecule and the Fc domain mediates immune effector functions to result in B-cell lysis *in vitro*. Data suggest that possible mechanisms of cell lysis include complement-dependent cytotoxicity and antibody-dependent, cell-mediated cytotoxicity.

12.2 Pharmacodynamics

In patients with CLL refractory to fludarabine and alemtuzumab, the median decrease in circulating CD19-positive B cells was 91% (n = 50) with the 8th infusion and 85% (n = 32) with the 12th infusion. The time to recovery of lymphocytes, including CD19-positive B cells, to normal levels has not been determined.

12.3 Pharmacokinetics

Pharmacokinetic data were obtained from 146 patients with refractory CLL who received a 300-mg initial dose followed by 7 weekly and 4 monthly infusions of 2,000 mg. The C_{max} and $AUC_{(0-\infty)}$ after the 8th infusion in Study 1 were approximately 40% and 60% higher than after the 4th infusion in Study 2. The mean volume of distribution at steady-state (V_{ss}) values ranged from 1.7 to 5.1 L. Ofatumumab is eliminated through both a target-independent route and a B cell-mediated route. Ofatumumab exhibited dose-dependent clearance in the dose range of 100 to 2,000 mg. Due to the depletion of B cells, the clearance of ofatumumab decreased substantially after subsequent infusions compared to the first infusion. The mean clearance between the 4th and 12th infusions was approximately 0.01 L/hr and exhibited large inter-subject variability with CV% greater than 50%. The mean $t_{1/2}$ between the 4th and 12th infusions was approximately 14 days (range: 2.3 to 61.5 days).

Special Populations: Cross-study analyses were performed on data from patients with a variety of conditions, including 162 patients with CLL, who received multiple infusions of ARZERRA as a single agent at doses ranging from 100 to 2,000 mg. The effects of various covariates (e.g., body size [weight, height, body surface area], age, gender, baseline creatinine clearance) on ofatumumab pharmacokinetics were assessed in a population pharmacokinetic analysis.

Body Weight: Volume of distribution and clearance increased with body weight. However, this increase was not clinically significant. No dosage adjustment is recommended based on body weight.

Age: Age did not significantly influence ofatumumab pharmacokinetics in patients ranging from 21 to 86 years of age. No pharmacokinetic data are available in pediatric patients.

Gender: Gender had a modest effect on ofatumumab pharmacokinetics (14% to 25% lower clearance and volume of distribution in female patients compared to male patients) in a cross-study population analysis (41% of the patients in this analysis were male and 59% were female). These effects are not considered clinically important, and no dosage adjustment is recommended.

Renal Impairment: Creatinine clearance at baseline did not have a clinically important effect on ofatumumab pharmacokinetics in patients with calculated creatinine clearance values ranging from 33 to 287 mL/min.

13 NONCLINICAL TOXICOLOGY

13.1 Carcinogenesis, Mutagenesis, Impairment of Fertility

No carcinogenicity or mutagenicity studies of ofatumumab have been conducted. In a repeat-dose toxicity study, no tumorigenic or unexpected mitogenic responses were noted in cynomolgus monkeys treated for 7 months with up to 3.5 times the human dose of ofatumumab. Effects on male and female fertility have not been evaluated in animal studies.

13.3 Reproductive and Developmental Toxicology

Pregnant cynomolgus monkeys dosed with 0.7 or 3.5 times the human dose of ofatumumab weekly during the period of organogenesis (gestation days 20 to 50) had no maternal toxicity or teratogenicity. Both dose levels of ofatumumab depleted circulating B cells in the dams, with signs of initial B cell recovery 50 days after the final dose. Following Caesarean section at gestational day 100, fetuses from ofatumumab-treated dams exhibited decreases in mean peripheral B-cell counts (decreased to approximately 10% of control values), splenic B-cell counts (decreased to approximately 15 to 20% of control values), and spleen weights (decreased by 15% for the low-dose and by 30% for the high-dose group, compared to control values). Fetuses from treated dams exhibiting anti-ofatumumab antibody responses had higher B cell counts and higher spleen weights compared to the fetuses from other treated dams, indicating partial recovery in those animals developing anti-ofatumumab antibodies. When compared to control animals, fetuses from treated dams in both dose groups had a 10% decrease in mean placental weights. A 15% decrease in mean thymus weight compared to the controls was also observed in fetuses from dams treated with 3.5 times the human dose of ofatumumab. The biological significance of decreased placental and thymic weights is unknown.

The kinetics of B-lymphocyte recovery and the potential long-term effects of perinatal B-cell depletion in offspring from ofatumumab-treated dams have not been studied in animals.

14 CLINICAL STUDIES

Study 1 was a single-arm, multicenter study in 154 patients with relapsed or refractory CLL. ARZERRA was administered by intravenous infusion according to the following schedule: 300 mg (Week 0), 2,000 mg weekly for 7 infusions (Weeks 1 through 7), and 2,000 mg every 4 weeks for 4 infusions (Weeks 12 through 24). Patients with CLL refractory to fludarabine and alemtuzumab (n = 59) comprised the efficacy population. Drug refractoriness was defined as failure to achieve at least a partial response to, or disease progression within 6 months of, the last dose of fludarabine or alemtuzumab. The main efficacy outcome was durable objective tumor response rate. Objective tumor responses were determined using the 1996 National Cancer Institute Working Group (NCIWG) Guidelines for CLL.

In patients with CLL refractory to fludarabine and alemtuzumab, the median age was 64 years (range: 41 to 86 years), 75% were male, and 95% were White. The median number of prior therapies was 5; 93% received prior alkylating agents, 59% received prior rituximab, and all received prior fludarabine and alemtuzumab. Eighty-eight percent of patients received at least 8 infusions of ARZERRA and 54% received 12 infusions.

The investigator-determined overall response rate in patients with CLL refractory to fludarabine and alemtuzumab was 42% (99% CI: 26, 60) with a median duration of response of 6.5 months (95% CI: 5.8, 8.3). There were no complete responses. Anti-tumor activity was also observed in additional patients in Study 1 and in a multicenter, open-label, dose-escalation study (Study 2) conducted in patients with relapsed or refractory CLL.

16 HOW SUPPLIED/STORAGE AND HANDLING

ARZERRA (ofatumumab) is a sterile, clear to opalescent, colorless, preservative-free liquid concentrate (20 mg/mL) for dilution and intravenous administration provided in single-use glass vials with a latex-free rubber stopper and an aluminum overseal. Each vial contains either 100 mg ofatumumab in 5 mL of solution or 1,000 mg ofatumumab in 50 mL of solution.

ARZERRA is available as follows:

Carton Contents	NDC
3 single-use 100 mg/5 mL vials with 2 in-line filter sets	Vial: NDC 0173-0821-02 Carton of 3 vials: NDC 0173-0821-33
1 single-use 1,000 mg/50 mL vial with 2 in-line filter sets	Vial and Carton: NDC 0173-0821-01

Store ARZERRA refrigerated between 2° to 8°C (36° to 46°F). Do not freeze. Vials should be protected from light.

17 PATIENT COUNSELING INFORMATION

Advise patients to contact a healthcare professional for any of the following:

- Signs and symptoms of infusion reactions including fever, chills, rash, or breathing problems within 24 hours of infusion *[see Warnings and Precautions (5.1) and Adverse Reactions (6.1)]*
- Bleeding, easy bruising, petechiae, pallor, worsening weakness, or fatigue *[see Warnings and Precautions (5.2)]*
- Signs of infections including fever and cough *[see Warnings and Precautions (5.2) and Adverse Reactions (6.1)]*
- New neurological symptoms such as confusion, dizziness or loss of balance, difficulty talking or walking, or vision problems *[see Warnings and Precautions (5.3)]*
- Symptoms of hepatitis including worsening fatigue or yellow discoloration of skin or eyes *[see Warnings and Precautions (5.4)]*
- New or worsening abdominal pain or nausea *[see Warnings and Precautions (5.5)]*
- Pregnancy or nursing *[see Use in Specific Populations (8.1, 8.3)]*

Advise patients of the need for:

- Periodic monitoring for blood counts *[see Warnings and Precautions (5.2)]*
- Avoiding vaccination with live viral vaccines *[see Warnings and Precautions (5.6)]*

Manufactured by:
GLAXO GROUP LIMITED
Greenford, Middlesex, UB6 0NN, United Kingdom
U.S. Lic. 1809
Distributed by:
GlaxoSmithKline
Research Triangle Park, NC 27709

September 2011
ARZ:6PI

AVANDAMET ℞

[ə-van' də-met]

(rosiglitazone maleate and metformin hydrochloride) Tablets

HIGHLIGHTS OF PRESCRIBING INFORMATION

These highlights do not include all the information needed to use AVANDAMET safely and effectively. See full prescribing information for AVANDAMET.

AVANDAMET (rosiglitazone maleate and metformin hydrochloride) Tablets
Initial U.S. Approval: 2002

WARNINGS

See full prescribing information for complete boxed warning.

Rosiglitazone maleate: **CONGESTIVE HEART FAILURE AND MYOCARDIAL INFARCTION**

- **Thiazolidinediones, including rosiglitazone, cause or exacerbate heart failure in some patients (5.2). After initiation of AVANDAMET, and after dose increases, observe patients carefully for signs and symptoms of heart failure (including excessive, rapid weight gain, dyspnea, and/or edema). If these signs and symptoms develop, the heart failure should be managed according to current standards of care. Furthermore, discontinuation or dose reduction must be considered. (5.2)**
- **AVANDAMET is not recommended in patients with symptomatic heart failure. Initiation of AVANDAMET in patients with established NYHA Class III or IV heart failure is contraindicated. (4, 5.2)**
- **A meta-analysis of 52 clinical trials (mean duration 6 months; 16,995 total patients), most of which compared rosiglitazone to placebo, showed rosiglitazone to be associated with a statistically significant increased risk of myocardial infarction. Three other trials (mean duration 46 months; 14,067 total patients), comparing rosiglitazone to some other approved oral antidiabetic agents or placebo, showed a statistically non-significant increased risk of myocardial infarction and a statistically non-significant decreased risk of death. There have been no clinical trials directly comparing cardiovascular risk of rosiglitazone and ACTOS® (pioglitazone, another thiazolidinedione), but in a separate trial, pioglitazone (when compared to placebo) did not show an increased risk of myocardial infarction or death. (5.3)**
- **Because of the potential increased risk of myocardial infarction, AVANDAMET is available only through a restricted distribution program called the AVANDIA-Rosiglitazone Medicines Access Program. Both prescribers and patients need to enroll in the program. To enroll, call 1-800-AVANDIA or visit www.AVANDIA.com. *[See Warnings and Precautions (5.4).]***

Metformin hydrochloride: **LACTIC ACIDOSIS**

- **Lactic acidosis can occur due to metformin accumulation. The risk increases with conditions such as sepsis, dehydration, excess alcohol intake, hepatic insufficiency, renal impairment and acute congestive heart failure. (5.1)**
- **Symptoms include malaise, myalgias, respiratory distress, increasing somnolence and nonspecific abdominal distress. Laboratory abnormalities include low pH, increased anion gap and elevated blood lactate. (5.1)**
- **If acidosis is suspected, discontinue AVANDAMET and hospitalize the patient immediately. (5.1)**

RECENT MAJOR CHANGES

Boxed Warning	02/2011
Indications and Usage (1)	02/2011
Dosage and Administration (2)	02/2011
Warnings and Precautions, Cardiac Failure (5.2)	02/2011

Warnings and Precautions, Major Adverse Cardiovascular Events (5.3) 02/2011
Warnings and Precautions, Rosiglitazone REMS Program (5.4) 05/2011
Warnings and Precautions, Fractures (5.9) 02/2011

INDICATIONS AND USAGE

AVANDAMET is a combination antidiabetic product containing a thiazolidinedione and a biguanide. After consultation with a healthcare professional who has considered and advised the patient of the risks and benefits of rosiglitazone, this drug is indicated as an adjunct to diet and exercise to improve glycemic control when treatment with both rosiglitazone and metformin is appropriate in adults with type 2 diabetes mellitus who either are:

- already taking rosiglitazone, or
- not already taking rosiglitazone and are unable to achieve glycemic control on other diabetes medications and, in consultation with their healthcare provider, have decided not to take pioglitazone (ACTOS) or pioglitazone-containing products (ACTOPLUS MET®, ACTOPLUS MET XR®, DUETACT®) for medical reasons. (1)

Other Important Limitations of Use:

- Should not be used in patients with type 1 diabetes or for the treatment of diabetic ketoacidosis. (1)
- Coadministration with insulin is not recommended. (1, 5.2, 5.3)

DOSAGE AND ADMINISTRATION

- Individualize the starting dose based on the patient's current regimen. (2.1)
- Dose increases should be accompanied by careful monitoring for adverse events related to fluid retention. (2.1)
- Give in divided doses with meals with gradual dose escalation to reduce the gastrointestinal side effects. (2.2)
- Do not exceed the maximum recommended daily dose of 8 mg rosiglitazone and 2,000 mg metformin. (2.3)
- Do not initiate if the patient exhibits clinical evidence of active liver disease or increased serum transaminase levels. (2.4)

DOSAGE FORMS AND STRENGTHS

Oval, film-coated tablets containing rosiglitazone/metformin hydrochloride: 2 mg/500 mg, 4 mg/500 mg, 2 mg/1,000 mg, and 4 mg/1,000 mg (3)

CONTRAINDICATIONS

- Initiation in patients with established NYHA Class III or IV heart failure. (4)
- Use in significant renal disease or renal dysfunction. (4)
- Use in acute or chronic metabolic acidosis. (4)
- Use in patients undergoing radiologic studies involving intravascular administration of iodinated contrast materials. (4, 5.1)

WARNINGS AND PRECAUTIONS

- Fluid retention, which may exacerbate or lead to heart failure, may occur. Combination use with insulin and use in congestive heart failure NYHA Class I and II may increase risk of other cardiovascular effects. (5.2)
- Increased risk of myocardial infarction has been observed in a meta-analysis of 52 clinical trials of rosiglitazone (incidence rate 0.4% versus 0.3%). (5.3)
- Coadministration with insulin is not recommended. (1, 5.2, 5.3)
- Assess renal function before starting therapy and at least annually. (5.1)
- Avoid use in patients with evidence of hepatic disease. (2.4, 5.1)
- Warn patients against excessive alcohol intake. (5.1)
- Promptly evaluate patients who develop laboratory abnormalities or clinical illness for evidence of ketoacidosis or lactic acidosis. (5.1)
- Dose-related edema (5.5), weight gain (5.6), and anemia (5.10) may occur.
- Macular edema has been reported. (5.8)
- Increased incidence of bone fracture. (5.9)
- Measure hematologic parameters annually. (5.10)

ADVERSE REACTIONS

The most common adverse reactions (≥10%) include nausea/vomiting, diarrhea, headache, and dyspepsia. (6.1)

To report SUSPECTED ADVERSE REACTIONS, contact GlaxoSmithKline at 1-888-825-5249 or FDA at 1-800-FDA-1088 or www.fda.gov/medwatch.

DRUG INTERACTIONS

- Inhibitors of CYP2C8 (e.g., gemfibrozil) may increase rosiglitazone levels. (7.1)
- Inducers of CYP2C8 (e.g., rifampin) may decrease rosiglitazone levels. (7.1)
- Cationic drugs eliminated by renal tubular secretion; use with caution. (7.2)

USE IN SPECIFIC POPULATIONS

- Do not use during pregnancy. No human or animal data. (8.1)
- Safety and effectiveness in children under 18 years have not been established. (8.4)
- Because reduced renal function is associated with increasing age, use with caution in elderly patients. (8.5)

See 17 for PATIENT COUNSELING INFORMATION and Medication Guide

Revised: 05/2011

FULL PRESCRIBING INFORMATION: CONTENTS*

*** Sections or subsections omitted from the full prescribing information are not listed**

FULL PRESCRIBING INFORMATION

WARNINGS

***Rosiglitazone maleate:* CONGESTIVE HEART FAILURE AND MYOCARDIAL INFARCTION**

- Thiazolidinediones, including rosiglitazone, cause or exacerbate congestive heart failure in some patients *[see Warnings and Precautions (5.2)]*. After initiation of AVANDAMET, and after dose increases, observe patients carefully for signs and symptoms of heart failure (including excessive, rapid weight gain, dyspnea, and/or edema). If these signs and symptoms develop, the heart failure should be managed according to current standards of care. Furthermore, discontinuation or dose reduction of AVANDAMET must be considered.
- AVANDAMET is not recommended in patients with symptomatic heart failure. Initiation of AVANDAMET in patients with established NYHA Class III or IV heart failure is contraindicated. *[See Contraindications (4) and Warnings and Precautions (5.2).]*
- A meta-analysis of 52 clinical trials (mean duration 6 months; 16,995 total patients), most of which compared rosiglitazone to placebo, showed rosiglitazone to be associated with an increased risk of myocardial infarction. Three other trials (mean duration 46 months; 14,067 total patients), comparing rosiglitazone to some other approved oral antidiabetic agents or placebo, showed a statistically non-significant increased risk of myocardial infarction, and a statistically non-significant decreased risk of death. There have been no clinical trials directly comparing cardiovascular risk of rosiglitazone and ACTOS® (pioglitazone, another thiazolidinedione), but in a separate trial, pioglitazone (when compared to placebo) did not show an increased risk of myocardial infarction or death. *[See Warnings and Precautions (5.3).]*
- Because of the potential increased risk of myocardial infarction, AVANDAMET is available only through a restricted distribution program called the AVANDIA-Rosiglitazone Medicines Access Program. Both prescribers and patients need to enroll in the program. To enroll, call 1-800-AVANDIA or visit www.AVANDIA.com. *[See Warnings and Precautions (5.4).]*

***Metformin hydrochloride:* LACTIC ACIDOSIS**

- Lactic acidosis is a rare, but serious complication that can occur due to metformin accumulation. The risk increases with conditions such as sepsis, dehydration, excess alcohol intake, hepatic insufficiency, renal impairment, and acute congestive heart failure. *[See Warnings and Precautions (5.1).]*
- Symptoms include malaise, myalgias, respiratory distress, increasing somnolence, and nonspecific abdominal distress. Laboratory abnormalities include low pH, increased anion gap and elevated blood lactate. *[See Warnings and Precautions (5.1).]*
- If acidosis is suspected, discontinue AVANDAMET and hospitalize the patient immediately *[see Warnings and Precautions (5.1)]*.

1 INDICATIONS AND USAGE

After consultation with a healthcare professional who has considered and advised the patient of the risks and benefits of rosiglitazone, AVANDAMET® is indicated as an adjunct to diet and exercise to improve glycemic control when treatment with both rosiglitazone and metformin is appropriate in adults with type 2 diabetes mellitus who either are:

- already taking rosiglitazone, or
- not already taking rosiglitazone and unable to achieve glycemic control on other diabetes medications and, in consultation with their healthcare provider, have decided not to take pioglitazone (ACTOS®) or pioglitazone-containing products (ACTOPLUS MET®, ACTOPLUS MET XR®, DUETACT®) for medical reasons.

Other Important Limitations of Use:

- Due to its mechanism of action, rosiglitazone is active only in the presence of endogenous insulin. Therefore, AVANDAMET should not be used in patients with type 1 diabetes.
- Coadministration of AVANDAMET with insulin is not recommended *[see Warnings and Precautions (5.2, 5.3)]*.

2 DOSAGE AND ADMINISTRATION

Prior to prescribing AVANDAMET, refer to *Indications and Usage (1)* for appropriate patient selection. Only prescribers enrolled in the AVANDIA-Rosiglitazone Medicines Access Program can prescribe AVANDAMET *[see Warnings and Precautions (5.4)]*.

2.1 Starting Dose

AVANDAMET is generally given in divided doses with meals.

All patients should start the rosiglitazone component of AVANDAMET at the lowest recommended dose. Further increases in the dose of rosiglitazone should be accompanied by careful monitoring for adverse events related to fluid retention *[see **Boxed Warning** and Warnings and Precautions (5.5)]*.

If therapy with a combination tablet containing rosiglitazone and metformin is considered appropriate for a patient with type 2 diabetes mellitus, then the selection of the dose of AVANDAMET should be based on the patient's current doses of rosiglitazone and/or metformin.

To switch to AVANDAMET for patients currently treated with metformin, the usual starting dose of AVANDAMET is 4 mg rosiglitazone (total daily dose) plus the dose of metformin already being taken (see Table 1).

To switch to AVANDAMET for patients currently treated with rosiglitazone, the usual starting dose of AVANDAMET is 1,000 mg metformin (total daily dose) plus the dose of rosiglitazone already being taken (see Table 1).

When switching from combination therapy of rosiglitazone plus metformin as separate tablets, the usual starting dose of AVANDAMET is the dose of rosiglitazone and metformin already being taken.

[See table 1 above]

2.2 Dose Titration

AVANDAMET is generally given in divided doses with meals, with gradual dose escalation. This reduces gastrointestinal side effects (largely due to metformin) and permits determination of the minimum effective dose for the individual patient.

Sufficient time should be given to assess adequacy of therapeutic response. FPG should be used initially to determine the therapeutic response to AVANDAMET. If additional glycemic control is needed, the daily dose of AVANDAMET may be increased by increments of 4 mg rosiglitazone and/or 500 mg metformin.

After an increase in metformin dosage, dose titration is recommended if patients are not adequately controlled after 1 to 2 weeks. After an increase in rosiglitazone dosage, dose titration is recommended if patients are not adequately controlled after 8 to 12 weeks.

2.3 Maximum Dose

The maximum recommended total daily dose of AVANDAMET is 8 mg rosiglitazone (taken as 4 mg twice daily) and 2,000 mg metformin (taken as 1,000 mg twice daily).

2.4 Specific Patient Populations

Renal Impairment: Any dosage adjustment should be based on a careful assessment of renal function. Generally, elderly, debilitated, and malnourished patients should not be titrated to the maximum dose of AVANDAMET. Monitoring of renal function is necessary to aid in prevention of metformin-associated lactic acidosis, particularly in the elderly *[see Warnings and Precautions (5.1)]*.

Hepatic Impairment: Liver enzymes should be measured prior to initiating treatment with AVANDAMET. Therapy with AVANDAMET should not be initiated if the patient exhibits clinical evidence of active liver disease or increased serum transaminase levels (ALT >2.5× upper limit of normal at start of therapy). After initiation of AVANDAMET, liver enzymes should be monitored periodically per the clinical judgment of the healthcare professional *[see Warnings and Precautions (5.7)] and Clinical Pharmacology (12.3)]*.

Geriatric: The initial and maintenance dosing of AVANDAMET should be conservative in patients with advanced age, due to the potential for decreased renal function in this population.

Pediatric: Safety and effectiveness of AVANDAMET in pediatric patients have not been established. AVANDAMET and rosiglitazone are not recommended for use in pediatric patients.

Pregnancy: AVANDAMET is not recommended for use in pregnancy.

Table 1. AVANDAMET Starting Dose for Patients Treated with Metformin and/or Rosiglitazone

PRIOR THERAPY	Usual AVANDAMET Starting Dose	
Total daily dose	Tablet strength	Number of tablets
Metformin[a]		
1,000 mg/day	2 mg/500 mg	1 tablet twice a day
2,000 mg/day	2 mg/1,000 mg	1 tablet twice a day
Rosiglitazone		
4 mg/day	2 mg/500 mg	1 tablet twice a day
8 mg/day	4 mg/500 mg	1 tablet twice a day

[a]For patients on doses of metformin between 1,000 and 2,000 mg/day, initiation of AVANDAMET requires individualization of therapy.

3 DOSAGE FORMS AND STRENGTHS

Each film-coated oval tablet contains rosiglitazone as the maleate and metformin hydrochloride as follows:

- 2 mg/500 mg – pale pink, debossed with gsk on one side and 2/500 on the other
- 4 mg/500 mg – orange, debossed with gsk on one side and 4/500 on the other
- 2 mg/1,000 mg – yellow, debossed with gsk on one side and 2/1000 on the other
- 4 mg/1,000 mg – pink, debossed with gsk on one side and 4/1000 on the other

4 CONTRAINDICATIONS

- Initiation in patients with established New York Heart Association (NYHA) Class III or IV heart failure *[see **Boxed Warning**]*.
- Use in patients with renal disease or renal dysfunction (e.g., as suggested by serum creatinine levels ≥1.5 mg/dL [males], ≥1.4 mg/dL [females], or abnormal creatinine clearance), which may also result from conditions such as cardiovascular collapse (shock), acute myocardial infarction, and septicemia *[see Warnings and Precautions (5.1)]*.
- Use in patients with acute or chronic metabolic acidosis, including diabetic ketoacidosis, with or without coma.
- Use in patients undergoing radiologic studies involving intravascular administration of iodinated contrast materials, because use of such products may result in acute alteration of renal function. AVANDAMET should be temporarily discontinued in these patients. *[See Warnings and Precautions (5.1).]*

5 WARNINGS AND PRECAUTIONS

5.1 Lactic Acidosis

Incidence and Management: Lactic acidosis is a rare, but serious, metabolic complication that can occur due to metformin accumulation during treatment with AVANDAMET; when it occurs, it is fatal in approximately 50% of cases. Lactic acidosis may also occur in association with a number of pathophysiologic conditions, including diabetes mellitus, and whenever there is significant tissue hypoperfusion and hypoxemia. Lactic acidosis is characterized by elevated blood lactate levels (>5 mmol/L), decreased blood pH, electrolyte disturbances with an increased anion gap, and an increased lactate/pyruvate ratio. When metformin is implicated as the cause of lactic acidosis, metformin plasma levels >5 mcg/mL are generally found.

The reported incidence of lactic acidosis in patients receiving metformin is very low (approximately 0.03 cases/1,000 patient years of exposure, with approximately 0.015 fatal cases/1,000 patient years of exposure). Reported cases have occurred primarily in diabetic patients with significant renal insufficiency, including both intrinsic renal disease and renal hypoperfusion, often in the setting of multiple concomitant medical/surgical problems and multiple concomitant medications. Patients with congestive heart failure requiring pharmacologic management, in particular those with unstable or acute congestive heart failure who are at risk of hypoperfusion and hypoxemia, are at increased risk of lactic acidosis. The risk of lactic acidosis increases with the degree of renal dysfunction and the patient's age. The risk of lactic acidosis may, therefore, be significantly decreased by regular monitoring of renal function in patients taking AVANDAMET and by use of the minimum effective dose of AVANDAMET. In particular, treatment of the elderly should be accompanied by careful monitoring of renal function. Treatment with AVANDAMET should not be initiated in patients ≥80 years of age unless measurement of creatinine clearance demonstrates that renal function is not reduced, as these patients are more susceptible to developing lactic acidosis. In addition, AVANDAMET should be promptly withheld in the presence of any condition associated with hypoxemia, dehydration, or sepsis. Because impaired hepatic function may significantly limit the ability to clear lactate, AVANDAMET should generally be avoided in patients with clinical or laboratory evidence of hepatic disease. Patients should be cautioned against excessive alcohol intake, either acute or chronic, when taking AVANDAMET, since alcohol potentiates the effects of metformin on lactate metabolism. In addition, AVANDAMET should be temporarily discontinued prior to any intravascular radiocontrast study and for any surgical procedure.

The onset of lactic acidosis often is subtle, and accompanied only by nonspecific symptoms such as malaise, myalgias, respiratory distress, increasing somnolence, and nonspecific abdominal distress. There may be associated hypothermia, hypotension, and resistant bradyarrhythmias with more marked acidosis. The patient and the patient's physician must be aware of the possible importance of such symptoms and the patient should be instructed to notify the physician immediately if they occur. AVANDAMET should be withdrawn until the situation is clarified. Serum electrolytes, ketones, blood glucose and, if indicated, blood pH, lactate levels, and even blood metformin levels may be useful. Once a patient is stabilized on any dose level of AVANDAMET, gastrointestinal symptoms, which are common during initiation of therapy, are unlikely to be drug related. Later occurrence of gastrointestinal symptoms could be due to lactic acidosis or other serious disease.

Levels of fasting venous plasma lactate above the upper limit of normal but less than 5 mmol/L in patients taking AVANDAMET do not necessarily indicate impending lactic acidosis and may be explainable by other mechanisms, such as poorly controlled diabetes or obesity, vigorous physical activity or technical problems in sample handling.

Lactic acidosis should be suspected in any diabetic patient with metabolic acidosis lacking evidence of ketoacidosis (ketonuria and ketonemia).

Lactic acidosis is a medical emergency that must be treated in a hospital setting. In a patient with lactic acidosis who is taking AVANDAMET, the drug should be discontinued immediately and general supportive measures promptly instituted. Because metformin is dialyzable (with a clearance of up to 170 mL/min under good hemodynamic conditions), prompt hemodialysis is recommended to correct the acidosis and remove the accumulated metformin. Such management often results in prompt reversal of symptoms and recovery *[see Contraindications (4)]*.

Factors That May Predispose Patients to Lactic Acidosis:

Assessment of Renal Function: Metformin is known to be substantially excreted by the kidney, and the risk of metformin accumulation and lactic acidosis increases with the degree of impairment of renal function. Thus, patients with serum creatinine levels above the upper limit of normal for their age should not receive AVANDAMET. In patients with advanced age, AVANDAMET should be carefully titrated to establish the minimum dose for adequate glycemic effect, because aging is associated with reduced renal function. *[See Dosage and Administration (2.4) and Use in Specific Populations (8.5).]*

Before initiation of therapy with AVANDAMET and at least annually thereafter, renal function should be assessed and verified as normal. In patients in whom development of renal dysfunction is anticipated, renal function should be assessed more frequently and AVANDAMET discontinued if evidence of renal impairment is present.

Medications That Affect Renal Function: Concomitant medication(s) that may affect renal function or result in significant hemodynamic change or may interfere with the disposition of metformin, such as cationic drugs that are eliminated by renal tubular secretion *[see Drug Interactions (7.2) and Clinical Pharmacology (12.4)]*, should be used with caution.

Hypoxic States: Cardiovascular collapse (shock) from whatever cause, acute congestive heart failure, acute myocardial infarction, and other conditions characterized by hypoxemia have been associated with lactic acidosis and may also cause prerenal azotemia. When such events occur in patients receiving AVANDAMET, the drug should be promptly discontinued.

Radiologic Studies With Intravascular Iodinated Contrast Materials: Intravascular contrast studies with iodinated materials can lead to acute alteration of renal function and have been associated with lactic acidosis in patients receiving metformin *[see Contraindications (4)]*. Therefore, in patients in whom any such study is planned, AVANDAMET should be temporarily discontinued at the time of or prior to the procedure, and withheld for 48 hours subsequent to the procedure and reinstituted only after renal function has been re-evaluated and found to be normal.

Surgical Procedures: Use of AVANDAMET should be temporarily suspended for any surgical procedure (except minor procedures not associated with restricted intake of food and fluids) and should not be restarted until the patient's oral intake has resumed and renal function has been evaluated as normal.

Alcohol Intake: Alcohol potentiates the effect of metformin on lactate metabolism. Patients, therefore, should be warned against excessive alcohol intake, acute or chronic, while receiving AVANDAMET.

Change in Clinical Status of Patients With Previously Controlled Diabetes: A patient with type 2 diabetes previously well-controlled on AVANDAMET who develops laboratory abnormalities or clinical illness (especially vague and poorly defined illness) should be evaluated promptly for evidence of ketoacidosis or lactic acidosis. Evaluation should include serum electrolytes and ketones, blood glucose and, if indicated, blood pH, lactate, pyruvate, and metformin levels. If acidosis of either form occurs, AVANDAMET must be stopped immediately and other appropriate corrective measures initiated.

[See also Warnings and Precautions (5.7).]

5.2 Cardiac Failure

Rosiglitazone, like other thiazolidinediones, alone or in combination with other antidiabetic agents, can cause fluid re-

tention, which may exacerbate or lead to heart failure. Patients should be observed for signs and symptoms of heart failure. If these signs and symptoms develop, the heart failure should be managed according to current standards of care. Furthermore, discontinuation or dose reduction of rosiglitazone must be considered *[see **Boxed Warning**]*.
Patients with congestive heart failure (CHF) NYHA Class I and II treated with rosiglitazone have an increased risk of cardiovascular events. A 52-week, double-blind, placebo-controlled echocardiographic trial was conducted in 224 patients with type 2 diabetes mellitus and NYHA Class I or II CHF (ejection fraction ≤45%) on background antidiabetic and CHF therapy. An independent committee conducted a blinded evaluation of fluid-related events (including congestive heart failure) and cardiovascular hospitalizations according to predefined criteria (adjudication). Separate from the adjudication, other cardiovascular adverse events were reported by investigators. Although no treatment difference in change from baseline of ejection fractions was observed, more cardiovascular adverse events were observed with rosiglitazone treatment compared to placebo during the 52-week trial. (See Table 2.)

Table 2. Emergent Cardiovascular Adverse Events in Patients With Congestive Heart Failure (NYHA Class I and II) Treated With Rosiglitazone or Placebo (in Addition to Background Antidiabetic and CHF Therapy)

Events	**Rosiglitazone**	**Placebo**
	N = 110 n (%)	N = 114 n (%)
Adjudicated		
Cardiovascular deaths	5 (5%)	4 (4%)
CHF worsening	7 (6%)	4 (4%)
– with overnight hospitalization	5 (5%)	4 (4%)
– without overnight hospitalization	2 (2%)	0 (0%)
New or worsening edema	28 (25%)	10 (9%)
New or worsening dyspnea	29 (26%)	19 (17%)
Increases in CHF medication	36 (33%)	20 (18%)
Cardiovascular hospitalization[a]	21 (19%)	15 (13%)
Investigator-reported, non-adjudicated		
Ischemic adverse events	10 (9%)	5 (4%)
– Myocardial infarction	5 (5%)	2 (2%)
– Angina	6 (5%)	3 (3%)

[a]Includes hospitalization for any cardiovascular reason.

Initiation of AVANDAMET in patients with established NYHA Class III or IV heart failure is contraindicated. AVANDAMET is not recommended in patients with symptomatic heart failure. *[See **Boxed Warning**.]*
Patients experiencing acute coronary syndromes have not been studied in controlled clinical trials. In view of the potential for development of heart failure in patients having an acute coronary event, initiation of AVANDAMET is not recommended for patients experiencing an acute coronary event, and discontinuation of AVANDAMET during this acute phase should be considered.
Patients with NYHA Class III and IV cardiac status (with or without CHF) have not been studied in controlled clinical trials. AVANDAMET is not recommended in patients with NYHA Class III and IV cardiac status.
Congestive Heart Failure During Coadministration of Rosiglitazone With Insulin: In trials in which rosiglitazone was added to insulin, rosiglitazone increased the risk of congestive heart failure. Coadministration of rosiglitazone and insulin is not recommended. *[See Indications and Usage (1) and Warnings and Precautions (5.3).]*
In 7 controlled, randomized, double-blind trials which had durations from 16 to 26 weeks and which were included in a meta-analysis[1]*[see Warnings and Precautions (5.3)]*, patients with type 2 diabetes mellitus were randomized to coadministration of rosiglitazone and insulin (N = 1,018) or insulin (N = 815). In these 7 trials, rosiglitazone was added to insulin. These trials included patients with long-standing diabetes (median duration of 12 years) and a high prevalence of pre-existing medical conditions, including peripheral neuropathy, retinopathy, ischemic heart disease, vascular disease, and congestive heart failure. The total number of patients with emergent congestive heart failure was 23 (2.3%) and 8 (1.0%) in the rosiglitazone plus insulin and insulin groups, respectively.
Heart Failure in Observational Studies of Elderly Diabetic Patients Comparing Rosiglitazone to Pioglitazone: Three observational studies[2-4] in elderly diabetic patients (age 65 years and older) found that rosiglitazone statistically significantly increased the risk of hospitalized heart failure compared to use of pioglitazone. One other observational study[5] in patients with a mean age of 54 years, which also included an analysis in a subpopulation of patients >65 years of age, found no statistically significant increase in emergency department visits or hospitalization for heart failure in patients treated with rosiglitazone compared to pioglitazone in the older subgroup.

5.3 Major Adverse Cardiovascular Events

Cardiovascular adverse events have been evaluated in a meta-analysis of 52 clinical trials, in long-term, prospective, randomized, controlled trials, and in observational studies.
Meta-Analysis of Major Adverse Cardiovascular Events in a Group of 52 Clinical Trials: A meta-analysis was conducted retrospectively to assess cardiovascular adverse events reported across 52 double-blind, randomized, controlled clinical trials (mean duration 6 months).[1] These trials had been conducted to assess glucose-lowering efficacy in type 2 diabetes. Prospectively planned adjudication of cardiovascular events did not occur in most of the trials. Some trials were placebo-controlled and some used active oral antidiabetic drugs as controls. Placebo-controlled trials included monotherapy trials (monotherapy with rosiglitazone versus placebo monotherapy) and add-on trials (rosiglitazone or placebo, added to sulfonylurea, metformin, or insulin). Active control trials included monotherapy trials (monotherapy with rosiglitazone versus sulfonylurea or metformin monotherapy) and add-on trials (rosiglitazone plus sulfonylurea or rosiglitazone plus metformin, versus sulfonylurea plus metformin). A total of 16,995 patients were included (10,039 in treatment groups containing rosiglitazone, 6,956 in comparator groups), with 5,167 patient-years of exposure to rosiglitazone and 3,637 patient-years of exposure to comparator. Cardiovascular events occurred more frequently for patients who received rosiglitazone than for patients who received comparators (see Table 3).

Table 3. Occurrence of Cardiovascular Events in a Meta-Analysis of 52 Clinical Trials

Event[a]	**Rosiglitazone (N=10,039) n (%)**	**Comparator (N=6,956) n (%)**
MACE (a composite of myocardial infarction, cardiovascular death, or stroke)	70 (0.7)	39 (0.6)
Myocardial Infarction	45 (0.4)	20 (0.3)
Cardiovascular Death	17 (0.2)	9 (0.1)
Stroke	18 (0.2)	16 (0.2)
All-cause Death	29 (0.3)	17 (0.2)

[a] Events are not exclusive: i.e., a patient with a cardiovascular death due to a myocardial infarction would be counted in 4 event categories (myocardial infarction; myocardial infarction, cardiovascular death, or stroke; cardiovascular death; all-cause death).

In this analysis, a statistically significant increased risk of myocardial infarction with rosiglitazone versus pooled comparators was observed. Analyses were performed using a composite of major adverse cardiovascular events (myocardial infarction, stroke, and cardiovascular death), referred to hereafter as MACE. Rosiglitazone had a statistically non-significant increased risk of MACE compared to the pooled comparators. A statistically significant increased risk of myocardial infarction and statistically non-significant increased risk of MACE with rosiglitazone was observed in the placebo-controlled trials. In the active-controlled trials, there was no increased risk of myocardial infarction or MACE. (See Figure 1 and Table 4.)

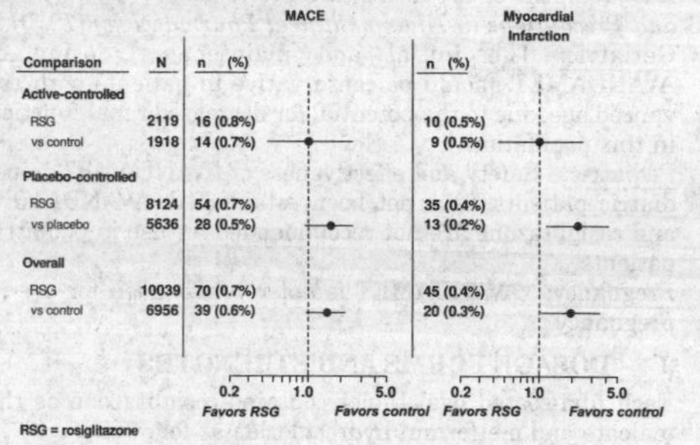

Figure 1. Forest Plot of Odds Ratios (95% Confidence Intervals) for MACE and Myocardial Infarction in the Meta-Analysis of 52 Clinical Trials

[See table 4 below]
Of the placebo-controlled trials in the meta-analysis, 7 trials had patients randomized to rosiglitazone plus insulin or insulin. There were more patients in the rosiglitazone plus insulin group compared to the insulin group with myocardial infarctions, MACE, cardiovascular deaths, and all-cause deaths (see Table 5). The total number of patients with stroke was 5 (0.5%) and 4 (0.5%) in the rosiglitazone plus insulin and insulin groups, respectively. The use of rosiglitazone in combination with insulin may increase the risk of myocardial infarction *[See Warnings and Precautions (5.1).]*
[See table 5 at top of next page]
Myocardial Infarction Events in Large, Long-Term, Prospective, Randomized, Controlled Trials of Rosiglitazone: Data from 3 large, long-term, prospective, randomized, controlled clinical trials of rosiglitazone were assessed separately from the meta-analysis.[6-8] These 3 trials included a total of 14,067 patients (treatment groups containing rosiglitazone N = 6,311; comparator groups N = 7,756), with patient-year exposure of 24,534 patient-years for rosiglitazone and 28,882 patient-years for comparator. Patient populations in the trials included patients with impaired glucose tolerance, patients with type 2 diabetes who were initiating oral agent monotherapy, and patients with type 2 diabetes who had failed monotherapy and were initiating dual oral agent therapy. Duration of follow-up exceeded 3 years in each trial.
In each of these trials, there was a statistically non-significant increase in the risk of myocardial infarction for rosiglitazone versus comparator medications.
In a long-term, randomized, placebo-controlled, 2×2 factorial trial intended to evaluate rosiglitazone, and separately ramipril (an angiotensin converting enzyme inhibitor [ACEI]), on progression to overt diabetes in 5,269 subjects with glucose intolerance, the incidence of myocardial infarction was higher in the subset of subjects who received rosiglitazone in combination with ramipril than among sub-

Table 4. Occurrence of MACE and Myocardial Infarction in a Meta-Analysis of 52 Clinical Trials by Trial Type

			MACE		**Myocardial Infarction**	
		N	n (%)	OR (95%CI)	n (%)	OR (95%CI)
Active-Controlled Trials	RSG	2,119	16 (0.8%)	1.05	10 (0.5%)	1.00
	Control	1,918	14 (0.7%)	(0.48, 2.34)	9 (0.5%)	(0.36, 2.82)
Placebo-Controlled Trials	RSG	8,124	54 (0.7%)	1.53	35 (0.4%)	2.23
	Placebo	5,636	28 (0.5%)	(0.94, 2.54)	13 (0.2%)	(1.14, 4.64)
Overall	RSG	10,039	70 (0.7%)	1.44	45 (0.4%)	1.8
	Control	6,956	39 (0.6%)	(0.95, 2.20)	20 (0.3%)	(1.03, 3.25)

RSG = rosiglitazone

jects who received ramipril alone but not in the subset of subjects who received rosiglitazone alone compared to placebo.[6] The higher incidence of myocardial infarction among subjects who received rosiglitazone in combination with ramipril was not confirmed in the two other large (total N = 8,798) long-term, randomized, active-controlled clinical trials conducted in patients with type 2 diabetes, in which 30% and 40% of patients in the two trials reported angiotensin-converting enzyme inhibitor use at baseline.[7,8]

There have been no adequately designed clinical trials directly comparing rosiglitazone to pioglitazone on cardiovascular risks. However, in a long-term, randomized, placebo-controlled cardiovascular outcomes trial comparing pioglitazone to placebo in patients with type 2 diabetes mellitus and prior macrovascular disease, pioglitazone was not associated with an increased risk of myocardial infarction or total mortality.[9]

The increased risk of myocardial infarction observed in the meta-analysis and large, long-term controlled clinical trials, and the increased risk of MACE observed in the meta-analysis described above, have not translated into a consistent finding of excess mortality from controlled clinical trials or observational studies. Clinical trials have not shown any difference between rosiglitazone and comparator medications in overall mortality or CV-related mortality.

Mortality in Observational Studies of Rosiglitazone Compared to Pioglitazone: Three observational studies in elderly diabetic patients (age 65 years and older) found that rosiglitazone statistically significantly increased the risk of all-cause mortality compared to use of pioglitazone.[2-4] One observational study[5] in patients with a mean age of 54 years found no difference in all-cause mortality between patients treated with rosiglitazone compared to pioglitazone and reported similar results in the subpopulation of patients >65 years of age. One additional small, prospective, observational study[10] found no statistically significant differences for CV mortality and all-cause mortality in patients treated with rosiglitazone compared to pioglitazone.

5.4 Rosiglitazone REMS (Risk Evaluation and Mitigation Strategy) Program

Because of the potential increased risk of myocardial infarction, AVANDAMET is available only through a restricted distribution program called the AVANDIA-Rosiglitazone Medicines Access Program *[see Indications and Usage (1)]*. Both prescribers and patients must enroll in the program to be able to prescribe or receive AVANDAMET, respectively. AVANDAMET will be available only from specially certified pharmacies participating in the program. As part of the program, prescribers will be educated about the potential increased risk of myocardial infarction and the need to limit the use of AVANDAMET to eligible patients. Prescribers will need to discuss with patients the risks and benefits of taking AVANDAMET. To enroll, call 1-800-AVANDIA or visit www.AVANDIA.com.

5.5 Edema

AVANDAMET should be used with caution in patients with edema. In a clinical trial in healthy volunteers who received rosiglitazone 8 mg once daily for 8 weeks, there was a statistically significant increase in median plasma volume compared to placebo. Since thiazolidinediones, including rosiglitazone, can cause fluid retention, which can exacerbate or lead to congestive heart failure, AVANDAMET should be used with caution in patients at risk for heart failure. Patients should be monitored for signs and symptoms of heart failure *[see **Boxed Warning**, Warnings and Precautions (5.2), and Patient Counseling Information (17.1)]*.

In controlled clinical trials of patients with type 2 diabetes, mild to moderate edema was reported in patients treated with rosiglitazone, and may be dose-related. Patients with ongoing edema were more likely to have adverse events associated with edema if started on combination therapy with insulin and rosiglitazone *[see Adverse Reactions (6.1)]*. The use of AVANDAMET in combination with insulin is not recommended. *[See Warnings and Precautions (5.2, 5.3).]*

5.6 Weight Gain

Dose-related weight gain was seen with rosiglitazone alone and rosiglitazone together with other hypoglycemic agents (see Table 6). No overall change in median weight was observed with AVANDAMET in drug-naïve patients. The mechanism of weight gain with rosiglitazone is unclear but probably involves a combination of fluid retention and fat accumulation.

[See table 6 above]

In a 4- to 6-year, monotherapy, comparative trial (ADOPT) in patients recently diagnosed with type 2 diabetes not previously treated with antidiabetic medication, the median weight change (25th, 75th percentiles) from baseline at 4 years was 3.5 kg (0.0, 8.1) for rosiglitazone, 2.0 kg (-1.0, 4.8) for glyburide, and -2.4 kg (-5.4, 0.5) for metformin.

In postmarketing experience with rosiglitazone alone or in combination with other hypoglycemic agents, there have been rare reports of unusually rapid increases in weight and increases in excess of that generally observed in clinical trials. Patients who experience such increases should be assessed for fluid accumulation and volume-related events such as excessive edema and congestive heart failure *[see **Boxed Warning**]*.

Table 5. Occurrence of Cardiovascular Events for Rosiglitazone in Combination With Insulin in a Meta-Analysis of 52 Clinical Trials

Event[a]	Rosiglitazone (N=1,018) (%)	Insulin (N = 815) (%)	OR (95% CI)
MACE (a composite of myocardial infarction, cardiovascular death, or stroke)	1.3	0.6	2.14 (0.70, 7.83)
Myocardial infarction	0.6	0.1	5.6 (0.67, 262.7)
Cardiovascular death	0.4	0.0	ND, (0.47, ∞)
All-cause death	0.6	0.2	2.19 (0.38, 22.61)

ND = not defined

[a] Events are not exclusive: i.e., a patient with a cardiovascular death due to a myocardial infarction would be counted in 4 event categories (myocardial infarction; myocardial infarction, cardiovascular death, or stroke; cardiovascular death; all-cause death).

Table 6. Weight Changes (kg) From Baseline at Endpoint During Clinical Trials [Median (25th, 75th, Percentile)]

Monotherapy

Duration	Control Group		Rosiglitazone 4 mg	Rosiglitazone 8 mg
26 weeks	Placebo	-0.9 (-2.8, 0.9) N = 210	1.0 (0.9, 3.6) N = 436	3.1 (1.1, 5.8) N = 439
52 weeks	Sulfonylurea	2.0 (0, 4.0) N = 173	2.0 (-0.6, 4.0) N = 150	2.6 (0, 5.3) N = 157

Combination Therapy

			Rosiglitazone + Control Therapy	
Duration	**Control Group**		**Rosiglitazone 4 mg**	**Rosiglitazone 8 mg**
24-26 weeks	Sulfonylurea	0 (-1.0, 1.3) N = 1,155	2.2 (0.5, 4.0) N = 613	3.5 (1.4, 5.9) N = 841
26 weeks	Metformin	-1.4 (-3.2, 0.2) N = 175	0.8 (-1.0, 2.6) N = 100	2.1 (0, 4.3) N = 184
26 weeks	Insulin	0.9 (-0.5, 2.7) N = 162	4.1 (1.4, 6.3) N = 164	5.4 (3.4, 7.3) N = 150

AVANDAMET + Insulin

Duration	Control Group		AVANDAMET + Insulin
24 weeks	Insulin	2.6 kg (0.3, 4.8) N = 145	3.3 kg (1.5, 6.0) N = 147

5.7 Hepatic Effects

Metformin: Since impaired hepatic function has been associated with some cases of lactic acidosis, AVANDAMET should generally be avoided in patients with clinical or laboratory evidence of hepatic disease.

Rosiglitazone: Liver enzymes should be measured prior to the initiation of therapy with AVANDAMET in all patients and periodically thereafter per the clinical judgment of the healthcare professional. Therapy with AVANDAMET should not be initiated in patients with increased baseline liver enzyme levels (ALT >2.5× upper limit of normal). Patients with mildly elevated liver enzymes (ALT levels ≤2.5× upper limit of normal) at baseline or during therapy with AVANDAMET should be evaluated to determine the cause of the liver enzyme elevation. Initiation of, or continuation of, therapy with AVANDAMET in patients with mild liver enzyme elevations should proceed with caution and include close clinical follow-up, including more frequent liver enzyme monitoring, to determine if the liver enzyme elevations resolve or worsen. If at any time ALT levels increase to >3× the upper limit of normal in patients on therapy with AVANDAMET, liver enzyme levels should be rechecked as soon as possible. If ALT levels remain >3× the upper limit of normal, therapy with AVANDAMET should be discontinued.

If any patient develops symptoms suggesting hepatic dysfunction, which may include unexplained nausea, vomiting, abdominal pain, fatigue, anorexia, and/or dark urine, liver enzymes should be checked. The decision whether to continue the patient on therapy with AVANDAMET should be guided by clinical judgment pending laboratory evaluations. If jaundice is observed, drug therapy should be discontinued.

In addition, if the presence of hepatic disease or hepatic dysfunction of sufficient magnitude to predispose to lactic acidosis is confirmed, therapy with AVANDAMET should be discontinued.

5.8 Macular Edema

Macular edema has been reported in postmarketing experience in some diabetic patients who were taking rosiglitazone or another thiazolidinedione. Some patients presented with blurred vision or decreased visual acuity, but some patients appear to have been diagnosed on routine ophthalmologic examination. Most patients had peripheral edema at the time macular edema was diagnosed. Some patients had improvement in their macular edema after discontinuation of their thiazolidinedione. Patients with diabetes should have regular eye exams by an ophthalmologist, per the Standards of Care of the American Diabetes Association. Additionally, any diabetic who reports any kind of visual symptom should be promptly referred to an ophthalmologist, regardless of the patient's underlying medications or other physical findings. *[See Adverse Reactions (6.3).]*

5.9 Fractures

In a 4- to 6-year comparative trial (ADOPT) of glycemic control with monotherapy in drug-naïve patients recently diagnosed with type 2 diabetes mellitus, an increased incidence of bone fracture was noted in female patients taking rosiglitazone. Over the 4- to 6-year period, the incidence of bone fracture in females was 9.3% (60/645) for rosiglitazone versus 3.5% (21/605) for glyburide and 5.1% (30/590) for metformin. This increased incidence was noted after the first year of treatment and persisted during the course of the trial. The majority of the fractures in the women who received rosiglitazone occurred in the upper arm, hand, and foot. These sites of fracture are different from those usually associated with postmenopausal osteoporosis (e.g., hip or spine). Other trials suggest that this risk may also apply to men, although the risk of fracture among women appears higher than that among men. The risk of fracture should be considered in the care of patients treated with rosiglitazone, and attention given to assessing and maintaining bone health according to current standards of care.

Table 7. Adverse Events (≥5% for Rosiglitazone Plus Metformin) Reported by Patients in 26-week Double-blind Clinical Trials of Rosiglitazone Added to Metformin Therapy

	Rosiglitazone + Metformin	Rosiglitazone	Placebo	Metformin
	N = 338	N = 2,526	N = 601	N = 225
Preferred term	%	%	%	%
Upper respiratory tract infection	16.0	9.9	8.7	8.9
Diarrhea	12.7	2.3	3.3	15.6
Injury	8.0	7.6	4.3	7.6
Anemia	7.1	1.9	0.7	2.2
Headache	6.5	5.9	5.0	8.9
Sinusitis	6.2	3.2	4.5	5.3
Fatigue	5.9	3.6	5.0	4.0
Back pain	5.0	4.0	3.8	4.0
Viral infection	5.0	3.2	4.0	3.6
Arthralgia	5.0	3.0	4.0	2.2

Table 8. On-Therapy Adverse Events (≥5 Events/100 Patient-Years [PY]) in Any Treatment Group Reported in a 4- to 6-Year Clinical Trial of Rosiglitazone as Monotherapy (ADOPT)

	Rosiglitazone	Glyburide	Metformin
	N = 1,456	N = 1,441	N = 1,454
	PY = 4,954	PY = 4,244	PY = 4,906
Nasopharyngitis	6.3	6.9	6.6
Back pain	5.1	4.9	5.3
Arthralgia	5.0	4.8	4.2
Hypertension	4.4	6.0	6.1
Upper respiratory tract infection	4.3	5.0	4.7
Hypoglycemia	2.9	13.0	3.4
Diarrhea	2.5	3.2	6.8

5.10 Hematologic Effects

Decreases in mean hemoglobin and hematocrit occurred in a dose-related fashion in adult patients treated with rosiglitazone *[see Adverse Reactions (6.2)]*. The observed changes may be related to the increased plasma volume observed with treatment with rosiglitazone and may be dose-related. The decrease in hemoglobin was seen more frequently in combination rosiglitazone and metformin therapy than in rosiglitazone therapy alone. Vitamin B_{12} deficiency may contribute to the observed reductions in hemoglobin *[see Warnings and Precautions (5.11)]*. Initial and periodic monitoring of hematologic parameters (e.g., hemoglobin/hematocrit and red blood cell indices) should be performed, at least on an annual basis.

5.11 Vitamin B12 Levels

In controlled clinical trials of metformin of 29 weeks' duration, a decrease to subnormal levels of previously normal serum vitamin B_{12} levels, without clinical manifestations, was observed in approximately 7% of patients. Such decrease, possibly due to interference with B_{12} absorption from the B_{12}-intrinsic factor complex, is, however, very rarely associated with anemia and appears to be rapidly reversible with discontinuation of metformin or vitamin B_{12} supplementation. Certain individuals (those with inadequate vitamin B_{12} or calcium intake or absorption) appear to be predisposed to developing subnormal vitamin B_{12} levels. In these patients, routine serum vitamin B_{12} measurements at 2- to 3-year intervals may be useful. Vitamin B_{12} deficiency should be excluded if megaloblastic anemia is suspected. *[See Warnings and Precautions (5.10).]*

5.12 Diabetes and Blood Glucose Control

Periodic fasting blood glucose and HbA1c measurements should be performed to monitor therapeutic response.

When a patient stabilized on any diabetic regimen is exposed to stress such as fever, trauma, infection, or surgery, a temporary loss of glycemic control may occur. At such times, it may be necessary to withhold AVANDAMET and temporarily administer insulin. AVANDAMET may be reinstituted after the acute episode is resolved.

Hypoglycemia does not occur in patients receiving metformin alone under usual circumstances of use but could occur when caloric intake is deficient, when strenuous exercise is not compensated by caloric supplementation, or during concomitant use with hypoglycemic agents (such as sulfonylureas or insulin) or ethanol. Elderly, debilitated or malnourished patients, and those with adrenal or pituitary insufficiency or alcohol intoxication are particularly susceptible to hypoglycemic effects. Hypoglycemia may be difficult to recognize in the elderly and in people who are taking β-adrenergic blocking drugs.

Patients receiving rosiglitazone in combination with other hypoglycemic agents may be at risk for hypoglycemia, and a reduction in the dose of the concomitant agent may be necessary.

5.13 Ovulation

Therapy with rosiglitazone, like other thiazolidinediones, may result in ovulation in some premenopausal anovulatory women. As a result, these patients may be at an increased risk for pregnancy while taking AVANDAMET *[see Use in Specific Populations (8.1)]*. Thus, adequate contraception in premenopausal women should be recommended. This possible effect has not been specifically investigated in clinical trials; therefore, the frequency of this occurrence is not known.

Although hormonal imbalance has been seen in preclinical studies *[see Nonclinical Toxicology (13.1)]*, the clinical significance of this finding is not known. If unexpected menstrual dysfunction occurs, the benefits of continued therapy with AVANDAMET should be reviewed.

6 ADVERSE REACTIONS

6.1 Clinical Trial Experience

Because clinical trials are conducted under widely varying conditions, adverse reaction rates observed in the clinical trials of a drug cannot be directly compared to rates in the clinical trials of another drug and may not reflect the rates observed in practice.

The incidence and types of adverse events reported in controlled, 26-week clinical trials of rosiglitazone administered in combination with metformin 2,500 mg/day in comparison to adverse reactions reported in association with rosiglitazone and metformin monotherapies are shown in Table 7. Overall, the types of adverse reactions without regard to causality reported when rosiglitazone was used in combination with metformin were similar to those reported during monotherapy with rosiglitazone.

[See table 7 above]

Reports of hypoglycemia in patients treated with rosiglitazone added to maximum metformin therapy in double-blind trials were more frequent (3.0%) than in patients treated with rosiglitazone (0.6%) or metformin monotherapies (1.3%) or placebo (0.2%). Overall, anemia and edema were generally mild to moderate in severity and usually did not require discontinuation of treatment with rosiglitazone.

Edema was reported in 4.8% of patients receiving rosiglitazone compared to 1.3% on placebo, and 2.2% on metformin monotherapy and 4.4% on rosiglitazone in combination with maximum doses of metformin.

Reports of anemia (7.1%) were greater in patients treated with rosiglitazone added to metformin compared to monotherapy with rosiglitazone. Lower pre-treatment hemoglobin/hematocrit levels in patients enrolled in the metformin and rosiglitazone combination therapy clinical trials may have contributed to the higher reporting rate of anemia in these trials *[see Adverse Reactions (6.2)]*.

Combination with Insulin: The incidence of hypoglycemia (confirmed by fingerstick blood glucose concentration ≤50 mg/dL) was 14% for patients on AVANDAMET plus insulin compared to 10% for patients on insulin monotherapy. The incidence of edema was 7% when insulin was added to AVANDAMET compared to 3% with insulin monotherapy. This trial excluded patients with pre-existing heart failure or new or worsening edema on AVANDAMET therapy. However, in 26-week double-blind, fixed-dose trials of rosiglitazone added to insulin, edema was reported with higher frequency (rosiglitazone in combination with insulin, 14.7%; insulin, 5.4%) *[see Warnings and Precautions (5.2)]*. In trials in which rosiglitazone was added to insulin, rosiglitazone increased the risk of congestive heart failure. The use of rosiglitazone in combination with insulin may increase the risk of myocardial infarction *[see Warnings and Precautions (5.2, 5.3)]*.

In a trial in which insulin was added to AVANDAMET, no myocardial ischemia was observed in the insulin group (N = 158), and no congestive heart failure was reported in either group. There was one myocardial ischemic event and one sudden death in the group receiving AVANDAMET plus insulin (N = 161). *[See Warnings and Precautions (5.2).]*

The incidence of anemia was 2% for AVANDAMET in combination with insulin compared to 1% for insulin monotherapy.

A long-term, 4- to 6-year trial (ADOPT) compared the use of rosiglitazone (n = 1,456), glyburide (n = 1,441), and metformin (n = 1,454) as monotherapy in patients recently diagnosed with type 2 diabetes who were not previously treated with antidiabetic medication. Table 8 presents adverse reactions without regard to causality; rates are expressed per 100 patient-years (PY) exposure to account for the differences in exposure to trial medication across the 3 treatment groups.

In ADOPT, fractures were reported in a greater number of women treated with rosiglitazone (9.3%, 2.7/100 patient-years) compared to glyburide (3.5%, 1.3/100 patient-years) or metformin (5.1%, 1.5/100 patient-years). The majority of the fractures in the women who received rosiglitazone were reported in the upper arm, hand, and foot. *[See Warnings and Precautions (5.9).]* The observed incidence of fractures for male patients was similar among the 3 treatment groups.

[See table 8 above]

6.2 Laboratory Abnormalities

Hematologic: Decreases in mean hemoglobin and hematocrit occurred in a dose-related fashion in adult patients treated with rosiglitazone (mean decreases in individual trials as much as 1.0 gram/dL hemoglobin and as much as 3.3% hematocrit). The changes occurred primarily during the first 3 months following initiation of rosiglitazone therapy or following an increase in rosiglitazone dose. The time course and magnitude of decreases were similar in patients treated with a combination of rosiglitazone and other hypoglycemic agents or monotherapy with rosiglitazone. Pretreatment levels of hemoglobin and hematocrit were lower in patients in metformin combination trials and may have contributed to the higher reporting rate of anemia. In a single trial in pediatric patients, decreases in hemoglobin and hematocrit (mean decreases of 0.29 g/dL and 0.95%, respectively) were reported with rosiglitazone. White blood cell counts also decreased slightly in adult patients treated with rosiglitazone. Decreases in hematologic parameters may be related to increased plasma volume observed with rosiglitazone treatment.

In controlled clinical trials of metformin of 29 weeks' duration, a decrease to subnormal levels of previously normal serum vitamin B_{12} levels, without clinical manifestations, was observed in approximately 7% of patients. Such a decrease, possibly due to interference with B_{12} absorption from the B_{12}-intrinsic factor complex, is, however, very rarely associated with anemia and appears to be rapidly reversible with discontinuation of metformin or vitamin B_{12} supplementation.

Lipids: Changes in serum lipids have been observed following treatment with rosiglitazone in adults *[see Clinical Pharmacology (12.2)]*.

Serum Transaminase Levels: In pre-approval clinical trials in 4,598 patients treated with rosiglitazone encompassing approximately 3,600 patient years of exposure, and in a long-term 4- to 6-year trial in 1,456 patients treated with rosiglitazone (4,954 patient-years exposure), there was no evidence of drug-induced hepatotoxicity.

In pre-approval controlled trials, 0.2% of patients treated with rosiglitazone had reversible elevations in ALT >3× the upper limit of normal compared to 0.2% on placebo and 0.5% on active comparators. The ALT elevations in patients treated with rosiglitazone were reversible. Hyperbilirubinemia was found in 0.3% of patients treated with rosiglitazone compared with 0.9% treated with placebo and 1% in patients treated with active comparators. In pre-approval clinical trials, there were no cases of idiosyncratic drug reactions leading to hepatic failure. *[See Warnings and Precautions (5.7).]*

In the 4- to 6-year ADOPT trial, patients treated with rosiglitazone (4,954 patient-years exposure), glyburide (4,244 patient-years exposure) or metformin (4,906 patient-years exposure) as monotherapy, had the same rate of ALT increase to >3× upper limit of normal (0.3 per 100 patient-years exposure).

6.3 Postmarketing Experience

In addition to adverse reactions reported from clinical trials, the events described below have been identified during post-approval use of AVANDAMET or its individual components. Because these events are reported voluntarily from a population of unknown size, it is not possible to reliably estimate their frequency or to always establish a causal relationship to drug exposure.

In patients receiving thiazolidinedione therapy, serious adverse events with or without a fatal outcome, potentially related to volume expansion (e.g., congestive heart failure, pulmonary edema, and pleural effusions) have been reported *[see* ***Boxed Warning*** *and Warnings and Precautions (5.2)]*.

There are postmarketing reports with rosiglitazone of hepatitis, hepatic enzyme elevations to 3 or more times the upper limit of normal, and hepatic failure with and without fatal outcome, although causality has not been established.

There are postmarketing reports with rosiglitazone of rash, pruritus, urticaria, angioedema, anaphylactic reaction, Stevens-Johnson syndrome, and new onset or worsening diabetic macular edema with decreased visual acuity *[see Warnings and Precautions (5.8)]*.

(See also GLUCOPHAGE® prescribing information.)

7 DRUG INTERACTIONS

7.1 Drugs Metabolized by Cytochrome P450

An inhibitor of CYP2C8 (e.g., gemfibrozil) may increase the AUC of rosiglitazone and an inducer of CYP2C8 (e.g., rifampin) may decrease the AUC of rosiglitazone. Therefore, if an inhibitor or an inducer of CYP2C8 is started or stopped during treatment with rosiglitazone, changes in diabetes treatment may be needed based upon clinical response. *[See Clinical Pharmacology (12.4).]*

7.2 Cationic Drugs

Although drug interactions for metformin with cationic drugs (e.g., amiloride, digoxin, morphine, procainamide, quinidine, quinine, ranitidine, triamterene, trimethoprim, and vancomycin) remain theoretical (except for cimetidine), careful patient monitoring and dose adjustment of AVANDAMET and/or the interfering drug is recommended in patients who are taking cationic medications that are excreted via the proximal renal tubular secretory system. *[See Warnings and Precautions (5.1) and Clinical Pharmacology (12.4).]*

7.3 Drugs That Produce Hyperglycemia

When drugs that produce hyperglycemia which may lead to loss of glycemic control are administered to a patient receiving AVANDAMET, the patient should be closely observed to maintain adequate glycemic control. *[See Clinical Pharmacology (12.4).]*

8 USE IN SPECIFIC POPULATIONS

8.1 Pregnancy

Pregnancy Category C.

All pregnancies have a background risk of birth defects, loss, or other adverse outcome regardless of drug exposure. This background risk is increased in pregnancies complicated by hyperglycemia and may be decreased with good metabolic control. It is essential for patients with diabetes or history of gestational diabetes to maintain good metabolic control before conception and throughout pregnancy. Careful monitoring of glucose control is essential in such patients. Most experts recommend that insulin monotherapy be used during pregnancy to maintain blood glucose levels as close to normal as possible. AVANDAMET should not be used during pregnancy.

Human Data: There are no adequate and well-controlled trials with AVANDAMET or its individual components in pregnant women. Rosiglitazone has been reported to cross the human placenta and be detectable in fetal tissue. The clinical significance of these findings is unknown.

Animal Studies: No animal studies have been conducted with AVANDAMET. The following data are based on findings in studies performed with rosiglitazone or metformin individually.

Rosiglitazone: There was no effect on implantation or the embryo with rosiglitazone treatment during early pregnancy in rats, but treatment during mid-late gestation was associated with fetal death and growth retardation in both rats and rabbits. Teratogenicity was not observed at doses up to 3 mg/kg in rats and 100 mg/kg in rabbits (approximately 20 and 75 times human AUC at the maximum recommended human daily dose of the rosiglitazone component of AVANDAMET, respectively). Rosiglitazone caused placental pathology in rats (3 mg/kg/day). Treatment of rats during gestation through lactation reduced litter size, neonatal viability, and postnatal growth, with growth retardation reversible after puberty. For effects on the placenta, embryo/fetus, and offspring, the no-effect dose was 0.2 mg/kg/day in rats and 15 mg/kg/day in rabbits. These no-effect levels are approximately 4 times human AUC at the maximum recommended human daily dose of the rosiglitazone component of AVANDAMET. Rosiglitazone reduced the number of uterine implantations and live offspring when juvenile female rats were treated at 40 mg/kg/day from 27 days of age through to sexual maturity (approximately 68 times human AUC at the maximum recommended daily dose). The no-effect level was 2 mg/kg/day (approximately 4 times human AUC at the maximum recommended daily dose). There was no effect on pre- or post-natal survival or growth.

Metformin: Metformin was not teratogenic in rats and rabbits at doses up to 600 mg/kg/day. This represents an exposure of about 2 and 6 times the maximum recommended human daily dose of 2,000 mg based on body surface area comparisons for rats and rabbits, respectively. Determination of fetal concentrations demonstrated a partial placental barrier to metformin.

8.2 Labor and Delivery

The effect of AVANDAMET or its components on labor and delivery in humans is unknown.

8.3 Nursing Mothers

No studies have been conducted with AVANDAMET. In studies performed with the individual components, both rosiglitazone-related material and metformin were detectable in milk from lactating rats. It is not known whether rosiglitazone or metformin is excreted in human milk. Because many drugs are excreted in human milk, AVANDAMET should not be administered to a nursing woman.

8.4 Pediatric Use

Safety and effectiveness of AVANDAMET in pediatric patients have not been established. AVANDAMET and rosiglitazone are not indicated for use in pediatric patients.

8.5 Geriatric Use

Metformin is known to be substantially excreted by the kidney and because the risk of serious adverse reactions to the drug is greater in patients with impaired renal function, AVANDAMET should only be used in patients with normal renal function *[see Contraindications (4), Warnings and Precautions (5.1), and Clinical Pharmacology (12.3)]*. Because reduced renal function is associated with increasing age, AVANDAMET should be used with caution in elderly patients. Care should be taken in dose selection and should be based on careful and regular monitoring of renal function. Generally, elderly patients should not be titrated to the maximum dose of AVANDAMET *[see Dosage and Administration (2.4) and Warnings and Precautions (5.1)]*.

10 OVERDOSAGE

Rosiglitazone: Limited data are available with regard to overdosage in humans. In clinical trials in volunteers, rosiglitazone has been administered at single oral doses of up to 20 mg and was well tolerated. In the event of an overdose, appropriate supportive treatment should be initiated as dictated by the patient's clinical status.

Metformin: Hypoglycemia has not been seen with ingestion of up to 85 grams of metformin, although lactic acidosis has occurred in such circumstances *[see Warnings and Precautions (5.1)]*. Metformin is dialyzable with a clearance of up to 170 mL/min under good hemodynamic conditions. Therefore, hemodialysis may be useful for removal of accumulated metformin from patients in whom metformin overdosage is suspected.

11 DESCRIPTION

AVANDAMET contains 2 oral antidiabetic drugs: rosiglitazone maleate and metformin hydrochloride.

Rosiglitazone maleate is an oral antidiabetic agent, which acts primarily by increasing insulin sensitivity. Rosiglitazone improves glycemic control while reducing circulating insulin levels. Rosiglitazone maleate is not chemically or functionally related to the sulfonylureas, the biguanides, or the alpha-glucosidase inhibitors. Chemically, rosiglitazone maleate is (±)-5-[[4-[2-(methyl-2-pyridinylamino)ethoxy]phenyl]methyl]-2,4-thiazolidinedione, (*Z*)-2-butenedioate (1:1) with a molecular weight of 473.52 (357.44 free base). The molecule has a single chiral center and is present as a racemate. Due to rapid interconversion, the enantiomers are functionally indistinguishable. The molecular formula is $C_{18}H_{19}N_3O_3S \cdot C_4H_4O_4$. Rosiglitazone maleate is a white to off-white solid with a melting point range of 122° to 123°C. The pK_a values of rosiglitazone maleate are 6.8 and 6.1. It is readily soluble in ethanol and a buffered aqueous solution with pH of 2.3; solubility decreases with increasing pH in the physiological range. The structural formula of rosiglitazone maleate is:

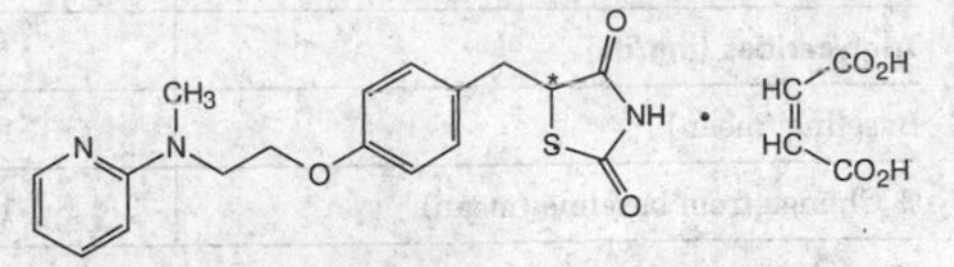

Metformin hydrochloride (N,N-dimethylimidodicarbonimidic diamide hydrochloride) is not chemically or pharmacologically related to any other classes of oral antidiabetic agents. Metformin hydrochloride is a white to off-white crystalline compound with a molecular formula of $C_4H_{11}N_5 \cdot HCl$ and a molecular weight of 165.63. Metformin hydrochloride is freely soluble in water and is practically insoluble in acetone, ether, and chloroform. The pK_a of metformin is 12.4. The pH of a 1% aqueous solution of metformin hydrochloride is 6.68. The structural formula of metformin hydrochloride is:

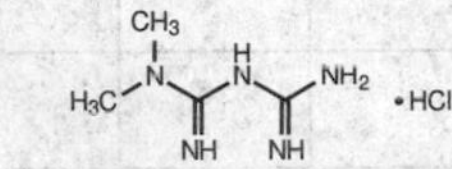

AVANDAMET is available for oral administration as film-coated tablets containing rosiglitazone maleate and metformin hydrochloride equivalent to: 2 mg rosiglitazone with 500 mg metformin hydrochloride (2 mg/500 mg), 4 mg rosiglitazone with 500 mg metformin hydrochloride (4 mg/500 mg), 2 mg rosiglitazone with 1,000 mg metformin hydrochloride (2 mg/1,000 mg), and 4 mg rosiglitazone with 1,000 mg metformin hydrochloride (4 mg/1,000 mg). Inactive ingredients are: Hypromellose 2910, lactose monohydrate, magnesium stearate, microcrystalline cellulose, polyethylene glycol 400, povidone 29-32, sodium starch glycolate, titanium dioxide, and 1 or more of the following: Red and yellow iron oxides.

12 CLINICAL PHARMACOLOGY

12.1 Mechanism of Action

AVANDAMET: AVANDAMET combines 2 antidiabetic agents with different mechanisms of action to improve glycemic control in patients with type 2 diabetes: Rosiglitazone, a member of the thiazolidinedione class, and metformin, a member of the biguanide class. Thiazolidinediones are insulin sensitizing agents that act primarily by enhancing peripheral glucose utilization, whereas biguanides act primarily by decreasing endogenous hepatic glucose production.

Rosiglitazone: Rosiglitazone improves glycemic control by improving insulin sensitivity. Rosiglitazone is a highly selective and potent agonist for the peroxisome proliferator–activated receptor-gamma (PPARγ). In humans, PPAR receptors are found in key target tissues for insulin action such as adipose tissue, skeletal muscle, and liver. Activation of PPARγ nuclear receptors regulates the transcription of insulin-responsive genes involved in the control of glucose production, transport, and utilization. In addition, PPARγ-responsive genes also participate in the regulation of fatty acid metabolism.

Insulin resistance is a common feature characterizing the pathogenesis of type 2 diabetes. The antidiabetic activity of rosiglitazone has been demonstrated in animal models of type 2 diabetes in which hyperglycemia and/or impaired glucose tolerance is a consequence of insulin resistance in target tissues. Rosiglitazone reduces blood glucose concentrations and reduces hyperinsulinemia in the ob/ob obese mouse, db/db diabetic mouse, and fa/fa fatty Zucker rat.

In animal models, the antidiabetic activity of rosiglitazone was shown to be mediated by increased sensitivity to insulin's action in the liver, muscle, and adipose tissue. Pharmacologic studies in animal models indicate that rosiglitazone

Table 9. Summary of Mean[a] Lipid Changes in a 32-Week Trial of AVANDAMET in Patients with Type 2 Diabetes Mellitus Who Have Inadequate Glycemic Control on Diet and Exercise

	AVANDAMET N[b] = 132	Rosiglitazone N[b] = 128	Metformin N[b] = 117
Total Cholesterol (mg/dL)			
Baseline (mean)	200.4	198.4	201.6
% Change from baseline (mean)	-2.2%	5.3%	-9.0%
LDL (mg/dL)			
Baseline (mean)	113.8	114.6	116.0
% Change from baseline (mean)	-0.2%	4.5%	-10.7%
HDL (mg/dL)			
Baseline (mean)	42.6	42.8	42.9
% Change from baseline (mean)	5.8%	3.1%	0.0%
Triglycerides (mg/dL)			
Baseline (mean)	180.3	166.6	175.7
% Change from baseline (mean)	-18.7%	-4.8%	-15.4%

[a]Data presented as geometric means throughout table.
[b]N = number of subjects with a baseline and end of treatment value.

Table 10. Mean (SD) Pharmacokinetic Parameters for Rosiglitazone and Metformin

Regimen	N	Pharmacokinetic Parameter			
		AUC_{0-inf} (ng.h/mL)	C_{max} (ng/mL)	T_{max}[a] (h)	$T_{½}$ (h)
Rosiglitazone					
A	25	1,442 (324)	242 (70)	0.95 (0.48-2.47)	4.26 (1.18)
B	25	1,398 (340)	254 (69)	0.57 (0.43-2.58)	3.95 (0.81)
C	24	349 (91)	63.0 (15.0)	0.57 (0.47-1.45)	3.87 (0.88)
Metformin					
A	25	7,116 (2,096)	1,106 (329)	2.97 (1.02-4.02)	3.46 (0.96)
B	25	7,413 (1,838)	1,135 (253)	2.50 (1.03-3.98)	3.36 (0.54)
C	24	6,945 (2,045)	1,080 (327)	2.97 (1.00-5.98)	3.35 (0.59)

[a]Median and range presented for T_{max}.
Regimen A = 4 mg/500 mg AVANDAMET; Regimen B = 4 mg rosiglitazone tablet + 500 mg metformin tablet; Regimen C = 1 mg/500 mg AVANDAMET

improves sensitivity to insulin in muscle and adipose tissue and inhibits hepatic gluconeogenesis. The expression of the insulin-regulated glucose transporter GLUT-4 was increased in adipose tissue. Rosiglitazone did not induce hypoglycemia in animal models of type 2 diabetes and/or impaired glucose tolerance.

Metformin: Metformin is an antidiabetic agent, which improves glucose tolerance in patients with type 2 diabetes, lowering both basal and postprandial plasma glucose. Its pharmacologic mechanisms of action are different from other classes of oral antidiabetic agents. Metformin decreases hepatic glucose production, decreases intestinal absorption of glucose, and increases peripheral glucose uptake and utilization. Unlike sulfonylureas, metformin does not produce hypoglycemia in either patients with type 2 diabetes or normal subjects except in special circumstances *[see Warnings and Precautions (5.12)]* and does not cause hyperinsulinemia. With metformin therapy, insulin secretion remains unchanged while fasting insulin levels and day-long plasma insulin response may actually decrease.

12.2 Pharmacodynamics

In all 26-week controlled trials, across the recommended dose range, rosiglitazone as monotherapy was associated with increases in total cholesterol, LDL-cholesterol and HDL-cholesterol and decreases in free fatty acids.

The lipid profiles of AVANDAMET as well as rosiglitazone and metformin monotherapies in patients who have inadequate glycemic control on diet and exercise are shown in Table 9.

[See table 9 above]

The pattern of LDL, HDL, and total cholesterol changes following therapy with rosiglitazone added to metformin was generally similar to those seen with rosiglitazone monotherapy, and a small decrease in mean triglycerides was observed with the combination therapy.

12.3 Pharmacokinetics

Absorption: *AVANDAMET:* In a bioequivalence and dose proportionality trial of AVANDAMET 4 mg/500 mg, both the rosiglitazone component and the metformin component were bioequivalent to coadministered 4 mg rosiglitazone tablet and 500 mg metformin tablet under fasted conditions (see Table 10). In this trial, dose proportionality of rosiglitazone in the combination formulations of 1 mg/500 mg and 4 mg/500 mg was demonstrated.

[See table 10 above]

Administration of AVANDAMET 4 mg/500 mg with food resulted in no change in overall exposure (AUC) for either rosiglitazone or metformin. However, there were decreases in C_{max} of both components (22% for rosiglitazone and 15% for metformin, respectively) and a delay in T_{max} of both components (1.5 hours for rosiglitazone and 0.5 hours for metformin, respectively). These changes are not likely to be clinically significant. The pharmacokinetics of both the rosiglitazone component and the metformin component of AVANDAMET when taken with food were similar to the pharmacokinetics of rosiglitazone and metformin when administered concomitantly as separate tablets with food.

Absorption: *Rosiglitazone:* The absolute bioavailability of rosiglitazone is 99%. Peak plasma concentrations are observed about 1 hour after dosing. Maximum plasma concentration (C_{max}) and the area under the curve (AUC) of rosiglitazone increase in a dose-proportional manner over the therapeutic dose range.

Absorption: *Metformin:* The absolute bioavailability of a 500 mg metformin tablet given under fasting conditions is approximately 50% to 60%. Trials using single oral doses of metformin tablets of 500 mg to 1,500 mg, and 850 mg to 2,550 mg, indicate that there is a lack of dose proportionality with increasing doses, which is due to decreased absorption rather than an alteration in elimination.

Distribution: *Rosiglitazone:* The mean (CV%) oral volume of distribution (V_{ss}/F) of rosiglitazone is approximately 17.6 (30%) liters, based on a population pharmacokinetic analysis. Rosiglitazone is approximately 99.8% bound to plasma proteins, primarily albumin.

Distribution: *Metformin:* The apparent volume of distribution (V/F) of metformin following single oral doses of 850 mg metformin averaged 654 ± 358 L. Metformin is negligibly bound to plasma proteins. Metformin partitions into erythrocytes, most likely as a function of time. At usual clinical doses and dosing schedules of metformin, steady-state plasma concentrations of metformin are reached within 24 to 48 hours and are generally <1 mcg/mL. During controlled clinical trials, maximum metformin plasma levels did not exceed 5 mcg/mL, even at maximum doses.

Metabolism and Excretion: *Rosiglitazone:* Rosiglitazone is extensively metabolized with no unchanged drug excreted in the urine. The major routes of metabolism were N-demethylation and hydroxylation, followed by conjugation with sulfate and glucuronic acid. All the circulating metabolites are considerably less potent than parent and, therefore, are not expected to contribute to the insulin-sensitizing activity of rosiglitazone. In vitro data demonstrate that rosiglitazone is predominantly metabolized by Cytochrome P450 (CYP) isoenzyme 2C8, with CYP2C9 contributing as a minor pathway. Following oral or intravenous administration of [^{14}C]rosiglitazone maleate, approximately 64% and 23% of the dose was eliminated in the urine and in the feces, respectively. The plasma half-life of [^{14}C]related material ranged from 103 to 158 hours. The elimination half-life is 3 to 4 hours and is independent of dose.

Metabolism and Excretion: *Metformin:* Intravenous single-dose trials in normal subjects demonstrate that metformin is excreted unchanged in the urine and does not undergo hepatic metabolism (no metabolites have been identified in humans) nor biliary excretion. Renal clearance is approximately 3.5 times greater than creatinine clearance which indicates that tubular secretion is the major route of metformin elimination. Following oral administration, approximately 90% of the absorbed drug is eliminated via the renal route within the first 24 hours, with a plasma elimination half-life of approximately 6.2 hours. In blood, the elimination half-life is approximately 17.6 hours, suggesting that the erythrocyte mass may be a compartment of distribution.

Special Populations: *Renal Impairment:* In subjects with decreased renal function (based on measured creatinine clearance), the plasma and blood half-life of metformin is prolonged and the renal clearance is decreased in proportion to the decrease in creatinine clearance *[see Warnings and Precautions (5.1) and GLUCOPHAGE prescribing information]*. Since metformin is contraindicated in patients with renal impairment, administration of AVANDAMET is contraindicated in these patients.

Hepatic Impairment: Unbound oral clearance of rosiglitazone was significantly lower in patients with moderate to severe liver disease (Child-Pugh Class B/C) compared to healthy subjects. As a result, unbound C_{max} and AUC_{0-inf} were increased 2- and 3-fold, respectively. Elimination half-life for rosiglitazone was about 2 hours longer in patients with liver disease, compared to healthy subjects. Therapy with AVANDAMET should not be initiated if the patient exhibits clinical evidence of active liver disease or increased serum transaminase levels (ALT >2.5× upper limit of normal) at baseline *[see Warnings and Precautions (5.7)]*.

No pharmacokinetic trials of metformin have been conducted in subjects with hepatic insufficiency.

Geriatric: Results of the population pharmacokinetics analysis (N = 716 <65 years; N = 331 ≥65 years) showed that age does not significantly affect the pharmacokinetics of rosiglitazone. However, limited data from controlled pharmacokinetic trials of metformin in healthy elderly subjects suggest that total plasma clearance of metformin is decreased, the half-life is prolonged, and C_{max} is increased, compared to healthy young subjects. From these data, it appears that the change in metformin pharmacokinetics with aging is primarily accounted for by a change in renal function *[see Use in Specific Populations (8.5) and GLUCOPHAGE prescribing information]*. Metformin treatment and therefore treatment with AVANDAMET should not be initiated in patients ≥80 years of age unless measurement of creatinine clearance demonstrates that renal function is not reduced *[see Dosage and Administration (2) and Warnings and Precautions (5.1)]*.

Gender: Results of the population pharmacokinetics analysis showed that the mean oral clearance of rosiglitazone in female patients (N = 405) was approximately 6% lower compared to male patients of the same body weight (N = 642). In rosiglitazone and metformin combination trials, efficacy was demonstrated with no gender differences in glycemic response.

Metformin pharmacokinetic parameters did not differ significantly between normal subjects and patients with type 2 diabetes when analyzed according to gender (males = 19, females = 16). Similarly, in controlled clinical trials in patients with type 2 diabetes, the antihyperglycemic effect of metformin tablets was comparable in males and females.

Race: Results of a population pharmacokinetic analysis including subjects of white, black, and other ethnic origins indicate that race has no influence on the pharmacokinetics of rosiglitazone.

No trials of metformin pharmacokinetic parameters according to race have been performed. In controlled clinical trials of metformin in patients with type 2 diabetes, the antihyperglycemic effect was comparable in whites (N = 249), blacks (N = 51), and Hispanics (N = 24).

Pediatric: No pharmacokinetic data from trials in pediatric subjects are available for AVANDAMET.

12.4 Drug-Drug Interactions

Rosiglitazone: *Drugs That Inhibit, Induce, or are Metabolized by Cytochrome P450:* In vitro drug metabolism studies suggest that rosiglitazone does not inhibit any of the major P450 enzymes at clinically relevant concentrations. In vitro data demonstrate that rosiglitazone is predominantly metabolized by CYP2C8, and to a lesser extent, 2C9. *[See Drug Interactions (7.1).]*

Rosiglitazone (4 mg twice daily) was shown to have no clinically relevant effect on the pharmacokinetics of nifedipine and oral contraceptives (ethinyl estradiol and norethindrone), which are predominantly metabolized by CYP3A4.

Gemfibrozil: Concomitant administration of gemfibrozil (600 mg twice daily), an inhibitor of CYP2C8, and rosiglitazone (4 mg once daily) for 7 days increased rosiglitazone AUC by 127%, compared to the administration of rosiglitazone (4 mg once daily) alone. Given the potential for dose-related adverse events with rosiglitazone, a decrease in the dose of rosiglitazone may be needed when gemfibrozil is introduced. *[See Drug Interactions (7.1).]*

Rifampin: Rifampin administration (600 mg once a day), an inducer of CYP2C8, for 6 days is reported to decrease rosiglitazone AUC by 66%, compared to the administration of rosiglitazone (8 mg) alone.[11] *[See Drug Interactions (7.1).]*

Metformin: *Cationic Drugs:* Cationic drugs (e.g., amiloride, digoxin, morphine, procainamide, quinidine, quinine, ranitidine, triamterene, trimethoprim, and vancomycin) that are eliminated by renal tubular secretion theoretically have the potential for interaction with metformin by competing for common renal tubular transport systems. Such interaction between metformin and oral cimetidine has been observed in normal healthy volunteers in both single- and multiple-dose, metformin-cimetidine drug interaction trials, with a 60% increase in peak metformin plasma and whole blood concentrations and a 40% increase in plasma and whole blood metformin AUC. There was no change in elimination half-life in the single-dose trial. Metformin had no effect on cimetidine pharmacokinetics. *[See Warnings and Precautions (5.1) and Drug Interactions (7.2).]*

Furosemide: A single-dose, metformin-furosemide drug interaction trial in healthy subjects demonstrated that pharmacokinetic parameters of both compounds were affected by coadministration. Furosemide increased the metformin plasma and blood C_{max} by 22% and blood AUC by 15%, without any significant change in metformin renal clearance. When administered with metformin, the C_{max} and AUC of furosemide were 31% and 12% smaller, respectively, than when administered alone, and the terminal half-life was decreased by 32%, without any significant change in furosemide renal clearance. No information is available about the interaction of metformin and furosemide when coadministered chronically.

Nifedipine: A single-dose, metformin-nifedipine drug interaction trial in normal healthy volunteers demonstrated that coadministration of nifedipine increased plasma metformin C_{max} and AUC by 20% and 9%, respectively, and increased the amount excreted in the urine. T_{max} and half-life were unaffected. Nifedipine appears to enhance the absorption of metformin. Metformin had minimal effects on nifedipine.

Table 11. Glycemic Parameters in a 26-Week Trial of Rosiglitazone Added to Metformin Therapy

	Metformin	Rosiglitazone 4 mg once daily + metformin	Rosiglitazone 8 mg once daily + metformin
N	113	116	110
FPG (mg/dL)			
Baseline (mean)	214	215	220
Change from baseline (mean)	6	-33	-48
Difference from metformin alone (adjusted mean)		-40[a]	-53[a]
% of patients with ≥30 mg/dL decrease from baseline	20%	45%	61%
HbA1c (%)			
Baseline (mean)	8.6	8.9	8.9
Change from baseline (mean)	0.5	-0.6	-0.8
Difference from metformin alone (adjusted mean)		-1.0[a]	-1.2[a]
% of patients with HbA1c ≥0.7% decrease from baseline	11%	45%	52%

[a]P <0.0001 compared to metformin.

Other: Certain drugs tend to produce hyperglycemia and may lead to loss of glycemic control. These drugs include thiazides and other diuretics, corticosteroids, phenothiazines, thyroid products, estrogens, oral contraceptives, phenytoin, nicotinic acid, sympathomimetics, calcium channel blocking drugs, and isoniazid.

In healthy volunteers, the pharmacokinetics of metformin and propranolol and metformin and ibuprofen were not affected when coadministered in single-dose interaction trials.

Metformin is negligibly bound to plasma proteins and is therefore, less likely to interact with highly protein-bound drugs such as salicylates, sulfonamides, chloramphenicol, and probenecid.

13 NONCLINICAL TOXICOLOGY

13.1 Carcinogenesis, Mutagenesis, Impairment of Fertility

No animal studies have been conducted with AVANDAMET. The following data are based on findings in studies performed with rosiglitazone or metformin individually.

Rosiglitazone: A 2-year carcinogenicity study was conducted in Charles River CD-1 mice at doses of 0.4, 1.5, and 6 mg/kg/day in the diet (highest dose equivalent to approximately 12 times human AUC at the maximum recommended human daily dose of the rosiglitazone component of AVANDAMET). Sprague-Dawley rats were dosed for 2 years by oral gavage at doses of 0.05, 0.3, and 2 mg/kg/day (highest dose equivalent to approximately 10 and 20 times human AUC at the maximum recommended human daily dose of the rosiglitazone component of AVANDAMET for male and female rats, respectively).

Rosiglitazone was not carcinogenic in the mouse. There was an increase in incidence of adipose hyperplasia in the mouse at doses ≥1.5 mg/kg/day (approximately 2 times human AUC at the maximum recommended human daily dose of the rosiglitazone component of AVANDAMET). In rats, there was a significant increase in the incidence of benign adipose tissue tumors (lipomas) at doses ≥0.3 mg/kg/day (approximately 2 times human AUC at the maximum recommended human daily dose of the rosiglitazone component of AVANDAMET). These proliferative changes in both species are considered due to the persistent pharmacological overstimulation of adipose tissue.

Rosiglitazone was not mutagenic or clastogenic in the in vitro bacterial assays for gene mutation, the in vitro chromosome aberration test in human lymphocytes, the in vivo mouse micronucleus test, and the in vivo/in vitro rat UDS assay. There was a small (about 2-fold) increase in mutation in the in vitro mouse lymphoma assay in the presence of metabolic activation.

Rosiglitazone had no effects on mating or fertility of male rats given up to 40 mg/kg/day (approximately 116 times human AUC at the maximum recommended human daily dose of the rosiglitazone component of AVANDAMET). Rosiglitazone altered estrous cyclicity (2 mg/kg/day) and reduced fertility (40 mg/kg/day) of female rats in association with lower plasma levels of progesterone and estradiol (approximately 20 and 200 times human AUC at the maximum recommended human daily dose of the rosiglitazone component of AVANDAMET, respectively). No such effects were noted at 0.2 mg/kg/day (approximately 3 times human AUC at the maximum recommended human daily dose of the rosiglitazone component of AVANDAMET). In juvenile rats dosed from 27 days of age through to sexual maturity (at up to 40 mg/kg/day), there was no effect on male reproductive performance, or on estrous cyclicity, mating performance or pregnancy incidence in females (approximately 68 times human AUC at the maximum recommended daily dose of rosiglitazone). In monkeys, rosiglitazone (0.6 and 4.6 mg/kg/day; approximately 3 and 15 times human AUC at the maximum recommended human daily dose of the rosiglitazone component of AVANDAMET, respectively) diminished the follicular phase rise in serum estradiol with consequential reduction in the luteinizing hormone surge, lower luteal phase progesterone levels, and amenorrhea. The mechanism for these effects appears to be direct inhibition of ovarian steroidogenesis.

Metformin: Long-term carcinogenicity studies have been performed in rats (dosing duration of 104 weeks) and mice (dosing duration of 91 weeks) at doses up to and including 900 mg/kg/day and 1,500 mg/kg/day, respectively. These doses are both approximately 4 times the maximum recommended human daily dose of 2,000 mg of the metformin component of AVANDAMET based on body surface area comparisons. No evidence of carcinogenicity with metformin was found in either male or female mice. Similarly, there was no tumorigenic potential observed with metformin in male rats. There was, however, an increased incidence of benign stromal uterine polyps in female rats treated with 900 mg/kg/day.

There was no evidence of mutagenic potential of metformin in the following in vitro tests: Ames test (*S. typhimurium*), gene mutation test (mouse lymphoma cells), or chromosomal aberrations test (human lymphocytes). Results in the in vivo mouse micronucleus test were also negative.

Fertility of male or female rats was unaffected by metformin when administrated at doses as high as 600 mg/kg/day, which is approximately 3 times the maximum recommended human daily dose of the metformin component of AVANDAMET based on body surface area comparisons.

13.2 Animal Toxicology

Heart weights were increased in mice (3 mg/kg/day), rats (5 mg/kg/day), and dogs (2 mg/kg/day) with rosiglitazone treatments (approximately 5, 22, and 2 times human AUC at the maximum recommended human daily dose of the rosiglitazone component of AVANDAMET, respectively). Effects in juvenile rats were consistent with those seen in adults. Morphometric measurement indicated that there was hypertrophy in cardiac ventricular tissues, which may be due to increased heart work as a result of plasma volume expansion.

14 CLINICAL STUDIES

AVANDAMET was not studied in patients previously treated with metformin monotherapy; however, the combination of rosiglitazone and metformin was compared to rosiglitazone and metformin monotherapies in clinical trials. Bioequivalence between AVANDAMET and coadministered rosiglitazone tablets and metformin tablets has been demonstrated *[see Clinical Pharmacology (12.3)]*.

A total of 670 patients with type 2 diabetes participated in two 26-week, randomized, double-blind, placebo/active-controlled trials designed to assess the efficacy of rosiglitazone in combination with metformin. Rosiglitazone, administered in either once-daily or twice-daily dosing regimens, was added to the therapy of patients who were inadequately controlled on 2.5 grams/day of metformin.

In one trial, patients inadequately controlled on 2.5 grams/day of metformin (mean baseline FPG 216 mg/dL and mean baseline HbA1c 8.8%) were randomized to receive rosiglitazone 4 mg once daily, rosiglitazone 8 mg once daily, or placebo in addition to metformin. A statistically significant improvement in FPG and HbA1c was observed in patients treated with the combinations of metformin and rosiglitazone 4 mg once daily and rosiglitazone 8 mg once daily, versus patients continued on metformin alone (see Table 11).

[See table 11 at top of previous page]

In a second 26-week trial, patients with type 2 diabetes inadequately controlled on 2.5 grams/day of metformin who were randomized to receive the combination of rosiglitazone 4 mg twice daily and metformin (N = 105) showed a statistically significant improvement in glycemic control with a mean treatment effect for FPG of -56 mg/dL and a mean treatment effect for HbA1c of -0.8% over metformin alone. The combination of metformin and rosiglitazone resulted in lower levels of FPG and HbA1c than either agent alone.

15 REFERENCES

1. Food and Drug Administration Briefing Document. Joint meeting of the Endocrinologic and Metabolic Drugs and Drug Safety and Risk Management Advisory Committees. July 13-14, 2010.
2. Winkelmayer WC, et al. Comparison of cardiovascular outcomes in elderly patients with diabetes who initiated rosiglitazone vs pioglitazone therapy. *Arch Intern Med* 2008;168(21):2368-2375.
3. Juurlink DN, et al. Adverse cardiovascular events during treatment with pioglitazone and rosiglitazone: population based cohort study. *BMJ* 2009; 339.
4. Graham DJ, et al. Risk of acute myocardial infarction, stroke, heart failure, and death in elderly medicare patients treated with rosiglitazone or pioglitazone. *JAMA* 2010;304:411-418.
5. Wertz DA, et al. Risk of cardiovascular events and all-cause mortality in patients with Thiazolidinediones in a managed-care population. *Circ Cardiovasc Qual Outcomes* 2010;3: 538-545.
6. DREAM Trial Investigators. Effect of rosiglitazone on the frequency of diabetes in patients with impaired glucose tolerance or impaired fasting glucose: a randomised controlled trial. *Lancet* 2006;368:1096-1105.
7. Kahn S, et al. Glycemic durability of rosiglitazone, metformin or glyburide monotherapy. *New England Journal of Medicine* 2006, 355:2427-2443.
8. Home P, et al. Rosiglitazone evaluated for cardiovascular outcomes in oral agent combination therapy for type 2 diabetes (RECORD): a multicenter, randomized, open-label trial. *Lancet* 2009, 373:2125-35.
9. Dormandy J et al. Secondary prevention of macrovascular events in patients with type 2 diabetes in the PROactive study (Prospective Pioglitazone Clinical Trial in Macrovascular Events): a randomized controlled trial. *Lancet* 2005, 366:1279-89.
10. Bilik D, et al. Thiazolidinediones, cardiovascular disease and cardiovascular mortality: translating research into action for diabetes (TRIAD). *Pharmocoepidemiol Drug Saf* 2010; 19: 715–721.
11. Park JY, Kim KA, Kang MH, et al. Effect of rifampin on the pharmacokinetics of rosiglitazone in healthy subjects. *Clin Pharmacol Ther* 2004;75:157-162.

16 HOW SUPPLIED/STORAGE AND HANDLING

Each film-coated oval tablet contains rosiglitazone as the maleate and metformin hydrochloride as follows:

2 mg/500 mg – pale pink, tablet, debossed with gsk on one side and 2/500 on the other.

4 mg/500 mg – orange, tablet, debossed with gsk on one side and 4/500 on the other.

2 mg/1,000 mg – yellow, tablet, debossed with gsk on one side and 2/1000 on the other.

4 mg/1,000 mg – pink, tablet, debossed with gsk on one side and 4/1000 on the other.

2 mg/500 mg bottles of 60: NDC 0173-0837-18
4 mg/500 mg bottles of 60: NDC 0173-0839-18
2 mg/1,000 mg bottles of 60: NDC 0173-0838-18
4 mg/1,000 mg bottles of 60: NDC 0173-0840-18

Store at 25°C (77°F); excursions permitted to 15° to 30°C (59° to 86°F). Dispense in a tight, light-resistant container.

17 PATIENT COUNSELING INFORMATION

See Medication Guide.

17.1 Patient Advice

There are multiple medications available to treat type 2 diabetes. The benefits and risks of each available diabetes medication should be taken into account when choosing a particular diabetes medication for a given patient.

Patients should be informed of the risks and benefits of AVANDAMET. AVANDAMET should only be taken by adults with type 2 diabetes who are already taking rosiglitazone, or who are not already taking rosiglitazone and are unable to achieve adequate glycemic control on other diabetes medications, and, in consultation with their healthcare provider, have decided not to take pioglitazone (ACTOS) or pioglitazone-containing medications (ACTOPLUS MET, ACTOPLUS MET XR, DUETACT) for medical reasons. Inform patients that they must be enrolled in the AVANDIA-Rosiglitazone Medicines Access Program in order to receive AVANDAMET.

Patients should be informed of the following:

- The risks of lactic acidosis, its symptoms, and conditions that predispose to its development, as noted in the WARNINGS and PRECAUTIONS sections, should be explained to patients. Patients should be advised to discontinue AVANDAMET immediately and to promptly notify their health practitioner if unexplained hyperventilation, myalgia, malaise, unusual somnolence, or other nonspecific symptoms occur. Once a patient is stabilized on any dose level of AVANDAMET, gastrointestinal symptoms, which are common during initiation of metformin therapy, are unlikely to be drug related. Later occurrence of gastrointestinal symptoms could be due to lactic acidosis or other serious disease.
- Avoid excessive alcohol intake, either acute or chronic, while receiving AVANDAMET.
- AVANDAMET is not recommended for patients with symptomatic heart failure.
- Results of a set of clinical trials suggest that treatment with AVANDAMET is associated with an increased risk for myocardial infarction (heart attack), especially in patients taking insulin. Clinical trials have not shown any difference between rosiglitazone and comparator medications in overall mortality or CV-related mortality.
- AVANDAMET is not recommended for patients who are taking insulin.
- Management of type 2 diabetes should include diet control. Caloric restriction, weight loss, and exercise are essential for the proper treatment of the diabetic patient because they help improve insulin sensitivity. This is important not only in the primary treatment of type 2 diabetes but also in maintaining the efficacy of drug therapy.
- It is important to adhere to dietary instructions and to regularly have blood glucose, glycosylated hemoglobin (HbA1c), renal function, and hematologic parameters tested. It can take 2 weeks to see a reduction in blood glucose and 2 to 3 months to see the full effect of AVANDAMET.
- Blood will be drawn to check their liver function prior to the start of therapy and periodically thereafter per the clinical judgment of the healthcare professional. Patients with unexplained symptoms of nausea, vomiting, abdominal pain, fatigue, anorexia, or dark urine should immediately report these symptoms to their physician.
- Patients who experience an unusually rapid increase in weight or edema or who develop shortness of breath or other symptoms of heart failure while on AVANDAMET should immediately report these symptoms to their physician.
- Therapy with AVANDAMET, like other thiazolidinediones, may result in ovulation in some premenopausal anovulatory women. As a result, these patients may be at an increased risk for pregnancy while taking AVANDAMET. Thus, adequate contraception in premenopausal women should be recommended. This possible effect has not been specifically investigated in clinical trials so the frequency of this occurrence is not known.

AVANDAMET and AVANDIA are registered trademarks of GlaxoSmithKline.

GLUCOPHAGE is a registered trademark of Merck Santé S.A.S. (an associate of Merck KGaA of Darmstadt, Germany; licensed to Bristol-Myers Squibb Company). ACTOS, ACTOPLUS MET, ACTOPLUS MET XR, and DUETACT are registered trademarks of Takeda Pharmaceutical Company Limited.

GlaxoSmithKline
Research Triangle Park, NC 27709

May 2011
AVM:20PI

MEDICATION GUIDE

AVANDAMET® (ah-VAN-duh-met)

(rosiglitazone maleate and metformin hydrochloride) Tablets

Read this Medication Guide carefully before you start taking AVANDAMET and each time you get a refill. There may be new information. This information does not take the place of talking with your doctor about your medical condition or your treatment. If you have any questions about AVANDAMET, ask your doctor or pharmacist.

What is the most important information I should know about AVANDAMET?

AVANDAMET is available only through the AVANDIA-Rosiglitazone Medicines Access Program. Both you and your doctor must be enrolled in the program so that you can get AVANDAMET. To enroll, you must:

- talk to your doctor,
- understand the risks and benefits of AVANDAMET, and
- agree to enroll in the program.

AVANDAMET may cause serious side effects, including:

New or worse heart failure

- Rosiglitazone, one of the medicines in AVANDAMET, can cause your body to keep extra fluid (fluid retention), which leads to swelling (edema) and weight gain. Extra body fluid can make some heart problems worse or lead to heart failure. Heart failure means your heart does not pump blood well enough.
- If you have severe heart failure, you cannot start AVANDAMET.
- If you have heart failure with symptoms (such as shortness of breath or swelling), even if these symptoms are not severe, AVANDAMET may not be right for you.

Call your doctor right away if you have any of the following:

- swelling or fluid retention, especially in the ankles or legs
- shortness of breath or trouble breathing, especially when you lie down
- an unusually fast increase in weight
- unusual tiredness

Myocardial Infarction ("Heart Attack")

Rosiglitazone, one of the medicines in AVANDAMET, may raise the risk of heart attack. The risk of having a heart attack may be higher in people who take AVANDAMET with insulin. Most people who take insulin should not also take AVANDAMET.

Symptoms of a heart attack can include the following:

- chest discomfort in the center of your chest that lasts for more than a few minutes, or that goes away or comes back
- chest discomfort that feels like uncomfortable pressure, squeezing, fullness or pain
- pain or discomfort in your arms, back, neck, jaw or stomach
- shortness of breath with or without chest discomfort
- breaking out in a cold sweat
- nausea or vomiting
- feeling lightheaded

Call your doctor or go to the nearest hospital emergency room right away if you think you are having a heart attack.

People with diabetes have a greater risk for heart problems. It is important to work with your doctor to manage other conditions, such as high blood pressure or high cholesterol.

Lactic acidosis

Metformin, one of the medicines in AVANDAMET, can cause a rare but serious condition called lactic acidosis (a build-up of an acid in the blood) that can cause death. Lactic acidosis is a medical emergency and must be treated in the hospital. Most people who have had lactic acidosis with metformin have other things that, combined with the metformin, led to the lactic acidosis. Tell your doctor if you have any of the following, because you have a higher chance for getting lactic acidosis with AVANDAMET if you:

- have kidney problems or your kidneys are affected by certain X-ray tests that use injectable dye. People with kidney problems should not take AVANDAMET.
- have liver problems
- drink alcohol very often, or drink a lot of alcohol in short-term "binge" drinking
- get dehydrated (lose a large amount of body fluids). This can happen if you are sick with a fever, vomiting or diarrhea. Dehydration can also happen when you sweat a lot with activity or exercise and do not drink enough fluids.
- have surgery
- have a heart attack, severe infection, or stroke
- are 80 years of age or older, and your kidneys are not working properly

The best way to keep from having a problem with lactic acidosis from metformin is to tell your doctor if you have any of the problems in the list above. Your doctor may decide to stop your AVANDAMET for a while if you have any of these things.

Lactic acidosis can be hard to diagnose early, because the early symptoms could seem like the symptoms of many other health problems besides lactic acidosis. You should call your doctor right away if you get the following symptoms, which could be signs of lactic acidosis:

- you feel very weak or tired
- you have unusual (not normal) muscle pain
- you have stomach pains
- you have trouble breathing
- you feel dizzy or lightheaded
- you have a slow or irregular heartbeat

AVANDAMET can have other serious side effects. Be sure to read the section below "What are possible side effects of AVANDAMET?".

What is AVANDAMET?

AVANDAMET contains two prescription medicines for treating diabetes, rosiglitazone maleate (AVANDIA) and metformin hydrochloride. AVANDAMET is used, with diet and exercise, to treat certain adults with type 2 ("adult-onset" or "non-insulin dependent") diabetes ("high blood sugar") who are:

- already taking rosiglitazone or rosiglitazone-containing products
- unable to control their blood sugar on other diabetes medicines, and after talking with their doctor have decided not to take pioglitazone (ACTOS) or pioglitazone-containing products (ACTOPLUS MET, ACTOPLUS MET XR, DUETACT)

Metformin works mainly by decreasing the production of sugar by your liver. Rosiglitazone helps your body respond better to its natural insulin and does not cause your body to make more insulin. These medicines work together to help control your blood sugar. AVANDAMET may be used alone or with other diabetes medicines.

AVANDAMET is not for people with type 1 diabetes mellitus or to treat a condition called diabetic ketoacidosis.

It is not known if AVANDAMET is safe and effective in children under 18 years old.

Who should not take AVANDAMET?

Do not take AVANDAMET if you:

- have kidney problems. Before you take AVANDAMET and while you take it, your doctor should test your blood to check for signs of kidney problems.
- have a condition known as metabolic acidosis, including diabetic ketoacidosis.
- are going to have an x-ray procedure with an injection of dyes (contrast agents) in your vein with a needle. Talk to your doctor about when to stop AVANDAMET and when to start it again.

Many people with heart failure should not start taking AVANDAMET. See "What should I tell my doctor before taking AVANDAMET?".

What should I tell my doctor before taking AVANDAMET?

Before starting AVANDAMET, ask your doctor about what the choices are for diabetes medicines, and what the expected benefits and possible risks are for you in particular.

Before taking AVANDAMET, tell your doctor about all your medical conditions, including if you:

- **have heart problems or heart failure**
- **have kidney problems**
- **have type 1 ("juvenile") diabetes or had diabetic ketoacidosis.** These conditions should be treated with insulin.
- **are going to have dye injected into a vein for an X-ray, CAT scan, heart study, or other type of scanning**
- **drink a lot of alcohol** (all the time or short binge drinking).
- **develop a serious condition such as a heart attack, severe infection, or a stroke.**
- **are 80 years old or older.** People who are over 80 years old should not take AVANDAMET unless their kidney function is checked and it is normal.
- **have a type of diabetic eye disease called macular edema** (swelling of the back of the eye).
- **have liver problems.** Your doctor should do blood tests to check your liver before you start taking AVANDAMET and during treatment as needed.
- **had liver problems while taking REZULIN®** (troglitazone), another medicine for diabetes.
- **are pregnant or plan to become pregnant.** AVANDAMET should not be used during pregnancy. It is not known if AVANDAMET can harm your unborn baby. You and your doctor should talk about the best way to control your diabetes during pregnancy. If you are a premenopausal woman (before the "change of life") who does not have regular monthly periods, AVANDAMET may increase your chances of becoming pregnant. Talk to your doctor about birth control choices while taking AVANDAMET. Tell your doctor right away if you become pregnant while taking AVANDAMET.
- **are breast-feeding or planning to breast-feed.** It is not known if AVANDAMET passes into breast milk. You should not use AVANDAMET while breast-feeding.

Tell your doctor about all the medicines you take including prescription and non-prescription medicines, vitamins or herbal supplements. AVANDAMET and certain other medicines can affect each other and may lead to serious side effects including high or low blood sugar, or heart problems. Your doctor may need to change your dose of AVANDAMET or your other medicines. Especially tell your doctor if you take:

- **insulin.**
- **any medicines for high blood pressure, high cholesterol or heart failure, or for prevention of heart disease or stroke.**

Know the medicines you take. Keep a list of all your medicines and show it to your doctor and pharmacist before you start a new medicine. They will tell you if it is alright to take AVANDAMET with other medicines.

How should I take AVANDAMET?

- Take AVANDAMET exactly as prescribed. Your doctor may need to change your dose until your blood sugar is better controlled.
- AVANDAMET should be taken by mouth and with meals.
- AVANDAMET may be prescribed alone or with other diabetes medicines. This will depend on how well your blood sugar is controlled.
- It can take 2 weeks for AVANDAMET to start lowering your blood sugar. It may take 2 to 3 months to see the full effect on your blood sugar level.
- If you miss a dose of AVANDAMET, take it as soon as you remember, unless it is time to take your next dose. Take your next dose at the usual time. Do not take double doses to make up for a missed dose.
- If you take too much AVANDAMET, call your doctor or poison control center right away.
- Test your blood sugar regularly as your doctor tells you.
- Diet and exercise can help your body use its blood sugar better. It is important to stay on your recommended diet, lose extra weight, and get regular exercise while taking AVANDAMET.
- Your doctor should do blood tests to check your liver and kidneys before you start AVANDAMET and during treatment as needed. Your doctor should also do regular blood sugar tests (for example, "A1C") to monitor your response to AVANDAMET.

There may be times when you will need to stop taking AVANDAMET for a short time. Tell your doctor if you:

- are sick with severe vomiting, diarrhea or fever, or if you drink a much lower amount of liquid than normal.
- are going to have dye injected into a vein for an X-ray, CAT scan, heart study or other type of scanning.
- plan to have surgery.

What should I avoid while taking AVANDAMET?

Do not drink a lot of alcohol while taking AVANDAMET. This means you should not "binge drink", and you should not drink a lot of alcohol on a regular basis. Drinking a lot of alcohol can increase the chance of getting lactic acidosis.

What are possible side effects of AVANDAMET?

AVANDAMET may cause serious side effects, including:

- **New or worse heart failure.** See "What is the most important information I should know about AVANDAMET?".
- **Heart attack.** See "What is the most important information I should know about AVANDAMET?".
- **Swelling (edema).** AVANDAMET can cause swelling due to fluid retention. See "What is the most important information I should know about AVANDAMET?".
- **Weight gain.** Rosiglitazone, one of the medicines in AVANDAMET, can cause weight gain that may be due to fluid retention or extra body fat. Metformin, the other medicine in AVANDAMET, can cause weight loss. There is little change in weight with AVANDAMET. Weight gain can be a serious problem for people with certain conditions including heart problems. See "What is the most important information I should know about AVANDAMET?"
- **Liver problems.** It is important for your liver to be working normally when you take AVANDAMET. Your doctor should do blood tests to check your liver before you start taking AVANDAMET and during treatment as needed. Call your doctor right away if you have unexplained symptoms such as:
  - nausea or vomiting
  - stomach pain
  - unusual or unexplained tiredness
  - loss of appetite
  - dark urine
  - yellowing of your skin or the whites of your eyes.
- **Macular edema** (a diabetic eye disease with swelling in the back of the eye). Tell your doctor right away if you have any changes in your vision. Your doctor should check your eyes regularly. Very rarely, some people have had vision changes due to swelling in the back of the eye while taking rosiglitazone, one of the medicines in AVANDAMET.
- **Fractures (broken bones),** usually in the hand, upper arm or foot. Talk to your doctor for advice on how to keep your bones healthy.
- **Low red blood cell count (anemia).**
- **Low blood sugar(hypoglycemia).** Lightheadedness, dizziness, shakiness or hunger may mean that your blood sugar is too low. This can happen if you skip meals, if you use another medicine that lowers blood sugar, or if you have certain medical problems. Call your doctor if low blood sugar levels are a problem for you.
- **Ovulation** (release of egg from an ovary in a woman) leading to pregnancy. Ovulation may happen in premenopausal women who do not have regular monthly periods. This can increase the chance of pregnancy. See "What should I tell my doctor before taking AVANDAMET?".

Common side effects of AVANDAMET include:

- **Diarrhea, nausea, and upset stomach.** These side effects usually happen during the first few weeks of treatment. Taking AVANDAMET with food can help lessen these side effects. If you have unusual or unexpected stomach problems, talk with your doctor. Stomach problems that start up later during treatment with AVANDAMET may be a sign of something more serious and should be discussed with your doctor.
- **Cold-like symptoms**
- **Headache**
- **Joint aches**
- **Dizziness**

Call your doctor for medical advice about side effects. You may report side effects to FDA at 1-800-FDA-1088.

How should I store AVANDAMET?

- Store AVANDAMET at room temperature, 59° to 86°F (15° to 30°C).
- Keep AVANDAMET in the container it comes in. Keep the container closed tightly.
- Safely, throw away AVANDAMET that is out of date or no longer needed.

Keep AVANDAMET and all medicines out of the reach of children.

General information about AVANDAMET

Medicines are sometimes prescribed for purposes other than those listed in a Medication Guide. Do not use AVANDAMET for a condition for which it was not prescribed. Do not give AVANDAMET to other people, even if they have the same symptoms you have. It may harm them.

This Medication Guide summarizes important information about AVANDAMET. If you would like more information, talk with your doctor. You can ask your doctor or pharmacist for information about AVANDAMET that is written for healthcare professionals. You can also find out more about AVANDAMET by calling 1-888-825-5249.

What are the ingredients in AVANDAMET?

Active Ingredients: Rosiglitazone maleate and metformin hydrochloride

Inactive Ingredients: Hypromellose 2910, lactose monohydrate, magnesium stearate, microcrystalline cellulose, polyethylene glycol 400, povidone 29-32, sodium starch glycolate, titanium dioxide, and 1 or more of the following: Red and yellow iron oxides.

Always check to make sure that the medicine you are taking is the correct one. AVANDAMET tablets are oval and look like this:

- 2 mg/500 mg – pale pink, with "gsk" on one side and "2/500" on the other.
- 4 mg/500 mg – orange, with "gsk" on one side and "4/500" on the other
- 2 mg/1,000 mg – yellow, with "gsk" on one side and "2/1000" on the other
- 4 mg/1,000 mg – pink, with "gsk" on one side and "4/1000" on the other

AVANDAMET and AVANDIA are registered trademarks of GlaxoSmithKline.

The other brands listed are trademarks of their respective owners and are not trademarks of GlaxoSmithKline. The makers of these brands are not affiliated with and do not endorse GlaxoSmithKline or its products.

This Medication Guide has been approved by the U.S. Food and Drug Administration.

GlaxoSmithKline
Research Triangle Park, NC 27709

May 2011
AVM:4MG

AVANDARYL® ℞

[ə-van' də-ril]
(rosiglitazone maleate and glimepiride)
Tablets

HIGHLIGHTS OF PRESCRIBING INFORMATION

These highlights do not include all the information needed to use AVANDARYL safely and effectively. See full prescribing information for AVANDARYL.

AVANDARYL (rosiglitazone maleate and glimepiride) Tablets

Initial U.S. Approval: 2005

WARNING: CONGESTIVE HEART FAILURE AND MYOCARDIAL INFARCTION

See full prescribing information for complete boxed warning.

- **Thiazolidinediones, including rosiglitazone, cause or exacerbate congestive heart failure in some patients (5.2). After initiation of AVANDARYL, and after dose increases, observe patients carefully for**

signs and symptoms of heart failure (including excessive, rapid weight gain, dyspnea, and/or edema). If these signs and symptoms develop, the heart failure should be managed according to current standards of care. Furthermore, discontinuation or dose reduction of AVANDARYL must be considered.

- **AVANDARYL is not recommended in patients with symptomatic heart failure. Initiation of AVANDARYL in patients with established NYHA Class III or IV heart failure is contraindicated. (4, 5.2)**
- **A meta-analysis of 52 clinical trials (mean duration 6 months; 16,995 total patients), most of which compared rosiglitazone to placebo, showed rosiglitazone to be associated with a statistically significant increased risk of myocardial infarction. Three other trials (mean duration 46 months; 14,067 total patients), comparing rosiglitazone to some other approved oral antidiabetic agents or placebo, showed a statistically non-significant increased risk of myocardial infarction and a statistically non-significant decreased risk of death. There have been no clinical trials directly comparing cardiovascular risk of rosiglitazone and ACTOS® (pioglitazone, another thiazolidinedione), but in a separate trial, pioglitazone (when compared to placebo) did not show an increased risk of myocardial infarction or death. (5.3)**
- **Because of the potential increased risk of myocardial infarction, AVANDARYL is available only through a restricted distribution program called the AVANDIA-Rosiglitazone Medicines Access Program. Both prescribers and patients need to enroll in the program. To enroll, call 1-800-AVANDIA or visit www.AVANDIA.com. *[See Warnings and Precautions (5.4).]***

RECENT MAJOR CHANGES

Boxed Warning	02/2011
Indications and Usage (1)	02/2011
Dosage and Administration (2)	02/2011
Warnings and Precautions, Cardiac Failure (5.2)	02/2011
Warnings and Precautions, Major Adverse Cardiovascular Events (5.3)	02/2011
Warnings and Precautions, Rosiglitazone REMS Program (5.4)	05/2011
Warnings and Precautions, Fractures (5.10)	02/2011

INDICATIONS AND USAGE

AVANDARYL is a combination antidiabetic product containing a thiazolidinedione and a sulfonylurea. After consultation with a healthcare professional who has considered and advised the patient of the risks and benefits of rosiglitazone, this drug is indicated as an adjunct to diet and exercise to improve glycemic control when treatment with both rosiglitazone and glimepiride is appropriate in adults with type 2 diabetes who either are:

- already taking rosiglitazone, or
- not already taking rosiglitazone and unable to achieve glycemic control on other diabetes medications and, in consultation with their healthcare provider, have decided not to take pioglitazone (ACTOS) or pioglitazone-containing products (ACTOPLUS MET®, ACTOPLUS MET XR®, DUETACT®) for medical reasons. (1)

Other Important Limitations of Use:

- Should not be used in patients with type 1 diabetes or for the treatment of diabetic ketoacidosis. (1, 4)
- Coadministration with insulin is not recommended. (1, 5.2, 5.3)

DOSAGE AND ADMINISTRATION

- Individualize the starting dose based on the patient's current regimen. (2.1)
- Dose increases should be accompanied by careful monitoring for adverse events related to fluid retention. (2.2)
- Do not exceed the maximum recommended daily dose of 8 mg rosiglitazone and 4 mg glimepiride. (2.3)
- Do not initiate if the patient exhibits clinical evidence of active liver disease or increased serum transaminase levels. (2.4)

DOSAGE FORMS AND STRENGTHS

Rounded triangular tablets containing rosiglitazone/glimepiride: 4 mg/1 mg, 4 mg/2 mg, 4 mg/4 mg, 8 mg/2 mg, and 8 mg/4 mg (3)

CONTRAINDICATIONS

- Initiation in patients with established NYHA Class III or IV heart failure. (4)

WARNINGS AND PRECAUTIONS

- One sulfonylurea has been shown to increase cardiovascular mortality; consider this risk when prescribing any sulfonylurea. (5.1)
- Fluid retention, which may exacerbate or lead to heart failure, may occur. Combination use with insulin and use in congestive heart failure NYHA Class I and II may increase risk of other cardiovascular effects. (5.2)
- Increased risk of myocardial infarction has been observed in a meta-analysis of 52 clinical trials of rosiglitazone (incidence rate 0.4% versus 0.3%). (5.3)
- Use with insulin is not recommended. (1, 5.2, 5.3)
- Severe hypoglycemia may occur. Use particular care in elderly or debilitated patients and those with adrenal, pituitary, renal or hepatic insufficiency. (5.5)
- Dose-related edema (5.6), weight gain (5.7), and anemia (5.11) may occur.
- Macular edema has been reported. (5.9)
- Increased incidence of bone fracture. (5.10)
- The glimepiride component may cause hemolytic anemia in patients with glucose 6-phosphate dehydrogenase (G6PD) deficiency. Consider a non-sulfonylurea alternative in these patients. (5.12)

ADVERSE REACTIONS

Common adverse reactions (≥5%) reported in clinical trials for AVANDARYL without regard to causality were headache, hypoglycemia, and nasopharyngitis. (6.1)

To report SUSPECTED ADVERSE REACTIONS, contact GlaxoSmithKline at 1-888-825-5249 or FDA at 1-800-FDA-1088 or www.fda.gov/medwatch.

DRUG INTERACTIONS

- Inhibitors of CYP2C8 (e.g., gemfibrozil) may increase rosiglitazone levels. (7.1)
- Inducers of CYP2C8 (e.g., rifampin) may decrease rosiglitazone levels. (7.1)
- Monitor patients for loss of control with drugs that cause hyperglycemia. (7.2)

USE IN SPECIFIC POPULATIONS

- Do not use during pregnancy. No human or animal data. (8.1)
- Safety and effectiveness in children under 18 years have not been established. (8.4)
- Elderly patients may be particularly susceptible to hypoglycemic effects. (8.5)

See 17 for PATIENT COUNSELING INFORMATION and Medication Guide

Revised: 05/2011

FULL PRESCRIBING INFORMATION: CONTENTS*

*** Sections or subsections omitted from the full prescribing information are not listed**

FULL PRESCRIBING INFORMATION

WARNING: CONGESTIVE HEART FAILURE AND MYOCARDIAL INFARCTION

- Thiazolidinediones, including rosiglitazone, cause or exacerbate congestive heart failure in some patients *[see Warnings and Precautions (5.2)]*. After initiation of AVANDARYL, and after dose increases, observe patients carefully for signs and symptoms of heart failure (including excessive, rapid weight gain, dyspnea, and/or edema). If these signs and symptoms develop, the heart failure should be managed according to current standards of care. Furthermore, discontinuation or dose reduction of AVANDARYL must be considered.
- AVANDARYL is not recommended in patients with symptomatic heart failure. Initiation of AVANDARYL in patients with established NYHA Class III or IV heart failure is contraindicated. *[See Contraindications (4) and Warnings and Precautions (5.2).]*
- A meta-analysis of 52 clinical trials (mean duration 6 months; 16,995 total patients), most of which compared rosiglitazone to placebo, showed rosiglitazone to be associated with an increased risk of myocardial infarction. Three other trials (mean duration 46 months; 14,067 total patients), comparing rosiglitazone to some other approved oral antidiabetic agents or placebo, showed a statistically non-significant increased risk of myocardial infarction, and a statistically non-significant decreased risk of death. There have been no clinical trials directly comparing cardiovascular risk of rosiglitazone and ACTOS® (pioglitazone, another thiazolidinedione), but in a separate trial, pioglitazone (when compared to placebo) did not show an increased risk of myocardial infarction or death. *[See Warnings and Precautions (5.3).]*
- Because of the potential increased risk of myocardial infarction, AVANDARYL is available only through a restricted distribution program called the AVANDIA-Rosiglitazone Medicines Access Program. Both prescribers and patients need to enroll in the program. To enroll, call 1-800-AVANDIA or visit www.AVANDIA.com. *[See Warnings and Precautions (5.4).]*

1 INDICATIONS AND USAGE

After consultation with a healthcare professional who has considered and advised the patient of the risks and benefits of rosiglitazone, AVANDARYL® is indicated as an adjunct to diet and exercise to improve glycemic control when treatment with both rosiglitazone and glimepiride is appropriate in adults with type 2 diabetes mellitus who either are:

- already taking rosiglitazone, or
- not already taking rosiglitazone and unable to achieve glycemic control on other diabetes medications and, in consultation with their healthcare provider, have decided not to take pioglitazone (ACTOS®) or pioglitazone-containing products (ACTOSPLUS MET®, ACTOPLUS MET XR®, DUETACT®) for medical reasons.

Other Important Limitations of Use:

- Due to its mechanism of action, rosiglitazone is active only in the presence of endogenous insulin. Therefore, AVANDARYL should not be used in patients with type 1 diabetes or for the treatment of diabetic ketoacidosis.
- Coadministration of AVANDARYL with insulin is not recommended *[see Warnings and Precautions (5.2, 5.3)]*.

2 DOSAGE AND ADMINISTRATION

Prior to prescribing AVANDARYL, refer to *Indications and Usage (1)* for appropriate patient selection. Only prescribers enrolled in the AVANDIA-Rosiglitazone Medicines Access Program can prescribe AVANDARYL *[see Warnings and Precautions (5.4)]*.

2.1 Starting Dose

The recommended starting dose is 4 mg/1 mg administered once daily with the first meal of the day. For adults already treated with a sulfonylurea or rosiglitazone, a starting dose of 4 mg/2 mg may be considered.

All patients should start the rosiglitazone component of AVANDARYL at the lowest recommended dose. Further increases in the dose of rosiglitazone should be accompanied by careful monitoring for adverse events related to fluid retention *[see **Boxed Warning** and Warnings and Precautions (5.6)]*.

When switching from combination therapy of rosiglitazone plus glimepiride as separate tablets, the usual starting dose of AVANDARYL is the dose of rosiglitazone and glimepiride already being taken.

2.2 Dose Titration

Dose increases should be individualized according to the glycemic response of the patient. Patients who may be more sensitive to glimepiride *[see Warnings and Precautions (5.5)]*, including the elderly, debilitated, or malnourished, and those with renal, hepatic, or adrenal insufficiency, should be carefully titrated to avoid hypoglycemia. If hypoglycemia occurs during up-titration of the dose or while maintained on therapy, a dosage reduction of the glimepiride component of AVANDARYL may be considered. Increases in the dose of rosiglitazone should be accompanied by careful monitoring for adverse events related to fluid retention *[see **Boxed Warning** and Warnings and Precautions (5.6)]*.

To switch to AVANDARYL for adults currently treated with rosiglitazone, dose titration of the glimepiride component of AVANDARYL is recommended if patients are not adequately controlled after 1 to 2 weeks. The glimepiride component may be increased in no more than 2 mg increments. After an increase in the dosage of the glimepiride component, dose titration of AVANDARYL is recommended if patients are not adequately controlled after 1 to 2 weeks.

To switch to AVANDARYL for adults currently treated with sulfonylurea, it may take 2 weeks to see a reduction in blood glucose and 2 to 3 months to see the full effect of the rosiglitazone component. Therefore, dose titration of the rosiglitazone component of AVANDARYL is recommended if patients are not adequately controlled after 8 to 12 weeks. Patients should be observed carefully (1 to 2 weeks) for hypoglycemia when being transferred from longer half-life sulfonylureas (e.g., chlorpropamide) to AVANDARYL due to potential overlapping of drug effect. After an increase in the dosage of the rosiglitazone component, dose titration of AVANDARYL is recommended if patients are not adequately controlled after 2 to 3 months.

2.3 Maximum Dose

The maximum recommended daily dose is 8 mg rosiglitazone and 4 mg glimepiride.

2.4 Specific Patient Populations

Elderly and Malnourished Patients and Those With Renal, Hepatic, or Adrenal Insufficiency: In elderly, debilitated, or malnourished patients, or in patients with renal, hepatic, or adrenal insufficiency, the starting dose, dose increments, and maintenance dosage of AVANDARYL should be conservative to avoid hypoglycemic reactions. *[See Warnings and Precautions (5.5) and Clinical Pharmacology (12.3).]*

Hepatic Impairment: Liver enzymes should be measured prior to initiating treatment with AVANDARYL. Therapy with AVANDARYL should not be initiated if the patient exhibits clinical evidence of active liver disease or increased serum transaminase levels (ALT >2.5× upper limit of normal at start of therapy). After initiation of AVANDARYL, liver enzymes should be monitored periodically per the clinical judgment of the healthcare professional. *[See Warnings and Precautions (5.8) and Clinical Pharmacology (12.3).]*

Pregnancy and Lactation: AVANDARYL should not be used during pregnancy or in nursing mothers.

Pediatric Use: Safety and effectiveness of AVANDARYL in pediatric patients have not been established. AVANDARYL and its components, rosiglitazone and glimepiride, are not recommended for use in pediatric patients.

3 DOSAGE FORMS AND STRENGTHS

Each rounded triangular tablet contains rosiglitazone maleate and glimepiride as follows:

- 4 mg/1 mg – yellow, gsk debossed on one side and 4/1 on the other.
- 4 mg/2 mg – orange, gsk debossed on one side and 4/2 on the other.
- 4 mg/4 mg – pink, gsk debossed on one side and 4/4 on the other.
- 8 mg/2 mg – pale pink, gsk debossed on one side and 8/2 on the other.
- 8 mg/4 mg – red, gsk debossed on one side and 8/4 on the other.

4 CONTRAINDICATIONS

Initiation of AVANDARYL in patients with established New York Heart Association (NYHA) Class III or IV heart failure is contraindicated *[see **Boxed Warning**]*.

5 WARNINGS AND PRECAUTIONS

5.1 Increased Risk of Cardiovascular Mortality for Sulfonylurea Drugs

The administration of oral hypoglycemic drugs has been reported to be associated with increased cardiovascular mortality as compared to treatment with diet alone or diet plus insulin. This warning is based on the trial conducted by the University Group Diabetes Program (UGDP), a long-term, prospective clinical trial designed to evaluate the effectiveness of glucose-lowering drugs in preventing or delaying vascular complications in patients with non-insulin-dependent diabetes. The trial involved 823 patients who were randomly assigned to one of four treatment groups (*Diabetes* 1970;19[Suppl. 2]:747-830). UGDP reported that patients treated for 5 to 8 years with diet plus a fixed dose of tolbutamide (1.5 grams per day) had a rate of cardiovascular mortality approximately 2½ times that of patients treated with diet alone. A significant increase in total mortality was not observed, but the use of tolbutamide was discontinued based on the increase in cardiovascular mortality, thus limiting the opportunity for the trial to show an increase in overall mortality. Despite controversy regarding the interpretation of these results, the findings of the UGDP trial provide an adequate basis for this warning. The patient should be informed of the potential risks and advantages of glimepiride-containing tablets and of alternative modes of therapy.

Although only one drug in the sulfonylurea class (tolbutamide) was included in this trial, it is prudent from a safety standpoint to consider that this warning may also apply to other oral hypoglycemic drugs in this class, in view of their close similarities in mode of action and chemical structure.

5.2 Cardiac Failure With Rosiglitazone

Rosiglitazone, like other thiazolidinediones, alone or in combination with other antidiabetic agents, can cause fluid retention, which may exacerbate or lead to heart failure. Patients should be observed for signs and symptoms of heart failure. If these signs and symptoms develop, the heart failure should be managed according to current standards of care. Furthermore, discontinuation or dose reduction of rosiglitazone must be considered *[see **Boxed Warning**]*.

Patients with congestive heart failure (CHF) NYHA Class I and II treated with rosiglitazone have an increased risk of cardiovascular events. A 52-week, double-blind, placebo-controlled echocardiographic trial was conducted in 224 patients with type 2 diabetes mellitus and NYHA Class I or II CHF (ejection fraction ≤45%) on background antidiabetic and CHF therapy. An independent committee conducted a blinded evaluation of fluid-related events (including congestive heart failure) and cardiovascular hospitalizations according to predefined criteria (adjudication). Separate from the adjudication, other cardiovascular adverse events were reported by investigators. Although no treatment difference in change from baseline of ejection fractions was observed, more cardiovascular adverse events were observed with rosiglitazone treatment compared to placebo during the 52-week trial. (See Table 1.)

Table 1. Emergent Cardiovascular Adverse Events in Patients With Congestive Heart Failure (NYHA Class I and II) Treated With Rosiglitazone or Placebo (in Addition to Background Antidiabetic and CHF Therapy)

Events	Rosiglitazone	Placebo
	N = 110 n (%)	N = 114 n (%)
Adjudicated		
Cardiovascular deaths	5 (5%)	4 (4%)
CHF worsening	7 (6%)	4 (4%)
– with overnight hospitalization	5 (5%)	4 (4%)
– without overnight hospitalization	2 (2%)	0 (0%)
New or worsening edema	28 (25%)	10 (9%)
New or worsening dyspnea	29 (26%)	19 (17%)
Increases in CHF medication	36 (33%)	20 (18%)
Cardiovascular hospitalization[a]	21 (19%)	15 (13%)
Investigator-reported, non-adjudicated		
Ischemic adverse events	10 (9%)	5 (4%)
– Myocardial infarction	5 (5%)	2 (2%)
– Angina	6 (5%)	3 (3%)

[a]Includes hospitalization for any cardiovascular reason.

Initiation of AVANDARYL in patients with established NYHA Class III or IV heart failure is contraindicated. AVANDARYL is not recommended in patients with symptomatic heart failure. *[See **Boxed Warning**.]*

Patients experiencing acute coronary syndromes have not been studied in controlled clinical trials. In view of the potential for development of heart failure in patients having an acute coronary event, initiation of AVANDARYL is not recommended for patients experiencing an acute coronary event, and discontinuation of AVANDARYL during this acute phase should be considered.

Patients with NYHA Class III and IV cardiac status (with or without CHF) have not been studied in controlled clinical trials. AVANDARYL is not recommended in patients with NYHA Class III and IV cardiac status.

Congestive Heart Failure During Coadministration of Rosiglitazone With Insulin: In trials in which rosiglitazone was added to insulin, rosiglitazone increased the risk of congestive heart failure. Coadministration of rosiglitazone and insulin is not recommended. *[See Indications and Usage (1) and Warnings and Precautions (5.3).]*

In 7 controlled, randomized, double-blind trials which had durations from 16 to 26 weeks and which were included in a meta-analysis[1] *[see Warnings and Precautions (5.3)]*, patients with type 2 diabetes mellitus were randomized to coadministration of rosiglitazone and insulin (N = 1,018) or insulin (N = 815). In these 7 trials, rosiglitazone was added to insulin. These trials included patients with long-standing diabetes (median duration of 12 years) and a high prevalence of pre-existing medical conditions, including peripheral neuropathy, retinopathy, ischemic heart disease, vascular disease, and congestive heart failure. The total number of patients with emergent congestive heart failure was 23 (2.3%) and 8 (1.0%) in the rosiglitazone plus insulin and insulin groups, respectively.

Heart Failure in Observational Studies of Elderly Diabetic Patients Comparing Rosiglitazone to Pioglitazone: Three observational studies[2-4] in elderly diabetic patients (age 65 years and older) found that rosiglitazone statistically significantly increased the risk of hospitalized heart failure compared to use of pioglitazone. One other observational study[5] in patients with a mean age of 54 years, which also included an analysis in a subpopulation of patients >65 years of age, found no statistically significant increase in emergency department visits or hospitalization for heart failure in patients treated with rosiglitazone compared to pioglitazone in the older subgroup.

5.3 Major Adverse Cardiovascular Events

Cardiovascular adverse events have been evaluated in a meta-analysis of 52 clinical trials, in long-term, prospective, randomized, controlled trials, and in observational studies.

Meta-Analysis of Major Adverse Cardiovascular Events in a Group of 52 Clinical Trials: A meta-analysis was conducted retrospectively to assess cardiovascular adverse events reported across 52 double-blind, randomized, controlled clinical trials (mean duration 6 months).[1] These trials had been conducted to assess glucose-lowering efficacy in type 2 diabetes. Prospectively planned adjudication of cardiovascular events did not occur in most of the trials. Some trials were placebo-controlled and some used active oral antidiabetic drugs as controls. Placebo-controlled trials included monotherapy trials (monotherapy with rosiglitazone versus placebo monotherapy) and add-on trials (rosiglitazone or placebo, added to sulfonylurea, metformin, or insulin). Active control trials included monotherapy trials (monotherapy with rosiglitazone versus sulfonylurea or metformin monotherapy) and add-on trials (rosiglitazone plus sulfonylurea or rosiglitazone plus metformin, versus sulfonylurea plus metformin). A total of 16,995 patients were included (10,039 in treatment groups containing rosiglitazone, 6,956 in comparator groups), with 5,167 patient-years of exposure to rosiglitazone and 3,637 patient-years of exposure to comparator. Cardiovascular events occurred more frequently for patients who received rosiglitazone than for patients who received comparators (see Table 2).

Table 2. Occurrence of Cardiovascular Events in a Meta-Analysis of 52 Clinical Trials

Event[a]	Rosiglitazone (N=10,039) n (%)	Comparator (N=6,956) n (%)
MACE (a composite of myocardial infarction, cardiovascular death, or stroke)	70 (0.7)	39 (0.6)
Myocardial Infarction	45 (0.4)	20 (0.3)
Cardiovascular Death	17 (0.2)	9 (0.1)
Stroke	18 (0.2)	16 (0.2)
All-cause Death	29 (0.3)	17 (0.2)

[a] Events are not exclusive: i.e., a patient with a cardiovascular death due to a myocardial infarction would be counted

Table 3. Occurrence of MACE and Myocardial Infarction in a Meta-Analysis of 52 Clinical Trials by Trial Type

			MACE		Myocardial Infarction	
		N	n (%)	OR (95%CI)	n (%)	OR (95%CI)
Active-Controlled Trials	RSG	2,119	16 (0.8%)	1.05	10 (0.5%)	1.00
	Control	1,918	14 (0.7%)	(0.48, 2.34)	9 (0.5%)	(0.36, 2.82)
Placebo-Controlled Trials	RSG	8,124	54 (0.7%)	1.53	35 (0.4%)	2.23
	Placebo	5,636	28 (0.5%)	(0.94, 2.54)	13 (0.2%)	(1.14, 4.64)
Overall	RSG	10,039	70 (0.7%)	1.44	45 (0.4%)	1.8
	Control	6,956	39 (0.6%)	(0.95, 2.20)	20 (0.3%)	(1.03, 3.25)

RSG = rosiglitazone

Table 4. Occurrence of Cardiovascular Events for Rosiglitazone in Combination With Insulin in a Meta-Analysis of 52 Clinical Trials

Event[a]	**Rosiglitazone (N=1,018) (%)**	**Insulin (N = 815) (%)**	OR (95% CI)
MACE (a composite of myocardial infarction, cardiovascular death, or stroke)	1.3	0.6	2.14 (0.70, 7.83)
Myocardial infarction	0.6	0.1	5.6 (0.67, 262.7)
Cardiovascular death	0.4	0.0	ND, (0.47, ∞)
All-cause death	0.6	0.2	2.19 (0.38, 22.61)

ND = not defined

[a] Events are not exclusive: i.e., a patient with a cardiovascular death due to a myocardial infarction would be counted in 4 event categories (myocardial infarction; myocardial infarction, cardiovascular death, or stroke; cardiovascular death; all-cause death).

in 4 event categories (myocardial infarction; myocardial infarction, cardiovascular death, or stroke; cardiovascular death; all-cause death).

In this analysis, a statistically significant increased risk of myocardial infarction with rosiglitazone versus pooled comparators was observed. Analyses were performed using a composite of major adverse cardiovascular events (myocardial infarction, stroke, and cardiovascular death), referred to hereafter as MACE. Rosiglitazone had a statistically non-significant increased risk of MACE compared to the pooled comparators. A statistically significant increased risk of myocardial infarction and statistically non-significant increased risk of MACE with rosiglitazone was observed in the placebo-controlled trials. In the active-controlled trials, there was no increased risk of myocardial infarction or MACE. (See Figure 1 and Table 3.)

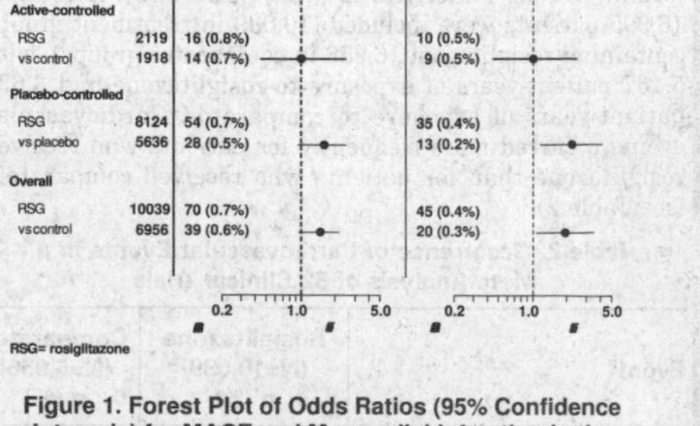

Figure 1. Forest Plot of Odds Ratios (95% Confidence Intervals) for MACE and Myocardial Infarction in the Meta-Analysis of 52 Clinical Trials

[See table 3 above]

Of the placebo-controlled trials in the meta-analysis, 7 trials had patients randomized to rosiglitazone plus insulin or insulin. There were more patients in the rosiglitazone plus insulin group compared to the insulin group with myocardial infarctions, MACE, cardiovascular deaths, and all-cause deaths (see Table 4). The total number of patients with stroke was 5 (0.5%) and 4 (0.5%) in the rosiglitazone plus insulin and insulin groups, respectively. The use of rosiglitazone in combination with insulin may increase the risk of myocardial infarction *[See Warnings and Precautions (5.1).]*

[See table 4 above]

Myocardial Infarction Events in Large, Long-Term, Prospective, Randomized, Controlled Trials of Rosiglitazone: Data from 3 large, long-term, prospective, randomized, controlled clinical trials of rosiglitazone were assessed separately from the meta-analysis.[6-8] These 3 trials included a total of 14,067 patients (treatment groups containing rosiglitazone N = 6,311; comparator groups N = 7,756), with patient-year exposure of 24,534 patient-years for rosiglitazone and 28,882 patient-years for comparator. Patient populations in the trials included patients with impaired glucose tolerance, patients with type 2 diabetes who were initiating oral agent monotherapy, and patients with type 2 diabetes who had failed monotherapy and were initiating dual oral agent therapy. Duration of follow-up exceeded 3 years in each trial.

In each of these trials, there was a statistically non-significant increase in the risk of myocardial infarction for rosiglitazone versus comparator medications.

In a long-term, randomized, placebo-controlled, 2x2 factorial trial intended to evaluate rosiglitazone, and separately ramipril (an angiotensin converting enzyme inhibitor [ACEI]), on progression to overt diabetes in 5,269 subjects with glucose intolerance, the incidence of myocardial infarction was higher in the subset of subjects who received rosiglitazone in combination with ramipril than among subjects who received ramipril alone but not in the subset of subjects who received rosiglitazone alone compared to placebo.[6] The higher incidence of myocardial infarction among subjects who received rosiglitazone in combination with ramipril was not confirmed in the two other large (total N = 8,798) long-term, randomized, active-controlled clinical trials conducted in patients with type 2 diabetes, in which 30% and 40% of patients in the two trials reported angiotensin-converting enzyme inhibitor use at baseline.[7,8]

There have been no adequately designed clinical trials directly comparing rosiglitazone to pioglitazone on cardiovascular risks. However, in a long-term, randomized, placebo-controlled cardiovascular outcomes trial comparing pioglitazone to placebo in patients with type 2 diabetes mellitus and prior macrovascular disease, pioglitazone was not associated with an increased risk of myocardial infarction or total mortality.[9]

The increased risk of myocardial infarction observed in the meta-analysis and large, long-term controlled clinical trials, and the increased risk of MACE observed in the meta-analysis described above, have not translated into a consistent finding of excess mortality from controlled clinical trials or observational studies. Clinical trials have not shown any difference between rosiglitazone and comparator medications in overall mortality or CV-related mortality.

Mortality in Observational Studies of Rosiglitazone Compared to Pioglitazone: Three observational studies in elderly diabetic patients (age 65 years and older) found that rosiglitazone statistically significantly increased the risk of all-cause mortality compared to use of ACTOS (pioglitazone).[2-4] One observational study[5] in patients with a mean age of 54 years found no difference in all-cause mortality between patients treated with rosiglitazone compared to ACTOS (pioglitazone) and reported similar results in the subpopulation of patients >65 years of age. One additional small, prospective, observational study[10] found no statistically significant differences for CV mortality and all-cause mortality in patients treated with rosiglitazone compared to ACTOS (pioglitazone).

5.4 Rosiglitazone REMS (Risk Evaluation and Mitigation Strategy) Program

Because of the potential increased risk of myocardial infarction, AVANDARYL is available only through a restricted distribution program called the AVANDIA-Rosiglitazone Medicines Access Program *[see Indications and Usage (1)]*. Both prescribers and patients must enroll in the program to be able to prescribe or receive AVANDARYL, respectively. AVANDARYL will be available only from specially certified pharmacies participating in the program. As part of the program, prescribers will be educated about the potential increased risk of myocardial infarction and the need to limit the use of AVANDARYL to eligible patients. Prescribers will need to discuss with patients the risks and benefits of taking AVANDARYL. To enroll, call 1-800-AVANDIA or visit www.AVANDIA.com.

5.5 Hypoglycemia

AVANDARYL is a combination tablet containing rosiglitazone and glimepiride, a sulfonylurea. All sulfonylurea drugs are capable of producing severe hypoglycemia. Proper patient selection, dosage, and instructions are important to avoid hypoglycemic episodes. Elderly patients are particularly susceptible to hypoglycemic action of glucose-lowering drugs. Debilitated or malnourished patients, and those with adrenal, pituitary, renal, or hepatic insufficiency are particularly susceptible to the hypoglycemic action of glucose-lowering drugs. A starting dose of 1 mg glimepiride, as contained in AVANDARYL 4 mg/1 mg, followed by appropriate dose titration is recommended in these patients. *[See Clinical Pharmacology (12.3).]* Hypoglycemia may be difficult to recognize in the elderly and in people who are taking beta-adrenergic blocking drugs or other sympatholytic agents. Hypoglycemia is more likely to occur when caloric intake is deficient, after severe or prolonged exercise, when alcohol is ingested, or when more than one glucose-lowering drug is used.

Patients receiving rosiglitazone in combination with a sulfonylurea may be at risk for hypoglycemia, and a reduction in the dose of the sulfonylurea may be necessary *[see Dosage and Administration (2.2)]*.

5.6 Edema

AVANDARYL should be used with caution in patients with edema. In a clinical trial in healthy volunteers who received 8 mg of rosiglitazone once daily for 8 weeks, there was a statistically significant increase in median plasma volume compared to placebo.

Since thiazolidinediones, including rosiglitazone, can cause fluid retention, which can exacerbate or lead to congestive heart failure, AVANDARYL should be used with caution in patients at risk for heart failure. Patients should be monitored for signs and symptoms of heart failure *[see **Boxed Warning**, Warnings and Precautions (5.2), and Patient Counseling Information (17.1)]*.

In controlled clinical trials of patients with type 2 diabetes, mild to moderate edema was reported in patients treated with rosiglitazone, and may be dose-related. Patients with ongoing edema were more likely to have adverse events associated with edema if started on combination therapy with insulin and rosiglitazone *[see Adverse Reactions (6.1)]*. The use of AVANDARYL in combination with insulin is not recommended*[see Warnings and Precautions (5.2, 5.3)]*.

5.7 Weight Gain

Dose-related weight gain was seen with AVANDARYL, rosiglitazone alone, and rosiglitazone together with other hypoglycemic agents (see Table 5). The mechanism of weight gain is unclear but probably involves a combination of fluid retention and fat accumulation.

[See table 5 at top of next page]

In a 4- to 6-year, monotherapy, comparative trial (ADOPT) in patients recently diagnosed with type 2 diabetes not previously treated with antidiabetic medication, the median weight change (25th, 75th percentiles) from baseline at 4 years was 3.5 kg (0.0, 8.1) for rosiglitazone, 2.0 kg (-1.0, 4.8) for glyburide, and -2.4 kg (-5.4, 0.5) for metformin.

In postmarketing experience with rosiglitazone alone or in combination with other hypoglycemic agents, there have been rare reports of unusually rapid increases in weight and increases in excess of that generally observed in clinical trials. Patients who experience such increases should be assessed for fluid accumulation and volume-related events such as excessive edema and congestive heart failure *[see **Boxed Warning**]*.

5.8 Hepatic Effects

With sulfonylureas, including glimepiride, there may be an elevation of liver enzyme levels in rare cases. In isolated instances, impairment of liver function (e.g., with cholestasis and jaundice), as well as hepatitis (which may also lead to liver failure) have been reported.

Liver enzymes should be measured prior to the initiation of therapy with AVANDARYL in all patients and periodically thereafter per the clinical judgment of the healthcare professional. Therapy with AVANDARYL should not be initiated in patients with increased baseline liver enzyme levels (ALT >2.5× upper limit of normal). Patients with mildly elevated liver enzymes (ALT levels ≤2.5× upper limit of normal) at baseline or during therapy with AVANDARYL should be evaluated to determine the cause of the liver enzyme elevation. Initiation of, or continuation of, therapy with AVANDARYL in patients with mild liver enzyme elevations should proceed with caution and include close clinical follow-up, including more frequent liver enzyme monitoring, to determine if the liver enzyme elevations resolve or worsen. If at any time ALT levels increase to >3× the upper limit of normal in patients on therapy with AVANDARYL, liver enzyme levels should be rechecked as soon as possible. If ALT levels remain >3× the upper limit of normal, therapy with AVANDARYL should be discontinued.

If any patient develops symptoms suggesting hepatic dysfunction, which may include unexplained nausea, vomiting, abdominal pain, fatigue, anorexia, and/or dark urine, liver enzymes should be checked. The decision whether to continue the patient on therapy with AVANDARYL should be guided by clinical judgment pending laboratory evaluations. If jaundice is observed, drug therapy should be discontinued.

5.9 Macular Edema

Macular edema has been reported in postmarketing experience in some diabetic patients who were taking rosiglitazone or another thiazolidinedione. Some patients presented with blurred vision or decreased visual acuity, but some patients appear to have been diagnosed on routine ophthalmologic examination. Most patients had peripheral edema at the time macular edema was diagnosed. Some patients had improvement in their macular edema after discontinuation of their thiazolidinedione. Patients with diabetes should have regular eye exams by an ophthalmologist, per the Standards of Care of the American Diabetes Association. Additionally, any diabetic who reports any kind of visual symptom should be promptly referred to an ophthalmologist, regardless of the patient's underlying medications or other physical findings. *[See Adverse Reactions (6.3).]*

5.10 Fractures

In a 4- to 6-year comparative trial (ADOPT) of glycemic control with monotherapy in drug-naïve patients recently diagnosed with type 2 diabetes mellitus, an increased incidence of bone fracture was noted in female patients taking rosiglitazone. Over the 4- to 6-year period, the incidence of bone fracture in females was 9.3% (60/645) for rosiglitazone versus 3.5% (21/605) for glyburide and 5.1% (30/590) for metformin. This increased incidence was noted after the first year of treatment and persisted during the course of the trial. The majority of the fractures in the women who received rosiglitazone occurred in the upper arm, hand, and foot. These sites of fracture are different from those usually associated with postmenopausal osteoporosis (e.g., hip or spine). Other trials suggest that this risk may also apply to men, although the risk of fracture among women appears higher than that among men. The risk of fracture should be considered in the care of patients treated with rosiglitazone, and attention given to assessing and maintaining bone health according to current standards of care.

5.11 Hematologic Effects

Decreases in hemoglobin and hematocrit occurred in a dose-related fashion in adult patients treated with rosiglitazone *[see Adverse Reactions (6.2)]*. The observed changes may be related to the increased plasma volume observed with treatment with rosiglitazone.

5.12 Hemolytic Anemia

Treatment of patients with glucose 6-phosphate dehydrogenase (G6PD) deficiency with sulfonylurea agents can lead to hemolytic anemia. Because glimepiride, a component of AVANDARYL, belongs to the class of sulfonylurea agents, caution should be used in patients with G6PD deficiency and a non-sulfonylurea alternative should be considered. In post-marketing experience, hemolytic anemia has also been reported in patients receiving sulfonylureas who did not have known G6PD deficiency *[see Adverse Reactions (6.1)]*.

5.13 Diabetes and Blood Glucose Control

When a patient stabilized on any antidiabetic regimen is exposed to stress such as fever, trauma, infection, or surgery, a temporary loss of glycemic control may occur. At such times, it may be necessary to withhold AVANDARYL and temporarily administer insulin. AVANDARYL may be reinstituted after the acute episode is resolved.

Periodic fasting glucose and HbA1c measurements should be performed to monitor therapeutic response.

Table 5. Weight Changes (kg) From Baseline at Endpoint During Clinical Trials [Median (25th, 75th, Percentile)]

Monotherapy

Duration	Control Group		Rosiglitazone 4 mg	Rosiglitazone 8 mg
26 weeks	Placebo	-0.9 (-2.8, 0.9) N = 210	1.0 (0.9, 3.6) N = 436	3.1 (1.1, 5.8) N = 439
52 weeks	Sulfonylurea	2.0 (0, 4.0) N = 173	2.0 (-0.6, 4.0) N = 150	2.6 (0, 5.3) N = 157

Combination Therapy

Duration	Control Group		Rosiglitazone + Control Therapy: Rosiglitazone 4 mg	Rosiglitazone + Control Therapy: Rosiglitazone 8 mg
24-26 weeks	Sulfonylurea	0 (-1.0, 1.3) N = 1,155	2.2 (0.5, 4.0) N = 613	3.5 (1.4, 5.9) N = 841
26 weeks	Metformin	-1.4 (-3.2, 0.2) N = 175	0.8 (-1.0, 2.6) N = 100	2.1 (0, 4.3) N = 184
26 weeks	Insulin	0.9 (-0.5, 2.7) N = 162	4.1 (1.4, 6.3) N = 164	5.4 (3.4, 7.3) N = 150

5.14 Ovulation

Therapy with rosiglitazone, like other thiazolidinediones, may result in ovulation in some premenopausal anovulatory women. As a result, these patients may be at an increased risk for pregnancy while taking rosiglitazone *[see Use in Specific Populations (8.1)]*. Thus, adequate contraception in premenopausal women should be recommended. This possible effect has not been specifically investigated in clinical trials; therefore the frequency of this occurrence is not known.

Although hormonal imbalance has been seen in preclinical studies *[see Nonclinical Toxicology (13.1)]*, the clinical significance of this finding is not known. If unexpected menstrual dysfunction occurs, the benefits of continued therapy with AVANDARYL should be reviewed.

6 ADVERSE REACTIONS

6.1 Clinical Trial Experience

Because clinical trials are conducted under widely varying conditions, adverse reaction rates observed in the clinical trials of a drug cannot be directly compared to rates in the clinical trials of another drug and may not reflect the rates observed in practice.

Trials utilizing rosiglitazone in combination with a sulfonylurea provide support for the use of AVANDARYL. Adverse event data from these trials, in addition to adverse events reported with the use of rosiglitazone and glimepiride therapy, are presented below.

Rosiglitazone: The most common adverse experiences with rosiglitazone monotherapy (≥5%) were upper respiratory tract infection, injury, and headache. Overall, the types of adverse experiences reported when rosiglitazone was added to a sulfonylurea were similar to those during monotherapy with rosiglitazone. In controlled combination therapy trials with sulfonylureas, mild to moderate hypoglycemic symptoms, which appear to be dose-related, were reported. Few patients were withdrawn for hypoglycemia (<1%) and few episodes of hypoglycemia were considered to be severe (<1%).

Events of anemia and edema tended to be reported more frequently at higher doses, and were generally mild to moderate in severity and usually did not require discontinuation of treatment with rosiglitazone.

Edema was reported by 4.8% of patients receiving rosiglitazone compared to 1.3% on placebo, and 1.0% on sulfonylurea monotherapy. The reporting rate of edema was higher for rosiglitazone 8 mg added to a sulfonylurea (12.4%) compared to other combinations, with the exception of insulin. Anemia was reported by 1.9% of patients receiving rosiglitazone compared to 0.7% on placebo, 0.6% on sulfonylurea monotherapy, and 2.3% on rosiglitazone in combination with a sulfonylurea. Overall, the types of adverse experiences reported when rosiglitazone was added to a sulfonylurea were similar to those during monotherapy with rosiglitazone.

In 26-week double-blind, fixed-dose trials, edema was reported with higher frequency in the rosiglitazone plus insulin combination trials (insulin, 5.4%; and rosiglitazone in combination with insulin, 14.7%). Reports of new onset or exacerbation of congestive heart failure occurred at rates of 1% for insulin alone, and 2% (4 mg) and 3% (8 mg) for insulin in combination with rosiglitazone *[see **Boxed Warning** and Warnings and Precautions (5.2)]*. The use of rosiglitazone in combination with insulin may increase the risk of myocardial infarction *[see Warnings and Precautions (5.3)]*.

Glimepiride: Hypoglycemia: The incidence of hypoglycemia with glimepiride, as documented by blood glucose values <60 mg/dL, ranged from 0.9% to 1.7% in 2 large, well-controlled, 1-year trials. In patients treated with glimepiride in US placebo-controlled trials (N = 746), adverse events, other than hypoglycemia, considered to be possibly or probably related to trial drug that occurred in more than 1% of patients included dizziness (1.7%), asthenia (1.6%), headache (1.5%), and nausea (1.1%).

Gastrointestinal Reactions: Vomiting, gastrointestinal pain, and diarrhea have been reported, but the incidence in placebo-controlled trials was less than 1%. In rare cases, there may be an elevation of liver enzyme levels. In isolated instances, impairment of liver function (e.g., with cholestasis and jaundice), as well as hepatitis, which may also lead to liver failure have been reported with sulfonylureas, including glimepiride.

Dermatologic Reactions: Allergic skin reactions, e.g., pruritus, erythema, urticaria, and morbilliform or maculopapular eruptions, occur in less than 1% of treated patients. These may be transient and may disappear despite continued use of glimepiride. If those hypersensitivity reactions persist or worsen, the drug should be discontinued. Porphyria cutanea tarda, photosensitivity reactions, and allergic vasculitis have been reported with sulfonylureas, including glimepiride.

Hematologic Reactions: Leukopenia, agranulocytosis, thrombocytopenia, hemolytic anemia *[see Warnings and Precautions (5.12)]*, aplastic anemia, and pancytopenia have been reported with sulfonylureas, including glimepiride.

Metabolic Reactions: Hepatic porphyria reactions and disulfiram-like reactions have been reported with sulfonylureas, including glimepiride. Cases of hyponatremia have been reported with glimepiride and all other sulfonylureas, most often in patients who are on other medications or have medical conditions known to cause hyponatremia or increase release of antidiuretic hormone. The syndrome of inappropriate antidiuretic hormone (SIADH) secretion has been reported with certain other sulfonylureas, including glimepiride, and it has been suggested that certain sulfonylureas may augment the peripheral (antidiuretic) action of ADH and/or increase release of ADH.

Other Reactions: Changes in accommodation and/or blurred vision may occur with the use of glimepiride. This is thought to be due to changes in blood glucose, and may be more pronounced when treatment is initiated. This condition is also seen in untreated diabetic patients, and may actually be reduced by treatment. In placebo-controlled trials of glimepiride, the incidence of blurred vision was placebo, 0.7%, and glimepiride, 0.4%.

Human Ophthalmology Data: Ophthalmic examinations were carried out in more than 500 subjects during long-term trials of glimepiride using the methodology of Taylor and West and Laties et al. No significant differences were seen between glimepiride and glyburide in the number of subjects with clinically important changes in visual acuity, intraocular tension, or in any of the 5 lens-related variables examined. Ophthalmic examinations were carried out during long-term trials using the method of Chylack et al. No significant or clinically meaningful differences were seen between glimepiride and glipizide with respect to cataract progression by subjective LOCS II grading and objective image analysis systems, visual acuity, intraocular pressure, and general ophthalmic examination *[see Nonclinical Toxicology (13.2)]*.

Long-Term Trial of Rosiglitazone as Monotherapy: A 4- to 6-year trial (ADOPT) compared the use of rosiglitazone (n = 1,456), glyburide (n = 1,441), and metformin (n = 1,454) as monotherapy in patients recently diagnosed with type 2 diabetes who were not previously treated with antidiabetic medication. Table 6 presents adverse reactions without regard to causality; rates are expressed per 100 patient-years (PY) exposure to account for the differences in exposure to trial medication across the 3 treatment groups.

In ADOPT, fractures were reported in a greater number of women treated with rosiglitazone (9.3%, 2.7/100 patient-years) compared to glyburide (3.5%, 1.3/100 patient-years) or metformin (5.1%, 1.5/100 patient-years). The majority of the fractures in the women who received rosiglitazone were reported in the upper arm, hand, and foot. *[See Warnings and Precautions (5.10).]* The observed incidence of fractures for male patients was similar among the 3 treatment groups.

Table 6. On-Therapy Adverse Events (≥5 Events/100 Patient-Years [PY]) in Any Treatment Group Reported in a 4- to 6-Year Clinical Trial of Rosiglitazone as Monotherapy (ADOPT)

	Rosiglitazone	Glyburide	Metformin
	N = 1,456	N = 1,441	N = 1,454
	PY = 4,954	PY = 4,244	PY = 4,906
Nasopharyngitis	6.3	6.9	6.6
Back pain	5.1	4.9	5.3
Arthralgia	5.0	4.8	4.2
Hypertension	4.4	6.0	6.1
Upper respiratory tract infection	4.3	5.0	4.7
Hypoglycemia	2.9	13.0	3.4
Diarrhea	2.5	3.2	6.8

6.2 Laboratory Abnormalities

Rosiglitazone: *Hematologic:* Decreases in mean hemoglobin and hematocrit occurred in a dose-related fashion in adult patients treated with rosiglitazone (mean decreases in individual trials as much as 1.0 g/dL hemoglobin and as much as 3.3% hematocrit). The changes occurred primarily during the first 3 months following initiation of therapy with rosiglitazone or following a dose increase in rosiglitazone. The time course and magnitude of decreases were similar in patients treated with a combination of rosiglitazone and other hypoglycemic agents or monotherapy with rosiglitazone. White blood cell counts also decreased slightly in adult patients treated with rosiglitazone. Decreases in hematologic parameters may be related to increased plasma volume observed with treatment with rosiglitazone.

Lipids: Changes in serum lipids have been observed following treatment with rosiglitazone in adults *[see Clinical Pharmacology (12.2)]*.

Serum Transaminase Levels: In pre-approval clinical trials in 4,598 patients treated with rosiglitazone encompassing approximately 3,600 patient-years of exposure, there was no evidence of drug-induced hepatotoxicity.

In pre-approval controlled trials, 0.2% of patients treated with rosiglitazone had reversible elevations in ALT >3× the upper limit of normal compared to 0.2% on placebo and 0.5% on active comparators. The ALT elevations in patients treated with rosiglitazone were reversible. Hyperbilirubinemia was found in 0.3% of patients treated with rosiglitazone compared with 0.9% treated with placebo and 1% in patients treated with active comparators. In pre-approval clinical trials, there were no cases of idiosyncratic drug reactions leading to hepatic failure. *[See Warnings and Precautions (5.8).]*

In the 4- to 6-year ADOPT trial, patients treated with rosiglitazone (4,954 patient-years exposure), glyburide (4,244 patient-years exposure) or metformin (4,906 patient-years exposure) as monotherapy had the same rate of ALT increase to >3× upper limit of normal (0.3 per 100 patient-years exposure).

6.3 Postmarketing Experience

In addition to adverse reactions reported from clinical trials, the events described below have been identified during post-approval use of AVANDARYL or its individual components. Because these events are reported voluntarily from a population of unknown size, it is not possible to reliably estimate their frequency or to always establish a causal relationship to drug exposure.

In patients receiving thiazolidinedione therapy, serious adverse events with or without a fatal outcome, potentially related to volume expansion (e.g., congestive heart failure, pulmonary edema, and pleural effusions) have been reported *[see **Boxed Warning** and Warnings and Precautions (5.2)]*.

There are postmarketing reports with rosiglitazone of hepatitis, hepatic enzyme elevations to 3 or more times the upper limit of normal, and hepatic failure with and without fatal outcome, although causality has not been established.

There are postmarketing reports with rosiglitazone of rash, pruritus, urticaria, angioedema, anaphylactic reaction, Stevens-Johnson syndrome, and new onset or worsening diabetic macular edema with decreased visual acuity *[see Warnings and Precautions (5.9)]*.

7 DRUG INTERACTIONS

7.1 Drugs Metabolized by Cytochrome P450

An inhibitor of CYP2C8 (e.g., gemfibrozil) may increase the AUC of rosiglitazone and an inducer of CYP2C8 (e.g., rifampin) may decrease the AUC of rosiglitazone. Therefore, if an inhibitor or an inducer of CYP2C8 is started or stopped during treatment with rosiglitazone, changes in diabetes treatment may be needed based upon clinical response. *[See Clinical Pharmacology (12.4).]*

A potential interaction between oral miconazole and oral hypoglycemic agents leading to severe hypoglycemia has been reported. Whether this interaction also occurs with the IV, topical, or vaginal preparations of miconazole is not known. Potential interactions of glimepiride with other drugs metabolized by cytochrome P450 2C9 also include phenytoin, diclofenac, ibuprofen, naproxen, and mefenamic acid. *[See Clinical Pharmacology (12.4).]*

7.2 Drugs That Produce Hyperglycemia

Certain drugs tend to produce hyperglycemia and may lead to loss of control. These drugs include the thiazides and other diuretics, corticosteroids, phenothiazines, thyroid products, estrogens, oral contraceptives, phenytoin, nicotinic acid, sympathomimetics, and isoniazid. When these drugs are administered to a patient receiving glimepiride, the patient should be closely observed for loss of control. When these drugs are withdrawn from a patient receiving glimepiride, the patient should be observed closely for hypoglycemia.

8 USE IN SPECIFIC POPULATIONS

8.1 Pregnancy

Pregnancy Category C.

All pregnancies have a background risk of birth defects, loss, or other adverse outcome regardless of drug exposure. This background risk is increased in pregnancies complicated by hyperglycemia and may be decreased with good metabolic control. It is essential for patients with diabetes or history of gestational diabetes to maintain good metabolic control before conception and throughout pregnancy. Careful monitoring of glucose control is essential in such patients. Most experts recommend that insulin monotherapy be used during pregnancy to maintain blood glucose levels as close to normal as possible. AVANDARYL should not be used during pregnancy.

Human Data: There are no adequate and well-controlled trials with AVANDARYL or its individual components in pregnant women. Rosiglitazone has been reported to cross the human placenta and be detectable in fetal tissue. The clinical significance of these findings is unknown.

Animal Studies: No animal studies have been conducted with AVANDARYL. The following data are based on findings in studies performed with rosiglitazone or glimepiride individually.

Rosiglitazone: There was no effect on implantation or the embryo with rosiglitazone treatment during early pregnancy in rats, but treatment during mid-late gestation was associated with fetal death and growth retardation in both rats and rabbits. Teratogenicity was not observed at doses up to 3 mg/kg in rats and 100 mg/kg in rabbits (approximately 20 and 75 times human AUC at the maximum recommended human daily dose, respectively). Rosiglitazone caused placental pathology in rats (3 mg/kg/day). Treatment of rats during gestation through lactation reduced litter size, neonatal viability, and postnatal growth, with growth retardation reversible after puberty. For effects on the placenta, embryo/fetus, and offspring, the no-effect dose was 0.2 mg/kg/day in rats and 15 mg/kg/day in rabbits. These no-effect levels are approximately 4 times human AUC at the maximum recommended human daily dose. Rosiglitazone reduced the number of uterine implantations and live offspring when juvenile female rats were treated at 40 mg/kg/day from 27 days of age through to sexual maturity (approximately 68 times human AUC at the maximum recommended daily dose). The no-effect level was 2 mg/kg/day (approximately 4 times human AUC at the maximum recommended daily dose). There was no effect on pre- or post-natal survival or growth.

Glimepiride: Glimepiride did not produce teratogenic effects in rats exposed orally up to 4,000 mg/kg body weight (approximately 4,000 times the maximum recommended human dose based on surface area) or in rabbits exposed up to 32 mg/kg body weight (approximately 60 times the maximum recommended human dose based on surface area). Glimepiride has been shown to be associated with intrauterine fetal death in rats when given in doses as low as 50 times the human dose based on surface area and in rabbits when given in doses as low as 0.1 times the human dose based on surface area. This fetotoxicity, observed only at doses inducing maternal hypoglycemia, has been similarly noted with other sulfonylureas, and is believed to be directly related to the pharmacologic (hypoglycemic) action of glimepiride.

In some studies in rats, offspring of dams exposed to high levels of glimepiride during pregnancy and lactation developed skeletal deformities consisting of shortening, thickening, and bending of the humerus during the postnatal period. Significant concentrations of glimepiride were observed in the serum and breast milk of the dams as well as in the serum of the pups. These skeletal deformations were determined to be the result of nursing from mothers exposed to glimepiride. Prolonged severe hypoglycemia (4 to 10 days) has been reported in neonates born to mothers who were receiving a sulfonylurea drug at the time of delivery. This has been reported more frequently with the use of agents with prolonged half-lives.

8.2 Labor and Delivery

The effect of AVANDARYL or its components on labor and delivery in humans is unknown.

8.3 Nursing Mothers

No trials have been conducted with AVANDARYL. It is not known whether rosiglitazone or glimepiride is excreted in human milk. Because many drugs are excreted in human milk, AVANDARYL should not be administered to a nursing woman.

Rosiglitazone: Drug-related material was detected in milk from lactating rats.

Glimepiride: In rat reproduction studies, significant concentrations of glimepiride were observed in the serum and breast milk of the dams, as well as in the serum of the pups. Although it is not known whether glimepiride is excreted in human milk, other sulfonylureas are excreted in human milk.

8.4 Pediatric Use

Safety and effectiveness of AVANDARYL in pediatric patients have not been established. AVANDARYL and its components, rosiglitazone and glimepiride, are not indicated for use in pediatric patients.

8.5 Geriatric Use

Rosiglitazone: Results of the population pharmacokinetic analysis showed that age does not significantly affect the pharmacokinetics of rosiglitazone *[see Clinical Pharmacology (12.3)]*. Therefore, no dosage adjustments are required for the elderly. In controlled clinical trials, no overall differences in safety and effectiveness between older (≥65 years) and younger (<65 years) patients were observed.

Glimepiride: In US clinical trials of glimepiride, 608 of 1,986 patients were 65 and older. No overall differences in safety or effectiveness were observed between these subjects and younger subjects, but greater sensitivity of some older individuals cannot be ruled out.

Comparison of glimepiride pharmacokinetics in type 2 diabetes patients ≤65 years (N = 49) and those >65 years (N = 42) was performed in a trial using a dosing regimen of 6 mg daily. There were no significant differences in glimepiride pharmacokinetics between the 2 age groups *[see Clinical Pharmacology (12.3)]*.

The drug is known to be substantially excreted by the kidney, and the risk of toxic reactions to this drug may be greater in patients with impaired renal function. Because elderly patients are more likely to have decreased renal function, care should be taken in dose selection, and it may be useful to monitor renal function.

Elderly patients are particularly susceptible to hypoglycemic action of glucose-lowering drugs. In elderly, debilitated, or malnourished patients, or in patients with renal, hepatic or adrenal insufficiency, the starting dose, dose increments, and maintenance dosage should be conservative based upon blood glucose levels prior to and after initiation of treatment to avoid hypoglycemic reactions. Hypoglycemia may be difficult to recognize in the elderly and in people who are taking beta-adrenergic blocking drugs or other sympatholytic agents *[see Dosage and Administration (2.4), Warnings and Precautions (5.5), and Clinical Pharmacology (12.3)]*.

10 OVERDOSAGE

Rosiglitazone: Limited data are available with regard to overdosage in humans. In clinical studies in volunteers, rosiglitazone has been administered at single oral doses of up to 20 mg and was well tolerated. In the event of an overdose, appropriate supportive treatment should be initiated as dictated by the patient's clinical status.

Glimepiride: Overdosage of sulfonylureas, including glimepiride, can produce hypoglycemia. Mild hypoglycemic symptoms without loss of consciousness or neurologic findings should be treated aggressively with oral glucose and adjustments in drug dosage and/or meal patterns. Close monitoring should continue until the physician is assured that the patient is out of danger. Severe hypoglycemic reactions with coma, seizure, or other neurological impairment occur infrequently, but constitute medical emergencies requiring immediate hospitalization. If hypoglycemic coma is diagnosed or suspected, the patient should be given a rapid IV injection of concentrated (50%) glucose solution. This should be followed by a continuous infusion of a more dilute (10%) glucose solution at a rate that will maintain the blood glucose level above 100 mg/dL. Patients should be closely monitored for a minimum of 24 to 48 hours, because hypoglycemia may recur after apparent clinical recovery.

11 DESCRIPTION

AVANDARYL contains 2 oral antidiabetic drugs used in the management of type 2 diabetes: rosiglitazone maleate and glimepiride.

Rosiglitazone maleate is an oral antidiabetic agent which acts primarily by increasing insulin sensitivity. Rosiglitazone maleate is not chemically or functionally related to the sulfonylureas, the biguanides, or the alpha-glucosidase inhibitors. Chemically, rosiglitazone maleate is (±)-5-[[4-[2-(methyl-2-pyridinylamino)ethoxy]phenyl] methyl]-2,4-thiazolidinedione, (*Z*)-2-butenedioate (1:1) with a molecular weight of 473.52 (357.44 free base). The molecule has a single chiral center and is present as a racemate. Due to rapid interconversion, the enantiomers are functionally indistinguishable. The molecular formula is $C_{18}H_{19}N_3O_3S \cdot C_4H_4O_4$. Rosiglitazone maleate is a white to off-white solid with a melting point range of 122° to 123°C. The pK_a values of rosiglitazone maleate are 6.8 and 6.1. It is readily soluble in ethanol and a buffered aqueous solution with pH of 2.3; solubility decreases with increasing pH in the physiological range. The structural formula of rosiglitazone maleate is:

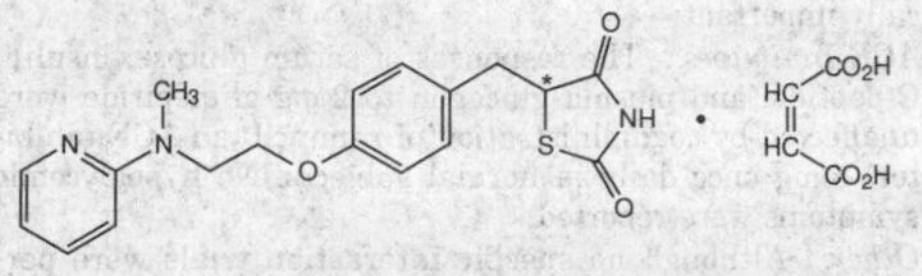

Glimepiride is an oral antidiabetic drug of the sulfonylurea class. Glimepiride is a white to yellowish-white, crystalline, odorless to practically odorless powder. Chemically, glimepiride is 1-[[p-[2-(3-ethyl-4-methyl-2-oxo-3-pyrroline-1-carboxamido)ethyl]phenyl]sulfonyl]-3-(trans-4-methylcyclohexyl)urea with a molecular weight of 490.62. The molecular formula for glimepiride is $C_{24}H_{34}N_4O_5S$. Glimepiride is practically insoluble in water. The structural formula of glimepiride is:

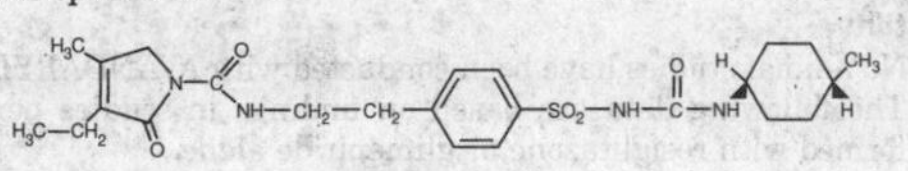

AVANDARYL is available for oral administration as tablets containing rosiglitazone maleate and glimepiride, respectively, in the following strengths (expressed as rosiglitazone maleate/glimepiride): 4 mg/1 mg, 4 mg/2 mg, 4 mg/4 mg, 8 mg/2 mg, and 8 mg/4 mg. Each tablet contains the following inactive ingredients: Hypromellose 2910, lactose monohydrate, macrogol (polyethylene glycol), magnesium stearate, microcrystalline cellulose, sodium starch glycolate, titanium dioxide, and 1 or more of the following: Yellow, red, or black iron oxides.

12 CLINICAL PHARMACOLOGY

12.1 Mechanism of Action

AVANDARYL combines 2 antidiabetic agents with different mechanisms of action to improve glycemic control in patients with type 2 diabetes: Rosiglitazone maleate, a member of the thiazolidinedione class, and glimepiride, a member of the sulfonylurea class. Thiazolidinediones are insulin-sensitizing agents that act primarily by enhancing peripheral glucose utilization, whereas sulfonylureas act primarily by stimulating release of insulin from functioning pancreatic beta cells.

Rosiglitazone: Rosiglitazone improves glycemic control by improving insulin sensitivity. Rosiglitazone is a highly selective and potent agonist for the peroxisome proliferator-activated receptor-gamma (PPARγ). In humans, PPAR receptors are found in key target tissues for insulin action such as adipose tissue, skeletal muscle, and liver. Activation of PPARγ nuclear receptors regulates the transcription of insulin-responsive genes involved in the control of glucose production, transport, and utilization. In addition, PPARγ-responsive genes also participate in the regulation of fatty acid metabolism.

Insulin resistance is a common feature characterizing the pathogenesis of type 2 diabetes. The antidiabetic activity of rosiglitazone has been demonstrated in animal models of type 2 diabetes in which hyperglycemia and/or impaired glucose tolerance is a consequence of insulin resistance in target tissues. Rosiglitazone reduces blood glucose concentrations and reduces hyperinsulinemia in the ob/ob obese mouse, db/db diabetic mouse, and fa/fa fatty Zucker rat.

In animal models, the antidiabetic activity of rosiglitazone was shown to be mediated by increased sensitivity to insulin's action in the liver, muscle, and adipose tissues. Pharmacologic studies in animal models indicate that rosiglitazone improves sensitivity to insulin in muscle and adipose tissue and inhibits hepatic gluconeogenesis. The expression of the insulin-regulated glucose transporter GLUT-4 was increased in adipose tissue. Rosiglitazone did not induce hypoglycemia in animal models of type 2 diabetes and/or impaired glucose tolerance.

Glimepiride: The primary mechanism of action of glimepiride in lowering blood glucose appears to be dependent on stimulating the release of insulin from functioning pancreatic beta cells. In addition, extrapancreatic effects may also play a role in the activity of sulfonylureas such as glimepiride. This is supported by both preclinical and clinical trials demonstrating that glimepiride administration can lead to increased sensitivity of peripheral tissues to insulin. These findings are consistent with the results of a long-term, randomized, placebo-controlled trial in which glimepiride therapy improved postprandial insulin/C-peptide responses and overall glycemic control without producing clinically meaningful increases in fasting insulin/C-peptide levels. However, as with other sulfonylureas, the mechanism by which glimepiride lowers blood glucose during long-term administration has not been clearly established.

12.2 Pharmacodynamics

The lipid profiles of rosiglitazone and glimepiride in a clinical trial of patients with inadequate glycemic control on diet and exercise were consistent with the known profile of each monotherapy. AVANDARYL was associated with increases in HDL and LDL (3% to 4% for each) and decreases in triglycerides (-4%), that were not considered to be clinically meaningful.

The pattern of LDL and HDL changes following therapy with rosiglitazone in patients previously treated with a sulfonylurea was generally similar to those seen with rosiglitazone in monotherapy. Rosiglitazone as monotherapy was associated with increases in total cholesterol, LDL, and HDL and decreases in free fatty acids. The changes in triglycerides during therapy with rosiglitazone were variable and were generally not statistically different from placebo or glyburide controls.

12.3 Pharmacokinetics

In a bioequivalence trial of AVANDARYL 4 mg/4 mg, the area under the curve (AUC) and maximum concentration (C_{max}) of rosiglitazone following a single dose of the combination tablet were bioequivalent to rosiglitazone 4 mg concomitantly administered with glimepiride 4 mg under fasted conditions. The AUC of glimepiride following a single fasted 4 mg/4 mg dose was equivalent to glimepiride concomitantly administered with rosiglitazone, while the C_{max} was 13% lower when administered as the combination tablet (see Table 7).

[See table 7 above]

Table 7. Pharmacokinetic Parameters for Rosiglitazone and Glimepiride (N = 28)

	Rosiglitazone		Glimepiride	
Parameter (Units)	**Regimen A**	**Regimen B**	**Regimen A**	**Regimen B**
$AUC_{0\text{-}inf}$ (ng.hr/mL)	1,259 (833-2,060)	1,253 (756-2,758)	1,052 (643-2,117)	1,101 (648 2,555)
$AUC_{0\text{-}t}$ (ng.hr/mL)	1,231 (810-2,019)	1,224 (744-2,654)	944 (511-1,898)	1,038 (606-2,337)
C_{max} (ng/mL)	257 (157-352)	251 (77.3-434)	151 (63.2-345)	173 (70.5-329)
T½ (hr)	3.53 (2.60-4.57)	3.54 (2.10-5.03)	7.63 (4.42-12.4)	5.08 (1.80-11.31)
T_{max} (hr)	1.00 (0.48-3.02)	0.98 (0.48-5.97)	3.02 (1.50-8.00)	2.53 (1.00-8.03)

AUC = area under the curve; C_{max} = maximum concentration; T½ = terminal half-life; T_{max} = time of maximum concentration.
Regimen A = AVANDARYL 4 mg/4 mg tablet; Regimen B = Concomitant dosing of a rosiglitazone 4 mg tablet AND a glimepiride 4 mg tablet.
Data presented as geometric mean (range), except T½ which is presented as arithmetic mean (range) and T_{max}, which is presented as median (range).

The rate and extent of absorption of both the rosiglitazone component and glimepiride component of AVANDARYL when taken with food were equivalent to the rate and extent of absorption of rosiglitazone and glimepiride when administered concomitantly as separate tablets with food.

Absorption: The AUC and C_{max} of glimepiride increased in a dose-proportional manner following administration of AVANDARYL 4 mg/1 mg, 4 mg/2 mg, and 4 mg/4 mg. Administration of AVANDARYL in the fed state resulted in no change in the overall exposure of rosiglitazone; however, the C_{max} of rosiglitazone decreased by 32% compared to the fasted state. There was an increase in both AUC (19%) and C_{max} (55%) of glimepiride in the fed state compared to the fasted state.

Rosiglitazone: The absolute bioavailability of rosiglitazone is 99%. Peak plasma concentrations are observed about 1 hour after dosing. The C_{max} and AUC of rosiglitazone increase in a dose-proportional manner over the therapeutic dose range.

Glimepiride: After oral administration, glimepiride is completely (100%) absorbed from the gastrointestinal tract. Trials with single oral doses in normal subjects and with multiple oral doses in patients with type 2 diabetes have shown significant absorption of glimepiride within 1 hour after administration and C_{max} at 2 to 3 hours.

Distribution: *Rosiglitazone:* The mean (CV%) oral volume of distribution (V_{ss}/F) of rosiglitazone is approximately 17.6 (30%) liters, based on a population pharmacokinetic analysis. Rosiglitazone is approximately 99.8% bound to plasma proteins, primarily albumin.

Glimepiride: After intravenous (IV) dosing in normal subjects, the volume of distribution (Vd) was 8.8 L (113 mL/kg), and the total body clearance (CL) was 47.8 mL/min. Protein binding was greater than 99.5%.

Metabolism and Excretion: *Rosiglitazone:* Rosiglitazone is extensively metabolized with no unchanged drug excreted in the urine. The major routes of metabolism were N-demethylation and hydroxylation, followed by conjugation with sulfate and glucuronic acid. All the circulating metabolites are considerably less potent than parent and, therefore, are not expected to contribute to the insulin-sensitizing activity of rosiglitazone. In vitro data demonstrate that rosiglitazone is predominantly metabolized by cytochrome P450 (CYP) isoenzyme 2C8, with CYP2C9 contributing as a minor pathway. Following oral or IV administration of [^{14}C]rosiglitazone maleate, approximately 64% and 23% of the dose was eliminated in the urine and in the feces, respectively. The plasma half-life of [^{14}C]related material ranged from 103 to 158 hours. The elimination half-life is 3 to 4 hours and is independent of dose.

Glimepiride: Glimepiride is completely metabolized by oxidative biotransformation after either an IV or oral dose. The major metabolites are the cyclohexyl hydroxy methyl derivative (M1) and the carboxyl derivative (M2). Cytochrome P450 2C9 has been shown to be involved in the biotransformation of glimepiride to M1. M1 is further metabolized to M2 by one or several cytosolic enzymes. M1, but not M2, possesses about ⅓ of the pharmacological activity as compared to its parent in an animal model; however, whether the glucose-lowering effect of M1 is clinically meaningful is not clear.

When [^{14}C]glimepiride was given orally, approximately 60% of the total radioactivity was recovered in the urine in 7 days and M1 (predominant) and M2 accounted for 80 to 90% of that recovered in the urine. Approximately 40% of the total radioactivity was recovered in feces and M1 and M2 (predominant) accounted for about 70% of that recovered in feces. No parent drug was recovered from urine or feces. After IV dosing in patients, no significant biliary excretion of glimepiride or its M1 metabolite has been observed.

Special Populations: No pharmacokinetic data are available for AVANDARYL in the following special populations. Information is provided for the individual components of AVANDARYL.

Gender: Rosiglitazone: Results of the population pharmacokinetics analysis showed that the mean oral clearance of rosiglitazone in female patients (N = 405) was approximately 6% lower compared to male patients of the same body weight (N = 642). Combination therapy with rosiglitazone and sulfonylureas improved glycemic control in both males and females with a greater therapeutic response observed in females. For a given body mass index (BMI), females tend to have a greater fat mass than males. Since the molecular target of rosiglitazone, PPARγ, is expressed in adipose tissues, this differentiating characteristic may account, at least in part, for the greater response to rosiglitazone in combination with sulfonylureas in females. Since therapy should be individualized, no dose adjustments are necessary based on gender alone.

Glimepiride: There were no differences between males and females in the pharmacokinetics of glimepiride when adjustment was made for differences in body weight.

Geriatric: Rosiglitazone: Results of the population pharmacokinetics analysis (N = 716 <65 years; N = 331 ≥65 years) showed that age does not significantly affect the pharmacokinetics of rosiglitazone.

Glimepiride: Comparison of glimepiride pharmacokinetics in type 2 diabetes patients 65 years and younger with those older than 65 years was performed in a trial using a dosing regimen of 6 mg daily. There were no significant differences in glimepiride pharmacokinetics between the 2 age groups. The mean AUC at steady state for the older patients was about 13% lower than that for the younger patients; the mean weight-adjusted clearance for the older patients was about 11% higher than that for the younger patients. *[See Use in Specific Populations (8.5).]*

Hepatic Impairment: Therapy with AVANDARYL should not be initiated if the patient exhibits clinical evidence of active liver disease or increased serum transaminase levels (ALT >2.5× upper limit of normal) at baseline *[see Warnings and Precautions (5.8)]*.

Rosiglitazone: Unbound oral clearance of rosiglitazone was significantly lower in patients with moderate to severe liver disease (Child-Pugh Class B/C) compared to healthy subjects. As a result, unbound C_{max} and AUC_{0-inf} were increased 2- and 3-fold, respectively. Elimination half-life for rosiglitazone was about 2 hours longer in patients with liver disease, compared to healthy subjects.

Glimepiride: No trials of glimepiride have been conducted in patients with hepatic insufficiency.

Race: Rosiglitazone: Results of a population pharmacokinetic analysis including subjects of white, black, and other ethnic origins indicate that race has no influence on the pharmacokinetics of rosiglitazone.

Glimepiride: No pharmacokinetic trials to assess the effects of race have been performed, but in placebo-controlled trials of glimepiride in patients with type 2 diabetes, the antihyperglycemic effect was comparable in whites (N = 536), blacks (N = 63), and Hispanics (N = 63).

Renal Impairment: Rosiglitazone: There are no clinically relevant differences in the pharmacokinetics of rosiglitazone in patients with mild to severe renal impairment or in hemodialysis-dependent patients compared to subjects with normal renal function.

Glimepiride: A single-dose glimepiride, open-label trial was conducted in 15 patients with renal impairment. Glimepiride (3 mg) was administered to 3 groups of patients with different levels of mean creatinine clearance (CL_{cr}); (Group I, CL_{cr} = 77.7 mL/min, N = 5), (Group II, CL_{cr} = 27.7 mL/min, N = 3), and (Group III, CL_{cr} = 9.4 mL/min, N = 7). Glimepiride was found to be well tolerated in all 3 groups. The results showed that glimepiride serum levels decreased as renal function decreased. However, M1 and M2 serum levels (mean AUC values) increased 2.3 and 8.6 times from Group I to Group III. The apparent terminal half-life (T½) for glimepiride did not change, while the half-lives for M1 and M2 increased as renal function decreased. Mean urinary excretion of M1 plus M2 as percent of dose, however, decreased (44.4%, 21.9%, and 9.3% for Groups I to III). A multiple-dose titration trial was also conducted in 16 type 2 diabetes patients with renal impairment using doses ranging from 1 to 8 mg daily for 3 months. The results were consistent with those observed after single doses. All patients with a CL_{cr} less than 22 mL/min had adequate control of their glucose levels with a dosage regimen of only 1 mg daily. The results from this trial suggest that a starting dose of 1 mg glimepiride, as contained in AVANDARYL 4 mg/1 mg, may be given to type 2 diabetes patients with kidney disease, and the dose may be titrated based on fasting glucose levels.

Pediatric: No pharmacokinetic data from trials in pediatric subjects are available for AVANDARYL.

Rosiglitazone: Pharmacokinetic parameters of rosiglitazone in pediatric patients were established using a population pharmacokinetic analysis with sparse data from 96 pediatric patients in a single pediatric clinical trial including 33 males and 63 females with ages ranging from 10 to 17 years (weights ranging from 35 to 178.3 kg). Population mean CL/F and V/F of rosiglitazone were 3.15 L/hr and 13.5 L, respectively. These estimates of CL/F and V/F were consistent with the typical parameter estimates from a prior adult population analysis.

Glimepiride: The pharmacokinetics of glimepiride (1 mg) were evaluated in a single-dose trial conducted in 30 type 2 diabetic patients (male = 7; female = 23) between ages 10 and 17 years. The mean AUC_{0-last} (338.8 ± 203.1 ng.hr/mL), C_{max} (102.4 ± 47.7 ng/mL), and T½ (3.1 ± 1.7 hours) were comparable to those previously reported in adults (AUC_{0-last} 315.2 ± 95.9 ng.hr/mL, C_{max} 103.2 ± 34.3 ng/mL, and T½ 5.3 ± 4.1 hours).

12.4 Drug-Drug Interactions

Single oral doses of glimepiride in 14 healthy adult subjects had no clinically significant effect on the steady-state pharmacokinetics of rosiglitazone. No clinically significant reductions in glimepiride AUC and C_{max} were observed after repeat doses of rosiglitazone (8 mg once daily) for 8 days in healthy adult subjects.

Rosiglitazone: *Drugs That Inhibit, Induce or are Metabolized by Cytochrome P450:* In vitro drug metabolism studies suggest that rosiglitazone does not inhibit any of the major P450 enzymes at clinically relevant concentrations. In vitro data demonstrate that rosiglitazone is predominantly metabolized by CYP2C8, and to a lesser extent, 2C9. *[See Drug Interactions (7.1).]*

Rosiglitazone (4 mg twice daily) was shown to have no clinically relevant effect on the pharmacokinetics of nifedipine and oral contraceptives (ethinyl estradiol and norethindrone), which are predominantly metabolized by CYP3A4.

Gemfibrozil: Concomitant administration of gemfibrozil (600 mg twice daily), an inhibitor of CYP2C8, and rosiglitazone (4 mg once daily) for 7 days increased rosiglitazone AUC by 127%, compared to the administration of rosiglitazone (4 mg once daily) alone. Given the potential for dose-related adverse events with rosiglitazone, a decrease in the dose of rosiglitazone may be needed when gemfibrozil is introduced *[see Drug Interactions (7.1)]*.

Rifampin: Rifampin administration (600 mg once a day), an inducer of CYP2C8, for 6 days is reported to decrease rosiglitazone AUC by 66%, compared to the administration of rosiglitazone (8 mg) alone *[see Drug Interactions (7.1)]*.[11]

Glyburide: Rosiglitazone (2 mg twice daily) taken concomitantly with glyburide (3.75 to 10 mg/day) for 7 days did not alter the mean steady-state 24-hour plasma glucose concentrations in diabetic patients stabilized on glyburide therapy. Repeat doses of rosiglitazone (8 mg once daily) for 8 days in healthy adult Caucasian subjects caused a decrease in glyburide AUC and C_{max} of approximately 30%. In Japanese subjects, glyburide AUC and C_{max} slightly increased following coadministration of rosiglitazone.

Digoxin: Repeat oral dosing of rosiglitazone (8 mg once daily) for 14 days did not alter the steady-state pharmacokinetics of digoxin (0.375 mg once daily) in healthy volunteers.

Warfarin: Repeat dosing with rosiglitazone had no clinically relevant effect on the steady-state pharmacokinetics of warfarin enantiomers.

Additional pharmacokinetic trials demonstrated no clinically relevant effect of acarbose, ranitidine, or metformin on the pharmacokinetics of rosiglitazone.

Glimepiride: The hypoglycemic action of sulfonylureas may be potentiated by certain drugs, including nonsteroidal anti-inflammatory drugs (NSAIDs) and other drugs that are highly protein bound, such as salicylates, sulfonamides, chloramphenicol, coumarins, probenecid, monoamine oxidase inhibitors, and beta-adrenergic blocking agents. When these drugs are administered to a patient receiving glimepiride, the patient should be observed closely for hypoglycemia. When these drugs are withdrawn from a patient receiving glimepiride, the patient should be observed closely for loss of glycemic control.

Certain drugs tend to produce hyperglycemia and may lead to loss of control. These drugs include the thiazides and other diuretics, corticosteroids, phenothiazines, thyroid products, estrogens, oral contraceptives, phenytoin, nicotinic acid, sympathomimetics, and isoniazid. When these drugs are administered to a patient receiving glimepiride, the patient should be closely observed for loss of control. When these drugs are withdrawn from a patient receiving glimepiride, the patient should be observed closely for hypoglycemia.

Drugs Metabolized by Cytochrome P450: A potential interaction between oral miconazole and oral hypoglycemic agents leading to severe hypoglycemia has been reported. Whether this interaction also occurs with the IV, topical, or vaginal preparations of miconazole is not known. There is a potential interaction of glimepiride with inhibitors (e.g., fluconazole) and inducers (e.g., rifampicin) of cytochrome P450 2C9.

Aspirin: Coadministration of aspirin (1 g three times daily) and glimepiride led to a 34% decrease in the mean glimepiride AUC and, therefore, a 34% increase in the mean CL/F. The mean C_{max} had a decrease of 4%. Blood glucose and serum C-peptide concentrations were unaffected and no hypoglycemic symptoms were reported.

H_2-Receptor Antagonists: Coadministration of either cimetidine (800 mg once daily) or ranitidine (150 mg twice daily) with a single 4-mg oral dose of glimepiride did not significantly alter the absorption and disposition of glimepiride, and no differences were seen in hypoglycemic symptomatology.

Beta-Blockers: Concomitant administration of propranolol (40 mg three times daily) and glimepiride significantly increased C_{max}, AUC, and T½ of glimepiride by 23%, 22%, and 15%, respectively, and it decreased CL/F by 18%. The recovery of M1 and M2 from urine, however, did not change. The pharmacodynamic responses to glimepiride were nearly identical in normal subjects receiving propranolol and placebo. Pooled data from clinical trials in patients with type 2 diabetes showed no evidence of clinically significant adverse interactions with uncontrolled concurrent administration of beta-blockers. However, if beta-blockers are used, caution should be exercised and patients should be warned about the potential for hypoglycemia.

Warfarin: Concomitant administration of glimepiride tablets (4 mg once daily) did not alter the pharmacokinetic characteristics of R- and S-warfarin enantiomers following administration of a single dose (25 mg) of racemic warfarin to healthy subjects. No changes were observed in warfarin plasma protein binding. Glimepiride treatment did result in a slight, but statistically significant, decrease in the pharmacodynamic response to warfarin. The reductions in mean area under the prothrombin time (PT) curve and maximum PT values during glimepiride treatment were very small (3.3% and 9.9%, respectively) and are unlikely to be clinically important.

ACE Inhibitors: The responses of serum glucose, insulin, C-peptide, and plasma glucagon to 2 mg glimepiride were unaffected by coadministration of ramipril (an ACE inhibitor) 5 mg once daily in normal subjects. No hypoglycemic symptoms were reported.

Other: Although no specific interaction trials were performed, pooled data from clinical trials showed no evidence of clinically significant adverse interactions with uncontrolled concurrent administration of aspirin and other salicylates, H_2-receptor antagonists, ACE inhibitors, calcium-channel blockers, estrogens, fibrates, NSAIDs, HMG CoA reductase inhibitors, sulfonamides, or thyroid hormone.

13 NONCLINICAL TOXICOLOGY

13.1 Carcinogenesis, Mutagenesis, Impairment of Fertility

No animal studies have been conducted with AVANDARYL. The following data are based on findings in studies performed with rosiglitazone or glimepiride alone.

Rosiglitazone: *Carcinogenesis:* A 2-year carcinogenicity study was conducted in Charles River CD-1 mice at doses of 0.4, 1.5, and 6 mg/kg/day in the diet (highest dose equivalent to approximately 12 times human AUC at the maximum recommended human daily dose). Sprague-Dawley rats were dosed for 2 years by oral gavage at doses of 0.05 mg/kg/day, 0.3 mg/kg/day, and 2 mg/kg/day (highest dose equivalent to approximately 10 and 20 times human AUC at the maximum recommended human daily dose for male and female rats, respectively).

Rosiglitazone was not carcinogenic in the mouse. There was an increase in incidence of adipose hyperplasia in the mouse at doses ≥1.5 mg/kg/day (approximately 2 times human AUC at the maximum recommended human daily dose). In rats, there was a significant increase in the incidence of benign adipose tissue tumors (lipomas) at doses ≥0.3 mg/kg/day (approximately 2 times human AUC at the maximum recommended human daily dose). These proliferative changes in both species are considered due to the persistent pharmacological overstimulation of adipose tissue.

Mutagenesis: Rosiglitazone was not mutagenic or clastogenic in the in vitro bacterial assays for gene mutation, the in vitro chromosome aberration test in human lymphocytes, the in vivo mouse micronucleus test, and the in vivo/in vitro rat UDS assay. There was a small (about 2-fold) increase in mutation in the in vitro mouse lymphoma assay in the presence of metabolic activation.

Impairment of Fertility: Rosiglitazone had no effects on mating or fertility of male rats given up to 40 mg/kg/day (approximately 116 times human AUC at the maximum recommended human daily dose). Rosiglitazone altered estrous cyclicity (2 mg/kg/day) and reduced fertility (40 mg/kg/day) of female rats in association with lower plasma levels of progesterone and estradiol (approximately 20 and 200 times human AUC at the maximum recommended human daily dose, respectively). No such effects were noted at 0.2 mg/kg/day (approximately 3 times human AUC at the maximum recommended human daily dose). In juvenile rats dosed from 27 days of age through to sexual maturity (at up to 40 mg/kg/day), there was no effect on male reproductive performance, or on estrous cyclicity, mating performance or pregnancy incidence in females (approximately 68 times human AUC at the maximum recommended daily dose). In monkeys, rosiglitazone (0.6 and 4.6 mg/kg/day; approximately 3 and 15 times human AUC at the maximum recommended human daily dose, respectively) diminished the follicular phase rise in serum estradiol with consequential reduction in the luteinizing hormone surge, lower luteal phase progesterone levels, and amenorrhea. The mechanism for these effects appears to be direct inhibition of ovarian steroidogenesis.

Glimepiride: *Carcinogenesis:* Studies in rats at doses of up to 5,000 parts per million (ppm) in complete feed (approximately 340 times the maximum recommended human dose, based on surface area) for 30 months showed no evidence of carcinogenesis. In mice, administration of glimepiride for 24 months resulted in an increase in benign pancreatic adenoma formation which was dose-related and is thought to be the result of chronic pancreatic stimulation. The no-effect dose for adenoma formation in mice in this study was 320 ppm in complete feed, or 46 to 54 mg/kg body weight/day. This is about 35 times the maximum human recommended dose based on surface area.

Mutagenesis: Glimepiride was non-mutagenic in a battery of in vitro and in vivo mutagenicity studies (Ames test, somatic cell mutation, chromosomal aberration, unscheduled DNA synthesis, mouse micronucleus test).

Impairment of Fertility: There was no effect of glimepiride on male mouse fertility in animals exposed up to 2,500 mg/kg body weight (>1,700 times the maximum recommended human dose based on surface area). Glimepiride had no effect on the fertility of male and female rats administered up to 4,000 mg/kg body weight (approximately 4,000 times the maximum recommended human dose based on surface area).

13.2 Animal Toxicology and/or Pharmacology

Rosiglitazone: Heart weights were increased in mice (3 mg/kg/day), rats (5 mg/kg/day), and dogs (2 mg/kg/day) with rosiglitazone treatments (approximately 5, 22, and 2 times human AUC at the maximum recommended human daily dose, respectively). Effects in juvenile rats were consistent with those seen in adults. Morphometric measurement indicated that there was hypertrophy in cardiac ventricular tissues, which may be due to increased heart work as a result of plasma volume expansion.

Glimepiride: Reduced serum glucose values and degranulation of the pancreatic beta cells were observed in beagle dogs exposed to glimepiride 320 mg/kg/day for 12 months (approximately 1,000 times the recommended human dose based on surface area). No evidence of tumor formation was observed in any organ. One female and one male dog developed bilateral subcapsular cataracts. Non-GLP studies indicated that glimepiride was unlikely to exacerbate cataract formation. Evaluation of the co-cataractogenic potential of glimepiride in several diabetic and cataract rat models was negative and there was no adverse effect of glimepiride on bovine ocular lens metabolism in organ culture *[see Adverse Reactions (6.1)]*.

14 CLINICAL STUDIES

The safety and efficacy of rosiglitazone added to a sulfonylurea have been studied in clinical trials in patients with type 2 diabetes inadequately controlled on sulfonylureas alone. No clinical trials have been conducted with the fixed-dose combination of AVANDARYL in patients inadequately controlled on a sulfonylurea or who have initially responded to rosiglitazone alone and require additional glycemic control.

A total of 3,457 patients with type 2 diabetes participated in ten 24- to 26-week randomized, double-blind, placebo/active-controlled trials and one 2-year double-blind, active-controlled trial in elderly patients designed to assess the efficacy and safety of rosiglitazone in combination with a sulfonylurea. Rosiglitazone 2 mg, 4 mg, or 8 mg daily, was administered either once daily (3 trials) or in divided doses twice daily (7 trials), to patients inadequately controlled on a submaximal or maximal dose of sulfonylurea.

In these trials, the combination of rosiglitazone 4 mg or 8 mg daily (administered as single or twice daily divided doses) and a sulfonylurea significantly reduced FPG and HbA1c compared to placebo plus sulfonylurea or further up-titration of the sulfonylurea. Table 8 shows pooled data for 8 trials in which rosiglitazone added to sulfonylurea was compared to placebo plus sulfonylurea.

[See table 8 above]

One of the 24- to 26-week trials included patients who were inadequately controlled on maximal doses of glyburide and switched to 4 mg of rosiglitazone daily as monotherapy; in this group, loss of glycemic control was demonstrated, as evidenced by increases in FPG and HbA1c.

Table 8. Glycemic Parameters in 24- to 26-Week Combination Trials of Rosiglitazone Plus Sulfonylurea

Twice Daily Divided Dosing (5 Trials)	**Sulfonylurea**	**Rosiglitazone 2 mg twice daily + sulfonylurea**	**Sulfonylurea**	**Rosiglitazone 4 mg twice daily + sulfonylurea**
N	397	497	248	346
FPG (mg/dL)				
Baseline (mean)	204	198	188	187
Change from baseline (mean)	11	-29	8	-43
Difference from sulfonylurea alone (adjusted mean)	—	-42[a]	—	-53[a]
% of patients with ≥30 mg/dL decrease from baseline	17%	49%	15%	61%
HbA1c (%)				
Baseline (mean)	9.4	9.5	9.3	9.6
Change from baseline (mean)	0.2	-1.0	0.0	-1.6
Difference from sulfonylurea alone (adjusted mean)	—	-1.1[a]	—	-1.4[a]
% of patients with ≥0.7% decrease from baseline	21%	60%	23%	75%
Once Daily Dosing (3 Trials)	**Sulfonylurea**	**Rosiglitazone 4 mg once daily + sulfonylurea**	**Sulfonylurea**	**Rosiglitazone 8 mg once daily + sulfonylurea**
N	172	172	173	176
FPG (mg/dL)				
Baseline (mean)	198	206	188	192
Change from baseline (mean)	17	-25	17	-43
Difference from sulfonylurea alone (adjusted mean)	—	-47[a]	—	-66[a]
% of patients with ≥30 mg/dL decrease from baseline	17%	48%	19%	55%
HbA1c (%)				
Baseline (mean)	8.6	8.8	8.9	8.9
Change from baseline (mean)	0.4	-0.5	0.1	-1.2
Difference from sulfonylurea alone (adjusted mean)	—	-0.9[a]	—	-1.4[a]
% of patients with ≥0.7% decrease from baseline	11%	36%	20%	68%

[a] P <0.0001 compared to sulfonylurea alone.

In a 2-year double-blind trial, elderly patients (aged 59 to 89 years) on half-maximal sulfonylurea (glipizide 10 mg twice daily) were randomized to the addition of rosiglitazone (N = 115, 4 mg once daily to 8 mg as needed) or to continued up-titration of glipizide (N = 110), to a maximum of 20 mg twice daily. Mean baseline FPG and HbA1c were 157 mg/dL and 7.72%, respectively, for the rosiglitazone plus glipizide arm and 159 mg/dL and 7.65%, respectively, for the glipizide up-titration arm. Loss of glycemic control (FPG ≥180 mg/dL) occurred in a significantly lower proportion of patients (2%) on rosiglitazone plus glipizide compared to patients in the glipizide up-titration arm (28.7%). About 78% of the patients on combination therapy completed the 2 years of therapy while only 51% completed on glipizide monotherapy. The effect of combination therapy on FPG and HbA1c was durable over the 2-year trial period, with patients achieving a mean of 132 mg/dL for FPG and a mean of 6.98% for HbA1c compared to no change on the glipizide arm.

15 REFERENCES

1. Food and Drug Administration Briefing Document. Joint meeting of the Endocrinologic and Metabolic Drugs and Drug Safety and Risk Management Advisory Committees. July 13-14, 2010.
2. Winkelmayer WC, et al. Comparison of cardiovascular outcomes in elderly patients with diabetes who initiated rosiglitazone vs pioglitazone therapy. *Arch Intern Med* 2008;168(21):2368-2375.
3. Juurlink DN, et al. Adverse cardiovascular events during treatment with pioglitazone and rosiglitazone: population based cohort study. *BMJ* 2009; 339.
4. Graham DJ, et al. Risk of acute myocardial infarction, stroke, heart failure, and death in elderly medicare patients treated with rosiglitazone or pioglitazone. *JAMA* 2010;304:411-418.
5. Wertz DA, et al. Risk of cardiovascular events and all-cause mortality in patients with Thiazolidinediones in a managed-care population. *Circ Cardiovasc Qual Outcomes* 2010;3: 538-545.
6. DREAM Trial Investigators. Effect of rosiglitazone on the frequency of diabetes in patients with impaired glucose tolerance or impaired fasting glucose: a randomised controlled trial. *Lancet* 2006;368:1096-1105.
7. Kahn S, et al. Glycemic durability of rosiglitazone, metformin or glyburide monotherapy. *New England Journal of Medicine* 2006, 355:2427-2443.
8. Home P, et al. Rosiglitazone evaluated for cardiovascular outcomes in oral agent combination therapy for type 2 diabetes (RECORD): a multicenter, randomized, open-label trial. *Lancet* 2009, 373:2125-35.
9. Dormandy J et al. Secondary prevention of macrovascular events in patients with type 2 diabetes in the PROactive study (Prospective Pioglitazone Clinical Trial in Macrovascular Events): a randomized controlled trial. *Lancet* 2005, 366:1279-89.
10. Bilik D, et al. Thiazolidinediones, cardiovascular disease and cardiovascular mortality: translating research into action for diabetes (TRIAD). *Pharmocoepidemiol Drug Saf* 2010; 19: 715–721.
11. Park JY, Kim KA, Kang MH, et al. Effect of rifampin on the pharmacokinetics of rosiglitazone in healthy subjects. *Clin Pharmacol Ther* 2004;75:157-162.

16 HOW SUPPLIED/STORAGE AND HANDLING

Each rounded triangular tablet contains rosiglitazone as the maleate and glimepiride as follows:

4 mg/1 mg – yellow, gsk debossed on one side and 4/1 on the other.

4 mg/2 mg – orange, gsk debossed on one side and 4/2 on the other.

4 mg/4 mg – pink, gsk debossed on one side and 4/4 on the other.

8 mg/2 mg – pale pink, gsk debossed on one side and 8/2 on the other.

8 mg/4 mg – red, gsk debossed on one side and 8/4 on the other.

4 mg/1 mg bottles of 30: NDC 0173-0841-13
4 mg/2 mg bottles of 30: NDC 0173-0842-13
4 mg/4 mg bottles of 30: NDC 0173-0843-13
8 mg/2 mg bottles of 30: NDC 0173-0844-13
8 mg/4 mg bottles of 30: NDC 0173-0845-13

Store at 25°C (77°F); excursions permitted to 15° to 30°C (59° to 86°F). Dispense in a tight, light-resistant container.

17 PATIENT COUNSELING INFORMATION

See Medication Guide.

17.1 Patient Advice

There are multiple medications available to treat type 2 diabetes. The benefits and risks of each available diabetes medication should be taken into account when choosing a particular diabetes medication for a given patient.

Patient should fully understand the risks and benefits of AVANDARYL. AVANDARYL should only be taken by adults with type 2 diabetes who are already taking rosiglitazone, or who are not already taking rosiglitazone and are unable to achieve adequate glycemic control on other diabetes medications, and, in consultation with their healthcare provider, have decided not to take pioglitazone (ACTOS) or pioglitazone-containing medications (ACTOPLUS MET, ACTOPLUS MET XR, DUETACT) for medical reasons. Inform patients that they must be enrolled in the AVANDIA-Rosiglitazone Medicines Access Program in order to receive AVANDARYL.

Patients should be informed of the following:

- AVANDARYL is not recommended in patients with symptomatic heart failure.
- Results of a set of clinical trials suggest that treatment with AVANDARYL is associated with an increased risk for myocardial infarction (heart attack), especially in patients taking insulin. Clinical trials have not shown any difference between rosiglitazone and comparator medications in overall mortality or CV-related mortality.
- AVANDARYL is not recommended for patients who are taking insulin.
- Management of type 2 diabetes should include diet control. Caloric restriction, weight loss, and exercise are essential for the proper treatment of the diabetic patient because they help improve insulin sensitivity. This is important not only in the primary treatment of type 2 diabetes, but also in maintaining the efficacy of drug therapy.
- It is important to adhere to dietary instructions and to regularly have blood glucose and glycosylated hemoglobin (HbA1c) tested. It can take 2 weeks to see a reduction in blood glucose and 2 to 3 months to see the full effect of AVANDARYL.
- The risks of hypoglycemia, its symptoms and treatment, and conditions that predispose to its development should be explained to patients and their family members.
- Blood will be drawn to check their liver function prior to the start of therapy and periodically thereafter per the clinical judgment of the healthcare professional. Patients with unexplained symptoms of nausea, vomiting, abdominal pain, fatigue, anorexia, or dark urine should immediately report these symptoms to their physician.
- Patients who experience an unusually rapid increase in weight or edema or who develop shortness of breath or other symptoms of heart failure while on AVANDARYL should immediately report these symptoms to their physician.
- AVANDARYL should be taken with the first meal of the day.
- Therapy with rosiglitazone, like other thiazolidinediones, may result in ovulation in some premenopausal anovulatory women. As a result, these patients may be at an increased risk for pregnancy while taking AVANDARYL. Thus, adequate contraception in premenopausal women should be recommended. This possible effect has not been specifically investigated in clinical trials so the frequency of this occurrence is not known.

AVANDARYL and AVANDIA are registered trademarks of GlaxoSmithKline. ACTOS, ACTOPLUS MET, ACTOPLUS MET XR, and DUETACT are registered trademarks of Takeda Pharmaceutical Company Limited.

GlaxoSmithKline
Research Triangle Park, NC 27709

May 2011
AVR:12PI

MEDICATION GUIDE

AVANDARYL® (ah-VAN-duh-ril)

(rosiglitazone maleate and glimepiride) Tablets

Read this Medication Guide carefully before you start taking AVANDARYL and each time you get a refill. There may be new information. This information does not take the place of talking with your doctor about your medical condition or your treatment. If you have any questions about AVANDARYL, ask your doctor or pharmacist.

What is the most important information I should know about AVANDARYL?

AVANDARYL is available only through the AVANDIA-Rosiglitazone Medicines Access Program. Both you and your doctor must be enrolled in the program so that you can get AVANDARYL. To enroll, you must:

- talk to your doctor,
- understand the risks and benefits of AVANDARYL, and
- agree to enroll in the program.

AVANDARYL may cause serious side effects, including:

New or worse heart failure

- Rosiglitazone, one of the two drugs that make up AVANDARYL, can cause your body to keep extra fluid (fluid retention), which leads to swelling (edema) and weight gain. Extra body fluid can make some heart problems worse or lead to heart failure. Heart failure means your heart does not pump blood well enough.
- If you have severe heart failure, you cannot start AVANDARYL.
- If you have heart failure with symptoms (such as shortness of breath or swelling), even if these symptoms are not severe, AVANDARYL may not be right for you.

Call your doctor right away if you have any of the following:

- swelling or fluid retention, especially in the ankles or legs
- shortness of breath or trouble breathing, especially when you lie down
- an unusually fast increase in weight
- unusual tiredness

Myocardial Infarction ("Heart Attack")

Rosiglitazone, one of the medicines in AVANDARYL, may raise the risk of heart attack. The risk of having a heart attack may be higher in people who take AVANDARYL with insulin. Most people who take insulin should not also take AVANDARYL.

Symptoms of a heart attack can include the following:

- chest discomfort in the center of your chest that lasts for more than a few minutes, or that goes away or comes back
- chest discomfort that feels like uncomfortable pressure, squeezing, fullness or pain
- pain or discomfort in your arms, back, neck, jaw or stomach
- shortness of breath with or without chest discomfort
- breaking out in a cold sweat
- nausea or vomiting
- feeling lightheaded

Call your doctor or go to the nearest hospital emergency room right away if you think you are having a heart attack.

People with diabetes have a greater risk for heart problems. It is important to work with your doctor to manage other conditions, such as high blood pressure or high cholesterol.

AVANDARYL can have other serious side effects. Be sure to read the section "What are possible side effects of AVANDARYL?".

What is AVANDARYL?

AVANDARYL contains 2 prescription medicines to treat diabetes, rosiglitazone maleate (AVANDIA) and glimepiride (AMARYL). AVANDARYL is used with diet and exercise to treat certain adults with type 2 ("adult-onset" or "non-insulin dependent") diabetes mellitus ("high blood sugar") who are:

- already taking rosiglitazone or rosiglitazone-containing products
- unable to control their blood sugar on other diabetes medicines, and after talking with their doctor have decided not to take pioglitazone (ACTOS) or pioglitazone-containing products (ACTOPLUS MET, ACTOPLUS MET XR, DUETACT)

Glimepiride can help your body release more of its own insulin. Rosiglitazone can help your body respond better to the insulin made in your body and does not cause your body to make more insulin. These medicines can work together to help control your blood sugar.

AVANDARYL is not for people with type 1 diabetes mellitus or to treat a condition called diabetic ketoacidosis.

It is not known if AVANDARYL is safe and effective in children under 18 years old.

Who should not take AVANDARYL?

Many people with heart failure should not start taking AVANDARYL (see "What should I tell my doctor before taking AVANDARYL?").

What should I tell my doctor before taking AVANDARYL?

Before starting AVANDARYL, ask your doctor about what the choices are for diabetes medicines and what the expected benefits and possible risks are for you in particular. Before taking AVANDARYL, tell your doctor about all your medical conditions, including if you:

- **have heart problems or heart failure.**
- **have type 1 ("juvenile") diabetes or had diabetic ketoacidosis.** These conditions should be treated with insulin and should not be treated with AVANDARYL.
- **have a type of diabetic eye disease called macular edema** (swelling of the back of the eye).
- **have liver problems.** Your doctor should do blood tests to check your liver before you start taking AVANDARYL and during treatment as needed.
- **had liver problems while taking REZULIN® (troglitazone), another medicine for diabetes.**
- **have kidney problems.** If people with kidney problems use AVANDARYL, they may need a lower dose of the medication.
- **have glucose 6-phosphate dehydrogenase (G6PD) deficiency.** This condition runs in families. People with G6PD deficiency who take glimepiride (one of the medicines in AVANDARYL) may develop hemolytic anemia (fast breakdown of red blood cells).
- **are pregnant or plan to become pregnant.** AVANDARYL should not be used during pregnancy. It is not known if AVANDARYL can harm your unborn baby. You and your doctor should talk about the best way to control your diabetes during pregnancy. If you are a premenopausal woman (before the "change of life") who does not have regular monthly periods, AVANDARYL may increase your chances of becoming pregnant. Talk to your doctor about birth control choices while taking AVANDARYL. Tell your doctor right away if you become pregnant while taking AVANDARYL.
- **are breast-feeding or planning to breast-feed.** It is not known if AVANDARYL passes into breast milk. You should not use AVANDARYL while breast-feeding.

Tell your doctor about all the medicines you take including prescription and non-prescription medicines, vitamins or herbal supplements. AVANDARYL and certain other medicines can affect each other and may lead to serious side effects including high or low blood sugar, or heart problems. Especially tell your doctor if you take:

- **insulin.**
- **any medicines for high blood pressure, high cholesterol or heart failure, or for prevention of heart disease or stroke.**

Know the medicines you take. Keep a list of all your medicines and show it to your doctor and pharmacist before you start a new medicine. They will tell you if it is alright to take AVANDARYL with other medicines.

How should I take AVANDARYL?

- Take AVANDARYL exactly as prescribed. Your doctor may need to change your dose until your blood sugar is better controlled.
- Take AVANDARYL by mouth one time each day with your first main meal.
- It usually takes a few days for AVANDARYL to start lowering your blood sugar. It may take 2 to 3 months to see the full effect on your blood sugar level.
- If you miss a dose of AVANDARYL, take it as soon as you remember unless it is time to take your next dose. Take your next dose at the usual time. Do not take double doses to make up for a missed dose.
- If you take too much AVANDARYL, call your doctor or poison control center right away.
- Test your blood sugar regularly as your doctor tells you.
- Your doctor should do blood tests to check your liver before you start AVANDARYL and during treatment as needed. Your doctor should also do regular blood sugar tests (for example, "A1c") to monitor your response to AVANDARYL.
- Call your doctor if you get sick, get injured, get an infection, or have surgery. AVANDARYL may not control your blood sugar levels during these times. Your doctor may need to stop AVANDARYL for a short time and give you insulin to control your blood sugar level.
- Diet and exercise can help your body use its blood sugar better. It is important to stay on your recommended diet, lose extra weight, and get regular exercise while taking AVANDARYL.

What are possible side effects of AVANDARYL?

AVANDARYL may cause serious side effects, including:

- **New or worse heart failure.** See "What is the most important information I should know about AVANDARYL?".
- **Heart attack.** See "What is the most important information I should know about AVANDARYL?".
- **Swelling (edema).** AVANDARYL can cause swelling due to fluid retention. See "What is the most important information I should know about AVANDARYL?".
- **Low blood sugar (hypoglycemia).** Lightheadedness, dizziness, shakiness or hunger may mean that your blood sugar is too low. This can happen if you skip meals, drink alcohol, use another medicine that lowers blood sugar, ex-

ercise (particularly hard or long), or if you have certain medical problems. Call your doctor if low blood sugar levels are a problem for you.
- **Weight gain.** Rosiglitazone, one of the medicines in AVANDARYL, can cause weight gain that may be due to fluid retention or extra body fat. Weight gain can be a serious problem for people with certain conditions including heart problems. See "What is the most important information I should know about AVANDARYL?".
- **Liver problems.** It is important for your liver to be working normally when you take AVANDARYL. Your doctor should do blood tests to check your liver before you start taking AVANDARYL and during treatment as needed. Call your doctor right away if you have unexplained symptoms such as:
  - nausea or vomiting
  - stomach pain
  - unusual or unexplained tiredness
  - loss of appetite
  - dark urine
  - yellowing of your skin or the whites of your eyes.
- **Macular edema** (a diabetic eye disease with swelling in the back of the eye). Tell your doctor right away if you have any changes in your vision. Your doctor should check your eyes regularly. Very rarely, some people have had vision changes due to swelling in the back of the eye while taking rosiglitazone, one of the medicines in AVANDARYL.
- **Fractures (broken bones)**, usually in the hand, upper arm or foot. Talk to your doctor for advice on how to keep your bones healthy.
- **Low red blood cell count (anemia).**
- **Ovulation** (release of egg from an ovary in women) leading to pregnancy. Ovulation may happen in premenopausal women who do not have regular monthly periods. This can increase the chance of pregnancy. See "What should I tell my doctor before taking AVANDARYL?".

The most common side effects with AVANDARYL include cold-like symptoms and headache.

Call your doctor for medical advice about side effects. You may report side effects to FDA at 1-800-FDA-1088.

How should I store AVANDARYL?
- Store AVANDARYL at room temperature, 59° to 86° F (15° to 30° C). Keep AVANDARYL in the container it comes in. Keep the container closed tightly.
- Safely, throw away AVANDARYL that is out of date or no longer needed.

Keep AVANDARYL and all medicines out of the reach of children.

General information about AVANDARYL

Medicines are sometimes prescribed for purposes other than those listed in a Medication Guide. Do not use AVANDARYL for a condition for which it was not prescribed. Do not give AVANDARYL to other people, even if they have the same symptoms you have. It may harm them.

This Medication Guide summarizes important information about AVANDARYL. If you would like more information, talk with your doctor. You can ask your doctor or pharmacist for information about AVANDARYL that is written for healthcare professionals. You can also find out more about AVANDARYL by calling 1-888-825-5249.

What are the ingredients in AVANDARYL?

Active Ingredients: Rosiglitazone maleate and glimepiride.

Inactive Ingredients: Hypromellose 2910, lactose monohydrate, macrogol (polyethylene glycol), magnesium stearate, microcrystalline cellulose, sodium starch glycolate, titanium dioxide, triacetin, and 1 or more of the following: Yellow, red, or black iron oxides.

Always check to make sure that the medicine you are taking is the correct one. AVANDARYL tablets are triangles with rounded corners and look like this:

4 mg/1 mg – yellow with "gsk" on one side and "4/1" on the other.

4 mg/2 mg – orange with "gsk" on one side and "4/2" on the other.

4 mg/4 mg – pink with "gsk" on one side and "4/4" on the other.

8 mg/2 mg – pale pink with "gsk" on one side and "8/2" on the other.

8 mg/4 mg – red with "gsk" on one side and "8/4" on the other.

AVANDARYL and AVANDIA are registered trademarks of GlaxoSmithKline.

The other brands listed are trademarks of their respective owners and are not trademarks of GlaxoSmithKline. The makers of these brands are not affiliated with and do not endorse GlaxoSmithKline or its products.

This Medication Guide has been approved by the U.S. Food and Drug Administration.

GlaxoSmithKline
Research Triangle Park, NC 27709

May 2011
AVR:4MG

AVANDIA® ℞

[ə-van′dē-ə]
(rosiglitazone maleate)
Tablets

HIGHLIGHTS OF PRESCRIBING INFORMATION
These highlights do not include all the information needed to use AVANDIA safely and effectively. See full prescribing information for AVANDIA.
AVANDIA (rosiglitazone maleate) Tablets
Initial U.S. Approval: 1999

WARNING: CONGESTIVE HEART FAILURE AND MYOCARDIAL INFARCTION

See full prescribing information for complete boxed warning.

- **Thiazolidinediones, including rosiglitazone, cause or exacerbate congestive heart failure in some patients (5.1). After initiation of AVANDIA, and after dose increases, observe patients carefully for signs and symptoms of heart failure (including excessive, rapid weight gain, dyspnea, and/or edema). If these signs and symptoms develop, the heart failure should be managed according to current standards of care. Furthermore, discontinuation or dose reduction of AVANDIA must be considered.**
- **AVANDIA is not recommended in patients with symptomatic heart failure. Initiation of AVANDIA in patients with established NYHA Class III or IV heart failure is contraindicated. (4, 5.1)**
- **A meta-analysis of 52 clinical trials (mean duration 6 months; 16,995 total patients), most of which compared AVANDIA to placebo, showed AVANDIA to be associated with a statistically significant increased risk of myocardial infarction. Three other trials (mean duration 46 months; 14,067 total patients), comparing AVANDIA to some other approved oral antidiabetic agents or placebo, showed a statistically non-significant increased risk of myocardial infarction and a statistically non-significant decreased risk of death. There have been no clinical trials directly comparing cardiovascular risk of AVANDIA and ACTOS® (pioglitazone, another thiazolidinedione), but in a separate trial, ACTOS (when compared to placebo) did not show an increased risk of myocardial infarction or death. (5.2)**
- **Because of the potential increased risk of myocardial infarction, AVANDIA is available only through a restricted distribution program called the AVANDIA-Rosiglitazone Medicines Access Program. Both prescribers and patients need to enroll in the program. To enroll, call 1-800-AVANDIA or visit www.AVANDIA.com. *[See Warnings and Precautions (5.3).]***

RECENT MAJOR CHANGES

Boxed Warning	02/2011
Indications and Usage (1)	02/2011
Dosage and Administration (2)	02/2011
Warnings and Precautions, Cardiac Failure (5.1)	02/2011
Warnings and Precautions, Major Adverse Cardiovascular Events (5.2)	02/2011
Warnings and Precautions, Rosiglitazone REMS Program (5.3)	05/2011
Warnings and Precautions, Fractures (5.8)	02/2011

INDICATIONS AND USAGE

AVANDIA is a thiazolidinedione antidiabetic agent. After consultation with a healthcare professional who has considered and advised the patient of the risks and benefits of AVANDIA, this drug is indicated as an adjunct to diet and exercise to improve glycemic control in adults with type 2 diabetes mellitus who either are:
- already taking AVANDIA, or
- not already taking AVANDIA and are unable to achieve adequate glycemic control on other diabetes medications, and, in consultation with their healthcare provider, have decided not to take pioglitazone (ACTOS) for medical reasons. (1)

Other Important Limitations of Use:
- AVANDIA should not be used in patients with type 1 diabetes mellitus or for the treatment of diabetic ketoacidosis. (1)
- Coadministration of AVANDIA and insulin is not recommended. (1, 5.1, 5.2)

DOSAGE AND ADMINISTRATION

- Start at 4 mg daily in single or divided doses; do not exceed 8 mg daily. (2)
- Dose increases should be accompanied by careful monitoring for adverse events related to fluid retention. (2)
- Do not initiate AVANDIA if the patient exhibits clinical evidence of active liver disease or increased serum transaminase levels. (2.1)

DOSAGE FORMS AND STRENGTHS

Pentagonal, film-coated tablets in the following strengths:
- 2 mg, 4 mg, and 8 mg (3)

CONTRAINDICATIONS

Initiation of AVANDIA in patients with established NYHA Class III or IV heart failure is contraindicated. (4)

WARNINGS AND PRECAUTIONS

- Fluid retention, which may exacerbate or lead to heart failure, may occur. Combination use with insulin and use in congestive heart failure NYHA Class I and II may increase risk of other cardiovascular effects. (5.1)
- Increased risk of myocardial infarction has been observed in a meta-analysis of 52 clinical trials (incidence rate 0.4% versus 0.3%). (5.2)
- Coadministration of AVANDIA and insulin is not recommended. (1, 5.1, 5.2)
- Dose-related edema (5.4), weight gain (5.5), and anemia (5.9) may occur.
- Macular edema has been reported. (5.7)
- Increased incidence of bone fracture. (5.8)

ADVERSE REACTIONS

Common adverse reactions (>5%) reported in clinical trials without regard to causality were upper respiratory tract infection, injury, and headache. (6.1)

To report SUSPECTED ADVERSE REACTIONS, contact GlaxoSmithKline at 1-888-825-5249 or FDA at 1-800-FDA-1088 or www.fda.gov/medwatch.

DRUG INTERACTIONS

Inhibitors of CYP2C8 (e.g., gemfibrozil) may increase rosiglitazone levels; inducers of CYP2C8 (e.g., rifampin) may decrease rosiglitazone levels. (7.1)

See 17 for PATIENT COUNSELING INFORMATION and Medication Guide

Revised: 05/2011

FULL PRESCRIBING INFORMATION: CONTENTS*

*** Sections or subsections omitted from the full prescribing information are not listed**

FULL PRESCRIBING INFORMATION

WARNING: CONGESTIVE HEART FAILURE AND MYOCARDIAL INFARCTION

- Thiazolidinediones, including rosiglitazone, cause or exacerbate congestive heart failure in some patients *[see Warnings and Precautions (5.1)]*. After initiation of AVANDIA, and after dose increases, observe patients carefully for signs and symptoms of heart failure (including excessive, rapid weight gain, dyspnea, and/or edema). If these signs and symptoms develop, the heart failure should be managed according to current standards of care. Furthermore, discontinuation or dose reduction of AVANDIA must be considered.
- AVANDIA is not recommended in patients with symptomatic heart failure. Initiation of AVANDIA in patients with established NYHA Class III or IV heart failure is contraindicated. *[See Contraindications (4) and Warnings and Precautions (5.1).]*
- A meta-analysis of 52 clinical trials (mean duration 6 months; 16,995 total patients), most of which compared AVANDIA to placebo, showed AVANDIA to be associated with a statistically significant increased risk of myocardial infarction. Three other trials (mean duration 46 months; 14,067 total patients), comparing AVANDIA to some other approved oral antidiabetic agents or placebo, showed a statistically non-significant increased risk of myocardial infarction, and a statistically non-significant decreased risk of death. There have been no clinical trials directly comparing cardiovascular risk of AVANDIA and ACTOS® (pioglitazone, another thiazolidinedione), but in a separate trial, pioglitazone (when compared to placebo) did not show an increased risk of myocardial infarction or death. *[See Warnings and Precautions (5.2).]*
- Because of the potential increased risk of myocardial infarction, AVANDIA is available only through a restricted distribution program called the AVANDIA-Rosiglitazone Medicines Access Program. Both prescribers and patients need to enroll in the program. To enroll, call 1-800-AVANDIA or visit www.AVANDIA.com. *[See Warnings and Precautions (5.3).]*

1 INDICATIONS AND USAGE

After consultation with a healthcare professional who has considered and advised the patient of the risks and benefits of AVANDIA®, this drug is indicated as an adjunct to diet and exercise to improve glycemic control in adults with type 2 diabetes mellitus who either are:
- already taking AVANDIA, or
- not already taking AVANDIA and are unable to achieve adequate glycemic control on other diabetes medications and, in consultation with their healthcare provider, have decided not to take pioglitazone (ACTOS®) for medical reasons.

Other Important Limitations of Use:
- Due to its mechanism of action, AVANDIA is active only in the presence of endogenous insulin. Therefore, AVANDIA should not be used in patients with type 1 diabetes mellitus or for the treatment of diabetic ketoacidosis.
- The coadministration of AVANDIA and insulin is not recommended *[see Warnings and Precautions (5.1)]*.

2 DOSAGE AND ADMINISTRATION

Prior to prescribing AVANDIA, refer to *Indications and Usage (1)* for appropriate patient selection. Only prescribers enrolled in the AVANDIA-Rosiglitazone Medicines Access Program can prescribe AVANDIA *[see Warnings and Precautions (5.3)]*.

AVANDIA may be administered at a starting dose of 4 mg either as a single daily dose or in 2 divided doses. For patients who respond inadequately following 8 to 12 weeks of treatment, as determined by reduction in fasting plasma glucose (FPG), the dose may be increased to 8 mg daily. Increases in the dose of AVANDIA should be accompanied by careful monitoring for adverse events related to fluid retention *[see Boxed Warning and Warnings and Precautions (5.1)]*. AVANDIA may be taken with or without food.

The total daily dose of AVANDIA should not exceed 8 mg. Patients receiving AVANDIA in combination with other hypoglycemic agents may be at risk for hypoglycemia, and a reduction in the dose of the concomitant agent may be necessary.

2.1 Specific Patient Populations

Renal Impairment: No dosage adjustment is necessary when AVANDIA is used as monotherapy in patients with renal impairment. Since metformin is contraindicated in such patients, concomitant administration of metformin and AVANDIA is also contraindicated in patients with renal impairment.

Hepatic Impairment: Liver enzymes should be measured prior to initiating treatment with AVANDIA. Therapy with AVANDIA should not be initiated if the patient exhibits clinical evidence of active liver disease or increased serum transaminase levels (ALT >2.5× upper limit of normal at start of therapy). After initiation of AVANDIA, liver enzymes should be monitored periodically per the clinical judgment of the healthcare professional. *[See Warnings and Precautions (5.6) and Clinical Pharmacology (12.3).]*

Pediatric: Data are insufficient to recommend pediatric use of AVANDIA *[see Use in Specific Populations (8.4)]*.

3 DOSAGE FORMS AND STRENGTHS

Pentagonal film-coated TILTAB® tablet contains rosiglitazone as the maleate as follows:
- 2 mg - pink, debossed with SB on one side and 2 on the other
- 4 mg - orange, debossed with SB on one side and 4 on the other
- 8 mg - red-brown, debossed with SB on one side and 8 on the other

4 CONTRAINDICATIONS

Initiation of AVANDIA in patients with established New York Heart Association (NYHA) Class III or IV heart failure is contraindicated *[see Boxed Warning]*.

5 WARNINGS AND PRECAUTIONS

5.1 Cardiac Failure

AVANDIA, like other thiazolidinediones, alone or in combination with other antidiabetic agents, can cause fluid retention, which may exacerbate or lead to heart failure. Patients should be observed for signs and symptoms of heart failure. If these signs and symptoms develop, the heart failure should be managed according to current standards of care. Furthermore, discontinuation or dose reduction of rosiglitazone must be considered *[see Boxed Warning]*.

Patients with congestive heart failure (CHF) NYHA Class I and II treated with AVANDIA have an increased risk of cardiovascular events. A 52-week, double-blind, placebo-controlled echocardiographic trial was conducted in 224 patients with type 2 diabetes mellitus and NYHA Class I or II CHF (ejection fraction ≤45%) on background antidiabetic and CHF therapy. An independent committee conducted a blinded evaluation of fluid-related events (including congestive heart failure) and cardiovascular hospitalizations according to predefined criteria (adjudication). Separate from the adjudication, other cardiovascular adverse events were reported by investigators. Although no treatment difference in change from baseline of ejection fractions was observed, more cardiovascular adverse events were observed following treatment with AVANDIA compared to placebo during the 52-week trial. (See Table 1.)

Table 1. Emergent Cardiovascular Adverse Events in Patients With Congestive Heart Failure (NYHA Class I and II) Treated With AVANDIA or Placebo (in Addition to Background Antidiabetic and CHF Therapy)

Events	AVANDIA	Placebo
	N = 110 n (%)	N = 114 n (%)
Adjudicated		
Cardiovascular deaths	5 (5%)	4 (4%)
CHF worsening	7 (6%)	4 (4%)
– with overnight hospitalization	5 (5%)	4 (4%)
– without overnight hospitalization	2 (2%)	0 (0%)
New or worsening edema	28 (25%)	10 (9%)
New or worsening dyspnea	29 (26%)	19 (17%)
Increases in CHF medication	36 (33%)	20 (18%)
Cardiovascular hospitalization[a]	21 (19%)	15 (13%)
Investigator-reported, non-adjudicated		
Ischemic adverse events	10 (9%)	5 (4%)
– Myocardial infarction	5 (5%)	2 (2%)
– Angina	6 (5%)	3 (3%)

[a] Includes hospitalization for any cardiovascular reason.

Initiation of AVANDIA in patients with established NYHA Class III or IV heart failure is contraindicated. AVANDIA is not recommended in patients with symptomatic heart failure. *[See Boxed Warning.]*

Patients experiencing acute coronary syndromes have not been studied in controlled clinical trials. In view of the potential for development of heart failure in patients having an acute coronary event, initiation of AVANDIA is not recommended for patients experiencing an acute coronary event, and discontinuation of AVANDIA during this acute phase should be considered.

Patients with NYHA Class III and IV cardiac status (with or without CHF) have not been studied in controlled clinical trials. AVANDIA is not recommended in patients with NYHA Class III and IV cardiac status.

Congestive Heart Failure During Coadministration of AVANDIA With Insulin: In trials in which AVANDIA was added to insulin, AVANDIA increased the risk of congestive heart failure. Coadministration of AVANDIA and insulin is not recommended. *[See Indications and Usage (1) and Warnings and Precautions (5.2).]*

In 7 controlled, randomized, double-blind trials which had durations from 16 to 26 weeks and which were included in a meta-analysis[1] *[see Warnings and Precautions (5.2)]*, patients with type 2 diabetes mellitus were randomized to coadministration of AVANDIA and insulin (N = 1,018) or insulin (N = 815). In these 7 trials, AVANDIA was added to insulin. These trials included patients with long-standing diabetes (median duration of 12 years) and a high prevalence of pre-existing medical conditions, including peripheral neuropathy, retinopathy, ischemic heart disease, vascular disease, and congestive heart failure. The total number of patients with emergent congestive heart failure was 23 (2.3%) and 8 (1.0%) in the AVANDIA plus insulin and insulin groups, respectively.

Heart Failure in Observational Studies of Elderly Diabetic Patients Comparing AVANDIA to ACTOS: Three observational studies[2-4] in elderly diabetic patients (age 65 years and older) found that AVANDIA statistically significantly increased the risk of hospitalized heart failure compared to use of ACTOS. One other observational study[5] in patients with a mean age of 54 years, which also included an analysis in a subpopulation of patients >65 years of age, found no statistically significant increase in emergency department visits or hospitalization for heart failure in patients treated with AVANDIA compared to ACTOS in the older subgroup.

5.2 Major Adverse Cardiovascular Events

Cardiovascular adverse events have been evaluated in a meta-analysis of 52 clinical trials, in long-term, prospective, randomized, controlled trials, and in observational studies.

Meta-Analysis of Major Adverse Cardiovascular Events in a Group of 52 Clinical Trials: A meta-analysis was conducted retrospectively to assess cardiovascular adverse events reported across 52 double-blind, randomized, controlled clinical trials (mean duration 6 months).[1] These trials had been conducted to assess glucose-lowering efficacy in type 2 diabetes. Prospectively planned adjudication of cardiovascular events did not occur in most of the trials. Some trials were placebo-controlled and some used active oral antidiabetic drugs as controls. Placebo-controlled trials included monotherapy trials (monotherapy with AVANDIA versus placebo monotherapy) and add-on trials (AVANDIA or placebo, added to sulfonylurea, metformin, or insulin). Active control trials included monotherapy trials (monotherapy with AVANDIA versus sulfonylurea or metformin monotherapy) and add-on trials (AVANDIA plus sulfonylurea or AVANDIA plus metformin, versus sulfonylurea plus metformin). A total of 16,995 patients were included (10,039 in treatment groups containing AVANDIA, 6,956 in comparator groups), with 5,167 patient-years of exposure to AVANDIA and 3,637 patient-years of exposure to comparator. Cardiovascular events occurred more frequently for patients who received AVANDIA than for patients who received comparators (see Table 2).

Table 2. Occurrence of Cardiovascular Events in a Meta-Analysis of 52 Clinical Trials

Event[a]	AVANDIA (Rosiglitazone) (N = 10,039) n (%)	Comparator (N = 6,956) n (%)
MACE (a composite of myocardial infarction, cardiovascular death, or stroke)	70 (0.7)	39 (0.6)
Myocardial Infarction	45 (0.4)	20 (0.3)
Cardiovascular Death	17 (0.2)	9 (0.1)
Stroke	18 (0.2)	16 (0.2)
All-cause Death	29 (0.3)	17 (0.2)

[a] Events are not exclusive: i.e., a patient with a cardiovascular death due to a myocardial infarction would be counted in 4 event categories (myocardial infarction; myocardial infarction, cardiovascular death, or stroke; cardiovascular death; all-cause death).

In this analysis, a statistically significant increased risk of myocardial infarction with AVANDIA versus pooled comparators was observed. Analyses were performed using a composite of major adverse cardiovascular events (myocardial infarction, stroke, and cardiovascular death), referred to hereafter as MACE. AVANDIA had a statistically nonsignificant increased risk of MACE compared to the pooled comparators. A statistically significant increased risk of myocardial infarction and statistically non significant increased risk of MACE with AVANDIA was observed in the placebo-controlled trials. In the active-controlled trials, there was no increased risk of myocardial infarction or MACE. (See Figure 1 and Table 3.)

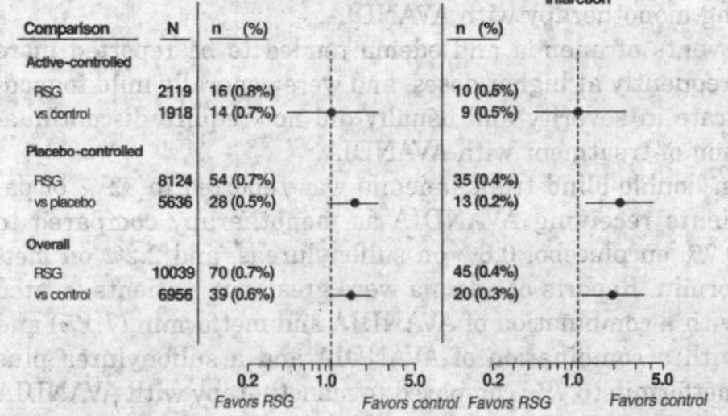

Figure 1. Forest Plot of Odds Ratios (95% Confidence Intervals) for MACE and Myocardial Infarction in the Meta-Analysis of 52 Clinical Trials

[See table 3 above]

Table 3. Occurrence of MACE and Myocardial Infarction in a Meta-Analysis of 52 Clinical Trials by Trial Type

			MACE		Myocardial Infarction	
		N	n (%)	OR (95%CI)	n (%)	OR (95%CI)
Active-Controlled Trials	RSG	2,119	16 (0.8%)	1.05	10 (0.5%)	1.00
	Control	1,918	14 (0.7%)	(0.48, 2.34)	9 (0.5%)	(0.36, 2.82)
Placebo-Controlled Trials	RSG	8,124	54 (0.7%)	1.53	35 (0.4%)	2.23
	Placebo	5,636	28 (0.5%)	(0.94, 2.54)	13 (0.2%)	(1.14, 4.64)
Overall	RSG	10,039	70 (0.7%)	1.44	45 (0.4%)	1.8
	Control	6,956	39 (0.6%)	(0.95, 2.20)	20 (0.3%)	(1.03, 3.25)

RSG = AVANDIA (rosiglitazone)

Of the placebo-controlled trials in the meta-analysis, 7 trials had patients randomized to AVANDIA plus insulin or insulin. There were more patients in the AVANDIA plus insulin group compared to the insulin group with myocardial infarctions, MACE, cardiovascular deaths, and all-cause deaths (see Table 4). The total number of patients with stroke was 5 (0.5%) and 4 (0.5%) in the AVANDIA plus insulin and insulin groups, respectively. The use of AVANDIA in combination with insulin may increase the risk of myocardial infarction.

[See table 4 above]

Table 4. Occurrence of Cardiovascular Events for AVANDIA in Combination With Insulin in a Meta-Analysis of 52 Clinical Trials

Event[a]	AVANDIA (Rosiglitazone) (N=1,018) (%)	Insulin (N = 815) (%)	OR (95% CI)
MACE (a composite of myocardial infarction, cardiovascular death, or stroke)	1.3	0.6	2.14 (0.70, 7.83)
Myocardial infarction	0.6	0.1	5.6 (0.67, 262.7)
Cardiovascular death	0.4	0.0	ND, (0.47, ∞)
All-cause death	0.6	0.2	2.19 (0.38, 22.61)

ND = not defined
[a] Events are not exclusive: i.e., a patient with a cardiovascular death due to a myocardial infarction would be counted in 4 event categories (myocardial infarction; myocardial infarction, cardiovascular death, or stroke; cardiovascular death; all-cause death).

Myocardial Infarction Events in Large, Long-Term, Prospective, Randomized, Controlled Trials of AVANDIA: Data from 3 large, long-term, prospective, randomized, controlled clinical trials of AVANDIA were assessed separately from the meta-analysis.[6-8] These 3 trials included a total of 14,067 patients (treatment groups containing AVANDIA N = 6,311; comparator groups N = 7,756), with patient-year exposure of 24,534 patient-years for AVANDIA and 28,882 patient years for comparator. Patient populations in the trials included patients with impaired glucose tolerance, patients with type 2 diabetes who were initiating oral agent monotherapy, and patients with type 2 diabetes who had failed monotherapy and were initiating dual oral agent therapy. Duration of follow-up exceeded 3 years in each trial.

In each of these trials, there was a statistically nonsignificant increase in the risk of myocardial infarction for AVANDIA versus comparator medications.

In a long-term, randomized, placebo-controlled, 2×2 factorial trial intended to evaluate AVANDIA, and separately ramipril (an angiotensin converting enzyme inhibitor [ACEI]), on progression to overt diabetes in 5,269 subjects with glucose intolerance, the incidence of myocardial infarction was higher in the subset of subjects who received AVANDIA in combination with ramipril than among subjects who received ramipril alone but not in the subset of subjects who received AVANDIA alone compared to placebo.[6] The higher incidence of myocardial infarction among subjects who received AVANDIA in combination with ramipril was not confirmed in the two other large (total N = 8,798) long-term, randomized, active-controlled clinical trials conducted in patients with type 2 diabetes, in which 30% and 40% of patients in the two trials reported angiotensin-converting enzyme inhibitor use at baseline.[7,8]

There have been no adequately designed clinical trials directly comparing AVANDIA to ACTOS (pioglitazone) on cardiovascular risks. However, in a long-term, randomized, placebo-controlled cardiovascular outcomes trial comparing ACTOS (pioglitazone) to placebo in patients with type 2 diabetes mellitus and prior macrovascular disease, ACTOS (pioglitazone) was not associated with an increased risk of myocardial infarction or total mortality.[9]

The increased risk of myocardial infarction observed in the meta-analysis and large, long-term controlled clinical trials, and the increased risk of MACE observed in the meta-analysis described above, have not translated into a consistent finding of excess mortality from controlled clinical trials or observational studies. Clinical trials have not shown any difference between AVANDIA and comparator medications in overall mortality or CV-related mortality.

Mortality in Observational Studies of AVANDIA Compared to ACTOS: Three observational studies in elderly diabetic patients (age 65 years and older) found that AVANDIA statistically significantly increased the risk of all-cause mortality compared to use of ACTOS.[2-4] One observational study[5] in patients with a mean age of 54 years found no difference in all-cause mortality between patients treated with AVANDIA compared to ACTOS and reported similar results in the subpopulation of patients >65 years of age. One additional small, prospective, observational study[10] found no statistically significant differences for CV mortality and all-cause mortality in patients treated with AVANDIA compared to ACTOS.

5.3 Rosiglitazone REMS (Risk Evaluation and Mitigation Strategy) Program

Because of the potential increased risk of myocardial infarction, AVANDIA is available only through a restricted distribution program called the AVANDIA-Rosiglitazone Medicines Access Program *[see Indications and Usage (1)]*. Both prescribers and patients must enroll in the program to be able to prescribe or receive AVANDIA, respectively. AVANDIA will be available only from specially certified pharmacies participating in the program. As part of the program, prescribers will be educated about the potential increased risk of myocardial infarction and the need to limit the use of AVANDIA to eligible patients. Prescribers will need to discuss with patients the risks and benefits of taking AVANDIA. To enroll, call 1-800-AVANDIA or visit www.AVANDIA.com.

5.4 Edema

AVANDIA should be used with caution in patients with edema. In a clinical trial in healthy volunteers who received 8 mg of AVANDIA once daily for 8 weeks, there was a statistically significant increase in median plasma volume compared to placebo.

Since thiazolidinediones, including rosiglitazone, can cause fluid retention, which can exacerbate or lead to congestive heart failure, AVANDIA should be used with caution in patients at risk for heart failure. Patients should be monitored for signs and symptoms of heart failure *[see Boxed Warning, Warnings and Precautions (5.1), and Patient Counseling Information (17)]*.

In controlled clinical trials of patients with type 2 diabetes, mild to moderate edema was reported in patients treated with AVANDIA, and may be dose related. Patients with ongoing edema were more likely to have adverse events associated with edema if started on combination therapy with insulin and AVANDIA *[see Adverse Reactions (6.1)]*.

5.5 Weight Gain

Dose-related weight gain was seen with AVANDIA alone and in combination with other hypoglycemic agents (Table 5). The mechanism of weight gain is unclear but probably involves a combination of fluid retention and fat accumulation.

In postmarketing experience, there have been reports of unusually rapid increases in weight and increases in excess of that generally observed in clinical trials. Patients who experience such increases should be assessed for fluid accumulation and volume-related events such as excessive edema and congestive heart failure *[see Boxed Warning]*.

[See table 5 at top of next page]

In a 4- to 6-year, monotherapy, comparative trial (ADOPT) in patients recently diagnosed with type 2 diabetes not previously treated with antidiabetic medication *[see Clinical Studies (14.1)]*, the median weight change (25th, 75th percentiles) from baseline at 4 years was 3.5 kg (0.0, 8.1) for AVANDIA, 2.0 kg (-1.0, 4.8) for glyburide, and -2.4 kg (-5.4, 0.5) for metformin.

In a 24-week trial in pediatric patients aged 10 to 17 years treated with AVANDIA 4 to 8 mg daily, a median weight gain of 2.8 kg (25th, 75th percentiles: 0.0, 5.8) was reported.

Table 5. Weight Changes (kg) From Baseline at Endpoint During Clinical Trials

Monotherapy	Duration	Control Group		AVANDIA 4 mg	AVANDIA 8 mg
			Median (25th, 75th percentile)	Median (25th, 75th percentile)	Median (25th, 75th percentile)
	26 weeks	placebo	-0.9 (-2.8, 0.9) N = 210	1.0 (-0.9, 3.6) N = 436	3.1 (1.1, 5.8) N = 439
	52 weeks	sulfonylurea	2.0 (0, 4.0) N = 173	2.0 (-0.6, 4.0) N = 150	2.6 (0, 5.3) N = 157
Combination therapy					
Sulfonylurea	24-26 weeks	sulfonylurea	0 (-1.0, 1.3) N = 1,155	2.2 (0.5, 4.0) N = 613	3.5 (1.4, 5.9) N = 841
Metformin	26 weeks	metformin	-1.4 (-3.2, 0.2) N = 175	0.8 (-1.0, 2.6) N = 100	2.1 (0, 4.3) N = 184
Insulin	26 weeks	insulin	0.9 (-0.5, 2.7) N = 162	4.1 (1.4, 6.3) N = 164	5.4 (3.4, 7.3) N = 150
Sulfonylurea + metformin	26 weeks	sulfonylurea + metformin	0.2 (-1.2, 1.6) N = 272	2.5 (0.8, 4.6) N = 275	4.5 (2.4, 7.3) N = 276

Table 6. Adverse Events (≥5% in Any Treatment Group) Reported by Patients in Short-Term[a] Double-Blind Clinical Trials With AVANDIA as Monotherapy

Preferred Term	AVANDIA Monotherapy	Placebo	Metformin	Sulfonylureas[b]
	N = 2,526	N = 601	N = 225	N = 626
	%	%	%	%
Upper respiratory tract infection	9.9	8.7	8.9	7.3
Injury	7.6	4.3	7.6	6.1
Headache	5.9	5.0	8.9	5.4
Back pain	4.0	3.8	4.0	5.0
Hyperglycemia	3.9	5.7	4.4	8.1
Fatigue	3.6	5.0	4.0	1.9
Sinusitis	3.2	4.5	5.3	3.0
Diarrhea	2.3	3.3	15.6	3.0
Hypoglycemia	0.6	0.2	1.3	5.9

[a] Short-term trials ranged from 8 weeks to 1 year.
[b] Includes patients receiving glyburide (N = 514), gliclazide (N = 91), or glipizide (N = 21).

5.6 Hepatic Effects

Liver enzymes should be measured prior to the initiation of therapy with AVANDIA in all patients and periodically thereafter per the clinical judgment of the healthcare professional. Therapy with AVANDIA should not be initiated in patients with increased baseline liver enzyme levels (ALT >2.5× upper limit of normal). Patients with mildly elevated liver enzymes (ALT levels ≤2.5× upper limit of normal) at baseline or during therapy with AVANDIA should be evaluated to determine the cause of the liver enzyme elevation. Initiation of, or continuation of, therapy with AVANDIA in patients with mild liver enzyme elevations should proceed with caution and include close clinical follow-up, including liver enzyme monitoring, to determine if the liver enzyme elevations resolve or worsen. If at any time ALT levels increase to >3× the upper limit of normal in patients on therapy with AVANDIA, liver enzyme levels should be rechecked as soon as possible. If ALT levels remain >3× the upper limit of normal, therapy with AVANDIA should be discontinued.

If any patient develops symptoms suggesting hepatic dysfunction, which may include unexplained nausea, vomiting, abdominal pain, fatigue, anorexia and/or dark urine, liver enzymes should be checked. The decision whether to continue the patient on therapy with AVANDIA should be guided by clinical judgment pending laboratory evaluations. If jaundice is observed, drug therapy should be discontinued. *[See Adverse Reactions (6.2, 6.3).]*

5.7 Macular Edema

Macular edema has been reported in postmarketing experience in some diabetic patients who were taking AVANDIA or another thiazolidinedione. Some patients presented with blurred vision or decreased visual acuity, but some patients appear to have been diagnosed on routine ophthalmologic examination. Most patients had peripheral edema at the time macular edema was diagnosed. Some patients had improvement in their macular edema after discontinuation of their thiazolidinedione. Patients with diabetes should have regular eye exams by an ophthalmologist, per the Standards of Care of the American Diabetes Association. Additionally, any diabetic who reports any kind of visual symptom should be promptly referred to an ophthalmologist, regardless of the patient's underlying medications or other physical findings. *[See Adverse Reactions (6.1).]*

5.8 Fractures

In a 4- to 6-year comparative trial (ADOPT) of glycemic control with monotherapy in drug-naïve patients recently diagnosed with type 2 diabetes mellitus, an increased incidence of bone fracture was noted in female patients taking AVANDIA. Over the 4- to 6-year period, the incidence of bone fracture in females was 9.3% (60/645) for AVANDIA versus 3.5% (21/605) for glyburide and 5.1% (30/590) for metformin. This increased incidence was noted after the first year of treatment and persisted during the course of the trial. The majority of the fractures in the women who received AVANDIA occurred in the upper arm, hand, and foot. These sites of fracture are different from those usually associated with postmenopausal osteoporosis (e.g., hip or spine). Other trials suggest that this risk may also apply to men, although the risk of fracture among women appears higher than that among men. The risk of fracture should be considered in the care of patients treated with AVANDIA, and attention given to assessing and maintaining bone health according to current standards of care.

5.9 Hematologic Effects

Decreases in mean hemoglobin and hematocrit occurred in a dose-related fashion in adult patients treated with AVANDIA *[see Adverse Reactions (6.2)]*. The observed changes may be related to the increased plasma volume observed with treatment with AVANDIA.

5.10 Diabetes and Blood Glucose Control

Patients receiving AVANDIA in combination with other hypoglycemic agents may be at risk for hypoglycemia, and a reduction in the dose of the concomitant agent may be necessary.

Periodic fasting blood glucose and HbA1c measurements should be performed to monitor therapeutic response.

5.11 Ovulation

Therapy with AVANDIA, like other thiazolidinediones, may result in ovulation in some premenopausal anovulatory women. As a result, these patients may be at an increased risk for pregnancy while taking AVANDIA *[see Use in Specific Populations (8.1)]*. Thus, adequate contraception in premenopausal women should be recommended. This possible effect has not been specifically investigated in clinical trials; therefore, the frequency of this occurrence is not known.

Although hormonal imbalance has been seen in preclinical studies *[see Nonclinical Toxicology (13.1)]*, the clinical significance of this finding is not known. If unexpected menstrual dysfunction occurs, the benefits of continued therapy with AVANDIA should be reviewed.

6 ADVERSE REACTIONS

6.1 Clinical Trial Experience

Adult: In clinical trials, approximately 9,900 patients with type 2 diabetes have been treated with AVANDIA.

Short-Term Trials of AVANDIA as Monotherapy and in Combination With Other Hypoglycemic Agents: The incidence and types of adverse events reported in short-term clinical trials of AVANDIA as monotherapy are shown in Table 6. [See table 6 above]

Overall, the types of adverse reactions without regard to causality reported when AVANDIA was used in combination with a sulfonylurea or metformin were similar to those during monotherapy with AVANDIA.

Events of anemia and edema tended to be reported more frequently at higher doses, and were generally mild to moderate in severity and usually did not require discontinuation of treatment with AVANDIA.

In double-blind trials, anemia was reported in 1.9% of patients receiving AVANDIA as monotherapy compared to 0.7% on placebo, 0.6% on sulfonylureas, and 2.2% on metformin. Reports of anemia were greater in patients treated with a combination of AVANDIA and metformin (7.1%) and with a combination of AVANDIA and a sulfonylurea plus metformin (6.7%) compared to monotherapy with AVANDIA or in combination with a sulfonylurea (2.3%). Lower pretreatment hemoglobin/hematocrit levels in patients enrolled in the metformin combination clinical trials may have contributed to the higher reporting rate of anemia in these trials *[see Adverse Reactions (6.2)]*.

In clinical trials, edema was reported in 4.8% of patients receiving AVANDIA as monotherapy compared to 1.3% on placebo, 1.0% on sulfonylureas, and 2.2% on metformin. The reporting rate of edema was higher for AVANDIA 8 mg in sulfonylurea combinations (12.4%) compared to other combinations, with the exception of insulin. Edema was reported in 14.7% of patients receiving AVANDIA in the insulin combination trials compared to 5.4% on insulin alone. Reports of new onset or exacerbation of congestive heart failure occurred at rates of 1% for insulin alone, and 2% (4 mg) and 3% (8 mg) for insulin in combination with AVANDIA *[see Boxed Warning and Warnings and Precautions (5.1)]*. The use of AVANDIA in combination with insulin may increase the risk of myocardial infarction *[see Warnings and Precautions (5.2)]*.

In controlled combination therapy trials with sulfonylureas, mild to moderate hypoglycemic symptoms, which appear to be dose related, were reported. Few patients were withdrawn for hypoglycemia (<1%) and few episodes of hypoglycemia were considered to be severe (<1%). Hypoglycemia was the most frequently reported adverse event in the fixed-dose insulin combination trials, although few patients withdrew for hypoglycemia (4 of 408 for AVANDIA plus insulin and 1 of 203 for insulin alone). Rates of hypoglycemia, confirmed by capillary blood glucose concentration ≤50 mg/dL, were 6% for insulin alone and 12% (4 mg) and 14% (8 mg) for insulin in combination with AVANDIA. *[See Warnings and Precautions (5.10).]*

Long-Term Trial of AVANDIA as Monotherapy: A 4- to 6-year trial (ADOPT) compared the use of AVANDIA (n = 1,456), glyburide (n = 1,441), and metformin (n = 1,454) as monotherapy in patients recently diagnosed with type 2 diabetes who were not previously treated with antidiabetic medication. Table 7 presents adverse reactions without regard to causality; rates are expressed per 100 patient-years (PY) exposure to account for the differences in exposure to trial medication across the 3 treatment groups.

In ADOPT, fractures were reported in a greater number of women treated with AVANDIA (9.3%, 2.7/100 patient-years) compared to glyburide (3.5%, 1.3/100 patient-years) or metformin (5.1%, 1.5/100 patient-years). The majority of the fractures in the women who received rosiglitazone were reported in the upper arm, hand, and foot. *[See Warnings and Precautions (5.8).]* The observed incidence of fractures for male patients was similar among the 3 treatment groups.

Table 7. On-Therapy Adverse Events (≥5 Events/100 Patient-Years [PY]) in Any Treatment Group Reported in a 4- to 6-Year Clinical Trial of AVANDIA as Monotherapy (ADOPT)

	AVANDIA	Glyburide	Metformin
	N = 1,456	N = 1,441	N = 1,454
	PY = 4,954	PY = 4,244	PY = 4,906
Nasopharyngitis	6.3	6.9	6.6
Back pain	5.1	4.9	5.3
Arthralgia	5.0	4.8	4.2
Hypertension	4.4	6.0	6.1
Upper respiratory tract infection	4.3	5.0	4.7
Hypoglycemia	2.9	13.0	3.4
Diarrhea	2.5	3.2	6.8

Pediatric: AVANDIA has been evaluated for safety in a single, active-controlled trial of pediatric patients with type 2 diabetes in which 99 were treated with AVANDIA and 101 were treated with metformin. The most common adverse reactions (>10%) without regard to causality for either AVANDIA or metformin were headache (17% versus 14%), nausea (4% versus 11%), nasopharyngitis (3% versus 12%), and diarrhea (1% versus 13%). In this trial, one case of diabetic ketoacidosis was reported in the metformin group. In addition, there were 3 patients in the rosiglitazone group who had FPG of ~300 mg/dL, 2+ ketonuria, and an elevated anion gap.

6.2 Laboratory Abnormalities

Hematologic: Decreases in mean hemoglobin and hematocrit occurred in a dose-related fashion in adult patients treated with AVANDIA (mean decreases in individual trials as much as 1.0 g/dL hemoglobin and as much as 3.3% hematocrit). The changes occurred primarily during the first 3 months following initiation of therapy with AVANDIA or following a dose increase in AVANDIA. The time course and magnitude of decreases were similar in patients treated with a combination of AVANDIA and other hypoglycemic agents or monotherapy with AVANDIA. Pre-treatment levels of hemoglobin and hematocrit were lower in patients in metformin combination trials and may have contributed to the higher reporting rate of anemia. In a single trial in pediatric patients, decreases in hemoglobin and hematocrit (mean decreases of 0.29 g/dL and 0.95%, respectively) were reported. Small decreases in hemoglobin and hematocrit have also been reported in pediatric patients treated with AVANDIA. White blood cell counts also decreased slightly in adult patients treated with AVANDIA. Decreases in hematologic parameters may be related to increased plasma volume observed with treatment with AVANDIA.

Lipids: Changes in serum lipids have been observed following treatment with AVANDIA in adults *[see Clinical Pharmacology (12.2)]*. Small changes in serum lipid parameters were reported in children treated with AVANDIA for 24 weeks.

Serum Transaminase Levels: In pre-approval clinical trials in 4,598 patients treated with AVANDIA (3,600 patient-years of exposure) and in a long-term 4- to 6-year trial in 1,456 patients treated with AVANDIA (4,954 patient-years exposure), there was no evidence of drug-induced hepatotoxicity.

In pre-approval controlled trials, 0.2% of patients treated with AVANDIA had elevations in ALT >3× the upper limit of normal compared to 0.2% on placebo and 0.5% on active comparators. The ALT elevations in patients treated with AVANDIA were reversible. Hyperbilirubinemia was found in 0.3% of patients treated with AVANDIA compared with 0.9% treated with placebo and 1% in patients treated with active comparators. In pre-approval clinical trials, there were no cases of idiosyncratic drug reactions leading to hepatic failure. *[See Warnings and Precautions (5.6).]*

Table 8. Week 24 FPG and HbA1c Change From Baseline Last-Observation-Carried Forward in Children With Baseline HbA1c >6.5%

	Naïve Patients		Previously-Treated Patients	
	Metformin	Rosiglitazone	Metformin	Rosiglitazone
	N = 40	N = 45	N = 43	N = 32
FPG (mg/dL)				
Baseline (mean)	170	165	221	205
Change from baseline (mean)	-21	-11	-33	-5
Adjusted treatment difference[a] (rosiglitazone–metformin)[b] (95% CI)		8 (-15, 30)		21 (-9, 51)
% of patients with ≥30 mg/dL decrease from baseline	43%	27%	44%	28%
HbA1c (%)				
Baseline (mean)	8.3	8.2	8.8	8.5
Change from baseline (mean)	-0.7	-0.5	-0.4	0.1
Adjusted treatment difference[a] (rosiglitazone–metformin)[b] (95% CI)		0.2 (-0.6, 0.9)		0.5 (-0.2, 1.3)
% of patients with ≥0.7% decrease from baseline	63%	52%	54%	31%

[a] Change from baseline means are least squares means adjusting for baseline HbA1c, gender, and region.
[b] Positive values for the difference favor metformin.

In the 4- to 6-year ADOPT trial, patients treated with AVANDIA (4,954 patient-years exposure), glyburide (4,244 patient-years exposure), or metformin (4,906 patient-years exposure), as monotherapy, had the same rate of ALT increase to >3× upper limit of normal (0.3 per 100 patient-years exposure).

6.3 Postmarketing Experience

In addition to adverse reactions reported from clinical trials, the events described below have been identified during post-approval use of AVANDIA. Because these events are reported voluntarily from a population of unknown size, it is not possible to reliably estimate their frequency or to always establish a causal relationship to drug exposure.

In patients receiving thiazolidinedione therapy, serious adverse events with or without a fatal outcome, potentially related to volume expansion (e.g., congestive heart failure, pulmonary edema, and pleural effusions) have been reported *[see Boxed Warning and Warnings and Precautions (5.1)]*.

There are postmarketing reports with AVANDIA of hepatitis, hepatic enzyme elevations to 3 or more times the upper limit of normal, and hepatic failure with and without fatal outcome, although causality has not been established.

There are postmarketing reports with AVANDIA of rash, pruritus, urticaria, angioedema, anaphylactic reaction, Stevens-Johnson syndrome, and new onset or worsening diabetic macular edema with decreased visual acuity *[see Warnings and Precautions (5.7)]*.

7 DRUG INTERACTIONS

7.1 CYP2C8 Inhibitors and Inducers

An inhibitor of CYP2C8 (e.g., gemfibrozil) may increase the AUC of rosiglitazone and an inducer of CYP2C8 (e.g., rifampin) may decrease the AUC of rosiglitazone. Therefore, if an inhibitor or an inducer of CYP2C8 is started or stopped during treatment with rosiglitazone, changes in diabetes treatment may be needed based upon clinical response. *[See Clinical Pharmacology (12.4).]*

8 USE IN SPECIFIC POPULATIONS

8.1 Pregnancy

Pregnancy Category C.

All pregnancies have a background risk of birth defects, loss, or other adverse outcome regardless of drug exposure. This background risk is increased in pregnancies complicated by hyperglycemia and may be decreased with good metabolic control. It is essential for patients with diabetes or history of gestational diabetes to maintain good metabolic control before conception and throughout pregnancy. Careful monitoring of glucose control is essential in such patients. Most experts recommend that insulin monotherapy be used during pregnancy to maintain blood glucose levels as close to normal as possible.

Human Data: Rosiglitazone has been reported to cross the human placenta and be detectable in fetal tissue. The clinical significance of these findings is unknown. There are no adequate and well-controlled trials in pregnant women. AVANDIA should not be used during pregnancy.

Animal Studies: There was no effect on implantation or the embryo with rosiglitazone treatment during early pregnancy in rats, but treatment during mid-late gestation was associated with fetal death and growth retardation in both rats and rabbits. Teratogenicity was not observed at doses up to 3 mg/kg in rats and 100 mg/kg in rabbits (approximately 20 and 75 times human AUC at the maximum recommended human daily dose, respectively). Rosiglitazone caused placental pathology in rats (3 mg/kg/day). Treatment of rats during gestation through lactation reduced litter size, neonatal viability, and postnatal growth, with growth retardation reversible after puberty. For effects on the placenta, embryo/fetus, and offspring, the no-effect dose was 0.2 mg/kg/day in rats and 15 mg/kg/day in rabbits. These no-effect levels are approximately 4 times human AUC at the maximum recommended human daily dose. Rosiglitazone reduced the number of uterine implantations and live offspring when juvenile female rats were treated at 40 mg/kg/day from 27 days of age through to sexual maturity (approximately 68 times human AUC at the maximum recommended daily dose). The no-effect level was 2 mg/kg/day (approximately 4 times human AUC at the maximum recommended daily dose). There was no effect on pre- or post-natal survival or growth.

8.2 Labor and Delivery

The effect of rosiglitazone on labor and delivery in humans is not known.

8.3 Nursing Mothers

Drug-related material was detected in milk from lactating rats. It is not known whether AVANDIA is excreted in human milk. Because many drugs are excreted in human milk, AVANDIA should not be administered to a nursing woman.

8.4 Pediatric Use

After placebo run-in including diet counseling, children with type 2 diabetes mellitus, aged 10 to 17 years and with a baseline mean body mass index (BMI) of 33 kg/m^2, were randomized to treatment with 2 mg twice daily of AVANDIA (n = 99) or 500 mg twice daily of metformin (n = 101) in a 24-week, double-blind clinical trial. As expected, FPG decreased in patients naïve to diabetes medication (n = 104) and increased in patients withdrawn from prior medication (usually metformin) (n = 90) during the run-in period. After at least 8 weeks of treatment, 49% of patients treated with AVANDIA and 55% of metformin-treated patients had their dose doubled if FPG >126 mg/dL. For the overall intent-to-treat population, at week 24, the mean change from baseline in HbA1c was -0.14% with AVANDIA and -0.49% with metformin. There was an insufficient number of patients in this trial to establish statistically whether these observed mean treatment effects were similar or different. Treatment effects differed for patients naïve to therapy with antidiabetic drugs and for patients previously treated with antidiabetic therapy (Table 8).

[See table 8 above]

Treatment differences depended on baseline BMI or weight such that the effects of AVANDIA and metformin appeared

more closely comparable among heavier patients. The median weight gain was 2.8 kg with rosiglitazone and 0.2 kg with metformin *[see Warnings and Precautions (5.5)]*. Fifty-four percent of patients treated with rosiglitazone and 32% of patients treated with metformin gained ≥2 kg, and 33% of patients treated with rosiglitazone and 7% of patients treated with metformin gained ≥5 kg on trial.
Adverse events observed in this trial are described in *Adverse Reactions (6.1)*.

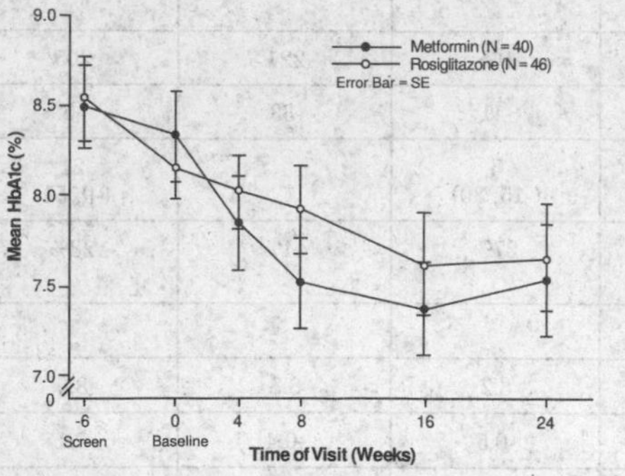

Figure 2. Mean HbA1c Over Time in a 24-Week Trial of AVANDIA and Metformin in Pediatric Patients — Drug Naïve Subgroup

8.5 Geriatric Use
Results of the population pharmacokinetic analysis showed that age does not significantly affect the pharmacokinetics of rosiglitazone *[see Clinical Pharmacology (12.3)]*. Therefore, no dosage adjustments are required for the elderly. In controlled clinical trials, no overall differences in safety and effectiveness between older (≥65 years) and younger (<65 years) patients were observed.

10 OVERDOSAGE
Limited data are available with regard to overdosage in humans. In clinical trials in volunteers, AVANDIA has been administered at single oral doses of up to 20 mg and was well-tolerated. In the event of an overdose, appropriate supportive treatment should be initiated as dictated by the patient's clinical status.

11 DESCRIPTION
AVANDIA (rosiglitazone maleate) is an oral antidiabetic agent which acts primarily by increasing insulin sensitivity. AVANDIA improves glycemic control while reducing circulating insulin levels.
Rosiglitazone maleate is not chemically or functionally related to the sulfonylureas, the biguanides, or the alpha-glucosidase inhibitors.
Chemically, rosiglitazone maleate is (±)-5-[[4-[2-(methyl-2-pyridinylamino)ethoxy]phenyl]methyl]-2,4-thiazolidinedione, (*Z*)-2-butenedioate (1:1) with a molecular weight of 473.52 (357.44 free base). The molecule has a single chiral center and is present as a racemate. Due to rapid interconversion, the enantiomers are functionally indistinguishable. The structural formula of rosiglitazone maleate is:

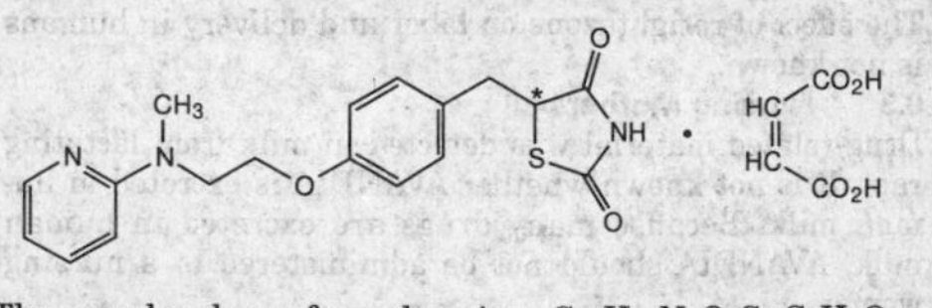

The molecular formula is $C_{18}H_{19}N_3O_3S \bullet C_4H_4O_4$. Rosiglitazone maleate is a white to off-white solid with a melting point range of 122° to 123°C. The pKa values of rosiglitazone maleate are 6.8 and 6.1. It is readily soluble in ethanol and a buffered aqueous solution with pH of 2.3; solubility decreases with increasing pH in the physiological range.
Each pentagonal film-coated TILTAB tablet contains rosiglitazone maleate equivalent to rosiglitazone, 2 mg, 4 mg, or 8 mg, for oral administration. Inactive ingredients are: Hypromellose 2910, lactose monohydrate, magnesium stearate, microcrystalline cellulose, polyethylene glycol 3000, sodium starch glycolate, titanium dioxide, triacetin, and 1 or more of the following: Synthetic red and yellow iron oxides and talc.

12 CLINICAL PHARMACOLOGY
12.1 Mechanism of Action
Rosiglitazone, a member of the thiazolidinedione class of antidiabetic agents, improves glycemic control by improving insulin sensitivity. Rosiglitazone is a highly selective and potent agonist for the peroxisome proliferator-activated receptor-gamma (PPARγ). In humans, PPAR receptors are found in key target tissues for insulin action such as adipose tissue, skeletal muscle, and liver. Activation of PPARγ nuclear receptors regulates the transcription of insulin-responsive genes involved in the control of glucose production, transport, and utilization. In addition, PPARγ-responsive genes also participate in the regulation of fatty acid metabolism.
Insulin resistance is a common feature characterizing the pathogenesis of type 2 diabetes. The antidiabetic activity of rosiglitazone has been demonstrated in animal models of type 2 diabetes in which hyperglycemia and/or impaired glucose tolerance is a consequence of insulin resistance in target tissues. Rosiglitazone reduces blood glucose concentrations and reduces hyperinsulinemia in the ob/ob obese mouse, db/db diabetic mouse, and fa/fa fatty Zucker rat.
In animal models, the antidiabetic activity of rosiglitazone was shown to be mediated by increased sensitivity to insulin's action in the liver, muscle, and adipose tissues. Pharmacological studies in animal models indicate that rosiglitazone inhibits hepatic gluconeogenesis. The expression of the insulin-regulated glucose transporter GLUT-4 was increased in adipose tissue. Rosiglitazone did not induce hypoglycemia in animal models of type 2 diabetes and/or impaired glucose tolerance.

12.2 Pharmacodynamics
Patients with lipid abnormalities were not excluded from clinical trials of AVANDIA. In all 26-week controlled trials, across the recommended dose range, AVANDIA as monotherapy was associated with increases in total cholesterol, LDL, and HDL and decreases in free fatty acids. These changes were statistically significantly different from placebo or glyburide controls (Table 9).
Increases in LDL occurred primarily during the first 1 to 2 months of therapy with AVANDIA and LDL levels remained elevated above baseline throughout the trials. In contrast, HDL continued to rise over time. As a result, the LDL/HDL ratio peaked after 2 months of therapy and then appeared to decrease over time. Because of the temporal nature of lipid changes, the 52-week glyburide-controlled trial is most pertinent to assess long-term effects on lipids. At baseline, week 26, and week 52, mean LDL/HDL ratios were 3.1, 3.2, and 3.0, respectively, for AVANDIA 4 mg twice daily. The corresponding values for glyburide were 3.2, 3.1, and 2.9. The differences in change from baseline between AVANDIA and glyburide at week 52 were statistically significant.
The pattern of LDL and HDL changes following therapy with AVANDIA in combination with other hypoglycemic agents were generally similar to those seen with AVANDIA in monotherapy.
The changes in triglycerides during therapy with AVANDIA were variable and were generally not statistically different from placebo or glyburide controls.
[See table 9 above]

Table 9. Summary of Mean Lipid Changes in 26-Week Placebo-Controlled and 52-Week Glyburide-Controlled Monotherapy Trials

	Placebo-Controlled Trials Week 26			Glyburide-Controlled Trial Week 26 and Week 52			
	Placebo	AVANDIA		Glyburide Titration		AVANDIA 8 mg	
		4 mg daily[a]	8 mg daily[a]	Wk 26	Wk 52	Wk 26	Wk 52
Free fatty acids							
N	207	428	436	181	168	166	145
Baseline (mean)	18.1	17.5	17.9	26.4	26.4	26.9	26.6
% Change from baseline (mean)	+0.2%	-7.8%	-14.7%	-2.4%	-4.7%	-20.8%	-21.5%
LDL							
N	190	400	374	175	160	161	133
Baseline (mean)	123.7	126.8	125.3	142.7	141.9	142.1	142.1
% Change from baseline (mean)	+4.8%	+14.1%	+18.6%	-0.9%	-0.5%	+11.9%	+12.1%
HDL							
N	208	429	436	184	170	170	145
Baseline (mean)	44.1	44.4	43.0	47.2	47.7	48.4	48.3
% Change from baseline (mean)	+8.0%	+11.4%	+14.2%	+4.3%	+8.7%	+14.0%	+18.5%

[a] Once daily and twice daily dosing groups were combined.

12.3 Pharmacokinetics
Maximum plasma concentration (C_{max}) and the area under the curve (AUC) of rosiglitazone increase in a dose-proportional manner over the therapeutic dose range (Table 10). The elimination half-life is 3 to 4 hours and is independent of dose.
[See table 10 above]

Table 10. Mean (SD) Pharmacokinetic Parameters for Rosiglitazone Following Single Oral Doses (N = 32)

Parameter	1 mg Fasting	2 mg Fasting	8 mg Fasting	8 mg Fed
$AUC_{0\text{-}inf}$ [ng•hr/mL]	358 (112)	733 (184)	2,971 (730)	2,890 (795)
C_{max} [ng/mL]	76 (13)	156 (42)	598 (117)	432 (92)
Half-life [hr]	3.16 (0.72)	3.15 (0.39)	3.37 (0.63)	3.59 (0.70)
CL/F[a] [L/hr]	3.03 (0.87)	2.89 (0.71)	2.85 (0.69)	2.97 (0.81)

[a] CL/F = Oral clearance.

<u>Absorption:</u> The absolute bioavailability of rosiglitazone is 99%. Peak plasma concentrations are observed about 1 hour after dosing. Administration of rosiglitazone with food resulted in no change in overall exposure (AUC), but there was an approximately 28% decrease in C_{max} and a delay in T_{max} (1.75 hours). These changes are not likely to be clinically significant; therefore, AVANDIA may be administered with or without food.
<u>Distribution:</u> The mean (CV%) oral volume of distribution (Vss/F) of rosiglitazone is approximately 17.6 (30%) liters, based on a population pharmacokinetic analysis. Rosiglitazone is approximately 99.8% bound to plasma proteins, primarily albumin.
<u>Metabolism:</u> Rosiglitazone is extensively metabolized with no unchanged drug excreted in the urine. The major routes of metabolism were N-demethylation and hydroxylation, followed by conjugation with sulfate and glucuronic acid. All

the circulating metabolites are considerably less potent than parent and, therefore, are not expected to contribute to the insulin-sensitizing activity of rosiglitazone.

In vitro data demonstrate that rosiglitazone is predominantly metabolized by Cytochrome P450 (CYP) isoenzyme 2C8, with CYP2C9 contributing as a minor pathway.

Excretion: Following oral or intravenous administration of [^{14}C]rosiglitazone maleate, approximately 64% and 23% of the dose was eliminated in the urine and in the feces, respectively. The plasma half-life of [^{14}C]related material ranged from 103 to 158 hours.

Population Pharmacokinetics in Patients With Type 2 Diabetes: Population pharmacokinetic analyses from 3 large clinical trials including 642 men and 405 women with type 2 diabetes (aged 35 to 80 years) showed that the pharmacokinetics of rosiglitazone are not influenced by age, race, smoking, or alcohol consumption. Both oral clearance (CL/F) and oral steady-state volume of distribution (Vss/F) were shown to increase with increases in body weight. Over the weight range observed in these analyses (50 to 150 kg), the range of predicted CL/F and Vss/F values varied by <1.7-fold and <2.3-fold, respectively. Additionally, rosiglitazone CL/F was shown to be influenced by both weight and gender, being lower (about 15%) in female patients.

Special Populations: *Geriatric:* Results of the population pharmacokinetic analysis (n = 716 <65 years; n = 331 ≥65 years) showed that age does not significantly affect the pharmacokinetics of rosiglitazone.

Gender: Results of the population pharmacokinetics analysis showed that the mean oral clearance of rosiglitazone in female patients (n = 405) was approximately 6% lower compared to male patients of the same body weight (n = 642).

As monotherapy and in combination with metformin, AVANDIA improved glycemic control in both males and females. In metformin combination trials, efficacy was demonstrated with no gender differences in glycemic response. In monotherapy trials, a greater therapeutic response was observed in females; however, in more obese patients, gender differences were less evident. For a given body mass index (BMI), females tend to have a greater fat mass than males. Since the molecular target PPARγ is expressed in adipose tissues, this differentiating characteristic may account, at least in part, for the greater response to AVANDIA in females. Since therapy should be individualized, no dose adjustments are necessary based on gender alone.

Hepatic Impairment: Unbound oral clearance of rosiglitazone was significantly lower in patients with moderate to severe liver disease (Child-Pugh Class B/C) compared to healthy subjects. As a result, unbound C_{max} and AUC_{0-inf} were increased 2- and 3-fold, respectively. Elimination half-life for rosiglitazone was about 2 hours longer in patients with liver disease, compared to healthy subjects.

Therapy with AVANDIA should not be initiated if the patient exhibits clinical evidence of active liver disease or increased serum transaminase levels (ALT >2.5× upper limit of normal) at baseline *[see Warnings and Precautions (5.6)]*.

Pediatric: Pharmacokinetic parameters of rosiglitazone in pediatric patients were established using a population pharmacokinetic analysis with sparse data from 96 pediatric patients in a single pediatric clinical trial including 33 males and 63 females with ages ranging from 10 to 17 years (weights ranging from 35 to 178.3 kg). Population mean CL/F and V/F of rosiglitazone were 3.15 L/hr and 13.5 L, respectively. These estimates of CL/F and V/F were consistent with the typical parameter estimates from a prior adult population analysis.

Renal Impairment: There are no clinically relevant differences in the pharmacokinetics of rosiglitazone in patients with mild to severe renal impairment or in hemodialysis-dependent patients compared to subjects with normal renal function. No dosage adjustment is therefore required in such patients receiving AVANDIA. Since metformin is contraindicated in patients with renal impairment, coadministration of metformin with AVANDIA is contraindicated in these patients.

Race: Results of a population pharmacokinetic analysis including subjects of Caucasian, black, and other ethnic origins indicate that race has no influence on the pharmacokinetics of rosiglitazone.

12.4 Drug-Drug Interactions

Drugs That Inhibit, Induce, or are Metabolized by Cytochrome P450: In vitro drug metabolism studies suggest that rosiglitazone does not inhibit any of the major P450 enzymes at clinically relevant concentrations. In vitro data demonstrate that rosiglitazone is predominantly metabolized by CYP2C8, and to a lesser extent, 2C9. AVANDIA (4 mg twice daily) was shown to have no clinically relevant effect on the pharmacokinetics of nifedipine and oral contraceptives (ethinyl estradiol and norethindrone), which are predominantly metabolized by CYP3A4.

Gemfibrozil: Concomitant administration of gemfibrozil (600 mg twice daily), an inhibitor of CYP2C8, and rosiglitazone (4 mg once daily) for 7 days increased rosiglitazone AUC by 127%, compared to the administration

Table 11. Glycemic Parameters in a 26-Week Placebo-Controlled Trial

	Placebo	AVANDIA		AVANDIA	
		4 mg once daily	2 mg twice daily	8 mg once daily	4 mg twice daily
	N = 173	N = 180	N = 186	N = 181	N = 187
FPG (mg/dL)					
Baseline (mean)	225	229	225	228	228
Change from baseline (mean)	8	-25	-35	-42	-55
Difference from placebo (adjusted mean)	–	-31[a]	-43[a]	-49[a]	-62[a]
% of patients with ≥30 mg/dL decrease from baseline	19%	45%	54%	58%	70%
HbA1c (%)					
Baseline (mean)	8.9	8.9	8.9	8.9	9.0
Change from baseline (mean)	0.8	0.0	-0.1	-0.3	-0.7
Difference from placebo (adjusted mean)	–	-0.8[a]	-0.9[a]	-1.1[a]	-1.5[a]
% of patients with ≥0.7% decrease from baseline	9%	28%	29%	39%	54%

[a]P <0.0001 compared to placebo.

of rosiglitazone (4 mg once daily) alone. Given the potential for dose-related adverse events with rosiglitazone, a decrease in the dose of rosiglitazone may be needed when gemfibrozil is introduced *[see Drug Interactions (7.1)]*.

Rifampin: Rifampin administration (600 mg once a day), an inducer of CYP2C8, for 6 days is reported to decrease rosiglitazone AUC by 66%, compared to the administration of rosiglitazone (8 mg) alone *[see Drug Interactions (7.1)]*.[11]

Glyburide: AVANDIA (2 mg twice daily) taken concomitantly with glyburide (3.75 to 10 mg/day) for 7 days did not alter the mean steady-state 24-hour plasma glucose concentrations in diabetic patients stabilized on glyburide therapy. Repeat doses of AVANDIA (8 mg once daily) for 8 days in healthy adult Caucasian subjects caused a decrease in glyburide AUC and C_{max} of approximately 30%. In Japanese subjects, glyburide AUC and C_{max} slightly increased following coadministration of AVANDIA.

Glimepiride: Single oral doses of glimepiride in 14 healthy adult subjects had no clinically significant effect on the steady-state pharmacokinetics of AVANDIA. No clinically significant reductions in glimepiride AUC and C_{max} were observed after repeat doses of AVANDIA (8 mg once daily) for 8 days in healthy adult subjects.

Metformin: Concurrent administration of AVANDIA (2 mg twice daily) and metformin (500 mg twice daily) in healthy volunteers for 4 days had no effect on the steady-state pharmacokinetics of either metformin or rosiglitazone.

Acarbose: Coadministration of acarbose (100 mg three times daily) for 7 days in healthy volunteers had no clinically relevant effect on the pharmacokinetics of a single oral dose of AVANDIA.

Digoxin: Repeat oral dosing of AVANDIA (8 mg once daily) for 14 days did not alter the steady-state pharmacokinetics of digoxin (0.375 mg once daily) in healthy volunteers.

Warfarin: Repeat dosing with AVANDIA had no clinically relevant effect on the steady-state pharmacokinetics of warfarin enantiomers.

Ethanol: A single administration of a moderate amount of alcohol did not increase the risk of acute hypoglycemia in type 2 diabetes mellitus patients treated with AVANDIA.

Ranitidine: Pretreatment with ranitidine (150 mg twice daily for 4 days) did not alter the pharmacokinetics of either single oral or intravenous doses of rosiglitazone in healthy volunteers. These results suggest that the absorption of oral rosiglitazone is not altered in conditions accompanied by increases in gastrointestinal pH.

13 NONCLINICAL TOXICOLOGY

13.1 Carcinogenesis, Mutagenesis, Impairment of Fertility

Carcinogenesis: A 2-year carcinogenicity study was conducted in Charles River CD-1 mice at doses of 0.4, 1.5, and 6 mg/kg/day in the diet (highest dose equivalent to approximately 12 times human AUC at the maximum recommended human daily dose). Sprague-Dawley rats were dosed for 2 years by oral gavage at doses of 0.05, 0.3, and 2 mg/kg/day (highest dose equivalent to approximately 10 and 20 times human AUC at the maximum recommended human daily dose for male and female rats, respectively).

Rosiglitazone was not carcinogenic in the mouse. There was an increase in incidence of adipose hyperplasia in the mouse at doses ≥1.5 mg/kg/day (approximately 2 times human AUC at the maximum recommended human daily dose). In rats, there was a significant increase in the incidence of benign adipose tissue tumors (lipomas) at doses ≥0.3 mg/kg/day (approximately 2 times human AUC at the maximum recommended human daily dose). These proliferative changes in both species are considered due to the persistent pharmacological overstimulation of adipose tissue.

Mutagenesis: Rosiglitazone was not mutagenic or clastogenic in the in vitro bacterial assays for gene mutation, the in vitro chromosome aberration test in human lymphocytes, the in vivo mouse micronucleus test, and the in vivo/in vitro rat UDS assay. There was a small (about 2-fold) increase in mutation in the in vitro mouse lymphoma assay in the presence of metabolic activation.

Impairment of Fertility: Rosiglitazone had no effects on mating or fertility of male rats given up to 40 mg/kg/day (approximately 116 times human AUC at the maximum recommended human daily dose). Rosiglitazone altered estrous cyclicity (2 mg/kg/day) and reduced fertility (40 mg/kg/day) of female rats in association with lower plasma levels of progesterone and estradiol (approximately 20 and 200 times human AUC at the maximum recommended human daily dose, respectively). No such effects were noted at 0.2 mg/kg/day (approximately 3 times human AUC at the maximum recommended human daily dose). In juvenile rats dosed from 27 days of age through to sexual maturity (at up to 40 mg/kg/day), there was no effect on male reproductive performance, or on estrous cyclicity, mating performance or pregnancy incidence in females (approximately 68 times human AUC at the maximum recommended human daily dose). In monkeys, rosiglitazone (0.6 and 4.6 mg/kg/day; approximately 3 and 15 times human AUC at the maximum recommended human daily dose, respectively) diminished the follicular phase rise in serum estradiol with consequential reduction in the luteinizing hormone surge, lower luteal phase progesterone levels, and amenorrhea. The mechanism for these effects appears to be direct inhibition of ovarian steroidogenesis.

13.2 Animal Toxicology

Heart weights were increased in mice (3 mg/kg/day), rats (5 mg/kg/day), and dogs (2 mg/kg/day) with rosiglitazone treatments (approximately 5, 22, and 2 times human AUC at the maximum recommended human daily dose, respectively). Effects in juvenile rats were consistent with those seen in adults. Morphometric measurement indicated that there was hypertrophy in cardiac ventricular tissues, which may be due to increased heart work as a result of plasma volume expansion.

14 CLINICAL STUDIES

14.1 Monotherapy

In clinical trials, treatment with AVANDIA resulted in an improvement in glycemic control, as measured by FPG and HbA1c, with a concurrent reduction in insulin and C-peptide. Postprandial glucose and insulin were also reduced. This is consistent with the mechanism of action of AVANDIA as an insulin sensitizer.

The maximum recommended daily dose is 8 mg. Dose-ranging trials suggested that no additional benefit was obtained with a total daily dose of 12 mg.

Short-Term Clinical Trials: A total of 2,315 patients with type 2 diabetes, previously treated with diet alone or antidiabetic medication(s), were treated with AVANDIA as monotherapy in 6 double-blind trials, which included two

Table 12. Glycemic Parameters in a 26-Week Combination Trial of AVANDIA Plus Metformin

	Metformin	AVANDIA 4 mg once daily + metformin	AVANDIA 8 mg once daily + metformin
	N = 113	N = 116	N = 110
FPG (mg/dL)			
Baseline (mean)	214	215	220
Change from baseline (mean)	6	-33	-48
Difference from metformin alone (adjusted mean)	–	-40[a]	-53[a]
% of patients with ≥30 mg/dL decrease from baseline	20%	45%	61%
HbA1c (%)			
Baseline (mean)	8.6	8.9	8.9
Change from baseline (mean)	0.5	-0.6	-0.8
Difference from metformin alone (adjusted mean)	–	-1.0[a]	-1.2[a]
% of patients with ≥0.7% decrease from baseline	11%	45%	52%

[a]*P* <0.0001 compared to metformin.

26-week placebo-controlled trials, one 52-week glyburide-controlled trial, and 3 placebo-controlled dose-ranging trials of 8 to 12 weeks duration. Previous antidiabetic medication(s) were withdrawn and patients entered a 2 to 4 week placebo run-in period prior to randomization.

Two 26-week, double-blind, placebo-controlled trials, in patients with type 2 diabetes (n = 1,401) with inadequate glycemic control (mean baseline FPG approximately 228 mg/dL [101 to 425 mg/dL] and mean baseline HbA1c 8.9% [5.2% to 16.2%]), were conducted. Treatment with AVANDIA produced statistically significant improvements in FPG and HbA1c compared to baseline and relative to placebo. Data from one of these trials are summarized in Table 11.

[See table 11 at top of previous page]

When administered at the same total daily dose, AVANDIA was generally more effective in reducing FPG and HbA1c when administered in divided doses twice daily compared to once daily doses. However, for HbA1c, the difference between the 4 mg once daily and 2 mg twice daily doses was not statistically significant.

Long-Term Clinical Trials: Long-term maintenance of effect was evaluated in a 52-week, double-blind, glyburide-controlled trial in patients with type 2 diabetes. Patients were randomized to treatment with AVANDIA 2 mg twice daily (N = 195) or AVANDIA 4 mg twice daily (N = 189) or glyburide (N = 202) for 52 weeks. Patients receiving glyburide were given an initial dosage of either 2.5 mg/day or 5.0 mg/day. The dosage was then titrated in 2.5 mg/day increments over the next 12 weeks, to a maximum dosage of 15.0 mg/day in order to optimize glycemic control. Thereafter, the glyburide dose was kept constant.

The median titrated dose of glyburide was 7.5 mg. All treatments resulted in a statistically significant improvement in glycemic control from baseline (Figure 3 and Figure 4). At the end of week 52, the reduction from baseline in FPG and HbA1c was -40.8 mg/dL and -0.53% with AVANDIA 4 mg twice daily; -25.4 mg/dL and -0.27% with AVANDIA 2 mg twice daily; and -30.0 mg/dL and -0.72% with glyburide. For HbA1c, the difference between AVANDIA 4 mg twice daily and glyburide was not statistically significant at week 52. The initial fall in FPG with glyburide was greater than with AVANDIA; however, this effect was less durable over time. The improvement in glycemic control seen with AVANDIA 4 mg twice daily at week 26 was maintained through week 52 of the trial.

[See figure 3 at top of next column]
[See figure 4 at top of next column]

Hypoglycemia was reported in 12.1% of glyburide-treated patients versus 0.5% (2 mg twice daily) and 1.6% (4 mg twice daily) of patients treated with AVANDIA. The improvements in glycemic control were associated with a mean weight gain of 1.75 kg and 2.95 kg for patients treated with 2 mg and 4 mg twice daily of AVANDIA, respectively, versus 1.9 kg in glyburide-treated patients. In patients treated with AVANDIA, C-peptide, insulin, pro-insulin, and pro-insulin split products were significantly reduced in a dose-ordered fashion, compared to an increase in the glyburide-treated patients.

A Diabetes Outcome Progression Trial (ADOPT) was a multicenter, double-blind, controlled trial (N = 4,351) conducted over 4 to 6 years to compare the safety and efficacy of AVANDIA, metformin, and glyburide monotherapy in patients recently diagnosed with type 2 diabetes mellitus (≤3

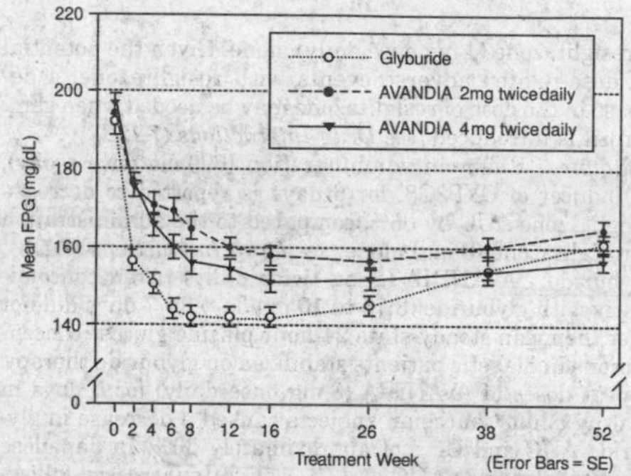

Figure 3. Mean FPG Over Time in a 52-Week Glyburide-Controlled Trial

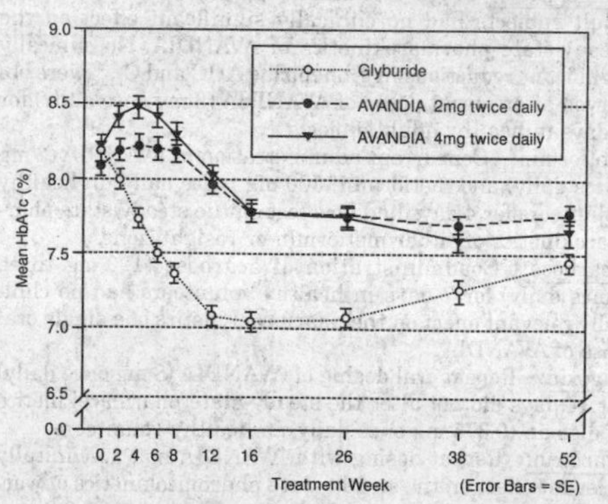

Figure 4. Mean HbA1c Over Time in a 52-Week Glyburide-Controlled Trial

years) inadequately controlled with diet and exercise. The mean age of patients in this trial was 57 years and the majority of patients (83%) had no known history of cardiovascular disease. The mean baseline FPG and HbA1c were 152 mg/dL and 7.4%, respectively. Patients were randomized to receive either AVANDIA 4 mg once daily, glyburide 2.5 mg once daily, or metformin 500 mg once daily, and doses were titrated to optimal glycemic control up to a maximum of 4 mg twice daily for AVANDIA, 7.5 mg twice daily for glyburide, and 1,000 mg twice daily for metformin. The primary efficacy outcome was time to consecutive FPG >180 mg/dL after at least 6 weeks of treatment at the maximum tolerated dose of study medication or time to inadequate glycemic control, as determined by an independent adjudication committee.

The cumulative incidence of the primary efficacy outcome at 5 years was 15% with AVANDIA, 21% with metformin, and 34% with glyburide (HR 0.68 [95% CI 0.55, 0.85] versus metformin, HR 0.37 [95% CI 0.30, 0.45] versus glyburide). Cardiovascular and adverse event data (including effects on body weight and bone fracture) from ADOPT for AVANDIA, metformin, and glyburide are described in *Warnings and Precautions (5.2, 5.5, and 5.8)* and *Adverse Reactions (6.1)*, respectively. As with all medications, efficacy results must be considered together with safety information to assess the potential benefit and risk for an individual patient.

14.2 Combination With Metformin or Sulfonylurea

The addition of AVANDIA to either metformin or sulfonylurea resulted in significant reductions in hyperglycemia compared to either of these agents alone. These results are consistent with an additive effect on glycemic control when AVANDIA is used as combination therapy.

Combination With Metformin: A total of 670 patients with type 2 diabetes participated in two 26-week, randomized, double-blind, placebo/active-controlled trials designed to assess the efficacy of AVANDIA in combination with metformin. AVANDIA, administered in either once daily or twice daily dosing regimens, was added to the therapy of patients who were inadequately controlled on a maximum dose (2.5 grams/day) of metformin.

In one trial, patients inadequately controlled on 2.5 grams/day of metformin (mean baseline FPG 216 mg/dL and mean baseline HbA1c 8.8%) were randomized to receive 4 mg of AVANDIA once daily, 8 mg of AVANDIA once daily, or placebo in addition to metformin. A statistically significant improvement in FPG and HbA1c was observed in patients treated with the combinations of metformin and 4 mg of AVANDIA once daily and 8 mg of AVANDIA once daily, versus patients continued on metformin alone (Table 12).

[See table 12 above]

In a second 26-week trial, patients with type 2 diabetes inadequately controlled on 2.5 grams/day of metformin who were randomized to receive the combination of AVANDIA 4 mg twice daily and metformin (N = 105) showed a statistically significant improvement in glycemic control with a mean treatment effect for FPG of -56 mg/dL and a mean treatment effect for HbA1c of -0.8% over metformin alone. The combination of metformin and AVANDIA resulted in lower levels of FPG and HbA1c than either agent alone.

Patients who were inadequately controlled on a maximum dose (2.5 grams/day) of metformin and who were switched to monotherapy with AVANDIA demonstrated loss of glycemic control, as evidenced by increases in FPG and HbA1c. In this group, increases in LDL and VLDL were also seen.

Combination With a Sulfonylurea: A total of 3,457 patients with type 2 diabetes participated in ten 24- to 26-week randomized, double-blind, placebo/active-controlled trials and one 2-year double-blind, active-controlled trial in elderly patients designed to assess the efficacy and safety of AVANDIA in combination with a sulfonylurea. AVANDIA 2 mg, 4 mg, or 8 mg daily was administered, either once daily (3 trials) or in divided doses twice daily (7 trials), to patients inadequately controlled on a submaximal or maximal dose of sulfonylurea.

In these trials, the combination of AVANDIA 4 mg or 8 mg daily (administered as single or twice daily divided doses) and a sulfonylurea significantly reduced FPG and HbA1c compared to placebo plus sulfonylurea or further up-titration of the sulfonylurea. Table 13 shows pooled data for 8 trials in which AVANDIA added to sulfonylurea was compared to placebo plus sulfonylurea.

[See table 13 at top of next page]

One of the 24- to 26-week trials included patients who were inadequately controlled on maximal doses of glyburide and switched to 4 mg of AVANDIA daily as monotherapy; in this group, loss of glycemic control was demonstrated, as evidenced by increases in FPG and HbA1c.

In a 2-year double-blind trial, elderly patients (aged 59 to 89 years) on half-maximal sulfonylurea (glipizide 10 mg twice daily) were randomized to the addition of AVANDIA (n = 115, 4 mg once daily to 8 mg as needed) or to continued up-titration of glipizide (n = 110), to a maximum of 20 mg twice daily. Mean baseline FPG and HbA1c were 157 mg/dL and 7.72%, respectively, for the AVANDIA plus glipizide arm and 159 mg/dL and 7.65%, respectively, for the glipizide up-titration arm. Loss of glycemic control (FPG ≥180 mg/dL) occurred in a significantly lower proportion of patients (2%) on AVANDIA plus glipizide compared to patients in the glipizide up-titration arm (28.7%). About 78% of the patients on combination therapy completed the 2 years of therapy while only 51% completed on glipizide monotherapy. The effect of combination therapy on FPG and HbA1c was durable over the 2-year trial period, with patients achieving a mean of 132 mg/dL for FPG and a mean of 6.98% for HbA1c compared to no change on the glipizide arm.

14.3 Combination With Sulfonylurea Plus Metformin

In two 24- to 26-week, double-blind, placebo-controlled, trials designed to assess the efficacy and safety of AVANDIA in combination with sulfonylurea plus metformin, AVANDIA 4 mg or 8 mg daily, was administered in divided doses twice daily, to patients inadequately controlled on submaximal (10 mg) and maximal (20 mg) doses of glyburide and maximal dose of metformin (2 g/day). A statistically significant improvement in FPG and HbA1c was observed in patients treated with the combinations of sulfonylurea plus metformin and 4 mg of AVANDIA and 8 mg of AVANDIA versus patients continued on sulfonylurea plus metformin, as shown in Table 14.

[See table 14 at top of next page]

15 REFERENCES

1. Food and Drug Administration Briefing Document. Joint meeting of the Endocrinologic and Metabolic Drugs and Drug Safety and Risk Management Advisory Committees. July 13-14, 2010.
2. Winkelmayer WC, et al. Comparison of cardiovascular outcomes in elderly patients with diabetes who initiated rosiglitazone vs pioglitazone therapy. *Arch Intern Med* 2008;168(21):2368-2375.
3. Juurlink DN, et al. Adverse cardiovascular events during treatment with pioglitazone and rosiglitazone: population based cohort study. *BMJ* 2009; 339.
4. Graham DJ, et al. Risk of acute myocardial infarction, stroke, heart failure, and death in elderly medicare patients treated with rosiglitazone or pioglitazone. *JAMA* 2010;304:411-418.
5. Wertz DA, et al. Risk of cardiovascular events and all-cause mortality in patients with Thiazolidinediones in a managed-care population. *Circ Cardiovasc Qual Outcomes* 2010;3: 538-545.
6. DREAM Trial Investigators. Effect of rosiglitazone on the frequency of diabetes in patients with impaired glucose tolerance or impaired fasting glucose: a randomised controlled trial. *Lancet* 2006;368:1096-1105.
7. Kahn S, et al. Glycemic durability of rosiglitazone, metformin or glyburide monotherapy. *New England Journal of Medicine* 2006, 355:2427-2443.
8. Home P, et al. Rosiglitazone evaluated for cardiovascular outcomes in oral agent combination therapy for type 2 diabetes (RECORD): a multicenter, randomized, open-label trial. *Lancet* 2009, 373:2125-35.
9. Dormandy J et al. Secondary prevention of macrovascular events in patients with type 2 diabetes in the PROactive study (Prospective Pioglitazone Clinical Trial in Macrovascular Events): a randomized controlled trial. *Lancet* 2005, 366:1279-89.
10. Bilik D, et al. Thiazolidinediones, cardiovascular disease and cardiovascular mortality: translating research into action for diabetes (TRIAD). *Pharmacoepidemiol Drug Saf* 2010; 19: 715–721.
11. Park JY, Kim KA, Kang MH, et al. Effect of rifampin on the pharmacokinetics of rosiglitazone in healthy subjects. *Clin Pharmacol Ther* 2004;75:157-162.

16 HOW SUPPLIED/STORAGE AND HANDLING

Each pentagonal film-coated TILTAB tablet contains rosiglitazone as the maleate as follows: 2 mg–pink, debossed with SB on one side and 2 on the other; 4 mg–orange, debossed with SB on one side and 4 on the other; 8 mg–red-brown, debossed with SB on one side and 8 on the other.

2 mg bottles of 60: NDC 0173-0834-18
4 mg bottles of 30: NDC 0173-0835-13
8 mg bottles of 30: NDC 0173-0836-13

Store at 25°C (77°F); excursions 15° to 30°C (59° to 86°F). Dispense in a tight, light-resistant container.

17 PATIENT COUNSELING INFORMATION

See Medication Guide.

17.1 Patient Advice

There are multiple medications available to treat type 2 diabetes. The benefits and risks of each available diabetes medication should be taken into account when choosing a particular diabetes medication for a given patient.

Patients should be informed of the risks and benefits of AVANDIA. AVANDIA should only be taken by adults with type 2 diabetes who are already taking AVANDIA, or who are not already taking AVANDIA and are unable to achieve adequate glycemic control on other diabetes medications, and, in consultation with their healthcare provider, have decided not to take pioglitazone (ACTOS) for medical reasons. Inform patients that they must be enrolled in the AVANDIA-Rosiglitazone Medicines Access Program in order to receive AVANDIA.

Patients should be informed of the following:

- AVANDIA is not recommended for patients with symptomatic heart failure.
- Results of a set of clinical trials suggest that treatment with AVANDIA is associated with an increased risk for myocardial infarction (heart attack), especially in patients taking insulin. Clinical trials have not shown any difference between AVANDIA and comparator medications in overall mortality or CV-related mortality.
- AVANDIA is not recommended for patients who are taking insulin.
- Management of type 2 diabetes should include diet control. Caloric restriction, weight loss, and exercise are essential for the proper treatment of the diabetic patient because they help improve insulin sensitivity. This is important not only in the primary treatment of type 2 diabetes, but in maintaining the efficacy of drug therapy.
- It is important to adhere to dietary instructions and to regularly have blood glucose and glycosylated hemoglobin tested. It can take 2 weeks to see a reduction in blood glucose and 2 to 3 months to see the full effect of AVANDIA.
- Blood will be drawn to check their liver function prior to the start of therapy and periodically thereafter per the clinical judgment of the healthcare professional. Patients with unexplained symptoms of nausea, vomiting, abdominal pain, fatigue, anorexia, or dark urine should immediately report these symptoms to their physician.
- Patients who experience an unusually rapid increase in weight or edema or who develop shortness of breath or other symptoms of heart failure while on AVANDIA should immediately report these symptoms to their physician.
- AVANDIA can be taken with or without meals.
- When using AVANDIA in combination with other hypoglycemic agents, the risk of hypoglycemia, its symptoms and treatment, and conditions that predispose to its development should be explained to patients and their family members.
- Therapy with AVANDIA, like other thiazolidinediones, may result in ovulation in some premenopausal anovulatory women. As a result, these patients may be at an increased risk for pregnancy while taking AVANDIA. Thus, adequate contraception in premenopausal women should be recommended. This possible effect has not been specifically investigated in clinical trials so the frequency of this occurrence is not known.

Table 13. Glycemic Parameters in 24- to 26-Week Combination Trials of AVANDIA Plus Sulfonylurea

Twice Daily Divided Dosing (5 Trials)	**Sulfonylurea**	**AVANDIA 2 mg twice daily + sulfonylurea**	**Sulfonylurea**	**AVANDIA 4 mg twice daily + sulfonylurea**
	N = 397	N = 497	N = 248	N = 346
FPG (mg/dL)				
Baseline (mean)	204	198	188	187
Change from baseline (mean)	11	-29	8	-43
Difference from sulfonylurea alone (adjusted mean)	–	-42[a]	–	-53[a]
% of patients with ≥30 mg/dL decrease from baseline	17%	49%	15%	61%
HbA1c (%)				
Baseline (mean)	9.4	9.5	9.3	9.6
Change from baseline (mean)	0.2	-1.0	0.0	-1.6
Difference from sulfonylurea alone (adjusted mean)	–	-1.1[a]	–	-1.4[a]
% of patients with ≥0.7% decrease from baseline	21%	60%	23%	75%
Once Daily Dosing (3 Trials)	**Sulfonylurea**	**AVANDIA 4 mg once daily + sulfonylurea**	**Sulfonylurea**	**AVANDIA 8 mg once daily + sulfonylurea**
	N = 172	N = 172	N = 173	N = 176
FPG (mg/dL)				
Baseline (mean)	198	206	188	192
Change from baseline (mean)	17	-25	17	-43
Difference from sulfonylurea alone (adjusted mean)	–	-47[a]	–	-66[a]
% of patients with ≥30 mg/dL decrease from baseline	17%	48%	19%	55%
HbA1c (%)				
Baseline (mean)	8.6	8.8	8.9	8.9
Change from baseline (mean)	0.4	-0.5	0.1	-1.2
Difference from sulfonylurea alone (adjusted mean)	–	-0.9[a]	–	-1.4[a]
% of patients with ≥0.7% decrease from baseline	11%	36%	20%	68%

[a] P <0.0001 compared to sulfonylurea alone.

AVANDIA and TILTAB are registered trademarks of GlaxoSmithKline. ACTOS is a registered trademark of Takeda Pharmaceutical Company Limited.

GlaxoSmithKline
Research Triangle Park, NC 27709

May 2011
AVD:30PI

MEDICATION GUIDE
AVANDIA® (ah-VAN-dee-a)
(rosiglitazone maleate) Tablets

Read this Medication Guide carefully before you start taking AVANDIA and each time you get a refill. There may be new information. This information does not take the place of talking with your doctor about your medical condition or your treatment. If you have any questions about AVANDIA, ask your doctor or pharmacist.

What is the most important information I should know about AVANDIA?

AVANDIA is available only through the AVANDIA-Rosiglitazone Medicines Access Program. Both you and your doctor must be enrolled in the program so that you can get AVANDIA. To enroll, you must:

- talk to your doctor,
- understand the risks and benefits of AVANDIA, and
- agree to enroll in the program.

AVANDIA may cause serious side effects, including:

New or worse heart failure

- AVANDIA can cause your body to keep extra fluid (fluid retention), which leads to swelling (edema) and weight

Table 14. Glycemic Parameters in a 26-Week Combination Trial of AVANDIA Plus Sulfonylurea and Metformin

	Sulfonylurea + metformin	AVANDIA 2 mg twice daily + sulfonylurea + metformin	AVANDIA 4 mg twice daily + sulfonylurea + metformin
	N = 273	N = 276	N = 277
FPG (mg/dL)			
Baseline (mean)	189	190	192
Change from baseline (mean)	14	-19	-40
Difference from sulfonylurea plus metformin (adjusted mean)	–	-30[a]	-52[a]
% of patients with ≥30 mg/dL decrease from baseline	16%	46%	62%
HbA1c (%)			
Baseline (mean)	8.7	8.6	8.7
Change from baseline (mean)	0.2	-0.4	-0.9
Difference from sulfonylurea plus metformin (adjusted mean)	–	-0.6[a]	-1.1[a]
% of patients with ≥0.7% decrease from baseline	16%	39%	63%

[a]P <0.0001 compared to placebo.

gain. Extra body fluid can make some heart problems worse or lead to heart failure. Heart failure means your heart does not pump blood well enough.
- If you have severe heart failure, you cannot start AVANDIA.
- If you have heart failure with symptoms (such as shortness of breath or swelling), even if these symptoms are not severe, AVANDIA may not be right for you.

Call your doctor right away if you have any of the following:
- swelling or fluid retention, especially in the ankles or legs
- shortness of breath or trouble breathing, especially when you lie down
- an unusually fast increase in weight
- unusual tiredness

Myocardial Infarction ("Heart Attack")

AVANDIA may raise the risk of a heart attack. The risk of having a heart attack may be higher in people who take AVANDIA with insulin. Most people who take insulin should not also take AVANDIA.

Symptoms of a heart attack can include the following:
- chest discomfort in the center of your chest that lasts for more than a few minutes, or that goes away or comes back
- chest discomfort that feels like uncomfortable pressure, squeezing, fullness or pain
- pain or discomfort in your arms, back, neck, jaw or stomach
- shortness of breath with or without chest discomfort
- breaking out in a cold sweat
- nausea or vomiting
- feeling lightheaded

Call your doctor or go to the nearest hospital emergency room right away if you think you are having a heart attack.

People with diabetes have a greater risk for heart problems. It is important to work with your doctor to manage other conditions, such as high blood pressure or high cholesterol. AVANDIA can have other serious side effects. Be sure to read the section below "What are possible side effects of AVANDIA?".

What is AVANDIA?

AVANDIA is a prescription medicine used with diet and exercise to treat certain adults with type 2 (adult-onset or non-insulin dependent) diabetes mellitus (high blood sugar) who are:
- already taking AVANDIA or
- unable to control their blood sugar on other diabetes medicines, and after talking with their doctor have decided not to take pioglitazone (ACTOS)

AVANDIA helps to control high blood sugar. AVANDIA may be used alone or with other diabetes medicines. AVANDIA can help your body respond better to insulin made in your body. AVANDIA does not cause your body to make more insulin.

AVANDIA is not for people with type 1 diabetes mellitus or to treat a condition called diabetic ketoacidosis.

It is not known if AVANDIA is safe and effective in children under 18 years old.

Who should not take AVANDIA?

Many people with heart failure should not start taking AVANDIA. See "What should I tell my doctor before taking AVANDIA?".

What should I tell my doctor before taking AVANDIA?

Before starting AVANDIA, ask your doctor about what the choices are for diabetes medicines, and what the expected benefits and possible risks are for you in particular.

Before taking AVANDIA, tell your doctor about all your medical conditions, including if you:
- **have heart problems or heart failure.**
- **have type 1 ("juvenile") diabetes or had diabetic ketoacidosis.** These conditions should be treated with insulin.
- **have a type of diabetic eye disease called macular edema** (swelling of the back of the eye).
- **have liver problems.** Your doctor should do blood tests to check your liver before you start taking AVANDIA and during treatment as needed.
- **had liver problems while taking REZULIN® (troglitazone), another medicine for diabetes.**
- **are pregnant or plan to become pregnant.** AVANDIA should not be used during pregnancy. It is not known if AVANDIA can harm your unborn baby. You and your doctor should talk about the best way to control your diabetes during pregnancy. If you are a premenopausal woman (before the "change of life") who does not have regular monthly periods, AVANDIA may increase your chances of becoming pregnant. Talk to your doctor about birth control choices while taking AVANDIA. Tell your doctor right away if you become pregnant while taking AVANDIA.
- **are breast-feeding or planning to breast-feed.** It is not known if AVANDIA passes into breast milk. You should not use AVANDIA while breast-feeding.

Tell your doctor about all the medicines you take including prescription and non-prescription medicines, vitamins or herbal supplements. AVANDIA and certain other medicines can affect each other and may lead to serious side effects including high or low blood sugar, or heart problems. Especially tell your doctor if you take:
- **insulin.**
- **any medicines for high blood pressure, high cholesterol or heart failure, or for prevention of heart disease or stroke.**

Know the medicines you take. Keep a list of your medicines and show it to your doctor and pharmacist before you start a new medicine. They will tell you if it is alright to take AVANDIA with other medicines.

How should I take AVANDIA?
- Take AVANDIA exactly as prescribed. Your doctor will tell you how many tablets to take and how often. The usual daily starting dose is 4 mg a day taken one time each day or 2 mg taken two times each day. Your doctor may need to adjust your dose until your blood sugar is better controlled.
- AVANDIA may be prescribed alone or with other diabetes medicines. This will depend on how well your blood sugar is controlled.
- Take AVANDIA with or without food.
- It can take 2 weeks for AVANDIA to start lowering blood sugar. It may take 2 to 3 months to see the full effect on your blood sugar level.
- If you miss a dose of AVANDIA, take it as soon as you remember, unless it is time to take your next dose. Take your next dose at the usual time. Do not take double doses to make up for a missed dose.
- If you take too much AVANDIA, call your doctor or poison control center right away.
- Test your blood sugar regularly as your doctor tells you.
- Diet and exercise can help your body use its blood sugar better. It is important to stay on your recommended diet, lose extra weight, and get regular exercise while taking AVANDIA.
- Your doctor should do blood tests to check your liver before you start AVANDIA and during treatment as needed. Your doctor should also do regular blood sugar tests (for example, "A1C") to monitor your response to AVANDIA.

What are possible side effects of AVANDIA?

AVANDIA may cause serious side effects including:
- **New or worse heart failure.** See "What is the most important information I should know about AVANDIA?".
- **Heart attack.** See "What is the most important information I should know about AVANDIA?".
- **Swelling (edema).** AVANDIA can cause swelling due to fluid retention. See "What is the most important information I should know about AVANDIA?".
- **Weight gain.** AVANDIA can cause weight gain that may be due to fluid retention or extra body fat. Weight gain can be a serious problem for people with certain conditions including heart problems. See "What is the most important information I should know about AVANDIA?".
- **Liver problems.** It is important for your liver to be working normally when you take AVANDIA. Your doctor should do blood tests to check your liver before you start taking AVANDIA and during treatment as needed. Call your doctor right away if you have unexplained symptoms such as:
  - nausea or vomiting
  - stomach pain
  - unusual or unexplained tiredness
  - loss of appetite
  - dark urine
  - yellowing of your skin or the whites of your eyes.
- **Macular edema** (a diabetic eye disease with swelling in the back of the eye). Tell your doctor right away if you have any changes in your vision. Your doctor should check your eyes regularly. Very rarely, some people have had vision changes due to swelling in the back of the eye while taking AVANDIA.
- **Fractures (broken bones),** usually in the hand, upper arm or foot. Talk to your doctor for advice on how to keep your bones healthy.
- **Low red blood cell count (anemia).**
- **Low blood sugar (hypoglycemia).** Lightheadedness, dizziness, shakiness or hunger may mean that your blood sugar is too low. This can happen if you skip meals, if you use another medicine that lowers blood sugar, or if you have certain medical problems. Call your doctor if low blood sugar levels are a problem for you.
- **Ovulation** (release of egg from an ovary in a woman) leading to pregnancy. Ovulation may happen in premenopausal women who do not have regular monthly periods. This can increase the chance of pregnancy. See "What should I tell my doctor before taking AVANDIA?".

The most common side effects of AVANDIA reported in clinical trials included cold-like symptoms and headache.

Call your doctor for medical advice about side effects. You may report side effects to FDA at 1-800-FDA-1088.

How should I store AVANDIA?
- Store AVANDIA at room temperature, 59° to 86°F (15° to 30°C). Keep AVANDIA in the container it comes in.
- Safely, throw away AVANDIA that is out of date or no longer needed.
- Keep AVANDIA and all medicines out of the reach of children.

General information about AVANDIA

Medicines are sometimes prescribed for purposes other than those listed in a Medication Guide. Do not use AVANDIA for a condition for which it was not prescribed. Do not give AVANDIA to other people, even if they have the same symptoms you have. It may harm them.

This Medication Guide summarizes important information about AVANDIA. If you would like more information, talk with your doctor. You can ask your doctor or pharmacist for information about AVANDIA that is written for healthcare professionals. You can also find out more about AVANDIA by calling 1-888-825-5249.

What are the ingredients in AVANDIA?

Active Ingredient: Rosiglitazone maleate.

Inactive Ingredients: Hypromellose 2910, lactose monohydrate, magnesium stearate, microcrystalline cellulose, polyethylene glycol 3000, sodium starch glycolate, titanium dioxide, triacetin, and 1 or more of the following: Synthetic red and yellow iron oxides and talc.

Always check to make sure that the medicine you are taking is the correct one. AVANDIA tablets are triangles with rounded corners and look like this:

2 mg – pink with "SB" on one side and "2" on the other.
4 mg – orange with "SB" on one side and "4" on the other.
8 mg – red-brown with "SB" on one side and "8" on the other.

AVANDIA is a registered trademark of GlaxoSmithKline. The other brands listed are trademarks of their respective owners and are not trademarks of GlaxoSmithKline. The makers of these brands are not affiliated with and do not endorse GlaxoSmithKline or its products.

This Medication Guide has been approved by the U.S. Food and Drug Administration.

GlaxoSmithKline
Research Triangle Park, NC 27709

May 2011
AVD:6MG

AVODART ℞

[*av'ō dart*]
(dutasteride)
Soft Gelatin Capsules

HIGHLIGHTS OF PRESCRIBING INFORMATION
These highlights do not include all the information needed to use AVODART safely and effectively. See full prescribing information for AVODART.
AVODART (dutasteride) Soft Gelatin Capsules
Initial U.S. Approval: 2001

RECENT MAJOR CHANGES

Warnings and Precautions, Evaluation for Other Urological Diseases (5.3)03/2012

INDICATIONS AND USAGE

AVODART is a 5 alpha-reductase inhibitor indicated for the treatment of symptomatic benign prostatic hyperplasia (BPH) in men with an enlarged prostate to: (1.1)
- improve symptoms,
- reduce the risk of acute urinary retention, and
- reduce the risk of the need for BPH-related surgery.

AVODART in combination with the alpha adrenergic antagonist, tamsulosin, is indicated for the treatment of symptomatic BPH in men with an enlarged prostate. (1.2)

Limitations of Use: AVODART is not approved for the prevention of prostate cancer. (1.3)

DOSAGE AND ADMINISTRATION

Monotherapy: 0.5 mg once daily. (2.1)

Combination with tamsulosin: 0.5 mg once daily and tamsulosin 0.4 mg once daily. (2.2)

Dosing considerations: Swallow whole. May take with or without food. (2)

DOSAGE FORMS AND STRENGTHS

0.5-mg soft gelatin capsules (3)

CONTRAINDICATIONS

- Pregnancy and women of childbearing potential. (4, 5.4, 8.1)
- Pediatric patients. (4)
- Patients with previously demonstrated, clinically significant hypersensitivity (e.g., serious skin reactions, angioedema) to AVODART or other 5 alpha-reductase inhibitors. (4)

WARNINGS AND PRECAUTIONS

- AVODART reduces serum prostate-specific antigen (PSA) concentration by approximately 50%. However, any confirmed increase in PSA while on AVODART may signal the presence of prostate cancer and should be evaluated, even if those values are still within the normal range for untreated men. (5.1)
- AVODART may increase the risk of high-grade prostate cancer. (5.2, 6.1)
- Prior to initiating treatment with AVODART, consideration should be given to other urological conditions that may cause similar symptoms. (5.3)
- Women who are pregnant or could become pregnant should not handle AVODART Capsules due to potential risk to a male fetus. (5.4, 8.1)
- Patients should not donate blood until 6 months after their last dose of AVODART. (5.5)

ADVERSE REACTIONS

The most common adverse reactions, reported in ≥1% of subjects treated with AVODART and more commonly than in subjects treated with placebo, are impotence, decreased libido, ejaculation disorders, and breast disorders. (6.1)

To report SUSPECTED ADVERSE REACTIONS, contact GlaxoSmithKline at 1-888-825-5249 or FDA at 1-800-FDA-1088 or www.fda.gov/medwatch.

DRUG INTERACTIONS

Use with caution in patients taking potent, chronic CYP3A4 enzyme inhibitors (e.g., ritonavir). (7)

See 17 for PATIENT COUNSELING INFORMATION and FDA-approved patient labeling

Revised: 04/2013

FULL PRESCRIBING INFORMATION: CONTENTS*

*** Sections or subsections omitted from the full prescribing information are not listed**

FULL PRESCRIBING INFORMATION

1 INDICATIONS AND USAGE

1.1 Monotherapy

AVODART® (dutasteride) Soft Gelatin Capsules are indicated for the treatment of symptomatic benign prostatic hyperplasia (BPH) in men with an enlarged prostate to:
- improve symptoms,
- reduce the risk of acute urinary retention (AUR), and
- reduce the risk of the need for BPH-related surgery.

1.2 Combination With Alpha Adrenergic Antagonist

AVODART in combination with the alpha adrenergic antagonist, tamsulosin, is indicated for the treatment of symptomatic BPH in men with an enlarged prostate.

1.3 Limitations of Use

AVODART is not approved for the prevention of prostate cancer.

2 DOSAGE AND ADMINISTRATION

The capsules should be swallowed whole and not chewed or opened, as contact with the capsule contents may result in irritation of the oropharyngeal mucosa. AVODART may be administered with or without food.

2.1 Monotherapy

The recommended dose of AVODART is 1 capsule (0.5 mg) taken once daily.

2.2 Combination With Alpha Adrenergic Antagonist

The recommended dose of AVODART is 1 capsule (0.5 mg) taken once daily and tamsulosin 0.4 mg taken once daily.

3 DOSAGE FORMS AND STRENGTHS

0.5-mg, opaque, dull yellow, gelatin capsules imprinted with "GX CE2" in red ink on one side.

4 CONTRAINDICATIONS

AVODART is contraindicated for use in:
- Pregnancy. In animal reproduction and developmental toxicity studies, dutasteride inhibited development of male fetus external genitalia. Therefore, AVODART may cause fetal harm when administered to a pregnant woman. If AVODART is used during pregnancy or if the patient becomes pregnant while taking AVODART, the patient should be apprised of the potential hazard to the fetus *[see Warnings and Precautions (5.4), Use in Specific Populations (8.1)]*.
- Women of childbearing potential *[see Warnings and Precautions (5.4), Use in Specific Populations (8.1)]*.
- Pediatric patients *[see Use in Specific Populations (8.4)]*.
- Patients with previously demonstrated, clinically significant hypersensitivity (e.g., serious skin reactions, angioedema) to AVODART or other 5 alpha-reductase inhibitors *[see Adverse Reactions (6.2)]*.

5 WARNINGS AND PRECAUTIONS

5.1 Effects on Prostate-Specific Antigen (PSA) and the Use of PSA in Prostate Cancer Detection

In clinical trials, AVODART reduced serum PSA concentration by approximately 50% within 3 to 6 months of treatment. This decrease was predictable over the entire range of PSA values in subjects with symptomatic BPH, although it may vary in individuals. AVODART may also cause decreases in serum PSA in the presence of prostate cancer. To interpret serial PSAs in men taking AVODART, a new PSA baseline should be established at least 3 months after starting treatment and PSA monitored periodically thereafter. Any confirmed increase from the lowest PSA value while on AVODART may signal the presence of prostate cancer and should be evaluated, even if PSA levels are still within the normal range for men not taking a 5 alpha-reductase inhibitor. Noncompliance with AVODART may also affect PSA test results.

To interpret an isolated PSA value in a man treated with AVODART for 3 months or more, the PSA value should be doubled for comparison with normal values in untreated men.The free-to-total PSA ratio (percent free PSA) remains constant, even under the influence of AVODART. If clinicians elect to use percent free PSA as an aid in the detection of prostate cancer in men receiving AVODART, no adjustment to its value appears necessary.

Coadministration of dutasteride and tamsulosin resulted in similar changes to serum PSA as dutasteride monotherapy.

5.2 Increased Risk of High-Grade Prostate Cancer

In men aged 50 to 75 years with a prior negative biopsy for prostate cancer and a baseline PSA between 2.5 ng/mL and 10.0 ng/mL taking AVODART in the 4-year Reduction by Dutasteride of Prostate Cancer Events (REDUCE) trial, there was an increased incidence of Gleason score 8-10 prostate cancer compared with men taking placebo (AVODART 1.0% versus placebo 0.5%) [see Indications and Usage (1.3), Adverse Reactions (6.1)]. In a 7-year placebo-controlled clinical trial with another 5 alpha-reductase inhibitor (finasteride 5 mg, PROSCAR), similar results for Gleason score 8-10 prostate cancer were observed (finasteride 1.8% versus placebo 1.1%).

5 alpha-reductase inhibitors may increase the risk of development of high-grade prostate cancer. Whether the effect of 5 alpha-reductase inhibitors to reduce prostate volume, or trial-related factors, impacted the results of these trials has not been established.

5.3 Evaluation for Other Urological Diseases

Prior to initiating treatment with AVODART, consideration should be given to other urological conditions that may cause similar symptoms. In addition, BPH and prostate cancer may coexist.

5.4 Exposure of Women—Risk to Male Fetus

AVODART Capsules should not be handled by a woman who is pregnant or who could become pregnant. Dutasteride is absorbed through the skin and could result in unintended fetal exposure. If a woman who is pregnant or who could become pregnant comes in contact with leaking dutasteride capsules, the contact area should be washed immediately with soap and water *[see Use in Specific Populations (8.1)]*.

5.5 Blood Donation

Men being treated with AVODART should not donate blood until at least 6 months have passed following their last dose. The purpose of this deferred period is to prevent administration of dutasteride to a pregnant female transfusion recipient.

5.6 Effect on Semen Characteristics

The effects of dutasteride 0.5 mg/day on semen characteristics were evaluated in normal volunteers aged 18 to 52 (n = 27 dutasteride, n = 23 placebo) throughout 52 weeks of treatment and 24 weeks of post-treatment follow-up. At 52 weeks, the mean percent reductions from baseline in total sperm count, semen volume, and sperm motility were 23%, 26%, and 18%, respectively, in the dutasteride group when adjusted for changes from baseline in the placebo group. Sperm concentration and sperm morphology were unaf-

Table 1. Adverse Reactions Reported in ≥1% of Subjects Over a 24-Month Period and More Frequently in the Group Receiving AVODART Than the Placebo Group (Randomized, Double-Blind, Placebo-Controlled Trials Pooled) by Time of Onset

Adverse Reaction	Adverse Reaction Time of Onset			
	Months 0–6	Months 7–12	Months 13–18	Months 19–24
AVODART (n) Placebo (n)	(n = 2,167) (n = 2,158)	(n = 1,901) (n = 1,922)	(n = 1,725) (n = 1,714)	(n = 1,605) (n = 1,555)
Impotence[a]				
AVODART	4.7%	1.4%	1.0%	0.8%
Placebo	1.7%	1.5%	0.5%	0.9%
Decreased libido[a]				
AVODART	3.0%	0.7%	0.3%	0.3%
Placebo	1.4%	0.6%	0.2%	0.1%
Ejaculation disorders[a]				
AVODART	1.4%	0.5%	0.5%	0.1%
Placebo	0.5%	0.3%	0.1%	0.0%
Breast disorders[b]				
AVODART	0.5%	0.8%	1.1%	0.6%
Placebo	0.2%	0.3%	0.3%	0.1%

[a]These sexual adverse reactions are associated with dutasteride treatment (including monotherapy and combination with tamsulosin). These adverse reactions may persist after treatment discontinuation. The role of dutasteride in this persistence is unknown.
[b]Includes breast tenderness and breast enlargement.

Table 2. Adverse Reactions Reported Over a 48-Month Period in ≥1% of Subjects and More Frequently in the Coadministration Therapy Group Than the Groups Receiving Monotherapy With AVODART or Tamsulosin (CombAT) by Time of Onset

Adverse Reaction	Adverse Reaction Time of Onset				
	Year 1		Year 2	Year 3	Year 4
	Months 0–6	Months 7–12			
Combination[a] AVODART Tamsulosin	(n = 1,610) (n = 1,623) (n = 1,611)	(n = 1,527) (n = 1,548) (n = 1,545)	(n = 1,428) (n = 1,464) (n = 1,468)	(n = 1,283) (n = 1,325) (n = 1,281)	(n = 1,200) (n = 1,200) (n = 1,112)
Ejaculation disorders[b,c]					
Combination	7.8%	1.6%	1.0%	0.5%	<0.1%
AVODART	1.0%	0.5%	0.5%	0.2%	0.3%
Tamsulosin	2.2%	0.5%	0.5%	0.2%	0.3%
Impotence[c,d]					
Combination	5.4%	1.1%	1.8%	0.9%	0.4%
AVODART	4.0%	1.1%	1.6%	0.6%	0.3%
Tamsulosin	2.6%	0.8%	1.0%	0.6%	1.1%
Decreased libido[c,e]					
Combination	4.5%	0.9%	0.8%	0.2%	0.0%
AVODART	3.1%	0.7%	1.0%	0.2%	0.0%
Tamsulosin	2.0%	0.6%	0.7%	0.2%	<0.1%
Breast disorders[f]					
Combination	1.1%	1.1%	0.8%	0.9%	0.6%
AVODART	0.9%	0.9%	1.2%	0.5%	0.7%
Tamsulosin	0.4%	0.4%	0.4%	0.2%	0.0%
Dizziness					
Combination	1.1%	0.4%	0.1%	<0.1%	0.2%
AVODART	0.5%	0.3%	0.1%	<0.1%	<0.1%
Tamsulosin	0.9%	0.5%	0.4%	<0.1%	0.0%

[a]Combination = AVODART 0.5 mg once daily plus tamsulosin 0.4 mg once daily.
[b]Includes anorgasmia, retrograde ejaculation, semen volume decreased, orgasmic sensation decreased, orgasm abnormal, ejaculation delayed, ejaculation disorder, ejaculation failure, and premature ejaculation.
[c]These sexual adverse reactions are associated with dutasteride treatment (including monotherapy and combination with tamsulosin). These adverse reactions may persist after treatment discontinuation. The role of dutasteride in this persistence is unknown.
[d]Includes erectile dysfunction and disturbance in sexual arousal.
[e]Includes libido decreased, libido disorder, loss of libido, sexual dysfunction, and male sexual dysfunction.
[f]Includes breast enlargement, gynecomastia, breast swelling, breast pain, breast tenderness, nipple pain, and nipple swelling.

fected. After 24 weeks of follow-up, the mean percent change in total sperm count in the dutasteride group remained 23% lower than baseline. While mean values for all semen parameters at all time-points remained within the normal ranges and did not meet predefined criteria for a clinically significant change (30%), 2 subjects in the dutasteride group had decreases in sperm count of greater than 90% from baseline at 52 weeks, with partial recovery at the 24-week follow-up. The clinical significance of dutasteride's effect on semen characteristics for an individual patient's fertility is not known.

6 ADVERSE REACTIONS

6.1 Clinical Trials Experience

Because clinical trials are conducted under widely varying conditions, adverse reaction rates observed in the clinical trials of a drug cannot be directly compared with rates in the clinical trial of another drug and may not reflect the rates observed in practice.

From clinical trials with AVODART as monotherapy or in combination with tamsulosin:

- The most common adverse reactions reported in subjects receiving AVODART were impotence, decreased libido, breast disorders (including breast enlargement and tenderness), and ejaculation disorders. The most common adverse reactions reported in subjects receiving combination therapy (AVODART plus tamsulosin) were impotence, decreased libido, breast disorders (including breast enlargement and tenderness), ejaculation disorders, and dizziness. Ejaculation disorders occurred significantly more in subjects receiving combination therapy (11%) compared with those receiving AVODART (2%) or tamsulosin (4%) as monotherapy.
- Trial withdrawal due to adverse reactions occurred in 4% of subjects receiving AVODART, and 3% of subjects receiving placebo in placebo-controlled trials with AVODART. The most common adverse reaction leading to trial withdrawal was impotence (1%).
- In the clinical trial evaluating the combination therapy, trial withdrawal due to adverse reactions occurred in 6% of subjects receiving combination therapy (AVODART plus tamsulosin) and 4% of subjects receiving AVODART or tamsulosin as monotherapy. The most common adverse reaction in all treatment arms leading to trial withdrawal was erectile dysfunction (1% to 1.5%).

Monotherapy: Over 4,300 male subjects with BPH were randomly assigned to receive placebo or 0.5-mg daily doses of AVODART in 3 identical 2-year, placebo-controlled, double-blind, Phase 3 treatment trials, each followed by a 2-year open-label extension. During the double-blind treatment period, 2,167 male subjects were exposed to AVODART, including 1,772 exposed for 1 year and 1,510 exposed for 2 years. When including the open-label extensions, 1,009 male subjects were exposed to AVODART for 3 years and 812 were exposed for 4 years. The population was aged 47 to 94 years (mean age: 66 years) and greater than 90% were Caucasian. Table 1 summarizes clinical adverse reactions reported in at least 1% of subjects receiving AVODART and at a higher incidence than subjects receiving placebo.

[See table 1 above]

Long-Term Treatment (Up to 4 Years): High-Grade Prostate Cancer: The REDUCE trial was a randomized, double-blind, placebo-controlled trial that enrolled 8,231 men aged 50 to 75 years with a serum PSA of 2.5 ng/mL to 10 ng/mL and a negative prostate biopsy within the previous 6 months. Subjects were randomized to receive placebo (N = 4,126) or 0.5-mg daily doses of AVODART (N = 4,105) for up to 4 years. The mean age was 63 years and 91% were Caucasian. Subjects underwent protocol-mandated scheduled prostate biopsies at 2 and 4 years of treatment or had "for-cause biopsies" at non-scheduled times if clinically indicated. There was a higher incidence of Gleason score 8-10 prostate cancer in men receiving AVODART (1.0%) compared with men on placebo (0.5%) *[see Indications and Usage (1.3), Warnings and Precautions (5.2)]*. In a 7-year placebo-controlled clinical trial with another 5 alpha-reductase inhibitor (finasteride 5 mg, PROSCAR), similar results for Gleason score 8-10 prostate cancer were observed (finasteride 1.8% versus placebo 1.1%).

No clinical benefit has been demonstrated in patients with prostate cancer treated with AVODART.

Reproductive and Breast Disorders: In the 3 pivotal placebo-controlled BPH trials with AVODART, each 4 years in duration, there was no evidence of increased sexual adverse reactions (impotence, decreased libido, and ejaculation disorder) or breast disorders with increased duration of treatment. Among these 3 trials, there was 1 case of breast cancer in the dutasteride group and 1 case in the placebo group. No cases of breast cancer were reported in any treatment group in the 4-year CombAT trial or the 4-year REDUCE trial.

The relationship between long-term use of dutasteride and male breast neoplasia is currently unknown.

Combination With Alpha-Blocker Therapy (CombAT): Over 4,800 male subjects with BPH were randomly assigned to receive 0.5-mg AVODART, 0.4-mg tamsulosin, or combination therapy (0.5-mg AVODART plus 0.4-mg tamsulosin) administered once daily in a 4-year double-blind trial. Overall, 1,623 subjects received monotherapy with AVODART; 1,611 subjects received monotherapy with tamsulosin; and 1,610 subjects received combination therapy. The population was aged 49 to 88 years (mean age: 66 years) and 88% were Caucasian. Table 2 summarizes adverse reactions reported in at least 1% of subjects in the combination group and at a higher incidence than subjects receiving monotherapy with AVODART or tamsulosin.

[See table 2 above]

Cardiac Failure: In CombAT, after 4 years of treatment, the incidence of the composite term cardiac failure in the combination therapy group (12/1,610; 0.7%) was higher than in either monotherapy group: AVODART, 2/1,623 (0.1%) and tamsulosin, 9/1,611 (0.6%). Composite cardiac failure was also examined in a separate 4-year placebo-controlled trial evaluating AVODART in men at risk for development of prostate cancer. The incidence of cardiac failure in subjects taking AVODART was 0.6% (26/4,105) compared with 0.4% (15/4,126) in subjects on placebo. A majority of subjects with cardiac failure in both trials had comorbidities associated with an increased risk of cardiac failure. Therefore, the clinical significance of the numerical imbalances in cardiac failure is unknown. No causal relationship between AVODART, alone or in combination with tamsulosin, and cardiac failure has been established. No imbalance was observed in the incidence of overall cardiovascular adverse events in either trial.

6.2 Postmarketing Experience

The following adverse reactions have been identified during post-approval use of AVODART. Because these reactions are reported voluntarily from a population of uncertain size, it is not always possible to reliably estimate their frequency or establish a causal relationship to drug exposure. These reactions have been chosen for inclusion due to a combination of their seriousness, frequency of reporting, or potential causal connection to AVODART.

Immune System Disorders: Hypersensitivity reactions, including rash, pruritus, urticaria, localized edema, serious skin reactions, and angioedema.

Neoplasms: Male breast cancer.

Psychiatric Disorders: Depressed mood.

Reproductive System and Breast Disorders: Testicular pain and testicular swelling.

7 DRUG INTERACTIONS

7.1 Cytochrome P450 3A Inhibitors

Dutasteride is extensively metabolized in humans by the CYP3A4 and CYP3A5 isoenzymes. The effect of potent CYP3A4 inhibitors on dutasteride has not been studied. Because of the potential for drug-drug interactions, use caution when prescribing AVODART to patients taking potent, chronic CYP3A4 enzyme inhibitors (e.g., ritonavir) *[see Clinical Pharmacology (12.3)]*.

7.2 Alpha Adrenergic Antagonists

The administration of AVODART in combination with tamsulosin or terazosin has no effect on the steady-state pharmacokinetics of either alpha adrenergic antagonist. The effect of administration of tamsulosin or terazosin on dutasteride pharmacokinetic parameters has not been evaluated.

7.3 Calcium Channel Antagonists

Coadministration of verapamil or diltiazem decreases dutasteride clearance and leads to increased exposure to dutasteride. The change in dutasteride exposure is not considered to be clinically significant. No dose adjustment is recommended *[see Clinical Pharmacology (12.3)]*.

7.4 Cholestyramine

Administration of a single 5-mg dose of AVODART followed 1 hour later by 12 g of cholestyramine does not affect the relative bioavailability of dutasteride *[see Clinical Pharmacology (12.3)]*.

7.5 Digoxin

AVODART does not alter the steady-state pharmacokinetics of digoxin when administered concomitantly at a dose of 0.5 mg/day for 3 weeks *[see Clinical Pharmacology (12.3)]*.

7.6 Warfarin

Concomitant administration of AVODART 0.5 mg/day for 3 weeks with warfarin does not alter the steady-state pharmacokinetics of the S- or R-warfarin isomers or alter the effect of warfarin on prothrombin time *[see Clinical Pharmacology (12.3)]*.

8 USE IN SPECIFIC POPULATIONS

8.1 Pregnancy

Pregnancy Category X. AVODART is contraindicated for use in women of childbearing potential and during pregnancy. AVODART is a 5 alpha-reductase inhibitor that prevents conversion of testosterone to dihydrotestosterone (DHT), a hormone necessary for normal development of male genitalia. In animal reproduction and developmental toxicity studies, dutasteride inhibited normal development of external genitalia in male fetuses. Therefore, AVODART may cause fetal harm when administered to a pregnant woman. If AVODART is used during pregnancy or if the patient becomes pregnant while taking AVODART, the patient should be apprised of the potential hazard to the fetus.

Abnormalities in the genitalia of male fetuses is an expected physiological consequence of inhibition of the conversion of testosterone to DHT by 5 alpha-reductase inhibitors. These results are similar to observations in male infants with genetic 5 alpha-reductase deficiency. Dutasteride is absorbed through the skin. To avoid potential fetal exposure, women who are pregnant or could become pregnant should not handle AVODART Soft Gelatin Capsules. If contact is made with leaking capsules, the contact area should be washed immediately with soap and water *[see Warnings and Precautions (5.4)]*. Dutasteride is secreted into semen. The highest measured semen concentration of dutasteride in treated men was 14 ng/mL. Assuming exposure of a 50-kg woman to 5 mL of semen and 100% absorption, the woman's dutasteride concentration would be about 0.0175 ng/mL. This concentration is more than 100 times less than concentrations producing abnormalities of male genitalia in animal studies. Dutasteride is highly protein bound in human semen (greater than 96%), which may reduce the amount of dutasteride available for vaginal absorption.

In an embryo-fetal development study in female rats, oral administration of dutasteride at doses 10 times less than the maximum recommended human dose (MRHD) of 0.5 mg daily resulted in abnormalities of male genitalia in the fetus (decreased anogenital distance at 0.05 mg/kg/day), nipple development, hypospadias, and distended preputial glands in male offspring (at all doses of 0.05, 2.5, 12.5, and 30 mg/kg/day). An increase in stillborn pups was observed at 111 times the MRHD, and reduced fetal body weight was observed at doses of about 15 times the MRHD (animal dose of 2.5 mg/kg/day). Increased incidences of skeletal variations considered to be delays in ossification associated with reduced body weight were observed at doses about 56 times the MRHD (animal dose of 12.5 mg/kg/day).

In a rabbit embryo-fetal study, doses 28- to 93-fold the MRHD (animal doses of 30, 100, and 200 mg/kg/day) were administered orally during the period of major organogenesis (gestation days 7 to 29) to encompass the late period of external genitalia development. Histological evaluation of the genital papilla of fetuses revealed evidence of feminization of the male fetus at all doses. A second embryo-fetal study in rabbits at 0.3- to 53-fold the expected clinical exposure (animal doses of 0.05, 0.4, 3.0, and 30 mg/kg/day) also produced evidence of feminization of the genitalia in male fetuses at all doses.

In an oral pre- and post-natal development study in rats, dutasteride doses of 0.05, 2.5, 12.5, or 30 mg/kg/day were administered. Unequivocal evidence of feminization of the genitalia (i.e., decreased anogenital distance, increased incidence of hypospadias, nipple development) of male offspring occurred at 14- to 90-fold the MRHD (animal doses of 2.5 mg/kg/day or greater). At 0.05-fold the expected clinical exposure (animal dose of 0.05 mg/kg/day), evidence of feminization was limited to a small, but statistically significant, decrease in anogenital distance. Animal doses of 2.5 to 30 mg/kg/day resulted in prolonged gestation in the parental females and a decrease in time to vaginal patency for female offspring and a decrease in prostate and seminal vesicle weights in male offspring. Effects on newborn startle response were noted at doses greater than or equal to 12.5 mg/kg/day. Increased stillbirths were noted at 30 mg/kg/day

In an embryo-fetal development study, pregnant rhesus monkeys were exposed intravenously to a dutasteride blood level comparable to the dutasteride concentration found in human semen. Dutasteride was administered on gestation days 20 to 100 at doses of 400, 780, 1,325, or 2,010 ng/day (12 monkeys/group). The development of male external genitalia of monkey offspring was not adversely affected. Reduction of fetal adrenal weights, reduction in fetal prostate weights, and increases in fetal ovarian and testis weights were observed at the highest dose tested in monkeys. Based on the highest measured semen concentration of dutasteride in treated men (14 ng/mL), these doses represent 0.8 to 16 times the potential maximum exposure of a 50-kg human female to 5 mL semen daily from a dutasteride-treated man, assuming 100% absorption. (These calculations are based on blood levels of parent drug which are achieved at 32 to 186 times the daily doses administered to pregnant monkeys on a ng/kg basis). Dutasteride is highly bound to proteins in human semen (greater than 96%), potentially reducing the amount of dutasteride available for vaginal absorption. It is not known whether rabbits or rhesus monkeys produce any of the major human metabolites.

Estimates of exposure multiples comparing animal studies to the MRHD for dutasteride are based on clinical serum concentration at steady state.

8.3 Nursing Mothers

AVODART is contraindicated for use in women of childbearing potential, including nursing women. It is not known whether dutasteride is excreted in human milk.

8.4 Pediatric Use

AVODART is contraindicated for use in pediatric patients. Safety and effectiveness in pediatric patients have not been established.

8.5 Geriatric Use

Of 2,167 male subjects treated with AVODART in 3 clinical trials, 60% were aged 65 years and older and 15% were aged 75 years and older. No overall differences in safety or efficacy were observed between these subjects and younger subjects. Other reported clinical experience has not identified differences in responses between the elderly and younger patients, but greater sensitivity of some older individuals cannot be ruled out *[see Clinical Pharmacology (12.3)]*.

8.6 Renal Impairment

No dose adjustment is necessary for AVODART in patients with renal impairment *[see Clinical Pharmacology (12.3)]*.

8.7 Hepatic Impairment

The effect of hepatic impairment on dutasteride pharmacokinetics has not been studied. Because dutasteride is extensively metabolized, exposure could be higher in hepatically impaired patients. However, in a clinical trial where 60 subjects received 5 mg (10 times the therapeutic dose) daily for 24 weeks, no additional adverse events were observed compared with those observed at the therapeutic dose of 0.5 mg *[see Clinical Pharmacology (12.3)]*.

10 OVERDOSAGE

In volunteer trials, single doses of dutasteride up to 40 mg (80 times the therapeutic dose) for 7 days have been administered without significant safety concerns. In a clinical trial, daily doses of 5 mg (10 times the therapeutic dose) were administered to 60 subjects for 6 months with no additional adverse effects to those seen at therapeutic doses of 0.5 mg.

There is no specific antidote for dutasteride. Therefore, in cases of suspected overdosage symptomatic and supportive treatment should be given as appropriate, taking the long half-life of dutasteride into consideration.

11 DESCRIPTION

AVODART is a synthetic 4-azasteroid compound that is a selective inhibitor of both the type 1 and type 2 isoforms of steroid 5 alpha-reductase, an intracellular enzyme that converts testosterone to DHT.

Dutasteride is chemically designated as (5α,17β)-N-{2,5 bis(trifluoromethyl)phenyl}-3-oxo-4-azaandrost-1-ene-17-carboxamide. The empirical formula of dutasteride is $C_{27}H_{30}F_6N_2O_2$, representing a molecular weight of 528.5 with the following structural formula:

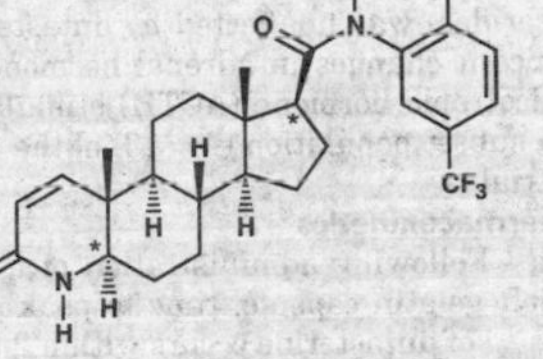

Dutasteride is a white to pale yellow powder with a melting point of 242° to 250°C. It is soluble in ethanol (44 mg/mL), methanol (64 mg/mL), and polyethylene glycol 400 (3 mg/mL), but it is insoluble in water.

Each AVODART Soft Gelatin Capsule, administered orally, contains 0.5 mg of dutasteride dissolved in a mixture of mono-di-glycerides of caprylic/capric acid and butylated hydroxytoluene. The inactive excipients in the capsule shell are ferric oxide (yellow), gelatin (from certified BSE-free bovine sources), glycerin, and titanium dioxide. The soft gelatin capsules are printed with edible red ink.

12 CLINICAL PHARMACOLOGY

12.1 Mechanism of Action

Dutasteride inhibits the conversion of testosterone to dihydrotestosterone (DHT). DHT is the androgen primarily responsible for the initial development and subsequent enlargement of the prostate gland. Testosterone is converted to DHT by the enzyme 5 alpha-reductase, which exists as 2 isoforms, type 1 and type 2. The type 2 isoenzyme is primarily active in the reproductive tissues, while the type 1 isoenzyme is also responsible for testosterone conversion in the skin and liver.

Dutasteride is a competitive and specific inhibitor of both type 1 and type 2 5 alpha-reductase isoenzymes, with which it forms a stable enzyme complex. Dissociation from this complex has been evaluated under in vitro and in vivo conditions and is extremely slow. Dutasteride does not bind to the human androgen receptor.

12.2 Pharmacodynamics

Effect on 5 Alpha-Dihydrotestosterone and Testosterone: The maximum effect of daily doses of dutasteride on the reduction of DHT is dose dependent and is observed within 1 to 2 weeks. After 1 and 2 weeks of daily dosing with dutasteride 0.5 mg, median serum DHT concentrations were reduced by 85% and 90%, respectively. In patients with BPH treated with dutasteride 0.5 mg/day for 4 years, the median decrease in serum DHT was 94% at 1 year, 93% at 2 years, and 95% at both 3 and 4 years. The median increase in serum testosterone was 19% at both 1 and 2 years, 26% at 3 years, and 22% at 4 years, but the mean and median levels remained within the physiologic range.

In patients with BPH treated with 5 mg/day of dutasteride or placebo for up to 12 weeks prior to transurethral resection of the prostate, mean DHT concentrations in prostatic tissue were significantly lower in the dutasteride group compared with placebo (784 and 5,793 pg/g, respectively, $P<0.001$). Mean prostatic tissue concentrations of testosterone were significantly higher in the dutasteride group compared with placebo (2,073 and 93 pg/g, respectively, $P<0.001$).

Adult males with genetically inherited type 2 5 alpha-reductase deficiency also have decreased DHT levels. These 5 alpha-reductase deficient males have a small prostate gland throughout life and do not develop BPH. Except for the associated urogenital defects present at birth, no other clinical abnormalities related to 5 alpha-reductase-deficiency have been observed in these individuals.

Effects on Other Hormones: In healthy volunteers, 52 weeks of treatment with dutasteride 0.5 mg/day (n = 26) resulted in no clinically significant change compared with placebo (n = 23) in sex hormone-binding globulin, estradiol, luteinizing hormone, follicle-stimulating hormone, thyroxine (free T4), and dehydroepiandrosterone. Statistically significant, baseline-adjusted mean increases compared with placebo were observed for total testosterone at 8 weeks (97.1 ng/dL, $P<0.003$) and thyroid-stimulating hormone at 52 weeks (0.4 mcIU/mL, $P<0.05$). The median percentage changes from baseline within the dutasteride group were 17.9% for testosterone at 8 weeks and 12.4% for thyroid-stimulating hormone at 52 weeks. After stopping dutasteride for 24 weeks, the mean levels of testosterone and thyroid-stimulating hormone had returned to baseline in the group of subjects with available data at the visit. In subjects with BPH treated with dutasteride in a large randomized, double-blind, placebo-controlled trial, there was a median percent increase in luteinizing hormone of 12% at 6 months and 19% at both 12 and 24 months.

Other Effects: Plasma lipid panel and bone mineral density were evaluated following 52 weeks of dutasteride 0.5 mg once daily in healthy volunteers. There was no change in bone mineral density as measured by dual energy x-ray absorptiometry compared with either placebo or baseline. In addition, the plasma lipid profile (i.e., total cholesterol, low density lipoproteins, high density lipoproteins, and triglycerides) was unaffected by dutasteride. No clinically significant changes in adrenal hormone responses to adrenocorticotropic hormone (ACTH) stimulation were observed in a subset population (n = 13) of the 1-year healthy volunteer trial.

12.3 Pharmacokinetics

Absorption: Following administration of a single 0.5-mg dose of a soft gelatin capsule, time to peak serum concentrations (T_{max}) of dutasteride occurs within 2 to 3 hours. Absolute bioavailability in 5 healthy subjects is approximately 60% (range: 40% to 94%). When the drug is administered with food, the maximum serum concentrations were reduced by 10% to 15%. This reduction is of no clinical significance.

Distribution: Pharmacokinetic data following single and repeat oral doses show that dutasteride has a large volume of distribution (300 to 500 L). Dutasteride is highly bound to plasma albumin (99.0%) and alpha-1 acid glycoprotein (96.6%).

In a trial of healthy subjects (n = 26) receiving dutasteride 0.5 mg/day for 12 months, semen dutasteride concentrations averaged 3.4 ng/mL (range: 0.4 to 14 ng/mL) at 12 months and, similar to serum, achieved steady-state concentrations at 6 months. On average, at 12 months 11.5% of serum dutasteride concentrations partitioned into semen.

Metabolism and Elimination: Dutasteride is extensively metabolized in humans. In vitro studies showed that dutasteride is metabolized by the CYP3A4 and CYP3A5 isoenzymes. Both of these isoenzymes produced the 4′-hydroxydutasteride, 6-hydroxydutasteride, and the 6,4′-dihydroxydutasteride metabolites. In addition, the 15-hydroxydutasteride metabolite was formed by CYP3A4. Dutasteride is not metabolized in vitro by human cytochrome P450 isoenzymes CYP1A2, CYP2A6, CYP2B6, CYP2C8, CYP2C9, CYP2C19, CYP2D6, and CYP2E1. In human serum following dosing to steady state, unchanged dutasteride, 3 major metabolites (4′-hydroxydutasteride, 1,2-dihydrodutasteride, and 6-hydroxydutasteride), and 2 minor metabolites (6,4′-dihydroxydutasteride and 15-hydroxydutasteride), as assessed by mass spectrometric response, have been detected. The absolute stereochemistry of the hydroxyl additions in the 6 and 15 positions is not known. In vitro, the 4′-hydroxydutasteride and 1,2-dihydrodutasteride metabolites are much less potent than dutasteride against both isoforms of human 5 alpha-reductase. The activity of 6β-hydroxydutasteride is comparable to that of dutasteride.

Dutasteride and its metabolites were excreted mainly in feces. As a percent of dose, there was approximately 5% unchanged dutasteride (~1% to ~15%) and 40% as dutasteride-related metabolites (~2% to ~90%). Only trace amounts of unchanged dutasteride were found in urine (<1%). Therefore, on average, the dose unaccounted for approximated 55% (range, 5% to 97%).

The terminal elimination half-life of dutasteride is approximately 5 weeks at steady state. The average steady-state serum dutasteride concentration was 40 ng/mL following 0.5 mg/day for 1 year. Following daily dosing, dutasteride serum concentrations achieve 65% of steady-state concentration after 1 month and approximately 90% after 3 months. Due to the long half-life of dutasteride, serum concentrations remain detectable (greater than 0.1 ng/mL) for up to 4 to 6 months after discontinuation of treatment.

Specific Populations: *Pediatric:* Dutasteride pharmacokinetics have not been investigated in subjects younger than 18 years.

Geriatric: No dose adjustment is necessary in the elderly. The pharmacokinetics and pharmacodynamics of dutasteride were evaluated in 36 healthy male subjects aged between 24 and 87 years following administration of a single 5-mg dose of dutasteride. In this single-dose trial, dutasteride half-life increased with age (approximately 170 hours in men aged 20 to 49 years, approximately 260 hours in men aged 50 to 69 years, and approximately 300 hours in men older than 70 years). Of 2,167 men treated with dutasteride in the 3 pivotal trials, 60% were age 65 and over and 15% were age 75 and over. No overall differences in safety or efficacy were observed between these patients and younger patients.

Gender: AVODART is contraindicated in pregnancy and women of childbearing potential and is not indicated for use in other women *[see Contraindications (4), Warnings and Precautions (5.1)]*. The pharmacokinetics of dutasteride in women have not been studied.

Race: The effect of race on dutasteride pharmacokinetics has not been studied.

Renal Impairment: The effect of renal impairment on dutasteride pharmacokinetics has not been studied. However, less than 0.1% of a steady-state 0.5-mg dose of dutasteride is recovered in human urine, so no adjustment in dosage is anticipated for patients with renal impairment.

Hepatic Impairment: The effect of hepatic impairment on dutasteride pharmacokinetics has not been studied. Because dutasteride is extensively metabolized, exposure could be higher in hepatically impaired patients.

Drug Interactions:

Cytochrome P450 Inhibitors: No clinical drug interaction trials have been performed to evaluate the impact of CYP3A enzyme inhibitors on dutasteride pharmacokinetics. However, based on in vitro data, blood concentrations of dutasteride may increase in the presence of inhibitors of CYP3A4/5 such as ritonavir, ketoconazole, verapamil, diltiazem, cimetidine, troleandomycin, and ciprofloxacin.

Dutasteride does not inhibit the in vitro metabolism of model substrates for the major human cytochrome P450 isoenzymes (CYP1A2, CYP2C9, CYP2C19, CYP2D6, and CYP3A4) at a concentration of 1,000 ng/mL, 25 times greater than steady-state serum concentrations in humans.

Alpha Adrenergic Antagonists: In a single-sequence, crossover trial in healthy volunteers, the administration of tamsulosin or terazosin in combination with AVODART had no effect on the steady-state pharmacokinetics of either alpha-adrenergic antagonist. Although the effect of administration of tamsulosin or terazosin on dutasteride pharmacokinetic parameters was not evaluated, the percent change in DHT concentrations was similar for AVODART alone compared with the combination treatment.

Calcium Channel Antagonists: In a population pharmacokinetics analysis, a decrease in clearance of dutasteride was noted when coadministered with the CYP3A4 inhibitors verapamil (-37%, n = 6) and diltiazem (-44%, n = 5). In contrast, no decrease in clearance was seen when amlodipine, another calcium channel antagonist that is not a CYP3A4 inhibitor, was coadministered with dutasteride (+7%, n = 4).

The decrease in clearance and subsequent increase in exposure to dutasteride in the presence of verapamil and diltiazem is not considered to be clinically significant. No dose adjustment is recommended.

Cholestyramine: Administration of a single 5-mg dose of AVODART followed 1 hour later by 12 g cholestyramine did not affect the relative bioavailability of dutasteride in 12 normal volunteers.

Digoxin: In a trial of 20 healthy volunteers, AVODART did not alter the steady-state pharmacokinetics of digoxin when administered concomitantly at a dose of 0.5 mg/day for 3 weeks.

Warfarin: In a trial of 23 healthy volunteers, 3 weeks of treatment with AVODART 0.5 mg/day did not alter the steady-state pharmacokinetics of the S- or R-warfarin isomers or alter the effect of warfarin on prothrombin time when administered with warfarin.

Other Concomitant Therapy: Although specific interaction trials were not performed with other compounds, approximately 90% of the subjects in the 3 randomized, double-blind, placebo-controlled safety and efficacy trials receiving AVODART were taking other medications concomitantly. No clinically significant adverse interactions could be attributed to the combination of AVODART and concurrent therapy when AVODART was coadministered with anti-hyperlipidemics, angiotensin-converting enzyme (ACE) inhibitors, beta-adrenergic blocking agents, calcium channel blockers, corticosteroids, diuretics, nonsteroidal anti-inflammatory drugs (NSAIDs), phosphodiesterase Type V inhibitors, and quinolone antibiotics.

13 NONCLINICAL TOXICOLOGY

13.1 Carcinogenesis, Mutagenesis, Impairment of Fertility

Carcinogenesis: A 2-year carcinogenicity study was conducted in B6C3F1 mice at doses of 3, 35, 250, and 500 mg/kg/day for males and 3, 35, and 250 mg/kg/day for females; an increased incidence of benign hepatocellular adenomas was noted at 250 mg/kg/day (290-fold the MRHD of a 0.5-mg daily dose) in female mice only. Two of the 3 major human metabolites have been detected in mice. The exposure to these metabolites in mice is either lower than in humans or is not known.

In a 2-year carcinogenicity study in Han Wistar rats, at doses of 1.5, 7.5, and 53 mg/kg/day in males and 0.8, 6.3, and 15 mg/kg/day in females, there was an increase in Leydig cell adenomas in the testes at 135-fold the MRHD (53 mg/kg/day and greater). An increased incidence of Leydig cell hyperplasia was present at 52-fold the MRHD (male rat doses of 7.5 mg/kg/day and greater). A positive correlation between proliferative changes in the Leydig cells and an increase in circulating luteinizing hormone levels has been demonstrated with 5 alpha-reductase inhibitors and is consistent with an effect on the hypothalamic-pituitary-testicular axis following 5 alpha-reductase inhibition. At tumorigenic doses, luteinizing hormone levels in rats were increased by 167%. In this study, the major human metabolites were tested for carcinogenicity at approximately 1 to 3 times the expected clinical exposure.

Mutagenesis: Dutasteride was tested for genotoxicity in a bacterial mutagenesis assay (Ames test), a chromosomal aberration assay in CHO cells, and a micronucleus assay in rats. The results did not indicate any genotoxic potential of the parent drug. Two major human metabolites were also negative in either the Ames test or an abbreviated Ames test.

Impairment of Fertility: Treatment of sexually mature male rats with dutasteride at 0.1- to 110-fold the MRHD (animal doses of 0.05, 10, 50, and 500 mg/kg/day for up to 31 weeks) resulted in dose- and time-dependent decreases in fertility; reduced cauda epididymal (absolute) sperm counts but not sperm concentration (at 50 and 500 mg/kg/day); reduced weights of the epididymis, prostate, and seminal vesicles; and microscopic changes in the male reproductive organs. The fertility effects were reversed by recovery week 6 at all doses, and sperm counts were normal at the end of a 14-week recovery period. The 5 alpha-reductase–related changes consisted of cytoplasmic vacuolation of tubular epithelium in the epididymides and decreased cytoplasmic content of epithelium, consistent with decreased secretory activity in the prostate and seminal vesicles. The microscopic changes were no longer present at recovery week 14 in the low-dose group and were partly recovered in the remaining treatment groups. Low levels of dutasteride (0.6 to 17 ng/mL) were detected in the serum of untreated female rats mated to males dosed at 10, 50, or 500 mg/kg/day for 29 to 30 weeks. In a fertility study in female rats, oral administration of dutasteride at doses of 0.05, 2.5, 12.5, and 30 mg/kg/day resulted in reduced litter size, increased embryo resorption, and feminization of male fetuses (decreased anogenital distance) at 2- to 10-fold the MRHD (animal doses of 2.5 mg/kg/day or greater). Fetal body weights were also reduced at less than 0.02-fold the MRHD in rats (0.5 mg/kg/day).

13.2 Animal Toxicology and/or Pharmacology

Central Nervous System Toxicology Studies: In rats and dogs, repeated oral administration of dutasteride resulted in some animals showing signs of non-specific, reversible, centrally-mediated toxicity without associated histopathological changes at exposures 425- and 315-fold the expected clinical exposure (of parent drug), respectively.

14 CLINICAL STUDIES

14.1 Monotherapy

AVODART 0.5 mg/day (n = 2,167) or placebo (n = 2,158) was evaluated in male subjects with BPH in three 2-year multicenter, placebo-controlled, double-blind trials, each with 2-year open-label extensions (n = 2,340). More than 90% of the trial population was Caucasian. Subjects were at least 50 years of age with a serum PSA ≥1.5 ng/mL and <10 ng/mL and BPH diagnosed by medical history and physical examination, including enlarged prostate (≥30 cc) and BPH symptoms that were moderate to severe according to the American Urological Association Symptom Index (AUA-SI). Most of the 4,325 subjects randomly assigned to receive either dutasteride or placebo completed 2 years of double-blind treatment (70% and 67%, respectively). Most of the 2,340 subjects in the trial extensions completed 2 additional years of open-label treatment (71%).

Effect on Symptom Scores: Symptoms were quantified using the AUA-SI, a questionnaire that evaluates urinary symptoms (incomplete emptying, frequency, intermittency, urgency, weak stream, straining, and nocturia) by rating on a 0 to 5 scale for a total possible score of 35, with higher numerical total symptom scores representing greater severity of symptoms. The baseline AUA-SI score across the 3 trials was approximately 17 units in both treatment groups. Subjects receiving dutasteride achieved statistically significant improvement in symptoms versus placebo by Month 3 in 1 trial and by Month 12 in the other 2 pivotal trials. At Month 12, the mean decrease from baseline in AUA-SI total symptom scores across the 3 trials pooled was -3.3 units for dutasteride and -2.0 units for placebo with a mean difference between the 2 treatment groups of -1.3 (range: -1.1 to -1.5 units in each of the 3 trials, P<0.001) and was consistent across the 3 trials. At Month 24, the mean decrease from baseline was -3.8 units for dutasteride and -1.7 units for placebo with a mean difference of -2.1 (range: -1.9 to -2.2 units in each of the 3 trials, P<0.001). See Figure 1. The improvement in BPH symptoms seen during the first 2 years of double-blind treatment was maintained throughout an additional 2 years of open-label extension trials.

These trials were prospectively designed to evaluate effects on symptoms based on prostate size at baseline. In men with prostate volumes ≥40 cc, the mean decrease was -3.8 units for dutasteride and -1.6 units for placebo, with a mean difference between the 2 treatment groups of -2.2 at Month 24. In men with prostate volumes <40 cc, the mean decrease was -3.7 units for dutasteride and -2.2 units for placebo, with a mean difference between the 2 treatment groups of -1.5 at Month 24.

Figure 1. AUA-SI Score[a] Change From Baseline (Randomized, Double-Blind, Placebo-Controlled Trials Pooled)

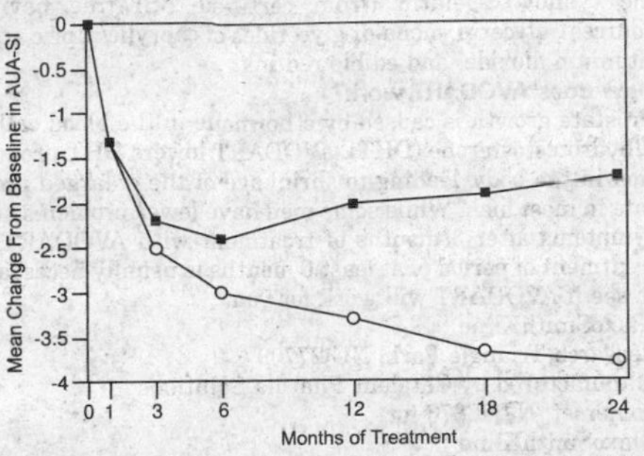

■ Placebo	n = 2,122	n = 2,123	n = 2,123	n = 2,123
○ Dutasteride	n = 2,122	n = 2,122	n = 2,122	n = 2,122

[a] AUA-SI score ranges from 0 to 35.

Effect on Acute Urinary Retention and the Need for BPH-Related Surgery: Efficacy was also assessed after 2 years of treatment by the incidence of AUR requiring catheterization and BPH-related urological surgical intervention. Compared with placebo, AVODART was associated with a statistically significantly lower incidence of AUR (1.8% for AVODART versus 4.2% for placebo, P<0.001; 57% reduction in risk, [95% CI: 38% to 71%]) and with a statistically significantly lower incidence of surgery (2.2% for AVODART versus 4.1% for placebo, P<0.001; 48% reduction in risk, [95% CI: 26% to 63%]). See Figures 2 and 3.

Figure 2. Percent of Subjects Developing Acute Urinary Retention Over a 24-Month Period (Randomized, Double-Blind, Placebo-Controlled Trials Pooled)

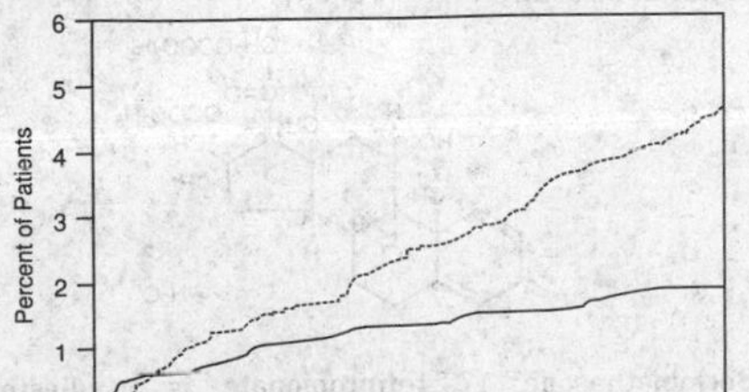

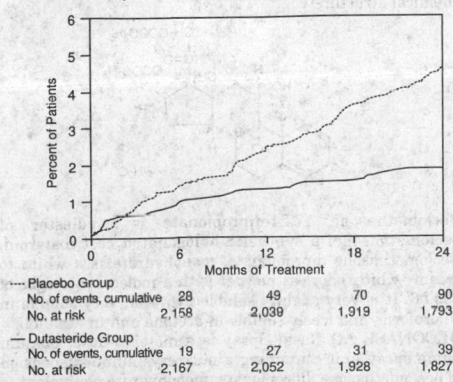

---- Placebo Group				
No. of events, cumulative	28	49	70	90
No. at risk	2,158	2,039	1,919	1,793
— Dutasteride Group				
No. of events, cumulative	19	27	31	39
No. at risk	2,167	2,052	1,928	1,827

[See figure 3 at top of next column]

Effect on Prostate Volume: A prostate volume of at least 30 cc measured by transrectal ultrasound was required for trial entry. The mean prostate volume at trial entry was approximately 54 cc.

Statistically significant differences (AVODART versus placebo) were noted at the earliest post-treatment prostate volume measurement in each trial (Month 1, Month 3, or Month 6) and continued through Month 24. At Month 12,

Figure 3. Percent of Subjects Having Surgery for Benign Prostatic Hyperplasia Over a 24-Month Period (Randomized, Double-Blind, Placebo-Controlled Trials Pooled)

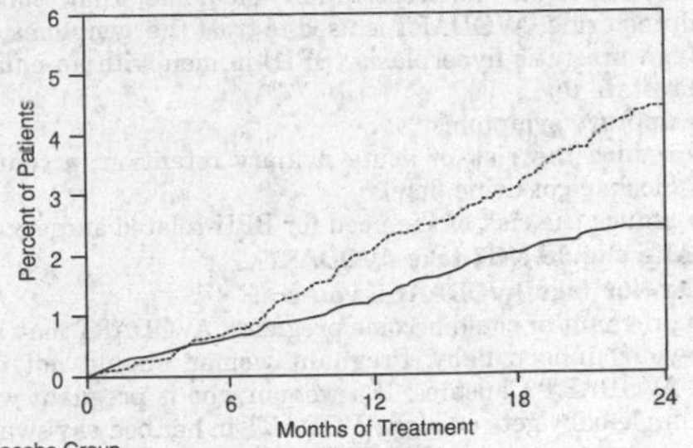

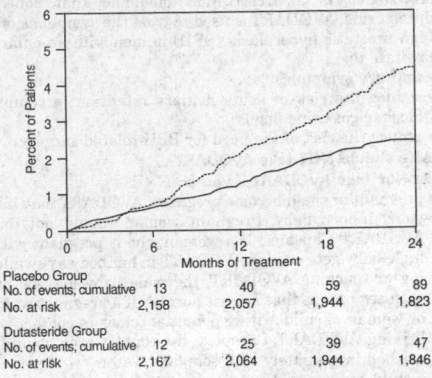

---- Placebo Group				
No. of events, cumulative	13	40	59	89
No. at risk	2,158	2,057	1,944	1,823
— Dutasteride Group				
No. of events, cumulative	12	25	39	47
No. at risk	2,167	2,064	1,944	1,846

the mean percent change in prostate volume across the 3 trials pooled was -24.7% for dutasteride and -3.4% for placebo; the mean difference (dutasteride minus placebo) was -21.3% (range: -21.0% to -21.6% in each of the 3 trials, P<0.001). At Month 24, the mean percent change in prostate volume across the 3 trials pooled was -26.7% for dutasteride and -2.2% for placebo with a mean difference of -24.5% (range: -24.0% to -25.1% in each of the 3 trials, P<0.001). See Figure 4. The reduction in prostate volume seen during the first 2 years of double-blind treatment was maintained throughout an additional 2 years of open-label extension trials.

Figure 4. Prostate Volume Percent Change From Baseline (Randomized, Double-Blind, Placebo-Controlled Trials Pooled)

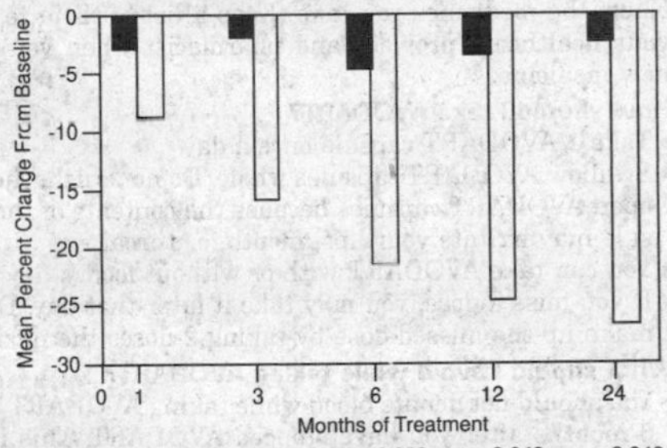

■ Placebo	n = 704	n = 645	n = 2,033	n = 2,043	n = 2,043
□ Dutasteride	n = 702	n = 630	n = 2,020	n = 2,027	n = 2,028

Effect on Maximum Urine Flow Rate: A mean peak urine flow rate (Q_{max}) of ≤15 mL/sec was required for trial entry. Q_{max} was approximately 10 mL/sec at baseline across the 3 pivotal trials.

Differences between the 2 groups were statistically significant from baseline at Month 3 in all 3 trials and were maintained through Month 12. At Month 12, the mean increase in Q_{max} across the 3 trials pooled was 1.6 mL/sec for AVODART and 0.7 mL/sec for placebo; the mean difference (dutasteride minus placebo) was 0.8 mL/sec (range: 0.7 to 1.0 mL/sec in each of the 3 trials, P<0.001). At Month 24, the mean increase in Q_{max} was 1.8 mL/sec for dutasteride and 0.7 mL/sec for placebo, with a mean difference of 1.1 mL/sec (range: 1.0 to 1.2 mL/sec in each of the 3 trials P<0.001). See Figure 5. The increase in maximum urine flow rate seen during the first 2 years of double-blind treatment was maintained throughout an additional 2 years of open-label extension trials.

[See figure 5 at top of next column]

Summary of Clinical Trials: Data from 3 large, well-controlled efficacy trials demonstrate that treatment with AVODART (0.5 mg once daily) reduces the risk of both AUR and BPH-related surgical intervention relative to placebo, improves BPH-related symptoms, decreases prostate volume, and increases maximum urinary flow rates. These data suggest that AVODART arrests the disease process of BPH in men with an enlarged prostate.

14.2 Combination With Alpha-Blocker Therapy (CombAT)

The efficacy of combination therapy (AVODART 0.5 mg/day plus tamsulosin 0.4 mg/day, n = 1,610) was compared with AVODART alone (n = 1,623) or tamsulosin alone (n = 1,611) in a 4-year multicenter, randomized, double-blind trial. Trial entry criteria were similar to the double-blind, placebo-controlled monotherapy efficacy trials described above in section 14.1. Eighty-eight percent (88%) of the enrolled trial population was Caucasian. Approximately 52%

Figure 5. Q_{max} Change From Baseline (Randomized, Double-Blind, Placebo-Controlled Trials Pooled)

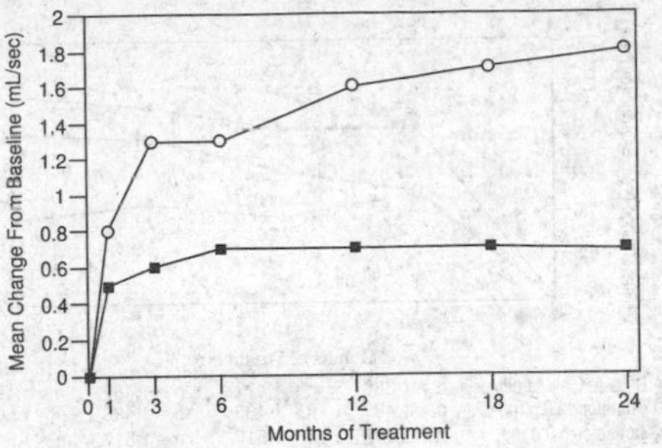

■ Placebo	n = 2,101	n = 2,105	n = 2,105	n = 2,105
○ Dutasteride	n = 2,103	n = 2,104	n = 2,104	n = 2,104

of subjects had previous exposure to 5 alpha-reductase inhibitor or alpha adrenergic antagonist treatment. Of the 4,844 subjects randomly assigned to receive treatment, 69% of subjects in the combination group, 67% in the group receiving AVODART, and 61% in the tamsulosin group completed 4 years of double-blind treatment.

Effect on Symptom Score: Symptoms were quantified using the first 7 questions of the International Prostate Symptom Score (IPSS) (identical to the AUA-SI). The baseline score was approximately 16.4 units for each treatment group. Combination therapy was statistically superior to each of the monotherapy treatments in decreasing symptom score at Month 24, the primary time point for this endpoint. At Month 24 the mean changes from baseline (±SD) in IPSS total symptom scores were -6.2 (±7.14) for combination, -4.9 (±6.81) for AVODART, and -4.3 (±7.01) for tamsulosin, with a mean difference between combination and AVODART of -1.3 units (P<0.001; [95% CI: -1.69, -0.86]), and between combination and tamsulosin of -1.8 units (P<0.001; [95% CI: -2.23, -1.40]). A significant difference was seen by Month 9 and continued through Month 48. At Month 48 the mean changes from baseline (±SD) in IPSS total symptom scores were -6.3 (±7.40) for combination, -5.3 (±7.14) for AVODART, and -3.8 (±7.74) for tamsulosin, with a mean difference between combination and AVODART of -0.96 units (P<0.001; [95% CI: -1.40, -0.52]), and between combination and tamsulosin of -2.5 units (P<0.001; [95% CI: -2.96, -2.07]). See Figure 6.

Figure 6. International Prostate Symptom Score Change From Baseline Over a 48-Month Period (Randomized, Double-Blind, Parallel Group Trial [CombAT Trial])

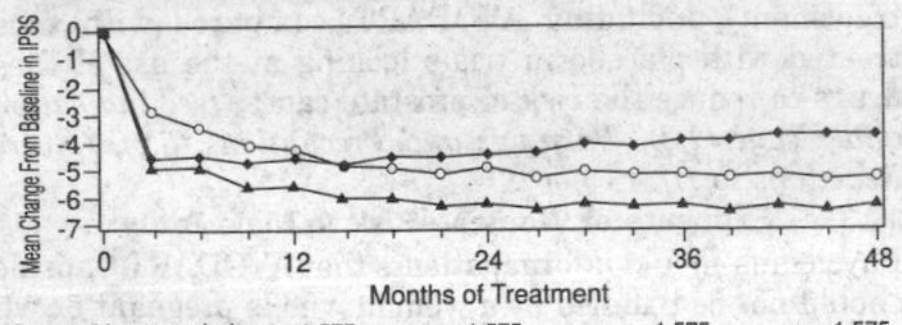

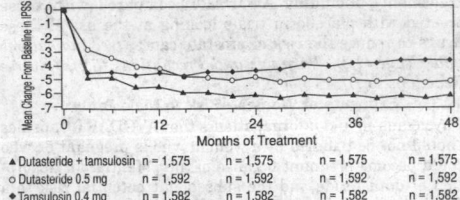

▲ Dutasteride + tamsulosin	n = 1,575	n = 1,575	n = 1,575	n = 1,575
○ Dutasteride 0.5 mg	n = 1,592	n = 1,592	n = 1,592	n = 1,592
◆ Tamsulosin 0.4 mg	n = 1,582	n = 1,582	n = 1,582	n = 1,582

Effect on Acute Urinary Retention or the Need for BPH-Related Surgery: After 4 years of treatment, combination therapy with AVODART and tamsulosin did not provide benefit over monotherapy with AVODART in reducing the incidence of AUR or BPH-related surgery.

Effect on Maximum Urine Flow Rate: The baseline Q_{max} was approximately 10.7 mL/sec for each treatment group. Combination therapy was statistically superior to each of the monotherapy treatments in increasing Q_{max} at Month 24, the primary time point for this endpoint. At Month 24, the mean increases from baseline (±SD) in Q_{max} were 2.4 (±5.26) mL/sec for combination, 1.9 (±5.10) mL/sec for AVODART, and 0.9 (±4.57) mL/sec for tamsulosin, with a mean difference between combination and AVODART of 0.5 mL/sec (P = 0.003; [95% CI: 0.17, 0.84]), and between combination and tamsulosin of 1.5 mL/sec (P<0.001; [95% CI: 1.19, 1.86]). This difference was seen by Month 6 and continued through Month 24. See Figure 7.

The additional improvement in Q_{max} of combination therapy over monotherapy with AVODART was no longer statistically significant at Month 48.

[See figure 7 at top of next column]

Effect on Prostate Volume: The mean prostate volume at trial entry was approximately 55 cc. At Month 24, the primary time point for this endpoint, the mean percent changes from baseline (±SD) in prostate volume were -26.9% (±22.57) for combination therapy, -28.0% (±24.88) for AVODART, and 0% (±31.14) for tamsulosin, with a mean difference between combination and AVODART of 1.1% (P = NS; [95% CI: -0.6, 2.8]), and between combination and tam-

Figure 7. Q_{max} Change From Baseline Over a 24-Month Period (Randomized, Double-Blind, Parallel Group Trial [CombAT Trial])

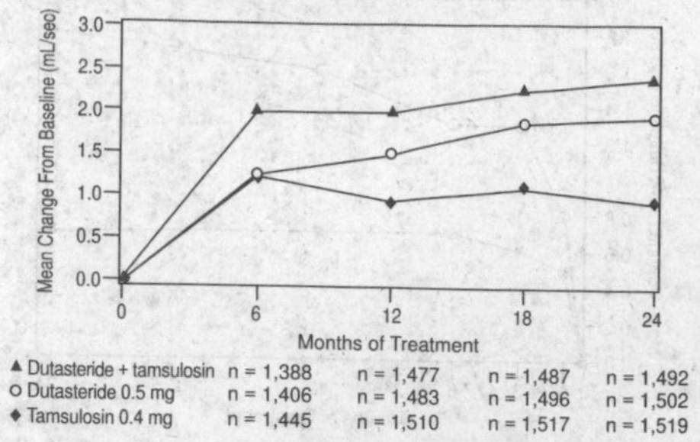

sulosin of -26.9% (P<0.001; [95% CI: -28.9, -24.9]). Similar changes were seen at Month 48: -27.3% (±24.91) for combination therapy, -28.0% (±25.74) for AVODART, and +4.6% (±35.45) for tamsulosin.

16 HOW SUPPLIED/STORAGE AND HANDLING

AVODART Soft Gelatin Capsules 0.5 mg are oblong, opaque, dull yellow, gelatin capsules imprinted with "GX CE2" with red edible ink on one side packaged in bottles of 30 (NDC 0173-0712-15) and 90 (NDC 0173-0712-04) with child-resistant closures.

Store at 25°C (77°F); excursions permitted to 15-30°C (59-86°F) [see USP Controlled Room Temperature].

Dutasteride is absorbed through the skin. AVODART Capsules should not be handled by women who are pregnant or who could become pregnant because of the potential for absorption of dutasteride and the subsequent potential risk to a developing male fetus *[see Warnings and Precautions (5.4)]*.

17 PATIENT COUNSELING INFORMATION

See FDA-approved patient labeling (Patient Information).

17.1 PSA Monitoring

Physicians should inform patients that AVODART reduces serum PSA levels by approximately 50% within 3 to 6 months of therapy, although it may vary for each individual. For patients undergoing PSA screening, increases in PSA levels while on treatment with AVODART may signal the presence of prostate cancer and should be evaluated by a healthcare provider *[see Warnings and Precautions (5.1)]*.

17.2 Increased Risk of High-Grade Prostate Cancer

Physicians should inform patients that there was an increase in high-grade prostate cancer in men treated with 5 alpha-reductase inhibitors (which are indicated for BPH treatment), including AVODART, compared with those treated with placebo in trials looking at the use of these drugs to reduce the risk of prostate cancer *[see Indications and Usage (1.3), Warnings and Precautions (5.2), Adverse Reactions (6.1)]*.

17.3 Exposure of Women—Risk to Male Fetus

Physicians should inform patients that AVODART Capsules should not be handled by a woman who is pregnant or who could become pregnant because of the potential for absorption of dutasteride and the subsequent potential risk to a developing male fetus. Dutasteride is absorbed through the skin and could result in unintended fetal exposure. If a pregnant woman or woman of childbearing potential comes in contact with leaking AVODART Capsules, the contact area should be washed immediately with soap and water *[see Warnings and Precautions (5.4), Use in Specific Populations (8.1)]*.

17.4 Blood Donation

Physicians should inform men treated with AVODART that they should not donate blood until at least 6 months following their last dose to prevent pregnant women from receiving dutasteride through blood transfusion *[see Warnings and Precautions (5.5)]*. Serum levels of dutasteride are detectable for 4 to 6 months after treatment ends *[see Clinical Pharmacology (12.3)]*.

GlaxoSmithKline
Research Triangle Park, NC 27709
Manufactured by Catalent Pharma Solutions
Somerset, NJ 08873 for
GlaxoSmithKline, Research Triangle Park, NC 27709

AVT:11PI

PHARMACIST-DETACH HERE AND GIVE INSTRUCTIONS TO PATIENT

PATIENT INFORMATION

AVODART® (av' ō dart)

(dutasteride) Capsules

AVODART is for use by men only.

Read this patient information before you start taking AVODART and each time you get a refill. There may be new information. This information does not take the place of talking with your healthcare provider about your medical condition or your treatment.

What is AVODART?

AVODART is a prescription medicine that contains dutasteride. AVODART is used to treat the symptoms of benign prostatic hyperplasia (BPH) in men with an enlarged prostate to:
- improve symptoms
- reduce the risk of acute urinary retention (a complete blockage of urine flow)
- reduce the risk of the need for BPH-related surgery

Who should NOT take AVODART?

Do Not Take AVODART if you are:
- pregnant or could become pregnant. AVODART may harm your unborn baby. Pregnant women should not touch AVODART Capsules. If a woman who is pregnant with a male baby gets enough AVODART in her body by swallowing or touching AVODART, the male baby may be born with sex organs that are not normal. If a pregnant woman or woman of childbearing potential comes in contact with leaking AVODART Capsules, the contact area should be washed immediately with soap and water.
- a child or a teenager.
- allergic to dutasteride or any of the ingredients in AVODART. See the end of this leaflet for a complete list of ingredients in AVODART.
- allergic to other 5 alpha-reductase inhibitors, for example, PROSCAR (finasteride) Tablets.

What should I tell my healthcare provider before taking AVODART?

Before you take AVODART, tell your healthcare provider if you:
- have liver problems

Tell your healthcare provider about all the medicines you take, including prescription and non-prescription medicines, vitamins, and herbal supplements. AVODART and other medicines may affect each other, causing side effects. AVODART may affect the way other medicines work, and other medicines may affect how AVODART works.

Know the medicines you take. Keep a list of them to show your healthcare provider and pharmacist when you get a new medicine.

How should I take AVODART?
- Take 1 AVODART capsule once a day.
- Swallow AVODART capsules whole. Do not crush, chew, or open AVODART capsules because the contents of the capsule may irritate your lips, mouth, or throat.
- You can take AVODART with or without food.
- If you miss a dose, you may take it later that day. Do not make up the missed dose by taking 2 doses the next day.

What should I avoid while taking AVODART?
- You should not donate blood while taking AVODART or for 6 months after you have stopped AVODART. This is important to prevent pregnant women from receiving AVODART through blood transfusions.

What are the possible side effects of AVODART?

AVODART may cause serious side effects, including:
- **Rare and serious allergic reactions, including:**
  - swelling of your face, tongue, or throat
  - serious skin reactions, such as skin peeling

Get medical help right away if you have these serious allergic reactions.
- **Higher chance of a more serious form of prostate cancer.**

The most common side effects of AVODART include:
- trouble getting or keeping an erection (impotence) [1]
- a decrease in sex drive (libido) [1]
- ejaculation problems[1]
- enlarged or painful breasts. If you notice breast lumps or nipple discharge, you should talk to your healthcare provider.

Depressed mood has been reported in patients receiving AVODART.

AVODART has been shown to reduce sperm count, semen volume, and sperm movement. However, the effect of AVODART on male fertility is not known.

Prostate-Specific Antigen (PSA) Test: Your healthcare provider may check you for other prostate problems, including prostate cancer before you start and while you take AVODART. A blood test called PSA (prostate-specific antigen) is sometimes used to see if you might have prostate cancer. AVODART will reduce the amount of PSA measured in your blood. Your healthcare provider is aware of this effect and can still use PSA to see if you might have prostate cancer. Increases in your PSA levels while on treatment with AVODART (even if the PSA levels are in the normal range) should be evaluated by your healthcare provider.

Tell your healthcare provider if you have any side effect that bothers you or that does not go away.

These are not all the possible side effects with AVODART. For more information, ask you healthcare provider or pharmacist.

Call your doctor for medical advice about side effects. You may report side effects to FDA at 1-800-FDA-1088.

[1]Some of these events may continue after you stop taking AVODART.

How should I store AVODART?
- Store AVODART Capsules at room temperature (59°F to 86°F or 15°C to 30°C).
- AVODART Capsules may become deformed and/or discolored if kept at high temperatures.
- Do not use AVODART if your capsules are deformed, discolored, or leaking.
- Safely throw away medicine that is no longer needed.

Keep AVODART and all medicines out of the reach of children.

Medicines are sometimes prescribed for purposes other than those listed in a patient leaflet. Do not use AVODART for a condition for which it was not prescribed. Do not give AVODART to other people, even if they have the same symptoms that you have. It may harm them.

This patient information leaflet summarizes the most important information about AVODART. If you would like more information, talk with your healthcare provider. You can ask your pharmacist or healthcare provider for information about AVODART that is written for health professionals.

For more information, go to www.AVODART.com or call 1-888-825-5249.

What are the ingredients in AVODART?

Active ingredient: dutasteride.

Inactive ingredients: butylated hydroxytoluene, ferric oxide (yellow), gelatin (from certified BSE-free bovine sources), glycerin, mono-di-glycerides of caprylic/capric acid, titanium dioxide, and edible red ink.

How does AVODART work?

Prostate growth is caused by a hormone in the blood called dihydrotestosterone (DHT). AVODART lowers DHT production in the body, leading to shrinkage of the enlarged prostate in most men. While some men have fewer problems and symptoms after 3 months of treatment with AVODART, a treatment of period of at least 6 months is usually necessary to see if AVODART will work for you.

GlaxoSmithKline
Research Triangle Park, NC 27709
Manufactured by Catalent Pharma Solutions
Somerset, NJ 08873 for
GlaxoSmithKline
Research Triangle Park, NC 27709

October 2012
AVT:8PIL

BECONASE AQ® ℞

[be'kō-nāz]

(beclomethasone dipropionate, monohydrate)

Nasal Spray, 42 mcg

For Intranasal Use Only.

SHAKE WELL BEFORE USE.

DESCRIPTION

Beclomethasone dipropionate, monohydrate, the active component of BECONASE AQ Nasal Spray, is an anti-inflammatory steroid having the chemical name 9-chloro-11β,17,21-trihydroxy-16β-methylpregna-1,4-diene-3,20-dione 17,21-dipropionate, monohydrate and the following chemical structure:

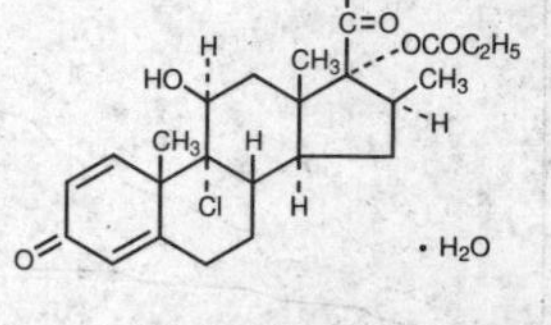

Beclomethasone 17,21-dipropionate is a diester of beclomethasone, a synthetic halogenated corticosteroid. Beclomethasone dipropionate, monohydrate is a white to creamy-white, odorless powder with a molecular weight of 539.06. It is very slightly soluble in water, very soluble in chloroform, and freely soluble in acetone and in ethanol.

BECONASE AQ Nasal Spray is a metered-dose, manual pump spray unit containing a microcrystalline suspension of beclomethasone dipropionate, monohydrate equivalent to 42 mcg of beclomethasone dipropionate, calculated on the dried basis, in an aqueous medium containing microcrystalline cellulose, carboxymethylcellulose sodium, dextrose, benzalkonium chloride, polysorbate 80, and 0.25% v/w phenylethyl alcohol. The pH through expiry is 5.0 to 6.8.

After initial priming (6 actuations), each actuation of the pump delivers from the nasal adapter 100 mg of suspension containing beclomethasone dipropionate, monohydrate equivalent to 42 mcg of beclomethasone dipropionate. If the pump is not used for 7 days, it should be primed until a fine spray appears. Each 25-g bottle of BECONASE AQ Nasal Spray provides 180 metered sprays.

CLINICAL PHARMACOLOGY

Mechanism of Action

Following topical administration, beclomethasone dipropionate produces anti-inflammatory and vasoconstrictor effects. The mechanisms responsible for the anti-inflammatory action of beclomethasone dipropionate are unknown. Corticosteroids have been shown to have a wide range of effects on multiple cell types (e.g., mast cells, eosinophils, neutrophils, macrophages, and lymphocytes) and mediators (e.g., histamine, eicosanoids, leukotrienes, and cytokines) involved in inflammation. The direct relationship of these findings to the effects of beclomethasone dipropionate on allergic rhinitis symptoms is not known.

Biopsies of nasal mucosa obtained during clinical studies showed no histopathologic changes when beclomethasone dipropionate was administered intranasally.

Beclomethasone dipropionate is a pro-drug with weak glucocorticoid receptor binding affinity. It is hydrolyzed via esterase enzymes to its active metabolite beclomethasone-17-monopropionate (B-17-MP), which has high topical anti-inflammatory activity.

Pharmacokinetics

Absorption: Beclomethasone dipropionate is sparingly soluble in water. When given by nasal inhalation in the form of an aqueous or aerosolized suspension, the drug is deposited primarily in the nasal passages. The majority of the drug is eventually swallowed. Following intranasal administration of aqueous beclomethasone dipropionate, the systemic absorption was assessed by measuring the plasma concentrations of its active metabolite B-17-MP, for which the absolute bioavailability following intranasal administration is 44% (43% of the administered dose came from the swallowed portion and only 1% of the total dose was bioavailable from the nose). The absorption of unchanged beclomethasone dipropionate following oral and intranasal dosing was undetectable (plasma concentrations <50 pg/mL).

Distribution: The tissue distribution at steady state for beclomethasone dipropionate is moderate (20 L) but more extensive for B-17-MP (424 L). There is no evidence of tissue storage of beclomethasone dipropionate or its metabolites. Plasma protein binding is moderately high (87%).

Metabolism: Beclomethasone dipropionate is cleared very rapidly from the systemic circulation by metabolism mediated via esterase enzymes that are found in most tissues. The main product of metabolism is the active metabolite (B-17-MP). Minor inactive metabolites, beclomethasone-21-monopropionate (B-21-MP) and beclomethasone (BOH), are also formed, but these contribute little to systemic exposure.

Elimination: The elimination of beclomethasone dipropionate and B-17-MP after intravenous administration are characterized by high plasma clearance (150 and 120 L/hour) with corresponding terminal elimination half-lives of 0.5 and 2.7 hours. Following oral administration of tritiated beclomethasone dipropionate, approximately 60% of the dose was excreted in the feces within 96 hours, mainly as free and conjugated polar metabolites. Approximately 12% of the dose was excreted as free and conjugated polar metabolites in the urine. The renal clearance of beclomethasone dipropionate and its metabolites is negligible.

Pharmacodynamics

The effects of beclomethasone dipropionate on hypothalamic-pituitary-adrenal (HPA) function have been evaluated in adult volunteers by other routes of administration. Studies with beclomethasone dipropionate by the intranasal route may demonstrate that there is more or that there is less absorption by this route of administration. There was no suppression of early morning plasma cortisol concentrations when beclomethasone dipropionate was administered in a dose of 1,000 mcg/day for 1 month as an oral aerosol or for 3 days by intramuscular injection. However, partial suppression of plasma cortisol concentrations was observed when beclomethasone dipropionate was administered in doses of 2,000 mcg/day either by oral aerosol or intramuscular injection. Immediate suppression of plasma cortisol concentrations was observed after single doses of 4,000 mcg of beclomethasone dipropionate. Suppression of HPA function (reduction of early morning plasma cortisol levels) has been reported in adult patients who received 1,600-mcg daily doses of oral beclomethasone dipropionate for 1 month. In clinical studies using beclomethasone dipropionate aerosol intranasally, there was no evidence of adrenal insufficiency. The effect of BECONASE AQ Nasal Spray on HPA function was not evaluated but would not be expected to differ from intranasal beclomethasone dipropionate aerosol.

In 1 study in children with asthma, the administration of inhaled beclomethasone at recommended daily doses for at least 1 year was associated with a reduction in nocturnal cortisol secretion. The clinical significance of this finding is not clear. It reinforces other evidence, however, that topical beclomethasone may be absorbed in amounts that can have systemic effects and that physicians should be alert for evidence of systemic effects, especially in chronically treated patients (see PRECAUTIONS).

INDICATIONS AND USAGE

BECONASE AQ Nasal Spray is indicated for the relief of the symptoms of seasonal or perennial allergic and nonallergic (vasomotor) rhinitis.

Results from 2 clinical trials have shown that significant symptomatic relief was obtained within 3 days. However, symptomatic relief may not occur in some patients for as long as 2 weeks. BECONASE AQ Nasal Spray should not be continued beyond 3 weeks in the absence of significant symptomatic improvement. BECONASE AQ Nasal Spray should not be used in the presence of untreated localized infection involving the nasal mucosa.

BECONASE AQ Nasal Spray is also indicated for the prevention of recurrence of nasal polyps following surgical removal.

Clinical studies have shown that treatment of the symptoms associated with nasal polyps may have to be continued for several weeks or more before a therapeutic result can be fully assessed. Recurrence of symptoms due to polyps can occur after stopping treatment, depending on the severity of the disease.

CONTRAINDICATIONS

Hypersensitivity to any of the ingredients of this preparation contraindicates its use.

WARNINGS

The replacement of a systemic corticosteroid with BECONASE AQ Nasal Spray can be accompanied by signs of adrenal insufficiency.

Careful attention must be given when patients previously treated for prolonged periods with systemic corticosteroids are transferred to BECONASE AQ Nasal Spray. This is particularly important in those patients who have associated asthma or other clinical conditions where too rapid a decrease in systemic corticosteroids may cause a severe exacerbation of their symptoms.

If recommended doses of intranasal beclomethasone are exceeded or if individuals are particularly sensitive or predisposed by virtue of recent systemic steroid therapy, symptoms of hypercorticism may occur, including very rare cases of menstrual irregularities, acneiform lesions, cataracts, and cushingoid features. If such changes occur, BECONASE AQ Nasal Spray should be discontinued slowly consistent with accepted procedures for discontinuing oral steroid therapy.

Persons who are using drugs that suppress the immune system are more susceptible to infections than healthy individuals. Chickenpox and measles, for example, can have a more serious or even fatal course in susceptible children or adults using corticosteroids. In children or adults who have not had these diseases or been properly immunized, particular care should be taken to avoid exposure. How the dose, route, and duration of corticosteroid administration affect the risk of developing a disseminated infection is not known. The contribution of the underlying disease and/or prior corticosteroid treatment to the risk is also not known. If exposed to chickenpox, prophylaxis with varicella zoster immune globulin (VZIG) may be indicated. If exposed to measles, prophylaxis with pooled intramuscular immunoglobulin (IG) may be indicated. (See the respective package inserts for complete VZIG and IG prescribing information.) If chickenpox develops, treatment with antiviral agents may be considered.

Avoid spraying in eyes.

PRECAUTIONS

General

Intranasal corticosteroids may cause a reduction in growth velocity when administered to pediatric patients (see PRECAUTIONS: Pediatric Use).

During withdrawal from oral corticosteroids, some patients may experience symptoms of withdrawal, e.g., joint and/or muscular pain, lassitude, and depression.

Rarely, immediate hypersensitivity reactions may occur after the intranasal administration of beclomethasone (see ADVERSE REACTIONS).

Rare instances of nasal septum perforation have been spontaneously reported.

Rare instances of wheezing, cataracts, glaucoma, and increased intraocular pressure have been reported following the intranasal use of beclomethasone dipropionate.

In clinical studies with beclomethasone dipropionate administered intranasally, the development of localized infections of the nose and pharynx with *Candida albicans* has occurred only rarely. When such an infection develops, it may require treatment with appropriate local therapy and discontinuation of treatment with BECONASE AQ Nasal Spray.

If persistent nasopharyngeal irritation occurs, it may be an indication for stopping BECONASE AQ Nasal Spray.

Beclomethasone dipropionate is absorbed into the circulation. Use of excessive doses of BECONASE AQ Nasal Spray may suppress HPA function.

Intranasal corticosteroids should be used with caution, if at all, in patients with active or quiescent tuberculous infections of the respiratory tract, untreated local or systemic fungal or bacterial infections, systemic viral or parasitic infections, or ocular herpes simplex.

For BECONASE AQ Nasal Spray to be effective in the treatment of nasal polyps, the spray must be able to enter the nose. Therefore, treatment of nasal polyps with BECONASE AQ Nasal Spray should be considered adjunctive therapy to surgical removal and/or the use of other medications that will permit effective penetration of BECONASE AQ Nasal Spray into the nose. Nasal polyps may recur after any form of treatment.

As with any long-term treatment, patients using BECONASE AQ Nasal Spray over several months or longer should be examined periodically for possible changes in the nasal mucosa.

Because of the inhibitory effect of corticosteroids on wound healing, patients who have experienced recent nasal septal ulcers, nasal surgery, or nasal trauma should not use a nasal corticosteroid until healing has occurred.

Although systemic effects have been minimal with recommended doses, this potential increases with excessive doses. Therefore, larger than recommended doses should be avoided.

Information for Patients

Patients being treated with BECONASE AQ Nasal Spray should receive the following information and instructions. This information is intended to aid them in the safe and effective use of this medication. It is not a disclosure of all possible adverse or intended effects.

Patients should use BECONASE AQ Nasal Spray at regular intervals since its effectiveness depends on its regular use. The patient should take the medication as directed. It is not acutely effective, and the prescribed dosage should not be increased. Instead, nasal vasoconstrictors or oral antihistamines may be needed until the effects of BECONASE AQ Nasal Spray are fully manifested. One to 2 weeks may pass before full relief is obtained. The patient should contact the physician if symptoms do not improve, if the condition worsens, or if sneezing or nasal irritation occurs.

For the proper use of BECONASE AQ Nasal Spray and to attain maximum improvement, the patient should read and follow carefully the patient's instructions accompanying the product.

Persons who are using immunosuppressant doses of corticosteroids should be warned to avoid exposure to chickenpox or measles. Patients should also be advised that if they are exposed, medical advice should be sought without delay.

Carcinogenesis, Mutagenesis, Impairment of Fertility

The carcinogenicity of beclomethasone dipropionate was evaluated in rats that were exposed for a total of 95 weeks, 13 weeks at inhalation doses up to 0.4 mg/kg and the remaining 82 weeks at combined oral and inhalation doses up to 2.4 mg/kg. There was no evidence of carcinogenicity in this study at the highest dose, approximately 60 times the maximum recommended daily intranasal dose in adults on a mg/m^2 basis or approximately 35 times the maximum recommended daily intranasal dose in children on a mg/m^2 basis.

Beclomethasone dipropionate did not induce gene mutation in bacterial cells or mammalian Chinese hamster ovary (CHO) cells in vitro. No significant clastogenic effect was seen in cultured CHO cells in vitro or in the mouse micronucleus test in vivo.

In rats, beclomethasone dipropionate caused decreased conception rates at an oral dose of 16 mg/kg (approximately 390 times the maximum recommended daily intranasal dose in adults on a mg/m^2 basis). There was no significant effect of beclomethasone dipropionate on fertility in rats at oral doses of 1.6 mg/kg (approximately 40 times the maximum recommended daily intranasal dose in adults on a mg/m^2 basis). Inhibition of the estrous cycle in dogs was observed following oral dosing at 0.5 mg/kg (approximately 40 times the maximum recommended daily intranasal dose in adults on a mg/m^2 basis). No inhibition of the estrous cycle in dogs was seen following 12 months' exposure at an estimated inhalation dose of 0.33 mg/kg (approximately 25 times the maximum recommended daily intranasal dose in adults on a mg/m^2 basis).

Pregnancy

Teratogenic Effects: Pregnancy Category C. Like other corticosteroids, beclomethasone dipropionate was teratogenic and embryocidal in the mouse and rabbit at a subcutaneous dose of 0.1 mg/kg in mice or 0.025 mg/kg in rabbits (approximately equal to the maximum recommended daily intranasal dose in adults on a mg/m^2 basis). No teratogenicity or embryocidal effects were seen in rats when exposed to an inhalation dose of 0.1 mg/kg plus oral doses of up to

10 mg/kg per day for a combined dose of 10.1 mg/kg (approximately 240 times the maximum recommended daily intranasal dose in adults on a mg/m^2 basis).

There are no adequate and well-controlled studies in pregnant women. Beclomethasone dipropionate should be used during pregnancy only if the potential benefit justifies the potential risk to the fetus.

Nonteratogenic Effects: Hypoadrenalism may occur in infants born of mothers receiving corticosteroids during pregnancy. Such infants should be carefully observed.

Nursing Mothers

It is not known whether beclomethasone dipropionate is excreted in human milk. Because other corticosteroids are excreted in human milk, caution should be exercised when BECONASE AQ Nasal Spray is administered to a nursing woman.

Pediatric Use

The safety and effectiveness of BECONASE AQ Nasal Spray have been established in children aged 6 years and above through evidence from extensive clinical use in adult and pediatric patients. The safety and effectiveness of BECONASE AQ Nasal Spray in children below 6 years of age have not been established.

Controlled clinical studies have shown that intranasal corticosteroids may cause a reduction in growth velocity in pediatric patients. This effect has been observed in the absence of laboratory evidence of HPA axis suppression, suggesting that growth velocity is a more sensitive indicator of systemic corticosteroid exposure in pediatric patients than some commonly used tests of HPA axis function. The long-term effects of this reduction in growth velocity associated with intranasal corticosteroids, including the impact on final adult height, are unknown. The potential for "catch-up" growth following discontinuation of treatment with intranasal corticosteroids has not been adequately studied. The growth of pediatric patients receiving intranasal corticosteroids, including BECONASE AQ Nasal Spray, should be monitored routinely (e.g., via stadiometry). The potential growth effects of prolonged treatment should be weighed against the clinical benefits obtained and the risks/benefits of treatment alternatives. To minimize the systemic effects of intranasal corticosteroids, including BECONASE AQ Nasal Spray, each patient should be titrated to the lowest dose that effectively controls his/her symptoms.

In a double-blind, controlled trial, 100 children between the ages of 6 and 9½ years with allergic rhinitis were randomized to receive aqueous intranasal beclomethasone dipropionate 168 mcg twice daily or placebo for 1 year. As measured by stadiometry, children who received beclomethasone dipropionate grew more slowly than those who received placebo. A difference in mean change in height was observed within 1 month of drug initiation. At the end of 12 months, the beclomethasone dipropionate-treated group had a growth velocity on average of 4.75 cm/year compared to 6.20 cm/year in the placebo group ($p<0.01$). While the placebo group had an expected distribution of growth velocity, approximately 50% of the beclomethasone dipropionate-treated children grew below the 10th percentile.

In children 7.3 years of age, the mean age of children in this study, the range for expected growth velocity is: boys – 3rd percentile = 4.1 cm/year, 50th percentile = 5.8 cm/year, and 97th percentile = 7.5 cm/year; girls – 3rd percentile = 4.3 cm/year, 50th percentile = 5.9 cm/year, and 97th percentile = 7.5 cm/year. The potential reversibility of the reduction in growth velocity was not studied. No significant differences were observed between the 2 groups for mean basal plasma cortisol or ACTH-stimulated plasma cortisol levels.

Geriatric Use

Clinical studies of BECONASE AQ Nasal Spray did not include sufficient numbers of subjects aged 65 and over to determine whether they respond differently from younger subjects. Other reported clinical experience has not identified differences in responses between the elderly and younger patients. In general, dose selection for an elderly patient should be cautious, starting at the low end of the dosing range, reflecting the greater frequency of decreased hepatic, renal, or cardiac function, and of concomitant disease or other drug therapy.

ADVERSE REACTIONS

In general, side effects in clinical studies have been primarily associated with irritation of the nasal mucous membranes.

Adverse reactions reported in controlled clinical trials and open studies in patients treated with BECONASE AQ Nasal Spray are described below.

Mild nasopharyngeal irritation following the use of beclomethasone aqueous nasal spray has been reported in up to 24% of patients treated, including occasional sneezing attacks (about 4%) occurring immediately following use of the spray. In patients experiencing these symptoms, none had to discontinue treatment. The incidence of transient irritation and sneezing was approximately the same in the group of patients who received placebo in these studies, implying that these complaints may be related to vehicle components of the formulation.

Fewer than 5 per 100 patients reported headache, nausea, or lightheadedness following the use of BECONASE AQ Nasal Spray. Fewer than 3 per 100 patients reported nasal stuffiness, nosebleeds, rhinorrhea, or tearing eyes.

Rare cases of ulceration of the nasal mucosa and instances of nasal septum perforation have been spontaneously reported (see PRECAUTIONS).

Reports of dryness and irritation of the nose and throat and unpleasant taste and smell have been received. There are rare reports of loss of taste and smell.

Rare instances of wheezing, cataracts, glaucoma, and increased intraocular pressure have been reported following the use of intranasal beclomethasone dipropionate (see PRECAUTIONS).

Rare cases of immediate and delayed hypersensitivity reactions, including anaphylactoid/anaphylactic reactions, urticaria, angioedema, rash, and bronchospasm, have been reported following the oral and intranasal inhalation of beclomethasone dipropionate.

Cases of growth suppression have been reported for intranasal corticosteroids, including BECONASE AQ (see PRECAUTIONS: Pediatric Use).

OVERDOSAGE

When used at excessive doses, systemic corticosteroid effects such as hypercorticism and adrenal suppression may appear. If such changes occur, BECONASE AQ Nasal Spray should be discontinued slowly consistent with accepted procedures for discontinuing oral steroid therapy. No deaths occurred when beclomethasone dipropionate was given as single oral doses of 3,000 mg/kg to mice (approximately 36,000 times the maximum recommended daily intranasal dose in adults on a mg/m^2 basis, or approximately 21,000 times the maximum recommended daily intranasal dose in children on a mg/m^2 basis) and 2,000 mg/kg to rats (approximately 48,000 times the maximum recommended daily intranasal dose in adults or approximately 29,000 times the maximum recommended daily intranasal dose in children on a mg/m^2 basis). One bottle of BECONASE AQ Nasal Spray contains beclomethasone dipropionate, monohydrate equivalent to 10.5 mg of beclomethasone dipropionate; therefore, acute overdosage is unlikely.

DOSAGE AND ADMINISTRATION

Adults and Children 12 Years of Age and Older

The usual dosage is 1 or 2 nasal inhalations (42 to 84 mcg) in each nostril twice a day (total dose, 168 to 336 mcg/day).

Children 6 to 12 Years of Age

Patients should be started with 1 nasal inhalation in each nostril twice daily; patients not adequately responding to 168 mcg or those with more severe symptoms may use 336 mcg (2 inhalations in each nostril). Once adequate control is achieved, the dosage should be decreased to 84 mcg (1 spray in each nostril) twice daily. BECONASE AQ Nasal Spray is *not* recommended for children below 6 years of age. The maximum total daily dosage should not exceed 2 sprays in each nostril twice daily (336 mcg/day).

In patients who respond to BECONASE AQ Nasal Spray, an improvement of the symptoms of seasonal or perennial rhinitis usually becomes apparent within a few days after the start of therapy with BECONASE AQ Nasal Spray. However, symptomatic relief may not occur in some patients for as long as 2 weeks. BECONASE AQ Nasal Spray should not be continued beyond 3 weeks in the absence of significant symptomatic improvement.

The therapeutic effects of corticosteroids, unlike those of decongestants, are not immediate. This should be explained to the patient in advance in order to ensure cooperation and continuation of treatment with the prescribed dosage regimen.

In the presence of excessive nasal mucous secretion or edema of the nasal mucosa, the drug may fail to reach the site of intended action. In such cases it is advisable to use a nasal vasoconstrictor during the first 2 to 3 days of therapy with BECONASE AQ Nasal Spray.

Directions for Use

Illustrated Patient's Instructions for Use accompany each package of BECONASE AQ Nasal Spray.

HOW SUPPLIED

BECONASE AQ Nasal Spray, 42 mcg is supplied in an amber glass bottle fitted with a metering atomizing pump and nasal adapter in a box of 1 (NDC 0173-0388-79) with patient's instructions for use. Each bottle contains 25 g of suspension and will provide 180 metered sprays.

The correct amount of medication in each spray cannot be assured after 180 sprays even though the bottle is not completely empty. The bottle should be discarded when the labeled number of actuations has been used.

Store between 15°and 30°C (59°and 86°F).

GlaxoSmithKline
Research Triangle Park, NC 27709
April 2005 RL-2182

Patient's Instructions for Use

PHARMACIST —DETACH HERE AND GIVE INSTRUCTIONS TO PATIENT

BECONASE AQ®
(beclomethasone dipropionate, monohydrate)
Nasal Spray, 42 mcg

For Intranasal Use Only. SHAKE WELL BEFORE USE.

Patient's Instructions for Use

Shake the suspension spray bottle well before using it. Read complete instructions carefully and use only as directed.

To Use:

1. Remove the safety clip and the plastic dust cap from the nasal applicator (Figure 1).

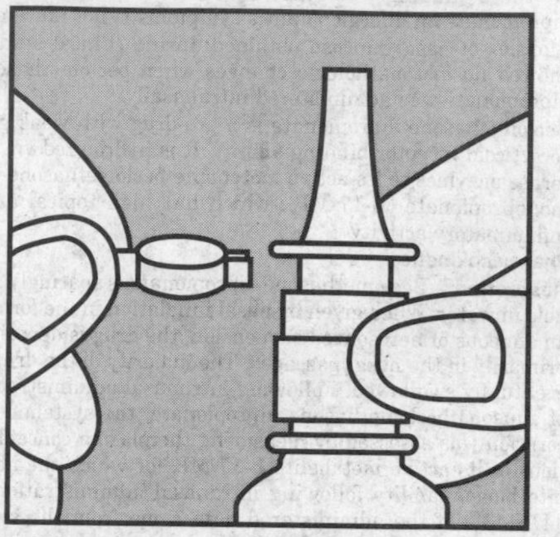

Figure 1

2. The very first time the spray is used, prime the pump into the air by pressing downward on the white collar, using your forefinger and middle finger while supporting the base of the bottle with your thumb. When you prime the pump for the first time, press down and release the pump 6 times or until a fine spray appears (Figure 2).

The pump is now ready for use. If the pump is not used for 7 days, prime until a fine spray appears.

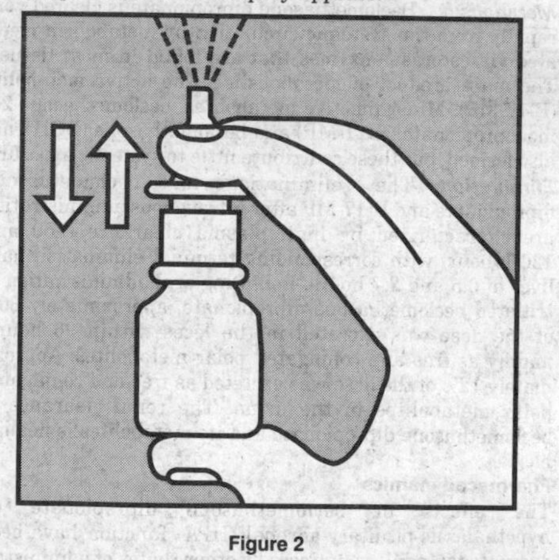

Figure 2

3. Gently blow your nose to clear your nostrils. Close 1 nostril. Tilt your head forward slightly and, keeping the bottle upright, carefully insert the nasal applicator into the other nostril (Figure 3).

[See figure 3 at top of next column]

4. For each spray, press firmly downward once on the white collar, using your forefinger and middle finger while supporting the base of the bottle with your thumb. Avoid spraying in eyes. Breathe gently inward through the nostril.

5. Breathe out through your mouth.

6. Repeat steps 5 through 7 in the other nostril.

7. Replace the plastic dust cap and safety clip.

8. DISCARD THE BOTTLE AFTER the date calculated by your doctor or pharmacist. The correct amount of medication in each spray cannot be assured after 180 sprays even though the bottle is not completely empty. Discard the bottle after 180 sprays. Before the discard date you should consult your doctor to see if a refill is needed. Do not take extra doses or stop taking BECONASE AQ Nasal Spray without consulting your doctor.

Cleansing: To clean the nasal applicator, remove the plastic dust cap and safety clip and then press gently upward on the white collar to free the nasal applicator. Wash the applicator and dust cap with cold water. Dry and replace with the plastic dust cap and safety clip back in position.

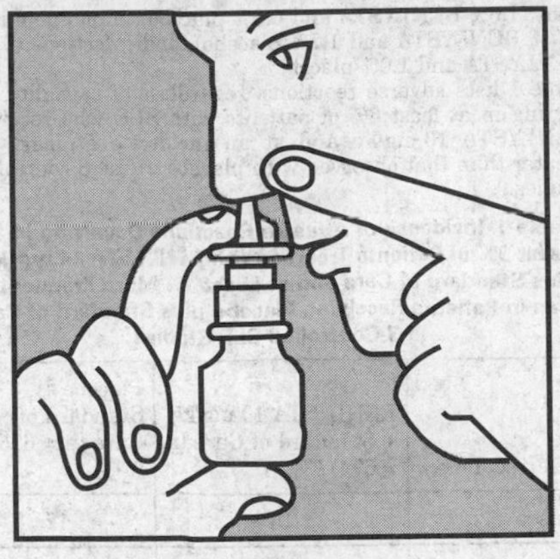

Figure 3

If the nasal applicator becomes blocked, remove the dust cap, unscrew the complete pump mechanism, and soak the pump in warm water for a few minutes. Rinse with cold water, dry, refit to bottle, and reprime the pump.

Caution: BECONASE AQ Nasal Spray is not intended to give rapid relief of your nasal symptoms. BECONASE AQ Nasal Spray controls the underlying disorders responsible for your attacks, so it is important that you use it regularly at the times recommended by your doctor. The full benefit of BECONASE AQ Nasal Spray may take a few days to develop.

Storage: Store between 15° and 30°C (59° and 86°F).

GlaxoSmithKline
Research Triangle Park, NC 27709
April 2005 RL-2182

BENLYSTA® ℞
(belimumab)
for injection, for intravenous use only

HIGHLIGHTS OF PRESCRIBING INFORMATION
These highlights do not include all the information needed to use BENLYSTA safely and effectively. See full prescribing information for BENLYSTA.
BENLYSTA® (belimumab)
for injection, for intravenous use only
Initial U.S. Approval: 2011

RECENT MAJOR CHANGES

Warning and Precautions (5.4) 03/2012

INDICATIONS AND USAGE

BENLYSTA is a B-lymphocyte stimulator (BLyS)-specific inhibitor indicated for the treatment of adult patients with active, autoantibody-positive, systemic lupus erythematosus who are receiving standard therapy. (1, 14)

Limitations of Use: The efficacy of BENLYSTA has not been evaluated in patients with severe active lupus nephritis or severe active central nervous system lupus (1). BENLYSTA has not been studied in combination with other biologics or intravenous cyclophosphamide (1). Use of BENLYSTA is not recommended in these situations.

DOSAGE AND ADMINISTRATION

- Recommended dosage regimen is 10 mg/kg at 2-week intervals for the first 3 doses and at 4-week intervals thereafter. Reconstitute, dilute and administer as an intravenous infusion only, over a period of 1 hour. (2.1)
- Consider administering premedication for prophylaxis against infusion reactions and hypersensitivity reactions (2.2)

DOSAGE FORMS AND STRENGTHS

Single-use vials of belimumab lyophilized powder:
- 120 mg per vial (3)
- 400 mg per vial (3)

CONTRAINDICATIONS

Previous anaphylaxis to belimumab. (4)

WARNINGS AND PRECAUTIONS

- Mortality: There were more deaths reported with BENLYSTA than with placebo during the controlled period of clinical trials. (5.1)
- Serious Infections: Serious and sometimes fatal infections have been reported in patients receiving immunosuppressive agents, including BENLYSTA. Use with caution in patients with chronic infections. Consider interrupting BENLYSTA therapy if patients develop a new infection during BENLYSTA treatment. (5.2)
- Hypersensitivity Reactions, Including Anaphylaxis: Serious and fatal reactions have been reported. BENLYSTA should be administered by healthcare providers prepared to manage anaphylaxis. Monitor patients during and for an appropriate period of time after administration of BENLYSTA. (2.2, 5.4)
- Depression: Depression and suicidality have been reported in BENLYSTA studies. Patients should be instructed to contact their healthcare provider if they experience new or worsening depression, suicidal thoughts or other mood changes. (5.6)
- Immunization: Live vaccines should not be given concurrently with BENLYSTA. (5.7)

ADVERSE REACTIONS

Common adverse reactions (≥5%) in clinical trials were: nausea, diarrhea, pyrexia, nasopharyngitis, bronchitis, insomnia, pain in extremity, depression, migraine, and pharyngitis. (6.1)

To report SUSPECTED ADVERSE REACTIONS, contact Human Genome Sciences, Inc. at 1-877-423-6597 or FDA at 1-800-FDA-1088 orwww.fda.gov/medwatch.

USE IN SPECIFIC POPULATIONS

- Pregnancy: Registry available. (8.1)

See 17 for PATIENT COUNSELING INFORMATION

Revised: 03/2012

FULL PRESCRIBING INFORMATION: CONTENTS*

*** Sections or subsections omitted from the full prescribing information are not listed**

FULL PRESCRIBING INFORMATION

1 INDICATIONS AND USAGE

BENLYSTA ® (belimumab) is indicated for the treatment of adult patients with active, autoantibody-positive, systemic lupus erythematosus (SLE) who are receiving standard therapy.

Limitations of Use

The efficacy of BENLYSTA has not been evaluated in patients with severe active lupus nephritis or severe active central nervous system lupus. BENLYSTA has not been studied in combination with other biologics or intravenous cyclophosphamide. Use of BENLYSTA is not recommended in these situations.

2 DOSAGE AND ADMINISTRATION

2.1 Dosage Schedule

BENLYSTA is for intravenous infusion **only** and must be reconstituted and diluted prior to administration *[see Dosage and Administration (2.3)]*. Do not administer as an intravenous push or bolus.

The recommended dosage regimen is 10 mg/kg at 2-week intervals for the first 3 doses and at 4-week intervals thereafter. Reconstitute, dilute and administer as an intravenous infusion only, over a period of 1 hour. The infusion rate may be slowed or interrupted if the patient develops an infusion reaction. The infusion must be discontinued immediately if the patient experiences a serious hypersensitivity reaction *[seeContraindications (4), Warnings and Precautions (5.4)]*.

2.2 Premedication Recommendations

Prior to dosing with BENLYSTA, consider administering premedication for prophylaxis against infusion reactions and hypersensitivity reactions. *[seeWarnings and Precautions (5.4, 5.5) and Adverse Reactions (6.1)]*.

2.3 Preparation of Solutions

BENLYSTA is provided as a lyophilized powder in a single-use vial for intravenous infusion only and should be reconstituted and diluted by a healthcare professional using aseptic technique as follows:

Reconstitution Instructions

1. Remove BENLYSTA from the refrigerator and allow to stand 10 to 15 minutes for the vial to reach room temperature.
2. Reconstitute the BENLYSTA powder with Sterile Water for Injection, USP, as follows. The reconstituted solution will contain a concentration of 80 mg/mL belimumab.
   - Reconstitute the 120 mg vial with 1.5 mL Sterile Water for Injection, USP.
   - Reconstitute the 400 mg vial with 4.8 mL Sterile Water for Injection, USP.
3. The stream of sterile water should be directed toward the side of the vial to minimize foaming. Gently swirl the vial for 60 seconds. Allow the vial to sit at room temperature during reconstitution, gently swirling the vial for 60 seconds every 5 minutes until the powder is dissolved. *Do not shake*. Reconstitution is typically complete within 10 to 15 minutes after the sterile water has been added, but it may take up to 30 minutes. Protect the reconstituted solution from sunlight.
4. If a mechanical reconstitution device (swirler) is used to reconstitute BENLYSTA, it should not exceed 500 rpm and the vial swirled for no longer than 30 minutes.
5. Once reconstitution is complete, the solution should be opalescent and colorless to pale yellow, and without particles. Small air bubbles, however, are expected and acceptable. **DilutionInstructions**
6. Dextrose intravenous solutions are incompatible with BENLYSTA. BENLYSTA should only be diluted in 0.9% Sodium Chloride Injection, USP. Dilute the reconstituted product to 250 mL in 0.9% Sodium Chloride Injection, USP (normal saline) for intravenous infusion. From a 250-mL infusion bag or bottle of normal saline, withdraw and discard a volume equal to the volume of the reconstituted solution of BENLYSTA required for the patient's dose. Then add the required volume of the reconstituted solution of BENLYSTA into the infusion bag or bottle. Gently invert the bag or bottle to mix the solution. Any unused solution in the vials must be discarded.
7. Parenteral drug products should be inspected visually for particulate matter and discoloration prior to administration, whenever solution and container permit. Discard the solution if any particulate matter or discoloration is observed.
8. The reconstituted solution of BENLYSTA, if not used immediately, should be stored protected from direct sunlight and refrigerated at 2° to 8°C (36° to 46°F). Solutions of BENLYSTA diluted in normal saline may be stored at 2° to 8°C (36° to 46°F) or room temperature. The total time from reconstitution of BENLYSTA to completion of infusion should not exceed 8 hours.
9. No incompatibilities between BENLYSTA and polyvinylchloride or polyolefin bags have been observed.

2.4 Administration Instructions

1. The diluted solution of BENLYSTA should be administered by intravenous infusion only, over a period of 1 hour.
2. BENLYSTA should be administered by healthcare providers prepared to manage anaphylaxis. *[seeWarnings and Precautions (5.4)]*
3. BENLYSTA should not be infused concomitantly in the same intravenous line with other agents. No physical or biochemical compatibility studies have been conducted to evaluate the coadministration of BENLYSTA with other agents.

3 DOSAGE FORMS AND STRENGTHS

Single-use vials of belimumab lyophilized powder for injection:
- 120 mg per vial
- 400 mg per vial

4 CONTRAINDICATIONS

BENLYSTA is contraindicated in patients who have had anaphylaxis with belimumab.

5 WARNINGS AND PRECAUTIONS

5.1 Mortality

There were more deaths reported with BENLYSTA than with placebo during the controlled period of the clinical trials. Out of 2133 patients in 3 clinical trials, a total of 14 deaths occurred during the placebo-controlled, double-blind treatment periods: 3/675 (0.4%), 5/673 (0.7%), 0/111 (0%), and 6/674 (0.9%) deaths in the placebo, BENLYSTA 1 mg/kg, BENLYSTA 4 mg/kg, and BENLYSTA 10 mg/kg groups, respectively. No single cause of death predominated. Etiologies included infection, cardiovascular disease and suicide.

5.2 Serious Infections

Serious and sometimes fatal infections have been reported in patients receiving immunosuppressive agents, including BENLYSTA. Physicians should exercise caution when considering the use of BENLYSTA in patients with chronic infections. Patients receiving any therapy for chronic infection should not begin therapy with BENLYSTA. Consider interrupting BENLYSTA therapy in patients who develop a new infection while undergoing treatment with BENLYSTA and monitor these patients closely.

In the controlled clinical trials, the overall incidence of infections was 71% in patients treated with BENLYSTA compared with 67% in patients who received placebo. The most frequent infections (>5% of patients receiving BENLYSTA) were upper respiratory tract infection, urinary tract infection, nasopharyngitis, sinusitis, bronchitis, and influenza. Serious infections occurred in 6.0% of patients treated with BENLYSTA and in 5.2% of patients who received placebo. The most frequent serious infections included pneumonia, urinary tract infection, cellulitis, and bronchitis. Infections leading to discontinuation of treatment occurred in 0.7% of patients receiving BENLYSTA and 1.0% of patients receiving placebo. Infections resulting in death occurred in 0.3% (4/1458) of patients treated with BENLYSTA and in 0.1% (1/675) of patients receiving placebo.

5.3 Malignancy

The impact of treatment with BENLYSTA on the development of malignancies is not known. In the controlled clinical trials, malignancies (including non-melanoma skin cancers) were reported in 0.4% of patients receiving BENLYSTA and 0.4% of patients receiving placebo. In the controlled clinical trials, malignancies, excluding non-melanoma skin cancers, were observed in 0.2% (3/1458) and 0.3% (2/675) of patients receiving BENLYSTA and placebo, respectively. As with other immunomodulating agents, the mechanism of action of BENLYSTA could increase the risk for the development of malignancies.

5.4 Hypersensitivity Reactions, Including Anaphylaxis

Hypersensitivity reactions, including anaphylaxis and death, have been reported in association with BENLYSTA. Delay in the onset of acute hypersensitivity reactions has been observed. Limited data suggest that patients with a history of multiple drug allergies or significant hypersensitivity may be at increased risk. In the controlled clinical trials, hypersensitivity reactions (occurring on the same day of infusion) were reported in 13% (191/1458) of patients receiving BENLYSTA and 11% (76/675) of patients receiving placebo. Anaphylaxis was observed in 0.6% (9/1458) of patients receiving BENLYSTA and 0.4% (3/675) of patients receiving placebo. Manifestations included hypotension, angioedema, urticaria or other rash, pruritus, and dyspnea. Due to overlap in signs and symptoms, it was not possible to distinguish between hypersensitivity reactions and infusion reactions in all cases *[see Warnings and Precautions (5.5)]*. Some patients (13%) received premedication, which may have mitigated or masked a hypersensitivity response; however, there is insufficient evidence to determine whether premedication diminishes the frequency or severity of hypersensitivity reactions.

BENLYSTA should be administered by healthcare providers prepared to manage anaphylaxis. In the event of a serious reaction, administration of BENLYSTA must be discontinued immediately and appropriate medical therapy administered. Patients should be monitored during and for an appropriate period of time after administration of BENLYSTA. Patients should be informed of the signs and symptoms of a hypersensitivity reaction and instructed to seek immediate medical care should a reaction occur.

5.5 Infusion Reactions

In the controlled clinical trials, adverse events associated with the infusion (occurring on the same day of the infusion) were reported in 17% (251/1458) of patients receiving BENLYSTA and 15% (99/675) of patients receiving placebo. Serious infusion reactions (excluding hypersensitivity reactions) were reported in 0.5% of patients receiving BENLYSTA and 0.4% of patients receiving placebo and included bradycardia, myalgia, headache, rash, urticaria, and hypotension. The most common infusion reactions (≥ 3% of patients receiving BENLYSTA) were headache, nausea, and skin reactions. Due to overlap in signs and symptoms, it was not possible to distinguish between hypersensitivity reactions and infusion reactions in all cases *[see Warnings and Precautions (5.4)]*. Some patients (13%) received premedication, which may have mitigated or masked an infusion reaction; however there is insufficient evidence to determine whether premedication diminishes the frequency or severity of infusion reactions *[seeAdverse Reactions (6.1)]*.

BENLYSTA should be administered by healthcare providers prepared to manage infusion reactions. The infusion rate may be slowed or interrupted if the patient develops an infusion reaction. Healthcare providers should be aware of the risk of hypersensitivity reactions, which may present as infusion reactions, and monitor patients closely.

5.6 Depression

In the controlled clinical trials, psychiatric events were reported more frequently with BENLYSTA (16%) than with placebo (12%), related primarily to depression-related events (6.3% BENLYSTA and 4.7% placebo), insomnia (6.0% BENLYSTA and 5.3% placebo), and anxiety (3.9% BENLYSTA and 2.8% placebo). Serious psychiatric events were reported in 0.8% of patients receiving BENLYSTA (0.6% and 1.2% with 1 and 10 mg/kg, respectively) and 0.4% of patients receiving placebo. Serious depression was reported in 0.4% (6/1458) of patients receiving BENLYSTA and 0.1% (1/675) of patients receiving placebo. Two suicides (0.1%) were reported in patients receiving BENLYSTA. The majority of patients who reported serious depression or suicidal behavior had a history of depression or other serious psychiatric disorders and most were receiving psychoactive medications. It is unknown if BENLYSTA treatment is associated with increased risk for these events.

Patients receiving BENLYSTA should be instructed to contact their healthcare provider if they experience new or worsening depression, suicidal thoughts, or other mood changes.

5.7 Immunization

Live vaccines should not be given for 30 days before or concurrently with BENLYSTA as clinical safety has not been established. No data are available on the secondary transmission of infection from persons receiving live vaccines to patients receiving BENLYSTA or the effect of BENLYSTA on new immunizations. Because of its mechanism of action, BENLYSTA may interfere with the response to immunizations.

5.8 Concomitant Use with Other Biologic Therapies or Intravenous Cyclophosphamide

BENLYSTA has not been studied in combination with other biologic therapies, including B-cell targeted therapies, or intravenous cyclophosphamide. Therefore, use of BENLYSTA is not recommended in combination with biologic therapies or intravenous cyclophosphamide.

6 ADVERSE REACTIONS

Because clinical trials are conducted under widely varying conditions, adverse reaction rates observed in the clinical trials of a drug cannot be directly compared with rates in the clinical trials of another drug and may not reflect the rates observed in practice.

The following have been observed with BENLYSTA and are discussed in detail in the Warnings and Precautions section:

- **Mortality**[see *Warnings and Precautions (5.1)]*
- **Serious Infections**[see *Warnings and Precautions (5.2)]*
- **Malignancy**[see *Warnings and Precautions (5.3)]*
- **Hypersensitivity Reactions, Including Anaphylaxis**[see *Warnings and Precautions (5.4)]*
- **Infusion reactions**[see *Warnings and Precautions (5.5)]*
- **Depression**[see *Warnings and Precautions (5.6)]*

6.1 Clinical Trials Experience

The data described below reflect exposure to BENLYSTA plus standard of care compared with placebo plus standard of care in 2133 patients in 3 controlled studies. Patients received BENLYSTA at doses of 1 mg/kg (N=673), 4 mg/kg (N=111; Trial 1 only), or 10 mg/kg (N=674) or placebo (N=675) intravenously over a 1-hour period on Days 0, 14, 28, and then every 28 days. In two of the studies (Trial 1 and Trial 3), treatment was given for 48 weeks, while in the other study (Trial 2) treatment was given for 72 weeks *[see Clinical Studies (14)]*. Because there was no apparent dose-related increase in the majority of adverse events observed with BENLYSTA, the safety data summarized below are presented for the 3 doses pooled, unless otherwise indicated; the adverse reaction table displays the results for the recommended dose of 10 mg/kg compared with placebo.

The population had a mean age of 39 (range 18 – 75), 94% were female, and 52% were Caucasian. In these trials, 93% of patients treated with BENLYSTA reported an adverse reaction compared with 92% treated with placebo.

The most common serious adverse reactions were serious infections (6.0% and 5.2% in the groups receiving BENLYSTA and placebo, respectively) [*see* Warnings and Precautions (5.2)].

The most commonly-reported adverse reactions, occurring in ≥5% of patients in clinical trials were nausea, diarrhea, pyrexia, nasopharyngitis, bronchitis, insomnia, pain in extremity, depression, migraine, and pharyngitis.

The proportion of patients who discontinued treatment due to any adverse reaction during the controlled clinical trials was 6.2% for patients receiving BENLYSTA and 7.1% for patients receiving placebo. The most common adverse reactions resulting in discontinuation of treatment (≥1% of patients receiving BENLYSTA or placebo) were infusion reactions (1.6% BENLYSTA and 0.9% placebo), lupus nephritis (0.7% BENLYSTA and 1.2% placebo), and infections (0.7% BENLYSTA and 1.0% placebo).

Table 1 lists adverse reactions, regardless of causality, occurring in at least 3% of patients with SLE who received BENLYSTA 10 mg/kg and at an incidence at least 1% greater than that observed with placebo in the 3 controlled studies.

Table 1. Incidence of Adverse Reactions Occurring in at Least 3% of Patients Treated With BENLYSTA 10 mg/kg Plus Standard of Care and at Least 1% More Frequently Than in Patients Receiving Placebo plus Standard of Care in 3 Controlled SLE Studies

Preferred Term	BENLYSTA 10 mg/kg + Standard of Care (n = 674) %	Placebo + Standard of Care (n = 675) %
Nausea	15	12
Diarrhea	12	9
Pyrexia	10	8
Nasopharyngitis	9	7
Bronchitis	9	5
Insomnia	7	5
Pain in extremity	6	4
Depression	5	4
Migraine	5	4
Pharyngitis	5	3
Cystitis	4	3
Leukopenia	4	2
Gastroenteritis viral	3	1

6.2 Immunogenicity

In Trials 2 and 3, anti-belimumab antibodies were detected in 4 of 563 (0.7%) patients receiving BENLYSTA 10 mg/kg and in 27 of 559 (4.8%) patients receiving BENLYSTA 1 mg/kg. The reported frequency for the group receiving 10 mg/kg may underestimate the actual frequency due to lower assay sensitivity in the presence of high drug concentrations. Neutralizing antibodies were detected in 3 patients receiving BENLYSTA 1 mg/kg. Three patients with anti-belimumab antibodies experienced mild infusion reactions of nausea, erythematous rash, pruritus, eyelid edema, headache, and dyspnea; none of the reactions was life-threatening. The clinical relevance of the presence of anti-belimumab antibodies is not known.

The data reflect the percentage of patients whose test results were positive for antibodies to belimumab in specific assays. The observed incidence of antibody positivity in an assay is highly dependent on several factors, including assay sensitivity and specificity, assay methodology, sample handling, timing of sample collection, concomitant medications, and underlying disease. For these reasons, comparison of the incidence of antibodies to belimumab with the incidence of antibodies to other products may be misleading.

6.3 Postmarketing Experience

The following adverse reactions have been identified during postapproval use of BENLYSTA. Because these reactions are reported voluntarily from a population of uncertain size, it is not always possible to reliably estimate their frequency or establish a causal relationship to drug exposure.

- Fatal anaphylaxis *[see Warnings and Precautions (5.4)]*.

7 DRUG INTERACTIONS

Formal drug interaction studies have not been performed with BENLYSTA. In clinical trials of patients with SLE, BENLYSTA was administered concomitantly with other drugs, including corticosteroids, antimalarials, immunomodulatory and immunosuppressive agents (including azathioprine, methotrexate, and mycophenolate), angiotensin pathway antihypertensives, HMG-CoA reductase inhibitors (statins), and NSAIDs without evidence of a clinically meaningful effect of these concomitant medications on belimumab pharmacokinetics. The effect of belimumab on the pharmacokinetics of other drugs has not been evaluated *[see Pharmacokinetics (12.3)]*.

8 USE IN SPECIFIC POPULATIONS

8.1 Pregnancy

Pregnancy Category C. There are no adequate and well-controlled clinical studies using BENLYSTA in pregnant women. Immunoglobulin G (IgG) antibodies, including BENLYSTA, can cross the placenta. Because animal reproduction studies are not always predictive of human response, BENLYSTA should be used during pregnancy only if the potential benefit to the mother justifies the potential risk to the fetus. Women of childbearing potential should use adequate contraception during treatment with BENLYSTA and for at least 4 months after the final treatment.

Nonclinical reproductive studies have been performed in pregnant cynomolgus monkeys receiving belimumab at doses of 0, 5 and 150 mg/kg by intravenous infusion (the high dose was approximately 9 times the anticipated maximum human exposure) every 2 weeks from gestation day 20 to 150. Belimumab was shown to cross the placenta. Belimumab was not associated with direct or indirect teratogenicity under the conditions tested. Fetal deaths were observed in 14%, 24% and 15% of pregnant females in the 0, 5 and 150 mg/kg groups, respectively. Infant deaths occurred with an incidence of 0%, 8% and 5%. The cause of fetal and infant deaths is not known. The relevance of these findings to humans is not known. Other treatment-related findings were limited to the expected reversible reduction of B cells in both dams and infants and reversible reduction of IgM in infant monkeys. B-cell numbers recovered after the cessation of belimumab treatment by about 1 year postpartum in adult monkeys and by 3 months of age in infant monkeys. IgM levels in infants exposed to belimumab in utero recovered by 6 months of age.

Pregnancy Registry: To monitor maternal-fetal outcomes of pregnant women exposed to BENLYSTA, a pregnancy registry has been established. Healthcare professionals are encouraged to register patients and pregnant women are encouraged to enroll themselves by calling 1-877-681-6296.

8.3 Nursing Mothers

It is not known whether BENLYSTA is excreted in human milk or absorbed systemically after ingestion. However, belimumab was excreted into the milk of cynomolgus monkeys. Because maternal antibodies are excreted in human breast milk, a decision should be made whether to discontinue breastfeeding or to discontinue the drug, taking into account the importance of breastfeeding to the infant and the importance of the drug to the mother.

8.4 Pediatric Use

Safety and effectiveness of BENLYSTA have not been established in children.

8.5 Geriatric Use

Clinical studies of BENLYSTA did not include sufficient numbers of subjects aged 65 or over to determine whether they respond differently from younger subjects. Use with caution in elderly patients.

8.6 Race

In Trial 2 and Trial 3, response rates for the primary endpoint were lower for black subjects in the BENLYSTA group relative to black subjects in the placebo group *[see Clinical Studies (14)]*. Use with caution in black/African-American patients.

10 OVERDOSAGE

There is no clinical experience with overdosage of BENLYSTA. Two doses of up to 20 mg/kg have been given by intravenous infusion to humans with no increase in incidence or severity of adverse reactions compared with doses of 1, 4, or 10 mg/kg.

11 DESCRIPTION

BENLYSTA (belimumab) is a human IgG1λ monoclonal antibody specific for soluble human B lymphocyte stimulator protein (BLyS, also referred to as BAFF and TNFSF13B). Belimumab has a molecular weight of approximately 147 kDa. Belimumab is produced by recombinant DNA technology in a mammalian cell expression system.

BENLYSTA is supplied as a sterile, white to off-white, preservative-free, lyophilized powder for intravenous infusion. Upon reconstitution with Sterile Water for Injection, USP, *[see Dosage and Administration (2.3)]* each single-use vial delivers 80 mg/mL belimumab in 0.16 mg/mL citric acid, 0.4 mg/mL polysorbate 80, 2.7 mg/mL sodium citrate, and 80 mg/mL sucrose, with a pH of 6.5.

12 CLINICAL PHARMACOLOGY

12.1 Mechanism of Action

BENLYSTA is a BLyS-specific inhibitor that blocks the binding of soluble BLyS, a B-cell survival factor, to its receptors on B cells. BENLYSTA does not bind B cells directly, but by binding BLyS, BENLYSTA inhibits the survival of B cells, including autoreactive B cells, and reduces the differentiation of B cells into immunoglobulin-producing plasma cells.

12.2 Pharmacodynamics

In Trial 1 and Trial 2 in which B cells were measured, treatment with BENLYSTA significantly reduced circulating CD19+, CD20+, naïve, and activated B cells, plasmacytoid cells, and the SLE B-cell subset at Week 52. Reductions in naïve and the SLE B-cell subset were observed as early as Week 8 and were sustained to Week 52. Memory cells increased initially and slowly declined toward baseline levels by Week 52. The clinical relevance of these effects on B cells has not been established.

Treatment with BENLYSTA led to reductions in IgG and anti-dsDNA, and increases in complement (C3 and C4). These changes were observed as early as Week 8 and were sustained through Week 52. The clinical relevance of normalizing these biomarkers has not been definitively established.

12.3 Pharmacokinetics

The pharmacokinetic parameters displayed in Table 2 are based on population parameter estimates which are specific to the 563 patients who received belimumab 10 mg/kg in Trials 2 and 3 *[see Clinical Studies (14)]*.

Table 2. Population Pharmacokinetic Parameters in Patients with SLE after Intravenous Infusion of BENLYSTA 10 mg/kg*

Pharmacokinetic Parameter	Population Estimates (n = 563)
Peak concentration (C_{max}, µg/mL)	313
Area under the curve ($AUC_{0-\infty}$, day•µg/mL)	3,083
Distribution half-life ($t_{½}$, days)	1.75
Terminal half-life ($t_{½}$, days)	19.4
Systemic clearance (CL, mL/day)	215
Volume of distribution (Vss, L)	5.29

* Intravenous infusions were administered at 2-week intervals for the first 3 doses and at 4-week intervals thereafter.

Drug Interactions: No formal drug interaction studies have been conducted with belimumab. Concomitant use of mycophenolate, azathioprine, methotrexate, antimalarials, NSAIDs, aspirin, and HMG-CoA reductase inhibitors did not significantly influence belimumab pharmacokinetics. Coadministration of steroids and angiotensin-converting enzyme (ACE) inhibitors resulted in an increase of systemic clearance of belimumab that was not clinically significant because the magnitude was well within the range of normal variability of clearance. The effect of belimumab on the pharmacokinetics of other drugs has not been evaluated.

Special Populations:

The following information is based on the population pharmacokinetic analysis.

Age: Age did not significantly influence belimumab pharmacokinetics in the study population, where the majority of subjects (70%) were between 18 and 45 years of age. No pharmacokinetic data are available in pediatric patients. Limited pharmacokinetic data are available for elderly patients as only 1.4% of the subjects included in the pharmacokinetic analysis were 65 years of age or older *[see Use in Specific Populations (8.5)]*.

Gender: Gender did not significantly influence belimumab pharmacokinetics in the largely (94%) female study population.

Race: Race did not significantly influence belimumab pharmacokinetics. The racial distribution was 53% white/Caucasian, 16% Asian, 16% Alaska native/American Indian, and 14% black/African-American.

Renal Impairment: No formal studies were conducted to examine the effects of renal impairment on the pharmacokinetics of belimumab. Belimumab has been studied in a limited number of patients with SLE and renal impairment (261 subjects with moderate renal impairment, creatinine clearance ≥30 and <60 mL/min; 14 subjects with severe renal impairment, creatinine clearance ≥15 and <30 mL/min). Although increases in creatinine clearance and proteinuria (>2 g/day) increased belimumab clearance, these effects were within the expected range of variability. Therefore, dosage adjustment in patients with renal impairment is not recommended.

Hepatic Impairment: No formal studies were conducted to examine the effects of hepatic impairment on the pharmacokinetics of belimumab. Belimumab has not been studied in patients with severe hepatic impairment. Baseline ALT and AST levels did not significantly influence belimumab pharmacokinetics.

13 NONCLINICAL TOXICOLOGY

13.1 Carcinogenesis, Mutagenesis, and Impairment of Fertility

Long-term animal studies have not been performed to evaluate the carcinogenic potential of belimumab. The mutagenic potential of belimumab was not evaluated.

Effects on male and female fertility have not been directly evaluated in animal studies.

14 CLINICAL STUDIES

The safety and effectiveness of BENLYSTA were evaluated in three randomized, double-blind, placebo-controlled studies involving 2133 patients with SLE according to the American College of Rheumatology criteria (Trial 1, 2, and 3). Patients with severe active lupus nephritis and severe active CNS lupus were excluded. Patients were on a stable standard of care SLE treatment regimen comprising any of the following (alone or in combination): corticosteroids, antimalarials, NSAIDs, and immunosuppressives. Use of other biologics and intravenous cyclophosphamide were not permitted.

Trial 1: BENLYSTA 1 mg/kg, 4 mg/kg, 10 mg/kg

Trial 1 enrolled 449 patients and evaluated doses of 1, 4, and 10 mg/kg BENLYSTA plus standard of care compared with placebo plus standard of care over 52 weeks in patients with SLE. Patients had to have a SELENA-SLEDAI score of ≥4 at baseline and a history of autoantibodies (anti-nuclear antibody (ANA) and/or anti-double-stranded DNA (anti-dsDNA), but 28% of the population was autoantibody negative at baseline. The co-primary endpoints were percent change in SELENA-SLEDAI score at Week 24 and time to first flare over 52 weeks. No significant differences between any of the BENLYSTA groups and the placebo group were observed. Exploratory analysis of this study identified a subgroup of patients (72%), who were autoantibody positive, in whom BENLYSTA appeared to offer benefit. The results of this study informed the design of Trials 2 and 3 and led to the selection of a target population and indication that is limited to autoantibody-positive SLE patients.

Trials 2 and 3: BENLYSTA 1 mg/kg and 10 mg/kg

Trials 2 and 3 were randomized, double-blind, placebo-controlled trials in patients with SLE that were similar in design except duration - Trial 2 was 76 weeks duration and Trial 3 was 52 weeks duration. Eligible patients had active SLE disease, defined as a SELENA-SLEDAI score ≥6, and positive autoantibody test results at screening. Patients were excluded from the study if they had ever received treatment with a B-cell targeted agent or if they were currently receiving other biologic agents. Intravenous cyclophosphamide was not permitted within the previous 6 months or during study. Trial 2 was conducted primarily in North America and Europe. Trial 3 was conducted in South America, Eastern Europe, Asia, and Australia.

Baseline concomitant medications included corticosteroids (Trial 2: 76%, Trial 3: 96%), immunosuppressives (Trial 2: 56%, Trial 3: 42%; including azathioprine, methotrexate and mycophenolate), and antimalarials (Trial 2: 63%, Trial 3: 67%). Most patients (>70%) were receiving 2 or more classes of SLE medications.

In Trial 2 and Trial 3, more than 50% of patients had 3 or more active organ systems at baseline. The most common active organ systems at baseline based on SELENA-SLEDAI were mucocutaneous (82% in both studies); immunology (Trial 2: 74%, Trial 3: 85%); and musculoskeletal (Trial 2: 73%, Trial 3: 59%). Less than 16% of patients had some degree of renal activity and less than 7% of patients had activity in the vascular, cardio-respiratory, or CNS systems.

At screening, patients were stratified by disease severity based on their SELENA-SLEDAI score (≤ 9 vs ≥10), proteinuria level (< 2 g/24 hr vs ≥ 2 g/24 hr), and race (African or Indigenous-American descent vs. other), and then randomly assigned to receive BENLYSTA 1 mg/kg, BENLYSTA 10 mg/kg, or placebo in addition to standard of care. The patients were administered study medication intravenously over a 1-hour period on Days 0, 14, 28, and then every 28 days for 48 weeks in Trial 3 and for 72 weeks in Trial 2.

The primary efficacy endpoint was a composite endpoint (SLE Responder Index or SRI) that defined response as meeting each of the following criteria at Week 52 compared with baseline:

- ≥ 4-point reduction in the SELENA-SLEDAI score, and
- no new British Isles Lupus Assessment Group (BILAG) A organ domain score or 2 new BILAG B organ domain scores, and
- no worsening (< 0.30-point increase) in Physician's Global Assessment (PGA) score.

The SRI uses the SELENA-SLEDAI score as an objective measure of reduction in global disease activity; the BILAG index to ensure no significant worsening in any specific organ system; and the PGA to ensure that improvements in disease activity are not accompanied by worsening of the patient's condition overall.

In both Trials 2 and 3, the proportion of SLE patients achieving an SRI response, as defined for the primary endpoint, was significantly higher in the BENLYSTA 10 mg/kg group than in the placebo group. The effect on the SRI was not consistently significantly different for the BENLYSTA 1 mg/kg group relative to placebo in both trials. The 1 mg/kg dose is not recommended. The trends in comparisons be-

Table 3. Clinical Response Rate in Patients with SLE After 52 Weeks of Treatment

Response*	Trial 2			Trial 3		
	Placebo + Standard of Care (n = 275)	BENLYSTA 1 mg/kg + Standard of Care (n = 271)	BENLYSTA 10 mg/kg + Standard of Care (n = 273)	Placebo + Standard of Care (n = 287)	BENLYSTA 1 mg/kg + Standard of Care† (n = 288)	BENLYSTA 10 mg/kg + Standard of Care (n = 290)
SLE Responder Index	34%	41% (p = 0.104)	43% (p = 0.021)	44%	51% (p = 0.013)	58% (p < 0.001)
Odds Ratio (95% CI) vs. placebo		1.3 (0.9, 1.9)	1.5 (1.1, 2.2)		1.6 (1.1, 2.2)	1.8 (1.3, 2.6)
Components of SLE Responder Index						
Percent of patients with reduction in SELENA-SLEDAI ≥4	36%	43%	47%	46%	53%	58%
Percent of patients with no worsening by BILAG index	65%	75%	69%	73%	79%	81%
Percent of patients with no worsening by PGA	63%	73%	69%	69%	79%	80%

* Patients dropping out of the study early or experiencing certain increases in background medication were considered as failures in these analyses. In both studies, a higher proportion of placebo patients were considered as failures for this reason as compared to the BENLYSTA groups.
† The 1 mg/kg dose is not recommended.

tween the treatment groups for the rates of response for the individual components of the endpoint were generally consistent with that of the SRI (Table 3). At Week 76 in Trial 2, the SRI response rate with BENLYSTA 10 mg/kg was not significantly different from that of placebo (39% and 32%, respectively).

[See table 3 above]

The reduction in disease activity seen in the SRI was related primarily to improvement in the most commonly involved organ systems namely, mucocutaneous, musculoskeletal, and immunology.

Effect in Black/African-American Patients:

Exploratory sub-group analyses of SRI response rate in patients of black race were performed. In Trial 2 and Trial 3 combined, the SRI response rate in black patients (N=148) in the BENLYSTA groups was less than that in the placebo group (22/50 or 44% for placebo, 15/48 or 31% for BENLYSTA 1 mg/kg, and 18/50 or 36% for BENLYSTA 10 mg/kg). In Trial 1, black patients (N = 106) in the BENLYSTA groups did not appear to have a different response than the rest of the study population. Although no definitive conclusions can be drawn from these subgroup analyses, caution should be used when considering BENLYSTA treatment in black/African-American SLE patients.

Effect on Concomitant Steroid Treatment:

In Trial 2 and Trial 3, 46% and 69% of patients, respectively, were receiving prednisone at doses > 7.5 mg/day at baseline. The proportion of patients able to reduce their average prednisone dose by at least 25% to ≤ 7.5 mg/day during Weeks 40 through 52 was not consistently significantly different for BENLYSTA relative to placebo in both trials. In Trial 2, 17% of patients receiving BENLYSTA 10 mg/kg and 19% of patients receiving BENLYSTA 1 mg/kg achieved this level of steroid reduction compared with 13% of patients receiving placebo. In Trial 3, 19%, 21%, and 12% of patients receiving BENLYSTA 10 mg/kg, BENLYSTA 1 mg/kg, and placebo, respectively, achieved this level of steroid reduction.

Effect on Severe SLE Flares:

The probability of experiencing a severe SLE flare, as defined by a modification of the SELENA Trial flare criteria which excluded severe flares triggered only by an increase of the SELENA-SLEDAI score to >12, was calculated for both Trials 2 and 3. The proportion of patients having at least 1 severe flare over 52 weeks was not consistently significantly different for BENLYSTA relative to placebo in both trials. In Trial 2, 18% of patients receiving BENLYSTA 10 mg/kg and 16% of patients receiving BENLYSTA 1 mg/kg had a severe flare compared with 24% of patients receiving placebo. In Trial 3, 14%, 18%, and 23% of patients receiving BENLYSTA 10 mg/kg, BENLYSTA 1 mg/kg and placebo, respectively, had a severe flare.

16 HOW SUPPLIED/STORAGE AND HANDLING

BENLYSTA is a sterile, preservative-free lyophilized powder for reconstitution, dilution, and intravenous infusion provided in single-use glass vials with a latex-free rubber stopper and a flip-off seal. Each 5-mL vial contains 120 mg of belimumab. Each 20-mL vial contains 400 mg of belimumab.

BENLYSTA is supplied as follows:

120 mg belimumab in a 5-mL single-use vial	NDC 49401-101-01
400 mg belimumab in a 20-mL single-use vial	NDC 49401-102-01

Store vials of BENLYSTA refrigerated between 2° to 8°C (36° to 46°F). Vials should be protected from light and stored in the original carton until use. *Do not freeze.* Avoid exposure to heat. Do not use beyond the expiration date.

17 PATIENT COUNSELING INFORMATION

See FDA-approved patient labeling (Medication Guide)

17.1 Advice for the Patient

Patients should be given the Medication Guide for BENLYSTA and provided an opportunity to read it prior to each treatment session. It is important that the patient's overall health be assessed at each infusion visit and any questions resulting from the patient's reading of the Medication Guide be discussed.

Mortality: Patients should be advised that more patients receiving BENLYSTA in the main clinical trials died than did patients receiving placebo treatment *[see Warnings and Precautions (5.1)]*.

Serious Infections: Patients should be advised that BENLYSTA may decrease their ability to fight infections. Patients should be asked if they have a history of chronic infections and if they are currently on any therapy for an infection *[see Warnings and Precautions (5.2)]*. Patients should be instructed to tell their healthcare provider if they develop signs or symptoms of an infection.

Hypersensitivity/Anaphylactic and Infusion Reactions: Educate patients on the signs and symptoms of anaphylaxis, including wheezing, difficulty breathing, peri-oral or lingual edema, and rash. Patients should be instructed to immediately tell their healthcare provider if they experience symptoms of an allergic reaction during or after the administration of BENLYSTA *[see Warnings and Precautions (5.4, 5.5)]*.

Depression: Patients should be instructed to contact their healthcare provider if they experience new or worsening depression, suicidal thoughts or other mood changes *[see Warnings and Precautions (5.6)]*.

Immunizations: Patients should be informed that they should not receive live vaccines while taking BENLYSTA. Response to vaccinations could be impaired by BENLYSTA *[see Warnings and Precautions (5.7)]*.

Pregnancy and Nursing Mothers: Patients should be informed that BENLYSTA has not been studied in pregnant women or nursing mothers so the effects of BENLYSTA on pregnant women or nursing infants are not known. Patients should be instructed to tell their healthcare provider if they are pregnant, become pregnant, or are thinking about becoming pregnant *[see Use in Specific Populations (8.1)]*. Patients should be instructed to tell their healthcare provider if they plan to breastfeed their infant *[see Use in Specific Populations (8.3)]*.

BENLYSTA is a registered trademark of Human Genome Sciences, Inc., used under license by GlaxoSmithKline.

Manufactured by:
Human Genome Sciences, Inc.
Rockville, Maryland 20850
US License No. 1820
Marketed by:
Human Genome Sciences, Inc.
Rockville, MD 20850
GlaxoSmithKline
Research Triangle Park, NC 27709

BEXXAR ℞

[bex'ar]

(tositumomab and iodine I 131 tositumomab)
Injection, for intravenous infusion

HIGHLIGHTS OF PRESCRIBING INFORMATION

These highlights do not include all the information needed to use BEXXAR safely and effectively. See full prescribing information for BEXXAR.

BEXXAR (tositumomab and iodine I 131 tositumomab) Injection, for intravenous infusion
Initial U.S. Approval: 2003

WARNING: SERIOUS ALLERGIC REACTIONS/ANAPHYLAXIS, PROLONGED AND SEVERE CYTOPENIAS, AND RADIATION EXPOSURE

See full prescribing information for complete boxed warning.

- **Serious Allergic Reactions: Immediately interrupt infusion and permanently discontinue the BEXXAR therapeutic regimen for serious allergic reactions (5.1)**
- **Prolonged and severe cytopenias occur in most patients. BEXXAR should not be administered to patients with >25% lymphoma marrow involvement, platelet count <100,000 cells/mm³, or neutrophil count <1,500 cells/mm³ (5.2, 6.1)**
- **Radiation Exposure: The BEXXAR therapeutic regimen is supplied only to certified healthcare professionals. Follow institutional radiation safety practices and applicable federal guidelines to minimize radiation exposure to household contacts and medical staff. (5.3)**

RECENT MAJOR CHANGES

Indications and Usage:
Rituximab-naïve Patients (1) Removed 08/2012

INDICATIONS AND USAGE

BEXXAR (tositumomab and Iodine I 131 tositumomab) is a CD20-directed radiotherapeutic antibody indicated for the treatment of patients with CD20-positive, relapsed or refractory, low-grade, follicular, or transformed non-Hodgkin's lymphoma who have progressed during or after rituximab therapy, including patients with rituximab-refractory non-Hodgkin's lymphoma. (1.1)

Determination of the effectiveness of the BEXXAR therapeutic regimen is based on overall response rates in patients whose disease is refractory to chemotherapy and rituximab. The effects of the BEXXAR therapeutic regimen on survival are not known. (1.1)

Important Limitation of Use

- BEXXAR therapeutic regimen is only indicated for a single course of treatment and is not indicated for a first-line treatment. (1.2)

DOSAGE AND ADMINISTRATION

The BEXXAR therapeutic regimen consists of a 2-part dosimetric step, followed 7 to 14 days later by a 2-part therapeutic step. (2.1)

DOSAGE FORMS AND STRENGTHS

- Tositumomab 225 mg solution (14 mg per mL), single use vial (3)
- Tositumomab 35 mg solution (14 mg per mL), single use vial (3)
- Iodine I 131 tositumomab solution containing 12-18 mCi Iodine-131 per vial (not less than 0.61 mCi per mL at calibration) and 2.0-6.1 mg tositumomab per vial (not less than 0.1 mg per mL), single use vial (3)
- Iodine I 131 tositumomab solution containing 112-168 mCi Iodine-131 per vial (not less than 5.6 mCi per mL at calibration) and 22-61 mg tositumomab per vial (not less than 1.1 mg per mL), single use vial (3)

CONTRAINDICATIONS

None (4)

WARNINGS AND PRECAUTIONS

- Secondary Malignancies: Hematological and non-hematological secondary malignancies have been reported. (5.4)
- Hypothyroidism: Thyroid-blocking medication is required prior to administration of the BEXXAR therapeutic regimen. Evaluate for clinical evidence of hypothyroidism and thyroid-stimulating hormone (TSH) level before treatment and annually thereafter. (5.5)
- Embryo-fetal Toxicity: Administration to a pregnant woman can cause embryo-fetal harm including severe, and possibly irreversible, neonatal hypothyroidism. Females and males of reproductive potential should use effective contraception to avoid pregnancy during treatment and for 12 months after the therapeutic dose. (5.6, 8.1, 8.7)

ADVERSE REACTIONS

The most common adverse reactions (≥25%) are neutropenia, thrombocytopenia, anemia, infections, infusion reactions, asthenia, fever, and nausea. (6)

To report SUSPECTED ADVERSE REACTIONS, contact GlaxoSmithKline at 1-888-825-5249 or FDA at 1-800-FDA-1088 or www.fda.gov/medwatch.

USE IN SPECIFIC POPULATIONS

- Nursing Mothers: Discontinue nursing. (8.3)

See 17 for PATIENT COUNSELING INFORMATION

Revised: 05/2013

FULL PRESCRIBING INFORMATION: CONTENTS*

*** Sections or subsections omitted from the full prescribing information are not listed**

FULL PRESCRIBING INFORMATION

WARNING: SERIOUS ALLERGIC REACTIONS (INCLUDING ANAPHYLAXIS), PROLONGED AND SEVERE CYTOPENIAS, AND RADIATION EXPOSURE

Serious Allergic Reactions (Including Anaphylaxis): Serious, including fatal, allergic reactions have occurred during or following administration of the BEXXAR therapeutic regimen. Have medications for the treatment of allergic reactions available for immediate use. Permanently discontinue the BEXXAR therapeutic regimen for serious allergic reactions and administer appropriate medical treatment *[see Warnings and Precautions (5.1)]*.

Prolonged and Severe Cytopenias: The BEXXAR therapeutic regimen resulted in severe and prolonged thrombocytopenia and neutropenia in more than 70% of the patients in clinical studies. The BEXXAR therapeutic regimen should not be administered to patients with greater than 25% lymphoma marrow involvement, platelet count less than 100,000 cells/mm^3 or neutrophil count less than 1,500 cells/mm^3 *[see Warnings and Precautions (5.2), Adverse Reactions (6.1)]*.

Radiation Exposure: The BEXXAR therapeutic regimen may be administered only under the supervision of physicians who are certified under or participating in the BEXXAR therapeutic regimen certification program and who are authorized under the Radioactive Materials License at their clinical site. Follow institutional radiation safety practices and applicable federal guidelines to minimize radiation exposure during handling and after administration of the BEXXAR therapeutic regimen *[see Warnings and Precautions (5.3)]*.

1 INDICATIONS AND USAGE

1.1 Relapsed or Refractory CD20-Positive, Non-Hodgkin's Lymphoma

The BEXXAR® therapeutic regimen (tositumomab and iodine I 131 tositumomab) is indicated for the treatment of patients with CD20-positive relapsed or refractory, low grade, follicular, or transformed non-Hodgkin's lymphoma who have progressed during or after rituximab therapy, including patients with rituximab-refractory non-Hodgkin's lymphoma.

Determination of the effectiveness of the BEXXAR therapeutic regimen is based on overall response rates in patients whose disease is refractory to chemotherapy and rituximab. The effects of the BEXXAR therapeutic regimen on survival are not known.

1.2 Important Limitations of Use

- The BEXXAR therapeutic regimen is only indicated for a single course of treatment.
- The safety and efficacy of additional courses of the BEXXAR therapeutic regimen have not been established.
- The BEXXAR therapeutic regimen is not indicated for first-line treatment of patients with CD20-positive non-Hodgkin's lymphoma.

2 DOSAGE AND ADMINISTRATION

The BEXXAR therapeutic regimen consists of 2 separate components (tositumomab and iodine I 131 tositumomab) administered in 2 separate steps (dosimetric dose and therapeutic dose) separated by 7 to 14 days.

Parenteral drug products should be inspected for particulate matter prior to administration, whenever solution and container permit *[see Description (11)]*.

2.1 Overview of Dosing Schedule

[See figure 1 at top of next column]

2.2 Recommended Dose

Dosimetric dose

1. Tositumomab 450 mg by intravenous infusion
2. I-131 tositumomab (5 mCi I-131 and 35 mg protein) by intravenous infusion

Figure 1
Dosing Schedule

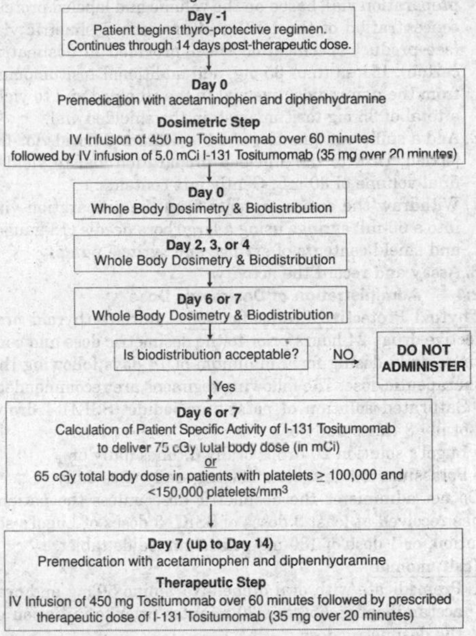

Day -1
Patient begins thyro-protective regimen.
Continues through 14 days post-therapeutic dose.
Day 0
Premedication with acetaminophen and diphenhydramine
Dosimetric Step
IV Infusion of 450 mg Tositumomab over 60 minutes
followed by IV infusion of 5.0 mCi I-131 Tositumomab (35 mg over 20 minutes)
Day 0
Whole Body Dosimetry & Biodistribution
Day 2, 3, or 4
Whole Body Dosimetry & Biodistribution
Day 6 or 7
Whole Body Dosimetry & Biodistribution
Is biodistribution acceptable?
NO
DO NOT ADMINISTER
Yes
Day 6 or 7
Calculation of Patient Specific Activity of I-131 Tositumomab
to deliver 75 cGy total body dose (in mCi)
or
65 cGy total body dose in patients with platelets ≥ 100,000 and
<150,000 platelets/mm3
Day 7 (up to Day 14)
Premedication with acetaminophen and diphenhydramine
Therapeutic Step
IV Infusion of 450 mg Tositumomab over 60 minutes followed by prescribed
therapeutic dose of I-131 Tositumomab (35 mg over 20 minutes)

Therapeutic dose (administered 7-14 days after dosimetric dose)

1. Tositumomab 450 mg by intravenous infusion
2. I-131 tositumomab (35 mg) by intravenous infusion. The iodine-131 dose is calculated based on 1) assessment of dosimetry and biodistribution obtained following the dosimetric dose, and 2) platelet counts obtained within 28 days prior to dosing.

If platelet counts are 150,000 platelets/mm^3 or greater:
The recommended dose (mCi) is the activity of Iodine-131 calculated to deliver 75 cGy total body irradiation

If platelet counts are 100,000 to 149,000 platelets/mm^3:
The recommended dose is the activity of Iodine-131 calculated to deliver 65 cGy total body irradiation

2.3 Preparation of Dosimetric Dose

TositumomabDosimetric Dose

1. Withdraw and discard 32 mL from a 50-mL bag 0.9% Sodium Chloride for Injection, USP.
2. Withdraw and transfer entire contents from each of the two 225-mg tositumomab vials (a total of 450 mg tositumomab in 32 mL) to remaining 18 mL in bag of 0.9% Sodium Chloride for Injection, USP to yield a final volume of 50 mL.
3. DO NOT SHAKE. Gently mix the solution by inverting/rotating the bag. The tositumomab solution is clear to opalescent, colorless to slightly yellow, and may contain white particulates.
4. Diluted tositumomab may be stored at 36°F to 46°F (2°C to 8°C) for 24 hours or at room temperature for 8 hours. Discard unused solution.

I-131 TositumomabDosimetric Dose

Required materials (not supplied):

- Lead shielding for preparation vial and syringe pump
- One sterile 30-mL preparation vial
- Two lead pots at room temperature

Method

1. Thaw contents (approximately 60 minutes) of I-131 tositumomab dosimetric vial at room temperature with appropriate lead shielding. Thawed undiluted I-131 tositumomab may be stored up to 8 hours at 36°F to 46°F (2°C to 8°C) or at room temperature.
2. Calculate the volume required for I-131 tositumomab activity of 5.0 mCi, based on the activity concentration of dosimetric vial (refer to product specification sheet provided in dosimetric carton).
3. Withdraw and transfer the calculated volume from I-131 tositumomab vial to the shielded preparation vial.
4. Assay preparation vial to confirm activity is 5.0 mCi (±10%) using a suitable radioactivity calibration system operated in accordance with the manufacturer's specifications and quality control for the measurement of Iodine-131.
    - If the preparation vial contains the calculated activity (±10%), proceed to step 5.
    - If the preparation vial does not contain the calculated activity (5 mCi ±10%), determine the activity concentration of the I-131 tositumomab based on the volume and the activity in the preparation vial. Add or subtract the appropriate volume of I-131 tositumomab to the preparation vial to achieve the desired activity of 5.0 mCi (±10%). Re-assay to confirm.

5. Calculate the amount of tositumomab in the shielded preparation vial, based on the volume and labeled protein concentration of the I-131 tositumomab dosimetric vial (see product specification sheet provided in dosimetric carton). If less than 35 mg, add additional tositumomab from the non-radioactive vial to the shielded vial to yield a total of 35 mg tositumomab in the shielded vial.
6. Add a sufficient quantity of 0.9% Sodium Chloride for Injection, USP to the shielded preparation vial to yield a final volume of 30 mL. Gently mix contents.
7. Withdraw the entire contents from the preparation vial into a 60-mL syringe using a large bore needle (18-gauge) and shield contents of syringe and syringe pump.
8. Assay and record the activity.

2.4 Administration of Dosimetric Dose

Thyroid Protective Pre-medication: Initiate thyroid protective drugs 24 hours prior to the dosimetric dose and continue daily dosing for a minimum of 14 days following the therapeutic dose. The following regimens are recommended:

- Saturated solution of potassium iodide (SSKI) 4 drops orally 3 times daily or
- Lugol's solution 20 drops orally 3 times daily or
- Potassium iodide tablets 130 mg orally once daily

Do not administer the dosimetric dose unless the patient has received at least 3 doses of SSKI, 3 doses of Lugol's solution, or 1 dose of 130-mg potassium iodide tablet.

Tositumomab

1. Premedicate with oral diphenhydramine 50 mg and oral acetaminophen 650 mg, 30 minutes prior to initiation of the dosimetric dose.
2. Administer 450 mg tositumomab in 50 mL 0.9% sodium chloride by intravenous infusion through a 0.22 micron in-line filter over 60 minutes (refer to *Site Training Manual* for diagram showing assembly of the infusion set components). Decrease the rate of infusion by 50% for mild to moderate infusion reactions. Discontinue for serious allergic reactions; interrupt for severe infusion reactions. If severe infusion reaction completely resolves, the infusion may be continued at 50% of the previous infusion rate.

I-131 Tositumomab

1. Attach the shielded syringe containing the I-131 tositumomab dose in a syringe pump to the intravenous line containing the in-line filter used in step 2 above. A change in filter can result in loss of up to 7% of the I-131 tositumomab dose.
2. Set syringe pump to deliver the entire dose of I-131 tositumomab over 20 minutes, immediately following completion of the tositumomab infusion. Decrease the rate of infusion by 50% for mild to moderate infusion reactions. Discontinue for serious allergic reactions; interrupt for severe infusion reactions. If severe infusion reaction completely resolves, the infusion may be continued at 50% of the previous infusion rate.
3. Upon completion of the I-131 tositumomab infusion, flush the IV line with 0.9% Sodium Chloride for Injection, USP.
4. Determine the combined residual activity of the syringe and infusion set components (stopcock, extension set, primary infusion set, and in-line filter set) by assaying these items in a suitable radioactivity calibration system immediately following completion of administration of all components of the dosimetric dose.
5. Calculate and record the dose delivered to the patient by subtracting the residual activity in the syringe and the infusion set components from the activity of I-131 tositumomab in the syringe prior to infusion.
6. Discard unused portion of Iodine I-131 tositumomab and infusion set components according to federal and state laws regarding radioactive and biohazardous waste.

2.5 Assessment of Dosimetry and Biodistribution

Additional copies of templates for recording dosimetry and calculation of the I-131 tositumomab therapeutic dose and the *Site Training Manual* may be obtained from the GlaxoSmithKline Wholesale Service Center (1-877-423-9927).

Obtain total body gamma camera counts and whole body images at the following timepoints:

1. Count 1 (Day 0): Within 1 hour following the end of the I-131 tositumomab infusion and prior to urination, obtain total body gamma camera count and whole body images.
2. Count 2 (Day 2, 3, or 4): Obtain total body gamma camera counts and whole body images, immediately following urination.
3. Count 3 (Day 6 or 7): Obtain total body gamma camera counts and whole body images, immediately following urination.

Verify that the expected biodistribution is present.

Assess Biodistribution: Determine total body residence time and examine whole body camera images done at Count 1 and Count 2. Examine image performed at Count 3 as needed to resolve ambiguities.

Expected biodistribution characteristics:

Count 1 (day of dosimetric dose)

- Most of the activity is in the blood pool (heart and major blood vessels). Uptake in normal liver and spleen is less than in the heart.

Count 2 (Day 2, 3, or 4) and Count 3 (Day 6 or 7)

- Activity in the blood pool decreases significantly. Decreased accumulation of activity in normal liver and spleen. Possible uptake present in thyroid, kidney, and urinary bladder with minimal uptake in the lungs. Possible increased intensity at known lymphoma sites.

Biodistribution is altered if any of the following is present:

Count 1:

- Blood pool is not visualized
- Diffuse, intense tracer uptake in the liver and/or spleen or uptake suggestive of urinary obstruction
- Diffuse uptake in normal lung greater than that of blood pool.

Count 2 and Count 3:

- Uptake is suggestive of urinary obstruction
- Diffuse uptake in normal lung which is greater than that of the blood pool
- Total body residence time is less than 50 hours
- Total body residence time is more than 150 hours.

2.6 Calculation of I-131 Therapeutic Dose

The therapeutic dose may be calculated manually using the total body residence time and activity hours (refer to the *Site Training Manual)*. The therapeutic dose may also be derived by using the GlaxoSmithKline BEXXAR therapeutic regimen Patient Management Templates (refer to the *Site Training Manual)*. For assistance with either manual or automated calculations call the GlaxoSmithKline Wholesale Service Center at 1-877-423-9927.

The following equation is used to calculate the activity of Iodine-131 required for delivery of the desired total body dose of radiation:

$$\text{Iodine-131 Activity (mCi)} = \frac{\text{Activity Hours (mCi hr)}}{\text{Residence Time (hr)}} \times \frac{\text{Desired Total Body Dose (65cGy or 75cGy)}}{\text{75cGy}}$$

2.7 Preparation of Therapeutic Dose

Tositumomab

A 450-mg dose of tositumomab should be prepared as previously described *[see Dosage and Administration (2.3)]*.

I-131 tositumomab

Required materials (not supplied):

- Lead shielding for preparation vial and syringe pump
- One sterile 50-mL preparation vial
- Two lead pots at room temperature.

Method

Thaw contents (approximately 60 minutes) of I-131 tositumomab therapeutic vial at room temperature with appropriate lead shielding. Thawed, undiluted I-131 tositumomab may be stored up to 8 hours at 36°F to 46°F (2°C to 8°C) or at room temperature. Do not freeze solutions of diluted I-131 tositumomab; store refrigerated until time of use.

1. Calculate the volume (see activity concentration on the product specification sheet provided with the therapeutic vial) of I-131 tositumomab activity required to deliver either 75cGy or 65cGy total body irradiation *[see Dosage and Administration (2.6)]*.
2. Withdraw and transfer the calculated volume from I-131 tositumomab vial to the shielded preparation vial.
3. Assay preparation vial to confirm calculated activity using a suitable radioactivity calibration system operated in accordance with the manufacturer's specifications and quality control for the measurement of Iodine-131.
   - If the assayed dose in the preparation vial contains the calculated activity (±10%), proceed to step 5.
   - If the assayed dose in the preparation vial does not contain the calculated activity (±10%), determine the activity concentration of I-131 tositumomab based on the volume and the activity in the preparation vial. Add or subtract the appropriate volume of I-131 tositumomab to the preparation vial to achieve the required I-131 tositumomab activity. Re-assay the preparation vial contents to confirm.
4. Calculate the amount of tositumomab in the shielded preparation vial, based on the volume and protein concentration of I-131 tositumomab (refer to product specification sheet for the vial in the therapeutic carton). If the amount of tositumomab in the preparation vial is less than 35 mg, add additional tositumomab from the non-radioactive 35-mg vial to the shielded preparation vial to yield a total of 35 mg tositumomab in the shielded vial.
5. Add a sufficient quantity of 0.9% Sodium Chloride for Injection, USP to the shielded preparation vial to yield a final volume of 30 mL. Gently mix contents.
6. Withdraw the entire contents from the shielded preparation vial into a 60-mL syringe using a large bore needle (18-gauge) and shield contents of syringe and syringe pump.
7. Assay and record activity.

2.8 Administration of Therapeutic Dose

Do not administer the therapeutic dose if biodistribution is altered *[see Dosage and Administration (2.5)]*.

Tositumomab

Premedicate with oral diphenhydramine 50 mg and oral acetaminophen 650 mg 30 minutes prior to initiation of the therapeutic dose.

Administer 450 mg tositumomab in 50 mL 0.9% sodium chloride by intravenous infusion through a 0.22 micron in-line filter over 60 minutes (refer to *Site Training Manual* for diagram showing assembly of the infusion set components). Decrease the rate of infusion by 50% for mild to moderate infusion reactions. Discontinue for serious allergic reactions; interrupt for severe infusion reactions. If severe infusion reaction completely resolves, the infusion may be continued at 50% of the previous infusion rate.

I-131 Tositumomab

Attach the shielded syringe containing the I-131 tositumomab therapeutic dose to the intravenous line containing the in-line filter used in step 2 above. **A change in filter can result in loss of up to 7% of the I-131 tositumomab dose.** Set syringe pump to deliver the entire dose of I-131 tositumomab over 20 minutes, immediately following completion of the tositumomab infusion. Decrease the rate of infusion by 50% for mild to moderate infusion reactions. Discontinue for serious allergic reactions; interrupt for severe infusion reactions. If severe infusion reaction completely resolves, the infusion may be continued at 50% of the previous infusion rate.

1. Upon completion of I-131 tositumomab infusion, flush the IV line with 0.9% Sodium Chloride for Injection, USP.
2. Determine the combined residual activity of the syringe and infusion set components (stopcock, extension set, primary infusion set and in-line filter set) by assaying these items in a suitable radioactivity calibration system immediately following completion of administration of all components of the therapeutic dose.
3. Calculate and record the dose delivered to the patient by subtracting the residual activity in the syringe and the infusion set components from the activity of I-131 tositumomab in the syringe prior to infusion.
4. Discard unused portion of Iodine I-131 tositumomab and infusion set components according to federal and state laws regarding radioactive and biohazardous waste.

2.9 Radiation Dosimetry

Estimations of radiation-absorbed doses for I-131 tositumomab were performed using sequential whole body images and the MIRDOSE 3 software program. Patients with apparent thyroid, stomach, or intestinal imaging were selected for organ dosimetry analyses. The estimated radiation-absorbed doses to organs and marrow from a course of the BEXXAR therapeutic regimen are presented in Table 1.

Table 1. Estimated Radiation-Absorbed Organ Doses

	The BEXXAR therapeutic regimen mGy/MBq Median	The BEXXAR therapeutic regimen mGy/MBq Range
Organ Regions of Interest (ROIs)		
Thyroid	2.71	1.4 - 6.2
Kidneys	1.96	1.5 - 2.5
Upper large intestine wall	1.34	0.8 - 1.7
Lower large intestine wall	1.30	0.8 - 1.6
Heart wall	1.25	0.5 - 1.8
Spleen	1.14	0.7 - 5.4
Testes	0.83	0.3 - 1.3
Liver	0.82	0.6 - 1.3
Lungs	0.79	0.5 - 1.1
Marrow space	0.65	0.5 - 1.1
Stomach wall	0.40	0.2 - 0.8
Whole Body ROIs		
Urine bladder wall	0.64	0.6 - 0.9
Bone surfaces	0.41	0.4 - 0.6

Pancreas	0.31	0.2 - 0.4
Gall bladder wall	0.29	0.2 - 0.3
Adrenals	0.28	0.2 - 0.3
Ovaries	0.25	0.2 - 0.3
Small intestine	0.23	0.2 - 0.3
Thymus	0.22	0.1 - 0.3
Uterus	0.20	0.2 - 0.2
Muscle	0.18	0.1 - 0.2
Breasts	0.16	0.1 - 0.2
Skin	0.13	0.1 - 0.2
Brain	0.13	0.1 - 0.2
Total body	0.24	0.2 - 0.3

3 DOSAGE FORMS AND STRENGTHS

Tositumomab 225-mg solution (14 mg per mL), single-use vial

Tositumomab 35-mg solution (14 mg per mL), single-use vial

I-131 tositumomab solution containing 12-18 mCi Iodine-131 per vial (not less than 20 mL containing not less than 0.61 mCi per mL at calibration) and 2.0-6.1 mg tositumomab per vial (not less than 0.1 mg per mL protein concentration), single-use vial

I-131 tositumomab solution containing 112-168 mCi Iodine-131 per vial (not less than 20 mL containing not less than 5.6 mCi per mL at calibration) and 22-61 mg tositumomab per vial (not less than 1.1 mg per mL protein concentration), single-use vial

4 CONTRAINDICATIONS

None

5 WARNINGS AND PRECAUTIONS

5.1 Serious Allergic Reactions, Including Anaphylaxis

The BEXXAR therapeutic regimen can cause severe, including fatal, allergic reactions *[see Adverse Reactions (6.1) and (6.3)]*. Premedicate with acetaminophen and diphenhydramine *[see Dosage and Administration (2.1), (2.4), and (2.8)]*. Have medications for the treatment of allergic reactions available for immediate use during administration. Signs and symptoms of severe allergic reactions may include fever, rigors or chills, sweating, hypotension, dyspnea, bronchospasm, and nausea during or within 48 hours of infusion. Immediately interrupt BEXXAR infusions for severe reactions and provide appropriate medical and supportive care measures. Permanently, discontinue the BEXXAR therapeutic regimen in patients who develop serious allergic reactions.

5.2 Prolonged and Severe Cytopenias

Patients receiving the BEXXAR therapeutic regimen experienced severe (NCI CTC grade 3-4) and prolonged neutropenia (63%), thrombocytopenia (53%), and anemia (29%) *[see Adverse Reactions (6.1)]*. The time to nadir was 4 to 7 weeks and the duration of cytopenias was approximately 30 days. Due to the variable nature of the onset of cytopenias, monitor patients with weekly complete blood counts for up to 12 weeks.

The BEXXAR therapeutic regimen should not be administered to patients with >25% lymphoma marrow involvement, platelet count <100,000 cells/mm^3, or neutrophil count <1,500 cells/mm^3.

5.3 Radiation Exposure

The BEXXAR therapeutic regimen contains Iodine-131. Follow institutional radiation safety practices and applicable federal guidelines to minimize radiation exposure during handling and after administration of the BEXXAR therapeutic regimen. Advise patients of the risks of radiation exposure of household contacts, pregnant women, and small children and of the steps to be taken to reduce these risks. The BEXXAR therapeutic regimen should be administered only by physicians enrolled in the certification program for dose calculation and administration of the BEXXAR therapeutic regimen. Further information regarding the BEXXAR therapeutic regimen certification program is available by phone at 1-877-423-9927.

5.4 Secondary Malignancies

Myelodysplastic syndrome (MDS) or acute leukemia may occur with the use of the BEXXAR therapeutic regimen and were reported in 10% of patients enrolled in clinical trials and 3% of patients enrolled in the expanded access program (median follow-up of 39 and 27 months, respectively). The median time to development of MDS or leukemia was 31 months *[see Adverse Reactions (6.1)]*.

Non-hematologic malignancies may occur with the use of the BEXXAR therapeutic regimen and were reported in 5% of patients enrolled in clinical trials or the expanded access program. In the absence of controlled studies, the relative risk of secondary malignancies in patients receiving the BEXXAR therapeutic regimen cannot be determined *[see Adverse Reactions (6.1)]*.

5.5 Hypothyroidism

The BEXXAR therapeutic regimen can cause hypothyroidism *[see Adverse Reactions (6.1)]*. Initiate thyroid-blocking medications at least 24 hours before administering the dosimetric dose and continue until 14 days after the therapeutic dose *[see Dosage and Administration (2.4)]*. The risk of hypothyroidism is likely to be increased in patients who do not complete the recommended thyroid-protective regimen. Evaluate for clinical evidence of hypothyroidism and thyroid-stimulating hormone (TSH) level before treatment and annually thereafter.

5.6 Embryo-fetal Toxicity

The BEXXAR therapeutic regimen can cause fetal harm when administered to a pregnant woman including severe, and possibly irreversible, neonatal hypothyroidism. Inform patients who are pregnant or become pregnant after the BEXXAR therapeutic regimen about the potential hazard to a fetus. Evaluate infants born to mothers treated with the BEXXAR therapeutic regimen during pregnancy for hypothyroidism at time of delivery and during the neonatal period *[see Use in Specific Populations (8.1)]*.

Males and females of reproductive potential should use effective contraception during treatment with the BEXXAR therapeutic regimen and for 12 months after the therapeutic dose *[see Use in Specific Populations (8.7)]*.

5.7 Excessive Radiation Exposure in Patients With Impaired Renal Function

There are no data regarding the safety of administration of the BEXXAR therapeutic regimen in patients with impaired renal function. Since the BEXXAR therapeutic regimen is primarily cleared through the kidneys, the rate of excretion of radiolabeled iodine is expected to be decreased in patients with impaired renal function or obstructive uropathy, which may result in increased patient exposure to I-131 tositumomab. *[See Use in Specific Populations (8.6), Clinical Pharmacology (12.3).]*

5.8 Immunization

The safety of immunization with live viral vaccines following administration of the BEXXAR therapeutic regimen and the ability of patients who have received the BEXXAR therapeutic regimen to generate a primary or anamnestic humoral response to any vaccine have not been studied. Do not administer live viral vaccines to patients recently treated with BEXXAR.

6 ADVERSE REACTIONS

The following serious adverse reactions are discussed in greater detail in other sections of the label:

- Serious Allergic Reactions, Including Anaphylaxis *[see Boxed Warning, Warnings and Precautions (5.1)]*
- Prolonged and Severe Cytopenias *[see Warnings and Precautions (5.2)]*
- Secondary malignancies *[see Warnings and Precautions (5.4)]*
- Hypothyroidism *[see Warnings and Precautions (5.5)]*

The most common adverse reactions in patients receiving the BEXXAR therapeutic regimen (per-patient incidence greater than 25%) were neutropenia, thrombocytopenia, anemia, infections (including pneumonia, bacteremia, septicemia, bronchitis, and skin infections), infusion reactions, asthenia, fever, and nausea *[see Boxed Warning, Warnings and Precautions (5.1, 5.2)]*.

The most common serious adverse reactions in patients receiving the BEXXAR therapeutic regimen were severe and prolonged cytopenias, infections (including pneumonia, bacteremia, septicemia, bronchitis, and skin infections), serious allergic reactions (including bronchospasm and angioedema), infusion reactions, and secondary leukemia and myelodysplastic syndrome *[see Boxed Warning, Warnings and Precautions (5.1, 5.2, 5.4)]*.

6.1 Clinical Trials Experience

Because clinical trials are conducted under widely varying conditions, adverse reaction rates observed in the clinical trials of a drug cannot be directly compared to rates in the clinical trials of another drug and may not reflect the rates observed in clinical practice.

The reported safety data reflects exposure to the BEXXAR therapeutic regimen in 230 patients with non-Hodgkin's lymphoma enrolled in 5 clinical trials using the recommended dose and schedule. Patients were followed for a median of 39 months; 79% were followed for at least 12 months for survival and selected adverse reactions. Patients had a median of 3 prior chemotherapy regimens, a median age of 55 years, and 60% were male. Twenty-seven percent (27%) had transformation to a higher grade histology; 29% had intermediate-grade histology, and 2% had high-grade histology (IWF); 68% had Ann Arbor stage IV disease. Patients enrolled in these studies were not permitted to have prior hematopoietic stem cell transplantation or irradiation to more than 25% of the marrow space.

Data on serious adverse reactions and human anti-mouse antibodies (HAMA) and TSH levels were obtained from an additional 765 patients enrolled in the expanded access program and used to supplement the characterization of delayed adverse reactions. Patients in the expanded access program had fewer prior chemotherapy regimens (2 versus 3) and a higher proportion had low-grade histology (77% versus 70%) compared to patients in clinical trials.

Table 2. Incidence of Non-Hematologic Adverse Reactions Occurring in ≥5% of Patients Treated With the BEXXAR Therapeutic Regimen (N = 230)

Body System Preferred Term	All Grades	Grade 3/4
Total	96%	48%
Body as a Whole	81%	12%
Asthenia	46%	2%
Fever	37%	2%
Infection[a]	21%	<1%
Pain	19%	1%
Chills	18%	1%
Headache	16%	0%
Abdominal pain	15%	3%
Back pain	8%	1%
Chest pain	7%	0%
Neck pain	6%	1%
Cardiovascular System	26%	3%
Hypotension	7%	1%
Vasodilatation	5%	0%
Digestive System	56%	9%
Nausea	36%	3%
Vomiting	15%	1%
Anorexia	14%	0%
Diarrhea	12%	0%
Constipation	6%	1%
Dyspepsia	6%	<1%
Endocrine System	7%	0%
Hypothyroidism	7%	0%
Metabolic and Nutritional Disorders	21%	3%
Peripheral edema	9%	0%
Weight loss	6%	<1%
Musculoskeletal System	23%	3%
Myalgia	13%	<1%
Arthralgia	10%	1%
Nervous System	26%	3%
Dizziness	5%	0%
Somnolence	5%	0%
Respiratory System	44%	8%
Cough increased	21%	1%
Pharyngitis	12%	0%
Dyspnea	11%	3%
Rhinitis	10%	0%
Pneumonia	6%	0%

Skin and Appendages	44%	5%
Rash	17%	<1%
Pruritus	10%	0%
Sweating	8%	<1%

[a] The COSTART term for infection includes a subset of infections (e.g., upper respiratory infection). Other types of infections are mapped to preferred terms (e.g., pneumonia and sepsis).

Table 3. Hematologic Toxicity[a] (N = 230)

Parameter	Values
Platelets	
Median nadir (cells/mm^3)	43,000
Per patient incidence[a] platelets <50,000/mm^3	53% (n = 123)
Median[b] duration of platelets <50,000/mm^3	32 days
Grade 3/4 without recovery to Grade 2, N (%)	16 (7%)
Per patient incidence[c] platelets <25,000/mm^3	21% (n = 47)
Absolute Neutrophil Count (ANC)	
Median nadir (cells/mm^3)	690
Per patient incidence[a] ANC <1,000 cells/mm^3	63% (n = 145)
Median[b] duration of ANC <1,000 cells/mm^3	31 days
Grade 3/4 without recovery to Grade 2, N (%)	15 (7%)
Per patient incidence[c] ANC <500 cells/mm^3	25% (n = 57)
Hemoglobin	
Median nadir (gm/dL)	10
Per patient incidence[a] <8 gm/dL	29% (n = 66)
Median[b]duration of hemoglobin <8.0 gm/dL	23 days
Grade 3/4 without recovery to Grade 2, N (%)	12 (5%)
Per patient incidence[c] hemoglobin <6.5 gm/dL	5% (n = 11)

[a] Grade 3/4 toxicity was assumed if patient was missing 2 or more weeks of hematology data between Week 5 and Week 9.

[b] Duration of Grade 3/4 of 1,000+ days (censored) was assumed for those patients with undocumented Grade 3/4 and no hematologic data on or after Week 9.

[c] Grade 4 toxicity was assumed if patient had documented Grade 3 toxicity and was missing 2 or more weeks of hematology data between Week 5 and Week 9.

Prolonged and Severe Cytopenias: The incidence and duration of severe cytopenias are shown in Table 3. Sixty-three (27%) patients received one or more hematologic supportive care measures following the therapeutic dose including G–CSF, epoetin alfa, platelet transfusions, and packed red blood cell transfusions. Twenty-eight (12%) patients experienced hemorrhagic adverse reactions.

Infections: One hundred and four patients (45%) patients experienced one or more infections. Twenty (9%) experienced serious infections including pneumonia, bacteremia, septicemia, bronchitis, and skin infections.

Allergic (Hypersensitivity) Reactions: Fourteen patients (6%) experienced one or more of the following adverse reactions: allergic reaction, facial edema, injection site hypersensitivity, anaphylactic reaction, laryngismus, and serum sickness.

Infusion-related Adverse Reactions: Infusion reactions including fever, rigors or chills, sweating, hypotension, dyspnea, bronchospasm, and nausea occurred during or within 48 hours of infusion. Sixty-seven patients (29%) experienced fever, rigors/chills, or sweating within 14 days following the dosimetric dose. All patients in the clinical studies received pretreatment with acetaminophen and an antihistamine.

Myelodysplastic Syndrome (MDS)/Secondary Leukemia: The incidence of MDS/secondary leukemia among the 230 patients included in the clinical studies was 10% (24/230), with a median follow-up of 39 months and a median time to development of 34 months. The cumulative incidence of MDS/secondary leukemia was 4.7% at 2 years and 15% at 5 years. The incidence of MDS/secondary leukemia among the 765 patients in the expanded access program was 3% (20/765), with a median follow-up of 27 months and a median time to development of 31 months. The cumulative incidence of MDS/secondary leukemia in this patient population was 1.6% at 2 years and 6% at 5 years.

Secondary Malignancies: Of the 995 patients in clinical studies and the expanded access programs, there were 65 secondary malignancies reported in 54 patients (5%) in clinical studies and the expanded access program. These included non–melanoma skin cancers (26), colorectal cancer (7), head and neck cancer (6), breast cancer (5), lung cancer (4), bladder cancer (4), melanoma (3), and gastric cancer (2).

Hypothyroidism: Of the 230 patients in the clinical studies, 203 patients did not have elevated TSH at study entry. Of these, 137 patients had at least one post-treatment TSH value available and were not taking thyroid hormonal treatment at study entry. With a median follow-up period of 46 months, the incidence of hypothyroidism (elevated TSH or initiation of thyroid replacement therapy) was 18% with a median time to development of 16 months. The cumulative incidences of hypothyroidism at 2 and 5 years in these 137 patients were 11% and 19%, respectively. Onset of hypothyroidism has occurred up to 90 months post-treatment. The cumulative incidence and median time to development of hypothyroidism were similar in the expanded access program.

6.2 Immunogenicity

There is a potential for immunogenicity with therapeutic proteins such as tositumomab. Serum samples from 989 chemotherapy-relapsed or refractory patients included in the clinical studies or the expanded access program were tested by an enzyme-linked immunosorbent assay (ELISA) that detects antibodies to the Fc portion of IgG_1 murine immunoglobulin. One percent of the patients (11/989) had a positive serology for HAMA prior to treatment. The post-treatment incidence of HAMA seropositivity is summarized in Table 4.

[See table 4 below]

In a study of 76 previously untreated patients with low-grade non-Hodgkin's lymphoma who received the BEXXAR therapeutic regimen, the incidence of conversion to HAMA seropositivity was 70%, with a median time to development of 27 days.

Immunogenicity assay results are highly dependent on several factors including assay sensitivity and specificity, assay methodology, sample handling, timing of sample collection, concomitant medications, and underlying disease. For these reasons, comparison of incidence of antibodies to BEXXAR with the incidence of antibodies to other products may be misleading.

6.3 Postmarketing Experience

The following adverse reactions have been identified during post-approval use of the BEXXAR therapeutic regimen. Because these reactions are reported voluntarily from a population of uncertain size, it is not always possible to reliably estimate their frequency or establish a causal relationship to drug exposure.

Immune system disorders: Hypersensitivity reactions including fatal anaphylaxis.

Nervous system disorders: Axonal neuropathy leading to quadriparesis.

7 DRUG INTERACTIONS

No formal drug-drug interaction studies have been conducted with tositumomab or I-131 tositumomab.

8 USE IN SPECIFIC POPULATIONS

8.1 Pregnancy

Pregnancy: Category D *[see Warnings and Precautions (5.6)]*: There are no studies of the BEXXAR therapeutic regimen in pregnant women or animals. Based on the transplacental passage of I-131, administration of the BEXXAR therapeutic regimen to a pregnant woman can cause fetal harm including severe and possibly irreversible neonatal hypothyroidism. Limited data suggest an increased risk of miscarriage up to a year following I-131 treatment.

Inform patients who are pregnant or become pregnant after the BEXXAR therapeutic regimen about the potential hazard to a fetus. Evaluate infants born to mothers treated with the BEXXAR therapeutic regimen for hypothyroidism at the time of delivery and during the neonatal period.

8.3 Nursing Mothers

Because immunoglobulins are secreted in human milk, it is expected that tositumomab would be present in human milk. Radiolabeled iodine is excreted in breast milk and may reach concentrations equal to or greater than maternal plasma concentrations. Because of the potential for serious adverse reactions in nursing infants from the BEXXAR therapeutic regimen, advise women to discontinue nursing or to consider alternative treatment, taking into account the importance of the BEXXAR therapeutic regimen to the mother.

8.4 Pediatric Use

The safety and effectiveness of the BEXXAR therapeutic regimen have not been established in children.

8.5 Geriatric Use

Clinical studies of the BEXXAR therapeutic regimen did not include sufficient numbers of subjects aged 65 years and older to determine whether they respond differently from younger subjects.

8.6 Renal Impairment

Use of the BEXXAR therapeutic regimen has not been studied in patients with renal impairment *[see Warnings and Precautions (5.6), Clinical Pharmacology (12.3)]*.

8.7 Females and Males of Reproductive Potential

Contraception: Females of reproductive potential should use effective contraception during treatment with the BEXXAR therapeutic regimen and for 12 months after treatment ends to avoid the embryo-fetal effects of the radioisotope and the risk of increased pregnancy loss during that time period.

The BEXXAR therapeutic regimen exposes the testes to radiation *[see Dosage and Administration (2.9)]*. Because of the potential for mutagenesis in male gametes, males of reproductive potential should use effective contraception during treatment with the BEXXAR therapeutic regimen and for 12 months after treatment ends.

Infertility: The BEXXAR therapeutic regimen results in radiation exposure of the ovaries and testes. Based on published studies examining patients treated with I-131, the BEXXAR therapeutic regimen may cause transient ovarian or testicular dysfunction. Radiation effects may persist for up to 12 months following treatment.

10 OVERDOSAGE

The maximum radiation activity of the I-131 component of the BEXXAR therapeutic regimen, administered to 4 patients, were doses calculated to deliver between 85 cGy and 88 cGy total body irradiation. The incidence of NCI Grade 4 cytopenias was increased in these 4 patients compared to patients who received the recommended therapeutic dose for the BEXXAR therapeutic regimen.

11 DESCRIPTION

The BEXXAR therapeutic regimen is composed of the monoclonal antibody tositumomab, and the radiolabeled monoclonal antibody, I-131 tositumomab.

Tositumomab is a murine IgG_{2a} lambda monoclonal antibody directed against the CD20 antigen, produced in mammalian cells. The approximate molecular weight of tositumomab is 150 kD.

Tositumomab is supplied as a sterile, pyrogen-free, clear to opalescent, colorless to slightly yellow, preservative-free solution that must be diluted before intravenous administration. The formulation contains 100 mg/mL maltose, 8.5 mg/mL sodium chloride, 1 mg/mL phosphate, 1 mg/mL potassium hydroxide, and Water for Injection, USP. The pH is approximately 7.2.

I-131 tositumomab is tositumomab covalently linked to Iodine-131. I-131 tositumomab is supplied as a sterile, clear, preservative-free liquid. The formulation for I-131 tositumomab contains 0.9 to 1.3 mg/mL ascorbic acid, 1 to 2 mg/mL maltose (dosimetric dose) or 9 to 15 mg/mL maltose (therapeutic dose), 4.4% to 6.6% (w/v) povidone, and 8.5 to 9.5 mg/mL sodium chloride. The pH is approximately 7.0.

Physical/Radiochemical Characteristics of Iodine-131: Iodine-131 decays with beta and gamma emissions with a physical half-life of 8.04 days. The principal beta emission has a mean energy of 191.6 keV, and the principal gamma emission has energy of 364.5 keV.

External Radiation: The specific gamma ray constant for Iodine-131 is 2.2 R/millicurie hour at 1 cm. Use a 2.55 cm thickness of Pb (to attenuate the radiation emitted by a factor of about 1,000) to minimize radiation exposure from this radionuclide.

The fraction of Iodine-131 radioactivity that remains in the vial × days after the date of calibration is $2^{-(x/8.04)}$. Physical decay is presented in Table 5.

Table 4. Incidence of HAMA Seropositivity Among Patients With Chemotherapy-refractory or Relapsed Non-Hodgkin's Lymphoma Receiving the BEXXAR Therapeutic Regimen

Chemotherapy-refractory or relapsed patients	Percent HAMA positive	Kaplan-Meier estimate of HAMA positivity		
		6 months	12 months	18 months
In clinical trials	23/219 (11%)	6%	17%	21%
In expanded-access program	57/569 (10%)	7%	12%	13%

Table 5. Physical Decay Chart: Iodine-131: Half-Life 8.04 Days

Days	Fraction Remaining
0[a]	1.000
1	0.917
2	0.842
3	0.772
4	0.708
5	0.650
6	0.596
7	0.547
8	0.502
9	0.460
10	0.422
11	0.387
12	0.355
13	0.326
14	0.299

[a] Calibration day.

12 CLINICAL PHARMACOLOGY

12.1 Mechanism of Action

Tositumomab binds specifically to an epitope within the extracellular domain of the CD20 molecule. The CD20 molecule is expressed on normal B lymphocytes (pre-B lymphocytes to mature B lymphocytes) and on B-cell non-Hodgkin's lymphomas. The CD20 molecule is not shed from the cell surface and is not internalized following antibody binding. The BEXXAR therapeutic regimen induces cell death by emitting ionizing radiation to CD20-expressing lymphocytes or neighboring cells. In addition to cell death mediated by the radioisotope, other possible mechanisms of action include antibody-dependent cellular cytotoxicity, complement-dependent cytotoxicity, and CD20-mediated apoptosis.

12.2 Pharmacodynamics

In two clinical studies (one in chemotherapy-naive patients and one in heavily pretreated patients), the administration of the BEXXAR therapeutic regimen resulted in sustained depletion of circulating CD20-positive cells. The assessment of circulating lymphocytes in these patients did not distinguish normal from malignant cells; consequently, recovery of normal B cell numbers was not directly assessed. At 7 weeks following treatment, the median number of circulating CD20-positive cells was zero (range: 0 to 490 cells/mm^3) with recovery beginning at approximately 12 weeks. At 6 months following treatment, 8 (14%) of 58 chemotherapy-naive patients and 6 (32%) of 19 heavily pretreated patients had CD20-positive cell counts below normal limits. There was no consistent effect of the BEXXAR therapeutic regimen on post-treatment serum IgG, IgA, or IgM levels.

12.3 Pharmacokinetics

A pharmacokinetic study of I-131 tositumomab determined that a 475-mg predose of unlabeled antibody decreased splenic targeting and increased the terminal half-life of the radiolabeled antibody. The median blood clearance following administration of 485 mg of tositumomab in 110 patients with non-Hodgkin's lymphomas was 68.2 mg/hr (range: 30.2 to 260.8 mg/hr). Patients with high tumor burden, splenomegaly, or bone marrow involvement were noted to have a larger volume of distribution, faster clearance, and shorter terminal half-life. The total body clearance, as measured by total body gamma camera counts, was dependent on the same factors noted for blood clearance. Patient-specific dosing, based on total body clearance, provided a consistent radiation dose despite variable pharmacokinetics, by allowing each patient's administered activity to be adjusted for individual patient variables. The median total body effective half-life, as measured by total body gamma camera counts, in 980 patients with non-Hodgkin's lymphoma was 67 hours (range: 28 to 115 hours).

Elimination of Iodine-131 occurs by decay (Table 5) and excretion in the urine. Five days following the dose, the whole body clearance was 67% of the injected dose. Ninety-eight percent (98%) of the clearance was accounted for in the urine.

13 NONCLINICAL TOXICOLOGY

13.1 Carcinogenesis, Mutagenesis, Impairment of Fertility

No long-term animal studies have been performed to establish the carcinogenic or mutagenic potential of the BEXXAR therapeutic regimen or to determine its effects on fertility in males or females. However, Iodine I-131 is a potential carcinogen and mutagen.

Administration of the BEXXAR therapeutic regimen exposes the testes and ovaries to radiation *[see Dosage and Administration (2.9)]*.

14 CLINICAL STUDIES

The clinical benefit of the BEXXAR therapeutic regimen was established in a single-arm clinical trial conducted in 40 patients with low-grade, transformed low-grade, or follicular large-cell lymphoma. Patients had a Karnofsky performance status of at least 60%, a granulocyte count of 1,500 cells/mm^3, a platelet count greater than or equal to 100,000/mm^3, less than or equal to 25% of the intratrabecular marrow space involved by lymphoma, and no evidence of progressive disease arising in a field irradiated with >3,500 cGy within one year of completion of irradiation.

This study enrolled 40 patients with low-grade or transformed low-grade or follicular large-cell lymphoma whose disease had not responded to, or had progressed following, at least 4 doses of rituximab therapy. The median age was 57 years (range: 35 to 78 years); the median time from diagnosis to protocol entry was 50 months (range: 12 to 170 months); and the median number of prior chemotherapy regimens was 4 (range: 1 to 11). Overall, 35 of the 40 patients were rituximab-refractory (defined as no response or a response of less than 6 months' duration following rituximab therapy).

The main outcome measure in Study was overall response rate as determined by an independent panel that reviewed patient records and radiologic studies (Table 6).

Table 6. Efficacy Outcomes for the BEXXAR Therapeutic Regimen

Response	n = 40
Overall Response	
Rate	68%
95% CI[a]	(51%, 81%)
Response Duration (months)	
Median	16
95% CI[a]	(10, NR[b])
Range	1+ to 38+
Complete Response[c]	
Rate	33%
95% CI[a]	(19%, 49%)
Complete Response[c] Response Duration (months)	
Median	NR[b]
95% CI[a]	(15, NR)
Range	4 to 38+

[a] CI = confidence interval
[b] NR = not reached, median duration of follow-up = 26 months
[c] Complete response rate = pathologic and clinical complete responses

The results of this study were supported by demonstration of durable objective responses in 4 single-arm studies enrolling 190 patients evaluable for efficacy with rituximab-naïve, follicular non-Hodgkin's lymphoma with or without transformation, who had relapsed following or were refractory to chemotherapy. In these studies, the overall response rates ranged from 47% to 64% and the median durations of response ranged from 12 to 18 months

16 HOW SUPPLIED/STORAGE AND HANDLING

The BEXXAR therapeutic regimen is supplied as 2 separate units: dosimetric step components and therapeutic step components. The components of the dosimetric step are shipped from separate sites; when ordering, ensure that the components are scheduled to arrive on the same day. Similarly, the components of the therapeutic step are shipped from separate sites; when ordering, ensure that the components are scheduled to arrive on the same day.

16.1 Dosimetric Dose Components

- A carton (NDC 0007-3260-31) containing 2 single-use 225-mg vials (NDC 0007-3260-01) and 1 single-use 35-mg vial (NDC 0007-3260-21) of tositumomab solution each at a nominal concentration of 14 mg/mL
- One single-use vial (NDC 0007-3261-01) containing not less than 20 mL of I-131 tositumomab solution at not less than protein and activity concentrations of 0.1 mg/mL and 0.61 mCi/mL (at calibration)

16.2 Therapeutic Dose Components

- A carton (NDC 0007-3260-36) containing 2 single-use 225-mg vials (NDC 0007-3260-01) and 1 single-use 35-mg vial (NDC 0007-3260-21) of tositumomab solution each at a nominal concentration of 14 mg/mL
- One or 2 single-use vials (NDC 0007-3262-01) each containing not less than 20 mL of I-131 tositumomab solution at not less than protein and activity concentrations of 1.1 mg/mL and 5.6 mCi/mL (at calibration)

16.3 Storage

Tositumomab: Store vials (including diluted vials) of tositumomab (35 mg and 225 mg) at 36°F to 46°F (2°C to 8°C). Protect from strong light. **Do not shake; do not freeze.** Diluted tositumomab solutions are stable for up to 24 hours when stored refrigerated and for up to 8 hours at room temperature. Discard unused portions.

I-131 tositumomab: Store vials of I-131 tositumomab in the original lead pot at a temperature of -4°F (-20°C) or below until thawed prior to administration.

Thawed dosimetric and therapeutic doses of I-131 tositumomab (including diluted vials) are stable for up to 8 hours at 36°F to 46°F (2°C to 8°C) or at room temperature. I-131 tositumomab does not contain a preservative. **Do not shake; do not freeze.** Discard unused portions according to federal and state laws regarding radioactive and biohazardous waste.

17 PATIENT COUNSELING INFORMATION

Advise patients:

- To take premedications, including thyroid-blocking agents as prescribed *[see Warnings and Precautions (5.5)]*.
- To contact a healthcare professional if they experience signs and symptoms of allergic reactions *[see Warnings and Precautions (5.1)]*.
- To report to a health care professional any signs of cytopenias (bleeding, easy bruising, petechiae or purpura, pallor, weakness or fatigue, or symptoms of infection such as fever) *[see Warnings and Precautions (5.2)]*.
- Of the need for frequent monitoring for up to 3 months after treatment, and the potential for persistent cytopenias beyond 3 months.
- Concerning the risk of radiation exposure to household contacts, pregnant women and small children from radioactive materials remaining in the patient's body following the BEXXAR therapeutic regimen. Provide patient-specific advice orally and in writing *[see Warnings and Precautions (5.3)]*.
- Of the need for life-long monitoring for hypothyroidism *[see Warnings and Precautions (5.5)]*.
- Who are pregnant that the BEXXAR therapeutic regimen can cause hypothyroidism in the infant *[see Warnings and Precautions (5.6), Use in Special Populations (8.7)]*.
- To check with their physicians before receiving live virus vaccinations *[see Warnings and Precautions (5.8)]*.
- Who are of reproductive potential to use effective contraceptive methods during treatment and for a minimum of 12 months following the BEXXAR therapeutic regimen *[see Use in Special Populations (8.7)]*.
- To discontinue nursing during and after the BEXXAR therapeutic regimen *[see Use in Special Populations (8.3)]*.

BEXXAR is a registered trademark of GlaxoSmithKline.
LUER-LOK is a trademark of Becton, Dickinson and Company.

Manufactured by **GlaxoSmithKline LLC**
Wilmington, DE 19808
U.S. Lic. 1727
Marketed by **GlaxoSmithKline**
Research Triangle Park, NC 27709

BXX:4PI

BOOSTRIX ℞

[boos' trix]

(Tetanus Toxoid, Reduced Diphtheria Toxoid and Acellular Pertussis Vaccine, Adsorbed)
Suspension for Intramuscular Injection

HIGHLIGHTS OF PRESCRIBING INFORMATION
These highlights do not include all the information needed to use BOOSTRIX safely and effectively. See full prescribing information for BOOSTRIX.
BOOSTRIX (Tetanus Toxoid, Reduced Diphtheria Toxoid and Acellular Pertussis Vaccine, Adsorbed)
Suspension for Intramuscular Injection
Initial U.S. Approval: 2005

INDICATIONS AND USAGE

BOOSTRIX is a vaccine indicated for active booster immunization against tetanus, diphtheria, and pertussis. BOOSTRIX is approved for use as a single dose in individuals 10 years of age and older. (1)

DOSAGE AND ADMINISTRATION

A single intramuscular injection (0.5 mL). (2.2)

DOSAGE FORMS AND STRENGTHS

Single-dose vials and prefilled syringes containing a 0.5-mL suspension for injection. (3)

CONTRAINDICATIONS

- Severe allergic reaction (e.g., anaphylaxis) after a previous dose of any tetanus toxoid-, diphtheria toxoid-, or pertussis antigen-containing vaccine or to any component of BOOSTRIX. (4.1)
- Encephalopathy (e.g., coma, decreased level of consciousness, prolonged seizures) within 7 days of administration of a previous pertussis antigen-containing vaccine. (4.2)

WARNINGS AND PRECAUTIONS

- BOOSTRIX is available in vials and 2 types of prefilled syringes. One type of prefilled syringe has a tip cap which may contain natural rubber latex. The other type has a tip cap and a rubber plunger which contain dry natural latex rubber. Use of these syringes may cause allergic reactions in latex-sensitive individuals. (5.1, 16)

- If Guillain-Barré syndrome occurred within 6 weeks of receipt of a prior vaccine containing tetanus toxoid, the risk of Guillain-Barré syndrome may be increased following a subsequent dose of tetanus toxoid-containing vaccine, including BOOSTRIX. (5.2)
- Syncope (fainting) can occur in association with administration of injectable vaccines, including BOOSTRIX. Procedures should be in place to avoid falling injury and to restore cerebral perfusion following syncope. (5.3)
- Progressive or unstable neurologic conditions are reasons to defer vaccination with a pertussis-containing vaccine, including BOOSTRIX. (5.4)
- Persons who experienced an Arthus-type hypersensitivity reaction following a prior dose of a tetanus toxoid-containing vaccine should not receive BOOSTRIX unless at least 10 years have elapsed since the last dose of a tetanus toxoid-containing vaccine. (5.5)

ADVERSE REACTIONS

- Common solicited adverse events (≥15%) in adolescents (10 to 18 years of age) were pain, redness, and swelling at the injection site, increase in arm circumference of injected arm, headache, fatigue, and gastrointestinal symptoms. (6.1)
- Common solicited adverse events (≥15%) in adults (19 to 64 years of age) were pain, redness, and swelling at the injection site, headache, fatigue, and gastrointestinal symptoms. (6.1)
- The most common solicited adverse event (≥15%) in the elderly (65 years of age and older) was pain at the injection site. (6.1)

To report SUSPECTED ADVERSE REACTIONS, contact GlaxoSmithKline at 1-888-825-5249 or VAERS at 1-800-822-7967 or www.vaers.hhs.gov.

DRUG INTERACTIONS

- In subjects 11 to 18 years of age, lower levels for antibodies to pertactin were observed when BOOSTRIX was administered concomitantly with meningococcal conjugate vaccine (serogroups A, C, Y, and W-135) as compared to BOOSTRIX administered first. (7.1)
- In subjects 19 to 64 years of age, lower levels for antibodies to FHA and pertactin were observed when BOOSTRIX was administered concomitantly with an inactivated influenza vaccine as compared to BOOSTRIX alone. (7.1)
- Do not mix BOOSTRIX with any other vaccine in the same syringe or vial. (7.1)

USE IN SPECIFIC POPULATIONS

- Safety and effectiveness of BOOSTRIX have not been established in pregnant women. (8.1)
- Register women who receive BOOSTRIX while pregnant in the pregnancy registry by calling 1-888-452-9622. (8.1)

See 17 for PATIENT COUNSELING INFORMATION

Revised: 02/2013

FULL PRESCRIBING INFORMATION: CONTENTS*

*** Sections or subsections omitted from the full prescribing information are not listed**

FULL PRESCRIBING INFORMATION

1 Indications and Usage

BOOSTRIX® is indicated for active booster immunization against tetanus, diphtheria, and pertussis. *BOOSTRIX is approved for use as a single dose in individuals 10 years of age and older.*

2 Dosage and Administration

2.1 Preparation for Administration

Shake vigorously to obtain a homogeneous, turbid, white suspension before administration. Do not use if resuspension does not occur with vigorous shaking. Parenteral drug products should be inspected visually for particulate matter and discoloration prior to administration, whenever solution and container permit. If either of these conditions exists, the vaccine should not be administered.

For the prefilled syringes, attach a sterile needle and administer intramuscularly.

For the vials, use a sterile needle and sterile syringe to withdraw the 0.5–mL dose and administer intramuscularly. Changing needles between drawing vaccine from a vial and injecting it into a recipient is not necessary unless the needle has been damaged or contaminated. Use a separate sterile needle and syringe for each individual.

Do not administer this product intravenously, intradermally, or subcutaneously.

2.2 Dose and Schedule

BOOSTRIX is administered as a single 0.5-mL intramuscular injection into the deltoid muscle of the upper arm.

There are no data to support repeat administration of BOOSTRIX.

Five years should elapse between the last dose of the recommended series of Diphtheria and Tetanus Toxoids and Acellular Pertussis Vaccine Adsorbed (DTaP) and/or Tetanus and Diphtheria Toxoids Adsorbed For Adult Use (Td) vaccine and the administration of BOOSTRIX.

2.3 Additional Dosing Information

Primary Series: The use of BOOSTRIX as a primary series or to complete the primary series for diphtheria, tetanus, or pertussis has not been studied.

Wound Management: If tetanus prophylaxis is needed for wound management, BOOSTRIX may be given if no previous dose of any Tetanus Toxoid, Reduced Diphtheria Toxoid and Acellular Pertussis Vaccine, Adsorbed (Tdap) has been administered.

3 Dosage Forms and Strengths

BOOSTRIX is a suspension for injection available in 0.5-mL single-dose vials and prefilled TIP-LOK® syringes.

4 Contraindications

4.1 Hypersensitivity

A severe allergic reaction (e.g., anaphylaxis) after a previous dose of any tetanus toxoid-, diphtheria toxoid-, or pertussis antigen-containing vaccine or any component of this vaccine is a contraindication to administration of BOOSTRIX *[see Description (11)]*. Because of the uncertainty as to which component of the vaccine might be responsible, none of the components should be administered. Alternatively, such individuals may be referred to an allergist for evaluation if immunization with any of these components is considered.

4.2 Encephalopathy

Encephalopathy (e.g., coma, decreased level of consciousness, prolonged seizures) within 7 days of administration of a previous dose of a pertussis antigen-containing vaccine that is not attributable to another identifiable cause is a contraindication to administration of any pertussis antigen-containing vaccine, including BOOSTRIX.

5 Warnings and Precautions

5.1 Latex

BOOSTRIX is available in vials and 2 types of prefilled syringes. One type of prefilled syringe has a tip cap which may contain natural rubber latex and a plunger which does not contain latex. The other type has a tip cap and a rubber plunger which contain dry natural latex rubber. Use of these syringes may cause allergic reactions in latex-sensitive individuals. The vial stopper does not contain latex. *[See How Supplied/Storage and Handling (16).]*

5.2 Guillain-Barré Syndrome and Brachial Neuritis

If Guillain-Barré syndrome occurred within 6 weeks of receipt of a prior vaccine containing tetanus toxoid, the risk of Guillain-Barré syndrome may be increased following a subsequent dose of tetanus toxoid-containing vaccine, including BOOSTRIX. A review by the Institute of Medicine (IOM) found evidence for a causal relationship between receipt of tetanus toxoid and both brachial neuritis and Guillain-Barré syndrome.[1]

5.3 Syncope

Syncope (fainting) can occur in association with administration of injectable vaccines, including BOOSTRIX. Syncope can be accompanied by transient neurological signs such as visual disturbance, paresthesia, and tonic-clonic limb movements. Procedures should be in place to avoid falling injury and to restore cerebral perfusion following syncope.

5.4 Progressive or Unstable Neurologic Disorders

Progressive or unstable neurologic conditions (e.g., cerebrovascular events and acute encephalopathic conditions) are reasons to defer vaccination with a pertussis-containing vaccine, including BOOSTRIX. It is not known whether administration of BOOSTRIX to persons with an unstable or progressive neurologic disorder might hasten manifestations of the disorder or affect the prognosis. Administration of BOOSTRIX to persons with an unstable or progressive neurologic disorder may result in diagnostic confusion between manifestations of the underlying illness and possible adverse effects of vaccination.

5.5 Arthus-Type Hypersensitivity

Persons who experienced an Arthus-type hypersensitivity reaction following a prior dose of a tetanus toxoid-containing vaccine usually have a high serum tetanus antitoxin level and should not receive BOOSTRIX or other tetanus toxoid-containing vaccines unless at least 10 years have elapsed since the last dose of tetanus toxoid-containing vaccine.

5.6 Altered Immunocompetence

As with any vaccine, if administered to immunosuppressed persons, including individuals receiving immunosuppressive therapy, the expected immune response may not be obtained.

5.7 Prevention and Management of Acute Allergic Reactions

Prior to administration, the healthcare provider should review the immunization history for possible vaccine sensitivity and previous vaccination-related adverse reactions to allow an assessment of benefits and risks. Epinephrine and other appropriate agents used for the control of immediate allergic reactions must be immediately available should an acute anaphylactic reaction occur.

6 Adverse Reactions

6.1 Clinical Trials Experience

Because clinical trials are conducted under widely varying conditions, adverse reaction rates observed in the clinical trials of a vaccine cannot be directly compared to rates in the clinical trials of another vaccine, and may not reflect the rates observed in practice. As with any vaccine, there is the possibility that broad use of BOOSTRIX could reveal adverse reactions not observed in clinical trials.

In clinical studies, 4,949 adolescents (10 to 18 years of age) and 4,076 adults (19 years of age and older) were vaccinated with a single dose of BOOSTRIX. Of these adolescents, 1,341 were vaccinated with BOOSTRIX in a coadministration study with meningococcal conjugate vaccine *[see Drug Interactions (7.1) and Clinical Studies (14.5)]*. Of these adults, 1,104 were 65 years of age and older *[see Clinical Studies (14.4)]*. A total of 860 adults19 years of age and older received concomitant vaccination with BOOSTRIX and influenza vaccines in a coadministration study *[see Drug Interactions (7.1) and Clinical Studies (14.5)]*. An additional 1,092 adolescents 10 to 18 years of age received a non-US formulation of BOOSTRIX (formulated to contain 0.5 mg aluminum per dose) in non-US clinical studies.

In a randomized, observer-blinded, controlled study in the US, 3,080 adolescents 10 to 18 years of age received a single dose of BOOSTRIX and 1,034 received the comparator Td vaccine, manufactured by MassBioLogics. There were no substantive differences in demographic characteristics between the vaccine groups. Among BOOSTRIX and comparator vaccine recipients, approximately 75% were 10 to 14 years of age and approximately 25% were 15 to 18 years of age. Approximately 98% of participants in this study had received the recommended series of 4 or 5 doses of either Diphtheria and Tetanus Toxoids and Pertussis Vaccine Adsorbed (DTwP) or a combination of DTwP and DTaP in childhood. Subjects were monitored for solicited adverse events using standardized diary cards (day 0-14). Unsolicited adverse events were monitored for the 31-day period following vaccination (day 0-30). Subjects were also monitored for 6 months post-vaccination for non-routine medical visits, visits to an emergency room, onset of new chronic illness, and serious adverse events. Information regarding late onset adverse events was obtained via a telephone call

6 months following vaccination. At least 97% of subjects completed the 6-month follow-up evaluation.

In a study conducted in Germany, BOOSTRIX was administered to 319 children 10 to 12 years of age previously vaccinated with 5 doses of acellular pertussis antigen-containing vaccines; 193 of these subjects had previously received 5 doses of INFANRIX® (Diphtheria and Tetanus Toxoids and Acellular Pertussis Vaccine Adsorbed). Adverse events were recorded on diary cards during the 15 days following vaccination. Unsolicited adverse events that occurred within 31 days of vaccination (day 0-30) were recorded on the diary card or verbally reported to the investigator. Subjects were monitored for 6 months post-vaccination for physician office visits, emergency room visits, onset of new chronic illness, and serious adverse events. The 6-month follow-up evaluation, conducted via telephone interview, was completed by 90% of subjects.

The US adult (19 to 64 years of age) study, a randomized, observer-blinded study, evaluated the safety of BOOSTRIX (N = 1,522) compared with ADACEL® (Tetanus Toxoid, Reduced Diphtheria Toxoid and Acellular Pertussis Vaccine Adsorbed) (N = 762), a Tdap vaccine manufactured by Sanofi Pasteur SA. Vaccines were administered as a single dose. There were no substantive differences in demographic characteristics between the vaccine groups. Subjects were monitored for solicited adverse events using standardized diary cards (day 0-14). Unsolicited adverse events were monitored for the 31-day period following vaccination (day 0-30). Subjects were also monitored for 6 months post-vaccination for serious adverse events, visits to an emergency room, hospitalizations, and onset of new chronic illness. Approximately 95% of subjects completed the 6-month follow-up evaluation.

The US elderly (65 years of age and older) study, a randomized, observer-blinded study, evaluated the safety of BOOSTRIX (N = 887) compared with DECAVAC® (Tetanus and Diphtheria Toxoids Adsorbed) (N = 445), a US-licensed Td vaccine, manufactured by Sanofi Pasteur SA. Vaccines were administered as a single dose. Among all vaccine recipients, the mean age was approximately 72 years; 54% were female and 95% were white. Subjects were monitored for solicited adverse events using standardized diary cards (day 0-3). Unsolicited adverse events were monitored for the 31-day period following vaccination (day 0-30). Subjects were also monitored for 6 months post-vaccination for serious adverse events. Approximately 99% of subjects completed the 6-month follow-up evaluation.

Solicited Adverse Events in the US Adolescent Study: Table 1 presents the solicited local adverse reactions and general adverse events within 15 days of vaccination with BOOSTRIX or Td vaccine for the total vaccinated cohort.

The primary safety endpoint was the incidence of grade 3 pain (spontaneously painful and/or prevented normal activity) at the injection site within 15 days of vaccination. Grade 3 pain was reported in 4.6% of those who received BOOSTRIX compared with 4.0% of those who received the Td vaccine. The difference in rate of grade 3 pain was within the pre-defined clinical limit for non-inferiority (upper limit of the 95% CI for the difference [BOOSTRIX minus Td] ≤4%).

Table 1. Rates of Solicited Local Adverse Reactions or General Adverse Events Within the 15-day[a] Post-Vaccination Period in Adolescents 10 to 18 Years of Age (Total Vaccinated Cohort)

	BOOSTRIX (N = 3,032) %	Td (N = 1,013) %
Local		
Pain, any[b]	75.3	71.7
Pain, grade 2 or 3[b]	51.2	42.5
Pain, grade 3[c]	4.6	4.0
Redness, any	22.5	19.8
Redness, >20 mm	4.1	3.9
Redness, ≥50 mm	1.7	1.6
Swelling, any	21.1	20.1
Swelling, >20 mm	5.3	4.9
Swelling, ≥50 mm	2.5	3.2
Arm circumference increase, >5 mm[d]	28.3	29.5
Arm circumference increase, >20 mm[d]	2.0	2.2
Arm circumference increase, >40 mm[d]	0.5	0.3
General		
Headache, any	43.1	41.5
Headache, grade 2 or 3[b]	15.7	12.7
Headache, grade 3	3.7	2.7
Fatigue, any	37.0	36.7
Fatigue, grade 2 or 3	14.4	12.9
Fatigue, grade 3	3.7	3.2
Gastrointestinal symptoms, any[e]	26.0	25.8
Gastrointestinal symptoms, grade 2 or 3[e]	9.8	9.7
Gastrointestinal symptoms, grade 3[e]	3.0	3.2
Fever, ≥99.5°F (37.5°C)[f]	13.5	13.1
Fever, >100.4°F (38.0°C)[f]	5.0	4.7
Fever, >102.2°F (39.0°C)[f]	1.4	1.0

Td = Tetanus and Diphtheria Toxoids Adsorbed For Adult Use manufactured by MassBioLogics.
N = Number of subjects in the total vaccinated cohort with local/general symptoms sheets completed.
Grade 2 = Local: painful when limb moved; General: interfered with normal activity.
Grade 3 = Local: spontaneously painful and/or prevented normal activity; General: prevented normal activity.
[a] Day of vaccination and the next 14 days.
[b] Statistically significantly higher (P <0.05) following BOOSTRIX as compared to Td vaccine.
[c] Grade 3 injection site pain following BOOSTRIX was not inferior to Td vaccine (upper limit of two-sided 95% CI for the difference [BOOSTRIX minus Td] in the percentage of subjects <4%).
[d] Mid-upper region of the vaccinated arm.
[e] Gastrointestinal symptoms included nausea, vomiting, diarrhea, and/or abdominal pain.
[f] Oral temperatures or axillary temperatures.

Unsolicited Adverse Events in the US Adolescent Study: The incidence of unsolicited adverse events reported in the 31 days after vaccination was comparable between the 2 groups (25.4% and 24.5% for BOOSTRIX and Td vaccine, respectively).

Solicited Adverse Events in the German Adolescent Study: Table 2 presents the rates of solicited local adverse reactions and fever within 15 days of vaccination for those subjects who had previously been vaccinated with 5 doses of INFANRIX. No cases of whole arm swelling were reported. Two individuals (2/193) reported large injection site swelling (range 110 to 200 mm diameter), in one case associated with grade 3 pain. Neither individual sought medical attention. These episodes were reported to resolve without sequelae within 5 days.

Table 2. Rates of Solicited Adverse Events Reported Within the 15-day[a] Post-Vaccination Period Following Administration of BOOSTRIX in Adolescents 10 to 12 Years of Age Who Had Previously Received 5 Doses of INFANRIX

	BOOSTRIX (N = 193) %
Pain, any	62.2
Pain, grade 2 or 3	33.2
Pain, grade 3	5.7
Redness, any	47.7
Redness, >20 mm	15.0
Redness, ≥50 mm	10.9
Swelling, any	38.9
Swelling, >20 mm	17.6
Swelling, ≥50 mm	14.0
Fever, ≥99.5°F (37.5°C)[b]	8.8
Fever, >100.4°F (38.0°C)[b]	4.1
Fever, >102.2°F (39.0°C)[b]	1.0

N = Number of subjects with local/general symptoms sheets completed.
Grade 2 = Painful when limb moved.
Grade 3 = Spontaneously painful and/or prevented normal activity.
[a]Day of vaccination and the next 14 days.
[b]Oral temperatures or axillary temperatures.

Solicited Adverse Events in the US Adult (19 to 64 Years of Age) Study: Table 3 presents solicited local adverse reactions and general adverse events within 15 days of vaccination with BOOSTRIX or the comparator Tdap vaccine for the total vaccinated cohort.

Table 3. Rates of Solicited Local Adverse Reactions or General Adverse Events Within the 15-day[a] Post-Vaccination Period in Adults 19 to 64 Years of Age (Total Vaccinated Cohort)

	BOOSTRIX (N = 1,480) %	Tdap (N = 741) %
Local		
Pain, any	61.0	69.2
Pain, grade 2 or 3	35.1	44.4
Pain, grade 3	1.6	2.3
Redness, any	21.1	27.1
Redness, >20 mm	4.0	6.2
Redness, ≥50 mm	1.6	2.3
Swelling, any	17.6	25.6
Swelling, >20 mm	3.9	6.3
Swelling, ≥50 mm	1.4	2.8
General		
Headache, any	30.1	31.0
Headache, grade 2 or 3	11.1	10.5
Headache, grade 3	2.2	1.5
Fatigue, any	28.1	28.9
Fatigue, grade 2 or 3	9.1	9.4
Fatigue, grade 3	2.5	1.2
Gastrointestinal symptoms, any[b]	15.9	17.5
Gastrointestinal symptoms, grade 2 or 3[b]	4.3	5.7
Gastrointestinal symptoms, grade 3[b]	1.2	1.3
Fever, ≥99.5°F (37.5°C)[c]	5.5	8.0
Fever, >100.4°F (38.0°C)[c]	1.0	1.5
Fever, >102.2°F (39.0°C)[c]	0.1	0.4

Tdap = Tetanus Toxoid, Reduced Diphtheria Toxoid and Acellular Pertussis Vaccine Adsorbed, a Tdap vaccine manufactured by Sanofi Pasteur SA.
N = Number of subjects in the total vaccinated cohort with local/general symptoms sheets completed.
Grade 2 = Local: painful when limb moved; General: interfered with normal activity.
Grade 3 = Local/General: prevented normal activity.
[a] Day of vaccination and the next 14 days.
[b] Gastrointestinal symptoms included nausea, vomiting, diarrhea, and/or abdominal pain.
[c] Oral temperatures.

Unsolicited Adverse Events in the US Adult (19 to 64 Years of Age) Study: The incidence of unsolicited adverse events reported in the 31 days after vaccination was comparable between the 2 groups (17.8% and 22.2% for BOOSTRIX and Tdap vaccine, respectively).

Solicited Adverse Events in the US Elderly (65 Years of Age and Older) Study: Table 4 presents solicited local adverse reactions and general adverse events within 4 days of vaccination with BOOSTRIX or the comparator Td vaccine for the total vaccinated cohort.

Table 4. Rates of Solicited Local Adverse Reactions or General Adverse Events Within 4 Days[a] of Vaccination in the Elderly 65 Years of Age and Older (Total Vaccinated Cohort)

	BOOSTRIX %	Td %
Local	(N = 882)	(N = 444)
Pain, any	21.5	27.7
Pain, grade 2 or 3	7.5	10.1
Pain, grade 3	0.2	0.7
Redness, any	10.8	12.6
Redness, >20 mm	1.4	2.5
Redness, ≥50 mm	0.6	0.9
Swelling, any	7.5	11.7

Swelling, >20 mm	2.2	3.4
Swelling, ≥50 mm	0.7	0.7
General	**(N = 882)**	**(N = 445)**
Fatigue, any	12.5	14.8
Fatigue, grade 2 or 3	2.5	2.9
Fatigue, grade 3	0.7	0.7
Headache, any	11.5	11.7
Headache, grade 2 or 3	1.9	2.2
Headache, grade 3	0.6	0.0
Gastrointestinal symptoms, any[b]	7.6	9.2
Gastrointestinal symptoms, grade 2 or 3[b]	1.7	1.8
Gastrointestinal symptoms, grade 3[b]	0.3	0.4
Fever, ≥99.5°F (37.5°C)[c]	2.0	2.5
Fever, >100.4°F (38.0°C)[c]	0.2	0.2
Fever, >102.2°F (39.0°C)[c]	0.0	0.0

Td = Tetanus and Diphtheria Toxoids Adsorbed, a US-licensed Td vaccine, manufactured by Sanofi Pasteur SA.
N = Number of subjects with a documented dose.
Grade 2 = Local: painful when limb moved; General: interfered with normal activity.
Grade 3 = Local/General: prevented normal activity.
[a] Day of vaccination and the next 3 days.
[b] Gastrointestinal symptoms included nausea, vomiting, diarrhea, and/or abdominal pain.
[c] Oral temperatures.

Unsolicited Adverse Events in the US Elderly (65 Years of Age and Older) Study: The incidence of unsolicited adverse events reported in the 31 days after vaccination was comparable between the 2 groups (17.1% and 14.4% for BOOSTRIX and Td vaccine, respectively).

Serious Adverse Events (SAEs): In the US and German adolescent safety studies, no serious adverse events were reported to occur within 31 days of vaccination. During the 6-month extended safety evaluation period, no serious adverse events that were of potential autoimmune origin or new onset and chronic in nature were reported to occur. In non-US adolescent studies in which serious adverse events were monitored for up to 37 days, one subject was diagnosed with insulin-dependent diabetes 20 days following administration of BOOSTRIX. No other serious adverse events of potential autoimmune origin or that were new onset and chronic in nature were reported to occur in these studies. In the US adult (19 to 64 years of age) study, serious adverse events were reported to occur during the entire study period (0-6 months) by 1.4% and 1.7% of subjects who received BOOSTRIX and the comparator Tdap vaccine, respectively. During the 6-month extended safety evaluation period, no serious adverse events of a neuroinflammatory nature or with information suggesting an autoimmune etiology were reported in subjects who received BOOSTRIX. In the US elderly (65 years of age and older) study, serious adverse events were reported to occur by 0.7% and 0.9% of subjects who received BOOSTRIX and the comparator Td vaccine, respectively, during the 31-day period after vaccination. Serious adverse events were reported to occur by 4.2% and 2.2% of subjects who received BOOSTRIX and the comparator Td vaccine, respectively, during the 6-month period after vaccination.

Concomitant Vaccination With Meningococcal Conjugate Vaccine in Adolescents: In a randomized study in the US, 1,341 adolescents (11 to 18 years of age) received either BOOSTRIX administered concomitantly with MENACTRA® (Meningococcal (Groups A, C, Y, and W-135) Polysaccharide Diphtheria Toxoid Conjugate Vaccine), (Sanofi Pasteur SA), or each vaccine administered separately 1 month apart *[see Drug Interactions (7.1) and Clinical Studies (14.5)]*. Safety was evaluated in 446 subjects who received BOOSTRIX administered concomitantly with meningococcal conjugate vaccine at different injection sites, 446 subjects who received BOOSTRIX followed by meningococcal conjugate vaccine 1 month later, and 449 subjects who received meningococcal conjugate vaccine followed by BOOSTRIX 1 month later. Solicited local adverse reactions and general adverse events were recorded on diary cards for 4 days (day 0-3) following each vaccination. Unsolicited adverse events were monitored for the 31-day period following each vaccination (day 0-30). Table 5 presents the percentages of subjects experiencing local reactions at the injection site for BOOSTRIX and solicited general events following BOOSTRIX. The incidence of unsolicited adverse events reported in the 31 days after any vaccination was similar following each dose of BOOSTRIX in all cohorts.
[See table 5 below]

6.2 Postmarketing Experience

In addition to reports in clinical trials, worldwide voluntary reports of adverse events received for BOOSTRIX in persons 10 years of age and older since market introduction of this vaccine are listed below. This list includes serious events or events which have causal connection to components of this or other vaccines or drugs. Because these events are reported voluntarily from a population of uncertain size, it is not possible to reliably estimate their frequency or establish a causal relationship to the vaccine.

Blood and Lymphatic System Disorders: Lymphadenitis, lymphadenopathy.

Immune System Disorders: Allergic reactions, including anaphylactic and anaphylactoid reactions.

Cardiac Disorders: Myocarditis.

General Disorders and Administration Site Conditions: Extensive swelling of the injected limb, injection site induration, injection site inflammation, injection site mass, injection site pruritus, injection site nodule, injection site warmth, injection site reaction.

Musculoskeletal and Connective Tissue Disorders: Arthralgia, back pain, myalgia.

Nervous System Disorders: Convulsions (with and without fever), encephalitis, facial palsy, loss of consciousness, paraesthesia, syncope.

Skin and Subcutaneous Tissue Disorders: Angioedema, exanthem, Henoch-Schönlein purpura, rash, urticaria.

Table 5. Rates of Solicited Local Adverse Reactions or General Adverse Events Reported Within the 4-day Post-Vaccination Period following Administration of BOOSTRIX in Individuals 11 to 18 Years of Age (Total Vaccinated Cohort)

	BOOSTRIX+MCV4[a] (N = 441) %	BOOSTRIX→MCV4[b] (N = 432-433) %	MCV4→BOOSTRIX[c] (N = 441) %
Local (at injection site for BOOSTRIX)			
Pain, any	70.1	70.4	47.8
Redness, any	22.7	25.7	17.9
Swelling, any	17.7	18.1	12.0
General (following administration of BOOSTRIX)			
Fatigue	34.0	32.1	20.4
Headache	34.0	30.7	17.0
Gastrointestinal symptoms[d]	15.2	14.5	7.7
Fever, ≥99.5°F (37.5°C)[e]	5.2	3.5	2.3

MCV4 = MENACTRA (Meningococcal (Groups A, C, Y, and W-135) Polysaccharide Diphtheria Toxoid Conjugate Vaccine), Sanofi Pasteur SA.
N = number of subjects in the total vaccinated cohort with local/general symptoms sheets completed.
[a] BOOSTRIX+MCV4 = concomitant vaccination with BOOSTRIX and MENACTRA.
[b] BOOSTRIX→MCV4 = BOOSTRIX followed by MCV4 1 month later.
[c] MCV4→BOOSTRIX = MCV4 followed by BOOSTRIX 1 month later.
[d] Gastrointestinal symptoms included nausea, vomiting, diarrhea, and/or abdominal pain.
[e] Oral temperatures.

7 Drug Interactions

7.1 Concomitant Vaccine Administration

BOOSTRIX was administered concomitantly with MENACTRA in a clinical study of subjects 11 to 18 years of age *[see Clinical Studies (14.5)]*. Post-vaccination geometric mean antibody concentrations (GMCs) to pertactin were lower following BOOSTRIX administered concomitantly with meningococcal conjugate vaccine compared to BOOSTRIX administered first. It is not known if the efficacy of BOOSTRIX is affected by the reduced response to pertactin.

BOOSTRIX was administered concomitantly with FLUARIX® (Influenza Virus Vaccine) in a clinical study of subjects 19 to 64 years of age *[see Clinical Studies (14.5)]*. Lower GMCs for antibodies to the pertussis antigens filamentous hemagglutinin (FHA) and pertactin were observed when BOOSTRIX was administered concomitantly with FLUARIX as compared with BOOSTRIX alone. It is not known if the efficacy of BOOSTRIX is affected by the reduced response to FHA and pertactin.

When BOOSTRIX is administered concomitantly with other injectable vaccines or Tetanus Immune Globulin, they should be given with separate syringes and at different injection sites. BOOSTRIX should not be mixed with any other vaccine in the same syringe or vial.

7.2 Immunosuppressive Therapies

Immunosuppressive therapies, including irradiation, antimetabolites, alkylating agents, cytotoxic drugs, and corticosteroids (used in greater than physiologic doses), may reduce the immune response to BOOSTRIX.

8 Use in Specific Populations

8.1 Pregnancy

Pregnancy Category B

A developmental toxicity study has been performed in female rats at a dose approximately 40 times the human dose (on a mL/kg basis) and revealed no evidence of harm to the fetus due to BOOSTRIX. Animal fertility studies have not been conducted with BOOSTRIX. There are no adequate and well-controlled studies in pregnant women. Because animal reproduction studies are not always predictive of human response, BOOSTRIX should be given to a pregnant woman only if clearly needed.

In a developmental toxicity study, the effect of BOOSTRIX on embryo-fetal and pre-weaning development was evaluated in pregnant rats. Animals were administered INFANRIX by intramuscular injection once prior to gestation and BOOSTRIX by intramuscular injection during the period of organogenesis (gestation days 6, 8, 11, and 15), 0.1 mL/rat/occasion (approximately 40-fold excess relative to the projected human dose of BOOSTRIX on a body weight basis). The antigens in INFANRIX are the same as those in BOOSTRIX, but INFANRIX is formulated with higher quantities of these antigens. No adverse effects on pregnancy, parturition, lactation parameters, and embryo-fetal or pre-weaning development were observed. There were no vaccine-related fetal malformations or other evidence of teratogenesis.

Pregnancy Registry: GlaxoSmithKline maintains a surveillance registry to collect data on pregnancy outcomes and newborn health status outcomes following vaccination with BOOSTRIX during pregnancy. Women who receive BOOSTRIX during pregnancy should be encouraged to contact GlaxoSmithKline directly or their healthcare provider should contact GlaxoSmithKline by calling 1-888-452-9622.

8.3 Nursing Mothers

It is not known whether BOOSTRIX is excreted in human milk. Because many drugs are excreted in human milk, caution should be exercised when BOOSTRIX is administered to a nursing woman.

8.4 Pediatric Use

BOOSTRIX is not indicated for use in children younger than 10 years of age. Safety and effectiveness of BOOSTRIX in this age group have not been established.

8.5 Geriatric Use

In clinical trials, 1,104 subjects 65 years of age and older received BOOSTRIX; of these subjects, 299 were 75 years of age and older. In the US elderly (65 years and older) study, immune responses to tetanus and diphtheria toxoids following BOOSTRIX were non-inferior to the comparator Td vaccine. Antibody responses to pertussis antigens following a single dose of BOOSTRIX in the elderly were non-inferior to those observed with INFANRIX administered as a 3-dose series in infants *[see Clinical Studies (14.4)]*. Solicited adverse events following BOOSTRIX were similar in frequency to those reported with the comparator Td vaccine *[see Adverse Reactions (6.1)]*.

Table 6. Antibody Responses to Tetanus and Diphtheria Toxoids Following BOOSTRIX Compared With Td Vaccine in Adolescents 10 to 18 Years of Age (ATP Cohort for Immunogenicity)

	N	% ≥0.1 IU/mL[a] (95% CI)	% ≥1.0 IU/mL[a] (95% CI)	% Booster Response[b] (95% CI)
Anti-Tetanus				
BOOSTRIX	2,469-2,516			
Pre-vaccination		97.7 (97.1, 98.3)	36.8 (34.9, 38.7)	–
Post-vaccination		100 (99.8, 100)[c]	99.5 (99.1, 99.7)[d]	89.7 (88.4, 90.8)[c]
Td	817-834			
Pre-vaccination		96.8 (95.4, 97.9)	39.9 (36.5, 43.4)	–
Post-vaccination		100 (99.6, 100)	99.8 (99.1, 100)	92.5 (90.5, 94.2)
Anti-Diphtheria				
BOOSTRIX	2,463-2,515			
Pre-vaccination		85.8 (84.3, 87.1)	17.1 (15.6, 18.6)	–
Post-vaccination		99.9 (99.7, 100)[c]	97.3 (96.6, 97.9)[d]	90.6 (89.4, 91.7)[c]
Td	814-834			
Pre-vaccination		84.8 (82.1, 87.2)	19.5 (16.9, 22.4)	–
Post-vaccination		99.9 (99.3, 100)	99.3 (98.4, 99.7)	95.9 (94.4, 97.2)

Td manufactured by MassBioLogics.
ATP = according-to-protocol; CI = Confidence Interval.
[a]Measured by ELISA.
[b]Booster response: In subjects with pre-vaccination <0.1 IU/mL, post-vaccination concentration ≥0.4 IU/mL. In subjects with pre-vaccination concentration ≥0.1 IU/mL, an increase of at least 4 times the pre-vaccination concentration.
[c]Seroprotection rate or booster response rate to BOOSTRIX was non-inferior to Td (upper limit of two-sided 95% CI on the difference for Td minus BOOSTRIX ≤10%).
[d]Non-inferiority criteria not prospectively defined for this endpoint.

11 Description

BOOSTRIX (Tetanus Toxoid, Reduced Diphtheria Toxoid and Acellular Pertussis Vaccine, Adsorbed) is a noninfectious, sterile, vaccine for intramuscular administration. It contains tetanus toxoid, diphtheria toxoid, and pertussis antigens (inactivated pertussis toxin [PT] and formaldehyde-treated filamentous hemagglutinin [FHA] and pertactin). The antigens are the same as those in INFANRIX, but BOOSTRIX is formulated with reduced quantities of these antigens.

Tetanus toxin is produced by growing *Clostridium tetani* in a modified Latham medium derived from bovine casein. The diphtheria toxin is produced by growing *Corynebacterium diphtheriae* in Fenton medium containing a bovine extract. The bovine materials used in these extracts are sourced from countries which the United States Department of Agriculture (USDA) has determined neither have nor are at risk of bovine spongiform encephalopathy (BSE). Both toxins are detoxified with formaldehyde, concentrated by ultrafiltration, and purified by precipitation, dialysis, and sterile filtration.

The acellular pertussis antigens (PT, FHA, and pertactin) are isolated from *Bordetella pertussis* culture grown in modified Stainer-Scholte liquid medium. PT and FHA are isolated from the fermentation broth; pertactin is extracted from the cells by heat treatment and flocculation. The antigens are purified in successive chromatographic and precipitation steps. PT is detoxified using glutaraldehyde and formaldehyde. FHA and pertactin are treated with formaldehyde.

Each antigen is individually adsorbed onto aluminum hydroxide. Each 0.5-mL dose is formulated to contain 5 Lf of tetanus toxoid, 2.5 Lf of diphtheria toxoid, 8 mcg of inactivated PT, 8 mcg of FHA, and 2.5 mcg of pertactin (69 kiloDalton outer membrane protein).

Tetanus and diphtheria toxoid potency is determined by measuring the amount of neutralizing antitoxin in previously immunized guinea pigs. The potency of the acellular pertussis components (inactivated PT and formaldehyde-treated FHA and pertactin) is determined by enzyme-linked immunosorbent assay (ELISA) on sera from previously immunized mice.

Each 0.5-mL dose contains aluminum hydroxide as adjuvant (not more than 0.39 mg aluminum by assay), 4.5 mg of sodium chloride, ≤100 mcg of residual formaldehyde, and ≤100 mcg of polysorbate 80 (Tween 80).

BOOSTRIX is available in vials and 2 types of prefilled syringes. One type of prefilled syringe has a tip cap which may contain natural rubber latex and a plunger which does not contain latex. The other type has a tip cap and a rubber plunger which contain dry natural latex rubber. The vial stopper does not contain latex. *[See How Supplied/Storage and Handling (16).]*

12 Clinical Pharmacology

12.1 Mechanism of Action

Tetanus: Tetanus is a condition manifested primarily by neuromuscular dysfunction caused by a potent exotoxin released by *C. tetani*. Protection against disease is due to the development of neutralizing antibodies to the tetanus toxin. A serum tetanus antitoxin level of at least 0.01 IU/mL, measured by neutralization assays, is considered the minimum protective level.[2] A level ≥0.1 IU/mL by ELISA has been considered as protective.

Diphtheria: Diphtheria is an acute toxin-mediated infectious disease caused by toxigenic strains of *C. diphtheriae*. Protection against disease is due to the development of neutralizing antibodies to the diphtheria toxin. A serum diphtheria antitoxin level of 0.01 IU/mL, measured by neutralization assays, is the lowest level giving some degree of protection; a level of 0.1 IU/mL by ELISA is regarded as protective.[3] Diphtheria antitoxin levels ≥1.0 IU/mL by ELISA have been associated with long-term protection.[3]

Pertussis: Pertussis (whooping cough) is a disease of the respiratory tract caused by *B. pertussis*. The role of the different components produced by *B. pertussis* in either the pathogenesis of, or the immunity to, pertussis is not well understood.

13 Nonclinical Toxicology

13.1 Carcinogenesis, Mutagenesis, Impairment of Fertility

BOOSTRIX has not been evaluated for carcinogenic or mutagenic potential, or for impairment of fertility.

14 Clinical Studies

The efficacy of the tetanus and diphtheria toxoid components of BOOSTRIX is based on the immunogenicity of the individual antigens compared to US-licensed vaccines using established serologic correlates of protection. The efficacy of the pertussis components of BOOSTRIX was evaluated by comparison of the immune response of adolescents and adults following a single dose of BOOSTRIX to the immune response of infants following a 3-dose primary series of INFANRIX. In addition, the ability of BOOSTRIX to induce a booster response to each of the antigens was evaluated.

14.1 Efficacy of INFANRIX

The efficacy of a 3-dose primary series of INFANRIX in infants has been assessed in 2 clinical studies: A prospective efficacy trial conducted in Germany employing a household contact study design and a double-blind, randomized, active Diphtheria and Tetanus Toxoids (DT)-controlled trial conducted in Italy sponsored by the National Institutes of Health (NIH) (for details see INFANRIX prescribing information). Serological data from a subset of infants immunized with INFANRIX in the household contact study were compared with the sera of adolescents and adults immunized with BOOSTRIX *[see Clinical Studies (14.2, 14.3)]*. In the household contact study, the protective efficacy of INFANRIX, in infants, against WHO-defined pertussis (21 days or more of paroxysmal cough with infection confirmed by culture and/or serologic testing) was calculated to be 89% (95% CI: 77%, 95%). When the definition of pertussis was expanded to include clinically milder disease, with infection confirmed by culture and/or serologic testing, the efficacy of INFANRIX against ≥7 days of any cough was 67% (95% CI: 52%, 78%) and against ≥7 days of paroxysmal cough was 81% (95% CI: 68%, 89%) (for details see INFANRIX prescribing information).

14.2 Immunological Evaluation in Adolescents

In a multicenter, randomized, controlled study conducted in the United States, the immune responses to each of the antigens contained in BOOSTRIX were evaluated in sera obtained approximately 1 month after administration of a single dose of vaccine to adolescent subjects (10 to 18 years of age). Of the subjects enrolled in this study, approximately 76% were 10 to 14 years of age and 24% were 15 to 18 years of age. Approximately 98% of participants in this study had received the recommended series of 4 or 5 doses of either DTwP or a combination of DTwP and DTaP in childhood. The racial/ethnic demographics were as follows: white 85.8%, black 5.7%, Hispanic 5.6%, Oriental 0.8%, and other 2.1%.

Response to Tetanus and Diphtheria Toxoids: The antibody responses to the tetanus and diphtheria toxoids of BOOSTRIX compared with Td vaccine are shown in Table 6. One month after a single dose, anti-tetanus and anti-diphtheria seroprotective rates (≥0.1 IU/mL by ELISA) and booster response rates were comparable between BOOSTRIX and the comparator Td vaccine.

[See table 6 above]

Response to Pertussis Antigens: The booster response rates of adolescents to the pertussis antigens are shown in Table 7. For each of the pertussis antigens the lower limit of the two-sided 95% CI for the percentage of subjects with a booster response exceeded the pre-defined lower limit of 80% for demonstration of an acceptable booster response.

Table 7. Booster Responses to the Pertussis Antigens Following BOOSTRIX in Adolescents 10 to 18 Years of Age (ATP Cohort for Immunogenicity)

	N	BOOSTRIX % Booster Response[a] (95% CI)
Anti-PT	2,677	84.5 (83.0, 85.9)
Anti-FHA	2,744	95.1 (94.2, 95.9)
Anti-pertactin	2,752	95.4 (94.5, 96.1)

ATP = according-to-protocol; CI = Confidence Interval.
[a]Booster response: In initially seronegative subjects (<5 EL.U./mL), post-vaccination antibody concentrations ≥20 EL.U./mL. In initially seropositive subjects with pre-vaccination antibody concentrations ≥5 EL.U./mL and <20 EL.U./mL, an increase of at least 4 times the pre-vaccination antibody concentration. In initially seropositive subjects with pre-vaccination antibody concentrations ≥20 EL.U./mL, an increase of at least 2 times the pre-vaccination antibody concentration.

The GMCs to each of the pertussis antigens 1 month following a single dose of BOOSTRIX in the US adolescent study (N = 2,941-2,979) were compared with the GMCs observed in infants following a 3-dose primary series of INFANRIX administered at 3, 4, and 5 months of age (N = 631-2,884). Table 8 presents the results for the total immunogenicity cohort in both studies (vaccinated subjects with serology data available for at least one pertussis antigen; the majority of subjects in the study of INFANRIX had anti-PT serology data only). These infants were a subset of those who formed the cohort for the German household contact study in which the efficacy of INFANRIX was demonstrated *[see Clinical Studies (14.1)]*. Although a serologic correlate of protection for pertussis has not been established, anti-PT, anti-FHA, and anti-pertactin antibody concentrations observed in adolescents 1 month after a single dose of BOOSTRIX were non-inferior to those observed in infants following a primary vaccination series with INFANRIX.

Table 8. Ratio of GMCs to Pertussis Antigens Following One Dose of BOOSTRIX in Adolescents 10 to 18 Years of Age Compared With 3 Doses of INFANRIX in Infants (Total Immunogenicity Cohort)

	GMC Ratio: BOOSTRIX/INFANRIX (95% CI)
Anti-PT	1.90 (1.82, 1.99)[a]
Anti-FHA	7.35 (6.85, 7.89)[a]

Anti-pertactin	4.19 (3.73, 4.71)[a]

GMC = geometric mean antibody concentration, measured in ELISA units; CI = Confidence Interval.

Number of subjects for BOOSTRIX GMC evaluation: Anti-PT = 2,941, anti-FHA = 2,979, and anti-pertactin = 2,978.

Number of subjects for INFANRIX GMC evaluation: Anti-PT = 2,884, anti-FHA = 685, and anti-pertactin = 631.

[a]GMC following BOOSTRIX was non-inferior to GMC following INFANRIX (lower limit of 95% CI for the GMC ratio of BOOSTRIX/INFANRIX >0.67).

14.3 Immunological Evaluation in Adults (19 to 64 Years of Age)

A multicenter, randomized, observer-blinded study, conducted in the United States, evaluated the immunogenicity of BOOSTRIX compared with the licensed comparator Tdap vaccine (Sanofi Pasteur SA). Vaccines were administered as a single dose to subjects (N = 2,284) who had not received a tetanus-diphtheria booster within 5 years. The immune responses to each of the antigens contained in BOOSTRIX were evaluated in sera obtained approximately 1 month after administration. Approximately 33% of patients were 19 to 29 years of age, 33% were 30 to 49 years of age and 34% were 50 to 64 years of age. Among subjects in the combined vaccine groups, 62% were female; 84% of subjects were white, 8% black, 1% Asian, and 7% were of other racial/ethnic groups.

Response to Tetanus and Diphtheria Toxoids: The antibody responses to the tetanus and diphtheria toxoids of BOOSTRIX compared with the comparator Tdap vaccine are shown in Table 9. One month after a single dose, anti-tetanus and anti-diphtheria seroprotective rates (≥0.1 IU/mL by ELISA) were comparable between BOOSTRIX and the comparator Tdap vaccine.

[See table 9 above]

Table 9. Antibody Responses to Tetanus and Diphtheria Toxoids Following One Dose of BOOSTRIX Compared With the Comparator Tdap Vaccine in Adults 19 to 64 Years of Age (ATP Cohort for Immunogenicity)

	N	% ≥0.1 IU/mL[a] (95% CI)	% ≥1.0 IU/mL[a] (95% CI)
Anti-Tetanus			
BOOSTRIX	1,445-1,447		
Pre-vaccination		95.9 (94.8, 96.9)	71.9 (69.5, 74.2)
Post-vaccination		99.6 (99.1, 99.8)[b]	98.3 (97.5, 98.9)[b]
Tdap	727-728		
Pre-vaccination		97.2 (95.8, 98.3)	74.7 (71.4, 77.8)
Post-vaccination		100 (95.5, 100)	99.3 (98.4, 99.8)
Anti-Diphtheria			
BOOSTRIX	1,440-1,444		
Pre-vaccination		85.2 (83.3, 87.0)	23.7 (21.5, 26.0)
Post-vaccination		98.2 (97.4, 98.8)[b]	87.9 (86.1, 89.5)[c]
Tdap	720-727		
Pre-vaccination		89.2 (86.7, 91.3)	26.5 (23.3, 29.9)
Post-vaccination		98.6 (97.5, 99.3)	92.0 (89.8, 93.9)

Tdap = Tetanus Toxoid, Reduced Diphtheria Toxoid and Acellular Pertussis Vaccine, Adsorbed manufactured by Sanofi Pasteur SA.
ATP = according-to-protocol; CI = Confidence Interval.
[a]Measured by ELISA.
[b]Seroprotection rates for BOOSTRIX were non-inferior to the comparator Tdap vaccine (lower limit of 95% CI on the difference of BOOSTRIX minus Tdap ≥-10%).
[c]Non-inferiority criteria not prospectively defined for this endpoint.

Response to Pertussis Antigens: Booster response rates to the pertussis antigens are shown in Table 10. For the FHA and pertactin antigens, the lower limit of the 95% CI for the booster responses exceeded the pre-defined limit of 80% demonstrating an acceptable booster response following BOOSTRIX. The PT antigen booster response lower limit of the 95% CI (74.9%) did not exceed the pre-defined limit of 80%.

Table 10. Booster Responses to the Pertussis Antigens Following One Dose of BOOSTRIX in Adults 19 to 64 Years of Age (ATP Cohort for Immunogenicity)

	N	BOOSTRIX % Booster Response[a] (95% CI)
Anti-PT	1,419	77.2 (74.9, 79.3)[b]
Anti-FHA	1,433	96.9 (95.8, 97.7)[c]
Anti-pertactin	1,441	93.2 (91.8, 94.4)[c]

ATP = according-to-protocol; CI = Confidence Interval.

[a]Booster response: In initially seronegative subjects (<5 EL.U./mL), post-vaccination antibody concentrations ≥20 EL.U./mL. In initially seropositive subjects with pre-vaccination antibody concentrations ≥5 EL.U./mL and <20 EL.U./mL, an increase of at least 4 times the pre-vaccination antibody concentration. In initially seropositive subjects with pre-vaccination antibody concentrations ≥20 EL.U./mL, an increase of at least 2 times the pre-vaccination antibody concentration.

[b]The PT antigen booster response lower limit of the 95% CI did not exceed the pre-defined limit of 80%.

[c]The FHA and pertactin antigens booster response lower limit of the 95% CI exceeded the pre-defined limit of 80%.

The GMCs to each of the pertussis antigens 1 month following a single dose of BOOSTRIX in the US adult (19 to 64 years of age) study were compared with the GMCs observed in infants following a 3-dose primary series of INFANRIX administered at 3, 4, and 5 months of age. Table 11 presents the results for the total immunogenicity cohort in both studies (vaccinated subjects with serology data available for at least one pertussis antigen). These infants were a subset of those who formed the cohort for the German household contact study in which the efficacy of INFANRIX was demonstrated *[see Clinical Studies (14.1)]*. Although a serologic correlate of protection for pertussis has not been established, anti-PT, anti-FHA, and anti-pertactin antibody concentrations observed in adults 1 month after a single dose of BOOSTRIX were non-inferior to those observed in infants following a primary vaccination series with INFANRIX.

Table 11. Ratio of GMCs to Pertussis Antigens Following One Dose of BOOSTRIX in Adults 19 to 64 Years of Age Compared With 3 Doses of INFANRIX in Infants (Total Immunogenicity Cohort)

	GMC Ratio: BOOSTRIX/INFANRIX (95% CI)
Anti-PT	1.39 (1.32, 1.47)[a]
Anti-FHA	7.46 (6.86, 8.12)[a]
Anti-pertactin	3.56 (3.10, 4.08)[a]

GMC = geometric mean antibody concentration; CI = Confidence Interval.

Number of subjects for BOOSTRIX GMC evaluation: Anti-PT = 1,460, anti-FHA = 1,472, and anti-pertactin = 1,473.

Number of subjects for INFANRIX GMC evaluation: Anti-PT = 2,884, anti-FHA = 685, and anti-pertactin = 631.

[a]BOOSTRIX was non-inferior to INFANRIX (lower limit of 95% CI for the GMC ratio of BOOSTRIX/INFANRIX ≥0.67).

14.4 Immunological Evaluation in the Elderly (65 Years of Age and Older)

The US elderly (65 years of age and older) study, a randomized, observer-blinded study, evaluated the immunogenicity of BOOSTRIX (N = 887) compared with a US-licensed comparator Td vaccine (N = 445) (Sanofi Pasteur SA). Vaccines were administered as a single dose to subjects who had not received a tetanus-diphtheria booster within 5 years. Among all vaccine recipients, the mean age was approximately 72 years of age; 54% were female and 95% were white. The immune responses to each of the antigens contained in BOOSTRIX were evaluated in sera obtained approximately 1 month after administration.

Response to Tetanus and Diphtheria Toxoids and Pertussis Antigens: Immune responses to tetanus and diphtheria toxoids and pertussis antigens were measured 1 month after administration of a single dose of BOOSTRIX or a comparator Td vaccine. Anti-tetanus and anti-diphtheria seroprotective rates (≥0.1 IU/mL) were comparable between BOOSTRIX and the comparator Td vaccine (Table 12).

Table 12. Immune Responses to Tetanus and Diphtheria Toxoids Following BOOSTRIX or Comparator Td Vaccine in the Elderly 65 Years of Age and Older (ATP Cohort for Immunogenicity)

	BOOSTRIX (N = 844-864)	Td (N = 430-439)
Anti-T		
% ≥0.1 IU/mL (95% CI)	96.8 (95.4, 97.8)[a]	97.5 (95.6, 98.7)
% ≥1.0 IU/mL (95% CI)	88.8 (86.5, 90.8)[a]	90.0 (86.8, 92.6)
Anti-D		
% ≥0.1 IU/mL (95% CI)	84.9 (82.3, 87.2)[a]	86.6 (83.0, 89.6)
% ≥1.0 IU/mL (95% CI)	52.0 (48.6, 55.4)[b]	51.2 (46.3, 56.0)

Td = Tetanus and Diphtheria Toxoids Adsorbed, a US-licensed Td vaccine, manufactured by Sanofi Pasteur SA.

ATP = according-to-protocol; CI = Confidence Interval.

[a]Seroprotection rates for BOOSTRIX were non-inferior to the comparator Td vaccine (lower limit of 95% CI on the difference of BOOSTRIX minus Td ≥-10%).

[b]Non-inferiority criteria not prospectively defined for this endpoint.

The GMCs to each of the pertussis antigens 1 month following a single dose of BOOSTRIX were compared with the GMCs of infants following a 3-dose primary series of INFANRIX administered at 3, 4, and 5 months of age. Table 13 presents the results for the total immunogenicity cohort in both studies (vaccinated subjects with serology data available for at least one pertussis antigen). These infants were a subset of those who formed the cohort for the German household contact study in which the efficacy of INFANRIX was demonstrated *[see Clinical Studies (14.1)]*. Although a serologic correlate of protection for pertussis has not been established, anti-PT, anti-FHA, and anti-pertactin antibody concentrations in the elderly (65 years of age and older) 1 month after a single dose of BOOSTRIX were non-inferior to those of infants following a primary vaccination series with INFANRIX.

Table 13. Ratio of GMCs to Pertussis Antigens Following One Dose of BOOSTRIX in the Elderly 65 Years of Age and Older Compared With 3 Doses of INFANRIX in Infants (Total Immunogenicity Cohort)

	GMC Ratio: BOOSTRIX/INFANRIX (95% CI)
Anti-PT	1.07 (1.00, 1.15)[a]
Anti-FHA	8.24 (7.45, 9.12)[a]
Anti-pertactin	0.93 (0.79, 1.10)[a]

GMC = geometric mean antibody concentration; CI = Confidence Interval.
Number of subjects for BOOSTRIX GMC evaluation: Anti-PT = 865, anti-FHA = 847, and anti-pertactin = 878.
Number of subjects for INFANRIX GMC evaluation: Anti-PT = 2,884, anti-FHA = 685, and anti-pertactin = 631.
[a]BOOSTRIX was non-inferior to INFANRIX (lower limit of 95% CI for the GMC ratio of BOOSTRIX/INFANRIX ≥0.67).

14.5 Concomitant Vaccine Administration

Concomitant Administration With Meningococcal Conjugate Vaccine: The concomitant use of BOOSTRIX and a tetravalent meningococcal (groups A, C, Y, and W-135) conjugate vaccine (Sanofi Pasteur SA) was evaluated in a randomized study in healthy adolescents 11 to 18 years of age. A total of 1,341 adolescents were vaccinated with BOOSTRIX. Of these, 446 subjects received BOOSTRIX administered concomitantly with meningococcal conjugate vaccine at different injection sites, 446 subjects received BOOSTRIX followed by meningococcal conjugate vaccine 1 month later, and 449 subjects received meningococcal conjugate vaccine followed by BOOSTRIX 1 month later. Immune responses to diphtheria and tetanus toxoids (% of subjects with anti-tetanus and anti-diphtheria antibodies ≥1.0 IU/mL by ELISA), pertussis antigens (booster responses and GMCs), and meningococcal antigens (vaccine responses) were measured 1 month (range 30 to 48 days) after concomitant or separate administration of BOOSTRIX and meningococcal conjugate vaccine. For BOOSTRIX given concomitantly with meningococcal conjugate vaccine compared to BOOSTRIX administered first, non-inferiority was demonstrated for all antigens, with the exception of the anti-pertactin GMC. The lower limit of the 95% CI for the GMC ratio was 0.54 for anti-pertactin (pre-specified limit ≥0.67). For the anti-pertactin booster response, non-inferiority was demonstrated. It is not known if the efficacy of BOOSTRIX is affected by the reduced response to pertactin.

There was no evidence that BOOSTRIX interfered with the antibody responses to the meningococcal antigens when measured by serum bactericidal assays (rSBA) when given concomitantly or sequentially (meningococcal conjugate vaccine followed by BOOSTRIX or BOOSTRIX followed by meningococcal conjugate vaccine.

Concomitant Administration With FLUARIX (Influenza Virus Vaccine): The concomitant use of BOOSTRIX and FLUARIX was evaluated in a multicenter, open-label, randomized, controlled study of 1,497 adults 19 to 64 years of age. In one group, subjects received BOOSTRIX and FLUARIX concurrently (n = 748). The other group received FLUARIX at the first visit, then 1 month later received BOOSTRIX (n = 749). Sera was obtained prior to and 1 month following concomitant or separate administration of BOOSTRIX and/or FLUARIX, as well as 1 month after the separate administration of FLUARIX.

Immune responses following concurrent administration of BOOSTRIX and FLUARIX were non-inferior to separate administration for diphtheria (seroprotection defined as ≥0.1 IU/mL), tetanus (seroprotection defined as ≥0.1 IU/mL and based on concentrations ≥1.0 IU/mL), pertussis toxin (PT) antigen (anti-PT GMC) and influenza antigens (percent of subjects with hemagglutination-inhibition [HI] antibody titer ≥1:40 and ≥4-fold rise in HI titer). Non-inferiority criteria were not met for the anti-pertussis antigens FHA and pertactin. The lower limit of the 95% CI of the GMC ratio was 0.64 for anti-FHA and 0.60 for anti-pertactin and the pre-specified limit was ≥0.67. It is not known if the efficacy of BOOSTRIX is affected by the reduced response to FHA and pertactin.

15 References

1. Institute of Medicine (IOM). Stratton KR, Howe CJ, Johnston RB, eds. *Adverse events associated with childhood vaccines. Evidence bearing on causality.* Washington, DC: National Academy Press; 1994.
2. Wassilak SGF, Roper MH, Kretsinger K, and Orenstein WA. Tetanus Toxoid. In: Plotkin SA, Orenstein WA, and Offit PA, eds. *Vaccines.* 5th ed. Saunders; 2008:805-839.
3. Vitek CR and Wharton M. Diphtheria Toxoid. In: Plotkin SA, Orenstein WA, and Offit PA, eds. *Vaccines.* 5th ed. Saunders; 2008:139-156.

16 How Supplied/Storage and Handling

BOOSTRIX is available in 0.5-mL single-dose vials and disposable prefilled TIP-LOK syringes (packaged without needles):
NDC 58160-842-01 Vial (contains no latex) in Package of 10: NDC 58160-842-11
NDC 58160-842-05 Syringe (tip cap may contain latex; plunger contains no latex) in Package of 1: NDC 58160-842-34
NDC 58160-842-43 Syringe (tip cap may contain latex; plunger contains no latex) in Package of 10: NDC 58160-842-52
NDC 58160-842-41 Syringe (tip cap and plunger contain latex) in Package of 10: NDC 58160-842-51
Store refrigerated between 2° and 8°C (36° and 46°F). Do not freeze. Discard if the vaccine has been frozen.

17 Patient Counseling Information

The patient, parent, or guardian should be:
- informed of the potential benefits and risks of immunization with BOOSTRIX.
- informed about the potential for adverse reactions that have been temporally associated with administration of BOOSTRIX or other vaccines containing similar components.
- instructed to report any adverse events to their healthcare provider.
- informed that safety and efficacy have not been established in pregnant women. Register women who receive BOOSTRIX while pregnant in the pregnancy registry by calling 1-888-452-9622.
- given the Vaccine Information Statements, which are required by the National Childhood Vaccine Injury Act of 1986 to be given prior to immunization. These materials are available free of charge at the Centers for Disease Control and Prevention (CDC) website (www.cdc.gov/vaccines).

BOOSTRIX, FLUARIX, INFANRIX, and TIP-LOK are registered trademarks of GlaxoSmithKline. The following are registered trademarks of their respective owners: ADACEL and DECAVAC/Sanofi Pasteur Limited; MENACTRA/Connaught Technology Corporation.
Manufactured by **GlaxoSmithKline Biologicals**
Rixensart, Belgium, US License 1617, and
Novartis Vaccines and Diagnostics GmbH
Marburg, Germany, US License 1754
Distributed by **GlaxoSmithKline**
Research Triangle Park, NC 27709

BTX:25PI

BREO ELLIPTA
(fluticasone furoate and vilanterol inhalation powder)

HIGHLIGHTS OF PRESCRIBING INFORMATION
These highlights do not include all the information needed to use the BREO ELLIPTA inhaler safely and effectively. See full prescribing information for BREO ELLIPTA.
BREO ELLIPTA(fluticasone furoate and vilanterol inhalation powder)
FOR ORAL INHALATION USE
Initial U.S. Approval: 2013

WARNING: ASTHMA-RELATED DEATH
See full prescribing information for complete boxed warning.
- **Long-acting beta$_2$-adrenergic agonists (LABA), such as vilanterol, one of the active ingredients in BREO ELLIPTA, increase the risk of asthma-related death. A placebo-controlled trial with another LABA (salmeterol) showed an increase in asthma-related deaths in subjects receiving salmeterol. This finding with salmeterol is considered a class effect of all LABA, including vilanterol. (5.1)**
- **The safety and efficacy of BREO ELLIPTA in patients with asthma have not been established. BREO ELLIPTA is not indicated for the treatment of asthma. (5.1)**

INDICATIONS AND USAGE

BREO ELLIPTA is a combination of fluticasone furoate, an inhaled corticosteroid (ICS), and vilanterol, a long-acting beta$_2$ adrenergic agonist (LABA), indicated for long-term, once-daily, maintenance treatment of airflow obstruction and for reducing exacerbations in patients with chronic obstructive pulmonary disease (COPD). (1)
Important limitations: Not indicated for relief of acute bronchospasm or for treatment of asthma. (1, 5.2)

DOSAGE AND ADMINISTRATION

- For oral inhalation only. (2)
- Maintenance treatment of COPD: 1 inhalation of BREO ELLIPTA 100 mcg/25 mcg once daily. (2)

DOSAGE FORMS AND STRENGTHS

Inhalation Powder. Inhaler containing 2 double-foil blister strips of powder formulation for oral inhalation. One strip contains fluticasone furoate 100 mcg per blister and the other contains vilanterol 25 mcg per blister. (3)

CONTRAINDICATIONS

Severe hypersensitivity to milk proteins or any ingredients. (4)

WARNINGS AND PRECAUTIONS

- LABA increase the risk of asthma-related death. (5.1)
- Do not initiate in acutely deteriorating COPD or to treat acute symptoms. (5.2)
- Do not use in combination with an additional medicine containing LABA because of risk of overdose. (5.3)
- *Candida albicans* infection of the mouth and pharynx may occur. Monitor patients periodically. Advise the patient to rinse his/her mouth without swallowing after inhalation to help reduce the risk. (5.4)
- Increased risk of pneumonia in patients with COPD taking BREO ELLIPTA. Monitor patients for signs and symptoms of pneumonia. (5.5)
- Potential worsening of infections (e.g., existing tuberculosis; fungal, bacterial, viral, or parasitic infection; ocular herpes simplex). Use with caution in patients with these infections. More serious or even fatal course of chickenpox or measles can occur in susceptible patients. (5.6)
- Risk of impaired adrenal function when transferring from systemic corticosteroids. Taper patients slowly from systemic corticosteroids if transferring to BREO ELLIPTA. (5.7)
- Hypercorticism and adrenal suppression may occur with very high dosages or at the regular dosage in susceptible individuals. If such changes occur, discontinue BREO ELLIPTA slowly. (5.8)
- If paradoxical bronchospasm occurs, discontinue BREO ELLIPTA and institute alternative therapy. (5.10)
- Use with caution in patients with cardiovascular disorders because of beta-adrenergic stimulation. (5.12)
- Assess for decrease in bone mineral density initially and periodically thereafter. (5.13)
- Close monitoring for glaucoma and cataracts is warranted. (5.14)
- Use with caution in patients with convulsive disorders, thyrotoxicosis, diabetes mellitus, and ketoacidosis. (5.15)
- Be alert to hypokalemia and hyperglycemia. (5.16)

ADVERSE REACTIONS

Most common adverse reactions (incidence ≥3%) are nasopharyngitis, upper respiratory tract infection, headache, and oral candidiasis. (6.1)
To report SUSPECTED ADVERSE REACTIONS, contact GlaxoSmithKline at 1-888-825-5249 or FDA at 1-800-FDA-1088 or www.fda.gov/medwatch.

DRUG INTERACTIONS

- Strong cytochrome P450 3A4 inhibitors (e.g., ketoconazole): Use with caution. May cause systemic corticosteroid and cardiovascular effects. (7.1)
- Monoamine oxidase inhibitors and tricyclic antidepressants: Use with extreme caution. May potentiate effect of vilanterol on vascular system. (7.2)
- Beta-blockers: Use with caution. May block bronchodilatory effects of beta-agonists and produce severe bronchospasm. (7.3)
- Diuretics: Use with caution. Electrocardiographic changes and/or hypokalemia associated with non–potassium-sparing diuretics may worsen with concomitant beta-agonists. (7.4)

USE IN SPECIFIC POPULATIONS

Hepatic impairment: Fluticasone furoate exposure may increase in patients with moderate or severe impairment. Monitor for systemic corticosteroid effects. (8.6, 12.3)
See 17 for PATIENT COUNSELING INFORMATION and Medication Guide

Revised: 05/2013

FULL PRESCRIBING INFORMATION: CONTENTS*

*** Sections or subsections omitted from the full prescribing information are not listed**

FULL PRESCRIBING INFORMATION

WARNING: ASTHMA-RELATED DEATH

Long-acting beta$_2$-adrenergic agonists (LABA) increase the risk of asthma-related death. Data from a large placebo-controlled US trial that compared the safety of another LABA (salmeterol) with placebo added to usual asthma therapy showed an increase in asthma-related deaths in subjects receiving salmeterol. This finding with salmeterol is considered a class effect of LABA, including vilanterol, an active ingredient in BREO™ ELLIPTA™ *[see Warnings and Precautions (5.1)]*.

The safety and efficacy of BREO ELLIPTA in patients with asthma have not been established. BREO ELLIPTA is not indicated for the treatment of asthma.

1 INDICATIONS AND USAGE

BREO ELLIPTA is a combination inhaled corticosteroid/long-acting beta$_2$-adrenergic agonist (ICS/LABA) indicated for the long-term, once-daily, maintenance treatment of airflow obstruction in patients with chronic obstructive pulmonary disease (COPD), including chronic bronchitis and/or emphysema. BREO ELLIPTA is also indicated to reduce exacerbations of COPD in patients with a history of exacerbations.

Important Limitations of Use: BREO ELLIPTA is NOT indicated for the relief of acute bronchospasm or for the treatment of asthma.

2 DOSAGE AND ADMINISTRATION

BREO ELLIPTA 100 mcg/25 mcg should be administered as 1 inhalation once daily by the orally inhaled route only. After inhalation, the patient should rinse his/her mouth with water without swallowing to help reduce the risk of oropharyngeal candidiasis.

BREO ELLIPTA should be taken at the same time every day. Do not use BREO ELLIPTA more than 1 time every 24 hours.

No dosage adjustment is required for geriatric patients, patients with hepatic impairment, or renally impaired patients *[see Clinical Pharmacology (12.3)]*.

3 DOSAGE FORMS AND STRENGTHS

Inhalation Powder. Disposable light grey and pale blue plastic inhaler containing 2 double-foil blister strips, each with 30 blisters containing powder intended for oral inhalation only. One strip contains fluticasone furoate (100 mcg per blister), and the other strip contains vilanterol (25 mcg per blister). An institutional pack containing 14 blisters per strip is also available.

4 CONTRAINDICATIONS

The use of BREO ELLIPTA is contraindicated in patients with severe hypersensitivity to milk proteins or who have demonstrated hypersensitivity to either fluticasone furoate, vilanterol, or any of the excipients *[see Warnings and Precautions (5.11), Description (11)]*.

5 WARNINGS AND PRECAUTIONS

5.1 Asthma-Related Death

- Data from a large placebo-controlled trial in subjects with asthma showed that LABA may increase the risk of asthma-related death. Data are not available to determine whether the rate of death in patients with COPD is increased by LABA.
- A 28-week, placebo-controlled, US trial comparing the safety of another LABA (salmeterol) with placebo, each added to usual asthma therapy, showed an increase in asthma-related deaths in subjects receiving salmeterol (13/13,176 in subjects treated with salmeterol vs 3/13,179 in subjects treated with placebo; relative risk: 4.37 [95% CI: 1.25, 15.34]). The increased risk of asthma-related death is considered a class effect of LABA, including vilanterol, one of the active ingredients in BREO ELLIPTA.
- No study adequate to determine whether the rate of asthma-related death is increased in subjects treated with BREO ELLIPTA has been conducted. The safety and efficacy of BREO ELLIPTA in patients with asthma have not been established. BREO ELLIPTA is not indicated for the treatment of asthma.

5.2 Deterioration of Disease and Acute Episodes

BREO ELLIPTA should not be initiated in patients during rapidly deteriorating or potentially life-threatening episodes of COPD. BREO ELLIPTA has not been studied in patients with acutely deteriorating COPD. The initiation of BREO ELLIPTA in this setting is not appropriate.

BREO ELLIPTA should not be used for the relief of acute symptoms, i.e., as rescue therapy for the treatment of acute episodes of bronchospasm. BREO ELLIPTA has not been studied in the relief of acute symptoms and extra doses should not be used for that purpose. Acute symptoms should be treated with an inhaled, short-acting beta$_2$-agonist.

When beginning treatment with BREO ELLIPTA, patients who have been taking oral or inhaled, short-acting beta$_2$-agonists on a regular basis (e.g., 4 times a day) should be instructed to discontinue the regular use of these drugs and to use them only for symptomatic relief of acute respiratory symptoms. When prescribing BREO ELLIPTA, the healthcare provider should also prescribe an inhaled, short-acting beta$_2$-agonist and instruct the patient on how it should be used. Increasing inhaled, short-acting beta$_2$-agonist use is a signal of deteriorating disease for which prompt medical attention is indicated.

COPD may deteriorate acutely over a period of hours or chronically over several days or longer. If BREO ELLIPTA no longer controls symptoms of bronchoconstriction; the patient's inhaled, short-acting, beta$_2$-agonist becomes less effective; or the patient needs more short-acting beta$_2$-agonist than usual, these may be markers of deterioration of disease. In this setting a re-evaluation of the patient and the COPD treatment regimen should be undertaken at once. Increasing the daily dose of BREO ELLIPTA beyond the recommended dose is not appropriate in this situation.

5.3 Excessive Use of BREO ELLIPTA and Use With Other Long-Acting Beta$_2$-Agonists

BREO ELLIPTA should not be used more often than recommended, at higher doses than recommended, or in conjunction with other medicines containing LABA, as an overdose may result. Clinically significant cardiovascular effects and fatalities have been reported in association with excessive use of inhaled sympathomimetic drugs. Patients using BREO ELLIPTA should not use another medicine containing a LABA (e.g., salmeterol, formoterol fumarate, arformoterol tartrate, indacaterol) for any reason.

5.4 Local Effects of Inhaled Corticosteroids

In clinical trials, the development of localized infections of the mouth and pharynx with *Candida albicans* has occurred in subjects treated with BREO ELLIPTA. When such an infection develops, it should be treated with appropriate local or systemic (i.e., oral) antifungal therapy while treatment with BREO ELLIPTA continues, but at times therapy with BREO ELLIPTA may need to be interrupted. Advise the patient to rinse his/her mouth without swallowing following inhalation to help reduce the risk of oropharyngeal candidiasis.

5.5 Pneumonia

An increase in the incidence of pneumonia has been observed in subjects with COPD receiving the fluticasone furoate/vilanterol combination, including BREO ELLIPTA 100 mcg/25 mcg, in clinical trials. There was also an increased incidence of pneumonias resulting in hospitalization. In some incidences these pneumonia events were fatal. Physicians should remain vigilant for the possible development of pneumonia in patients with COPD as the clinical features of such infections overlap with the symptoms of COPD exacerbations.

In replicate 12-month trials in 3,255 subjects with COPD who had experienced a COPD exacerbation in the previous year, there was a higher incidence of pneumonia reported in subjects receiving the fluticasone furoate/vilanterol combination (50 mcg/25 mcg: 6% [48 of 820 subjects]; 100 mcg/25 mcg: 6% [51 of 806 subjects]; or 200 mcg/25 mcg: 7% [55 of 811 subjects]) than in subjects receiving vilanterol 25 mcg (3% [27 of 818 subjects]). There was no fatal pneumonia in subjects receiving vilanterol or fluticasone furoate/vilanterol 50 mcg/25 mcg. There was fatal pneumonia in 1 subject receiving fluticasone furoate/vilanterol 100 mcg/25 mcg and in 7 subjects receiving fluticasone furoate/vilanterol 200 mcg/25 mcg (less than 1% for each treatment group).

5.6 Immunosuppression

Persons who are using drugs that suppress the immune system are more susceptible to infections than healthy individuals. Chickenpox and measles, for example, can have a more serious or even fatal course in susceptible children or adults using corticosteroids. In such children or adults who have not had these diseases or been properly immunized, particular care should be taken to avoid exposure. How the dose, route, and duration of corticosteroid administration affect the risk of developing a disseminated infection is not known. The contribution of the underlying disease and/or prior corticosteroid treatment to the risk is also not known. If a patient is exposed to chickenpox, prophylaxis with varicella zoster immune globulin (VZIG) may be indicated. If a patient is exposed to measles, prophylaxis with pooled intramuscular immunoglobulin (IG) may be indicated. (See the respective package inserts for complete VZIG and IG prescribing information.) If chickenpox develops, treatment with antiviral agents may be considered.

Inhaled corticosteroids should be used with caution, if at all, in patients with active or quiescent tuberculosis infections of the respiratory tract; systemic fungal, bacterial, viral, or parasitic infections; or ocular herpes simplex.

5.7 Transferring Patients From Systemic Corticosteroid Therapy

Particular care is needed for patients who have been transferred from systemically active corticosteroids to inhaled corticosteroids because deaths due to adrenal insufficiency have occurred in patients with asthma during and after transfer from systemic corticosteroids to less systemically available inhaled corticosteroids. After withdrawal from systemic corticosteroids, a number of months are required for recovery of hypothalamic-pituitary-adrenal (HPA) function.

Patients who have been previously maintained on 20 mg or more of prednisone (or its equivalent) may be most susceptible, particularly when their systemic corticosteroids have been almost completely withdrawn. During this period of HPA suppression, patients may exhibit signs and symptoms of adrenal insufficiency when exposed to trauma, surgery, or infection (particularly gastroenteritis) or other conditions associated with severe electrolyte loss. Although BREO ELLIPTA may control COPD symptoms during these episodes, in recommended doses it supplies less than normal physiological amount of glucocorticoid systemically and does NOT provide the mineralocorticoid activity that is necessary for coping with these emergencies.

During periods of stress or a severe COPD exacerbation, patients who have been withdrawn from systemic corticosteroids should be instructed to resume oral corticosteroids (in large doses) immediately and to contact their physicians for further instruction. These patients should also be instructed to carry a warning card indicating that they may need supplementary systemic corticosteroids during periods of stress or severe COPD exacerbation.

Patients requiring oral corticosteroids should be weaned slowly from systemic corticosteroid use after transferring to BREO ELLIPTA. Prednisone reduction can be accomplished by reducing the daily prednisone dose by 2.5 mg on a weekly basis during therapy with BREO ELLIPTA. Lung function (mean forced expiratory volume in 1 second [FEV$_1$]), beta-agonist use, and COPD symptoms should be carefully monitored during withdrawal of oral corticosteroids. In addition, patients should be observed for signs and symptoms of adrenal insufficiency, such as fatigue, lassitude, weakness, nausea and vomiting, and hypotension.

Transfer of patients from systemic corticosteroid therapy to BREO ELLIPTA may unmask allergic conditions previously suppressed by the systemic corticosteroid therapy (e.g., rhinitis, conjunctivitis, eczema, arthritis, eosinophilic conditions).

During withdrawal from oral corticosteroids, some patients may experience symptoms of systemically active corticosteroid withdrawal (e.g., joint and/or muscular pain, lassitude, and depression) despite maintenance or even improvement of respiratory function.

5.8 Hypercorticism and Adrenal Suppression

Inhaled fluticasone furoate is absorbed into the circulation and can be systemically active. Effects of fluticasone furoate on the HPA axis are not observed with the therapeutic dose of BREO ELLIPTA. However, exceeding the recommended dosage or coadministration with a strong cytochrome P450 3A4 (CYP3A4) inhibitor may result in HPA dysfunction *[see Warnings and Precautions (5.9), Drug Interactions (7.1)].*

Because of the possibility of significant systemic absorption of inhaled corticosteroids in sensitive patients, patients treated with BREO ELLIPTA should be observed carefully for any evidence of systemic corticosteroid effects. Particular care should be taken in observing patients postoperatively or during periods of stress for evidence of inadequate adrenal response.

It is possible that systemic corticosteroid effects such as hypercorticism and adrenal suppression (including adrenal crisis) may appear in a small number of patients who are sensitive to these effects. If such effects occur, BREO ELLIPTA should be reduced slowly, consistent with accepted procedures for reducing systemic corticosteroids, and other treatments for management of COPD symptoms should be considered.

5.9 Drug Interactions With Strong Cytochrome P450 3A4 Inhibitors

Caution should be exercised when considering the coadministration of BREO ELLIPTA with long-term ketoconazole and other known strong CYP3A4 inhibitors (e.g., ritonavir, clarithromycin, conivaptan, indinavir, itraconazole, lopinavir, nefazodone, nelfinavir, saquinavir, telithromycin, troleandomycin, voriconazole) because increased systemic corticosteroid and increased cardiovascular adverse effects may occur *[see Drug Interactions (7.1), Clinical Pharmacology (12.3)].*

5.10 Paradoxical Bronchospasm

As with other inhaled medicines, BREO ELLIPTA can produce paradoxical bronchospasm, which may be life threatening. If paradoxical bronchospasm occurs following dosing with BREO ELLIPTA, it should be treated immediately with an inhaled, short-acting bronchodilator; BREO ELLIPTA should be discontinued immediately; and alternative therapy should be instituted.

5.11 Hypersensitivity Reactions

Hypersensitivity reactions may occur after administration of BREO ELLIPTA. There have been reports of anaphylactic reactions in patients with severe milk protein allergy after inhalation of other powder products containing lactose; therefore, patients with severe milk protein allergy should not take BREO ELLIPTA *[see Contraindications (4)].*

5.12 Cardiovascular Effects

Vilanterol, like other beta$_2$-agonists, can produce a clinically significant cardiovascular effect in some patients as measured by increases in pulse rate, systolic or diastolic blood pressure, and also cardiac arrhythmias, such as supraventricular tachycardia and extrasystoles. If such effects occur, BREO ELLIPTA may need to be discontinued. In addition, beta-agonists have been reported to produce electrocardiographic changes, such as flattening of the T wave, prolongation of the QTc interval, and ST segment depression, although the clinical significance of these findings is unknown. In healthy subjects, large doses of inhaled fluticasone furoate/vilanterol (4 times the recommended dose of vilanterol, representing a 12-fold higher systemic exposure than seen in patients with COPD) have been associated with clinically significant prolongation of the QTc interval, which has the potential for producing ventricular arrhythmias. Therefore, BREO ELLIPTA, like other sympathomimetic amines, should be used with caution in patients with cardiovascular disorders, especially coronary insufficiency, cardiac arrhythmias, and hypertension.

5.13 Reduction in Bone Mineral Density

Decreases in bone mineral density (BMD) have been observed with long-term administration of products containing inhaled corticosteroids. The clinical significance of small changes in BMD with regard to long-term consequences such as fracture is unknown. Patients with major risk factors for decreased bone mineral content, such as prolonged immobilization, family history of osteoporosis, postmenopausal status, tobacco use, advanced age, poor nutrition, or chronic use of drugs that can reduce bone mass (e.g., anticonvulsants, oral corticosteroids) should be monitored and treated with established standards of care. Since patients with COPD often have multiple risk factors for reduced BMD, assessment of BMD is recommended prior to initiating BREO ELLIPTA and periodically thereafter. If significant reductions in BMD are seen and BREO ELLIPTA is still considered medically important for that patient's COPD therapy, use of medicine to treat or prevent osteoporosis should be strongly considered.

In replicate 12-month trials in 3,255 subjects with COPD, bone fractures were reported by 2% of subjects receiving the fluticasone furoate/vilanterol combination (50 mcg/25 mcg: 2% [14 of 820 subjects]; 100 mcg/25 mcg: 2% [19 of 806 subjects]; or 200 mcg/25 mcg: 2% [14 of 811 subjects]) than in subjects receiving vilanterol 25 mcg alone (less than 1% [8 of 818 subjects]).

5.14 Glaucoma and Cataracts

Glaucoma, increased intraocular pressure, and cataracts have been reported in patients with COPD following the long-term administration of inhaled corticosteroids. Therefore, close monitoring is warranted in patients with a change in vision or with a history of increased intraocular pressure, glaucoma, and/or cataracts.

In replicate 12-month trials in 3,255 subjects with COPD, similar incidences of ocular effects (including glaucoma and cataracts) were reported in subjects receiving the fluticasone furoate/vilanterol combination (50 mcg/25 mcg: less than 1% [7 of 820 subjects]; 100 mcg/25 mcg: 1% [12 of 806 subjects]; 200 mcg/25 mcg: less than 1% [7 of 811 subjects]) as those receiving vilanterol 25 mcg alone (1% [9 of 818 subjects]).

5.15 Coexisting Conditions

BREO ELLIPTA, like all medicines containing sympathomimetic amines, should be used with caution in patients with convulsive disorders or thyrotoxicosis and in those who are unusually responsive to sympathomimetic amines. Doses of the related beta$_2$-adrenoceptor agonist albuterol, when administered intravenously, have been reported to aggravate preexisting diabetes mellitus and ketoacidosis.

5.16 Hypokalemia and Hyperglycemia

Beta-adrenergic agonist medicines may produce significant hypokalemia in some patients, possibly through intracellular shunting, which has the potential to produce adverse cardiovascular effects. The decrease in serum potassium is usually transient, not requiring supplementation. Beta-agonist medications may produce transient hyperglycemia in some patients. In 4 clinical trials of 6- and 12-month duration evaluating BREO ELLIPTA in subjects with COPD, there was no evidence of a treatment effect on serum glucose or potassium.

6 ADVERSE REACTIONS

LABA, such as vilanterol, one of the active ingredients in BREO ELLIPTA, increase the risk of asthma-related death. BREO ELLIPTA is not indicated for the treatment of asthma. *[See Boxed Warnings and Warnings and Precautions (5.1).]*

Systemic and local corticosteroid use may result in the following:

- Increased risk of pneumonia in COPD *[see Warnings and Precautions (5.5)]*
- Increased risk for decrease in bone mineral density *[see Warnings and Precautions (5.13)]*

6.1 Clinical Trials Experience

Because clinical trials are conducted under widely varying conditions, adverse reaction rates observed in the clinical trials of a drug cannot be directly compared with rates in the clinical trials of another drug and may not reflect the rates observed in practice.

The clinical program for BREO ELLIPTA included 7,700 subjects with COPD in two 6-month lung function trials, two 12-month exacerbation trials, and 6 other trials of shorter duration. A total of 2,034 subjects have received at least 1 dose of BREO ELLIPTA 100 mcg/25 mcg, and 1,087 subjects have received higher doses of fluticasone furoate/vilanterol. The safety data described below are based on the confirmatory 6-month and 12-month trials. Adverse reactions observed in the other trials were similar to those observed in the confirmatory trials.

6-Month Trials: The incidence of adverse reactions associated with BREO ELLIPTA in Table 1 is based on 2 placebo-controlled, 6-month clinical trials (Trials 1 and 2; n = 1,224 and n = 1,030, respectively). Of the 2,254 subjects, 70% were male and 84% were Caucasian. They had a mean age of 62 years and an average smoking history of 44 pack years, with 54% identified as current smokers. At screening, the mean postbronchodilator percent predicted FEV$_1$ was 48% (range: 14% to 87%), the mean postbronchodilator FEV$_1$/forced vital capacity (FVC) ratio was 47% (range: 17% to 88%), and the mean percent reversibility was 14% (range: -41% to 152%).

Subjects received 1 inhalation once daily of the following: BREO ELLIPTA 100 mcg/25 mcg, fluticasone furoate/vilanterol 50 mcg/25 mcg, fluticasone furoate/vilanterol 200 mcg/25 mcg, fluticasone furoate 100 mcg, fluticasone furoate 200 mcg, vilanterol 25 mcg, or placebo.

[See table 1 above]

Table 1. Adverse Reactions With ≥3% Incidence and More Common Than Placebo With BREO ELLIPTA in Subjects With Chronic Obstructive Pulmonary Disease

Adverse Event	BREO ELLIPTA 100 mcg/25 mcg (n = 410) %	Vilanterol 25 mcg (n = 408) %	Fluticasone Furoate 100 mcg (n = 410) %	Placebo (n = 412) %
Infections and infestations				
Nasopharyngitis	9	10	8	8
Upper respiratory tract infection	7	5	4	3
Oropharyngeal candidiasis[a]	5	2	3	2
Nervous system disorders				
Headache	7	9	7	5

[a] Includes terms oral candidiasis, oropharyngeal candidiasis, candidiasis, and oropharyngitis fungal.

12-Month Trials: Long-term safety data is based on two 12-month trials (Trials 3 and 4; n = 1,633 and n = 1,622, respectively). Trials 3 and 4 included 3,255 subjects, of which 57% were male and 85% were Caucasian. They had a mean age of 64 years and an average smoking history of 46 pack years, with 44% identified as current smokers. At screening, the mean postbronchodilator percent predicted FEV$_1$ was 45% (range: 12% to 91%), and the mean postbronchodilator FEV$_1$/FVC ratio was 46% (range: 17% to 81%), indicating that the subject population had moderate to very severely impaired airflow obstruction. Subjects received 1 inhalation once daily of the following: BREO ELLIPTA 100 mcg/25 mcg, fluticasone furoate/vilanterol 50 mcg/25 mcg, fluticasone furoate/vilanterol 200 mcg/25 mcg, or vilanterol 25 mcg. In addition to the events shown in Table 1, adverse reactions occurring in greater than or equal to 3% of the subjects treated with BREO ELLIPTA (N = 806) for 12 months included COPD, back pain, pneumonia *[see Warnings and Precautions (5.5)]*, bronchitis, sinusitis, cough, oropharyngeal pain, arthralgia, hypertension, influenza, pharyngitis, diarrhea, peripheral edema, and pyrexia.

7 DRUG INTERACTIONS

7.1 Inhibitors of Cytochrome P450 3A4

Fluticasone furoate and vilanterol, the individual components of BREO ELLIPTA, are both substrates of CYP3A4. Concomitant administration of the potent CYP3A4 inhibitor ketoconazole increases the systemic exposure to fluticasone furoate and vilanterol. Caution should be exercised when considering the coadministration of BREO ELLIPTA with long-term ketoconazole and other known strong CYP3A4 inhibitors (e.g., ritonavir, clarithromycin, conivaptan, indinavir, itraconazole, lopinavir, nefazodone, nelfinavir, saquinavir, telithromycin, troleandomycin, voriconazole) *[see Warnings and Precautions (5.9) and Clinical Pharmacology (12.3)].*

7.2 Monoamine Oxidase Inhibitors and Tricyclic Antidepressants

Vilanterol, like other beta$_2$-agonists, should be administered with extreme caution to patients being treated with monoamine oxidase inhibitors, tricyclic antidepressants, or drugs known to prolong the QTc interval or within 2 weeks of discontinuation of such agents, because the effect of adrenergic agonists on the cardiovascular system may be potentiated by these agents. Drugs that are known to prolong the QTc interval have an increased risk of ventricular arrhythmias.

7.3 Beta-Adrenergic Receptor Blocking Agents

Beta-blockers not only block the pulmonary effect of beta-agonists, such as vilanterol, a component of BREO ELLIPTA, but may produce severe bronchospasm in patients with reversible obstructive airways disease. Therefore, patients with COPD should not normally be treated with beta-blockers. However, under certain circumstances, there may be no acceptable alternatives to the use of beta-adrenergic blocking agents for these patients; cardioselective beta-blockers could be considered, although they should be administered with caution.

7.4 Non–Potassium-Sparing Diuretics

The electrocardiographic changes and/or hypokalemia that may result from the administration of non–potassium-sparing diuretics (such as loop or thiazide diuretics) can be acutely worsened by beta-agonists, especially when the recommended dose of the beta-agonist is exceeded. Although the clinical significance of these effects is not known, caution is advised in the coadministration of beta-agonists with non–potassium-sparing diuretics.

8 USE IN SPECIFIC POPULATIONS

8.1 Pregnancy

Teratogenic Effects: Pregnancy Category C. There are no adequate and well-controlled trials with BREO ELLIPTA in pregnant women. Corticosteroids and beta$_2$-agonists have been shown to be teratogenic in laboratory animals when administered systemically at relatively low dosage levels. Because animal studies are not always predictive of human response, BREO ELLIPTA should be used during pregnancy only if the potential benefit justifies the potential risk to the fetus. Women should be advised to contact their physicians if they become pregnant while taking BREO ELLIPTA.

Fluticasone Furoate and Vilanterol: There was no evidence of teratogenic interactions between fluticasone furoate and vilanterol in rats at approximately 9 and 40 times, respectively, the maximum recommended human daily inhalation dose (MRHDID) in adults (on a mcg/m^2 basis at maternal inhaled doses of fluticasone furoate and vilanterol, alone or in combination, up to approximately 95 mcg/kg/day).

Fluticasone Furoate: There were no teratogenic effects in rats and rabbits at approximately 9 and 2 times, respectively, the MRHDID in adults (on a mcg/m^2 basis at maternal inhaled doses up to 91 and 8 mcg/kg/day in rats and rabbits, respectively). There were no effects on perinatal and postnatal development in rats at approximately 3 times the MRHDID in adults (on a mcg/m^2 basis at maternal doses up to 27 mcg/kg/day).

Vilanterol: There were no teratogenic effects in rats and rabbits at approximately 13,000 and 160 times, respectively, the MRHDID in adults (on a mcg/m^2 basis at maternal inhaled doses up to 33,700 mcg/kg/day in rats and on an AUC basis at maternal inhaled doses up to 591 mcg/kg/day in rabbits). However, fetal skeletal variations were observed in rabbits at approximately 1,000 times the MRHDID in adults (on an AUC basis at maternal inhaled or subcutaneous doses of 5,740 or 300 mcg/kg/day, respectively). The skeletal variations included decreased or absent ossification in cervical vertebral centrum and metacarpals. There were no effects on perinatal and postnatal development in rats at approximately 3,900 times the MRHDID in adults (on a mcg/m^2 basis at maternal oral doses up to 10,000 mcg/kg/day).

Nonteratogenic Effects: Hypoadrenalism may occur in infants born of mothers receiving corticosteroids during pregnancy. Such infants should be carefully monitored.

8.2 Labor and Delivery

There are no adequate and well-controlled human trials that have investigated the effects of BREO ELLIPTA during labor and delivery.

Because beta-agonists may potentially interfere with uterine contractility, BREO ELLIPTA should be used during labor only if the potential benefit justifies the potential risk.

8.3 Nursing Mothers

It is not known whether fluticasone furoate or vilanterol are excreted in human breast milk. However, other corticosteroids and beta$_2$-agonists have been detected in human milk. Since there are no data from controlled trials on the use of BREO ELLIPTA by nursing mothers, caution should be exercised when it is administered to a nursing woman.

8.4 Pediatric Use

BREO ELLIPTA is not indicated for use in children. The safety and efficacy in pediatric patients have not been established.

8.5 Geriatric Use

Based on available data, no adjustment of the dosage of BREO ELLIPTA in geriatric patients is necessary, but greater sensitivity in some older individuals cannot be ruled out.

Clinical trials of BREO ELLIPTA for COPD included 2,508 subjects aged 65 and older and 564 subjects aged 75 and older. No overall differences in safety or effectiveness were observed between these subjects and younger subjects, and other reported clinical experience has not identified differences in responses between the elderly and younger subjects.

8.6 Hepatic Impairment

Fluticasone furoate systemic exposure increased by up to 3-fold in subjects with hepatic impairment compared with healthy subjects. Hepatic impairment had no effect on vilanterol systemic exposure. Use BREO ELLIPTA with caution in patients with moderate or severe hepatic impairment. Monitor patients for corticosteroid-related side effects *[see Clinical Pharmacology (12.3)]*.

8.7 Renal Impairment

There were no significant increases in either fluticasone furoate or vilanterol exposure in subjects with severe renal impairment (CrCl<30 mL/min) compared with healthy subjects. No dosage adjustment is required in patients with renal impairment *[see Clinical Pharmacology (12.3)]*.

10 OVERDOSAGE

No human overdosage data has been reported for BREO ELLIPTA.

BREO ELLIPTA contains both fluticasone furoate and vilanterol; therefore, the risks associated with overdosage for the individual components described below apply to BREO ELLIPTA.

10.1 Fluticasone Furoate

Because of low systemic bioavailability (15.2%) and an absence of acute drug-related systemic findings in clinical trials, overdosage of fluticasone furoate is unlikely to require any treatment other than observation. If used at excessive doses for prolonged periods, systemic effects such as hypercorticism may occur *[see Warnings and Precautions (5.8)]*.

Single- and repeat-dose trials of fluticasone furoate at doses of 50 to 4,000 mcg have been studied in human subjects. Decreases in mean serum cortisol were observed at dosages of 500 mcg or higher given once daily for 14 days.

10.2 Vilanterol

The expected signs and symptoms with overdosage of vilanterol are those of excessive beta-adrenergic stimulation and/or occurrence or exaggeration of any of the signs and symptoms of beta-adrenergic stimulation (e.g., angina, hypertension or hypotension, tachycardia with rates up to 200 beats/min, arrhythmias, nervousness, headache, tremor, seizures, muscle cramps, dry mouth, palpitation, nausea, dizziness, fatigue, malaise, insomnia, hyperglycemia, hypokalemia, metabolic acidosis). As with all inhaled sympathomimetic medicines, cardiac arrest and even death may be associated with an overdose of vilanterol.

Treatment of overdosage consists of discontinuation of BREO ELLIPTA together with institution of appropriate symptomatic and/or supportive therapy. The judicious use of a cardioselective beta-receptor blocker may be considered, bearing in mind that such medicine can produce bronchospasm. Cardiac monitoring is recommended in cases of overdosage.

11 DESCRIPTION

BREO ELLIPTA is a combination of fluticasone furoate (an ICS) and vilanterol (a LABA).

One active component of BREO ELLIPTA is fluticasone furoate, a synthetic trifluorinated corticosteroid having the chemical name (6α,11β,16α,17α)-6,9-difluoro-17-{[(fluoromethyl)thio]carbonyl}-11-hydroxy-16-methyl-3-oxoandrosta-1,4-dien-17-yl 2-furancarboxylate and the following chemical structure:

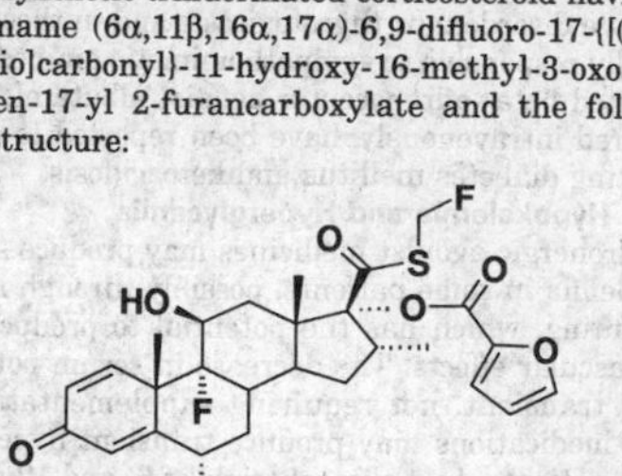

Fluticasone furoate is a white powder with a molecular weight of 538.6, and the empirical formula is $C_{27}H_{29}F_3O_6S$. It is practically insoluble in water.

The other active component of BREO ELLIPTA is vilanterol trifenatate, a LABA with the chemical name triphenylacetic acid-4-{(1R)-2-[(6-{2-[2,6-dicholorobenzyl)oxy]ethoxy}hexyl)amino]-1-hydroxyethyl}-2-(hydroxymethyl)phenol (1:1) and the following chemical structure:

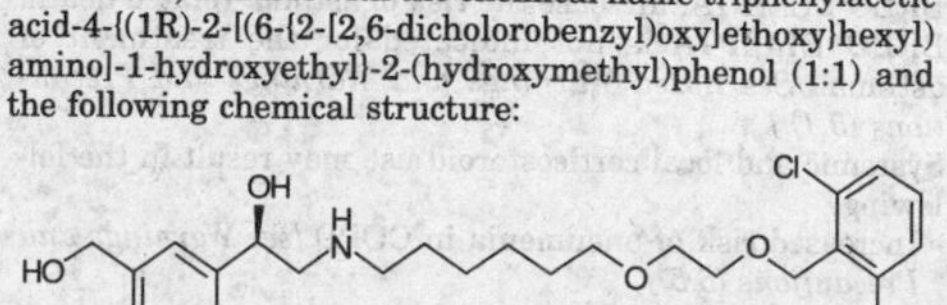

Vilanterol trifenatate is a white powder with a molecular weight of 774.8, and the empirical formula is $C_{24}H_{33}Cl_2NO_5C_{20}H_{16}O_2$. It is practically insoluble in water.

BREO ELLIPTA is a light grey and pale blue plastic inhaler containing 2 double-foil blister strips. Each blister on one strip contains a white powder mix of micronized fluticasone furoate (100 mcg) and lactose monohydrate (12.4 mg), and each blister on the other strip contains a white powder mix of micronized vilanterol trifenatate (40 mcg equivalent to 25 mcg of vilanterol), magnesium stearate (125 mcg), and lactose monohydrate (12.34 mg). The lactose monohydrate contains milk proteins. After the inhaler is activated, the powder within both blisters is exposed and ready for dispersion into the airstream created by the patient inhaling through the mouthpiece.

Under standardized in vitro test conditions, BREO ELLIPTA delivers 92 mcg of fluticasone furoate and 22 mcg of vilanterol per blister when tested at a flow rate of 60 L/min for 4 seconds.

In adult subjects with obstructive lung disease and severely compromised lung function (COPD with FEV$_1$/FVC less than 70% and FEV$_1$ less than 30% predicted or FEV$_1$ less than 50% predicted plus chronic respiratory failure), mean peak inspiratory flow through the ELLIPTA inhaler was 66.5 L/min (range: 43.5 to 81.0 L/min).

The actual amount of drug delivered to the lung will depend on patient factors, such as inspiratory flow profile.

12 CLINICAL PHARMACOLOGY

12.1 Mechanism of Action

BREO ELLIPTA: Since BREO ELLIPTA contains both fluticasone furoate and vilanterol, the mechanisms of action described below for the individual components apply to BREO ELLIPTA. These drugs represent 2 different classes of medications (a synthetic corticosteroid and a LABA) that have different effects on clinical and physiological indices.

Fluticasone Furoate: Fluticasone furoate is a synthetic trifluorinated corticosteroid with anti-inflammatory activity. Fluticasone furoate has been shown in vitro to exhibit a binding affinity for the human glucocorticoid receptor that is approximately 29.9 times that of dexamethasone and 1.7 times that of fluticasone propionate. The clinical relevance of these in vitro findings is unknown. The precise mechanism through which fluticasone furoate affects COPD symptoms is not known. Corticosteroids have been shown to have a wide range of actions on multiple cell types (e.g., mast cells, eosinophils, neutrophils, macrophages, lymphocytes) and mediators (e.g., histamine, eicosanoids, leukotrienes, cytokines) involved in inflammation. Specific effects of fluticasone furoate demonstrated in in vitro and in vivo models included activation of the glucocorticoid response element, inhibition of pro-inflammatory transcription factors such as NFkB, and inhibition of antigen-induced lung eosinophilia in sensitized rats.

Vilanterol: Vilanterol is a LABA. In vitro tests have shown the functional selectivity of vilanterol was similar to salmeterol. The clinical relevance of this in vitro finding is unknown.

Although beta$_2$-receptors are the predominant adrenergic receptors in bronchial smooth muscle and beta$_1$-receptors are the predominant receptors in the heart, there are also beta$_2$-receptors in the human heart comprising 10% to 50% of the total beta-adrenergic receptors. The precise function of these receptors has not been established, but they raise the possibility that even highly selective beta$_2$-agonists may have cardiac effects.

The pharmacologic effects of beta$_2$-adrenoceptor agonist drugs, including vilanterol, are at least in part attributable to stimulation of intracellular adenyl cyclase, the enzyme that catalyzes the conversion of adenosine triphosphate (ATP) to cyclic-3',5'-adenosine monophosphate (cyclic AMP). Increased cyclic AMP levels cause relaxation of bronchial smooth muscle and inhibition of release of mediators of immediate hypersensitivity from cells, especially from mast cells.

12.2 Pharmacodynamics

Cardiovascular Effects: *Healthy Subjects:* QTc interval prolongation was studied in a double-blind, multiple dose, placebo- and positive-controlled crossover study in 85 healthy volunteers. The maximum mean (95% upper confidence bound) difference in QTcF from placebo after baseline-correction was 4.9 (7.5) milliseconds and 9.6 (12.2) milliseconds seen 30 minutes after dosing for fluticasone furoate /vilanterol 200mcg/25 mcg and fluticasone furoate/vilanterol 800 mcg/100 mcg, respectively.

A dose-dependent increase in heart rate was also observed. The maximum mean (95% upper confidence bound) difference in heart rate from placebo after baseline-correction was 7.8 (9.4) beats/min and 17.1 (18.7) beats/min seen 10 minutes after dosing for fluticasone furoate/vilanterol 200 mcg/25 mcg and fluticasone furoate/vilanterol 800 mcg/100 mcg, respectively.

Chronic Obstructive Pulmonary Disease: In 4 clinical trials of 6- and 12-month duration, there was no evidence of a treatment effect on heart rate, QTcF, or blood pressure in subjects with COPD given combination doses of fluticasone furoate (50, 100, or 200 mcg)/vilanterol 25 mcg, the individual components of fluticasone furoate or vilanterol alone, or placebo *[see Clinical Studies (14)]*.

HPA Axis Effects: *Healthy Subjects:* Inhaled fluticasone furoate at repeat doses up to 400 mcg was not associated with statistically significant decreases in serum or urinary cortisol in healthy subjects. Decreases in serum and urine cortisol levels were observed at fluticasone furoate exposures several-fold higher than exposures observed at the therapeutic dose.

Chronic Obstructive Pulmonary Disease: In a trial with subjects with COPD, treatment with fluticasone furoate/vilanterol (50 mcg/25 mcg, 100 mcg/25 mcg, and 200 mcg/25 mcg), vilanterol 25 mcg, and fluticasone furoate (100 and 200 mcg) for 6 months did not affect 24-hour urinary cortisol excretion. A separate trial with subjects with COPD demonstrated no effects on serum cortisol after 28 days of treatment with fluticasone furoate/vilanterol (50 mcg/25 mcg, 100 mcg/25 mcg, and 200 mcg/25 mcg).

12.3 Pharmacokinetics

Linear pharmacokinetics was observed for fluticasone furoate (200 to 800 mcg) and vilanterol (25 to 100 mcg). On repeated once-daily inhalation administration, steady state of fluticasone furoate and vilanterol plasma concentrations was achieved after 6 days, and the accumulation was up to 2.6-fold for fluticasone furoate and 2.4-fold for vilanterol as compared with single dose.

Absorption: *Fluticasone Furoate:* Fluticasone furoate plasma levels may not predict therapeutic effect. Peak plasma concentrations are reached within 0.5 to 1 hour. Absolute bioavailability of fluticasone furoate when administrated by inhalation was 15.2%, primarily due to absorption of the inhaled portion of the dose delivered to the lung. Oral bioavailability from the swallowed portion of the dose is low (approximately 1.3%) due to extensive first-pass metabolism. Systemic exposure (AUC) in subjects with COPD was 46% lower than observed in healthy subjects.

Vilanterol: Vilanterol plasma levels may not predict therapeutic effect. Peak plasma concentrations are reached within 10 minutes following inhalation. Absolute bioavailability of vilanterol when administrated by inhalation was 27.3%, primarily due to absorption of the inhaled portion of the dose delivered to the lung. Oral bioavailability from the swallowed portion of the dose of vilanterol is low (less than 2%) due to extensive first-pass metabolism. Systemic exposure in subjects with COPD was 24% higher than observed in healthy subjects.

Distribution: *Fluticasone Furoate:* Following intravenous administration to healthy subjects, the mean volume of distribution at steady state was 661 L. Binding of fluticasone furoate to human plasma proteins was high (99.6%).

Vilanterol: Following intravenous administration to healthy subjects, the mean volume of distribution at steady state was 165 L. Binding of vilanterol to human plasma proteins was 93.9%.

Metabolism: *Fluticasone Furoate:* Fluticasone furoate is cleared from systemic circulation principally by hepatic metabolism via CYP3A4 to metabolites with significantly reduced corticosteroid activity. There was no in vivo evidence for cleavage of the furoate moiety resulting in the formation of fluticasone.

Vilanterol: Vilanterol is mainly metabolized, principally via CYP3A4, to a range of metabolites with significantly reduced β_1- and β_2-agonist activity.

Elimination: *Fluticasone Furoate:* Fluticasone furoate and its metabolites are eliminated primarily in the feces, accounting for approximately 101% and 90% of the orally and intravenously administered dose, respectively. Urinary excretion accounted for approximately 1% and 2% of the orally and intravenously administered doses, respectively. Following repeat-dose inhaled administration, the plasma elimination phase half-life averaged 24 hours.

Vilanterol: Following oral administration, vilanterol was eliminated mainly by metabolism followed by excretion of metabolites in urine and feces (approximately 70% and 30% of the recovered radioactive dose, respectively). The effective half-life for accumulation of vilanterol, as determined from inhalation administration of multiple doses of vilanterol 25 mcg, is 21.3 hours in subjects with COPD.

Special Populations: The effect of renal and hepatic impairment and other intrinsic factors on the pharmacokinetics of fluticasone furoate and vilanterol is shown in Figure 1.

[See figure at top of next column]

Race: Systemic exposure ($AUC_{(0-24)}$) to inhaled fluticasone furoate 200 mcg was 27% to 49% higher in healthy subjects of Japanese, Korean, and Chinese heritage compared with Caucasian subjects. Similar differences were observed for subjects with COPD (Figure 1). However, there is no evidence that this higher exposure to fluticasone furoate results in clinically relevant effects on urinary cortisol excretion or on efficacy in these racial groups.

There was no effect of race on the pharmacokinetics of vilanterol in subjects with COPD.

Hepatic Impairment: Fluticasone Furoate: Following repeat dosing of fluticasone furoate/vilanterol 200 mcg/25 mcg (100 mcg/12.5 mcg in the severe impairment group) for 7 days, there was an increase of 34%, 83%, and 75% in fluticasone furoate systemic exposure (AUC) in subjects with mild, moderate, and severe hepatic impairment, respectively, compared with healthy subjects (see Figure 1).

Figure 1. Impact of Intrinsic Factors on the Pharmacokinetics (PK) of Fluticasone Furoate and Vilanterol Following Administration as Fluticasone Furoate/Vilanterol Combination

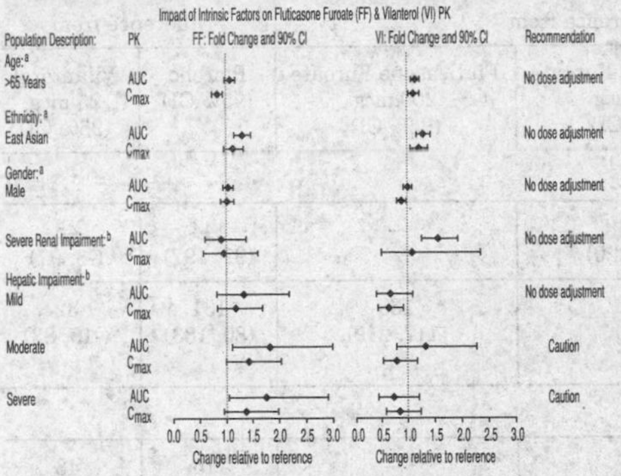

[a]Age, gender, and ethnicity comparison for BREO ELLIPTA (fluticasone furoate/vilanterol 100 mcg/25 mcg) in subjects with COPD.

[b]Renal groups (fluticasone furoate/vilanterol 200 mcg/25 mcg) and hepatic groups (fluticasone furoate/vilanterol 200 mcg/25 mcg or fluticasone furoate/vilanterol 100 mcg/12.5 mcg) compared with healthy control group.

In subjects with moderate hepatic impairment receiving fluticasone furoate/vilanterol 200 mcg/25 mcg, mean serum cortisol (0 to 24 hours) was reduced by 34% (95% CI: 11%, 51%) compared with healthy subjects. In subjects with severe hepatic impairment receiving fluticasone furoate/vilanterol 100 mcg/12.5 mcg, mean serum cortisol (0 to 24 hours) was increased by 14% (95% CI: -16%, 55%) compared with healthy subjects. Patients with moderate to severe hepatic disease should be closely monitored.

Vilanterol: Hepatic impairment had no effect on vilanterol systemic exposure (C_{max} and $AUC_{(0-24)}$ on Day 7) following repeat-dose administration of fluticasone furoate/vilanterol 200 mcg/25 mcg (100 mcg/12.5 mcg in the severe impairment group) for 7 days (see Figure 1).

There were no additional clinically relevant effects of the fluticasone furoate/vilanterol combinations on heart rate or serum potassium in subjects with mild or moderate hepatic impairment (vilanterol 25 mcg combination) or with severe hepatic impairment (vilanterol 12.5 mcg combination) compared with healthy subjects.

Renal Impairment: Fluticasone furoate systemic exposure was not increased and vilanterol systemic exposure ($AUC_{(0-24)}$) was 56% higher in subjects with severe renal impairment compared with healthy subjects (see Figure 1). There was no evidence of greater corticosteroid or beta-agonist class-related systemic effects (assessed by serum cortisol, heart rate, and serum potassium) in subjects with severe renal impairment compared with healthy subjects.

Drug Interactions: There were no clinically relevant differences in the pharmacokinetics or pharmacodynamics of either fluticasone furoate or vilanterol when administered in combination compared with administration alone. The potential for fluticasone furoate and vilanterol to inhibit or induce metabolic enzymes and transporter systems is negligible at low inhalation doses.

Inhibitors of Cytochrome P450 3A4: The exposure (AUC) of fluticasone furoate and vilanterol were 36% and 65% higher, respectively, when coadministered with ketoconazole 400 mg compared with placebo (see Figure 2). The increase in fluticasone furoate exposure was associated with a 27% reduction in weighted mean serum cortisol (0 to 24 hours). The increase in vilanterol exposure was not associated with an increase in beta-agonist–related systemic effects on heart rate or blood potassium.

Figure 2. Impact of Coadministered Drugs[a] on the Pharmacokinetics (PK) of Fluticasone Furoate and Vilanterol Following Administration as Fluticasone Furoate/Vilanterol Combination or Vilanterol Coadministered With a Long-Acting Muscarinic Antagonist

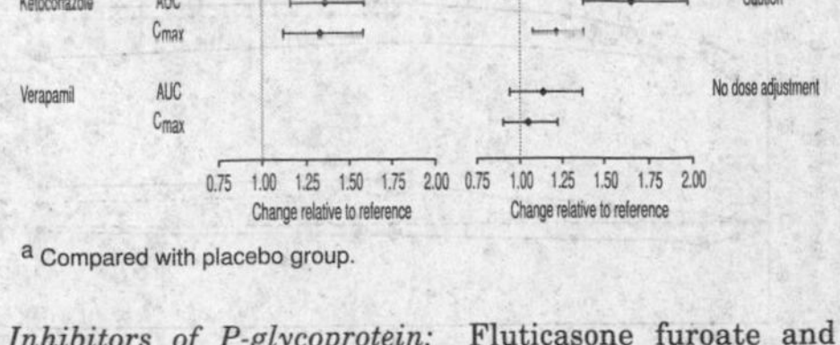

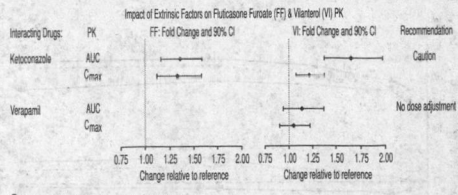

[a] Compared with placebo group.

Inhibitors of P-glycoprotein: Fluticasone furoate and vilanterol are both substrates of P-glycoprotein (P-gp). Coadministration of repeat-dose (240 mg once daily) verapamil (a potent P-gp inhibitor and moderate CYP3A4 inhibitor) did not affect the vilanterol C_{max} or AUC in healthy subjects (see Figure 2). Drug interaction trials with a specific P-gp inhibitor and fluticasone furoate have not been conducted.

13 NONCLINICAL TOXICOLOGY

13.1 Carcinogenesis, Mutagenesis, Impairment of Fertility

BREO ELLIPTA: No studies of carcinogenicity, mutagenicity, or impairment of fertility were conducted with BREO ELLIPTA; however, studies are available for the individual components, fluticasone furoate and vilanterol, as described below.

Fluticasone Furoate: Fluticasone furoate produced no treatment-related increases in the incidence of tumors in 2-year inhalation studies in rats and mice at inhaled doses up to 9 and 19 mcg/kg/day, respectively (approximately equal to the MRHDID in adults on a mcg/m^2 basis).

Fluticasone furoate did not induce gene mutation in bacteria or chromosomal damage in a mammalian cell mutation test in mouse lymphoma L5178Y cells in vitro. There was also no evidence of genotoxicity in the in vivo micronucleus test in rats.

No evidence of impairment of fertility was observed in male and female rats at inhaled fluticasone furoate doses up to 29 and 91 mcg/kg/day, respectively (approximately 3 and 9 times, respectively, the MRHDID in adults on a mcg/m^2 basis).

Vilanterol: In a 2-year carcinogenicity study in mice, vilanterol caused a statistically significant increase in ovarian tubulostromal adenomas in females at an inhalation dose of 29,500 mcg/kg/day (approximately 8,750 times the MRHDID in adults on an AUC basis). No increase in tumors was seen at an inhalation dose of 615 mcg/kg/day (approximately 530 times the MRHDID in adults on an AUC basis).

In a 2-year carcinogenicity study in rats, vilanterol caused statistically significant increases in mesovarian leiomyomas in females and shortening of the latency of pituitary tumors at inhalation doses greater than or equal to 84.4 mcg/kg/day (greater than or equal to approximately 45 times the MRHDID in adults on an AUC basis). No tumors were seen at an inhalation dose of 10.5 mcg/kg/day (approximately 2 times the MRHDID in adults on an AUC basis).

These tumor findings in rodents are similar to those reported previously for other beta-adrenergic agonist drugs. The relevance of these findings to human use is unknown.

Vilanterol tested negative in the following genotoxicity assays: the in vitro Ames assay, in vivo rat bone marrow micronucleus assay, in vivo rat unscheduled DNA synthesis (UDS) assay, and in vitro Syrian hamster embryo (SHE) cell assay. Vilanterol tested equivocal in the in vitro mouse lymphoma assay.

No evidence of impairment of fertility was observed in reproductive studies conducted in male and female rats at inhaled vilanterol doses up to 31,500 and 37,100 mcg/kg/day, respectively (approximately 12,000 and 14,000 times, respectively, the MRHDID in adults on a mcg/m^2 basis).

14 CLINICAL STUDIES

The safety and efficacy of BREO ELLIPTA were evaluated in 7,700 subjects with COPD. The development program included 4 confirmatory trials of 6- and 12-months' duration, three 12-week active comparator trials, and dose-ranging trials of shorter duration. The efficacy of BREO ELLIPTA is based primarily on the dose-ranging trials and the 4 confirmatory trials described below.

14.1 Dose-Ranging Trials

Dose selection for BREO ELLIPTA for COPD was based on dose-ranging trials for the individual components, vilanterol and fluticasone furoate, in patients with COPD and asthma. **BREO ELLIPTA 100 mcg/25 mcg is not indicated for asthma.**

Vilanterol: Dose selection for vilanterol in COPD was supported by a 28-day, randomized, double-blind, placebo-controlled, parallel-group trial evaluating 5 doses of vilanterol (3 to 50 mcg) or placebo dosed in the morning in 602 patients with COPD. Results demonstrated dose-related increases in FEV_1 compared with placebo at Day 1 and Day 28 (Figure 3).

[See figure 3 at top of next column]

The differences in trough FEV_1 on Day 28 from placebo for the 3-, 6.25-, 12.5-, 25-, and 50-mcg doses were 92 mL (95% CI: 39, 144), 98 mL (95% CI: 46, 150), 110 mL (95% CI: 57, 162), 137 mL (95% CI: 85, 190), and 165 mL (95% CI: 112, 217), respectively. These results supported the evaluation of vilanterol 25 mcg in the confirmatory COPD trials.

Dose-ranging trials in subjects with asthma evaluated doses from 3 to 50 mcg and 12.5 mcg once-daily versus 6.25 mcg twice-daily dosing frequency. The results supported the selection of the vilanterol 25 mcg once-daily dose for further evaluation in the confirmatory COPD trials.

Fluticasone Furoate: Eight doses of fluticasone furoate ranging from 25 to 800 mcg once daily were evaluated in 3 randomized, double-blind, placebo-controlled, 8-week trials in subjects with asthma. A dose-related increase in trough FEV_1 at Week 8 was seen for doses from 25 to 200 mcg with

Table 2. Least Squares Mean Change From Baseline in Weighted Mean FEV1 (0-4 h) and Trough FEV1 at 6 Months

Treatment	N	Weighted Mean FEV_1 (0-4 h)[a] (mL)			Trough FEV_1[b] (mL)	
		Difference from			Difference from	
		Placebo (95% CI)	Fluticasone Furoate 100 mcg (95% CI)	Fluticasone Furoate 200 mcg (95% CI)	Placebo (95% CI)	Vilanterol 25 mcg (95% CI)
Trial 1						
BREO ELLIPTA 100 mcg/25 mcg	204	214 (161, 266)	168 (116, 220)	—	144 (91, 197)	45 (-8, 97)
Fluticasone furoate/ vilanterol 200 mcg/25 mcg	205	209 (157, 261)	—	168 (117, 219)	131 (80, 183)	32 (-19, 83)
Trial 2						
BREO ELLIPTA 100 mcg/25 mcg	206	173 (123, 224)	120 (70, 170)	—	115 (60, 169)	48 (-6, 102)

[a] At Day 168.
[b] At Day 169.

Figure 3. Least Squares (LS) Mean Difference From Placebo in Post-Dose Serial FEV1 (0-24 h, mL) on Days 1 and 28

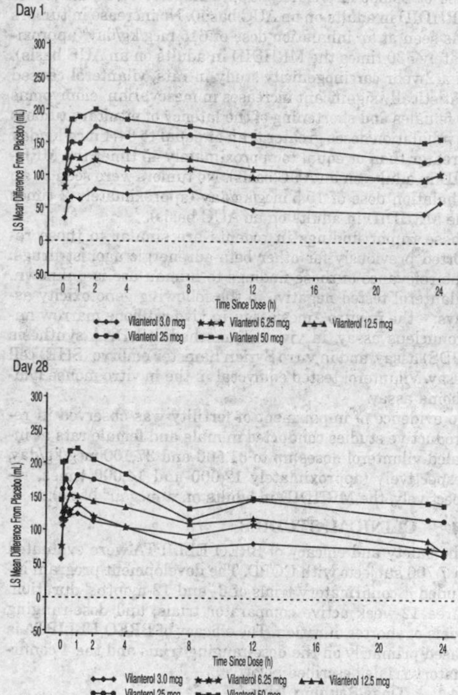

no consistent additional benefit for doses above 200 mcg. To evaluate dosing frequency, a separate trial compared fluticasone furoate 200 mcg once-daily, fluticasone furoate 100 mcg twice-daily, fluticasone propionate 100 mcg twice-daily, and fluticasone propionate 200 mcg twice-daily. The results supported the selection of the once-daily dosing frequency.

Based on the dose-ranging trials in asthma and COPD, once-daily doses of fluticasone furoate/vilanterol 50 mcg/25 mcg, 100 mcg/25 mcg, and 200 mcg/25 mcg were evaluated in the confirmatory COPD trials.

14.2 Confirmatory Trials

The clinical development program for BREO ELLIPTA included 4 confirmatory trials in subjects with COPD designed to evaluate the efficacy of BREO ELLIPTA on lung function (Trials 1 and 2) and exacerbations (Trials 3 and 4).

Lung Function: Trials 1 and 2 were 24-week, randomized, double-blind, placebo-controlled trials designed to evaluate the efficacy of BREO ELLIPTA on lung function in subjects with COPD. In Trial 1, subjects were randomized to BREO ELLIPTA 100 mcg/25 mcg, fluticasone furoate/vilanterol 200 mcg/25 mcg, fluticasone furoate 100 mcg, fluticasone furoate 200 mcg, vilanterol 25 mcg, and placebo. In Trial 2, subjects were randomized to BREO ELLIPTA 100 mcg/25 mcg, fluticasone furoate/vilanterol 50 mcg/25 mcg, fluticasone furoate 100 mcg, vilanterol 25 mcg, and placebo. All treatments were administered as 1 inhalation once daily.

Of the 2,254 patients, 70% were male and 84% were Caucasian. They had a mean age of 62 years and an average smoking history of 44 pack years, with 54% identified as current smokers. At screening, the mean postbronchodilator percent predicted FEV_1 was 48% (range: 14% to 87%), mean postbronchodilator FEV_1/FVC ratio was 47% (range: 17% to 88%), and the mean percent reversibility was 14% (range: -41% to 152%).

The co-primary efficacy variables in both trials were weighted mean FEV_1 (0 to 4 hours) postdose on Day 168 and change from baseline in trough FEV_1 on Day 169 (the mean of the FEV_1 values obtained 23 and 24 hours after the final dose on Day 168). The weighted mean comparison of the fluticasone furoate/vilanterol combination with fluticasone furoate was assessed to evaluate the contribution of vilanterol to BREO ELLIPTA. The trough FEV_1 comparison of the fluticasone furoate/vilanterol combination with vilanterol was assessed to evaluate the contribution of fluticasone furoate to BREO ELLIPTA.

BREO ELLIPTA 100 mcg/25 mcg demonstrated a larger increase in the weighted mean FEV_1 (0 to 4 hours) relative to placebo and fluticasone furoate 100 mcg at Day 168 (Table 2).

[See table 2 above]

Serial spirometric evaluations were performed pre-dose and up to 4 hours after dosing. Results from Trial 1 at Day 1 and Day 168 are shown in Figure 4. Similar results were seen in Trial 2 (not shown).

Figure 4. Raw Mean Change From Baseline in Post-Dose Serial FEV1 (0-4 h, mL) on Days 1 and 168

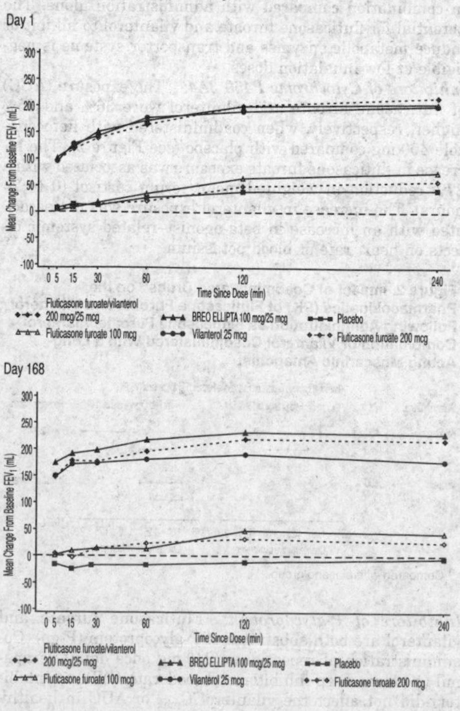

The second co-primary variable was change from baseline in trough FEV_1 following the final treatment day. At Day 169, both Trials 1 and 2 demonstrated significant increases in trough FEV_1 for all strengths of the fluticasone furoate/vilanterol combination compared with placebo (Table 2). The comparison of BREO ELLIPTA 100 mcg/25 mcg with vilanterol did not achieve statistical significance (Table 2).

Trials 1 and 2 evaluated FEV_1 as a secondary endpoint. Peak FEV_1 was defined as the maximum postdose FEV_1 recorded within 4 hours after the first dose of trial medicine on Day 1 (measurements recorded at 5, 15, and 30 minutes and 1, 2, and 4 hours). In both trials, differences in mean change from baseline in peak FEV_1 were observed for the groups receiving fluticasone furoate/vilanterol 100 mcg/25 mcg compared with placebo (152 and 139 mL, respectively). The median time to onset, defined as a 100-mL increase from baseline in FEV_1, was 16 minutes in subjects receiving fluticasone furoate/vilanterol 100 mcg/25 mcg.

Exacerbations: Trials 3 and 4 were randomized, double-blind, 52-week trials designed to evaluate the effect of BREO ELLIPTA on the rate of moderate and severe COPD exacerbations. All patients were treated with fluticasone propionate/salmeterol 250 mcg/50 mcg twice daily during a 4-week run-in period prior to being randomly assigned to 1 of the following treatment groups: BREO ELLIPTA 100 mcg/25 mcg, fluticasone furoate/vilanterol 50 mcg/25 mcg, fluticasone furoate/vilanterol 200 mcg/25 mcg, or vilanterol 25 mcg.

The primary efficacy variable in both trials was the annual rate of moderate/severe exacerbations. The comparison of the fluticasone furoate/vilanterol combination with vilanterol was assessed to evaluate the contribution of fluticasone furoate to BREO ELLIPTA. In these 2 trials, exacerbations were defined as worsening of 2 or more major symptoms (dyspnea, sputum volume, and sputum purulence) or worsening of any 1 major symptom together with any 1 of the following minor symptoms: sore throat, colds (nasal discharge and/or nasal congestion), fever without other cause, and increased cough or wheeze for at least 2 consecutive days. COPD exacerbations were considered to be of moderate severity if treatment with systemic corticosteroids and/or antibiotics was required and were considered to be severe if hospitalization was required.

Trials 3 and 4 included 3,255 subjects, of which 57% were male and 85% were Caucasian. They had a mean age of 64 years and an average smoking history of 46 pack years, with 44% identified as current smokers. At screening, the mean postbronchodilator percent predicted FEV_1 was 45% (range: 12% to 91%), and mean postbronchodilator FEV_1/FVC ratio was 46% (range: 17% to 81%), indicating that the subject population had moderate to very severely impaired airflow obstruction. The mean percent reversibility was 15% (range: -65% to 313%).

Patients treated with BREO ELLIPTA 100 mcg/25 mcg had a lower annual rate of moderate/severe COPD exacerbations compared with vilanterol in both trials (Table 3).

[See table 3 at top of next page]

16 HOW SUPPLIED/STORAGE AND HANDLING

BREO ELLIPTA is supplied as a disposable light grey and pale blue plastic inhaler containing 2 double-foil strips, each with 30 blisters. The inhaler is packaged within a moisture-protective foil tray with a desiccant and a peelable lid (NDC 0173-0859-10).

BREO ELLIPTA is also supplied in an institutional pack as a disposable light grey and pale blue plastic inhaler containing 2 double-foil strips, each with 14 blisters. It is packaged within a moisture-protective foil tray with a desiccant and a peelable lid (NDC 0173-0859-14).

Store at room temperature between 68°F and 77°F (20°C and 25°C); excursions permitted from 59° to 86°F (15° to 30°C) [See USP Controlled Room Temperature]. Store in a dry place away from direct heat or sunlight. Keep out of reach of children.

BREO ELLIPTA should be stored inside the unopened moisture-protective foil tray and only removed from the tray immediately before initial use. Discard BREO ELLIPTA 6 weeks after opening the foil tray or when the counter reads "0" (after all blisters have been used), whichever comes first. The inhaler is not reusable. Do not attempt to take the inhaler apart.

17 PATIENT COUNSELING INFORMATION

See FDA-approved patient labeling (Medication Guide and Instructions for Use)

17.1 Asthma-Related Death

Patients should be informed that LABA, such as vilanterol, one of the active ingredients in BREO ELLIPTA, increase the risk of asthma-related death. BREO ELLIPTA is not indicated for the treatment of asthma.

17.2 Not for Acute Symptoms

BREO ELLIPTA is not meant to relieve acute symptoms of COPD and extra doses should not be used for that purpose. Acute symptoms should be treated with a rescue inhaler such as albuterol. The physician should provide the patient with such medicine and instruct the patient in how it should be used.

Patients should be instructed to notify their physicians immediately if they experience any of the following:
- Symptoms get worse
- Need for more inhalations than usual of their rescue inhaler
- Significant decrease in lung function as outlined by the physician

Patients should not stop therapy with BREO ELLIPTA without physician/provider guidance since symptoms may recur after discontinuation.

17.3 Do Not Use Additional Long-Acting Beta$_2$-Agonists

When patients are prescribed BREO ELLIPTA, other medicines containing a LABA should not be used.

17.4 Risks Associated With Corticosteroid Therapy

Local Effects: Patients should be advised that localized infections with *Candida albicans* occurred in the mouth and pharynx in some patients. If oropharyngeal candidiasis develops, it should be treated with appropriate local or systemic (i.e., oral) antifungal therapy while still continuing therapy with BREO ELLIPTA, but at times therapy with BREO ELLIPTA may need to be temporarily interrupted under close medical supervision. Rinsing the mouth without swallowing after inhalation is advised to help reduce the risk of thrush.

Pneumonia: Patients with COPD who have received BREO ELLIPTA have a higher risk of pneumonia and should be instructed to contact their healthcare providers if they develop symptoms of pneumonia (e.g., fever, chills, change in sputum color, increase in breathing problems).

Immunosuppression: Patients who are on immunosuppressant doses of corticosteroids should be warned to avoid exposure to chickenpox or measles and, if exposed, to consult their physicians without delay. Patients should be informed of potential worsening of existing tuberculosis, fungal, bacterial, viral, or parasitic infections, or ocular herpes simplex.

Hypercorticism and Adrenal Suppression: Patients should be advised that BREO ELLIPTA may cause systemic corticosteroid effects of hypercorticism and adrenal suppression. Additionally, patients should be instructed that deaths due to adrenal insufficiency have occurred during and after transfer from systemic corticosteroids.

Reduction in Bone Mineral Density: Patients who are at an increased risk for decreased BMD should be advised that the use of corticosteroids may pose an additional risk.

Ocular Effects: Long-term use of inhaled corticosteroids may increase the risk of some eye problems (cataracts or glaucoma); regular eye examinations should be considered.

17.5 Risks Associated With Beta-Agonist Therapy

Patients should be informed of adverse effects associated with beta$_2$-agonists, such as palpitations, chest pain, rapid heart rate, tremor, or nervousness.

BREO and ELLIPTA are trademarks of GlaxoSmithKline.

BREO ELLIPTA was developed in collaboration with Theravance.

GlaxoSmithKline
Research Triangle Park, NC 27709

BRE:1PI

Table 3. Moderate and Severe Chronic Obstructive Pulmonary Disease Exacerbations

Treatment	N	Mean Annual Rate (exacerbations/year)	Ratio vs Vilanterol	95% CI
Trial 3				
Fluticasone furoate/vilanterol 200 mcg/25 mcg	409	0.79	0.69	(0.56, 0.85)
BREO ELLIPTA 100 mcg/ 25 mcg	403	0.90	0.79	(0.64, 0.97)
Fluticasone furoate/vilanterol 50 mcg/25 mcg	412	0.92	0.81	(0.66, 0.99)
Vilanterol 25 mcg	409	1.14	—	—
Trial 4				
Fluticasone furoate/vilanterol 200 mcg/25 mcg	402	0.90	0.85	(0.70, 1.04)
BREO ELLIPTA 100 mcg/ 25 mcg	403	0.70	0.66	(0.54, 0.81)
Fluticasone furoate/vilanterol 50 mcg/25 mcg	408	0.92	0.87	(0.72, 1.06)
Vilanterol 25 mcg	409	1.05	—	—

Medication Guide

BREO™ ELLIPTA™ (*BREE-oh ee-LIP-ta*)

(fluticasone furoate and vilanterol inhalation powder)

Read the Medication Guide that comes with BREO ELLIPTA before you start using it and each time you get a refill. There may be new information. This Medication Guide does not take the place of talking to your healthcare provider about your medical condition or treatment.

What is the most important information I should know about BREO ELLIPTA?

BREO ELLIPTA is only approved for use in chronic obstructive pulmonary disease (COPD). BREO ELLIPTA is NOT approved for use in asthma.

BREO ELLIPTA can cause serious side effects, including:
- **People with asthma who take long-acting beta$_2$-adrenergic agonist (LABA) medicines, such as vilanterol (one of the medicines in BREO ELLIPTA), have an increased risk of death from asthma problems.** It is not known whether fluticasone furoate, the other medicine in BREO ELLIPTA, reduces the risk of death from asthma problems seen with LABA medicines.
- **It is not known if LABA medicines, such as vilanterol (one of the medicines in BREO ELLIPTA), increase the risk of death in people with COPD.**
- **Call your healthcare provider if breathing problems worsen over time while using BREO ELLIPTA.** You may need different treatment.
- **Get emergency medical care if:**
  - **your breathing problems worsen quickly**
  - **you use your rescue inhaler, but it does not relieve your breathing problems.**

What is BREO ELLIPTA?

BREO ELLIPTA combines an inhaled corticosteroid (ICS) medicine, fluticasone furoate, and a LABA medicine, vilanterol.
- ICS medicines, such as fluticasone furoate (one of the medicines in BREO ELLIPTA), help to decrease inflammation in the lungs. Inflammation in the lungs can lead to breathing problems.
- LABA medicines, such as vilanterol (one of the medicines in BREO ELLIPTA), help the muscles around the airways in your lungs stay relaxed to prevent symptoms such as wheezing, cough, chest tightness, and shortness of breath. These symptoms can happen when the muscles around the airways tighten. This makes it hard to breathe.

BREO ELLIPTA is used for COPD. COPD is a chronic lung disease that includes chronic bronchitis, emphysema, or both. BREO ELLIPTA is a prescription medicine that is used long term as 1 inhalation 1 time each day to improve symptoms of COPD for better breathing and to reduce the number of flare-ups (the worsening of your COPD symptoms for several days).
- **BREO ELLIPTA is not for use to treat sudden symptoms of COPD.** Always have a rescue inhaler (an inhaled, short-acting bronchodilator) with you to treat sudden symptoms. If you do not have a rescue inhaler, contact your healthcare provider to have one prescribed for you.
- **BREO ELLIPTA is not for the treatment of asthma. It is not known if BREO ELLIPTA is safe and effective in people with asthma.**
- BREO ELLIPTA should not be used in children. It is not known if BREO ELLIPTA is safe and effective in children.

Who should not use BREO ELLIPTA?

Do not use BREO ELLIPTA if you:
- have a severe allergy to milk proteins. Ask your healthcare provider if you are not sure.
- are allergic to fluticasone furoate, vilanterol, or any of the ingredients in BREO ELLIPTA. See "What are the ingredients in BREO ELLIPTA?" below for a complete list of ingredients.

What should I tell my healthcare provider before using BREO ELLIPTA?

Tell your healthcare provider about all of your health conditions, including if you:
- have heart problems
- have high blood pressure
- have seizures
- have thyroid problems
- have diabetes
- have liver problems
- have weak bones (osteoporosis)
- have an immune system problem
- have eye problems such as glaucoma or cataracts
- are allergic to any of the ingredients in BREO ELLIPTA, any other medicines, or food products. See "What are the ingredients in BREO ELLIPTA?" below for a complete list of ingredients.
- have any type of viral, bacterial, or fungal infection
- are exposed to chickenpox or measles or been around anyone who has chickenpox or measles
- have any other medical conditions
- are pregnant or planning to become pregnant. It is not known if BREO ELLIPTA may harm your unborn baby.
- are breastfeeding. It is not known if the medicines in BREO ELLIPTA pass into your milk and if they can harm your baby.

Tell your healthcare provider about all the medicines you take, including prescription and non-prescription medicines, vitamins, and herbal supplements. BREO ELLIPTA and certain other medicines may interact with each other. This may cause serious side effects. Especially, tell your healthcare provider if you take antifungal or anti-HIV medicines.

Know the medicines you take. Keep a list of them to show your healthcare provider and pharmacist when you get a new medicine.

How should I use BREO ELLIPTA?

Read the step-by-step instructions for using BREO ELLIPTA at the end of this Medication Guide.
- **Do not** use BREO ELLIPTA unless your healthcare provider has taught you how to use the inhaler and you understand how to use it correctly.
- Use BREO ELLIPTA exactly as prescribed. **Do not** use BREO ELLIPTA more often than prescribed.
- Use 1 inhalation of BREO ELLIPTA 1 time each day. Use BREO ELLIPTA at the same time each day.
- If you miss a dose of BREO ELLIPTA, take it as soon as you remember. Do not take more than 1 inhalation per day. Take your next dose at your usual time. Do not take 2 doses at one time.
- If you take too much BREO ELLIPTA, call your healthcare provider and get medical help right away if you have any unusual symptoms, such as worsening shortness of breath, chest pain, increased heart rate, or shakiness.
- **Do not use other medicines that contain a LABA for any reason.** Ask your healthcare provider or pharmacist if any of your other medicines are LABA medicines.
- Do not stop using BREO ELLIPTA unless told to do so by your healthcare provider because your symptoms might get worse. Your healthcare provider will change your medicines as needed.
- **BREO ELLIPTA does not relieve sudden symptoms.** Always have a rescue inhaler with you to treat sudden symptoms. If you do not have a rescue inhaler, call your healthcare provider to have one prescribed for you.
- Call your healthcare provider or get medical care right away if:
  - your breathing problems get worse
  - you need to use your rescue inhaler more often than usual
  - your rescue inhaler does not work as well to relieve your symptoms
  - you need to use 4 or more inhalations of your rescue inhaler in 24 hours for 2 or more days in a row
  - you use 1 whole canister of your rescue inhaler in 8 weeks

What are the possible side effects with BREO ELLIPTA?

BREO ELLIPTA can cause serious side effects, including:
- **See "What is the most important information I should know about BREO ELLIPTA?"**
- **pneumonia.** People with COPD have a higher chance of getting pneumonia. BREO ELLIPTA may increase the chance of getting pneumonia. Call your healthcare provider if you notice any of the following symptoms:
  - increase in mucus (sputum) production
  - change in mucus color
  - fever
  - chills

  - increased cough
  - increased breathing problems
- **thrush (fungal infection) in mouth and throat.** You may develop a yeast infection (*Candida albicans*) in your mouth or throat. Rinse your mouth with water without swallowing after using BREO ELLIPTA to help prevent thrush in your mouth and throat.
- **serious allergic reactions.** Call your healthcare provider or get emergency medical care if you get any of the following symptoms of a serious allergic reaction:
  - rash
  - hives
  - swelling of the face, mouth, and tongue
  - breathing problems
- **sudden breathing problems immediately after inhaling your medicine**
- **effects on heart**
  - increased blood pressure
  - a fast and/or irregular heartbeat
  - chest pain
- **effects on nervous system**
  - tremor
  - nervousness
- **reduced adrenal function (adrenal insufficiency).** Adrenal insufficiency is a condition in which the adrenal glands do not make enough steroid hormones. This can happen when you stop taking oral corticosteroid medicines (such as prednisone) and start taking a medicine containing an inhaled corticosteroid (such as BREO ELLIPTA). When your body is under stress from fever, trauma (such as a car accident), infection, surgery, or worse COPD symptoms, adrenal insufficiency can get worse and may cause death. Symptoms of adrenal insufficiency include:
  - feeling tired (fatigue)
  - lack of energy
  - weakness
  - nausea and vomiting
  - low blood pressure
- **changes in laboratory blood values (sugar, potassium)**
- **weakened immune system and increased chance of getting infections (immunosuppression)**
- **bone thinning or weakness (osteoporosis)**
- **eye problems including glaucoma and cataracts.** You should have regular eye exams while using BREO ELLIPTA.

Common side effects of BREO ELLIPTA include:
- runny nose and sore throat
- upper respiratory tract infection
- headache
- thrush in the mouth and/or throat. Rinse your mouth without swallowing after use to help prevent this.

Tell your healthcare provider about any side effect that bothers you or that does not go away.

These are not all the side effects with BREO ELLIPTA. Ask your healthcare provider or pharmacist for more information.

Call your doctor for medical advice about side effects. You may report side effects to FDA at 1-800-FDA-1088.

How do I store BREO ELLIPTA?
- Store BREO ELLIPTA at room temperature between 68°F and 77°F (20°C and 25°C). Keep in a dry place away from heat and sunlight.
- Store BREO ELLIPTA in the unopened foil tray and only open when ready for use.
- Safely throw away BREO ELLIPTA in the trash 6 weeks after you open the foil tray or when the counter reads "0", whichever comes first. Write the date you open the tray on the label on the inhaler.
- **Keep BREO ELLIPTA and all medicines out of the reach of children.**

General Information about BREO ELLIPTA

Medicines are sometimes prescribed for purposes not mentioned in a Medication Guide. Do not use BREO ELLIPTA for a condition for which it was not prescribed. Do not give your BREO ELLIPTA to other people, even if they have the same condition that you have. It may harm them.

This Medication Guide summarizes the most important information about BREO ELLIPTA. If you would like more information, talk with your healthcare provider or pharmacist. You can ask your healthcare provider or pharmacist for information about BREO ELLIPTA that was written for healthcare professionals.

For more information about BREO ELLIPTA, call 1-888-825-5249 or visit our website at www.myBREO.com.

What are the ingredients in BREO ELLIPTA?

Active ingredients: fluticasone furoate, vilanterol

Inactive ingredients: lactose monohydrate (contains milk proteins), magnesium stearate

Instructions for Use

For Oral Inhalation Only.

Read this before you start:
- **If you open and close the cover without inhaling the medicine, you will lose the dose.**
- **The lost dose will be securely held inside the inhaler, but it will no longer be available to be inhaled.**
- **It is not possible to accidentally take a double dose or an extra dose in one inhalation.**

Your BREO ELLIPTA inhaler

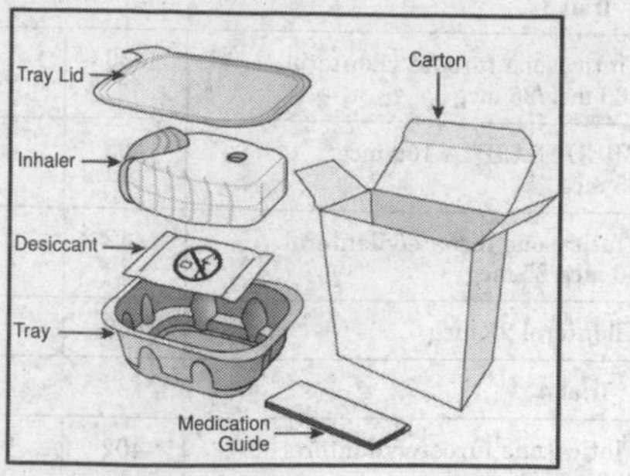

How to use your inhaler
- BREO ELLIPTA comes in a foil tray.
- Peel back the lid to open the tray. See Figure A.
- The tray contains a desiccant to reduce moisture. Do not eat or inhale. Throw it away in the household trash out of reach of children and pets. See Figure B.

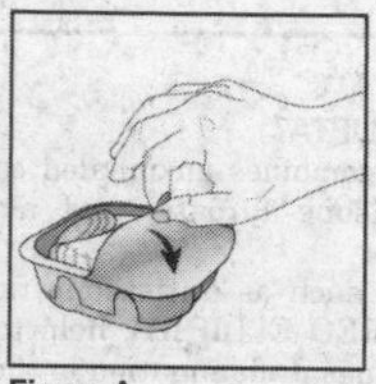

Figure A

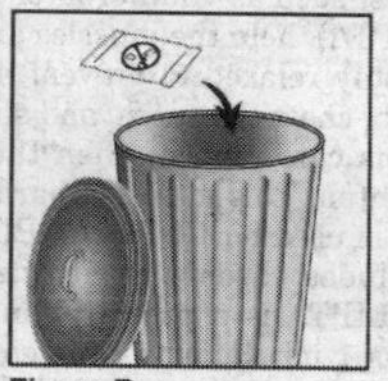

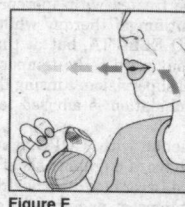

Figure B

Important Notes:
- Your inhaler contains 30 doses (14 doses if you have a sample or institutional pack).
- Each time you open the cover of the inhaler fully (you will hear a clicking sound), a dose is ready to be inhaled. This is shown by a decrease in the number on the counter.
- If you open and close the cover without inhaling the medicine, you will lose the dose. The lost dose will be held in the inhaler, but it will no longer be available to be inhaled. It is not possible to accidentally take a double dose or an extra dose in one inhalation.
- **Do not** open the cover of the inhaler until you are ready to use it. To avoid wasting doses after the inhaler is ready, **do not** close the cover until after you have inhaled the medicine.
- Write the "Tray opened" and "Discard" dates on the inhaler label. The "Discard" date is 6 weeks from the date you open the tray.

Check the counter. See Figure C.

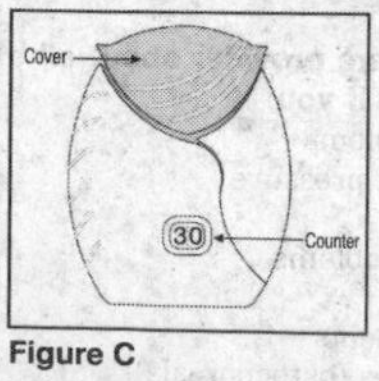

Figure C

- Before the inhaler is used for the first time, the counter should show the number 30 (14 if you have a sample or institutional pack). This is the number of doses in the inhaler.
- Each time you open the cover, you prepare 1 dose of medicine.
- The counter counts down by 1 each time you open the cover.

Prepare your dose:

Wait to open the cover until you are ready to take your dose.

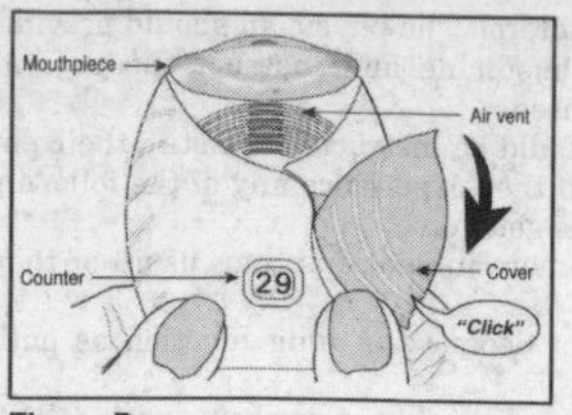

Figure D

Step 1. Open the cover of the inhaler. See Figure D.
- Slide the cover down to expose the mouthpiece. You should hear a "click." The counter will count down by 1 number. You do not need to shake this kind of inhaler. **Your inhaler is now ready to use.**
- If the counter does not count down as you hear the click, the inhaler will not deliver the medicine. Call your healthcare provider or pharmacist if this happens.

Figure E

Step 2. Breathe out. See Figure E.
- While holding the inhaler away from your mouth, breathe out (exhale) fully. Do not breathe out into the mouthpiece.

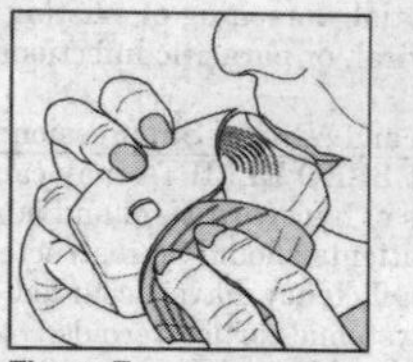

Figure F

Step 3. Inhale your medicine. See Figure F.
- Put the mouthpiece between your lips, and close your lips firmly around it. Your lips should fit over the curved shape of the mouthpiece.
- Take one long, steady, deep breath in through your mouth. **Do not** breathe in through your nose.

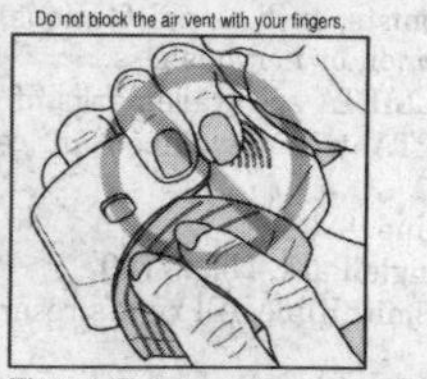

Figure G

- Do not block the air vent with your fingers. **See Figure G.**

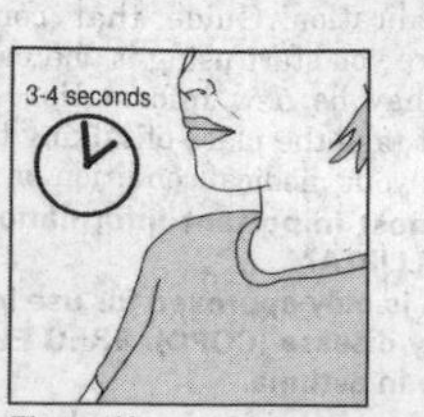

Figure H

- **Remove the inhaler from your mouth and hold your breath for about 3 to 4 seconds** (or as long as comfortable for you). **See Figure H.**

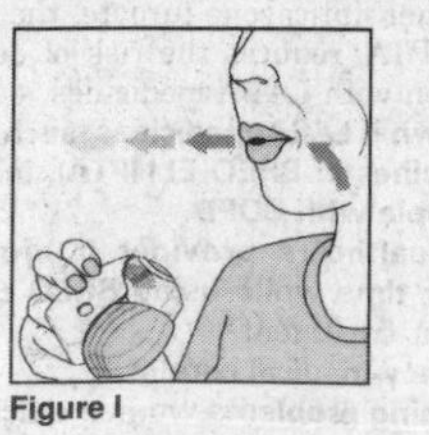

Figure I

Step 4. Breathe out slowly and gently. See Figure I.

- You may not taste or feel the medicine, even when you are using the inhaler correctly.
- **Do not** take another dose from the inhaler even if you do not feel or taste the medicine.

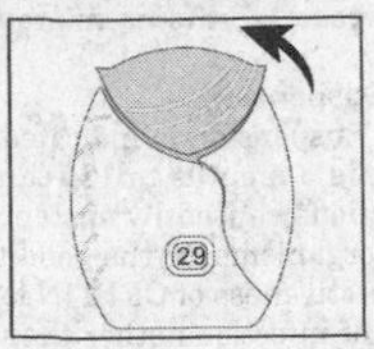

Figure J

Step 5. Close the inhaler. See Figure J.
- You can clean the mouthpiece if needed, using a dry tissue, before you close the cover. Routine cleaning is not required.
- Slide the cover up and over the mouthpiece as far as it will go.

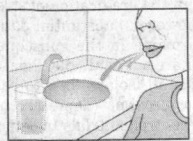

Figure K

Step 6. Rinse your mouth. See Figure K.
- Rinse your mouth with water after you have used the inhaler and spit the water out. **Do not** swallow the water.

Important Note: When should you get a refill?

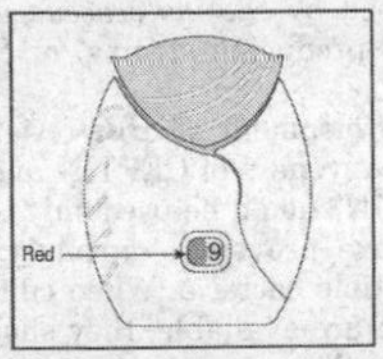

Figure L

- **When you have less than 10 doses remaining** in your inhaler, the left half of the counter shows red as a reminder to get a refill. **See Figure L.**
- After you have inhaled the last dose, the counter will show "0" and will be empty.
- Throw the empty inhaler away in your household trash out of reach of children and pets.

If you have questions about BREO ELLIPTA or how to use your inhaler, call GlaxoSmithKline (GSK) at 1-888-825-5249 or visit www.myBREO.com.

This Medication Guide has been approved by the U.S. Food and Drug Administration.

BREO and ELLIPTA are trademarks of GlaxoSmithKline.

BREO ELLIPTA was developed in collaboration with Theravance.

GlaxoSmithKline
Research Triangle Park, NC 27709

May 2013
BRE:1MG

CEFTIN® Tablets ℞

[sĕf' tin]

(cefuroxime axetil tablets)

CEFTIN® for Oral Suspension ℞

(cefuroxime axetil powder for oral suspension)

To reduce the development of drug-resistant bacteria and maintain the effectiveness of CEFTIN and other antibacterial drugs, CEFTIN should be used only to treat or prevent infections that are proven or strongly suspected to be caused by bacteria.

DESCRIPTION

CEFTIN Tablets and CEFTIN for Oral Suspension contain cefuroxime as cefuroxime axetil. CEFTIN is a semisynthetic, broad-spectrum cephalosporin antibiotic for oral administration.

Chemically, cefuroxime axetil, the 1-(acetyloxy) ethyl ester of cefuroxime, is (*RS*)-1-hydroxyethyl (6*R*,7*R*)-7-[2-(2-furyl)glyoxyl-amido]-3-(hydroxymethyl)-8-oxo-5-thia-1-azabicyclo[4.2.0]-oct-2-ene-2-carboxylate, 7^2-(*Z*)-(*O*-methyloxime), 1-acetate 3-carbamate. Its molecular formula is $C_{20}H_{22}N_4O_{10}S$, and it has a molecular weight of 510.48.

Cefuroxime axetil is in the amorphous form and has the following structural formula:

Table 1. Postprandial Pharmacokinetics of Cefuroxime Administered as CEFTIN Tablets to Adults[a]

Dose[b] (Cefuroxime Equivalent)	Peak Plasma Concentration (mcg/mL)	Time of Peak Plasma Concentration (hr)	Mean Elimination Half-life (hr)	AUC (mcg•hr/mL)
125 mg	2.1	2.2	1.2	6.7
250 mg	4.1	2.5	1.2	12.9
500 mg	7.0	3.0	1.2	27.4
1,000 mg	13.6	2.5	1.3	50.0

[a]Mean values of 12 healthy adult volunteers.
[b]Drug administered immediately after a meal.

Table 2. Postprandial Pharmacokinetics of Cefuroxime Administered as CEFTIN for Oral Suspension to Pediatric Patients[a]

Dose[b] (Cefuroxime Equivalent)	n	Peak Plasma Concentration (mcg/mL)	Time of Peak Plasma Concentration (hr)	Mean Elimination Half-life (hr)	AUC (mcg•hr/mL)
10 mg/kg	8	3.3	3.6	1.4	12.4
15 mg/kg	12	5.1	2.7	1.9	22.5
20 mg/kg	8	7.0	3.1	1.9	32.8

[a]Mean age = 23 months.
[b]Drug administered with milk or milk products.

Table 3. Pharmacokinetics of Cefuroxime Administered as 250 mg/5 mL or 2 × 125 mg/5 mL CEFTIN for Oral Suspension to Adults[a] With Food

Dose (Cefuroxime Equivalent)	Peak Plasma Concentration (mcg/mL)	Time of Peak Plasma Concentration (hr)	Mean Elimination Half-life (hr)	AUC (mcg•hr/mL)
250 mg/5 mL	2.23	3	1.40	8.92
2 × 125 mg/5 mL	2.37	3	1.44	9.75

[a]Mean values of 18 healthy adult volunteers.

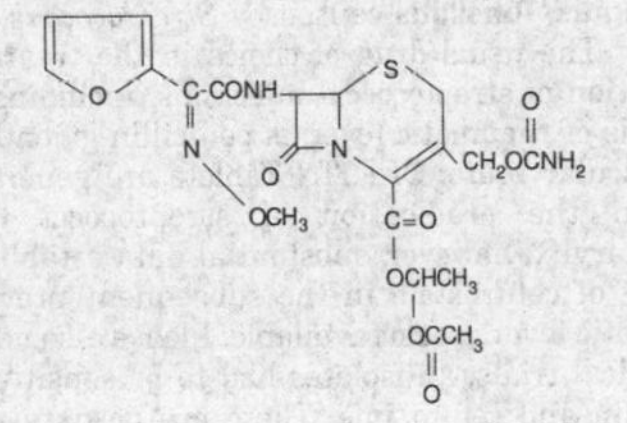

CEFTIN Tablets are film-coated and contain the equivalent of 250 or 500 mg of cefuroxime as cefuroxime axetil. CEFTIN Tablets contain the inactive ingredients colloidal silicon dioxide, croscarmellose sodium, hydrogenated vegetable oil, hypromellose, methylparaben, microcrystalline cellulose, propylene glycol, propylparaben, sodium benzoate, sodium lauryl sulfate, and titanium dioxide.

CEFTIN for Oral Suspension, when reconstituted with water, provides the equivalent of 125 mg or 250 mg of cefuroxime (as cefuroxime axetil) per 5 mL of suspension. CEFTIN for Oral Suspension contains the inactive ingredients acesulfame potassium, aspartame, povidone K30, stearic acid, sucrose, tutti-frutti flavoring, and xanthan gum.

CLINICAL PHARMACOLOGY

Absorption and Metabolism

After oral administration, cefuroxime axetil is absorbed from the gastrointestinal tract and rapidly hydrolyzed by nonspecific esterases in the intestinal mucosa and blood to cefuroxime. Cefuroxime is subsequently distributed throughout the extracellular fluids. The axetil moiety is metabolized to acetaldehyde and acetic acid.

Pharmacokinetics

Approximately 50% of serum cefuroxime is bound to protein. Serum pharmacokinetic parameters for CEFTIN Tablets and CEFTIN for Oral Suspension are shown in Tables 1 and 2.

[See table 1 above]
[See table 2 above]

Comparative Pharmacokinetic Properties

A 250 mg/5 mL-dose of CEFTIN Suspension is bioequivalent to 2 times 125 mg/5 mL-dose of CEFTIN Suspension when administered with food (see Table 3). **CEFTIN for Oral Suspension was not bioequivalent to CEFTIN Tablets when tested in healthy adults. The tablet and powder for oral suspension formulations are NOT substitutable on a milligram-per-milligram basis.** The area under the curve for the suspension averaged 91% of that for the tablet, and the peak plasma concentration for the suspension averaged 71% of the peak plasma concentration of the tablets. Therefore, the safety and effectiveness of both the tablet and oral suspension formulations had to be established in separate clinical trials.

[See table 3 above]

Food Effect on Pharmacokinetics

Absorption of the tablet is greater when taken after food (absolute bioavailability of CEFTIN Tablets increases from 37% to 52%). Despite this difference in absorption, the clinical and bacteriologic responses of patients were independent of food intake at the time of tablet administration in 2 studies where this was assessed.

All pharmacokinetic and clinical effectiveness and safety studies in pediatric patients using the suspension formulation were conducted in the fed state. No data are available on the absorption kinetics of the suspension formulation when administered to fasted pediatric patients.

Renal Excretion

Cefuroxime is excreted unchanged in the urine; in adults, approximately 50% of the administered dose is recovered in the urine within 12 hours. The pharmacokinetics of cefuroxime in the urine of pediatric patients have not been studied at this time. Until further data are available, the renal pharmacokinetic properties of cefuroxime axetil established in adults should not be extrapolated to pediatric patients.

Because cefuroxime is renally excreted, the serum half-life is prolonged in patients with reduced renal function. In a study of 20 elderly patients (mean age = 83.9 years) having a mean creatinine clearance of 34.9 mL/min, the mean serum elimination half-life was 3.5 hours. Despite the lower elimination of cefuroxime in geriatric patients, dosage adjustment based on age is not necessary (see PRECAUTIONS: Geriatric Use).

Microbiology

The in vivo bactericidal activity of cefuroxime axetil is due to cefuroxime's binding to essential target proteins and the resultant inhibition of cell-wall synthesis.

Cefuroxime has bactericidal activity against a wide range of common pathogens, including many beta-lactamase-producing strains. Cefuroxime is stable to many bacterial beta-lactamases, especially plasmid-mediated enzymes that are commonly found in enterobacteriaceae.

Cefuroxime has been demonstrated to be active against most strains of the following microorganisms both in vitro and in clinical infections as described in the INDICATIONS AND USAGE (see INDICATIONS AND USAGE).

Aerobic Gram-Positive Microorganisms

Staphylococcus aureus (including beta-lactamase-producing strains)
Streptococcus pneumoniae
Streptococcus pyogenes

Aerobic Gram-Negative Microorganisms

Escherichia coli
Haemophilus influenzae (including beta-lactamase-producing strains)
Haemophilus parainfluenzae
Klebsiella pneumoniae
Moraxella catarrhalis (including beta-lactamase-producing strains)
Neisseria gonorrhoeae (including beta-lactamase-producing strains)

Spirochetes

Borrelia burgdorferi

Cefuroxime has been shown to be active in vitro against most strains of the following microorganisms; however, the clinical significance of these findings is unknown.

Cefuroxime exhibits in vitro minimum inhibitory concentrations (MICs) of 4.0 mcg/mL or less (systemic susceptible breakpoint) against most (≥90%) strains of the following microorganisms; however, the safety and effectiveness of cefuroxime in treating clinical infections due to these microorganisms have not been established in adequate and well-controlled trials.

Aerobic Gram-Positive Microorganisms

Staphylococcus epidermidis
Staphylococcus saprophyticus
Streptococcus agalactiae

NOTE: *Listeria monocytogenes* and certain strains of enterococci, e.g., *Enterococcus faecalis* (formerly *Streptococcus faecalis*), are resistant to cefuroxime. Methicillin-resistant staphylococci are resistant to cefuroxime.

Aerobic Gram-Negative Microorganisms

Morganella morganii
Proteus inconstans
Proteus mirabilis
Providencia rettgeri

NOTE: *Pseudomonas* spp., *Campylobacter* spp., *Acinetobacter calcoaceticu* , *Legionella* spp., and most strains of *Serratia* spp. and *Proteus vulgaris* are resistant to most first- and second-generation cephalosporins. Some strains of *Morganella morganii*, *Enterobacter cloacae*, and *Citrobacter* spp. have been shown by in vitro tests to be resistant to cefuroxime and other cephalosporins.

Anaerobic Microorganisms

Peptococcus niger

NOTE: Most strains of *Clostridium difficile* and *Bacteroides fragilis* are resistant to cefuroxime.

Susceptibility Tests

Dilution Techniques

Quantitative methods that are used to determine MICs provide reproducible estimates of the susceptibility of bacteria to antimicrobial compounds. One such standardized procedure uses a standardized dilution method[1] (broth, agar, or microdilution) or equivalent with cefuroxime powder. The MIC values obtained should be interpreted according to the following criteria:

MIC (mcg/mL)	Interpretation
≤4	(S) Susceptible
8-16	(I) Intermediate
≥32	(R) Resistant

A report of "Susceptible" indicates that the pathogen, if in the blood, is likely to be inhibited by usually achievable concentrations of the antimicrobial compound in blood. A report of "Intermediate" indicates that inhibitory concentrations of the antibiotic may be achieved if high dosage is used or if the infection is confined to tissues or fluids in which high antibiotic concentrations are attained. This category also provides a buffer zone that prevents small, uncontrolled technical factors from causing major discrepancies in interpretation. A report of "Resistant" indicates that usually achievable concentrations of the antimicrobial compound in the blood are unlikely to be inhibitory and that other therapy should be selected.

Standardized susceptibility test procedures require the use of laboratory control microorganisms. Standard cefuroxime powder should give the following MIC values:

Microorganism	MIC (mcg/mL)
Escherichia coli ATCC 25922	2-8
Staphylococcus aureus ATCC 29213	0.5-2

Diffusion Techniques

Quantitative methods that require measurement of zone diameters provide estimates of the susceptibility of bacteria to antimicrobial compounds. One such standardized procedure[2] that has been recommended (for use with disks) to test the susceptibility of microorganisms to cefuroxime uses the 30-mcg cefuroxime disk. Interpretation involves correlation of the diameter obtained in the disk test with the MIC for cefuroxime.

Reports from the laboratory providing results of the standard single-disk susceptibility test with a 30-mcg cefuroxime disk should be interpreted according to the following criteria:

Zone Diameter (mm)	Interpretation
≥23	(S) Susceptible
15-22	(I) Intermediate
≤14	(R) Resistant

Interpretation should be as stated above for results using dilution techniques.

As with standard dilution techniques, diffusion methods require the use of laboratory control microorganisms. The 30-mcg cefuroxime disk provides the following zone diameters in these laboratory test quality control strains:

Microorganism	Zone Diameter (mm)
Escherichia coli ATCC 25922	20-26
Staphylococcus aureus ATCC 25923	27-35

INDICATIONS AND USAGE

NOTE: CEFTIN TABLETS AND CEFTIN FOR ORAL SUSPENSION ARE NOT BIOEQUIVALENT AND ARE NOT SUBSTITUTABLE ON A MILLIGRAM-PER-MILLIGRAM BASIS *(SEE CLINICAL PHARMACOLOGY)*.

CEFTIN Tablets

CEFTIN Tablets are indicated for the treatment of patients with mild to moderate infections caused by susceptible strains of the designated microorganisms in the conditions listed below:

1. **Pharyngitis/Tonsillitis** caused by *Streptococcus pyogenes*.
   NOTE: The usual drug of choice in the treatment and prevention of streptococcal infections, including the prophylaxis of rheumatic fever, is penicillin given by the intramuscular route. CEFTIN Tablets are generally effective in the eradication of streptococci from the nasopharynx; however, substantial data establishing the efficacy of cefuroxime in the subsequent prevention of rheumatic fever are not available. Please also note that in all clinical trials, all isolates had to be sensitive to both penicillin and cefuroxime. There are no data from adequate and well-controlled trials to demonstrate the effectiveness of cefuroxime in the treatment of penicillin-resistant strains of *Streptococcus pyogenes*.
2. **Acute Bacterial Otitis Media** caused by *Streptococcus pneumoniae*, *Haemophilus influenzae* (including beta-lactamase-producing strains), *Moraxella catarrhalis* (including beta-lactamase-producing strains), or *Streptococcus pyogenes*.
3. **Acute Bacterial Maxillary Sinusitis** caused by *Streptococcus pneumoniae* or *Haemophilus influenzae* (non-beta-lactamase-producing strains only) *(see CLINICAL STUDIES)*.
   NOTE: In view of the insufficient numbers of isolates of beta-lactamase-producing strains of *Haemophilus influenzae* and *Moraxella catarrhalis* that were obtained from clinical trials with CEFTIN Tablets for patients with acute bacterial maxillary sinusitis, it was not possible to adequately evaluate the effectiveness of CEFTIN Tablets for sinus infections known, suspected, or considered potentially to be caused by beta-lactamase-producing *Haemophilus influenzae* or *Moraxella catarrhalis*.
4. **Acute Bacterial Exacerbations of Chronic Bronchitis and Secondary Bacterial Infections of Acute Bronchitis** caused by *Streptococcus pneumoniae*, *Haemophilus influenzae* (beta-lactamase negative strains), or *Haemophilus parainfluenzae* (beta-lactamase negative strains) *(see DOSAGE AND ADMINISTRATION and CLINICAL STUDIES)*.
5. **Uncomplicated Skin and Skin-Structure Infections** caused by *Staphylococcus aureus* (including beta-lactamase-producing strains) or *Streptococcus pyogenes*.
6. **Uncomplicated Urinary Tract Infections** caused by *Escherichia coli* or *Klebsiella pneumoniae*.
7. **Uncomplicated Gonorrhea**, urethral and endocervical, caused by penicillinase-producing and non-penicillinase-producing strains of *Neisseria gonorrhoeae* and uncomplicated gonorrhea, rectal, in females, caused by non-penicillinase-producing strains of *Neisseria gonorrhoeae*.
8. **Early Lyme Disease (erythema migrans)** caused by *Borrelia burgdorferi*.

CEFTIN for Oral Suspension

CEFTIN for Oral Suspension is indicated for the treatment of pediatric patients 3 months to 12 years of age with mild to moderate infections caused by susceptible strains of the designated microorganisms in the conditions listed below. The safety and effectiveness of CEFTIN for Oral Suspension in the treatment of infections other than those specifically listed below have not been established either by adequate and well-controlled trials or by pharmacokinetic data with which to determine an effective and safe dosing regimen.

1. **Pharyngitis/Tonsillitis** caused by *Streptococcus pyogenes*.
   NOTE: The usual drug of choice in the treatment and prevention of streptococcal infections, including the prophylaxis of rheumatic fever, is penicillin given by the intramuscular route. CEFTIN for Oral Suspension is generally effective in the eradication of streptococci from the nasopharynx; however, substantial data establishing the efficacy of cefuroxime in the subsequent prevention of rheumatic fever are not available. Please also note that in all clinical trials, all isolates had to be sensitive to both penicillin and cefuroxime. There are no data from adequate and well-controlled trials to demonstrate the effectiveness of cefuroxime in the treatment of penicillin-resistant strains of *Streptococcus pyogenes*.
2. **Acute Bacterial Otitis Media** caused by *Streptococcus pneumoniae*, *Haemophilus influenzae* (including beta-lactamase-producing strains), *Moraxella catarrhalis* (including beta-lactamase-producing strains), or *Streptococcus pyogenes*.
3. **Impetigo** caused by *Staphylococcus aureus* (including beta-lactamase-producing strains) or *Streptococcus pyogenes*.

To reduce the development of drug-resistant bacteria and maintain the effectiveness of CEFTIN and other antibacterial drugs, CEFTIN should be used only to treat or prevent infections that are proven or strongly suspected to be caused by susceptible bacteria. When culture and susceptibility information are available, they should be considered in selecting or modifying antibacterial therapy. In the absence of such data, local epidemiology and susceptibility patterns may contribute to the empiric selection of therapy.

CONTRAINDICATIONS

CEFTIN products are contraindicated in patients with known allergy to the cephalosporin group of antibiotics.

WARNINGS

CEFTIN TABLETS AND CEFTIN FOR ORAL SUSPENSION ARE NOT BIOEQUIVALENT AND ARE THEREFORE NOT SUBSTITUTABLE ON A MILLIGRAM-PER-MILLIGRAM BASIS (SEE CLINICAL PHARMACOLOGY).

BEFORE THERAPY WITH CEFTIN PRODUCTS IS INSTITUTED, CAREFUL INQUIRY SHOULD BE MADE TO DETERMINE WHETHER THE PATIENT HAS HAD PREVIOUS HYPERSENSITIVITY REACTIONS TO CEFTIN PRODUCTS, OTHER CEPHALOSPORINS, PENICILLINS, OR OTHER DRUGS. IF THIS PRODUCT IS TO BE GIVEN TO PENICILLIN-SENSITIVE PATIENTS, CAUTION SHOULD BE EXERCISED BECAUSE CROSS-HYPERSENSITIVITY AMONG BETA-LACTAM ANTIBIOTICS HAS BEEN CLEARLY DOCUMENTED AND MAY OCCUR IN UP TO 10% OF PATIENTS WITH A HISTORY OF PENICILLIN ALLERGY. IF A CLINICALLY SIGNIFICANT ALLERGIC REACTION TO CEFTIN PRODUCTS OCCURS, DISCONTINUE THE DRUG AND INSTITUTE APPROPRIATE THERAPY. SERIOUS ACUTE HYPERSENSITIVITY REACTIONS MAY REQUIRE TREATMENT WITH EPINEPHRINE AND OTHER EMERGENCY MEASURES, INCLUDING OXYGEN, INTRAVENOUS FLUIDS, INTRAVENOUS ANTIHISTAMINES, CORTICOSTEROIDS, PRESSOR AMINES, AND AIRWAY MANAGEMENT, AS CLINICALLY INDICATED.

Clostridium difficile associated diarrhea (CDAD) has been reported with use of nearly all antibacterial agents, including CEFTIN, and may range in severity from mild diarrhea to fatal colitis. Treatment with antibacterial agents alters the normal flora of the colon leading to overgrowth of *C. difficile*.

C. difficile produces toxins A and B which contribute to the development of CDAD. Hypertoxin producing strains of *C. difficile* cause increased morbidity and mortality, as these infections can be refractory to antimicrobial therapy and may require colectomy. CDAD must be considered in all patients who present with diarrhea following antibiotic use. Careful medical history is necessary since CDAD has been reported to occur over2o months after the administration of antibacterial agents.

If CDAD is suspected or confirmed, ongoing antibiotic use not directed against *C. difficile* may need to be discontinued.

Appropriate fluid and electrolyte management, protein supplementation, antibiotic treatment of *C. difficile*, and surgical evaluation should be instituted as clinically indicated.

PRECAUTIONS

General

As with other broad-spectrum antibiotics, prolonged administration of cefuroxime axetil may result in overgrowth of nonsusceptible microorganisms. If superinfection occurs during therapy, appropriate measures should be taken.

Cephalosporins, including cefuroxime axetil, should be given with caution to patients receiving concurrent treatment with potent diuretics because these diuretics are suspected of adversely affecting renal function.

Cefuroxime axetil, as with other broad-spectrum antibiotics, should be prescribed with caution in individuals with a history of colitis. The safety and effectiveness of cefuroxime axetil have not been established in patients with gastrointestinal malabsorption. Patients with gastrointestinal malabsorption were excluded from participating in clinical trials of cefuroxime axetil.

Cephalosporins may be associated with a fall in prothrombin activity. Those at risk include patients with renal or hepatic impairment or poor nutritional state, as well as patients receiving a protracted course of antimicrobial therapy, and patients previously stabilized on anticoagulant therapy. Prothrombin time should be monitored in patients at risk and exogenous Vitamin K administered as indicated.

Prescribing CEFTIN in the absence of a proven or strongly suspected bacterial infection or a prophylactic indication is unlikely to provide benefit to the patient and increases the risk of the development of drug-resistant bacteria.

Diarrhea is a common problem caused by antibiotics which usually ends when the antibiotic is discontinued. Sometimes after starting treatment with antibiotics, patients can develop watery and bloody stools (with or without stomach cramps and fever) even as late as 2 or more months after having taken the last dose of the antibiotic. If this occurs, patients should contact their physician as soon as possible.

Information for Patients/Caregivers (Pediatric)

Phenylketonurics

CEFTIN for Oral Suspension 125 mg/5 mL contains phenylalanine 11.8 mg per 5 mL (1 teaspoonful) constituted suspension. CEFTIN for Oral Suspension 250 mg/5 mL contains phenylalanine 25.2 mg per 5 mL (1 teaspoonful) constituted suspension.

1. During clinical trials, the tablet was tolerated by pediatric patients old enough to swallow the cefuroxime axetil tablet whole. The crushed tablet has a strong, persistent, bitter taste and should not be administered to pediatric patients in this manner. Pediatric patients who cannot swallow the tablet whole should receive the oral suspension.
2. Discontinuation of therapy due to taste and/or problems of administering this drug occurred in 1.4% of pediatric patients given the oral suspension. Complaints about taste (which may impair compliance) occurred in 5% of pediatric patients.
3. Patients should be counseled that antibacterial drugs, including CEFTIN, should only be used to treat bacterial infections. They do not treat viral infections (e.g., the common cold). When CEFTIN is prescribed to treat a bacterial infection, patients should be told that although it is common to feel better early in the course of therapy, the medication should be taken exactly as directed. Skipping doses or not completing the full course of therapy may: (1) decrease the effectiveness of the immediate treatment, and (2) increase the likelihood that bacteria will develop resistance and will not be treatable by CEFTIN or other antibacterial drugs in the future.

Drug/Laboratory Test Interactions

A false-positive reaction for glucose in the urine may occur with copper reduction tests (Benedict's or Fehling's solution or with CLINITEST® tablets), but not with enzyme-based tests for glycosuria (e.g., CLINISTIX®). As a false-negative result may occur in the ferricyanide test, it is recommended that either the glucose oxidase or hexokinase method be used to determine blood/plasma glucose levels in patients receiving cefuroxime axetil. The presence of cefuroxime does not interfere with the assay of serum and urine creatinine by the alkaline picrate method.

Drug/Drug Interactions

Concomitant administration of probenecid with cefuroxime axetil tablets increases the area under the serum concentration versus time curve by 50%. The peak serum cefuroxime concentration after a 1.5-g single dose is greater when taken with 1 g of probenecid (mean = 14.8 mcg/mL) than without probenecid (mean = 12.2 mcg/mL).

Drugs that reduce gastric acidity may result in a lower bioavailability of CEFTIN compared with that of fasting state and tend to cancel the effect of postprandial absorption.

In common with other antibiotics, cefuroxime axetil may affect the gut flora, leading to lower estrogen reabsorption and reduced efficacy of combined oral estrogen/progesterone contraceptives.

Carcinogenesis, Mutagenesis, Impairment of Fertility

Although lifetime studies in animals have not been performed to evaluate carcinogenic potential, no mutagenic activity was found for cefuroxime axetil in a battery of bacterial mutation tests. Positive results were obtained in an in vitro chromosome aberration assay; however, negative results were found in an in vivo micronucleus test at doses up to 1.5 g/kg. Reproduction studies in rats at doses up to 1,000 mg/kg/day (9 times the recommended maximum human dose based on mg/m²) have revealed no impairment of fertility.

Pregnancy

Teratogenic Effects

Pregnancy Category B. Reproduction studies have been performed in mice at doses up to 3,200 mg/kg/day (14 times the recommended maximum human dose based on mg/m²) and in rats at doses up to 1,000 mg/kg/day (9 times the recommended maximum human dose based on mg/m²) and have revealed no evidence of impaired fertility or harm to the fetus due to cefuroxime axetil. There are, however, no adequate and well-controlled studies in pregnant women. Because animal reproduction studies are not always predictive of human response, this drug should be used during pregnancy only if clearly needed.

Labor and Delivery

Cefuroxime axetil has not been studied for use during labor and delivery.

Nursing Mothers

Because cefuroxime is excreted in human milk, consideration should be given to discontinuing nursing temporarily during treatment with cefuroxime axetil.

Pediatric Use

The safety and effectiveness of CEFTIN have been established for pediatric patients aged 3 months to 12 years for acute bacterial maxillary sinusitis based upon its approval in adults. Use of CEFTIN in pediatric patients is supported by pharmacokinetic and safety data in adults and pediatric patients, and by clinical and microbiological data from adequate and well-controlled studies of the treatment of acute bacterial maxillary sinusitis in adults and of acute otitis media with effusion in pediatric patients. It is also supported by postmarketing adverse events surveillance *(see CLINICAL PHARMACOLOGY, INDICATIONS AND USAGE, ADVERSE REACTIONS, DOSAGE AND ADMINISTRATION, and CLINICAL STUDIES).*

Geriatric Use

Of the total number of subjects who received cefuroxime axetil in 20 clinical studies of CEFTIN, 375 were 65 and older while 151 were 75 and older. No overall differences in safety or effectiveness were observed between these subjects and younger adult subjects.The geriatric patients reported somewhat fewer gastrointestinal events and less frequent vaginal candidiasis compared with patients aged 12 to 64 years old; however, no clinically significant differences were reported between the elderly and younger adult patients. Other reported clinical experience has not identified differences in responses between the elderly and younger adult patients.

ADVERSE REACTIONS

CEFTIN TABLETS IN CLINICAL TRIALS

Multiple-Dose Dosing Regimens

7 to 10 Days Dosing

Using multiple doses of cefuroxime axetil tablets, 912 patients were treated with cefuroxime axetil (125 to 500 mg twice daily). There were no deaths or permanent disabilities thought related to drug toxicity. Twenty (2.2%) patients discontinued medication due to adverse events thought by the investigators to be possibly, probably, or almost certainly related to drug toxicity. Seventeen (85%) of the 20 patients who discontinued therapy did so because of gastrointestinal disturbances, including diarrhea, nausea, vomiting, and abdominal pain. The percentage of cefuroxime axetil tablet-treated patients who discontinued study drug because of adverse events was very similar at daily doses of 1,000, 500, and 250 mg (2.3%, 2.1%, and 2.2%, respectively). However, the incidence of gastrointestinal adverse events increased with the higher recommended doses.

The following adverse events were thought by the investigators to be possibly, probably, or almost certainly related to cefuroxime axetil tablets in multiple-dose clinical trials (n = 912 cefuroxime axetil-treated patients).

Table 4. Adverse Reactions--CEFTIN Tablets

Multiple-Dose Dosing Regimens--Clinical Trials

Incidence ≥1%	Diarrhea/loose stools 3.7% Nausea/vomiting 3.0% Transient elevation in AST 2.0% Transient elevation in ALT 1.6% Eosinophilia 1.1% Transient elevation in LDH 1.0%
Incidence <1% but >0.1%	Abdominal pain Abdominal cramps Flatulence Indigestion Headache Vaginitis Vulvar itch Rash Hives Itch Dysuria Chills Chest pain Shortness of breath Mouth ulcers Swollen tongue Sleepiness Thirst Anorexia Positive Coombs test

5-Day Experience (see CLINICAL STUDIES)

In clinical trials using CEFTIN in a dose of 250 mg twice daily in the treatment of secondary bacterial infections of acute bronchitis, 399 patients were treated for 5 days and 402 patients were treated for 10 days. No difference in the occurrence of adverse events was found between the 2 regimens.

In Clinical Trials for Early Lyme Disease With 20 Days Dosing

Two multicenter trials assessed cefuroxime axetil tablets 500 mg twice a day for 20 days. The most common drug-related adverse experiences were diarrhea (10.6% of patients), Jarisch-Herxheimer reaction (5.6%), and vaginitis (5.4%). Other adverse experiences occurred with frequencies comparable to those reported with 7 to 10 days dosing.

Single Dose Regimen for Uncomplicated Gonorrhea

In clinical trials using a single dose of cefuroxime axetil tablets, 1,061 patients were treated with the recommended dosage of cefuroxime axetil (1,000 mg) for the treatment of uncomplicated gonorrhea. There were no deaths or permanent disabilities thought related to drug toxicity in these studies.

The following adverse events were thought by the investigators to be possibly, probably, or almost certainly related to cefuroxime axetil in 1,000-mg single-dose clinical trials of cefuroxime axetil tablets in the treatment of uncomplicated gonorrhea conducted in the United States.

Table 5. Adverse Reactions--CEFTIN Tablets

1-g Single-Dose Regimen for Uncomplicated Gonorrhea—Clinical Trials

Incidence ≥1%	Nausea/vomiting 6.8% Diarrhea 4.2%
Incidence <1% but >0.1%	Abdominal pain Dyspepsia Erythema Rash Pruritus Vaginal candidiasis Vaginal itch Vaginal discharge Headache Dizziness Somnolence Muscle cramps Muscle stiffness Muscle spasm of neck Tightness/pain in chest Bleeding/pain in urethra Kidney pain Tachycardia Lockjaw-type reaction

CEFTIN FOR ORAL SUSPENSION IN CLINICAL TRIALS

In clinical trials using multiple doses of cefuroxime axetil powder for oral suspension, pediatric patients (96.7% of whom were younger than 12 years of age) were treated with the recommended dosages of cefuroxime axetil (20 to 30 mg/kg/day divided twice a day up to a maximum dose of 500 or 1,000 mg/day, respectively). There were no deaths or permanent disabilities in any of the patients in these studies. Eleven US patients (1.2%) discontinued medication due to adverse events thought by the investigators to be possibly, probably, or almost certainly related to drug toxicity. The discontinuations were primarily for gastrointestinal disturbances, usually diarrhea or vomiting. During clinical trials, discontinuation of therapy due to the taste and/or problems with administering this drug occurred in 13 (1.4%) pediatric patients enrolled at centers in the United States.

The following adverse events were thought by the investigators to be possibly, probably, or almost certainly related to cefuroxime axetil for oral suspension in multiple-dose clinical trials (n = 931 cefuroxime axetil-treated US patients).

Table 6. Adverse Reactions—CEFTIN for Oral Suspension Multiple-Dose Dosing Regimens—Clinical Trials

Incidence ≥1%	Diarrhea/loose stools 8.6% Dislike of taste 5.0% Diaper rash 3.4% Nausea/vomiting 2.6%
Incidence <1% but >0.1%	Abdominal pain Flatulence Gastrointestinal infection Candidiasis Vaginal irritation Rash Hyperactivity Irritable behavior Eosinophilia Positive direct Coombs test Elevated liver enzymes Viral illness Upper respiratory infection Sinusitis Cough Urinary tract infection Joint swelling Arthralgia Fever Ptyalism

POSTMARKETING EXPERIENCE WITH CEFTIS

In addition to adverse events reported during clinical trials, the following events have been identified during clinical practice in patients treated with CEFTIN Tablets or with CEFTIN for Oral Suspension and were reported spontaneously. Data are generally insufficient to allow an estimate of incidence or to establish causation.

General

The following hypersensitivity reactions have been reported: Anaphylaxis, angioedema, pruritus, rash, serum sickness-like reaction, urticaria.

Gastrointestinal

Pseudomembranous colitis *(see WARNINGS)*.

Hematologic

Hemolytic anemia, leukopenia, pancytopenia, thrombocytopenia, and increased prothrombin time.

Hepatic

Hepatic impairment including hepatitis and cholestasis, jaundice.

Neurologic

Seizure.

Skin

Erythema multiforme, Stevens-Johnson syndrome, toxic epidermal necrolysis.

Urologic

Renal dysfunction.

CEPHALOSPORIN-CLASS ADVERSE REACTIONS

In addition to the adverse reactions listed above that have been observed in patients treated with cefuroxime axetil, the following adverse reactions and altered laboratory tests have been reported for cephalosporin-class antibiotics: Toxic nephropathy, aplastic anemia, hemorrhage, increased BUN, increased creatinine, false-positive test for urinary glucose, increased alkaline phosphatase, neutropenia, elevated bilirubin, and agranulocytosis.

Several cephalosporins have been implicated in triggering seizures, particularly in patients with renal impairment when the dosage was not reduced *(see DOSAGE AND ADMINISTRATION and OVERDOSAGE)*. If seizures associated with drug therapy occur, the drug should be discontinued. Anticonvulsant therapy can be given if clinically indicated.

OVERDOSAGE

Overdosage of cephalosporins can cause cerebral irritation leading to convulsions. Serum levels of cefuroxime can be reduced by hemodialysis and peritoneal dialysis.

DOSAGE AND ADMINISTRATION

NOTE: CEFTIN TABLETS AND CEFTIN FOR ORAL SUSPENSION ARE NOT BIOEQUIVALENT AND ARE NOT SUBSTITUTABLE ON A MILLIGRAM-PER-MILLIGRAM BASIS ***(SEE CLINICAL PHARMACOLOGY).***

Table 7. CEFTIN Tablets

(May be administered without regard to meals.)

Population/Infection	Dosage	Duration (days)
Adolescents and Adults (13 years and older)		
Pharyngitis/tonsillitis	250 mg b.i.d.	10
Acute bacterial maxillary sinusitis	250 mg b.i.d.	10
Acute bacterial exacerbations of chronic bronchitis	250 or 500 mg b.i.d.	10[a]
Secondary bacterial infections of acute bronchitis	250 or 500 mg b.i.d.	5-10
Uncomplicated skin and skin-structure infections	250 or 500 mg b.i.d.	10
Uncomplicated urinary tract infections	250 mg b.i.d.	7-10
Uncomplicated gonorrhea	1,000 mg once	single dose
Early Lyme disease	500 mg b.i.d.	20
Pediatric Patients (who can swallow tablets whole)		
Acute otitis media	250 mg b.i.d.	10
Acute bacterial maxillary sinusitis	250 mg b.i.d.	10

[a]The safety and effectiveness of CEFTIN administered for less than 10 days in patients with acute exacerbations of chronic bronchitis have not been established.

CEFTIN for Oral Suspension

CEFTIN for Oral Suspension may be administered to pediatric patients ranging in age from 3 months to 12 years, according to dosages in Table 8:

Table 8. CEFTIN for Oral Suspension

(Must be administered with food. Shake well each time before using.)

Population/ Infection	Dosage	Daily Maximum Dose	Duration (days)
Pediatric Patients (3 months to 12 years)			
Pharyngitis/ tonsillitis	20 mg/kg/day divided b.i.d.	500 mg	10
Acute otitis media	30 mg/kg/day divided b.i.d.	1,000 mg	10
Acute bacterial maxillary sinusitis	30 mg/kg/day divided b.i.d.	1,000 mg	10
Impetigo	30 mg/kg/day divided b.i.d.	1,000 mg	10

Patients With Renal Failure

The safety and efficacy of cefuroxime axetil in patients with renal failure have not been established. Since cefuroxime is renally eliminated, its half-life will be prolonged in patients with renal failure.

Directions for Mixing CEFTIN for Oral Suspension

Prepare a suspension at the time of dispensing as follows:

1. Shake the bottle to loosen the powder.
2. Remove the cap.
3. Add the total amount of water for reconstitution (see Table 9) and replace the cap.
4. Invert the bottle and vigorously rock the bottle from side to side so that water rises through the powder.
5. Once the sound of the powder against the bottle disappears, turn the bottle upright and vigorously shake it in a diagonal direction.

Table 9. Amount of Water Required for Reconstitution of Labeled Volumes of CEFTIN for Oral Suspension

CEFTIN for Oral Suspension	Labeled Volume After Reconstitution	Amount of Water Required for Reconstitution
125 mg/5 mL	100 mL	37 mL
250 mg/5 mL	50 mL	19 mL
	100 mL	35 mL

NOTE: SHAKE THE ORAL SUSPENSION WELL BEFORE EACH USE. Replace cap securely after each opening. Store the reconstituted suspension between 2° and 8°C (36° and 46°F) (in a refrigerator). DISCARD AFTER 10 DAYS.

HOW SUPPLIED

CEFTIN Tablets

CEFTIN Tablets, 250 mg of cefuroxime (as cefuroxime axetil), are white, capsule-shaped, film-coated tablets engraved with "GX ES7" on one side and blank on the other side as follows:

20 Tablets/Bottle NDC 0173-0387-00

CEFTIN Tablets, 500 mg of cefuroxime (as cefuroxime axetil), are white, capsule-shaped, film-coated tablets engraved with "GX EG2" on one side and blank on the other side as follows:

20 Tablets/Bottle NDC 0173-0394-00

Store the tablets between 15° and 30°C (59° and 86°F). Replace cap securely after each opening.

CEFTIN for Oral Suspension

CEFTIN for Oral Suspension is provided as dry, white to off-white, tutti-frutti-flavored powder. When reconstituted as directed, CEFTIN for Oral Suspension provides the equivalent of 125 mg or 250 mg of cefuroxime (as cefuroxime axetil) per 5 mL of suspension. It is supplied in amber glass bottles as follows:

125 mg/5 mL:

100-mL Suspension NDC 0173-0740-00

250 mg/5 mL:

50-mL Suspension NDC 0173-0741-10

100-mL Suspension NDC 0173-0741-00

Before reconstitution, store dry powder between 2° and 30°C (36° and 86°F).

After reconstitution, immediately store suspension between 2° and 8°C (36° and 46°F), in a refrigerator. DISCARD AFTER 10 DAYS.

CLINICAL STUDIES

Ceftin Tablets

Acute Bacterial Maxillary Sinusitis

One adequate and well-controlled study was performed in patients with acute bacterial maxillary sinusitis. In this study each patient had a maxillary sinus aspirate collected by sinus puncture before treatment was initiated for presumptive acute bacterial sinusitis. All patients had to have radiographic and clinical evidence of acute maxillary sinusitis. As shown in the following summary of the study, the general clinical effectiveness of CEFTIN Tablets was comparable to an oral antimicrobial agent that contained a specific beta-lactamase inhibitor in treating acute maxillary sinusitis. However, sufficient microbiology data were obtained to demonstrate the effectiveness of CEFTIN Tablets in treating acute bacterial maxillary sinusitis due only to *Streptococcus pneumoniae* or non-beta-lactamase-producing *Haemophilus influenzae*. An insufficient number of beta-lactamase-producing *Haemophilus influenzae* and *Moraxella catarrhalis* isolates were obtained in this trial to adequately evaluate the effectiveness of CEFTIN Tablets in the treatment of acute bacterial maxillary sinusitis due to these 2 organisms.

This study enrolled 317 adult patients, 132 patients in the United States and 185 patients in South America. Patients were randomized in a 1:1 ratio to cefuroxime axetil 250 mg twice daily or an oral antimicrobial agent that contained a specific beta-lactamase inhibitor. An intent-to-treat analysis of the submitted clinical data yielded the following results:

[See table 10 at top of next page]

In this trial and in a supporting maxillary puncture trial, 15 evaluable patients had non-beta-lactamase-producing *Haemophilus influenzae* as the identified pathogen. Ten (10) of these 15 patients (67%) had their pathogen (non-beta-lactamase-producing *Haemophilus influenzae*) eradicated. Eighteen (18) evaluable patients had *Streptococcus pneumoniae* as the identified pathogen. Fifteen (15) of these 18 patients (83%) had their pathogen (*Streptococcus pneumoniae*) eradicated.

Safety

The incidence of drug-related gastrointestinal adverse events was statistically significantly higher in the control arm (an oral antimicrobial agent that contained a specific beta-lactamase inhibitor) versus the cefuroxime axetil arm (12% versus 1%, respectively; $P<.001$), particularly drug-related diarrhea (8% versus 1%, respectively; $P = .001$).

Early Lyme Disease

Two adequate and well-controlled studies were performed in patients with early Lyme disease. In these studies all patients had to present with physician-documented erythema migrans, with or without systemic manifestations of infection. Patients were randomized in a 1:1 ratio to a 20-day course of treatment with cefuroxime axetil 500 mg twice daily or doxycycline 100 mg 3 times daily. Patients were assessed at 1 month posttreatment for success in treating early Lyme disease (Part I) and at 1 year posttreatment for success in preventing the progression to the sequelae of late Lyme disease (Part II).

A total of 355 adult patients (181 treated with cefuroxime axetil and 174 treated with doxycycline) were enrolled in the 2 studies. In order to objectively validate the clinical diagnosis of early Lyme disease in these patients, 2 ap-

Table 10. Clinical Effectiveness of CEFTIN Tablets Compared to Beta-Lactamase Inhibitor-Containing Control Drug in the Treatment of Acute Bacterial Maxillary Sinusitis

	US Patients[a]		South American Patients[b]	
	CEFTIN (n = 49)	Control (n = 43)	CEFTIN (n = 87)	Control (n = 89)
Clinical success (cure + improvement)	65%	53%	77%	74%
Clinical cure	53%	44%	72%	64%
Clinical improvement	12%	9%	5%	10%

[a] 95% Confidence interval around the success difference [-0.08, +0.32].
[b] 95% Confidence interval around the success difference [-0.10, +0.16].

Table 11. Clinical Effectiveness of CEFTIN Tablets Compared to Doxycycline in the Treatment of Early Lyme Disease

	Part I (1 Month Posttreatment)[a]		Part II (1 Year Posttreatment)[b]	
	CEFTIN (n = 125)	Doxycycline (n = 108)	CEFTIN (n = 105[c])	Doxycycline (n = 83[c])
Satisfactory clinical outcome[d]	91%	93%	84%	87%
Clinical cure/success	72%	73%	73%	73%
Clinical improvement	19%	19%	10%	13%

[a] 95% confidence interval around the satisfactory difference for Part I (-0.08, +0.05).
[b] 95% confidence interval around the satisfactory difference for Part II (-0.13, +0.07).
[c] n's include patients assessed as unsatisfactory clinical outcomes (failure + recurrence) in Part I (CEFTIN - 11 [5 failure, 6 recurrence]; doxycycline - 8 [6 failure, 2 recurrence]).
[d] Satisfactory clinical outcome includes cure + improvement (Part I) and success + improvement (Part II).

Table 12. Clinical Effectiveness of CEFTIN Tablets 250 mg Twice Daily in Secondary Bacterial Infections of Acute Bronchitis: Comparison of 5 Versus 10 Days' Treatment Duration

	CAE-516 and CAE-517[a]		CAEA4001 and CAEA4002[b]	
	5 Day (n = 127)	10 Day (n = 139)	5 Day (n = 173)	10 Day (n = 192)
Clinical success (cure + improvement)	80%	87%	84%	82%
Clinical cure	61%	70%	73%	72%
Clinical improvement	19%	17%	11%	10%

[a] 95% Confidence interval around the success difference [-0.164, +0.029].
[b] 95% Confidence interval around the success difference [-0.061, +0.103].

proaches were used: 1) blinded expert reading of photographs, when available, of the pretreatment erythema migrans skin lesion; and 2) serologic confirmation (using enzyme-linked immunosorbent assay [ELISA] and immunoblot assay ["Western" blot]) of the presence of antibodies specific to *Borrelia burgdorferi*, the etiologic agent of Lyme disease. By these procedures, it was possible to confirm the physician diagnosis of early Lyme disease in 281 (79%) of the 355 study patients. The efficacy data summarized below are specific to this "validated" patient subset, while the safety data summarized below reflect the entire patient population for the 2 studies.

Analysis of the submitted clinical data for evaluable patients in the "validated" patient subset yielded the following results:

[See table 11 above]

CEFTIN and doxycycline were effective in prevention of the development of sequelae of late Lyme disease.

Safety

Drug-related adverse events affecting the skin were reported significantly more frequently by patients treated with doxycycline than by patients treated with cefuroxime axetil (12% versus 3%, respectively; $P = .002$), primarily reflecting the statistically significantly higher incidence of drug-related photosensitivity reactions in the doxycycline arm versus the cefuroxime axetil arm (9% versus 0%, respectively; $P<.001$). While the incidence of drug-related gastrointestinal adverse events was similar in the 2 treatment groups (cefuroxime axetil - 13%; doxycycline - 11%), the incidence of drug-related diarrhea was statistically significantly higher in the cefuroxime axetil arm versus the doxycycline arm (11% versus 3%, respectively; $P = .005$).

Secondary Bacterial Infections of Acute Bronchitis

Four randomized, controlled clinical studies were performed comparing 5 days versus 10 days of CEFTIN for the treatment of patients with secondary bacterial infections of acute bronchitis. These studies enrolled a total of 1,253 patients (CAE-516 n = 360; CAE-517 n = 177; CAEA4001 n = 362; CAEA4002 n = 354). The protocols for CAE-516 and CAE-517 were identical and compared CEFTIN 250 mg twice daily for 5 days, CEFTIN 250 mg twice daily for 10 days, and AUGMENTIN® 500 mg 3 times daily for 10 days. These 2 studies were conducted simultaneously. CAEA4001 and CAEA4002 compared CEFTIN 250 mg twice daily for 5 days, CEFTIN 250 mg twice daily for 10 days, and CECLOR® 250 mg 3 times daily for 10 days. They were otherwise identical to CAE-516 and CAE-517 and were conducted over the following 2 years. Patients were required to have polymorphonuclear cells present on the Gram stain of their screening sputum specimen, but isolation of a bacterial pathogen from the sputum culture was not required for inclusion. The following table demonstrates the results of the clinical outcome analysis of the pooled studies CAE-516/CAE-517 and CAEA4001/CAEA4002, respectively:

[See table 12 above]

The response rates for patients who were both clinically and bacteriologically evaluable were consistent with those reported for the clinically evaluable patients.

Safety

In these clinical trials, 399 patients were treated with CEFTIN for 5 days and 402 patients with CEFTIN for 10 days. No difference in the occurrence of adverse events was observed between the 2 regimens.

REFERENCES

1. National Committee for Clinical Laboratory Standards. *Methods for Dilution Antimicrobial Susceptibility Tests for Bacteria that Grow Aerobically*. 3rd ed. Approved Standard NCCLS Document M7-A3, Vol. 13, No. 25. Villanova, Pa: NCCLS; 1993.
2. National Committee for Clinical Laboratory Standards. *Performance Standards for Antimicrobial Disk Susceptibility Tests*. 4th ed. Approved Standard NCCLS Document M2-A4, Vol. 10, No. 7. Villanova, Pa: NCCLS; 1990.

CEFTIN and AUGMENTIN are registered trademarks of GlaxoSmithKline.
CLINITEST and CLINISTIX are registered trademarks of Ames Division, Miles Laboratories, Inc.

GlaxoSmithKline
Research Triangle Park, NC 27709

January 2010 CFT:1PI

CERVARIX ℞

[*cer-va-rix*]
[Human Papillomavirus Bivalent (Types 16 and 18) Vaccine, Recombinant]
Suspension for Intramuscular Injection

HIGHLIGHTS OF PRESCRIBING INFORMATION
These highlights do not include all the information needed to use CERVARIX safely and effectively. See full prescribing information for CERVARIX.
CERVARIX [Human Papillomavirus Bivalent (Types 16 and 18) Vaccine, Recombinant]
Suspension for Intramuscular Injection
Initial U.S. Approval: 2009

INDICATIONS AND USAGE

CERVARIX is a vaccine indicated for the prevention of the following diseases caused by oncogenic human papillomavirus (HPV) types 16 and 18:
- cervical cancer,
- cervical intraepithelial neoplasia (CIN) grade 2 or worse and adenocarcinoma *in situ*, and
- cervical intraepithelial neoplasia (CIN) grade 1. (1.1)

CERVARIX is approved for use in females 9 through 25 years of age.
Limitations of Use and Effectiveness (1.2)
- CERVARIX does not provide protection against disease due to all HPV types. (14.3)
- CERVARIX has not been demonstrated to provide protection against disease from vaccine and non-vaccine HPV types to which a woman has previously been exposed through sexual activity. (14.2)

DOSAGE AND ADMINISTRATION

Three doses (0.5-mL each) by intramuscular injection according to the following schedule: 0, 1, and 6 months. (2.2)

DOSAGE FORMS AND STRENGTHS

Single-dose prefilled syringes containing a 0.5-mL suspension for injection. (3)

CONTRAINDICATIONS

Severe allergic reactions (e.g., anaphylaxis) to any component of CERVARIX. (4)

WARNINGS AND PRECAUTIONS

- Because vaccinees may develop syncope, sometimes resulting in falling with injury, observation for 15 minutes after administration is recommended. Syncope, sometimes associated with tonic-clonic movements and other seizure-like activity, has been reported following vaccination with CERVARIX. When syncope is associated with tonic-clonic movements, the activity is usually transient and typically responds to restoring cerebral perfusion by maintaining a supine or Trendelenburg position. (5.1)
- CERVARIX is available in 2 types of prefilled syringes. One type of prefilled syringe has a tip cap which may contain natural rubber latex. The other type has a tip cap and a rubber plunger which contain dry natural latex rubber. Use of these syringes may cause allergic reactions in latex-sensitive individuals. (5.2, 16)

ADVERSE REACTIONS

- Most common local adverse reactions in ≥20% of subjects were pain, redness, and swelling at the injection site. (6.1)
- Most common general adverse events in ≥20% of subjects were fatigue, headache, myalgia, gastrointestinal symptoms, and arthralgia. (6.1)

To report SUSPECTED ADVERSE REACTIONS, contact GlaxoSmithKline at 1-888-825-5249 or VAERS at 1-800-822-7967 or www.vaers.hhs.gov

DRUG INTERACTIONS

Do not mix CERVARIX with any other vaccine in the same syringe or vial. (7.1)

USE IN SPECIFIC POPULATIONS

- Safety has not been established in pregnant women. Register women who receive CERVARIX while pregnant in the pregnancy registry by calling 1-888-452-9622. (8.1)
- Immunocompromised individuals may have a reduced immune response to CERVARIX. (8.6)

See 17 for PATIENT COUNSELING INFORMATION and FDA-approved patient labeling

Revised: 08/2012

FULL PRESCRIBING INFORMATION: CONTENTS*

*** Sections or subsections omitted from the full prescribing information are not listed**

FULL PRESCRIBING INFORMATION

1 INDICATIONS AND USAGE

1.1 Indications

CERVARIX® is indicated for the prevention of the following diseases caused by oncogenic human papillomavirus (HPV) types 16 and 18 *[see Clinical Studies (14)]*:
- cervical cancer,
- cervical intraepithelial neoplasia (CIN) grade 2 or worse and adenocarcinoma *in situ*, and
- cervical intraepithelial neoplasia (CIN) grade 1.

CERVARIX is approved for use in females 9 through 25 years of age.

1.2 Limitations of Use and Effectiveness

CERVARIX does not provide protection against disease due to all HPV types *[see Clinical Studies (14.3)]*.

CERVARIX has not been demonstrated to provide protection against disease from vaccine and non-vaccine HPV types to which a woman has previously been exposed through sexual activity *[see Clinical Studies (14.2)]*.

Females should continue to adhere to recommended cervical cancer screening procedures *[see Patient Counseling Information (17)]*.

Vaccination with CERVARIX may not result in protection in all vaccine recipients.

2 DOSAGE AND ADMINISTRATION

2.1 Preparation for Administration

Shake syringe well before withdrawal and use. Parenteral drug products should be inspected visually for particulate matter and discoloration prior to administration, whenever solution and container permit. If either of these conditions exists, the vaccine should not be administered. With thorough agitation, CERVARIX is a homogeneous, turbid, white suspension. Do not administer if it appears otherwise.

Attach a sterile needle and administer intramuscularly.

Do not administer this product intravenously, intradermally, or subcutaneously.

2.2 Dose and Schedule

Immunization with CERVARIX consists of 3 doses of 0.5-mL each, by intramuscular injection according to the following schedule: 0, 1, and 6 months. The preferred site of administration is the deltoid region of the upper arm.

3 DOSAGE FORMS AND STRENGTHS

CERVARIX is a suspension for intramuscular injection available in 0.5-mL single-dose prefilled TIP-LOK® syringes.

4 CONTRAINDICATIONS

Severe allergic reactions (e.g., anaphylaxis) to any component of CERVARIX *[see Description (11)]*.

5 WARNINGS AND PRECAUTIONS

5.1 Syncope

Because vaccinees may develop syncope, sometimes resulting in falling with injury, observation for 15 minutes after administration is recommended. Syncope, sometimes associated with tonic-clonic movements and other seizure-like activity, has been reported following vaccination with CERVARIX. When syncope is associated with tonic-clonic movements, the activity is usually transient and typically responds to restoring cerebral perfusion by maintaining a supine or Trendelenburg position.

5.2 Latex

CERVARIX is available in 2 types of prefilled syringes. One type of prefilled syringe has a tip cap which may contain natural rubber latex and a plunger which does not contain latex. The other type has a tip cap and a rubber plunger which contain dry natural latex rubber. Use of these syringes may cause allergic reactions in latex-sensitive individuals. *[See How Supplied / Storage and Handling (16).]*

5.3 Preventing and Managing Allergic Vaccine Reactions

Prior to administration, the healthcare provider should review the immunization history for possible vaccine hypersensitivity and previous vaccination-related adverse reactions to allow an assessment of benefits and risks. Appropriate medical treatment and supervision should be readily available in case of anaphylactic reactions following administration of CERVARIX.

6 ADVERSE REACTIONS

The most common local adverse reactions (≥20% of subjects) were pain, redness, and swelling at the injection site.

The most common general adverse events (≥20% of subjects) were fatigue, headache, myalgia, gastrointestinal symptoms, and arthralgia.

6.1 Clinical Studies Experience

Because clinical trials are conducted under widely varying conditions, adverse reaction rates observed in the clinical trials of a vaccine cannot be directly compared with rates in the clinical trials of another vaccine, and may not reflect the rates observed in practice. There is the possibility that broad use of CERVARIX could reveal adverse reactions not observed in clinical trials.

Studies in Females 9 Through 25 Years of Age: The safety of CERVARIX was evaluated by pooling data from controlled and uncontrolled clinical trials involving 23,952 females 9 through 25 years of age in the pre-licensure clinical development program. In these studies, 13,024 females (9 through 25 years of age) received at least one dose of CERVARIX and 10,928 females received at least one dose of a control [Hepatitis A Vaccine containing 360 EL.U. (10 through 14 years of age), Hepatitis A Vaccine containing 720 EL.U. (15 through 25 years of age), or $Al(OH)_3$ (500 mcg, 15 through 25 years of age)].

Data on solicited local and general adverse events were collected by subjects or parents using standardized diary cards for 7 consecutive days following each vaccine dose (i.e., day of vaccination and the next 6 days). Unsolicited adverse events were recorded with diary cards for 30 days following each vaccination (day of vaccination and 29 subsequent days). Parents and/or subjects were also asked at each study visit about the occurrence of any adverse events and instructed to immediately report serious adverse events throughout the study period. These studies were conducted in North America, Latin America, Europe, Asia, and Australia. Overall, the majority of subjects were white (59.5%), followed by Asian (25.9%), Hispanic (8.5%), black (3.4%), and other racial/ethnic groups (2.7%).

Solicited Adverse Events: The reported frequencies of solicited local injection site reactions (pain, redness, and swelling) and general adverse events (fatigue, fever, gastrointestinal symptoms, headache, arthralgia, myalgia, and urticaria) within 7 days after vaccination in females 9 through 25 years of age are presented in Table 1. An analysis of solicited local injection site reactions by dose is presented in Table 2. Local reactions were reported more frequently with CERVARIX when compared with the control groups; in ≥76% of recipients of CERVARIX, these local reactions were mild to moderate in intensity. Compared with dose 1, pain was reported less frequently after doses 2 and 3 of CERVARIX, in contrast to redness and swelling where there was a small increased incidence. There was no increase in the frequency of general adverse events with successive doses.

[See table 1 below]

[See table 2 at top of next page]

Table 1. Rates of Solicited Local Adverse Reactions and General Adverse Events in Females 9 Through 25 Years of Age Within 7 Days of Vaccination (Total Vaccinated Cohort[a])

	CERVARIX (9-25 yrs) %	HAV 720[b] (15-25 yrs) %	HAV 360[c] (10-14 yrs) %	$Al(OH)_3$ Control[d] (15-25 yrs) %
Local Adverse Reaction	**N = 6,669**	**N = 3,079**	**N = 1,027**	**N = 549**
Pain	91.9	78.0	64.2	87.2
Redness	48.4	27.6	25.2	24.4
Swelling	44.3	19.8	17.3	21.3
General Adverse Event	**N = 6,670**	**N = 3,079**	**N = 1,027**	**N = 549**
Fatigue	54.6	53.7	42.3	53.6
Headache	53.4	51.3	45.2	61.4
GI[e]	27.9	27.3	24.6	32.8
Fever (≥99.5°F)	12.9	10.9	16.0	13.5
Rash	9.5	8.4	6.7	10.0
	N = 6,119	**N = 3,079**	**N = 1,027**	—
Myalgia[f]	48.8	44.9	33.1	—
Arthralgia[f]	20.7	17.9	19.9	—
Urticaria[f]	7.2	7.9	5.4	—

[a]Total vaccinated cohort included subjects with at least one documented dose (N).
[b]HAV 720 = Hepatitis A Vaccine control group [720 EL.U. of antigen and 500 mcg $Al(OH)_3$].
[c]HAV 360 = Hepatitis A Vaccine control group [360 EL.U. of antigen and 250 mcg of $Al(OH)_3$].
[d]$Al(OH)_3$ Control = control containing 500 mcg $Al(OH)_3$.
[e]GI = Gastrointestinal symptoms, including nausea, vomiting, diarrhea, and/or abdominal pain.
[f]Adverse events solicited in a subset of subjects.

The pattern of solicited local adverse reactions and general adverse events following administration of CERVARIX was similar between the age cohorts (9 through 14 years and 15 through 25 years).

Unsolicited Adverse Events: The frequency of unsolicited adverse events that occurred within 30 days of vaccination (≥1% for CERVARIX and greater than any of the control groups) in females 9 through 25 years of age are presented in Table 3.

[See table 3 above]

New Onset Autoimmune Diseases (NOADs): The pooled safety database, which included controlled and uncontrolled trials which enrolled females 9 through 25 years of age, was searched for new medical conditions indicative of potential new onset autoimmune diseases. Overall, the incidence of potential NOADs, as well as NOADs, in the group receiving CERVARIX was 0.8% (96/12,772) and comparable to the pooled control group (0.8%, 87/10,730) during the 4.3 years of follow-up (Table 4).

In the largest randomized, controlled trial (Study 2) which enrolled females 15 through 25 years of age and which included active surveillance for potential NOADs, the incidence of potential NOADs and NOADs was 0.8% among subjects who received CERVARIX (78/9,319) and 0.8% among subjects who received Hepatitis A Vaccine [720 EL.U. of antigen and 500 mcg $Al(OH)_3$] control (77/9,325).

Table 4. Incidence of New Medical Conditions Indicative of Potential New Onset Autoimmune Disease and New Onset Autoimmune Disease Throughout the Follow-up Period Regardless of Causality in Females 9 Through 25 Years of Age (Total Vaccinated Cohort[a])

	CERVARIX N = 12,772	Pooled Control Group[b] N = 10,730
	n (%)[c]	n (%)[c]
Total Number of Subjects With at Least One Medical Condition	96 (0.8)	87 (0.8)
Arthritis[d]	9 (0.1)	4 (0.0)
Celiac disease	2 (0.0)	5 (0.0)
Dermatomyositis	0 (0.0)	1 (0.0)
Diabetes mellitus insulin-dependent (Type 1 or unspecified)	5 (0.0)	5 (0.0)
Erythema nodosum	3 (0.0)	0 (0.0)
Hyperthyroidism[e]	15 (0.1)	15 (0.1)
Hypothyroidism[f]	30 (0.2)	28 (0.3)
Inflammatory bowel disease[g]	8 (0.1)	4 (0.0)
Multiple sclerosis	4 (0.0)	1 (0.0)
Myelitis transverse	1 (0.0)	0 (0.0)
Optic neuritis/Optic neuritis retrobulbar	3 (0.0)	1 (0.0)
Psoriasis[h]	8 (0.1)	11 (0.1)
Raynaud's phenomenon	0 (0.0)	1 (0.0)
Rheumatoid arthritis	4 (0.0)	3 (0.0)
Systemic lupus erythematosus[i]	2 (0.0)	3 (0.0)
Thrombocytopenia[j]	1 (0.0)	1 (0.0)
Vasculitis[k]	1 (0.0)	3 (0.0)
Vitiligo	2 (0.0)	2 (0.0)

[a]Total vaccinated cohort included subjects with at least one documented dose (N).
[b]Pooled Control Group = Hepatitis A Vaccine control group [720 EL.U. of antigen and 500 mcg $Al(OH)_3$], Hepatitis A Vaccine control group [360 EL.U. of antigen and 250 mcg of $Al(OH)_3$], and a control containing 500 mcg $Al(OH)_3$.
[c]n (%): number and percentage of subjects with medical condition.
[d]Term includes reactive arthritis and arthritis.
[e]Term includes Basedow's disease, goiter, and hyperthyroidism.
[f]Term includes thyroiditis, autoimmune thyroiditis, and hypothyroidism.
[g]Term includes colitis ulcerative, Crohn's disease, proctitis ulcerative, and inflammatory bowel disease.
[h]Term includes psoriatic arthropathy, nail psoriasis, guttate psoriasis, and psoriasis.
[i]Term includes systemic lupus erythematosus and cutaneous lupus erythematosus.
[j]Term includes idiopathic thrombocytopenic purpura and thrombocytopenia.
[k]Term includes leukocytoclastic vasculitis and vasculitis.

Table 2. Rates of Solicited Local Adverse Reactions in Females 9 Through 25 Years of Age by Dose Within 7 Days of Vaccination (Total Vaccinated Cohort[a])

	CERVARIX (9-25 yrs) %			HAV 720[b] (15-25 yrs) %			HAV 360[c] (10-14 yrs) %			$Al(OH)_3$ Control[d] (15-25 yrs) %		
	Post-Dose			Post-Dose			Post-Dose			Post-Dose		
	1	2	3	1	2	3	1	2	3	1	2	3
N	6,653	6,428	6,168	3,070	2,919	2,758	1,027	1,021	1,011	546	521	500
Pain	87.0	76.4	78.5	65.6	54.4	56.1	48.5	38.5	36.9	79.1	66.8	72.4
Pain, Grade 3[e]	7.5	5.6	7.7	2.0	1.4	2.0	0.8	0.2	1.6	9.0	6.0	8.6
Redness	28.4	30.1	35.7	16.6	15.2	16.1	15.6	13.3	12.1	11.5	11.5	15.6
Redness, >50 mm	0.2	0.5	1.0	0.1	0.1	0.0	0.1	0.2	0.1	0.2	0.0	0.0
Swelling	22.8	25.5	32.7	10.5	9.4	10.5	9.4	8.6	7.6	10.3	10.4	12.0
Swelling, >50 mm	1.1	1.0	1.3	0.2	0.2	0.2	0.4	0.3	0.0	0.0	0.0	0.0

[a]Total vaccinated cohort included subjects with at least one documented dose (N).
[b]HAV 720 = Hepatitis A Vaccine control group [720 EL.U. of antigen and 500 mcg $Al(OH)_3$].
[c]HAV 360 = Hepatitis A Vaccine control group [360 EL.U. of antigen and 250 mcg of $Al(OH)_3$].
[d]$Al(OH)_3$ Control = control containing 500 mcg $Al(OH)_3$.
[e]Defined as spontaneously painful or pain that prevented normal daily activities.

Table 3. Rates of Unsolicited Adverse Events in Females 9 Through 25 Years of Age Within 30 Days of Vaccination (≥1% For CERVARIX and Greater Than HAV 720, HAV 360, or $Al(OH)_3$ Control) (Total Vaccinated Cohort[a])

	CERVARIX % N = 6,893	HAV 720[b] % N = 3,186	HAV 360[c] % N = 1,032	$Al(OH)_3$Control[d] % N = 581
Headache	5.2	7.6	3.3	9.3
Nasopharyngitis	3.7	3.4	5.9	3.3
Influenza	3.1	5.6	1.3	1.9
Pharyngolaryngeal pain	2.9	2.7	2.2	2.2
Dizziness	2.2	2.6	1.5	3.1
Upper respiratory infection	2.0	1.3	6.7	1.5
Chlamydia infection	1.9	4.4	0.0	0.0
Dysmenorrhea	1.9	2.3	1.9	4.0
Pharyngitis	1.4	1.8	2.2	0.5
Injection site bruising	1.4	1.8	0.7	1.5
Vaginal infection	1.3	2.2	0.1	0.9
Injection site pruritus	1.3	0.5	0.6	0.2
Back pain	1.1	1.3	0.7	3.1
Urinary tract infection	1.0	1.4	0.3	1.2

[a]Total vaccinated cohort included subjects with at least one dose administered (N).
[b]HAV 720 = Hepatitis A Vaccine control group [720 EL.U. of antigen and 500 mcg $Al(OH)_3$].
[c]HAV 360 = Hepatitis A Vaccine control group [360 EL.U. of antigen and 250 mcg of $Al(OH)_3$].
[d]$Al(OH)_3$ Control = control containing 500 mcg $Al(OH)_3$.

Serious Adverse Events: In the pooled safety database, inclusive of controlled and uncontrolled studies, which enrolled females 9 through 72 years of age, 5.3% (864/16,381) of subjects who received CERVARIX and 5.9% (814/13,811) of subjects who received control reported at least one serious adverse event, without regard to causality, during the entire follow-up period (up to 7.4 years).

Among females 9 through 25 years of age enrolled in these clinical studies, 6.3% of subjects who received CERVARIX and 7.2% of subjects who received the control reported at least one serious adverse event during the entire follow-up period (up to 7.4 years).

Deaths: In completed and ongoing studies which enrolled 57,323 females 9 through 72 years of age, 37 deaths were reported during the 7.4 years of follow-up: 20 in subjects who received CERVARIX (0.06%, 20/33,623) and 17 in subjects who received control (0.07%, 17/23,700). Causes of death among subjects were consistent with those reported in adolescent and adult female populations. The most common causes of death were motor vehicle accident (5 subjects who received CERVARIX; 5 subjects who received control) and suicide (2 subjects who received CERVARIX; 5 subjects who received control), followed by neoplasm (3 subjects who received CERVARIX; 2 subjects who received control), autoimmune disease (3 subjects who received CERVARIX; 1 subject who received control), infectious disease (3 subjects who received CERVARIX; 1 subject who received control), homicide (2 subjects who received CERVARIX; 1 subject who received control), cardiovascular disorders (2 subjects who received CERVARIX), and death of unknown cause (2 subjects who received control). Among females 10 through 25 years of age, 31 deaths were reported (0.05%, 16/29,467 of subjects who received CERVARIX and 0.07%, 15/20,192 of subjects who received control).

6.2 Postmarketing Experience

In addition to reports in clinical trials, worldwide voluntary reports of adverse events received for CERVARIX since market introduction (2007) are listed below. This list includes serious events or events which have suspected causal association to CERVARIX. Because these events are reported voluntarily from a population of uncertain size, it is not always possible to reliably estimate their frequency or establish a causal relationship to vaccination.

Blood and Lymphatic System Disorders: Lymphadenopathy.

Immune System Disorders: Allergic reactions (including anaphylactic and anaphylactoid reactions), angioedema, erythema multiforme.

Nervous System Disorders: Syncope or vasovagal responses to injection (sometimes accompanied by tonic-clonic movements).

7 DRUG INTERACTIONS

7.1 Concomitant Vaccine Administration

There are no data to assess the concomitant use of CERVARIX with other vaccines.

Do not mix CERVARIX with any other vaccine in the same syringe or vial.

7.2 Hormonal Contraceptives

Among 7,693 subjects 15 through 25 years of age in Study 2 (CERVARIX, N = 3,821 or Hepatitis A Vaccine 720 EL.U., N = 3,872) who used hormonal contraceptives for a mean of 2.8 years, the observed efficacy of CERVARIX was similar to that observed among subjects who did not report use of hormonal contraceptives.

7.3 Immunosuppressive Therapies

Immunosuppressive therapies, including irradiation, antimetabolites, alkylating agents, cytotoxic drugs, and corticosteroids (used in greater than physiologic doses), may reduce the immune response to CERVARIX *[see Use in Specific Populations (8.6)]*.

8 USE IN SPECIFIC POPULATIONS

8.1 Pregnancy

Pregnancy Category B

Reproduction studies have been performed in rats at a dose approximately 47 times the human dose (on a mg/kg basis) and revealed no evidence of impaired fertility or harm to the fetus due to CERVARIX. There are, however, no adequate and well-controlled studies in pregnant women. Because animal reproduction studies are not always predictive of human response, this drug should be used during pregnancy only if clearly needed.

Non-Clinical Studies: An evaluation of the effect of CERVARIX on embryo-fetal, pre- and post-natal development was conducted using rats. One group of rats was administered CERVARIX 30 days prior to gestation and during the period of organogenesis (gestation days 6, 8, 11, and 15). A second group of rats was administered saline at 30 days prior to gestation followed by CERVARIX on days 6, 8, 11, and 15 of gestation. Two additional groups of rats received either saline or adjuvant following the same dosing regimen. CERVARIX was administered at 0.1 mL/rat/occasion (approximately 47-fold excess relative to the projected human dose on a mg/kg basis) by intramuscular injection. No adverse effects on mating, fertility, pregnancy, parturition, lactation, or embryo-fetal, pre- and post-natal development were observed. There were no vaccine-related fetal malformations or other evidence of teratogenesis.

Clinical Studies: *Overall Outcomes:* In clinical studies, pregnancy testing was performed prior to each vaccine administration and vaccination was discontinued if a subject had a positive pregnancy test. In all clinical trials, subjects were instructed to take precautions to avoid pregnancy until 2 months after the last vaccination. During pre-licensure clinical development, a total of 7,276 pregnancies were reported among 3,696 females receiving CERVARIX and 3,580 females receiving a control (Hepatitis A Vaccine 360 EL.U., Hepatitis A Vaccine 720 EL.U., or 500 mcg $Al(OH)_3$). The overall proportions of pregnancy outcomes were similar between treatment groups. The majority of women gave birth to normal infants (62.2% and 62.6% of recipients of CERVARIX and control, respectively). Other outcomes included spontaneous abortion (11.0% and 10.8% of recipients of CERVARIX and control, respectively), elective termination (5.8% and 6.1% of recipients of CERVARIX and control, respectively), abnormal infant other than congenital anomaly (2.8% and 3.2% of recipients of CERVARIX and control, respectively), and premature birth (2.0% and 1.7% of recipients of CERVARIX and control, respectively). Other outcomes (congenital anomaly, stillbirth, ectopic pregnancy, and therapeutic abortion) were reported less frequently in 0.1% to 0.8% of pregnancies in both groups.

Outcomes Around Time of Vaccination: Sub-analyses were conducted to describe pregnancy outcomes in 761 women [N = 396 for CERVARIX and N = 365 pooled control, HAV 360 EL.U., HAV 720 EL.U., and 500 mcg $Al(OH)_3$] who had their last menstrual period within 30 days prior to, or 45 days after a vaccine dose and for whom pregnancy outcome was known. The majority of women gave birth to normal infants (65.2% and 69.3% of recipients of CERVARIX and control, respectively). Spontaneous abortion was reported in a total of 11.7% of subjects (13.6% of recipients of CERVARIX and 9.6% of control recipients) and elective termination was reported in a total of 9.7% of subjects (9.9% of recipients of CERVARIX and 9.6% of control recipients). Abnormal infant other than congenital anomaly was reported in a total of 4.9% of subjects (5.1% of recipients of CERVARIX and 4.7% of control recipients) and premature birth was reported in a total of 2.5% of subjects (2.5% of both groups). Other outcomes (congenital anomaly, stillbirth, ectopic pregnancy, and therapeutic abortion) were reported in 0.3% to 1.8% of pregnancies among recipients of CERVARIX and in 0.3% to 1.4% of pregnancies among control recipients.

It is not known whether the observed numerical imbalance in spontaneous abortions in pregnancies which occurred around the time of vaccination is due to a vaccine-related effect.

Pregnancy Registry: GlaxoSmithKline maintains a surveillance registry to collect data on pregnancy outcomes and newborn health status outcomes following vaccination with CERVARIX during pregnancy. Women who receive CERVARIX during pregnancy should be encouraged to contact GlaxoSmithKline directly or their healthcare provider should contact GlaxoSmithKline by calling 1-888-452-9622.

8.3 Nursing Mothers

In non-clinical studies in rats, serological data suggest a transfer of anti-HPV-16 and anti-HPV-18 antibodies via milk during lactation in rats. Excretion of vaccine-induced antibodies in human milk has not been studied for CERVARIX. Because many drugs are excreted in human milk, caution should be exercised when CERVARIX is administered to a nursing woman.

8.4 Pediatric Use

Safety and effectiveness in pediatric patients younger than 9 years of age have not been established. The safety and effectiveness of CERVARIX have been evaluated in 1,275 subjects 9 through 14 years of age and 6,362 subjects 15 through 17 years of age. *[See Adverse Reactions (6.1) and Clinical Studies (14.5).]*

8.5 Geriatric Use

Clinical studies of CERVARIX did not include sufficient numbers of subjects 65 years of age and older to determine whether they respond differently from younger subjects. CERVARIX is not approved for use in subjects 65 years of age and older.

8.6 Immunocompromised Individuals

The immune response to CERVARIX may be diminished in immunocompromised individuals *[see Drug Interactions (7.3)]*.

11 DESCRIPTION

CERVARIX [Human Papillomavirus Bivalent (Types 16 and 18) Vaccine, Recombinant] is a non-infectious recombinant, AS04-adjuvanted vaccine that contains recombinant L1 protein, the major antigenic protein of the capsid, of oncogenic HPV types 16 and 18. The L1 proteins are produced in separate bioreactors using the recombinant Baculovirus expression vector system in a serum-free culture media composed of chemically-defined lipids, vitamins, amino acids, and mineral salts. Following replication of the L1 encoding recombinant Baculovirus in *Trichoplusia ni* insect cells, the L1 protein accumulates in the cytoplasm of the cells. The L1 proteins are released by cell disruption and purified by a series of chromatographic and filtration methods. Assembly of the L1 proteins into virus-like particles (VLPs) occurs at the end of the purification process. The purified, non-infectious VLPs are then adsorbed on to aluminum (as hydroxide salt). The adjuvant system, AS04, is composed of 3-*O*-desacyl-4′-monophosphoryl lipid A (MPL) adsorbed on to aluminum (as hydroxide salt).

CERVARIX is prepared by combining the adsorbed VLPs of each HPV type together with the AS04 adjuvant system in sodium chloride, sodium dihydrogen phosphate dihydrate, and Water for Injection.

CERVARIX is a sterile suspension for intramuscular injection. Each 0.5-mL dose is formulated to contain 20 mcg of HPV type 16 L1 protein, 20 mcg of HPV type 18 L1 protein, 50 mcg of the 3-*O*-desacyl-4′-monophosphoryl lipid A (MPL), and 0.5 mg of aluminum hydroxide. Each dose also contains 4.4 mg of sodium chloride and 0.624 mg of sodium dihydrogen phosphate dihydrate. Each dose may also contain residual amounts of insect cell and viral protein (<40 ng) and bacterial cell protein (<150 ng) from the manufacturing process. CERVARIX does not contain a preservative.

CERVARIX is available in 2 types of prefilled syringes. One type of prefilled syringe has a tip cap which may contain natural rubber latex and a plunger which does not contain latex. The other type has a tip cap and a rubber plunger which contain dry natural latex rubber. *[See How Supplied/Storage and Handling (16).]*

12 CLINICAL PHARMACOLOGY

12.1 Mechanism of Action

Animal studies suggest that the efficacy of L1 VLP vaccines may be mediated by the development of IgG neutralizing antibodies directed against HPV-L1 capsid proteins generated as a result of vaccination.

13 NONCLINICAL TOXICOLOGY

13.1 Carcinogenesis, Mutagenesis, Impairment of Fertility

CERVARIX has not been evaluated for its carcinogenic or mutagenic potential. Vaccination of female rats with CERVARIX, at doses shown to be significantly immunogenic in the rat, had no effect on fertility.

14 CLINICAL STUDIES

Cervical intraepithelial neoplasia (CIN) grade 2 and 3 lesions or cervical adenocarcinoma *in situ* (AIS) are the immediate and necessary precursors of squamous cell carcinoma and adenocarcinoma of the cervix, respectively. Their detection and removal has been shown to prevent cancer. Therefore, CIN2/3 and AIS (precancerous lesions) serve as surrogate markers for the prevention of cervical cancer. In clinical studies to evaluate the efficacy of CERVARIX, the endpoints were cases of CIN2/3 and AIS associated with HPV-16, HPV-18, and other oncogenic HPV types. Persistent infection with HPV-16 and HPV-18 that lasts for 12 months was also an endpoint.

The efficacy of CERVARIX to prevent histopathologically-confirmed CIN2/3 or AIS was assessed in 2 double-blind, randomized, controlled clinical studies that enrolled a total of 19,778 females 15 through 25 years of age.

Study 1 (HPV 001) enrolled women who were negative for oncogenic HPV DNA (HPV types 16, 18, 31, 33, 35, 39, 45, 51, 52, 56, 58, 59, 66, and 68) in cervical samples, seronegative for HPV-16 and HPV-18 antibodies and had normal cytology. This represents a population presumed "naïve" without current HPV infection at the time of vaccination and without prior exposure to either HPV-16 or HPV-18. Subjects were enrolled in an extended follow-up study (Study 1 extension [HPV 007]) to evaluate the long-term efficacy, immunogenicity, and safety. These subjects have been followed for up to 6.4 years.

In Study 2 (HPV 008), women were vaccinated regardless of baseline HPV DNA status, serostatus or cytology. This study reflects a population of women naïve (without current infection and without prior exposure) or non-naïve (with current infection and/or with prior exposure) to HPV. Before vaccination, cervical samples were assessed for oncogenic HPV DNA (HPV types 16, 18, 31, 33, 35, 39, 45, 51, 52, 56, 58, 59, 66, and 68) and serostatus of HPV-16 and HPV-18 antibodies.

In both studies, testing for oncogenic HPV types was conducted using SPF_{10}-$LiPA_{25}$ PCR to detect HPV DNA in archived biopsy samples.

14.1 Prophylactic Efficacy Against HPV Types 16 and 18

Study 2: A randomized, double-blind, controlled clinical trial was conducted in which 18,665 healthy females 15 through 25 years of age received CERVARIX or Hepatitis A Vaccine control on a 0-, 1-, and 6-month schedule. Among subjects, 54.8% of subjects were white, 31.5% Asian, 7.1% Hispanic, 3.7% black, and 2.9% were of other racial/ethnic groups.

In this study, women were randomized and vaccinated regardless of baseline HPV DNA status, serostatus or cytology. Women with HPV-16 or HPV-18 DNA present in baseline cervical samples (HPV DNA positive) at study entry were considered currently infected with that specific HPV type. If HPV DNA was not detected by PCR, women were considered HPV DNA negative. Additionally, cervical samples were assessed for cytologic abnormalities and serologic testing was performed for anti-HPV-16 and anti-HPV-18 serum antibodies at baseline. Women with anti-HPV serum antibodies present were considered to have prior exposure to HPV and characterized as seropositive. Women seropositive for HPV-16 or HPV-18 but DNA negative for that specific serotype were considered as having cleared a previous natural infection. Women without antibodies to HPV-16 and HPV-18 were characterized as seronegative. Before vaccination, 73.6% of subjects were naïve (without current infection [DNA negative] and without prior exposure [seronegative]) to HPV-16 and/or HPV-18.

Efficacy endpoints included histological evaluation of precancerous and dysplastic lesions (CIN grade 1, grade 2, or grade 3), and AIS. The mean follow-up after the first dose was approximately 39 months. Virological endpoints (HPV DNA in cervical samples detected by PCR) included 12-month persistent infection (defined as at least 2 positive specimens for the same HPV type over a minimum interval of 10 months).

The according to protocol (ATP) cohort for efficacy analyses for HPV-16 and/or HPV-18 included all subjects who received 3 doses of vaccine, for whom efficacy endpoint measures were available and who were HPV-16 and/or HPV-18 DNA negative and seronegative at baseline and HPV-16 and/or HPV-18 DNA negative at month 6 for the HPV type considered in the analysis. Case counting for the ATP cohort started on day 1 after the third dose of vaccine. This cohort included women who had normal or low-grade cytology (cytological abnormalities including atypical squamous cells of undetermined significance [ASC-US] or low grade squamous intraepithelial lesions [LSIL]) at baseline and excluded women with high-grade cytology.

The total vaccinated cohort (TVC) for each efficacy analysis included all subjects who received at least one dose of the vaccine, for whom efficacy endpoint measures were available, irrespective of their HPV DNA status, cytology, and serostatus at baseline. This cohort included women with or without current HPV infection and/or prior exposure. Case counting for the TVC started on day 1 after the first dose. The TVC naïve is a subset of the TVC that had normal cytology, and were HPV DNA negative for 14 oncogenic HPV types and seronegative for HPV-16 and HPV-18 at baseline. CERVARIX was efficacious in the prevention of precancerous lesions or AIS associated with HPV-16 or HPV-18 (Table 5).

[See table 5 above]

Table 5. Efficacy of CERVARIX Against Histopathological Lesions Associated With HPV-16 or HPV-18 in Females 15 Through 25 Years of Age (According to Protocol Cohort[a]) (Study 2)

	CERVARIX		Control[b]		% Efficacy (96.1% CI)[c]
	N	Number of Cases	N	Number of Cases	
CIN2/3 or AIS	7,344	4	7,312	56	92.9 (79.9, 98.3)
CIN1/2/3 or AIS	7,344	8	7,312	96	91.7 (82.4, 96.7)

CI = Confidence Interval.

[a]Subjects (including women who had normal cytology, ASC-US, or LSIL at baseline) who received 3 doses of vaccine and were HPV DNA negative and seronegative at baseline and HPV DNA negative at month 6 for the corresponding HPV type (N). The mean follow-up was approximately 35 months.

[b]Hepatitis A Vaccine control group [720 EL.U. of antigen and 500 mcg $Al(OH)_3$].

[c]The 96.1% confidence interval reflected in this final analysis results from statistical adjustment for the previously conducted interim analysis.

Since CIN3 or AIS represents a more immediate precursor to cervical cancer, cases of CIN3 or AIS associated with HPV-16 or HPV-18 were evaluated. In the ATP cohort, CERVARIX was efficacious in the prevention of CIN3 or AIS associated with HPV-16 or HPV-18 (vaccine efficacy = 80.0% [96.1% CI: 0.3, 98.1]).

Subjects who were already infected with one vaccine HPV type (16 or 18) prior to vaccination were protected from precancerous lesions or AIS and infection caused by the other vaccine HPV type.

Efficacy of CERVARIX against 12-month persistent infection with HPV-16 or HPV-18 was also evaluated. In the ATP cohort, CERVARIX reduced the incidence of 12-month persistent infection with HPV-16 and/or HPV-18 by 91.4% (96.1% CI: 86.1, 95.0).

Immune response following natural infection does not reliably confer protection against future infections. Among subjects who received 3 doses of CERVARIX and who were seropositive at baseline and DNA negative for HPV-16 or HPV-18 at baseline and month 6, CERVARIX reduced the incidence of 12-month persistent infection by 95.8% (96.1% CI: 72.4, 99.9). However, the number of cases of CIN2/3 or AIS was too few to determine efficacy against histopathological endpoints in this population.

Study 1 and Study 1 Extension: In a second double-blind, randomized, controlled study (Study 1), the efficacy of CERVARIX in the prevention of HPV-16 or HPV-18 incident and persistent infections was compared with aluminum hydroxide control in 1,113 females 15 through 25 years of age. The population was naïve to current oncogenic HPV infection or prior exposure to HPV-16 and HPV-18 at the time of vaccination (total cohort). A total of 776 subjects were enrolled in the extended follow-up study (Study 1 Extension) to evaluate the long-term efficacy, immunogenicity, and safety of CERVARIX. These subjects have been followed for up to 6.4 years.

In Study 1 and Study 1 Extension, with up to 6.4 years of follow-up (mean 5.9 years), in naïve females 15 through 25 years of age, efficacy against CIN2/3 or AIS associated with HPV-16 or HPV-18 was 100% (98.67% CI: 28.4, 100). Efficacy against 12-month persistent infection with HPV-16 or HPV-18 was 100% (98.67% CI: 74.4, 100). The confidence interval reflected in this final analysis results from statistical adjustment for analyses previously conducted.

14.2 Efficacy Against HPV Types 16 and 18, Regardless of Current Infection or Prior Exposure to HPV-16 or HPV-18

Study 2: The study included women regardless of HPV DNA status (current infection) and serostatus (prior exposure) to vaccine types, HPV-16 or HPV-18 at baseline. Efficacy analyses included lesions arising among women regardless of baseline DNA status and serostatus, including HPV infections present at first vaccination and those from infections acquired after dose 1. In this population which includes naïve (without current infection and prior exposure) and non-naïve women, CERVARIX was efficacious in the prevention of precancerous lesions or AIS associated with HPV-16 or HPV-18 (Table 6).

However, among women HPV DNA positive regardless of serostatus at baseline, there was no clear evidence of efficacy against precancerous lesions or AIS associated with HPV-16 or HPV-18 (Table 6).

[See table 6 above]

Table 6. Efficacy of CERVARIX Against Disease Associated With HPV-16 or HPV-18 in Females 15 Through 25 Years of Age, Regardless of Current or Prior Exposure to Vaccine HPV Types (Study 2)

	CERVARIX		Control		% Efficacy (96.1% CI)[b]
	N	Number of Cases[a]	N	Number of Cases[a]	
CIN2/3 or AIS					
Prophylactic Efficacy[c]	5,449	3	5,436	85	96.5 (89.0, 99.4)
HPV-16 or HPV-18 DNA Positive at Baseline[d]	641	90	592	92	--
Regardless of Current Infection or Prior Exposure to HPV-16 or HPV-18[e]	8,667	107	8,682	240	55.5[f] (43.2, 65.3)
CIN2/3 or AIS					
Prophylactic Efficacy[c]	5,449	1	5,436	63	98.4 (90.4, 100)
HPV-16 or HPV-18 DNA Positive at Baseline[d]	641	74	592	73	--
Regardless of Current Infection or Prior Exposure to HPV-16 or HPV-18[e]	8,667	82	8,682	174	52.8[f] (37.5, 64.7)
CIN3 or AIS					
Prophylactic Efficacy[c]	5,449	0	5,436	13	100 (64.7, 100)
HPV-16 or HPV-18 DNA Positive at Baseline[d]	641	41	592	38	--
Regardless of Current Infection or Prior Exposure to HPV-16 or HPV-18[e]	8,667	43	8,682	65	33.6[f] (-1.1, 56.9)

CI = Confidence Interval.

Table does not include disease due to non-vaccine HPV types.

[a]Cases = Histopathological cases associated with HPV-16 and/or HPV-18.

[b]The 96.1% confidence interval reflected in this final analysis results from statistical adjustment for the previously conducted interim analysis.

[c]TVC naïve: includes all vaccinated subjects (who received at least one dose of vaccine) who had normal cytology, were HPV DNA negative for 14 oncogenic HPV types, and seronegative for HPV-16 and HPV-18 at baseline (N). Case counting started on day 1 after the first dose.

[d]TVC subset: includes all vaccinated subjects (who received at least one dose of vaccine) who were HPV DNA positive for HPV-16 or HPV-18 irrespective of serostatus at baseline (N). Case counting started on day 1 after the first dose.

[e]TVC: includes all vaccinated subjects (who received at least one dose of vaccine) irrespective of HPV DNA status and serostatus at baseline (N). Case counting started on day 1 after the first dose.

[f]Observed vaccine efficacy includes the prophylactic efficacy of CERVARIX and the impact of CERVARIX on the course of infections present at first vaccination.

14.3 Efficacy Against Cervical Disease Irrespective of HPV Type, Regardless of Current or Prior Infection with Vaccine or Non-Vaccine HPV Types

Study 2: The impact of CERVARIX against the overall burden of HPV-related cervical disease results from a combination of prophylactic efficacy against, and disease contribution of, HPV-16, HPV-18, and non-vaccine HPV types.

In the population naïve to oncogenic HPV (TVC naïve), CERVARIX reduced the overall incidence of CIN1/2/3 or AIS, CIN2/3 or AIS, and CIN3 or AIS regardless of the HPV DNA type in the lesion (Table 7). In the population of women naïve and non-naïve (TVC), vaccine efficacy against CIN1/2/3 or AIS, CIN2/3 or AIS, and CIN3 or AIS was demonstrated in all women regardless of HPV DNA type in the lesion (Table 7).

[See table 7 at top of next page]

In exploratory analyses, CERVARIX reduced definitive cervical therapy procedures (includes loop electrosurgical excision procedure [LEEP], cold-knife Cone, and laser procedures) by 24.7% (96.1% CI: 7.4, 38.9) in the TVC and by 68.8% (96.1% CI: 50.0, 81.2) in the TVC naïve.

To assess reductions in disease caused by non-vaccine HPV types, two analyses were conducted combining 12 non-vaccine oncogenic HPV types, including and excluding lesions in which HPV-16 or HPV-18 were also detected. In these analyses, among females who received 3 doses of CERVARIX and were DNA negative for the specific HPV type at baseline and month 6, CERVARIX reduced the incidence of CIN2/3 or AIS by 54.0% (96.1% CI: 34.0, 68.4) and 37.4% (96.1% CI: 7.4, 58.2), respectively.

Post-hoc analyses, adjusted for multiplicity, were conducted to assess the impact of CERVARIX on CIN2/3 or AIS due to specific non-vaccine HPV types. The ATP cohort for these analyses included all subjects irrespective of serostatus who received 3 doses of CERVARIX and were DNA negative for the specific HPV type at baseline and month 6. These post-hoc analyses were also conducted in the TVC naïve population. In analyses including lesions in which HPV-16 or HPV-18 were also detected, vaccine efficacy in prevention of CIN2/3 or AIS associated with HPV-31 was 92.0% (99.7% CI: 49.0, 99.8) and 100% (99.7% CI: 62.3, 100), respectively. In analyses excluding lesions in which HPV-16 or HPV-18 were detected, vaccine efficacy in prevention of CIN2/3 or AIS associated with HPV-31 was 89.4% (99.7% CI: 29.0, 99.7) and 100% (99.7% CI: 36.3, 100), respectively.

14.4 Immunogenicity

The minimum anti-HPV titer that confers protective efficacy has not been determined.

The antibody response to HPV-16 and HPV-18 was measured using a type-specific binding ELISA (developed by

Table 7. Efficacy of CERVARIX in Prevention of CIN or AIS Irrespective of Any HPV Type in Females 15 Through 25 Years of Age, Regardless of Current or Prior Infection with Vaccine or Non-Vaccine Types (Study 2)

	CERVARIX		Control		% Efficacy (96.1% CI)[a]
	N	Number of Cases	N	Number of Cases	
CIN1/2/3 or AIS					
Prophylactic Efficacy[b]	5,449	106	5,436	211	50.1 (35.9, 61.4)
Irrespective of HPV DNA at Baseline[c]	8,667	451	8,682	577	21.7 (10.7, 31.4)
CIN2/3 or AIS					
Prophylactic Efficacy[b]	5,449	33	5,436	110	70.2 (54.7, 80.9)
Irrespective of HPV DNA at Baseline[c]	8,667	224	8,682	322	30.4 (16.4, 42.1)
CIN3 or AIS					
Prophylactic Efficacy[b]	5,449	3	5,436	23	87.0 (54.9, 97.7)
Irrespective of HPV DNA at Baseline[c]	8,667	77	8,682	116	33.4 (9.1, 51.5)

CI = Confidence Interval.
[a]The 96.1% confidence interval reflected in this final analysis results from statistical adjustment for the previously conducted interim analysis.
[b]TVC naïve: includes all vaccinated subjects (who received at least one dose of vaccine) who had normal cytology, were HPV DNA negative for 14 oncogenic HPV types (including HPV-16 and HPV-18), and seronegative for HPV-16 and HPV-18 at baseline (N). Case counting started on day 1 after the first dose.
[c]TVC: includes all vaccinated subjects (who received at least one dose of vaccine) irrespective of HPV DNA status and serostatus at baseline (N). Case counting started on day 1 after the first dose.

Table 8. Summary of Anti-HPV Geometric Mean Titers (GMTs) for HPV-16 and HPV-18 at Month 7 for Initially Seronegative Females 15 Through 25 Years of Age (According to Protocol Cohort for Immunogenicity[a]) (Study 2)

Antibody Assay	N	CERVARIX GMT (95% CI)	N	Control GMT (95% CI)
ELISA[b] (EL.U./mL)				
Anti-HPV-16	865	9,206.5 (8,609.4, 9,845.1)	740	4.4 (4.2, 4.6)
Anti-HPV-18	930	4,741.3 (4,452.2, 5,049.1)	772	3.8 (3.6, 3.9)
PBNA[c] (ED_{50})				
Anti-HPV-16	46	27,364.8 (19,780.1, 37,857.9)	44	20.0 (20.0, 20.0)
Anti-HPV-18	46	9,052 (6,851.8, 11,960.5)	44	20.0 (20.0, 20.0)

[a]Subjects who received 3 doses of vaccine for whom assay results were available for at least one post-vaccination antibody measurement (N). Subjects who acquired either HPV-16 or HPV-18 infection during the study were excluded.
[b]Enzyme linked immunosorbent assay (assay cut-off 8 EL.U./mL for anti-HPV-16 antibody and 7 EL.U./mL for anti-HPV-18 antibody).
[c]Pseudovirion-based neutralization assay (assay cut-off 40 ED_{50} for both anti-HPV-16 antibody and anti-HPV-18 antibody).

GlaxoSmithKline) and a pseudovirion-based neutralization assay (PBNA). In a subset of subjects tested for HPV-16 and HPV-18, the ELISA has been shown to correlate with the PBNA. The scales for these assays are unique to each HPV type and each assay, thus, comparison between HPV types or assays is not appropriate.

Duration of Immune Response: The duration of immunity following a complete schedule of immunization with CERVARIX has not been established. In Study 1 and Study 1 Extension, the immune response against HPV-16 and HPV-18 was evaluated for up to 76 months post-dose 1, in females 15 through 25 years of age. Vaccine-induced geometric mean titers (GMTs) for both HPV-16 and HPV-18 peaked at month 7 and thereafter reached a plateau that was sustained from month 18 up to month 76. At all timepoints, >98% of subjects were seropositive for both HPV-16 (≥8 EL.U./mL, the limit of detection) and HPV-18 (≥7 EL.U./mL, the limit of detection) by ELISA.

In Study 2, GMTs for ELISA and PBNA one month post dose 3 were measured (Table 8). The ATP cohort for immunogenicity included all evaluable subjects for whom data concerning immunogenicity endpoint measures were available. These included subjects for whom assay results were available for antibodies against at least one vaccine type. Subjects who acquired either HPV-16 or HPV-18 infection during the trial were excluded. Of subjects seronegative at baseline, 99.5% were seropositive for anti-HPV-16 and anti-HPV-18 antibodies at month 7 post-vaccination.

[See table 8 above]

14.5 Bridging of Efficacy from Women to Adolescent Girls

The immunogenicity of CERVARIX was evaluated in 3 clinical studies involving 1,275 girls 9 through 14 years of age who received at least one dose of CERVARIX.

Study 3 (HPV 013) was a double-blind, randomized, controlled study in which 1,035 subjects received CERVARIX and 1,032 subjects received a Hepatitis A Vaccine 360 EL.U. as the control vaccine with a subset of subjects evaluated for immunogenicity. All initially seronegative subjects in the group who received CERVARIX were seropositive after vaccination, i.e., had levels of antibody greater than the limit of detection of the assay to both HPV-16 (≥8 EL.U./mL) and HPV-18 (≥7 EL.U./mL) antigens. The GMTs for anti-HPV-16 and anti-HPV-18 antibodies in initially seronegative subjects are presented in Table 9.

[See table 9 at top of next page]

In Study 4 (HPV 012), the immunogenicity of CERVARIX administered to girls 10 through 14 years of age was compared to that in females 15 through 25 years of age. The immune response in girls 10 through 14 years of age measured one month post-dose 3 was non-inferior to that seen in females 15 through 25 years of age for both HPV-16 and HPV-18 antigens (Table 10).

[See table 10 at top of next page]

In Study 5, a post-hoc analysis compared the immunogenicity of CERVARIX administered to girls 9 through 14 years of age (n = 68) to that in females 15 through 25 years of age (n = 114). In these initially seronegative subjects, the immune response in girls 9 through 14 years of age measured one month post-dose 3 was non-inferior to that observed in females 15 through 25 years of age for both HPV-16 and HPV-18 antigens [lower limit of the 2-sided 95% CI for the GMT ratio (9-14 year olds/15-25 year olds) was >0.5]. The GMTs for anti-HPV-16 and anti-HPV-18 antibodies at month 7 were 22,261.3 EL.U./mL and 7,398.8 EL.U./mL, respectively, in girls 9 through 14 years of age and 10,322.0 EL.U./mL and 4,261.5 EL.U./mL, respectively, in females 15 through 25 years of age.

Based on these immunogenicity data, the efficacy of CERVARIX is inferred in girls 9 through 14 years of age.

16 HOW SUPPLIED/STORAGE AND HANDLING

CERVARIX is available in 0.5-mL single-dose disposable prefilled TIP-LOK syringes (packaged without needles):

NDC 58160-830-05 Syringe (tip cap may contain latex; plunger contains no latex) in Package of 1: NDC 58160-830-34

NDC 58160-830-43 Syringe (tip cap may contain latex; plunger contains no latex) in Package of 10: NDC 58160-830-52

NDC 58160-830-32 Syringe (tip cap and plunger contain latex) in Package of 1: NDC 58160-830-32

NDC 58160-830-41 Syringe (tip cap and plunger contain latex) in Package of 5: NDC 58160-830-46

Store refrigerated between 2° and 8°C (36° and 46°F). Do not freeze. Discard if the vaccine has been frozen. Upon storage, a fine, white deposit with a clear, colorless supernatant may be observed. This does not constitute a sign of deterioration.

17 PATIENT COUNSELING INFORMATION

See FDA-approved patient labeling.

17.1 Patient Advice

Provide the Vaccine Information Statements prior to immunization. These are required by the National Childhood Vaccine Injury Act of 1986 and are available free of charge at the Centers for Disease Control and Prevention (CDC) website (www.cdc.gov/vaccines).

Inform the patient, parent, or guardian:

- Vaccination does not substitute for routine cervical cancer screening. Women who receive CERVARIX should continue to undergo cervical cancer screening per standard of care.
- CERVARIX does not protect against disease from HPV types to which a woman has previously been exposed through sexual activity.
- Since syncope has been reported following vaccination in young females, sometimes resulting in falling with injury, observation for 15 minutes after administration is recommended.
- Information regarding potential benefits and risks associated with vaccination.
- Report any adverse events to their healthcare provider.
- Safety has not been established in pregnant women. CERVARIX is not recommended for use in pregnant women or women planning to become pregnant during the vaccination course. Register women who receive CERVARIX while pregnant in the pregnancy registry by calling 1-888-452-9622.

CERVARIX and TIP-LOK are registered trademarks of GlaxoSmithKline.

Manufactured by **GlaxoSmithKline Biologicals**
Rixensart, Belgium, US License 1617
Distributed by **GlaxoSmithKline**
Research Triangle Park, NC 27709

CRX:8PI

PATIENT INFORMATION

CERVARIX® (SERV-ah-rix)

[Human Papillomavirus Bivalent (Types 16 and 18) Vaccine, Recombinant]

Read this Patient Information carefully before getting CERVARIX. You (the person getting CERVARIX) will need 3 doses of the vaccine. Read this information before each dose of CERVARIX. This information does not take the place of talking with your healthcare provider about CERVARIX.

What is CERVARIX?

CERVARIX is a vaccine given by injection (shot) to girls and women 9 through 25 years of age.

- CERVARIX helps protect against cervical cancer and precancers caused by human papillomavirus (HPV) types 16 and 18.
- There are many types of HPV but only certain types cause cervical cancer. HPV types 16 and 18 are the 2 most common types of HPV that lead to cervical cancer and precancers.

Table 9. Geometric Mean Titers (GMTs) at Months 7 and 18 for Initially Seronegative Females 10 Through 14 Years of Age (According To Protocol Cohort for Immunogenicity[a]) (Study 3)

Age Group	Anti-HPV-16 Antibodies GMT EL.U./mL (95% CI)			Anti-HPV-18 Antibodies GMT EL.U./mL (95% CI)		
	N	Month 7	Month 18	N	Month 7	Month 18
10-14 years of age	556-619	19,882.0 (18,626.7, 21,221.9)	3,888.8 (3,605.0, 4,195.0)	562-628	8,262.0 (7,725.0, 8,836.2)	1,539.4 (1,418.8, 1,670.3)

[a]Subjects who received 3 doses of vaccine for whom assay results were available for at least one post-vaccination antibody measurement (N).

Table 10. Geometric Mean Titers (GMTs) and Seropositivity Rates at Month 7 for Initially Seronegative Females 10 Through 14 Years of Age Compared to 15 Through 25 Years of Age (According To Protocol Cohort for Immunogenicity[a]) (Study 4)

Antibody Assay	10-14 Years of Age			15-25 Years of Age		
	N	GMT[b] EL.U./mL (95% CI)	SeropositivityRate[c] %	N	GMT[b] EL.U./mL (95% CI)	SeropositivityRate[c] %
Anti-HPV-16	143	17,272.5 (15,117.9, 19,734.1)	100	118	7,438.9 (6,324.6, 8,749.6)	100
Anti-HPV-18	141	6,863.8 (5,976.3, 7,883.0)	100	116	3,070.1 (2,600.0, 3,625.4)	100

[a]Subjects who received 3 doses of vaccine for whom assay results were available for at least one post-vaccination antibody measurement (N).
[b]Non-inferiority based on the upper limit of the 2-sided 95% CI for the GMT ratio (15-25 year olds/10-14 year olds) was <2.
[c]Non-inferiority based on the upper limit of the 2-sided 95% CI for the difference between the seropositivity rates for 10-14 year olds and 15-25 year olds was <10%.

- Abnormal Pap smear results can indicate the presence of precancers. Some precancers can lead to cervical cancer.
- CERVARIX is not a treatment for HPV.
- You can not get HPV diseases from CERVARIX.

What important information should I know about CERVARIX?

- You should continue to get routine cervical cancer screening (such as a Pap smear).
- CERVARIX may not fully protect everyone who gets the vaccine.
- Not all cervical cancers are caused by the HPV types CERVARIX protects against. CERVARIX will not protect against diseases from all HPV types.
- CERVARIX will not protect against HPV types that you already have.

Who should not get CERVARIX?

You should not get CERVARIX if you have or have had:
- an allergic reaction to a previous dose of CERVARIX.
- an allergy to any of the ingredients in CERVARIX (listed below).

What should I tell my healthcare provider before getting CERVARIX?

Tell your healthcare provider about all your health conditions, including if you:
- have had an allergic reaction after a previous dose of CERVARIX.
- have an allergy to latex.
- have a weakened immune system.
- are taking any other medicine or have recently gotten any other vaccine.
- have a fever over 100°F (37.8°C).
- are pregnant or are planning to get pregnant during the time period of the 3 shots. CERVARIX is not recommended for use in pregnant women.

Pregnancy Registry: If you are vaccinated during pregnancy, there is a registry. The purpose of the registry is to collect safety information about the health of you and your baby. Contact the registry as soon as you become aware of the pregnancy or ask your healthcare provider to contact the registry for you. You or your healthcare provider can get information and enroll in the registry by calling 1-888-452-9622.

Your healthcare provider will decide if you should get CERVARIX.

How is CERVARIX given?

CERVARIX is given as an injection (shot) in a muscle in your arm.

You will need a total of 3 shots as follows:
- First dose: given at a time decided by you and your healthcare provider
- Second dose: given 1 month after the first dose
- Third dose: given 6 months after the first dose

Fainting may occur, sometimes resulting in falling with injury, especially in young females. Your healthcare provider may ask you to sit or lie down for 15 minutes after you get CERVARIX. Some people who faint may shake or become stiff. If this happens, it may require evaluation or treatment by your healthcare provider.

Make sure you get all 3 doses on time for the best protection. If you miss a scheduled dose, talk to your healthcare provider.

What are the possible side effects of CERVARIX?

The most common side effects of CERVARIX are:
- pain, redness, and swelling where you got the shot
- feeling tired
- headache
- muscle aches
- nausea, vomiting, diarrhea, and stomach pain
- joint aches

Other possible side effects include:
- swollen glands (neck, armpit, or groin).

Call your healthcare provider or seek medical treatment immediately if you develop hives, difficulty breathing, or swelling of the throat, because these may be signs of a severe allergic reaction.

Tell your healthcare provider about these or any other side effects that concern you. For a more complete list of side effects, ask your healthcare provider.

What are the ingredients in CERVARIX?

CERVARIX contains proteins of HPV types 16 and 18. The vaccine also contains 3-*O*-desacyl-4′-monophosphoryl lipid A (MPL), aluminum hydroxide, sodium chloride, and sodium dihydrogen phosphate dehydrate.

CERVARIX contains no preservatives.

This is a summary of information about CERVARIX. If you would like more information, please talk with your healthcare provider or visit www.cervarix.com.

CERVARIX is a registered trademark of GlaxoSmithKline.

Manufactured by **GlaxoSmithKline Biologicals**
Rixensart, Belgium, US License 1617
Distributed by **GlaxoSmithKline**
Research Triangle Park, NC 27709

July 2011
CRX:2PIL

COREG® ℞

[*kor' eg*]
(carvedilol)
tablets

HIGHLIGHTS OF PRESCRIBING INFORMATION
These highlights do not include all the information needed to use COREG safely and effectively. See full prescribing information for COREG.
COREG® (carvedilol) tablets
Initial U.S. Approval: 1995

RECENT MAJOR CHANGES

Warnings and Precautions, Major Surgery (5.9)	October 2010
Warnings and Precautions, Intraoperative Floppy Iris Syndrome (5.14)	January 2011

INDICATIONS AND USAGE

COREG is an alpha/beta-adrenergic blocking agent indicated for the treatment of:
- Mild to severe chronic heart failure (1.1)
- Left ventricular dysfunction following myocardial infarction in clinically stable patients (1.2)
- Hypertension (1.3)

DOSAGE AND ADMINISTRATION

Take with food. Individualize dosage and monitor during up-titration. (2)
- Heart failure: Start at 3.125 mg twice daily and increase to 6.25, 12.5, and then 25 mg twice daily over intervals of at least 2 weeks. Maintain lower doses if higher doses are not tolerated. (2.1)
- Left ventricular dysfunction following myocardial infarction: Start at 6.25 mg twice daily and increase to 12.5 mg then 25 mg twice daily after intervals of 3 to 10 days. A lower starting dose or slower titration may be used. (2.2)
- Hypertension: Start at 6.25 mg twice daily and increase if needed for blood pressure control to 12.5 mg then 25 mg twice daily over intervals of 1 to 2 weeks. (2.3)

DOSAGE FORMS AND STRENGTHS

Tablets: 3.125, 6.25, 12.5, 25 mg (3)

CONTRAINDICATIONS

- Bronchial asthma or related bronchospastic conditions (4)
- Second- or third-degree AV block (4)
- Sick sinus syndrome (4)
- Severe bradycardia (unless permanent pacemaker in place) (4)
- Patients in cardiogenic shock or decompensated heart failure requiring the use of IV inotropic therapy. (4)
- Severe hepatic impairment (2.4, 4)
- History of serious hypersensitivity reaction (e.g., Stevens-Johnson syndrome, anaphylactic reaction, angioedema) to any component of this medication or other medications containing carvedilol. (4)

WARNINGS AND PRECAUTIONS

- Acute exacerbation of coronary artery disease upon cessation of therapy: Do not abruptly discontinue. (5.1)
- Bradycardia, hypotension, worsening heart failure/fluid retention may occur. Reduce the dose as needed. (5.2, 5.3, 5.4)
- Non-allergic bronchospasm (e.g., chronic bronchitis and emphysema): Avoid β-blockers. (4) However, if deemed necessary, use with caution and at lowest effective dose. (5.5)
- Diabetes: Monitor glucose as β-blockers may mask symptoms of hypoglycemia or worsen hyperglycemia. (5.6)

ADVERSE REACTIONS

Most common adverse events (6.1):
- Heart failure and left ventricular dysfunction following myocardial infarction (≥10%): Dizziness, fatigue, hypotension, diarrhea, hyperglycemia, asthenia, bradycardia, weight increase
- Hypertension (≥5%): Dizziness

To report SUSPECTED ADVERSE REACTIONS, contact GlaxoSmithKline at 1-888-825-5249 or FDA at 1-800-FDA-1088 or www.fda.gov/medwatch.

DRUG INTERACTIONS

- CYP P450 2D6 enzyme inhibitors may increase and rifampin may decrease carvedilol levels. (7.1, 7.5)
- Hypotensive agents (e.g., reserpine, MAO inhibitors, clonidine) may increase the risk of hypotension and/or severe bradycardia. (7.2)
- Cyclosporine or digoxin levels may increase. (7.3, 7.4)
- Both digitalis glycosides and β-blockers slow atrioventricular conduction and decrease heart rate. Concomitant use can increase the risk of bradycardia. (7.4)
- Amiodarone may increase carvedilol levels resulting in further slowing of the heart rate or cardiac conduction. (7.6)
- Verapamil- or diltiazem-type calcium channel blockers may affect ECG and/or blood pressure. (7.7)
- Insulin and oral hypoglycemics action may be enhanced. (7.8)

See 17 for PATIENT COUNSELING INFORMATION and FDA-approved patient labeling

Revised: 07/2011

FULL PRESCRIBING INFORMATION: CONTENTS*

*** Sections or subsections omitted from the full prescribing information are not listed**

FULL PRESCRIBING INFORMATION

1 INDICATIONS AND USAGE

1.1 Heart Failure

COREG is indicated for the treatment of mild-to-severe chronic heart failure of ischemic or cardiomyopathic origin, usually in addition to diuretics, ACE inhibitors, and digitalis, to increase survival and, also, to reduce the risk of hospitalization *[see Drug Interactions (7.4) and Clinical Studies (14.1)]*.

1.2 Left Ventricular Dysfunction Following Myocardial Infarction

COREG is indicated to reduce cardiovascular mortality in clinically stable patients who have survived the acute phase of a myocardial infarction and have a left ventricular ejection fraction of ≤40% (with or without symptomatic heart failure) *[see Clinical Studies (14.2)]*.

1.3 Hypertension

COREG is indicated for the management of essential hypertension *[see Clinical Studies 14.3, Clinical Studies (14.4)]*. It can be used alone or in combination with other antihypertensive agents, especially thiazide-type diuretics *[see Drug Interactions (7.2)]*.

2 DOSAGE AND ADMINISTRATION

COREG should be taken with food to slow the rate of absorption and reduce the incidence of orthostatic effects.

2.1 Heart Failure

DOSAGE MUST BE INDIVIDUALIZED AND CLOSELY MONITORED BY A PHYSICIAN DURING UP-TITRATION. Prior to initiation of COREG, it is recommended that fluid retention be minimized. The recommended starting dose of COREG is 3.125 mg twice daily for 2 weeks. If tolerated, patients may have their dose increased to 6.25, 12.5, and 25 mg twice daily over successive intervals of at least 2 weeks. Patients should be maintained on lower doses if higher doses are not tolerated. A maximum dose of 50 mg twice daily has been administered to patients with mild-to-moderate heart failure weighing over 85 kg (187 lbs).

Patients should be advised that initiation of treatment and (to a lesser extent) dosage increases may be associated with transient symptoms of dizziness or lightheadedness (and rarely syncope) within the first hour after dosing. During these periods, patients should avoid situations such as driving or hazardous tasks, where symptoms could result in injury. Vasodilatory symptoms often do not require treatment, but it may be useful to separate the time of dosing of COREG from that of the ACE inhibitor or to reduce temporarily the dose of the ACE inhibitor. The dose of COREG should not be increased until symptoms of worsening heart failure or vasodilation have been stabilized.

Fluid retention (with or without transient worsening heart failure symptoms) should be treated by an increase in the dose of diuretics.

The dose of COREG should be reduced if patients experience bradycardia (heart rate <55 beats/minute).

Episodes of dizziness or fluid retention during initiation of COREG can generally be managed without discontinuation of treatment and do not preclude subsequent successful titration of, or a favorable response to, carvedilol.

2.2 Left Ventricular Dysfunction Following Myocardial Infarction

DOSAGE MUST BE INDIVIDUALIZED AND MONITORED DURING UP-TITRATION. Treatment with COREG may be started as an inpatient or outpatient and should be started after the patient is hemodynamically stable and fluid retention has been minimized. It is recommended that COREG be started at 6.25 mg twice daily and increased after 3 to 10 days, based on tolerability, to 12.5 mg twice daily, then again to the target dose of 25 mg twice daily. A lower starting dose may be used (3.125 mg twice daily) and/or the rate of up-titration may be slowed if clinically indicated (e.g., due to low blood pressure or heart rate, or fluid retention). Patients should be maintained on lower doses if higher doses are not tolerated. The recommended dosing regimen need not be altered in patients who received treatment with an IV or oral β-blocker during the acute phase of the myocardial infarction.

2.3 Hypertension

DOSAGE MUST BE INDIVIDUALIZED. The recommended starting dose of COREG is 6.25 mg twice daily. If this dose is tolerated, using standing systolic pressure measured about 1 hour after dosing as a guide, the dose should be maintained for 7 to 14 days, and then increased to 12.5 mg twice daily if needed, based on trough blood pressure, again using standing systolic pressure one hour after dosing as a guide for tolerance. This dose should also be maintained for 7 to 14 days and can then be adjusted upward to 25 mg twice daily if tolerated and needed. The full antihypertensive effect of COREG is seen within 7 to 14 days. Total daily dose should not exceed 50 mg.

Concomitant administration with a diuretic can be expected to produce additive effects and exaggerate the orthostatic component of carvedilol action.

2.4 Hepatic Impairment

COREG should not be given to patients with severe hepatic impairment *[see Contraindications (4)]*.

3 DOSAGE FORMS AND STRENGTHS

The white, oval, film-coated tablets are available in the following strengths: 3.125 mg–engraved with 39 and SB, 6.25 mg–engraved with 4140 and SB, 12.5 mg–engraved with 4141 and SB, and 25 mg–engraved with 4142 and SB.

4 CONTRAINDICATIONS

COREG is contraindicated in the following conditions:

- Bronchial asthma or related bronchospastic conditions. Deaths from status asthmaticus have been reported following single doses of COREG.
- Second- or third-degree AV block
- Sick sinus syndrome
- Severe bradycardia (unless a permanent pacemaker is in place)
- Patients with cardiogenic shock or who have decompensated heart failure requiring the use of intravenous inotropic therapy. Such patients should first be weaned from intravenous therapy before initiating COREG.
- Patients with severe hepatic impairment
- Patients with a history of a serious hypersensitivity reaction (e.g., Stevens-Johnson syndrome, anaphylactic reaction, angioedema) to any component of this medication or other medications containing carvedilol.

5 WARNINGS AND PRECAUTIONS

5.1 Cessation of Therapy

Patients with coronary artery disease, who are being treated with COREG, should be advised against abrupt discontinuation of therapy. Severe exacerbation of angina and the occurrence of myocardial infarction and ventricular arrhythmias have been reported in angina patients following the abrupt discontinuation of therapy with β-blockers. The last 2 complications may occur with or without preceding exacerbation of the angina pectoris. As with other β-blockers, when discontinuation of COREG is planned, the patients should be carefully observed and advised to limit physical activity to a minimum. COREG should be discontinued over 1 to 2 weeks whenever possible. If the angina worsens or acute coronary insufficiency develops, it is recommended that COREG be promptly reinstituted, at least temporarily. Because coronary artery disease is common and may be unrecognized, it may be prudent not to discontinue therapy with COREG abruptly even in patients treated only for hypertension or heart failure.

5.2 Bradycardia

In clinical trials, COREG caused bradycardia in about 2% of hypertensive patients, 9% of heart failure patients, and 6.5% of myocardial infarction patients with left ventricular dysfunction. If pulse rate drops below 55 beats/minute, the dosage should be reduced.

5.3 Hypotension

In clinical trials of primarily mild-to-moderate heart failure, hypotension and postural hypotension occurred in 9.7% and syncope in 3.4% of patients receiving COREG compared to 3.6% and 2.5% of placebo patients, respectively. The risk for these events was highest during the first 30 days of dosing, corresponding to the up-titration period and was a cause for discontinuation of therapy in 0.7% of patients receiving COREG, compared to 0.4% of placebo patients. In a long-term, placebo-controlled trial in severe heart failure (COPERNICUS), hypotension and postural hypotension occurred in 15.1% and syncope in 2.9% of heart failure patients receiving COREG compared to 8.7% and 2.3% of placebo patients, respectively. These events were a cause for discontinuation of therapy in 1.1% of patients receiving COREG, compared to 0.8% of placebo patients.

Postural hypotension occurred in 1.8% and syncope in 0.1% of hypertensive patients, primarily following the initial dose or at the time of dose increase and was a cause for discontinuation of therapy in 1% of patients.

In the CAPRICORN study of survivors of an acute myocardial infarction, hypotension or postural hypotension occurred in 20.2% of patients receiving COREG compared to 12.6% of placebo patients. Syncope was reported in 3.9% and 1.9% of patients, respectively. These events were a cause for discontinuation of therapy in 2.5% of patients receiving COREG, compared to 0.2% of placebo patients.

Starting with a low dose, administration with food, and gradual up-titration should decrease the likelihood of syncope or excessive hypotension *[see Dosage and Administration (2.1, 2.2, 2.3)]*. During initiation of therapy, the patient should be cautioned to avoid situations such as driving or hazardous tasks, where injury could result should syncope occur.

5.4 Heart Failure/Fluid Retention

Worsening heart failure or fluid retention may occur during up-titration of carvedilol. If such symptoms occur, diuretics should be increased and the carvedilol dose should not be advanced until clinical stability resumes *[see Dosage and Administration (2)]*. Occasionally it is necessary to lower the carvedilol dose or temporarily discontinue it. Such episodes do not preclude subsequent successful titration of, or a favorable response to, carvedilol. In a placebo-controlled trial of patients with severe heart failure, worsening heart failure during the first 3 months was reported to a similar degree with carvedilol and with placebo. When treatment was maintained beyond 3 months, worsening heart failure was reported less frequently in patients treated with carvedilol than with placebo. Worsening heart failure observed during long-term therapy is more likely to be related to the patients' underlying disease than to treatment with carvedilol.

5.5 Non-allergic Bronchospasm

Patients with bronchospastic disease (e.g., chronic bronchitis and emphysema) should, in general, not receive β-blockers. COREG may be used with caution, however, in patients who do not respond to, or cannot tolerate, other antihypertensive agents. It is prudent, if COREG is used, to use the smallest effective dose, so that inhibition of endogenous or exogenous β-agonists is minimized.

In clinical trials of patients with heart failure, patients with bronchospastic disease were enrolled if they did not require oral or inhaled medication to treat their bronchospastic disease. In such patients, it is recommended that carvedilol be used with caution. The dosing recommendations should be followed closely and the dose should be lowered if any evidence of bronchospasm is observed during up-titration.

5.6 Glycemic Control in Type 2 Diabetes

In general, β-blockers may mask some of the manifestations of hypoglycemia, particularly tachycardia. Nonselective β-blockers may potentiate insulin-induced hypoglycemia and delay recovery of serum glucose levels. Patients subject to spontaneous hypoglycemia, or diabetic patients receiving insulin or oral hypoglycemic agents, should be cautioned about these possibilities.

In heart failure patients with diabetes, carvedilol therapy may lead to worsening hyperglycemia, which responds to intensification of hypoglycemic therapy. It is recommended that blood glucose be monitored when carvedilol dosing is initiated, adjusted, or discontinued. Studies designed to examine the effects of carvedilol on glycemic control in patients with diabetes and heart failure have not been conducted.

In a study designed to examine the effects of carvedilol on glycemic control in a population with mild-to-moderate hypertension and well-controlled type 2 diabetes mellitus, carvedilol had no adverse effect on glycemic control, based on HbA1c measurements *[see Clinical Studies (14.4)]*.

5.7 Peripheral Vascular Disease

β-blockers can precipitate or aggravate symptoms of arterial insufficiency in patients with peripheral vascular disease. Caution should be exercised in such individuals.

5.8 Deterioration of Renal Function

Rarely, use of carvedilol in patients with heart failure has resulted in deterioration of renal function. Patients at risk appear to be those with low blood pressure (systolic blood pressure <100 mm Hg), ischemic heart disease and diffuse vascular disease, and/or underlying renal insufficiency. Renal function has returned to baseline when carvedilol was stopped. In patients with these risk factors it is recommended that renal function be monitored during up-titration of carvedilol and the drug discontinued or dosage reduced if worsening of renal function occurs.

5.9 Major Surgery

Chronically administered beta-blocking therapy should not be routinely withdrawn prior to major surgery; however, the impaired ability of the heart to respond to reflex adrenergic stimuli may augment the risks of general anesthesia and surgical procedures.

5.10 Thyrotoxicosis

β-adrenergic blockade may mask clinical signs of hyperthyroidism, such as tachycardia. Abrupt withdrawal of β-blockade may be followed by an exacerbation of the symptoms of hyperthyroidism or may precipitate thyroid storm.

5.11 Pheochromocytoma

In patients with pheochromocytoma, an α-blocking agent should be initiated prior to the use of any β-blocking agent. Although carvedilol has both α- and β-blocking pharmacologic activities, there has been no experience with its use in this condition. Therefore, caution should be taken in the administration of carvedilol to patients suspected of having pheochromocytoma.

5.12 Prinzmetal's Variant Angina

Agents with non-selective β-blocking activity may provoke chest pain in patients with Prinzmetal's variant angina. There has been no clinical experience with carvedilol in these patients although the α-blocking activity may prevent such symptoms. However, caution should be taken in the administration of carvedilol to patients suspected of having Prinzmetal's variant angina.

5.13 Risk of Anaphylactic Reaction

While taking β-blockers, patients with a history of severe anaphylactic reaction to a variety of allergens may be more reactive to repeated challenge, either accidental, diagnostic, or therapeutic. Such patients may be unresponsive to the usual doses of epinephrine used to treat allergic reaction.

5.14 Intraoperative Floppy Iris Syndrome

Intraoperative Floppy Iris Syndrome (IFIS) has been observed during cataract surgery in some patients treated with alpha-1 blockers (COREG is an alpha/beta blocker). This variant of small pupil syndrome is characterized by the combination of a flaccid iris that billows in response to intraoperative irrigation currents, progressive intraoperative miosis despite preoperative dilation with standard mydriatic drugs, and potential prolapse of the iris toward the phacoemulsification incisions. The patient's ophthalmologist should be prepared for possible modifications to the surgical technique, such as utilization of iris hooks, iris dilator rings, or viscoelastic substances. There does not appear to be a benefit of stopping alpha-1 blocker therapy prior to cataract surgery.

6 ADVERSE REACTIONS

6.1 Clinical Studies Experience

COREG has been evaluated for safety in patients with heart failure (mild, moderate, and severe), in patients with left ventricular dysfunction following myocardial infarction and in hypertensive patients. The observed adverse event profile was consistent with the pharmacology of the drug and the health status of the patients in the clinical trials. Adverse events reported for each of these patient populations are provided below. Excluded are adverse events considered too general to be informative, and those not reasonably associated with the use of the drug because they were associated with the condition being treated or are very common in the treated population. Rates of adverse events were generally similar across demographic subsets (men and women, elderly and non-elderly, blacks and non-blacks).

Heart Failure

COREG has been evaluated for safety in heart failure in more than 4,500 patients worldwide of whom more than 2,100 participated in placebo-controlled clinical trials. Approximately 60% of the total treated population in placebo-controlled clinical trials received COREG for at least 6 months and 30% received COREG for at least 12 months. In the COMET trial, 1,511 patients with mild-to-moderate heart failure were treated with COREG for up to 5.9 years (mean 4.8 years). Both in US clinical trials in mild-to-moderate heart failure that compared COREG in daily doses up to 100 mg (n = 765) to placebo (n = 437), and in a multinational clinical trial in severe heart failure (COPERNICUS) that compared COREG in daily doses up to 50 mg (n = 1,156) with placebo (n = 1,133), discontinuation rates for adverse experiences were similar in carvedilol and placebo patients. In placebo-controlled clinical trials, the only cause of discontinuation >1%, and occurring more often on carvedilol was dizziness (1.3% on carvedilol, 0.6% on placebo in the COPERNICUS trial).

Table 1 shows adverse events reported in patients with mild-to-moderate heart failure enrolled in US placebo-controlled clinical trials, and with severe heart failure enrolled in the COPERNICUS trial. Shown are adverse events that occurred more frequently in drug-treated patients than placebo-treated patients with an incidence of >3% in patients treated with carvedilol regardless of causality. Median study medication exposure was 6.3 months for both carvedilol and placebo patients in the trials of mild-to-moderate heart failure, and 10.4 months in the trial of severe heart failure patients. The adverse event profile of COREG observed in the long-term COMET study was generally similar to that observed in the US Heart Failure Trials.

[See table 1 above]

Table 1. Adverse Events (%) Occurring More Frequently With COREG Than With Placebo in Patients With Mild-to-Moderate Heart Failure (HF) Enrolled in US Heart Failure Trials or in Patients With Severe Heart Failure in the COPERNICUS Trial (Incidence >3% in Patients Treated With Carvedilol, Regardless of Causality)

	Mild-to-Moderate HF		Severe HF	
	COREG	Placebo	COREG	Placebo
	(n = 765)	(n = 437)	(n = 1,156)	(n = 1,133)
Body as a Whole				
Asthenia	7	7	11	9
Fatigue	24	22	—	—
Digoxin level increased	5	4	2	1
Edema generalized	5	3	6	5
Edema dependent	4	2	—	—
Cardiovascular				
Bradycardia	9	1	10	3
Hypotension	9	3	14	8
Syncope	3	3	8	5
Angina pectoris	2	3	6	4
Central Nervous System				
Dizziness	32	19	24	17
Headache	8	7	5	3
Gastrointestinal				
Diarrhea	12	6	5	3
Nausea	9	5	4	3
Vomiting	6	4	1	2
Metabolic				
Hyperglycemia	12	8	5	3
Weight increase	10	7	12	11
BUN increased	6	5	—	—
NPN increased	6	5	—	—
Hypercholesterolemia	4	3	1	1
Edema peripheral	2	1	7	6
Musculoskeletal				
Arthralgia	6	5	1	1
Respiratory				
Cough increased	8	9	5	4
Rales	4	4	4	2
Vision				
Vision abnormal	5	2	—	—

Cardiac failure and dyspnea were also reported in these studies, but the rates were equal or greater in patients who received placebo.

The following adverse events were reported with a frequency of >1% but ≤3% and more frequently with COREG in either the US placebo-controlled trials in patients with mild-to-moderate heart failure, or in patients with severe heart failure in the COPERNICUS trial.

Incidence >1% to ≤3%

Body as a Whole: Allergy, malaise, hypovolemia, fever, leg edema.

Cardiovascular: Fluid overload, postural hypotension, aggravated angina pectoris, AV block, palpitation, hypertension.

Central and Peripheral Nervous System: Hypesthesia, vertigo, paresthesia.

Gastrointestinal: Melena, periodontitis.

Liver and Biliary System: SGPT increased, SGOT increased.

Metabolic and Nutritional: Hyperuricemia, hypoglycemia, hyponatremia, increased alkaline phosphatase, glycosuria, hypervolemia, diabetes mellitus, GGT increased, weight loss, hyperkalemia, creatinine increased.

Musculoskeletal: Muscle cramps.

Platelet, Bleeding and Clotting: Prothrombin decreased, purpura, thrombocytopenia.

Psychiatric: Somnolence.

Reproductive, male: Impotence.

Special Senses: Blurred vision.

Urinary System: Renal insufficiency, albuminuria, hematuria.

Left Ventricular Dysfunction Following Myocardial Infarction

COREG has been evaluated for safety in survivors of an acute myocardial infarction with left ventricular dysfunction in the CAPRICORN trial which involved 969 patients who received COREG and 980 who received placebo. Approximately 75% of the patients received COREG for at least 6 months and 53% received COREG for at least 12 months. Patients were treated for an average of 12.9 months and 12.8 months with COREG and placebo, respectively.

The most common adverse events reported with COREG in the CAPRICORN trial were consistent with the profile of the drug in the US heart failure trials and the COPERNICUS trial. The only additional adverse events reported in CAPRICORN in >3% of the patients and more commonly on carvedilol were dyspnea, anemia, and lung edema. The following adverse events were reported with a frequency of >1% but ≤3% and more frequently with COREG: Flu syndrome, cerebrovascular accident, peripheral vascular disorder, hypotonia, depression, gastrointestinal pain, arthritis, and gout. The overall rates of discontinuations due to adverse events were similar in both groups of patients. In this database, the only cause of discontinuation >1%, and occurring more often on carvedilol was hypotension (1.5% on carvedilol, 0.2% on placebo).

Hypertension

COREG has been evaluated for safety in hypertension in more than 2,193 patients in US clinical trials and in 2,976 patients in international clinical trials. Approximately 36% of the total treated population received COREG for at least 6 months. Most adverse events reported during therapy with COREG were of mild to moderate severity. In US controlled clinical trials directly comparing COREG in doses up to 50 mg (n = 1,142) to placebo (n = 462), 4.9% of patients receiving COREG discontinued for adverse events versus 5.2% of placebo patients. Although there was no overall difference in discontinuation rates, discontinuations were more common in the carvedilol group for postural hypotension (1% versus 0). The overall incidence of adverse events in US placebo-controlled trials increased with increasing dose of COREG. For individual adverse events this could only be distinguished for dizziness, which increased in frequency from 2% to 5% as total daily dose increased from 6.25 mg to 50 mg.

Table 2 shows adverse events in US placebo-controlled clinical trials for hypertension that occurred with an incidence of≥1% regardless of causality, and that were more frequent in drug-treated patients than placebo-treated patients.

Table 2. Adverse Events (%) Occurring in US Placebo-Controlled Hypertension Trials (Incidence ≥1%, Regardless of Causality)*

	COREG (n = 1,142)	Placebo (n = 462)
Cardiovascular		
Bradycardia	2	—
Postural hypotension	2	—
Peripheral edema	1	—
Central Nervous System		
Dizziness	6	5
Insomnia	2	1
Gastrointestinal		
Diarrhea	2	1
Hematologic		
Thrombocytopenia	1	—
Metabolic		
Hypertriglyceridemia	1	—

* Shown are events with rate >1% rounded to nearest integer.

Dyspnea and fatigue were also reported in these studies, but the rates were equal or greater in patients who received placebo.

The following adverse events not described above were reported as possibly or probably related to COREG in worldwide open or controlled trials with COREG in patients with hypertension or heart failure.

Incidence >0.1% to ≤1%

Cardiovascular: Peripheral ischemia, tachycardia.

Central and Peripheral Nervous System: Hypokinesia.

Gastrointestinal: Bilirubinemia, increased hepatic enzymes (0.2% of hypertension patients and 0.4% of heart failure patients were discontinued from therapy because of increases in hepatic enzymes) *[see Adverse Reactions (6.2)]*.

Psychiatric: Nervousness, sleep disorder, aggravated depression, impaired concentration, abnormal thinking, paroniria, emotional lability.

Respiratory System: Asthma *[see Contraindications (4)]*.

Reproductive, male: Decreased libido.

Skin and Appendages: Pruritus, rash erythematous, rash maculopapular, rash psoriaform, photosensitivity reaction.

Special Senses: Tinnitus.

Urinary System: Micturition frequency increased.

Autonomic Nervous System: Dry mouth, sweating increased.

Metabolic and Nutritional: Hypokalemia, hypertriglyceridemia.

Hematologic: Anemia, leukopenia.

The following events were reported in ≤0.1% of patients and are potentially important: Complete AV block, bundle branch block, myocardial ischemia, cerebrovascular disorder, convulsions, migraine, neuralgia, paresis, anaphylactoid reaction, alopecia, exfoliative dermatitis, amnesia, GI hemorrhage, bronchospasm, pulmonary edema, decreased hearing, respiratory alkalosis, increased BUN, decreased HDL, pancytopenia, and atypical lymphocytes.

6.2 Laboratory Abnormalities

Reversible elevations in serum transaminases (ALT or AST) have been observed during treatment with COREG. Rates of transaminase elevations (2- to 3-times the upper limit of normal) observed during controlled clinical trials have generally been similar between patients treated with COREG and those treated with placebo. However, transaminase elevations, confirmed by rechallenge, have been observed with COREG. In a long-term, placebo-controlled trial in severe heart failure, patients treated with COREG had lower values for hepatic transaminases than patients treated with placebo, possibly because improvements in cardiac function induced by COREG led to less hepatic congestion and/or improved hepatic blood flow.

COREG has not been associated with clinically significant changes in serum potassium, total triglycerides, total cholesterol, HDL cholesterol, uric acid, blood urea nitrogen, or creatinine. No clinically relevant changes were noted in fasting serum glucose in hypertensive patients; fasting serum glucose was not evaluated in the heart failure clinical trials.

6.3 Postmarketing Experience

The following adverse reactions have been identified during post-approval use of COREG. Because these reactions are reported voluntarily from a population of uncertain size, it is not always possible to reliably estimate their frequency or establish a causal relationship to drug exposure.

Blood and Lymphatic System Disorders: Aplastic anemia.

Immune System Disorders: Hypersensitivity (e.g., anaphylactic reactions, angioedema, urticaria).

Renal and Urinary Disorders: Urinary incontinence.

Respiratory, Thoracic and Mediastinal Disorders: Interstitial pneumonitis.

Skin and Subcutaneous Tissue Disorders: Stevens-Johnson syndrome, toxic epidermal necrolysis, erythema multiforme.

7 DRUG INTERACTIONS

7.1 CYP2D6 Inhibitors and Poor Metabolizers

Interactions of carvedilol with potent inhibitors of CYP2D6 isoenzyme (such as quinidine, fluoxetine, paroxetine, and propafenone) have not been studied, but these drugs would be expected to increase blood levels of the R(+) enantiomer of carvedilol *[seeClinical Pharmacology (12.3)]*. Retrospective analysis of side effects in clinical trials showed that poor 2D6 metabolizers had a higher rate of dizziness during up-titration, presumably resulting from vasodilating effects of the higher concentrations of the α-blocking R(+) enantiomer.

7.2 Hypotensive Agents

Patients taking both agents with β-blocking properties and a drug that can deplete catecholamines (e.g., reserpine and monoamine oxidase inhibitors) should be observed closely for signs of hypotension and/or severe bradycardia.

Concomitant administration of clonidine with agents with β-blocking properties may potentiate blood-pressure- and heart-rate-lowering effects. When concomitant treatment with agents with β-blocking properties and clonidine is to be terminated, the β-blocking agent should be discontinued first. Clonidine therapy can then be discontinued several days later by gradually decreasing the dosage.

7.3 Cyclosporine

Modest increases in mean trough cyclosporine concentrations were observed following initiation of carvedilol treatment in 21 renal transplant patients suffering from chronic vascular rejection. In about 30% of patients, the dose of cyclosporine had to be reduced in order to maintain cyclosporine concentrations within the therapeutic range, while in the remainder no adjustment was needed. On the average for the group, the dose of cyclosporine was reduced about 20% in these patients. Due to wide interindividual variability in the dose adjustment required, it is recommended that cyclosporine concentrations be monitored closely after initiation of carvedilol therapy and that the dose of cyclosporine be adjusted as appropriate.

7.4 Digitalis Glycosides

Both digitalis glycosides and β-blockers slow atrioventricular conduction and decrease heart rate. Concomitant use can increase the risk of bradycardia. Digoxin concentrations are increased by about 15% when digoxin and carvedilol are administered concomitantly. Therefore, increased monitoring of digoxin is recommended when initiating, adjusting, or discontinuing COREG *[see Clinical Pharmacology (12.5)]*.

7.5 Inducers/Inhibitors of Hepatic Metabolism

Rifampin reduced plasma concentrations of carvedilol by about 70% *[see Clinical Pharmacology (12.5)]*. Cimetidine increased AUC by about 30% but caused no change in C_{max} *[see Clinical Pharmacology (12.5)]*.

7.6 Amiodarone

Amiodarone, and its metabolite desethyl amiodarone, inhibitors of CYP2C9 and P-glycoprotein, increased concentrations of the S(-)-enantiomer of carvedilol by at least 2-fold *[see Clinical Pharmacology (12.5)]*. The concomitant administration of amiodarone or other CYP2C9 inhibitors such as fluconazole with COREG may enhance the β-blocking properties of carvedilol resulting in further slowing of the heart rate or cardiac conduction. Patients should be observed for signs of bradycardia or heart block, particularly when one agent is added to pre-existing treatment with the other.

7.7 Calcium Channel Blockers

Conduction disturbance (rarely with hemodynamic compromise) has been observed when COREG is co-administered with diltiazem. As with other agents with β-blocking properties, if COREG is to be administered with calcium channel blockers of the verapamil or diltiazem type, it is recommended that ECG and blood pressure be monitored.

7.8 Insulin or Oral Hypoglycemics

Agents with β-blocking properties may enhance the blood-sugar-reducing effect of insulin and oral hypoglycemics. Therefore, in patients taking insulin or oral hypoglycemics, regular monitoring of blood glucose is recommended *[see Warnings and Precautions (5.6)]*.

7.9 Anesthesia

If treatment with COREG is to be continued perioperatively, particular care should be taken when anesthetic agents which depress myocardial function, such as ether, cyclopropane, and trichloroethylene, are used *[see Overdosage (10)]*.

8 USE IN SPECIFIC POPULATIONS

8.1 Pregnancy

Pregnancy Category C. Studies performed in pregnant rats and rabbits given carvedilol revealed increased post-implantation loss in rats at doses of 300 mg/kg/day (50 times the maximum recommended human dose [MRHD] as mg/m^2) and in rabbits at doses of 75 mg/kg/day (25 times the MRHD as mg/m^2). In the rats, there was also a decrease in fetal body weight at the maternally toxic dose of 300 mg/kg/day (50 times the MRHD as mg/m^2), which was accompanied by an elevation in the frequency of fetuses with delayed skeletal development (missing or stunted 13th rib). In rats the no-observed-effect level for developmental toxicity was 60 mg/kg/day (10 times the MRHD as mg/m^2); in rabbits it was 15 mg/kg/day (5 times the MRHD as mg/m^2). There are no adequate and well-controlled studies in pregnant women. COREG should be used during pregnancy only if the potential benefit justifies the potential risk to the fetus.

8.3 Nursing Mothers

It is not known whether this drug is excreted in human milk. Studies in rats have shown that carvedilol and/or its metabolites (as well as other β-blockers) cross the placental barrier and are excreted in breast milk. There was increased mortality at one week post-partum in neonates from rats treated with 60 mg/kg/day (10 times the MRHD as mg/m^2) and above during the last trimester through day 22 of lactation. Because many drugs are excreted in human milk and because of the potential for serious adverse reactions in nursing infants from β-blockers, especially bradycardia, a decision should be made whether to discontinue nursing or to discontinue the drug, taking into account the importance of the drug to the mother. The effects of other α- and β-blocking agents have included perinatal and neonatal distress.

8.4 Pediatric Use

Effectiveness of COREG in patients younger than 18 years of age has not been established.

In a double-blind trial, 161 children (mean age 6 years, range 2 months to 17 years; 45% less than 2 years old) with chronic heart failure [NYHA class II-IV, left ventricular ejection fraction <40% for children with a systemic left ventricle (LV), and moderate-severe ventricular dysfunction qualitatively by echo for those with a systemic ventricle that was not an LV] who were receiving standard background treatment were randomized to placebo or to 2 dose levels of carvedilol. These dose levels produced placebo-corrected heart rate reduction of 4-6 heart beats per minute, indicative of β-blockade activity. Exposure appeared to be lower in pediatric subjects than adults. After 8 months of follow-up, there was no significant effect of treatment on clinical outcomes. Adverse reactions in this trial that occurred in greater than 10% of patients treated with COREG and at twice the rate of placebo-treated patients included chest pain (17% versus 6%), dizziness (13% versus 2%), and dyspnea (11% versus 0%).

8.5 Geriatric Use

Of the 765 patients with heart failure randomized to COREG in US clinical trials, 31% (235) were 65 years of age or older, and 7.3% (56) were 75 years of age or older. Of the 1,156 patients randomized to COREG in a long-term, placebo-controlled trial in severe heart failure, 47% (547) were 65 years of age or older, and 15% (174) were 75 years of age or older. Of 3,025 patients receiving COREG in heart failure trials worldwide, 42% were 65 years of age or older. Of the 975 myocardial infarction patients randomized to COREG in the CAPRICORN trial, 48% (468) were 65 years of age or older, and 11% (111) were 75 years of age or older. Of the 2,065 hypertensive patients in US clinical trials of efficacy or safety who were treated with COREG, 21% (436) were 65 years of age or older. Of 3,722 patients receiving COREG in hypertension clinical trials conducted worldwide, 24% were 65 years of age or older.

With the exception of dizziness in hypertensive patients (incidence 8.8% in the elderly versus 6% in younger patients), no overall differences in the safety or effectiveness (see Figures 2 and 4) were observed between the older subjects and younger subjects in each of these populations. Similarly, other reported clinical experience has not identified differences in responses between the elderly and younger subjects, but greater sensitivity of some older individuals cannot be ruled out.

10 OVERDOSAGE

Overdosage may cause severe hypotension, bradycardia, cardiac insufficiency, cardiogenic shock, and cardiac arrest. Respiratory problems, bronchospasms, vomiting, lapses of consciousness, and generalized seizures may also occur.

The patient should be placed in a supine position and, where necessary, kept under observation and treated under intensive-care conditions. Gastric lavage or pharmacologically induced emesis may be used shortly after ingestion. The following agents may be administered:

for excessive bradycardia: Atropine, 2 mg IV.

to support cardiovascular function: Glucagon, 5 to 10 mg IV rapidly over 30 seconds, followed by a continuous infusion of 5 mg/hour; sympathomimetics (dobutamine, isoprenaline, adrenaline) at doses according to body weight and effect.

If peripheral vasodilation dominates, it may be necessary to administer adrenaline or noradrenaline with continuous monitoring of circulatory conditions. For therapy-resistant bradycardia, pacemaker therapy should be performed. For bronchospasm, β-sympathomimetics (as aerosol or IV) or aminophylline IV should be given. In the event of seizures, slow IV injection of diazepam or clonazepam is recommended.

NOTE: In the event of severe intoxication where there are symptoms of shock, treatment with antidotes must be continued for a sufficiently long period of time consistent with the 7- to 10-hour half-life of carvedilol.

Cases of overdosage with COREG alone or in combination with other drugs have been reported. Quantities ingested in some cases exceeded 1,000 milligrams. Symptoms experienced included low blood pressure and heart rate. Standard supportive treatment was provided and individuals recovered.

11 DESCRIPTION

Carvedilol is a nonselective β-adrenergic blocking agent with α_1-blocking activity. It is (±)-1-(Carbazol-4-yloxy)-3-[[2-(o-methoxyphenoxy)ethyl]amino]-2-propanol. Carvedilol is a racemic mixture with the following structure:

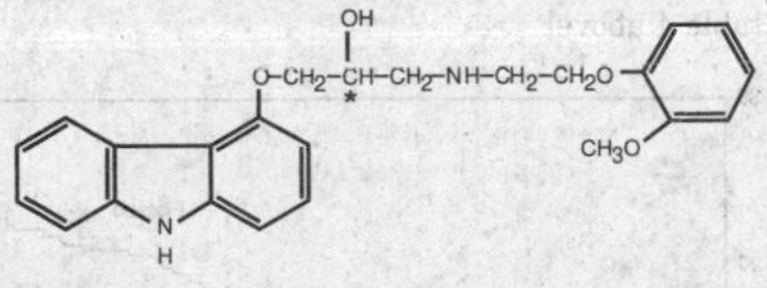

COREG is a white, oval, film-coated tablet containing 3.125 mg, 6.25 mg, 12.5 mg, or 25 mg of carvedilol. The 6.25 mg, 12.5 mg, and 25 mg tablets are TILTAB® tablets. Inactive ingredients consist of colloidal silicon dioxide, crospovidone, hypromellose, lactose, magnesium stearate, polyethylene glycol, polysorbate 80, povidone, sucrose, and titanium dioxide.

Carvedilol is a white to off-white powder with a molecular weight of 406.5 and a molecular formula of $C_{24}H_{26}N_2O_4$. It is freely soluble in dimethylsulfoxide; soluble in methylene chloride and methanol; sparingly soluble in 95% ethanol and isopropanol; slightly soluble in ethyl ether; and practically insoluble in water, gastric fluid (simulated, TS, pH 1.1), and intestinal fluid (simulated, TS without pancreatin, pH 7.5).

12 CLINICAL PHARMACOLOGY

12.1 Mechanism of Action

COREG is a racemic mixture in which nonselective β-adrenoreceptor blocking activity is present in the S(-) enantiomer and α_1-adrenergic blocking activity is present in both R(+) and S(-) enantiomers at equal potency. COREG has no intrinsic sympathomimetic activity.

12.2 Pharmacodynamics

Heart Failure

The basis for the beneficial effects of COREG in heart failure is not established.

Two placebo-controlled studies compared the acute hemodynamic effects of COREG to baseline measurements in 59 and 49 patients with NYHA class II-IV heart failure receiving diuretics, ACE inhibitors, and digitalis. There were significant reductions in systemic blood pressure, pulmonary artery pressure, pulmonary capillary wedge pressure, and heart rate. Initial effects on cardiac output, stroke volume index, and systemic vascular resistance were small and variable.

These studies measured hemodynamic effects again at 12 to 14 weeks. COREG significantly reduced systemic blood pressure, pulmonary artery pressure, right atrial pressure, systemic vascular resistance, and heart rate, while stroke volume index was increased.

Among 839 patients with NYHA class II-III heart failure treated for 26 to 52 weeks in 4 US placebo-controlled trials, average left ventricular ejection fraction (EF) measured by radionuclide ventriculography increased by 9 EF units (%) in patients receiving COREG and by 2 EF units in placebo patients at a target dose of 25-50 mg twice daily. The effects of carvedilol on ejection fraction were related to dose. Doses of 6.25 mg twice daily, 12.5 mg twice daily, and 25 mg twice daily were associated with placebo-corrected increases in EF of 5 EF units, 6 EF units, and 8 EF units, respectively; each of these effects were nominally statistically significant.

Left Ventricular Dysfunction Following Myocardial Infarction

The basis for the beneficial effects of COREG in patients with left ventricular dysfunction following an acute myocardial infarction is not established.

Hypertension

The mechanism by which β-blockade produces an antihypertensive effect has not been established.

β-adrenoreceptor blocking activity has been demonstrated in animal and human studies showing that carvedilol (1) reduces cardiac output in normal subjects; (2) reduces exercise- and/or isoproterenol-induced tachycardia; and (3) reduces reflex orthostatic tachycardia. Significant β-adrenoreceptor blocking effect is usually seen within 1 hour of drug administration.

α_1-adrenoreceptor blocking activity has been demonstrated in human and animal studies, showing that carvedilol (1) attenuates the pressor effects of phenylephrine; (2) causes vasodilation; and (3) reduces peripheral vascular resistance. These effects contribute to the reduction of blood pressure and usually are seen within 30 minutes of drug administration.

Due to the α_1-receptor blocking activity of carvedilol, blood pressure is lowered more in the standing than in the supine position, and symptoms of postural hypotension (1.8%), including rare instances of syncope, can occur. Following oral administration, when postural hypotension has occurred, it has been transient and is uncommon when COREG is administered with food at the recommended starting dose and titration increments are closely followed *[see Dosage and Administration (2)]*.

In hypertensive patients with normal renal function, therapeutic doses of COREG decreased renal vascular resistance with no change in glomerular filtration rate or renal plasma flow. Changes in excretion of sodium, potassium, uric acid, and phosphorus in hypertensive patients with normal renal function were similar after COREG and placebo.

COREG has little effect on plasma catecholamines, plasma aldosterone, or electrolyte levels, but it does significantly reduce plasma renin activity when given for at least 4 weeks. It also increases levels of atrial natriuretic peptide.

12.3 Pharmacokinetics

COREG is rapidly and extensively absorbed following oral administration, with absolute bioavailability of approximately 25% to 35% due to a significant degree of first-pass metabolism. Following oral administration, the apparent mean terminal elimination half-life of carvedilol generally ranges from 7 to 10 hours. Plasma concentrations achieved are proportional to the oral dose administered. When administered with food, the rate of absorption is slowed, as evidenced by a delay in the time to reach peak plasma levels, with no significant difference in extent of bioavailability. Taking COREG with food should minimize the risk of orthostatic hypotension.

Carvedilol is extensively metabolized. Following oral administration of radiolabelled carvedilol to healthy volunteers, carvedilol accounted for only about 7% of the total radioactivity in plasma as measured by area under the curve (AUC). Less than 2% of the dose was excreted unchanged in the urine. Carvedilol is metabolized primarily by aromatic ring oxidation and glucuronidation. The oxidative metabolites are further metabolized by conjugation via glucuronidation and sulfation. The metabolites of carvedilol are excreted primarily via the bile into the feces. Demethylation and hydroxylation at the phenol ring produce 3 active metabolites with β-receptor blocking activity. Based on preclinical studies, the 4'-hydroxyphenyl metabolite is approximately 13 times more potent than carvedilol for β-blockade. Compared to carvedilol, the 3 active metabolites exhibit weak vasodilating activity. Plasma concentrations of the active metabolites are about one-tenth of those observed for carvedilol and have pharmacokinetics similar to the parent.

Carvedilol undergoes stereoselective first-pass metabolism with plasma levels of R(+)-carvedilol approximately 2 to 3 times higher than S(-)-carvedilol following oral administration in healthy subjects. The mean apparent terminal elimination half-lives for R(+)-carvedilol range from 5 to 9 hours compared with 7 to 11 hours for the S(-)-enantiomer.

The primary P450 enzymes responsible for the metabolism of both R(+) and S(-)-carvedilol in human liver microsomes were CYP2D6 and CYP2C9 and to a lesser extent CYP3A4, 2C19, 1A2, and 2E1. CYP2D6 is thought to be the major enzyme in the 4'- and 5'-hydroxylation of carvedilol, with a potential contribution from 3A4. CYP2C9 is thought to be of primary importance in the O-methylation pathway of S(-)-carvedilol.

Carvedilol is subject to the effects of genetic polymorphism with poor metabolizers of debrisoquin (a marker for cytochrome P450 2D6) exhibiting 2- to 3-fold higher plasma concentrations of R(+)-carvedilol compared to extensive metabolizers. In contrast, plasma levels of S(-)-carvedilol are increased only about 20% to 25% in poor metabolizers, indicating this enantiomer is metabolized to a lesser extent by cytochrome P450 2D6 than R(+)-carvedilol. The pharmacokinetics of carvedilol do not appear to be different in poor metabolizers of S-mephenytoin (patients deficient in cytochrome P450 2C19).

Carvedilol is more than 98% bound to plasma proteins, primarily with albumin. The plasma-protein binding is independent of concentration over the therapeutic range. Carvedilol is a basic, lipophilic compound with a steady-state volume of distribution of approximately 115 L, indicating substantial distribution into extravascular tissues. Plasma clearance ranges from 500 to 700 mL/min.

12.4 Specific Populations

Heart Failure

Steady-state plasma concentrations of carvedilol and its enantiomers increased proportionally over the 6.25 to 50 mg dose range in patients with heart failure. Compared to healthy subjects, heart failure patients had increased mean AUC and C_{max} values for carvedilol and its enantiomers, with up to 50% to 100% higher values observed in 6 patients with NYHA class IV heart failure. The mean apparent terminal elimination half-life for carvedilol was similar to that observed in healthy subjects.

Geriatric

Plasma levels of carvedilol average about 50% higher in the elderly compared to young subjects.

Hepatic Impairment

Compared to healthy subjects, patients with severe liver impairment (cirrhosis) exhibit a 4- to 7-fold increase in carvedilol levels. Carvedilol is contraindicated in patients with severe liver impairment.

Renal Impairment

Although carvedilol is metabolized primarily by the liver, plasma concentrations of carvedilol have been reported to be increased in patients with renal impairment. Based on mean AUC data, approximately 40% to 50% higher plasma concentrations of carvedilol were observed in hypertensive patients with moderate to severe renal impairment compared to a control group of hypertensive patients with normal renal function. However, the ranges of AUC values were similar for both groups. Changes in mean peak plasma levels were less pronounced, approximately 12% to 26% higher in patients with impaired renal function.

Consistent with its high degree of plasma protein-binding, carvedilol does not appear to be cleared significantly by hemodialysis.

12.5 Drug-Drug Interactions

Since carvedilol undergoes substantial oxidative metabolism, the metabolism and pharmacokinetics of carvedilol may be affected by induction or inhibition of cytochrome P450 enzymes.

Amiodarone

In a pharmacokinetic study conducted in 106 Japanese patients with heart failure, coadministration of small loading and maintenance doses of amiodarone with carvedilol resulted in at least a 2-fold increase in the steady-state trough concentrations of S(-)-carvedilol *[see Drug Interactions (7.6)]*.

Cimetidine

In a pharmacokinetic study conducted in 10 healthy male subjects, cimetidine (1,000 mg/day) increased the steady-state AUC of carvedilol by 30% with no change in C_{max} *[see Drug Interactions (7.5)]*.

Table 3. Results of COMET

End point	Carvedilol N = 1,511	Metoprolol N = 1,518	Hazard ratio	(95% CI)
All-cause mortality	34%	40%	0.83	0.74 – 0.93
Mortality + all hospitalization	74%	76%	0.94	0.86 – 1.02
Cardiovascular death	30%	35%	0.80	0.70 – 0.90
Sudden death	14%	17%	0.81	0.68 – 0.97
Death due to circulatory failure	11%	13%	0.83	0.67 – 1.02
Death due to stroke	0.9%	2.5%	0.33	0.18 – 0.62

Table 4. Results of COPERNICUS Trial in Patients With Severe Heart Failure

End point	Placebo (N = 1,133)	Carvedilol (N = 1,156)	Hazard ratio (95% CI)	% Reduction	Nominal p value
Mortality	190	130	0.65 (0.52 – 0.81)	35	0.00013
Mortality + all hospitalization	507	425	0.76 (0.67 – 0.87)	24	0.00004
Mortality + CV hospitalization	395	314	0.73 (0.63 – 0.84)	27	0.00002
Mortality + HF hospitalization	357	271	0.69 (0.59 – 0.81)	31	0.000004

Cardiovascular = CV; Heart failure = HF.

Digoxin

Following concomitant administration of carvedilol (25 mg once daily) and digoxin (0.25 mg once daily) for 14 days, steady-state AUC and trough concentrations of digoxin were increased by 14% and 16%, respectively, in 12 hypertensive patients *[see Drug Interactions (7.4)]*.

Glyburide

In 12 healthy subjects, combined administration of carvedilol (25 mg once daily) and a single dose of glyburide did not result in a clinically relevant pharmacokinetic interaction for either compound.

Hydrochlorothiazide

A single oral dose of carvedilol 25 mg did not alter the pharmacokinetics of a single oral dose of hydrochlorothiazide 25 mg in 12 patients with hypertension. Likewise, hydrochlorothiazide had no effect on the pharmacokinetics of carvedilol.

Rifampin

In a pharmacokinetic study conducted in 8 healthy male subjects, rifampin (600 mg daily for 12 days) decreased the AUC and C_{max} of carvedilol by about 70% *[see Drug Interactions (7.5)]*.

Torsemide

In a study of 12 healthy subjects, combined oral administration of carvedilol 25 mg once daily and torsemide 5 mg once daily for 5 days did not result in any significant differences in their pharmacokinetics compared with administration of the drugs alone.

Warfarin

Carvedilol (12.5 mg twice daily) did not have an effect on the steady-state prothrombin time ratios and did not alter the pharmacokinetics of R(+)- and S(-)-warfarin following concomitant administration with warfarin in 9 healthy volunteers.

13 NONCLINICAL TOXICOLOGY

13.1 Carcinogenesis, Mutagenesis, Impairment of Fertility

In 2-year studies conducted in rats given carvedilol at doses up to 75 mg/kg/day (12 times the MRHD when compared on a mg/m^2 basis) or in mice given up to 200 mg/kg/day (16 times the MRHD on a mg/m^2 basis), carvedilol had no carcinogenic effect.

Carvedilol was negative when tested in a battery of genotoxicity assays, including the Ames and the CHO/HGPRT assays for mutagenicity and the in vitro hamster micronucleus and in vivo human lymphocyte cell tests for clastogenicity.

At doses ≥200 mg/kg/day (≥32 times the MRHD as mg/m^2) carvedilol was toxic to adult rats (sedation, reduced weight gain) and was associated with a reduced number of successful matings, prolonged mating time, significantly fewer corpora lutea and implants per dam, and complete resorption of 18% of the litters. The no-observed-effect dose level for overt toxicity and impairment of fertility was 60 mg/kg/day (10 times the MRHD as mg/m^2).

14 CLINICAL STUDIES

14.1 Heart Failure

A total of 6,975 patients with mild to severe heart failure were evaluated in placebo-controlled studies of carvedilol.

Mild-to-Moderate Heart Failure

Carvedilol was studied in 5 multicenter, placebo-controlled studies, and in 1 active-controlled study (COMET study) involving patients with mild-to-moderate heart failure.

Four US multicenter, double-blind, placebo-controlled studies enrolled 1,094 patients (696 randomized to carvedilol) with NYHA class II-III heart failure and ejection fraction≤0.35. The vast majority were on digitalis, diuretics, and an ACE inhibitor at study entry. Patients were assigned to the studies based upon exercise ability. An Australia-New Zealand double-blind, placebo-controlled study enrolled 415 patients (half randomized to carvedilol) with less severe heart failure. All protocols excluded patients expected to undergo cardiac transplantation during the 7.5 to 15 months of double-blind follow-up. All randomized patients had tolerated a 2-week course on carvedilol 6.25 mg twice daily.

In each study, there was a primary end point, either progression of heart failure (1 US study) or exercise tolerance (2 US studies meeting enrollment goals and the Australia-New Zealand study). There were many secondary end points specified in these studies, including NYHA classification, patient and physician global assessments, and cardiovascular hospitalization. Other analyses not prospectively planned included the sum of deaths and total cardiovascular hospitalizations. In situations where the primary end points of a trial do not show a significant benefit of treatment, assignment of significance values to the other results is complex, and such values need to be interpreted cautiously.

The results of the US and Australia-New Zealand trials were as follows:

Slowing Progression of Heart Failure: One US multicenter study (366 subjects) had as its primary end point the sum of cardiovascular mortality, cardiovascular hospitalization, and sustained increase in heart failure medications. Heart failure progression was reduced, during an average follow-up of 7 months, by 48% (p = 0.008).

In the Australia-New Zealand study, death and total hospitalizations were reduced by about 25% over 18 to 24 months. In the 3 largest US studies, death and total hospitalizations were reduced by 19%, 39%, and 49%, nominally statistically significant in the last 2 studies. The Australia-New Zealand results were statistically borderline.

Functional Measures: None of the multicenter studies had NYHA classification as a primary end point, but all such studies had it as a secondary end point. There was at least a trend toward improvement in NYHA class in all studies. Exercise tolerance was the primary end point in 3 studies; in none was a statistically significant effect found.

Subjective Measures: Health-related quality of life, as measured with a standard questionnaire (a primary end point in 1 study), was unaffected by carvedilol. However, patients' and investigators' global assessments showed significant improvement in most studies.

Mortality: Death was not a pre-specified end point in any study, but was analyzed in all studies. Overall, in these 4 US trials, mortality was reduced, nominally significantly so in 2 studies.

COMET Trial

In this double-blind trial, 3,029 patients with NYHA class II-IV heart failure (left ventricular ejection fraction≤35%) were randomized to receive either carvedilol (target dose: 25 mg twice daily) or immediate-release metoprolol tartrate (target dose: 50 mg twice daily). The mean age of the patients was approximately 62 years, 80% were males, and the mean left ventricular ejection fraction at baseline was 26%. Approximately 96% of the patients had NYHA class II or III heart failure. Concomitant treatment included diuretics (99%), ACE inhibitors (91%), digitalis (59%), aldosterone antagonists (11%), and "statin" lipid-lowering agents (21%). The mean duration of follow-up was 4.8 years. The mean dose of carvedilol was 42 mg per day.

The study had 2 primary end points: All-cause mortality and the composite of death plus hospitalization for any reason. The results of COMET are presented in Table 3 below. All-cause mortality carried most of the statistical weight and was the primary determinant of the study size. All-cause mortality was 34% in the patients treated with carvedilol and was 40% in the immediate-release metoprolol group (p = 0.0017; hazard ratio = 0.83, 95%CI 0.74-0.93). The effect on mortality was primarily due to a reduction in cardiovascular death. The difference between the 2 groups with respect to the composite end point was not significant (p = 0.122). The estimated mean survival was 8.0 years with carvedilol and 6.6 years with immediate-release metoprolol.

[See table 3 above]

It is not known whether this formulation of metoprolol at any dose or this low dose of metoprolol in any formulation has any effect on survival or hospitalization in patients with heart failure. Thus, this trial extends the time over which carvedilol manifests benefits on survival in heart failure, but it is not evidence that carvedilol improves outcome over the formulation of metoprolol (TOPROL-XL®) with benefits in heart failure.

Severe Heart Failure (COPERNICUS)

In a double-blind study (COPERNICUS), 2,289 patients with heart failure at rest or with minimal exertion and left ventricular ejection fraction <25% (mean 20%), despite digitalis (66%), diuretics (99%), and ACE inhibitors (89%) were randomized to placebo or carvedilol. Carvedilol was titrated from a starting dose of 3.125 mg twice daily to the maximum tolerated dose or up to 25 mg twice daily over a minimum of 6 weeks. Most subjects achieved the target dose of 25 mg. The study was conducted in Eastern and Western Europe, the United States, Israel, and Canada. Similar numbers of subjects per group (about 100) withdrew during the titration period.

The primary end point of the trial was all-cause mortality, but cause-specific mortality and the risk of death or hospitalization (total, cardiovascular [CV], or heart failure [HF]) were also examined. The developing trial data were followed by a data monitoring committee, and mortality analyses were adjusted for these multiple looks. The trial was stopped after a median follow-up of 10 months because of an observed 35% reduction in mortality (from 19.7% per patient year on placebo to 12.8% on carvedilol, hazard ratio 0.65, 95% CI 0.52 – 0.81, p = 0.0014, adjusted) (see Figure 1). The results of COPERNICUS are shown in Table 4.

[See table 4 above]

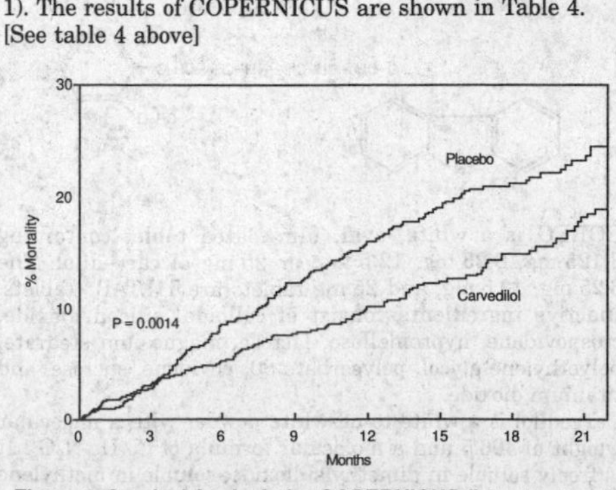

Figure 1. Survival Analysis for COPERNICUS (intent-to-treat)

The effect on mortality was principally the result of a reduction in the rate of sudden death among patients without worsening heart failure.

Patients' global assessments, in which carvedilol-treated patients were compared to placebo, were based on pre-specified, periodic patient self-assessments regarding whether clinical status post-treatment showed improvement, worsening or no change compared to baseline. Patients treated with carvedilol showed significant improvements in global assessments compared with those treated with placebo in COPERNICUS.

The protocol also specified that hospitalizations would be assessed. Fewer patients on COREG than on placebo were hospitalized for any reason (372 versus 432, p = 0.0029), for cardiovascular reasons (246 versus 314, p = 0.0003), or for worsening heart failure (198 versus 268, p = 0.0001).

COREG had a consistent and beneficial effect on all-cause mortality as well as the combined end points of all-cause mortality plus hospitalization (total, CV, or for heart failure) in the overall study population and in all subgroups examined, including men and women, elderly and non-elderly, blacks and non-blacks, and diabetics and non-diabetics (see Figure 2).

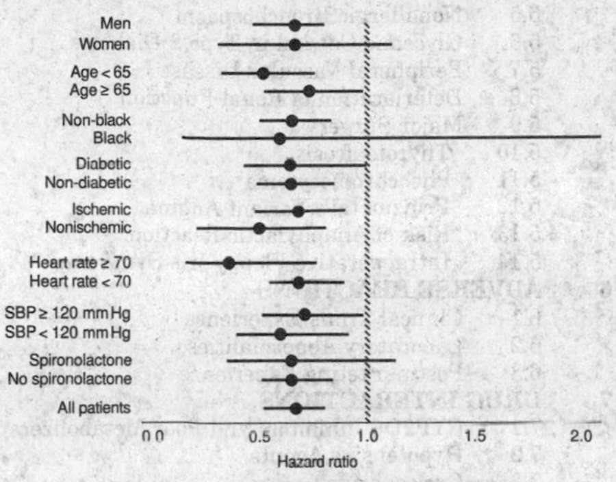

Figure 2. Effects on Mortality for Subgroups in COPERNICUS

14.2 Left Ventricular Dysfunction Following Myocardial Infarction

CAPRICORN was a double-blind study comparing carvedilol and placebo in 1,959 patients with a recent myocardial infarction (within 21 days) and left ventricular ejection fraction of ≤40%, with (47%) or without symptoms of heart failure. Patients given carvedilol received 6.25 mg twice daily, titrated as tolerated to 25 mg twice daily. Patients had to have a systolic blood pressure >90 mm Hg, a sitting heart rate >60 beats/minute, and no contraindication to β-blocker use. Treatment of the index infarction included aspirin (85%), IV or oral β-blockers (37%), nitrates (73%), heparin (64%), thrombolytics (40%), and acute angioplasty (12%). Background treatment included ACE inhibitors or angiotensin receptor blockers (97%), anticoagulants (20%), lipid-lowering agents (23%), and diuretics (34%). Baseline population characteristics included an average age of 63 years, 74% male, 95% Caucasian, mean blood pressure 121/74 mm Hg, 22% with diabetes, and 54% with a history of hypertension. Mean dosage achieved of carvedilol was 20 mg twice daily; mean duration of follow-up was 15 months.

All-cause mortality was 15% in the placebo group and 12% in the carvedilol group, indicating a 23% risk reduction in patients treated with carvedilol (95% CI 2-40%, p = 0.03), as shown in Figure 3. The effects on mortality in various subgroups are shown in Figure 4. Nearly all deaths were cardiovascular (which were reduced by 25% by carvedilol), and most of these deaths were sudden or related to pump failure (both types of death were reduced by carvedilol). Another study end point, total mortality and all-cause hospitalization, did not show a significant improvement.

There was also a significant 40% reduction in fatal or nonfatal myocardial infarction observed in the group treated with carvedilol (95% CI 11% to 60%, p = 0.01). A similar reduction in the risk of myocardial infarction was also observed in a meta-analysis of placebo-controlled trials of carvedilol in heart failure.

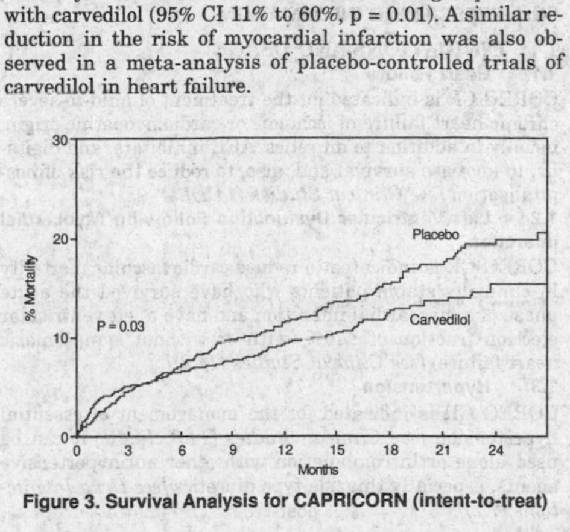

Figure 3. Survival Analysis for CAPRICORN (intent-to-treat)

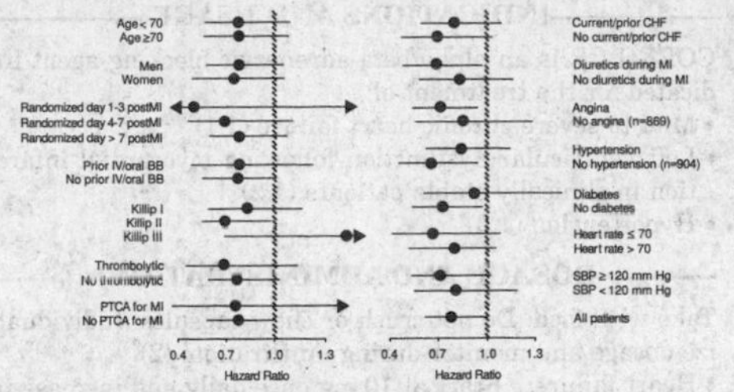

Figure 4. Effects on Mortality for Subgroups in CAPRICORN

14.3 Hypertension

COREG was studied in 2 placebo-controlled trials that utilized twice-daily dosing, at total daily doses of 12.5 to 50 mg. In these and other studies, the starting dose did not exceed 12.5 mg. At 50 mg/day, COREG reduced sitting trough (12-hour) blood pressure by about 9/5.5 mm Hg; at 25 mg/day the effect was about 7.5/3.5 mm Hg. Comparisons of trough to peak blood pressure showed a trough to peak ratio for blood pressure response of about 65%. Heart rate fell by about 7.5 beats/minute at 50 mg/day. In general, as is true for other β-blockers, responses were smaller in black than non-black patients. There were no age- or gender-related differences in response.

The peak antihypertensive effect occurred 1 to 2 hours after a dose. The dose-related blood pressure response was accompanied by a dose-related increase in adverse effects *[see Adverse Reactions (6)]*.

14.4 Hypertension With Type 2 Diabetes Mellitus

In a double blind study (GEMINI), COREG, added to an ACE inhibitor or angiotensin receptor blocker, was evaluated in a population with mild-to-moderate hypertension and well-controlled type 2 diabetes mellitus. The mean HbA1c at baseline was 7.2%. COREG was titrated to a mean dose of 17.5 mg twice daily and maintained for 5 months. COREG had no adverse effect on glycemic control, based on HbA1c measurements (mean change from baseline of 0.02%, 95% CI -0.06 to 0.10, p = NS) *[see Warnings and Precautions (5.6)]*.

16 HOW SUPPLIED/STORAGE AND HANDLING

The white, oval, film-coated tablets are available in the following strengths: 3.125 mg–engraved with 39 and SB, in bottles of 100; 6.25 mg–engraved with 4140 and SB, in bottles of 100; 12.5 mg–engraved with 4141 and SB, in bottles of 100; 25 mg–engraved with 4142 and SB, in bottles of 100. The 6.25 mg, 12.5 mg, and 25 mg tablets are TILTAB tablets.

- 3.125 mg 100's: NDC 0007-4139-20
- 6.25 mg 100's: NDC 0007-4140-20
- 12.5 mg 100's: NDC 0007-4141-20
- 25 mg 100's: NDC 0007-4142-20

Store below 30°C (86°F). Protect from moisture. Dispense in a tight, light-resistant container.

17 PATIENT COUNSELING INFORMATION

See FDA-Approved Patient Labeling.

17.1 Patient Advice

Patients taking COREG should be advised of the following:
- Patients should take COREG with food.
- Patients should not interrupt or discontinue using COREG without a physician's advice.
- Patients with heart failure should consult their physician if they experience signs or symptoms of worsening heart failure such as weight gain or increasing shortness of breath.
- Patients may experience a drop in blood pressure when standing, resulting in dizziness and, rarely, fainting. Patients should sit or lie down when these symptoms of lowered blood pressure occur.
- If experiencing dizziness or fatigue, patients should avoid driving or hazardous tasks.
- Patients should consult a physician if they experience dizziness or faintness, in case the dosage should be adjusted.
- Diabetic patients should report any changes in blood sugar levels to their physician.
- Contact lens wearers may experience decreased lacrimation.

17.2 FDA-Approved Patient Labeling

Patient labeling is provided as a tear-off leaflet at the end of this full prescribing information.

COREG, COREG CR, and TILTAB are registered trademarks of GlaxoSmithKline.

TOPROL-XL is a registered trademark of the AstraZeneca group of companies.

Manufactured for
GlaxoSmithKline
Research Triangle Park, NC 27709
Manufactured by
Patheon Puerto Rico, Inc.
Manati, PR 00674 USA

July 2011
CRG:22PI

PHARMACIST-DETACH HERE AND GIVE INSTRUCTIONS TO PATIENT

PATIENT INFORMATION
COREG® (Co-REG)
Carvedilol Tablets

Read the Patient Information that comes with COREG before you start taking it and each time you get a refill. There may be new information. This information does not take the place of talking with your doctor about your medical condition or your treatment. If you have any questions about COREG, ask your doctor or pharmacist.

What is COREG?

COREG is a prescription medicine that belongs to a group of medicines called "beta-blockers". COREG is used, often with other medicines, for the following conditions:
- To treat patients with certain types of heart failure
- To treat patients who had a heart attack that worsened how well the heart pumps
- To treat patients with high blood pressure (hypertension)

COREG is not approved for use in children under 18 years of age.

Who should not take COREG?

Do not take COREG if you:
- Have severe heart failure and are hospitalized in the intensive care unit or require certain intravenous medications that help support circulation (inotropic medications)
- Are prone to asthma or other breathing problems
- Have a slow heartbeat or a heart that skips a beat (irregular heartbeat)
- Have liver problems
- Are allergic to any of the ingredients in COREG. The active ingredient is carvedilol. See the end of this leaflet for a list of all the ingredients in COREG.

What should I tell my doctor before taking COREG?

Tell your doctor about all of your medical conditions, including if you:
- Have asthma or other lung problems (such as bronchitis or emphysema)
- Have problems with blood flow in your feet and legs (peripheral vascular disease) COREG can make some of your symptoms worse.
- Have diabetes
- Have thyroid problems
- Have a condition called pheochromocytoma
- Have had severe allergic reactions
- Are pregnant or trying to become pregnant. It is not known if COREG is safe for your unborn baby. You and your doctor should talk about the best way to control your high blood pressure during pregnancy.
- Are breastfeeding. It is not known if COREG passes into your breast milk. You should not breastfeed while using COREG.
- Are scheduled for surgery and will be given anesthetic agents
- Are scheduled for cataract surgery and have taken or are currently taking COREG.
- Are taking prescription or non-prescription medicines, vitamins, and herbal supplements. COREG and certain other medicines can affect each other and cause serious side effects. COREG may affect the way other medicines work. Also, other medicines may affect how well COREG works.

Keep a list of all the medicines you take. Show this list to your doctor and pharmacist before you start a new medicine.

How should I take COREG?

It is important for you to take your medicine every day as directed by your doctor. If you stop taking COREG suddenly, you could have chest pain and/or a heart attack. If your doctor decides that you should stop taking COREG, your doctor may slowly lower your dose over a period of time before stopping it completely.
- Take COREG exactly as prescribed. Your doctor will tell you how many tablets to take and how often. In order to minimize possible side effects, your doctor might begin with a low dose and then slowly increase the dose.
- **Do not stop taking COREG and do not change the amount of COREG you take without talking to your doctor.**
- Tell your doctor if you gain weight or have trouble breathing while taking COREG.
- Take COREG with food.
- If you miss a dose of COREG, take your dose as soon as you remember, unless it is time to take your next dose. Take your next dose at the usual time. Do not take 2 doses at the same time.
- If you take too much COREG, call your doctor or poison control center right away.

What should I avoid while taking COREG?
- COREG can cause you to feel dizzy, tired, or faint. Do not drive a car, use machinery, or do anything that needs you to be alert if you have these symptoms.

What are possible side effects of COREG?

- Low blood pressure (which may cause dizziness or fainting when you stand up). If these happen, sit or lie down right away and tell your doctor.
- **Tiredness.** If you feel tired or dizzy you should not drive, use machinery, or do anything that needs you to be alert.
- Slow heartbeat.
- Changes in your blood sugar. If you have diabetes, tell your doctor if you have any changes in your blood sugar levels.
- COREG may hide some of the symptoms of low blood sugar, especially a fast heartbeat.
- COREG may mask the symptoms of hyperthyroidism (overactive thyroid).
- Worsening of severe allergic reactions.
- Rare but serious allergic reactions (including hives or swelling of the face, lips, tongue, and/or throat that may cause difficulty in breathing or swallowing) have happened in patients who were on COREG. These reactions can be life-threatening.

Other side effects of COREG include shortness of breath, weight gain, diarrhea, and fewer tears or dry eyes that become bothersome if you wear contact lenses.

Call your doctor if you have any side effects that bother you or don't go away.

How should I store COREG?

- Store COREG at less than 86°F (30°C). Keep the tablets dry.
- Safely, throw away COREG that is out of date or no longer needed.
- Keep COREG and all medicines out of the reach of children.

General Information about COREG

Medicines are sometimes prescribed for conditions other than those described in patient information leaflets. Do not use COREG for a condition for which it was not prescribed. Do not give COREG to other people, even if they have the same symptoms you have. It may harm them.

This leaflet summarizes the most important information about COREG. If you would like more information, talk with your doctor. You can ask your doctor or pharmacist for information about COREG that is written for healthcare professionals. You can also find out more about COREG by visiting the website www.COREG.com or calling 1-888-825-5249. This call is free.

What are the ingredients in COREG?

Active Ingredient: Carvedilol.

Inactive Ingredients: Colloidal silicon dioxide, crospovidone, hypromellose, lactose, magnesium stearate, polyethylene glycol, polysorbate 80, povidone, sucrose, and titanium dioxide.

Carvedilol tablets come in the following strengths: 3.125 mg, 6.25 mg, 12.5 mg, 25 mg.

What is high blood pressure (hypertension)?

Blood pressure is the force of blood in your blood vessels when your heart beats and when your heart rests. You have high blood pressure when the force is too much. High blood pressure makes the heart work harder to pump blood through the body and causes damage to blood vessels. COREG can help your blood vessels relax so your blood pressure is lower. Medicines that lower blood pressure may lower your chance of having a stroke or heart attack.

COREG is a registered trademark of GlaxoSmithKline.

Manufactured for
GlaxoSmithKline
Research Triangle Park, NC 27709
Manufactured by
Patheon Puerto Rico, Inc.
Manati, PR 00674 USA

January 2011
CRG:4PIL

COREG CR® ℞

[kor' eg]
(carvedilol phosphate)
Extended-release Capsules

HIGHLIGHTS OF PRESCRIBING INFORMATION

These highlights do not include all the information needed to use COREG CR safely and effectively. See full prescribing information for COREG CR.

COREG CR® (carvedilol phosphate) Extended-release Capsules

Initial U.S. Approval: 1995

RECENT MAJOR CHANGES

Warnings and Precautions, Major Surgery (5.9)	October 2010
Warnings and Precautions, Intraoperative Floppy Iris Syndrome (5.14)	January 2011

INDICATIONS AND USAGE

COREG CR is an alpha/beta-adrenergic blocking agent indicated for the treatment of:

- Mild to severe chronic heart failure (1.1)
- Left ventricular dysfunction following myocardial infarction in clinically stable patients (1.2)
- Hypertension (1.3)

DOSAGE AND ADMINISTRATION

Take with food. Do not crush or chew capsules. Individualize dosage and monitor during up-titration. (2)

- Heart failure: Start at 10 mg once daily and increase to 20, 40, and then 80 mg once daily over intervals of at least 2 weeks. Maintain lower doses if higher doses are not tolerated. (2.1)
- Left ventricular dysfunction following myocardial infarction: Start at 20 mg once daily and increase to 40 mg then 80 mg once daily after intervals of 3 to 10 days. A lower starting dose or slower titration may be used. (2.2)
- Hypertension: Start at 20 mg once daily and increase if needed for blood pressure control to 40 mg then 80 mg once daily over intervals of 1 to 2 weeks. (2.3)
- Elderly patients (> 65 years of age): When switching from higher doses of immediate-release carvedilol to COREG CR, a lower starting dose should be considered to reduce the risk of hypotension and syncope. (2.5)

DOSAGE FORMS AND STRENGTHS

Capsules: 10, 20, 40, 80 mg (3)

CONTRAINDICATIONS

- Bronchial asthma or related bronchospastic conditions (4)
- Second- or third-degree AV block (4)
- Sick sinus syndrome (4)
- Severe bradycardia (unless permanent pacemaker in place) (4)
- Patients in cardiogenic shock or decompensated heart failure requiring the use of IV inotropic therapy. (4)
- Severe hepatic impairment (2.4, 4)
- History of serious hypersensitivity reaction (e.g., Stevens-Johnson syndrome, anaphylactic reaction, angioedema) to carvedilol or any of the components of COREG CR. (4)

WARNINGS AND PRECAUTIONS

- Acute exacerbation of coronary artery disease upon cessation of therapy: Do not abruptly discontinue. (5.1)
- Bradycardia, hypotension, worsening heart failure/fluid retention may occur. Reduce the dose as needed. (5.2, 5.3, 5.4)
- Non-allergic bronchospasm (e.g., chronic bronchitis and emphysema): Avoid β-blockers. (4) However, if deemed necessary, use with caution and at lowest effective dose. (5.5)
- Diabetes: Monitor glucose as β-blockers may mask symptoms of hypoglycemia or worsen hyperglycemia. (5.6)

ADVERSE REACTIONS

The safety profile of COREG CR was similar to that observed for immediate-release carvedilol. Most common adverse events seen with immediate-release carvedilol. (6.1):

- Heart failure and left ventricular dysfunction following myocardial infarction (≥10%): Dizziness, fatigue, hypotension, diarrhea, hyperglycemia, asthenia, bradycardia, weight increase
- Hypertension (≥5%): Dizziness

To report SUSPECTED ADVERSE REACTIONS, contact GlaxoSmithKline at 1-888-825-5249 or FDA at 1-800-FDA-1088 or www.fda.gov/medwatch.

DRUG INTERACTIONS

- CYP P450 2D6 enzyme inhibitors may increase and rifampin may decrease carvedilol levels. (7.1)
- Hypotensive agents (e.g., reserpine, MAO inhibitors, clonidine) may increase the risk of hypotension and/or severe bradycardia. (7.2)
- Cyclosporine or digoxin levels may increase. (7.3, 7.4)
- Both digitalis glycosides and β-blockers slow atrioventricular conduction and decrease heart rate. Concomitant use can increase the risk of bradycardia. (7.4)
- Amiodarone may increase carvedilol levels resulting in further slowing of the heart rate or cardiac conduction. (7.6)
- Verapamil- or diltiazem-type calcium channel blockers may affect ECG and/or blood pressure. (7.7)
- Insulin and oral hypoglycemics action may be enhanced. (7.8)

See 17 for PATIENT COUNSELING INFORMATION and FDA-approved patient labeling

Revised: 08/2011

FULL PRESCRIBING INFORMATION: CONTENTS*

*** Sections or subsections omitted from the full prescribing information are not listed**

FULL PRESCRIBING INFORMATION

1 INDICATIONS AND USAGE

1.1 Heart Failure

COREG CR is indicated for the treatment of mild-to-severe chronic heart failure of ischemic or cardiomyopathic origin, usually in addition to diuretics, ACE inhibitors, and digitalis, to increase survival and, also, to reduce the risk of hospitalization *[see Clinical Studies (14.1)]*.

1.2 Left Ventricular Dysfunction Following Myocardial Infarction

COREG CR is indicated to reduce cardiovascular mortality in clinically stable patients who have survived the acute phase of a myocardial infarction and have a left ventricular ejection fraction of ≤40% (with or without symptomatic heart failure) *[see Clinical Studies (14.2)]*.

1.3 Hypertension

COREG CR is indicated for the management of essential hypertension *[see Clinical Studies (14.3, 14.4)]*. It can be used alone or in combination with other antihypertensive agents, especially thiazide-type diuretics *[see Drug Interactions (7.2)]*.

2 DOSAGE AND ADMINISTRATION

COREG CR is an extended-release capsule intended for once-daily administration. Patients controlled with immediate-release carvedilol tablets alone or in combination with other medications may be switched to COREG CR extended-release capsules based on the total daily doses shown in Table 1.

Table 1. Dosing Conversion

Daily Dose of Immediate-Release Carvedilol Tablets	Daily Dose of COREG CR Capsules*
6.25 mg (3.125 mg twice daily)	10 mg once daily
12.5 mg (6.25 mg twice daily)	20 mg once daily
25 mg (12.5 mg twice daily)	40 mg once daily
50 mg (25 mg twice daily)	80 mg once daily

* When switching from carvedilol 12.5 mg or 25 mg twice daily, a starting dose of COREG CR 20 mg or 40 mg once daily, respectively, may be warranted for elderly patients or those at increased risk of hypotension, dizziness, or syncope. Subsequent titration to higher doses should, as appropriate, be made after an interval of at least 2 weeks.

COREG CR should be taken once daily in the morning with food. COREG CR should be swallowed as a whole capsule. COREG CR and/or its contents should not be crushed, chewed, or taken in divided doses.

Alternative Administration: The capsules may be carefully opened and the beads sprinkled over a spoonful of applesauce. The applesauce should not be warm because it could affect the modified-release properties of this formulation. The mixture of drug and applesauce should be consumed immediately in its entirety. The drug and applesauce mixture should not be stored for future use. Absorption of the beads sprinkled on other foods has not been tested.

2.1 Heart Failure

DOSAGE MUST BE INDIVIDUALIZED AND CLOSELY MONITORED BY A PHYSICIAN DURING UP-TITRATION. Prior to initiation of COREG CR, it is recommended that fluid retention be minimized. The recommended starting dose of COREG CR is 10 mg once daily for 2 weeks. Patients who tolerate a dose of 10 mg once daily may have their dose increased to 20, 40, and 80 mg over successive intervals of at least 2 weeks. Patients should be maintained on lower doses if higher doses are not tolerated. Patients should be advised that initiation of treatment and (to a lesser extent) dosage increases may be associated with transient symptoms of dizziness or lightheadedness (and rarely syncope) within the first hour after dosing. Thus during these periods they should avoid situations such as driving or hazardous tasks, where symptoms could result in injury. Vasodilatory symptoms often do not require treatment, but it may be useful to separate the time of dosing of COREG CR from that of the ACE inhibitor or to reduce temporarily the dose of the ACE inhibitor. The dose of COREG CR should not be increased until symptoms of worsening heart failure or vasodilation have been stabilized.

Fluid retention (with or without transient worsening heart failure symptoms) should be treated by an increase in the dose of diuretics.

The dose of COREG CR should be reduced if patients experience bradycardia (heart rate <55 beats/minute).

Episodes of dizziness or fluid retention during initiation of COREG CR can generally be managed without discontinuation of treatment and do not preclude subsequent successful titration of, or a favorable response to, COREG CR.

2.2 Left Ventricular Dysfunction Following Myocardial Infarction

DOSAGE MUST BE INDIVIDUALIZED AND MONITORED DURING UP-TITRATION. Treatment with COREG CR may be started as an inpatient or outpatient and should be started after the patient is hemodynamically stable and fluid retention has been minimized. It is recommended that COREG CR be started at 20 mg once daily and increased after 3 to 10 days, based on tolerability, to 40 mg once daily, then again to the target dose of 80 mg once daily. A lower starting dose may be used (10 mg once daily) and/or the rate of up-titration may be slowed if clinically indicated (e.g., due to low blood pressure or heart rate, or fluid retention). Patients should be maintained on lower doses if higher doses are not tolerated. The recommended dosing regimen need not be altered in patients who received treatment with an IV or oral β-blocker during the acute phase of the myocardial infarction.

2.3 Hypertension

DOSAGE MUST BE INDIVIDUALIZED. The recommended starting dose of COREG CR is 20 mg once daily. If this dose is tolerated, using standing systolic pressure measured about one hour after dosing as a guide, the dose should be maintained for 7 to 14 days, and then increased to 40 mg once daily if needed, based on trough blood pressure, again using standing systolic pressure one hour after dosing as a guide for tolerance. This dose should also be maintained for 7 to 14 days and can then be adjusted upward to 80 mg once daily if tolerated and needed. Although not specifically studied, it is anticipated the full antihypertensive effect of COREG CR would be seen within 7 to 14 days as had been demonstrated with immediate-release carvedilol. Total daily dose should not exceed 80 mg.

Concomitant administration with a diuretic can be expected to produce additive effects and exaggerate the orthostatic component of COREG CR action.

2.4 Hepatic Impairment

COREG CR should not be given to patients with severe hepatic impairment *[see Contraindications (4)]*.

2.5 Geriatric Use

When switching elderly patients (65 years of age or older) who are taking the higher doses of immediate-release carvedilol tablets (25 mg twice daily) to COREG CR, a lower starting dose (40 mg) of COREG CR is recommended to minimize the potential for dizziness, syncope, or hypotension *[see Dosage and Administration (2)]*. Patients who have switched and who tolerate COREG CR should, as appropriate, have their dose increased to after an interval of at least 2 weeks *[see Use in Specific Populations (8.5)]*.

3 DOSAGE FORMS AND STRENGTHS

The hard gelatin capsules are filled with white to off-white microparticles and are available in the following strengths:

- 10 mg – white and green capsule shell printed with GSK COREG CR and 10 mg
- 20 mg – white and yellow capsule shell printed with GSK COREG CR and 20 mg
- 40 mg – yellow and green capsule shell printed with GSK COREG CR and 40 mg
- 80 mg – white capsule shell printed with GSK COREG CR and 80 mg

4 CONTRAINDICATIONS

COREG CR is contraindicated in the following conditions:

- Bronchial asthma or related bronchospastic conditions. Deaths from status asthmaticus have been reported following single doses of immediate-release carvedilol.
- Second- or third-degree AV block
- Sick sinus syndrome
- Severe bradycardia (unless a permanent pacemaker is in place)
- Patients with cardiogenic shock or who have decompensated heart failure requiring the use of intravenous inotropic therapy. Such patients should first be weaned from intravenous therapy before initiating COREG CR.
- Patients with severe hepatic impairment
- Patients with a history of a serious hypersensitivity reaction (e.g., Stevens-Johnson syndrome, anaphylactic reaction, angioedema) to carvedilol or any of the components of COREG CR.

5 WARNINGS AND PRECAUTIONS

In clinical trials of COREG CR in patients with hypertension (338 subjects) and in patients with left ventricular dysfunction following a myocardial infarction or heart failure (187 subjects), the profile of adverse events observed with carvedilol phosphate was generally similar to that observed with the administration of immediate-release carvedilol. Therefore, the information included within this section is based on data from controlled clinical trials with COREG CR as well as immediate-release carvedilol.

5.1 Cessation of Therapy

Patients with coronary artery disease, who are being treated with COREG CR, should be advised against abrupt discontinuation of therapy. Severe exacerbation of angina and the occurrence of myocardial infarction and ventricular arrhythmias have been reported in angina patients following the abrupt discontinuation of therapy with β-blockers. The last 2 complications may occur with or without preceding exacerbation of the angina pectoris. As with other β-blockers, when discontinuation of COREG CR is planned, the patients should be carefully observed and advised to limit physical activity to a minimum. COREG CR should be discontinued over 1 to 2 weeks whenever possible. If the angina worsens or acute coronary insufficiency develops, it is recommended that COREG CR be promptly reinstituted, at least temporarily. Because coronary artery disease is common and may be unrecognized, it may be prudent not to discontinue therapy with COREG CR abruptly even in patients treated only for hypertension or heart failure.

5.2 Bradycardia

In clinical trials with immediate-release carvedilol, bradycardia was reported in about 2% of hypertensive patients, 9% of heart failure patients, and 6.5% of myocardial infarction patients with left ventricular dysfunction. Bradycardia was reported in 0.5% of patients receiving COREG CR in a study of heart failure patients and myocardial infarction patients with left ventricular dysfunction. There were no reports of bradycardia in the clinical trial of COREG CR in hypertension. However, if pulse rate drops below 55 beats/minute, the dosage of COREG CR should be reduced.

5.3 Hypotension

In clinical trials of primarily mild-to-moderate heart failure with immediate-release carvedilol, hypotension and postural hypotension occurred in 9.7% and syncope in 3.4% of patients receiving carvedilol compared to 3.6% and 2.5% of placebo patients, respectively. The risk for these events was highest during the first 30 days of dosing, corresponding to the up-titration period and was a cause for discontinuation of therapy in 0.7% of carvedilol patients, compared to 0.4% of placebo patients. In a long-term, placebo-controlled trial in severe heart failure (COPERNICUS), hypotension and postural hypotension occurred in 15.1% and syncope in 2.9% of heart failure patients receiving carvedilol compared to 8.7% and 2.3% of placebo patients, respectively. These events were a cause for discontinuation of therapy in 1.1% of carvedilol patients, compared to 0.8% of placebo patients.

In a trial comparing heart failure patients switched to COREG CR or maintained on immediate-release carvedilol, there was a 2-fold increase in the combined incidence of hypotension, syncope or dizziness in elderly patients (> 65 years) switched from the highest dose of carvedilol (25 mg twice daily) to COREG CR 80 mg once daily *[see Dosage and Administration (2), Use in Specific Populations (8.5)]*.

In the clinical trial of COREG CR in hypertensive patients, syncope was reported in 0.3% of patients receiving COREG CR compared to 0% of patients receiving placebo. There were no reports of postural hypotension in this trial. Postural hypotension occurred in 1.8% and syncope in 0.1% of hypertensive patients receiving immediate-release carvedilol, primarily following the initial dose or at the time of dose increase and was a cause for discontinuation of therapy in 1% of patients.

In the CAPRICORN study of survivors of an acute myocardial infarction with left ventricular dysfunction, hypotension or postural hypotension occurred in 20.2% of patients receiving carvedilol compared to 12.6% of placebo patients. Syncope was reported in 3.9% and 1.9% of patients, respectively. These events were a cause for discontinuation of therapy in 2.5% of patients receiving carvedilol, compared to 0.2% of placebo patients.

Starting with a low dose, administration with food, and gradual up-titration should decrease the likelihood of syncope or excessive hypotension *[see Dosage and Administration (2.1, 2.2, 2.3)]*. During initiation of therapy, the patient should be cautioned to avoid situations such as driving or hazardous tasks, where injury could result should syncope occur.

5.4 Heart Failure/Fluid Retention

Worsening heart failure or fluid retention may occur during up-titration of carvedilol. If such symptoms occur, diuretics should be increased and the dose of COREG CR should not be advanced until clinical stability resumes *[see Dosage and Administration (2)]*. Occasionally it is necessary to lower the dose of COREG CR or temporarily discontinue it. Such episodes do not preclude subsequent successful titration of, or a favorable response to, COREG CR. In a placebo-controlled trial of patients with severe heart failure, worsening heart failure during the first 3 months was reported to a similar degree with immediate-release carvedilol and with placebo. When treatment was maintained beyond 3 months, worsening heart failure was reported less frequently in patients treated with carvedilol than with placebo. Worsening heart failure observed during long-term therapy is more likely to be related to the patients' underlying disease than to treatment with carvedilol.

5.5 Nonallergic Bronchospasm

Patients with bronchospastic disease (e.g., chronic bronchitis and emphysema) should, in general, not receive β-blockers. COREG CR may be used with caution, however, in patients who do not respond to, or cannot tolerate, other antihypertensive agents. It is prudent, if COREG CR is used, to use the smallest effective dose, so that inhibition of endogenous or exogenous β-agonists is minimized.

In clinical trials of patients with heart failure, patients with bronchospastic disease were enrolled if they did not require oral or inhaled medication to treat their bronchospastic disease. In such patients, it is recommended that COREG CR be used with caution. The dosing recommendations should be followed closely and the dose should be lowered if any evidence of bronchospasm is observed during up-titration.

5.6 Glycemic Control in Type 2 Diabetes

In general, β-blockers may mask some of the manifestations of hypoglycemia, particularly tachycardia. Nonselective β-blockers may potentiate insulin-induced hypoglycemia and delay recovery of serum glucose levels. Patients subject to spontaneous hypoglycemia, or diabetic patients receiving insulin or oral hypoglycemic agents, should be cautioned about these possibilities.

In heart failure patients with diabetes, carvedilol therapy may lead to worsening hyperglycemia, which responds to in-

Table 2. Adverse Events (%) Occurring More Frequently With Immediate-Release Carvedilol Than With Placebo in Patients With Mild-to-Moderate Heart Failure (HF) Enrolled in US Heart Failure Trials or in Patients With Severe Heart Failure in the COPERNICUS Trial (Incidence >3% in Patients Treated With Carvedilol, Regardless of Causality)

	Mild-to-Moderate HF		Severe HF	
	Carvedilol (n = 765)	Placebo (n = 437)	Carvedilol (n = 1,156)	Placebo (n = 1,133)
Body as a Whole				
Asthenia	7	7	11	9
Fatigue	24	22	—	—
Digoxin level increased	5	4	2	1
Edema generalized	5	3	6	5
Edema dependent	4	2	—	—
Cardiovascular				
Bradycardia	9	1	10	3
Hypotension	9	3	14	8
Syncope	3	3	8	5
Angina pectoris	2	3	6	4
Central Nervous System				
Dizziness	32	19	24	17
Headache	8	7	5	3
Gastrointestinal				
Diarrhea	12	6	5	3
Nausea	9	5	4	3
Vomiting	6	4	1	2
Metabolic				
Hyperglycemia	12	8	5	3
Weight increase	10	7	12	11
BUN increased	6	5	—	—
NPN increased	6	5	—	—
Hypercholesterolemia	4	3	1	1
Edema peripheral	2	1	7	6
Musculoskeletal				
Arthralgia	6	5	1	1
Respiratory				
Cough increased	8	9	5	4
Rales	4	4	4	2
Vision				
Vision abnormal	5	2	—	—

tensification of hypoglycemic therapy. It is recommended that blood glucose be monitored when dosing with COREG CR is initiated, adjusted, or discontinued. Studies designed to examine the effects of carvedilol on glycemic control in patients with diabetes and heart failure have not been conducted.

In a study designed to examine the effects of immediate-release carvedilol on glycemic control in a population with mild-to-moderate hypertension and well-controlled type 2 diabetes mellitus, carvedilol had no adverse effect on glycemic control, based on HbA1c measurements *[see Clinical Studies (14.4)]*.

5.7 Peripheral Vascular Disease

β-blockers can precipitate or aggravate symptoms of arterial insufficiency in patients with peripheral vascular disease. Caution should be exercised in such individuals.

5.8 Deterioration of Renal Function

Rarely, use of carvedilol in patients with heart failure has resulted in deterioration of renal function. Patients at risk appear to be those with low blood pressure (systolic blood pressure <100 mm Hg), ischemic heart disease and diffuse vascular disease, and/or underlying renal insufficiency. Renal function has returned to baseline when carvedilol was stopped. In patients with these risk factors it is recommended that renal function be monitored during up-titration of COREG CR and the drug discontinued or dosage reduced if worsening of renal function occurs.

5.9 Major Surgery

Chronically administered beta-blocking therapy should not be routinely withdrawn prior to major surgery; however, the impaired ability of the heart to respond to reflex adrenergic stimuli may augment the risks of general anesthesia and surgical procedures.

5.10 Thyrotoxicosis

β-adrenergic blockade may mask clinical signs of hyperthyroidism, such as tachycardia. Abrupt withdrawal of β-blockade may be followed by an exacerbation of the symptoms of hyperthyroidism or may precipitate thyroid storm.

5.11 Pheochromocytoma

In patients with pheochromocytoma, an α-blocking agent should be initiated prior to the use of any β-blocking agent. Although carvedilol has both α- and β-blocking pharmacologic activities, there has been no experience with its use in this condition. Therefore, caution should be taken in the administration of carvedilol to patients suspected of having pheochromocytoma.

5.12 Prinzmetal's Variant Angina

Agents with non-selective β-blocking activity may provoke chest pain in patients with Prinzmetal's variant angina. There has been no clinical experience with carvedilol in these patients although the α-blocking activity may prevent such symptoms. However, caution should be taken in the administration of COREG CR to patients suspected of having Prinzmetal's variant angina.

5.13 Risk of Anaphylactic Reaction

While taking β-blockers, patients with a history of severe anaphylactic reaction to a variety of allergens may be more reactive to repeated challenge, either accidental, diagnostic, or therapeutic. Such patients may be unresponsive to the usual doses of epinephrine used to treat allergic reaction.

5.14 Intraoperative Floppy Iris Syndrome

Intraoperative Floppy Iris Syndrome (IFIS) has been observed during cataract surgery in some patients treated with alpha-1 blockers (COREG CR is an alpha/beta blocker). This variant of small pupil syndrome is characterized by the combination of a flaccid iris that billows in response to intraoperative irrigation currents, progressive intraoperative miosis despite preoperative dilation with standard mydriatic drugs, and potential prolapse of the iris toward the phacoemulsification incisions. The patient's ophthalmologist should be prepared for possible modifications to the surgical technique, such as utilization of iris hooks, iris dilator rings, or viscoelastic substances. There does not appear to be a benefit of stopping alpha-1 blocker therapy prior to cataract surgery.

6 ADVERSE REACTIONS

6.1 Clinical Trials Experience

Carvedilol has been evaluated for safety in patients with heart failure (mild, moderate, and severe), in patients with left ventricular dysfunction following myocardial infarction, and in hypertensive patients. The observed adverse event profile was consistent with the pharmacology of the drug and the health status of the patients in the clinical trials. Adverse events reported for each of these patient populations reflecting the use of either COREG CR or immediate-release carvedilol are provided below. Excluded are adverse events considered too general to be informative, and those not reasonably associated with the use of the drug because they were associated with the condition being treated or are very common in the treated population. Rates of adverse events were generally similar across demographic subsets (men and women, elderly and non-elderly, blacks and non-blacks). COREG CR has been evaluated for safety in a 4-week (2 weeks of immediate-release carvedilol and 2 weeks of COREG CR) clinical study (n = 187) which included 157 patients with stable mild, moderate, or severe chronic heart failure and 30 patients with left ventricular dysfunction following acute myocardial infarction. The profile of adverse events observed with COREG CR in this small, short-term study was generally similar to that observed with immediate-release carvedilol. Differences in safety would not be expected based on the similarity in plasma levels for COREG CR and immediate-release carvedilol.

Heart Failure

The following information describes the safety experience in heart failure with immediate-release carvedilol.

Carvedilol has been evaluated for safety in heart failure in more than 4,500 patients worldwide of whom more than 2,100 participated in placebo-controlled clinical trials. Approximately 60% of the total treated population in placebo-controlled clinical trials received carvedilol for at least 6 months and 30% received carvedilol for at least 12 months. In the COMET trial, 1,511 patients with mild-to-moderate heart failure were treated with carvedilol for up to 5.9 years (mean 4.8 years). Both in US clinical trials in mild-to-moderate heart failure that compared carvedilol in daily doses up to 100 mg (n = 765) to placebo (n = 437), and in a multinational clinical trial in severe heart failure (COPERNICUS) that compared carvedilol in daily doses up to 50 mg (n = 1,156) with placebo (n = 1,133), discontinuation rates for adverse experiences were similar in carvedilol and placebo patients. In placebo-controlled clinical trials, the only cause of discontinuation >1%, and occurring more often on carvedilol was dizziness (1.3% on carvedilol, 0.6% on placebo in the COPERNICUS trial).

Table 2 shows adverse events reported in patients with mild-to-moderate heart failure enrolled in US placebo-controlled clinical trials, and with severe heart failure enrolled in the COPERNICUS trial. Shown are adverse events that occurred more frequently in drug-treated patients than placebo-treated patients with an incidence of >3% in patients treated with carvedilol regardless of causality. Median study medication exposure was 6.3 months for both carvedilol and placebo patients in the trials of mild-to-moderate heart failure, and 10.4 months in the trial of severe heart failure patients. The adverse event profile of carvedilol observed in the long-term COMET study was generally similar to that observed in the US Heart Failure Trials.

[See table 2 at top of previous page]

Cardiac failure and dyspnea were also reported in these studies, but the rates were equal or greater in patients who received placebo.

The following adverse events were reported with a frequency of >1% but ≤3% and more frequently with carvedilol in either the US placebo-controlled trials in patients with mild-to-moderate heart failure, or in patients with severe heart failure in the COPERNICUS trial.

Incidence >1% to ≤3%

Body as a Whole: Allergy, malaise, hypovolemia, fever, leg edema.

Cardiovascular: Fluid overload, postural hypotension, aggravated angina pectoris, AV block, palpitation, hypertension.

Central and Peripheral Nervous System: Hypesthesia, vertigo, paresthesia.

Gastrointestinal: Melena, periodontitis.

Liver and Biliary System: SGPT increased, SGOT increased.

Metabolic and Nutritional: Hyperuricemia, hypoglycemia, hyponatremia, increased alkaline phosphatase, glycosuria, hypervolemia, diabetes mellitus, GGT increased, weight loss, hyperkalemia, creatinine increased.

Musculoskeletal: Muscle cramps.

Platelet, Bleeding and Clotting: Prothrombin decreased, purpura, thrombocytopenia.

Psychiatric: Somnolence.

Reproductive, male: Impotence.

Special Senses: Blurred vision.

Urinary System: Renal insufficiency, albuminuria, hematuria.

Left Ventricular Dysfunction Following Myocardial Infarction

The following information describes the safety experience in left ventricular dysfunction following acute myocardial infarction with immediate-release carvedilol.

Carvedilol has been evaluated for safety in survivors of an acute myocardial infarction with left ventricular dysfunction in the CAPRICORN trial which involved 969 patients who received carvedilol and 980 who received placebo. Approximately 75% of the patients received carvedilol for at least 6 months and 53% received carvedilol for at least 12 months. Patients were treated for an average of 12.9 months and 12.8 months with carvedilol and placebo, respectively.

The most common adverse events reported with carvedilol in the CAPRICORN trial were consistent with the profile of the drug in the US heart failure trials and the COPERNICUS trial. The only additional adverse events reported in CAPRICORN in >3% of the patients and more commonly on carvedilol were dyspnea, anemia, and lung edema. The following adverse events were reported with a frequency of >1% but ≤3% and more frequently with carvedilol: Flu syndrome, cerebrovascular accident, peripheral vascular disorder, hypotonia, depression, gastrointestinal pain, arthritis, and gout. The overall rates of discontinuations due to adverse events were similar in both groups of patients. In this database, the only cause of discontinuation >1%, and occurring more often on carvedilol was hypotension (1.5% on carvedilol, 0.2% on placebo).

Hypertension

COREG CR was evaluated for safety in an 8-week double-blind trial in 337 subjects with essential hypertension. The profile of adverse events observed with COREG CR was generally similar to that observed with immediate-release carvedilol. The overall rates of discontinuations due to adverse events were similar between COREG CR and placebo.

Table 3. Adverse Events (%) Occurring More Frequently With COREG CR Than With Placebo in Patients With Hypertension (Incidence ≥1% in Patients Treated With Carvedilol, Regardless of Causality)

	COREG CR (n = 253)	Placebo (n = 84)
Nasopharyngitis	4	0
Dizziness	2	1
Nausea	2	0
Edema peripheral	2	1
Nasal congestion	1	0
Paresthesia	1	0
Sinus congestion	1	0
Diarrhea	1	0
Insomnia	1	0

The following information describes the safety experience in hypertension with immediate-release carvedilol.

Carvedilol has been evaluated for safety in hypertension in more than 2,193 patients in US clinical trials and in 2,976 patients in international clinical trials. Approximately 36% of the total treated population received carvedilol for at least 6 months. In general, carvedilol was well tolerated at doses up to 50 mg daily. Most adverse events reported during carvedilol therapy were of mild to moderate severity. In US controlled clinical trials directly comparing carvedilol monotherapy in doses up to 50 mg (n = 1,142) to placebo (n = 462), 4.9% of carvedilol patients discontinued for adverse events versus 5.2% of placebo patients. Although there was no overall difference in discontinuation rates, discontinuations were more common in the carvedilol group for postural hypotension (1% versus 0). The overall incidence of adverse events in US placebo-controlled trials was found to increase with increasing dose of carvedilol. For individual adverse events this could only be distinguished for dizziness, which increased in frequency from 2% to 5% as total daily dose increased from 6.25 mg to 50 mg as single or divided doses. Table 4 shows adverse events in US placebo-controlled clinical trials for hypertension that occurred with an incidence of ≥1% regardless of causality, and that were more frequent in drug-treated patients than placebo-treated patients.

Table 4. Adverse Events (% Occurrence) in US Placebo-Controlled Hypertension Trials With Immediate-Release Carvedilol (Incidence ≥1% in Patients Treated With Carvedilol, Regardless of Causality)*

	Carvedilol (n = 1,142)	Placebo (n = 462)
Cardiovascular		
Bradycardia	2	—
Postural hypotension	2	—
Peripheral edema	1	—
Central Nervous System		
Dizziness	6	5
Insomnia	2	1
Gastrointestinal		
Diarrhea	2	1
Hematologic		
Thrombocytopenia	1	—
Metabolic		
Hypertriglyceridemia	1	—

* Shown are events with rate >1% rounded to nearest integer.

Dyspnea and fatigue were also reported in these studies, but the rates were equal or greater in patients who received placebo.

The following adverse events not described above were reported as possibly or probably related to carvedilol in worldwide open or controlled trials with carvedilol in patients with hypertension or heart failure.

Incidence >0.1% to ≤1%

Cardiovascular: Peripheral ischemia, tachycardia.

Central and Peripheral Nervous System: Hypokinesia.

Gastrointestinal: Bilirubinemia, increased hepatic enzymes (0.2% of hypertension patients and 0.4% of heart failure patients were discontinued from therapy because of increases in hepatic enzymes) *[see Adverse Reactions (6.2)]*.

Psychiatric: Nervousness, sleep disorder, aggravated depression, impaired concentration, abnormal thinking, paroniria, emotional lability.

Respiratory System: Asthma *[see Contraindications (4)]*.

Reproductive, male: Decreased libido.

Skin and Appendages: Pruritus, rash erythematous, rash maculopapular, rash psoriaform, photosensitivity reaction.

Special Senses: Tinnitus.

Urinary System: Micturition frequency increased.

Autonomic Nervous System: Dry mouth, sweating increased.

Metabolic and Nutritional: Hypokalemia, hypertriglyceridemia.

Hematologic: Anemia, leukopenia.

The following events were reported in ≤0.1% of patients and are potentially important: Complete AV block, bundle branch block, myocardial ischemia, cerebrovascular disorder, convulsions, migraine, neuralgia, paresis, anaphylactoid reaction, alopecia, exfoliative dermatitis, amnesia, GI hemorrhage, bronchospasm, pulmonary edema, decreased hearing, respiratory alkalosis, increased BUN, decreased HDL, pancytopenia, and atypical lymphocytes.

6.2 Laboratory Abnormalities

Reversible elevations in serum transaminases (ALT or AST) have been observed during treatment with carvedilol. Rates of transaminase elevations (2- to 3-times the upper limit of normal) observed during controlled clinical trials have generally been similar between patients treated with carvedilol and those treated with placebo. However, transaminase elevations, confirmed by rechallenge, have been observed with carvedilol. In a long-term, placebo-controlled trial in severe heart failure, patients treated with carvedilol had lower values for hepatic transaminases than patients treated with placebo, possibly because carvedilol-induced improvements in cardiac function led to less hepatic congestion and/or improved hepatic blood flow.

Carvedilol therapy has not been associated with clinically significant changes in serum potassium, total triglycerides, total cholesterol, HDL cholesterol, uric acid, blood urea nitrogen, or creatinine. No clinically relevant changes were noted in fasting serum glucose in hypertensive patients; fasting serum glucose was not evaluated in the heart failure clinical trials.

6.3 Postmarketing Experience

The following adverse reactions have been identified during post-approval use of COREG® or COREG CR. Because these reactions are reported voluntarily from a population of uncertain size, it is not always possible to reliably estimate their frequency or establish a causal relationship to drug exposure.

Blood and Lymphatic System Disorders: Aplastic anemia.

Immune System Disorders: Hypersensitivity (e.g., anaphylactic reactions, angioedema, urticaria).

Renal and Urinary Disorders: Urinary incontinence.

Respiratory, Thoracic and Mediastinal Disorders: Interstitial pneumonitis.

Skin and Subcutaneous Tissue Disorders: Stevens-Johnson syndrome, toxic epidermal necrolysis, erythema multiforme.

7 DRUG INTERACTIONS

7.1 CYP2D6 Inhibitors and Poor Metabolizers

Interactions of carvedilol with potent inhibitors of CYP2D6 isoenzyme (such as quinidine, fluoxetine, paroxetine, and propafenone) have not been studied, but these drugs would be expected to increase blood levels of the R(+) enantiomer of carvedilol *[see Clinical Pharmacology (12.3)]*. Retrospective analysis of side effects in clinical trials showed that poor 2D6 metabolizers had a higher rate of dizziness during up-titration, presumably resulting from vasodilating effects of the higher concentrations of the α-blocking R(+) enantiomer.

7.2 Hypotensive Agents

Patients taking both agents with β-blocking properties and a drug that can deplete catecholamines (e.g., reserpine and monoamine oxidase inhibitors) should be observed closely for signs of hypotension and/or severe bradycardia.

Concomitant administration of clonidine with agents with β-blocking properties may potentiate blood-pressure- and heart-rate-lowering effects. When concomitant treatment with agents with β-blocking properties and clonidine is to be terminated, the β-blocking agent should be discontinued first. Clonidine therapy can then be discontinued several days later by gradually decreasing the dosage.

7.3 Cyclosporine

Modest increases in mean trough cyclosporine concentrations were observed following initiation of carvedilol treatment in 21 renal transplant patients suffering from chronic vascular rejection. In about 30% of patients, the dose of cyclosporine had to be reduced in order to maintain cyclosporine concentrations within the therapeutic range, while in the remainder no adjustment was needed. On the average for the group, the dose of cyclosporine was reduced about 20% in these patients. Due to wide interindividual variability in the dose adjustment required, it is recommended that cyclosporine concentrations be monitored closely after initiation of carvedilol therapy and that the dose of cyclosporine be adjusted as appropriate.

7.4 Digitalis Glycosides

Both digitalis glycosides and β-blockers slow atrioventricular conduction and decrease heart rate. Concomitant use can increase the risk of bradycardia. Digoxin concentrations are increased by about 15% when digoxin and carvedilol are administered concomitantly. Therefore, increased monitoring of digoxin is recommended when initiating, adjusting, or discontinuing COREG CR *[see Clinical Pharmacology (12.5)]*.

7.5 Inducers/Inhibitors of Hepatic Metabolism

Rifampin reduced plasma concentrations of carvedilol by about 70% *[see Clinical Pharmacology (12.5)]*. Cimetidine increased area under the curve (AUC) by about 30% but caused no change in C_{max} *[see Clinical Pharmacology (12.5)]*.

7.6 Amiodarone

Amiodarone, and its metabolite desethyl amiodarone, inhibitors of CYP2C9 and P-glycoprotein, increased concentrations of the S(-) enantiomer of carvedilol by at least 2-fold *[see Clinical Pharmacology (12.5)]*. The concomitant administration of amiodarone or other CYP2C9 inhibitors such as fluconazole with COREG CR may enhance the β-blocking properties of carvedilol resulting in further slowing of the heart rate or cardiac conduction. Patients should be observed for signs of bradycardia or heart block, particularly when one agent is added to pre-existing treatment with the other.

7.7 Calcium Channel Blockers

Conduction disturbance (rarely with hemodynamic compromise) has been observed when carvedilol is co-administered with diltiazem. As with other agents with β-blocking properties, if COREG CR is to be administered orally with calcium channel blockers of the verapamil or diltiazem type, it is recommended that ECG and blood pressure be monitored.

7.8 Insulin or Oral Hypoglycemics

Agents with β-blocking properties may enhance the blood-sugar-reducing effect of insulin and oral hypoglycemics. Therefore, in patients taking insulin or oral hypoglycemics, regular monitoring of blood glucose is recommended *[see Warnings and Precautions (5.6)]*.

7.9 Proton Pump Inhibitors

There is no clinically meaningful increase in AUC and C_{max} with concomitant administration of carvedilol extended-release capsules with pantoprazole.

7.10 Anesthesia

If treatment with COREG CR is to be continued perioperatively, particular care should be taken when anesthetic agents which depress myocardial function, such as ether, cyclopropane, and trichloroethylene, are used *[see Overdosage (10)]*.

8 USE IN SPECIFIC POPULATIONS

8.1 Pregnancy

Pregnancy Category C. Studies performed in pregnant rats and rabbits given carvedilol revealed increased post-implantation loss in rats at doses of 300 mg/kg/day (50 times the maximum recommended human dose [MRHD] as mg/m^2) and in rabbits at doses of 75 mg/kg/day (25 times the MRHD as mg/m^2). In the rats, there was also a decrease in fetal body weight at the maternally toxic dose of 300 mg/kg/day (50 times the MRHD as mg/m^2), which was accompanied by an elevation in the frequency of fetuses with delayed skeletal development (missing or stunted 13th rib). In rats the no-observed-effect level for developmental toxicity was 60 mg/kg/day (10 times the MRHD as mg/m^2); in rabbits it was 15 mg/kg/day (5 times the MRHD as mg/m^2). There are no adequate and well-controlled studies in pregnant women. COREG CR should be used during pregnancy only if the potential benefit justifies the potential risk to the fetus.

8.3 Nursing Mothers

It is not known whether this drug is excreted in human milk. Studies in rats have shown that carvedilol and/or its metabolites (as well as other β-blockers) cross the placental barrier and are excreted in breast milk. There was increased mortality at one week post partum in neonates from rats treated with 60 mg/kg/day (10 times the MRHD as mg/m^2) and above during the last trimester through day 22 of lactation. Because many drugs are excreted in human milk and because of the potential for serious adverse reactions in nursing infants from β-blockers, especially bradycardia, a decision should be made whether to discontinue nursing or to discontinue the drug, taking into account the importance of the drug to the mother. The effects of other α- and β-blocking agents have included perinatal and neonatal distress.

8.4 Pediatric Use

Effectiveness of carvedilol in patients younger than 18 years of age has not been established.

In a double-blind trial, 161 children (mean age 6 years, range 2 months to 17 years; 45% younger than 2 years old) with chronic heart failure [NYHA class II-IV, left ventricular ejection fraction <40% for children with a systemic left ventricle (LV), and moderate-severe ventricular dysfunction qualitatively by echo for those with a systemic ventricle that was not an LV] who were receiving standard background treatment were randomized to placebo or to 2 dose levels of carvedilol. These dose levels produced placebo-corrected heart rate reduction of 4-6 heart beats per minute, indicative of β-blockade activity. Exposure appeared to be lower in pediatric subjects than adults. After 8 months of follow-up, there was no significant effect of treatment on clinical outcomes. Adverse reactions in this trial that occurred in greater than 10% of patients treated with immediate-release carvedilol and at twice the rate of placebo-treated patients included chest pain (17% versus 6%), dizziness (13% versus 2%), and dyspnea (11% versus 0%).

8.5 Geriatric Use

The initial clinical studies of COREG CR in patients with hypertension, heart failure, and left ventricular dysfunction following myocardial infarction did not include sufficient numbers of subjects 65 years of age or older to determine whether they respond differently from younger patients.

A randomized study (n = 405) comparing mild to severe heart failure patients switched to COREG CR or maintained on immediate-release carvedilol included 220 patients who were 65 years of age or older. In this elderly subgroup, the combined incidence of dizziness, hypotension, or syncope was 24% (18/75) in patients switched from the highest dose of immediate-release carvedilol (25 mg twice daily) to the highest dose of COREG CR (80 mg once daily) compared to 11% (4/36) in patients maintained on immediate-release carvedilol (25 mg twice daily). When switching from the higher doses of immediate-release carvedilol to COREG CR, a lower starting dose is recommended for elderly patients *[see Dosage and Administration (2.5)]*.

The following information is available for trials with immediate-release carvedilol. Of the 765 patients with heart failure randomized to carvedilol in US clinical trials, 31% (235) were 65 years of age or older, and 7.3% (56) were 75 years of age or older. Of the 1,156 patients randomized to carvedilol in a long-term, placebo-controlled trial in severe heart failure, 47% (547) were 65 years of age or older, and 15% (174) were 75 years of age or older. Of 3,025 patients receiving carvedilol in heart failure trials worldwide, 42% were 65 years of age or older. Of the 975 myocardial infarction patients randomized to carvedilol in the CAPRICORN trial, 48% (468) were 65 years of age or older, and 11% (111) were 75 years of age or older. Of the 2,065 hypertensive patients in US clinical trials of efficacy or safety who were treated with carvedilol, 21% (436) were 65 years of age or older. Of 3,722 patients receiving immediate-release carvedilol in hypertension clinical trials conducted worldwide, 24% were 65 years of age or older.

With the exception of dizziness in hypertensive patients (incidence 8.8% in the elderly versus 6% in younger patients), no overall differences in the safety or effectiveness (see Figures 2 and 4) were observed between the older subjects and younger subjects in each of these populations. Similarly, other reported clinical experience has not identified differences in responses between the elderly and younger subjects, but greater sensitivity of some older individuals cannot be ruled out.

10 OVERDOSAGE

Overdosage may cause severe hypotension, bradycardia, cardiac insufficiency, cardiogenic shock, and cardiac arrest. Respiratory problems, bronchospasms, vomiting, lapses of consciousness, and generalized seizures may also occur.

The patient should be placed in a supine position and, where necessary, kept under observation and treated under intensive-care conditions. Gastric lavage or pharmacologically induced emesis may be used shortly after ingestion. The following agents may be administered:

for excessive bradycardia: atropine, 2 mg IV.

to support cardiovascular function: glucagon, 5 to 10 mg IV rapidly over 30 seconds, followed by a continuous infusion of 5 mg/hour; sympathomimetics (dobutamine, isoprenaline, adrenaline) at doses according to body weight and effect.

If peripheral vasodilation dominates, it may be necessary to administer adrenaline or noradrenaline with continuous monitoring of circulatory conditions. For therapy-resistant bradycardia, pacemaker therapy should be performed. For bronchospasm, β-sympathomimetics (as aerosol or IV) or aminophylline IV should be given. In the event of seizures, slow IV injection of diazepam or clonazepam is recommended.

NOTE: In the event of severe intoxication where there are symptoms of shock, treatment with antidotes must be continued for a sufficiently long period of time consistent with the 7- to 10-hour half-life of carvedilol.

There is no experience of overdosage with COREG CR. Cases of overdosage with carvedilol alone or in combination with other drugs have been reported. Quantities ingested in some cases exceeded 1,000 milligrams. Symptoms experienced included low blood pressure and heart rate. Standard supportive treatment was provided and individuals recovered.

11 DESCRIPTION

Carvedilol phosphate is a nonselective β-adrenergic blocking agent with α_1-blocking activity. It is (*2RS*)-1-(*9H*-Carbazol-4-yloxy)-3-[[2-(2-methoxyphenoxy)ethyl]amino]propan-2-ol phosphate salt (1:1) hemihydrate. It is a racemic mixture with the following structure:

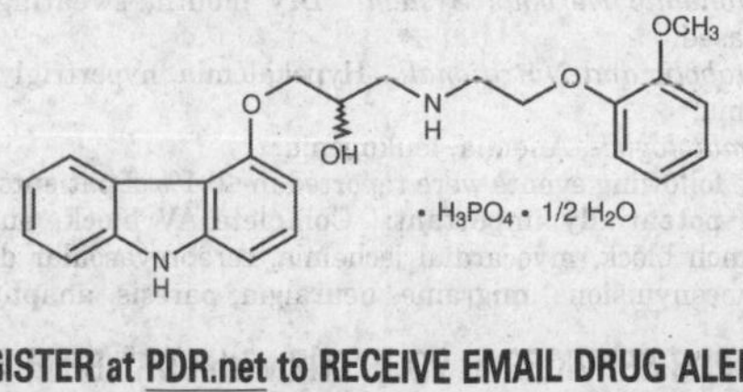

Carvedilol phosphate is a white to almost-white solid with a molecular weight of 513.5 (406.5 carvedilol free base) and a molecular formula of $C_{24}H_{26}N_2O_4 \bullet H_3PO_4 \bullet 1/2\ H_2O$.

COREG CR is available for once-a-day administration as controlled-release oral capsules containing 10, 20, 40, or 80 mg carvedilol phosphate. COREG CR hard gelatin capsules are filled with carvedilol phosphate immediate-release and controlled-release microparticles that are drug-layered and then coated with methacrylic acid copolymers. Inactive ingredients include crospovidone, hydrogenated castor oil, hydrogenated vegetable oil, magnesium stearate, methacrylic acid copolymers, microcrystalline cellulose, and povidone.

12 CLINICAL PHARMACOLOGY

12.1 Mechanism of Action

Carvedilol is a racemic mixture in which nonselective β-adrenoreceptor blocking activity is present in the S(-) enantiomer and α_1-adrenergic blocking activity is present in both R(+) and S(-) enantiomers at equal potency. Carvedilol has no intrinsic sympathomimetic activity.

12.2 Pharmacodynamics

Heart Failure and Left Ventricular Dysfunction Following Myocardial Infarction

The basis for the beneficial effects of carvedilol in patients with heart failure and in patients with left ventricular dysfunction following an acute myocardial infarction is not known. The concentration-response relationship for β_1-blockade following administration of COREG CR is equivalent (±20%) to immediate-release carvedilol tablets.

Hypertension

The mechanism by which β-blockade produces an antihypertensive effect has not been established.

β-adrenoreceptor blocking activity has been demonstrated in animal and human studies showing that carvedilol (1) reduces cardiac output in normal subjects; (2) reduces exercise- and/or isoproterenol-induced tachycardia; and (3) reduces reflex orthostatic tachycardia. Significant β-adrenoreceptor blocking effect is usually seen within 1 hour of drug administration.

α_1-adrenoreceptor blocking activity has been demonstrated in human and animal studies, showing that carvedilol (1) attenuates the pressor effects of phenylephrine; (2) causes vasodilation; and (3) reduces peripheral vascular resistance. These effects contribute to the reduction of blood pressure and usually are seen within 30 minutes of drug administration.

Due to the α_1-receptor blocking activity of carvedilol, blood pressure is lowered more in the standing than in the supine position, and symptoms of postural hypotension (1.8%), including rare instances of syncope, can occur. Following oral administration, when postural hypotension has occurred, it has been transient and is uncommon when immediate-release carvedilol is administered with food at the recommended starting dose and titration increments are closely followed *[see Dosage and Administration (2)]*.

In a randomized, double-blind, placebo-controlled trial, the β_1-blocking effect of COREG CR, as measured by heart rate response to submaximal bicycle ergometry, was shown to be equivalent to that observed with immediate-release carvedilol at steady state in adult patients with essential hypertension.

In hypertensive patients with normal renal function, therapeutic doses of carvedilol decreased renal vascular resistance with no change in glomerular filtration rate or renal plasma flow. Changes in excretion of sodium, potassium, uric acid, and phosphorus in hypertensive patients with normal renal function were similar after carvedilol and placebo.

Carvedilol has little effect on plasma catecholamines, plasma aldosterone, or electrolyte levels, but it does significantly reduce plasma renin activity when given for at least 4 weeks. It also increases levels of atrial natriuretic peptide.

12.3 Pharmacokinetics

Absorption

Carvedilol is rapidly and extensively absorbed following oral administration of immediate-release carvedilol tablets, with an absolute bioavailability of approximately 25% to 35% due to a significant degree of first-pass metabolism. COREG CR extended-release capsules have approximately 85% of the bioavailability of immediate-release carvedilol tablets. For corresponding dosages *[see Dosage and Administration (2)]*, the exposure (AUC, C_{max}, trough concentration) of carvedilol as COREG CR extended-release capsules is equivalent to those of immediate-release carvedilol tablets when both are administered with food. The absorption of carvedilol from COREG CR is slower and more prolonged compared to the immediate-release carvedilol tablet with peak concentrations achieved approximately 5 hours after administration. Plasma concentrations of carvedilol increase in a dose-proportional manner over the dosage range of COREG CR 10 to 80 mg. Within-subject and between-subject variability for AUC and C_{max} is similar for COREG CR and immediate-release carvedilol.

Effect of Food
Administration of COREG CR with a high-fat meal resulted in increases (~20%) in AUC and C_{max} compared to COREG CR administered with a standard meal. Decreases in AUC (27%) and C_{max} (43%) were observed when COREG CR was administered in the fasted state compared to administration after a standard meal. COREG CR should be taken with food.
In a study with adult subjects, sprinkling the contents of the COREG CR capsule on applesauce did not appear to have a significant effect on overall exposure (AUC) compared to administration of the intact capsule following a standard meal but did result in a decrease in C_{max} (18%).
Distribution
Carvedilol is more than 98% bound to plasma proteins, primarily with albumin. The plasma-protein binding is independent of concentration over the therapeutic range. Carvedilol is a basic, lipophilic compound with a steady-state volume of distribution of approximately 115 L, indicating substantial distribution into extravascular tissues.
Metabolism and Excretion
Carvedilol is extensively metabolized. Following oral administration of radiolabelled carvedilol to healthy volunteers, carvedilol accounted for only about 7% of the total radioactivity in plasma as measured by AUC. Less than 2% of the dose was excreted unchanged in the urine. Carvedilol is metabolized primarily by aromatic ring oxidation and glucuronidation. The oxidative metabolites are further metabolized by conjugation via glucuronidation and sulfation. The metabolites of carvedilol are excreted primarily via the bile into the feces. Demethylation and hydroxylation at the phenol ring produce 3 active metabolites with β-receptor blocking activity. Based on preclinical studies, the 4′-hydroxyphenyl metabolite is approximately 13 times more potent than carvedilol for β-blockade.
Compared to carvedilol, the 3 active metabolites exhibit weak vasodilating activity. Plasma concentrations of the active metabolites are about one-tenth of those observed for carvedilol and have pharmacokinetics similar to the parent.
Carvedilol undergoes stereoselective first-pass metabolism with plasma levels of R(+)-carvedilol approximately 2 to 3 times higher than S(-)-carvedilol following oral administration of COREG CR in healthy subjects. Apparent clearance is 90 L/h and 213 L/h for R(+)- and S(-)-carvedilol, respectively.
The primary P450 enzymes responsible for the metabolism of both R(+) and S(-)-carvedilol in human liver microsomes were CYP2D6 and CYP2C9 and to a lesser extent CYP3A4, 2C19, 1A2, and 2E1. CYP2D6 is thought to be the major enzyme in the 4′- and 5′-hydroxylation of carvedilol, with a potential contribution from 3A4. CYP2C9 is thought to be of primary importance in the O-methylation pathway of S(-)-carvedilol.
Carvedilol is subject to the effects of genetic polymorphism with poor metabolizers of debrisoquin (a marker for cytochrome P450 2D6) exhibiting 2- to 3-fold higher plasma concentrations of R(+)-carvedilol compared to extensive metabolizers. In contrast, plasma levels of S(-)-carvedilol are increased only about 20% to 25% in poor metabolizers, indicating this enantiomer is metabolized to a lesser extent by cytochrome P450 2D6 than R(+)-carvedilol. The pharmacokinetics of carvedilol do not appear to be different in poor metabolizers of S-mephenytoin (patients deficient in cytochrome P450 2C19).

12.4 Specific Populations
Heart Failure
Following administration of immediate-release carvedilol tablets, steady-state plasma concentrations of carvedilol and its enantiomers increased proportionally over the dose range in patients with heart failure. Compared to healthy subjects, heart failure patients had increased mean AUC and C_{max} values for carvedilol and its enantiomers, with up to 50% to 100% higher values observed in 6 patients with NYHA class IV heart failure. The mean apparent terminal elimination half-life for carvedilol was similar to that observed in healthy subjects.
For corresponding dose levels *[see Dosage and Administration (2)]*, the steady-state pharmacokinetics of carvedilol (AUC, C_{max}, trough concentrations) observed after administration of COREG CR to chronic heart failure patients (mild, moderate, and severe) were similar to those observed after administration of immediate-release carvedilol tablets.
Hypertension
For corresponding dose levels *[see Dosage and Administration (2)]*, the pharmacokinetics (AUC, C_{max}, and trough concentrations) observed with administration of COREG CR were equivalent (±20%) to those observed with immediate-release carvedilol tablets following repeat dosing in patients with essential hypertension.
Geriatric
Plasma levels of carvedilol average about 50% higher in the elderly compared to young subjects after administration of immediate-release carvedilol.
Hepatic Impairment
No studies have been performed with COREG CR in patients with hepatic impairment. Compared to healthy subjects, patients with severe liver impairment (cirrhosis) exhibit a 4- to 7-fold increase in carvedilol levels. Carvedilol is contraindicated in patients with severe liver impairment.
Renal Impairment
No studies have been performed with COREG CR in patients with renal impairment. Although carvedilol is metabolized primarily by the liver, plasma concentrations of carvedilol have been reported to be increased in patients with renal impairment after dosing with immediate-release carvedilol. Based on mean AUC data, approximately 40% to 50% higher plasma concentrations of carvedilol were observed in hypertensive patients with moderate to severe renal impairment compared to a control group of hypertensive patients with normal renal function. However, the ranges of AUC values were similar for both groups. Changes in mean peak plasma levels were less pronounced, approximately 12% to 26% higher in patients with impaired renal function. Consistent with its high degree of plasma protein binding, carvedilol does not appear to be cleared significantly by hemodialysis.

12.5 Drug-Drug Interactions
Since carvedilol undergoes substantial oxidative metabolism, the metabolism and pharmacokinetics of carvedilol may be affected by induction or inhibition of cytochrome P450 enzymes.
The following drug interaction studies were performed with immediate-release carvedilol tablets.
Amiodarone
In a pharmacokinetic study conducted in 106 Japanese patients with heart failure, coadministration of small loading and maintenance doses of amiodarone with carvedilol resulted in at least a 2-fold increase in the steady-state trough concentrations of S(-)-carvedilol *[see Drug Interactions (7.6)]*.
Cimetidine
In a pharmacokinetic study conducted in 10 healthy male subjects, cimetidine (1,000 mg/day) increased the steady-state AUC of carvedilol by 30% with no change in C_{max} *[see Drug Interactions (7.5)]*.
Digoxin
Following concomitant administration of carvedilol (25 mg once daily) and digoxin (0.25 mg once daily) for 14 days, steady-state AUC and trough concentrations of digoxin were increased by 14% and 16%, respectively, in 12 hypertensive patients *[see Drug Interactions (7.4)]*.
Glyburide
In 12 healthy subjects, combined administration of carvedilol (25 mg once daily) and a single dose of glyburide did not result in a clinically relevant pharmacokinetic interaction for either compound.
Hydrochlorothiazide
A single oral dose of carvedilol 25 mg did not alter the pharmacokinetics of a single oral dose of hydrochlorothiazide 25 mg in 12 patients with hypertension. Likewise, hydrochlorothiazide had no effect on the pharmacokinetics of carvedilol.
Rifampin
In a pharmacokinetic study conducted in 8 healthy male subjects, rifampin (600 mg daily for 12 days) decreased the AUC and C_{max} of carvedilol by about 70% *[see Drug Interactions (7.5)]*.
Torsemide
In a study of 12 healthy subjects, combined oral administration of carvedilol 25 mg once daily and torsemide 5 mg once daily for 5 days did not result in any significant differences in their pharmacokinetics compared with administration of the drugs alone.
Warfarin
Carvedilol (12.5 mg twice daily) did not have an effect on the steady-state prothrombin time ratios and did not alter the pharmacokinetics of R(+)- and S(-)-warfarin following concomitant administration with warfarin in 9 healthy volunteers.

13 NONCLINICAL TOXICOLOGY

13.1 Carcinogenesis, Mutagenesis, Impairment of Fertility
In 2-year studies conducted in rats given carvedilol at doses up to 75 mg/kg/day (12 times the MRHD when compared on a mg/m² basis) or in mice given up to 200 mg/kg/day (16 times the MRHD on a mg/m² basis), carvedilol had no carcinogenic effect.
Carvedilol was negative when tested in a battery of genotoxicity assays, including the Ames and the CHO/HGPRT assays for mutagenicity and the in vitro hamster micronucleus and in vivo human lymphocyte cell tests for clastogenicity.
At doses ≥200 mg/kg/day (≥32 times the MRHD as mg/m²) carvedilol was toxic to adult rats (sedation, reduced weight gain) and was associated with a reduced number of successful matings, prolonged mating time, significantly fewer corpora lutea and implants per dam, and complete resorption of 18% of the litters. The no-observed-effect dose level for overt toxicity and impairment of fertility was 60 mg/kg/day (10 times the MRHD as mg/m²).

14 CLINICAL STUDIES

Support for the use of COREG CR extended-release capsules for the treatment of mild-to-severe heart failure and for patients with left ventricular dysfunction following myocardial infarction is based on the equivalence of pharmacokinetic and pharmacodynamic (β_1-blockade) parameters between COREG CR and immediate-release carvedilol *[see Clinical Pharmacology (12.2, 12.3)]*.
The clinical trials performed with immediate-release carvedilol in heart failure and left ventricular dysfunction following myocardial infarction are presented below.

14.1 Heart Failure
A total of 6,975 patients with mild-to-severe heart failure were evaluated in placebo-controlled and active-controlled studies of immediate-release carvedilol.
Mild-to-Moderate Heart Failure
Carvedilol was studied in 5 multicenter, placebo-controlled studies, and in 1 active-controlled study (COMET study) involving patients with mild-to-moderate heart failure.
Four US multicenter, double-blind, placebo-controlled studies enrolled 1,094 patients (696 randomized to carvedilol) with NYHA class II-III heart failure and ejection fraction ≤0.35. The vast majority were on digitalis, diuretics, and an ACE inhibitor at study entry. Patients were assigned to the studies based upon exercise ability. An Australia-New Zealand double-blind, placebo-controlled study enrolled 415 patients (half randomized to immediate-release carvedilol) with less severe heart failure. All protocols excluded patients expected to undergo cardiac transplantation during the 7.5 to 15 months of double-blind follow-up. All randomized patients had tolerated a 2-week course on immediate-release carvedilol 6.25 mg twice daily.
In each study, there was a primary end point, either progression of heart failure (1 US study) or exercise tolerance (2 US studies meeting enrollment goals and the Australia-New Zealand study). There were many secondary end points specified in these studies, including NYHA classification, patient and physician global assessments, and cardiovascular hospitalization. Other analyses not prospectively planned included the sum of deaths and total cardiovascular hospitalizations. In situations where the primary end points of a trial do not show a significant benefit of treatment, assignment of significance values to the other results is complex, and such values need to be interpreted cautiously.
The results of the US and Australia-New Zealand trials were as follows:
Slowing Progression of Heart Failure: One US multicenter study (366 subjects) had as its primary end point the sum of cardiovascular mortality, cardiovascular hospitalization, and sustained increase in heart failure medications. Heart failure progression was reduced, during an average follow-up of 7 months, by 48% ($p = 0.008$).
In the Australia-New Zealand study, death and total hospitalizations were reduced by about 25% over 18 to 24 months. In the 3 largest US studies, death and total hospitalizations were reduced by 19%, 39%, and 49%, nominally statistically significant in the last 2 studies. The Australia-New Zealand results were statistically borderline.
Functional Measures: None of the multicenter studies had NYHA classification as a primary end point, but all such studies had it as a secondary end point. There was at least a trend toward improvement in NYHA class in all studies. Exercise tolerance was the primary end point in 3 studies; in none was a statistically significant effect found.
Subjective Measures: Health-related quality of life, as measured with a standard questionnaire (a primary end point in 1 study), was unaffected by carvedilol. However, patients' and investigators' global assessments showed significant improvement in most studies.
Mortality: Death was not a pre-specified end point in any study, but was analyzed in all studies. Overall, in these 4 US trials, mortality was reduced, nominally significantly so in 2 studies.
The COMET Trial
In this double-blind trial, 3,029 patients with NYHA class II-IV heart failure (left ventricular ejection fraction ≤35%) were randomized to receive either carvedilol (target dose: 25 mg twice daily) or immediate-release metoprolol tartrate (target dose: 50 mg twice daily). The mean age of the patients was approximately 62 years, 80% were males, and the mean left ventricular ejection fraction at baseline was 26%. Approximately 96% of the patients had NYHA class II or III heart failure. Concomitant treatment included diuretics (99%), ACE inhibitors (91%), digitalis (59%), aldosterone antagonists (11%), and "statin" lipid-lowering agents (21%). The mean duration of follow-up was 4.8 years. The mean dose of carvedilol was 42 mg per day.

Table 5. Results of COMET

End point	Carvedilol N = 1,511	Metoprolol N = 1,518	Hazard ratio	(95% CI)
All-cause mortality	34%	40%	0.83	0.74 – 0.93
Mortality + all hospitalization	74%	76%	0.94	0.86 – 1.02
Cardiovascular death	30%	35%	0.80	0.70 – 0.90
Sudden death	14%	17%	0.81	0.68 – 0.97
Death due to circulatory failure	11%	13%	0.83	0.67 – 1.02
Death due to stroke	0.9%	2.5%	0.33	0.18 – 0.62

Table 6. Results of COPERNICUS Trial in Patients With Severe Heart Failure

End point	Placebo (N = 1,133)	Carvedilol (N = 1,156)	Hazard ratio (95% CI)	% Reduction	Nominal p value
Mortality	190	130	0.65 (0.52 – 0.81)	35	0.00013
Mortality + all hospitalization	507	425	0.76 (0.67 – 0.87)	24	0.00004
Mortality + CV hospitalization	395	314	0.73 (0.63 – 0.84)	27	0.00002
Mortality + HF hospitalization	357	271	0.69 (0.59 – 0.81)	31	0.000004

Cardiovascular = CV; Heart failure = HF

The study had 2 primary end points: all-cause mortality and the composite of death plus hospitalization for any reason. The results of COMET are presented in Table 5 below. All-cause mortality carried most of the statistical weight and was the primary determinant of the study size. All-cause mortality was 34% in the patients treated with carvedilol and was 40% in the immediate-release metoprolol group (p = 0.0017; hazard ratio = 0.83, 95% CI 0.74–0.93). The effect on mortality was primarily due to a reduction in cardiovascular death. The difference between the 2 groups with respect to the composite end point was not significant (p = 0.122). The estimated mean survival was 8.0 years with carvedilol and 6.6 years with immediate-release metoprolol.

[See table 5 above]

It is not known whether this formulation of metoprolol at any dose or this low dose of metoprolol in any formulation has any effect on survival or hospitalization in patients with heart failure. Thus, this trial extends the time over which carvedilol manifests benefits on survival in heart failure, but it is not evidence that carvedilol improves outcome over the formulation of metoprolol (TOPROL-XL®) with benefits in heart failure.

Severe Heart Failure (COPERNICUS)

In a double-blind study, 2,289 patients with heart failure at rest or with minimal exertion and left ventricular ejection fraction <25% (mean 20%), despite digitalis (66%), diuretics (99%), and ACE inhibitors (89%) were randomized to placebo or carvedilol. Carvedilol was titrated from a starting dose of 3.125 mg twice daily to the maximum tolerated dose or up to 25 mg twice daily over a minimum of 6 weeks. Most subjects achieved the target dose of 25 mg. The study was conducted in Eastern and Western Europe, the United States, Israel, and Canada. Similar numbers of subjects per group (about 100) withdrew during the titration period.

The primary end point of the trial was all-cause mortality, but cause-specific mortality and the risk of death or hospitalization (total, cardiovascular [CV], or heart failure [HF]) were also examined. The developing trial data were followed by a data monitoring committee, and mortality analyses were adjusted for these multiple looks. The trial was stopped after a median follow-up of 10 months because of an observed 35% reduction in mortality (from 19.7% per patient year on placebo to 12.8% on carvedilol, hazard ratio 0.65, 95% CI 0.52 – 0.81, p = 0.0014, adjusted) (see Figure 1). The results of COPERNICUS are shown in Table 6.

[See table 6 above]

[See figure 1 at top of next column]

The effect on mortality was principally the result of a reduction in the rate of sudden death among patients without worsening heart failure.

Patients' global assessments, in which carvedilol-treated patients were compared to placebo, were based on pre-specified, periodic patient self-assessments regarding whether clinical status post-treatment showed improvement, worsening, or no change compared to baseline. Patients treated with carvedilol showed significant improvements in global assessments compared with those treated with placebo in COPERNICUS.

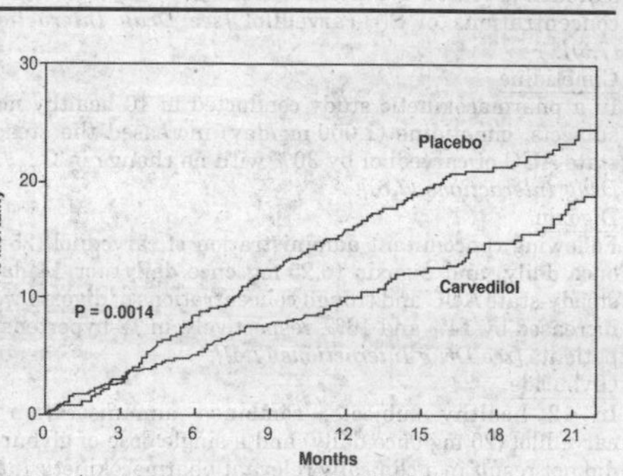

Figure 1. Survival Analysis for COPERNICUS (intent-to-treat)

The protocol also specified that hospitalizations would be assessed. Fewer patients on immediate-release carvedilol than on placebo were hospitalized for any reason (372 versus 432, p = 0.0029), for cardiovascular reasons (246 versus 314, p = 0.0003), or for worsening heart failure (198 versus 268, p = 0.0001).

Immediate-release carvedilol had a consistent and beneficial effect on all-cause mortality as well as the combined end points of all-cause mortality plus hospitalization (total, CV, or for heart failure) in the overall study population and in all subgroups examined, including men and women, elderly and non-elderly, blacks and non-blacks, and diabetics and non-diabetics (see Figure 2).

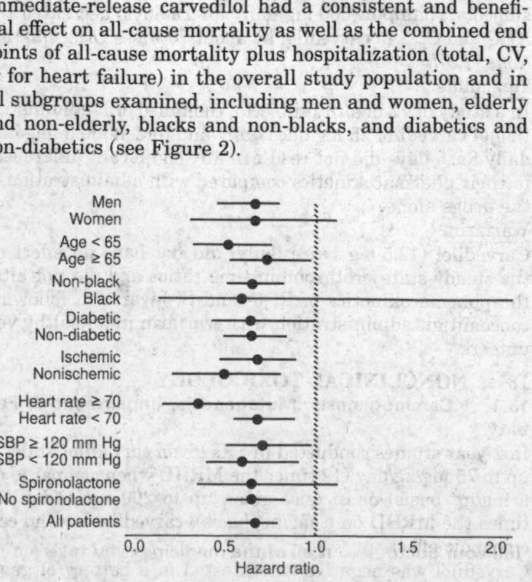

Figure 2. Effects on Mortality for Subgroups in COPERNICUS

Although the clinical trials used twice-daily dosing, clinical pharmacologic and pharmacokinetic data provide a reasonable basis for concluding that once-daily dosing with COREG CR should be adequate in the treatment of heart failure.

14.2 Left Ventricular Dysfunction Following Myocardial Infarction

CAPRICORN was a double-blind study comparing carvedilol and placebo in 1,959 patients with a recent myocardial infarction (within 21 days) and left ventricular ejection fraction of ≤40%, with (47%) or without symptoms of heart failure. Patients given carvedilol received 6.25 mg twice daily, titrated as tolerated to 25 mg twice daily. Patients had to have a systolic blood pressure >90 mm Hg, a sitting heart rate >60 beats/minute, and no contraindication to β-blocker use. Treatment of the index infarction included aspirin (85%), IV or oral β-blockers (37%), nitrates (73%), heparin (64%), thrombolytics (40%), and acute angioplasty (12%). Background treatment included ACE inhibitors or angiotensin receptor blockers (97%), anticoagulants (20%), lipid-lowering agents (23%), and diuretics (34%). Baseline population characteristics included an average age of 63 years, 74% male, 95% Caucasian, mean blood pressure 121/74 mm Hg, 22% with diabetes, and 54% with a history of hypertension. Mean dosage achieved of carvedilol was 20 mg twice daily; mean duration of follow-up was 15 months.

All-cause mortality was 15% in the placebo group and 12% in the carvedilol group, indicating a 23% risk reduction in patients treated with carvedilol (95% CI 2% to 40%, p = 0.03), as shown in Figure 3. The effects on mortality in various subgroups are shown in Figure 4. Nearly all deaths were cardiovascular (which were reduced by 25% by carvedilol), and most of these deaths were sudden or related to pump failure (both types of death were reduced by carvedilol). Another study end point, total mortality and all-cause hospitalization, did not show a significant improvement.

There was also a significant 40% reduction in fatal or non-fatal myocardial infarction observed in the group treated with carvedilol (95% CI 11% to 60%, p = 0.01). A similar reduction in the risk of myocardial infarction was also observed in a meta-analysis of placebo-controlled trials of carvedilol in heart failure.

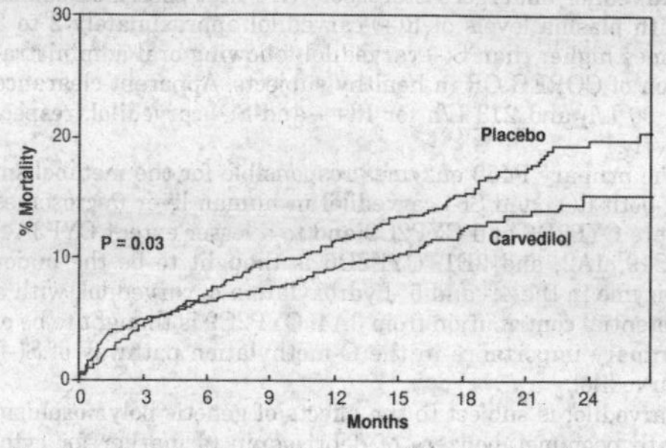

Figure 3. Survival Analysis for CAPRICORN (intent-to-treat)

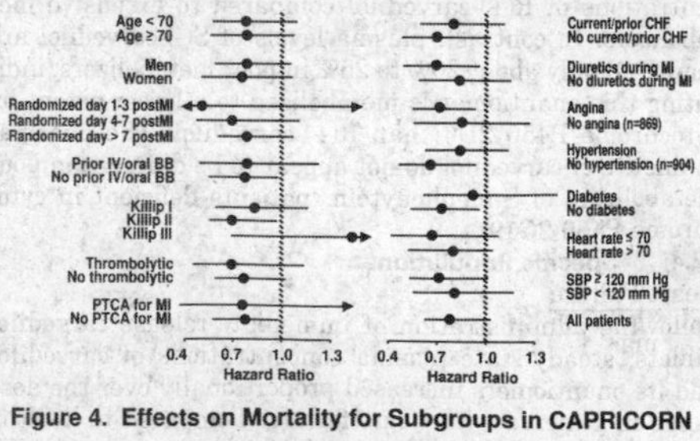

Figure 4. Effects on Mortality for Subgroups in CAPRICORN

Although the clinical trials used twice-daily dosing, clinical pharmacologic and pharmacokinetic data provide a reasonable basis for concluding that once-daily dosing with COREG CR should be adequate in the treatment of left ventricular dysfunction following myocardial infarction.

14.3 Hypertension

A double-blind, randomized, placebo-controlled, 8-week trial evaluated the blood pressure lowering effects of COREG CR 20 mg, 40 mg, and 80 mg once daily in 338 patients with essential hypertension (sitting diastolic blood pressure [DBP] ≥90 and ≤109 mm Hg). Of 337 evaluable patients, a total of 273 patients (81%) completed the study. Of the 64 (19%) patients withdrawn from the study, 10 (3%) were due to adverse events, 10 (3%) were due to lack of efficacy; the remaining 44 (13%) withdrew for other reasons. The mean age of the patients was approximately 53 years, 66% were male, and the mean sitting systolic blood pressure (SBP) and DBP at baseline were 150 mm Hg and 99 mm Hg, respectively. Dose titration occurred at 2-week intervals.

Statistically significant reductions in blood pressure as measured by 24-hour ambulatory blood pressure monitoring (ABPM) were observed with each dose of COREG CR compared to placebo. Placebo-subtracted mean changes from baseline in mean SBP/DBP were -6.1/-4.0 mm Hg, -9.4/-7.6 mm Hg, and -11.8/-9.2 mm Hg for COREG CR 20 mg, 40 mg, and 80 mg, respectively. Placebo-subtracted mean changes from baseline in mean trough (average of hours 20-24) SBP/DBP were -3.3/-2.8 mm Hg, -4.9/-5.2 mm Hg, and -8.4/-7.4 mm Hg for COREG CR 20 mg, 40 mg, and 80 mg, respectively. The placebo-corrected trough to peak (3-7 hr) ratio was approximately 0.6 for COREG CR 80 mg. In this study, assessments of 24-hour ABPM monitoring demonstrated statistically significant blood pressure reductions with COREG CR throughout the dosing period (Figure 5).

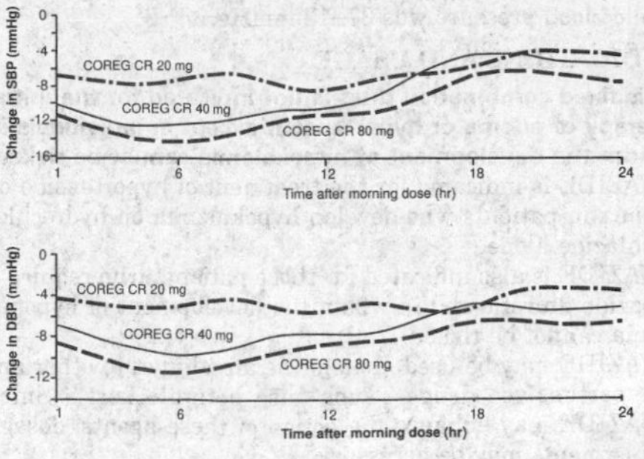

Lines smoothed using locally weighted regression smoothing methodology.

Figure 5. Changes from Baseline in Systolic Blood Pressure and Diastolic Blood Pressure Measured by 24-Hour ABPM

Immediate-release carvedilol was studied in 2 placebo-controlled trials that utilized twice-daily dosing, at total daily doses of 12.5 to 50 mg. In these and other studies, the starting dose did not exceed 12.5 mg. At 50 mg/day, COREG reduced sitting trough (12-hour) blood pressure by about 9/5.5 mm Hg; at 25 mg/day the effect was about 7.5/3.5 mm Hg. Comparisons of trough-to-peak blood pressure showed a trough-to-peak ratio for blood pressure response of about 65%. Heart rate fell by about 7.5 beats/minute at 50 mg/day. In general, as is true for other β-blockers, responses were smaller in black than non-black patients. There were no age- or gender-related differences in response. The dose-related blood pressure response was accompanied by a dose-related increase in adverse effects *[see Adverse Reactions (6)]*.

14.4 Hypertension With Type 2 Diabetes Mellitus

In a double-blind study (GEMINI), carvedilol, added to an ACE inhibitor or angiotensin receptor blocker, was evaluated in a population with mild-to-moderate hypertension and well-controlled type 2 diabetes mellitus. The mean HbA1c at baseline was 7.2%. COREG was titrated to a mean dose of 17.5 mg twice daily and maintained for 5 months. COREG had no adverse effect on glycemic control, based on HbA1c measurements (mean change from baseline of 0.02%, 95% CI -0.06 to 0.10, p = NS) *[see Warnings and Precautions (5.6)]*.

16 HOW SUPPLIED/STORAGE AND HANDLING

The hard gelatin capsules are available in the following strengths:

- 10 mg – white and green capsule shell printed with GSK COREG CR and 10 mg
- 20 mg – white and yellow capsule shell printed with GSK COREG CR and 20 mg
- 40 mg – yellow and green capsule shell printed with GSK COREG CR and 40 mg
- 80 mg – white capsule shell printed with GSK COREG CR and 80 mg
- 10 mg 30's: NDC 0007-3370-13
- 20 mg 30's: NDC 0007-3371-13
- 40 mg 30's: NDC 0007-3372-13
- 80 mg 30's: NDC 0007-3373-13

Store at 25°C (77°F); excursions 15° to 30°C (59° to 86°F). Dispense in a tight, light-resistant container.

17 PATIENT COUNSELING INFORMATION

See FDA Approved Patient Labeling (17.2).

17.1 Patient Advice

Patients taking COREG CR should be advised of the following:

- Patients should not interrupt or discontinue using COREG CR without a physician's advice.
- Patients with heart failure should consult their physician if they experience signs or symptoms of worsening heart failure such as weight gain or increasing shortness of breath.
- Patients may experience a drop in blood pressure when standing, resulting in dizziness and, rarely, fainting. Patients should sit or lie down when these symptoms of lowered blood pressure occur.
- If experiencing dizziness or fatigue, patients should avoid driving or hazardous tasks.
- Patients should consult a physician if they experience dizziness or faintness, in case the dosage should be adjusted.
- Patients should not crush or chew COREG CR capsules.
- Patients should take COREG CR with food.
- Diabetic patients should report any changes in blood sugar levels to their physician.
- Contact lens wearers may experience decreased lacrimation.

17.2 FDA-Approved Patient Labeling

Patient labeling is provided as a tear-off leaflet at the end of this full prescribing information.

COREG CR and COREG are registered trademarks of GlaxoSmithKline.

TOPROL-XL is a registered trademark of the AstraZeneca group of companies.

GlaxoSmithKline
Research Triangle Park, NC 27709

August 2011
CCR:16PI

PHARMACIST-DETACH HERE AND GIVE INSTRUCTIONS TO PATIENT

PATIENT INFORMATION LEAFLET

COREG CR® (Co-REG)

(carvedilol phosphate) Extended-release Capsules

Read the Patient Information that comes with COREG CR before you start taking it and each time you get a refill. There may be new information. This information does not take the place of talking with your doctor about your medical condition or your treatment. If you have any questions about COREG CR, ask your doctor or pharmacist.

What is the most important information I should know about COREG CR?

It is important for you to take your medicine every day as directed by your doctor. If you stop taking COREG CR suddenly, you could have chest pain and a heart attack. If your doctor decides that you should stop taking COREG CR, your doctor may slowly lower your dose over time before stopping it completely.

What is COREG CR?

COREG CR is a prescription medicine that belongs to a group of medicines called "beta-blockers". COREG CR is used, often with other medicines, for the following conditions:

- to treat patients with certain types of heart failure
- to treat patients who had a heart attack that worsened how well the heart pumps
- to treat patients with high blood pressure (hypertension)

COREG CR is not approved for use in children under 18 years of age.

Who should not take COREG CR?

Do not take COREG CR if you:

- have severe heart failure and require certain intravenous medicines that help support circulation.
- have asthma or other breathing problems.
- have a slow heartbeat or certain conditions that cause your heart to skip a beat (irregular heartbeat).
- have liver problems.
- are allergic to any of the ingredients in COREG CR. *See "What are the ingredients in COREG CR?"*

What should I tell my doctor before taking COREG CR?

Tell your doctor about all of your medical conditions, including if you:

- have asthma or other lung problems (such as bronchitis or emphysema).
- have problems with blood flow in your feet and legs (peripheral vascular disease). COREG CR can make some of your symptoms worse.
- have diabetes.
- have thyroid problems.
- have a condition called pheochromocytoma.
- have had severe allergic reactions.
- are scheduled for surgery and will be given anesthetic agents.
- are scheduled for cataract surgery and have taken or are currently taking COREG CR.
- are pregnant or trying to become pregnant. It is not known if COREG CR is safe for your unborn baby. You and your doctor should talk about the best way to control your high blood pressure during pregnancy.
- are breastfeeding. It is not known if COREG CR passes into your breast milk. You should not breastfeed while using COREG CR.

Tell your doctor about all of the medicines you take including prescription and non-prescription medicines, vitamins, and herbal supplements. COREG CR and certain other medicines can affect each other and cause serious side effects. COREG CR may affect the way other medicines work. Also, other medicines may affect how well COREG CR works.

Know the medicines you take. Keep a list of your medicines and show it to your doctor and pharmacist before you start a new medicine.

How should I take COREG CR?

- Take COREG CR exactly as prescribed. Take COREG CR **one** time each day with food. **It is important that you take COREG CR only one time each day.** To lessen possible side effects, your doctor might begin with a low dose and then slowly increase the dose.
- Swallow COREG CR capsules whole. Do not chew or crush COREG CR capsules.
- If you have trouble swallowing COREG CR whole:
  - The capsule may be carefully opened and the beads sprinkled over a spoonful of applesauce which should be eaten right away. The applesauce should not be warm.
  - Do not sprinkle beads on foods other than applesauce.
- **Do not stop taking COREG CR and do not change the amount of COREG CR you take without talking to your doctor.**
- If you miss a dose of COREG CR, take your dose as soon as you remember, unless it is time to take your next dose. Take your next dose at the usual time. Do not take 2 doses at the same time.
- If you take too much COREG CR, call your doctor or poison control center right away.

What should I avoid while taking COREG CR?

COREG CR can cause you to feel dizzy, tired, or faint. Do not drive a car, use machinery, or do anything that needs you to be alert if you have these symptoms.

What are possible side effects of COREG CR?

Serious side effects of COREG CR include:

- **chest pain and heart attack if you suddenly stop taking COREG CR.** *See "What is the most important information I should know about COREG CR?"*
- **slow heart beat.**
- **low blood pressure (which may cause dizziness or fainting when you stand up).** If these happen, sit or lie down, and tell your doctor right away.
- **worsening heart failure.** Tell your doctor right away if you have signs and symptoms that your heart failure may be worse, such as weight gain or increased shortness of breath.
- **changes in your blood sugar. If you have diabetes, tell your doctor if you have any changes in your blood sugar levels.**
- masking (hiding) the symptoms of low blood sugar, especially a fast heartbeat.
- **new or worsening symptoms of peripheral vascular disease.**
  - leg pain that happens when you walk, but goes away when you rest
  - no feeling (numbness) in your legs or feet while you are resting
  - cold legs or feet
- masking the symptoms of hyperthyroidism (overactive thyroid), such as a fast heartbeat.
- **worsening of severe allergic reactions.** Medicines to treat a severe allergic reaction may not work as well while you are taking COREG CR.
- **rare but serious allergic reactions** (including hives or swelling of the face, lips, tongue, and/or throat that may cause difficulty in breathing or swallowing) have happened in patients who were on COREG or COREG CR. These reactions can be life-threatening. In some cases, these reactions happened in patients who had been on COREG before taking COREG CR.

Common side effects of COREG CR include shortness of breath, weight gain, diarrhea, and tiredness. If you wear contact lenses, you may have fewer tears or dry eyes that can become bothersome.

Call your doctor if you have any side effects that bother you or don't go away.

How should I store COREG CR?

Store COREG CR at less than 86°F (30°C).

Safely throw away COREG CR that is out of date or no longer needed.

Keep COREG CR and all medicines out of the reach of children.

General information about COREG CR

Medicines are sometimes prescribed for conditions other than those described in patient information leaflets. Do not use COREG CR for a condition for which it was not prescribed. Do not give COREG CR to other people, even if they have the same symptoms you have. It may harm them.

This leaflet summarizes the most important information about COREG CR. If you would like more information, talk with your doctor. You can ask your doctor or pharmacist for information about COREG CR that is written for healthcare professionals. You can also find out more about COREG CR by visiting the website www.COREGCR.com or calling 1-888-825-5249. This call is free.

What are the ingredients in COREG CR?

Active ingredient: carvedilol phosphate

Inactive ingredients: crospovidone, hydrogenated castor oil, hydrogenated vegetable oil, magnesium stearate, methacrylic acid copolymers, microcrystalline cellulose, and povidone

COREG CR capsules come in the following strengths: 10 mg, 20 mg, 40 mg, 80 mg.

What is high blood pressure (hypertension)? Blood pressure is the force of blood in your blood vessels when your heart beats and when your heart rests. You have high blood pressure when the force is too much. High blood pressure makes the heart work harder to pump blood through the body and causes damage to blood vessels. COREG CR can help your blood vessels relax so your blood pressure is lower. Medicines that lower blood pressure may lower your chance of having a stroke or heart attack.

COREG CR and COREG are registered trademarks of GlaxoSmithKline.

GlaxoSmithKline
Research Triangle Park, NC 27709

January 2011
CCR:5PIL

DYAZIDE® ℞
[dī′ ə-zīd]
(hydrochlorothiazide/triamterene)
Capsules

DESCRIPTION

Each capsule of DYAZIDE (hydrochlorothiazide and triamterene) for oral use, with opaque red cap and opaque white body, contains hydrochlorothiazide 25 mg and triamterene 37.5 mg, and is imprinted with the product name DYAZIDE and SB. Hydrochlorothiazide is a diuretic/antihypertensive agent and triamterene is an antikaliuretic agent.

Hydrochlorothiazide is slightly soluble in water. It is soluble in dilute ammonia, dilute aqueous sodium hydroxide, and dimethylformamide. It is sparingly soluble in methanol.

Hydrochlorothiazide is 6-chloro-3,4-dihydro-2H-1, 2, 4-benzothiadiazine-7-sulfonamide 1,1-dioxide, and its structural formula is:

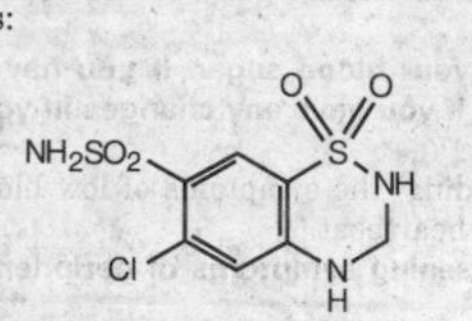

At 50°C, triamterene is practically insoluble in water (less than 0.1%). It is soluble in formic acid, sparingly soluble in methoxyethanol, and very slightly soluble in alcohol.

Triamterene is 2, 4, 7-triamino-6-phenylpteridine and its structural formula is:

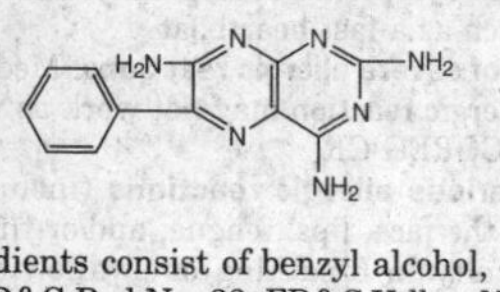

Inactive ingredients consist of benzyl alcohol, cetylpyridinium chloride, D&C Red No. 33, FD&C Yellow No. 6, gelatin, glycine, lactose, magnesium stearate, microcrystalline cellulose, povidone, polysorbate 80, sodium starch glycolate, titanium dioxide, and trace amounts of other inactive ingredients.

Capsules of DYAZIDE meet Drug Release Test 3 as published in the current USP monograph for Triamterene and Hydrochlorothiazide Capsules.

CLINICAL PHARMACOLOGY

DYAZIDE is a diuretic/antihypertensive drug product that combines natriuretic and antikaliuretic effects. Each component complements the action of the other. The hydrochlorothiazide component blocks the reabsorption of sodium and chloride ions, and thereby increases the quantity of sodium traversing the distal tubule and the volume of water excreted. A portion of the additional sodium presented to the distal tubule is exchanged there for potassium and hydrogen ions. With continued use of hydrochlorothiazide and depletion of sodium, compensatory mechanisms tend to increase this exchange and may produce excessive loss of potassium, hydrogen, and chloride ions. Hydrochlorothiazide also decreases the excretion of calcium and uric acid, may increase the excretion of iodide, and may reduce glomerular filtration rate. The exact mechanism of the antihypertensive effect of hydrochlorothiazide is not known.

The triamterene component of DYAZIDE exerts its diuretic effect on the distal renal tubule to inhibit the reabsorption of sodium in exchange for potassium and hydrogen ions. Its natriuretic activity is limited by the amount of sodium reaching its site of action. Although it blocks the increase in this exchange that is stimulated by mineralocorticoids (chiefly aldosterone), it is not a competitive antagonist of aldosterone and its activity can be demonstrated in adrenalectomized rats and patients with Addison's disease. As a result, the dose of triamterene required is not proportionally related to the level of mineralocorticoid activity, but is dictated by the response of the individual patients, and the kaliuretic effect of concomitantly administered drugs. By inhibiting the distal tubular exchange mechanism, triamterene maintains or increases the sodium excretion and reduces the excess loss of potassium, hydrogen and chloride ions induced by hydrochlorothiazide. As with hydrochlorothiazide, triamterene may reduce glomerular filtration and renal plasma flow. Via this mechanism it may reduce uric acid excretion although it has no tubular effect on uric acid reabsorption or secretion. Triamterene does not affect calcium excretion. No predictable antihypertensive effect has been demonstrated for triamterene.

Duration of diuretic activity and effective dosage range of the hydrochlorothiazide and triamterene components of DYAZIDE are similar. Onset of diuresis with DYAZIDE takes place within 1 hour, peaks at 2 to 3 hours and tapers off during the subsequent 7 to 9 hours.

DYAZIDE is well absorbed.

Upon administration of a single oral dose to fasted normal male volunteers, the following mean pharmacokinetic parameters were determined:

[See table below]

where $AUC_{(0-48)}$, C_{max}, T_{max} and Ae represent area under the plasma concentration versus time plot, maximum plasma concentration, time to reach C_{max}, and amount excreted in urine over 48 hours.

	$AUC_{(0-48)}$ ng*hrs/mL (± SD)	C_{max} ng/mL (± SD)	Median T_{max} Hrs	Ae Mg (± SD)
Triamterene	148.7 (87.9)	46.4 (29.4)	1.1	2.7 (1.4)
hydroxytriamterene sulfate	1,865 (471)	720 (364)	1.3	19.7 (6.1)
hydrochlorothiazide	834 (177)	135.1 (35.7)	2.0	14.3 (3.8)

A capsule of DYAZIDE is bioequivalent to a single-entity 25 mg hydrochlorothiazide tablet and 37.5 mg triamterene capsule used in the double-blind clinical trial below (see Clinical Trials).

In a limited study involving 12 subjects, coadministration of DYAZIDE with a high-fat meal resulted in: (1) an increase in the mean bioavailability of triamterene by about 67% (90% confidence interval = 0.99, 1.90), p-hydroxytriamterene sulfate by about 50% (90% confidence interval = 1.06, 1.77), hydrochlorothiazide by about 17% (90% confidence interval = 0.90, 1.34); (2) increases in the peak concentrations of triamterene and p-hydroxytriamterene; and (3) a delay of up to 2 hours in the absorption of the active constituents.

CLINICAL TRIALS

A placebo-controlled, double-blind trial was conducted to evaluate the efficacy of DYAZIDE. This trial demonstrated that DYAZIDE (25 mg hydrochlorothiazide/37.5 mg triamterene) was effective in controlling blood pressure while reducing the incidence of hydrochlorothiazide-induced hypokalemia. This trial involved 636 patients with mild to moderate hypertension controlled by hydrochlorothiazide 25 mg daily and who had hypokalemia (serum potassium <3.5 mEq/L) secondary to the hydrochlorothiazide. Patients were randomly assigned to 4 weeks' treatment with once-daily regimens of 25 mg hydrochlorothiazide plus placebo, or 25 mg hydrochlorothiazide combined with one of the following doses of triamterene: 25 mg, 37.5 mg, 50 mg, or 75 mg.

Blood pressure and serum potassium were monitored at baseline and throughout the trial. All five treatment groups had similar mean blood pressure and serum potassium concentrations at baseline (mean systolic blood pressure range: 137±14 mmHg to 140±16 mmHg; mean diastolic blood pressure range: 86±9 mmHg to 88±8 mmHg; mean serum potassium range: 2.3 to 3.4 mEq/L with the majority of patients having values between 3.1 and 3.4 mEq/L).

While all triamterene regimens reversed hypokalemia, at week 4 the 37.5 mg regimen proved optimal compared with the other tested regimens. On this regimen, 81% of the patients had a significant ($p<0.05$) reversal of hypokalemia vs. 59% of patients on the placebo/hydrochlorothiazide regimen. The mean serum potassium concentration on 37.5 mg triamterene went from 3.2±0.2 mEq/L at baseline to 3.7±0.3 mEq/L at week 4, a significantly greater ($p<0.05$) improvement than that achieved with placebo/hydrochlorothiazide (i.e., 3.2±0.2 mEq/L at baseline and 3.5±0.4 mEq/L at week 4). Also, 51% of patients in the 37.5 mg triamterene group had an increase in serum potassium of ≥0.5 mEq/L at week 4 vs. 33% in the placebo group. The 37.5 mg triamterene/25 mg hydrochlorothiazide regimen also maintained control of blood pressure; mean supine systolic blood pressure at week 4 was 138±21 mmHg while mean supine diastolic blood pressure was 87±13 mmHg.

INDICATIONS AND USAGE

This fixed combination drug is not indicated for the initial therapy of edema or hypertension except in individuals in whom the development of hypokalemia cannot be risked.

DYAZIDE is indicated for the treatment of hypertension or edema in patients who develop hypokalemia on hydrochlorothiazide alone.

DYAZIDE is also indicated for those patients who require a thiazide diuretic and in whom the development of hypokalemia cannot be risked.

DYAZIDE may be used alone or as an adjunct to other antihypertensive drugs, such as beta-blockers. Since DYAZIDE may enhance the action of these agents, dosage adjustments may be necessary.

Usage in Pregnancy

The routine use of diuretics in an otherwise healthy woman is inappropriate and exposes mother and fetus to unnecessary hazard. Diuretics do not prevent development of toxemia of pregnancy, and there is no satisfactory evidence that they are useful in the treatment of developed toxemia. Edema during pregnancy may arise from pathological causes or from the physiologic and mechanical consequences of pregnancy. Diuretics are indicated in pregnancy when edema is due to pathologic causes, just as they are in the absence of pregnancy. Dependent edema in pregnancy resulting from restriction of venous return by the expanded uterus is properly treated through elevation of the lower extremities and use of support hose; use of diuretics to lower intravascular volume in this case is illogical and unnecessary. There is hypervolemia during normal pregnancy which is harmful to neither the fetus nor the mother (in the absence of cardiovascular disease), but which is associated with edema, including generalized edema in the majority of pregnant women. If this edema produces discomfort, increased recumbency will often provide relief. In rare instances this edema may cause extreme discomfort which is not relieved by rest. In these cases a short course of diuretics may provide relief and may be appropriate.

CONTRAINDICATIONS

Antikaliuretic Therapy and Potassium Supplementation

DYAZIDE should not be given to patients receiving other potassium-sparing agents such as spironolactone, amiloride, or other formulations containing triamterene. Concomitant potassium-containing salt substitutes should also not be used.

Potassium supplementation should not be used with DYAZIDE except in severe cases of hypokalemia. Such concomitant therapy can be associated with rapid increases in serum potassium levels. If potassium supplementation is used, careful monitoring of the serum potassium level is necessary.

Impaired Renal Function

DYAZIDE is contraindicated in patients with anuria, acute and chronic renal insufficiency or significant renal impairment.

Hypersensitivity

Hypersensitivity to either drug in the preparation or to other sulfonamide-derived drugs is a contraindication.

Hyperkalemia

DYAZIDE should not be used in patients with preexisting elevated serum potassium.

WARNINGS

> **Hyperkalemia:** Abnormal elevation of serum potassium levels (greater than or equal to 5.5 mEq/liter) can occur with all potassium-sparing diuretic combinations, including DYAZIDE. Hyperkalemia is more likely to occur in patients with renal impairment and diabetes (even without evidence of renal impairment), and in the elderly or severely ill. Since uncorrected hyperkalemia may be fatal, serum potassium levels must be monitored at frequent intervals especially in patients first receiving DYAZIDE, when dosages are changed or with any illness that may influence renal function.

If hyperkalemia is suspected (warning signs include paresthesias, muscular weakness, fatigue, flaccid paralysis of the extremities, bradycardia, and shock), an electrocardiogram (ECG) should be obtained. However, it is important to monitor serum potassium levels because hyperkalemia may not be associated with ECG changes.

If hyperkalemia is present, DYAZIDE should be discontinued immediately and a thiazide alone should be substituted. If the serum potassium exceeds 6.5 mEq/liter more vigorous therapy is required. The clinical situation dictates the procedures to be employed. These include the intravenous administration of calcium chloride solution, sodium bicarbonate solution, and/or the oral or parenteral administration of glucose with a rapid-acting insulin preparation. Cationic exchange resins such as sodium polystyrene sulfonate may be orally or rectally administered. Persistent hyperkalemia may require dialysis.

The development of hyperkalemia associated with potassium-sparing diuretics is accentuated in the presence of renal impairment (see CONTRAINDICATIONS section). Patients with mild renal functional impairment should not receive this drug without frequent and continuing monitoring of serum electrolytes. Cumulative drug effects may be observed in patients with impaired renal function. The renal clearances of hydrochlorothiazide and the pharmacologically active metabolite of triamterene, the sulfate ester of hydroxytriamterene, have been shown to be reduced and the plasma levels increased following administration of DYAZIDE to elderly patients and patients with impaired renal function.

Hyperkalemia has been reported in diabetic patients with the use of potassium-sparing agents even in the absence of apparent renal impairment. Accordingly, serum electrolytes must be frequently monitored if DYAZIDE is used in diabetic patients.

Metabolic or Respiratory Acidosis

Potassium-sparing therapy should also be avoided in severely ill patients in whom respiratory or metabolic acidosis may occur. Acidosis may be associated with rapid elevations in serum potassium levels. If DYAZIDE is employed, frequent evaluations of acid/base balance and serum electrolytes are necessary.

Acute Myopia and Secondary Angle-Closure Glaucoma

Hydrochlorothiazide, a sulfonamide, can cause an idiosyncratic reaction, resulting in acute transient myopia and acute angle-closure glaucoma. Symptoms include acute onset of decreased visual acuity or ocular pain and typically occur within hours to weeks of drug initiation. Untreated acute angle-closure glaucoma can lead to permanent vision loss. The primary treatment is to discontinue hydrochlorothiazide as rapidly as possible. Prompt medical or surgical treatments may need to be considered if the intraocular pressure remains uncontrolled. Risk factors for developing acute angle-closure glaucoma may include a history of sulfonamide or penicillin allergy.

PRECAUTIONS

Diabetes

Caution should be exercised when administering DYAZIDE to patients with diabetes, since thiazides may cause hyperglycemia, glycosuria, and alter insulin requirements in diabetes. Also, diabetes mellitus may become manifest during thiazide administration.

Impaired Hepatic Function

Thiazides should be used with caution in patients with impaired hepatic function. They can precipitate hepatic coma in patients with severe liver disease. Potassium depletion induced by the thiazide may be important in this connection. Administer DYAZIDE cautiously and be alert for such early signs of impending coma as confusion, drowsiness, and tremor; if mental confusion increases discontinue DYAZIDE for a few days. Attention must be given to other factors that may precipitate hepatic coma, such as blood in the gastrointestinal tract or preexisting potassium depletion.

Hypokalemia

Hypokalemia is uncommon with DYAZIDE; but, should it develop, corrective measures should be taken such as potassium supplementation or increased intake of potassium-rich foods. Institute such measures cautiously with frequent determinations of serum potassium levels, especially in patients receiving digitalis or with a history of cardiac arrhythmias. If serious hypokalemia (serum potassium less than 3.0 mEq/L) is demonstrated by repeat serum potassium determinations, DYAZIDE should be discontinued and potassium chloride supplementation initiated. Less serious hypokalemia should be evaluated with regard to other coexisting conditions and treated accordingly.

Electrolyte Imbalance

Electrolyte imbalance, often encountered in such conditions as heart failure, renal disease or cirrhosis of the liver, may also be aggravated by diuretics and should be considered during therapy with DYAZIDE when using high doses for prolonged periods or in patients on a salt-restricted diet. Serum determinations of electrolytes should be performed, and are particularly important if the patient is vomiting excessively or receiving fluids parenterally. Possible fluid and electrolyte imbalance may be indicated by such warning signs as: dry mouth, thirst, weakness, lethargy, drowsiness, restlessness, muscle pain or cramps, muscular fatigue, hypotension, oliguria, tachycardia, and gastrointestinal symptoms.

Hypochloremia

Although any chloride deficit is generally mild and usually does not require specific treatment except under extraordinary circumstances (as in liver disease or renal disease), chloride replacement may be required in the treatment of metabolic alkalosis. Dilutional hyponatremia may occur in edematous patients in hot weather; appropriate therapy is water restriction, rather than administration of salt, except in rare instances when the hyponatremia is life threatening. In actual salt depletion, appropriate replacement is the therapy of choice.

Renal Stones

Triamterene has been found in renal stones in association with the other usual calculus components. DYAZIDE should be used with caution in patients with a history of renal stones.

Laboratory Tests

Serum Potassium

The normal adult range of serum potassium is 3.5 to 5.0 mEq per liter with 4.5 mEq often being used for a reference point. If hypokalemia should develop, corrective measures should be taken such as potassium supplementation or increased dietary intake of potassium-rich foods.

Institute such measures cautiously with frequent determinations of serum potassium levels. Potassium levels persistently above 6 mEq per liter require careful observation and treatment. Serum potassium levels do not necessarily indicate true body potassium concentration. A rise in plasma pH may cause a decrease in plasma potassium concentration and an increase in the intracellular potassium concentration. Discontinue corrective measures for hypokalemia immediately if laboratory determinations reveal an abnormal elevation of serum potassium.

Discontinue DYAZIDE and substitute a thiazide diuretic alone until potassium levels return to normal.

Serum Creatinine and BUN

DYAZIDE may produce an elevated blood urea nitrogen level, creatinine level or both. This apparently is secondary to a reversible reduction of glomerular filtration rate or a depletion of intravascular fluid volume (prerenal azotemia) rather than renal toxicity; levels usually return to normal when DYAZIDE is discontinued. If azotemia increases, discontinue DYAZIDE. Periodic BUN or serum creatinine determinations should be made, especially in elderly patients and in patients with suspected or confirmed renal insufficiency.

Serum PBI

Thiazide may decrease serum PBI levels without sign of thyroid disturbance.

Parathyroid Function

Thiazides should be discontinued before carrying out tests for parathyroid function. Calcium excretion is decreased by thiazides.

Pathologic changes in the parathyroid glands with hypercalcemia and hypophosphatemia have been observed in a few patients on prolonged thiazide therapy. The common complications of hyperparathyroidism such as bone resorption and peptic ulceration have not been seen.

Drug Interactions

Angiotensin-converting Enzyme Inhibitors

Potassium-sparing agents should be used with caution in conjunction with angiotensin-converting enzyme (ACE) inhibitors due to an increased risk of hyperkalemia.

Oral Hypoglycemic Drugs

Concurrent use with chlorpropamide may increase the risk of severe hyponatremia.

Nonsteroidal Anti-inflammatory Drugs

A possible interaction resulting in acute renal failure has been reported in a few patients on DYAZIDE when treated with indomethacin, a nonsteroidal anti-inflammatory agent. Caution is advised in administering nonsteroidal anti-inflammatory agents with DYAZIDE.

Lithium

Lithium generally should not be given with diuretics because they reduce its renal clearance and increase the risk of lithium toxicity. Read circulars for lithium preparations before use of such concomitant therapy with DYAZIDE.

Surgical Considerations

Thiazides have been shown to decrease arterial responsiveness to norepinephrine (an effect attributed to loss of sodium). This diminution is not sufficient to preclude effectiveness of the pressor agent for therapeutic use. Thiazides have also been shown to increase the paralyzing effect of nondepolarizing muscle relaxants such as tubocurarine (an effect attributed to potassium loss); consequently caution should be observed in patients undergoing surgery.

Other Considerations

Concurrent use of hydrochlorothiazide with amphotericin B or corticosteroids or corticotropin (ACTH) may intensify electrolyte imbalance, particularly hypokalemia, although the presence of triamterene minimizes the hypokalemic effect.

Thiazides may add to or potentiate the action of other antihypertensive drugs. See INDICATIONS AND USAGE for concomitant use with other antihypertensive drugs.

The effect of oral anticoagulants may be decreased when used concurrently with hydrochlorothiazide; dosage adjustments may be necessary.

DYAZIDE may raise the level of blood uric acid; dosage adjustments of antigout medication may be necessary to control hyperuricemia and gout.

The following agents given together with triamterene may promote serum potassium accumulation and possibly result in hyperkalemia because of the potassium-sparing nature of triamterene, especially in patients with renal insufficiency: blood from blood bank (may contain up to 30 mEq of potassium per liter of plasma or up to 65 mEq per liter of whole blood when stored for more than 10 days); low-salt milk (may contain up to 60 mEq of potassium per liter); potassium-containing medications (such as parenteral penicillin G potassium); salt substitutes (most contain substantial amounts of potassium).

Exchange resins, such as sodium polystyrene sulfonate, whether administered orally or rectally, reduce serum potassium levels by sodium replacement of the potassium; fluid retention may occur in some patients because of the increased sodium intake.

Chronic or overuse of laxatives may reduce serum potassium levels by promoting excessive potassium loss from the intestinal tract; laxatives may interfere with the potassium-retaining effects of triamterene.

The effectiveness of methenamine may be decreased when used concurrently with hydrochlorothiazide because of alkalinization of the urine.

Drug/Laboratory Test Interactions

Triamterene and quinidine have similar fluorescence spectra; thus, DYAZIDE will interfere with the fluorescent measurement of quinidine.

Carcinogenesis, Mutagenesis, Impairment of Fertility

Carcinogenesis

Long-term studies have not been conducted with DYAZIDE (the triamterene/hydrochlorothiazide combination), or with triamterene alone.

Hydrochlorothiazide

Two-year feeding studies in mice and rats, conducted under the auspices of the National Toxicology Program (NTP), treated mice and rats with doses of hydrochlorothiazide up to 600 and 100 mg/kg/day, respectively. On a body-weight basis, these doses are 600 times (in mice) and 100 times (in rats) the Maximum Recommended Human Dose (MRHD) for the hydrochlorothiazide component of DYAZIDE at 50 mg/day (or 1.0 mg/kg/day based on 50 kg individuals). On the basis of body-surface area, these doses are 56 times (in mice) and 21 times (in rats) the MRHD. These studies uncovered no evidence of carcinogenic potential of hydrochlorothiazide in rats or female mice, but there was equivocal evidence of hepatocarcinogenicity in male mice.

Mutagenesis

Studies of the mutagenic potential of DYAZIDE (the triamterene/hydrochlorothiazide combination), or of triamterene alone have not been performed.

Hydrochlorothiazide

Hydrochlorothiazide was not genotoxic in in vitro assays using strains TA 98, TA 100, TA 1535, TA 1537 and TA 1538 of *Salmonella typhimurium* (the Ames test); in the Chinese Hamster Ovary (CHO) test for chromosomal aberrations; or in in vivo assays using mouse germinal cell chromosomes, Chinese hamster bone marrow chromosomes, and the *Drosophila* sex-linked recessive lethal trait gene. Positive test results were obtained in the in vitro CHO Sister Chromatid Exchange (clastogenicity) test, and in the mouse Lymphoma Cell (mutagenicity) assays, using concentrations of hydrochlorothiazide of 43 to 1300 mcg/mL. Positive test results were also obtained in the *Aspergillus nidulans* nondisjunction assay, using an unspecified concentration of hydrochlorothiazide.

Impairment of Fertility

Studies of the effects of DYAZIDE (the triamterene/hydrochlorothiazide combination), or of triamterene alone on animal reproductive function have not been conducted.

Hydrochlorothiazide

Hydrochlorothiazide had no adverse effects on the fertility of mice and rats of either sex in studies wherein these species were exposed, via their diet, to doses of up to 100 and 4 mg/kg/day, respectively, prior to mating and throughout gestation. Corresponding multiples of the MRHD are 100 (mice) and 4 (rats) on the basis of body-weight and 9.4 (mice) and 0.8 (rats) on the basis of body-surface area.

Pregnancy: Category C
Teratogenic Effects
DYAZIDE
Animal reproduction studies to determine the potential for fetal harm by DYAZIDE have not been conducted. However, a One Generation Study in the rat approximated composition of DYAZIDE by using a 1:1 ratio of triamterene to hydrochlorothiazide (30:30 mg/kg/day); there was no evidence of teratogenicity at those doses which were, on a body-weight basis, 15 and 30 times, respectively, the MRHD, and on the basis of body-surface area, 3.1 and 6.2 times, respectively, the MRHD.
The safe use of DYAZIDE in pregnancy has not been established since there are no adequate and well-controlled studies with DYAZIDE in pregnant women. DYAZIDE should be used during pregnancy only if the potential benefit justifies the risk to the fetus.
Triamterene
Reproduction studies have been performed in rats at doses as high as 20 times the MRHD on the basis of body-weight, and 6 times the human dose on the basis of body-surface area without evidence of harm to the fetus due to triamterene.
Because animal reproduction studies are not always predictive of human response, this drug should be used during pregnancy only if clearly needed.
Hydrochlorothiazide
Hydrochlorothiazide was orally administered to pregnant mice and rats during respective periods of major organogenesis at doses up to 3,000 and 1,000 mg/kg/day, respectively. At these doses, which are multiples of the MRHD equal to 3,000 for mice and 1,000 for rats, based on body-weight, and equal to 282 for mice and 206 for rats, based on body-surface area, there was no evidence of harm to the fetus.
There are, however, no adequate and well-controlled studies in pregnant women. Because animal reproduction studies are not always predictive of human response, this drug should be used during pregnancy only if clearly needed.
Nonteratogenic Effects
Thiazides and triamterene have been shown to cross the placental barrier and appear in cord blood. The use of thiazides and triamterene in pregnant women requires that the anticipated benefit be weighed against possible hazards to the fetus. These hazards include fetal or neonatal jaundice, pancreatitis, thrombocytopenia, and possible other adverse reactions which have occurred in the adult.
Nursing Mothers
Thiazides and triamterene in combination have not been studied in nursing mothers. Triamterene appears in animal milk; this may occur in humans. Thiazides are excreted in human breast milk. If use of the combination drug product is deemed essential, the patient should stop nursing.
Pediatric Use
Safety and effectiveness in pediatric patients have not been established.

ADVERSE REACTIONS

Adverse effects are listed in decreasing order of severity.
Hypersensitivity
Anaphylaxis, rash, urticaria, subacute cutaneous lupus erythematosus-like reactions, photosensitivity.
Cardiovascular
Arrhythmia, postural hypotension.
Metabolic
Diabetes mellitus, hyperkalemia, hypokalemia, hyponatremia, acidosis, hypercalcemia, hyperglycemia, glycosuria, hyperuricemia, hypochloremia.
Gastrointestinal
Jaundice and/or liver enzyme abnormalities, pancreatitis, nausea and vomiting, diarrhea, constipation, abdominal pain.
Renal
Acute renal failure (one case of irreversible renal failure has been reported), interstitial nephritis, renal stones composed primarily of triamterene, elevated BUN, and serum creatinine, abnormal urinary sediment.
Hematologic
Leukopenia, thrombocytopenia and purpura, megaloblastic anemia.
Musculoskeletal
Muscle cramps.
Central Nervous System
Weakness, fatigue, dizziness, headache, dry mouth.
Miscellaneous
Impotence, sialadenitis.
Thiazides alone have been shown to cause the following additional adverse reactions:
Central Nervous System
Paresthesias, vertigo.
Ophthalmic
Xanthopsia, transient blurred vision.
Respiratory
Allergic pneumonitis, pulmonary edema, respiratory distress.
Other
Necrotizing vasculitis, exacerbation of lupus.
Hematologic
Aplastic anemia, agranulocytosis, hemolytic anemia.
Neonate and infancy
Thrombocytopenia and pancreatitis–rarely, in newborns whose mothers have received thiazides during pregnancy.
Skin
Erythema multiforme including Stevens-Johnson syndrome, exfoliative dermatitis including toxic epidermal necrolysis.

DOSAGE AND ADMINISTRATION

The usual dose of DYAZIDE is one or two capsules given once daily, with appropriate monitoring of serum potassium and of the clinical effect (see WARNINGS, Hyperkalemia).

OVERDOSAGE

Electrolyte imbalance is the major concern (see WARNINGS section). Symptoms reported include: polyuria, nausea, vomiting, weakness, lassitude, fever, flushed face, and hyperactive deep tendon reflexes. If hypotension occurs, it may be treated with pressor agents such as levarterenol to maintain blood pressure. Carefully evaluate the electrolyte pattern and fluid balance. Induce immediate evacuation of the stomach through emesis or gastric lavage. There is no specific antidote.
Reversible acute renal failure following ingestion of 50 tablets of a product containing a combination of 50 mg triamterene and 25 mg hydrochlorothiazide has been reported. Although triamterene is largely protein-bound (approximately 67%), there may be some benefit to dialysis in cases of overdosage.

HOW SUPPLIED

Capsules containing 25 mg hydrochlorothiazide and 37.5 mg triamterene, in bottles of 1,000 capsules; in Patient-Pak™ unit-of-use bottles of 100.
They are supplied as follows:
NDC 0007-3650-22–in Patient-Pak™ unit-of-use bottles of 100.
NDC 0007-3650-30–bottles of 1,000.
Store at controlled room temperature 20° to 25°C (68° to 77°F); excursions permitted to 15° to 30°C (59° to 86°F). Protect from light. Dispense in a tight, light-resistant container.
GlaxoSmithKline
Research Triangle Park, NC 27709
DYAZIDE is a registered trademark of GlaxoSmithKline.

February 2011
DYZ:74PI

ENGERIX-B ℞

[in' jə-rix]
[Hepatitis B Vaccine (Recombinant)]
Suspension for Intramuscular Injection

HIGHLIGHTS OF PRESCRIBING INFORMATION
These highlights do not include all the information needed to use ENGERIX-B safely and effectively. See full prescribing information for ENGERIX-B.
ENGERIX-B [Hepatitis B Vaccine (Recombinant)]
Suspension for Intramuscular Injection
Initial U.S. Approval: 1989

RECENT MAJOR CHANGES

Warnings and Precautions, Syncope (5.2)	03/2012
Warnings and Precautions, Multiple Sclerosis (5.8)	10/2011

INDICATIONS AND USAGE

ENGERIX-B is a vaccine indicated for immunization against infection caused by all known subtypes of hepatitis B virus. (1)

DOSAGE AND ADMINISTRATION

- ENGERIX-B is administered by intramuscular injection. (2.2)
- Persons from birth through 19 years of age: A series of 3 doses (0.5 mL each) given on a 0-, 1-, 6-month schedule. (2.3)
- Persons 20 years of age and older: A series of 3 doses (1 mL each) given on a 0-, 1-, 6-month schedule. (2.3)
- Adults on hemodialysis: A series of 4 doses (2 mL each) given as a single 2-mL dose or as two 1-mL doses on a 0-, 1-, 2-, 6-month schedule. (2.3)

DOSAGE FORMS AND STRENGTHS

- ENGERIX-B is a sterile suspension available in the following presentations:
- 0.5-mL (10 mcg) single-dose vials and prefilled syringes (3)
- 1-mL (20 mcg) single-dose vials and prefilled syringes (3)

CONTRAINDICATIONS

Severe allergic reaction (e.g., anaphylaxis) after a previous dose of any hepatitis B-containing vaccine, or to any component of ENGERIX-B, including yeast. (4)

WARNINGS AND PRECAUTIONS

- ENGERIX-B is available in vials and 2 types of prefilled syringes. One type of prefilled syringe has a tip cap which may contain natural rubber latex. The other type has a tip cap and a rubber plunger which contain dry natural latex rubber. Use of these syringes may cause allergic reactions in latex-sensitive individuals. (5.1, 16)
- Syncope (fainting) can occur in association with administration of injectable vaccines, including ENGERIX-B. Procedures should be in place to avoid falling injury and to restore cerebral perfusion following syncope. (5.2)
- Apnea following intramuscular vaccination has been observed in some infants born prematurely. Decisions about when to administer an intramuscular vaccine, including ENGERIX-B, to infants born prematurely should be based on consideration of the infant's medical status, and the potential benefits and possible risks of vaccination. (5.4)

ADVERSE REACTIONS

The most common solicited adverse events were injection-site soreness (22%) and fatigue (14%). (6.1)
To report SUSPECTED ADVERSE REACTIONS, contact GlaxoSmithKline at 1-888-825-5249 or VAERS at 1-800-822-7967 or www.vaers.hhs.gov .

DRUG INTERACTIONS

Do not mix ENGERIX-B with any other vaccine or product in the same syringe or vial. (7.1)

USE IN SPECIFIC POPULATIONS

- Safety and effectiveness of ENGERIX-B have not been established in pregnant women and nursing mothers. ENGERIX-B should only be given to a pregnant woman if clearly needed. (8.1, 8.3)
- Antibody responses are lower in persons older than 60 years of age than in younger adults. (8.5)

See 17 for PATIENT COUNSELING INFORMATION
Revised: 07/2012

FULL PRESCRIBING INFORMATION: CONTENTS*

*** Sections or subsections omitted from the full prescribing information are not listed**

FULL PRESCRIBING INFORMATION

1 INDICATIONS AND USAGE

ENGERIX-B® is indicated for immunization against infection caused by all known subtypes of hepatitis B virus.

2 DOSAGE AND ADMINISTRATION

2.1 Preparation for Administration

Shake well before use. With thorough agitation, ENGERIX-B is a homogeneous, turbid white suspension. Do not administer if it appears otherwise. Parenteral drug products should be inspected visually for particulate matter and discoloration prior to administration, whenever solution and container permit. If either of these conditions exists, the vaccine should not be administered.

For the prefilled syringes, attach a sterile needle and administer intramuscularly.

For the vials, use a sterile needle and sterile syringe to withdraw the vaccine dose and administer intramuscularly. Changing needles between drawing vaccine from a vial and injecting it into a recipient is not necessary unless the needle has been damaged or contaminated. Use a separate sterile needle and syringe for each individual.

2.2 Administration

ENGERIX-B should be administered by intramuscular injection. The preferred administration site is the anterolateral aspect of the thigh for infants younger than 1 year and the deltoid muscle in older children (whose deltoid is large enough for an intramuscular injection) and adults. ENGERIX-B should not be administered in the gluteal region; such injections may result in suboptimal response.

ENGERIX-B may be administered subcutaneously to persons at risk of hemorrhage (e.g., hemophiliacs). However, hepatitis B vaccines administered subcutaneously are known to result in a lower antibody response. Additionally, when other aluminum-adsorbed vaccines have been administered subcutaneously, an increased incidence of local reactions including subcutaneous nodules has been observed. Therefore, subcutaneous administration should be used only in persons who are at risk of hemorrhage with intramuscular injections.

Do not administer intravenously or intradermally.

2.3 Recommended Dose and Schedule

Persons From Birth Through 19 Years of Age: Primary immunization for infants (born of hepatitis B surface antigen [HBsAg]-negative or HBsAg-positive mothers), children (birth through 10 years of age), and adolescents (11 through 19 years of age) consists of a series of 3 doses (0.5 mL each) given on a 0-, 1-, and 6-month schedule.

Persons 20 Years of Age and Older: Primary immunization for persons 20 years of age and older consists of a series of 3 doses (1 mL each) given on a 0-, 1-, and 6-month schedule.

Adults on Hemodialysis: Primary immunization consists of a series of 4 doses (2 mL each) given as a single 2-mL dose or two 1-mL doses on a 0-, 1-, 2-, and 6-month schedule. In hemodialysis patients, antibody response is lower than in healthy persons and protection may persist only as long as antibody levels remain above 10 mIU/mL. Therefore, the need for booster doses should be assessed by annual antibody testing. A 2-mL booster dose (as a single 2-mL dose or two 1-mL doses) should be given when antibody levels decline below 10 mIU/mL.[1] *[See Clinical Studies (14.2).]*

Table 1. Recommended Dosage and Administration Schedules

Group	Dose[a]	Schedules
Infants born of:		
HBsAg-negative mothers	0.5 mL	0, 1, 6 months
HBsAg-positive mothers[b]	0.5 mL	0, 1, 6 months
Children:		
Birth through 10 years of age	0.5 mL	0, 1, 6 months
Adolescents:		
11 through 19 years of age	0.5 mL	0, 1, 6 months
Adults:		
20 years of age and older	1 mL	0, 1, 6 months
Adults on hemodialysis	2 mL[c]	0, 1, 2, 6 months

HBsAg = Hepatitis B surface antigen
[a]0.5 mL (10 mcg); 1 mL (20 mcg).
[b]Infants born to HBsAg-positive mothers should also receive hepatitis B immune globulin (HBIG) *[see Dosage and Administration (2.5)]*.
[c]Given as a single 2-mL dose or as two 1-mL doses.

2.4 Alternate Dosing Schedules

There are alternate dosing and administration schedules which may be used for specific populations (e.g., neonates born of hepatitis B–infected mothers, persons who have or might have been recently exposed to the virus, and travelers to high-risk areas) (Table 2). For some of these alternate schedules, an additional dose at 12 months is recommended for prolonged maintenance of protective titers.

Table 2. Alternate Dosage and Administration Schedules

Group	Dose[a]	Schedules
Infants born of:		
HBsAg-positive mothers[b]	0.5 mL	0, 1, 2, 12 months
Children		
Birth through 10 years of age	0.5 mL	0, 1, 2, 12 months
5 through 10 years of age	0.5 mL	0, 12, 24 months[c]
Adolescents:		
11 through 16 years of age	0.5 mL	0, 12, 24 months[c]
11 through 19 years of age	1 mL	0, 1, 6 months
11 through 19 years of age	1 mL	0, 1, 2, 12 months
Adults:		
20 years of age and older	1 mL	0, 1, 2, 12 months

HBsAg = Hepatitis B surface antigen
[a]0.5 mL (10 mcg); 1 mL (20 mcg).
[b]Infants born to HBsAg-positive mothers should also receive hepatitis B immune globulin (HBIG) *[see Dosage and Administration (2.5)]*.
[c]For children and adolescents for whom an extended administration schedule is acceptable based on risk of exposure.

2.5 Booster Vaccinations

Whenever administration of a booster dose is appropriate, the dose of ENGERIX-B is 0.5 mL for children 10 years of age and younger and 1 mL for persons 11 years of age and older. Studies have demonstrated a substantial increase in antibody titers after booster vaccination with ENGERIX-B. See Section 2.2 for information on booster vaccination for adults on hemodialysis.

2.6 Known or Presumed Exposure to Hepatitis B Virus

Persons with known or presumed exposure to the hepatitis B virus (e.g., neonates born of infected mothers, persons who experienced percutaneous or permucosal exposure to the virus) should be given hepatitis B immune globulin (HBIG) in addition to ENGERIX-B in accordance with Advisory Committee on Immunization Practices recommendations and with the package insert for HBIG. ENGERIX-B can be given on either dosing schedule (0, 1, and 6 months or 0, 1, 2, and 12 months).

3 DOSAGE FORMS AND STRENGTHS

ENGERIX-B is a sterile suspension available in the following presentations:

- 0.5-mL (10 mcg) single-dose vials and prefilled TIP-LOK® syringes
- 1-mL (20 mcg) single-dose vials and prefilled TIP-LOK syringes

[See Description (11) and How Supplied/Storage and Handling (16).]

4 CONTRAINDICATIONS

Severe allergic reaction (e.g., anaphylaxis) after a previous dose of any hepatitis B-containing vaccine, or to any component of ENGERIX-B, including yeast, is a contraindication to administration of ENGERIX-B *[see Description (11) and How Supplied/Storage and Handling (16)]*.

5 WARNINGS AND PRECAUTIONS

5.1 Latex

ENGERIX-B is available in vials and 2 types of prefilled syringes. One type of prefilled syringe has a tip cap which may contain natural rubber latex. The other type has a tip cap and a rubber plunger which contain dry natural latex rubber. Use of these syringes may cause allergic reactions in latex-sensitive individuals. The vial stopper does not contain latex. *[See How Supplied/Storage and Handling (16).]*

5.2 Syncope

Syncope (fainting) can occur in association with administration of injectable vaccines, including ENGERIX-B. Syncope can be accompanied by transient neurological signs such as visual disturbance, paresthesia, and tonic-clonic limb movements. Procedures should be in place to avoid falling injury and to restore cerebral perfusion following syncope.

5.3 Infants Weighing Less Than 2,000 g

Hepatitis B vaccine should be deferred for infants weighing <2,000 g if the mother is documented to be HBsAg negative at the time of the infant's birth. Vaccination can commence at chronological age 1 month or hospital discharge. Infants weighing <2,000 g born to HBsAg-positive mothers or mothers of unknown HBsAg status should receive vaccine and hepatitis B immune globulin (HBIG) within 12 hours if HBsAg status cannot be determined; the birth dose should not be counted as the first dose in the vaccine series and it should be followed with a full 3-dose standard regimen (total of 4 doses).[2] *[See Dosage and Administration (2).]*

5.4 Apnea in Premature Infants

Apnea following intramuscular vaccination has been observed in some infants born prematurely. Decisions about when to administer an intramuscular vaccine, including ENGERIX-B, to infants born prematurely should be based on consideration of the infant's medical status, and the potential benefits and possible risks of vaccination. For ENGERIX-B, this assessment should include consideration of the mother's hepatitis B antigen status and the high probability of maternal transmission of hepatitis B virus to infants born of mothers who are HBsAg positive if vaccination is delayed.

5.5 Preventing and Managing Allergic Vaccine Reactions

Prior to immunization, the healthcare provider should review the immunization history for possible vaccine sensitivity and previous vaccination-related adverse reactions to allow an assessment of benefits and risks. Epinephrine and other appropriate agents used for the control of immediate allergic reactions must be immediately available should an acute anaphylactic reaction occur. *[See Contraindications (4).]*

5.6 Moderate or Severe Acute Illness

To avoid diagnostic confusion between manifestations of an acute illness and possible vaccine adverse effects, vaccination with ENGERIX-B should be postponed in persons with moderate or severe acute febrile illness unless they are at immediate risk of hepatitis B infection (e.g., infants born of HBsAg -positive mothers).

5.7 Altered Immunocompetence

Immunocompromised persons may have a diminished immune response to ENGERIX-B, including individuals receiving immunosuppressant therapy.

5.8 Multiple Sclerosis

Results from 2 clinical studies indicate that there is no association between hepatitis B vaccination and the development of multiple sclerosis,3 and that vaccination with hepatitis B vaccine does not appear to increase the short-term risk of relapse in multiple sclerosis.4

5.9 Limitations of Vaccine Effectiveness

Hepatitis B has a long incubation period. ENGERIX-B may not prevent hepatitis B infection in individuals who had an unrecognized hepatitis B infection at the time of vaccine administration. Additionally, it may not prevent infection in individuals who do not achieve protective antibody titers.

6 ADVERSE REACTIONS

6.1 Clinical Trials Experience

Because clinical trials are conducted under widely varying conditions, adverse reaction rates observed in the clinical trials of a vaccine cannot be directly compared to rates in the clinical trials of another vaccine and may not reflect the rates observed in practice.

The most common solicited adverse events were injection site soreness (22%) and fatigue (14%).

In 36 clinical studies, a total of 13,495 doses of ENGERIX-B were administered to 5,071 healthy adults and children who were initially seronegative for hepatitis B markers, and healthy neonates. All subjects were monitored for 4 days post-administration. Frequency of adverse events tended to decrease with successive doses of ENGERIX-B.

Using a symptom checklist, the most frequently reported adverse events were injection site soreness (22%) and fatigue (14%). Other events are listed below. Parent or guardian completed forms for children and neonates. Neonatal checklist did not include headache, fatigue, or dizziness.

Incidence 1% to 10% of Injections: *Nervous System Disorders:* Dizziness, headache.

General Disorders and Administration Site Conditions: Fever (>37.5°C), injection site erythema, injection site induration, injection site swelling.

Incidence <1% of Injections: *Infections and Infestations:* Upper respiratory tract illnesses.

Blood and Lymphatic System Disorders: Lymphadenopathy.

Metabolism and Nutrition Disorders: Anorexia.

Psychiatric Disorders: Agitation, insomnia.

Nervous System Disorders: Somnolence, tingling.

Vascular Disorders: Flushing, hypotension.

Gastrointestinal Disorders: Abdominal pain/cramps, constipation, diarrhea, nausea, vomiting.

Skin and Subcutaneous Tissue Disorders: Erythema, petechiae, pruritus, rash, sweating, urticaria.

Musculoskeletal and Connective Tissue Disorders: Arthralgia, back pain, myalgia, pain/stiffness in arm, shoulder, or neck.

General Disorders and Administration Site Conditions: Chills, influenza-like symptoms, injection site ecchymosis, injection site pain, injection site pruritus, irritability, malaise, weakness.

6.2 Postmarketing Experience

In addition to reports in clinical trials, worldwide voluntary reports of adverse events received for ENGERIX-B since market introduction (1990) are listed below. This list includes serious adverse events or events which have a suspected causal connection to components of ENGERIX-B.

The following adverse events have been identified during postapproval use of ENGERIX-B. Because these events are reported voluntarily from a population of unknown size, it is not always possible to reliably estimate their frequency or establish a causal relationship to the vaccine.

Infections and Infestations: Herpes zoster, meningitis.

Blood and Lymphatic System Disorders: Thrombocytopenia.

Immune System Disorders: Allergic reaction, anaphylactoid reaction, anaphylaxis. An apparent hypersensitivity syndrome (serum sickness-like) of delayed onset has been reported days to weeks after vaccination, including: arthralgia/arthritis (usually transient), fever, and dermatologic reactions such as urticaria, erythema multiforme, ecchymoses, and erythema nodosum.

Nervous System Disorders: Encephalitis, encephalopathy, migraine, multiple sclerosis, neuritis, neuropathy including hypoesthesia, paresthesia, Guillain-Barré syndrome and Bell's palsy, optic neuritis, paralysis, paresis, seizures, syncope, transverse myelitis.

Eye Disorders: Conjunctivitis, keratitis, visual disturbances.

Ear and Labyrinth Disorders: Earache, tinnitus, vertigo.

Cardiac Disorders: Palpitations, tachycardia.

Vascular Disorders: Vasculitis.

Respiratory, Thoracic and Mediastinal Disorders: Apnea, bronchospasm including asthma-like symptoms.

Gastrointestinal Disorders: Dyspepsia.

Skin and Subcutaneous Tissue Disorders: Alopecia, angioedema, eczema, erythema multiforme including Stevens-Johnson syndrome, erythema nodosum, lichen planus, purpura.

Musculoskeletal and Connective Tissue Disorders: Arthritis, muscular weakness.

General Disorders and Administration Site Conditions: Injection site reaction.

Investigations: Abnormal liver function tests.

7 DRUG INTERACTIONS

7.1 Concomitant Administration With Vaccines and Immune Globulin

ENGERIX-B may be administered concomitantly with immune globulin.

When concomitant administration of other vaccines or immune globulin is required, they should be given with different syringes and at different injection sites. Do not mix ENGERIX-B with any other vaccine or product in the same syringe or vial.

8 USE IN SPECIFIC POPULATIONS

8.1 Pregnancy

Pregnancy Category C

Animal reproduction studies have not been conducted with ENGERIX-B. It is also not known whether ENGERIX-B can cause fetal harm when administered to a pregnant woman or can affect reproduction capacity. ENGERIX-B should be given to a pregnant woman only if clearly needed.

8.3 Nursing Mothers

It is not known whether ENGERIX-B is excreted in human milk. Because many drugs are excreted in human milk, caution should be exercised when ENGERIX-B is administered to a nursing woman.

8.4 Pediatric Use

Safety and effectiveness of ENGERIX-B have been established in all pediatric age groups. Maternally transferred antibodies do not interfere with the active immune response to the vaccine. *[See Adverse Reactions (6) and Clinical Studies (14.1, 14.3, 14.4).]*

8.5 Geriatric Use

Clinical studies of ENGERIX-B used for licensure did not include sufficient numbers of subjects 65 years of age and older to determine whether they respond differently from younger subjects. However, in later studies it has been shown that a diminished antibody response and seroprotective levels can be expected in persons older than 60 years of age.[5]

11 DESCRIPTION

ENGERIX-B [Hepatitis B Vaccine (Recombinant)] is a sterile suspension of noninfectious hepatitis B virus surface antigen (HBsAg) for intramuscular administration. It contains purified surface antigen of the virus obtained by culturing genetically engineered *Saccharomycescerevisiae* cells, which carry the surface antigen gene of the hepatitis B virus. The HBsAg expressed in the cells is purified by several physicochemical steps and formulated as a suspension of the antigen adsorbed on aluminum hydroxide. The procedures used to manufacture ENGERIX-B result in a product that contains no more than 5% yeast protein.

Each 0.5-mL pediatric/adolescent dose contains 10 mcg of HBsAg adsorbed on 0.25 mg aluminum as aluminum hydroxide.

Each 1-mL adult dose contains 20 mcg of HBsAg adsorbed on 0.5 mg aluminum as aluminum hydroxide.

ENGERIX-B contains the following excipients: Sodium chloride (9 mg/mL) and phosphate buffers (disodium phosphate dihydrate, 0.98 mg/mL; sodium dihydrogen phosphate dihydrate, 0.71 mg/mL).

ENGERIX-B is available in vials and 2 types of prefilled syringes. One type of prefilled syringe has a tip cap which may contain natural rubber latex. The other type has a tip cap and a rubber plunger which contain dry natural latex rubber. The vial stopper does not contain latex. *[See How Supplied/Storage and Handling (16).]*

ENGERIX-B is formulated without preservatives.

12 CLINICAL PHARMACOLOGY

12.1 Mechanism of Action

Infection with hepatitis B virus can have serious consequences including acute massive hepatic necrosis and chronic active hepatitis. Chronically infected persons are at increased risk for cirrhosis and hepatocellular carcinoma.

Antibody concentrations ≥10 mIU/mL against HBsAg are recognized as conferring protection against hepatitis B virus infection.[1] Seroconversion is defined as antibody titers ≥1 mIU/mL.

13 NONCLINICAL TOXICOLOGY

13.1 Carcinogenesis, Mutagenesis, Impairment of Fertility

ENGERIX-B has not been evaluated for carcinogenic or mutagenic potential, or for impairment of fertility.

14 CLINICAL STUDIES

14.1 Efficacy in Neonates

Protective efficacy with ENGERIX-B has been demonstrated in a clinical trial in neonates at high risk of hepatitis B infection.[6,7] Fifty-eight neonates born of mothers who were both HBsAg-positive and hepatitis B "e" antigen (HBeAg)-positive were given ENGERIX-B (10 mcg/0.5 mL) at 0, 1, and 2 months, without concomitant hepatitis B immune globulin (HBIG). Two infants became chronic carriers in the 12-month follow-up period after initial inoculation. Assuming an expected carrier rate of 70%, the protective efficacy rate against the chronic carrier state during the first 12 months of life was 95%.

14.2 Efficacy and Immunogenicity in Specific Populations

Homosexual Men: ENGERIX-B (20 mcg/1 mL) given at 0, 1, and 6 months was evaluated in homosexual men 16 to 59 years of age. Four of 244 subjects became infected with hepatitis B during the period prior to completion of the 3-dose immunization schedule. No additional subjects became infected during the 18-month follow-up period after completion of the immunization course.

Adults with Chronic Hepatitis C: In a clinical trial of 67 adults 25 to 67 years of age with chronic hepatitis C, ENGERIX-B (20 mcg/1 mL) was given at 0, 1, and 6 months. Of the subjects assessed at month 7 (N = 31), 100% responded with seroprotective titers. The geometric mean antibody titer (GMT) was 1,260 mIU/mL (95% Confidence Interval [CI]: 709, 2,237).

Adults on Hemodialysis: Hemodialysis patients given hepatitis B vaccines respond with lower titers, which remain at protective levels for shorter durations than in normal subjects. In a clinical trial of 56 adults who had been on hemodialysis for a mean period of 56 months, ENGERIX-B (40 mcg/2 mL given as two 1-mL doses) was given at 0, 1, 2, and 6 months. Two months after the fourth dose, 67% (29/43) of patients had seroprotective antibody levels (≥10 mIU/mL) and the GMT among seroconverters was 93 mIU/mL.

14.3 Immunogenicity in Neonates

In clinical studies, neonates were given ENGERIX-B (10 mcg/0.5 mL) at 0, 1, and 6 months or at 0, 1, and 2 months of age. The immune response to vaccination was evaluated in sera obtained one month after the third dose of ENGERIX-B.

Among infants administered ENGERIX-B at 0, 1, and 6 months, 100% of evaluable subjects (N = 52) seroconverted by month 7. The GMT was 713 mIU/mL. Of these, 97% had seroprotective levels (≥10 mIU/mL).

Among infants enrolled (N = 381) to receive ENGERIX-B at 0, 1, and 2 months of age, 96% had seroprotective levels (≥10 mIU/mL) by month 4. The GMT among seroconverters (N = 311) (antibody titer ≥1 mIU/mL) was 210 mIU/mL. A subset of these children received a fourth dose of ENGERIX-B at 12 months of age. One month following this dose, seroconverters (N = 126) had a GMT of 2,941 mIU/mL.

14.4 Immunogenicity in Children and Adults

Persons 6 Months Through 10 Years of Age: In clinical trials, children (N = 242) 6 months through 10 years of age were given ENGERIX-B (10 mcg/0.5 mL) at 0, 1, and 6 months. One to 2 months after the third dose, the seroprotection rate was 98% and the GMT of seroconverters was 4,023 mIU/mL.

Persons 5 Through 16 Years of Age: In a separate clinical trial including both children and adolescents 5 through 16 years of age, ENGERIX-B (10 mcg/0.5 mL) was administered at 0, 1, and 6 months (N = 181) or 0, 12, and 24 months (N = 161). Immediately before the third dose of vaccine, seroprotection was achieved in 92.3% of subjects vaccinated on the 0-, 1-, and 6-month schedule and 88.8% of subjects on the 0-, 12-, and 24-month schedule (GMT: 117.9 mIU/mL versus 162.1 mIU/mL, respectively, $P = 0.18$). One month following the third dose, seroprotection was achieved in 99.5% of children vaccinated on the 0-, 1-, and 6-month schedule compared to 98.1% of those on the 0-, 12-, and 24-month schedule. GMTs were higher ($P = 0.02$) for children receiving vaccine on the 0-, 1-, and 6-month schedule compared to those on the 0-, 12-, and 24-month schedule (5,687.4 mIU/mL versus 3,158.7 mIU/mL, respectively).

Persons 11 Through 19 Years of Age: In clinical trials with healthy adolescent subjects 11 through 19 years of age, ENGERIX-B (10 mcg/0.5 mL) given at 0, 1, and 6 months produced a seroprotection rate of 97% at month 8 (N = 119) with a GMT of 1,989 mIU/mL (N = 118, 95% CI: 1,318, 3,020). Immunization with ENGERIX-B (20 mcg/1 mL) at 0, 1, and 6 months produced a seroprotection rate of 99% at month 8 (N = 122) with a GMT of 7,672 mIU/mL (N = 122, 95% CI: 5,248, 10,965).

Persons 16 Through 65 Years of Age: Clinical trials in healthy adult and adolescent subjects (16 through 65 years of age) have shown that following a course of 3 doses of ENGERIX-B (20 mcg/1 mL) given at 0, 1, and 6 months, the seroprotection (antibody titers ≥10 mIU/mL) rate for all individuals was 79% at month 6 (5 months after second dose) and 96% at month 7 (1 month after third dose); the GMT for seroconverters was 2,204 mIU/mL at month 7 (N = 110).

An alternate 3-dose schedule (20 mcg/1 mL given at 0, 1, and 2 months) designed for certain populations (e.g., individuals who have or might have been recently exposed to the virus and travelers to high-risk areas) was also evaluated. At month 3 (1 month after third dose), 99% of all individuals were seroprotected and remained protected through month 12. On the alternate schedule, a fourth dose of ENGERIX-B (20 mcg/1 mL) at 12 months produced a GMT of 9,163 mIU/mL at month 13 (1 month after fourth dose) (N = 373).

Persons 40 Years of Age and Older: Among subjects 40 years of age and older given ENGERIX-B (20 mcg/1 mL) at 0, 1, and 6 months, the seroprotection rate 1 month after the third dose was 88% and the GMT for seroconverters was 610 mIU/mL (N = 50). In adults older than 40 years of age, ENGERIX-B produced anti-HBsAg antibody titers that were lower than those in younger adults.

14.5 Interchangeability With Other Hepatitis B Vaccines

A controlled study (N = 48) demonstrated that completion of a course of immunization with 1 dose of ENGERIX-B (20 mcg/1 mL) at month 6 following 2 doses of RECOMBIVAX HB® (10 mcg) at months 0 and 1 produced a similar GMT (4,077 mIU/mL) to immunization with 3 doses of RECOMBIVAX HB (10 mcg) at months 0, 1, and 6 (GMT: 2,654 mIU/mL). Thus, ENGERIX-B can be used to complete a vaccination course initiated with RECOMBIVAX HB.[8]

15 REFERENCES

1. Centers for Disease Control and Prevention. Hepatitis B. In: Atkinson W, Wolfe C, Humiston S, Nelson R, eds. *Epidemiology and Prevention of Vaccine-Preventable Diseases*. 6th ed. Atlanta, GA: Public Health Foundation; 2000:207-229.
2. Centers for Disease Control and Prevention. A Comprehensive Immunization Strategy to Eliminate Transmission of Hepatitis B Virus Infection in the United States. Recommendations of the Advisory Committee on Immunization Practices (ACIP). Part 1: Immunization of Infants, Children, and Adolescents, MMWR 2005;54(RR-16);1-23.
3. Ascherio A, Zhang SM, Hernán MA, et al. Hepatitis B vaccination and the risk of multiple sclerosis. *N Engl J Med.* 2001;344(5):327-332.
4. Confavreux C, Suissa S, Saddier P, et al. Vaccination and the risk of relapse in multiple sclerosis. *N Engl J Med.* 2001-344(5):319-326.
5. Centers for Disease Control and Prevention. A Comprehensive Immunization Strategy to Eliminate Transmission of Hepatitis B Virus Infection in the United States. Recommendations of the Advisory Committee on Immunization Practices (ACIP). Part 2: Immunization of Adults, MMWR 2006;55(RR-16);1-25.
6. André FE, Safary A. Clinical experience with a yeast-derived hepatitis B vaccine. In: Zuckerman AJ, ed. *Viral Hepatitis and Liver Disease*. New York, NY: Alan R Liss, Inc.; 1988:1025-1030.
7. Poovorawan Y, Sanpavat S, Pongpunlert W, et al. Protective efficacy of a recombinant DNA hepatitis B vaccine in neonates of HBe antigen-positive mothers. *JAMA.* 1989;261(22):3278-3281.
8. Bush LM, Moonsammy GI, Boscia JA. Evaluation of initiating a hepatitis B vaccination schedule with one vaccine and completing it with another. *Vaccine.* 1991;9(11):807-809.

16 HOW SUPPLIED/STORAGE AND HANDLING

ENGERIX-B is available in single-dose vials and prefilled disposable TIP-LOK syringes (packaged without needles) (Preservative Free Formulation):

10 mcg/0.5 mL Pediatric/Adolescent Dose

NDC 58160-820-01 Vial (contains no latex) in Package of 10: NDC 58160-820-11

NDC 58160-820-43 Syringe (tip cap may contain latex) in Package of 10: NDC 58160-820-52

20 mcg/mL Adult Dose

NDC 58160-821-01 Vial (contains no latex) in Package of 10: NDC 58160-821-11

NDC 58160-821-05 Syringe (tip cap may contain latex) in Package of 1: NDC 58160-821-34

NDC 58160-821-43 Syringe (tip cap may contain latex) in Package of 5: NDC 58160-821-48

NDC 58160-821-43 Syringe (tip cap may contain latex) in Package of 10: NDC 58160-821-52

NDC 58160-821-32 Syringe (tip cap and plunger contain latex) in Package of 1: NDC 58160-821-32

NDC 58160-821-31 Syringe (tip cap and plunger contain latex) in Package of 5: NDC 58160-821-46

Store refrigerated between 2° and 8°C (36° and 46°F). Do not freeze; discard if product has been frozen. Do not dilute to administer.

17 PATIENT COUNSELING INFORMATION

- Inform vaccine recipients and parents or guardians of the potential benefits and risks of immunization with ENGERIX-B.
- Emphasize, when educating vaccine recipients and parents or guardians regarding potential side effects, that ENGERIX-B contains non-infectious purified HBsAg and cannot cause hepatitis B infection.
- Instruct vaccine recipients and parents or guardians to report any adverse events to their healthcare provider.
- Give vaccine recipients and parents or guardians the Vaccine Information Statements, which are required by the National Childhood Vaccine Injury Act of 1986 to be given prior to immunization. These materials are available free of charge at the Centers for Disease Control and Prevention (CDC) website (www.cdc.gov/vaccines).

ENGERIX-B and TIP-LOK are registered trademarks of GlaxoSmithKline. RECOMBIVAX HB is a registered trademark of Merck & Co.

Manufactured by **GlaxoSmithKline Biologicals**
Rixensart, Belgium, US License No. 1617
Distributed by **GlaxoSmithKline**
Research Triangle Park, NC 27709

ENG:51PI

EPIVIR-HBV® ℞
[ĕp'ə-vir]
(lamivudine)
Tablets

EPIVIR-HBV® ℞
(lamivudine)
Oral Solution

WARNING

LACTIC ACIDOSIS AND SEVERE HEPATOMEGALY WITH STEATOSIS, INCLUDING FATAL CASES, HAVE BEEN REPORTED WITH THE USE OF NUCLEOSIDE ANALOGUES ALONE OR IN COMBINATION, INCLUDING LAMIVUDINE AND OTHER ANTIRETROVIRALS (SEE WARNINGS).

HUMAN IMMUNODEFICIENCY VIRUS (HIV) COUNSELING AND TESTING SHOULD BE OFFERED TO ALL PATIENTS BEFORE BEGINNING EPIVIR-HBV AND PERIODICALLY DURING TREATMENT (SEE WARNINGS), BECAUSE EPIVIR-HBV TABLETS AND ORAL SOLUTION CONTAIN A LOWER DOSE OF THE SAME ACTIVE INGREDIENT (LAMIVUDINE) AS EPIVIR® TABLETS AND ORAL SOLUTION USED TO TREAT HIV INFECTION. IF TREATMENT WITH EPIVIR-HBV IS PRESCRIBED FOR CHRONIC HEPATITIS B FOR A PATIENT WITH UNRECOGNIZED OR UNTREATED HIV INFECTION, RAPID EMERGENCE OF HIV RESISTANCE IS LIKELY BECAUSE OF SUBTHERAPEUTIC DOSE AND INAPPROPRIATE MONOTHERAPY.

SEVERE ACUTE EXACERBATIONS OF HEPATITIS B HAVE BEEN REPORTED IN PATIENTS WHO HAVE DISCONTINUED ANTI-HEPATITIS B THERAPY (INCLUDING EPIVIR-HBV). HEPATIC FUNCTION SHOULD BE MONITORED CLOSELY WITH BOTH CLINICAL AND LABORATORY FOLLOW-UP FOR AT LEAST SEVERAL MONTHS IN PATIENTS WHO DISCONTINUE ANTI-HEPATITIS B THERAPY. IF APPROPRIATE, INITIATION OF ANTI-HEPATITIS B THERAPY MAY BE WARRANTED (SEE WARNINGS).

DESCRIPTION

EPIVIR-HBV is a brand name for lamivudine, a synthetic nucleoside analogue with activity against hepatitis B virus (HBV) and HIV. Lamivudine was initially developed for the treatment of HIV infection as EPIVIR. Please see the complete prescribing information for EPIVIR Tablets and Oral Solution for additional information. The chemical name of lamivudine is (2R,cis)-4-amino-1-(2-hydroxymethyl-1,3-oxathiolan-5-yl)-(1H)-pyrimidin-2-one. Lamivudine is the (-)enantiomer of a dideoxy analogue of cytidine. Lamivudine has also been referred to as (-)2′,3′-dideoxy, 3′-thiacytidine. It has a molecular formula of $C_8H_{11}N_3O_3S$ and a molecular weight of 229.3. It has the following structural formula:

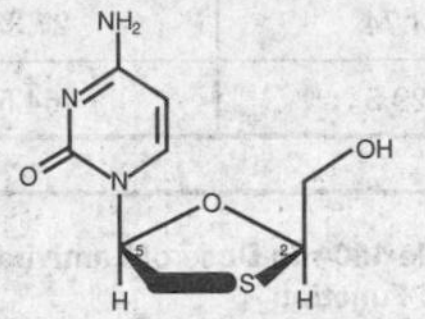

Lamivudine is a white to off-white crystalline solid with a solubility of approximately 70 mg/mL in water at 20°C.

EPIVIR-HBV Tablets are for oral administration. Each tablet contains 100 mg of lamivudine and the inactive ingredients hypromellose, macrogol 400, magnesium stearate, microcrystalline cellulose, polysorbate 80, red iron oxide, sodium starch glycolate, titanium dioxide, and yellow iron oxide.

EPIVIR-HBV Oral Solution is for oral administration. One milliliter (1 mL) of EPIVIR-HBV Oral Solution contains 5 mg of lamivudine (5 mg/mL) in an aqueous solution and the inactive ingredients artificial strawberry and banana flavors, citric acid (anhydrous), methylparaben, propylene glycol, propylparaben, sodium citrate (dihydrate), and sucrose (200 mg).

MICROBIOLOGY

Mechanism of Action:

Lamivudine is a synthetic nucleoside analogue. Intracellularly, lamivudine is phosphorylated to its active 5′-triphosphate metabolite, lamivudine triphosphate, 3TC-TP. Incorporation of the monophosphate form into viral DNA by HBV reverse transcriptase results in DNA chain termination. 3TC-TP also inhibits the RNA- and DNA-dependent DNA polymerase activities of HIV-1 reverse transcriptase (RT). 3TC-TP is a weak inhibitor of mammalian α, β, and γ-DNA polymerases.

Antiviral Activity:

Activity of lamivudine against HBV in cell culture was assessed in HBV DNA-transfected 2.2.15 cells, HB611 cells, and infected human primary hepatocytes. EC_{50} values (the concentration of drug needed to reduce the level of extracellular HBV DNA by 50%) varied from 0.01 μM (2.3 ng/mL) to 5.6 μM (1.3 mcg/mL) depending upon the duration of exposure of cells to lamivudine, the cell model system, and the protocol used. See the EPIVIR package insert for information regarding activity of lamivudine against HIV.

Resistance:

Lamivudine-resistant isolates were identified in patients with virologic breakthrough, defined when using solution hybridization assay as the detection of HBV DNA in serum on 2 or more occasions after failing to detect HBV DNA on 2 or more occasions and defined when using PCR assay as a >1 $\log_{10}$ (10-fold) increase in serum HBV DNA from nadir during treatment in a patient who had an initial virologic response.

Lamivudine-resistant HBV isolates develop M204V/I substitutions in the YMDD motif of the catalytic domain of the viral reverse transcriptase. M204V/I substitutions are frequently accompanied by other substitutions (V173L, L180M) which enhance the level of lamivudine resistance or act as compensatory mutations improving replication efficiency. Other substitutions detected in lamivudine-resistant HBV isolates include L80I and A181T.

In 4 controlled clinical trials in adults with HBeAg-positive chronic hepatitis B virus infection (CHB), YMDD-mutant HBV was detected in 81 of 335 patients receiving lamivudine 100 mg once daily for 52 weeks. The prevalence of YMDD substitutions was less than 10% in each of these trials for patients studied at 24 weeks and increased to an average of 24% (range in 4 studies: 16% to 32%) at 52 weeks. In limited data from a long-term follow-up trial in patients who continued 100 mg/day lamivudine after one of these studies, YMDD substitutions further increased from 18% (10 of 57) at 1 year to 41% (20 of 49), 53% (27 of 51), and 69% (31 of 45) after 2, 3, and 4 years of treatment, respectively. Over the 5-year treatment period, the proportion of patients who developed YMDD-mutant HBV at any time was 69% (40 of 58).

In a controlled trial in pediatric patients, YMDD-mutant HBV was detected in 31 of 166 (19%) patients receiving lamivudine for 52 weeks. For a subgroup who remained on lamivudine therapy in a follow-up study, YMDD mutations increased from 24% (29 of 121) at 12 months to 59% (68 of 115) at 24 months and 64% (66 of 103) at 36 months of lamivudine treatment.

In a controlled study, treatment-naive patients with HBeAg-positive CHB were treated with lamivudine or lamivudine plus adefovir dipivoxil combination therapy. Following 104 weeks of therapy, YMDD-mutant HBV was detected in 7 of 40 (18%) patients receiving combination therapy compared with 15 of 35 (43%) patients receiving lamivudine-only therapy. In another controlled study, combination therapy was evaluated in adult patients with HBeAg-positive CHB who had YMDD-mutant HBV and diminished clinical and virologic response to lamivudine. Following 52 weeks of lamivudine plus adefovir dipivoxil combination therapy (n = 46) or lamivudine-only therapy (n = 49), YMDD-mutant HBV was detected less frequently in patients receiving combination therapy, 62% vs 96%.

A published study suggested that the rates of lamivudine resistance in patients treated for HBeAg-negative CHB appear to be more variable (0% to 27% at 1 year and 10% to 56% at 2 years).

Cross-Resistance:

HBV: HBV containing lamivudine resistance-associated substitutions (rtL180M, rtM204I, rtM204V, rtL180M + rtM204V, rtV173L + rtL180M + rtM204V) retain susceptibility to adefovir dipivoxil but have reduced susceptibility to entecavir (30 fold) and telbivudine (>100 fold). The lamivudine resistance-associated substitution rtA181T results in diminished response to adefovir and telbivudine. Similarly, HBV with entecavir resistance-associated substitutions (I169T/M250V and T184G/S202I) have >1,000-fold reductions in susceptibility to lamivudine.

HIV: In studies of HIV-1-infected patients who received lamivudine monotherapy or combination therapy with lamivudine plus zidovudine for at least 12 weeks, HIV-1 isolates with reduced susceptibility in cell culture to lamivudine were detected in most patients (see WARNINGS).

CLINICAL PHARMACOLOGY

Pharmacokinetics in Adults:

The pharmacokinetic properties of lamivudine have been studied as single and multiple oral doses ranging from 5 to 600 mg per day administered to HBV-infected patients.

The pharmacokinetic properties of lamivudine have also been studied in asymptomatic, HIV-infected adult patients after administration of single intravenous (IV) doses ranging from 0.25 to 8 mg/kg, as well as single and multiple (twice-daily regimen) oral doses ranging from 0.25 to 10 mg/kg.

Absorption and Bioavailability: Lamivudine was rapidly absorbed after oral administration in HBV-infected patients and in healthy subjects. Following single oral doses of 100 mg, the peak serum lamivudine concentration (C_{max}) in HBV-infected patients (steady state) and healthy subjects (single dose) was 1.28 ± 0.56 mcg/mL and 1.05 ± 0.32 mcg/mL (mean ± SD), respectively, which occurred between 0.5 and 2 hours after administration. The area under the plasma concentration versus time curve ($AUC_{[0\text{-}24\ hr]}$) following 100 mg lamivudine oral single and repeated daily doses to steady state was 4.3 ± 1.4 (mean ± SD) and 4.7 ± 1.7 mcg•hr/mL, respectively. The relative bioavailability of the tablet and solution were then demonstrated in healthy subjects. Although the solution demonstrated a slightly higher peak serum concentration (C_{max}), there was no significant difference in systemic exposure (AUC∞) between the solution and the tablet. Therefore, the solution and the tablet may be used interchangeably.

After oral administration of lamivudine once daily to HBV-infected adults, the AUC and C_{max} increased in proportion to dose over the range from 5 mg to 600 mg once daily.

The 100-mg tablet was administered orally to 24 healthy subjects on 2 occasions, once in the fasted state and once with food (standard meal: 967 kcal; 67 grams fat, 33 grams protein, 58 grams carbohydrate). There was no significant difference in systemic exposure (AUC∞) in the fed and fasted states; therefore, EPIVIR-HBV Tablets and Oral Solution may be administered with or without food.

Lamivudine was rapidly absorbed after oral administration in HIV-infected patients. Absolute bioavailability in 12 adult patients was 86% ± 16% (mean ± SD) for the 150-mg tablet and 87% ± 13% for the 10-mg/mL oral solution.

Distribution: The apparent volume of distribution after IV administration of lamivudine to 20 asymptomatic HIV-infected patients was 1.3 ± 0.4 L/kg, suggesting that lamivudine distributes into extravascular spaces. Volume of distribution was independent of dose and did not correlate with body weight.

Binding of lamivudine to human plasma proteins is low (<36%) and independent of dose. In vitro studies showed that over the concentration range of 0.1 to 100 mcg/mL, the amount of lamivudine associated with erythrocytes ranged from 53% to 57% and was independent of concentration.

Table 1. Pharmacokinetic Parameters (Mean ± SD) Dose-Normalized to a Single 100-mg Oral Dose of Lamivudine in Patients With Varying Degrees of Renal Function

Parameter	Creatinine Clearance Criterion (Number of Subjects)		
	≥80 mL/min (n = 9)	20-59 mL/min (n = 8)	<20 mL/min (n = 6)
Creatinine clearance (mL/min)	97 (range 82-117)	39 (range 25-49)	15 (range 13-19)
C_{max} (mcg/mL)	1.31 ± 0.35	1.85 ± 0.40	1.55 ± 0.31
AUC∞ (mcg•hr/mL)	5.28 ± 1.01	14.67 ± 3.74	27.33 ± 6.56
Cl/F (mL/min)	326.4 ± 63.8	120.1 ± 29.5	64.5 ± 18.3

Table 2. Pharmacokinetic Parameters (Mean ± SD) Dose-Normalized to a Single 100-mg Dose of Lamivudine in 3 Groups of Subjects With Normal or Impaired Hepatic Function

Parameter	Normal (n = 8)	Impairment[a]	
		Moderate (n = 8)	Severe (n = 8)
C_{max} (mcg/mL)	0.92 ± 0.31	1.06 ± 0.58	1.08 ± 0.27
AUC∞ (mcg•hr/mL)	3.96 ± 0.58	3.97 ± 1.36	4.30 ± 0.63
T_{max} (hr)	1.3 ± 0.8	1.4 ± 0.8	1.4 ± 1.2
Cl/F (mL/min)	424.7 ± 61.9	456.9 ± 129.8	395.2 ± 51.8
Clr (mL/min)	279.2 ± 79.2	323.5 ± 100.9	216.1 ± 58.0

[a] Hepatic impairment assessed by aminopyrine breath test.

Metabolism: Metabolism of lamivudine is a minor route of elimination. In man, the only known metabolite of lamivudine is the trans-sulfoxide metabolite. In 9 healthy subjects receiving 300 mg of lamivudine as single oral doses, a total of 4.2% (range 1.5% to 7.5%) of the dose was excreted as the trans-sulfoxide metabolite in the urine, the majority of which was excreted in the first 12 hours.

Serum concentrations of the trans-sulfoxide metabolite have not been determined.

Elimination: The majority of lamivudine is eliminated unchanged in urine by active organic cationic secretion. In 9 healthy subjects given a single 300-mg oral dose of lamivudine, renal clearance was 199.7 ± 56.9 mL/min (mean ± SD). In 20 HIV-infected patients given a single IV dose, renal clearance was 280.4 ± 75.2 mL/min (mean ± SD), representing 71% ± 16% (mean ± SD) of total clearance of lamivudine.

In most single-dose studies in HIV- or HBV-infected patients or healthy subjects with serum sampling for 24 hours after dosing, the observed mean elimination half-life ($t_{1/2}$) ranged from 5 to 7 hours. In HIV-infected patients, total clearance was 398.5 ± 69.1 mL/min (mean ± SD). Oral clearance and elimination half-life were independent of dose and body weight over an oral dosing range from 0.25 to 10 mg/kg.

Special Populations:

Adults With Impaired Renal Function: The pharmacokinetic properties of lamivudine have been determined in healthy subjects and in subjects with impaired renal function, with and without hemodialysis (Table 1).

[See table 1 above]

Exposure (AUC∞), C_{max}, and half-life increased with diminishing renal function (as expressed by creatinine clearance). Apparent total oral clearance (Cl/F) of lamivudine decreased as creatinine clearance decreased. T_{max} was not significantly affected by renal function. Based on these observations, it is recommended that the dosage of lamivudine be modified in patients with renal impairment (see DOSAGE AND ADMINISTRATION).

Hemodialysis increases lamivudine clearance from a mean of 64 to 88 mL/min; however, the length of time of hemodialysis (4 hours) was insufficient to significantly alter mean lamivudine exposure after a single-dose administration. Continuous ambulatory peritoneal dialysis and automated peritoneal dialysis have negligible effects on lamivudine clearance. Therefore, it is recommended, following correction of dose for creatinine clearance, that no additional dose modification be made after routine hemodialysis or peritoneal dialysis.

It is not known whether lamivudine can be removed by continuous (24-hour) hemodialysis.

The effect of renal impairment on lamivudine pharmacokinetics in pediatric patients with chronic hepatitis B is not known.

Adults With Impaired Hepatic Function: The pharmacokinetic properties of lamivudine have been determined in adults with impaired hepatic function (Table 2). Patients were stratified by severity of hepatic functional impairment.

[See table 2 above]

Pharmacokinetic parameters were not altered by diminishing hepatic function. Therefore, no dose adjustment for lamivudine is required for patients with impaired hepatic function. Safety and efficacy of EPIVIR-HBV have not been established in the presence of decompensated liver disease (see PRECAUTIONS).

Post-Hepatic Transplant: Fourteen HBV-infected patients received liver transplant following lamivudine therapy and completed pharmacokinetic assessments at enrollment, 2 weeks after 100-mg once-daily dosing (pre-transplant), and 3 months following transplant; there were no significant differences in pharmacokinetic parameters. The overall exposure of lamivudine is primarily affected by renal dysfunction; consequently, transplant patients with reduced renal function had generally higher exposure than patients with normal renal function. Safety and efficacy of EPIVIR-HBV have not been established in this population (see PRECAUTIONS).

Pediatric Patients: Lamivudine pharmacokinetics were evaluated in a 28-day dose-ranging study in 53 pediatric patients with chronic hepatitis B. Patients aged 2 to 12 years were randomized to receive lamivudine 0.35 mg/kg twice daily, 3 mg/kg once daily, 1.5 mg/kg twice daily, or 4 mg/kg twice daily. Patients aged 13 to 17 years received lamivudine 100 mg once daily. Lamivudine was rapidly absorbed (T_{max} 0.5 to 1 hour). In general, both C_{max} and exposure (AUC) showed dose proportionality in the dosing range studied. Weight-corrected oral clearance was highest at age 2 and declined from 2 to 12 years, where values were then similar to those seen in adults. A dose of 3 mg/kg given once daily produced a steady-state lamivudine AUC (mean 5,953 ng•hr/mL ± 1,562 SD) similar to that associated with a dose of 100 mg/day in adults.

Gender: There are no significant gender differences in lamivudine pharmacokinetics.

Race: There are no significant racial differences in lamivudine pharmacokinetics.

Drug Interactions:

Multiple doses of lamivudine and a single dose of interferon were coadministered to 19 healthy male subjects in a pharmacokinetics study. Results indicated a small (10%) reduction in lamivudine AUC, but no change in interferon pharmacokinetic parameters when the 2 drugs were given in combination. All other pharmacokinetic parameters (C_{max}, T_{max}, and $t_{1/2}$) were unchanged. There was no significant pharmacokinetic interaction between lamivudine and interferon alfa in this study.

Lamivudine and zidovudine were coadministered to 12 asymptomatic HIV-positive adult patients in a single-center, open-label, randomized, crossover study. No significant differences were observed in AUC∞ or total clearance for lamivudine or zidovudine when the 2 drugs were administered together. Coadministration of lamivudine with zidovudine resulted in an increase of 39% ± 62% (mean ± SD) in C_{max} of zidovudine.

Lamivudine and trimethoprim/sulfamethoxazole (TMP/SMX) were coadministered to 14 HIV-positive patients in a single-center, open-label, randomized, crossover study. Each patient received treatment with a single 300-mg dose of lamivudine and TMP 160 mg/SMX 800 mg once a day for 5 days with concomitant administration of lamivudine 300 mg with the fifth dose in a crossover design. Coadministration of TMP/SMX with lamivudine resulted in an increase of 44% ± 23% (mean ± SD) in lamivudine AUC∞, a decrease of 29% ± 13% in lamivudine oral clearance, and a decrease of 30% ± 36% in lamivudine renal clearance. The pharmacokinetic properties of TMP and SMX were not altered by coadministration with lamivudine (see PRECAUTIONS: Drug Interactions).

Lamivudine and zalcitabine may inhibit the intracellular phosphorylation of one another. Therefore, use of lamivudine in combination with zalcitabine is not recommended.

INDICATIONS AND USAGE

EPIVIR-HBV is indicated for the treatment of chronic hepatitis B associated with evidence of hepatitis B viral replication and active liver inflammation. This indication is based on 1-year histologic and serologic responses in adult patients with compensated chronic hepatitis B, and more limited information from a study in pediatric patients ages 2 to 17 years (see Description of Clinical Studies below).

The following point should be considered when initiating therapy with EPIVIR-HBV:

- Due to high rates of resistance development in treated patients, initiation of lamivudine treatment should only be considered when the use of an alternative antiviral agent with a higher genetic barrier to resistance is not available or appropriate.

Description of Clinical Studies:

Adults: The safety and efficacy of EPIVIR-HBV were evaluated in 4 controlled studies in 967 patients with compensated chronic hepatitis B. All patients were 16 years of age or older and had chronic hepatitis B virus infection (serum HBsAg-positive for at least 6 months) accompanied by evidence of HBV replication (serum HBeAg-positive and positive for serum HBV DNA, as measured by a research solution-hybridization assay) and persistently elevated ALT levels and/or chronic inflammation on liver biopsy compatible with a diagnosis of chronic viral hepatitis. Three of these studies provided comparisons of EPIVIR-HBV 100 mg once daily versus placebo, and results of these comparisons are summarized below.

- Study 1 was a randomized, double-blind study of EPIVIR-HBV 100 mg once daily versus placebo for 52 weeks followed by a 16-week no-treatment period in treatment-naive US patients.
- Study 2 was a randomized, double-blind, 3-arm study that compared EPIVIR-HBV 25 mg once daily versus EPIVIR-HBV 100 mg once daily versus placebo for 52 weeks in Asian patients.
- Study 3 was a randomized, partially-blind, 3-arm study conducted primarily in North America and Europe in patients who had ongoing evidence of active chronic hepatitis B despite previous treatment with interferon alfa. The study compared EPIVIR-HBV 100 mg once daily for 52 weeks, followed by either EPIVIR-HBV 100 mg or matching placebo once daily for 16 weeks (Arm 1), versus placebo once daily for 68 weeks (Arm 2). (A third arm using a combination of interferon and lamivudine is not presented here because there was not sufficient information to evaluate this regimen.)

Principal endpoint comparisons for the histologic and serologic outcomes in lamivudine (100 mg daily) and placebo recipients in placebo-controlled studies are shown in the following tables.

[See table 3 at top of next page]

[See table 4 at top of next page]

Normalization of serum ALT levels was more frequent with lamivudine treatment compared with placebo in Studies 1-3.

The majority of lamivudine-treated patients showed a decrease of HBV DNA to below the assay limit early in the course of therapy. However, reappearance of assay-detectable HBV DNA during lamivudine treatment was observed in approximately one third of patients after this initial response.

Pediatrics: The safety and efficacy of EPIVIR-HBV were evaluated in a double-blind clinical trial in 286 patients ranging from 2 to 17 years of age, who were randomized (2:1) to receive 52 weeks of lamivudine (3 mg/kg once daily to a maximum of 100 mg once daily) or placebo. All patients had compensated chronic hepatitis B accompanied by evidence of hepatitis B virus replication (positive serum HBeAg and positive for serum HBV DNA by a research branched-chain DNA assay) and persistently elevated serum ALT levels. The combination of loss of HBeAg and reduction of HBV DNA to below the assay limit of the research assay, evaluated at Week 52, was observed in 23% of lamivudine subjects and 13% of placebo subjects. Normalization of serum ALT was achieved and maintained to Week 52 more frequently in patients treated with EPIVIR-HBV compared with placebo (55% versus 13%). As in the adult controlled trials, most lamivudine-treated subjects had decreases in HBV DNA below the assay limit early in treatment, but about one third of subjects with this initial response had reappearance of assay-detectable HBV DNA during treatment. Adolescents (ages 13 to 17 years) showed less evidence of treatment effect than younger children.

CONTRAINDICATIONS

EPIVIR-HBV Tablets and EPIVIR-HBV Oral Solution are contraindicated in patients with previously demonstrated clinically significant hypersensitivity to any of the components of the products.

WARNINGS

Lactic Acidosis/Severe Hepatomegaly With Steatosis:
Lactic acidosis and severe hepatomegaly with steatosis, including fatal cases, have been reported with the use of nucleoside analogues alone or in combination, including lamivudine and other antiretrovirals. A majority of these cases have been in women. Obesity and prolonged nucleoside exposure may be risk factors. Most of these reports have described patients receiving nucleoside analogues for treatment of HIV infection, but there have been reports of lactic acidosis in patients receiving lamivudine for hepatitis B. Particular caution should be exercised when administering EPIVIR or EPIVIR-HBV to any patient with known risk factors for liver disease; however, cases have also been reported in patients with no known risk factors. Treatment with EPIVIR or EPIVIR-HBV should be suspended in any patient who develops clinical or laboratory findings suggestive of lactic acidosis or pronounced hepatotoxicity (which may include hepatomegaly and steatosis even in the absence of marked transaminase elevations).

Important Differences Between Lamivudine-Containing Products, HIV Testing, and Risk of Emergence of Resistant HIV:
EPIVIR-HBV Tablets and Oral Solution contain a lower dose of the same active ingredient (lamivudine) as EPIVIR Tablets and Oral Solution, COMBIVIR® (lamivudine/zidovudine) Tablets, EPZICOM® (abacavir sulfate and lamivudine) Tablets, and TRIZIVIR® (abacavir, lamivudine, and zidovudine) Tablets used to treat HIV infection. The formulation and dosage of lamivudine in EPIVIR-HBV are not appropriate for patients dually infected with HBV and HIV. If a decision is made to administer lamivudine to such patients, the higher dosage indicated for HIV therapy should be used as part of an appropriate combination regimen, and the prescribing information for EPIVIR, COMBIVIR, EPZICOM, or TRIZIVIR as well as for EPIVIR-HBV should be consulted. HIV counseling and testing should be offered to all patients before beginning EPIVIR-HBV and periodically during treatment because of the risk of rapid emergence of resistant HIV and limitation of treatment options if EPIVIR-HBV is prescribed to treat chronic hepatitis B in a patient who has unrecognized or untreated HIV infection or acquires HIV infection during treatment.

Posttreatment Exacerbations of Hepatitis:
Clinical and laboratory evidence of exacerbations of hepatitis have occurred after discontinuation of EPIVIR-HBV (these have been primarily detected by serum ALT elevations, in addition to the re-emergence of HBV DNA commonly observed after stopping treatment; see Table 7 for more information regarding frequency of posttreatment ALT elevations). Although most events appear to have been self-limited, fatalities have been reported in some cases. The causal relationship to discontinuation of lamivudine treatment is unknown. Patients should be closely monitored with both clinical and laboratory follow-up for at least several months after stopping treatment. There is insufficient evidence to determine whether re-initiation of therapy alters the course of posttreatment exacerbations of hepatitis.

Pancreatitis:
Pancreatitis has been reported in patients receiving lamivudine, particularly in HIV-infected pediatric patients with prior nucleoside exposure.

PRECAUTIONS

General:
Patients should be assessed before beginning treatment with EPIVIR-HBV by a physician experienced in the management of chronic hepatitis B.

Emergence of Resistance-Associated HBV Mutations:
In controlled clinical trials, YMDD-mutant HBV were detected in patients with on-lamivudine re-appearance of HBV DNA after an initial decline below the solution-hybridization assay limit (see MICROBIOLOGY: Drug Resistance). These mutations can be detected by a research assay and have been associated with reduced susceptibility to lamivudine in vitro. Lamivudine-treated patients (adult and pediatric) with YMDD-mutant HBV at 52 weeks showed diminished treatment responses in comparison to lamivudine-treated patients without evidence of YMDD mutations, including lower rates of HBeAg seroconversion and HBeAg loss (no greater than placebo recipients), more frequent return of positive HBV DNA by solution-hybridization or branched-chain DNA assay, and more frequent ALT elevations. In the controlled trials, when patients developed YMDD-mutant HBV, they had a rise in HBV DNA and ALT from their own previous on-treatment levels. Progression of hepatitis B, including death, has been reported in some patients with YMDD-mutant HBV, including patients from the liver transplant setting and from other clinical trials. In clinical practice, monitoring of ALT and HBV DNA levels during lamivudine treatment may aid in treatment decisions if emergence of viral mutants is suspected.

Table 3. Histologic Response at Week 52 Among Adult Patients Receiving EPIVIR-HBV 100 mg Once Daily or Placebo

	Study 1		Study 2		Study 3	
Assessment	EPIVIR-HBV (n = 62)	Placebo (n = 63)	EPIVIR-HBV (n = 131)	Placebo (n = 68)	EPIVIR-HBV (n = 110)	Placebo (n = 54)
Improvement[a]	55%	25%	56%	26%	56%	26%
No Improvement	27%	59%	36%	62%	25%	54%
Missing Data	18%	16%	8%	12%	19%	20%

[a] Improvement was defined as a ≥2-point decrease in the Knodell Histologic Activity Index (HAI)[1] at Week 52 compared with pretreatment HAI. Patients with missing data at baseline were excluded.

Table 4. HBeAg Seroconversion[a] at Week 52 Among Adult Patients Receiving EPIVIR-HBV 100 mg Once Daily or Placebo

	Study 1		Study 2		Study 3	
Seroconversion	EPIVIR-HBV (n = 63)	Placebo (n = 69)	EPIVIR-HBV (n = 140)	Placebo (n = 70)	EPIVIR-HBV (n = 108)	Placebo (n = 53)
Responder	17%	6%	16%	4%	15%	13%
Nonresponder	67%	78%	80%	91%	69%	68%
Missing Data	16%	16%	4%	4%	17%	19%

[a] Three-component seroconversion was defined as Week 52 values showing loss of HBeAg, gain of HBeAb, and reduction of HBV DNA to below the solution-hybridization assay limit. Subjects with negative baseline HBeAg or HBV DNA assay were excluded from the analysis.

Limitations of Populations Studied:
Safety and efficacy of EPIVIR-HBV have not been established in patients with decompensated liver disease or organ transplants; pediatric patients <2 years of age; patients dually infected with HBV and HCV, hepatitis delta, or HIV; or other populations not included in the principal phase III controlled studies. There are no studies in pregnant women and no data regarding effect on vertical transmission, and appropriate infant immunizations should be used to prevent neonatal acquisition of HBV.

Assessing Patients During Treatment:
Patients should be monitored regularly during treatment by a physician experienced in the management of chronic hepatitis B. The safety and effectiveness of treatment with EPIVIR-HBV beyond 1 year have not been established. During treatment, combinations of such events such as return of persistently elevated ALT, increasing levels of HBV DNA over time after an initial decline below assay limit, progression of clinical signs or symptoms of hepatic disease, and/or worsening of hepatic necroinflammatory findings may be considered as potentially reflecting loss of therapeutic response. Such observations should be taken into consideration when determining the advisability of continuing therapy with EPIVIR-HBV.

The optimal duration of treatment, the durability of HBeAg seroconversions occurring during treatment, and the relationship between treatment response and long-term outcomes such as hepatocellular carcinoma or decompensated cirrhosis are not known.

Patients With Impaired Renal Function:
Reduction of the dosage of EPIVIR-HBV is recommended for patients with impaired renal function (see CLINICAL PHARMACOLOGY and DOSAGE AND ADMINISTRATION).

Information for Patients:
A Patient Package Insert (PPI) for EPIVIR-HBV is available for patient information.

Patients should remain under the care of a physician while taking EPIVIR-HBV. They should discuss any new symptoms or concurrent medications with their physician.

Patients should be advised that EPIVIR-HBV is not a cure for hepatitis B, that the long-term treatment benefits of EPIVIR-HBV are unknown at this time, and, in particular, that the relationship of initial treatment response to outcomes such as hepatocellular carcinoma and decompensated cirrhosis is unknown. Patients should be informed that deterioration of liver disease has occurred in some cases when treatment was discontinued. Patients should be advised to discuss any changes in regimen with their physician.

Patients should be informed that emergence of resistant hepatitis B virus and worsening of disease can occur during treatment, and they should promptly report any new symptoms to their physician.

Patients should be counseled on the importance of testing for HIV to avoid inappropriate therapy and development of resistant HIV, and HIV counseling and testing should be offered before starting EPIVIR-HBV and periodically during therapy. Patients should be advised that EPIVIR-HBV Tablets and EPIVIR-HBV Oral Solution contain a lower dose of the same active ingredient (lamivudine) as EPIVIR Tablets, EPIVIR Oral Solution, COMBIVIR Tablets, EPZICOM Tablets, and TRIZIVIR Tablets. EPIVIR-HBV should not be taken concurrently with EPIVIR, COMBIVIR, EPZICOM, or TRIZIVIR (see WARNINGS). Patients infected with both HBV and HIV who are planning to change their HIV treatment regimen to a regimen that does not include EPIVIR, COMBIVIR, EPZICOM, or TRIZIVIR should discuss continued therapy for hepatitis B with their physician.

Patients should be advised that treatment with EPIVIR-HBV has not been shown to reduce the risk of transmission of HBV to others through sexual contact or blood contamination (see Pregnancy section).

Diabetic patients should be advised that each 20-mL dose of EPIVIR-HBV Oral Solution contains 4 grams of sucrose.

Drug Interactions:
Lamivudine is predominantly eliminated in the urine by active organic cationic secretion. The possibility of interactions with other drugs administered concurrently should be considered, particularly when their main route of elimination is active renal secretion via the organic cationic transport system (e.g., trimethoprim).

TMP 160 mg/SMX 800 mg once daily has been shown to increase lamivudine exposure (AUC) by 44% (see CLINICAL PHARMACOLOGY). No change in dose of either drug is recommended. There is no information regarding the effect on lamivudine pharmacokinetics of higher doses of TMP/SMX such as those used to treat *Pneumocystis carinii* pneumonia. No data are available regarding interactions with other drugs that have renal clearance mechanisms similar to that of lamivudine.

Lamivudine and zalcitabine may inhibit the intracellular phosphorylation of one another. Therefore, use of lamivudine in combination with zalcitabine is not recommended.

Carcinogenesis, Mutagenesis, and Impairment of Fertility:
Lamivudine long-term carcinogenicity studies in mice and rats showed no evidence of carcinogenic potential at exposures up to 34 times (mice) and 200 times (rats) those ob-

served in humans at the recommended therapeutic dose for chronic hepatitis B. Lamivudine was not active in a microbial mutagenicity screen or an in vitro cell transformation assay, but showed weak in vitro mutagenic activity in a cytogenetic assay using cultured human lymphocytes and in the mouse lymphoma assay. However, lamivudine showed no evidence of in vivo genotoxic activity in the rat at oral doses of up to 2,000 mg/kg producing plasma levels of 60 to 70 times those in humans at the recommended dose for chronic hepatitis B. In a study of reproductive performance, lamivudine administered to rats at doses up to 4,000 mg/kg/day, producing plasma levels 80 to 120 times those in humans, revealed no evidence of impaired fertility and no effect on the survival, growth, and development to weaning of the offspring.

Pregnancy:

Pregnancy Category C. Reproduction studies have been performed in rats and rabbits at orally administered doses up to 4,000 mg/kg/day and 1,000 mg/kg/day, respectively, producing plasma levels up to approximately 60 times that for the adult HBV dose. No evidence of teratogenicity due to lamivudine was observed. Evidence of early embryolethality was seen in the rabbit at exposure levels similar to those observed in humans, but there was no indication of this effect in the rat at exposures up to 60 times that in humans. Studies in pregnant rats and rabbits showed that lamivudine is transferred to the fetus through the placenta. There are no adequate and well-controlled studies in pregnant women. Because animal reproductive toxicity studies are not always predictive of human response, lamivudine should be used during pregnancy only if the potential benefits outweigh the risks.

Lamivudine has not been shown to affect the transmission of HBV from mother to infant, and appropriate infant immunizations should be used to prevent neonatal acquisition of HBV.

Pregnancy Registry: To monitor maternal-fetal outcomes of pregnant women exposed to lamivudine, a Pregnancy Registry has been established. Physicians are encouraged to register patients by calling 1-800-258-4263.

Nursing Mothers:

A study in lactating rats administered 45 mg/kg of lamivudine showed that lamivudine concentrations in milk were slightly greater than those in plasma. Lamivudine is also excreted in human milk. Samples of breast milk obtained from 20 mothers receiving lamivudine monotherapy (300 mg twice daily) or combination therapy (150 mg lamivudine twice daily and 300 mg zidovudine twice daily) had measurable concentrations of lamivudine.

Because of the potential for serious adverse reactions in nursing infants, **mothers should be instructed not to breastfeed if they are receiving lamivudine.**

Pediatric Use:

HBV: Safety and efficacy of lamivudine for treatment of chronic hepatitis B in children have been studied in pediatric patients from 2 to 17 years of age in a controlled clinical trial (see CLINICAL PHARMACOLOGY, INDICATIONS AND USAGE, and DOSAGE AND ADMINISTRATION).

Safety and efficacy in pediatric patients <2 years of age have not been established.

HIV: See the complete prescribing information for EPIVIR Tablets and Oral Solution for additional information on pharmacokinetics of lamivudine in HIV-infected children.

Geriatric Use:

Clinical studies of EPIVIR-HBV did not include sufficient numbers of subjects aged 65 and over to determine whether they respond differently from younger subjects. In general, dose selection for an elderly patient should be cautious, reflecting the greater frequency of decreased hepatic, renal, or cardiac function, and of concomitant disease or other drug therapy. In particular, because lamivudine is substantially excreted by the kidney and elderly patients are more likely to have decreased renal function, renal function should be monitored and dosage adjustments should be made accordingly (see PRECAUTIONS: Patients with Impaired Renal Function and DOSAGE AND ADMINISTRATION).

ADVERSE REACTIONS

Several serious adverse events reported with lamivudine (lactic acidosis and severe hepatomegaly with steatosis, posttreatment exacerbations of hepatitis B, pancreatitis, and emergence of viral mutants associated with reduced drug susceptibility and diminished treatment response) are also described in WARNINGS and PRECAUTIONS.

Clinical Trials In Chronic Hepatitis B:

Adults: Selected clinical adverse events observed with a ≥5% frequency during therapy with EPIVIR-HBV compared with placebo are listed in Table 5. Frequencies of specified laboratory abnormalities during therapy with EPIVIR-HBV compared with placebo are listed in Table 6.

Table 5. Selected Clinical Adverse Events (≥5% Frequency) in 3 Placebo-Controlled Clinical Trials in Adults During Treatment[a] (Studies 1-3)

Adverse Event	EPIVIR-HBV (n = 332)	Placebo (n = 200)
Non-site Specific		
Malaise and fatigue	24%	28%
Fever or chills	7%	9%
Ear, Nose, and Throat		
Ear, nose, and throat infections	25%	21%
Sore throat	13%	8%
Gastrointestinal		
Nausea and vomiting	15%	17%
Abdominal discomfort and pain	16%	17%
Diarrhea	14%	12%
Musculoskeletal		
Myalgia	14%	17%
Arthralgia	7%	5%
Neurological		
Headache	21%	21%
Skin		
Skin rashes	5%	5%

[a] Includes patients treated for 52 to 68 weeks.

Table 6. Frequencies of Specified Laboratory Abnormalities in 3 Placebo-Controlled Trials in Adults During Treatment[a] (Studies 1-3)

Test (Abnormal Level)	Patients With Abnormality/ Patients With Observations	
	EPIVIR-HBV	Placebo
ALT >3 × baseline[b]	37/331 (11%)	26/199 (13%)
Albumin <2.5 g/dL	0/331 (0%)	2/199 (1%)
Amylase >3 × baseline	2/259 (<1%)	4/167 (2%)
Serum Lipase ≥2.5 × ULN[c]	19/189 (10%)	9/127 (7%)
CPK ≥7 × baseline	31/329 (9%)	9/198 (5%)
Neutrophils <750/mm^3	0/331 (0%)	1/199 (<1%)
Platelets <50,000/mm^3	10/272 (4%)	5/168 (3%)

[a] Includes patients treated for 52 to 68 weeks.
[b] See *Table 7* for posttreatment ALT values.
[c] Includes observations during and after treatment in the 2 placebo-controlled trials that collected this information.
ULN = Upper limit of normal.

In patients followed for up to 16 weeks after discontinuation of treatment, posttreatment ALT elevations were observed more frequently in patients who had received EPIVIR-HBV than in patients who had received placebo. A comparison of ALT elevations between Weeks 52 and 68 in patients who discontinued EPIVIR-HBV at Week 52 and patients in the same studies who received placebo throughout the treatment course is shown in Table 7.

Table 7. Posttreatment ALT Elevations in 2 Placebo-Controlled Studies in Adults With No-Active-Treatment Follow-up (Studies 1 and 3)

Abnormal Value	Patients With ALT Elevation/Patients With Observations[a]	
	EPIVIR-HBV	Placebo
ALT ≥2 × baseline value	37/137 (27%)	22/116 (19%)
ALT ≥3 × baseline value[b]	29/137 (21%)	9/116 (8%)
ALT ≥2 × baseline value and absolute ALT >500 IU/L	21/137 (15%)	8/116 (7%)
ALT ≥2 × baseline value; and bilirubin >2 × ULN and ≥2 × baseline value	1/137 (0.7%)	1/116 (0.9%)

[a] Each patient may be represented in one or more category.
[b] Comparable to a Grade 3 toxicity in accordance with modified WHO criteria.
ULN = Upper limit of normal.

Lamivudine in Patients With HIV:

In HIV-infected patients, safety information reflects a higher dose of lamivudine (150 mg b.i.d.) than the dose used to treat chronic hepatitis B in HIV-negative patients. In clinical trials using lamivudine as part of a combination regimen for treatment of HIV infection, several clinical adverse events occurred more often in lamivudine-containing treatment arms than in comparator arms. These included nasal signs and symptoms (20% vs. 11%), dizziness (10% vs. 4%), and depressive disorders (9% vs. 4%). Pancreatitis was observed in 9 of the 2,613 adult patients (<0.5%) who received EPIVIR in controlled clinical trials. Laboratory abnormalities reported more often in lamivudine-containing arms included neutropenia and elevations of liver function tests (also more frequent in lamivudine-containing arms for a retrospective analysis of HIV/HBV dually infected patients in one study), and amylase elevations. Please see the complete prescribing information for EPIVIR Tablets and Oral Solution for more information.

Pediatric Patients With Hepatitis B:

Most commonly observed adverse events in the pediatric trials were similar to those in adult trials; in addition, respiratory symptoms (cough, bronchitis, and viral respiratory infections) were reported in both lamivudine and placebo recipients. Posttreatment transaminase elevations were observed in some patients followed after cessation of lamivudine.

Pediatric Patients With HIV Infection:

In early open-label studies of lamivudine in children with HIV, peripheral neuropathy and neutropenia were reported, and pancreatitis was observed in 14% to 15% of patients.

Observed During Clinical Practice:

The following events have been identified during post-approval use of lamivudine in clinical practice. Because they are reported voluntarily from a population of unknown size, estimates of frequency cannot be made. These events have been chosen for inclusion due to either their seriousness, frequency of reporting, potential causal connection to lamivudine, or a combination of these factors. Postmarketing experience with lamivudine at this time is largely limited to use in HIV-infected patients.

Digestive: Stomatitis.
Endocrine and Metabolic: Hyperglycemia.
General: Weakness.
Hemic and Lymphatic: Anemia (including pure red cell aplasia and severe anemias progressing on therapy), lymphadenopathy, splenomegaly.
Hepatic and Pancreatic: Lactic acidosis and steatosis, pancreatitis, posttreatment exacerbation of hepatitis *(see WARNINGS and PRECAUTIONS)*.
Hypersensitivity: Anaphylaxis, urticaria.
Musculoskeletal: Rhabdomyolysis.
Nervous: Paresthesia, peripheral neuropathy.
Respiratory: Abnormal breath sounds/wheezing.
Skin: Alopecia, pruritus, rash.

OVERDOSAGE

There is no known antidote for EPIVIR-HBV. One case of an adult ingesting 6 g of EPIVIR was reported; there were no clinical signs or symptoms noted and hematologic tests remained normal. Because a negligible amount of lamivudine was removed via (4-hour) hemodialysis, continuous ambulatory peritoneal dialysis, and automated peritoneal dialysis, it is not known if continuous hemodialysis would provide clinical benefit in a lamivudine overdose event. If overdose occurs, the patient should be monitored, and standard supportive treatment applied as required.

DOSAGE AND ADMINISTRATION

Adults:

The recommended oral dose of EPIVIR-HBV for treatment of chronic hepatitis B in adults is 100 mg once daily (see paragraph below and WARNINGS). Safety and effectiveness of treatment beyond 1 year have not been established and the optimum duration of treatment is not known (see PRECAUTIONS).

The formulation and dosage of lamivudine in EPIVIR-HBV are not appropriate for patients dually infected with HBV and HIV. If lamivudine is administered to such patients, the higher dosage indicated for HIV therapy should be used as part of an appropriate combination regimen, and the prescribing information for EPIVIR as well as EPIVIR-HBV should be consulted.

Pediatric Patients:

The recommended oral dose of EPIVIR-HBV for pediatric patients 2 to 17 years of age with chronic hepatitis B is 3 mg/kg once daily up to a maximum daily dose of 100 mg. Safety and effectiveness of treatment beyond 1 year have not been established and the optimum duration of treatment is not known (see PRECAUTIONS).

EPIVIR-HBV is available in a 5-mg/mL oral solution when a liquid formulation is needed. (Please see information above regarding distinctions between different lamivudine-containing products.)

Dose Adjustment:

It is recommended that doses of EPIVIR-HBV be adjusted in accordance with renal function (Table 8) (see CLINICAL PHARMACOLOGY: Special Populations).

Table 8. Adjustment of Adult Dosage of EPIVIR-HBV in Accordance With Creatinine Clearance

Creatinine Clearance (mL/min)	Recommended Dosage of EPIVIR-HBV
≥50	100 mg once daily
30-49	100 mg first dose, then 50 mg once daily
15-29	100 mg first dose, then 25 mg once daily
5-14	35 mg first dose, then 15 mg once daily
<5	35 mg first dose, then 10 mg once daily

No additional dosing of EPIVIR-HBV is required after routine (4-hour) hemodialysis or peritoneal dialysis.

Although there are insufficient data to recommend a specific dose adjustment of EPIVIR-HBV in pediatric patients with renal impairment, a dose reduction should be considered.

HOW SUPPLIED

EPIVIR-HBV Tablets, 100 mg, are butterscotch-colored, film-coated, biconvex, capsule-shaped tablets imprinted with "GX CG5" on one side.

Bottles of 60 tablets (NDC 0173-0662-00) with child-resistant closures.

Store at 25°C (77°F), excursions permitted to 15° to 30°C (59° to 86°F) [see USP Controlled Room Temperature].

EPIVIR-HBV Oral Solution, a clear, colorless to pale yellow, strawberry-banana-flavored liquid, contains 5 mg of lamivudine in each 1 mL in plastic bottles of 240 mL.

Bottles of 240 mL (NDC 0173-0663-00) with child-resistant closures. This product does not require reconstitution.

Store at controlled room temperature of 20° to 25°C (68° to 77°F) (see USP) in tightly closed bottles.

REFERENCES

1. Knodell RG, Ishak KG, Black WC, et al. Formulation and application of a numerical scoring system for assessing histological activity in asymptomatic chronic active hepatitis. *Hepatology*. 1982;1:431-435.

EPIVIR-HBV is a registered trademark of GlaxoSmithKline.

The other brands listed are trademarks of their respective owners and are not trademarks of GlaxoSmithKline. The makers of these brands are not affiliated with and do not endorse GlaxoSmithKline or its products.

GlaxoSmithKline
Research Triangle Park, NC 27709
Manufactured under agreement from
Shire Pharmaceuticals Group plc
Basingstoke, UK

January 2011
EPH: 2PI

PHARMACIST-DETACH HERE AND GIVE INSTRUCTIONS TO PATIENT

PATIENT INFORMATION

EPIVIR-HBV® (lamivudine) Tablets
EPIVIR-HBV® (lamivudine) Oral Solution

Please read this information before you start taking EPIVIR-HBV (pronounced EP-i-veer h-b-v). Re-read it each time you get your prescription, in case some information has changed. **This information does not take the place of careful discussions with your doctor when you start this medication and at checkups. Stay under a doctor's care when you take EPIVIR-HBV and do not change or stop treatment without first talking with your doctor.**

What is EPIVIR-HBV?

EPIVIR-HBV is the brand name of a product that contains lamivudine, a drug used to treat chronic hepatitis B in patients with actively growing virus and liver inflammation. Hepatitis B can cause damage to cells in the liver. Eventually, this can scar the liver.

The lamivudine in EPIVIR-HBV can reduce the ability of the hepatitis B virus to multiply and infect new liver cells. It may help to lower the amount of hepatitis B virus in your body. EPIVIR-HBV contains a lower dose of lamivudine than the dose in EPIVIR®, COMBIVIR®, EPZICOM®, and TRIZIVIR®.

Why should I consider HIV testing before starting treatment with EPIVIR-HBV?

Your doctor or healthcare provider should offer you counseling and testing for HIV infection (sometimes called the AIDS virus) before treatment for hepatitis B is started with EPIVIR-HBV, and periodically during treatment. EPIVIR-HBV Tablets and EPIVIR-HBV Oral Solution contain a lower dose of the medicine than other lamivudine-containing drugs, such as EPIVIR, COMBIVIR, EPZICOM, and TRIZIVIR which are used to treat HIV. Treatment with EPIVIR-HBV in HIV-infected patients may cause the HIV virus to be less treatable with lamivudine and some other drugs.

If I am HIV-positive, can I take EPIVIR-HBV?

People who have both chronic hepatitis B and HIV should not take EPIVIR-HBV. EPIVIR-HBV Tablets and EPIVIR-HBV Oral Solution contain a lower dose of the same drug (lamivudine) as EPIVIR Tablets, EPIVIR Oral Solution, COMBIVIR Tablets, EPZICOM Tablets, and TRIZIVIR Tablets. If you have both hepatitis B and HIV, make sure that your doctor or healthcare provider is aware that you have both infections. If you are prescribed lamivudine as part of your combination treatment for HIV, you should use only the products and doses that are intended for treatment of HIV infection, because the lower dose of lamivudine in EPIVIR-HBV could cause the HIV virus to be less responsive to treatment. If you are planning to change your HIV treatment to a regimen that does not include EPIVIR, COMBIVIR, EPZICOM, or TRIZIVIR, you should first discuss this change with your doctor or healthcare provider.

Does EPIVIR-HBV cure hepatitis B infection?

EPIVIR-HBV is not a cure for hepatitis B. In studies comparing EPIVIR-HBV with placebo (an inactive sugar pill) for 1 year, more people treated with EPIVIR-HBV had reductions in liver inflammation. It is not known whether EPIVIR-HBV will reduce the risk of getting liver cancer or cirrhosis that may be caused by the hepatitis B virus.

In studies, some patients developed hepatitis B viruses that are resistant to EPIVIR-HBV. These patients generally had less benefit from treatment with EPIVIR-HBV. Some patients have had worsening of hepatitis after resistant virus appears. The long-term importance of a resistant virus is not known.

What happens if I stop taking EPIVIR-HBV?

After stopping treatment with EPIVIR-HBV, some patients have had symptoms or blood tests showing that their hepatitis has gotten worse. Therefore, your doctor should check your health, which may include blood tests, for at least several months after stopping treatment with EPIVIR-HBV. Tell your doctor right away about any new or unusual symptoms that you notice after stopping treatment.

Who should not take EPIVIR-HBV?

You should not take EPIVIR-HBV if you have or may have HIV infection (sometimes called the AIDS virus). EPIVIR-HBV does not contain an appropriate dose of lamivudine for treatment of HIV infection, and using EPIVIR-HBV could cause the HIV virus to become less treatable with lamivudine and some other drugs.

You should not take EPIVIR-HBV if you are also taking EPIVIR, COMBIVIR, EPZICOM, or TRIZIVIR. These drugs all contain lamivudine.

You should not take EPIVIR-HBV if you have had an allergic reaction to lamivudine.

EPIVIR-HBV has not been studied in children less than 2 years old.

Can pregnant women and nursing mothers take EPIVIR-HBV?

There are no studies of EPIVIR-HBV in pregnant women. If you are pregnant or if you become pregnant while taking EPIVIR-HBV, notify your doctor or healthcare provider immediately.

EPIVIR-HBV has not been shown to prevent the spread of the hepatitis B virus from mother to infant.

It is not known whether lamivudine is passed to the infant in breast milk. If there is lamivudine in the breast milk, this could cause side effects in nursing infants. Mothers should not breastfeed while taking EPIVIR-HBV or other forms of lamivudine.

How should I take EPIVIR-HBV?

Your doctor will tell you how much EPIVIR-HBV to take. The usual dose is 1 EPIVIR-HBV Tablet orally (by mouth) once a day. Your doctor may prescribe a lower dose if you have problems with your kidneys. EPIVIR-HBV may be taken with food or on an empty stomach. To help you remember to take your EPIVIR-HBV as prescribed, you should try to take EPIVIR-HBV at the same time each day. You must not skip doses or stop treatment without first talking with your doctor or healthcare provider. A strawberry-banana-flavored liquid of EPIVIR-HBV is available for patients who need a liquid.

If you miss your regular time for taking your dose, but then remember it during that same day, take your missed dose immediately. Then, take your next dose at the regularly scheduled time the following day. Do **not** take 2 doses of EPIVIR-HBV at once to make up for missing a dose. If you are not sure what to do if you miss taking your medication, check with your doctor or healthcare provider for further instructions.

EPIVIR-HBV can usually be taken with many other medications; however, be sure to tell your doctor or healthcare provider about all medications (including over-the-counter and prescription drugs) that you are taking. EPIVIR-HBV Tablets and EPIVIR-HBV Oral Solution contain a lower dose of the same drug (lamivudine) as EPIVIR Tablets, EPIVIR Oral Solution, COMBIVIR Tablets, EPZICOM Tablets, and TRIZIVIR Tablets; therefore, EPIVIR-HBV should not be taken together with EPIVIR, COMBIVIR, EPZICOM, or TRIZIVIR.

You should talk to your doctor about any changes in your treatment.

What are the possible side effects of EPIVIR-HBV?

You should stay under the care of a doctor during treatment so you can be checked for possible serious side effects. Serious side effects such as inflammation of the pancreas can occur with EPIVIR-HBV. Lactic acid buildup in the body and an enlarged liver have been reported with EPIVIR-HBV; this is not common but can result in death.

Hepatitis B virus sometimes becomes resistant to EPIVIR-HBV during treatment, and some people have had tests showing that their hepatitis was getting worse around the time the virus became resistant. Some people also have worsening of hepatitis after stopping EPIVIR-HBV. You should discuss any change in treatment with your doctor.

In studies, the most common side effects seen during treatment with EPIVIR-HBV were ear, nose, and throat infections; malaise and fatigue (feeling tired and run down); headache; abdominal discomfort and pain; nausea and vomiting; diarrhea; muscle pain; sore throat; joint pain; fever or chills; and skin rash.

This list of possible side effects is not complete. Your doctor or pharmacist can discuss with you a more complete list of possible side effects with EPIVIR-HBV. Talk to your doctor right away about any side effects or other unusual symptoms that occur when taking EPIVIR-HBV.

Does EPIVIR-HBV reduce the risk of passing hepatitis B to others?

No, EPIVIR-HBV has not been shown to reduce the risk of passing hepatitis B to others through sexual contact or exposure to infected blood. EPIVIR-HBV also has not been shown to reduce the risk of a mother passing hepatitis B to her baby.

What previous or current medical problems or conditions should I discuss with my doctor or healthcare provider?

Talk to your doctor or healthcare provider if:

- You have HIV infection.
- You are pregnant or if you become pregnant while taking EPIVIR-HBV.
- You are breastfeeding.
- You have diabetes. Each 20 mL dose (100 mg) of EPIVIR-HBV Oral Solution contains 4 grams of sucrose.

Also talk to your doctor or healthcare provider about:

- Problems with your blood counts.
- Problems with your muscles.
- Problems with your kidneys.
- Problems with your pancreas.
- Any side effects or unusual symptoms during treatment.

How should I store EPIVIR-HBV Tablets and Oral Solution?

EPIVIR-HBV Tablets and Oral Solution should be stored at room temperature. They do not require refrigeration. **Keep EPIVIR-HBV and all medicines out of the reach of children.**

Other Information

This medication is prescribed for a particular condition. Do not use it for any other condition or give it to anybody else. For more complete information about EPIVIR-HBV ask your doctor or pharmacist. You can also ask to read the longer information leaflet that is written for health professionals.

Keep EPIVIR-HBV and all medicines out of the reach of children. In case of overdose, get medical help or contact a Poison Control Center right away.

EPIVIR-HBV is a registered trademark of GlaxoSmithKline.

The other brands listed are trademarks of their respective owners and are not trademarks of GlaxoSmithKline. The makers of these brands are not affiliated with and do not endorse GlaxoSmithKline or its products.

GlaxoSmithKline
Research Triangle Park, NC 27709
Manufactured under agreement from
Shire Pharmaceuticals Group plc
Basingstoke, UK

January 2011
EPH: 2PIL

FLOLAN® ℞

[flō'lan]
(epoprostenol sodium)
for Injection

DESCRIPTION

FLOLAN (epoprostenol sodium) for Injection is a sterile sodium salt formulated for intravenous (IV) administration. Each vial of FLOLAN contains epoprostenol sodium equivalent to either 0.5 mg (500,000 ng) or 1.5 mg (1,500,000 ng) epoprostenol, 3.76 mg glycine, 2.93 mg sodium chloride, and 50 mg mannitol. Sodium hydroxide may have been added to adjust pH.

Table 1. Hemodynamics During Chronic Administration of FLOLAN in Patients With Idiopathic or Heritable PAH

	Baseline		Mean Change from Baseline at End of Treatment Period*	
Hemodynamic Parameter	FLOLAN (N = 52)	Standard Therapy (N = 54)	FLOLAN (N = 48)	Standard Therapy (N = 41)
CI (L/min/m²)	2.0	2.0	0.3†	-0.1
PAPm (mm Hg)	60	60	-5†	1
PVR (Wood U)	16	17	-4†	1
SAPm (mm Hg)	89	91	-4	-3
SV (mL/beat)	44	43	6†	-1
TPR (Wood U)	20	21	-5†	1

* At 8 weeks: FLOLAN N = 10, conventional therapy N = 11 (N is the number of patients with hemodynamic data).
At 12 weeks: FLOLAN N = 38, conventional therapy N = 30 (N is the number of patients with hemodynamic data).
† Denotes statistically significant difference between FLOLAN and conventional therapy groups.
CI = cardiac index, PAPm = mean pulmonary arterial pressure, PVR = pulmonary vascular resistance, SAPm = mean systemic arterial pressure, SV = stroke volume, TPR = total pulmonary resistance.

Epoprostenol (PGI_2, PGX, prostacyclin), a metabolite of arachidonic acid, is a naturally occurring prostaglandin with potent vasodilatory activity and inhibitory activity of platelet aggregation.

Epoprostenol is (5Z,9α,11α,13E,15S)-6,9-epoxy-11,15-dihydroxyprosta-5,13-dien-1-oic acid.

Epoprostenol sodium has a molecular weight of 374.45 and a molecular formula of $C_{20}H_{31}NaO_5$. The structural formula is:

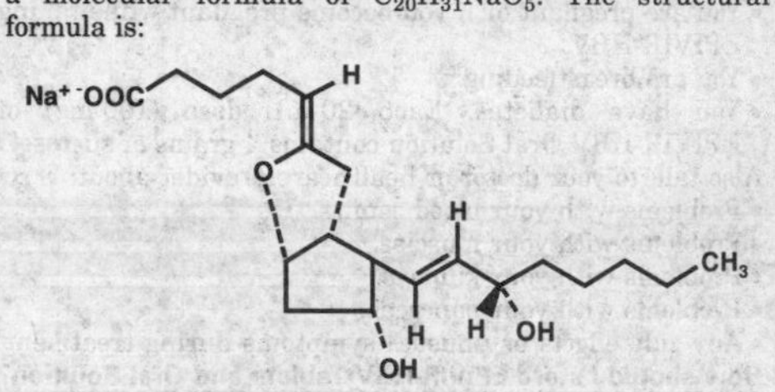

FLOLAN is a white to off-white powder that must be reconstituted with STERILE DILUENT for FLOLAN. STERILE DILUENT for FLOLAN is supplied in glass vials containing 50 mL of 94 mg glycine, 73.3 mg sodium chloride, sodium hydroxide (added to adjust pH), and Water for Injection, USP.

The reconstituted solution of FLOLAN has a pH of 10.2 to 10.8 and is increasingly unstable at a lower pH.

CLINICAL PHARMACOLOGY

General

Epoprostenol has 2 major pharmacological actions: (1) direct vasodilation of pulmonary and systemic arterial vascular beds, and (2) inhibition of platelet aggregation. In animals, the vasodilatory effects reduce right- and left-ventricular afterload and increase cardiac output and stroke volume. The effect of epoprostenol on heart rate in animals varies with dose. At low doses, there is vagally mediated bradycardia, but at higher doses, epoprostenol causes reflex tachycardia in response to direct vasodilation and hypotension. No major effects on cardiac conduction have been observed. Additional pharmacologic effects of epoprostenol in animals include bronchodilation, inhibition of gastric acid secretion, and decreased gastric emptying.

Pharmacokinetics

Epoprostenol is rapidly hydrolyzed at neutral pH in blood and is also subject to enzymatic degradation. Animal studies using tritium-labeled epoprostenol have indicated a high clearance (93 mL/kg/min), small volume of distribution (357 mL/kg), and a short half-life (2.7 minutes). During infusions in animals, steady-state plasma concentrations of tritium-labeled epoprostenol were reached within 15 minutes and were proportional to infusion rates.

No available chemical assay is sufficiently sensitive and specific to assess the in vivo human pharmacokinetics of epoprostenol. The in vitro half-life of epoprostenol in human blood at 37°C and pH 7.4 is approximately 6 minutes; therefore, the in vivo half-life of epoprostenol in humans is expected to be no greater than 6 minutes. The in vitro pharmacologic half-life of epoprostenol in human plasma, based on inhibition of platelet aggregation, was similar for males (n = 954) and females (n = 1,024).

Tritium-labeled epoprostenol has been administered to humans in order to identify the metabolic products of epoprostenol. Epoprostenol is metabolized to 2 primary metabolites: 6-keto-$PGF_{1\alpha}$ (formed by spontaneous degradation) and 6,15-diketo-13,14-dihydro-$PGF_{1\alpha}$ (enzymatically formed), both of which have pharmacological activity orders of magnitude less than epoprostenol in animal test systems. The recovery of radioactivity in urine and feces over a 1-week period was 82% and 4% of the administered dose, respectively. Fourteen additional minor metabolites have been isolated from urine, indicating that epoprostenol is extensively metabolized in humans.

CLINICAL TRIALS IN PULMONARY ARTERIAL HYPERTENSION (PAH)

Acute Hemodynamic Effects

Acute intravenous infusions of FLOLAN for up to 15 minutes in patients with idiopathic or heritable PAH or PAH associated with scleroderma spectrum of diseases (PAH/SSD) produce dose-related increases in cardiac index (CI) and stroke volume (SV) and dose-related decreases in pulmonary vascular resistance (PVR), total pulmonary resistance (TPR), and mean systemic arterial pressure (SAPm). The effects of FLOLAN on mean pulmonary artery pressure (PAPm) were variable and minor.

Chronic Infusion in Idiopathic or Heritable PAH

Hemodynamic Effects

Chronic continuous infusions of FLOLAN in patients with idiopathic or heritable PAH were studied in 2 prospective, open, randomized trials of 8 and 12 weeks' duration comparing FLOLAN plus conventional therapy to conventional therapy alone. Dosage of FLOLAN was determined as described in DOSAGE AND ADMINISTRATION and averaged 9.2 ng/kg/min at study's end. Conventional therapy varied among patients and included some or all of the following: anticoagulants in essentially all patients; oral vasodilators, diuretics, and digoxin in one half to two thirds of patients; and supplemental oxygen in about half the patients. Except for 2 New York Heart Association (NYHA) functional Class II patients, all patients were either functional Class III or Class IV. As results were similar in the 2 studies, the pooled results are described. Chronic hemodynamic effects were generally similar to acute effects. Increases in CI, SV, and arterial oxygen saturation and decreases in PAPm, mean right atrial pressure (RAPm), TPR, and systemic vascular resistance (SVR) were observed in patients who received FLOLAN chronically compared to those who did not. Table 1 illustrates the treatment-related hemodynamic changes in these patients after 8 or 12 weeks of treatment.

[See table 1 above]

These hemodynamic improvements appeared to persist when FLOLAN was administered for at least 36 months in an open, nonrandomized study.

Clinical Effects

Statistically significant improvement was observed in exercise capacity, as measured by the 6-minute walk test in patients receiving continuous intravenous FLOLAN plus conventional therapy (N = 52) for 8 or 12 weeks compared to those receiving conventional therapy alone (N = 54). Improvements were apparent as early as the first week of therapy. Increases in exercise capacity were accompanied by statistically significant improvement in dyspnea and fatigue, as measured by the Chronic Heart Failure Questionnaire and the Dyspnea Fatigue Index.

Survival was improved in NYHA functional Class III and Class IV patients with idiopathic or heritable PAH treated with FLOLAN for 12 weeks in a multicenter, open, randomized, parallel study. At the end of the treatment period, 8 of 40 (20%) patients receiving conventional therapy alone died, whereas none of the 41 patients receiving FLOLAN died (p = 0.003).

Chronic Infusion in PAH/Scleroderma Spectrum of Diseases (SSD)

Hemodynamic Effects

Chronic continuous infusions of FLOLAN in patients with PAH/SSD were studied in a prospective, open, randomized trial of 12 weeks' duration comparing FLOLAN plus conventional therapy (N = 56) to conventional therapy alone (N = 55). Except for 5 NYHA functional Class II patients, all patients were either functional Class III or Class IV. Dosage of FLOLAN was determined as described in DOSAGE AND ADMINISTRATION and averaged 11.2 ng/kg/min at study's end. Conventional therapy varied among patients and included some or all of the following: anticoagulants in essentially all patients, supplemental oxygen and diuretics in two thirds of the patients, oral vasodilators in 40% of the patients, and digoxin in a third of the patients. A statistically significant increase in CI, and statistically significant decreases in PAPm, RAPm, PVR, and SAPm after 12 weeks of treatment were observed in patients who received FLOLAN chronically compared to those who did not. Table 2 illustrates the treatment-related hemodynamic changes in these patients after 12 weeks of treatment.

[See table 2 at top of next page]

Clinical Effects

Statistically significant improvement was observed in exercise capacity, as measured by the 6-minute walk, in patients receiving continuous intravenous FLOLAN plus conventional therapy for 12 weeks compared to those receiving conventional therapy alone. Improvements were apparent in some patients at the end of the first week of therapy. Increases in exercise capacity were accompanied by statistically significant improvements in dyspnea and fatigue, as measured by the Borg Dyspnea Index and Dyspnea Fatigue Index. At week 12, NYHA functional class improved in 21 of 51 (41%) patients treated with FLOLAN compared to none of the 48 patients treated with conventional therapy alone. However, more patients in both treatment groups (28/51 [55%] with FLOLAN and 35/48 [73%] with conventional therapy alone) showed no change in functional class, and 2/51 (4%) with FLOLAN and 13/48 (27%) with conventional therapy alone worsened. Of the patients randomized, NYHA functional class data at 12 weeks were not available for 5 patients treated with FLOLAN and 7 patients treated with conventional therapy alone.

No statistical difference in survival over 12 weeks was observed in PAH/SSD patients treated with FLOLAN as compared to those receiving conventional therapy alone. At the end of the treatment period, 4 of 56 (7%) patients receiving FLOLAN died, whereas 5 of 55 (9%) patients receiving conventional therapy alone died.

No controlled clinical trials with FLOLAN have been performed in patients with pulmonary hypertension associated with other diseases.

INDICATIONS AND USAGE

FLOLAN is indicated for the treatment of pulmonary arterial hypertension (WHO Group I) to improve exercise capacity. Studies establishing effectiveness included predominantly patients with NYHA Functional Class III-IV symptoms and etiologies of idiopathic or heritable PAH or PAH associated with connective tissue diseases.

CONTRAINDICATIONS

A large study evaluating the effect of FLOLAN on survival in NYHA Class III and IV patients with congestive heart failure due to severe left ventricular systolic dysfunction was terminated after an interim analysis of 471 patients revealed a higher mortality in patients receiving FLOLAN plus conventional therapy than in those receiving conventional therapy alone. The chronic use of FLOLAN in patients with congestive heart failure due to severe left ventricular systolic dysfunction is therefore contraindicated.

Some patients with pulmonary hypertension have developed pulmonary edema during dose initiation, which may be associated with pulmonary veno-occlusive disease. FLOLAN should not be used chronically in patients who develop pulmonary edema during dose initiation.

FLOLAN is also contraindicated in patients with known hypersensitivity to the drug or to structurally related compounds.

WARNINGS

FLOLAN must be reconstituted only as directed using STERILE DILUENT for FLOLAN. FLOLAN must not be reconstituted or mixed with any other parenteral medications or solutions prior to or during administration.

Abrupt Withdrawal

Abrupt withdrawal (including interruptions in drug delivery) or sudden large reductions in dosage of FLOLAN may result in symptoms associated with rebound pulmonary hypertension, including dyspnea, dizziness, and asthenia. In clinical trials, one Class III patient's death was judged attributable to the interruption of FLOLAN. Avoid abrupt withdrawal.

Sepsis

See ADVERSE REACTIONS: Adverse Events Attributable to the Drug Delivery System.

PRECAUTIONS

General

FLOLAN should be used only by clinicians experienced in the diagnosis and treatment of pulmonary hypertension. Carefully establish the diagnosis of idiopathic or heritable PAH or PAH/CTD.

FLOLAN is a potent pulmonary and systemic vasodilator. Initiate FLOLAN in a setting with adequate personnel and equipment for physiologic monitoring and emergency care. Dose initiation has been performed during right heart catheterization and without cardiac catheterization. During dose initiation, asymptomatic increases in pulmonary artery pressure coincident with increases in cardiac output occurred rarely. In such cases, consider dose reduction, but such an increase does not imply that chronic treatment is contraindicated.

FLOLAN is a potent inhibitor of platelet aggregation. Therefore, expect an increased risk for hemorrhagic complications, particularly for patients with other risk factors for bleeding (see PRECAUTIONS: Drug Interactions).

During chronic use, deliver FLOLAN continuously on an ambulatory basis through a permanent indwelling central venous catheter. Unless contraindicated, administer anticoagulant therapy to patients receiving FLOLAN to reduce the risk of pulmonary thromboembolism or systemic embolism through a patent foramen ovale. To reduce the risk of infection, use aseptic technique in the reconstitution and administration of FLOLAN and in routine catheter care. Because FLOLAN is metabolized rapidly, even brief interruptions in the delivery of FLOLAN may result in symptoms associated with rebound pulmonary hypertension including dyspnea, dizziness, and asthenia. Intravenous therapy with FLOLAN will likely be needed for prolonged periods, possibly years, so consider the patient's ability to accept and care for a permanent intravenous catheter and infusion pump.

Based on clinical trials, the acute hemodynamic response to FLOLAN did not correlate well with improvement in exercise tolerance or survival during chronic use of FLOLAN. Adjust dosage of FLOLAN during chronic use at the first sign of recurrence or worsening of symptoms attributable to pulmonary hypertension or the occurrence of adverse events associated with FLOLAN (see DOSAGE AND ADMINISTRATION). Following dosage adjustments, monitor standing and supine blood pressure and heart rate closely for several hours.

Information for Patients

Patients receiving FLOLAN should receive the following information. **FLOLAN must be reconstituted only with STERILE DILUENT for FLOLAN.** FLOLAN is infused continuously through a permanent indwelling central venous catheter via a small, portable infusion pump. Thus, therapy with FLOLAN requires commitment by the patient to drug reconstitution, drug administration, and care of the permanent central venous catheter. Patients must adhere to sterile technique in preparing the drug and in the care of the catheter, and even brief interruptions in the delivery of FLOLAN may result in rapid symptomatic deterioration. A patient's decision to receive FLOLAN should be based upon the understanding that there is a high likelihood that therapy with FLOLAN will be needed for prolonged periods, possibly years. The patient's ability to accept and care for a permanent intravenous catheter and infusion pump should also be carefully considered.

Drug Interactions

Additional reductions in blood pressure may occur when FLOLAN is administered with diuretics, antihypertensive agents, or other vasodilators. When other antiplatelet agents or anticoagulants are used concomitantly, there is the potential for FLOLAN to increase the risk of bleeding. However, patients receiving infusions of FLOLAN in clinical trials were maintained on anticoagulants without evidence of increased bleeding. In clinical trials, FLOLAN was used with digoxin, diuretics, anticoagulants, oral vasodilators, and supplemental oxygen.

In a pharmacokinetic substudy in patients with congestive heart failure receiving furosemide or digoxin in whom therapy with FLOLAN was initiated, apparent oral clearance values for furosemide (n = 23) and digoxin (n = 30) were decreased by 13% and 15%, respectively, on the second day of therapy and had returned to baseline values by day 87. The change in furosemide clearance value is not likely to be clinically significant. However, patients on digoxin may show elevations of digoxin concentrations after initiation of therapy with FLOLAN, which may be clinically significant in patients prone to digoxin toxicity.

Table 2. Hemodynamics During Chronic Administration of FLOLAN in Patients With PAH/SSD

Hemodynamic Parameter	Baseline: FLOLAN (N = 56)	Baseline: Conventional Therapy (N = 55)	Mean Change from Baseline at 12 Weeks: FLOLAN (N = 50)	Mean Change from Baseline at 12 Weeks: Conventional Therapy (N = 48)
CI (L/min/m^2)	1.9	2.2	0.5*	-0.1
PAPm (mm Hg)	51	49	-5*	1
RAPm (mm Hg)	13	11	-1*	1
PVR (Wood U)	14	11	-5*	1
SAPm (mm Hg)	93	89	-8*	-1

* Denotes statistically significant difference between FLOLAN and conventional therapy groups (N is the number of patients with hemodynamic data).

CI = cardiac index, PAPm = mean pulmonary arterial pressure, RAPm = mean right arterial pressure, PVR = pulmonary vascular resistance, SAPm = mean systemic arterial pressure.

Carcinogenesis, Mutagenesis, Impairment of Fertility

Long-term studies in animals have not been performed to evaluate carcinogenic potential. A micronucleus test in rats revealed no evidence of mutagenicity. The Ames test and DNA elution tests were also negative, although the instability of epoprostenol makes the significance of these tests uncertain. Fertility was not impaired in rats given FLOLAN by subcutaneous injection at doses up to 100 mcg/kg/day (600 mcg/m^2/day, 2.5 times the recommended human dose [4.6 ng/kg/min or 245.1 mcg/m^2/day, IV] based on body surface area).

Pregnancy

Pregnancy Category B. Reproductive studies have been performed in pregnant rats and rabbits at doses up to 100 mcg/kg/day (600 mcg/m^2/day in rats, 2.5 times the recommended human dose, and 1,180 mcg/m^2/day in rabbits, 4.8 times the recommended human dose based on body surface area) and have revealed no evidence of impaired fertility or harm to the fetus due to FLOLAN. There are, however, no adequate and well-controlled studies in pregnant women. Because animal reproduction studies are not always predictive of human response, this drug should be used during pregnancy only if clearly needed.

Labor and Delivery

The use of FLOLAN during labor, vaginal delivery, or cesarean section has not been adequately studied in humans.

Nursing Mothers

It is not known whether this drug is excreted in human milk. Because many drugs are excreted in human milk, caution should be exercised when FLOLAN is administered to a nursing woman.

Pediatric Use

Safety and effectiveness in pediatric patients have not been established.

Geriatric Use

Clinical studies of FLOLAN in pulmonary hypertension did not include sufficient numbers of subjects aged 65 and over to determine whether they respond differently from younger patients. Other reported clinical experience has not identified differences in responses between the elderly and younger patients. In general, dose selection for an elderly patient should be cautious, usually starting at the low end of the dosing range, reflecting the greater frequency of decreased hepatic, renal, or cardiac function and of concomitant disease or other drug therapy.

ADVERSE REACTIONS

During clinical trials, adverse events were classified as follows: (1) adverse events during dose initiation and escalation, (2) adverse events during chronic dosing, and (3) adverse events associated with the drug delivery system.

Adverse Events During Dose Initiation and Escalation

During early clinical trials, FLOLAN was increased in 2-ng/kg/min increments until the patients developed symptomatic intolerance. The most common adverse events and the adverse events that limited further increases in dose were generally related to vasodilation, the major pharmacologic effect of FLOLAN. The most common dose-limiting adverse events (occurring in ≥1% of patients) were nausea, vomiting, headache, hypotension, and flushing, but also include chest pain, anxiety, dizziness, bradycardia, dyspnea, abdominal pain, musculoskeletal pain, and tachycardia. Table 3 lists the adverse events reported during dose initiation and escalation in decreasing order of frequency.

Table 3. Adverse Events During Dose Initiation and Escalation

Adverse Events Occurring in ≥1% of Patients	FLOLAN (n = 391)
Flushing	58%
Headache	49%
Nausea/vomiting	32%
Hypotension	16%
Anxiety, nervousness, agitation	11%
Chest pain	11%
Dizziness	8%
Bradycardia	5%
Abdominal pain	5%
Musculoskeletal pain	3%
Dyspnea	2%
Back pain	2%
Sweating	1%
Dyspepsia	1%
Hypesthesia/paresthesia	1%
Tachycardia	1%

Adverse Events During Chronic Administration

Interpretation of adverse events is complicated by the clinical features of PAH, which are similar to some of the pharmacologic effects of FLOLAN (e.g., dizziness, syncope). Adverse events which may be related to the underlying disease include dyspnea, fatigue, chest pain, edema, hypoxia, right ventricular failure, and pallor. Several adverse events, on the other hand, can clearly be attributed to FLOLAN. These include hypotension, bradycardia, tachycardia, pulmonary edema, bleeding at various sites, thrombocytopenia, headache, abdominal pain, pain (unspecified), sweating, rash, arthralgia, jaw pain, flushing, diarrhea, nausea and vomiting, flu-like symptoms, anxiety/nervousness, and agitation. In addition, chest pain, fatigue, and pallor have been reported during FLOLAN therapy, and a role for the drug in these events cannot be excluded.

Adverse Events During Chronic Administration for Idiopathic or Heritable PAH

In an effort to separate the adverse effects of the drug from the adverse effects of the underlying disease, Table 4 lists adverse events that occurred at a rate at least 10% greater on FLOLAN in controlled trials.

Table 4. Adverse Events Regardless of Attribution Occurring in Patients With Idiopathic or Heritable PAH With ≥10% Difference Between FLOLAN and Conventional Therapy Alone

Adverse Event	FLOLAN (n = 52)	Conventional Therapy (n = 54)
Occurrence More Common With FLOLAN		
General		
Chills/fever/sepsis/flu-like symptoms	25%	11%
Cardiovascular		
Tachycardia	35%	24%
Flushing	42%	2%

Gastrointestinal		
Diarrhea	37%	6%
Nausea/vomiting	67%	48%
Musculoskeletal		
Jaw pain	54%	0%
Myalgia	44%	31%
Nonspecific musculoskeletal pain	35%	15%
Neurological		
Anxiety/nervousness/tremor	21%	9%
Dizziness	83%	70%
Headache	83%	33%
Hypesthesia, hyperesthesia, paresthesia	12%	2%

Thrombocytopenia has been reported during uncontrolled clinical trials in patients receiving FLOLAN.

Adverse Events During Chronic Administration for PAH/SSD

In an effort to separate the adverse effects of the drug from the adverse effects of the underlying disease, Table 5 lists adverse events that occurred at a rate at least 10% greater on FLOLAN in the controlled trial.

Table 5. Adverse Events Regardless of Attribution Occurring in Patients with PAH/SSD With ≥10% Difference Between FLOLAN and Conventional Therapy Alone

Adverse Event	FLOLAN (n = 56)	Conventional Therapy (n = 55)
Occurrence More Common With FLOLAN		
Cardiovascular		
Flushing	23%	0%
Hypotension	13%	0%
Gastrointestinal		
Anorexia	66%	47%
Nausea/vomiting	41%	16%
Diarrhea	50%	5%
Musculoskeletal		
Jaw pain	75%	0%
Pain/neck pain/arthralgia	84%	65%
Neurological		
Headache	46%	5%
Skin and Appendages		
Skin ulcer	39%	24%
Eczema/rash/urticaria	25%	4%

Although the relationship to FLOLAN administration has not been established, pulmonary embolism has been reported in several patients taking FLOLAN and there have been reports of hepatic failure.

Adverse Events Attributable to the Drug Delivery System

Chronic infusions of FLOLAN are delivered using a small, portable infusion pump through an indwelling central venous catheter. During controlled PAH trials of up to 12 weeks' duration, the local infection rate was about 18%, and the rate for pain was about 11%. During long-term follow-up, sepsis was reported at a rate of 0.3 infections/patient per year in patients treated with FLOLAN. This rate was higher than reported in patients using chronic indwelling central venous catheters to administer parenteral nutrition, but lower than reported in oncology patients using these catheters. Malfunctions in the delivery system resulting in an inadvertent bolus of or a reduction in FLOLAN were associated with symptoms related to excess or insufficient FLOLAN, respectively (see ADVERSE REACTIONS: Adverse Events During Chronic Administration).

Observed During Clinical Practice

In addition to adverse reactions reported from clinical trials, the following events have been identified during post-approval use of FLOLAN. Because they are reported voluntarily from a population of unknown size, estimates of frequency cannot be made. These events have been chosen for inclusion due to a combination of their seriousness, frequency of reporting, or potential causal connection to FLOLAN.

Blood and Lymphatic

Anemia, hypersplenism, pancytopenia, splenomegaly.

Endocrine and Metabolic

Hyperthyroidism.

OVERDOSAGE

Signs and symptoms of excessive doses of FLOLAN during clinical trials are the expected dose-limiting pharmacologic effects of FLOLAN, including flushing, headache, hypotension, tachycardia, nausea, vomiting, and diarrhea. Treatment will ordinarily require dose reduction of FLOLAN.

One patient with PAH/CTD accidentally received 50 mL of an unspecified concentration of FLOLAN. The patient vomited and became unconscious with an initially unrecordable blood pressure. FLOLAN was discontinued and the patient regained consciousness within seconds. In clinical practice, fatal occurrences of hypoxemia, hypotension, and respiratory arrest have been reported following overdosage of FLOLAN.

Single intravenous doses of FLOLAN at 10 and 50 mg/kg (2,703 and 27,027 times the recommended acute phase human dose based on body surface area) were lethal to mice and rats, respectively. Symptoms of acute toxicity were hypoactivity, ataxia, loss of righting reflex, deep slow breathing, and hypothermia.

DOSAGE AND ADMINISTRATION

Important Note

FLOLAN must be reconstituted only with STERILE DILUENT for FLOLAN. Do not dilute reconstituted solutions of FLOLAN or administer with other parenteral solutions or medications (see WARNINGS).

Dosage

Administer continuous chronic infusion of FLOLAN through a central venous catheter. Temporary peripheral intravenous infusion may be used until central access is established. Initiate chronic infusion of FLOLAN at 2 ng/kg/min and increase in increments of 2 ng/kg/min every 15 minutes or longer until dose-limiting pharmacologic effects are elicited or until a tolerance limit to the drug is established or further increases in the infusion rate are not clinically warranted (see Dosage Adjustments). If dose-limiting pharmacologic effects occur, then decrease the infusion rate until FLOLAN is tolerated. In clinical trials, the most common dose-limiting adverse events were nausea, vomiting, hypotension, sepsis, headache, abdominal pain, or respiratory disorder (most treatment-limiting adverse events were not serious). If the initial infusion rate of 2 ng/kg/min is not tolerated, identify a lower dose that is tolerated by the patient.

In the controlled 12-week trial in PAH/SSD, for example, the dose increased from a mean starting dose of 2.2 ng/kg/min. During the first 7 days of treatment, the dose was increased daily to a mean dose of 4.1 ng/kg/min on day 7 of treatment. At the end of week 12, the mean dose was 11.2 ng/kg/min. The mean incremental increase was 2 to 3 ng/kg/min every 3 weeks.

Dosage Adjustments

Base changes in the chronic infusion rate on persistence, recurrence, or worsening of the patient's symptoms of pulmonary hypertension and the occurrence of adverse events due to excessive doses of FLOLAN. In general, expect increases in dose from the initial chronic dose.

Consider increments in dose if symptoms of PAH persist or recur Increase the infusion by 1- to 2-ng/kg/min increments at intervals sufficient to allow assessment of clinical response; these intervals should be at least 15 minutes. In clinical trials, incremental increases in dose occurred at intervals of 24 to 48 hours or longer. Following establishment of a new chronic infusion rate, observe the patient, and monitor standing and supine blood pressure and heart rate for several hours to ensure that the new dose is tolerated. During chronic infusion, the occurrence of dose-limiting pharmacological events may necessitate a decrease in infusion rate, but the adverse event may occasionally resolve without dosage adjustment. Make dosage decreases gradually in 2-ng/kg/min decrements every 15 minutes or longer until the dose-limiting effects resolve. Avoid abrupt withdrawal of FLOLAN or sudden large reductions in infusion rates. Except in life-threatening situations (e.g., unconsciousness, collapse, etc.), adjust infusion rates of FLOLAN only under the direction of a physician.

In patients receiving lung transplants, doses of FLOLAN were tapered after the initiation of cardiopulmonary bypass.

Administration

FLOLAN is administered by continuous intravenous infusion via a central venous catheter using an ambulatory infusion pump. During initiation of treatment, FLOLAN may be administered peripherally.

The ambulatory infusion pump used to administer FLOLAN should: (1) be small and lightweight, (2) be able to adjust infusion rates in 2-ng/kg/min increments, (3) have occlusion, end-of-infusion, and low-battery alarms, (4) be accurate to ±6% of the programmed rate, and (5) be positive pressure-driven (continuous or pulsatile) with intervals between pulses not exceeding 3 minutes at infusion rates used to deliver FLOLAN. The reservoir should be made of polyvinyl chloride, polypropylene, or glass. The infusion pump used in the most recent clinical trials was the CADD-1 HFX 5100 (SIMS Deltec). A 60-inch microbore non-DEHP extension set with proximal antisyphon valve, low priming volume (0.9 mL), and in-line 0.22 micron filter was used during clinical trials.

To avoid interruptions in drug delivery, the patient should have access to a backup infusion pump and intravenous infusion sets. Consider a multi-lumen catheter if other intravenous therapies are routinely administered.

To facilitate extended use at ambient temperatures exceeding 25°C (77°F), a cold pouch with frozen gel packs was used in clinical trials (see DOSAGE AND ADMINISTRATION: Storage and Stability). The cold pouches and gel packs used in clinical trials were obtained from Palco Labs, Palo Alto, California. Any cold pouch used must be capable of maintaining the temperature of reconstituted FLOLAN between 2° and 8°C for 12 hours.

Reconstitution

FLOLAN is stable only when reconstituted with STERILE DILUENT for FLOLAN. FLOLAN must not be reconstituted or mixed with any other parenteral medications or solutions prior to or during administration.

Select a concentration for the solution of FLOLAN that is compatible with the infusion pump being used with respect to minimum and maximum flow rates, reservoir capacity, and the infusion pump criteria listed above. When administered chronically, prepare FLOLAN in a drug delivery reservoir appropriate for the infusion pump with a total reservoir volume of at least 100 mL, using 2 vials of STERILE DILUENT for FLOLAN for use during a 24-hour period. Table 6 gives directions for preparing several different concentrations of FLOLAN.

Table 6. Reconstitution and Dilution Instructions

To make 100 mL of solution with Final Concentration (ng/mL) of:	Directions:
3,000 ng/mL	Dissolve contents of one 0.5-mg vial with 5 mL of STERILE DILUENT for FLOLAN. Withdraw 3 mL and add to sufficient STERILE DILUENT for FLOLAN to make a total of 100 mL.
5,000 ng/mL	Dissolve contents of one 0.5-mg vial with 5 mL of STERILE DILUENT for FLOLAN. Withdraw entire vial contents and add sufficient STERILE DILUENT for FLOLAN to make a total of 100 mL.
10,000 ng/mL	Dissolve contents of two 0.5-mg vials each with 5 mL of STERILE DILUENT for FLOLAN. Withdraw entire vial contents and add sufficient STERILE DILUENT for FLOLAN to make a total of 100 mL.
15,000 ng/mL*	Dissolve contents of one 1.5-mg vial with 5 mL of STERILE DILUENT for FLOLAN. Withdraw entire vial contents and add sufficient STERILE DILUENT for FLOLAN to make a total of 100 mL.

* Higher concentrations may be required for patients who receive FLOLAN long-term.

Generally, 3,000 ng/mL and 10,000 ng/mL are satisfactory concentrations to deliver between 2 to 16 ng/kg/min in adults. Infusion rates may be calculated using the following formula:

Infusion Rate (mL/hr) = [Dose (ng/kg/min) × Weight (kg) × 60 min/hr]
Final Concentration (ng/mL)

Tables 7 through 10 provide infusion delivery rates for doses up to 16 ng/kg/min based upon patient weight, drug delivery rate, and concentration of the solution of FLOLAN to be used. These tables may be used to select the most appropriate concentration of FLOLAN that will result in an infusion rate between the minimum and maximum flow rates of the infusion pump and that will allow the desired duration of infusion from a given reservoir volume. Higher infusion rates, and therefore, more concentrated solutions may be necessary with long-term administration of FLOLAN.

[See table 7 at top of next page]
[See table 8 at top of next page]
[See table 9 at top of next page]
[See table 10 at top of next page]

Storage and Stability

Unopened vials of FLOLAN are stable until the date indicated on the package when stored at 15° to 25°C (59° to 77°F) and protected from light in the carton. Unopened vials of STERILE DILUENT for FLOLAN are stable until the date indicated on the package when stored at 15° to 25°C (59° to 77°F).

Prior to use, reconstituted solutions of FLOLAN must be protected from light and must be refrigerated at 2° to 8°C (36° to 46°F) if not used immediately. **Do not freeze recon-**

Table 7. Infusion Rates for FLOLAN at a Concentration of 3,000 ng/mL

Patient Weight (kg)	Dose or Drug Delivery Rate (ng/kg/min) 2	4	6	8	10	12	14	16
	Infusion Delivery Rate (mL/h)							
10	---	---	1.2	1.6	2.0	2.4	2.8	3.2
20	---	1.6	2.4	3.2	4.0	4.8	5.6	6.4
30	1.2	2.4	3.6	4.8	6.0	7.2	8.4	9.6
40	1.6	3.2	4.8	6.4	8.0	9.6	11.2	12.8
50	2.0	4.0	6.0	8.0	10.0	12.0	14.0	16.0
60	2.4	4.8	7.2	9.6	12.0	14.4	16.8	19.2
70	2.8	5.6	8.4	11.2	14.0	16.8	19.6	22.4
80	3.2	6.4	9.6	12.8	16.0	19.2	22.4	25.6
90	3.6	7.2	10.8	14.4	18.0	21.6	25.2	28.8
100	4.0	8.0	12.0	16.0	20.0	24.0	28.0	32.0

Table 8. Infusion Rates for FLOLAN at a Concentration of 5,000 ng/mL

Patient Weight (kg)	Dose or Drug Delivery Rate (ng/kg/min) 2	4	6	8	10	12	14	16
	Infusion Delivery Rate (mL/h)							
10	---	---	---	1.0	1.2	1.4	1.7	1.9
20	---	1.0	1.4	1.9	2.4	2.9	3.4	3.8
30	---	1.4	2.2	2.9	3.6	4.3	5.0	5.8
40	1.0	1.9	2.9	3.8	4.8	5.8	6.7	7.7
50	1.2	2.4	3.6	4.8	6.0	7.2	8.4	9.6
60	1.4	2.9	4.3	5.8	7.2	8.6	10.1	11.5
70	1.7	3.4	5.0	6.7	8.4	10.1	11.8	13.4
80	1.9	3.8	5.8	7.7	9.6	11.5	13.4	15.4
90	2.2	4.3	6.5	8.6	10.8	13.0	15.1	17.3
100	2.4	4.8	7.2	9.6	12.0	14.4	16.8	19.2

Table 9. Infusion Rates for FLOLAN at a Concentration of 10,000 ng/mL

Patient Weight (kg)	Dose or Drug Delivery Rate (ng/kg/min) 4	6	8	10	12	14	16
	Infusion Delivery Rate (mL/h)						
20	---	---	1.0	1.2	1.4	1.7	1.9
30	---	1.1	1.4	1.8	2.2	2.5	2.9
40	1.0	1.4	1.9	2.4	2.9	3.4	3.8
50	1.2	1.8	2.4	3.0	3.6	4.2	4.8
60	1.4	2.2	2.9	3.6	4.3	5.0	5.8
70	1.7	2.5	3.4	4.2	5.0	5.9	6.7
80	1.9	2.9	3.8	4.8	5.8	6.7	7.7
90	2.2	3.2	4.3	5.4	6.5	7.6	8.6
100	2.4	3.6	4.8	6.0	7.2	8.4	9.6

Table 10. Infusion Rates for FLOLAN at a Concentration of 15,000 ng/mL

Patient Weight (kg)	Dose or Drug Delivery Rate (ng/kg/min) 4	6	8	10	12	14	16
	Infusion Delivery Rate (mL/h)						
30	---	---	1.0	1.2	1.4	1.7	1.9
40	---	1.0	1.3	1.6	1.9	2.2	2.6
50	---	1.2	1.6	2.0	2.4	2.8	3.2
60	1.0	1.4	1.9	2.4	2.9	3.4	3.8
70	1.1	1.7	2.2	2.8	3.4	3.9	4.5
80	1.3	1.9	2.6	3.2	3.8	4.5	5.1
90	1.4	2.2	2.9	3.6	4.3	5.0	5.8
100	1.6	2.4	3.2	4.0	4.8	5.6	6.4

stituted solutions of FLOLAN. Discard any reconstituted solution that has been frozen. Discard any reconstituted solution if it has been refrigerated for more than 48 hours.
During use, a single reservoir of reconstituted solution of FLOLAN can be administered at room temperature for a total duration of 8 hours, or it can be used with a cold pouch and administered up to 24 hours with the use of 2 frozen 6-oz gel packs in a cold pouch. When stored or in use, insulate reconstituted FLOLAN from temperatures greater than 25°C (77°F) and less than 0°C (32°F), and do not expose to direct sunlight.

Use at Room Temperature
Prior to use at room temperature, 15° to 25°C (59° to 77°F), reconstituted solutions of FLOLAN may be stored refrigerated at 2° to 8°C (36° to 46°F) for no longer than 40 hours. When administered at room temperature, reconstituted solutions may be used for no longer than 8 hours. This 48-hour period allows the patient to reconstitute a 2-day supply (200 mL) of FLOLAN. Each 100-mL daily supply may be divided into 3 equal portions. Two of the portions are stored refrigerated at 2° to 8°C (36° to 46°F) until they are used.

Use with a Cold Pouch
Prior to infusion with the use of a cold pouch, solutions may be stored refrigerated at 2° to 8°C (36° to 46°F) for up to 24 hours. When a cold pouch is employed during the infusion, reconstituted solutions of FLOLAN may be used for no longer than 24 hours. Change gel packs every 12 hours. Reconstituted solutions may be kept at 2° to 8°C (36° to 46°F), either in refrigerated storage or in a cold pouch or a combination of the two, for no more than 48 hours.
Inspect parenteral drug products for particulate matter and discoloration prior to administration whenever solution and container permit. If either occurs, do not administer.

HOW SUPPLIED

FLOLAN for Injection is supplied as a sterile freeze-dried powder in 17-mL flint glass vials with gray butyl rubber closures, individually packaged in a carton.
17-mL vial containing epoprostenol sodium equivalent to 0.5 mg (500,000 ng), carton of 1 (NDC 0173-0517-00).
17-mL vial containing epoprostenol sodium equivalent to 1.5 mg (1,500,000 ng), carton of 1 (NDC 0173-0519-00).
Store the vials of FLOLAN at 15° to 25°C (59° to 77°F). Protect from light.
The STERILE DILUENT for FLOLAN is supplied in flint glass vials containing 50-mL diluent with fluororesin-faced butyl rubber closures.
50-mL of STERILE DILUENT for FLOLAN, tray of 2 vials (NDC 0173-0518-01).
Store the vials of STERILE DILUENT for FLOLAN at 15° to 25°C (59° to 77°F). DO NOT FREEZE.
GlaxoSmithKline
Research Triangle Park, NC 27709

March 2011
FLL:2PI

FLONASE® ℞

[flō'nāz]
(fluticasone propionate)
Nasal Spray, 50 mcg
For Intranasal Use Only. SHAKE GENTLY BEFORE USE.

DESCRIPTION

Fluticasone propionate, the active component of FLONASE Nasal Spray, is a synthetic corticosteroid having the chemical name *S*-(fluoromethyl)6α,9-difluoro-11β-17-dihydroxy-16α-methyl-3-oxoandrosta-1,4-diene-17β-carbothioate, 17-propionate and the following chemical structure:

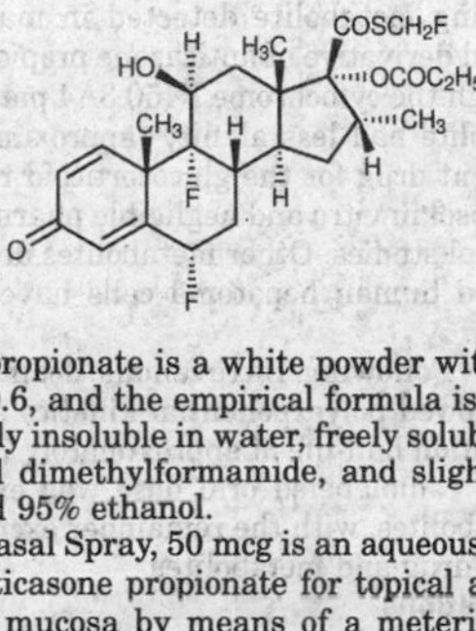

Fluticasone propionate is a white powder with a molecular weight of 500.6, and the empirical formula is $C_{25}H_{31}F_3O_5S$. It is practically insoluble in water, freely soluble in dimethyl sulfoxide and dimethylformamide, and slightly soluble in methanol and 95% ethanol.
FLONASE Nasal Spray, 50 mcg is an aqueous suspension of microfine fluticasone propionate for topical administration to the nasal mucosa by means of a metering, atomizing spray pump. FLONASE Nasal Spray also contains microcrystalline cellulose and carboxymethylcellulose sodium, dextrose, 0.02% w/w benzalkonium chloride, polysorbate 80, and 0.25% w/w phenylethyl alcohol, and has a pH between 5 and 7.
It is necessary to prime the pump before first use or after a period of non-use (1 week or more). After initial priming (6 actuations), each actuation delivers 50 mcg of fluticasone propionate in 100 mg of formulation through the nasal adapter. Each 16-g bottle of FLONASE Nasal Spray provides 120 metered sprays. After 120 metered sprays, the amount of fluticasone propionate delivered per actuation may not be consistent and the unit should be discarded.

CLINICAL PHARMACOLOGY

Mechanism of Action
Fluticasone propionate is a synthetic trifluorinated corticosteroid with anti-inflammatory activity. In vitro dose response studies on a cloned human glucocorticoid receptor system involving binding and gene expression afforded 50% responses at 1.25 and 0.17 nM concentrations, respectively. Fluticasone propionate was 3-fold to 5-fold more potent than dexamethasone in these assays. Data from the McKenzie vasoconstrictor assay in man also support its potent glucocorticoid activity.
In preclinical studies, fluticasone propionate revealed progesterone-like activity similar to the natural hormone. However, the clinical significance of these findings in relation to the low plasma levels (see Pharmacokinetics) is not known.
The precise mechanism through which fluticasone propionate affects allergic rhinitis symptoms is not known. Corticosteroids have been shown to have a wide range of effects on multiple cell types (e.g., mast cells, eosinophils, neutrophils, macrophages, and lymphocytes) and mediators (e.g., histamine, eicosanoids, leukotrienes, and cytokines) involved in inflammation. In 7 trials in adults, FLONASE Nasal Spray has decreased nasal mucosal eosinophils in 66% (35% for placebo) of patients and basophils in 39% (28% for placebo) of patients. The direct relationship of these findings to long-term symptom relief is not known.
FLONASE Nasal Spray, like other corticosteroids, is an agent that does not have an immediate effect on allergic symptoms. A decrease in nasal symptoms has been noted in some patients 12 hours after initial treatment with FLONASE Nasal Spray. Maximum benefit may not be reached for several days. Similarly, when corticosteroids are discontinued, symptoms may not return for several days.

Pharmacokinetics
Absorption: The activity of FLONASE Nasal Spray is due to the parent drug, fluticasone propionate. Indirect calculations indicate that fluticasone propionate delivered by the intranasal route has an absolute bioavailability averaging less than 2%. After intranasal treatment of patients with allergic rhinitis for 3 weeks, fluticasone propionate plasma concentrations were above the level of detection (50 pg/mL) only when recommended doses were exceeded and then only in occasional samples at low plasma levels. Due to the low

bioavailability by the intranasal route, the majority of the pharmacokinetic data was obtained via other routes of administration. Studies using oral dosing of radiolabeled drug have demonstrated that fluticasone propionate is highly extracted from plasma and absorption is low. Oral bioavailability is negligible, and the majority of the circulating radioactivity is due to an inactive metabolite.

Distribution: Following intravenous administration, the initial disposition phase for fluticasone propionate was rapid and consistent with its high lipid solubility and tissue binding. The volume of distribution averaged 4.2 L/kg.

The percentage of fluticasone propionate bound to human plasma proteins averaged 91% with no obvious concentration relationship. Fluticasone propionate is weakly and reversibly bound to erythrocytes and freely equilibrates between erythrocytes and plasma. Fluticasone propionate is not significantly bound to human transcortin.

Metabolism: The total blood clearance of fluticasone propionate is high (average, 1,093 mL/min), with renal clearance accounting for less than 0.02% of the total. The only circulating metabolite detected in man is the 17β-carboxylic acid derivative of fluticasone propionate, which is formed through the cytochrome P450 3A4 pathway. This inactive metabolite had less affinity (approximately 1/2,000) than the parent drug for the glucocorticoid receptor of human lung cytosol in vitro and negligible pharmacological activity in animal studies. Other metabolites detected in vitro using cultured human hepatoma cells have not been detected in man.

Elimination: Following intravenous dosing, fluticasone propionate showed polyexponential kinetics and had a terminal elimination half-life of approximately 7.8 hours. Less than 5% of a radiolabeled oral dose was excreted in the urine as metabolites, with the remainder excreted in the feces as parent drug and metabolites.

Special Populations

Fluticasone propionate nasal spray was not studied in any special populations, and no gender-specific pharmacokinetic data have been obtained.

Drug Interactions

Fluticasone propionate is a substrate of cytochrome P450 3A4. Coadministration of fluticasone propionate and the highly potent cytochrome P450 3A4 inhibitor ritonavir is not recommended based upon a multiple-dose, crossover drug interaction study in 18 healthy subjects. Fluticasone propionate aqueous nasal spray (200 mcg once daily) was coadministered for 7 days with ritonavir (100 mg twice daily). Plasma fluticasone propionate concentrations following fluticasone propionate aqueous nasal spray alone were undetectable (<10 pg/mL) in most subjects, and when concentrations were detectable, peak levels (C_{max}) averaged 11.9 pg/mL (range, 10.8 to 14.1 pg/mL) and $AUC_{(0-\tau)}$ averaged 8.43 pg•hr/mL (range, 4.2 to 18.8 pg•hr/mL). Fluticasone propionate C_{max} and $AUC_{(0-\tau)}$ increased to 318 pg/mL (range, 110 to 648 pg/mL) and 3,102.6 pg•hr/mL (range, 1,207.1 to 5,662.0 pg•hr/mL), respectively, after coadministration of ritonavir with fluticasone propionate aqueous nasal spray. This significant increase in plasma fluticasone propionate exposure resulted in a significant decrease (86%) in plasma cortisol area under the plasma concentration versus time curve (AUC).

Caution should be exercised when other potent cytochrome P450 3A4 inhibitors are coadministered with fluticasone propionate. In a drug interaction study, coadministration of orally inhaled fluticasone propionate (1,000 mcg) and ketoconazole (200 mg once daily) resulted in increased fluticasone propionate exposure and reduced plasma cortisol AUC, but had no effect on urinary excretion of cortisol.

In another multiple-dose drug interaction study, coadministration of orally inhaled fluticasone propionate (500 mcg twice daily) and erythromycin (333 mg 3 times daily) did not affect fluticasone propionate pharmacokinetics.

Pharmacodynamics

In a trial to evaluate the potential systemic and topical effects of FLONASE Nasal Spray on allergic rhinitis symptoms, the benefits of comparable drug blood levels produced by FLONASE Nasal Spray and oral fluticasone propionate were compared. The dosages used were 200 mcg of FLONASE Nasal Spray, the nasal spray vehicle (plus oral placebo), and 5 and 10 mg of oral fluticasone propionate (plus nasal spray vehicle) per day for 14 days. Plasma levels were undetectable in the majority of patients after intranasal dosing, but present at low levels in the majority after oral dosing. FLONASE Nasal Spray was significantly more effective in reducing symptoms of allergic rhinitis than either the oral fluticasone propionate or the nasal vehicle. This trial demonstrated that the therapeutic effect of FLONASE Nasal Spray can be attributed to the topical effects of fluticasone propionate.

In another trial, the potential systemic effects of FLONASE Nasal Spray on the hypothalamic-pituitary-adrenal (HPA) axis were also studied in allergic patients. FLONASE Nasal Spray given as 200 mcg once daily or 400 mcg twice daily was compared with placebo or oral prednisone 7.5 or 15 mg given in the morning. FLONASE Nasal Spray at either dosage for 4 weeks did not affect the adrenal response to 6-hour cosyntropin stimulation, while both dosages of oral prednisone significantly reduced the response to cosyntropin.

CLINICAL TRIALS

A total of 13 randomized, double-blind, parallel-group, multicenter, vehicle placebo-controlled clinical trials were conducted in the United States in adults and pediatric patients (4 years of age and older) to investigate regular use of FLONASE Nasal Spray in patients with seasonal or perennial allergic rhinitis. The trials included 2,633 adults (1,439 men and 1,194 women) with a mean age of 37 (range, 18 to 79 years). A total of 440 adolescents (405 boys and 35 girls), mean age of 14 (range, 12 to 17 years), and 500 children (325 boys and 175 girls), mean age of 9 (range, 4 to 11 years) were also studied. The overall racial distribution was 89% white, 4% black, and 7% other. These trials evaluated the total nasal symptom scores (TNSS) that included rhinorrhea, nasal obstruction, sneezing, and nasal itching in known allergic patients who were treated for 2 to 24 weeks. Subjects treated with FLONASE Nasal Spray exhibited significantly greater decreases in TNSS than vehicle placebo-treated patients. Nasal mucosal basophils and eosinophils were also reduced at the end of treatment in adult studies; however, the clinical significance of this decrease is not known.

There were no significant differences between fluticasone propionate regimens whether administered as a single daily dose of 200 mcg (two 50-mcg sprays in each nostril) or as 100 mcg (one 50-mcg spray in each nostril) twice daily in 6 clinical trials. A clear dose response could not be identified in clinical trials. In 1 trial, 200 mcg/day was slightly more effective than 50 mcg/day during the first few days of treatment; thereafter, no difference was seen.

Two randomized, double-blind, parallel-group, multicenter, vehicle placebo-controlled 28-day trials were conducted in the United States in 732 patients (243 given FLONASE) 12 years of age and older to investigate "as-needed" use of FLONASE Nasal Spray (200 mcg) in patients with seasonal allergic rhinitis. Patients were instructed to take the study medication only on days when they thought they needed the medication for symptom control, not to exceed 2 sprays per nostril on any day, and not more than once daily. "As-needed" use was prospectively defined as average use of study medication no more than 75% of study days. Average use of study medications was 57% to 70% of days for all treatment arms. The studies demonstrated significantly greater reduction in TNSS (sum of nasal congestion, rhinorrhea, sneezing, and nasal itching) with FLONASE Nasal Spray 200 mcg compared to placebo. The relative difference in efficacy with as-needed use as compared to regularly administered doses was not studied.

Three randomized, double-blind, parallel-group, vehicle placebo-controlled trials were conducted in 1,191 patients to investigate regular use of FLONASE Nasal Spray in patients with perennial nonallergic rhinitis. These trials evaluated the patient-rated TNSS (nasal obstruction, postnasal drip, rhinorrhea) in patients treated for 28 days of double-blind therapy and in 1 of the 3 trials for 6 months of open-label treatment. Two of these trials demonstrated that patients treated with FLONASE Nasal Spray at a dosage of 100 mcg twice daily exhibited statistically significant decreases in TNSS compared with patients treated with vehicle.

Individualization of Dosage

Patients should use FLONASE Nasal Spray at regular intervals for optimal effect.

Adult patients may be started on a 200-mcg once-daily regimen (two 50-mcg sprays in each nostril once daily). An alternative 200-mcg/day dosage regimen can be given as 100 mcg twice daily (one 50-mcg spray in each nostril twice daily).

Individual patients will experience a variable time to onset and different degree of symptom relief. In 4 randomized, double-blind, vehicle placebo-controlled, parallel-group allergic rhinitis studies and 2 studies of patients in an outdoor "park" setting (park studies), a decrease in nasal symptoms in treated subjects compared to placebo was shown to occur as soon as 12 hours after treatment with a 200-mcg dose of FLONASE Nasal Spray. Maximum effect may take several days. Regular-use patients who have responded may be able to be maintained (after 4 to 7 days) on 100 mcg/day (1 spray in each nostril once daily).

Some patients (12 years of age and older) with seasonal allergic rhinitis may find as-needed use of FLONASE Nasal Spray (not to exceed 200 mcg daily) effective for symptom control (see CLINICAL TRIALS). Greater symptom control may be achieved with scheduled regular use. Efficacy of as-needed use of FLONASE Nasal Spray has not been studied in pediatric patients under 12 years of age with seasonal allergic rhinitis, or patients with perennial allergic or nonallergic rhinitis.

Pediatric patients (4 years of age and older) should be started with 100 mcg (1 spray in each nostril once daily). Treatment with 200 mcg (2 sprays in each nostril once daily or 1 spray in each nostril twice daily) should be reserved for pediatric patients not adequately responding to 100 mcg daily. Once adequate control is achieved, the dosage should be decreased to 100 mcg (1 spray in each nostril) daily.

Maximum total daily doses should not exceed 2 sprays in each nostril (total dose, 200 mcg/day). There is no evidence that exceeding the recommended dose is more effective.

INDICATIONS AND USAGE

FLONASE Nasal Spray is indicated for the management of the nasal symptoms of seasonal and perennial allergic and nonallergic rhinitis in adults and pediatric patients 4 years of age and older.

Safety and effectiveness of FLONASE Nasal Spray in children below 4 years of age have not been adequately established.

CONTRAINDICATIONS

FLONASE Nasal Spray is contraindicated in patients with a hypersensitivity to any of its ingredients.

WARNINGS

The replacement of a systemic corticosteroid with a topical corticosteroid can be accompanied by signs of adrenal insufficiency, and in addition some patients may experience symptoms of withdrawal, e.g., joint and/or muscular pain, lassitude, and depression. Patients previously treated for prolonged periods with systemic corticosteroids and transferred to topical corticosteroids should be carefully monitored for acute adrenal insufficiency in response to stress. In those patients who have asthma or other clinical conditions requiring long-term systemic corticosteroid treatment, too rapid a decrease in systemic corticosteroids may cause a severe exacerbation of their symptoms.

The concomitant use of intranasal corticosteroids with other inhaled corticosteroids could increase the risk of signs or symptoms of hypercorticism and/or suppression of the HPA axis.

A drug interaction study in healthy subjects has shown that ritonavir (a highly potent cytochrome P450 3A4 inhibitor) can significantly increase plasma fluticasone propionate exposure, resulting in significantly reduced serum cortisol concentrations (see CLINICAL PHARMACOLOGY: Drug Interactions and PRECAUTIONS: Drug Interactions). During postmarketing use, there have been reports of clinically significant drug interactions in patients receiving fluticasone propionate and ritonavir, resulting in systemic corticosteroid effects including Cushing syndrome and adrenal suppression. Therefore, coadministration of fluticasone propionate and ritonavir is not recommended unless the potential benefit to the patient outweighs the risk of systemic corticosteroid side effects.

Persons who are using drugs that suppress the immune system are more susceptible to infections than healthy individuals. Chickenpox and measles, for example, can have a more serious or even fatal course in susceptible children or adults using corticosteroids. In children or adults who have not had these diseases or been properly immunized, particular care should be taken to avoid exposure. How the dose, route, and duration of corticosteroid administration affect the risk of developing a disseminated infection is not known. The contribution of the underlying disease and/or prior corticosteroid treatment to the risk is also not known. If exposed to chickenpox, prophylaxis with varicella zoster immune globulin (VZIG) may be indicated. If exposed to measles, prophylaxis with pooled intramuscular immunoglobulin (IG) may be indicated. (See the respective package inserts for complete VZIG and IG prescribing information.) If chickenpox develops, treatment with antiviral agents may be considered.

Avoid spraying in eyes.

PRECAUTIONS

General

Intranasal corticosteroids may cause a reduction in growth velocity when administered to pediatric patients (see PRECAUTIONS: Pediatric Use).

Rarely, immediate hypersensitivity reactions or contact dermatitis may occur after the administration of FLONASE Nasal Spray. Rare instances of wheezing, nasal septum perforation, cataracts, glaucoma, and increased intraocular pressure have been reported following the intranasal application of corticosteroids, including fluticasone propionate.

Use of excessive doses of corticosteroids may lead to signs or symptoms of hypercorticism and/or suppression of HPA function.

Although systemic effects have been minimal with recommended doses of FLONASE Nasal Spray, potential risk increases with larger doses. Therefore, larger than recommended doses of FLONASE Nasal Spray should be avoided.

When used at higher than recommended doses or in rare individuals at recommended doses, systemic corticosteroid effects such as hypercorticism and adrenal suppression may appear. If such changes occur, the dosage of FLONASE

Nasal Spray should be discontinued slowly consistent with accepted procedures for discontinuing oral corticosteroid therapy.

In clinical studies with fluticasone propionate administered intranasally, the development of localized infections of the nose and pharynx with *Candida albicans* has occurred only rarely. When such an infection develops, it may require treatment with appropriate local therapy and discontinuation of treatment with FLONASE Nasal Spray. Patients using FLONASE Nasal Spray over several months or longer should be examined periodically for evidence of *Candida* infection or other signs of adverse effects on the nasal mucosa.

Intranasal corticosteroids should be used with caution, if at all, in patients with active or quiescent tuberculous infections of the respiratory tract; untreated local or systemic fungal or bacterial infections; systemic viral or parasitic infections; or ocular herpes simplex.

Because of the inhibitory effect of corticosteroids on wound healing, patients who have experienced recent nasal septal ulcers, nasal surgery, or nasal trauma should not use a nasal corticosteroid until healing has occurred.

Information for Patients

Patients being treated with FLONASE Nasal Spray should receive the following information and instructions. This information is intended to aid them in the safe and effective use of this medication. It is not a disclosure of all possible adverse or intended effects.

Patients should be warned to avoid exposure to chickenpox or measles and, if exposed, to consult their physician without delay.

Patients should use FLONASE Nasal Spray at regular intervals for optimal effect. Some patients (12 years of age and older) with seasonal allergic rhinitis may find as-needed use of 200 mcg once daily effective for symptom control (see CLINICAL TRIALS).

A decrease in nasal symptoms may occur as soon as 12 hours after starting therapy with FLONASE Nasal Spray. Results in several clinical trials indicate statistically significant improvement within the first day or two of treatment; however, the full benefit of FLONASE Nasal Spray may not be achieved until treatment has been administered for several days. The patient should not increase the prescribed dosage but should contact the physician if symptoms do not improve or if the condition worsens.

For the proper use of FLONASE Nasal Spray and to attain maximum improvement, the patient should read and follow carefully the patient's instructions accompanying the product.

Drug Interactions

Fluticasone propionate is a substrate of cytochrome P450 3A4. A drug interaction study with fluticasone propionate aqueous nasal spray in healthy subjects has shown that ritonavir (a highly potent cytochrome P450 3A4 inhibitor) can significantly increase plasma fluticasone propionate exposure, resulting in significantly reduced serum cortisol concentrations (see CLINICAL PHARMACOLOGY: Drug Interactions). During postmarketing use, there have been reports of clinically significant drug interactions in patients receiving fluticasone propionate and ritonavir, resulting in systemic corticosteroid effects including Cushing syndrome and adrenal suppression. Therefore, coadministration of fluticasone propionate and ritonavir is not recommended unless the potential benefit to the patient outweighs the risk of systemic corticosteroid side effects.

In a placebo-controlled crossover study in 8 healthy volunteers, coadministration of a single dose of orally inhaled fluticasone propionate (1,000 mcg; 5 times the maximum daily intranasal dose) with multiple doses of ketoconazole (200 mg) to steady state resulted in increased plasma fluticasone propionate exposure, a reduction in plasma cortisol AUC, and no effect on urinary excretion of cortisol. Caution should be exercised when FLONASE Nasal Spray is coadministered with ketoconazole and other known potent cytochrome P450 3A4 inhibitors.

Carcinogenesis, Mutagenesis, Impairment of Fertility

Fluticasone propionate demonstrated no tumorigenic potential in mice at oral doses up to 1,000 mcg/kg (approximately 20 times the maximum recommended daily intranasal dose in adults and approximately 10 times the maximum recommended daily intranasal dose in children on a mcg/m^2 basis) for 78 weeks or in rats at inhalation doses up to 57 mcg/kg (approximately 2 times the maximum recommended daily intranasal dose in adults and approximately equivalent to the maximum recommended daily intranasal dose in children on a mcg/m^2 basis) for 104 weeks.

Fluticasone propionate did not induce gene mutation in prokaryotic or eukaryotic cells in vitro. No significant clastogenic effect was seen in cultured human peripheral lymphocytes in vitro or in the mouse micronucleus test.

No evidence of impairment of fertility was observed in reproductive studies conducted in male and female rats at subcutaneous doses up to 50 mcg/kg (approximately 2 times the maximum recommended daily intranasal dose in adults on a mcg/m^2 basis). Prostate weight was significantly reduced at a subcutaneous dose of 50 mcg/kg.

Overall Adverse Experiences With >3% Incidence on Fluticasone Propionate in Controlled Clinical Trials With FLONASE Nasal Spray in Patients ≥4 Years With Seasonal or Perennial Allergic Rhinitis

Adverse Experience	Vehicle Placebo (n = 758) %	FLONASE 100 mcg Once Daily (n = 167) %	FLONASE 200 mcg Once Daily (n = 782) %
Headache	14.6	6.6	16.1
Pharyngitis	7.2	6.0	7.8
Epistaxis	5.4	6.0	6.9
Nasal burning/nasal irritation	2.6	2.4	3.2
Nausea/vomiting	2.0	4.8	2.6
Asthma symptoms	2.9	7.2	3.3
Cough	2.8	3.6	3.8

Pregnancy

Teratogenic Effects: Pregnancy Category C. Subcutaneous studies in the mouse and rat at 45 and 100 mcg/kg, respectively (approximately equivalent to and 4 times, respectively, the maximum recommended daily intranasal dose in adults on a mcg/m^2 basis), revealed fetal toxicity characteristic of potent corticosteroid compounds, including embryonic growth retardation, omphalocele, cleft palate, and retarded cranial ossification.

In the rabbit, fetal weight reduction and cleft palate were observed at a subcutaneous dose of 4 mcg/kg (less than the maximum recommended daily intranasal dose in adults on a mcg/m^2 basis). However, no teratogenic effects were reported at oral doses up to 300 mcg/kg (approximately 25 times the maximum recommended daily intranasal dose in adults on a mcg/m^2 basis) of fluticasone propionate to the rabbit. No fluticasone propionate was detected in the plasma in this study, consistent with the established low bioavailability following oral administration (see CLINICAL PHARMACOLOGY).

Fluticasone propionate crossed the placenta following oral administration of 100 mcg/kg to rats and 300 mcg/kg to rabbits (approximately 4 and 25 times, respectively, the maximum recommended daily intranasal dose in adults on a mcg/m^2 basis).

There are no adequate and well-controlled studies in pregnant women. Fluticasone propionate should be used during pregnancy only if the potential benefit justifies the potential risk to the fetus.

Experience with oral corticosteroids since their introduction in pharmacologic, as opposed to physiologic, doses suggests that rodents are more prone to teratogenic effects from corticosteroids than humans. In addition, because there is a natural increase in corticosteroid production during pregnancy, most women will require a lower exogenous corticosteroid dose and many will not need corticosteroid treatment during pregnancy.

Nursing Mothers

It is not known whether fluticasone propionate is excreted in human breast milk. However, other corticosteroids have been detected in human milk. Subcutaneous administration to lactating rats of 10 mcg/kg of tritiated fluticasone propionate (less than the maximum recommended daily intranasal dose in adults on a mcg/m^2 basis) resulted in measurable radioactivity in the milk. Since there are no data from controlled trials on the use of intranasal fluticasone propionate by nursing mothers, caution should be exercised when FLONASE Nasal Spray is administered to a nursing woman.

Pediatric Use

Six hundred fifty (650) patients aged 4 to 11 years and 440 patients aged 12 to 17 years were studied in US clinical trials with fluticasone propionate nasal spray. The safety and effectiveness of FLONASE Nasal Spray in children below 4 years of age have not been established.

Controlled clinical studies have shown that intranasal corticosteroids may cause a reduction in growth velocity in pediatric patients. This effect has been observed in the absence of laboratory evidence of HPA axis suppression, suggesting that growth velocity is a more sensitive indicator of systemic corticosteroid exposure in pediatric patients than some commonly used tests of HPA axis function. The long-term effects of this reduction in growth velocity associated with intranasal corticosteroids, including the impact on final adult height, are unknown. The potential for "catch-up" growth following discontinuation of treatment with intranasal corticosteroids has not been adequately studied. The growth of pediatric patients receiving intranasal corticosteroids, including FLONASE Nasal Spray, should be monitored routinely (e.g., via stadiometry). The potential growth effects of prolonged treatment should be weighed against the clinical benefits obtained and the risks/benefits of treatment alternatives. To minimize the systemic effects of intranasal corticosteroids, including FLONASE Nasal Spray, each patient should be titrated to the lowest dose that effectively controls his/her symptoms.

A 1-year placebo-controlled clinical growth study was conducted in 150 pediatric patients (ages 3 to 9 years) to assess the effect of FLONASE Nasal Spray (single daily dose of 200 mcg, the maximum approved dose) on growth velocity. From the primary population of 56 patients receiving FLONASE Nasal Spray and 52 receiving placebo, the point estimate for growth velocity with FLONASE Nasal Spray was 0.14 cm/year lower than that noted with placebo (95% confidence interval ranging from 0.54 cm/year lower than placebo to 0.27 cm/year higher than placebo). Thus, no statistically significant effect on growth was noted compared to placebo. No evidence of clinically relevant changes in HPA axis function or bone mineral density was observed as assessed by 12-hour urinary cortisol excretion and dual energy x-ray absorptiometry, respectively.

The potential for FLONASE Nasal Spray to cause growth suppression in susceptible patients or when given at higher doses cannot be ruled out.

Geriatric Use

A limited number of patients 65 years of age and older (n = 129) or 75 years of age and older (n = 11) have been treated with FLONASE Nasal Spray in US and non-US clinical trials. While the number of patients is too small to permit separate analysis of efficacy and safety, the adverse reactions reported in this population were similar to those reported by younger patients.

ADVERSE REACTIONS

In controlled US studies, more than 3,300 patients with seasonal allergic, perennial allergic, or perennial nonallergic rhinitis received treatment with intranasal fluticasone propionate. In general, adverse reactions in clinical studies have been primarily associated with irritation of the nasal mucous membranes, and the adverse reactions were reported with approximately the same frequency by patients treated with the vehicle itself. The complaints did not usually interfere with treatment. Less than 2% of patients in clinical trials discontinued because of adverse events; this rate was similar for vehicle placebo and active comparators.

Systemic corticosteroid side effects were not reported during controlled clinical studies up to 6 months' duration with FLONASE Nasal Spray. If recommended doses are exceeded, however, or if individuals are particularly sensitive or taking FLONASE Nasal Spray in conjunction with administration of other corticosteroids, symptoms of hypercorticism, e.g., Cushing syndrome, could occur.

The following incidence of common adverse reactions (>3%, where incidence in fluticasone propionate-treated subjects exceeded placebo) is based upon 7 controlled clinical trials in which 536 patients (57 girls and 108 boys aged 4 to 11 years, 137 female and 234 male adolescents and adults) were treated with FLONASE Nasal Spray 200 mcg once daily over 2 to 4 weeks and 2 controlled clinical trials in which 246 patients (119 female and 127 male adolescents and adults) were treated with FLONASE Nasal Spray 200 mcg once daily over 6 months. Also included in the table are adverse events from 2 studies in which 167 children (45 girls and 122 boys aged 4 to 11 years) were treated with FLONASE Nasal Spray 100 mcg once daily for 2 to 4 weeks. [See table above]

Other adverse events that occurred in ≤3% but ≥1% of patients and that were more common with fluticasone propionate (with uncertain relationship to treatment) included: blood in nasal mucus, runny nose, abdominal pain, diarrhea, fever, flu-like symptoms, aches and pains, dizziness, bronchitis.

Observed During Clinical Practice

In addition to adverse events reported from clinical trials, the following events have been identified during postapproval use of intranasal fluticasone propionate in clinical practice. Because they are reported voluntarily from a population of unknown size, estimates of frequency cannot be made. These events have been chosen for inclusion due to either their seriousness, frequency of reporting, or causal connection to fluticasone propionate or a combination of these factors.

General: Hypersensitivity reactions, including angioedema, skin rash, edema of the face and tongue, pruritus, urticaria, bronchospasm, wheezing, dyspnea, and anaphylaxis/anaphylactoid reactions, which in rare instances were severe.
Ear, Nose, and Throat: Alteration or loss of sense of taste and/or smell and, rarely, nasal septal perforation, nasal ulcer, sore throat, throat irritation and dryness, cough, hoarseness, and voice changes.
Eye: Dryness and irritation, conjunctivitis, blurred vision, glaucoma, increased intraocular pressure, and cataracts.
Cases of growth suppression have been reported for intranasal corticosteroids, including FLONASE (see PRECAUTIONS: Pediatric Use).

OVERDOSAGE

Chronic overdosage may result in signs/symptoms of hypercorticism (see PRECAUTIONS). Intranasal administration of 2 mg (10 times the recommended dose) of fluticasone propionate twice daily for 7 days to healthy human volunteers was well tolerated. Single oral doses up to 16 mg have been studied in human volunteers with no acute toxic effects reported. Repeat oral doses up to 80 mg daily for 10 days in volunteers and repeat oral doses up to 10 mg daily for 14 days in patients were well tolerated. Adverse reactions were of mild or moderate severity, and incidences were similar in active and placebo treatment groups. Acute overdosage with this dosage form is unlikely since 1 bottle of FLONASE Nasal Spray contains approximately 8 mg of fluticasone propionate.
The oral and subcutaneous median lethal doses in mice and rats were >1,000 mg/kg (>20,000 and >41,000 times, respectively, the maximum recommended daily intranasal dose in adults and >10,000 and >20,000 times, respectively, the maximum recommended daily intranasal dose in children on a mg/m^2 basis).

DOSAGE AND ADMINISTRATION

Patients should use FLONASE Nasal Spray at regular intervals for optimal effect.

Adults

The recommended starting dosage in **adults** is 2 sprays (50 mcg of fluticasone propionate each) in each nostril once daily (total daily dose, 200 mcg). The same dosage divided into 100 mcg given twice daily (e.g., 8 a.m. and 8 p.m.) is also effective. After the first few days, patients may be able to reduce their dosage to 100 mcg (1 spray in each nostril) once daily for maintenance therapy. Some patients (12 years of age and older) with seasonal allergic rhinitis may find as-needed use of 200 mcg once daily effective for symptom control (see CLINICAL TRIALS). Greater symptom control may be achieved with scheduled regular use.

Adolescents and Children (4 Years of Age and Older)

Patients should be started with 100 mcg (1 spray in each nostril once daily). Patients not adequately responding to 100 mcg may use 200 mcg (2 sprays in each nostril). Once adequate control is achieved, the dosage should be decreased to 100 mcg (1 spray in each nostril) daily.
The maximum total daily dosage should not exceed 2 sprays in each nostril (200 mcg/day) (see CLINICAL TRIALS: Individualization of Dosage)
FLONASE Nasal Spray is not recommended for children under 4 years of age.

Directions for Use

Illustrated patient's instructions for proper use accompany each package of FLONASE Nasal Spray.

HOW SUPPLIED

FLONASE Nasal Spray, 50 mcg is supplied in an amber glass bottle fitted with a white metering atomizing pump, white nasal adapter, and green dust cover in a box of 1 (NDC 0173-0453-01) with patient's instructions for use. Each bottle contains a net fill weight of 16 g and will provide 120 actuations. Each actuation delivers 50 mcg of fluticasone propionate in 100 mg of formulation through the nasal adapter. The correct amount of medication in each spray cannot be assured after 120 sprays even though the bottle is not completely empty. The bottle should be discarded when the labeled number of actuations has been used.

Store between 4° and 30°C (39° and 86°F).

GlaxoSmithKline
Research Triangle Park, NC 27709

August 2007 FLN:1PI

[See figure at top of next column]

Flonase®
(fluticasone propionate)
Nasal Spray, 50 mcg

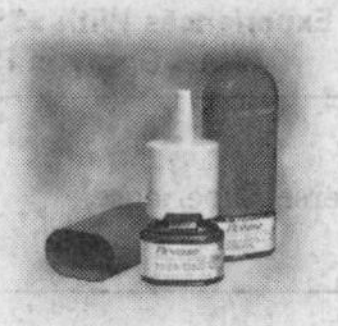

Please read this leaflet carefully before you start to take your medicine. It provides a summary of information on your medicine.
For further information ask your doctor or pharmacist.

WHAT YOU SHOULD KNOW ABOUT RHINITIS

Rhinitis is a word that means inflammation of the lining of the nose. If you suffer from rhinitis, your nose becomes stuffy and runny. Rhinitis can also make your nose itchy, and you may sneeze a lot. Rhinitis can be caused by allergies to pollen, animals, molds, or other materials—or it may have a nonallergic cause.

WHAT YOU SHOULD KNOW ABOUT FLONASE NASAL SPRAY

Your doctor has prescribed FLONASE Nasal Spray, a medicine that can help treat your rhinitis. FLONASE Nasal Spray contains fluticasone propionate, which is a synthetic corticosteroid. Corticosteroids are natural substances found in the body that help fight inflammation. When you spray FLONASE into your nose, it helps to reduce the symptoms of allergic reactions and the stuffiness, runniness, itching, and sneezing that can bother you.

THINGS TO REMEMBER ABOUT FLONASE NASAL SPRAY

1. Shake gently before using.
2. Use your nasal spray as directed by your doctor. The directions are on the pharmacy label.
3. Keep your nasal spray **out of the reach of children.**

BEFORE USING YOUR NASAL SPRAY

- If you are pregnant (or intending to become pregnant),
- If you are breastfeeding a baby,
- If you are allergic to FLONASE Nasal Spray or any other nasal corticosteroid,
- If you are taking a medicine containing ritonavir (commonly used to treat HIV infection or AIDS),

TELL YOUR DOCTOR BEFORE STARTING TO TAKE THIS MEDICINE. In some circumstances, this medicine may not be suitable and your doctor may wish to give you a different medicine. Make sure that your doctor knows what other medicines you are taking.

USING YOUR NASAL SPRAY

- Follow the instructions shown in the rest of this leaflet. If you have any problems, tell your doctor or pharmacist.
- It is important that you use it as directed by your doctor. The pharmacist's label will usually tell you what dose to take and how often. If it doesn't, or you are not sure, ask your doctor or pharmacist.

DOSAGE

- For **ADULTS**, the usual starting dosage is ***2 sprays in each nostril once daily***. Sometimes your doctor may recommend using 1 spray in each nostril twice a day (morning and evening). You should not use more than a total of 2 sprays in each nostril daily. After you have begun to feel better, 1 spray in each nostril daily may be adequate for you.
  For **ADOLESCENTS and CHILDREN** (4 years of age and older), the usual starting dosage is ***1 spray in each nostril once daily***. Sometimes your doctor may recommend using 2 sprays in each nostril daily. Then, after you have begun to feel better, 1 spray in each nostril daily may be adequate for you.
- DO NOT use more of your medicine or take it more often than your doctor advises.
- FLONASE may begin to work within 12 hours of the first dose, but it takes several days of regular use to reach its greatest effect. It is important that you use FLONASE Nasal Spray as prescribed by your doctor. Best results will be obtained by using the spray on a regular basis. If symptoms disappear, contact your doctor for further instructions.
- If you also have itchy, watery eyes, you should tell your doctor. You may be given an additional medicine to treat your eyes. Be careful not to confuse them, particularly if the second medicine is an eye drop.
- If you miss a dose, just take your regularly scheduled next dose when it is due. DO NOT DOUBLE the dose.

HOW TO USE YOUR NASAL SPRAY

Read the complete instructions carefully and use only as directed.

BEFORE USING

1. Shake the bottle gently and then remove the dust cover (Figure 1).

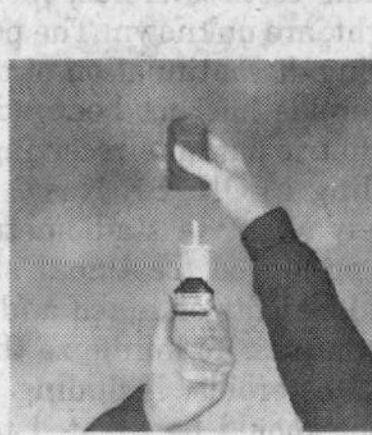

Figure 1

2. It is necessary to prime the pump into the air the first time it is used, or when you have not used it for a week or more. To prime the pump, hold the bottle as shown with the nasal applicator pointing away from you and with your forefinger and middle finger on either side of the nasal applicator and your thumb underneath the bottle. When you prime the pump for the first time, press down and release the pump 6 times (Figure 2). The pump is now ready for use. If the pump is not used for 7 days, prime until a fine spray appears.

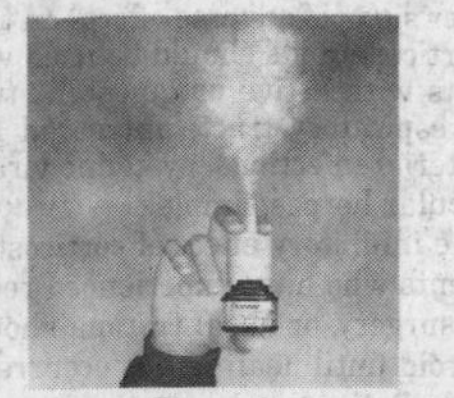

Figure 2

USING THE SPRAY

3. Blow your nose to clear your nostrils.
4. Close one nostril. Tilt your head forward slightly and, keeping the bottle upright, carefully insert the nasal applicator into the other nostril (Figure 3).

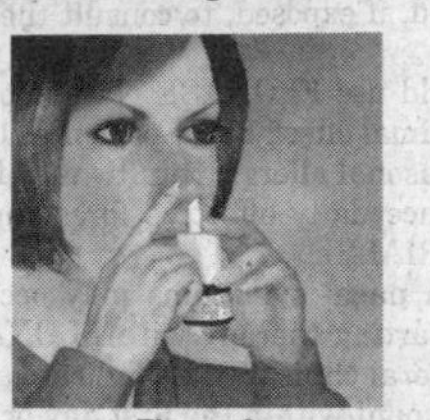

Figure 3

5. Start to breathe in through your nose, and WHILE BREATHING IN press firmly and quickly down once on the applicator to release the spray. To get a full actuation, use your forefinger and middle finger to spray while supporting the base of the bottle with your thumb. Avoid spraying in eyes. Breathe gently inwards through the nostril (Figure 4).

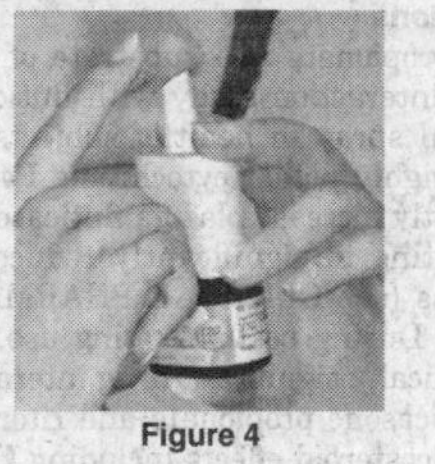

Figure 4

6. Breathe out through your mouth.
7. If a second spray is required in that nostril, repeat steps 4 through 6.
8. Repeat steps 4 through 7 in the other nostril.
9. Wipe the nasal applicator with a clean tissue and replace the dust cover (Figure 5).

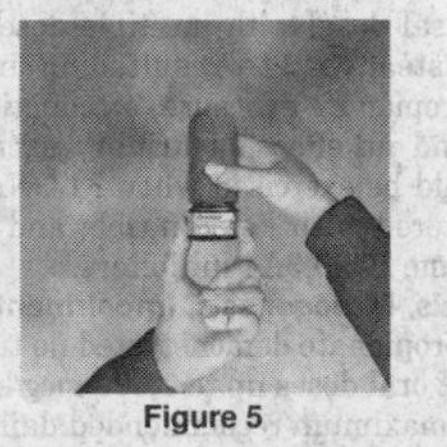

Figure 5

10. Do not use this bottle for more than the labeled number of sprays even though the bottle is not completely empty. Before you throw the bottle away, you should consult your doctor to see if a refill is needed. Do not take extra doses or stop taking FLONASE Nasal Spray without consulting your doctor.

CLEANING

Your nasal spray should be cleaned at least once a week. To do this:

1. Remove the dust cover and then gently pull upwards to free the nasal applicator.
2. Wash the applicator and dust cover under warm tap water. Allow to dry at room temperature, then place the applicator and dust cover back on the bottle.
3. If the nasal applicator becomes blocked, it can be removed as above and left to soak in warm water. Rinse

with cold tap water, dry, and refit. **Do not try to unblock the nasal applicator by inserting a pin or other sharp object.**

STORING YOUR NASAL SPRAY

- Keep your FLONASE Nasal Spray **out of the reach of children.**
- Avoid spraying in eyes.
- Store between 4° and 30°C (39° and 86°F).
- Do not use your FLONASE Nasal Spray after the date shown as "EXP" on the label or box.

REMEMBER: This medicine has been prescribed for you by your doctor. DO NOT give this medicine to anyone else.

FURTHER INFORMATION

This leaflet does not contain the complete information about your medicine. *If you have any questions, or are not sure about something, then you should ask your doctor or pharmacist.*

You may want to read this leaflet again. Please DO NOT THROW IT AWAY until you have finished your medicine.

GlaxoSmithKline
Research Triangle Park, NC 27709

July 2003 RL-2019

FLOVENT DISKUS 50 mcg ℞

[flō'vent]
(fluticasone propionate inhalation powder, 50 mcg)

FLOVENT DISKUS 100 mcg ℞

(fluticasone propionate inhalation powder, 100 mcg)

FLOVENT DISKUS 250 mcg ℞

(fluticasone propionate inhalation powder, 250 mcg)
FOR ORAL INHALATION

HIGHLIGHTS OF PRESCRIBING INFORMATION
These highlights do not include all the information needed to use FLOVENT DISKUS safely and effectively. See full prescribing information for FLOVENT DISKUS.
FLOVENT DISKUS 50 mcg
(fluticasone propionate inhalation powder, 50 mcg)
FLOVENT DISKUS 100 mcg
(fluticasone propionate inhalation powder, 100 mcg)
FLOVENT DISKUS 250 mcg
(fluticasone propionate inhalation powder, 250 mcg)
FOR ORAL INHALATION
Initial U.S. Approval: 1994

INDICATIONS AND USAGE

FLOVENT DISKUS is an inhaled corticosteroid indicated for:

- Maintenance treatment of asthma as prophylactic therapy in patients 4 years and older. (1)
- Treatment of asthma for patients requiring oral corticosteroid therapy. (1)

FLOVENT DISKUS is NOT indicated for the relief of acute bronchospasm. (1)

DOSAGE AND ADMINISTRATION

For oral inhalation only. Dosing is based on prior asthma therapy. (2)

Previous Therapy	Recommended Starting Dosage	Highest Recommended Dosage
Patients aged ≥12 years		
Bronchodilators alone	100 mcg twice daily	500 mcg twice daily
Inhaled corticosteroids	100-250 mcg twice daily	500 mcg twice daily
Oral corticosteroids	500-1,000 mcg twice daily	1,000 mcg twice daily
Patients aged 4-11 years	50 mcg twice daily	100 mcg twice daily

DOSAGE FORMS AND STRENGTHS

Inhalation powder with 50, 100, or 250 mcg per actuation. (3)

CONTRAINDICATIONS

- Primary treatment of status asthmaticus or acute episodes of asthma requiring intensive measures. (4)
- Severe hypersensitivity to milk proteins. (4)

WARNINGS AND PRECAUTIONS

- Localized infections: *Candida albicans* infection of the mouth and pharynx. Monitor patients periodically for signs of adverse effects on the oral cavity. Advise patients to rinse mouth following inhalation. (5.1)
- Immunosuppression: Potential worsening of existing tuberculosis; fungal, bacterial, viral, or parasitic infection; or ocular herpes simplex. More serious or even fatal course of chickenpox or measles in susceptible patients. Use caution in patients with above because of the potential for worsening of these infections. (5.3)
- Transferring patients from systemic corticosteroids: Risk of impaired adrenal function when transferring from oral steroids. Taper patients slowly from systemic corticosteroids if transferring to FLOVENT DISKUS. (5.4)
- Hypercorticism and adrenal suppression: May occur with very high dosages or at the regular dosage in susceptible individuals. If such changes occur, discontinue FLOVENT DISKUS slowly. (5.5)
- Hypersensitivity reactions, including anaphylaxis, may occur after administration of FLOVENT DISKUS. Discontinue FLOVENT DISKUS if such reactions occur. (4, 5.6)
- Effect on growth: Monitor growth of pediatric patients. (5.8)
- Glaucoma and cataracts: Close monitoring is warranted. (5.9)

ADVERSE REACTIONS

Most common adverse reactions (incidence >3%) include upper respiratory tract infection or inflammation, throat irritation, sinusitis, rhinitis, oral candidiasis, nausea and vomiting, gastrointestinal discomfort, fever, cough, bronchitis, and headache. (6.1)

To report SUSPECTED ADVERSE REACTIONS, contact GlaxoSmithKline at 1-888-825-5249 or FDA at 1-800-FDA-1088 or www.fda.gov/medwatch.

DRUG INTERACTIONS

Use with strong cytochrome P450 3A4 inhibitors such as ritonavir and ketoconazole is not recommended. Systemic corticosteroid effects may occur. (7.1, 7.2)

USE IN SPECIFIC POPULATIONS

Hepatic impairment: Monitor patients for signs of increased drug exposure. (8.6)

See 17 for PATIENT COUNSELING INFORMATION and FDA-approved patient labeling

Revised: 01/2012

FULL PRESCRIBING INFORMATION: CONTENTS*

*** Sections or subsections omitted from the full prescribing information are not listed**

FULL PRESCRIBING INFORMATION

1 INDICATIONS AND USAGE

FLOVENT® DISKUS® is indicated for the maintenance treatment of asthma as prophylactic therapy in patients 4 years and older. It is also indicated for patients requiring oral corticosteroid therapy for asthma. Many of these patients may be able to reduce or eliminate their requirement for oral corticosteroids over time.

FLOVENT DISKUS is NOT indicated for the relief of acute bronchospasm.

2 DOSAGE AND ADMINISTRATION

FLOVENT DISKUS should be administered by the orally inhaled route only in patients 4 years and older. Individual patients will experience a variable time to onset and degree of symptom relief. Maximum benefit may not be achieved for 1 to 2 weeks or longer after starting treatment.

After asthma stability has been achieved, it is always desirable to titrate to the lowest effective dosage to reduce the possibility of side effects. For patients who do not respond adequately to the starting dosage after 2 weeks of therapy, higher dosages may provide additional asthma control. The safety and efficacy of FLOVENT DISKUS when administered in excess of recommended dosages have not been established.

The recommended starting dosage and the highest recommended dosage of FLOVENT DISKUS, based on prior asthma therapy, are listed in Table 1.

Table 1. Recommended Dosages of FLOVENT DISKUS

NOTE: In all patients, it is desirable to titrate to the lowest effective dosage once asthma stability is achieved.

Previous Therapy	Recommended Starting Dosage	Highest Recommended Dosage
Adult and adolescent patients (aged ≥12 years)		
Bronchodilators alone	100 mcg twice daily	500 mcg twice daily
Inhaled corticosteroids	100-250 mcg twice daily[a]	500 mcg twice daily
Oral corticosteroids[b]	500-1,000 mcg twice daily[c]	1,000 mcg twice daily
Pediatric patients (aged 4-11 years)[d]	50 mcg twice daily[a]	100 mcg twice daily

[a]Starting dosages above 100 mcg twice daily for adult and adolescent patients and 50 mcg twice daily for pediatric patients aged 4 to 11 years may be considered for patients with poorer asthma control or those who have previously required doses of inhaled corticosteroids that are in the higher range for the specific agent.

[b]For patients currently receiving chronic oral corticosteroid therapy, prednisone should be reduced no faster than 2.5 to 5 mg/day on a weekly basis beginning after at least 1 week of therapy with FLOVENT DISKUS. Patients should be carefully monitored for signs of asthma instability, including serial objective measures of airflow, and for signs of adrenal insufficiency *[see Warnings and Precautions (5.4)]*. Once prednisone reduction is complete, the dosage of FLOVENT DISKUS should be reduced to the lowest effective dosage.

[c]The choice of starting dosage should be made on the basis of individual patient assessment. A controlled clinical study of 111 oral corticosteroid-dependent patients with asthma showed few significant differences between the 2 doses of FLOVENT DISKUS on safety and efficacy endpoints. However, inability to decrease the dose of oral corticosteroids further during corticosteroid reduction may be indicative of the need to increase the dose of fluticasone propionate up to the maximum of 1,000 mcg twice daily.

[d]Because individual responses may vary, pediatric patients previously maintained on other inhaled corticosteroids may require dosage adjustments upon transfer to FLOVENT DISKUS.

3 DOSAGE FORMS AND STRENGTHS

FLOVENT DISKUS is an inhalation powder. Each actuation delivers 46, 94, or 229 mcg of fluticasone propionate from the DISKUS® inhalation unit. FLOVENT DISKUS is supplied as a disposable orange inhalation unit containing 60 blisters of powder formulation packaged in a plastic-coated, moisture-protective foil pouch. An institutional pack containing 28 blisters is also available.

4 CONTRAINDICATIONS

The use of FLOVENT DISKUS is contraindicated in the following conditions:

- Primary treatment of status asthmaticus or other acute episodes of asthma where intensive measures are required *[see Warnings and Precautions (5.2)]*.
- Severe hypersensitivity to milk proteins *[see Warnings and Precautions (5.6), Adverse Reactions (6.2), Description (11)]*.

5 WARNINGS AND PRECAUTIONS

5.1 Local Effects

In clinical studies, the development of localized infections of the mouth and pharynx with *Candida albicans* has occurred in patients treated with FLOVENT DISKUS. When such an infection develops, it should be treated with appropriate local or systemic (i.e., oral antifungal) therapy while treatment with FLOVENT DISKUS continues, but at times therapy with FLOVENT DISKUS may need to be interrupted. Patients should rinse the mouth after inhalation of FLOVENT DISKUS *[see Adverse Reactions (6.1)]*.

5.2 Acute Asthma Episodes

FLOVENT DISKUS is not to be regarded as a bronchodilator and is not indicated for rapid relief of bronchospasm. Patients should be instructed to contact their physicians immediately when episodes of asthma that are not responsive to bronchodilators occur during the course of treatment with FLOVENT DISKUS. During such episodes, patients may require therapy with oral corticosteroids.

5.3 Immunosuppression

Persons who are using drugs that suppress the immune system are more susceptible to infections than healthy individuals. Chickenpox and measles, for example, can have a more serious or even fatal course in susceptible children or adults using corticosteroids. In such children or adults who have not had these diseases or been properly immunized, particular care should be taken to avoid exposure. How the dose, route, and duration of corticosteroid administration affect the risk of developing a disseminated infection is not known. The contribution of the underlying disease and/or prior corticosteroid treatment to the risk is also not known. If exposed to chickenpox, prophylaxis with varicella zoster immune globulin (VZIG) may be indicated. If exposed to measles, prophylaxis with pooled intramuscular immunoglobulin (IG) may be indicated. (See the respective package inserts for complete VZIG and IG prescribing information.) If chickenpox develops, treatment with antiviral agents may be considered.

Because of the potential for worsening infections, inhaled corticosteroids should be used with caution, if at all, in patients with active or quiescent tuberculosis infection of the respiratory tract; untreated systemic fungal, bacterial, viral or parasitic infections; or ocular herpes simplex.

5.4 Transferring Patients From Systemic Corticosteroid Therapy

Particular care is needed for patients who have been transferred from systemically active corticosteroids to inhaled corticosteroids because deaths due to adrenal insufficiency have occurred in patients with asthma during and after transfer from systemic corticosteroids to less systemically available inhaled corticosteroids. After withdrawal from systemic corticosteroids, a number of months are required for recovery of hypothalamic-pituitary-adrenal (HPA) function.

Patients requiring oral corticosteroids should be weaned slowly from systemic corticosteroid use after transferring to FLOVENT DISKUS. In a clinical trial of 111 patients, prednisone reduction was accomplished by reducing the daily prednisone dose by 2.5 mg on a weekly basis during transfer to FLOVENT DISKUS. Successive reduction of prednisone dose was allowed only when lung function; symptoms; and as-needed, short-acting beta-agonist use were better than or comparable to that seen before initiation of prednisone dose reduction. Lung function (forced expiratory volume in 1 second [FEV_1] or morning peak expiratory flow [AM PEF]), beta-agonist use, and asthma symptoms should be carefully monitored during withdrawal of oral corticosteroids. In addition to monitoring asthma signs and symptoms, patients should be observed for signs and symptoms of adrenal insufficiency such as fatigue, lassitude, weakness, nausea and vomiting, and hypotension.

Patients who have been previously maintained on 20 mg or more per day of prednisone (or its equivalent) may be most susceptible, particularly when their systemic corticosteroids have been almost completely withdrawn. During this period of HPA suppression, patients may exhibit signs and symptoms of adrenal insufficiency when exposed to trauma, surgery, or infection (particularly gastroenteritis) or other conditions associated with severe electrolyte loss. Although inhaled corticosteroids may provide control of asthma symptoms during these episodes, in recommended doses they supply less than normal physiological amounts of glucocorticoid (cortisol) systemically and do NOT provide the mineralocorticoid activity that is necessary for coping with these emergencies.

During periods of stress or a severe asthma attack, patients who have been withdrawn from systemic corticosteroids should be instructed to resume oral corticosteroids immediately and to contact their physicians for further instruction. These patients should also be instructed to carry a warning card indicating that they may need supplementary systemic corticosteroids during periods of stress or a severe asthma attack.

Transfer of patients from systemic corticosteroid therapy to FLOVENT DISKUS may unmask conditions previously suppressed by the systemic corticosteroid therapy, e.g., rhinitis, conjunctivitis, eczema, arthritis, and eosinophilic conditions. Some patients may experience symptoms of systemically active corticosteroid withdrawal, e.g., joint and/or muscular pain, lassitude, and depression, despite maintenance or even improvement of respiratory function.

5.5 Hypercorticism and Adrenal Suppression

Fluticasone propionate will often help control asthma symptoms with less suppression of HPA function than therapeutically equivalent oral doses of prednisone. Since fluticasone propionate is absorbed into the circulation and can be systemically active at higher doses, the beneficial effects of FLOVENT DISKUS in minimizing HPA dysfunction may be expected only when recommended dosages are not exceeded and individual patients are titrated to the lowest effective dose. A relationship between plasma levels of fluticasone propionate and inhibitory effects on stimulated cortisol production has been shown after 4 weeks of treatment with fluticasone propionate. Since individual sensitivity to effects on cortisol production exists, physicians should consider this information when prescribing FLOVENT DISKUS.

Because of the possibility of systemic absorption of inhaled corticosteroids, patients treated with FLOVENT DISKUS should be observed carefully for any evidence of systemic corticosteroid effects. Particular care should be taken in observing patients postoperatively or during periods of stress for evidence of inadequate adrenal response.

It is possible that systemic corticosteroid effects such as hypercorticism and adrenal suppression (including adrenal crisis) may appear in a small number of patients, particularly when FLOVENT DISKUS is administered at higher than recommended doses over prolonged periods of time. If such effects occur, the dosage of FLOVENT DISKUS should be reduced slowly, consistent with accepted procedures for reducing systemic corticosteroids and for management of asthma.

5.6 Hypersensitivity Reactions, Including Anaphylaxis

Hypersensitivity reactions, including anaphylaxis, angioedema, urticaria, and bronchospasm, may occur after administration of FLOVENT DISKUS. There have been reports of anaphylactic reactions in patients with severe milk protein allergy; therefore, patients with severe milk protein allergy should not take FLOVENT DISKUS *[see Contraindications (4)]*.

5.7 Reduction in Bone Mineral Density

Decreases in bone mineral density (BMD) have been observed with long-term administration of products containing inhaled corticosteroids. The clinical significance of small changes in BMD with regard to long-term outcomes is unknown. Patients with major risk factors for decreased bone mineral content, such as prolonged immobilization, family history of osteoporosis, postmenopausal status, tobacco use, advanced age, poor nutrition, or chronic use of drugs that can reduce bone mass (e.g., anticonvulsants, oral corticosteroids) should be monitored and treated with established standards of care.

5.8 Effect on Growth

Orally inhaled corticosteroids may cause a reduction in growth velocity when administered to pediatric patients *[see Use in Specific Populations (8.4)]*. Monitor the growth of pediatric patients receiving FLOVENT DISKUS routinely (e.g., via stadiometry). To minimize the systemic effects of orally inhaled corticosteroids, including FLOVENT DISKUS, titrate each patient's dose to the lowest dosage that effectively controls his/her symptoms.

5.9 Glaucoma and Cataracts

Glaucoma, increased intraocular pressure, and cataracts have been reported in patients following the long-term administration of inhaled corticosteroids, including fluticasone propionate. Therefore, close monitoring is warranted in patients with a change in vision or with a history of increased intraocular pressure, glaucoma, and/or cataracts.

5.10 Paradoxical Bronchospasm

As with other inhaled medications, bronchospasm may occur with an immediate increase in wheezing after dosing. If bronchospasm occurs following dosing with FLOVENT DISKUS, it should be treated immediately with a fast-acting inhaled bronchodilator. Treatment with FLOVENT DISKUS should be discontinued immediately and alternative therapy instituted.

5.11 Drug Interactions With Strong Cytochrome P450 3A4 Inhibitors

The use of strong cytochrome P450 3A4 (CYP3A4) inhibitors (e.g., ritonavir, atazanavir, clarithromycin, indinavir, itraconazole, nefazodone, nelfinavir, saquinavir, ketoconazole, telithromycin) with FLOVENT DISKUS is not recommended because increased systemic corticosteroid adverse effects may occur *[see Drug Interactions (7.1), Clinical Pharmacology (12.3)]*.

5.12 Eosinophilic Conditions and Churg-Strauss Syndrome

In rare cases, patients on inhaled fluticasone propionate may present with systemic eosinophilic conditions. Some of these patients have clinical features of vasculitis consistent with Churg-Strauss syndrome, a condition that is often treated with systemic corticosteroid therapy. These events usually, but not always, have been associated with the reduction and/or withdrawal of oral corticosteroid therapy following the introduction of fluticasone propionate. Cases of serious eosinophilic conditions have also been reported with other inhaled corticosteroids in this clinical setting. Physicians should be alert to eosinophilia, vasculitic rash, worsening pulmonary symptoms, cardiac complications, and/or neuropathy presenting in their patients. A causal relationship between fluticasone propionate and these underlying conditions has not been established.

6 ADVERSE REACTIONS

Systemic and local corticosteroid use may result in the following:

- *Candida albicans* infection *[see Warnings and Precautions (5.1)]*
- Immunosuppression *[see Warnings and Precautions (5.3)]*
- Hypercorticism and adrenal suppression *[see Warnings and Precautions (5.5)]*
- Reduction in bone mineral density *[see Warnings and Precautions (5.7)]*
- Growth effects *[see Warnings and Precautions (5.8)]*
- Glaucoma and cataracts *[see Warnings and Precautions (5.9)]*

6.1 Clinical Trials Experience

Because clinical trials are conducted under widely varying conditions, adverse reaction rates observed in the clinical trials of a drug cannot be directly compared with rates in the clinical trials of another drug and may not reflect the rates observed in practice.

The incidence of common adverse reactions in Table 2 is based upon 7 placebo-controlled US clinical trials in which 1,176 pediatric, adolescent, and adult patients (466 females and 710 males) previously treated with as-needed bronchodilators and/or inhaled corticosteroids were treated twice daily for up to 12 weeks with FLOVENT DISKUS (doses of 50 to 500 mcg) or placebo.

[See table 2 at top of next page]

Table 2 includes all events (whether considered drug-related or nondrug-related by the investigator) that occurred at a rate of over 3% in any of the groups treated with FLOVENT DISKUS and were more common than in the placebo group. Less than 2% of patients discontinued from the studies because of adverse reactions. The average duration of exposure was 73 to 79 days in the active treatment groups compared with 56 days in the placebo group.

Additional Adverse Reactions: Other adverse reactions not previously listed, whether considered drug-related or not by the investigators, that were reported more frequently by patients with asthma treated with FLOVENT DISKUS compared with patients treated with placebo include the following: palpitations; soft tissue injuries; contusions and hematomas; wounds and lacerations; burns; poisoning and toxicity; pressure-induced disorders; hoarseness/dysphonia; epistaxis; ear, nose, throat, and tonsil signs and symptoms; ear, nose, and throat polyps; allergic ear, nose, and throat disorders; throat constriction; fluid disturbances; weight gain; appetite disturbances; keratitis and conjunctivitis; blepharoconjunctivitis; gastrointestinal signs and symptoms; oral ulcerations; dental discomfort and pain; oral erythema and rashes; mouth and tongue disorders; oral discomfort and pain; tooth decay; cholecystitis; arthralgia and articular rheumatism; muscle cramps and spasms; musculoskeletal inflammation; dizziness; sleep disorders; migraines; paralysis of cranial nerves; edema and swelling; bacterial infections; fungal infections; mobility disorders; mood disorders; bacterial reproductive infections; photodermatitis; dermatitis and dermatosis; viral skin infections; eczema; pruritus; acne and folliculitis; urinary infections.

Three (3) of the 7 placebo-controlled US clinical trials were pediatric studies. A total of 592 patients 4 to 11 years were treated with FLOVENT DISKUS (dosages of 50 or 100 mcg twice daily) or placebo; an additional 174 patients 4 to 11 years received FLOVENT® ROTADISK® (fluticasone propionate inhalation powder) at the same doses. There were no clinically relevant differences in the pattern or severity of adverse events in children compared with those reported in adults.

In the first 16 weeks of a 52-week clinical trial in adult patients with asthma who previously required oral corticosteroids (daily doses of 5 to 40 mg oral prednisone), the effects of FLOVENT DISKUS 500 mcg twice daily (n = 41) and 1,000 mcg twice daily (n = 36) were compared with placebo (n = 34) for the frequency of reported adverse events. The average duration of exposure for patients taking FLOVENT DISKUS was 105 days compared with 75 days for placebo. Adverse events, whether or not considered drug related by the investigators, reported in more than 5 patients in the group taking FLOVENT DISKUS and that occurred more frequently with FLOVENT DISKUS than with placebo are shown below (percent FLOVENT DISKUS and percent placebo).

Ear, Nose, and Throat: Hoarseness/dysphonia (9% and 0%), nasal congestion/blockage (16% and 0%), oral candidiasis (31% and 21%), rhinitis (13% and 9%), sinusitis/sinus infection (33% and 12%), throat irritation (10% and 9%), and upper respiratory tract infection (31% and 24%).

Gastrointestinal: Nausea and vomiting (9% and 0%).

Lower Respiratory: Cough (9% and 3%) and viral respiratory infections (9% and 6%).

Musculoskeletal: Arthralgia and articular rheumatism (17% and 3%) and muscle pain (12% and 0%).

Non-Site Specific: Malaise and fatigue (16% and 9%) and pain (10% and 3%).

Skin: Pruritus (6% and 0%) and skin rashes (8% and 3%).

6.2 Postmarketing Experience

In addition to adverse reactions reported from clinical trials, the following adverse reactions have been identified during postmarketing use of fluticasone propionate. Because these reactions are reported voluntarily from a population of uncertain size, it is not always possible to reliably estimate their frequency or establish a causal relationship to drug exposure. These events have been chosen for inclusion due to either their seriousness, frequency of reporting, or causal connection to fluticasone propionate or a combination of these factors.

Ear, Nose, and Throat: Aphonia, facial and oropharyngeal edema, and throat soreness.

Endocrine and Metabolic: Cushingoid features, growth velocity reduction in children/adolescents, hyperglycemia, and osteoporosis.

Eye: Cataracts.

Immune System Disorders: Immediate and delayed hypersensitivity reactions, including anaphylaxis, rash, angioedema, and bronchospasm, have been reported. Anaphylactic reactions in patients with severe milk protein allergy have been reported.

Psychiatry: Agitation, aggression, anxiety, depression, and restlessness. Behavioral changes, including hyperactivity and irritability, have been reported very rarely and primarily in children.

Respiratory: Asthma exacerbation, bronchospasm, chest tightness, dyspnea, immediate bronchospasm, pneumonia, and wheeze.

Skin: Contusions and ecchymoses.

Eosinophilic Conditions: In rare cases, patients on inhaled fluticasone propionate may present with systemic eosinophilic conditions, with some patients presenting with clinical features of vasculitis consistent with Churg-Strauss syndrome, a condition that is often treated with systemic corticosteroid therapy. These events usually, but not always, have been associated with the reduction and/or withdrawal of oral corticosteroid therapy following the introduction of fluticasone propionate *[see Warnings and Precautions (5.12)]*.

7 DRUG INTERACTIONS

7.1 Strong Cytochrome P450 3A4 Inhibitors

Fluticasone propionate is a substrate of CYP3A4. The use of strong CYP3A4 inhibitors (e.g., ritonavir, atazanavir, clarithromycin, indinavir, itraconazole, nefazodone, nelfinavir, saquinavir, ketoconazole, telithromycin) with FLOVENT DISKUS is not recommended because increased systemic corticosteroid adverse effects may occur.

A drug interaction study with fluticasone propionate aqueous nasal spray in healthy subjects has shown that ritonavir (a strong CYP3A4 inhibitor) can significantly increase plasma fluticasone propionate concentration, resulting in significantly reduced serum cortisol concentrations *[see Clinical Pharmacology (12.3)]*. During postmarketing use, there have been reports of clinically significant drug interactions in patients receiving fluticasone propionate and ritonavir, resulting in systemic corticosteroid effects including

Table 2. Adverse Reactions With >3% Incidence in US Controlled Clinical Trials With FLOVENT DISKUS in Patients With Asthma Previously Receiving Bronchodilators and/or Inhaled Corticosteroids

Adverse Event	FLOVENT DISKUS 50 mcg Twice Daily (n = 178) %	FLOVENT DISKUS 100 mcg Twice Daily (n = 305) %	FLOVENT DISKUS 250 mcg Twice Daily (n = 86) %	FLOVENT DISKUS 500 mcg Twice Daily (n = 64) %	Placebo (n = 543) %
Ear, nose, and throat					
Upper respiratory tract infection	20	18	21	14	16
Throat irritation	13	13	3	22	8
Sinusitis/sinus infection	9	10	6	6	6
Upper respiratory inflammation	5	5	0	5	3
Rhinitis	4	3	1	2	2
Oral candidiasis	<1	9	6	5	7
Gastrointestinal					
Nausea and vomiting	8	4	1	2	4
Gastrointestinal discomfort and pain	4	3	2	2	3
Viral gastrointestinal infection	4	3	3	5	1
Non-site specific					
Fever	7	7	1	2	4
Viral infection	2	2	0	5	2
Lower respiratory					
Viral respiratory infection	4	5	1	2	4
Cough	3	5	1	5	4
Bronchitis	2	3	0	8	1
Neurological					
Headache	12	12	2	14	7
Musculoskeletal and trauma					
Muscle injury	2	0	1	5	1
Musculoskeletal pain	4	3	2	5	2
Injury	2	<1	0	5	<1

Cushing syndrome and adrenal suppression. Therefore, coadministration of fluticasone propionate and ritonavir is not recommended unless the potential benefit to the patient outweighs the risk of systemic corticosteroid side effects.

Coadministration of orally inhaled fluticasone propionate (1,000 mcg) and ketoconazole (200 mg once daily) resulted in a 1.9-fold increase in plasma fluticasone propionate exposure and a 45% decrease in plasma cortisol area under the curve (AUC), but had no effect on urinary excretion of cortisol. Coadministration of fluticasone propionate and ketoconazole is not recommended unless the potential benefit to the patient outweighs the risk of systemic corticosteroid side effects.

8 USE IN SPECIFIC POPULATIONS

8.1 Pregnancy

Pregnancy Category C: There are no adequate and well-controlled studies with FLOVENT DISKUS in pregnant women. FLOVENT DISKUS should be used during pregnancy only if the potential benefit justifies the potential risk to the fetus.

Teratogenic Effects: Subcutaneous studies in the mouse and rat at doses approximately 0.1 and 0.4, respectively, times the maximum recommended human daily inhalation dose (MRHD) in adults on a mg/m^2 basis revealed fetal toxicity characteristic of potent corticosteroid compounds, including embryonic growth retardation, omphalocele, cleft palate, and retarded cranial ossification.

In the rabbit, fetal weight reduction and cleft palate were observed at a subcutaneous dose approximately 0.03 times the MRHD in adults on a mg/m^2 basis. However, no teratogenic effects were reported at oral doses up to approximately 2 times the MRHD in adults on a mg/m^2 basis. No fluticasone propionate was detected in the plasma in this study, consistent with the established low bioavailability following oral administration *[see Clinical Pharmacology (12.3)]*.

Experience with oral corticosteroids since their introduction in pharmacologic, as opposed to physiologic, doses suggests that rodents are more prone to teratogenic effects from corticosteroids than humans. In addition, because there is a natural increase in corticosteroid production during pregnancy, most women will require a lower exogenous corticosteroid dose and many will not need corticosteroid treatment during pregnancy.

8.3 Nursing Mothers

It is not known whether fluticasone propionate is excreted in human breast milk. However, other corticosteroids have been detected in human milk. Subcutaneous administration to lactating rats of tritiated fluticasone propionate at a dose approximately 0.04 times the MRHD in adults on a mg/m^2 basis resulted in measurable radioactivity in milk.

Since there are no data from controlled trials on the use of FLOVENT DISKUS by nursing mothers, caution should be exercised when FLOVENT DISKUS is administered to a nursing woman.

8.4 Pediatric Use

The safety and effectiveness of FLOVENT DISKUS in children 4 years and older have been established *[see Adverse Reactions (6.1), Clinical Pharmacology (12.3), Clinical Studies (14.2)]*. The safety and effectiveness of FLOVENT DISKUS in children younger than 4 years have not been established.

Effects on Growth: Orally inhaled corticosteroids may cause a reduction in growth velocity when administered to pediatric patients. A reduction of growth velocity in children or teenagers may occur as a result of poorly controlled asthma or from use of corticosteroids including inhaled corticosteroids. The effects of long-term treatment of children and adolescents with inhaled corticosteroids, including fluticasone propionate, on final adult height are not known. Controlled clinical studies have shown that inhaled corticosteroids may cause a reduction in growth in pediatric patients. In these studies, the mean reduction in growth velocity was approximately 1 cm/year (range: 0.3 to 1.8 cm/year) and appears to depend upon dose and duration of exposure. This effect was observed in the absence of laboratory evidence of HPA axis suppression, suggesting that growth velocity is a more sensitive indicator of systemic corticosteroid exposure in pediatric patients than some commonly used tests of HPA axis function. The long-term effects of this reduction in growth velocity associated with orally inhaled corticosteroids, including the impact on final adult height, are unknown. The potential for "catch-up" growth following discontinuation of treatment with orally inhaled corticosteroids has not been adequately studied. The effects on growth velocity of treatment with orally inhaled corticosteroids for over 1 year, including the impact on final adult height, are unknown. The growth of children and adolescents receiving orally inhaled corticosteroids, including FLOVENT DISKUS, should be monitored routinely (e.g., via stadiometry). The potential growth effects of prolonged treatment should be weighed against the clinical benefits obtained and the risks associated with alternative therapies. To minimize the systemic effects of orally inhaled corticosteroids, including FLOVENT DISKUS, each patient should be titrated to the lowest dose that effectively controls his/her symptoms.

A 52-week placebo-controlled study to assess the potential growth effects of fluticasone propionate inhalation powder (FLOVENT ROTADISK) at 50 and 100 mcg twice daily was conducted in the US in 325 prepubescent children (244 males and 81 females) aged 4 to 11 years. The mean growth velocities at 52 weeks observed in the intent-to-treat population were 6.32 cm/year in the placebo group (n = 76), 6.07 cm/year in the 50-mcg group (n = 98), and 5.66 cm/year in the 100-mcg group (n = 89). An imbalance in the proportion of children entering puberty between groups and a higher dropout rate in the placebo group due to poorly controlled asthma may be confounding factors in interpreting these data. A separate subset analysis of children who remained prepubertal during the study revealed growth rates at 52 weeks of 6.10 cm/year in the placebo group (n = 57), 5.91 cm/year in the 50-mcg group (n = 74), and 5.67 cm/year in the 100-mcg group (n = 79). In children aged 8.5 years, the mean age of children in this study, the range for expected growth velocity is: boys – 3rd percentile = 3.8 cm/year, 50th percentile = 5.4 cm/year, and 97th percentile = 7.0 cm/year; girls – 3rd percentile = 4.2 cm/year, 50th percentile = 5.7 cm/year, and 97th percentile = 7.3 cm/year. The clinical significance of these growth data is not certain.

8.5 Geriatric Use

Safety data have been collected on 280 patients (FLOVENT DISKUS n = 83, FLOVENT ROTADISK n = 197) 65 years or older and 33 patients (FLOVENT DISKUS n = 14, FLOVENT ROTADISK n = 19) 75 years or older who have been treated with fluticasone propionate inhalation powder in US and non-US clinical trials. No overall differences in safety or effectiveness were observed between these patients and younger patients, and other reported clinical experience has not identified differences in responses between the elderly and younger patients, but greater sensitivity of some older individuals cannot be ruled out.

8.6 Hepatic Impairment

Formal pharmacokinetic studies using FLOVENT DISKUS have not been conducted in patients with hepatic impairment. Since fluticasone propionate is predominantly cleared by hepatic metabolism, impairment of liver function may lead to accumulation of fluticasone propionate in plasma. Therefore, patients with hepatic disease should be closely monitored.

8.7 Renal Impairment

Formal pharmacokinetic studies using FLOVENT DISKUS have not been conducted in patients with renal impairment.

10 OVERDOSAGE

Chronic overdosage may result in signs/symptoms of hypercorticism *[see Warnings and Precautions (5.5)]*. Inhalation by healthy volunteers of a single dose of 4,000 mcg of fluticasone propionate inhalation powder or single doses of 1,760 or 3,520 mcg of fluticasone propionate CFC inhalation aerosol was well tolerated. Doses of 1,320 mcg administered to healthy human volunteers twice daily for 7 to 15 days were also well tolerated. Repeat oral doses up to 80 mg daily for 10 days in healthy volunteers and repeat oral doses up to 20 mg daily for 42 days in patients were well tolerated. Adverse reactions were of mild or moderate severity, and incidences were similar in active and placebo treatment groups. No deaths were seen in mice given an oral dose of 1,000 mg/kg (approximately 2,000 and 9,600 times the MRHD in adults and children aged 4 to 11 years, respectively, on a mg/m^2 basis). No deaths were seen in rats given an oral dose of 1,000 mg/kg (approximately 4,100 and 19,000 times the MRHD in adults and children aged 4 to 11 years, respectively, on a mg/m^2 basis).

11 DESCRIPTION

The active component of FLOVENT DISKUS 50 mcg, FLOVENT DISKUS 100 mcg, and FLOVENT DISKUS 250 mcg is fluticasone propionate, a corticosteroid having the chemical name *S*-(fluoromethyl) 6α,9-difluoro-11β,17-dihydroxy-16α-methyl-3-oxoandrosta-1,4-diene-17β-carbothioate, 17-propionate and the following chemical structure:

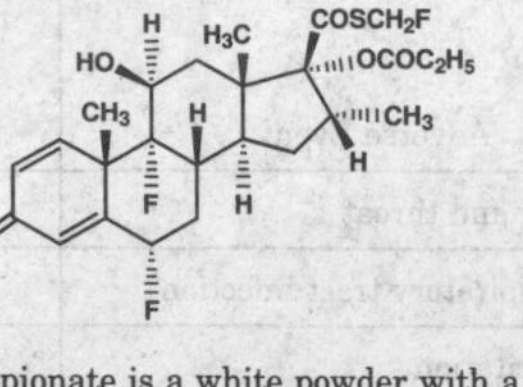

Fluticasone propionate is a white powder with a molecular weight of 500.6, and the empirical formula is $C_{25}H_{31}F_3O_5S$. It is practically insoluble in water, freely soluble in dimethyl sulfoxide and dimethylformamide, and slightly soluble in methanol and 95% ethanol.

FLOVENT DISKUS 50 mcg, FLOVENT DISKUS 100 mcg, and FLOVENT DISKUS 250 mcg are specially designed plastic inhalation delivery systems containing a double-foil blister strip of a powder formulation of fluticasone propionate intended for oral inhalation only. The DISKUS inhalation unit, which is the delivery component, is an integral part of the drug product. Each blister on the double-foil strip within the unit contains 50, 100, or 250 mcg of microfine fluticasone propionate in 12.5 mg of formulation containing lactose (which contains milk proteins). After a blister containing medication is opened by activating the DISKUS, the medication is dispersed into the airstream created by the patient inhaling through the mouthpiece.

Under standardized in vitro test conditions, FLOVENT DISKUS delivers 46, 94, or 229 mcg of fluticasone propionate from FLOVENT DISKUS 50 mcg, FLOVENT DISKUS 100 mcg, or FLOVENT DISKUS 250 mcg, respectively, when tested at a flow rate of 60 L/min for 2 seconds. In adult patients with obstructive lung disease and severely compromised lung function (FEV_1 20% to 30% of predicted), mean peak inspiratory flow (PIF) through a DISKUS was 82.4 L/min (range: 46.1 to 115.3 L/min). In children with asthma 4 and 8 years old, mean PIF through FLOVENT DISKUS was 70 and 104 L/min, respectively (range: 48 to 123 L/min).

The actual amount of drug delivered to the lung may depend on patient factors, such as inspiratory flow profile.

12 CLINICAL PHARMACOLOGY

12.1 Mechanism of Action

Fluticasone propionate is a synthetic trifluorinated corticosteroid with potent anti-inflammatory activity. In vitro assays using human lung cytosol preparations have established fluticasone propionate as a human glucocorticoid receptor agonist with an affinity 18 times greater than dexamethasone, almost twice that of beclomethasone-17-monopropionate (BMP), the active metabolite of beclomethasone dipropionate, and over 3 times that of budesonide. Data from the McKenzie vasoconstrictor assay in man are consistent with these results. The clinical significance of these findings is unknown.

Inflammation is an important component in the pathogenesis of asthma. Corticosteroids have been shown to inhibit multiple cell types (e.g., mast cells, eosinophils, basophils, lymphocytes, macrophages, neutrophils) and mediator production or secretion (e.g., histamine, eicosanoids, leukotrienes, cytokines) involved in the asthmatic response. These anti-inflammatory actions of corticosteroids contribute to their efficacy in asthma.

Though effective for the treatment of asthma, corticosteroids do not affect asthma symptoms immediately. Individual patients will experience a variable time to onset and degree of symptom relief. Maximum benefit may not be achieved for 1 to 2 weeks or longer after starting treatment. When corticosteroids are discontinued, asthma stability may persist for several days or longer.

Studies in patients with asthma have shown a favorable ratio between topical anti-inflammatory activity and systemic corticosteroid effects with recommended doses of orally inhaled fluticasone propionate. This is explained by a combination of a relatively high local anti-inflammatory effect, negligible oral systemic bioavailability (<1%), and the minimal pharmacological activity of the only metabolite detected in man.

12.2 Pharmacodynamics

In clinical trials with fluticasone propionate inhalation powder using dosages up to and including 250 mcg twice daily, occasional abnormal short cosyntropin tests (peak serum cortisol <18 mcg/dL assessed by radioimmunoassay) were noted both in patients receiving fluticasone propionate and in patients receiving placebo. The incidence of abnormal tests at 500 mcg twice daily was greater than placebo. In a 2-year study carried out with the DISKHALER® inhalation device in 64 patients with mild, persistent asthma (mean FEV_1 91% of predicted) randomized to fluticasone propionate 500 mcg twice daily or placebo, no patient receiving fluticasone propionate had an abnormal response to 6-hour cosyntropin infusion (peak serum cortisol <18 mcg/dL). With a peak cortisol threshold <35 mcg/dL, 1 patient receiving fluticasone propionate (4%) had an abnormal response at 1 year; repeat testing at 18 months and 2 years was normal. Another patient receiving fluticasone propionate (5%) had an abnormal response at 2 years. No patient on placebo had an abnormal response at 1 or 2 years.

In a placebo-controlled clinical study conducted in patients aged 4 to 11 years, a 30-minute cosyntropin stimulation test was performed in 41 patients after 12 weeks of dosing with 50 or 100 mcg twice daily of fluticasone propionate via the DISKUS device. One patient receiving fluticasone propionate via DISKUS had a prestimulation plasma cortisol concentration <5 mcg/dL, and 2 patients had a rise in cortisol of <7 mcg/dL. However, all poststimulation values were >18 mcg/dL.

The potential systemic effects of inhaled fluticasone propionate on the HPA axis were also studied in patients with asthma. Fluticasone propionate given by inhalation aerosol at dosages of 220, 440, 660, or 880 mcg twice daily was compared with placebo or oral prednisone 10 mg given once daily for 4 weeks. For most patients, the ability to increase cortisol production in response to stress, as assessed by 6-hour cosyntropin stimulation, remained intact with inhaled fluticasone propionate treatment. No patient had an abnormal response (peak serum cortisol <18 mcg/dL) after dosing with placebo or fluticasone propionate 220 mcg twice daily. For patients treated with 440, 660, and 880 mcg twice daily, 10%, 16%, and 12%, respectively, had an abnormal response as compared with 29% of patients treated with prednisone.

12.3 Pharmacokinetics

Absorption: Fluticasone propionate acts locally in the lung; therefore, plasma levels do not predict therapeutic effect. Studies using oral dosing of labeled and unlabeled drug have demonstrated that the oral systemic bioavailability of fluticasone propionate is negligible (<1%), primarily due to incomplete absorption and presystemic metabolism in the gut and liver. In contrast, the majority of the fluticasone propionate delivered to the lung is systemically absorbed. The absolute bioavailability of fluticasone propionate from the DISKUS device in healthy volunteers averages 7.8%.

Peak steady-state fluticasone propionate plasma concentrations in adult patients with asthma (N = 11) ranged from undetectable to 266 pg/mL after a 500-mcg twice-daily dosage of fluticasone propionate inhalation powder using the DISKUS device. The mean fluticasone propionate plasma concentration was 110 pg/mL.

Distribution: Following intravenous administration, the initial disposition phase for fluticasone propionate was rapid and consistent with its high lipid solubility and tissue binding. The volume of distribution averaged 4.2 L/kg.

The percentage of fluticasone propionate bound to human plasma proteins averages 99%. Fluticasone propionate is weakly and reversibly bound to erythrocytes and is not significantly bound to human transcortin.

Metabolism: The total clearance of fluticasone propionate is high (average, 1,093 mL/min), with renal clearance accounting for less than 0.02% of the total. The only circulating metabolite detected in man is the 17β-carboxylic acid derivative of fluticasone propionate, which is formed through the CYP3A4 pathway. This metabolite had less affinity (approximately 1/2,000) than the parent drug for the corticosteroid receptor of human lung cytosol in vitro and negligible pharmacological activity in animal studies. Other metabolites detected in vitro using cultured human hepatoma cells have not been detected in man.

Elimination: Following intravenous dosing, fluticasone propionate showed polyexponential kinetics and had a terminal elimination half-life of approximately 7.8 hours. Less than 5% of a radiolabeled oral dose was excreted in the urine as metabolites, with the remainder excreted in the feces as parent drug and metabolites.

Specific Populations: *Gender:* Full pharmacokinetic profiles were obtained from 9 female and 16 male patients given 500 mcg twice daily. No overall differences in fluticasone propionate pharmacokinetics were observed.

Pediatrics: In a clinical study conducted in patients aged 4 to 11 years with mild to moderate asthma, fluticasone propionate concentrations were obtained in 61 patients at 20 and 40 minutes after dosing with 50 and 100 mcg twice daily of fluticasone propionate inhalation powder using the DISKUS. Plasma concentrations were low and ranged from undetectable (about 80% of the plasma samples) to 88 pg/mL. Mean peak fluticasone propionate plasma concentrations at the 50- and 100-mcg dose levels were 5 and 8 pg/mL, respectively.

Hepatic and Renal Impairment: Formal pharmacokinetic studies using FLOVENT DISKUS have not been conducted in patients with hepatic or renal impairment. However, since fluticasone propionate is predominantly cleared by hepatic metabolism, impairment of liver function may lead to accumulation of fluticasone propionate in plasma. Therefore, patients with hepatic disease should be closely monitored.

Drug Interactions: *Ritonavir:* Fluticasone propionate is a substrate of CYP3A4. Coadministration of fluticasone propionate and the strong CYP3A4 inhibitor ritonavir is not recommended based upon a multiple-dose, crossover drug interaction study in 18 healthy subjects. Fluticasone propionate aqueous nasal spray (200 mcg once daily) was coadministered for 7 days with ritonavir (100 mg twice daily). Plasma fluticasone propionate concentrations following fluticasone propionate aqueous nasal spray alone were undetectable (<10 pg/mL) in most subjects, and when concentrations were detectable, peak levels (C_{max}) averaged 11.9 pg/mL (range: 10.8 to 14.1 pg/mL) and $AUC_{(0-\tau)}$ averaged 8.43 pg•hr/mL (range: 4.2 to 18.8 pg•hr/mL). Fluticasone propionate C_{max} and $AUC_{(0-\tau)}$ increased to 318 pg/mL (range: 110 to 648 pg/mL) and 3,102.6 pg•hr/mL (range: 1,207.1 to 5,662.0 pg•hr/mL), respectively, after coadministration of ritonavir with fluticasone propionate aqueous nasal spray. This significant increase in plasma fluticasone propionate concentration resulted in a significant decrease (86%) in serum cortisol AUC.

Ketoconazole: In a placebo-controlled, crossover study in 8 healthy adult volunteers, coadministration of a single dose of orally inhaled fluticasone propionate (1,000 mcg) with multiple doses of ketoconazole (200 mg) to steady state resulted in increased plasma fluticasone propionate exposure, a reduction in plasma cortisol AUC, and no effect on urinary excretion of cortisol.

Following orally inhaled fluticasone propionate alone, $AUC_{(2\text{-last})}$ averaged 1.559 ng•hr/mL (range: 0.555 to 2.906 ng•hr/mL) and $AUC_{(2-\infty)}$ averaged 2.269 ng•hr/mL (range: 0.836 to 3.707 ng•hr/mL). Fluticasone propionate $AUC_{(2\text{-last})}$ and $AUC_{(2-\infty)}$ increased to 2.781 ng•hr/mL (range: 2.489 to 8.486 ng•hr/mL) and 4.317 ng•hr/mL (range: 3.256 to 9.408 ng•hr/mL), respectively, after coadministration of ketoconazole with orally inhaled fluticasone propionate. This increase in plasma fluticasone propionate concentration resulted in a decrease (45%) in serum cortisol AUC.

Erythromycin: In a multiple-dose drug interaction study, coadministration of orally inhaled fluticasone propionate (500 mcg twice daily) and erythromycin (333 mg 3 times daily) did not affect fluticasone propionate pharmacokinetics.

13 NONCLINICAL TOXICOLOGY

13.1 Carcinogenesis, Mutagenesis, Impairment of Fertility

Fluticasone propionate demonstrated no tumorigenic potential in mice at oral doses up to 1,000 mcg/kg (approximately 2 and 10 times the MRHD in adults and children aged 4 to 11 years, respectively, on a mg/m^2 basis) for 78 weeks or in rats at inhalation doses up to 57 mcg/kg (approximately 0.2 times and approximately equivalent to the MRHD in adults and children aged 4 to 11 years, respectively, on a mg/m^2 basis) for 104 weeks.

Fluticasone propionate did not induce gene mutation in prokaryotic or eukaryotic cells in vitro. No significant clastogenic effect was seen in cultured human peripheral lymphocytes in vitro or in the in vivo mouse micronucleus test.

No evidence of impairment of fertility was observed in reproductive studies conducted in male and female rats at subcutaneous doses up to 50 mcg/kg (approximately 0.2 times the MRHD in adults on a mg/m^2 basis). Prostate weight was significantly reduced at a subcutaneous dose of 50 mcg/kg.

13.2 Animal Toxicology and/or Pharmacology

Reproductive Toxicology: Subcutaneous studies in the mouse and rat at 45 and 100 mcg/kg (approximately 0.1 and 0.4 times the MRHD in adults on a mg/m^2 basis, respectively) revealed fetal toxicity characteristic of potent corticosteroid compounds, including embryonic growth retardation, omphalocele, cleft palate, and retarded cranial ossification.

In the rabbit, fetal weight reduction and cleft palate were observed at a subcutaneous dose of 4 mcg/kg (approximately 0.03 times the MRHD in adults on a mg/m^2 basis). However, no teratogenic effects were reported at oral doses up to 300 mcg/kg (approximately 2 times the MRHD in adults on a mg/m^2 basis) of fluticasone propionate. No fluticasone propionate was detected in the plasma in this study, consistent with the established low bioavailability following oral administration *[see Clinical Pharmacology (12.3)]*.

Fluticasone propionate crossed the placenta following subcutaneous administration to mice and rats and oral administration to rabbits.

14 CLINICAL STUDIES

14.1 Adult and Adolescent Patients 12 Years and Older

Four randomized, double-blind, parallel-group, placebo-controlled, US clinical trials were conducted in 1,036 adult and adolescent patients (aged ≥12 years) with asthma to assess the efficacy and safety of FLOVENT DISKUS in the treatment of asthma. Fixed dosages of 100, 250, and 500 mcg twice daily were compared with placebo to provide information about appropriate dosing to cover a range of asthma severity. Patients in these studies included those inadequately controlled with bronchodilators alone and those already maintained on daily inhaled corticosteroids. All doses were delivered by inhalation of the contents of 1 or 2 blisters from FLOVENT DISKUS twice daily.

Figures 1 through 4 display results of pulmonary function tests (mean percent change from baseline in FEV_1 prior to AM dose) for 3 recommended dosages of FLOVENT DISKUS (100, 250, and 500 mcg twice daily) and placebo from the four 12-week trials in adolescents and adults. These trials used predetermined criteria for lack of efficacy (indicators of worsening asthma), resulting in withdrawal of more patients in the placebo group. Therefore, pulmonary function results at Endpoint (the last evaluable FEV_1 result, including most patients' lung function data) are also displayed. Pulmonary function, as determined by percent change from baseline in FEV_1 at recommended dosages of FLOVENT DISKUS improved significantly compared with placebo by the first week of treatment, and improvement was maintained for up to 1 year or more.

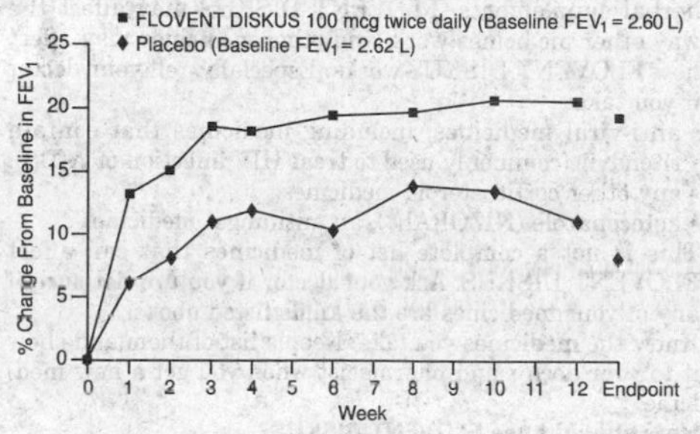

Figure 1. A 12-Week Clinical Trial Evaluating FLOVENT DISKUS 100 mcg Twice Daily in Adolescents and Adults Receiving Bronchodilators Alone

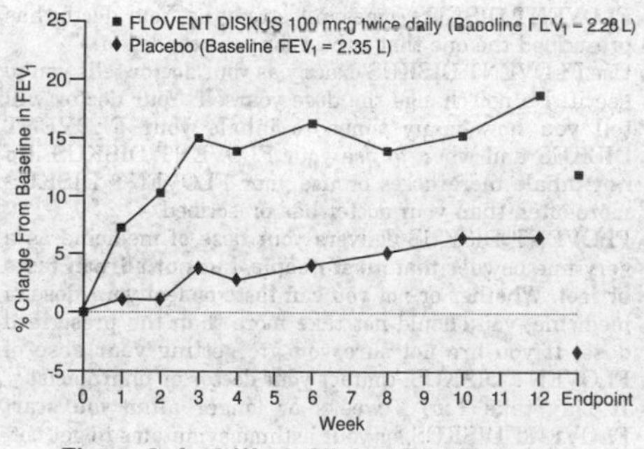

Figure 2. A 12-Week Clinical Trial Evaluating FLOVENT DISKUS 100 mcg Twice Daily in Adolescents and Adults Receiving Inhaled Corticosteroids

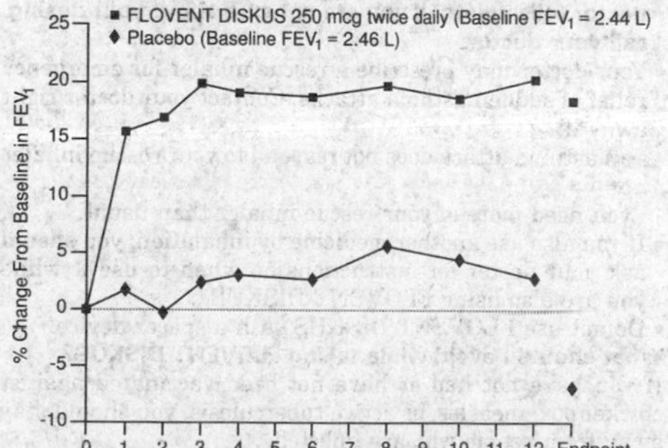

Figure 3. A 12-Week Clinical Trial Evaluating FLOVENT DISKUS 250 mcg Twice Daily in Adolescents and Adults Receiving Inhaled Corticosteroids or Bronchodilators Alone

[See figure 4 at top of next column]

In all 4 efficacy trials, measures of pulmonary function (FEV_1) were statistically significantly improved as compared with placebo at all twice-daily doses. Patients on all dosages of FLOVENT DISKUS were also less likely to discontinue study participation due to asthma deterioration (as defined by predetermined criteria for lack of efficacy in-

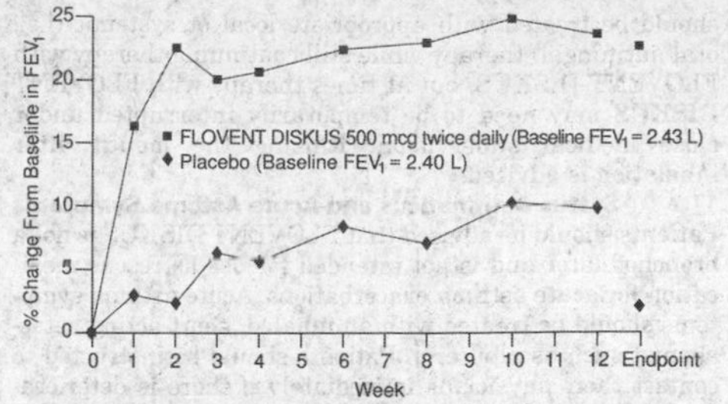

Figure 4. A 12-Week Clinical Trial Evaluating FLOVENT DISKUS 500 mcg Twice Daily in Adolescents and Adults Receiving Inhaled Corticosteroids or Bronchodilators Alone

cluding lung function and patient-recorded variables such as AM PEF, albuterol use, and nighttime awakenings due to asthma) compared with placebo.

In a clinical trial of 111 patients with severe asthma requiring chronic oral prednisone therapy (average baseline daily prednisone dose was 14 mg), fluticasone propionate given by inhalation powder at doses of 500 and 1,000 mcg twice daily was evaluated. Both doses enabled a statistically significantly larger percentage of patients to wean from oral prednisone as compared with placebo (75% of the patients on 500 mcg twice daily and 89% of the patients on 1,000 mcg twice daily as compared with 9% of patients on placebo). Accompanying the reduction in oral corticosteroid use, patients treated with fluticasone propionate had significantly improved lung function and fewer asthma symptoms as compared with the placebo group.

14.2 Pediatric Patients Aged 4 to 11 Years

A 12-week, placebo-controlled clinical trial was conducted in 437 pediatric patients (177 received FLOVENT DISKUS), approximately half of whom were receiving inhaled corticosteroids at baseline. In this study, doses of fluticasone propionate inhalation powder 50 and 100 mcg twice daily significantly improved FEV_1 (15% and 18% change from baseline at Endpoint, respectively) compared with placebo (7% change). AM PEF was also significantly improved with doses of fluticasone propionate 50 and 100 mcg twice daily (26% and 27% change from baseline at Endpoint, respectively) compared with placebo (14% change). In this study, patients on active treatment were significantly less likely to discontinue treatment due to asthma deterioration (as defined by predetermined criteria for lack of efficacy including lung function and patient recorded variables such as AM PEF, albuterol use, and nighttime awakenings due to asthma).

Two other 12-week placebo-controlled clinical trials were conducted in 504 pediatric patients with asthma, approximately half of whom were receiving inhaled corticosteroids at baseline. In these studies, FLOVENT DISKUS was efficacious at doses of 50 and 100 mcg twice daily when compared with placebo on major endpoints including lung function and symptom scores. Pulmonary function improved significantly compared with placebo by the first week of treatment, and patients treated with FLOVENT DISKUS were also less likely to discontinue study participation due to asthma deterioration. One hundred ninety-two (192) patients received FLOVENT DISKUS for up to 1 year during an open-label extension. Data from this open-label extension suggested that lung function improvements could be maintained up to 1 year.

16 HOW SUPPLIED/STORAGE AND HANDLING

FLOVENT DISKUS 50 mcg (NDC 0173-0600-02), FLOVENT DISKUS 100 mcg (NDC 0173-0602-02), and FLOVENT DISKUS 250 mcg (NDC 0173-0601-02) are each supplied as a disposable orange inhalation unit containing 60 blisters of powder formulation packaged in a plastic-coated, moisture-protective foil pouch in a carton of 1.

FLOVENT DISKUS 100 mcg (NDC 0173-0602-00) and FLOVENT DISKUS 250 mcg (NDC 0173-0601-00) are also each supplied in an institutional pack of 1 disposable orange inhalation unit containing 28 blisters of powder formulation packaged in a plastic-coated, moisture-protective foil pouch in a carton of 1.

Store at controlled room temperature (see USP), 20° to 25°C (68° to 77°F) in a dry place away from direct heat or sunlight. Keep out of reach of children. The DISKUS inhalation device is not reusable. FLOVENT DISKUS should be discarded 6 weeks (50-mcg strength) or 2 months (100- and 250-mcg strengths) after removal from the moisture-protective foil pouch or after all blisters have been used (when the dose indicator reads "0"), whichever comes first. Do not attempt to take the device apart.

17 PATIENT COUNSELING INFORMATION

See FDA-Approved patient labeling (Patient Information).

17.1 Oral Candidiasis

Patients should be advised that localized infections with *Candida albicans* have occurred in the mouth and pharynx in some patients. If oropharyngeal candidiasis develops, it should be treated with appropriate local or systemic (i.e., oral antifungal) therapy while still continuing therapy with FLOVENT DISKUS, but at times therapy with FLOVENT DISKUS may need to be temporarily interrupted under close medical supervision. Rinsing the mouth after inhalation is advised.

17.2 Status Asthmaticus and Acute Asthma Symptoms

Patients should be advised that FLOVENT DISKUS is not a bronchodilator and is not intended for use as rescue medication for acute asthma exacerbations. Acute asthma symptoms should be treated with an inhaled, short-acting beta$_2$-agonist such as albuterol. Patients should be instructed to contact their physicians immediately if there is deterioration of their asthma.

17.3 Immunosuppression

Patients who are on immunosuppressant doses of corticosteroids should be warned to avoid exposure to chickenpox or measles and if they are exposed to consult their physicians without delay. Patients should be informed of potential worsening of existing tuberculosis, fungal, bacterial, viral, or parasitic infections, or ocular herpes simplex.

17.4 Hypercorticism and Adrenal Suppression

Patients should be advised that FLOVENT DISKUS may cause systemic corticosteroid effects of hypercorticism and adrenal suppression. Additionally, patients should be instructed that deaths due to adrenal insufficiency have occurred during and after transfer from systemic corticosteroids. Patients should taper slowly from systemic corticosteroids if transferring to FLOVENT DISKUS.

17.5 Hypersensitivity Reactions, Including Anaphylaxis

Patients should be advised that hypersensitivity reactions, including anaphylaxis, angioedema, urticaria, and bronchospasm, may occur after administration of FLOVENT DISKUS. Patients should discontinue FLOVENT DISKUS if such reactions occur. There have been reports of anaphylactic reactions in patients with severe milk protein allergy; therefore, patients with severe milk protein allergy should not take FLOVENT DISKUS.

17.6 Reduction in Bone Mineral Density

Patients who are at an increased risk for decreased BMD should be advised that the use of corticosteroids may pose an additional risk.

17.7 Reduced Growth Velocity

Patients should be informed that orally inhaled corticosteroids, including FLOVENT DISKUS, may cause a reduction in growth velocity when administered to pediatric patients. Physicians should closely follow the growth of children and adolescents taking corticosteroids by any route.

17.8 Ocular Effects

Long-term use of inhaled corticosteroids may increase the risk of some eye problems (cataracts or glaucoma); regular eye examinations should be considered.

17.9 Use Daily for Best Effect

Patients should use FLOVENT DISKUS at regular intervals as directed. Individual patients will experience a variable time to onset and degree of symptom relief and the full benefit may not be achieved until treatment has been administered for 1 to 2 weeks or longer. Patients should not increase the prescribed dosage but should contact their physicians if symptoms do not improve or if the condition worsens. Patients should be instructed not to stop use of FLOVENT DISKUS abruptly. Patients should contact their physicians immediately if they discontinue use of FLOVENT DISKUS.

GlaxoSmithKline
Research Triangle Park, NC 27709

September 2011
FLD:6PI

Patient Information

FLOVENT®*[flō' vent]* DISKUS® 50 mcg
(fluticasone propionate inhalation powder, 50 mcg)
FLOVENT® DISKUS® 100 mcg
(fluticasone propionate inhalation powder, 100 mcg)
FLOVENT® DISKUS® 250 mcg
(fluticasone propionate inhalation powder, 250 mcg)
FOR ORAL INHALATION ONLY

Read this Patient Information before you start to use FLOVENT DISKUS and each time you get a refill. There may be new information. This information does not take the place of talking with your doctor about your medical condition or your treatment.

What is FLOVENT DISKUS?

FLOVENT DISKUS is an inhaled prescription corticosteroid medicine for the long-term treatment of asthma in people aged 4 and older.

- FLOVENT DISKUS helps to prevent symptoms of asthma
- FLOVENT DISKUS does not treat the sudden symptoms of an asthma attack, such as wheezing, cough, shortness of breath, and chest pain or tightness. **Always have a fast-acting bronchodilator medicine (rescue inhaler) with you to treat sudden symptoms.**

It is not known if FLOVENT DISKUS is safe and effective in children younger than 4 years of age.

Who should not use FLOVENT DISKUS?

Do not use FLOVENT DISKUS

- to treat sudden symptoms of asthma. **FLOVENT DISKUS is not a rescue inhaler and should not be used to give you fast relief from your asthma attack.** Always use a rescue inhaler, such as albuterol, during a sudden asthma attack.
- if you have severe allergy to milk proteins or fluticasone propionate. Ask your doctor if you are not sure.

What should I tell my doctor before taking FLOVENT DISKUS?

Before you use FLOVENT DISKUS, tell your doctor if you:

- have liver problems.
- have been exposed to chickenpox or measles.
- have any other medical conditions.
- are pregnant or planning to become pregnant. It is not known if FLOVENT DISKUS will harm your unborn baby. Talk to your doctor if you are pregnant or plan to become pregnant.
- are breast-feeding or plan to breast-feed. It is not known if FLOVENT DISKUS passes into your breast milk. You and your doctor should decide if you should use FLOVENT DISKUS while you breast-feed.

Tell your doctor about all the medicines you take including prescription and non-prescription medicines, vitamins, and herbal supplements. FLOVENT DISKUS may affect the way other medicines work, and other medicines may affect how FLOVENT DISKUS works. Especially, tell your doctor if you take:

- anti-viral medicines, including medicines that contain ritonavir (commonly used to treat HIV infection or AIDS).
- any other corticosteroid medicines.
- ketoconazole (NIZORAL®), an antifungal medicine.

This is not a complete list of medicines that can affect FLOVENT DISKUS. Ask your doctor if you are not sure if any of your medicines are the kinds listed above.

Know the medicines you take. Keep a list of them and show it to your doctor and pharmacist when you get a new medicine.

How should I use FLOVENT DISKUS?

- Read the detailed Instructions for Use at the end of this leaflet.
- An adult should always watch a child use FLOVENT DISKUS to make sure that it is used correctly, as instructed by your doctor.
- FLOVENT DISKUS comes in 3 strengths. Your doctor has prescribed the one that is best for your condition.
- Use FLOVENT DISKUS exactly as your doctor tells you to use it. Do not change the dose yourself. Your doctor will tell you how many times to inhale your FLOVENT DISKUS and when to use your FLOVENT DISKUS. **Do not** inhale more doses or use your FLOVENT DISKUS more often than your doctor has prescribed.
- FLOVENT DISKUS delivers your dose of medicine as a very fine powder **that most people, but not all, can taste or feel.** Whether or not you can taste or feel your dose of medicine, you should not take more than the prescribed dose. If you are not sure you are getting your dose of FLOVENT DISKUS, contact your doctor or pharmacist.
- It may take 1 to 2 weeks or longer after you start FLOVENT DISKUS for your asthma symptoms to get better. You must use FLOVENT DISKUS regularly. **Do not stop using FLOVENT DISKUS, even if you are feeling better, unless your doctor tells you to.**
- If you miss a dose, just take your next dose at your regular time. **Do not take 2 doses at the same time unless your doctor tells you to. If you are not sure about your dosing, call your doctor.**
- Your doctor may prescribe a rescue inhaler for emergency relief of sudden asthma attacks. Contact your doctor right away if:
  - an asthma attack does not respond to your rescue inhaler or
  - you need more of your rescue inhaler than usual.
- If you also use another medicine by inhalation, you should ask your doctor for instructions on when to use it while you are also using FLOVENT DISKUS.
- Do not use FLOVENT DISKUS with a spacer device.

What should I avoid while taking FLOVENT DISKUS?

If you have not had or have not been vaccinated against chickenpox, measles, or active tuberculosis, you should stay away from people who are infected.

What are the possible side effects of FLOVENT DISKUS?

FLOVENT DISKUS can cause serious side effects, including:

- **fungal infection (thrush) in your mouth and throat.** Tell your doctor if you have any redness or white-colored coating in your mouth.
- **decreased ability to fight infections.** Symptoms of infection may include: fever, pain, aches, chills, feeling tired, nausea and vomiting. Tell your doctor about any signs of infection while you use FLOVENT DISKUS.
- **decreased adrenal function (adrenal insufficiency).** Symptoms of decreased adrenal function include tiredness, weakness, nausea and vomiting, and low blood pressure. Decreased adrenal function can lead to death.
- **allergic reaction (anaphylaxis).** Call your doctor and stop FLOVENT DISKUS right away if you have any symptoms of an allergic reaction:

• swelling of the face, throat, and tongue	• rash
• hives	• breathing problems

- **lower bone mineral density.** This may be a problem for people who already have a higher chance of low bone density (osteoporosis).
- **slow growth in children.** The growth of children using FLOVENT DISKUS should be checked regularly.
- **eye problems including glaucoma and cataracts.** Tell your doctor about any vision changes while using FLOVENT DISKUS. Your doctor may tell you to have your eyes checked.
- **increased wheezing (bronchospasm).** Increased wheezing can happen right away after using FLOVENT DISKUS. Always have a rescue inhaler with you to treat sudden wheezing.

Call your doctor right away if you have any of the serious side effects listed above or if you have worsening lung symptoms.

The most common side effects of FLOVENT DISKUS include:

• a cold or upper respiratory tract infection	• fever
• throat irritation	• headache
• nausea and vomiting	

Tell your doctor if you have any side effects that bother you or that do not go away. These are not all the possible side effects of FLOVENT DISKUS. For more information ask your doctor or pharmacist.

Call your doctor for medical advice about side effects. You may report side effects to FDA at 1-800-FDA-1088 or 1-800-332-1088.

How should I store FLOVENT DISKUS?

Store FLOVENT DISKUS at room temperature between 68°F to 77°F (20°C to 25°C). Store FLOVENT DISKUS in a dry place away from heat and sunlight.

FLOVENT DISKUS is not reusable. Safely throw away medicine that is out of date or no longer needed.

Do not try to take FLOVENT DISKUS apart.

Keep FLOVENT DISKUS and all medicines out of the reach of children.

General information about the safe and effective use of FLOVENT DISKUS.

Medicines are sometimes prescribed for purposes other than those listed in a Patient Information leaflet. Do not use FLOVENT DISKUS for a condition for which it was not prescribed. Do not give FLOVENT DISKUS to other people, even if they have the same symptoms that you have. It may harm them.

This Patient Information leaflet summarizes the most important information about FLOVENT DISKUS. If you would like more information, talk with your healthcare provider. You can ask your pharmacist or doctor for information about FLOVENT DISKUS that is written for health professionals.

For more information go to www.floventdiskus.com or call 1-888-825-5249.

What are the ingredients in FLOVENT DISKUS?

Active ingredient: fluticasone propionate (microfine)
Inactive ingredient: lactose (which contains milk proteins)

Instructions for Using FLOVENT DISKUS

The parts of your FLOVENT DISKUS

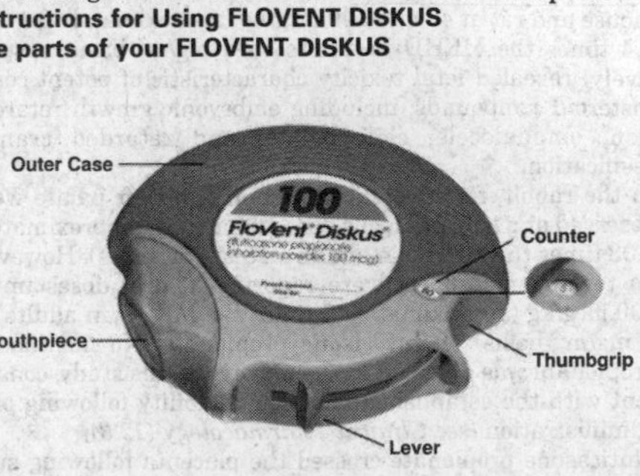

Figure 1

The counter shows you how many doses are left. The counter number will count down each time you use FLOVENT DISKUS. After you have used 55 doses (23 doses from the sample and institutional packs), the numbers 5 to 0 will show in **red** to warn you that there are only a few doses left (see Figure 1).

Using your FLOVENT DISKUS

- Take FLOVENT DISKUS out of the moisture-protective foil pouch just before you use it for the first time. Safely throw away the foil pouch.
- FLOVENT DISKUS will be in the closed position. Write the "Pouch opened" and "Use by" dates in the blank lines on the label (see Figure 1). The "Use by" date for FLOVENT DISKUS 50 mcg is 6 weeks from the date you opened the pouch. The "Use by" date for FLOVENT DISKUS 100 mcg and FLOVENT DISKUS 250 mcg is 2 months from the date you opened the pouch.

Read the following steps before using FLOVENT DISKUS and follow them at each use. If you have any questions, ask your doctor or pharmacist.

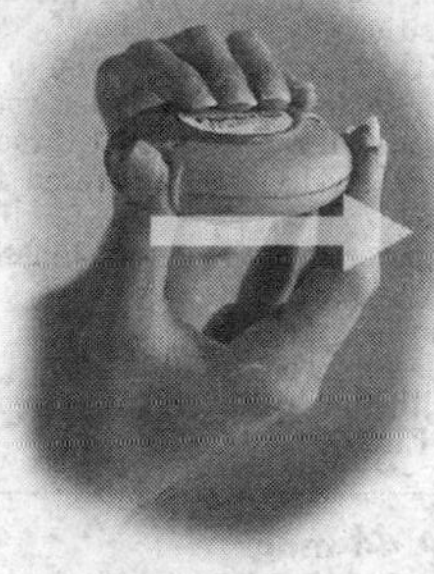

Figure 2

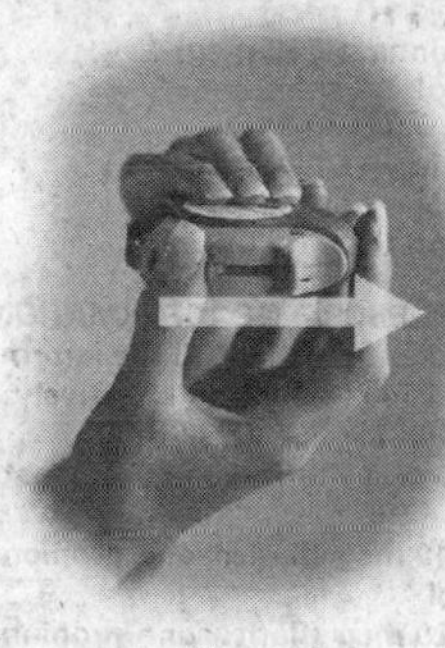

Figure 3

1. Open

Hold FLOVENT DISKUS in one hand and put the thumb of your other hand on the thumbgrip. Push your thumb away from you as far as it will go until the mouthpiece shows and snaps into place (see Figure 2).

2. Click

Hold FLOVENT DISKUS in a level, flat position with the mouthpiece towards you. Slide the lever away from you as far as it will go until it clicks (see Figure 3). The number on the dose counter will count down by 1. FLOVENT DISKUS is now ready to use.

To avoid releasing a dose by mistake before you are ready to inhale:

- **Do not close FLOVENT DISKUS.**
- **Do not tilt FLOVENT DISKUS.**
- **Do not play with the lever.**
- **Do not slide the lever more than once.**

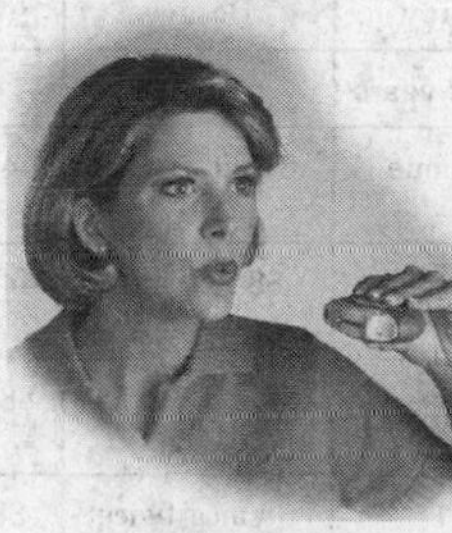

Figure 4

[See figure 5 at top of next column]

3. Inhale

Before you inhale your dose of FLOVENT DISKUS, breathe out as far as you can while you hold FLOVENT DISKUS level and away from your mouth (see Figure 4). **Never breathe out into the FLOVENT DISKUS mouthpiece.**

Put the mouthpiece to your lips (see Figure 5). Breathe in quickly and deeply through FLOVENT DISKUS. Do not breathe in through your nose.

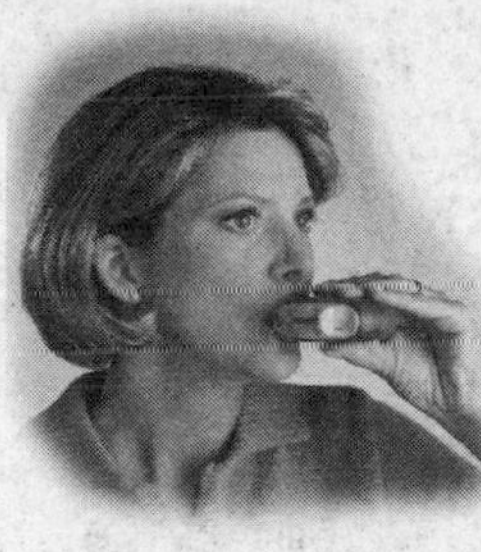

Figure 5

Remove FLOVENT DISKUS from your mouth. Hold your breath for about 10 seconds, or for as long as is comfortable. Breathe out slowly.

Rinse your mouth with water after inhaling the medicine. Spit out the water. Do not swallow it.

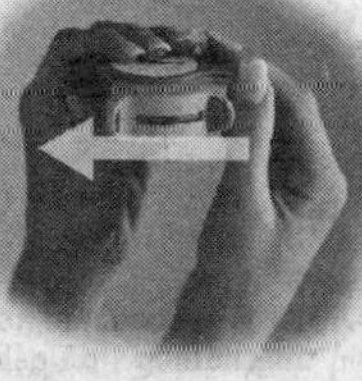

Figure 6

4. Close FLOVENT DISKUS when you are finished taking a dose. Put your thumb on the thumbgrip and slide it back towards you as far as it will go (see Figure 6). FLOVENT DISKUS will click shut. The lever will automatically return to its original position.

FLOVENT DISKUS is now ready for you to take your next scheduled dose in about 12 hours. When you are ready for your next dose, you will repeat steps 1 through 4.

FLOVENT and DISKUS are registered trademarks of GlaxoSmithKline.

NIZORAL is a registered trademark of Janssen Pharmaceutica.

GlaxoSmithKline
Research Triangle Park, NC 27709

September 2011 FLD:5PIL

Patient Information

FLOVENT® *[flō' vent]* DISKUS® 50 mcg
(fluticasone propionate inhalation powder, 50 mcg)
FLOVENT® DISKUS® 100 mcg
(fluticasone propionate inhalation powder, 100 mcg)
FLOVENT® DISKUS® 250 mcg
(fluticasone propionate inhalation powder, 250 mcg)
FOR ORAL INHALATION

Read this Patient Information before you start to use FLOVENT DISKUS and each time you get a refill. There may be new information. This information does not take the place of talking with your doctor about your medical condition or your treatment.

What is FLOVENT DISKUS?

FLOVENT DISKUS is an inhaled prescription corticosteroid medicine for the long-term treatment of asthma in people aged 4 and older.

- FLOVENT DISKUS helps to prevent symptoms of asthma
- FLOVENT DISKUS does not treat the sudden symptoms of an asthma attack, such as wheezing, cough, shortness of breath, and chest pain or tightness. **Always have a fast-acting bronchodilator medicine (rescue inhaler) with you to treat sudden symptoms.**

It is not known if FLOVENT DISKUS is safe and effective in children younger than 4 years of age.

Who should not use FLOVENT DISKUS?

Do not use FLOVENT DISKUS

- to treat sudden symptoms of asthma. **FLOVENT DISKUS is not a rescue inhaler and should not be used to give you fast relief from your asthma attack.** Always use a rescue inhaler, such as albuterol, during a sudden asthma attack.
- if you have severe allergy to milk proteins or fluticasone propionate. Ask your doctor if you are not sure.

What should I tell my doctor before taking FLOVENT DISKUS?

Before you use FLOVENT DISKUS, tell your doctor if you:

- have liver problems.
- have been exposed to chickenpox or measles.
- have any other medical conditions.
- are pregnant or planning to become pregnant. It is not known if FLOVENT DISKUS will harm your unborn baby. Talk to your doctor if you are pregnant or plan to become pregnant.
- are breast-feeding or plan to breast-feed. It is not known if FLOVENT DISKUS passes into your breast milk. You and your doctor should decide if you should use FLOVENT DISKUS while you breast-feed.

Tell your doctor about all the medicines you take including prescription and non-prescription medicines, vitamins, and herbal supplements. FLOVENT DISKUS may affect the way other medicines work, and other medicines may affect how FLOVENT DISKUS works. Especially, tell your doctor if you take:

- anti-viral medicines, including medicines that contain ritonavir (commonly used to treat HIV infection or AIDS).
- any other corticosteroid medicines.
- ketoconazole (NIZORAL®), an antifungal medicine.

This is not a complete list of medicines that can affect FLOVENT DISKUS. Ask your doctor if you are not sure if any of your medicines are the kinds listed above.

Know the medicines you take. Keep a list of them and show it to your doctor and pharmacist when you get a new medicine.

How should I use FLOVENT DISKUS?

- Read the detailed Instructions for Use at the end of this leaflet.
- An adult should always watch a child use FLOVENT DISKUS to make sure that it is used correctly, as instructed by your doctor.
- FLOVENT DISKUS comes in 3 strengths. Your doctor has prescribed the one that is best for your condition.
- Use FLOVENT DISKUS exactly as your doctor tells you to use it. Do not change the dose yourself. Your doctor will tell you how many times to inhale your FLOVENT DISKUS and when to use your FLOVENT DISKUS. **Do not** inhale more doses or use your FLOVENT DISKUS more often than your doctor has prescribed.
- FLOVENT DISKUS delivers your dose of medicine as a very fine powder **that most people, but not all, can taste or feel.** Whether or not you can taste or feel your dose of medicine, you should not take more than the prescribed dose. If you are not sure you are getting your dose of FLOVENT DISKUS, contact your doctor or pharmacist.
- It may take 1 to 2 weeks or longer after you start FLOVENT DISKUS for your asthma symptoms to get better. You must use FLOVENT DISKUS regularly. **Do not stop using FLOVENT DISKUS, even if you are feeling better, unless your doctor tells you to.**
- If you miss a dose, just take your next dose at your regular time. **Do not take 2 doses at the same time unless your doctor tells you to. If you are not sure about your dosing, call your doctor.**
- Your doctor may prescribe a rescue inhaler for emergency relief of sudden asthma attacks. Contact your doctor right away if:
  - ◦ an asthma attack does not respond to your rescue inhaler or
  - ◦ you need more of your rescue inhaler than usual.
- If you also use another medicine by inhalation, you should ask your doctor for instructions on when to use it while you are also using FLOVENT DISKUS.
- Do not use FLOVENT DISKUS with a spacer device.

What should I avoid while taking FLOVENT DISKUS?

If you have not had or have not been vaccinated against chickenpox, measles, or active tuberculosis, you should stay away from people who are infected.

What are the possible side effects of FLOVENT DISKUS?

FLOVENT DISKUS can cause serious side effects, including:

- **fungal infection (thrush) in your mouth and throat.** Tell your doctor if you have any redness or white-colored coating in your mouth.
- **decreased ability to fight infections.** Symptoms of infection may include: fever, pain, aches, chills, feeling tired, nausea and vomiting. Tell your doctor about any signs of infection while you use FLOVENT DISKUS.
- **decreased adrenal function (adrenal insufficiency).** Symptoms of decreased adrenal function include tiredness, weakness, nausea and vomiting, and low blood pressure. Decreased adrenal function can lead to death.
- **allergic reaction (anaphylaxis).** Call your doctor and stop FLOVENT DISKUS right away if you have any symptoms of an allergic reaction:

• swelling of the face, throat, and tongue	• rash
• hives	• breathing problems

- **lower bone mineral density.** This may be a problem for people who already have a higher chance of low bone density (osteoporosis).
- **slow growth in children.** The growth of children using FLOVENT DISKUS should be checked regularly.
- **eye problems including glaucoma and cataracts.** Tell your doctor about any vision changes while using FLOVENT DISKUS. Your doctor may tell you to have your eyes checked.

- **increased wheezing (bronchospasm).** Increased wheezing can happen right away after using FLOVENT DISKUS. Always have a rescue inhaler with you to treat sudden wheezing.

Call your doctor right away if you have any of the serious side effects listed above or if you have worsening lung symptoms.

The most common side effects of FLOVENT DISKUS include:

- a cold or upper respiratory tract infection
- fever
- throat irritation
- headache
- nausea and vomiting

Tell your doctor if you have any side effects that bother you or that do not go away. These are not all the possible side effects of FLOVENT DISKUS. For more information ask your doctor or pharmacist.

Call your doctor for medical advice about side effects. You may report side effects to FDA at 1-800-FDA-1088 or 1-800-332-1088.

How should I store FLOVENT DISKUS?

Store FLOVENT DISKUS at room temperature between 68°F to 77°F (20°C to 25°C). Store FLOVENT DISKUS in a dry place away from heat and sunlight.

FLOVENT DISKUS is not reusable. Safely throw away medicine that is out of date or no longer needed.

Do not try to take FLOVENT DISKUS apart.

Keep FLOVENT DISKUS and all medicines out of the reach of children.

General information about the safe and effective use of FLOVENT DISKUS.

Medicines are sometimes prescribed for purposes other than those listed in a Patient Information leaflet. Do not use FLOVENT DISKUS for a condition for which it was not prescribed. Do not give FLOVENT DISKUS to other people, even if they have the same symptoms that you have. It may harm them.

This Patient Information leaflet summarizes the most important information about FLOVENT DISKUS. If you would like more information, talk with your healthcare provider. You can ask your pharmacist or doctor for information about FLOVENT DISKUS that is written for health professionals.

For more information go to www.floventdiskus.com or call 1-888-825-5249.

What are the ingredients in FLOVENT DISKUS?

Active ingredient: fluticasone propionate (microfine)

Inactive ingredient: lactose (which contains milk proteins)

Instructions for Using FLOVENT DISKUS

The parts of your FLOVENT DISKUS

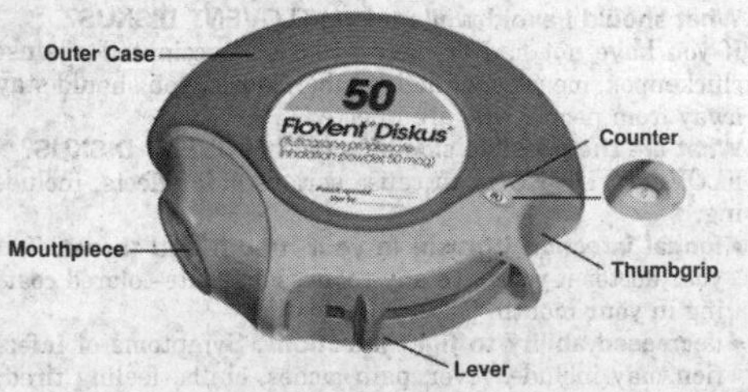

Figure 1

The counter shows you how many doses are left. The counter number will count down each time you use FLOVENT DISKUS. After you have used 55 doses (23 doses from the sample and institutional packs), the numbers 5 to 0 will show in **red** to warn you that there are only a few doses left (see Figure 1).

Using your FLOVENT DISKUS

- Take FLOVENT DISKUS out of the moisture-protective foil pouch just before you use it for the first time. Safely throw away the foil pouch.
- FLOVENT DISKUS will be in the closed position. Write the "Pouch opened" and "Use by" dates in the blank lines on the label (see Figure 1). The "Use by" date for FLOVENT DISKUS 50 mcg is 6 weeks from the date you opened the pouch. The "Use by" date for FLOVENT DISKUS 100 mcg and FLOVENT DISKUS 250 mcg is 2 months from the date you opened the pouch.

Read the following steps before using FLOVENT DISKUS and follow them at each use. If you have any questions, ask your doctor or pharmacist.

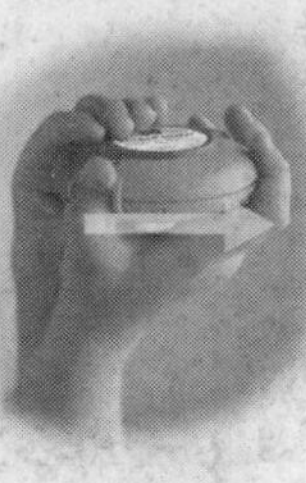

Figure 2

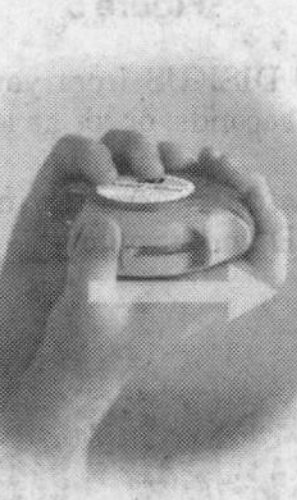

Figure 3

1. Open

Hold FLOVENT DISKUS in one hand and put the thumb of your other hand on the thumbgrip. Push your thumb away from you as far as it will go until the mouthpiece shows and snaps into place (see Figure 2).

2. Click

Hold FLOVENT DISKUS in a level, flat position with the mouthpiece towards you. Slide the lever away from you as far as it will go until it clicks (see Figure 3). The number on the dose counter will count down by 1. FLOVENT DISKUS is now ready to use.

To avoid releasing a dose by mistake before you are ready to inhale:

- **Do not close FLOVENT DISKUS.**
- **Do not tilt FLOVENT DISKUS.**
- **Do not play with the lever.**
- **Do not slide the lever more than once.**

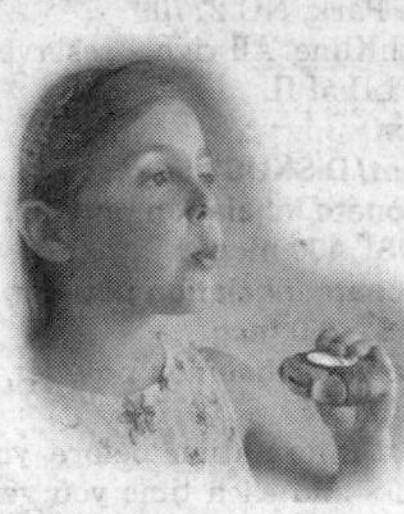

Figure 4

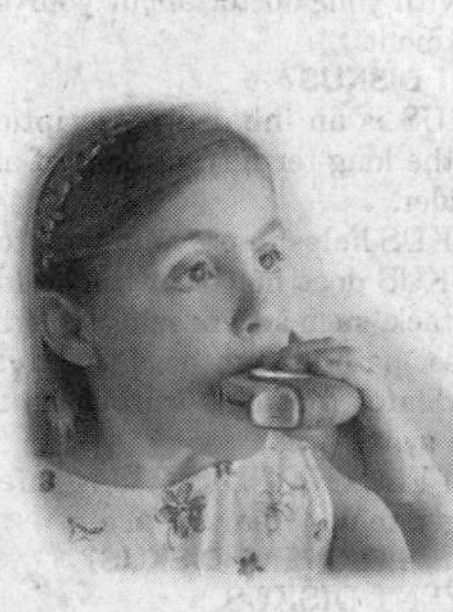

Figure 5

3. Inhale

Before you inhale your dose of FLOVENT DISKUS, breathe out as far as you can while you hold FLOVENT DISKUS level and away from your mouth (see Figure 4). **Never breathe out into the FLOVENT DISKUS mouthpiece.**

Put the mouthpiece to your lips (see Figure 5). Breathe in quickly and deeply through FLOVENT DISKUS. Do not breathe in through your nose.

Remove FLOVENT DISKUS from your mouth. Hold your breath for about 10 seconds, or for as long as is comfortable. Breathe out slowly.

Rinse your mouth with water after inhaling the medicine. Spit out the water. Do not swallow it.

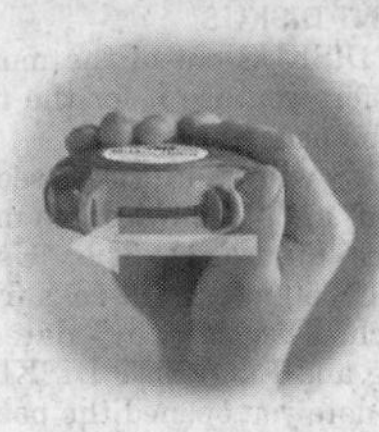

Figure 6

4. Close FLOVENT DISKUS when you are finished taking a dose. Put your thumb on the thumbgrip and slide it back towards you as far as it will go (see Figure 6). FLOVENT DISKUS will click shut. The lever will automatically return to its original position.

FLOVENT DISKUS is now ready for you to take your next scheduled dose in about 12 hours. When you are ready for your next dose, you will repeat steps 1 through 4.

FLOVENT and DISKUS are registered trademarks of GlaxoSmithKline.

NIZORAL is a registered trademark of Janssen Pharmaceutica.

GlaxoSmithKline
Research Triangle Park, NC 27709

September 2011 FLD:5PIL

FLOVENT HFA 44 mcg ℞

[flō′ vent]

(fluticasone propionate 44 mcg)
Inhalation Aerosol

FLOVENT HFA 110 mcg ℞

(fluticasone propionate 110 mcg)
Inhalation Aerosol

FLOVENT HFA 220 mcg ℞

(fluticasone propionate 220 mcg)
Inhalation Aerosol
For Oral Inhalation Only

HIGHLIGHTS OF PRESCRIBING INFORMATION

These highlights do not include all the information needed to use FLOVENT HFA safely and effectively. See full prescribing information for FLOVENT HFA.

FLOVENT HFA 44 mcg (fluticasone propionate 44 mcg) Inhalation Aerosol
FLOVENT HFA 110 mcg (fluticasone propionate 110 mcg) Inhalation Aerosol
FLOVENT HFA 220 mcg (fluticasone propionate 220 mcg) Inhalation Aerosol
FOR ORAL INHALATION ONLY
Initial U.S. Approval: 1994

INDICATIONS AND USAGE

FLOVENT HFA is an inhaled corticosteroid indicated for:

- Maintenance treatment of asthma as prophylactic therapy in patients aged 4 years and older. (1)
- Treatment of asthma for patients requiring oral corticosteroid therapy. (1)

FLOVENT HFA is NOT indicated for the relief of acute bronchospasm. (1)

DOSAGE AND ADMINISTRATION

For oral inhalation only. Dosing is based on prior asthma therapy. (2)

Previous Therapy	Recommended Starting Dosage	Highest Recommended Dosage
Patients aged ≥12 years		
Bronchodilators alone	88 mcg twice daily	440 mcg twice daily
Inhaled corticosteroids	88-220 mcg twice daily	440 mcg twice daily
Oral corticosteroids	440 mcg twice daily	880 mcg twice daily
Patients aged 4-11 years	88 mcg twice daily	88 mcg twice daily

DOSAGE FORMS AND STRENGTHS

Inhalation aerosol with 44, 110, or 220 mcg per actuation. (3)

CONTRAINDICATIONS

- Primary treatment of status asthmaticus or acute episodes of asthma requiring intensive measures. (4)
- Hypersensitivity to any ingredient. (4)

WARNINGS AND PRECAUTIONS

- Localized infections: *Candida albicans* infection of the mouth and pharynx. Monitor patients periodically for signs of adverse effects on the oral cavity. Advise patients to rinse mouth following inhalation. (5.1)
- Immunosuppression: Potential worsening of existing tuberculosis; fungal, bacterial, viral, or parasitic infection; or ocular herpes simplex. More serious or even fatal course of chickenpox or measles in susceptible patients. Use caution in patients with above because of the potential for worsening of these infections. (5.3)
- Transferring patients from systemic corticosteroids: Risk of impaired adrenal function when transferring from oral steroids. Taper patients slowly from systemic corticosteroids if transferring to FLOVENT HFA. (5.4)
- Hypercorticism and adrenal suppression: May occur with very high dosages or at the regular dosage in susceptible individuals. If such changes occur, discontinue FLOVENT HFA slowly. (5.5)
- Hypersensitivity reactions, including anaphylaxis, may occur after administration of FLOVENT HFA. Discontinue FLOVENT HFA if such reactions occur. (4, 5.6)
- Decreases in bone mineral density: Assess bone mineral density initially and periodically thereafter in patients at risk. (5.7)
- Effect on growth: Monitor growth of pediatric patients. (5.8)
- Glaucoma and cataracts: Close monitoring is warranted. (5.9)

ADVERSE REACTIONS

Most common adverse reactions (incidence >3%) include upper respiratory tract infection or inflammation, throat irritation, sinusitis, dysphonia, candidiasis, cough, bronchitis, and headache. (6.1)

To report SUSPECTED ADVERSE REACTIONS, contact GlaxoSmithKline at 1-888-825-5249 or FDA at 1-800-FDA-1088 or www.fda.gov/medwatch

DRUG INTERACTIONS

Use with strong cytochrome P450 3A4 inhibitors such as ritonavir and ketoconazole is not recommended. Systemic corticosteroid effects may occur. (7.1)

USE IN SPECIFIC POPULATIONS

Hepatic impairment: Monitor patients for signs of increased drug exposure. (8.6)

See 17 for PATIENT COUNSELING INFORMATION and FDA-approved patient labeling

Revised: 01/2012

FULL PRESCRIBING INFORMATION: CONTENTS*

*** Sections or subsections omitted from the full prescribing information are not listed**

FULL PRESCRIBING INFORMATION

1 INDICATIONS AND USAGE

FLOVENT® HFA Inhalation Aerosol is indicated for the maintenance treatment of asthma as prophylactic therapy in patients aged 4 years and older. It is also indicated for patients requiring oral corticosteroid therapy for asthma. Many of these patients may be able to reduce or eliminate their requirement for oral corticosteroids over time.

FLOVENT HFA Inhalation Aerosol is NOT indicated for the relief of acute bronchospasm.

2 DOSAGE AND ADMINISTRATION

FLOVENT HFA should be administered by the orally inhaled route only in patients aged 4 years and older. Individual patients will experience a variable time to onset and degree of symptom relief. Maximum benefit may not be achieved for 1 to 2 weeks or longer after starting treatment. After asthma stability has been achieved, it is always desirable to titrate to the lowest effective dosage to reduce the possibility of side effects. For patients who do not respond adequately to the starting dosage after 2 weeks of therapy, higher dosages may provide additional asthma control. The safety and efficacy of FLOVENT HFA when administered in excess of recommended dosages have not been established.

The recommended starting dosage and the highest recommended dosage of FLOVENT HFA, based on prior asthma therapy, are listed in Table 1.

Table 1. Recommended Dosages of FLOVENT HFA Inhalation Aerosol

NOTE: In all patients, it is desirable to titrate to the lowest effective dosage once asthma stability is achieved.

Previous Therapy	Recommended Starting Dosage	Highest Recommended Dosage
Adult and adolescent patients (aged ≥12 years)		
Bronchodilators alone	88 mcg twice daily	440 mcg twice daily
Inhaled corticosteroids	88-220 mcg twice daily[a]	440 mcg twice daily
Oral corticosteroids[b]	440 mcg twice daily	880 mcg twice daily
Pediatric patients (aged 4-11 years)[c]	88 mcg twice daily	88 mcg twice daily

[a] Starting dosages above 88 mcg twice daily may be considered for patients with poorer asthma control or those who have previously required doses of inhaled corticosteroids that are in the higher range for the specific agent.

[b] For patients currently receiving chronic oral corticosteroid therapy, prednisone should be reduced no faster than 2.5 to 5 mg/day on a weekly basis beginning after at least 1 week of therapy with FLOVENT HFA. Patients should be carefully monitored for signs of asthma instability, including serial objective measures of airflow, and for signs of adrenal insufficiency *[see Warnings and Precautions (5.4)]*. Once prednisone reduction is complete, the dosage of FLOVENT HFA should be reduced to the lowest effective dosage.

[c] Recommended pediatric dosage is 88 mcg twice daily regardless of prior therapy. A valved holding chamber and face mask may be used to deliver FLOVENT HFA to young patients.

FLOVENT HFA should be primed before using for the first time by releasing 4 test sprays into the air away from the face, shaking well for 5 seconds before each spray. In cases where the inhaler has not been used for more than 7 days or when it has been dropped, prime the inhaler again by shaking well for 5 seconds and releasing 1 test spray into the air away from the face.

3 DOSAGE FORMS AND STRENGTHS

FLOVENT HFA is an inhalation aerosol. Each actuation delivers 44, 110, or 220 mcg of fluticasone propionate from the actuator. FLOVENT HFA 44 mcg is supplied in 10.6-g pressurized aluminum canisters, and FLOVENT HFA 110 mcg and FLOVENT HFA 220 mcg are supplied in 12-g pressurized aluminum canisters. Each canister contains 120 metered inhalations and is fitted with a counter and a dark orange oral actuator with a peach strapcap.

4 CONTRAINDICATIONS

The use of FLOVENT HFA is contraindicated in the following conditions:

- Primary treatment of status asthmaticus or other acute episodes of asthma where intensive measures are required *[see Warnings and Precautions (5.2)]*
- Hypersensitivity to any of the ingredients of FLOVENT HFA contraindicates their use *[see Warnings and Precautions (5.6), Adverse Reactions (6.2), Description (11)]*

5 WARNINGS AND PRECAUTIONS

5.1 Local Effects

In clinical studies, the development of localized infections of the mouth and pharynx with *Candida albicans* has occurred in patients treated with FLOVENT HFA. When such an infection develops, it should be treated with appropriate local or systemic (i.e., oral antifungal) therapy while treatment with FLOVENT HFA continues, but at times therapy with FLOVENT HFA may need to be interrupted. Patients should rinse the mouth after inhalation of FLOVENT HFA *[see Adverse Reactions (6.1)]*.

5.2 Acute Asthma Episodes

FLOVENT HFA is not to be regarded as a bronchodilator and is not indicated for rapid relief of bronchospasm. Patients should be instructed to contact their physicians immediately when episodes of asthma that are not responsive to bronchodilators occur during the course of treatment with FLOVENT HFA. During such episodes, patients may require therapy with oral corticosteroids.

5.3 Immunosuppression

Persons who are using drugs that suppress the immune system are more susceptible to infections than healthy individuals. Chickenpox and measles, for example, can have a more serious or even fatal course in susceptible children or adults using corticosteroids. In such children or adults who have not had these diseases or been properly immunized, particular care should be taken to avoid exposure. How the dose, route, and duration of corticosteroid administration affect the risk of developing a disseminated infection is not known. The contribution of the underlying disease and/or prior corticosteroid treatment to the risk is also not known. If a patient is exposed to chickenpox, prophylaxis with varicella zoster immune globulin (VZIG) may be indicated. If a patient is exposed to measles, prophylaxis with pooled intramuscular immunoglobulin (IG) may be indicated. (See the respective package inserts for complete VZIG and IG prescribing information.) If chickenpox develops, treatment with antiviral agents may be considered.

Because of the potential for worsening infections, inhaled corticosteroids should be used with caution, if at all, in patients with active or quiescent tuberculosis infection of the respiratory tract; untreated systemic fungal, bacterial, viral, or parasitic infections; or ocular herpes simplex.

5.4 Transferring Patients From Systemic Corticosteroid Therapy

Particular care is needed for patients who have been transferred from systemically active corticosteroids to inhaled corticosteroids because deaths due to adrenal insufficiency have occurred in patients with asthma during and after transfer from systemic corticosteroids to less systemically available inhaled corticosteroids. After withdrawal from systemic corticosteroids, a number of months are required for recovery of hypothalamic-pituitary-adrenal (HPA) function.

Patients requiring oral corticosteroids should be weaned slowly from systemic corticosteroid use after transferring to FLOVENT HFA. In a clinical trial of 168 patients, prednisone reduction was successfully accomplished by reducing the daily prednisone dose on a weekly basis following initiation of treatment with FLOVENT HFA. Successive reduction of prednisone dose was allowed only when lung function, symptoms, and as-needed short-acting beta-agonist use were better than or comparable to that seen before initiation of prednisone dose reduction. Lung function (forced expiratory volume in 1 second [FEV_1] or morning peak expiratory flow [AM PEF]), beta-agonist use, and asthma symptoms should be carefully monitored during withdrawal of oral corticosteroids. In addition to monitoring asthma signs and symptoms, patients should be observed for signs

Table 2. Adverse Reactions With >3% Incidence in US Controlled Clinical Trials With FLOVENT HFA in Patients Aged 12 Years and Older With Asthma Previously Receiving Bronchodilators and/or Inhaled Corticosteroids

Adverse Event	FLOVENT HFA 88 mcg Twice Daily (n = 203) %	FLOVENT HFA 220 mcg Twice Daily (n = 204) %	FLOVENT HFA 440 mcg Twice Daily (n = 202) %	Placebo (n = 203) %
Ear, nose, and throat				
Upper respiratory tract infection	18	16	16	14
Throat irritation	8	8	10	5
Upper respiratory inflammation	2	5	5	1
Sinusitis/sinus infection	6	7	4	3
Hoarseness/dysphonia	2	3	6	<1
Gastrointestinal				
Candidiasis mouth/throat & non-site specific	4	2	5	<1
Lower respiratory				
Cough	4	6	4	5
Bronchitis	2	2	6	5
Neurological				
Headache	11	7	5	6

and symptoms of adrenal insufficiency such as fatigue, lassitude, weakness, nausea and vomiting, and hypotension.

Patients who have been previously maintained on 20 mg or more per day of prednisone (or its equivalent) may be most susceptible, particularly when their systemic corticosteroids have been almost completely withdrawn. During this period of HPA suppression, patients may exhibit signs and symptoms of adrenal insufficiency when exposed to trauma, surgery, or infection (particularly gastroenteritis) or other conditions associated with severe electrolyte loss. Although inhaled corticosteroids may provide control of asthma symptoms during these episodes, in recommended doses they supply less than normal physiological amounts of glucocorticoid (cortisol) systemically and do NOT provide the mineralocorticoid activity that is necessary for coping with these emergencies.

During periods of stress or a severe asthma attack, patients who have been withdrawn from systemic corticosteroids should be instructed to resume oral corticosteroids immediately and to contact their physicians for further instruction. These patients should also be instructed to carry a warning card indicating that they may need supplementary systemic corticosteroids during periods of stress or a severe asthma attack.

Transfer of patients from systemic corticosteroid therapy to FLOVENT HFA may unmask conditions previously suppressed by the systemic corticosteroid therapy (e.g., rhinitis, conjunctivitis, eczema, arthritis, eosinophilic conditions). Some patients may experience symptoms of systemically active corticosteroid withdrawal (e.g., joint and/or muscular pain, lassitude, and depression, despite maintenance or even improvement of respiratory function).

5.5 Hypercorticism and Adrenal Suppression

Fluticasone propionate will often help control asthma symptoms with less suppression of HPA function than therapeutically equivalent oral doses of prednisone. Since fluticasone propionate is absorbed into the circulation and can be systemically active at higher doses, the beneficial effects of FLOVENT HFA in minimizing HPA dysfunction may be expected only when recommended dosages are not exceeded and individual patients are titrated to the lowest effective dose. A relationship between plasma levels of fluticasone propionate and inhibitory effects on stimulated cortisol production has been shown after 4 weeks of treatment with fluticasone propionate. Since individual sensitivity to effects on cortisol production exists, physicians should consider this information when prescribing FLOVENT HFA.

Because of the possibility of systemic absorption of inhaled corticosteroids, patients treated with FLOVENT HFA should be observed carefully for any evidence of systemic corticosteroid effects. Particular care should be taken in observing patients postoperatively or during periods of stress for evidence of inadequate adrenal response.

It is possible that systemic corticosteroid effects such as hypercorticism and adrenal suppression (including adrenal crisis) may appear in a small number of patients, particularly when FLOVENT HFA is administered at higher than recommended doses over prolonged periods of time. If such effects occur, the dosage of FLOVENT HFA should be reduced slowly, consistent with accepted procedures for reducing systemic corticosteroids and for management of asthma.

5.6 Hypersensitivity Reactions, Including Anaphylaxis

Hypersensitivity reactions, including anaphylaxis, angioedema, urticaria, and bronchospasm, may occur after administration of FLOVENT HFA *[see Contraindications (4)]*.

5.7 Reduction in Bone Mineral Density

Decreases in bone mineral density (BMD) have been observed with long-term administration of products containing inhaled corticosteroids. The clinical significance of small changes in BMD with regard to long-term outcomes is unknown. Patients with major risk factors for decreased bone mineral content, such as prolonged immobilization, family history of osteoporosis, postmenopausal status, tobacco use, advanced age, poor nutrition, or chronic use of drugs that can reduce bone mass (e.g., anticonvulsants, oral corticosteroids), should be monitored and treated with established standards of care.

5.8 Effect on Growth

Orally inhaled corticosteroids may cause a reduction in growth velocity when administered to pediatric patients *[see Use in Specific Populations (8.4)]*. Monitor the growth of pediatric patients receiving FLOVENT HFA routinely (e.g., via stadiometry). To minimize the systemic effects of orally inhaled corticosteroids, including FLOVENT HFA, titrate each patient's dosage to the lowest dosage that effectively controls his/her symptoms *[see Dosage and Administration (2)]*.

5.9 Glaucoma and Cataracts

Glaucoma, increased intraocular pressure, and cataracts have been reported in patients following the long-term administration of inhaled corticosteroids, including fluticasone propionate. Therefore, close monitoring is warranted in patients with a change in vision or with a history of increased intraocular pressure, glaucoma, and/or cataracts.

5.10 Paradoxical Bronchospasm

As with other inhaled medications, bronchospasm may occur with an immediate increase in wheezing after dosing. If bronchospasm occurs following dosing with FLOVENT HFA, it should be treated immediately with a fast-acting inhaled bronchodilator. Treatment with FLOVENT HFA should be discontinued immediately and alternative therapy instituted.

5.11 Drug Interactions With Strong Cytochrome P450 3A4 Inhibitors

The use of strong cytochrome P450 3A4 (CYP3A4) inhibitors (e.g., ritonavir, atazanavir, clarithromycin, indinavir, itraconazole, nefazodone, nelfinavir, saquinavir, ketoconazole, telithromycin) with FLOVENT HFA is not recommended because increased systemic corticosteroid adverse effects may occur *[see Drug Interactions (7.1), Clinical Pharmacology (12.3)]*.

5.12 Eosinophilic Conditions and Churg-Strauss Syndrome

In rare cases, patients on inhaled fluticasone propionate may present with systemic eosinophilic conditions. Some of these patients have clinical features of vasculitis consistent with Churg-Strauss syndrome, a condition that is often treated with systemic corticosteroid therapy. These events usually, but not always, have been associated with the reduction and/or withdrawal of oral corticosteroid therapy following the introduction of fluticasone propionate. Cases of serious eosinophilic conditions have also been reported with other inhaled corticosteroids in this clinical setting. Physicians should be alert to eosinophilia, vasculitic rash, worsening pulmonary symptoms, cardiac complications, and/or neuropathy presenting in their patients. A causal relationship between fluticasone propionate and these underlying conditions has not been established.

6 ADVERSE REACTIONS

Systemic and local corticosteroid use may result in the following:

- *Candida albicans* infection *[see Warnings and Precautions (5.1)]*
- Immunosuppression *[see Warnings and Precautions (5.3)]*
- Hypercorticism and adrenal suppression *[see Warnings and Precautions (5.5)]*
- Reduction in bone mineral density *[see Warnings and Precautions (5.7)]*
- Growth effects *[see Warnings and Precautions (5.8)]*
- Glaucoma and cataracts *[see Warnings and Precautions (5.9)]*

6.1 Clinical Trials Experience

Because clinical trials are conducted under widely varying conditions, adverse reaction rates observed in the clinical trials of a drug cannot be directly compared with rates in the clinical trials of another drug and may not reflect the rates observed in practice.

The incidence of common adverse reactions in Table 2 is based upon 2 placebo-controlled US clinical trials in which 812 adult and adolescent patients (457 females and 355 males) previously treated with as-needed bronchodilators and/or inhaled corticosteroids were treated twice daily for up to 12 weeks with 2 inhalations of FLOVENT HFA 44 mcg Inhalation Aerosol, FLOVENT HFA 110 mcg Inhalation Aerosol, FLOVENT HFA 220 mcg Inhalation Aerosol (dosages of 88, 220, or 440 mcg twice daily), or placebo.

[See table 2 above]

Table 2 includes all events (whether considered drug-related or nondrug-related by the investigator) that occurred at a rate of over 3% in any of the groups treated with FLOVENT HFA and were more common than in the placebo group. Less than 2% of patients discontinued from the studies because of adverse reactions. The average duration of exposure was 73 to 76 days in the active treatment groups compared with 60 days in the placebo group.

Additional Adverse Reactions: Other adverse reactions not previously listed, whether considered drug-related or not by the investigators, that were reported more frequently by patients with asthma treated with FLOVENT HFA compared with patients treated with placebo include the following: rhinitis, rhinorrhea/post-nasal drip, nasal sinus disorders, laryngitis, diarrhea, viral gastrointestinal infections, dyspeptic symptoms, gastrointestinal discomfort and pain, hyposalivation, musculoskeletal pain, muscle pain, muscle stiffness/tightness/rigidity, dizziness, migraines, fever, viral infections, pain, chest symptoms, viral skin infections, muscle injuries, soft tissue injuries, urinary infections.

Fluticasone propionate inhalation aerosol (440 or 880 mcg twice daily) was administered for 16 weeks to 168 patients with asthma requiring oral corticosteroids (Study 3). Adverse reactions not included above, but reported by more than 3 patients in either group treated with FLOVENT HFA and more commonly than in the placebo group included nausea and vomiting, arthralgia and articular rheumatism, and malaise and fatigue.

In 2 long-term studies (26 and 52 weeks), the pattern of adverse reactions in patients treated with FLOVENT HFA at dosages up to 440 mcg twice daily was similar to that observed in the 12-week studies. There were no new and/or unexpected adverse reactions with long-term treatment.

Pediatric Patients Aged 4 to 11 Years: FLOVENT HFA has been evaluated for safety in 56 pediatric patients who received 88 mcg twice daily for 4 weeks. Types of adverse reactions in these pediatric patients were generally similar to those observed in adults and adolescents.

6.2 Postmarketing Experience

In addition to adverse reactions reported from clinical trials, the following adverse reactions have been identified during postmarketing use of fluticasone propionate. Because these reactions are reported voluntarily from a population of uncertain size, it is not always possible to reliably estimate their frequency or establish a causal relationship to drug exposure. These events have been chosen for inclusion due to either their seriousness, frequency of reporting, or causal connection to fluticasone propionate or a combination of these factors.

Ear, Nose, and Throat: Aphonia, facial and oropharyngeal edema, and throat soreness and irritation.

Endocrine and Metabolic: Cushingoid features, growth velocity reduction in children/adolescents, hyperglycemia, osteoporosis, and weight gain.

Eye: Cataracts.

Gastrointestinal Disorders: Dental caries and tooth discoloration.

Psychiatry: Agitation, aggression, anxiety, depression, and restlessness. Behavioral changes, including hyperactivity and irritability, have been reported very rarely and primarily in children.

Immune System Disorders: Immediate and delayed hypersensitivity reactions, including urticaria, anaphylaxis, rash, and angioedema and bronchospasm, have been reported.

Respiratory: Asthma exacerbation, chest tightness, cough, dyspnea, immediate and delayed bronchospasm, paradoxical bronchospasm, pneumonia, and wheeze.

Skin: Contusions, cutaneous hypersensitivity reactions, ecchymoses, and pruritus.

Eosinophilic Conditions: In rare cases, patients on inhaled fluticasone propionate may present with systemic eosinophilic conditions, with some patients presenting with clinical features of vasculitis consistent with Churg-Strauss syndrome, a condition that is often treated with systemic corticosteroid therapy. These events usually, but not always, have been associated with the reduction and/or withdrawal of oral corticosteroid therapy following the introduction of fluticasone propionate *[see Warnings and Precautions (5.12)]*.

7 DRUG INTERACTIONS

7.1 Strong Cytochrome P450 3A4 Inhibitors

Fluticasone propionate is a substrate of CYP3A4. The use of strong CYP3A4 inhibitors (e.g., ritonavir, atazanavir, clarithromycin, indinavir, itraconazole, nefazodone, nelfinavir, saquinavir, ketoconazole, telithromycin) with FLOVENT HFA is not recommended because increased systemic corticosteroid adverse effects may occur.

A drug interaction study with fluticasone propionate aqueous nasal spray in healthy subjects has shown that ritonavir (a strong CYP3A4 inhibitor) can significantly increase plasma fluticasone propionate concentration, resulting in significantly reduced serum cortisol concentrations *[see Clinical Pharmacology (12.3)]*. During postmarketing use, there have been reports of clinically significant drug interactions in patients receiving fluticasone propionate and ritonavir, resulting in systemic corticosteroid effects including Cushing's syndrome and adrenal suppression. Therefore, coadministration of fluticasone propionate and ritonavir is not recommended unless the potential benefit to the patient outweighs the risk of systemic corticosteroid side effects.

Coadministration of orally inhaled fluticasone propionate (1,000 mcg) and ketoconazole (200 mg once daily) resulted in a 1.9-fold increase in plasma fluticasone propionate exposure and a 45% decrease in plasma cortisol area under the curve (AUC), but had no effect on urinary excretion of cortisol. Coadministration of fluticasone propionate and ketoconazole is not recommended unless the potential benefit to the patient outweighs the risk of systemic corticosteroid side effects.

8 USE IN SPECIFIC POPULATIONS

8.1 Pregnancy

Pregnancy Category C. There are no adequate and well-controlled studies with FLOVENT HFA in pregnant women. FLOVENT HFA should be used during pregnancy only if the potential benefit justifies the potential risk to the fetus.

Teratogenic Effects: Subcutaneous studies in mice at a dose approximately 0.1 times the maximum recommended human daily inhalation dose (MRHD) in adults on a mg/m^2 basis and in the rat at a dose approximately 0.5 times the MRHD in adults on a mg/m^2 basis revealed fetal toxicity characteristic of potent corticosteroid compounds, including embryonic growth retardation, omphalocele, cleft palate, and retarded cranial ossification.

In rabbits, fetal weight reduction and cleft palate were observed at a subcutaneous dose approximately 0.04 times the MRHD in adults on a mg/m^2 basis. However, no teratogenic effects were reported at oral doses up to approximately 3 times the MRHD in adults on a mg/m^2 basis. No fluticasone propionate was detected in the plasma in this study, consistent with the established low bioavailability following oral administration *[see Clinical Pharmacology (12.3)]*.

Experience with oral corticosteroids since their introduction in pharmacologic, as opposed to physiologic, doses suggests that rodents are more prone to teratogenic effects from corticosteroids than humans. In addition, because there is a natural increase in corticosteroid production during pregnancy, most women will require a lower exogenous corticosteroid dose and many will not need corticosteroid treatment during pregnancy.

8.3 Nursing Mothers

It is not known whether fluticasone propionate is excreted in human breast milk. However, other corticosteroids have been detected in human milk. Subcutaneous administration to lactating rats of tritiated fluticasone propionate (approximately 0.05 times the MRHD in adults on a mg/m^2 basis) resulted in measurable radioactivity in milk.

Since there are no data from controlled trials on the use of FLOVENT HFA by nursing mothers, caution should be exercised when FLOVENT HFA is administered to a nursing woman.

8.4 Pediatric Use

The safety and effectiveness of FLOVENT HFA in children 4 years and older have been established *[see Adverse Reactions (6.1), Clinical Pharmacology (12.3), Clinical Studies (14.2)]*. The safety and effectiveness of FLOVENT HFA in children younger than 4 years have not been established. Use of FLOVENT HFA in patients aged 4 to 11 years is supported by evidence from adequate and well-controlled studies in adults and adolescents 12 years and older, pharmacokinetic studies in patients aged 4 to 11 years, established

Table 3. In Vitro Medication Delivery Through AeroChamber Plus Valved Holding Chamber With a Face Mask

Age	Face Mask	Flow Rate (L/min)	Holding Time (seconds)	Mean Medication Delivery Through AeroChamber Plus VHC (mcg/actuation)	Body Weight 50th Percentile (kg)[a]	Medication Delivered per Actuation (mcg/kg)[b]
6 to 12 Months	Small	4.9	0	8.3	7.5-9.9	0.8-1.1
			2	6.7		0.7-0.9
			5	7.5		0.8-1.0
			10	7.5		0.8-1.0
2 to 5 Years	Small	8.0	0	7.3	12.3-18.0	0.4-0.6
			2	6.8		0.4-0.6
			5	6.7		0.4-0.5
			10	7.7		0.4-0.6
2 to 5 Years	Medium	8.0	0	7.8	12.3-18.0	0.4-0.6
			2	7.7		0.4-0.6
			5	8.1		0.5-0.7
			10	9.0		0.5-0.7
>5 Years	Medium	12.0	0	12.3	18.0	0.7
			2	11.8		0.7
			5	12.0		0.7
			10	10.1		0.6

[a] Centers for Disease Control growth charts, developed by the National Center for Health Statistics in collaboration with the National Center for Chronic Disease Prevention and Health Promotion (2000). Ranges correspond to the average of the 50th percentile weight for boys and girls at the ages indicated.

[b] A single inhalation of FLOVENT HFA in a 70-kg adult without use of a valved holding chamber and face mask delivers approximately 44 mcg, or 0.6 mcg/kg.

efficacy of fluticasone propionate formulated as FLOVENT® DISKUS® (fluticasone propionate inhalation powder) and FLOVENT® ROTADISK® (fluticasone propionate inhalation powder) in patients aged 4 to 11 years, and supportive findings with FLOVENT HFA in a study conducted in patients aged 4 to 11 years.

Effects on Growth: Orally inhaled corticosteroids may cause a reduction in growth velocity when administered to pediatric patients. A reduction of growth velocity in children or teenagers may occur as a result of poorly controlled asthma or from use of corticosteroids including inhaled corticosteroids. The effects of long-term treatment of children and adolescents with inhaled corticosteroids, including fluticasone propionate, on final adult height are not known. Controlled clinical studies have shown that inhaled corticosteroids may cause a reduction in growth in pediatric patients. In these studies, the mean reduction in growth velocity was approximately 1 cm/year (range: 0.3 to 1.8 cm/year) and appears to depend upon dose and duration of exposure. This effect was observed in the absence of laboratory evidence of HPA axis suppression, suggesting that growth velocity is a more sensitive indicator of systemic corticosteroid exposure in pediatric patients than some commonly used tests of HPA axis function. The long-term effects of this reduction in growth velocity associated with orally inhaled corticosteroids, including the impact on final adult height, are unknown. The potential for "catch-up" growth following discontinuation of treatment with orally inhaled corticosteroids has not been adequately studied. The effects on growth velocity of treatment with orally inhaled corticosteroids for over 1 year, including the impact on final adult height, are unknown. The growth of children and adolescents receiving orally inhaled corticosteroids, including FLOVENT HFA, should be monitored routinely (e.g., via stadiometry). The potential growth effects of prolonged treatment should be weighed against the clinical benefits obtained and the risks associated with alternative therapies. To minimize the systemic effects of orally inhaled corticosteroids, including FLOVENT HFA, each patient should be titrated to the lowest dose that effectively controls his/her symptoms.

Since a cross study comparison in adolescent and adult patients (aged 12 years and older) indicated that systemic exposure of inhaled fluticasone propionate from FLOVENT HFA would be higher than exposure from FLOVENT ROTADISK, results from a study to assess the potential growth effects of FLOVENT ROTADISK in pediatric patients (aged 4 to 11 years) are provided.

A 52-week placebo-controlled study to assess the potential growth effects of fluticasone propionate inhalation powder (FLOVENT ROTADISK) at 50 and 100 mcg twice daily was conducted in the US in 325 prepubescent children (244 males and 81 females) aged 4 to 11 years. The mean growth velocities at 52 weeks observed in the intent-to-treat population were 6.32 cm/year in the placebo group (n = 76), 6.07 cm/year in the 50-mcg group (n = 98), and 5.66 cm/year in the 100-mcg group (n = 89). An imbalance in the proportion of children entering puberty between groups and a higher dropout rate in the placebo group due to poorly controlled asthma may be confounding factors in interpreting these data. A separate subset analysis of children who remained prepubertal during the study revealed growth rates at 52 weeks of 6.10 cm/year in the placebo group (n = 57), 5.91 cm/year in the 50-mcg group (n = 74), and 5.67 cm/year in the 100-mcg group (n = 79). In children aged 8.5 years, the mean age of children in this study, the range for expected growth velocity is: boys – 3rd percentile = 3.8 cm/year, 50th percentile = 5.4 cm/year, and 97th percentile = 7.0 cm/year; girls – 3rd percentile = 4.2 cm/year, 50th percentile = 5.7 cm/year, and 97th percentile = 7.3 cm/year.

The clinical significance of these growth data is not certain. Physicians should closely follow the growth of children and adolescents taking corticosteroids by any route, and weigh the benefits of corticosteroid therapy against the possibility of growth suppression if growth appears slowed. Patients should be maintained on the lowest dose of inhaled corticosteroid that effectively controls their asthma.

Children Younger Than 4 Years: *Pharmacokinetics: [see Clinical Pharmacology (12.3)].*

Pharmacodynamics: A 12-week, double-blind, placebo-controlled, parallel-group study was conducted in children with asthma aged 1 to less than 4 years. Twelve-hour overnight urinary cortisol excretion after a 12-week treatment period with 88 mcg of FLOVENT HFA twice daily (n = 73) and with placebo (n = 42) were calculated. The mean and median change from baseline in urine cortisol over 12 hours were -0.7 and 0.0 mcg for FLOVENT HFA and 0.3 and -0.2 mcg for placebo, respectively.

In a 1-way crossover study in children aged 6 to less than 12 months with reactive airways disease (N = 21), serum cortisol was measured over a 12-hour dosing period. Patients received placebo treatment for a 2-week period followed by a 4-week treatment period with 88 mcg of FLOVENT HFA twice daily with an AeroChamber Plus® Valved Holding Chamber (VHC) with face mask. The geometric mean ratio of serum cortisol over 12 hours ($AUC_{0\text{-}12\ hr}$) following FLOVENT HFA (n = 16) versus placebo (n = 18) was 0.95 (95% CI: 0.72, 1.27).

Safety: FLOVENT HFA administered as 88 mcg twice daily has been evaluated for safety in 239 pediatric patients aged 1 to less than 4 years in a 12-week, double-blind, placebo-controlled study. Treatments were administered with an AeroChamber Plus VHC with face mask. In pediatric patients aged 1 to less than 4 years receiving FLOVENT HFA, the following events occurred with a frequency greater than 3% and more frequently than in pediatric patients who received placebo, regardless of causality assessment: pyrexia, nasopharyngitis, upper respiratory tract infection, vomiting, otitis media, diarrhea, bronchitis, pharyngitis, and viral infection.

FLOVENT HFA administered as 88 mcg twice daily has also been evaluated for safety in 23 pediatric patients aged 6 to 12 months in an open-label placebo-controlled study. Treatments were administered with an AeroChamber Plus VHC with face mask for 2 weeks with placebo followed by 4 weeks with active drug. There was no discernable difference in the types of adverse events reported between patients receiving placebo compared to the active drug.

In Vitro Testing of Dose Delivery With Holding Chambers: In vitro dose characterization studies were performed to evaluate the delivery of FLOVENT HFA via holding chambers with attached face masks. The studies were conducted with 2 different holding chambers (AeroChamber Plus VHC and AeroChamber Z-STAT Plus™ VHC) and face masks (small and medium size) at inspiratory flow rates of 4.9, 8.0, and 12.0 L/min in combination with holding times of 0, 2, 5, and 10 seconds. The flow rates were selected to be representative of inspiratory flow rates of children aged 6 to 12 months, 2 to 5 years, and over 5 years, respectively. The mean delivered dose of fluticasone propionate through the holding chambers with face masks was lower than the 44 mcg of fluticasone propionate delivered directly from the actuator mouthpiece. The results were similar through both holding chambers (see Table 3 for data for the AeroChamber Plus VHC). The fine particle fraction (approximately 1 to 5 µm) across the flow rates used in these studies was 70% to 84% of the delivered dose, consistent with the removal of the coarser fraction by the holding chamber. In contrast, the fine particle fraction for FLOVENT HFA delivered without a holding chamber typically represents 42% to 55% of the delivered dose measured at the standard flow rate of 28.3 L/min. These data suggest that, on a per kilogram basis, young children receive a comparable dose of fluticasone propionate when delivered via a holding chamber and face mask as adults do without their use.

[See table 3 at top of previous page]

8.5 Geriatric Use

Of the total number of patients treated with FLOVENT HFA in US and non-US clinical trials, 173 were 65 years or older, 19 of which were 75 years or older. No overall differences in safety or effectiveness were observed between these patients and younger patients, and other reported clinical experience has not identified differences in responses between the elderly and younger patients, but greater sensitivity of some older individuals cannot be ruled out.

8.6 Hepatic Impairment

Formal pharmacokinetic studies using FLOVENT HFA have not been conducted in patients with hepatic impairment. Since fluticasone propionate is predominantly cleared by hepatic metabolism, impairment of liver function may lead to accumulation of fluticasone propionate in plasma. Therefore, patients with hepatic disease should be closely monitored.

8.7 Renal Impairment

Formal pharmacokinetic studies using FLOVENT HFA have not been conducted in patients with renal impairment.

10 OVERDOSAGE

Chronic overdosage may result in signs/symptoms of hypercorticism *[see Warnings and Precautions (5.5)]*. Inhalation by healthy volunteers of a single dose of 1,760 or 3,520 mcg of fluticasone propionate CFC inhalation aerosol was well tolerated. Doses of 1,320 mcg administered to healthy human volunteers twice daily for 7 to 15 days were also well tolerated. Repeat oral doses up to 80 mg daily for 10 days in healthy volunteers and repeat oral doses up to 20 mg daily for 42 days in patients were well tolerated. Adverse reactions were of mild or moderate severity, and incidences were similar in active and placebo treatment groups.

No deaths were seen in mice given an oral dose of 1,000 mg/kg (approximately 2,300 and 11,000 times the MRHD for adults and children aged 4 to 11 years, respectively, on a mg/m^2 basis). No deaths were seen in rats given an oral dose of 1,000 mg/kg (approximately 4,600 and 22,000 times the MRHD in adults and children aged 4 to 11 years, respectively, on a mg/m^2 basis).

11 DESCRIPTION

The active component of FLOVENT HFA 44 mcg Inhalation Aerosol, FLOVENT HFA 110 mcg Inhalation Aerosol, and FLOVENT HFA 220 mcg Inhalation Aerosol is fluticasone propionate, a corticosteroid having the chemical name *S*-(fluoromethyl) 6α,9-difluoro-11β,17-dihydroxy-16α-methyl-3-oxoandrosta-1,4-diene-17β-carbothioate, 17-propionate and the following chemical structure:

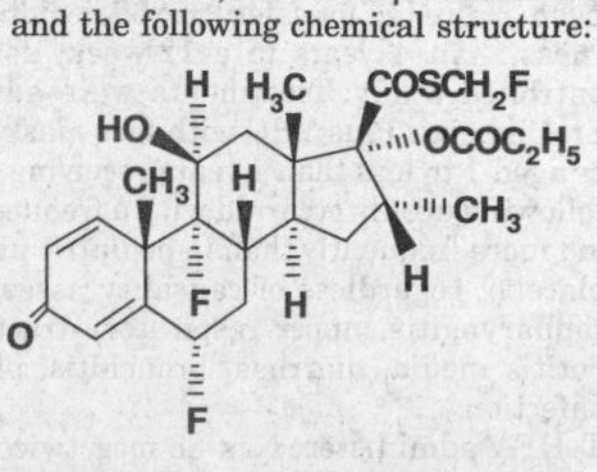

Fluticasone propionate is a white powder with a molecular weight of 500.6, and the empirical formula is $C_{25}H_{31}F_3O_5S$. It is practically insoluble in water, freely soluble in dimethyl sulfoxide and dimethylformamide, and slightly soluble in methanol and 95% ethanol.

FLOVENT HFA 44 mcg Inhalation Aerosol, FLOVENT HFA 110 mcg Inhalation Aerosol, and FLOVENT HFA 220 mcg Inhalation Aerosol are pressurized metered-dose aerosol units fitted with a counter. FLOVENT HFA is intended for oral inhalation only. Each unit contains a microcrystalline suspension of fluticasone propionate (micronized) in propellant HFA-134a (1,1,1,2-tetrafluoroethane). It contains no other excipients.

After priming, each actuation of the inhaler delivers 50, 125, or 250 mcg of fluticasone propionate in 60 mg of suspension (for the 44-mcg product) or in 75 mg of suspension (for the 110- and 220-mcg products) from the valve. Each actuation delivers 44, 110, or 220 mcg of fluticasone propionate from the actuator. The actual amount of drug delivered to the lung may depend on patient factors, such as the coordination between the actuation of the device and inspiration through the delivery system.

Each 10.6-g canister (44 mcg) and each 12-g canister (110 and 220 mcg) provides 120 inhalations.

FLOVENT HFA should be primed before using for the first time by releasing 4 test sprays into the air away from the face, shaking well for 5 seconds before each spray. In cases where the inhaler has not been used for more than 7 days or when it has been dropped, prime the inhaler again by shaking well for 5 seconds and releasing 1 test spray into the air away from the face.

This product does not contain any chlorofluorocarbon (CFC) as the propellant.

12 CLINICAL PHARMACOLOGY

12.1 Mechanism of Action

Fluticasone propionate is a synthetic trifluorinated corticosteroid with potent anti-inflammatory activity. In vitro assays using human lung cytosol preparations have established fluticasone propionate as a human glucocorticoid receptor agonist with an affinity 18 times greater than dexamethasone, almost twice that of beclomethasone-17-monopropionate (BMP), the active metabolite of beclomethasone dipropionate, and over 3 times that of budesonide. Data from the McKenzie vasoconstrictor assay in man are consistent with these results. The clinical significance of these findings is unknown.

Inflammation is an important component in the pathogenesis of asthma. Corticosteroids have been shown to inhibit multiple cell types (e.g., mast cells, eosinophils, basophils, lymphocytes, macrophages, neutrophils) and mediator production or secretion (e.g., histamine, eicosanoids, leukotrienes, cytokines) involved in the asthmatic response. These anti-inflammatory actions of corticosteroids contribute to their efficacy in asthma.

Though effective for the treatment of asthma, corticosteroids do not affect asthma symptoms immediately. Individual patients will experience a variable time to onset and degree of symptom relief. Maximum benefit may not be achieved for 1 to 2 weeks or longer after starting treatment. When corticosteroids are discontinued, asthma stability may persist for several days or longer.

Studies in patients with asthma have shown a favorable ratio between topical anti-inflammatory activity and systemic corticosteroid effects with recommended doses of orally inhaled fluticasone propionate. This is explained by a combination of a relatively high local anti-inflammatory effect, negligible oral systemic bioavailability (less than 1%), and the minimal pharmacological activity of the only metabolite detected in man.

12.2 Pharmacodynamics

Serum cortisol concentrations, urinary excretion of cortisol, and urine 6-β-hydroxycortisol excretion collected over 24 hours in 24 healthy subjects following 8 inhalations of fluticasone propionate HFA 44, 110, and 220 mcg decreased with increasing dose. However, in patients with asthma treated with 2 inhalations of fluticasone propionate HFA 44, 110, and 220 mcg twice daily for at least 4 weeks, differences in serum cortisol $AUC_{(0-12\ hr)}$ (n = 65) and 24-hour urinary excretion of cortisol (n = 47) compared with placebo were not related to dose and generally not significant. In the study with healthy volunteers, the effect of propellant was also evaluated by comparing results following the 220-mcg strength inhaler containing HFA 134a propellant with the same strength of inhaler containing CFC 11/12 propellant. A lesser effect on the HPA axis with the HFA formulation was observed for serum cortisol, but not urine cortisol and 6-betahydroxy cortisol excretion. In addition, in a crossover study of children with asthma aged 4 to 11 years (N = 40), 24-hour urinary excretion of cortisol was not affected after a 4-week treatment period with 88 mcg of fluticasone propionate HFA twice daily compared with urinary excretion after the 2-week placebo period. The ratio (95% CI) of urinary excretion of cortisol over 24 hours following fluticasone propionate HFA versus placebo was 0.987 (0.796, 1.223).

The potential systemic effects of fluticasone propionate HFA on the HPA axis were also studied in patients with asthma. Fluticasone propionate given by inhalation aerosol at dosages of 440 or 880 mcg twice daily was compared with placebo in oral corticosteroid-dependent patients with asthma (range of mean dose of prednisone at baseline: 13 to 14 mg/day) in a 16-week study. Consistent with maintenance treatment with oral corticosteroids, abnormal plasma cortisol responses to short cosyntropin stimulation (peak plasma cortisol less than 18 mcg/dL) were present at baseline in the majority of patients participating in this study (69% of patients later randomized to placebo and 72% to 78% of patients later randomized to fluticasone propionate HFA). At week 16, 8 patients (73%) on placebo compared with 14 (54%) and 13 (68%) patients receiving fluticasone propionate HFA (440 and 880 mcg twice daily, respectively) had post-stimulation cortisol levels of less than 18 mcg/dL.

12.3 Pharmacokinetics

Absorption: Fluticasone propionate acts locally in the lung; therefore, plasma levels do not predict therapeutic effect. Studies using oral dosing of labeled and unlabeled drug have demonstrated that the oral systemic bioavailability of fluticasone propionate is negligible (less than 1%), primarily due to incomplete absorption and presystemic metabolism in the gut and liver. In contrast, the majority of the fluticasone propionate delivered to the lung is systemically absorbed.

Distribution: Following intravenous administration, the initial disposition phase for fluticasone propionate was rapid and consistent with its high lipid solubility and tissue binding. The volume of distribution averaged 4.2 L/kg.

The percentage of fluticasone propionate bound to human plasma proteins averages 99%. Fluticasone propionate is weakly and reversibly bound to erythrocytes and is not significantly bound to human transcortin.

Metabolism: The total clearance of fluticasone propionate is high (average, 1,093 mL/min), with renal clearance accounting for less than 0.02% of the total. The only circulating metabolite detected in man is the 17β-carboxylic acid derivative of fluticasone propionate, which is formed through the CYP 3A4 pathway. This metabolite had less affinity (approximately 1/2,000) than the parent drug for the corticosteroid receptor of human lung cytosol in vitro and negligible pharmacological activity in animal studies. Other metabolites detected in vitro using cultured human hepatoma cells have not been detected in man.

Elimination: Following intravenous dosing, fluticasone propionate showed polyexponential kinetics and had a terminal elimination half-life of approximately 7.8 hours. Less than 5% of a radiolabeled oral dose was excreted in the urine as metabolites, with the remainder excreted in the feces as parent drug and metabolites.

Specific Populations: *Gender:* No significant difference in clearance (CL/F) of fluticasone propionate was observed.

Pediatrics: A population pharmacokinetic analysis was performed for FLOVENT HFA using steady-state data from 4 controlled clinical trials and single-dose data from 1 controlled clinical trial. The combined cohort for analysis included 269 patients (161 males and 108 females) with asthma aged 6 months to 66 years who received treatment with FLOVENT HFA. Most of these subjects (n = 215) were treated with FLOVENT HFA 44 mcg given as 88 mcg twice daily. FLOVENT HFA was delivered using an AeroChamber Plus VHC with a face mask to patients aged less than 4 years. Data from adult patients with asthma following FLOVENT HFA 110 mcg given as 220 mcg twice daily (n = 15) and following FLOVENT HFA 220 mcg given as 440 mcg twice daily (n = 17) at steady state were also included. Data for 22 patients came from a single-dose crossover study of 264 mcg (6 doses of FLOVENT HFA 44 mcg) with and without AeroChamber Plus VHC in children with asthma aged 4 to 11 years.

Stratification of exposure data following FLOVENT HFA 88 mcg by age and study indicated that systemic exposure to fluticasone propionate at steady state was similar in children aged 6 to less than 12 months, children aged 1 to less than 4 years, and adults and adolescents aged 12 years and older. Exposure was lower in children aged 4 to 11 years, who did not use a VHC, as shown in Table 4.

[See table 4 at top of next page]

The lower exposure to fluticasone propionate in children aged 4 to 11 years who did not use a VHC may reflect the inability to coordinate actuation and inhalation of the metered-dose inhaler. The impact of the use of a VHC on exposure to fluticasone propionate in patients aged 4 to 11 years was evaluated in a single-dose crossover study with FLOVENT HFA 44 mcg given as 264 mcg. In this study, use of a VHC increased systemic exposure to fluticasone propionate (Table 5), possibly correcting for the inability to coordinate actuation and inhalation.

[See table 5 at top of next page]

There was a dose-related increase in systemic exposure in patients aged 12 years and older receiving higher doses of fluticasone propionate (220 and 440 mcg twice daily). The $AUC_{0-\tau}$ in pg•hr/mL was 358 (95% CI: 272, 473) and 640 (95% CI: 477, 858), and C_{max} in pg/mL was 47.3 (95% CI: 37, 61) and 87 (95% CI: 68, 112) following fluticasone propionate 220 and 440 mcg, respectively.

Hepatic and Renal Impairment: Formal pharmacokinetic studies using FLOVENT HFA have not been conducted in patients with hepatic or renal impairment. However, since fluticasone propionate is predominantly cleared by hepatic metabolism, impairment of liver function may lead to accumulation of fluticasone propionate in plasma. Therefore, patients with hepatic disease should be closely monitored.
Race: No significant difference in clearance (CL/F) of fluticasone propionate in Caucasian, African-American, Asian, or Hispanic populations was observed.
Drug Interactions: *Ritonavir:* Fluticasone propionate is a substrate of CYP3A4. Coadministration of fluticasone propionate and the strong CYP3A4 inhibitor ritonavir is not recommended based upon a multiple-dose, crossover drug interaction study in 18 healthy subjects. Fluticasone propionate aqueous nasal spray (200 mcg once daily) was coadministered for 7 days with ritonavir (100 mg twice daily). Plasma fluticasone propionate concentrations following fluticasone propionate aqueous nasal spray alone were undetectable (less than 10 pg/mL) in most subjects, and when concentrations were detectable, peak levels (C_{max}) averaged 11.9 pg/mL (range: 10.8 to 14.1 pg/mL) and $AUC_{(0-\tau)}$ averaged 8.43 pg•hr/mL (range: 4.2 to 18.8 pg•hr/mL). Fluticasone propionate C_{max} and $AUC_{(0-\tau)}$ increased to 318 pg/mL (range: 110 to 648 pg/mL) and 3,102.6 pg•hr/mL (range: 1,207.1 to 5,662.0 pg•hr/mL), respectively, after coadministration of ritonavir with fluticasone propionate aqueous nasal spray. This significant increase in plasma fluticasone propionate exposure resulted in a significant decrease (86%) in serum cortisol AUC.
Ketoconazole: In a placebo-controlled, crossover study in 8 healthy adult volunteers, coadministration of a single dose of orally inhaled fluticasone propionate (1,000 mcg) with multiple doses of ketoconazole (200 mg) to steady state resulted in increased plasma fluticasone propionate exposure, a reduction in plasma cortisol AUC, and no effect on urinary excretion of cortisol.
Following orally inhaled fluticasone propionate alone, $AUC_{(2\text{-last})}$ averaged 1.559 ng•hr/mL (range: 0.555 to 2.906 ng•hr/mL) and $AUC_{(2\text{-}\infty)}$ averaged 2.269 ng•hr/mL (range: 0.836 to 3.707 ng•hr/mL). Fluticasone propionate $AUC_{(2\text{-last})}$ and $AUC_{(2\text{-}\infty)}$ increased to 2.781 ng•hr/mL (range: 2.489 to 8.486 ng•hr/mL) and 4.317 ng•hr/mL (range: 3.256 to 9.408 ng•hr/mL), respectively, after coadministration of ketoconazole with orally inhaled fluticasone propionate. This increase in plasma fluticasone propionate concentration resulted in a decrease (45%) in serum cortisol AUC.
Erythromycin: In a multiple-dose drug interaction study, coadministration of orally inhaled fluticasone propionate (500 mcg twice daily) and erythromycin (333 mg 3 times daily) did not affect fluticasone propionate pharmacokinetics.

13 NONCLINICAL TOXICOLOGY

13.1 Carcinogenesis, Mutagenesis, Impairment of Fertility

Fluticasone propionate demonstrated no tumorigenic potential in mice at oral doses up to 1,000 mcg/kg (approximately 2 and 10 times the MRHD in adults and children aged 4 to 11 years, respectively, on a mg/m^2 basis) for 78 weeks or in rats at inhalation doses up to 57 mcg/kg (approximately 0.3 times and approximately equivalent to the MRHD in adults and children aged 4 to 11 years, respectively, on a mg/m^2 basis) for 104 weeks.
Fluticasone propionate did not induce gene mutation in prokaryotic or eukaryotic cells in vitro. No significant clastogenic effect was seen in cultured human peripheral lymphocytes in vitro or in the in vivo mouse micronucleus test.
No evidence of impairment of fertility was observed in reproductive studies conducted in male and female rats at subcutaneous doses up to 50 mcg/kg (approximately 0.2 times the MRHD in adults on a mg/m^2 basis). Prostate weight was significantly reduced at a subcutaneous dose of 50 mcg/kg.

13.2 Animal Toxicology and/or Pharmacology

Reproductive Toxicology: Subcutaneous studies in mice and rats at 45 and 100 mcg/kg (approximately 0.1 and 0.5 times the MRHD in adults on a mg/m^2 basis, respectively) revealed fetal toxicity characteristic of potent corticosteroid compounds, including embryonic growth retardation, omphalocele, cleft palate, and retarded cranial ossification.
In rabbits, fetal weight reduction and cleft palate were observed at a subcutaneous dose of 4 mcg/kg (approximately 0.04 times the MRHD in adults on a mg/m^2 basis). However, no teratogenic effects were reported at oral doses up to 300 mcg/kg (approximately 3 times the MRHD in adults on a mg/m^2 basis) of fluticasone propionate. No fluticasone propionate was detected in the plasma in this study, consistent with the established low bioavailability following oral administration *[see Clinical Pharmacology (12.3)]*.
Fluticasone propionate crossed the placenta following subcutaneous administration to mice and rats and oral administration to rabbits.
In animals and humans, propellant HFA-134a was found to be rapidly absorbed and rapidly eliminated, with an elimination half-life of 3 to 27 minutes in animals and 5 to 7 minutes in humans. Time to maximum plasma concentration (T_{max}) and mean residence time are both extremely short, leading to a transient appearance of HFA-134a in the blood with no evidence of accumulation.
Propellant HFA-134a is devoid of pharmacological activity except at very high doses in animals (i.e., 380 to 1,300 times the maximum human exposure based on comparisons of AUC values), primarily producing ataxia, tremors, dyspnea, or salivation. These events are similar to effects produced by the structurally related CFCs, which have been used extensively in metered-dose inhalers.

Table 4. Systemic Exposure to Fluticasone Propionate Following FLOVENT HFA 88 mcg Twice Daily

Age	Valved Holding Chamber	N	$AUC_{0-\tau}$, pg•hr/mL (95% CI)	C_{max}, pg/mL (95% CI)
6 to <12 Months	Yes	17	141 (88, 227)	19 (13, 29)
1 to <4 Years	Yes	164	143 (131, 157)	20 (18, 21)
4 to 11 Years	No	14	68 (48, 97)	11 (8, 16)
≥12 Years	No	20	149 (106, 210)	20 (15, 27)

Table 5. Systemic Exposure to Fluticasone Propionate Following a Single Dose of FLOVENT HFA 264 mcg

Age	Valved Holding Chamber	N	$AUC_{(0-\infty)}$, pg•hr/mL (95% CI)	C_{max}, pg/mL (95% CI)
4 to 11 Years	Yes	22	373 (297, 468)	61 (51, 73)
4 to 11 Years	No	21	141 (111, 178)	23 (19, 28)

14 CLINICAL STUDIES

14.1 Adult and Adolescent Patients Aged 12 Years and Older

Three randomized, double-blind, parallel-group, placebo-controlled, US clinical trials were conducted in 980 adult and adolescent patients (aged 12 years and older) with asthma to assess the efficacy and safety of FLOVENT HFA in the treatment of asthma. Fixed dosages of 88, 220, and 440 mcg twice daily (each dose administered as 2 inhalations of the 44-, 110-, and 220-mcg strengths, respectively) and 880 mcg twice daily (administered as 4 inhalations of the 220-mcg strength) were compared with placebo to provide information about appropriate dosing to cover a range of asthma severity. Patients in these studies included those inadequately controlled with bronchodilators alone (Study 1), those already receiving inhaled corticosteroids (Study 2), and those requiring oral corticosteroid therapy (Study 3). In all 3 studies, patients (including placebo-treated patients) were allowed to use VENTOLIN® (albuterol, USP) Inhalation Aerosol as needed for relief of acute asthma symptoms. In Studies 1 and 2, other maintenance asthma therapies were discontinued.
Study 1 enrolled 397 patients with asthma inadequately controlled on bronchodilators alone. FLOVENT HFA was evaluated at dosages of 88, 220, and 440 mcg twice daily for 12 weeks. Baseline FEV_1 values were similar across groups (mean 67% of predicted normal). All 3 dosages of FLOVENT HFA demonstrated a statistically significant improvement in lung function as measured by improvement in AM predose FEV_1 compared with placebo. This improvement was observed after the first week of treatment, and was maintained over the 12-week treatment period.
At Endpoint (last observation), mean change from baseline in AM pre-dose percent predicted FEV_1 was greater in all 3 groups treated with FLOVENT HFA (9.0% to 11.2%) compared with the placebo group (3.4%). The mean differences between the groups treated with FLOVENT HFA 88, 220, and 440 mcg and the placebo group were statistically significant, and the corresponding 95% confidence intervals were (2.2%, 9.2%), (2.8%, 9.9%), and (4.3%, 11.3%), respectively.
Figure 1 displays results of pulmonary function tests (mean percent change from baseline in FEV_1 prior to AM dose) for the recommended starting dosage of FLOVENT HFA (88 mcg twice daily) and placebo from Study 1. This trial used predetermined criteria for lack of efficacy (indicators of worsening asthma), resulting in withdrawal of more patients in the placebo group. Therefore, pulmonary function results at Endpoint (the last evaluable FEV_1 result, including most patients' lung function data) are also displayed.
[See figure 1 at top of next column]
In Study 2, FLOVENT HFA at dosages of 88, 220, and 440 mcg twice daily was evaluated over 12 weeks of treatment in 415 patients with asthma who were already receiving an inhaled corticosteroid at a daily dose within its recommended dose range in addition to as-needed albuterol. Baseline FEV_1 values were similar across groups (mean 65% to 66% of predicted normal). All 3 dosages of FLOVENT HFA demonstrated a statistically significant improvement

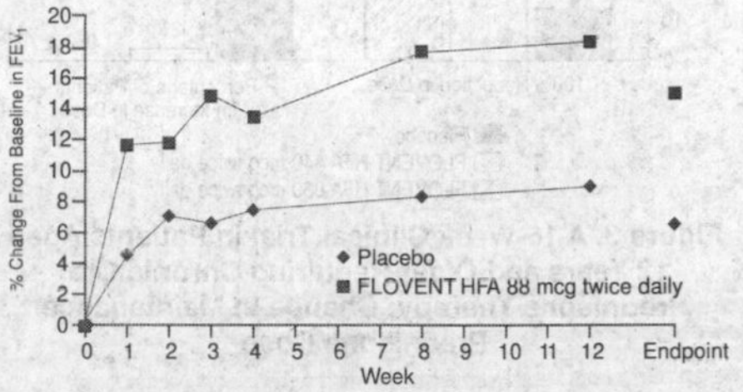

Figure 1. A 12-Week Clinical Trial in Patients Aged 12 Years and Older Inadequately Controlled on Bronchodilators Alone: Mean Percent Change From Baseline in FEV_1 Prior to AM Dose (Study 1)

in lung function, as measured by improvement in FEV_1, compared with placebo. This improvement was observed after the first week of treatment and was maintained over the 12-week treatment period. Discontinuations from the study for lack of efficacy (defined by a pre-specified decrease in FEV_1 or PEF, or an increase in use of VENTOLIN or night time awakenings requiring treatment with VENTOLIN) were lower in the groups treated with FLOVENT HFA (6% to 11%) compared with placebo (50%).
At Endpoint (last observation), mean change from baseline in AM pre-dose percent predicted FEV_1 was greater in all 3 groups treated with FLOVENT HFA (2.2% to 4.6%) compared with the placebo group (-8.3%). The mean differences between the groups treated with FLOVENT HFA 88, 220, and 440 mcg and the placebo group were statistically significant, and the corresponding 95% confidence intervals were (7.1%, 13.8%), (8.2%, 14.9%), and (9.6%, 16.4%), respectively.
Figure 2 displays the mean percent change from baseline in FEV_1 from Week 1 through Week 12. This study also used predetermined criteria for lack of efficacy, resulting in withdrawal of more patients in the placebo group; therefore, pulmonary function results at Endpoint are also displayed.

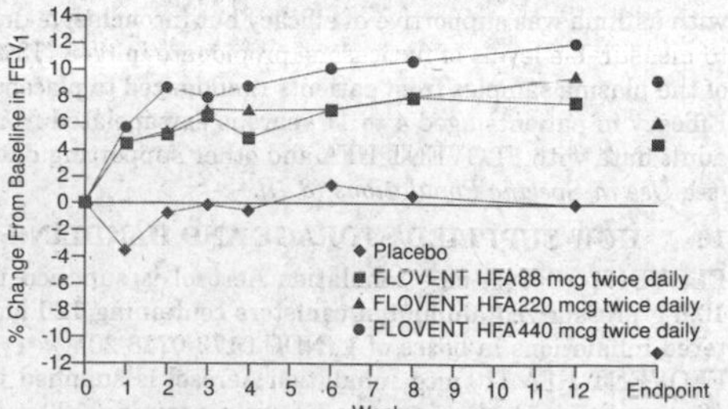

Figure 2. A 12-Week Clinical Trial in Patients Aged 12 Years and Older Already Receiving Daily Inhaled Corticosteroids: Mean Percent Change From Baseline in FEV_1 Prior to AM Dose (Study 2)

In both studies, use of VENTOLIN, AM and PM PEF, and asthma symptom scores showed numerical improvement with FLOVENT HFA compared with placebo.
Study 3 enrolled 168 patients with asthma requiring oral prednisone therapy (average baseline daily prednisone dose ranged from 13 to 14 mg). FLOVENT HFA at dosages of 440 and 880 mcg twice daily was evaluated over a 16-week treatment period. Baseline FEV_1 values were similar across groups (mean 59% to 62% of predicted normal). Over the

course of the study, patients treated with either dosage of FLOVENT HFA required a statistically significantly lower mean daily oral prednisone dose (6 mg) compared with placebo-treated patients (15 mg). Both dosages of FLOVENT HFA enabled a larger percentage of patients (59% and 56% in the groups treated with FLOVENT HFA 440 and 880 mcg, respectively, twice daily) to eliminate oral prednisone as compared with placebo (13%) (see Figure 3). There was no efficacy advantage of FLOVENT HFA 880 mcg twice daily compared with 440 mcg twice daily. Accompanying the reduction in oral corticosteroid use, patients treated with either dosage of FLOVENT HFA had statistically significantly improved lung function, fewer asthma symptoms, and less use of VENTOLIN Inhalation Aerosol compared with the placebo-treated patients.

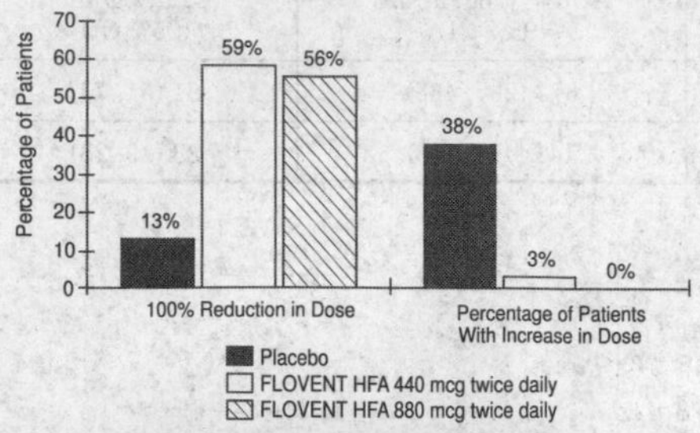

Figure 3. A 16-Week Clinical Trial in Patients Aged 12 Years and Older Requiring Chronic Oral Prednisone Therapy: Change in Maintenance Prednisone Dose

Two long-term safety studies (Study 4 and Study 5) of ≥6 months' duration were conducted in 507 adult and adolescent patients with asthma. Study 4 was designed to monitor the safety of 2 doses of FLOVENT HFA, while Study 5 compared fluticasone propionate HFA with fluticasone propionate CFC. Study 4 enrolled 182 patients who were treated daily with low to high doses of inhaled corticosteroids, beta-agonists (short-acting [as needed or regularly scheduled] or long-acting), theophylline, inhaled cromolyn or nedocromil sodium, leukotriene receptor antagonists, or 5-lipoxygenase inhibitors at baseline. FLOVENT HFA at dosages of 220 and 440 mcg twice daily was evaluated over a 26-week treatment period in 89 and 93 patients, respectively. Study 5 enrolled 325 patients who were treated daily with moderate to high doses of inhaled corticosteroids, with or without concurrent use of salmeterol or albuterol, at baseline. Fluticasone propionate HFA at a dosage of 440 mcg twice daily and fluticasone propionate CFC at a dosage of 440 mcg twice daily were evaluated over a 52-week treatment period in 163 and 162 patients, respectively. Baseline FEV_1 values were similar across groups (mean 81% to 84% of predicted normal). Throughout the 52-week treatment period, asthma control was maintained with both formulations of fluticasone propionate compared with baseline. In both studies, none of the patients were withdrawn due to lack of efficacy.

14.2 Pediatric Patients Aged 4 to 11 Years

A 12-week clinical trial conducted in 241 pediatric patients with asthma was supportive of efficacy but inconclusive due to measurable levels of fluticasone propionate in 6/48 (13%) of the plasma samples from patients randomized to placebo. Efficacy in patients aged 4 to 11 years is extrapolated from adult data with FLOVENT HFA and other supporting data *[see Use in Specific Populations (8.4)]*.

16 HOW SUPPLIED/STORAGE AND HANDLING

FLOVENT HFA 44 mcg Inhalation Aerosol is supplied in 10.6-g pressurized aluminum canisters containing 120 metered inhalations in boxes of 1 (NDC 0173-0718-20).

FLOVENT HFA 110 mcg Inhalation Aerosol is supplied in 12-g pressurized aluminum canisters containing 120 metered inhalations in boxes of 1 (NDC 0173-0719-20).

FLOVENT HFA 220 mcg Inhalation Aerosol is supplied in 12-g pressurized aluminum canisters containing 120 metered inhalations in boxes of 1 (NDC 0173-0720-20).

Each canister is fitted with a counter and a dark orange oral actuator with a peach strapcap packaged within a plastic-coated, moisture-protective foil pouch and patient's instructions. The moisture-protective foil pouch also contains a desiccant that should be discarded when the pouch is opened.

The dark orange actuator supplied with FLOVENT HFA should not be used with any other product canisters, and actuators from other products should not be used with a FLOVENT HFA canister.

The correct amount of medication in each inhalation cannot be assured after the counter reads 000, even though the canister is not completely empty and will continue to operate. The inhaler should be discarded when the counter reads 000.

Keep out of reach of children. Avoid spraying in eyes.

Contents Under Pressure: Do not puncture. Do not use or store near heat or open flame. Exposure to temperatures above 120°F may cause bursting. Never throw into fire or incinerator.

Store at 25°C (77°F); excursions permitted from 15° to 30°C (59° to 86°F). Store the inhaler with the mouthpiece down. For best results, the inhaler should be at room temperature before use. SHAKE WELL BEFORE USING.

FLOVENT HFA does not contain CFCs as the propellant.

17 PATIENT COUNSELING INFORMATION

See FDA-approved patient labeling (Patient Information and Instructions for Use).

17.1 Oral Candidiasis

Patients should be advised that localized infections with *Candida albicans* have occurred in the mouth and pharynx in some patients. If oropharyngeal candidiasis develops, it should be treated with appropriate local or systemic (i.e., oral antifungal) therapy while still continuing therapy with FLOVENT HFA, but at times therapy with FLOVENT HFA may need to be temporarily interrupted under close medical supervision. Rinsing the mouth after inhalation is advised.

17.2 Status Asthmaticus and Acute Asthma Symptoms

Patients should be advised that FLOVENT HFA is not a bronchodilator and is not intended for use as rescue medication for acute asthma exacerbations. Acute asthma symptoms should be treated with an inhaled, short-acting $beta_2$-agonist such as albuterol. Patients should be instructed to contact their physicians immediately if there is deterioration of their asthma.

17.3 Immunosuppression

Patients who are on immunosuppressant doses of corticosteroids should be warned to avoid exposure to chickenpox or measles and if they are exposed to consult their physicians without delay. Patients should be informed of potential worsening of existing tuberculosis, fungal, bacterial, viral, or parasitic infections, or ocular herpes simplex.

17.4 Hypercorticism and Adrenal Suppression

Patients should be advised that FLOVENT HFA may cause systemic corticosteroid effects of hypercorticism and adrenal suppression. Additionally, patients should be instructed that deaths due to adrenal insufficiency have occurred during and after transfer from systemic corticosteroids. Patients should taper slowly from systemic corticosteroids if transferring to FLOVENT HFA.

17.5 Hypersensitivity Reactions, Including Anaphylaxis

Patients should be advised that hypersensitivity reactions including anaphylaxis, angioedema, urticaria, and bronchospasm may occur after administration of FLOVENT HFA. Patients should discontinue FLOVENT HFA if such reactions occur.

17.6 Reduction in Bone Mineral Density

Patients who are at an increased risk for decreased BMD should be advised that the use of corticosteroids may pose an additional risk.

17.7 Reduced Growth Velocity

Patients should be informed that orally inhaled corticosteroids, including FLOVENT HFA, may cause a reduction in growth velocity when administered to pediatric patients. Physicians should closely follow the growth of children and adolescents taking corticosteroids by any route.

17.8 Ocular Effects

Long-term use of inhaled corticosteroids may increase the risk of some eye problems (cataracts or glaucoma); regular eye examinations should be considered.

17.9 Use Daily for Best Effect

Patients should use FLOVENT HFA at regular intervals as directed. Individual patients will experience a variable time to onset and degree of symptom relief and the full benefit may not be achieved until treatment has been administered for 1 to 2 weeks or longer. Patients should not increase the prescribed dosage but should contact their physicians if symptoms do not improve or if the condition worsens. Patients should be instructed not to stop use of FLOVENT HFA abruptly. Patients should contact their physicians immediately if they discontinue use of FLOVENT HFA.

DISKUS, FLOVENT, ROTADISK, and VENTOLIN are registered trademarks of GlaxoSmithKline.

AeroChamber Plus is a registered trademark and AeroChamber Z-STAT Plus is a trademark of Monaghan Medical Corp. or an affiliate of Monaghan Medical Corp.

GlaxoSmithKline

Research Triangle Park, NC 27709

January 2012

FLH:4PI

PHARMACIST—DETACH HERE AND GIVE LEAFLET TO PATIENT

Patient Information

FLOVENT® *[flō' vent]* HFA 44 mcg
(fluticasone propionate 44 mcg)
Inhalation Aerosol
FLOVENT® HFA 110 mcg
(fluticasone propionate 110 mcg)
Inhalation Aerosol
FLOVENT® HFA 220 mcg
(fluticasone propionate 220 mcg)
Inhalation Aerosol
FOR ORAL INHALATION ONLY

Read this leaflet carefully before you start to use FLOVENT HFA Inhalation Aerosol.

Keep this leaflet because it has important summary information about FLOVENT HFA. This leaflet does not contain all the information about your medicine. If you have any questions or are not sure about something, you should ask your doctor or pharmacist.

Read the new leaflet that comes with each refill of your prescription because there may be new information.

What is FLOVENT HFA?

FLOVENT HFA contains a medicine called fluticasone propionate, which is a synthetic corticosteroid. Corticosteroids are natural substances found in the body that help fight inflammation. Corticosteroids are used to treat asthma because they reduce airway inflammation.

FLOVENT HFA is used to treat asthma in patients 4 years and older. When inhaled regularly, FLOVENT HFA also helps to prevent symptoms of asthma.

FLOVENT HFA comes in 3 strengths. Your doctor has prescribed the one that is best for your condition.

Who should not use FLOVENT HFA?

Do not use FLOVENT HFA if you:

- are allergic to any of the ingredients in FLOVENT HFA or other inhaled corticosteroids. See "What are the ingredients in FLOVENT HFA?" below.
- have an acute asthma attack or status asthmaticus. **FLOVENT HFA is not a bronchodilator and should not be used to give you fast relief from your breathing problems during an asthma attack.** Always use a short-acting bronchodilator (rescue medicine), such as albuterol inhaler, during a sudden asthma attack. You must take FLOVENT HFA at regular times as recommended by your doctor, and not as an emergency medicine.

What should I tell my doctor before taking FLOVENT HFA?

Tell your doctor if you:

- have liver problems.
- have been exposed to chickenpox or measles.
- have any other medical conditions.
- are pregnant or planning to become pregnant. It is not known if FLOVENT HFA will harm your unborn baby.
- are breastfeeding a baby. It is not known if FLOVENT HFA passes into your breast milk.

Tell your doctor about all the medicines you take including prescription and non-prescription medicines, vitamins, and herbal supplements. FLOVENT HFA may affect the way other medicines work, and other medicines may affect how FLOVENT HFA works. Especially, tell your doctor if you take:

- a medicine containing ritonavir (commonly used to treat HIV infection or AIDS). The anti-HIV medicines NORVIR® (ritonavir capsules) Soft Gelatin, NORVIR (ritonavir oral solution), and KALETRA® (lopinavir/ritonavir) tablets contain ritonavir.
- any other corticosteroid medicines.
- ketoconazole (NIZORAL®), an antifungal medicine.

How should I use FLOVENT HFA?

1. It is important that you inhale each dose as your doctor has prescribed. The prescription label provided by your pharmacist will usually tell you what dose to take and how often. If it doesn't or if you aren't sure, ask your doctor or pharmacist. DO NOT inhale more doses or use your FLOVENT HFA more often than your doctor has prescribed.
2. It may take 1 to 2 weeks or longer for this medicine to work, and it is very important that you use it regularly. **Do not stop taking FLOVENT HFA, even if you are feeling better, unless your doctor tells you to.**
3. If you miss a dose, just take your next scheduled dose when it is due. **Do not double the dose.**
4. Your doctor may prescribe additional medicine (such as fast-acting bronchodilators) for emergency relief if a sudden asthma attack occurs. Contact your doctor if:
   - an asthma attack does not respond to the additional medicine or
   - you need more of the additional medicine than usual.
5. If you also use another medicine by inhalation, you should ask your doctor for instructions on when to use it while you are also using FLOVENT HFA.
6. Children should use FLOVENT HFA with an adult's help, as instructed by the child's healthcare provider. A valved holding chamber (a kind of spacer) and face mask may be used to deliver FLOVENT HFA to young patients.

What should I avoid while taking FLOVENT HFA?
If you have not had or not been vaccinated against chickenpox, measles, or active tuberculosis, you should stay away from people who are infected.

What are the possible side effects of FLOVENT HFA?
FLOVENT HFA can cause serious side effects, including:
- **fungal infections (thrush) in your mouth and throat.** Tell your doctor if you have any redness or white-colored coating in your mouth
- **decreased ability to fight infections.** Symptoms of infection may include: fever, pain, aches, chills, feeling tired, nausea and vomiting. Tell your doctor about any signs of infection while you use FLOVENT HFA.
- **decreased adrenal function (adrenal insufficiency).** Symptoms of decreased adrenal function include tiredness, weakness, nausea and vomiting, and low blood pressure. Decreased adrenal function can lead to death
- **allergic reaction (anaphylaxis).** Call your doctor and stop FLOVENT HFA right away if you have any symptoms of an allergic reaction:
- swelling of the face, throat and tongue
- hives
- rash
- breathing problems
- **lower bone mineral density.** This may be a problem for people who already have a higher chance of low bone density (osteoporosis).
- **slow growth in children.** The growth of children using FLOVENT HFA should be checked regularly.
- **eye problems including glaucoma and cataracts.** Tell your doctor about any vision changes while using FLOVENT HFA. Your doctor may tell you to have your eyes checked.
- **increased wheezing (bronchospasm).** Increased wheezing can happen right away after using FLOVENT HFA. Always have a rescue inhaler with you to treat sudden wheezing.

Tell your doctor right away if you have any of the serious side effects listed above or if you have worsening lung symptoms.

The most common side effects of FLOVENT HFA include:
- a cold or upper respiratory tract infection
- throat irritation
- headache
- fever
- diarrhea
- ear infection

Tell your doctor if you have any side effects that bother you or that do not go away. These are not all the possible side effects of FLOVENT HFA. For more information ask your doctor or pharmacist.

Call your doctor for medical advice about side effects. You may report side effects to FDA at 1-800-FDA-1088 or 1-800-332-1088.

How should I store FLOVENT HFA?
Store FLOVENT HFA at room temperature between 59°and 86°F (15°-30°C). Store the inhaler with the mouthpiece down. For best results, the inhaler should be at room temperature before use.

Keep FLOVENT HFA and all medicines out of the reach of children.

This Patient Information leaflet summarizes the most important information about FLOVENT HFA. If you would like more information, talk with your healthcare provider. You can ask your pharmacist or doctor for information about FLOVENT HFA that is written for health professionals. You can also contact the company that makes FLOVENT HFA (toll free) at 1-888-825-5249.

What are the ingredients in FLOVENT HFA?
Active ingredient: fluticasone propionate (micronized)
Inactive ingredient: propellant HFA-134a

Instructions for Using FLOVENT HFA

The parts of your FLOVENT HFA
There are 2 main parts to your FLOVENT HFA inhaler—the metal canister that holds the medicine and the dark orange plastic actuator that sprays the medicine from the canister (see Figure 1).
[See figure 1 at top of next column]
The canister has a counter to show how many sprays of medicine you have left. The number shows through a window in the back of the actuator. The counter starts at 124. The number will count down by 1 each time you spray the inhaler. The counter will stop counting at 000.

Never try to change the numbers or take the counter off the metal canister. The counter cannot be reset, and it is permanently attached to the canister.

The mouthpiece of the actuator is covered by a cap. A strap on this cap keeps it attached to the actuator.

Do not use the actuator with a canister of medicine from any other inhaler. And do not use a FLOVENT HFA canister with an actuator from any other inhaler.

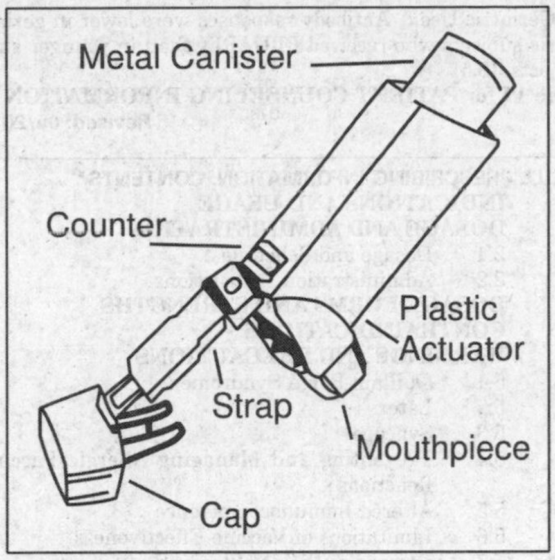

Figure 1

Using your FLOVENT HFA
- The inhaler should be at room temperature before you use it.
- Take your FLOVENT HFA inhaler out of the moisture-protective foil pouch just before you use it for the first time. Safely throw away the foil pouch and the drying packet that comes inside the pouch.
- **Priming the inhaler:**
Before you use FLOVENT HFA for the first time, you must prime the inhaler so that you will get the right amount of medicine when you use it. To prime the inhaler, take the cap off the mouthpiece and shake the inhaler well for 5 seconds. Then spray the inhaler into the air away from your face. **Avoid spraying in eyes.** Shake and spray the inhaler like this 3 more times to finish priming it. The counter should now read 120.
You must prime the inhaler again if you have not used it in more than 7 days or if you drop it. Take the cap off the mouthpiece and shake the inhaler well for 5 seconds. Then spray it 1 time into the air away from your face.
- If a child needs help using the inhaler, an adult should help the child use the inhaler with or without a valved holding chamber, which may also be attached to a face mask. The adult should follow the instructions that came with the valved holding chamber. An adult should watch a child use the inhaler to be sure it is used correctly.

Read the following 7 steps before using FLOVENT HFA and follow them at each use. If you have any questions, ask your doctor or pharmacist.

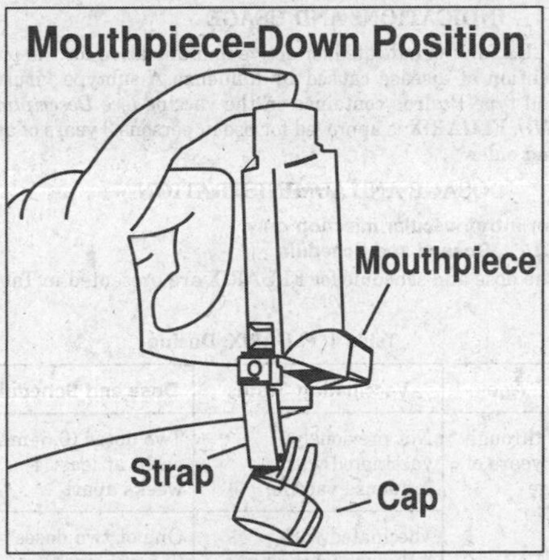

Figure 2

1. **Take the cap off the mouthpiece of the actuator** (see Figure 2). Look inside the mouthpiece for foreign objects, and take out any you see.
Make sure the canister fits firmly in the actuator.
Shake the inhaler well for 5 seconds.
2. Hold the inhaler with the mouthpiece down (see Figure 2). **Breathe out through your mouth** and push as much air from your lungs as you can. Put the mouthpiece in your mouth and close your lips around it.
3. Push the top of the canister all the way down while you breathe in deeply and slowly through your mouth (see Figure 3).
Right after the spray comes out, take your finger off the canister. After you have breathed in all the way, take the inhaler out of your mouth and close your mouth.
4. **Hold your breath as long as you can,** up to 10 seconds. Then breathe normally.
5. **Wait about 30 seconds and shake the inhaler well** for 5 seconds. Repeat steps 2 through 4.
6. After you finish taking this medicine, rinse your mouth with water. Spit out the water. Do not swallow it.
7. Put the cap back on the mouthpiece after each time you use the inhaler. Make sure it snaps firmly into place.

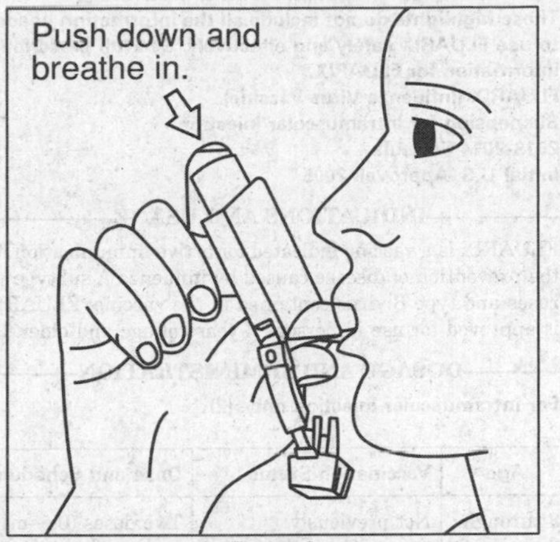

Figure 3

Cleaning your FLOVENT HFA
Clean the inhaler at least once a week after your evening dose. It is important to keep the canister and plastic actuator clean so the medicine will not build-up and block the spray.

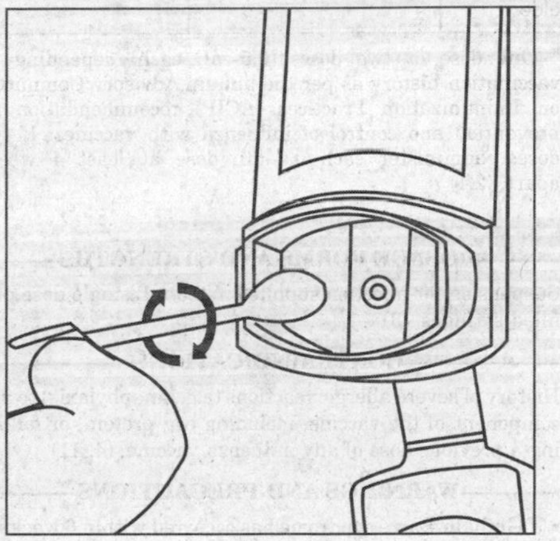
Figure 4

1. Take the cap off the mouthpiece. The strap on the cap will stay attached to the actuator. Do not take the canister out of the plastic actuator.
2. Use a clean cotton swab dampened with water to clean the small circular opening where the medicine sprays out of the canister. Gently twist the swab in a circular motion to take off any medicine (see Figure 4). Repeat with a new swab dampened with water to take off any medicine still at the opening.
3. Wipe the inside of the mouthpiece with a clean tissue dampened with water. Let the actuator air-dry overnight.
4. Put the cap back on the mouthpiece after the actuator has dried.

Replacing your FLOVENT HFA
- **When the counter reads 020,** you should refill your prescription or ask your doctor if you need a refill of your prescription.
- **When the counter reads 000,** throw the inhaler away. You should not keep using the inhaler because you will not receive the right amount of medicine.
- **Do not use the inhaler** after the expiration date, which is on the packaging it comes in.

FLOVENT is a registered trademark of GlaxoSmithKline. The other brands listed are trademarks of their respective owners and are not trademarks of GlaxoSmithKline. The makers of these brands are not affiliated with and do not endorse GlaxoSmithKline or its products.

GlaxoSmithKline
Research Triangle Park, NC 27709

November 2010
FLH:2PIL

FLUARIX ℞
[flū'-a-rix]
(Influenza Virus Vaccine)
Suspension for Intramuscular Injection
2013-2014 Formula

HIGHLIGHTS OF PRESCRIBING INFORMATION
These highlights do not include all the information needed to use FLUARIX safely and effectively. See full prescribing information for FLUARIX.
FLUARIX (Influenza Virus Vaccine)
Suspension for Intramuscular Injection
2013-2014 Formula
Initial U.S. Approval: 2005

INDICATIONS AND USAGE

FLUARIX is a vaccine indicated for active immunization for the prevention of disease caused by influenza A subtype viruses and type B virus contained in the vaccine. FLUARIX is approved for use in persons 3 years of age and older. (1)

DOSAGE AND ADMINISTRATION

For intramuscular injection only. (2)

Age	Vaccination Status	Dose and Schedule
3 through 8 years of age	Not previously vaccinated with influenza vaccine	Two doses (0.5–mL each) at least 4 weeks apart (2.1)
	Vaccinated with influenza vaccine in a previous season	One or two doses[a] (0.5–mL each) (2.1)
9 years of age and older	Not applicable	One 0.5–mL dose (2.1)

[a] One dose or two doses (0.5–mL each) depending on vaccination history as per the annual Advisory Committee on Immunization Practices (ACIP) recommendation on prevention and control of influenza with vaccines. If two doses, administer each 0.5–mL dose at least 4 weeks apart. (2.1)

DOSAGE FORMS AND STRENGTHS

Suspension for injection supplied in 0.5-mL single-dose prefilled syringes. (3)

CONTRAINDICATIONS

History of severe allergic reactions (e.g., anaphylaxis) to any component of the vaccine, including egg protein, or following a previous dose of any influenza vaccine. (4, 11)

WARNINGS AND PRECAUTIONS

- If Guillain-Barré syndrome has occurred within 6 weeks of receipt of a prior influenza vaccine, the decision to give FLUARIX should be based on potential benefits and risks. (5.1)
- The tip caps of the prefilled syringes of FLUARIX may contain natural rubber latex which may cause allergic reactions in latex-sensitive individuals. (5.2)
- Syncope (fainting) can occur in association with administration of injectable vaccines, including FLUARIX. Procedures should be in place to avoid falling injury and to restore cerebral perfusion following syncope. (5.3)

ADVERSE REACTIONS

- In adults, the most common (≥10%) local and general adverse events were pain and redness at the injection site, muscle aches, fatigue, and headache. (6.1)
- In children 5 years through 17 years of age, the most common (≥10%) local and general adverse events were similar to those in adults but also included swelling at the injection site. (6.1)
- In children 3 years through 4 years of age, the most common (≥10%) local and general adverse events were pain, redness, and swelling at the injection site, irritability, loss of appetite, and drowsiness. (6.1)

To report SUSPECTED ADVERSE REACTIONS, contact GlaxoSmithKline at 1-888-825-5249 or VAERS at 1-800-822-7967 or www.vaers.hhs.gov.

USE IN SPECIFIC POPULATIONS

- Safety and effectiveness of FLUARIX have not been established in pregnant women or nursing mothers. (8.1, 8.3)
- Register women who receive FLUARIX while pregnant in the pregnancy registry by calling 1-888-452-9622. (8.1)
- In a clinical study of children younger than 3 years of age, antibody titers were lower after FLUARIX than after an active comparator. (8.4)
- Geriatric Use: Antibody responses were lower in geriatric subjects who received FLUARIX than in younger subjects. (8.5)

See 17 for PATIENT COUNSELING INFORMATION
Revised: 05/2013

FULL PRESCRIBING INFORMATION: CONTENTS*

*** Sections or subsections omitted from the full prescribing information are not listed**

FULL PRESCRIBING INFORMATION

1 INDICATIONS AND USAGE

FLUARIX® is indicated for active immunization for the prevention of disease caused by influenza A subtype viruses and type B virus contained in the vaccine *[see Description (11)]*. FLUARIX is approved for use in persons 3 years of age and older.

2 DOSAGE AND ADMINISTRATION

For intramuscular injection only.

2.1 Dosage and Schedule

The dose and schedule for FLUARIX are presented in Table 1.

Table 1. FLUARIX: Dosing

Age	Vaccination Status	Dose and Schedule
3 through 8 years of age	Not previously vaccinated with influenza vaccine	Two doses (0.5–mL each) at least 4 weeks apart
	Vaccinated with influenza vaccine in a previous season	One or two doses[a] (0.5–mL each)
9 years of age and older	Not applicable	One 0.5–mL dose

[a] One dose or two doses (0.5– mL each) depending on vaccination history as per the annual Advisory Committee on Immunization Practices (ACIP) recommendation on prevention and control of influenza with vaccines. If two doses, administer each 0.5– mL dose 4 weeks apart.

2.2 Administration Instructions

Shake well before administration. Parenteral drug products should be inspected visually for particulate matter and discoloration prior to administration, whenever solution and container permit. If either of these conditions exists, the vaccine should not be administered.

Attach a sterile needle to the prefilled syringe and administer intramuscularly.

The preferred site for intramuscular injection is the deltoid muscle of the upper arm. Do not inject in the gluteal area or areas where there may be a major nerve trunk.

Do not administer this product intravenously, intradermally, or subcutaneously.

3 DOSAGE FORMS AND STRENGTHS

FLUARIX is a suspension for injection. Each 0.5-mL dose is supplied in single-dose prefilled TIP–LOK® syringes.

4 CONTRAINDICATIONS

Do not administer FLUARIX to anyone with a history of severe allergic reactions (e.g., anaphylaxis) to any component of the vaccine, including egg protein, or following a previous administration of any influenza vaccine *[see Description (11)]*.

5 WARNINGS AND PRECAUTIONS

5.1 Guillain-Barré Syndrome

If Guillain–Barré syndrome (GBS) has occurred within 6 weeks of receipt of a prior influenza vaccine, the decision to give FLUARIX should be based on careful consideration of the potential benefits and risks.

The 1976 swine influenza vaccine was associated with an increased frequency of GBS. Evidence for a causal relation of GBS with subsequent vaccines prepared from other influenza viruses is inconclusive. If influenza vaccine does pose a risk, it is probably slightly more than one additional case/one million persons vaccinated.

5.2 Latex

The tip caps of the prefilled syringes of FLUARIX may contain natural rubber latex which may cause allergic reactions in latex–sensitive individuals.

5.3 Syncope

Syncope (fainting) can occur in association with administration of injectable vaccines, including FLUARIX. Syncope can be accompanied by transient neurological signs such as visual disturbance, paresthesia, and tonic-clonic limb movements. Procedures should be in place to avoid falling injury and to restore cerebral perfusion following syncope.

5.4 Preventing and Managing Allergic Vaccine Reactions

Prior to administration, the healthcare provider should review the immunization history for possible vaccine sensitivity and previous vaccination–related adverse reactions. Appropriate medical treatment and supervision must be available to manage possible anaphylactic reactions following administration of FLUARIX.

5.5 Altered Immunocompetence

If FLUARIX is administered to immunosuppressed persons, including individuals receiving immunosuppressive therapy, the immune response may be lower than in immunocompetent persons.

5.6 Limitations of Vaccine Effectiveness

Vaccination with FLUARIX may not protect all susceptible individuals.

5.7 Persons at Risk of Bleeding

As with other intramuscular injections, FLUARIX should be given with caution in individuals with bleeding disorders such as hemophilia or on anticoagulant therapy, to avoid the risk of hematoma following the injection.

6 ADVERSE REACTIONS

6.1 Clinical Trials Experience

Because clinical trials are conducted under widely varying conditions, adverse reaction rates observed in the clinical trials of a vaccine cannot be directly compared to rates in the clinical trials of another vaccine, and may not reflect the rates observed in practice. There is the possibility that broad use of FLUARIX could reveal adverse reactions not observed in clinical trials.

Adults: In adults, the most common (≥10%) local adverse reactions and general adverse events observed with FLUARIX were pain and redness at the injection site, muscle aches, fatigue, and headache.

FLUARIX has been administered to 10,317 adults 18 through 64 years of age and 606 subjects 65 years of age and older in 4 clinical trials.

One of the 4 clinical trials was a randomized, double-blind, placebo-controlled study that evaluated a total of 952 subjects: FLUARIX (N = 760) and placebo (N = 192). The population was 18 through 64 years of age (mean 39.1), 54% were female and 80% were white. Solicited events were collected for 4 days (day of vaccination and the next 3 days) (Table 2). Unsolicited events that occurred within 21 days of vaccination (day 0-20) were recorded using diary cards supplemented by spontaneous reports and a medical history as reported by subjects.

Table 2. Incidence of Solicited Local Adverse Reactions or General Adverse Events Within 4 Days[a] of Vaccination in Adults 18 Through 64 Years of Age[b] (Total Vaccinated Cohort)

	FLUARIX N = 760 %	Placebo N = 192 %
Local Adverse Reactions		
Pain	55	12
Redness	18	10
Swelling	9	6
General Adverse Events		
Muscle aches	23	12
Fatigue	20	18
Headache	19	21
Arthralgia	6	6
Shivering	3	3
Fever ≥100.4°F (38.0°C)	2	2

Total vaccinated cohort for safety included all vaccinated subjects for whom safety data were available.
[a] 4 days included day of vaccination and the subsequent 3 days.
[b] NCT00100399.

Unsolicited adverse events that occurred in ≥1% of recipients of FLUARIX and at a rate greater than placebo included upper respiratory tract infection (3.9% versus 2.6%), nasopharyngitis (2.5% versus 1.6%), nasal congestion (2.2% versus 2.1%), diarrhea (1.6% versus 0%), influenza-like illness (1.6% versus 0.5%), vomiting (1.4% versus 0%), and dysmenorrhea (1.3% versus 1.0%).
A randomized, single-blind, active-controlled US study evaluated subjects randomized to receive FLUARIX (N = 917) or FLUZONE (N = 910), a US–licensed trivalent, inactivated influenza virus vaccine (Sanofi Pasteur SA) stratified by age: 18 through 64 years and 65 years of age and older. In the overall population, 59% of subjects were female and 91% were white. Solicited events were collected using diary cards for 4 days (day of vaccination and the next 3 days) (Table 3). Unsolicited events that occurred within 21 days of vaccination (day 0-20) were recorded using diary cards.
[See table 3 above]
Unsolicited adverse events that occurred in ≥1% of all recipients of FLUARIX or the comparator influenza vaccine in the 21-day post-vaccination period included headache (2.8% versus 2.3%), back pain (1.5% versus 0.4%), pain in extremity (1.2% versus 0.7%), pharyngolaryngeal pain (1.2% versus 0.9%), cough (1.1% versus 0.9%), fatigue (1.1% versus 0.7%), nasopharyngitis (1.0% versus 1.3%), nausea (0.4% versus 1.0%), arthralgia (0.3% versus 1.0%), and injection site pruritus (0.2% versus 1.0%).
A double-blind, placebo-controlled study in subjects 18 through 64 years of age randomized (2:1) to receive FLUARIX (N = 5,103) or placebo (N = 2,549) was conducted to evaluate the efficacy of FLUARIX. In the total population, 60% were female and 99.9% were white. In a subset (FLUARIX [N = 305] and placebo [N = 155]), unsolicited events that occurred within 21 days of vaccination (day 0-20) were recorded on diary cards. The percentage of subjects reporting at least one unsolicited event was similar among the groups (24.3% for FLUARIX and 22.6% for placebo). Unsolicited adverse events that occurred in ≥1% of recipients of FLUARIX and at a rate greater than placebo included injection site pain (5.2% versus 1.3%), dysmenorrhea (1.3% versus 0.6%), and migraine (1.0% versus 0.0%).
Incidence of Adverse Events Reported in ≥1% of Subjects in Non-US Clinical Trials: The following additional adverse events have been observed in adults in non-US clinical trials with FLUARIX. No adverse events were observed at an incidence of >10%.
General Disorders and Administration Site Conditions: Injection site ecchymosis, injection site induration, malaise.
Infections and Infestations: Rhinitis.
Musculoskeletal and Connective Tissue Disorders: Musculoskeletal pain, neck pain.
Skin and Subcutaneous Tissue Disorders: Sweating.
Serious Adverse Events: In the 4 clinical trials in adults (N = 10,923), there was a single case of anaphylaxis reported with FLUARIX (<0.01%).
Children: In children 5 years through 17 years of age, the most common (≥10%) local and general adverse events were similar to those in adults but also included swelling at the injection site. In children 3 years through 4 years of age, the most common (≥10%) local and general adverse events included pain, redness, and swelling at the injection site, irritability, loss of appetite, and drowsiness.
A single-blind, active-controlled US study evaluated subjects 6 months through 17 years of age who received FLUARIX (N = 2,081) or FLUZONE (N = 1,173), a US–licensed trivalent, inactivated influenza virus vaccine (Sanofi Pasteur SA) (Study 005). Children 6 months through 8 years of age with no history of influenza vaccination received 2 doses approximately 28 days apart. Children 6 months through 8 years of age with a history of influenza vaccination and children 9 years of age and older received 1 dose. Children 6 months through 35 months of age received 0.25 mL of FLUARIX or comparator influenza vaccine, and children 3 years of age and older received 0.5 mL of FLUARIX or comparator influenza vaccine.
Study subjects were 6 months through 17 years of age and 49% were female; 68% were white, 18% were black, 3% were Asian, and 11% were of other racial/ethnic groups.
Solicited local and general adverse events were collected using diary cards for 4 days (day of vaccination and the next 3 days). Unsolicited adverse events that occurred within 28 days of vaccination (day 0-27) after the first vaccination in all subjects and 21 days (day 0-20) after the second vaccination in unprimed subjects were recorded using diary cards.
The frequencies of solicited adverse events for children 3 years through 4 years of age and for children 5 years through 17 years of age were similar for FLUARIX and the comparator vaccine (Table 4).
[See table 4 above]

Table 3. Incidence of Solicited Local Adverse Reactions or General Adverse Events in Adults Within 4 Days[a] of Vaccination With FLUARIX or Comparator Influenza Vaccine by Age Group[b] (Total Vaccinated Cohort)

	18 Through 64 Years of Age		65 Years of Age and Older	
	FLUARIX N = 315 %	Comparator Influenza Vaccine N = 314 %	FLUARIX N = 601-602 %	Comparator Influenza Vaccine N = 596 %
Local Adverse Reactions				
Pain	48	53	19	18
Redness	13	16	11	13
Swelling	9	11	6	9
General Adverse Events				
Fatigue	21	18	9	10
Headache	20	21	8	8
Muscle aches	16	13	7	7
Arthralgia	9	9	6	5
Shivering	3	5	2	2
Fever ≥99.5°F (37.5°C)	3	1	2	1

Total vaccinated cohort for safety included all vaccinated subjects for whom safety data were available.
[a] 4 days included day of vaccination and the subsequent 3 days.
[b] NCT00197288.

Table 4. Incidence of Solicited Local Adverse Reactions or General Adverse Events Within 4 Days[a] of First Vaccination With FLUARIX or Comparator Influenza Vaccine by Age Group in Children 3 Through 17 Years of Age[b]

	3 Through 4 Years of Age		5 Through 17 Years of Age	
	FLUARIX N = 350 %	Comparator Influenza Vaccine N = 341 %	FLUARIX N = 1,348 %	Comparator Influenza Vaccine N = 451 %
Local Adverse Reactions				
Pain	35	38	56	56
Redness	23	20	18	16
Swelling	14	13	14	13
General Adverse Events				
Irritability	21	22	–	–
Loss of appetite	13	15	–	–
Drowsiness	13	20	–	–
Fever ≥99.5°F (37.5°C)	7	8	4	3
Muscle aches	–	–	29	29
Fatigue	–	–	20	19
Headache	–	–	15	16
Arthralgia	–	–	6	6
Shivering	–	–	3	4

[a] 4 days included day of vaccination and the subsequent 3 days.
[b] NCT00383123.

Table 5. Attack Rates and Vaccine Efficacy Against Culture-Confirmed Influenza A and/or B in Adults 18 Through 64 Years of Age[a] (Total Vaccinated Cohort)

		Attack Rates (n/N)		Vaccine Efficacy		
	N	N	%	%	LL	UL
Antigenically Matched Strains[b]						
FLUARIX	5,103	49	1.0	66.9[c]	51.9	77.4
Placebo	2,549	74	2.9	–	–	–
All Culture-Confirmed Influenza (Matched, Unmatched, and Untyped)[d]						
FLUARIX	5,103	63	1.2	61.6[c]	46.0	72.8
Placebo	2,549	82	3.2	–	–	–

[a] NCT00363870.
[b] There were no vaccine matched culture-confirmed cases of A/New Caledonia/20/1999 (H1N1) or B/Malaysia/2506/2004 influenza strains with FLUARIX or placebo.
[c] Vaccine efficacy for FLUARIX exceeded a pre-defined threshold of 35% for the lower limit of the 2-sided 95% CI.
[d] Of the 22 additional cases, 18 were unmatched and 4 were untyped; 15 of the 22 cases were A (H3N2) (11 cases with FLUARIX and 4 cases with placebo).

Table 6. Rates With HI Titers ≥1:40 and Rates of Seroconversion to Each Antigen Following FLUARIX or Placebo (21 Days After Vaccination) in Adults 18 Through 64 Years of Age[a] (ATP Cohort)

	FLUARIX[b] N = 745 % (95% CI)		Placebo N = 190 % (95% CI)	
% With HI Titers ≥1:40	**Pre-vaccination**	**Post-vaccination**	**Pre-vaccination**	**Post-vaccination**
A/New Caledonia/20/99 (H1N1)	54.8 (51.1, 58.4)	96.6 (95.1, 97.8)	52.1 (44.8, 59.4)	51.1 (43.7, 58.4)
A/Wyoming/3/2003 (H3N2)	68.7 (65.3, 72)	99.1 (98.1, 99.6)	65.3 (58, 72)	65.3 (58, 72)
B/Jiangsu/10/2003	49.5 (45.9, 53.2)	98.8 (97.7, 99.4)	48.9 (41.6, 56.3)	51.1 (43.7, 58.4)
Seroconversion[c]	**Post-vaccination**		**Post-vaccination**	
A/New Caledonia/20/99 (H1N1)	59.6 (56, 63.1)		0 (0, 1.9)	
A/Wyoming/3/2003 (H3N2)	61.9 (58.3, 65.4)		1.1 (0.1, 3.8)	
B/Jiangsu/10/2003	77.6 (74.4, 80.5)		1.1 (0.1, 3.8)	

HI = hemagglutination-inhibition; ATP = according–to–protocol; CI = Confidence Interval.
ATP cohort for immunogenicity included subjects for whom assay results were available after vaccination for at least one study vaccine antigen.
[a] NCT00100399.
[b]Results obtained following vaccination with FLUARIX manufactured for the 2004-2005 season.
[c]Seroconversion defined as at least a 4-fold increase in serum titers of HI antibodies to ≥1:40.

In children who received a second dose of FLUARIX or the comparator vaccine, the incidences of adverse events following the second dose were similar to those observed after the first dose.

Unsolicited adverse events that occurred in ≥1% of recipients of FLUARIX 6 months through 17 years of age included upper respiratory tract infection (5.5%), pyrexia (4.8%), cough (4.7%), vomiting (3.2%), headache (2.8%), rhinorrhea (2.7%), diarrhea (2.5%), pharyngolaryngeal pain (2.4%), nasopharyngitis (2.3%), otitis media (2.0%), nasal congestion (1.8%), upper abdominal pain (1.4%), and upper respiratory tract congestion (1.0%). The incidences of these events were similar in recipients of the comparator vaccine.

6.2 Postmarketing Experience

Worldwide voluntary reports of adverse events received for FLUARIX since market introduction of this vaccine are listed below. This list includes serious events or events which have causal connection to FLUARIX. Because these events are reported voluntarily from a population of uncertain size, it is not always possible to reliably estimate their frequency or establish a causal relationship to the vaccine.

Blood and Lymphatic System Disorders: Lymphadenopathy.

Cardiac Disorders: Tachycardia.

Ear and Labyrinth Disorders: Vertigo.

Eye Disorders: Conjunctivitis, eye irritation, eye pain, eye redness, eye swelling, eyelid swelling.

Gastrointestinal Disorders: Abdominal pain or discomfort, nausea, swelling of the mouth, throat, and/or tongue.

General Disorders and Administration Site Conditions: Asthenia, chest pain, chills, feeling hot, injection site mass, injection site reaction, injection site warmth, body aches.

Immune System Disorders: Anaphylactic reaction including shock, anaphylactoid reaction, hypersensitivity, serum sickness.

Infections and Infestations: Injection site abscess, injection site cellulitis, pharyngitis, rhinitis, tonsillitis.

Musculoskeletal and Connective Tissue Disorders: Pain in extremity.

Nervous System Disorders: Convulsion, dizziness, encephalomyelitis, facial palsy, facial paresis, Guillain-Barré syndrome, hypoesthesia, myelitis, neuritis, neuropathy, paresthesia, syncope.

Respiratory, Thoracic, and Mediastinal Disorders: Asthma, bronchospasm, cough, dyspnea, respiratory distress, stridor.

Skin and Subcutaneous Tissue Disorders: Angioedema, erythema, erythema multiforme, facial swelling, pruritus, rash, Stevens-Johnson syndrome, urticaria.

Vascular Disorders: Henoch-Schönlein purpura, vasculitis.

6.3 Adverse Events Associated With Influenza Vaccines

Immediate and presumably allergic reactions (e.g., hives, angioedema, allergic asthma, and systemic anaphylaxis) rarely occur after influenza vaccination. These reactions probably result from hypersensitivity to certain vaccine components, such as residual egg protein. Although FLUARIX contains only a limited quantity of egg protein, this protein can induce immediate hypersensitivity reactions among persons who have severe egg allergy *[see Contraindications (4)]*.

Neurological disorders temporally associated with influenza vaccination such as encephalopathy, optic neuritis/neuropathy, partial facial paralysis, and brachial plexus neuropathy have been reported.

Microscopic polyangitis (vasculitis) has been reported temporally associated with influenza vaccination.

7 DRUG INTERACTIONS

7.1 Concomitant Vaccine Administration

FLUARIX should not be mixed with any other vaccine in the same syringe or vial.

There are insufficient data to assess the concurrent administration of FLUARIX with other vaccines. When concomitant administration of other vaccines is required, the vaccines should be administered at different injection sites.

7.2 Immunosuppressive Therapies

Immunosuppressive therapies, including irradiation, antimetabolites, alkylating agents, cytotoxic drugs, and corticosteroids (used in greater than physiologic doses), may reduce the immune response to FLUARIX.

8 USE IN SPECIFIC POPULATIONS

8.1 Pregnancy

Pregnancy Category B

A reproductive and developmental toxicity study has been performed in female rats at a dose approximately 56 times the human dose (on a mg/kg basis) and revealed no evidence of impaired female fertility or harm to the fetus due to FLUARIX. There are, however, no adequate and well-controlled studies in pregnant women. Because animal reproduction studies are not always predictive of human response, FLUARIX should be given to a pregnant woman only if clearly needed.

In a reproductive and developmental toxicity study, the effect of FLUARIX on embryo-fetal and pre-weaning development was evaluated in pregnant rats. Animals were administered FLUARIX by intramuscular injection once prior to gestation, and during the period of organogenesis (gestation days 6, 8, 11, and 15), 0.1 mL/rat/occasion (approximately 56-fold excess relative to the projected human dose on a body weight basis). No adverse effects on mating, female fertility, pregnancy, parturition, lactation parameters, and embryo-fetal or pre-weaning development were observed. There were no vaccine-related fetal malformations or other evidence of teratogenesis.

Pregnancy Registry: GlaxoSmithKline maintains a surveillance registry to collect data on pregnancy outcomes and newborn health status outcomes following vaccination with FLUARIX during pregnancy. Women who receive FLUARIX during pregnancy should be encouraged to contact GlaxoSmithKline directly or their healthcare provider should contact GlaxoSmithKline by calling 1-888-452-9622.

8.3 Nursing Mothers

It is not known whether FLUARIX is excreted in human milk. Because many drugs are excreted in human milk, caution should be exercised when FLUARIX is administered to a nursing woman.

8.4 Pediatric Use

The immune response to FLUARIX has been evaluated in children 6 months through 4 years of age. In a randomized, controlled study, serum hemagglutination-inhibition (HI) antibody titers were lower in children 6 months through 35 months of age compared to a US-licensed vaccine. Based on these data, FLUARIX is not approved for use in children younger than 3 years of age. Immune responses in children 3 years through 4 years of age receiving FLUARIX or a US-licensed vaccine have been evaluated *[see Clinical Studies (14.2)]*. Safety has been evaluated in children 6 months through 17 years of age. The frequencies of solicited and unsolicited adverse events for children 3 years through 4 years of age and for children 5 years through 17 years of age were similar for FLUARIX and the comparator vaccine *[see Adverse Reactions (6.1)]*.

8.5 Geriatric Use

A randomized, single-blind, active-controlled study evaluated immunological non–inferiority in a cohort of subjects 65 years of age and older who received FLUARIX (N = 606) or another US–licensed trivalent, inactivated influenza virus vaccine (N = 604) (Sanofi Pasteur SA). In subjects receiving FLUARIX or the comparator vaccine, geometric mean antibody titers post-vaccination were lower in geriatric subjects than in younger subjects (18 through 64 years of age). FLUARIX was non–inferior to the comparator vaccine for each of the 3 influenza strains based on mean antibody titers and seroconversion rates. *[See Clinical Studies (14.2).]* Solicited local and general adverse events were similar for FLUARIX and the comparator vaccine among geriatric subjects (Table 3). For both vaccines, the frequency of solicited events in subjects 65 years of age and older was lower than in younger subjects (Table 3). *[See Adverse Reactions (6.1).]*

11 DESCRIPTION

FLUARIX, Influenza Virus Vaccine, for intramuscular injection, is a sterile colorless and slightly opalescent suspension. FLUARIX is a vaccine prepared from influenza viruses propagated in embryonated chicken eggs. Each of the influenza viruses is produced and purified separately. After harvesting the virus-containing fluids, each influenza virus is concentrated and purified by zonal centrifugation using a linear sucrose density gradient solution containing detergent to disrupt the viruses. Following dilution, the vaccine is further purified by diafiltration. Each influenza virus solution is inactivated by the consecutive effects of sodium deoxycholate and formaldehyde leading to the production of a "split virus." Each split inactivated virus is then suspended in sodium phosphate-buffered isotonic sodium chloride solution. The vaccine is formulated from the 3 split inactivated virus solutions.

FLUARIX has been standardized according to USPHS requirements for the 2013–2014 influenza season and is formulated to contain 45 micrograms (mcg) hemagglutinin (HA) per 0.5-mL dose, in the recommended ratio of 15 mcg HA of each of the following 3 strains: A/Christchurch/16/2010 NIB–74XP (H1N1) (an A/California/7/2009–like virus), A/Texas/50/2012 NYMC X-223A (H3N2) (an A/Victoria/361/2011-like virus), and B/Massachusetts/2/2012 NYMC BX-51B.

FLUARIX is formulated without preservatives. FLUARIX does not contain thimerosal. Each 0.5-mL dose also contains octoxynol-10 (TRITON® X-100) ≤0.085 mg, α-tocopheryl hydrogen succinate ≤0.1 mg, and polysorbate 80 (Tween 80) ≤0.415 mg. Each dose may also contain residual amounts of hydrocortisone ≤0.0016 mcg, gentamicin sulfate ≤0.15 mcg, ovalbumin ≤0.05 mcg, formaldehyde ≤5 mcg, and sodium deoxycholate ≤50 mcg from the manufacturing process.

The tip caps of the prefilled syringes of FLUARIX may contain natural rubber latex; the plungers are not made with natural rubber latex.

12 CLINICAL PHARMACOLOGY

12.1 Mechanism of Action

Influenza illness and its complications follow infection with influenza viruses. Global surveillance of influenza identifies yearly antigenic variants. For example, since 1977, antigenic variants of influenza A (H1N1 and H3N2) viruses and influenza B viruses have been in global circulation. Specific levels of hemagglutination-inhibition (HI) antibody titer post-vaccination with inactivated influenza virus vaccines have not been correlated with protection from influenza illness but the HI antibody titers have been used as a measure of vaccine activity. In some human challenge studies, HI antibody titers of ≥1:40 have been associated with protection from influenza illness in up to 50% of subjects.[1,2] Antibody against one influenza virus type or subtype confers little or no protection against another virus. Furthermore, antibody to one antigenic variant of influenza virus might not protect against a new antigenic variant of the same type or subtype. Frequent development of antigenic variants through antigenic drift is the virological basis for seasonal epidemics and the reason for the usual incorporation of one or more new strains in each year's influenza vaccine. Therefore, inactivated influenza vaccines are standardized to contain the hemagglutinins of strains (i.e., typically 2 type A and 1 type B), representing the influenza viruses likely to circulate in the United States in the upcoming winter.

Annual revaccination is recommended because immunity declines during the year after vaccination, and because circulating strains of influenza virus change from year to year.[3]

13 NONCLINICAL TOXICOLOGY

13.1 Carcinogenesis, Mutagenesis, Impairment of Fertility

FLUARIX has not been evaluated for carcinogenic or mutagenic potential, or for impairment of fertility.

14 CLINICAL STUDIES

14.1 Efficacy Against Culture-Confirmed Influenza

The efficacy of FLUARIX was evaluated in a randomized, double-blind, placebo-controlled study conducted in 2 European countries during the 2006-2007 influenza season. Efficacy of FLUARIX, containing A/New Caledonia/20/1999 (H1N1), A/Wisconsin/67/2005 (H3N2), and B/Malaysia/2506/2004 influenza strains, was defined as the prevention of culture-confirmed influenza A and/or B cases, for vaccine antigenically matched strains, compared with placebo. Healthy subjects 18 through 64 years of age (mean 39.9 years) were randomized (2:1) to receive FLUARIX (N = 5,103) or placebo (N = 2,549) and monitored for influenza-like illnesses (ILI) starting 2 weeks post-vaccination and lasting for approximately 7 months. In the overall population, 60% of subjects were female and 99.9% were white. Culture-confirmed influenza was assessed by active and passive surveillance of ILI. Influenza-like illness was defined as at least one general symptom (fever ≥100°F and/or myalgia) and at least one respiratory symptom (cough and/or sore throat). After an episode of ILI, nose and throat swab samples were collected for analysis; attack rates and vaccine efficacy were calculated (Table 5).

[See table 5 at top of previous page]

Table 7. Immune Responses 21 Days After Vaccination With FLUARIX Compared With Comparator Influenza Vaccine in Adults 18 Years of Age and Older[a] (ATP Cohort)

	FLUARIX N = 858-866 (95% CI)		Comparator Influenza Vaccine N = 846-854 (95% CI)	
GMTs	**Pre-vaccination**	**Post-vaccination**	**Pre-vaccination**	**Post-vaccination**
Anti-H1	27.9 (25.6, 30.5)	138.0 (125.2, 152.1)	29.1 (26.6, 31.7)	92.0 (84.5, 100.3)
Anti-H3	16.3 (15.1, 17.6)	121.6 (110.5, 133.7)	16.5 (15.4, 17.6)	114.0 (104.4, 124.5)
Anti-B	47.7 (44.1, 51.6)	231.9 (215.4, 249.6)	54.1 (49.9, 58.6)	273.7 (253.4, 295.7)
Seroconversion[b]	**% (95% CI) Post-vaccination**		**% (95% CI) Post-vaccination**	
A/New Caledonia/20/99 (H1N1)	45.7 (42.3, 49.1)		33.8 (30.6, 37.1)	
A/New York/55/2004 (H3N2)	67.1 (63.9, 70.3)		65.5 (62.2, 68.7)	
B/Jiangsu/10/2003	52.7 (49.3, 56.1)		53.8 (50.4, 57.2)	

Comparator influenza vaccine manufactured by Sanofi Pasteur SA.
ATP = according–to–protocol; GMT = geometric mean antibody titer; CI = Confidence Interval;
H1 = A/New Caledonia/20/99 (H1N1); H3 = A/New York/55/2004 (H3N2) for FLUARIX and A/California/7/2004 (H3N2) for comparator influenza vaccine; B = B/Jiangsu/10/2003.
ATP cohort included all eligible and evaluable subjects with results of at least one serological assay.
[a] NCT00197288.
[b] Seroconversion defined as at least a 4-fold increase in serum titers of HI antibodies to ≥1:40.

Table 8. Rates With HI Titers ≥1:40 and Rates of Seroconversion to Each Antigen Following FLUARIX or Comparator Influenza Vaccine in Children 3 Through 4 Years of Age[a] (ATP Cohort)

	FLUARIX[b] % (95% CI)		Comparator Influenza Vaccine[c] % (95% CI)	
% with HI titers ≥1:40	**Pre-vaccination N = 220**	**Post-vaccination N = 220**	**Pre-vaccination N = 220**	**Post-vaccination N = 221**
A/New Caledonia	17.3 (12.5, 22.9)	81.8 (76.1, 86.7)	20.5 (15.3, 26.4)	85.5 (80.2, 89.9)
A/Wisconsin	59.5 (52.7, 66.1)	88.2 (83.2, 92.1)	55.5 (48.6, 62.1)	93.7 (89.6, 96.5)
B/Malaysia	13.6 (9.4, 18.9)	55.0 (48.2, 61.7)	11.8 (7.9, 16.8)	58.4 (51.6, 64.9)
Seroconversion[d]	**Post-vaccination**		**Post-vaccination**	
A/New Caledonia	72.7 (66.3, 78.5)		72.3 (65.9, 78.1)	
A/Wisconsin	70.9 (64.4, 76.8)		70.5 (64.0, 76.4)	
B/Malaysia	53.2 (46.4, 59.9)		55.5 (48.6, 62.1)	

HI = hemagglutination inhibition; ATP = according-to-protocol; CI = Confidence Interval.
[a] NCT00383123.
[b] Results obtained following vaccination with FLUARIX manufactured for the 2006–2007 season.
[c] US– licensed trivalent, inactivated influenza virus vaccine (Sanofi Pasteur SA) without preservative manufactured for the 2006-2007 season.
[d] Seroconversion defined as at least a 4-fold increase in serum titers of HI antibodies to ≥1:40.

In a post-hoc, exploratory analysis by age, vaccine efficacy (against culture-confirmed influenza A and/or B cases, for vaccine antigenically matched strains) in subjects 18 through 49 years of age was 73.4% (95% CI: 59.3, 82.8) [number of influenza cases: FLUARIX (n = 35/3,602) and placebo (n = 66/1,810)]. In subjects 50 through 64 years of age, vaccine efficacy was 13.8% (95% CI: –137.0, 66.3) [number of influenza cases: FLUARIX (n = 14/1,501) and placebo (n = 8/739)]. As the study lacked statistical power to evaluate efficacy within age subgroups, the clinical significance of these results is unknown.

14.2 Immunological Evaluation

Adults: In a randomized, double-blind, placebo-controlled study conducted in healthy subjects 18 through 64 years of age (mean 39.1 years) in the United States, the immune responses to each of the antigens contained in FLUARIX were evaluated in sera obtained 21 days after administration of FLUARIX (N = 745) and were compared to those following administration of a placebo vaccine (N = 190). In the overall population, 54% of subjects were female and 80% were white. For each of the influenza antigens, the percentage of subjects who achieved seroconversion, defined as at least a 4–fold increase in serum hemagglutination-inhibition (HI) titer over baseline to ≥1:40 following vaccination, and the percentage of subjects who achieved HI titers of ≥1:40 are presented in Table 6. The lower limit of the 2-sided 95% CI for the percentage of subjects who achieved seroconversion or an HI titer of ≥1:40 exceeded the pre-defined lower limits of 40% and 70%, respectively.

[See table 6 at top of previous page]

Non-Inferiority Study: In a randomized, single-blind, active-controlled US study, immunological non-inferiority of

FLUARIX (N = 923) was compared with FLUZONE (N = 922), a US–licensed trivalent, inactivated influenza virus vaccine (Sanofi Pasteur SA). Subjects 18 through 64 years and 65 years of age and older were evaluated for immune responses to each of the vaccine antigens 21 days following vaccination *[see Use in Specific Populations (8.5)]*. In the overall population, 59% of subjects were female and 91% were white. The co-primary immunogenicity endpoints were geometric mean titers (GMTs) of serum HI antibodies and the percentage of subjects who achieved seroconversion, defined as at least a 4-fold increase in serum HI titer over baseline to ≥1:40, following vaccination. The primary immunogenicity analyses were performed on the According-to-Protocol (ATP) cohort which included all eligible and evaluable subjects with results of at least one serological assay. For each of the influenza antigens, the GMTs and the percentage of subjects who achieved seroconversion are presented in Table 7. FLUARIX was non-inferior to the comparator influenza vaccine based on antibody GMTs (upper limit of the 2-sided 95% CI for the GMT ratio [comparator influenza vaccine/FLUARIX] ≤1.5) and seroconversion rates (upper limit of the 2-sided 95% CI on difference of the comparator influenza vaccine minus FLUARIX ≤10%).

[See table 7 at top of previous page]

Children: The immune response of FLUARIX was compared to FLUZONE, a US–licensed trivalent, inactivated influenza virus vaccine (Sanofi Pasteur SA), in a single-blind, randomized study in a subset of children 6 months through 4 years of age (Study 005). The immune responses to each of the antigens contained in FLUARIX formulated for the 2006-2007 season were evaluated in sera obtained after 1 or 2 doses of FLUARIX (N = 426) and were compared to those following administration of the comparator influenza vaccine (N = 445). Further details on the clinical study design and demographic information have been previously described *[see Adverse Reactions (6.1)]*.

Non-inferiority of the immune response for FLUARIX to comparator influenza vaccine for subjects 6 months through 4 years of age was not demonstrated mainly due to lower antibody response to FLUARIX compared to the comparator influenza vaccine in subjects 6 months through 35 months of age. In subjects 3 years through 4 years of age, FLUARIX met at least one of the pre-specified criteria for demonstration of non-inferiority (GMT and seroconversion rate) for the influenza A strains but not for the influenza B strain. Seroconversion rates and the percentage of subjects with HI titers ≥1:40 were analyzed as secondary endpoints. In subjects 3 years through 4 years of age, the lower limit of the 95% Confidence Interval of the seroconversion rate for FLUARIX or the comparator influenza vaccine exceeded 40% for all 3 strains; also in this age group, the lower limit of the 95% Confidence Interval of the rate with HI titer ≥1:40 for FLUARIX or the comparator influenza vaccine exceeded 70% for both A strains (Table 8).

[See table 8 at top of previous page]

15 REFERENCES

1. Hannoun C, Megas F, Piercy J. Immunogenicity and protective efficacy of influenza vaccination. *Virus Res.* 2004;103:133-138.
2. Hobson D, Curry RL, Beare AS, et al. The role of serum haemagglutination-inhibiting antibody in protection against challenge infection with influenza A2 and B viruses. *J Hyg Camb.* 1972;70:767-777.
3. Centers for Disease Control and Prevention. Prevention and Control of Influenza with Vaccines: Recommendations of the Advisory Committee on Immunization Practices (ACIP). *MMWR* 2010;59(RR–8):1-62.

16 HOW SUPPLIED/STORAGE AND HANDLING

FLUARIX is supplied in 0.5-mL single-dose prefilled TIP–LOK syringes (packaged without needles).

NDC 58160-880-41 Syringe in Package of 10: , NDC 58160-880-52

Store refrigerated between 2° and 8°C (36° and 46°F). Do not freeze. Discard if the vaccine has been frozen. Store in the original package to protect from light.

17 PATIENT COUNSELING INFORMATION

Provide the following information to the vaccine recipient or guardian:

- Inform of the potential benefits and risks of immunization with FLUARIX.
- Educate regarding potential side effects, emphasizing that: (1) FLUARIX contains non–infectious killed viruses and cannot cause influenza and (2) FLUARIX is intended to provide protection against illness due to influenza viruses only, and cannot provide protection against all respiratory illness.
- Instruct to report any adverse events to their healthcare provider.
- Inform that safety and efficacy have not been established in pregnant women. Register women who receive FLUARIX while pregnant in the pregnancy registry by calling 1-888-452-9622.
- Give the Vaccine Information Statements, which are required by the National Childhood Vaccine Injury Act of 1986 to be given prior to immunization. These materials are available free of charge at the Centers for Disease Control and Prevention (CDC) website (www.cdc.gov/vaccines).
- Instruct that annual revaccination is recommended.

FLUARIX and TIP–LOK are registered trademarks of GlaxoSmithKline. FLUZONE is a registered trademark of Sanofi Pasteur Limited. TRITON is a registered trademark of Union Carbide Chemicals & Plastics Technology Corp.

Manufactured by **GlaxoSmithKline Biologicals**, Dresden, Germany,
a branch of **SmithKline Beecham Pharma GmbH & Co. KG**, Munich, Germany

Licensed by **GlaxoSmithKline Biologicals**, Rixensart, Belgium, US License 1617

Distributed by **GlaxoSmithKline**, Research Triangle Park, NC 27709

FLX:16PI

FLUARIX QUADRIVALENT ℞

(Influenza Virus Vaccine)
Suspension for Intramuscular Injection

HIGHLIGHTS OF PRESCRIBING INFORMATION

These highlights do not include all the information needed to use FLUARIX QUADRIVALENT safely and effectively. See full prescribing information for FLUARIX QUADRIVALENT.

FLUARIX QUADRIVALENT (Influenza Virus Vaccine)
Suspension for Intramuscular Injection
2013-2014 Formula
Initial U.S. Approval: 2012

INDICATIONS AND USAGE

FLUARIX QUADRIVALENT is a vaccine indicated for active immunization for the prevention of disease caused by influenza A subtype viruses and type B viruses contained in the vaccine. FLUARIX QUADRIVALENT is approved for use in persons 3 years of age and older. (1)

DOSAGE AND ADMINISTRATION

For intramuscular injection only. (2)

Age	Vaccination Status	Dose and Schedule
3 through 8 years of age	Not previously vaccinated with influenza vaccine	Two doses (0.5-mL each) at least 4 weeks apart (2.1)
	Vaccinated with influenza vaccine in a previous season	One or two doses[a] (0.5-mL each) (2.1)
9 years of age and older	Not applicable	One 0.5-mL dose (2.1)

[a]One dose or two doses (0.5-mL each) depending on vaccination history as per the annual Advisory Committee on Immunization Practices (ACIP) recommendation on prevention and control of influenza with vaccines. If two doses, administer each 0.5-mL dose at least 4 weeks apart. (2.1)

DOSAGE FORMS AND STRENGTHS

Suspension for injection supplied in 0.5-mL single-dose prefilled syringes. (3)

CONTRAINDICATIONS

History of severe allergic reactions (e.g., anaphylaxis) to any component of the vaccine, including egg protein, or following a previous dose of any influenza vaccine. (4, 11)

WARNINGS AND PRECAUTIONS

- If Guillain-Barré syndrome has occurred within 6 weeks of receipt of a prior influenza vaccine, the decision to give FLUARIX QUADRIVALENT should be based on careful consideration of potential benefits and risks. (5.1)
- The tip caps of the prefilled syringes of FLUARIX QUADRIVALENT may contain natural rubber latex which may cause allergic reactions in latex-sensitive individuals. (5.2)
- Syncope (fainting) can occur in association with administration of injectable vaccines, including FLUARIX QUADRIVALENT. Procedures should be in place to avoid falling injury and to restore cerebral perfusion following syncope. (5.3)

ADVERSE REACTIONS

- In adults, the most common (≥10%) injection site adverse reaction was pain (36%); the most common systemic adverse events were muscle aches (16%), headache (16%), and fatigue (16%). (6.1)
- In children 3 through17 years of age, the injection site adverse reactions were pain (44%), redness (23%), and swelling (19%). (6.1)
- In children 3 through 5 years of age, the most common (≥10%) systemic adverse events were drowsiness (17%), irritability (17%), and loss of appetite (16%); in children 6 through 17 years of age, the most common systemic adverse events were fatigue (20%), muscle aches (18%), headache (16%), arthralgia (10%), and gastrointestinal symptoms (10%). (6.1)

To report SUSPECTED ADVERSE REACTIONS, contact GlaxoSmithKline at 1-888-825-5249 or VAERS at 1-800-822-7967 or www.vaers.hhs.gov.

USE IN SPECIFIC POPULATIONS

- Safety and effectiveness of FLUARIX QUADRIVALENT have not been established in pregnant women or nursing mothers. (8.1, 8.3)
- Register women who receive FLUARIX QUADRIVALENT while pregnant in the pregnancy registry by calling 1-888-452-9622. (8.1)
- Geriatric Use: Antibody responses were lower in geriatric subjects who received FLUARIX QUADRIVALENT than in younger subjects. (8.5)

See 17 for PATIENT COUNSELING INFORMATION

Revised: 05/2013

FULL PRESCRIBING INFORMATION: CONTENTS*

*** Sections or subsections omitted from the full prescribing information are not listed**

FULL PRESCRIBING INFORMATION

1 INDICATIONS AND USAGE

FLUARIX® QUADRIVALENT is indicated for active immunization for the prevention of disease caused by influenza A subtype viruses and type B viruses contained in the vaccine *[see Description (11)]*. FLUARIX QUADRIVALENT is approved for use in persons 3 years of age and older.

2 DOSAGE AND ADMINISTRATION

For intramuscular injection only.

2.1 Dosage and Schedule

The dose and schedule for FLUARIX QUADRIVALENT are presented in Table 1.

Table 1. FLUARIX QUADRIVALENT: Dosing

Age	Vaccination Status	Dose and Schedule
3 through 8 years of age	Not previously vaccinated with influenza vaccine	Two doses (0.5-mL each) at least 4 weeks apart
	Vaccinated with influenza vaccine in a previous season	One or two doses[a] (0.5-mL each)
9 years of age and older	Not applicable	One 0.5-mL dose

[a]One dose or two doses (0.5-mL each) depending on vaccination history as per the annual Advisory Committee on Immunization Practices (ACIP) recommendation on prevention and control of influenza with vaccines. If two doses, administer each 0.5-mL dose 4 weeks apart.

2.2 Administration Instructions

Shake well before administration. Parenteral drug products should be inspected visually for particulate matter and discoloration prior to administration, whenever solution and container permit. If either of these conditions exists, the vaccine should not be administered.

Attach a sterile needle to the prefilled syringe and administer intramuscularly.

The preferred site for intramuscular injection is the deltoid muscle of the upper arm. Do not inject in the gluteal area or areas where there may be a major nerve trunk.

Do not administer this product intravenously, intradermally, or subcutaneously.

3 DOSAGE FORMS AND STRENGTHS

FLUARIX QUADRIVALENT is a suspension for injection. Each 0.5-mL dose is supplied in single-dose prefilled TIP–LOK® syringes.

4 CONTRAINDICATIONS

Do not administer FLUARIX QUADRIVALENT to anyone with a history of severe allergic reactions (e.g., anaphylaxis) to any component of the vaccine, including egg protein, or following a previous administration of any influenza vaccine *[see Description (11)]*.

5 WARNINGS AND PRECAUTIONS

5.1 Guillain-Barré Syndrome

If Guillain–Barré syndrome (GBS) has occurred within 6 weeks of receipt of a prior influenza vaccine, the decision to give FLUARIX QUADRIVALENT should be based on careful consideration of the potential benefits and risks.

The 1976 swine influenza vaccine was associated with an increased frequency of GBS. Evidence for a causal relation of GBS with subsequent vaccines prepared from other influenza viruses is inconclusive. If influenza vaccine does pose a risk, it is probably slightly more than one additional case/one million persons vaccinated.

5.2 Latex

The tip caps of the prefilled syringes of FLUARIX QUADRIVALENT may contain natural rubber latex which may cause allergic reactions in latex-sensitive individuals.

5.3 Syncope

Syncope (fainting) can occur in association with administration of injectable vaccines, including FLUARIX QUADRIVALENT. Syncope can be accompanied by transient neurological signs such as visual disturbance, paresthesia, and tonic-clonic limb movements. Procedures should be in place to avoid falling injury and to restore cerebral perfusion following syncope.

5.4 Preventing and Managing Allergic Vaccine Reactions

Prior to administration, the healthcare provider should review the immunization history for possible vaccine sensitivity and previous vaccination–related adverse reactions. Appropriate medical treatment and supervision must be available to manage possible anaphylactic reactions following administration of FLUARIX QUADRIVALENT.

5.5 Altered Immunocompetence

If FLUARIX QUADRIVALENT is administered to immunosuppressed persons, including individuals receiving immunosuppressive therapy, the immune response may be lower than in immunocompetent persons.

Table 2. FLUARIX QUADRIVALENT: Incidence of Solicited Local Adverse Reactions and Systemic Adverse Events Within 7 Days[a] of Vaccination in Adults[b] (Total Vaccinated Cohort)

	FLUARIX QUADRIVALENT[c] N = 3,011-3,015 %	Trivalent Influenza Vaccine (TIV)	
		TIV-1 (B Victoria)[d] N = 1,003 %	TIV-2 (B Yamagata)[e] N = 607 %
Local			
Pain	36	37	31
Redness	2	2	2
Swelling	2	2	1
Systemic			
Muscle aches	16	19	16
Headache	16	16	13
Fatigue	16	18	15
Arthralgia	8	10	9
Gastrointestinal symptoms[f]	7	7	6
Shivering	4	5	4
Fever ≥99.5°F (37.5°C)	2	1	2

Total vaccinated cohort for safety included all vaccinated subjects for whom safety data were available.

[a] 7 days included day of vaccination and the subsequent 6 days.

[b] Study 1: NCT01204671.

[c] Contained the same composition as FLUARIX (trivalent formulation) manufactured for the 2010-2011 season and an additional influenza type B virus of Yamagata lineage.

[d] Contained the same composition as FLUARIX manufactured for the 2010-2011 season (2 influenza A subtype viruses and an influenza type B virus of Victoria lineage).

[e] Contained the same 2 influenza A subtype viruses as FLUARIX manufactured for the 2010-2011 season and an influenza type B virus of Yamagata lineage.

[f] Gastrointestinal symptoms included nausea, vomiting, diarrhea, and/or abdominal pain.

5.6 Limitations of Vaccine Effectiveness

Vaccination with FLUARIX QUADRIVALENT may not protect all susceptible individuals.

5.7 Persons at Risk of Bleeding

As with other intramuscular injections, FLUARIX QUADRIVALENT should be given with caution in individuals with bleeding disorders such as hemophilia or on anticoagulant therapy, to avoid the risk of hematoma following the injection.

6 ADVERSE REACTIONS

The safety experience with FLUARIX (trivalent influenza vaccine) is relevant to FLUARIX QUADRIVALENT because both vaccines are manufactured using the same process and have overlapping compositions *[see Description (11)]*.

6.1 Clinical Trials Experience

In adults who received FLUARIX QUADRIVALENT, the most common (≥10%) injection site adverse reaction was pain (36%). The most common (≥10%) systemic adverse events were muscle aches (16%), headache (16%), and fatigue (16%).

In children 3 through 17 years of age who received FLUARIX QUADRIVALENT, injection site adverse reactions were pain (44%), redness (23%), and swelling (19%). In children 3 through 5 years of age, the most common (≥10%) systemic adverse events were drowsiness (17%), irritability (17%), and loss of appetite (16%); in children 6 through 17 years of age, the most common systemic adverse events were fatigue (20%), muscle aches (18%), headache (16%), arthralgia (10%), and gastrointestinal symptoms (10%).

Because clinical trials are conducted under widely varying conditions, adverse reaction rates observed in the clinical trials of a vaccine cannot be directly compared to rates in the clinical trials of another vaccine, and may not reflect the rates observed in practice. There is the possibility that broad use of FLUARIX QUADRIVALENT could reveal adverse reactions not observed in clinical trials.

FLUARIX QUADRIVALENT in Adults: Study 1 was a randomized, double-blind (2 arms) and open-label (one arm), active-controlled, safety, and immunogenicity study. In this study, subjects received FLUARIX QUADRIVALENT (N = 3,036) or one of two formulations of comparator trivalent influenza vaccine (FLUARIX, TIV-1, N = 1,010 or TIV-2, N = 610), each containing an influenza type B virus that corresponded to one of the two type B viruses in FLUARIX QUADRIVALENT (a type B virus of the Victoria lineage or a type B virus of the Yamagata lineage). The population was 18 years of age and older (mean age 58 years) and 57% were female; 69% were White, 27% were Asian, and 4% were of other racial/ethnic groups. Solicited events were collected for 7 days (day of vaccination and the next 6 days). The frequencies of solicited adverse events are shown in Table 2.

[See table 2 above]

Unsolicited events occurring within 21 days of vaccination (day 0-20) were reported in 13%, 14%, and 15% of subjects who received FLUARIX QUADRIVALENT, TIV-1, or TIV-2, respectively. The unsolicited adverse reactions that occurred most frequently (≥0.1% for FLUARIX QUADRIVALENT) included dizziness, injection site hematoma, injection site pruritus, and rash. Serious adverse events occurring within 21 days of vaccination were reported in 0.5%, 0.6%, and 0.2% of subjects who received FLUARIX QUADRIVALENT, TIV-1, or TIV-2, respectively.

FLUARIX QUADRIVALENT in Children: Study 2 was a randomized, double-blind, active-controlled, safety, and immunogenicity study. In this study, subjects received FLUARIX QUADRIVALENT (N = 915) or one of two formulations of comparator trivalent influenza vaccine (FLUARIX, TIV-1, N = 912 or TIV-2, N = 911), each containing an influenza type B virus that corresponded to one of the two type B viruses in FLUARIX QUADRIVALENT (a type B virus of the Victoria lineage or a type B virus of the Yamagata lineage). Subjects were 3 through 17 years of age and 52% were male; 56% were White, 29% were Asian, 12% were Black, and 3% were of other racial/ethnic groups. Children 3 through 8 years of age with no history of influenza vaccination received 2 doses approximately 28 days apart. Children 3 through 8 years of age with a history of influenza vaccination and children 9 years of age and older received one dose. Solicited local adverse reactions and systemic adverse events were collected using diary cards for 7 days (day of vaccination and the next 6 days). The frequencies of solicited adverse events are shown in Table 3.

[See table 3 at top of next page]

In children who received a second dose of FLUARIX QUADRIVALENT, TIV-1, or TIV-2, the incidences of adverse events following the second dose were generally lower than those observed after the first dose.

Unsolicited adverse events occurring within 28 days of any vaccination were reported in 31%, 33%, and 34% of subjects who received FLUARIX QUADRIVALENT, TIV-1, or TIV-2,

Table 3. FLUARIX QUADRIVALENT: Incidence of Solicited Local Adverse Reactions and Systemic Adverse Events Within 7 Days[a] After First Vaccination in Children 3 Through 17 Years of Age[b] (Total Vaccinated Cohort)

	FLUARIX QUADRIVALENT[c] %	Trivalent Influenza Vaccine (TIV)	
		TIV-1 (B Victoria)[d] %	TIV-2 (B Yamagata)[e] %
3 Through 17 Years of Age			
Local	N = 903	N = 901	N = 905
Pain[f]	44	42	40
Redness	23	21	21
Swelling	19	17	15
3 Through 5 Years of Age			
Systemic	N = 291	N = 314	N = 279
Drowsiness	17	12	14
Irritability	17	13	14
Loss of appetite	16	8	10
Fever ≥99.5°F (37.5°C)	9	9	8
6 Through 17 Years of Age			
Systemic	N = 613	N = 588	N = 626
Fatigue	20	19	16
Muscle aches	18	16	16
Headache	16	19	15
Arthralgia	10	9	7
Gastrointestinal symptoms[g]	10	10	7
Shivering	6	4	5
Fever ≥99.5°F (37.5°C)	6	9	6

Total vaccinated cohort for safety included all vaccinated subjects for whom safety data were available.
[a] 7 days included day of vaccination and the subsequent 6 days.
[b] Study 2: NCT01196988.
[c] Contained the same composition as FLUARIX (trivalent formulation) manufactured for the 2010-2011 season and an additional influenza type B virus of Yamagata lineage.
[d] Contained the same composition as FLUARIX manufactured for the 2010-2011 season (2 influenza A subtype viruses and an influenza type B virus of Victoria lineage).
[e] Contained the same 2 influenza A subtype viruses as FLUARIX manufactured for the 2010-2011 season and an influenza type B virus of Yamagata lineage.
[f] Percentage of subjects with pain by age subgroup: 39%, 38%, and 37% for FLUARIX QUADRIVALENT, TIV-1, and TIV-2, respectively, in children 3 through 8 years of age and 52%, 50%, and 46% for FLUARIX QUADRIVALENT, TIV-1, and TIV-2, respectively, in children 9 through 17 years of age.
[g] Gastrointestinal symptoms included nausea, vomiting, diarrhea, and/or abdominal pain.

respectively. The unsolicited adverse reactions that occurred most frequently (≥0.1% for FLUARIX QUADRIVALENT) included injection site pruritus and rash. Serious adverse events occurring within 28 days of any vaccination were reported in 0.1%, 0.1%, and 0.1% of subjects who received FLUARIX QUADRIVALENT, TIV-1, or TIV-2, respectively.

FLUARIX (Trivalent Formulation): FLUARIX has been administered to 10,317 adults 18 through 64 years of age, 606 subjects 65 years of age and older, and 2,115 children 6 months through 17 years of age in clinical trials. The incidence of solicited adverse events in each age group is shown in Tables 4 and 5.

[See table 4 at top of next page]

[See table 5 at top of next page]

In children who received a second dose of FLUARIX or the comparator vaccine, the incidences of adverse events following the second dose were similar to those observed after the first dose.

Serious Adverse Events: In the 4 clinical trials in adults (N = 10,923), there was a single case of anaphylaxis within one day following administration of FLUARIX (<0.01%).

6.2 Postmarketing Experience

Beyond those events reported above in the clinical trials for FLUARIX QUADRIVALENT or FLUARIX, the following adverse events have been spontaneously reported during postapproval use of FLUARIX (trivalent influenza vaccine). This list includes serious events or events which have causal connection to FLUARIX. Because these events are reported voluntarily from a population of uncertain size, it is not always possible to reliably estimate their frequency or establish a causal relationship to the vaccine.

Blood and Lymphatic System Disorders: Lymphadenopathy.

Cardiac Disorders: Tachycardia.

Ear and Labyrinth Disorders: Vertigo.

Eye Disorders: Conjunctivitis, eye irritation, eye pain, eye redness, eye swelling, eyelid swelling.

Gastrointestinal Disorders: Abdominal pain or discomfort, swelling of the mouth, throat, and/or tongue.

General Disorders and Administration Site Conditions: Asthenia, chest pain, feeling hot, injection site mass, injection site reaction, injection site warmth, body aches.

Immune System Disorders: Anaphylactic reaction including shock, anaphylactoid reaction, hypersensitivity, serum sickness.

Infections and Infestations: Injection site abscess, injection site cellulitis, pharyngitis, rhinitis, tonsillitis.

Nervous System Disorders: Convulsion, encephalomyelitis, facial palsy, facial paresis, Guillain-Barré syndrome, hypoesthesia, myelitis, neuritis, neuropathy, paresthesia, syncope.

Respiratory, Thoracic, and Mediastinal Disorders: Asthma, bronchospasm, dyspnea, respiratory distress, stridor.

Skin and Subcutaneous Tissue Disorders: Angioedema, erythema, erythema multiforme, facial swelling, pruritus, Stevens-Johnson syndrome, sweating, urticaria.

Vascular Disorders: Henoch-Schönlein purpura, vasculitis.

7 DRUG INTERACTIONS

7.1 Concomitant Vaccine Administration

FLUARIX QUADRIVALENT should not be mixed with any other vaccine in the same syringe or vial.

There are insufficient data to assess the concurrent administration of FLUARIX QUADRIVALENT with other vaccines. When concomitant administration of other vaccines is required, the vaccines should be administered at different injection sites.

7.2 Immunosuppressive Therapies

Immunosuppressive therapies, including irradiation, antimetabolites, alkylating agents, cytotoxic drugs, and corticosteroids (used in greater than physiologic doses), may reduce the immune response to FLUARIX QUADRIVALENT.

8 USE IN SPECIFIC POPULATIONS

8.1 Pregnancy

Pregnancy Category B

A reproductive and developmental toxicity study has been performed in female rats at doses approximately 80 times the human dose (on a mg/kg basis) and revealed no evidence of impaired female fertility or harm to the fetus due to FLUARIX QUADRIVALENT. There are, however, no adequate and well-controlled studies in pregnant women. Because animal reproduction studies are not always predictive of human response, FLUARIX QUADRIVALENT should be given to a pregnant woman only if clearly needed.

In a reproductive and developmental toxicity study, the effect of FLUARIX QUADRIVALENT on embryo-fetal and pre-weaning development was evaluated in rats. Animals were administered FLUARIX QUADRIVALENT by intramuscular injection twice prior to gestation, during the period of organogenesis (gestation days 3, 8, 11, and 15), and during lactation (day 7), 0.2 mL/rat/occasion (approximately 80-fold excess relative to the projected human dose on a body weight basis). No adverse effects on mating, female fertility, pregnancy, parturition, lactation parameters, and embryo-fetal or pre-weaning development were observed. There were no vaccine-related fetal malformations or other evidence of teratogenesis.

Pregnancy Registry: GlaxoSmithKline maintains a surveillance registry to collect data on pregnancy outcomes and newborn health status outcomes following vaccination with FLUARIX QUADRIVALENT during pregnancy. Women who receive FLUARIX QUADRIVALENT during pregnancy should be encouraged to contact GlaxoSmithKline directly or their healthcare provider should contact GlaxoSmithKline by calling 1-888-452-9622.

8.3 Nursing Mothers

It is not known whether FLUARIX QUADRIVALENT is excreted in human milk. Because many drugs are excreted in human milk, caution should be exercised when FLUARIX QUADRIVALENT is administered to a nursing woman.

8.4 Pediatric Use

Safety and effectiveness of FLUARIX QUADRIVALENT in children younger than 3 years of age have not been established.

Safety and immunogenicity of FLUARIX QUADRIVALENT in children 3 through 17 years of age have been evaluated *[see Adverse Reactions (6.1) and Clinical Studies (14.3)]*.

8.5 Geriatric Use

In a randomized, double-blind (2 arms) and open-label (one arm), active-controlled study, immunogenicity and safety were evaluated in a cohort of subjects 65 years of age and older who received FLUARIX QUADRIVALENT (N = 1,517); 469 of these subjects were 75 years of age and older. In subjects 65 years of age and older, the geometric mean antibody titers post-vaccination and seroconversion rates were lower than in younger subjects (18 through 64 years of age) and the frequencies of solicited and unsolicited adverse events were generally lower than in younger subjects.

11 DESCRIPTION

FLUARIX QUADRIVALENT, Influenza Virus Vaccine, for intramuscular injection, is a sterile colorless and slightly opalescent suspension. FLUARIX QUADRIVALENT is prepared from influenza viruses propagated in embryonated chicken eggs. Each of the influenza viruses is produced and purified separately. After harvesting the virus-containing fluids, each influenza virus is concentrated and purified by zonal centrifugation using a linear sucrose density gradient solution containing detergent to disrupt the viruses. Following dilution, the vaccine is further purified by diafiltration. Each influenza virus solution is inactivated by the consecutive effects of sodium deoxycholate and formaldehyde leading to the production of a "split virus." Each split inactivated virus is then suspended in sodium phosphate-buffered isotonic sodium chloride solution. Each vaccine is formulated from the split inactivated virus solutions.

FLUARIX QUADRIVALENT is standardized according to United States Public Health Service requirements for the 2013-2014 influenza season and is formulated to contain 60 micrograms (mcg) hemagglutinin (HA) per 0.5-mL dose, in the recommended ratio of 15 mcg HA of each of the following 4 influenza virus strains: A/Christchurch/16/2010 NIB-74XP (H1N1) (an A/California/7/2009-like virus), A/Texas/50/2012 NYMC X-223A (H3N2) (an A/Victoria/361/2011-like virus), B/Massachusetts/2/2012 NYMC BX-51B, and B/Brisbane/60/2008.

FLUARIX QUADRIVALENT is formulated without preservatives. FLUARIX QUADRIVALENT does not contain thimerosal. Each 0.5-mL dose also contains octoxynol-10 (TRITON® X-100) ≤0.115 mg, α-tocopheryl hydrogen succinate ≤0.135 mg, and polysorbate 80 (Tween 80) ≤0.550 mg. Each dose may also contain residual amounts of hydrocortisone ≤0.0016 mcg, gentamicin sulfate ≤0.15 mcg, ovalbumin ≤0.05 mcg, formaldehyde ≤5 mcg, and sodium deoxycholate ≤65 mcg from the manufacturing process.

The tip caps of the prefilled syringes of FLUARIX QUADRIVALENT may contain natural rubber latex; the plungers are not made with natural rubber latex.

12 CLINICAL PHARMACOLOGY

12.1 Mechanism of Action

Influenza illness and its complications follow infection with influenza viruses. Global surveillance of influenza identifies yearly antigenic variants. Since 1977, antigenic variants of influenza A (H1N1 and H3N2) viruses and influenza B viruses have been in global circulation.

Public health authorities give annual influenza vaccine composition recommendations. Inactivated influenza vaccines are standardized to contain the hemagglutinins of influenza viruses representing the virus types or subtypes likely to circulate in the United States during the influenza season. Two influenza type B virus lineages (Victoria and Yamagata) are of public health importance because they have co-circulated since 2001. FLUARIX (trivalent influenza vaccine) contains 2 influenza A subtype viruses and one influenza type B virus.

Specific levels of hemagglutination-inhibition (HI) antibody titer post-vaccination with inactivated influenza virus vaccines have not been correlated with protection from influenza illness but the HI antibody titers have been used as a measure of vaccine activity. In some human challenge studies, HI antibody titers of ≥1:40 have been associated with protection from influenza illness in up to 50% of subjects.[1,2] Antibody against one influenza virus type or subtype confers little or no protection against another virus. Furthermore, antibody to one antigenic variant of influenza virus might not protect against a new antigenic variant of the same type or subtype. Frequent development of antigenic variants through antigenic drift is the virological basis for seasonal epidemics and the reason for the usual replacement of one or more influenza viruses in each year's influenza vaccine.

Annual revaccination is recommended because immunity declines during the year after vaccination, and because circulating strains of influenza virus change from year to year.[3]

13 NONCLINICAL TOXICOLOGY

13.1 Carcinogenesis, Mutagenesis, Impairment of Fertility

FLUARIX QUADRIVALENT have not been evaluated for carcinogenic or mutagenic potential. Vaccination of female rats with FLUARIX QUADRIVALENT, at doses shown to be immunogenic in the rat, had no effect on fertility.

14 CLINICAL STUDIES

14.1 Efficacy Against Culture-Confirmed Influenza

The efficacy experience with FLUARIX is relevant to FLUARIX QUADRIVALENT because both vaccines are manufactured using the same process and have overlapping compositions *[see Description (11)]*.

The efficacy of FLUARIX was evaluated in a randomized, double-blind, placebo-controlled study conducted in 2 European countries during the 2006-2007 influenza season. Efficacy of FLUARIX, containing A/New Caledonia/20/1999 (H1N1), A/Wisconsin/67/2005 (H3N2), and B/Malaysia/2506/2004 influenza virus strains, was defined as the prevention of culture-confirmed influenza A and/or B cases, for vaccine antigenically matched strains, compared with placebo. Healthy subjects 18 through 64 years of age (mean age 40 years) were randomized (2:1) to receive FLUARIX (N = 5,103) or placebo (N = 2,549) and monitored for influenza-like illnesses (ILI) starting 2 weeks post-vaccination and lasting for approximately 7 months. In the overall population, 60% of subjects were female and 99.9% were White. Culture-confirmed influenza was assessed by active and passive surveillance of ILI. Influenza-like illness was defined as at least one general symptom (fever ≥100°F and/or myalgia) and at least one respiratory symptom (cough and/or sore throat). After an episode of ILI, nose and throat swab samples were collected for analysis; attack rates and vaccine efficacy were calculated (Table 6).

[See table 6 at top of next page]

In a post-hoc, exploratory analysis by age, vaccine efficacy (against culture-confirmed influenza A and/or B cases, for vaccine antigenically matched strains) in subjects 18 through 49 years of age was 73.4% (95% CI: 59.3, 82.8) [number of influenza cases: FLUARIX (n = 35/3,602) and placebo (n = 66/1,810)]. In subjects 50 through 64 years of age, vaccine efficacy was 13.8% (95% CI: –137.0, 66.3) [number of influenza cases: FLUARIX (n = 14/1,501) and placebo (n = 8/739)]. As the study lacked statistical power to evaluate efficacy within age subgroups, the clinical significance of these results is unknown.

14.2 Immunological Evaluation of FLUARIX QUADRIVALENT in Adults

Study 1 was a randomized, double-blind (2 arms) and open-label (one arm), active-controlled, safety, immunogenicity,

Table 4. FLUARIX (Trivalent Formulation): Incidence of Solicited Local Adverse Reactions and Systemic Adverse Events Within 4 Days[a] of Vaccination in Adults (Total Vaccinated Cohort)

	Study 3[b]		Study 4[c]	
	18 Through 64 Years of Age		65 Years of Age and Older	
	FLUARIX N = 760 %	Placebo N = 192 %	FLUARIX N = 601-602 %	Comparator N = 596 %
Local				
Pain	55	12	19	18
Redness	18	10	11	13
Swelling	9	6	6	9
Systemic				
Muscle aches	23	12	7	7
Fatigue	20	18	9	10
Headache	19	21	8	8
Arthralgia	6	6	6	5
Shivering	3	3	2	2
Fever ≥100.4°F (38.0°C)	2	2	–	–
Fever ≥99.5°F (37.5°C)	–	–	2	1

Total vaccinated cohort for safety included all vaccinated subjects for whom safety data were available.
[a] 4 days included day of vaccination and the subsequent 3 days.
[b] Study 3 was a randomized, double-blind, placebo-controlled, safety, and immunogenicity study (NCT00100399).
[c] Study 4 was a randomized, single-blind, active-controlled, safety, and immunogenicity study (NCT00197288). The active control was Fluzone, a US-licensed trivalent, inactivated influenza virus vaccine (Sanofi Pasteur SA).

Table 5. FLUARIX (Trivalent Formulation): Incidence of Solicited Local Adverse Reactions and Systemic Adverse Events Within 4 Days[a] of First Vaccination in Children 3 Through 17 Years of Age[b] (Total Vaccinated Cohort)

	3 Through 4 Years of Age		5 Through 17 Years of Age	
	FLUARIX N = 350 %	Comparator N = 341 %	FLUARIX N = 1,348 %	Comparator N = 451 %
Local				
Pain	35	38	56	56
Redness	23	20	18	16
Swelling	14	13	14	13
Systemic				
Irritability	21	22	–	–
Loss of appetite	13	15	–	–
Drowsiness	13	20	–	–
Fever ≥99.5°F (37.5°C)	7	8	4	3
Muscle aches	–	–	29	29
Fatigue	–	–	20	19
Headache	–	–	15	16
Arthralgia	–	–	6	6
Shivering	–	–	3	4

Total vaccinated cohort for safety included all vaccinated subjects for whom safety data were available.
[a] 4 days included day of vaccination and the subsequent 3 days.
[b] Study 6 was a single-blind, active-controlled, safety, and immunogenicity US study (NCT00383123). The active control was Fluzone, a US-licensed trivalent, inactivated influenza virus vaccine (Sanofi Pasteur SA).

Table 6. FLUARIX (Trivalent Formulation): Attack Rates and Vaccine Efficacy Against Culture-Confirmed Influenza A and/or B in Adults (Total Vaccinated Cohort)

		Attack Rates (n/N)		Vaccine Efficacy		
	N	N	%	%	LL	UL
Antigenically Matched Strains[a]						
FLUARIX	5,103	49	1.0	66.9[b]	51.9	77.4
Placebo	2,549	74	2.9	–	–	–
All Culture-Confirmed Influenza (Matched, Unmatched, and Untyped)[c]						
FLUARIX	5,103	63	1.2	61.6[b]	46.0	72.8
Placebo	2,549	82	3.2	–	–	–

[a] There were no vaccine matched culture-confirmed cases of A/New Caledonia/20/1999 (H1N1) or B/Malaysia/2506/2004 influenza virus strains with FLUARIX or placebo.
[b] Vaccine efficacy for FLUARIX exceeded a pre-defined threshold of 35% for the lower limit of the 2-sided 95% CI.
[c] Of the 22 additional cases, 18 were unmatched and 4 were untyped; 15 of the 22 cases were A (H3N2) (11 cases with FLUARIX and 4 cases with placebo).

Table 7. FLUARIX QUADRIVALENT: Immune Responses to Each Antigen 21 Days After Vaccination in Adults (ATP Cohort for Immunogenicity)

	FLUARIX QUADRIVALENT[a]	Trivalent Influenza Vaccine (TIV)	
		TIV-1 (B Victoria)[b]	TIV-2 (B Yamagata)[c]
GMTs	N = 1,809 (95% CI)	N = 608 (95% CI)	N = 534 (95% CI)
A/California/7/2009 (H1N1)	201.1 (188.1, 215.1)	218.4 (194.2, 245.6)	213.0 (187.6, 241.9)
A/Victoria/210/2009 (H3N2)	314.7 (296.8, 333.6)	298.2 (268.4, 331.3)	340.4 (304.3, 380.9)
B/Brisbane/60/2008 (Victoria lineage)	404.6 (386.6, 423.4)	393.8 (362.7, 427.6)	258.5 (234.6, 284.8)
B/Brisbane/3/2007 (Yamagata lineage)	601.8 (573.3, 631.6)	386.6 (351.5, 425.3)	582.5 (534.6, 634.7)
Seroconversion[d]	N = 1,801 % (95% CI)	N = 605 % (95% CI)	N = 530 % (95% CI)
A/California/7/2009 (H1N1)	77.5 (75.5, 79.4)	77.2 (73.6, 80.5)	80.2 (76.5, 83.5)
A/Victoria/210/2009 (H3N2)	71.5 (69.3, 73.5)	65.8 (61.9, 69.6)	70.0 (65.9, 73.9)
B/Brisbane/60/2008 (Victoria lineage)	58.1 (55.8, 60.4)	55.4 (51.3, 59.4)	47.5 (43.2, 51.9)
B/Brisbane/3/2007 (Yamagata lineage)	61.7 (59.5, 64.0)	45.6 (41.6, 49.7)	59.1 (54.7, 63.3)

ATP = according–to–protocol; GMT = geometric mean antibody titer; CI = Confidence Interval.
ATP cohort for immunogenicity included subjects for whom assay results were available after vaccination for at least one study vaccine antigen.
[a] Contained the same composition as FLUARIX (trivalent formulation) manufactured for the 2010-2011 season and an additional influenza type B virus of Yamagata lineage.
[b] Contained the same composition as FLUARIX manufactured for the 2010-2011 season (2 influenza A subtype viruses and an influenza type B virus of Victoria lineage).
[c] Contained the same 2 influenza A subtype viruses as FLUARIX manufactured for the 2010-2011 season and an influenza type B virus of Yamagata lineage.
[d] Seroconversion defined as a pre-vaccination HI titer of <1:10 with a post-vaccination titer ≥1:40 or at least a 4-fold increase in serum titers of HI antibodies to ≥1:40.

and non-inferiority study. In this study, subjects received FLUARIX QUADRIVALENT (N = 1,809) or one of two formulations of comparator trivalent influenza vaccine (FLUARIX, TIV-1, N = 608 or TIV-2, N = 534), each containing an influenza type B virus that corresponded to one of the two type B viruses in FLUARIX QUADRIVALENT (a type B virus of the Victoria lineage or a type B virus of the Yamagata lineage). Subjects 18 years of age and older (mean age 58 years) were evaluated for immune responses to each of the vaccine antigens 21 days following vaccination. In the overall population, 57% of subjects were female; 69% were White, 27% were Asian, and 4% were of other racial/ethnic groups.

The immunogenicity endpoints were geometric mean antibody titers (GMTs) of serum hemagglutination-inhibition (HI) antibodies adjusted for baseline, and the percentage of subjects who achieved seroconversion, defined as a pre-vaccination HI titer of <1:10 with a post-vaccination titer ≥1:40 or at least a 4–fold increase in serum HI antibody titer over baseline to ≥1:40 following vaccination, performed on the According-to-Protocol (ATP) cohort for whom immunogenicity assay results were available after vaccination. FLUARIX QUADRIVALENT was non–inferior to both TIVs based on adjusted GMTs (upper limit of the 2–sided 95% CI for the GMT ratio [TIV/FLUARIX QUADRIVALENT] ≤1.5) and seroconversion rates (upper limit of the 2–sided 95% CI on difference of the TIV minus FLUARIX QUADRIVALENT ≤10%). The antibody response to influenza B strains contained in FLUARIX QUADRIVALENT was higher than the antibody response after vaccination with a TIV containing an influenza B strain from a different lineage. There was no evidence that the addition of the second B strain resulted in immune interference to other strains included in the vaccine (Table 7).

[See table 7 above]

14.3 Immunological Evaluation of FLUARIX QUADRIVALENT in Children

Study 2 was a randomized, double-blind, active-controlled, safety, immunogenicity, and non-inferiority study. In this study, subjects received FLUARIX QUADRIVALENT (N = 791) or one of two formulations of comparator trivalent influenza vaccine (FLUARIX, TIV-1, N = 819 or TIV-2, N = 801), each containing an influenza type B virus that corresponded to one of the two type B viruses in FLUARIX QUADRIVALENT (a type B virus of the Victoria lineage or a type B virus of the Yamagata lineage). In children 3 through 17 years of age, immune responses to each of the vaccine antigens were evaluated in sera 28 days following 1 or 2 doses. In the overall population, 52% of subjects were male; 56% were White, 29% were Asian, 12% were Black, and 3% were of other racial/ethnic groups.

The immunogenicity endpoints were geometric mean antibody titers (GMTs) adjusted for baseline, and the percentage of subjects who achieved seroconversion, defined as a pre-vaccination HI titer of <1:10 with a post-vaccination titer ≥1:40 or at least a 4–fold increase in serum HI titer over baseline to ≥1:40, following vaccination, performed on the According-to-Protocol (ATP) cohort for whom immunogenicity assay results were available after vaccination. FLUARIX QUADRIVALENT was non-inferior to both TIVs based on adjusted GMTs (upper limit of the 2–sided 95% CI for the GMT ratio [TIV/FLUARIX QUADRIVALENT] ≤1.5) and seroconversion rates (upper limit of the 2–sided 95% CI on difference of the TIV minus FLUARIX QUADRIVALENT ≤10%). The antibody response to influenza B strains contained in FLUARIX QUADRIVALENT was higher than the antibody response after vaccination with a TIV containing an influenza B strain from a different lineage. There was no evidence that the addition of the second B strain resulted in immune interference to other strains included in the vaccine (Table 8).

[See table 8 at top of next page]

15 REFERENCES

1. Hannoun C, Megas F, Piercy J. Immunogenicity and protective efficacy of influenza vaccination. *Virus Res.* 2004;103:133-138.
2. Hobson D, Curry RL, Beare AS, et al. The role of serum haemagglutination-inhibiting antibody in protection against challenge infection with influenza A2 and B viruses. *J Hyg Camb.* 1972;70:767-777.
3. Centers for Disease Control and Prevention. Prevention and Control of Influenza with Vaccines: Recommendations of the Advisory Committee on Immunization Practices (ACIP). *MMWR* 2010;59(RR-8):1-62.

16 HOW SUPPLIED/STORAGE AND HANDLING

NDC 58160-900-41 Syringe in Package of 10: NDC 58160-900-52

Store refrigerated between 2° and 8°C (36° and 46°F). Do not freeze. Discard if the vaccine has been frozen. Store in the original package to protect from light.

17 PATIENT COUNSELING INFORMATION

Provide the following information to the vaccine recipient or guardian:

- Inform of the potential benefits and risks of immunization with FLUARIX QUADRIVALENT.
- Educate regarding potential side effects, emphasizing that: (1) FLUARIX QUADRIVALENT contain non–infectious killed viruses and cannot cause influenza and (2) FLUARIX QUADRIVALENT are intended to provide protection against illness due to influenza viruses only, and cannot provide protection against all respiratory illness.
- Instruct to report any adverse events to their healthcare provider.
- Inform that safety and efficacy have not been established in pregnant women. Register women who receive FLUARIX QUADRIVALENT while pregnant in the pregnancy registry by calling 1-888-452-9622.
- Give the Vaccine Information Statements, which are required by the National Childhood Vaccine Injury Act of 1986 prior to each immunization. These materials are available free of charge at the Centers for Disease Control and Prevention (CDC) website (www.cdc.gov/vaccines).
- Instruct that annual revaccination is recommended.

Table 8. FLUARIX QUADRIVALENT: Immune Responses to Each Antigen 28 Days After Last Vaccination in Children 3 Through 17 Years of Age (ATP Cohort for Immunogenicity)

	FLUARIX QUADRIVALENT[a]	Trivalent Influenza Vaccine (TIV)	
		TIV-1 (B Victoria)[b]	TIV-2 (B Yamagata)[c]
GMTs	N = 791 (95% CI)	N = 818 (95% CI)	N = 801 (95% CI)
A/California/7/2009 (H1N1)	386.2 (357.3, 417.4)	433.2 (401.0, 468.0)	422.3 (390.5, 456.5)
A/Victoria/210/2009 (H3N2)	228.8 (215.0, 243.4)	227.3 (213.3, 242.3)	234.0 (219.1, 249.9)
B/Brisbane/60/2008 (Victoria lineage)	244.2 (227.5, 262.1)	245.6 (229.2, 263.2)	88.4 (81.5, 95.8)
B/Brisbane/3/2007 (Yamagata lineage)	569.6 (533.6, 608.1)	224.7 (207.9, 242.9)	643.3 (603.2, 686.1)
Seroconversion[d]	N = 790 % (95% CI)	N = 818 % (95% CI)	N = 800 % (95% CI)
A/California/7/2009 (H1N1)	91.4 (89.2, 93.3)	89.9 (87.6, 91.8)	91.6 (89.5, 93.5)
A/Victoria/210/2009 (H3N2)	72.3 (69.0, 75.4)	70.7 (67.4, 73.8)	71.9 (68.6, 75.0)
B/Brisbane/60/2008 (Victoria lineage)	70.0 (66.7, 73.2)	68.5 (65.2, 71.6)	29.6 (26.5, 32.9)
B/Brisbane/3/2007 (Yamagata lineage)	72.5 (69.3, 75.6)	37.0 (33.7, 40.5)	70.8 (67.5, 73.9)

ATP = according–to–protocol; GMT = geometric mean antibody titer; CI = Confidence Interval.
ATP cohort for immunogenicity included subjects for whom assay results were available after vaccination for at least one study vaccine antigen.
[a] Contained the same composition as FLUARIX (trivalent formulation) manufactured for the 2010-2011 season and an additional influenza type B virus of Yamagata lineage.
[b] Contained the same composition as FLUARIX manufactured for the 2010-2011 season (2 influenza A subtype viruses and an influenza type B virus of Victoria lineage).
[c] Contained the same 2 influenza A subtype viruses as FLUARIX manufactured for the 2010-2011 season and an influenza B virus of Yamagata lineage.
[d] Seroconversion defined as a pre-vaccination HI titer of <1:10 with a post-vaccination titer ≥1:40 or at least a 4-fold increase in serum titers of HI antibodies to ≥1:40.

FLUARIX and TIP–LOK are registered trademarks of GlaxoSmithKline. FLUZONE is a registered trademark of Sanofi Pasteur Limited. TRITON is a registered trademark of Union Carbide Chemicals & Plastics Technology Corp.
Manufactured by **GlaxoSmithKline Biologicals**, Dresden, Germany,
a branch of **SmithKline Beecham Pharma GmbH & Co. KG**, Munich, Germany
Licensed by **GlaxoSmithKline Biologicals**, Rixensart, Belgium, US License 1617
Distributed by **GlaxoSmithKline**, Research Triangle Park, NC 27709

FLQ:2PI

FLULAVAL ℞

[flū' la-val]
(Influenza Virus Vaccine)
Suspension for Intramuscular Injection
2013-2014 Formula

HIGHLIGHTS OF PRESCRIBING INFORMATION
These highlights do not include all the information needed to use FLULAVAL safely and effectively. See full prescribing information for FLULAVAL.
FLULAVAL (Influenza Virus Vaccine)
Suspension for Intramuscular Injection
2013-2014 Formula
Initial U.S. Approval: 2006

RECENT MAJOR CHANGES

Indications and Usage (1)	08/2013
Dosage and Administration (2.1)	08/2013

INDICATIONS AND USAGE

- FLULAVAL is a vaccine indicated for active immunization for the prevention of disease caused by influenza A subtype viruses and type B virus contained in the vaccine. FLULAVAL is approved for use in persons 3 years of age and older. (1)

DOSAGE AND ADMINISTRATION

For intramuscular injection only. (2)

Age	Vaccination Status	Dose and Schedule
3 through 8 years of age	Not previously vaccinated with influenza vaccine	Two doses (0.5–mL each) at least 4 weeks apart (2.1)
	Vaccinated with influenza vaccine in a previous season	One or two doses[a] (0.5–mL each) (2.1)
9 years of age and older	Not applicable	One 0.5–mL dose (2.1)

[a] One dose or two doses (0.5-mL each) depending on vaccination history as per the annual Advisory Committee on Immunization Practices (ACIP) recommendation on prevention and control of influenza with vaccines. If two doses administer each 0.5 mL dose at least 4 weeks apart. (2.1)

DOSAGE FORMS AND STRENGTHS

Suspension for injection in 5-mL multi-dose vials containing ten 0.5 mL doses. (3)

CONTRAINDICATIONS

History of severe allergic reactions (e.g., anaphylaxis) to any component of the vaccine, including egg protein, or following a previous dose of any influenza vaccine. (4, 11)

WARNINGS AND PRECAUTIONS

- If Guillain-Barré syndrome has occurred within 6 weeks of receipt of a prior influenza vaccine, the decision to give FLULAVAL should be based on careful consideration of the potential benefits and risks. (5.1)
- Syncope (fainting) can occur in association with administration of injectable vaccines, including FLULAVAL. Procedures should be in place to avoid falling injury and to restore cerebral perfusion following syncope. (5.2)

ADVERSE REACTIONS

- In adults, the most common (≥10%) solicited local adverse reactions were pain (51%), redness (13%), and/or swelling (11%); the most common solicited systemic adverse events were fatigue (20%), headache (18%), and muscle aches/arthralgia (18%). (6.1)
- In children 3 through 17 years of age, the most common (≥10%) solicited local adverse reaction was pain (56%). (6.1)
- In children 3 through 4 years of age, the most common (≥10%) solicited systemic adverse events were irritability (25%), drowsiness (19%), and loss of appetite (16%). (6.1)
- In children 5 through 17 years of age, the most common (≥10%) solicited systemic adverse events were muscle aches (24%), headache (17%), and fatigue (17%). (6.1)

To report SUSPECTED ADVERSE REACTIONS, contact GlaxoSmithKline at 1-888-825-5249 or VAERS at 1-800-822-7967 or www.vaers.hhs.gov.

USE IN SPECIFIC POPULATIONS

- Safety and effectiveness of FLULAVAL have not been established in pregnant women or nursing mothers. (8.1, 8.3)
- Register women who receive FLULAVAL while pregnant in the pregnancy registry by calling 1-888-452-9622. (8.1)
- Geriatric Use: Antibody responses were lower in geriatric subjects who received FLULAVAL than in younger subjects. (8.5)

See 17 for PATIENT COUNSELING INFORMATION
Revised: 08/2013

FULL PRESCRIBING INFORMATION: CONTENTS*

*** Sections or subsections omitted from the full prescribing information are not listed**

FULL PRESCRIBING INFORMATION

1 INDICATIONS AND USAGE

FLULAVAL® is indicated for active immunization for the prevention of disease caused by influenza A subtype viruses and type B virus contained in the vaccine. FLULAVAL is approved for use in persons 3 years of age and older.

2 DOSAGE AND ADMINISTRATION

For intramuscular injection only.

2.1 Dosage and Schedule

The dose and schedule for FLULAVAL are presented in Table 1.

Table 2. FLULAVAL: Incidence of Solicited Local Adverse Reactions and Systemic Adverse Events Within 4 Days[a] of Vaccination in Adults (Total Vaccinated Cohort)

	Percentage of Subjects Reporting Event					
	Study 1[b] 18 Through 64 Years of Age		Study 2[b] 50 Years of Age and Older		Study 3[b] 18 Through 49 Years of Age	
	FLULAVAL N = 721	Comparator[c] N = 279	FLULAVAL N = 610	Comparator[c] N = 615	FLULAVAL N = 3,783	Placebo N = 3,828
Local Adverse Reactions						
Pain	24	31	25	32	51	14
Redness	11	10	10	11	13	6
Swelling	10	10	7	9	11	3
Systemic Adverse Events						
Headache	18	17	11	12	18	19
Fatigue	17	15	12	13	20	18
Muscle achesd[d]	13	16	11	10	18	10
Fever (≥99.5°F)	11	10	1	1	3	1
Malaise	10	10	6	7	9	6
Sore throat	9	9	5	6	9	9
Reddened eyes	6	5	4	7	7	6
Cough	6	7	5	6	8	7
Chills	5	2	3	6	4	4
Chest tightness	3	1	2	2	3	3
Facial swelling	1	1	1	2	1	1

Total vaccinated cohort for safety included all vaccinated subjects for whom safety data were available.
[a] 4 days included day of vaccination and the subsequent 3 days.
[b] Study 1: NCT01389479; Study 2: NCT00232947; Study 3: NCT00216242.
[c] US–licensed trivalent, inactivated influenza virus vaccine (manufactured by Sanofi Pasteur SA).
[d] For Study 2 and Study 3, includes muscle aches and arthralgia.

Age	Vaccination Status	Dose and Schedule
3 through 8 years of age	Not previously vaccinated with influenza vaccine	Two doses (0.5–mL each) at least 4 weeks apart
	Vaccinated with influenza vaccine in a previous season	One or two doses[a] (0.5–mL each)
9 years of age and older	Not applicable	One 0.5–mL dose

[a] One dose or two doses (0.5–mL each) depending on vaccination history as per the annual Advisory Committee on Immunization Practices (ACIP) recommendation on prevention and control of influenza with vaccines. If two doses administer each 0.5–mL dose at least 4 weeks apart.

2.2 Administration Instructions

Shake the multi-dose vial vigorously each time before withdrawing a dose of vaccine. Parenteral drug products should be inspected visually for particulate matter and discoloration prior to administration, whenever solution and container permit. If either of these conditions exists, the vaccine should not be administered.

Use a sterile needle and sterile syringe to withdraw the 0.5–mL dose from the multi-dose vial and administer intramuscularly. A sterile syringe with a needle bore no larger than 23 gauge is recommended for administration. It is recommended that small syringes (0.5-mL or 1-mL) be used to minimize any product loss. Use a separate sterile needle and syringe for each dose withdrawn from the multi-dose vial.

The preferred site for intramuscular injection is the deltoid muscle of the upper arm. Do not inject in the gluteal area or areas where there may be a major nerve trunk.

Between uses, return the multi-dose vial to the recommended storage conditions, between 2° and 8°C (36° and 46°F). Do not freeze. Discard if the vaccine has been frozen. Once entered, a multi-dose vial, and any residual contents, should be discarded after 28 days.

Do not administer this product intravenously, intradermally, or subcutaneously.

3 DOSAGE FORMS AND STRENGTHS

FLULAVAL is a suspension for injection available in 5-mL multi-dose vials containing ten 0.5 mL doses.

4 CONTRAINDICATIONS

Do not administer FLULAVAL to anyone with a history of severe allergic reactions (e.g., anaphylaxis) to any component of the vaccine, including egg protein, or following a previous dose of any influenza vaccine.

5 WARNINGS AND PRECAUTIONS

5.1 Guillain-Barré Syndrome

If Guillain-Barré syndrome (GBS) has occurred within 6 weeks of receipt of a prior influenza vaccine, the decision to give FLULAVAL should be based on careful consideration of the potential benefits and risks.

The 1976 swine influenza vaccine was associated with an elevated risk of GBS. Evidence for a causal relation of GBS with other influenza vaccines is inconclusive; if an excess risk exists, it is probably slightly more than one additional case/one million persons vaccinated.

5.2 Syncope

Syncope (fainting) can occur in association with administration of injectable vaccines, including FLULAVAL. Syncope can be accompanied by transient neurological signs such as visual disturbance, paresthesia, and tonic-clonic limb movements. Procedures should be in place to avoid falling injury and to restore cerebral perfusion following syncope.

5.3 Preventing and Managing Allergic Vaccine Reactions

Prior to administration, the healthcare provider should review the immunization history for possible vaccine sensitivity and previous vaccination-related adverse reactions. Appropriate medical treatment and supervision must be available to manage possible anaphylactic reactions following administration of FLULAVAL.

5.4 Altered Immunocompetence

If FLULAVAL is administered to immunosuppressed persons, including individuals receiving immunosuppressive therapy, the immune response may be lower than in immunocompetent persons.

5.5 Limitations of Vaccine Effectiveness

Vaccination with FLULAVAL may not protect all susceptible individuals.

5.6 Persons at Risk of Bleeding

As with other intramuscular injections, FLULAVAL should be given with caution in individuals with bleeding disorders such as hemophilia or on anticoagulant therapy to avoid the risk of hematoma following the injection.

6 ADVERSE REACTIONS

6.1 Clinical Trials Experience

In adults who received FLULAVAL, the most common (≥10%) solicited local adverse reactions were pain (51%), redness (13%), and swelling (11%); the most common (≥10%) solicited systemic adverse events were fatigue (20%), headache (18%), and muscle aches/arthralgia (18%).

In children 3 through 17 years of age who received FLULAVAL, the most common (≥10%) solicited local adverse reaction was pain (56%). In children 3 through 4 years of age, the most common (≥10%) solicited systemic adverse events were irritability (25%), drowsiness (19%), and loss of appetite (16%). In children 5 through 17 years of age, the most common (≥10%) systemic adverse events were muscle aches (24%), headache (17%), and fatigue (17%).

Because clinical trials are conducted under widely varying conditions, adverse reaction rates observed in the clinical trials of a vaccine cannot be directly compared to rates in the clinical trials of another vaccine, and may not reflect the rates observed in practice. There is the possibility that broad use of FLULAVAL could reveal adverse reactions not observed in clinical trials.

FLULAVAL in Adults: Safety data was obtained from 3 randomized, controlled trials, one of which was a placebo-controlled efficacy study. In these trials, 9,836 subjects were randomized to receive either FLULAVAL (5,114 subjects in the safety analysis), FLUZONE, a US–licensed trivalent, inactivated influenza virus vaccine, manufactured by Sanofi Pasteur SA (894 subjects in the safety analysis), or placebo (3,828 subjects in the safety analysis), intramuscularly. In these studies, solicited events were collected for 4 days (i.e., 30 minutes post-vaccination through the next 3 days). Unsolicited adverse events that occurred within 22 days of vaccination (day 0–21) were recorded based on spontaneous reports or in response to queries about changes in health status.

Study 1 (Immunogenicity): Safety information was collected in a randomized, controlled US study. This study included 1,000 adults 18 through 64 years of age who were randomized to receive FLULAVAL (N = 721) or a US–licensed trivalent, inactivated influenza virus vaccine (N = 279). Among recipients of FLULAVAL, 57% were female; 91% of subjects were white and 9% were of other racial/ethnic groups. The mean age of subjects was 38 years; 80% were 18 through 49 years of age and 20% were 50 through 64 years of age.

Study 2 (Immunogenicity Non-Inferiority): Safety information was collected in a randomized, double-blind, active-controlled US study. The study included 1,225 adults ≥50 years of age randomized to receive FLULAVAL (N = 610) or a US–licensed trivalent, inactivated influenza virus vaccine (N = 615). In the total population, 57% were female; 95% of subjects were white and 5% were of other racial/ethnic groups. The mean age of subjects was 66 years (46% were 50 through 64 years of age, 41% were 65 through 79 years of age, and 13% were ≥80 years of age).

Study 3 (Efficacy): Safety information was collected in a double-blind, placebo-controlled US study. The study included 7,658 adults 18 through 49 years of age randomized to receive FLULAVAL (N = 3,807) or placebo (N = 3,851). In the total population, 61% were female; 84% of subjects were white, 10% black, 2% Asian, and 4% were of other racial/ethnic groups. The mean age of subjects was 33 years.

Solicited Adverse Events: Solicited local adverse reactions and systemic adverse events collected for 4 days (day of vaccination and the next 3 days) are presented in Table 2.

[See table 2 above]

Unsolicited Adverse Events: The incidence of unsolicited adverse events in the 21 days post-vaccination was comparable for FLULAVAL and the active comparator in Study 1 (16% and 15%, respectively) and in Study 2 (18% and 21%, respectively). In Study 3, the incidence of unsolicited adverse events was comparable for the groups (21% for FLULAVAL and 19% for placebo).

Unsolicited adverse events defined as reported with FLULAVAL in >1.0% of subjects are described as follows: Study 1: Cough, headache, and pharyngolaryngeal pain; Study 2: Diarrhea, headache, and nasopharyngitis; and Study 3: Pharyngolaryngeal pain, headache, fatigue, cough, injection site pain, upper respiratory tract infection, musculoskeletal pain, nasopharyngitis, injection site erythema and discomfort.

Serious Adverse Events (SAEs): In Study 1, no SAEs were reported. In Study 2, 3% of subjects receiving FLULAVAL and 3% of subjects receiving the active comparator reported SAEs. In Study 3, 1% of subjects receiving FLULAVAL and 1% of subjects receiving placebo reported SAEs. In the 3 clinical trials, the rates of SAEs were comparable between groups and none of the SAEs were considered related to vaccination.

FLULAVAL in Children: *Study 4 (Immunogenicity Non-Inferiority):* An observer-blind, active-controlled US study evaluated subjects 3 through 17 years of age who received FLULAVAL (N = 1,055) or FLUZONE (N = 1,061), a US–licensed trivalent, inactivated influenza virus vaccine, manufactured by Sanofi Pasteur SA. In the overall population, 53% were male; 78% of subjects were White, 12% were Black, 2% were Asian, and 8% were of other racial/ethnic groups. The mean age of subjects was 8 years. Children 3 through 8 years of age with no history of influenza vaccination received 2 doses approximately 28 days apart. Children 3 through 8 years of age with a history of influenza vaccination and children 9 years of age and older received one dose. Solicited local adverse reactions and systemic adverse events were collected for 4 days (day of vaccination and the next 3 days) (Table 3).

Table 3. FLULAVAL: Incidence of Solicited Local Adverse Reactions and Systemic Adverse Events Within 4 Days[a] of First Vaccination in Children 3 Through 17 Years of Age[b] (Total Vaccinated Cohort)

	FLULAVAL %	Active Comparator[c] %
	3 Through 17 Years of Age	
Local Adverse Reactions	N = 1,042	N = 1,026
Pain	56	53
Redness	4	5
Swelling	4	5
	3 Through 4 Years of Age	
Systemic Adverse Events	N = 293	N = 279
Irritability	25	27
Drowsiness	19	19
Loss of appetite	16	13
Fever ≥100.4°F (38.0°C)	5	3
	5 Through 17 Years of Age	
Systemic Adverse Events	N = 750	N = 747
Muscle aches	24	23
Headache	17	15
Fatigue	17	17
Arthralgia	8	10
Shivering	6	5
Fever ≥100.4°F (38.0°C)	5	4

Total vaccinated cohort for safety included all vaccinated subjects for whom safety data were available.
[a] 4 days included day of vaccination and the subsequent 3 days.
[b] Study 4: NCT00980005.
[c] US–licensed trivalent, inactivated influenza virus vaccine (manufactured by Sanofi Pasteur SA).

In children who received a second dose of FLULAVAL or the comparator vaccine, the incidences of adverse events following the second dose were generally lower than those observed after the first dose.

The incidence of unsolicited adverse events that occurred within 28 days (day 0-27) of any vaccination reported in subjects who received FLULAVAL (N = 1,055) or FLUZONE (N = 1,061) was 40% and 37%, respectively. The unsolicited adverse events that occurred most frequently (≥0.1% of subjects for FLULAVAL) and considered possibly related to vaccination included diarrhea, influenza-like illness, injection site hematoma, injection site rash, injection site warmth, rash, upper abdominal pain, and vomiting. The rates of SAEs were comparable between groups (0.9% and 0.6% for FLULAVAL and the comparator, respectively); none of the SAEs were considered related to vaccination.

6.2 Postmarketing Experience

In addition to reports in clinical trials, the following adverse events have been identified during postapproval use of FLULAVAL. Because these events are reported voluntarily from a population of uncertain size, it is not always possible to reliably estimate their incidence rate or establish a causal relationship to the vaccine. Adverse events described here are included because: a) they represent reactions which are known to occur following immunizations generally or influenza immunizations specifically; b) they are potentially serious; or c) the frequency of reporting.

Blood and Lymphatic System Disorders: Lymphadenopathy.
Eye Disorders: Eye pain, photophobia.
Gastrointestinal Disorders: Dysphagia.
General Disorders and Administration Site Conditions: Chest pain, injection site inflammation, asthenia, injection site rash, abnormal gait, injection site bruising, injection site sterile abscess.
Immune System Disorders: Allergic including anaphylaxis, angioedema.
Infections and Infestations: Rhinitis, laryngitis, cellulitis.
Musculoskeletal and Connective Tissue Disorders: Muscle weakness, arthritis.

Table 4. FLULAVAL QUADRIVALENT: Influenza Attack Rates and Vaccine Efficacy Against Influenza A and/or B in Children 3 Through 8 Years of Age[a] (According to Protocol Cohort for Efficacy)

	N[b]	n[c]	Influenza Attack Rate % (n/N)	Vaccine Efficacy % (CI)
All RT-PCR-Positive Influenza				
FLULAVAL QUADRIVALENT	2,379	58	2.4	55.4[d] (95% CI: 39.1, 67.3)
HAVRIX[e]	2,398	128	5.3	–
All Culture-Confirmed Influenza[f]				
FLULAVAL QUADRIVALENT	2,379	50	2.1	55.9 (97.5% CI: 35.4, 69.9)
HAVRIX[e]	2,398	112	4.7	–
Antigenically Matched Culture-Confirmed Influenza				
FLULAVAL QUADRIVALENT	2,379	31	1.3	45.1[g] (97.5% CI: 9.3, 66.8)
HAVRIX[e]	2,398	56	2.3	–

CI = Confidence Interval; RT-PCR = reverse transcriptase polymerase chain reaction.
[a] Study 5: NCT01218308.
[b] According to protocol cohort for efficacy included subjects who met all eligibility criteria, were successfully contacted at least once post-vaccination, and complied with the protocol-specified efficacy criteria.
[c] Number of influenza cases.
[d] Vaccine efficacy for FLULAVAL QUADRIVALENT met the pre-defined criterion of >30% for the lower limit of the 2-sided 95% CI.
[e] Hepatitis A Vaccine used as a control vaccine.
[f] Of 162 culture-confirmed influenza cases, 108 (67%) were antigenically typed (87 matched; 21 unmatched); 54 (33%) could not be antigenically typed [but were typed by RT-PCR and nucleic acid sequence analysis: 5 cases A (H1N1) (5 with HAVRIX), 47 cases A (H3N2) (10 with FLULAVAL QUADRIVALENT, 37 with HAVRIX), and 2 cases B Victoria (2 with HAVRIX)].
[g] Since only 67% of cases could be typed, the clinical significance of this result is unknown.

Nervous System Disorders: Dizziness, paresthesia, hypoesthesia, hypokinesia, tremor, somnolence, syncope, Guillain Barré syndrome, convulsions/seizures, facial or cranial nerve paralysis, encephalopathy, limb paralysis.
Psychiatric Disorders: Insomnia.
Respiratory, Thoracic, and Mediastinal Disorders: Dyspnea, dysphonia, bronchospasm, throat tightness.
Skin and Subcutaneous Tissue Disorders: Urticaria, pruritus, sweating.
Vascular Disorders: Flushing, pallor.

7 DRUG INTERACTIONS

7.1 Concomitant Administration With Other Vaccines

FLULAVAL should not be mixed with any other vaccine in the same syringe or vial.

There are insufficient data to assess the concomitant administration of FLULAVAL with other vaccines. When concomitant administration of other vaccines is required, the vaccines should be administered at different injection sites.

7.2 Immunosuppressive Therapies

Immunosuppressive therapies, including irradiation, antimetabolites, alkylating agents, cytotoxic drugs, and corticosteroids (used in greater than physiologic doses), may reduce the immune response to FLULAVAL.

8 USE IN SPECIFIC POPULATIONS

8.1 Pregnancy

Pregnancy Category B

A reproductive and developmental toxicity study has been performed in female rats at a dose 40-fold the human dose (on a mg/kg basis) and showed no evidence of impaired female fertility or harm to the fetus due to FLULAVAL. There are, however, no adequate and well-controlled studies in pregnant women. Because animal reproduction studies are not always predictive of human response, FLULAVAL should be given to a pregnant woman only if clearly needed.

In a reproductive and developmental toxicity study, the effect of FLULAVAL on embryo-fetal and pre-weaning development was evaluated in pregnant rats. Animals were administered FLULAVAL by intramuscular injection once prior to gestation, and during the period of organogenesis (gestation days 6, 8, 11, and 15), 0.1 mL/dose/rat (approximately 40-fold higher than the projected human dose on a body weight basis). No adverse effects on mating, female fertility, pregnancy, parturition, lactation parameters, and embryo-fetal or pre-weaning development were observed. There were no vaccine-related fetal malformations or other evidence of teratogenesis.

Pregnancy Registry: GlaxoSmithKline maintains a surveillance registry to collect data on pregnancy outcomes and newborn health status outcomes following vaccination with FLULAVAL during pregnancy. Women who receive FLULAVAL during pregnancy should be encouraged to contact GlaxoSmithKline directly or their healthcare provider should contact GlaxoSmithKline by calling 1-888-452-9622.

8.3 Nursing Mothers

It is not known whether FLULAVAL is excreted in human milk. Because many drugs are excreted in human milk, caution should be exercised when FLULAVAL is administered to a nursing woman.

8.4 Pediatric Use

Safety and effectiveness of FLULAVAL in children younger than 3 years of age have not been established.

Safety and immunogenicity of FLULAVAL in children 3 through 17 years of age have been evaluated *[see Adverse Reactions (6.1) and Clinical Studies (14)]*.

8.5 Geriatric Use

In clinical trials, there were 330 subjects 65 years of age and older who received FLULAVAL; 142 of these subjects were 75 years of age and older. Hemagglutination inhibition antibody responses were lower in geriatric subjects than younger subjects after administration of FLULAVAL. *[See Clinical Studies (14.2).]* Solicited adverse events were similar in frequency to those reported in younger subjects *[see Adverse Reactions (6.1)]*.

11 DESCRIPTION

FLULAVAL, Influenza Virus Vaccine, for intramuscular injection, is a trivalent, split-virion, inactivated influenza virus vaccine prepared from virus propagated in the allantoic cavity of embryonated hens' eggs. Each of the influenza viruses is produced and purified separately. The virus is inactivated with ultraviolet light treatment followed by formaldehyde treatment, purified by centrifugation, and disrupted with sodium deoxycholate.

FLULAVAL is a sterile, translucent to whitish opalescent suspension in a phosphate-buffered saline solution that may sediment slightly. The sediment resuspends upon shaking to form a homogeneous suspension.

FLULAVAL has been standardized according to USPHS requirements for the 2013–2014 influenza season and is formulated to contain 45 micrograms (mcg) hemagglutinin (HA) per 0.5-mL dose in the recommended ratio of 15 mcg HA of each of the following 3 strains: A/California/7/2009 NYMC X–179A (H1N1), A/Texas/50/2012 NYMC X-223A (H3N2) (an A/Victoria/361/2011-like virus), and B/Massachusetts/2/2012 NYMC BX-51B.

Thimerosal, a mercury derivative, is added as a preservative. Each 0.5-mL dose contains 50 mcg thimerosal (<25 mcg mercury). Each 0.5-mL dose may also contain residual amounts of ovalbumin (≤0.3 mcg), formaldehyde (≤25 mcg), and sodium deoxycholate (≤50 mcg) from the manufacturing process. Antibiotics are not used in the manufacture of this vaccine.

The vial stoppers are not made with natural rubber latex.

Table 5. FLULAVAL QUADRIVALENT: Incidence of Adverse Outcomes Associated With RT-PCR-Positive Influenza in Children 3 Through 8 Years of Age[a] (Total Vaccinated Cohort)[b]

	FLULAVAL QUADRIVALENT N = 2,584			HAVRIX[c] N = 2,584		
Adverse Outcome[d]	**Number of Events**	**Number of Subjects[e]**	**%**	**Number of Events**	**Number of Subjects[e]**	**%**
Fever >102.2°F/39.0°C	16[f]	15	0.6	51[f]	50	1.9
Shortness of breath	0	0	0	5	5	0.2
Pneumonia	0	0	0	3	3	0.1
Wheezing	1	1	0	1	1	0
Bronchitis	1	1	0	1	1	0
Pulmonary congestion	0	0	0	1	1	0
Acute otitis media	0	0	0	1	1	0
Bronchiolitis	0	0	0	0	0	0
Croup	0	0	0	0	0	0
Encephalitis	0	0	0	0	0	0
Myocarditis	0	0	0	0	0	0
Myositis	0	0	0	0	0	0
Seizure	0	0	0	0	0	0

[a] Study 5: NCT01218308.
[b] Total vaccinated cohort included all vaccinated subjects for whom data were available.
[c] Hepatitis A Vaccine used as a control vaccine.
[d] In subjects who presented with more than one adverse outcome, each outcome was counted in the respective category.
[e] Number of subjects presenting with at least one event in each group.
[f] One subject in each group had sequential influenza due to influenza type A and type B viruses.

12 CLINICAL PHARMACOLOGY

12.1 Mechanism of Action

Influenza illness and its complications follow infection with influenza viruses. Global surveillance of influenza identifies yearly antigenic variants. Since 1977, antigenic variants of influenza A (H1N1 and H3N2) viruses and influenza B viruses have been in global circulation.

Specific levels of hemagglutination inhibition (HI) antibody titer post-vaccination with inactivated influenza virus vaccines have not been correlated with protection from influenza illness but the antibody titers have been used as a measure of vaccine activity. In some human challenge studies, antibody titers of ≥1:40 have been associated with protection from influenza illness in up to 50% of subjects.[1,2] Antibody against one influenza virus type or subtype confers little or no protection against another virus. Furthermore, antibody to one antigenic variant of influenza virus might not protect against a new antigenic variant of the same type or subtype. Frequent development of antigenic variants through antigenic drift is the virological basis for seasonal epidemics and the reason for the usual change of one or more new strains in each year's influenza vaccine. Therefore, inactivated influenza vaccines are standardized to contain the hemagglutinins of strains (i.e., typically 2 type A and 1 type B), representing the influenza viruses likely to circulate in the United States in the upcoming winter.

Annual revaccination is recommended because immunity declines during the year after vaccination, and because circulating strains of influenza virus change from year to year.[3]

13 NONCLINICAL TOXICOLOGY

13.1 Carcinogenesis, Mutagenesis, Impairment of Fertility

FLULAVAL has not been evaluated for carcinogenic or mutagenic potential. Vaccination of female rats with FLULAVAL, at doses shown to be immunogenic in the rat, had no effect on fertility.

14 CLINICAL STUDIES

The effectiveness of FLULAVAL was demonstrated based on clinical endpoint efficacy data for FLULAVAL QUADRIVALENT (Influenza Virus Vaccine), clinical endpoint efficacy data for FLULAVAL, and on an evaluation of serum HI antibody responses to FLULAVAL. FLULAVAL QUADRIVALENT, an inactivated influenza virus vaccine that contains the hemagglutinins of two influenza A subtype viruses and two influenza type B viruses, is manufactured according to the same process as FLULAVAL.

14.1 Efficacy Against Influenza

Efficacy Trial in Children: The efficacy of FLULAVAL QUADRIVALENT was evaluated in Study 5, a randomized, observer-blind, non-influenza vaccine-controlled study conducted in 3 countries in Asia, 3 in Latin America, and 2 in the Middle East/Europe during the 2010-2011 influenza season. Healthy subjects 3 through 8 years of age were randomized (1:1) to receive FLULAVAL QUADRIVALENT (N = 2,584), containing A/California/7/2009 (H1N1), A/Victoria/210/2009 (H3N2), B/Brisbane/60/2008 (Victoria lineage), and B/Florida/4/2006 (Yamagata lineage) influenza strains, or HAVRIX® (Hepatitis A Vaccine) (N = 2,584), as a control vaccine. Children with no history of influenza vaccination received 2 doses of FLULAVAL QUADRIVALENT or HAVRIX approximately 28 days apart. Children with a history of influenza vaccination received one dose of FLULAVAL QUADRIVALENT or HAVRIX. In the overall population, 52% were male; 60% were Asian, 5% were White, and 35% were of other racial/ethnic groups. The mean age of subjects was 5 years.

Efficacy of FLULAVAL QUADRIVALENT was assessed for the prevention of reverse transcriptase polymerase chain reaction (RT-PCR)-positive influenza A and/or B disease presenting as influenza-like illness (ILI). ILI was defined as a temperature ≥100°F in the presence of at least one of the following symptoms on the same day: cough, sore throat, runny nose, or nasal congestion. Subjects with ILI (monitored by passive and active surveillance for approximately 6 months) had nasal and throat swabs collected and tested for influenza A and/or B by RT-PCR. All RT-PCR-positive specimens were further tested in cell culture. Vaccine efficacy was calculated based on the ATP cohort for efficacy (Table 4).

[See table 4 at top of previous page]

In an exploratory analysis by age, vaccine efficacy against RT-PCR-positive influenza A and/or B disease presenting as ILI was evaluated in subjects 3 through 4 years of age and 5 through 8 years of age; vaccine efficacy was 35.3% (95% CI: –1.3, 58.6) and 67.7% (95% CI: 49.7, 79.2), respectively. As the study lacked statistical power to evaluate efficacy within age subgroups, the clinical significance of these results is unknown.

As a secondary objective in the study, subjects with RT-PCR-positive influenza A and/or B were prospectively classified based on the presence of adverse outcomes that have been associated with influenza infection (defined as fever >102.2°F/39.0°C, physician-verified shortness of breath, pneumonia, wheezing, bronchitis, bronchiolitis, pulmonary congestion, croup and/or acute otitis media, and/or physician-diagnosed serious extra-pulmonary complications, including myositis, encephalitis, seizure and/or myocarditis).

The risk reduction of fever >102.2°F/39.0°C associated with RT-PCR-positive influenza was 71.0% (95% CI: 44.8, 84.8) based on the ATP cohort for efficacy [FLULAVAL QUADRIVALENT (n = 12/2,379); HAVRIX (n = 41/2,398)]. The other pre-specified adverse outcomes had too few cases to calculate a risk reduction. The incidence of these adverse outcomes is presented in Table 5.

[See table 5 above]

Efficacy Trial in Adults: The efficacy of FLULAVAL was evaluated in a randomized, double-blind, placebo-controlled study conducted in the United States during the 2005-2006 and 2006-2007 influenza seasons (Study 3). Efficacy of FLULAVAL was defined as the prevention of culture-confirmed influenza A and/or B cases, for vaccine antigenically matched strains, compared with placebo. Healthy subjects 18 through 49 years of age were randomized (1:1); a total of 3,783 subjects received FLULAVAL and 3,828 subjects received placebo *[see Adverse Reactions (6.1)]*. Subjects were monitored for influenza-like illnesses (ILI) starting 2 weeks post-vaccination and for duration of approximately 7 months thereafter. Culture-confirmed influenza was assessed by active and passive surveillance of ILI. Influenza-like illness was defined as illness sufficiently severe to limit daily activity and including cough, and at least one of the following: Fever >99.9°F, nasal congestion or runny nose, sore throat, muscle aches or arthralgia, headache, feverishness or chills. After an episode of ILI, nose and throat swab samples were collected for analysis; attack rates and vaccine efficacy were calculated using the per protocol cohort (Table 6). Of note, the 1.2% attack rate in the placebo group for culture-confirmed, antigenically matched strains was lower than expected, contributing to a wide confidence interval for the estimate of vaccine efficacy.

Table 6. FLULAVAL: Influenza Attack Rates and Vaccine Efficacy Against Culture-Confirmed Influenza in Adults 18 Through 49 Years of Age[a] (Per Protocol Cohort)

			Influenza Attack Rates	Vaccine Efficacy	
	N[b]	**n[c]**	**% (n/N)**	**%**	**97.5% CI Lower Limit**
Antigenically Matched Strains					
FLULAVAL	3,714	23	0.6	46.3	9.8[d]
Placebo	3,768	45	1.2	–	–
All Culture-Confirmed Influenza (Matched, Unmatched, and Untyped)					
FLULAVAL	3,714	30	0.8	49.3	20.3
Placebo	3,768	60	1.6	–	–

CI = Confidence Interval.
[a] Study 3: NCT00216242.
[b] Per Protocol Cohort for efficacy included subjects with no protocol deviations considered to compromise efficacy data.
[c] Number of influenza cases.
[d] Lower limit of the one-sided 97.5% CI for vaccine efficacy against influenza due to antigenically matched strains was less than the pre-defined success criterion of ≥35%.

14.2 Immunological Evaluation

Adults: Study 1 was a randomized, blinded, active-controlled US study performed in healthy adults 18 through 64 years of age (N = 1,000). A total of 721 subjects received FLULAVAL, and 279 received a US–licensed trivalent, inactivated influenza virus vaccine, FLUZONE (manufactured by Sanofi Pasteur SA), intramuscularly; 959 subjects had complete serological data and no major protocol deviations *[see Adverse Reactions (6.1)]*.

Analyses of immunogenicity (Table 7) were performed for each hemagglutinin (HA) antigen contained in the vaccine: 1) assessment of the lower bounds of 2–sided 95% confidence intervals for the proportion of subjects with HI antibody titers of ≥1:40 after vaccination, and 2) assessment of the lower bounds of 2-sided 95% confidence intervals for rates of seroconversion (defined as a 4–fold increase in post-vaccination HI antibody titer from pre-vaccination titer ≥1:10, or an increase in titer from <1:10 to ≥1:40). The pre-specified success criteria for HI titer ≥1:40 was 70% and for seroconversion rate was 40%. The lower limit of the 2-sided 95% CI for the percentage of subjects who achieved an HI titer of ≥1:40 exceeded the pre-defined criteria for the A strains. The lower limit of the 2-sided 95% CI for the percentage of subjects who achieved seroconversion exceeded the pre-defined criteria for all 3 strains.

Table 7. Immune Responses to Each Antigen 21 Days After Vaccination With FLULAVAL[a] in Adults 18 Through 64 Years of Age (Per Protocol Cohort)[b]

	FLULAVAL N = 692 % of Subjects (95% CI)	
HI titers ≥1:40	**Pre-vaccination**	**Post-vaccination**
A/New Caledonia/20/99 (H1N1)	24.6	96.5 (94.9, 97.8)
A/Wyoming/03/03 (H3N2)	58.7	98.7 (97.6, 99.4)
B/Jiangsu/10/03	5.4	62.9 (59.1, 66.5)
Seroconversion[c] to:		
A/New Caledonia/20/99 (H1N1)	85.6 (82.7, 88.1)	
A/Wyoming/03/03 (H3N2)	79.3 (76.1, 82.3)	
B/Jiangsu/10/03	58.4 (54.6, 62.1)	

HI – hemagglutination inhibition; CI = Confidence Interval.
[a] Results obtained following vaccination with FLULAVAL manufactured for the 2004–2005 season.
[b] Per Protocol Cohort for immunogenicity included subjects with complete pre- and post-dose HI titer data and no major protocol deviations.
[c] Seroconversion defined as a 4–fold increase in post-vaccination HI antibody titer from pre-vaccination titer ≥1:10, or an increase in titer from <1:10 to ≥1:40.

Study 2 (Immunogenicity Non-Inferiority): In a randomized, double-blind, active-controlled US study, immunological non-inferiority of FLULAVAL was compared with a US–licensed trivalent, inactivated influenza virus vaccine, FLUZONE, manufactured by Sanofi Pasteur SA. A total of 1,225 adults ≥50 years of age and older in stable health were randomized to receive FLULAVAL or the comparator vaccine intramuscularly *[see Adverse Reactions (6.1)]*.

Analyses of immunogenicity were performed for each HA antigen contained in the vaccines: 1) assessment of the lower bounds of 2–sided 95% confidence intervals for the geometric mean antibody titer (GMT) ratio (FLULAVAL/comparator), and 2) assessment of the lower bounds of 2–sided 95% confidence intervals for seroconversion rates (defined as a 4–fold increase in post-vaccination HI antibody titer from pre-vaccination titer ≥1:10, or an increase in titer from <1:10 to ≥1:40). Non-inferiority of FLULAVAL to the comparator vaccine was established for all 6 co-primary endpoints (Table 8). Within each age stratum, immunogenicity results were similar between the groups.

[See table 8 above]

Children: In Stud 4, the immune response of FLULAVAL (N = 987) was compared to FLUZONE, a US–licensed trivalent, inactivated influenza virus vaccine (N = 979), manufactured by Sanofi Pasteur SA, in an observer-blind, randomized study in children 3 through 17 years of age. The immune responses to each of the antigens contained in FLULAVAL formulated for the 2009-2010 season were evaluated in sera obtained after one or 2 doses of FLULAVAL and were compared to those following the comparator influenza vaccine *[see Adverse Reactions (6.1)]*.

The non-inferiority endpoints were geometric mean antibody titers (GMTs) adjusted for baseline, and the percentage of subjects who achieved seroconversion, defined as at least a 4–fold increase in serum HI titer over baseline to ≥1:40, following vaccination, performed on the According–to–Protocol (ATP) cohort. FLULAVAL was non-inferior to the comparator influenza for all strains based on adjusted GMTs and seroconversion rates (Table 9).

[See table 9 above]

Table 8. Immune Responses to Each Antigen 21 Days After Vaccination With FLULAVAL Versus Comparator Influenza Vaccine in Adults 50 Years of Age and Older[a] (Per Protocol Cohort)[b]

	FLULAVAL N = 592	Active Comparator[c] N = 595	
GMTs Against	**GMT (95% CI)**	**GMT (95% CI)**	**GMT Ratio[d] (95% CI)**
A/New Caledonia/20/99 (H1N1)	113.4 (104.7, 122.8)	110.2 (101.8, 119.3)	1.03 (0.92, 1.15)
A/New York/55/04 (H3N2)	223.9 (199.5, 251.3)	214.6 (191.3, 240.7)	1.04 (0.89, 1.23)
B/Jiangsu/10/03	82.3 (74.7, 90.6)	97.1 (88.2, 106.8)	0.85 (0.74, 0.97)
Seroconversion[e] to:	**% of Subjects (95% CI)**	**% of Subjects (95% CI)**	**Difference in Seroconversion Rates[f] (95% CI)**
A/New Caledonia/20/99 (H1N1)	34 (30.0, 37.6)	32 (28.3, 35.9)	2 (-3.7, 7.0)
A/New York/55/04 (H3N2)	83 (80.3, 86.3)	82 (78.4, 84.6)	1 (-2.6, 6.1)
B/Jiangsu/10/03	53 (49.0, 57.1)	56 (51.6, 59.6)	-3 (-8.3, 3.1)

GMT = geometric mean antibody titer; CI = Confidence Interval.
[a] Results obtained following vaccination with influenza vaccines manufactured for the 2005–2006 season.
[b] Per Protocol Cohort for immunogenicity included subjects with complete pre- and post-dose HI titer data and no major protocol deviations.
[c] US–licensed trivalent, inactivated influenza virus vaccine (manufactured by Sanofi Pasteur SA).
[d] FLULAVAL met non–inferiority criteria based on GMTs (lower limit of 2–sided 95% CI for GMT ratio [FLULAVAL/comparator vaccine] ≥0.67).
[e] Seroconversion defined as a 4–fold increase in post-vaccination HI antibody titer from pre-vaccination titer ≥1:10, or an increase in titer from <1:10 to ≥1:40.
[f] FLULAVAL met non–inferiority criteria based on seroconversion rates (lower limit of 2–sided 95% CI for difference of FLULAVAL minus the comparator vaccine ≥–10%).

Table 9. Immune Responses to Each Antigen 28 Days After Last Vaccination With FLULAVAL Versus Comparator Influenza Vaccine in Children 3 Through 17 Years of Age[a] (According to Protocol Cohort for Immunogenicity)[b]

	FLULAVAL	Active Comparator[c]	
GMTs Against	**N = 987 (95% CI)**	**N = 979 (95% CI)**	**GMT Ratio[d] (95% CI)**
A/Brisbane (H1N1)	320.9 (298.3, 345.2)	329.4 (306.8, 353.7)	1.03 (0.94, 1.13)
A/Uruguay (H3N2)	414.7 (386.5, 444.9)	451.9 (423.8, 481.8)	1.05 (0.96, 1.13)
B/Brisbane	213.7 (198.5, 230.1)	200.2 (186.1, 215.3)	0.93 (0.85, 1.02)
Seroconversion[e] to:	**N = 987 % (95% CI)**	**N = 978 % (95% CI)**	**Difference in Seroconversion Rate[f] (95% CI)**
A/Brisbane (H1N1)	59.8 (56.6, 62.9)	58.2 (55.0, 61.3)	-1.6 (-5.9, 2.8)
A/Uruguay (H3N2)	68.2 (65.2, 71.1)	66.2 (63.1, 69.1)	-2.0 (-6.1, 2.1)
B/Brisbane	81.1 (78.5, 83.5)	78.6 (75.9, 81.2)	-2.4 (-6.0, 1.1)

GMT = geometric mean antibody titer; CI = Confidence Interval.
[a] Results obtained following vaccination with influenza vaccines formulated for the 2009-2010 season.
[b] According to protocol cohort for immunogenicity included all evaluable subjects for whom assay results were available after vaccination for at least one study vaccine antigen.
[c] US–licensed trivalent, inactivated influenza virus vaccine (Sanofi Pasteur SA).
[d] FLULAVAL met non–inferiority criteria based on GMTs (upper limit of 2–sided 95% CI for GMT ratio [comparator vaccine/FLULAVAL] ≤1.5).
[e] Seroconversion defined as a 4–fold increase in post-vaccination HI antibody titer from pre-vaccination titer ≥1:10, or an increase in titer from <1:10 to ≥1:40.
[f] FLULAVAL met non–inferiority criteria based on seroconversion rates (upper limit of 2–sided 95% CI for difference of the comparator vaccine minus FLULAVAL ≤10%).

15 REFERENCES

1. Hannoun C, Megas F, Piercy J. Immunogenicity and protective efficacy of influenza vaccination. *Virus Res* 2004;103:133-138.
2. Hobson D, Curry RL, Beare AS, et al. The role of serum haemagglutination-inhibiting antibody in protection against challenge infection with influenza A2 and B viruses. *J Hyg Camb* 1972;70:767-777.
3. Centers for Disease Control and Prevention. Prevention and control of influenza with vaccines: Recommendations of the Advisory Committee on Immunization Practices (ACIP). *MMWR* 2010;59(RR-8):1-62.

16 HOW SUPPLIED/STORAGE AND HANDLING

FLULAVAL is supplied in a 5-mL multi-dose vial containing 10 doses (0.5-mL each).

NDC 19515-890-02 Vial (containing 10 doses) in Package of 1: NDC 19515-890-07

Once entered, a multi-dose vial should be discarded after 28 days. Store refrigerated between 2° and 8°C (36° and 46°F). Do not freeze. Discard if the vaccine has been frozen. Store in the original package to protect from light.

17 PATIENT COUNSELING INFORMATION

Provide the following information to the vaccine recipient or guardian:

- Inform of the potential benefits and risks of immunization with FLULAVAL.
- Educate regarding potential side effects, emphasizing that: (1) FLULAVAL contains non-infectious killed viruses and cannot cause influenza, and (2) FLULAVAL is intended to provide protection against illness due to influenza viruses only, and cannot provide protection against all respiratory illness.
- Instruct to report any adverse events to their healthcare provider.
- Inform that safety and efficacy have not been established in pregnant women. Register women who receive FLULAVAL while pregnant in the pregnancy registry by calling 1-888-452-9622.
- Give the Vaccine Information Statements, which are required by the National Childhood Vaccine Injury Act of 1986 prior to immunization. These materials are available free of charge at the Centers for Disease Control and Prevention (CDC) website (www.cdc.gov/vaccines).
- Instruct that annual revaccination is recommended.

FLULAVAL and HAVRIX are registered trademarks of GlaxoSmithKline. FLUZONE is a registered trademark of Sanofi Pasteur Limited.

Manufactured by **ID Biomedical Corporation of Quebec**
Quebec City, QC, Canada, US License 1739
Distributed by **GlaxoSmithKline**
Research Triangle Park, NC 27709

FLV:12PI

FLULAVAL QUADRIVALENT ℞

(Influenza Virus Vaccine)
Suspension for Intramuscular Injection
2013-2014 Formula

HIGHLIGHTS OF PRESCRIBING INFORMATION

These highlights do not include all the information needed to use FLULAVAL QUADRIVALENT safely and effectively. See full prescribing information for FLULAVAL QUADRIVALENT.

FLULAVAL QUADRIVALENT (Influenza Virus Vaccine)
Suspension for Intramuscular Injection
2013-2014 Formula
Initial U.S. Approval: 2013

INDICATIONS AND USAGE

FLULAVAL QUADRIVALENT is a vaccine indicated for active immunization for the prevention of disease caused by influenza A subtype viruses and type B viruses contained in the vaccine. FLULAVAL QUADRIVALENT is approved for use in persons 3 years of age and older. (1)

DOSAGE AND ADMINISTRATION

For intramuscular injection only. (2)

Age	Vaccination Status	Dose and Schedule
3 through 8 years of age	Not previously vaccinated with influenza vaccine	Two doses (0.5–mL each) at least 4 weeks apart (2.1)
	Vaccinated with influenza vaccine in a previous season	One or two doses[a] (0.5–mL each) (2.1)
9 years of age and older	Not applicable	One 0.5–mL dose (2.1)

[a] One dose or two doses (0.5–mL each) depending on vaccination history as per the annual Advisory Committee on Immunization Practices (ACIP) recommendation on prevention and control of influenza with vaccines. If two doses, administer each 0.5–mL dose at least 4 weeks apart. (2.1)

DOSAGE FORMS AND STRENGTHS

Suspension for injection in 5-mL multi-dose vials containing ten 0.5–mL doses. (3)

CONTRAINDICATIONS

History of severe allergic reactions (e.g., anaphylaxis) to any component of the vaccine, including egg protein, or following a previous dose of any influenza vaccine. (4, 11)

WARNINGS AND PRECAUTIONS

- If Guillain-Barré syndrome has occurred within 6 weeks of receipt of a prior influenza vaccine, the decision to give FLULAVAL QUADRIVALENT should be based on careful consideration of the potential benefits and risks. (5.1)
- Syncope (fainting) can occur in association with administration of injectable vaccines, including FLULAVAL QUADRIVALENT. Procedures should be in place to avoid falling injury and to restore cerebral perfusion following syncope. (5.2)

ADVERSE REACTIONS

- In adults, the most common (≥10%) solicited local adverse reaction was pain (60%); most common solicited systemic adverse events were muscle aches (26%), headache (22%), fatigue (22%), and arthralgia (15%). (6.1)
- In children 3 through 17 years of age, the most common (≥10%) solicited local adverse reaction was pain (65%). (6.1)
- In children 3 through 4 years of age, the most common (≥10%) solicited systemic adverse events were irritability (26%), drowsiness (21%), and loss of appetite (17%). (6.1)
- In children 5 through 17 years of age, the most common (≥10%) solicited systemic adverse events were muscle aches (29%), fatigue (22%), headache (22%), arthralgia (13%), and gastrointestinal symptoms (10%). (6.1)

To report SUSPECTED ADVERSE REACTIONS, contact GlaxoSmithKline at 1-888-825-5249 or VAERS at 1-800-822-7967 or www.vaers.hhs.gov

USE IN SPECIFIC POPULATIONS

- Safety and effectiveness of FLULAVAL QUADRIVALENT have not been established in pregnant women or nursing mothers. (8.1, 8.3)
- Register women who receive FLULAVAL QUADRIVALENT while pregnant in the pregnancy registry by calling 1-888-452-9622. (8.1)
- Geriatric Use: Antibody responses were lower in geriatric subjects who received FLULAVAL QUADRIVALENT than in younger subjects. (8.5)

See 17 for PATIENT COUNSELING INFORMATION

Revised: 08/2013

FULL PRESCRIBING INFORMATION: CONTENTS*

*** Sections or subsections omitted from the full prescribing information are not listed**

FULL PRESCRIBING INFORMATION

1 INDICATIONS AND USAGE

FLULAVAL® QUADRIVALENT is indicated for active immunization for the prevention of disease caused by influenza A subtype viruses and type B viruses contained in the vaccine. FLULAVAL QUADRIVALENT is approved for use in persons 3 years of age and older.

2 DOSAGE AND ADMINISTRATION

For intramuscular injection only.

2.1 Dosage and Schedule

The dose and schedule for FLULAVAL QUADRIVALENT are presented in Table 1.

Table 1. FLULAVAL QUADRIVALENT: Dosing

Age	Vaccination Status	Dose and Schedule
3 through 8 years of age	Not previously vaccinated with influenza vaccine	Two doses (0.5–mL each) at least 4 weeks apart
	Vaccinated with influenza vaccine in a previous season	One or two doses[a] (0.5–mL each)
9 years of age and older	Not applicable	One 0.5–mL dose

[a] One dose or two doses (0.5–mL each) depending on vaccination history as per the annual Advisory Committee on Immunization Practices (ACIP) recommendation on prevention and control of influenza with vaccines. If two doses, administer each 0.5–mL dose at least 4 weeks apart.

2.2 Administration Instructions

Shake the multi-dose vial vigorously each time before withdrawing a dose of vaccine. Parenteral drug products should be inspected visually for particulate matter and discoloration prior to administration, whenever solution and container permit. If either of these conditions exists, the vaccine should not be administered.

Use a sterile needle and sterile syringe to withdraw the 0.5–mL dose from the multi-dose vial and administer intramuscularly. A sterile syringe with a needle bore no larger than 23 gauge is recommended for administration. It is recommended that small syringes (0.5–mL or 1–mL) be used to minimize any product loss. Use a separate sterile needle and syringe for each dose withdrawn from the multi-dose vial.

The preferred site for intramuscular injection is the deltoid muscle of the upper arm. Do not inject in the gluteal area or areas where there may be a major nerve trunk.

Between uses, return the multi-dose vial to the recommended storage conditions, between 2° and 8°C (36° and 46°F). Do not freeze. Discard if the vaccine has been frozen. Once entered, a multi-dose vial, and any residual contents, should be discarded after 28 days.

3 DOSAGE FORMS AND STRENGTHS

FLULAVAL QUADRIVALENT is a suspension for injection available in 5–mL multi-dose vials containing ten 0.5–mL doses.

4 CONTRAINDICATIONS

Do not administer FLULAVAL QUADRIVALENT to anyone with a history of severe allergic reactions (e.g., anaphylaxis) to any component of the vaccine, including egg protein, or following a previous dose of any influenza vaccine *[see Description (11)]*.

5 WARNINGS AND PRECAUTIONS

5.1 Guillain-Barré Syndrome

If Guillain-Barré syndrome (GBS) has occurred within 6 weeks of receipt of a prior influenza vaccine, the decision to give FLULAVAL QUADRIVALENT should be based on careful consideration of the potential benefits and risks.

The 1976 swine influenza vaccine was associated with an elevated risk of GBS. Evidence for a causal relation of GBS with other influenza vaccines is inconclusive; if an excess risk exists, it is probably slightly more than one additional case/one million persons vaccinated.

5.2 Syncope

Syncope (fainting) can occur in association with administration of injectable vaccines, including FLULAVAL QUADRIVALENT. Syncope can be accompanied by transient neurological signs such as visual disturbance, paresthesia, and tonic-clonic limb movements. Procedures should be in place to avoid falling injury and to restore cerebral perfusion following syncope.

5.3 Preventing and Managing Allergic Vaccine Reactions

Prior to administration, the healthcare provider should review the immunization history for possible vaccine sensitivity and previous vaccination-related adverse reactions. Appropriate medical treatment and supervision must be available to manage possible anaphylactic reactions following administration of FLULAVAL QUADRIVALENT.

5.4 Altered Immunocompetence

If FLULAVAL QUADRIVALENT is administered to immunosuppressed persons, including individuals receiving immunosuppressive therapy, the immune response may be lower than in immunocompetent persons.

5.5 Limitations of Vaccine Effectiveness

Vaccination with FLULAVAL QUADRIVALENT may not protect all susceptible individuals.

5.6 Persons at Risk of Bleeding

As with other intramuscular injections, FLULAVAL QUADRIVALENT should be given with caution in individuals with bleeding disorders such as hemophilia or on anticoagulant therapy to avoid the risk of hematoma following the injection.

6 ADVERSE REACTIONS

6.1 Clinical Trials Experience

In adults who received FLULAVAL QUADRIVALENT, the most common (≥10%) solicited local adverse reaction was pain (60%); the most common (≥10%) solicited systemic adverse events were muscle aches (26%), headache (22%), fatigue (22%), and arthralgia (15%).

In children 3 through 17 years of age who received FLULAVAL QUADRIVALENT, the most common (≥10%) solicited local adverse reaction was pain (65%). In children 3 through 4 years of age, the most common (≥10%) solicited systemic adverse events were irritability (26%), drowsiness (21%), and loss of appetite (17%). In children 5 through 17 years of age, the most common (≥10%) systemic adverse events were muscle aches (29%), fatigue (22%), headache (22%), arthralgia (13%), and gastrointestinal symptoms (10%).

Because clinical trials are conducted under widely varying conditions, adverse reaction rates observed in the clinical trials of a vaccine cannot be directly compared to rates in the clinical trials of another vaccine, and may not reflect the rates observed in practice. There is the possibility that broad use of FLULAVAL QUADRIVALENT could reveal adverse reactions not observed in clinical trials.

FLULAVAL QUADRIVALENT has been administered to 1,384 adults 18 years of age and older and 3,516 pediatric subjects 3 through 17 years of age in 4 clinical trials.

FLULAVAL QUADRIVALENT in Adults: Study 1 was a randomized, double-blind, active-controlled, safety and immunogenicity study. In this study, subjects received FLULAVAL QUADRIVALENT (N = 1,272), or one of two formulations of a comparator trivalent influenza vaccine (FLULAVAL, TIV-1, N = 213 or TIV-2, N = 218), each containing an influenza type B virus that corresponded to one of the two B viruses in FLULAVAL QUADRIVALENT (a type B virus of the Victoria lineage or a type B virus of the Yamagata lineage). The population was 18 years of age and older (mean age 50 years) and 61% were female; 61% of subjects were White, 3% were Black, 1% were Asian, and 35% were of other racial/ethnic groups. Solicited adverse events were collected for 7 days (day of vaccination and the next 6 days). The incidence of local adverse reactions and systemic adverse events occurring within 7 days of vaccination in adults are shown in Table 2.

[See table 2 above]

Table 2. FLULAVAL QUADRIVALENT: Incidence of Solicited Local Adverse Reactions and Systemic Adverse Events Within 7 Days[a] of Vaccination in Adults 18 Years of Age and Older[b] (Total Vaccinated Cohort)

	FLULAVAL QUADRIVALENT[c] N = 1,260 %	Trivalent Influenza Vaccine (TIV) TIV-1 (B Victoria)[d] N = 208 %	TIV-2 (B Yamagata)[e] N = 216 %
Local Adverse Reactions			
Pain	60	45	41
Swelling	3	1	4
Redness	2	3	1
Systemic Adverse Events			
Muscle aches	26	25	19
Headache	22	20	23
Fatigue	22	22	17
Arthralgia	15	17	15
Gastrointestinal symptoms[f]	9	10	7
Shivering	9	8	6
Fever ≥100.4°F (38.0°C)	2	1	1

Total vaccinated cohort for safety included all vaccinated subjects for whom safety data were available.
[a]7 days included day of vaccination and the subsequent 6 days.
[b]Study 1: NCT01196975.
[c]Contained two A strains and two B strains, one of Victoria lineage and one of Yamagata lineage.
[d]Contained two A strains and a B strain of Victoria lineage.
[e]Contained the same two A strains as FLULAVAL and a B strain of Yamagata lineage.
[f]Gastrointestinal symptoms included nausea, vomiting, diarrhea, and/or abdominal pain.

Unsolicited adverse events occurring within 21 days of vaccination were reported in 19%, 23%, and 23% of subjects who received FLULAVAL QUADRIVALENT (N = 1,272), TIV-1 (B Victoria) (N = 213), or TIV-2 (B Yamagata) (N = 218), respectively. The unsolicited adverse events that occurred most frequently (≥1% for FLULAVAL QUADRIVALENT) included nasopharyngitis, upper respiratory tract infection, headache, cough and oropharyngeal pain. Serious adverse events occurring within 21 days of vaccination were reported in 0.4%, 0%, and 0% of subjects who received FLULAVAL QUADRIVALENT, TIV-1 (B Victoria), or TIV-2 (B Yamagata), respectively.

FLULAVAL QUADRIVALENT in Children: Study 2 was a randomized, double-blind, active-controlled study. In this study, subjects received FLULAVAL QUADRIVALENT (N = 932), or one of two formulations of a comparator trivalent influenza vaccine [FLUARIX® (Influenza Virus Vaccine), TIV-1, N = 929 or TIV-2, N = 932], each containing an influenza type B virus that corresponded to one of the two B viruses in FLULAVAL QUADRIVALENT (a type B virus of the Victoria lineage or a type B virus of the Yamagata lineage). The population was 3 through 17 years of age (mean age 9 years) and 53% were male; 65% were White, 13% were Asian, 9% were Black, and 13% were of other racial/ethnic groups. Children 3 through 8 years of age with no history of influenza vaccination received 2 doses approximately 28 days apart. Children 3 through 8 years of age with a history of influenza vaccination and children 9 years of age and older received one dose. Solicited local adverse reactions and systemic adverse events were collected for 7 days (day of vaccination and the next 6 days). The incidence of local adverse reactions and systemic adverse events occurring within 7 days of vaccination in children are shown in Table 3.

Table 3. FLULAVAL QUADRIVALENT: Incidence of Solicited Local Adverse Reactions and Systemic Adverse Events Within 7 Days[a] of First Vaccination in Children 3 Through 17 Years of Age[b] (Total Vaccinated Cohort)

	FLULAVAL QUADRIVALENT[c] %	Trivalent Influenza Vaccine (TIV) TIV-1 (B Victoria)[d] %	TIV-2 (B Yamagata)[e] %
		3 Through 17 Years of Age	
Local Adverse Reactions	N = 913	N = 911	N = 915
Pain	65	55	56
Swelling	6	3	4
Redness	5	3	4
		3 Through 4 Years of Age	
Systemic Adverse Events	N = 185	N = 187	N = 189
Irritability	26	17	22
Drowsiness	21	20	23
Loss of appetite	17	16	13
Fever ≥100.4°F (38.0°C)	5	6	4

(Table continued on next page)

[See table 3 above and on next page]

In children who received a second dose of FLULAVAL QUADRIVALENT, FLUARIX TIV-1 (B Victoria), or TIV-2 (B Yamagata), the incidences of adverse events following the second dose were generally lower than those observed after the first dose.

Unsolicited adverse events occurring within 28 days of vaccination were reported in 30%, 31% and 30% of subjects who received FLULAVAL QUADRIVALENT (N = 932), FLUARIX TIV-1 (B Victoria) (N = 929), or TIV-2 (B Yamagata) (N = 932), respectively. The unsolicited adverse events that occurred most frequently (≥1% for FLULAVAL QUADRIVALENT) included vomiting, pyrexia, bronchitis, nasopharyngitis, pharyngitis, upper respiratory tract infection, headache, cough, oropharyngeal pain, and rhinorrhea. Serious adverse events occurring within 28 days of any vaccination were reported in 0.1%, 0.2%, and 0.2% of subjects who received FLULAVAL QUADRIVALENT, FLUARIX TIV-1 (B Victoria), or TIV-2 (B Yamagata), respectively.

Study 3 was a randomized, observer-blind, non-influenza vaccine-controlled study evaluating the efficacy of FLULAVAL QUADRIVALENT. The study included subjects 3 through 8 years of age who received FLULAVAL QUADRIVALENT (N = 2,584) or HAVRIX® (Hepatitis A Vaccine) (N = 2,584), as a control vaccine. Children with no history of influenza vaccination received 2 doses of FLULAVAL QUADRIVALENT or HAVRIX approximately 28 days apart. Children with a history of influenza vaccination received one dose of FLULAVAL QUADRIVALENT or HAVRIX. In the overall population, 52% were male; 60% were Asian, 5% were White, and 35% were of other racial/ethnic groups. The mean age of subjects was 5 years. Solicited local adverse reactions and systemic adverse events were collected for 7 days (day of vaccination and the next 6 days). The incidence of local adverse reactions and systemic adverse events occurring within 7 days of vaccination in children are shown in Table 4.

Table 3 *(cont.)*. FLULAVAL QUADRIVALENT: Incidence of Solicited Local Adverse Reactions and Systemic Adverse Events Within 7 Days[a] of First Vaccination in Children 3 Through 17 Years of Age[b] (Total Vaccinated Cohort)

	FLULAVAL QUADRIVALENT[c] %	Trivalent Influenza Vaccine (TIV) TIV-1 (B Victoria)[d] %	Trivalent Influenza Vaccine (TIV) TIV-2 (B Yamagata)[e] %
	5 Through 17 Years of Age		
Systemic Adverse Events	N = 727	N = 724	N = 725
Muscle aches	29	25	25
Fatigue	22	24	23
Headache	22	22	20
Arthralgia	13	12	11
Gastrointestinal symptoms[f]	10	10	9
Shivering	7	7	7
Fever ≥100.4°F (38.0°C)	2	4	3

Total vaccinated cohort for safety included all vaccinated subjects for whom safety data were available.
[a] 7 days included day of vaccination and the subsequent 6 days.
[b] Study 2: NCT01198756.
[c] Contained two A strains and two B strains, one of Victoria lineage and one of Yamagata lineage.
[d] Contained two A strains and a B strain of Victoria lineage.
[e] Contained the same two A strains as FLUARIX and a B strain of Yamagata lineage.
[f] Gastrointestinal symptoms included nausea, vomiting, diarrhea, and/or abdominal pain.

Table 4. FLULAVAL QUADRIVALENT: Incidence of Solicited Local Adverse Reactions and Systemic Adverse Events Within 7 Days[a] of First Vaccination in Children 3 Through 8 Years of Age[b] (Total Vaccinated Cohort)

	FLULAVAL QUADRIVALENT %	HAVRIX[c] %
	3 Through 8 Years of Age	
Local Adverse Reactions	N = 2,546	N = 2,551
Pain	39	28
Swelling	1	0.3
Redness	0.4	0.2
	3 Through 4 Years of Age	
Systemic Adverse Events	N = 898	N = 895
Loss of appetite	9	8
Irritability	8	8
Drowsiness	8	7
Fever ≥100.4°F (38.0°C)	4	4
	5 Through 8 Years of Age	
Systemic Adverse Events	N = 1,648	N = 1,654
Muscle aches	12	10
Headache	11	11
Fatigue	8	7
Arthralgia	6	5
Gastrointestinal symptoms[d]	6	6
Shivering	3	3
Fever ≥100.4°F (38.0°C)	3	3

Total vaccinated cohort for safety included all vaccinated subjects for whom safety data were available.
[a] 7 days included day of vaccination and the subsequent 6 days.
[b] Study 3: NCT01218308.
[c] Hepatitis A Vaccine used as a control vaccine.
[d] Gastrointestinal symptoms included nausea, vomiting, diarrhea, and/or abdominal pain.

In children who received a second dose of FLULAVAL QUADRIVALENT or HAVRIX, the incidences of adverse events following the second dose were generally lower than those observed after the first dose.

The frequency of unsolicited adverse events occurring within 28 days of vaccination was similar in both groups (33% for both FLULAVAL QUADRIVALENT and HAVRIX). The unsolicited adverse events that occurred most frequently (≥1% for FLULAVAL QUADRIVALENT) included diarrhea, pyrexia, gastroenteritis, nasopharyngitis, upper respiratory tract infection, varicella, cough, and rhinorrhea. Serious adverse events occurring within 28 days of any vaccination were reported in 0.7% of subjects who received FLULAVAL QUADRIVALENT and in 0.2% of subjects who received HAVRIX.

6.2 Postmarketing Experience

There are no postmarketing data available for FLULAVAL QUADRIVALENT. The following adverse events have been spontaneously reported during postapproval use of FLULAVAL (trivalent influenza vaccine). Because these events are reported voluntarily from a population of uncertain size, it is not always possible to reliably estimate their incidence rate or establish a causal relationship to the vaccine. Adverse events described here are included because: a) they represent reactions which are known to occur following immunizations generally or influenza immunizations specifically; b) they are potentially serious; or c) the frequency of reporting.

Blood and Lymphatic System Disorders: Lymphadenopathy

Eye Disorders: Eye pain, photophobia

Gastrointestinal Disorders: Dysphagia, vomiting

General Disorders and Administration Site Conditions: Chest pain, injection site inflammation, asthenia, injection site rash, influenza-like symptoms, abnormal gait, injection site bruising, injection site sterile abscess.

Immune System Disorders: Allergic reactions including anaphylaxis, angioedema

Infections and Infestations: Rhinitis, laryngitis, cellulitis

Musculoskeletal and Connective Tissue Disorders: Muscle weakness, arthritis

Nervous System Disorders: Dizziness, paresthesia, hypoesthesia, hypokinesia, tremor, somnolence, syncope, Guillain-Barré syndrome, convulsions/seizures, facial or cranial nerve paralysis, encephalopathy, limb paralysis

Psychiatric Disorders: Insomnia

Respiratory, Thoracic, and Mediastinal Disorders: Dyspnea, dysphonia, bronchospasm, throat tightness

Skin and Subcutaneous Tissue Disorders: Urticaria, localized or generalized rash, pruritus, sweating

Vascular Disorders: Flushing, pallor

7 DRUG INTERACTIONS

7.1 Concomitant Administration With Other Vaccines

FLULAVAL QUADRIVALENT should not be mixed with any other vaccine in the same syringe or vial.

There are insufficient data to assess the concomitant administration of FLULAVAL QUADRIVALENT with other vaccines. When concomitant administration of other vaccines is required, the vaccines should be administered at different injection sites.

7.2 Immunosuppressive Therapies

Immunosuppressive therapies, including irradiation, antimetabolites, alkylating agents, cytotoxic drugs, and corticosteroids (used in greater than physiologic doses), may reduce the immune response to FLULAVAL QUADRIVALENT.

8 USE IN SPECIFIC POPULATIONS

8.1 Pregnancy

Pregnancy Category B

A reproductive and developmental toxicity study has been performed in female rats at a dose 80-fold the human dose (on a mg/kg basis) and showed no evidence of impaired female fertility or harm to the fetus due to FLULAVAL QUADRIVALENT. There are, however, no adequate and well-controlled studies in pregnant women. Because animal reproduction studies are not always predictive of human response, FLULAVAL QUADRIVALENT should be given to a pregnant woman only if clearly needed.

In a reproductive and developmental toxicity study, the effect of FLULAVAL QUADRIVALENT on embryo-fetal and pre-weaning development was evaluated in rats. Animals were administered FLULAVAL QUADRIVALENT by intramuscular injection twice prior to gestation, during the period of organogenesis (gestation days 3, 8, 11, and 15), and during lactation (day 7), 0.2 mL/dose/rat (80-fold higher than the projected human dose on a body weight basis). No adverse effects on mating, female fertility, pregnancy, parturition, lactation parameters, and embryo-fetal or pre-weaning development were observed. There were no vaccine-related fetal malformations or other evidence of teratogenesis.

Pregnancy Registry:

GlaxoSmithKline maintains a surveillance registry to collect data on pregnancy outcomes and newborn health status outcomes following vaccination with FLULAVAL QUADRIVALENT during pregnancy. Women who receive FLULAVAL QUADRIVALENT during pregnancy should be encouraged to contact GlaxoSmithKline directly or their healthcare provider should contact GlaxoSmithKline by calling 1-888-452-9622.

8.3 Nursing Mothers

It is not known whether FLULAVAL QUADRIVALENT is excreted in human milk. Because many drugs are excreted in human milk, caution should be exercised when FLULAVAL QUADRIVALENT is administered to a nursing woman.

8.4 Pediatric Use

Safety and effectiveness of FLULAVAL QUADRIVALENT in children younger than 3 years of age have not been established.

Safety and immunogenicity of FLULAVAL QUADRIVALENT in children 3 through 17 years of age have been evaluated *[see Adverse Reactions (6.1) and Clinical Studies (14.2)]*.

8.5 Geriatric Use

In a randomized, double-blind, active-controlled study, immunogenicity and safety were evaluated in a cohort of subjects 65 years of age and older who received FLULAVAL QUADRIVALENT (N = 397); approximately one-third of these subjects were 75 years of age and older. In subjects 65 years of age and older, the geometric mean antibody titers post-vaccination and seroconversion rates were lower than in younger subjects (18 to 64 years of age) and the frequencies of solicited and unsolicited adverse events were generally lower than in younger subjects *[see Adverse Reactions (6.1) and Clinical Studies (14.2)]*.

11 DESCRIPTION

FLULAVAL QUADRIVALENT, Influenza Virus Vaccine, for intramuscular injection, is a quadrivalent, split-virion, inactivated influenza virus vaccine prepared from virus propagated in the allantoic cavity of embryonated hens' eggs. Each of the influenza viruses is produced and purified separately. The virus is inactivated with ultraviolet light treatment followed by formaldehyde treatment, purified by centrifugation, and disrupted with sodium deoxycholate.

FLULAVAL QUADRIVALENT is a sterile, translucent to whitish opalescent suspension in a phosphate-buffered saline solution that may sediment slightly. The sediment resuspends upon shaking to form a homogeneous suspension.

FLULAVAL QUADRIVALENT has been standardized according to USPHS requirements for the 2013–2014 influenza season and is formulated to contain 60 micrograms (mcg) hemagglutinin (HA) per 0.5–mL dose in the recommended ratio of 15 mcg HA of each of the following 4 viruses (two A strains and two B strains): A/California/7/2009 NYMC X–179A (H1N1), A/Texas/50/2012 NYMC X–223A (H3N2) (an A/Victoria/361/2011–like virus), B/Massachusetts/2/2012 NYMC BX–51B, and B/Brisbane/60/2008.

Thimerosal, a mercury derivative, is added as a preservative. Each 0.5-mL dose contains 50 mcg thimerosal

(<25 mcg mercury), α-tocopheryl hydrogen succinate (≤320 mcg), and polysorbate 80 (≤887 mcg). Each 0.5-mL dose may also contain residual amounts of ovalbumin (≤0.3 mcg), formaldehyde (≤25 mcg), and sodium deoxycholate (≤50 mcg) from the manufacturing process. Antibiotics are not used in the manufacture of this vaccine.
The vial stoppers are not made with natural rubber latex.

12 CLINICAL PHARMACOLOGY

12.1 Mechanism of Action

Influenza illness and its complications follow infection with influenza viruses. Global surveillance of influenza identifies yearly antigenic variants. Since 1977, antigenic variants of influenza A (H1N1 and H3N2) viruses and influenza B viruses have been in global circulation.
Public health authorities recommend influenza vaccine strains annually. Inactivated influenza vaccines are standardized to contain the hemagglutinins of strains representing the influenza viruses likely to circulate in the United States during the influenza season. Two B strain lineages (Victoria and Yamagata) are of public health importance because they have co-circulated since 2001. FLULAVAL (trivalent influenza vaccine) contains only two influenza A subtype viruses and one influenza type B virus. In 6 of the last 11 seasons, the most predominant circulating influenza B lineage was not included in the annual trivalent vaccine. Quadrivalent vaccines, such as FLULAVAL QUADRIVALENT, contain two influenza A subtype viruses and two influenza type B viruses (one of the Victoria lineage and one of the Yamagata lineage).
Specific levels of hemagglutination inhibition (HI) antibody titer post-vaccination with inactivated influenza virus vaccines have not been correlated with protection from influenza illness but the antibody titers have been used as a measure of vaccine activity. In some human challenge studies, antibody titers of ≥1:40 have been associated with protection from influenza illness in up to 50% of subjects.[1,2]
Antibody against one influenza virus type or subtype confers little or no protection against another virus. Furthermore, antibody to one antigenic variant of influenza virus might not protect against a new antigenic variant of the same type or subtype. Frequent development of antigenic variants through antigenic drift is the virological basis for seasonal epidemics and the reason for the usual change of one or more new strains in each year's influenza vaccine.
Annual revaccination is recommended because immunity declines during the year after vaccination, and because circulating strains of influenza virus change from year to year.[3]

13 NONCLINICAL TOXICOLOGY

13.1 Carcinogenesis, Mutagenesis, Impairment of Fertility

FLULAVAL QUADRIVALENT has not been evaluated for carcinogenic or mutagenic potential. Vaccination of female rats with FLULAVAL QUADRIVALENT, at doses shown to be immunogenic in the rat, had no effect on fertility.

14 CLINICAL STUDIES

14.1 Efficacy Against Influenza

The efficacy of FLULAVAL QUADRIVALENT was evaluated in Study 3, a randomized, observer-blind, non-influenza vaccine-controlled study conducted in 3 countries in Asia, 3 in Latin America, and 2 in the Middle East/Europe during the 2010-2011 influenza season. Healthy subjects 3 through 8 years of age were randomized (1:1) to receive FLULAVAL QUADRIVALENT (N = 2,584), containing A/California/7/2009 (H1N1), A/Victoria/210/2009 (H3N2), B/Brisbane/60/2008 (Victoria lineage), and B/Florida/4/2006 (Yamagata lineage) influenza strains, or HAVRIX (N = 2,584), as a control vaccine. Children with no history of influenza vaccination received 2 doses of FLULAVAL QUADRIVALENT or HAVRIX approximately 28 days apart. Children with a history of influenza vaccination received one dose of FLULAVAL QUADRIVALENT or HAVRIX *[see Adverse Reactions (6.1)]*.
Efficacy of FLULAVAL QUADRIVALENT was assessed for the prevention of reverse transcriptase polymerase chain reaction (RT-PCR)-positive influenza A and/or B disease presenting as influenza-like illness (ILI). ILI was defined as a temperature ≥100°F in the presence of at least one of the following symptoms on the same day: cough, sore throat, runny nose, or nasal congestion. Subjects with ILI (monitored by passive and active surveillance for approximately 6 months) had nasal and throat swabs collected and tested for influenza A and/or B by RT-PCR. All RT-PCR-positive specimens were further tested in cell culture. Vaccine efficacy was calculated based on the ATP cohort for efficacy (Table 5).
[See table 5 above]
In an exploratory analysis by age, vaccine efficacy against RT-PCR-positive influenza A and/or B disease presenting as ILI was evaluated in subjects 3 through 4 years of age and 5 through 8 years of age; vaccine efficacy was 35.3% (95% CI: −1.3, 58.6) and 67.7% (95% CI: 49.7, 79.2), respectively. As the study lacked statistical power to evaluate efficacy within age subgroups, the clinical significance of these results is unknown.
As a secondary objective in the study, subjects with RT-PCR-positive influenza A and/or B were prospectively classified based on the presence of adverse outcomes that have been associated with influenza infection (defined as fever >102.2°F/39.0°C, physician-verified shortness of breath, pneumonia, wheezing, bronchitis, bronchiolitis, pulmonary congestion, croup and/or acute otitis media, and/or physician-diagnosed serious extra-pulmonary complications, including myositis, encephalitis, seizure and/or myocarditis).
The risk reduction of fever >102.2°F/39.0°C associated with RT-PCR-positive influenza was 71.0% (95% CI: 44.8, 84.8) based on the ATP cohort for efficacy [FLULAVAL

Table 5. FLULAVAL QUADRIVALENT: Influenza Attack Rates and Vaccine Efficacy Against Influenza A and/or B in Children 3 Through 8 Years of Age[a] (According to Protocol Cohort for Efficacy)

	N[b]	n[c]	Influenza Attack Rate % (n/N)	Vaccine Efficacy % (CI)
All RT-PCR-Positive Influenza				
FLULAVAL QUADRIVALENT	2,379	58	2.4	55.4[d] (95% CI: 39.1, 67.3)
HAVRIX[e]	2,398	128	5.3	–
All Culture-Confirmed Influenza[f]				
FLULAVAL QUADRIVALENT	2,379	50	2.1	55.9 (97.5% CI: 35.4, 69.9)
HAVRIX[e]	2,398	112	4.7	–
Antigenically Matched Culture-Confirmed Influenza				
FLULAVAL QUADRIVALENT	2,379	31	1.3	45.1[g] (97.5% CI: 9.3, 66.8)
HAVRIX[e]	2,398	56	2.3	–

CI = Confidence Interval; RT-PCR = reverse transcriptase polymerase chain reaction.
[a] Study 3: NCT01218308.
[b] According to protocol cohort for efficacy included subjects who met all eligibility criteria, were successfully contacted at least once post-vaccination, and complied with the protocol-specified efficacy criteria.
[c] Number of influenza cases.
[d] Vaccine efficacy for FLULAVAL QUADRIVALENT met the pre-defined criterion of >30% for the lower limit of the 2-sided 95% CI.
[e] Hepatitis A Vaccine used as a control vaccine.
[f] Of 162 culture-confirmed influenza cases, 108 (67%) were antigenically typed (87 matched; 21 unmatched); 54 (33%) could not be antigenically typed [but were typed by RT-PCR and nucleic acid sequence analysis: 5 cases A (H1N1) (5 with HAVRIX), 47 cases A (H3N2) (10 with FLULAVAL QUADRIVALENT; 37 with HAVRIX), and 2 cases B Victoria (2 with HAVRIX)].
[g] Since only 67% of cases could be typed, the clinical significance of this result is unknown.

Table 6. FLULAVAL QUADRIVALENT: Incidence of Adverse Outcomes Associated With RT-PCR-Positive Influenza in Children 3 Through 8 Years of Age[a] (Total Vaccinated Cohort)[b]

	FLULAVAL QUADRIVALENT N = 2,584			HAVRIX[c] N = 2,584		
Adverse Outcome[d]	**Number of Events**	**Number of Subjects[e]**	**%**	**Number of Events**	**Number of Subjects[e]**	**%**
Fever >102.2°F/39.0°C	16[f]	15	0.6	51[f]	50	1.9
Shortness of breath	0	0	0	5	5	0.2
Pneumonia	0	0	0	3	3	0.1
Wheezing	1	1	0	1	1	0
Bronchitis	1	1	0	1	1	0
Pulmonary congestion	0	0	0	1	1	0
Acute otitis media	0	0	0	1	1	0
Bronchiolitis	0	0	0	0	0	0
Croup	0	0	0	0	0	0
Encephalitis	0	0	0	0	0	0
Myocarditis	0	0	0	0	0	0
Myositis	0	0	0	0	0	0
Seizure	0	0	0	0	0	0

[a]Study 3: NCT01218308.
[b] Total vaccinated cohort included all vaccinated subjects for whom data were available.
[c]Hepatitis A Vaccine used as a control vaccine.
[d]In subjects who presented with more than one adverse outcome, each outcome was counted in the respective category.
[e]Number of subjects presenting with at least one event in each group.
[f]One subject in each group had sequential influenza due to influenza type A and type B viruses.

Table 7. Non-inferiority of FLULAVAL QUADRIVALENT Relative to Trivalent Influenza Vaccine (TIV) 21 Days Post-Vaccination in Adults 18 Years of Age and Older[a] (According to Protocol Cohort for Immunogenicity)[b]

	FLULAVAL QUADRIVALENT[c]	TIV-1 (B Victoria)[d]	TIV-2 (B Yamagata)[e]
Geometric Mean Titers Against	**N = 1,245-1,246 (95% CI)**	**N = 204 (95% CI)**	**N = 210-211 (95% CI)**
A/California/7/2009 (H1N1)	204.6[f] (190.4, 219.9)	176.0 (149.1, 207.7)	149.0 (122.9, 180.7)
A/Victoria/210/2009 (H3N2)	125.4[f] (117.4, 133.9)	147.5 (124.1, 175.2)	141.0 (118.1, 168.3)
B/Brisbane/60/2008 (Victoria lineage)	177.7[f] (167.8, 188.1)	135.9 (118.1, 156.5)	71.9 (61.3, 84.2)
B/Florida/4/2006 (Yamagata lineage)	399.7[f] (378.1, 422.6)	176.9 (153.8, 203.5)	306.6 (266.2, 353.3)

CI = Confidence Interval.
[a] Study 1: NCT01196975.
[b] According to protocol cohort for immunogenicity included all evaluable subjects for whom assay results were available after vaccination for at least one study vaccine antigen.
[c] Containing A/California/07/2009 (H1N1), A/Victoria/210/2009 (H3N2), B/Florida/04/2006 (Yamagata lineage), and B/Brisbane/60/2008 (Victoria lineage)
[d] Containing A/California/07/2009 (H1N1), A/Victoria/210/2009 (H3N2), and B/Brisbane/60/2008 (Victoria lineage)
[e] Containing A/California/07/2009 (H1N1), A/Victoria/210/2009 (H3N2), and B/Florida/04/2006 (Yamagata lineage).
[f] Non–inferior to both TIVs based on adjusted GMTs [upper limit of the 2–sided 95% CI for the GMT ratio (TIV/FLULAVAL QUADRIVALENT) ≤1.5]; superior to TIV-1 (B Victoria) with respect to the B strain of Yamagata lineage and to TIV-2 (B Yamagata) with respect to the B strain of Victoria lineage based on adjusted GMTs [lower limit of the 2–sided 95% CI for the GMT ratio (FLULAVAL QUADRIVALENT/TIV) >1.5].

Table 8. Non-inferiority of FLULAVAL QUADRIVALENT Relative to Trivalent Influenza Vaccine (TIV) at 28 Days Post-Vaccination in Children 3 Through 17 Years of Age[a] (According to Protocol Cohort for Immunogenicity)[b]

	FLULAVAL QUADRIVALENT[c]	TIV-1 (B Victoria)[d]	TIV-2 (B Yamagata)[e]
Geometric Mean Titers Against	**N = 878 (95% CI)**	**N = 871 (95% CI)**	**N = 877-878 (95% CI)**
A/California/7/2009 (H1N1)	362.7[f] (335.3, 392.3)	429.1 (396.5, 464.3)	420.2 (388.8, 454.0)
A/Victoria/210/2009 (H3N2)	143.7[f] (134.2, 153.9)	139.6 (130.5, 149.3)	151.0 (141.0, 161.6)
B/Brisbane/60/2008 (Victoria lineage)	250.5[f] (230.8, 272.0)	245.4 (226.9, 265.4)	68.1 (61.9, 74.9)
B/Florida/4/2006 (Yamagata lineage)	512.5[f] (477.6, 549.9)	197.0 (180.7, 214.8)	579.0 (541.2, 619.3)
Seroconversion[g] to:	**N = 876 % (95% CI)**	**N = 870 % (95% CI)**	**N = 876-877 % (95% CI)**
A/California/7/2009 (H1N1)	84.4[f] (81.8, 86.7)	86.8 (84.3, 89.0)	85.5 (83.0, 87.8)
A/Victoria/210/2009 (H3N2)	70.1[f] (66.9, 73.1)	67.8 (64.6, 70.9)	69.6 (66.5, 72.7)
B/Brisbane/60/2008 (Victoria lineage)	74.5[f] (71.5, 77.4)	71.5 (68.4, 74.5)	29.9 (26.9, 33.1)
B/Florida/4/2006 (Yamagata lineage)	75.2[f] (72.2, 78.1)	41.3 (38.0, 44.6)	73.4 (70.4, 76.3)

CI = Confidence Interval.
[a] Study 2: NCT01198756.
[b] According to protocol cohort for immunogenicity included all evaluable subjects for whom assay results were available after vaccination for at least one study vaccine antigen.
[c] Containing A/California/07/2009 (H1N1), A/Victoria/210/2009 (H3N2), B/Florida/04/2006 (Yamagata lineage), and B/Brisbane/60/2008 (Victoria lineage).
[d] Containing A/California/07/2009 (H1N1), A/Victoria/210/2009 (H3N2), and B/Brisbane/60/2008 (Victoria lineage).
[e] Containing A/California/07/2009 (H1N1), A/Victoria/210/2009 (H3N2), and B/Florida/04/2006 (Yamagata lineage).
[f] Non–inferior to both TIVs based on adjusted GMTs [upper limit of the 2-sided 95% CI for the GMT ratio (TIV/FLULAVAL QUADRIVALENT) ≤1.5] and seroconversion rates (upper limit of the 2–sided 95% CI on difference of the TIV minus FLULAVAL QUADRIVALENT ≤10%); superior to TIV-1 (B Victoria) with respect to the B strain of Yamagata lineage and to TIV-2 (B Yamagata) with respect to the B strain of Victoria lineage based on adjusted GMTs [lower limit of the 2–sided 95% CI for the GMT ratio (FLULAVAL QUADRIVALENT/TIV) >1.5] and seroconversion rates (lower limit of the 2–sided 95% CI on difference of FLULAVAL QUADRIVALENT minus the TIV >10%).
[g] Seroconversion defined as a 4–fold increase in post-vaccination antibody titer from pre-vaccination titer ≥1:10, or an increase in titer from <1:10 to ≥1:40.

QUADRIVALENT (n = 12/2,379); HAVRIX (n = 41/2,398)]. The other pre-specified adverse outcomes had too few cases to calculate a risk reduction. The incidence of these adverse outcomes is presented in Table 6.
[See table 6 at top of previous page]

14.2 Immunological Evaluation

Adults: Study 1 was a randomized, double-blind, active-controlled, safety and immunogenicity study conducted in subjects 18 years of age and older. In this study, subjects received FLULAVAL QUADRIVALENT (N = 1,246), or one of two formulations of a comparator trivalent influenza vaccine (FLULAVAL, TIV-1, N = 204 or TIV-2, N = 211), each containing an influenza type B virus that corresponded to one of the two B viruses in FLULAVAL QUADRIVALENT (a type B virus of the Victoria lineage or a type B virus of the Yamagata lineage) *[see Adverse Reactions (6.1)]*.

Immune responses, specifically hemagglutination inhibition (HI) antibody titers to each virus strain in the vaccine, were evaluated in sera obtained 21 days after administration of FLULAVAL QUADRIVALENT or the comparators. The immunogenicity endpoint was geometric mean antibody titers (GMTs) adjusted for baseline, performed on the According-to-Protocol (ATP) cohort for whom immunogenicity assay results were available after vaccination. FLULAVAL QUADRIVALENT was non–inferior to both TIVs based on adjusted GMTs (Table 7). The antibody response to influenza B strains contained in FLULAVAL QUADRIVALENT was higher than the antibody response after vaccination with a TIV containing an influenza B strain from a different lineage. There was no evidence that the addition of the second B strain resulted in immune interference to other strains included in the vaccine (Table 7).
[See table 7 above]

Children: Study 2 was a randomized, double-blind, active-controlled study conducted in children 3 through 17 years of age. In this study, subjects received FLULAVAL QUADRIVALENT (N = 878), or one of two formulations of a comparator trivalent influenza vaccine (FLUARIX, TIV-1, N = 871 or TIV-2 N = 878), each containing an influenza type B virus that corresponded to one of the two B viruses in FLULAVAL QUADRIVALENT (a type B virus of the Victoria lineage or a type B virus of the Yamagata lineage) *[see Adverse Reactions (6.1)]*.

Immune responses, specifically HI antibody titers to each virus strain in the vaccine, were evaluated in sera obtained 28 days following one or 2 doses of FLULAVAL QUADRIVALENT or the comparators. The immunogenicity endpoints were GMTs adjusted for baseline, and the percentage of subjects who achieved seroconversion, defined as at least a 4–fold increase in serum HI titer over baseline to ≥1:40, following vaccination, performed on the ATP cohort. FLULAVAL QUADRIVALENT was non-inferior to both TIVs based on adjusted GMTs and seroconversion rates (Table 8). The antibody response to influenza B strains contained in FLULAVAL QUADRIVALENT was higher than the antibody response after vaccination with a TIV containing an influenza B strain from a different lineage. There was no evidence that the addition of the second B strain resulted in immune interference to other strains included in the vaccine (Table 8).
[See table 8 above]

15 REFERENCES

1. Hannoun C, Megas F, Piercy J. Immunogenicity and protective efficacy of influenza vaccination. *Virus Res* 2004;103:133-138.
2. Hobson D, Curry RL, Beare AS, et al. The role of serum haemagglutination-inhibiting antibody in protection against challenge infection with influenza A2 and B viruses. *J Hyg Camb* 1972;70:767-777.
3. Centers for Disease Control and Prevention. Prevention and control of influenza with vaccines: Recommendations of the Advisory Committee on Immunization Practices (ACIP). *MMWR* 2010;59(RR-8):1-62.

16 HOW SUPPLIED/STORAGE AND HANDLING

FLULAVAL QUADRIVALENT is supplied in a 5-mL multi-dose vial containing 10 doses (0.5 mL each).

NDC 19515-895-01 Vial (containing 10 doses) in Package of 1: NDC 19515-895-11

Once entered, a multi-dose vial should be discarded after 28 days. Store refrigerated between 2° and 8°C (36° and 46°F). Do not freeze. Discard if the vaccine has been frozen. Store in the original package to protect from light.

17 PATIENT COUNSELING INFORMATION

Provide the following information to the vaccine recipient or guardian:
- Inform of the potential benefits and risks of immunization with FLULAVAL QUADRIVALENT.
- Educate regarding potential side effects, emphasizing that (1) FLULAVAL QUADRIVALENT contains non-infectious killed viruses and cannot cause influenza, and (2) FLULAVAL QUADRIVALENT is intended to provide protection against illness due to influenza viruses only, and cannot provide protection against all respiratory illness.
- Instruct to report any adverse events to their healthcare provider.
- Inform that safety and efficacy have not been established in pregnant women. Register women who receive FLULAVAL QUADRIVALENT while pregnant in the pregnancy registry by calling 1-888-452-9622.
- Give the Vaccine Information Statements, which are required by the National Childhood Vaccine Injury Act of

1986 prior to immunization. These materials are available free of charge at the Centers for Disease Control and Prevention (CDC) website (www.cdc.gov/vaccines).

- Instruct that annual revaccination is recommended.

FLUARIX, FLULAVAL, and HAVRIX are registered trademarks of GlaxoSmithKline.

Manufactured by **ID Biomedical Corporation of Quebec**
Quebec City, QC, Canada, US License 1739
Distributed by **GlaxoSmithKline**
Research Triangle Park, NC 27709

FVQ.1PI

HAVRIX ℞

[hav' rix]
(Hepatitis A Vaccine)
Suspension for Intramuscular Injection

HIGHLIGHTS OF PRESCRIBING INFORMATION
These highlights do not include all the information needed to use HAVRIX safely and effectively. See full prescribing information for HAVRIX.
HAVRIX (Hepatitis A Vaccine)
Suspension for Intramuscular Injection
Initial U.S. Approval: 1995

INDICATIONS AND USAGE

HAVRIX is a vaccine indicated for active immunization against disease caused by hepatitis A virus (HAV). HAVRIX is approved for use in persons 12 months of age or older. Primary immunization should be administered at least 2 weeks prior to expected exposure to HAV. (1)

DOSAGE AND ADMINISTRATION

- HAVRIX is administered by intramuscular injection. (2.2)
- Children and adolescents: A single 0.5-mL dose and a 0.5-mL booster dose administered between 6 to 12 months later. (2.3)
- Adults: A single 1-mL dose and a 1-mL booster dose administered between 6 to 12 months later. (2.3)

DOSAGE FORMS AND STRENGTHS

- Suspension for injection available in the following presentations:
- 0.5-mL single-dose vials and prefilled syringes. (3)
- 1-mL single-dose vials and prefilled syringes. (3)

CONTRAINDICATIONS

Severe allergic reaction (e.g., anaphylaxis) after a previous dose of any hepatitis A-containing vaccine, or to any component of HAVRIX, including neomycin. (4)

WARNINGS AND PRECAUTIONS

- HAVRIX is available in vials and 2 types of prefilled syringes. One type of prefilled syringe has a tip cap which may contain natural rubber latex. The other type has a tip cap and a rubber plunger which contain dry natural latex rubber. Use of these syringes may cause allergic reactions in latex-sensitive individuals. (5.1, 16)
- Syncope (fainting) can occur in association with administration of injectable vaccines, including HAVRIX. Procedures should be in place to avoid falling injury and to restore cerebral perfusion following syncope. (5.2)

ADVERSE REACTIONS

- In studies of adults and children 2 years of age and older, the most common solicited adverse events were injection-site soreness (56% of adults and 21% of children) and headache (14% of adults and less than 9% of children). (6.1)
- In studies of children 11 to 25 months of age, the most frequently reported solicited local reactions were pain (32%) and redness (29%). Common solicited general adverse events were irritability (42%), drowsiness (28%), and loss of appetite (28%). (6.1)

To report SUSPECTED ADVERSE REACTIONS, contact GlaxoSmithKline at 1-888-825-5249 or VAERS at 1-800-822-7967 or www.vaers.hhs.gov.

DRUG INTERACTIONS

Do not mix HAVRIX with any other vaccine or product in the same syringe or vial. (7.1)

USE IN SPECIFIC POPULATIONS

Safety and effectiveness of HAVRIX have not been established in pregnant women and nursing mothers. (8.1)

See 17 for PATIENT COUNSELING INFORMATION

Revised: 06/2013

FULL PRESCRIBING INFORMATION: CONTENTS*

*** Sections or subsections omitted from the full prescribing information are not listed**

FULL PRESCRIBING INFORMATION

1 INDICATIONS AND USAGE

HAVRIX® is indicated for active immunization against disease caused by hepatitis A virus (HAV). HAVRIX is approved for use in persons 12 months of age and older. Primary immunization should be administered at least 2 weeks prior to expected exposure to HAV.

2 DOSAGE AND ADMINISTRATION

2.1 Preparation for Administration

Shake well before use. With thorough agitation, HAVRIX is a homogeneous, turbid, white suspension. Do not administer if it appears otherwise. Parenteral drug products should be inspected visually for particulate matter and discoloration prior to administration, whenever solution and container permit. If either of these conditions exists, the vaccine should not be administered.

For the prefilled syringes, attach a sterile needle and administer intramuscularly.

For the vials, use a sterile needle and sterile syringe to withdraw the vaccine dose and administer intramuscularly. Changing needles between drawing vaccine from a vial and injecting it into a recipient is not necessary unless the needle has been damaged or contaminated. Use a separate sterile needle and syringe for each individual.

2.2 Administration

HAVRIX should be administered by intramuscular injection only. HAVRIX should not be administered in the gluteal region; such injections may result in suboptimal response.

Do not administer this product intravenously, intradermally, or subcutaneously.

2.3 Recommended Dose and Schedule

Children and Adolescents: Primary immunization for children and adolescents (12 months through 18 years of age) consists of a single 0.5-mL dose and a 0.5-mL booster dose administered anytime between 6 and 12 months later. The preferred sites for intramuscular injections are the anterolateral aspect of the thigh in young children or the deltoid muscle of the upper arm in older children.

Adults: Primary immunization for adults consists of a single 1-mL dose and a 1-mL booster dose administered anytime between 6 and 12 months later. In adults, the injection should be given in the deltoid region.

3 DOSAGE FORMS AND STRENGTHS

Suspension for injection available in the following presentations:

- 0.5-mL single-dose vials and prefilled TIP-LOK® syringes.
- 1-mL single-dose vials and prefilled TIP-LOK syringes. *[See How Supplied/Storage and Handling (16).]*

4 CONTRAINDICATIONS

Severe allergic reaction (e.g., anaphylaxis) after a previous dose of any hepatitis A-containing vaccine, or to any component of HAVRIX, including neomycin, is a contraindication to administration of HAVRIX *[see Description (11)]*.

5 WARNINGS AND PRECAUTIONS

5.1 Latex

HAVRIX is available in vials and 2 types of prefilled syringes. One type of prefilled syringe has a tip cap which may contain natural rubber latex. The other type has a tip cap and a rubber plunger which contain dry natural latex rubber. Use of these syringes may cause allergic reactions in latex-sensitive individuals. The vial stopper does not contain latex. *[See How Supplied/Storage and Handling (16).]*

5.2 Syncope

Syncope (fainting) can occur in association with administration of injectable vaccines, including HAVRIX. Syncope can be accompanied by transient neurological signs such as visual disturbance, paresthesia, and tonic-clonic limb movements. Procedures should be in place to avoid falling injury and to restore cerebral perfusion following syncope.

5.3 Preventing and Managing Allergic Vaccine Reactions

Appropriate medical treatment and supervision must be available to manage possible anaphylactic reactions following administration of the vaccine *[see Contraindications (4)]*.

5.4 Altered Immunocompetence

Immunocompromised persons may have a diminished immune response to HAVRIX, including individuals receiving immunosuppressant therapy.

5.5 Limitations of Vaccine Effectiveness

Hepatitis A virus has a relatively long incubation period (15 to 50 days). HAVRIX may not prevent hepatitis A infection in individuals who have an unrecognized hepatitis A infection at the time of vaccination. Additionally, vaccination with HAVRIX may not protect all individuals.

6 ADVERSE REACTIONS

6.1 Clinical Trials Experience

Because clinical trials are conducted under widely varying conditions, adverse reaction rates observed in the clinical trials of a vaccine cannot be directly compared to rates in the clinical trials of another vaccine, and may not reflect the rates observed in practice.

The safety of HAVRIX has been evaluated in 61 clinical trials involving approximately 37,000 individuals receiving doses of 360 EL.U. (n = 21,928 in 3- or 4-dose schedule), 720 EL.U. (n = 12,274 in 2- or 3-dose schedule), or 1440 EL.U. (n = 2,782 in 2- or 3-dose schedule).

Of solicited adverse events in clinical trials of adults, who received HAVRIX 1440 EL.U., and children (2 years of age and older), who received either HAVRIX 360 EL.U. or 720 EL.U., the most frequently reported was injection-site soreness (56% of adults and 21% of children); less than 0.5% of soreness was reported as severe. Headache was reported by 14% of adults and less than 9% of children. Other solicited and unsolicited events occurring during clinical trials are listed below.

Incidence 1% to 10% of Injections: *Metabolism and Nutrition Disorders:* Anorexia.

Gastrointestinal Disorders: Nausea.

General Disorders and Administration Site Conditions: Fatigue, fever >99.5°F (37.5°C), induration, redness, and swelling of the injection site; malaise.

Incidence <1% of Injections: *Infections and Infestations:* Pharyngitis, upper respiratory tract infections.

Blood and Lymphatic System Disorders: Lymphadenopathy.

Psychiatric Disorders: Insomnia.

Nervous System Disorders: Dysgeusia, hypertonia.

Eye Disorders: Photophobia.

Ear and Labyrinth Disorders: Vertigo.

Gastrointestinal Disorders: Abdominal pain, diarrhea, vomiting.

Skin and Subcutaneous Tissue Disorders: Pruritus, rash, urticaria.

Musculoskeletal and Connective Tissue Disorders: Arthralgia, myalgia.

General Disorders and Administration Site Conditions: Injection site hematoma.

Investigations: Creatine phosphokinase increased.

Coadministration Studies of HAVRIX in Children 11 to 25 Months of Age: In 4 studies, 3,152 children 11 to 25 months of age received at least one dose of HAVRIX 720 EL.U. administered alone or concomitantly with other routine childhood vaccinations *[see Clinical Studies (14.2, 14.5)]*. The studies included HAV 210 (N = 1,084), HAV 232 (N = 394), HAV 220 (N = 433), and HAV 231 (N = 1,241).

In the largest of these studies (HAV 231) conducted in the US, 1,241 children 15 months of age were randomized to receive: Group 1) HAVRIX alone; Group 2) HAVRIX concomitantly with measles, mumps, and rubella (MMR) vaccine

Table 1. Solicited Local Adverse Reactions and General Adverse Events Occurring Within 4 Days of Vaccination[a] in Children 15 to 24 Months of Age With HAVRIX Administered Alone or Concomitantly With MMR and Varicella Vaccines (TVC)

	Group 1 HAVRIX Dose 1 %	Group 2 HAVRIX+ MMR+V[b] Dose 1 %	Group 1 HAVRIX Dose 2 %	Group 2 HAVRIX Dose 2 %
Local (at injection site for HAVRIX)				
N	298	411	272	373
Pain, any	23.8	23.6	24.3	30.3
Redness, any	20.1	20.0	22.8	23.9
Swelling, any	8.7	10.2	9.6	9.9
General				
N	300	417	271	375
Irritability, any	33.3	43.9	31.0	27.2
Irritability, grade 3	0.3	1.9	1.5	0.3
Drowsiness, any	22.3	35.3	21.0	20.8
Drowsiness, grade 3	1.0	2.2	1.1	0.0
Loss of appetite, any	18.3	26.1	19.9	20.5
Loss of appetite, grade 3	1.0	1.4	0.4	0.3
Fever ≥100.6°F (38.1°C)	3.0	4.8	3.3	2.7
Fever ≥101.5°F (38.6°C)	2.0	2.6	1.8	1.6
Fever ≥102.4°F (39.1°C)	0.7	0.7	0.4	1.1

Total vaccinated cohort (TVC) = all subjects who received at least one dose of vaccine.
N = number of subjects who received at least one dose of vaccine and for whom diary card information was available.
Grade 3: drowsiness defined as prevented normal daily activities; irritability/fussiness defined as crying that could not be comforted/prevented normal daily activities; loss of appetite defined as no eating at all.
[a] Within 4 days of vaccination defined as day of vaccination and the next 3 days.
[b] MMR = measles, mumps, and rubella vaccine; V = varicella vaccine.

(manufactured by Merck and Co.) and varicella vaccine (manufactured by Merck and Co.); or Group 3) MMR and varicella vaccines. Subjects in Group 3 who received MMR and varicella vaccines received the first dose of HAVRIX 42 days later. A second dose of HAVRIX was administered to all subjects 6 to 9 months after the first dose of HAVRIX. Solicited local adverse reactions and general events were recorded by parents/guardians on diary cards for 4 days (days 0 to 3) after vaccination. Unsolicited adverse events were recorded on the diary card for 31 days after vaccination. Telephone follow-up was conducted 6 months after the last vaccination to inquire about serious adverse events, new onset chronic illnesses and medically significant events. A total of 1,035 children completed the 6-month follow-up. Among subjects in all groups combined, 53% were male; 69% of subjects were white, 16% were Hispanic, 9% were black and 6% were other racial/ethnic groups.

Percentages of subjects with solicited local adverse reactions and general adverse events following HAVRIX administered alone (Group 1) or concomitantly with MMR and varicella vaccines (Group 2) are presented in Table 1. The solicited adverse events from the 3 additional coadministration studies conducted with HAVRIX were comparable to those from Study HAV 231.

[See table 1 above]

Serious Adverse Events in Children 11 to 25 Months of Age: Among these 4 studies, 0.9% (29/3,152) of subjects reported a serious adverse event within the 31-day period following vaccination with HAVRIX. Among subjects administered HAVRIX alone 1.0% (13/1,332) reported a serious adverse event. Among subjects who received HAVRIX concomitantly with other childhood vaccines, 0.9% (8/909) reported a serious adverse event. In these 4 studies, there were 4 reports of seizure within 31 days post-vaccination: these occurred 2, 9, and 27 days following the first dose of HAVRIX administered alone and 12 days following the second dose of HAVRIX. In one subject who received INFANRIX and Hib conjugate vaccine followed by HAVRIX 6 weeks later, bronchial hyperreactivity and respiratory distress were reported on the day of administration of HAVRIX alone.

6.2 Postmarketing Experience

In addition to reports in clinical trials, worldwide voluntary reports of adverse events received for HAVRIX since market introduction of this vaccine are listed below. This list includes serious adverse events or events which have a suspected causal connection to components of HAVRIX or other vaccines or drugs. Because these events are reported voluntarily from a population of uncertain size, it is not always possible to reliably estimate their frequency or establish a causal relationship to the vaccine.

Infections and Infestations: Rhinitis.

Blood and Lymphatic System Disorders: Thrombocytopenia.

Immune System Disorders: Anaphylactic reaction, anaphylactoid reaction, serum sickness–like syndrome.

Nervous System Disorders: Convulsion, dizziness, encephalopathy, Guillain-Barré syndrome, hypoesthesia, multiple sclerosis, myelitis, neuropathy, paresthesia, somnolence, syncope.

Vascular Disorders: Vasculitis.

Respiratory, Thoracic, and Mediastinal Disorders: Dyspnea.

Hepatobiliary Disorders: Hepatitis, jaundice.

Skin and Subcutaneous Tissue Disorders: Angioedema, erythema multiforme, hyperhidrosis.

Congenital, Familial, and Genetic Disorders: Congenital anomaly.

Musculoskeletal and Connective Tissue Disorders: Musculoskeletal stiffness.

General Disorders and Administration Site Conditions: Chills, influenza-like symptoms, injection site reaction, local swelling.

7 DRUG INTERACTIONS

7.1 Concomitant Administration With Vaccines and Immune Globulin

In clinical studies HAVRIX was administered concomitantly with the following vaccines *[see Adverse Reactions (6.1) and Clinical Studies (14.5)]*:

- INFANRIX (DTaP);
- Hib conjugate vaccine;
- pneumococcal 7-valent conjugate vaccine;
- MMR vaccine;
- varicella vaccine.

HAVRIX may be administered concomitantly with immune globulin.

When concomitant administration of other vaccines or immune globulin is required, they should be given with different syringes and at different injection sites. Do not mix HAVRIX with any other vaccine or product in the same syringe or vial.

7.2 Immunosuppressive Therapies

Immunosuppressive therapies, including irradiation, antimetabolites, alkylating agents, cytotoxic drugs, and corticosteroids (used in greater than physiologic doses), may reduce the immune response to HAVRIX.

8 USE IN SPECIFIC POPULATIONS

8.1 Pregnancy

Pregnancy Category C

Animal reproduction studies have not been conducted with HAVRIX. It is also not known whether HAVRIX can cause fetal harm when administered to a pregnant woman or can affect reproduction capacity. HAVRIX should be given to a pregnant woman only if clearly needed.

8.3 Nursing Mothers

It is not known whether HAVRIX is excreted in human milk. Because many drugs are excreted in human milk, caution should be exercised when HAVRIX is administered to a nursing woman.

8.4 Pediatric Use

The safety and effectiveness of HAVRIX, doses of 360 EL.U. or 720 EL.U., have been evaluated in more than 22,000 subjects 1 year to 18 years of age.

The safety and effectiveness of HAVRIX have not been established in subjects younger than 12 months of age.

8.5 Geriatric Use

Clinical studies of HAVRIX did not include sufficient numbers of subjects 65 years of age and older to determine whether they respond differently from younger subjects. Other reported clinical experience has not identified differences in overall safety between these subjects and younger adult subjects.

8.6 Hepatic Impairment

Subjects with chronic liver disease had a lower antibody response to HAVRIX than healthy subjects *[see Clinical Studies (14.3)]*.

11 DESCRIPTION

HAVRIX (Hepatitis A Vaccine) is a sterile suspension of inactivated virus for intramuscular administration. The virus (strain HM175) is propagated in MRC-5 human diploid cells. After removal of the cell culture medium, the cells are lysed to form a suspension. This suspension is purified through ultrafiltration and gel permeation chromatography procedures. Treatment of this lysate with formalin ensures viral inactivation. Viral antigen activity is referenced to a standard using an enzyme linked immunosorbent assay (ELISA), and is therefore expressed in terms of ELISA Units (EL.U.).

Each 1-mL adult dose of vaccine contains 1440 EL.U. of viral antigen, adsorbed on 0.5 mg of aluminum as aluminum hydroxide.

Each 0.5-mL pediatric dose of vaccine contains 720 EL.U. of viral antigen, adsorbed onto 0.25 mg of aluminum as aluminum hydroxide.

HAVRIX contains the following excipients: Amino acid supplement (0.3% w/v) in a phosphate-buffered saline solution and polysorbate 20 (0.05 mg/mL). From the manufacturing process, HAVRIX also contains residual MRC-5 cellular proteins (not more than 5 mcg/mL), formalin (not more than 0.1 mg/mL), and neomycin sulfate (not more than 40 ng/mL), an aminoglycoside antibiotic included in the cell growth media.

HAVRIX is formulated without preservatives.

HAVRIX is available in vials and 2 types of prefilled syringes. One type of prefilled syringe has a tip cap which may contain natural rubber latex. The other type has a tip cap and a rubber plunger which contain dry natural latex rubber. The vial stopper does not contain latex. *[See How Supplied/Storage and Handling (16).]*

12 CLINICAL PHARMACOLOGY

12.1 Mechanism of Action

The hepatitis A virus belongs to the picornavirus family. It is one of several hepatitis viruses that cause systemic disease with pathology in the liver.

The incubation period for hepatitis A averages 28 days (range: 15 to 50 days).[1] The course of hepatitis A infection is extremely variable, ranging from asymptomatic infection to icteric hepatitis and death.

The presence of antibodies to HAV confers protection against hepatitis A infection. However, the lowest titer needed to confer protection has not been determined.

13 NONCLINICAL TOXICOLOGY

13.1 Carcinogenesis, Mutagenesis, Impairment of Fertility

HAVRIX has not been evaluated for its carcinogenic potential, mutagenic potential, or potential for impairment of fertility.

14 CLINICAL STUDIES

14.1 Pediatric Effectiveness Studies

Protective efficacy with HAVRIX has been demonstrated in a double-blind, randomized controlled study in school children (age 1 to 16 years) in Thailand who were at high risk of HAV infection. A total of 40,119 children were randomized to be vaccinated with either HAVRIX 360 EL.U. or ENGERIX-B 10 mcg at 0, 1, and 12 months. Of these, 19,037 children received 2 doses of HAVRIX (0 and 1 months) and 19,120 children received 2 doses of control vaccine, ENGERIX-B (0 and 1 months). A total of 38,157 children entered surveillance at day 138 and were observed for an additional 8 months. Using the protocol-defined endpoint (≥2 days absence from school, ALT level >45 U/mL, and a positive result in the HAVAB-M test), 32 cases of clinical hepatitis A occurred in the control group. In the HAVRIX group, 2 cases were identified. These 2 cases were mild in terms of both biochemical and clinical indices of hepatitis A disease. Thus the calculated efficacy rate for prevention of clinical hepatitis A was 94% (95% Confidence Interval [CI]: 74, 98).

In outbreak investigations occurring in the trial, 26 clinical cases of hepatitis A (of a total of 34 occurring in the trial) occurred. No cases occurred in vaccinees who received HAVRIX.

Using additional virological and serological analyses post hoc, the efficacy of HAVRIX was confirmed. Up to 3 additional cases of mild clinical illness may have occurred in vaccinees. Using available testing, these illnesses could neither be proven nor disproven to have been caused by HAV. By including these as cases, the calculated efficacy rate for prevention of clinical hepatitis A would be 84% (95% CI: 60, 94).

14.2 Immunogenicity in Children and Adolescents

Immune Response to HAVRIX 720 EL.U./0.5 mL at 11 to 25 Months of Age (Study HAV 210): In this prospective, open-label, multicenter study, 1,084 children were administered study vaccine in one of 5 groups:

(1) Children 11 to 13 months of age who received HAVRIX on a 0- and 6-month schedule;

(2) Children 15 to 18 months of age who received HAVRIX on a 0- and 6-month schedule;

(3) Children 15 to 18 months of age who received HAVRIX coadministered with INFANRIX and Haemophilus b (Hib) conjugate vaccine (no longer US-licensed) at month 0 and HAVRIX at month 6;

(4) Children 15 to 18 months of age who received INFANRIX coadministered with Hib conjugate vaccine at month 0 and HAVRIX at months 1 and 7;

(5) Children 23 to 25 months of age who received HAVRIX on a 0- and 6-month schedule.

Among subjects in all groups, 52% were male; 61% of subjects were white, 9% were black, 3% were Asian, and 27% were other racial/ethnic groups. The anti-hepatitis A antibody vaccine responses and GMTs, calculated on responders for groups 1, 2, and 5 are presented in Table 2. Vaccine response rates were similar among the 3 age groups that received HAVRIX. One month after the second dose of HAVRIX, the GMT in each of the younger age groups (11 to 13 and 15 to 18 months of age) was shown to be similar to that achieved in the 23 to 25 months of age group.

Table 2. Anti-Hepatitis A Immune Response Following 2 Doses of HAVRIX 720 EL.U./0.5 mL Administered 6 Months Apart in Children Given the First Dose of HAVRIX at 11 to 13 Months of Age, 15 to 18 Months of Age, or 23 to 25 Months of Age

Age group	N	Vaccine Response		GMT (mIU/mL)
		%	95% CI	
11-13 months (Group 1)	218	99	97, 100	1,461[a]
15-18 months (Group 2)	200	100	98, 100	1,635[a]
23-25 months (Group 5)	211	100	98, 100	1,911

Vaccine response = Seroconversion (anti-HAV ≥15 mIU/mL [lower limit of antibody measurement by assay]) in children initially seronegative or at least the maintenance of the pre-vaccination anti-HAV concentration in initially seropositive children.

CI = Confidence Interval; GMT = Geometric mean antibody titer.

[a] Calculated on vaccine responders one month post-dose 2. GMTs in children 11 to 13 months of age and 15 to 18 months of age were non-inferior (similar) to the GMT in children 23 to 25 months of age (i.e., the lower limit of the two-sided 95% CI on the GMT ratio for Group 1/Group 5 and for Group 2/Group 5 were both ≥0.5).

In 3 additional clinical studies (HAV 232, HAV 220, and HAV 231), children received either 2 doses of HAVRIX alone or the first dose of HAVRIX concomitantly administered with other routinely recommended US-licensed vaccines followed by a second dose of HAVRIX. After the second dose of HAVRIX, there was no evidence for interference with the anti-HAV response in the children who received concomitantly administered vaccines compared to those who received HAVRIX alone. *[See Adverse Reactions (6.1) and Clinical Studies (14.5).]*

Immune Response to HAVRIX 360 EL.U. Among Individuals 2 to 18 Years of Age: In 6 clinical studies, 762 subjects 2 to 18 years of age received 2 doses of HAVRIX (360 EL.U.) given 1 month apart (GMT ranged from 197 to 660 mIU/mL). Ninety-nine percent of subjects seroconverted following 2 doses. When a third dose of HAVRIX 360 EL.U. was administered 6 months following the initial dose, all subjects were seropositive (anti-HAV ≥20 mIU/mL) 1 month following the third dose, with GMTs rising to a range of 3,388 to 4,643 mIU/mL. In 1 study in which children were followed for an additional 6 months, all subjects remained seropositive.

Immune Response to HAVRIX 720 EL.U./0.5 mL Among Individuals 2 to 19 Years of Age: In 4 clinical studies, 314 children and adolescents ranging from 2 to 19 years of age were immunized with 2 doses of HAVRIX 720 EL.U./0.5 mL given 6 months apart. One month after the first dose, seroconversion (anti-HAV ≥20 mIU/mL [lower limit of antibody measurement by assay]) ranged from 96.8% to 100%, with GMTs of 194 mIU/mL to 305 mIU/mL. In studies in which sera were obtained 2 weeks following the initial dose, seroconversion ranged from 91.6% to 96.1%. One month following the booster dose at month 6, all subjects were seropositive, with GMTs ranging from 2,495 mIU/mL to 3,644 mIU/mL.

In an additional study in which the booster dose was delayed until 1 year following the initial dose, 95.2% of the subjects were seropositive just prior to administration of the booster dose. One month later, all subjects were seropositive, with a GMT of 2,657 mIU/mL.

14.3 Immunogenicity in Adults

More than 400 healthy adults 18 to 50 years of age in 3 clinical studies were given a single 1440 EL.U. dose of HAVRIX. All subjects were seronegative for hepatitis A antibodies at baseline. Specific humoral antibodies against HAV were elicited in more than 96% of subjects when measured 1 month after vaccination. By day 15, 80% to 98% of vaccinees had already seroconverted (anti-HAV ≥20 mIU/mL [lower limit of antibody measurement by assay]). GMTs of seroconverters ranged from 264 to 339 mIU/mL at day 15 and increased to a range of 335 to 637 mIU/mL by 1 month following vaccination.

The GMTs obtained following a single dose of HAVRIX are at least several times higher than that expected following receipt of immune globulin.

In a clinical study using 2.5 to 5 times the standard dose of immune globulin (standard dose = 0.02 to 0.06 mL/kg), the GMT in recipients was 146 mIU/mL at 5 days post-administration, 77 mIU/mL at month 1, and 63 mIU/mL at month 2.

In 2 clinical trials in which a booster dose of 1440 EL.U. was given 6 months following the initial dose, 100% of vaccinees (n = 269) were seropositive 1 month after the booster dose, with GMTs ranging from 3,318 mIU/mL to 5,925 mIU/mL. The titers obtained from this additional dose approximate those observed several years after natural infection.

In a subset of vaccinees (n = 89), a single dose of HAVRIX 1440 EL.U. elicited specific anti-HAV neutralizing antibodies in more than 94% of vaccinees when measured 1 month after vaccination. These neutralizing antibodies persisted until month 6. One hundred percent of vaccinees had neutralizing antibodies when measured 1 month after a booster dose given at month 6.

Immunogenicity of HAVRIX was studied in subjects with chronic liver disease of various etiologies. 189 healthy adults and 220 adults with either chronic hepatitis B (n = 46), chronic hepatitis C (n = 104), or moderate chronic liver disease of other etiology (n = 70) were vaccinated with HAVRIX 1440 EL.U. on a 0- and 6-month schedule. The last group consisted of alcoholic cirrhosis (n = 17), autoimmune hepatitis (n = 10), chronic hepatitis/cryptogenic cirrhosis (n = 9), hemochromatosis (n = 2), primary biliary cirrhosis (n = 15), primary sclerosing cholangitis (n = 4), and unspecified (n = 13). At each time point, geometric mean antibody titers (GMTs) were lower for subjects with chronic liver disease than for healthy subjects. At month 7, the GMTs ranged from 478 mIU/mL (chronic hepatitis C) to 1,245 mIU/mL (healthy). One month after the first dose, seroconversion rates in adults with chronic liver disease were lower than in healthy adults. However, 1 month after the booster dose at month 6, seroconversion rates were similar in all groups; rates ranged from 94.7% to 98.1%. The relevance of these data to the duration of protection afforded by HAVRIX is unknown.

In subjects with chronic liver disease, local injection site reactions with HAVRIX were similar among all 4 groups, and no serious adverse events attributed to the vaccine were reported in subjects with chronic liver disease.

14.4 Duration of Immunity

The duration of immunity following a complete schedule of immunization with HAVRIX has not been established.

14.5 Immune Response to Concomitantly Administered Vaccines

In 3 clinical studies HAVRIX was administered concomitantly with other routinely recommended US-licensed vaccines: Study HAV 232: Diphtheria and tetanus toxoids and acellular pertussis vaccine adsorbed (INFANRIX, DTaP) and Haemophilus b (Hib) conjugate vaccine (tetanus toxoid conjugate) (manufactured by sanofi pasteur SA); Study HAV 220: Pneumococcal 7-valent conjugate vaccine (PCV-7) (manufactured by Pfizer), and Study HAV 231: MMR and varicella vaccines. *[See Adverse Reactions (6.1).]*

Concomitant Administration With DTaP and Hib Conjugate Vaccine (Study HAV 232): In this US multicenter study, 468 subjects, children 15 months of age were randomized to receive: Group 1) HAVRIX coadministered with INFANRIX and Hib conjugate vaccine (n = 127); Group 2) INFANRIX and Hib conjugate vaccine alone followed by a first dose of HAVRIX one month later (n = 132); or Group 3) HAVRIX alone (n = 135). All subjects received a second dose of HAVRIX alone 6 to 9 months following the first dose. Among subjects in all groups combined, 53% were male; 64% of subjects were white, 12% were black, 6% were Hispanic, and 18% were other racial/ethnic groups.

There was no evidence for reduced antibody response to diphtheria and tetanus toxoids (percentage of subjects with antibody levels ≥0.1 mIU/mL to each antigen), pertussis antigens (percentage of subjects with seroresponse, antibody concentrations ≥5 EL.U./mL in seronegative subjects or post-vaccination antibody concentration ≥2 times the pre-vaccination antibody concentration in seropositive subjects, and GMTs), or Hib (percentage of subjects with antibody levels ≥1 mcg/mL to polyribosyl-ribitol phosphate, PRP) when HAVRIX was administered concomitantly with INFANRIX and Hib conjugate vaccine (Group 1) relative to INFANRIX and Hib conjugate vaccine administered together (Group 2).

Concomitant Administration With Pneumococcal 7-Valent Conjugate Vaccine (Study HAV 220): In this US multicenter study, 433 children 15 months of age were randomized to receive: Group 1) HAVRIX coadministered with PCV-7 vaccine (n = 137); Group 2) HAVRIX administered alone (n = 147); or Group 3) PCV-7 vaccine administered alone (n = 149) followed by a first dose of HAVRIX one month later. All subjects received a second dose of HAVRIX 6 to 9 months after the first dose. Among subjects in all groups combined, 53% were female; 61% of subjects were white, 16% were Hispanic, 15% were black, and 8% were other racial/ethnic groups.

There was no evidence for reduced antibody response to PCV-7 (GMC to each serotype) when HAVRIX was administered concomitantly with PCV-7 vaccine (Group 1) relative to PCV-7 administered alone (Group 3).

Concomitant Administration With MMR and Varicella Vaccines (Study HAV 231): In a US multicenter study, there was no evidence for interference in the immune response to MMR and varicella vaccines (the percentage of subjects with pre-specified seroconversion/seroresponse levels) administered at 15 months of age concomitantly with HAVRIX relative to the response when MMR and varicella vaccines are administered without HAVRIX. *[See Adverse Reactions (6.1).]*

15 REFERENCES

1. Centers for Disease Control and Prevention. Prevention of hepatitis A through active or passive immunization: Recommendations of the Immunization Practices Advisory Committee (ACIP). *MMWR* 2006;55(RR-7):1-23.

16 HOW SUPPLIED/STORAGE AND HANDLING

HAVRIX is available in single-dose vials (contain no latex) and prefilled disposable TIP-LOK syringes (may contain latex) (packaged without needles) (Preservative Free Formulation):

720 EL.U./0.5 mL

NDC 58160-825-01 Vial (contains no latex) in Package of 10: NDC 58160-825-11

NDC 58160-825-43 Syringe (tip cap may contain latex) in Package of 10: NDC 58160-825-52

NDC 58160-825-41 Syringe (tip cap and plunger contain latex) in Package of 10: NDC 58160-825-51

1440 EL.U./mL

NDC 58160-826-01 Vial (contains no latex) in Package of 10: NDC 58160-826-11

NDC 58160-826-05 Syringe (tip cap may contain latex) in Package of 1: NDC 58160-826-34

NDC 58160-826-43 Syringe (tip cap may contain latex) in Package of 5: NDC 58160-826-48

NDC 58160-826-43 Syringe (tip cap may contain latex) in Package of 10: NDC 58160-826-52

NDC 58160-826-32 Syringe (tip cap and plunger contain latex) in Package of 1: NDC 58160-826-32

NDC 58160-826-41 Syringe (tip cap and plunger contain latex) in Package of 5: NDC 58160-826-46
Store refrigerated between 2° and 8°C (36° and 46°F). Do not freeze. Discard if the vaccine has been frozen. Do not dilute to administer.

17 PATIENT COUNSELING INFORMATION

- Inform vaccine recipients and parents or guardians of the potential benefits and risks of immunization with HAVRIX.
- Emphasize, when educating vaccine recipients and parents or guardians regarding potential side effects, that HAVRIX contains non-infectious killed viruses and cannot cause hepatitis A infection.
- Instruct vaccine recipients and parents or guardians to report any adverse events to their healthcare provider.
- Give vaccine recipients and parents or guardians the Vaccine Information Statements, which are required by the National Childhood Vaccine Injury Act of 1986 to be given prior to immunization. These materials are available free of charge at the Centers for Disease Control and Prevention (CDC) website (www.cdc.gov/vaccines).

HAVRIX, ENGERIX-B, INFANRIX, and TIP-LOK are registered trademarks of GlaxoSmithKline.
Manufactured by **GlaxoSmithKline Biologicals**
Rixensart, Belgium, US License No. 1617
Distributed by **GlaxoSmithKline**
Research Triangle Park, NC 27709

HVX:40PI

HYCAMTIN® ℞

[hī-kam' tin]
(topotecan)
Capsules

HIGHLIGHTS OF PRESCRIBING INFORMATION
These highlights do not include all the information needed to use HYCAMTIN safely and effectively. See full prescribing information for HYCAMTIN.
HYCAMTIN® (topotecan) Capsules
Initial U.S. Approval: 1996

> **WARNING: Bone Marrow Suppression**
> ***See full prescribing information for complete boxed warning***
> **HYCAMTIN should be administered only to patients with baseline neutrophil counts of ≥1,500 cells/mm³ and a platelet count ≥100,000 cells/mm³. In order to assess the occurrence of bone marrow suppression, blood cell counts should be monitored.**

RECENT MAJOR CHANGES

Contraindications (4)	10/2011
Warnings and Precautions, Pregnancy (5.4)	10/2011

INDICATIONS AND USAGE

HYCAMTIN is a topoisomerase inhibitor indicated for treatment of patients with relapsed small cell lung cancer. (1)

DOSAGE AND ADMINISTRATION

- 2.3 mg/m²/day orally once daily for 5 consecutive days repeated every 21 days. (2)
- See dose modification guidelines for patients with bone marrow toxicity or Grade 3 or 4 diarrhea. (2.3)

DOSAGE FORMS AND STRENGTHS

0.25 mg and 1 mg capsules. (3)

CONTRAINDICATIONS

- History of severe hypersensitivity reactions (e.g., anaphylactoid reactions) to topotecan or to any of its ingredients. (4)
- Severe bone marrow depression. (4)

WARNINGS AND PRECAUTIONS

- Bone marrow suppression. HYCAMTIN should be administered only to patients with adequate bone marrow reserves. Peripheral blood counts should be monitored. (5.1) Dose may need to be adjusted. (2.3)
- Topotecan-induced neutropenia can lead to neutropenic colitis. (5.1)
- Diarrhea, including severe diarrhea requiring hospitalization, has been reported during treatment with HYCAMTIN capsules. (5.2) Dose may need to be adjusted. (2.3)
- HYCAMTIN has been associated with reports of interstitial lung disease, some of which have been fatal. (5.3)
- Pregnancy: Can cause fetal harm. Advise women of potential risk to the fetus. (5.4, 8.1)

ADVERSE REACTIONS

The most common Grade 3 or 4 hematologic adverse reactions with HYCAMTIN capsules were neutropenia (61%), anemia (25%), and thrombocytopenia (37%). The most common (≥10%) non-hematologic adverse reactions (all grades) were nausea (27%), diarrhea (14%), vomiting (19%), fatigue (11%), and alopecia (10%).

To report SUSPECTED ADVERSE REACTIONS, contact GlaxoSmithKline at 1-888-825-5249 or FDA at 1-800-FDA-1088 or www.fda.gov/medwatch.

DRUG INTERACTIONS

- Patients should be carefully monitored for adverse reactions when HYCAMTIN capsules are administered with a drug known to inhibit ABCG2 (BCRP) or ABCB1 (P-glycoprotein). (7.1)

USE IN SPECIFIC POPULATIONS

- Geriatric use: Among patients who received HYCAMTIN capsules in 4 thoracic cancer studies, drug-related diarrhea was more frequent in patients ≥65 years of age (28%) compared to those <65 years of age (19%). (5.2) (6.1)
- Nursing Mothers: Discontinue nursing when receiving HYCAMTIN. (8.3)

See 17 for PATIENT COUNSELING INFORMATION and FDA-approved patient labeling

Revised: 10/2011

FULL PRESCRIBING INFORMATION: CONTENTS*

*** Sections or subsections omitted from the full prescribing information are not listed**

FULL PRESCRIBING INFORMATION

> **WARNING: Bone Marrow Suppression**
> **HYCAMTIN should be administered only to patients with baseline neutrophil counts of ≥1,500 cells/mm³ and a platelet count ≥100,000 cells/mm³. In order to assess the occurrence of bone marrow suppression, blood cell counts should be monitored.**

1 INDICATIONS AND USAGE

HYCAMTIN capsules are indicated for the treatment of relapsed small cell lung cancer in patients with a prior complete or partial response and who are at least 45 days from the end of first-line chemotherapy.

2 DOSAGE AND ADMINISTRATION

2.1 Recommended Dosing

The recommended dose of HYCAMTIN capsules is 2.3 mg/m²/day once daily for 5 consecutive days repeated every 21 days. Round the calculated oral daily dose to the nearest 0.25 mg, and prescribe the minimum number of 1 mg and 0.25 mg capsules. The same number of capsules should be prescribed for each of the 5 dosing days.

HYCAMTIN capsules may be taken with or without food. The capsules must be swallowed whole and must not be chewed, crushed, or divided. If your patient vomits after taking the dose of HYCAMTIN, the patient should not take a replacement dose.

2.2 Adjustment of Dose in Special Populations

Renal Function Impairment

No dosage adjustment of HYCAMTIN capsules appears to be required for treating patients with mild renal impairment (CLcr = 50-80 mL/min). A dose adjustment of HYCAMTIN capsules to 1.8 mg/m²/day is predicted to adjust the area under the curve (AUC) to the normal range for patients with moderate renal impairment (CLcr = 30-49 mL/min). Insufficient data are available in patients with severe renal impairment (CLcr <30 mL/min) to provide a dosage recommendation for HYCAMTIN capsules *[see Use in Specific Populations (8.6)]*.

2.3 Dose Modification Guidelines

Patients should not be treated with subsequent courses of HYCAMTIN until neutrophils recover to >1,000 cells/mm³, platelets recover to >100,000 cells/mm³, and hemoglobin levels recover to ≥9.0 g/dL (with transfusion if necessary).

For patients who experience severe neutropenia (neutrophils <500 cells/mm³ associated with fever or infection or lasting for 7 days or more) or neutropenia (neutrophils 500 to 1,000 cells/mm³ lasting beyond day 21 of the treatment course), the HYCAMTIN capsules dose should be reduced by 0.4 mg/m²/day for subsequent courses. Doses should be similarly reduced if the platelet count falls below 25,000 cells/mm³.

For patients who experience Grade 3 or 4 diarrhea, the HYCAMTIN capsules dose should be reduced by 0.4 mg/m²/day for subsequent courses *[see Warnings and Precautions (5.2)]*. Patients with Grade 2 diarrhea may need to follow the same dose modification guidelines.

3 DOSAGE FORMS AND STRENGTHS

HYCAMTIN capsules contain topotecan hydrochloride expressed as topotecan free base. The 0.25 mg capsules are opaque white to yellowish-white and imprinted with HYCAMTIN and 0.25 mg. The 1 mg capsules are opaque pink and imprinted with HYCAMTIN and 1 mg.

4 CONTRAINDICATIONS

HYCAMTIN is contraindicated in patients who have a history of severe hypersensitivity reactions (e.g., anaphylactoid reactions) to topotecan or to any of its ingredients. HYCAMTIN should not be used in patients with severe bone marrow depression.

5 WARNINGS AND PRECAUTIONS

5.1 Bone Marrow Suppression

Bone marrow suppression (primarily neutropenia) is a dose-limiting toxicity of HYCAMTIN. Neutropenia is not cumulative over time. The following data on myelosuppression are based on an integrated safety database from 4 thoracic malignancy studies (N = 682) using HYCAMTIN capsules at 2.3 mg/m²/day for 5 consecutive days. The median day for neutrophil, red blood cell, and platelet nadirs occurred on day 15.

Neutropenia

Grade 4 neutropenia (<500 cells/mm³) occurred in 32% of patients with a median duration of 7 days and was most common during course 1 of treatment (20% of patients). Infection, sepsis, and febrile neutropenia occurred in 17%, 2%, and 4% of patients, respectively. Death due to sepsis occurred in 1% of patients. Pancytopenia has been reported. Topotecan-induced neutropenia can lead to neutropenic colitis. Fatalities due to neutropenic colitis have been reported. In patients presenting with fever, neutropenia, and a compatible pattern of abdominal pain, the possibility of neutropenic colitis should be considered. *[See Dosage and Administration (2.3).]*

Thrombocytopenia

Grade 4 thrombocytopenia (<10,000 cells/mm³) occurred in 6% of patients, with a median duration of 3 days.

Anemia

Grade 3 or 4 anemia (<8 g/dL) occurred in 25% of patients.

Monitoring of Bone Marrow Function

HYCAMTIN should be administered only in patients with adequate bone marrow reserves, including a baseline neutrophil count of ≥1,500 cells/mm^3 and a platelet count ≥100,000 cells/mm^3. Frequent monitoring of peripheral blood cell counts should be instituted during treatment with HYCAMTIN.

5.2 Diarrhea

Diarrhea, including severe diarrhea requiring hospitalization, has been reported during treatment with HYCAMTIN capsules. Diarrhea related to HYCAMTIN capsules can occur at the same time as drug-related neutropenia and its sequelae. Communication with patients prior to drug administration regarding these side effects and proactive management of early and all signs and symptoms of diarrhea is important. Treatment-related diarrhea is associated with significant morbidity and may be life-threatening. Should diarrhea occur during treatment with HYCAMTIN capsules, physicians are advised to aggressively manage diarrhea. Clinical guidelines describing the aggressive management of diarrhea include specific recommendations on patient communication and awareness, recognition of early warning signs, use of anti-diarrheals and antibiotics, changes in fluid intake and diet, and need for hospitalization.

Of the 682 patients who received HYCAMTIN capsules in the 4 thoracic cancer studies, the overall incidence of drug-related diarrhea was 22%, including 4% with Grade 3 and 0.4% with Grade 4. Drug-related diarrhea was more frequent in patients ≥65 years of age (28%) compared to those <65 years of age (19%). *[See Adverse Reactions (6.1) and Use in Specific Populations (8.5).]*

5.3 Interstitial Lung Disease

HYCAMTIN has been associated with reports of interstitial lung disease (ILD), some of which have been fatal *[see Adverse Reactions (6.2)]*. Underlying risk factors include history of ILD, pulmonary fibrosis, lung cancer, thoracic exposure to radiation, and use of pneumotoxic drugs and/or colony stimulating factors. Patients should be monitored for pulmonary symptoms indicative of interstitial lung disease (e.g., cough, fever, dyspnea, and/or hypoxia), and HYCAMTIN should be discontinued if a new diagnosis of ILD is confirmed.

5.4 Pregnancy

Pregnancy Category D

HYCAMTIN can cause fetal harm when administered to a pregnant woman. Topotecan caused embryolethality, fetotoxicity, and teratogenicity in rats and rabbits when administered during organogenesis. There are no adequate and well controlled studies of HYCAMTIN in pregnant women. If this drug is used during pregnancy, or if a patient becomes pregnant while taking this drug, the patient should be apprised of the potential hazard to the fetus *[see Use in Specific Populations, Pregnancy (8.1)]*.

5.5 Drug Interactions

P-glycoprotein inhibitors (e.g., cyclosporine A, elacridar, ketoconazole, ritonavir, and saquinavir) can cause significant increases in topotecan exposure. The concomitant use of P-glycoprotein inhibitors with HYCAMTIN capsules should be avoided. *[See Drug Interactions (7.1).]*

6 ADVERSE REACTIONS

6.1 Clinical Trials Experience

The safety of HYCAMTIN capsules has been evaluated in 682 patients with thoracic cancer (3 recurrent small cell lung cancer [SCLC] studies and 1 recurrent non-small cell lung cancer [NSCLC] study) who received at least one dose of HYCAMTIN capsules. Because clinical trials are conducted under widely varying conditions, adverse reaction rates observed in the clinical trials of a drug cannot be directly compared to rates in the clinical trials of another drug and may not reflect the rates observed in practice.

Table 1 describes the hematologic and non-hematologic adverse reactions in recurrent SCLC patients treated with HYCAMTIN capsules plus best supportive care (BSC) and in the overall thoracic cancer patient population.

[See table 1 above]

Table 1. Incidence (≥5%) of Adverse Reactions in Small Cell Lung Cancer Patients Treated With HYCAMTIN Capsules Plus BSC and in 4 Thoracic Cancer Studies

	HYCAMTIN Capsules + BSC (N = 70)			HYCAMTIN Capsules Thoracic Cancer Population (N = 682)		
Adverse Reaction	**All Grades (%)**	**Grade 3 (%)**	**Grade 4 (%)**	**All Grades (%)**	**Grade 3 (%)**	**Grade 4 (%)**
Hematologic						
Anemia	94	15	10	98	18	7
Leukopenia	90	25	16	86	29	15
Neutropenia	91	28	33	83	24	32
Thrombocytopenia	81	30	7	81	29	6
Non-hematologic						
Nausea	27	1	0	33	3	0
Diarrhea	14	4	1	22	4	0.4
Vomiting	19	1	0	21	3	0.4
Alopecia	10	0	0	20	0.1	0
Fatigue	11	0	0	19	4	0.1
Anorexia	7	0	0	14	2	0
Asthenia	3	0	0	7	2	0
Pyrexia	7	1	0	5	1	1

BSC = Best Supportive Care.
N = total number of patients treated.
Adverse reactions were graded using NCI Common Toxicity Criteria.

Diarrhea Adverse Reactions

Of the 70 patients who received HYCAMTIN capsules plus BSC, the incidence of drug-related diarrhea was 14%, with 4% Grade 3 and 1% Grade 4.

In the 682 patients who received HYCAMTIN capsules in the 4 thoracic cancer studies, the incidence of drug-related diarrhea was 22%, with 4% Grade 3 and 0.4% Grade 4. The overall incidence of drug-related diarrhea was more frequent in patients ≥65 years of age (28%, n = 225) with 10% Grade 1, 9% Grade 2, 7% Grade 3, and 1% Grade 4 compared to those <65 years of age (19%, n = 457) with 7% Grade 1, 9% Grade 2, 3% Grade 3, and 0% Grade 4. The incidence of Grade 3 or 4 diarrhea proximate (within 5 days) to Grade 3 or 4 neutropenia events in the HYCAMTIN capsules treatment group was 5%. The median time to onset of Grade 2 or worse diarrhea was 9 days in the HYCAMTIN capsules group.

Deaths Occurring Within 30 Days Following the Last Dose of Study Medication

In the 682 patients who received HYCAMTIN capsules in the 4 thoracic cancer studies, 39 deaths occurred within 30 days after the last dose of study medication for a reason other than progressive disease; 13 of these deaths were attributed to hematologic toxicity, 5 were attributed to nonhematologic toxicity, and 21 were attributed to other causes. One patient death (68 years of age) was attributed to treatment-related diarrhea and one death (68 years of age) attributed diarrhea as a contributory event; both patients received HYCAMTIN capsules.

In addition to the adverse reactions listed previously, the following adverse reactions have been reported with HYCAMTIN for Injection:

- Incidence >10%: Febrile neutropenia, abdominal pain, stomatitis, constipation.
- Incidence 1 to 10%: Sepsis, hypersensitivity (including rash), hyperbilirubinemia, malaise.

6.2 Postmarketing Experience

There is no postmarketing experience with HYCAMTIN capsules. The following adverse reactions have been identified during post-approval use of HYCAMTIN for Injection. Because these reactions are reported voluntarily from a population of uncertain size, it is not always possible to reliably estimate their frequency or establish a causal relationship to drug exposure.

Blood and lymphatic system disorders: Severe bleeding (in association with thrombocytopenia).

Immune system disorders: Allergic manifestations, anaphylactoid reactions.

Respiratory, thoracic, and mediastinal disorders: Interstitial lung disease.

Gastrointestinal disorders: Abdominal pain potentially associated with neutropenic colitis *[see Warnings and Precautions (5.1)]*.

Skin and subcutaneous tissue disorders: Angioedema, severe dermatitis, severe pruritus.

7 DRUG INTERACTIONS

7.1 Drugs That Inhibit Drug Efflux Transporters

Topotecan is a substrate for both ABCB1 [P-glycoprotein (P-gp)] and ABCG2 (BCRP). Elacridar (inhibitor of ABCB1 and ABCG2) administered with HYCAMTIN capsules increased topotecan exposure to approximately 2.5-fold of control. Cyclosporine A (inhibitor of ABCB1, ABCC1 [MRP-1], and CYP3A4) with HYCAMTIN capsules increased topotecan exposure to 2- to 3-fold of control. Patients should be carefully monitored for adverse reactions when HYCAMTIN capsules are administered with a drug known to inhibit these transporters. *[See Clinical Pharmacology (12.3).]*

7.2 Effects of Topotecan on Drug Metabolizing Enzymes

In vitro inhibition studies using marker substrates known to be metabolized by human cytochromes P450 (CYP1A2, CYP2A6, CYP2C8/9, CYP2C19, CYP2D6, CYP2E, CYP3A, or CYP4A) or dihydropyrimidine dehydrogenase indicate that the activities of these enzymes were not altered by topotecan. Enzyme inhibition by topotecan has not been evaluated in vivo.

7.3 Effects of Other Drugs on Topotecan Pharmacokinetics

The pharmacokinetics of topotecan were generally unchanged when coadministered with ranitidine.

8 USE IN SPECIFIC POPULATIONS

8.1 Pregnancy

Pregnancy Category D. *[See Warnings and Precautions (5.4).]*

HYCAMTIN can cause fetal harm when administered to a pregnant woman. In rabbits, an IV dose of 0.10 mg/kg/day (about equal to the clinical IV dose on a mg/m^2 basis) given on days 6 through 20 of gestation caused maternal toxicity, embryolethality, and reduced fetal body weight. In the rat, an IV dose of 0.23 mg/kg/day (about equal to the clinical IV dose on a mg/m^2 basis) given for 14 days before mating through gestation day 6 caused fetal resorption, microphthalmia, pre-implant loss, and mild maternal toxicity. An IV dose of 0.10 mg/kg/day (about half the clinical IV dose on a mg/m^2 basis) given to rats on days 6 through 17 of gestation caused an increase in post-implantation mortality. This dose also caused an increase in total fetal malformations. The most frequent malformations were of the eye (microphthalmia, anophthalmia, rosette formation of the retina, coloboma of the retina, ectopic orbit), brain (dilated lateral and third ventricles), skull, and vertebrae.

There are no adequate and well controlled studies of HYCAMTIN in pregnant women. If this drug is used during pregnancy, or if a patient becomes pregnant while taking this drug, the patient should be apprised of the potential hazard to the fetus.

8.3 Nursing Mothers

Rats excrete high concentrations of topotecan into milk. Lactating female rats given 4.72 mg/m^2 IV (about twice the clinical dose on a mg/m^2 basis) excreted topotecan into milk at concentrations up to 48-fold higher than those in plasma. It is not known whether the drug is excreted in human milk. Because many drugs are excreted in human milk, and because of the potential for serious adverse reactions in nursing infants from HYCAMTIN, discontinue breastfeeding when women are receiving HYCAMTIN.

8.4 Pediatric Use

Safety and effectiveness in pediatric patients have not been established.

8.5 Geriatric Use

Of the 682 patients with thoracic cancer in 4 clinical studies who received HYCAMTIN capsules, 33% (n = 225) were 65 years of age and older, while 4.8% (n = 33) were 75 years of age and older. Treatment-related diarrhea was more frequent in patients ≥65 years of age (28%) compared to those <65 years of age (19%). *[See Warnings and Precautions (5.2) and Adverse Reactions (6.1).]* Among patients ≥65 years of age, those receiving HYCAMTIN capsules plus BSC showed a survival benefit compared to those receiving BSC alone.

There were no apparent differences in the pharmacokinetics of topotecan in elderly patients with creatinine clearance of ≥60 mL/minute *[see Clinical Pharmacology (12.3)]*.

This drug is known to be excreted by the kidney, and the risk of toxic reactions to this drug may be greater in patients with impaired renal function *[see Dosage and Administration (2.2)]*.

8.6 Renal Impairment

A cross-study analysis of data collected from 217 patients with advanced solid tumors indicated that exposure ($AUC_{0-\infty}$) to topotecan lactone, the pharmacologically active moiety, was 10% and 20% higher in patients with mild renal (CLcr = 50-80 mL/min) and moderate renal (CLcr = 30-49 mL/min) impairment, respectively, than in patients with normal renal function (CLcr >80 mL/min) *[see Dosage and Administration (2.2)]*.

8.7 Hepatic Impairment

In a population pharmacokinetic analysis involving oral topotecan administered at doses of 0.15-2.7 mg/m^2/day to 118 cancer patients, the pharmacokinetics of total topotecan did not differ significantly based on patient serum bilirubin, ALT, or AST. No dosage adjustment appeared to be required for patients with impaired hepatic function (serum bilirubin of >1.5 mg/dL).

10 OVERDOSAGE

There is no known antidote for overdosage with HYCAMTIN capsules. The primary anticipated complication of overdosage would consist of hematological toxicity. The patient should be observed closely for bone marrow suppression, and supportive measures (such as the prophylactic use of G-CSF and/or antibiotic therapy) should be considered.

11 DESCRIPTION

Topotecan hydrochloride is a semi-synthetic derivative of camptothecin and is an anti-tumor drug with topoisomerase I-inhibitory activity.

The chemical name for topotecan hydrochloride is (*S*)-10-[(dimethylamino)methyl]-4-ethyl-4,9-dihydroxy-1*H*-pyrano[3′,4′:6,7] indolizino [1,2-*b*]quinoline-3,14-(4*H*,12*H*)-dione monohydrochloride. It has the molecular formula $C_{23}H_{23}N_3O_5$•HCl and a molecular weight of 457.9. It is soluble in water and melts with decomposition at 213° to 218°C.

Topotecan hydrochloride has the following structural formula:

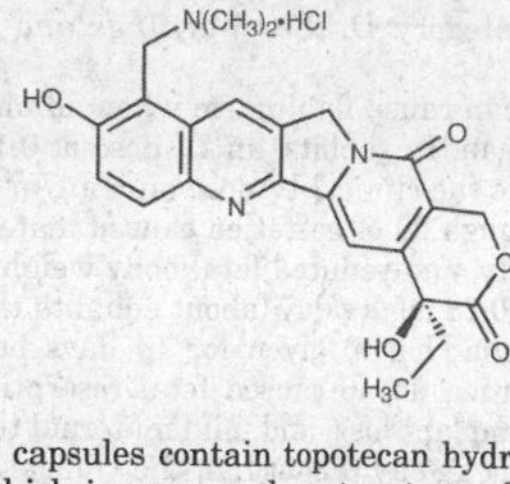

HYCAMTIN capsules contain topotecan hydrochloride, the content of which is expressed as topotecan free base. The major excipients are hydrogenated vegetable oil, glyceryl monostearate, gelatin, and titanium dioxide. The capsules are imprinted with edible black ink. The 1 mg capsules also contain red iron oxide.

12 CLINICAL PHARMACOLOGY

12.1 Mechanism of Action

Topoisomerase I relieves torsional strain in DNA by inducing reversible single strand breaks. Topotecan binds to the topoisomerase I-DNA complex and prevents religation of these single strand breaks. The cytotoxicity of topotecan is thought to be due to double strand DNA damage produced during DNA synthesis, when replication enzymes interact with the ternary complex formed by topotecan, topoisomerase I, and DNA. Mammalian cells cannot efficiently repair these double strand breaks.

12.2 Pharmacodynamics

The dose-limiting toxicity of topotecan is leukopenia. White blood cell count decreases with increasing topotecan dose or topotecan AUC. There is a correlation between topotecan lactone AUC day 1 and percent decrease of leukocytes.

12.3 Pharmacokinetics

The pharmacokinetics of HYCAMTIN capsules after oral administration have been evaluated in cancer patients following doses of 1.2 to 3.1 mg/m^2 administered daily for 5 days. Topotecan exhibits biexponential pharmacokinetics with a mean terminal half-life of 3 to 6 hours. Total exposure (AUC) increases approximately proportionally with dose. Plasma protein binding of topotecan is about 35%.

Absorption

Topotecan is rapidly absorbed with peak plasma concentrations occurring between 1 to 2 hours following oral administration. The oral bioavailability of topotecan was about 40%. Following a high-fat meal, the extent of exposure was similar in the fed and fasted states, while t_{max} was delayed from 1.5 to 3 hours (topotecan lactone) and from 3 to 4 hours (total topotecan), respectively. HYCAMTIN capsules can be given without regard to food.

Following coadministration of the ABCG2 (BCRP) and ABCB1 (P-gp) inhibitor elacridar (GF120918) at 100 to 1,000 mg doses with oral topotecan, the $AUC_{0-\infty}$ of topotecan lactone and total topotecan increased approximately 2.5-fold.

Administration of oral cyclosporine A (15 mg/kg), an inhibitor of transporters ABCB1 (P-gp) and ABCC1 (MRP-1) as well as the metabolizing enzyme CYP3A4, within 4 hours of oral topotecan increased the dose-normalized AUC_{0-24} of topotecan lactone and total topotecan to 2.0- to 3-fold of control. *[See Drug Interactions (7.1).]*

Metabolism and Elimination

Topotecan undergoes a reversible pH-dependent hydrolysis of its lactone moiety; it is the lactone form that is pharmacologically active. At pH ≤4, the lactone is exclusively present, whereas the ring-opened hydroxy-acid form predominates at physiologic pH. The mean metabolite:parent AUC ratio was <10% for total topotecan and topotecan lactone.

In a mass balance study in 4 patients with advanced solid tumors, the overall recovery of drug-related material following 5 daily doses of topotecan was 57% of the administered oral dose. In the urine, 20% of the oral administered dose was excreted as total topotecan and 2% was excreted as N-desmethyl topotecan *[see Use in Specific Populations (8.6)]*. Fecal elimination of total topotecan accounted for 33% while fecal elimination of N-desmethyl topotecan was 1.5%. Overall, the N-desmethyl metabolite contributed a mean of <6% (range 4 to 8%) of the total drug-related material accounted for in the urine and feces. O-glucuronides of both topotecan and N-desmethyl topotecan have been identified in the urine.

Age, Gender, and Race

A cross-study analysis in 217 patients with advanced solid tumors indicated that age and gender did not significantly affect the pharmacokinetics of oral topotecan. There are insufficient data to determine an effect of race on pharmacokinetics of oral topotecan.

13 NONCLINICAL TOXICOLOGY

13.1 Carcinogenesis, Mutagenesis, Impairment of Fertility

Carcinogenicity testing of topotecan has not been done. Nevertheless, topotecan is known to be genotoxic to mammalian cells and is a probable carcinogen. Topotecan was mutagenic to L5178Y mouse lymphoma cells and clastogenic to cultured human lymphocytes with and without metabolic activation. It was also clastogenic to mouse bone marrow. Topotecan did not cause mutations in bacterial cells.

Topotecan given to female rats prior to mating at a dose of 1.4 mg/m^2 IV (about 3/5th of the oral clinical dose on a mg/m^2 basis) caused superovulation possibly related to inhibition of follicular atresia. This dose given to pregnant female rats also caused increased pre-implantation loss. Studies in dogs given 0.4 mg/m^2 IV (about 1/6th the oral clinical dose on a mg/m^2 basis) of topotecan daily for a month suggest that treatment may cause an increase in the incidence of multinucleated spermatogonial giant cells in the testes. Topotecan may impair fertility in women and men.

14 CLINICAL STUDIES

14.1 Small Cell Lung Cancer

HYCAMTIN capsules were studied in patients with relapsed SCLC in a randomized, comparative, open label trial. The patients were prior responders (complete or partial) to first-line chemotherapy, were not considered candidates for standard intravenous chemotherapy, and had relapsed at least 45 days from the end of first-line chemotherapy. Seventy-one patients were randomized to HYCAMTIN capsules (2.3 mg/m^2/day administered for 5 consecutive days repeated every 21 days) and Best Supportive Care (BSC) and 70 patients were randomized to BSC alone. The primary objective was to compare the overall survival between the 2 treatment arms. Patients in the HYCAMTIN capsules plus BSC group received a median of 4 courses (range 1 to 10) and maintained a median dose intensity of HYCAMTIN capsules, 3.77 mg/m^2/week. The median patient age in the HYCAMTIN capsules plus BSC arm and the BSC alone treatment arm was 60 years and 58 years while the percentage of patients ≥65 years of age was 34% and 29%, respectively. All but 1 patient were Caucasian. The HYCAMTIN capsules plus BSC treatment arm included 68% of patients with extensive disease and 28% with liver metastasis. In the BSC alone arm, 61% of patients had extensive disease and 20% had liver metastases. Both treatment arms recruited 73% males. In the HYCAMTIN capsules plus BSC arm, 18% of patients had prior carboplatin and 62% had prior cisplatin. In the BSC alone arm, 26% of patients had prior carboplatin and 51% had prior cisplatin.

The HYCAMTIN capsules plus BSC arm showed a statistically significant improvement in overall survival compared with the BSC alone arm (Log-rank p = 0.0104). Survival results are shown in Table 2 and Figure 1.

Table 2. Overall Survival in Small Cell Lung Cancer Patients With HYCAMTIN Capsules Plus BSC Compared With BSC Alone

	Treatment Group	
	HYCAMTIN Capsules + BSC (N = 71)	BSC (N = 70)
Median (weeks) (95% CI)	25.9 (18.3, 31.6)	13.9 (11.1, 18.6)
Hazard ratio (95% CI)	0.64 (0.45, 0.90)	
Log-rank p-value	0.0104	

BSC = Best Supportive Care.
N = total number of patients randomized.
CI = Confidence Interval.

Figure 1. Kaplan-Meier Estimates for Survival

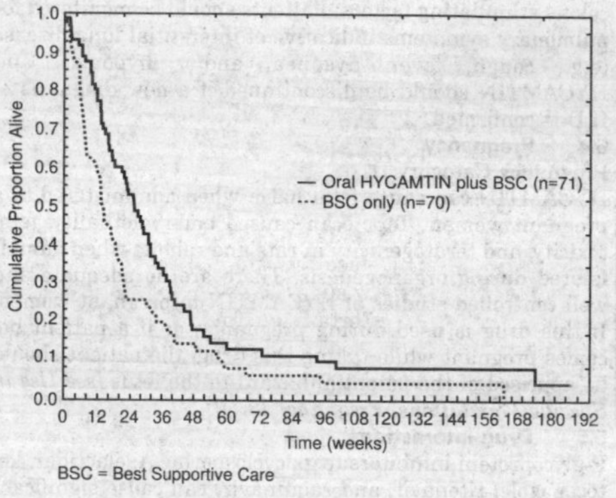

BSC = Best Supportive Care

15 REFERENCES

1. The National Institute for Occupational Safety and Health. NIOSH Alert. Preventing Occupational Exposures to Antineoplastic and Other Hazardous Drugs in Health Care Settings. Available at: www.cdc.gov/niosh/docs/2004-165/ Accessed October 2, 2007.
2. Occupational Safety and Health Administration. Controlling Occupational Exposure to Hazardous Drugs. OSHA Technical Manual, TED 1-0.15A. Section VI: Chapter 2. Available at: www.osha.gov/dts/osta/otm/otm_vi/otm_vi_2.html Accessed October 2, 2007.
3. American Society of Health-System Pharmacists. ASHP Guidelines on Handling Hazardous Drugs. *Am J Health-Syst Pharm.* 2006;63:1172-1193.
4. Polovich, M., White, J.M., Kelleher, L.O., eds. *Chemotherapy and Biotherapy Guidelines and Recommendations for Practice.* 2nd ed. Pittsburgh, PA: Oncology Nursing Society: 2005.

16 HOW SUPPLIED/STORAGE AND HANDLING

The 0.25 mg HYCAMTIN capsules are opaque white to yellowish-white imprinted with HYCAMTIN and 0.25 mg and are available in bottles of 10: NDC 0007-4205-11.

The 1 mg HYCAMTIN capsules are opaque pink imprinted with HYCAMTIN and 1 mg and are available in bottles of 10: NDC 0007-4207-11.

Store refrigerated 2° to 8°C (36° to 46°F). Store the bottles protected from light in the original outer cartons.

Procedures for proper handling and disposal of anticancer drugs should be used. Several guidelines on this subject have been published.[1-4]

HYCAMTIN capsules should not be opened or crushed. Direct contact of the capsule contents with the skin or mucous membranes should be avoided. If such contacts occur, wash thoroughly with soap and water or wash the eyes immediately with gently flowing water for at least 15 minutes. Consult the healthcare provider in case of a skin reaction or if the drug gets in the eyes.

17 PATIENT COUNSELING INFORMATION

See FDA-approved patient labeling (17.4).

17.1 Bone Marrow Suppression

Patients should be informed that HYCAMTIN decreases blood cell counts such as white blood cells, platelets, and red blood cells. Patients who develop fever or other signs of infection such as chills, cough, or burning pain on urination while on therapy should notify their physician promptly. Patients should be told that frequent blood tests will be performed while taking HYCAMTIN to monitor for the occurrence of bone marrow suppression.

17.2 Pregnancy

Patients should be advised to use effective contraceptive measures to prevent pregnancy and to avoid breastfeeding during treatment with HYCAMTIN.

17.3 Diarrhea

Patients should be informed that HYCAMTIN capsules cause diarrhea which may be severe in some cases. Patients should be told how to manage and/or prevent diarrhea and to inform their physician if severe diarrhea occurs during treatment with HYCAMTIN capsules.

17.4 FDA-Approved Patient Labeling

See separate leaflet.

HYCAMTIN is a registered trademark of GlaxoSmithKline.

GlaxoSmithKline
Research Triangle Park, NC 27709

October 2011
HYC:5PI

PATIENT INFORMATION
HYCAMTIN® (hi-CAM-tin)
(topotecan) Capsules

Read the Patient Information that comes with HYCAMTIN capsules before you start taking it and each time you get a refill. There may be new information. This information does not take the place of talking with your healthcare provider about your medical condition or treatment.

What is the most important information I should know about taking HYCAMTIN capsules?

HYCAMTIN capsules can cause serious side effects:

Decreased blood counts. Taking HYCAMTIN affects your bone marrow and can cause a severe decrease in your blood cell counts (bone marrow suppression) - neutrophils (a type of white blood cell important in fighting bacterial infections), red blood cells (blood cells that carry oxygen to the tissues), and platelets (important for clotting and control of bleeding).

- You should have blood tests regularly to check your blood counts. A decrease in neutrophils (neutropenia) may affect how your body fights infection.
- Your healthcare provider will tell you if your blood counts are too low before you begin treatment with HYCAMTIN.
- Your dose of HYCAMTIN may need to be changed or stopped until your blood counts recover enough after each cycle of treatment.
- Call your healthcare provider right away if you get any of the following signs of infection:
  - fever (temperature of 100.5°F or greater)
  - chills
  - cough
  - burning or pain on urination
- Tell your healthcare provider about any abnormal bleeding or bruising.

Diarrhea. Diarrhea may occur from taking HYCAMTIN capsules, and may be serious enough that you must be treated in the hospital. Tell your healthcare provider right away if you have:

- diarrhea with fever
- diarrhea 3 or more times a day
- diarrhea with stomach-area pain or cramps

See "What are the possible side effects of HYCAMTIN capsules?"

What are HYCAMTIN capsules?

HYCAMTIN capsules are prescription medicines you take by mouth. HYCAMTIN capsules are used to treat a certain type of lung cancer called small cell lung cancer.

HYCAMTIN capsules may be right for you if:

- your cancer responded to your first chemotherapy
- your cancer came back at least 45 days after you finished your last dose of chemotherapy

It is not known if HYCAMTIN is safe and effective in children.

Who should not take HYCAMTIN capsules?

Do not take HYCAMTIN capsules if:

- you are allergic to anything in HYCAMTIN capsules. See the end of this leaflet for a complete list of ingredients in HYCAMTIN capsules.
- the results of your last blood test show blood counts that are too low. Your healthcare provider will tell you.

What else should I tell my healthcare provider before taking HYCAMTIN capsules?

Before you take HYCAMTIN capsules, tell your healthcare provider if you:

- are pregnant or may become pregnant. HYCAMTIN capsules may harm your unborn baby. You should not become pregant while you are taking HYCAMTIN capsules.
- are breastfeeding or plan to breastfeed. It is not known if HYCAMTIN passes into your breast milk or if it can harm your baby. You and your healthcare provider should decide if you will take HYCAMTIN or breast feed. You should not do both.
- **Tell your healthcare provider about all the medicines you take,** including prescription and non-prescription medicines, vitamins, and herbal supplements. HYCAMTIN capsules and other medicines may affect each other causing side effects. Especially tell your healthcare provider if you are taking cyclosporine (SANDIMMUNE®, GENGRAF®, NEORAL®), ketoconazole (NIZORAL®, EXTINA®), ritonavir (NORVIR®, KALETRA®), saquinavir (INVIRASE®).
- Know your medicines. Keep a list of your medicines and show it to your healthcare provider and pharmacist when you get a new medicine.

How should I take HYCAMTIN capsules?

- **Take HYCAMTIN capsules exactly as your doctor prescribes them.**
- Your healthcare provider may want you to take both 1 mg and 0.25 mg capsules together to make up your complete dose. You must be able to tell the difference between the capsules. The 1 mg capsule is a pink color and the 0.25 mg capsule is a white to yellowish-white color.
- Take HYCAMTIN capsules once a day for 5 days in a row. This treatment will normally be repeated every 3 weeks (a treatment cycle). Your healthcare provider will decide how long you will take HYCAMTIN capsules.
- Swallow HYCAMTIN capsules whole with water. Do not open, chew, or crush HYCAMTIN capsules. HYCAMTIN capsules may be taken with or without food.
- If any of the HYCAMTIN capsules are broken or leaking, do not touch them with your bare hands. Carefully dispose of the capsules, and then wash your hands well with soap and water.
- If you get any of the contents of HYCAMTIN capsules on your skin or in your eyes, do the following:
  - Wash the area of skin well with soap and water right away,
  - Wash your eyes right away with gently flowing water for at least 15 minutes.
  - Call your healthcare provider if you get a skin reaction or if you get the medicine in your eyes.
- If you take too much HYCAMTIN, contact your healthcare provider right away.
- If you forget to take HYCAMTIN at any time, do not double the dose to make up for a forgotten dose. Wait and take the next scheduled dose. Let your healthcare provider know that you missed a dose.
- If you vomit after taking your HYCAMTIN, do not take another dose on the same day. Let your healthcare provider know right away that you have vomited.

What should I avoid while taking HYCAMTIN capsules?

HYCAMTIN may make you feel drowsy or sleepy both during and for several days after treatment. If you feel tired or weak, do not drive and do not use heavy tools or operate machinery.

What are the possible side effects of HYCAMTIN capsules?

HYCAMTIN can cause serious side effects including:

- See "What is the most important information I should know about HYCAMTIN capsules?"
- Lung problems that can cause death. Tell your healthcare provider right away if you have **new or worse** symptoms of coughing, fever, shortness of breath, or problems breathing. Your healthcare provider may tell you to stop taking HYCAMTIN capsules.

The following side effects have been reported in patients taking HYCAMTIN capsules:

- stomach problems such as nausea (feeling sick) and vomiting
- tiredness
- hair loss
- weakness

Tell your healthcare provider if you have any side effect that bothers you or does not go away. Your healthcare provider may change your dose of HYCAMTIN to a dose that is better for you or may stop your treatment with HYCAMTIN for a while. This can help reduce the side effects and may keep them from getting worse. Let your healthcare provider know if this helps or does not help your side effects.

These are not all of the possible side effects of HYCAMTIN capsules. For more information, ask your doctor or pharmacist.

Call your doctor for medical advice about side effects. You may report side effects to FDA at 1-800-FDA-1088.

How should I store HYCAMTIN capsules?

- Store HYCAMTIN capsules in a refrigerator between 36° to 46°F (2° and 8°C).
- Keep the bottle of HYCAMTIN capsules in the carton that it comes in to protect it from light.
- Dispose of HYCAMTIN capsules that are out of date or no longer needed.
- **Keep HYCAMTIN capsules and all other medicines out of the reach of children.**

What are the ingredients in HYCAMTIN capsules?

Active Ingredient: Topotecan

Inactive Ingredients: Hydrogenated vegetable oil, glyceryl monostearate, gelatin, and titanium dioxide. The 1 mg capsules also contain red iron oxide. The capsules are imprinted with edible black ink.

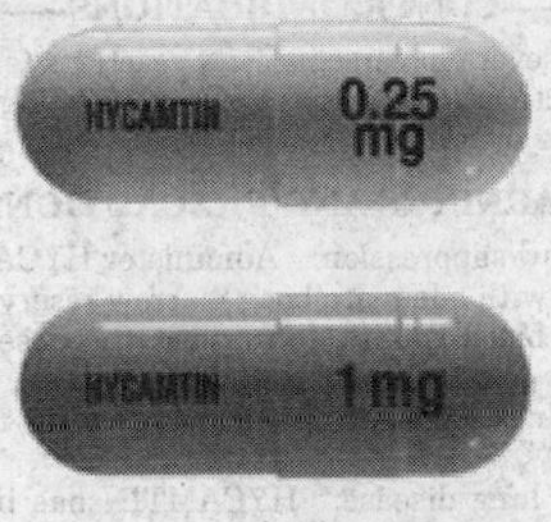

(capsules shown larger than actual size)

General information about HYCAMTIN capsules

Medicines are sometimes prescribed for conditions that are not mentioned in Patient Information leaflets. Only your doctor knows what treatment is best for you. Do not use HYCAMTIN capsules for a condition for which it was not prescribed by your healthcare provider. Do not give HYCAMTIN capsules to other people, even if they have the same condition that you have. It may harm them.

This leaflet summarizes the most important information about HYCAMTIN capsules. If you would like more information, talk with your healthcare provider. You can ask your pharmacist or healthcare provider for information about HYCAMTIN capsules that is written for health professionals. For more information you can call toll-free 1-888-825-5249 or visit www.gsk.com.

This patient information leaflet has been approved by the US Food and Drug Administration.

HYCAMTIN is a registered trademark of GlaxoSmithKline.

The following are registered trademarks of their respective owners: GENGRAF, KALETRA, and NORVIR/Abbott Laboratories; INVIRASE/Genentech; NIZORAL/Janssen Pharmaceuticals; NEORAL and SANDIMMUNE/Novartis Pharmaceuticals Corporation; EXTINA/Stiefel Laboratories.

GlaxoSmithKline
Research Triangle Park, NC 27709

October 2011
HYC:5PIL

HYCAMTIN® ℞

[hī-kam'tin]
(topotecan hydrochloride)
for Injection

HIGHLIGHTS OF PRESCRIBING INFORMATION

These highlights do not include all the information needed to use HYCAMTIN safely and effectively. See full prescribing information for HYCAMTIN.

HYCAMTIN® (topotecan hydrochloride) for Injection
Initial U.S. Approval: 1996

> **WARNING: BONE MARROW SUPPRESSION**
> ***See full prescribing information for complete boxed warning***
> **Do not give HYCAMTIN to patients with baseline neutrophil counts less than 1,500 cells/mm³. In order to monitor the occurrence of bone marrow suppression, primarily neutropenia, which may be severe and result in infection and death, monitor peripheral blood cell counts frequently on all patients receiving HYCAMTIN. (5.1)**

INDICATIONS AND USAGE

HYCAMTIN for Injection is a topoisomerase inhibitor indicated for:

- metastatic carcinoma of the ovary after failure of initial or subsequent chemotherapy. (1)
- small cell lung cancer sensitive disease after failure of first-line chemotherapy. (1)
- combination therapy with cisplatin for stage IV-B, recurrent, or persistent carcinoma of the cervix which is not amenable to curative treatment with surgery and/or radiation therapy. (1)

DOSAGE AND ADMINISTRATION

- Ovarian cancer and small cell lung cancer: 1.5mg/m^2 by intravenous infusion over 30 minutes daily for 5 consecutive days, starting on day one of a 21-day course. (2.1)
- Cervical cancer: 0.75mg/m^2 by intravenous infusion over 30 minutes on days 1, 2, and 3 followed by cisplatin 50mg/m^2 by intravenous infusion on day 1 repeated every 21 days. (2.2)

See Dosage Modification Guidelines for patients with neutropenia or reduced platelets. (2.1, 2.2)
See Dosage Adjustment in Renal Impairment. (2.3)

DOSAGE FORMS AND STRENGTHS

4-mg (free base) single-dose vial. (3)

CONTRAINDICATIONS

- History of severe hypersensitivity reactions (e.g., anaphylactoid reactions) to topotecan or any of its ingredients (4)
- Severe bone marrow depression (4)

WARNINGS AND PRECAUTIONS

- Bone marrow suppression: Administer HYCAMTIN only to patients with adequate bone marrow reserves. Monitor peripheral blood counts and adjust the dose if needed. (5.1)
- Topotecan-induced neutropenia can lead to neutropenic colitis. (5.2)
- Interstitial lung disease: HYCAMTIN has been associated with reports of interstitial lung disease. Monitor patients for symptoms and discontinue HYCAMTIN if the diagnosis is confirmed. (5.3)
- Pregnancy: Can cause fetal harm. Advise women of potential risk to the fetus. (5.4, 8.1)

ADVERSE REACTIONS

Ovarian and small cell lung cancer:

- The most common hematologic adverse reactions were: neutropenia (97%), leukopenia (97%), anemia (89%), and thrombocytopenia (69%). (6.1)
- The most common (>25%) non-hematologic adverse reactions (all grades) were: nausea, alopecia, vomiting, sepsis or pyrexia/infection with neutropenia, diarrhea, constipation, fatigue, and pyrexia. (6.1)

Cervical cancer (HYCAMTIN plus cisplatin):

- The most common hematologic adverse reactions (all grades) were: anemia (94%), leukopenia (91%), neutropenia (89%), and thrombocytopenia (74%). (6.1)
- The most common (>25%) non-hematologic adverse reactions (all grades) were: pain, nausea, vomiting, and infection/febrile neutropenia. (6.1)

To report SUSPECTED ADVERSE REACTIONS, contact GlaxoSmithKline at 1-888-825-5249 or FDA at 1-800-FDA-1088 or www.fda.gov/medwatch.

DRUG INTERACTIONS

- Do not initiate G-CSF until 24 hours after completion of treatment with HYCAMTIN. Concomitant administration can prolong duration of neutropenia. (7)
- Greater myelosuppression is likely to be seen when used in combination with other cytotoxic agents. (7)

USE IN SPECIFIC POPULATIONS

- Nursing Mothers: Discontinue nursing when receiving HYCAMTIN. (8.3)

See 17 for PATIENT COUNSELING INFORMATION

Revised: 04/2010

FULL PRESCRIBING INFORMATION: CONTENTS*

*** Sections or subsections omitted from the full prescribing information are not listed**

FULL PRESCRIBING INFORMATION

WARNING: BONE MARROW SUPPRESSION

Do not give HYCAMTIN to patients with baseline neutrophil counts less than 1,500 cells/mm^3. In order to monitor the occurrence of bone marrow suppression, primarily neutropenia, which may be severe and result in infection and death, monitor peripheral blood counts frequently on all patients receiving HYCAMTIN *[see Warnings and Precautions (5.1)]*.

1 INDICATIONS AND USAGE

HYCAMTIN is indicated for the treatment of:

- metastatic carcinoma of the ovary after failure of initial or subsequent chemotherapy.
- small cell lung cancer sensitive disease after failure of first-line chemotherapy. In clinical studies submitted to support approval, sensitive disease was defined as disease responding to chemotherapy but subsequently progressing at least 60 days (in the Phase 3 study) or at least 90 days (in the Phase 2 studies) after chemotherapy *[see Clinical Studies (14)]*.

HYCAMTIN in combination with cisplatin is indicated for the treatment of:

- stage IV-B, recurrent, or persistent carcinoma of the cervix which is not amenable to curative treatment with surgery and/or radiation therapy.

2 DOSAGE AND ADMINISTRATION

Prior to administration of the first course of HYCAMTIN, patients must have a baseline neutrophil count of >1,500 cells/mm^3 and a platelet count of >100,000 cells/mm^3.

2.1 Ovarian Cancer and Small Cell Lung Cancer

Recommended Dosage:

- The recommended dose of HYCAMTIN is 1.5 mg/m^2 by intravenous infusion over 30 minutes daily for 5 consecutive days, starting on day 1 of a 21-day course.
- In the absence of tumor progression, a minimum of 4 courses is recommended because tumor response may be delayed. The median time to response in 3 ovarian clinical trials was 9 to 12 weeks, and median time to response in 4 small cell lung cancer trials was 5 to 7 weeks.

Dosage Modification Guidelines:

- In the event of severe neutropenia (defined as <500 cells/mm^3) during any course, reduce the dose by 0.25 mg/m^2 (to 1.25 mg/m^2) for subsequent courses.
- Alternatively, in the event of severe neutropenia, administer G-CSF (granulocyte-colony stimulating factor) following the subsequent course (before resorting to dose reduction) starting from day 6 of the course (24 hours after completion of topotecan administration).
- In the event the platelet count falls below 25,000 cells/mm^3, reduce doses by 0.25 mg/m^2 (to 1.25 mg/m^2) for subsequent courses.

2.2 Cervical Cancer

Recommended Dosage:

The recommended dose of HYCAMTIN is 0.75 mg/m^2 by intravenous infusion over 30 minutes daily on days 1, 2, and 3; followed by cisplatin 50 mg/m^2 by intravenous infusion on day 1 repeated every 21 days (a 21-day course).

Dosage Modification Guidelines:

Dosage adjustments for subsequent courses of HYCAMTIN in combination with cisplatin are specific for each drug. See manufacturer's prescribing information for cisplatin administration and hydration guidelines and for cisplatin dosage adjustment in the event of hematologic toxicity.

- In the event of severe febrile neutropenia (defined as <500 cells/mm^3 with temperature of 38.0°C or 100.4°F), reduce the dose of HYCAMTIN to 0.60 mg/m^2 for subsequent courses.
- Alternatively, in the event of severe febrile neutropenia, administer G-CSF following the subsequent course (before resorting to dose reduction) starting from day 4 of the course (24 hours after completion of administration of HYCAMTIN).
- If febrile neutropenia occurs despite the use of G-CSF, reduce the dose of HYCAMTIN to 0.45 mg/m^2 for subsequent courses.
- In the event the platelet count falls below 25,000 cells/mm^3, reduce doses to 0.60 mg/m^2 for subsequent courses.

2.3 Dosage Adjustment in Specific Populations

Renal Impairment:

No dosage adjustment of HYCAMTIN appears to be required for patients with mild renal impairment (Cl_{cr} 40 to 60 mL/min.). Dosage adjustment of HYCAMTIN to 0.75 mg/m^2 is recommended for patients with moderate renal impairment (20 to 39 mL/min.). Insufficient data are available in patients with severe renal impairment to provide a dosage recommendation for HYCAMTIN *[see Use in Specific Populations (8.6) and Clinical Pharmacology (12.3)]*.

HYCAMTIN in combination with cisplatin for the treatment of cervical cancer should only be initiated in patients with serum creatinine ≤1.5 mg/dL. In the clinical trial, cisplatin was discontinued for a serum creatinine >1.5 mg/dL. Insufficient data are available regarding continuing monotherapy with HYCAMTIN after cisplatin discontinuation in patients with cervical cancer.

2.4 Instructions for Handling, Preparation and Intravenous Adminstration

Handling:

HYCAMTIN is a cytotoxic anticancer drug. Prepare HYCAMTIN under a vertical laminar flow hood while wearing gloves and protective clothing. If HYCAMTIN solution contacts the skin, wash the skin immediately and thoroughly with soap and water. If HYCAMTIN contacts mucous membranes, flush thoroughly with water.

Use procedures for proper handling and disposal of anticancer drugs. Several guidelines on this subject have been published.[1-4]

Preparation and Administration:

Each 4-mg vial of HYCAMTIN is reconstituted with 4 mL Sterile Water for Injection. Then the appropriate volume of the reconstituted solution is diluted in either 0.9% Sodium Chloride Intravenous Infusion or 5% Dextrose Intravenous Infusion prior to administration.

Stability:

Unopened vials of HYCAMTIN are stable until the date indicated on the package when stored between 20° and 25°C (68° and 77°F) [see USP] and protected from light in the original package. Because the vials contain no preservative, contents should be used immediately after reconstitution.

Reconstituted vials of HYCAMTIN diluted for infusion are stable at approximately 20° to 25°C (68° to 77°F) and ambient lighting conditions for 24 hours.

3 DOSAGE FORMS AND STRENGTHS

4-mg (free base) single-dose vial, light yellow to greenish powder.

4 CONTRAINDICATIONS

HYCAMTIN is contraindicated in patients who have a history of severe hypersensitivity reactions (e.g., anaphylactoid reactions) to topotecan or to any of its ingredients. HYCAMTIN should not be used in patients with severe bone marrow depression.

5 WARNINGS AND PRECAUTIONS

5.1 Bone Marrow Suppression

Bone marrow suppression (primarily neutropenia) is the dose-limiting toxicity of HYCAMTIN. Neutropenia is not cumulative over time. In ovarian cancer, the overall treatment-related death rate was 1%. In the comparative study in small cell lung cancer, however, the treatment-related death rates were 5% for HYCAMTIN and 4% for CAV (cyclophosphamide-doxorubicin-vincristine).

Neutropenia:

- Ovarian and small cell lung cancer experience: Grade 4 neutropenia (<500 cells/mm^3) was most common during course 1 of treatment (60% of patients) and occurred in 39% of all courses, with a median duration of 7 days. The nadir neutrophil count occurred at a median of 12 days. Therapy-related sepsis or febrile neutropenia occurred in 23% of patients, and sepsis was fatal in 1%. Pancytopenia has been reported.
- Cervical cancer experience: Grade 3 and grade 4 neutropenia affected 26% and 48% of patients, respectively.

Thrombocytopenia:

- Ovarian and small cell lung cancer experience: Grade 4 thrombocytopenia (<25,000/mm^3) occurred in 27% of patients and in 9% of courses, with a median duration of 5 days and platelet nadir at a median of 15 days. Platelet transfusions were given to 15% of patients in 4% of courses.

- Cervical cancer experience: Grade 3 and grade 4 thrombocytopenia affected 26% and 7% of patients, respectively.

Anemia:

- Ovarian and small cell lung cancer experience: Grade 3/4 anemia (<8 g/dL) occurred in 37% of patients and in 14% of courses. Median nadir was at day 15. Transfusions were needed in 52% of patients in 22% of courses.
- Cervical cancer experience: Grade 3 and grade 4 anemia affected 34% and 6% of patients, respectively.

Monitoring of Bone Marrow Function:

Administer HYCAMTIN only in patients with adequate bone marrow reserves, including baseline neutrophil count of at least 1,500 cells/mm^3 and platelet count at least 100,000/mm^3. Monitor peripheral blood counts frequently during treatment with HYCAMTIN. Do not treat patients with subsequent courses of HYCAMTIN until neutrophils recover to >1,000 cells/mm^3, platelets recover to >100,000 cells/mm^3, and hemoglobin levels recover to 9.0 g/dL (with transfusion if necessary). Severe myelotoxicity has been reported when HYCAMTIN is used in combination with cisplatin *[see Drug Interactions (7.1)]*.

5.2 Neutropenic Colitis

Topotecan-induced neutropenia can lead to neutropenic colitis. Fatalities due to neutropenic colitis have been reported in clinical trials with HYCAMTIN. In patients presenting with fever, neutropenia, and a compatible pattern of abdominal pain, consider the possibility of neutropenic colitis.

5.3 Interstitial Lung Disease

HYCAMTIN has been associated with reports of interstitial lung disease (ILD), some of which have been fatal *[see Adverse Reactions (6.2)]*. Underlying risk factors include history of ILD, pulmonary fibrosis, lung cancer, thoracic exposure to radiation, and use of pneumotoxic drugs and/or colony stimulating factors. Monitor patients for pulmonary symptoms indicative of interstitial lung disease (e.g., cough, fever, dyspnea, and/or hypoxia), and discontinue HYCAMTIN if a new diagnosis of ILD is confirmed.

5.4 Pregnancy

Pregnancy Category D

HYCAMTIN can cause fetal harm when administered to a pregnant woman.

Topotecan caused embryolethality, fetotoxicity, and teratogenicity in rats and rabbits when administered during organogenesis. There are no adequate and well controlled studies of HYCAMTIN in pregnant women. If this drug is used during pregnancy, or if a patient becomes pregnant while receiving HYCAMTIN, the patient should be apprised of the potential hazard to the fetus. *[see Use in Specific Populations, Pregnancy (8.1)]*.

5.5 Inadvertent Extravasation

Inadvertent extravasation with HYCAMTIN has been observed, most reactions have been mild but severe cases have been reported.

6 ADVERSE REACTIONS

6.1 Clinical Trials Experience

Because clinical trials are conducted under widely varying conditions, adverse reaction rates observed in the clinical trials of a drug cannot be directly compared to rates in the clinical trials of another drug and may not reflect the rates observed in practice.

Ovarian Cancer and Small Cell Lung Cancer:

Data in the following section are based on the combined experience of 453 patients with metastatic ovarian carcinoma, and 426 patients with small cell lung cancer treated with HYCAMTIN. Table 1 lists the principal hematologic adverse reactions and Table 2 lists non-hematologic adverse reactions occurring in at least 15% of patients.

Table 1. Hematologic Adverse Reactions Experienced in ≥15% Ovarian Cancer and Small Cell Lung Cancer Patients Receiving HYCAMTIN

Hematologic Adverse Reaction	Patients (n = 879) % Incidence
Neutropenia	
<1,500 cells/mm^3	97
<500 cells/mm^3	78
Leukopenia	
<3,000 cells/mm^3	97
<1,000 cells/mm^3	32
Thrombocytopenia	
<75,000/mm^3	69
<25,000/mm^3	27
Anemia	
<10 g/dL	89
<8 g/dL	37

Table 2. Non-hematologic Adverse Reactions Experienced by ≥15% of Ovarian Cancer and Small Cell Lung Cancer Patients Receiving HYCAMTIN

Non-hematologic Adverse Reaction	Percentage of Patients with Adverse Reaction (879 Patients)		
	All Grades	Grade 3	Grade 4
Infections and infestations			
Sepsis or pyrexia/ infection with neutropenia [a]	43	NR	23
Metabolism and nutrition disorders			
Anorexia	19	2	<1
Nervous system disorders			
Headache	18	1	<1
Respiratory, thoracic, and mediastinal disorders			
Dyspnea	22	5	3
Coughing	15	1	0
Gastrointestinal disorders			
Nausea	64	7	1
Vomiting	45	4	1
Diarrhea	32	3	1
Constipation	29	2	1
Abdominal pain	22	2	2
Stomatitis	18	1	<1
Skin and subcutaneous tissue disorders			
Alopecia	49	NA	NA
Rash[b]	16	1	0
General disorders and administrative site conditions			
Fatigue	29	5	0
Pyrexia	28	1	<1
Pain[c]	23	2	1
Asthenia	25	4	2

NA = Not applicable

NR = Not reported separately

[a] Does not include Grade 1 sepsis or pyrexia.

[b] Rash also includes pruritus, rash erythematous, urticaria, dermatitis, bullous eruption, and maculopapular rash.

[c] Pain includes body pain, back pain, and skeletal pain.

Nervous System Disorders:

Paresthesia occurred in 7% of patients but was generally grade 1.

Hepatobiliary Disorders:

Grade 1 transient elevations in hepatic enzymes occurred in 8% of patients. Greater elevations, grade 3/4, occurred in 4%. Grade 3/4 elevated bilirubin occurred in <2% of patients.

Table 3 shows the grade 3/4 hematologic and major non-hematologic adverse reactions in the topotecan/paclitaxel comparator trial in ovarian cancer.

Table 3. Adverse Reactions Experienced by ≥5% of Ovarian Cancer Patients Randomized to Receive HYCAMTIN or Paclitaxel

Adverse Reaction	HYCAMTIN (n = 112)	Paclitaxel (n = 114)
Hematologic Grade 3/4	**%**	**%**
Grade 4 neutropenia (<500 cells/mm^3)	80	21
Grade 3/4 anemia (Hgb <8 g/dL)	41	6
Grade 4 thrombocytopenia (<25,000 plts/mm^3)	27	3
Pyrexia/Grade 4 neutropenia	23	4
Non-hematologic Grade 3/4	**%**	**%**
Infections and infestations		
Documented sepsis[a]	5	2
Respiratory, thoracic, and mediastinal disorders		
Dyspnea	6	5
Gastrointestinal disorders		
Abdominal pain	5	4
Constipation	5	0
Diarrhea	6	1
Intestinal obstruction	5	4
Nausea	10	2
Vomiting	10	3
General disorders and administrative site conditions		
Fatigue	7	6
Asthenia	5	3
Pain[b]	5	7

[a] Death related to sepsis occurred in 2% of patients receiving HYCAMTIN, and 0% of patients receiving paclitaxel.

[b] Pain includes body pain, skeletal pain, and back pain.

Table 4 shows the grade 3/4 hematologic and major non-hematologic adverse reactions in the topotecan/CAV comparator trial in small cell lung cancer.

Table 4. Adverse Reactions Experienced by ≥5% of Small Cell Lung Cancer Patients Randomized to Receive HYCAMTIN or CAV

Adverse Reaction	HYCAMTIN (n = 107)	CAV (n = 104)
Hematologic Grade 3/4	**%**	**%**
Grade 4 neutropenia (<500 cells/mm^3)	70	72
Grade 3/4 anemia (Hgb <8 g/dL)	42	20
Grade 4 thrombocytopenia (<25,000 plts/mm^3)	29	5
Pyrexia/Grade 4 neutropenia	28	26
Non-hematologic Grade 3/4	**%**	**%**
Infections and infestations		
Documented sepsis[a]	5	5
Respiratory, thoracic, and mediastinal disorders		
Dyspnea	9	14
Pneumonia	8	6
Gastrointestinal disorders		
Abdominal pain	6	4
Nausea	8	6
General disorders and administrative site conditions		
Fatigue	6	10
Asthenia	9	7
Pain[b]	5	7

[a] Death related to sepsis occurred in 3% of patients receiving HYCAMTIN, and 1% of patients receiving CAV.

[b] Pain includes body pain, skeletal pain, and back pain.

Cervical Cancer:

In the comparative trial with HYCAMTIN plus cisplatin versus cisplatin in patients with cervical cancer, the most common dose-limiting adverse reaction was myelosuppression. Table 5 shows the hematologic adverse reactions and Table 6 shows the non-hematologic adverse reactions in patients with cervical cancer.

Table 5. Hematologic Adverse Reactions in Patients with Cervical Cancer Treated with HYCAMTIN Plus Cisplatin or Cisplatin Monotherapy[a]

Hematologic Adverse Reaction	HYCAMTIN Plus Cisplatin (n = 140)	Cisplatin (n = 144)
Anemia		
All grades (Hgb <12 g/dL)	131 (94%)	130 (90%)
Grade 3 (Hgb <8-6.5 g/dL)	47 (34%)	28 (19%)
Grade 4 (Hgb <6.5 g/dL)	9 (6%)	5 (3%)
Leukopenia		
All grades (<3,800 cells/mm^3)	128 (91%)	43 (30%)
Grade 3 (<2,000-1,000 cells/mm^3)	58 (41%)	1 (1%)
Grade 4 (<1,000 cells/mm^3)	35 (25%)	0 (0%)
Neutropenia		
All grades (<2,000 cells/mm^3)	125 (89%)	28 (19%)
Grade 3 (<1,000-500 cells/mm^3)	36 (26%)	1 (1%)
Grade 4 (<500 cells/mm^3)	67 (48%)	1 (1%)
Thrombocytopenia		
All grades (<130,000 cells/mm^3)	104 (74%)	21 (15%)
Grade 3 (<50,000-10,000 cells/mm^3)	36 (26%)	5 (3%)
Grade 4 (<10,000 cells/mm^3)	10 (7%)	0 (0%)

[a] Includes patients who were eligible and treated.

Table 6. Non-hematologic Adverse Reactions Experienced by ≥5% of Patients with Cervical Cancer Treated with HYCAMTIN Plus Cisplatin or Cisplatin Monotherapy[a]

Adverse Reaction	HYCAMTIN Plus Cisplatin (n = 140)			Cisplatin (n = 144)		
	All Grades[b]	Grade 3	Grade 4	All Grades[b]	Grade 3	Grade 4
General disorders and administrative site conditions						
Constitutional[c]	96 (69%)	11 (8%)	0	89 (62%)	17 (12%)	0
Pain[d]	82 (59%)	28 (20%)	3 (2%)	72 (50%)	18 (13%)	5 (3%)
Gastrointestinal disorders						
Vomiting	56 (40%)	20 (14%)	2 (1%)	53 (37%)	13 (9%)	0
Nausea	77 (55%)	18 (13%)	2 (1%)	79 (55%)	13 (9%)	0
Stomatitis-pharyngitis	8 (6%)	1 (<1%)	0	0	0	0
Other	88 (63%)	16 (11%)	4 (3%)	80 (56%)	12 (8%)	3 (2%)
Dermatology	67 (48%)	1 (<1%)	0	29 (20%)	0	0
Metabolic-Laboratory	55 (39%)	13 (9%)	7 (5%)	44 (31%)	14 (10%)	1 (<1%)
Genitourinary	51 (36%)	9 (6%)	9 (6%)	49 (34%)	7 (5%)	7 (5%)
Nervous system disorders						
Neuropathy	4 (3%)	1 (<1%)	0	3 (2%)	1 (<1%)	0
Other	49 (35%)	3 (2%)	1 (<1%)	43 (30%)	7 (5%)	2 (1%)
Infection-febrile neutropenia	39 (28%)	21 (15%)	5 (4%)	26 (18%)	11 (8%)	0
Cardiovascular	35 (25%)	7 (5%)	6 (4%)	22 (15%)	8 (6%)	3 (2%)
Hepatic	34 (24%)	5 (4%)	2 (1%)	23 (16%)	2 (1%)	0
Pulmonary	24 (17%)	4 (3%)	0	23 (16%)	5 (3%)	3 (2%)
Vascular disorders						
Hemorrhage	21 (15%)	8 (6%)	1 (<1%)	20 (14%)	3 (2%)	1 (<1%)
Coagulation	8 (6%)	4 (3%)	3 (2%)	10 (7%)	7 (5%)	0
Musculoskeletal	19 (14%)	3 (2%)	0	7 (5%)	1 (<1%)	1 (<1%)
Allergy-Immunology	8 (6%)	2 (1%)	1 (<1%)	4 (3%)	0	1 (<1%)
Endocrine	8 (6%)	0	0	4 (3%)	2 (1%)	0
Sexual reproduction function	7 (5%)	0	0	10 (7%)	1 (<1%)	0
Ocular-visual	7 (5%)	0	0	7 (5%)	1 (<1%)	0

Data were collected using NCI Common Toxicity Criteria, v. 2.0.

[a] Includes patients who were eligible and treated.

[b] Grades 1 through 4 only. There were 3 patients who experienced grade 5 deaths with investigator-designated attribution. One was a grade 5 hemorrhage in which the drug-related thrombocytopenia aggravated the event. A second patient experienced bowel obstruction, cardiac arrest, pleural effusion and respiratory failure which were not treatment related but probably aggravated by treatment. A third patient experienced a pulmonary embolism and adult respiratory distress syndrome, the latter was indirectly treatment-related.

[c] Constitutional includes fatigue (lethargy, malaise, asthenia), fever (in the absence of neutropenia), rigors, chills, sweating, and weight gain or loss.

[d] Pain includes abdominal pain or cramping, arthralgia, bone pain, chest pain (non-cardiac and non-pleuritic), dysmenorrhea, dyspareunia, earache, headache, hepatic pain, myalgia, neuropathic pain, pain due to radiation, pelvic pain, pleuritic pain, rectal or perirectal pain, and tumor pain.

[See table 6 above]

6.2 Postmarketing Experience

In addition to adverse reactions reported from clinical trials or listed in other sections of the prescribing information, the following reactions have been identified during post-marketing use of HYCAMTIN. Because they are reported voluntarily from a population of unknown size, estimates of frequency cannot be made. These reactions have been chosen for inclusion due to a combination of their seriousness, frequency of reporting, or potential causal connection to HYCAMTIN.

Blood and Lymphatic System Disorders:
Severe bleeding (in association with thrombocytopenia) *[see Warnings and Precautions (5.1)]*.

Immune System Disorders:
Allergic manifestations; Anaphylactoid reactions.

Gastrointestinal Disorders:
Abdominal pain potentially associated with neutropenic colitis *[see Warnings and Precautions (5.2)]*.

Pulmonary Disorders:
Interstitial lung disease *[see Warnings and Precautions (5.3)]*.

Skin and Subcutaneous Tissue Disorders:
Angioedema, severe dermatitis, severe pruritus.

General Disorders and Administrative Site Conditions:
Inadvertant extravastation *[see Warnings and Precautions (5.5)]*.

7 DRUG INTERACTIONS

G-CSF: Concomitant administration of G-CSF can prolong the duration of neutropenia, so if G-CSF is to be used, do not initiat it until day 6 of the course of therapy, 24 hours after completion of treatment with HYCAMTIN.

Platinum and Other Cytotoxic Agents: Myelosuppression was more severe when HYCAMTIN, at a dose of 1.25 mg/m^2/day for 5 days, was given in combination with cisplatin at a dose of 50 mg/m^2 in Phase 1 studies. In one study, 1 of 3 patients had severe neutropenia for 12 days and a second patient died with neutropenic sepsis.

Greater myelosuppression is also likely to be seen when HYCAMTIN is used in combination with other cytotoxic agents, thereby necessitating a dose reduction. However, when combining HYCAMTIN with platinum agents (e.g., cisplatin or carboplatin), a distinct sequence-dependent interaction on myelosuppression has been reported. Coadministration of a platinum agent on day 1 of dosing with HYCAMTIN required lower doses of each agent compared to coadministration on day 5 of the dosing schedule for HYCAMTIN.

For information on the pharmacokinetics, efficacy, safety, and dosing of HYCAMTIN at a dose of 0.75 mg/m^2/day on days 1, 2, and 3 in combination with cisplatin 50 mg/m^2 on day 1 for cervical cancer, *see Dosage and Administration (2), Adverse Reactions (6), Clinical Pharmacology (12.3), and Clinical Studies (14).*

8 USE IN SPECIFIC POPULATIONS

8.1 Pregnancy

Pregnancy Category D [see Warnings and Precautions (5.3)].
HYCAMTIN can cause fetal harm when administered to a pregnant woman. In rabbits, a dose of 0.10 mg/kg/day (about equal to the clinical dose on a mg/m^2 basis) given on days 6 through 20 of gestation caused maternal toxicity, embryolethality, and reduced fetal body weight. In the rat, a dose of 0.23 mg/kg/day (about equal to the clinical dose on a mg/m^2 basis) given for 14 days before mating through gestation day 6 caused fetal resorption, microphthalmia, preimplant loss, and mild maternal toxicity. A dose of 0.10 mg/kg/day (about half the clinical dose on a mg/m^2 basis) given to rats on days 6 through 17 of gestation caused an increase in post-implantation mortality. This dose also caused an increase in total fetal malformations. The most frequent malformations were of the eye (microphthalmia, anophthalmia, rosette formation of the retina, coloboma of the retina, ectopic orbit), brain (dilated lateral and third ventricles), skull, and vertebrae.

There are no adequate and well controlled studies of HYCAMTIN in pregnant women. If this drug is used during pregnancy, or if a patient becomes pregnant while receiving HYCAMTIN, the patient should be apprised of the potential hazard to the fetus. *[see Warnings and Precautions (5.4)]*

8.3 Nursing Mothers

Rats excrete high concentrations of topotecan into milk. Lactating female rats given 4.72 mg/m^2 IV (about twice the clinical dose on a mg/m^2 basis) excreted topotecan into milk at concentrations up to 48-fold higher than those in plasma. It is not known whether the drug is excreted in human milk. Because many drugs are excreted in human milk and because of the potential for serious adverse reactions in nursing infants from HYCAMTIN, discontinue breastfeeding when women are receiving HYCAMTIN.

8.4 Pediatric Use

Safety and effectiveness in pediatric patients have not been established.

8.5 Geriatric Use

Of the 879 patients with metastatic ovarian cancer or small cell lung cancer in clinical studies of HYCAMTIN, 32% (n = 281) were 65 years of age and older, while 3.8% (n = 33) were 75 years of age and older. Of the 140 patients with stage IV-B, relapsed, or refractory cervical cancer in clinical studies of HYCAMTIN who received HYCAMTIN plus cisplatin in the randomized clinical trial, 6% (n = 9) were 65 years of age and older, while 3% (n = 4) were 75 years of age and older. No overall differences in effectiveness or safety were observed between these patients and younger adult patients, and other reported clinical experience has not identified differences in responses between the elderly and younger adult patients, but greater sensitivity of some older individuals cannot be ruled out.

There were no apparent differences in the pharmacokinetics of topotecan in elderly patients, once the age-related decrease in renal function was considered *[see Clinical Pharmacology (12.3)].*

This drug is known to be substantially excreted by the kidney, and the risk of toxic reactions to this drug may be greater in patients with impaired renal function. Because elderly patients are more likely to have decreased renal function, care should be taken in dose selection, and it may be useful to monitor renal function *[see Dosage and Administration (2.3)]*.

8.6 Renal Impairment

No dosage adjustment of HYCAMTIN appears to be required for patients with mild renal impairment (Cl_{cr} 40 to 60 mL/min.). Dosage reduction is recommended for patients with moderate renal impairment (Cl_{cr} 20 to 39 mL/min.). Insufficient data are available in patients with severe renal impairment to provide a dosage recommendation for HYCAMTIN. *[see Dosage and Administration (2.3) and Clinical Pharmacology (12.3)]*.

10 OVERDOSAGE

There is no known antidote for overdosage with HYCAMTIN. The primary anticipated complication of overdosage would consist of bone marrow suppression.

One patient on a single-dose regimen of 17.5 mg/m^2 given on day 1 of a 21-day cycle had received a single dose of 35 mg/m^2. This patient experienced severe neutropenia (nadir of 320/mm^3) 14 days later but recovered without incident.

Observe patients closely for bone marrow suppression, and supportive measures (such as the prophylactic use of G-CSF and/or antibiotic therapy).

11 DESCRIPTION

HYCAMTIN (topotecan hydrochloride) is a semi-synthetic derivative of camptothecin and is an anti-tumor drug with topoisomerase I-inhibitory activity.

HYCAMTIN for Injection is supplied as a sterile lyophilized, buffered, light yellow to greenish powder available in single-dose vials. Each vial contains topotecan hydrochloride equivalent to 4 mg of topotecan as free base. The reconstituted solution ranges in color from yellow to yellow-green and is intended for administration by intravenous infusion. Inactive ingredients are mannitol, 48 mg, and tartaric acid, 20 mg. Hydrochloric acid and sodium hydroxide may be used to adjust the pH. The solution pH ranges from 2.5 to 3.5.

The chemical name for topotecan hydrochloride is (*S*)-10-[(dimethylamino)methyl]-4-ethyl-4,9-dihydroxy-1*H*-pyrano [3′,4′:6,7] indolizino [1,2-*b*]quinoline-3,14-(4*H*,12*H*)-dione monohydrochloride. It has the molecular formula $C_{23}H_{23}N_3O_5{\bullet}HCl$ and a molecular weight of 457.9.

Topotecan hydrochloride has the following structural formula:

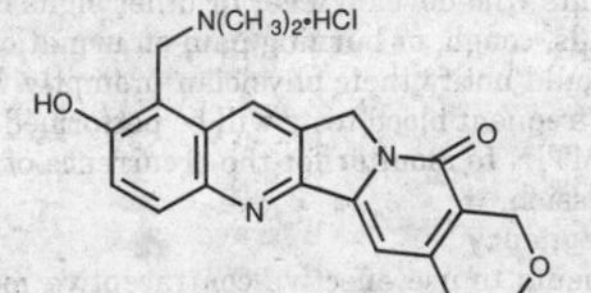

It is soluble in water and melts with decomposition at 213° to 218°C.

12 CLINICAL PHARMACOLOGY

12.1 Mechanism of Action

Topoisomerase I relieves torsional strain in DNA by inducing reversible single strand breaks. Topotecan binds to the topoisomerase I-DNA complex and prevents religation of these single strand breaks. The cytotoxicity of topotecan is thought to be due to double strand DNA damage produced during DNA synthesis, when replication enzymes interact with the ternary complex formed by topotecan, topoisomerase I, and DNA. Mammalian cells cannot efficiently repair these double strand breaks.

12.2 Pharmacodynamics

The dose-limiting toxicity of topotecan is leukopenia. White blood cell count decreases with increasing topotecan dose or topotecan AUC. When topotecan is administered at a dose of 1.5 mg/m^2/day for 5 days, an 80% to 90% decrease in white blood cell count at nadir is typically observed after the first cycle of therapy.

12.3 Pharmacokinetics

The pharmacokinetics of topotecan have been evaluated in cancer patients following doses of 0.5 to 1.5 mg/m^2 administered as a 30-minute infusion. Topotecan exhibits multiexponential pharmacokinetics with a terminal half-life of 2 to 3 hours. Total exposure (AUC) is approximately dose-proportional.

Distribution:

Binding of topotecan to plasma proteins is about 35%.

Metabolism:

Topotecan undergoes a reversible pH dependent hydrolysis of its lactone moiety; it is the lactone form that is pharmacologically active. At pH ≤4, the lactone is exclusively present, whereas the ring-opened hydroxy-acid form predominates at physiologic pH. In vitro studies in human liver microsomes indicate topotecan is metabolized to an N-demethylated metabolite. The mean metabolite:parent AUC ratio was about 3% for total topotecan and topotecan lactone following IV administration.

Excretion:

Renal clearance is an important determinant of topotecan elimination.

In a mass balance/excretion study in 4 patients with solid tumors, the overall recovery of total topotecan and its N-desmethyl metabolite in urine and feces over 9 days averaged 73.4 ± 2.3% of the administered IV dose. Mean values of 50.8 ± 2.9% as total topotecan and 3.1 ± 1.0% as N-desmethyl topotecan were excreted in the urine following IV administration. Fecal elimination of total topotecan accounted for 17.9 ± 3.6% while fecal elimination of N-desmethyl topotecan was 1.7 ± 0.6%. An O-glucuronidation metabolite of topotecan and N-desmethyl topotecan has been identified in the urine. These metabolites, topotecan-O-glucuronide and N-desmethyl topotecan-O-glucuronide, were less than 2% of the administered dose.

Effect of Gender:

The overall mean topotecan plasma clearance in male patients was approximately 24% higher than that in female patients, largely reflecting difference in body size.

Effect of Age:

Topotecan pharmacokinetics have not been specifically studied in an elderly population, but population pharmacokinetic analysis in female patients did not identify age as a significant factor. Decreased renal clearance, which is common in the elderly, is a more important determinant of topotecan clearance *[see Dosage and Administration (2.3) and Use in Specific Populations (8.6)]*.

Effect of Race:

The effect of race on topotecan pharmacokinetics has not been studied.

Effect of Renal Impairment:

In patients with mild renal impairment (creatinine clearance of 40 to 60 mL/min.), topotecan plasma clearance was decreased to about 67% of the value in patients with normal renal function. In patients with moderate renal impairment (Cl_{cr} of 20 to 39 mL/min.), topotecan plasma clearance was reduced to about 34% of the value in control patients, with an increase in half-life. Mean half-life, estimated in 3 renally impaired patients, was about 5.0 hours. Dosage adjustment is recommended for these patients *[see Dosage and Administration (2.3)]*.

Effect of Hepatic Impairment:

Plasma clearance in patients with hepatic impairment (serum bilirubin levels between 1.7 and 15.0 mg/dL) was decreased to about 67% of the value in patients without hepatic impairment. Topotecan half-life increased slightly, from 2.0 hours to 2.5 hours, but these hepatically impaired patients tolerated the usual recommended topotecan dosage regimen.

Drug Interactions:

Pharmacokinetic studies of the interaction of topotecan with concomitantly administered medications have not been formally investigated.

In vitro inhibition studies using marker substrates known to be metabolized by human P450 CYP1A2, CYP2A6, CYP2C8/9, CYP2C19, CYP2D6, CYP2E, CYP3A, or CYP4A or dihydropyrimidine dehydrogenase indicate that the activities of these enzymes were not altered by topotecan. Enzyme inhibition by topotecan has not been evaluated in vivo.

Cisplatin:

Administration of cisplatin (60 or 75 mg/m^2 on day 1) before topotecan (0.75 mg/m^2/day on days 1 to 5) in 9 patients with ovarian cancer had no significant effect on the C_{max} and AUC of total topotecan.

Topotecan had no effect on the pharmacokinetics of free platinum in 15 patients with ovarian cancer who were administered cisplatin 50 mg/m^2 (n = 9) or 75 mg/m^2 (n = 6) on day 2 after paclitaxel 110 mg/m^2 on day 1 before topotecan 0.3 mg/m^2 IV daily on days 2-6. Topotecan had no effect on dose-normalized (60 mg/m^2) C_{max} values of free platinum in 13 patients with ovarian cancer who were administered 60 mg/m^2 (n = 10) or 75 mg/m^2 (n = 3) cisplatin on day 1 before topotecan 0.75 mg/m^2 IV daily on days 1 to 5.

No pharmacokinetic data are available following topotecan (0.75 mg/m^2/day for 3 consecutive days) and cisplatin (50 mg/m^2/day on day 1) in patients with cervical cancer.

Myelosuppression was more severe when HYCAMTIN was given in combination with cisplatin. *[see Drug Interactions (7)]*.

13 NONCLINICAL TOXICOLOGY

13.1 Carcinogenesis, Mutagenesis, Impairment of Fertility

Carcinogenicity testing of topotecan has not been performed. Topotecan is known to be genotoxic to mammalian cells and is a probable carcinogen. Topotecan was mutagenic to L5178Y mouse lymphoma cells and clastogenic to cultured human lymphocytes with and without metabolic activation. It was also clastogenic to mouse bone marrow. Topotecan did not cause mutations in bacterial cells.

Topotecan given to female rats prior to mating at a dose of 1.4 mg/m^2 IV (about equal to the clinical dose on a mg/m^2 basis) caused superovulation possibly related to inhibition of follicular atresia. This dose given to pregnant female rats also caused increased pre-implantation loss. Studies in dogs given 0.4 mg/m^2 IV (about 1/4th the clinical dose on a mg/m^2 basis) of topotecan daily for a month suggest that treatment may cause an increase in the incidence of multinucleated spermatogonial giant cells in the testes. Topotecan may impair fertility in women and men.

14 CLINICAL STUDIES

14.1 Ovarian Cancer

HYCAMTIN was studied in 2 clinical trials of 223 patients given topotecan with metastatic ovarian carcinoma. All patients had disease that had recurred on, or was unresponsive to, a platinum-containing regimen. Patients in these 2 studies received an initial dose of 1.5 mg/m^2 given by intravenous infusion over 30 minutes for 5 consecutive days, starting on day 1 of a 21-day course.

One study was a randomized trial of 112 patients treated with HYCAMTIN (1.5 mg/m^2/day × 5 days starting on day 1 of a 21-day course) and 114 patients treated with paclitaxel (175 mg/m^2 over 3 hours on day 1 of a 21-day course). All patients had recurrent ovarian cancer after a platinum-containing regimen or had not responded to at least 1 prior platinum-containing regimen. Patients who did not respond to the study therapy, or who progressed, could be given the alternative treatment.

Response rates, response duration, and time to progression are shown in Table 7.

Table 7. Efficacy of HYCAMTIN Versus Paclitaxel in Ovarian Cancer

Parameter	HYCAMTIN (n = 112)	Paclitaxel (n = 114)
Complete response rate	5%	3%
Partial response rate	16%	11%
Overall response rate	21%	14%
95% Confidence interval	13 to 28%	8 to 20%
(*P*-value)	(0.20)	
Response duration[a] (weeks)	n = 23	n = 16
Median	25.9	21.6
95% Confidence interval	22.1 to 32.9	16.0 to 34.0
hazard-ratio (HYCAMTIN:paclitaxel) (*P*-value)	0.78 (0.48)	
Time to progression (weeks)		
Median	18.9	14.7
95% Confidence interval	12.1 to 23.6	11.9 to 18.3
hazard-ratio (HYCAMTIN:paclitaxel) (*P*-value)	0.76 (0.07)	
Survival (weeks)		
Median	63.0	53.0
95% Confidence interval	46.6 to 71.9	42.3 to 68.7
hazard-ratio (HYCAMTIN:paclitaxel) (*P*-value)	0.97 (0.87)	

[a] The calculation for duration of response was based on the interval between first response and time to progression.

The median time to response was 7.6 weeks (range 3.1 to 21.7) with HYCAMTIN compared to 6.0 weeks (range 2.4 to 18.1) with paclitaxel. Consequently, the efficacy of HYCAMTIN may not be achieved if patients are withdrawn from treatment prematurely.

In the crossover phase, 8 of 61 (13%) patients who received HYCAMTIN after paclitaxel had a partial response and 5 of 49 (10%) patients who received paclitaxel after HYCAMTIN had a response (2 complete responses).

Table 9. Percentage of Patients With Symptom Improvement[a]: HYCAMTIN Versus CAV in Patients With Small Cell Lung Cancer

Symptom	HYCAMTIN (n = 107)		CAV (n = 104)	
	n[b]	(%)	n[b]	(%)
Shortness of breath	68	(28)	61	(7)
Interference with daily activity	67	(27)	63	(11)
Fatigue	70	(23)	65	(9)
Hoarseness	40	(33)	38	(13)
Cough	69	(25)	61	(15)
Insomnia	57	(33)	53	(19)
Anorexia	56	(32)	57	(16)
Chest pain	44	(25)	41	(17)
Hemoptysis	15	(27)	12	(33)

[a] Defined as improvement sustained over at least 2 courses compared to baseline.
[b] Number of patients with baseline and at least 1 post-baseline assessment.

HYCAMTIN was active in ovarian cancer patients who had developed resistance to platinum-containing therapy, defined as tumor progression while on, or tumor relapse within 6 months after completion of, a platinum-containing regimen. One complete and 6 partial responses were seen in 60 patients, for a response rate of 12%. In the same study, there were no complete responders and 4 partial responders on the paclitaxel arm, for a response rate of 7%.

HYCAMTIN was also studied in an open-label, non-comparative trial in 111 patients with recurrent ovarian cancer after treatment with a platinum-containing regimen, or who had not responded to 1 prior platinum-containing regimen. The response rate was 14% (95% CI = 7% to 20%). The median duration of response was 22 weeks (range 4.6 to 41.9 weeks). The time to progression was 11.3 weeks (range 0.7 to 72.1 weeks). The median survival was 67.9 weeks (range 1.4 to 112.9 weeks).

14.2 Small Cell Lung Cancer

HYCAMTIN was studied in 426 patients with recurrent or progressive small cell lung cancer in 1 randomized, comparative study and in 3 single-arm studies.

Randomized Comparative Study:

In a randomized, comparative, Phase 3 trial, 107 patients were treated with HYCAMTIN (1.5 mg/m^2/day × 5 days starting on day 1 of a 21-day course) and 104 patients were treated with CAV (1,000 mg/m^2 cyclophosphamide, 45 mg/m^2 doxorubicin, 2 mg vincristine administered sequentially on day 1 of a 21-day course). All patients were considered sensitive to first-line chemotherapy (responders who then subsequently progressed ≥60 days after completion of first-line therapy). A total of 77% of patients treated with HYCAMTIN and 79% of patients treated with CAV received platinum/etoposide with or without other agents as first-line chemotherapy.

Response rates, response duration, time to progression, and survival are shown in Table 8.

Table 8. Efficacy of HYCAMTIN Versus CAV (cyclophosphamide-doxorubicin-vincristine) in Small Cell Lung Cancer Patients Sensitive to First-Line Chemotherapy

Parameter	HYCAMTIN (n = 107)	CAV (n = 104)
Complete response rate	0%	1%
Partial response rate	24%	17%
Overall response rate	24%	18%
Difference in overall response rates	6%	
95% Confidence interval of the difference	(−6 to 18%)	
Response duration[a] (weeks)	n = 26	n = 19
Median	14.4	15.3
95% Confidence interval	13.1 to 18.0	13.1 to 23.1
hazard-ratio (HYCAMTIN:CAV) (95% CI)	1.42 (0.73 to 2.76)	
(*P*-value)	(0.30)	
Time to progression (weeks)		
Median	13.3	12.3
95% Confidence interval	11.4 to 16.4	11.0 to 14.1
hazard-ratio (HYCAMTIN:CAV) (95% CI)	0.92 (0.69 to 1.22)	
(*P*-value)	(0.55)	
Survival (weeks)		
Median	25.0	24.7
95% Confidence interval	20.6 to 29.6	21.7 to 30.3
hazard-ratio (HYCAMTIN:CAV) (95% CI)	1.04 (0.78 to 1.39)	
(*P*-value)	(0.80)	

[a] The calculation for duration of response was based on the interval between first response and time to progression.

The time to response was similar in both arms: HYCAMTIN median of 6 weeks (range 2.4 to 15.7) versus CAV median 6 weeks (range 5.1 to 18.1).

Changes on a disease-related symptom scale in patients who received HYCAMTIN or who received CAV are presented in Table 9. It should be noted that not all patients had all symptoms, nor did all patients respond to all questions. Each symptom was rated on a 4-category scale with an improvement defined as a change in 1 category from baseline sustained over 2 courses. Limitations in interpretation of the rating scale and responses preclude formal statistical analysis.

[See table 9 above]

Single-Arm Studies:

HYCAMTIN was also studied in 3 open-label, non-comparative trials in a total of 319 patients with recurrent or progressive small cell lung cancer after treatment with first-line chemotherapy. In all 3 studies, patients were stratified as either sensitive (responders who then subsequently progressed ≥90 days after completion of first-line therapy) or refractory (no response to first-line chemotherapy or who responded to first-line therapy and then progressed within 90 days of completing first-line therapy). Response rates ranged from 11% to 31% for sensitive patients and 2% to 7% for refractory patients. Median time to progression and median survival were similar in all 3 studies and the comparative study.

14.3 Cervical Cancer

In a comparative trial, 147 eligible women were randomized to HYCAMTIN (0.75 mg/m^2/day IV over 30 minutes × 3 consecutive days starting on day 1 of a 21-day course) plus cisplatin (50 mg/m^2 on day 1) and 146 eligible women were randomized to cisplatin (50 mg/m^2 IV on day 1 of a 21-day course). All patients had histologically confirmed Stage IV-B, recurrent, or persistent carcinoma of the cervix considered not amenable to curative treatment with surgery and/or radiation. Fifty-six percent (56%) of patients treated with HYCAMTIN plus cisplatin and 56% of patients treated with cisplatin had received prior cisplatin with or without other agents as first-line chemotherapy.

Median survival of eligible patients receiving HYCAMTIN plus cisplatin was 9.4 months (95% CI: 7.9 to 11.9) compared to 6.5 months (95% CI: 5.8 to 8.8) among patients randomized to cisplatin alone with a log rank *P*-value of 0.033 (significance level was 0.044 after adjusting for the interim analysis). The unadjusted hazard ratio for overall survival was 0.76 (95% CI: 0.59 to 0.98).

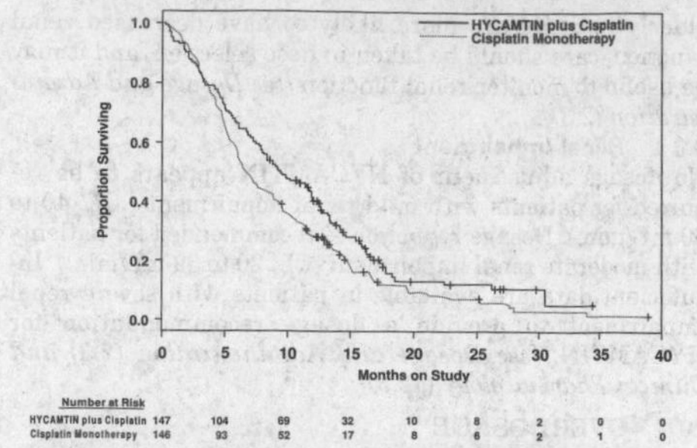

Figure 1. Overall Survival Curves Comparing HYCAMTIN plus Cisplatin versus Cisplatin Monotherapy in Cervical Cancer Patients

15 REFERENCES

1. Preventing Occupational Exposures to Antineoplastic and Other Hazardous Drugs in Health Care Settings. NIOSH Alert 2004-165.
2. OSHA Technical Manual, TED 1-0.15A, Section VI: Chapter 2. Controlling Occupational Exposure to Hazardous Drugs. OSHA, 1999. http://www.osha.gov/dts/osta/otm/otm_vi/otm_vi_2.html
3. American Society of Health-System Pharmacists. ASHP Guidelines on Handling Hazardous Drugs. *Am J Health-Syst Pharm*. 2006;63:1172-1193.
4. Polovich M, White JM, Kelleher LO (eds.) 2005. Chemotherapy and Biotherapy Guidelines and Recommendations for Practice. (2nd ed) Pittsburgh, PA: Oncology Nursing Society.

16 HOW SUPPLIED/STORAGE AND HANDLING

HYCAMTIN for Injection is supplied in 4-mg (free base) single-dose vials.

NDC 0007-4201-01 (package of 1)
NDC 0007-4201-05 (package of 5)

Storage: Store the vials protected from light in the original cartons at controlled room temperature between 20° and 25°C (68° and 77°F) [see USP].

17 PATIENT COUNSELING INFORMATION

17.1 Bone Marrow Suppression

Inform patients that HYCAMTIN decreases blood cell counts such as white blood cells, platelets, and red blood cells. Patients who develop fever or other signs of infection such as chills, cough, or burning pain on urination while on therapy should notify their physician promptly. Inform patients that frequent blood tests will be performed while taking HYCAMTIN to monitor for the occurrence of bone marrow suppression.

17.2 Pregnancy

Advise patients to use effective contraceptive measures to prevent pregnancy and to avoid breastfeeding during treatment with HYCAMTIN.

17.3 Asthenia and Fatigue

Inform patients that HYCAMTIN may cause asthenia or fatigue. If these symptoms occur, caution should be observed when driving or operating machinery.

GlaxoSmithKline
Research Triangle Park, NC 27709

April 2010
HYJ:20PI

IMITREX ℞

[ĭm′ĭ-trĕx]

(sumatriptan succinate)
Injection
For Subcutaneous Use

HIGHLIGHTS OF PRESCRIBING INFORMATION

These highlights do not include all the information needed to use IMITREX safely and effectively. See full prescribing information for IMITREX.

IMITREX (sumatriptan succinate) Injection
For Subcutaneous Use
Initial U.S. Approval: 1992

INDICATIONS AND USAGE

IMITREX is a serotonin (5-HT$_{1B/1D}$) receptor agonist (triptan) indicated for:

- Acute treatment of migraine with or without aura in adults (1)
- Acute treatment of cluster headache in adults (1)

Limitations of Use:

- Use only if a clear diagnosis of migraine or cluster headache has been established. (1)
- Not indicated for the prevention of migraine attacks. (1)

DOSAGE AND ADMINISTRATION

- For subcutaneous use only. (2.1)
- Acute treatment of migraine: 1- to 6-mg Single dose. (2.1)
- Acute treatment of cluster headache: 6-mg Single dose. (2.1)
- Maximum dose in a 24-hour period: 12 mg, Separate doses by at least 1 hour. (2.1)
- Patients receiving doses other than 4 or 6 mg: Use the 6-mg single-dose vial. (2.3)

DOSAGE FORMS AND STRENGTHS

- Injection: 4- and 6-mg single-dose prefilled syringe cartridges for use with IMITREX STATdose Pen (3)
- Injection: 6-mg single-dose vial (3)

CONTRAINDICATIONS

- Coronary artery disease or coronary vasospasm (4)
- Wolff-Parkinson-White syndrome or other cardiac accessory conduction pathway disorders (4)
- History of stroke, transient ischemic attack, or hemiplegic or basilar migraine (4)
- Peripheral vascular disease (4)
- Ischemic bowel disease (4)
- Uncontrolled hypertension (4)
- Recent (within 24 hours) use of another 5-HT_1 agonist (e.g., another triptan) or of an ergotamine-containing medication (4)
- Concurrent or recent (past 2 weeks) use of monoamine oxidase-A inhibitor (4)
- Known hypersensitivity to sumatriptan (4)
- Severe hepatic impairment (4)

WARNINGS AND PRECAUTIONS

- Myocardial ischemia/infarction and Prinzmetal's angina: Perform cardiac evaluation in patients with multiple cardiovascular risk factors. (5.1)
- Arrhythmias: Discontinue IMITREX if occurs. (5.2)
- Chest/throat/neck/jaw pain, tightness, pressure, or heaviness: Generally not associated with myocardial ischemia; evaluate for coronary artery disease in patients at high risk. (5.3)
- Cerebral hemorrhage, subarachnoid hemorrhage, and stroke: Discontinue IMITREX if occurs. (5.4)
- Gastrointestinal ischemia and infarction events, peripheral vasospastic reactions: Discontinue IMITREX if occurs. (5.5)
- Medication overuse headache: Detoxification may be necessary. (5.6)
- Serotonin syndrome: Discontinue IMITREX if occurs. (5.7)
- Increase in blood pressure: Monitor blood pressure. (5.8)
- Anaphylactic/anaphylactoid reactions: Discontinue IMITREX if occurs. (5.9)
- Seizures: Use with caution in patients with epilepsy or a lowered seizure threshold. (5.10)

ADVERSE REACTIONS

Most common adverse reactions (≥5% and > placebo) were injection site reactions, tingling, dizziness/vertigo, warm/hot sensation, burning sensation, feeling of heaviness, pressure sensation, flushing, feeling of tightness, and numbness. (6.1)

To report SUSPECTED ADVERSE REACTIONS, contact GlaxoSmithKline at 1-888-825-5249 or FDA at 1-800-FDA-1088 or www.fda.gov/medwatch

USE IN SPECIFIC POPULATIONS

- Pregnancy: Based on animal data, may cause fetal harm (8.1)
- Geriatric use: A cardiovascular evaluation is recommended in those who have other cardiovascular risk factors prior to receiving IMITREX. (8.5)

See 17 for PATIENT COUNSELING INFORMATION and FDA-approved patient labeling

Revised: 10/2012

FULL PRESCRIBING INFORMATION: CONTENTS*

*** Sections or subsections omitted from the full prescribing information are not listed**

FULL PRESCRIBING INFORMATION

1 INDICATIONS AND USAGE

IMITREX® Injection is indicated in adults for (1) the acute treatment of migraine, with or without aura, and (2) the acute treatment of cluster headache.

Limitations of Use:

- Use only if a clear diagnosis of migraine or cluster headache has been established.
- If a patient has no response to the first migraine attack treated with IMITREX, reconsider the diagnosis of migraine before IMITREX is administered to treat any subsequent attacks.
- IMITREX is not indicated for the prevention of migraine attacks.

2 DOSAGE AND ADMINISTRATION

2.1 Dosing Information

The maximum single recommended adult dose of IMITREX Injection for the acute treatment of migraine or cluster headache is 6 mg injected subcutaneously. For the treatment of migraine, if side effects are dose limiting, lower doses (1 to 5 mg) may be used *[see Clinical Studies (14.1)]*. For the treatment of cluster headache, the efficacy of lower doses has not been established.

The maximum cumulative dose that may be given in 24 hours is 12 mg, two 6-mg injections separated by at least 1 hour. A second 6-mg dose should only be considered if some response to a first injection was observed.

2.2 Administration Using the IMITREX STATdose Pen®

An autoinjector device (IMITREX STATdose Pen) is available for use with 4- and 6-mg prefilled syringe cartridges. With this device, the needle penetrates approximately 1/4 inch (5 to 6 mm). The injection is intended to be given subcutaneously, and intramuscular or intravascular delivery must be avoided. Instruct patients on the proper use of IMITREX STATdose Pen and direct them to use injection sites with an adequate skin and subcutaneous thickness to accommodate the length of the needle.

2.3 Administration of Doses of IMITREX Other Than 4 or 6 mg

In patients receiving doses other than 4 or 6 mg, use the 6-mg single-dose vial; do not use the IMITREX STATdose Pen. Visually inspect the vial for particulate matter and discoloration before administration. Do not use if particulates and discolorations are noted.

3 DOSAGE FORMS AND STRENGTHS

- Injection: 4- and 6-mg single-dose prefilled syringe cartridges for use with the IMITREX STATdose Pen
- Injection: 6-mg single-dose vial

4 CONTRAINDICATIONS

IMITREX Injection is contraindicated in patients with:

- Ischemic coronary artery disease (CAD) (angina pectoris, history of myocardial infarction, or documented silent ischemia) or coronary artery vasospasm, including Prinzmetal's angina *[see Warnings and Precautions (5.1)]*.
- Wolff-Parkinson-White syndrome or arrhythmias associated with other cardiac accessory conduction pathway disorders *[see Warnings and Precautions (5.2)]*.
- History of stroke or transient ischemic attack (TIA) because these patients are at a higher risk of stroke *[see Warnings and Precautions (5.4)]*.
- History of hemiplegic or basilar migraine.
- Peripheral vascular disease *[see Warnings and Precautions (5.5)]*.
- Ischemic bowel disease *[see Warnings and Precautions (5.5)]*.
- Uncontrolled hypertension *[see Warnings and Precautions (5.8)]*.
- Recent (i.e., within 24 hours) use of ergotamine-containing medication, ergot-type medication (such as dihydroergotamine or methysergide), or another 5-hydroxytryptamine$_1$ (5 HT_1) agonist *[see Drug Interactions (7.1, 7.3)]*.
- Concurrent administration of an MAO-A inhibitor or recent (within 2 weeks) use of an MAO-A inhibitor *[see Drug Interactions (7.2) and Clinical Pharmacology (12.3)]*.
- Known hypersensitivity to sumatriptan *[see Warnings and Precautions (5.9) and Adverse Reactions (6.2)]*.
- Severe hepatic impairment *[see Clinical Pharmacology (12.3)]*.

5 WARNINGS AND PRECAUTIONS

5.1 Myocardial Ischemia, Myocardial Infarction, and Prinzmetal's Angina

The use of IMITREX Injection is contraindicated in patients with ischemic or vasospastic CAD. There have been rare reports of serious cardiac adverse reactions, including acute myocardial infarction, occurring within a few hours following administration of IMITREX Injection. Some of these reactions occurred in patients without known CAD. 5-HT_1 agonists, including IMITREX Injection, may cause coronary artery vasospasm (Prinzmetal's angina), even in patients without a history of CAD.

Perform a cardiovascular evaluation in triptan-naive patients who have multiple cardiovascular risk factors (e.g., increased age, diabetes, hypertension, smoking, obesity, strong family history of CAD) prior to receiving IMITREX Injection. If there is evidence of CAD or coronary artery vasospasm, IMITREX Injection is contraindicated. For patients with multiple cardiovascular risk factors who have a negative cardiovascular evaluation, consider administering the first dose of IMITREX Injection in a medically supervised setting and performing an electrocardiogram (ECG) immediately following IMITREX Injection. For such patients, consider periodic cardiovascular evaluation in intermittent long-term users of IMITREX Injection.

Evaluate patients with signs or symptoms suggestive of angina following IMITREX Injection for the presence of CAD or Prinzmetal's angina before receiving additional doses of IMITREX Injection.

5.2 Arrhythmias

Life-threatening disturbances of cardiac rhythm, including ventricular tachycardia and ventricular fibrillation leading to death, have been reported within a few hours following the administration of 5-HT_1 agonists. Discontinue IMITREX Injection if these disturbances occur. IMITREX Injection is contraindicated in patients with Wolff-Parkinson-White syndrome or arrhythmias associated with other cardiac accessory conduction pathway disorders.

5.3 Chest, Throat, Neck, and/or Jaw Pain/Tightness/Pressure

As with other 5-HT_1 agonists, sensations of tightness, pain, pressure, and heaviness in the precordium, throat, neck, and jaw commonly occur after treatment with IMITREX Injection and are usually non-cardiac in origin. However, perform a cardiac evaluation if these patients are at high cardiac risk. The use of IMITREX Injection is contraindicated in patients shown to have CAD and those with Prinzmetal's variant angina.

5.4 Cerebrovascular Events

Cerebral hemorrhage, subarachnoid hemorrhage, and stroke have occurred in patients treated with 5-HT_1 agonists, and some have resulted in fatalities. In a number of cases, it appears possible that the cerebrovascular events were primary, the 5-HT_1 agonist having been administered in the incorrect belief that the symptoms experienced were a consequence of migraine when they were not. Also, patients with migraine may be at increased risk of certain cerebrovascular events (e.g., stroke, hemorrhage, TIA). Discontinue IMITREX Injection if a cerebrovascular event occurs.

As with other acute migraine therapies, before treating headaches in patients not previously diagnosed as migraineurs, and in migraineurs who present with atypical symptoms, exclude other potentially serious neurological conditions. IMITREX Injection is contraindicated in patients with a history of stroke or TIA.

5.5 Other Vasospasm Reactions

5-HT_1 agonists, including IMITREX Injection, may cause non-coronary vasospastic reactions, such as peripheral vascular ischemia, gastrointestinal vascular ischemia and infarction (presenting with abdominal pain and bloody diarrhea), splenic infarction, and Raynaud's syndrome. Until further evaluation, IMITREX Injection is contraindicated in patients who experience symptoms or signs suggestive of non-coronary vasospasm reaction following the use of any 5-HT_1 agonist.

Reports of transient and permanent blindness and significant partial vision loss have been reported with the use of 5-HT_1 agonists. Since visual disorders may be part of a migraine attack, a causal relationship between these events and the use of 5-HT_1 agonists have not been clearly established.

5.6 Medication Overuse Headache

Overuse of acute migraine drugs (e.g., ergotamine, triptans, opioids, combination of drugs for 10 or more days per month) may lead to exacerbation of headache (medication overuse headache). Medication overuse headache may present as migraine-like daily headaches, or as a marked increase in frequency of migraine attacks. Detoxification of patients, including withdrawal of the overused drugs, and treatment of withdrawal symptoms (which often includes a transient worsening of headache) may be necessary.

5.7 Serotonin Syndrome

Serotonin syndrome may occur with triptans, including IMITREX Injection, particularly during coadministration with selective serotonin reuptake inhibitors (SSRIs), serotonin norepinephrine reuptake inhibitors (SNRIs), tricyclic antidepressants (TCAs), and MAO inhibitors *[see Drug Interactions (7.4)]*. Serotonin syndrome symptoms may include mental status changes (e.g., agitation, hallucinations, coma), autonomic instability (e.g., tachycardia, labile blood pressure, hyperthermia), neuromuscular aberrations (e.g., hyperreflexia, incoordination), and/or gastrointestinal symptoms (e.g., nausea, vomiting, diarrhea). The onset of symptoms usually occurs within minutes to hours of receiving a new or a greater dose of a serotonergic medication. Discontinue IMITREX Injection if serotonin syndrome is suspected.

5.8 Increase in Blood Pressure

Significant elevation in blood pressure, including hypertensive crisis with acute impairment of organ systems, has been reported on rare occasions in patients treated with 5-HT_1 agonists, including patients without a history of hypertension. Monitor blood pressure in patients treated with IMITREX. IMITREX Injection is contraindicated in patients with uncontrolled hypertension.

5.9 Anaphylactic/Anaphylactoid Reactions

Anaphylactic/anaphylactoid reactions have occurred in patients receiving sumatriptan. Such reactions can be life threatening or fatal. In general, anaphylactic reactions to drugs are more likely to occur in individuals with a history of sensitivity to multiple allergens. IMITREX Injection is contraindicated in patients with prior serious anaphylactic reaction.

5.10 Seizures

Seizures have been reported following administration of sumatriptan. Some have occurred in patients with either a history of seizures or concurrent conditions predisposing to seizures. There are also reports in patients where no such predisposing factors are apparent. IMITREX Injection should be used with caution in patients with a history of epilepsy or conditions associated with a lowered seizure threshold.

6 ADVERSE REACTIONS

The following adverse reactions are discussed in more detail in other sections of the labeling:

- Myocardial ischemia, myocardial infarction, and Prinzmetal's angina *[see Warnings and Precautions (5.1)]*
- Arrhythmias *[see Warnings and Precautions (5.2)]*
- Chest, throat, neck, and/or jaw pain/tightness/pressure *[see Warnings and Precautions (5.3)]*
- Cerebrovascular events *[see Warnings and Precautions (5.4)]*
- Other vasospasm reactions *[see Warnings and Precautions (5.5)]*
- Medication overuse headache *[see Warnings and Precautions (5.6)]*
- Serotonin syndrome *[see Warnings and Precautions (5.7)]*
- Increase in blood pressure *[see Warnings and Precautions (5.8)]*
- Anaphylactic/anaphylactoid reactions *[see Warnings and Precautions (5.9)]*
- Seizures *[see Warnings and Precautions (5.10)]*

6.1 Clinical Trials Experience

Because clinical trials are conducted under widely varying conditions, adverse reaction rates observed in the clinical trials of a drug cannot be directly compared with rates in the clinical trials of another drug and may not reflect the rates observed in practice.

Migraine Headache: Table 1 lists adverse reactions that occurred in 2 US placebo-controlled clinical trials in migraine subjects *[Studies 2 and 3, see Clinical Studies (14.1)]* following either a single 6-mg dose of IMITREX Injection or placebo. Only reactions that occurred at a frequency of 2% or more in groups treated with IMITREX Injection 6 mg and that occurred at a frequency greater than the placebo group are included in Table 1.

Table 1. Adverse Reactions Reported by at Least 2% of Subjects and at a Greater Frequency Than Placebo in 2 Placebo-Controlled Migraine Clinical Trials (Studies 2 and 3)[a]

	Percent of Subjects Reporting	
	IMITREX Injection 6 mg Subcutaneous (n = 547)	Placebo (n = 370)
Atypical sensations	42	9
Tingling	14	3
Warm/hot sensation	11	4
Burning sensation	7	<1
Feeling of heaviness	7	1
Pressure sensation	7	2
Feeling of tightness	5	<1
Numbness	5	2
Feeling strange	2	<1
Tight feeling in head	2	<1
Cardiovascular		
Flushing	7	2
Chest discomfort	5	1
Tightness in chest	3	<1
Pressure in chest	2	<1
Ear, nose, and throat		
Throat discomfort	3	<1
Discomfort: nasal cavity/sinuses	2	<1
Injection site reaction[b]	59	24
Miscellaneous		
Jaw discomfort	2	0
Musculoskeletal		
Weakness	5	<1
Neck pain/stiffness	5	<1
Myalgia	2	<1
Neurological		
Dizziness/vertigo	12	4
Drowsiness/sedation	3	2
Headache	2	<1
Skin		
Sweating	2	1

[a] The sum of the percentages cited is greater than 100% because subjects may have experienced more than 1 type of adverse reaction. Only reactions that occurred at a frequency of 2% or more in groups treated with IMITREX Injection and occurred at a frequency greater than the placebo groups are included.

[b] Includes injection site pain, stinging/burning, swelling, erythema, bruising, bleeding.

The incidence of adverse reactions in controlled clinical trials was not affected by gender or age of the subjects. There were insufficient data to assess the impact of race on the incidence of adverse reactions.

Cluster Headache: In the controlled clinical trials assessing the efficacy of IMITREX Injection as a treatment for cluster headache *[Studies 4 and 5, see Clinical Studies (14.2)]*, no new significant adverse reactions were detected that had not already been identified in trials of IMITREX in subjects with migraine.

Overall, the frequency of adverse reactions reported in the trials of cluster headache was generally lower than in the migraine trials. Exceptions include reports of paresthesia (5% IMITREX, 0% placebo), nausea and vomiting (4% IMITREX, 0% placebo), and bronchospasm (1% IMITREX, 0% placebo).

Other Adverse Reactions: In the paragraphs that follow, the frequencies of less commonly reported adverse reactions are presented. Reaction frequencies were calculated as the number of subjects reporting a reaction divided by the total number of subjects (N = 6,218) exposed to subcutaneous IMITREX Injection. All reported reactions are included except those already listed in the previous table. Reactions are further classified within body system categories and enumerated in order of decreasing frequency using the following definitions: frequent are defined as those occurring in at least 1/100 subjects, infrequent are those occurring in 1/100 to 1/1,000 subjects, and rare are those occurring in fewer than 1/1,000 subjects.

Cardiovascular: Infrequent were hypertension, hypotension, bradycardia, tachycardia, palpitations, and syncope. Rare was arrhythmia.

Gastrointestinal: Frequent was abdominal discomfort.

Musculoskeletal: Frequent were muscle cramps.

Neurological: Frequent was anxiety. Infrequent were mental confusion, euphoria, agitation, tremor. Rare were myoclonia, sleep disturbance, and dystonia.

Respiratory: Infrequent was dyspnea.

Skin: Infrequent were erythema, pruritus, and skin rashes.

Miscellaneous: Infrequent was "serotonin agonist effect".

Adverse Events Observed With Other Formulations of IMITREX: The following adverse events occurred in clinical trials with IMITREX® Tablets and IMITREX® Nasal Spray. Because the reports include events observed in open and uncontrolled trials, the role of IMITREX in their causation cannot be reliably determined. All reported events are included except those already listed, those too general to be informative, and those not reasonably associated with the use of the drug.

Cardiovascular: Angina, cerebrovascular lesion, heart block, peripheral cyanosis, phlebitis, thrombosis.

Gastrointestinal: Abdominal distention and colitis.

Neurological: Convulsions, hallucinations, syncope, suicide, and twitching.

Miscellaneous: Edema, hypersensitivity, swelling of extremities, and swelling of face.

6.2 Postmarketing Experience

The following adverse reactions have been identified during postapproval use of IMITREX Tablets, IMITREX Nasal Spray, and IMITREX Injection. Because these reactions are reported voluntarily from a population of uncertain size, it is not always possible to reliably estimate their frequency or establish a causal relationship to drug exposure. These reactions have been chosen for inclusion due to either their seriousness, frequency of reporting, or causal connection to IMITREX or a combination of these factors.

Blood: Hemolytic anemia, pancytopenia, thrombocytopenia.

Ear, Nose, and Throat: Deafness.

Eye: Ischemic optic neuropathy, retinal artery occlusion, retinal vein thrombosis.

Neurological: Central nervous system vasculitis, cerebrovascular accident, serotonin syndrome, subarachnoid hemorrhage.

Non-Site Specific: Angioedema, cyanosis, temporal arteritis.

Skin: Exacerbation of sunburn, hypersensitivity reactions (allergic vasculitis, erythema, pruritus, rash, shortness of breath, urticaria), photosensitivity. Following subcutaneous administration of IMITREX, pain, redness, stinging, induration, swelling, contusion, subcutaneous bleeding, and, on rare occasions, lipoatrophy (depression in the skin) or lipohypertrophy (enlargement or thickening of tissue) have been reported.

Urogenital: Acute renal failure.

7 DRUG INTERACTIONS

7.1 Ergot-Containing Drugs

Ergot-containing drugs have been reported to cause prolonged vasospastic reactions. Because these effects may be additive, use of ergotamine-containing or ergot-type medications (like dihydroergotamine or methysergide) and IMITREX Injection within 24 hours of each other is contraindicated.

7.2 Monoamine Oxidase-A Inhibitors

MAO-A inhibitors increase systemic exposure by 2-fold. Therefore, the use of IMITREX Injection in patients receiving MAO-A inhibitors is contraindicated *[see Clinical Pharmacology (12.3)]*.

7.3 Other 5-HT_1 Agonists

Because their vasospastic effects may be additive, coadministration of IMITREX Injection and other 5-HT_1 agonists (e.g., triptans) within 24 hours of each other is contraindicated.

7.4 Selective Serotonin Reuptake Inhibitors/Serotonin Norepinephrine Reuptake Inhibitors and Serotonin Syndrome

Cases of serotonin syndrome have been reported during coadministration of triptans and SSRIs, or SNRIs, SNRIs, TCAs, and MAO inhibitors *[see Warnings and Precautions (5.7)]*.

8 USE IN SPECIFIC POPULATIONS

8.1 Pregnancy

Pregnancy Category C: There are no adequate and well-controlled trials of IMITREX Injection in pregnant women. IMITREX Injection should be used during pregnancy only if the potential benefit justifies the potential risk to the fetus.

When sumatriptan was administered intravenously to pregnant rabbits daily throughout the period of organogenesis, embryolethality was observed at doses at or close to those producing maternal toxicity. These doses were less than the maximum recommended human dose (MRHD) of 12 mg/day on a mg/m^2 basis. Oral administration of sumatriptan to rabbits during organogenesis was associated with increased incidences of fetal vascular and skeletal abnormalities. The highest no-effect dose for these effects was 15 mg/kg/day. The intravenous administration of sumatriptan to pregnant rats throughout organogenesis at doses that are approximately 10 times the MRHD on a mg/m^2 basis, did not produce evidence of embryolethality. The subcutaneous administration of sumatriptan to pregnant rats prior to and throughout pregnancy did not produce evidence of embryolethality or teratogenicity.

8.3 Nursing Mothers

It is not known whether sumatriptan is excreted in human breast milk following subcutaneous administration. Because many drugs are excreted in human milk, and because of the potential for serious adverse reactions in nursing infants from IMITREX, a decision should be made whether to discontinue nursing or to discontinue the drug, taking into account the importance of the drug to the mother.

8.4 Pediatric Use

Safety and effectiveness of IMITREX Injection in pediatric patients under 18 years of age have not been established; therefore, IMITREX Injection is not recommended for use in patients under 18 years of age.

Two controlled clinical trials evaluated IMITREX Nasal Spray (5 to 20 mg) in 1,248 adolescent migraineurs aged 12 to 17 years who treated a single attack. The trials did not establish the efficacy of IMITREX Nasal Spray compared with placebo in the treatment of migraine in adolescents. Adverse reactions observed in these clinical trials were similar in nature to those reported in clinical trials in adults.

Five controlled clinical trials (2 single-attack trials, 3 multiple-attack trials) evaluating oral IMITREX (25 to 100 mg) in pediatric subjects aged 12 to 17 years enrolled a total of 701 adolescent migraineurs. These trials did not establish the efficacy of oral IMITREX compared with placebo in the treatment of migraine in adolescents. Adverse reactions observed in these clinical trials were similar in nature to those reported in clinical trials in adults. The frequency of all adverse reactions in these subjects appeared to be both dose- and age-dependent, with younger subjects reporting reactions more commonly than older adolescents.

Postmarketing experience documents that serious adverse reactions have occurred in the pediatric population after use of subcutaneous, oral, and/or intranasal IMITREX. These reports include reactions similar in nature to those reported rarely in adults, including stroke, visual loss, and death. A myocardial infarction has been reported in a 14-year-old male following the use of oral IMITREX; clinical signs occurred within 1 day of drug administration. Since clinical data to determine the frequency of serious adverse reactions in pediatric patients who might receive subcutaneous, oral, or intranasal IMITREX are not presently available, the use of IMITREX in patients under 18 years of age is not recommended.

8.5 Geriatric Use

Clinical trials of IMITREX Injection did not include sufficient numbers of subjects aged 65 and over to determine whether they respond differently from younger subjects. Other reported clinical experience has not identified differences in responses between the elderly and younger subjects. In general, dose selection for an elderly patient should be cautious, usually starting at the low end of the dosing range, reflecting the greater frequency of decreased hepatic, renal, or cardiac function and of concomitant disease or other drug therapy.

A cardiovascular evaluation is recommended for geriatric patients who have other cardiovascular risk factors (e.g., diabetes, hypertension, smoking, obesity, strong family history of CAD) prior to receiving IMITREX Injection *[see Warnings and Precautions (5.1)]*.

10 OVERDOSAGE

No gross overdoses in clinical practice have been reported. Coronary vasospasm was observed after intravenous administration of IMITREX Injection *[see Contraindications (4)]*. Overdoses would be expected from animal data (dogs at 0.1 g/kg, rats at 2 g/kg) to possibly cause convulsions, tremor, inactivity, erythema of the extremities, reduced respiratory rate, cyanosis, ataxia, mydriasis, injection site reactions (desquamation, hair loss, and scab formation), and paralysis.

The elimination half-life of sumatriptan is about 2 hours *[see Clinical Pharmacology (12.3)]*, and therefore monitoring of patients after overdose with IMITREX Injection should continue for at least 10 hours or while symptoms or signs persist.

It is unknown what effect hemodialysis or peritoneal dialysis has on the serum concentrations of sumatriptan.

11 DESCRIPTION

IMITREX Injection contains sumatriptan succinate, a selective 5-$HT_{1B/1D}$ receptor agonist. Sumatriptan succinate is chemically designated as 3-[2-(dimethylamino)ethyl]-N-methyl-indole-5-methanesulfonamide succinate (1:1), and it has the following structure:

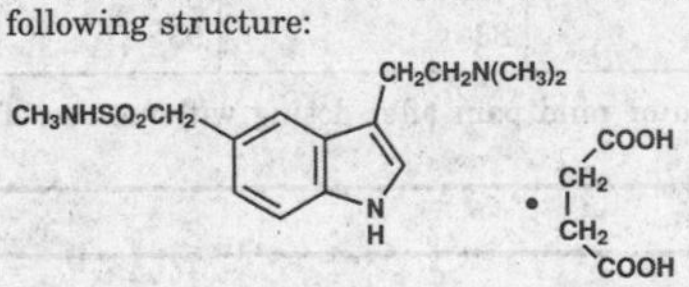

The empirical formula is $C_{14}H_{21}N_3O_2S \bullet C_4H_6O_4$, representing a molecular weight of 413.5. Sumatriptan succinate is a white to off-white powder that is readily soluble in water and in saline.

IMITREX Injection is a clear, colorless to pale yellow, sterile, nonpyrogenic solution for subcutaneous injection. Each 0.5 mL of IMITREX Injection 8 mg/mL solution contains 4 mg of sumatriptan (base) as the succinate salt and 3.8 mg of sodium chloride, USP in Water for Injection, USP. Each 0.5 mL of IMITREX Injection 12 mg/mL solution contains 6 mg of sumatriptan (base) as the succinate salt and 3.5 mg of sodium chloride, USP in Water for Injection, USP. The pH range of both solutions is approximately 4.2 to 5.3. The osmolality of both injections is 291 mOsmol.

12 CLINICAL PHARMACOLOGY

12.1 Mechanism of Action

Sumatriptan binds with high affinity to human cloned 5-HT_{1B}/$_{1D}$ receptors. IMITREX presumably exerts its therapeutic effects in the treatment of migraine headache by binding to 5-HT_{1B}/$_{1D}$ receptors located on intracranial blood vessels and sensory nerves of the trigeminal system.

Current theories proposed to explain the etiology of migraine headache suggest that symptoms are due to local cranial vasodilatation and/or to the release of sensory neuropeptides (including substance P and calcitonin gene-related peptide) through nerve endings in the trigeminal system. The therapeutic activity of IMITREX for the treatment of migraine and cluster headaches is thought to be due to the agonist effects at the 5-$HT_{1B/1D}$ receptors on intracranial blood vessels (including the arterio-venous anastomoses) and sensory nerves of the trigeminal system, which result in cranial vessel constriction and inhibition of pro-inflammatory neuropeptide release.

12.2 Pharmacodynamics

Blood Pressure: Significant elevation in blood pressure, including hypertensive crisis, has been reported in patients with and without a history of hypertension *[see Warnings and Precautions (5.8)]*.

Peripheral (Small) Arteries: In healthy volunteers (N = 18), a trial evaluating the effects of sumatriptan on peripheral (small vessel) arterial reactivity failed to detect a clinically significant increase in peripheral resistance.

Heart Rate: Transient increases in blood pressure observed in some subjects in clinical trials carried out during sumatriptan's development as a treatment for migraine were not accompanied by any clinically significant changes in heart rate.

12.3 Pharmacokinetics

Absorption and Bioavailability: The bioavailability of sumatriptan via subcutaneous site injection to 18 healthy male subjects was 97% ± 16% of that obtained following intravenous injection.

After a single 6-mg subcutaneous manual injection into the deltoid area of the arm in 18 healthy males (age: 24 ± 6 years, weight: 70 kg), the maximum serum concentration (C_{max}) of sumatriptan was (mean ± standard deviation) 74 ± 15 ng/mL and the time to peak concentration (T_{max}) was 12 minutes after injection (range: 5 to 20 minutes). In this trial, the same dose injected subcutaneously in the thigh gave a C_{max} of 61 ± 15 ng/mL by manual injection versus 52 ± 15 ng/mL by autoinjector techniques. The T_{max} or amount absorbed was not significantly altered by either the site or technique of injection.

Distribution: Protein binding, determined by equilibrium dialysis over the concentration range of 10 to 1,000 ng/mL, is low, approximately 14% to 21%. The effect of sumatriptan on the protein binding of other drugs has not been evaluated.

Following a 6-mg subcutaneous injection into the deltoid area of the arm in 9 males (mean age: 33 years, mean weight: 77 kg) the volume of distribution central compartment of sumatriptan was 50 ± 8 liters and the distribution half–life was 15 ± 2 minutes.

Metabolism: In vitro studies with human microsomes suggest that sumatriptan is metabolized by MAO, predominantly the A isoenzyme. Most of a radiolabeled dose of sumatriptan excreted in the urine is the major metabolite indole acetic acid (IAA) or the IAA glucuronide, both of which are inactive.

Elimination: After a single 6-mg subcutaneous dose, 22% ± 4% was excreted in the urine as unchanged sumatriptan and 38% ± 7% as the IAA metabolite.

Following a 6 mg subcutaneous injection into the deltoid area of the arm, the systemic clearance of sumatriptan was 1,194 ± 149 mL/min and the terminal half-life was 115 ± 19 minutes.

Special Populations: *Age*: The pharmacokinetics of sumatriptan in the elderly (mean age: 72 years, 2 males and 4 females) and in subjects with migraine (mean age: 38 years, 25 males and 155 females) were similar to that in healthy male subjects (mean age: 30 years).

Renal Impairment: The effect of renal impairment on the pharmacokinetics of sumatriptan has not been examined.

Hepatic Impairment: The effect of mild to moderate hepatic disease on the pharmacokinetics of subcutaneously administered sumatriptan has been evaluated. There were no significant differences in the pharmacokinetics of subcutaneously administered sumatriptan in moderately hepatically impaired subjects compared with healthy controls. The pharmacokinetics of subcutaneously administered sumatriptan in patients with severe hepatic impairment has not been studied. The use of IMITREX Injection in this population is contraindicated *[see Contraindications (4)]*.

Race: The systemic clearance and C_{max} of sumatriptan were similar in black (n = 34) and Caucasian (n = 38) healthy male subjects.

Drug Interaction Studies: *Monoamine Oxidase-A Inhibitors:* In a trial of 14 healthy females, pretreatment with an MAO-A inhibitor decreased the clearance of sumatriptan, resulting in a 2-fold increase in the area under the sumatriptan plasma concentration-time curve (AUC), corresponding to a 40% increase in elimination half-life.

13 NONCLINICAL TOXICOLOGY

13.1 Carcinogenesis, Mutagenesis, Impairment of Fertility

Carcinogenesis: In carcinogenicity studies, rats and mice were given sumatriptan by oral gavage. Mice were dosed for 78 weeks and rats were dosed for 104 weeks. Average exposures achieved in mice receiving the highest dose were approximately 110 times the exposure attained in humans after the maximum recommended single dose of 6 mg. The highest dose to rats was approximately 260 times the maximum single dose of 6 mg on a mg/m2 basis. There was no evidence of an increase in tumors in either species related to sumatriptan administration.

Mutagenesis: Sumatriptan was not mutagenic in the presence or absence of metabolic activation when tested in 2 gene mutation assays (the Ames test and the in vitro mammalian Chinese hamster V79/HGPRT assay). It was not clastogenic in 2 cytogenetics assays (the in vitro human lymphocyte assay and the in vivo rat micronucleus assay).

Impairment of Fertility: A fertility study (Segment I) by the subcutaneous route, during which male and female rats were dosed daily with sumatriptan prior to and throughout the mating period, has shown no evidence of impaired fertility at doses equivalent to approximately 100 times the maximum recommended single human dose of 6 mg on a mg/m^2 basis. However, following oral administration, a treatment-related decrease in fertility, secondary to a decrease in mating, was seen for rats treated with 50 and 500 mg/kg/day. The no-effect dose for this finding was approximately 8 times the maximum recommended single human dose of 6 mg on a mg/m^2 basis. It is not clear whether the problem is associated with the treatment of males or females or both.

13.2 Animal Toxicology and/or Pharmacology

Corneal Opacities: Dogs receiving oral sumatriptan developed corneal opacities and defects in the corneal epithelium. Corneal opacities were seen at the lowest dosage tested, 2 mg/kg/day, and were present after 1 month of treatment. Defects in the corneal epithelium were noted in a 60-week study. Earlier examinations for these toxicities were not conducted and no-effect doses were not established; however, the relative exposure at the lowest dose tested was approximately 5 times the human exposure after a 100-mg oral dose or 3 times the human exposure after a 6-mg subcutaneous dose.

Melanin Binding: In rats with a single subcutaneous dose (0.5 mg/kg) of radiolabeled sumatriptan, the elimination half-life of radioactivity from the eye was 15 days, suggesting that sumatriptan and its metabolites bind to the melanin of the eye. The clinical significance of this binding is unknown.

14 CLINICAL STUDIES

14.1 Migraine

In controlled clinical trials enrolling more than 1,000 subjects during migraine attacks who were experiencing mod-

Table 2. Proportion of Subjects With Migraine Relief and Incidence of Adverse Events by Time and by IMITREX Dose in Study 1

Dose of IMITREX Injection	Percent Subjects With Relief[a]				Adverse Events Incidence (%)
	at 10 Minutes	at 30 Minutes	at 1 Hour	at 2 Hours	
Placebo	5	15	24	21	55
1 mg	10	40	43	40	63
2 mg	7	23	57	43	63
3 mg	17	47	57	60	77
4 mg	13	37	50	57	80
6 mg	10	63	73	70	83
8 mg	23	57	80	83	93

[a] Relief is defined as the reduction of moderate or severe pain to no or mild pain after dosing without use of rescue medication.

Table 3. Proportion of Subjects With Pain Relief and Relief of Migraine Symptoms After 1 and 2 Hours of Treatment in Studies 2 and 3

1-Hour Data	Study 2		Study 3	
	Placebo (n = 190)	IMITREX 6 mg (n = 384)	Placebo (n = 180)	IMITREX 6 mg (n = 350)
Subjects with pain relief (grade 0/1)	18%	70%[a]	26%	70%[a]
Subjects with no pain	5%	48%[a]	13%	49%[a]
Subjects without nausea	48%	73%[a]	50%	73%[a]
Subjects without photophobia	23%	56%[a]	25%	58%[a]
Subjects with little or no clinical disability[b]	34%	76%[a]	34%	76%[a]
2-Hour Data	Study 2		Study 3	
	Placebo[c]	IMITREX 6 mg[d]	Placebo[c]	IMITREX 6 mg[d]
Subjects with pain relief (grade 0/1)	31%	81%[a]	39%	82%[a]
Subjects with no pain	11%	63%[a]	19%	65%[a]
Subjects without nausea	56%	82%[a]	63%	81%[a]
Subjects without photophobia	31%	72%[a]	35%	71%[a]
Subjects with little or no clinical disability[b]	42%	85%[a]	49%	84%[a]

[a] $P < 0.05$ versus placebo.
[b] A successful outcome in terms of clinical disability was defined prospectively as ability to work mildly impaired or ability to work and function normally.
[c] Includes subjects that may have received an additional placebo injection 1 hour after the initial injection.
[d] Includes subjects that may have received an additional 6 mg of IMITREX Injection 1 hour after the initial injection.

Table 4. Proportion of Subjects With Cluster Headache Relief by Time in Studies 4 and 5

	Study 4		Study 5	
	Placebo (n = 39)	IMITREX 6 mg (n = 39)	Placebo (n = 88)	IMITREX 6 mg (n = 92)
Subjects with pain relief (no/mild)				
5 Minutes post-injection	8%	21%	7%	23%[a]
10 Minutes post-injection	10%	49%[a]	25%	49%[a]
15 m inutes post-injection	26%	74%[a]	35%	75%[a]

[a] $P < 0.05$.
(n = Number of headaches treated.)

erate or severe pain and 1 or more of the symptoms enumerated in Table 3, onset of relief began as early as 10 minutes following a 6-mg IMITREX Injection. Lower doses of IMITREX Injection may also prove effective, although the proportion of subjects obtaining adequate relief was decreased and the latency to that relief is greater with lower doses.

In Study 1, 6 different doses of IMITREX Injection (n = 30 each group) were compared with placebo (n = 62), in a single-attack, parallel-group design, the dose response relationship was found to be as shown in Table 2.

[See table 2 above]

In 2 randomized, placebo-controlled clinical trials of IMITREX Injection 6 mg in 1,104 subjects with moderate or severe migraine pain (Studies 2 and 3), the onset of relief was less than 10 minutes. Headache relief, as defined by a reduction in pain from severe or moderately severe to mild or no headache, was achieved in 70% of the subjects within 1 hour of a single 6-mg subcutaneous dose of IMITREX Injection. Approximately 82% and 65% of subjects treated with IMITREX 6 mg had headache relief and were pain free within 2 hours, respectively.

Table 3 shows the 1- and 2-hour efficacy results for IMITREX Injection 6 mg in Studies 2 and 3.

[See table 3 above]

IMITREX Injection also relieved photophobia, phonophobia (sound sensitivity), nausea, and vomiting associated with migraine attacks. Similar efficacy was seen when subjects self-administered IMITREX Injection using the IMITREX STATdose Pen.

The efficacy of IMITREX Injection was unaffected by whether or not the migraine was associated with aura, duration of attack, gender or age of the subject, or concomitant use of common migraine prophylactic drugs (e.g., beta-blockers).

14.2 Cluster Headache

The efficacy of IMITREX Injection in the acute treatment of cluster headache was demonstrated in 2 randomized, double-blind, placebo-controlled, 2-period crossover trials (Studies 4 and 5). Subjects aged 21 to 65 years were enrolled and were instructed to treat a moderate to very severe headache within 10 minutes of onset. Headache relief was defined as a reduction in headache severity to mild or no pain. In both trials, the proportion of individuals gaining relief at 10 or 15 minutes was significantly greater among subjects receiving 6 mg of IMITREX Injection compared with those who received placebo (see Table 4).

[See table 4 above]

An estimate of the cumulative probability of a subject with a cluster headache obtaining relief after being treated with either IMITREX Injection or placebo is presented in Figure 1.

Figure 1. Time to Relief of Cluster Headache from Time of Injection[a]

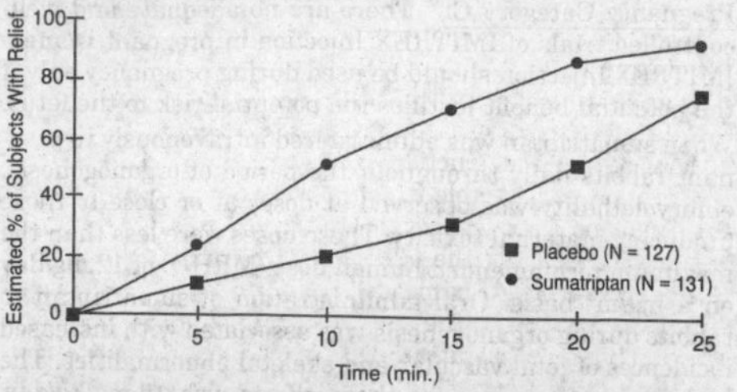

[a] The figure uses Kaplan-Meier (product limit) Survivorship Plot. Subjects taking rescue medication were censored at 15 minutes.

The plot was constructed with data from subjects who either experienced relief or did not require (request) rescue medication within a period of 2 hours following treatment. As a consequence, the data in the plot are derived from only a subset of the 258 headaches treated (rescue medication was required in 52 of the 127 placebo-treated headaches and 18 of the 131 headaches treated with IMITREX Injection).

Other data suggest that treatment with IMITREX Injection is not associated with an increase in early recurrence of headache and has little effect on the incidence of later-occurring headaches (i.e., those occurring after 2, but before 18 or 24 hours).

16 HOW SUPPLIED/STORAGE AND HANDLING

IMITREX Injection contains sumatriptan (base) as the succinate salt and is supplied as a clear, colorless to pale yellow, sterile, nonpyrogenic solution as follows:

Prefilled Syringe and/or Autoinjector Pen: Each pack contains a Patient Information and Patients Instructions for Use leaflet.

- IMITREX STATdose System®, 4 mg, containing 1 IMITREX STATdose Pen, 2 prefilled single-dose syringe cartridges, and 1 carrying case (NDC 0173-0739-00).
- IMITREX STATdose System, 6 mg, containing 1 IMITREX STATdose Pen, 2 prefilled single-dose syringe cartridges, and 1 carrying case (NDC 0173-0479-00).
- Two 4-mg single-dose prefilled syringe cartridges for use with IMITREX STATdose System (NDC 0173-0739-02).
- Two 6-mg single-dose prefilled syringe cartridges for use with IMITREX STATdose System (NDC 0173-0478-00).

Single-Dose Vial:

- IMITREX Injection single-dose vial (6 mg/0.5 mL) in cartons containing 5 vials (NDC 0173-0449-02).

Store between 2° and 30°C (36° and 86°F). Protect from light.

17 PATIENT COUNSELING INFORMATION

See FDA-approved patient labeling (Patient Information and Instructions for Use).

17.1 Risk of Myocardial Ischemia and/or Infarction, Prinzmetal's Angina, Other Vasospasm-Related Events, Arrhythmias, and Cerebrovascular Events

Inform patients that IMITREX Injection may cause serious cardiovascular side effects such as myocardial infarction or stroke. Although serious cardiovascular events can occur without warning symptoms, patients should be alert for the signs and symptoms of chest pain, shortness of breath, irregular heartbeat, significant rise in blood pressure, weakness, and slurring of speech and should ask for medical advice when observing any indicative sign or symptoms. Patients should be apprised of the importance of this follow-up *[see Warnings and Precautions (5.1, 5.2, 5.4, 5.5, 5.8)]*.

17.2 Anaphylactic/Anaphylactoid Reactions

Inform patients that anaphylactic/anaphylactoid reactions have occurred in patients receiving IMITREX Injection. Such reactions can be life threatening or fatal. In general, anaphylactic reactions to drugs are more likely to occur in individuals with a history of sensitivity to multiple allergens *[see Warnings and Precautions (5.9)]*.

17.3 Medication Overuse Headache

Inform patients that use of acute migraine drugs for 10 or more days per month may lead to an exacerbation of headache and encourage patients to record headache frequency and drug use (e.g., by keeping a headache diary) *[see Warnings and Precautions (5.6)]*.

17.4 Pregnancy

Inform patients that IMITREX Injection should not be used during pregnancy unless the potential benefit justifies the potential risk to the fetus *[see Use in Specific Populations (8.1)]*.

17.5 Nursing Mothers

Advise patients to notify their healthcare provider if they are breastfeeding or plan to breastfeed *[see Use in Specific Populations (8.3)]*.

17.6 Ability To Perform Complex Tasks

Since migraines or treatment with IMITREX Injection may cause somnolence and dizziness, instruct patients to evaluate their ability to perform complex tasks during migraine attacks and after administration of IMITREX Injection.

17.7 Serotonin Syndrome

Patients should be cautioned about the risk of serotonin syndrome with the use of IMITREX Injection or other triptans, particularly during combined use with SSRIs, SNRIs, TCAs, and MAO inhibitors *[see Warnings and Precautions (5.7) and Drug Interactions (7.4)]*.

17.8 How to Use IMITREX Injection

Provide patients instruction on the proper use of IMITREX Injection if they are able to self-administer IMITREX Injection in medically unsupervised situation.

Inform patients that the needle in the IMITREX STATdose Pen penetrates approximately 1/4 of an inch (5 to 6 mm). Inform patients that the injection is intended to be given subcutaneously and intramuscular or intravascular delivery should be avoided. Instruct patients to use injection sites with an adequate skin and subcutaneous thickness to accommodate the length of the needle.

IMITREX, IMITREX STATdose Pen, and IMITREX STATdose System are registered trademarks of GlaxoSmithKline.

GlaxoSmithKline
Research Triangle Park, NC 27709

IMJ:4PI

Patient Information
IMITREX® (IM-i-trex)
(sumatriptansuccinate)
Injection

Read this Patient Information before you start taking IMITREX and each time you get a refill. There may be new information. This information does not take the place of talking with your healthcare provider about your medical condition or treatment.

What is the most important information I should know about IMITREX?

IMITREX can cause serious side effects, including:

Heart attack and other heart problems. Heart problems may lead to death.

Stop taking IMITREX and get emergency medical help right away if you have any of the following symptoms of a heart attack:

- discomfort in the center of your chest that lasts for more than a few minutes, or that goes away and comes back
- severe tightness, pain, pressure, or heaviness in your chest, throat, neck, or jaw
- pain or discomfort in your arms, back, neck, jaw, or stomach
- shortness of breath with or without chest discomfort
- breaking out in a cold sweat
- nausea or vomiting
- feeling lightheaded

IMITREX is not for people with risk factors for heart disease unless a heart exam is done and shows no problem. You have a higher risk for heart disease if you:

- have high blood pressure
- have high cholesterol levels
- smoke
- are overweight
- have diabetes
- have a family history of heart disease

What is IMITREX?

IMITREX is a prescription medicine used to treat acute migraine headaches with or without aura and acute cluster headaches in adults who have been diagnosed with migraine or cluster headaches.

IMITREX is not used to treat other types of headaches such as hemiplegic (that make you unable to move on one side of your body) or basilar (rare form of migraine with aura) migraines.

IMITREX is not used to prevent or decrease the number of migraine or cluster headaches you have.

It is not known if IMITREX is safe and effective in children under 18 years of age.

Who should not take IMITREX?

Do not take IMITREX if you have:

- heart problems or a history of heart problems
- narrowing of blood vessels to your legs, arms, stomach, or kidney (peripheral vascular disease)
- uncontrolled high blood pressure
- hemiplegic migraines or basilar migraines. If you are not sure if you have these types of migraines, ask your healthcare provider.
- had a stroke, transient ischemic attacks (TIAs), or problems with your blood circulation
- taken any of the following medicines in the last 24 hours:
  - almotriptan (AXERT®)
  - eletriptan (RELPAX®)
  - frovatriptan (FROVA®)
  - naratriptan (AMERGE®)
  - rizatriptan (MAXALT®, MAXALT-MLT®)
  - sumatriptan and naproxen (TREXIMET®)
  - ergotamines (CAFERGOT®, ERGOMAR®, MIGERGOT®)
  - dihydroergotamine (D.H.E. 45®, MIGRANAL®)

Ask your healthcare provider if you are not sure if your medicine is listed above.
- an allergy to sumatriptan or any of the ingredients in IMITREX. See the end of this leaflet for a complete list of ingredients in IMITREX.

What should I tell my healthcare provider before taking IMITREX?

Before you take IMITREX, tell your healthcare provider about all of your medical conditions, including if you:

- have high blood pressure
- have high cholesterol
- have diabetes
- smoke
- are overweight
- have heart problems or family history of heart problems or stroke
- have liver problems
- have had epilepsy or seizures
- are not using effective birth control
- become pregnant while taking IMITREX
- are breastfeeding or plan to breastfeed. IMITREX passes into your breast milk and may harm your baby. Talk with your healthcare provider about the best way to feed your baby if you take IMITREX.

Tell your healthcare provider about all the medicines you take, including prescription and nonprescription medicines, vitamins, and herbal supplements.

Using IMITREX with certain other medicines can affect each other, causing serious side effects.

Especially tell your healthcare provider if you take antidepressant medicines called:

- selective serotonin reuptake inhibitors (SSRIs)
- serotonin norepinephrine reuptake inhibitors (SNRIs)
- tricyclic antidepressants (TCAs)
- monoamine oxidase inhibitors (MAOIs)

Ask your healthcare provider or pharmacist for a list of these medicines if you are not sure.

Know the medicines you take. Keep a list of them to show your healthcare provider or pharmacist when you get a new medicine.

How should I take IMITREX?

- Certain people should take their first dose of IMITREX in their healthcare provider's office or in another medical setting. Ask your healthcare provider if you should take your first dose in a medical setting.
- Use IMITREX exactly as your healthcare provider tells you to use it.
- Your healthcare provider may change your dose. Do not change your dose without first talking with your healthcare provider.
- For adults, the usual dose is a single injection given just below the skin.
- You should give an injection as soon as the symptoms of your headache start, but it may be given at any time during a migraine attack.
- If you did not get any relief after the first injection, do not give a second injection without first talking with your healthcare provider.
- You can take a second injection 1 hour after the first injection, but not sooner, if your headache came back after your first injection.
- Do not take more than 12 mg in a 24–hour period.
- If you use too much IMITREX, call your healthcare provider or go to the nearest hospital emergency room right away.
- You should write down when you have headaches and when you take IMITREX so you can talk with your healthcare provider about how IMITREX is working for you.

What should I avoid while taking IMITREX?

IMITREX can cause dizziness, weakness, or drowsiness. If you have these symptoms, do not drive a car, use machinery, or do anything where you need to be alert.

What are the possible side effects of IMITREX?

IMITREX may cause serious side effects. See "What is the most important information I should know about IMITREX?"

These serious side effects include:

- changes in color or sensation in your fingers and toes (Raynaud's syndrome)
- stomach and intestinal problems (gastrointestinal and colonic ischemic events). Symptoms of gastrointestinal and colonic ischemic events include:
  - sudden or severe stomach pain
  - stomach pain after meals
  - weight loss
  - nausea or vomiting
  - constipation or diarrhea
  - bloody diarrhea
  - fever
- problems with blood circulation to your legs and feet (peripheral vascular ischemia). Symptoms of peripheral vascular ischemia include:
  - cramping and pain in your legs or hips
  - feeling of heaviness or tightness in your leg muscles
  - burning or aching pain in your feet or toes while resting
  - numbness, tingling, or weakness in your legs
  - cold feeling or color changes in 1 or both legs or feet
- medication overuse headaches. Some people who use too many IMITREX injections may have worse headaches (medication overuse headache). If your headaches get worse, your healthcare provider may decide to stop your treatment with IMITREX.
- serotonin syndrome. Serotonin syndrome is a rare but serious problem that can happen in people using IMITREX, especially if IMITREX is used with anti–depressant medicines called SSRIs or SNRIs.

  Call your healthcare provider right away if you have any of the following symptoms of serotonin syndrome:
  - mental changes such as seeing things that are not there (hallucinations), agitation, or coma
  - fast heartbeat
  - changes in blood pressure
  - high body temperature
  - tight muscles
  - trouble walking
- seizures. Seizures have happened in people taking IMITREX who have never had seizures before. Talk with your healthcare provider about your chance of having seizures while you take IMITREX.

The most common side effects of IMITREX include:

- pain or redness at your injection site
- tingling or numbness in your fingers or toes
- dizziness
- warm, hot, burning feeling to your face (flushing)
- discomfort or stiffness in your neck
- feeling weak, drowsy, or tired

Tell your healthcare provider if you have any side effect that bothers you or that does not go away.

These are not all the possible side effects of IMITREX. For more information, ask your healthcare provider or pharmacist.

Call your doctor for medical advice about side effects. You may report side effects to FDA at 1-800-FDA-1088.

How should I store IMITREX Injection?

- Store IMITREX between 36°F to 86°F (2°C to 30°C).
- Store your medicine away from light.
- Keep your medicine in the packaging or carrying case provided with it.

Keep IMITREX and all medicines out of the reach of children.

General information about the safe and effective use of IMITREX

Medicines are sometimes prescribed for purposes other than those listed in Patient Information leaflets. Do not use IMITREX for a condition for which it was not prescribed. Do not give IMITREX to other people, even if they have the same symptoms you have. It may harm them.

This Patient Information leaflet summarizes the most important information about IMITREX. If you would like more information, talk with your healthcare provider. You can ask your healthcare provider or pharmacist for information about IMITREX that is written for healthcare professionals. For more information, go to www.gsk.com or call 1-888-825-5249.

What are the ingredients in IMITREX Injection?

Active ingredient: sumatriptan succinate

Inactive ingredients: sodium chloride, water for injection

This Patient Information and Instructions for Use has been approved by the U.S. Food and Drug Administration.

IMITREX, AMERGE, TREXIMET are registered trademarks of GlaxoSmithKline. The other brands listed are trademarks of their respective owners and are not trademarks of GlaxoSmithKline. The makers of these brands are not affiliated with and do not endorse GlaxoSmithKline or its products.

GlaxoSmithKline
Research Triangle Park, NC 27709

October 2012
IMJ:3PPI

IMITREX® ℞
[ĭm'ĭ-trĕx]
(sumatriptan)
Nasal Spray

DESCRIPTION

IMITREX (sumatriptan) Nasal Spray contains sumatriptan, a selective 5-hydroxytryptamine$_1$ receptor subtype agonist. Sumatriptan is chemically designated as 3-[2-(dimethylamino)ethyl]-N-methyl-1H-indole-5-methanesulfonamide, and it has the following structure:

Table 1. Percentage of Patients With Headache Response (No or Mild Pain) 2 Hours Following Treatment

	Placebo	IMITREX Nasal Spray 5 mg	IMITREX Nasal Spray 10 mg	IMITREX Nasal Spray 20 mg
Study 1	25% (n = 63)	49%[a] (n = 121)	46%[a] (n = 112)	64%[abc] (n = 118)
Study 2	25% (n = 138)	Not applicable	44%[a] (n = 273)	55%[ab] (n = 277)
Study 3	35% (n = 100)	Not applicable	54%[a] (n = 106)	63%[a] (n = 202)
Study 4	29% (n = 112)	Not applicable	43% (n = 106)	62%[ab] (n = 215)
Study 5[d]	36% (n = 198)	45%[a] (n = 296)	53%[a] (n = 291)	60%[ac] (n = 286)

[a]*P*<0.05 in comparison with placebo.
[b]*P*<0.05 in comparison with 10 mg.
[c]*P*<0.05 in comparison with 5 mg.
[d]Data are for attack 1 only of multiattack study for comparison.

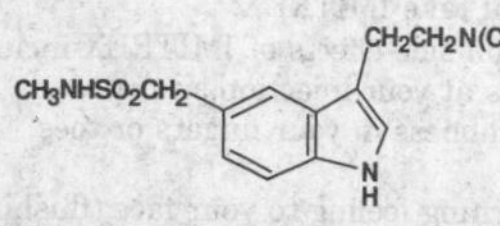

The empirical formula is $C_{14}H_{21}N_3O_2S$, representing a molecular weight of 295.4. Sumatriptan is a white to off-white powder that is readily soluble in water and in saline. Each IMITREX Nasal Spray contains 5 or 20 mg of sumatriptan in a 100-µL unit dose aqueous buffered solution containing monobasic potassium phosphate NF, anhydrous dibasic sodium phosphate USP, sulfuric acid NF, sodium hydroxide NF, and purified water USP. The pH of the solution is approximately 5.5. The osmolality of the solution is 372 or 742 mOsmol for the 5- and 20-mg IMITREX Nasal Spray, respectively.

CLINICAL PHARMACOLOGY

Mechanism of Action

Sumatriptan is an agonist for a vascular 5-hydroxytryptamine$_1$ receptor subtype (probably a member of the 5-HT_{1D} family) having only a weak affinity for 5-HT_{1A}, 5-HT_{5A}, and 5-HT_7 receptors and no significant affinity (as measured using standard radioligand binding assays) or pharmacological activity at 5-HT_2, 5-HT_3, or 5-HT_4 receptor subtypes or at alpha$_1$-, alpha$_2$-, or beta-adrenergic; dopamine$_1$; dopamine$_2$; muscarinic; or benzodiazepine receptors.

The vascular 5-HT_1 receptor subtype that sumatriptan activates is present on cranial arteries in both dog and primate, on the human basilar artery, and in the vasculature of human dura mater and mediates vasoconstriction. This action in humans correlates with the relief of migraine headache. In addition to causing vasoconstriction, experimental data from animal studies show that sumatriptan also activates 5-HT_1 receptors on peripheral terminals of the trigeminal nerve innervating cranial blood vessels. Such an action may contribute to the antimigrainous effect of sumatriptan in humans.

In the anesthetized dog, sumatriptan selectively reduces the carotid arterial blood flow with little or no effect on arterial blood pressure or total peripheral resistance. In the cat, sumatriptan selectively constricts the carotid arteriovenous anastomoses while having little effect on blood flow or resistance in cerebral or extracerebral tissues.

Pharmacokinetics

In a study of 20 female volunteers, the mean maximum concentration following a 5- and 20-mg intranasal dose was 5 and 16 ng/mL, respectively. The mean C_{max} following a 6-mg subcutaneous injection is 71 ng/mL (range: 49 to 110 ng/mL). The mean C_{max} is 18 ng/mL (range: 7 to 47 ng/mL) following oral dosing with 25 mg and 51 ng/mL (range: 28 to 100 ng/mL) following oral dosing with 100 mg of sumatriptan. In a study of 24 male volunteers, the bioavailability relative to subcutaneous injection was low, approximately 17%, primarily due to presystemic metabolism and partly due to incomplete absorption.

Protein binding, determined by equilibrium dialysis over the concentration range of 10 to 1,000 ng/mL, is low, approximately 14% to 21%. The effect of sumatriptan on the protein binding of other drugs has not been evaluated, but would be expected to be minor, given the low rate of protein binding. The mean volume of distribution after subcutaneous dosing is 2.7 L/kg and the total plasma clearance is approximately 1,200 mL/min.

The elimination half-life of sumatriptan administered as a nasal spray is approximately 2 hours, similar to the half-life seen after subcutaneous injection. Only 3% of the dose is excreted in the urine as unchanged sumatriptan; 42% of the dose is excreted as the major metabolite, the indole acetic acid analogue of sumatriptan.

Clinical and pharmacokinetic data indicate that administration of two 5-mg doses, 1 dose in each nostril, is equivalent to administration of a single 10-mg dose in 1 nostril.

Special Populations

Renal Impairment: The effect of renal impairment on the pharmacokinetics of sumatriptan has not been examined, but little clinical effect would be expected as sumatriptan is largely metabolized to an inactive substance.

Hepatic Impairment: The effect of hepatic disease on the pharmacokinetics of subcutaneously and orally administered sumatriptan has been evaluated, but the intranasal dosage form has not been studied in hepatic impairment. There were no statistically significant differences in the pharmacokinetics of subcutaneously administered sumatriptan in hepatically impaired patients compared with healthy controls. However, the liver plays an important role in the presystemic clearance of orally administered sumatriptan. In 1 small study involving oral sumatriptan in hepatically impaired patients (N = 8) matched for sex, age, and weight with healthy subjects, the hepatically impaired patients had an approximately 70% increase in AUC and C_{max} and a T_{max} 40 minutes earlier compared with the healthy subjects. The bioavailability of nasally absorbed sumatriptan following intranasal administration, which would not undergo first-pass metabolism, should not be altered in hepatically impaired patients. The bioavailability of the swallowed portion of the intranasal sumatriptan dose has not been determined, but would be increased in these patients. The swallowed intranasal dose is small, however, compared with the usual oral dose, so that its impact should be minimal.

Age: The pharmacokinetics of oral sumatriptan in the elderly (mean age: 72 years, 2 males and 4 females) and in patients with migraine (mean age: 38 years, 25 males and 155 females) were similar to that in healthy male subjects (mean age: 30 years). Intranasal sumatriptan has not been evaluated for age differences (see PRECAUTIONS: Geriatric Use).

Race: The systemic clearance and C_{max} of sumatriptan were similar in black (n = 34) and Caucasian (n = 38) healthy male subjects. Intranasal sumatriptan has not been evaluated for race differences.

Drug Interactions

Monoamine Oxidase Inhibitors: Treatment with monoamine oxidase inhibitors (MAOIs) generally leads to an increase of sumatriptan plasma levels (see CONTRAINDICATIONS and PRECAUTIONS).

MAOI interaction studies have not been performed with intranasal sumatriptan. Due to gut and hepatic metabolic first-pass effects, the increase of systemic exposure after coadministration of an MAO-A inhibitor with oral sumatriptan is greater than after coadministration of the MAOI with subcutaneous sumatriptan. The effects of an MAOI on systemic exposure after intranasal sumatriptan would be expected to be greater than the effect after subcutaneous sumatriptan but smaller than the effect after oral sumatriptan because only swallowed drug would be subject to first-pass effects.

In a study of 14 healthy females, pretreatment with an MAO-A inhibitor decreased the clearance of subcutaneous sumatriptan. Under the conditions of this experiment, the result was a 2-fold increase in the area under the sumatriptan plasma concentration × time curve (AUC), corresponding to a 40% increase in elimination half-life. This interaction was not evident with an MAO-B inhibitor.

A small study evaluating the effect of pretreatment with an MAO-A inhibitor on the bioavailability from a 25-mg oral sumatriptan tablet resulted in an approximately 7-fold increase in systemic exposure.

Xylometazoline: An in vivo drug interaction study indicated that 3 drops of xylometazoline (0.1% w/v), a decongestant, administered 15 minutes prior to a 20-mg nasal dose of sumatriptan did not alter the pharmacokinetics of sumatriptan.

CLINICAL TRIALS

The efficacy of IMITREX Nasal Spray in the acute treatment of migraine headaches was demonstrated in 8, randomized, double-blind, placebo-controlled studies, of which 5 used the recommended dosing regimen and used the marketed formulation. Patients enrolled in these 5 studies were predominately female (86%) and Caucasian (95%), with a mean age of 41 (range of 18 to 65). Patients were instructed to treat a moderate to severe headache. Headache response, defined as a reduction in headache severity from moderate or severe pain to mild or no pain, was assessed up to 2 hours after dosing. Associated symptoms such as nausea, photophobia, and phonophobia were also assessed. Maintenance of response was assessed for up to 24 hours postdose. A second dose of IMITREX Nasal Spray or other medication was allowed 2 to 24 hours after the initial treatment for recurrent headache. The frequency and time to use of these additional treatments were also determined. In all studies, doses of 10 and 20 mg were compared with placebo in the treatment of 1 to 3 migraine attacks. Patients received doses as a single spray into 1 nostril. In 2 studies, a 5-mg dose was also evaluated.

In all 5 trials utilizing the market formulation and recommended dosage regimen, the percentage of patients achieving headache response 2 hours after treatment was significantly greater among patients receiving IMITREX Nasal Spray at all doses (with one exception) compared with those who received placebo. In 4 of the 5 studies, there was a statistically significant greater percentage of patients with headache response at 2 hours in the 20-mg group when compared with the lower dose groups (5 and 10 mg). There were no statistically significant differences between the 5- and 10-mg dose groups in any study. The results from the 5 controlled clinical trials are summarized in Table 1. Note that, in general, comparisons of results obtained in studies conducted under different conditions by different investigators with different samples of patients are ordinarily unreliable for purposes of quantitative comparison.

[See table 1 above]

The estimated probability of achieving an initial headache response over the 2 hours following treatment is depicted in Figure 1.

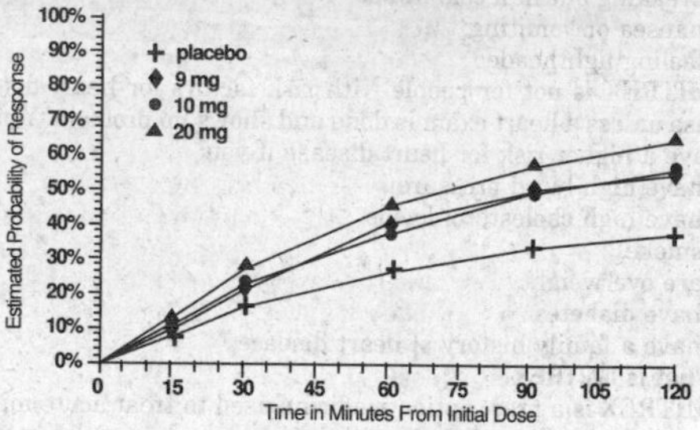

Figure 1. Estimated Probability of Achieving Initial Headache Response Within 120 Minutes[a]

[a]The figure shows the probability over time of obtaining headache response (no or mild pain) following treatment with intranasal sumatriptan. The averages displayed are based on pooled data from the 5 clinical controlled trials providing evidence of efficacy. Kaplan-Meier plot with patients not achieving response within 120 minutes censored to 120 minutes.

For patients with migraine-associated nausea, photophobia, and phonophobia at baseline, there was a lower incidence of these symptoms at 2 hours following administration of IMITREX Nasal Spray compared with placebo.

Two to 24 hours following the initial dose of study treatment, patients were allowed to use additional treatment for pain relief in the form of a second dose of study treatment or other medication. The estimated probability of patients taking a second dose or other medication for migraine over the 24 hours following the initial dose of study treatment is summarized in Figure 2.

[See figure 2 at top of next column]

There is evidence that doses above 20 mg do not provide a greater effect than 20 mg. There was no evidence to suggest that treatment with sumatriptan was associated with an increase in the severity of recurrent headaches. The efficacy of IMITREX Nasal Spray was unaffected by presence of aura; duration of headache prior to treatment; gender, age, or weight of the patient; or concomitant use of common migraine prophylactic drugs (e.g., beta-blockers, calcium channel blockers, tricyclic antidepressants). There were insufficient data to assess the impact of race on efficacy.

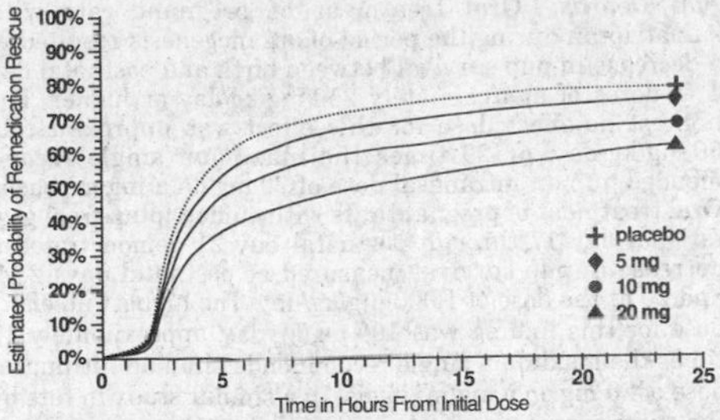

Figure 2. The Estimated Probability of Patients Taking a Second Dose or Other Medication for Migraine Over the 24 Hours Following the Initial Dose of Study Treatment[a]

[a]Kaplan-Meier plot based on data obtained in the 3 clinical controlled trials providing evidence of efficacy with patients not using additional treatments censored to 24 hours. Plot also includes patients who had no response to the initial dose. No remedication was allowed within 2 hours postdose.

INDICATIONS AND USAGE

IMITREX Nasal Spray is indicated for the acute treatment of migraine attacks with or without aura in adults.

IMITREX Nasal Spray is not intended for the prophylactic therapy of migraine or for use in the management of hemiplegic or basilar migraine (see CONTRAINDICATIONS). Safety and effectiveness of IMITREX Nasal Spray have not been established for cluster headache, which is present in an older, predominantly male population.

CONTRAINDICATIONS

IMITREX Nasal Spray should not be given to patients with history, symptoms, or signs of ischemic cardiac, cerebrovascular, or peripheral vascular syndromes. In addition, patients with other significant underlying cardiovascular diseases should not receive IMITREX Nasal Spray. Ischemic cardiac syndromes include, but are not limited to, angina pectoris of any type (e.g., stable angina of effort, vasospastic forms of angina such as the Prinzmetal variant), all forms of myocardial infarction, and silent myocardial ischemia. Cerebrovascular syndromes include, but are not limited to, strokes of any type as well as transient ischemic attacks. Peripheral vascular disease includes, but is not limited to, ischemic bowel disease (see WARNINGS).

Because IMITREX Nasal Spray may increase blood pressure, it should not be given to patients with uncontrolled hypertension.

Concurrent administration of MAO-A inhibitors or use within 2 weeks of discontinuation of MAO-A inhibitor therapy is contraindicated (see CLINICAL PHARMACOLOGY: Drug Interactions and PRECAUTIONS: Drug Interactions).

IMITREX Nasal Spray and any ergotamine-containing or ergot-type medication (like dihydroergotamine or methysergide) should not be used within 24 hours of each other, nor should IMITREX Nasal Spray and another 5-HT$_1$ agonist.

IMITREX Nasal Spray should not be administered to patients with hemiplegic or basilar migraine.

IMITREX Nasal Spray is contraindicated in patients with hypersensitivity to sumatriptan or any of its components.

IMITREX Nasal Spray is contraindicated in patients with severe hepatic impairment.

WARNINGS

IMITREX Nasal Spray should only be used where a clear diagnosis of migraine headache has been established.

Risk of Myocardial Ischemia and/or Infarction and Other Adverse Cardiac Events

Sumatriptan should not be given to patients with documented ischemic or vasospastic coronary artery disease (CAD) (see CONTRAINDICATIONS). It is strongly recommended that sumatriptan not be given to patients in whom unrecognized CAD is predicted by the presence of risk factors (e.g., hypertension, hypercholesterolemia, smoker, obesity, diabetes, strong family history of CAD, female with surgical or physiological menopause, male over 40 years of age) unless a cardiovascular evaluation provides satisfactory clinical evidence that the patient is reasonably free of coronary artery and ischemic myocardial disease or other significant underlying cardiovascular disease. The sensitivity of cardiac diagnostic procedures to detect cardiovascular disease or predisposition to coronary artery vasospasm is modest, at best. If, during the cardiovascular evaluation, the patient's medical history or electrocardiographic investigations reveal findings indicative of, or consistent with, coronary artery vasospasm or myocardial ischemia, sumatriptan should not be administered (see CONTRAINDICATIONS).

For patients with risk factors predictive of CAD, who are determined to have a satisfactory cardiovascular evaluation, it is strongly recommended that administration of the first dose of sumatriptan nasal spray take place in the setting of a physician's office or similar medically staffed and equipped facility unless the patient has previously received sumatriptan. Because cardiac ischemia can occur in the absence of clinical symptoms, consideration should be given to obtaining an electrocardiogram (ECG) during the interval immediately following the first dose in these patients with risk factors.

It is recommended that patients who are intermittent long-term users of sumatriptan and who have or acquire risk factors predictive of CAD, as described above, undergo periodic interval cardiovascular evaluation as they continue to use sumatriptan.

The systematic approach described above is intended to reduce the likelihood that patients with unrecognized cardiovascular disease will be inadvertently exposed to sumatriptan.

Drug-Associated Cardiac Events and Fatalities

Serious adverse cardiac events, including acute myocardial infarction, life-threatening disturbances of cardiac rhythm, and death have been reported within a few hours following the administration of IMITREX® (sumatriptan succinate) Injection or IMITREX® (sumatriptan succinate) Tablets. Considering the extent of use of sumatriptan in patients with migraine, the incidence of these events is extremely low.

The fact that sumatriptan can cause coronary vasospasm, that some of these events have occurred in patients with no prior cardiac disease history and with documented absence of CAD, and the close proximity of the events to sumatriptan use support the conclusion that some of these cases were caused by the drug. In many cases, however, where there has been known underlying coronary artery disease, the relationship is uncertain.

Premarketing Experience WithSumatriptan: Among approximately 4,000 patients with migraine who participated in premarketing controlled and uncontrolled clinical trials of sumatriptan nasal spray, 1 patient experienced an asymptomatic subendocardial infarction possibly subsequent to a coronary vasospastic event.

Of 6,348 patients with migraine who participated in premarketing controlled and uncontrolled clinical trials of oral sumatriptan, 2 experienced clinical adverse events shortly after receiving oral sumatriptan that may have reflected coronary vasospasm. Neither of these adverse events was associated with a serious clinical outcome.

Among the more than 1,900 patients with migraine who participated in premarketing controlled clinical trials of subcutaneous sumatriptan, there were 8 patients who sustained clinical events during or shortly after receiving sumatriptan that may have reflected coronary artery vasospasm. Six of these 8 patients had ECG changes consistent with transient ischemia, but without accompanying clinical symptoms or signs. Of these 8 patients, 4 had either findings suggestive of CAD or risk factors predictive of CAD prior to study enrollment.

Postmarketing Experience WithSumatriptan: Serious cardiovascular events, some resulting in death, have been reported in association with the use of IMITREX Injection or IMITREX Tablets. The uncontrolled nature of postmarketing surveillance, however, makes it impossible to determine definitively the proportion of the reported cases that were actually caused by sumatriptan or to reliably assess causation in individual cases. On clinical grounds, the longer the latency between the administration of IMITREX and the onset of the clinical event, the less likely the association is to be causative. Accordingly, interest has focused on events beginning within 1 hour of the administration of IMITREX.

Cardiac events that have been observed to have onset within 1 hour of sumatriptan administration include: coronary artery vasospasm, transient ischemia, myocardial infarction, ventricular tachycardia and ventricular fibrillation, cardiac arrest, and death.

Some of these events occurred in patients who had no findings of CAD and appear to represent consequences of coronary artery vasospasm. However, among domestic reports of serious cardiac events within 1 hour of sumatriptan administration, almost all of the patients had risk factors predictive of CAD and the presence of significant underlying CAD was established in most cases (see CONTRAINDICATIONS).

Drug-Associated Cerebrovascular Events and Fatalities

Cerebral hemorrhage, subarachnoid hemorrhage, stroke, and other cerebrovascular events have been reported in patients treated with oral or subcutaneous sumatriptan, and some have resulted in fatalities. The relationship of sumatriptan to these events is uncertain. In a number of cases, it appears possible that the cerebrovascular events were primary, sumatriptan having been administered in the incorrect belief that the symptoms experienced were a consequence of migraine when they were not. As with other acute migraine therapies, before treating headaches in patients not previously diagnosed as migraineurs, and in migraineurs who present with atypical symptoms, care should be taken to exclude other potentially serious neurological conditions. It should also be noted that patients with migraine may be at increased risk of certain cerebrovascular events (e.g., cerebrovascular accident, transient ischemic attack).

Other Vasospasm-Related Events

Sumatriptan may cause vasospastic reactions other than coronary artery vasospasm. Both peripheral vascular ischemia and colonic ischemia with abdominal pain and bloody diarrhea have been reported. Very rare reports of transient and permanent blindness and significant partial vision loss have been reported with the use of sumatriptan. Visual disorders may also be part of a migraine attack.

Serotonin Syndrome

Serotonin syndrome may occur with triptans, including IMITREX, particularly during combined use with selective serotonin reuptake inhibitors (SSRIs) or serotonin norepinephrine reuptake inhibitors (SNRIs). Serotonin syndrome symptoms may include mental status changes (e.g., agitation, hallucinations, coma), autonomic instability (e.g., tachycardia, labile blood pressure, hyperthermia), neuromuscular aberrations (e.g., hyperreflexia, incoordination), and/or gastrointestinal symptoms (e.g., nausea, vomiting, diarrhea). The onset of symptoms can occur within minutes to hours of receiving a new or a greater dose of a serotonergic medication. Treatment with IMITREX should be discontinued if serotonin syndrome is suspected.

Increase in Blood Pressure

Significant elevation in blood pressure, including hypertensive crisis, has been reported on rare occasions in patients with and without a history of hypertension. Sumatriptan is contraindicated in patients with uncontrolled hypertension (see CONTRAINDICATIONS). Sumatriptan should be administered with caution to patients with controlled hypertension as transient increases in blood pressure and peripheral vascular resistance have been observed in a small proportion of patients.

Local Irritation

Of the 3,378 patients using the nasal spray (5-, 10-, or 20-mg doses) on 1 or 2 occasions in controlled clinical studies, approximately 5% noted irritation in the nose and throat. Irritative symptoms such as burning, numbness, paresthesia, discharge, and pain or soreness were noted to be severe in about 1% of patients treated. The symptoms were transient and in approximately 60% of the cases, the symptoms resolved in less than 2 hours. Limited examinations of the nose and throat did not reveal any clinically noticeable injury in these patients.

The consequences of extended and repeated use of IMITREX Nasal Spray on the nasal and/or respiratory mucosa have not been systematically evaluated in patients. No increase in the incidence of local irritation was observed in patients using IMITREX Nasal Spray repeatedly for up to 1 year.

In inhalation studies in rats dosed daily for up to 1 month at exposures as low as one half the maximum daily human exposure (based on dose per surface area of nasal cavity), epithelial hyperplasia (with and without keratinization) and squamous metaplasia were observed in the larynx at all doses tested. These changes were partially reversible after a 2-week drug-free period. When dogs were dosed daily with various formulations by intranasal instillation for up to 13 weeks at exposures of 2 to 4 times the maximum daily human exposure (based on dose per surface area of nasal cavity), respiratory and nasal mucosa exhibited evidence of epithelial hyperplasia, focal squamous metaplasia, granulomata, bronchitis, and fibrosing alveolitis. A no-effect dose was not established. The changes observed in both species are not considered to be signs of either preneoplastic or neoplastic transformation.

Local effects on nasal and respiratory tissues after chronic intranasal dosing in animals have not been studied.

Concomitant Drug Use

In patients taking MAO-A inhibitors, sumatriptan plasma levels attained after treatment with recommended doses are 2-fold (following subcutaneous administration) to 7-fold (following oral administration) higher than those obtained under other conditions. Accordingly, the coadministration of IMITREX Nasal Spray and an MAO-A inhibitor is contraindicated (see CLINICAL PHARMACOLOGY and CONTRAINDICATIONS).

Hypersensitivity

Hypersensitivity (anaphylaxis/anaphylactoid) reactions have occurred on rare occasions in patients receiving sumatriptan. Such reactions can be life threatening or fatal. In general, hypersensitivity reactions to drugs are more likely to occur in individuals with a history of sensitivity to multiple allergens (see CONTRAINDICATIONS).

PRECAUTIONS

General

Chest discomfort and jaw or neck tightness have been reported infrequently following the administration of

IMITREX Nasal Spray and have also been reported following use of IMITREX Tablets. Chest, jaw, or neck tightness is relatively common after administration of IMITREX Injection. Only rarely have these symptoms been associated with ischemic ECG changes. However, because sumatriptan may cause coronary artery vasospasm, patients who experience signs or symptoms suggestive of angina following sumatriptan should be evaluated for the presence of CAD or a predisposition to Prinzmetal variant angina before receiving additional doses of sumatriptan, and should be monitored electrocardiographically if dosing is resumed and similar symptoms recur. Similarly, patients who experience other symptoms or signs suggestive of decreased arterial flow, such as ischemic bowel syndrome or Raynaud syndrome, following sumatriptan should be evaluated for atherosclerosis or predisposition to vasospasm (see WARNINGS).

IMITREX Nasal Spray should also be administered with caution to patients with diseases that may alter the absorption, metabolism, or excretion of drugs, such as impaired hepatic or renal function.

There have been rare reports of seizure following administration of sumatriptan. Sumatriptan should be used with caution in patients with a history of epilepsy or conditions associated with a lowered seizure threshold.

Care should be taken to exclude other potentially serious neurologic conditions before treating headache in patients not previously diagnosed with migraine headache or who experience a headache that is atypical for them. There have been rare reports where patients received sumatriptan for severe headaches that were subsequently shown to have been secondary to an evolving neurologic lesion (see WARNINGS).

For a given attack, if a patient does not respond to the first dose of sumatriptan, the diagnosis of migraine headache should be reconsidered before administration of a second dose.

Overuse

Overuse of acute migraine drugs (e.g., ergotamine, triptans, opioids, or a combination of drugs for 10 or more days per month) may lead to exacerbation of headache (medication overuse headache). Medication overuse headache may present as migraine-like daily headaches, or as a marked increase in frequency of migraine attacks. Detoxification of patients, including withdrawal of the overused drugs, and treatment of withdrawal symptoms (which often includes a transient worsening of headache) may be necessary. Migraine patients should be informed about the risks of medication overuse and encouraged to record headache frequency and drug use.

Information for Patients

See PATIENT INFORMATION at the end of this labeling for the text of the separate leaflet provided for patients.

Patients should be cautioned about the risk of serotonin syndrome with the use of sumatriptan or other triptans, especially during combined use with SSRIs or SNRIs.

Laboratory Tests

No specific laboratory tests are recommended for monitoring patients prior to and/or after treatment with sumatriptan.

Drug Interactions

Selective Serotonin Reuptake Inhibitors/Serotonin Norepinephrine Reuptake Inhibitors and Serotonin Syndrome: Cases of life-threatening serotonin syndrome have been reported during combined use of SSRIs or SNRIs and triptans (see WARNINGS).

Ergot-Containing Drugs: Ergot-containing drugs have been reported to cause prolonged vasospastic reactions. Because there is a theoretical basis that these effects may be additive, use of ergotamine-containing or ergot-type medications (like dihydroergotamine or methysergide) and sumatriptan within 24 hours of each other should be avoided (see CONTRAINDICATIONS).

Monoamine Oxidase-A Inhibitors: MAO-A inhibitors reduce sumatriptan clearance, significantly increasing systemic exposure. Therefore, the use of IMITREX Nasal Spray in patients receiving MAO-A inhibitors is contraindicated (see CLINICAL PHARMACOLOGY and CONTRAINDICATIONS).

Drug/Laboratory Test Interactions

IMITREX Nasal Spray is not known to interfere with commonly employed clinical laboratory tests.

Carcinogenesis, Mutagenesis, Impairment of Fertility

Carcinogenesis: In carcinogenicity studies, rats and mice were given sumatriptan by oral gavage (rats: 104 weeks) or drinking water (mice: 78 weeks). Average exposures achieved in mice receiving the highest dose (target dose of 160 mg/kg/day) were approximately 184 times the exposure attained in humans after the maximum recommended single intranasal dose of 20 mg. The highest dose administered to rats (160 mg/kg/day, reduced from 360 mg/kg/day during week 21) was approximately 78 times the maximum recommended single intranasal dose of 20 mg on a mg/m^2 basis. There was no evidence of an increase in tumors in either species related to sumatriptan administration. Local effects on nasal and respiratory tissue after chronic intranasal dosing in animals have not been evaluated (see WARNINGS).

Mutagenesis: Sumatriptan was not mutagenic in the presence or absence of metabolic activation when tested in 2 gene mutation assays (the Ames test and the in vitro mammalian Chinese hamster V79/HGPRT assay). In 2 cytogenetics assays (the in vitro human lymphocyte assay and the in vivo rat micronucleus assay) sumatriptan was not associated with clastogenic activity.

Impairment of Fertility: In a study in which male and female rats were dosed daily with oral sumatriptan prior to and throughout the mating period, there was a treatment-related decrease in fertility secondary to a decrease in mating in animals treated with 50 and 500 mg/kg/day. The highest no-effect dose for this finding was 5 mg/kg/day, or approximately twice the maximum recommended single human intranasal dose of 20 mg on a mg/m^2 basis. It is not clear whether the problem is associated with treatment of the males or females or both combined. In a similar study by the subcutaneous route there was no evidence of impaired fertility at 60 mg/kg/day, the maximum dose tested, which is equivalent to approximately 29 times the maximum recommended single human intranasal dose of 20 mg on a mg/m^2 basis. Fertility studies, in which sumatriptan was administered by the intranasal route, were not conducted.

Pregnancy

Pregnancy Category C. In reproductive toxicity studies in rats and rabbits, oral treatment with sumatriptan was associated with embryolethality, fetal abnormalities, and pup mortality. When administered by the intravenous route to rabbits, sumatriptan has been shown to be embryolethal. Reproductive toxicity studies for sumatriptan by the intranasal route have not been conducted.

There are no adequate and well-controlled studies in pregnant women. Therefore, IMITREX Nasal Spray should be used during pregnancy only if the potential benefit justifies the potential risk to the fetus. In assessing this information, the following findings should be considered.

Embryolethality: When given orally or intravenously to pregnant rabbits daily throughout the period of organogenesis, sumatriptan caused embryolethality at doses at or close to those producing maternal toxicity. In the oral studies this dose was 100 mg/kg/day, and in the intravenous studies this dose was 2.0 mg/kg/day. The mechanism of the embryolethality is not known. The highest no-effect dose for embryolethality by the oral route was 50 mg/kg/day, which is approximately 48 times the maximum single recommended human intranasal dose of 20 mg on a mg/m^2 basis. By the intravenous route, the highest no-effect dose was 0.75 mg/kg/day, or approximately 0.7 times the maximum single recommended human intranasal dose of 20 mg on a mg/m^2 basis.

The intravenous administration of sumatriptan to pregnant rats throughout organogenesis at 12.5 mg/kg/day, the maximum dose tested, did not cause embryolethality. This dose is approximately 6 times the maximum single recommended human intranasal dose of 20 mg on a mg/m^2 basis. Additionally, in a study in rats given subcutaneous sumatriptan daily, prior to and throughout pregnancy, at 60 mg/kg/day, the maximum dose tested, there was no evidence of increased embryo/fetal lethality. This dose is equivalent to approximately 29 times the maximum recommended single human intranasal dose of 20 mg on a mg/m^2 basis.

Teratogenicity: Oral treatment of pregnant rats with sumatriptan during the period of organogenesis resulted in an increased incidence of blood vessel abnormalities (cervicothoracic and umbilical) at doses of approximately 250 mg/kg/day or higher. The highest no-effect dose was approximately 60 mg/kg/day, which is approximately 29 times the maximum single recommended human intranasal dose of 20 mg on a mg/m^2 basis. Oral treatment of pregnant rabbits with sumatriptan during the period of organogenesis resulted in an increased incidence of cervicothoracic vascular and skeletal abnormalities. The highest no-effect dose for these effects was 15 mg/kg/day, or approximately 14 times the maximum single recommended human intranasal dose of 20 mg on a mg/m^2 basis.

A study in which rats were dosed daily with oral sumatriptan prior to and throughout gestation demonstrated embryo/fetal toxicity (decreased body weight, decreased ossification, increased incidence of rib variations) and an increased incidence of a syndrome of malformations (short tail/short body and vertebral disorganization) at 500 mg/kg/day. The highest no-effect dose was 50 mg/kg/day, or approximately 24 times the maximum single recommended human intranasal dose of 20 mg on a mg/m^2 basis. In a study in rats dosed daily with subcutaneous sumatriptan prior to and throughout pregnancy, at a dose of 60 mg/kg/day, the maximum dose tested, there was no evidence of teratogenicity. This dose is equivalent to approximately 29 times the maximum recommended single human intranasal dose of 20 mg on a mg/m^2 basis.

Pup Deaths: Oral treatment of pregnant rats with sumatriptan during the period of organogenesis resulted in a decrease in pup survival between birth and postnatal day 4 at doses of approximately 250 mg/kg/day or higher. The highest no-effect dose for this effect was approximately 60 mg/kg/day, or 29 times the maximum single recommended human intranasal dose of 20 mg on a mg/m^2 basis. Oral treatment of pregnant rats with sumatriptan from gestational day 17 through postnatal day 21 demonstrated a decrease in pup survival measured at postnatal days 2, 4, and 20 at the dose of 1,000 mg/kg/day. The highest no-effect dose for this finding was 100 mg/kg/day, approximately 49 times the maximum single recommended human intranasal dose of 20 mg on a mg/m^2 basis. In a similar study in rats by the subcutaneous route there was no increase in pup death at 81 mg/kg/day, the highest dose tested, which is equivalent to 40 times the maximum single recommended human intranasal dose of 20 mg on a mg/m^2 basis.

Nursing Mothers

Sumatriptan is excreted in human breast milk following subcutaneous administration. Infant exposure to sumatriptan can be minimized by avoiding breastfeeding for 12 hours after treatment with IMITREX Nasal Spray.

Pediatric Use

Safety and effectiveness of IMITREX Nasal Spray in pediatric patients under 18 years of age have not been established; therefore, IMITREX Nasal Spray is not recommended for use in patients under 18 years of age.

Two controlled clinical trials evaluated sumatriptan nasal spray (5 to 20 mg) in 1,248 adolescent migraineurs aged 12 to 17 years who treated a single attack. The studies did not establish the efficacy of sumatriptan nasal spray compared with placebo in the treatment of migraine in adolescents. Adverse events observed in these clinical trials were similar in nature to those reported in clinical trials in adults.

Five controlled clinical trials (2 single attack studies, 3 multiple attack studies) evaluating oral sumatriptan (25 to 100 mg) in pediatric patients aged 12 to 17 years enrolled a total of 701 adolescent migraineurs. These studies did not establish the efficacy of oral sumatriptan compared with placebo in the treatment of migraine in adolescents. Adverse events observed in these clinical trials were similar in nature to those reported in clinical trials in adults. The frequency of all adverse events in these patients appeared to be both dose- and age-dependent, with younger patients reporting events more commonly than older adolescents.

Postmarketing experience documents that serious adverse events have occurred in the pediatric population after use of subcutaneous, oral, and/or intranasal sumatriptan. These reports include events similar in nature to those reported rarely in adults, including stroke, visual loss, and death. A myocardial infarction has been reported in a 14-year-old male following the use of oral sumatriptan; clinical signs occurred within 1 day of drug administration. Since clinical data to determine the frequency of serious adverse events in pediatric patients who might receive injectable, oral, or intranasal sumatriptan are not presently available, the use of sumatriptan in patients aged younger than 18 years is not recommended.

Geriatric Use

The use of sumatriptan in elderly patients is not recommended because elderly patients are more likely to have decreased hepatic function, they are at higher risk for CAD, and blood pressure increases may be more pronounced in the elderly (see WARNINGS).

ADVERSE REACTIONS

Serious cardiac events, including some that have been fatal, have occurred following the use of IMITREX Injection or Tablets. These events are extremely rare and most have been reported in patients with risk factors predictive of CAD. Events reported have included coronary artery vasospasm, transient myocardial ischemia, myocardial infarction, ventricular tachycardia, and ventricular fibrillation (see CONTRAINDICATIONS, WARNINGS, and PRECAUTIONS).

Significant hypertensive episodes, including hypertensive crises, have been reported on rare occasions in patients with or without a history of hypertension (see WARNINGS).

Incidence in Controlled Clinical Trials

Among 3,653 patients treated with IMITREX Nasal Spray in active- and placebo-controlled clinical trials, less than 0.4% of patients withdrew for reasons related to adverse events. Table 2 lists adverse events that occurred in worldwide placebo-controlled clinical trials in 3,419 migraineurs. The events cited reflect experience gained under closely monitored conditions of clinical trials in a highly selected patient population. In actual clinical practice or in other clinical trials, these frequency estimates may not apply, as the conditions of use, reporting behavior, and the kinds of patients treated may differ.

Only events that occurred at a frequency of 1% or more in the IMITREX Nasal Spray 20-mg treatment group and were more frequent in that group than in the placebo group are included in Table 2.

[See table 2 above]
Phonophobia also occurred in more than 1% of patients but was more frequent on placebo.
IMITREX Nasal Spray is generally well tolerated. Across all doses, most adverse reactions were mild and transient and did not lead to long-lasting effects. The incidence of adverse events in controlled clinical trials was not affected by gender, weight, or age of the patients; use of prophylactic medications; or presence of aura. There were insufficient data to assess the impact of race on the incidence of adverse events.

Other Events Observed in Association With the Administration of IMITREX Nasal Spray
In the paragraphs that follow, the frequencies of less commonly reported adverse clinical events are presented. Because the reports include events observed in open and uncontrolled studies, the role of IMITREX Nasal Spray in their causation cannot be reliably determined. Furthermore, variability associated with adverse event reporting, the terminology used to describe adverse events, etc., limit the value of the quantitative frequency estimates provided. Event frequencies are calculated as the number of patients who used IMITREX Nasal Spray (5, 10, or 20 mg in controlled and uncontrolled trials) and reported an event divided by the total number of patients (N = 3,711) exposed to IMITREX Nasal Spray. All reported events are included except those already listed in the previous table, those too general to be informative, and those not reasonably associated with the use of the drug. Events are further classified within body system categories and enumerated in order of decreasing frequency using the following definitions: infrequent adverse events are those occurring in 1/100 to 1/1,000 patients and rare adverse events are those occurring in fewer than 1/1,000 patients.
Atypical Sensations: Infrequent were tingling, warm/hot sensation, numbness, pressure sensation, feeling strange, feeling of heaviness, feeling of tightness, paresthesia, cold sensation, and tight feeling in head. Rare were dysesthesia and prickling sensation.
Cardiovascular: Infrequent were flushing and hypertension (see WARNINGS), palpitations, tachycardia, changes in ECG, and arrhythmia (see WARNINGS and PRECAUTIONS). Rare were abdominal aortic aneurysm, hypotension, bradycardia, pallor, and phlebitis.
Chest Symptoms: Infrequent were chest tightness, chest discomfort, and chest pressure/heaviness (see PRECAUTIONS: General).
Ear, Nose, and Throat: Infrequent were disturbance of hearing and ear infection. Rare were otalgia and Meniere disease.
Endocrine and Metabolic: Infrequent was thirst. Rare were galactorrhea, hypothyroidism, and weight loss.
Eye: Infrequent were irritation of eyes and visual disturbance.
Gastrointestinal: Infrequent were abdominal discomfort, diarrhea, dysphagia, and gastroesophageal reflux. Rare were constipation, flatulence/eructation, hematemesis, intestinal obstruction, melena, gastroenteritis, colitis, hemorrhage of gastrointestinal tract, and pancreatitis.
Mouth and Teeth: Infrequent was disorder of mouth and tongue (e.g., burning of tongue, numbness of tongue, dry mouth).
Musculoskeletal: Infrequent were neck pain/stiffness, backache, weakness, joint symptoms, arthritis, and myalgia. Rare were muscle cramps, tetany, intervertebral disc disorder, and muscle stiffness.
Neurological: Infrequent were drowsiness/sedation, anxiety, sleep disturbances, tremors, syncope, shivers, chills, depression, agitation, sensation of lightness, and mental confusion. Rare were difficulty concentrating, hunger, lacrimation, memory disturbances, monoplegia/diplegia, apathy, disturbance of smell, disturbance of emotions, dysarthria, facial pain, intoxication, stress, decreased appetite, difficulty coordinating, euphoria, and neoplasm of pituitary.
Respiratory: Infrequent were dyspnea and lower respiratory tract infection. Rare was asthma.
Skin: Infrequent were rash/skin eruption, pruritus, and erythema. Rare were herpes, swelling of face, sweating, and peeling of skin.
Urogenital: Infrequent were dysuria, disorder of breasts, and dysmenorrhea. Rare were endometriosis and increased urination.
Miscellaneous: Infrequent were cough, edema, and fever. Rare were hypersensitivity, swelling of extremities, voice disturbances, difficulty in walking, and lymphadenopathy.

Other Events Observed in the Clinical Development of IMITREX
The following adverse events occurred in clinical trials with IMITREX Injection and IMITREX Tablets. Because the reports include events observed in open and uncontrolled studies, the role of IMITREX in their causation cannot be reliably determined. All reported events are included except those already listed, those too general to be informative, and those not reasonably associated with the use of the drug.

Table 2. Treatment-Emergent Adverse Events Reported by at Least 1% of Patients in Controlled Migraine Trials

Adverse Event Type	Placebo (n = 704)	Percent of Patients Reporting IMITREX 5 mg (n = 496)	IMITREX 10 mg (n = 1,007)	IMITREX 20 mg (n = 1,212)
Atypical sensations				
Burning sensation	0.1%	0.4%	0.6%	1.4%
Ear, nose, and throat				
Disorder/discomfort of nasal cavity/sinuses	2.4%	2.8%	2.5%	3.8%
Throat discomfort	0.9%	0.8%	1.8%	2.4%
Gastrointestinal				
Nausea and/or vomiting	11.3%	12.2%	11.0%	13.5%
Neurological				
Bad/unusual taste	1.7%	13.5%	19.3%	24.5%
Dizziness/vertigo	0.9%	1.0%	1.7%	1.4%

Breasts: Breast swelling; cysts, lumps, and masses of breasts; nipple discharge; primary malignant breast neoplasm; and tenderness.
Cardiovascular: Abnormal pulse, angina, atherosclerosis, cerebral ischemia, cerebrovascular lesion, heart block, peripheral cyanosis, pulsating sensations, Raynaud syndrome, thrombosis, transient myocardial ischemia, various transient ECG changes (nonspecific ST or T wave changes, prolongation of PR or QTc intervals, sinus arrhythmia, nonsustained ventricular premature beats, isolated junctional ectopic beats, atrial ectopic beats, delayed activation of the right ventricle), and vasodilation.
Ear, Nose, and Throat: Allergic rhinitis; ear, nose, and throat hemorrhage; external otitis; feeling of fullness in the ear(s); hearing disturbances; hearing loss; nasal inflammation; sensitivity to noise; sinusitis; tinnitus; and upper respiratory inflammation.
Endocrine and Metabolic: Dehydration; endocrine cysts, lumps, and masses; elevated thyrotropin stimulating hormone (TSH) levels; fluid disturbances; hyperglycemia; hypoglycemia; polydipsia; and weight gain.
Eye: Accommodation disorders, blindness and low vision, conjunctivitis, disorders of sclera, external ocular muscle disorders, eye edema and swelling, eye itching, eye hemorrhage, eye pain, keratitis, mydriasis, and vision alterations.
Gastrointestinal: Abdominal distention, dental pain, disturbances of liver function tests, dyspeptic symptoms, feelings of gastrointestinal pressure, gallstones, gastric symptoms, gastritis, gastrointestinal pain, hypersalivation, hyposalivation, oral itching and irritation, peptic ulcer, retching, salivary gland swelling, and swallowing disorders.
Hematological Disorders: Anemia.
Injection Site Reaction
Miscellaneous: Contusions, fluid retention, hematoma, hypersensitivity to various agents, jaw discomfort, miscellaneous laboratory abnormalities, overdose, "serotonin agonist effect," and speech disturbance.
Musculoskeletal: Acquired musculoskeletal deformity, arthralgia and articular rheumatitis, muscle atrophy, muscle tiredness, musculoskeletal inflammation, need to flex calf muscles, rigidity, tightness, and various joint disturbances (pain, stiffness, swelling, ache).
Neurological: Aggressiveness, bradylogia, cluster headache, convulsions, detachment, disturbances of taste, drug abuse, dystonia, facial paralysis, globus hystericus, hallucinations, headache, heat sensitivity, hyperesthesia, hysteria, increased alertness, malaise/fatigue, migraine, motor dysfunction, myoclonia, neuralgia, neurotic disorders, paralysis, personality change, phobia, photophobia, psychomotor disorders, radiculopathy, raised intracranial pressure, relaxation, stinging sensations, transient hemiplegia, simultaneous hot and cold sensations, suicide, tickling sensations, twitching, and yawning.
Pain and Other Pressure Sensations: Chest pain, neck tightness/pressure, throat/jaw pain/tightness/pressure, and pain (location specified).
Respiratory: Breathing disorders, bronchitis, diseases of the lower respiratory tract, hiccoughs, and influenza.
Skin: Dry/scaly skin, eczema, seborrheic dermatitis, skin nodules, skin tenderness, tightness of skin, and wrinkling of skin.
Urogenital: Abortion, abnormal menstrual cycle, bladder inflammation, hematuria, inflammation of fallopian tubes, intermenstrual bleeding, menstruation symptoms, micturition disorders, renal calculus, urethritis, urinary frequency, and urinary infections.

Postmarketing Experience (Reports for Subcutaneous or Oral Sumatriptan)
The following section enumerates potentially important adverse events that have occurred in clinical practice and that have been reported spontaneously to various surveillance systems. The events enumerated represent reports arising from both domestic and nondomestic use of oral or subcutaneous dosage forms of sumatriptan. The events enumerated include all except those already listed in the ADVERSE REACTIONS section above or those too general to be informative. Because the reports cite events reported spontaneously from worldwide postmarketing experience, frequency of events and the role of sumatriptan in their causation cannot be reliably determined. It is assumed, however, that systemic reactions following sumatriptan use are likely to be similar regardless of route of administration.
Blood: Hemolytic anemia, pancytopenia, thrombocytopenia.
Cardiovascular: Atrial fibrillation, cardiomyopathy, colonic ischemia (see WARNINGS), Prinzmetal variant angina, pulmonary embolism, shock, thrombophlebitis.
Ear, Nose, and Throat: Deafness.
Eye: Ischemic optic neuropathy, retinal artery occlusion, retinal vein thrombosis, loss of vision.
Gastrointestinal: Ischemic colitis with rectal bleeding (see WARNINGS), xerostomia.
Hepatic: Elevated liver function tests.
Neurological: Central nervous system vasculitis, cerebrovascular accident, dysphasia, serotonin syndrome, subarachnoid hemorrhage.
Non-Site Specific: Angioneurotic edema, cyanosis, death (see WARNINGS), temporal arteritis.
Psychiatry: Panic disorder.
Respiratory: Bronchospasm in patients with and without a history of asthma.
Skin: Exacerbation of sunburn, hypersensitivity reactions (allergic vasculitis, erythema, pruritus, rash, shortness of breath, urticaria; in addition, severe anaphylaxis/anaphylactoid reactions have been reported [see WARNINGS]), photosensitivity.
Urogenital: Acute renal failure.

DRUG ABUSE AND DEPENDENCE

One clinical study with IMITREX (sumatriptan succinate) Injection enrolling 12 patients with a history of substance abuse failed to induce subjective behavior and/or physiologic response ordinarily associated with drugs that have an established potential for abuse.

OVERDOSAGE

In clinical trials, the highest single doses of IMITREX Nasal Spray administered without significant adverse effects were 40 mg to 12 volunteers and 40 mg to 85 migraine patients, which is twice the highest single recommended dose. In addition, 12 volunteers were administered a total daily dose of 60 mg (20 mg 3 times daily) for 3.5 days without significant adverse events.
Overdose in animals has been fatal and has been heralded by convulsions, tremor, paralysis, inactivity, ptosis, erythema of the extremities, abnormal respiration, cyanosis, ataxia, mydriasis, salivation, and lacrimation. The elimination half-life of sumatriptan is about 2 hours (see CLINICAL PHARMACOLOGY), and therefore monitoring of patients after overdose with IMITREX Nasal Spray should continue for at least 10 hours or while symptoms or signs persist. It is unknown what effect hemodialysis or peritoneal dialysis has on the serum concentrations of sumatriptan.

DOSAGE AND ADMINISTRATION

In controlled clinical trials, single doses of 5, 10, or 20 mg of IMITREX Nasal Spray administered into 1 nostril were effective for the acute treatment of migraine in adults. A greater proportion of patients had headache response following a 20-mg dose than following a 5- or 10-mg dose (see CLINICAL TRIALS). Individuals may vary in response to doses of IMITREX Nasal Spray. The choice of dose should therefore be made on an individual basis, weighing the possible benefit of the 20-mg dose with the potential for a greater risk of adverse events. A 10-mg dose may be achieved by the administration of a single 5-mg dose in each nostril. There is evidence that doses above 20 mg do not provide a greater effect than 20 mg.
If the headache returns, the dose may be repeated once after 2 hours, not to exceed a total daily dose of 40 mg. The safety of treating an average of more than 4 headaches in a 30-day period has not been established.

HOW SUPPLIED

IMITREX Nasal Spray 5 mg (NDC 0173-0524-00) and 20 mg (NDC 0173-0523-00) are each supplied in boxes of 6 nasal spray devices. Each unit dose spray supplies 5 and 20 mg, respectively, of sumatriptan.

Store between 36° and 86°F (2° and 30°C). Protect from light.

ANIMAL TOXICOLOGY

Corneal Opacities

Dogs receiving oral sumatriptan developed corneal opacities and defects in the corneal epithelium. Corneal opacities were seen at the lowest dosage tested, 2 mg/kg/day, and were present after 1 month of treatment. Defects in the corneal epithelium were noted in a 60-week study. Earlier examinations for these toxicities were not conducted and no-effect doses were not established; however, the relative exposure at the lowest dose tested was approximately 5 times the human exposure after a 100-mg oral dose or 3 times the human exposure after a 6-mg subcutaneous dose or 22 times the human exposure after a single 20-mg intranasal dose. There is evidence of alterations in corneal appearance on the first day of intranasal dosing to dogs. Changes were noted at the lowest dose tested, which was approximately 2 times the maximum single human intranasal dose of 20 mg on a mg/m^2 basis.

GlaxoSmithKline
Research Triangle Park, NC 27709

March 2012
IMN:3PI

PATIENT INFORMATION

The following wording is contained in a separate leaflet provided for patients.

Patient Information
IMITREX® (IM-i-trex)
(sumatriptan)
Nasal Spray

Read this Patient Information before you start using IMITREX Nasal Spray and each time you get a refill. There may be new information. This information does not take the place of talking with your healthcare provider about your medical condition or treatment.

What is the most important information I should know about IMITREX Nasal Spray?

IMITREX Nasal Spray can cause serious side effects, including:

Heart attack and other heart problems. Heart problems may lead to death.

Stop taking IMITREX Nasal Spray and get emergency medical help right away if you have any of the following symptoms of a heart attack:
- discomfort in the center of your chest that lasts for more than a few minutes, or that goes away and comes back
- chest pain or chest discomfort that feels like heavy pressure, squeezing, or fullness
- pain or discomfort in your arms, back, neck, jaw, or stomach
- shortness of breath with or without chest discomfort
- breaking out in a cold sweat
- nausea or vomiting
- feeling lightheaded

IMITREX Nasal Spray is not for people with risk factors for heart disease unless a heart exam is done and shows no problem. You have a higher risk for heart disease if you:
- have high blood pressure
- have high cholesterol levels
- smoke
- are overweight
- have diabetes
- have a family history of heart disease
- are a female who has gone through menopause
- are a male over age 40

Serotonin syndrome. Serotonin syndrome is a serious and life-threatening problem that can happen in people using IMITREX Nasal Spray, especially if IMITREX Nasal Spray is used with anti-depressant medicines called selective serotonin reuptake inhibitors (SSRIs) or selective norepinephrine reuptake inhibitors (SNRIs).

Ask your healthcare provider or pharmacist for a list of these medicines if you are not sure.

Call your healthcare provider right away if you have any of the following symptoms of serotonin syndrome:
- mental changes such as seeing things that are not there (hallucinations), agitation, or coma
- fast heartbeat
- changes in blood pressure
- high body temperature
- tight muscles
- trouble walking
- nausea, vomiting, or diarrhea

What is IMITREX Nasal Spray?

IMITREX Nasal Spray is a prescription medicine used to treat acute migraine headaches with or without aura in adults.

IMITREX Nasal Spray is not used to prevent or decrease the number of migraine headaches you have.

IMITREX Nasal Spray is not used to treat other types of headaches such as hemiplegic migraines (that make you unable to move on one side of your body) or basilar migraines (rare form of migraine with aura).

It is not known if IMITREX Nasal Spray is safe and effective to treat cluster headaches.

It is not known if IMITREX Nasal Spray is safe and effective in children under 18 years of age.

Who should not use IMITREX Nasal Spray?

Do not use IMITREX Nasal Spray if you have:
- heart problems or a history of heart problems
- narrowing of blood vessels to your legs, arms, stomach, or kidney (peripheral vascular disease)
- uncontrolled high blood pressure
- severe liver problems
- hemiplegic migraines or basilar migraines. If you are not sure if you have these types of migraines, ask your healthcare provider.
- had a stroke, transient ischemic attacks (TIAs), or problems with your blood circulation
- taken any of the following medicines in the last 24 hours:
  - almotriptan (AXERT®)
  - eletriptan (RELPAX®)
  - frovatriptan (FROVA®)
  - naratriptan (AMERGE®)
  - rizatriptan (MAXALT®, MAXALT-MLT®)
  - sumatriptan and naproxen (TREXIMET®)
  - ergotamines (CAFERGOT®, ERGOMAR®, MIGERGOT®)
  - dihydroergotamine (D.H.E. 45®, MIGRANAL®)

Ask your doctor if you are not sure if your medicine is listed above.
- an allergy to sumatriptan or any of the ingredients in IMITREX Nasal Spray. See the end of this leaflet for a complete list of ingredients in IMITREX Nasal Spray.

What should I tell my healthcare provider before taking IMITREX Nasal Spray?

Before you use IMITREX Nasal Spray, tell your healthcare provider about all of your medical conditions, including if you:
- have high blood pressure
- have high cholesterol
- have diabetes
- smoke
- are overweight
- are a female who has gone through menopause
- have heart disease or a family history of heart disease or stroke
- have kidney problems
- have liver problems
- have had epilepsy or seizures
- are not using effective birth control
- are pregnant or plan to become pregnant. It is not known if IMITREX Nasal Spray will harm your unborn baby.
- become pregnant while taking IMITREX Nasal Spray
- are breastfeeding or plan to breastfeed. IMITREX Nasal Spray passes into your breast milk and may harm your baby. Talk with your healthcare provider about the best way to feed your baby if you use IMITREX Nasal Spray.

Tell your healthcare provider about all the medicines you take, including prescription and nonprescription medicines, vitamins, and herbal supplements.

IMITREX Nasal Spray and other medicines may affect each other, causing side effects.

Especially tell your healthcare provider if you take anti-depressant medicines called:
- selective serotonin reuptake inhibitors (SSRIs)
- serotonin norepinephrine reuptake inhibitors (SNRIs)
- monoamine oxidase inhibitors (MAOIs)

Ask your healthcare provider or pharmacist for a list of these medicines if you are not sure.

Know the medicines you take. Keep a list of them to show your healthcare provider or pharmacist when you get a new medicine.

How should I use IMITREX Nasal Spray?

Before using IMITREX Nasal Spray, read the Instructions for Use at the end of the Patient Information leaflet.
- Certain people should take their first dose of IMITREX Nasal Spray in their healthcare provider's office or in another medical setting. Ask your healthcare provider if you should take your first dose in a medical setting.
- Use IMITREX Nasal Spray exactly as your healthcare provider tells you to use it.
- Your healthcare provider may change your dose. Do not change your dose without first talking with your healthcare provider.
- If you do not get any relief after your first nasal spray, do not use a second nasal spray without first talking with your healthcare provider.
- If your headache comes back after the first nasal spray or you only get some relief from your headache, you can use a second nasal spray 2 hours after the first nasal spray.
- Do not take more than a total of 40 mg of IMITREX Nasal Spray in a 24-hour period.
- It is not known how using IMITREX Nasal Spray for a long time affects the nose and throat.
- Some people who use too much IMITREX Nasal Spray may have worse headaches (medication overuse headache). If your headaches get worse, your healthcare provider may decide to stop your treatment with IMITREX Nasal Spray.
- If you use too much IMITREX Nasal Spray, call your healthcare provider or go to the nearest hospital emergency room right away.
- You should write down when you have headaches and when you take IMITREX Nasal Spray so you can talk with your healthcare provider about how IMITREX Nasal Spray is working for you.

What should I avoid while taking IMITREX Nasal Spray?

IMITREX Nasal Spray can cause dizziness, weakness, or drowsiness. If you have these symptoms, do not drive a car, use machinery, or do anything where you need to be alert.

What are the possible side effects of IMITREX Nasal Spray?

IMITREX Nasal Spray may cause serious side effects. See "What is the most important information I should know about IMITREX Nasal Spray?"

These serious side effects include:
- changes in color or sensation in your fingers and toes (Raynaud's syndrome)
- stomach and intestinal problems (gastrointestinal and colonic ischemic events). Symptoms of gastrointestinal and colonic ischemic events include:
  - sudden or severe stomach pain
  - stomach pain after meals
  - weight loss
  - nausea or vomiting
  - constipation or diarrhea
  - bloody diarrhea
  - fever
- problems with blood circulation to your legs and feet (peripheral vascular ischemia). Symptoms of peripheral vascular ischemia include:
  - cramping and pain in your legs or hips
  - feeling of heaviness or tightness in your leg muscles
  - burning or aching pain in your feet or toes while resting
  - numbness, tingling, or weakness in your legs
  - cold feeling or color changes in 1 or both legs or feet
- shortness of breath or wheezing
- hives (itchy bumps); swelling of your tongue, mouth, or throat

The most common side effects of IMITREX Nasal Spray include:
- dizziness
- warm, hot, burning feeling to your face (flushing)
- discomfort of your neck, throat, or nose
- unusual or bad taste in your mouth
- feeling weak, drowsy, or tired
- sensitivity to loud noises

Tell your healthcare provider if you have any side effect that bothers you or that does not go away.

These are not all the possible side effects of IMITREX Nasal Spray. For more information, ask your healthcare provider or pharmacist.

Call your doctor for medical advice about side effects. You may report side effects to FDA at 1-800-FDA-1088.

How should I store IMITREX Nasal Spray?
- Store between 36°F to 86°F (2°C to 30°C).
- Store your medicine away from light.

Keep IMITREX Nasal Spray and all medicines out of the reach of children.

General information about the safe and effective use of IMITREX Nasal Spray.

Medicines are sometimes prescribed for purposes other than those listed in Patient Information leaflets. Do not use IMITREX Nasal Spray for a condition for which it was not prescribed. Do not give IMITREX Nasal Spray to other people, even if they have the same symptoms you have. It may harm them.

This Patient Information leaflet summarizes the most important information about IMITREX Nasal Spray. If you would like more information, talk with your healthcare provider. You can ask your healthcare provider or pharmacist for information about IMITREX Nasal Spray that is written for healthcare professionals.

For more information, go to www.gsk.com or call 1-888-825-5249.

What are the ingredients in IMITREX Nasal Spray?

Active ingredient: sumatriptan

Inactive ingredients: monobasic potassium phosphate NF, anhydrous dibasic sodium phosphate USP, sulfuric acid NF, sodium hydroxide NF, and purified water USP.

imitrex, AMERGE, and TREXIMET are registered trademarks of GlaxoSmithKline. The other brands listed are trademarks of their respective owners and are not trademarks of GlaxoSmithKline. The makers of these brands are not affiliated with and do not endorse GlaxoSmithKline or its products.

This Patient Information has been approved by the U.S. Food and Drug Administration.

GlaxoSmithKline
Research Triangle Park, NC 27709

March 2012
IMN:3PIL

IMITREX® ℞

[ĭm′ĭ-trĕx]
(sumatriptansuccinate)
Tablets

DESCRIPTION

IMITREX Tablets contain sumatriptan (as the succinate), a selective 5-hydroxytryptamine$_1$ receptor subtype agonist. Sumatriptan succinate is chemically designated as 3-[2-(dimethylamino)ethyl] N-methyl-indole-5-methanesulfonamide succinate (1:1), and it has the following structure:

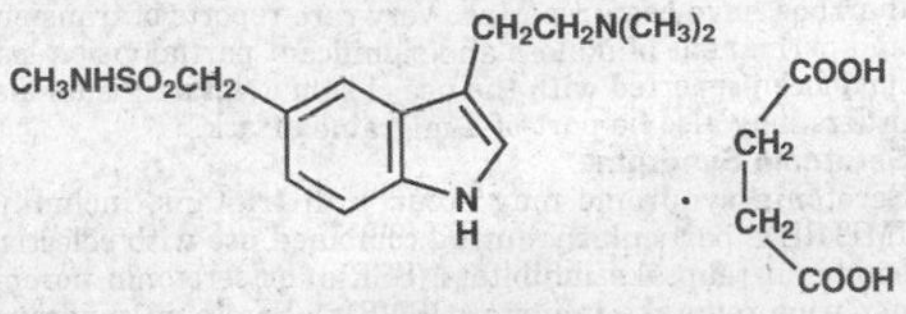

The empirical formula is $C_{14}H_{21}N_3O_2S \bullet C_4H_6O_4$, representing a molecular weight of 413.5. Sumatriptan succinate is a white to off-white powder that is readily soluble in water and in saline. Each IMITREX Tablet for oral administration contains 35, 70, or 140 mg of sumatriptan succinate equivalent to 25, 50, or 100 mg of sumatriptan, respectively. Each tablet also contains the inactive ingredients croscarmellose sodium, dibasic calcium phosphate, magnesium stearate, microcrystalline cellulose, and sodium bicarbonate. Each 100-mg tablet also contains hypromellose, iron oxide, titanium dioxide, and triacetin.

CLINICAL PHARMACOLOGY

Mechanism of Action

Sumatriptan is an agonist for a vascular 5-hydroxytryptamine$_1$ receptor subtype (probably a member of the 5-HT_{1D} family) having only a weak affinity for 5-HT_{1A}, 5-HT_{5A}, and 5-HT_7 receptors and no significant affinity (as measured using standard radioligand binding assays) or pharmacological activity at 5-HT_2, 5-HT_3, or 5-HT_4 receptor subtypes or at alpha$_1$-, alpha$_2$-, or beta-adrenergic; dopamine$_1$; dopamine$_2$; muscarinic; or benzodiazepine receptors.

The vascular 5-HT_1 receptor subtype that sumatriptan activates is present on cranial arteries in both dog and primate, on the human basilar artery, and in the vasculature of human dura mater and mediates vasoconstriction. This action in humans correlates with the relief of migraine headache. In addition to causing vasoconstriction, experimental data from animal studies show that sumatriptan also activates 5-HT_1 receptors on peripheral terminals of the trigeminal nerve innervating cranial blood vessels. Such an action may also contribute to the antimigrainous effect of sumatriptan in humans.

In the anesthetized dog, sumatriptan selectively reduces the carotid arterial blood flow with little or no effect on arterial blood pressure or total peripheral resistance. In the cat, sumatriptan selectively constricts the carotid arteriovenous anastomoses while having little effect on blood flow or resistance in cerebral or extracerebral tissues.

Pharmacokinetics

The mean maximum concentration following oral dosing with 25 mg is 18 ng/mL (range: 7 to 47 ng/mL) and 51 ng/mL (range: 28 to 100 ng/mL) following oral dosing with 100 mg of sumatriptan. This compares with a C_{max} of 5 and 16 ng/mL following dosing with a 5- and 20-mg intranasal dose, respectively. The mean C_{max} following a 6-mg subcutaneous injection is 71 ng/mL (range: 49 to 110 ng/mL). The bioavailability is approximately 15%, primarily due to presystemic metabolism and partly due to incomplete absorption. The C_{max} is similar during a migraine attack and during a migraine-free period, but the T_{max} is slightly later during the attack, approximately 2.5 hours compared to 2.0 hours. When given as a single dose, sumatriptan displays dose proportionality in its extent of absorption (area under the curve [AUC]) over the dose range of 25 to 200 mg, but the C_{max} after 100 mg is approximately 25% less than expected (based on the 25-mg dose).

A food effect study involving administration of IMITREX Tablets 100 mg to healthy volunteers under fasting conditions and with a high-fat meal indicated that the C_{max} and AUC were increased by 15% and 12%, respectively, when administered in the fed state.

Plasma protein binding is low (14% to 21%). The effect of sumatriptan on the protein binding of other drugs has not been evaluated, but would be expected to be minor, given the low rate of protein binding. The apparent volume of distribution is 2.4 L/kg.

The elimination half-life of sumatriptan is approximately 2.5 hours. Radiolabeled ^{14}C-sumatriptan administered orally is largely renally excreted (about 60%) with about 40% found in the feces. Most of the radiolabeled compound excreted in the urine is the major metabolite, indole acetic acid (IAA), which is inactive, or the IAA glucuronide. Only 3% of the dose can be recovered as unchanged sumatriptan.

In vitro studies with human microsomes suggest that sumatriptan is metabolized by monoamine oxidase (MAO), predominantly the A isoenzyme, and inhibitors of that enzyme may alter sumatriptan pharmacokinetics to increase systemic exposure. No significant effect was seen with an MAO-B inhibitor (see CONTRAINDICATIONS, WARNINGS, and PRECAUTIONS: Drug Interactions).

Special Populations

Renal Impairment: The effect of renal impairment on the pharmacokinetics of sumatriptan has not been examined, but little clinical effect would be expected as sumatriptan is largely metabolized to an inactive substance.

Hepatic Impairment: The liver plays an important role in the presystemic clearance of orally administered sumatriptan. Accordingly, the bioavailability of sumatriptan following oral administration may be markedly increased in patients with liver disease. In 1 small study of hepatically impaired patients (N = 8) matched for sex, age, and weight with healthy subjects, the hepatically impaired patients had an approximately 70% increase in AUC and C_{max} and a T_{max} 40 minutes earlier compared to the healthy subjects (see DOSAGE AND ADMINISTRATION).

Age: The pharmacokinetics of oral sumatriptan in the elderly (mean age: 72 years, 2 males and 4 females) and in patients with migraine (mean age: 38 years, 25 males and 155 females) were similar to that in healthy male subjects (mean age: 30 years) (see PRECAUTIONS: Geriatric Use).

Gender: In a study comparing females to males, no pharmacokinetic differences were observed between genders for AUC, C_{max}, T_{max}, and half-life.

Race: The systemic clearance and C_{max} of sumatriptan were similar in black (N = 34) and Caucasian (N = 38) healthy male subjects.

Drug Interactions

Monoamine Oxidase Inhibitors: Treatment with MAO-A inhibitors generally leads to an increase of sumatriptan plasma levels (see CONTRAINDICATIONS and PRECAUTIONS).

Due to gut and hepatic metabolic first-pass effects, the increase of systemic exposure after coadministration of an MAO-A inhibitor with oral sumatriptan is greater than after coadministration of the monoamine oxidase inhibitors (MAOI) with subcutaneous sumatriptan. In a study of 14 healthy females, pretreatment with an MAO-A inhibitor decreased the clearance of subcutaneous sumatriptan. Under the conditions of this experiment, the result was a 2-fold increase in the area under the sumatriptan plasma concentration × time curve (AUC), corresponding to a 40% increase in elimination half-life. This interaction was not evident with an MAO-B inhibitor.

A small study evaluating the effect of pretreatment with an MAO-A inhibitor on the bioavailability from a 25-mg oral sumatriptan tablet resulted in an approximately 7-fold increase in systemic exposure.

Alcohol: Alcohol consumed 30 minutes prior to sumatriptan ingestion had no effect on the pharmacokinetics of sumatriptan.

CLINICAL STUDIES

The efficacy of IMITREX Tablets in the acute treatment of migraine headaches was demonstrated in 3, randomized, double-blind, placebo-controlled studies. Patients enrolled in these 3 studies were predominately female (87%) and Caucasian (97%), with a mean age of 40 years (range, 18 to 65 years). Patients were instructed to treat a moderate to severe headache. Headache response, defined as a reduction in headache severity from moderate or severe pain to mild or no pain, was assessed up to 4 hours after dosing. Associated symptoms such as nausea, photophobia, and phonophobia were also assessed. Maintenance of response was assessed for up to 24 hours postdose. A second dose of IMITREX Tablets or other medication was allowed 4 to 24 hours after the initial treatment for recurrent headache. Acetaminophen was offered to patients in Studies 2 and 3 beginning at 2 hours after initial treatment if the migraine pain had not improved or worsened. Additional medications were allowed 4 to 24 hours after the initial treatment for recurrent headache or as rescue in all 3 studies. The frequency and time to use of these additional treatments were also determined. In all studies, doses of 25, 50, and 100 mg were compared to placebo in the treatment of migraine attacks. In 1 study, doses of 25, 50, and 100 mg were also compared to each other.

In all 3 trials, the percentage of patients achieving headache response 2 and 4 hours after treatment was significantly greater among patients receiving IMITREX Tablets at all doses compared to those who received placebo. In 1 of the 3 studies, there was a statistically significant greater percentage of patients with headache response at 2 and 4 hours in the 50- or 100-mg group when compared to the 25-mg dose groups. There were no statistically significant differences between the 50- and 100-mg dose groups in any study. The results from the 3 controlled clinical trials are summarized in Table 1.

Comparisons of drug performance based upon results obtained in different clinical trials are never reliable. Because studies are conducted at different times, with different samples of patients, by different investigators, employing different criteria and/or different interpretations of the same criteria, under different conditions (dose, dosing regimen, etc.), quantitative estimates of treatment response and the timing of response may be expected to vary considerably from study to study.

[See table 1 above]

Table 1. Percentage of Patients With Headache Response (No or Mild Pain) 2 and 4 Hours Following Treatment

	Placebo 2 hr 4 hr	IMITREX Tablets 25 mg 2 hr 4 hr	IMITREX Tablets 50 mg 2 hr 4 hr	IMITREX Tablets 100 mg 2 hr 4 hr
Study 1	27% 38% (N = 94)	52%[a] 67%[a] (N = 298)	61%[ab] 78%[ab] (N = 296)	62%[ab] 79%[ab] (N = 296)
Study 2	26% 38% (N = 65)	52%[a] 70%[a] (N = 66)	50%[a] 68%[a] (N = 62)	56%[a] 71%[a] (N = 66)
Study 3	17% 19% (N = 47)	52%[a] 65%[a] (N = 48)	54%[a] 72%[a] (N = 46)	57%[a] 78%[a] (N = 46)

[a] $P<0.05$ in comparison with placebo.
[b] $P<0.05$ in comparison with 25 mg.

The estimated probability of achieving an initial headache response over the 4 hours following treatment is depicted in Figure 1.

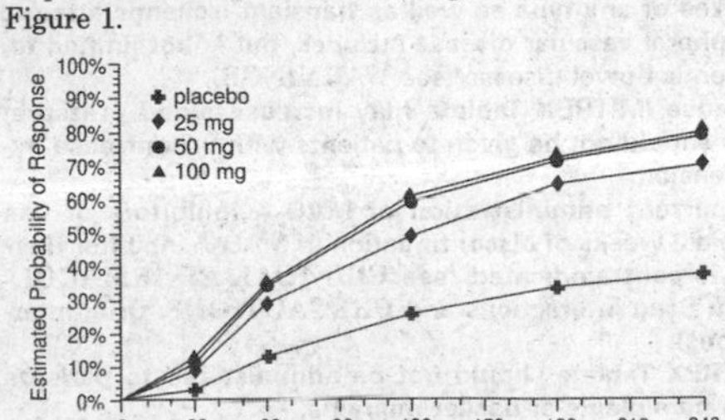

Figure 1. Estimated Probability of Achieving Initial Headache Response Within 240 Minutes[a]

[a] The figure shows the probability over time of obtaining headache response (no or mild pain) following treatment with sumatriptan. The averages displayed are based on pooled data from the 3 clinical controlled trials providing evidence of efficacy. Kaplan-Meier plot with patients not achieving response and/or taking rescue within 240 minutes censored to 240 minutes.

For patients with migraine-associated nausea, photophobia, and/or phonophobia at baseline, there was a lower incidence of these symptoms at 2 hours (Study 1) and at 4 hours (Studies 1, 2, and 3) following administration of IMITREX Tablets compared to placebo.

As early as 2 hours in Studies 2 and 3 or 4 hours in Study 1, through 24 hours following the initial dose of study treatment, patients were allowed to use additional treatment for pain relief in the form of a second dose of study treatment or other medication. The estimated probability of patients taking a second dose or other medication for migraine over the 24 hours following the initial dose of study treatment is summarized in Figure 2.

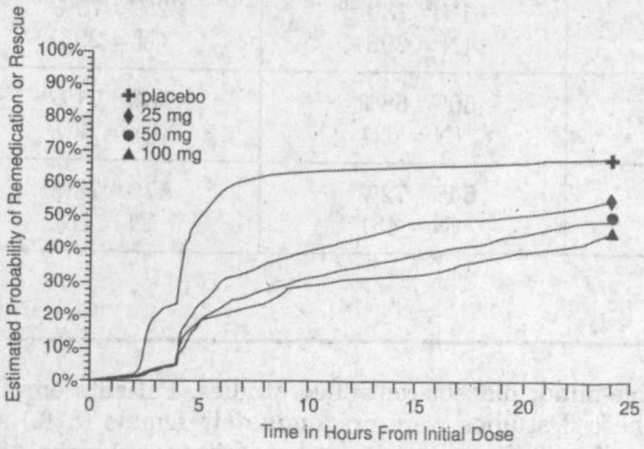

Figure 2. The Estimated Probability of Patients Taking a Second Dose or Other Medication for Migraine Over the 24 Hours Following the Initial Dose of Study Treatment[a]

[a]Kaplan-Meier plot based on data obtained in the 3 clinical controlled trials providing evidence of efficacy with patients not using additional treatments censored to 24 hours. Plot also includes patients who had no response to the initial dose. No remedication was allowed within 2 hours postdose.

There is evidence that doses above 50 mg do not provide a greater effect than 50 mg. There was no evidence to suggest that treatment with sumatriptan was associated with an increase in the severity of recurrent headaches. The efficacy of IMITREX Tablets was unaffected by presence of aura; duration of headache prior to treatment; gender, age, or weight of the patient; relationship to menses; or concomitant use of common migraine prophylactic drugs (e.g., beta-blockers, calcium channel blockers, tricyclic antidepressants). There were insufficient data to assess the impact of race on efficacy.

INDICATIONS AND USAGE

IMITREX Tablets are indicated for the acute treatment of migraine attacks with or without aura in adults.

IMITREX Tablets are not intended for the prophylactic therapy of migraine or for use in the management of hemiplegic or basilar migraine (see CONTRAINDICATIONS). Safety and effectiveness of IMITREX Tablets have not been established for cluster headache, which is present in an older, predominantly male population.

CONTRAINDICATIONS

IMITREX Tablets should not be given to patients with history, symptoms, or signs of ischemic cardiac, cerebrovascular, or peripheral vascular syndromes. In addition, patients with other significant underlying cardiovascular diseases should not receive IMITREX Tablets. Ischemic cardiac syndromes include, but are not limited to, angina pectoris of any type (e.g., stable angina of effort, vasospastic forms of angina such as the Prinzmetal variant), all forms of myocardial infarction, and silent myocardial ischemia. Cerebrovascular syndromes include, but are not limited to, strokes of any type as well as transient ischemic attacks. Peripheral vascular disease includes, but is not limited to, ischemic bowel disease (see WARNINGS).

Because IMITREX Tablets may increase blood pressure, they should not be given to patients with uncontrolled hypertension.

Concurrent administration of MAO-A inhibitors or use within 2 weeks of discontinuation of MAO-A inhibitor therapy is contraindicated (see CLINICAL PHARMACOLOGY: Drug Interactions and PRECAUTIONS: Drug Interactions).

IMITREX Tablets should not be administered to patients with hemiplegic or basilar migraine.

IMITREX Tablets and any ergotamine-containing or ergot-type medication (like dihydroergotamine or methysergide) should not be used within 24 hours of each other, nor should IMITREX and another 5-HT_1 agonist.

IMITREX Tablets are contraindicated in patients with hypersensitivity to sumatriptan or any of their components.

IMITREX Tablets are contraindicated in patients with severe hepatic impairment.

WARNINGS

IMITREX Tablets should only be used where a clear diagnosis of migraine headache has been established.

Risk of Myocardial Ischemia and/or Infarction and Other Adverse Cardiac Events

Sumatriptan should not be given to patients with documented ischemic or vasospastic coronary artery disease (CAD) (see CONTRAINDICATIONS). It is strongly recommended that sumatriptan not be given to patients in whom unrecognized CAD is predicted by the presence of risk factors (e.g., hypertension, hypercholesterolemia, smoker, obesity, diabetes, strong family history of CAD, female with surgical or physiological menopause, male over 40 years of age) unless a cardiovascular evaluation provides satisfactory clinical evidence that the patient is reasonably free of coronary artery and ischemic myocardial disease or other significant underlying cardiovascular disease. The sensitivity of cardiac diagnostic procedures to detect cardiovascular disease or predisposition to coronary artery vasospasm is modest, at best. If, during the cardiovascular evaluation, the patient's medical history or electrocardiographic investigations reveal findings indicative of, or consistent with, coronary artery vasospasm or myocardial ischemia, sumatriptan should not be administered (see CONTRAINDICATIONS).

For patients with risk factors predictive of CAD, who are determined to have a satisfactory cardiovascular evaluation, it is strongly recommended that administration of the first dose of sumatriptan tablets take place in the setting of a physician's office or similar medically staffed and equipped facility unless the patient has previously received sumatriptan. Because cardiac ischemia can occur in the absence of clinical symptoms, consideration should be given to obtaining on the first occasion of use an electrocardiogram (ECG) during the interval immediately following IMITREX Tablets in these patients with risk factors.

It is recommended that patients who are intermittent long-term users of sumatriptan and who have or acquire risk factors predictive of CAD, as described above, undergo periodic interval cardiovascular evaluation as they continue to use sumatriptan.

The systematic approach described above is intended to reduce the likelihood that patients with unrecognized cardiovascular disease will be inadvertently exposed to sumatriptan.

Drug-Associated Cardiac Events and Fatalities

Serious adverse cardiac events, including acute myocardial infarction, life-threatening disturbances of cardiac rhythm, and death have been reported within a few hours following the administration of IMITREX® (sumatriptan succinate) Injection or IMITREX Tablets. Considering the extent of use of sumatriptan in patients with migraine, the incidence of these events is extremely low.

The fact that sumatriptan can cause coronary vasospasm, that some of these events have occurred in patients with no prior cardiac disease history and with documented absence of CAD, and the close proximity of the events to sumatriptan use support the conclusion that some of these cases were caused by the drug. In many cases, however, where there has been known underlying coronary artery disease, the relationship is uncertain.

Premarketing Experience WithSumatriptan: Of 6,348 patients with migraine who participated in premarketing controlled and uncontrolled clinical trials of oral sumatriptan, 2 experienced clinical adverse events shortly after receiving oral sumatriptan that may have reflected coronary vasospasm. Neither of these adverse events was associated with a serious clinical outcome.

Among the more than 1,900 patients with migraine who participated in premarketing controlled clinical trials of subcutaneous sumatriptan, there were 8 patients who sustained clinical events during or shortly after receiving sumatriptan that may have reflected coronary artery vasospasm. Six of these 8 patients had ECG changes consistent with transient ischemia, but without accompanying clinical symptoms or signs. Of these 8 patients, 4 had either findings suggestive of CAD or risk factors predictive of CAD prior to study enrollment.

Among approximately 4,000 patients with migraine who participated in premarketing controlled and uncontrolled clinical trials of sumatriptan nasal spray, 1 patient experienced an asymptomatic subendocardial infarction possibly subsequent to a coronary vasospastic event.

Postmarketing Experience WithSumatriptan: Serious cardiovascular events, some resulting in death, have been reported in association with the use of IMITREX Injection or IMITREX Tablets. The uncontrolled nature of postmarketing surveillance, however, makes it impossible to determine definitively the proportion of the reported cases that were actually caused by sumatriptan or to reliably assess causation in individual cases. On clinical grounds, the longer the latency between the administration of IMITREX and the onset of the clinical event, the less likely the association is to be causative. Accordingly, interest has focused on events beginning within 1 hour of the administration of IMITREX.

Cardiac events that have been observed to have onset within 1 hour of sumatriptan administration include: coronary artery vasospasm, transient ischemia, myocardial infarction, ventricular tachycardia and ventricular fibrillation, cardiac arrest, and death.

Some of these events occurred in patients who had no findings of CAD and appear to represent consequences of coronary artery vasospasm. However, among domestic reports of serious cardiac events within 1 hour of sumatriptan administration, almost all of the patients had risk factors predictive of CAD and the presence of significant underlying CAD was established in most cases (see CONTRAINDICATIONS).

Drug-Associated Cerebrovascular Events and Fatalities

Cerebral hemorrhage, subarachnoid hemorrhage, stroke, and other cerebrovascular events have been reported in patients treated with oral or subcutaneous sumatriptan, and some have resulted in fatalities. The relationship of sumatriptan to these events is uncertain. In a number of cases, it appears possible that the cerebrovascular events were primary, sumatriptan having been administered in the incorrect belief that the symptoms experienced were a consequence of migraine when they were not. As with other acute migraine therapies, before treating headaches in patients not previously diagnosed as migraineurs, and in migraineurs who present with atypical symptoms, care should be taken to exclude other potentially serious neurological conditions. It should also be noted that patients with migraine may be at increased risk of certain cerebrovascular events (e.g., cerebrovascular accident, transient ischemic attack).

Other Vasospasm-Related Events

Sumatriptan may cause vasospastic reactions other than coronary artery vasospasm. Both peripheral vascular ischemia and colonic ischemia with abdominal pain and bloody diarrhea have been reported. Very rare reports of transient and permanent blindness and significant partial vision loss have been reported with the use of sumatriptan. Visual disorders may also be part of a migraine attack.

Serotonin Syndrome

Serotonin syndrome may occur with triptans, including IMITREX, particularly during combined use with selective serotonin reuptake inhibitors (SSRIs) or serotonin norepinephrine reuptake inhibitors (SNRIs). Serotonin syndrome symptoms may include mental status changes (e.g., agitation, hallucinations, coma), autonomic instability (e.g., tachycardia, labile blood pressure, hyperthermia), neuromuscular aberrations (e.g., hyperreflexia, incoordination), and/or gastrointestinal symptoms (e.g., nausea, vomiting, diarrhea). The onset of symptoms can occur within minutes to hours of receiving a new or a greater dose of a serotonergic medication. Treatment with IMITREX should be discontinued if serotonin syndrome is suspected.

Increase in Blood Pressure

Significant elevation in blood pressure, including hypertensive crisis, has been reported on rare occasions in patients with and without a history of hypertension. Sumatriptan is contraindicated in patients with uncontrolled hypertension (see CONTRAINDICATIONS). Sumatriptan should be administered with caution to patients with controlled hypertension as transient increases in blood pressure and peripheral vascular resistance have been observed in a small proportion of patients.

Concomitant Drug Use

In patients taking MAO-A inhibitors, sumatriptan plasma levels attained after treatment with recommended doses are 7-fold higher following oral administration than those obtained under other conditions. Accordingly, the coadministration of IMITREX Tablets and an MAO-A inhibitor is contraindicated (see CLINICAL PHARMACOLOGY and CONTRAINDICATIONS).

Hypersensitivity

Hypersensitivity (anaphylaxis/anaphylactoid) reactions have occurred on rare occasions in patients receiving sumatriptan. Such reactions can be life threatening or fatal. In general, hypersensitivity reactions to drugs are more likely to occur in individuals with a history of sensitivity to multiple allergens (see CONTRAINDICATIONS).

PRECAUTIONS

General

Chest discomfort and jaw or neck tightness have been reported following use of IMITREX Tablets and have also been reported infrequently following administration of IMITREX® (sumatriptan) Nasal Spray. Chest, jaw, or neck tightness is relatively common after administration of IMITREX Injection. Only rarely have these symptoms been associated with ischemic ECG changes. However, because sumatriptan may cause coronary artery vasospasm, patients who experience signs or symptoms suggestive of angina following sumatriptan should be evaluated for the presence of CAD or a predisposition to Prinzmetal variant angina before receiving additional doses of sumatriptan, and should be monitored electrocardiographically if dosing is resumed and similar symptoms recur. Similarly, patients who experience other symptoms or signs suggestive of decreased arterial flow, such as ischemic bowel syndrome or Raynaud syndrome following sumatriptan should be evaluated for atherosclerosis or predisposition to vasospasm (see WARNINGS).

IMITREX should also be administered with caution to patients with diseases that may alter the absorption, metabolism, or excretion of drugs, such as impaired hepatic or renal function.

There have been rare reports of seizure following administration of sumatriptan. Sumatriptan should be used with caution in patients with a history of epilepsy or conditions associated with a lowered seizure threshold.

Care should be taken to exclude other potentially serious neurologic conditions before treating headache in patients not previously diagnosed with migraine headache or who experience a headache that is atypical for them. There have been rare reports where patients received sumatriptan for severe headaches that were subsequently shown to have been secondary to an evolving neurologic lesion (see WARNINGS).

For a given attack, if a patient does not respond to the first dose of sumatriptan, the diagnosis of migraine should be reconsidered before administration of a second dose.

Overuse

Overuse of acute migraine drugs (e.g., ergotamine, triptans, opioids, or a combination of drugs for 10 or more days per month) may lead to exacerbation of headache (medication overuse headache). Medication overuse headache may present as migraine-like daily headaches, or as a marked increase in frequency of migraine attacks. Detoxification of patients, including withdrawal of the overused drugs, and treatment of withdrawal symptoms (which often includes a transient worsening of headache) may be necessary. Migraine patients should be informed about the risks of medication overuse and encouraged to record headache frequency and drug use.

Information for Patients

See PATIENT INFORMATION at the end of this labeling for the text of the separate leaflet provided for patients.

Patients should be cautioned about the risk of serotonin syndrome with the use of sumatriptan or other triptans, especially during combined use with SSRIs or SNRIs.

Laboratory Tests

No specific laboratory tests are recommended for monitoring patients prior to and/or after treatment with sumatriptan.

Drug Interactions

Selective Serotonin Reuptake Inhibitors/Serotonin Norepinephrine Reuptake Inhibitors and Serotonin Syndrome: Cases of life-threatening serotonin syndrome have been reported during combined use of SSRIs or SNRIs and triptans (see WARNINGS).

Ergot-Containing Drugs: Ergot-containing drugs have been reported to cause prolonged vasospastic reactions. Because there is a theoretical basis that these effects may be additive, use of ergotamine-containing or ergot-type medications (like dihydroergotamine or methysergide) and sumatriptan within 24 hours of each other should be avoided (see CONTRAINDICATIONS).

Monoamine Oxidase-A Inhibitors: MAO-A inhibitors reduce sumatriptan clearance, significantly increasing systemic exposure. Therefore, the use of IMITREX Tablets in patients receiving MAO-A inhibitors is contraindicated (see CLINICAL PHARMACOLOGY and CONTRAINDICATIONS).

Drug/Laboratory Test Interactions

IMITREX Tablets are not known to interfere with commonly employed clinical laboratory tests.

Carcinogenesis, Mutagenesis, Impairment of Fertility

Carcinogenesis: In carcinogenicity studies, rats and mice were given sumatriptan by oral gavage (rats: 104 weeks) or drinking water (mice: 78 weeks). Average exposures achieved in mice receiving the highest dose (target dose of 160 mg/kg/day) were approximately 40 times the exposure attained in humans after the maximum recommended single oral dose of 100 mg. The highest dose administered to rats (160 mg/kg/day, reduced from 360 mg/kg/day during week 21) was approximately 15 times the maximum recommended single human oral dose of 100 mg on a mg/m^2 basis. There was no evidence of an increase in tumors in either species related to sumatriptan administration.

Mutagenesis: Sumatriptan was not mutagenic in the presence or absence of metabolic activation when tested in 2 gene mutation assays (the Ames test and the in vitro mammalian Chinese hamster V79/HGPRT assay). In 2 cytogenetics assays (the in vitro human lymphocyte assay and the in vivo rat micronucleus assay) sumatriptan was not associated with clastogenic activity.

Impairment of Fertility: In a study in which male and female rats were dosed daily with oral sumatriptan prior to and throughout the mating period, there was a treatment-related decrease in fertility secondary to a decrease in mating in animals treated with 50 and 500 mg/kg/day. The highest no-effect dose for this finding was 5 mg/kg/day, or approximately one half of the maximum recommended single human oral dose of 100 mg on a mg/m^2 basis. It is not clear whether the problem is associated with treatment of the males or females or both combined. In a similar study by the subcutaneous route there was no evidence of impaired fertility at 60 mg/kg/day, the maximum dose tested, which is equivalent to approximately 6 times the maximum recommended single human oral dose of 100 mg on a mg/m^2 basis.

Pregnancy

Pregnancy Category C. In reproductive toxicity studies in rats and rabbits, oral treatment with sumatriptan was associated with embryolethality, fetal abnormalities, and pup mortality. When administered by the intravenous route to rabbits, sumatriptan has been shown to be embryolethal. There are no adequate and well-controlled studies in pregnant women. Therefore, IMITREX should be used during pregnancy only if the potential benefit justifies the potential risk to the fetus. In assessing this information, the following findings should be considered.

Embryolethality: When given orally or intravenously to pregnant rabbits daily throughout the period of organogenesis, sumatriptan caused embryolethality at doses at or close to those producing maternal toxicity. In the oral studies this dose was 100 mg/kg/day, and in the intravenous studies this dose was 2.0 mg/kg/day. The mechanism of the embryolethality is not known. The highest no-effect dose for embryolethality by the oral route was 50 mg/kg/day, which is approximately 9 times the maximum single recommended human oral dose of 100 mg on a mg/m^2 basis. By the intravenous route, the highest no-effect dose was 0.75 mg/kg/day, or approximately one tenth of the maximum single recommended human oral dose of 100 mg on a mg/m^2 basis.

The intravenous administration of sumatriptan to pregnant rats throughout organogenesis at 12.5 mg/kg/day, the maximum dose tested, did not cause embryolethality. This dose is equivalent to the maximum single recommended human oral dose of 100 mg on a mg/m^2 basis. Additionally, in a study in rats given subcutaneous sumatriptan daily prior to and throughout pregnancy at 60 mg/kg/day, the maximum dose tested, there was no evidence of increased embryo/fetal lethality. This dose is equivalent to approximately 6 times the maximum recommended single human oral dose of 100 mg on a mg/m^2 basis.

Teratogenicity: Oral treatment of pregnant rats with sumatriptan during the period of organogenesis resulted in an increased incidence of blood vessel abnormalities (cervicothoracic and umbilical) at doses of approximately 250 mg/kg/day or higher. The highest no-effect dose was approximately 60 mg/kg/day, which is approximately 6 times the maximum single recommended human oral dose of 100 mg on a mg/m^2 basis. Oral treatment of pregnant rabbits with sumatriptan during the period of organogenesis resulted in an increased incidence of cervicothoracic vascular and skeletal abnormalities. The highest no-effect dose for these effects was 15 mg/kg/day, or approximately 3 times the maximum single recommended human oral dose of 100 mg on a mg/m^2 basis.

A study in which rats were dosed daily with oral sumatriptan prior to and throughout gestation demonstrated embryo/fetal toxicity (decreased body weight, decreased ossification, increased incidence of rib variations) and an increased incidence of a syndrome of malformations (short tail/short body and vertebral disorganization) at 500 mg/kg/day. The highest no-effect dose was 50 mg/kg/day, or approximately 5 times the maximum single recommended human oral dose of 100 mg on a mg/m^2 basis. In a study in rats dosed daily with subcutaneous sumatriptan prior to and throughout pregnancy, at a dose of 60 mg/kg/day, the maximum dose tested, there was no evidence of teratogenicity. This dose is equivalent to approximately 6 times the maximum recommended single human oral dose of 100 mg on a mg/m$_2$ basis.

Pup Deaths: Oral treatment of pregnant rats with sumatriptan during the period of organogenesis resulted in a decrease in pup survival between birth and postnatal day 4 at doses of approximately 250 mg/kg/day or higher. The highest no-effect dose for this effect was approximately 60 mg/kg/day, or 6 times the maximum single recommended human oral dose of 100 mg on a mg/m^2 basis.

Oral treatment of pregnant rats with sumatriptan from gestational day 17 through postnatal day 21 demonstrated a decrease in pup survival measured at postnatal days 2, 4, and 20 at the dose of 1,000 mg/kg/day. The highest no-effect dose for this finding was 100 mg/kg/day, approximately 10 times the maximum single recommended human oral dose of 100 mg on a mg/m^2 basis. In a similar study in rats by the subcutaneous route there was no increase in pup death at 81 mg/kg/day, the highest dose tested, which is equivalent to 8 times the maximum single recommended human oral dose of 100 mg on a mg/m^2 basis.

Nursing Mothers

Sumatriptan is excreted in human breast milk following subcutaneous administration. Infant exposure to sumatriptan can be minimized by avoiding breastfeeding for 12 hours after treatment with IMITREX Tablets.

Pediatric Use

Safety and effectiveness of IMITREX Tablets in pediatric patients under 18 years of age have not been established; therefore, IMITREX Tablets are not recommended for use in patients under 18 years of age.

Two controlled clinical trials evaluating sumatriptan nasal spray (5 to 20 mg) in pediatric patients aged 12 to 17 years enrolled a total of 1,248 adolescent migraineurs who treated a single attack. The studies did not establish the efficacy of sumatriptan nasal spray compared to placebo in the treatment of migraine in adolescents. Adverse events observed in these clinical trials were similar in nature to those reported in clinical trials in adults.

Five controlled clinical trials (2 single attack studies, 3 multiple attack studies) evaluating oral sumatriptan (25 to 100 mg) in pediatric patients aged 12 to 17 years enrolled a total of 701 adolescent migraineurs. These studies did not establish the efficacy of oral sumatriptan compared to placebo in the treatment of migraine in adolescents. Adverse events observed in these clinical trials were similar in nature to those reported in clinical trials in adults. The frequency of all adverse events in these patients appeared to be both dose- and age-dependent, with younger patients reporting events more commonly than older adolescents.

Postmarketing experience documents that serious adverse events have occurred in the pediatric population after use of subcutaneous, oral, and/or intranasal sumatriptan. These reports include events similar in nature to those reported rarely in adults, including stroke, visual loss, and death. A myocardial infarction has been reported in a 14-year-old male following the use of oral sumatriptan; clinical signs occurred within 1 day of drug administration. Since clinical data to determine the frequency of serious adverse events in pediatric patients who might receive injectable, oral, or intranasal sumatriptan are not presently available, the use of sumatriptan in patients aged younger than 18 years is not recommended.

Geriatric Use

The use of sumatriptan in elderly patients is not recommended because elderly patients are more likely to have decreased hepatic function, they are at higher risk for CAD, and blood pressure increases may be more pronounced in the elderly (see WARNINGS).

ADVERSE REACTIONS

Serious cardiac events, including some that have been fatal, have occurred following the use of IMITREX Injection or Tablets. These events are extremely rare and most have been reported in patients with risk factors predictive of CAD. Events reported have included coronary artery vasospasm, transient myocardial ischemia, myocardial infarction, ventricular tachycardia, and ventricular fibrillation (see CONTRAINDICATIONS, WARNINGS, and PRECAUTIONS).

Significant hypertensive episodes, including hypertensive crises, have been reported on rare occasions in patients with or without a history of hypertension (see WARNINGS).

Incidence in Controlled Clinical Trials

Table 2 lists adverse events that occurred in placebo-controlled clinical trials in patients who took at least 1 dose of study drug. Only events that occurred at a frequency of 2% or more in any group treated with IMITREX Tablets and were more frequent in that group than in the placebo group are included in Table 2. The events cited reflect experience gained under closely monitored conditions of clinical trials in a highly selected patient population. In actual clinical practice or in other clinical trials, these frequency estimates may not apply, as the conditions of use, reporting behavior, and the kinds of patients treated may differ.

[See table 2 at top of next page]

Other events that occurred in more than 1% of patients receiving IMITREX Tablets and at least as often on placebo included nausea and/or vomiting, migraine, headache, hyposalivation, dizziness, and drowsiness/sleepiness.

IMITREX Tablets are generally well tolerated. Across all doses, most adverse reactions were mild and transient and did not lead to long-lasting effects. The incidence of adverse events in controlled clinical trials was not affected by gender or age of the patients. There were insufficient data to assess the impact of race on the incidence of adverse events.

Other Events Observed in Association With the Administration of IMITREX Tablets

In the paragraphs that follow, the frequencies of less commonly reported adverse clinical events are presented. Because the reports include events observed in open and uncontrolled studies, the role of IMITREX Tablets in their causation cannot be reliably determined. Furthermore, variability associated with adverse event reporting, the terminology used to describe adverse events, etc., limit the value of quantitative frequency estimates provided. Event frequencies are calculated as the number of patients who used IMITREX Tablets (25, 50, or 100 mg) and reported an event divided by the total number of patients (N = 6,348) exposed to IMITREX Tablets. All reported events are included except those already listed in the previous table, those too general to be informative, and those not reasonably associated with the use of the drug. Events are further classified within body system categories and enumerated in order of decreasing frequency using the following defini-

Table 2. Treatment Emergent Adverse Events Reported by at Least 2% of Patients in Controlled Migraine Trials[a]

Adverse Event Type	Percent of Patients Reporting			
	Placebo (N = 309)	IMITREX 25 mg (N = 417)	IMITREX 50 mg (N = 771)	IMITREX 100 mg (N = 437)
Atypical sensations	4%	5%	6%	6%
Paresthesia (all types)	2%	3%	5%	3%
Sensation warm/cold	2%	3%	2%	3%
Pain and other pressure sensations	4%	6%	6%	8%
Chest - pain/tightness/pressure and/or heaviness	1%	1%	2%	2%
Neck/throat/jaw - pain/ tightness/pressure	<1%	<1%	2%	3%
Pain - location specified	1%	2%	1%	1%
Other - pressure/tightness/ heaviness	2%	1%	1%	3%
Neurological				
Vertigo	<1%	<1%	<1%	2%
Other				
Malaise/fatigue	<1%	2%	2%	3%

[a]Events that occurred at a frequency of 2% or more in the group treated with IMITREX Tablets and that occurred more frequently in that group than the placebo group.

tions: frequent adverse events are defined as those occurring in at least 1/100 patients, infrequent adverse events are those occurring in 1/100 to 1/1,000 patients, and rare adverse events are those occurring in fewer than 1/1,000 patients.

Atypical Sensations: Frequent were burning sensation and numbness. Infrequent was tight feeling in head. Rare were dysesthesia.

Cardiovascular: Frequent were palpitations, syncope, decreased blood pressure, and increased blood pressure. Infrequent were arrhythmia, changes in ECG, hypertension, hypotension, pallor, pulsating sensations, and tachycardia. Rare were angina, atherosclerosis, bradycardia, cerebral ischemia, cerebrovascular lesion, heart block, peripheral cyanosis, thrombosis, transient myocardial ischemia, and vasodilation.

Ear, Nose, and Throat: Frequent were sinusitis, tinnitus; allergic rhinitis; upper respiratory inflammation; ear, nose, and throat hemorrhage; external otitis; hearing loss; nasal inflammation; and sensitivity to noise. Infrequent were hearing disturbances and otalgia. Rare was feeling of fullness in the ear(s).

Endocrine and Metabolic: Infrequent was thirst. Rare were elevated thyrotropin stimulating hormone (TSH) levels; galactorrhea; hyperglycemia; hypoglycemia; hypothyroidism; polydipsia; weight gain; weight loss; endocrine cysts, lumps, and masses; and fluid disturbances.

Eye: Rare were disorders of sclera, mydriasis, blindness and low vision, visual disturbances, eye edema and swelling, eye irritation and itching, accommodation disorders, external ocular muscle disorders, eye hemorrhage, eye pain, and keratitis and conjunctivitis.

Gastrointestinal: Frequent were diarrhea and gastric symptoms. Infrequent were constipation, dysphagia, and gastroesophageal reflux. Rare were gastrointestinal bleeding, hematemesis, melena, peptic ulcer, gastrointestinal pain, dyspeptic symptoms, dental pain, feelings of gastrointestinal pressure, gastritis, gastroenteritis, hypersalivation, abdominal distention, oral itching and irritation, salivary gland swelling, and swallowing disorders.

Hematological Disorders: Rare was anemia.

Musculoskeletal: Frequent was myalgia. Infrequent was muscle cramps. Rare were tetany; muscle atrophy, weakness, and tiredness; arthralgia and articular rheumatitis; acquired musculoskeletal deformity; muscle stiffness, tightness, and rigidity; and musculoskeletal inflammation.

Neurological: Frequent were phonophobia and photophobia. Infrequent were confusion, depression, difficulty concentrating, disturbance of smell, dysarthria, euphoria, facial pain, heat sensitivity, incoordination, lacrimation, monoplegia, sleep disturbance, shivering, syncope, and tremor. Rare were aggressiveness, apathy, bradylogia, cluster headache, convulsions, decreased appetite, drug abuse, dystonic reaction, facial paralysis, hallucinations, hunger, hyperesthesia, hysteria, increased alertness, memory disturbance, neuralgia, paralysis, personality change, phobia, radiculopathy, rigidity, suicide, twitching, agitation, anxiety, depressive disorders, detachment, motor dysfunction, neurotic disorders, psychomotor disorders, taste disturbances, and raised intracranial pressure.

Respiratory: Frequent was dyspnea. Infrequent was asthma. Rare were hiccoughs, breathing disorders, cough, and bronchitis.

Skin: Frequent was sweating. Infrequent were erythema, pruritus, rash, and skin tenderness. Rare were dry/scaly skin, tightness of skin, wrinkling of skin, eczema, seborrheic dermatitis, and skin nodules.

Breasts: Infrequent was tenderness. Rare were nipple discharge; breast swelling; cysts, lumps, and masses of breasts; and primary malignant breast neoplasm.

Urogenital: Infrequent were dysmenorrhea, increased urination, and intermenstrual bleeding. Rare were abortion and hematuria, urinary frequency, bladder inflammation, micturition disorders, urethritis, urinary infections, menstruation symptoms, abnormal menstrual cycle, inflammation of fallopian tubes, and menstrual cycle symptoms.

Miscellaneous: Frequent was hypersensitivity. Infrequent were fever, fluid retention, and overdose. Rare were edema, hematoma, lymphadenopathy, speech disturbance, voice disturbances, contusions.

Other Events Observed in the Clinical Development of IMITREX

The following adverse events occurred in clinical trials with IMITREX Injection and IMITREX Nasal Spray. Because the reports include events observed in open and uncontrolled studies, the role of IMITREX in their causation cannot be reliably determined. All reported events are included except those already listed, those too general to be informative, and those not reasonably associated with the use of the drug.

Atypical Sensations: Feeling strange, prickling sensation, tingling, and hot sensation.

Cardiovascular: Abdominal aortic aneurysm, abnormal pulse, flushing, phlebitis, Raynaud syndrome, and various transient ECG changes (nonspecific ST or T wave changes, prolongation of PR or QTc intervals, sinus arrhythmia, nonsustained ventricular premature beats, isolated junctional ectopic beats, atrial ectopic beats, delayed activation of the right ventricle).

Chest Symptoms: Chest discomfort.

Endocrine and Metabolic: Dehydration.

Ear, Nose, and Throat: Disorder/discomfort nasal cavity and sinuses, ear infection, Meniere disease, and throat discomfort.

Eye: Vision alterations.

Gastrointestinal: Abdominal discomfort, colitis, disturbance of liver function tests, flatulence/eructation, gallstones, intestinal obstruction, pancreatitis, and retching.

Injection Site Reaction

Miscellaneous: Difficulty in walking, hypersensitivity to various agents, jaw discomfort, miscellaneous laboratory abnormalities, "serotonin agonist effect," swelling of the extremities, and swelling of the face.

Mouth and Teeth: Disorder of mouth and tongue (e.g., burning of tongue, numbness of tongue, dry mouth).

Musculoskeletal: Arthritis, backache, intervertebral disc disorder, neck pain/stiffness, need to flex calf muscles, and various joint disturbances (pain, stiffness, swelling, ache).

Neurological: Bad/unusual taste, chills, diplegia, disturbance of emotions, sedation, globus hystericus, intoxication, myoclonia, neoplasm of pituitary, relaxation, sensation of lightness, simultaneous hot and cold sensations, stinging sensations, stress, tickling sensations, transient hemiplegia, and yawning.

Respiratory: Influenza and diseases of the lower respiratory tract and lower respiratory tract infection.

Skin: Skin eruption, herpes, and peeling of the skin.

Urogenital: Disorder of breasts, endometriosis, and renal calculus.

Postmarketing Experience (Reports for Subcutaneous or Oral Sumatriptan)

The following section enumerates potentially important adverse events that have occurred in clinical practice and that have been reported spontaneously to various surveillance systems. The events enumerated represent reports arising from both domestic and nondomestic use of oral or subcutaneous dosage forms of sumatriptan. The events enumerated include all except those already listed in the ADVERSE REACTIONS section above or those too general to be informative. Because the reports cite events reported spontaneously from worldwide postmarketing experience, frequency of events and the role of sumatriptan in their causation cannot be reliably determined. It is assumed, however, that systemic reactions following sumatriptan use are likely to be similar regardless of route of administration.

Blood: Hemolytic anemia, pancytopenia, thrombocytopenia.

Cardiovascular: Atrial fibrillation, cardiomyopathy, colonic ischemia (see WARNINGS), Prinzmetal variant angina, pulmonary embolism, shock, thrombophlebitis.

Ear, Nose, and Throat: Deafness.

Eye: Ischemic optic neuropathy, retinal artery occlusion, retinal vein thrombosis, loss of vision.

Gastrointestinal: Ischemic colitis with rectal bleeding (see WARNINGS), xerostomia.

Hepatic: Elevated liver function tests.

Neurological: Central nervous system vasculitis, cerebrovascular accident, dysphasia, serotonin syndrome, subarachnoid hemorrhage.

Non-Site Specific: Angioneurotic edema, cyanosis, death (see WARNINGS), temporal arteritis.

Psychiatry: Panic disorder.

Respiratory: Bronchospasm in patients with and without a history of asthma.

Skin: Exacerbation of sunburn, hypersensitivity reactions (allergic vasculitis, erythema, pruritus, rash, shortness of breath, urticaria; in addition, severe anaphylaxis/anaphylactoid reactions have been reported [see WARNINGS]), photosensitivity.

Urogenital: Acute renal failure.

DRUG ABUSE AND DEPENDENCE

One clinical study with IMITREX Injection enrolling 12 patients with a history of substance abuse failed to induce subjective behavior and/or physiologic response ordinarily associated with drugs that have an established potential for abuse.

OVERDOSAGE

Patients (N = 670) have received single oral doses of 140 to 300 mg without significant adverse effects. Volunteers (N = 174) have received single oral doses of 140 to 400 mg without serious adverse events.

Overdose in animals has been fatal and has been heralded by convulsions, tremor, paralysis, inactivity, ptosis, erythema of the extremities, abnormal respiration, cyanosis, ataxia, mydriasis, salivation, and lacrimation. The elimination half-life of sumatriptan is approximately 2.5 hours (see CLINICAL PHARMACOLOGY), and therefore monitoring of patients after overdose with IMITREX Tablets should continue for at least 12 hours or while symptoms or signs persist.

It is unknown what effect hemodialysis or peritoneal dialysis has on the serum concentrations of sumatriptan.

DOSAGE AND ADMINISTRATION

In controlled clinical trials, single doses of 25, 50, or 100 mg of IMITREX Tablets were effective for the acute treatment of migraine in adults. There is evidence that doses of 50 and 100 mg may provide a greater effect than 25 mg (see CLINICAL TRIALS). There is also evidence that doses of 100 mg do not provide a greater effect than 50 mg. Individuals may vary in response to doses of IMITREX Tablets. The choice of dose should therefore be made on an individual basis, weighing the possible benefit of a higher dose with the potential for a greater risk of adverse events.

If the headache returns or the patient has a partial response to the initial dose, the dose may be repeated after 2 hours, not to exceed a total daily dose of 200 mg. If a headache returns following an initial treatment with IMITREX Injection, additional single IMITREX Tablets (up to 100 mg/day) may be given with an interval of at least 2 hours between tablet doses. The safety of treating an average of more than 4 headaches in a 30-day period has not been established.

Because of the potential of MAO-A inhibitors to cause unpredictable elevations in the bioavailability of oral sumatriptan, their combined use is contraindicated (see CONTRAINDICATIONS).

Hepatic disease/functional impairment may also cause unpredictable elevations in the bioavailability of orally administered sumatriptan. Consequently, if treatment is deemed advisable in the presence of liver disease, the maximum single dose should in general not exceed 50 mg (see CLINICAL PHARMACOLOGY for the basis of this recommendation).

HOW SUPPLIED

IMITREX Tablets, 25, 50, and 100 mg of sumatriptan (base) as the succinate.

IMITREX Tablets, 25 mg are white, triangular-shaped, film-coated tablets debossed with "I" on one side and"25" on the other in blister packs of 9 tablets (NDC 0173-0735-00).

IMITREX Tablets, 50 mg are white, triangular-shaped, film-coated tablets debossed with "IMITREX 50" on one side and a chevron shape (^) on the other in blister packs of 9 tablets (NDC 0173-0736-01).

IMITREX Tablets, 100 mg, are pink, triangular-shaped, film-coated tablets debossed with "IMITREX 100" on one side and a chevron shape (^) on the other in blister packs of 9 tablets (NDC 0173-0737-01).

Store between 36° and 86°F (2° and 30°C).

ANIMAL TOXICOLOGY

Corneal Opacities

Dogs receiving oral sumatriptan developed corneal opacities and defects in the corneal epithelium. Corneal opacities were seen at the lowest dosage tested, 2 mg/kg/day, and were present after 1 month of treatment. Defects in the corneal epithelium were noted in a 60-week study. Earlier examinations for these toxicities were not conducted and no-effect doses were not established; however, the relative exposure at the lowest dose tested was approximately 5 times the human exposure after a 100-mg oral dose. There is evidence of alterations in corneal appearance on the first day of intranasal dosing to dogs. Changes were noted at the lowest dose tested, which was approximately one half the maximum single human oral dose of 100 mg on a mg/m^2 basis.

GlaxoSmithKline
Research Triangle Park, NC 27709

March 2012
IMT:3PI

PATIENT INFORMATION

The following wording is contained in a separate leaflet provided for patients.

Patient Information
IMITREX® (IM-i-trex)
(sumatriptansuccinate)
Tablets

Read this Patient Information before you start taking IMITREX and each time you get a refill. There may be new information. This information does not take the place of talking with your healthcare provider about your medical condition or treatment.

What is the most important information I should know about IMITREX?

IMITREX can cause serious side effects, including:

Heart attack and other heart problems. Heart problems may lead to death.

Stop taking IMITREX and get emergency medical help right away if you have any of the following symptoms of a heart attack:
- discomfort in the center of your chest that lasts for more than a few minutes, or that goes away and comes back
- chest pain or chest discomfort that feels like heavy pressure, squeezing, or fullness
- pain or discomfort in your arms, back, neck, jaw, or stomach
- shortness of breath with or without chest discomfort
- breaking out in a cold sweat
- nausea or vomiting
- feeling lightheaded

IMITREX is not for people with risk factors for heart disease unless a heart exam is done and shows no problem. You have a higher risk for heart disease if you:
- have high blood pressure
- have high cholesterol levels
- smoke
- are overweight
- have diabetes
- have a family history of heart disease
- are a female who has gone through menopause
- are a male over age 40

Serotonin syndrome. Serotonin syndrome is a serious and life-threatening problem that can happen in people taking IMITREX, especially if IMITREX is used with antidepressant medicines called selective serotonin reuptake inhibitors (SSRIs) or selective norepinephrine reuptake inhibitors (SNRIs).

Ask your healthcare provider or pharmacist for a list of these medicines if you are not sure.

Call your healthcare provider right away if you have any of the following symptoms of serotonin syndrome:
- mental changes such as seeing things that are not there (hallucinations), agitation, or coma
- fast heartbeat
- changes in blood pressure
- high body temperature
- tight muscles
- trouble walking
- nausea, vomiting, or diarrhea

What is IMITREX?

IMITREX is a prescription medicine used to treat acute migraine headaches with or without aura in adults.

IMITREX is not used to prevent or decrease the number of migraine headaches you have.

IMITREX is not used to treat other types of headaches such as hemiplegic (that make you unable to move on one side of your body) or basilar migraines (rare form of migraine with aura).

It is not known if IMITREX is safe and effective to treat cluster headaches.

It is not known if IMITREX is safe and effective in children under 18 years of age.

Who should not take IMITREX?

Do not take IMITREX if you have:
- heart problems or a history of heart problems
- narrowing of blood vessels to your legs, arms, stomach, or kidney (peripheral vascular disease)
- uncontrolled high blood pressure
- severe liver problems
- hemiplegic migraines or basilar migraines. If you are not sure if you have these types of migraines, ask your healthcare provider.
- had a stroke, transient ischemic attacks (TIAs), or problems with your blood circulation
- taken any of the following medicines in the last 24 hours:
  - almotriptan (AXERT®)
  - eletriptan (RELPAX®)
  - frovatriptan (FROVA®)
  - naratriptan (AMERGE®)
  - rizatriptan (MAXALT®, MAXALT-MLT®)
  - sumatriptan and naproxen (TREXIMET®)
  - ergotamines (CAFERGOT®, ERGOMAR®, MIGERGOT®)
  - dihydroergotamine (D.H.E. 45®, MIGRANAL®)

Ask your doctor if you are not sure if your medicine is listed above.
- an allergy to sumatriptan or any of the ingredients in IMITREX. See the end of this leaflet for a complete list of ingredients in IMITREX.

What should I tell my healthcare provider before taking IMITREX?

Before you take IMITREX, tell your healthcare provider about all of your medical conditions, including if you:
- have high blood pressure
- have high cholesterol
- have diabetes
- smoke
- are overweight
- are a female who has gone through menopause
- have heart disease or a family history of heart disease or stroke
- have kidney problems
- have liver problems
- have had epilepsy or seizures
- are not using effective birth control
- are pregnant or plan to become pregnant. It is not known if IMITREX will harm your unborn baby.
- become pregnant while taking IMITREX
- are breastfeeding or plan to breastfeed. IMITREX passes into your breast milk and may harm your baby. Talk with your healthcare provider about the best way to feed your baby if you take IMITREX.

Tell your healthcare provider about all the medicines you take, including prescription and nonprescription medicines, vitamins, and herbal supplements.

IMITREX and other medicines may affect each other, causing side effects.

Especially tell your healthcare provider if you take antidepressant medicines called:
- selective serotonin reuptake inhibitors (SSRIs)
- serotonin norepinephrine reuptake inhibitors (SNRIs)
- monoamine oxidase inhibitors (MAOIs)

Ask your healthcare provider or pharmacist for a list of these medicines if you are not sure.

Know the medicines you take. Keep a list of them to show your healthcare provider or pharmacist when you get a new medicine.

How should I take IMITREX?
- Certain people should take their first dose of IMITREX in their healthcare provider's office or in another medical setting. Ask your healthcare provider if you should take your first dose in a medical setting.
- Take IMITREX exactly as your healthcare provider tells you to take it.
- Your healthcare provider may change your dose. Do not change your dose without first talking to your healthcare provider.
- Take IMITREX with water or other liquids.
- If you do not get any relief after your first IMITREX tablet, do not take a second tablet without first talking with your healthcare provider.
- If your headache comes back or you only get some relief from your headache, you can take a second tablet 2 hours after the first tablet.
- Do not take more than a total of 200 mg of IMITREX tablets in a 24-hour period.
- Some people who take too many IMITREX tablets may have worse headaches (medication overuse headache). If your headaches get worse, your healthcare provider may decide to stop your treatment with IMITREX.
- If you take too much IMITREX, call your healthcare provider or go to the nearest hospital emergency room right away.
- You should write down when you have headaches and when you take IMITREX so you can talk with your healthcare provider about how IMITREX is working for you.

What should I avoid while taking IMITREX?

IMITREX can cause dizziness, weakness, or drowsiness. If you have these symptoms, do not drive a car, use machinery, or do anything where you need to be alert.

What are the possible side effects of IMITREX?

IMITREX may cause serious side effects. See "What is the most important information I should know about IMITREX?"

These serious side effects include:
- changes in color or sensation in your fingers and toes (Raynaud's syndrome)
- stomach and intestinal problems (gastrointestinal and colonic ischemic events). Symptoms of gastrointestinal and colonic ischemic events include:
  - sudden or severe stomach pain
  - stomach pain after meals
  - weight loss
  - nausea or vomiting
  - constipation or diarrhea
  - bloody diarrhea
  - fever
- problems with blood circulation to your legs and feet (peripheral vascular ischemia). Symptoms of peripheral vascular ischemia include:
  - cramping and pain in your legs or hips
  - feeling of heaviness or tightness in your leg muscles
  - burning or aching pain in your feet or toes while resting
  - numbness, tingling, or weakness in your legs
  - cold feeling or color changes in 1 or both legs or feet
- shortness of breath or wheezing
- hives (itchy bumps); swelling of your tongue, mouth, or throat

The most common side effects of IMITREX include:
- tingling or numbness in your fingers or toes
- dizziness
- warm, hot, burning feeling to your face (flushing)
- feeling weak, drowsy, or tired

Tell your healthcare provider if you have any side effect that bothers you or that does not go away.

These are not all the possible side effects of IMITREX. For more information, ask your healthcare provider or pharmacist.

Call your doctor for medical advice about side effects. You may report side effects to FDA at 1-800-FDA-1088.

How should I store IMITREX Tablets?

Store IMITREX between 36°F to 86°F (2°C to 30°C).

Keep IMITREX and all medicines out of the reach of children.

General information about the safe and effective use of IMITREX.

Medicines are sometimes prescribed for purposes other than those listed in Patient Information leaflets. Do not use IMITREX for a condition for which it was not prescribed. Do not give IMITREX to other people, even if they have the same symptoms you have. It may harm them.

This Patient Information leaflet summarizes the most important information about IMITREX. If you would like more information, talk with your healthcare provider. You can ask your healthcare provider or pharmacist for information about IMITREX that is written for healthcare professionals. For more information, go to www.gsk.com or call 1-888-825-5249.

What are the ingredients in IMITREX Tablets?

Active ingredient: sumatriptan succinate

Inactive ingredients: croscarmellose sodium, dibasic calcium phosphate, magnesium stearate, microcrystalline cellulose, and sodium bicarbonate

100-mg tablets also contain hypromellose, iron oxide, titanium dioxide, and triacetin.

imitrex, AMERGE, and TREXIMET are registered trademarks of GlaxoSmithKline. The other brands listed are trademarks of their respective owners and are not trademarks of GlaxoSmithKline. The makers of these brands are not affiliated with and do not endorse GlaxoSmithKline or its products.

This Patient Information has been approved by the U.S. Food and Drug Administration.

GlaxoSmithKline
Research Triangle Park, NC 27709

March 2012
IMT:3PIL

INFANRIX ℞

[in' fan-rix]

(Diphtheria and Tetanus Toxoids and Acellular Pertussis Vaccine Adsorbed)
Suspension for Intramuscular Injection

HIGHLIGHTS OF PRESCRIBING INFORMATION

These highlights do not include all the information needed to use INFANRIX safely and effectively. See full prescribing information for INFANRIX.

INFANRIX (Diphtheria and Tetanus Toxoids and Acellular Pertussis Vaccine Adsorbed)
Suspension for Intramuscular Injection
Initial U.S. Approval: 1997

RECENT MAJOR CHANGES

Warnings and Precautions, Syncope (5.3) 03/2012

INDICATIONS AND USAGE

INFANRIX is a vaccine indicated for active immunization against diphtheria, tetanus, and pertussis as a 5-dose series in infants and children 6 weeks to 7 years of age. (1)

DOSAGE AND ADMINISTRATION

A 0.5-mL intramuscular injection given as a 5-dose series: (2.2)

- One dose each at 2, 4, and 6 months of age.
- One booster dose at 15 to 20 months of age and another booster dose at 4 to 6 years of age.

DOSAGE FORMS AND STRENGTHS

Single-dose vials and prefilled syringes containing a 0.5-mL suspension for injection. (3)

CONTRAINDICATIONS

- Severe allergic reaction (e.g., anaphylaxis) after a previous dose of any diphtheria toxoid, tetanus toxoid, or pertussis-containing vaccine, or to any component of INFANRIX. (4.1)
- Encephalopathy within 7 days of administration of a previous pertussis-containing vaccine. (4.2)
- Progressive neurologic disorders. (4.3)

WARNINGS AND PRECAUTIONS

- If Guillain-Barré syndrome occurs within 6 weeks of receipt of a prior vaccine containing tetanus toxoid, the decision to give INFANRIX should be based on potential benefits and risks. (5.1)
- INFANRIX is available in vials and 2 types of prefilled syringes. One type of prefilled syringe has a tip cap which may contain natural rubber latex. The other type has a tip cap and a rubber plunger which contain dry natural latex rubber. Use of these syringes may cause allergic reactions in latex sensitive individuals. (5.2, 16)
- Syncope (fainting) can occur in association with administration of injectable vaccines, including INFANRIX. Procedures should be in place to avoid falling injury and to restore cerebral perfusion following syncope. (5.3)
- If temperature ≥105°F, collapse or shock-like state, or persistent, inconsolable crying lasting ≥3 hours have occurred within 48 hours after receipt of a pertussis-containing vaccine, or if seizures have occurred within 3 days after receipt of a pertussis-containing vaccine, the decision to give INFANRIX should be based on potential benefits and risks. (5.4)
- For children at higher risk for seizures, an antipyretic may be administered at the time of vaccination with INFANRIX. (5.5)
- Apnea following intramuscular vaccination has been observed in some infants born prematurely. Decisions about when to administer an intramuscular vaccine, including INFANRIX, to infants born prematurely should be based on consideration of the individual infant's medical status, and the potential benefits and possible risks of vaccination. (5.6)

ADVERSE REACTIONS

Rates of injection site reactions (pain, redness, swelling) ranged from 10% to 53%, depending on reaction and dose number, and were highest following doses 4 and 5. Fever was common (20% to 30%) following doses 1-3. Other common solicited adverse events were drowsiness, irritability/fussiness, and loss of appetite, reported in approximately 15% to 60% of subjects, depending on event and dose number. (6.1)

To report SUSPECTED ADVERSE REACTIONS, contact GlaxoSmithKline at 1-888-825-5249 or VAERS at 1-800-822-7967 or www.vaers.hhs.gov.

DRUG INTERACTIONS

Do not mix INFANRIX with any other vaccine in the same syringe or vial. (7.1)

See 17 for PATIENT COUNSELING INFORMATION

Revised: 07/2012

FULL PRESCRIBING INFORMATION: CONTENTS*

*** Sections or subsections omitted from the full prescribing information are not listed**

FULL PRESCRIBING INFORMATION

1 INDICATIONS AND USAGE

INFANRIX® is indicated for active immunization against diphtheria, tetanus, and pertussis as a 5-dose series in infants and children 6 weeks to 7 years of age (prior to seventh birthday).

2 DOSAGE AND ADMINISTRATION

2.1 Preparation for Administration

Shake vigorously to obtain a homogeneous, turbid, white suspension. Do not use if resuspension does not occur with vigorous shaking. Parenteral drug products should be inspected visually for particulate matter and discoloration prior to administration, whenever solution and container permit. If either of these conditions exists, the vaccine should not be administered.

For the prefilled syringes, attach a sterile needle and administer intramuscularly.

For the vials, use a sterile needle and sterile syringe to withdraw the 0.5-mL dose and administer intramuscularly. Changing needles between drawing vaccine from a vial and injecting it into a recipient is not necessary unless the needle has been damaged or contaminated. Use a separate sterile needle and syringe for each individual.

Do not administer this product intravenously, intradermally, or subcutaneously.

2.2 Dose and Schedule

A 0.5-mL dose of INFANRIX is approved for intramuscular administration in infants and children 6 weeks to 7 years of age (prior to the seventh birthday) as a 5-dose series. The series consists of a primary immunization course of 3 doses administered at 2, 4, and 6 months of age (at intervals of 4 to 8 weeks), followed by 2 booster doses, administered at 15 to 20 months of age and at 4 to 6 years of age. The first dose may be given as early as 6 weeks of age.

The preferred administration site is the anterolateral aspect of the thigh for most infants younger than 12 months of age and the deltoid muscle of the upper arm for most children 12 months of age to 7 years of age.

2.3 Use of INFANRIX With Other DTaP Vaccines

Sufficient data are not available on the safety and effectiveness of interchanging INFANRIX and Diphtheria and Tetanus Toxoids and Acellular Pertussis (DTaP) vaccines from different manufacturers for successive doses of the DTaP vaccination series. Because the pertussis antigen components of INFANRIX and PEDIARIX® [Diphtheria and Tetanus Toxoids and Acellular Pertussis Adsorbed, Hepatitis B (Recombinant) and Inactivated Poliovirus Vaccine] are the same, INFANRIX may be used to complete a DTaP vaccination series initiated with PEDIARIX.

2.4 Additional Dosing Information

If any recommended dose of pertussis vaccine cannot be given *[see Contraindications (4.2, 4.3) and Warnings and Precautions (5.5)]*, Diphtheria and Tetanus Toxoids Adsorbed (DT) For Pediatric Use should be given according to its prescribing information.

3 DOSAGE FORMS AND STRENGTHS

INFANRIX is a suspension for injection available in 0.5-mL single-dose vials and prefilled TIP-LOK® syringes.

4 CONTRAINDICATIONS

4.1 Hypersensitivity

Severe allergic reaction (e.g., anaphylaxis) after a previous dose of any diphtheria toxoid, tetanus toxoid, or pertussis-containing vaccine, or to any component of INFANRIX is a contraindication *[see Description (11)]*. Because of the uncertainty as to which component of the vaccine might be responsible, no further vaccination with any of these components should be given. Alternatively, such individuals may be referred to an allergist for evaluation if immunization with any of these components is being considered.

4.2 Encephalopathy

Encephalopathy (e.g., coma, decreased level of consciousness, prolonged seizures) within 7 days of administration of a previous dose of a pertussis-containing vaccine that is not attributable to another identifiable cause is a contraindication to administration of any pertussis-containing vaccine, including INFANRIX.

4.3 Progressive Neurologic Disorder

Progressive neurologic disorder, including infantile spasms, uncontrolled epilepsy, or progressive encephalopathy is a contraindication to administration of any pertussis-containing vaccine, including INFANRIX. Pertussis vaccine should not be administered to individuals with these conditions until a treatment regimen has been established and the condition has stabilized.

5 WARNINGS AND PRECAUTIONS

5.1 Guillain-Barré Syndrome

If Guillain-Barré syndrome occurs within 6 weeks of receipt of a prior vaccine containing tetanus toxoid, the decision to give any tetanus toxoid-containing vaccine, including INFANRIX, should be based on careful consideration of the potential benefits and possible risks. When a decision is made to withhold tetanus toxoid, other available vaccines should be given, as indicated.

5.2 Latex

INFANRIX is available in vials and 2 types of prefilled syringes. One type of prefilled syringe has a tip cap which may contain natural rubber latex and a plunger which does not contain latex. The other type has a tip cap and a rubber plunger which contain dry natural latex rubber. Use of these syringes may cause allergic reactions in latex sensitive individuals. The vial stopper does not contain latex. *[See How Supplied/Storage and Handling (16).]*

5.3 Syncope

Syncope (fainting) can occur in association with administration of injectable vaccines, including INFANRIX. Syncope can be accompanied by transient neurological signs such as visual disturbance, paresthesia, and tonic-clonic limb movements. Procedures should be in place to avoid falling injury and to restore cerebral perfusion following syncope.

5.4 Adverse Events Following Prior Pertussis Vaccination

If any of the following events occur in temporal relation to receipt of a pertussis-containing vaccine, the decision to give any pertussis-containing vaccine, including INFANRIX, should be based on careful consideration of the potential benefits and possible risks:

- Temperature of ≥40.5°C (105°F) within 48 hours not due to another identifiable cause;
- Collapse or shock-like state (hypotonic-hyporesponsive episode) within 48 hours;
- Persistent, inconsolable crying lasting ≥3 hours, occurring within 48 hours;

Seizures with or without fever occurring within 3 days.

5.5 Children at Risk for Seizures

For children at higher risk for seizures than the general population, an appropriate antipyretic may be administered at the time of vaccination with a pertussis-containing vaccine, including INFANRIX, and for the ensuing 24 hours to reduce the possibility of post-vaccination fever.

5.6 Apnea in Premature Infants

Apnea following intramuscular vaccination has been observed in some infants born prematurely. Decisions about when to administer an intramuscular vaccine, including INFANRIX, to infants born prematurely should be based on consideration of the individual infant's medical status, and the potential benefits and possible risks of vaccination.

5.7 Preventing and Managing Allergic Vaccine Reactions

Prior to administration, the healthcare provider should review the patient's immunization history for possible vaccine hypersensitivity. Epinephrine and other appropriate agents used for the control of immediate allergic reactions must be immediately available should an acute anaphylactic reaction occur.

6 ADVERSE REACTIONS

6.1 Clinical Trials Experience

Because clinical trials are conducted under widely varying conditions, adverse reaction rates observed in the clinical trials of a vaccine cannot be directly compared to rates in the clinical trials of another vaccine and may not reflect the rates observed in practice. There is the possibility that broad use of INFANRIX could reveal adverse reactions not observed in clinical trials.

Approximately 95,000 doses of INFANRIX have been administered in clinical studies. In these studies, 29,243 infants have received INFANRIX in primary series studies, 6,081 children have received a fourth consecutive dose of INFANRIX, 1,764 children have received a fifth consecutive dose of INFANRIX, and 559 children have received a dose of INFANRIX following 3 doses of PEDIARIX.

Solicited Adverse Events: In a US study, 335 infants received INFANRIX, ENGERIX-B® [Hepatitis B Vaccine (Recombinant)], inactivated poliovirus vaccine (IPV, Sanofi Pasteur SA), Haemophilus b (Hib) conjugate vaccine (Wyeth Pharmaceuticals Inc.), and pneumococcal 7-valent conjugate (PCV7) vaccine (Wyeth Pharmaceuticals Inc.) concomitantly at separate sites. All vaccines were administered at 2, 4, and 6 months of age. Data on solicited local reactions and general adverse events were collected by parents using standardized diary cards for 4 consecutive days following each vaccine dose (i.e., day of vaccination and the next 3 days) (Table 1). Among subjects, 69% were White, 16% were Hispanic, 8% were Black, 4% were Asian, and 2% were of other racial/ethnic groups.

Table 1. Solicited Local Reactions and General Adverse Events (%) Occurring Within 4 Days of Vaccination[a] With Separate Concomitant Administration of INFANRIX, ENGERIX-B, IPV, Haemophilus b (Hib) Conjugate Vaccine, and Pneumococcal Conjugate Vaccine (PCV7) (Modified Intent To Treat Cohort)

	INFANRIX, ENGERIX-B, IPV, Hib Vaccine, & PCV7		
	Dose 1	Dose 2	Dose 3
Local[b]			
N	335	323	315
Pain, any	31.9	30.0	29.8
Pain, grade 2 or 3	9.0	8.7	8.9
Pain, grade 3	2.7	1.5	1.3
Redness, any	18.2	32.8	39.0
Redness, >20 mm	0.3	0.0	1.9
Swelling, any	9.6	20.4	24.8
Swelling, >20 mm	0.6	0.0	1.3
General			
N	333	321	311
Fever[c] (≥100.4°F)	19.8	30.2	23.8
Fever[c] (>101.3°F)	4.5	9.7	5.8
Fever[c] (>102.2°F)	0.3	3.1	2.3
Fever[c] (>103.1°F)	0.0	0.3	0.3
N	335	323	315
Drowsiness, any	54.0	48.3	38.4
Drowsiness, grade 2 or 3	17.6	12.4	11.1
Drowsiness, grade 3	3.6	0.6	1.9
Irritability/ Fussiness, any	61.5	61.6	56.5
Irritability/ Fussiness, grade 2 or 3	19.4	21.1	19.4
Irritability/ Fussiness, grade 3	3.9	3.4	3.2
Loss of appetite, any	27.8	26.6	23.8
Loss of appetite, grade 2 or 3	5.1	3.4	5.4
Loss of appetite, grade 3	0.6	0.3	0.0

Hib conjugate vaccine and PCV7 manufactured by Wyeth Pharmaceuticals Inc. IPV manufactured by Sanofi Pasteur SA.

Modified intent to treat cohort = all vaccinated subjects for whom safety data were available.

N = number of infants for whom at least one symptom sheet was completed; for fever, numbers exclude missing temperature recordings or tympanic measurements.

Grade 2: pain defined as cried/protested on touch; drowsiness defined as interfered with normal daily activities; irritability/fussiness defined as crying more than usual/interfered with normal daily activities; loss of appetite defined as eating less than usual/interfered with normal daily activities.

Grade 3: pain defined as cried when limb was moved/ spontaneously painful; drowsiness defined as prevented normal daily activities; irritability/fussiness defined as crying that could not be comforted/prevented normal daily activities; loss of appetite defined as no eating at all.

[a]Within 4 days of vaccination defined as day of vaccination and the next 3 days.

[b]Local reactions at the injection site for INFANRIX.

[c]Axillary temperatures increased by 1°C and oral temperatures increased by 0.5°C to derive equivalent rectal temperature.

In a US study, the safety of a booster dose of INFANRIX was evaluated in children 15 to 18 months of age whose previous 3 DTaP doses were with INFANRIX (N = 251) or PEDIARIX (N = 559). Vaccines administered concurrently with the fourth dose of INFANRIX included measles, mumps, and rubella (MMR) vaccine (Merck & Co., Inc.), varicella vaccine (Merck & Co., Inc.), pneumococcal 7-valent conjugate (PCV7) vaccine (Wyeth Pharmaceuticals Inc.), and any US-licensed Hib conjugate vaccine; these were given concomitantly in 13.2%, 6.3%, 37.4%, and 41.2% of subjects, respectively. Data on solicited adverse events were collected by parents using standardized diary cards for 4 consecutive days following each vaccine dose (i.e., day of vaccination and the next 3 days) (Table 2). Among subjects, 85% were White, 6% were Hispanic, 6% were Black, 1% were Asian, and 2% were of other racial/ethnic groups.

Table 2. Solicited Local Reactions and General Adverse Events (%) Occurring Within 4 Days of Vaccination[a] With INFANRIX Administered as the Fourth Dose Following 3 Previous Doses of INFANRIX or PEDIARIX (Total Vaccinated Cohort)

	Group Primed With INFANRIX[b] N = 247	Group Primed With PEDIARIX[c] N = 553
Local[d]		
Pain, any	44.5	48.3
Pain, grade 2 or 3	19.0	18.6
Pain, grade 3	3.6	3.4
Redness, any	48.2	49.9
Redness, >20 mm	6.1	6.0
Swelling, any	32.8	32.7
Swelling, >20 mm	3.6	5.2
Increase in mid-thigh circumference, any	33.2	26.2
Increase in mid-thigh circumference, >40 mm	0.0	1.3
General		
Fever[e] (>99.5°F)	8.9	15.4
Fever[e] (>100.4°F)	4.5	6.7
Fever[e] (>101.3°F)	2.0	2.0
Drowsiness, any	35.6	31.3
Drowsiness, grade 2 or 3	9.3	6.7
Drowsiness, grade 3	2.4	1.3
Irritability, any	52.2	53.9
Irritability, grade 2 or 3	18.2	19.7
Irritability, grade 3	3.2	1.4
Loss of appetite, any	24.7	23.3
Loss of appetite, grade 2 or 3	5.3	4.9
Loss of appetite, grade 3	2.4	0.5

Total Vaccinated Cohort = all subjects who received a dose of study vaccine.

N = number of subjects for whom at least one symptom sheet was completed.

Grade 2: pain defined as cried/protested on touch; drowsiness defined as interfered with normal daily activities; irritability defined as crying more than usual/ interfered with normal daily activities; loss of appetite defined as eating less than usual/no effect on normal daily activities.

Grade 3: pain defined as cried when limb was moved/ spontaneously painful; drowsiness defined as prevented normal daily activities; irritability defined as crying that could not be comforted/prevented normal daily activities; loss of appetite defined as eating less than usual/ interfered with normal daily activities.

[a]Within 4 days of vaccination defined as day of vaccination and the next 3 days.

[b]Received INFANRIX, ENGERIX-B, IPV (Sanofi Pasteur SA), PCV7 vaccine (Wyeth Pharmaceuticals Inc.), and Hib conjugate vaccine (Wyeth Pharmaceuticals Inc.) at 2, 4, and 6 months of age.

[c]Received PEDIARIX, PCV7 vaccine (Wyeth Pharmaceuticals Inc.), and Hib conjugate vaccine (Wyeth Pharmaceuticals Inc.) at 2, 4, and 6 months of age or PCV7 vaccine 2 weeks later.

[d] Local reactions at the injection site for INFANRIX.

[e]Axillary temperatures.

In a US study, the safety of a fifth consecutive dose of INFANRIX coadministered at separate sites with a fourth dose of IPV (Sanofi Pasteur SA) and a second dose of MMR vaccine (Merck & Co., Inc.) was evaluated in 1,053 children 4 to 6 years of age. Data on solicited adverse events were collected by parents using standardized diary cards for 4 consecutive days following each vaccine dose (i.e., day of vaccination and the next 3 days) (Table 3). Among subjects, 43% were White, 18% Hispanic, 15% Asian, 7% Black, and 17% were of other racial/ethnic groups.

Table 3. Solicited Local Reactions and General Adverse Events (%) Occurring Within 4 Days of Vaccination[a] With a Fifth Consecutive Dose of INFANRIX When Coadministered With IPV and MMR Vaccine (Total Vaccinated Cohort)

Local[b]	**N = 1,039-1,043**
Pain, any	53.3
Pain, grade 2 or 3[c]	12.0
Pain, grade 3[c]	0.6
Redness, any	36.6
Redness, ≥50 mm	20.0
Redness, ≥110 mm	4.1
Arm circumference increase, any	37.8
Arm circumference increase, >20 mm	7.4
Arm circumference increase, >30 mm	3.2

Table 4. Selected Adverse Events Occurring Within 48 Hours Following Vaccination With INFANRIX or Whole-Cell DTP in Italian Infants at 2, 4, or 6 Months of Age

Event	INFANRIX (N = 13,761 Doses)		Whole-Cell DTP Vaccine (N = 13,520 Doses)	
	Number	Rate/1,000 Doses	Number	Rate/1,000 Doses
Fever (≥104°F)[ab]	5	0.36	32	2.4
Hypotonic-hyporesponsive episode[c]	0	0	9	0.67
Persistent crying ≥3 hours[a]	6	0.44	54	4.0
Seizures[d]	1[e]	0.07	3[f]	0.22

[a] P <0.001.
[b] Rectal temperatures.
[c] P = 0.002.
[d] Not statistically significant at P <0.05.
[e] Maximum rectal temperature within 72 hours of vaccination = 103.1°F.
[f] Maximum rectal temperature within 72 hours of vaccination = 99.5°F, 101.3°F, and 102.2°F.

Swelling, any	27.0
Swelling, ≥50 mm	11.5
Swelling, ≥110 mm	1.8
General	**N = 993-1,036**
Drowsiness, any	17.5
Drowsiness, grade 3[d]	0.8
Fever, ≥99.5°F	14.8
Fever, >100.4°F	4.4
Fever, >102.2°F	1.1
Fever, >104°F	0.0
Loss of appetite, any	16.0
Loss of appetite, grade 3[e]	0.6

IPV manufactured by Sanofi Pasteur SA. MMR vaccine manufactured by Merck & Co., Inc.
Total Vaccinated Cohort = all vaccinated subjects for whom safety data were available.
N = number of children with evaluable data for the events listed.
[a] Within 4 days of vaccination defined as day of vaccination and the next 3 days.
[b] Local reactions at the injection site for INFANRIX.
[c] Grade 2 defined as painful when the limb was moved; Grade 3 defined as preventing normal daily activities.
[d] Grade 3 defined as preventing normal daily activities.
[e] Grade 3 defined as not eating at all.

In the US booster immunization studies in which INFANRIX was administered as the fourth or fifth dose in the DTaP series following previous doses with INFANRIX or PEDIARIX, large swelling reactions of the limb injected with INFANRIX were assessed.

In the fourth dose study, a large swelling reaction was defined as injection site swelling with a diameter of >50 mm, a >50 mm increase in the mid-thigh circumference compared to the pre-vaccination measurement, and/or any diffuse swelling that interfered with or prevented daily activities. The overall incidence of large swelling reactions occurring within 4 days (Day 0-Day 3) following INFANRIX was 2.3%.

In the fifth dose study, a large swelling reaction was defined as swelling that involved >50% of the injected upper arm length and that was associated with a >30 mm increase in mid-upper arm circumference within 4 days following vaccination. The incidence of large swelling reactions following the fifth consecutive dose of INFANRIX was 1.0%.

Less Common and Serious General Adverse Events: Selected adverse events reported from a double-blind, randomized Italian clinical efficacy trial involving 4,696 children administered INFANRIX or 4,678 children administered whole-cell DTP vaccine (DTwP) (manufactured by Connaught Laboratories, Inc.) as a 3-dose primary series are shown in Table 4. The incidence of rectal temperature ≥104°F, hypotonic-hyporesponsive episodes and persistent crying ≥3 hours following administration of INFANRIX was significantly less than that following administration of whole-cell DTP vaccine.

[See table 4 above]

In a German safety study that enrolled 22,505 infants (66,867 doses of INFANRIX administered as a 3-dose primary series at 3, 4, and 5 months of age), all subjects were monitored for unsolicited adverse events that occurred within 28 days following vaccination using report cards. In a subset of subjects (N = 2,457), these cards were standardized diaries which solicited specific adverse events that occurred within 8 days of each vaccination in addition to unsolicited adverse events which occurred from enrollment until approximately 30 days following the third vaccination. Cards from the whole cohort were returned at subsequent visits and were supplemented by spontaneous reporting by parents and a medical history after the first and second doses of vaccine. In the subset of 2,457, adverse events following the third dose of vaccine were reported via standardized diaries and spontaneous reporting at a follow-up visit. Adverse events in the remainder of the cohort were reported via report cards which were returned by mail approximately 28 days after the third dose of vaccine. Adverse events (rates per 1,000 doses) occurring within 7 days following any of the first 3 doses included: unusual crying (0.09), febrile seizure (0.0), afebrile seizure (0.13), and hypotonic-hyporesponsive episodes (0.01).

6.2 Postmarketing Experience

In addition to reports in clinical trials, worldwide voluntary reports of adverse events received for INFANRIX since market introduction are listed below. This list includes serious events and events which have a plausible causal connection to INFANRIX. These adverse events were reported voluntarily from a population of uncertain size; therefore, it is not always possible to reliably estimate their frequency or establish a causal relationship to vaccination.

Infections and Infestations: Bronchitis, cellulitis, respiratory tract infection.

Blood and Lymphatic System Disorders: Lymphadenopathy, thrombocytopenia.

Immune System Disorders: Anaphylactic reaction, hypersensitivity.

Nervous System Disorders: Encephalopathy, headache, hypotonia, syncope.

Ear and Labyrinth Disorders: Ear pain.

Cardiac Disorders: Cyanosis.

Respiratory, Thoracic, and Mediastinal Disorders: Apnea, cough.

Skin and Subcutaneous Tissue Disorders: Angioedema, erythema, pruritus, rash, urticaria.

General Disorders and Administration Site Conditions: Fatigue, injection site induration, injection site reaction, Sudden Infant Death Syndrome.

7 DRUG INTERACTIONS

7.1 Concomitant Vaccine Administration

In clinical trials, INFANRIX was given concomitantly with Hib conjugate vaccine, pneumococcal 7-valent conjugate vaccine, hepatitis B vaccine, IPV, and the second dose of MMR vaccine *[see Adverse Reactions (6.1) and Clinical Studies (14.3)]*.

When INFANRIX is administered concomitantly with other injectable vaccines, they should be given with separate syringes. INFANRIX should not be mixed with any other vaccine in the same syringe or vial.

7.2 Immunosuppressive Therapies

Immunosuppressive therapies, including irradiation, antimetabolites, alkylating agents, cytotoxic drugs, and corticosteroids (used in greater than physiologic doses), may reduce the immune response to INFANRIX.

8 USE IN SPECIFIC POPULATIONS

8.1 Pregnancy

Pregnancy Category C

Animal reproduction studies have not been conducted with INFANRIX. It is also not known whether INFANRIX can cause fetal harm when administered to a pregnant woman or can affect reproduction capacity.

8.4 Pediatric Use

Safety and effectiveness of INFANRIX in infants younger than 6 weeks of age and children 7 to 16 years of age have not been established. INFANRIX is not approved for use in these age groups.

11 DESCRIPTION

INFANRIX (Diphtheria and Tetanus Toxoids and Acellular Pertussis Vaccine Adsorbed) is a noninfectious, sterile vaccine for intramuscular administration. Each 0.5-mL dose is formulated to contain 25 Lf of diphtheria toxoid, 10 Lf of tetanus toxoid, 25 mcg of inactivated pertussis toxin (PT), 25 mcg of filamentous hemagglutinin (FHA), and 8 mcg of pertactin (69 kiloDalton outer membrane protein).

The diphtheria toxin is produced by growing *Corynebacterium diphtheriae* in Fenton medium containing a bovine extract. Tetanus toxin is produced by growing *Clostridium tetani* in a modified Latham medium derived from bovine casein. The bovine materials used in these extracts are sourced from countries which the United States Department of Agriculture (USDA) has determined neither have nor present an undue risk for bovine spongiform encephalopathy (BSE). Both toxins are detoxified with formaldehyde, concentrated by ultrafiltration, and purified by precipitation, dialysis, and sterile filtration.

The acellular pertussis antigens (PT, FHA, and pertactin) are isolated from *Bordetella pertussis* culture grown in modified Stainer-Scholte liquid medium. PT and FHA are isolated from the fermentation broth; pertactin is extracted from the cells by heat treatment and flocculation. The antigens are purified in successive chromatographic and precipitation steps. PT is detoxified using glutaraldehyde and formaldehyde. FHA and pertactin are treated with formaldehyde.

Diphtheria and tetanus toxoids and pertussis antigens (PT, FHA, and pertactin) are individually adsorbed onto aluminum hydroxide.

Diphtheria and tetanus toxoid potency is determined by measuring the amount of neutralizing antitoxin in previously immunized guinea pigs. The potency of the acellular pertussis components (PT, FHA, and pertactin) is determined by enzyme-linked immunosorbent assay (ELISA) on sera from previously immunized mice.

Each 0.5-mL dose contains aluminum hydroxide as adjuvant (not more than 0.625 mg aluminum by assay) and 4.5 mg of sodium chloride. Each dose also contains ≤100 mcg of residual formaldehyde and ≤100 mcg of polysorbate 80 (Tween 80).

INFANRIX is available in vials and 2 types of prefilled syringes. One type of prefilled syringe has a tip cap which may contain natural rubber latex and a plunger which does not contain latex. The other type has a tip cap and a rubber plunger which contain dry natural latex rubber. The vial stopper does not contain latex. *[See How Supplied/Storage and Handling (16).]*

INFANRIX is formulated without preservatives.

12 CLINICAL PHARMACOLOGY

12.1 Mechanism of Action

Diphtheria: Diphtheria is an acute toxin-mediated infectious disease caused by toxigenic strains of *C. diphtheriae*. Protection against disease is due to the development of neutralizing antibodies to the diphtheria toxin. A serum diphtheria antitoxin level of 0.01 IU/mL is the lowest level giving some degree of protection; a level of 0.1 IU/mL is regarded as protective.[1]

Tetanus: Tetanus is an acute toxin-mediated infectious disease caused by a potent exotoxin released by *C. tetani*. Protection against disease is due to the development of neutralizing antibodies to the tetanus toxin. A serum tetanus antitoxin level of at least 0.01 IU/mL, measured by neutralization assays, is considered the minimum protective level.[2,3] A level of 0.1 IU/mL is considered protective.[4]

Pertussis: Pertussis (whooping cough) is a disease of the respiratory tract caused by *B. pertussis*. The role of the different components produced by *B. pertussis* in either the pathogenesis of, or the immunity to, pertussis is not well understood. There is no well established serological correlate of protection for pertussis.

13 NONCLINICAL TOXICOLOGY

13.1 Carcinogenesis, Mutagenesis, Impairment of Fertility

INFANRIX has not been evaluated for carcinogenic or mutagenic potential, or for impairment of fertility.

14 CLINICAL STUDIES

14.1 Diphtheria and Tetanus

Efficacy of diphtheria toxoid used in INFANRIX was determined on the basis of immunogenicity studies. A VERO cell toxin neutralizing test confirmed the ability of infant sera (N = 45), obtained one month after a 3-dose primary series, to neutralize diphtheria toxin. Levels of diphtheria antitoxin ≥0.01 IU/mL were achieved in 100% of the sera tested. Efficacy of tetanus toxoid used in INFANRIX was determined on the basis of immunogenicity studies. An in vivo mouse neutralization assay confirmed the ability of infant sera (N = 45), obtained one month after a 3-dose primary series, to neutralize tetanus toxin. Levels of tetanus antitoxin ≥0.01 IU/mL were achieved in 100% of the sera tested.

14.2 Pertussis

Efficacy of a 3-dose primary series of INFANRIX has been assessed in 2 clinical studies.

A double-blind, randomized, active Diphtheria and Tetanus Toxoids (DT)-controlled trial conducted in Italy assessed the absolute protective efficacy of INFANRIX when administered at 2, 4, and 6 months of age. The population used in the primary analysis of the efficacy of INFANRIX included 4,481 infants vaccinated with INFANRIX and 1,470 DT vaccinees. The mean length of follow-up was 17 months, beginning 30 days after the third dose of vaccine. After 3 doses, the absolute protective efficacy of INFANRIX against WHO-defined typical pertussis (21 days or more of paroxysmal cough with infection confirmed by culture and/or serologic testing) was 84% (95% CI: 76, 89). When the definition of pertussis was expanded to include clinically milder disease with respect to type and duration of cough, with infection confirmed by culture and/or serologic testing, the efficacy of INFANRIX was calculated to be 71% (95% CI: 60, 78) against >7 days of any cough and 73% (95% CI: 63, 80) against ≥14 days of any cough. Vaccine efficacy after 3 doses and with no booster dose in the second year of life was assessed in 2 subsequent follow-up periods. A follow-up period from 24 months to a mean age of 33 months was conducted in a partially unblinded cohort (children who received DT were offered pertussis vaccine and those who declined were retained in the study cohort). During this period, the efficacy of INFANRIX against WHO-defined pertussis was 78% (95% CI: 62, 87). During the third follow-up period which was conducted in an unblinded manner among children from 3 to 6 years of age, the efficacy of INFANRIX against WHO-defined pertussis was 86% (95% CI: 79, 91). Thus, protection against pertussis in children administered 3 doses of INFANRIX in infancy was sustained to 6 years of age.

A prospective efficacy trial was also conducted in Germany employing a household contact study design. In preparation for this study, 3 doses of INFANRIX were administered at 3, 4, and 5 months of age to more than 22,000 children living in 6 areas of Germany in a safety and immunogenicity study. Infants who did not participate in the safety and immunogenicity study could have received a DTwP vaccine or DT vaccine. Index cases were identified by spontaneous presentation to a physician. Households with at least one other member (i.e., besides index case) aged 6 through 47 months were enrolled. Household contacts of index cases were monitored for incidence of pertussis by a physician who was blinded to the vaccination status of the household. Calculation of vaccine efficacy was based on attack rates of pertussis in household contacts classified by vaccination status. Of the 173 household contacts who had not received a pertussis vaccine, 96 developed WHO-defined pertussis, as compared with 7 of 112 contacts vaccinated with INFANRIX. The protective efficacy of INFANRIX was calculated to be 89% (95% CI: 77, 95), with no indication of waning of protection up until the time of the booster vaccination. The average age of infants vaccinated with INFANRIX at the end of follow-up in this trial was 13 months (range 6 to 25 months). When the definition of pertussis was expanded to include clinically milder disease, with infection confirmed by culture and/or serologic testing, the efficacy of INFANRIX against ≥7 days of any cough was 67% (95% CI: 52, 78) and against ≥7 days of paroxysmal cough was 81% (95% CI: 68, 89). The corresponding efficacy of INFANRIX against ≥14 days of any cough or paroxysmal cough were 73% (95% CI: 59, 82) and 84% (95% CI: 71, 91), respectively.

Pertussis Immune Response to INFANRIX Administered as a 3-Dose Primary Series: The immune responses to each of the 3 pertussis antigens contained in INFANRIX were evaluated in sera obtained 1 month after the third dose of vaccine in each of 3 studies (schedule of administration: 2, 4, and 6 months of age in the Italian efficacy study and one US study; 3, 4, and 5 months of age in the German efficacy study). One month after the third dose of INFANRIX, the response rates to each pertussis antigen were similar in all 3 studies. Thus, although a serologic correlate of protection for pertussis has not been established, the antibody responses to these 3 pertussis antigens (PT, FHA, and pertactin) in a US population were similar to those achieved in 2 populations in which efficacy of INFANRIX was demonstrated.

14.3 Immune Response to Concomitantly Administered Vaccines

In a US study, INFANRIX was given concomitantly, at separate sites, with Hib conjugate vaccine (Sanofi Pasteur SA) at 2, 4, and 6 months of age. Subjects also received ENGERIX-B and oral poliovirus vaccine (OPV). One month after the third dose of Hib conjugate vaccine, 90% of 72 infants had anti-PRP (polyribosyl-ribitol-phosphate) ≥1.0 mcg/mL.

In a US study, INFANRIX was given concomitantly, at separate sites, with ENGERIX-B, IPV (Sanofi Pasteur SA), pneumococcal 7-valent conjugate (PCV7), and Hib conjugate vaccines (Wyeth Pharmaceuticals Inc.) at 2, 4, and 6 months of age. Immune responses were measured in sera obtained approximately one month after the third dose of vaccines. Among 121 subjects who had not received a birth dose of hepatitis B vaccine, 99.2% had anti-HBsAg (hepatitis B surface antigen) ≥10 mIU/mL following the third dose of ENGERIX-B. Among 153 subjects, 100% had anti-poliovirus 1, 2, and 3, ≥1:8 following the third dose of IPV. Although serological correlates for protection have not been established for the pneumococcal serotypes, a threshold level of ≥0.3 mcg/mL was evaluated. Following the third dose of PCV7 vaccine, 91.8% to 99.4% of subjects (N = 146-156) had anti-pneumococcal polysaccharide ≥0.3 mcg/mL for serotypes 4, 9V, 14, 18C, 19F, and 23F, and 73.0% had a level ≥0.3 mcg/mL for serotype 6B.

15 REFERENCES

1. Vitek CR and Wharton M. Diphtheria Toxoid. In: Plotkin SA, Orenstein WA, and Offit PA, eds. *Vaccines.* 5th ed. Saunders; 2008:139-156.
2. Wassilak SGF, Roper MH, Kretsinger K, and Orenstein WA. Tetanus Toxoid. In: Plotkin SA, Orenstein WA, and Offit PA, eds. *Vaccines.* 5th ed. Saunders; 2008:805-839.
3. Department of Health and Human Services, Food and Drug Administration. Biological products; Bacterial vaccines and toxoids; Implementation of efficacy review; Proposed rule. *Federal Register* December 13, 1985;50(240):51002-51117.
4. Centers for Disease Control and Prevention. General Recommendations on Immunization. Recommendations of the Advisory Committee on Immunization Practices (ACIP). *MMWR* 2006;55(RR-15):1-48.

16 HOW SUPPLIED/STORAGE AND HANDLING

INFANRIX is available in 0.5-mL single-dose vials and disposable prefilled TIP-LOK syringes (packaged without needles):

NDC 58160-810-01 Vial (contains no latex) in Package of 10: NDC 58160-810-11

NDC 58160-810-43 Syringe (tip cap may contain latex; plunger contains no latex) in Package of 10: NDC 58160-810-52

NDC 58160-810-41 Syringe (tip cap and plunger contain latex) in Package of 10: NDC 58160-810-51

Store refrigerated between 2° and 8°C (36° and 46°F). Do not freeze. Discard if the vaccine has been frozen.

17 PATIENT COUNSELING INFORMATION

The parent or guardian should be:

- informed of the potential benefits and risks of immunization with INFANRIX, and of the importance of completing the immunization series.
- informed about the potential for adverse reactions that have been temporally associated with administration of INFANRIX or other vaccines containing similar components.
- instructed to report any adverse events to their healthcare provider.
- given the Vaccine Information Statements, which are required by the National Childhood Vaccine Injury Act of 1986 to be given prior to immunization. These materials are available free of charge at the Centers for Disease Control and Prevention (CDC) website (www.cdc.gov/vaccines).

ENGERIX-B, INFANRIX, PEDIARIX, and TIP-LOK are registered trademarks of GlaxoSmithKline.

Manufactured by **GlaxoSmithKline Biologicals**
Rixensart, Belgium, US License 1617
Novartis Vaccines and Diagnostics GmbH
Marburg, Germany, US License 1754
Distributed by **GlaxoSmithKline**
Research Triangle Park, NC 27709

INF:24PI

JALYN ℞

[JAY-LIN]

(dutasteride and tamsulosin hydrochloride) Capsules

HIGHLIGHTS OF PRESCRIBING INFORMATION
These highlights do not include all the information needed to use JALYN safely and effectively. See full prescribing information for JALYN.
JALYN (dutasteride and tamsulosin hydrochloride) Capsules
Initial U.S. Approval: 2010

RECENT MAJOR CHANGES

Contraindications (4)	04/2013
Warnings and Precautions, Intraoperative Floppy Iris Syndrome (5.9)	04/2013

INDICATIONS AND USAGE

JALYN is a combination of dutasteride, a 5 alpha-reductase inhibitor, and tamsulosin, an alpha adrenergic antagonist, indicated for the treatment of symptomatic benign prostatic hyperplasia (BPH) in men with an enlarged prostate. (1.1)

Limitations of Use: Dutasteride-containing products, including JALYN, are not approved for the prevention of prostate cancer. (1.2)

DOSAGE AND ADMINISTRATION

- Take one capsule daily approximately 30 minutes after the same meal each day. (2)
- Swallow capsule whole. (2)

DOSAGE FORMS AND STRENGTHS

0.5 mg dutasteride and 0.4 mg tamsulosin hydrochloride. (3)

CONTRAINDICATIONS

- Pregnancy and women of childbearing potential. (4, 5.6, 8.1)
- Pediatric patients. (4)
- Patients with previously demonstrated, clinically significant hypersensitivity (e.g., serious skin reactions, angioedema, urticaria, pruritus, respiratory symptoms) to dutasteride, other 5 alpha-reductase inhibitors, tamsulosin, or any component of JALYN. (4)

WARNINGS AND PRECAUTIONS

- Orthostatic hypotension and/or syncope can occur. Advise patients of symptoms related to postural hypotension and to avoid situations where injury could result if syncope occurs. (5.1)
- Do not use JALYN with other alpha adrenergic antagonists, as this may increase the risk of hypotension. (5.2)
- JALYN reduces serum prostate-specific antigen (PSA) concentration by approximately 50%. However, any confirmed increase in PSA while on JALYN may signal the presence of prostate cancer and should be evaluated, even if those values are still within the normal range for untreated men. (5.3)
- Do not use JALYN with strong inhibitors of cytochrome P450 (CYP) 3A4 (e.g., ketoconazole). Use caution in combination with moderate CYP3A4 inhibitors (e.g., erythromycin) or strong (e.g., paroxetine) or moderate CYP2D6 inhibitors, or known poor metabolizers of CYP2D6. Concomitant use with known inhibitors can cause a marked increase in drug exposure. (5.2, 7.1, 12.3)
- Exercise caution with concomitant use of PDE-5 inhibitors, as this may increase the risk of hypotension. (5.2)
- Drugs that contain dutasteride, including JALYN, may increase the risk of high-grade prostate cancer. (5.4, 6.1)
- Prior to initiating treatment with JALYN, consideration should be given to other urological conditions that may cause similar symptoms. (5.5)
- Women who are pregnant or could become pregnant should not handle JALYN Capsules due to potential risk to a male fetus. (5.6, 8.1)
- Advise patients about the possibility and seriousness of priapism. (5.7)
- Patients should not donate blood until 6 months after their last dose of JALYN. (5.8)
- Intraoperative Floppy Iris Syndrome has been observed during cataract surgery after alpha adrenergic antagonist exposure. Advise patients considering cataract surgery to tell their ophthalmologist that they take or have taken JALYN Capsules. (5.9)
- Exercise caution with concomitant use of warfarin. (5.2, 7.4. 12.3)

ADVERSE REACTIONS

The most common adverse reactions, reported in ≥1% of subjects treated with coadministered dutasteride and tamsulosin are ejaculation disorders, impotence, decreased libido, dizziness, and breast disorders. (6.1)

To report SUSPECTED ADVERSE REACTIONS, contact GlaxoSmithKline at 1-888-825-5249 or FDA at 1-800-FDA-1088 or www.fda.gov/medwatch.

See 17 for PATIENT COUNSELING INFORMATION and FDA-approved patient labeling

Revised: 04/2013

FULL PRESCRIBING INFORMATION: CONTENTS*

*** Sections or subsections omitted from the full prescribing information are not listed**

FULL PRESCRIBING INFORMATION

1 INDICATIONS AND USAGE

1.1 Benign Prostatic Hyperplasia (BPH) Treatment

JALYN™ (dutasteride and tamsulosin hydrochloride) Capsules are indicated for the treatment of symptomatic BPH in men with an enlarged prostate.

1.2 Limitations of Use

Dutasteride-containing products, including JALYN, are not approved for the prevention of prostate cancer.

2 DOSAGE AND ADMINISTRATION

The recommended dosage of JALYN is 1 capsule (0.5 mg dutasteride and 0.4 mg tamsulosin hydrochloride) taken once daily approximately 30 minutes after the same meal each day.

The capsules should be swallowed whole and not chewed or opened. Contact with the contents of the JALYN capsule may result in irritation of the oropharyngeal mucosa.

3 DOSAGE FORMS AND STRENGTHS

JALYN Capsules, containing 0.5 mg dutasteride and 0.4 mg tamsulosin hydrochloride, are oblong, hard-shell capsules with a brown body and an orange cap imprinted with "GS 7CZ" in black ink.

4 CONTRAINDICATIONS

JALYN is contraindicated for use in:

- Pregnancy. In animal reproduction and developmental toxicity studies, dutasteride inhibited development of male fetus external genitalia. Therefore, JALYN may cause fetal harm when administered to a pregnant woman. If JALYN is used during pregnancy, or if the patient becomes pregnant while taking JALYN, the patient should be apprised of the potential hazard to the fetus *[see Warnings and Precautions (5.6), Use in Specific Populations (8.1)]*.
- Women of childbearing potential *[see Warnings and Precautions (5.6), Use in Specific Populations (8.1)]*.
- Pediatric patients *[see Use in Specific Populations (8.4)]*.
- Patients with previously demonstrated, clinically significant hypersensitivity (e.g., serious skin reactions, angioedema, urticaria, pruritus, respiratory symptoms) to dutasteride, other 5 alpha-reductase inhibitors, tamsulosin, or any other component of JALYN *[see Adverse Reactions (6.2)]*.

5 WARNINGS AND PRECAUTIONS

5.1 Orthostatic Hypotension

As with other alpha adrenergic antagonists, orthostatic hypotension (postural hypotension, dizziness, and vertigo) may occur in patients treated with tamsulosin-containing products, including JALYN, and can result in syncope. Patients starting treatment with JALYN should be cautioned to avoid situations where syncope could result in an injury *[see Adverse Reactions (6.1)]*.

5.2 Drug-Drug Interactions

Strong Inhibitors of CYP3A4: Tamsulosin-containing products, including JALYN, should not be coadministered with strong CYP3A4 inhibitors (e.g., ketoconazole) as this can significantly increase tamsulosin exposure *[see Drug Interactions (7.1), Clinical Pharmacology (12.3)]*.

Inhibitors of CYP2D6 and Moderate Inhibitors of CYP3A4: Tamsulosin-containing products, including JALYN, should be used with caution when coadministered with moderate inhibitors of CYP3A4 (e.g., erythromycin), strong (e.g., paroxetine) or moderate (e.g., terbinafine) inhibitors of CYP2D6, or in patients known to be poor metabolizers of CYP2D6, as there is a potential for significant increase in tamsulosin exposure *[see Drug Interactions (7.1), Clinical Pharmacology (12.3)]*.

Cimetidine: Caution is advised when tamsulosin-containing products, including JALYN, are coadministered with cimetidine *[see Drug Interactions (7.1), Clinical Pharmacology (12.3)]*.

Other Alpha Adrenergic Antagonists: Tamsulosin-containing products, including JALYN, should not be coadministered with other alpha adrenergic antagonists because of the increased risk of symptomatic hypotension.

Phosphodiesterase-5 Inhibitors (PDE-5 Inhibitors): Caution is advised when alpha adrenergic antagonist-containing products, including JALYN, are coadministered with PDE-5 inhibitors. Alpha adrenergic antagonists and PDE-5 inhibitors are both vasodilators that can lower blood pressure. Concomitant use of these 2 drug classes can potentially cause symptomatic hypotension.

Warfarin: Caution should be exercised with concomitant administration of warfarin and tamsulosin-containing products, including JALYN *[see Drug Interactions (7.4), Clinical Pharmacology (12.3)]*.

5.3 Effects on Prostate-Specific Antigen (PSA) and the Use of PSA in Prostate Cancer Detection

Coadministration of dutasteride with tamsulosin resulted in similar changes to serum PSA as with dutasteride monotherapy.

In clinical trials, dutasteride reduced serum PSA concentration by approximately 50% within 3 to 6 months of treatment. This decrease was predictable over the entire range of PSA values in patients with symptomatic BPH, although it may vary in individuals. Dutasteride-containing treatment, including JALYN, may also cause decreases in serum PSA in the presence of prostate cancer. To interpret serial PSAs in men treated with a dutasteride-containing product, including JALYN, a new baseline PSA should be established at least 3 months after starting treatment and PSA monitored periodically thereafter. Any confirmed increase from the lowest PSA value while on a dutasteride-containing treatment, including JALYN, may signal the presence of prostate cancer and should be evaluated, even if PSA levels are still within the normal range for men not taking a 5 alpha-reductase inhibitor. Noncompliance with JALYN may also affect PSA test results.

To interpret an isolated PSA value in a man treated with JALYN, for 3 months or more, the PSA value should be doubled for comparison with normal values in untreated men.

The free-to-total PSA ratio (percent free PSA) remains constant, even under the influence of dutasteride. If clinicians elect to use percent free PSA as an aid in the detection of prostate cancer in men receiving JALYN, no adjustment to its value appears necessary.

5.4 Increased Risk of High-Grade Prostate Cancer

In men aged 50 to 75 years with a prior negative biopsy for prostate cancer and a baseline PSA between 2.5 ng/mL and 10.0 ng/mL taking dutasteride in the 4-year Reduction by Dutasteride of Prostate Cancer Events (REDUCE) trial, there was an increased incidence of Gleason score 8-10 prostate cancer compared with men taking placebo (dutasteride 1.0% versus placebo 0.5%) [see Indications and Usage (1.2), Adverse Reactions (6.1)]. In a 7-year placebo-controlled clinical trial with another 5 alpha-reductase inhibitor (finasteride 5 mg, PROSCAR®), similar results for Gleason score 8-10 prostate cancer were observed (finasteride 1.8% versus placebo 1.1%).

5 alpha-reductase inhibitors may increase the risk of development of high-grade prostate cancer. Whether the effect of 5 alpha-reductase inhibitors to reduce prostate volume or trial-related factors impacted the results of these trials has not been established.

5.5 Evaluation for Other Urological Diseases

Prior to initiating treatment with JALYN, consideration should be given to other urological conditions that may cause similar symptoms. In addition, BPH and prostate cancer may coexist.

5.6 Exposure of Women—Risk to Male Fetus

JALYN Capsules should not be handled by a woman who is pregnant or who could become pregnant. Dutasteride is absorbed through the skin and could result in unintended fetal exposure. If a woman who is pregnant or could become pregnant comes in contact with a leaking capsule, the contact area should be washed immediately with soap and water *[see Use in Specific Populations (8.1)]*.

5.7 Priapism

Priapism (persistent painful penile erection unrelated to sexual activity) has been associated (probably less than 1 in 50,000) with the use of alpha-adrenergic antagonists, including tamsulosin, which is a component of JALYN. Because this condition can lead to permanent impotence if not properly treated, patients should be advised about the seriousness of the condition.

5.8 Blood Donation

Men being treated with a dutasteride-containing product, including JALYN, should not donate blood until at least 6 months have passed following their last dose. The purpose of this deferred period is to prevent administration of dutasteride to a pregnant female transfusion recipient.

5.9 Intraoperative Floppy Iris Syndrome

Intraoperative Floppy Iris Syndrome (IFIS) has been observed during cataract surgery in some patients on or previously treated with alpha adrenergic antagonists, including tamsulosin, which is a component of JALYN.

Most reports were in patients taking the alpha adrenergic antagonist when IFIS occurred, but in some cases, the alpha adrenergic antagonist had been stopped prior to surgery. In most of these cases, the alpha adrenergic antagonist had been stopped recently prior to surgery (2 to 14 days), but in a few cases, IFIS was reported after the patients had been off the alpha adrenergic antagonist for a longer period (5 weeks to 9 months). IFIS is a variant of small pupil syndrome and is characterized by the combination of a flaccid iris that billows in response to intraoperative irrigation currents, progressive intraoperative miosis despite preoperative dilation with standard mydriatic drugs, and potential prolapse of the iris toward the phacoemulsification incisions. The patient's ophthalmologist should be prepared for possible modifications to their surgical technique, such as the utilization of iris hooks, iris dilator rings, or viscoelastic substances.

IFIS may increase the risk of eye complications during and after the operation. The benefit of stopping alpha adrenergic antagonist therapy prior to cataract surgery has not been established. The initiation of therapy with tamsulosin in patients for whom cataract surgery is scheduled is not recommended.

5.10 Sulfa Allergy

In patients with sulfa allergy, allergic reaction to tamsulosin has been rarely reported. If a patient reports a serious or life-threatening sulfa allergy, caution is warranted when administering tamsulosin-containing products, including JALYN.

5.11 Effect on Semen Characteristics

Dutasteride: The effects of dutasteride 0.5 mg/day on semen characteristics were evaluated in normal volunteers aged 18 to 52 (n = 27 dutasteride, n = 23 placebo) throughout 52 weeks of treatment and 24 weeks of post-treatment follow-up. At 52 weeks, the mean percent reductions from baseline in total sperm count, semen volume, and sperm motility were 23%, 26%, and 18%, respectively, in the dutasteride group when adjusted for changes from baseline in the placebo group. Sperm concentration and sperm morphology were unaffected. After 24 weeks of follow-up, the mean percent change in total sperm count in the dutasteride group remained 23% lower than baseline. While mean values for all semen parameters at all time-points remained within the normal ranges and did not meet predefined criteria for a clinically significant change (30%), 2 subjects in the dutasteride group had decreases in sperm count of greater than 90% from baseline at 52 weeks, with partial recovery at the 24-week follow-up. The clinical significance of dutasteride's effect on semen characteristics for an individual patient's fertility is not known.

Tamsulosin: The effects of tamsulosin hydrochloride on sperm counts or sperm function have not been evaluated.

6 ADVERSE REACTIONS

6.1 Clinical Trials Experience

There have been no clinical trials conducted with JALYN; however, the clinical efficacy and safety of coadministered dutasteride and tamsulosin, which are individual components of JALYN, have been evaluated in a multicenter, randomized, double-blind, parallel group trial (the Combination with Alpha-Blocker Therapy, or CombAT, trial). Because clinical trials are conducted under widely varying conditions, adverse reaction rates observed in the clinical trials of a drug cannot be directly compared with rates in the clinical trial of another drug and may not reflect the rates observed in practice.

- The most common adverse reactions reported in subjects receiving coadministered dutasteride and tamsulosin were impotence, decreased libido, breast disorders (including breast enlargement and tenderness), ejaculation disorders, and dizziness. Ejaculation disorders occurred significantly more in subjects receiving coadministration therapy (11%) compared with those receiving dutasteride (2%) or tamsulosin (4%) as monotherapy.
- Trial withdrawal due to adverse reactions occurred in 6% of subjects receiving coadministered dutasteride and tamsulosin, and in 4% of subjects receiving dutasteride or tamsulosin as monotherapy. The most common adverse reaction in all treatment arms leading to trial withdrawal was erectile dysfunction (1% to 1.5%).

In the CombAT trial, over 4,800 male subjects with BPH were randomly assigned to receive 0.5 mg dutasteride, 0.4 mg tamsulosin hydrochloride, or coadministration therapy (0.5 mg dutasteride and 0.4 mg tamsulosin hydrochloride) administered once daily in a 4-year double-blind trial. Overall, 1,623 subjects received monotherapy with dutasteride; 1,611 subjects received monotherapy with tamsulosin; and 1,610 subjects received coadministration therapy. The population was aged 49 to 88 years (mean age: 66 years) and 88% were Caucasian. Table 1 summarizes adverse reactions reported in at least 1% of subjects receiving coadminstration therapy and at a higher incidence than subjects receiving either dutasteride or tamsulosin as monotherapy.

[See table 1 above]

Table 1. Adverse Reactions Reported Over a 48-Month Period in ≥1% of Subjects and More Frequently in the Coadministration Therapy Group Than the Dutasteride or Tamsulosin Monotherapy Group (CombAT) by Time of Onset

Adverse Reaction	Adverse Reaction Time of Onset				
	Year 1		Year 2	Year 3	Year 4
	Months 0–6	Months 7–12			
Coadministration[a]	(n = 1,610)	(n = 1,527)	(n = 1,428)	(n = 1,283)	(n = 1,200)
Dutasteride	(n = 1,623)	(n = 1,548)	(n = 1,464)	(n = 1,325)	(n = 1,200)
Tamsulosin	(n = 1,611)	(n = 1,545)	(n = 1,468)	(n = 1,281)	(n = 1,112)
Ejaculation disorders[b,c]					
Coadministration	7.8%	1.6%	1.0%	0.5%	<0.1%
Dutasteride	1.0%	0.5%	0.5%	0.2%	0.3%
Tamsulosin	2.2%	0.5%	0.5%	0.2%	0.3%
Impotence[c,d]					
Coadministration	5.4%	1.1%	1.8%	0.9%	0.4%
Dutasteride	4.0%	1.1%	1.6%	0.6%	0.3%
Tamsulosin	2.6%	0.8%	1.0%	0.6%	1.1%
Decreased libido[c,e]					
Coadministration	4.5%	0.9%	0.8%	0.2%	0.0%
Dutasteride	3.1%	0.7%	1.0%	0.2%	0.0%
Tamsulosin	2.0%	0.6%	0.7%	0.2%	<0.1%
Breast disorders[f]					
Coadministration	1.1%	1.1%	0.8%	0.9%	0.6%
Dutasteride	0.9%	0.9%	1.2%	0.5%	0.7%
Tamsulosin	0.4%	0.4%	0.4%	0.2%	0.0%
Dizziness					
Coadministration	1.1%	0.4%	0.1%	<0.1%	0.2%
Dutasteride	0.5%	0.3%	0.1%	<0.1%	<0.1%
Tamsulosin	0.9%	0.5%	0.4%	<0.1%	0.0%

[a]Coadministration = AVODART® 0.5 mg once daily plus tamsulosin 0.4 mg once daily.

[b]Includes anorgasmia, retrograde ejaculation, semen volume decreased, orgasmic sensation decreased, orgasm abnormal, ejaculation delayed, ejaculation disorder, ejaculation failure, and premature ejaculation.

[c]These sexual adverse reactions are associated with dutasteride treatment (including monotherapy and combination with tamsulosin). These adverse reactions may persist after treatment discontinuation. The role of dutasteride in this persistence is unknown.

[d]Includes erectile dysfunction and disturbance in sexual arousal.

[e]Includes libido decreased, libido disorder, loss of libido, sexual dysfunction, and male sexual dysfunction.

[f]Includes breast enlargement, gynecomastia, breast swelling, breast pain, breast tenderness, nipple pain, and nipple swelling.

Cardiac Failure: In CombAT, after 4 years of treatment, the incidence of the composite term cardiac failure in the coadministration group (12/1,610; 0.7%) was higher than in either monotherapy group: dutasteride, 2/1,623 (0.1%) and tamsulosin, 9/1,611 (0.6%). Composite cardiac failure was also examined in a separate 4-year placebo-controlled trial evaluating dutasteride in men at risk for development of prostate cancer. The incidence of cardiac failure in subjects taking dutasteride was 0.6% (26/4,105) compared with 0.4% (15/4,126) in subjects on placebo. A majority of subjects with cardiac failure in both trials had comorbidities associated with an increased risk of cardiac failure. Therefore, the clinical significance of the numerical imbalances in cardiac failure is unknown. No causal relationship between dutasteride, alone or coadministered with tamsulosin, and cardiac failure has been established. No imbalance was observed in the incidence of overall cardiovascular adverse events in either trial.

Additional information regarding adverse reactions in placebo-controlled trials with dutasteride or tamsulosin monotherapy follows:

Dutasteride:

Long-Term Treatment (Up to 4 Years): High-Grade Prostate Cancer: The REDUCE trial was a randomized, double-blind, placebo-controlled trial that enrolled 8,231 men aged 50 to 75 years with a serum PSA of 2.5 ng/mL to 10 ng/mL and a negative prostate biopsy within the previous 6 months. Subjects were randomized to receive placebo (N = 4,126) or 0.5-mg daily doses of dutasteride (N = 4,105) for up to 4 years. The mean age was 63 years and 91% were Caucasian. Subjects underwent protocol-mandated scheduled prostate biopsies at 2 and 4 years of treatment or had "for-cause biopsies" at non-scheduled times if clinically indicated. There was a higher incidence of Gleason score 8-10 prostate cancer in men receiving dutasteride (1.0%) compared with men on placebo (0.5%) *[see Indications and Usage (1.2), Warnings and Precautions (5.4)]*. In a 7-year placebo-controlled clinical trial with another 5 alpha-reductase inhibitor (finasteride 5 mg, PROSCAR), similar results for Gleason score 8-10 prostate cancer were observed (finasteride 1.8% versus placebo 1.1%).

No clinical benefit has been demonstrated in patients with prostate cancer treated with dutasteride.

Reproductive and Breast Disorders: In the 3 pivotal placebo-controlled BPH trials with dutasteride, each 4 years in duration, there was no evidence of increased sexual adverse reactions (impotence, decreased libido, and ejaculation disorder) or breast disorders with increased duration of treatment. Among these 3 trials, there was 1 case of breast cancer in the dutasteride group and 1 case in the placebo group. No cases of breast cancer were reported in any treatment group in the 4-year CombAT trial or the 4-year REDUCE trial.

The relationship between long-term use of dutasteride and male breast neoplasia is currently unknown.

Tamsulosin: According to the tamsulosin prescribing information, in two 13-week treatment trials with tamsulosin monotherapy, adverse reactions occurring in at least 2% of subjects receiving 0.4 mg tamsulosin hydrochloride and at an incidence higher than in subjects receiving placebo were: infection, asthenia, back pain, chest pain, somnolence, insomnia, rhinitis, pharyngitis, cough increased, sinusitis, and diarrhea.

Signs and Symptoms of Orthostasis: According to the tamsulosin prescribing information, in clinical trials with tamsulosin monotherapy, a positive orthostatic test result was observed in 16% (81/502) of subjects receiving 0.4 mg tamsulosin hydrochloride versus 11% (54/493) of subjects receiving placebo. Because orthostasis was detected more frequently in the tamsulosin-treated subjects than in placebo recipients, there is a potential risk of syncope *[see Warnings and Precaution (5.1)]*.

6.2 Postmarketing Experience

The following adverse reactions have been identified during post-approval use of the individual components of JALYN. Because these reactions are reported voluntarily from a population of uncertain size, it is not always possible to reliably estimate their frequency or establish a causal relationship to drug exposure. These reactions have been chosen for inclusion due to a combination of their seriousness, frequency of reporting, or potential causal connection to drug exposure.

Dutasteride:

Immune System Disorders: Hypersensitivity reactions, including rash, pruritus, urticaria, localized edema, serious skin reactions, and angioedema.

Neoplasms: Male breast cancer.

Psychiatric Disorders: Depressed mood.

Reproductive System and Breast Disorders: Testicular pain and testicular swelling.

Tamsulosin:

Immune System Disorders: Hypersensitivity reactions, including rash, urticaria, pruritus, angioedema, and respiratory problems have been reported with positive rechallenge in some cases.

Cardiac Disorders: Palpitations, dyspnea, atrial fibrillation, arrhythmia, and tachycardia.

Skin Disorders: Skin desquamation, including Stevens-Johnson syndrome.

Gastrointestinal Disorders: Constipation, vomiting.

Reproductive System and Breast Disorders: Priapism.

Vascular Disorders: Hypotension.

Ophthalmologic Disorders: During cataract surgery, a variant of small pupil syndrome known as Intraoperative floppy iris syndrome (IFIS) associated with alpha adrenergic antagonist therapy *[see Warnings and Precautions (5.9)]*.

7 DRUG INTERACTIONS

There have been no drug interaction trials using JALYN. The following sections reflect information available for the individual components.

7.1 Cytochrome P450 3A Inhibitors

Dutasteride: Dutasteride is extensively metabolized in humans by the CYP3A4 and CYP3A5 isoenzymes. The effect of potent CYP3A4 inhibitors on dutasteride has not been studied. Because of the potential for drug-drug interactions, use caution when prescribing a dutasteride-containing product, including JALYN, to patients taking potent, chronic CYP3A4 enzyme inhibitors (e.g., ritonavir) *[see Clinical Pharmacology (12.3)]*.

Tamsulosin: *Strong and Moderate Inhibitors of CYP3A4 or CYP2D6:* Tamsulosin is extensively metabolized, mainly by CYP3A4 or CYP2D6.

Concomitant treatment with ketoconazole (a strong inhibitor of CYP3A4) resulted in increases in the C_{max} and AUC of tamsulosin by factors of 2.2 and 2.8, respectively. Concomitant treatment with paroxetine (a strong inhibitor of CYP2D6) resulted in increases in the C_{max} and AUC of tamsulosin by factors of 1.3 and 1.6, respectively. A similar increase in exposure is expected in poor metabolizers (PM) of CYP2D6 as compared to extensive metabolizers (EM). Since CYP2D6 PMs cannot be readily identified and the potential for significant increase in tamsulosin exposure exists when tamsulosin 0.4 mg is coadministered with strong CYP3A4 inhibitors in CYP2D6 PMs, tamsulosin 0.4 mg capsules should not be used in combination with strong inhibitors of CYP3A4 (e.g., ketoconazole). The effects of coadministration of both a CYP3A4 and a CYP2D6 inhibitor with tamsulosin have not been evaluated. However, there is a potential for significant increase in tamsulosin exposure when tamsulosin 0.4 mg is coadministered with a combination of both CYP3A4 and CYP2D6 inhibitors *[see Warnings and Precautions (5.2), Clinical Pharmacology (12.3)]*.

Cimetidine: Treatment with cimetidine resulted in a moderate increase in tamsulosin hydrochloride AUC (44%) *[see Warnings and Precautions (5.2), Clinical Pharmacology (12.3)].*

7.2 Warfarin

Dutasteride: Concomitant administration of dutasteride 0.5 mg/day for 3 weeks with warfarin does not alter the steady-state pharmacokinetics of the S- or R-warfarin isomers or alter the effect of warfarin on prothrombin time *[see Clinical Pharmacology (12.3)].*

Tamsulosin: A definitive drug-drug interaction trial between tamsulosin hydrochloride and warfarin was not conducted. Results from limited in vitro and in vivo studies are inconclusive. Caution should be exercised with concomitant administration of warfarin and tamsulosin-containing products, including JALYN *[see Warnings and Precautions (5.2), Clinical Pharmacology (12.3)].*

7.3 Nifedipine, Atenolol, Enalapril

Tamsulosin: Dosage adjustments are not necessary when tamsulosin is administered concomitantly with nifedipine, atenolol, or enalapril *[see Clinical Pharmacology (12.3)].*

7.4 Digoxin and Theophylline

Dutasteride: Dutasteride does not alter the steady-state pharmacokinetics of digoxin when administered concomitantly at a dose of 0.5 mg/day for 3 weeks *[see Clinical Pharmacology (12.3)].*

Tamsulosin: Dosage adjustments are not necessary when tamsulosin is administered concomitantly with digoxin or theophylline *[see Clinical Pharmacology (12.3)].*

7.5 Furosemide

Tamsulosin: Tamsulosin had no effect on the pharmacodynamics (excretion of electrolytes) of furosemide. While furosemide produced an 11% to 12% reduction in tamsulosin hydrochloride C_{max} and AUC, these changes are expected to be clinically insignificant and do not require adjustment of the dose of tamsulosin *[see Clinical Pharmacology (12.3)].*

7.6 Calcium Channel Antagonists

Dutasteride: Coadministration of verapamil or diltiazem decreases dutasteride clearance and leads to increased exposure to dutasteride. The change in dutasteride exposure is not considered to be clinically significant. No dosage adjustment of dutasteride is recommended *[see Clinical Pharmacology (12.3)].*

7.7 Cholestyramine

Dutasteride: Administration of a single 5-mg dose of dutasteride followed 1 hour later by a 12-g dose of cholestyramine does not affect the relative bioavailability of dutasteride *[see Clinical Pharmacology (12.3)].*

8 USE IN SPECIFIC POPULATIONS

8.1 Pregnancy

Pregnancy Category X. There are no adequate and well-controlled studies in pregnant women with JALYN or its individual components.

Dutasteride: Dutasteride is contraindicated for use in women of childbearing potential and during pregnancy. Dutasteride is a 5 alpha-reductase inhibitor that prevents conversion of testosterone to dihydrotestosterone (DHT), a hormone necessary for normal development of male genitalia. In animal reproduction and developmental toxicity studies, dutasteride inhibited normal development of external genitalia in male fetuses. Therefore, dutasteride may cause fetal harm when administered to a pregnant woman. If dutasteride is used during pregnancy or if the patient becomes pregnant while taking dutasteride, the patient should be apprised of the potential hazard to the fetus.

Abnormalities in the genitalia of male fetuses is an expected physiological consequence of inhibition of the conversion of testosterone to DHT by 5 alpha-reductase inhibitors. These results are similar to observations in male infants with genetic 5 alpha-reductase deficiency. Dutasteride is absorbed through the skin. To avoid potential fetal exposure, women who are pregnant or could become pregnant should not handle dutasteride-containing capsules, including JALYN Capsules. If contact is made with leaking capsules, the contact area should be washed immediately with soap and water *[see Warnings and Precautions (5.6)].* Dutasteride is secreted into semen. The highest measured semen concentration of dutasteride in treated men was 14 ng/mL. Assuming exposure of a 50-kg woman to 5 mL of semen and 100% absorption, the woman's dutasteride concentration would be about 0.0175 ng/mL. This concentration is more than 100 times less than concentrations producing abnormalities of male genitalia in animal studies. Dutasteride is highly protein bound in human semen (greater than 96%), which may reduce the amount of dutasteride available for vaginal absorption.

In an embryo-fetal development study in female rats, oral administration of dutasteride at doses 10 times less than the maximum recommended human dose (MRHD) of 0.5 mg daily resulted in abnormalities of male genitalia in the fetus (decreased anogenital distance at 0.05 mg/kg/day), nipple development, hypospadias, and distended preputial glands in male offspring (at all doses of 0.05, 2.5, 12.5, and 30 mg/kg/day). An increase in stillborn pups was observed at 111 times the MRHD, and reduced fetal body weight was observed at doses of about 15 times the MRHD (animal dose of 2.5 mg/kg/day). Increased incidences of skeletal variations considered to be delays in ossification associated with reduced body weight were observed at doses at about 56 times the MRHD (animal dose of 12.5 mg/kg/day).

In a rabbit embryo-fetal study, doses 28- to 93-fold the MRHD (animal doses of 30, 100, and 200 mg/kg/day) were administered orally during the period of major organogenesis (gestation days 7 to 29) to encompass the late period of external genitalia development. Histological evaluation of the genital papilla of fetuses revealed evidence of feminization of the male fetus at all doses. A second embryo-fetal study in rabbits at 0.3- to 53-fold the expected clinical exposure (animal doses of 0.05, 0.4, 3.0, and 30 mg/kg/day) also produced evidence of feminization of the genitalia in male fetuses at all doses.

In an oral pre- and post-natal development study in rats, dutasteride doses of 0.05, 2.5, 12.5, or 30 mg/kg/day were administered. Unequivocal evidence of feminization of the genitalia (i.e., decreased anogenital distance, increased incidence of hypospadias, nipple development) of male offspring occurred at 14- to 90-fold the MRHD (animal doses of 2.5 mg/kg/day or greater). At 0.05-fold the expected clinical exposure (animal dose of 0.05 mg/kg/day), evidence of feminization was limited to a small, but statistically significant, decrease in anogenital distance. Animal doses of 2.5 to 30 mg/kg/day resulted in prolonged gestation in the parental females and a decrease in time to vaginal patency for female offspring and a decrease in prostate and seminal vesicle weights in male offspring. Effects on newborn startle response were noted at doses greater than or equal to 12.5 mg/kg/day. Increased stillbirths were noted at 30 mg/kg/day.

In an embryo-fetal development study, pregnant rhesus monkeys were exposed intravenously to a dutasteride blood level comparable to the dutasteride concentration found in human semen. Dutasteride was administered on gestation days 20 to 100 at doses of 400, 780, 1,325, or 2,010 ng/day (12 monkeys/group). The development of male external genitalia of monkey offspring was not adversely affected. Reduction of fetal adrenal weights, reduction in fetal prostate weights, and increases in fetal ovarian and testis weights were observed at the highest dose tested in monkeys. Based on the highest measured semen concentration of dutasteride in treated men (14 ng/mL), these doses represent 0.8 to 16 times the potential maximum exposure of a 50-kg human female to 5 mL semen daily from a dutasteride-treated man, assuming 100% absorption. (These calculations are based on blood levels of parent drug which are achieved at 32 to 186 times the daily doses administered to pregnant monkeys on a ng/kg basis). Dutasteride is highly bound to proteins in human semen (greater than 96%), potentially reducing the amount of dutasteride available for vaginal absorption. It is not known whether rabbits or rhesus monkeys produce any of the major human metabolites.

Estimates of exposure multiples comparing animal studies to the MRHD for dutasteride are based on clinical serum concentration at steady state.

Tamsulosin: Administration of tamsulosin to pregnant female rats at dose levels up to approximately 50 times the human therapeutic AUC exposure (animal dose of 300 mg/kg/day) revealed no evidence of harm to the fetus. Administration of tamsulosin hydrochloride to pregnant rabbits at dose levels up to 50 mg/kg/day produced no evidence of fetal harm. However, because of the effect of dutasteride on the fetus, JALYN is contraindicated for use in pregnant women. Estimates of exposure multiples comparing animal studies to the MRHD for tamsulosin are based on AUC.

8.3 Nursing Mothers

JALYN is contraindicated for use in women of childbearing potential, including nursing women. It is not known whether dutasteride or tamsulosin is excreted in human milk.

8.4 Pediatric Use

JALYN is contraindicated for use in pediatric patients. Safety and effectiveness of JALYN in pediatric patients have not been established.

8.5 Geriatric Use

Of 1,610 male subjects treated with coadministered dutasteride and tamsulosin in the CombAT trial, 58% of enrolled subjects were aged 65 years and older and 13% of enrolled subjects were aged 75 years and older. No overall differences in safety or efficacy were observed between these subjects and younger subjects but greater sensitivity of some older individuals cannot be ruled out *[see Clinical Pharmacology (12.3)].*

8.6 Renal Impairment

The effect of renal impairment on dutasteride and tamsulosin pharmacokinetics has not been studied using JALYN. Because no dosage adjustment is necessary for dutasteride or tamsulosin in patients with moderate-to-severe renal impairment ($10 \leq CL_{cr} < 30$ mL/min/1.73 m^2), no dosage adjustment is necessary for JALYN in patients with moderate-to-severe renal impairment. However, patients with end-stage renal disease (CL_{cr}<10 mL/min/1.73 m^2) have not been studied *[see Clinical Pharmacology (12.3)].*

8.7 Hepatic Impairment

The effect of hepatic impairment on dutasteride and tamsulosin pharmacokinetics has not been studied using JALYN. The following text reflects information available for the individual components.

Dutasteride: The effect of hepatic impairment on dutasteride pharmacokinetics has not been studied. Because dutasteride is extensively metabolized, exposure could be higher in hepatically impaired patients. However, in a clinical trial where 60 subjects received 5 mg (10 times the therapeutic dose) daily for 24 weeks, no additional adverse events were observed compared with those observed at the therapeutic dose of 0.5 mg *[see Clinical Pharmacology (12.3)].*

Tamsulosin: Patients with moderate hepatic impairment do not require an adjustment in tamsulosin dosage. Tamsulosin has not been studied in patients with severe hepatic impairment *[see Clinical Pharmacology (12.3)].*

10 OVERDOSAGE

No data are available with regard to overdosage with JALYN. The following text reflects information available for the individual components.

Dutasteride: In volunteer trials, single doses of dutasteride up to 40 mg (80 times the therapeutic dose) for 7 days have been administered without significant safety concerns. In a clinical trial, daily doses of 5 mg (10 times the therapeutic dose) were administered to 60 subjects for 6 months with no additional adverse effects to those seen at therapeutic doses of 0.5 mg.

There is no specific antidote for dutasteride. Therefore, in cases of suspected overdosage symptomatic and supportive treatment should be given as appropriate, taking the long half-life of dutasteride into consideration.

Tamsulosin: Should overdosage of tamsulosin lead to hypotension *[see Warnings and Precautions (5.1), Adverse Reactions (6.1)]*, support of the cardiovascular system is of first importance. Restoration of blood pressure and normalization of heart rate may be accomplished by keeping the patient in the supine position. If this measure is inadequate, then administration of intravenous fluids should be considered. If necessary, vasopressors should then be used and renal function should be monitored and supported as needed. Laboratory data indicate that tamsulosin is 94% to 99% protein bound; therefore, dialysis is unlikely to be of benefit.

11 DESCRIPTION

JALYN (dutasteride and tamsulosin hydrochloride) Capsules contain dutasteride (a selective inhibitor of both the type 1 and type 2 isoforms of steroid 5 alpha-reductase, an intracellular enzyme that converts testosterone to DHT and tamsulosin (an antagonist of alpha$_{1A}$-adrenoceptors in the prostate). Each JALYN Capsule contains the following:

- One dutasteride oblong, opaque, dull-yellow soft gelatin capsule, containing 0.5 mg of dutasteride dissolved in a mixture of butylated hydroxytoluene and mono-diglycerides of caprylic/capric acid. The inactive ingredients in the soft-gelatin capsule shell are ferric oxide (yellow), gelatin (from certified BSE-free bovine sources), glycerin, and titanium dioxide.
- Tamsulosin hydrochloride white to off-white pellets, containing 0.4 mg tamsulosin hydrochloride and the inactive ingredients: methacrylic acid copolymer dispersion, microcrystalline cellulose, talc, and triethyl citrate.

The above components are encapsulated in a hard-shell capsule made with the inactive ingredients of carrageenan, FD&C yellow 6, hypromellose, iron oxide red, potassium chloride, titanium dioxide, and imprinted with "GS 7CZ" in black ink.

Dutasteride: Dutasteride is a synthetic 4-azasteroid compound chemically designated as (5α,17β)-N-{2,5 bis(trifluoromethyl)phenyl}-3-oxo-4-azaandrost-1-ene-17-carboxamide. The empirical formula of dutasteride is $C_{27}H_{30}F_6N_2O_2$, representing a molecular weight of 528.5 with the following structural formula:

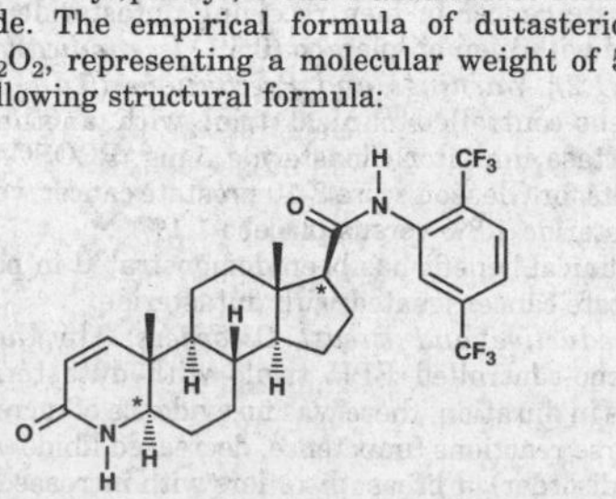

Dutasteride is a white to pale yellow powder with a melting point of 242° to 250°C. It is soluble in ethanol (44 mg/mL), methanol (64 mg/mL), and polyethylene glycol 400 (3 mg/mL), but it is insoluble in water.

Tamsulosin: Tamsulosin hydrochloride is a synthetic compound chemically designated as (-)-(*R*)-5-[2-[[2-(*o*-Ethoxyphenoxy)ethyl]amino]propyl]-2-methoxybenzenesulfonamide, monohydrochloride.

The empirical formula of tamsulosin hydrochloride is $C_{20}H_{28}N_2O_5S \bullet HCl$. The molecular weight of tamsulosin hydrochloride is 444.97. Its structural formula is:

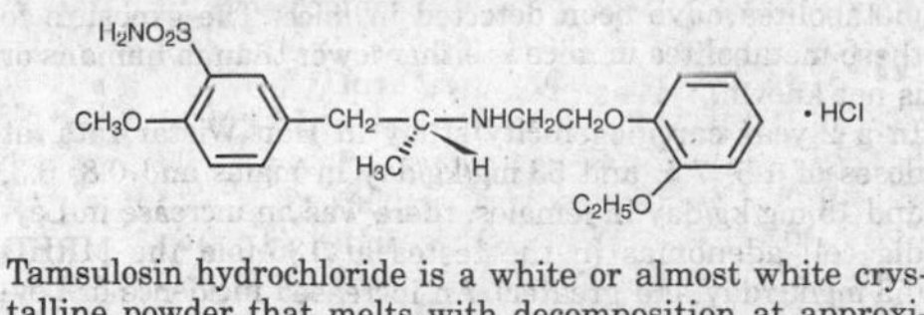

Tamsulosin hydrochloride is a white or almost white crystalline powder that melts with decomposition at approximately 234°C. It is sparingly soluble in water and slightly soluble in methanol, ethanol, acetone, and ethyl acetate.

12 CLINICAL PHARMACOLOGY

12.1 Mechanism of Action

JALYN is a combination of 2 drugs with different mechanisms of action to improve symptoms in patients with BPH: dutasteride, a 5 alpha-reductase inhibitor, and tamsulosin, an antagonist of $alpha_{1A}$-adrenoreceptors.

Dutasteride: Dutasteride inhibits the conversion of testosterone to DHT. DHT is the androgen primarily responsible for the initial development and subsequent enlargement of the prostate gland. Testosterone is converted to DHT by the enzyme 5 alpha-reductase, which exists as 2 isoforms, type 1 and type 2. The type 2 isoenzyme is primarily active in the reproductive tissues, while the type 1 isoenzyme is also responsible for testosterone conversion in the skin and liver.

Dutasteride is a competitive and specific inhibitor of both type 1 and type 2 5 alpha-reductase isoenzymes, with which it forms a stable enzyme complex. Dissociation from this complex has been evaluated under in vitro and in vivo conditions and is extremely slow. Dutasteride does not bind to the human androgen receptor.

Tamsulosin: Smooth muscle tone is mediated by the sympathetic nervous stimulation of $alpha_1$-adrenoceptors, which are abundant in the prostate, prostatic capsule, prostatic urethra, and bladder neck. Blockade of these adrenoceptors can cause smooth muscles in the bladder neck and prostate to relax, resulting in an improvement in urine flow rate and a reduction in symptoms of BPH.

Tamsulosin, an $alpha_1$-adrenoceptor blocking agent, exhibits its selectivity for $alpha_1$-receptors in the human prostate. At least 3 discrete $alpha_1$-adrenoceptor subtypes have been identified: $alpha_{1A}$, $alpha_{1B}$, and $alpha_{1D}$; their distribution differs between human organs and tissue. Approximately 70% of the $alpha_1$-receptors in human prostate are of the $alpha_{1A}$ subtype. Tamsulosin is not intended for use as an antihypertensive.

12.2 Pharmacodynamics

Dutasteride: *Effect on 5 Alpha-Dihydrotestosterone and Testosterone:* The maximum effect of daily doses of dutasteride on the reduction of DHT is dose-dependent and is observed within 1 to 2 weeks. After 1 and 2 weeks of daily dosing with dutasteride 0.5 mg, median serum DHT concentrations were reduced by 85% and 90%, respectively. In patients with BPH treated with dutasteride 0.5 mg/day for 4 years, the median decrease in serum DHT was 94% at 1 year, 93% at 2 years, and 95% at both 3 and 4 years. The median increase in serum testosterone was 19% at both 1 and 2 years, 26% at 3 years, and 22% at 4 years, but the mean and median levels remained within the physiologic range.

In patients with BPH treated with 5 mg/day of dutasteride or placebo for up to 12 weeks prior to transurethral resection of the prostate, mean DHT concentrations in prostatic tissue were significantly lower in the dutasteride group compared with placebo (784 and 5,793 pg/g, respectively, $P<0.001$). Mean prostatic tissue concentrations of testosterone were significantly higher in the dutasteride group compared with placebo (2,073 and 93 pg/g, respectively, $P<0.001$).

Adult males with genetically inherited type 2 5 alpha-reductase deficiency also have decreased DHT levels. These 5 alpha-reductase deficient males have a small prostate gland throughout life and do not develop BPH. Except for the associated urogenital defects present at birth, no other clinical abnormalities related to 5 alpha-reductase deficiency have been observed in these individuals.

Effects on Other Hormones: In healthy volunteers, 52 weeks of treatment with dutasteride 0.5 mg/day (n = 26) resulted in no clinically significant change compared with placebo (n = 23) in sex hormone-binding globulin, estradiol, luteinizing hormone, follicle-stimulating hormone, thyroxine (free T4), and dehydroepiandrosterone. Statistically significant, baseline-adjusted mean increases compared with placebo were observed for total testosterone at 8 weeks (97.1 ng/dL, $P<0.003$) and thyroid-stimulating hormone at 52 weeks (0.4 mcIU/mL, $P<0.05$). The median percentage changes from baseline within the dutasteride group were 17.9% for testosterone at 8 weeks and 12.4% for thyroid-stimulating hormone at 52 weeks. After stopping dutasteride for 24 weeks, the mean levels of testosterone and thyroid-stimulating hormone had returned to baseline in the group of subjects with available data at the visit. In subjects with BPH treated with dutasteride in a large randomized, double-blind, placebo-controlled trial, there was a median percent increase in luteinizing hormone of 12% at 6 months and 19% at both 12 and 24 months.

Other Effects: Plasma lipid panel and bone mineral density were evaluated following 52 weeks of dutasteride 0.5 mg once daily in healthy volunteers. There was no change in bone mineral density as measured by dual energy x-ray absorptiometry compared with either placebo or baseline. In addition, the plasma lipid profile (i.e., total cholesterol, low density lipoproteins, high density lipoproteins, and triglycerides) was unaffected by dutasteride. No clinically significant changes in adrenal hormone responses to adrenocorticotropic hormone (ACTH) stimulation were observed in a subset population (n = 13) of the 1-year healthy volunteer trial.

12.3 Pharmacokinetics

The pharmacokinetics of dutasteride and tamsulosin from JALYN are comparable to the pharmacokinetics of dutasteride and tamsulosin when administered separately.

Absorption: The pharmacokinetic parameters of dutasteride and tamsulosin observed after administration of JALYN in a single dose, randomized, 3-period partial cross-over trial are summarized in Table 2 below.

Table 2. Arithmetic Means (SD) of Serum Dutasteride and Tamsulosin in Single-Dose Pharmacokinetic Parameters Under Fed Conditions

Component	N	$AUC_{(0-t)}$ (ng hr/mL)	C_{max} (ng/mL)	T_{max} (hr)[a]	$t_{1/2}$ (hr)
Dutasteride	92	39.6 (23.1)	2.14 (0.77)	3.00 (1.00-10.00)	
Tamsulosin	92	187.2 (95.7)	11.3 (4.44)	6.00 (2.00-24.00)	13.5 (3.92)[b]

[a] Median (range).
[b] N = 91.

[See table 2 above]

Dutasteride: Following administration of a single 0.5-mg dose of a soft gelatin capsule, time to peak absolute bioavailability in 5 healthy subjects is approximately 60% (range: 40% to 94%).

Tamsulosin: Absorption of tamsulosin is essentially complete (>90%) following oral administration of 0.4-mg tamsulosin hydrochloride capsules under fasting conditions. Tamsulosin exhibits linear kinetics following single and multiple dosing, with achievement of steady-state concentrations by the fifth day of once-daily dosing.

Effect of Food: Food does not affect the pharmacokinetics of dutasteride following administration of JALYN. However, a mean 30% decrease in tamsulosin C_{max} was observed when JALYN was administered with food, similar to that seen when tamsulosin monotherapy was administered under fed versus fasting conditions.

Distribution: *Dutasteride:* Pharmacokinetic data following single and repeat oral doses show that dutasteride has a large volume of distribution (300 to 500 L). Dutasteride is highly bound to plasma albumin (99.0%) and alpha-1 acid glycoprotein (96.6%).

In a trial of healthy subjects (n = 26) receiving dutasteride 0.5 mg/day for 12 months, semen dutasteride concentrations averaged 3.4 ng/mL (range: 0.4 to 14 ng/mL) at 12 months and, similar to serum, achieved steady-state concentrations at 6 months. On average, at 12 months 11.5% of serum dutasteride concentrations partitioned into semen.

Tamsulosin: The mean steady-state apparent volume of distribution of tamsulosin after intravenous administration to 10 healthy male adults was 16 L, which is suggestive of distribution into extracellular fluids in the body.

Tamsulosin is extensively bound to human plasma proteins (94% to 99%), primarily alpha-1 acid glycoprotein (AAG), with linear binding over a wide concentration range (20 to 600 ng/mL). The results of 2-way in vitro studies indicate that the binding of tamsulosin to human plasma proteins is not affected by amitriptyline, diclofenac, glyburide, simvastatin plus simvastatin-hydroxy acid metabolite, warfarin, diazepam, or propranolol. Likewise, tamsulosin had no effect on the extent of binding of these drugs.

Metabolism: *Dutasteride:* Dutasteride is extensively metabolized in humans. In vitro studies showed that dutasteride is metabolized by the CYP3A4 and CYP3A5 isoenzymes. Both of these isoenzymes produced the 4'-hydroxydutasteride, 6-hydroxydutasteride, and the 6,4'-dihydroxydutasteride metabolites. In addition, the 15-hydroxydutasteride metabolite was formed by CYP3A4. Dutasteride is not metabolized in vitro by human cytochrome P450 isoenzymes CYP1A2, CYP2A6, CYP2B6, CYP2C8, CYP2C9, CYP2C19, CYP2D6, and CYP2E1. In human serum following dosing to steady state, unchanged dutasteride, 3 major metabolites (4'-hydroxydutasteride, 1,2-dihydrodutasteride, and 6-hydroxydutasteride), and 2 minor metabolites (6,4'-dihydroxydutasteride and 15-hydroxydutasteride), as assessed by mass spectrometric response, have been detected. The absolute stereochemistry of the hydroxyl additions in the 6 and 15 positions is not known. In vitro, the 4'-hydroxydutasteride and 1,2-dihydrodutasteride metabolites are much less potent than dutasteride against both isoforms of human 5α-reductase. The activity of 6β-hydroxydutasteride is comparable to that of dutasteride.

Tamsulosin: There is no enantiomeric bioconversion from tamsulosin [R(-) isomer] to the S(+) isomer in humans. Tamsulosin is extensively metabolized by cytochrome P450 enzymes in the liver and less than 10% of the dose is excreted in urine unchanged. However, the pharmacokinetic profile of the metabolites in humans has not been established. In vitro studies indicate that CYP3A4 and CYP2D6 are involved in metabolism of tamsulosin as well as some minor participation of other CYP isoenzymes. Inhibition of hepatic drug metabolizing enzymes may lead to increased exposure to tamsulosin *[see Drug Interactions (7.2)]*. The metabolites of tamsulosin undergo extensive conjugation to glucuronide or sulfate prior to renal excretion.

Incubations with human liver microsomes showed no evidence of clinically significant metabolic interactions between tamsulosin and amitriptyline, albuterol, glyburide, and finasteride. However, results of the in vitro testing of the tamsulosin interaction with diclofenac and warfarin were equivocal.

Excretion: *Dutasteride:* Dutasteride and its metabolites were excreted mainly in feces. As a percent of dose, there was approximately 5% unchanged dutasteride (approximately 1% to approximately 15%) and 40% as dutasteride-related metabolites (~2% to ~90%). Only trace amounts of unchanged dutasteride were found in urine (<1%). Therefore, on average, the dose unaccounted for approximated 55% (range: 5% to 97%). The terminal elimination half-life of dutasteride is approximately 5 weeks at steady state. The average steady-state serum dutasteride concentration was 40 ng/mL following 0.5 mg/day for 1 year. Following daily dosing, dutasteride serum concentrations achieve 65% of steady-state concentration after 1 month and approximately 90% after 3 months. Due to the long half-life of dutasteride, serum concentrations remain detectable (greater than 0.1 ng/mL) for up to 4 to 6 months after discontinuation of treatment.

Tamsulosin: On administration of the radiolabeled dose of tamsulosin to 4 healthy volunteers, 97% of the administered radioactivity was recovered, with urine (76%) representing the primary route of excretion compared to feces (21%) over 168 hours.

Following intravenous or oral administration of an immediate-release formulation, the elimination half-life of tamsulosin in plasma ranges from 5 to 7 hours. Because of absorption rate-controlled pharmacokinetics with tamsulosin hydrochloride capsules, the apparent half-life of tamsulosin is approximately 9 to 13 hours in healthy volunteers and 14 to 15 hours in the target population.

Tamsulosin undergoes restrictive clearance in humans, with a relatively low systemic clearance (2.88 L/hr).

Specific Populations: *Pediatric:* The pharmacokinetics of dutasteride and tamsulosin administered together have not been investigated in subjects younger than 18 years.

Geriatric: Dutasteride and tamsulosin pharmacokinetics using JALYN have not been studied in geriatric patients. The following text reflects information for the individual components.

Dutasteride: No dosage adjustment is necessary in the elderly. The pharmacokinetics and pharmacodynamics of dutasteride were evaluated in 36 healthy male subjects aged between 24 and 87 years following administration of a single 5-mg dose of dutasteride. In this single-dose trial, dutasteride half-life increased with age (approximately 170 hours in men aged 20 to 49 years, approximately 260 hours in men aged 50 to 69 years, and approximately 300 hours in men older than 70 years).

Tamsulosin: Cross-study comparison of tamsulosin overall exposure (AUC) and half-life indicate that the pharmacokinetic disposition of tamsulosin may be slightly prolonged in geriatric males compared with young, healthy male volunteers. Intrinsic clearance is independent of tamsulosin binding to AAG, but diminishes with age, resulting in a 40% overall higher exposure (AUC) in subjects aged 55 to 75 years compared with subjects aged 20 to 32 years.

Gender: Dutasteride: Dutasteride is contraindicated in pregnancy and women of childbearing potential and is not indicated for use in other women *[see Contraindications (4), Warnings and Precautions (5.6)]*. The pharmacokinetics of dutasteride in women have not been studied.

Tamsulosin: Tamsulosin is not indicated for use in women. No information is available on the pharmacokinetics of tamsulosin in women.

Race: The effect of race on pharmacokinetics of dutasteride and tamsulosin administered together or separately has not been studied.

Renal Impairment: The effect of renal impairment on dutasteride and tamsulosin pharmacokinetics has not been studied using JALYN. The following text reflects information for the individual components.

Dutasteride: The effect of renal impairment on dutasteride pharmacokinetics has not been studied. However, less than 0.1% of a steady-state 0.5-mg dose of dutasteride is recovered in human urine, so no adjustment in dosage is anticipated for patients with renal impairment.

Tamsulosin: The pharmacokinetics of tamsulosin have been compared in 6 subjects with mild-moderate ($30 \leq CL_{cr}$ <70 mL/min/1.73 m^2) or moderate-severe ($10 \leq CL_{cr}$ <30 mL/min/1.73 m^2) renal impairment and 6 normal subjects (CL_{cr} >90 mL/min/1.73 m^2). While a change in the overall plasma concentration of tamsulosin was observed as the result of altered binding to AAG, the unbound (active) concentration of tamsulosin, as well as the intrinsic clearance, remained relatively constant. Therefore, patients with renal impairment do not require an adjustment in tamsulosin dosing. However, patients with end-stage renal disease (CL_{cr} <10 mL/min/1.73 m^2) have not been studied.

Hepatic Impairment: The effect of hepatic impairment on dutasteride and tamsulosin pharmacokinetics has not been studied using JALYN. The following text reflects information available for the individual components.

Dutasteride: The effect of hepatic impairment on dutasteride pharmacokinetics has not been studied. Because dutasteride is extensively metabolized, exposure could be higher in hepatically impaired patients.

Tamsulosin: The pharmacokinetics of tamsulosin have been compared in 8 subjects with moderate hepatic impairment (Child-Pugh classification: Grades A and B) and 8 normal subjects. While a change in the overall plasma concentration of tamsulosin was observed as the result of altered binding to AAG, the unbound (active) concentration of tamsulosin does not change significantly with only a modest (32%) change in intrinsic clearance of unbound tamsulosin. Therefore, patients with moderate hepatic impairment do not require an adjustment in tamsulosin dosage. Tamsulosin has not been studied in patients with severe hepatic impairment.

Drug Interactions: There have been no drug interaction studies using JALYN. The following text reflects information available for the individual components.

Cytochrome P450 Inhibitors: Dutasteride: No clinical drug interaction trials have been performed to evaluate the impact of CYP3A enzyme inhibitors on dutasteride pharmacokinetics. However, based on in vitro data, blood concentrations of dutasteride may increase in the presence of inhibitors of CYP3A4/5 such as ritonavir, ketoconazole, verapamil, diltiazem, cimetidine, troleandomycin, and ciprofloxacin.

Dutasteride does not inhibit the in vitro metabolism of model substrates for the major human cytochrome P450 isoenzymes (CYP1A2, CYP2C9, CYP2C19, CYP2D6, and CYP3A4) at a concentration of 1,000 ng/mL, 25 times greater than steady-state serum concentrations in humans.

Tamsulosin: Strong and Moderate Inhibitors of CYP3A4 or CYP2D6: The effects of ketoconazole (a strong inhibitor of CYP3A4) at 400 mg once daily for 5 days on the pharmacokinetics of a single tamsulosin hydrochloride capsule 0.4 mg dose was investigated in 24 healthy volunteers (age range: 23 to 47 years). Concomitant treatment with ketoconazole resulted in increases in the C_{max} and AUC of tamsulosin by factors of 2.2 and 2.8, respectively. The effects of concomitant administration of a moderate CYP3A4 inhibitor (e.g., erythromycin) on the pharmacokinetics of tamsulosin have not been evaluated.

The effects of paroxetine (a strong inhibitor of CYP2D6) at 20 mg once daily for 9 days on the pharmacokinetics of a single tamsulosin capsule 0.4 mg dose was investigated in 24 healthy volunteers (age range: 23 to 47 years). Concomitant treatment with paroxetine resulted in increases in the C_{max} and AUC of tamsulosin by factors of 1.3 and 1.6, respectively. A similar increase in exposure is expected in poor metabolizers (PM) of CYP2D6 as compared to extensive metabolizers (EM). A fraction of the population (about 7% of Caucasians and 2% of African-Americans) are CYP2D6 PMs. Since CYP2D6 PMs cannot be readily identified and the potential for significant increase in tamsulosin exposure exists when tamsulosin 0.4 mg is coadministered with strong CYP3A4 inhibitors in CYP2D6 PMs, tamsulosin 0.4 mg capsules should not be used in combination with strong inhibitors of CYP3A4 (e.g., ketoconazole).

The effects of concomitant administration of a moderate CYP2D6 inhibitor (e.g., terbinafine) on the pharmacokinetics of tamsulosin have not been evaluated.

The effects of co-administration of both a CYP3A4 and a CYP2D6 inhibitor with tamsulosin capsules have not been evaluated. However, there is a potential for significant increase in tamsulosin exposure when tamsulosin 0.4 mg is coadministered with a combination of both CYP3A4 and CYP2D6 inhibitors.

Cimetidine: The effects of cimetidine at the highest recommended dose (400 mg every 6 hours for 6 days) on the pharmacokinetics of a single tamsulosin capsule 0.4 mg dose was investigated in 10 healthy volunteers (age range: 21 to 38 years). Treatment with cimetidine resulted in a significant decrease (26%) in the clearance of tamsulosin hydrochloride, which resulted in a moderate increase in tamsulosin hydrochloride AUC (44%).

Alpha Adrenergic Antagonists: Dutasteride: In a single-sequence, crossover trial in healthy volunteers, the administration of tamsulosin or terazosin in combination with dutasteride had no effect on the steady-state pharmacokinetics of either alpha-adrenergic antagonist. Although the effect of administration of tamsulosin or terazosin on dutasteride pharmacokinetic parameters was not evaluated, the percent change in DHT concentrations was similar for dutasteride, alone or in combination with tamsulosin or terazosin.

Warfarin: Dutasteride: In a trial of 23 healthy volunteers, 3 weeks of treatment with dutasteride 0.5 mg/day did not alter the steady-state pharmacokinetics of the S- or R-warfarin isomers or alter the effect of warfarin on prothrombin time when administered with warfarin.

Tamsulosin: A definitive drug-drug interaction trial between tamsulosin and warfarin was not conducted. Results from limited in vitro and in vivo studies are inconclusive. Therefore, caution should be exercised with concomitant administration of warfarin and tamsulosin.

Nifedipine, Atenolol, Enalapril: Tamsulosin: In 3 trials in hypertensive subjects (age range: 47 to 79 years) whose blood pressure was controlled with stable doses of nifedipine extended-release, atenolol, or enalapril for at least 3 months, tamsulosin hydrochloride capsules 0.4 mg for 7 days followed by tamsulosin hydrochloride capsules 0.8 mg for another 7 days (n = 8 per trial) resulted in no clinically significant effects on blood pressure and pulse rate compared with placebo (n = 4 per trial). Therefore, dosage adjustments are not necessary when tamsulosin is administered concomitantly with nifedipine extended-release, atenolol, or enalapril.

Digoxin and Theophylline: Dutasteride: In a trial of 20 healthy volunteers, dutasteride did not alter the steady-state pharmacokinetics of digoxin when administered concomitantly at a dose of 0.5 mg/day for 3 weeks.

Tamsulosin: In 2 trials in healthy volunteers (n = 10 per trial; age range: 19 to 39 years) receiving tamsulosin capsules 0.4 mg/day for 2 days, followed by tamsulosin capsules 0.8 mg/day for 5 to 8 days, single intravenous doses of digoxin 0.5 mg or theophylline 5 mg/kg resulted in no change in the pharmacokinetics of digoxin or theophylline. Therefore, dosage adjustments are not necessary when a tamsulosin capsule is administered concomitantly with digoxin or theophylline.

Furosemide: Tamsulosin: The pharmacokinetic and pharmacodynamic interaction between tamsulosin hydrochloride capsules 0.8 mg/day (steady-state) and furosemide 20 mg intravenously (single dose) was evaluated in 10 healthy volunteers (age range: 21 to 40 years). Tamsulosin had no effect on the pharmacodynamics (excretion of electrolytes) of furosemide. While furosemide produced an 11% to 12% reduction in tamsulosin C_{max} and AUC, these changes are expected to be clinically insignificant and do not require dose adjustment for tamsulosin.

Calcium Channel Antagonists: Dutasteride: In a population pharmacokinetics analysis, a decrease in clearance of dutasteride was noted when coadministered with the CYP3A4 inhibitors verapamil (-37%, n = 6) and diltiazem (-44%, n = 5). In contrast, no decrease in clearance was seen when amlodipine, another calcium channel antagonist that is not a CYP3A4 inhibitor, was coadministered with dutasteride (+7%, n = 4). The decrease in clearance and subsequent increase in exposure to dutasteride in the presence of verapamil and diltiazem is not considered to be clinically significant. No dosage adjustment is recommended.

Cholestyramine: Dutasteride: Administration of a single 5-mg dose of dutasteride followed 1 hour later by 12 g cholestyramine did not affect the relative bioavailability of dutasteride in 12 normal volunteers.

13 NONCLINICAL TOXICOLOGY

13.1 Carcinogenesis, Mutagenesis, Impairment of Fertility

No non-clinical studies have been conducted with JALYN. The following information is based on studies performed with dutasteride or tamsulosin.

Carcinogenesis:

Dutasteride: A 2-year carcinogenicity study was conducted in B6C3F1 mice at doses of 3, 35, 250, and 500 mg/kg/day for males and 3, 35, and 250 mg/kg/day for females; an increased incidence of benign hepatocellular adenomas was noted at 250 mg/kg/day (290-fold the MRHD of a 0.5-mg daily dose) in female mice only. Two of the 3 major human metabolites have been detected in mice. The exposure to these metabolites in mice is either lower than in humans or is not known.

In a 2-year carcinogenicity study in Han Wistar rats, at doses of 1.5, 7.5, and 53 mg/kg/day in males and 0.8, 6.3, and 15 mg/kg/day in females, there was an increase in Leydig cell adenomas in the testes at 135-fold the MRHD (53 mg/kg/day and greater). An increased incidence of Leydig cell hyperplasia was present at 52-fold the MRHD (male rat doses of 7.5 mg/kg/day and greater). A positive correlation between proliferative changes in the Leydig cells and an increase in circulating luteinizing hormone levels has been demonstrated with 5 alpha-reductase inhibitors and is consistent with an effect on the hypothalamic-pituitary-testicular axis following 5 alpha-reductase inhibition. At tumorigenic doses, luteinizing hormone levels in rats were increased by 167%. In this study, the major human metabolites were tested for carcinogenicity at approximately 1 to 3 times the expected clinical exposure.

Tamsulosin: In a rat carcinogenicity assay, no increases in tumor incidence was observed in rats administered up to 3 times the MRHD of 0.8 mg/day (based on AUC of animal doses up to 43 mg/kg/day in males and up to 52 mg/kg/day in females), with the exception of a modest increase in the frequency of mammary gland fibroadenomas in female rats receiving doses of 5.4 mg/kg or greater.

In a carcinogenicity assay, mice were administered up to 8 times the MRHD of tamsulosin (oral doses up to 127 mg/kg/day in males and 158 mg/kg/day in females). There were no significant tumor findings in male mice. Female mice treated for 2 years with the 2 highest doses of 45 and 158 mg/kg/day had statistically significant increases in the incidence of mammary gland fibroadenomas (P<0.0001) and adenocarcinomas.

The increased incidences of mammary gland neoplasms in female rats and mice were considered secondary to tamsulosin-induced hyperprolactinemia. It is not known if tamsulosin elevates prolactin in humans. The relevance for human risk of the findings of prolactin-mediated endocrine tumors in rodents is not known.

Mutagenesis:

Dutasteride: Dutasteride was tested for genotoxicity in a bacterial mutagenesis assay (Ames test), a chromosomal aberration assay in CHO cells, and a micronucleus assay in rats. The results did not indicate any genotoxic potential of the parent drug. Two major human metabolites were also negative in either the Ames test or an abbreviated Ames test.

Tamsulosin: Tamsulosin produced no evidence of mutagenic potential in vitro in the Ames reverse mutation test, mouse lymphoma thymidine kinase assay, unscheduled DNA repair synthesis assay, and chromosomal aberration assays in CHO cells or human lymphocytes. There were no mutagenic effects in the in vivo sister chromatid exchange and mouse micronucleus assay.

Impairment of Fertility:

Dutasteride: Treatment of sexually mature male rats with dutasteride at 0.1- to 110-fold the MRHD (animal doses of 0.05, 10, 50, and 500 mg/kg/day for up to 31 weeks) resulted in dose- and time-dependent decreases in fertility; reduced cauda epididymal (absolute) sperm counts but not sperm concentration (at 50 and 500 mg/kg/day); reduced weights of the epididymis, prostate, and seminal vesicles; and microscopic changes in the male reproductive organs. The fertility effects were reversed by recovery week 6 at all doses, and sperm counts were normal at the end of a 14-week recovery period. The 5 alpha-reductase–related changes consisted of cytoplasmic vacuolation of tubular epithelium in the epididymides and decreased cytoplasmic content of epithelium, consistent with decreased secretory activity in the prostate and seminal vesicles. The microscopic changes were no longer present at recovery week 14 in the low-dose group and were partly recovered in the remaining treatment groups. Low levels of dutasteride (0.6 to 17 ng/mL) were detected in the serum of untreated female rats mated to males dosed at 10, 50, or 500 mg/kg/day for 29 to 30 weeks.

In a fertility study in female rats, oral administration of dutasteride at doses of 0.05, 2.5, 12.5, and 30 mg/kg/day resulted in reduced litter size, increased embryo resorption and feminization of male fetuses (decreased anogenital distance) at 2- to 10-fold the MRHD (animal doses of 2.5 mg/kg/day or greater). Fetal body weights were also reduced at less than 0.02-fold the MRHD in rats (0.5 mg/kg/day).

Tamsulosin: Studies in rats revealed significantly reduced fertility in males at approximately 50 times the MRHD based on AUC (single or multiple daily doses of 300 mg/kg/day of tamsulosin hydrochloride). The mechanism of decreased fertility in male rats is considered to be an effect of the compound on the vaginal plug formation possibly due to changes of semen content or impairment of ejaculation. The effects on fertility were reversible showing improvement by 3 days after a single dose and 4 weeks after multiple dosing. Effects on fertility in males were completely reversed within nine weeks of discontinuation of multiple dosing. Multiple doses of 0.2 and 16 times the MRHD (animal doses of 10 and 100 mg/kg/day tamsulosin hydrochloride) did not significantly alter fertility in male rats. Effects of tamsulosin on sperm counts or sperm function have not been evaluated.

Studies in female rats revealed significant reductions in fertility after single or multiple dosing with 300 mg/kg/day of the R-isomer or racemic mixture of tamsulosin hydrochloride, respectively. In female rats, the reductions in fertility after single doses were considered to be associated with impairments in fertilization. Multiple dosing with 10 or 100 mg/kg/day of the racemic mixture did not significantly alter fertility in female rats.

Estimates of exposure multiples comparing animal studies to the MRHD for dutasteride are based on clinical serum concentration at steady state.

Estimates of exposure multiples comparing animal studies to the MRHD for tamsulosin are based on AUC.

13.2 Animal Toxicology and/or Pharmacology

Central Nervous System Toxicology Studies:

Dutasteride: In rats and dogs, repeated oral administration of dutasteride resulted in some animals showing signs of non-specific, reversible, centrally-mediated toxicity without associated histopathological changes at exposures 425- and 315-fold the expected clinical exposure (of parent drug), respectively.

14 CLINICAL STUDIES

The trial supporting the efficacy of JALYN was a 4-year multicenter, randomized, double-blind, parallel-group trial (CombAT trial) investigating the efficacy of the coadministration of dutasteride 0.5 mg/day and tamsulosin hydrochloride 0.4 mg/day (n = 1,610) compared with dutasteride alone (n = 1,623) or tamsulosin alone (n = 1,611). Subjects were at least 50 years of age with a serum PSA ≥1.5 ng/mL and <10 ng/mL and BPH diagnosed by medical history and physical examination, including enlarged prostate (≥30 cc) and BPH symptoms that were moderate to severe according to the International Prostate Symptom Score (IPSS). Eighty-eight percent (88%) of the enrolled trial population was Caucasian. Approximately 52% of subjects had previous exposure to 5 alpha-reductase inhibitor or alpha adrenergic antagonist treatment. Of the 4,844 subjects randomly assigned to receive treatment, 69% of subjects in the coadministration group, 67% in the dutasteride group, and 61% in the tamsulosin group completed 4 years of double-blind treatment.

Effect on Symptom Score: Symptoms were quantified using the first 7 questions of the International Prostate Symptom Score (IPSS). The baseline score was approximately 16.4 units for each treatment group. Coadministration therapy was statistically superior to each of the monotherapy treatments in decreasing symptom score at Month 24, the primary time point for this endpoint. At Month 24, the mean changes from baseline (±SD) in IPSS total symptom scores were -6.2 (±7.14) for the coadministration group, -4.9 (±6.81) for dutasteride, and -4.3 (±7.01) for tamsulosin, with a mean difference between coadministration and dutasteride of -1.3 units (P<0.001; [95% CI: -1.69, -0.86]), and between coadministration and tamsulosin of -1.8 units (P<0.001; [95% CI: -2.23, -1.40]). A significant difference was seen by Month 9 and continued through Month 48. At Month 48 the mean changes from baseline (±SD) in IPSS total symptom scores were -6.3 (±7.40) for coadministration, -5.3 (±7.14) for dutasteride, and -3.8 (±7.74) for tamsulosin, with a mean difference between coadministration and dutasteride of -0.96 units (P<0.001; [95% CI: -1.40, -0.52]), and between coadministration and tamsulosin of -2.5 units (P<0.001; [95% CI: -2.96, -2.07]). See Figure 1.

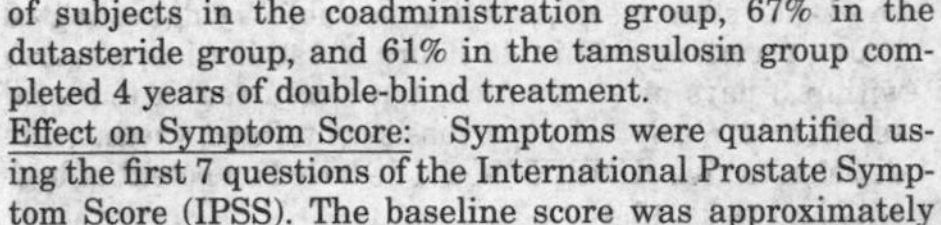

Figure 1. International Prostate Symptom Score Change From Baseline Over a 48-Month Period (Randomized, Double-Blind, Parallel-Group Trial [CombAT Trial])

Effect on Acute Urinary Retention or the Need for BPH-Related Surgery: After 4 years of treatment, coadministration therapy with dutasteride and tamsulosin did not provide benefit over dutasteride monotherapy in reducing the incidence of AUR or BPH-related surgery.

In separate 2-year randomized, double-blind trials, compared with placebo, dutasteride monotherapy was associated with a statistically significantly lower incidence of AUR (1.8% for dutasteride versus 4.2% for placebo; 57% reduction in risk) and with a statistically significantly lower incidence of BPH-related surgery (2.2% for dutasteride versus. 4.1% for placebo; 48% reduction in risk).

Effect on Maximum Urine Flow Rate: The baseline Q_{max} was approximately 10.7 mL/sec for each treatment group. Coadministration therapy was statistically superior to each of the monotherapy treatments in increasing Q_{max} at Month 24, the primary time point for this endpoint. At Month 24, the mean increases from baseline (±SD) in Q_{max} were 2.4 (±5.26) mL/sec for coadministration group, 1.9 (±5.10) mL/sec for dutasteride, and 0.9 (±4.57) mL/sec for tamsulosin, with a mean difference between coadministration and dutasteride of 0.5 mL/sec (P = 0.003; [95% CI: 0.17, 0.84]), and between coadministration and tamsulosin of 1.5 mL/sec (P<0.001; [95% CI: 1.19, 1.86]). This difference was seen by Month 6 and continued through Month 24. See Figure 2.

The additional improvement in Q_{max} of coadministration therapy over dutasteride monotherapy was no longer statistically significant at Month 48.

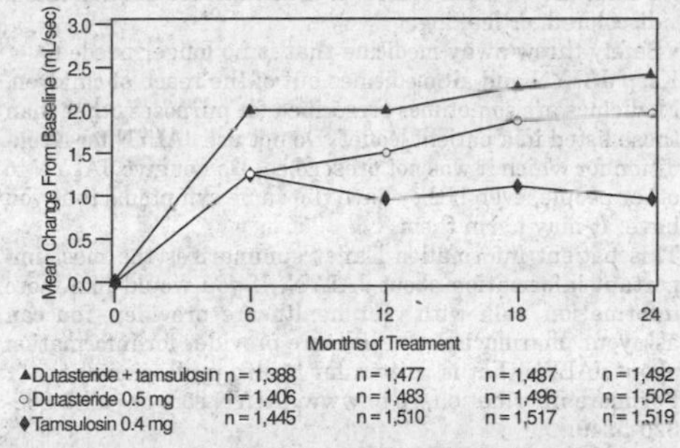

Figure 2. Q-max Change From Baseline Over a 24-Month Period (Randomized, Double-Blind, Parallel-Group Trial [CombAT Trial])

Effect on Prostate Volume: The mean prostate volume at trial entry was approximately 55 cc. At Month 24, the primary time point for this endpoint, the mean percent changes from baseline (±SD) in prostate volume were -26.9% (±22.57) for coadministration therapy, -28.0% (±24.88) for dutasteride, and 0% (±31.14) for tamsulosin, with a mean difference between coadministration and dutasteride of 1.1% (P = NS; [95% CI: -0.6, 2.8]), and between coadministration and tamsulosin of -26.9% (P<0.001; [95% CI: -28.9, -24.9]). Similar changes were seen at Month 48: -27.3% (±24.91) for coadministration therapy, -28.0% (±25.74) for dutasteride, and +4.6% (±35.45) for tamsulosin.

16 HOW SUPPLIED/STORAGE AND HANDLING

JALYN Capsules, containing 0.5 mg dutasteride and 0.4 mg tamsulosin hydrochloride, are oblong hard-shell capsules with a brown body and an orange cap imprinted with "GS 7CZ" in black ink. They are available in bottles with child-resistant closures as follows:

Bottle of 30 (NDC 0173-0809-13).

Bottle of 90 (NDC 0173-0809-59).

Store at 25°C (77°F); excursions permitted 15° to 30°C (59° to 86°F). [see USP Controlled Room Temperature]. Capsules may become deformed and/or discolored if kept at high temperatures.

Dutasteride is absorbed through the skin. JALYN Capsules should not be handled by women who are pregnant or who could become pregnant because of the potential for absorption of dutasteride and the subsequent potential risk to a developing male fetus *[see Warnings and Precautions (5.6)]*.

17 PATIENT COUNSELING INFORMATION

See FDA-approved patient labeling (Patient Information)

17.1 Orthostatic Hypotension

Physicians should inform patients about the possible occurrence of symptoms related to orthostatic hypotension, such as dizziness and vertigo, and the potential risk of syncope when taking JALYN. Patients starting treatment with JALYN should be cautioned to avoid situations where injury could result should syncope occur (e.g., driving, operating machinery, performing hazardous tasks). Patients should sit or lie down at the first signs of orthostatic hypotension *[see Warnings and Precautions (5.1)]*.

17.2 PSA Monitoring

Physicians should inform patients that JALYN reduces serum PSA levels by approximately 50% within 3 to 6 months of therapy, although it may vary for each individual. For patients undergoing PSA screening, increases in PSA levels while on treatment with JALYN may signal the presence of prostate cancer and should be evaluated by a healthcare provider *[see Warnings and Precautions (5.3)]*.

17.3 Risk of High-Grade Prostate Cancer

Physicians should inform patients that there was an increase in high-grade prostate cancer in men treated with 5 alpha-reductase inhibitors (which are indicated for BPH treatment), including dutasteride, which is a component of JALYN, compared with those treated with placebo in trials looking at the use of these drugs to reduce the risk of prostate cancer *[see Indications and Usage (1.2), Warnings and Precautions (5.4), Adverse Reactions (6.1)]*.

17.4 Exposure of Women—Risk to Male Fetus

Physicians should inform patients that JALYN Capsules should not be handled by a woman who is pregnant or who could become pregnant because of the potential for absorption of dutasteride and the subsequent potential risk to a developing male fetus. Dutasteride is absorbed through the skin and could result in unintended fetal exposure. If a pregnant woman or woman of childbearing potential comes in contact with leaking JALYN Capsules, the contact area should be washed immediately with soap and water *[see Warnings and Precautions (5.6), Use in Specific Populations (8.1)]*.

17.5 Instructions for Use

JALYN Capsules should be swallowed whole and not chewed, crushed, or opened. JALYN Capsules may become deformed and/or discolored if kept at high temperatures. If this occurs, capsules should not be used.

17.6 Priapism

Physicians should inform patients about the possibility of priapism as a result of treatment with JALYN or other alpha adrenergic antagonist-containing medications. Patients should be informed that this reaction is extremely rare, but can lead to permanent erectile dysfunction if not brought to immediate medical attention *[see Warnings and Precautions (5.7)]*.

17.7 Blood Donation

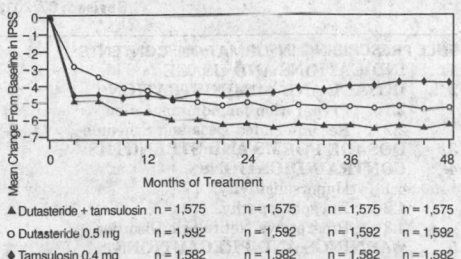

Physicians should inform men treated with JALYN that they should not donate blood until at least 6 months following their last dose to prevent pregnant women from receiving dutasteride through blood transfusion *[see Warnings and Precautions (5.8)]*. Serum levels of dutasteride are detectable for 4 to 6 months after treatment ends *[see Clinical Pharmacology (12.3)]*.

17.8 Intraoperative Floppy Iris Syndrome (IFIS)

Physicians should advise patients considering cataract surgery to tell their ophthalmologist that they take or have taken JALYN, an alpha adrenergic antagonist-containing product *[see Warnings and Precautions (5.9)]*.

JALYN and AVODART are trademarks of GlaxoSmithKline. The other brands listed are trademarks of their respective owners and are not trademarks of GlaxoSmithKline. The makers of these brands are not affiliated with and do not endorse GlaxoSmithKline or its products.

Jointly Manufactured by
Catalent Pharma Solutions
F-67930 Beinheim, France
D-73614 Schorndorf, Germany
and
Rottendorf Pharma GmbH
D-59320 Ennigerloh, Germany
Distributed by
GlaxoSmithKline
Research Triangle Park, NC 27709

JLN:7PI

PHARMACIST—DETACH HERE AND GIVE INSTRUCTIONS TO PATIENT

PATIENT INFORMATION

JALYN™ [JAY-lin]

(dutasteride and tamsulosin hydrochloride)

Capsules

JALYN is for use by men only.

Read this patient information before you start taking JALYN and each time you get a refill. There may be new information. This information does not take the place of talking with your healthcare provider about your medical condition or your treatment.

What is JALYN?

JALYN is a prescription medicine that contains 2 medicines: dutasteride and tamsulosin. JALYN is used to treat the symptoms of benign prostatic hyperplasia (BPH) in men with an enlarged prostate.

Who should not take JALYN?

Do Not Take JALYN if you are:

- pregnant or could become pregnant. JALYN may harm your unborn baby. Pregnant women should not touch JALYN Capsules. If a woman who is pregnant with a male baby gets enough JALYN in her body by swallowing or touching JALYN, the male baby may be born with sex organs that are not normal. If a pregnant woman or woman of childbearing potential comes in contact with leaking JALYN Capsules, the contact area should be washed immediately with soap and water.

- a child or teenager.
- allergic to dutasteride, tamsulosin, or any of the ingredients in JALYN. See the end of this leaflet for a complete list of ingredients in JALYN.
- taking another medicine that contains an alpha-blocker.
- allergic to other 5 alpha-reductase inhibitors, for example, PROSCAR® (finasteride) Tablets.

What should I tell my healthcare provider before taking JALYN?

Before you take JALYN, tell your healthcare provider if you:

- have a history of low blood pressure
- take medicines to treat high blood pressure
- plan to have cataract surgery
- have liver problems
- are allergic to sulfa medications
- have any other medical conditions

Tell your healthcare provider about all the medicines you take, including prescription and non-prescription medicines, vitamins, and herbal supplements. JALYN and other medicines may affect each other, causing side effects. JALYN may affect the way other medicines work, and other medicines may affect how JALYN works.

Know the medicines you take. Keep a list of them to show your healthcare provider and pharmacist when you get a new medicine.

How should I take JALYN?

- Take JALYN exactly as your healthcare provider tells you to take it.
- Swallow JALYN Capsules whole. Do not crush, chew, or open JALYN Capsules because the contents of the capsule may irritate your lips, mouth, or throat.
- Take your JALYN 1 time each day, about 30 minutes after the same meal every day. For example, you may take JALYN 30 minutes after dinner every day.
- If you miss a dose, you can take it later that same day, 30 minutes after a meal. Do not take 2 JALYN capsules in the same day. If you stop or forget to take JALYN for several days, talk with your healthcare provider before starting again.
- If you take too much JALYN, call your healthcare provider or go to the nearest hospital emergency room right away.

What should I avoid while taking JALYN?

- Avoid driving, operating machinery, or other dangerous activities when starting treatment with JALYN until you know how JALYN affects you. JALYN can cause a sudden drop in your blood pressure, especially at the start of treatment. A sudden drop in blood pressure may cause you to faint, feel dizzy or lightheaded.
- You should not donate blood while taking JALYN or for 6 months after you have stopped JALYN. This is important to prevent pregnant women from receiving JALYN through blood transfusions.

What are the possible side effects of JALYN?

JALYN may cause serious side effects, including:

- **Decreased blood pressure.** JALYN may cause a sudden drop in your blood pressure upon standing from a sitting or lying position, especially at the start of treatment. Symptoms of low blood pressure may include:
- fainting
- dizziness
- feeling lightheaded
- **Rare and serious allergic reactions, including:**
- swelling of your face, tongue, or throat
- difficulty breathing
- serious skin reactions, such as skin peeling

Get medical help right away if you have these serious allergic reactions.

- **Higher chance of a more serious form of prostate cancer.**
- **Eye problems during cataract surgery.** During cataract surgery, a condition called intraoperative floppy iris syndrome (IFIS) can happen if you take or have taken JALYN in the past. If you need to have cataract surgery, tell your surgeon if you take or have taken JALYN.
- **A painful erection that will not go away.** Rarely, JALYN can cause a painful erection (priapism), which cannot be relieved by having sex. If this happens, get medical help right away. If priapism is not treated, there could be lasting damage to your penis, including not being able to have an erection.

The most common side effects of JALYN include:

- ejaculation problems[1]
- trouble getting or keeping an erection (impotence)[1]
- a decrease in sex drive (libido)[1]
- dizziness
- enlarged or painful breasts. If you notice breast lumps or nipple discharge, you should talk to your healthcare provider.
- runny nose

[1]Some of these events may continue after you stop taking JALYN.

Depressed mood has been reported in patients receiving dutasteride, an ingredient of JALYN.

Dutasteride, an ingredient of JALYN, has been shown to reduce sperm count, semen volume, and sperm movement. However, the effect of JALYN on male fertility is not known.

Prostate-Specific Antigen (PSA) Test: Your healthcare provider may check you for other prostate problems, including prostate cancer before you start and while you take JALYN. A blood test called PSA (prostate-specific antigen) is sometimes used to see if you might have prostate cancer. JALYN will reduce the amount of PSA measured in your blood. Your healthcare provider is aware of this effect and can still use PSA to see if you might have prostate cancer. Increases in your PSA levels while on treatment with JALYN (even if the PSA levels are in the normal range) should be evaluated by your healthcare provider.

Tell your healthcare provider if you have any side effect that bothers you or that does not go away.

These are not all the possible side effects with JALYN. For more information, ask your healthcare provider or pharmacist.

Call your doctor for medical advice about side effects. You may report side effects to FDA at 1-800-FDA-1088.

How should I store JALYN?

- Store JALYN Capsules at room temperature (59° to 86°F or 15° to 30°C).
- JALYN Capsules may become deformed and/or discolored if kept at high temperatures.
- Do not use or touch JALYN if your capsules are deformed, discolored, or leaking.
- Safely throw away medicine that is no longer needed.

Keep JALYN and all medicines out of the reach of children. Medicines are sometimes prescribed for purposes other than those listed in a patient leaflet. Do not use JALYN for a condition for which it was not prescribed. Do not give JALYN to other people, even if they have the same symptoms that you have. It may harm them.

This patient information leaflet summarizes the most important information about JALYN. If you would like more information, talk with your healthcare provider. You can ask your pharmacist or healthcare provider for information about JALYN that is written for health professionals.

For more information, go to www.JALYN.com or call 1-888-825-5249.

What are the ingredients in JALYN?

Active ingredients: dutasteride and tamsulosin hydrochloride

Inactive ingredients: black ink, butylated hydroxytoluene, carrageenan, FD&C yellow 6, ferric oxide (yellow), gelatin (from certified BSE-free bovine sources), glycerin, hypromellose, iron oxide red, methacrylic acid copolymer dispersion, microcrystalline cellulose, mono-di-glycerides of caprylic/capric acid, potassium chloride, talc, titanium dioxide, and triethyl citrate.

How does JALYN work?

JALYN contains 2 medications, dutasteride and tamsulosin. These 2 medications work in different ways to improve symptoms of BPH. Dutasteride shrinks the enlarged prostate and tamsulosin relaxes muscles in the prostate and neck of the bladder. These 2 medications, when used together, can improve symptoms of BPH better than either medication when used alone.

JALYN is a registered trademark of GlaxoSmithKline.

The other brands listed are trademarks of their respective owners and are not trademarks of GlaxoSmithKline. The makers of these brands are not affiliated with and do not endorse GlaxoSmithKline or its products.

Jointly Manufactured by
Catalent Pharma Solutions
F-67930 Beinheim, France
D-73614 Schorndorf, Germany
and
Rottendorf Pharma GmbH
D-59320 Ennigerloh, Germany
Distributed by
GlaxoSmithKline
Research Triangle Park, NC 27709

April 2013
JLN:6PIL

KINRIX ℞

[kin' rix]

(Diphtheria and Tetanus Toxoids and Acellular Pertussis Adsorbed and Inactivated Poliovirus Vaccine) Suspension for Intramuscular Injection

HIGHLIGHTS OF PRESCRIBING INFORMATION

These highlights do not include all the information needed to use KINRIX safely and effectively. See full prescribing information for KINRIX.

KINRIX (Diphtheria and Tetanus Toxoids and Acellular Pertussis Adsorbed and Inactivated Poliovirus Vaccine) Suspension for Intramuscular Injection

Initial U.S. Approval: 2008

RECENT MAJOR CHANGES

Warnings and Precautions, Syncope (5.3) 03/2012

INDICATIONS AND USAGE

A single dose of KINRIX is indicated for active immunization against diphtheria, tetanus, pertussis, and poliomyelitis as the fifth dose in the diphtheria, tetanus, and acellular pertussis (DTaP) vaccine series and the fourth dose in the inactivated poliovirus vaccine (IPV) series in children 4 through 6 years of age whose previous DTaP vaccine doses have been with INFANRIX and/or PEDIARIX for the first three doses and INFANRIX for the fourth dose. (1)

DOSAGE AND ADMINISTRATION

A single intramuscular injection (0.5 mL). (2.2)

DOSAGE FORMS AND STRENGTHS

Single-dose vials and prefilled syringes containing a 0.5-mL suspension for injection. (3)

CONTRAINDICATIONS

- Severe allergic reaction (e.g., anaphylaxis) after a previous dose of any diphtheria toxoid, tetanus toxoid, pertussis- or poliovirus-containing vaccine, or to any component of KINRIX, including neomycin and polymyxin B. (4.1)
- Encephalopathy within 7 days of administration of a previous pertussis-containing vaccine. (4.2)
- Progressive neurologic disorders. (4.3)

WARNINGS AND PRECAUTIONS

- If Guillain-Barré syndrome occurs within 6 weeks of receipt of a prior vaccine containing tetanus toxoid, the decision to give KINRIX should be based on potential benefits and risks. (5.1)
- KINRIX is available in vials and 2 types of prefilled syringes. One type of prefilled syringe has a tip cap which may contain natural rubber latex. The other type has a tip cap and a rubber plunger which contain dry natural latex rubber. Use of these syringes may cause allergic reactions in latex sensitive individuals. (5.2, 16)
- Syncope (fainting) can occur in association with administration of injectable vaccines, including KINRIX. Procedures should be in place to avoid falling injury and to restore cerebral perfusion following syncope. (5.3)
- If adverse events (i.e., temperature ≥105°F, collapse or shock-like state, persistent, inconsolable crying lasting ≥3 hours, occurring within 48 hours of vaccination; seizures within 3 days of vaccination) have occurred in temporal relation to receipt of a pertussis-containing vaccine, the decision to give KINRIX should be based on potential benefits and risks. (5.4)
- For children at higher risk for seizures, an antipyretic may be administered at the time of vaccination with KINRIX. (5.5)

ADVERSE REACTIONS

- The most frequently reported solicited local reaction (>50%) was injection site pain. Other common solicited local reactions (≥25%) were redness, increase in arm circumference, and swelling. (6.1)
- Common solicited general adverse events (≥15%) were drowsiness, fever (≥99.5°F), and loss of appetite. (6.1)

To report SUSPECTED ADVERSE REACTIONS, contact GlaxoSmithKline at 1-888-825-5249 or VAERS at 1-800-822-7967 or www.vaers.hhs.gov.

DRUG INTERACTIONS

Do not mix KINRIX with any other vaccine in the same syringe or vial. (7.1)

See 17 for PATIENT COUNSELING INFORMATION

Revised: 07/2012

FULL PRESCRIBING INFORMATION: CONTENTS*

*** Sections or subsections omitted from the full prescribing information are not listed**

FULL PRESCRIBING INFORMATION

1 INDICATIONS AND USAGE

A single dose of KINRIX® is indicated for active immunization against diphtheria, tetanus, pertussis, and poliomyelitis as the fifth dose in the diphtheria, tetanus, and acellular pertussis (DTaP) vaccine series and the fourth dose in the inactivated poliovirus vaccine (IPV) series in children 4 through 6 years of age whose previous DTaP vaccine doses have been with INFANRIX® (Diphtheria and Tetanus Toxoids and Acellular Pertussis Vaccine Adsorbed) and/or PEDIARIX® [Diphtheria and Tetanus Toxoids and Acellular Pertussis Adsorbed, Hepatitis B (Recombinant) and Inactivated Poliovirus Vaccine] for the first three doses and INFANRIX for the fourth dose.

2 DOSAGE AND ADMINISTRATION

2.1 Preparation for Administration

Shake vigorously to obtain a homogeneous, turbid, white suspension. Do not use if resuspension does not occur with vigorous shaking. Parenteral drug products should be inspected visually for particulate matter and discoloration prior to administration, whenever solution and container permit. If either of these conditions exists, the vaccine should not be administered.

For the prefilled syringes, attach a sterile needle and administer intramuscularly.

For the vials, use a sterile needle and sterile syringe to withdraw the 0.5-mL dose and administer intramuscularly. Changing needles between drawing vaccine from a vial and injecting it into a recipient is not necessary unless the needle has been damaged or contaminated. Use a separate sterile needle and syringe for each individual.

Do not administer this product intravenously, intradermally, or subcutaneously.

2.2 Recommended Dose and Schedule

KINRIX is to be administered as a 0.5-mL dose by intramuscular injection. The preferred site of administration is the deltoid muscle of the upper arm. Do not administer this product intravenously, intradermally, or subcutaneously.

KINRIX may be used for the fifth dose in the DTaP immunization series and the fourth dose in the IPV immunization series in children 4 through 6 years of age (prior to the seventh birthday) whose previous DTaP vaccine doses have been with INFANRIX and/or PEDIARIX for the first three doses and INFANRIX for the fourth dose *[see Indications and Usage (1)]*.

3 DOSAGE FORMS AND STRENGTHS

KINRIX is a suspension for injection available in 0.5-mL single-dose vials and prefilled TIP LOK® syringes.

4 CONTRAINDICATIONS

4.1 Hypersensitivity

Severe allergic reaction (e.g., anaphylaxis) after a previous dose of any diphtheria toxoid, tetanus toxoid, pertussis- or poliovirus-containing vaccine, or to any component of KINRIX, including neomycin and polymyxin B, is a contraindication to administration of KINRIX *[see Description (11)]*. Because of the uncertainty as to which component of the vaccine might be responsible, no further vaccination with any of these components should be given. Alternatively, such individuals may be referred to an allergist for evaluation if immunization with any of these components is considered.

4.2 Encephalopathy

Encephalopathy (e.g., coma, decreased level of consciousness, prolonged seizures) within 7 days of administration of a previous dose of a pertussis-containing vaccine that is not attributable to another identifiable cause is a contraindication to administration of any pertussis-containing vaccine, including KINRIX.

4.3 Progressive Neurologic Disorder

Progressive neurologic disorder, including infantile spasms, uncontrolled epilepsy, or progressive encephalopathy is a contraindication to administration of any pertussis-containing vaccine, including KINRIX. Pertussis vaccine should not be administered to individuals with such conditions until a treatment regimen has been established and the condition has stabilized.

5 WARNINGS AND PRECAUTIONS

5.1 Guillain-Barré Syndrome

If Guillain-Barré syndrome occurs within 6 weeks of receipt of a prior vaccine containing tetanus toxoid, the decision to give any tetanus toxoid-containing vaccine, including KINRIX, should be based on careful consideration of the potential benefits and possible risks. When a decision is made to withhold tetanus toxoid, other available vaccines should be given, as indicated.

5.2 Latex

KINRIX is available in vials and 2 types of prefilled syringes. One type of prefilled syringe has a tip cap which may contain natural rubber latex and a plunger which does not contain latex. The other type has a tip cap and a rubber plunger which contain dry natural latex rubber. Use of these syringes may cause allergic reactions in latex sensitive individuals. The vial stopper does not contain latex. *[See How Supplied/Storage and Handling (16).]*

5.3 Syncope

Syncope (fainting) can occur in association with administration of injectable vaccines, including KINRIX. Syncope can be accompanied by transient neurological signs such as visual disturbance, paresthesia, and tonic-clonic limb movements. Procedures should be in place to avoid falling injury and to restore cerebral perfusion following syncope.

5.4 Adverse Events Following Prior Pertussis Vaccination

If any of the following events occur in temporal relation to receipt of a pertussis-containing vaccine, the decision to give any pertussis-containing vaccine, including KINRIX, should be based on careful consideration of the potential benefits and possible risks:

- Temperature of ≥40.5°C (105°F) within 48 hours not due to another identifiable cause;
- Collapse or shock-like state (hypotonic-hyporesponsive episode) within 48 hours;
- Persistent, inconsolable crying lasting ≥3 hours, occurring within 48 hours;
- Seizures with or without fever occurring within 3 days.

When a decision is made to withhold pertussis vaccination, other available vaccines should be given, as indicated.

5.5 Children at Risk for Seizures

For children at higher risk for seizures than the general population, an appropriate antipyretic may be administered at the time of vaccination with a pertussis-containing vaccine, including KINRIX, and for the ensuing 24 hours to reduce the possibility of post-vaccination fever.

5.6 Preventing and Managing Allergic Vaccine Reactions

Prior to administration, the healthcare provider should review the patient's immunization history for possible vaccine sensitivity and previous vaccination-related adverse reactions to allow an assessment of benefits and risks. Epinephrine and other appropriate agents used for the control of immediate allergic reactions must be immediately available should an acute anaphylactic reaction occur.

6 ADVERSE REACTIONS

6.1 Clinical Trials Experience

Because clinical trials are conducted under widely varying conditions, adverse reaction rates observed in the clinical trials of a vaccine cannot be directly compared with rates in the clinical trials of another vaccine, and may not reflect the rates observed in practice.

A total of 3,537 children were vaccinated with a single dose of KINRIX in 3 clinical trials. Of these, 381 children received a non-US formulation of KINRIX (containing ≤2.5 mg 2-phenoxyethanol per dose as preservative). The primary study (Study 048), conducted in the United States, was a randomized, controlled clinical trial in which children 4 to 6 years of age were vaccinated with KINRIX (N = 3,156) or control vaccines (INFANRIX and IPOL® vaccine [IPV, Sanofi Pasteur SA]; N = 1,053) as a fifth DTaP vaccine dose following 4 doses of INFANRIX and as a fourth IPV dose following 3 doses of IPOL. Subjects also received the second dose of US-licensed measles, mumps, and rubella (MMR) vaccine (Merck & Co., Inc.) administered concomitantly, at separate sites.

Data on adverse events were collected by parents/guardians using standardized forms for 4 consecutive days following vaccination with KINRIX or control vaccines (i.e., day of vaccination and the next 3 days). The reported frequencies of solicited local reactions and general adverse events in Study 048 are presented in Table 1.

In 3 studies (Study 046, 047, and 048), children were monitored for unsolicited adverse events, including serious adverse events, that occurred in the 31-day period following vaccination and in 2 studies (Study 047 and 048), parents/guardians were actively queried about changes in the child's health status, including the occurrence of serious adverse events, through 6 months post-vaccination.

Table 1. Percentage of Children 4 to 6 Years of Age Reporting Solicited Local Reactions or General Adverse Events Within 4 Days of Vaccination[a] With KINRIX or Separate Concomitant Administration of INFANRIX and IPV When Coadministered With MMR Vaccine (Study 048) (Total Vaccinated Cohort)

	KINRIX	INFANRIX + IPV
Local[b]	**N = 3,121-3,128**	**N = 1,039-1,043**
Pain, any	57.0[c]	53.3
Pain, grade 2 or 3[d]	13.7	12.0
Pain, grade 3[d]	1.6[c]	0.6
Redness, any	36.6	36.6
Redness, ≥50 mm	17.6	20.0
Redness, ≥110 mm	2.9	4.1
Arm circumference increase, any	36.0	37.8
Arm circumference increase, >20 mm	6.9	7.4
Arm circumference increase, >30 mm	2.4	3.2
Swelling, any	26.0	27.0
Swelling, ≥50 mm	10.2	11.5
Swelling, ≥110 mm	1.4	1.8
General	**N = 3,037-3,120**	**N = 993-1,036**
Drowsiness, any	19.1	17.5
Drowsiness, grade 3[e]	0.8	0.8
Fever, ≥99.5°F	16.0	14.8
Fever, >100.4°F	6.5[c]	4.4
Fever, >102.2°F	1.1	1.1
Fever, >104°F	0.1	0.0
Loss of appetite, any	15.5	16.0
Loss of appetite, grade 3[f]	0.8	0.6

IPV manufactured by Sanofi Pasteur SA. MMR vaccine manufactured by Merck & Co., Inc.

Total Vaccinated Cohort = all vaccinated subjects for whom safety data were available.

N = number of children with evaluable data for the events listed.

[a] Within 4 days of vaccination defined as day of vaccination and the next 3 days.

[b]Local reactions at the injection site for KINRIX or INFANRIX.

[c]Statistically higher than comparator group (P <0.05).

[d]Grade 2 defined as painful when the limb was moved; Grade 3 defined as preventing normal daily activities.

[e] Grade 3 defined as preventing normal daily activities.

[f] Grade 3 defined as not eating at all.

In Study 048, KINRIX was non-inferior to INFANRIX with regard to swelling that involved >50% of the injected upper arm length and that was associated with a >30 mm increase in mid-upper arm circumference within 4 days following vaccination (upper limit of two-sided 95% Confidence Interval for difference in percentage of KINRIX [0.6%, n = 20] minus INFANRIX [1.0%, n = 11] ≤2%).

Serious Adverse Events: Within the 31-day period following study vaccination in 3 studies (Study 046, 047, and 048), in which all subjects received concomitant MMR vaccine (US-licensed MMR vaccine [Merck & Co., Inc.] in Study 047 and 048; non-US-licensed MMR vaccine in Study 046), 3 subjects (0.1% [3/3,537]) who received KINRIX reported serious adverse events (dehydration and hypernatremia; cerebrovascular accident; dehydration and gastroenteritis) and 4 subjects (0.3% [4/1,434]) who received INFANRIX and IPV (Sanofi Pasteur SA) reported serious adverse events (cellulitis; constipation; foreign body trauma; fever without identified etiology).

6.2 Postmarketing Experience

In addition to reports in clinical trials, the following adverse events, for which a causal relationship to components of KINRIX is plausible, have been reported since market introduction of DTaP-IPV manufactured by GlaxoSmithKline outside the U.S. Because these events are reported voluntarily from a population of uncertain size, it is not always possible to reliably estimate their frequency or establish a causal relationship to vaccination.

General Disorders and Administration Site Conditions: Injection site vesicles.
Nervous System Disorders: Syncope.
Skin and Subcutaneous Tissue Disorders: Pruritus.
Additional adverse events reported following postmarketing use of INFANRIX, for which a causal relationship to vaccination is plausible, are: Allergic reactions, including anaphylactoid reactions, anaphylaxis, angioedema, and urticaria, apnea, collapse or shock-like state (hypotonic-hyporesponsive episode), convulsions (with or without fever), lymphadenopathy, and thrombocytopenia.

7 DRUG INTERACTIONS

7.1 Concomitant Vaccine Administration

In clinical trials, KINRIX was administered concomitantly with the second dose of MMR vaccine *[see Clinical Studies (14)]*.
Data are not available on concomitant use of KINRIX and varicella vaccine.
When KINRIX is administered concomitantly with other injectable vaccines, they should be given with separate syringes. KINRIX should not be mixed with any other vaccine in the same syringe or vial.

7.2 Immunosuppressive Therapies

Immunosuppressive therapies, including irradiation, antimetabolites, alkylating agents, cytotoxic drugs, and corticosteroids (used in greater than physiologic doses), may reduce the immune response to KINRIX.

8 USE IN SPECIFIC POPULATIONS

8.1 Pregnancy

Pregnancy Category C
Animal reproduction studies have not been conducted with KINRIX. It is also not known whether KINRIX can cause fetal harm when administered to a pregnant woman or can affect reproduction capacity.

8.4 Pediatric Use

Safety and effectiveness of KINRIX in children younger than 4 years of age and children 7 to 16 years of age have not been evaluated. KINRIX is not approved for use in persons in these age groups.

11 DESCRIPTION

KINRIX (Diphtheria and Tetanus Toxoids and Acellular Pertussis Adsorbed and Inactivated Poliovirus Vaccine) is a noninfectious, sterile vaccine for intramuscular administration. Each 0.5-mL dose is formulated to contain 25 Lf of diphtheria toxoid, 10 Lf of tetanus toxoid, 25 mcg of inactivated pertussis toxin (PT), 25 mcg of filamentous hemagglutinin (FHA), 8 mcg of pertactin (69 kiloDalton outer membrane protein), 40 D-antigen Units (DU) of Type 1 poliovirus (Mahoney), 8 DU of Type 2 poliovirus (MEF-1), and 32 DU of Type 3 poliovirus (Saukett). The diphtheria, tetanus, and pertussis components of KINRIX are the same as those in INFANRIX and PEDIARIX and the poliovirus component is the same as that in PEDIARIX.
The diphtheria toxin is produced by growing *Corynebacterium diphtheriae* in Fenton medium containing a bovine extract. Tetanus toxin is produced by growing *Clostridium tetani* in a modified Latham medium derived from bovine casein. The bovine materials used in these extracts are sourced from countries which the United States Department of Agriculture (USDA) has determined neither have nor are at risk of bovine spongiform encephalopathy (BSE). Both toxins are detoxified with formaldehyde, concentrated by ultrafiltration, and purified by precipitation, dialysis, and sterile filtration.
The acellular pertussis antigens (PT, FHA, and pertactin) are isolated from *Bordetella pertussis* culture grown in modified Stainer-Scholte liquid medium. PT and FHA are isolated from the fermentation broth; pertactin is extracted from the cells by heat treatment and flocculation. The antigens are purified in successive chromatographic and precipitation steps. PT is detoxified using glutaraldehyde and formaldehyde. FHA and pertactin are treated with formaldehyde.
Diphtheria and tetanus toxoids and pertussis antigens (inactivated PT, FHA, and pertactin) are individually adsorbed onto aluminum hydroxide.
The inactivated poliovirus component of KINRIX is an enhanced potency component. Each of the 3 strains of poliovirus is individually grown in VERO cells, a continuous line of monkey kidney cells, cultivated on microcarriers. Calf serum and lactalbumin hydrolysate are used during VERO cell culture and/or virus culture. Calf serum is sourced from countries the USDA has determined neither have nor are at risk of BSE. After clarification, each viral suspension is purified by ultrafiltration, diafiltration, and successive chromatographic steps, and inactivated with formaldehyde. The 3 purified viral strains are then pooled to form a trivalent concentrate.
Diphtheria and tetanus toxoid potency is determined by measuring the amount of neutralizing antitoxin in previously immunized guinea pigs. The potency of the acellular pertussis components (inactivated PT, FHA, and pertactin)

Table 2. Pre-Vaccination Antibody Levels and Post-Vaccination[a] Antibody Responses Following KINRIX Compared With Separate Concomitant Administration of INFANRIX and IPV in Children 4 to 6 Years of Age When Coadministered With MMR Vaccine (Study 048) (ATP Cohort for Immunogenicity)

	KINRIX	INFANRIX + IPV
	N = 787-851	N = 237-262
Anti-Diphtheria Toxoid		
Pre-vaccination % ≥0.1 IU/mL (95% CI)[b]	87.7 (85.3, 89.9)	85.5 (80.6, 89.5)
Post-vaccination % ≥0.1 IU/mL (95% CI)[b]	100 (99.6, 100)	100 (98.6, 100)
% Booster Response (95% CI)[c]	99.5 (98.8, 99.9)[d]	100 (98.6, 100)
Anti-Tetanus Toxoid		
Pre-vaccination % ≥0.1 IU/mL (95% CI)[b]	87.8 (85.4, 90.0)	88.2 (83.6, 91.8)
Post-vaccination % ≥0.1 IU/mL (95% CI)[b]	100 (99.6, 100)	100 (98.6, 100)
% Booster Response (95% CI)[c]	96.7 (95.2, 97.8)[d]	93.9 (90.2, 96.5)
Anti-PT		
% Booster Response (95% CI)[e]	92.2 (90.2, 94.0)[d]	92.6 (88.7, 95.5)
Anti-FHA		
% Booster Response (95% CI)[e]	95.4 (93.7, 96.7)[d]	96.2 (93.1, 98.1)
Anti-Pertactin		
% Booster Response (95% CI)[e]	97.8 (96.5, 98.6)[d]	96.9 (94.1, 98.7)
Anti-Poliovirus 1		
Pre-vaccination % ≥1:8 (95% CI)[b]	88.3 (85.9, 90.4)	85.1 (80.1, 89.2)
Post-vaccination % ≥1:8 (95% CI)[b]	99.9 (99.3, 100)	100 (98.5, 100)
Post-vaccination GMT (95% CI)	2,127 (1,976, 2,290)[f]	1,685 (1,475, 1,925)
Anti-Poliovirus 2		
Pre-vaccination % ≥1:8 (95% CI)[b]	91.8 (89.7, 93.6)	87.0 (82.3, 90.8)
Post-vaccination % ≥1:8 (95% CI)[b]	100 (99.6, 100)	100 (98.5, 100)
Post-vaccination GMT (95% CI)	2,265 (2,114, 2,427)[f]	1,818 (1,606, 2,057)
Anti-Poliovirus 3		
Pre-vaccination % ≥1:8 (95% CI)[b]	84.7 (82.0, 87.0)	85.0 (80.1, 89.1)
Post-vaccination % ≥1:8 (95% CI)[b]	100 (99.5, 100)	100 (98.5, 100)
Post-vaccination GMT (95% CI)	3,588 (3,345, 3,849)[f]	3,365 (2,961, 3,824)

IPV manufactured by Sanofi Pasteur SA. MMR vaccine manufactured by Merck & Co., Inc.
ATP = according-to-protocol; CI = Confidence Interval; GMT = geometric mean antibody titer
N = number of subjects with available results.
[a] One month blood sampling, range 31 to 48 days.
[b] Seroprotection defined as anti-diphtheria toxoid and anti-tetanus toxoid antibody concentrations ≥0.1 IU/mL by ELISA and as anti-poliovirus Type 1, Type 2, and Type 3 antibody titer ≥1:8 by micro-neutralization assay for poliovirus.
[c] Booster response: In subjects with pre-vaccination <0.1 IU/mL, post-vaccination concentration ≥0.4 IU/mL. In subjects with pre-vaccination concentration ≥0.1 IU/mL, an increase of at least 4 times the pre-vaccination concentration.
[d] KINRIX was non-inferior to INFANRIX + IPV based on booster response rates (upper limit of two-sided 95% CI on the difference of INFANRIX + IPV minus KINRIX ≤10%).
[e] Booster response: In subjects with pre-vaccination <5 EL.U./mL, post-vaccination concentration ≥20 EL.U./mL. In subjects with pre-vaccination ≥5 EL.U./mL and <20 EL.U./mL, an increase of at least 4 times the pre-vaccination concentration. In subjects with pre-vaccination ≥20 EL.U./mL, an increase of at least 2 times the pre-vaccination concentration.
[f] KINRIX was non-inferior to INFANRIX + IPV based on post-vaccination anti-poliovirus antibody GMTs adjusted for baseline titer (upper limit of two-sided 95% CI for the GMT ratio [INFANRIX + IPV:KINRIX] ≤1.5).

is determined by enzyme-linked immunosorbent assay (ELISA) on sera from previously immunized mice. The potency of the inactivated poliovirus component is determined by using the D-antigen ELISA and by a poliovirus neutralizing cell culture assay on sera from previously immunized rats.
Each 0.5-mL dose contains aluminum hydroxide as adjuvant (not more than 0.6 mg aluminum by assay) and 4.5 mg of sodium chloride. Each dose also contains ≤100 mcg of residual formaldehyde and ≤100 mcg of polysorbate 80 (Tween 80). Neomycin sulfate and polymyxin B are used in the poliovirus vaccine manufacturing process and may be present in the final vaccine at ≤0.05 ng neomycin and ≤0.01 ng polymyxin B per dose.
KINRIX is available in vials and 2 types of prefilled syringes. One type of prefilled syringe has a tip cap which may contain natural rubber latex and a plunger which does not contain latex. The other type has a tip cap and a rubber plunger which contain dry natural latex rubber. The vial stopper does not contain latex. *[See How Supplied/Storage and Handling (16).]*
KINRIX does not contain a preservative.

12 CLINICAL PHARMACOLOGY

12.1 Mechanism of Action

Diphtheria: Diphtheria is an acute toxin-mediated infectious disease caused by toxigenic strains of *C. diphtheriae*. Protection against disease is due to the development of neutralizing antibodies to the diphtheria toxin. A serum diphtheria antitoxin level of 0.01 IU/mL is the lowest level giving some degree of protection; a level of 0.1 IU/mL is regarded as protective.[1]
Tetanus: Tetanus is an acute toxin-mediated disease caused by a potent exotoxin released by *C. tetani*. Protection against disease is due to the development of neutralizing antibodies to the tetanus toxin. A serum tetanus antitoxin level of at least 0.01 IU/mL, measured by neutralization assays, is considered the minimum protective level.[2,3] A level of ≥0.1 IU/mL is considered protective.[4]
Pertussis: Pertussis (whooping cough) is a disease of the respiratory tract caused by *B. pertussis*. The role of the different components produced by *B. pertussis* in either the pathogenesis of, or the immunity to, pertussis is not well understood. There is no well established serological correlate of protection for pertussis. The efficacy of the pertussis component of KINRIX was determined in clinical trials of INFANRIX administered as a 3-dose series in infants (see INFANRIX prescribing information).
Poliomyelitis: Poliovirus is an enterovirus that belongs to the picornavirus family. Three serotypes of poliovirus have been identified (Types 1, 2, and 3). Neutralizing antibodies against the 3 poliovirus serotypes are recognized as conferring protection against poliomyelitis disease.[5]

13 NONCLINICAL TOXICOLOGY

13.1 Carcinogenesis, Mutagenesis, Impairment of Fertility

KINRIX has not been evaluated for carcinogenic or mutagenic potential, or for impairment of fertility.

14 CLINICAL STUDIES

14.1 Immunological Evaluation

In a US multicenter study (Study 048), 4,209 children were randomized in a 3:1 ratio to receive either KINRIX or INFANRIX and IPV (Sanofi Pasteur SA) administered concomitantly at separate sites. Subjects also received MMR vaccine (Merck & Co., Inc.) administered concomitantly at a separate site. Subjects were children 4 through 6 years of age who previously received 4 doses of INFANRIX, 3 doses of IPV, and 1 dose of MMR vaccine. Among subjects in both vaccine groups combined, 49.6% were female; 45.6% of subjects were White, 18.8% Hispanic, 13.6% Asian, 7.0% Black, and 15.0% were of other racial/ethnic groups.

Levels of antibodies to the diphtheria, tetanus, pertussis (PT, FHA, and pertactin), and poliovirus antigens were measured in sera obtained immediately prior to vaccination and 1 month (range 31 to 48 days) after vaccination (Table 2). The co-primary immunogenicity endpoints were anti-diphtheria toxoid, anti-tetanus toxoid, anti-PT, anti-FHA, and anti-pertactin booster responses, and anti-poliovirus Type 1, Type 2, and Type 3 geometric mean antibody titers (GMTs) 1 month after vaccination. KINRIX was shown to be non-inferior to INFANRIX and IPV administered separately, in terms of booster responses to DTaP antigens and post-vaccination GMTs for anti-poliovirus antibodies (Table 2).

[See table 2 at top of previous page]

14.2 Concomitant Vaccine Administration

In a US study (Study 047), among recipients of DTaP-IPV (same formulation as KINRIX but also containing 2-phenoxyethanol) and the second dose of MMR vaccine (Merck & Co., Inc.) who had pre-vaccination sera tested for antibodies to measles, mumps, and rubella (N = 175-181), 99% of subjects were seropositive for antibodies to measles, mumps, and rubella prior to vaccination.

15 REFERENCES

1. Vitek CR and Wharton M. Diphtheria Toxoid. In: Plotkin SA, Orenstein WA, and Offit PA, eds. *Vaccines*. 5th ed. Saunders; 2008:139-156.
2. Wassilak SGF, Roper MH, Kretsinger K, and Orenstein WA. Tetanus Toxoid. In: Plotkin SA, Orenstein WA, and Offit PA, eds. *Vaccines*. 5th ed. Saunders; 2008:805-839.
3. Department of Health and Human Services, Food and Drug Administration. Biological products; Bacterial vaccines and toxoids; Implementation of efficacy review; Proposed rule. *Federal Register* December 13, 1985;50(240):51002-51117.
4. Centers for Disease Control and Prevention. General Recommendations on Immunization. Recommendations of the Advisory Committee on Immunization Practices (ACIP). *MMWR* 2006;55(RR-15):1-48.
5. Sutter RW, Pallansch MA, Sawyer LA, et al. Defining surrogate serologic tests with respect to predicting protective vaccine efficacy: Poliovirus vaccination. In: Williams JC, Goldenthal KL, Burns DL, Lewis Jr BP, eds. Combined vaccines and simultaneous administration. Current issues and perspectives. New York, NY: The New York Academy of Sciences; 1995:289-299.

16 HOW SUPPLIED/STORAGE AND HANDLING

KINRIX is available in 0.5-mL single-dose vials and disposable prefilled TIP-LOK syringes (packaged without needles):

NDC 58160-812-01 Vial (contains no latex) in Package of 10: NDC 58160-812-11

NDC 58160-812-43 Syringe (tip cap may contain latex; plunger contains no latex) in Package of 10: NDC 58160-812-52

NDC 58160-812-41 Syringe (tip cap and plunger contain latex) in Package of 5: NDC 58160-812-46

NDC 58160-812-41 Syringe (tip cap and plunger contain latex) in Package of 10: NDC 58160-812-51

Store refrigerated between 2° and 8°C (36° and 46°F). Do not freeze. Discard if the vaccine has been frozen.

17 PATIENT COUNSELING INFORMATION

Parents or guardians should be:

- informed of the potential benefits and risks of immunization with KINRIX.
- informed about the potential for adverse reactions that have been temporally associated with administration of KINRIX or other vaccines containing similar components.
- instructed to report any adverse events to their healthcare provider.
- given the Vaccine Information Statements, which are required by the National Childhood Vaccine Injury Act of 1986 to be given prior to immunization. These materials are available free of charge at the Centers for Disease Control and Prevention (CDC) website (www.cdc.gov/vaccines).

INFANRIX, KINRIX, PEDIARIX, and TIP-LOK are registered trademarks of GlaxoSmithKline. IPOL is a registered trademark of Sanofi Pasteur Limited.

Manufactured by **GlaxoSmithKline Biologicals**
Rixensart, Belgium, US License 1617, and
Novartis Vaccines and Diagnostics GmbH
Marburg, Germany, US License 1754
Distributed by **GlaxoSmithKline**
Research Triangle Park, NC 27709

KNX:9PI

LAMICTAL ℞
[la-mĭk' tal]
(lamotrigine)
Tablets

LAMICTAL ℞
(lamotrigine)
Chewable Dispersible Tablets

LAMICTAL ODT ℞
(lamotrigine)
Orally Disintegrating Tablets

HIGHLIGHTS OF PRESCRIBING INFORMATION
These highlights do not include all the information needed to use LAMICTAL safely and effectively. See full prescribing information for LAMICTAL.
LAMICTAL (lamotrigine) Tablets
LAMICTAL (lamotrigine) Chewable Dispersible Tablets
LAMICTAL ODT (lamotrigine) Orally Disintegrating Tablets
Initial U.S. Approval: 1994

WARNING: SERIOUS SKIN RASHES
See full prescribing information for complete boxed warning.
Cases of life-threatening serious rashes, including Stevens-Johnson syndrome, toxic epidermal necrolysis, and/or rash-related death, have been caused by LAMICTAL. The rate of serious rash is greater in pediatric patients than in adults. Additional factors that may increase the risk of rash include (5.1):
- **coadministration with valproate**
- **exceeding recommended initial dose of LAMICTAL**
- **exceeding recommended dose escalation of LAMICTAL**

Benign rashes are also caused by LAMICTAL; however, it is not possible to predict which rashes will prove to be serious or life threatening. LAMICTAL should be discontinued at the first sign of rash, unless the rash is clearly not drug related. (5.1)

INDICATIONS AND USAGE

LAMICTAL is an antiepileptic drug (AED) indicated for:
Epilepsy—adjunctive therapy in patients ≥2 years of age: (1.1)
- partial seizures
- primary generalized tonic-clonic seizures
- generalized seizures of Lennox-Gastaut syndrome

Epilepsy—monotherapy in patients ≥16 years of age: conversion to monotherapy in patients with partial seizures who are receiving treatment with carbamazepine, phenobarbital, phenytoin, primidone, or valproate as the single AED. (1.1)

Bipolar Disorder in patients ≥18 years of age: maintenance treatment of Bipolar I Disorder to delay the time to occurrence of mood episodes in patients treated for acute mood episodes with standard therapy. (1.2)

DOSAGE AND ADMINISTRATION

- Dosing is based on concomitant medications, indication, and patient age. (2.2, 2.4)
- To avoid an increased risk of rash, the recommended initial dose and subsequent dose escalations should not be exceeded. LAMICTAL Starter Kits and LAMICTAL ODT Patient Titration Kits are available for the first 5 weeks of treatment. (2.1, 16)
- Do not restart LAMICTAL in patients who discontinued due to rash unless the potential benefits clearly outweigh the risks. (2.1)
- Adjustments to maintenance doses will in most cases be required in patients starting or stopping estrogen-containing oral contraceptives. (2.1, 5.8)
- LAMICTAL should be discontinued over a period of at least 2 weeks (approximately 50% reduction per week). (2.1, 5.9)

Epilepsy
- Adjunctive therapy—See Table 1 for patients >12 years of age and Tables 2 and 3 for patients 2 to 12 years. (2.2)
- Conversion to monotherapy—See Table 4. (2.3)

Bipolar Disorder: See Tables 5 and 6. (2.4)

DOSAGE FORMS AND STRENGTHS

Tablets: 25 mg, 100 mg, 150 mg, and 200 mg scored. (3.1, 16)
Chewable Dispersible Tablets: 2 mg, 5 mg, and 25 mg. (3.2, 16)
Orally Disintegrating Tablets: 25 mg, 50 mg, 100 mg, and 200 mg. (3.3, 16)

CONTRAINDICATIONS

Hypersensitivity to the drug or its ingredients. (Boxed Warning, 4)

WARNINGS AND PRECAUTIONS

- Life-threatening serious rash and/or rash-related death may result. (Boxed Warning, 5.1)
- Fatal or life-threatening hypersensitivity reaction: Multiorgan hypersensitivity reactions, also known as Drug Reaction with Eosinophilia and Systemic Symptoms (DRESS), may be fatal or life threatening. Early signs may include rash, fever, and lymphadenopathy. These reactions may be associated with other organ involvement, such as hepatitis, hepatic failure, blood dyscrasias, or acute multiorgan failure. LAMICTAL should be discontinued if alternate etiology for this reaction is not found. (5.2)
- Blood dyscrasias (e.g., neutropenia, thrombocytopenia, pancytopenia): May occur, either with or without an associated hypersensitivity syndrome. (5.3)
- Suicidal behavior and ideation. (5.4)
- Clinical worsening, emergence of new symptoms, and suicidal ideation/behaviors may be associated with treatment of bipolar disorder. Patients should be closely monitored, particularly early in treatment or during dosage changes. (5.5)
- Aseptic meningitis reported in pediatric and adult patients. (5.6)
- Medication errors involving LAMICTAL have occurred. In particular the names LAMICTAL or lamotrigine can be confused with names of other commonly used medications. Medication errors may also occur between the different formulations of LAMICTAL. (3.4, 5.7, 16, 17.10)

ADVERSE REACTIONS

- Most common adverse reactions (incidence ≥10%) in adult epilepsy clinical studies were dizziness, headache, diplopia, ataxia, nausea, blurred vision, somnolence, rhinitis, and rash. Additional adverse reactions (incidence ≥10%) reported in children in epilepsy clinical studies included vomiting, infection, fever, accidental injury, pharyngitis, abdominal pain, and tremor. (6.1)
- Most common adverse reactions (incidence >5%) in adult bipolar clinical studies were nausea, insomnia, somnolence, back pain, fatigue, rash, rhinitis, abdominal pain, and xerostomia. (6.1)

To report SUSPECTED ADVERSE REACTIONS, contact GlaxoSmithKline at 1-888-825-5249 or FDA at 1-800-FDA-1088 or www.fda.gov/medwatch.

DRUG INTERACTIONS

- Valproate increases lamotrigine concentrations more than 2-fold. (7, 12.3)
- Carbamazepine, phenytoin, phenobarbital, and primidone decrease lamotrigine concentrations by approximately 40%. (7, 12.3)
- Oral estrogen-containing contraceptives and rifampin also decrease lamotrigine concentrations by approximately 50%. (7, 12.3)

USE IN SPECIFIC POPULATIONS

- Hepatic impairment: Dosage adjustments required. (2.1)
- Healthcare professionals can enroll patients in the Lamotrigine Pregnancy Registry (1-800-336-2176). Patients can enroll themselves in the North American Antiepileptic Drug Pregnancy Registry (1-888-233-2334). (8.1)
- Efficacy of LAMICTAL, used as adjunctive treatment for partial seizures, was not demonstrated in a small, randomized, double-blind, placebo-controlled study in very young pediatric patients (1 to 24 months). (8.4)

See 17 for PATIENT COUNSELING INFORMATION and Medication Guide

Revised: 09/2012

FULL PRESCRIBING INFORMATION: CONTENTS*

*** Sections or subsections omitted from the full prescribing information are not listed**

FULL PRESCRIBING INFORMATION

WARNING: SERIOUS SKIN RASHES

LAMICTAL® can cause serious rashes requiring hospitalization and discontinuation of treatment. The incidence of these rashes, which have included Stevens-Johnson syndrome, is approximately 0.8% (8 per 1,000) in pediatric patients (2 to 16 years of age) receiving LAMICTAL as adjunctive therapy for epilepsy and 0.3% (3 per 1,000) in adults on adjunctive therapy for epilepsy. In clinical trials of bipolar and other mood disorders, the rate of serious rash was 0.08% (0.8 per 1,000) in adult patients receiving LAMICTAL as initial monotherapy and 0.13% (1.3 per 1,000) in adult patients receiving LAMICTAL as adjunctive therapy. In a prospectively followed cohort of 1,983 pediatric patients (2 to 16 years of age) with epilepsy taking adjunctive LAMICTAL, there was 1 rash-related death. In worldwide postmarketing experience, rare cases of toxic epidermal necrolysis and/or rash-related death have been reported in adult and pediatric patients, but their numbers are too few to permit a precise estimate of the rate.

Other than age, there are as yet no factors identified that are known to predict the risk of occurrence or the severity of rash caused by LAMICTAL. There are suggestions, yet to be proven, that the risk of rash may also be increased by (1) coadministration of LAMICTAL with valproate (includes valproic acid and divalproex sodium), (2) exceeding the recommended initial dose of LAMICTAL, or (3) exceeding the recommended dose escalation for LAMICTAL. However, cases have occurred in the absence of these factors. Nearly all cases of life-threatening rashes caused by LAMICTAL have occurred within 2 to 8 weeks of treatment initiation. However, isolated cases have occurred after prolonged treatment (e.g., 6 months). Accordingly, duration of therapy cannot be relied upon as means to predict the potential risk heralded by the first appearance of a rash.

Although benign rashes are also caused by LAMICTAL, it is not possible to predict reliably which rashes will prove to be serious or life threatening. Accordingly, LAMICTAL should ordinarily be discontinued at the first sign of rash, unless the rash is clearly not drug related. Discontinuation of treatment may not prevent a rash from becoming life threatening or permanently disabling or disfiguring *[see Warnings and Precautions (5.1)]*.

1 INDICATIONS AND USAGE

1.1 Epilepsy

Adjunctive Therapy: LAMICTAL is indicated as adjunctive therapy for the following seizure types in patients ≥2 years of age:
- partial seizures
- primary generalized tonic-clonic seizures
- generalized seizures of Lennox-Gastaut syndrome

Monotherapy: LAMICTAL is indicated for conversion to monotherapy in adults (≥16 years of age) with partial seizures who are receiving treatment with carbamazepine, phenytoin, phenobarbital, primidone, or valproate as the single antiepileptic drug (AED).

Safety and effectiveness of LAMICTAL have not been established (1) as initial monotherapy; (2) for conversion to monotherapy from AEDs other than carbamazepine, phenytoin, phenobarbital, primidone, or valproate; or (3) for simultaneous conversion to monotherapy from 2 or more concomitant AEDs.

1.2 Bipolar Disorder

LAMICTAL is indicated for the maintenance treatment of Bipolar I Disorder to delay the time to occurrence of mood episodes (depression, mania, hypomania, mixed episodes) in adults (≥18 years of age) treated for acute mood episodes with standard therapy. The effectiveness of LAMICTAL in the acute treatment of mood episodes has not been established.

The effectiveness of LAMICTAL as maintenance treatment was established in 2 placebo-controlled trials in patients with Bipolar I Disorder as defined by DSM-IV *[see Clinical Studies (14.2)]*. The physician who elects to prescribe LAMICTAL for periods extending beyond 16 weeks should periodically re-evaluate the long-term usefulness of the drug for the individual patient.

2 DOSAGE AND ADMINISTRATION

2.1 General Dosing Considerations

Rash: There are suggestions, yet to be proven, that the risk of severe, potentially life-threatening rash may be increased by (1) coadministration of LAMICTAL with valproate, (2) exceeding the recommended initial dose of LAMICTAL, or (3) exceeding the recommended dose escalation for LAMICTAL. However, cases have occurred in the absence of these factors *[see Boxed Warning]*. Therefore, it is important that the dosing recommendations be followed closely.

The risk of nonserious rash may be increased when the recommended initial dose and/or the rate of dose escalation of LAMICTAL is exceeded and in patients with a history of allergy or rash to other AEDs.

LAMICTAL Starter Kits and LAMICTAL® ODT™ Patient Titration Kits provide LAMICTAL at doses consistent with the recommended titration schedule for the first 5 weeks of treatment, based upon concomitant medications, for patients with epilepsy (>12 years of age) and Bipolar I Disorder (≥18 years of age) and are intended to help reduce the potential for rash. The use of LAMICTAL Starter Kits and LAMICTAL ODT Patient Titration Kits is recommended for appropriate patients who are starting or restarting LAMICTAL *[see How Supplied/Storage and Handling (16)]*.

It is recommended that LAMICTAL not be restarted in patients who discontinued due to rash associated with prior treatment with lamotrigine, unless the potential benefits clearly outweigh the risks. If the decision is made to restart a patient who has discontinued lamotrigine, the need to restart with the initial dosing recommendations should be assessed. The greater the interval of time since the previous dose, the greater consideration should be given to restarting with the initial dosing recommendations. If a patient has discontinued lamotrigine for a period of more than 5 half-lives, it is recommended that initial dosing recommendations and guidelines be followed. The half-life of lamotrigine is affected by other concomitant medications *[see Clinical Pharmacology (12.3)]*.

LAMICTAL Added to Drugs Known to Induce or Inhibit Glucuronidation: Drugs other than those listed in the Clinical Pharmacology section *[see Clinical Pharmacology (12.3)]* have not been systematically evaluated in combination with lamotrigine. Because lamotrigine is metabolized predominantly by glucuronic acid conjugation, drugs that are known to induce or inhibit glucuronidation may affect the apparent clearance of lamotrigine and doses of LAMICTAL may require adjustment based on clinical response.

Target Plasma Levels for Patients With Epilepsy or Bipolar Disorder: A therapeutic plasma concentration range has not been established for lamotrigine. Dosing of LAMICTAL should be based on therapeutic response *[see Clinical Pharmacology (12.3)]*.

Women Taking Estrogen-Containing Oral Contraceptives: *Starting LAMICTAL in Women Taking Estrogen-Containing Oral Contraceptives:* Although estrogen-containing oral contraceptives have been shown to increase the clearance of lamotrigine *[see Clinical Pharmacology (12.3)]*, no adjustments to the recommended dose-escalation guidelines for LAMICTAL should be necessary solely based on the use of estrogen-containing oral contraceptives. Therefore, dose escalation should follow the recommended guidelines for initiating adjunctive therapy with LAMICTAL based on the concomitant AED or other concomitant medications (see Table 1 or Table 5). See below for adjustments to maintenance doses of LAMICTAL in women taking estrogen-containing oral contraceptives.

Adjustments to the Maintenance Dose of LAMICTAL in Women Taking Estrogen-Containing Oral Contraceptives:

(1) Taking Estrogen-Containing Oral Contraceptives: For women not taking carbamazepine, phenytoin, phenobarbital, primidone, or other drugs such as rifampin that induce lamotrigine glucuronidation *[see Drug Interactions (7), Clinical Pharmacology (12.3)]*, the maintenance dose of LAMICTAL will in most cases need to be increased, by as much as 2-fold over the recommended target maintenance dose, to maintain a consistent lamotrigine plasma level *[see Clinical Pharmacology (12.3)]*.

(2) Starting Estrogen-Containing Oral Contraceptives: In women taking a stable dose of LAMICTAL and not taking carbamazepine, phenytoin, phenobarbital, primidone, or other drugs such as rifampin that induce lamotrigine glucuronidation *[see Drug Interactions (7), Clinical Pharmacology (12.3)]*, the maintenance dose will in most cases need to be increased by as much as 2-fold to maintain a consistent lamotrigine plasma level. The dose increases should begin at the same time that the oral contraceptive is introduced and continue, based on clinical response, no more rapidly than 50 to 100 mg/day every week. Dose increases should not exceed the recommended rate (see Table 1 or Table 5) unless lamotrigine plasma levels or clinical response support larger increases. Gradual transient increases in lamotrigine plasma levels may occur during the week of inactive hormonal preparation ("pill-free" week), and these increases will be greater if dose increases are made in the days before or during the week of inactive hormonal preparation. Increased lamotrigine plasma levels could result in additional adverse reactions, such as dizziness, ataxia, and diplopia. If adverse reactions attributable to LAMICTAL consistently occur during the "pill-free" week, dose adjustments to the overall maintenance dose may be necessary. Dose adjustments limited to the "pill-free" week are not recommended. For women taking LAMICTAL in addition to carbamazepine, phenytoin, phenobarbital, primidone, or other drugs such as rifampin that induce lamotrigine glucuronidation *[see Drug Interactions (7), Clinical Pharmacology (12.3)]*, no adjustment to the dose of LAMICTAL should be necessary.

(3) Stopping Estrogen-Containing Oral Contraceptives: For women not taking carbamazepine, phenytoin, phenobarbital, primidone, or other drugs such as rifampin that induce lamotrigine glucuronidation *[see Drug Interactions (7), Clinical Pharmacology (12.3)]*, the maintenance dose of LAMICTAL will in most cases need to be decreased by as much as 50% in order to maintain a consistent lamotrigine plasma level. The decrease in dose of LAMICTAL should not exceed 25% of the total daily dose per week over a 2-week period, unless clinical response or lamotrigine plasma levels indicate otherwise *[see Clinical Pharmacology (12.3)]*. For women taking LAMICTAL in addition to carbamazepine, phenytoin, phenobarbital, primidone, or other drugs such as rifampin that induce lamotrigine glucuronidation *[see Drug Interactions (7), Clinical Pharmacology (12.3)]*, no adjustment to the dose of LAMICTAL should be necessary.

Women and Other Hormonal Contraceptive Preparations or Hormone Replacement Therapy: The effect of other hormonal contraceptive preparations or hormone replacement therapy on the pharmacokinetics of lamotrigine has not been systematically evaluated. It has been reported that ethinylestradiol, not progestogens, increased the clearance of lamotrigine up to 2-fold, and the progestin-only pills had no effect on lamotrigine plasma levels. Therefore, adjustments to the dosage of LAMICTAL in the presence of progestogens alone will likely not be needed.

Patients With Hepatic Impairment: Experience in patients with hepatic impairment is limited. Based on a clinical pharmacology study in 24 patients with mild, moderate,

Table 1. Escalation Regimen for LAMICTAL in Patients Over 12 Years of Age With Epilepsy

	For Patients TAKING Valproate[a]	For Patients NOT TAKING Carbamazepine, Phenytoin, Phenobarbital, Primidone,[b] or Valproate[a]	For Patients TAKING Carbamazepine, Phenytoin, Phenobarbital, or Primidone[b] and NOT TAKING Valproate[a]
Weeks 1 and 2	**25 mg every *other* day**	**25 mg every day**	**50 mg/day**
Weeks 3 and 4	**25 mg every day**	**50 mg/day**	**100 mg/day** (in 2 divided doses)
Week 5 onwards to maintenance	Increase by 25 to 50 mg/day every 1 to 2 weeks	Increase by 50 mg/day every 1 to 2 weeks	Increase by 100 mg/day every 1 to 2 weeks.
Usual maintenance dose	**100 to 200 mg/day with valproate alone** **100 to 400 mg/day with valproate and other drugs that induce glucuronidation** (in 1 or 2 divided doses)	**225 to 375 mg/day** (in 2 divided doses)	**300 to 500 mg/day** (in 2 divided doses)

[a]Valproate has been shown to inhibit glucuronidation and decrease the apparent clearance of lamotrigine *[see Drug Interactions (7), Clinical Pharmacology (12.3)]*.
[b]These drugs induce lamotrigine glucuronidation and increase clearance *[see Drug Interactions (7), Clinical Pharmacology (12.3)]*. Other drugs that have similar effects include estrogen-containing oral contraceptives *[see Drug Interactions (7), Clinical Pharmacology (12.3)]*. Dosing recommendations for oral contraceptives can be found in General Dosing Considerations *[see Dosage and Administration (2.1)]*. Patients on rifampin, or other drugs that induce lamotrigine glucuronidation and increase clearance, should follow the same dosing titration/maintenance regimen as that used with anticonvulsants that have this effect.

Table 2. Escalation Regimen for LAMICTAL in Patients 2 to 12 Years of Age With Epilepsy

	For Patients TAKING Valproate[a]	For Patients NOT TAKING Carbamazepine, Phenytoin, Phenobarbital, Primidone,[b] or Valproate[a]	For Patients TAKING Carbamazepine, Phenytoin, Phenobarbital, or Primidone[b] and NOT TAKING Valproate[a]
Weeks 1 and 2	**0.15 mg/kg/day** in 1 or 2 divided doses, rounded down to the nearest whole tablet (see Table 3 for weight-based dosing guide)	**0.3 mg/kg/day** in 1 or 2 divided doses, rounded down to the nearest whole tablet	**0.6 mg/kg/day** in 2 divided doses, rounded down to the nearest whole tablet
Weeks 3 and 4	**0.3 mg/kg/day** in 1 or 2 divided doses, rounded down to the nearest whole tablet (see Table 3 for weight-based dosing guide)	**0.6 mg/kg/day** in 2 divided doses, rounded down to the nearest whole tablet	**1.2 mg/kg/day** in 2 divided doses, rounded down to the nearest whole tablet
Week 5 onwards to maintenance	The dose should be increased every 1 to 2 weeks as follows: calculate 0.3 mg/kg/day, round this amount down to the nearest whole tablet, and add this amount to the previously administered daily dose	The dose should be increased every 1 to 2 weeks as follows: calculate 0.6 mg/kg/day, round this amount down to the nearest whole tablet, and add this amount to the previously administered daily dose	The dose should be increased every 1 to 2 weeks as follows: calculate 1.2 mg/kg/day, round this amount down to the nearest whole tablet, and add this amount to the previously administered daily dose
Usual maintenance dose	**1 to 5 mg/kg/day**(maximum 200 mg/day in 1 or 2 divided doses) **1 to 3 mg/kg/day** with valproate alone	**4.5 to 7.5 mg/kg/day** (maximum 300 mg/day in 2 divided doses)	**5 to 15 mg/kg/day** (maximum 400 mg/day in 2 divided doses)
Maintenance dose in patients less than 30 kg	May need to be increased by as much as 50%, based on clinical response	May need to be increased by as much as 50%, based on clinical response	May need to be increased by as much as 50%, based on clinical response

Note: Only whole tablets should be used for dosing.
[a]Valproate has been shown to inhibit glucuronidation and decrease the apparent clearance of lamotrigine *[see Drug Interactions (7), Clinical Pharmacology (12.3)]*.
[b]These drugs induce lamotrigine glucuronidation and increase clearance *[see Drug Interactions (7), Clinical Pharmacology (12.3)]*. Other drugs that have similar effects include estrogen-containing oral contraceptives *[see Drug Interactions (7), Clinical Pharmacology (12.3)]*. Dosing recommendations for oral contraceptives can be found in General Dosing Considerations *[see Dosage and Administration (2.1)]*. Patients on rifampin, or other drugs that induce lamotrigine glucuronidation and increase clearance, should follow the same dosing titration/maintenance regimen as that used with anticonvulsants that have this effect.

and severe liver impairment *[see Use in Specific Populations (8.6), Clinical Pharmacology (12.3)]*, the following general recommendations can be made. No dosage adjustment is needed in patients with mild liver impairment. Initial, escalation, and maintenance doses should generally be reduced by approximately 25% in patients with moderate and severe liver impairment without ascites and 50% in patients with severe liver impairment with ascites. Escalation and maintenance doses may be adjusted according to clinical response.

Patients With Renal Impairment: Initial doses of LAMICTAL should be based on patients' concomitant medications (see Tables 1-3 or Table 5); reduced maintenance doses may be effective for patients with significant renal impairment *[see Use in Specific Populations (8.7), Clinical Pharmacology (12.3)]*. Few patients with severe renal impairment have been evaluated during chronic treatment with LAMICTAL. Because there is inadequate experience in this population, LAMICTAL should be used with caution in these patients.

Discontinuation Strategy: *Epilepsy:* For patients receiving LAMICTAL in combination with other AEDs, a re-evaluation of all AEDs in the regimen should be considered if a change in seizure control or an appearance or worsening of adverse reactions is observed.
If a decision is made to discontinue therapy with LAMICTAL, a step-wise reduction of dose over at least 2 weeks (approximately 50% per week) is recommended unless safety concerns require a more rapid withdrawal *[see Warnings and Precautions (5.9)]*.
Discontinuing carbamazepine, phenytoin, phenobarbital, primidone, or other drugs such as rifampin that induce lamotrigine glucuronidation should prolong the half-life of lamotrigine; discontinuing valproate should shorten the half-life of lamotrigine.
Bipolar Disorder: In the controlled clinical trials, there was no increase in the incidence, type, or severity of adverse reactions following abrupt termination of LAMICTAL. In clinical trials in patients with Bipolar Disorder, 2 patients experienced seizures shortly after abrupt withdrawal of LAMICTAL. However, there were confounding factors that may have contributed to the occurrence of seizures in these bipolar patients. Discontinuation of LAMICTAL should involve a step-wise reduction of dose over at least 2 weeks (approximately 50% per week) unless safety concerns require a more rapid withdrawal *[see Warnings and Precautions (5.9)]*.

2.2 Epilepsy – Adjunctive Therapy

This section provides specific dosing recommendations for patients greater than 12 years of age and patients 2 to 12 years of age. Within each of these age-groups, specific dosing recommendations are provided depending upon concomitant AED or other concomitant medications (Table 1 for patients greater than 12 years of age and Table 2 for patients 2 to 12 years of age). A weight-based dosing guide for patients 2 to 12 years of age on concomitant valproate is provided in Table 3.
Patients Over 12 Years of Age: Recommended dosing guidelines are summarized in Table 1.
[See table 1 above]
Patients 2 to 12 Years of Age: Recommended dosing guidelines are summarized in Table 2.
Smaller starting doses and slower dose escalations than those used in clinical trials are recommended because of the suggestion that the risk of rash may be decreased by smaller starting doses and slower dose escalations. Therefore, maintenance doses will take longer to reach in clinical practice than in clinical trials. It may take several weeks to months to achieve an individualized maintenance dose. Maintenance doses in patients weighing less than 30 kg, regardless of age or concomitant AED, may need to be increased as much as 50%, based on clinical response.
The smallest available strength of LAMICTAL Chewable Dispersible Tablets is 2 mg, and only whole tablets should be administered. If the calculated dose cannot be achieved using whole tablets, the dose should be rounded down to the nearest whole tablet *[see How Supplied/Storage and Handling (16) and Medication Guide]*.
[See table 2 above]

Table 3. The Initial Weight-Based Dosing Guide for Patients 2 to 12 Years of Age Taking Valproate (Weeks 1 to 4) With Epilepsy

If the patient's weight is		Give this daily dose, using the most appropriate combination of LAMICTAL 2-mg and 5-mg tablets	
Greater than	And less than	Weeks 1 and 2	Weeks 3 and 4
6.7 kg	14 kg	2 mg every *other* day	2 mg every day
14.1 kg	27 kg	2 mg every day	4 mg every day
27.1 kg	34 kg	4 mg every day	8 mg every day
34.1 kg	40 kg	5 mg every day	10 mg every day

Usual Adjunctive Maintenance Dose for Epilepsy: The usual maintenance doses identified in Tables 1 and 2 are derived from dosing regimens employed in the placebo-controlled adjunctive studies in which the efficacy of LAMICTAL was established. In patients receiving multidrug regimens employing carbamazepine, phenytoin, phenobarbital, or primidone **without valproate**, maintenance doses of adjunctive LAMICTAL as high as 700 mg/day have been used. In patients receiving **valproate alone**, maintenance doses of adjunctive LAMICTAL as high as 200 mg/day have been used. The advantage of using doses above those recommended in Tables 1 through 4 has not been established in controlled trials.

Table 5. Escalation Regimen for LAMICTAL for Patients With Bipolar Disorder

	For Patients TAKING Valproate[a]	For Patients NOT TAKING Carbamazepine, Phenytoin, Phenobarbital, Primidone,[b] or Valproate[a]	For Patients TAKING Carbamazepine, Phenytoin, Phenobarbital, or Primidone[b] and NOT TAKING Valproate[a]
Weeks 1 and 2	25 mg every *other* day	25 mg daily	50 mg daily
Weeks 3 and 4	25 mg daily	50 mg daily	100 mg daily, in divided doses
Week 5	50 mg daily	100 mg daily	200 mg daily, in divided doses
Week 6	100 mg daily	200 mg daily	300 mg daily, in divided doses
Week 7	100 mg daily	200 mg daily	up to 400 mg daily, in divided doses

[a]Valproate has been shown to inhibit glucuronidation and decrease the apparent clearance of lamotrigine *[see Drug Interactions (7), Clinical Pharmacology (12.3)]*.
[b]These drugs induce lamotrigine glucuronidation and increase clearance *[see Drug Interactions (7), Clinical Pharmacology (12.3)]*. Other drugs that have similar effects include estrogen-containing oral contraceptives *[see Drug Interactions (7), Clinical Pharmacology (12.3)]*. Dosing recommendations for oral contraceptives can be found in General Dosing Considerations *[see Dosage and Administration (2.1)]*. Patients on rifampin, or other drugs that induce lamotrigine glucuronidation and increase clearance, should follow the same dosing titration/maintenance regimen as that used with anticonvulsants that have this effect.

Table 6. Dosage Adjustments to LAMICTAL for Patients With Bipolar Disorder Following Discontinuation of Psychotropic Medications

	Discontinuation of Psychotropic Drugs (excluding Carbamazepine, Phenytoin, Phenobarbital, Primidone,[b] or Valproate[a])	After Discontinuation of Valproate[a]	After Discontinuation of Carbamazepine, Phenytoin, Phenobarbital, or Primidone[b]
		Current dose of LAMICTAL (mg/day) 100	Current dose of LAMICTAL (mg/day) 400
Week 1	Maintain current dose of LAMICTAL	150	400
Week 2	Maintain current dose of LAMICTAL	200	300
Week 3 onward	Maintain current dose of LAMICTAL	200	200

[a]Valproate has been shown to inhibit glucuronidation and decrease the apparent clearance of lamotrigine *[see Drug Interactions (7), Clinical Pharmacology (12.3)]*.
[b]These drugs induce lamotrigine glucuronidation and increase clearance *[see Drug Interactions (7), Clinical Pharmacology (12.3)]*. Other drugs that have similar effects include estrogen-containing oral contraceptives *[see Drug Interactions (7), Clinical Pharmacology (12.3)]*. Dosing recommendations for oral contraceptives can be found in General Dosing Considerations *[see Dosage and Administration (2.1)]*. Patients on rifampin, or other drugs that induce lamotrigine glucuronidation and increase clearance, should follow the same dosing titration/maintenance regimen as that used with anticonvulsants that have this effect.

2.3 Epilepsy – Conversion From Adjunctive Therapy to Monotherapy

The goal of the transition regimen is to effect the conversion to monotherapy with LAMICTAL under conditions that ensure adequate seizure control while mitigating the risk of serious rash associated with the rapid titration of LAMICTAL.

The recommended maintenance dose of LAMICTAL as monotherapy is 500 mg/day given in 2 divided doses.

To avoid an increased risk of rash, the recommended initial dose and subsequent dose escalations of LAMICTAL should not be exceeded *[see Boxed Warning]*.

Conversion From Adjunctive Therapy With Carbamazepine, Phenytoin, Phenobarbital, or Primidone to Monotherapy With LAMICTAL: After achieving a dose of 500 mg/day of LAMICTAL according to the guidelines in Table 1, the concomitant AED should be withdrawn by 20% decrements each week over a 4-week period. The regimen for the withdrawal of the concomitant AED is based on experience gained in the controlled monotherapy clinical trial.

Conversion From Adjunctive Therapy With Valproate to Monotherapy With LAMICTAL: The conversion regimen involves 4 steps outlined in Table 4.

Table 4. Conversion From Adjunctive Therapy With Valproate to Monotherapy With LAMICTAL in Patients ≥16 Years of Age With Epilepsy

	LAMICTAL	Valproate
Step 1	Achieve a dose of 200 mg/day according to guidelines in Table 1 (if not already on 200 mg/day).	Maintain previous stable dose.
Step 2	Maintain at 200 mg/day.	Decrease to 500 mg/day by decrements no greater than 500 mg/day/week and then maintain the dose of 500 mg/day for 1 week.
Step 3	Increase to 300 mg/day and maintain for 1 week.	Simultaneously decrease to 250 mg/day and maintain for 1 week.
Step 4	Increase by 100 mg/day every week to achieve maintenance dose of 500 mg/day.	Discontinue.

Conversion From Adjunctive Therapy With Antiepileptic Drugs Other Than Carbamazepine, Phenytoin, Phenobarbital, Primidone, or Valproate to Monotherapy With LAMICTAL: No specific dosing guidelines can be provided for conversion to monotherapy with LAMICTAL with AEDs other than carbamazepine, phenobarbital, phenytoin, primidone, or valproate.

2.4 Bipolar Disorder

The goal of maintenance treatment with LAMICTAL is to delay the time to occurrence of mood episodes (depression, mania, hypomania, mixed episodes) in patients treated for acute mood episodes with standard therapy. The target dose of LAMICTAL is 200 mg/day (100 mg/day in patients taking valproate, which decreases the apparent clearance of lamotrigine, and 400 mg/day in patients not taking valproate and taking either carbamazepine, phenytoin, phenobarbital, primidone, or other drugs such as rifampin that increase the apparent clearance of lamotrigine). In the clinical trials, doses up to 400 mg/day as monotherapy were evaluated; however, no additional benefit was seen at 400 mg/day compared with 200 mg/day *[see Clinical Studies (14.2)]*. Accordingly, doses above 200 mg/day are not recommended. Treatment with LAMICTAL is introduced, based on concurrent medications, according to the regimen outlined in Table 5. If other psychotropic medications are withdrawn following stabilization, the dose of LAMICTAL should be adjusted. For patients discontinuing valproate, the dose of LAMICTAL should be doubled over a 2-week period in equal weekly increments (see Table 6). For patients discontinuing carbamazepine, phenytoin, phenobarbital, primidone, or other drugs such as rifampin that induce lamotrigine glucuronidation, the dose of LAMICTAL should remain constant for the first week and then should be decreased by half over a 2-week period in equal weekly decrements (see Table 6). The dose of LAMICTAL may then be further adjusted to the target dose (200 mg) as clinically indicated.

If other drugs are subsequently introduced, the dose of LAMICTAL may need to be adjusted. In particular, the introduction of valproate requires reduction in the dose of LAMICTAL *[see Drug Interactions (7), Clinical Pharmacology (12.3)]*.

To avoid an increased risk of rash, the recommended initial dose and subsequent dose escalations of LAMICTAL should not be exceeded *[see Boxed Warning]*.

[See table 5 above]

[See table 6 above]

The benefit of continuing treatment in patients who had been stabilized in an 8- to 16-week open-label phase with LAMICTAL was established in 2 randomized, placebo-controlled clinical maintenance trials *[see Clinical Studies (14.2)]*. However, the optimal duration of treatment with LAMICTAL has not been established. Thus, patients should be periodically reassessed to determine the need for maintenance treatment.

2.5 Administration of LAMICTAL Chewable Dispersible Tablets

LAMICTAL Chewable Dispersible Tablets may be swallowed whole, chewed, or dispersed in water or diluted fruit juice. If the tablets are chewed, consume a small amount of water or diluted fruit juice to aid in swallowing.

To disperse LAMICTAL Chewable Dispersible Tablets, add the tablets to a small amount of liquid (1 teaspoon, or enough to cover the medication). Approximately 1 minute later, when the tablets are completely dispersed, swirl the solution and consume the entire quantity immediately. *No attempt should be made to administer partial quantities of the dispersed tablets.*

2.6 Administration of LAMICTAL ODT Orally Disintegrating Tablets

LAMICTAL ODT Orally Disintegrating Tablets should be placed onto the tongue and moved around in the mouth. The tablet will disintegrate rapidly, can be swallowed with or without water, and can be taken with or without food.

3 DOSAGE FORMS AND STRENGTHS

3.1 Tablets

25 mg, white, scored, shield-shaped tablets debossed with "LAMICTAL" and "25."

100 mg, peach, scored, shield-shaped tablets debossed with "LAMICTAL" and "100."

150 mg, cream, scored, shield-shaped tablets debossed with "LAMICTAL" and "150."

200 mg, blue, scored, shield-shaped tablets debossed with "LAMICTAL" and "200."

3.2 Chewable Dispersible Tablets

2 mg, white to off-white, round tablets debossed with "LTG" over "2."

5 mg, white to off-white, caplet-shaped tablets debossed with "GX CL2."

25 mg, white, super elliptical-shaped tablets debossed with "GX CL5."

3.3 Orally Disintegrating Tablets

25 mg, white to off-white, round, flat-faced, radius edge, tablets debossed with "LMT" on one side and "25" on the other side.

50 mg, white to off-white, round, flat-faced, radius edge, tablets debossed with "LMT" on one side and "50" on the other side.

100 mg, white to off-white, round, flat-faced, radius edge, tablets debossed with "LAMICTAL" on one side and "100" on the other side.

200 mg, white to off-white, round, flat-faced, radius edge, tablets debossed with "LAMICTAL" on one side and "200" on the other side.

3.4 Potential Medication Errors

Patients should be strongly advised to visually inspect their tablets to verify that they are receiving LAMICTAL as well as the correct formulation of LAMICTAL each time they fill their prescription. Depictions of the LAMICTAL Tablets,

Chewable Dispersible Tablets, and Orally Disintegrating Tablets can be found in the Medication Guide that accompanies the product.

4 CONTRAINDICATIONS

LAMICTAL is contraindicated in patients who have demonstrated hypersensitivity to the drug or its ingredients *[see Boxed Warning, Warnings and Precautions (5.1, 5.2)]*.

5 WARNINGS AND PRECAUTIONS

5.1 Serious Skin Rashes

[see Boxed Warning]

Pediatric Population: The incidence of serious rash associated with hospitalization and discontinuation of LAMICTAL in a prospectively followed cohort of pediatric patients (2 to 16 years of age) with epilepsy receiving adjunctive therapy was approximately 0.8% (16 of 1,983). When 14 of these cases were reviewed by 3 expert dermatologists, there was considerable disagreement as to their proper classification. To illustrate, one dermatologist considered none of the cases to be Stevens-Johnson syndrome; another assigned 7 of the 14 to this diagnosis. There was 1 rash-related death in this 1,983-patient cohort. Additionally, there have been rare cases of toxic epidermal necrolysis with and without permanent sequelae and/or death in US and foreign postmarketing experience.

There is evidence that the inclusion of valproate in a multidrug regimen increases the risk of serious, potentially life-threatening rash in pediatric patients. In pediatric patients who used valproate concomitantly, 1.2% (6 of 482) experienced a serious rash compared with 0.6% (6 of 952) patients not taking valproate.

Adult Population: Serious rash associated with hospitalization and discontinuation of LAMICTAL occurred in 0.3% (11 of 3,348) of adult patients who received LAMICTAL in premarketing clinical trials of epilepsy. In the bipolar and other mood disorders clinical trials, the rate of serious rash was 0.08% (1 of 1,233) of adult patients who received LAMICTAL as initial monotherapy and 0.13% (2 of 1,538) of adult patients who received LAMICTAL as adjunctive therapy. No fatalities occurred among these individuals. However, in worldwide postmarketing experience, rare cases of rash-related death have been reported, but their numbers are too few to permit a precise estimate of the rate.

Among the rashes leading to hospitalization were Stevens-Johnson syndrome, toxic epidermal necrolysis, angioedema, and those associated with multiorgan hypersensitivity *[see Warnings and Precautions (5.2)]*.

There is evidence that the inclusion of valproate in a multidrug regimen increases the risk of serious, potentially life-threatening rash in adults. Specifically, of 584 patients administered LAMICTAL with valproate in epilepsy clinical trials, 6 (1%) were hospitalized in association with rash; in contrast, 4 (0.16%) of 2,398 clinical trial patients and volunteers administered LAMICTAL in the absence of valproate were hospitalized.

Patients With History of Allergy or Rash to Other Antiepileptic Drugs: The risk of nonserious rash may be increased when the recommended initial dose and/or the rate of dose escalation of LAMICTAL is exceeded and in patients with a history of allergy or rash to other AEDs.

5.2 Multiorgan Hypersensitivity Reactions and Organ Failure

Multiorgan hypersensitivity reactions, also known as Drug Reaction with Eosinophilia and Systemic Symptoms (DRESS), have occurred with LAMICTAL. Some have been fatal or life threatening. DRESS typically, although not exclusively, presents with fever, rash, and/or lymphadenopathy in association with other organ system involvement, such as hepatitis, nephritis, hematologic abnormalities, myocarditis, or myositis, sometimes resembling an acute viral infection. Eosinophilia is often present. This disorder is variable in its expression, and other organ systems not noted here may be involved.

Fatalities associated with acute multiorgan failure and various degrees of hepatic failure have been reported in 2 of 3,796 adult patients and 4 of 2,435 pediatric patients who received LAMICTAL in epilepsy clinical trials. Rare fatalities from multiorgan failure have also been reported in postmarketing use.

Isolated liver failure without rash or involvement of other organs has also been reported with LAMICTAL.

It is important to note that early manifestations of hypersensitivity (e.g., fever, lymphadenopathy) may be present even though a rash is not evident. If such signs or symptoms are present, the patient should be evaluated immediately. LAMICTAL should be discontinued if an alternative etiology for the signs or symptoms cannot be established.

Prior to initiation of treatment with LAMICTAL, the patient should be instructed that a rash or other signs or symptoms (e.g., fever, lymphadenopathy) may herald a serious medical event and that the patient should report any such occurrence to a physician immediately.

Table 7. Risk by Indication for Antiepileptic Drugs in the Pooled Analysis

Indication	Placebo Patients With Events Per 1,000 Patients	Drug Patients With Events Per 1,000 Patients	Relative Risk: Incidence of Events in Drug Patients/ Incidence in Placebo Patients	Risk Difference: Additional Drug Patients With Events Per 1,000 Patients
Epilepsy	1.0	3.4	3.5	2.4
Psychiatric	5.7	8.5	1.5	2.9
Other	1.0	1.8	1.9	0.9
Total	2.4	4.3	1.8	1.9

5.3 Blood Dyscrasias

There have been reports of blood dyscrasias that may or may not be associated with multiorgan hypersensitivity (also known as DRESS) *[see Warnings and Precautions (5.2)]*. These have included neutropenia, leukopenia, anemia, thrombocytopenia, pancytopenia, and, rarely, aplastic anemia and pure red cell aplasia.

5.4 Suicidal Behavior and Ideation

AEDs, including LAMICTAL, increase the risk of suicidal thoughts or behavior in patients taking these drugs for any indication. Patients treated with any AED for any indication should be monitored for the emergence or worsening of depression, suicidal thoughts or behavior, and/or any unusual changes in mood or behavior.

Pooled analyses of 199 placebo-controlled clinical trials (monotherapy and adjunctive therapy) of 11 different AEDs showed that patients randomized to 1 of the AEDs had approximately twice the risk (adjusted Relative Risk 1.8, 95% CI:1.2, 2.7) of suicidal thinking or behavior compared to patients randomized to placebo. In these trials, which had a median treatment duration of 12 weeks, the estimated incidence of suicidal behavior or ideation among 27,863 AED-treated patients was 0.43%, compared to 0.24% among 16,029 placebo-treated patients, representing an increase of approximately 1 case of suicidal thinking or behavior for every 530 patients treated. There were 4 suicides in drug-treated patients in the trials and none in placebo-treated patients, but the number of events is too small to allow any conclusion about drug effect on suicide.

The increased risk of suicidal thoughts or behavior with AEDs was observed as early as 1 week after starting treatment with AEDs and persisted for the duration of treatment assessed. Because most trials included in the analysis did not extend beyond 24 weeks, the risk of suicidal thoughts or behavior beyond 24 weeks could not be assessed.

The risk of suicidal thoughts or behavior was generally consistent among drugs in the data analyzed. The finding of increased risk with AEDs of varying mechanism of action and across a range of indications suggests that the risk applies to all AEDs used for any indication. The risk did not vary substantially by age (5 to 100 years) in the clinical trials analyzed.

Table 7 shows absolute and relative risk by indication for all evaluated AEDs.

[See table 7 above]

The relative risk for suicidal thoughts or behavior was higher in clinical trials for epilepsy than in clinical trials for psychiatric or other conditions, but the absolute risk differences were similar for the epilepsy and psychiatric indications.

Anyone considering prescribing LAMICTAL or any other AED must balance the risk of suicidal thoughts or behavior with the risk of untreated illness. Epilepsy and many other illnesses for which AEDs are prescribed are themselves associated with morbidity and mortality and an increased risk of suicidal thoughts and behavior. Should suicidal thoughts and behavior emerge during treatment, the prescriber needs to consider whether the emergence of these symptoms in any given patient may be related to the illness being treated.

Patients, their caregivers, and families should be informed that AEDs increase the risk of suicidal thoughts and behavior and should be advised of the need to be alert for the emergence or worsening of the signs and symptoms of depression, any unusual changes in mood or behavior, or the emergence of suicidal thoughts, behavior, or thoughts about self-harm. Behaviors of concern should be reported immediately to healthcare providers.

5.5 Use in Patients With Bipolar Disorder

Acute Treatment of Mood Episodes: Safety and effectiveness of LAMICTAL in the acute treatment of mood episodes have not been established.

Children and Adolescents (less than 18 years of age): Safety and effectiveness of LAMICTAL in patients below the age of 18 years with mood disorders have not been established *[see Suicidal Behavior and Ideation (5.4)]*.

Clinical Worsening and Suicide Risk Associated With Bipolar Disorder: Patients with bipolar disorder may experience worsening of their depressive symptoms and/or the emergence of suicidal ideation and behaviors (suicidality) whether or not they are taking medications for bipolar disorder. Patients should be closely monitored for clinical worsening (including development of new symptoms) and suicidality, especially at the beginning of a course of treatment or at the time of dose changes.

In addition, patients with a history of suicidal behavior or thoughts, those patients exhibiting a significant degree of suicidal ideation prior to commencement of treatment, and young adults are at an increased risk of suicidal thoughts or suicide attempts and should receive careful monitoring during treatment *[see Suicidal Behavior and Ideation (5.4)]*.

Consideration should be given to changing the therapeutic regimen, including possibly discontinuing the medication, in patients who experience clinical worsening (including development of new symptoms) and/or the emergence of suicidal ideation/behavior especially if these symptoms are severe, abrupt in onset, or were not part of the patient's presenting symptoms.

Prescriptions for LAMICTAL should be written for the smallest quantity of tablets consistent with good patient management in order to reduce the risk of overdose. Overdoses have been reported for LAMICTAL, some of which have been fatal *[see Overdosage (10.1)]*.

5.6 Aseptic Meningitis

Therapy with LAMICTAL increases the risk of developing aseptic meningitis. Because of the potential for serious outcomes of untreated meningitis due to other causes, patients should also be evaluated for other causes of meningitis and treated as appropriate.

Postmarketing cases of aseptic meningitis have been reported in pediatric and adult patients taking LAMICTAL for various indications. Symptoms upon presentation have included headache, fever, nausea, vomiting, and nuchal rigidity. Rash, photophobia, myalgia, chills, altered consciousness, and somnolence were also noted in some cases. Symptoms have been reported to occur within 1 day to one and a half months following the initiation of treatment. In most cases, symptoms were reported to resolve after discontinuation of LAMICTAL. Re-exposure resulted in a rapid return of symptoms (from within 30 minutes to 1 day following re-initiation of treatment) that were frequently more severe. Some of the patients treated with LAMICTAL who developed aseptic meningitis had underlying diagnoses of systemic lupus erythematosus or other autoimmune diseases. Cerebrospinal fluid (CSF) analyzed at the time of clinical presentation in reported cases was characterized by a mild-to-moderate pleocytosis, normal glucose levels, and mild-to-moderate increase in protein. CSF white blood cell count differentials showed a predominance of neutrophils in a majority of the cases, although a predominance of lymphocytes was reported in approximately one third of the cases. Some patients also had new onset of signs and symptoms of involvement of other organs (predominantly hepatic and renal involvement), which may suggest that in these cases the aseptic meningitis observed was part of a hypersensitivity reaction *[see Warnings and Precautions (5.2)]*.

5.7 Potential Medication Errors

Medication errors involving LAMICTAL have occurred. In particular, the names LAMICTAL or lamotrigine can be confused with the names of other commonly used medications. Medication errors may also occur between the different formulations of LAMICTAL. To reduce the potential of medication errors, write and say LAMICTAL clearly. Depictions of the LAMICTAL Tablets, Chewable Dispersible Tablets, and Orally Disintegrating Tablets can be found in the Medication Guide that accompanies the product to highlight the distinctive markings, colors, and shapes that serve to identify the different presentations of the drug and thus may help reduce the risk of medication errors. To avoid the medication error of using the wrong drug or formulation, patients should be strongly advised to visually inspect their tablets to verify that they are LAMICTAL, as well as the correct formulation of LAMICTAL, each time they fill their prescription.

5.8 Concomitant Use With Oral Contraceptives

Some estrogen-containing oral contraceptives have been shown to decrease serum concentrations of lamotrigine *[see*

Clinical Pharmacology (12.3)]. **Dosage adjustments will be necessary in most patients who start or stop estrogen-containing oral contraceptives while taking LAMICTAL***[see Dosage and Administration (2.1)]*. During the week of inactive hormone preparation ("pill-free" week) of oral contraceptive therapy, plasma lamotrigine levels are expected to rise, as much as doubling at the end of the week. Adverse reactions consistent with elevated levels of lamotrigine, such as dizziness, ataxia, and diplopia, could occur.

5.9 Withdrawal Seizures

As with other AEDs, LAMICTAL should not be abruptly discontinued. In patients with epilepsy there is a possibility of increasing seizure frequency. In clinical trials in patients with Bipolar Disorder, 2 patients experienced seizures shortly after abrupt withdrawal of LAMICTAL; however, there were confounding factors that may have contributed to the occurrence of seizures in these bipolar patients. Unless safety concerns require a more rapid withdrawal, the dose of LAMICTAL should be tapered over a period of at least 2 weeks (approximately 50% reduction per week) *[see Dosage and Administration (2.1)]*.

5.10 Status Epilepticus

Valid estimates of the incidence of treatment-emergent status epilepticus among patients treated with LAMICTAL are difficult to obtain because reporters participating in clinical trials did not all employ identical rules for identifying cases. At a minimum, 7 of 2,343 adult patients had episodes that could unequivocally be described as status epilepticus. In addition, a number of reports of variably defined episodes of seizure exacerbation (e.g., seizure clusters, seizure flurries) were made.

5.11 Sudden Unexplained Death in Epilepsy (SUDEP)

During the premarketing development of LAMICTAL, 20 sudden and unexplained deaths were recorded among a cohort of 4,700 patients with epilepsy (5,747 patient-years of exposure).

Some of these could represent seizure-related deaths in which the seizure was not observed, e.g., at night. This represents an incidence of 0.0035 deaths per patient-year. Although this rate exceeds that expected in a healthy population matched for age and sex, it is within the range of estimates for the incidence of sudden unexplained deaths in patients with epilepsy not receiving LAMICTAL (ranging from 0.0005 for the general population of patients with epilepsy, to 0.004 for a recently studied clinical trial population similar to that in the clinical development program for LAMICTAL, to 0.005 for patients with refractory epilepsy). Consequently, whether these figures are reassuring or suggest concern depends on the comparability of the populations reported upon to the cohort receiving LAMICTAL and the accuracy of the estimates provided. Probably most reassuring is the similarity of estimated SUDEP rates in patients receiving LAMICTAL and those receiving other AEDs, chemically unrelated to each other, that underwent clinical testing in similar populations. Importantly, that drug is chemically unrelated to LAMICTAL. This evidence suggests, although it certainly does not prove, that the high SUDEP rates reflect population rates, not a drug effect.

5.12 Addition of LAMICTAL to a Multidrug Regimen That Includes Valproate

Because valproate reduces the clearance of lamotrigine, the dosage of lamotrigine in the presence of valproate is less than half of that required in its absence.

5.13 Binding in the Eye and Other Melanin-Containing Tissues

Because lamotrigine binds to melanin, it could accumulate in melanin-rich tissues over time. This raises the possibility that lamotrigine may cause toxicity in these tissues after extended use. Although ophthalmological testing was performed in 1 controlled clinical trial, the testing was inadequate to exclude subtle effects or injury occurring after long-term exposure. Moreover, the capacity of available tests to detect potentially adverse consequences, if any, of lamotrigine's binding to melanin is unknown *[see Clinical Pharmacology (12.2)]*.

Accordingly, although there are no specific recommendations for periodic ophthalmological monitoring, prescribers should be aware of the possibility of long-term ophthalmologic effects.

5.14 Laboratory Tests

The value of monitoring plasma concentrations of lamotrigine in patients treated with LAMICTAL has not been established. Because of the possible pharmacokinetic interactions between lamotrigine and other drugs including AEDs (see Table 15), monitoring of the plasma levels of lamotrigine and concomitant drugs may be indicated, particularly during dosage adjustments. In general, clinical judgment should be exercised regarding monitoring of plasma levels of lamotrigine and other drugs and whether or not dosage adjustments are necessary.

6 ADVERSE REACTIONS

The following adverse reactions are described in more detail in the *Warnings and Precautions* section of the label:

- Serious skin rashes *[see Warnings and Precautions (5.1)]*
- Multiorgan hypersensitivity reactions and organ failure *[see Warnings and Precautions (5.2)]*
- *Blood dyscrasias [see Warnings and Precautions (5.3)]*
- *Suicidal behavior and ideation [see Warnings and Precautions (5.4)]*
- Aseptic meningitis *[see Warnings and Precautions (5.6)]*
- Withdrawal seizures *[see Warnings and Precautions(5.9)]*
- Status epilepticus *[see Warnings and Precautions(5.10)]*
- Sudden unexplained death in epilepsy *[see Warnings and Precautions(5.11)]*

6.1 Clinical Trials

Because clinical trials are conducted under widely varying conditions, adverse reaction rates observed in the clinical trials of a drug cannot be directly compared with rates in the clinical trials of another drug and may not reflect the rates observed in practice.

LAMICTAL has been evaluated for safety in patients with epilepsy and in patients with Bipolar I Disorder. Adverse reactions reported for each of these patient populations are provided below. Excluded are adverse reactions considered too general to be informative and those not reasonably attributable to the use of the drug.

Epilepsy: *Most Common Adverse Reactions in All Clinical Studies: Adjunctive Therapy in Adults With Epilepsy:* The most commonly observed (≥5% for LAMICTAL and more common on drug than placebo) adverse reactions seen in association with LAMICTAL during adjunctive therapy in adults and not seen at an equivalent frequency among placebo-treated patients were: dizziness, ataxia, somnolence, headache, diplopia, blurred vision, nausea, vomiting, and rash. Dizziness, diplopia, ataxia, blurred vision, nausea, and vomiting were dose-related. Dizziness, diplopia, ataxia, and blurred vision occurred more commonly in patients receiving carbamazepine with LAMICTAL than in patients receiving other AEDs with LAMICTAL. Clinical data suggest a higher incidence of rash, including serious rash, in patients receiving concomitant valproate than in patients not receiving valproate *[see Warnings and Precautions (5.1)]*.

Approximately 11% of the 3,378 adult patients who received LAMICTAL as adjunctive therapy in premarketing clinical trials discontinued treatment because of an adverse reaction. The adverse reactions most commonly associated with discontinuation were rash (3.0%), dizziness (2.8%), and headache (2.5%).

In a dose-response study in adults, the rate of discontinuation of LAMICTAL for dizziness, ataxia, diplopia, blurred vision, nausea, and vomiting was dose-related.

Monotherapy in Adults With Epilepsy: The most commonly observed (≥5% for LAMICTAL and more common on drug than placebo) adverse reactions seen in association with the use of LAMICTAL during the monotherapy phase of the controlled trial in adults not seen at an equivalent rate in the control group were vomiting, coordination abnormality, dyspepsia, nausea, dizziness, rhinitis, anxiety, insomnia, infection, pain, weight decrease, chest pain, and dysmenorrhea. The most commonly observed (≥5% for LAMICTAL and more common on drug than placebo) adverse reactions associated with the use of LAMICTAL during the conversion to monotherapy (add-on) period, not seen at an equivalent frequency among low-dose valproate-treated patients, were dizziness, headache, nausea, asthenia, coordination abnormality, vomiting, rash, somnolence, diplopia, ataxia, accidental injury, tremor, blurred vision, insomnia, nystagmus, diarrhea, lymphadenopathy, pruritus, and sinusitis.

Approximately 10% of the 420 adult patients who received LAMICTAL as monotherapy in premarketing clinical trials discontinued treatment because of an adverse reaction. The adverse reactions most commonly associated with discontinuation were rash (4.5%), headache (3.1%), and asthenia (2.4%).

Adjunctive Therapy in Pediatric Patients With Epilepsy: The most commonly observed (≥5% for LAMICTAL and more common on drug than placebo) adverse reactions seen in association with the use of LAMICTAL as adjunctive treatment in pediatric patients 2 to 16 years of age and not seen at an equivalent rate in the control group were infection, vomiting, rash, fever, somnolence, accidental injury, dizziness, diarrhea, abdominal pain, nausea, ataxia, tremor, asthenia, bronchitis, flu syndrome, and diplopia.

In 339 patients 2 to 16 years of age with partial seizures or generalized seizures of Lennox-Gastaut syndrome, 4.2% of patients on LAMICTAL and 2.9% of patients on placebo discontinued due to adverse reactions. The most commonly reported adverse reaction that led to discontinuation of LAMICTAL was rash.

Approximately 11.5% of the 1,081 pediatric patients 2 to 16 years of age who received LAMICTAL as adjunctive therapy in premarketing clinical trials discontinued treatment because of an adverse reaction. The adverse reactions most commonly associated with discontinuation were rash (4.4%), reaction aggravated (1.7%), and ataxia (0.6%).

Controlled Adjunctive Clinical Studies in Adults With Epilepsy: Table 8 lists treatment-emergent adverse reactions that occurred in at least 2% of adult patients with epilepsy treated with LAMICTAL in placebo-controlled trials and were numerically more common in the patients treated with LAMICTAL. In these studies, either LAMICTAL or placebo was added to the patient's current AED therapy. Adverse reactions were usually mild to moderate in intensity.

Table 8. Treatment-Emergent Adverse Reaction Incidence in Placebo-Controlled Adjunctive Trials in Adult Patients With Epilepsy[a] (Adverse reactions in at least 2% of patients treated with LAMICTAL and numerically more frequent than in the placebo group.)

Body System/Adverse Reaction	Percent of Patients Receiving Adjunctive LAMICTAL (n = 711)	Percent of Patients Receiving Adjunctive Placebo (n = 419)
Body as a whole		
Headache	29	19
Flu syndrome	7	6
Fever	6	4
Abdominal pain	5	4
Neck pain	2	1
Reaction aggravated (seizure exacerbation)	2	1
Digestive		
Nausea	19	10
Vomiting	9	4
Diarrhea	6	4
Dyspepsia	5	2
Constipation	4	3
Anorexia	2	1
Musculoskeletal		
Arthralgia	2	0
Nervous		
Dizziness	38	13
Ataxia	22	6
Somnolence	14	7
Incoordination	6	2
Insomnia	6	2
Tremor	4	1
Depression	4	3
Anxiety	4	3
Convulsion	3	1
Irritability	3	2
Speech disorder	3	0
Concentration disturbance	2	1
Respiratory		
Rhinitis	14	9
Pharyngitis	10	9
Cough increased	8	6
Skin and appendages		
Rash	10	5
Pruritus	3	2
Special senses		
Diplopia	28	7
Blurred vision	16	5
Vision abnormality	3	1
Urogenital		
Female patients only	(n = 365)	(n = 207)
Dysmenorrhea	7	6
Vaginitis	4	1
Amenorrhea	2	1

[a]Patients in these adjunctive studies were receiving 1 to 3 of the following concomitant AEDs (carbamazepine, phenytoin, phenobarbital, or primidone) in addition to LAMICTAL or placebo. Patients may have reported multiple adverse reactions during the study or at discontinuation; thus, patients may be included in more than one category.

In a randomized, parallel study comparing placebo and 300 and 500 mg/day of LAMICTAL, some of the more common drug-related adverse reactions were dose-related (see Table 9).

Table 9. Dose-Related Adverse Reactions From a Randomized, Placebo-Controlled Adjunctive Trial in Adults With Epilepsy

Adverse Reaction	Percent of Patients Experiencing Adverse Reactions		
	Placebo (n = 73)	LAMICTAL 300 mg (n = 71)	LAMICTAL 500 mg (n = 72)
Ataxia	10	10	28[ab]
Blurred vision	10	11	25[ab]
Diplopia	8	24[a]	49[ab]
Dizziness	27	31	54[ab]
Nausea	11	18	25[a]
Vomiting	4	11	18[a]

[a]Significantly greater than placebo group ($P<0.05$).
[b]Significantly greater than group receiving LAMICTAL 300 mg ($P<0.05$).

The overall adverse reaction profile for LAMICTAL was similar between females and males, and was independent of age. Because the largest non-Caucasian racial subgroup was only 6% of patients exposed to LAMICTAL in placebo-controlled trials, there are insufficient data to support a statement regarding the distribution of adverse reaction reports by race. Generally, females receiving either LAMICTAL as adjunctive therapy or placebo were more likely to report adverse reactions than males. The only adverse reaction for which the reports on LAMICTAL were greater than 10% more frequent in females than males (without a corresponding difference by gender on placebo) was dizziness (difference = 16.5%). There was little difference between females and males in the rates of discontinuation of LAMICTAL for individual adverse reactions.

Controlled Monotherapy Trial in Adults With Partial Seizures: Table 10 lists treatment-emergent adverse reactions that occurred in at least 5% of patients with epilepsy treated with monotherapy with LAMICTAL in a double-blind trial following discontinuation of either concomitant carbamazepine or phenytoin not seen at an equivalent frequency in the control group.

Table 10. Treatment-Emergent Adverse Reaction Incidence in Adults With Partial Seizures in a Controlled Monotherapy Trial[a] (Adverse reactions in at least 5% of patients treated with LAMICTAL and numerically more frequent than in the valproate group.)

Body System/ Adverse Reaction	Percent of Patients Receiving LAMICTAL as Monotherapy[b] (n = 43)	Percent of Patients Receiving Low-Dose Valproate[c] Monotherapy (n = 44)
Body as a whole		
Pain	5	0
Infection	5	2
Chest pain	5	2
Digestive		
Vomiting	9	0
Dyspepsia	7	2
Nausea	7	2
Metabolic and nutritional		
Weight decrease	5	2
Nervous		
Coordination abnormality	7	0
Dizziness	7	0
Anxiety	5	0
Insomnia	5	2
Respiratory		
Rhinitis	7	2
Urogenital (female patients only)	(n = 21)	(n = 28)
Dysmenorrhea	5	0

[a]Patients in these studies were converted to LAMICTAL or valproate monotherapy from adjunctive therapy with carbamazepine or phenytoin. Patients may have reported multiple adverse reactions during the study; thus, patients may be included in more than one category.
[b]Up to 500 mg/day.
[c]1,000 mg/day.

Adverse reactions that occurred with a frequency of less than 5% and greater than 2% of patients receiving LAMICTAL and numerically more frequent than placebo were:

Body as a Whole: Asthenia, fever.

Digestive: Anorexia, dry mouth, rectal hemorrhage, peptic ulcer.

Metabolic and Nutritional: Peripheral edema.

Nervous System: Amnesia, ataxia, depression, hypesthesia, libido increase, decreased reflexes, increased reflexes, nystagmus, irritability, suicidal ideation.

Respiratory: Epistaxis, bronchitis, dyspnea.

Skin and Appendages: Contact dermatitis, dry skin, sweating.

Special Senses: Vision abnormality.

Incidence in Controlled Adjunctive Trials in Pediatric Patients With Epilepsy: Table 11 lists adverse reactions that occurred in at least 2% of 339 pediatric patients with partial seizures or generalized seizures of Lennox-Gastaut syndrome, who received LAMICTAL up to 15 mg/kg/day or a maximum of 750 mg/day. Reported adverse reactions were classified using COSTART terminology.

Table 11. Treatment-Emergent Adverse Reaction Incidence in Placebo-Controlled Adjunctive Trials in Pediatric Patients With Epilepsy (Adverse reactions in at least 2% of patients treated with LAMICTAL and numerically more frequent than in the placebo group.)

Body System/ Adverse Reaction	Percent of Patients Receiving LAMICTAL (n = 168)	Percent of Patients Receiving Placebo (n = 171)
Body as a whole		
Infection	20	17
Fever	15	14
Accidental injury	14	12
Abdominal pain	10	5
Asthenia	8	4
Flu syndrome	7	6
Pain	5	4
Facial edema	2	1
Photosensitivity	2	0
Cardiovascular		
Hemorrhage	2	1
Digestive		
Vomiting	20	16
Diarrhea	11	9
Nausea	10	2
Constipation	4	2
Dyspepsia	2	1
Hemic and lymphatic		
Lymphadenopathy	2	1
Metabolic and nutritional		
Edema	2	0
Nervous system		
Somnolence	17	15
Dizziness	14	4
Ataxia	11	3
Tremor	10	1
Emotional lability	4	2
Gait abnormality	4	2
Thinking abnormality	3	2
Convulsions	2	1
Nervousness	2	1
Vertigo	2	1
Respiratory		
Pharyngitis	14	11
Bronchitis	7	5
Increased cough	7	6
Sinusitis	2	1
Bronchospasm	2	1
Skin		
Rash	14	12
Eczema	2	1
Pruritus	2	1
Special senses		
Diplopia	5	1
Blurred vision	4	1
Visual abnormality	2	0
Urogenital		
Male and female patients		
Urinary tract infection	3	0

Bipolar Disorder: The most commonly observed (≥5%) treatment-emergent adverse reactions seen in association with the use of LAMICTAL as monotherapy (100 to 400 mg/day) in adult patients (≥18 years of age) with Bipolar Disorder in the 2 double-blind, placebo-controlled trials of 18 months' duration, and numerically more frequent than in placebo-treated patients are included in Table 12. Adverse reactions that occurred in at least 5% of patients and were numerically more common during the dose-escalation phase of LAMICTAL in these trials (when patients may have been receiving concomitant medications) compared with the monotherapy phase were: headache (25%), rash (11%), dizziness (10%), diarrhea (8%), dream abnormality (6%), and pruritus (6%).

During the monotherapy phase of the double-blind, placebo-controlled trials of 18 months' duration, 13% of 227 patients who received LAMICTAL (100 to 400 mg/day), 16% of 190 patients who received placebo, and 23% of 166 patients who received lithium discontinued therapy because of an adverse reaction. The adverse reactions which most commonly led to discontinuation of LAMICTAL were rash (3%) and mania/hypomania/mixed mood adverse reactions (2%). Approximately 16% of 2,401 patients who received LAMICTAL (50 to 500 mg/day) for Bipolar Disorder in premarketing trials discontinued therapy because of an adverse reaction, most commonly due to rash (5%) and mania/hypomania/mixed mood adverse reactions (2%).

The overall adverse reaction profile for LAMICTAL was similar between females and males, between elderly and nonelderly patients, and among racial groups.

Table 12. Treatment-Emergent Adverse Reaction Incidence in 2 Placebo-Controlled Trials in Adults With Bipolar I Disorder[a] (Adverse reactions in at least 5% of patients treated with LAMICTAL as monotherapy and numerically more frequent than in the placebo group.)

Body System/ Adverse Reaction	Percent of Patients Receiving LAMICTAL (n = 227)	Percent of Patients Receiving Placebo (n = 190)
General		
Back pain	8	6
Fatigue	8	5
Abdominal pain	6	3
Digestive		
Nausea	14	11
Constipation	5	2
Vomiting	5	2
Nervous System		
Insomnia	10	6
Somnolence	9	7
Xerostomia (dry mouth)	6	4
Respiratory		
Rhinitis	7	4
Exacerbation of cough	5	3
Pharyngitis	5	4
Skin		
Rash (nonserious)[b]	7	5

[a]Patients in these studies were converted to LAMICTAL (100 to 400 mg/day) or placebo monotherapy from add-on therapy with other psychotropic medications. Patients may have reported multiple adverse reactions during the study; thus, patients may be included in more than one category.
[b]In the overall bipolar and other mood disorders clinical trials, the rate of serious rash was 0.08% (1 of 1,233) of adult patients who received LAMICTAL as initial monotherapy and 0.13% (2 of 1,538) of adult patients who received LAMICTAL as adjunctive therapy *[see Warnings and Precautions (5.1)]*.

These adverse reactions were usually mild to moderate in intensity. Other reactions that occurred in 5% or more patients but equally or more frequently in the placebo group included: dizziness, mania, headache, infection, influenza, pain, accidental injury, diarrhea, and dyspepsia.

Adverse reactions that occurred with a frequency of less than 5% and greater than 1% of patients receiving LAMICTAL and numerically more frequent than placebo were:

General: Fever, neck pain.

Cardiovascular: Migraine.

Digestive: Flatulence.

Metabolic and Nutritional: Weight gain, edema.

Musculoskeletal: Arthralgia, myalgia.

Table 13. Established and Other Potentially Significant Drug Interactions

Concomitant Drug	Effect on Concentration of Lamotrigine or Concomitant Drug	Clinical Comment
Estrogen-containing oral contraceptive preparations containing 30 mcg ethinylestradiol and 150 mcg levonorgestrel	↓ lamotrigine	Decreased lamotrigine levels approximately 50%.
	↓ levonorgestrel	Decrease in levonorgestrel component by 19%.
Carbamazepine (CBZ) and CBZ epoxide	↓ lamotrigine ? CBZ epoxide	Addition of carbamazepine decreases lamotrigine concentration approximately 40%. May increase CBZ epoxide levels
Phenobarbital/primidone	↓ lamotrigine	Decreased lamotrigine concentration approximately 40%.
Phenytoin (PHT)	↓ lamotrigine	Decreased lamotrigine concentration approximately 40%.
Rifampin	↓ lamotrigine	Decreased lamotrigine AUC approximately 40%.
Valproate	↑ lamotrigine	Increased lamotrigine concentrations slightly more than 2-fold.
	? valproate	Decreased valproate concentrations an average of 25% over a 3-week period then stabilized in healthy volunteers; no change in controlled clinical trials in epilepsy patients.

↓= Decreased (induces lamotrigine glucuronidation).
↑= Increased (inhibits lamotrigine glucuronidation).
? = Conflicting data.

Nervous System: Amnesia, depression, agitation, emotional lability, dyspraxia, abnormal thoughts, dream abnormality, hypoesthesia.
Respiratory: Sinusitis.
Urogenital: Urinary frequency.
Adverse Reactions Following Abrupt Discontinuation: In the 2 maintenance trials, there was no increase in the incidence, severity, or type of adverse reactions in Bipolar Disorder patients after abruptly terminating therapy with LAMICTAL. In clinical trials in patients with Bipolar Disorder, 2 patients experienced seizures shortly after abrupt withdrawal of LAMICTAL. However, there were confounding factors that may have contributed to the occurrence of seizures in these bipolar patients *[see Warnings and Precautions (5.9)]*.
Mania/Hypomania/Mixed Episodes: During the double-blind, placebo-controlled clinical trials in Bipolar I Disorder in which patients were converted to monotherapy with LAMICTAL (100 to 400 mg/day) from other psychotropic medications and followed for up to 18 months, the rates of manic or hypomanic or mixed mood episodes reported as adverse reactions were 5% for patients treated with LAMICTAL (n = 227), 4% for patients treated with lithium (n = 166), and 7% for patients treated with placebo (n = 190). In all bipolar controlled trials combined, adverse reactions of mania (including hypomania and mixed mood episodes) were reported in 5% of patients treated with LAMICTAL (n = 956), 3% of patients treated with lithium (n = 280), and 4% of patients treated with placebo (n = 803).

6.2 Other Adverse Reactions Observed in All Clinical Trials

LAMICTAL has been administered to 6,694 individuals for whom complete adverse reaction data was captured during all clinical trials, only some of which were placebo controlled. During these trials, all adverse reactions were recorded by the clinical investigators using terminology of their own choosing. To provide a meaningful estimate of the proportion of individuals having adverse reactions, similar types of adverse reactions were grouped into a smaller number of standardized categories using modified COSTART dictionary terminology. The frequencies presented represent the proportion of the 6,694 individuals exposed to LAMICTAL who experienced an event of the type cited on at least one occasion while receiving LAMICTAL. All reported adverse reactions are included except those already listed in the previous tables or elsewhere in the labeling, those too general to be informative, and those not reasonably associated with the use of the drug.
Adverse reactions are further classified within body system categories and enumerated in order of decreasing frequency using the following definitions: *frequent* adverse reactions are defined as those occurring in at least 1/100 patients; *infrequent* adverse reactions are those occurring in 1/100 to 1/1,000 patients; *rare* adverse reactions are those occurring in fewer than 1/1,000 patients.
Body as a Whole: *Infrequent:* Allergic reaction, chills, and malaise.
Cardiovascular System: *Infrequent:* Flushing, hot flashes, hypertension, palpitations, postural hypotension, syncope, tachycardia, and vasodilation.
Dermatological: *Infrequent:* Acne, alopecia, hirsutism, maculopapular rash, skin discoloration, and urticaria. *Rare:* Angioedema, erythema, exfoliative dermatitis, fungal dermatitis, herpes zoster, leukoderma, multiforme erythema, petechial rash, pustular rash, Stevens-Johnson syndrome, and vesiculobullous rash.
Digestive System: *Infrequent:* Dysphagia, eructation, gastritis, gingivitis, increased appetite, increased salivation, liver function tests abnormal, and mouth ulceration. *Rare:* Gastrointestinal hemorrhage, glossitis, gum hemorrhage, gum hyperplasia, hematemesis, hemorrhagic colitis, hepatitis, melena, stomach ulcer, stomatitis, and tongue edema.
Endocrine System: *Rare:* Goiter and hypothyroidism.
Hematologic and Lymphatic System: *Infrequent:* Ecchymosis and leukopenia. *Rare:* Anemia, eosinophilia, fibrin decrease, fibrinogen decrease, iron deficiency anemia, leukocytosis, lymphocytosis, macrocytic anemia, petechia, and thrombocytopenia.
Metabolic and Nutritional Disorders: *Infrequent:* Aspartate transaminase increased. *Rare:* Alcohol intolerance, alkaline phosphatase increase, alanine transaminase increase, bilirubinemia, general edema, gamma glutamyl transpeptidase increase, and hyperglycemia.
Musculoskeletal System: *Infrequent:* Arthritis, leg cramps, myasthenia, and twitching. *Rare:* Bursitis, muscle atrophy, pathological fracture, and tendinous contracture.
Nervous System: *Frequent:* Confusion and paresthesia. *Infrequent:* Akathisia, apathy, aphasia, central nervous system (CNS) depression, depersonalization, dysarthria, dyskinesia, euphoria, hallucinations, hostility, hyperkinesia, hypertonia, libido decreased, memory decrease, mind racing, movement disorder, myoclonus, panic attack, paranoid reaction, personality disorder, psychosis, sleep disorder, stupor, and suicidal ideation. *Rare:* Choreoathetosis, delirium, delusions, dysphoria, dystonia, extrapyramidal syndrome, faintness, grand mal convulsions, hemiplegia, hyperalgesia, hyperesthesia, hypokinesia, hypotonia, manic depression reaction, muscle spasm, neuralgia, neurosis, paralysis, and peripheral neuritis.
Respiratory System: *Infrequent:* Yawn. *Rare:* Hiccup and hyperventilation.
Special Senses: *Frequent:* Amblyopia. *Infrequent:* Abnormality of accommodation, conjunctivitis, dry eyes, ear pain, photophobia, taste perversion, and tinnitus. *Rare:* Deafness, lacrimation disorder, oscillopsia, parosmia, ptosis, strabismus, taste loss, uveitis, and visual field defect.
Urogenital System: *Infrequent:* Abnormal ejaculation, hematuria, impotence, menorrhagia, polyuria, and urinary incontinence. *Rare:* Acute kidney failure, anorgasmia, breast abscess, breast neoplasm, creatinine increase, cystitis, dysuria, epididymitis, female lactation, kidney failure, kidney pain, nocturia, urinary retention, and urinary urgency.

6.3 Postmarketing Experience

The following adverse events (not listed above in clinical trials or other sections of the prescribing information) have been identified during postapproval use of LAMICTAL. Because these events are reported voluntarily from a population of uncertain size, it is not always possible to reliably estimate their frequency or establish a causal relationship to drug exposure.
Blood and Lymphatic: Agranulocytosis, hemolytic anemia, lymphadenopathy not associated with hypersensitivity disorder.
Gastrointestinal: Esophagitis.
Hepatobiliary Tract and Pancreas: Pancreatitis.
Immunologic: Lupus-like reaction, vasculitis.
Lower Respiratory: Apnea.
Musculoskeletal: Rhabdomyolysis has been observed in patients experiencing hypersensitivity reactions.
Neurology: Exacerbation of Parkinsonian symptoms in patients with pre-existing Parkinson's disease, tics.
Non-site Specific: Progressive immunosuppression.

7 DRUG INTERACTIONS

Significant drug interactions with lamotrigine are summarized in Table 13. Additional details of these drug interaction studies are provided in the Clinical Pharmacology section *[see Clinical Pharmacology (12.3)]*.
[See table 13 above]

8 USE IN SPECIFIC POPULATIONS

8.1 Pregnancy

Teratogenic Effects: Pregnancy Category C. No evidence of teratogenicity was found in mice, rats, or rabbits when lamotrigine was orally administered to pregnant animals during the period of organogenesis at doses up to 1.2, 0.5, and 1.1 times, respectively, on a mg/m^2 basis, the highest usual human maintenance dose (i.e., 500 mg/day). However, maternal toxicity and secondary fetal toxicity producing reduced fetal weight and/or delayed ossification were seen in mice and rats, but not in rabbits at these doses. Teratology studies were also conducted using bolus intravenous administration of the isethionate salt of lamotrigine in rats and rabbits. In rat dams administered an intravenous dose at 0.6 times the highest usual human maintenance dose, the incidence of intrauterine death without signs of teratogenicity was increased.
A behavioral teratology study was conducted in rats dosed during the period of organogenesis. At day 21 postpartum, offspring of dams receiving 5 mg/kg/day or higher displayed a significantly longer latent period for open field exploration and a lower frequency of rearing. In a swimming maze test performed on days 39 to 44 postpartum, time to completion was increased in offspring of dams receiving 25 mg/kg/day. These doses represent 0.1 and 0.5 times the clinical dose on a mg/m^2 basis, respectively.
Lamotrigine did not affect fertility, teratogenesis, or postnatal development when rats were dosed prior to and during mating, and throughout gestation and lactation at doses equivalent to 0.4 times the highest usual human maintenance dose on a mg/m^2 basis.
When pregnant rats were orally dosed at 0.1, 0.14, or 0.3 times the highest human maintenance dose (on a mg/m^2 basis) during the latter part of gestation (days 15 to 20), maternal toxicity and fetal death were seen. In dams, food consumption and weight gain were reduced, and the gestation period was slightly prolonged (22.6 vs. 22.0 days in the control group). Stillborn pups were found in all 3 drug-treated groups with the highest number in the high-dose group. Postnatal death was also seen, but only in the 2 highest doses, and occurred between days 1 and 20. Some of these deaths appear to be drug-related and not secondary to the maternal toxicity. A no-observed-effect level (NOEL) could not be determined for this study.
Although lamotrigine was not found to be teratogenic in the above studies, lamotrigine decreases fetal folate concentrations in rats, an effect known to be associated with teratogenesis in animals and humans. There are no adequate and well-controlled studies in pregnant women. Because animal reproduction studies are not always predictive of human response, this drug should be used during pregnancy only if the potential benefit justifies the potential risk to the fetus.
Non-Teratogenic Effects: As with other AEDs, physiological changes during pregnancy may affect lamotrigine concentrations and/or therapeutic effect. There have been reports of decreased lamotrigine concentrations during pregnancy and restoration of pre-partum concentrations after delivery. Dosage adjustments may be necessary to maintain clinical response.
Pregnancy Exposure Registry: To provide information regarding the effects of in utero exposure to LAMICTAL, physicians are advised to recommend that pregnant patients taking LAMICTAL enroll in the North American Antiepileptic Drug (NAAED) Pregnancy Registry. This can be done by calling the toll-free number 1-888-233-2334,

and must be done by patients themselves. Information on the registry can also be found at the website http://www.aedpregnancyregistry.org/.
Physicians are also encouraged to register patients in the Lamotrigine Pregnancy Registry; enrollment in this registry must be done prior to any prenatal diagnostic tests and **before fetal outcome is known. Physicians** can obtain information by calling the Lamotrigine Pregnancy Registry at 1-800-336-2176 (toll-free).

8.2 Labor and Delivery
The effect of LAMICTAL on labor and delivery in humans is unknown.

8.3 Nursing Mothers
Lamotrigine is present in milk from lactating women taking LAMICTAL. Data from multiple small studies indicate that lamotrigine plasma levels in human milk-fed infants have been reported to be as high as 50% of the maternal serum levels. Neonates and young infants are at risk for high serum levels because maternal serum and milk levels can rise to high levels postpartum if lamotrigine dosage has been increased during pregnancy but not later reduced to the pre-pregnancy dosage. Lamotrigine exposure is further increased due to the immaturity of the infant glucuronidation capacity needed for drug clearance. Events including apnea, drowsiness, and poor sucking have been reported in infants who have been human milk-fed by mothers using lamotrigine; whether or not these events were caused by lamotrigine is unknown. Human milk-fed infants should be closely monitored for adverse events resulting from lamotrigine. Measurement of infant serum levels should be performed to rule out toxicity if concerns arise. Human milk-feeding should be discontinued in infants with lamotrigine toxicity. Caution should be exercised when LAMICTAL is administered to a nursing woman.

8.4 Pediatric Use
LAMICTAL is indicated for adjunctive therapy in patients ≥2 years of age for partial seizures, the generalized seizures of Lennox-Gastaut syndrome, and primary generalized tonic-clonic seizures.
Safety and efficacy of LAMICTAL, used as adjunctive treatment for partial seizures, were not demonstrated in a small randomized, double-blind, placebo-controlled, withdrawal study in very young pediatric patients (1 to 24 months of age). LAMICTAL was associated with an increased risk for infectious adverse reactions (LAMICTAL 37%, placebo 5%), and respiratory adverse reactions (LAMICTAL 26%, placebo 5%). Infectious adverse reactions included bronchiolitis, bronchitis, ear infection, eye infection, otitis externa, pharyngitis, urinary tract infection, and viral infection. Respiratory adverse reactions included nasal congestion, cough, and apnea.
Safety and effectiveness in patients below the age of 18 years with Bipolar Disorder have not been established.

8.5 Geriatric Use
Clinical studies of LAMICTAL for epilepsy and in Bipolar Disorder did not include sufficient numbers of subjects 65 years of age and over to determine whether they respond differently from younger subjects or exhibit a different safety profile than that of younger patients. In general, dose selection for an elderly patient should be cautious, usually starting at the low end of the dosing range, reflecting the greater frequency of decreased hepatic, renal, or cardiac function, and of concomitant disease or other drug therapy.

8.6 Patients With Hepatic Impairment
Experience in patients with hepatic impairment is limited. Based on a clinical pharmacology study in 24 patients with mild, moderate, and severe liver impairment *[see Clinical Pharmacology (12.3)]*, the following general recommendations can be made. No dosage adjustment is needed in patients with mild liver impairment. Initial, escalation, and maintenance doses should generally be reduced by approximately 25% in patients with moderate and severe liver impairment without ascites and 50% in patients with severe liver impairment with ascites. Escalation and maintenance doses may be adjusted according to clinical response *[see Dosage and Administration (2.1)]*.

8.7 Patients With Renal Impairment
Lamotrigine is metabolized mainly by glucuronic acid conjugation, with the majority of the metabolites being recovered in the urine. In a small study comparing a single dose of lamotrigine in patients with varying degrees of renal impairment with healthy volunteers, the plasma half-life of lamotrigine was significantly longer in the patients with renal impairment *[see Clinical Pharmacology (12.3)]*.
Initial doses of LAMICTAL should be based on patients' AED regimens; reduced maintenance doses may be effective for patients with significant renal impairment. Few patients with severe renal impairment have been evaluated during chronic treatment with LAMICTAL. Because there is inadequate experience in this population, LAMICTAL should be used with caution in these patients *[see Dosage and Administration (2.1)]*.

10 OVERDOSAGE

10.1 Human Overdose Experience
Overdoses involving quantities up to 15 g have been reported for LAMICTAL, some of which have been fatal. Overdose has resulted in ataxia, nystagmus, increased seizures, decreased level of consciousness, coma, and intraventricular conduction delay.

10.2 Management of Overdose
There are no specific antidotes for lamotrigine. Following a suspected overdose, hospitalization of the patient is advised. General supportive care is indicated, including frequent monitoring of vital signs and close observation of the patient. If indicated, emesis should be induced; usual precautions should be taken to protect the airway. It should be kept in mind that lamotrigine is rapidly absorbed *[see Clinical Pharmacology (12.3)]*. It is uncertain whether hemodialysis is an effective means of removing lamotrigine from the blood. In 6 renal failure patients, about 20% of the amount of lamotrigine in the body was removed by hemodialysis during a 4-hour session. A Poison Control Center should be contacted for information on the management of overdosage of LAMICTAL.

11 DESCRIPTION

LAMICTAL (lamotrigine), an AED of the phenyltriazine class, is chemically unrelated to existing AEDs. Its chemical name is 3,5-diamino-6-(2,3-dichlorophenyl)-*as*-triazine, its molecular formula is $C_9H_7N_5Cl_2$, and its molecular weight is 256.09. Lamotrigine is a white to pale cream-colored powder and has a pK_a of 5.7. Lamotrigine is very slightly soluble in water (0.17 mg/mL at 25°C) and slightly soluble in 0.1 M HCl (4.1 mg/mL at 25°C). The structural formula is:

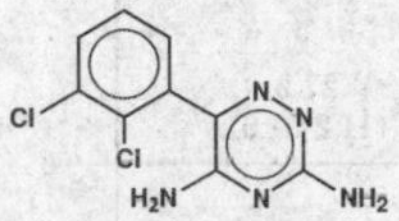

LAMICTAL Tablets are supplied for oral administration as 25 mg (white), 100 mg (peach), 150 mg (cream), and 200 mg (blue) tablets. Each tablet contains the labeled amount of lamotrigine and the following inactive ingredients: lactose; magnesium stearate; microcrystalline cellulose; povidone; sodium starch glycolate; FD&C Yellow No. 6 Lake (100-mg tablet only); ferric oxide, yellow (150-mg tablet only); and FD&C Blue No. 2 Lake (200-mg tablet only).
LAMICTAL Chewable Dispersible Tablets are supplied for oral administration. The tablets contain 2 mg (white), 5 mg (white), or 25 mg (white) of lamotrigine and the following inactive ingredients: blackcurrant flavor, calcium carbonate, low-substituted hydroxypropylcellulose, magnesium aluminum silicate, magnesium stearate, povidone, saccharin sodium, and sodium starch glycolate.
LAMICTAL ODT Orally Disintegrating Tablets are supplied for oral administration. The tablets contain 25 mg (white to off-white), 50 mg (white to off-white), 100 mg (white to off-white), or 200 mg (white to off-white) of lamotrigine and the following inactive ingredients: artificial cherry flavor, crospovidone, ethylcellulose, magnesium stearate, mannitol, polyethylene, and sucralose.
LAMICTAL ODT Orally Disintegrating Tablets are formulated using technologies (Microcaps® and AdvaTab®) designed to mask the bitter taste of lamotrigine and achieve a rapid dissolution profile. Tablet characteristics including flavor, mouth-feel, after-taste, and ease of use were rated as favorable in a study of 108 healthy volunteers.

12 CLINICAL PHARMACOLOGY

12.1 Mechanism of Action
The precise mechanism(s) by which lamotrigine exerts its anticonvulsant action are unknown. In animal models designed to detect anticonvulsant activity, lamotrigine was effective in preventing seizure spread in the maximum electroshock (MES) and pentylenetetrazol (scMet) tests, and prevented seizures in the visually and electrically evoked after-discharge (EEAD) tests for antiepileptic activity. Lamotrigine also displayed inhibitory properties in the kindling model in rats both during kindling development and in the fully kindled state. The relevance of these models to human epilepsy, however, is not known.
One proposed mechanism of action of lamotrigine, the relevance of which remains to be established in humans, involves an effect on sodium channels. In vitro pharmacological studies suggest that lamotrigine inhibits voltage-sensitive sodium channels, thereby stabilizing neuronal membranes and consequently modulating presynaptic transmitter release of excitatory amino acids (e.g., glutamate and aspartate).
Although the relevance for human use is unknown, the following data characterize the performance of lamotrigine in receptor binding assays. Lamotrigine had a weak inhibitory effect on the serotonin $5\text{-}HT_3$ receptor (IC_{50} = 18 μM). It does not exhibit high affinity binding (IC_{50}>100 μM) to the following neurotransmitter receptors: adenosine A_1 and A_2; adrenergic α_1, α_2, and β; dopamine D_1 and D_2; γ-aminobutyric acid (GABA) A and B; histamine H_1; kappa opioid; muscarinic acetylcholine; and serotonin $5\text{-}HT_2$. Studies have failed to detect an effect of lamotrigine on dihydropyridine-sensitive calcium channels. It had weak effects at sigma opioid receptors (IC_{50} = 145 μM). Lamotrigine did not inhibit the uptake of norepinephrine, dopamine, or serotonin (IC_{50}>200 μM) when tested in rat synaptosomes and/or human platelets in vitro.
Effect of Lamotrigine on N-Methyl d-Aspartate-Receptor Mediated Activity: Lamotrigine did not inhibit N-methyl d-aspartate (NMDA)-induced depolarizations in rat cortical slices or NMDA-induced cyclic GMP formation in immature rat cerebellum, nor did lamotrigine displace compounds that are either competitive or noncompetitive ligands at this glutamate receptor complex (CNQX, CGS, TCHP). The IC_{50} for lamotrigine effects on NMDA-induced currents (in the presence of 3 μM of glycine) in cultured hippocampal neurons exceeded 100 μM.
The mechanisms by which lamotrigine exerts its therapeutic action in Bipolar Disorder have not been established.

12.2 Pharmacodynamics
Folate Metabolism: In vitro, lamotrigine inhibited dihydrofolate reductase, the enzyme that catalyzes the reduction of dihydrofolate to tetrahydrofolate. Inhibition of this enzyme may interfere with the biosynthesis of nucleic acids and proteins. When oral daily doses of lamotrigine were given to pregnant rats during organogenesis, fetal, placental, and maternal folate concentrations were reduced. Significantly reduced concentrations of folate are associated with teratogenesis *[see Use in Specific Populations (8.1)]*. Folate concentrations were also reduced in male rats given repeated oral doses of lamotrigine. Reduced concentrations were partially returned to normal when supplemented with folinic acid.
Accumulation in Kidneys: Lamotrigine accumulated in the kidney of the male rat, causing chronic progressive nephrosis, necrosis, and mineralization. These findings are attributed to α-2 microglobulin, a species- and sex-specific protein that has not been detected in humans or other animal species.
Melanin Binding: Lamotrigine binds to melanin-containing tissues, e.g., in the eye and pigmented skin. It has been found in the uveal tract up to 52 weeks after a single dose in rodents.
Cardiovascular: In dogs, lamotrigine is extensively metabolized to a 2-N-methyl metabolite. This metabolite causes dose-dependent prolongations of the PR interval, widening of the QRS complex, and, at higher doses, complete AV conduction block. Similar cardiovascular effects are not anticipated in humans because only trace amounts of the 2-N-methyl metabolite (<0.6% of lamotrigine dose) have been found in human urine *[see Clinical Pharmacology (12.3)]*. However, it is conceivable that plasma concentrations of this metabolite could be increased in patients with a reduced capacity to glucuronidate lamotrigine (e.g., in patients with liver disease).

12.3 Pharmacokinetics
The pharmacokinetics of lamotrigine have been studied in patients with epilepsy, healthy young and elderly volunteers, and volunteers with chronic renal failure. Lamotrigine pharmacokinetic parameters for adult and pediatric patients and healthy normal volunteers are summarized in Tables 14 and 16.
[See table 14 at top of next page]
Absorption: Lamotrigine is rapidly and completely absorbed after oral administration with negligible first-pass metabolism (absolute bioavailability is 98%). The bioavailability is not affected by food. Peak plasma concentrations occur anywhere from 1.4 to 4.8 hours following drug administration. The lamotrigine chewable/dispersible tablets were found to be equivalent, whether they were administered as dispersed in water, chewed and swallowed, or swallowed as whole, to the lamotrigine compressed tablets in terms of rate and extent of absorption. In terms of rate and extent of absorption, lamotrigine orally disintegrating tablets whether disintegrated in the mouth or swallowed whole with water were equivalent to the lamotrigine compressed tablets swallowed with water.
Dose Proportionality: In healthy volunteers not receiving any other medications and given single doses, the plasma concentrations of lamotrigine increased in direct proportion to the dose administered over the range of 50 to 400 mg. In 2 small studies (n = 7 and 8) of patients with epilepsy who were maintained on other AEDs, there also was a linear relationship between dose and lamotrigine plasma concentrations at steady state following doses of 50 to 350 mg twice daily.
Distribution: Estimates of the mean apparent volume of distribution (Vd/F) of lamotrigine following oral administration ranged from 0.9 to 1.3 L/kg. Vd/F is independent of dose and is similar following single and multiple doses in both patients with epilepsy and in healthy volunteers.
Protein Binding: Data from in vitro studies indicate that lamotrigine is approximately 55% bound to human plasma proteins at plasma lamotrigine concentrations from 1 to 10 mcg/mL (10 mcg/mL is 4 to 6 times the trough plasma concentration observed in the controlled efficacy trials). Be-

Table 14. Mean[a] Pharmacokinetic Parameters in Healthy Volunteers and Adult Patients With Epilepsy

Adult Study Population	Number of Subjects	T_{max}: Time of Maximum Plasma Concentration (hr)	$t_{1/2}$: Elimination Half-life (hr)	Cl/F: Apparent Plasma Clearance (mL/min/kg)
Healthy volunteers taking no other medications:				
Single-dose LAMICTAL	179	2.2 (0.25-12.0)	32.8 (14.0-103.0)	0.44 (0.12-1.10)
Multiple-dose LAMICTAL	36	1.7 (0.5-4.0)	25.4 (11.6-61.6)	0.58 (0.24-1.15)
Healthy volunteers taking valproate:				
Single-dose LAMICTAL	6	1.8 (1.0-4.0)	48.3 (31.5-88.6)	0.30 (0.14-0.42)
Multiple-dose LAMICTAL	18	1.9 (0.5-3.5)	70.3 (41.9-113.5)	0.18 (0.12-0.33)
Patients with epilepsy taking valproate only:				
Single-dose LAMICTAL	4	4.8 (1.8-8.4)	58.8 (30.5-88.8)	0.28 (0.16-0.40)
Patients with epilepsy taking carbamazepine, phenytoin, phenobarbital, or primidone[b] plus valproate:				
Single-dose LAMICTAL	25	3.8 (1.0-10.0)	27.2 (11.2-51.6)	0.53 (0.27-1.04)
Patients with epilepsy taking carbamazepine, phenytoin, phenobarbital, or primidone:[b]				
Single-dose LAMICTAL	24	2.3 (0.5-5.0)	14.4 (6.4-30.4)	1.10 (0.51-2.22)
Multiple-dose LAMICTAL	17	2.0 (0.75-5.93)	12.6 (7.5-23.1)	1.21 (0.66-1.82)

[a]The majority of parameter means determined in each study had coefficients of variation between 20% and 40% for half-life and Cl/F and between 30% and 70% for T_{max}. The overall mean values were calculated from individual study means that were weighted based on the number of volunteers/patients in each study. The numbers in parentheses below each parameter mean represent the range of individual volunteer/patient values across studies.

[b]Carbamazepine, phenobarbital, phenytoin, and primidone have been shown to increase the apparent clearance of lamotrigine. Estrogen-containing oral contraceptives and other drugs such as rifampin that induce lamotrigine glucuronidation have also been shown to increase the apparent clearance of lamotrigine *[see Drug Interactions (7)]*.

cause lamotrigine is not highly bound to plasma proteins, clinically significant interactions with other drugs through competition for protein binding sites are unlikely. The binding of lamotrigine to plasma proteins did not change in the presence of therapeutic concentrations of phenytoin, phenobarbital, or valproate. Lamotrigine did not displace other AEDs (carbamazepine, phenytoin, phenobarbital) from protein-binding sites.

Metabolism: Lamotrigine is metabolized predominantly by glucuronic acid conjugation; the major metabolite is an inactive 2-N-glucuronide conjugate. After oral administration of 240 mg of ^{14}C-lamotrigine (15 µCi) to 6 healthy volunteers, 94% was recovered in the urine and 2% was recovered in the feces. The radioactivity in the urine consisted of unchanged lamotrigine (10%), the 2-N-glucuronide (76%), a 5-N-glucuronide (10%), a 2-N-methyl metabolite (0.14%), and other unidentified minor metabolites (4%).

Enzyme Induction: The effects of lamotrigine on the induction of specific families of mixed-function oxidase isozymes have not been systematically evaluated.

Following multiple administrations (150 mg twice daily) to normal volunteers taking no other medications, lamotrigine induced its own metabolism, resulting in a 25% decrease in $t_{1/2}$ and a 37% increase in Cl/F at steady state compared with values obtained in the same volunteers following a single dose. Evidence gathered from other sources suggests that self-induction by lamotrigine may not occur when lamotrigine is given as adjunctive therapy in patients receiving enzyme-inducing drugs such as carbamazepine, phenytoin, phenobarbital, primidone, or drugs such as rifampin that induce lamotrigine glucuronidation *[see Drug Interactions (7)]*.

Elimination: The elimination half-life and apparent clearance of lamotrigine following administration of LAMICTAL to adult patients with epilepsy and healthy volunteers is summarized in Table 14. Half-life and apparent oral clearance vary depending on concomitant AEDs.

Drug Interactions: The apparent clearance of lamotrigine is affected by the coadministration of certain medications *[see Warnings and Precautions (5.8, 5.12), Drug Interactions (7)]*.

The net effects of drug interactions with LAMICTAL are summarized in Tables 13 and 15, followed by details of the drug interaction studies below.

Table 15. Summary of Drug Interactions With LAMICTAL

Drug	Drug Plasma Concentration With Adjunctive LAMICTAL[a]	Lamotrigine Plasma Concentration With Adjunctive Drugs[b]
Oral contraceptives (e.g., ethinylestradiol/ levonorgestrel)[c]	↔[d]	↓
Bupropion	Not assessed	↔
Carbamazepine (CBZ)	↔	↓
CBZ epoxide[e]	?	
Felbamate	Not assessed	↔
Gabapentin	Not assessed	↔
Levetiracetam	↔	↔
Lithium	↔	Not assessed
Olanzapine	↔	↔[f]
Oxcarbazepine	↔	↔
10-monohydroxy oxcarbazepine metabolite[g]	↔	
Phenobarbital/primidone	↔	↓
Phenytoin (PHT)	↔	↓
Pregabalin	↔	↔
Rifampin	Not assessed	↓
Topiramate	↔[h]	↔
Valproate	↓	↑
Valproate + PHT and/or CBZ	Not assessed	↔
Zonisamide	Not assessed	↔

[a]From adjunctive clinical trials and volunteer studies.

[b]Net effects were estimated by comparing the mean clearance values obtained in adjunctive clinical trials and volunteer studies.

[c]The effect of other hormonal contraceptive preparations or hormone replacement therapy on the pharmacokinetics of lamotrigine has not been systematically evaluated in clinical trials, although the effect may be similar to that seen with the ethinylestradiol/levonorgestrel combinations.

[d]Modest decrease in levonorgestrel.

[e]Not administered, but an active metabolite of carbamazepine.

[f]Slight decrease, not expected to be clinically relevant.

[g]Not administered, but an active metabolite of oxcarbazepine.

[h]Slight increase, not expected to be clinically relevant.

↔ = No significant effect.

? = Conflicting data.

Estrogen-Containing Oral Contraceptives: In 16 female volunteers, an oral contraceptive preparation containing 30 mcg ethinylestradiol and 150 mcg levonorgestrel increased the apparent clearance of lamotrigine (300 mg/day) by approximately 2-fold with mean decreases in AUC of 52% and in C_{max} of 39%. In this study, trough serum lamotrigine concentrations gradually increased and were approximately 2-fold higher on average at the end of the week of the inactive hormone preparation compared with trough lamotrigine concentrations at the end of the active hormone cycle.

Gradual transient increases in lamotrigine plasma levels (approximate 2-fold increase) occurred during the week of inactive hormone preparation ("pill-free" week) for women not also taking a drug that increased the clearance of lamotrigine (carbamazepine, phenytoin, phenobarbital, primidone, or other drugs such as rifampin that induce lamotrigine glucuronidation *[see Drug Interactions (7)]*). The increase in lamotrigine plasma levels will be greater if the dose of LAMICTAL is increased in the few days before or during the "pill-free"week. Increases in lamotrigine plasma levels could result in dose-dependent adverse reactions.

In the same study, coadministration of LAMICTAL (300 mg/day) in 16 female volunteers did not affect the pharmacokinetics of the ethinylestradiol component of the oral contraceptive preparation. There were mean decreases in the AUC and C_{max} of the levonorgestrel component of 19% and 12%, respectively. Measurement of serum progesterone indicated that there was no hormonal evidence of ovulation in any of the 16 volunteers, although measurement of serum FSH, LH, and estradiol indicated that there was some loss of suppression of the hypothalamic-pituitary-ovarian axis.

The effects of doses of LAMICTAL other than 300 mg/day have not been systematically evaluated in controlled clinical trials.

The clinical significance of the observed hormonal changes on ovulatory activity is unknown. However, the possibility of decreased contraceptive efficacy in some patients cannot be excluded. Therefore, patients should be instructed to promptly report changes in their menstrual pattern (e.g., break-through bleeding).

Dosage adjustments may be necessary for women receiving estrogen-containing oral contraceptive preparations *[see Dosage and Administration (2.1)]*.

Other Hormonal Contraceptives or Hormone Replacement Therapy: The effect of other hormonal contraceptive preparations or hormone replacement therapy on the pharmacokinetics of lamotrigine has not been systematically evaluated. It has been reported that ethinylestradiol, not progestogens, increased the clearance of lamotrigine up to 2-fold, and the progestin-only pills had no effect on lamotrigine plasma levels. Therefore, adjustments to the dosage of LAMICTAL in the presence of progestogens alone will likely not be needed.

Bupropion: The pharmacokinetics of a 100-mg single dose of LAMICTAL in healthy volunteers (n = 12) were not changed by coadministration of bupropion sustained-release formulation (150 mg twice daily) starting 11 days before LAMICTAL.

Carbamazepine: LAMICTAL has no appreciable effect on steady-state carbamazepine plasma concentration. Limited clinical data suggest there is a higher incidence of dizziness, diplopia, ataxia, and blurred vision in patients receiving carbamazepine with lamotrigine than in patients receiving other AEDs with lamotrigine *[see Adverse Reactions (6.1)]*. The mechanism of this interaction is unclear. The effect of lamotrigine on plasma concentrations of carbamazepine-epoxide is unclear. In a small subset of patients (n = 7) studied in a placebo-controlled trial, lamotrigine had no effect on carbamazepine-epoxide plasma concentrations, but in a small, uncontrolled study (n = 9), carbamazepine-epoxide levels increased.

The addition of carbamazepine decreases lamotrigine steady-state concentrations by approximately 40%.

Felbamate: In a study of 21 healthy volunteers, coadministration of felbamate (1,200 mg twice daily) with lamotrigine (100 mg twice daily for 10 days) appeared to have no clinically relevant effects on the pharmacokinetics of lamotrigine.

Folate Inhibitors: Lamotrigine is a weak inhibitor of dihydrofolate reductase. Prescribers should be aware of this action when prescribing other medications that inhibit folate metabolism.

Gabapentin: Based on a retrospective analysis of plasma levels in 34 patients who received lamotrigine both with and without gabapentin, gabapentin does not appear to change the apparent clearance of lamotrigine.

Levetiracetam: Potential drug interactions between levetiracetam and lamotrigine were assessed by evaluating serum concentrations of both agents during placebo-controlled clinical trials. These data indicate that lamotrigine does not influence the pharmacokinetics of levetiracetam and that levetiracetam does not influence the pharmacokinetics of lamotrigine.

Lithium: The pharmacokinetics of lithium were not altered in healthy subjects (n = 20) by coadministration of lamotrigine (100 mg/day) for 6 days.

Olanzapine: The AUC and C_{max} of olanzapine were similar following the addition of olanzapine (15 mg once daily) to lamotrigine (200 mg once daily) in healthy male volunteers (n = 16) compared with the AUC and C_{max} in healthy male volunteers receiving olanzapine alone (n = 16).

In the same study, the AUC and C_{max} of lamotrigine were reduced on average by 24% and 20%, respectively, following the addition of olanzapine to lamotrigine in healthy male volunteers compared with those receiving lamotrigine alone. This reduction in lamotrigine plasma concentrations is not expected to be clinically relevant.

Oxcarbazepine: The AUC and C_{max} of oxcarbazepine and its active 10-monohydroxy oxcarbazepine metabolite were not significantly different following the addition of oxcarbazepine (600 mg twice daily) to lamotrigine (200 mg once daily) in healthy male volunteers (n = 13) compared with healthy male volunteers receiving oxcarbazepine alone (n = 13).

In the same study, the AUC and C_{max} of lamotrigine were similar following the addition of oxcarbazepine (600 mg twice daily) to LAMICTAL in healthy male volunteers compared with those receiving LAMICTAL alone. Limited clinical data suggest a higher incidence of headache, dizziness, nausea, and somnolence with coadministration of lamotrigine and oxcarbazepine compared with lamotrigine alone or oxcarbazepine alone.

Phenobarbital, Primidone: The addition of phenobarbital or primidone decreases lamotrigine steady-state concentrations by approximately 40%.

Phenytoin: Lamotrigine has no appreciable effect on steady-state phenytoin plasma concentrations in patients with epilepsy. The addition of phenytoin decreases lamotrigine steady-state concentrations by approximately 40%.

Pregabalin: Steady-state trough plasma concentrations of lamotrigine were not affected by concomitant pregabalin (200 mg 3 times daily) administration. There are no pharmacokinetic interactions between lamotrigine and pregabalin.

Rifampin: In 10 male volunteers, rifampin (600 mg/day for 5 days) significantly increased the apparent clearance of a single 25-mg dose of lamotrigine by approximately 2-fold (AUC decreased by approximately 40%).

Topiramate: Topiramate resulted in no change in plasma concentrations of lamotrigine. Administration of lamotrigine resulted in a 15% increase in topiramate concentrations.

Valproate: When lamotrigine was administered to healthy volunteers (n = 18) receiving valproate, the trough steady-state valproate plasma concentrations decreased by an average of 25% over a 3-week period, and then stabilized. However, adding lamotrigine to the existing therapy did not cause a change in valproate plasma concentrations in either adult or pediatric patients in controlled clinical trials.

The addition of valproate increased lamotrigine steady-state concentrations in normal volunteers by slightly more than 2-fold. In one study, maximal inhibition of lamotrigine clearance was reached at valproate doses between 250 and 500 mg/day and did not increase as the valproate dose was further increased.

Zonisamide: In a study of 18 patients with epilepsy, coadministration of zonisamide (200 to 400 mg/day) with lamotrigine (150 to 500 mg/day for 35 days) had no significant effect on the pharmacokinetics of lamotrigine.

Known Inducers or Inhibitors of Glucuronidation: Drugs other than those listed above have not been systematically evaluated in combination with lamotrigine. Since lamotrigine is metabolized predominately by glucuronic acid conjugation, drugs that are known to induce or inhibit glucuronidation may affect the apparent clearance of lamotrigine and doses of lamotrigine may require adjustment based on clinical response.

Other: Results of in vitro experiments suggest that clearance of lamotrigine is unlikely to be reduced by concomitant administration of amitriptyline, clonazepam, clozapine, fluoxetine, haloperidol, lorazepam, phenelzine, risperidone, sertraline, or trazodone.

Results of in vitro experiments suggest that lamotrigine does not reduce the clearance of drugs eliminated predominantly by CYP2D6.

Table 16. Mean Pharmacokinetic Parameters in Pediatric Patients With Epilepsy

Pediatric Study Population	Number of Subjects	T_{max} (hr)	$t_{1/2}$ (hr)	Cl/F (mL/min/kg)
Ages 10 months-5.3 years				
Patients taking carbamazepine, phenytoin, phenobarbital, or primidone[a]	10	3.0 (1.0-5.9)	7.7 (5.7-11.4)	3.62 (2.44-5.28)
Patients taking AEDs with no known effect on the apparent clearance of lamotrigine	7	5.2 (2.9-6.1)	19.0 (12.9-27.1)	1.2 (0.75-2.42)
Patients taking valproate only	8	2.9 (1.0-6.0)	44.9 (29.5-52.5)	0.47 (0.23-0.77)
Ages 5-11 years				
Patients taking carbamazepine, phenytoin, phenobarbital, or primidone[a]	7	1.6 (1.0-3.0)	7.0 (3.8-9.8)	2.54 (1.35-5.58)
Patients taking carbamazepine, phenytoin, phenobarbital, or primidone[a] plus valproate	8	3.3 (1.0-6.4)	19.1 (7.0-31.2)	0.89 (0.39-1.93)
Patients taking valproate only[b]	3	4.5 (3.0-6.0)	65.8 (50.7-73.7)	0.24 (0.21-0.26)
Ages 13-18 years				
Patients taking carbamazepine, phenytoin, phenobarbital, or primidone[a]	11	[c]	[c]	1.3
Patients taking carbamazepine, phenytoin, phenobarbital, or primidone[a] plus valproate	8	[c]	[c]	0.5
Patients taking valproate only	4	[c]	[c]	0.3

[a]Carbamazepine, phenobarbital, phenytoin, and primidone have been shown to increase the apparent clearance of lamotrigine. Estrogen-containing oral contraceptives and rifampin have also been shown to increase the apparent clearance of lamotrigine *[see Drug Interactions (7)]*.

[b]Two subjects were included in the calculation for mean T_{max}.

[c]Parameter not estimated.

Special Populations: *Patients With Renal Impairment:* Twelve volunteers with chronic renal failure (mean creatinine clearance: 13 mL/min, range: 6 to 23) and another 6 individuals undergoing hemodialysis were each given a single 100-mg dose of lamotrigine. The mean plasma half-lives determined in the study were 42.9 hours (chronic renal failure), 13.0 hours (during hemodialysis), and 57.4 hours (between hemodialysis) compared with 26.2 hours in healthy volunteers. On average, approximately 20% (range: 5.6 to 35.1) of the amount of lamotrigine present in the body was eliminated by hemodialysis during a 4-hour session *[see Dosage and Administration (2.1)]*.

Hepatic Disease: The pharmacokinetics of lamotrigine following a single 100-mg dose of lamotrigine were evaluated in 24 subjects with mild, moderate, and severe hepatic impairment (Child-Pugh Classification system) and compared with 12 subjects without hepatic impairment. The patients with severe hepatic impairment were without ascites (n = 2) or with ascites (n = 5). The mean apparent clearances of lamotrigine in patients with mild (n = 12), moderate (n = 5), severe without ascites (n = 2), and severe with ascites (n = 5) liver impairment were 0.30 ± 0.09, 0.24 ± 0.1, 0.21 ± 0.04, and 0.15 ± 0.09 mL/min/kg, respectively, as compared with 0.37 ± 0.1 mL/min/kg in the healthy controls. Mean half-lives of lamotrigine in patients with mild, moderate, severe without ascites, and severe with ascites hepatic impairment were 46 ± 20, 72 ± 44, 67 ± 11, and 100 ± 48 hours, respectively, as compared with 33 ± 7 hours in healthy controls *[see Dosage and Administration (2.1)]*.

Age: Pediatric Patients: The pharmacokinetics of lamotrigine following a single 2-mg/kg dose were evaluated in 2 studies of pediatric patients (n = 29 for patients 10 months to 5.9 years of age and n = 26 for patients 5 to 11 years of age). Forty-three patients received concomitant therapy with other AEDs and 12 patients received lamotrigine as monotherapy. Lamotrigine pharmacokinetic parameters for pediatric patients are summarized in Table 16.

Population pharmacokinetic analyses involving patients 2 to 18 years of age demonstrated that lamotrigine clearance was influenced predominantly by total body weight and concurrent AED therapy. The oral clearance of lamotrigine was higher, on a body weight basis, in pediatric patients than in adults. Weight-normalized lamotrigine clearance was higher in those subjects weighing less than 30 kg, compared with those weighing greater than 30 kg. Accordingly, patients weighing less than 30 kg may need an increase of as much as 50% in maintenance doses, based on clinical response, as compared with subjects weighing more than 30 kg being administered the same AEDs *[see Dosage and Administration (2.2)]*. These analyses also revealed that, after accounting for body weight, lamotrigine clearance was not significantly influenced by age. Thus, the same weight-adjusted doses should be administered to children irrespective of differences in age. Concomitant AEDs which influence lamotrigine clearance in adults were found to have similar effects in children.

[See table 16 above]

Elderly: The pharmacokinetics of lamotrigine following a single 150-mg dose of LAMICTAL were evaluated in 12 elderly volunteers between the ages of 65 and 76 years (mean creatinine clearance = 61 mL/min, range: 33 to 108 mL/min). The mean half-life of lamotrigine in these subjects was 31.2 hours (range: 24.5 to 43.4 hours), and the mean clearance was 0.40 mL/min/kg (range: 0.26 to 0.48 mL/min/kg).

Gender: The clearance of lamotrigine is not affected by gender. However, during dose escalation of LAMICTAL in one clinical trial in patients with epilepsy on a stable dose of valproate (n = 77), mean trough lamotrigine concentrations, unadjusted for weight, were 24% to 45% higher (0.3 to 1.7 mcg/mL) in females than in males.

Race: The apparent oral clearance of lamotrigine was 25% lower in non-Caucasians than Caucasians.

13 NONCLINICAL TOXICOLOGY

13.1 Carcinogenesis, Mutagenesis, Impairment of Fertility

No evidence of carcinogenicity was seen in 1 mouse study or 2 rat studies following oral administration of lamotrigine for up to 2 years at maximum tolerated doses (30 mg/kg/day for mice and 10 to 15 mg/kg/day for rats, doses that are equivalent to 90 mg/m^2 and 60 to 90 mg/m^2, respectively). Steady-state plasma concentrations ranged from 1 to 4 mcg/mL in the mouse study and 1 to 10 mcg/mL in the rat study. Plasma concentrations associated with the recommended human doses of 300 to 500 mg/day are generally in the range of 2 to 5 mcg/mL, but concentrations as high as 19 mcg/mL have been recorded.

Lamotrigine was not mutagenic in the presence or absence of metabolic activation when tested in 2 gene mutation assays (the Ames test and the in vitro mammalian mouse lymphoma assay). In 2 cytogenetic assays (the in vitro human lymphocyte assay and the in vivo rat bone marrow assay), lamotrigine did not increase the incidence of structural or numerical chromosomal abnormalities.

No evidence of impairment of fertility was detected in rats given oral doses of lamotrigine up to 2.4 times the highest usual human maintenance dose of 8.33 mg/kg/day or 0.4 times the human dose on a mg/m^2 basis. The effect of lamotrigine on human fertility is unknown.

14 CLINICAL STUDIES

14.1 Epilepsy

Monotherapy With LAMICTAL in Adults With Partial Seizures Already Receiving Treatment With Carbamazepine, Phenytoin, Phenobarbital, or Primidone as the Single Antiepileptic Drug: The effectiveness of monotherapy with LAMICTAL was established in a multicenter, double-blind clinical trial enrolling 156 adult outpatients with partial seizures. The patients experienced at least 4 simple partial, complex partial, and/or secondarily generalized seizures during each of 2 consecutive 4-week periods while receiving carbamazepine or phenytoin monotherapy during baseline. LAMICTAL (target dose of 500 mg/day) or valproate (1,000 mg/day) was added to either carbamazepine or phenytoin monotherapy over a 4-week period. Patients were then converted to monotherapy with LAMICTAL or valproate during the next 4 weeks, then continued on monotherapy for an additional 12-week period.

Study endpoints were completion of all weeks of study treatment or meeting an escape criterion. Criteria for escape relative to baseline were: (1) doubling of average monthly seizure count, (2) doubling of highest consecutive 2-day seizure frequency, (3) emergence of a new seizure type (defined as a seizure that did not occur during the 8-week baseline) that is more severe than seizure types that occur during study treatment, or (4) clinically significant prolongation of generalized tonic-clonic seizures. The primary efficacy variable was the proportion of patients in each treatment group who met escape criteria.

The percentages of patients who met escape criteria were 42% (32/76) in the group receiving LAMICTAL and 69% (55/80) in the valproate group. The difference in the percentage of patients meeting escape criteria was statistically significant ($P = 0.0012$) in favor of LAMICTAL. No differences in efficacy based on age, sex, or race were detected.

Patients in the control group were intentionally treated with a relatively low dose of valproate; as such, the sole objective of this study was to demonstrate the effectiveness and safety of monotherapy with LAMICTAL, and cannot be interpreted to imply the superiority of LAMICTAL to an adequate dose of valproate.

Adjunctive Therapy With LAMICTAL in Adults With Partial Seizures: The effectiveness of LAMICTAL as adjunctive therapy (added to other AEDs) was established in 3 multicenter, placebo-controlled, double-blind clinical trials in 355 adults with refractory partial seizures. The patients had a history of at least 4 partial seizures per month in spite of receiving one or more AEDs at therapeutic concentrations and, in 2 of the studies, were observed on their established AED regimen during baselines that varied between 8 to 12 weeks. In the third, patients were not observed in a prospective baseline. In patients continuing to have at least 4 seizures per month during the baseline, LAMICTAL or placebo was then added to the existing therapy. In all 3 studies, change from baseline in seizure frequency was the primary measure of effectiveness. The results given below are for all partial seizures in the intent-to-treat population (all patients who received at least one dose of treatment) in each study, unless otherwise indicated. The median seizure frequency at baseline was 3 per week while the mean at baseline was 6.6 per week for all patients enrolled in efficacy studies.

One study (n = 216) was a double-blind, placebo-controlled, parallel trial consisting of a 24-week treatment period. Patients could not be on more than 2 other anticonvulsants and valproate was not allowed. Patients were randomized to receive placebo, a target dose of 300 mg/day of LAMICTAL, or a target dose of 500 mg/day of LAMICTAL. The median reductions in the frequency of all partial seizures relative to baseline were 8% in patients receiving placebo, 20% in patients receiving 300 mg/day of LAMICTAL, and 36% in patients receiving 500 mg/day of LAMICTAL. The seizure frequency reduction was statistically significant in the 500-mg/day group compared with the placebo group, but not in the 300-mg/day group.

A second study (n = 98) was a double-blind, placebo-controlled, randomized, crossover trial consisting of two 14-week treatment periods (the last 2 weeks of which consisted of dose tapering) separated by a 4-week washout period. Patients could not be on more than 2 other anticonvulsants and valproate was not allowed. The target dose of LAMICTAL was 400 mg/day. When the first 12 weeks of the treatment periods were analyzed, the median change in seizure frequency was a 25% reduction on LAMICTAL compared with placebo ($P<0.001$).

The third study (n = 41) was a double-blind, placebo-controlled, crossover trial consisting of two 12-week treatment periods separated by a 4-week washout period. Patients could not be on more than 2 other anticonvulsants. Thirteen patients were on concomitant valproate; these patients received 150 mg/day of LAMICTAL. The 28 other patients had a target dose of 300 mg/day of LAMICTAL. The median change in seizure frequency was a 26% reduction on LAMICTAL compared with placebo ($P<0.01$).

No differences in efficacy based on age, sex, or race, as measured by change in seizure frequency, were detected.

Adjunctive Therapy With LAMICTAL in Pediatric Patients With Partial Seizures: The effectiveness of LAMICTAL as adjunctive therapy in pediatric patients with partial seizures was established in a multicenter, double-blind, placebo-controlled trial in 199 patients 2 to 16 years of age (n = 98 on LAMICTAL, n = 101 on placebo). Following an 8-week baseline phase, patients were randomized to 18 weeks of treatment with LAMICTAL or placebo added to their current AED regimen of up to 2 drugs. Patients were dosed based on body weight and valproate use. Target doses were designed to approximate 5 mg/kg/day for patients taking valproate (maximum dose: 250 mg/day) and 15 mg/kg/day for the patients not taking valproate (maximum dose: 750 mg/day). The primary efficacy endpoint was percentage change from baseline in all partial seizures. For the intent-to-treat population, the median reduction of all partial seizures was 36% in patients treated with LAMICTAL and 7% on placebo, a difference that was statistically significant ($P<0.01$).

Adjunctive Therapy With LAMICTAL in Pediatric and Adult Patients With Lennox-Gastaut Syndrome: The effectiveness of LAMICTAL as adjunctive therapy in patients with Lennox-Gastaut syndrome was established in a multicenter, double-blind, placebo-controlled trial in 169 patients 3 to 25 years of age (n = 79 on LAMICTAL, n = 90 on placebo). Following a 4-week single-blind, placebo phase, patients were randomized to 16 weeks of treatment with LAMICTAL or placebo added to their current AED regimen of up to 3 drugs. Patients were dosed on a fixed-dose regimen based on body weight and valproate use. Target doses were designed to approximate 5 mg/kg/day for patients taking valproate (maximum dose: 200 mg/day) and 15 mg/kg/day for patients not taking valproate (maximum dose: 400 mg/day). The primary efficacy endpoint was percentage change from baseline in major motor seizures (atonic, tonic, major myoclonic, and tonic-clonic seizures). For the intent-to-treat population, the median reduction of major motor seizures was 32% in patients treated with LAMICTAL and 9% on placebo, a difference that was statistically significant ($P<0.05$). Drop attacks were significantly reduced by LAMICTAL (34%) compared with placebo (9%), as were tonic-clonic seizures (36% reduction versus 10% increase for LAMICTAL and placebo, respectively).

Adjunctive Therapy With LAMICTAL in Pediatric and Adult Patients With Primary Generalized Tonic-Clonic Seizures: The effectiveness of LAMICTAL as adjunctive therapy in patients with primary generalized tonic-clonic seizures was established in a multicenter, double-blind, placebo-controlled trial in 117 pediatric and adult patients ≥2 years (n = 58 on LAMICTAL, n = 59 on placebo). Patients with at least 3 primary generalized tonic-clonic seizures during an 8-week baseline phase were randomized to 19 to 24 weeks of treatment with LAMICTAL or placebo added to their current AED regimen of up to 2 drugs. Patients were dosed on a fixed-dose regimen, with target doses ranging from 3 mg/kg/day to 12 mg/kg/day for pediatric patients and from 200 mg/day to 400 mg/day for adult patients based on concomitant AED.

The primary efficacy endpoint was percentage change from baseline in primary generalized tonic-clonic seizures. For the intent-to-treat population, the median percent reduction of primary generalized tonic-clonic seizures was 66% in patients treated with LAMICTAL and 34% on placebo, a difference that was statistically significant ($P = 0.006$).

14.2 Bipolar Disorder

The effectiveness of LAMICTAL in the maintenance treatment of Bipolar I Disorder was established in 2 multicenter, double-blind, placebo-controlled studies in adult patients who met DSM-IV criteria for Bipolar I Disorder. Study 1 enrolled patients with a current or recent (within 60 days) depressive episode as defined by DSM-IV and Study 2 included patients with a current or recent (within 60 days) episode of mania or hypomania as defined by DSM-IV. Both studies included a cohort of patients (30% of 404 patients in Study 1 and 28% of 171 patients in Study 2) with rapid cycling Bipolar Disorder (4 to 6 episodes per year).

In both studies, patients were titrated to a target dose of 200 mg of LAMICTAL, as add-on therapy or as monotherapy, with gradual withdrawal of any psychotropic medications during an 8- to 16-week open-label period. Overall 81% of 1,305 patients participating in the open-label period were receiving 1 or more other psychotropic medications, including benzodiazepines, selective serotonin reuptake inhibitors (SSRIs), atypical antipsychotics (including olanzapine), valproate, or lithium, during titration of LAMICTAL. Patients with a CGI-severity score of 3 or less maintained for at least 4 continuous weeks, including at least the final week on monotherapy with LAMICTAL, were randomized to a placebo-controlled, double-blind treatment period for up to 18 months. The primary endpoint was TIME (time to intervention for a mood episode or one that was emerging, time to discontinuation for either an adverse event that was judged to be related to Bipolar Disorder, or for lack of efficacy). The mood episode could be depression, mania, hypomania, or a mixed episode.

In Study 1, patients received double-blind monotherapy with LAMICTAL 50 mg/day (n = 50), LAMICTAL 200 mg/day (n = 124), LAMICTAL 400 mg/day (n = 47), or placebo (n = 121). LAMICTAL (200- and 400-mg/day treatment groups combined) was superior to placebo in delaying the time to occurrence of a mood episode. Separate analyses of the 200- and 400-mg/day dose groups revealed no added benefit from the higher dose.

In Study 2, patients received double-blind monotherapy with LAMICTAL (100 to 400 mg/day, n = 59), or placebo (n = 70). LAMICTAL was superior to placebo in delaying time to occurrence of a mood episode. The mean dose of LAMICTAL was about 211 mg/day.

Although these studies were not designed to separately evaluate time to the occurrence of depression or mania, a combined analysis for the 2 studies revealed a statistically significant benefit for LAMICTAL over placebo in delaying the time to occurrence of both depression and mania, although the finding was more robust for depression.

16 HOW SUPPLIED/STORAGE AND HANDLING

LAMICTAL (lamotrigine) Tablets

25 mg, white, scored, shield-shaped tablets debossed with "LAMICTAL" and "25", bottles of 100 (NDC 0173-0633-02). Store at 25°C (77°F); excursions permitted to 15-30°C (59-86°F) [see USP Controlled Room Temperature] in a dry place.

100 mg, peach, scored, shield-shaped tablets debossed with "LAMICTAL" and "100", bottles of 100 (NDC 0173-0642-55).
150 mg, cream, scored, shield-shaped tablets debossed with "LAMICTAL" and "150", bottles of 60 (NDC 0173-0643-60).
200 mg, blue, scored, shield-shaped tablets debossed with "LAMICTAL" and "200", bottles of 60 (NDC 0173-0644-60).
Store at 25°C (77°F); excursions permitted to 15-30°C (59-86°F) [see USP Controlled Room Temperature] in a dry place and protect from light.

LAMICTAL (lamotrigine) Starter Kit for Patients Taking Valproate (Blue Kit)

25 mg, white, scored, shield-shaped tablets debossed with "LAMICTAL" and "25", blisterpack of 35 tablets (NDC 0173-0633-10).

Store at 25°C (77°F); excursions permitted to 15-30°C (59-86°F) [see USP Controlled Room Temperature] in a dry place.

LAMICTAL (lamotrigine) Starter Kit for Patients Taking Carbamazepine, Phenytoin, Phenobarbital, or Primidone and Not Taking Valproate (Green Kit)

25 mg, white, scored, shield-shaped tablets debossed with "LAMICTAL" and "25" and 100 mg, peach, scored, shield-shaped tablets debossed with "LAMICTAL" and "100", blisterpack of 98 tablets (84/25-mg tablets and 14/100-mg tablets) (NDC 0173-0817-28).

Store at 25°C (77°F); excursions permitted to 15-30°C (59-86°F) [see USP Controlled Room Temperature] in a dry place and protect from light.

LAMICTAL (lamotrigine) Starter Kit for Patients Not Taking Carbamazepine, Phenytoin, Phenobarbital, Primidone, or Valproate (Orange Kit)

25 mg, white, scored, shield-shaped tablets debossed with "LAMICTAL" and "25" and 100 mg, peach, scored, shield-shaped tablets debossed with "LAMICTAL" and "100", blisterpack of 49 tablets (42/25-mg tablets and 7/100-mg tablets) (NDC 0173-0594-02).

Store at 25°C (77°F); excursions permitted to 15-30°C (59-86°F) [see USP Controlled Room Temperature] in a dry place and protect from light.

LAMICTAL (lamotrigine) Chewable Dispersible Tablets

2 mg, white to off-white, round tablets debossed with "LTG" over "2", bottles of 30 (NDC 0173-0699-00). ORDER DIRECTLY FROM GlaxoSmithKline 1-800-334-4153.
5 mg, white to off-white, caplet-shaped tablets debossed with "GX CL2", bottles of 100 (NDC 0173-0526-00).
25 mg, white, super elliptical-shaped tablets debossed with "GX CL5", bottles of 100 (NDC 0173-0527-00).
Store at 25°C (77°F); excursions permitted to 15-30°C (59-86°F) [see USP Controlled Room Temperature] in a dry place.

LAMICTAL ODT (lamotrigine) Orally Disintegrating Tablets

25 mg, white to off-white, round, flat-faced, radius edge, tablets debossed with "LMT" on one side and "25" on the other, Maintenance Packs of 30 (NDC 0173-0772-02).
50 mg, white to off-white, round, flat-faced, radius edge, tablets debossed with "LMT" on one side and "50" on the other, Maintenance Packs of 30 (NDC 0173-0774-02).
100 mg, white to off-white, round, flat-faced, radius edge, tablets debossed with "LAMICTAL" on one side and "100" on the other, Maintenance Packs of 30 (NDC 0173-0776-02).
200 mg, white to off-white, round, flat-faced, radius edge, tablets debossed with "LAMICTAL" on one side and "200" on the other, Maintenance Packs of 30 (NDC 0173-0777-02).
Store between 20°C to 25°C (68°F to 77°F); with excursions permitted between 15°C and 30°C (59°F and 86°F).

LAMICTAL ODT (lamotrigine) Patient Titration Kit for Patients Taking Valproate (Blue ODT Kit)

25 mg, white to off-white, round, flat-faced, radius edge, tablets debossed with "LMT" on one side and "25" on the other, and 50 mg, white to off-white, round, flat-faced, radius edge, tablets debossed with "LMT" on one side and "50" on the other, blisterpack of 28 tablets (21/25-mg tablets and 7/50-mg tablets) (NDC 0173-0779-00).

LAMICTAL ODT (lamotrigine) Patient Titration Kit for Patients Taking Carbamazepine, Phenytoin, Phenobarbital, or Primidone and Not Taking Valproate (Green ODT Kit)

50 mg, white to off-white, round, flat-faced, radius edge, tablets debossed with "LMT" on one side and "50" on the other, and 100 mg, white to off-white, round, flat-faced, ra-

dius edge, tablets debossed with "LAMICTAL" on one side and "100" on the other, blisterpack of 56 tablets (42/50-mg tablets and 14/100-mg tablets) (NDC 0173-0780-00).

LAMICTAL ODT (lamotrigine) Patient Titration Kit for Patients Not Taking Carbamazepine, Phenytoin, Phenobarbital, Primidone, or Valproate (Orange ODT Kit)
25 mg, white to off-white, round, flat-faced, radius edge, tablets debossed with "LMT" on one side and "25" on the other, 50 mg, white to off-white, round, flat-faced, radius edge, tablets debossed with "LMT" on one side and "50" on the other, and 100 mg, white to off-white, round, flat-faced, radius edge, tablets debossed with "LAMICTAL" on one side and "100" on the other, blisterpack of 35 (14/25-mg tablets, 14/50-mg tablets, and 7/100-mg tablets) (NDC 0173-0778-00).

Store between 20°C to 25°C (68°F to 77°F); with excursions permitted between 15°C and 30°C (59°F and 86°F).

Blisterpacks: If the product is dispensed in a blisterpack, the patient should be advised to examine the blisterpack before use and not use if blisters are torn, broken, or missing.

17 PATIENT COUNSELING INFORMATION

See FDA-approved patient labeling (Medication Guide).

17.1 Rash
Prior to initiation of treatment with LAMICTAL, the patient should be instructed that a rash or other signs or symptoms of hypersensitivity (e.g., fever, lymphadenopathy) may herald a serious medical event and that the patient should report any such occurrence to a physician immediately.

17.2 Multiorgan Hypersensitivity Reactions, Blood Dyscrasias, and Organ Failure
Patients should be instructed that multiorgan hypersensitivity reactions and acute multiorgan failure may occur with LAMICTAL. Isolated organ failure or isolated blood dyscrasias without evidence of multiorgan hypersensitivity may also occur. Patients should contact their physician immediately if they experience any signs or symptoms of these conditions *[see Warnings and Precautions (5.2, 5.3)]*.

17.3 Suicidal Thinking and Behavior
Patients, their caregivers, and families should be counseled that AEDs, including LAMICTAL, may increase the risk of suicidal thoughts and behavior and should be advised of the need to be alert for the emergence or worsening of symptoms of depression, any unusual changes in mood or behavior, or the emergence of suicidal thoughts, behavior, or thoughts about self-harm. Behaviors of concern should be reported immediately to healthcare providers.

17.4 Worsening of Seizures
Patients should be advised to notify their physician if worsening of seizure control occurs.

17.5 Central Nervous System Adverse Effects
Patients should be advised that LAMICTAL may cause dizziness, somnolence, and other symptoms and signs of CNS depression. Accordingly, they should be advised neither to drive a car nor to operate other complex machinery until they have gained sufficient experience on LAMICTAL to gauge whether or not it adversely affects their mental and/or motor performance.

17.6 Pregnancy and Nursing
Patients should be advised to notify their physicians if they become pregnant or intend to become pregnant during therapy. Patients should be advised to notify their physicians if they intend to breastfeed or are breastfeeding an infant.
Patients should also be encouraged to enroll in the NAAED Pregnancy Registry if they become pregnant. This registry is collecting information about the safety of antiepileptic drugs during pregnancy. To enroll, patients can call the toll-free number 1-888-233-2334 *[see Use in Specific Populations (8.1)]*.
Patients who intend to breastfeed should be informed that LAMICTAL is present in breast milk and that they should monitor their child for potential adverse effects of this drug. Benefits and risks of continuing breastfeeding should be discussed with the patient.

17.7 Oral Contraceptive Use
Women should be advised to notify their physician if they plan to start or stop use of oral contraceptives or other female hormonal preparations. Starting estrogen-containing oral contraceptives may significantly decrease lamotrigine plasma levels and stopping estrogen-containing oral contraceptives (including the "pill-free" week) may significantly increase lamotrigine plasma levels *[see Warnings and Precautions (5.8), Clinical Pharmacology (12.3)]*. Women should also be advised to promptly notify their physician if they experience adverse reactions or changes in menstrual pattern (e.g., break-through bleeding) while receiving LAMICTAL in combination with these medications.

17.8 Discontinuing LAMICTAL
Patients should be advised to notify their physician if they stop taking LAMICTAL for any reason and not to resume LAMICTAL without consulting their physician.

17.9 Aseptic Meningitis
Patients should be advised that LAMICTAL may cause aseptic meningitis. Patients should be advised to notify their physician immediately if they develop signs and symptoms of meningitis such as headache, fever, nausea, vomiting, stiff neck, rash, abnormal sensitivity to light, myalgia, chills, confusion, or drowsiness while taking LAMICTAL.

17.10 Potential Medication Errors
Medication errors involving LAMICTAL have occurred. In particular the names LAMICTAL or lamotrigine can be confused with the names of other commonly used medications. Medication errors may also occur between the different formulations of LAMICTAL. To reduce the potential of medication errors, write and say LAMICTAL clearly. Depictions of the LAMICTAL Tablets, Chewable Dispersible Tablets, and Orally Disintegrating Tablets can be found in the Medication Guide that accompanies the product to highlight the distinctive markings, colors, and shapes that serve to identify the different presentations of the drug and thus may help reduce the risk of medication errors. **To avoid a medication error of using the wrong drug or formulation, patients should be strongly advised to visually inspect their tablets to verify that they are LAMICTAL, as well as the correct formulation of LAMICTAL, each time they fill their prescription** *[see Dosage Forms and Strengths (3.1, 3.2, 3.3), How Supplied/Storage and Handling (16)]*.

LAMICTAL is a registered trademark of GlaxoSmithKline.
Microcaps and AdvaTab are registered trademarks of Eurand, Inc.

GlaxoSmithKline
Research Triangle Park, NC 27709

LAMICTAL Tablets and Chewable Dispersible Tablets are manufactured by
DSM Pharmaceuticals, Inc., Greenville, NC 27834 or
GlaxoSmithKline, Research Triangle Park, NC 27709
LAMICTAL Orally Disintegrating Tablets are manufactured by
Eurand, Inc., Vandalia, OH 45377

LMT:8PI

MEDICATION GUIDE
LAMICTAL® (la-MIK-tal)
(lamotrigine)
Tablets and Chewable Dispersible Tablets
LAMICTAL® ODT™
(lamotrigine)
Orally Disintegrating Tablets

Read this Medication Guide before you start taking LAMICTAL and each time you get a refill. There may be new information. This information does not take the place of talking with your healthcare provider about your medical condition or treatment. If you have questions about LAMICTAL, ask your healthcare provider or pharmacist.

What is the most important information I should know about LAMICTAL?

1. LAMICTAL may cause a serious skin rash that may cause you to be hospitalized or even cause death.
There is no way to tell if a mild rash will become more serious. A serious skin rash can happen at any time during your treatment with LAMICTAL, but is more likely to happen within the first 2 to 8 weeks of treatment. Children between 2 to 16 years of age have a higher chance of getting this serious skin rash while taking LAMICTAL.
The risk of getting a serious skin rash is higher if you:
- take LAMICTAL while taking valproate [DEPAKENE® (valproic acid) or DEPAKOTE® (divalproex sodium)]
- take a higher starting dose of LAMICTAL than your healthcare provider prescribed
- increase your dose of LAMICTAL faster than prescribed.

Call your healthcare provider right away if you have any of the following:
- **a skin rash**
- **blistering or peeling of your skin**
- **hives**
- **painful sores in your mouth or around your eyes**

These symptoms may be the first signs of a serious skin reaction. A healthcare provider should examine you to decide if you should continue taking LAMICTAL.

2. Other serious reactions, including serious blood problems or liver problems. LAMICTAL can also cause other types of allergic reactions or serious problems that may affect organs and other parts of your body like your liver or blood cells. You may or may not have a rash with these types of reactions. Call your healthcare provider right away if you have any of these symptoms:
- fever
- frequent infections
- severe muscle pain
- swelling of your face, eyes, lips, or tongue
- swollen lymph glands
- unusual bruising or bleeding
- weakness, fatigue
- yellowing of your skin or the white part of your eyes

3. Like other antiepileptic drugs, LAMICTAL may cause suicidal thoughts or actions in a very small number of people, about 1 in 500.

Call a healthcare provider right away if you have any of these symptoms, especially if they are new, worse, or worry you:
- thoughts about suicide or dying
- attempt to commit suicide
- new or worse depression
- new or worse anxiety
- feeling agitated or restless
- panic attacks
- trouble sleeping (insomnia)
- new or worse irritability
- acting aggressive, being angry, or violent
- acting on dangerous impulses
- an extreme increase in activity and talking (mania)
- other unusual changes in behavior or mood

Do not stop LAMICTAL without first talking to a healthcare provider.
- Stopping LAMICTAL suddenly can cause serious problems.
- Suicidal thoughts or actions can be caused by things other than medicines. If you have suicidal thoughts or actions, your healthcare provider may check for other causes.

How can I watch for early symptoms of suicidal thoughts and actions?
- Pay attention to any changes, especially sudden changes, in mood, behaviors, thoughts, or feelings.
- Keep all follow-up visits with your healthcare provider as scheduled.
- Call your healthcare provider between visits as needed, especially if you are worried about symptoms.

4. LAMICTAL may rarely cause aseptic meningitis, a serious inflammation of the protective membrane that covers the brain and spinal cord.

Call your healthcare provider right away if you have any of the following symptoms:
- headache
- fever
- nausea
- vomiting
- stiff neck
- rash
- unusual sensitivity to light
- muscle pains
- chills
- confusion
- drowsiness

Meningitis has many causes other than LAMICTAL, which your doctor would check for if you developed meningitis while taking LAMICTAL.

LAMICTAL can have other serious side effects. For more information ask your healthcare provider or pharmacist. Tell your healthcare provider if you have any side effect that bothers you. Be sure to read the section below entitled "What are the possible side effects of LAMICTAL?"

5. Patients prescribed LAMICTAL have sometimes been given the wrong medicine because many medicines have names similar to LAMICTAL, so always check that you receive LAMICTAL.
Taking the wrong medication can cause serious health problems. When your healthcare provider gives you a prescription for LAMICTAL:
- Make sure you can read it clearly.
- Talk to your pharmacist to check that you are given the correct medicine.
- Each time you fill your prescription, check the tablets you receive against the pictures of the tablets below.
  These pictures show the distinct wording, colors, and shapes of the tablets that help to identify the right strength of LAMICTAL Tablets, Chewable Dispersible Tablets, and Orally Disintegrating Tablets. Immediately call your pharmacist if you receive a LAMICTAL tablet that does not look like one of the tablets shown below, as you may have received the wrong medication.

[See first table at top of next page]

LAMICTAL (lamotrigine) Chewable Dispersible Tablets
[See second table at top of next page]

LAMICTAL ODT (lamotrigine) Orally Disintegrating Tablets
[See third table at top of next page]

What is LAMICTAL?
LAMICTAL is a prescription medicine used:
1. together with other medicines to treat certain types of seizures (partial seizures, primary generalized tonic-clonic seizures, generalized seizures of Lennox-Gastaut syndrome) in people 2 years or older.
2. alone when changing from other medicines used to treat partial seizures in people 16 years or older.
3. for the long-term treatment of Bipolar I Disorder to lengthen the time between mood episodes in people 18 years or older who have been treated for mood episodes with other medicine.

It is not known if LAMICTAL is safe or effective in children or teenagers under the age of 18 with mood disorders such as bipolar disorder or depression.

LAMICTAL (lamotrigine) Tablets

25 mg, white
Imprinted with
LAMICTAL 25

100 mg, peach
Imprinted with
LAMICTAL 100

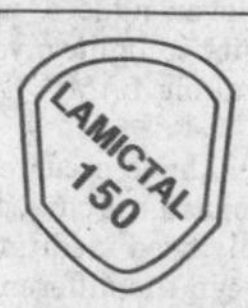

150 mg, cream
Imprinted with
LAMICTAL 150

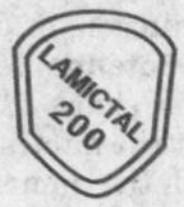

200 mg, blue
Imprinted with
LAMICTAL 200

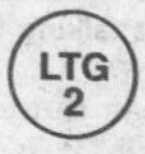

2 mg, white
Imprinted with
LTG 2

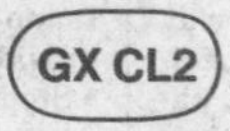

5 mg, white
Imprinted with
GX CL2

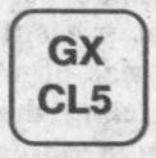

25 mg, white
Imprinted with
GX CL5

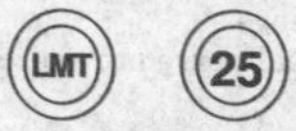

25 mg, white to
off-white
Imprinted with LMT
on one side
25 on the other

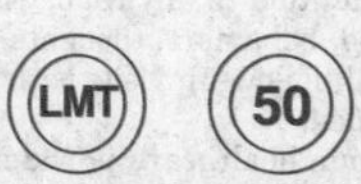

50 mg, white to off-white
Imprinted with
LMT on one side
50 on the other

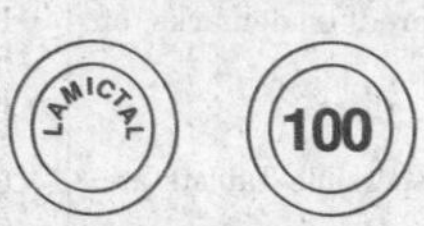

100 mg, white to off-white
Imprinted with
LAMICTAL on one side
100 on the other

200 mg, white to off-white
Imprinted with
LAMICTAL on one side
200 on the other

It is not known if LAMICTAL is safe or effective when used alone as the first treatment of seizures in adults.

Who should not take LAMICTAL?

You should not take LAMICTAL if you have had an allergic reaction to lamotrigine or to any of the inactive ingredients in LAMICTAL. See the end of this leaflet for a complete list of ingredients in LAMICTAL.

What should I tell my healthcare provider before taking LAMICTAL?

Before taking LAMICTAL, tell your healthcare provider about all of your medical conditions, including if you:

- have had a rash or allergic reaction to another antiseizure medicine.
- have or have had depression, mood problems or suicidal thoughts or behavior.
- have had aseptic meningitis after taking LAMICTAL or LAMICTAL XR (lamotrigine).
- are taking oral contraceptives (birth control pills) or other female hormonal medicines. Do not start or stop taking birth control pills or other female hormonal medicine until you have talked with your healthcare provider. Tell your healthcare provider if you have any changes in your menstrual pattern such as breakthrough bleeding. Stopping these medicines may cause side effects (such as dizziness, lack of coordination, or double vision). Starting these medicines may lessen how well LAMICTAL works.
- are pregnant or plan to become pregnant. It is not known if LAMICTAL will harm your unborn baby. If you become pregnant while taking LAMICTAL, talk to your healthcare provider about registering with the North American Antiepileptic Drug Pregnancy Registry. You can enroll in this registry by calling 1-888-233-2334. The purpose of this registry is to collect information about the safety of antiepileptic drugs during pregnancy.
- are breastfeeding. LAMICTAL passes into breast milk and may cause side effects in a breastfed baby. If you breastfeed while taking LAMICTAL, watch your baby closely for trouble breathing, episodes of temporarily stopping breathing, sleepiness, or poor sucking. Call your baby's healthcare provider right away if you see any of these problems. Talk to your healthcare provider about the best way to feed your baby if you take LAMICTAL.

Tell your healthcare provider about all the medicines you take or if you are planning to take a new medicine, including prescription and non-prescription medicines, vitamins, and herbal supplements. If you use LAMICTAL with certain other medicines, they can affect each other, causing side effects.

How should I take LAMICTAL?

- Take LAMICTAL exactly as prescribed.
- Your healthcare provider may change your dose. Do not change your dose without talking to your healthcare provider.
- Do not stop taking LAMICTAL without talking to your healthcare provider. Stopping LAMICTAL suddenly may cause serious problems. For example, if you have epilepsy and you stop taking LAMICTAL suddenly, you may get seizures that do not stop. Talk with your healthcare provider about how to stop LAMICTAL slowly.
- If you miss a dose of LAMICTAL, take it as soon as you remember. If it is almost time for your next dose, just skip the missed dose. Take the next dose at your regular time. **Do not take two doses at the same time.**
- You may not feel the full effect of LAMICTAL for several weeks.
- If you have epilepsy, tell your healthcare provider if your seizures get worse or if you have any new types of seizures.
- Swallow LAMICTAL tablets whole.
- If you have trouble swallowing LAMICTAL tablets, tell your healthcare provider because there may be another form of LAMICTAL you can take.
- LAMICTAL ODT should be placed on the tongue and moved around the mouth. The tablet will rapidly disintegrate, can be swallowed with or without water, and can be taken with or without food.
- LAMICTAL Chewable Dispersible tablets may be swallowed whole, chewed, or mixed in water or diluted fruit juice. If the tablets are chewed, drink a small amount of water or diluted fruit juice to help in swallowing. To break up LAMICTAL Chewable Dispersible tablets, add the tablets to a small amount of liquid (1 teaspoon, or enough to cover the medicine) in a glass or spoon. Wait at least 1 minute or until the tablets are completely broken up, mix the solution together and take the whole amount right away.
- If you receive LAMICTAL in a blisterpack, examine the blisterpack before use. Do not use if blisters are torn, broken, or missing.

What should I avoid while taking LAMICTAL?

Do not drive a car or operate complex, hazardous machinery until you know how LAMICTAL affects you.

What are possible side effects of LAMICTAL?

- See "What is the most important information I should know about LAMICTAL?"

Common side effects of LAMICTAL include:

• dizziness	• tremor
• headache	• rash
• blurred or double vision	• fever
• lack of coordination	• abdominal pain
• sleepiness	• back pain
• nausea, vomiting	• tiredness
• insomnia	• dry mouth

Tell your healthcare provider about any side effect that bothers you or that does not go away.

These are not all the possible side effects of LAMICTAL. For more information, ask your healthcare provider or pharmacist.

Call your doctor for medical advice about side effects. You may report side effects to FDA at 1-800-FDA-1088.

How should I store LAMICTAL?

- Store LAMICTAL at room temperature between 68°F to 77°F (20°C to 25°C).
- **Keep LAMICTAL and all medicines out of the reach of children.**

General information about LAMICTAL

Medicines are sometimes prescribed for purposes other than those listed in a Medication Guide. Do not use LAMICTAL for a condition for which it was not prescribed. Do not give LAMICTAL to other people, even if they have the same symptoms you have. It may harm them.

This Medication Guide summarizes the most important information about LAMICTAL. If you would like more information, talk with your healthcare provider. You can ask your healthcare provider or pharmacist for information about LAMICTAL that is written for healthcare professionals.

For more information, go to www.lamictal.com or call 1-888-825-5249.

What are the ingredients in LAMICTAL?

LAMICTAL Tablets

Active ingredient: lamotrigine.

Inactive ingredients: lactose; magnesium stearate, microcrystalline cellulose, povidone, sodium starch glycolate, FD&C Yellow No. 6 Lake (100 mg tablet only), ferric oxide, yellow (150 mg tablet only), and FD&C Blue No. 2 Lake (200 mg tablet only).

LAMICTAL Chewable Dispersible Tablets

Active ingredient: lamotrigine.

Inactive ingredients: blackcurrant flavor, calcium carbonate, low-substituted hydroxypropylcellulose, magnesium aluminum silicate, magnesium stearate, povidone, saccharin sodium, and sodium starch glycolate.

LAMICTAL ODT Orally Disintegrating Tablets

Active ingredient: lamotrigine

Inactive ingredients: artificial cherry flavor, crospovidone, ethylcellulose, magnesium stearate, mannitol, polyethylene, and sucralose.

This Medication Guide has been approved by the U.S. Food and Drug Administration.

LAMICTAL is a registered trademark of GlaxoSmithKline. DEPAKENE and DEPAKOTE are registered trademarks of Abbott Laboratories.

GlaxoSmithKline
Research Triangle Park, NC 27709

LAMICTAL Tablets and Chewable Dispersible Tablets are manufactured by
DSM Pharmaceuticals, Inc.,
Greenville, NC 27834 or
GlaxoSmithKline
Research Triangle Park, NC 27709

LAMICTAL Orally Disintegrating Tablets are manufactured by
Eurand, Inc., Vandalia, OH 45377

December 2011
LMT:7MG

LAMICTAL XR ℞

[la-mik' tal]
(lamotrigine)
Extended-Release Tablets

HIGHLIGHTS OF PRESCRIBING INFORMATION

These highlights do not include all the information needed to use LAMICTAL XR safely and effectively. See full prescribing information for LAMICTAL XR.

LAMICTAL XR (lamotrigine) Extended-Release Tablets
Initial U.S. Approval: 1994

WARNING: SERIOUS SKIN RASHES

See full prescribing information for complete boxed warning.

Cases of life-threatening serious rashes, including Stevens-Johnson syndrome and toxic epidermal necrolysis, and/or rash-related death have been caused by lamotrigine. The rate of serious rash is greater in pediatric patients than in adults. Additional factors that may increase the risk of rash include (5.1):

- **coadministration with valproate**
- **exceeding recommended initial dose of LAMICTAL XR**
- **exceeding recommended dose escalation for LAMICTAL XR**

Benign rashes are also caused by lamotrigine; however, it is not possible to predict which rashes will prove to be serious or life threatening. LAMICTAL XR should be discontinued at the first sign of rash, unless the rash is clearly not drug related. (5.1)

INDICATIONS AND USAGE

LAMICTAL XR is an antiepileptic drug (AED) indicated for:
- adjunctive therapy for primary generalized tonic-clonic (PGTC) seizures and partial onset seizures with or without secondary generalization in patients ≥13 years of age (1.1)
- conversion to monotherapy in patients ≥13 years of age with partial seizures who are receiving treatment with a single AED (1.2)
- Limitation of use: Safety and effectiveness in patients less than 13 years of age have not been established. (1.3)

DOSAGE AND ADMINISTRATION

- Do not exceed the recommended initial dosage and subsequent dose escalation. (2.1)
- Initiation of adjunctive therapy and conversion to monotherapy requires slow titration dependent on concomitant AEDs; the prescriber must refer to the appropriate algorithm in Dosage and Administration (2.2, 2.3)
  - Adjunct therapy target therapeutic dose range is 200 to 600 mg daily and is dependent on concomitant AEDs. (2.2)
  - Conversion to monotherapy: Target therapeutic dosage range is 250 to 300 mg daily. (2.3)
- Conversion from immediate-release lamotrigine to LAMICTAL XR: The initial dose of LAMICTAL XR should match the total daily dose of the immediate-release lamotrigine. Patients should be closely monitored for seizure control after conversion. (2.4)
- Do not restart LAMICTAL XR in patients who discontinued due to rash unless the potential benefits clearly outweigh the risks. (2.1, 5.1)
- Adjustments to maintenance doses are likely in patients starting or stopping estrogen-containing oral contraceptives. (2.1, 5.7)
- Discontinuation: Taper over a period of at least 2 weeks (approximately 50% dose reduction per week). (2.1, 5.8)

DOSAGE FORMS AND STRENGTHS

Extended-Release Tablets: 25 mg, 50 mg, 100 mg, 200 mg, 250 mg, and 300 mg. (3.1, 16)

CONTRAINDICATIONS

Hypersensitivity to the drug or its ingredients. (Boxed Warning, 4)

WARNINGS AND PRECAUTIONS

- Life-threatening serious rash and/or rash-related death: Discontinue at the first sign of rash, unless the rash is clearly not drug related. (Boxed Warning, 5.1)
- Fatal or life-threatening hypersensitivity reaction: Multiorgan hypersensitivity reactions, also known as Drug Reaction with Eosinophilia and Systemic Symptoms (DRESS), may be fatal or life threatening. Early signs may include rash, fever, and lymphadenopathy. These reactions may be associated with other organ involvement, such as hepatitis, hepatic failure, blood dyscrasias, or acute multiorgan failure. LAMICTAL XR should be discontinued if alternate etiology for this reaction is not found. (5.2)
- Blood dyscrasias (e.g., neutropenia, thrombocytopenia, pancytopenia): May occur, either with or without an associated hypersensitivity syndrome. Monitor for signs of anemia, unexpected infection, or bleeding. (5.3)
- Suicidal behavior and ideation: Monitor for suicidal thoughts or behaviors. (5.4)
- Aseptic meningitis: Monitor for signs of meningitis. (5.5)
- Medication errors due to product name confusion: Strongly advise patients to visually inspect tablets to verify the received drug is correct. (3.2, 5.6, 16, 17.10)

ADVERSE REACTIONS

- Most common adverse reactions with use as adjunctive therapy (treatment difference between LAMICTAL XR and placebo >4%) are dizziness, tremor/intention tremor, vomiting, and diplopia. (6.1)
- Most common adverse reactions with use as monotherapy were similar to those seen with previous studies conducted with immediate-release lamotrigine and LAMICTAL XR. (6.1)

To report SUSPECTED ADVERSE REACTIONS, contact GlaxoSmithKline at 1-888-825-5249 or FDA at 1-800-FDA-1088 or www.fda.gov/medwatch.

DRUG INTERACTIONS

- Valproate increases lamotrigine concentrations more than 2-fold. (7, 12.3)
- Carbamazepine, phenytoin, phenobarbital, and primidone decrease lamotrigine concentrations by approximately 40%. (7, 12.3)
- Estrogen-containing oral contraceptives and rifampin also decrease lamotrigine concentrations by approximately 50%. (7, 12.3)

USE IN SPECIFIC POPULATIONS

- Pregnancy: Based on animal data may cause fetal harm. Pregnancy registry available. (8.1)
- Hepatic impairment: Dosage adjustments required in patients with moderate and severe liver impairment. (2.1, 8.6)
- Renal impairment: Reduced maintenance doses may be effective for patients with significant renal impairment. (2.1, 8.7)

See 17 for PATIENT COUNSELING INFORMATION and Medication Guide

Revised: 10/2012

FULL PRESCRIBING INFORMATION: CONTENTS*

*** Sections or subsections omitted from the full prescribing information are not listed**

FULL PRESCRIBING INFORMATION

WARNING: SERIOUS SKIN RASHES

LAMICTAL® XR™ can cause serious rashes requiring hospitalization and discontinuation of treatment. The incidence of these rashes, which have included Stevens-Johnson syndrome, is approximately 0.8% (8 per 1,000) in pediatric patients (aged 2 to 16 years) receiving immediate-release lamotrigine as adjunctive therapy for epilepsy and 0.3% (3 per 1,000) in adults on adjunctive therapy for epilepsy. In a prospectively followed cohort of 1,983 pediatric patients (aged 2 to 16 years) with epilepsy taking adjunctive immediate-release lamotrigine, there was 1 rash-related death. LAMICTAL XR is not approved for patients less than 13 years of age. In worldwide postmarketing experience, rare cases of toxic epidermal necrolysis and/or rash-related death have been reported in adult and pediatric patients, but their numbers are too few to permit a precise estimate of the rate.

The risk of serious rash caused by treatment with LAMICTAL XR is not expected to differ from that with immediate-release lamotrigine. However, the relatively limited treatment experience with LAMICTAL XR makes it difficult to characterize the frequency and risk of serious rashes caused by treatment with LAMICTAL XR.

Other than age, there are as yet no factors identified that are known to predict the risk of occurrence or the severity of rash caused by LAMICTAL XR. There are suggestions, yet to be proven, that the risk of rash may also be increased by (1) coadministration of LAMICTAL XR with valproate (includes valproic acid and divalproex sodium), (2) exceeding the recommended initial dose of LAMICTAL XR, or (3) exceeding the recommended dose escalation for LAMICTAL XR. However, cases have occurred in the absence of these factors.

Nearly all cases of life-threatening rashes caused by immediate-release lamotrigine have occurred within 2 to 8 weeks of treatment initiation. However, isolated cases have occurred after prolonged treatment (e.g., 6 months). Accordingly, duration of therapy cannot be relied upon as means to predict the potential risk heralded by the first appearance of a rash.

Although benign rashes are also caused by LAMICTAL XR, it is not possible to predict reliably which rashes will prove to be serious or life threatening. Accordingly, LAMICTAL XR should ordinarily be discontinued at the first sign of rash, unless the rash is clearly not drug related. Discontinuation of treatment may not prevent a rash from becoming life threatening or permanently disabling or disfiguring *[see Warnings and Precautions (5.1)]*.

1 INDICATIONS AND USAGE

1.1 Adjunctive Therapy

LAMICTAL XR is indicated as adjunctive therapy for primary generalized tonic-clonic (PGTC) seizures and partial onset seizures with or without secondary generalization in patients ≥13 years of age.

1.2 Monotherapy

LAMICTAL XR is indicated for conversion to monotherapy in patients ≥13 years of age with partial seizures who are receiving treatment with a single antiepileptic drug (AED). Safety and effectiveness of LAMICTAL XR have not been established (1) as initial monotherapy or (2) for simultaneous conversion to monotherapy from two or more concomitant AEDs.

1.3 Limitation of Use

Safety and effectiveness of LAMICTAL XR for use in patients less than 13 years of age have not been established.

2 DOSAGE AND ADMINISTRATION

LAMICTAL XR Extended-Release Tablets are taken once daily, with or without food. Tablets must be swallowed whole and must not be chewed, crushed, or divided.

2.1 General Dosing Considerations

Rash: There are suggestions, yet to be proven, that the risk of severe, potentially life-threatening rash may be in-

Table 1. Escalation Regimen for LAMICTAL XR in Patients ≥13 Years of Age

	For Patients TAKING Valproate[a]	For Patients NOT TAKING Carbamazepine, Phenytoin, Phenobarbital, Primidone,[b] or Valproate[a]	For Patients TAKING Carbamazepine, Phenytoin, Phenobarbital, or Primidone[b] and NOT TAKING Valproate[a]
Weeks 1 and 2	25 mg every *other* day	25 mg every day	50 mg every day
Weeks 3 and 4	25 mg every day	50 mg every day	100 mg every day
Week 5	50 mg every day	100 mg every day	200 mg every day
Week 6	100 mg every day	150 mg every day	300 mg every day
Week 7	150 mg every day	200 mg every day	400 mg every day
Maintenance range (week 8 and onward)	200 to 250 mg every day[c]	300 to 400 mg every day[c]	400 to 600 mg every day[c]

[a]Valproate has been shown to inhibit glucuronidation and decrease the apparent clearance of lamotrigine *[see Drug Interactions (7), Clinical Pharmacology (12.3)]*.
[b]These drugs induce lamotrigine glucuronidation and increase clearance *[see Drug Interactions (7), Clinical Pharmacology (12.3)]*. Other drugs that have similar effects include estrogen-containing oral contraceptives *[see Drug Interactions (7), Clinical Pharmacology (12.3)]*. Dosing recommendations for oral contraceptives can be found in General Dosing Considerations *[see Dosage and Administration (2.1)]*. Patients on rifampin, or other drugs that induce lamotrigine glucuronidation and increase clearance, should follow the same dosing titration/maintenance regimen as that used with anticonvulsants that have this effect.
[c]Dose increases at week 8 or later should not exceed 100 mg daily at weekly intervals.

creased by (1) coadministration of LAMICTAL XR with valproate, (2) exceeding the recommended initial dose of LAMICTAL XR, or (3) exceeding the recommended dose escalation for LAMICTAL XR. However, cases have occurred in the absence of these factors *[see Boxed Warning]*. Therefore, it is important that the dosing recommendations be followed closely.
The risk of nonserious rash may be increased when the recommended initial dose and/or the rate of dose escalation for LAMICTAL XR is exceeded and in patients with a history of allergy or rash to other AEDs.
LAMICTAL XR Patient Titration Kits provide LAMICTAL XR at doses consistent with the recommended titration schedule for the first 5 weeks of treatment, based upon concomitant medications, for patients with partial onset seizures and are intended to help reduce the potential for rash. The use of LAMICTAL XR Patient Titration Kits is recommended for appropriate patients who are starting or restarting LAMICTAL XR *[see How Supplied/Storage and Handling (16)]*.
It is recommended that LAMICTAL XR not be restarted in patients who discontinued due to rash associated with prior treatment with lamotrigine, unless the potential benefits clearly outweigh the risks. If the decision is made to restart a patient who has discontinued LAMICTAL XR, the need to restart with the initial dosing recommendations should be assessed. The greater the interval of time since the previous dose, the greater consideration should be given to restarting with the initial dosing recommendations. If a patient has discontinued lamotrigine for a period of more than 5 half-lives, it is recommended that initial dosing recommendations and guidelines be followed. The half-life of lamotrigine is affected by other concomitant medications *[see Clinical Pharmacology (12.3)]*.
LAMICTAL XR Added to Drugs Known to Induce or Inhibit Glucuronidation: Drugs other than those listed in the Clinical Pharmacology section *[see Clinical Pharmacology (12.3)]* have not been systematically evaluated in combination with lamotrigine. Because lamotrigine is metabolized predominantly by glucuronic acid conjugation, drugs that are known to induce or inhibit glucuronidation may affect the apparent clearance of lamotrigine and doses of LAMICTAL XR may require adjustment based on clinical response.
Target Plasma Levels: A therapeutic plasma concentration range has not been established for lamotrigine. Dosing of LAMICTAL XR should be based on therapeutic response *[see Clinical Pharmacology (12.3)]*.
Women Taking Estrogen-Containing Oral Contraceptives: *Starting LAMICTAL XR in Women Taking Estrogen-Containing Oral Contraceptives:* Although estrogen-containing oral contraceptives have been shown to increase the clearance of lamotrigine *[see Clinical Pharmacology (12.3)]*, no adjustments to the recommended dose-escalation guidelines for LAMICTAL XR should be necessary solely based on the use of estrogen-containing oral contraceptives. Therefore, dose escalation should follow the recommended guidelines for initiating adjunctive therapy with LAMICTAL XR based on the concomitant AED or other concomitant medications (see Table 1). See below for adjustments to maintenance doses of LAMICTAL XR in women taking estrogen-containing oral contraceptives.
Adjustments to the Maintenance Dose of LAMICTAL XR in Women Taking Estrogen-Containing Oral Contraceptives:
(1) Taking Estrogen-Containing Oral Contraceptives: For women not taking carbamazepine, phenytoin, phenobarbital, primidone, or other drugs such as rifampin that induce lamotrigine glucuronidation *[see Drug Interactions (7), Clinical Pharmacology (12.3)]*, the maintenance dose of LAMICTAL XR will in most cases need to be increased by as much as 2-fold over the recommended target maintenance dose to maintain a consistent lamotrigine plasma level *[see Clinical Pharmacology (12.3)]*.
(2) Starting Estrogen-Containing Oral Contraceptives: In women taking a stable dose of LAMICTAL XR and not taking carbamazepine, phenytoin, phenobarbital, primidone, or other drugs such as rifampin that induce lamotrigine glucuronidation *[see Drug Interactions (7), Clinical Pharmacology (12.3)]*, the maintenance dose will in most cases need to be increased by as much as 2-fold to maintain a consistent lamotrigine plasma level. The dose increases should begin at the same time that the oral contraceptive is introduced and continue, based on clinical response, no more rapidly than 50 to 100 mg/day every week. Dose increases should not exceed the recommended rate (see Table 1) unless lamotrigine plasma levels or clinical response support larger increases. Gradual transient increases in lamotrigine plasma levels may occur during the week of inactive hormonal preparation (pill-free week), and these increases will be greater if dose increases are made in the days before or during the week of inactive hormonal preparation. Increased lamotrigine plasma levels could result in additional adverse reactions, such as dizziness, ataxia, and diplopia. If adverse reactions attributable to LAMICTAL XR consistently occur during the pill-free week, dose adjustments to the overall maintenance dose may be necessary. Dose adjustments limited to the pill-free week are not recommended. For women taking LAMICTAL XR in addition to carbamazepine, phenytoin, phenobarbital, primidone, or other drugs such as rifampin that induce lamotrigine glucuronidation *[see Drug Interactions (7), Clinical Pharmacology (12.3)]*, no adjustment to the dose of LAMICTAL XR should be necessary.
(3) Stopping Estrogen-Containing Oral Contraceptives: For women not taking carbamazepine, phenytoin, phenobarbital, primidone, or other drugs such as rifampin that induce lamotrigine glucuronidation *[see Drug Interactions (7), Clinical Pharmacology (12.3)]*, the maintenance dose of LAMICTAL XR will in most cases need to be decreased by as much as 50% in order to maintain a consistent lamotrigine plasma level. The decrease in dose of LAMICTAL XR should not exceed 25% of the total daily dose per week over a 2-week period, unless clinical response or lamotrigine plasma levels indicate otherwise *[see Clinical Pharmacology (12.3)]*. For women taking LAMICTAL XR in addition to carbamazepine, phenytoin, phenobarbital, primidone, or other drugs such as rifampin that induce lamotrigine glucuronidation *[see Drug Interactions (7), Clinical Pharmacology (12.3)]*, no adjustment to the dose of LAMICTAL XR should be necessary.
Women and Other Hormonal Contraceptive Preparations or Hormone Replacement Therapy: The effect of other hormonal contraceptive preparations or hormone replacement therapy on the pharmacokinetics of lamotrigine has not been systematically evaluated. It has been reported that ethinylestradiol, not progestogens, increased the clearance of lamotrigine up to 2-fold, and the progestin-only pills had no effect on lamotrigine plasma levels. Therefore, adjustments to the dosage of LAMICTAL XR in the presence of progestogens alone will likely not be needed.
Patients With Hepatic Impairment: Experience in patients with hepatic impairment is limited. Based on a clinical pharmacology study in 24 patients with mild, moderate, and severe liver impairment *[see Use in Specific Populations (8.6), Clinical Pharmacology (12.3)]*, the following general recommendations can be made. No dosage adjustment is needed in patients with mild liver impairment. Initial, escalation, and maintenance doses should generally be reduced by approximately 25% in patients with moderate and severe liver impairment without ascites and 50% in patients with severe liver impairment with ascites. Escalation and maintenance doses may be adjusted according to clinical response.
Patients With Renal Impairment: Initial doses of LAMICTAL XR should be based on patients' concomitant medications (see Table 1); reduced maintenance doses may be effective for patients with significant renal impairment *[see Use in Specific Populations (8.7), Clinical Pharmacology (12.3)]*. Few patients with severe renal impairment have been evaluated during chronic treatment with immediate-release lamotrigine. Because there is inadequate experience in this population, LAMICTAL XR should be used with caution in these patients.
Discontinuation Strategy: For patients receiving LAMICTAL XR in combination with other AEDs, a re-evaluation of all AEDs in the regimen should be considered if a change in seizure control or an appearance or worsening of adverse reactions is observed.
If a decision is made to discontinue therapy with LAMICTAL XR, a step-wise reduction of dose over at least 2 weeks (approximately 50% per week) is recommended unless safety concerns require a more rapid withdrawal *[see Warnings and Precautions (5.8)]*.
Discontinuing carbamazepine, phenytoin, phenobarbital, primidone, or other drugs such as rifampin that induce lamotrigine glucuronidation should prolong the half-life of lamotrigine; discontinuing valproate should shorten the half-life of lamotrigine.

2.2 Adjunctive Therapy for Primary Generalized Tonic-Clonic and Partial Onset Seizures

This section provides specific dosing recommendations for patients ≥13 years of age. Specific dosing recommendations are provided depending upon concomitant AED or other concomitant medications.
[See table 1 above]

2.3 Conversion From Adjunctive Therapy to Monotherapy

The goal of the transition regimen is to attempt to maintain seizure control while mitigating the risk of serious rash associated with the rapid titration of LAMICTAL XR.
The recommended maintenance dosage range of LAMICTAL XR as monotherapy is 250 to 300 mg given once daily.
The recommended initial dose and subsequent dose escalations for LAMICTAL XR should not be exceeded *[see Boxed Warning]*.
Conversion From Adjunctive Therapy With Carbamazepine, Phenytoin, Phenobarbital, or Primidone to Monotherapy With LAMICTAL XR: After achieving a dosage of 500 mg/day of LAMICTAL XR using the guidelines in Table 1, the concomitant enzyme-inducing AED should be withdrawn by 20% decrements each week over a 4-week period. Two weeks after completion of withdrawal of the enzyme-inducing AED, the dosage of LAMICTAL XR may be decreased no faster than 100 mg/day each week to achieve the monotherapy maintenance dosage range of 250 to 300 mg/day.
The regimen for the withdrawal of the concomitant AED is based on experience gained in the controlled monotherapy clinical trial using immediate-release lamotrigine.
Conversion From Adjunctive Therapy With Valproate to Monotherapy With LAMICTAL XR: The conversion regimen involves the 4 steps outlined in Table 2.

Table 2. Conversion From Adjunctive Therapy With Valproate to Monotherapy With LAMICTAL XR in Patients ≥13 Years of Age With Epilepsy

	LAMICTAL XR	Valproate
Step 1	Achieve a dosage of 150 mg/day according to guidelines in Table 1.	Maintain established stable dose.
Step 2	Maintain at 150 mg/day.	Decrease dosage by decrements no greater than 500 mg/day/week to 500 mg/day and then maintain for 1 week.

Step 3	Increase to 200 mg/day.	Simultaneously decrease to 250 mg/day and maintain for 1 week.
Step 4	Increase to 250 or 300 mg/day.	Discontinue.

Conversion From Adjunctive Therapy With Antiepileptic Drugs Other Than Carbamazepine, Phenytoin, Phenobarbital, Primidone, or Valproate to Monotherapy With LAMICTAL XR: After achieving a dosage of 250 to 300 mg/day of LAMICTAL XR using the guidelines in Table 1, the concomitant AED should be withdrawn by 20% decrements each week over a 4-week period. No adjustment to the monotherapy dose of LAMICTAL XR is needed.

2.4 Conversion From Immediate-Release Lamotrigine Tablets to LAMICTAL XR

Patients may be converted directly from immediate-release lamotrigine to LAMICTAL XR Extended-Release Tablets. The initial dose of LAMICTAL XR should match the total daily dose of immediate-release lamotrigine. However, some subjects on concomitant enzyme-inducing agents may have lower plasma levels of lamotrigine on conversion and should be monitored *[see Clinical Pharmacology (12.3)]*.

Following conversion to LAMICTAL XR, all patients (but especially those on drugs that induce lamotrigine glucuronidation) should be closely monitored for seizure control *[see Drug Interactions (7)]*. Depending on the therapeutic response after conversion, the total daily dose may need to be adjusted within the recommended dosing instructions (Table 1).

3 DOSAGE FORMS AND STRENGTHS

3.1 Extended-Release Tablets

25 mg, yellow with white center, round, biconvex, film-coated tablets printed with "LAMICTAL" and "XR 25."

50 mg, green with white center, round, biconvex, film-coated tablets printed with "LAMICTAL" and "XR 50."

100 mg, orange with white center, round, biconvex, film-coated tablets printed with "LAMICTAL" and "XR 100."

200 mg, blue with white center, round, biconvex, film-coated tablets printed with "LAMICTAL" and "XR 200."

250 mg, purple with white center, caplet-shaped, film-coated tablets printed with "LAMICTAL" and "XR 250."

300 mg, gray with white center, caplet-shaped, film-coated tablets printed with "LAMICTAL" and "XR 300."

3.2 Potential Medication Errors

Patients should be strongly advised to visually inspect their tablets to verify that they are receiving LAMICTAL XR, as opposed to other medications, and that they are receiving the correct formulation of lamotrigine each time they fill their prescription. Depictions of the LAMICTAL XR tablets can be found in the Medication Guide.

4 CONTRAINDICATIONS

LAMICTAL XR is contraindicated in patients who have demonstrated hypersensitivity (e.g., rash, angioedema, acute urticaria, extensive pruritus, mucosal ulceration) to the drug or its ingredients *[see Boxed Warning, Warnings and Precautions (5.1, 5.2)]*.

5 WARNINGS AND PRECAUTIONS

5.1 Serious Skin Rashes

The risk of serious rash caused by treatment with LAMICTAL XR is not expected to differ from that with immediate-release lamotrigine *[see Boxed Warning]*. However, the relatively limited treatment experience with LAMICTAL XR makes it difficult to characterize the frequency and risk of serious rashes caused by treatment with LAMICTAL XR.

Pediatric Population: The incidence of serious rash associated with hospitalization and discontinuation of immediate-release lamotrigine in a prospectively followed cohort of pediatric patients (aged 2 to 16 years) with epilepsy receiving adjunctive therapy with immediate-release lamotrigine was approximately 0.8% (16 of 1,983). When 14 of these cases were reviewed by 3 expert dermatologists, there was considerable disagreement as to their proper classification. To illustrate, one dermatologist considered none of the cases to be Stevens-Johnson syndrome; another assigned 7 of the 14 to this diagnosis. There was 1 rash-related death in this 1,983-patient cohort. Additionally, there have been rare cases of toxic epidermal necrolysis with and without permanent sequelae and/or death in US and foreign postmarketing experience.

There is evidence that the inclusion of valproate in a multidrug regimen increases the risk of serious, potentially life-threatening rash in pediatric patients. In pediatric patients who used valproate concomitantly, 1.2% (6 of 482) experienced a serious rash compared with 0.6% (6 of 952) patients not taking valproate.

LAMICTAL XR is not approved in patients less than 13 years of age.

Table 3. Risk by Indication for Antiepileptic Drugs in the Pooled Analysis

Indication	Placebo Patients With Events per 1,000 Patients	Drug Patients With Events per 1,000 Patients	Relative Risk: Incidence of Events in Drug Patients/ Incidence in Placebo Patients	Risk Difference: Additional Drug Patients With Events per 1,000 Patients
Epilepsy	1.0	3.4	3.5	2.4
Psychiatric	5.7	8.5	1.5	2.9
Other	1.0	1.8	1.9	0.9
Total	2.4	4.3	1.8	1.9

Adult Population: Serious rash associated with hospitalization and discontinuation of immediate-release lamotrigine occurred in 0.3% (11 of 3,348) of adult patients who received immediate-release lamotrigine in premarketing clinical trials of epilepsy. In worldwide postmarketing experience, rare cases of rash-related death have been reported, but their numbers are too few to permit a precise estimate of the rate.

Among the rashes leading to hospitalization were Stevens-Johnson syndrome, toxic epidermal necrolysis, angioedema, and those associated with multiorgan hypersensitivity *[see Warnings and Precautions (5.2)]*.

There is evidence that the inclusion of valproate in a multidrug regimen increases the risk of serious, potentially life-threatening rash in adults. Specifically, of 584 patients administered immediate-release lamotrigine with valproate in epilepsy clinical trials, 6 (1%) were hospitalized in association with rash; in contrast, 4 (0.16%) of 2,398 clinical trial patients and volunteers administered immediate-release lamotrigine in the absence of valproate were hospitalized.

Patients With History of Allergy or Rash to Other Antiepileptic Drugs: The risk of nonserious rash may be increased when the recommended initial dose and/or the rate of dose escalation for LAMICTAL XR is exceeded and in patients with a history of allergy or rash to other AEDs.

5.2 Multiorgan Hypersensitivity Reactions and Organ Failure

Multiorgan hypersensitivity reactions, also known as Drug Reaction with Eosinophilia and Systemic Symptoms (DRESS), have occurred with LAMICTAL. Some have been fatal or life threatening. DRESS typically, although not exclusively, presents with fever, rash, and/or lymphadenopathy in association with other organ system involvement, such as hepatitis, nephritis, hematologic abnormalities, myocarditis, or myositis, sometimes resembling an acute viral infection. Eosinophilia is often present. This disorder is variable in its expression and other organ systems not noted here may be involved.

Fatalities associated with acute multiorgan failure and various degrees of hepatic failure have been reported in 2 of 3,796 adult patients and 4 of 2,435 pediatric patients who received LAMICTAL in epilepsy clinical trials. Rare fatalities from multiorgan failure have also been reported in postmarketing use.

Isolated liver failure without rash or involvement of other organs has also been reported with LAMICTAL.

It is important to note that early manifestations of hypersensitivity (e.g., fever, lymphadenopathy) may be present even though a rash is not evident. If such signs or symptoms are present, the patient should be evaluated immediately. LAMICTAL XR should be discontinued if an alternative etiology for the signs or symptoms cannot be established.

Prior to initiation of treatment with LAMICTAL XR, the patient should be instructed that a rash or other signs or symptoms of hypersensitivity (e.g., fever, lymphadenopathy) may herald a serious medical event and that the patient should report any such occurrence to a physician immediately.

5.3 Blood Dyscrasias

There have been reports of blood dyscrasias with immediate-release lamotrigine that may or may not be associated with multiorgan hypersensitivity (also known as DRESS) *[see Warnings and Precautions (5.2)]*. These have included neutropenia, leukopenia, anemia, thrombocytopenia, pancytopenia, and, rarely, aplastic anemia and pure red cell aplasia.

5.4 Suicidal Behavior and Ideation

AEDs, including LAMICTAL XR, increase the risk of suicidal thoughts or behavior in patients taking these drugs for any indication. Patients treated with any AED for any indication should be monitored for the emergence or worsening of depression, suicidal thoughts or behavior, and/or any unusual changes in mood or behavior.

Pooled analyses of 199 placebo-controlled clinical trials (monotherapy and adjunctive therapy) of 11 different AEDs showed that patients randomized to 1 of the AEDs had approximately twice the risk (adjusted Relative Risk 1.8, 95% CI:1.2, 2.7) of suicidal thinking or behavior compared to patients randomized to placebo. In these trials, which had a median treatment duration of 12 weeks, the estimated incidence of suicidal behavior or ideation among 27,863 AED-treated patients was 0.43%, compared to 0.24% among 16,029 placebo-treated patients, representing an increase of approximately 1 case of suicidal thinking or behavior for every 530 patients treated. There were 4 suicides in drug-treated patients in the trials and none in placebo-treated patients, but the number of events is too small to allow any conclusion about drug effect on suicide.

The increased risk of suicidal thoughts or behavior with AEDs was observed as early as 1 week after starting treatment with AEDs and persisted for the duration of treatment assessed. Because most trials included in the analysis did not extend beyond 24 weeks, the risk of suicidal thoughts or behavior beyond 24 weeks could not be assessed.

The risk of suicidal thoughts or behavior was generally consistent among drugs in the data analyzed. The finding of increased risk with AEDs of varying mechanism of action and across a range of indications suggests that the risk applies to all AEDs used for any indication. The risk did not vary substantially by age (5 to 100 years) in the clinical trials analyzed.

Table 3 shows absolute and relative risk by indication for all evaluated AEDs.

[See table 3 above]

The relative risk for suicidal thoughts or behavior was higher in clinical trials for epilepsy than in clinical trials for psychiatric or other conditions, but the absolute risk differences were similar for the epilepsy and psychiatric indications.

Anyone considering prescribing LAMICTAL XR or any other AED must balance the risk of suicidal thoughts or behavior with the risk of untreated illness. Epilepsy and many other illnesses for which AEDs are prescribed are themselves associated with morbidity and mortality and an increased risk of suicidal thoughts and behavior. Should suicidal thoughts and behavior emerge during treatment, the prescriber needs to consider whether the emergence of these symptoms in any given patient may be related to the illness being treated.

Patients, their caregivers, and families should be informed that AEDs increase the risk of suicidal thoughts and behavior and should be advised of the need to be alert for the emergence or worsening of the signs and symptoms of depression; any unusual changes in mood or behavior; or the emergence of suicidal thoughts, behavior, or thoughts about self-harm. Behaviors of concern should be reported immediately to healthcare providers.

5.5 Aseptic Meningitis

Therapy with lamotrigine increases the risk of developing aseptic meningitis. Because of the potential for serious outcomes of untreated meningitis due to other causes, patients should also be evaluated for other causes of meningitis and treated as appropriate.

Postmarketing cases of aseptic meningitis have been reported in pediatric and adult patients taking lamotrigine for various indications. Symptoms upon presentation have included headache, fever, nausea, vomiting, and nuchal rigidity. Rash, photophobia, myalgia, chills, altered consciousness, and somnolence were also noted in some cases. Symptoms have been reported to occur within 1 day to one and a half months following the initiation of treatment. In most cases, symptoms were reported to resolve after discontinuation of lamotrigine. Re-exposure resulted in a rapid return of symptoms (from within 30 minutes to 1 day following re-initiation of treatment) that were frequently more severe. Some of the patients treated with LAMICTAL who developed aseptic meningitis had underlying diagnoses of systemic lupus erythematosus or other autoimmune diseases.

Cerebrospinal fluid (CSF) analyzed at the time of clinical presentation in reported cases was characterized by a mild to moderate pleocytosis, normal glucose levels, and mild to moderate increase in protein. CSF white blood cell count differentials showed a predominance of neutrophils in a majority of the cases, although a predominance of lymphocytes was reported in approximately one third of the cases. Some patients also had new onset of signs and symptoms of involvement of other organs (predominantly hepatic and renal involvement), which may suggest that in these cases the aseptic meningitis observed was part of a hypersensitivity reaction *[see Warnings and Precautions (5.2)]*.

5.6 Potential Medication Errors

Medication errors involving LAMICTAL have occurred. In particular, the names LAMICTAL or lamotrigine can be confused with the names of other commonly used medications. Medication errors may also occur between the different formulations of LAMICTAL. To reduce the potential of medication errors, write and say LAMICTAL XR clearly. Depictions of the LAMICTAL XR Extended-Release Tablets can be found in the Medication Guide. Each LAMICTAL XR tablet has a distinct color and white center, and is printed with "LAMICTAL XR" and the tablet strength. These distinctive features serve to identify the different presentations of the drug and thus may help reduce the risk of medication errors. LAMICTAL XR is supplied in round, unit-of-use bottles with orange caps containing 30 tablets. The label on the bottle includes a depiction of the tablets that further communicates to patients and pharmacists that the medication is LAMICTAL XR and the specific tablet strength included in the bottle. The unit-of-use bottle with a distinctive orange cap and distinctive bottle label features serves to identify the different presentations of the drug and thus may help to reduce the risk of medication errors. To avoid the medication error of using the wrong drug or formulation, patients should be strongly advised to visually inspect their tablets to verify that they are LAMICTAL XR each time they fill their prescription.

5.7 Concomitant Use With Oral Contraceptives

Some estrogen-containing oral contraceptives have been shown to decrease serum concentrations of lamotrigine *[see Clinical Pharmacology (12.3)]*. **Dosage adjustments will be necessary in most patients who start or stop estrogen-containing oral contraceptives while taking LAMICTAL XR***[see Dosage and Administration (2.1)]*. During the week of inactive hormone preparation (pill-free week) of oral contraceptive therapy, plasma lamotrigine levels are expected to rise, as much as doubling at the end of the week. Adverse reactions consistent with elevated levels of lamotrigine, such as dizziness, ataxia, and diplopia, could occur.

5.8 Withdrawal Seizures

As with other AEDs, LAMICTAL XR should not be abruptly discontinued. In patients with epilepsy there is a possibility of increasing seizure frequency. Unless safety concerns require a more rapid withdrawal, the dose of LAMICTAL XR should be tapered over a period of at least 2 weeks (approximately 50% reduction per week) *[see Dosage and Administration (2.1)]*.

5.9 Status Epilepticus

Valid estimates of the incidence of treatment-emergent status epilepticus among patients treated with immediate-release lamotrigine are difficult to obtain because reporters participating in clinical trials did not all employ identical rules for identifying cases. At a minimum, 7 of 2,343 adult patients had episodes that could unequivocally be described as status epilepticus. In addition, a number of reports of variably defined episodes of seizure exacerbation (e.g., seizure clusters, seizure flurries) were made.

5.10 Sudden Unexplained Death in Epilepsy

During the premarketing development of immediate-release lamotrigine, 20 sudden and unexplained deaths were recorded among a cohort of 4,700 patients with epilepsy (5,747 patient-years of exposure).

Some of these could represent seizure-related deaths in which the seizure was not observed, e.g., at night. This represents an incidence of 0.0035 deaths per patient-year. Although this rate exceeds that expected in a healthy population matched for age and sex, it is within the range of estimates for the incidence of sudden unexplained death in patients with epilepsy not receiving lamotrigine (ranging from 0.0005 for the general population of patients with epilepsy, to 0.004 for a recently studied clinical trial population similar to that in the clinical development program for immediate-release lamotrigine, to 0.005 for patients with refractory epilepsy). Consequently, whether these figures are reassuring or suggest concern depends on the comparability of the populations reported upon to the cohort receiving immediate-release lamotrigine and the accuracy of the estimates provided. Probably most reassuring is the similarity of estimated sudden unexplained death in epilepsy (SUDEP) rates in patients receiving immediate-release lamotrigine and those receiving other AEDs, chemically unrelated to each other, that underwent clinical testing in similar populations. Importantly, that drug is chemically unrelated to lamotrigine. This evidence suggests, although it certainly does not prove, that the high SUDEP rates reflect population rates, not a drug effect.

5.11 Addition of LAMICTAL XR to a Multidrug Regimen That Includes Valproate

Because valproate reduces the clearance of lamotrigine, the dosage of lamotrigine in the presence of valproate is less than half of that required in its absence *[see Dosage and Administration (2.1, 2.2), Drug Interactions (7)]*.

5.12 Binding in the Eye and Other Melanin-Containing Tissues

Because lamotrigine binds to melanin, it could accumulate in melanin-rich tissues over time. This raises the possibility that lamotrigine may cause toxicity in these tissues after extended use. Although ophthalmological testing was performed in 1 controlled clinical trial, the testing was inadequate to exclude subtle effects or injury occurring after long-term exposure. Moreover, the capacity of available tests to detect potentially adverse consequences, if any, of lamotrigine binding to melanin is unknown *[see Clinical Pharmacology (12.2)]*.

Accordingly, although there are no specific recommendations for periodic ophthalmological monitoring, prescribers should be aware of the possibility of long-term ophthalmologic effects.

5.13 Laboratory Tests

Plasma Concentrations of Lamotrigine: The value of monitoring plasma concentrations of lamotrigine in patients treated with LAMICTAL XR has not been established. Because of the possible pharmacokinetic interactions between lamotrigine and other drugs, including AEDs (see Table 6), monitoring of the plasma levels of lamotrigine and concomitant drugs may be indicated, particularly during dosage adjustments. In general, clinical judgment should be exercised regarding monitoring of plasma levels of lamotrigine and other drugs and whether or not dosage adjustments are necessary.

Effect on Leukocytes: Treatment with LAMICTAL XR caused an increased incidence of subnormal (below the reference range) values in some hematology analytes (e.g., total white blood cells, monocytes). The treatment effect (LAMICTAL XR % - Placebo %) incidence of subnormal counts was 3% for total white blood cells and 4% for monocytes.

6 ADVERSE REACTIONS

The following adverse reactions are described in more detail in the *Warnings and Precautions* section of the label:

- Serious skin rashes *[see Warnings and Precautions (5.1)]*
- Multiorgan hypersensitivity reactions and organ failure *[see Warnings and Precautions (5.2)]*
- Blood dyscrasias *[see Warnings and Precautions (5.3)]*
- Suicidal behavior and ideation *[see Warnings and Precautions (5.4)]*
- Aseptic meningitis *[see Warnings and Precautions (5.5)]*
- Withdrawal seizures *[see Warnings and Precautions (5.8)]*
- Status epilepticus *[see Warnings and Precautions (5.9)]*
- Sudden unexplained death in epilepsy *[see Warnings and Precautions (5.10)]*

6.1 Clinical Trial Experience With LAMICTAL XR for Treatment of Primary Generalized Tonic-Clonic and Partial Onset Seizures

Most Common Adverse Reactions in Clinical Studies: *Adjunctive Therapy in Patients With Epilepsy:* Because clinical trials are conducted under widely varying conditions, adverse reaction rates observed in the clinical trials of a drug cannot be directly compared with rates in the clinical trials of another drug and may not reflect the rates observed in practice.

LAMICTAL XR has been evaluated for safety in patients ≥13 years of age with PGTC and partial onset seizures. The most commonly observed adverse reactions in these 2 double-blind, placebo-controlled trials of adjunctive therapy with LAMICTAL XR were, in order of decreasing incidence (treatment difference between LAMICTAL XR and placebo ≥4%): dizziness, tremor/intention tremor, vomiting, and diplopia.

In these 2 trials, adverse reactions led to withdrawal of 4 (2%) patients in the group receiving placebo and 10 (5%) patients in the group receiving LAMICTAL XR. Dizziness was the most common reason for withdrawal in the group receiving LAMICTAL XR (5 patients [3%]). The next most common adverse reactions leading to withdrawal in 2 patients each (1%) were rash, headache, nausea, and nystagmus.

Table 4 displays the incidence of adverse reactions in these two 19-week, double-blind, placebo-controlled studies of patients with PGTC and partial onset seizures.

Table 4. Adverse Reaction Incidence in Double-Blind, Placebo-Controlled Adjunctive Trials of Patients With Epilepsy (Adverse Reactions ≥2% of Patients Treated With LAMICTAL XR and Numerically More Frequent Than in the Placebo Group)

Body System/Adverse Reaction	LAMICTAL XR (n = 190) %	Placebo (n = 195) %
Ear and labyrinth disorders		
Vertigo	3	<1
Eye disorders		
Diplopia	5	<1
Vision blurred	3	2
Gastrointestinal disorders		
Nausea	7	4
Vomiting	6	3
Diarrhea	5	3
Constipation	2	<1
Dry mouth	2	1
General disorders and administration site conditions		
Asthenia and fatigue	6	4
Infections and infestations		
Sinusitis	2	1
Metabolic and nutritional disorders		
Anorexia	3	2
Musculoskeletal and connective tissue disorder		
Myalgia	2	0
Nervous system		
Dizziness	14	6
Tremor and intention tremor	6	1
Somnolence	5	3
Cerebellar coordination and balance disorder	3	0
Nystagmus	2	<1
Psychiatric disorders		
Depression	3	<1
Anxiety	3	0
Respiratory, thoracic, and mediastinal disorders		
Pharyngolaryngeal pain	3	2
Vascular disorder		
Hot flush	2	0

Note: In these trials the incidence of nonserious rash was 2% for LAMICTAL XR and 3% for placebo. In clinical trials evaluating immediate-release lamotrigine, the rate of serious rash was 0.3% in adults on adjunctive therapy for epilepsy *[see Boxed Warning]*.

Adverse reactions were also analyzed to assess the incidence of the onset of an event in the titration period, and in the maintenance period, and if adverse reactions occurring in the titration phase persisted in the maintenance phase. The incidence for many adverse reactions caused by treatment with LAMICTAL XR was increased relative to placebo (i.e., treatment difference between LAMICTAL XR and placebo ≥2%) in either the titration or maintenance phases of the study. During the titration phase, an increased incidence (shown in descending order of % treatment difference) was observed for diarrhea, nausea, vomiting, somnolence, vertigo, myalgia, hot flush, and anxiety. During the maintenance phase, an increased incidence was observed for dizziness, tremor, and diplopia. Some adverse reactions developing in the titration phase were notable for persisting (>7 days) into the maintenance phase. These "persistent" adverse reactions included somnolence and dizziness.

There were inadequate data to evaluate the effect of dose and/or concentration on the incidence of adverse reactions because, although patients were randomized to different target doses based upon concomitant AED, the plasma exposure was expected to be generally similar among all patients receiving different doses. However, in a randomized, parallel study comparing placebo and 300 and 500 mg/day of immediate-release lamotrigine, the incidence of the most common adverse reactions (≥5%) such as ataxia, blurred vision, diplopia, and dizziness were dose related. Less common adverse reactions (<5%) were not assessed for dose-response relationships.

Monotherapy in Patients With Epilepsy: Adverse reactions observed in this study were generally similar to those observed and attributed to drug in adjunctive and monotherapy immediate-release lamotrigine and adjunctive LAMICTAL XR placebo-controlled studies. Only 2 adverse events, nasopharyngitis and upper respiratory tract infection, were observed at a rate of ≥3% and not reported at a similar rate in previous studies. Because this study did not include a placebo control group, causality could not be established *[see Clinical Studies (14.3)]*.

6.2 Other Adverse Reactions Observed During the Clinical Development of Immediate-Release Lamotrigine

All reported reactions are included except those already listed in the previous tables or elsewhere in the labeling, those too general to be informative, and those not reasonably associated with the use of the drug.

Adjunctive Therapy in Adults With Epilepsy: In addition to the adverse reactions reported above from the development of LAMICTAL XR, the following adverse reactions with an uncertain relationship to lamotrigine were reported during the clinical development of immediate-release lamotrigine for treatment of epilepsy in adults. These reactions occurred in ≥2% of patients receiving immediate-release lamotrigine and more frequently than in the placebo group.

Body as a Whole: Headache, flu syndrome, fever, neck pain.

Musculoskeletal: Arthralgia.

Nervous: Insomnia, convulsion, irritability, speech disorder, concentration disturbance.

Respiratory: Pharyngitis, cough increased.

Skin and Appendages: Rash, pruritus.

Urogenital (female patients only): Vaginitis, amenorrhea, dysmenorrhea.

Monotherapy in Adults With Epilepsy: In addition to the adverse reactions reported above from the development of LAMICTAL XR, the following adverse reactions with an uncertain relationship to lamotrigine were reported during the clinical development of immediate-release lamotrigine for treatment of epilepsy in adults. These reactions occurred in >2% of patients receiving immediate-release lamotrigine and more frequently than in the placebo group.

Body as a Whole: Chest pain.

Digestive: Rectal hemorrhage, peptic ulcer.

Metabolic and Nutritional: Weight decrease, peripheral edema.

Nervous: Hypesthesia, libido increase, decreased reflexes.

Respiratory: Epistaxis, dyspnea.

Skin and Appendages: Contact dermatitis, dry skin, sweating.

Special Senses: Vision abnormality.

Urogenital (female patients only): Dysmenorrhea.

Other Clinical Trial Experience: Immediate-release lamotrigine has been administered to 6,694 individuals for whom complete adverse reaction data was captured during all clinical trials, only some of which were placebo controlled.

Adverse reactions are further classified within body system categories and enumerated in order of decreasing frequency using the following definitions: *frequent* adverse reactions are defined as those occurring in at least 1/100 patients; *infrequent* adverse reactions are those occurring in 1/100 to 1/1,000 patients; *rare* adverse reactions are those occurring in fewer than 1/1,000 patients.

Cardiovascular System: *Infrequent:* Hypertension, palpitations, postural hypotension, syncope, tachycardia, vasodilation.

Dermatological: *Infrequent:* Acne, alopecia, hirsutism, maculopapular rash, urticaria. *Rare:* Leukoderma, multiforme erythema, petechial rash, pustular rash.

Digestive System: *Infrequent:* Dysphagia, liver function tests abnormal, mouth ulceration. *Rare:* Gastrointestinal hemorrhage, hemorrhagic colitis, hepatitis, melena and stomach ulcer.

Endocrine System: *Rare:* Goiter, hypothyroidism.

Hematologic and Lymphatic System: *Infrequent:* Ecchymosis, leukopenia. *Rare:* Anemia, eosinophilia, fibrin decrease, fibrinogen decrease, iron deficiency anemia, leukocytosis, lymphocytosis, macrocytic anemia, petechia, thrombocytopenia.

Metabolic and Nutritional Disorders: *Infrequent:* Aspartate transaminase increased. *Rare:* Alcohol intolerance, alkaline phosphatase increase, alanine transaminase increase, bilirubinemia, gamma glutamyl transpeptidase increase, hyperglycemia.

Musculoskeletal System: *Rare:* Muscle atrophy, pathological fracture, tendinous contracture.

Nervous System: *Frequent:* Confusion. *Infrequent:* Akathisia, apathy, aphasia, depersonalization, dysarthria, dyskinesia, euphoria, hallucinations, hostility, hyperkinesia, hypertonia, libido decreased, memory decrease, mind racing, movement disorder, myoclonus, panic attack, paranoid reaction, personality disorder, psychosis, stupor. *Rare:* Choreoathetosis, delirium, delusions, dysphoria, dystonia, extrapyramidal syndrome, hemiplegia, hyperalgesia, hyperesthesia, hypokinesia, hypotonia, manic depression reaction, neuralgia, paralysis, peripheral neuritis.

Respiratory System: *Rare:* Hiccup, hyperventilation.

Special Senses: *Frequent:* Amblyopia. *Infrequent:* Abnormality of accommodation, conjunctivitis, dry eyes, ear pain, photophobia, taste perversion, tinnitus. *Rare:* Deafness, lacrimation disorder, oscillopsia, parosmia, ptosis, strabismus, taste loss, uveitis, visual field defect.

Urogenital System: *Infrequent:* Abnormal ejaculation, hematuria, impotence, menorrhagia, polyuria, urinary incontinence. *Rare:* Acute kidney failure, breast neoplasm, creatinine increase, female lactation, kidney failure, kidney pain, nocturia, urinary retention, urinary urgency.

6.3 Postmarketing Experience With Immediate-Release Lamotrigine

The following adverse events (not listed above in clinical trials or other sections of the prescribing information) have been identified during postapproval use of immediate-release lamotrigine. Because these events are reported voluntarily from a population of uncertain size, it is not always possible to reliably estimate their frequency or establish a causal relationship to drug exposure.

Blood and Lymphatic: Agranulocytosis, hemolytic anemia, lymphadenopathy not associated with hypersensitivity disorder.

Gastrointestinal: Esophagitis.

Hepatobiliary Tract and Pancreas: Pancreatitis.

Immunologic: Lupus-like reaction, vasculitis.

Lower Respiratory: Apnea.

Musculoskeletal: Rhabdomyolysis has been observed in patients experiencing hypersensitivity reactions.

Neurology: Exacerbation of Parkinsonian symptoms in patients with pre-existing Parkinson's disease, tics.

Non-site Specific: Progressive immunosuppression.

7 DRUG INTERACTIONS

Significant drug interactions with lamotrigine are summarized in Table 5. Additional details of these drug interaction studies, which were conducted using immediate-release lamotrigine, are provided in the Clinical Pharmacology section *[see Clinical Pharmacology (12.3)]*.

Table 5. Established and Other Potentially Significant Drug Interactions

Concomitant Drug	Effect on Concentration of Lamotrigine or Concomitant Drug	Clinical Comment
Estrogen-containing oral contraceptive preparations containing 30 mcg ethinylestradiol and 150 mcg levonorgestrel	↓ lamotrigine	Decreased lamotrigine levels approximately 50%.
	↓ levonorgestrel	Decrease in levonorgestrel component by 19%.
Carbamazepine and carbamazepine epoxide	↓ lamotrigine ? CBZ epoxide	Addition of carbamazepine decreases lamotrigine concentration approximately 40%. May increase carbamazepine epoxide levels.
Phenobarbital/primidone	↓ lamotrigine	Decreased lamotrigine concentration approximately 40%.
Phenytoin	↓ lamotrigine	Decreased lamotrigine concentration approximately 40%.
Rifampin	↓ lamotrigine	Decreased lamotrigine AUC approximately 40%.
Valproate	↑ lamotrigine ? valproate	Increased lamotrigine concentrations slightly more than 2-fold. Decreased valproate concentrations an average of 25% over a 3-week period then stabilized in healthy volunteers; no change in controlled clinical trials in epilepsy patients.

↓ = Decreased (induces lamotrigine glucuronidation).
↑ = Increased (inhibits lamotrigine glucuronidation).
? = Conflicting data.

[See table 5 above]

8 USE IN SPECIFIC POPULATIONS

8.1 Pregnancy

As with other AEDs, physiological changes during pregnancy may affect lamotrigine concentrations and/or therapeutic effect. There have been reports of decreased lamotrigine concentrations during pregnancy and restoration of pre-partum concentrations after delivery. Dosage adjustments may be necessary to maintain clinical response.

Pregnancy Category C.

There are no adequate and well-controlled studies in pregnant women. In animal studies, lamotrigine was developmentally toxic at doses lower than those administered clinically. LAMICTAL XR should be used during pregnancy only if the potential benefit justifies the potential risk to the fetus.

When lamotrigine was administered to pregnant mice, rats, or rabbits during the period of organogenesis (oral doses of up to 125, 25, and 30 mg/kg, respectively), reduced fetal body weight and increased incidences of fetal skeletal variations were seen in mice and rats at doses that were also maternally toxic. The no-effect doses for embryo-fetal developmental toxicity in mice, rats, and rabbits (75, 6.25, and 30 mg/kg, respectively) are similar to (mice and rabbits) or less than the human dose of 400 mg/day on a body surface area (mg/m^2) basis.

In a study in which pregnant rats were administered lamotrigine (oral doses of 5 or 25 mg/kg) during the period of organogenesis and offspring were evaluated postnatally, behavioral abnormalities were observed in exposed offspring at both doses. The lowest effect dose for developmental neurotoxicity in rats is less than the human dose of 400 mg/day on a mg/m^2 basis. Maternal toxicity was observed at the higher dose tested.

When pregnant rats were administered lamotrigine (oral doses of 5, 10, or 20 mg/kg) during the latter part of gestation, increased offspring mortality (including stillbirths) was seen at all doses. The lowest effect dose for peri/postnatal developmental toxicity in rats is less than the human dose of 400 mg/day on a mg/m^2 basis. Maternal toxicity was observed at the 2 highest doses tested.

Lamotrigine decreases fetal folate concentrations in rat, an effect known to be associated with adverse pregnancy outcomes in animals and humans.

Pregnancy Registry: To provide information regarding the effects of in utero exposure to LAMICTAL XR, physicians are advised to recommend that pregnant patients taking LAMICTAL XR enroll in the North American Antiepileptic Drug (NAAED) Pregnancy Registry. This can be done by calling the toll-free number 1-888-233-2334, and must be done by patients themselves. Information on the registry can also be found at the website http://www.aedpregnancyregistry.org.

8.2 Labor and Delivery

The effect of LAMICTAL XR on labor and delivery in humans is unknown.

8.3 Nursing Mothers

Lamotrigine is present in milk from lactating women taking LAMICTAL XR. Data from multiple small studies indicate that lamotrigine plasma levels in human milk-fed infants have been reported to be as high as 50% of the maternal serum levels. Neonates and young infants are at risk for high serum levels because maternal serum and milk levels can rise to high levels postpartum if lamotrigine dosage has been increased during pregnancy but not later reduced to the pre-pregnancy dosage. Lamotrigine exposure is further increased due to the immaturity of the infant glucuronidation capacity needed for drug clearance. Events including apnea, drowsiness, and poor sucking have been reported in infants who have been human milk-fed by mothers using lamotrigine; whether or not these events were caused by lamotrigine is unknown. Human milk-fed infants should be closely monitored for adverse events resulting from lamotrigine. Measurement of infant serum levels should be performed to rule out toxicity if concerns arise. Human milk-feeding should be discontinued in infants with lamotrigine toxicity. Caution should be exercised when LAMICTAL XR is administered to a nursing woman.

8.4 Pediatric Use

LAMICTAL XR is indicated as adjunctive therapy for PGTC and partial onset seizures with or without secondary generalization in patients ≥13 years of age. Safety and effectiveness of LAMICTAL XR for any use in patients less than 13 years of age have not been established.

Immediate-release lamotrigine is indicated for adjunctive therapy in patients ≥2 years of age for partial seizures, the generalized seizures of Lennox-Gastaut syndrome, and PGTC seizures.

Safety and efficacy of immediate-release lamotrigine, used as adjunctive treatment for partial seizures, were not demonstrated in a small, randomized, double-blind, placebo-controlled withdrawal study in very young pediatric patients (aged 1 to 24 months). Immediate-release lamotrigine was associated with an increased risk for infectious adverse reactions (lamotrigine 37%, placebo 5%), and respiratory adverse reactions (lamotrigine 26%, placebo 5%). Infectious adverse reactions included bronchiolitis, bronchitis, ear infection, eye infection, otitis externa, pharyngitis, urinary tract infection, and viral infection. Respiratory adverse reactions included nasal congestion, cough, and apnea.

In a juvenile animal study in which lamotrigine (oral doses of 5, 15, or 30 mg/kg) was administered to young rats (postnatal days 7 to 62), decreased viability and growth were seen at the highest dose tested and long-term behavioral abnormalities (decreased locomotor activity, increased reactivity, and learning deficits in animals tested as adults) were observed at the 2 highest doses. The no-effect dose for adverse effects on neurobehavioral development is less than the human dose of 400 mg/day on a mg/m^2 basis.

8.5 Geriatric Use

Clinical studies of LAMICTAL XR for epilepsy did not include sufficient numbers of subjects aged 65 years and over to determine whether they respond differently from younger subjects or exhibit a different safety profile than that of younger patients. In general, dose selection for an elderly patient should be cautious, usually starting at the low end of the dosing range, reflecting the greater frequency of decreased hepatic, renal, or cardiac function, and of concomitant disease or other drug therapy.

8.6 Patients With Hepatic Impairment

Experience in patients with hepatic impairment is limited. Based on a clinical pharmacology study with immediate-release lamotrigine in 24 patients with mild, moderate, and severe liver impairment *[see Clinical Pharmacology (12.3)]*, the following general recommendations can be made. No dosage adjustment is needed in patients with mild liver impairment. Initial, escalation, and maintenance doses should generally be reduced by approximately 25% in patients with moderate and severe liver impairment without ascites and 50% in patients with severe liver impairment with ascites. Escalation and maintenance doses may be adjusted according to clinical response *[see Dosage and Administration (2.1)]*.

8.7 Patients With Renal Impairment

Lamotrigine is metabolized mainly by glucuronic acid conjugation, with the majority of the metabolites being recovered in the urine. In a small study comparing a single dose of immediate-release lamotrigine in patients with varying degrees of renal impairment with healthy volunteers, the plasma half-life of lamotrigine was approximately twice as long in the patients with significant renal impairment *[see Clinical Pharmacology (12.3)]*.

Initial doses of LAMICTAL XR should be based on patients' AED regimens; reduced maintenance doses may be effective for patients with significant renal impairment. Few patients with severe renal impairment have been evaluated during chronic treatment with lamotrigine. Because there is inadequate experience in this population, LAMICTAL XR should be used with caution in these patients *[see Dosage and Administration (2.1)]*.

10 OVERDOSAGE

10.1 Human Overdose Experience

Overdoses involving quantities up to 15 g have been reported for immediate-release lamotrigine, some of which have been fatal. Overdose has resulted in ataxia, nystagmus, increased seizures, decreased level of consciousness, coma, and intraventricular conduction delay.

10.2 Management of Overdose

There are no specific antidotes for lamotrigine. Following a suspected overdose, hospitalization of the patient is advised. General supportive care is indicated, including frequent monitoring of vital signs and close observation of the patient. If indicated, emesis should be induced; usual precautions should be taken to protect the airway. It is uncertain whether hemodialysis is an effective means of removing lamotrigine from the blood. In 6 renal failure patients, about 20% of the amount of lamotrigine in the body was removed by hemodialysis during a 4-hour session. A Poison Control Center should be contacted for information on the management of overdosage of LAMICTAL XR.

11 DESCRIPTION

LAMICTAL XR (lamotrigine), an AED of the phenyltriazine class, is chemically unrelated to existing AEDs. Its chemical name is 3,5-diamino-6-(2,3-dichlorophenyl)-*as*-triazine, its molecular formula is $C_9H_7N_5Cl_2$, and its molecular weight is 256.09. Lamotrigine is a white to pale cream-colored powder and has a pK$_a$ of 5.7. Lamotrigine is very slightly soluble in water (0.17 mg/mL at 25°C) and slightly soluble in 0.1 M HCl (4.1 mg/mL at 25°C). The structural formula is:

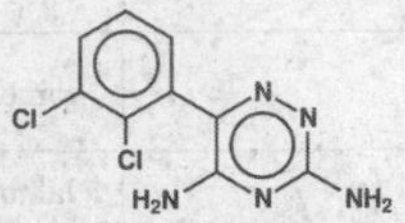

LAMICTAL XR Extended-Release Tablets are supplied for oral administration as 25-mg (yellow with white center), 50-mg (green with white center), 100-mg (orange with white center), 200-mg (blue with white center), 250-mg (purple with white center), and 300-mg (gray with white center) tablets. Each tablet contains the labeled amount of lamotrigine and the following inactive ingredients: glycerol monostearate, hypromellose, lactose monohydrate; magnesium stearate; methacrylic acid copolymer dispersion, polyethylene glycol 400, polysorbate 80, silicon dioxide (25- and 50-mg tablets only), titanium dioxide, triethyl citrate, carmine (250-mg tablet only), iron oxide black (50-, 250-, and 300-mg tablets only), iron oxide yellow (25-, 50-, and 100-mg tablets only), iron oxide red (100-mg tablet only), FD&C Blue No. 2 Aluminum Lake (200- and 250-mg tablets only). Tablets are printed with edible black ink.

LAMICTAL XR Extended-Release Tablets contain a modified-release eroding formulation as the core. The tablets are coated with a clear enteric coat and have an aperture drilled through the coats on both faces of the tablet (DiffCORE™) to enable a controlled release of drug in the acidic environment of the stomach. The combination of this and the modified-release core are designed to control the dissolution rate of lamotrigine over a period of approximately 12 to 15 hours, leading to a gradual increase in serum lamotrigine levels.

12 CLINICAL PHARMACOLOGY

12.1 Mechanism of Action

The precise mechanism(s) by which lamotrigine exerts its anticonvulsant action is unknown. In animal models designed to detect anticonvulsant activity, lamotrigine was effective in preventing seizure spread in the maximum electroshock and pentylenetetrazol tests, and prevented seizures in the visually and electrically evoked after-discharge tests for antiepileptic activity. Lamotrigine also displayed inhibitory properties in a kindling model in rats both during kindling development and in the fully kindled state. The relevance of these models to human epilepsy, however, is not known.

One proposed mechanism of action of lamotrigine, the relevance of which remains to be established in humans, involves an effect on sodium channels. In vitro pharmacological studies suggest that lamotrigine inhibits voltage-sensitive sodium channels, thereby stabilizing neuronal membranes and consequently modulating presynaptic transmitter release of excitatory amino acids (e.g., glutamate and aspartate).

Effect of Lamotrigine on N-Methyl d-Aspartate-Receptor Mediated Activity: Lamotrigine did not inhibit N-methyl d-aspartate (NMDA)-induced depolarizations in rat cortical slices or NMDA-induced cyclic GMP formation in immature rat cerebellum, nor did lamotrigine displace compounds that are either competitive or noncompetitive ligands at this glutamate receptor complex (CNQX, CGS, TCHP). The IC$_{50}$ for lamotrigine effects on NMDA-induced currents (in the presence of 3 μM of glycine) in cultured hippocampal neurons exceeded 100 μM.

12.2 Pharmacodynamics

Folate Metabolism: In vitro, lamotrigine inhibited dihydrofolate reductase, the enzyme that catalyzes the reduction of dihydrofolate to tetrahydrofolate. Inhibition of this enzyme may interfere with the biosynthesis of nucleic acids and proteins. When oral daily doses of lamotrigine were given to pregnant rats during organogenesis, fetal, placental, and maternal folate concentrations were reduced. Significantly reduced concentrations of folate are associated with teratogenesis *[see Use in Specific Populations (8.1)]*. Folate concentrations were also reduced in male rats given repeated oral doses of lamotrigine. Reduced concentrations were partially returned to normal when supplemented with folinic acid.

Cardiovascular: In dogs, lamotrigine is extensively metabolized to a 2-N-methyl metabolite. This metabolite causes dose-dependent prolongation of the PR interval, widening of the QRS complex, and, at higher doses, complete AV conduction block. Similar cardiovascular effects are not anticipated in humans because only trace amounts of the 2-N-methyl metabolite (<0.6% of lamotrigine dose) have been found in human urine *[see Clinical Pharmacology (12.3)]*. However, it is conceivable that plasma concentrations of this metabolite could be increased in patients with a reduced capacity to glucuronidate lamotrigine (e.g., in patients with liver disease, patients taking concomitant medications that inhibit glucuronidation).

12.3 Pharmacokinetics

In comparison to immediate-release lamotrigine, the plasma lamotrigine levels following administration of LAMICTAL XR are not associated with any significant changes in trough plasma concentrations, and are characterized by lower peaks, longer time to peaks, and lower peak-to-trough fluctuation, as described in detail below.

Absorption: Lamotrigine is absorbed after oral administration with negligible first-pass metabolism. The bioavailability of lamotrigine is not affected by food.

In an open-label, crossover study of 44 subjects with epilepsy receiving concomitant AEDs, the steady-state pharmacokinetics of lamotrigine were compared following administration of equivalent total doses of LAMICTAL XR given once daily with those of lamotrigine immediate-release given twice daily. In this study, the median time to peak concentration (T_{max}) following administration of LAMICTAL XR was 4 to 6 hours in patients taking carbamazepine, phenytoin, phenobarbital, or primidone; 9 to 11 hours in patients taking valproate; and 6 to 10 hours in patients taking AEDs other than carbamazepine, phenytoin, phenobarbital, primidone, or valproate. In comparison, the median T_{max} following administration of immediate-release lamotrigine was between 1 and 1.5 hours.

The steady-state trough concentrations for extended-release lamotrigine were similar to or higher than those of immediate-release lamotrigine depending on concomitant AED (Table 6). A mean reduction in the lamotrigine C_{max} by 11% to 29% was observed for LAMICTAL XR compared to immediate-release lamotrigine, resulting in a decrease in the peak-to-trough fluctuation in serum lamotrigine concentrations. However, in some subjects receiving enzyme-inducing AEDs, a reduction in C_{max} of 44% to 77% was observed. The degree of fluctuation was reduced by 17% in patients taking enzyme-inducing AEDs; 34% in patients taking valproate; and 37% in patients taking AEDs other than carbamazepine, phenytoin, phenobarbital, primidone, or valproate. LAMICTAL XR and immediate-release lamotrigine regimens were similar with respect to area under the curve (AUC, a measure of the extent of bioavailability) for patients receiving AEDs other than those known to induce the metabolism of lamotrigine. The relative bioavailability of extended-release lamotrigine was approximately 21% lower than immediate-release lamotrigine in subjects receiving enzyme-inducing AEDs. However, a reduction in exposure of up to 70% was observed in some subjects in this group when they switched to LAMICTAL XR. Therefore, doses may need to be adjusted in some subjects based on therapeutic response.

Table 6. Steady-State Bioavailability of LAMICTAL XR Relative to Immediate-Release Lamotrigine at Equivalent Daily Doses (Ratio of Extended-Release to Immediate-Release 90% CI)

Concomitant Antiepileptic Drug	AUC (0-24ss)	C_{max}	C_{min}
Enzyme-inducing antiepileptic drugs[a]	0.79 (0.69, 0.90)	0.71 (0.61, 0.82)	0.99 (0.89, 1.09)
Valproate	0.94 (0.81, 1.08)	0.88 (0.75, 1.03)	0.99 (0.88, 1.10)
Antiepileptic drugs other than enzyme-inducing antiepileptic drugs[a] or valproate	1.00 (0.88, 1.14)	0.89 (0.78, 1.03)	1.14 (1.03, 1.25)

[a] Enzyme-inducing antiepileptic drugs include carbamazepine, phenytoin, phenobarbital, and primidone.

Dose Proportionality: In healthy volunteers not receiving any other medications and given LAMICTAL XR once daily, the systemic exposure to lamotrigine increased in direct proportion to the dose administered over the range of 50 to 200 mg. At doses between 25 and 50 mg, the increase was less than dose proportional, with a 2-fold increase in dose resulting in an approximately 1.6-fold increase in systemic exposure.

Distribution: Estimates of the mean apparent volume of distribution (Vd/F) of lamotrigine following oral administration ranged from 0.9 to 1.3 L/kg. Vd/F is independent of dose and is similar following single and multiple doses in both patients with epilepsy and in healthy volunteers.

Protein Binding: Data from in vitro studies indicate that lamotrigine is approximately 55% bound to human plasma proteins at plasma lamotrigine concentrations from 1 to 10 mcg/mL (10 mcg/mL is 4 to 6 times the trough plasma concentration observed in the controlled efficacy trials). Because lamotrigine is not highly bound to plasma proteins, clinically significant interactions with other drugs through competition for protein binding sites are unlikely. The binding of lamotrigine to plasma proteins did not change in the presence of therapeutic concentrations of phenytoin, phenobarbital, or valproate. Lamotrigine did not displace other AEDs (carbamazepine, phenytoin, phenobarbital) from protein-binding sites.

Metabolism: Lamotrigine is metabolized predominantly by glucuronic acid conjugation; the major metabolite is an inactive 2-N-glucuronide conjugate. After oral administration of 240 mg of ^{14}C-lamotrigine (15 µCi) to 6 healthy volunteers, 94% was recovered in the urine and 2% was recovered in the feces. The radioactivity in the urine consisted of unchanged lamotrigine (10%), the 2-N-glucuronide (76%), a 5-N-glucuronide (10%), a 2-N-methyl metabolite (0.14%), and other unidentified minor metabolites (4%).

Enzyme Induction: The effects of lamotrigine on the induction of specific families of mixed-function oxidase isozymes have not been systematically evaluated.

Following multiple administrations (150 mg twice daily) to normal volunteers taking no other medications, lamotrigine induced its own metabolism, resulting in a 25% decrease in t½ and a 37% increase in CL/F at steady state compared with values obtained in the same volunteers following a single dose. Evidence gathered from other sources suggests that self-induction by lamotrigine may not occur when lamotrigine is given as adjunctive therapy in patients receiving enzyme-inducing drugs such as carbamazepine, phenytoin, phenobarbital, primidone, or other drugs such as rifampin that induce lamotrigine glucuronidation *[see Drug Interactions (7)]*.

Elimination: The elimination half-life and apparent clearance of lamotrigine following oral administration of immediate-release lamotrigine to adult patients with epilepsy and healthy volunteers is summarized in Table 7. Half-life and apparent clearance vary depending on concomitant AEDs.

Since the half-life of lamotrigine following administration of single doses of immediate-release lamotrigine is comparable to that observed following administration of LAMICTAL XR, similar changes in the half-life of lamotrigine would be expected for LAMICTAL XR.

[See table 7 above]

Drug Interactions: The apparent clearance of lamotrigine is affected by the coadministration of certain medications *[see Warnings and Precautions (5.7, 5.11), Drug Interactions (7)]*.

The net effects of drug interactions with lamotrigine are summarized in Table 8. Details of the drug interaction studies, which were done using immediate-release lamotrigine, are provided in Table 8.

Table 7. Mean[a] Pharmacokinetic Parameters of Immediate-Release Lamotrigine in Healthy Volunteers and Adult Patients With Epilepsy

Adult Study Population	Number of Subjects	t½: Elimination Half-life (hr)	CL/F: Apparent Plasma Clearance (mL/min/kg)
Healthy volunteers taking no other medications:			
Single-dose lamotrigine	179	32.8 (14.0-103.0)	0.44 (0.12-1.10)
Multiple-dose lamotrigine	36	25.4 (11.6-61.6)	0.58 (0.24-1.15)
Healthy volunteers taking valproate:			
Single-dose lamotrigine	6	48.3 (31.5-88.6)	0.30 (0.14-0.42)
Multiple-dose lamotrigine	18	70.3 (41.9-113.5)	0.18 (0.12-0.33)
Patients with epilepsy taking valproate only:			
Single-dose lamotrigine	4	58.8 (30.5-88.8)	0.28 (0.16-0.40)
Patients with epilepsy taking carbamazepine, phenytoin, phenobarbital, or primidone[b] plus valproate:			
Single-dose lamotrigine	25	27.2 (11.2-51.6)	0.53 (0.27-1.04)
Patients with epilepsy taking carbamazepine, phenytoin, phenobarbital, or primidone:[b]			
Single-dose lamotrigine	24	14.4 (6.4-30.4)	1.10 (0.51-2.22)
Multiple-dose lamotrigine	17	12.6 (7.5-23.1)	1.21 (0.66-1.82)

[a]The majority of parameter means determined in each study had coefficients of variation between 20% and 40% for half-life and CL/F and between 30% and 70% for T_{max}. The overall mean values were calculated from individual study means that were weighted based on the number of volunteers/patients in each study. The numbers in parentheses below each parameter mean represent the range of individual volunteer/patient values across studies.

[b]Carbamazepine, phenobarbital, phenytoin, and primidone have been shown to increase the apparent clearance of lamotrigine. Estrogen-containing oral contraceptives and other drugs such as rifampin that induce lamotrigine glucuronidation have also been shown to increase the apparent clearance of lamotrigine *[see Drug Interactions (7)]*.

Table 8. Summary of Drug Interactions With Lamotrigine

Drug	Drug Plasma Concentration With Adjunctive Lamotrigine[a]	Lamotrigine Plasma Concentration With Adjunctive Drugs[b]
Oral contraceptives (e.g., ethinylestradiol/levonorgestrel[c])	↔[d]	↓
Bupropion	Not assessed	↔
Carbamazepine	↔	↓
Carbamazepine epoxide[e]	?	
Felbamate	Not assessed	↔
Gabapentin	Not assessed	↔
Levetiracetam	↔	↔
Lithium	↔	Not assessed
Olanzapine	↔	↔[f]
Oxcarbazepine	↔	↔
10-monohydroxy oxcarbazepine metabolite[g]	↔	
Phenobarbital/primidone	↔	↓
Phenytoin	↔	↓
Pregabalin	↔	↔
Rifampin	Not assessed	↓
Topiramate	↔[h]	↔
Valproate	↓	↑
Valproate + phenytoin and/or carbamazepine	Not assessed	↔
Zonisamide	Not assessed	↔

[a]From adjunctive clinical trials and volunteer studies.

[b]Net effects were estimated by comparing the mean clearance values obtained in adjunctive clinical trials and volunteer studies.

[c]The effect of other hormonal contraceptive preparations or hormone replacement therapy on the pharmacokinetics of lamotrigine has not been systematically evaluated in clinical trials, although the effect may be similar to that seen with the ethinylestradiol/levonorgestrel combinations.

[d]Modest decrease in levonorgestrel.

[e]Not administered, but an active metabolite of carbamazepine.

[f]Slight decrease, not expected to be clinically relevant.

[g]Not administered, but an active metabolite of oxcarbazepine.

[h]Slight increase, not expected to be clinically relevant.

↔ = No significant effect.

? = Conflicting data.

Estrogen-Containing Oral Contraceptives: In 16 female volunteers, an oral contraceptive preparation containing 30 mcg ethinylestradiol and 150 mcg levonorgestrel increased the apparent clearance of lamotrigine (300 mg/day) by approximately 2-fold with mean decreases in AUC of 52% and in C_{max} of 39%. In this study, trough serum lamotrigine concentrations gradually increased and were approximately 2-fold higher on average at the end of the week of the inactive hormone preparation compared with trough lamotrigine concentrations at the end of the active hormone cycle.

Gradual transient increases in lamotrigine plasma levels (approximate 2-fold increase) occurred during the week of inactive hormone preparation (pill-free week) for women not also taking a drug that increased the clearance of lamotrigine (carbamazepine, phenytoin, phenobarbital, primidone, or other drugs such as rifampin that induce lamotrigine glucuronidation) *[see Drug Interactions (7)]*. The increase in lamotrigine plasma levels will be greater if the dose of LAMICTAL XR is increased in the few days before or during the pill-free week. Increases in lamotrigine plasma levels could result in dose-dependent adverse reactions.

In the same study, coadministration of lamotrigine (300 mg/day) in 16 female volunteers did not affect the pharmacokinetics of the ethinylestradiol component of the oral contraceptive preparation. There were mean decreases in the AUC and C_{max} of the levonorgestrel component of 19% and 12%, respectively. Measurement of serum progesterone indicated that there was no hormonal evidence of ovulation in any of the 16 volunteers, although measurement of serum FSH, LH, and estradiol indicated that there was some loss of suppression of the hypothalamic-pituitary-ovarian axis.

The effects of doses of lamotrigine other than 300 mg/day have not been systematically evaluated in controlled clinical trials.

The clinical significance of the observed hormonal changes on ovulatory activity is unknown. However, the possibility of decreased contraceptive efficacy in some patients cannot be excluded. Therefore, patients should be instructed to promptly report changes in their menstrual pattern (e.g., break-through bleeding).

Dosage adjustments may be necessary for women receiving estrogen-containing oral contraceptive preparations *[see Dosage and Administration (2.1)]*.

Other Hormonal Contraceptives or Hormone Replacement Therapy: The effect of other hormonal contraceptive preparations or hormone replacement therapy on the pharmacokinetics of lamotrigine has not been systematically evaluated. It has been reported that ethinylestradiol, not progestogens, increased the clearance of lamotrigine up to 2-fold, and the progestin-only pills had no effect on lamotrigine plasma levels. Therefore, adjustments to the dosage of LAMICTAL XR in the presence of progestogens alone will likely not be needed.

Bupropion: The pharmacokinetics of a 100-mg single dose of lamotrigine in healthy volunteers (n = 12) were not changed by coadministration of bupropion sustained-release formulation (150 mg twice daily) starting 11 days before lamotrigine.

Carbamazepine: Lamotrigine has no appreciable effect on steady-state carbamazepine plasma concentration. Limited clinical data suggest there is a higher incidence of dizziness, diplopia, ataxia, and blurred vision in patients receiving carbamazepine with lamotrigine than in patients receiving other AEDs with lamotrigine *[see Adverse Reactions (6.1)]*.

The mechanism of this interaction is unclear. The effect of lamotrigine on plasma concentrations of carbamazepine-epoxide is unclear. In a small subset of patients (n = 7) studied in a placebo-controlled trial, lamotrigine had no effect on carbamazepine-epoxide plasma concentrations, but in a small, uncontrolled study (n = 9), carbamazepine-epoxide levels increased.

The addition of carbamazepine decreases lamotrigine steady-state concentrations by approximately 40%.

Esomeprazole: In a study of 30 subjects, coadministration of LAMICTAL XR with esomeprazole resulted in no significant change in lamotrigine levels and a small decrease in T_{max}. The levels of gastric pH were not altered compared with pre-lamotrigine dosing.

Felbamate: In a study of 21 healthy volunteers, coadministration of felbamate (1,200 mg twice daily) with lamotrigine (100 mg twice daily for 10 days) appeared to have no clinically relevant effects on the pharmacokinetics of lamotrigine.

Folate Inhibitors: Lamotrigine is a weak inhibitor of dihydrofolate reductase. Prescribers should be aware of this action when prescribing other medications that inhibit folate metabolism.

Gabapentin: Based on a retrospective analysis of plasma levels in 34 patients who received lamotrigine both with and without gabapentin, gabapentin does not appear to change the apparent clearance of lamotrigine.

Levetiracetam: Potential drug interactions between levetiracetam and lamotrigine were assessed by evaluating serum concentrations of both agents during placebo-controlled clinical trials. These data indicate that lamotrigine does not influence the pharmacokinetics of levetiracetam and that levetiracetam does not influence the pharmacokinetics of lamotrigine.

Lithium: The pharmacokinetics of lithium were not altered in healthy subjects (n = 20) by coadministration of lamotrigine (100 mg/day) for 6 days.

Olanzapine: The AUC and C_{max} of olanzapine were similar following the addition of olanzapine (15 mg once daily) to lamotrigine (200 mg once daily) in healthy male volunteers (n = 16) compared with the AUC and C_{max} in healthy male volunteers receiving olanzapine alone (n = 16).

In the same study, the AUC and C_{max} of lamotrigine were reduced on average by 24% and 20%, respectively, following the addition of olanzapine to lamotrigine in healthy male volunteers compared with those receiving lamotrigine alone. This reduction in lamotrigine plasma concentrations is not expected to be clinically relevant.

Oxcarbazepine: The AUC and C_{max} of oxcarbazepine and its active 10-monohydroxy oxcarbazepine metabolite were not significantly different following the addition of oxcarbazepine (600 mg twice daily) to lamotrigine (200 mg once daily) in healthy male volunteers (n = 13) compared with healthy male volunteers receiving oxcarbazepine alone (n = 13).

In the same study, the AUC and C_{max} of lamotrigine were similar following the addition of oxcarbazepine (600 mg twice daily) to lamotrigine in healthy male volunteers compared with those receiving lamotrigine alone. Limited clinical data suggest a higher incidence of headache, dizziness, nausea, and somnolence with coadministration of lamotrigine and oxcarbazepine compared with lamotrigine alone or oxcarbazepine alone.

Phenobarbital, Primidone: The addition of phenobarbital or primidone decreases lamotrigine steady-state concentrations by approximately 40%.

Phenytoin: Lamotrigine has no appreciable effect on steady-state phenytoin plasma concentrations in patients with epilepsy. The addition of phenytoin decreases lamotrigine steady-state concentrations by approximately 40%.

Pregabalin: Steady-state trough plasma concentrations of lamotrigine were not affected by concomitant pregabalin (200 mg 3 times daily) administration. There are no pharmacokinetic interactions between lamotrigine and pregabalin.

Rifampin: In 10 male volunteers, rifampin (600 mg/day for 5 days) significantly increased the apparent clearance of a single 25-mg dose of lamotrigine by approximately 2-fold (AUC decreased by approximately 40%).

Topiramate: Topiramate resulted in no change in plasma concentrations of lamotrigine. Administration of lamotrigine resulted in a 15% increase in topiramate concentrations.

Valproate: When lamotrigine was administered to healthy volunteers (n = 18) receiving valproate, the trough steady-state valproate plasma concentrations decreased by an average of 25% over a 3-week period, and then stabilized. However, adding lamotrigine to the existing therapy did not cause a change in valproate plasma concentrations in either adult or pediatric patients in controlled clinical trials.

The addition of valproate increased lamotrigine steady-state concentrations in normal volunteers by slightly more than 2-fold. In one study, maximal inhibition of lamotrigine clearance was reached at valproate doses between 250 and 500 mg/day and did not increase as the valproate dose was further increased.

Zonisamide: In a study of 18 patients with epilepsy, coadministration of zonisamide (200 to 400 mg/day) with lamotrigine (150 to 500 mg/day for 35 days) had no significant effect on the pharmacokinetics of lamotrigine.

Known Inducers or Inhibitors of Glucuronidation: Drugs other than those listed above have not been systematically evaluated in combination with lamotrigine. Since lamotrigine is metabolized predominately by glucuronic acid conjugation, drugs that are known to induce or inhibit glucuronidation may affect the apparent clearance of lamotrigine, and doses of LAMICTAL XR may require adjustment based on clinical response.

Other: Results of in vitro experiments suggest that clearance of lamotrigine is unlikely to be reduced by concomitant administration of amitriptyline, clonazepam, clozapine, fluoxetine, haloperidol, lorazepam, phenelzine, risperidone, sertraline, or trazodone.

Results of in vitro experiments suggest that lamotrigine does not reduce the clearance of drugs eliminated predominantly by CYP2D6.

Special Populations: *Patients With Renal Impairment:* Twelve volunteers with chronic renal failure (mean creatinine clearance: 13 mL/min, range: 6 to 23) and another 6 individuals undergoing hemodialysis were each given a single 100 mg dose of immediate-release lamotrigine. The mean plasma half-lives determined in the study were 42.9 hours (chronic renal failure), 13.0 hours (during hemodialysis), and 57.4 hours (between hemodialysis) compared with 26.2 hours in healthy volunteers. On average, approximately 20% (range: 5.6 to 35.1) of the amount of lamotrigine present in the body was eliminated by hemodialysis during a 4-hour session *[see Dosage and Administration (2.1)]*.

Hepatic Disease: The pharmacokinetics of lamotrigine following a single 100-mg dose of immediate-release lamotrigine were evaluated in 24 subjects with mild, moderate, and severe hepatic impairment (Child-Pugh Classification system) and compared with 12 subjects without hepatic impairment. The patients with severe hepatic impairment were without ascites (n = 2) or with ascites (n = 5). The mean apparent clearances of lamotrigine in patients with mild (n = 12), moderate (n = 5), severe without ascites (n = 2), and severe with ascites (n = 5) liver impairment were 0.30 ± 0.09, 0.24 ± 0.1, 0.21 ± 0.04, and 0.15 ± 0.09 mL/min/kg, respectively, as compared with 0.37 ± 0.1 mL/min/kg in the healthy controls. Mean half-lives of lamotrigine in patients with mild, moderate, severe without ascites, and severe with ascites hepatic impairment were 46 ± 20, 72 ± 44, 67 ± 11, and 100 ± 48 hours, respectively, as compared with 33 ± 7 hours in healthy controls *[see Dosage and Administration (2.1)]*.

Elderly: The pharmacokinetics of lamotrigine following a single 150-mg dose of immediate-release lamotrigine were evaluated in 12 elderly volunteers between the ages of 65 and 76 years (mean creatinine clearance: 61 mL/min, range: 33 to 108 mL/min). The mean half-life of lamotrigine in these subjects was 31.2 hours (range: 24.5 to 43.4 hours), and the mean clearance was 0.40 mL/min/kg (range: 0.26 to 0.48 mL/min/kg).

Gender: The clearance of lamotrigine is not affected by gender. However, during dose escalation of immediate-release lamotrigine in one clinical trial in patients with epilepsy on a stable dose of valproate (n = 77), mean trough lamotrigine concentrations, unadjusted for weight, were 24% to 45% higher (0.3 to 1.7 mcg/mL) in females than in males.

Race: The apparent oral clearance of lamotrigine was 25% lower in non-Caucasians than Caucasians.

Pediatric Patients: Safety and effectiveness of LAMICTAL XR for use in patients less than 13 years of age have not been established.

13 NONCLINICAL TOXICOLOGY

13.1 Carcinogenesis, Mutagenesis, Impairment of Fertility

No evidence of carcinogenicity was seen in mouse or rat following oral administration of lamotrigine for up to 2 years at doses up to 30 mg/kg/day and 10 to 15 mg/kg/day in mouse and rat, respectively. The highest doses tested are less than the human dose of 400 mg/day on a body surface area (mg/m^2) basis.

Lamotrigine was negative in in vitro gene mutation (Ames and mouse lymphoma *tk*) assays and in clastogenicity (in vitro human lymphocyte and in vivo rat bone marrow) assays.

No evidence of impaired fertility was detected in rats given oral doses of lamotrigine up to 20 mg/kg/day. The highest dose tested is less than the human dose of 400 mg/day on a mg/m^2 basis.

14 CLINICAL STUDIES

14.1 Adjunctive Therapy for Primary Generalized Tonic-Clonic Seizures

The effectiveness of LAMICTAL XR as adjunctive therapy was established in PGTC seizures in a 19-week, international, multicenter, double-blind, randomized, placebo-controlled study in 143 patients 13 years of age and older (n = 70 on LAMICTAL XR and n = 73 on placebo). Patients with at least 3 PGTC seizures during an 8-week baseline phase were randomized to 19 weeks of treatment with LAMICTAL XR or placebo added to their current AED regimen of up to 2 drugs. Patients were dosed on a fixed-dose regimen, with target doses ranging from 200 to 500 mg/day of LAMICTAL XR based on concomitant AED(s) (target dose = 200 mg for valproate, 300 mg for AEDs not altering plasma lamotrigine levels, and 500 mg for enzyme-inducing AEDs).

The primary efficacy endpoint was percent change from baseline in PGTC seizure frequency during the double-blind treatment phase. For the intent-to-treat population, the median percent reduction in PGTC seizure frequency was 75% in patients treated with LAMICTAL XR and 32% in patients treated with placebo, a difference that was statistically significant, defined as a 2-sided P value ≥0.05.

Figure 1 presents the percentage of patients (X-axis) with a percent reduction in PGTC seizure frequency (responder rate) from baseline through the entire treatment period at least as great as that represented on the Y-axis. A positive value on the Y-axis indicates an improvement from baseline (i.e., a decrease in seizure frequency), while a negative value indicates a worsening from baseline (i.e., an increase in seizure frequency). Thus, in a display of this type, a curve for an effective treatment is shifted to the left of the curve for placebo. The proportion of patients achieving any particular level of reduction in PGTC seizure frequency was consistently higher for the group treated with LAMICTAL XR compared with the placebo group. For example, 70% of patients randomized to LAMICTAL XR experienced a 50% or greater reduction in PGTC seizure frequency, compared with 32% of patients randomized to placebo. Patients with an increase in seizure frequency >100% are represented on the Y-axis as equal to or greater than -100%.

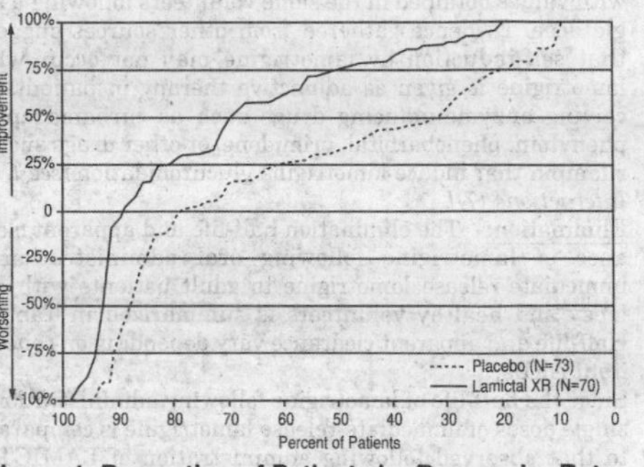

Figure 1. Proportion of Patients by Responder Rate for LAMICTAL XR and Placebo Group (Primary Generalized Tonic-Clonic Seizures Study)

14.2 Adjunctive Therapy for Partial Onset Seizures

The effectiveness of immediate-release lamotrigine as adjunctive therapy was initially established in 3 pivotal, multicenter, placebo-controlled, double-blind clinical trials in 355 adults with refractory partial onset seizures.

The effectiveness of LAMICTAL XR as adjunctive therapy in partial onset seizures, with or without secondary generalization, was established in a 19-week, multicenter, double-blind, placebo-controlled trial in 236 patients 13 years of age and older (approximately 93% of patients were aged 16 to 65 years). Approximately 36% were from the U.S. and approximately 64% were from other countries including Argentina, Brazil, Chile, Germany, India, Korea, Russian Federation, and Ukraine. Patients with at least 8 partial onset seizures during an 8-week prospective baseline phase (or 4-week prospective baseline coupled with a 4-week historical baseline documented with seizure diary data) were randomized to treatment with LAMICTAL XR (n = 116) or placebo (n = 120) added to their current regimen of 1 or 2 AEDs. Approximately half of the patients were taking 2 concomitant AEDs at baseline. Target doses ranged from 200 to 500 mg/day of LAMICTAL XR based on concomitant AED (target dose = 200 mg for valproate, 300 mg for AEDs not altering plasma lamotrigine, and 500 mg for enzyme-inducing AEDs). The median partial seizure frequency per week at baseline was 2.3 for LAMICTAL XR and 2.1 for placebo.

The primary endpoint was the median percent change from baseline in partial onset seizure frequency during the entire double-blind treatment phase. The median percent reductions in weekly partial onset seizures were 47% in patients treated with LAMICTAL XR and 25% on placebo, a difference that was statistically significant, defined as a 2-sided P value ≤0.05.

Figure 2 presents the percentage of patients (X-axis) with a percent reduction in partial seizure frequency (responder rate) from baseline through the entire treatment period at least as great as that represented on the Y-axis. The proportion of patients achieving any particular level of reduction in partial seizure frequency was consistently higher for the group treated with LAMICTAL XR compared with the placebo group. For example, 44% of patients randomized to LAMICTAL XR experienced a 50% or greater reduction in partial seizure frequency compared with 21% of patients randomized to placebo.

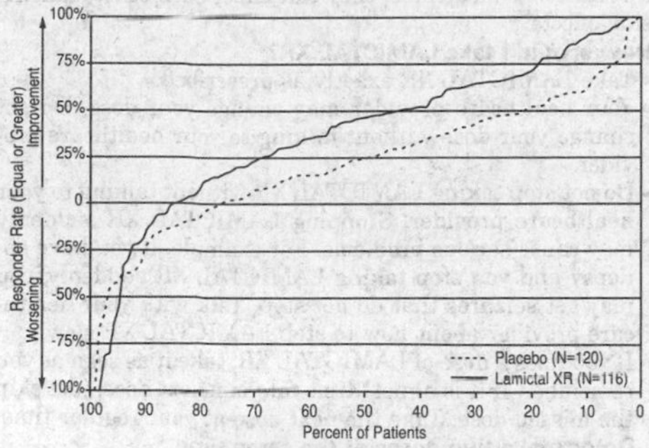

Figure 2. Proportion of Patients by Responder Rate for LAMICTAL XR and Placebo Group (Partial Onset Seizure Study)

14.3 Conversion to Monotherapy for Partial Onset Seizures

The effectiveness of LAMICTAL XR as monotherapy for partial onset seizures was established in a historical-control trial in 223 adults with partial seizures. The historical control methodology is described in a publication by French, et al. *[see References (15)]*. Briefly, in this study, patients were randomized to ultimately receive either LAMICTAL XR 300 mg or 250 mg once a day, and their responses were compared to those of a historical control group. The historical control consisted of a pooled analysis of the control groups from 8 studies of similar design, which utilized a subtherapeutic dose of an AED as a comparator. Statistical superiority to the historical control was considered to be demonstrated if the upper 95% confidence interval for the proportion of patients meeting escape criteria in patients receiving LAMICTAL XR remained below the lower 95% prediction interval of 65.3% derived from the historical control data.

In this study, patients ≥13 years of age experienced at least 4 partial seizures during an 8-week baseline period with at least 2 seizures occurring during each of 2 consecutive 4-week periods while receiving valproate or a non–enzyme-inducing AED. LAMICTAL XR was added to either valproate or a non–enzyme-inducing AED over a 6- to 7-week period followed by the gradual withdrawal of the background AED. Patients were then continued on monotherapy with LAMICTAL XR for 12 weeks. The escape criteria were one or more of the following: (1) doubling of average monthly seizure count during any 28 consecutive days, (2) doubling of highest consecutive 2-day seizure frequency during the entire treatment phase, (3) emergence of a new seizure type compared to baseline (4) clinically significant prolongation of generalized tonic-clonic seizures or worsening of seizure considered by the investigator to require intervention. These criteria were similar to those in the 8 controlled trials from which the historical control group was constituted.

The upper 95% confidence limits of the proportion of subjects meeting escape criteria (40.2% at 300 mg/day and 44.5% at 250 mg/day) were below the threshold of 65.3% derived from the historical control data.

Although the study population was not fully comparable to the historical controlled population and the study was not fully blinded, numerous sensitivity analyses supported the primary results. Efficacy was further supported by the established effectiveness of the immediate-release formulation as monotherapy.

15 REFERENCES

1. French JA, Wang S, Warnock B, Temkin N. Historical control monotherapy design in the treatment of epilepsy. *Epilepsia*. 2010; 51(10):1936-1943.

16 HOW SUPPLIED/STORAGE AND HANDLING

LAMICTAL XR (lamotrigine) Extended-Release Tablets

25 mg, yellow with a white center, round, biconvex, film-coated tablets printed on one face in black ink with "LAMICTAL" and "XR 25", unit-of-use bottles of 30 with orange caps (NDC 0173-0754-00).

50 mg, green with a white center, round, biconvex, film-coated tablets printed on one face in black ink with "LAMICTAL" and "XR 50", unit-of-use bottles of 30 with orange caps (NDC 0173-0755-00).

100 mg, orange with a white center, round, biconvex, film-coated tablets printed on one face in black ink with "LAMICTAL" and "XR 100", unit-of-use bottles of 30 with orange caps (NDC 0173-0756-00).

200 mg, blue with a white center, round, biconvex, film-coated tablets printed on one face in black ink with "LAMICTAL" and "XR 200", unit-of-use bottles of 30 with orange caps (NDC 0173-0757-00).

250 mg, purple with a white center, caplet-shaped, film-coated tablets printed on one face in black ink with "LAMICTAL" and "XR 250", unit-of-use bottles of 30 with orange caps (NDC 0173-0781-00).

300 mg, gray with a white center, caplet-shaped, film-coated tablets printed on one face in black ink with "LAMICTAL" and "XR 300", unit-of-use bottles of 30 with orange caps (NDC 0173-0761-00).

LAMICTAL XR (lamotrigine) Patient Titration Kit for Patients Taking Valproate (Blue XR Kit)

25 mg, yellow with a white center, round, biconvex, film-coated tablets printed on one face in black ink with "LAMICTAL" and "XR 25" and 50 mg, green with a white center, round, biconvex, film-coated tablets printed on one face in black ink with "LAMICTAL" and "XR 50"; blisterpack of 21/25-mg tablets and 7/50-mg tablets (NDC 0173-0758-00).

LAMICTAL XR (lamotrigine) Patient Titration Kit for Patients Taking Carbamazepine, Phenytoin, Phenobarbital, or Primidone, and Not Taking Valproate (Green XR Kit)

50 mg, green with a white center, round, biconvex, film-coated tablets printed on one face in black ink with "LAMICTAL" and "XR 50"; 100 mg, orange with a white center, round, biconvex, film-coated tablets printed on one face in black ink with "LAMICTAL" and "XR 100"; and 200 mg, blue with a white center, round, biconvex, film-coated tablets printed on one face in black ink with "LAMICTAL" and "XR 200"; blisterpack of 14/50-mg tablets, 14/100-mg tablets, and 7/200-mg tablets (NDC 0173-0759-00).

LAMICTAL XR (lamotrigine) Patient Titration Kit for Patients Not Taking Carbamazepine, Phenytoin, Phenobarbital, Primidone, or Valproate (Orange XR Kit)

25 mg, yellow with a white center, round, biconvex, film-coated tablets printed on one face in black ink with "LAMICTAL" and "XR 25"; 50 mg, green with a white center, round, biconvex, film-coated tablets printed on one face in black ink with "LAMICTAL" and "XR 50"; and 100 mg, orange with a white center, round, biconvex, film-coated tablets printed on one face in black ink with "LAMICTAL" and "XR 100"; blisterpack of 14/25-mg tablets, 14/50 mg tablets, and 7/100-mg tablets (NDC 0173-0760-00).

Storage: Store at 25°C (77°F); excursions permitted to 15-30°C (59-86°F) [see USP Controlled Room Temperature].

17 PATIENT COUNSELING INFORMATION

See FDA-approved patient labeling (Medication Guide).

17.1 Rash

Prior to initiation of treatment with LAMICTAL XR, the patient should be instructed that a rash or other signs or symptoms of hypersensitivity (e.g., fever, lymphadenopathy) may herald a serious medical event and that the patient should report any such occurrence to a physician immediately.

17.2 Multiorgan Hypersensitivity Reactions, Blood Dyscrasias, and Organ Failure

Patients should be instructed that multiorgan hypersensitivity reactions and acute multiorgan failure may occur with LAMICTAL. Isolated organ failure or isolated blood dyscrasias without evidence of multiorgan hypersensitivity may also occur. Patients should contact their physician immediately if they experience any signs or symptoms of these conditions *[see Warnings andPrecautions (5.2, 5.3)]*.

17.3 Suicidal Thinking and Behavior

Patients, their caregivers, and families should be counseled that AEDs, including LAMICTAL XR, may increase the risk of suicidal thoughts and behavior and should be advised of the need to be alert for the emergence or worsening of symptoms of depression; any unusual changes in mood or behavior; or the emergence of suicidal thoughts, behavior, or thoughts about self-harm. Behaviors of concern should be reported immediately to healthcare providers.

17.4 Worsening of Seizures

Patients should be advised to notify their physicians if worsening of seizure control occurs.

17.5 Central Nervous System Adverse Effects

Patients should be advised that LAMICTAL XR may cause dizziness, somnolence, and other symptoms and signs of central nervous system depression. Accordingly, they should be advised neither to drive a car nor to operate other complex machinery until they have gained sufficient experience on LAMICTAL XR to gauge whether or not it adversely affects their mental and/or motor performance.

17.6 Pregnancy and Nursing

Patients should be advised to notify their physicians if they become pregnant or intend to become pregnant during therapy. Patients should be advised to notify their physicians if they intend to breastfeed or are breastfeeding an infant.

Patients should also be encouraged to enroll in the NAAED Pregnancy Registry if they become pregnant. This registry is collecting information about the safety of antiepileptic drugs during pregnancy. To enroll, patients can call the toll-free number 1-888-233-2334 *[see Use in Specific Populations (8.1)]*.

Patients who intend to breastfeed should be informed that LAMICTAL XR is present in breast milk and that they should monitor their child for potential adverse effects of this drug. Benefits and risks of continuing breastfeeding should be discussed with the patient.

17.7 Oral Contraceptive Use

Women should be advised to notify their physicians if they plan to start or stop use of oral contraceptives or other female hormonal preparations. Starting estrogen-containing oral contraceptives may significantly decrease lamotrigine plasma levels and stopping estrogen-containing oral contraceptives (including the pill-free week) may significantly increase lamotrigine plasma levels *[see Warnings and Precautions (5.7), Clinical Pharmacology (12.3)]*. Women should also be advised to promptly notify their physicians if they experience adverse reactions or changes in menstrual pattern (e.g., break-through bleeding) while receiving LAMICTAL XR in combination with these medications.

17.8 Discontinuing LAMICTAL XR

Patients should be advised to notify their physicians if they stop taking LAMICTAL XR for any reason and not to resume LAMICTAL XR without consulting their physicians.

17.9 Aseptic Meningitis

Patients should be advised that LAMICTAL XR may cause aseptic meningitis. Patients should be advised to notify their physicians immediately if they develop signs and symptoms of meningitis such as headache, fever, nausea, vomiting, stiff neck, rash, abnormal sensitivity to light, myalgia, chills, confusion, or drowsiness while taking LAMICTAL XR.

17.10 Potential Medication Errors

Medication errors involving LAMICTAL have occurred. In particular the names LAMICTAL or lamotrigine can be confused with the names of other commonly used medications. Medication errors may also occur between the different formulations of LAMICTAL. To reduce the potential of medication errors, write and say LAMICTAL XR clearly. Depictions of the LAMICTAL XR Extended-Release Tablets can be found in the Medication Guide. Each LAMICTAL XR tablet has a distinct color and white center, and is printed with "LAMICTAL XR" and the tablet strength. These distinctive features serve to identify the different presentations of the drug and thus may help reduce the risk of medication errors. LAMICTAL XR is supplied in round, unit-of-use bottles with orange caps containing 30 tablets. The label on the bottle includes a depiction of the tablets that further communicates to patients and pharmacists that the medication is LAMICTAL XR and the specific tablet strength included in the bottle. The unit-of-use bottle with a distinctive orange cap and distinctive bottle label features serves to identify the different presentations of the drug and thus may help to reduce the risk of medication errors. **To avoid a medication error of using the wrong drug or formulation, patients should be strongly advised to visually inspect their tablets to verify that they are LAMICTAL XR each time they fill their prescription and to immediately talk to their doctor/pharmacist if they receive a LAMICTAL XR tablet without a white center and without "LAMICTAL XR" and the strength printed on the tablet as they may have received the wrong medication** *[see Dosage Forms and Strengths (3), How Supplied/Storage and Handling (16)]*.

LAMICTAL XR and DiffCORE are trademarks of GlaxoSmithKline.

GlaxoSmithKline
Research Triangle Park, NC 27709

LXR:13PI

MEDICATION GUIDE
LAMICTAL® (la-MIK-tal) XR™
(lamotrigine)
Extended-Release Tablets

Read this Medication Guide before you start taking LAMICTAL XR and each time you get a refill. There may be new information. This information does not take the place of talking with your healthcare provider about your medical condition or treatment. If you have questions about LAMICTAL XR, ask your healthcare provider or pharmacist.

What is the most important information I should know about LAMICTAL XR?

1. LAMICTAL XR may cause a serious skin rash that may cause you to be hospitalized or even cause death.

There is no way to tell if a mild rash will become more serious. A serious skin rash can happen at any time during your treatment with LAMICTAL XR, but is more likely to happen within the first 2 to 8 weeks of treatment. Children between 2 to 16 years of age have a higher chance of getting this serious skin rash while taking LAMICTAL XR. LAMICTAL XR is not approved for use in children less than 13 years old.

The risk of getting a serious skin rash is higher if you:

- take LAMICTAL XR while taking valproate [DEPAKENE® (valproic acid) or DEPAKOTE® (divalproex sodium)].
- take a higher starting dose of LAMICTAL XR than your healthcare provider prescribed.
- increase your dose of LAMICTAL XR faster than prescribed.

Call your healthcare provider right away if you have any of the following:

- **a skin rash**
- **blistering or peeling of your skin**
- **hives**
- **painful sores in your mouth or around your eyes**

These symptoms may be the first signs of a serious skin reaction. A healthcare provider should examine you to decide if you should continue taking LAMICTAL XR.

2. Other serious reactions, including serious blood problems or liver problems. LAMICTAL XR can also cause other types of allergic reactions or serious problems that may affect organs and other parts of your body like your liver or blood cells. You may or may not have a rash with these types of reactions. Call your healthcare provider right away if you have any of these symptoms:

- fever
- frequent infections
- severe muscle pain
- swelling of your face, eyes, lips, or tongue
- swollen lymph glands
- unusual bruising or bleeding
- weakness, fatigue
- yellowing of your skin or the white part of your eyes

3. Like other antiepileptic drugs, LAMICTAL XR may cause suicidal thoughts or actions in a very small number of people, about 1 in 500.

Call a healthcare provider right away if you have any of these symptoms, especially if they are new, worse, or worry you:

- thoughts about suicide or dying
- attempt to commit suicide
- new or worse depression
- new or worse anxiety
- feeling agitated or restless
- panic attacks
- trouble sleeping (insomnia)
- new or worse irritability
- acting aggressive, being angry, or violent
- acting on dangerous impulses
- an extreme increase in activity and talking (mania)
- other unusual changes in behavior or mood

Do not stop LAMICTAL XR without first talking to a healthcare provider.

- Stopping LAMICTAL XR suddenly can cause serious problems.
- Suicidal thoughts or actions can be caused by things other than medicines. If you have suicidal thoughts or actions, your healthcare provider may check for other causes.

How can I watch for early symptoms of suicidal thoughts and actions?

- Pay attention to any changes, especially sudden changes, in mood, behaviors, thoughts, or feelings.
- Keep all follow-up visits with your healthcare provider as scheduled.
- Call your healthcare provider between visits as needed, especially if you are worried about symptoms.

4. LAMICTAL XR may rarely cause aseptic meningitis, a serious inflammation of the protective membrane that covers the brain and spinal cord.

Call your healthcare provider right away if you have any of the following symptoms:

- headache
- fever
- nausea
- vomiting
- stiff neck
- rash
- unusual sensitivity to light
- muscle pains
- chills
- confusion
- drowsiness

Meningitis has many causes other than LAMICTAL XR, which your doctor would check for if you developed meningitis while taking LAMICTAL XR.

LAMICTAL XR can have other serious side effects . For more information ask your healthcare provider or pharmacist. Tell your healthcare provider if you have any side effect that bothers you. Be sure to read the section below entitled "What are the possible side effects of LAMICTAL XR?"

5. Patients prescribed LAMICTAL have sometimes been given the wrong medicine because many medicines have names similar to LAMICTAL, so always check that you receive LAMICTAL XR.

Taking the wrong medication can cause serious health problems. When your healthcare provider gives you a prescription for LAMICTAL XR:

- Make sure you can read it clearly.
- Talk to your pharmacist to check that you are given the correct medicine.
- Each time you fill your prescription, check the tablets you receive against the pictures of the tablets below.

These pictures show the distinct wording, colors, and shapes of the tablets that help to identify the right strength of LAMICTAL XR. Immediately call your pharmacist if you receive a LAMICTAL XR tablet that does not look like one of the tablets shown below, as you may have received the wrong medication.

LAMICTAL XR (lamotrigine) Extended-Release Tablets

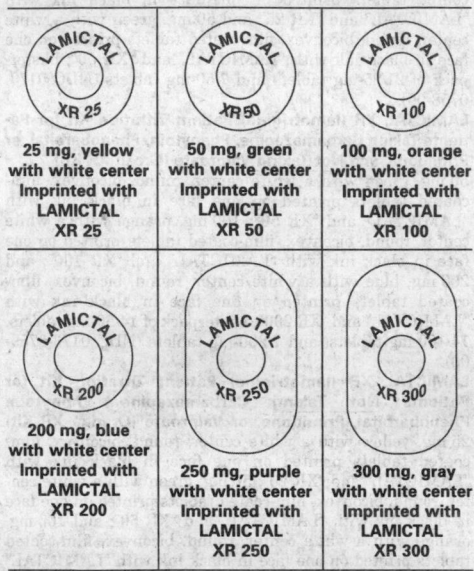

 **25 mg, yellow with white center Imprinted with LAMICTAL XR 25**	 **50 mg, green with white center Imprinted with LAMICTAL XR 50**	 **100 mg, orange with white center Imprinted with LAMICTAL XR 100**
 **200 mg, blue with white center Imprinted with LAMICTAL XR 200**	 **250 mg, purple with white center Imprinted with LAMICTAL XR 250**	 **300 mg, gray with white center Imprinted with LAMICTAL XR 300**

What is LAMICTAL XR?

LAMICTAL XR is a prescription medicine used:

- together with other medicines to treat primary generalized tonic-clonic seizures and partial onset seizures in people 13 years or older.
- alone when changing from other medicines used to treat partial seizures in people 13 years or older.
  It is not known if LAMICTAL XR is safe or effective in children under the age of 13. Other forms of LAMICTAL can be used in children 2 to 12 years.

Who should not take LAMICTAL XR?

You should not take LAMICTAL XR if you have had an allergic reaction to lamotrigine or to any of the inactive ingredients in LAMICTAL XR. See the end of this leaflet for a complete list of ingredients in LAMICTAL XR.

What should I tell my healthcare provider before taking LAMICTAL XR?

Before taking LAMICTAL XR, tell your healthcare provider about all of your medical conditions, including if you:

- have had a rash or allergic reaction to another antiseizure medicine.
- have or have had depression, mood problems, or suicidal thoughts or behavior.
- have had aseptic meningitis after taking LAMICTAL (lamotrigine) or LAMICTAL XR.
- are taking oral contraceptives (birth control pills) or other female hormonal medicines. Do not start or stop taking birth control pills or other female hormonal medicine until you have talked with your healthcare provider. Tell your healthcare provider if you have any changes in your menstrual pattern such as breakthrough bleeding. Stopping these medicines may cause side effects (such as dizziness, lack of coordination, or double vision). Starting these medicines may lessen how well LAMICTAL XR works.
- are pregnant or plan to become pregnant. It is not known if LAMICTAL XR will harm your unborn baby. If you become pregnant while taking LAMICTAL XR, talk to your healthcare provider about registering with the North American Antiepileptic Drug Pregnancy Registry. You can enroll in this registry by calling 1-888-233-2334. The purpose of this registry is to collect information about the safety of antiepileptic drugs during pregnancy.
- are breastfeeding. LAMICTAL XR passes into breast milk and may cause side effects in a breastfed baby. If you breastfeed while taking LAMICTAL XR, watch your baby closely for trouble breathing, episodes of temporarily stopping breathing, sleepiness, or poor sucking. Call your baby's healthcare provider right away if you see any of these problems. Talk to your healthcare provider about the best way to feed your baby if you take LAMICTAL XR.

Tell your healthcare provider about all the medicines you take or if you are planning to take a new medicine, including prescription and non-prescription medicines, vitamins, and herbal supplements. If you use LAMICTAL XR with certain other medicines, they can affect each other, causing side effects.

How should I take LAMICTAL XR?

- Take LAMICTAL XR exactly as prescribed.
- Your healthcare provider may change your dose. Do not change your dose without talking to your healthcare provider.
- Do not stop taking LAMICTAL XR without talking to your healthcare provider. Stopping LAMICTAL XR suddenly may cause serious problems. For example, if you have epilepsy and you stop taking LAMICTAL XR suddenly, you may get seizures that do not stop. Talk with your healthcare provider about how to stop LAMICTAL XR slowly.
- If you miss a dose of LAMICTAL XR, take it as soon as you remember. If it is almost time for your next dose, just skip the missed dose. Take the next dose at your regular time. **Do not take two doses at the same time.**
- You may not feel the full effect of LAMICTAL XR for several weeks.
- If you have epilepsy, tell your healthcare provider if your seizures get worse or if you have any new types of seizures.
- LAMICTAL XR can be taken with or without food.
- Do not chew, crush, or divide LAMICTAL XR.
- Swallow LAMICTAL XR tablets whole.
- If you have trouble swallowing LAMICTAL XR tablets, tell your healthcare provider because there may be another form of LAMICTAL you can take.
- If you receive LAMICTAL XR in a blisterpack, examine the blisterpack before use. Do not use if blisters are torn, broken, or missing.

What should I avoid while taking LAMICTAL XR?

Do not drive a car or operate complex, hazardous machinery until you know how LAMICTAL XR affects you.

What are possible side effects of LAMICTAL XR?

- See "What is the most important information I should know about LAMICTAL XR?" Common side effects of LAMICTAL XR include:
- dizziness
- tremor
- double vision
- nausea
- vomiting
- trouble with balance and coordination
- anxiety

Other common side effects that have been reported with another form of LAMICTAL include headache, sleepiness, blurred vision, runny nose, and rash.

Tell your healthcare provider about any side effect that bothers you or that does not go away.

These are not all the possible side effects of LAMICTAL XR. For more information, ask your healthcare provider or pharmacist.

Call your doctor for medical advice about side effects. You may report side effects to FDA at 1-800-FDA-1088.

How should I store LAMICTAL XR?

- Store LAMICTAL XR at room temperature between 59°F to 86°F (15°C to 30°C).
- **Keep LAMICTAL XR and all medicines out of the reach of children.**

General information about LAMICTAL XR

Medicines are sometimes prescribed for purposes other than those listed in a Medication Guide. Do not use LAMICTAL XR for a condition for which it was not prescribed. Do not give LAMICTAL XR to other people, even if they have the same symptoms you have. It may harm them.

This Medication Guide summarizes the most important information about LAMICTAL XR. If you would like more information, talk with your healthcare provider. You can ask your healthcare provider or pharmacist for information about LAMICTAL XR that is written for healthcare professionals.

For more information, go to www.lamictalxr.com or call 1-888-825-5249.

What are the ingredients in LAMICTAL XR?

Active ingredient: lamotrigine.

Inactive ingredients: glycerol monostearate, hypromellose, lactose monohydrate, magnesium stearate, methacrylic acid copolymer dispersion, polyethylene glycol 400, polysorbate 80, silicon dioxide (25 mg and 50 mg tablets only), titanium dioxide, triethyl citrate, carmine (250 mg tablet only), iron oxide black (50 mg, 250 mg, and 300 mg tablets only), iron oxide yellow (25 mg, 50 mg, and 100 mg tablets only), iron oxide red (100 mg tablet only), FD&C Blue No. 2 Aluminum Lake (200 mg and 250 mg tablets only). Tablets are printed with edible black ink.

This Medication Guide has been approved by the U.S. Food and Drug Administration.

LAMICTAL XR is a trademark of GlaxoSmithKline.
DEPAKENE and DEPAKOTE are registered trademarks of Abbott Laboratories.
GlaxoSmithKline
Research Triangle Park, NC 27709

December 2011
LXR:10MG

LOVAZA® ℞

[lō-vā' zā]

(omega-3-acid ethyl esters)
Capsules, for oral use

HIGHLIGHTS OF PRESCRIBING INFORMATION
These highlights do not include all the information needed to use LOVAZA safely and effectively. See full prescribing information for LOVAZA.
LOVAZA® (omega-3-acid ethyl esters) Capsules, for oral use
Initial U.S. Approval: 2004

RECENT MAJOR CHANGES

Indications and Usage, Limitations of Use (1)	06/2013
Warnings and Precautions, Recurrent Atrial Fibrillation or Flutter (5.3)	08/2012

INDICATIONS AND USAGE

LOVAZA is a combination of ethyl esters of omega 3 fatty acids, principally EPA and DHA, indicated as an adjunct to diet to reduce triglyceride (TG) levels in adult patients with severe (≥500 mg/dL) hypertriglyceridemia. (1)

Limitations of Use:

- The effect of LOVAZA on the risk for pancreatitis in patients with severe hypertriglyceridemia has not been determined. (1)
- The effect of LOVAZA on cardiovascular mortality and morbidity in patients with severe hypertriglyceridemia has not been determined. (1)

DOSAGE AND ADMINISTRATION

- The daily dose of LOVAZA is 4 grams per day taken as a single 4-gram dose (4 capsules) or as two 2-gram doses (2 capsules given twice daily). (2)
- Patients should be advised to swallow LOVAZA capsules whole. Do not break open, crush, dissolve or chew LOVAZA. (2)

DOSAGE FORMS AND STRENGTHS

Capsules: 1-gram (3)

CONTRAINDICATIONS

LOVAZA is contraindicated in patients with known hypersensitivity (e.g., anaphylactic reaction) to LOVAZA or any of its components. (4)

WARNINGS AND PRECAUTIONS

- In patients with hepatic impairment, monitor ALT and AST levels periodically during therapy. (5.1)
- LOVAZA may increase levels of LDL. Monitor LDL levels periodically during therapy. (5.1)
- Use with caution in patients with known hypersensitivity to fish and/or shellfish. (5.2)
- There is a possible association between LOVAZA and more frequent recurrences of symptomatic atrial fibrillation or flutter in patients with paroxysmal or persistent atrial fibrillation, particularly within the first months of initiating therapy. (5.3)

ADVERSE REACTIONS

The most common adverse reactions (incidence >3% and greater than placebo) were eructation, dyspepsia, and taste perversion. (6)

To report SUSPECTED ADVERSE REACTIONS, contact GlaxoSmithKline at 1-888-825-5249 or FDA at 1-800-FDA-1088 or www.fda.gov/medwatch

DRUG INTERACTIONS

Omega-3-acids may prolong bleeding time. Patients taking LOVAZA and an anticoagulant or other drug affecting coagulation (e.g., anti-platelet agents) should be monitored periodically. (7.1)

USE IN SPECIFIC POPULATIONS

- Pregnancy: Use during pregnancy only if the potential benefit justifies the potential risk to the fetus. (8.1)

See 17 for PATIENT COUNSELING INFORMATION and FDA-approved patient labeling

Revised: 06/2013

FULL PRESCRIBING INFORMATION: CONTENTS*

*** Sections or subsections omitted from the full prescribing information are not listed**

FULL PRESCRIBING INFORMATION

1 INDICATIONS AND USAGE

LOVAZA® (omega-3-acid ethyl esters) is indicated as an adjunct to diet to reduce triglyceride (TG) levels in adult patients with severe (≥500 mg/dL) hypertriglyceridemia.

Usage Considerations: Patients should be placed on an appropriate lipid-lowering diet before receiving LOVAZA and should continue this diet during treatment with LOVAZA.

Laboratory studies should be done to ascertain that the lipid levels are consistently abnormal before instituting LOVAZA therapy. Every attempt should be made to control serum lipids with appropriate diet, exercise, weight loss in obese patients, and control of any medical problems such as diabetes mellitus and hypothyroidism that are contributing to the lipid abnormalities. Medications known to exacerbate hypertriglyceridemia (such as beta blockers, thiazides, estrogens) should be discontinued or changed if possible prior to consideration of triglyceride-lowering drug therapy.

Limitations of Use:

The effect of LOVAZA on the risk for pancreatitis in patients with severe hypertriglyceridemia has not been determined.

The effect of LOVAZA on cardiovascular mortality and morbidity in patients with severe hypertriglyceridemia has not been determined.

2 DOSAGE AND ADMINISTRATION

- Assess triglyceride levels carefully before initiating therapy. Identify other causes (e.g., diabetes mellitus, hypothyroidism, or medications) of high triglyceride levels and manage as appropriate. *[see Indications and Usage (1)]*.
- Patients should be placed on an appropriate lipid-lowering diet before receiving LOVAZA, and should continue this diet during treatment with LOVAZA. In clinical studies, LOVAZA was administered with meals.

The daily dose of LOVAZA is 4 grams per day. The daily dose may be taken as a single 4-gram dose (4 capsules) or as two 2-gram doses (2 capsules given twice daily).

Patients should be advised to swallow LOVAZA capsules whole. Do not break open, crush, dissolve or chew LOVAZA.

3 DOSAGE FORMS AND STRENGTHS

LOVAZA (omega-3-acid ethyl esters) capsules are supplied as 1-gram transparent soft-gelatin capsules filled with light-yellow oil and bearing the designation LOVAZA.

4 CONTRAINDICATIONS

LOVAZA is contraindicated in patients with known hypersensitivity (e.g., anaphylactic reaction) to LOVAZA or any of its components.

5 WARNINGS AND PRECAUTIONS

5.1 Monitoring: Laboratory Tests

In patients with hepatic impairment, alanine aminotransferase (ALT) and aspartate aminotransferase (AST) levels should be monitored periodically during therapy with LOVAZA. In some patients, increases in ALT levels without a concurrent increase in AST levels were observed.

In some patients, LOVAZA increases LDL-C levels. LDL-C levels should be monitored periodically during therapy with LOVAZA.

Laboratory studies should be performed periodically to measure the patient's TG levels during therapy with LOVAZA.

5.2 Fish Allergy

LOVAZA contains ethyl esters of omega-3 fatty acids (EPA and DHA) obtained from the oil of several fish sources. It is not known whether patients with allergies to fish and/or shellfish, are at increased risk of an allergic reaction to LOVAZA. LOVAZA should be used with caution in patients with known hypersensitivity to fish and/or shellfish.

5.3 Recurrent Atrial Fibrillation (AF) or Flutter

In a double-blind, placebo-controlled trial of 663 patients with symptomatic paroxysmal AF (n=542) or persistent AF (n=121), recurrent AF or flutter was observed in patients randomized to LOVAZA who received 8 grams/day for 7 days and 4 grams/day thereafter for 23 weeks at a higher rate relative to placebo. Patients in this trial had median baseline triglycerides of 127 mg/dL, had no substantial structural heart disease, were taking no anti-arrhythmic therapy (rate control permitted), and were in normal sinus rhythm at baseline.

At 24 weeks, in the paroxysmal AF stratum, there were 129 (47%) first recurrent symptomatic AF or flutter events on placebo and 141 (53%) on LOVAZA [primary endpoint, HR 1.19; 95% CI 0.93, 1.35]. In the persistent AF stratum, there were 19 (35%) events on placebo and 34 (52%) events on LOVAZA [HR 1.63; 95% CI 0.91, 2.18]. For both strata combined, the HR was 1.25; 95% CI 1.00, 1.40. Although the clinical significance of these results is uncertain, there is a possible association between LOVAZA and more frequent recurrences of symptomatic atrial fibrillation or flutter in patients with paroxysmal or persistent atrial fibrillation, particularly within the first 2 to 3 months of initiating therapy.

LOVAZA is not indicated for the treatment of AF or flutter.

6 ADVERSE REACTIONS

6.1 Clinical Trials Experience

Because clinical trials are conducted under widely varying conditions, adverse reaction rates observed in the clinical trials of a drug cannot be directly compared to rates in the clinical trials of another drug and may not reflect the rates observed in practice.

Adverse reactions reported in at least 3% and at a greater rate than placebo for patients treated with LOVAZA based on pooled data across 23 clinical studies are listed in Table 1.

Table 1. Adverse Reactions Occurring at Incidence ≥3% and Greater than Placebo in Clinical Studies of LOVAZA

	LOVAZA (N = 655)		Placebo (N = 370)	
Adverse Reaction[a]	**n**	**%**	**n**	**%**
Eructation	29	4	5	1
Dyspepsia	22	3	6	2
Taste perversion	27	4	1	<1

[a] Studies included subjects with HTG and severe HTG.

Additional adverse reactions from clinical studies are listed below:

Digestive System: Constipation, gastrointestinal disorder and vomiting.

Metabolic and Nutritional Disorders: Increased ALT and increased AST.

Skin: Pruritus and rash.

6.2 Postmarketing Experience

In addition to adverse reactions reported from clinical trials, the events described below have been identified during post-approval use of LOVAZA. Because these events are reported voluntarily from a population of unknown size, it is not possible to reliably estimate their frequency or to always establish a causal relationship to drug exposure.

The following events have been reported: anaphylactic reaction, hemorrhagic diathesis.

7 DRUG INTERACTIONS

7.1 Anticoagulants or Other Drugs Affecting Coagulation

Some studies with omega-3-acids demonstrated prolongation of bleeding time. The prolongation of bleeding time reported in these studies has not exceeded normal limits and did not produce clinically significant bleeding episodes. Clinical studies have not been done to thoroughly examine the effect of LOVAZA and concomitant anticoagulants. Patients receiving treatment with LOVAZA and an anticoagulant or other drug affecting coagulation (e.g., anti-platelet agents) should be monitored periodically.

Table 2. Median Baseline and Percent Change From Baseline in Lipid Parameters in Patients with Very High TG Levels (≥500 mg/dL)

Parameter	LOVAZA N = 42		Placebo N = 42		Difference
	BL	% Change	BL	% Change	
TG	816	-44.9	788	+6.7	-51.6
Non-HDL-C	271	-13.8	292	-3.6	-10.2
TC	296	-9.7	314	-1.7	-8.0
VLDL-C	175	-41.7	175	-0.9	-40.8
HDL-C	22	+9.1	24	0.0	+9.1
LDL-C	89	+44.5	108	-4.8	+49.3

BL = Baseline (mg/dL); % Change = Median Percent Change from Baseline; Difference = LOVAZA Median % Change – Placebo Median % Change

8 USE IN SPECIFIC POPULATIONS

8.1 Pregnancy

Pregnancy Category C: There are no adequate and well-controlled studies in pregnant women. It is unknown whether LOVAZA can cause fetal harm when administered to a pregnant woman or can affect reproductive capacity. LOVAZA should be used during pregnancy only if the potential benefit to the patient justifies the potential risk to the fetus.

Animal Data

Omega-3-acid ethyl esters have been shown to have an embryocidal effect in pregnant rats when given in doses resulting in exposures 7 times the recommended human dose of 4 grams/day based on a body surface area comparison.

In female rats given oral gavage doses of 100, 600, and 2,000 mg/kg/day beginning 2 weeks prior to mating and continuing through gestation and lactation, no adverse effects were observed in the high dose group (5 times human systemic exposure following an oral dose of 4 grams/day based on body surface area comparison).

In pregnant rats given oral gavage doses of 1,000, 3,000, and 6,000 mg/kg/day from gestation day 6 through 15, no adverse effects were observed (14 times human systemic exposure following an oral dose of 4 grams/day based on a body surface area comparison).

In pregnant rats given oral gavage doses of 100, 600, and 2,000 mg/kg/day from gestation day 14 through lactation day 21, no adverse effects were seen at 2,000 mg/kg/day (5 times the human systemic exposure following an oral dose of 4 grams/day based on a body surface area comparison). However, decreased live births (20% reduction) and decreased survival to postnatal day 4 (40% reduction) were observed in a dose-ranging study using higher doses of 3,000 mg/kg/day (7 times the human systemic exposure following an oral dose of 4 grams/day based on a body surface area comparison).

In pregnant rabbits given oral gavage doses of 375, 750, and 1,500 mg/kg/day from gestation day 7 through 19, no findings were observed in the fetuses in groups given 375 mg/kg/day (2 times human systemic exposure following an oral dose of 4 grams/day based on a body surface area comparison). However, at higher doses, evidence of maternal toxicity was observed (4 times human systemic exposure following an oral dose of 4 grams/day based on a body surface area comparison).

8.3 Nursing Mothers

Studies with omega-3-acid ethyl esters have demonstrated excretion in human milk. The effect of this excretion on the infant of a nursing mother is unknown; caution should be exercised when LOVAZA is administered to a nursing mother. An animal study in lactating rats given oral gavage ^{14}C-ethyl EPA demonstrated that drug levels were 6 to 14 times higher in milk than in plasma.

8.4 Pediatric Use

Safety and effectiveness in pediatric patients have not been established.

8.5 Geriatric Use

A limited number of patients older than 65 years were enrolled in the clinical studies of LOVAZA. Safety and efficacy findings in subjects older than 60 years did not appear to differ from those of subjects younger than 60 years.

9 DRUG ABUSE AND DEPENDENCE

LOVAZA does not have any known drug abuse or withdrawal effects.

11 DESCRIPTION

LOVAZA, a lipid-regulating agent, is supplied as a liquid-filled gel capsule for oral administration. Each 1-gram capsule of LOVAZA contains at least 900 mg of the ethyl esters of omega-3 fatty acids sourced from fish oils. These are predominantly a combination of ethyl esters of eicosapentaenoic acid (EPA - approximately 465 mg) and docosahexaenoic acid (DHA - approximately 375 mg).

The empirical formula of EPA ethyl ester is $C_{22}H_{34}O_2$, and the molecular weight of EPA ethyl ester is 330.51. The structural formula of EPA ethyl ester is:

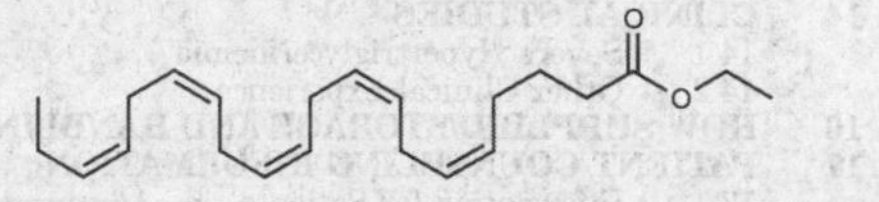

The empirical formula of DHA ethyl ester is $C_{24}H_{36}O_2$, and the molecular weight of DHA ethyl ester is 356.55. The structural formula of DHA ethyl ester is:

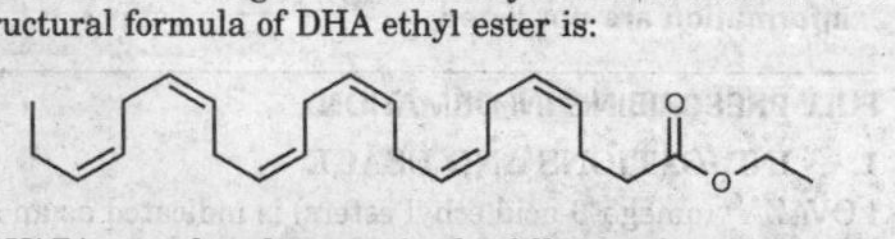

LOVAZA capsules also contain the following inactive ingredients: 4 mg α-tocopherol (in a carrier of soybean oil), and gelatin, glycerol, and purified water (components of the capsule shell).

12 CLINICAL PHARMACOLOGY

12.1 Mechanism of Action

The mechanism of action of LOVAZA is not completely understood. Potential mechanisms of action include inhibition of acyl-CoA:1,2-diacylglycerol acyltransferase, increased mitochondrial and peroxisomal β-oxidation in the liver, decreased lipogenesis in the liver, and increased plasma lipoprotein lipase activity. LOVAZA may reduce the synthesis of triglycerides in the liver because EPA and DHA are poor substrates for the enzymes responsible for TG synthesis, and EPA and DHA inhibit esterification of other fatty acids.

12.3 Pharmacokinetics

In healthy volunteers and in patients with hypertriglyceridemia, EPA and DHA were absorbed when administered as ethyl esters orally. Omega-3-acids administered as ethyl esters (LOVAZA) induced significant, dose-dependent increases in serum phospholipid EPA content, though increases in DHA content were less marked and not dose-dependent when administered as ethyl esters.

Specific Populations

Age

Uptake of EPA and DHA into serum phospholipids in subjects treated with LOVAZA was independent of age (<49 years versus ≥49 years).

Gender

Females tended to have more uptake of EPA into serum phospholipids than males. The clinical significance of this is unknown.

Pediatric

Pharmacokinetics of LOVAZA have not been studied.

Renal or Hepatic Impairment

LOVAZA has not been studied in patients with renal or hepatic impairment.

Drug-Drug Interactions

Simvastatin

In a 14-day study of 24 healthy adult subjects, daily co-administration of simvastatin 80 mg with LOVAZA 4 grams did not affect the extent (AUC) or rate (C_{max}) of exposure to simvastatin or the major active metabolite, beta-hydroxy simvastatin at steady state.

Atorvastatin

In a 14-day study of 50 healthy adult subjects, daily co-administration of atorvastatin 80 mg with LOVAZA 4 grams did not affect AUC or C_{max} of exposure to atorvastatin, 2-hydroxyatorvastatin, or 4-hydroxyatorvastatin at steady state.

Rosuvastatin

In a 14-day study of 48 healthy adult subjects, daily co-administration of rosuvastatin 40 mg with LOVAZA 4 grams did not affect AUC or C_{max} of exposure to rosuvastatin at steady state.

In vitro studies using human liver microsomes indicated that clinically significant cytochrome P450 mediated inhibition by EPA/DHA combinations are not expected in humans.

13 NONCLINICAL TOXICOLOGY

13.1 Carcinogenesis, Mutagenesis, Impairment of Fertility

In a rat carcinogenicity study with oral gavage doses of 100, 600, and 2,000 mg/kg/day, males were treated with omega-3-acid ethyl esters for 101 weeks and females for 89 weeks without an increased incidence of tumors (up to 5 times human systemic exposures following an oral dose of 4 grams/day based on a body surface area comparison). Standard lifetime carcinogenicity bioassays were not conducted in mice.

Omega-3-acid ethyl esters were not mutagenic or clastogenic with or without metabolic activation in the bacterial mutagenesis (Ames) test with *Salmonella typhimurium* and *Escherichia coli* or in the chromosomal aberration assay in Chinese hamster V79 lung cells or human lymphocytes. Omega-3-acid ethyl esters were negative in the in vivo mouse micronucleus assay.

In a rat fertility study with oral gavage doses of 100, 600, and 2,000 mg/kg/day, males were treated for 10 weeks prior to mating and females were treated for 2 weeks prior to and throughout mating, gestation, and lactation. No adverse effect on fertility was observed at 2,000 mg/kg/day (5 times human systemic exposure following an oral dose of 4 grams/day based on a body surface area comparison).

14 CLINICAL STUDIES

14.1 Severe Hypertriglyceridemia

The effects of LOVAZA 4 grams per day were assessed in 2 randomized, placebo-controlled, double-blind, parallel-group studies of 84 adult patients (42 on LOVAZA, 42 on placebo) with very high triglyceride levels. Patients whose baseline triglyceride levels were between 500 and 2,000 mg/dL were enrolled in these 2 studies of 6 and 16 weeks duration. The median triglyceride and LDL-C levels in these patients were 792 mg/dL and 100 mg/dL, respectively. Median HDL-C level was 23.0 mg/dL.

The changes in the major lipoprotein lipid parameters for the groups receiving LOVAZA or placebo are shown in Table 2.

[See table 2 above]

LOVAZA 4 grams per day reduced median TG, VLDL-C, and non-HDL-C levels and increased median HDL-C from baseline relative to placebo. Treatment with LOVAZA to reduce very high TG levels may result in elevations in LDL-C and non-HDL-C in some individuals. Patients should be monitored to ensure that the LDL-C level does not increase excessively.

The effect of LOVAZA on the risk of pancreatitis in patients with severe hypertriglyceridemia has not been determined.

The effect of LOVAZA on cardiovascular mortality and morbidity in patients with severe hypertriglyceridemia has not been determined.

14.2 Other Clinical Experience

The effects of LOVAZA 4 grams per day as add-on therapy to treatment with simvastatin were evaluated in a randomized, placebo-controlled, double-blind, parallel-group study of 254 adult patients (122 on LOVAZA and 132 on placebo) with persistent high triglycerides (200 to 499 mg/dL) despite simvastatin therapy. Patients were treated with open-label simvastatin 40 mg per day for 8 weeks prior to randomization to control their LDL-C to no greater than 10% above NCEP ATP III goal and remained on this dose throughout the study. Following 8 weeks of open-label treatment with simvastatin, patients were randomized to either LOVAZA 4 grams per day or placebo for an additional 8 weeks with simvastatin co-therapy. The median baseline triglyceride and LDL-C levels in these patients were 268 mg/dL and 89 mg/dL, respectively. Median baseline non-HDL-C and HDL-C levels were 138 mg/dL and 45 mg/dL, respectively.

The changes in the major lipoprotein lipid parameters for the groups receiving LOVAZA plus simvastatin or placebo plus simvastatin are shown in Table 3.

[See table 3 at top of next page]

LOVAZA 4 grams per day significantly reduced non-HDL-C, TG, TC, VLDL-C, and Apo-B levels and increased HDL-C and LDL-C from baseline relative to placebo.

16 HOW SUPPLIED/STORAGE AND HANDLING

LOVAZA (omega-3-acid ethyl esters) capsules are supplied as 1-gram transparent soft-gelatin capsules filled with light-yellow oil and bearing the designation LOVAZA.

Bottles of 120: NDC 0173-0783-02

Store at 25°C (77°F); excursions permitted to 15° to 30°C (59° to 86°F) [see USP Controlled Room Temperature]. Do not freeze. Keep out of reach of children.

17 PATIENT COUNSELING INFORMATION

See FDA-approved patient labeling (17.2).

17.1 Information for Patients

- LOVAZA should be used with caution in patients with known sensitivity or allergy to fish and/or shellfish *[see Warnings and Precautions (5.2)]*.
- Patients should be advised that use of lipid-regulating agents does not reduce the importance of adhering to diet *[see Dosage and Administration (2)]*.
- Patients should be advised not to alter LOVAZA capsules in any way and to ingest intact capsules only *[see Dosage and Administration (2)]*.
- Instruct patients to take LOVAZA as prescribed. If a dose is missed, patients should take it as soon as they remember. However, if they miss one day of LOVAZA, they should not double the dose when they take it.

17.2 FDA-Approved Patient Labeling

Patient labeling is provided as a tear-off leaflet at the end of this full prescribing information.

Manufactured for GlaxoSmithKline by:
Catalent Pharma Solutions
St. Petersburg, FL 33716

Distributed by:
GlaxoSmithKline
Research Triangle Park, NC 27709

LOVAZA is a registered trademark of the GlaxoSmithKline group of companies.

LVZ:10PI

PHARMACIST-DETACH HERE AND GIVE INSTRUCTIONS TO PATIENT

PATIENT INFORMATION
LOVAZA® (lō-vā-zā)
(omega-3-acid ethyl esters)
Capsules

Read this Patient Information before you start taking LOVAZA, and each time you get a refill. There may be new information. This information does not take the place of talking with your doctor about your medical condition or your treatment.

What is LOVAZA?

LOVAZA is a prescription medicine used along with a low fat and low cholesterol diet to lower very high triglyceride (fat) levels in adults.

It is not known if LOVAZA changes your risk of having inflammation of your pancreas (pancreatitis).

It is not known if LOVAZA prevents you from having a heart attack or stroke.

It is not known if LOVAZA is safe and effective in children.

Who should not take LOVAZA?

Do not take LOVAZA if you are allergic to omega-3-acid ethyl esters or any of the ingredients in LOVAZA. See the end of this leaflet for a complete list of ingredients in LOVAZA.

What should I tell my doctor before taking LOVAZA?

Before you take LOVAZA, tell your doctor if you:

- have diabetes.
- have a low thyroid problem (hypothyroidism).
- have a liver problem.
- have a pancreas problem.
- have a certain heart rhythm problem called atrial fibrillation or flutter.
- are allergic to fish or shellfish. It is not known if people who are allergic to fish or shellfish are also allergic to LOVAZA.
- are pregnant or plan to become pregnant. It is not known if LOVAZA will harm your unborn baby.
- are breastfeeding or plan to breastfeed. LOVAZA can pass into your breast milk. You and your doctor should decide if you will take LOVAZA or breastfeed.

Tell your doctor about all the medicines you take, including prescription and non-prescription medicine, vitamins, and herbal supplements.

LOVAZA can interact with certain other medicines that you are taking. Using LOVAZA with medicines that affect blood clotting (anticoagulants or blood thinners) may cause serious side effects.

Know the medicines you take. Keep a list of them to show your doctor and pharmacist when you get a new medicine.

How should I take LOVAZA?

- Take LOVAZA exactly as your doctor tells you to take it.
- You should not take more than 4 capsules of LOVAZA each day. Either take all 4 capsules at one time, or 2 capsules two times a day.

Table 3. Response to the Addition of LOVAZA 4 grams per day to Ongoing Simvastatin 40 mg per day Therapy in Patients with High Triglycerides (200 to 499 mg/dL)

Parameter	LOVAZA + Simvastatin N = 122			Placebo + Simvastatin N = 132			Difference	P-Value
	BL	EOT	Median % Change	BL	EOT	Median % Change		
Non-HDL-C	137	123	-9.0	141	134	-2.2	-6.8	<0.0001
TG	268	182	-29.5	271	260	-6.3	-23.2	<0.0001
TC	184	172	-4.8	184	178	-1.7	-3.1	<0.05
VLDL-C	52	37	-27.5	52	49	-7.2	-20.3	<0.05
Apo-B	86	80	-4.2	87	85	-1.9	-2.3	<0.05
HDL-C	46	48	+3.4	43	44	-1.2	+4.6	<0.05
LDL-C	91	88	+0.7	88	85	-2.8	+3.5	=0.05

BL = Baseline (mg/dL); EOT = End of Treatment (mg/dL); Median % Change = Median Percent Change from Baseline; Difference = LOVAZA Median % Change – Placebo Median % Change

- Do not change your dose or stop LOVAZA without talking to your doctor.
- Take LOVAZA with or without food.
- Take LOVAZA capsules whole. Do not break, crush, dissolve, or chew LOVAZA capsules before swallowing. If you cannot swallow LOVAZA capsules whole, tell your doctor. You may need a different medicine.
- Your doctor may start you on a diet that is low in saturated fat, cholesterol, carbohydrates, and low in added sugars before giving you LOVAZA. Stay on this diet while taking LOVAZA.
- Your doctor should do blood tests to check your triglyceride, bad cholesterol and liver function levels while you take LOVAZA.

What are the possible side effects of LOVAZA?

LOVAZA may cause serious side effects, including:

- increases in the results of blood tests used to check your liver function (ALT and AST) and your bad cholesterol levels (LDL-C).
- increases in the frequency of a heart rhythm problem (atrial fibrillation or flutter) may especially happen in the first few months of taking LOVAZA if you already have that problem.

The most common side effects of LOVAZA include:

- burping
- upset stomach
- a change in your sense of taste.

Talk to your doctor if you have a side effect that bothers you or does not go away.

These are not all the possible side effects of LOVAZA. For more information, ask your doctor or pharmacist.

Call your doctor for medical advice about side effects. You may report side effects to FDA at 1-800-FDA-1088.

How should I store LOVAZA?

- Store LOVAZA at room temperature between 68°F to 77°F (20°C to 25°C).
- Do not freeze LOVAZA.
- Safely throw away medicine that is out of date or no longer needed.

Keep LOVAZA and all medicines out of the reach of children.

General information about the safe and effective use of LOVAZA

Medicines are sometimes prescribed for purposes other than those listed in a Patient Information leaflet. Do not use LOVAZA for a condition for which it was not prescribed. Do not give LOVAZA to other people, even if they have the same symptoms you have. It may harm them.

This Patient Information Leaflet summarizes the most important information about LOVAZA. If you would like more information, talk with your doctor. You can ask your doctor or pharmacist for information about LOVAZA that is written for health professionals.

For more information go to www.LOVAZA.com or call 1-888-825-5249.

What are the ingredients in LOVAZA?

Active Ingredient: omega-3-acid ethyl esters, mostly EPA and DHA

Inactive Ingredients: alpha-tocopherol (in soybean oil), gelatin, glycerol, purified water.

This patient labeling has been approved by the U.S. Food and Drug Administration.

Manufactured for GlaxoSmithKline by:
Catalent Pharma Solutions
St. Petersburg, FL 33716

Distributed by:
GlaxoSmithKline
Research Triangle Park, NC 27709

June 2013
LVZ:8PIL

MALARONE ℞
[mal'ə-rōn]
(atovaquone and proguanil hydrochloride)
Tablets

MALARONE ℞
(atovaquone and proguanil hydrochloride)
Pediatric Tablets

HIGHLIGHTS OF PRESCRIBING INFORMATION

These highlights do not include all the information needed to use MALARONE safely and effectively. See full prescribing information for MALARONE.

MALARONE (atovaquone and proguanil hydrochloride) Tablets

MALARONE (atovaquone and proguanil hydrochloride) Pediatric Tablets

Initial U.S. Approval: 2000

INDICATIONS AND USAGE

MALARONE is an antimalarial indicated for:

- prophylaxis of *Plasmodium falciparum* malaria, including in areas where chloroquine resistance has been reported. (1.1)
- treatment of acute, uncomplicated *P. falciparum* malaria. (1.2)

DOSAGE AND ADMINISTRATION

- MALARONE should be taken with food or a milky drink.

Prophylaxis (2.1):

- Start prophylaxis 1 or 2 days before entering a malaria-endemic area and continue daily during the stay and for 7 days after return.
- Adults: One adult strength tablet per day.
- Pediatric Patients: Dosage based on body weight (see Table 1).

Treatment (2.2):

- Adults: Four adult strength tablets as a single daily dose for 3 days.
- Pediatric Patients: Dosage based on body weight (see Table 2).

Renal Impairment (2.3):

- Do not use for prophylaxis of malaria in patients with severe renal impairment.
- Use with caution for treatment of malaria in patients with severe renal impairment.

DOSAGE FORMS AND STRENGTHS

- Tablets (adult strength): 250 mg atovaquone and 100 mg proguanil hydrochloride. (3)
- Pediatric Tablets: 62.5 mg atovaquone and 25 mg proguanil hydrochloride. (3)

CONTRAINDICATIONS

- Known serious hypersensitivity reactions to atovaquone or proguanil hydrochloride or any component of the formulation. (4.1)
- Prophylaxis of *P. falciparum* malaria in patients with severe renal impairment (creatinine clearance <30 mL/min). (4.2)

WARNINGS AND PRECAUTIONS

- Atovaquone absorption may be reduced in patients with diarrhea or vomiting. If used in patients who are vomiting, parasitemia should be closely monitored and the use of an antiemetic considered. In patients with severe or persistent diarrhea or vomiting, alternative antimalarial therapy may be required. (5.1)
- In mixed *P. falciparum* and *Plasmodium vivax* infection, *P. vivax* relapse occurred commonly when patients were treated with MALARONE alone. (5.2)
- In the event of recrudescent *P. falciparum* infections after treatment or prophylaxis failure, patients should be treated with a different blood schizonticide. (5.2)
- Elevated liver laboratory tests and cases of hepatitis and hepatic failure requiring liver transplantation have been reported with prophylactic use. (5.3)
- MALARONE has not been evaluated for the treatment of cerebral malaria or other severe manifestations of complicated malaria. Patients with severe malaria are not candidates for oral therapy. (5.4)

ADVERSE REACTIONS

- Prophylaxis: common adverse reactions (4%) in adults were diarrhea, dreams, oral ulcers, and headache; these events occurred in a similar or lower proportion of subjects receiving MALARONE than an active comparator. Common adverse reactions (5%) in pediatric patients included abdominal pain, headache, cough, and vomiting. (6.1)
- Treatment: common adverse reactions (5%) in adolescents and adults were abdominal pain, nausea, vomiting, headache, diarrhea, asthenia, anorexia, and dizziness. Common adverse reactions (6%) in pediatric patients included vomiting, pruritus, and diarrhea. (6.1)

To report SUSPECTED ADVERSE REACTIONS, contact GlaxoSmithKline at 1-888-825-5249 or FDA at 1-800-FDA-1088 or www.fda.gov/medwatch

DRUG INTERACTIONS

- Administration with rifampin or rifabutin is known to reduce atovaquone concentrations; concomitant use with MALARONE is not recommended. (7.1)
- Proguanil may potentiate anticoagulant effect of warfarin and other coumarin-based anticoagulants. Caution advised when initiating or withdrawing MALARONE in patients on anticoagulants; coagulation tests should be closely monitored. (7.2)
- Tetracycline may reduce atovaquone concentrations; parasitemia should be closely monitored. (7.3)

USE IN SPECIFIC POPULATIONS

- Caution should be exercised when administered to a nursing woman as proguanil is excreted into human milk. (8.3)
- Renal impairment: contraindicated for prophylaxis of *P. falciparum* malaria in patients with severe renal impairment (8.6).

See 17 for PATIENT COUNSELING INFORMATION

Revised: 06/2013

FULL PRESCRIBING INFORMATION: CONTENTS*

*** Sections or subsections omitted from the full prescribing information are not listed**

FULL PRESCRIBING INFORMATION

1 INDICATIONS AND USAGE

1.1 Prevention of Malaria

MALARONE® is indicated for the prophylaxis of *Plasmodium falciparum* malaria, including in areas where chloroquine resistance has been reported.

1.2 Treatment of Malaria

MALARONE is indicated for the treatment of acute, uncomplicated *P. falciparum* malaria. MALARONE has been shown to be effective in regions where the drugs chloroquine, halofantrine, mefloquine, and amodiaquine may have unacceptable failure rates, presumably due to drug resistance.

2 DOSAGE AND ADMINISTRATION

The daily dose should be taken at the same time each day with food or a milky drink. In the event of vomiting within 1 hour after dosing, a repeat dose should be taken.

MALARONE may be crushed and mixed with condensed milk just prior to administration to patients who may have difficulty swallowing tablets.

2.1 Prevention of Malaria

Start prophylactic treatment with MALARONE 1 or 2 days before entering a malaria–endemic area and continue daily during the stay and for 7 days after return.

Adults: One MALARONE Tablet (adult strength = 250 mg atovaquone/100 mg proguanil hydrochloride) per day.

Pediatric Patients: The dosage for prevention of malaria in pediatric patients is based upon body weight (Table 1).

Table 1. Dosage for Prevention of Malaria in Pediatric Patients

Weight (kg)	Atovaquone/ Proguanil HCl Total Daily Dose	Dosage Regimen
11-20	62.5 mg/25 mg	1 MALARONE Pediatric Tablet daily
21-30	125 mg/50 mg	2 MALARONE Pediatric Tablets as a single daily dose
31-40	187.5 mg/75 mg	3 MALARONE Pediatric Tablets as a single daily dose
>40	250 mg/100 mg	1 MALARONE Tablet (adult strength) as a single daily dose

2.2 Treatment of Acute Malaria

Adults: Four MALARONE Tablets (adult strength; total daily dose 1 g atovaquone/400 mg proguanil hydrochloride) as a single daily dose for 3 consecutive days.

Pediatric Patients: The dosage for treatment of acute malaria in pediatric patients is based upon body weight (Table 2).

Table 2. Dosage for Treatment of Acute Malaria in Pediatric Patients

Weight (kg)	Atovaquone/ Proguanil HCl Total Daily Dose	Dosage Regimen
5-8	125 mg/50 mg	2 MALARONE Pediatric Tablets daily for 3 consecutive days
9-10	187.5 mg/75 mg	3 MALARONE Pediatric Tablets daily for 3 consecutive days
11-20	250 mg/100 mg	1 MALARONE Tablet (adult strength) daily for 3 consecutive days
21-30	500 mg/200 mg	2 MALARONE Tablets (adult strength) as a single daily dose for 3 consecutive days
31-40	750 mg/300 mg	3 MALARONE Tablets (adult strength) as a single daily dose for 3 consecutive days
>40	1 g/400 mg	4 MALARONE Tablets (adult strength) as a single daily dose for 3 consecutive days

2.3 Renal Impairment

Do not use MALARONE for malaria prophylaxis in patients with severe renal impairment (creatinine clearance <30 mL/min) *[see Contraindications (4.2)]*. Use with caution for the treatment of malaria in patients with severe renal impairment, only if the benefits of the 3-day treatment regimen outweigh the potential risks associated with increased drug exposure. No dosage adjustments are needed in patients with mild (creatinine clearance 50 to 80 mL/min) or moderate (creatinine clearance 30 to 50 mL/min) renal impairment. *[See Clinical Pharmacology (12.3).]*

3 DOSAGE FORMS AND STRENGTHS

Each MALARONE Tablet (adult strength) contains 250 mg atovaquone and 100 mg proguanil hydrochloride. MALARONE Tablets are pink, film–coated, round, biconvex tablets engraved with "GX CM3" on one side.

Each MALARONE Pediatric Tablet contains 62.5 mg atovaquone and 25 mg proguanil hydrochloride. MALARONE Pediatric Tablets are pink, film–coated, round, biconvex tablets engraved with "GX CG7" on one side.

4 CONTRAINDICATIONS

4.1 Hypersensitivity

MALARONE is contraindicated in individuals with known hypersensitivity reactions (e.g., anaphylaxis, erythema multiforme or Stevens-Johnson syndrome, angioedema, vasculitis) to atovaquone or proguanil hydrochloride or any component of the formulation.

4.2 Severe Renal Impairment

MALARONE is contraindicated for prophylaxis of *P. falciparum* malaria in patients with severe renal impairment (creatinine clearance <30 mL/min) because of pancytopenia in patients with severe renal impairment treated with proguanil *[see Use in Specific Populations (8.6), and Clinical Pharmacology (12.3)]*.

5 WARNINGS AND PRECAUTIONS

5.1 Vomiting and Diarrhea

Absorption of atovaquone may be reduced in patients with diarrhea or vomiting. If MALARONE is used in patients who are vomiting, parasitemia should be closely monitored and the use of an antiemetic considered. *[See Dosage and Administration (2).]* Vomiting occurred in up to 19% of pediatric patients given treatment doses of MALARONE. In the controlled clinical trials, 15.3% of adults received an antiemetic when they received atovaquone/proguanil and 98.3% of these patients were successfully treated. In patients with severe or persistent diarrhea or vomiting, alternative antimalarial therapy may be required.

5.2 Relapse of Infection

In mixed *P. falciparum* and *Plasmodium vivax* infections, *P. vivax* parasite relapse occurred commonly when patients were treated with MALARONE alone.

In the event of recrudescent *P. falciparum* infections after treatment with MALARONE or failure of chemoprophylaxis with MALARONE, patients should be treated with a different blood schizonticide.

5.3 Hepatotoxicity

Elevated liver laboratory tests and cases of hepatitis and hepatic failure requiring liver transplantation have been reported with prophylactic use of MALARONE.

5.4 Severe or Complicated Malaria

MALARONE has not been evaluated for the treatment of cerebral malaria or other severe manifestations of complicated malaria, including hyperparasitemia, pulmonary edema, or renal failure. Patients with severe malaria are not candidates for oral therapy.

6 ADVERSE REACTIONS

6.1 Clinical Trials Experience

Because clinical trials are conducted under widely varying conditions, adverse reaction rates observed in the clinical trials of a drug cannot be directly compared to rates in the clinical trials of another drug and may not reflect the rates observed in practice.

Because MALARONE contains atovaquone and proguanil hydrochloride, the type and severity of adverse reactions associated with each of the compounds may be expected. The lower prophylactic doses of MALARONE were better tolerated than the higher treatment doses.

Prophylaxis of *P. falciparum* Malaria: In 3 clinical trials (2 of which were placebo–controlled) 381 adults (mean age 31 years) received MALARONE for the prophylaxis of malaria; the majority of adults were black (90%) and 79% were male. In a clinical trial for the prophylaxis of malaria, 125 pediatric patients (mean age 9 years) received MALARONE; all subjects were black and 52% were male. Adverse experiences reported in adults and pediatric patients, considered attributable to therapy, occurred in similar proportions of subjects receiving MALARONE or placebo in all studies. Prophylaxis with MALARONE was discontinued prematurely due to a treatment–related adverse experience in 3 of 381 (0.8%) adults and 0 of 125 pediatric patients.

In a placebo–controlled study of malaria prophylaxis with MALARONE involving 330 pediatric patients (aged 4 to 14 years) in Gabon, a malaria–endemic area, the safety profile of MALARONE was consistent with that observed in the earlier prophylactic studies in adults and pediatric patients. The most common treatment–emergent adverse events with MALARONE were abdominal pain (13%), headache (13%), and cough (10%). Abdominal pain (13% vs. 8%) and vomiting (5% vs. 3%) were reported more often with MALARONE than with placebo. No patient withdrew from the study due to an adverse experience with MALARONE. No routine laboratory data were obtained during this study.

Non–immune travelers visiting a malaria–endemic area received MALARONE (n = 1,004) for prophylaxis of malaria in 2 active-controlled clinical trials. In one study (n = 493), the mean age of subjects was 33 years and 53% were male; 90% of subjects were white, 6% of subjects were black and the remaining were of other racial/ethnic groups. In the other study (n = 511), the mean age of subjects was 36 years and 51% were female; the majority of subjects (97%) were white. Adverse experiences occurred in a similar or lower proportion of subjects receiving MALARONE than an active comparator (Table 3). Fewer neuropsychiatric adverse experiences occurred in subjects who received MALARONE than mefloquine. Fewer gastrointestinal adverse experiences occurred in subjects receiving MALARONE than chloroquine/proguanil. Compared with active comparator drugs, subjects receiving MALARONE had fewer adverse experiences overall that were attributed to prophylactic therapy (Table 3). Prophylaxis with MALARONE was discontinued prematurely due to a treatment–related adverse experience in 7 of 1,004 travelers.

[See table 3 above]

Table 3. Adverse Experiences in Active-Controlled Clinical Trials of MALARONE for Prophylaxis of P. falciparum Malaria

	Percent of Subjects With Adverse Experiences[a] (Percent of Subjects With Adverse Experiences Attributable to Therapy)							
	Study 1				Study 2			
	MALARONE n = 493 (28 days)[b]		Mefloquine n = 483 (53 days)[b]		MALARONE n = 511 (26 days)[b]		Chloroquine plus Proguanil n = 511 (49 days)[b]	
Diarrhea	38	(8)	36	(7)	34	(5)	39	(7)
Nausea	14	(3)	20	(8)	11	(2)	18	(7)
Abdominal pain	17	(5)	16	(5)	14	(3)	22	(6)
Headache	12	(4)	17	(7)	12	(4)	14	(4)
Dreams	7	(7)	16	(14)	6	(4)	7	(3)
Insomnia	5	(3)	16	(13)	4	(2)	5	(2)
Fever	9	(<1)	11	(1)	8	(<1)	8	(<1)
Dizziness	5	(2)	14	(9)	7	(3)	8	(4)
Vomiting	8	(1)	10	(2)	8	(0)	14	(2)
Oral ulcers	9	(6)	6	(4)	5	(4)	7	(5)
Pruritus	4	(2)	5	(2)	3	(1)	2	(<1)
Visual difficulties	2	(2)	5	(3)	3	(2)	3	(2)
Depression	<1	(<1)	5	(4)	<1	(<1)	1	(<1)
Anxiety	1	(<1)	5	(4)	<1	(<1)	1	(<1)
Any adverse experience	64	(30)	69	(42)	58	(22)	66	(28)
Any neuropsychiatric event	20	(14)	37	(29)	16	(10)	20	(10)
Any GI event	49	(16)	50	(19)	43	(12)	54	(20)

[a]Adverse experiences that started while receiving active study drug.
[b] Mean duration of dosing based on recommended dosing regimens.

In a third active–controlled study, MALARONE (n = 110) was compared with chloroquine/proguanil (n = 111) for the prophylaxis of malaria in 221 non-immune pediatric patients (2 to 17 years of age). The mean duration of exposure was 23 days for MALARONE, 46 days for chloroquine, and 43 days for proguanil, reflecting the different recommended dosage regimens for these products. Fewer patients treated with MALARONE reported abdominal pain (2% vs. 7%) or nausea (<1% vs. 7%) than children who received chloroquine/proguanil. Oral ulceration (2% vs. 2%), vivid dreams (2% vs. <1%), and blurred vision (0% vs. 2%) occurred in similar proportions of patients receiving either MALARONE or chloroquine/proguanil, respectively. Two patients discontinued prophylaxis with chloroquine/proguanil due to adverse events, while none of those receiving MALARONE discontinued due to adverse events.

Treatment of Acute, Uncomplicated *P. falciparum* Malaria: In 7 controlled trials, 436 adolescents and adults received MALARONE for treatment of acute, uncomplicated *P. falciparum* malaria. The range of mean ages of subjects was 26 to 29 years; 79% of subjects were male. In these studies, 48% of subjects were classified as other racial/ethnic groups, primarily Asian; 42% of subjects were black and the remaining subjects were white. Attributable adverse experiences that occurred in 5% of patients were abdominal pain (17%), nausea (12%), vomiting (12%), headache (10%), diarrhea (8%), asthenia (8%), anorexia (5%), and dizziness (5%). Treatment was discontinued prematurely due to an adverse experience in 4 of 436 (0.9%) adolescents and adults treated with MALARONE.

In 2 controlled trials, 116 pediatric patients (weighing 11 to 40 kg) (mean age 7 years) received MALARONE for the treatment of malaria. The majority of subjects were black (72%); 28% were of other racial/ethnic groups, primarily Asian. Attributable adverse experiences that occurred in 5% of patients were vomiting (10%) and pruritus (6%). Vomiting occurred in 43 of 319 (13%) pediatric patients who did not have symptomatic malaria but were given treatment doses of MALARONE for 3 days in a clinical trial. The design of this clinical trial required that any patient who vomited be withdrawn from the trial. Among pediatric patients with symptomatic malaria treated with MALARONE, treatment was discontinued prematurely due to an adverse experience in 1 of 116 (0.9%).

In a study of 100 pediatric patients (5 to <11 kg body weight) who received MALARONE for the treatment of uncomplicated *P. falciparum* malaria, only diarrhea (6%) occurred in 5% of patients as an adverse experience attributable to MALARONE. In 3 patients (3%), treatment was discontinued prematurely due to an adverse experience.

Abnormalities in laboratory tests reported in clinical trials were limited to elevations of transaminases in malaria patients being treated with MALARONE. The frequency of these abnormalities varied substantially across trials of treatment and were not observed in the randomized portions of the prophylaxis trials.

One active-controlled trial evaluated the treatment of malaria in Thai adults (n = 182); the mean age of subjects was 26 years (range 15 to 63 years); 80% of subjects were male. Early elevations of ALT and AST occurred more frequently in patients treated with MALARONE (n = 91) compared to patients treated with an active control, mefloquine (n = 91). On Day 7, rates of elevated ALT and AST with MALARONE and mefloquine (for patients who had normal baseline levels of these clinical laboratory parameters) were ALT 26.7% vs. 15.6%; AST 16.9% vs. 8.6%, respectively. By Day 14 of this 28–day study, the frequency of transaminase elevations equalized across the 2 groups.

6.2 Postmarketing Experience

In addition to adverse events reported from clinical trials, the following events have been identified during postmarketing use of MALARONE. Because they are reported voluntarily from a population of unknown size, estimates of frequency cannot be made. These events have been chosen for inclusion due to a combination of their seriousness, frequency of reporting, or potential causal connection to MALARONE.

Blood and Lymphatic System Disorders: Neutropenia and anemia. Pancytopenia in patients with severe renal impairment treated with proguanil *[see Contraindications (4.2)]*.

Immune System Disorders: Allergic reactions including anaphylaxis, angioedema, and urticaria, and vasculitis.

Nervous System Disorders: Seizures and psychotic events (such as hallucinations); however, a causal relationship has not been established.

Gastrointestinal Disorders: Stomatitis.

Hepatobiliary Disorders: Elevated liver laboratory tests, hepatitis, cholestasis; hepatic failure requiring transplant has been reported.

Skin and Subcutaneous Tissue Disorders: Photosensitivity, rash, erythema multiforme, and Stevens-Johnson syndrome.

7 DRUG INTERACTIONS

7.1 Rifampin/Rifabutin

Concomitant administration of rifampin or rifabutin is known to reduce atovaquone concentrations *[see Clinical Pharmacology (12.3)]*. The concomitant administration of MALARONE and rifampin or rifabutin is not recommended.

7.2 Anticoagulants

Proguanil may potentiate the anticoagulant effect of warfarin and other coumarin-based anticoagulants. The mechanism of this potential drug interaction has not been established. Caution is advised when initiating or withdrawing malaria prophylaxis or treatment with MALARONE in patients on continuous treatment with coumarin-based anticoagulants. When these products are administered concomitantly, coagulation tests should be closely monitored.

7.3 Tetracycline

Concomitant treatment with tetracycline has been associated with a reduction in plasma concentrations of atovaquone *[see Clinical Pharmacology (12.3)]*. Parasitemia should be closely monitored in patients receiving tetracycline.

7.4 Metoclopramide

While antiemetics may be indicated for patients receiving MALARONE, metoclopramide may reduce the bioavailability of atovaquone and should be used only if other antiemetics are not available *[see Clinical Pharmacology (12.3)]*.

7.5 Indinavir

Concomitant administration of atovaquone and indinavir did not result in any change in the steady–state AUC and C_{max} of indinavir but resulted in a decrease in the C_{trough} of indinavir *[see Clinical Pharmacology (12.3)]*. Caution should be exercised when prescribing atovaquone with indinavir due to the decrease in trough concentrations of indinavir.

8 USE IN SPECIFIC POPULATIONS

8.1 Pregnancy

Pregnancy Category C

Atovaquone: Atovaquone was not teratogenic and did not cause reproductive toxicity in rats at doses up to 1,000 mg/kg/day corresponding to maternal plasma concentrations up to 7.3 times the estimated human exposure during treatment of malaria based on AUC. In rabbits, atovaquone caused adverse fetal effects and maternal toxicity at a dose of 1,200 mg/kg/day corresponding to plasma concentrations that were approximately 1.3 times the estimated human exposure during treatment of malaria based on AUC. Adverse fetal effects in rabbits, including decreased fetal body lengths and increased early resorptions and post-implantation losses, were observed only in the presence of maternal toxicity.

In a pre- and post-natal study in rats, atovaquone did not produce adverse effects in offspring at doses up to 1,000 mg/kg/day corresponding to AUC exposures of approximately 7.3 times the estimated human exposure during treatment of malaria.

Proguanil: A pre- and post-natal study in Sprague-Dawley rats revealed no adverse effects at doses up to 16 mg/kg/day of proguanil hydrochloride (up to 0.04-times the average human exposure based on AUC). Pre- and post-natal studies of proguanil in animals at exposures similar to or greater than those observed in humans have not been conducted.

Atovaquone and Proguanil: The combination of atovaquone and proguanil hydrochloride was not teratogenic in pregnant rats at atovaquone:proguanil hydrochloride (50:20 mg/kg/day) corresponding to plasma concentrations up to 1.7 and 0.1 times, respectively, the estimated human exposure during treatment of malaria based on AUC. In pregnant rabbits, the combination of atovaquone and proguanil hydrochloride was not teratogenic or embryotoxic to rabbit fetuses at atovaquone:proguanil hydrochloride (100:40 mg/kg/day) corresponding to plasma concentrations of approximately 0.3 and 0.5 times, respectively, the estimated human exposure during treatment of malaria based on AUC.

There are no adequate and well-controlled studies of atovaquone and/or proguanil hydrochloride in pregnant women. MALARONE should be used during pregnancy only if the potential benefit justifies the potential risk to the fetus.

Falciparum malaria carries a higher risk of morbidity and mortality in pregnant women than in the general population. Maternal death and fetal loss are both known complications of falciparum malaria in pregnancy. In pregnant women who must travel to malaria–endemic areas, personal protection against mosquito bites should always be employed in addition to antimalarials. *[See Patient Counseling Information (17).]*

The proguanil component of MALARONE acts by inhibiting the parasitic dihydrofolate reductase *[see Clinical Pharmacology (12.1)]*. However, there are no clinical data indicating that folate supplementation diminishes drug efficacy. For women of childbearing age receiving folate supplements to prevent neural tube birth defects, such supplements may be continued while taking MALARONE.

8.3 Nursing Mothers

It is not known whether atovaquone is excreted into human milk. In a rat study, atovaquone concentrations in the milk were 30% of the concurrent atovaquone concentrations in the maternal plasma.

Proguanil is excreted into human milk in small quantities. Caution should be exercised when MALARONE is administered to a nursing woman.

8.4 Pediatric Use

Prophylaxis of Malaria: Safety and effectiveness have not been established in pediatric patients who weigh less than 11 kg. The efficacy and safety of MALARONE have been established for the prophylaxis of malaria in controlled trials involving pediatric patients weighing 11 kg or more *[see Clinical Studies (14.1)]*.

Treatment of Malaria: Safety and effectiveness have not been established in pediatric patients who weigh less than 5 kg. The efficacy and safety of MALARONE for the treatment of malaria have been established in controlled trials involving pediatric patients weighing 5 kg or more *[see Clinical Studies (14.2)]*.

8.5 Geriatric Use

Clinical trials of MALARONE did not include sufficient numbers of subjects aged 65 years and older to determine whether they respond differently from younger subjects. In general, dose selection for an elderly patient should be cautious, reflecting the greater frequency of decreased hepatic, renal, or cardiac function, the higher systemic exposure to cycloguanil, and the greater frequency of concomitant disease or other drug therapy. *[See Clinical Pharmacology (12.3).]*

8.6 Renal Impairment

Do not use MALARONE for malaria prophylaxis in patients with severe renal impairment (creatinine clearance <30 mL/min). Use with caution for the treatment of malaria in patients with severe renal impairment, only if the benefits of the 3-day treatment regimen outweigh the potential risks associated with increased drug exposure. No dosage adjustments are needed in patients with mild (creatinine clearance 50 to 80 mL/min) or moderate (creatinine clearance 30 to 50 mL/min) renal impairment. *[See Clinical Pharmacology (12.3).]*

8.7 Hepatic Impairment

No dosage adjustments are needed in patients with mild or moderate hepatic impairment *[see Clinical Pharmacology (12.3)]*. No trials have been conducted in patients with severe hepatic impairment.

10 OVERDOSAGE

There is no information on overdoses of MALARONE substantially higher than the doses recommended for treatment.

There is no known antidote for atovaquone, and it is currently unknown if atovaquone is dialyzable. Overdoses up to 31,500 mg of atovaquone have been reported. In one such patient who also took an unspecified dose of dapsone, methemoglobinemia occurred. Rash has also been reported after overdose.

Overdoses of proguanil hydrochloride as large as 1,500 mg have been followed by complete recovery, and doses as high as 700 mg twice daily have been taken for over 2 weeks without serious toxicity. Adverse experiences occasionally associated with proguanil hydrochloride doses of 100 to 200 mg/day, such as epigastric discomfort and vomiting, would be likely to occur with overdose. There are also reports of reversible hair loss and scaling of the skin on the palms and/or soles, reversible aphthous ulceration, and hematologic side effects.

11 DESCRIPTION

MALARONE (atovaquone and proguanil hydrochloride) Tablets (adult strength) and MALARONE (atovaquone and proguanil hydrochloride) Pediatric Tablets, for oral administration, contain a fixed–dose combination of the antimalarial agents atovaquone and proguanil hydrochloride.

The chemical name of atovaquone is *trans*-2-[4-(4-chlorophenyl)cyclohexyl]-3-hydroxy-1,4-naphthalenedione. Atovaquone is a yellow crystalline solid that is practically insoluble in water. It has a molecular weight of 366.84 and the molecular formula $C_{22}H_{19}ClO_3$. The compound has the following structural formula:

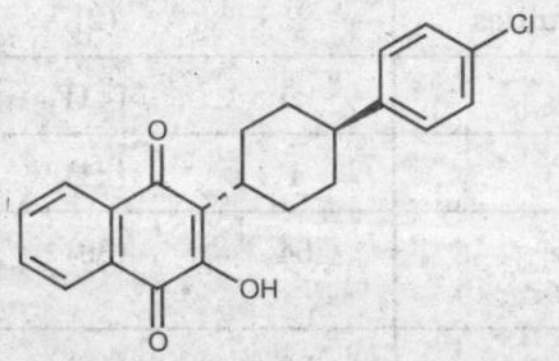

The chemical name of proguanil hydrochloride is 1-(4-chlorophenyl)-5-isopropyl-biguanide hydrochloride. Proguanil hydrochloride is a white crystalline solid that is sparingly soluble in water. It has a molecular weight of 290.22 and the molecular formula $C_{11}H_{16}ClN_5 \bullet HCl$. The compound has the following structural formula:

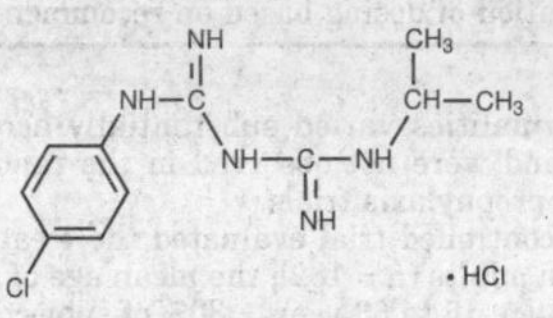

Each MALARONE Tablet (adult strength) contains 250 mg of atovaquone and 100 mg of proguanil hydrochloride and each MALARONE Pediatric Tablet contains 62.5 mg of atovaquone and 25 mg of proguanil hydrochloride. The inactive ingredients in both tablets are low–substituted hydroxypropyl cellulose, magnesium stearate, microcrystalline cellulose, poloxamer 188, povidone K30, and sodium starch glycolate. The tablet coating contains hypromellose, polyethylene glycol 400, polyethylene glycol 8000, red iron oxide, and titanium dioxide.

12 CLINICAL PHARMACOLOGY

12.1 Mechanism of Action

The constituents of MALARONE, atovaquone and proguanil hydrochloride, interfere with 2 different pathways involved in the biosynthesis of pyrimidines required for nucleic acid replication. Atovaquone is a selective inhibitor of parasite mitochondrial electron transport. Proguanil hydrochloride primarily exerts its effect by means of the metabolite cycloguanil, a dihydrofolate reductase inhibitor. Inhibition of dihydrofolate reductase in the malaria parasite disrupts deoxythymidylate synthesis.

12.2 Pharmacodynamics

No trials of the pharmacodynamics of MALARONE have been conducted.

12.3 Pharmacokinetics

Absorption: Atovaquone is a highly lipophilic compound with low aqueous solubility. The bioavailability of atovaquone shows considerable inter–individual variability. Dietary fat taken with atovaquone increases the rate and extent of absorption, increasing AUC 2 to 3 times and C_{max} 5 times over fasting. The absolute bioavailability of the tablet formulation of atovaquone when taken with food is 23%. MALARONE Tablets should be taken with food or a milky drink.

Distribution: Atovaquone is highly protein bound (>99%) over the concentration range of 1 to 90 mcg/mL. A population pharmacokinetic analysis demonstrated that the apparent volume of distribution of atovaquone (V/F) in adult and pediatric patients after oral administration is approximately 8.8 L/kg.

Proguanil is 75% protein bound. A population pharmacokinetic analysis demonstrated that the apparent V/F of proguanil in adult and pediatric patients >15 years of age with body weights from 31 to 110 kg ranged from 1,617 to 2,502 L. In pediatric patients 15 years of age with body weights from 11 to 56 kg, the V/F of proguanil ranged from 462 to 966 L.

In human plasma, the binding of atovaquone and proguanil was unaffected by the presence of the other.

Metabolism: In a study where ^{14}C–labeled atovaquone was administered to healthy volunteers, greater than 94% of the dose was recovered as unchanged atovaquone in the feces over 21 days. There was little or no excretion of atovaquone in the urine (less than 0.6%). There is indirect evidence that atovaquone may undergo limited metabolism; however, a specific metabolite has not been identified. Between 40% to 60% of proguanil is excreted by the kidneys. Proguanil is metabolized to cycloguanil (primarily via CYP2C19) and 4-chlorophenylbiguanide. The main routes of elimination are hepatic biotransformation and renal excretion.

Elimination: The elimination half–life of atovaquone is about 2 to 3 days in adult patients.

The elimination half–life of proguanil is 12 to 21 hours in both adult patients and pediatric patients, but may be longer in individuals who are slow metabolizers.

A population pharmacokinetic analysis in adult and pediatric patients showed that the apparent clearance (CL/F) of both atovaquone and proguanil are related to the body weight. The values CL/F for both atovaquone and proguanil in subjects with body weight 11 kg are shown in Table 4.

Table 4. Apparent Clearance for Atovaquone and Proguanil in Patients as a Function of Body Weight

	Atovaquone		Proguanil	
Body Weight	N	CL/F (L/hr) Mean ± SD[a] (range)	N	CL/F (L/hr) Mean ± SD[a] (range)
11-20 kg	159	1.34 ± 0.63 (0.52-4.26)	146	29.5 ± 6.5 (10.3-48.3)
21-30 kg	117	1.87 ± 0.81 (0.52-5.38)	113	40.0 ± 7.5 (15.9-62.7)
31-40 kg	95	2.76 ± 2.07 (0.97-12.5)	91	49.5 ± 8.30 (25.8-71.5)
>40 kg	368	6.61 ± 3.92 (1.32-20.3)	282	67.9 ± 19.9 (14.0-145)

[a] SD = standard deviation.

The pharmacokinetics of atovaquone and proguanil in patients with body weight below 11 kg have not been adequately characterized.

Pediatrics: The pharmacokinetics of proguanil and cycloguanil are similar in adult patients and pediatric patients. However, the elimination half–life of atovaquone is shorter in pediatric patients (1 to 2 days) than in adult patients (2 to 3 days). In clinical trials, plasma trough concentrations of atovaquone and proguanil in pediatric patients weighing 5 to 40 kg were within the range observed in adults after dosing by body weight.

Geriatrics: In a single–dose study, the pharmacokinetics of atovaquone, proguanil, and cycloguanil were compared in 13 elderly subjects (age 65 to 79 years) to 13 younger subjects (age 30 to 45 years). In the elderly subjects, the extent of systemic exposure (AUC) of cycloguanil was increased (point estimate = 2.36, 90% CI = 1.70, 3.28). T_{max} was longer in elderly subjects (median 8 hours) compared with younger subjects (median 4 hours) and average elimination half–life was longer in elderly subjects (mean 14.9 hours) compared with younger subjects (mean 8.3 hours).

Renal Impairment: In patients with mild renal impairment (creatinine clearance 50 to 80 mL/min), oral clearance and/or AUC data for atovaquone, proguanil, and cycloguanil are within the range of values observed in patients with normal renal function (creatinine clearance >80 mL/min). In patients with moderate renal impairment (creatinine clearance 30 to 50 mL/min), mean oral clearance for proguanil was reduced by approximately 35% compared with patients with normal renal function (creatinine clearance >80 mL/min) and the oral clearance of atovaquone was comparable between patients with normal renal function and mild renal impairment. No data exist on the use of MALARONE for long-term prophylaxis (over 2 months) in individuals with moderate renal failure. In patients with severe renal impairment (creatinine clearance <30 mL/min), atovaquone C_{max} and AUC are reduced but the elimination half–lives for proguanil and cycloguanil are prolonged, with corresponding increases in AUC, resulting in the potential of drug accumulation and toxicity with repeated dosing *[see Contraindications (4.2)]*.

Hepatic Impairment: In a single–dose study, the pharmacokinetics of atovaquone, proguanil, and cycloguanil were compared in 13 subjects with hepatic impairment (9 mild, 4 moderate, as indicated by the Child–Pugh method) to 13 subjects with normal hepatic function. In subjects with mild or moderate hepatic impairment as compared to healthy subjects, there were no marked differences (<50%) in the rate or extent of systemic exposure of atovaquone. However, in subjects with moderatehepatic impairment, the elimination half–life of atovaquone was increased (point estimate = 1.28, 90% CI = 1.00 to 1.63). Proguanil AUC, C_{max}, and its elimination half-life increased in subjects with mild hepatic impairment when compared to healthy subjects (Table 5). Also, the proguanil AUC and its elimination half-life increased in subjects with moderate hepatic impairment when compared to healthy subjects. Consistent with the increase in proguanil AUC, there were marked decreases in the systemic exposure of cycloguanil (C_{max} and AUC) and an increase in its elimination half–life in subjcets with mild hepatic impairment when compared to healthy volunteers (Table 5). There were few measurable cycloguanil concentrations in subjects with moderate hepatic impairment. The pharmacokinetics of atovaquone, proguanil, and cycloguanil after administration of MALARONE have not been studied in patients with severe hepatic impairment.

[See table 5 above]

Table 5. Point Estimates (90% CI) for Proguanil and Cycloguanil Parameters in Subjects With Mild and Moderate Hepatic Impairment Compared to Healthy Volunteers

Parameter	Comparison	Proguanil	Cycloguanil
$AUC_{(0\text{-inf})}$[a]	mild:healthy	1.96 (1.51, 2.54)	0.32 (0.22, 0.45)
C_{max}[a]	mild:healthy	1.41 (1.16, 1.71)	0.35 (0.24, 0.50)
$t_{1/2}$[b]	mild:healthy	1.21 (0.92, 1.60)	0.86 (0.49, 1.48)
$AUC_{(0\text{-inf})}$[a]	moderate:healthy	1.64 (1.14, 2.34)	ND
C_{max}[a]	moderate:healthy	0.97 (0.69, 1.36)	ND
$t_{1/2}$[b]	moderate:healthy	1.46 (1.05, 2.05)	ND

ND = not determined due to lack of quantifiable data.
[a] Ratio of geometric means.
[b]Mean difference.

Drug Interactions: There are no pharmacokinetic interactions between atovaquone and proguanil at the recommended dose.

Atovaquone is highly protein bound (>99%) but does not displace other highly protein–bound drugs in vitro.

Proguanil is metabolized primarily by CYP2C19. Potential pharmacokinetic interactions between proguanil or cycloguanil and other drugs that are CYP2C19 substrates or inhibitors are unknown.

Rifampin / Rifabutin: Concomitant administration of rifampin orrifabutin is known to reduce atovaquone concentrations by approximately 50% and 34%, respectively. The mechanisms of these interactions are unknown.

Tetracycline: Concomitant treatment with tetracycline has been associated with approximately a 40% reduction in plasma concentrations of atovaquone.

Metoclopramide: Concomitant treatment with metoclopramide has been associated with decreased bioavailability of atovaquone.

Indinavir: Concomitant administration of atovaquone (750 mg twice daily with food for 14 days) and indinavir (800 mg three times daily without food for 14 days) did not result in any change in the steady–state AUC and C_{max} of indinavir but resulted in a decrease in the C_{trough} of indinavir (23% decrease [90% CI = 8%, 35%]).

12.4 Microbiology

Activity *In Vitro* and *In Vivo*: Atovaquone and cycloguanil (an active metabolite of proguanil) are active against the erythrocytic and exoerythrocytic stages of *Plasmodium* spp. Enhanced efficacy of the combination compared to either atovaquone or proguanil hydrochloride alone was demonstrated in clinical trials in both immune and non-immune patients *[see Clinical Studies (14.1, 14.2)]*.

Drug Resistance: Strains of *P. falciparum* with decreased susceptibility to atovaquone or proguanil/cycloguanil alone can be selected in vitro or in vivo. The combination of atovaquone and proguanil hydrochloride may not be effective for treatment of recrudescent malaria that develops after prior therapy with the combination.

13 NONCLINICAL TOXICOLOGY

13.1 Carcinogenesis, Mutagenesis, Impairment of Fertility

Genotoxicity studies have not been performed with atovaquone in combination with proguanil. Effects of MALARONE on male and female reproductive performance are unknown.

Atovaquone: A 24–month carcinogenicity study in CD rats was negative for neoplasms at doses up to 500 mg/kg/day corresponding to approximately 54 times the average steady-state plasma concentrations in humans during prophylaxis of malaria. In CD-1 mice, a 24–month study showed treatment–related increases in incidence of hepatocellular adenoma and hepatocellular carcinoma at all doses tested (50, 100, and 200 mg/kg/day) which correlated with at least 15 times the average steady–state plasma concentrations in humans during prophylaxis of malaria.

Atovaquone was negative with or without metabolic activation in the Ames *Salmonella* mutagenicity assay, the Mouse Lymphoma mutagenesis assay, and the Cultured Human Lymphocyte cytogenetic assay. No evidence of genotoxicity was observed in the in vivo Mouse Micronucleus assay.

Atovaquone did not impair fertility in male and female rats at doses up to 1,000 mg/kg/day corresponding to plasma exposures of approximately 7.3 times the estimated human exposure during treatment of malaria based on AUC.

Proguanil: No evidence of a carcinogenic effect was observed in 24–month studies conducted in CD-1 mice at doses up to 16 mg/kg/day corresponding to 1.5 times the average human plasma exposure during prophylaxis of malaria based on AUC, and in Wistar Hannover rats at doses up 20 mg/kg/day corresponding to 1.1 times the average human plasma exposure during prophylaxis of malaria based on AUC.

Proguanil was negative with or without metabolic activation in the Ames *Salmonella* mutagenicity assay and the Mouse Lymphoma mutagenesis assay. No evidence of genotoxicity was observed in the in vivo Mouse Micronucleus assay.

Cycloguanil, the active metabolite of proguanil, was also negative in the Ames test, but was positive in the Mouse Lymphoma assay and the Mouse Micronucleus assay. These positive effects with cycloguanil, a dihydrofolate reductase inhibitor, were significantly reduced or abolished with folinic acid supplementation.

A fertility study in Sprague-Dawley rats revealed no adverse effects at doses up to 16 mg/kg/day of proguanil hydrochloride (up to 0.04-times the average human exposure during treatment of malaria based on AUC). Fertility studies of proguanil in animals at exposures similar to or greater than those observed in humans have not been conducted.

13.2 Animal Toxicology and/or Pharmacology

Fibrovascular proliferation in the right atrium, pyelonephritis, bone marrow hypocellularity, lymphoid atrophy, and gastritis/enteritis were observed in dogs treated with proguanil hydrochloride for 6 months at a dose of 12 mg/kg/day (approximately 3.9 times the recommended daily human dose for malaria prophylaxis on a mg/m^2 basis). Bile duct hyperplasia, gall bladder mucosal atrophy, and interstitial pneumonia were observed in dogs treated with proguanil hydrochloride for 6 months at a dose of 4 mg/kg/day (approximately 1.3 times the recommended daily human dose for malaria prophylaxis on a mg/m^2 basis). Mucosal hyperplasia of the cecum and renal tubular basophilia were observed in rats treated with proguanil hydrochloride for 6 months at a dose of 20 mg/kg/day (approximately 1.6 times the recommended daily human dose for malaria prophylaxis on a mg/m^2 basis). Adverse heart, lung, liver, and gall bladder effects observed in dogs and kidney effects observed in rats were not shown to be reversible.

14 CLINICAL STUDIES

14.1 Prevention of P. falciparum Malaria

MALARONE was evaluated for prophylaxis of *P. falciparum* malaria in 5 clinical trials in malaria–endemic areas and in 3 active–controlled trials in non–immune travelers to malaria–endemic areas.

Three placebo–controlled trials of 10 to 12 weeks' duration were conducted among residents of malaria–endemic areas in Kenya, Zambia, and Gabon. The mean age of subjects was 30 (range 17–55), 32 (range 16–64), and 10 (range 5–16) years, respectively. Of a total of 669 randomized patients (including 264 pediatric patients 5 to 16 years of age), 103 were withdrawn for reasons other than falciparum malaria or drug–related adverse events (55% of these were lost to follow–up and 45% were withdrawn for protocol violations). The results are listed in Table 6.

Table 6. Prevention of Parasitemia[a] in Placebo Controlled Clinical Trials of MALARONE for Prophylaxis of P. falciparum Malaria in Residents of Malaria Endemic Areas

	MALARONE	Placebo
Total number of patients randomized	326	343
Failed to complete study	57	46
Developed parasitemia (*P. falciparum*)	2	92

[a] Free of parasitemia during the 10 to 12-week period of prophylactic therapy.

In another study, 330 Gabonese pediatric patients (weighing 13 to 40 kg, and aged 4 to 14 years) who had received successful open–label radical cure treatment with artesunate, were randomized to receive either MALARONE (dosage based on body weight) or placebo in a double–blind fashion for 12 weeks. Blood smears were obtained weekly and any time malaria was suspected. Nineteen of the 165 children given MALARONE and 18 of 165 patients given placebo withdrew from the study for reasons other than parasitemia (primary reason was lost to follow-up). One out of 150 evaluable patients (<1%) who received MALARONE developed *P. falciparum* parasitemia while receiving prophylaxis with MALARONE compared with 31 (22%) of the 144 evaluable placebo recipients.

In a 10–week study in 175 South African subjects who moved into malaria–endemic areas and were given prophylaxis with 1 MALARONE Tablet daily, parasitemia developed in 1 subject who missed several doses of medication. Since no placebo control was included, the incidence of malaria in this study was not known.

Two active-controlled trials were conducted in non–immune travelers who visited a malaria–endemic area. The mean duration of travel was 18 days (range 2 to 38 days). Of a total of 1,998 randomized patients who received MALARONE or controlled drug, 24 discontinued from the study before follow-up evaluation 60 days after leaving the endemic area. Nine of these were lost to follow-up, 2 withdrew because of an adverse experience, and 13 were discontinued for other reasons. These trials were not large enough to allow for statements of comparative efficacy. In addition, the true exposure rate to *P. falciparum* malaria in both trials is unknown. The results are listed in Table 7.

[See table 7 at top of next page]

A third randomized, open–label study was conducted which included 221 otherwise healthy pediatric patients (weighing 11 kg and 2 to 17 years of age) who were at risk of contracting malaria by traveling to an endemic area. The mean duration of travel was 15 days (range 1 to 30 days). Prophylaxis with MALARONE (n = 110, dosage based on body weight) began 1 or 2 days before entering the endemic area and lasted until 7 days after leaving the area. A control group (n = 111) received prophylaxis with chloroquine/proguanil dosed according to WHO guidelines. No cases of malaria occurred in either group of children. However, the study was not large enough to allow for statements of comparative efficacy. In addition, the true exposure rate to *P. falciparum* malaria in this study is unknown.

Causal Prophylaxis: In separate trials with small numbers of volunteers, atovaquone and proguanil hydrochloride were independently shown to have causal prophylactic activity directed against liver–stage parasites of *P. falciparum*. Six patients given a single dose of atovaquone 250 mg 24 hours prior to malaria challenge were protected from developing malaria, whereas all 4 placebo–treated patients developed malaria.

Table 7. Prevention of Parasitemia[a] in Active-Controlled Clinical Trials of MALARONE for Prophylaxis of P. falciparum Malaria in Non-Immune Travelers

	MALARONE	Mefloquine	Chloroquine plus Proguanil
Total number of randomized patients who received study drug	1,004	483	511
Failed to complete study	14	6	4
Developed parasitemia (*P. falciparum*)	0	0	3

[a] Free of parasitemia during the period of prophylactic therapy.

Table 8. Parasitological Response in 8 Clinical Trials of MALARONE for Treatment of P. falciparum Malaria

	MALARONE[a]		Comparator		
Study Site	Evaluable Patients (n)	% Sensitive Response[b]	Drug(s)	Evaluable Patients (n)	% Sensitive Response[b]
Brazil	74	98.6%	Quinine and tetracycline	76	100.0%
Thailand	79	100.0%	Mefloquine	79	86.1%
France[c]	21	100.0%	Halofantrine	18	100.0%
Kenya[c,d]	81	93.8%	Halofantrine	83	90.4%
Zambia	80	100.0%	Pyrimethamine/ sulfadoxine (P/S)	80	98.8%
Gabon[c]	63	98.4%	Amodiaquine	63	81.0%
Philippines	54	100.0%	Chloroquine (Cq) Cq and P/S	23 32	30.4% 87.5%
Peru	19	100.0%	Chloroquine P/S	13 7	7.7% 100.0%

[a] MALARONE = 1,000 mg atovaquone and 400 mg proguanil hydrochloride (or equivalent based on body weight for patients weighing 40 kg) once daily for 3 days.
[b] Elimination of parasitemia with no recurrent parasitemia during follow–up for 28 days.
[c] Patients hospitalized only for acute care. Follow–up conducted in outpatients.
[d] Study in pediatric patients 3 to 12 years of age.

During the 4 weeks following cessation of prophylaxis in clinical trial participants who remained in malaria–endemic areas and were available for evaluation, malaria developed in 24 of 211 (11.4%) subjects who took placebo and 9 of 328 (2.7%) who took MALARONE. While new infections could not be distinguished from recrudescent infections, all but 1 of the infections in patients treated with MALARONE occurred more than 15 days after stopping therapy. The single case occurring on day 8 following cessation of therapy with MALARONE probably represents a failure of prophylaxis with MALARONE.
The possibility that delayed cases of *P. falciparum* malaria may occur some time after stopping prophylaxis with MALARONE cannot be ruled out. Hence, returning travelers developing febrile illnesses should be investigated for malaria.

14.2 Treatment of Acute, Uncomplicated P. falciparum Malaria Infections

In 3 phase II clinical trials, atovaquone alone, proguanil hydrochloride alone, and the combination of atovaquone and proguanil hydrochloride were evaluated for the treatment of acute, uncomplicated malaria caused by *P. falciparum*. Among 156 evaluable patients, the parasitological cure rate (elimination of parasitemia with no recurrent parasitemia during follow–up for 28 days) was 59/89 (66%) with atovaquone alone, 1/17 (6%) with proguanil hydrochloride alone, and 50/50 (100%) with the combination of atovaquone and proguanil hydrochloride.
MALARONE was evaluated for treatment of acute, uncomplicated malaria caused by *P. falciparum* in 8 phase III randomized, open-label, controlled clinical trials (N = 1,030 enrolled in both treatment groups). The mean age of subjects was 27 years and 16% were children 12 years of age; 74% of subjects were male. Evaluable patients included those whose outcome at 28 days was known. Among 471 evaluable patients treated with the equivalent of 4 MALARONE Tablets once daily for 3 days, 464 had a sensitive response (elimination of parasitemia with no recurrent parasitemia during follow–up for 28 days) (Table 8). Seven patients had a response of RI resistance (elimination of parasitemia but with recurrent parasitemia between 7 and 28 days after starting treatment). In these trials, the response to treatment with MALARONE was similar to treatment with the comparator drug in 4 trials.

[See table 8 above]
When these 8 trials were pooled and 2 additional trials evaluating MALARONE alone (without a comparator arm) were added to the analysis, the overall efficacy (elimination of parasitemia with no recurrent parasitemia during follow–up for 28 days) in 521 evaluable patients was 98.7%.
The efficacy of MALARONE in the treatment of the erythrocytic phase of nonfalciparum malaria was assessed in a small number of patients. Of the 23 patients in Thailand infected with *P. vivax* and treated with atovaquone/proguanil hydrochloride 1,000 mg/400 mg daily for 3 days, parasitemia cleared in 21 (91.3%) at 7 days. Parasite relapse occurred commonly when *P. vivax* malaria was treated with MALARONE alone. Relapsing malarias including *P. vivax* and *P. ovale* require additional treatment to prevent relapse.
The efficacy of MALARONE in treating acute uncomplicated *P. falciparum* malaria in children weighing 5 and <11 kg was examined in an open–label, randomized trial conducted in Gabon. Patients received either MALARONE (2 or 3 MALARONE Pediatric Tablets once daily depending upon body weight) for 3 days (n = 100) or amodiaquine (10 mg/kg/day) for 3 days (n = 100). In this study, the MALARONE Tablets were crushed and mixed with condensed milk just prior to administration. An adequate clinical response (elimination of parasitemia with no recurrent parasitemia during follow–up for 28 days) was obtained in 95% (87/92) of the evaluable pediatric patients who received MALARONE and in 53% (41/78) of those evaluable who received amodiaquine. A response of RI resistance (elimination of parasitemia but with recurrent parasitemia between 7 and 28 days after starting treatment) was noted in 3% and 40% of the patients, respectively. Two cases of RIII resistance (rising parasite count despite therapy) were reported in the patients receiving MALARONE. There were 4 cases of RIII in the amodiaquine arm.

16 HOW SUPPLIED/STORAGE AND HANDLING

MALARONE Tablets, containing 250 mg atovaquone and 100 mg proguanil hydrochloride.

- Bottle of 100 tablets with child-resistant closure (NDC 0173-0675-01).
- Unit Dose Pack of 24 (NDC 0173-0675-02).

MALARONE Pediatric Tablets, containing 62.5 mg atovaquone and 25 mg proguanil hydrochloride.

- Bottle of 100 tablets with child-resistant closure (NDC 0173-0676-01).

Storage Conditions: Store at 25°C (77°F). Temperature excursions are permitted to 15° to 30°C (59° to 86°F) (see USP Controlled Room Temperature).

17 PATIENT COUNSELING INFORMATION

Patients should be instructed:

- to take MALARONE at the same time each day with food or a milky drink.
- to take a repeat dose of MALARONE if vomiting occurs within 1 hour after dosing.
- to take a dose as soon as possible if a dose is missed, then return to their normal dosing schedule. However, if a dose is skipped, the patient should not double the next dose.
- that rare serious adverse events such as hepatitis, severe skin reactions, neurological, and hematological events have been reported when MALARONE was used for the prophylaxis or treatment of malaria.
- to consult a healthcare professional regarding alternative forms of prophylaxis if prophylaxis with MALARONE is prematurely discontinued for any reason.
- that protective clothing, insect repellents, and bednets are important components of malaria prophylaxis.
- that no chemoprophylactic regimen is 100% effective; therefore, patients should seek medical attention for any febrile illness that occurs during or after return from a malaria–endemic area and inform their healthcare professional that they may have been exposed to malaria.
- that falciparum malaria carries a higher risk of death and serious complications in pregnant women than in the general population. Pregnant women anticipating travel to malarious areas should discuss the risks and benefits of such travel with their physicians.

GlaxoSmithKline
Research Triangle Park, NC 27709

MLR:6PI

MENHIBRIX ℞

(Meningococcal Groups C and Y and Haemophilus b Tetanus Toxoid Conjugate Vaccine)
Solution for Intramuscular Injection

HIGHLIGHTS OF PRESCRIBING INFORMATION
These highlights do not include all the information needed to use MENHIBRIX safely and effectively. See full prescribing information for MENHIBRIX.
MENHIBRIX (Meningococcal Groups C and Y and Haemophilus b Tetanus Toxoid Conjugate Vaccine)
Solution for Intramuscular Injection
Initial U.S. Approval: 2012

INDICATIONS AND USAGE

MENHIBRIX is a vaccine indicated for active immunization to prevent invasive disease caused by *Neisseria meningitidis* serogroups C and Y and *Haemophilus influenzae* type b. MENHIBRIX is approved for use in children 6 weeks of age through 18 months of age. (1)

DOSAGE AND ADMINISTRATION

Four doses (0.5 mL each) by intramuscular injection at 2, 4, 6, and 12 through 15 months of age. The first dose may be given as early as 6 weeks of age. The fourth dose may be given as late as 18 months of age. (2.3)

DOSAGE FORMS AND STRENGTHS

Solution for injection supplied as a single-dose vial of lyophilized vaccine to be reconstituted with the accompanying vial of saline diluent. A single dose after reconstitution is 0.5 mL. (3)

CONTRAINDICATIONS

Severe allergic reaction (e.g., anaphylaxis) after a previous dose of any meningococcal-, *H. influenzae* type b-, or tetanus toxoid-containing vaccine or any component of MENHIBRIX. (4)

WARNINGS AND PRECAUTIONS

- If Guillain-Barré syndrome has occurred within 6 weeks of receipt of a prior vaccine containing tetanus toxoid, the decision to give any tetanus toxoid-containing vaccine, including MENHIBRIX, should be based on consideration of the potential benefits and possible risks. (5.1)
- Syncope (fainting) can occur in association with administration of injectable vaccines, including MENHIBRIX. Procedures should be in place to avoid falling injury and to restore cerebral perfusion following syncope. (5.2)
- Apnea following intramuscular vaccination has been observed in some infants born prematurely. Decisions about when to administer an intramuscular vaccine, including MENHIBRIX, to infants born prematurely should be

based on consideration of the individual infant's medical status, and the potential benefits and possible risks of vaccination. (5.3)

ADVERSE REACTIONS

Rates of local injection site pain, redness, and swelling ranged from 15% to 46% depending on reaction and specific dose in schedule. Commonly reported systemic events included irritability (62% to 71%), drowsiness (49% to 63%), loss of appetite (30% to 34%), and fever (11% to 26%) (specific rate depended on the event and dose in the schedule). (6.1)

To report SUSPECTED ADVERSE REACTIONS, contact GlaxoSmithKline at 1-888-825-5249 or VAERS at 1-800-822-7967 or www.vaers.hhs.gov.

DRUG INTERACTIONS

Do not mix MENHIBRIX with any other vaccine in the same syringe or vial. (7.1)

See 17 for PATIENT COUNSELING INFORMATION

Revised: 06/2012

FULL PRESCRIBING INFORMATION: CONTENTS*

*** Sections or subsections omitted from the full prescribing information are not listed**

FULL PRESCRIBING INFORMATION

1 INDICATIONS AND USAGE

MENHIBRIX® is indicated for active immunization to prevent invasive disease caused by *Neisseria meningitidis* serogroups C and Y and *Haemophilus influenzae* type b. MENHIBRIX is approved for use in children 6 weeks of age through 18 months of age.

2 DOSAGE AND ADMINISTRATION

2.1 Reconstitution

MENHIBRIX is to be reconstituted only with the accompanying saline diluent. The reconstituted vaccine should be a clear and colorless solution. Parenteral drug products should be inspected visually for particulate matter and discoloration prior to administration, whenever solution and container permit. If either of these conditions exists, the vaccine should not be administered.

[See figures 1 through 4 above]

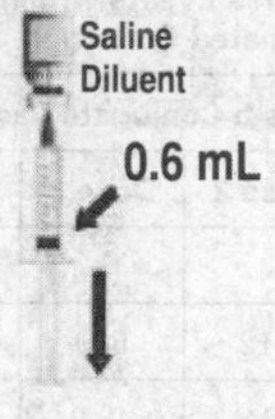

Figure 1. Cleanse both vial stoppers. Withdraw 0.6 mL of saline from diluent vial.

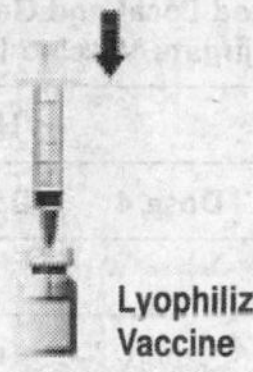

Figure 2. Transfer saline diluent into the lyophilized vaccine vial.

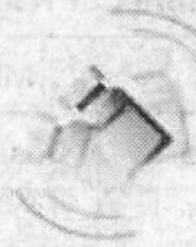

Figure 3. Shake the vial well.

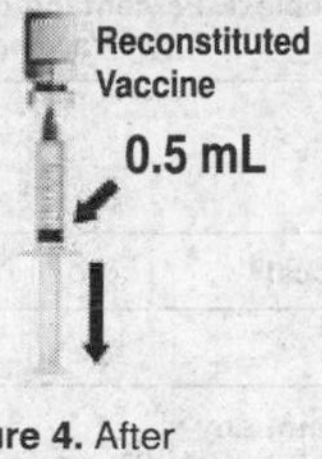

Figure 4. After reconstitution, withdraw 0.5 mL of reconstituted vaccine and administer **intramuscularly.**

2.2 Administration

For intramuscular use only. Do not administer this product intravenously, intradermally, or subcutaneously.

After reconstitution, administer MENHIBRIX immediately. Use a separate sterile needle and sterile syringe for each individual. The preferred administration site is the anterolateral aspect of the thigh for most infants younger than 1 year of age. In older children, the deltoid muscle is usually large enough for an intramuscular injection.

2.3 Dose and Schedule

A 4-dose series, with each 0.5-mL dose given by intramuscular injection at 2, 4, 6, and 12 through 15 months of age. The first dose may be given as early as 6 weeks of age. The fourth dose may be given as late as 18 months of age.

3 DOSAGE FORMS AND STRENGTHS

MENHIBRIX is a solution for injection supplied as a single-dose vial of lyophilized vaccine to be reconstituted with the accompanying vial of saline diluent. A single dose after reconstitution is 0.5 mL.

4 CONTRAINDICATIONS

Severe allergic reaction (e.g., anaphylaxis) after a previous dose of any meningococcal-, *H. influenzae* type b-, or tetanus toxoid-containing vaccine or any component of this vaccine is a contraindication to administration of MENHIBRIX *[see Description (11)]*.

5 WARNINGS AND PRECAUTIONS

5.1 Guillain-Barré Syndrome

If Guillain-Barré syndrome has occurred within 6 weeks of receipt of a prior vaccine containing tetanus toxoid, the decision to give any tetanus toxoid-containing vaccine, including MENHIBRIX, should be based on consideration of the potential benefits and possible risks.

5.2 Syncope

Syncope (fainting) can occur in association with administration of injectable vaccines, including MENHIBRIX. Syncope can be accompanied by transient neurological signs such as visual disturbance, paresthesia, and tonic-clonic limb movements. Procedures should be in place to avoid falling injury and to restore cerebral perfusion following syncope.

5.3 Apnea in Premature Infants

Apnea following intramuscular vaccination has been observed in some infants born prematurely. Decisions about when to administer an intramuscular vaccine, including MENHIBRIX, to infants born prematurely should be based on consideration of the individual infant's medical status, and the potential benefits and possible risks of vaccination.

5.4 Preventing and Managing Allergic Vaccine Reactions

Prior to administration, the healthcare provider should review the patient's immunization history for possible vaccine hypersensitivity. Epinephrine and other appropriate agents used for the control of immediate allergic reactions must be immediately available should an acute anaphylactic reaction occur.

5.5 Altered Immunocompetence

Safety and effectiveness of MENHIBRIX in immunosuppressed children have not been evaluated. If MENHIBRIX is administered to immunosuppressed children, including children receiving immunosuppressive therapy, the expected immune response may not be obtained.

5.6 Tetanus Immunization

Immunization with MENHIBRIX does not substitute for routine tetanus immunization.

6 ADVERSE REACTIONS

6.1 Clinical Trials Experience

Because clinical trials are conducted under widely varying conditions, adverse reaction rates observed in the clinical trials of a vaccine cannot be directly compared with rates in the clinical trials of another vaccine, and may not reflect the rates observed in practice. There is the possibility that broad use of MENHIBRIX could reveal adverse reactions not observed in clinical trials.

A total of 7,521 infants received at least one dose of MENHIBRIX in 6 clinical studies.[1-6] In 5 of these studies, 6,686 children received 4 consecutive doses of MENHIBRIX.[2-6] Across all studies, approximately half of participants were female; 50% were white, 41% were Hispanic, 4% were black, 1% were Asian and 4% were of other racial/ethnic groups.

Two randomized, controlled, pivotal trials enrolled participants to receive 4 doses of MENHIBRIX or a monovalent Haemophilus b Conjugate (Hib) vaccine, administered at 2, 4, 6, and 12 to 15 months of age (Study 009/010[5] and Study 011/012[6]). Together, these trials evaluated safety in 8,571 infants who received at least one dose of MENHIBRIX (N = 6,414) or Hib vaccine (N = 2,157).[5,6]

In Study 009/010[5], conducted in the United States, Australia, and Mexico, 4,180 infants were randomized 3:1 to receive MENHIBRIX or a control US-licensed Hib vaccine. Safety data are available for 3,136 infants who received MENHIBRIX and 1,044 infants who received a control Haemophilus b Conjugate Vaccine (Tetanus Toxoid Conjugate) (PRP-T, manufactured by Sanofi Pasteur SA) at 2, 4, and 6 months of age. For dose 4 administered at 12 to 15 months of age, safety data are available for 2,769 toddlers who received MENHIBRIX and 923 toddlers who received a control Haemophilus b Conjugate Vaccine (Meningococcal Protein Conjugate) (PRP-OMP, manufactured by Merck and Co., Inc.). With doses 1, 2, and 3 of MENHIBRIX or PRP-T, infants concomitantly received PEDIARIX® [Diphtheria and Tetanus Toxoids and Acellular Pertussis Adsorbed, Hepatitis B (Recombinant) and Inactivated Poliovirus Vaccine] and Pneumococcal 7-valent Conjugate Vaccine (Diphtheria CRM_{197} Protein) (PCV7, manufactured by Wyeth Pharmaceuticals, Inc.). With dose 4 of MENHIBRIX or PRP-OMP, toddlers concomitantly received PCV7, Measles, Mumps, and Rubella Virus Vaccine Live (MMR, manufactured by Merck & Co., Inc.), and Varicella Virus Vaccine Live (manufactured by Merck & Co., Inc.).

Data on solicited adverse events were collected by parents/guardians using standardized forms for 4 consecutive days following vaccination with MENHIBRIX or control Hib vaccine (i.e., day of vaccination and the next 3 days).[5] Children were monitored for unsolicited adverse events that occurred in the 31-day period following vaccination and were monitored for serious adverse events, new onset chronic disease, rash, and conditions prompting emergency department visits or physician office visits during the entire study period (6 months following the last vaccine administered). Among participants in both groups, 66% were from the United States, 19% were from Mexico, and 14% were from Australia. Forty-eight percent of participants were female; 64% were white, 22% were Hispanic, 6% were black, 1% were Asian, and 7% were of other racial/ethnic groups.

In the second pivotal study (Study 011/012[6]), conducted in the United States and Mexico and evaluating the same vaccines and vaccination schedule, participants were monitored for serious adverse events, new onset chronic disease, rash, and conditions prompting emergency department visits during the entire study period (6 months following the last vaccine administered). Among participants in both groups, 30% were from the United States and 70% were from Mexico.

In addition to the pivotal studies, safety data are available from 4 studies which either did not include a fourth dose of MENHIBRIX[1], used a dosing regimen not approved in the United States[2,3], or incorporated a comparator vaccine which was not licensed in the United States.[4] In these studies, participants were monitored for unsolicited adverse events and serious adverse events occurring in the 31–day period following vaccination. In 2 of these studies[3,4], participants were monitored for serious adverse events, new onset chronic disease, rash, and conditions prompting emergency department visits or physician office visits through 6 months after the last vaccination.

Solicited Adverse Events: The reported frequencies of solicited local and systemic adverse events from US participants in Study 009/010 are presented in Table 1.[5] Because of differences in reported rates of solicited adverse events between US and non-US participants, only the solicited adverse event data in US participants are presented. Among the US participants included in Table 1, 48% were female; 76% were white, 10% were black, 4% were Hispanic, 2% were Asian, and 8% were of other racial/ethnic groups.

Table 1. Percentage of US Children from Study 009/010 With Solicited Local and General Adverse Events within 4 Days of Vaccinationa With MENHIBRIX or Haemophilus b Conjugate Vaccine (Total Vaccinated Cohort)

	MENHIBRIX[b]				Haemophilus b Conjugate Vaccine[b,c]			
	Dose 1	Dose 2	Dose 3	Dose 4	Dose 1	Dose 2	Dose 3	Dose 4
Local[d]								
N	2,009	1,874	1,725	1,533	659	612	569	492
Pain, any	46.2	44.6	41.4	42.1	61.6	52.8	49.9	50.4
Pain, grade 3[e]	3.7	3.3	2.3	1.6	11.4	5.1	3.0	5.3
Redness, any	20.6	31.0	35.5	34.6	27.9	33.7	42.2	46.7
Redness, >30 mm	0.1	0.3	0.1	0.7	1.8	0.3	0.4	1.2
Swelling, any	14.7	20.4	23.8	25.4	20.5	20.8	28.6	31.7
Swelling, >30 mm	0.5	0.3	0.3	0.6	1.5	0.2	0.4	0.8
Systemic								
N	2,008-2,009	1,871	1,723	1,535-1,536	659	609-610	569	493-494
Irritability	67.5	70.8	65.8	62.1	76.9	75.1	65.4	66.1
Irritability, grade 3[f]	3.7	4.8	3.3	2.5	7.4	5.6	4.2	4.3
Drowsiness, any	62.8	57.7	49.5	48.7	66.9	61.8	52.4	48.5
Drowsiness, grade 3[g]	2.7	3.2	1.7	2.1	2.7	2.6	1.4	2.0
Loss of appetite, any	33.8	32.1	30.1	32.1	37.6	33.6	30.2	32.5
Loss of appetite, grade 3[h]	0.5	0.7	0.5	1.1	0.3	0.7	1.1	2.2
Fever, ≥100.4F[i]	18.9	25.9	23.0	11.0	21.4	28.2	23.7	12.6
Fever, ≥102.2F[i]	1.1	1.9	3.2	1.5	0.9	2.6	2.8	2.0
Fever, >104F[i]	0.0	0.1	0.3	0.3	0.0	0.0	0.4	0.2

Total Vaccinated Cohort = all participants who received at least one dose of either vaccine.
N = number of participants who completed the symptom sheet for a given symptom at the specified dose.
[a]Within 4 days of vaccination defined as day of vaccination and the next 3 days.
[b]Co-administered with PEDIARIXand PCV7 at doses 1, 2, 3 and PCV7, MMR and varicella vaccines at dose 4.
[c]US-licensed monovalent Haemophilus b Conjugate Vaccine manufactured by Sanofi Pasteur SA for doses 1, 2, and 3 (PRP-T) and by Merck & Co., Inc for dose 4 (PRP-OMP).
[d]Local reactions at the injection site for MENHIBRIX or Haemophilus b Conjugate Vaccine.
[e]Cried when limb was moved/spontaneously painful.
[f]Crying that could not be comforted/prevented normal daily activities.
[g]Prevented normal daily activities.
[h]Not eating at all.
[i]Across both treatment groups, 54%, 56%, and 59% of participants had temperatures measured rectally following doses 1, 2, and 3, respectively; 45%, 44%, and 40% of participants had temperatures measured by the axillary route for doses 1, 2, and 3, respectively. For dose 4, >90% of participants had temperatures measured via the axillary route.

[See table 1 above]
The reported rates of some solicited adverse events in participants from Australia and Mexico varied from those in the United States.[5] For example, in Australia, pain after dose 1 was reported in 28.4% of participants who received MENHIBRIX and 33.3% of control participants, while in Mexico pain after dose 1 was reported in 73.7% of participants who received MENHIBRIX and 79.4% of control participants. Fever after dose 1 was reported in 10.4% of participants who received MENHIBRIX and 10.7% of control participants in Australia, while it was reported in 44.0% of participants who received MENHIBRIX and 35.7% of control participants in Mexico. The reported incidences of pain and fever in US participants after dose 1 are provided in Table 1.

Unsolicited Adverse Events: Among participants who received MENHIBRIX or Hib control vaccine co-administered with US-licensed vaccines at 2, 4, 6 and 12 to 15 months of age[1,3-5], the incidence of unsolicited adverse events reported within the 31-day period following study vaccination (doses 1, 2, and 3) was comparable between MENHIBRIX (61.9%; 2,578/4,166) and PRP-T (62.5%; 1,042/1,666). The incidence of unsolicited adverse events reported within the 31-day period following dose 4 was also comparable between MENHIBRIX (42.5%; 1,541/3,630) and PRP-OMP (41.4%; 520/1,257).

Serious Adverse Events: Following doses 1, 2, and 3[1,3-6], 1.8% (137/7,444) of participants who received MENHIBRIX and 2.1% (59/2,779) of participants who received PRP-T reported at least one serious adverse event within the 31-day period. Up to 6 months following the last vaccine administered (doses 1, 2, and 3) or until administration of dose 4[3-6], 4.8% (365/7,362) of participants who received MENHIBRIX and 5.0% (134/2,697) of participants in the PRP-T group reported at least one serious adverse event.

Following dose 4[3-6], 0.5% (35/6,640) of participants who received MENHIBRIX and 0.5% (12/2,267) of participants who received PRP-OMP reported at least one serious adverse event within the 31-day period. Up to 6 months following the last vaccine administered (dose 4), 2.5% (165/6,640) of participants who received MENHIBRIX and 2.0% (46/2,267) of participants who received PRP-OMP reported at least one serious adverse event.

6.2 Postmarketing Experience

The following adverse events have been spontaneously reported during post-approval use of HIBERIX® (Haemophilus b Conjugate Vaccine [Tetanus Toxoid Conjugate]) in the United States and other countries. These events are relevant because the Haemophilus b capsular polysaccharide tetanus toxoid conjugate is included as a component antigen in both MENHIBRIX and HIBERIX. Because these events are reported voluntarily from a population of uncertain size, it is not possible to reliably estimate their frequency or to establish a causal relationship to vaccine exposure.

The following adverse events were included based on one or more of the following factors: seriousness, frequency of reporting, or strength of evidence for a causal relationship to HIBERIX.

General Disorders and Administration Site Conditions: Extensive swelling of the vaccinated limb, injection site induration.

Immune System Disorders: Allergic reactions (including anaphylactic and anaphylactoid reactions), angioedema.

Nervous System Disorders: Convulsions (with or without fever), hypotonic-hyporesponsive episode, somnolence, syncope or vasovagal responses to injection.

Respiratory, Thoracic, and Mediastinal Disorders: Apnea.

Skin and Subcutaneous Tissue Disorders: Rash, urticaria.

7 DRUG INTERACTIONS

7.1 Concomitant Vaccine Administration

In clinical studies, MENHIBRIX was administered concomitantly with routinely recommended pediatric US-licensed vaccines *[see Adverse Reactions (6.1) and Clinical Studies (14.2)]*.

If MENHIBRIX is administered concomitantly with other injectable vaccines, they should be given with separate syringes and at different injection sites. MENHIBRIX should not be mixed with any other vaccine in the same syringe or vial.

7.2 Interference With Laboratory Tests

Haemophilus b capsular polysaccharide derived from Haemophilus b Conjugate Vaccines has been detected in the urine of some vaccinees.[7] Urine antigen detection may not have a diagnostic value in suspected disease due to *H. influenza* type b within 1 to 2 weeks after receipt of a *H. influenza* type b-containing vaccine, including MENHIBRIX.

7.3 Immunosuppressive Therapies

Immunosuppressive therapies, including irradiation, antimetabolites, alkylating agents, cytotoxic drugs, and corticosteroids (used in greater than physiologic doses), may reduce the immune response to MENHIBRIX.

8 USE IN SPECIFIC POPULATIONS

8.1 Pregnancy

Pregnancy Category C

Animal reproduction studies have not been conducted with MENHIBRIX. It is also not known whether MENHIBRIX can cause fetal harm when administered to a pregnant woman or can affect reproduction capacity.

8.4 Pediatric Use

Safety and effectiveness of MENHIBRIX in children younger than 6 weeks of age and in children 19 months to 16 years of age have not been established.

11 DESCRIPTION

MENHIBRIX (Meningococcal Groups C and Y and Haemophilus b Tetanus Toxoid Conjugate Vaccine), for intramuscular injection, is supplied as a sterile, lyophilized powder which is reconstituted at the time of use with the accompanying saline diluent. MENHIBRIX contains *Neisseria meningitidis* serogroup C and Y capsular polysaccharide antigens and Haemophilus b capsular polysaccharide (polyribosyl-ribitol-phosphate [PRP]). The *Neisseria meningitidis* C strain and Y strain are grown in semi-synthetic media and undergo heat inactivation and purification. The PRP is a high molecular weight polymer prepared from the *Haemophilus influenzae* type b strain 20,752 grown in a synthetic medium that undergoes heat inactivation and purification. The tetanus toxin, prepared from *Clostridium tetani* grown in a semi-synthetic medium, is detoxified with formaldehyde and purified. Each capsular polysaccharide is individually covalently bound to the inactivated tetanus toxoid. After purification, the conjugate is lyophilized in the presence of sucrose as a stabilizer. The diluent for MENHIBRIX is a sterile saline solution (0.9% sodium chloride) supplied in vials.

When MENHIBRIX is reconstituted with the accompanying saline diluent, each 0.5-mL dose is formulated to contain 5 mcg of purified *Neisseria meningitidis* C capsular polysaccharide conjugated to approximately 5 mcg of tetanus toxoid, 5 mcg of purified *Neisseria meningitidis* Y capsular polysaccharide conjugated to approximately 6.5 mcg of tetanus toxoid, and 2.5 mcg of purified Haemophilus b capsular polysaccharide conjugated to approximately 6.25 mcg of tetanus toxoid. Each dose also contains 96.8 mcg of Tris (trometamol)-HCl, 12.6 mg of sucrose, and ≤0.72 mcg of residual formaldehyde. MENHIBRIX does not contain preservatives. The vial stoppers do not contain latex.

12 CLINICAL PHARMACOLOGY

12.1 Mechanism of Action

Neisseria meningitidis: The presence of bactericidal anticapsular meningococcal antibodies has been associated with protection from invasive meningococcal disease.[8] MENHIBRIX induces production of bactericidal antibodies specific to the capsular polysaccharides of serogroups C and Y.

Haemophilus influenzae type b: Specific levels of antibodies to PRP (anti-PRP) have been shown to correlate with protection against invasive disease due to *H. influenzae* type b. Based on data from passive antibody studies[9] and a clinical efficacy study with unconjugated *Haemophilus* b polysaccharide vaccine[10], an anti-PRP concentration of 0.15 mcg/mL has been accepted as a minimal protective level. Data from an efficacy study with unconjugated *Haemophilus* b polysaccharide vaccine indicate that an anti-PRP concentration of ≥1.0 mcg/mL predicts protection through at least a 1-year period.[11,12] These antibody levels have been used to evaluate the effectiveness of *H. influenzae* type b-containing vaccines, including MENHIBRIX.

13 NONCLINICAL TOXICOLOGY

13.1 Carcinogenesis, Mutagenesis, Impairment of Fertility

MENHIBRIX has not been evaluated for carcinogenic or mutagenic potential, or for impairment of fertility.

14 CLINICAL STUDIES

14.1 Immunological Evaluation

In Study 009/010[5] the immune response to MENHIBRIX and control vaccines was evaluated in a subset of US participants. In this clinical study, MENHIBRIX and Hib control vaccines were administered concomitantly with routinely recommended US-licensed vaccines *[see Adverse Reactions (6.1)]*. Among participants in the ATP immunogenicity cohort for both vaccine groups combined, 47% were female; 81% of participants were white, 8% were black, 4% were Hispanic, 1% were Asian, and 6% were of other racial/ethnic groups.

Study objectives included evaluation of *N. meningitidis* serogroups C (MenC) and Y (MenY) as measured by serum bactericidal assay using human complement (hSBA) and antibodies to PRP as measured by enzyme-linked immunosorbent assay (ELISA) in sera obtained approximately one month (range 21 to 48 days) after dose 3 of MENHIBRIX or PRP-T and approximately 6 weeks (range 35 to 56 days) after dose 4 of MENHIBRIX or PRP-OMP. The hSBA-MenC and hSBA-MenY geometric mean antibody titers (GMTs) and the percentage of participants with hSBA-MenC and hSBA-MenY levels ≥1:8 are presented in Table 2. Anti-PRP geometric mean antibody concentrations (GMCs) and the percentage of participants with anti-PRP levels ≥0.15 mcg/mL and ≥1.0 mcg/mL are presented in Table 3.

Table 2. Bactericidal Antibody Responses FollowingMENHIBRIX (One Month After Dose 3 and 6 Weeks After Dose 4) in US Children Vaccinated at 2, 4, 6, and 12 to 15 Months of Age (ATP Cohort for Immunogenicity)

	MENHIBRIX Post-Dose 3	MENHIBRIX Post-Dose 4
hSBA-MenC	N = 491	N = 331
% ≥1:8 95% CI	98.8 97.4, 99.6	98.5[a] 96.5, 99.5
GMT 95% CI	968 864, 1084	2040 1746, 2383
hSBA-MenY	N = 481	N = 342
% ≥1:8 95% CI	95.8 93.7, 97.4	98.8[a] 97.0, 99.7
GMT 95% CI	237 206, 272	1390 1205, 1602

ATP = according to protocol; CI = confidence interval; GMT = geometric mean antibody titer.

N = number of US children eligible for inclusion in the ATP immunogenicity cohort for whom serological results were available for the post-dose 3 and post-dose 4 immunological evaluations.

[a]Acceptance criteria were met (lower limit of 95% CI for the percentage of participants with hSBA-MenC and hSBA-MenY titers ≥1:8 ≥90% following 4 doses).

Table 3. Comparison of anti-PRP Responses FollowingMENHIBRIX or Haemophilus b Conjugate Vaccine[a] (One Month After Dose 3 and 6 Weeks After Dose 4) in US Children Vaccinated at 2, 4, 6, and 12 to 15 Months of Age (ATP Cohort for Immunogenicity)

	Post-Dose 3		Post-Dose 4	
	MENHIBRIX	PRP-T	MENHIBRIX	PRP-OMP
Anti-PRP	N = 518	N – 171	N = 361	N = 126
% ≥0.15 mcg/mL 95% CI	100 99.3, 100	98.2 95.0, 99.6	100 99.0, 100	100 97.1, 100
% ≥1.0 mcg/mL 95% CI	96.3[b] 94.3, 97.8	91.2 85.9, 95.0	99.2[b] 97.6, 99.8	99.2 95.7, 100
GMC (mcg/mL) 95% CI	11.0 10.0, 12.1	6.5 5.3, 7.9	34.9 30.7, 39.6	20.2 16.4, 24.9

ATP = according to protocol; anti-PRP = antibody concentrations to *H. influenzae* capsular polysaccharide; CI = confidence interval; GMC = geometric mean antibody concentration.

N = number of US children eligible for inclusion in the ATP immunogenicity cohort for whom serological results were available for the post-dose 3 and post-dose 4 immunological evaluations.

[a]US-licensed monovalent Haemophilus b Conjugate Vaccine for doses 1, 2, and 3 (PRP-T) and for dose 4 (PRP-OMP).

[b]Non-inferiority was demonstrated (lower limit of 95% CI on the group difference of MENHIBRIX minus Haemophilus b Conjugate Vaccine ≥-10%).

[See table 3 above]

14.2 Concomitant Vaccine Administration

In participants who received MENHIBRIX concomitantly with PEDIARIX and PCV7 at 2, 4, and 6 months of age, there was no evidence for reduced antibody response to pertussis antigens (GMC to pertussis toxin, filamentous hemagglutinin, and pertactin), diphtheria toxoid (antibody levels ≥0.1 IU/mL), tetanus toxoid (antibody levels ≥0.1 IU/mL), poliovirus types 1, 2, and 3 (neutralizing antibody levels ≥1:8 to each virus), hepatitis B (anti-hepatitis B surface antigen ≥10 mIU/mL) or PCV7 (antibody levels ≥0.2 mcg/mL and GMC to each serotype) relative to the response in control participants administered PRP-T concomitantly with PEDIARIX and PCV7. The immune responses to PEDIARIX[3,5] and PCV7[3] were evaluated one month following dose 3.

There was no evidence for interference in the immune response to MMR and varicella vaccines (initially seronegative participants with anti-measles ≥200 mIU/mL, anti-mumps ≥51 ED_{50}, anti-rubella ≥10 IU/mL, and anti-varicella ≥1:40) administered at 12 to 15 months of age concomitantly with MENHIBRIX and PCV7 relative to these vaccines administered concomitantly with PRP-OMP and PCV7.[4,5] The immune responses to MMR and varicella vaccines were evaluated 6 weeks post-vaccination. Data are insufficient to evaluate potential interference when a fourth PCV7 dose is administered concomitantly with MENHIBRIX at 12 to 15 months of age.

15 References

All NCT numbers are as noted in the National Library of Medicine clinical trial database (see www.clinicaltrials.gov).

1. NCT00127855 (001).
2. NCT00129116 (003/004).
3. NCT00129129 (005/006).
4. NCT00134719 (007/008).
5. NCT00289783 (009/010).
6. NCT00345579/NCT00345683 (011/012).
7. Rothstein EP, Madore DV, Girone JAC, et al. Comparison of antigenuria after immunization with three *Haemophilus influenzae* type b conjugate vaccines. *Pediatr Infect Dis J* 1991;10:311-314.
8. Goldschneider I, Gotschlich EC, Artenstein MS. Human immunity to the meningococcus. I. The role of humoral antibodies. *J Exp Med* 1969;129:1307-1326.
9. Robbins JB, Parke JC, Schneerson R, et al. Quantitative measurement of "natural" and immunization-induced *Haemophilus influenzae* type b capsular polysaccharide antibodies. *Pediatr Res* 1973;7:103-110.
10. Peltola H, Käythy H, Sivonen A, et al. *Haemophilus influenzae* type b capsular polysaccharide vaccine in children: A double-blind field study of 100,000 vaccinees 3 months to 5 years of age in Finland. *Pediatrics* 1977;60:730-737.
11. Käythy H, Peltola H, Karanko V, et al. The protective level of serum antibodies to the capsular polysaccharide of *Haemophilus influenzae* type b. *J Infect Dis* 1983;147:1100.
12. Anderson P. The protective level of serum antibodies to the capsular polysaccharide of *Haemophilus influenzae* type b. *J Infect Dis* 1984;149:1034.

16 HOW SUPPLIED/STORAGE AND HANDLING

MENHIBRIX is available in single-dose vials of lyophilized vaccine, accompanied by vials containing 0.85 mL of saline diluent (packaged without syringes or needles).

Supplied as package of 10 doses (NDC 58160-801-11):
NDC 58160-809-01 Vial of lyophilized vaccine in Package of 10: NDC 58160-809-05
NDC 58160-813-01 Vial of saline diluent in Package of 10: NDC 58160-813-05

16.1 Storage Before Reconstitution

Lyophilized vaccine vials: Store refrigerated between 2° and 8°C (36° and 46°F). Protect vials from light.

Diluent: Store refrigerated or at controlled room temperature between 2° and 25°C (36° and 77°F). Do not freeze. Discard if the diluent has been frozen.

16.2 Storage After Reconstitution

After reconstitution, administer MENHIBRIX immediately. Do not freeze. Discard if the vaccine has been frozen.

17 PATIENT COUNSELING INFORMATION

- Inform parents or guardians of the potential benefits and risks of immunization with MENHIBRIX, and of the importance of completing the immunization series.
- Inform parents or guardians about the potential for adverse reactions that have been temporally associated with administration of MENHIBRIX or other vaccines containing similar components.
- Instruct parents or guardians to report any adverse events to their healthcare provider.
- Give parents or guardians the Vaccine Information Statements, which are required by the National Childhood Vaccine Injury Act of 1986 to be given prior to immunization. These materials are available free of charge at the Centers for Disease Control and Prevention (CDC) website (www.cdc.gov/vaccines).

HIBERIX, MENHIBRIX, and PEDIARIX are registered trademarks of GlaxoSmithKline.

Manufactured by **GlaxoSmithKline Biologicals**
Rixensart, Belgium, US License 1617, and
Distributed by **GlaxoSmithKline**
Research Triangle Park, NC 27709

MNX:1PI

MEKINIST ℞
(trametinib)
tablets, for oral use

HIGHLIGHTS OF PRESCRIBING INFORMATION
These highlights do not include all the information needed to use MEKINIST safely and effectively. See full prescribing information for MEKINIST.
MEKINIST (trametinib) tablets, for oral use
Initial U.S. Approval: 2013

INDICATIONS AND USAGE

MEKINIST is a kinase inhibitor indicated for the treatment of patients with unresectable or metastatic melanoma with BRAF V600E or V600K mutations as detected by an FDA-approved test. (1)

Limitation of use: MEKINIST is not indicated for the treatment of patients who have received prior BRAF-inhibitor therapy. (1)

DOSAGE AND ADMINISTRATION

- Confirm the presence of BRAF V600E or V600K mutation in tumor specimens prior to initiation of treatment with MEKINIST. (2.1)
- The recommended dose is 2 mg orally once daily taken at least 1 hour before or at least 2 hours after a meal. (2.2)

DOSAGE FORMS AND STRENGTHS

Tablets: 0.5 mg, 1 mg, and 2 mg. (3)

CONTRAINDICATIONS

None. (4)

WARNINGS AND PRECAUTIONS

- Cardiomyopathy: Re-assess LVEF after one month of treatment, and evaluate approximately every 2 to 3 months thereafter. (5.1)
- Retinal Pigment Epithelial Detachment (RPED): Perform ophthalmologic evaluation for any visual disturbances. Withhold MEKINIST if RPED is diagnosed and discontinue if no improvement after 3 weeks. (5.2)
- Retinal Vein Occlusion (RVO): Discontinue MEKINIST. (5.3)
- Interstitial Lung Disease (ILD): Withhold MEKINIST for new or progressive unexplained pulmonary symptoms or findings, such as cough, dyspnea, hypoxia, or infiltrates. Permanently discontinue MEKINIST for treatment-related ILD or pneumonitis. (5.4)
- Serious Skin Toxicity: Monitor for skin toxicities and for secondary infections. Discontinue for intolerable Grade 2, or Grade 3 or 4 rash not improving within 3 weeks despite interruption of MEKINIST. (5.5)
- Embryofetal Toxicity: Can cause fetal harm. Advise females of reproductive potential of potential risk to the fetus. (5.6, 8.1, 8.6)

ADVERSE REACTIONS

Most common adverse reactions (≥20%) for MEKINIST include rash, diarrhea, and lymphedema. (6.1)

To report SUSPECTED ADVERSE REACTIONS, contact GlaxoSmithKline at 1-888-825-5249 or FDA at 1-800-FDA-1088 or www.fda.gov/medwatch.

USE IN SPECIFIC POPULATIONS

- Nursing Mothers: Discontinue drug or nursing. (8.3)
- Females and Males of Reproductive Potential: Counsel female patients on pregnancy planning and prevention. May impair fertility. (8.6)

See 17 for PATIENT COUNSELING INFORMATION and FDA-approved patient labeling

Revised: 05/2013

FULL PRESCRIBING INFORMATION: CONTENTS*

*** Sections or subsections omitted from the full prescribing information are not listed**

FULL PRESCRIBING INFORMATION

1 INDICATIONS AND USAGE

MEKINIST™ is indicated for the treatment of patients with unresectable or metastatic melanoma with BRAF V600E or V600K mutations, as detected by an FDA-approved test *[see Clinical Studies (14.1)]*.

Limitation of use: MEKINIST is not indicated for treatment of patients who have received prior BRAF-inhibitor therapy *[see Clinical Studies (14.2)]*.

2 DOSAGE AND ADMINISTRATION

2.1 Patient Selection

Select patients for treatment of unresectable or metastatic melanoma with MEKINIST based on presence of BRAF V600E or V600K mutation in tumor specimens *[see Clinical Studies (14.1)]*. Information on FDA-approved tests for the detection of BRAF V600 mutations in melanoma is available at: http://www.fda.gov/CompanionDiagnostics.

2.2 Recommended Dosing

The recommended dose is 2 mg orally once daily until disease progression or unacceptable toxicity. Take at least 1 hour before or 2 hours after a meal. Do not take a missed dose within 12 hours of the next dose.

2.3 Dose Modifications

[See table 1 above]

Table 1. Recommended Dose Modifications for MEKINIST

Target Organ	Adverse Reaction[a]	Dose Modification
Cutaneous	Grade 2 rash	Reduce dose of MEKINIST by 0.5 mg <u>or</u> discontinue MEKINIST in patients taking MEKINIST 1 mg daily
	Intolerable Grade 2 rash that does not improve within 3 weeks following dose reduction Grade 3 or 4 rash	Withhold MEKINIST for up to 3 weeks If improved within 3 weeks, resume MEKINIST at a lower dose (reduced by 0.5 mg) <u>or</u> discontinue MEKINIST in patients taking MEKINIST 1 mg daily
	Intolerable Grade 2, or Grade 3 or 4 rash that does not improve within 3 weeks despite interruption of dosing of MEKINIST	Permanently discontinue MEKINIST
Cardiac	Asymptomatic, absolute decrease in LVEF of 10% <u>or</u> greater from baseline <u>and</u> is below institutional lower limits of normal (LLN) from pretreatment value	Withhold MEKINIST for up to 4 weeks
	Asymptomatic, absolute decrease in LVEF of 10% or greater from baseline <u>and</u> is below LLN that improves to normal LVEF value within 4 weeks following interruption of MEKINIST	If improved within 4 weeks, resume MEKINIST at a lower dose (reduced by 0.5 mg) <u>or</u> discontinue MEKINIST in patients taking MEKINIST 1 mg daily
	Symptomatic congestive heart failure Absolute decrease in LVEF of greater than 20% from baseline that is below LLN Absolute decrease in LVEF of 10% <u>or</u> greater from baseline and is below LLN that does not improve to normal LVEF value within 4 weeks following interruption of MEKINIST	Permanently discontinue MEKINIST
Ocular	Grade 2-3 retinal pigment epithelial detachments (RPED)	Withhold MEKINIST for up to 3 weeks
	Grade 2-3 RPED that improves to Grade 0-1 within 3 weeks	If improved within 3 weeks, resume MEKINIST at a lower dose (reduced by 0.5 mg) <u>or</u> discontinue MEKINIST in patients taking MEKINIST 1 mg daily
	Retinal vein occlusion Grade 2-3 RPED that does not improve to at least Grade 1 within 3 weeks	Permanently discontinue MEKINIST
Pulmonary	Interstitial lung disease/pneumonitis	Permanently discontinue MEKINIST
Other	Grade 3 adverse reaction	Withhold MEKINIST for up to 3 weeks
	If Grade 3 adverse reaction improves to Grade 0-1 following interruption of MEKINIST within 3 weeks	Reduce dose of MEKINIST by 0.5 mg <u>or</u> discontinue MEKINIST in patients taking MEKINIST 1 mg daily
	Grade 4 adverse reaction Grade 3 adverse reaction that does not improve to Grade 0-1 within 3 weeks	Permanently discontinue MEKINIST

[a] Note: The intensity of clinical adverse events graded by the National Cancer Institute Common Terminology Criteria for Adverse Events (CTCAE) version 4.0.

3 DOSAGE FORMS AND STRENGTHS

0.5 mg Tablets: Yellow, modified oval, biconvex, film-coated tablets with 'GS' debossed on one face and 'TFC' on the opposing face.

1 mg Tablets: White, round, biconvex, film-coated tablets with 'GS' debossed on one face and 'LHE' on the opposing face.

2 mg Tablets: Pink, round, biconvex, film-coated tablets with 'GS' debossed on one face and 'HMJ' on the opposing face.

4 CONTRAINDICATIONS

None.

5 WARNINGS AND PRECAUTIONS

5.1 Cardiomyopathy

In Trial 1, cardiomyopathy [defined as cardiac failure, left ventricular dysfunction, or decreased left ventricular ejection fraction (LVEF)] occurred in 7% (14/211) of patients treated with MEKINIST; no chemotherapy-treated patient in Trial 1 developed cardiomyopathy. The median time to onset of cardiomyopathy in patients treated with MEKINIST was 63 days (range: 16 to 156 days); cardiomyopathy was identified within the first month of treatment with MEKINIST in five of these 14 patients. Four percent of patients in Trial 1 required discontinuation (4/211) and/or dose reduction (7/211) of MEKINIST. Cardiomyopathy resolved in 10 of these 14 (71%) patients.

Across clinical trials of MEKINIST at the recommended dose (N = 329), 11% of patients developed evidence of cardiomyopathy (decrease in LVEF below institutional lower limits of normal with an absolute decrease in LVEF ≥10% below baseline) and 5% demonstrated a decrease in LVEF below institutional lower limits of normal with an absolute decrease in LVEF of ≥20% below baseline.

Assess LVEF by echocardiogram or multigated acquisition (MUGA) scan before initiation of MEKINIST, one month after initiation of MEKINIST, and then at 2- to 3-month intervals while on treatment. Withhold treatment if absolute LVEF value decreases by 10% from pre-treatment values and is less than the lower limit of normal. Permanently discontinue MEKINIST for symptomatic cardiomyopathy or persistent, asymptomatic LVEF dysfunction that does not resolve within 4 weeks *[see Dosage and Administration (2.3)]*.

5.2 Retinal Pigment Epithelial Detachment (RPED)

Retinal pigment epithelial detachments (RPED) can occur during treatment with MEKINIST. In Trial 1, where ophthalmologic examinations including retinal evaluation were performed pretreatment and at regular intervals during treatment, one patient (0.5%) receiving MEKINIST developed RPED and no cases of RPED were identified in chemotherapy-treated patients. Across all clinical trials of MEKINIST, the incidence of RPED was 0.8% (14/1749).

Retinal detachments were often bilateral and multifocal, occurring in the macular region of the retina. RPED led to reduction in visual acuity that resolved after a median of 11.5 days (range: 3 to 71 days) following the interruption of dosing with MEKINIST, although Ocular Coherence Tomography (OCT) abnormalities persisted beyond a month in at least several cases.

Perform ophthalmological evaluation at any time a patient reports visual disturbances and compare to baseline, if available. Withhold MEKINIST if RPED is diagnosed. If resolution of the RPED is documented on repeat ophthalmological evaluation within 3 weeks, resume MEKINIST at a reduced dose *[see Dosage and Administration (2.3)]*.

5.3 Retinal Vein Occlusion (RVO)

Across all clinical trials of MEKINIST, the incidence of RVO was 0.2% (4/1749). An RVO may lead to macular edema, decreased visual function, neovascularization, and glaucoma. Urgently (within 24 hours) perform ophthalmological evaluation for patient-reported loss of vision or other visual disturbances. Permanently discontinue MEKINIST in patients with documented retinal vein occlusion *[see Dosage and Administration (2.3)]*.

5.4 Interstitial Lung Disease

In clinical trials of MEKINIST at the recommended dose (N = 329), interstitial lung disease (ILD) or pneumonitis occurred in 1.8% of patients. In Trial 1, 2.4% (5/211) of patients treated with MEKINIST developed ILD or pneumonitis; all five patients required hospitalization. The median time to first presentation of ILD or pneumonitis was 160 days (range: 60 to 172 days).

Withhold MEKINIST in patients presenting with new or progressive pulmonary symptoms and findings including cough, dyspnea, hypoxia, pleural effusion, or infiltrates, pending clinical investigations. Permanently discontinue MEKINIST for patients diagnosed with treatment-related ILD or pneumonitis.

5.5 Serious Skin Toxicity

In Trial 1, the overall incidence of skin toxicity including rash, dermatitis, acneiform rash, palmar-plantar erythrodysesthesia syndrome, and erythema was 87% in patients treated with MEKINIST and 13% in chemotherapy-treated patients. Severe skin toxicity occurred in 12% of patients treated with MEKINIST. Skin toxicity requiring hospitalization occurred in 6% of patients treated with MEKINIST, most commonly for secondary infections of the skin requiring intravenous antibiotics or severe skin toxicity without secondary infection. In comparison, no patients treated with chemotherapy required hospitalization for severe skin toxicity or infections of the skin. The median time to onset of skin toxicity in patients treated with MEKINIST was 15 days (range: 1 to 221 days) and median time to resolution of skin toxicity was 48 days (range: 1 to 282 days). Reductions in the dose of MEKINIST were required in 12% and permanent discontinuation of MEKINIST was required in 1% of patients with skin toxicity.

Monitor patients receiving MEKINIST for skin toxicities and for secondary infections *[see Dosage and Administration (2.3)]*.

5.6 Embryofetal Toxicity

Based on its mechanism of action, MEKINIST can cause fetal harm when administered to a pregnant woman. MEKINIST was embryotoxic and abortifacient in rabbits at doses greater than or equal to those resulting in exposures approximately 0.3 times the human exposure at the recommended clinical dose. If this drug is used during pregnancy, or if the patient becomes pregnant while taking this drug, the patient should be apprised of the potential hazard to a fetus. *[See Use in Specific Populations (8.1).]*

Advise female patients of reproductive potential to use highly effective contraception during treatment with MEKINIST and for 4 months after treatment. Advise patients to contact their healthcare provider if they become pregnant, or if pregnancy is suspected, while taking MEKINIST. *[See Use in Specific Populations (8.1, 8.6).]*

6 ADVERSE REACTIONS

The following adverse reactions are discussed in greater detail in another section of the label:

- Cardiomyopathy *[see Warnings and Precautions (5.1)]*
- Retinal pigment epithelial detachment *[see Warnings and Precautions (5.2)]*
- Retinal vein occlusion *[see Warnings and Precautions (5.3)]*
- Interstitial lung disease *[see Warnings and Precautions (5.4)]*
- Serious skin toxicity *[see Warnings and Precautions (5.5)]*

6.1 Clinical Trials Experience

Because clinical trials are conducted under widely varying conditions, adverse reaction rates observed in the clinical trials of a drug cannot be directly compared to rates in the clinical trials of another drug and may not reflect the rates observed in practice.

The data described in the Warnings and Precautions section and below reflect exposure to MEKINIST in 329 patients including 107 (33%) exposed for greater than or equal to 6 months and 30 (9%) exposed for greater than or equal to one year. MEKINIST was studied in open-label, single-arm trials (N = 118) or in an open-label, randomized, active-controlled trial (N = 211). The median age was 54, 60% were male, >99% were white, and all patients had metastatic melanoma. All patients received 2 mg once-daily doses of MEKINIST. The incidence of RPED and RVO are obtained from the 1,749 patients from all clinical trials with MEKINIST.

Table 2 presents adverse reactions identified from analyses of Trial 1, *[see Clinical Studies (14.1)]* a randomized, open-label trial of patients with BRAF V600E or V600K mutation-positive melanoma receiving MEKINIST (N = 211) 2 mg orally once daily or chemotherapy (N = 99) [either dacarbazine 1,000 mg/m^2 every 3 weeks or paclitaxel 175 mg/m^2 every 3 weeks]. Patients with abnormal LVEF, history of acute coronary syndrome within 6 months, or current evidence of Class II or greater congestive heart failure (New York Heart Association) were excluded from Trial 1. The median duration of treatment with MEKINIST was 4.3 months. In Trial 1, 9% of patients receiving MEKINIST experienced adverse reactions resulting in permanent discontinuation of trial medication. The most common adverse reactions resulting in permanent discontinuation of MEKINIST were decreased left ventricular ejection fraction (LVEF), pneumonitis, renal failure, diarrhea, and rash. Adverse reactions led to dose reductions in 27% of patients treated with MEKINIST. Rash and decreased LVEF were the most common reasons cited for dose reductions of MEKINIST.

[See table 2 above]

Table 2. Selected Adverse Reactions Occurring in ≥10% of Patients Receiving MEKINIST and at a Higher Incidence than in the Control Arm[a]

Adverse Reactions	MEKINIST (N = 211)		Chemotherapy (N = 99)	
	All Grades[b]	Grades 3 and 4[c]	All Grades[b]	Grades 3 and 4[c]
Skin and subcutaneous tissue disorders				
Rash	57	8	10	0
Dermatitis acneiform	19	<1	1	0
Dry skin	11	0	0	0
Pruritus	10	2	1	0
Paronychia	10	0	1	0
Gastrointestinal disorders				
Diarrhea	43	0	16	2
Stomatitis[d]	15	2	2	0
Abdominal pain[e]	13	1	5	1
Vascular disorders				
Lymphedema[f]	32	1	4	0
Hypertension	15	12	7	3
Hemorrhage[g]	13	<1	0	0

[a]Events included are higher in the trametinib arm compared with chemotherapy by ≥5% in overall incidence or by ≥2% Grade 3-4 adverse reactions higher in trametinib arm compared with chemotherapy.
[b] National Cancer Institute Common Terminology Criteria for Adverse Events, version 4.0.
[c] Grade 4 adverse reactions were limited to rash (n = 1) in trametinib arm and diarrhea (n = 1) in the chemotherapy arm.
[d] Includes the following terms: stomatitis, aphthous stomatitis, mouth ulceration, and mucosal inflammation.
[e] Includes the following terms: abdominal pain, abdominal pain lower, abdominal pain upper, and abdominal tenderness.
[f] Includes the following terms: lymphodema, edema, and peripheral edema.
[g] Includes the following terms: epistaxis, gingival bleeding, hematochezia, rectal hemorrhage, melena, vaginal hemorrhage, hemorrhoidal hemorrhage, hematuria, and conjunctival hemorrhage.

Other clinically important adverse reactions observed in ≤10% of patients (N = 329) treated with MEKINIST were:

Nervous System Disorders: Dizziness, dysgeusia.
Ocular Disorders: Vision blurred, dry eye.
Infections and Infestations: Folliculitis, rash pustular, cellulitis.
Cardiac Disorders: Bradycardia.
Gastrointestinal Disorders: Xerostomia.
Musculoskeletal and Connective Tissue Disorders: Rhabdomyolysis.

[See table 3 above]

Table 3. Percent-Patient Incidence of Laboratory Abnormalities Occurring at a Higher Incidence in Patients Treated With MEKINIST in Trial 1 [Between Arm Difference of ≥5% (All Grades) or ≥2% (Grades 3 or 4)[a]]

Preferred Term	MEKINIST (N = 211)		Chemotherapy (N = 99)	
	All Grades	Grades 3 and 4	All Grades	Grades 3 and 4
Increased Aspartate aminotransferase (AST)	60	2	16	1
Increased Alanine aminotransferase (ALT)	39	3	20	3
Hypoalbuminemia	42	2	23	1
Anemia	38	2	26	3
Increased Alkaline phosphatase	24	2	18	3

[a]No Grade 4 events were reported in either treatment arm.

7 DRUG INTERACTIONS

No formal clinical studies have been conducted to evaluate human cytochrome P450 (CYP) enzyme-mediated drug interactions with trametinib *[see Clinical Pharmacology (12.3)]*.

8 USE IN SPECIFIC POPULATIONS

8.1 Pregnancy

Pregnancy Category D

Risk Summary: MEKINIST can cause fetal harm when administered to a pregnant woman. Trametinib was embryotoxic and abortifacient in rabbits at doses greater than or equal to those resulting in exposures approximately 0.3 times the human exposure at the recommended clinical dose. If this drug is used during pregnancy, or if the patient becomes pregnant while taking this drug, the patient should be apprised of the potential hazard to the fetus *[see Warnings and Precautions (5.6)]*.

Animal Data: In reproductive toxicity studies, administration of trametinib to rats during the period of organogenesis resulted in decreased fetal weights at doses greater than or equal to 0.031 mg/kg/day (approximately 0.3 times the human exposure based on AUC at the recommended dose). In rats, at a dose resulting in exposures 1.8-fold higher than the human exposure at the recommended dose, there was maternal toxicity and an increase in post-implantation loss. In pregnant rabbits, administration of trametinib during the period of organogenesis resulted in decreased fetal body weight and increased incidence of variations in ossification at doses greater than or equal to 0.039 mg/kg/day (approximately 0.08 times the human exposure at the recommended dose based on AUC). In rabbits administered trametinib at 0.15 mg/kg/day (approximately 0.3 times the human exposure at the recommended dose based on AUC) there was an increase in post-implantation loss, including total loss of pregnancy, compared to control animals.

8.3 Nursing Mothers

It is not known whether this drug is present in human milk. Because many drugs are present in human milk and because of the potential for serious adverse reactions in nursing infants from MEKINIST, a decision should be made whether to discontinue nursing or to discontinue the drug taking into account the importance of the drug to the mother.

8.4 Pediatric Use

The safety and effectiveness of MEKINIST have not been established in pediatric patients.

8.5 Geriatric Use

Clinical studies of MEKINIST did not include sufficient numbers of subjects aged 65 and over to determine whether they respond differently from younger subjects. In Trial 1, 49 patients (23%) were 65 years of age and older, and 9 patients (4%) were 75 years of age and older.

8.6 Females and Males of Reproductive Potential

Contraception: *Females*

MEKINIST can cause fetal harm when administered during pregnancy. Advise female patients of reproductive potential to use highly effective contraception during treatment and for 4 months after treatment. Advise patients to contact their healthcare provider if they become pregnant, or if pregnancy is suspected, while taking MEKINIST *[see Use in Specific Populations (8.1)]*.

Infertility: *Females*

Trametinib may impair fertility in female patients *[see Nonclinical Toxicology (13.1)]*.

8.7 Hepatic Impairment

No formal clinical study has been conducted to evaluate the effect of hepatic impairment on the pharmacokinetics of trametinib. No dose adjustment is recommended in patients with mild hepatic impairment based on a population pharmacokinetic analysis *[see Clinical Pharmacology (12.3)]*.

The appropriate dose of MEKINIST has not been established in patients with moderate or severe hepatic impairment.

8.8 Renal Impairment

No formal clinical study has been conducted to evaluate the effect of renal impairment on the pharmacokinetics of trametinib. No dose adjustment is recommended in patients with mild or moderate renal impairment based on a population pharmacokinetic analysis *[see Clinical Pharmacology (12.3)]*. The appropriate dose of MEKINIST has not been established in patients with severe renal impairment.

10 OVERDOSAGE

There were no reported cases of inadvertent overdosage with MEKINIST. The highest doses of MEKINIST evaluated in clinical trials were 4 mg orally once daily and 10 mg administered orally once daily on two consecutive days followed by 3 mg once daily. In seven patients treated on one of these two schedules, there were two cases of retinal pigment epithelial detachments for an incidence of 28%. Since trametinib is highly bound to plasma proteins, hemodialysis is likely to be ineffective in the treatment of overdose with MEKINIST.

11 DESCRIPTION

Trametinib dimethyl sulfoxide is a kinase inhibitor. The chemical name is acetamide, N-[3-[3-cyclopropyl-5-[(2-fluoro-4- iodophenyl)amino]-3,4,6,7-tetrahydro-6,8-dimethyl- 2,4,7-trioxopyrido[4,3-d]pyrimidin-1(2H)-yl]phenyl]-, compound with 1,1'-sulfinylbis[methane] (1:1). It has a molecular formula $C_{26}H_{23}FIN_5O_4 \bullet C_2H_6OS$ with a molecular mass of 693.53. Trametinib dimethyl sulfoxide has the following chemical structure:

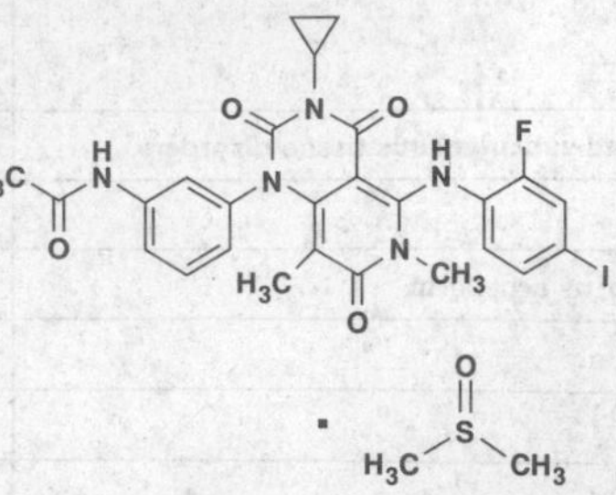

Trametinib dimethyl sulfoxide is a white to almost white powder. It is practically insoluble in the pH range of 2 to 8 in aqueous media.

MEKINIST (trametinib) Tablets are supplied as 0.5-mg, 1-mg, and 2-mg tablets for oral administration. Each 0.5-mg tablet contains 0.5635 mg trametinib dimethyl sulfoxide equivalent to 0.5 mg of trametinib non-solvated parent. Each 1-mg tablet contains 1.127 mg trametinib dimethyl sulfoxide equivalent to 1 mg of trametinib non-solvated parent. Each 2-mg tablet contains 2.254 mg trametinib dimethyl sulfoxide equivalent to 2 mg of trametinib non-solvated parent.

The inactive ingredients of MEKINIST Tablets are: **Tablet Core:** mannitol, microcrystalline cellulose, hypromellose, croscarmellose sodium, magnesium stearate (vegetable source), sodium lauryl sulfate, colloidal silicon dioxide. **Coating:** hypromellose, titanium dioxide, polyethylene glycol, polysorbate 80 (2-mg tablets), iron oxide yellow (0.5-mg tablets), iron oxide red (2-mg tablets).

12 CLINICAL PHARMACOLOGY

12.1 Mechanism of Action

Trametinib is a reversible inhibitor of mitogen-activated extracellular signal regulated kinase 1 (MEK1) and MEK2 activation and of MEK1 and MEK2 kinase activity. MEK proteins are upstream regulators of the extracellular signal-related kinase (ERK) pathway, which promotes cellular proliferation. BRAF V600E mutations result in constitutive activation of the BRAF pathway which includes MEK1 and MEK2. Trametinib inhibits BRAF V600 mutation-positive melanoma cell growth in vitro and in vivo.

12.2 Pharmacodynamics

Administration of 1 mg and 2 mg trametinib to patients with BRAF V600 mutation-positive melanoma resulted in dose-dependent changes in tumor biomarkers including inhibition of phosphorylated ERK, inhibition of Ki67 (a marker of cell proliferation), and increases in p27 (a marker of apoptosis).

12.3 Pharmacokinetics

The pharmacokinetics (PK) of trametinib were characterized following single- and repeat-oral administration in patients with solid tumors and BRAF V600 mutation-positive metastatic melanoma.

Absorption: After oral administration, the median time to achieve peak plasma concentrations (T_{max}) is 1.5 hours post-dose. The mean absolute bioavailability of a single 2-mg oral dose of trametinib tablet is 72%. The increase in C_{max} was dose proportional after a single dose of 0.125 to 10 mg while the increase in AUC was greater than dose proportional. After repeat doses of 0.125 to 4 mg daily, both C_{max} and AUC increase proportionally with dose. Inter-subject variability in AUC and C_{max} at steady state is 22% and 28%, respectively.

Administration of a single dose of trametinib with a high-fat, high-calorie meal decreased AUC by 24%, C_{max} by 70%, and delayed T_{max} by approximately 4 hours as compared to fasted conditions *[see Dosage and Administration (2.2)]*.

Distribution: Trametinib is 97.4% bound to human plasma proteins. The apparent volume of distribution (V_c/F) is 214 L.

Metabolism: Trametinib is metabolized predominantly via deacetylation alone or with mono-oxygenation or in combination with glucuronidation biotransformation pathways in vitro. Deacetylation is likely mediated by hydrolytic enzymes, such as carboxyl-esterases or amidases.

Following a single dose of [^{14}C]-trametinib, approximately 50% of circulating radioactivity is represented as the parent compound. However, based on metabolite profiling after repeat dosing of trametinib, ≥75% of drug-related material in plasma is the parent compound.

Elimination: The estimated elimination half-life based on the population PK model is 3.9 to 4.8 days. The apparent clearance is 4.9 L/h.

Following oral administration of [^{14}C]-trametinib, >80% of excreted radioactivity was recovered in the feces while <20% of excreted radioactivity was recovered in the urine with <0.1% of the excreted dose as parent.

Specific Populations: Based on a population pharmacokinetic analysis, age, gender, and body weight do not have a clinically important effect on the exposure of trametinib. There are insufficient data to evaluate potential differences in the exposure of trametinib by race or ethnicity.

Hepatic Impairment: Based on a population pharmacokinetic analysis in 64 patients with mild hepatic impairment (total bilirubin ≤ULN and AST >ULN or total bilirubin >1.0-1.5 × ULN and any AST), mild hepatic impairment has no clinically important effect on the systemic exposure of trametinib. The pharmacokinetics of trametinib have not been studied in patients with moderate or severe hepatic impairment *[see Use in Specific Populations (8.7)]*.

Renal Impairment: As renal excretion of trametinib is low (<20%), renal impairment is unlikely to have a clinically important effect on the exposure of trametinib. Based on a population PK analysis in 223 patients with mild renal impairment (GFR 60 to 89 mL/min/1.73 m^2) and 35 patients with moderate renal impairment (GFR 30 to 59 mL/min/1.73 m^2), mild and moderate renal impairment have no clinically important effects on the systemic exposure of trametinib. The PK of trametinib have not been studied in patients with severe renal impairment *[see Use in Specific Populations (8.8)]*.

Pediatrics: No studies have been conducted to evaluate the pharmacokinetics of trametinib in pediatric patients.

Drug Interactions: No formal drug interaction studies have been conducted with trametinib. Trametinib is not a substrate of CYP enzymes or efflux transporters P-gp or BCRP in vitro.

Based on in vitro studies, trametinib is not an inhibitor of CYP450 including CYP1A2, CYP2A6, CYP2B6, CYP2C9, CYP2C19, CYP2D6, and CYP3A4 or of transporters including OATP1B1, OATP1B3, P-gp, and BCRP at a clinically relevant systemic concentration of 0.04 μM. Trametinib is an inhibitor of CYP2C8 in vitro.

Trametinib is an inducer of CYP3A4 in vitro. Based on cross-study comparisons, oral administration of trametinib 2 mg once daily with everolimus (sensitive CYP3A4 substrate) 5 mg once daily, had no clinically important effect on the AUC and C_{max} of everolimus.

13 NONCLINICAL TOXICOLOGY

13.1 Carcinogenesis, Mutagenesis, Impairment of Fertility

Carcinogenicity studies with trametinib have not been conducted. Trametinib was not genotoxic in studies evaluating reverse mutations in bacteria, chromosomal aberrations in mammalian cells, and micronuclei in the bone marrow of rats.

Trametinib may impair fertility in humans. In female rats given trametinib for up to 13 weeks, increased follicular cysts and decreased corpora lutea were observed at doses ≥0.016 mg/kg/day (approximately 0.3 times the human exposure at the recommended dose based on AUC). In rat and dog toxicity studies up to 13 weeks in duration, there were no treatment effects observed on male reproductive tissues *[see Use in Specific Populations (8.6)]*.

14 CLINICAL STUDIES

14.1 BRAF V600E or V600K Mutation-Positive Metastatic Melanoma

The safety and efficacy of MEKINIST were evaluated in an international, multi-center, randomized (2:1), open label, active-controlled trial (Trial 1) in 322 patients with BRAF V600E or V600K mutation-positive, unresectable or metastatic melanoma. Patients were not permitted to have more than one prior chemotherapy regimen for advanced or metastatic disease; prior treatment with a BRAF inhibitor or MEK inhibitor was not permitted. The primary efficacy outcome measure was progression-free survival (PFS). Patients were randomized to receive MEKINIST 2 mg orally once daily (N = 214) or chemotherapy (N = 108) consisting of either dacarbazine 1,000 mg/m^2 intravenously every 3 weeks or paclitaxel 175 mg/m^2 intravenously every 3 weeks. Treatment continued until disease progression or unacceptable toxicity. Randomization was stratified according to prior use of chemotherapy for advanced or metastatic disease (yes versus no) and lactate dehydrogenase level (normal versus greater than upper limit of normal). Tumor tissue was evaluated for BRAF mutations at a central testing site using a clinical trial assay. Tumor samples from 289 patients (196 patients treated with MEKINIST and 93 chemotherapy-treated patients) were also tested retrospectively using an FDA-approved companion diagnostic test, THxID™-BRAF assay.

The median age for randomized patients was 54 years, 54% were male, >99% were white, and all patients had baseline ECOG performance status of 0 or 1. Most patients had metastatic disease (94%), were Stage M1c (64%), had elevated LDH (36%), no history of brain metastasis (97%), and received no prior chemotherapy for advanced or metastatic disease (66%). The distribution of BRAF V600 mutations was BRAF V600E (87%), V600K (12%), or both (<1%). The median durations of follow-up prior to initiation of alternative treatment were 4.9 months for patients treated with MEKINIST and 3.1 months for patients treated with chemotherapy. Fifty-one (47%) patients crossed over from the chemotherapy arm at the time of disease progression to receive MEKINIST.

Trial 1 demonstrated a statistically significant increase in progression-free survival in the patients treated with MEKINIST. Table 4 and Figure 1 summarize the PFS results.

Table 4. Investigator-Assessed Progression-Free Survival and Confirmed Objective Response Results

	MEKINIST N = 214	Chemotherapy N = 108
PFS		
Number of Events (%)	117 (55%)	77 (71%)
Progressive Disease	107 (50%)	70 (65%)
Death	10 (5%)	7 (6%)
Median, months (95% CI)	4.8 (4.3, 4.9)	1.5 (1.4, 2.7)
HR[a] (95% CI)	0.47 (0.34, 0.65)	
*P*value (log-rank test)	*P*<0.0001	
Confirmed Tumor Responses		
Objective Response Rate	22%	8%
(95% CI)	(17, 28)	(4, 15)
CR, n (%)	4 (2%)	0
PR, n (%)	43 (20%)	9 (8%)
Duration of Response		
Median, months (95% CI)	5.5 (4.1, 5.9)	NR (3.5, NR)

[a] Pike estimator.

CI = confidence interval; CR = complete response; HR = Hazard Ratio; NR = Not reached, PFS = Progression-free Survival; PR = partial response.

Figure 1. Kaplan-Meier Curves of Investigator-Assessed Progression-Free Survival (ITT population)

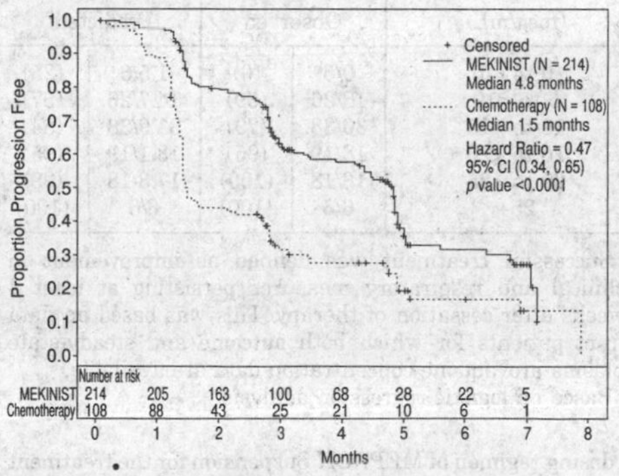

In supportive analyses based on independent radiologic review committee assessment, the PFS results were consistent with those of the primary efficacy analysis.

14.2 Lack of Clinical Activity in Metastatic Melanoma Following BRAF Inhibitor Therapy

The clinical activity of MEKINIST was evaluated in a single-arm, multicenter, international trial (Trial 2) in 40 patients with BRAF V600E or V600K mutation-positive, unresectable or metastatic melanoma who had received prior treatment with a BRAF inhibitor. All patients received MEKINIST at a dose of 2 mg orally once daily until disease progression or unacceptable toxicity.

The median age was 58 years, 63% were male, all were white, 98% had baseline ECOG PS of 0 or 1, and the distribution of BRAF V600 mutations was V600E (83%), V600K (10%), and the remaining patients had multiple V600 mutations (5%), or unknown mutational status (2%). No patient in Trial 2 achieved a confirmed partial or complete response as determined by the clinical investigators.

16 HOW SUPPLIED/STORAGE AND HANDLING

0.5 mg Tablets: Yellow, modified oval, biconvex, film-coated tablets with 'GS' debossed on one face and 'TFC' on the opposing face and are available in bottles of 30 (NDC 0173-0849-13).

1 mg Tablets: White, round, biconvex, film-coated tablets with 'GS' debossed on one face and 'LHE' on the opposing face and are available in bottles of 30 (NDC 0173-0858-13).

2 mg Tablets: Pink, round, biconvex, film-coated tablets with 'GS' debossed on one face and 'HMJ' on the opposing face and are available in bottles of 30 (NDC 0173-0848-13).

Store refrigerated at 2° to 8°C (36° to 46°F). Do not freeze. Dispense in original bottle. Do not remove desiccant. Protect from moisture and light. Do not place medication in pill boxes.

17 PATIENT COUNSELING INFORMATION

See FDA-approved patient labeling (Patient Information).

Inform patients of the following:

- Evidence of BRAF V600E or V600K mutation within the tumor specimen is necessary to identify patients for whom treatment with MEKINIST is indicated *[see Dosage and Administration (2.1)]*.
- MEKINIST can cause cardiomyopathy. Advise patients to immediately report any signs or symptoms of heart failure to their healthcare provider. *[See Warnings and Precautions (5.1).]*
- MEKINIST causes severe visual disturbances that can lead to blindness. Advise patients to contact their healthcare provider if they experience any changes in their vision. *[See Warnings and Precautions (5.2, 5.3).]*
- MEKINIST can cause interstitial lung disease (or pneumonitis). Advise patients to contact their healthcare provider as soon as possible if they experience dyspnea. *[See Warnings and Precautions (5.4).]*
- MEKINIST often causes skin toxicities including acneiform rash. Advise patients to contact their healthcare provider for progressive or intolerable rash. *[See Warnings and Precautions (5.5).]*
- MEKINIST causes hypertension. Advise patients that they need to undergo blood pressure monitoring and to contact their healthcare provider if they develop symptoms of hypertension.
- MEKINIST often causes diarrhea which may be severe in some cases. Inform patients of the need to contact their healthcare provider if severe diarrhea occurs during treatment.
- MEKINIST should be taken at least 1 hour before or at least 2 hours after a meal.
- MEKINIST can cause fetal harm if taken during pregnancy. Instruct female patients to use highly effective contraception during treatment and for 4 months after treatment. Advise patients to contact their healthcare provider if they become pregnant, or if pregnancy is suspected, while taking MEKINIST [*see Use in Specific Populations (8.1, 8.6)*].
- Nursing infants may experience serious adverse reactions if the mother is taking MEKINIST. Advise lactating mothers to discontinue nursing while taking MEKINIST *[see Use in Specific Populations (8.3)]*.

MEKINIST is a trademark of GlaxoSmithKline.

THxID BRAF™ assay is a trademark of bioMerieux.

GlaxoSmithKline
Research Triangle Park, NC 27709

MKN:1PI

Patient Information

MEKINIST™ (MEK-in-ist)
(trametinib)
tablets

What is MEKINIST?

MEKINIST is a prescription medicine used to treat people with a type of skin cancer called melanoma:

- that has spread to other parts of the body or cannot be removed by surgery, and
- that has a certain type of abnormal "BRAF" gene

MEKINIST should not be used to treat people who have received a BRAF inhibitor for treatment of their melanoma.

Your healthcare provider will perform a test to make sure that MEKINIST is right for you.

It is not known if MEKINIST is safe and effective in children.

What should I tell my healthcare provider before taking MEKINIST?

Before you take MEKINIST, tell your healthcare provider if you:

- have heart problems
- have lung or breathing problems
- have eye problems
- have high blood pressure (hypertension)
- have liver or kidney problems
- have any other medical conditions
- are pregnant or plan to become pregnant. MEKINIST can harm your unborn baby.
    - Women who may become pregnant should use effective birth control (contraception) during treatment with MEKINIST and for 4 months after stopping treatment. Talk to your healthcare provider about birth control methods that may be right for you. Tell your healthcare provider right away if you become pregnant during treatment with MEKINIST.
- are breastfeeding or plan to breastfeed. It is not known if MEKINIST passes into your breast milk. You and your healthcare provider should decide if you will take MEKINIST or breastfeed. You should not do both.

Tell your healthcare provider about all the medicines you take, including prescription and over-the-counter medicines, vitamins, and herbal supplements.

Know the medicines you take. Keep a list of them to show your healthcare provider and pharmacist when you get a new medicine.

How should I take MEKINIST?

- Take MEKINIST exactly as your healthcare provider tells you to take it. Do not change your dose or stop MEKINIST unless your healthcare provider tells you.
- Take MEKINIST one time a day.
- Take MEKINIST 1 hour before or 2 hours after meals.
- If you miss a dose, take it as soon as you remember. If it is within 12 hours of your next scheduled dose, skip the missed dose. Just take the next dose at your regular time.
- If you take too much MEKINIST, call your healthcare provider or go to the nearest hospital emergency room right away.

What are the possible side effects of MEKINIST?

MEKINIST may cause serious side effects, including:

- **heart problems, including heart failure.** Your healthcare provider should check your heart function before you start taking MEKINIST and during treatment. Signs and symptoms of heart problems may include:
    - feeling like your heart is pounding or racing
    - shortness of breath
    - swelling of your ankles and feet
    - feeling lightheaded
- **eye problems.** MEKINIST can cause eye problems including blindness. Tell your healthcare provider right away if you get these symptoms of eye problems:
    - blurred vision, loss of vision, or other vision changes
    - see color dots
    - halo (seeing blurred outline around objects)
- **lung or breathing problems.** Tell your healthcare provider if you have any new or worsening symptoms of lung or breathing problems, including:
    - shortness of breath
    - cough
- **skin rash.** Rash is the most common side effect of MEKINIST and in some cases can be severe and can result in admission to the hospital if severe. Tell your healthcare provider if you get any of the following symptoms:
    - skin rash
    - acne
    - redness, swelling, peeling, or tenderness of hands or feet
    - skin redness

The most common side effects of MEKINIST include:

- diarrhea
- swelling of the face, arms, or legs

MEKINIST can cause new or worsening high blood pressure (hypertension). Your healthcare provider should check your blood pressure during treatment with MEKINIST. Tell your healthcare provider if you develop high blood pressure, your blood pressure worsens, or you have severe headache, lightheadedness, or dizziness.

Tell your healthcare provider if you have any side effect that bothers you or that does not go away.

These are not all the possible side effects of MEKINIST. For more information, ask your healthcare provider or pharmacist.

Call your doctor for medical advice about side effects. You may report side effects to FDA at 1-800-FDA-1088.

How should I store MEKINIST?

- Store MEKINIST in the refrigerator between 36°F to 46°F (2°C to 8°C). Do not freeze.
- Keep MEKINIST dry and away from moisture.
- The bottle of MEKINIST contains a desiccant packet to help keep your medicine dry. Do not throw away the desiccant packet.
- Keep MEKINIST in its original bottle. Do not place tablets in a pill box.
- Safely throw away MEKINIST that is out of date or no longer needed.

Keep MEKINIST and all medicine out of the reach of children.

General information about MEKINIST

Medicines are sometimes prescribed for purposes other than those listed in a Patient Information Leaflet. Do not use MEKINIST for a condition for which it was not prescribed. Do not give MEKINIST to other people, even if they have the same symptoms that you have. It may harm them.

You can ask your healthcare provider or pharmacist for information about MEKINIST that is written for health professionals.

For more information, go to www.MEKINIST.com or call 1-888-825-5249.

What are the ingredients in MEKINIST?

Active ingredient: trametinib

Inactive ingredients:

Tablet Core: mannitol, microcrystalline cellulose, hypromellose, croscarmellose sodium, magnesium stearate (vegetable source), sodium lauryl sulfate, colloidal silicon dioxide. Tablet Coating: hypromellose, titanium dioxide, polyethylene glycol, polysorbate 80 (2-mg tablets), iron oxide yellow (0.5-mg tablets), iron oxide red (2-mg tablets).

This Patient Information has been approved by the U.S. Food and Drug Administration.

MEKINIST is a trademark of GlaxoSmithKline.

GlaxoSmithKline
Research Triangle Park, NC 27709

Issued: May 2013
MKN:1PIL

MEPRON® ℞
(atovaquone)
Suspension

DESCRIPTION

MEPRON (atovaquone) is an antiprotozoal agent. The chemical name of atovaquone is *trans*-2-[4-(4-chlorophenyl)cyclohexyl]-3-hydroxy-1,4-naphthalenedione. Atovaquone is a yellow crystalline solid that is practically insoluble in water. It has a molecular weight of 366.84 and the molecular formula $C_{22}H_{19}ClO_3$. The compound has the following structural formula:

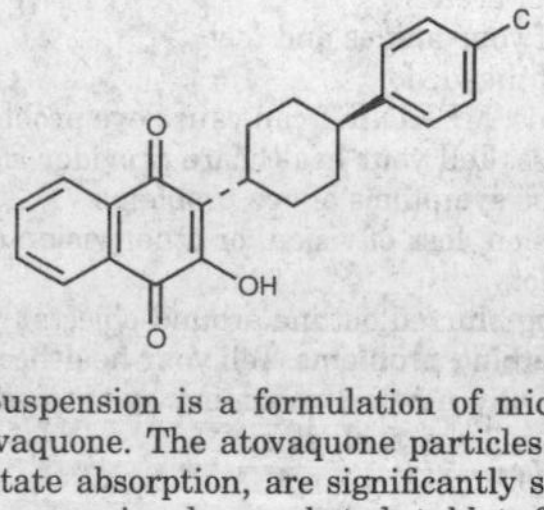

MEPRON Suspension is a formulation of micro-fine particles of atovaquone. The atovaquone particles, reduced in size to facilitate absorption, are significantly smaller than those in the previously marketed tablet formulation. MEPRON Suspension is for oral administration and is bright yellow with a citrus flavor. Each teaspoonful (5 mL) contains 750 mg of atovaquone and the inactive ingredients benzyl alcohol, flavor, poloxamer 188, purified water, saccharin sodium, and xanthan gum.

MICROBIOLOGY

Mechanism of Action

Atovaquone is a hydroxy-1,4-naphthoquinone, an analog of ubiquinone, with antipneumocystis activity. The mechanism of action against *Pneumocystis jiroveci* has not been fully elucidated. In *Plasmodium* species, the site of action appears to be the cytochrome bc_1 complex (Complex III). Several metabolic enzymes are linked to the mitochondrial electron transport chain via ubiquinone. Inhibition of electron transport by atovaquone will result in indirect inhibition of these enzymes. The ultimate metabolic effects of such blockade may include inhibition of nucleic acid and ATP synthesis.

Activity In Vitro

Several laboratories, using different in vitro methodologies, have shown the IC_{50} (50% inhibitory concentration) of atovaquone against rat *P. jiroveci* to be in the range of 0.1 to 3.0 mcg/mL.

Drug Resistance

Phenotypic resistance to atovaquone in vitro has not been demonstrated for *P. jiroveci*. However, in 2 patients who developed *Pneumocystis carinii* pneumonia (PCP) after prophylaxis with atovaquone, DNA sequence analysis identified mutations in the predicted amino acid sequence of *P. jiroveci* cytochrome b (a likely target site for atovaquone). The clinical significance of this is unknown.

CLINICAL PHARMACOLOGY

Pharmacokinetics

Absorption

Atovaquone is a highly lipophilic compound with low aqueous solubility. The bioavailability of atovaquone is highly dependent on formulation and diet. The suspension formulation provides an approximately 2-fold increase in atovaquone bioavailability in the fasting or fed state compared to the previously marketed tablet formulation. The absolute bioavailability of a 750-mg dose of MEPRON Suspension administered under fed conditions in 9 HIV-infected (CD4 >100 cells/mm^3) volunteers was 47% ± 15%. In the same study, the bioavailability of a 750-mg dose of the previously marketed tablet formulation was 23% ± 11%. Administering atovaquone with food enhances its absorption by approximately 2 fold. In one study, 16 healthy volunteers received a single dose of 750 mg MEPRON Suspension after an overnight fast and following a standard breakfast (23 g fat: 610 kCal). The mean (±SD) area under the concentration-time curve (AUC) values were 324 ± 115 and 801 ± 320 hr•mcg/mL under fasting and fed conditions, respectively, representing a 2.6 ± 1.0-fold increase. The effect of food (23 g fat: 400 kCal) on plasma atovaquone concentrations was also evaluated in a multiple-dose, randomized, crossover study in 19 HIV-infected volunteers (CD4 <200 cells/mm^3) receiving daily doses of 500 mg MEPRON Suspension. AUC was 280 ± 114 hr•mcg/mL when atovaquone was administered with food as compared to 169 ± 77 hr•mcg/mL under fasting conditions. Maximum plasma atovaquone concentration (C_{max}) was 15.1 ± 6.1 and 8.8 ± 3.7 mcg/mL when atovaquone was administered with food and under fasting conditions, respectively.

Dose Proportionality

Plasma atovaquone concentrations do not increase proportionally with dose. When MEPRON Suspension was administered with food at dosage regimens of 500 mg once daily, 750 mg once daily, and 1,000 mg once daily, average steady-state plasma atovaquone concentrations were 11.7 ± 4.8, 12.5 ± 5.8, and 13.5 ± 5.1 mcg/mL, respectively. The corresponding C_{max} concentrations were 15.1 ± 6.1, 15.3 ± 7.6, and 16.8 ± 6.4 mcg/mL. When MEPRON Suspension was administered to 5 HIV-infected volunteers at a dose of 750 mg twice daily, the average steady-state plasma atovaquone concentration was 21.0 ± 4.9 mcg/mL and C_{max} was 24.0 ± 5.7 mcg/mL. The minimum plasma atovaquone concentration (C_{min}) associated with the 750-mg twice-daily regimen was 16.7 ± 4.6 mcg/mL.

Distribution

Following the intravenous administration of atovaquone, the volume of distribution at steady state (Vd_{ss}) was 0.60 ± 0.17 L/kg (n = 9). Atovaquone is extensively bound to plasma proteins (99.9%) over the concentration range of 1 to 90 mcg/mL. In 3 HIV-infected children who received 750 mg atovaquone as the tablet formulation 4 times daily for 2 weeks, the cerebrospinal fluid concentrations of atovaquone were 0.04, 0.14, and 0.26 mcg/mL, representing less than 1% of the plasma concentration.

Elimination

The plasma clearance of atovaquone following intravenous (IV) administration in 9 HIV-infected volunteers was 10.4 ± 5.5 mL/min (0.15 ± 0.09 mL/min/kg). The half-life of atovaquone was 62.5 ± 35.3 hours after IV administration and ranged from 67.0 ± 33.4 to 77.6 ± 23.1 hours across studies following administration of MEPRON Suspension. The half-life of atovaquone is long due to presumed enterohepatic cycling and eventual fecal elimination. In a study where ^{14}C-labelled atovaquone was administered to healthy volunteers, greater than 94% of the dose was recovered as unchanged atovaquone in the feces over 21 days. There was little or no excretion of atovaquone in the urine (less than 0.6%). There is indirect evidence that atovaquone may undergo limited metabolism; however, a specific metabolite has not been identified.

Special Populations

Pediatrics

In a study of MEPRON Suspension in 27 HIV-infected, asymptomatic infants and children between 1 month and 13 years of age, the pharmacokinetics of atovaquone were age dependent. These patients were dosed once daily with food for 12 days. The average steady-state plasma atovaquone concentrations in the 24 patients with available concentration data are shown in Table 1.

Table 1. Average Steady-State Plasma Atovaquone Concentrations in Pediatric Patients

	Dose of MEPRON Suspension		
	10 mg/kg	30 mg/kg	45 mg/kg
Age	Average C_{ss} in mcg/mL (mean ± SD)		
1-3 months	5.9 (n = 1)	27.8 ± 5.8 (n = 4)	——
>3-24 months	5.7 ± 5.1 (n = 4)	9.8 ± 3.2 (n = 4)	15.4 ± 6.6 (n = 4)
>2-13 years	16.8 ± 6.4 (n = 4)	37.1 ± 10.9 (n = 3)	——

Hepatic/Renal Impairment

The pharmacokinetics of atovaquone have not been studied in patients with hepatic or renal impairment.

Drug Interactions

Rifampin

In a study with 13 HIV-infected volunteers, the oral administration of rifampin 600 mg every 24 hours with MEPRON Suspension 750 mg every 12 hours resulted in a 52% ± 13% decrease in the average steady-state plasma atovaquone concentration and a 37% ± 42% increase in the average steady-state plasma rifampin concentration. The half-life of atovaquone decreased from 82 ± 36 hours when administered without rifampin to 50 ± 16 hours with rifampin. Rifabutin, another rifamycin, is structurally similar to rifampin and may possibly have some of the same drug interactions as rifampin. No interaction trials have been conducted with MEPRON and rifabutin.

Trimethoprim/Sulfamethoxazole (TMP-SMX)

The possible interaction between atovaquone and TMP-SMX was evaluated in 6 HIV-infected adult volunteers as part of a larger multiple-dose, dose-escalation, and chronic dosing study of MEPRON Suspension. In this crossover study, MEPRON Suspension 500 mg once daily, or TMP-SMX tablets (160 mg trimethoprim and 800 mg sulfamethoxazole) twice daily, or the combination were administered with food to achieve steady state. No difference was observed in the average steady-state plasma atovaquone concentration after coadministration with TMP-SMX. Coadministration of MEPRON with TMP-SMX resulted in a 17% and 8% decrease in average steady-state concentrations of trimethoprim and sulfamethoxazole in plasma, respectively. This effect is minor and would not be expected to produce clinically significant events.

Zidovudine

Data from 14 HIV-infected volunteers who were given atovaquone tablets 750 mg every 12 hours with zidovudine 200 mg every 8 hours showed a 24% ± 12% decrease in zidovudine apparent oral clearance, leading to a 35% ± 23% increase in plasma zidovudine AUC. The glucuronide metabolite:parent ratio decreased from a mean of 4.5 when zidovudine was administered alone to 3.1 when zidovudine was administered with atovaquone tablets. This effect is minor and would not be expected to produce clinically significant events. Zidovudine had no effect on atovaquone pharmacokinetics.

Relationship Between Plasma Atovaquone Concentration and Clinical Outcome

In a comparative study of atovaquone tablets with TMP-SMX for oral treatment of mild-to-moderate *PCP* (see INDICATIONS AND USAGE), where AIDS patients received 750 mg atovaquone tablets 3 times daily for 21 days, the mean steady-state atovaquone concentration was 13.9 ± 6.9 mcg/mL (n = 133). Analysis of these data established a relationship between plasma atovaquone concentration and successful treatment. This is shown in Table 2.

Table 2. Relationship Between Plasma Atovaquone Concentration and Successful Treatment

Steady-State Plasma Atovaquone Concentrations (mcg/mL)	Successful Treatment[a] No. Successes/No. in Group (%) Observed		Predicted[b]	
0 to <5	0/6	(0)	1.5/6	(25)
5 to <10	18/26	(69)	14.7/26	(57)
10 to <15	30/38	(79)	31.9/38	(84)
15 to <20	18/19	(95)	18.1/19	(95)
20 to <25	18/18	(100)	17.8/18	(99)
25+	6/6	(100)	6/6	(100)

[a] Successful treatment was defined as improvement in clinical and respiratory measures persisting at least 4 weeks after cessation of therapy. This was based on data from patients for which both outcome and steady-state plasma atovaquone concentration data are available.

[b] Based on logistic regression analysis.

A dosing regimen of MEPRON Suspension for the treatment of mild-to-moderate PCP has been selected to achieve average plasma atovaquone concentrations of approximately 20 mcg/mL, because this plasma concentration was previously shown to be well tolerated and associated with the highest treatment success rates (Table 2). In an open-label PCP treatment study with MEPRON Suspension, dosing regimens of 1,000 mg once daily, 750 mg twice daily, 1,500 mg once daily, and 1,000 mg twice daily were explored. The average steady-state plasma atovaquone concentration achieved at the 750-mg twice-daily dose given with meals was 22.0 ± 10.1 mcg/mL (n = 18).

INDICATIONS AND USAGE

MEPRON Suspension is indicated for the prevention of *Pneumocystis jiroveci* pneumonia in patients who are intolerant to trimethoprim-sulfamethoxazole (TMP-SMX).

MEPRON Suspension is also indicated for the acute oral treatment of mild-to-moderate PCP in patients who are intolerant to TMP-SMX.

Prevention of PCP

The indication for prevention of PCP is based on the results of 2 clinical trials comparing MEPRON Suspension to dapsone or aerosolized pentamidine in HIV-infected adult and adolescent patients at risk of PCP (CD4 <200 cells/mm^3 or a prior episode of PCP) and intolerant to TMP-SMX.

Dapsone Comparative Study

This randomized, open-label trial enrolled a total of 1,057 patients at 48 study centers. Patients were randomized to receive 1,500 mg MEPRON Suspension once daily (n = 536) or 100 mg dapsone once daily (n = 521). Median follow-up was 24 months. Patients randomized to the dapsone arm who were seropositive for *Toxoplasma gondii* and had a CD4 count <100 cells/mm^3 also received pyrimethamine and folinic acid. PCP event rates are shown in Table 3. There was no significant difference in mortality rates between the groups.

Aerosolized Pentamidine Comparative Study

This randomized, open-label trial enrolled a total of 549 patients at 35 study centers. Patients were randomized to receive 1,500 mg MEPRON Suspension once daily (n = 175), 750 mg MEPRON Suspension once daily (n = 188), or 300 mg aerosolized pentamidine once monthly (n = 186). Median follow-up was 11.3 months. The results of the PCP event rates appear in Table 3. There were no significant differences in mortality rates among the groups.

[See table 3 above]

Table 3. Confirmed or Presumed/Probable PCP Events (As-Treated Analysis)[a]

	Study 115-211		Study 115-213		
Assessment	Atovaquone 1,500 mg/day (n = 527)	Dapsone 100 mg/day (n = 510)	Atovaquone 750 mg/day (n = 188)	Atovaquone 1,500 mg/day (n = 172)	Aerosolized Pentamidine 300 mg/month (n = 169)
%	15	19	23	18	17
Relative Risk[b] (CI)[c]	0.77 (0.57, 1.04)		1.47 (0.86, 2.50)	1.14 (0.63, 2.06)	

[a]Those events occurring during or within 30 days of stopping assigned treatment.
[b]Relative risk <1 favors atovaquone and values >1 favor comparator. These trials were designed to show superiority of atovaquone to the comparator. This was not shown.
[c]The confidence level of the interval for the dapsone comparative study was 95% and for the pentamidine comparative study was 97.5%.
An analysis of all PCP events (intent-to-treat analysis) showed results similar to those above.

Treatment of PCP

The indication for treatment of mild-to-moderate PCP is based on the results of comparative pharmacokinetic studies of the suspension and tablet formulations (see CLINICAL PHARMACOLOGY) and clinical efficacy studies of the tablet formulation which established a relationship between plasma atovaquone concentration and successful treatment. The results of a randomized, double-blind trial comparing MEPRON to TMP-SMX in AIDS patients with mild-to-moderate PCP (defined in the study protocol as an alveolar-arterial oxygen diffusion gradient [(A-a)DO_2][1]≤45 mm Hg and PaO_2≥60 mm Hg on room air) and a randomized trial comparing MEPRON to IV pentamidine isethionate in patients with mild-to-moderate PCP intolerant to trimethoprim or sulfa-antimicrobials are summarized below:

TMP-SMX Comparative Study

This double-blind, randomized trial initiated in 1990 was designed to compare the safety and efficacy of MEPRON to that of TMP-SMX for the treatment of AIDS patients with histologically confirmed PCP. Only patients with mild-to-moderate PCP were eligible for enrollment.

A total of 408 patients were enrolled into the trial at 37 study centers. Eighty-six patients without histologic confirmation of PCP were excluded from the efficacy analyses. Of the 322 patients with histologically confirmed PCP, 160 were randomized to receive MEPRON and 162 to TMP-SMX.

Study participants randomized to treatment with MEPRON were to receive 750 mg MEPRON (three 250-mg tablets) 3 times daily for 21 days and those randomized to TMP-SMX were to receive 320 mg TMP plus 1,600 mg SMX 3 times daily for 21 days.

Therapy success was defined as improvement in clinical and respiratory measures persisting at least 4 weeks after cessation of therapy. Therapy failures included lack of response, treatment discontinuation due to an adverse experience, and unevaluable.

There was a significant difference (*P = 0.03*) in mortality rates between the treatment groups. Among the 322 patients with confirmed PCP, 13 of 160 (8%) patients treated with MEPRON and 4 of 162 (2.5%) patients receiving TMP-SMX died during the 21-day treatment course or 8-week follow-up period. In the intent-to-treat analysis for all 408 randomized patients, there were 16 (8%) deaths in the arm treated with MEPRON and 7 (3.4%) deaths in the TMP-SMX arm (*P* = 0.051). Of the 13 patients treated with MEPRON who died, 4 died of PCP and 5 died with a combination of bacterial infections and PCP; bacterial infections did not appear to be a factor in any of the 4 deaths among TMP-SMX-treated patients.

A correlation between plasma atovaquone concentrations and death was demonstrated; in general, patients with lower plasma concentrations were more likely to die. For those patients for whom day 4 plasma atovaquone concentration data are available, 5 (63%) of the 8 patients with concentrations <5 mcg/mL died during participation in the study. However, only 1 (2.0%) of the 49 patients with day 4 plasma atovaquone concentrations ≥5 mcg/mL died.

Sixty-two percent of patients on MEPRON and 64% of patients on TMP-SMX were classified as protocol-defined therapy successes (Table 4).

[See table 4 above]

Table 4. Outcome of Treatment for PCP-Positive Patients Enrolled in the TMP-SMX Comparative Study

	Number of Patients (% of Total)				
Outcome of Therapy[a]	MEPRON (n = 160)		TMP-SMX (n = 162)		*P* Value
Therapy success	99	(62)	103	(64)	0.75
Therapy failure					
-Lack of response	28	(17)	10	(6)	<0.01
-Adverse experience	11	(7)	33	(20)	<0.01
-Unevaluable	22	(14)	16	(10)	0.28
Required alternate PCP therapy during study	55	(34)	55	(34)	0.95

[a] As defined by the protocol and described in study description above.

The failure rate due to lack of response was significantly larger for patients receiving MEPRON while the failure rate due to adverse experiences was significantly larger for patients receiving TMP-SMX.

There were no significant differences in the effect of either treatment on additional indicators of response (i.e., arterial blood gas measurements, vital signs, serum LDH levels, clinical symptoms, and chest radiographs).

Pentamidine Comparative Study

This unblinded, randomized trial initiated in 1991 was designed to compare the safety and efficacy of MEPRON to that of pentamidine for the treatment of histologically confirmed mild or moderate PCP in AIDS patients. Approximately 80% of the patients either had a history of intolerance to trimethoprim or sulfa-antimicrobials (the primary therapy group) or were experiencing intolerance to TMP-SMX with treatment of an episode of PCP at the time of enrollment in the study (the salvage treatment group).

Patients randomized to MEPRON were to receive 750 mg atovaquone (three 250-mg tablets) 3 times daily for 21 days and those randomized to pentamidine isethionate were to receive a 3- to 4-mg/kg single IV infusion daily for 21 days.

A total of 174 patients were enrolled into the trial at 22 study centers. Thirty-nine patients without histologic confirmation of PCP were excluded from the efficacy analyses. Of the 135 patients with histologically confirmed PCP, 70 were randomized to receive MEPRON and 65 to pentamidine. One hundred and ten (110) of these were in the primary therapy group and 25 were in the salvage therapy group. One patient in the primary therapy group randomized to receive pentamidine did not receive study medication.

There was no difference in mortality rates between the treatment groups. Among the 135 patients with confirmed PCP, 10 of 70 (14%) patients randomized to MEPRON and 9 of 65 (14%) patients randomized to pentamidine died during the 21-day treatment course or 8-week follow-up period. In the intent-to-treat analysis for all randomized patients, there were 11 (12.5%) deaths in the arm treated with MEPRON and 12 (14%) deaths in the pentamidine arm. For those patients for whom day 4 plasma atovaquone concentrations are available, 3 of 5 (60%) patients with concentrations <5 mcg/mL died during participation in the study. However, only 2 of 21 (9%) patients with day 4 plasma concentrations ≥5 mcg/mL died.

The therapeutic outcomes for the 134 patients who received study medication in this trial are presented in Table 5.

[See table 5 above]

Table 5. Outcome of Treatment for PCP-Positive Patients Enrolled in the Pentamidine Comparative Study

	Primary Treatment					Salvage Treatment				
Outcome of Therapy	MEPRON (n = 56)		Pentamidine (n = 53)		*P* Value	MEPRON (n = 14)		Pentamidine (n = 11)		*P* Value
Therapy success	32	(57%)	21	(40%)	0.09	13	(93%)	7	(64%)	0.14
Therapy failure										
-Lack of response	16	(29%)	9	(17%)	0.18	0		0		—
-Adverse experience	2	(3.6%)	19	(36%)	<0.01	0		3	(27%)	0.07
-Unevaluable	6	(11%)	4	(8%)	0.75	1	(7%)	1	(9%)	1.00
Required alternate PCP therapy during study	19	(34%)	29	(55%)	0.04	0		4	(36%)	0.03

CONTRAINDICATIONS

MEPRON Suspension is contraindicated for patients who develop or have a history of potentially life-threatening allergic reactions to any of the components of the formulation.

WARNINGS

Clinical experience with MEPRON for the treatment of PCP has been limited to patients with mild-to-moderate PCP ([(A-a)DO_2][1] ≤45 mm Hg). Treatment of more severe episodes of PCP has not been systematically studied with this agent. Also, the efficacy of MEPRON in patients who are failing therapy with TMP-SMX has not been systematically studied.

PRECAUTIONS

General

Absorption of orally administered MEPRON is limited but can be significantly increased when the drug is taken with food. Plasma atovaquone concentrations have been shown to correlate with the likelihood of successful treatment and survival. Therefore, parenteral therapy with other agents should be considered for patients who have difficulty taking MEPRON with food (see CLINICAL PHARMACOLOGY). Gastrointestinal disorders may limit absorption of orally administered drugs. Patients with these disorders also may not achieve plasma concentrations of atovaquone associated with response to therapy in controlled trials.

Based upon the spectrum of in vitro antimicrobial activity, atovaquone is not effective therapy for concurrent pulmonary conditions such as bacterial, viral, or other fungal pneumonia or mycobacterial diseases. Clinical deterioration in patients may be due to infections with other pathogens, as well as progressive PCP. All patients with acute PCP

Table 6. Treatment-Limiting Adverse Experiences in the Dapsone Comparative PCP Prevention Study

Treatment-Limiting Adverse Experience	Percentage of Patients with Treatment-Limiting Adverse Experience			
	All Patients		Patients Not Taking Either Drug at Enrollment	
	MEPRON 1,500 mg/day (n = 536)	Dapsone 100 mg/day (n = 521)	MEPRON 1,500 mg/day (n = 238)	Dapsone 100 mg/day (n = 249)
Any event	24.4	25.9	20.2	43.4
Rash	6.3	8.8	7.6	16.1
Nausea	4.1	0.6	2.5	0.8
Diarrhea	3.2	0.2	2.1	0.4
Vomiting	2.2	0.6	1.3	0.8
Allergic reaction	1.1	2.9	0.8	4.8
Fever	0.6	2.9	0	5.6
Anemia	0	1.5	0	2.0

Table 7. Treatment-Emergent Adverse Experiences in the Aerosolized Pentamidine Comparative PCP Prevention Study

Treatment-Emergent Adverse Experience	Percentage of Patients with Treatment-Emergent Adverse Experience		
	MEPRON 1,500 mg/day (n = 175)	MEPRON 750 mg/day (n = 188)	Aerosolized Pentamidine (n = 186)
Diarrhea	42	42	35
Rash	39	46	28
Headache	28	31	22
Nausea	26	32	23
Cough increased	25	25	31
Fever	25	31	18
Rhinitis	24	18	17
Asthenia	22	31	31
Infection	22	18	19
Abdominal pain	20	21	20
Dyspnea	15	21	16
Vomiting	15	22	11
Patients discontinuing therapy due to an adverse experience	25	16	7
Patients reporting at least 1 adverse experience	98	96	89

should be carefully evaluated for other possible causes of pulmonary disease and treated with additional agents as appropriate.

Rare cases of hepatitis, elevated liver function tests and one case of fatal liver failure have been reported in patients treated with atovaquone. A causal relationship between atovaquone use and these events could not be established because of numerous confounding medical conditions and concomitant drug therapies. (See ADVERSE REACTIONS.)

If it is necessary to treat patients with severe hepatic impairment, caution is advised and administration should be closely monitored.

Information for Patients

The importance of taking the prescribed dose of MEPRON should be stressed. Patients should be instructed to take their daily doses of MEPRON with meals, as the presence of food will significantly improve the absorption of the drug.

Drug Interactions

Atovaquone is highly bound to plasma protein (>99.9%). Therefore, caution should be used when administering MEPRON concurrently with other highly plasma protein-bound drugs with narrow therapeutic indices, as competition for binding sites may occur. The extent of plasma protein binding of atovaquone in human plasma is not affected by the presence of therapeutic concentrations of phenytoin (15 mcg/mL), nor is the binding of phenytoin affected by the presence of atovaquone.

Rifampin

Coadministration of rifampin and MEPRON Suspension results in a significant decrease in average steady-state plasma atovaquone concentrations (see CLINICAL PHARMACOLOGY: Drug Interactions). Alternatives to rifampin should be considered during the course of PCP treatment with MEPRON.

Rifabutin, another rifamycin, is structurally similar to rifampin and may possibly have some of the same drug interactions as rifampin. No interaction trials have been conducted with MEPRON and rifabutin.

Drug/Laboratory Test Interactions

It is not known if MEPRON interferes with clinical laboratory test or assay results.

Carcinogenesis, Mutagenesis, Impairment of Fertility

Carcinogenicity studies in rats were negative; 24-month studies in mice showed treatment-related increases in incidence of hepatocellular adenoma and hepatocellular carcinoma at all doses tested which ranged from 1.4 to 3.6 times the average steady-state plasma concentrations in humans during acute treatment of *PCP*. Atovaquone was negative with or without metabolic activation in the Ames *Salmonella* mutagenicity assay, the Mouse Lymphoma mutagenesis assay, and the Cultured Human Lymphocyte cytogenetic assay. No evidence of genotoxicity was observed in the in vivo Mouse Micronucleus assay.

Pregnancy

Pregnancy Category C. Atovaquone was not teratogenic and did not cause reproductive toxicity in rats at plasma concentrations up to 2 to 3 times the estimated human exposure. Atovaquone caused maternal toxicity in rabbits at plasma concentrations that were approximately one half the estimated human exposure. Mean fetal body lengths and weights were decreased and there were higher numbers of early resorption and post-implantation loss per dam. It is not clear whether these effects were caused by atovaquone directly or were secondary to maternal toxicity. Concentrations of atovaquone in rabbit fetuses averaged 30% of the concurrent maternal plasma concentrations. In a separate study in rats given a single ^{14}C-radiolabelled dose, concentrations of radiocarbon in rat fetuses were 18% (middle gestation) and 60% (late gestation) of concurrent maternal plasma concentrations. There are no adequate and well-controlled studies in pregnant women. MEPRON should be used during pregnancy only if the potential benefit justifies the potential risk to the fetus.

Nursing Mothers

It is not known whether atovaquone is excreted into human milk. Because many drugs are excreted into human milk, caution should be exercised when MEPRON is administered to a nursing woman. In a rat study, atovaquone concentrations in the milk were 30% of the concurrent atovaquone concentrations in the maternal plasma.

Pediatric Use

Evidence of safety and effectiveness in pediatric patients has not been established. A relationship between plasma atovaquone concentrations and successful treatment of PCP has been established in adults (see Table 2). In a study of MEPRON Suspension in 27 HIV-infected, asymptomatic infants and children between 1 month and 13 years of age, the pharmacokinetics of atovaquone were age-dependent (see CLINICAL PHARMACOLOGY: Special Populations). No drug-related treatment-limiting adverse events were observed in the pharmacokinetic study.

Geriatric Use

Clinical studies of MEPRON did not include sufficient numbers of subjects aged 65 and over to determine whether they respond differently from younger subjects. Other reported clinical experience has not identified differences in responses between the elderly and younger patients. In general, dose selection for an elderly patient should be cautious, reflecting the greater frequency of decreased hepatic, renal, or cardiac function, and of concomitant disease or other drug therapy.

ADVERSE REACTIONS

Because many patients who participated in clinical trials with MEPRON had complications of advanced HIV disease, it was often difficult to distinguish adverse events caused by MEPRON from those caused by underlying medical conditions. There were no life-threatening or fatal adverse experiences caused by MEPRON.

PCP Prevention Studies

In the dapsone comparative study of MEPRON Suspension, adverse experience data were collected only for treatment-limiting events. Among the entire population (n = 1,057), treatment-limiting events occurred at similar frequencies in patients treated with MEPRON Suspension or dapsone (Table 6). Among patients who were taking neither dapsone nor atovaquone at enrollment (n = 487), treatment-limiting events occurred in 43% of patients treated with dapsone and 20% of patients treated with MEPRON Suspension (P <0.001). In both populations, the type of treatment-limiting events differed between the 2 treatment arms. Hypersensitivity reactions (rash, fever, allergic reaction) and anemia were more common in patients treated with dapsone, while gastrointestinal events (nausea, diarrhea, and vomiting) were more common in patients treated with MEPRON Suspension.

[See table 6 above]

Table 7 summarizes the clinical adverse experiences reported by ≥20% of patients in any group in the aerosolized pentamidine comparative study of MEPRON Suspension (n = 549), regardless of attribution. The incidence of adverse experiences at the recommended dose was similar to that seen with aerosolized pentamidine. Rash was the only individual adverse experience that occurred significantly more commonly in patients treated with both dosages of MEPRON Suspension (39% to 46%) than in patients treated with aerosolized pentamidine (28%). Among patients treated with MEPRON Suspension, there was no evidence of a dose-related increase in the incidence of adverse experiences. Treatment-limiting adverse experiences occurred less often in patients treated with aerosolized pentamidine (7%) than in patients treated with 1,500 mg MEPRON Suspension once daily (25%, $P \leq 0.001$) or 750 mg MEPRON Suspension once daily (16%, P = 0.004). The most common adverse experiences requiring discontinuation of dosing in the group receiving 1,500 mg MEPRON Suspension once daily were rash (6%), diarrhea (4%), and nausea (3%). The most common adverse experience requiring discontinuation of dosing in the group receiving aerosolized pentamidine was bronchospasm (2%).

[See table 7 above]

Other events occurring in ≥10% of the patients receiving the recommended dose of MEPRON included sweating, flu syndrome, pain, sinusitis, pruritus, insomnia, depression, and myalgia. Bronchospasm occurred more frequently in patients receiving aerosolized pentamidine (11%) than in patients receiving MEPRON 1,500 mg/day (4%) and MEPRON 750 mg/day (2%).

Neither MEPRON nor aerosolized pentamidine was associated with a substantial change from baseline values in any measured laboratory parameter, nor were there any significant differences in any measured laboratory parameter between MEPRON and aerosolized pentamidine. Some patients had laboratory abnormalities considered serious by the investigator or that contributed to discontinuation of therapy.

PCP Treatment Studies

Table 8 summarizes all the clinical adverse experiences reported by ≥5% of the study population during the TMP-SMX comparative study of MEPRON (n = 408), regardless of attribution. The incidence of adverse experiences with MEPRON Suspension at the recommended dose was similar to that seen with the tablet formulation of atovaquone.

Table 8. Treatment-Emergent Adverse Experiences in the TMP-SMX Comparative PCP Treatment Study

Treatment-Emergent Adverse Experience	Percentage of Patients with Treatment-Emergent Adverse Experience	
	MEPRON (n = 203)	TMP-SMX (n = 205)
Rash (including maculopapular)	23	34
Nausea	21	44
Diarrhea	19	7
Headache	16	22
Vomiting	14	35
Fever	14	25
Insomnia	10	9
Asthenia	8	8
Pruritus	5	9
Monilia, oral	5	10
Abdominal pain	4	7
Constipation	3	17
Dizziness	3	8
Patients discontinuing therapy due to an adverse experience	9	24
Patients reporting at least 1 adverse experience	63	65

Although an equal percentage of patients receiving MEPRON and TMP-SMX reported at least 1 adverse experience, more patients receiving TMP-SMX required discontinuation of therapy due to an adverse event. Twenty-four percent of patients receiving TMP-SMX were prematurely discontinued from therapy due to an adverse experience versus 9% of patients receiving MEPRON. Four percent of patients receiving MEPRON had therapy discontinued due to development of rash. The majority of cases of rash among patients receiving MEPRON were mild and did not require the discontinuation of dosing. The only other clinical adverse experience that led to premature discontinuation of dosing of MEPRON by more than 1 patient was vomiting (<1%). The most common adverse experience requiring discontinuation of dosing in the TMP-SMX group was rash (8%).

Laboratory test abnormalities reported for ≥5% of the study population during the treatment period are summarized in Table 9. Two percent of patients treated with MEPRON and 7% of patients treated with TMP-SMX had therapy prematurely discontinued due to elevations in ALT/AST. In general, patients treated with MEPRON developed fewer abnormalities in measures of hepatocellular function (ALT, AST, alkaline phosphatase) or amylase values than patients treated with TMP-SMX.

Table 9. Treatment-Emergent Laboratory Test Abnormalities in the TMP-SMX Comparative PCP Treatment Study

Laboratory Test Abnormality	Percentage of Patients Developing a Laboratory Test Abnormality	
	MEPRON	TMP-SMX
Anemia (Hgb<8.0 g/dL)	6	7
Neutropenia (ANC<750 cells/mm^3)	3	9
Elevated ALT (>5 × ULN)	6	16
Elevated AST (>5 × ULN)	4	14
Elevated alkaline phosphatase (>2.5 × ULN)	8	6
Elevated amylase (>1.5 × ULN)	7	12
Hyponatremia (<0.96 × LLN)	7	26

ULN = upper limit of normal range.
LLN = lower limit of normal range.

Table 10 summarizes the clinical adverse experiences reported by ≥5% of the primary therapy study population (n = 144) during the comparative trial of MEPRON and intravenous pentamidine, regardless of attribution. A slightly lower percentage of patients who received MEPRON reported occurrence of adverse events than did those who received pentamidine (63% vs 72%). However, only 7% of patients discontinued treatment with MEPRON due to adverse events, while 41% of patients who received pentamidine discontinued treatment for this reason (*P*<0.001). Of the 5 patients who discontinued therapy with MEPRON, 3 reported rash (4%). Rash was not severe in any patient. No other reason for discontinuation of MEPRON was cited more than once. The most frequently cited reasons for discontinuation of pentamidine therapy were hypoglycemia (11%) and vomiting (9%).

Table 10. Treatment-Emergent Adverse Experiences in the Pentamidine Comparative PCP Treatment Study (Primary Therapy Group)

Treatment-Emergent Adverse Experience	Percentage of Patients with Treatment-Emergent Adverse Experience	
	MEPRON (n = 73)	Pentamidine (n = 71)
Fever	40	25
Nausea	22	37
Rash	22	13
Diarrhea	21	31
Insomnia	19	14
Headache	18	28
Vomiting	14	17
Cough	14	1
Abdominal pain	10	11
Pain	10	10
Sweat	10	3
Monilia, oral	10	3
Asthenia	8	14
Dizziness	8	14
Anxiety	7	10
Anorexia	7	10
Sinusitis	7	6
Dyspepsia	5	10
Rhinitis	5	7
Taste perversion	3	13
Hypoglycemia	1	15
Hypotension	1	10
Patients discontinuing therapy due to an adverse experience	7	41
Patients reporting at least 1 adverse experience	63	72

Laboratory test abnormalities reported in ≥5% of patients in the pentamidine comparative study are presented in Table 11. Laboratory abnormality was reported as the reason for discontinuation of treatment in 2 of 73 patients who received MEPRON. One patient (1%) had elevated creatinine and BUN levels and 1 patient (1%) had elevated amylase levels. Laboratory abnormalities were the sole or contributing factor in 14 patients who prematurely discontinued pentamidine therapy. In the 71 patients who received pentamidine, laboratory parameters most frequently reported as reasons for discontinuation were hypoglycemia (11%), elevated creatinine levels (6%), and leukopenia (4%).

Table 11. Treatment-Emergent Laboratory Test Abnormalities in the Pentamidine Comparative PCP Treatment Study

Laboratory Test Abnormality	Percentage of Patients Developing a Laboratory Test Abnormality	
	MEPRON	Pentamidine
Anemia (Hgb<8.0 g/dL)	4	9
Neutropenia (ANC<750 cells/mm^3)	5	9
Hyponatremia (<0.96 × LLN)	10	10
Hyperkalemia (>1.18 × ULN)	0	5
Alkaline phosphatase (>2.5 × ULN)	5	2
Hyperglycemia (>1.8 × ULN)	9	13
Elevated AST (>5 × ULN)	0	5
Elevated amylase (>1.5 × ULN)	8	4
Elevated creatinine (>1.5 × ULN)	0	7

ULN = upper limit of normal range.
LLN = lower limit of normal range.

Postmarketing Experience

In addition to adverse events reported from clinical trials, the following events have been identified during post-approval use of MEPRON. Because they are reported voluntarily from a population of unknown size, estimates of frequency cannot be made. These events have been chosen for inclusion due to a combination of their seriousness, frequency of reporting, or potential causal connection to MEPRON.

Blood and Lymphatic System Disorders

Methemoglobinemia, thrombocytopenia.

Immune System Disorders

Hypersensitivity reactions including angioedema, bronchospasm, throat tightness, and urticaria.

Eye Disorders

Vortex keratopathy.

Gastrointestinal Disorders

Pancreatitis.

Hepatobiliary Disorders

Rare cases of hepatitis, and one case of fatal liver failure have been reported with atovaquone usage.

Skin and Subcutaneous Tissue Disorders
Erythema multiforme, Stevens-Johnson syndrome, and skin desquamation have been reported in patients receiving multiple drug therapy including atovaquone.
Renal and Urinary Disorders
Acute renal impairment.

OVERDOSAGE

There is no known antidote for atovaquone, and it is currently unknown if atovaquone is dialyzable. The median lethal dose is higher than the maximum oral dose tested in mice and rats (1,825 mg/kg/day). Overdoses up to 31,500 mg of atovaquone have been reported. In 1 such patient who also took an unspecified dose of dapsone, methemoglobinemia occurred. Rash has also been reported after overdose.

DOSAGE AND ADMINISTRATION

Dosage

Prevention of PCP: Adults and Adolescents (13 to 16 Years)
The recommended oral dose is 1,500 mg (10 mL) once daily administered with a meal.
Treatment of Mild-to-Moderate PCP: Adults and Adolescents (13 to 16 Years)
The recommended oral dose is 750 mg (5 mL) administered with meals twice daily for 21 days (total daily dose 1,500 mg).
Note: Failure to administer MEPRON Suspension with meals may result in lower plasma atovaquone concentrations and may limit response to therapy (see CLINICAL PHARMACOLOGY and PRECAUTIONS).

Administration

Foil Pouch
Open pouch by removing tab at perforation and tear at notch. Take entire contents by mouth. Can be discharged into a dosing spoon or cup or directly into the mouth.
Bottle
SHAKE BOTTLE GENTLY BEFORE USING.

HOW SUPPLIED

MEPRON Suspension (bright yellow, citrus flavored) containing 750 mg atovaquone in each teaspoonful (5 mL).
Bottle of 210 mL with child-resistant cap (NDC 0173-0665-18).
Store at 15° to 25°C (59° to 77°F). DO NOT FREEZE. Dispense in tight container as defined in USP.
5-mL child-resistant foil pouch - unit dose pack of 42 (NDC 0173-0547-00).
Store at 15° to 25°C (59° to 77°F). DO NOT FREEZE.
[1] $(A\text{-}a)DO_2 = [(713 \times FiO_2) - (PaCO_2/0.8)] - PaO_2$ (mm Hg)
GlaxoSmithKline
Research Triangle Park, NC 27709

March 2013
MPR:2PI

PEDIARIX ℞

[pēd'ē-ə-rix]
[Diphtheria and Tetanus Toxoids and Acellular Pertussis Adsorbed, Hepatitis B (Recombinant) and Inactivated Poliovirus Vaccine]
Suspension for Intramuscular Injection

HIGHLIGHTS OF PRESCRIBING INFORMATION
These highlights do not include all the information needed to use PEDIARIX safely and effectively. See full prescribing information for PEDIARIX.
PEDIARIX [Diphtheria and Tetanus Toxoids and Acellular Pertussis Adsorbed, Hepatitis B (Recombinant) and Inactivated Poliovirus Vaccine]
Suspension for Intramuscular Injection
Initial U.S. Approval: 2002

RECENT MAJOR CHANGES

Warnings and Precautions, Syncope (5.4) 03/2012

INDICATIONS AND USAGE

PEDIARIX is a vaccine indicated for active immunization against diphtheria, tetanus, pertussis, infection caused by all known subtypes of hepatitis B virus, and poliomyelitis. PEDIARIX is approved for use as a three-dose series in infants born of hepatitis B surface antigen (HBsAg)-negative mothers. PEDIARIX may be given as early as 6 weeks of age through 6 years of age (prior to the 7th birthday). (1)

DOSAGE AND ADMINISTRATION

Three doses (0.5 mL each) by intramuscular injection at 2, 4, and 6 months of age. (2.2)

DOSAGE FORMS AND STRENGTHS

Single-dose prefilled syringes containing a 0.5-mL suspension for injection. (3)

CONTRAINDICATIONS

- Severe allergic reaction (e.g., anaphylaxis) after a previous dose of any diphtheria toxoid, tetanus toxoid, pertussis, hepatitis B, or poliovirus-containing vaccine, or to any component of PEDIARIX. (4.1)
- Encephalopathy within 7 days of administration of a previous pertussis-containing vaccine. (4.2)
- Progressive neurologic disorders. (4.3)

WARNINGS AND PRECAUTIONS

- In clinical trials, PEDIARIX was associated with higher rates of fever, relative to separately administered vaccines. (5.1)
- If Guillain-Barré syndrome occurs within 6 weeks of receipt of a prior vaccine containing tetanus toxoid, the decision to give PEDIARIX should be based on potential benefits and risks. (5.2)
- PEDIARIX is available in 2 types of prefilled syringes. One type of prefilled syringe has a tip cap which may contain natural rubber latex. The other type has a tip cap and a rubber plunger which contain dry natural latex rubber. Use of these syringes may cause allergic reactions in latex sensitive individuals. (5.3, 16)
- Syncope (fainting) can occur in association with administration of injectable vaccines, including PEDIARIX. Procedures should be in place to avoid falling injury and to restore cerebral perfusion following syncope. (5.4)
- If specified adverse events (i.e., temperature ≥105°F, collapse or shock-like state, or inconsolable crying lasting ≥3 hours, within 48 hours after vaccination; seizures within 3 days after vaccination) have occurred following a pertussis-containing vaccine, the decision to give PEDIARIX should be based on potential benefits and risks. (5.5)
- For children at higher risk for seizures, an antipyretic may be administered at the time of vaccination with PEDIARIX. (5.6)
- Apnea following intramuscular vaccination has been observed in some infants born prematurely. Decisions about when to administer an intramuscular vaccine, including PEDIARIX, to infants born prematurely should be based on consideration of the individual infant's medical status, and the potential benefits and possible risks of vaccination. (5.7)

ADVERSE REACTIONS

Common solicited adverse events following any dose (≥25%) included local injection site reactions (pain, redness, and swelling), fever (≥100.4°F), drowsiness, irritability/fussiness and loss of appetite. (6.1)
To report SUSPECTED ADVERSE REACTIONS, contact GlaxoSmithKline at 1-888-825-5249 or VAERS at 1-800-822-7967 or www.vaers.hhs.gov

DRUG INTERACTIONS

Do not mix PEDIARIX with any other vaccine in the same syringe or vial. (7.1)
See 17 for PATIENT COUNSELING INFORMATION
Revised: 08/2012

FULL PRESCRIBING INFORMATION: CONTENTS*

*** Sections or subsections omitted from the full prescribing information are not listed**

FULL PRESCRIBING INFORMATION

1 INDICATIONS AND USAGE

PEDIARIX® is indicated for active immunization against diphtheria, tetanus, pertussis, infection caused by all known subtypes of hepatitis B virus, and poliomyelitis. PEDIARIX is approved for use as a three-dose series in infants born of hepatitis B surface antigen (HBsAg)-negative mothers. PEDIARIX may be given as early as 6 weeks of age through 6 years of age (prior to the 7th birthday).

2 DOSAGE AND ADMINISTRATION

2.1 Preparation for Administration

Shake vigorously to obtain a homogeneous, turbid, white suspension. Do not use if resuspension does not occur with vigorous shaking. Parenteral drug products should be inspected visually for particulate matter and discoloration prior to administration, whenever solution and container permit. If either of these conditions exists, the vaccine should not be administered.
Attach a sterile needle and administer intramuscularly.
The preferred administration site is the anterolateral aspect of the thigh for children younger than 1 year. In older children, the deltoid muscle is usually large enough for an intramuscular injection. The vaccine should not be injected in the gluteal area or areas where there may be a major nerve trunk. Gluteal injections may result in suboptimal hepatitis B immune response.
Do not administer this product intravenously, intradermally, or subcutaneously.

2.2 Recommended Dose and Schedule

Immunization with PEDIARIX consists of 3 doses of 0.5 mL each, by intramuscular injection, at 2, 4, and 6 months of age (at intervals of 6 to 8 weeks, preferably 8 weeks). The first dose may be given as early as 6 weeks of age. Three doses of PEDIARIX constitute a primary immunization course for diphtheria, tetanus, pertussis, and poliomyelitis and the complete vaccination course for hepatitis B.

2.3 Modified Schedules in Previously Vaccinated Children

Children Previously Vaccinated With Diphtheria and Tetanus Toxoids and Acellular Pertussis Vaccine Adsorbed (DTaP): PEDIARIX may be used to complete the first 3 doses of the DTaP series in children who have received 1 or 2 doses of INFANRIX® (Diphtheria and Tetanus Toxoids and Acellular Pertussis Vaccine Adsorbed), manufactured by GlaxoSmithKline, identical to the DTaP component of PEDIARIX *[see Description (11)]* and are also scheduled to receive the other vaccine components of PEDIARIX. Data are not available on the safety and effectiveness of using PEDIARIX following one or more doses of a DTaP vaccine from a different manufacturer.
Children Previously Vaccinated With Hepatitis B Vaccine: PEDIARIX may be used to complete the hepatitis B vaccination series following 1 or 2 doses of another hepatitis B vaccine (monovalent or as part of a combination vaccine), including vaccines from other manufacturers, in children born of HBsAg-negative mothers who are also scheduled to receive the other vaccine components of PEDIARIX.
A 3-dose series of PEDIARIX may be administered to infants born of HBsAg-negative mothers and who received a dose of hepatitis B vaccine at or shortly after birth. However, data are limited regarding the safety of PEDIARIX in such infants *[see Adverse Reactions (6.1)]*. There are no data to support the use of a 3-dose series of PEDIARIX in infants who have previously received more than one dose of hepatitis B vaccine.
Children Previously Vaccinated With Inactivated Poliovirus Vaccine (IPV): PEDIARIX may be used to complete the first 3 doses of the IPV series in children who have received 1 or 2 doses of IPV from a different manufacturer and are also scheduled to receive the other vaccine components of PEDIARIX.

2.4 Booster Immunization Following PEDIARIX

Children who have received a 3-dose series with PEDIARIX should complete the DTaP and IPV series according to the recommended schedule.[1] Because the pertussis antigens contained in INFANRIX and KINRIX® (Diphtheria and Tetanus Toxoids and Acellular Pertussis Adsorbed and Inactivated Poliovirus Vaccine), manufactured by GlaxoSmithKline, are the same as those in PEDIARIX, these children should receive INFANRIX as their fourth dose of DTaP and either INFANRIX or KINRIX as their fifth dose of DTaP, according to the respective prescribing information for these vaccines. KINRIX or another manufacturer's IPV may be used to complete the 4-dose IPV series according to the respective prescribing information.

3 DOSAGE FORMS AND STRENGTHS

PEDIARIX is a suspension for injection available in 0.5-mL single-dose prefilled TIP-LOK® syringes.

4 CONTRAINDICATIONS

4.1 Hypersensitivity

A severe allergic reaction (e.g., anaphylaxis) after a previous dose of any diphtheria toxoid-, tetanus toxoid-, pertussis antigen-, hepatitis B-, or poliovirus-containing vaccine or any component of this vaccine, including yeast, neomycin, and polymyxin B, is a contraindication to administration of PEDIARIX *[see Description (11)]*.

4.2 Encephalopathy

Encephalopathy (e.g., coma, decreased level of consciousness, prolonged seizures) within 7 days of administration of a previous dose of a pertussis-containing vaccine that is not attributable to another identifiable cause is a contraindication to administration of any pertussis-containing vaccine, including PEDIARIX.

4.3 Progressive Neurologic Disorder

Progressive neurologic disorder, including infantile spasms, uncontrolled epilepsy, or progressive encephalopathy is a contraindication to administration of any pertussis-containing vaccine, including PEDIARIX. PEDIARIX should not be administered to individuals with such conditions until the neurologic status is clarified and stabilized.

5 WARNINGS AND PRECAUTIONS

5.1 Fever

In clinical trials, administration of PEDIARIX in infants was associated with higher rates of fever, relative to separately administered vaccines *[see Adverse Reactions (6.1)]*.

5.2 Guillain-Barré Syndrome

If Guillain-Barré syndrome occurs within 6 weeks of receipt of a prior vaccine containing tetanus toxoid, the decision to give PEDIARIX or any vaccine containing tetanus toxoid should be based on careful consideration of the potential benefits and possible risks.

5.3 Latex

PEDIARIX is available in 2 types of prefilled syringes. One type of prefilled syringe has a tip cap which may contain natural rubber latex and a plunger which does not contain latex. The other type has a tip cap and a rubber plunger which contain dry natural latex rubber. Use of these syringes may cause allergic reactions in latex sensitive individuals. *[See How Supplied/Storage and Handling (16).]*

5.4 Syncope

Syncope (fainting) can occur in association with administration of injectable vaccines, including PEDIARIX. Syncope can be accompanied by transient neurological signs such as visual disturbance, paresthesia, and tonic- clonic limb movements. Procedures should be in place to avoid falling injury and to restore cerebral perfusion following syncope.

5.5 Adverse Events Following Prior Pertussis Vaccination

If any of the following events occur in temporal relation to receipt of a vaccine containing a pertussis component, the decision to give any pertussis-containing vaccine, including PEDIARIX, should be based on careful consideration of the potential benefits and possible risks:

- Temperature of ≥40.5oC (105oF) within 48 hours not due to another identifiable cause;
- Collapse or shock-like state (hypotonic-hyporesponsive episode) within 48 hours;
- Persistent, inconsolable crying lasting ≥3 hours, occurring within 48 hours;
- Seizures with or without fever occurring within 3 days.

5.6 Children at Risk for Seizures

For children at higher risk for seizures than the general population, an appropriate antipyretic may be administered at the time of vaccination with a vaccine containing a pertussis component, including PEDIARIX, and for the ensuing 24 hours to reduce the possibility of post-vaccination fever.

5.7 Apnea in Premature Infants

Apnea following intramuscular vaccination has been observed in some infants born prematurely. Decisions about when to administer an intramuscular vaccine, including PEDIARIX, to infants born prematurely should be based on consideration of the individual infant's medical status, and the potential benefits and possible risks of vaccination.

5.8 Preventing and Managing Allergic Vaccine Reactions

Prior to administration, the healthcare provider should review the immunization history for possible vaccine sensitivity and previous vaccination-related adverse reactions to allow an assessment of benefits and risks. Epinephrine and other appropriate agents used for the control of immediate allergic reactions must be immediately available should an acute anaphylactic reaction occur.

Table 1. Percentage of Infants With Solicited Local Reactions or General Adverse Events Within 4 Days of Vaccination[a] at 2, 4, and 6 Months of Age With PEDIARIX Administered Concomitantly With Hib Conjugate Vaccine and 7-valent Pneumococcal Conjugate Vaccine (PCV7) or With Separate Concomitant Administration of INFANRIX, ENGERIX-B, IPV, Hib Conjugate Vaccine, and PCV7 (Modified Intent To Treat Cohort)

	PEDIARIX, Hib Vaccine, & PCV7			INFANRIX, ENGERIX-B, IPV, Hib Vaccine, & PCV7		
	Dose 1	**Dose 2**	**Dose 3**	**Dose 1**	**Dose 2**	**Dose 3**
Local[b]						
N	**671**	**653**	**648**	**335**	**323**	**315**
Pain, any	36.1	36.1	31.2	31.9	30.0	29.8
Pain, grade 2 or 3	11.5	10.9	10.6	9.0	8.7	8.9
Pain, grade 3	2.4	2.5	1.7	2.7	1.5	1.3
Redness, any	24.9[c]	37.2	40.1	18.2	32.8	39.0
Redness, >5 mm	6.0[c]	9.6[c]	12.7[c]	1.8	5.9	7.3
Redness, >20 mm	0.9	1.2[c]	2.8	0.3	0.0	1.9
Swelling, any	17.3[c]	26.5[c]	28.7	9.6	20.4	24.8
Swelling, >5 mm	5.8[c]	9.6[c]	9.3[c]	1.8	5.0	4.1
Swelling, >20 mm	1.9	2.5[c]	3.1	0.6	0.0	1.3
General						
N	**667**	**644**	**645**	**333**	**321**	**311**
Fever[d], ≥100.4°F	27.9[c]	38.8[c]	33.5[c]	19.8	30.2	23.8
Fever[d], >101.3°F	7.0	14.1[c]	8.8	4.5	9.7	5.8
Fever[d], >102.2°F	2.2[c]	3.6	3.4	0.3	3.1	2.3
Fever[d], >103.1°F	0.4	1.4	1.1	0.0	0.3	0.3
Fever[d], M.A.	1.2[c]	0.2	0.8	0.0	0.6	0.0
N	**671**	**653**	**648**	**335**	**323**	**315**
Drowsiness, any	57.2	51.6	40.9	54.0	48.3	38.4
Drowsiness, grade 2 or 3	15.8	13.8	11.4	17.6	12.4	11.1
Drowsiness, grade 3	2.5	1.2	0.9	3.6	0.6	1.9
Irritability/Fussiness, any	60.5	64.9	61.1	61.5	61.6	56.5
Irritability/Fussiness, grade 2 or 3	19.8	27.9[c]	25.2[c]	19.4	21.1	19.4
Irritability/Fussiness, grade 3	3.4	4.4	3.5	3.9	3.4	3.2
Loss of appetite, any	30.4	30.6	26.2	27.8	26.6	23.8
Loss of appetite, grade 2 or 3	6.6	7.8[c]	5.9	5.1	3.4	5.4
Loss of appetite, grade 3	0.7	0.3	0.2	0.6	0.3	0.0

Hib conjugate vaccine (Wyeth Pharmaceuticals Inc.; no longer licensed in the US); PCV7 (Wyeth Pharmaceuticals Inc.); IPV (Sanofi Pasteur SA).

Modified intent to treat cohort = all vaccinated subjects for whom safety data were available.

N = number of infants for whom at least one symptom sheet was completed; for fever, numbers exclude missing temperature recordings or tympanic measurements.

M.A. = medically attended (a visit to or from medical personnel).

Grade 2 defined as sufficiently discomforting to interfere with daily activities.

Grade 3 defined as preventing normal daily activities.

[a] Within 4 days of vaccination defined as day of vaccination and the next 3 days.

[b] Local reactions at the injection site for PEDIARIX or INFANRIX.

[c] Rate significantly higher in the group that received PEDIARIX compared to separately administered vaccines [*P* value <0.05 (2-sided Fisher Exact test) or the 95% CI on the difference between groups (Separate minus PEDIARIX) does not include 0].

[d] Axillary temperatures increased by 1°C and oral temperatures increased by 0.5°C to derive equivalent rectal temperature.

6 ADVERSE REACTIONS

6.1 Clinical Trials Experience

Because clinical trials are conducted under widely varying conditions, adverse event rates observed in the clinical trials of a vaccine cannot be directly compared to rates in the clinical trials of another vaccine, and may not reflect the rates observed in practice.

A total of 23,849 doses of PEDIARIX have been administered to 8,088 infants who received one or more doses as part of the 3-dose series during 14 clinical studies. Common adverse events that occurred in ≥25% of subjects following any dose of PEDIARIX included local injection site reactions (pain, redness, and swelling), fever, drowsiness, irritability/fussiness, and loss of appetite. In comparative studies (including the German and US studies described below), administration of PEDIARIX was associated with higher rates of fever relative to separately administered vaccines *[see Warnings and Precautions (5.1)]*. The prevalence of fever was highest on the day of vaccination and the day following vaccination. More than 96% of episodes of fever resolved within the 4-day period following vaccination (i.e., the period including the day of vaccination and the next 3 days).

In the largest of the 14 studies, conducted in Germany, safety data were available for 4,666 infants who received PEDIARIX administered concomitantly at separate sites with 1 of 4 *Haemophilusinfluenzae* type b (Hib) conjugate vaccines (GlaxoSmithKline [licensed in the US only for booster immunization], Wyeth Pharmaceuticals Inc. [no longer licensed in the US], Sanofi Pasteur SA [US-licensed], or Merck & Co, Inc. [US-licensed]) at 3, 4, and 5 months of age and for 768 infants in the control group that received separate US-licensed vaccines (INFANRIX, Hib conjugate vaccine [Sanofi Pasteur SA], and oral poliovirus vaccine [OPV] [Wyeth Pharmaceuticals, Inc.; no longer licensed in the US]). In this study, information on adverse events that occurred within 30 days following vaccination was collected. More than 95% of study participants were white.

In a US study, the safety of PEDIARIX administered to 673 infants was compared to the safety of separately administered INFANRIX, ENGERIX-B® [Hepatitis B Vaccine (Recombinant)], and IPV (Sanofi Pasteur SA) in 335 infants. In both groups, infants received Hib conjugate vaccine (Wyeth Pharmaceuticals Inc.; no longer licensed in the US) and 7-valent pneumococcal conjugate vaccine (Wyeth Pharmaceuticals Inc.) concomitantly at separate sites. All vaccines were administered at 2, 4, and 6 months of age. Data on solicited local reactions and general adverse events were collected by parents using standardized diary cards for 4 consecutive days following each vaccine dose (i.e., day of vaccination and the next 3 days). Telephone follow-up was

Table 2. Percentage of Infants With Seizures (With or Without Fever) Within 8 Days of Vaccination and Medically-Attended Fever Within 4 Days of Vaccination With PEDIARIX Compared With Historical Controls

	PEDIARIX			Historical DTaP Controls			Difference (PEDIARIX–DTaP Controls)
	N	n	% (95% CI)	N	n	% (95% CI)	% (95% CI)
All seizures (with or without fever)							
Dose 1, Days 0-7	40,000	7	0.02 (0.01, 0.04)	39,232	6	0.02 (0.01, 0.03)	0.00 (-0.02, 0.02)
Dose 2, Days 0-7	40,000	3	0.01 (0.00, 0.02)	37,405	4	0.01 (0.00, 0.03)	0.00 (-0.02, 0.01)
Dose 3, Days 0-7	40,000	6	0.02 (0.01, 0.03)	40,000	5	0.01 (0.00, 0.03)	0.00 (-0.01, 0.02)
Total doses	120,000	16	0.01 (0.01, 0.02)	116,637	15	0.01 (0.01, 0.02)	0.00 (-0.01, 0.01)
Medically-attended fever[a]							
Dose 1, Days 0-3	7,500	14	0.19 (0.11, 0.30)	7,500	14	0.19 (0.11, 0.30)	0.00 (-0.14, 0.14)
Dose 2, Days 0-3	7,500	25	0.33 (0.22, 0.48)	7,500	15	0.20 (0.11, 0.33)	0.13 (-0.03, 0.30)
Dose 3, Days 0-3	7,500	21	0.28 (0.17, 0.43)	7,500	19	0.25 (0.15, 0.39)	0.03 (-0.14, 0.19)
Total doses	22,500	60	0.27 (0.20, 0.34)	22,500	48	0.21 (0.16, 0.28)	0.05 (-0.01, 0.14)

DTaP – any US-licensed DTaP vaccine. Infants received 7-valent pneumococcal conjugate vaccine (Wyeth Pharmaceuticals Inc.) concomitantly with each dose of PEDIARIX or DTaP. Other US-licensed vaccines were administered according to routine practices at the study sites.
N = number of subjects in the given cohort.
n = number of subjects with events reported in the given cohort.
[a] Medically-attended fever defined as fever ≥100.4°F that resulted in hospitalization, an emergency department visit, or an outpatient visit.

conducted 1 month and 6 months after the third vaccination to inquire about serious adverse events. At the 6-month follow-up, information also was collected on new onset of chronic illnesses. A total of 638 subjects who received PEDIARIX and 313 subjects who received INFANRIX, ENGERIX-B, and IPV completed the 6-month follow-up. Among subjects in both study groups combined, 69% were white, 18% were Hispanic, 7% were black, 3% were Oriental, and 3% were of other racial/ethnic groups.

Solicited Adverse Events: Data on solicited local reactions and general adverse events from the US safety study are presented in Table 1. This study was powered to evaluate fever >101.3°F following dose 1. The rate of fever ≥100.4°F following each dose was significantly higher in the group that received PEDIARIX compared to separately administered vaccines. Other statistically significant differences between groups in rates of fever, as well as other solicited adverse events, are noted in Table 1. Medical attention (a visit to or from medical personnel) for fever within 4 days following vaccination was sought in the group who received PEDIARIX for 8 infants after the first dose (1.2%), 1 infant following the second dose (0.2%), and 5 infants following the third dose (0.8%) (Table 1). Following dose 2, medical attention for fever was sought for 2 infants (0.6%) who received separately administered vaccines (Table 1). Among infants who had a medical visit for fever within 4 days following vaccination, 9 of 14 who received PEDIARIX and 1 of 2 who received separately administered vaccines, had one or more diagnostic studies performed to evaluate the cause of fever.
[See table 1 at top of previous page]

Serious Adverse Events: Within 30 days following any dose of vaccine in the US safety study in which all subjects received concomitant Hib and pneumococcal conjugate vaccines, 7 serious adverse events were reported in 7 subjects (1% [7/673]) who received PEDIARIX (1 case each of pyrexia, gastroenteritis, and culture negative clinical sepsis and 4 cases of bronchiolitis) and 5 serious adverse events were reported in 4 subjects (1% [4/335]) who received INFANRIX, ENGERIX-B, and IPV (uteropelvic junction obstruction and testicular atrophy in one subject and 3 cases of bronchiolitis).

Deaths: In 14 clinical trials, 5 deaths were reported among 8,088 (0.06%) recipients of PEDIARIX and 1 death was reported among 2,287 (0.04%) recipients of comparator vaccines. Causes of death in the group that received PEDIARIX included 2 cases of Sudden Infant Death Syndrome (SIDS) and one case of each of the following: convulsive disorder, congenital immunodeficiency with sepsis, and neuroblastoma. One case of SIDS was reported in the comparator group. The rate of SIDS among all recipients of PEDIARIX across the 14 trials was 0.25/1,000. The rate of SIDS observed for recipients of PEDIARIX in the German safety study was 0.2/1,000 infants (reported rate of SIDS in Germany in the latter part of the 1990s was 0.7/1,000 newborns). The reported rate of SIDS in the United States from 1990 to 1994 was 1.2/1,000 live births. By chance alone, some cases of SIDS can be expected to follow receipt of pertussis-containing vaccines.

Onset of Chronic Illnesses: In the US safety study in which all subjects received concomitant Hib and pneumococcal conjugate vaccines, 21 subjects (3%) who received PEDIARIX and 14 subjects (4%) who received INFANRIX, ENGERIX-B, and IPV reported new onset of a chronic illness during the period from 1 to 6 months following the last dose of study vaccines. Among the chronic illnesses reported in the subjects who received PEDIARIX, there were 4 cases of asthma and 1 case each of diabetes mellitus and chronic neutropenia. There were 4 cases of asthma in subjects who received INFANRIX, ENGERIX-B, and IPV.

Seizures: In the German safety study over the entire study period, 6 subjects in the group that received PEDIARIX (N = 4,666) reported seizures. Two of these subjects had a febrile seizure, 1 of whom also developed afebrile seizures. The remaining 4 subjects had afebrile seizures, including 2 with infantile spasms. Two subjects reported seizures within 7 days following vaccination (1 subject had both febrile and afebrile seizures, and 1 subject had afebrile seizures), corresponding to a rate of 0.22 seizures per 1,000 doses (febrile seizures 0.07 per 1,000 doses, afebrile seizures 0.14 per 1,000 doses). No subject who received concomitant INFANRIX, Hib vaccine, and OPV (N = 768) reported seizures. In a separate German study that evaluated the safety of INFANRIX in 22,505 infants who received 66,867 doses of INFANRIX administered as a 3-dose primary series, the rate of seizures within 7 days of vaccination with INFANRIX was 0.13 per 1,000 doses (febrile seizures 0.0 per 1,000 doses, afebrile seizures 0.13 per 1,000 doses).

Over the entire study period in the US safety study in which all subjects received concomitant Hib and pneumococcal conjugate vaccines, 4 subjects in the group that received PEDIARIX (N = 673) reported seizures. Three of these subjects had a febrile seizure and 1 had an afebrile seizure. Over the entire study period, 2 subjects in the group that received INFANRIX, ENGERIX-B, and IPV (N = 335) reported febrile seizures. There were no afebrile seizures in this group. No subject in either study group had seizures within 7 days following vaccination.

Other Neurological Events of Interest: No cases of hypotonic-hyporesponsiveness or encephalopathy were reported in either the German or US safety studies.

Safety of PEDIARIX After a Previous Dose of Hepatitis B Vaccine: Limited data are available on the safety of administering PEDIARIX after a previous dose of hepatitis B vaccine. In 2 separate studies, 160 Moldovan infants and 96 US infants, respectively, received 3 doses of PEDIARIX following 1 previous dose of hepatitis B vaccine. Neither study was designed to detect significant differences in rates of adverse events associated with PEDIARIX administered after a previous dose of hepatitis B vaccine compared to PEDIARIX administered without a previous dose of hepatitis B vaccine.

6.2 Postmarketing Safety Surveillance Study

In a safety surveillance study conducted at a health maintenance organization in the US, infants who received one or more doses of PEDIARIX from approximately mid-2003 through mid-2005 were compared to age-, gender-, and area-matched historical controls who received one or more doses of separately administered US-licensed DTaP vaccine from 2002 through approximately mid-2003. Only infants who received 7-valent pneumococcal conjugate vaccine (Wyeth Pharmaceuticals Inc.) concomitantly with PEDIARIX or DTaP vaccine were included in the cohorts. Other US-licensed vaccines were administered according to routine practices at the study sites, but concomitant administration with PEDIARIX or DTaP was not a criterion for inclusion in the cohorts. A birth dose of hepatitis B vaccine had been administered routinely to infants in the historical DTaP control cohort, but not to infants who received PEDIARIX. For each of Doses 1-3, a random sample of 40,000 infants who received PEDIARIX was compared to the historical DTaP control cohort for the incidence of seizures (with or without fever) during the 8-day period following vaccination. For each dose, random samples of 7,500 infants in each cohort were also compared for the incidence of medically-attended fever (fever ≥100.4°F that resulted in hospitalization, an emergency department visit, or an outpatient visit) during the 4-day period following vaccination. Possible seizures and medical visits plausibly related to fever were identified by searching automated inpatient and outpatient data files. Medical record reviews of identified events were conducted to verify the occurrence of seizures or medically-attended fever. The incidence of verified seizures and medically-attended fever from this study are presented in Table 2.
[See table 2 above]

6.3 Postmarketing Spontaneous Reports for PEDIARIX

In addition to reports in clinical trials, worldwide voluntary reports of adverse events received for PEDIARIX since market introduction of this vaccine are listed below. This list includes serious adverse events or events which have a suspected causal connection to components of PEDIARIX. Because these events are reported voluntarily from a population of uncertain size, it is not possible to reliably estimate their frequency or establish a causal relationship to vaccine exposure.

Cardiac Disorders: Cyanosis.

Gastrointestinal Disorders: Diarrhea, vomiting.

General Disorders and Administration Site Conditions: Fatigue, injection site cellulitis, injection site induration, injection site itching, injection site nodule/lump, injection site reaction, injection site vesicles, injection site warmth, limb pain, limb swelling.

Immune System Disorders: Anaphylactic reaction, anaphylactoid reaction, hypersensitivity.

Infections and Infestations: Upper respiratory tract infection.

Investigations: Abnormal liver function tests.

Nervous System Disorders: Bulging fontanelle, depressed level of consciousness, encephalitis, hypotonia, hypotonic-hyporesponsive episode, lethargy, somnolence, syncope.

Psychiatric Disorders: Crying, insomnia, nervousness, restlessness, screaming, unusual crying.

Respiratory, Thoracic, and Mediastinal Disorders: Apnea, cough, dyspnea.

Skin and Subcutaneous Tissue Disorders: Angioedema, erythema, rash, urticaria.

Vascular Disorders: Pallor, petechiae.

6.4 Postmarketing Spontaneous Reports for INFANRIX and/or ENGERIX-B

Worldwide voluntary reports of adverse events received for INFANRIX and/or ENGERIX-B in children younger than 7 years of age but not already reported for PEDIARIX are listed below. This list includes serious adverse events or events which have a suspected causal connection to components of INFANRIX and/or ENGERIX-B. Because these events are reported voluntarily from a population of uncertain size, it is not possible to reliably estimate their frequency or establish a causal relationship to vaccine exposure.

Blood and Lymphatic System Disorders: Idiopathic thrombocytopenic purpura[1,2], lymphadenopathy[1], thrombocytopenia[1,2].

Gastrointestinal Disorders: Abdominal pain[2], intussusception[1,2], nausea[2].

General Disorders and Administration Site Conditions: Asthenia[2], malaise[2].

Hepatobiliary Disorders: Jaundice[2].

Immune System Disorders: Anaphylactic shock[1], serum sickness–like disease[2].

Musculoskeletal and Connective Tissue Disorders: Arthralgia[2], arthritis[2], muscular weakness[2], myalgia[2].
Nervous System Disorders: Encephalopathy[1], headache[1], meningitis[2], neuritis[2], neuropathy[2], paralysis[2].
Skin and Subcutaneous Tissue Disorders: Alopecia[2], erythema multiforme[2], lichen planus[2], pruritus[1,2], Stevens Johnson syndrome[1].
Vascular Disorders: Vasculitis[2].

[1]Following INFANRIX (licensed in the United States in 1997).
[2]Following ENGERIX-B (licensed in the United States in 1989).

7 DRUG INTERACTIONS

7.1 Concomitant Vaccine Administration

Immune responses following concomitant administration of PEDIARIX, Hib conjugate vaccine (Wyeth Pharmaceuticals Inc.; no longer licensed in the US), and 7-valent pneumococcal conjugate vaccine (Wyeth Pharmaceuticals Inc.) were evaluated in a clinical trial *[see Clinical Studies (14.3)]*.
When PEDIARIX is administered concomitantly with other injectable vaccines, they should be given with separate syringes and at different injection sites. PEDIARIX should not be mixed with any other vaccine in the same syringe or vial.

7.2 Immunosuppressive Therapies

Immunosuppressive therapies, including irradiation, antimetabolites, alkylating agents, cytotoxic drugs, and corticosteroids (used in greater than physiologic doses), may reduce the immune response to PEDIARIX.

8 USE IN SPECIFIC POPULATIONS

8.1 Pregnancy

Pregnancy Category C
Animal reproduction studies have not been conducted with PEDIARIX. It is not known whether PEDIARIX can cause fetal harm when administered to a pregnant woman or if PEDIARIX can affect reproduction capacity.

8.4 Pediatric Use

Safety and effectiveness of PEDIARIX were established in the age group 6 weeks through 6 months on the basis of clinical studies *[see Adverse Reactions (6.1) and Clinical Studies (14.1, 14.2)]*. Safety and effectiveness of PEDIARIX in the age group 7 months through 6 years are supported by evidence in infants 6 weeks through 6 months of age. Safety and effectiveness of PEDIARIX in infants younger than 6 weeks of age and children 7 to 16 years of age have not been evaluated.

11 DESCRIPTION

PEDIARIX [Diphtheria and Tetanus Toxoids and Acellular Pertussis Adsorbed, Hepatitis B (Recombinant) and Inactivated Poliovirus Vaccine] is a noninfectious, sterile vaccine for intramuscular administration. Each 0.5-mL dose is formulated to contain 25 Lf of diphtheria toxoid, 10 Lf of tetanus toxoid, 25 mcg of inactivated pertussis toxin (PT), 25 mcg of filamentous hemagglutinin (FHA), 8 mcg of pertactin (69 kiloDalton outer membrane protein), 10 mcg of HBsAg, 40 D-antigen Units (DU) of Type 1 poliovirus (Mahoney), 8 DU of Type 2 poliovirus (MEF-1), and 32 DU of Type 3 poliovirus (Saukett). The diphtheria, tetanus, and pertussis components are the same as those in INFANRIX and KINRIX. The hepatitis B surface antigen is the same as that in ENGERIX-B.
The diphtheria toxin is produced by growing *Corynebacterium diphtheriae* in Fenton medium containing a bovine extract. Tetanus toxin is produced by growing *Clostridium tetani* in a modified Latham medium derived from bovine casein. The bovine materials used in these extracts are sourced from countries which the United States Department of Agriculture (USDA) has determined neither have nor present an undue risk for bovine spongiform encephalopathy (BSE). Both toxins are detoxified with formaldehyde, concentrated by ultrafiltration, and purified by precipitation, dialysis, and sterile filtration.
The acellular pertussis antigens (PT, FHA, and pertactin) are isolated from *Bordetella pertussis* culture grown in modified Stainer-Scholte liquid medium. PT and FHA are isolated from the fermentation broth; pertactin is extracted from the cells by heat treatment and flocculation. The antigens are purified in successive chromatographic and precipitation steps. PT is detoxified using glutaraldehyde and formaldehyde. FHA and pertactin are treated with formaldehyde.
The hepatitis B surface antigen is obtained by culturing genetically engineered *Saccharomycescerevisiae* cells, which carry the surface antigen gene of the hepatitis B virus, in synthetic medium. The surface antigen expressed in the *S. cerevisiae* cells is purified by several physiochemical steps, which include precipitation, ion exchange chromatography, and ultrafiltration.
The inactivated poliovirus component is an enhanced potency component. Each of the 3 strains of poliovirus is individually grown in VERO cells, a continuous line of monkey kidney cells, cultivated on microcarriers. Calf serum and lactalbumin hydrolysate are used during VERO cell culture and/or virus culture. Calf serum is sourced from countries the USDA has determined neither have nor present an undue risk for BSE. After clarification, each viral suspension is purified by ultrafiltration, diafiltration, and successive chromatographic steps, and inactivated with formaldehyde. The 3 purified viral strains are then pooled to form a trivalent concentrate.
Diphtheria and tetanus toxoids and pertussis antigens (inactivated PT, FHA, and pertactin) are individually adsorbed onto aluminum hydroxide. The hepatitis B component is adsorbed onto aluminum phosphate.
Diphtheria and tetanus toxoid potency is determined by measuring the amount of neutralizing antitoxin in previously immunized guinea pigs. The potency of the acellular pertussis component (inactivated PT, FHA, and pertactin) is determined by enzyme-linked immunosorbent assay (ELISA) on sera from previously immunized mice. Potency of the hepatitis B component is established by HBsAg ELISA. The potency of the inactivated poliovirus component is determined by using the D-antigen ELISA and by a poliovirus neutralizing cell culture assay on sera from previously immunized rats.
Each 0.5-mL dose contains aluminum salts as adjuvant (not more than 0.85 mg aluminum by assay) and 4.5 mg of sodium chloride. Each dose also contains ≤100 mcg of residual formaldehyde and ≤100 mcg of polysorbate 80 (Tween 80).
Neomycin sulfate and polymyxin B are used in the poliovirus vaccine manufacturing process and may be present in the final vaccine at ≤0.05 ng neomycin and ≤0.01 ng polymyxin B per dose. The procedures used to manufacture the HBsAg antigen result in a product that contains ≤5% yeast protein.
PEDIARIX is available in 2 types of prefilled syringes. One type of prefilled syringe has a tip cap which may contain natural rubber latex and a plunger which does not contain latex. The other type has a tip cap and a rubber plunger which contain dry natural latex rubber. *[See How Supplied/ Storage and Handling (16).]*
PEDIARIX is formulated without preservatives.

12 CLINICAL PHARMACOLOGY

12.1 Mechanism of Action

Diphtheria: Diphtheria is an acute toxin-mediated infectious disease caused by toxigenic strains of *C. diphtheriae*. Protection against disease is due to the development of neutralizing antibodies to the diphtheria toxin. A serum diphtheria antitoxin level of 0.01 IU/mL is the lowest level giving some degree of protection; a level of 0.1 IU/mL is regarded as protective.[2]
Tetanus: Tetanus is an acute toxin-mediated disease caused by a potent exotoxin released by *C. tetani*. Protection against disease is due to the development of neutralizing antibodies to the tetanus toxin. A serum tetanus antitoxin level of at least 0.01 IU/mL, measured by neutralization assays, is considered the minimum protective level.[3,4] A level ≥0.1 IU/mL is considered protective.[5]
Pertussis: Pertussis (whooping cough) is a disease of the respiratory tract caused by *B. pertussis*. The role of the different components produced by *B. pertussis* in either the pathogenesis of, or the immunity to, pertussis is not well understood. There is no established serological correlate of protection for pertussis.
Hepatitis B: Infection with hepatitis B virus can have serious consequences including acute massive hepatic necrosis and chronic active hepatitis. Chronically infected persons are at increased risk for cirrhosis and hepatocellular carcinoma.
Antibody concentrations ≥10 mIU/mL against HBsAg are recognized as conferring protection against hepatitis B virus infection.[6]
Poliomyelitis: Poliovirus is an enterovirus that belongs to the picornavirus family. Three serotypes of poliovirus have been identified (Types 1, 2, and 3). Poliovirus neutralizing antibodies confer protection against poliomyelitis disease.[7]

13 NONCLINICAL TOXICOLOGY

13.1 Carcinogenesis, Mutagenesis, Impairment of Fertility

PEDIARIX has not been evaluated for carcinogenic or mutagenic potential, or for impairment of fertility.

14 CLINICAL STUDIES

The efficacy of PEDIARIX is based on the immunogenicity of the individual antigens compared to licensed vaccines. Serological correlates of protection exist for the diphtheria, tetanus, hepatitis B, and poliovirus components. The efficacy of the pertussis component, which does not have a well established correlate of protection, was determined in clinical trials of INFANRIX.

14.1 Efficacy of INFANRIX

Efficacy of a 3-dose primary series of INFANRIX has been assessed in 2 clinical studies.
A double-blind, randomized, active Diphtheria and Tetanus Toxoids (DT)-controlled trial conducted in Italy, sponsored by the National Institutes of Health (NIH), assessed the absolute protective efficacy of INFANRIX when administered at 2, 4, and 6 months of age. The population used in the primary analysis of the efficacy of INFANRIX included 4,481 infants vaccinated with INFANRIX and 1,470 DT vaccinees. After 3 doses, the absolute protective efficacy of INFANRIX against WHO-defined typical pertussis (21 days or more of paroxysmal cough with infection confirmed by culture and/or serologic testing) was 84% (95% CI: 76%, 89%). When the definition of pertussis was expanded to include clinically milder disease, with infection confirmed by culture and/or serologic testing, the efficacy of INFANRIX was 71% (95% CI: 60%, 78%) against >7 days of any cough and 73% (95% CI: 63%, 80%) against ≥14 days of any cough. A longer unblinded follow-up period showed that after 3 doses and with no booster dose in the second year of life, the efficacy of INFANRIX against WHO-defined pertussis was 86% (95% CI: 79%, 91%) among children followed to 6 years of age. For details see INFANRIX prescribing information.
A prospective efficacy trial was also conducted in Germany employing a household contact study design. In this study, the protective efficacy of INFANRIX administered to infants at 3, 4, and 5 months of age, against WHO-defined pertussis was 89% (95% CI: 77%, 95%). When the definition of pertussis was expanded to include clinically milder disease, with infection confirmed by culture and/or serologic testing, the efficacy of INFANRIX against ≥7 days of any cough was 67% (95% CI: 52%, 78%) and against ≥7 days of paroxysmal cough was 81% (95% CI: 68%, 89%). For details see INFANRIX prescribing information.

14.2 Immunological Evaluation of PEDIARIX

In a US multicenter study, infants were randomized to 1 of 3 groups: (1) a combination vaccine group that received PEDIARIX concomitantly with Hib conjugate vaccine (Wyeth Pharmaceuticals Inc.; no longer licensed in the US) and US-licensed 7-valent pneumococcal conjugate vaccine (Wyeth Pharmaceuticals Inc.); (2) a separate vaccine group that received US-licensed INFANRIX, ENGERIX-B, and IPV (Sanofi Pasteur SA) concomitantly with the same Hib and pneumococcal conjugate vaccines; and (3) a staggered vaccine group that received PEDIARIX concomitantly with the same Hib conjugate vaccine but with the same pneumococcal conjugate vaccine administered 2 weeks later. The schedule of administration was 2, 4, and 6 months of age. Infants either did not receive a dose of hepatitis B vaccine prior to enrollment or were permitted to receive one dose of hepatitis B vaccine administered at least 30 days prior to enrollment. For the separate vaccine group, ENGERIX-B was not administered at 4 months of age to subjects who received a dose of hepatitis B vaccine prior to enrollment. Among subjects in all 3 vaccine groups combined, 84% were white, 7% were Hispanic, 6% were black, 0.7% were Oriental, and 2.4% were of other racial/ethnic groups.
The immune responses to the pertussis (PT, FHA, and pertactin), diphtheria, tetanus, poliovirus, and hepatitis B antigens were evaluated in sera obtained one month (range 20 to 60 days) after the third dose of PEDIARIX or INFANRIX. Geometric mean antibody concentrations (GMCs) adjusted for pre-vaccination values for PT, FHA, and pertactin and the seroprotection rates for diphtheria, tetanus, and the polioviruses among subjects who received PEDIARIX in the combination vaccine group were shown to be non-inferior to those achieved following separately administered vaccines (Table 3).
Because of differences in the hepatitis B vaccination schedule among subjects in the study, no clinical limit for non-inferiority was pre-defined for the hepatitis B immune response. However, in a previous US study, non-inferiority of PEDIARIX relative to separately administered INFANRIX, ENGERIX-B, and an oral poliovirus vaccine, with respect to the hepatitis B immune response was demonstrated.

Table 3. Antibody Responses Following PEDIARIX as Compared to Separate Concomitant Administration of INFANRIX, ENGERIX-B, and IPV (One Month[a] After Administration of Dose 3) in Infants Vaccinated at 2, 4, and 6 Months of Age When Administered Concomitantly With Hib Conjugate Vaccine and Pneumococcal Conjugate Vaccine (PCV7)

	PEDIARIX, Hib Vaccine, & PCV7	INFANRIX, ENGERIX-B, IPV, Hib Vaccine, & PCV7
	(N = 164-168)	(N = 141-155)
Anti-Diphtheria Toxoid % ≥0.1 IU/mL[b]	99.4	98.7
Anti-Tetanus Toxoid % ≥0.1 IU/mL[b]	100	98.1

Anti-PT		
% VR[c]	98.7	95.1
GMC[b]	48.1	28.6
Anti-FHA		
% VR[c]	98.7	96.5
GMC[b]	111.9	97.6
Anti-Pertactin		
% VR[c]	91.7	95.1
GMC[b]	95.3	80.6
Anti-Polio 1		
% ≥1:8[b,d]	100	100
Anti-Polio 2		
% ≥1:8[b,d]	100	100
Anti-Polio 3		
% ≥1:8[b,d]	100	100
	(N = 114-128)	**(N = 111-121)**
Anti-HBsAg[e]		
% ≥10 mIU/mL[f]	97.7	99.2
GMC (mIU/mL)[f]	1032.1	614.5

Hib conjugate vaccine (Wyeth Pharmaceuticals Inc.; no longer licensed in the US); PCV7 (Wyeth Pharmaceuticals Inc.); IPV (Sanofi Pasteur SA).
Assay methods used: ELISA for anti-diphtheria, anti-tetanus, anti-PT, anti-FHA, anti-pertactin, and anti-HBsAg; micro-neutralization for anti-polio (1, 2, and 3).
VR = vaccine response: In initially seronegative infants, appearance of antibodies (concentration ≥5 EL.U./mL); in initially seropositive infants, at least maintenance of pre-vaccination concentration.
GMC = geometric mean antibody concentration. GMCs are adjusted for pre-vaccination levels.
[a] One month blood sampling, range 20 to 60 days.
[b] Seroprotection rate or GMC for PEDIARIX not inferior to separately administered vaccines [upper limit of 90% CI on GMC ratio (separate vaccine group/combination vaccine group) <1.5 for anti-PT, anti-FHA, and anti-pertactin, and upper limit of 95% CI for the difference in seroprotection rates (separate vaccine group minus combination vaccine group) <10% for diphtheria and tetanus and <5% for the 3 polioviruses]. GMCs are adjusted for pre-vaccination levels.
[c] The upper limit of 95% CI for differences in vaccine response rates (separate vaccine group minus combination group) was 0.31, 1.52, and 9.46 for PT, FHA, and pertactin, respectively. No clinical limit defined for non-inferiority.
[d] Poliovirus neutralizing antibody titer.
[e] Subjects who received a previous dose of hepatitis B vaccine were excluded from the analysis of hepatitis B seroprotection rates and GMCs presented in the table.
[f] No clinical limit defined for non-inferiority.

14.3 Concomitant Vaccine Administration

In a US multicenter study *[see Clinical Studies (14.2)]*, there was no evidence for interference with the immune responses to PEDIARIX when administered concomitantly with 7-valent pneumococcal conjugate vaccine (Wyeth Pharmaceuticals Inc.) relative to 2 weeks prior.

Anti-PRP (Hib polyribosyl-ribitol-phosphate) seroprotection rates and GMCs of pneumococcal antibodies one month (range 20 to 60 days) after the third dose of vaccines for the combination vaccine group and the separate vaccine group from the US multicenter study *[see Clinical Studies (14.2)]*, are presented in Table 4.

Table 4. Anti-PRP Seroprotection Rates and GMCs (mcg/mL) of Pneumococcal Antibodies One Month[a] Following the Third Dose of Hib Conjugate Vaccine and Pneumococcal Conjugate Vaccine (PCV7) Administered Concomitantly With PEDIARIX or With INFANRIX, ENGERIX-B, and IPV

	PEDIARIX, Hib Vaccine, & PCV7	INFANRIX, ENGERIX-B, IPV, Hib Vaccine, & PCV7
	(N = 161-168)	**(N = 146-156)**
	% (95% CI)	**% (95% CI)**
Anti-PRP ≥0.15 mcg/mL	100 (97.8, 100)	99.4 (96.5, 100)
Anti-PRP ≥1.0 mcg/mL	95.8 (91.6, 98.3)	91.0 (85.3, 95.0)
	GMC (95% CI)	**GMC (95% CI)**
Pneumococcal Serotype		
4	1.7 (1.5, 2.0)	2.1 (1.8, 2.4)
6B	0.8 (0.7, 1.0)	0.7 (0.5, 0.9)
9V	1.6 (1.4, 1.8)	1.6 (1.4, 1.9)
14	4.7 (4.0, 5.4)	6.3 (5.4, 7.4)
18C	2.6 (2.3, 3.0)	3.0 (2.5, 3.5)
19F	1.1 (1.0, 1.3)	1.1 (0.9, 1.2)
23F	1.5 (1.2, 1.8)	1.8 (1.5, 2.3)

Hib conjugate vaccine (Wyeth Pharmaceuticals Inc.; no longer licensed in the US); PCV7 (Wyeth Pharmaceuticals Inc.); IPV (Sanofi Pasteur SA).
Assay method used: ELISA for anti-PRP and 7 pneumococcal serotypes.
GMC = geometric mean antibody concentration.
[a] One month blood sampling, range 20 to 60 days.

15 REFERENCES

1. Centers for Disease Control and Prevention. Recommended immunization schedules for persons aged 0-18 years—United States, 2010. *MMWR* 2010;58(51&52).
2. Vitek CR and Wharton M. Diphtheria Toxoid. In: Plotkin SA, Orenstein WA, and Offit PA, eds. *Vaccines*. 5th ed. Saunders;2008:139-156.
3. Wassilak SGF, Roper MH, Kretsinger K, and Orenstein WA. Tetanus Toxoid. In: Plotkin SA, Orenstein WA, and Offit PA, eds. *Vaccines*. 5th ed. Saunders;2008:805-839.
4. Department of Health and Human Services, Food and Drug Administration. Biological products; Bacterial vaccines and toxoids; Implementation of efficacy review; Proposed rule. *Federal Register* December 13, 1985;50(240):51002-51117.
5. Centers for Disease Control and Prevention. General Recommendations on Immunization. Recommendations of the Advisory Committee on Immunization Practices (ACIP). *MMWR* 2006;55(RR-15):1-48.
6. Ambrosch F, Frisch-Niggemeyer W, Kremsner P, et al. Persistence of vaccine-induced antibodies to hepatitis B surface antigen and the need for booster vaccination in adult subjects. *Postgrad Med J* 1987;63(Suppl. 2):129-135.
7. Sutter RW, Pallansch MA, Sawyer LA, et al. Defining surrogate serologic tests with respect to predicting protective vaccine efficacy: Poliovirus vaccination. In: Williams JC, Goldenthal KL, Burns DL, Lewis Jr BP, eds. Combined vaccines and simultaneous administration. Current issues and perspectives. New York, NY: The New York Academy of Sciences; 1995:289-299.

16 HOW SUPPLIED/STORAGE AND HANDLING

PEDIARIX is available in 0.5 mL single-dose disposable prefilled TIP-LOK syringes (packaged without needles):
NDC 58160-811-43 Syringe (tip cap may contain latex; plunger contains no latex) in Package of 10: NDC 58160-811-52
NDC 58160-811-41 Syringe (tip cap and plunger contain latex) in Package of 10: NDC 58160-811-51
Store refrigerated between 2° and 8°C (36° and 46°F). Do not freeze. Discard if the vaccine has been frozen.

17 PATIENT COUNSELING INFORMATION

The parent or guardian should be:
- informed of the potential benefits and risks of immunization with PEDIARIX, and of the importance of completing the immunization series.
- informed about the potential for adverse reactions that have been temporally associated with administration of PEDIARIX or other vaccines containing similar components.
- instructed to report any adverse events to their healthcare provider.
- given the Vaccine Information Statements, which are required by the National Childhood Vaccine Injury Act of 1986 to be given prior to immunization. These materials are available free of charge at the Centers for Disease Control and Prevention (CDC) website (www.cdc.gov/nip).

PEDIARIX, INFANRIX, KINRIX, TIP-LOK, and ENGERIX-B are registered trademarks of GlaxoSmithKline.

Manufactured by **GlaxoSmithKline Biologicals**
Rixensart, Belgium, US License 1617, and
Novartis Vaccines and Diagnostics GmbH
Marburg, Germany, US License 1754

Distributed by **GlaxoSmithKline**
Research Triangle Park, NC 27709

PDX:21PI

POTIGA ℂ
(ezogabine)
Tablets

HIGHLIGHTS OF PRESCRIBING INFORMATION
These highlights do not include all the information needed to use POTIGA safely and effectively. See full prescribing information for POTIGA.
POTIGA (ezogabine) Tablets, CV
Initial U.S. Approval: 2011

INDICATIONS AND USAGE

POTIGA is a potassium channel opener indicated as adjunctive treatment of partial-onset seizures in patients aged 18 years and older. (1)

DOSAGE AND ADMINISTRATION

- Administer in 3 divided doses daily, with or without food. (2)
- The initial dosage should be 100 mg 3 times daily (300 mg per day) for 1 week. (2)
- Titrate to maintenance dosage by increasing the dosage at weekly intervals by no more than 150 mg per day. (2)
- Optimize effective dosage between 200 mg 3 times daily (600 mg per day) to 400 mg 3 times daily (1,200 mg per day). (2)
- In controlled clinical trials, 400 mg 3 times daily (1,200 mg per day) showed limited improvement compared to 300 mg 3 times daily (900 mg per day) with an increase in adverse reactions and discontinuations. (2)
- When discontinuing POTIGA, reduce the dosage gradually over a period of at least 3 weeks. (2, 5.6)
- Dosing adjustments are required for geriatric patients and patients with moderate to severe renal or hepatic impairment (2)

DOSAGE FORMS AND STRENGTHS

Tablets: 50 mg, 200 mg, 300 mg, and 400 mg. (3)

CONTRAINDICATIONS

None. (4)

WARNINGS AND PRECAUTIONS

- Urinary retention: Patients should be carefully monitored for urologic symptoms. (5.1)
- Neuropsychiatric symptoms: Monitor for confusional state, psychotic symptoms, and hallucinations. (5.2)
- Dizziness and somnolence: Monitor for dizziness and somnolence. (5.3)
- QT prolongation: QT interval should be monitored in patients taking concomitant medications known to increase the QT interval or with certain heart conditions. (5.4)
- Suicidal behavior and ideation: Monitor for suicidal thoughts or behaviors. (5.5)

ADVERSE REACTIONS

The most common adverse reactions (incidence ≥4% and approximately twice placebo) are dizziness, somnolence, fatigue, confusional state, vertigo, tremor, abnormal coordination, diplopia, disturbance in attention, memory impairment, asthenia, blurred vision, gait disturbance, aphasia, dysarthria, and balance disorder. (6.1)
To report SUSPECTED ADVERSE REACTIONS, contact GlaxoSmithKline at 1-888-825-5249 or FDA at 1-800-FDA-1088 or www.fda.gov/medwatch.

DRUG INTERACTIONS

- Ezogabine plasma levels may be reduced by concomitant administration of phenytoin or carbamazepine. An increase in dosage of POTIGA should be considered when adding phenytoin or carbamazepine. (7.1)
- N-acetyl metabolite of ezogabine may inhibit renal clearance of digoxin, a P-glycoprotein substrate. Monitor digoxin levels. (7.2)

USE IN SPECIFIC POPULATIONS

- Pregnancy: Based on animal data, may cause fetal harm. Pregnancy registry available. (8.1)
- Pediatric use: Safety and effectiveness in patients under 18 years of age have not been established. (8.4)

See 17 for PATIENT COUNSELING INFORMATION and Medication Guide

Revised: 06/2013

FULL PRESCRIBING INFORMATION: CONTENTS*

FULL PRESCRIBING INFORMATION

1 INDICATIONS AND USAGE

POTIGA™ is indicated as adjunctive treatment of partial-onset seizures in patients aged 18 years and older.

2 DOSAGE AND ADMINISTRATION

The initial dosage should be 100 mg 3 times daily (300 mg per day). The dosage should be increased gradually at weekly intervals by no more than 50 mg 3 times daily (increase in the daily dose of no more than 150 mg per day) up to a maintenance dosage of 200 mg to 400 mg 3 times daily (600 mg to 1,200 mg per day), based on individual patient response and tolerability. This information is summarized in Table 1 under General Dosing. In the controlled clinical trials, 400 mg 3 times daily showed limited evidence of additional improvement in seizure reduction, but an increase in adverse events and discontinuations, compared to the 300 mg 3 times daily dosage. The safety and efficacy of doses greater than 400 mg 3 times daily (1,200 mg per day) have not been examined in controlled trials.

No adjustment in dosage is required for patients with mild renal or hepatic impairment (see General Dosing, Table 1). Dosage adjustment is required in patients with moderate and greater renal or hepatic impairment (see Dosing in Specific Populations, Table 1).

POTIGA should be given orally in 3 equally divided doses daily, with or without food.

POTIGA Tablets should be swallowed whole.

If POTIGA is discontinued, the dosage should be gradually reduced over a period of at least 3 weeks, unless safety concerns require abrupt withdrawal.

[See table 1 above]

Table 1. Dosing Recommendations

Specific Population	Initial Dose	Titration	Maximum Dose
General Dosing			
General population (including patients with mild renal or hepatic impairment)	100 mg 3 times daily (300 mg per day)	Increase by no more than 50 mg 3 times daily, at weekly intervals	400 mg 3 times daily (1,200 mg per day)
Dosing in Specific Populations			
Geriatrics (patients >65 years)	50 mg 3 times daily (150 mg per day)	Increase by no more than 50 mg 3 times daily, at weekly intervals	250 mg 3 times daily (750 mg per day)
Renal impairment (patients with CrCL <50 mL per min or end-stage renal disease on dialysis)	50 mg 3 times daily (150 mg per day)		200 mg 3 times daily (600 mg per day)
Hepatic impairment (patients with Child-Pugh 7-9)	50 mg 3 times daily (150 mg per day)		250 mg 3 times daily (750 mg per day)
Hepatic impairment (patients with Child-Pugh >9)	50 mg 3 times daily (150 mg per day)		200 mg 3 times daily (600 mg per day)

Table 2. Major Neuro-Psychiatric Symptoms in Placebo-Controlled Epilepsy Trials

Adverse Reaction	Number (%) With Adverse Reaction		Number (%) Discontinuing	
	POTIGA (n = 813)	Placebo (n = 427)	POTIGA (n = 813)	Placebo (n = 427)
Confusional state	75 (9%)	11 (3%)	32 (4%)	4 (<1%)
Psychosis	9 (1%)	0	6 (<1%)	0
Hallucinations[a]	14 (2%)	2 (<1%)	6 (<1%)	0

[a]Hallucinations includes visual, auditory, and mixed hallucinations.

3 DOSAGE FORMS AND STRENGTHS

50 mg, purple, round, film-coated tablets debossed with "RTG 50" on one side.

200 mg, yellow, oblong, film-coated tablets debossed with "RTG-200" on one side.

300 mg, green, oblong, film-coated tablets debossed with "RTG-300" on one side.

400 mg, purple, oblong, film-coated tablets debossed with "RTG-400" on one side.

4 CONTRAINDICATIONS

None.

5 WARNINGS AND PRECAUTIONS

5.1 Urinary Retention

POTIGA caused urinary retention in clinical trials. Urinary retention was generally reported within the first 6 months of treatment, but was also observed later. Urinary retention was reported as an adverse event in 29 of 1,365 (approximately 2%) patients treated with POTIGA in the open-label and placebo-controlled epilepsy database *[see Clinical Studies (14)]*. Of these 29 patients, 5 (17%) required catheterization, with post-voiding residuals of up to 1,500 mL. POTIGA was discontinued in 4 patients who required catheterization. Following discontinuation, these 4 patients were able to void spontaneously; however, 1 of the 4 patients continued intermittent self-catheterization. A fifth patient continued treatment with POTIGA and was able to void spontaneously after catheter removal. Hydronephrosis occurred in 2 patients, one of whom had associated renal function impairment that resolved upon discontinuation of POTIGA. Hydronephrosis was not reported in placebo patients.

In the placebo-controlled epilepsy trials, "urinary retention," "urinary hesitation," and "dysuria" were reported in 0.9%, 2.2%, and 2.3% of patients on POTIGA, respectively, and in 0.5%, 0.9%, and 0.7% of patients on placebo, respectively.

Because of the increased risk of urinary retention on POTIGA, urologic symptoms should be carefully monitored. Closer monitoring is recommended for patients who have other risk factors for urinary retention (e.g., benign prostatic hyperplasia [BPH]), patients who are unable to communicate clinical symptoms (e.g., cognitively impaired patients), or patients who use concomitant medications that may affect voiding (e.g., anticholinergics). In these patients, a comprehensive evaluation of urologic symptoms prior to and during treatment with POTIGA may be appropriate.

5.2 Neuro-Psychiatric Symptoms

Confusional state, psychotic symptoms, and hallucinations were reported more frequently as adverse reactions in patients treated with POTIGA than in those treated with placebo in placebo-controlled epilepsy trials (see Table 2). Discontinuations resulting from these reactions were more common in the drug-treated group (see Table 2). These effects were dose-related and generally appeared within the first 8 weeks of treatment. Half of the patients in the controlled trials who discontinued POTIGA due to hallucinations or psychosis required hospitalization. Approximately two-thirds of patients with psychosis in controlled trials had no prior psychiatric history. The psychiatric symptoms in the vast majority of patients in both controlled and open-label trials resolved within 7 days of discontinuation of POTIGA. Rapid titration at greater than the recommended doses appeared to increase the risk of psychosis and hallucinations.

[See table 2 above]

5.3 Dizziness and Somnolence

POTIGA causes dose-related increases in dizziness and somnolence *[see Adverse Reactions (6.1)]*. In placebo-controlled trials in patients with epilepsy, dizziness was reported in 23% of patients treated with POTIGA and 9% of patients treated with placebo. Somnolence was reported in 22% of patients treated with POTIGA and 12% of patients treated with placebo. In these trials 6% of patients on POTIGA and 1.2% on placebo discontinued treatment because of dizziness; 3% of patients on POTIGA and <1.0% on placebo discontinued because of somnolence.

Most of these adverse reactions were mild to moderate in intensity and occurred during the titration phase. For those patients continued on POTIGA, dizziness and somnolence appeared to diminish with continued use.

5.4 QT Interval Effect

A study of cardiac conduction showed that POTIGA produced a mean 7.7-msec QT prolongation in healthy volunteers titrated to 400 mg 3 times daily. The QT-prolonging effect occurred within 3 hours. The QT interval should be monitored when POTIGA is prescribed with medicines known to increase QT interval and in patients with known prolonged QT interval, congestive heart failure, ventricular hypertrophy, hypokalemia, or hypomagnesemia *[see Clinical Pharmacology (12.2)]*.

5.5 Suicidal Behavior and Ideation

Antiepileptic drugs (AEDs), including POTIGA, increase the risk of suicidal thoughts or behavior in patients taking these drugs for any indication. Patients treated with any AED for any indication should be monitored for the emergence or worsening of depression, suicidal thoughts or behavior, and/or any unusual changes in mood or behavior.

Pooled analyses of 199 placebo-controlled clinical trials (mono- and adjunctive-therapy) of 11 different AEDs showed that patients randomized to one of the AEDs had approximately twice the risk (adjusted relative risk 1.8, 95% confidence interval [CI]: 1.2, 2.7) of suicidal thinking or behavior compared to patients randomized to placebo. In these trials, which had a median treatment duration of 12 weeks, the estimated incidence of suicidal behavior or ideation among 27,863 AED-treated patients was 0.43% compared to 0.24% among 16,029 placebo-treated patients, representing an increase of approximately 1 case of suicidal thinking or behavior for every 530 patients treated. There were 4 suicides in drug-treated patients in the trials and none in placebo-treated patients, but the number is too small to allow any conclusion about drug effect on suicide.

The increased risk of suicidal thoughts or behavior with AEDs was observed as early as 1 week after starting treatment with AEDs and persisted for the duration of treatment

Table 3. Risk of Suicidal Thoughts or Behaviors by Indication for Antiepileptic Drugs in the Pooled Analysis

Indication	Placebo Patients With Events per 1,000 Patients	Drug Patients With Events per 1,000 Patients	Relative Risk: Incidence of Events in Drug Patients/ Incidence in Placebo Patients	Risk Difference: Additional Drug Patients With Events per 1,000 Patients
Epilepsy	1.0	3.4	3.5	2.4
Psychiatric	5.7	8.5	1.5	2.9
Other	1.0	1.8	1.9	0.9
Total	2.4	4.3	1.8	1.9

Table 4. Adverse Reaction Incidence in Placebo-Controlled Adjunctive Trials in Adult Patients With Partial Onset Seizures (Adverse reactions in at least 2% of patients treated with POTIGA in any treatment group and numerically more frequent than in the placebo group.)

Body System/Adverse Reaction	Placebo	POTIGA			
		600 mg/day	900 mg/day	1,200 mg/day	All
	(N = 427) %	(N = 281) %	(N = 273) %	(N = 259) %	(N = 813) %
Eye					
Diplopia	2	8	6	7	7
Blurred vision	2	2	4	10	5
Gastrointestinal					
Nausea	5	6	6	9	7
Constipation	1	1	4	5	3
Dyspepsia	2	3	2	3	2
General					
Fatigue	6	16	15	13	15
Asthenia	2	4	6	4	5
Infections and infestations					
Influenza	2	4	1	5	3
Investigations					
Weight increased	1	2	3	3	3
Nervous system					
Dizziness	9	15	23	32	23
Somnolence	12	15	25	27	22
Memory impairment	3	3	6	9	6
Tremor	3	3	10	12	8
Vertigo	2	8	8	9	8
Abnormal coordination	3	5	5	12	7
Disturbance in attention	<1	6	6	7	6
Gait disturbance	1	2	5	6	4
Aphasia	<1	1	3	7	4
Dysarthria	<1	4	2	8	4
Balance disorder	<1	3	3	5	4
Paresthesia	2	3	2	5	3
Amnesia	<1	<1	3	3	2
Dysphasia	<1	1	1	3	2
Psychiatric					
Confusional state	3	4	8	16	9
Anxiety	2	3	2	5	3
Disorientation	<1	<1	<1	5	2
Psychotic disorder	0	0	<1	2	<1
Renal and urinary					
Dysuria	<1	1	2	4	2
Urinary hesitation	<1	2	1	4	2
Hematuria	<1	2	1	2	2
Chromaturia	<1	<1	2	3	2

assessed. Because most trials included in the analysis did not extend beyond 24 weeks, the risk of suicidal thoughts or behavior beyond 24 weeks could not be assessed.

The risk of suicidal thoughts or behavior was generally consistent among drugs in the data analyzed. The finding of increased risk with AEDs of varying mechanism of action and across a range of indications suggests that the risk applies to all AEDs used for any indication. The risk did not vary substantially by age (5 to 100 years) in the clinical trials analyzed.

Table 3 shows absolute and relative risk by indication for all evaluated AEDs.

[See table 3 above]

The relative risk for suicidal thoughts or behavior was higher in clinical trials in patients with epilepsy than in clinical trials in patients with psychiatric or other conditions, but the absolute risk differences were similar for epilepsy and psychiatric indications.

Anyone considering prescribing POTIGA or any other AED must balance this risk with the risk of untreated illness. Epilepsy and many other illnesses for which AEDs are prescribed are themselves associated with morbidity and mortality and an increased risk of suicidal thoughts and behavior. Should suicidal thoughts and behavior emerge during treatment, the prescriber needs to consider whether the emergence of these symptoms in any given patient may be related to the illness being treated.

Patients, their caregivers, and families should be informed that AEDs increase the risk of suicidal thoughts and behavior and should be advised of the need to be alert for the emergence or worsening of the signs and symptoms of depression; any unusual changes in mood or behavior; or the emergence of suicidal thoughts, behavior, or thoughts about self-harm. Behaviors of concern should be reported immediately to healthcare providers.

5.6 Withdrawal Seizures

As with all AEDs, when POTIGA is discontinued, it should be withdrawn gradually when possible to minimize the potential of increased seizure frequency *[see Dosage and Administration (2)]*. The dosage of POTIGA should be reduced over a period of at least 3 weeks, unless safety concerns require abrupt withdrawal.

6 ADVERSE REACTIONS

The following adverse reactions are described in more detail in the *Warnings and Precautions* section of the label:

- Urinary retention *[see Warnings and Precautions (5.1)]*
- Neuro-psychiatric symptoms *[see Warnings and Precautions (5.2)]*
- Dizziness and somnolence *[see Warnings and Precautions (5.3)]*
- QT interval effect *[see Warnings and Precautions (5.4)]*
- Suicidal behavior and ideation *[see Warnings and Precautions (5.5)]*
- Withdrawal seizures *[see Warnings and Precautions (5.6)]*

6.1 Clinical Trials Experience

Because clinical trials are conducted under widely varying conditions and for varying durations, adverse reaction frequencies observed in the clinical trials of a drug cannot be directly compared with frequencies in the clinical trials of another drug and may not reflect the frequencies observed in practice.

POTIGA was administered as adjunctive therapy to 1,365 patients with epilepsy in all controlled and uncontrolled clinical studies during the premarketing development. A total of 801 patients were treated for at least 6 months, 585 patients were treated for 1 year or longer, and 311 patients were treated for at least 2 years.

Adverse Reactions Leading to Discontinuation in All Controlled Clinical Studies: In the 3 randomized, double-blind, placebo-controlled studies, 199 of 813 patients (25%) receiving POTIGA and 45 of 427 patients (11%) receiving placebo discontinued treatment because of adverse reactions. The most common adverse reactions leading to withdrawal in patients receiving POTIGA were dizziness (6%), confusional state (4%), fatigue (3%), and somnolence (3%).

Common Adverse Reactions in All Controlled Clinical Studies: Overall, the most frequently reported adverse reactions in patients receiving POTIGA (≥4% and occurring approximately twice the placebo rate) were dizziness (23%), somnolence (22%), fatigue (15%), confusional state (9%), vertigo (8%), tremor (8%), abnormal coordination (7%), diplopia (7%), disturbance in attention (6%), memory impairment (6%), asthenia (5%), blurred vision (5%), gait disturbance (4%), aphasia (4%), dysarthria (4%), and balance disorder (4%). In most cases the reactions were of mild or moderate intensity.

[See table 4 above]

Other adverse reactions reported in these 3 studies in <2% of patients treated with POTIGA and numerically greater than placebo were increased appetite, hallucinations, myoclonus, peripheral edema, hypokinesia, dry mouth, dysphagia, hyperhydrosis, urinary retention, malaise, and increased liver enzymes.

Most of the adverse reactions appear to be dose related (especially those classified as psychiatric and nervous system symptoms), including dizziness, somnolence, confusional state, tremor, abnormal coordination, memory impairment, blurred vision, gait disturbance, aphasia, balance disorder, constipation, dysuria, and chromaturia.

POTIGA was associated with dose-related weight gain, with mean weight increasing by 0.2 kg, 1.2 kg, 1.6 kg, and 2.7 kg in the placebo, 600 mg per day, 900 mg per day, and 1,200 mg per day groups, respectively.

Additional Adverse Reactions Observed During All Phase 2 and 3 Clinical Trials: Following is a list of adverse reactions reported by patients treated with POTIGA during all clinical trials: rash, nystagmus, dyspnea, leukopenia, muscle spasms, alopecia, nephrolithiasis, syncope, neutropenia, thrombocytopenia, euphoric mood, renal colic, coma, encephalopathy.

Comparison of Gender, Age, and Race: The overall adverse reaction profile of POTIGA was similar for females and males.

There are insufficient data to support meaningful analyses of adverse reactions by age or race. Approximately 86% of the population studied was Caucasian, and 0.8% of the population was older than 65 years.

7 DRUG INTERACTIONS

7.1 Antiepileptic Drugs

The potentially significant interactions between POTIGA and concomitant AEDs are summarized in Table 5.

[See table 5 at top of next page]

7.2 Digoxin

Data from an *in vitro* study showed that the N-acetyl metabolite of ezogabine (NAMR) inhibited P-glycoprotein–mediated transport of digoxin in a concentration-dependent manner, indicating that NAMR may inhibit renal clearance of digoxin. Administration of POTIGA at therapeutic doses may increase digoxin serum concentrations. Serum levels of digoxin should be monitored *[see Clinical Pharmacology (12.3)]*.

7.3 Alcohol
Alcohol increased systemic exposure to POTIGA. Patients should be advised of possible worsening of ezogabine's general dose-related adverse reactions if they take POTIGA with alcohol *[see Clinical Pharmacology (12.3)]*.

7.4 Laboratory Tests
Ezogabine has been shown to interfere with clinical laboratory assays of both serum and urine bilirubin, which can result in falsely elevated readings.

8 USE IN SPECIFIC POPULATIONS

8.1 Pregnancy
Pregnancy Category C. There are no adequate and well-controlled studies in pregnant women. POTIGA should be used during pregnancy only if the potential benefit justifies the potential risk to the fetus.

In animal studies, doses associated with maternal plasma exposures (AUC) to ezogabine and its major circulating metabolite, NAMR, similar to or below those expected in humans at the maximum recommended human dose (MRHD) of 1,200 mg per day produced developmental toxicity when administered to pregnant rats and rabbits. The maximum doses evaluated were limited by maternal toxicity (acute neurotoxicity).

Treatment of pregnant rats with ezogabine (oral doses of up to 46 mg/kg/day) throughout organogenesis increased the incidences of fetal skeletal variations. The no-effect dose for embryo-fetal toxicity in rats (21 mg/kg/day) was associated with maternal plasma exposures (AUC) to ezogabine and NAMR less than those in humans at the MRHD. Treatment of pregnant rabbits with ezogabine (oral doses of up to 60 mg/kg/day) throughout organogenesis resulted in decreased fetal body weights and increased incidences of fetal skeletal variations. The no-effect dose for embryo-fetal toxicity in rabbits (12 mg/kg/day) was associated with maternal plasma exposures to ezogabine and NAMR less than those in humans at the MRHD.

Administration of ezogabine (oral doses of up to 61.9 mg/kg/day) to rats throughout pregnancy and lactation resulted in increased pre- and postnatal mortality, decreased body weight gain, and delayed reflex development in the offspring. The no-effect dose for pre- and postnatal developmental effects in rats (17.8 mg/kg/day) was associated with maternal plasma exposures to ezogabine and NAMR less than those in humans at the MRHD.

Pregnancy Registry: To provide information regarding the effects of *in utero* exposure to POTIGA, physicians are advised to recommend that pregnant patients taking POTIGA enroll in the North American Antiepileptic Drug (NAAED) Pregnancy Registry. This can be done by calling the toll-free number 1-888-233-2334, and must be done by patients themselves. Information on the registry can also be found at the website www.aedpregnancyregistry.org.

8.2 Labor and Delivery
The effects of POTIGA on labor and delivery in humans are unknown.

8.3 Nursing Mothers
It is not known whether ezogabine is excreted in human milk. However, ezogabine and/or its metabolites are present in the milk of lactating rats. Because of the potential for serious adverse reactions in nursing infants from POTIGA, a decision should be made whether to discontinue nursing or to discontinue the drug, taking into account the importance of the drug to the mother.

8.4 Pediatric Use
The safety and effectiveness of POTIGA in patients under 18 years of age have not been established.

In juvenile animal studies, increased sensitivity to acute neurotoxicity and urinary bladder toxicity was observed in young rats compared to adults. In studies in which rats were dosed starting on postnatal day 7, ezogabine-related mortality, clinical signs of neurotoxicity, and renal and urinary tract toxicities were observed at doses ≥2 mg/kg/day. The no-effect level was associated with plasma ezogabine exposures (AUC) less than those expected in human adults at the MRHD of 1,200 mg per day. In studies in which dosing began on postnatal day 28, acute central nervous system effects, but no apparent renal or urinary tract effects, were observed at doses of up to 30 mg/kg/day. These doses were associated with plasma ezogabine exposures less than those achieved clinically at the MRHD.

8.5 Geriatric Use
There were insufficient numbers of elderly patients enrolled in partial-onset seizure controlled trials (n = 8 patients on ezogabine) to determine the safety and efficacy of POTIGA in this population. Dosage adjustment is recommended in patients aged 65 years and older *[see Dosage and Administration (2), Clinical Pharmacology (12.3)]*.

POTIGA may cause urinary retention. Elderly men with symptomatic BPH may be at increased risk for urinary retention.

8.6 Patients With Renal Impairment
Dosage adjustment is recommended for patients with creatinine clearance <50 mL/min or patients with end-stage renal disease (ESRD) receiving dialysis treatments *[see Dosage and Administration (2), Clinical Pharmacology (12.3)]*.

8.7 Patients With Hepatic Impairment
No dosage adjustment is required for patients with mild hepatic impairment.

In patients with moderate or severe hepatic impairment, the initial and maintenance dosage of POTIGA should be reduced *[see Dosage and Administration (2), Clinical Pharmacology (12.3)]*.

Table 5. Significant Interactions Between POTIGA and Concomitant Antiepileptic Drugs

AED	Dose of AED (mg/day)	Dose of POTIGA (mg/day)	Influence of POTIGA on AED	Influence of AED on POTIGA	Dosage Adjustment
Carbamazepine[a,b]	600-2,400	300-1,200	None	31% decrease in AUC, 23% decrease in C_{max}	consider an increase in dosage of POTIGA when adding carbamazepine[c]
Phenytoin[a,b]	120-600	300-1,200	None	34% decrease in AUC, 18% decrease in C_{max}	consider an increase in dosage of POTIGA when adding phenytoin[c]

[a] Based on results of a Phase 2 study.
[b] Inducer for uridine 5′-diphosphate (UDP)-glucuronyltransferases (UGTs).
[c] A decrease in dosage of POTIGA should be considered when carbamazepine or phenytoin is discontinued.
[See Clinical Pharmacology (12.3)]

9 DRUG ABUSE AND DEPENDENCE

9.1 Controlled Substance
POTIGA is a Schedule V controlled substance.

9.2 Abuse
A human abuse potential study was conducted in recreational sedative-hypnotic abusers (n = 36) in which single oral doses of ezogabine (300 mg [n = 33], 600 mg [n = 34], 900 mg [n =6]), the sedative-hypnotic alprazolam (1.5 mg and 3.0 mg), and placebo were administered. Euphoria-type subjective responses to the 300-mg and 600-mg doses of ezogabine were statistically different from placebo but statistically indistinguishable from those produced by either dose of alprazolam. Adverse events reported following administration of single oral doses of 300 mg, 600 mg, and 900 mg ezogabine given without titration included euphoric mood (18%, 21%, and 33%, respectively; 8% from placebo), hallucination (0%, 0%, and 17%, respectively; 0% from placebo) and somnolence (18%, 15%, and 67%, respectively; 15% from placebo).

In Phase 1 clinical studies, healthy individuals who received oral ezogabine (200 mg to 1,650 mg) reported euphoria (8.5%), feeling drunk (5.5%), hallucination (5.1%), disorientation (1.7%), and feeling abnormal (1.5%).

In the 3 randomized, double-blind, placebo-controlled Phase 2 and 3 clinical studies, patients with partial seizures who received oral ezogabine (300 mg to 1,200 mg) reported euphoric mood (0.5%) and feeling drunk (0.9%), while those who received placebo did not report either adverse event (0%).

9.3 Dependence
In a 28-day physical dependence study in which rats received daily ezogabine administration, abrupt drug discontinuation produced behavioral changes that included piloerection, increases in high step gait, and tremors, compared to vehicle-treated animals. These data show that ezogabine produces a withdrawal syndrome indicative of physical dependence.

10 OVERDOSAGE

10.1 Signs, Symptoms, and Laboratory Findings
There is limited experience of overdose with POTIGA. Total daily doses of POTIGA over 2,500 mg were reported during clinical trials. In addition to adverse reactions seen at therapeutic doses, symptoms reported with POTIGA overdose included agitation, aggressive behavior, and irritability. There were no reported sequelae.

In an abuse potential study, cardiac arrhythmia (asystole or ventricular tachycardia) occurred in 2 volunteers within 3 hours of receiving a single 900-mg dose of POTIGA. The arrhythmias spontaneously resolved and both volunteers recovered without sequelae.

10.2 Management of Overdose
There is no specific antidote for overdose with POTIGA. In the event of overdose, standard medical practice for the management of any overdose should be used. An adequate airway, oxygenation, and ventilation should be ensured; monitoring of cardiac rhythm and vital sign measurement is recommended. A certified poison control center should be contacted for updated information on the management of overdose with POTIGA.

11 DESCRIPTION
The chemical name of ezogabine is N-[2-amino-4-(4-fluorobenzylamino)-phenyl] carbamic acid ethyl ester, and it has the following structure:

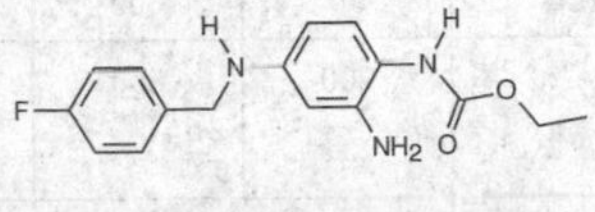

The empirical formula is $C_{16}H_{18}FN_3O_2$, representing a molecular weight of 303.3. Ezogabine is a white to slightly colored, odorless, tasteless, crystalline powder. At room temperature, ezogabine is practically insoluble in aqueous media at pH values above 4, while the solubility is higher in polar organic solvents. At gastric pH, ezogabine is sparingly soluble in water (about 16 g/L). The pKa is approximately 3.7 (basic).

POTIGA is supplied for oral administration as 50-mg, 200-mg, 300-mg, and 400-mg film-coated immediate-release tablets. Each tablet contains the labeled amount of ezogabine and the following inactive ingredients: carmine (50-mg and 400-mg tablets), croscarmellose sodium, FD&C Blue No. 2 (50-mg, 300-mg, and 400-mg tablets), hypromellose, iron oxide yellow (200–mg and 300-mg tablets), lecithin, magnesium stearate, microcrystalline cellulose, polyvinyl alcohol, talc, titanium dioxide, and xanthan gum.

12 CLINICAL PHARMACOLOGY

12.1 Mechanism of Action
The mechanism by which ezogabine exerts its therapeutic effects has not been fully elucidated. *In vitro* studies indicate that ezogabine enhances transmembrane potassium currents mediated by the KCNQ (Kv7.2 to 7.5) family of ion channels. By activating KCNQ channels, ezogabine is thought to stabilize the resting membrane potential and reduce brain excitability. *In vitro* studies suggest that ezogabine may also exert therapeutic effects through augmentation of GABA-mediated currents.

12.2 Pharmacodynamics
The QTc prolongation risk of POTIGA was evaluated in healthy subjects. In a randomized, double-blind, active- and placebo-controlled parallel-group study, 120 healthy subjects (40 in each group) were administered POTIGA titrated up to the final dose of 400 mg 3 times daily, placebo, and placebo and moxifloxacin (on day 22). After 22 days of dosing, the maximum mean (upper 1-sided, 95% CI) increase of baseline- and placebo-adjusted QTc interval based on Fridericia correction method (QTcF) was 7.7 msec (11.9 msec) and was observed at 3 hours after dosing in subjects who achieved 1,200 mg per day. No effects on heart rate, PR, or QRS intervals were noted.

Patients who are prescribed POTIGA with medicines known to increase QT interval or who have known prolonged QT interval, congestive heart failure, ventricular hypertrophy, hypokalemia, or hypomagnesemia should be observed closely *[see Warnings and Precautions (5.4)]*.

12.3 Pharmacokinetics
The pharmacokinetic profile is approximately linear in daily doses between 600 mg and 1,200 mg in patients with epilepsy, with no unexpected accumulation following repeated administration. The pharmacokinetics of ezogabine are similar in healthy volunteers and patients with epilepsy.

Absorption: After both single and multiple oral doses, ezogabine is rapidly absorbed with median time to maximum plasma concentration (T_{max}) values generally between 0.5 and 2 hours. Absolute oral bioavailability of ezogabine relative to an intravenous dose of ezogabine is approximately 60%. High-fat food does not affect the extent to which ezogabine is absorbed based on plasma AUC values, but it increases peak concentration (C_{max}) by approximately 38% and delays T_{max} by 0.75 hour.

POTIGA can be taken with or without food.

Distribution: Data from *in vitro* studies indicate that ezogabine and NAMR are approximately 80% and 45% bound to plasma protein, respectively. Clinically significant interactions with other drugs through displacement from proteins are not anticipated. The steady-state volume of dis-

Table 6. Interactions Between POTIGA and Concomitant Antiepileptic Drugs

AED	Dose of AED (mg/day)	Dose of POTIGA (mg/day)	Influence of POTIGA on AED	Influence of AED on POTIGA	Dosage Adjustment
Carbamazepine[a,b]	600-2,400	300-1,200	None	31% decrease in AUC, 23% decrease in C_{max}, 28% increase in clearance	consider an increase in dosage of POTIGA when adding carbamazepine[c]
Phenytoin[a,b]	120-600	300-1,200	None	34% decrease in AUC, 18% decrease in C_{max}, 33% increase in clearance	consider an increase in dosage of POTIGA when adding phenytoin[c]
Topiramate[a]	250-1,200	300-1,200	None	None	None
Valproate[a]	750-2,250	300-1,200	None	None	None
Phenobarbital	90	600	None	None	None
Lamotrigine	200	600	18% decrease in AUC, 22% increase in clearance	None	None
Others[d]			None	None	None

[a]Based on results of a Phase 2 study.
[b]Inducer for uridine 5′-diphosphate (UDP)-glucuronyltransferases (UGTs).
[c]A decrease in dose of POTIGA should be considered when carbamazepine or phenytoin is discontinued.
[d]Zonisamide, valproic acid, clonazepam, gabapentin, levetiracetam, oxcarbazepine, phenobarbital, pregabalin, topiramate, clobazam, and lamotrigine, based on a population pharmacokinetic analysis using pooled data from Phase 3 clinical trials.

tribution of ezogabine is 2 to 3 L/kg following intravenous dosing, suggesting that ezogabine is well distributed in the body.

Metabolism: Ezogabine is extensively metabolized primarily via glucuronidation and acetylation in humans. A substantial fraction of the ezogabine dose is converted to inactive N-glucuronides, the predominant circulating metabolites in humans. Ezogabine is also metabolized to NAMR that is also subsequently glucuronidated. NAMR has antiepileptic activity, but it is less potent than ezogabine in animal seizure models. Additional minor metabolites of ezogabine are an N-glucoside of ezogabine and a cyclized metabolite believed to be formed from NAMR. *In vitro* studies using human biomaterials showed that the N-acetylation of ezogabine was primarily carried out by NAT2, while glucuronidation was primarily carried out by UGT1A4, with contributions by UGT1A1, UGT1A3, and UGT1A9.

In vitro studies showed no evidence of oxidative metabolism of ezogabine or NAMR by cytochrome P450 enzymes. Coadministration of ezogabine with medications that are inhibitors or inducers of cytochrome P450 enzymes is therefore unlikely to affect the pharmacokinetics of ezogabine or NAMR.

Elimination: Results of a mass balance study suggest that renal excretion is the major route of elimination for ezogabine and NAMR. About 85% of the dose was recovered in the urine, with the unchanged parent drug and NAMR accounting for 36% and 18% of the administered dose, respectively, and the total N-glucuronides of ezogabine and NAMR accounting for 24% of the administered dose. Approximately 14% of the radioactivity was recovered in the feces, with unchanged ezogabine accounting for 3% of the total dose. Average total recovery in both urine and feces within 240 hours after dosing is approximately 98%.

Ezogabine and its N-acetyl metabolite have similar elimination half-lives ($t_{1/2}$) of 7 to 11 hours. The clearance of ezogabine following intravenous dosing was approximately 0.4 to 0.6 L/hr/kg. Ezogabine is actively secreted into the urine.

Specific Populations: *Race:* No study has been conducted to investigate the impact of race on pharmacokinetics of ezogabine. A population pharmacokinetic analysis comparing Caucasians and non-Caucasians (predominately African American and Hispanic patients) showed no significant pharmacokinetic difference. No adjustment of the ezogabine dose for race is recommended.

Gender: The impact of gender on the pharmacokinetics of ezogabine was examined following a single dose of POTIGA to healthy young (aged 21 to 40 years) and elderly (aged 66 to 82 years) subjects. The AUC values were approximately 20% higher in young females compared to young males and approximately 30% higher in elderly females compared to elderly males. The C_{max} values were approximately 50% higher in young females compared to young males and approximately 100% higher in elderly females compared to elderly males. There was no gender difference in weight-normalized clearance. Overall, no adjustment of the dosage of POTIGA is recommended based on gender.

Pediatric Patients: The pharmacokinetics of ezogabine in pediatric patients have not been investigated.

Geriatric: The impact of age on the pharmacokinetics of ezogabine was examined following a single dose of ezogabine to healthy young (aged 21 to 40 years) and elderly (aged 66 to 82 years) subjects. Systemic exposure (AUC) of ezogabine was approximately 40% to 50% higher and terminal half-life was prolonged by approximately 30% in the elderly compared to the younger subjects. The peak concentration (C_{max}) was similar to that observed in younger subjects. A dosage reduction in the elderly is recommended *[see Dosage and Administration (2), Use in Specific Populations (8.5)]*.

Renal Impairment: The pharmacokinetics of ezogabine were studied following a single 100-mg dose of POTIGA in subjects with normal (CrCL >80 ml/min), mild (CrCL ≥50 to <80 mL/min), moderate (CrCL ≥30 to <50 mL/min), or severe renal impairment (CrCL <30 mL/min) (n = 6 in each cohort) and in subjects with ESRD requiring hemodialysis (n = 6). The ezogabine AUC was increased by approximately 30% in patients with mild renal impairment and doubled in patients with moderate impairment to ESRD (CrCL <50 mL/min) relative to healthy subjects. Similar increases in NAMR exposure were observed in the various degrees of renal impairment. The effect of hemodialysis on ezogabine clearance has not been established. Dosage reduction is recommended for patients with creatinine clearance <50 mL/min and for patients with ESRD receiving dialysis *[see Dosage and Administration (2), Use in Specific Populations (8.6)]*.

Hepatic Impairment: The pharmacokinetics of ezogabine were studied following a single 100-mg dose of POTIGA in subjects with normal, mild (Child-Pugh score 5 to 6), moderate (Child-Pugh score 7 to 9), or severe hepatic (Child-Pugh score >9) impairment (n = 6 in each cohort). Relative to healthy subjects, ezogabine AUC was not affected by mild hepatic impairment, but was increased by approximately 50% in subjects with moderate hepatic impairment and doubled in subjects with severe hepatic impairment. There was an increase of approximately 30% in exposure to NAMR in patients with moderate to severe impairment. Dosage reduction is recommended for patients with moderate and severe hepatic impairment *[see Dosage and Administration (2), Use in Specific Populations (8.7)]*.

Drug Interactions: *In vitro* studies using human liver microsomes indicated that ezogabine does not inhibit enzyme activity for CYP1A2, CYP2A6, CYP2C8, CYP2C9, CYP2C19, CYP2D6, CYP2E1, and CYP3A4/5. Inhibition of CYP2B6 by ezogabine has not been evaluated. In addition, *in vitro* studies in human primary hepatocytes showed that ezogabine and NAMR did not induce CYP1A2 or CYP3A4/5 activity. Therefore, ezogabine is unlikely to affect the pharmacokinetics of substrates of the major cytochrome P450 isoenzymes through inhibition or induction mechanisms.

Ezogabine is neither a substrate nor an inhibitor of P-glycoprotein, an efflux transporter. NAMR is a P-glycoprotein inhibitor. Data from an *in vitro* study showed that NAMR inhibited P-glycoprotein–mediated transport of digoxin in a concentration-dependent manner, indicating that NAMR may inhibit renal clearance of digoxin. Administration of POTIGA at therapeutic doses may increase digoxin serum concentrations *[see Drug Interactions (7.2)]*.

Interactions with Antiepileptic Drugs: The interactions between POTIGA and concomitant AEDs are summarized in Table 6.

[See table 6 above]

Oral Contraceptives: In one study examining the potential interaction between ezogabine (150 mg 3 times daily for 3 days) and the combination oral contraceptive norgestrel/ethinyl estradiol (0.3 mg/0.03 mg) tablets in 20 healthy females, no significant alteration in the pharmacokinetics of either drug was observed.

In a second study examining the potential interaction of repeated ezogabine dosing (250 mg 3 times daily for 14 days) and the combination oral contraceptive norethindrone/ethinyl estradiol (1 mg/0.035 mg) tablets in 25 healthy females, no significant alteration in the pharmacokinetics of either drug was observed.

Alcohol: In a healthy volunteer study, the coadministration of ethanol 1g/kg (5 standard alcohol drinks) over 20 minutes and ezogabine (200 mg) resulted in an increase in the ezogabine C_{max} and AUC by 23% and 37%, respectively *[see Drug Interactions (7.3)]*.

13 NONCLINICAL TOXICOLOGY

13.1 Carcinogenesis, Mutagenesis, Impairment of Fertility

Carcinogenesis: In a one-year neonatal mouse study of ezogabine (2 single-dose oral administrations of up to 96 mg/kg on postnatal days 8 and 15), a dose-related increase in the frequency of lung neoplasms (bronchioalveolar carcinoma and/or adenoma) was observed in treated males. No evidence of carcinogenicity was observed in rats following oral administration of ezogabine (oral gavage doses of up to 50 mg/kg/day) for 2 years. Plasma exposure (AUC) to ezogabine at the highest doses tested was less than that in humans at the maximum recommended human dose (MRHD) of 1,200 mg per day.

Mutagenesis: Highly purified ezogabine was negative in the *in vitro* Ames assay, the *in vitro* Chinese hamster ovary (CHO) *Hprt* gene mutation assay, and the *in vivo* mouse micronucleus assay. Ezogabine was positive in the *in vitro* chromosomal aberration assay in human lymphocytes. The major circulating metabolite of ezogabine, NAMR, was negative in the *in vitro* Ames assay, but positive in the *in vitro* chromosomal aberration assay in CHO cells.

Impairment of Fertility: Ezogabine had no effect on fertility, general reproductive performance, or early embryonic development when administered to male and female rats at doses of up to 46.4 mg/kg/day (associated with a plasma ezogabine exposure [AUC] less than that in humans at the MRHD) prior to and during mating, and continuing in females through gestation day 7.

14 CLINICAL STUDIES

The efficacy of POTIGA as adjunctive therapy in partial-onset seizures was established in 3 multicenter, randomized, double-blind, placebo-controlled studies in 1,239 adult patients. The primary endpoint consisted of the percent change in seizure frequency from baseline in the double-blind treatment phase.

Patients enrolled in the studies had partial onset seizures with or without secondary generalization and were not adequately controlled with 1 to 3 concomitant AEDs, with or without concomitant vagus nerve stimulation. More than 75% of patients were taking 2 or more concomitant AEDs. During an 8-week baseline period, patients experienced at least 4 partial onset seizures per 28 days on average with no seizure-free period exceeding 3 to 4 weeks. Patients had a mean duration of epilepsy of 22 years. Across the 3 studies, the median baseline seizure frequency ranged from 8 to 12 seizures per month. The criteria for statistical significance was $P<0.05$.

Patients were randomized to the total daily maintenance dosages of 600 mg per day, 900 mg per day, or 1,200 mg per day, each administered in 3 equally divided doses. During the titration phase of all 3 studies, treatment was initiated at 300 mg per day (100 mg 3 times per day) and increased in weekly increments of 150 mg per day to the target maintenance dosage.

Figure 1 shows the median percent reduction in 28-day seizure frequency (baseline to double-blind phase) as compared with placebo across all 3 studies. A statistically significant effect was observed with POTIGA at doses of 600 mg per day (Study 1), at 900 mg per day (Studies 1 and 3), and at 1,200 mg per day (Studies 2 and 3).

[See figure 1 at top of next page]

Figure 2 shows changes from baseline in the 28-day total partial seizure frequency by category for patients treated with POTIGA and placebo in an integrated analysis across the 3 clinical trials. Patients in whom the seizure frequency increased are shown at left as "worse." Patients in whom the seizure frequency decreased are shown in five categories.

Figure 1. Median Percent Reduction From Baseline in Seizure Frequency per 28 Days by Dose

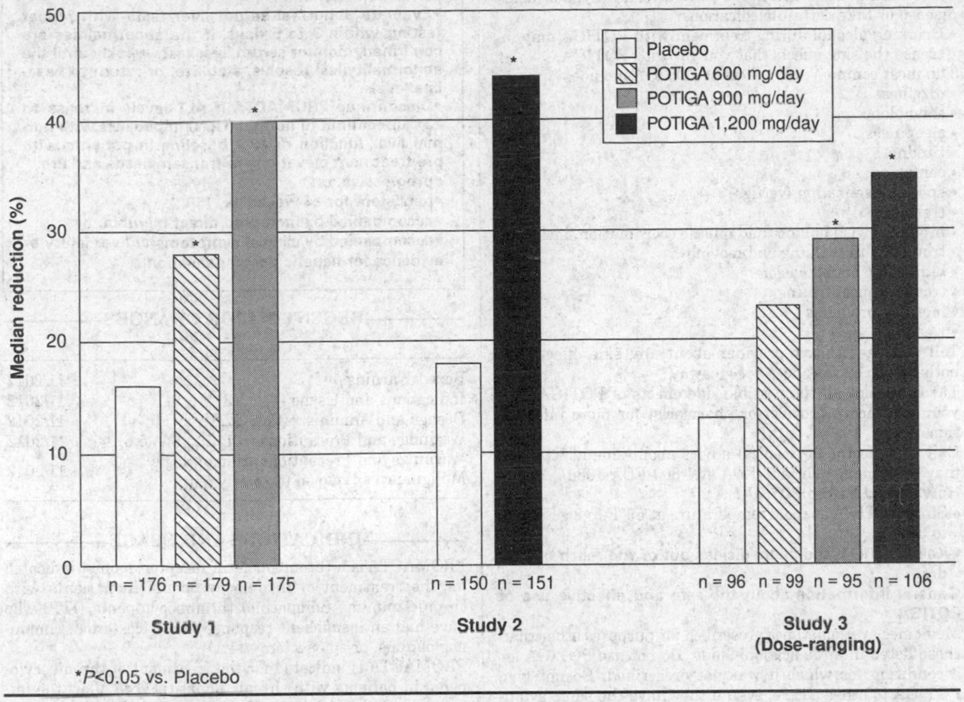

Figure 2. Proportion of Patients by Category of Seizure Response for POTIGA and Placebo Across All Three Double-blind Trials

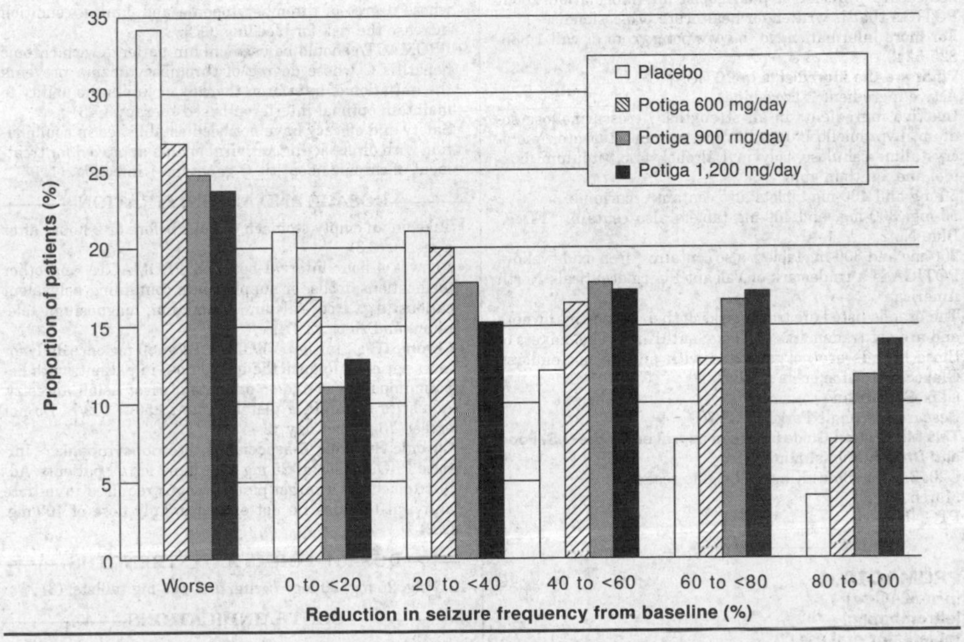

[See figure 2 above]

16 HOW SUPPLIED/STORAGE AND HANDLING

POTIGA is supplied as film-coated immediate-release tablets for oral administration containing 50 mg, 200 mg, 300 mg, or 400 mg of ezogabine in the following packs:

50-mg Tablets: purple, round, film-coated tablets debossed with "RTG 50" on one side in bottles of 90 tablets with desiccant (NDC 0173-0810-59).

200-mg Tablets: yellow, oblong, film-coated tablets debossed with "RTG-200" on one side in bottles of 90 tablets with desiccant (NDC 0173-0812-59).

300-mg Tablets: green, oblong, film-coated tablets debossed with "RTG-300" on one side in bottles of 90 tablets with desiccant (NDC 0173-0813-59).

400-mg Tablets: purple, oblong, film-coated tablets debossed with "RTG-400" on one side in bottles of 90 tablets with desiccant (NDC 0173-0814-59).

Store at 25°C (77°F); excursions permitted to 15°-30°C (59°-86°F) [See USP Controlled Room Temperature.]

17 PATIENT COUNSELING INFORMATION

See FDA-approved patient labeling (Medication Guide).

17.1 Urinary Retention

Patients should be informed that POTIGA can cause urinary retention (including urinary hesitation and dysuria). If patients experience any symptoms of urinary retention, inability to urinate, and/or pain with urination, they should be instructed to seek immediate medical assistance *[see Warnings and Precautions (5.1)]*. For patients who cannot reliably report symptoms of urinary retention (for example, patients with cognitive impairment), urologic consultation may be helpful.

17.2 Psychiatric Symptoms

Patients should be informed that POTIGA can cause psychiatric symptoms such as confusional state, disorientation, hallucinations, and other symptoms of psychosis. Patients and their caregivers should be instructed to notify their physicians if they experience psychotic symptoms *[see Warnings and Precautions (5.2)]*.

17.3 Central Nervous System Effects

Patients should be informed that POTIGA may cause dizziness, somnolence, memory impairment, abnormal coordination/balance, disturbance in attention, and ophthalmological effects such as diplopia or blurred vision. Patients taking POTIGA should be advised not to drive, operate complex machinery, or engage in other hazardous activities until they have become accustomed to any such effects associated with POTIGA *[see Warnings and Precautions (5.3)]*.

17.4 Suicidal Thinking and Behavior

Patients, their caregivers, and families should be informed that AEDs, including POTIGA, may increase the risk of suicidal thoughts and behavior and should be advised of the need to be alert for the emergence or worsening of symptoms of depression, any unusual changes in mood or behavior, or the emergence of suicidal thoughts, behavior, or thoughts about self-harm. Behaviors of concern should be reported immediately to healthcare providers *[see Warnings and Precautions (5.5)]*.

17.5 Pregnancy

Patients should be advised to notify their physicians if they become pregnant or intend to become pregnant during therapy. Patients should be advised to notify their physicians if they intend to breastfeed or are breastfeeding an infant.

Patients should be encouraged to enroll in the NAAED Pregnancy Registry if they become pregnant. This registry collects information about the safety of AEDs during pregnancy. To enroll, patients can call the toll-free number 1-888-233-2334 *[see Use in Specific Populations (8.1)]*.

POTIGA is a trademark of Valeant Pharmaceuticals North America.

GlaxoSmithKline
Research Triangle Park, NC 27709

June 2013
PTG:6PI

MEDICATION GUIDE

POTIGA™ (po-TEE-ga) Tablets, CV
(ezogabine)

Read this Medication Guide before you start taking POTIGA and each time you get a refill. There may be new information. This Medication Guide does not take the place of talking to your healthcare provider about your medical condition or treatment. If you have questions about POTIGA, ask your healthcare provider or pharmacist.

What is the most important information I should know about POTIGA?

Do not stop POTIGA without first talking to a healthcare provider. Stopping POTIGA suddenly can cause serious problems. Stopping POTIGA suddenly can cause you to have more seizures more often.

1. POTIGA can make it hard for you to urinate (empty your bladder) and may cause you to be unable to urinate. Call your healthcare provider right away if you:
- are unable to start urinating
- have trouble emptying your bladder
- have a weak urine stream
- have pain with urination

2. POTIGA can cause mental (psychiatric) problems, including:
- confusion
- new or worse aggressive behavior, hostility, anger, or irritability
- new or worse psychosis (hearing or seeing things that are not real)
- being suspicious or distrustful (believing things that are not true)
- other unusual or extreme changes in behavior or mood

Tell your healthcare provider right away if you have any new or worsening mental problems while using POTIGA.

3. Like other antiepileptic drugs, POTIGA may cause suicidal thoughts or actions in a very small number of people, about 1 in 500.

Call a healthcare provider right away if you have any of these symptoms, especially if they are new, worse, or worry you:
- thoughts about suicide or dying
- attempt to commit suicide
- new or worse depression
- new or worse anxiety
- feeling agitated or restless
- panic attacks
- trouble sleeping (insomnia)
- new or worse irritability
- acting aggressive, being angry, or violent
- acting on dangerous impulses
- an extreme increase in activity and talking (mania)
- other unusual changes in behavior or mood

Suicidal thoughts or actions can be caused by things other than medicines. If you have suicidal thoughts or actions, your healthcare provider may check for other causes.

How can I watch for early symptoms of suicidal thoughts and actions?

- Pay attention to any changes, especially sudden changes, in mood, behaviors, thoughts, or feelings.
- Keep all follow-up visits with your healthcare provider as scheduled.

Call your healthcare provider between visits as needed, especially if you are worried about symptoms.

Do not stop POTIGA without first talking to a healthcare provider.

Stopping POTIGA suddenly can cause serious problems. Stopping POTIGA suddenly can cause you to have more seizures more often.

What is POTIGA?

POTIGA is a prescription medicine that is used with other medicines to treat partial onset seizures in people with epilepsy who are 18 years of age or older.

POTIGA is a controlled substance (CV) because it can be abused or lead to drug dependence. Keep your POTIGA in a safe place to protect it from theft. Never give your POTIGA to anyone else because it may harm them. Selling or giving away this medicine is against the law.

It is not known if POTIGA is safe and effective in children under 18 years of age.

What should I tell my healthcare provider before taking POTIGA?

Before you take POTIGA, tell your healthcare provider if you:

- have trouble urinating
- have an enlarged prostate
- have or have had depression, mood problems, or suicidal thoughts or behavior
- have heart problems, including a condition called long QT Syndrome, or have low potassium or magnesium in your blood
- have liver problems
- have kidney problems
- drink alcohol
- have any other medical conditions
- are pregnant or plan to become pregnant. It is not known if POTIGA will harm your unborn baby.
  - If you become pregnant while taking POTIGA, talk to your healthcare provider about registering with the North American Antiepileptic Drug Pregnancy Registry. The purpose of this registry is to collect information about the safety of medicines used to treat seizures during pregnancy. You can enroll in this registry by calling 1-888-233-2334.
- are breastfeeding or plan to breastfeed. It is not known if POTIGA passes into your breast milk. Talk to your healthcare provider about the best way to feed your baby if you take POTIGA. You and your healthcare provider should decide if you will take POTIGA or breastfeed. You should not do both.

Tell your healthcare provider about all the medicines you take, including prescription and non-prescription medicines, vitamins, and herbal supplements. Taking POTIGA with certain other medicines can affect each other, causing side effects. **Especially tell your healthcare provider if you take:**

- digoxin (LANOXIN®)
- phenytoin (DILANTIN®, PHENYTEK®)
- carbamazepine (CARBATROL®, TEGRETOL®, TEGRETOL®-XR, EQUETRO®, EPITOL®)

Know the medicines you take. Keep a list of them to show your doctor and pharmacist when you get a new medicine.

- Take POTIGA exactly as your healthcare provider tells you to take it. Your healthcare provider will tell you how much POTIGA to take and when to take it.
- Your healthcare provider may change your dose of POTIGA. Do not change your dose without talking to your healthcare provider.
- POTIGA can be taken with or without food.
- Swallow POTIGA Tablets whole. Do not break, crush, dissolve, or chew POTIGA tablets before swallowing.
- Talk to your doctor about what to do if you miss one or more doses of POTIGA.
- If you take too much POTIGA, call your local Poison Control Center or go to the nearest hospital emergency room right away.

What should I avoid while taking POTIGA?

Do not drive, operate machinery, or do other dangerous activities until you know how POTIGA affects you. POTIGA can cause dizziness, sleepiness, double-vision, and blurred vision.

What are the possible side effects of POTIGA?

POTIGA may cause serious side effects, including:

- See "What is the most important information I should know about POTIGA?"

Dizziness and sleepiness. These symptoms can increase when your dose of POTIGA is increased. See "What should I avoid while taking POTIGA?"

Changes in your heart rhythm and the electrical activity of your heart. Your healthcare provider should monitor your heart during treatment if you have a certain type of heart disease or take certain medications.

- Drinking alcohol during treatment with POTIGA may increase the side effects that you get with POTIGA.

The most common side effects of POTIGA include:

- dizziness
- somnolence
- sleepiness
- tiredness
- confusion
- spinning sensation (vertigo)
- tremor
- problems with balance and muscle coordination, including trouble with walking and moving
- blurred or double vision
- trouble concentrating
- memory problems
- weakness

Tell your healthcare provider about any side effect that bothers you or that does not go away.

These are not all the possible side effects of POTIGA. Ask your healthcare provider or pharmacist for more information.

Call your doctor for medical advice about side effects. You may report side effects to FDA at 1-800-FDA-1088.

How should I store POTIGA?

- Store POTIGA at room temperature at 59°F to 86°F (15°C to 30°C).
- **Keep POTIGA and all medicines out of the reach of children.**

General information about the safe and effective use of POTIGA.

Medicines are sometimes prescribed for purposes other than those listed in a Medication Guide. Do not use POTIGA for a condition for which it was not prescribed. Do not give POTIGA to other people, even if they have the same symptoms you have. It may harm them.

This Medication Guide summarizes the most important information about POTIGA. If you would like more information, talk with your healthcare provider. You can ask your healthcare provider or pharmacist for information about POTIGA that is written for healthcare professionals.

For more information, go to www.potiga.com or call 1-888-825-5249.

What are the ingredients in POTIGA?

Active ingredient: ezogabine.

Inactive ingredients in all strengths: croscarmellose sodium, hypromellose, lecithin, magnesium stearate, microcrystalline cellulose, polyvinyl alcohol, talc, titanium dioxide, and xanthan gum.

50-mg and 400-mg tablets also contain: carmine.

50-mg, 300-mg, and 400-mg tablets also contain: FD&C Blue No 2.

200-mg and 300-mg tablets also contain: iron oxide yellow.

POTIGA is a trademark of Valeant Pharmaceuticals North America.

The brands listed are trademarks of their respective owners and are not trademarks of GlaxoSmithKline. The makers of these brands are not affiliated with and do not endorse GlaxoSmithKline or its products.

GlaxoSmithKline
Research Triangle Park, NC 27709

This Medication Guide has been approved by the U.S. Food and Drug Administration.

March 2012
PTG:4MG

PROMACTA ℞

[pro-MAC-ta]
(eltrombopag)
tablets, for oral use

HIGHLIGHTS OF PRESCRIBING INFORMATION

These highlights do not include all the information needed to use PROMACTA safely and effectively. See full prescribing information for PROMACTA.

PROMACTA (eltrombopag) tablets, for oral use
Initial U.S. Approval: 2008

WARNING: RISK FOR HEPATOTOXICITY

See full prescribing information for complete boxed warning

PROMACTA may cause hepatotoxicity. PROMACTA, in combination with interferon and ribavirin in patients with chronic hepatitis C, may increase the risk of hepatic decompensation. (5.1, 5.2)

•Measure serum alanineaminotransferase (ALT), aspartate aminotransferase (AST), and bilirubin prior to initiation of PROMACTA, every 2 weeks during the dose adjustment phase, and monthly following establishment of a stable dose. If bilirubin is elevated, perform fractionation.

•Evaluate abnormal serum liver tests with repeat testing within 3 to 5 days. If the abnormalities are confirmed, monitor serum liver tests weekly until the abnormality(ies) resolve, stabilize, or return to baseline levels.

•Discontinue PROMACTA if ALT levels increase to ≥3× upper limit of normal (ULN) in patients with normal liver function or ≥3× baseline in patients with pre-treatment elevations in transaminases and are:

•progressive, or

•persistent for ≥4 weeks, or

•accompanied by increased direct bilirubin, or

•accompanied by clinical symptoms of liver injury or evidence for hepatic decompensation.

RECENT MAJOR CHANGES

Boxed Warning	11/2012
Indications and Usage (1.2, 1.3)	11/2012
Dosage and Administration (2.2)	11/2012
Warnings and Precautions (5.1, 5.2, 5.4, 5.6)	11/2012
Warnings and Precautions, Hematologic Malignancies removal (formerly 5.4)	11/2012

INDICATIONS AND USAGE

PROMACTA is a thrombopoietin receptor agonist indicated for the treatment of thrombocytopenia in patients with chronic immune (idiopathic) thrombocytopenia (ITP) who have had an insufficient response to corticosteroids, immunoglobulins, or splenectomy. (1.1)

PROMACTA is indicated for the treatment of thrombocytopenia in patients with chronic hepatitis C to allow the initiation and maintenance of interferon-based therapy. (1.2)

Limitations of Use:

- PROMACTA should not be used to normalize platelet counts. (1.3)
- PROMACTA should be used only in patients with ITP whose degree of thrombocytopenia and clinical condition increase the risk for bleeding. (1.3)
- PROMACTA should be used only in patients with chronic hepatitis C whose degree of thrombocytopenia prevents the initiation of interferon therapy or limits the ability to maintain optimal interferon-based therapy. (1.3)
- Safety and efficacy have not been established in combination with direct acting antiviral agents approved for treatment of chronic hepatitis C genotype 1 infection. (1.3)

DOSAGE AND ADMINISTRATION

- Take on an empty stomach (1 hour before or 2 hours after a meal). (2.3)
- Allow a 4-hour interval between PROMACTA and other medications, foods, or supplements containing polyvalent cations (e.g., iron, calcium, aluminum, magnesium, selenium, and zinc). (2.3)
- **Chronic ITP:** Initiate PROMACTA at 50 mg once daily for most patients. Reduce the initial dose in patients with hepatic impairment and/or patients of East Asian ancestry. Adjust to maintain a platelet count ≥50 × 109/L. Do not exceed 75 mg per day. (2.1)
- **Chronic Hepatitis C-associated thrombocytopenia:** Initiate PROMACTA at 25 mg once daily for all patients. Adjust to achieve a target platelet count required to initiate antiviral therapy. Do not exceed a daily dose of 100 mg. (2.2)

DOSAGE FORMS AND STRENGTHS

12.5 mg, 25 mg, 50 mg, 75 mg, and 100 mg tablets. (3)

CONTRAINDICATIONS

None. (4)

WARNINGS AND PRECAUTIONS

- Hepatotoxicity: Monitor liver function before and during therapy. (5.1)
- Hepatic decompensation in patients with chronic hepatitis C: Monitor patients with low albumin levels or with MELD score ≥10 at baseline. (5.2)
- Thrombotic/thromboembolic complications: Portal vein thrombosis has been reported in patients with chronic liver disease receiving PROMACTA. Monitor platelet counts regularly. (5.4)

ADVERSE REACTIONS

- The most common adverse reactions in ITP patients (≥3% and greater than placebo) were: nausea, diarrhea, upper respiratory tract infection, vomiting, increased ALT, myalgia, urinary tract infection, oropharyngeal pain, increased AST, pharyngitis, back pain, influenza, paresthesia, and rash. (6.1)

- The most common adverse reactions in thrombocytopenic patients with chronic hepatitis C (≥10% and greater than placebo) were: anemia, pyrexia, fatigue, headache, nausea, diarrhea, decreased appetite, influenza-like illness, asthenia, insomnia, cough, pruritus, chills, myalgia, alopecia, and peripheral edema. (6.1)

To report SUSPECTED ADVERSE REACTIONS, contact GlaxoSmithKline at 1-888-825-5249 or FDA at 1-800-FDA-1088 or www.fda.gov/medwatch.

DRUG INTERACTIONS

PROMACTA must not be taken within 4 hours of any medications or products containing polyvalent cations such as antacids, dairy products, and mineral supplements. (7.1)

USE IN SPECIFIC POPULATIONS

- Pregnancy: Based on animal data, PROMACTA may cause fetal harm. (8.1)
- Nursing Mothers: A decision should be made to discontinue PROMACTA or nursing, taking into account the importance of PROMACTA to the mother. (8.3)
- Reduce the initial dose in chronic ITP patients with hepatic impairment. (8.6)

See 17 for PATIENT COUNSELING INFORMATION and Medication Guide

Revised: 11/2012

FULL PRESCRIBING INFORMATION: CONTENTS*

*** Sections or subsections omitted from the full prescribing information are not listed**

FULL PRESCRIBING INFORMATION

WARNING: RISK FOR HEPATOTOXICITY

PROMACTA may cause hepatotoxicity. PROMACTA, in combination with interferon and ribavirin in patients with chronic hepatitis C, may increase the risk of hepatic decompensation *[see Warnings and Precautions (5.1, 5.2)].*

- **Measure serum alanineaminotransferase (ALT), aspartate aminotransferase (AST), and bilirubin prior to initiation of PROMACTA, every 2 weeks during the dose adjustment phase, and monthly following establishment of a stable dose. If bilirubin is elevated, perform fractionation.**
- **Evaluate abnormal serum liver tests with repeat testing within 3 to 5 days. If the abnormalities are confirmed, monitor serum liver tests weekly until the abnormality(ies) resolve, stabilize, or return to baseline levels.**
- **Discontinue PROMACTA if ALT levels increase to ≥3× the upper limit of normal (ULN) in patients with normal liver function or ≥3× baseline in patients with pre-treatment elevations in transaminases and are:**
  - **progressive, or**
  - **persistent for ≥4 weeks, or**
  - **accompanied by increased direct bilirubin, or**
  - **accompanied by clinical symptoms of liver injury or evidence for hepatic decompensation.**

1 INDICATIONS AND USAGE

1.1 Treatment of Thrombocytopenia in Patients with Chronic ITP

PROMACTA® is indicated for the treatment of thrombocytopenia in patients with chronic immune (idiopathic) thrombocytopenia (ITP) who have had an insufficient response to corticosteroids, immunoglobulins, or splenectomy.

1.2 Treatment of Thrombocytopenia in Patients with Hepatitis C Infection

PROMACTA is indicated for the treatment of thrombocytopenia in patients with chronic hepatitis C to allow the initiation and maintenance of interferon-based therapy.

1.3 Limitations of Use

- PROMACTA should not be used to normalize platelet counts.
- PROMACTA should be used only in patients with ITP whose degree of thrombocytopenia and clinical condition increase the risk for bleeding.
- PROMACTA should be used only in patients with chronic hepatitis C whose degree of thrombocytopenia prevents the initiation of interferon-based therapy or limits the ability to maintain interferon-based therapy.
- Safety and efficacy have not been established in combination with direct acting antiviral agents approved for treatment of chronic hepatitis C genotype 1 infection.

2 DOSAGE AND ADMINISTRATION

2.1 Chronic Immune (Idiopathic) Thrombocytopenia

Use the lowest dose of PROMACTA to achieve and maintain a platelet count greater than or equal to 50×10^9/L as necessary to reduce the risk for bleeding. Dose adjustments are based upon the platelet count response. Do not use PROMACTA to normalize platelet counts *[see Warnings and Precautions (5.4)]*. In clinical trials, platelet counts generally increased within 1 to 2 weeks after starting PROMACTA and decreased within 1 to 2 weeks after discontinuing PROMACTA *[see Clinical Studies (14.1)]*.

Initial Dose Regimen: Initiate PROMACTA at a dose of 50 mg once daily, except in patients who are of East Asian ancestry (such as Chinese, Japanese, Taiwanese, or Korean) or who have mild to severe hepatic impairment (Child-Pugh Class A, B, C).

For ITP patients of East Asian ancestry, initiate PROMACTA at a reduced dose of 25 mg once daily *[see Use in Specific Populations (8.8) and Clinical Pharmacology (12.3)]*.

For ITP patients with mild, moderate, or severe hepatic impairment (Child-Pugh Class A, B, C), initiate PROMACTA at a reduced dose of 25 mg once daily *[see Use in Specific Populations (8.6) and Clinical Pharmacology (12.3)]*.

For ITP patients of East Asian ancestry with hepatic impairment (Child-Pugh Class A, B, C), consider initiating PROMACTA at a reduced dose of 12.5 mg once daily *[see Clinical Pharmacology (12.3)]*.

Monitoring and Dose Adjustment: After initiating PROMACTA, adjust the dose to achieve and maintain a platelet count greater than or equal to 50×10^9/L as necessary to reduce the risk for bleeding. Do not exceed a dose of 75 mg daily. Monitor clinical hematology and liver tests regularly throughout therapy with PROMACTA and modify the dosage regimen of PROMACTA based on platelet counts as outlined in Table 1. During therapy with PROMACTA, assess CBCs with differentials (including platelet counts) weekly until a stable platelet count has been achieved. Obtain CBCs with differentials (including platelet counts) monthly thereafter.

Table 1. Dose Adjustments of PROMACTA in Adults With Chronic Immune (Idiopathic) Thrombocytopenia

Platelet Count Result	Dose Adjustment or Response
$<50 \times 10^9$/L following at least 2 weeks of PROMACTA	Increase daily dose by 25 mg to a maximum of 75 mg/day. For patients taking 12.5 mg once daily, increase the dose to 25 mg daily before increasing the dose amount by 25 mg.
$\geq 200 \times 10^9$/L to $\leq 400 \times 10^9$/L at any time	Decrease the daily dose by 25 mg. Wait 2 weeks to assess the effects of this and any subsequent dose adjustments.
$>400 \times 10^9$/L	Stop PROMACTA; increase the frequency of platelet monitoring to twice weekly. Once the platelet count is $<150 \times 10^9$/L, reinitiate therapy at a daily dose reduced by 25 mg. For patients taking 25 mg once daily, reinitiate therapy at a daily dose of 12.5 mg.
$>400 \times 10^9$/L after 2 weeks of therapy at lowest dose of PROMACTA	Discontinue PROMACTA.

In ITP patients with hepatic impairment (Child-Pugh Class A, B, C), after initiating PROMACTA or after any subsequent dosing increase, wait 3 weeks before increasing the dose.

Modify the dosage regimen of concomitant ITP medications, as medically appropriate, to avoid excessive increases in platelet counts during therapy with PROMACTA. Do not administer more than one dose of PROMACTA within any 24-hour period.

Discontinuation: Discontinue PROMACTA if the platelet count does not increase to a level sufficient to avoid clinically important bleeding after 4 weeks of therapy with PROMACTA at the maximum daily dose of 75 mg. Excessive platelet count responses, as outlined in Table 1, or important liver test abnormalities also necessitate discontinuation of PROMACTA *[see Warnings and Precautions (5.1)]*.

2.2 Chronic Hepatitis C-Associated Thrombocytopenia

Use the lowest dose of PROMACTA to achieve and maintain a platelet count necessary to initiate and maintain antiviral therapy with pegylated interferon and ribavirin . Dose adjustments are based upon the platelet count response. Do not use PROMACTA to normalize platelet counts *[see Warnings and Precautions (5.4)]*. In clinical trials, platelet counts generally began to rise within the first week of treatment with PROMACTA *[see Clinical Studies (14.2)]*.

Initial Dose Regimen: Initiate PROMACTA at a dose of 25 mg once daily.

Monitoring and Dose Adjustment: Adjust the dose of PROMACTA in 25 mg increments every 2 weeks as necessary to achieve the target platelet count required to initiate antiviral therapy. Monitor platelet counts every week prior to starting antiviral therapy.

During antiviral therapy, adjust the dose of PROMACTA to avoid dose reductions of peginterferon . Monitor CBCs with differentials (including platelet counts) weekly during antiviral therapy until a stable platelet count is achieved. Monitor platelet counts monthly thereafter. Do not exceed a dose of 100 mg daily. Monitor clinical hematology and liver tests regularly throughout therapy with PROMACTA.

For specific dosage instructions for peginterferon or ribavirin, refer to their respective prescribing information.

Table 2. Dose Adjustments of PROMACTA In Adults With Chronic Hepatitis C

Platelet Count Result	Dose Adjustment or Response
<50 × 109/L following at least 2 weeks of PROMACTA	Increase daily dose by 25 mg to a maximum of 100 mg/day.
≥200 × 109/L to ≤400 × 109/L at any time	Decrease the daily dose by 25 mg. Wait 2 weeks to assess the effects of this and any subsequent dose adjustments.

>400 × 109/L	Stop PROMACTA; increase the frequency of platelet monitoring to twice weekly. Once the platelet count is <150 × 109/L, reinitiate therapy at a daily dose reduced by 25 mg. For patients taking 25 mg once daily, reinitiate therapy at a daily dose of 12.5 mg.
>400 × 109/L after 2 weeks of therapy at lowest dose of PROMACTA	Discontinue PROMACTA.

Discontinuation: The prescribing information for pegylated interferon and ribavirin include recommendations for antiviral treatment discontinuation for treatment futility. Refer to pegylated interferon and ribavirin prescribing information for discontinuation recommendations for antiviral treatment futility.

PROMACTA should be discontinued when antiviral therapy is discontinued. Excessive platelet count responses, as outlined in Table 2, or important liver test abnormalities also necessitate discontinuation of PROMACTA *[see Warnings and Precautions (5.1)]*.

2.3 Administration

Take PROMACTA on an empty stomach (1 hour before or 2 hours after a meal) *[see Clinical Pharmacology (12.3)]*.

Allow at least a 4-hour interval between PROMACTA and other medications (e.g., antacids), calcium-rich foods (e.g., dairy products and calcium fortified juices), or supplements containing polyvalent cations such as iron, calcium, aluminum, magnesium, selenium, and zinc *[see Drug Interactions (7.1)]*.

3 DOSAGE FORMS AND STRENGTHS

- 12.5 mg tablets — round, biconvex, white, film-coated tablets debossed with GS MZ1 and 12.5 on one side. Each tablet, for oral administration, contains eltrombopag olamine, equivalent to 12.5 mg of eltrombopag free acid.
- 25 mg tablets — round, biconvex, orange, film-coated tablets debossed with GS NX3 and 25 on one side. Each tablet, for oral administration, contains eltrombopag olamine, equivalent to 25 mg of eltrombopag free acid.
- 50 mg tablets — round, biconvex, blue, film-coated tablets debossed with GS UFU and 50 on one side. Each tablet, for oral administration, contains eltrombopag olamine, equivalent to 50 mg of eltrombopag free acid.
- 75 mg tablets — round, biconvex, pink, film-coated tablets debossed with GS FFS and 75 on one side. Each tablet, for oral administration, contains eltrombopag olamine, equivalent to 75 mg of eltrombopag free acid.
- 100 mg tablets — round, biconvex, green, film-coated tablets debossed with GS 1L5 and 100 on one side. Each tablet, for oral administration, contains eltrombopag olamine, equivalent to 100 mg of eltrombopag free acid.

4 CONTRAINDICATIONS

None.

5 WARNINGS AND PRECAUTIONS

5.1 Hepatotoxicity

PROMACTA may cause hepatotoxicity. In the controlled clinical trials in chronic ITP, one patient experienced Grade 4 (NCI Common Terminology Criteria for Adverse Events [NCI CTCAE] toxicity scale) elevations in serum liver test values during therapy with PROMACTA, worsening of underlying cardiopulmonary disease, and death. One patient in the placebo group experienced a Grade 4 liver test abnormality. Overall, serum liver test abnormalities (predominantly Grade 2 or less in severity) were reported in 11% and 7% of the PROMACTA and placebo groups, respectively. In the 3 controlled chronic ITP trials, four patients (1%) treated with PROMACTA and three patients in the placebo group (2%) discontinued treatment due to hepatobiliary laboratory abnormalities. Seven of the patients treated with PROMACTA in the controlled trials with hepatobiliary laboratory abnormalities were re-exposed to PROMACTA in the extension trial. Six of these patients again experienced liver test abnormalities (predominantly Grade 1) resulting in discontinuation of PROMACTA in one patient. In the extension chronic ITP trial, one additional patient had PROMACTA discontinued due to liver test abnormalities (≤Grade 3).

In 2 controlled clinical trials in patients with chronic hepatitis C and thrombocytopenia, ALT or AST ≥3× ULN was reported in 34% and 38% of the PROMACTA and placebo groups, respectively. Most patients receiving PROMACTA in combination with peginterferon / ribavirin therapy will experience indirect hyperbilirubinemia . Overall, total bilirubin ≥1.5 × ULN was reported in 76% and 50% of patients receiving PROMACTA and placebo, respectively.

Measure serum ALT, AST, and bilirubin prior to initiation of PROMACTA, every 2 weeks during the dose adjustment phase, and monthly following establishment of a stable dose. If bilirubin is elevated, perform fractionation. Evaluate abnormal serum liver tests with repeat testing within 3 to 5 days. If the abnormalities are confirmed, monitor serum liver tests weekly until the abnormality(ies) resolve, stabilize, or return to baseline levels. Discontinue PROMACTA if ALT levels increase to ≥3× ULN in patients with normal liver function or ≥3× baseline in patients with pre-treatment elevations in transaminasesand are:

- progressive, or
- persistent for ≥4 weeks, or
- accompanied by increased direct bilirubin, or
- accompanied by clinical symptoms of liver injury or evidence for hepatic decompensation.

Reinitiating treatment with PROMACTA is not recommended. If the potential benefit for reinitiating treatment with PROMACTA is considered to outweigh the risk for hepatotoxicity, then cautiously reintroduce PROMACTA and measure serum liver tests weekly during the dose adjustment phase. If liver tests abnormalities persist, worsen or recur, then permanently discontinue PROMACTA.

5.2 Hepatic Decompensation in Patients with Chronic Hepatitis C

Chronic hepatitis C patients with cirrhosis may be at risk of hepatic decompensation and death when treated with alfainterferons . In 2 controlled clinical trials in patients with chronic hepatitis C and thrombocytopenia, ascites and encephalopathy were reported more frequently for PROMACTA (7%) than placebo (4%). Patients with low albumin levels (<3.5 g/dL) or Model for End-Stage Liver Disease (MELD) score ≥10 at baseline had a greater risk of hepatic decompensation. Patients with these characteristics should be closely monitored for signs and symptoms of hepatic decompensation. Refer to alfa interferon prescribing information for discontinuation recommendations. PROMACTA should be discontinued if antiviral therapy is discontinued for hepatic decompensation.

5.3 Bone Marrow Reticulin Formation and Risk for Bone Marrow Fibrosis

PROMACTA may increase the risk for development or progression of reticulin fiber deposition within the bone marrow. In the extension trial in chronic ITP, 151 patients have had bone marrow biopsies evaluated for increased reticulin and collagen fiber deposition. Bone marrow biopsies taken after 1 year of therapy showed predominantly myelofibrosis (MF) Grade 1 or less in 140/151 (93%) of patients. There were 11/151 (7%) of patients with MF Grade 2. Four patients had collagen deposition reported. One patient with a pre-existing MF Grade 1 developed a MF Grade 2 and subsequently discontinued treatment with PROMACTA. Clinical trials have not demonstrated clinical consequences to date. If new or worsening blood morphological abnormalities or cytopenias occur, consider a bone marrow biopsy including staining for fibrosis.

5.4 Thrombotic/Thromboembolic Complications

In 2 controlled clinical trials in patients with chronic hepatitis C and thrombocytopenia, 3% (31/955) treated with PROMACTA experienced a thrombotic event compared to 1% (5/484) on placebo. The majority of events were of the portal venous system (1% in patients treated with PROMACTA versus <1% for placebo).

Thrombotic/thromboembolic complications may result from increases in platelet counts with PROMACTA. Reported thrombotic/thromboembolic complications included both venous and arterial events and were observed at low and at normal platelet counts.

Consider the potential for an increased risk of thromboembolism when administering PROMACTA to patients with known risk factors for thromboembolism (e.g., Factor V Leiden, ATIII deficiency, antiphospholipid syndrome, chronic liver disease). To minimize the risk for thrombotic/thromboembolic complications, do not use PROMACTA in an attempt to normalize platelet counts. Follow the dose adjustment guidelines to achieve and maintain target platelet counts *[see Dosage and Administration (2.1, 2.2)]*.

In a controlled trial in non-ITP thrombocytopenic patients with chronic liver disease undergoing elective invasive procedures (N = 292), the risk of thrombotic events was increased in patients treated with 75 mg PROMACTA once daily. Seven thrombotic complications (six patients) were reported in the group that received PROMACTA and three thrombotic complications were reported in the placebo group (two patients). All of the thrombotic complications reported in the group that received PROMACTA were portal vein thrombosis (PVT). Symptoms of PVT included abdominal pain, nausea, vomiting, and diarrhea. Five of the six patients in the group that received PROMACTA experienced a thrombotic complication within 30 days of completing treatment with PROMACTA and at a platelet count above 200×10^9/L. The risk of portal venous thrombosis was increased in thrombocytopenic patients with chronic liver disease treated with 75 mg PROMACTA once daily for 2 weeks in preparation for invasive procedures.

5.5 Laboratory Monitoring

Complete Blood Counts (CBCs): Obtain CBCs with differentials (including platelet counts) weekly during the dose adjustment phase of therapy with PROMACTA and then monthly following establishment of a stable dose of PROMACTA. Obtain CBCs with differentials (including platelet counts) weekly for at least 4 weeks following discontinuation of PROMACTA. *[See Dosage and Administration (2.1, 2.2) and Warnings and Precautions (5.3).]*

Liver Tests: Monitor serum liver tests (ALT, AST, and bilirubin) prior to initiation of PROMACTA, every 2 weeks during the dose adjustment phase, and monthly following establishment of a stable dose. PROMACTA inhibits UGT1A1 and OATP1B1, which may lead to indirect hyperbilirubinemia. If bilirubin is elevated, perform fractionation. If abnormal levels are detected, repeat the tests within 3 to 5 days. If the abnormalities are confirmed, monitor serum liver tests weekly until the abnormality(ies) resolve, stabilize, or return to baseline levels. Discontinue PROMACTA for the development of important liver test abnormalities *[see Warnings and Precautions (5.1)]*.

5.6 Cataracts

In the 3 controlled clinical trials in chronic ITP, cataracts developed or worsened in 15 (7%) patients who received 50 mg PROMACTA daily and 8 (7%) placebo-group patients. In the extension trial, cataracts developed or worsened in 4% of patients who underwent ocular examination prior to therapy with PROMACTA. In the 2 controlled clinical trials in patients with chronic hepatitis C and thrombocytopenia, cataracts developed or worsened in 8% patients treated with PROMACTA and 5% patients treated with placebo.

Cataracts were observed in toxicology studies of eltrombopag in rodents *[see Nonclinical Toxicology (13.2)]*. Perform a baseline ocular examination prior to administration of PROMACTA and, during therapy with PROMACTA, regularly monitor patients for signs and symptoms of cataracts.

6 ADVERSE REACTIONS

The following serious adverse reactions associated with PROMACTA are described in other sections.

- Hepatotoxicity *[see Warnings and Precautions (5.1)]*
- Hepatic Decompensation in Patients With Chronic Hepatitis C *[see Warnings and Precautions (5.2)]*
- Bone Marrow Reticulin Formation and Risk for Bone Marrow Fibrosis *[see Warnings and Precautions (5.3)]*
- Thrombotic/Thromboembolic Complications *[see Warnings and Precautions (5.4)]*
- Cataracts *[see Warnings and Precautions (5.6)]*

6.1 Clinical Trials Experience

Because clinical trials are conducted under widely varying conditions, adverse reaction rates observed in the clinical trials of a drug cannot be directly compared to rates in the clinical trials of another drug and may not reflect the rates observed in practice.

Chronic Immune (Idiopathic) Thrombocytopenia: In clinical trials, hemorrhage was the most common serious adverse reaction and most hemorrhagic reactions followed discontinuation of PROMACTA. Other serious adverse reactions included liver test abnormalities and thrombotic/thromboembolic complications *[see Warnings and Precautions (5.1, 5.4)]*.

The data described below reflect exposure of PROMACTA to 446 patients with chronic ITP aged 18 to 85, of whom 65% were female across the ITP clinical development program including 3 placebo-controlled trials. PROMACTA was administered to 277 patients for at least 6 months and 202 patients for at least 1 year.

Table 3 presents the most common adverse drug reactions (experienced by ≥3% of patients receiving PROMACTA) from the 3 placebo-controlled trials, with a higher incidence in PROMACTA versus placebo.

Table 3. Adverse Reactions (≥3%) from Three Placebo-Controlled Trials in Adults With Chronic Immune (Idiopathic) Thrombocytopenia

Adverse Reaction	PROMACTA 50mg n = 241 (%)	Placebo n = 128 (%)
Nausea	9	3
Diarrhea	9	7
Upper respiratory tract infection	7	6
Vomiting	6	<1
Increased ALT	5	3
Myalgia	5	2
Urinary tract infection	5	3
Oropharyngeal pain	4	3

Increased AST	4	2
Pharyngitis	4	2
Back pain	3	2
Influenza	3	2
Paresthesia	3	2
Rash	3	2

In the 3 controlled clinical chronic ITP trials, alopecia, musculoskeletal pain, blood alkaline phosphatase increased, and dry mouth were the adverse reactions reported in 2% of patients treated with PROMACTA and in no patients who received placebo.

Among 299 patients with chronic ITP who received PROMACTA in the single-arm extension trial, the adverse reactions occurred in a pattern similar to that seen in the placebo-controlled trials. Table 4 presents the most common treatment-related adverse reactions (experienced by ≥3% of patients receiving PROMACTA) from the extension trial.

Table 4. Treatment-Related Adverse Reactions (≥3%) from Extension Trial in Adults With Chronic Immune (Idiopathic) Thrombocytopenia

Adverse Reaction	PROMACTA 50mg n = 299 (%)
Headache	10
Hyperbilirubinemia	6
ALT increased	6
Cataract	5
AST increased	4
Fatigue	4
Nausea	4

In a placebo-controlled trial of PROMACTA in non-ITP thrombocytopenic patients with chronic liver disease, six patients in the PROMACTA group and one patient in the placebo group developed portal vein thromboses *[see Warnings and Precautions (5.4)]*.

Chronic Hepatitis C-Associated Thrombocytopenia: In the 2 placebo-controlled trials, 955 patients with chronic hepatitis C-associated thrombocytopenia received PROMACTA. Table 5 presents the most common adverse drug reactions (experienced by ≥10% of patients receiving PROMACTA compared to placebo).

Table 5. Adverse Reactions (≥10% and Greater than Placebo) from Two Placebo-Controlled Trials in Adults With Chronic Hepatitis C

Adverse Reaction	PROMACTA + Peginterferon/ Ribavirin n = 955 (%)	Placebo + Peginterferon/ Ribavirin n = 484 (%)
Anemia	40	35
Pyrexia	30	24
Fatigue	28	23
Headache	21	20
Nausea	19	14
Diarrhea	19	11
Decreased appetite	18	14
Influenza-like illness	18	16
Asthenia	16	13
Insomnia	16	15
Cough	15	12
Pruritus	15	13
Chills	14	9
Myalgia	12	10
Alopecia	10	6
Peripheral edema	10	5

In the 2 controlled clinical trials in patients with chronic hepatitis C, hyperbilirubinemia was also reported (8% for PROMACTA versus 3% for placebo).

7 DRUG INTERACTIONS

In vitro, CYP1A2, CYP2C8, UDP-glucuronosyltransferase (UGT)1A1 and UGT1A3 are involved in the metabolism of eltrombopag. *In vitro*, eltrombopag inhibits the following metabolic or transporter systems: CYP2C8, CYP2C9, UGT1A1, UGT1A3, UGT1A4, UGT1A6, UGT1A9, UGT2B7, UGT2B15, OATP1B1 and breast cancer resistance protein (BCRP) *[see Clinical Pharmacology (12.3)]*.

7.1 Polyvalent Cations (Chelation)

Eltrombopag chelates polyvalent cations (such as iron, calcium, aluminum, magnesium, selenium, and zinc) in foods, mineral supplements, and antacids. In a clinical trial, administration of PROMACTA with a polyvalent cation-containing antacid decreased plasma eltrombopag systemic exposure by approximately 70% *[see Clinical Pharmacology (12.3)]*.

PROMACTA must not be taken within 4 hours of any medications or products containing polyvalent cations such as antacids, dairy products, and mineral supplements to avoid significant reduction in PROMACTA absorption due to chelation *[see Dosage and Administration (2.3)]*.

7.2 Transporters

Co-administration of PROMACTA with the OATP1B1 and BCRP substrate, rosuvastatin, to healthy adult subjects increased plasma rosuvastatin $AUC_{0-\infty}$ by 55% and C_{max} by 103% *[see Clinical Pharmacology (12.3)]*.

Use caution when concomitantly administering PROMACTA and drugs that are substrates of OATP1B1 [e.g., atorvastatin, bosentan, ezetimibe, fluvastatin, glyburide, olmesartan, pitavastatin, pravastatin, rosuvastatin, repaglinide, rifampin, simvastatin acid, SN-38 (active metabolite of irinotecan), valsartan] or BCRP (e.g., imatinib, irinotecan, lapatinib, methotrexate, mitoxantrone, rosuvastatin, sulfasalazine, topotecan). Monitor patients closely for signs and symptoms of excessive exposure to the drugs that are substrates of OATP1B1 or BCRP and consider reduction of the dose of these drugs, if appropriate. In clinical trials with PROMACTA, a dose reduction of rosuvastatin by 50% was recommended.

7.3 Lopinavir/ritonavir

In a drug interaction trial, co-administration of PROMACTA with lopinavir/ritonavir (LPV/RTV) decreased plasma eltrombopag exposure by 17% *[see Clinical Pharmacology (12.3)]*. No dose adjustment is recommended when PROMACTA is co-administered with LPV/RTV. Drug interactions with other HIV protease inhibitors have not been evaluated.

7.4 Peginterferon Alfa 2a/b Therapy

Co-administration of peginterferon alfa 2a (PEGASYS®) or 2b (PEGINTRON®) did not affect eltrombopag exposure in 2 randomized, double-blind, placebo-controlled trials with adult patients with chronic hepatitis C *[see Clinical Pharmacology (12.3)]*.

8 USE IN SPECIFIC POPULATIONS

8.1 Pregnancy

Pregnancy Category C

There are no adequate and well-controlled studies of eltrombopag use in pregnancy. In animal reproduction and developmental toxicity studies, there was evidence of embryolethality and reduced fetal weights at maternally toxic doses. PROMACTA should be used in pregnancy only if the potential benefit to the mother justifies the potential risk to the fetus.

Pregnancy Registry: A pregnancy registry has been established to collect information about the effects of PROMACTA during pregnancy. Physicians are encouraged to register pregnant patients, or pregnant women may enroll themselves in the PROMACTA pregnancy registry by calling 1-888-825-5249.

In an early embryonic development study, female rats received oral eltrombopag at doses of 10, 20, or 60 mg/kg/day (0.8, 2, and 6 times, respectively, the human clinical exposure based on AUC in ITP patients at 75 mg/day and 0.3, 1, and 3 times, respectively, the human clinical exposure based on AUC in chronic hepatitis C patients at 100 mg/day). Increased pre- and post-implantation loss and reduced fetal weight were observed at the highest dose which also caused maternal toxicity.

Eltrombopag was administered orally to pregnant rats at 10, 20, or 60 mg/kg/day (0.8, 2, and 6 times, respectively, the human clinical exposure based on AUC in ITP patients at 75 mg/day and 0.3, 1, and 3 times, respectively, the human clinical exposure based on AUC in chronic hepatitis C patients at 100 mg/day). Decreased fetal weights (6% to 7%) and a slight increase in the presence of cervical ribs were observed at the highest dose which also caused maternal toxicity. However, no evidence of major structural malformations was observed.

Pregnant rabbits were treated with oral eltrombopag doses of 30, 80, or 150 mg/kg/day (0.04, 0.3, and 0.5 times, respectively, the human clinical exposure based on AUC in ITP patients at 75 mg/day and 0.02, 0.1, and 0.3 times, respectively, the human clinical exposure based on AUC in chronic hepatitis C patients at 100 mg/day). No evidence of fetotoxicity, embryolethality, or teratogenicity was observed.

In a pre- and post-natal developmental toxicity study in pregnant rats (F0), no adverse effects on maternal reproductive function or on the development of the offspring (F1) were observed at doses up to 20 mg/kg/day (2 times the human clinical exposure based on AUC in ITP patients at 75 mg/day and similar to the human clinical exposure based on AUC in chronic hepatitis C patients at 100 mg/day). Eltrombopag was detected in the plasma of offspring (F1). The plasma concentrations in pups increased with dose following administration of drug to the F0 dams.

8.3 Nursing Mothers

It is not known whether eltrombopag is excreted in human milk. Because many drugs are excreted in human milk and because of the potential for serious adverse reactions in nursing infants from PROMACTA, a decision should be made whether to discontinue nursing or to discontinue PROMACTA taking into account the importance of PROMACTA to the mother.

8.4 Pediatric Use

The safety and efficacy of PROMACTA in pediatric patients have not been established.

8.5 Geriatric Use

Of the 106 patients in 2 randomized clinical trials of PROMACTA 50 mg in chronic ITP, 22% were 65 years of age and over, while 9% were 75 years of age and over. In the 2 randomized clinical trials of PROMACTA in patients with chronic hepatitis C and thrombocytopenia, 7% were 65 years of age and over, while fewer than 1% were 75 years of age and over. No overall differences in safety or effectiveness were observed between these patients and younger patients in the placebo-controlled trials, but greater sensitivity of some older individuals cannot be ruled out.

8.6 Hepatic Impairment

Hepatic impairment influences the exposure of PROMACTA *[see Clinical Pharmacology (12.3)]*.

A reduction in the initial dose of PROMACTA in patients with chronic ITP is recommended for patients with hepatic impairment (Child-Pugh Class A, B, C) *[see Dosage and Administration (2.1) and Warnings and Precautions (5.1)]*. No dosage adjustment is necessary for HCV patients with hepatic impairment *[see Clinical Pharmacology (12.3)]*.

8.7 Renal Impairment

No adjustment in the initial PROMACTA dose is needed for patients with renal impairment *[see Clinical Pharmacology (12.3)]*. Closely monitor patients with impaired renal function when administering PROMACTA.

8.8 Ethnicity

Patients of East Asian ethnicity (i.e., Japanese, Chinese, Taiwanese, and Korean) exhibit higher eltrombopag exposures. A reduction in the initial dose of PROMACTA is recommended for ITP patients of East Asian ancestry and patients of East Asian ancestry with hepatic impairment (Child-Pugh Class A, B, C) *[see Dosage and Administration (2.1)]*. No dose reduction is needed in patients of East Asian ethnicity with chronic hepatitis C *[see Clinical Pharmacology (12.3)]*.

10 OVERDOSAGE

In the event of overdose, platelet counts may increase excessively and result in thrombotic/thromboembolic complications.

In one report, a subject who ingested 5,000 mg of PROMACTA had a platelet count increase to a maximum of 929×10^9/L at 13 days following the ingestion. The patient also experienced rash, bradycardia, ALT/AST elevations, and fatigue. The patient was treated with gastric lavage, oral lactulose, intravenous fluids, omeprazole, atropine, furosemide, calcium, dexamethasone, and plasmapheresis; however, the abnormal platelet count and liver test abnormalities persisted for 3 weeks. After 2 months follow-up, all events had resolved without sequelae.

In case of an overdose, consider oral administration of a metal cation-containing preparation, such as calcium, aluminum, or magnesium preparations to chelate eltrombopag and thus limit absorption. Closely monitor platelet counts. Reinitiate treatment with PROMACTA in accordance with dosing and administration recommendations *[see Dosage and Administration (2.1, 2.2)]*.

11 DESCRIPTION

PROMACTA (eltrombopag) Tablets contain eltrombopag olamine, a small molecule thrombopoietin (TPO) receptor agonist for oral administration. Eltrombopag interacts with the transmembrane domain of the TPO receptor (also known as cMpl) leading to increased platelet production. Each tablet contains eltrombopag olamine in the amount equivalent to 12.5 mg, 25 mg, 50 mg, 75 mg, or 100 mg of eltrombopag free acid.

Eltrombopag olamine is a biphenyl hydrazone. The chemical name for eltrombopag olamine is 3'-{(2Z)-2-[1-(3,4-dimethylphenyl)-3-methyl-5-oxo-1,5-dihydro-4H-pyrazol-4-ylidene]hydrazino}-2'-hydroxy-3-biphenylcarboxylic acid - 2-aminoethanol (1:2). It has the molecular formula $C_{25}H_{22}N_4O_4 \bullet 2(C_2H_7NO)$. The molecular weight is 564.65 for eltrombopag olamine and 442.5 for eltrombopag free acid. Eltrombopag olamine has the following structural formula:

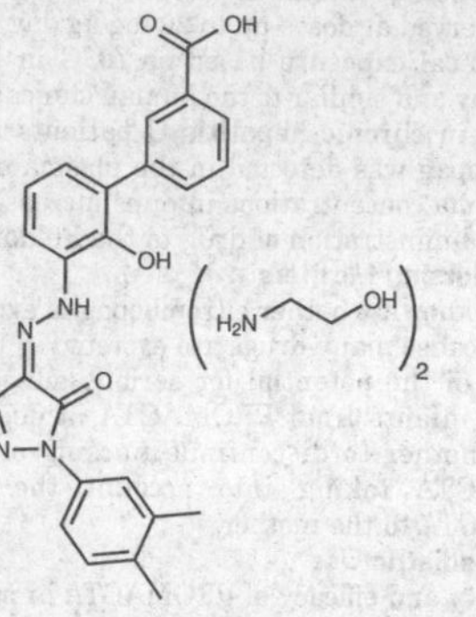

Eltrombopag olamine is practically insoluble in aqueous buffer across a pH range of 1 to 7.4, and is sparingly soluble in water.

The inactive ingredients of PROMACTA are: **Tablet Core:** magnesium stearate, mannitol, microcrystalline cellulose, povidone, and sodium starch glycolate. **Coating:** hypromellose, polyethylene glycol 400, titanium dioxide, polysorbate 80 (12.5 mg tablet), FD&C Yellow No. 6 aluminum lake (25 mg tablet), FD&C Blue No. 2 aluminum lake (50 mg tablet), Iron Oxide Red and Iron Oxide Black (75 mg tablet), or Iron Oxide Yellow and Iron Oxide Black (100 mg tablet).

12 CLINICAL PHARMACOLOGY

12.1 Mechanism of Action

Eltrombopag is an orally bioavailable, small-molecule TPO-receptor agonist that interacts with the transmembrane domain of the human TPO-receptor and initiates signaling cascades that induce proliferation and differentiation of megakaryocytes from bone marrow progenitor cells.

12.3 Pharmacokinetics

Absorption: Eltrombopag is absorbed with a peak concentration occurring 2 to 6 hours after oral administration. Based on urinary excretion and biotransformation products eliminated in feces, the oral absorption of drug-related material following administration of a single 75 mg solution dose was estimated to be at least 52%.

An open-label, randomized, crossover trial was conducted to assess the effect of food on the bioavailability of eltrombopag. A standard high-fat breakfast significantly decreased plasma eltrombopag $AUC_{0-\infty}$ by approximately 59% and C_{max} by 65% and delayed t_{max} by 1 hour. The calcium content of this meal may have also contributed to this decrease in exposure.

Distribution: The concentration of eltrombopag in blood cells is approximately 50% to 79% of plasma concentrations based on a radiolabel study. *In vitro* studies suggest that eltrombopag is highly bound to human plasma proteins (>99%). Eltrombopag is a substrate of BCRP, but is not a substrate for P-glycoprotein (P-gp) or OATP1B1.

Metabolism: Absorbed eltrombopag is extensively metabolized, predominantly through pathways including cleavage, oxidation, and conjugation with glucuronic acid, glutathione, or cysteine. *In vitro* studies suggest that CYP1A2 and CYP2C8 are responsible for the oxidative metabolism of eltrombopag. UGT1A1 and UGT1A3 are responsible for the glucuronidation of eltrombopag.

Elimination: The predominant route of eltrombopag excretion is via feces (59%), and 31% of the dose is found in the urine. Unchanged eltrombopag in feces accounts for approximately 20% of the dose; unchanged eltrombopag is not detectable in urine. The plasma elimination half-life of eltrombopag is approximately 21 to 32 hours in healthy subjects and 26 to 35 hours in ITP patients.

Drug Interactions: *Polyvalent Cation-containing Antacids:* In a clinical trial, co-administration of 75 mg of PROMACTA with a polyvalent cation-containing antacid (1,524 mg aluminum hydroxide, 1,425 mg magnesium carbonate, and sodium alginate) to 26 healthy adult subjects decreased plasma eltrombopag $AUC_{0-\infty}$ and C_{max} by approximately 70%. The contribution of sodium alginate to this interaction is not known.

Cytochrome P450 Enzymes (CYPs): In a clinical trial, PROMACTA 75 mg once daily was administered for 7 days to 24 healthy male subjects did not show inhibition or induction of the metabolism of a combination of probe substrates for CYP1A2 (caffeine), CYP2C19 (omeprazole), CYP2C9 (flurbiprofen), or CYP3A4 (midazolam) in humans. Probe substrates for CYP2C8 were not evaluated in this trial.

Rosuvastatin: In a clinical trial, co-administration of 75 mg of PROMACTA once daily for 5 days with a single 10 mg dose of the OATP1B1 and BCRP substrate, rosuvastatin to 39 healthy adult subjects increased plasma rosuvastatin $AUC_{0-\infty}$ by 55% and C_{max} by 103%.

Lopinavir/Ritonavir: In a clinical trial, co-administration of repeat dose lopinavir 400 mg /ritonavir 100 mg twice daily with a single dose of PROMACTA 100 mg to 40 healthy adult subjects decreased plasma eltrombopag $AUC_{0-\infty}$ by 17%.

Pegylated Interferon alfa-2a + Ribavirin and Pegylated Interferon alfa-2b + Ribavirin: The pharmacokinetics of eltrombopag in both the presence and absence of pegylated interferon alfa 2a and 2b therapy were evaluated using a population pharmacokinetic analysis in 635 patients with chronic hepatitis C. The population PK model estimates of clearance indicate no significant difference in eltrombopag clearance in the presence of pegylated interferon alfa plus ribavirin therapy.

In vitro Studies: Eltrombopag is an inhibitor of CYP2C8 and CYP2C9 *in vitro* . Eltrombopag is an inhibitor of UGT1A1, UGT1A3, UGT1A4, UGT1A6, UGT1A9, UGT2B7, and UGT2B15 *in vitro* . Eltrombopag is an inhibitor of the organic anion transporting polypeptide OATP1B1 and BCRP *in vitro* .

Specific Populations: *Ethnicity:* Based on two population PK analyses of eltrombopag concentrations in ITP and chronic hepatitis C patients, East Asian (i.e., Japanese, Chinese, Taiwanese, and Korean) subjects exhibited 50 to 55% higher eltrombopag plasma concentrations compared to non-East Asian subjects *[see Dosage and Administration (2.1, 2.2)]*.

An approximately 40% higher systemic eltrombopag exposure in healthy African-American subjects was noted in at least one clinical pharmacology trial. The effect of African-American ethnicity on exposure and related safety and efficacy of eltrombopag has not been established.

Hepatic Impairment: In a pharmacokinetic trial, the disposition of a single 50 mg dose of PROMACTA in patients with mild, moderate, and severe hepatic impairment was compared to subjects with normal hepatic function. The degree of hepatic impairment was based on Child-Pugh score. Plasma eltrombopag $AUC_{0-\infty}$ was 41% higher in patients with mild hepatic impairment (Child-Pugh Class A) compared to subjects with normal hepatic function. Plasma eltrombopag $AUC_{0-\infty}$ was approximately 2-fold higher in patients with moderate (Child-Pugh Class B) and severe hepatic impairment (Child-Pugh Class C). The half-life of eltrombopag was prolonged 2-fold in these patients. This clinical trial did not evaluate protein binding effects.

Chronic Liver Disease: A population PK analysis in thrombocytopenic patients with chronic liver disease following repeat doses of eltrombopag demonstrated that mild hepatic impairment resulted in an 87% to 110% higher plasma eltrombopag $AUC_{(0-\tau)}$ and patients with moderate hepatic impairment had approximately 141% to 240% higher plasma eltrombopag $AUC_{(0-\tau)}$ values compared to patients with normal hepatic function. The half-life of eltrombopag was prolonged 3-fold in patients with mild hepatic impairment and 4-fold in patients with moderate hepatic impairment. This clinical trial did not evaluate protein binding effects.

Chronic Hepatitis C: A population PK in 28 healthy adults and 635 patients with chronic hepatitis C demonstrated that patients with chronic hepatitis C treated with PROMACTA had higher plasma $AUC_{(0-\tau)}$ values as compared to healthy subjects, and $AUC_{(0-\tau)}$ increased with increasing Child-Pugh score. Patients with chronic hepatitis C and mild hepatic impairment had approximately 100% to 144% higher plasma $AUC_{(0-\tau)}$ compared with healthy subjects. This clinical trial did not evaluate protein binding effects.

Renal Impairment: The disposition of a single 50 mg dose of PROMACTA in patients with mild (creatinine clearance (CrCl) of 50 to 80 mL/min), moderate (CrCl of 30 to 49 mL/min), and severe (CrCl less than 30 mL/min) renal impairment was compared to subjects with normal renal function. Average total plasma eltrombopag $AUC_{0-\infty}$ was 32% to 36% lower in subjects with mild to moderate renal impairment and 60% lower in subjects with severe renal impairment compared with healthy subjects. The effect of renal impairment on unbound (active) eltrombopag exposure has not been assessed.

12.6 Assessment of Risk of QT/QTc Prolongation

There is no indication of a QT/QTc prolonging effect of PROMACTA at doses up to 150 mg daily for 5 days. The effects of PROMACTA at doses up to 150 mg daily for 5 days (supratherapeutic doses) on the QT/QTc interval was evaluated in a double-blind, randomized, placebo- and positive-controlled (moxifloxacin 400 mg, single oral dose) crossover trial in healthy adult subjects. Assay sensitivity was confirmed by significant QTc prolongation by moxifloxacin.

13 NONCLINICAL TOXICOLOGY

13.1 Carcinogenesis, Mutagenesis, Impairment of Fertility

Eltrombopag does not stimulate platelet production in rats, mice, or dogs because of unique TPO receptor specificity. Data from these animals do not fully model effects in humans.

Eltrombopag was not carcinogenic in mice at doses up to 75 mg/kg/day or in rats at doses up to 40 mg/kg/day (exposures up to 4 times the human clinical exposure based on AUC in ITP patients at 75 mg/day and 2 times the human clinical exposure based on AUC in chronic hepatitis C patients at 100 mg/day).

Eltrombopag was not mutagenic or clastogenic in a bacterial mutation assay or in 2 *in vivo* assays in rats (micronucleus and unscheduled DNA synthesis, 10 times the human clinical exposure based on C_{max} in ITP patients at 75 mg/day and 7 times the human clinical exposure based on C_{max} in chronic hepatitis C patients at 100 mg/day). In the *in vitro* mouse lymphoma assay, eltrombopag was marginally positive (<3-fold increase in mutation frequency).

Eltrombopag did not affect female fertility in rats at doses up to 20 mg/kg/day (2 times the human clinical exposure based on AUC in ITP patients at 75 mg/day and similar to the human clinical exposure based on AUC in chronic hepatitis C patients at 100 mg/day). Eltrombopag did not affect male fertility in rats at doses up to 40 mg/kg/day, the highest dose tested (3 times the human clinical exposure based on AUC in ITP patients at 75 mg/day and 2 times the human clinical exposure based on AUC in chronic hepatitis C patients at 100 mg/day).

13.2 Animal Pharmacology/Toxicology

Eltrombopag is phototoxic *in vitro*. There was no evidence of *in vivo* cutaneous or ocular phototoxicity in rodents.

Treatment-related cataracts were detected in rodents in a dose- and time-dependent manner. At ≥6 times the human clinical exposure based on AUC in ITP patients at 75 mg/day and 3 times the human clinical exposure based on AUC in chronic hepatitis C patients at 100 mg/day, cataracts were observed in mice after 6 weeks and in rats after 28 weeks of dosing. At ≥4 times the human clinical exposure based on AUC in ITP patients at 75 mg/day and 2 times the human clinical exposure based on AUC in chronic hepatitis C patients at 100 mg/day, cataracts were observed in mice after 13 weeks and in rats after 39 weeks of dosing *[see Warnings and Precautions (5.6)]*.

Renal tubular toxicity was observed in studies up to 14 days in duration in mice and rats at exposures that were generally associated with morbidity and mortality. Tubular toxicity was also observed in a 2-year oral carcinogenicity study in mice at doses of 25, 75, and 150 mg/kg/day. The exposure at the lowest dose was 1.2 times the human clinical exposure based on AUC in ITP patients at 75 mg/day and 0.6 times the human clinical exposure based on AUC in chronic hepatitis C patients at 100 mg/day. No similar effects were observed in mice after 13 weeks at exposures greater than those associated with renal changes in the 2-year study, suggesting that this effect is both dose- and time-dependent.

14 CLINICAL STUDIES

14.1 Chronic ITP

The efficacy and safety of PROMACTA in adult patients with chronic ITP were evaluated in 3 randomized, double-blind, placebo-controlled trials and in an open-label extension trial.

Trials 1 and 2: In trials 1 and 2, patients who had completed at least one prior ITP therapy and who had a platelet count $<30 \times 10^9$/L were randomized to receive either PROMACTA or placebo daily for up to 6 weeks, followed by 6 weeks off therapy. During the trials, PROMACTA or placebo was discontinued if the platelet count exceeded 200×10^9/L. The primary efficacy endpoint was response rate, defined as a shift from a baseline platelet count of $<30 \times 10^9$/L to $\geq 50 \times 10^9$/L at any time during the treatment period.

The median age of the patients was 50 years and 60% were female. Approximately 70% of the patients had received at least 2 prior ITP therapies (predominantly corticosteroids, immunoglobulins, rituximab, cytotoxic therapies, danazol, and azathioprine) and 40% of the patients had undergone splenectomy. The median baseline platelet counts (approximately 18×10^9/L) were similar among all treatment groups.

Trial 1 randomized 114 patients (2:1) to PROMACTA 50 mg or placebo. Trial 2 randomized 117 patients (1:1:1:1) among placebo or 1 of 3 dose regimens of PROMACTA, 30 mg, 50 mg, or 75 mg each administered daily.

Table 6 shows for each trial the primary efficacy outcomes for the placebo groups and the patient groups who received the 50 mg daily regimen of PROMACTA.

Table 6. Trials 1 and 2 Platelet Count Response (≥50 × 10^9/L) Rates in Adults With Chronic Immune (Idiopathic) Thrombocytopenia

Trial	PROMACTA 50 mg Daily	Placebo
1	43/73 (59%)[a]	6/37 (16%)
2	19/27 (70%)[a]	3/27 (11%)

[a]*P* value <0.001 for PROMACTA versus placebo.

The platelet count response to PROMACTA was similar among patients who had or had not undergone splenectomy. In general, increases in platelet counts were detected 1 week following initiation of PROMACTA and the maximum response was observed after 2 weeks of therapy. In the placebo and 50 mg dose groups of PROMACTA, the trial drug was discontinued due to an increase in platelet counts to >200 × 10^9/L in 3% and 27% of the patients, respectively. The median duration of treatment with the 50 mg dose of PROMACTA was 42 days in Trial 1 and 43 days in Trial 2. Of 7 patients who underwent hemostatic challenges, additional ITP medications were required in 3 of 3 placebo group patients and 0 of 4 patients treated with PROMACTA. Surgical procedures accounted for most of the hemostatic challenges. Hemorrhage requiring transfusion occurred in one placebo group patient and no patients treated with PROMACTA.

Trial 3: In this trial, 197 patients were randomized (2:1) to receive either PROMACTA 50 mg once daily (n = 135) or placebo (n = 62) for 6 months, during which time the dose of PROMACTA could be adjusted based on individual platelet counts. Patients were allowed to taper or discontinue concomitant ITP medications after being treated with PROMACTA for 6 weeks. Patients were permitted to receive rescue treatments at any time during the trial as clinically indicated. The primary endpoint was the odds of achieving a platelet count ≥50 × 10^9/L and ≤400 × 10^9/L for patients receiving PROMACTA relative to placebo and was based on patient response profiles throughout the 6-month treatment period.

The median age of the patients treated with PROMACTA and placebo was 47 years and 52.5 years, respectively. Approximately half of the patients treated with PROMACTA and placebo (47% and 50%, respectively) were receiving concomitant ITP medication (predominantly corticosteroids) at randomization and had baseline platelet counts 15 × 10^9/L (50% and 48%, respectively). A similar percentage of patients treated with PROMACTA and placebo (37% and 34%, respectively) had a prior splenectomy.

In 134 patients who completed 26 weeks of treatment, a sustained platelet response (platelet count ≥50 × 10^9/L and ≤400 × 10^9/L for 6 out of the last 8 weeks of the 26-week treatment period in the absence of rescue medication at any time) was achieved by 60% of patients treated with PROMACTA, compared to 10% of patients treated with placebo (splenectomized patients: PROMACTA 51%, placebo 8%; non-splenectomized patients: PROMACTA 66%, placebo 11%). The proportion of responders in the PROMACTA treatment group was between 37% and 56% compared to 7% and 19% in the placebo treatment group for all on-therapy visits. Patients treated with PROMACTA were significantly more likely to achieve a platelet count between 50 × 10^9/L and 400 × 10^9/L during the entire 6-month treatment period compared to those patients treated with placebo.

Outcomes of treatment are presented in Table 7 for all patients enrolled in the trial.

Table 7. Outcomes of Treatment from Trial 3 in Adults With Chronic Immune (Idiopathic) Thrombocytopenia

Outcome	PROMACTA N = 135	Placebo N = 62
Mean number of weeks with platelet counts ≥50 × 109/L	11.3	2.4
Requiring rescue therapy, n (%)	24 (18)	25 (40)

Among 94 patients receiving other ITP therapy at baseline, 37 (59%) of 63 patients in the PROMACTA group and 10 (32%) of 31 patients in the placebo group discontinued concomitant therapy at some time during the trial.

Extension Trial: Patients who completed any prior clinical trial with PROMACTA were enrolled in an open-label, single-arm trial in which attempts were made to decrease the dose or eliminate the need for any concomitant ITP medications. PROMACTA was administered to 299 patients; 249 completed 6 months, 210 patients completed 12 months, and 138 patients completed 24 months of therapy. The median baseline platelet count was 19 × 10^9/L prior to administration of PROMACTA.

Table 8. Trials 1 and 2 Sustained Virologic Response in Adults With Chronic Hepatitis C

	Trial 1[a]		Trial 2[b]	
Pre-antiviral Treatment Phase	N = 715		N = 805	
% Patients who achieved target platelet counts and initiated antiviral therapyc	95%		94%	
Antiviral Treatment Phase	**PROMACTA N = 450 %**	**Placebo N = 232 %**	**PROMACTA N = 506 %**	**Placebo N = 253 %**
Overall SVR[d]	23	14	19	13
HCV Genotype 2,3	35	24	34	25
HCV Genotype 1,4,6	18	10	13	7

[a] PROMACTA given in combination with peginterferon alfa-2a (180 mcg once weekly for 48 weeks for genotypes 1/4/6; 24 weeks for genotype 2 or 3) plus ribavirin (800 to 1,200 mg daily in 2 divided doses orally).
[b] PROMACTA given in peginterferon alfa-2b (1.5 mcg/kg once weekly for 48 weeks for genotypes 1/4/6; 24 weeks for genotype 2 or 3) plus ribavirin (800 to 1,400 mg daily in 2 divided doses orally).
[c] Target platelet count was ≥90 × 10^9 /L for Trial 1 and ≥100 × 10^9 /L for Trial 2.
[d]*P* value <0.05 for PROMACTA versus placebo.

14.2 Chronic Hepatitis C-Associated Thrombocytopenia

The efficacy and safety of PROMACTA for the treatment of thrombocytopenia in adult patients with chronic hepatitis C were evaluated in 2 randomized, double-blind, placebo-controlled trials. Trial 1 utilized peginterferon alfa-2a (PEGASYS®) plus ribavirin for antiviral treatment and Trial 2 utilized peginterferon alfa-2b (PEGINTRON®) plus ribavirin. In both trials, patients with a platelet count of <75 × 10^9/L were enrolled and stratified by platelet count, screening HCV RNA, and HCV genotype. Patients were excluded if they had evidence of decompensated liver disease with Child-Pugh score > 6 (class B and C), history of ascites, or hepatic encephalopathy. The median age of the patients in both trials was 52 years, 63% were male, and 74% were Caucasian. Sixty-nine percent of patients had HCV genotypes 1, 4, 6 with the remainder genotypes 2 and 3. Approximately 30% of patients had been previously treated with interferon and ribavirin. The majority of patients (90%) had bridging fibrosis and cirrhosis, as indicated by noninvasive testing. A similar proportion (95%) of patients in both treatment groups had Child-Pugh level A (score 5-6) at baseline. A similar proportion of patients (2%) in both treatment groups had baseline international normalized ratio (INR) > 1.7. Median baseline platelet counts (approximately 60 × 10^9/L) were similar in both treatment groups. The trials consisted of two phases – a pre-antiviral treatment phase and an antiviral treatment phase. In the pre-antiviral treatment phase, patients received open-label PROMACTA to increase the platelet count to a threshold of ≥90 × 10^9/L for Trial 1 and ≥100 × 10^9/L for Trial 2. PROMACTA was administered at an initial dose of 25 mg once daily for 2 weeks and increased in 25 mg increments over 2 to 3 week periods to achieve the optimal platelet count to initiate antiviral therapy. The maximal time patients could receive open-label PROMACTA was 9 weeks. If threshold platelet counts were achieved, patients were randomized (2:1) to the same dose of PROMACTA at the end of the pre-treatment phase or to placebo. PROMACTA was administered in combination with pegylated interferon and ribavirin per their respective prescribing information for up to 48 weeks.

The primary efficacy endpoint for both trials was sustained virologic response (SVR) defined as the percentage of patients with undetectable HCV-RNA at 24 weeks after completion of antiviral treatment. The median time to achieve the target platelet count ≥90 × 10^9/L was approximately 2 weeks. Ninety-five percent of patients were able to initiate antiviral therapy.

In both trials, a significantly greater proportion of patients treated with PROMACTA achieved SVR (see Table 8). The improvement in the proportion of patients who achieved SVR was consistent across subgroups based on baseline platelet count (<50 × 10^9/L versus ≥50 × 10^9/L). In patients with high baseline viral loads (≥800,000), the SVR rate was 18% (82/452) for PROMACTA versus 8% (20/239) for placebo.

[See table 8 above]

The majority of patients treated with PROMACTA (76%) maintained a platelet count ≥50 × 10^9/L compared to 19% for placebo. A greater proportion of patients on PROMACTA did not require any antiviral dose reduction as compared to placebo (45% versus 27%).

16 HOW SUPPLIED/STORAGE AND HANDLING

- The 12.5 mg tablets are round, biconvex, white, film-coated tablets debossed with GS MZ1 and 12.5 on one side and are available in bottles of 30: NDC 0007-4643-13.
- The 25 mg tablets are round, biconvex, orange, film-coated tablets debossed with GS NX3 and 25 on one side and are available in bottles of 30: NDC 0007-4640-13.
- The 50 mg tablets are round, biconvex, blue, film-coated tablets debossed with GS UFU and 50 on one side and are available in bottles of 30: NDC 0007-4641-13.
- The 75 mg tablets are round, biconvex, pink, film-coated tablets debossed with GS FFS and 75 on one side and are available in bottles of 30: NDC 0007-4642-13.
- The 100 mg tablets are round, biconvex, green, film-coated tablets debossed with GS 1L5 and 100 on one side and are available in bottles of 30: NDC 0007-4644-13. This product contains a desiccant.

Store at room temperature between 20°C and 25°C (68°F to 77°F); excursions permitted to 15° to 30°C (59° to 86°F) [see USP Controlled Room Temperature]. Do not remove desiccant if present. Dispense in original bottle.

17 PATIENT COUNSELING INFORMATION

See FDA-approved patient labeling (Medication Guide).

Prior to treatment, patients should fully understand and be informed of the following risks and considerations for PROMACTA:

- For patients with ITP, therapy with PROMACTA is administered to achieve and maintain a platelet count ≥50 × 10^9/L as necessary to reduce the risk for bleeding.
- For patients with chronic hepatitis C, therapy with PROMACTA is administered to achieve and maintain a platelet count necessary to initiate and maintain antiviral therapy with pegylated interferon and ribavirin.
- Therapy with PROMACTA may be associated with hepatobiliary laboratory abnormalities.
- Advise patients with chronic hepatitis C and cirrhosis that they may be at risk for hepatic decompensation when receiving alfa interferon therapy.
- Advise patients that they should report any of the following signs and symptoms of liver problems to their healthcare provider right away.
  - yellowing of the skin or the whites of the eyes (jaundice)
  - unusual darkening of the urine
  - unusual tiredness
  - right upper stomach area pain
- Advise patients that thrombocytopenia and risk of bleeding may reoccur upon discontinuing PROMACTA, particularly if PROMACTA is discontinued while the patient is on anticoagulants or antiplatelet agents.
- Advise patients that too much PROMACTA may result in excessive platelet counts and a risk for thrombotic/thromboembolic complications.
- Advise patients that during therapy with PROMACTA, they should continue to avoid situations or medications that may increase the risk for bleeding.
- Advise patients to have a baseline ocular examination prior to administration of PROMACTA and be monitored for signs and symptoms of cataracts during therapy.
- Advise patients to keep at least a 4-hour interval between PROMACTA and foods, mineral supplements, and antacids which contain polyvalent cations such as iron, calcium, aluminum, magnesium, selenium, and zinc.

PROMACTA is a registered trademark of GlaxoSmithKline.

The following are registered trademarks of their respective owners: PEGASYS/Hoffmann-La Roche Inc.; PEGINTRON/Schering Corporation; FibroSURE/Laboratory Corporation of America Holdings.

GlaxoSmithKline
Research Triangle Park, NC 27709

November 2012
PRM:5PI

MEDICATION GUIDE
PROMACTA®(pro-MAC-ta)
(eltrombopag)
Tablets

Read this Medication Guide before you start taking PROMACTA and each time you get a refill. There may be new information. This Medication Guide does not take the place of talking with your healthcare provider about your medical condition or treatment.

What is the most important information I should know about PROMACTA?

PROMACTA can cause serious side effects, including:

- **Liver problems.** PROMACTA may damage your liver and cause serious illness and death. You must have blood tests to check your liver before you start taking PROMACTA and during treatment with PROMACTA. Your healthcare provider will order these blood tests. In some cases PROMACTA treatment may need to be stopped. Tell your healthcare provider right away if you have any of these signs and symptoms of liver problems:
  - yellowing of the skin or the whites of the eyes (jaundice)
  - unusual darkening of the urine
  - unusual tiredness
  - right upper stomach area pain
  - confusion
  - swelling of the stomach area (abdomen)

Your risk of developing liver problems may be increased if you have chronic hepatitis C virus with cirrhosis, and take PROMACTA with interferon and ribavirin treatment.

See "What are the possible side effects of PROMACTA?" for other side effects of PROMACTA.

What is PROMACTA?

PROMACTA is a prescription medicine used to treat low blood platelet counts in adults with:

- chronic immune (idiopathic) thrombocytopenia (ITP), when other medicines to treat your ITP or surgery to remove the spleen have not worked well enough.
- chronic hepatitis C virus (HCV) infection before and during treatment with interferon.

PROMACTA is used to try to raise your platelet count in order to lower your risk for bleeding. PROMACTA is not used to make your platelet count normal.

PROMACTA is for treatment of certain people with low platelet counts caused by chronic ITP or chronic HCV, not low platelet counts caused by other conditions or diseases.

It is not known if PROMACTA is safe and effective when used with other antiviral medicines which are approved to treat chronic hepatitis C.

It is not known if PROMACTA is safe and effective in children.

What should I tell my healthcare provider before taking PROMACTA?

Before you take PROMACTA, tell your healthcare provider if you:

- have liver or kidney problems
- have or had a blood clot
- have a history of cataracts
- have had surgery to remove your spleen (splenectomy)
- have a bone marrow problem
- have bleeding problems
- are Asian and you are of Chinese, Japanese, Taiwanese, or Korean ancestry, you may need a lower dose of PROMACTA.
- have any other medical conditions
- are pregnant or plan to become pregnant. It is not known if PROMACTA will harm an unborn baby.

  Pregnancy Registry: There is a registry for women who become pregnant during treatment with PROMACTA. If you become pregnant, consider this registry. The purpose of the registry is to collect safety information about the health of you and your baby. Contact the registry as soon as you become aware of the pregnancy, or ask your healthcare provider to contact the registry for you. You and your healthcare provider can get information and enroll in the registry by calling 1-888-825-5249.
- are breastfeeding or plan to breastfeed. It is not known if PROMACTA passes into your breast milk. You and your healthcare provider should decide whether you will take PROMACTA or breastfeed. You should not do both.

Tell your healthcare provider about all the medicines you take, including prescription and non-prescription medicines, vitamins, and herbal supplements. PROMACTA may affect the way certain medicines work. Certain other medicines may affect the way PROMACTA works.

Especially tell your healthcare provider if you take:

- certain medicines used to treat high cholesterol, called "statins".
- a blood thinner medicine.

Certain medicines may keep PROMACTA from working correctly. Take PROMACTA either 4 hours before or 4 hours after taking these products:

- antacids used to treat stomach ulcers or heartburn.
- multivitamins or products that contain iron, calcium, aluminum, magnesium, selenium, and zinc which may be found in mineral supplements.

Ask your healthcare provider if you are not sure if your medicine is one that is listed above.

Know the medicines you take. Keep a list of them and show it to your healthcare provider and pharmacist when you get a new medicine.

How should I take PROMACTA?

- Take PROMACTA exactly as your healthcare provider tells you. Do not stop taking PROMACTA without talking with your healthcare provider first. Do not change your dose or schedule for taking PROMACTA unless your healthcare provider tells you to change it.
- Take PROMACTA on an empty stomach, either 1 hour before or 2 hours after eating food.
- Take PROMACTA at least 4 hours before or 4 hours after eating dairy products and calcium fortified juices.
- If you miss a dose of PROMACTA, wait and take your next scheduled dose. Do not take more than one dose of PROMACTA in one day.
- If you take too much PROMACTA, you may have a higher risk of serious side effects. Call your healthcare provider right away.
- Your healthcare provider will check your platelet count every week and change your dose of PROMACTA as needed. This will happen every week until your healthcare provider decides that your dose of PROMACTA can stay the same. After that, you will need to have blood tests every month. When you stop taking PROMACTA, you will need to have blood tests for at least 4 weeks to check if your platelet count drops too low.
- Tell your healthcare provider about any bruising or bleeding that happens while you take and after you stop taking PROMACTA.

What should I avoid while taking PROMACTA?

Avoid situations and medicines that may increase your risk of bleeding.

What are the possible side effects of PROMACTA?

PROMACTA may cause serious side effects, including:

- See **"What is the most important information I should know about PROMACTA?"**
- **Bone marrow changes (increased reticulin and possible bone marrow fibrosis).** Long-term use of PROMACTA may cause changes in your bone marrow. These changes may lead to abnormal blood cells or your body making less blood cells. The mild form of these bone marrow changes is called "increased reticulin" which may progress to a more severe form called "fibrosis". The mild form may cause no problems while the severe form may cause life-threatening blood problems. Signs of bone marrow changes may show up as abnormal results in your blood tests. Your healthcare provider will decide if abnormal blood test results mean that you should have bone marrow tests or if you should stop taking PROMACTA.
- **High platelet counts and higher risk for blood clots.** Your risk of getting a blood clot is increased if your platelet count is too high during treatment with PROMACTA. Your risk of getting a blood clot may also be increased during treatment with PROMACTA if you have normal or low platelet counts. You may have severe problems or die from some forms of blood clots, such as clots that travel to the lungs or that cause heart attacks or strokes. Your healthcare provider will check your blood platelet counts, and change your dose or stop PROMACTA if your platelet counts get too high. Tell your healthcare provider right away if you have signs and symptoms of a blood clot in the leg, such as swelling, pain, or tenderness in your leg.

  People with chronic liver disease may be at risk for a type of blood clot in the stomach area. Stomach area pain may be a symptom of this type of blood clot.
- **New or worsened cataracts (a clouding of the lens in the eye).** New or worsened cataracts have happened in people taking PROMACTA. Your healthcare provider will check your eyes before and during your treatment with PROMACTA. Tell your healthcare provider about any changes in your eyesight while taking PROMACTA.

The most common side effects of PROMACTA when used to treat chronic ITP are:

- nausea
- diarrhea
- upper respiratory tract infection. Symptoms may include runny nose, stuffy nose, and sneezing
- vomiting
- muscle aches
- urinary tract infections. Symptoms may include frequent or urgent need to urinate, low fever in some people, pain or burning with urination
- pain or swelling (inflammation) in your throat or mouth (oropharyngeal pain and pharyngitis)
- abnormal liver function tests
- back pain
- "flu" like symptoms (influenza) including fever, headache, tiredness, cough, sore throat, and body aches
- skin tingling, itching, or burning
- rash

The most common side effects when PROMACTA is used in combination with other medicines to treat chronic HCV are:

- low red blood cell count (anemia)
- fever
- tiredness
- headache
- nausea
- diarrhea
- decreased appetite
- "flu" like symptoms (influenza) including fever, headache, tiredness, cough, sore throat, and body aches
- feeling weak
- trouble sleeping
- cough
- itching
- chills
- muscle aches
- hair loss
- swelling in your ankles, feet, and legs

Tell your healthcare provider if you have any side effect that bothers you or that does not go away. These are not all the possible side effects of PROMACTA. For more information, ask your healthcare provider or pharmacist.

Call your doctor for medical advice about side effects. You may report side effects to FDA at 1-800-FDA-1088.

How should I store PROMACTA Tablets?

- Store at room temperature between 68°F to 77°F (20°C to 25°C).
- Keep PROMACTA tightly closed in the bottle given to you.
- The PROMACTA bottle may contain a desiccant pack to help keep your medicine dry. Do not remove the desiccant pack from the bottle.
- **Keep PROMACTA and all medicines out of the reach of children.**

General information about the safe and effective use of PROMACTA

Medicines are sometimes prescribed for purposes other than those listed in a Medication Guide. Do not use PROMACTA for a condition for which it was not prescribed. Do not give PROMACTA to other people even if they have the same symptoms that you have. It may harm them.

This Medication Guide summarizes the most important information about PROMACTA. If you would like more information, talk with your healthcare provider. You can ask your healthcare provider or pharmacist for information about PROMACTA that is written for healthcare professionals.

For more information, go to www.PROMACTA.com or call toll-free 1-888-825-5249.

What are the ingredients in PROMACTA?

Active ingredient: eltrombopag olamine.

Inactive ingredients:

- Tablet Core: magnesium stearate, mannitol, microcrystalline cellulose, povidone, and sodium starch glycolate.
- Coating: hypromellose, polyethylene glycol 400, titanium dioxide, polysorbate 80 (12.5 mg tablet), and FD&C Yellow No. 6 aluminum lake (25 mg tablet), FD&C Blue No. 2 aluminum lake (50 mg tablet), Iron Oxide Red and Iron Oxide Black (75 mg tablet), or Iron Oxide Yellow and Iron Oxide Black (100 mg tablet).

This Medication Guide has been approved by the U.S. Food and Drug Administration.

PROMACTA is a registered trademark of GlaxoSmithKline.
GlaxoSmithKline
Research Triangle Park, NC 27709

Revised: November 2012
PRM:6MG

RAXIBACUMAB INJECTION ℞
for intravenous use

HIGHLIGHTS OF PRESCRIBING INFORMATION
These highlights do not include all the information needed to use RAXIBACUMAB safely and effectively. See full prescribing information for RAXIBACUMAB.
RAXIBACUMAB injection, for intravenous use
Initial U.S. Approval: 2012

INDICATIONS AND USAGE

Raxibacumab is indicated for the treatment of adult and pediatric patients with inhalational anthrax due to *Bacillus anthracis* in combination with appropriate antibacterial drugs, and for prophylaxis of inhalational anthrax when alternative therapies are not available or are not appropriate. (1)

Limitations of Use:

- The effectiveness of raxibacumab is based solely on efficacy studies in animal models of inhalational anthrax. (1.2, 14.1)
- There have been no studies of raxibacumab in the pediatric population. Dosing in pediatric patients was derived using a population PK approach. (1.2, 8.4)
- Raxibacumab does not cross the blood-brain barrier and does not prevent or treat meningitis. Raxibacumab should be used in combination with appropriate antibacterial drugs. (1.2)

DOSAGE AND ADMINISTRATION

- Premedicate with diphenhydramine. (5.1)
- Dilute and administer as an intravenous infusion over 2 hours and 15 minutes. (2.2)
  - Adults: 40 mg/kg raxibacumab. (2.1)
  - Pediatrics greater than 50 kg: 40 mg/kg raxibacumab. (2.2)
  - Pediatrics greater than 15 kg to 50 kg: 60 mg/kg raxibacumab. (2.2)
  - Pediatrics 15 kg or less: 80 mg/kg raxibacumab. (2.2)

DOSAGE FORMS AND STRENGTHS

Single-use vial contains 1,700 mg/34 mL (50 mg/mL) raxibacumab solution. (3)

CONTRAINDICATIONS

None. (4)

WARNINGS AND PRECAUTIONS

Infusion reactions may occur. Premedicate with diphenhydramine. Slow or interrupt infusion and administer treatment based on severity of the reaction. (5.1)

ADVERSE REACTIONS

Common adverse reactions in healthy adult subjects (≥1.5%) were: rash, pain in extremity, pruritus, and somnolence. (6.1)

To report SUSPECTED ADVERSE REACTIONS, contact GlaxoSmithKline at 1-888-825-5249 or FDA at 1-800-FDA-1088 or www.fda.gov/medwatch.

USE IN SPECIFIC POPULATIONS

- Nursing Mothers: Caution should be exercised when administered to a nursing woman. (8.3)
- Pediatric Use: Safety and effectiveness in children <16 years of age not studied. (8.4)

See 17 for PATIENT COUNSELING INFORMATION

Revised: 08/2013

FULL PRESCRIBING INFORMATION: CONTENTS*

*** Sections or subsections omitted from the full prescribing information are not listed**

FULL PRESCRIBING INFORMATION

1 INDICATIONS AND USAGE

1.1 Inhalational Anthrax

Raxibacumab is indicated for the treatment of adult and pediatric patients with inhalational anthrax due to *Bacillus anthracis* in combination with appropriate antibacterial drugs. Raxibacumab is also indicated for prophylaxis of inhalational anthrax when alternative therapies are not available or are not appropriate.

1.2 Limitations of Use

The effectiveness of raxibacumab is based solely on efficacy studies in animal models of inhalational anthrax. It is not ethical or feasible to conduct controlled clinical trials with intentional exposure of humans to anthrax. *[See Clinical Studies (14.1).]*

Safety and pharmacokinetics (PK) of raxibacumab have been studied in adult healthy volunteers. There have been no studies of safety or PK of raxibacumab in the pediatric population. A population PK approach was used to derive dosing regimens that are predicted to provide pediatric patients with exposure comparable to the observed exposure in adults. *[See Use in Specific Populations (8.4).]*

Raxibacumab binds to the protective antigen (PA) of *B. anthracis*; it does not have direct antibacterial activity. Raxibacumab does not cross the blood-brain barrier and does not prevent or treat meningitis. Raxibacumab should be used in combination with appropriate antibacterial drugs.

2 DOSAGE AND ADMINISTRATION

2.1 Dose and Schedule for Adults

Administer raxibacumab as a single dose of 40 mg/kg intravenously over 2 hours and 15 minutes after dilution in 0.9% Sodium Chloride Injection, USP (normal saline) to a final volume of 250 mL. Administer 25 to 50 mg diphenhydramine within 1 hour prior to raxibacumab infusion to reduce the risk of infusion reactions. Diphenhydramine route of administration (oral or IV) should be based on the temporal proximity to the start of raxibacumab infusion. *[See Warnings and Precautions (5.1) and Adverse Reactions (6.1).]*

2.2 Dose and Schedule for Pediatric Patients

The recommended dose for pediatric patients is based on weight as shown in Table 1 below.

Table 1. Recommended Pediatric Dose

Pediatric Body Weight	Pediatric Dose
Greater than 50 kg	40 mg/kg
Greater than 15 kg to 50 kg	60 mg/kg
15 kg or less	80 mg/kg

Premedicate with diphenhydramine within 1 hour prior to raxibacumab infusion. Diphenhydramine route of administration (oral or IV) should be based on the temporal proximity to the start of raxibacumab infusion. Infuse raxibacumab over 2 hours and 15 minutes. No pediatric patients were studied during the development of raxibacumab. The dosing recommendations in Table 1 above are derived from simulations designed to match the observed adult exposure to raxibacumab at a 40 mg/kg dose. *[See Use in Specific Populations (8.4).]*

2.3 Preparation for Administration

The recommended dose of raxibacumab is weight-based, given as an intravenous infusion after dilution in a compatible solution to a final volume of 250 mL (adults and children 50 kg or heavier) or to a volume indicated based on the child's weight (see Table 2). Dilute raxibacumab using one of the following compatible solutions:

- 0.9% Sodium Chloride Injection, USP
- 0.45% Sodium Chloride Injection, USP

Keep vials in their cartons prior to preparation of an infusion solution to protect raxibacumab from light. Raxibacumab vials contain no preservative.

[See table 2 above]

Table 2. Raxibacumab Dose, Diluents, Infusion Volume and Rate by Body Weight

	Preparation			Administration	
Body Weight (kg)	Dose (mg/kg)	Total Infusion Volume (mL)	Type of Diluent	Infusion rate (mL/hr) First 20 minutes	Infusion rate (mL/hr) Remaining infusion
1 or less	80	7	0.45% or 0.9% NaCl	0.5	3.5
1.1 to 2		15		1	7
2.1 to 3		20		1.2	10
3.1 to 4.9		25		1.5	12
5 to 10		50		3	25
11 to 15		100	0.9% NaCl	6	50
16 to 30	60	100		6	50
31 to 40		250		15	125
41 to 50		250		15	125
Greater than 50 or adult	40	250		15	125

Preparation: Follow the steps below to prepare the raxibacumab intravenous infusion solution.

1. Calculate the milligrams of raxibacumab injection by multiplying the recommended mg/kg dose in Table 2 by patient weight in kilograms.
2. Calculate the required volume in milliliters of raxibacumab injection needed for the dose by dividing the calculated dose in milligrams (step 1) by the concentration, 50 mg/mL. Each single-use vial allows delivery of 34 mL raxibacumab.

Based on the total infusion volume selected in Table 2, prepare either a syringe or infusion bag as appropriate following the steps below.

Syringe Preparation

3. Select an appropriate size syringe for the total volume of infusion to be administered, as described in Table 2.
4. Using the selected syringe, withdraw the volume of raxibacumab as calculated in step 2.
5. Withdraw an appropriate amount of compatible solution to prepare a total volume infusion syringe as specified in Table 2.
6. Gently mix the solution. Do not shake.
7. Discard any unused portion remaining in the raxibacumab vial(s).
8. The prepared solution is stable for 8 hours stored at room temperature.

Infusion Bag Preparation

3. Select appropriate size bag of compatible solution (see compatible solutions listed above), withdraw a volume of solution from the bag equal to the calculated volume in milliliters of raxibacumab in step 2 above. Discard the solution that was withdrawn from the bag.
4. Withdraw the required volume of raxibacumab injection from the raxibacumab vial(s).
5. Transfer the required volume of raxibacumab injection to the selected infusion bag (step 3). Gently invert the bag to mix the solution. Do not shake.
6. Discard any unused portion remaining in the raxibacumab vial(s).
7. The prepared solution is stable for 8 hours stored at room temperature.

Parenteral drug products should be inspected visually for particulate matter and discoloration prior to administration, whenever solution and container permit. Discard the solution if particulate matter is present or color is abnormal. *[See Description (11).]*

Administration: Administer the infusion solution as described in Table 2. The rate of infusion may be slowed or interrupted if the subject develops any signs of adverse reactions, including infusion-associated symptoms.

3 DOSAGE FORMS AND STRENGTHS

Raxibacumab is available as a single-use vial which contains 1,700 mg/34 mL (50 mg/mL) raxibacumab injection *[see Description (11)]*.

4 CONTRAINDICATIONS

None.

5 WARNINGS AND PRECAUTIONS

5.1 Infusion Reactions

Infusion-related reactions were reported during administration of raxibacumab in clinical trials including reports of rash, urticaria, and pruritus. If these reactions occur, slow or interrupt raxibacumab infusion and administer appropriate treatment based on severity of the reaction.

Table 3. Adverse Reactions Reported in ≥1.5% of Healthy Adult Subjects Exposed to Raxibacumab 40 mg/kg IV

Preferred Term	Placebo N = 80 (%)	Single dose raxibacumab N = 283 (%)	Double dose raxibacumab ≥4 months apart N = 20 (%)	Double dose raxibacumab 2 weeks apart N = 23 (%)	Total raxibacumab subjects N = 326 (%)
Rash/Rash erythematous/Rash papular	1 (1.3)	9 (3.2)	0	0	9 (2.8)
Pain in extremity	1 (1.3)	7 (2.5)	0	0	7 (2.1)
Pruritus	0	7 (2.5)	0	0	7 (2.1)
Somnolence	0	4 (1.4)	0	1 (4.3)	5 (1.5)

Premedicate with diphenhydramine within 1 hour prior to administering raxibacumab to reduce the risk of infusion reactions *[see Dosage and Administration (2.1) and Adverse Reactions (6.1)]*.

6 ADVERSE REACTIONS

6.1 Clinical Trials Experience

Because clinical trials are conducted under widely varying conditions, adverse reaction rates observed in the clinical trials of a drug cannot be directly compared with rates in the clinical trials of another drug and may not reflect the rates observed in practice. The safety of raxibacumab has been studied only in healthy volunteers. It has not been studied in patients with inhalational anthrax.

The safety of raxibacumab has been evaluated in 326 healthy subjects treated with a dose of 40 mg/kg in 3 clinical trials: a drug interaction study with ciprofloxacin (study 1), a repeat-dose study of 20 subjects with the second raxibacumab dose administered ≥4 months after the first dose (study 2), and a placebo-controlled study evaluating single doses with a subset of subjects receiving 2 raxibacumab doses 14 days apart (study 3). Raxibacumab was administered to 86 healthy subjects in study 1. In study 3, 240 healthy subjects received raxibacumab (217 received 1 dose and 23 received 2 doses) and 80 subjects received placebo.

The overall safety of raxibacumab was evaluated as an integrated summary of these 3 clinical trials. Of 326 raxibacumab subjects, 283 received single doses, 23 received 2 doses 14 days apart, and 20 received 2 doses more than 4 months apart. The subjects were 18 to 88 years of age, 53% female, 74% Caucasian, 17% Black/African American, 6% Asian, and 15% Hispanic.

Adverse Reactions Leading to Discontinuation of Raxibacumab Infusion

Four subjects (1.2%) had their infusion of raxibacumab discontinued for adverse reactions: 2 subjects (neither of whom received diphenhydramine premedication) due to urticaria (mild), and 1 subject each discontinued for clonus (mild) and dyspnea (moderate).

Most Frequently Reported Adverse Reactions

The most frequently reported adverse reactions were rash, pain in extremity, pruritus, and somnolence.

[See table 3 above]

Rashes

For all subjects exposed to raxibacumab in clinical trials, the rate of rash was 2.8% (9/326) compared with 1.3% (1/80) placebo subjects. Mild to moderate infusion-related rashes were reported in 22.2% (6/27) of subjects who did not receive diphenhydramine premedication compared to 3.3% (2/61) of subjects who were premedicated with diphenhydramine in the ciprofloxacin/raxibacumab combination study (study 1). In the placebo-controlled raxibacumab study where all subjects received diphenhydramine (study 3), the rate of rash was 2.5% in both placebo- and raxibacumab-treated subjects.

Less Common Adverse Reactions

Clinically significant adverse reactions that were reported in <1.5% of subjects exposed to raxibacumab and at rates higher than in placebo subjects are listed below:

- *Blood and lymphatic system*: anemia, leukopenia, lymphadenopathy
- *Cardiac disorders*: palpitations
- *Ear and labyrinth*: vertigo
- *General disorders and administration site*: fatigue, infusion site pain, peripheral edema
- *Investigations*: blood amylase increased, blood creatine phosphokinase increased, prothombin time prolonged
- *Musculoskeletal and connective tissue*: back pain, muscle spasms
- *Nervous system*: syncope vasovagal
- *Psychiatric*: insomnia
- *Vascular*: flushing, hypertension

Immunogenicity

The development of anti-raxibacumab antibodies was evaluated in all subjects receiving single and double doses of raxibacumab in studies 1, 2, and 3. Immunogenic responses against raxibacumab were not detected in any raxibacumab-treated human subjects following single or repeat doses of raxibacumab.

The incidence of antibody formation is highly dependent on the sensitivity and specificity of the immunogenicity assay. Additionally, the observed incidence of any antibody positivity in an assay is highly dependent on several factors, including assay sensitivity and specificity, assay methodology, sample handling, timing of sample collection, concomitant medications, and underlying disease. For these reasons, comparison of the incidence of antibodies to raxibacumab with the incidence of antibodies to other products may be misleading.

7 DRUG INTERACTIONS

7.1 Ciprofloxacin

Co-administration of 40 mg/kg raxibacumab IV with IV or oral ciprofloxacin in human subjects did not alter the PK of either ciprofloxacin or raxibacumab *[see Clinical Pharmacology (12.3)]*.

8 USE IN SPECIFIC POPULATIONS

8.1 Pregnancy

Pregnancy Category B

A single embryonic-fetal development study was conducted in pregnant, healthy New Zealand White rabbits administered 2 intravenous doses of raxibacumab up to 120 mg/kg (3 times the human dose on a mg/kg basis) on gestation days 7 and 14. No evidence of harm to the pregnant dam or the fetuses due to raxibacumab was observed. C_{max} values in rabbits after dosing with 120 mg/kg were 3,629 mcg/mL and 4,337 mcg/mL after the first and second dose of raxibacumab, respectively; these are more than 3 and 4 times the mean C_{max} values in humans. Estimates of exposure (AUC) were not generated in the embryo-fetal rabbit study. No adequate and well-controlled studies in pregnant women were conducted. Because animal reproduction studies are not always predictive of human response, raxibacumab should be used during pregnancy only if clearly needed.

8.3 Nursing Mothers

Raxibacumab has not been evaluated in nursing women. Although human immunoglobulins are excreted in human milk, published data suggest that neonatal consumption of human milk does not result in substantial absorption of these maternal immunoglobulins into circulation. Inform a nursing woman that the effects of local gastrointestinal and systemic exposure to raxibacumab on nursing infant are unknown.

8.4 Pediatric Use

As in adults, the effectiveness of raxibacumab in pediatric patients is based solely on efficacy studies in animal models of inhalational anthrax. As exposure of healthy children to raxibacumab is not ethical, a population PK approach was used to derive dosing regimens that are predicted to provide pediatric patients with exposure comparable to the observed exposure in adults receiving 40 mg/kg. The dose for pediatric patients is based on weight. *[See Dosage and Administration (2.2).]*

There have been no studies of safety or PK of raxibacumab in the pediatric population.

8.5 Geriatric Use

Clinical studies of raxibacumab did not include sufficient numbers of subjects aged 65 years and older to determine whether they respond differently from younger subjects. Of the total number of subjects in clinical studies of raxibacumab, 6.4% (21/326) were 65 years and older, while 1.5% (5/326) were 75 years and older. However, no alteration of dosing is needed for patients ≥65 years of age *[see Clinical Pharmacology (12.3)]*.

10 OVERDOSAGE

There is no clinical experience with overdosage of raxibacumab. In case of overdosage, monitor patients for any signs or symptoms of adverse effects.

11 DESCRIPTION

Raxibacumab is a human IgG1λ monoclonal antibody that binds the PA component of *B. anthracis* toxin. Raxibacumab has a molecular weight of approximately 146 kilodaltons. Raxibacumab is produced by recombinant DNA technology in a murine cell expression system.

Raxibacumab is supplied as a sterile, liquid formulation in single-dose vials for intravenous infusion. Each vial contains 50 mg/mL raxibacumab in citric acid (0.13 mg/mL), glycine (18 mg/mL), polysorbate 80 [0.2 mg/mL (w/v)], sodium citrate (2.8 mg/mL), and sucrose (10 mg/mL), with a pH of 6.5. Each vial contains a minimum of 35.1 mL filled into a 50 mL vial (to allow delivery of 1700 mg/34 mL). Raxibacumab is a clear to opalescent, colorless to pale yellow, liquid.

12 CLINICAL PHARMACOLOGY

12.1 Mechanism of Action

Raxibacumab is a monoclonal antibody that binds the PA of *B. anthracis[see Clinical Pharmacology (12.4)].*

12.3 Pharmacokinetics

The PK of raxibacumab are linear over the dose range of 1 to 40 mg/kg following single IV dosing in humans; raxibacumab was not tested at doses higher than 40 mg/kg in humans. Following single IV administration of raxibacumab 40 mg/kg in healthy, male and female human subjects, the mean C_{max} and AUC_{inf} were 1,020.3 ± 140.6 mcg/mL and 1,5845.8 ± 4,333.5 mcg•day/mL, respectively. Mean raxibacumab steady-state volume of distribution was greater than plasma volume, suggesting some tissue distribution. Clearance values were much smaller than the glomerular filtration rate indicating that there is virtually no renal clearance of raxibacumab.

Because the effectiveness of raxibacumab cannot be tested in humans, a comparison of raxibacumab exposures achieved in healthy human subjects to those observed in animal models of inhalational anthrax in therapeutic efficacy studies is necessary to support the dosage regimen of 40 mg/kg IV as a single dose for the treatment of inhalational anthrax in humans. Humans achieve similar or greater systemic exposure (C_{max} and AUC_{inf}) to raxibacumab following a single 40 mg/kg IV dose compared with New Zealand White rabbits and cynomolgus macaques receiving the same dosage regimen.

Effects of Gender, Age, and Race

Raxibacumab PK were evaluated via a population PK analysis using serum samples from 322 healthy subjects who received a single 40 mg/kg IV dose across 3 clinical trials. Based on this analysis, gender (female versus male), race (non-Caucasian versus Caucasian), or age (elderly versus young) had no meaningful effects on the PK parameters for raxibacumab.

Raxibacumab PK have not been evaluated in children *[see Dosage and Administration (2.2) and Use in Specific Populations (8.4)]*.

Repeat Dosing

Although raxibacumab is intended for single dose administration, the PK of raxibacumab following a second administration of 40 mg/kg IV given 14 days after the first 40 mg/kg IV dose was assessed in 23 healthy subjects (study 3). The mean raxibacumab concentration at 28 days after the second dose was approximately twice the mean raxibacumab concentration at 14 days following the first dose. In the human study assessing the immunogenicity of raxibacumab (study 2), 20 healthy subjects who had initially received a single dose of raxibacumab 40 mg/kg IV received a second 40 mg/kg IV dose at ≥4 months following their first dose. No statistically significant differences in mean estimates of AUC_{inf}, CL, or half-life of raxibacumab between the 2 doses administered ≥4 months apart were observed. The mean C_{max} following the second dose was 15% lower than the C_{max} following the first dose.

Ciprofloxacin Interaction Study

In an open-label study evaluating the effect of raxibacumab on ciprofloxacin PK in healthy adult male and female subjects (study 1), the administration of 40 mg/kg raxibacumab IV following ciprofloxacin IV infusion or ciprofloxacin oral tablet ingestion did not alter the PK of ciprofloxacin administered PO and/or IV. Likewise, ciprofloxacin did not alter the PK of raxibacumab *[see Drug Interactions (7.1)]*.

12.4 Microbiology

Mechanism of Action

Raxibacumab is a monoclonal antibody that binds free PA with an affinity equilibrium dissociation constant (Kd) of 2.78 ± 0.9 nM. Raxibacumab inhibits the binding of PA to its cellular receptors, preventing the intracellular entry of the anthrax lethal factor and edema factor, the enzymatic toxin components responsible for the pathogenic effects of anthrax toxin.

Activity In Vitro and In Vivo

Raxibacumab binds in vitro to PA from the Ames, Vollum, and Sterne strains of *B. anthracis*. Raxibacumab binds to an epitope on PA that is conserved across reported strains of *B. anthracis*.

In vivo studies in rats suggest that raxibacumab neutralizes the toxicity due to lethal toxin, as animals slowly infused with lethal toxin (a combination of PA + lethal factor) survived 7 days following administration. The median time to death in control rats was 16 hours. Similar observations were noted in animal efficacy studies in rabbits and monkeys challenged with *B. anthracis* spores by the inhalational route. PA was detected in animals following exposure to *B. anthracis* spores. PA levels rose and then fell to undetectable levels in animals that responded to treatment and survived, whereas levels continued to rise in animals that failed treatment and died or were euthanized because of poor clinical condition. *[See Clinical Studies (14.1).]*

13 NONCLINICAL TOXICOLOGY

13.1 Carcinogenesis, Mutagenesis, Impairment of Fertility

Carcinogenicity, genotoxicity, and fertility studies have not been conducted with raxibacumab.

13.2 Animal Toxicology

Healthy cynomolgus macaques administered 3 intravenous doses or 3 subcutaneous doses of 40 mg/kg raxibacumab once every 12 days, or a single intramuscular dose (40 mg/kg) of raxibacumab, showed no adverse effects, including no effects up to 120 days post-dosing.

Studies with raxibacumab in rabbit, cynomolgus macaque, and human donor tissues showed no cross reactivity with brain.

Anthrax infected rabbits and monkeys administered an intravenous injection of raxibacumab (40 mg/kg) at time of PA toxemia reproducibly showed greater severity of central nervous system (CNS) lesions (bacteria, inflammation, hemorrhage, and necrosis) in non-surviving animals compared to dead placebo control animals, with no difference in mean time to death from spore challenge. The raxibacumab monoclonal antibody appears unable to penetrate the CNS until compromise of the blood brain barrier (BBB) during the later stages of anthrax infection. The most severe brain lesions in rabbits were associated with bacteria and raxibacumab tissue binding in a similar pattern as endogenous IgG antibody that leaked across the compromised BBB. No dose/exposure-response relationship for brain histopathology was identified. Surviving rabbits and monkeys at the end of the 28 day studies showed no microscopic evidence of CNS lesions. CNS toxicity was not observed in healthy monkeys administered raxibacumab (40 mg/kg) or in GLP combination treatment studies with antibacterials in rabbits (levofloxacin) or in monkeys (ciprofloxacin) at any time.

14 CLINICAL STUDIES

Because it is not feasible or ethical to conduct controlled clinical trials in humans with inhalational anthrax, the effectiveness of raxibacumab for therapeutic treatment of inhalational anthrax is based on efficacy studies in rabbits and monkeys. Raxibacumab effectiveness has not been studied in humans. Because the animal efficacy studies are conducted under widely varying conditions, the survival rates observed in the animal studies cannot be directly compared between studies and may not reflect the rates observed in clinical practice.

The efficacy of raxibacumab for treatment of inhalational anthrax was studied in a monkey model (study 2) and a rabbit model (studies 3 and 4) of inhalational anthrax disease. These 3 studies tested raxibacumab efficacy compared to placebo. Another study in a rabbit model (study 1) evaluated the efficacy of raxibacumab in combination with an antibacterial drug relative to the antibacterial drug alone. Studies were randomized and blinded.

The animals were challenged with aerosolized *B. anthracis* spores (Ames strain) at 200×LD_{50} to achieve 100% mortality if untreated. In rabbit study 1, treatment was delayed until 84 hours after spore challenge. In monkey study 2, study treatment commenced at the time of a positive serum electrochemiluminescence (ECL) assay for *B. anthracis* PA. The mean time between spore challenge and initiation of study treatment was 42 hours. In rabbit studies 3 and 4, sustained elevation of body temperature above baseline for 2 hours or a positive result on serum ECL assay for PA served as the trigger for initiation of study treatment. The mean time between spore challenge and initiation of study treatment was 28 hours post-exposure. Efficacy in all therapeutic studies in animals was determined based on survival at the end of the study. Most study animals (88% to 100%) were bacteremic and had a positive ECL assay for PA prior to treatment in all 4 studies.

14.1 Treatment of Inhalational Anthrax in Combination with Antibacterial Drug

The efficacy of raxibacumab administered with levofloxacin as treatment of animals with systemic anthrax disease (84 hours after spore challenge) was evaluated in New Zealand White rabbits (study 1). The dose of levofloxacin was chosen to yield a comparable exposure to that achieved by the recommended doses in humans. Levofloxacin and raxibacumab PK in this study were unaffected by product co-administration. Forty-two percent of challenged animals survived to treatment. Treatment with antibacterial drug plus raxibacumab resulted in 82% survival compared to 65% survival in rabbits treated with antibacterial drug alone, $P = 0.0874$ (see Table 4).

[See table 4 above]

Table 4. Survival Rates in NZW Rabbits in Combination Therapy Study, All Treated Animals

	NZW Rabbits (35 days)[a] Study 1		
	Number (%) Survivors	*P* value[b]	95% CI[c] Levo vs Levo + Raxibacumab
Antibacterial drug alone	24/37 (65%)	-	-
Antibacterial drug + Raxibacumab 40 mg/kg IV single dose	32/39 (82%)	0.0874	(-2.4, 36.7)

[a] Survival assessed 28 days after last dose of levofloxacin.
[b] *P* value based on a two-sided likelihood ratio chi-square test.
[c] 95% confidence interval based on normal approximation.

14.2 Postexposure Prophylaxis/Early Treatment of Inhalational Anthrax

Monkey study 2 and rabbit studies 3 and 4 evaluated treatment with raxibacumab alone at an earlier time point after exposure than rabbit study 1. Treatment with raxibacumab alone resulted in a statistically significant dose-dependent improvement in survival relative to placebo when administered at the time of initial manifestations of anthrax disease in the rabbit and monkey infection models (see Table 5). Raxibacumab at 40 mg/kg IV single dose was superior to placebo in the rabbit and monkey studies in the all treated and the bacteremic animal analysis populations. All surviving animals developed toxin-neutralizing antibodies.

[See table 5 above]

Table 5. Survival Rates in Animals Treated with Raxibacumab, All Treated Animals

	Cynomolgus Macaques at 28 days[a] Study 2			NZW Rabbits at 14 days[b] Study 3			NZW Rabbits at 28 days[a] Study 4		
	Number (%) Survivors	*P* value[c]	95% CI[d]	Number (%) Survivors	*P* value[c]	95% CI[d]	Number (%) Survivors	*P* value[c]	95% CI[d]
Placebo	0/12			0/17			0/24		
20 mg/kg raxibacumab	7/14 (50%)	0.0064	(19.3, 73.7)	5/18 (28%)	0.0455	(6.6, 52.5)	-		
40 mg/kg raxibacumab	9/14 (64%)	0.0007	(31.6, 84.7)	8/18 (44%)	0.0029	(21.3, 66.7)	11/24 (46%)	0.0002	(27.0, 66.1)

[a] Survival measured at 28 days after spore challenge.
[b] Survival measured at 14 days after spore challenge.
[c] *P* value based on two-sided Fisher's exact test for comparisons between raxibacumab and placebo.
[d] 95% CIs are exact confidence intervals for the difference between raxibacumab and placebo.

In other animal studies evaluating antibacterial drug alone and raxibacumab-antibacterial drug combination, the efficacy of an antibacterial drug alone (levofloxacin in rabbits and ciprofloxacin in monkeys) was very high (95-100%) when given at the initial manifestations of inhalational anthrax disease. The timing of treatment was similar to that reported for studies 2, 3, and 4 above.

In another study, rabbits were exposed to 100×LD_{50} *B. anthracis* spores and administered raxibacumab at a single dose of 40 mg/kg at the time of exposure, 12 hours, 24 hours, or 36 hours after exposure. Survival was 12/12 (100%) in animals treated at time of exposure or 12 hours, but decreased to 6/12 (50%) and 5/12 (42%) at 24 hours and 36 hours, respectively.

16 HOW SUPPLIED/STORAGE AND HANDLING

Raxibacumab is supplied in single-use vials containing 1,700 mg/34 mL (50 mg/mL) raxibacumab injection and is available in the following packaging configuration:

Single Unit Carton: Contains one (1) single-use vial of raxibacumab 1,700 mg/34 mL (deliverable) (NDC 49401 104-01).

Raxibacumab must be refrigerated at 2° to 8°C (36° to 46°F). DO NOT FREEZE. Protect the vial from exposure to light, prior to use. Brief exposure to light, as with normal use, is acceptable. Store vial in original carton until time of use.

17 PATIENT COUNSELING INFORMATION

See FDA-approved patient labeling (Patient Information).

17.1 Efficacy Based on Animal Models

Inform patients that the efficacy of raxibacumab is based solely on efficacy studies demonstrating a survival benefit in animals and that the effectiveness of raxibacumab has not been tested in humans with anthrax. The safety of raxibacumab has been tested in healthy adults, but no safety data are available in children or pregnant women. Limited data are available in geriatric patients *[see Use in Specific Populations (8.5)]*.

17.2 Pregnancy and Nursing Mothers

Inform patients that raxibacumab has not been studied in pregnant women or nursing mothers so the effects of raxibacumab on pregnant women or nursing infants are not known. Instruct patients to tell their healthcare professional if they are pregnant, become pregnant, or are thinking about becoming pregnant. Instruct patients to tell their healthcare professional if they plan to breastfeed their infant. *[See Use in Specific Populations (8.1, 8.3).]*

17.3 Infusion Reactions

Infusion-related reactions were reported during administration of raxibacumab in clinical trials, including reports of rash, urticaria, and pruritus.

Prophylactic administration of diphenhydramine is recommended within 1 hour prior to administering raxibacumab. Diphenhydramine route of administration (oral or IV) should be based on the temporal proximity to the start of raxibacumab infusion.

Manufactured by
Human Genome Sciences, Inc.
(a subsidiary of GlaxoSmithKline)
Rockville, MD 20850
U.S. License No. 1820
Marketed by
GlaxoSmithKline
Research Triangle Park, NC 27709

RXB:3PI

PATIENT INFORMATION

RAXIBACUMAB (rack-see-BACK-u-mab)

Injection Solution for IV use

What is RAXIBACUMAB?

- RAXIBACUMAB is a prescription medicine used along with antibiotic medicines to treat people with inhalational anthrax. Raxibacumab can also be used to prevent anthrax disease when there are no other treatment options.
- The effectiveness of RAXIBACUMAB has been studied only in animals with inhalational anthrax. There have been no studies in people who have inhalational anthrax.
- The safety of RAXIBACUMAB was studied in healthy adults. There have been no studies of raxibacumab in children 16 years of age and younger.
- RAXIBACUMAB is not used for prevention or treatment of anthrax meningitis.

Before you receive RAXIBACUMAB, tell your healthcare provider about all of your medical conditions, including if you are:

- allergic to any of the ingredients in raxibacumab. See the end of this leaflet for a list of the ingredients in RAXIBACUMAB.
- allergic to diphenhydramine (Benadryl®).
- pregnant or planning to become pregnant. It is not known if RAXIBACUMAB will harm your unborn baby.
- breastfeeding or plan to breastfeed. It is not known if RAXIBACUMAB passes into your breast milk. You and your healthcare provider should decide if you will receive RAXIBACUMAB or breastfeed.

Tell your healthcare provider about all the medicines you take, including prescription and non-prescription medicines, vitamins, and herbal supplements.

How will I receive RAXIBACUMAB?

- You will be given 1 dose of RAXIBACUMAB by a healthcare provider through a vein (IV or intravenous infusion). It takes about 2 hours to give you the full dose of medicine.
- Your healthcare provider should give you a medicine called diphenhydramine (Benadryl®) before you receive RAXIBACUMAB to help reduce your chances of developing a skin reaction from RAXIBACUMAB. Benadryl may be given to you to take by mouth or through a vein.
- Benadryl may make you sleepy, and you should use caution if you will be driving or operating equipment.

What are the possible side effects of RAXIBACUMAB?

RAXIBACUMAB may cause serious side effects, including:

- **infusion reactions.** Tell your healthcare provider right away if you have rash, hives, or itching while receiving RAXIBACUMAB.

The most common side effects of RAXIBACUMAB include rash, pain in your arms or legs, itchiness, and sleepiness.

Tell your healthcare provider if you have any side effect that bothers you or that does not go away. These are not all the possible side effects of RAXIBACUMAB. For more information, ask your healthcare provider.

Call your healthcare provider for medical advice about side effects. You may report side effects to FDA at 1-800-FDA-1088. **For more information go to dailymed.nlm.nih.gov.**

General information about the safe and effective use of RAXIBACUMAB.

- This patient information leaflet summarizes the most important information about RAXIBACUMAB. If you would like more information, talk to your healthcare provider. You can ask your pharmacist or healthcare provider for information about RAXIBACUMAB that is written for health professionals.

What are the ingredients in RAXIBACUMAB?

Active ingredient: RAXIBACUMAB

Inactive ingredients: citric acid, glycine, polysorbate 80, sodium citrate, and sucrose

Manufactured by: Human Genome Sciences, Inc. (a subsidiary of GlaxoSmithKline), Rockville, MD 20850

Marketed by: GlaxoSmithKline, Research Triangle Park, NC 27709

For more information, go to www.gsk.com or call 1-888-825-5249.

This Patient Information has been approved by the U.S. Food and Drug Administration.

Issued: December 2012

RXB:1PIL

RELENZA ℞

[rə-lin'zə]

(zanamivir)

Inhalation Powder, for oral inhalation

HIGHLIGHTS OF PRESCRIBING INFORMATION

These highlights do not include all the information needed to use RELENZA safely and effectively. See full prescribing information for RELENZA.

RELENZA (zanamivir) Inhalation Powder, for oral inhalation

Initial U.S. Approval: 1999

RECENT MAJOR CHANGES

Contraindications (4) 12/2011

INDICATIONS AND USAGE

RELENZA, an influenza neuraminidase inhibitor, is indicated for:

Treatment of influenza in patients aged 7 years and older who have been symptomatic for no more than 2 days. (1.1)

Prophylaxis of influenza in patients aged 5 years and older. (1.2)

Important Limitations on Use of RELENZA:

Not recommended for treatment or prophylaxis of influenza in:

- Individuals with underlying airways disease. (5.1)

Not proven effective for:

- Treatment in individuals with underlying airways disease. (1.3)
- Prophylaxis in nursing home residents. (1.3)

Not a substitute for annual influenza vaccination. (1.3)

Consider available information on influenza drug susceptibility patterns and treatment effects when deciding whether to use RELENZA. (1.3)

DOSAGE AND ADMINISTRATION

Indication	Dose
Treatment of Influenza (2.2)	10 mg twice daily for 5 days
Prophylaxis: (2.3)	
Household Setting	10 mg once daily for 10 days
Community Outbreaks	10 mg once daily for 28 days

Note: The 10-mg dose is provided by 2 inhalations (one 5-mg blister per inhalation). (2.1)

DOSAGE FORMS AND STRENGTHS

Blister for oral inhalation: 5 mg. Four 5-mg blisters of powder on a ROTADISK® for oral inhalation via DISKHALER®. Packaged in carton containing 5 ROTADISKs (total of 10 doses) and 1 DISKHALER inhalation device. (3)

CONTRAINDICATIONS

Do not use in patients with history of allergic reaction to any ingredient of RELENZA, including lactose milk proteins. (4)

WARNINGS AND PRECAUTIONS

- **Bronchospasm:** Serious, sometimes fatal, cases have occurred. Not recommended in individuals with underlying airways disease. Discontinue RELENZA if bronchospasm or decline in respiratory function develops. (5.1)
- **Allergic Reactions:** Discontinue RELENZA and initiate appropriate treatment if an allergic reaction occurs or is suspected. (5.2)
- **Neuropsychiatric Events:** Patients with influenza, particularly pediatric patients, may be at an increased risk of seizures, confusion, or abnormal behavior early in their illness. Monitor for signs of abnormal behavior. (5.3)
- **High-risk Underlying Medical Conditions:** Safety and effectiveness have not been demonstrated in these patients. (5.4)

ADVERSE REACTIONS

The most common adverse events reported in >1.5% of patients treated with RELENZA and more commonly than in patients treated with placebo are:

- **Treatment Studies – sinusitis, dizziness.**
- **Prophylaxis Studies – fever and/or chills, arthralgia and articular rheumatism. (6.1)**

To report SUSPECTED ADVERSE REACTIONS, contact GlaxoSmithKline at 1-888-825-5249 or FDA at 1-800-FDA-1088 or www.fda.gov/medwatch.

DRUG INTERACTIONS

Live attenuated influenza vaccine, intranasal (7):

- Do not administer until 48 hours following cessation of RELENZA.
- Do not administer RELENZA until 2 weeks following administration of the live attenuated influenza vaccine, unless medically indicated.

See 17 for PATIENT COUNSELING INFORMATION and FDA-approved patient labeling

Revised: 12/2011

FULL PRESCRIBING INFORMATION: CONTENTS*

*** Sections or subsections omitted from the full prescribing information are not listed**

FULL PRESCRIBING INFORMATION

1 INDICATIONS AND USAGE

1.1 Treatment of Influenza

RELENZA® (zanamivir) Inhalation Powder is indicated for treatment of uncomplicated acute illness due to influenza A and B virus in adults and pediatric patients aged 7 years and older who have been symptomatic for no more than 2 days.

1.2 Prophylaxis of Influenza

RELENZA is indicated for prophylaxis of influenza in adults and pediatric patients aged 5 years and older.

1.3 Important Limitations on Use of RELENZA

- RELENZA is not recommended for treatment or prophylaxis of influenza in individuals with underlying airways disease (such as asthma or chronic obstructive pulmonary disease) due to risk of serious bronchospasm *[see Warnings and Precautions (5.1)]*.
- RELENZA has not been proven effective for treatment of influenza in individuals with underlying airways disease.
- RELENZA has not been proven effective for prophylaxis of influenza in the nursing home setting.
- RELENZA is not a substitute for early influenza vaccination on an annual basis as recommended by the Centers for Disease Control's Immunization Practices Advisory Committee.
- Influenza viruses change over time. Emergence of resistance mutations could decrease drug effectiveness. Other factors (for example, changes in viral virulence) might also diminish clinical benefit of antiviral drugs. Prescribers should consider available information on influenza drug susceptibility patterns and treatment effects when deciding whether to use RELENZA.
- There is no evidence for efficacy of zanamivir in any illness caused by agents other than influenza virus A and B.
- Patients should be advised that the use of RELENZA for treatment of influenza has not been shown to reduce the risk of transmission of influenza to others.

2 DOSAGE AND ADMINISTRATION

2.1 Dosing Considerations

- RELENZA is for administration to the respiratory tract by *oral inhalation only*, using the DISKHALER device provided *[see Warnings and Precautions (5.6)]*.
- The 10-mg dose is provided by 2 inhalations (one 5-mg blister per inhalation).
- Patients should be instructed in the use of the delivery system. Instructions should include a demonstration whenever possible. If RELENZA is prescribed for children, it should be used only under adult supervision and instruction, and the supervising adult should first be instructed by a healthcare professional *[see Patient Counseling Information (17.4)]*.
- Patients scheduled to use an inhaled bronchodilator at the same time as RELENZA should use their bronchodilator before taking RELENZA *[see Patient Counseling Information (17.2)]*.

2.2 Treatment of Influenza

- The recommended dose of RELENZA for treatment of influenza in adults and pediatric patients aged 7 years and older is 10 mg twice daily (approximately 12 hours apart) for 5 days.
- Two doses should be taken on the first day of treatment whenever possible provided there is at least 2 hours between doses.
- On subsequent days, doses should be about 12 hours apart (e.g., morning and evening) at approximately the same time each day.
- The safety and efficacy of repeated treatment courses have not been studied.

2.3 Prophylaxis of Influenza

Household Setting:

- The recommended dose of RELENZA for prophylaxis of influenza in adults and pediatric patients aged 5 years and older in a household setting is 10 mg once daily for 10 days.
- The dose should be administered at approximately the same time each day.
- There are no data on the effectiveness of prophylaxis with RELENZA in a household setting when initiated more than 1.5 days after the onset of signs or symptoms in the index case.

Community Outbreaks:

- The recommended dose of RELENZA for prophylaxis of influenza in adults and adolescents in a community setting is 10 mg once daily for 28 days.
- The dose should be administered at approximately the same time each day.
- There are no data on the effectiveness of prophylaxis with RELENZA in a community outbreak when initiated more than 5 days after the outbreak was identified in the community.
- The safety and effectiveness of prophylaxis with RELENZA have not been evaluated for longer than 28 days' duration.

3 DOSAGE FORMS AND STRENGTHS

Blister for oral inhalation: 5 mg. Four 5-mg blisters of powder on a ROTADISK for oral inhalation via DISKHALER. Packaged in carton containing 5 ROTADISKs (total of 10 doses) and 1 DISKHALER inhalation device *[see How Supplied/Storage and Handling (16)]*.

4 CONTRAINDICATIONS

Do not use in patients with history of allergic reaction to any ingredient of RELENZA including milk proteins *[see Warnings and Precautions (5.2), Description (11)]*.

5 WARNINGS AND PRECAUTIONS

5.1 Bronchospasm

RELENZA is not recommended for treatment or prophylaxis of influenza in individuals with underlying airways disease (such as asthma or chronic obstructive pulmonary disease).

Serious cases of bronchospasm, including fatalities, have been reported during treatment with RELENZA in patients with and without underlying airways disease. Many of these cases were reported during postmarketing and causality was difficult to assess.

RELENZA should be discontinued in any patient who develops bronchospasm or decline in respiratory function; immediate treatment and hospitalization may be required.

Some patients without prior pulmonary disease may also have respiratory abnormalities from acute respiratory infection that could resemble adverse drug reactions or increase patient vulnerability to adverse drug reactions.

Bronchospasm was documented following administration of zanamivir in 1 of 13 patients with mild or moderate asthma (but without acute influenza-like illness) in a Phase I study. In a Phase III study in patients with acute influenza-like illness superimposed on underlying asthma or chronic obstructive pulmonary disease, 10% (24 of 244) of patients on zanamivir and 9% (22 of 237) on placebo experienced a greater than 20% decline in FEV_1 following treatment for 5 days.

If use of RELENZA is considered for a patient with underlying airways disease, the potential risks and benefits should be carefully weighed. If a decision is made to prescribe RELENZA for such a patient, this should be done only under conditions of careful monitoring of respiratory function, close observation, and appropriate supportive care including availability of fast-acting bronchodilators.

5.2 Allergic Reactions

Allergic-like reactions, including oropharyngeal edema, serious skin rashes, and anaphylaxis have been reported in postmarketing experience with RELENZA. RELENZA should be stopped and appropriate treatment instituted if an allergic reaction occurs or is suspected.

5.3 Neuropsychiatric Events

Influenza can be associated with a variety of neurologic and behavioral symptoms which can include events such as seizures, hallucinations, delirium, and abnormal behavior, in some cases resulting in fatal outcomes. These events may occur in the setting of encephalitis or encephalopathy but can occur without obvious severe disease.

There have been postmarketing reports (mostly from Japan) of delirium and abnormal behavior leading to injury in patients with influenza who were receiving neuraminidase inhibitors, including RELENZA. Because these events were reported voluntarily during clinical practice, estimates of frequency cannot be made, but they appear to be uncommon based on usage data for RELENZA. These events were reported primarily among pediatric patients and often had an abrupt onset and rapid resolution. The contribution of RELENZA to these events has not been established. Patients with influenza should be closely monitored for signs of abnormal behavior. If neuropsychiatric symptoms occur, the risks and benefits of continuing treatment should be evaluated for each patient.

5.4 Limitations of Populations Studied

Safety and efficacy have not been demonstrated in patients with high-risk underlying medical conditions. No information is available regarding treatment of influenza in patients with any medical condition sufficiently severe or unstable to be considered at imminent risk of requiring inpatient management.

5.5 Bacterial Infections

Serious bacterial infections may begin with influenza-like symptoms or may coexist with or occur as complications during the course of influenza. RELENZA has not been shown to prevent such complications.

5.6 Importance of Proper Route of Administration

RELENZA Inhalation Powder must not be made into an extemporaneous solution for administration by nebulization or mechanical ventilation. There have been reports of hospitalized patients with influenza who received a solution made with RELENZA Inhalation Powder administered by nebulization or mechanical ventilation, including a fatal case where it was reported that the lactose in this formulation obstructed the proper functioning of the equipment. RELENZA Inhalation Powder must only be administered using the device provided *[see Dosage and Administration (2.1)]*.

5.7 Importance of Proper Use of DISKHALER

Effective and safe use of RELENZA requires proper use of the DISKHALER to inhale the drug. Prescribers should carefully evaluate the ability of young children to use the delivery system if use of RELENZA is considered *[see Use in Specific Populations (8.4)]*.

6 ADVERSE REACTIONS

See Warnings and Precautions for information about risk of serious adverse events such as bronchospasm (5.1) and allergic-like reactions (5.2), and for safety information in patients with underlying airways disease (5.1).

6.1 Clinical Trials Experience

Because clinical trials are conducted under widely varying conditions, adverse reaction rates observed in the clinical trials of a drug cannot be directly compared with rates in the clinical trials of another drug and may not reflect the rates observed in practice.

The placebo used in clinical studies consisted of inhaled lactose powder, which is also the vehicle for the active drug; therefore, some adverse events occurring at similar frequencies in different treatment groups could be related to lactose vehicle inhalation.

Treatment of Influenza: *Clinical Trials in Adults and Adolescents:* Adverse events that occurred with an incidence ≥1.5% in treatment studies are listed in Table 1. This table shows adverse events occurring in patients aged ≥12 years receiving RELENZA 10 mg inhaled twice daily, RELENZA in all inhalation regimens, and placebo inhaled twice daily (where placebo consisted of the same lactose vehicle used in RELENZA).

Table 1. Summary of Adverse Events ≥1.5% Incidence During Treatment in Adults and Adolescents

Adverse Event	RELENZA		Placebo (Lactose Vehicle) (n = 1,520)
	10 mg b.i.d. **Inhaled** (n = 1,132)	All Dosing Regimens[a] (n = 2,289)	
Body as a whole			
Headaches	2%	2%	3%
Digestive			
Diarrhea	3%	3%	4%
Nausea	3%	3%	3%
Vomiting	1%	1%	2%
Respiratory			
Nasal signs and symptoms	2%	3%	3%
Bronchitis	2%	2%	3%
Cough	2%	2%	3%
Sinusitis	3%	2%	2%
Ear, nose, and throat infections	2%	1%	2%
Nervous system			
Dizziness	2%	1%	<1%

[a] Includes studies where RELENZA was administered intranasally (6.4 mg 2 to 4 times per day in addition to inhaled preparation) and/or inhaled more frequently (q.i.d.) than the currently recommended dose.

Additional adverse reactions occurring in less than 1.5% of patients receiving RELENZA included malaise, fatigue, fever, abdominal pain, myalgia, arthralgia, and urticaria.

The most frequent laboratory abnormalities in Phase III treatment studies included elevations of liver enzymes and CPK, lymphopenia, and neutropenia. These were reported in similar proportions of zanamivir and lactose vehicle placebo recipients with acute influenza-like illness.

Clinical Trials in Pediatric Patients: Adverse events that occurred with an incidence ≥1.5% in children receiving treatment doses of RELENZA in 2 Phase III studies are listed in Table 2. This table shows adverse events occurring in pediatric patients aged 5 to 12 years receiving RELENZA 10 mg inhaled twice daily and placebo inhaled twice daily (where placebo consisted of the same lactose vehicle used in RELENZA).

Table 2. Summary of Adverse Events ≥1.5% Incidence During Treatment in Pediatric Patients[a]

Adverse Event	RELENZA 10 mg b.i.d. Inhaled (n = 291)	Placebo (Lactose Vehicle) (n = 318)
Respiratory		
Ear, nose, and throat infections	5%	5%
Ear, nose, and throat hemorrhage	<1%	2%
Asthma	<1%	2%
Cough	<1%	2%
Digestive		
Vomiting	2%	3%
Diarrhea	2%	2%
Nausea	<1%	2%

[a] Includes a subset of patients receiving RELENZA for treatment of influenza in a prophylaxis study.

In 1 of the 2 studies described in Table 2, some additional information is available from children (aged 5 to 12 years) without acute influenza-like illness who received an investigational prophylaxis regimen of RELENZA; 132 children received RELENZA and 145 children received placebo. Among these children, nasal signs and symptoms (zanamivir 20%, placebo 9%), cough (zanamivir 16%, placebo 8%), and throat/tonsil discomfort and pain (zanamivir 11%, placebo 6%) were reported more frequently with RELENZA than placebo. In a subset with chronic pulmonary disease, lower respiratory adverse events (described as asthma, cough, or viral respiratory infections which could include influenza-like symptoms) were reported in 7 of 7 zanamivir recipients and 5 of 12 placebo recipients.

Prophylaxis of Influenza: *Family/Household Prophylaxis Studies:* Adverse events that occurred with an incidence of ≥1.5% in the 2 prophylaxis studies are listed in Table 3. This table shows adverse events occurring in patients aged ≥5 years receiving RELENZA 10 mg inhaled once daily for 10 days.

Table 3. Summary of Adverse Events ≥1.5% Incidence During 10-Day Prophylaxis Studies in Adults, Adolescents, and Children[a]

Adverse Event	Contact Cases	
	RELENZA (n = 1,068)	Placebo (n = 1,059)
Lower respiratory		
Viral respiratory infections	13%	19%
Cough	7%	9%
Neurologic		
Headaches	13%	14%
Ear, nose, and throat		
Nasal signs and symptoms	12%	12%
Throat and tonsil discomfort and pain	8%	9%
Nasal inflammation	1%	2%
Musculoskeletal		
Muscle pain	3%	3%
Endocrine and metabolic		
Feeding problems (decreased or increased appetite and anorexia)	2%	2%
Gastrointestinal		
Nausea and vomiting	1%	2%
Non-site specific		
Malaise and fatigue	5%	5%
Temperature regulation disturbances (fever and/or chills)	5%	4%

[a] In prophylaxis studies, symptoms associated with influenza-like illness were captured as adverse events; subjects were enrolled during a winter respiratory season during which time any symptoms that occurred were captured as adverse events.

Community Prophylaxis Studies: Adverse events that occurred with an incidence of ≥1.5% in 2 prophylaxis studies are listed in Table 4. This table shows adverse events occurring in patients aged ≥5 years receiving RELENZA 10 mg inhaled once daily for 28 days.

Table 4. Summary of Adverse Events ≥1.5% Incidence During 28-Day Prophylaxis Studies in Adults, Adolescents, and Children[a]

Adverse Event	RELENZA (n = 2,231)	Placebo (n = 2,239)
Neurologic		
Headaches	24%	26%
Ear, nose, and throat		
Throat and tonsil discomfort and pain	19%	20%
Nasal signs and symptoms	12%	13%
Ear, nose, and throat infections	2%	2%
Lower respiratory		
Cough	17%	18%
Viral respiratory infections	3%	4%
Musculoskeletal		
Muscle pain	8%	8%
Musculoskeletal pain	6%	6%
Arthralgia and articular rheumatism	2%	<1%
Endocrine and metabolic		
Feeding problems (decreased or increased appetite and anorexia)	4%	4%
Gastrointestinal		
Nausea and vomiting	2%	3%
Diarrhea	2%	2%
Non-site specific		
Temperature regulation disturbances (fever and/or chills)	9%	10%
Malaise and fatigue	8%	8%

[a] In prophylaxis studies, symptoms associated with influenza-like illness were captured as adverse events; subjects were enrolled during a winter respiratory season during which time any symptoms that occurred were captured as adverse events.

6.2 Postmarketing Experience

In addition to adverse events reported from clinical trials, the following events have been identified during postmarketing use of zanamivir (RELENZA). Because they are reported voluntarily from a population of unknown size, estimates of frequency cannot be made. These events have been chosen for inclusion due to a combination of their seriousness, frequency of reporting, or potential causal connection to zanamivir (RELENZA).

Allergic Reactions: Allergic or allergic-like reaction, including oropharyngeal edema *[see Warnings and Precautions (5.2)]*.

Psychiatric: Delirium, including symptoms such as altered level of consciousness, confusion, abnormal behavior, delusions, hallucinations, agitation, anxiety, nightmares *[see Warnings and Precautions (5.3)]*.

Cardiac: Arrhythmias, syncope.

Neurologic: Seizures. Vasovagal-like episodes have been reported shortly following inhalation of zanamivir.

Respiratory: Bronchospasm, dyspnea *[see Warnings and Precautions (5.1)]*.

Skin: Facial edema; rash, including serious cutaneous reactions (e.g., erythema multiforme, Stevens-Johnson syndrome, toxic epidermal necrolysis); urticaria *[see Warnings and Precautions (5.2)]*.

7 DRUG INTERACTIONS

Zanamivir is not a substrate nor does it affect cytochrome P450 (CYP) isoenzymes (CYP1A1/2, 2A6, 2C9, 2C18, 2D6, 2E1, and 3A4) in human liver microsomes. No clinically significant pharmacokinetic drug interactions are predicted based on data from in vitro studies.

The concurrent use of RELENZA with live attenuated influenza vaccine (LAIV) intranasal has not been evaluated. However, because of potential interference between these products, LAIV should not be administered within 2 weeks before or 48 hours after administration of RELENZA, unless medically indicated. The concern about possible interference arises from the potential for antiviral drugs to inhibit replication of live vaccine virus.

Trivalent inactivated influenza vaccine can be administered at any time relative to use of RELENZA *[see Clinical Pharmacology (12.4)]*.

8 USE IN SPECIFIC POPULATIONS

8.1 Pregnancy

Pregnancy Category C. There are no adequate and well-controlled studies of zanamivir in pregnant women. Zanamivir should be used during pregnancy only if the potential benefit justifies the potential risk to the fetus.

Embryo/fetal development studies were conducted in rats (dosed from days 6 to 15 of pregnancy) and rabbits (dosed from days 7 to 19 of pregnancy) using the same IV doses (1, 9, and 90 mg/kg/day). Pre- and post-natal developmental studies were performed in rats (dosed from day 16 of pregnancy until litter day 21 to 23). No malformations, maternal toxicity, or embryotoxicity were observed in pregnant rats or rabbits and their fetuses. Because of insufficient blood sampling timepoints in rat and rabbit reproductive toxicity studies, AUC values were not available. In a subchronic study in rats at the 90 mg/kg/day IV dose, the AUC values were greater than 300 times the human exposure at the proposed clinical dose.

An additional embryo/fetal study, in a different strain of rat, was conducted using subcutaneous administration of zanamivir, 3 times daily, at doses of 1, 9, or 80 mg/kg during days 7 to 17 of pregnancy. There was an increase in the incidence rates of a variety of minor skeleton alterations and variants in the exposed offspring in this study. Based on AUC measurements, the 80 mg/kg dose produced an exposure greater than 1,000 times the human exposure at the proposed clinical dose. However, in most instances, the individual incidence rate of each skeletal alteration or variant remained within the background rates of the historical occurrence in the strain studied.

Zanamivir has been shown to cross the placenta in rats and rabbits. In these animals, fetal blood concentrations of zanamivir were significantly lower than zanamivir concentrations in the maternal blood.

8.3 Nursing Mothers

Studies in rats have demonstrated that zanamivir is excreted in milk. However, nursing mothers should be instructed that it is not known whether zanamivir is excreted in human milk. Because many drugs are excreted in human milk, caution should be exercised when RELENZA is administered to a nursing mother.

8.4 Pediatric Use

Treatment of Influenza: Safety and effectiveness of RELENZA for treatment of influenza have not been assessed in pediatric patients younger than 7 years, but were studied in a Phase III treatment study in pediatric patients, where 471 children aged 5 to 12 years received zanamivir or placebo *[see Clinical Studies (14.1)]*. Adolescents were included in the 3 principal Phase III adult treatment studies. In these studies, 67 patients were aged 12 to 16 years. No definite differences in safety and efficacy were observed between these adolescent patients and young adults.

In a Phase I study of 16 children aged 6 to 12 years with signs and symptoms of respiratory disease, 4 did not produce a measurable peak inspiratory flow rate (PIFR) through the DISKHALER (3 with no adequate inhalation on request, 1 with missing data), 9 had measurable PIFR on each of 2 inhalations, and 3 achieved measurable PIFR on only 1 of 2 inhalations. Neither of two 6-year-olds and one of two 7-year-olds produced measurable PIFR. Overall, 8 of the 16 children (including all those younger than 8 years) either did not produce measurable inspiratory flow through the DISKHALER or produced peak inspiratory flow rates below the 60 L/min considered optimal for the device under standardized in vitro testing; lack of measurable flow rate was related to low or undetectable serum concentrations *[see Clinical Pharmacology (12.3), Clinical Studies (14.1)]*. Prescribers should carefully evaluate the ability of young children to use the delivery system if prescription of RELENZA is considered.

Prophylaxis of Influenza: The safety and effectiveness of RELENZA for prophylaxis of influenza have been studied in 4 Phase III studies where 273 children aged 5 to 11 years and 239 adolescents aged 12 to 16 years received RELENZA. No differences in safety and effectiveness were observed between pediatric and adult subjects *[see Clinical Studies (14.2)]*.

8.5 Geriatric Use

Of the total number of patients in 6 clinical studies of RELENZA for treatment of influenza, 59 patients were aged 65 years and older, while 24 patients were aged 75 years and older. Of the total number of patients in 4 clinical studies of RELENZA for prophylaxis of influenza in households and community settings, 954 patients were aged 65 years and older, while 347 patients were aged 75 years and older. No overall differences in safety or effectiveness were observed between these patients and younger patients, and other reported clinical experience has not identified differences in responses between the elderly and younger patients, but greater sensitivity of some older individuals cannot be ruled out. Elderly patients may need assistance with use of the device.

In 2 additional studies of RELENZA for prophylaxis of influenza in the nursing home setting, efficacy was not demonstrated *[see Indications and Usage (1.3)]*.

10 OVERDOSAGE

There have been no reports of overdosage from administration of RELENZA.

11 DESCRIPTION

The active component of RELENZA is zanamivir. The chemical name of zanamivir is 5-(acetylamino)-4-[(aminoiminomethyl)-amino]-2,6-anhydro-3,4,5-trideoxy-D-glycero-D-galacto-non-2-enonic acid. It has a molecular formula of $C_{12}H_{20}N_4O_7$ and a molecular weight of 332.3. It has the following structural formula:

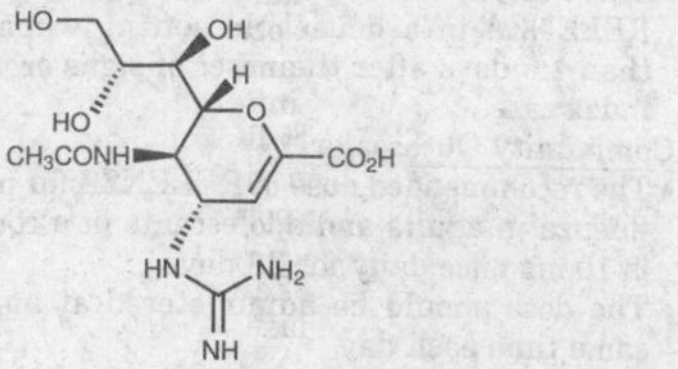

Zanamivir is a white to off-white powder for oral inhalation with a solubility of approximately 18 mg/mL in water at 20°C.

RELENZA is for administration to the respiratory tract by oral inhalation only. Each RELENZA ROTADISK contains 4 regularly spaced double-foil blisters with each blister containing a powder mixture of 5 mg of zanamivir and 20 mg of lactose (which contains milk proteins). The contents of each blister are inhaled using a specially designed breath-activated plastic device for inhaling powder called the DISKHALER. After a RELENZA ROTADISK is loaded into the DISKHALER, a blister that contains medication is pierced and the zanamivir is dispersed into the air stream created when the patient inhales through the mouthpiece. The amount of drug delivered to the respiratory tract will depend on patient factors such as inspiratory flow. Under standardized in vitro testing, RELENZA ROTADISK delivers 4 mg of zanamivir from the DISKHALER device when tested at a pressure drop of 3 kPa (corresponding to a flow rate of about 62 to 65 L/min) for 3 seconds.

12 CLINICAL PHARMACOLOGY

12.1 Mechanism of Action

Zanamivir is an antiviral drug *[see Clinical Pharmacology (12.4)]*.

12.3 Pharmacokinetics

Absorption and Bioavailability: Pharmacokinetic studies of orally inhaled zanamivir indicate that approximately 4% to 17% of the inhaled dose is systemically absorbed. The peak serum concentrations ranged from 17 to 142 ng/mL within 1 to 2 hours following a 10 mg dose. The area under the serum concentration versus time curve (AUC_{∞}) ranged from 111 to 1,364 ng•hr/mL.

Distribution: Zanamivir has limited plasma protein binding (<10%).

Metabolism: Zanamivir is renally excreted as unchanged drug. No metabolites have been detected in humans.

Elimination: The serum half-life of zanamivir following administration by oral inhalation ranges from 2.5 to 5.1 hours. It is excreted unchanged in the urine with excretion of a single dose completed within 24 hours. Total clearance ranges from 2.5 to 10.9 L/hr. Unabsorbed drug is excreted in the feces.

Impaired Hepatic Function: The pharmacokinetics of zanamivir have not been studied in patients with impaired hepatic function.

Impaired Renal Function: After a single intravenous dose of 4 mg or 2 mg of zanamivir in volunteers with mild/moderate or severe renal impairment, respectively, significant decreases in renal clearance (and hence total clearance: normals 5.3 L/hr, mild/moderate 2.7 L/hr, and severe 0.8 L/hr; median values) and significant increases in half-life (normals 3.1 hr, mild/moderate 4.7 hr, and severe 18.5 hr; median values) and systemic exposure were observed. Safety and efficacy have not been documented in the presence of severe renal insufficiency. Due to the low systemic bioavailability of zanamivir following oral inhalation, no dosage adjustments are necessary in patients with renal impairment. However, the potential for drug accumulation should be considered.

Pediatric Patients: The pharmacokinetics of zanamivir were evaluated in pediatric patients with signs and symptoms of respiratory illness. Sixteen patients, aged 6 to 12 years, received a single dose of 10 mg zanamivir dry powder via DISKHALER. Five patients had either undetectable zanamivir serum concentrations or had low drug concentrations (8.32 to 10.38 ng/mL) that were not detectable after 1.5 hours. Eleven patients had C_{max} median values of 43 ng/mL (range: 15 to 74) and AUC_{∞} median values of 167 ng•hr/mL (range: 58 to 279). Low or undetectable serum concentrations were related to lack of measurable PIFR in individual patients *[see Use in Specific Populations (8.4), Clinical Studies (14.1)]*.

Geriatric Patients: The pharmacokinetics of zanamivir have not been studied in patients older than 65 years *[see Use in Specific Populations (8.5)]*.

Gender, Race, and Weight: In a population pharmacokinetic analysis in patient studies, no clinically significant differences in serum concentrations and/or pharmacokinetic parameters (V/F, CL/F, ka, AUC_{0-3}, C_{max}, T_{max}, CLr, and % excreted in urine) were observed when demographic variables (gender, age, race, and weight) and indices of infection (laboratory evidence of infection, overall symptoms, symptoms of upper respiratory illness, and viral titers) were considered. There were no significant correlations between measures of systemic exposure and safety parameters.

12.4 Microbiology

Mechanism of Action: Zanamivir is an inhibitor of influenza virus neuraminidase affecting release of viral particles.

Antiviral Activity: The antiviral activity of zanamivir against laboratory and clinical isolates of influenza virus was determined in cell culture assays. The concentrations of zanamivir required for inhibition of influenza virus were highly variable depending on the assay method used and virus isolate tested. The 50% and 90% effective concentrations (EC_{50} and EC_{90}) of zanamivir were in the range of 0.005 to 16.0 µM and 0.005 to >100 µM, respectively (1 µM = 0.33 mcg/mL). The relationship between the cell culture inhibition of influenza virus by zanamivir and the inhibition of influenza virus replication in humans has not been established.

Resistance: Influenza viruses with reduced susceptibility to zanamivir have been selected in cell culture by multiple passages of the virus in the presence of increasing concentrations of the drug. Genetic analysis of these viruses showed that the reduced susceptibility in cell culture to zanamivir is associated with mutations that result in amino acid changes in the viral neuraminidase or viral hemagglutinin or both. Resistance mutations selected in cell culture which result in neuraminidase amino acid substitutions include E119G/A/D and R292K. Mutations selected in cell culture in hemagglutinin include: K68R, G75E, E114K, N145S, S165N, S186F, N199S, and K222T.

In an immunocompromised patient infected with influenza B virus, a variant virus emerged after treatment with an investigational nebulized solution of zanamivir for 2 weeks. Analysis of this variant showed a hemagglutinin substitution (T198I) which resulted in a reduced affinity for human cell receptors, and a substitution in the neuraminidase active site (R152K) which reduced the enzyme's activity to zanamivir by 1,000-fold. Insufficient information is available to characterize the risk of emergence of zanamivir resistance in clinical use.

Cross-Resistance: Cross-resistance has been observed between some zanamivir-resistant and some oseltamivir-resistant influenza virus mutants generated in cell culture. However, some of the in cell culture zanamivir-induced resistance mutations, E119G/A/D and R292K, occurred at the same neuraminidase amino acid positions as in the clinical isolates resistant to oseltamivir, E119V and R292K. No studies have been performed to assess risk of emergence of cross-resistance during clinical use.

Influenza Vaccine Interaction Study: An interaction study (n = 138) was conducted to evaluate the effects of zanamivir (10 mg once daily) on the serological response to a single dose of trivalent inactivated influenza vaccine, as measured by hemagglutination inhibition titers. There was no difference in hemagglutination inhibition antibody titers at 2 weeks and 4 weeks after vaccine administration between zanamivir and placebo recipients.

Influenza Challenge Studies: Antiviral activity of zanamivir was supported for infection with influenza A virus, and to a more limited extent for infection with influenza B virus, by Phase I studies in volunteers who received intranasal inoculations of challenge strains of influenza virus, and received an intranasal formulation of zanamivir or placebo starting before or shortly after viral inoculation.

13 NONCLINICAL TOXICOLOGY

13.1 Carcinogenesis, Mutagenesis, Impairment of Fertility

Carcinogenesis: In 2-year carcinogenicity studies conducted in rats and mice using a powder formulation administered through inhalation, zanamivir induced no statistically significant increases in tumors over controls. The maximum daily exposures in rats and mice were approximately 23 to 25 and 20 to 22 times, respectively, greater than those in humans at the proposed clinical dose based on AUC comparisons.

Mutagenesis: Zanamivir was not mutagenic in in vitro and in vivo genotoxicity assays which included bacterial mutation assays in *S. typhimurium* and *E. coli*, mammalian mutation assays in mouse lymphoma, chromosomal aberration assays in human peripheral blood lymphocytes, and the in vivo mouse bone marrow micronucleus assay.

Impairment of Fertility: The effects of zanamivir on fertility and general reproductive performance were investigated in male (dosed for 10 weeks prior to mating, and throughout mating, gestation/lactation, and shortly after weaning) and female rats (dosed for 3 weeks prior to mating through Day 19 of pregnancy, or Day 21 post partum) at IV doses 1, 9, and 90 mg/kg/day. Zanamivir did not impair mating or fertility of male or female rats, and did not affect the sperm of treated male rats. The reproductive performance of the F1 generation born to female rats given zanamivir was not affected. Based on a subchronic study in rats at a 90 mg/kg/day IV dose, AUC values ranged between 142 and 199 mcg•hr/mL (>300 times the human exposure at the proposed clinical dose).

14 CLINICAL STUDIES

14.1 Treatment of Influenza

Adults and Adolescents: The efficacy of RELENZA 10 mg inhaled twice daily for 5 days in the treatment of influenza has been evaluated in placebo-controlled studies conducted in North America, the Southern Hemisphere, and Europe during their respective influenza seasons. The magnitude of treatment effect varied between studies, with possible relationships to population-related factors including amount of symptomatic relief medication used.

Populations Studied: The principal Phase III studies enrolled 1,588 patients aged 12 years and older (median age 34 years, 49% male, 91% Caucasian), with uncomplicated influenza-like illness within 2 days of symptom onset. Influenza was confirmed by culture, hemagglutination inhibition antibodies, or investigational direct tests. Of 1,164 patients with confirmed influenza, 89% had influenza A and 11% had influenza B. These studies served as the principal basis for efficacy evaluation, with more limited Phase II studies providing supporting information where necessary. Following randomization to either zanamivir or placebo (inhaled lactose vehicle), all patients received instruction and supervision by a healthcare professional for the initial dose.

Principal Results: The definition of time to improvement in major symptoms of influenza included no fever and self-assessment of "none" or "mild" for headache, myalgia, cough, and sore throat. A Phase II and a Phase III study conducted in North America (total of over 600 influenza-positive patients) suggested up to 1 day of shortening of median time to this defined improvement in symptoms in patients receiving zanamivir compared with placebo, although statistical significance was not reached in either of these studies. In a study conducted in the Southern Hemisphere (321 influenza-positive patients), a 1.5-day difference in median time to symptom improvement was observed. Additional evidence of efficacy was provided by the European study.

Other Findings: There was no consistent difference in treatment effect in patients with influenza A compared with influenza B; however, these trials enrolled smaller numbers of patients with influenza B and thus provided less evidence in support of efficacy in influenza B.

In general, patients with lower temperature (e.g., 38.2°C or less) or investigator-rated as having less severe symptoms at entry derived less benefit from therapy.

No consistent treatment effect was demonstrated in patients with underlying chronic medical conditions, including respiratory or cardiovascular disease *[see Warnings and Precautions (5.4)]*.

No consistent differences in rate of development of complications were observed between treatment groups.

Some fluctuation of symptoms was observed after the primary study endpoint in both treatment groups.

Pediatric Patients: The efficacy of RELENZA 10 mg inhaled twice daily for 5 days in the treatment of influenza in pediatric patients has been evaluated in a placebo-controlled study conducted in North America and Europe, enrolling 471 patients, aged 5 to 12 years (55% male, 90% Caucasian), within 36 hours of symptom onset. Of 346 patients with confirmed influenza, 65% had influenza A and 35% had influenza B. The definition of time to improvement included no fever and parental assessment of no or mild cough and absent/minimal muscle and joint aches or pains, sore throat, chills/feverishness, and headache. Median time to symptom improvement was 1 day shorter in patients receiving zanamivir compared with placebo. No consistent differences in rate of development of complications were observed between treatment groups. Some fluctuation of symptoms was observed after the primary study endpoint in both treatment groups.

Although this study was designed to enroll children aged 5 to 12 years, the product is indicated only for children aged 7 years and older. This evaluation is based on the combination of lower estimates of treatment effect in 5- and 6-year-olds compared with the overall study population, and evidence of inadequate inhalation through the DISKHALER in a pharmacokinetic study *[see Use in Specific Populations (8.4), Clinical Pharmacology (12.3)]*.

14.2 Prophylaxis of Influenza

The efficacy of RELENZA in preventing naturally occurring influenza illness has been demonstrated in 2 post-exposure prophylaxis studies in households and 2 seasonal prophylaxis studies during community outbreaks of influenza. The primary efficacy endpoint in these studies was the incidence of symptomatic, laboratory-confirmed influenza, defined as the presence of 2 or more of the following symptoms: oral temperature ≥100°F/37.8°C or feverishness, cough, headache, sore throat, and myalgia; and laboratory confirmation of influenza A or B by culture, PCR, or seroconversion (defined as a 4-fold increase in convalescent antibody titer from baseline).

Household Prophylaxis Studies: Two studies assessed post-exposure prophylaxis in household contacts of an index case. Within 1.5 days of onset of symptoms in an index case, each household (including all family members aged ≥5 years) was randomized to RELENZA 10 mg inhaled once daily or placebo inhaled once daily for 10 days. In the first study only, each index case was randomized to RELENZA 10 mg inhaled twice daily for 5 days or inhaled placebo twice daily for 5 days. In this study, the proportion of households with at least 1 new case of symptomatic laboratory-confirmed influenza was reduced from 19.0% (32 of 168 households) for the placebo group to 4.1% (7 of 169 households) for the group receiving RELENZA.

In the second study, index cases were not treated. The incidence of symptomatic laboratory-confirmed influenza was reduced from 19.0% (46 of 242 households) for the placebo group to 4.1% (10 of 245 households) for the group receiving RELENZA.

Seasonal Prophylaxis Studies: Two seasonal prophylaxis studies assessed RELENZA 10 mg inhaled once daily versus placebo inhaled once daily for 28 days during community outbreaks. The first study enrolled subjects aged 18 years or older (mean age 29 years) from 2 university communities. The majority of subjects were unvaccinated (86%). In this study, the incidence of symptomatic laboratory-confirmed influenza was reduced from 6.1% (34 of 554) for the placebo group to 2.0% (11 of 553) for the group receiving RELENZA. The second seasonal prophylaxis study enrolled subjects aged 12 to 94 years (mean age 60 years) with 56% of them older than 65 years. Sixty-seven percent of the subjects were vaccinated. In this study, the incidence of symptomatic laboratory-confirmed influenza was reduced from 1.4% (23 of 1,685) for the placebo group to 0.2% (4 of 1,678) for the group receiving RELENZA.

16 HOW SUPPLIED/STORAGE AND HANDLING

RELENZA is supplied in a circular double-foil pack (a ROTADISK) containing 4 blisters of the drug. Five ROTADISKs are packaged in a white polypropylene tube. The tube is packaged in a carton with 1 blue and gray DISKHALER inhalation device (NDC 0173-0681-01).

Store at 25°C (77°F); excursions permitted to 15° to 30°C (59° to 86°F) (see USP Controlled Room Temperature). Keep out of reach of children. Do not puncture any RELENZA ROTADISK blister until taking a dose using the DISKHALER.

17 PATIENT COUNSELING INFORMATION

See FDA-approved patient labeling (Patient Information and Instructions for Use).

17.1 Bronchospasm

Patients should be advised of the risk of bronchospasm, especially in the setting of underlying airways disease, and should stop RELENZA and contact their physician if they experience increased respiratory symptoms during treatment such as worsening wheezing, shortness of breath, or other signs or symptoms of bronchospasm*[see Warnings and Precautions (5.1)]*. If a decision is made to prescribe RELENZA for a patient with asthma or chronic obstructive pulmonary disease, the patient should be made aware of the risks and should have a fast-acting bronchodilator available.

17.2 Concomitant Bronchodilator Use

Patients scheduled to take inhaled bronchodilators at the same time as RELENZA should be advised to use their bronchodilators before taking RELENZA.

17.3 Neuropsychiatric Events

Patients with influenza (the flu), particularly children and adolescents, may be at an increased risk of seizures, confusion, or abnormal behavior early in their illness. These events may occur after beginning RELENZA or may occur when flu is not treated. These events are uncommon but may result in accidental injury to the patient. Therefore, patients should be observed for signs of unusual behavior and a healthcare professional should be contacted immediately if the patient shows any signs of unusual behavior *[see Warnings and Precautions (5.3)]*.

17.4 Instructions for Use

Patients should be instructed in use of the delivery system. Instructions should include a demonstration whenever possible. For the proper use of RELENZA, the patient should read and follow carefully the accompanying Instructions for Use.

If RELENZA is prescribed for children, it should be used only under adult supervision and instruction, and the supervising adult should first be instructed by a healthcare professional *[see Dosage and Administration (2.1)]*.

17.5 Risk of Influenza Transmission to Others

Patients should be advised that the use of RELENZA for treatment of influenza has not been shown to reduce the risk of transmission of influenza to others.

RELENZA, DISKHALER, and ROTADISK are registered trademarks of GlaxoSmithKline.

GlaxoSmithKline
Research Triangle Park, NC 27709

December 2011
RLZ:9PI

Patient Information

RELENZA® (zanamivir) Inhalation Powder

This leaflet contains important patient information about RELENZA (zanamivir) Inhalation Powder, and should be read completely before beginning treatment. It does not, however, take the place of discussions with your healthcare provider about your medical condition or your treatment. This summary does not list all benefits and risks of RELENZA. The medication described here can only be prescribed and dispensed by a licensed healthcare provider, who has information about your medical condition and more information about the drug, including how to take it, what to expect, and potential side effects. If you have any questions about RELENZA, talk with your healthcare provider.

What is RELENZA?

RELENZA (ruh-LENS-uh) is a medicine for the treatment of influenza (flu, infection caused by influenza virus) and for reducing the chance of getting the flu in community and household settings. It belongs to a group of medicines called neuraminidase inhibitors. These medications attack the influenza virus and prevent it from spreading inside your body. RELENZA treats the cause of influenza at its source, rather than simply masking the symptoms.

Important Safety Information About RELENZA

Some patients have had bronchospasm (wheezing) or serious breathing problems when they used RELENZA. Many but not all of these patients had previous asthma or chronic obstructive pulmonary disease. RELENZA has not been shown to shorten the duration of influenza in people with these diseases. Because of the risk of side effects and because it has not been shown to help them, RELENZA is not recommended for people with chronic respiratory disease such as asthma or chronic obstructive pulmonary disease.

If you develop worsening respiratory symptoms such as wheezing or shortness of breath, stop using RELENZA and contact your healthcare provider right away.

If you have chronic respiratory disease such as asthma and chronic obstructive pulmonary disease and your healthcare provider has prescribed RELENZA, you should have a fast-acting, inhaled bronchodilator available for your use. If you are scheduled to use an inhaled bronchodilator at the same time as RELENZA, use the inhaled bronchodilator **before** using RELENZA.

Read the rest of this leaflet for more information about side effects and risks.

Other kinds of infections can appear like influenza or occur along with influenza, and need different kinds of treatment. Contact your healthcare provider if you feel worse or develop new symptoms during or after treatment, or if your influenza symptoms do not start to get better.

Who should not take RELENZA?

RELENZA is not recommended for people who have chronic lung disease such as asthma or chronic obstructive pulmonary disease. RELENZA has not been shown to shorten the duration of influenza in people with these diseases, and some people have had serious side effects of bronchospasm and worsening lung function. (See the section of this Patient Information entitled **"Important Safety Information About RELENZA."**)

You should not take RELENZA if you are allergic to zanamivir or any other ingredient of RELENZA. Also tell your healthcare provider if you have any type of chronic condition including lung or heart disease, if you are allergic to any other medicines, milk proteins or other food products, or if you are pregnant.

RELENZA was not effective in reducing the chance of getting the flu in 2 studies in nursing home patients.

RELENZA does not treat flu-like illness that is not caused by influenza virus.

Who should consider taking RELENZA?

Adult and pediatric patients at least 7 years of age who have influenza symptoms that appeared within the previous day or two. Typical symptoms of influenza include sudden onset of fever, cough, headache, fatigue, muscular weakness, and sore throat.

RELENZA can also help reduce the chance of getting the flu in adults and children at least 5 years of age who have a higher chance of getting the flu because they spend time with someone who has the flu. RELENZA can also reduce the chance of getting the flu if there is a flu outbreak in the community.

The use of RELENZA for the treatment of flu has not been shown to reduce the risk of spreading the virus to others.

Can I take other medications with RELENZA?

RELENZA has been shown to have an acceptable safety profile when used as labeled, with minimal risk of drug interactions. Your healthcare provider may recommend taking other medications, including over-the-counter medications, to reduce fever or other symptoms while you are taking RELENZA. Before starting treatment, make sure that your healthcare provider knows if you are taking other medicines. If you are scheduled to use an inhaled bronchodilator at the same time as RELENZA, you should use the inhaled bronchodilator **before** using RELENZA.

Before taking RELENZA, please let your healthcare provider know if you received live attenuated influenza vaccine (FLUMIST®) intranasal in the past 2 weeks.

How and when should I take RELENZA?

RELENZA is packaged in medicine disks called ROTADISKS® and is inhaled by mouth using a delivery device called a DISKHALER®. Each ROTADISK contains 4 blisters. Each blister contains 5 mg of active drug and 20 mg of lactose powder (which contains milk proteins).

You should receive a demonstration on how to use RELENZA in the DISKHALER from a healthcare provider. Before taking RELENZA, read the "Patient Instructions for Use." Make sure that you understand these instructions and talk to your healthcare provider if you have any questions. Children who use RELENZA should always be supervised by an adult who understands how to use RELENZA. Proper use of the DISKHALER to inhale the drug is necessary for safe and effective use of RELENZA.

If you have the flu the usual dose for treatment is 2 inhalations of RELENZA (1 blister per inhalation) twice daily (in the morning and evening) for 5 days. It is important that you begin your treatment with RELENZA as soon as possible from the first appearance of your flu symptoms. Take 2 doses on the first day of treatment whenever possible if there are at least 2 hours between doses.

To reduce the chance of getting the flu, the usual dose is 2 inhalations of RELENZA (1 blister per inhalation) once daily for 10 or 28 days as prescribed by your healthcare provider.

Never share RELENZA with anyone, even if they have the same symptoms. If you feel worse or develop new symptoms during treatment with RELENZA, or if your flu symptoms do not start to get better, stop using the medicine and contact your healthcare provider.

What if I miss a dose?

If you forget to take your medicine at any time, take the missed dose as soon as you remember, except if it is near the next dose (within 2 hours). Then continue to take RELENZA at the usual times. You do not need to take a double dose. If you have missed several doses, inform your healthcare provider and follow the advice given to you.

What are important or common possible side effects of taking RELENZA?

Some patients have had breathing problems while taking RELENZA. This can be very serious and need treatment right away. Most of the patients who had this problem had asthma or chronic obstructive pulmonary disease, but some did not. If you have trouble breathing or have wheezing after your dose of RELENZA, stop taking RELENZA and get medical attention.

In studies, the most common side effects with RELENZA have been headaches; diarrhea; nausea; vomiting; nasal irritation; bronchitis; cough; sinusitis; ear, nose, and throat infections; and dizziness. Other side effects that have been reported, but were not as common, include rashes and allergic reactions, some of which were severe.

People with influenza (the flu), particularly children and adolescents, may be at an increased risk of seizures, confusion, or abnormal behavior early in their illness. These events may occur after beginning RELENZA or may occur when flu is not treated. These events are uncommon but may result in accidental injury to the patient. Therefore, patients should be observed for signs of unusual behavior and a healthcare professional should be contacted immediately if the patient shows any signs of unusual behavior.

If you are not feeling well when you take RELENZA, you may faint or become lightheaded after inhaling RELENZA. You should sit down in a relaxed position before inhaling the dose of RELENZA, and you should only hold your breath for as long as is comfortable after inhaling the dose.

If you are not feeling well, you are advised to have someone with you while you are inhaling the dose of RELENZA.

This list of side effects is not complete. Your healthcare provider or pharmacist can discuss with you a more complete list of possible side effects with RELENZA. Talk to your healthcare provider promptly about any side effects you have.

Please refer to the section entitled **"Important Safety Information About RELENZA"** for additional information.

Should I get a flu shot?

RELENZA is not a substitute for a flu shot. You should receive an annual flu shot according to guidelines on immunization practices that your healthcare provider can share with you.

What if I am pregnant or nursing?

If you are pregnant or planning to become pregnant while taking RELENZA, talk to your healthcare provider before taking this medication. RELENZA is normally not recommended for use during pregnancy or nursing, as the effects on the unborn child or nursing infant are unknown.

How and where should I store RELENZA?

RELENZA should be stored at room temperature below 77°F (25°C). RELENZA is not in a childproof container. Keep RELENZA out of the reach of children. Discard the DISKHALER after finishing your treatment.

INSTRUCTIONS FOR USE

RELENZA®
(ZANAMIVIR) INHALATION POWDER

IMPORTANT: Read Step-by-Step Instructions before using the DISKHALER®.

Be sure to take the dose your healthcare provider has prescribed.

BEFORE YOU START:

Please read the entire Patient Information leaflet for important information about the effects of RELENZA including the section "Important Safety Information About RELENZA" for information about the risk of breathing difficulties.

If RELENZA is prescribed for a child, dosing should be supervised by an adult who understands how to use RELENZA and has been instructed in its use by a healthcare provider.

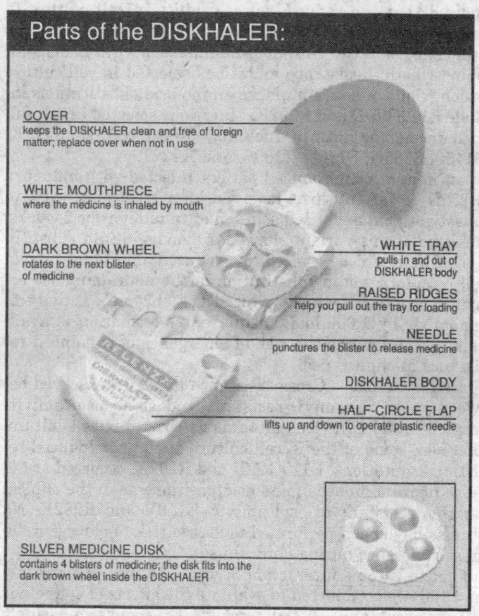

Step-by-step instructions for using the DISKHALER®

Step A: Load the medicine into the DISKHALER

1. Start by pulling off the blue cover.
2. **Always check inside the mouthpiece to make sure it is clear before each use. If foreign objects are in the mouthpiece, they could be inhaled and cause serious harm.**
3. Pull the white mouthpiece by the edges to extend the white tray all the way.
4. Once the white tray is extended all the way, find the raised ridges on each side of it. Press in these ridges, both sides at the same time, and **pull the whole white tray out of the DISKHALER body.**
5. Place one silver medicine disk onto the dark brown wheel, flat side up. The four silver blisters on the underside of the medicine disk will drop neatly into the four holes in the wheel.
6. Push in the white tray as far as it will go. Now the DISKHALER is loaded with medicine.

[See figure at top of next column]

Step B: Puncture the blister

Be sure to keep the DISKHALER level.

The DISKHALER punctures one blister of medicine at a time so you can inhale the right amount. It does not matter which blister you start with. Check to make sure that the silver foil is unbroken.

1. Be sure to keep the DISKHALER level so the medicine does not spill out.
2. Locate the half-circle flap with the name "RELENZA" on top of the DISKHALER.

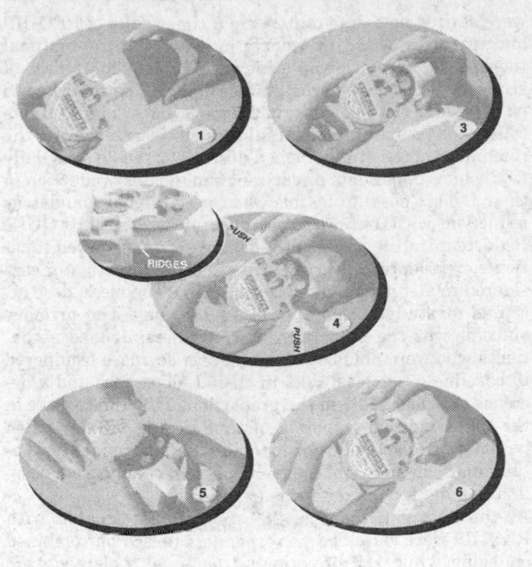

3. Lift this flap from the outer edge until it cannot go any farther. Flap must be **straight up** for the plastic needle to puncture both the **top** and **bottom** of the silver medicine disk inside.
4. Keeping the DISKHALER level, click the flap down into place.

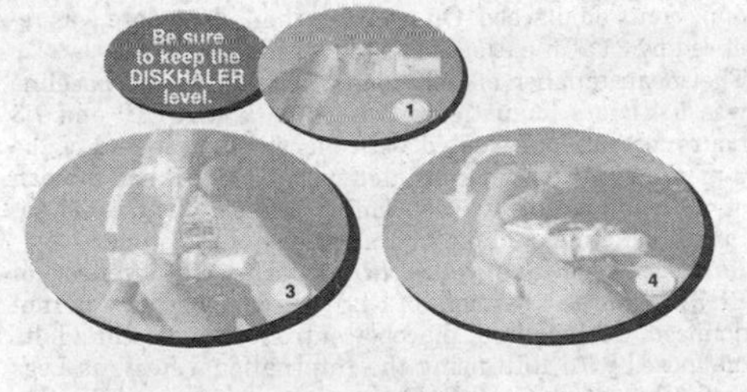

Step C: Inhale

1. Before putting the white mouthpiece into your mouth, breathe all the way out (exhale).
   Then put the white mouthpiece into your mouth. Be sure to keep the DISKHALER level so the medicine does not spill out.
2. Close your lips firmly around the mouthpiece. Be sure not to cover the small holes on either side of it.
3. Breathe in through your mouth steadily and as deeply as you can. Your breath pulls the medicine into your airways and lungs.
4. Hold your breath for a few seconds to help RELENZA stay in your lungs where it can work.

To take another inhalation, move to the next blister by following Step D below.

Once you've inhaled the number of blisters prescribed by your healthcare provider, replace the cover until your next dose.

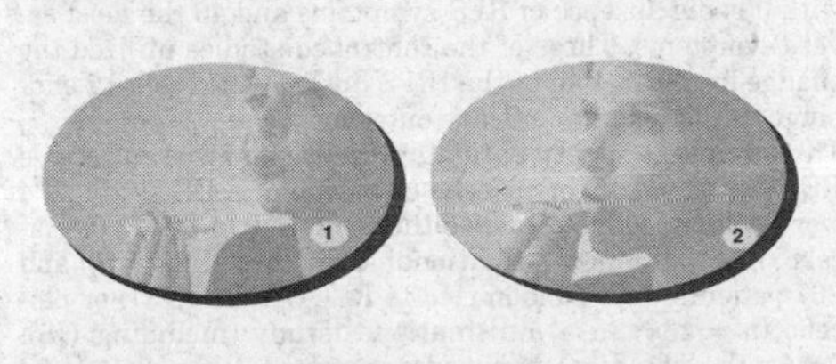

Step D: Move the medicine disk to the next blister

1. **Pull** the mouthpiece to extend the white tray, without removing it.
2. Then **push** it back until it clicks. This pull-push motion rotates the medicine disk to the next blister.
3. To take your next inhalation, repeat Steps B and C.

If all 4 blisters in the medicine disk have been used, you are ready to start a new medicine disk (see Step A). Check to make sure that the silver foil is unbroken each time you are ready to puncture the next blister.

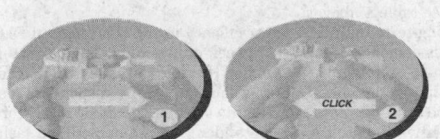

IMPORTANT INSTRUCTIONS

Read this entire leaflet before using RELENZA. Even if you have had a previous prescription for RELENZA, read this leaflet to see if any information has changed.

If you have the flu, the usual dose is 2 inhalations twice daily. To reduce the chance of getting the flu, the usual dose is 2 inhalations once daily. However, you must take the number of inhalations your healthcare provider has prescribed.

If you feel worse or develop new symptoms during or after treatment, or if your flu symptoms do not start to improve, stop using the medicine and contact your healthcare provider.

Keep out of reach of children.

Always check inside the mouthpiece to make sure it is clear before each use. If foreign objects are in the mouthpiece, they could be inhaled and cause serious harm.

Always replace the cover after each use.

Throw away the DISKHALER after treatment is completed.

This DISKHALER is for use only with RELENZA. Do not use the RELENZA DISKHALER device with FLOVENT® (fluticasone propionate) and do not use RELENZA with the FLOVENT DISKHALER device.

Store at 25°C (77°F); excursions permitted to 15° to 30°C (59° to 86°F) (see USP Controlled Room Temperature).

REMEMBER: This medicine has been prescribed for you by your healthcare provider. DO NOT give this medicine to anyone else.

RELENZA, FLOVENT, ROTADISK, and DISKHALER are registered trademarks of GlaxoSmithKline.

FLUMIST is a registered trademark of MedImmune, Inc.

GlaxoSmithKline
Research Triangle Park, NC 27709

December 2011
RLZ: 5PIL

REQUIP® ℞

[*rē′kwip*]
(ropinirole tablets)
Patient Information Included

DESCRIPTION

REQUIP (ropinirole) is an orally administered non-ergoline dopamine agonist. It is the hydrochloride salt of 4-[2-(dipropylamino)ethyl]-1,3-dihydro-2H-indol-2-one monohydrochloride and has an empirical formula of $C_{16}H_{24}N_2O \bullet HCl$. The molecular weight is 296.84 (260.38 as the free base).

The structural formula is:

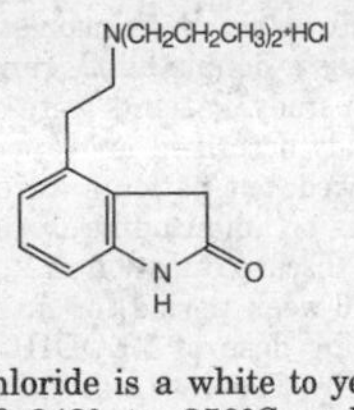

Ropinirole hydrochloride is a white to yellow solid with a melting range of 243° to 250°C and a solubility of 133 mg/mL in water.

Each pentagonal film-coated TILTAB® tablet with beveled edges contains 0.29 mg, 0.57 mg, 1.14 mg, 2.28 mg, 3.42 mg, 4.56 mg, or 5.70 mg ropinirole hydrochloride equivalent to ropinirole, 0.25 mg, 0.5 mg, 1 mg, 2 mg, 3 mg, 4 mg, or 5 mg. Inactive ingredients consist of: croscarmellose sodium, hydrous lactose, magnesium stearate, microcrystalline cellulose, and one or more of the following: carmine, FD&C Blue No. 2 aluminum lake, FD&C Yellow No. 6 aluminum lake, hypromellose, iron oxides, polyethylene glycol, polysorbate 80, titanium dioxide.

CLINICAL PHARMACOLOGY

Mechanism of Action

REQUIP is a non-ergoline dopamine agonist with high relative in vitro specificity and full intrinsic activity at the D_2 and D_3 dopamine receptor subtypes, binding with higher affinity to D_3 than to D_2 or D_4 receptor subtypes.

Ropinirole has moderate in vitro affinity for opioid receptors. Ropinirole and its metabolites have negligible in vitro affinity for dopamine D_1, 5-HT_1, 5-HT_2, benzodiazepine, GABA, muscarinic, alpha$_1$-, alpha$_2$-, and beta-adrenoreceptors.

Parkinson's Disease: The precise mechanism of action of REQUIP as a treatment for Parkinson's disease is unknown, although it is believed to be due to stimulation of postsynaptic dopamine D_2-type receptors within the caudate-putamen in the brain. This conclusion is supported by studies that show that ropinirole improves motor function in various animal models of Parkinson's disease. In particular, ropinirole attenuates the motor deficits induced by lesioning the ascending nigrostriatal dopaminergic pathway with the neurotoxin 1-methyl-4-phenyl-1,2,3,6-tetrahydropyridine (MPTP) in primates. The relevance of D_3 receptor binding in Parkinson's disease is unknown.

Restless Legs Syndrome (RLS): The precise mechanism of action of REQUIP as a treatment for Restless Legs Syndrome (also known as Ekbom Syndrome) is unknown. Although the pathophysiology of RLS is largely unknown, neuropharmacological evidence suggests primary dopaminergic system involvement. Positron emission tomographic (PET) studies suggest that a mild striatal presynaptic dopaminergic dysfunction may be involved in the pathogenesis of RLS.

Clinical Pharmacology Studies

In healthy normotensive subjects, single oral doses of REQUIP in the range 0.01 to 2.5 mg had little or no effect on supine blood pressure and pulse rates. Upon standing, REQUIP caused decreases in systolic and diastolic blood pressure at doses above 0.25 mg. In some subjects, these changes were associated with the emergence of orthostatic symptoms, bradycardia, and, in one case, transient sinus arrest with syncope. With repeat dosing and slow titration up to 4 mg once daily in healthy volunteers, postural hypotension or hypotension-related adverse events were noted in 13% of subjects on REQUIP and none of the subjects on placebo.

The mechanism of postural hypotension induced by REQUIP is presumed to be due to a D_2-mediated blunting of the noradrenergic response to standing and subsequent decrease in peripheral vascular resistance. Nausea is a common concomitant symptom of orthostatic signs and symptoms.

At oral doses as low as 0.2 mg, REQUIP suppressed serum prolactin concentrations in healthy male volunteers.

REQUIP had no dose-related effect on ECG wave form and rhythm in young, healthy, male volunteers in the range of 0.01 to 2.5 mg.

REQUIP had no dose- or exposure-related effect on mean QT intervals in healthy male and female volunteers titrated to doses up to 4 mg/day. The effect of REQUIP on QT intervals at higher exposures achieved either due to drug interactions or at doses used in Parkinson's disease has not been systematically evaluated.

Pharmacokinetics

Absorption, Distribution, Metabolism, and Elimination: The pharmacokinetics of ropinirole are similar in Parkinson's disease patients and patients with Restless Legs Syndrome. Ropinirole is rapidly absorbed after oral administration, reaching peak concentration in approximately 1-2 hours. In clinical studies, over 88% of a radiolabeled dose was recovered in urine and the absolute bioavailability was 55%, indicating a first-pass effect. Relative bioavailability from a tablet compared to an oral solution is 85%. Food does not affect the extent of absorption of ropinirole, although its T_{max} is increased by 2.5 hours and its C_{max} is decreased by approximately 25% when the drug is taken with a high-fat meal. The clearance of ropinirole after oral administration to patients is 47 L/hr (cv = 45%) and its elimination half-life is approximately 6 hours. Ropinirole is extensively metabolized by the liver to inactive metabolites and displays linear kinetics over the therapeutic dosing range of 1 to 8 mg 3 times daily. Steady-state concentrations are expected to be achieved within 2 days of dosing. Accumulation upon multiple dosing is predictive from single dosing.

Ropinirole is widely distributed throughout the body, with an apparent volume of distribution of 7.5 L/kg (cv = 32%). It is up to 40% bound to plasma proteins and has a blood-to-plasma ratio of 1:1.

The major metabolic pathways are N-despropylation and hydroxylation to form the inactive N-despropyl and hydroxy metabolites. In vitro studies indicate that the major cytochrome P_{450} isozyme involved in the metabolism of ropinirole is CYP1A2, an enzyme known to be stimulated by smoking and omeprazole, and inhibited by, for example, fluvoxamine, mexiletine, and the older fluoroquinolones such as ciprofloxacin and norfloxacin. The N-despropyl metabolite is converted to carbamyl glucuronide, carboxylic acid, and N-despropyl hydroxy metabolites. The hydroxy metabolite of ropinirole is rapidly glucuronidated. Less than 10% of the administered dose is excreted as unchanged drug in urine. N-despropyl ropinirole is the predominant metabolite found in urine (40%), followed by the carboxylic acid metabolite (10%), and the glucuronide of the hydroxy metabolite (10%).

P_{450} Interaction: In vitro metabolism studies showed that CYP1A2 was the major enzyme responsible for the metabolism of ropinirole. Inhibitors or inducers of this enzyme have been shown to alter its clearance when coadministered with ropinirole. Therefore, if therapy with a drug known to be a potent inhibitor of CYP1A2 is stopped or started during treatment with REQUIP, adjustment of the dose of REQUIP may be required.

Table 1. Mean Change in IRLS Score and Percent Responders on CGI-I

	REQUIP	Placebo	p-value
Mean Change in IRLS score at Week 12			
US study	-13.5	-9.8	p<0.0001
Multinational study (excluding US)	-11.0	-8.0	p=0.0036
Multinational study (including US)	-11.2	-8.7	p=0.0197
Percent responders on CGI-I at Week 12			
US study	73.3%	56.5%	p=0.0006
Multinational study (excluding US)	53.4%	40.9%	p=0.0416
Multinational study (including US)	59.5%	39.6%	p=0.0010

Population Subgroups

Because therapy with REQUIP is initiated at a low dose and gradually titrated upward according to clinical tolerability to obtain the optimum therapeutic effect, adjustment of the initial dose based on gender, weight, or age is not necessary.

Age: Oral clearance of ropinirole is reduced by 15% in patients above 65 years of age compared to younger patients. Dosage adjustment is not necessary in the elderly (above 65 years), as the dose of ropinirole is to be individually titrated to clinical response.

Gender: Female and male patients showed similar oral clearance.

Race: The influence of race on the pharmacokinetics of ropinirole has not been evaluated.

Cigarette Smoking: Smoking is expected to increase the clearance of ropinirole since CYP1A2 is known to be induced by smoking. In a study in patients with RLS, smokers (n = 7) had an approximate 30% lower C_{max} and a 38% lower AUC than did nonsmokers (n = 11), when those parameters were normalized for dose.

Renal Impairment: Based on population pharmacokinetic analysis, no difference was observed in the pharmacokinetics of ropinirole in patients with moderate renal impairment (creatinine clearance between 30 to 50 mL/min.) compared to an age-matched population with creatinine clearance above 50 mL/min. Therefore, no dosage adjustment is necessary in moderately renally impaired patients. The use of REQUIP in patients with severe renal impairment has not been studied.

The effect of hemodialysis on drug removal is not known, but because of the relatively high apparent volume of distribution of ropinirole (525 L), the removal of the drug by hemodialysis is unlikely.

Hepatic Impairment: The pharmacokinetics of ropinirole have not been studied in hepatically impaired patients. These patients may have higher plasma levels and lower clearance of the drug than patients with normal hepatic function. The drug should be titrated with caution in this population.

Other Diseases: Population pharmacokinetic analysis revealed no change in the oral clearance of ropinirole in patients with concomitant diseases such as hypertension, depression, osteoporosis/arthritis, and insomnia compared to patients with Parkinson's disease only.

Clinical Trials

Parkinson's Disease: The effectiveness of REQUIP in the treatment of Parkinson's disease was evaluated in a multinational drug development program consisting of 11 randomized, controlled trials. Four were conducted in patients with early Parkinson's disease and no concomitant levodopa (L-dopa), and 7 were conducted in patients with advanced Parkinson's disease with concomitant L-dopa.

Among these 11 studies, 3 placebo-controlled studies provide the most persuasive evidence of ropinirole's effectiveness in the management of patients with Parkinson's disease who were and were not receiving concomitant L-dopa. Two of these 3 trials enrolled patients with early Parkinson's disease (without L-dopa) and 1 enrolled patients receiving L-dopa.

In these studies a variety of measures were used to assess the effects of treatment (e.g., the Unified Parkinson's Disease Rating Scale [UPDRS], Clinical Global Impression [CGI] scores, patient diaries recording time "on" and "off," and tolerability of L-dopa dose reductions).

In both studies of early Parkinson's disease (without L-dopa) patients, the motor component (Part III) of the UPDRS was the primary outcome assessment. The UPDRS is a 4-part multi-item rating scale intended to evaluate mentation (Part I), activities of daily living (Part II), motor performance (Part III), and complications of therapy (Part IV). Part III of the UPDRS contains 14 items designed to assess the severity of the cardinal motor findings in patients with Parkinson's disease (e.g., tremor, rigidity, bradykinesia, postural instability, etc.) scored for different body regions and has a maximum (worst) score of 108. Responders were defined as patients with at least a 30% reduction in the Part III score.

In the study of advanced Parkinson's disease (with L-dopa) patients, both reduction in percent awake time spent"off" and the ability to reduce the daily use of L-dopa were assessed as a combined endpoint and individually.

Studies in Patients With Early Parkinson's Disease (Without L-dopa): One early therapy study was a 12-week multicenter study in which 63 patients (41 on REQUIP) with idiopathic Parkinson's disease receiving concomitant anti-Parkinson medication (but not L-dopa) were randomized to either REQUIP or placebo. Patients had a mean disease duration of approximately 2 years. Patients were eligible for enrollment if they presented with bradykinesia and at least tremor, rigidity, or postural instability. In addition, they must have been classified as Hoehn & Yahr Stage I-IV. This scale, ranging from I = unilateral involvement with minimal impairment to V = confined to wheelchair or bed, is a standard instrument used for staging patients with Parkinson's disease. The primary outcome measure in this trial was the proportion of patients experiencing a decrease (compared to baseline) of at least 30% in the UPDRS motor score.

Patients were titrated for up to 10 weeks, starting at 0.5 mg twice daily, with weekly increments of 0.5 mg twice daily to a maximum of 5 mg twice daily. Once patients reached their maximally tolerated dose (or 5 mg twice daily), they were maintained on that dose through 12 weeks. The mean dose achieved by patients at study endpoint was 7.4 mg/day. At the end of 12 weeks, 71% of patients treated with REQUIP were responders, compared with 41% of patients in the placebo group (p = 0.021).

Statistically significant differences between the percentage of responders on REQUIP compared to placebo were seen after 8 weeks of treatment.

In addition, the mean percentage improvement from baseline in the Total Motor Score was 43% in patients treated with REQUIP compared with 21% in patients treated with placebo (p = 0.018).

Statistically significant differences in UPDRS motor score between REQUIP and placebo were seen after 2 weeks of treatment.

The median daily dose at which a 30% reduction in UPDRS motor score was sustained was 4 mg.

The second trial in early Parkinson's disease (without L-dopa) patients was a double-blind, randomized, placebo-controlled, 6-month study. Patients were essentially similar to those in the study described above; concomitant use of selegiline was allowed, but patients were not permitted to use anticholinergics or amantadine during the study. Patients had a mean disease duration of 2 years and limited (not more than a 6-week period) or no prior exposure to L-dopa. The starting dose of REQUIP in this trial was 0.25 mg 3 times daily. The dose was titrated at weekly intervals by increments of 0.25 mg 3 times daily to a dose of 1 mg 3 times daily. Further titrations at weekly intervals were at increments of 0.5 mg 3 times daily up to a dose of 3 mg 3 times daily, and then weekly at increments of 1 mg 3 times daily. Patients were to be titrated to a dose of at least 1.5 mg 3 times daily and then to their maximally tolerated dose, up to a maximum of 8 mg 3 times daily. The mean dose attained in patients at study endpoint was 15.7 mg/day.

The primary measure of effectiveness was the mean percent reduction (improvement) from baseline in the UPDRS Motor Score. In this study 241 patients were enrolled. At the end of the 6-month study, patients treated with REQUIP had 22% improvement in motor score, compared with a 4% worsening in the placebo group (p<0.001).

Statistically significant differences in UPDRS motor score improvement between REQUIP and placebo were seen after 12 weeks of treatment.

Study in Patients With Advanced Parkinson's Disease (With L-dopa): This double-blind, randomized, placebo-controlled, 6-month trial evaluated 148 patients (Hoehn & Yahr II-IV) who were not adequately controlled on L-dopa. Patients in this study had a mean disease duration of approximately 9 years, had been exposed to L-dopa for approximately 7 years, and had experienced "on-off" periods with L-dopa therapy. Patients previously receiving stable doses of selegiline, amantadine, and/or anticholinergic agents could continue on these agents during the study. Patients were started at a dose of 0.25 mg 3 times daily of REQUIP and titrated upward by weekly intervals until an optimal therapeutic response was achieved. The maximum dose of study medication was 8 mg 3 times daily. All patients had to be titrated to at least a dose of 2.5 mg 3 times daily. Patients could then be maintained on this dose level or higher for the remainder of the study. Once a dose of 2.5 mg 3 times daily was achieved, patients underwent a mandatory reduction in their L-dopa dose, to be followed by additional mandatory reductions with continued escalation of the dose of REQUIP. Reductions in the dosage of L-dopa were also allowed if patients experienced adverse events that the investigator considered related to dopaminergic therapy. The mean dose attained at study endpoint was 16.3 mg/day. The primary outcome was the proportion of responders, defined as patients who were able both to achieve a decrease (compared to baseline) of at least 20% in their L-dopa dose and a decrease of at least 20% in the proportion of the time awake in the "off" condition (a period of time during the day when patients are particularly immobile), as determined by patient diary. In addition, the mean percent change from baseline in daily L-dopa dose was examined.

At the end of 6 months, 28% of patients treated with REQUIP were classified as responders (based on combined endpoint) while 11% of patients treated with placebo were responders (p = 0.02). Based on the protocol-mandated reductions in L-dopa dosage with escalating doses of REQUIP, patients treated with REQUIP had a 19.4% mean reduction in L-dopa dose while patients treated with placebo had a 3% reduction (p<0.001). L-dopa dosage reduction was also allowed during the study if dyskinesias or other dopaminergic effects occurred. Overall, reduction of L-dopa dose was sustained in 87% of patients treated with REQUIP and in 57% of patients on placebo. On average, the L-dopa dose was reduced by 31% in patients treated with REQUIP.

The mean number of "off" hours per day during baseline was 6.4 hours for patients treated with REQUIP and 7.3 hours for patients treated with placebo. At the end of the 6-month study, patients treated with REQUIP had a mean of 4.9 hours per day of "off" time, while placebo-treated patients had a mean of 6.4 hours per day of "off" time.

Restless Legs Syndrome (RLS): The effectiveness of REQUIP in the treatment of RLS was demonstrated in randomized, double-blind, placebo-controlled studies in adults diagnosed with RLS using the International Restless Legs Syndrome Study Group diagnostic criteria (see INDICATIONS AND USAGE). Patients were required to have a history of a minimum of 15 RLS episodes/month during the previous month and a total score of ≥15 on the International RLS Rating Scale (IRLS scale) at baseline. Patients with RLS secondary to other conditions (e.g., pregnancy, renal failure, and anemia) were excluded. All studies employed flexible dosing, with patients initiating therapy at 0.25 mg REQUIP once daily. Patients were titrated based on clinical response and tolerability over 7 weeks to a maximum of 4 mg once daily. All doses were taken between 1 and 3 hours before bedtime.

A variety of measures were used to assess the effects of treatment, including the IRLS Scale and Clinical Global Impression-Global Improvement (CGI-I) scores. The IRLS Scale contains 10 items designed to assess the severity of sensory and motor symptoms, sleep disturbance, daytime somnolence, and impact on activities of daily living and mood associated with RLS. The range of scores is 0 to 40, with 0 being absence of RLS symptoms and 40 the most severe symptoms. Three of the controlled studies utilized the change from baseline in the IRLS Scale at the week 12 endpoint as the primary efficacy outcome.

Three hundred eighty patients were randomized to receive REQUIP (n = 187) or placebo (n = 193) in a US study; 284 were randomized to receive either REQUIP (n = 146) or placebo (n = 138) in a multinational study (excluding US); and 267 patients were randomized to REQUIP (n = 131) or placebo (n = 136) in a multinational study (including US). Across the 3 studies, the mean duration of RLS was 16 to 22 years (range of 0 to 65 years), mean age was approximately 54 years (range of 18 to 79 years), and approximately 61% were women. The mean dose at week 12 was approximately 2 mg/day for the 3 studies.

In all 3 studies, a statistically significant difference between the treatment group receiving REQUIP and the treatment group receiving placebo was observed at week 12 for both the mean change from baseline in the IRLS Scale total score and the percentage of patients rated as responders (much improved or very much improved) on the CGI-I (see Table 1).

[See table 1 above]

Long-term maintenance of efficacy in the treatment of RLS was demonstrated in a 36-week study. Following a 24-week single-blind treatment phase (flexible doses of REQUIP of 0.25 to 4 mg once daily), patients who were responders (defined as a decrease of >6 points on the IRLS Scale total score relative to baseline) were randomized in double-blind fashion to placebo or continuation of REQUIP for an additional

12 weeks. Relapse was defined as an increase of at least 6 points on the IRLS Scale total score to a total score of at least 15, or withdrawal due to lack of efficacy. For patients who were responders at week 24, the mean dose of ropinirole was 2 mg (range 0.25 to 4 mg). Patients continued on REQUIP demonstrated a significantly lower relapse rate compared with patients randomized to placebo (32.6% vs 57.8%, p = 0.0156).

INDICATIONS AND USAGE

Parkinson's Disease

REQUIP is indicated for the treatment of the signs and symptoms of idiopathic Parkinson's disease.

The effectiveness of REQUIP was demonstrated in randomized, controlled trials in patients with early Parkinson's disease who were not receiving concomitant L-dopa therapy as well as in patients with advanced disease on concomitant L-dopa (see CLINICAL PHARMACOLOGY: Clinical Trials).

Restless Legs Syndrome

REQUIP is indicated for the treatment of moderate-to-severe primary Restless Legs Syndrome (RLS).

Key diagnostic criteria for RLS are: an urge to move the legs usually accompanied or caused by uncomfortable and unpleasant leg sensations; symptoms begin or worsen during periods of rest or inactivity such as lying or sitting; symptoms are partially or totally relieved by movement such as walking or stretching at least as long as the activity continues; and symptoms are worse or occur only in the evening or night. Difficulty falling asleep may frequently be associated with moderate-to-severe RLS.

CONTRAINDICATIONS

REQUIP is contraindicated for patients known to have hypersensitivity reaction (including urticaria, angioedema, rash, pruritus) to ropinirole or to any of the excipients.

WARNINGS

Falling Asleep During Activities of Daily Living

Patients treated with REQUIP have reported falling asleep while engaged in activities of daily living, including the operation of motor vehicles, which sometimes resulted in accidents. Although many of these patients reported somnolence while on REQUIP, some perceived that they had no warning signs such as excessive drowsiness, and believed that they were alert immediately prior to the event. Some of these events have been reported as late as 1 year after initiation of treatment.

In controlled clinical trials, somnolence was a common occurrence in patients receiving REQUIP and is more frequent in Parkinson's disease (up to 40% REQUIP, 6% placebo) than in Restless Legs Syndrome (12% REQUIP, 6% placebo). Many clinical experts believe that falling asleep while engaged in activities of daily living always occurs in a setting of preexisting somnolence, although patients may not give such a history. For this reason, prescribers should continually reassess patients for drowsiness or sleepiness, especially since some of the events occur well after the start of treatment. Prescribers should also be aware that patients may not acknowledge drowsiness or sleepiness until directly questioned about drowsiness or sleepiness during specific activities.

Before initiating treatment with REQUIP, patients should be advised of the potential to develop drowsiness and specifically asked about factors that may increase the risk with REQUIP such as concomitant sedating medications, the presence of sleep disorders (other than Restless Legs Syndrome), and concomitant medications that increase ropinirole plasma levels (e.g., ciprofloxacin—see PRECAUTIONS: Drug Interactions). If a patient develops significant daytime sleepiness or episodes of falling asleep during activities that require active participation (e.g., conversations, eating, etc.), REQUIP should ordinarily be discontinued. (See DOSAGE AND ADMINISTRATION for guidance in discontinuing REQUIP.) If a decision is made to continue REQUIP, patients should be advised to not drive and to avoid other potentially dangerous activities. There is insufficient information to establish that dose reduction will eliminate episodes of falling asleep while engaged in activities of daily living.

Syncope

Syncope, sometimes associated with bradycardia, was observed in association with ropinirole in both Parkinson's disease patients and RLS patients. In the 2 double-blind, placebo-controlled studies of REQUIP in patients with Parkinson's disease who were not being treated with L-dopa, 11.5% (18 of 157) of patients on REQUIP had syncope compared to 1.4% (2 of 147) of patients on placebo. Most of these cases occurred more than 4 weeks after initiation of therapy with REQUIP, and were usually associated with a recent increase in dose.

Of 208 patients being treated with both L-dopa and REQUIP in placebo-controlled advanced Parkinson's disease trials, there were reports of syncope in 6 (2.9%) compared to 2 of 120 (1.7%) of placebo/L-dopa patients.

In patients with RLS, of 496 patients treated with REQUIP in 12-week placebo-controlled trials, there were reports of syncope in 5 (1.0%) compared with 1 of 500 (0.2%) patients treated with placebo.

Because the studies of REQUIP excluded patients with significant cardiovascular disease, it is not known to what extent the estimated incidence figures apply to either Parkinson's disease or RLS patients in clinical practice. Therefore, patients with severe cardiovascular disease should be treated with caution.

Two of 47 Parkinson's disease patient volunteers enrolled in phase 1 studies had syncope following a 1-mg dose. In 2 studies in RLS patients that used a forced titration regimen and orthostatic challenge with intensive blood pressure monitoring, 1 of 55 RLS patients treated with REQUIP compared with 0 of 27 patients receiving placebo reported syncope. In phase 1 studies including 110 healthy volunteers, 1 patient developed hypotension, bradycardia, and sinus arrest of 26 seconds accompanied by syncope; the patient recovered spontaneously without intervention. One other healthy volunteer reported syncope.

Symptomatic Hypotension

Dopamine agonists, in clinical studies and clinical experience, appear to impair the systemic regulation of blood pressure, with resulting postural hypotension, especially during dose escalation. Parkinson's disease patients, in addition, appear to have an impaired capacity to respond to a postural challenge. For these reasons, Parkinson's patients being treated with dopaminergic agonists ordinarily (1) require careful monitoring for signs and symptoms of postural hypotension, especially during dose escalation, and (2) should be informed of this risk (see PRECAUTIONS: Information for Patients).

Although the clinical trials were not designed to systematically monitor blood pressure, there were individual reported cases of postural hypotension in early Parkinson's disease (without L-dopa) in patients treated with REQUIP. Most of these cases occurred more than 4 weeks after initiation of therapy with REQUIP and were usually associated with a recent increase in dose.

In 12-week placebo-controlled trials of patients with RLS, the adverse event orthostatic hypotension was reported by 4 of 496 patients (0.8%) treated with REQUIP compared with 2 of 500 patients (0.4%) receiving placebo.

In two phase 2 studies in patients with RLS that used a forced-titration regimen and orthostatic challenges with intensive blood pressure monitoring, 14 of 55 patients (25%) receiving REQUIP experienced an adverse event of hypotension or postural hypotension. As described above, one additional patient was noted to have an episode of vasovagal syncope (although no blood pressure recording was documented). None of the 27 patients receiving placebo had a similar adverse event. In these studies, 11 of the 55 patients (20%) receiving REQUIP and 3 of the 26 patients (12%) who had post-dose blood pressure assessments following placebo, experienced an orthostatic blood pressure decrease of at least 40 mm Hg systolic and/or at least 20 mm Hg diastolic; not all of these changes were associated with clinical symptoms. Except for its forced nature these studies used a similar titration schedule as those in the phase 3 efficacy trials.

In phase 1 studies of REQUIP that included 110 healthy volunteers, 9 subjects had documented symptomatic postural hypotension. These episodes appeared mainly at doses above 0.8 mg and these doses are higher than the starting doses recommended for either Parkinson's disease patients or RLS patients. In 8 of these 9 individuals, the hypotension was accompanied by bradycardia, but did not develop into syncope (see Syncope subsection). None of these events resulted in death or hospitalization.

One of 47 Parkinson's disease patient volunteers enrolled in phase 1 studies had documented hypotension following a 2-mg dose on 2 occasions.

Hallucinations

In double-blind, placebo-controlled, early-therapy studies in patients with Parkinson's disease who were not treated with L-dopa, 5.2% (8 of 157) of patients treated with REQUIP reported hallucinations, compared to 1.4% of patients on placebo (2 of 147). Among those patients receiving both REQUIP and L-dopa in advanced Parkinson's disease (with L-dopa) studies, 10.1% (21 of 208) were reported to experience hallucinations, compared to 4.2% (5 of 120) of patients treated with placebo and L-dopa.

Hallucinations were of sufficient severity to cause discontinuation of treatment in 1.3% of the early Parkinson's disease (without L-dopa) patients and 1.9% of the advanced Parkinson's disease (with L-dopa) patients, compared to 0% and 1.7% of placebo patients, respectively.

In patients with RLS, hallucinations were reported by 0% of patients treated with REQUIP (0 of 496) compared with 0.2% of patients who received placebo (1 of 500) in the 12-week placebo-controlled trials; in premarketing long-term open-label studies, 0.5% of patients reported hallucinations during therapy with REQUIP (2 of 390) but did not discontinue treatment and symptoms resolved.

PRECAUTIONS

General

Dyskinesia: REQUIP may potentiate the dopaminergic side effects of L-dopa and may cause and/or exacerbate preexisting dyskinesia in patients treated with L-dopa for Parkinson's disease. Decreasing the dose of L-dopa may ameliorate this side effect.

Renal Impairment: No dosage adjustment is needed in patients with mild to moderate renal impairment (creatinine clearance of 30 to 50 mL/min). The use of REQUIP in patients with severe renal impairment has not been studied.

Hepatic Impairment: The pharmacokinetics of ropinirole have not been studied in patients with hepatic impairment. Since patients with hepatic impairment may have higher plasma levels and lower clearance, REQUIP should be titrated with caution in these patients.

Events Reported With Dopaminergic Therapy: Withdrawal-Emergent Hyperpyrexia and Confusion: Although not reported with REQUIP, a symptom complex resembling the neuroleptic malignant syndrome (characterized by elevated temperature, muscular rigidity, altered consciousness, and autonomic instability), with no other obvious etiology, has been reported in association with rapid dose reduction, withdrawal of, or changes in anti-Parkinsonian therapy.

Fibrotic Complications: Cases of retroperitoneal fibrosis, pulmonary infiltrates, pleural effusion, pleural thickening, pericarditis, and cardiac valvulopathy have been reported in some patients treated with ergot-derived dopaminergic agents. While these complications may resolve when the drug is discontinued, complete resolution does not always occur.

Although these adverse events are believed to be related to the ergoline structure of these compounds, whether other, nonergot-derived dopamine agonists can cause them is unknown.

A small number of reports have been received of possible fibrotic complications, including pleural effusion, pleural fibrosis, interstitial lung disease, and cardiac valvulopathy, in the development program and postmarketing experience for REQUIP. While the evidence is not sufficient to establish a causal relationship between REQUIP and these fibrotic complications, a contribution of REQUIP cannot be completely ruled out in rare cases.

Melanoma: Epidemiologic studies have shown that patients with Parkinson's disease have a higher risk (2- to approximately 6-fold higher) of developing melanoma than the general population. Whether the increased risk observed was due to Parkinson's disease or other factors, such as drugs used to treat Parkinson's disease, is unclear.

For the reasons stated above, patients and providers are advised to monitor for melanomas frequently and on a regular basis when using REQUIP for *any* indication. Ideally, periodic skin examinations should be performed by appropriately qualified individuals (e.g., dermatologists).

Augmentation and Rebound in RLS: Reports in the literature indicate treatment of RLS with dopaminergic medications can result in a worsening of symptoms in the early morning hours, referred to as rebound. Augmentation has also been described during therapy for RLS. Augmentation refers to the earlier onset of symptoms in the evening (or even the afternoon), increase in symptoms, and spread of symptoms to involve other extremities. The controlled trials of REQUIP in patients with RLS excluded patients with augmentation and rebound and were generally not of sufficient duration to capture these phenomena. The frequency of augmentation and/or rebound after longer use of REQUIP and the appropriate management of these events, have not been evaluated in controlled clinical trials.

Retinal Pathology: Albino Rats: Retinal degeneration was observed in albino rats in the 2-year carcinogenicity study at all doses tested (equivalent to 0.6 to 20 times the maximum recommended human dose on a mg/m^2 basis), but was statistically significant at the highest dose (50 mg/kg/day). Additional studies to further evaluate the specific pathology (e.g., loss of photoreceptor cells) have not been performed. Similar changes were not observed in a 2-year carcinogenicity study in albino mice or in rats or monkeys treated for 1 year. The potential significance of this effect in humans has not been established, but cannot be disregarded because disruption of a mechanism that is universally present in vertebrates (e.g., disk shedding) may be involved.

Human: In order to evaluate the effect of REQUIP in humans, ocular electroretinogram (ERG) assessments were conducted during a 2-year, double-blind, multicenter, flexible dose, L-dopa controlled clinical study of REQUIP in patients with Parkinson's disease. A total of 156 patients (78 on ropinirole, mean dose 11.9 mg/day and 78 on L-dopa, mean dose 555.2 mg/day) were evaluated for evidence of retinal dysfunction through electroretinograms. There was no clinically meaningful difference between the treatment groups in retinal function over the duration of the study.

Binding to Melanin: REQUIP binds to melanin-containing tissues (i.e., eyes, skin) in pigmented rats. After a single dose, long-term retention of drug was demonstrated, with a half-life in the eye of 20 days. It is not known if REQUIP accumulates in these tissues over time.

Information for Patients

Physicians should instruct their patients to read the Patient Information leaflet before starting therapy with REQUIP and to reread it upon prescription renewal for new information regarding the use of REQUIP.

Patients should be instructed to take REQUIP only as prescribed. If a dose is missed, patients should be advised not to double their next dose.

REQUIP can be taken with or without food. Patients may be advised that taking REQUIP with food may reduce the occurrence of nausea. However, this has not been established in controlled clinical trials.

Patients should be advised that they may develop postural (orthostatic) hypotension with or without symptoms such as dizziness, nausea, syncope, and sometimes sweating. Hypotension and/or orthostatic symptoms may occur more frequently during initial therapy or with an increase in dose at any time (cases have been seen after weeks of treatment). Accordingly, patients should be cautioned against rising rapidly after sitting or lying down, especially if they have been doing so for prolonged periods, and especially at the initiation of treatment with REQUIP.

Patients should be alerted to the potential sedating effects associated with REQUIP, including somnolence and the possibility of falling asleep while engaged in activities of daily living. Since somnolence is a frequent adverse event with potentially serious consequences, patients should neither drive a car nor engage in other potentially dangerous activities until they have gained sufficient experience with REQUIP to gauge whether or not it affects their mental and/or motor performance adversely. Patients should be advised that if increased somnolence or episodes of falling asleep during activities of daily living (e.g., watching television, passenger in a car, etc.) are experienced at any time during treatment, they should not drive or participate in potentially dangerous activities until they have contacted their physician.

Because of possible additive effects, caution should be advised when patients are taking other sedating medications or alcohol in combination with REQUIP and when taking concomitant medications that increase plasma levels of ropinirole (e.g., ciprofloxacin).

Because of the possible additive sedative effects, caution should also be used when patients are taking alcohol or other CNS depressants (e.g., benzodiazepines, antipsychotics, antidepressants, etc.) in combination with REQUIP.

Patients should be informed they may experience hallucinations (unreal visions, sounds, or sensations) while taking REQUIP. These were uncommon in patients taking REQUIP for Restless Legs Syndrome. The risk is greater in patients with Parkinson's disease; the elderly are at greater risk than younger patients with Parkinson's disease; and the risk is greater in patients who are taking REQUIP with L-dopa, or taking higher doses of REQUIP.

Impulse Control Symptoms Including Compulsive Behaviors: There have been reports of patients experiencing intense urges to gamble, increased sexual urges, and other intense urges and the inability to control these urges while taking one or more of the medications that increase central dopaminergic tone, that are generally used for the treatment of Parkinson's disease or Restless Legs Syndrome, including REQUIP. Although it is not proven that the medications caused these events, these urges were reported to have stopped in some cases when the dose was reduced or the medication was stopped. Prescribers should ask patients about the development of new or increased gambling urges, sexual urges or other urges while being treated with REQUIP. Patients should inform their physician if they experience new or increased gambling urges, increased sexual urges or other intense urges while taking REQUIP. Physicians should consider dose reduction or stopping the medication if a patient develops such urges while taking REQUIP.

Because of the possibility that ropinirole may be excreted in breast milk, patients should be advised to notify their physicians if they intend to breastfeed or are breastfeeding an infant.

Because ropinirole has been shown to have adverse effects on embryo-fetal development, including teratogenic effects, in animals, and because experience in humans is limited, patients should be advised to notify their physician if they become pregnant or intend to become pregnant during therapy (see PRECAUTIONS: Pregnancy).

Drug Interactions

P_{450} Interaction: In vitro metabolism studies showed that CYP1A2 was the major enzyme responsible for the metabolism of ropinirole. There is thus the potential for substrates or inhibitors of this enzyme when coadministered with ropinirole to alter its clearance. Therefore, if therapy with a drug known to be a potent inhibitor of CYP1A2 is stopped or started during treatment with REQUIP, adjustment of the dose of REQUIP may be required.

L-dopa: Coadministration of carbidopa + l-dopa (SINEMET® 10/100 mg twice daily) with ropinirole (2 mg 3 times daily) had no effect on the steady-state pharmacokinetics of ropinirole (n = 28 patients). Oral administration of REQUIP 2 mg 3 times daily increased mean steady state C_{max} of l-dopa by 20%, but its AUC was unaffected (n = 23 patients).

Digoxin: Coadministration of REQUIP (2 mg 3 times daily) with digoxin (0.125 to 0.25 mg once daily) did not alter the steady-state pharmacokinetics of digoxin in 10 patients.

Theophylline: Administration of theophylline (300 mg twice daily, a substrate of CYP1A2) did not alter the steady-state pharmacokinetics of ropinirole (2 mg 3 times daily) in 12 patients with Parkinson's disease. Ropinirole (2 mg 3 times daily) did not alter the pharmacokinetics of theophylline (5 mg/kg IV) in 12 patients with Parkinson's disease.

Ciprofloxacin: Coadministration of ciprofloxacin (500 mg twice daily), an inhibitor of CYP1A2, with ropinirole (2 mg 3 times daily) increased ropinirole AUC by 84% on average and C_{max} by 60% (n = 12 patients).

Estrogens: Population pharmacokinetic analysis revealed that estrogens (mainly ethinylestradiol: intake 0.6 to 3 mg over 4-month to 23-year period) reduced the oral clearance of ropinirole by 36% in 16 patients. Dosage adjustment may not be needed for REQUIP in patients on estrogen therapy because patients must be carefully titrated with ropinirole to tolerance or adequate effect. However, if estrogen therapy is stopped or started during treatment with REQUIP, then adjustment of the dose of REQUIP may be required.

Dopamine Antagonists: Since ropinirole is a dopamine agonist, it is possible that dopamine antagonists such as neuroleptics (phenothiazines, butyrophenones, thioxanthenes) or metoclopramide may diminish the effectiveness of REQUIP. Patients with major psychotic disorders treated with neuroleptics should only be treated with dopamine agonists if the potential benefits outweigh the risks.

Population analysis showed that commonly administered drugs, e.g., selegiline, amantadine, tricyclic antidepressants, benzodiazepines, ibuprofen, thiazides, antihistamines, and anticholinergics, did not affect the oral clearance of ropinirole.

Carcinogenesis, Mutagenesis, Impairment of Fertility

Two-year carcinogenicity studies were conducted in Charles River CD-1 mice at doses of 5, 15, and 50 mg/kg/day and in Sprague-Dawley rats at doses of 1.5, 15, and 50 mg/kg/day (top doses equivalent to 10 and 20 times, respectively, the maximum recommended human dose (MRHD) of 24 mg/day on a mg/m^2 basis). In the male rat, there was a significant increase in testicular Leydig cell adenomas at all doses tested, i.e., ≥1.5 mg/kg (0.6 times the MRHD on a mg/m^2 basis). This finding is of questionable significance because the endocrine mechanisms believed to be involved in the production of Leydig cell hyperplasia and adenomas in rats are not relevant to humans. In the female mouse, there was an increase in benign uterine endometrial polyps at a dose of 50 mg/kg/day (10 times the MRHD on a mg/m^2 basis).

Ropinirole was not mutagenic or clastogenic in the in vitro Ames test, the in vitro chromosome aberration test in human lymphocytes, the in vitro mouse lymphoma (L1578Y cells) assay, and the in vivo mouse micronucleus test.

When administered to female rats prior to and during mating and throughout pregnancy, ropinirole caused disruption of implantation at doses of 20 mg/kg/day (8 times the MRHD on a mg/m^2 basis) or greater. This effect is thought to be due to the prolactin-lowering effect of ropinirole. In humans, chorionic gonadotropin, not prolactin, is essential for implantation. In rat studies using low doses (5 mg/kg) during the prolactin-dependent phase of early pregnancy (gestation days 0 to 8), ropinirole did not affect female fertility at dosages up to 100 mg/kg/day (40 times the MRHD on a mg/m^2 basis). No effect on male fertility was observed in rats at dosages up to 125 mg/kg/day (50 times the MRHD on a mg/m^2 basis).

Pregnancy

Pregnancy Category C. In animal reproduction studies, ropinirole has been shown to have adverse effects on embryo-fetal development, including teratogenic effects. Ropinirole given to pregnant rats during organogenesis (20 mg/kg on gestation days 6 and 7 followed by 20, 60, 90, 120, or 150 mg/kg on gestation days 8 through 15) resulted in decreased fetal body weight at 60 mg/kg/day, increased fetal death at 90 mg/kg/day, and digital malformations at 150 mg/kg/day (24, 36, and 60 times the MRHD on a mg/m^2 basis, respectively). The combined administration of ropinirole (10 mg/kg/day, 8 times the MRHD on a mg/m^2 basis) and L-dopa (250 mg/kg/day) to pregnant rabbits during organogenesis produced a greater incidence and severity of fetal malformations (primarily digit defects) than were seen in the offspring of rabbits treated with L-dopa alone. No indication of an effect on development of the conceptus was observed in rabbits when a maternally toxic dose of ropinirole was administered alone (20 mg/kg/day, 16 times the MRHD on a mg/m^2 basis). In a perinatal-postnatal study in rats, 10 mg/kg/day (4 times the MRHD on a mg/m^2 basis) of ropinirole impaired growth and development of nursing offspring and altered neurological development of female offspring.

There are no adequate and well-controlled studies using REQUIP in pregnant women. REQUIP should be used during pregnancy only if the potential benefit outweighs the potential risk to the fetus.

Nursing Mothers

REQUIP inhibits prolactin secretion in humans and could potentially inhibit lactation.

Studies in rats have shown that REQUIP and/or its metabolite(s) is excreted in breast milk. It is not known whether this drug is excreted in human milk. Because many drugs are excreted in human milk and because of the potential for serious adverse reactions in nursing infants from REQUIP, a decision should be made whether to discontinue nursing or to discontinue the drug, taking into account the importance of the drug to the mother.

Pediatric Use

Safety and effectiveness in the pediatric population have not been established.

ADVERSE REACTIONS

Parkinson's Disease

During the premarketing development of REQUIP, patients received REQUIP either without L-dopa (early Parkinson's disease studies) or as concomitant therapy with L-dopa (advanced Parkinson's disease studies). Because these 2 populations may have differential risks for various adverse events, this section will, in general, present adverse event data for these 2 populations separately.

Early Parkinson's Disease (Without L-dopa): The most commonly observed adverse events (>5%) in the double-blind, placebo-controlled early Parkinson's disease trials associated with the use of REQUIP (n = 157) not seen at an equivalent frequency among the placebo-treated patients (n = 147) were, in order of decreasing incidence: nausea, dizziness, somnolence, headache, vomiting, syncope, fatigue, dyspepsia, viral infection, constipation, pain, increased sweating, asthenia, dependent/leg edema, orthostatic symptoms, abdominal pain, pharyngitis, confusion, hallucinations, urinary tract infections, and abnormal vision.

Approximately 24% of 157 patients treated with REQUIP who participated in the double-blind, placebo-controlled early Parkinson's disease (without l-dopa) trials discontinued treatment due to adverse events compared to 13% of 147 patients who received placebo. The adverse events most commonly causing discontinuation of treatment by patients treated with REQUIP were: nausea (6.4%), dizziness (3.8%), aggravated Parkinson's disease (1.3%), hallucinations (1.3%), somnolence (1.3%), vomiting (1.3%), and headache (1.3%). Of these, hallucinations appear to be dose-related. While other adverse events leading to discontinuation may be dose-related, the titration design utilized in these trials precluded an adequate assessment of the dose response. For example, in the larger of the 2 trials described in CLINICAL PHARMACOLOGY: Clinical Trials, the difference in the rate of discontinuations emerged only after 10 weeks of treatment, suggesting, although not proving, that the effect could be related to dose.

Adverse Event Incidence in Controlled Clinical Studies: Table 2 lists treatment-emergent adverse events that occurred in ≥2% of patients with early Parkinson's disease (without l-dopa) treated with REQUIP participating in the double-blind, placebo-controlled studies and were numerically more common in the group treated with REQUIP. In these studies, either REQUIP or placebo was used as early therapy (i.e., without l-dopa).

The prescriber should be aware that these figures cannot be used to predict the incidence of adverse events in the course of usual medical practice where patient characteristics and other factors differ from those that prevailed in the clinical studies. Similarly, the cited frequencies cannot be compared with figures obtained from other clinical investigations involving different treatments, uses, and investigators. However, the cited figures do provide the prescribing physician with some basis for estimating the relative contribution of drug and non-drug factors to the adverse-events incidence rate in the population studied.

Table 2. Treatment-Emergent Adverse Event* Incidence in Double-Blind, Placebo-Controlled Early Parkinson's Disease (Without l-dopa) Trials (Events ≥2% of Patients Treated With REQUIP and Numerically More Frequent Than the Placebo Group)

Adverse Experience	REQUIP (n = 157) (%)	Placebo (n = 147) (%)
Autonomic nervous system		
Flushing	3	1
Dry mouth	5	3

Increased sweating	6	4
Body as a whole		
Asthenia	6	1
Chest pain	4	2
Dependent edema	6	3
Leg edema	7	1
Fatigue	11	4
Malaise	3	1
Pain	8	4
Cardiovascular general		
Hypertension	5	3
Hypotension	2	0
Orthostatic symptoms	6	5
Syncope	12	1
Central/peripheral nervous system		
Dizziness	40	22
Hyperkinesia	2	1
Hypesthesia	4	2
Vertigo	2	0
Gastrointestinal system		
Abdominal pain	6	3
Anorexia	4	1
Dyspepsia	10	5
Flatulence	3	1
Nausea	60	22
Vomiting	12	7
Heart rate/rhythm		
Extrasystoles	2	1
Atrial fibrillation	2	0
Palpitation	3	2
Tachycardia	2	0
Metabolic/nutritional		
Increased alkaline phosphatase	3	1
Psychiatric		
Amnesia	3	1
Impaired concentration	2	0
Confusion	5	1
Hallucination	5	1
Somnolence	40	6
Yawning	3	0
Reproductive male		
Impotence	3	1
Resistance mechanism		
Viral infection	11	3
Respiratory system		
Bronchitis	3	1
Dyspnea	3	0
Pharyngitis	6	4
Rhinitis	4	3
Sinusitis	4	3
Urinary system		
Urinary tract infection	5	4
Vascular extracardiac		
Peripheral ischemia	3	0
Vision		
Eye abnormality	3	1
Abnormal vision	6	3
Xerophthalmia	2	0

*Patients may have reported multiple adverse experiences during the study or at discontinuation; thus, patients may be included in more than one category.

Other events reported by 1% or more of early Parkinson's disease (without L-dopa) patients treated with REQUIP, but that were equally or more frequent in the placebo group, were: headache, upper respiratory infection, insomnia, arthralgia, tremor, back pain, anxiety, dyskinesias, aggravated Parkinsonism, depression, falls, myalgia, leg cramps, paresthesias, nervousness, diarrhea, arthritis, hot flushes, weight loss, rash, cough, hyperglycemia, muscle spasm, arthrosis, abnormal dreams, dystonia, increased salivation, bradycardia, gout, basal cell carcinoma, gingivitis, hematuria, and rigors.

Among the treatment-emergent adverse events in patients treated with REQUIP, hallucinations appear to be dose-related.

The incidence of adverse events was not materially different between women and men.

Advanced Parkinson's Disease (With L-dopa): The most commonly observed adverse events (>5%), in the double-blind, placebo-controlled advanced Parkinson's disease (with l-dopa) trials associated with the use of REQUIP (n = 208) as an adjunct to l-dopa not seen at an equivalent frequency among the placebo-treated patients (n = 120) were, in order of decreasing incidence: dyskinesias, nausea, dizziness, aggravated Parkinsonism, somnolence, headache, insomnia, injury, hallucinations, falls, abdominal pain, upper respiratory infection, confusion, increased sweating, vomiting, viral infection, increased drug level, arthralgia, tremor, anxiety, urinary tract infection, constipation, dry mouth, pain, hypokinesia, and paresthesia.

Approximately 24% of 208 patients who received REQUIP in the double-blind, placebo-controlled advanced Parkinson's disease (with l-dopa) trials discontinued treatment due to adverse events compared to 18% of 120 patients who received placebo. The events most commonly (≥1%) causing discontinuation of treatment by patients treated with REQUIP were: dizziness (2.9%), dyskinesias (2.4%), vomiting (2.4%), confusion (2.4%), nausea (1.9%), hallucinations (1.9%), anxiety (1.9%), and increased sweating (1.4%). Of these, hallucinations and dyskinesias appear to be dose-related.

Adverse Event Incidence in Controlled Clinical Studies: Table 3 lists treatment-emergent adverse events that occurred in ≥2% of patients with advanced Parkinson's disease (with l-dopa) treated with REQUIP who participated in the double-blind, placebo-controlled studies and were numerically more common in the group treated with REQUIP. In these studies, either REQUIP or placebo was used as an adjunct to l-dopa. Adverse events were usually mild or moderate in intensity.

The prescriber should be aware that these figures cannot be used to predict the incidence of adverse events in the course of usual medical practice where patient characteristics and other factors differ from those that prevailed in the clinical studies. Similarly, the cited frequencies cannot be compared with figures obtained from other clinical investigations involving different treatments, uses, and investigators. However, the cited figures do provide the prescribing physician with some basis for estimating the relative contribution of drug and non-drug factors to the adverse events incidence rate in the population studied.

Table 3. Treatment-Emergent Adverse Event* Incidence in Double-Blind, Placebo-Controlled Advanced Parkinson's Disease (With L-dopa) Trials (Events ≥2% of Patients Treated With REQUIP and Numerically More Frequent Than the Placebo Group)

Adverse Experience	REQUIP (n = 208) (%)	Placebo (n = 120) (%)
Autonomic nervous system		
Dry mouth	5	1
Increased sweating	7	2
Body as a whole		
Increased drug level	7	3
Pain	5	3
Cardiovascular general		
Hypotension	2	1
Syncope	3	2
Central/peripheral nervous system		
Dizziness	26	16
Dyskinesia	34	13
Falls	10	7
Headache	17	12
Hypokinesia	5	4
Paresis	3	0
Paresthesia	5	3
Tremor	6	3
Gastrointestinal system		
Abdominal pain	9	8
Constipation	6	3
Diarrhea	5	3
Dysphagia	2	1
Flatulence	2	1
Nausea	30	18
Increased saliva	2	1
Vomiting	7	4
Metabolic/nutritional		
Weight decrease	2	1
Musculoskeletal system		
Arthralgia	7	5
Arthritis	3	1
Psychiatric		
Amnesia	5	1
Anxiety	6	3
Confusion	9	2
Abnormal dreaming	3	2
Hallucinations	10	4
Nervousness	5	3
Somnolence	20	8
Red blood cell		
Anemia	2	0
Resistance mechanism		
Upper respiratory tract infection	9	8
Respiratory system		
Dyspnea	3	2
Urinary system		
Pyuria	2	1
Urinary incontinence	2	1
Urinary tract infection	6	3
Vision		
Diplopia	2	1

*Patients may have reported multiple adverse experiences during the study or at discontinuation; thus, patients may be included in more than one category.

Other events reported by 1% or more of patients treated with both REQUIP and L-dopa, but equally or more frequent in the placebo/L-dopa group, were: myocardial infarction, orthostatic symptoms, virus infections, asthenia, dyspepsia, myalgia, back pain, depression, leg cramps, fatigue, rhinitis, chest pain, hematuria, vertigo, tinnitus, leg edema, hot flushes, abnormal gait, hyperkinesia, and pharyngitis.

Among the treatment-emergent adverse events in patients treated with REQUIP, hallucinations and dyskinesias appear to be dose-related.

Restless Legs Syndrome

The most commonly observed adverse events (>5%) in the 12-week double-blind, placebo-controlled trials in the treatment of Restless Legs Syndrome with REQUIP (n = 496) and at least twice the rate for placebo-treated patients (n = 500) were, in order of decreasing incidence: nausea, somnolence, vomiting, dizziness, and fatigue (see Table 4). Occurrences of nausea in clinical trials were generally mild to moderate in intensity (see also DOSAGE AND ADMINISTRATION: General Dosing Considerations).

Approximately 5% of 496 patients treated with REQUIP who participated in the double-blind, placebo-controlled trials in the treatment of RLS discontinued treatment due to adverse events compared to 4% of 500 patients who received placebo. The adverse events most commonly causing discontinuation of treatment by patients treated with REQUIP were: nausea (1.6%), dizziness (0.8 %), and headache (0.8%).

Adverse Event Incidence in Controlled Clinical Studies: Table 4 lists treatment-emergent adverse events that occurred in ≥2% of patients with RLS treated with REQUIP participating in the 12-week double-blind, placebo-controlled studies and were numerically more common in the group treated with REQUIP.

The prescriber should be aware that these figures cannot be used to predict the incidence of adverse events in the course of usual medical practice where patient characteristics and other factors differ from those that prevailed in the clinical studies. Similarly, the cited frequencies cannot be compared with figures obtained from other clinical investigations involving different treatments, uses, and investigators. However, the cited figures do provide the prescribing physician with some basis for estimating the relative contribution of drug and non-drug factors to the adverse-events incidence rate in the population studied.

Table 4. Treatment-Emergent Adverse Event Incidence in Double-Blind, Placebo-Controlled RLS Trials (Events ≥2% of Patients Treated With REQUIP and Numerically More Frequent Than the Placebo Group)

Adverse Experience	REQUIP (n = 496) (%)	Placebo (n = 500) (%)
Ear and labyrinth disorders		
Vertigo	2	1
Gastrointestinal disorders		
Nausea	40	8
Vomiting	11	2
Diarrhea	5	3
Dyspepsia	4	3
Dry mouth	3	2
Abdominal pain upper	3	1
General disorders and administration site conditions		
Fatigue	8	4
Edema peripheral	2	1
Infections and infestations		
Nasopharyngitis	9	8
Influenza	3	2
Musculoskeletal and connective tissue disorders		
Arthralgia	4	3
Muscle cramps	3	2
Pain in extremity	3	2
Nervous system disorders		
Somnolence	12	6
Dizziness	11	5

Paresthesia	3	1
Respiratory, thoracic, and mediastinal disorders		
Cough	3	2
Nasal congestion	2	1
Skin and subcutaneous tissue disorders		
Hyperhidrosis	3	1

Other events reported by 2% or more of patients treated with REQUIP, but equally or more frequent in the placebo group, were headache, insomnia, restless legs syndrome, upper respiratory tract infection, back pain, and sinusitis.

Other Adverse Events Observed During All Phase 2/3 Clinical Trials for Parkinson's Disease

REQUIP has been administered to 1,599 individuals in clinical trials. During these trials, all adverse events were recorded by the clinical investigators using terminology of their own choosing. To provide a meaningful estimate of the proportion of individuals having adverse events, similar types of events were grouped into a smaller number of standardized categories using modified WHOART dictionary terminology. These categories are used in the listing below. The frequencies presented represent the proportion of the 1,599 individuals exposed to REQUIP who experienced events of the type cited on at least 1 occasion while receiving REQUIP. All reported events that occurred at least twice (or once for serious or potentially serious events), except those already listed above, trivial events, and terms too vague to be meaningful, are included without regard to determination of a causal relationship to REQUIP, except that events very unlikely to be drug-related have been deleted.

Events are further classified within body system categories and enumerated in order of decreasing frequency using the following definitions: frequent adverse events are defined as those occurring in at least 1/100 patients and infrequent adverse events are those occurring in 1/100 to 1/1,000 patients and rare events are those occurring in fewer than 1/1,000 patients.

Body as a Whole: ***Infrequent:*** Cellulitis, peripheral edema, fever, influenza-like symptoms, enlarged abdomen, precordial chest pain, and generalized edema. ***Rare:*** Ascites.

Cardiovascular: ***Infrequent:*** Cardiac failure, bradycardia, tachycardia, supraventricular tachycardia, angina pectoris, bundle branch block, cardiac arrest, cardiomegaly, aneurysm, mitral insufficiency. ***Rare:*** Ventricular tachycardia.

Central/Peripheral Nervous System: ***Frequent:*** Neuralgia. ***Infrequent:*** Involuntary muscle contractions, hypertonia, dysphonia, abnormal coordination, extrapyramidal disorder, migraine, choreoathetosis, coma, stupor, aphasia, convulsions, hypotonia, peripheral neuropathy, paralysis. ***Rare:*** Grand mal convulsions, hemiparesis, hemiplegia.

Endocrine: ***Infrequent:*** Hypothyroidism, gynecomastia, hyperthyroidism. ***Rare:*** Goiter, SIADH.

Gastrointestinal: ***Infrequent:*** Increased hepatic enzymes, bilirubinemia, cholecystitis, cholelithiasis colitis, dysphagia, periodontitis, fecal incontinence, gastroesophageal reflux, hemorrhoids, toothache, eructation, gastritis, esophagitis, hiccups, diverticulitis, duodenal ulcer, gastric ulcer, melena, duodenitis, gastrointestinal hemorrhage, glossitis, rectal hemorrhage, pancreatitis, stomatitis and ulcerative stomatitis, tongue edema. ***Rare:*** Biliary pain, hemorrhagic gastritis, hematemesis, salivary duct obstruction.

Hematologic: ***Infrequent:*** Purpura, thrombocytopenia, hematoma, Vitamin B12 deficiency, hypochromic anemia, eosinophilia, leukocytosis, leukopenia, lymphocytosis, lymphopenia, lymphedema.

Metabolic/Nutritional: ***Frequent:*** Increased BUN. ***Infrequent:*** Hypoglycemia, increased alkaline phosphatase, increased LDH, weight increase, hyperphosphatemia, hyperuricemia, diabetes mellitus, glycosuria, hypokalemia, hypercholesterolemia, hyperkalemia, acidosis, hyponatremia, thirst, increased CPK, dehydration. ***Rare:*** Hypochloremia.

Musculoskeletal: ***Infrequent:*** Aggravated arthritis, tendonitis, osteoporosis, bursitis, polymyalgia rheumatica, muscle weakness, skeletal pain, torticollis. ***Rare:*** Dupuytren's contracture requiring surgery.

Neoplasm: ***Infrequent:*** Malignant breast neoplasm. ***Rare:*** Bladder carcinoma, benign brain neoplasm, esophageal carcinoma, malignant laryngeal neoplasm, lipoma, rectal carcinoma, uterine neoplasm.

Psychiatric: ***Infrequent:*** Increased libido, agitation, apathy, impaired concentration, depersonalization, paranoid reaction, personality disorder, euphoria, delirium, dementia, delusion, emotional lability, decreased libido, manic reaction, somnambulism, aggressive reaction, neurosis. ***Rare:*** Suicide attempt.

Genitourinary: ***Infrequent:*** Amenorrhea, vaginal hemorrhage, penile disorder, prostatic disorder, balanoposthitis, epididymitis, perineal pain, dysuria, micturition frequency, albuminuria, nocturia, polyuria, renal calculus. ***Rare:*** Breast enlargement, mastitis, uterine hemorrhage, ejaculation disorder, Peyronie's disease, pyelonephritis, acute renal failure, uremia.

Resistance Mechanism: ***Infrequent:*** Herpes zoster, otitis media, sepsis, abscess, herpes simplex, fungal infection, genital moniliasis.

Respiratory: ***Infrequent:*** Asthma, epistaxis, laryngitis, pleurisy, pulmonary edema.

Skin/Appendage: ***Infrequent:*** Pruritus, dermatitis, eczema, skin ulceration, alopecia, skin hypertrophy, skin discoloration, urticaria, fungal dermatitis, furunculosis, hyperkeratosis, photosensitivity reaction, psoriasis, maculopapular rash, psoriaform rash, seborrhea.

Special Senses: ***Infrequent:*** Tinnitus, earache, decreased hearing, abnormal lacrimation, conjunctivitis, blepharitis, glaucoma, abnormal accommodation, blepharospasm, eye pain, photophobia. ***Rare:*** Scotoma.

Vascular Extracardiac: ***Infrequent:*** Varicose veins, phlebitis, peripheral gangrene. ***Rare:*** Limb embolism, pulmonary embolism, gangrene, subarachnoid hemorrhage, deep thrombophlebitis, leg thrombophlebitis, thrombosis.

Falling Asleep During Activities of Daily Living: Patients treated with REQUIP have reported falling asleep while engaged in activities of daily living, including operation of a motor vehicle which sometimes resulted in accidents (see bolded WARNING).

Other Adverse Events Observed During Phase 2/3 Clinical Trials for RLS

REQUIP has been administered to 911 individuals in clinical trials. During these trials, all adverse events were recorded by the clinical investigators using terminology of their own choosing. To provide a meaningful estimate of the proportion of individuals having adverse events, similar types of events were grouped into a smaller number of standardized categories using MedDRA dictionary terminology. These categories are used in the listing below. The frequencies presented represent the proportion of the 911 individuals exposed to REQUIP who experienced events of the type cited on at least one occasion while receiving REQUIP. All reported events that occurred at least twice (or once for serious or potentially serious events), except those already listed, trivial events, and terms too vague to be meaningful, are included without regard to determination of a causal relationship to REQUIP, except that events very unlikely to be drug-related have been deleted.

Events are further classified within body system categories and enumerated in order of decreasing frequency using the following definitions: frequent adverse events are defined as those occurring in at least 1/100 patients and infrequent adverse events are those occurring in 1/100 to 1/1,000 patients.

Blood and Lymphatic System Disorders: ***Infrequent:*** Anemia, lymphadenopathy.

Cardiac Disorders: ***Frequent:*** Palpitations. ***Infrequent:*** Acute coronary syndrome, angina pectoris, angina unstable, bradycardia, cardiac failure, cardiovascular disorder, coronary artery disease, myocardial infarction, sick sinus syndrome, tachycardia.

Congenital, Familial, and Genetic Disorders: ***Infrequent:*** Pigmented nevus.

Ear and Labyrinth Disorders: ***Infrequent:*** Ear pain, middle ear effusion, tinnitus.

Endocrine Disorders: ***Infrequent:*** Goiter, hypothyroidism.

Eye Disorders: ***Infrequent:*** Blepharitis, conjunctival hemorrhage, conjunctivitis, eye irritation, eye pain, keratoconjunctivitis sicca, vision blurred, visual acuity reduced, visual disturbance.

Gastrointestinal Disorders: ***Frequent:*** Abdominal pain, constipation, gastroesophageal reflux disease, stomach discomfort, toothache. ***Infrequent:*** Abdominal adhesions, abdominal discomfort, abdominal distension, abdominal pain lower, duodenal ulcer, dysphagia, eructation, flatulence, gastric disorder, gastric hemorrhage, gastric polyps, gastric ulcer, gastritis, gastrointestinal pain, hematemesis, hemorrhoids, hiatus hernia, intestinal obstruction, irritable bowel syndrome, loose stools, mouth ulceration, pancreatitis acute, peptic ulcer, rectal hemorrhage, reflux esophagitis.

General Disorders and Administration Site Conditions: ***Frequent:*** Asthenia, chest pain, influenza-like illness, rigors. ***Infrequent:*** Chest discomfort, feeling cold, feeling hot, hunger, lethargy, malaise, edema, pain, pyrexia.

Hepatobiliary Disorders: ***Infrequent:*** Cholecystitis, cholelithiasis, ischemic hepatitis.

Immune System Disorders: ***Infrequent:*** Hypersensitivity.

Infections and Infestations: ***Frequent:*** Bronchitis, gastroenteritis, gastroenteritis viral, lower respiratory tract infection, rhinitis, tooth abscess, urinary tract infection. ***Infrequent:*** Appendicitis, bacterial infection, bladder infection, bronchitis acute, candidiasis, cellulitis, cystitis, diarrhea infectious, diverticulitis, ear infection, folliculitis, fungal infection, gastrointestinal infection, herpes simplex, infected cyst, laryngitis, localized infection, mastitis, otitis externa, otitis media, pharyngitis, pneumonia, postoperative infection, respiratory tract infection, tonsillitis, tooth infection, vaginal candidiasis, vaginal infection, vaginal mycosis, viral infection, viral upper respiratory tract infection, wound infection.

Injury, Poisoning, and Procedural Complications: ***Infrequent:*** Concussion, lower limb fracture, post procedural hemorrhage, road traffic accident.

Investigations: ***Infrequent:*** Blood cholesterol increased, blood iron decreased, blood pressure increased, blood urine present, hemoglobin decreased, heart rate increased, protein urine present, weight decreased, weight increased.

Metabolism and Nutrition Disorders: ***Infrequent:*** Anorexia, decreased appetite, diabetes mellitus non-insulin-dependent, fluid retention, gout, hypercholesterolemia.

Musculoskeletal and Connective Tissue Disorders: ***Frequent:*** Muscle spasms, musculoskeletal stiffness, myalgia, neck pain, osteoarthritis, tendonitis. ***Infrequent:*** Arthritis, aseptic necrosis bone, bone pain, bone spur, bursitis, groin pain, intervertebral disc degeneration, intervertebral disc protrusion, joint stiffness, joint swelling, localized osteoarthritis, monoarthritis, muscle contracture, muscle tightness, muscle twitching, osteoporosis, rotator cuff syndrome, sacroiliitis, synovitis.

Neoplasms Benign, Malignant, and Unspecified: ***Infrequent:*** Anaplastic thyroid cancer, angiomyolipoma, basal cell carcinoma, breast cancer, gastric cancer, gastrointestinal stromal tumor, malignant melanoma, prostate cancer, skin papilloma, squamous cell carcinoma, uterine leiomyoma.

Nervous System Disorders: ***Frequent:*** Hypoesthesia, migraine. ***Infrequent:*** Amnesia, aphasia, ataxia, balance disorder, benign intracranial hypertension, burning sensation, carpal tunnel syndrome, disturbance in attention, dizziness postural, dysgeusia, dyskinesia, head discomfort, hyperesthesia, hypersomnia, lethargy, loss of consciousness, memory impairment, migraine with aura, migraine without aura, neuralgia, sciatica, sedation, sinus headache, sleep apnea syndrome, syncope vasovagal, tension headache, transient ischemic attack, tremor.

Psychiatric Disorders: ***Frequent:*** Anxiety, depression, irritability, sleep disorder. ***Infrequent:*** Abnormal dreams, agitation, bruxism, confusional state, depressed mood, disorientation, early morning awakening, libido decreased, loss of libido, mood swings, nervousness, nightmare, panic attack, stress symptoms, tension.

Renal and Urinary Disorders: ***Infrequent:*** Dysuria, hematuria, hypertonic bladder, micturition disorder, nephrolithiasis, nocturia, pollakiuria, proteinuria, urinary retention.

Reproductive System and Breast Disorders: ***Frequent:*** Erectile dysfunction. ***Infrequent:*** Breast cyst, dysmenorrhea, menorrhagia, pelvic peritoneal adhesions, postmenopausal hemorrhage, premenstrual syndrome, prostatitis.

Respiratory, Thoracic and Mediastinal Disorders: ***Frequent:*** Asthma, pharyngolaryngeal pain. ***Infrequent:*** Dry throat, dyspnea, epistaxis, hemoptysis, hoarseness, interstitial lung disease, nasal mucosal disorder, nasal polyps, respiratory tract congestion, rhinorrhea, sinus congestion, sneezing, wheezing, yawning.

Skin and Subcutaneous Tissue Disorders: ***Frequent:*** Night sweats, rash. ***Infrequent:*** Acne, actinic keratosis, alopecia, cold sweat, dermatitis, dermatitis allergic, dermatitis contact, eczema, exanthem, face edema, photosensitivity reaction, pruritus, psoriasis, rash pruritic, skin lesion, urticaria.

Vascular Disorders: ***Frequent:*** Hot flush, hypertension, hypotension. ***Infrequent:*** Atherosclerosis, circulatory collapse, flushing, hematoma, thrombosis, varicose vein.

Postmarketing Reports

The following adverse events (not listed above in clinical trials or other sections of the prescribing information) have been identified during postapproval use of ropinirole. Because these events are reported voluntarily from a population of uncertain size, it is not always possible to reliably estimate their frequency or establish a causal relationship to drug exposure.

Immune Systems Disorders: Hypersensitivity reactions (including urticaria, angioedema, rash, and pruritus).

Psychiatric Disorders: Impulse control symptoms, pathological gambling, increased libido including hypersexuality.

DRUG ABUSE AND DEPENDENCE

Controlled Substance Class

REQUIP is not a controlled substance.

Physical and Psychological Dependence

Animal studies and human clinical trials with REQUIP did not reveal any potential for drug-seeking behavior or physical dependence.

OVERDOSAGE

In the Parkinson's disease program, there have been patients who accidentally or intentionally took more than their prescribed dose of ropinirole. The largest overdose reported in the Parkinson's disease clinical trials was 435 mg taken over a 7-day period (62.1 mg/day). Of patients who received a dose greater than 24 mg/day, reported symptoms included adverse events commonly reported during dopaminergic therapy (nausea, dizziness), as well as visual hallucinations, hyperhidrosis, claustrophobia, chorea, palpitations, asthenia, and nightmares. Additional symptoms reported for doses of 24 mg or less or for overdoses of unknown amount included vomiting, increased coughing, fatigue, syncope, vasovagal syncope, dyskinesia, agitation, chest pain, orthostatic hypotension, somnolence, and confusional state.

Overdose Management

It is anticipated that the symptoms of overdose with REQUIP will be related to its dopaminergic activity. General supportive measures are recommended. Vital signs should be maintained, if necessary. Removal of any unabsorbed material (e.g., by gastric lavage) should be considered.

DOSAGE AND ADMINISTRATION

General Dosing Considerations for Parkinson's Disease and RLS

REQUIP can be taken with or without food. Patients may be advised that taking REQUIP with food may reduce the occurrence of nausea. However, this has not been established in controlled clinical trials.

If a significant interruption in therapy with REQUIP has occurred, retitration of therapy may be warranted.

Geriatric Use: Pharmacokinetic studies demonstrated a reduced clearance of ropinirole in the elderly (see CLINICAL PHARMACOLOGY). Dose adjustment is not necessary since the dose is individually titrated to clinical response.

Renal Impairment: The pharmacokinetics of ropinirole were not altered in patients with moderate renal impairment (see CLINICAL PHARMACOLOGY). Therefore, no dosage adjustment is necessary in patients with moderate renal impairment. The use of REQUIP in patients with severe renal impairment has not been studied.

Hepatic Impairment: The pharmacokinetics of ropinirole have not been studied in patients with hepatic impairment. Since patients with hepatic impairment may have higher plasma levels and lower clearance, REQUIP should be titrated with caution in these patients.

Dosing for Parkinson's Disease

In all clinical studies, dosage was initiated at a subtherapeutic level and gradually titrated to therapeutic response. The dosage should be increased to achieve a maximum therapeutic effect, balanced against the principal side effects of nausea, dizziness, somnolence, and dyskinesia.

The recommended starting dose for Parkinson's disease is 0.25 mg 3 times daily. Based on individual patient response, dosage should then be titrated with weekly increments as described in Table 5. After week 4, if necessary, daily dosage may be increased by 1.5 mg/day on a weekly basis up to a dose of 9 mg/day, and then by up to 3 mg/day weekly to a total dose of 24 mg/day. Doses greater than 24 mg/day have not been tested in clinical trials.

Table 5. Ascending-Dose Schedule of REQUIP for Parkinson's Disease

Week	Dosage	Total Daily Dose
1	0.25 mg 3 times daily	0.75 mg
2	0.5 mg 3 times daily	1.5 mg
3	0.75 mg 3 times daily	2.25 mg
4	1 mg 3 times daily	3 mg

When REQUIP is administered as adjunct therapy to L-dopa, the concurrent dose of L-dopa may be decreased gradually as tolerated. L-dopa dosage reduction was allowed during the advanced Parkinson's disease (with L-dopa) study if dyskinesias or other dopaminergic effects occurred. Overall, reduction of L-dopa dose was sustained in 87% of patients treated with REQUIP and in 57% of patients on placebo. On average the L-dopa dose was reduced by 31% in patients treated with REQUIP.

REQUIP for Parkinson's disease patients should be discontinued gradually over a 7-day period. The frequency of administration should be reduced from 3 times daily to twice daily for 4 days. For the remaining 3 days, the frequency should be reduced to once daily prior to complete withdrawal of REQUIP.

Dosing for Restless Legs Syndrome

In all clinical trials, the dose for REQUIP was initiated at 0.25 mg once daily, 1 to 3 hours before bedtime. Patients were titrated based on clinical response and tolerability.

The recommended adult starting dosage for RLS is 0.25 mg once daily, 1 to 3 hours before bedtime. After 2 days, the dosage can be increased to 0.5 mg once daily and to 1 mg once daily at the end of the first week of dosing, then as shown in Table 6 as needed to achieve efficacy. For RLS, the safety and effectiveness of doses greater than 4 mg once daily have not been established.

Table 6. Dose Titration Schedule for RLS

Day/Week	Dosage to be taken once daily, 1 to 3 hours before bedtime
Days 1 and 2	0.25 mg
Days 3-7	0.5 mg
Week 2	1 mg
Week 3	1.5 mg
Week 4	2 mg
Week 5	2.5 mg
Week 6	3 mg
Week 7	4 mg

In clinical trials of patients being treated for RLS with doses up to 4 mg once daily, REQUIP was discontinued without a taper.

HOW SUPPLIED

Tablets

Each pentagonal film-coated TILTAB® tablet with beveled edges contains ropinirole hydrochloride equivalent to the labeled amount of ropinirole as follows:

0.25 mg: white tablets imprinted with "SB" and "4890" in bottles of 100 (NDC 0007-4890-20).

0.5 mg: yellow tablets imprinted with "SB" and "4891" in bottles of 100 (NDC 0007-4891-20).

1 mg: green tablets imprinted with "SB" and "4892" in bottles of 100 (NDC 0007-4892-20).

2 mg: pale yellowish-pink tablets imprinted with "SB" and "4893" in bottles of 100 (NDC 0007-4893-20).

3 mg: pale to moderate reddish-purple tablets, imprinted with "SB" and"4895" in bottles of 100 (NDC 0007-4895-20).

4 mg: pale brown tablets imprinted with "SB" and "4896" in bottles of 100 (NDC 0007-4896-20).

5 mg: blue tablets imprinted with "SB" and "4894" in bottles of 100 (NDC 0007-4894-20).

STORAGE: Protect from light and moisture. Close container tightly after each use.

Store at controlled room temperature 20°-25°C (68°-77°F) [see USP].

GlaxoSmithKline
Research Triangle Park, NC 27709

REQUIP and TILTAB are registered trademarks of GlaxoSmithKline.

SINEMET is a registered trademark of Merck & Co., Inc.

May 2009
REP:3PI

PHARMACIST DETACH HERE AND GIVE INSTRUCTIONS TO PATIENT

PATIENT INFORMATION

REQUIP® (ropinirole tablets)

If you have Restless Legs Syndrome (RLS, also known as Ekbom Syndrome), read this side

Read this information completely before you start taking REQUIP. Read the information each time you get more medicine. There may be new information. This leaflet provides a summary about REQUIP. It does not include everything there is to know about your medicine. This information should not take the place of discussions with your doctor about your medical condition or REQUIP.

What is REQUIP?

REQUIP is a prescription medicine to treat moderate-to-severe primary Restless Legs Syndrome. It is sometimes used to treat Parkinson's disease. Having one of these conditions does not mean you have or will develop the other.

What is the most important information I should know about REQUIP?

- Patients with RLS should take REQUIP differently than patients with Parkinson's disease (see **How should I take REQUIP for RLS?** for the recommended dosing for RLS). A lower dose of REQUIP is generally needed for patients with RLS, and is taken once daily before bedtime.
- There are known side effects of REQUIP. If you fall asleep or feel very sleepy while doing normal activities such as driving, faint, feel dizzy, nauseated, or sweaty when you stand up from sitting or lying down, you should talk with your doctor (see **What are the possible side effects of REQUIP?**).
- Before starting REQUIP, be sure to tell your doctor if you are taking any medicines that make you drowsy.

Unusual urges: Some patients taking REQUIP or REQUIP XL get urges to behave in a way unusual for them. Examples of this are an unusual urge to gamble or increased sexual urges and behaviors. If you notice or your family notices that you are developing any unusual behaviors, talk to your healthcare provider.

Who should not take REQUIP?

You should not take REQUIP if you are allergic to the active ingredient ropinirole or to any of the inactive ingredients. Your doctor and pharmacist have a list of the inactive ingredients.

What should I tell my doctor?

Be sure to tell your doctor if:

- you are pregnant or plan to become pregnant.
- you are breastfeeding.
- you have daytime sleepiness from a sleep disorder other than RLS or have unexpected sleepiness or periods of sleep while taking REQUIP.
- you are taking any other prescription or over-the-counter medicines. Some of these medicines may increase your chances of getting side effects while taking REQUIP.
- you start or stop taking other medicines while you are taking REQUIP. This may increase your chances of getting side effects.
- you start or stop smoking while you are taking REQUIP. Smoking may decrease the treatment effect of REQUIP.
- you feel dizzy, nauseated, sweaty, or faint when you stand up from sitting or lying down.
- you drink alcoholic beverages. This may increase your chances of becoming drowsy or sleepy while taking REQUIP.

How should I take REQUIP for RLS?

- Be sure to take REQUIP exactly as directed by your doctor or healthcare provider.
- The usual way to take REQUIP is once in the evening, 1 to 3 hours before bedtime.
- Your doctor will start you on a low dose of REQUIP. Your doctor may change the dose until you are taking the amount of medicine that is right for you to control your symptoms.
- **If you miss your dose, do not double your next dose.** Take only your usual dose 1 to 3 hours before your next bedtime.
- Contact your doctor, if you stop taking REQUIP for any reason. Do not restart without consulting your doctor.
- You can take REQUIP with or without food. Taking REQUIP with food may decrease the chances of feeling nauseated.

What are the possible side effects of REQUIP?

- Most people who take REQUIP tolerate it well. The most commonly reported side effects in people taking REQUIP for RLS are nausea, vomiting, dizziness, and drowsiness or sleepiness. You should be careful until you know if REQUIP affects your ability to remain alert while doing normal daily activities, and you should watch for the development of significant daytime sleepiness or episodes of falling asleep. It is possible that you could fall asleep while doing normal activities such as driving a car, doing physical tasks, or using hazardous machinery while taking REQUIP. Your chances of falling asleep while doing normal activities while taking REQUIP are greater if you are taking other medicines that cause drowsiness.
- When you start taking REQUIP or when you increase your dose, you may feel dizzy, nauseated, sweaty or faint, when first standing up from sitting or lying down. Therefore, do not stand up quickly after sitting or lying down, particularly if you have been sitting or lying down for a long period of time. Take a minute sitting on the edge of the bed or chair before you get up.
- Hallucinations (unreal sounds, visions, or sensations) have been reported in patients taking REQUIP. These were uncommon in patients taking REQUIP for RLS. The risk is greater in patients with Parkinson's disease who are elderly, taking REQUIP with L-dopa, or taking higher doses of REQUIP than recommended for RLS.

Some patients taking REQUIP get urges to behave in a way unusual for them. Examples of this are an unusual urge to gamble or increased sexual urges and behaviors. If you notice or your family notices that you are developing any unusual behaviors, talk to your healthcare provider.

This is not a complete list of side effects and should not take the place of discussions with your healthcare providers. Your doctor or pharmacist can give you a more complete list of possible side effects.

Call your healthcare provider for medical advice about side effects. You may report side effects to FDA at 1-800-FDA-1088.

Other Information about REQUIP

- Studies of people with Parkinson's disease show that they may be at an increased risk of developing melanoma, a form of skin cancer, when compared to people without Parkinson's disease. It is not known if this problem is associated with Parkinson's disease or the medicines used to treat Parkinson's disease. REQUIP is one of the medicines used to treat Parkinson's disease, therefore, patients being treated with REQUIP should have periodic skin examinations.
- Take REQUIP exactly as your doctor prescribes it.
- Do not share REQUIP with other people, even if they have the same symptoms you have.
- Keep REQUIP out of the reach of children.

- Store REQUIP at room temperature out of direct sunlight.
- Keep REQUIP in a tightly closed container.

This leaflet summarizes important information about REQUIP. Medicines are sometimes prescribed for purposes other than those listed in this leaflet. Do not take REQUIP for a condition for which it was not prescribed. For more information, talk with your doctor or pharmacist. They can give you information about REQUIP that is written for healthcare professionals.

PATIENT INFORMATION

REQUIP® (ropinirole tablets)

If you have Parkinson's disease, read this side

Read this information completely before you start taking REQUIP. Read the information each time you get more medicine. There may be new information. This leaflet provides a summary about REQUIP. It does not include everything there is to know about your medicine. This information should not take the place of discussions with your doctor about your medical condition or REQUIP.

What is REQUIP?

REQUIP is a prescription medicine used to treat Parkinson's disease. It is also used to treat moderate-to-severe primary Restless Legs Syndrome. Having one of these conditions does not mean you have or will develop the other.

What is the most important information I should know about REQUIP?

- Patients with Parkinson's disease should take REQUIP differently than patients with Restless Legs Syndrome (see **How should I take REQUIP for Parkinson's disease?**). For Parkinson's disease, a higher dose of REQUIP is generally needed, and is taken more frequently throughout the day.
- There are known side effects of REQUIP (see **What are the possible side effects of REQUIP?**).
- If you fall asleep or feel very sleepy while doing normal activities such as driving, faint, feel dizzy, nauseated, or sweaty when you stand up from sitting or lying down, you should talk with your doctor.
- Hallucinations (unreal visions, sounds, or sensations) have been reported in patients taking REQUIP. The risk is greater in patients with Parkinson's disease who are elderly, taking REQUIP with L-dopa or taking higher doses of REQUIP. If these occur, you should discuss them with your doctor.
- REQUIP may make some of the side effects of L-dopa worse. REQUIP may cause uncontrolled sudden movements or make such movements you already have worse or more frequent. You should notify your doctor in such a case as dosage adjustments to your anti-Parkinson's medications may be necessary.
- Before starting REQUIP, be sure to tell your doctor if you are taking any medicines that make you drowsy.

Unusual urges: Some patients taking REQUIP or REQUIP XL get urges to behave in a way unusual for them. Examples of this are an unusual urge to gamble or increased sexual urges and behaviors. If you notice or your family notices that you are developing any unusual behaviors, talk to your healthcare provider.

Who should not take REQUIP?

You should not take REQUIP if you are allergic to the active ingredient ropinirole or to any of the inactive ingredients. Your doctor and pharmacist have a list of the inactive ingredients.

What should I tell my doctor?

Be sure to tell your doctor if:

- you are pregnant or plan to become pregnant.
- you are breastfeeding.
- you have daytime sleepiness from a sleep disorder or have unexpected sleepiness or periods of sleep while taking REQUIP.
- you are taking any other prescription or over-the-counter medicines. Some of these medicines may increase your chances of getting side effects while taking REQUIP.
- you start or stop taking other medicines while you are taking REQUIP. This may increase your chances of getting side effects.
- you start or stop smoking while you are taking REQUIP. Smoking may decrease the treatment effect of REQUIP.
- you feel dizzy, nauseated, sweaty, or faint when you first stand up from sitting or lying down.
- you drink alcoholic beverages. This may increase your chances of becoming drowsy or sleepy while taking REQUIP.

How should I take REQUIP for Parkinson's disease?

- Be sure to take your REQUIP exactly as directed by your doctor or healthcare provider.
- Three times a day is the usual way to take REQUIP for Parkinson's disease.
- Your doctor will start you on a low dose of REQUIP. Your doctor will change the dose until you are taking the right amount of medicine to control your symptoms. It may take several weeks before you reach a dose that controls your symptoms.
- **If you miss a dose, do not double your next dose.**
- Contact your doctor, if you stop taking REQUIP for any reason. Do not restart without consulting your doctor.
- Your doctor may prescribe REQUIP alone or add REQUIP to medicine that you are already taking for Parkinson's disease.
- You can take REQUIP with or without food. Taking REQUIP with food may decrease the chances of feeling nauseated.

What are the possible side effects of REQUIP?

- Most people who take REQUIP tolerate it well. The most commonly reported side effects in people taking REQUIP are nausea, headache, dizziness, drowsiness or sleepiness.
- You should be careful until you know if REQUIP affects your ability to remain alert while doing normal daily activities, and you should watch for the development of significant daytime sleepiness or episodes of falling asleep. It is possible that you could fall asleep while doing normal activities such as driving a car, doing physical tasks, or using hazardous machinery while taking REQUIP. Your chances of falling asleep while doing normal activities while taking REQUIP are greater if you are taking other medicines that cause drowsiness.
- When you start taking REQUIP or when you increase your dose, you may feel dizzy, nauseated, sweaty or faint, when first standing up from sitting or lying down. Therefore, do not stand up quickly after sitting or lying down, particularly if you have been sitting or lying down for a long period of time. Take a minute sitting on the edge of the bed or chair before you get up.
- Hallucinations (unreal visions, sounds, or sensations) have been reported in patients taking REQUIP. The risk is greater in patients with Parkinson's disease who are elderly, taking REQUIP with L-dopa, or taking higher amounts of REQUIP.
- If you are taking L-dopa for Parkinson's disease, REQUIP may make some of the side effects of L-dopa worse. REQUIP may cause uncontrolled sudden movements or make such movements you already have worse or more frequent.

Some patients taking REQUIP get urges to behave in a way unusual for them. Examples of this are an unusual urge to gamble or increased sexual urges and behaviors. If you notice or your family notices that you are developing any unusual behaviors, talk to your healthcare provider.

This is not a complete list of side effects and should not take the place of discussions with your healthcare providers. Your doctor or pharmacist can give you a more complete list of possible side effects.

Call your healthcare provider for medical advice about side effects. You may report side effects to FDA at 1-800-FDA-1088.

Other Information about REQUIP

- Studies of people with Parkinson's disease show that they may be at an increased risk of developing melanoma, a form of skin cancer, when compared to people without Parkinson's disease. It is not known if this problem is associated with Parkinson's disease or the medicines used to treat Parkinson's disease, therefore, patients being treated with REQUIP should have periodic skin examinations.
- Take REQUIP exactly as your doctor prescribes it.
- Do not share REQUIP with other people, even if they have the same symptoms you have.
- Keep REQUIP out of the reach of children.
- Store REQUIP at room temperature out of direct sunlight.
- Keep REQUIP in a tightly closed container.

This leaflet summarizes important information about REQUIP. Medicines are sometimes prescribed for purposes other than those listed in this leaflet. Do not take REQUIP for a condition for which it was not prescribed. For more information, talk with your doctor or pharmacist. They can give you information about REQUIP that is written for healthcare professionals.

GlaxoSmithKline
Research Triangle Park, NC 27709

April 2009
REP:2PIL

REQUIP XL ℞

[rē' kwip]

(ropinirole extended-release tablets)

HIGHLIGHTS OF PRESCRIBING INFORMATION

These highlights do not include all the information needed to use REQUIP XL safely and effectively. See full prescribing information for REQUIP XL.

REQUIP XL (ropinirole extended-release tablets)

Initial U.S. Approval: 1997

INDICATIONS AND USAGE

REQUIP XL is an orally administered, non-ergoline dopamine agonist indicated for the treatment of signs and symptoms of idiopathic Parkinson's disease. (1.1)

DOSAGE AND ADMINISTRATION

- REQUIP XL tablets are taken once daily, with or without food. Tablets must be swallowed whole and must not be chewed, crushed, or divided. (2.1)
- The starting dose is 2 mg taken once daily for 1 to 2 weeks, followed by increases of 2 mg/day at 1 week or longer intervals as appropriate, depending on therapeutic response and tolerability, up to a maximally recommended dose of 24 mg/day. Patients should be assessed for therapeutic response and tolerability at a minimal interval of 1 week or longer after each dose increment. Caution should be exercised during dose titration because too rapid a rate of titration can lead to dose selection that does not provide additional benefit, but that increases the risk of adverse reactions. (2.2, 14.2)
- Patients may be switched directly from immediate-release ropinirole to REQUIP XL. The initial switching dose of REQUIP XL should most closely match the total daily dose of immediate-release ropinirole, see Table 1. (2.3)
- If REQUIP XL must be discontinued, it should be tapered gradually over a 7-day period. (2.2)

DOSAGE FORMS AND STRENGTHS

Tablets: 2 mg, 4 mg, 6 mg, 8 mg, and 12 mg (3)

CONTRAINDICATIONS

None (4)

WARNINGS AND PRECAUTIONS

- Falling asleep during activities of daily living may occur, including the operation of motor vehicles, which sometimes resulted in accidents. Sudden onset of sleep may occur without apparent warning or daytime drowsiness. Sedating medications (such as alcohol or CNS depressants), the presence of sleeping disorders, or other medications that increase plasma levels of ropinirole, may increase the risk of somnolence or falling asleep while engaged in activities of daily living. Before initiating treatment, patients should be advised of the potential of sudden onset of sleep or to develop drowsiness and asked about risk factors they may have. If a patient develops sudden onset of sleep during activities that require active participation (e.g., conversations, eating, etc.) and/or cannot avoid high-risk activities in the future, REQUIP XL should ordinarily be discontinued. (5.1)
- Syncope, sometimes associated with bradycardia, may occur. (5.2)
- Symptomatic hypotension (including postural/orthostatic hypotension) may occur, especially during dose escalation. (5.3)
- Elevation of blood pressure and changes in heart rate may occur. (5.4)
- Hallucination may occur. (5.5)
- Dyskinesia may be caused or exacerbated. Decreasing the L-dopa dose may lessen or eliminate this side effect. (5.6)

ADVERSE REACTIONS

- Most common adverse reactions (incidence ≥5% and greater than placebo) in advanced Parkinson's disease with concomitant L-dopa were dyskinesia, nausea, dizziness, hallucination, somnolence, abdominal pain/discomfort, and orthostatic hypotension. (6.1)
- Most common adverse reactions (incidence ≥5%) in early Parkinson's disease without L-dopa were nausea, somnolence, abdominal pain/discomfort, dizziness, headache, and constipation. (6.1)

To report SUSPECTED ADVERSE REACTIONS, contact GlaxoSmithKline at 1-888-825-5249 or FDA at 1-800-FDA-1088 or www.fda.gov/medwatch.

DRUG INTERACTIONS

- CYP1A2 is the major enzyme responsible for the metabolism of ropinirole. Thus inhibitors (e.g., ciprofloxacin, fluvoxamine) or inducers (e.g., omeprazole or smoking) of CYP1A2 may alter the clearance of ropinirole. Adjustment of dosage of REQUIP XL may be required. (7.1)
- Higher doses of estrogens, usually associated with hormone replacement therapy (HRT), reduced oral clearance of ropinirole. Starting or stopping HRT treatment may require adjustment of dosage of REQUIP XL. (7.3)
- Dopamine antagonists, such as neuroleptics (e.g., phenothiazines, butyrophenones, thioxanthenes) or metoclopramide, may diminish effectiveness of ropinirole. (7.4)

USE IN SPECIFIC POPULATIONS

Pregnancy: REQUIP XL should be used during pregnancy only if the potential benefit outweighs the potential risk to the fetus. (8.1)

See 17 for PATIENT COUNSELING INFORMATION and FDA-approved patient labeling

Revised: 12/2012

FULL PRESCRIBING INFORMATION: CONTENTS*

*** Sections or subsections omitted from the full prescribing information are not listed**

FULL PRESCRIBING INFORMATION

1 INDICATIONS AND USAGE

1.1 Parkinson's Disease

REQUIP XL® (ropinirole extended-release tablets) is indicated for the treatment of the signs and symptoms of idiopathic Parkinson's disease.

2 DOSAGE AND ADMINISTRATION

2.1 General Dosing Considerations

- REQUIP XL extended-release tablets are taken once daily, with or without food. Taking REQUIP XL with food may reduce the occurrence of nausea; this has not been established in controlled clinical trials *[see Clinical Pharmacology (12.3)]*.
- Tablets must be swallowed whole and must not be chewed, crushed, or divided.
- If a significant interruption in therapy with REQUIP XL has occurred, retitration of therapy may be warranted.

2.2 Dosing for Parkinson's Disease

The starting dose is 2 mg taken once daily for 1 to 2 weeks, followed by increases of 2 mg/day at 1-week or longer intervals as appropriate, depending on therapeutic response and tolerability, up to a maximally recommended dose of 24 mg/day.

In clinical trials, dosage was initiated at 2 mg/day and gradually titrated based on individual therapeutic response and tolerability. Doses greater than 24 mg/day have not been studied in clinical trials. Patients should be assessed for therapeutic response and tolerability at a minimal interval of 1 week or longer after each dose increment. Caution should be exercised during dose titration because too rapid a rate of titration may lead to dose selection that may not provide additional benefit, but that may increase the risk of adverse reactions *[see Clinical Studies (14.2)]*. Due to the flexible dosing design used in clinical studies, specific dose response information could not be determined.

When REQUIP XL is administered as adjunct therapy to L-dopa, the concurrent dose of L-dopa may be decreased gradually as tolerated. In the placebo-controlled advanced Parkinson's disease study, the L-dopa dose was reduced once patients reached a dose of REQUIP XL of 8 mg/day. Overall, L-dopa dose reduction was sustained in 93% of patients treated with REQUIP XL and in 72% of patients on placebo. On average the L-dopa dose was reduced by 34% in patients treated with REQUIP XL *[see Clinical Studies (14)]*.

REQUIP XL should be discontinued gradually over a 7-day period.

2.3 Switching From Immediate-Release Ropinirole Tablets to REQUIP XL

Patients may be switched directly from immediate-release ropinirole to REQUIP XL tablets. The initial dose of REQUIP XL should most closely match the total daily dose of the immediate-release formulation of REQUIP, as shown in Table 1.

Table 1. Conversion from Immediate-Release REQUIP to REQUIP XL

Immediate-Release Ropinirole Tablets Total Daily Dose (mg)	REQUIP XL Tablets Total Daily Dose (mg)
0.75 to 2.25	2
3 to 4.5	4
6	6
7.5 to 9	8
12	12
15 to 18	16
21	20
24	24

Following conversion to REQUIP XL, the dose may be adjusted depending on therapeutic response and tolerability *[see Dosage and Administration (2.2)]*.

3 DOSAGE FORMS AND STRENGTHS

- 2 mg, pink, biconvex, capsule-shaped, film-coated, tablets debossed with "GS" and "3V2"
- 4 mg, light brown, biconvex, capsule-shaped, film-coated, tablets debossed with "GS" and "WXG"
- 6 mg, white, biconvex, capsule-shaped, film-coated, tablets debossed with "GS" and "11F"
- 8 mg, red, biconvex, capsule-shaped, film-coated, tablets debossed with "GS" and "5CC"
- 12 mg, green, biconvex, capsule-shaped, film-coated, tablets debossed with "GS" and "YX7"

4 CONTRAINDICATIONS

None.

5 WARNINGS AND PRECAUTIONS

5.1 Falling Asleep During Activities of Daily Living

Patients treated with ropinirole have reported falling asleep while engaged in activities of daily living, including the operation of motor vehicles, which sometimes resulted in accidents. Although many of these patients reported somnolence while on ropinirole, some perceived that they had no warning signs such as excessive drowsiness, and believed that they were alert immediately prior to the event. Some of these events have been reported more than 1 year after initiation of treatment.

Among the 613 patients who received REQUIP XL in clinical trials, there were 5 cases of sudden onset of sleep and 2 cases of motor vehicle accident in which it is not known if falling asleep was a contributing factor.

During the 6-month trial in advanced Parkinson's disease, somnolence was reported in 7% (14 of 202) of patients receiving REQUIP XL compared with 4% (7 of 191) of patients receiving placebo. During the 36-week trial in early Parkinson's disease, somnolence was reported in 11% (16 of 140) of patients receiving REQUIP XL compared with 15% (22 of 149) of patients receiving the immediate-release formulation of REQUIP *[see Adverse Reactions (6)]*. However, because dose-response was not systematically studied with REQUIP XL, the occurrence of somnolence at the highest recommended doses may be higher than these reported frequencies *[see Adverse Reactions (6)]*.

Many clinical experts believe that falling asleep while engaged in activities of daily living always occurs in a setting of preexisting somnolence, although patients may not give such a history. For this reason, prescribers should continually reassess patients for drowsiness or sleepiness, especially since some of the events occur well after the start of treatment. Prescribers should also be aware that patients may not acknowledge drowsiness or sleepiness until directly questioned about drowsiness or sleepiness during specific activities.

Before initiating treatment with REQUIP XL, patients should be advised of the potential to develop drowsiness and specifically asked about factors that may increase the risk with REQUIP XL such as concomitant sedating medications, the presence of sleep disorders, and concomitant medications that increase ropinirole plasma levels (e.g., ciprofloxacin) *[see Drug Interactions (7.1)]*. If a patient develops significant daytime sleepiness or episodes of falling asleep during activities that require active participation (e.g., driving a motor vehicle, conversations, eating, etc.), REQUIP XL should ordinarily be discontinued *[see Dosage and Administration for guidance in discontinuing REQUIP XL (2.2)]*. If a decision is made to continue REQUIP XL, patients should be advised to not drive and to avoid other potentially dangerous activities. There is insufficient information to establish that dose reduction will eliminate episodes of falling asleep while engaged in activities of daily living.

5.2 Syncope

Syncope, sometimes associated with bradycardia, was observed during treatment with ropinirole in Parkinson's disease patients.

In a placebo-controlled study involving patients with advanced Parkinson's disease, syncope occurred in 2 of the 202 patients (1%) who received REQUIP XL, and in none of the 191 patients who received placebo.

Because the study of REQUIP XL excluded patients with significant cardiovascular disease, it is not known to what extent the estimated incidence figure applies to patients with Parkinson's disease in clinical practice. Therefore, patients with significant cardiovascular disease should be treated with caution.

5.3 Hypotension

Dopamine agonists, in clinical studies and clinical experience, appear to impair the systemic regulation of blood pressure, with resulting postural hypotension, especially during dose escalation. In addition, patients with Parkinson's disease appear to have an impaired capacity to respond to a postural challenge. For these reasons, patients being treated with dopaminergic agonists ordinarily (1) require careful monitoring for signs and symptoms of postural hypotension, especially during dose escalation, and (2) should be informed of this risk *[see Patient Counseling Information (17.2)]*.

In a placebo-controlled trial involving patients with advanced Parkinson's disease, hypotension was reported as an adverse event in 5 of 202 patients (2%) receiving REQUIP XL and in none of the 191 patients receiving placebo. Orthostatic hypotension was reported as an adverse event in 5% of patients receiving REQUIP XL, and in 1% of placebo recipients.

An analysis of the randomized, double-blinded, placebo-controlled study in advanced Parkinson's disease was conducted using a variety of adverse event terms possibly suggestive of hypotension, including hypotension, orthostatic hypotension, dizziness, vertigo, and blood pressure decreased. This analysis showed a higher incidence of these events with REQUIP XL (7%, 15 of 202) vs. placebo (3%, 6 of 191). This increased incidence was observed in a setting in which patients were very carefully titrated, and patients with clinically relevant cardiovascular disease or symptomatic orthostatic hypotension at baseline had been excluded from this study.

Orthostatic vital signs (semi-supine to standing) were monitored throughout the study in the advanced Parkinson's disease study and changes related to REQUIP XL (compared with placebo) from baseline were assessed.

The frequency of any orthostatic hypotension at any time during the study was 38% for REQUIP XL vs. 31% for placebo for mild to moderate systolic blood pressure decrements (≥20 mm Hg), 63% for REQUIP XL vs. 58% for placebo for mild to moderate diastolic blood pressure decrements (≥10 mm Hg), 10% for REQUIP XL vs. 7% for placebo for severe diastolic blood pressure decrements (≥20 mm Hg), and 23% for REQUIP XL vs. 19% for placebo for mild to moderate combined systolic and diastolic blood pressure decrements.

Significant decrements in blood pressure unrelated to standing were also reported in some patients taking REQUIP XL. In the semi-supine position, the frequency was 10% for REQUIP XL vs. 8% for placebo for severe systolic blood pressure decrease (≥40 mm Hg), and was 25% for REQUIP XL vs. 21% for placebo for severe diastolic blood pressure decrease (≥20 mm Hg).

The increased incidence for hypotension and/or orthostatic hypotension was observed in both the titration and maintenance phases and in some cases persisted into the maintenance period after developing in the titration phase.

5.4 Elevation of Blood Pressure and Changes in Heart Rate

In the placebo-controlled study in advanced Parkinson's disease, there were no clear effects of REQUIP XL on average changes in blood pressure or heart rate compared with placebo. However, there was an increased incidence of patients treated with REQUIP XL who met various outlier criteria, as described below.

In the semi-supine position, the frequency was 8% for REQUIP XL vs. 5% for placebo for severe systolic blood pressure increase (≥40 mm Hg). In the standing position, the frequency was 9% for REQUIP XL vs. 6% for placebo for severe systolic blood pressure increase (≥40 mm Hg).

In the semi-supine position, the frequency was 23% for REQUIP XL vs. 18% for placebo for moderate pulse increase (≥15 beats/minute), and 19% for REQUIP XL vs. 17% for placebo for moderate pulse decrease (≥15 beats/minute). In the standing position, the frequency was 2% for REQUIP XL vs. <1% for placebo for severe pulse increase (≥30 beats/minute), and 24% for REQUIP XL vs. 19% for placebo for moderate pulse decrease (≥15 beats/minute).

The increased incidence for various elevations of systolic and/or diastolic blood pressure and/or changes in pulse was observed in both the titration and maintenance phases as well as persisting into the maintenance period after developing in the titration phase.

Elevation of blood pressure and/or changes in heart rate in patients taking REQUIP XL should be considered when treating patients with cardiovascular disease.

5.5 Hallucination

In the double-blind, placebo-controlled, advanced Parkinson's disease trial 8% (17 of 202) of patients receiving REQUIP XL reported hallucination compared with 2% (4 of 191) patients receiving placebo. Hallucination led to discontinuation of treatment in 2% (4 of 202) of patients on REQUIP XL and 1% (2 of 191) of patients on placebo.

The incidence of hallucination is increased in patients over age 65. Coadministration of entacapone and L-dopa with ropinirole may also increase the risk of hallucination. In a placebo-controlled clinical trial, hallucination occurred in 0 of 43 patients taking entacapone plus L-dopa, in 9 of 155 patients taking REQUIP XL plus L-dopa (6%), and in 7 of 47 patients taking entacapone with REQUIP XL plus L-dopa (15%).

5.6 Dyskinesia

REQUIP XL may potentiate the dopaminergic side effects of L-dopa and may cause and/or exacerbate preexisting dyskinesia in patients treated with L-dopa for Parkinson's disease. Decreasing the dose of a dopaminergic drug may ameliorate this side effect.

5.7 Major Psychotic Disorders

Patients with a major psychotic disorder should ordinarily not be treated with REQUIP XL because of the risk of exacerbating the psychosis. In addition, many treatments for psychosis may decrease the effectiveness of REQUIP XL *[see Drug Interactions (7.4)]*.

5.8 Events Reported With Dopaminergic Therapy

Withdrawal-Emergent Hyperpyrexia and Confusion: Although not reported during the clinical development of ropinirole, a symptom complex resembling the neuroleptic malignant syndrome (characterized by elevated temperature, muscular rigidity, altered consciousness, and autonomic instability), with no other obvious etiology, has been reported in association with rapid dose reduction, withdrawal of, or changes in dopaminergic therapy. Therefore, it is recommended that the dose be tapered at the end of treatment with REQUIP XL as a prophylactic measure *[see Dosage and Administration (2.2)]*.

Fibrotic Complications: Cases of retroperitoneal fibrosis, pulmonary infiltrates, pleural effusion, pleural thickening, pericarditis, and cardiac valvulopathy have been reported in some patients treated with ergot-derived dopaminergic agents. While these complications may resolve when the drug is discontinued, complete resolution does not always occur.

Although these adverse reactions are believed to be related to the ergoline structure of these compounds, whether other, nonergot-derived dopamine agonists, such as REQUIP or REQUIP XL, can cause them is unknown.

A small number of reports have been received of possible fibrotic complications, including pleural effusion, pleural fibrosis, interstitial lung disease, and cardiac valvulopathy, in the development program and postmarketing experience for ropinirole. In the clinical development program (N = 613), 2 patients treated with REQUIP XL had pleural effusion. While the evidence is not sufficient to establish a causal relationship between ropinirole and these fibrotic complications, a contribution of ropinirole cannot be completely ruled out in rare cases.

Melanoma: Some epidemiologic studies have shown that patients with Parkinson's disease have a higher risk (perhaps 2- to 4-fold higher) of developing melanoma than the general population. Whether the observed increased risk was due to Parkinson's disease or other factors, such as drugs used to treat Parkinson's disease, was unclear. Ropinirole is one of the dopamine agonists used to treat Parkinson's disease. Although ropinirole has not been associated with an increased risk of melanoma specifically, its potential role as a risk factor has not been systematically studied. In the clinical development program (N = 613), one patient treated with REQUIP XL and also levodopa/carbidopa developed melanoma. Patients using REQUIP XL should be made aware of these results and undergo periodic dermatologic screening.

5.9 Retinal Pathology

Human: Because of observations made in albino rats (see below), ocular electroretinogram (ERG) assessments were conducted during a 2-year, double-blind, multicenter, flexible-dose, l-dopa controlled clinical study of immediate-release ropinirole in patients with Parkinson's disease. A total of 156 patients (78 on immediate-release ropinirole, mean dose 11.9 mg/day and 78 on l-dopa, mean dose 555.2 mg/day) were evaluated for evidence of retinal dysfunction through electroretinograms. There was no clinically meaningful difference between the treatment groups in retinal function over the duration of the study.

Albino Rats: Retinal degeneration was observed in albino rats in the 2-year carcinogenicity study at all doses tested (equivalent to 0.6 to 20 times the maximum recommended human dose (MRHD) of 24 mg/day on a mg/m^2 basis), but was statistically significant at the highest dose (50 mg/kg/day). Retinal degeneration was not observed in pigmented rats after 3 months in a 2-year carcinogenicity study in albino mice, or in 1-year studies in monkeys or albino rats. The potential significance of this effect for humans has not been established, but cannot be disregarded because disruption of a mechanism that is universally present in vertebrates (e.g., disk shedding) may be involved.

5.10 Binding to Melanin

Ropinirole binds to melanin-containing tissues (i.e., eyes, skin) in pigmented rats. After a single dose, long-term retention of drug was demonstrated, with a half-life in the eye of 20 days.

6 ADVERSE REACTIONS

The following adverse reactions are described in more detail in the *Warnings and Precautions* section of the label:

- Falling asleep during activities of daily living (5.1)
- Syncope (5.2)
- Symptomatic hypotension, hypotension, postural/orthostatic hypotension (5.3)
- Elevation of blood pressure and changes in heart rate (5.4)
- Hallucination (5.5)
- Dyskinesia (5.6)
- Major psychotic disorders (5.7)
- Events with dopaminergic therapy (5.8)
- Retinal pathology (5.9)

6.1 Clinical Trial Experience

Because clinical trials are conducted under widely varying conditions, adverse reaction rates observed in the clinical trials of a drug cannot be directly compared with rates in the clinical trials of another drug (or of another development program of a different formulation of the same drug) and may not reflect the rates observed in practice.

During the premarketing development of REQUIP XL, patients with advanced Parkinson's disease received REQUIP XL or placebo as adjunctive therapy in 1 clinical trial. In a second trial, patients with early Parkinson's disease were treated with REQUIP XL or the immediate-release formulation of REQUIP without L-dopa.

Advanced Parkinson's Disease (With L-dopa): The most commonly observed adverse reactions (≥5% and numerically greater than placebo) in the 24-week, double-blind, placebo-controlled trial for the treatment of advanced Parkinson's disease during treatment with REQUIP XL were, in order of decreasing incidence: dyskinesia, nausea, dizziness, hallucination, somnolence, abdominal pain/discomfort, and orthostatic hypotension.

Approximately 6% of 202 patients treated with REQUIP XL discontinued treatment due to adverse event(s) compared with 5% of 191 patients who received placebo. The adverse event most commonly causing discontinuation of treatment with REQUIP XL was hallucination (2%).

Table 2 lists adverse reactions that occurred with a frequency of at least 2% (and were numerically greater than placebo) in patients with advanced Parkinson's disease treated with REQUIP XL who participated in the 26-week, double-blind, placebo-controlled study. In this study, either REQUIP XL or placebo was used as an adjunct to L -dopa. Adverse reactions were generally mild or moderate in intensity.

Table 2. Treatment-Emergent Adverse Reaction Incidence in a Double-Blind, Placebo-Controlled Trial in Advanced Stage Parkinson's Disease (With L-dopa) (Events ≥2% of Patients Treated with REQUIP XL and >% with Placebo)

Body System/Adverse Reaction	REQUIP XL (n = 202) %	Placebo (n = 191) %
Ear and labyrinth disorders		
Vertigo	4	2
Gastrointestinal disorders		
Nausea	11	4
Constipation	4	2
Abdominal pain/discomfort	6	3
Diarrhea	3	2
Dry mouth	2	<1
General disorders		
Edema peripheral	4	1
Injury, poisoning, and procedural complications		
Fall*	2	1
Musculoskeletal and connective tissue disorders		
Back pain	3	2
Nervous system disorders		
Dyskinesia*	13	3
Dizziness	8	3
Somnolence	7	4
Psychiatric disorders		
Hallucination	8	2
Anxiety	2	1
Vascular disorders		
Orthostatic hypotension	5	1
Hypotension	2	0
Hypertension*	3	2

*Dose-related.

Although this study was not designed for optimally characterizing dose-related adverse reactions, there was a suggestion (based upon comparison of incidence of adverse reactions across dose ranges for REQUIP XL and placebo) that the incidence for dyskinesia, hypertension, and fall was dose-related to REQUIP XL.

The incidence for many adverse reactions with REQUIP XL treatment was increased relative to placebo (i.e., REQUIP XL % - Placebo % = treatment difference ≥2%) in either the titration or maintenance phases of the study. During the titration phase, an increased incidence (shown in descending order of % treatment difference) was observed for dyskinesia, nausea, abdominal pain/discomfort, orthostatic hypotension, dizziness, vertigo, hypertension, peripheral edema, and dry mouth. During the maintenance phase, an increased incidence was observed for dyskinesia, nausea, dizziness, hallucination, somnolence, fall, hypertension, abnormal dreams, constipation, chest pain, bronchitis, and nasopharyngitis. Some adverse reactions developing in the titration phase persisted (≥7 days) into the maintenance phase. These "persistent" adverse reactions included dyskinesia, hallucination, orthostatic hypotension, and dry mouth.

The incidence of adverse reactions was not clearly different between women and men.

Early Parkinson's Disease (Without L-dopa): The most commonly observed adverse reactions (≥5%) in the 36-week early Parkinson's disease trial during treatment with REQUIP XL were, in order of decreasing incidence: nausea (19%), somnolence (11%), abdominal pain/discomfort (7%), dizziness (6%), headache (6%), and constipation (5%). The type of adverse reactions and the frequency (i.e. incidence) with which they occurred were generally similar over the whole treatment period in this study of early Parkinson's disease patients who were initially treated with REQUIP XL or the immediate-release formulation of REQUIP and subsequently crossed over to treatment with the other formulation.

During the titration phase, an increased incidence with REQUIP XL compared with the immediate-release formulation of REQUIP (i.e., REQUIP XL % - REQUIP IR % = treatment difference ≥2%), shown in descending order of % treatment difference, was observed for: constipation, hallucination, vertigo, abdominal pain/discomfort, nausea, vomiting, fall, headache, diarrhea, pyrexia, and flatulence. During the maintenance phase, an increased incidence was observed for fall, myalgia, and sleep disorder. Several adverse reactions developing in the titration phase persisted

(≥7 days) into the maintenance phase. These "persistent" adverse reactions included: constipation, hallucination, muscle spasms, flatulence, insomnia, sleep disorder, abdominal pain/discomfort, cough, and nasopharyngitis.

6.2 Adverse Reactions Observed During the Clinical Development of the Immediate-Release Formulation of REQUIP for Parkinson's Disease (Advanced and Early)

Because clinical trials are conducted under widely varying conditions, adverse reaction rates observed in the clinical trials of a drug cannot be directly compared to rates in the clinical trials of another drug (or of another development program of a different formulation of the same drug) and may not reflect the rates observed in practice.

In patients with advanced Parkinson's disease who were treated with the immediate-release formulation of REQUIP, the most common adverse reactions (≥5% treatment difference from placebo; presented in order of decreasing treatment difference frequency) were dyskinesia (21%), somnolence (12%), nausea (12%), dizziness (10%), confusion (7%), hallucinations (6%), headache (5%), and increased sweating (5%). In patients with early Parkinson's disease who were treated with the immediate-release formulation of REQUIP, the most common adverse reactions (≥5% treatment difference from placebo; presented in order of decreasing treatment difference frequency) were nausea (38%), somnolence (34%), dizziness (18%), syncope (11%), viral infection (8%), fatigue (7%), leg edema (6%), asthenia (5%), and dyspepsia (5%).

7 DRUG INTERACTIONS

7.1 P450 Interaction

In vitro metabolism studies showed that CYP1A2 is the major enzyme responsible for the metabolism of ropinirole. There is thus the potential for inducers or inhibitors of this enzyme to alter the clearance of ropinirole. Therefore, if therapy with a drug known to be a potent inducer or inhibitor of CYP1A2 is stopped or started during treatment with ropinirole, adjustment of the dose of ropinirole may be required.

Coadministration of ciprofloxacin, an inhibitor of CYP1A2, with immediate-release ropinirole increased the AUC of ropinirole by 84% on average and C_{max} by 60% *[see Clinical Pharmacology (12.3)]*.

Cigarette smoking is expected to increase the clearance of ropinirole since CYP1A2 is known to be induced by smoking. In one study in patients with Restless Legs Syndrome, cigarette smokers had an approximate 30% lower C_{max} and a 38% lower AUC than did nonsmokers, when those parameters were normalized for dose.

There is no evidence of interaction between ropinirole and other CYP1A2 substrates (e.g., theophylline).

Ropinirole and its circulating metabolites do not inhibit or induce P450 enzymes; therefore, ropinirole is unlikely to affect the pharmacokinetics of other drugs by a P450 mechanism *[see Clinical Pharmacology (12.3)]*.

7.2 L-dopa

Coadministration of carbidopa + L-dopa (SINEMET®) with immediate-release ropinirole had no effect on the steady-state pharmacokinetics of ropinirole. Oral administration of immediate-release ropinirole increased mean steady-state C_{max} of L-dopa by 20%, but its AUC was unaffected *[see Clinical Pharmacology (12.3)]*.

7.3 Estrogens

Population pharmacokinetic analysis revealed that higher doses of estrogens (usually associated with hormone replacement therapy [HRT]) reduced the oral clearance of ropinirole by approximately 35%. Dosage adjustment is not needed for initiating REQUIP XL in patients on estrogen therapy because patients are individually titrated with REQUIP XL to tolerance or adequate effect. If estrogen therapy is stopped or started during treatment with REQUIP XL, then adjustment of the dose of REQUIP XL may be required.

7.4 Dopamine Antagonists

Since ropinirole is a dopamine agonist, it is possible that dopamine antagonists such as neuroleptics (e.g., phenothiazines, butyrophenones, thioxanthenes) or metoclopramide may diminish the effectiveness of REQUIP XL. Patients with a history or presence of major psychotic disorders should be treated with dopamine agonists only if the potential benefits outweigh the risks.

8 USE IN SPECIFIC POPULATIONS

8.1 Pregnancy

Pregnancy Category C. There are no adequate and well-controlled studies using ropinirole in pregnant women. REQUIP XL should be used during pregnancy only if the potential benefit outweighs the potential risk to the fetus.

In animal reproduction studies, ropinirole has been shown to have adverse effects on embryo-fetal development, including teratogenic effects. Treatment of pregnant rats with ropinirole during organogenesis resulted in decreased fetal body weight, increased fetal death, and digital malformations at 24, 36, and 60 times the MRHD, respectively. The combined administration of ropinirole at 8 times the MRHD and a clinically relevant dose of L-dopa to pregnant rabbits during organogenesis produced a greater incidence and severity of fetal malformations (primarily digit defects) than were seen in the offspring of rabbits treated with L-dopa alone. In a perinatal-postnatal study in rats, impaired growth and development of nursing offspring and altered neurological development of female offspring were observed when dams were treated with 4 times the MRHD.

8.3 Nursing Mothers

Ropinirole inhibits prolactin secretion in humans and could potentially inhibit lactation.

Ropinirole has been detected in the milk of lactating rats. Although many drugs are excreted in human milk, transfer of ropinirole into human milk has not been demonstrated. Due to the potential for serious adverse reactions in nursing infants, a decision should be made whether to discontinue nursing or to discontinue the drug, taking into account the importance of ropinirole to the mother.

8.4 Pediatric Use

Safety and effectiveness in the pediatric population have not been established.

8.5 Geriatric Use

Dosage adjustment is not necessary in the elderly (above 65 years), as the dose of REQUIP XL is to be individually titrated to clinical response *[see Clinical Pharmacology (12.3)]*. Pharmacokinetic studies conducted in patients demonstrated that oral clearance of ropinirole is reduced by 15% in patients above 65 years of age compared to younger patients.

Of the total number of patients who participated in clinical trials of REQUIP XL for Parkinson's disease, 387 patients were 65 and over and 107 patients were 75 and over. Among patients receiving REQUIP XL, hallucination was more common in elderly subjects (10%) compared with non-elderly subjects (2%). The incidence of overall adverse events increased with increasing age for both patients receiving REQUIP XL and placebo.

8.6 Renal Impairment

No dosage adjustment of ropinirole is needed in patients with moderate renal impairment (creatinine clearance of 30 to 50 mL/min). The use of ropinirole in patients with severe renal impairment has not been studied.

8.7 Hepatic Impairment

The pharmacokinetics of ropinirole have not been studied in patients with hepatic impairment. Since patients with hepatic impairment may have higher plasma levels and lower clearance, ropinirole should be titrated with caution in these patients.

9 DRUG ABUSE AND DEPENDENCE

9.1 Controlled Substance

Ropinirole is not a controlled substance.

9.3 Dependence

Animal studies and human clinical trials with ropinirole did not reveal any potential for drug-seeking behavior or physical dependence.

10 OVERDOSAGE

10.1 Human Overdose Experience

In the Parkinson's disease program, there have been patients who accidentally or intentionally took more than their prescribed dose of ropinirole. The largest overdose reported with immediate-release ropinirole in clinical trials was 435 mg taken over a 7-day period (62.1 mg/day). Of patients who received a dose greater than 24 mg/day, reported symptoms included adverse events commonly reported during dopaminergic therapy (nausea, dizziness), as well as visual hallucination, hyperhidrosis, claustrophobia, chorea, palpitations, asthenia, and nightmares. Additional symptoms reported for doses of 24 mg or less or for overdoses of unknown amount included vomiting, increased coughing, fatigue, syncope, vasovagal syncope, dyskinesia, agitation, chest pain, orthostatic hypotension, somnolence, and confusional state.

10.2 Overdose Management

The symptoms of overdose with ropinirole are generally related to its dopaminergic activity; these symptoms may be alleviated by appropriate treatment with dopamine antagonists such as neuroleptics or metoclopramide. General supportive measures are recommended. Vital signs should be maintained, if necessary. Removal of any unabsorbed material (e.g., by gastric lavage) may be considered.

11 DESCRIPTION

REQUIP (ropinirole) is an orally administered non-ergoline dopamine agonist. It is supplied as the hydrochloride salt of ropinirole 4-[2-(dipropylamino)ethyl]-1,3-dihydro-2H-indol-2-one and has an empirical formula of $C_{16}H_{24}N_2O \cdot HCl$. The molecular weight is 296.84 (260.38 as the free base).

The structural formula is:

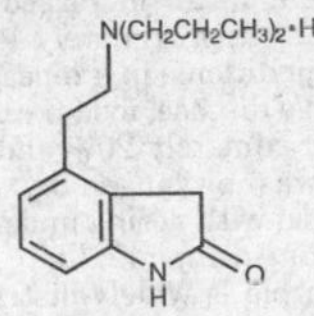

Ropinirole hydrochloride is a white to yellow solid with a melting range of 243° to 250°C and a solubility of 133 mg/mL in water.

REQUIP XL extended-release tablets are formulated as a three-layered tablet with a central, active-containing, slow-release layer, and 2 placebo outer layers acting as barrier layers which control the surface area available for drug release. Each biconvex, capsule-shaped tablet contains 2.28 mg, 4.56 mg, 6.84 mg, 9.12 mg, or 13.68 mg ropinirole hydrochloride equivalent to ropinirole 2 mg, 4 mg, 6 mg, 8 mg, or 12 mg, respectively. Inactive ingredients consist of carboxymethylcellulose sodium, colloidal silicon dioxide, glyceryl behenate, hydrogenated castor oil, hypromellose, lactose monohydrate, magnesium stearate, maltodextrin, mannitol, povidone, and one or more of the following: FD&C Yellow No. 6 aluminum lake, FD&C Blue No. 2 aluminum lake, ferric oxides (black, red, yellow), polyethylene glycol 400, titanium dioxide.

12 CLINICAL PHARMACOLOGY

12.1 Mechanism of Action

Ropinirole is a non-ergoline dopamine agonist with high relative in vitro specificity and full intrinsic activity at the D_2 and D_3 dopamine receptor subtypes, binding with higher affinity to D_3 than to D_2 or D_4 receptor subtypes.

Ropinirole has moderate in vitro affinity for opioid receptors. Ropinirole and its metabolites have negligible in vitro affinity for dopamine D_1, 5-HT_1, 5-HT_2, benzodiazepine, GABA, muscarinic, alpha$_1$-, alpha$_2$-, and beta-adrenoreceptors.

The precise mechanism of action of ropinirole as a treatment for Parkinson's disease is unknown, although it is believed to be due to stimulation of postsynaptic dopamine D_2-type receptors within the caudate-putamen in the brain. This conclusion is supported by studies that show that ropinirole improves motor function in various animal models of Parkinson's disease. In particular, ropinirole attenuates the motor deficits induced by lesioning the ascending nigrostriatal dopaminergic pathway with the neurotoxin 1-methyl-4-phenyl-1,2,3,6-tetrahydropyridine (MPTP) in primates. The relevance of D_3 receptor binding in Parkinson's disease is unknown.

12.2 Pharmacodynamics

Clinical experience with dopamine agonists, including ropinirole, suggests an association with impaired ability to regulate blood pressure with resulting postural hypotension, especially during dose escalation. In some subjects in clinical trials, blood pressure changes were associated with the emergence of orthostatic symptoms, bradycardia, and, in one case in a healthy volunteer, transient sinus arrest with syncope.

The mechanism of postural hypotension induced by ropinirole is presumed to be due to a D_2-mediated blunting of the noradrenergic response to standing and subsequent decrease in peripheral vascular resistance. Nausea is a common concomitant symptom of orthostatic signs and symptoms.

At oral doses as low as 0.2 mg, ropinirole suppressed serum prolactin concentrations in healthy male volunteers.

Immediate-release ropinirole had no dose-related effect on ECG wave form and rhythm in young, healthy, male volunteers in the range of 0.01 to 2.5 mg. Immediate-release ropinirole had no dose- or exposure-related effect on mean QT intervals in healthy male and female volunteers titrated to doses up to 4 mg/day. The effect of ropinirole on QTc intervals at higher exposures achieved either due to drug interactions, hepatic impairment, or at higher doses has not been systematically evaluated.

12.3 Pharmacokinetics

Absorption: In clinical studies with immediate-release ropinirole, over 88% of a radiolabeled dose was recovered in urine, and the absolute bioavailability was 45% to 55%, indicating approximately 50% first-pass effect.

Ropinirole displayed linear kinetics up to doses of 24 mg/day (8 mg immediate-release, 3 times a day). Increase in systemic exposure of ropinirole following oral administration of 2 to 12 mg of REQUIP XL was approximately dose-proportional. For REQUIP XL, steady-state concentrations of ropinirole are expected to be achieved within 4 days of dosing.

Relative bioavailability of REQUIP XL extended-release tablets compared with immediate-release tablets was approximately 100%. In a repeat-dose study in patients with Parkinson's disease using REQUIP XL 8 mg, the dose-normalized $AUC_{(0-24)}$ and C_{min} for REQUIP XL and immediate-release ropinirole were similar. Dose-normalized C_{max} was, on average, 12% lower for REQUIP XL than for the immediate-release formulation and the median time-to-peak concentration was 6 to 10 hours. In a single-dose study, administration of REQUIP XL to healthy volunteers with food (i.e., high-fat meal) increased AUC by approximately 30% and C_{max} by approximately 44%, compared with dosing under fasted conditions. In a repeat-dose study in patients with Parkinson's disease, food (i.e., high-fat meal) increased AUC by approximately 20% and C_{max} by approximately 44%; T_{max} was prolonged by 3 hours (median prolongation) compared with dosing under fasted conditions *[see Dosage and Administration (2.1)]*.

Distribution: Ropinirole is widely distributed throughout the body, with an apparent volume of distribution of 7.5 L/kg (cv = 32%). It is up to 40% bound to plasma proteins and has a blood-to-plasma ratio of 1:1.

Metabolism: Ropinirole is extensively metabolized by the liver. The major metabolic pathways are N-despropylation and hydroxylation to form the inactive N-despropyl metabolite and hydroxy metabolites. The N-despropyl metabolite is converted to carbamyl glucuronide, carboxylic acid, and N-despropyl hydroxy metabolites. The hydroxy metabolite of ropinirole is rapidly glucuronidated.

In vitro studies indicate that the major cytochrome P450 isozyme involved in the metabolism of ropinirole is CYP1A2, an enzyme known to be induced by smoking and omeprazole, and inhibited by, for example, fluvoxamine, mexiletine, and the older fluoroquinolones such as ciprofloxacin and norfloxacin.

Elimination: The clearance of ropinirole after oral administration to patients is 47 L/hr (cv = 45%) and its elimination half-life is approximately 6 hours. Less than 10% of the administered dose is excreted as unchanged drug in urine. N-despropyl ropinirole is the predominant metabolite found in urine (40%), followed by the carboxylic acid metabolite (10%), and the glucuronide of the hydroxy metabolite (10%).

Drug Interactions: *Ciprofloxacin:* Coadministration of ciprofloxacin (500 mg twice daily), an inhibitor of CYP1A2, with immediate-release ropinirole (2 mg 3 times daily) increased ropinirole AUC by 84% on average and C_{max} by 60% (n = 12 patients).

Digoxin: Coadministration of immediate-release ropinirole (2 mg 3 times daily) with digoxin (0.125 to 0.25 mg once daily) did not alter the steady-state pharmacokinetics of digoxin in 10 patients.

Theophylline: Administration of theophylline (300 mg twice daily, a substrate of CYP1A2) did not alter the steady-state pharmacokinetics of immediate-release ropinirole (2 mg 3 times daily) in 12 patients with Parkinson's disease. Immediate-release ropinirole (2 mg 3 times daily) did not alter the pharmacokinetics of theophylline (5 mg/kg IV) in 12 patients with Parkinson's disease.

L-dopa: Coadministration of carbidopa + l-dopa (SINEMET 10/100 mg twice daily) with immediate-release ropinirole (2 mg 3 times daily) had no effect on the steady-state pharmacokinetics of ropinirole (n = 28 patients). Oral administration of immediate-release ropinirole 2 mg 3 times daily increased mean steady-state C_{max} of l-dopa by 20%, but its AUC was unaffected (n = 23 patients).

Estrogens: Population pharmacokinetic analysis revealed that higher doses of estrogens (usually associated with hormone replacement therapy [HRT]) reduced the oral clearance of ropinirole by approximately 35%.

Commonly Administered Drugs: Population analysis showed that commonly administered drugs, e.g., selegiline, amantadine, tricyclic antidepressants, benzodiazepines, ibuprofen, thiazides, antihistamines, and anticholinergics, did not affect the oral clearance of ropinirole.

Population Subgroups: Because therapy with REQUIP XL is initiated at a low dose and gradually titrated upward according to clinical tolerability to obtain the optimum therapeutic effect, adjustment of the initial dose based on gender, weight, or age is not necessary.

Age: Oral clearance of ropinirole is reduced by approximately 15% in patients above 65 years of age compared with younger patients. Dosage adjustment is not necessary in the elderly (above 65 years), as the dose of ropinirole is individually titrated to clinical response.

Gender: Female and male patients showed similar oral clearance.

Race: The influence of race on the pharmacokinetics of ropinirole has not been evaluated.

Renal Impairment: Based on population pharmacokinetic analysis, no difference was observed in the pharmacokinetics of ropinirole in patients with moderate renal impairment (creatinine clearance between 30 to 50 mL/min) compared with an age-matched population with creatinine clearance above 50 mL/min. Therefore, no dosage adjustment is necessary in patients with moderate renal impairment. The use of ropinirole in patients with severe renal impairment has not been studied.

The effect of hemodialysis on ropinirole clearance is not known, but because of the relatively high apparent volume of distribution of ropinirole (7.5 L/kg), significant removal of ropinirole by hemodialysis is unlikely.

Hepatic Impairment: The pharmacokinetics of ropinirole have not been studied in patients with hepatic impairment. These patients may have higher plasma levels and lower clearance of ropinirole than patients with normal hepatic function. REQUIP XL should be titrated with caution in this population.

Other Diseases: Population pharmacokinetic analysis revealed no change in the oral clearance of ropinirole in patients with concomitant diseases such as hypertension, depression, osteoporosis/arthritis, and insomnia compared with patients who had Parkinson's disease only.

13 NONCLINICAL TOXICOLOGY

13.1 Carcinogenesis, Mutagenesis, Impairment of Fertility

Two-year carcinogenicity studies were conducted in Charles River CD-1 mice at doses of 5, 15, and 50 mg/kg/day and in Sprague-Dawley rats at doses of 1.5, 15, and 50 mg/kg/day (top doses which, based on mg/m^2, are equivalent to 10 and 20 times, respectively, the MRHD of 24 mg/day). In the male rat, there was a significant increase in testicular Leydig cell adenomas at all doses tested, i.e., ≥1.5 mg/kg (0.6 times the MRHD on a mg/m^2 basis). This finding is of questionable significance because the endocrine mechanisms believed to be involved in the production of Leydig cell hyperplasia and adenomas in rats are not relevant to humans. In the female mouse, there was an increase in benign uterine endometrial polyps at a dose of 50 mg/kg/day (10 times the MRHD on a mg/m^2 basis).

Ropinirole was not mutagenic or clastogenic in the in vitro Ames test, the in vitro chromosome aberration test in human lymphocytes, the in vitro mouse lymphoma (L1578Y cells) assay, and the in vivo mouse micronucleus test.

When administered to female rats prior to and during mating and throughout pregnancy, ropinirole caused disruption of implantation at doses of 20 mg/kg/day (8 times the MRHD on a mg/m^2 basis) or greater. This effect is thought to be due to the prolactin-lowering effect of ropinirole. In humans, chorionic gonadotropin, not prolactin, is essential for implantation. In rat studies using low doses (5 mg/kg) during the prolactin-dependent phase of early pregnancy (gestation days 0 to 8), ropinirole did not affect female fertility at dosages up to 100 mg/kg/day (40 times the MRHD on a mg/m^2 basis). No effect on male fertility was observed in rats at dosages up to 125 mg/kg/day (50 times the MRHD on a mg/m^2 basis).

14 CLINICAL STUDIES

The effectiveness of the immediate-release formulation of ropinirole (REQUIP tablets) in the treatment of early and advanced Parkinson's disease was initially established in 3 randomized, double-blind, placebo-controlled trials.

The effectiveness of REQUIP XL in the treatment of Parkinson's disease was supported by 2 randomized, double-blind, multicenter clinical trials and clinical pharmacokinetic considerations. One trial conducted in advanced Parkinson's disease patients compared REQUIP XL with placebo as adjunctive therapy to L-dopa. A second trial compared REQUIP XL with REQUIP tablets in early phase Parkinson's disease patients not receiving L-dopa.

In these studies a variety of measures were used to assess the effects of treatment (e.g., patient diaries recording time "on" and "off," tolerability of L-dopa dose reductions, and the Unified Parkinson's Disease Rating Scale [UPDRS] scores). The UPDRS is a multi-item rating scale evaluating mentation (Part I), activities of daily living (Part II), motor performance (Part III), and complications of therapy (Part IV). Part III of the UPDRS contains 14 items designed to assess the severity of the cardinal motor findings in patients with Parkinson's disease (e.g., tremor, rigidity, bradykinesia, postural instability, etc.) scored for different body regions and has a maximum (worst) score of 108.

14.1 Study in Patients With Advanced Parkinson's Disease (With L-dopa)

The effectiveness of REQUIP XL as adjunctive therapy to L-dopa in patients with Parkinson's disease was established in a randomized, double-blind, placebo-controlled, parallel group, 24-week clinical trial in 393 patients (Hoehn & Yahr criteria Stages II-IV) who were not adequately controlled by L-dopa therapy. Patients were allowed to be on concomitant selegiline, amantadine, anticholinergics, and catechol-O-methyltransferase (COMT) inhibitors provided the doses were stable for at least 4 weeks prior to screening and throughout the trial. The primary efficacy endpoint evaluated was the mean change from baseline in total awake time spent "off".

Patients in this study had a mean disease duration of 8.6 years, a mean duration of exposure to L-dopa of 6.5 years, had experienced a minimum of 3 hours awake time "off" with a baseline average of approximately 7 hours awake time "off", and had a mean baseline UPDRS motor score of approximately 30 points with similar mean data in each treatment group. The mean baseline dose of L-dopa in the group receiving REQUIP XL was 824 mg/day and 776 mg/day for the placebo group. Patients initiated treatment at 2 mg/day for 1 week followed by increases of 2 mg/day at weekly intervals to a minimum dose of 6 mg/day. The following week, the REQUIP XL total daily dose could be further increased (based upon therapeutic response and tolerability) to 8 mg/day. Once a daily dose of 8 mg/day was reached, the background L-dopa dosage was reduced. Thereafter, the daily dose could be increased by up to 4 mg/day approximately every 2 weeks until an optimal dose was achieved (based upon therapeutic response and tolerability). The mean dose of REQUIP XL at the end of Week 24 was 18.8 mg/day. Dose titrations were based upon the degree of symptom control, planned L-dopa dosage reduction, and/or tolerability. The maximal allowed daily dosage for REQUIP XL was 24 mg/day.

The primary efficacy endpoint was mean change from baseline in total awake time spent "off" at Week 24. At baseline the mean total awake time spent "off" was approximately 7 hours in each treatment group. At Week 24, the total awake time spent "off", on average, had decreased by approximately 2 hours in the group receiving REQUIP XL and by approximately half an hour in the placebo group. The adjusted mean difference in total awake time spent "off" between REQUIP XL and placebo was -1.7 hours, which was statistically significant (ANCOVA, p< 0.0001). Results for this endpoint showing the statistical superiority of REQUIP XL over Placebo are presented in Table 3.

Table 3. Change from Baseline in Total Awake Time Spent "Off" at Week 24

	REQUIP XL (n = 201)	Placebo (n = 190)
Mean "Off" time at Baseline (hours)	7.0	7.0
Mean Change from Baseline in "Off" time (hours)	-2.1	-0.4

The difference between groups in favor of REQUIP XL, with regard to a decrease in total "off" hours, was primarily related to an increase in total "on" hours without troublesome dyskinesia. Patients treated with REQUIP XL had a mean reduction in L-dopa dose of 278 mg/day (34%) while patients treated with placebo had a mean reduction of 164 mg/day (21%). In patients who reduced their L-dopa dose, reduction was sustained in 93% of patients treated with REQUIP XL and in 72% of patients treated with placebo (p<0.001).

14.2 Study in Patients With Early Parkinson's Disease (Without L-dopa)

A 36-week multicenter, double-blind, titration/3-period maintenance, cross-over study compared the efficacy of REQUIP XL with the immediate-release formulation of REQUIP (IR) in 161 patients with early phase Parkinson's disease (Hoehn & Yahr Stages I-III) with limited prior exposure to L-dopa or dopamine agonists. Eligible subjects were randomized (1:1:1:1) to 4 treatment sequences (2 were titrated on REQUIP IR and 2 on REQUIP XL). The REQUIP IR titration was slower in rate than that of the REQUIP XL. Patients were titrated, during the 12-week titration period, to their optimal dosage, based upon tolerance and therapeutic response. This was followed by 3 consecutive 8-week maintenance periods, during which patients were either maintained on the prior formulation or switched to the alternative formulation. All switches were performed overnight by using the approximately equivalent doses of ropinirole. The primary efficacy endpoint was the change of UPDRS motor score within each maintenance period.

Patients in all 4 groups started out with similar UPDRS motor scores (about 21) at baseline. All 4 groups exhibited similar improvement in UPDRS total motor scores from baseline until the completion of the titration phase, with a change in score of about -9 observed for the groups started on REQUIP IR and of about -10 for the groups started on REQUIP XL. No difference was observed between groups when switches were made between identical formulations or between different formulations. This suggests therapeutic dosage equivalence between REQUIP IR and REQUIP XL formulations.

The optimal daily dose at the end of the titration period for patients on REQUIP IR was substantially lower (mean 7 mg) compared to the dose at the end of the titration period for patients on REQUIP XL (mean 18 mg). In this study, the marked difference in the final optimal dosages suggests that the higher doses afforded no additional benefit when compared to the lower doses *[see Dosage and Administration (2)]*.

16 HOW SUPPLIED/STORAGE AND HANDLING

Each biconvex, capsule-shaped, film-coated tablet contains ropinirole hydrochloride equivalent to the labeled amount of ropinirole as follows:

- 2 mg: pink tablets debossed with "GS" and "3V2", in bottles of 30 (NDC 0007–4885–13) and 90 (NDC 0007-4885-59).

- 4 mg: light brown tablets debossed with "GS" and "WXG", in bottles of 30 (NDC 0007–4887–13) and 90 (NDC 0007-4887-59).
- 6 mg: white tablets debossed with "GS" and "11F", in bottles of 30 (NDC 0007-4883-13).
- 8 mg: red tablets debossed with "GS" and "5CC", in bottles of 30 (NDC 0007–4888–13) and 90 (NDC 0007-4888-59).
- 12 mg: green tablets debossed with "GS" and "YX7", in bottles of 30 (NDC 0007-4882-13).

Storage: Store at 25°C (77°F), excursions permitted to 15-30°C (59-86°F) [see USP Controlled Room Temperature]. Dispense in a tight, light-resistant container as defined in the USP.

17 PATIENT COUNSELING INFORMATION

See FDA-approved patient labeling (Patient Information).

Physicians should instruct their patients to read the Patient Information leaflet before starting therapy with REQUIP XL and to reread it upon prescription renewal for new information regarding the use of REQUIP XL.

17.1 Dosing Instructions

- Patients should be instructed to take REQUIP XL only as prescribed. If a dose is missed, patients should be advised not to double their next dose.
- REQUIP XL can be taken with or without food. Taking REQUIP XL with food may reduce the occurrence of nausea *[see Dosage and Administration (2.1)]*.
- REQUIP XL tablets should be swallowed whole. They should not be chewed, crushed, or divided *[see Dosage and Administration (2.1)]*.
- Ropinirole is the active ingredient that is in both REQUIP XL and REQUIP tablets (the immediate-release formulation). Ask your patient if they are taking another medication containing ropinirole.

17.2 Postural (Orthostatic) Hypotension

Patients should be advised that they may develop postural (orthostatic) hypotension with or without symptoms such as dizziness, nausea, syncope, and sometimes sweating. Hypotension and/or orthostatic symptoms may occur more frequently during initial therapy or with an increase in dose at any time (cases have been seen after weeks of treatment). Accordingly, patients should be cautioned against standing up rapidly after sitting or lying down, especially if they have been doing so for prolonged periods, and especially at the initiation of treatment with REQUIP XL *[see Warnings and Precautions (5.2, 5.3)]*.

17.3 Elevation of Blood Pressure and Changes in Heart Rate

Patients should be alerted to the possibility of increases in blood pressure during treatment with REQUIP XL. Exacerbation of hypertension may occur. Medication dose adjustment may be necessary if elevation of blood pressure is sustained over multiple evaluations. Patients with cardiovascular disease, who may not tolerate marked changes in heart rate, should also be alerted to the possibility that they may experience significant increases or decreases in heart rate during treatment with REQUIP XL *[see Warnings and Precautions (5.4)]*.

17.4 Sedating Effects

Patients should be alerted to the potential sedating effects caused by REQUIP XL, including somnolence and the possibility of falling asleep while engaged in activities of daily living. Since somnolence is a frequent adverse reaction with potentially serious consequences, patients should neither drive a car nor engage in other potentially dangerous activities until they have gained sufficient experience with REQUIP XL to gauge whether or not it affects their mental and/or motor performance adversely. Patients should be advised that if increased somnolence or episodes of falling asleep during activities of daily living (e.g., conversations, eating, driving a motor vehicle, etc.) are experienced at any time during treatment, they should not drive or participate in potentially dangerous activities until they have contacted their physician.

Because of possible additive effects, caution should be advised when patients are taking other sedating medications, alcohol, or other CNS depressants (e.g., benzodiazepines, antipsychotics, antidepressants, etc.) in combination with REQUIP XL or when taking concomitant medications that increase plasma levels of ropinirole (e.g., ciprofloxacin) *[see Warnings and Precautions (5.1)]*.

17.5 Hallucination

Patients should be informed they may experience hallucinations (unreal visions, sounds, or sensations) while taking ropinirole. The elderly are at greater risk than younger patients with Parkinson's disease; and the risk is greater in patients who are taking ropinirole with L-dopa or taking higher doses of ropinirole, and may also be further increased in patients taking any other drugs that increase dopaminergic tone *[see Warnings and Precautions (5.5)]*.

17.6 Impulse Control Symptoms, Including Compulsive Behaviors

There have been reports of patients experiencing intense urges to gamble, increased sexual urges, and other intense urges and the inability to control these urges while taking one or more of the medications that increase central dopaminergic tone, that are generally used for the treatment of Parkinson's disease or Restless Legs Syndrome, including ropinirole. In the clinical development program (N = 613), 6 patients treated with REQUIP XL exhibited compulsive behaviors consisting of pathological gambling and/or hypersexuality. Although it is not proven that the medications caused these events, these urges were reported to have stopped in some cases when the dose was reduced or the medication was stopped. Prescribers should ask patients about the development of new or increased gambling urges, sexual urges or other urges while being treated with REQUIP XL. Patients should inform their physician if they experience new or increased gambling urges, increased sexual urges or other intense urges while taking REQUIP XL. Physicians should consider dose reduction or stopping the medication if a patient develops such urges while taking REQUIP XL.

17.7 Nursing Mothers

Because of the possibility that ropinirole may be excreted in breast milk, a decision should be made whether to discontinue nursing or to discontinue the drug, taking into account the importance of the drug to the mother *[see Use in Specific Populations (8.3)]*.

Patients should be advised that ropinirole could inhibit lactation, as ropinirole inhibits prolactin secretion.

17.8 Pregnancy

Because ropinirole has been shown to have adverse effects on embryo-fetal development, including teratogenic effects, in animals, and because experience in humans is limited, patients should be advised to notify their physician if they become pregnant or intend to become pregnant during therapy *[see Use in Specific Populations (8.1)]*.

REQUIP XL is a registered trademark of GlaxoSmithKline.
SINEMET is a registered trademark of Merck & Co., Inc.
GlaxoSmithKline
Research Triangle Park, NC 27709

RXL:5PI

PATIENT INFORMATION
REQUIP® (RE-qwip) (ropinirole tablets)
REQUIP XL® (RE-qwip)
(ropinirole extended-release tablets)

IF YOU HAVE PARKINSON'S DISEASE, READ THIS SIDE
IF YOU HAVE RESTLESS LEGS SYNDROME, READ THE OTHER SIDE

IMPORTANT NOTE: REQUIP XL has not been studied in Restless Legs Syndrome (RLS) and is not approved for the treatment of RLS. However, an immediate-release form of ropinirole (REQUIP) is approved for the treatment of RLS (see other side of this leaflet).

Read this information completely before you start taking REQUIP or REQUIP XL. Read the information each time you get more medicine. There may be new information. This leaflet provides a summary about REQUIP and REQUIP XL. It does not include everything there is to know about your medicine. This information should not take the place of discussions with your healthcare provider about your medical condition or treatment with REQUIP or REQUIP XL.

What are REQUIP and REQUIP XL?

REQUIP is a short-acting prescription medicine containing ropinirole (usually taken 3 times a day) used to treat Parkinson's disease. It is also used to treat a condition called Restless Legs Syndrome.

REQUIP XL is a long-acting prescription medicine containing ropinirole (taken once a day) used to treat Parkinson's disease.

You should not be taking more than one medicine containing ropinirole. Inform your physician if you are taking any other medicine containing ropinirole.

REQUIP and REQUIP XL have not been studied in children.

What is the most important information I should know about REQUIP and REQUIP XL?

REQUIP and REQUIP XL can cause serious side effects including:

- **Falling asleep during normal activities.** You may fall asleep while doing normal activities such as driving a car, doing physical tasks, or using hazardous machinery while taking REQUIP or REQUIP XL. You may suddenly fall asleep without being drowsy or without warning. This may result in having accidents. Your chances of falling asleep while doing normal activities while taking REQUIP or REQUIP XL are greater if you take other medicines that cause drowsiness. Tell your healthcare provider right away if this happens. Before starting REQUIP or REQUIP XL, be sure to tell your healthcare provider if you take any medicines that make you drowsy.
- **Changes in blood pressure.** REQUIP and REQUIP XL can decrease or increase your blood pressure. Lowering of your blood pressure is of special concern. If you faint, feel dizzy, nauseated, or sweaty when you stand up from sitting or lying down, this may mean that your blood pressure is decreased. If you notice this, you should contact your healthcare provider. Also, when changing position from lying down or sitting to standing up, you should do it carefully and slowly. Lowering of your blood pressure can happen especially when you start taking REQUIP or REQUIP XL or when your dose is increased.
- **Fainting.** Fainting can occur, and sometimes your heart rate may be decreased. This can happen especially when you start taking REQUIP or REQUIP XL or your dose is increased. Tell your healthcare provider if you faint or feel dizzy.
- **Hallucinations** (unreal visions, sounds, or sensations) can occur in patients taking REQUIP or REQUIP XL. The chances of having hallucinations are higher in patients with Parkinson's disease who are elderly, taking REQUIP or REQUIP XL with other Parkinson's disease drugs, or taking higher doses of REQUIP or REQUIP XL. If you have hallucinations, talk with your healthcare provider.
- **Uncontrolled sudden movements.** REQUIP or REQUIP XL may cause uncontrolled sudden movements or make such movements you already have worse or more frequent. Tell your healthcare provider if this happens. The doses of your anti-Parkinson's medicines may need to be changed.

Unusual urges. Some patients taking REQUIP or REQUIP XL get urges to behave in a way unusual for them. Examples of this are an unusual urge to gamble or increased sexual urges and behaviors. If you notice or your family notices that you are developing any unusual behaviors, talk to your healthcare provider.

See "What are the possible side effects of REQUIP and REQUIP XL?"

What should I tell my healthcare provider before taking REQUIP or REQUIP XL?

Be sure to tell your healthcare provider if you:

- have daytime sleepiness from a sleep disorder or have unexpected or unpredictable sleepiness or periods of sleep.
- are taking any other prescription or over-the-counter medicines. Some of these medicines may increase your chances of getting side effects while taking REQUIP or REQUIP XL.
- start or stop taking other medicines while you are taking REQUIP or REQUIP XL. This may increase your chances of getting side effects.
- start or stop smoking while you are taking REQUIP or REQUIP XL. Smoking may decrease the treatment effect of REQUIP or REQUIP XL.
- feel dizzy, nauseated, sweaty, or faint when you first stand up from sitting or lying down.
- drink alcoholic beverages. This may increase your chances of becoming drowsy or sleepy while taking REQUIP or REQUIP XL.
- have high or low blood pressure.
- are pregnant or plan to become pregnant. REQUIP and REQUIP XL should only be used during pregnancy if needed.
- are breastfeeding. It is not known if REQUIP or REQUIP XL passes into your breast milk. Talk to your healthcare provider to decide whether you will breastfeed or take REQUIP or REQUIP XL.
- are allergic to any of the ingredients in REQUIP or REQUIP XL. See the end of this Patient Information leaflet for a complete list of the ingredients in REQUIP and REQUIP XL.

How should I take REQUIP or REQUIP XL for Parkinson's disease?

- Take REQUIP or REQUIP XL exactly as directed by your healthcare provider.
- Do not suddenly stop taking REQUIP or REQUIP XL without talking to your healthcare provider. If you stop this medicine suddenly, you may develop fever, confusion, or severe muscle stiffness.
- Before starting REQUIP or REQUIP XL, you should talk to your healthcare provider about what to do if you miss a dose. If you have missed the previous dose and it is time for your next dose, **do not double the dose.**
- Your healthcare provider will start you on a low dose of REQUIP or REQUIP XL. Your healthcare provider will change the dose until you are taking the right amount of medicine to control your symptoms. **It may take several weeks before you reach a dose that controls your symptoms.**

If you are taking REQUIP:

- REQUIP tablets are usually taken 3 times each day for Parkinson's disease.

If you are taking REQUIP XL:

- Take REQUIP XL tablets 1 time each day for Parkinson's disease, preferably at or around the same time of day.
- Swallow REQUIP XL tablets whole. Do not chew, crush, or split REQUIP XL tablets.

If you are taking either REQUIP or REQUIP XL:

- Contact your healthcare provider if you stop taking REQUIP or REQUIP XL for any reason. Do not restart without talking with your healthcare provider.

- Your healthcare provider may prescribe REQUIP or REQUIP XL alone, or add REQUIP or REQUIP XL to medicine that you are already taking for Parkinson's disease.
- You should not substitute REQUIP for REQUIP XL or REQUIP XL for REQUIP without talking with your healthcare provider.
- You can take REQUIP or REQUIP XL with or without food. If you experience nausea you may try taking REQUIP or REQUIP XL with food.

What are the possible side effects of REQUIP and REQUIP XL?

Serious side effects in people taking REQUIP and REQUIP XL are described in the section "REQUIP and REQUIP XL can cause serious side effects including" and include:

- Falling asleep during normal activities
- Changes in blood pressure
- Fainting
- Hallucinations
- Uncontrolled sudden movements

Some patients taking REQUIP or REQUIP XL get urges to behave in a way unusual for them. Examples of this are an unusual urge to gamble or increased sexual urges and behaviors. If you notice or your family notices that you are developing any unusual behaviors, talk to your healthcare provider.

You should be careful until you know if REQUIP or REQUIP XL affects your ability to remain alert while doing normal daily activities, driving a car, operating machinery, or working at heights. You should also watch for the development of significant daytime sleepiness or episodes of falling asleep.

Common side effects in people taking REQUIP and REQUIP XL include:

- Fainting
- Sleepiness
- Hallucinations
- Dizziness
- Nausea or vomiting
- Uncontrolled sudden movements
- Leg swelling
- Fatigue
- Headache
- Upset stomach
- Increased sweating

This is not a complete list of side effects and should not take the place of discussions with your healthcare providers. Your healthcare provider or pharmacist can give you a more complete list of possible side effects.

Call your healthcare provider for medical advice about side effects. You may report side effects to FDA at 1-800-FDA-1088.

How should I store REQUIP and REQUIP XL?

- Store REQUIP tablets between 68°-77°F (20°-25°C).
- Store REQUIP XL tablets between 59°-86°F (15°-30°C).
- Store REQUIP or REQUIP XL at room temperature out of direct sunlight.
- Keep REQUIP or REQUIP XL in a tightly closed container.
- Keep REQUIP or REQUIP XL out of the reach of children.

Other Information about REQUIP and REQUIP XL:

- Do not share REQUIP or REQUIP XL with other people, even if they have the same symptoms you have.
- Studies of people with Parkinson's disease show that they may be at an increased risk of developing melanoma, a form of skin cancer, when compared to people without Parkinson's disease. It is not known if this problem is associated with Parkinson's disease or the medicines used to treat Parkinson's disease. REQUIP and REQUIP XL are two of the medicines used to treat Parkinson's disease; therefore, patients being treated with REQUIP or REQUIP XL should have periodic skin examinations.

This patient information leaflet summarizes the most important information about REQUIP and REQUIP XL for Parkinson's disease. Medicines are sometimes prescribed for purposes other than those listed in this leaflet. Do not take REQUIP or REQUIP XL for a condition for which it was not prescribed. For more information, talk with your healthcare provider or pharmacist. They can give you information about REQUIP and REQUIP XL that is written for healthcare professionals. For more information call 1-888-825-5249 (toll-free) or visit www.requipxl.com.

What are the ingredients in REQUIP and REQUIP XL?

The following ingredients are in REQUIP:

Active ingredient: ropinirole (as ropinirole hydrochloride)

Inactive ingredients: croscarmellose sodium, hydrous lactose, magnesium stearate, microcrystalline cellulose, and one or more of the following: carmine, FD&C Blue No. 2 aluminum lake, FD&C Yellow No. 6 aluminum lake, hypromellose, iron oxides, polyethylene glycol, polysorbate 80, titanium dioxide.

The following ingredients are in REQUIP XL:

Active ingredient: ropinirole (as ropinirole hydrochloride)

Inactive ingredients: carboxymethylcellulose sodium, colloidal silicon dioxide, glycerol behenate, hydrogenated castor oil, hypromellose, lactose monohydrate, magnesium stearate, maltodextrin, mannitol, povidone, and one or more of the following: FD&C Yellow No. 6 aluminum lake, FD&C Blue No. 2 aluminum lake, ferric oxides (black, red, yellow), polyethylene glycol 400, titanium dioxide.

PATIENT INFORMATION

REQUIP® (RE-qwip)

(ropinirole tablets)

IF YOU HAVE RESTLESS LEGS SYNDROME (RLS), READ THIS SIDE

IF YOU HAVE PARKINSON'S DISEASE, READ THE OTHER SIDE

Read this information completely before you start taking REQUIP. Read the information each time you get more medicine. There may be new information. This leaflet provides a summary about REQUIP. It does not include everything there is to know about your medicine. This information should not take the place of discussions with your healthcare provider about your medical condition or treatment with REQUIP.

Patients with RLS should take REQUIP differently than patients with Parkinson's disease (see **How should I take REQUIP for RLS?** for the recommended dosing for RLS). A lower dose of REQUIP is generally needed for patients with RLS, and is taken once daily before bedtime.

What is the most important information I should know about REQUIP?

REQUIP can cause serious side effects including:

- **Falling asleep during normal activities.** You may fall asleep while doing normal activities such as driving a car, doing physical tasks, or using hazardous machinery while taking REQUIP. You may suddenly fall asleep without being drowsy or without warning. This may result in having accidents. Your chances of falling asleep while doing normal activities while taking REQUIP are greater if you take other medicines that cause drowsiness. Tell your healthcare provider right away if this happens. Before starting REQUIP, be sure to tell your healthcare provider if you take any medicines that make you drowsy.
- **Decrease in blood pressure.** REQUIP can decrease your blood pressure. Lowering of your blood pressure is of special concern. If you faint, feel dizzy, nauseated, or sweaty when you stand up from sitting or lying down, this may mean that your blood pressure is decreased. If you notice this, you should contact your healthcare provider. Also, when changing position from lying down or sitting to standing up, you should do it carefully and slowly. Lowering of your blood pressure can happen especially when you start taking REQUIP or when your dose is increased.
- **Fainting.** Fainting can occur, and sometimes your heart rate may be decreased. This can happen especially when you start taking REQUIP or your dose is increased. Tell your healthcare provider if you faint or feel dizzy.
- **Hallucinations** (unreal visions, sounds, or sensations) can occur in patients taking REQUIP. If you have hallucinations, talk with your healthcare provider.

Unusual urges. Some patients taking REQUIP get urges to behave in a way unusual for them. Examples of this are an unusual urge to gamble or increased sexual urges and behaviors. If you notice or your family notices that you are developing any unusual behaviors, talk to your healthcare provider.

See "What are the possible side effects of REQUIP?"

What is REQUIP?

REQUIP is a prescription medicine containing ropinirole used to treat moderate-to-severe primary Restless Legs Syndrome. It is also used to treat Parkinson's disease. Having one of these conditions does not mean you have or will develop the other.

REQUIP has not been studied in children.

What should I tell my healthcare provider before taking REQUIP?

Be sure to tell your healthcare provider if you:

- have daytime sleepiness from a sleep disorder or have unexpected or unpredictable sleepiness or periods of sleep.
- are taking any other prescription or over-the-counter medicines. Some of these medicines may increase your chances of getting side effects while taking REQUIP.
- start or stop taking other medicines while you are taking REQUIP. This may increase your chances of getting side effects.
- start or stop smoking while you are taking REQUIP. Smoking may decrease the treatment effect of REQUIP.
- feel dizzy, nauseated, sweaty, or faint when you first stand up from sitting or lying down.
- drink alcoholic beverages. This may increase your chances of becoming drowsy or sleepy while taking REQUIP.
- have high or low blood pressure.
- are pregnant or plan to become pregnant. REQUIP should only be used during pregnancy if needed.
- are breastfeeding. It is not known if REQUIP passes into your breast milk. Talk to your healthcare provider to decide whether you will breastfeed or take REQUIP.
- are allergic to any of the ingredients in REQUIP. See the end of this Patient Information leaflet for a complete list of the ingredients in REQUIP.

How should I take REQUIP for RLS?

- Take REQUIP exactly as directed by your healthcare provider.
- The usual way to take REQUIP is once in the evening, 1 to 3 hours before bedtime.
- Your healthcare provider will start you on a low dose of REQUIP. Your healthcare provider may change the dose until you are taking the right amount of medicine to control your symptoms.
- **If you miss your dose, do not double your next dose.** Take only your usual dose 1 to 3 hours before your next bedtime.
- Contact your healthcare provider if you stop taking REQUIP for any reason. Do not restart without consulting your healthcare provider.
- You can take REQUIP with or without food. Taking REQUIP with food may decrease the chances of feeling nauseated.

What are the possible side effects of REQUIP?

Serious side effects in people taking REQUIP are described in the section "REQUIP can cause serious side effects including" and include:

- Falling asleep during normal activities
- Decrease in blood pressure
- Fainting
- Hallucinations

Some patients taking REQUIP get urges to behave in a way unusual for them. Examples of this are an unusual urge to gamble or increased sexual urges and behaviors. If you notice or your family notices that you are developing any unusual behaviors, talk to your healthcare provider.

You should be careful until you know if REQUIP affects your ability to remain alert while doing normal daily activities, driving a car, operating machinery, or working at heights. You should also watch for the development of significant daytime sleepiness or episodes of falling asleep.

Common side effects in people taking REQUIP include:

- Nausea or vomiting
- Sleepiness or drowsiness
- Dizziness
- Fatigue

This is not a complete list of side effects and should not take the place of discussions with your healthcare providers. Your healthcare provider or pharmacist can give you a more complete list of possible side effects.

Call your healthcare provider for medical advice about side effects. You may report side effects to FDA at 1-800-FDA-1088.

How should I store REQUIP?

- Store REQUIP tablets between 68°-77°F (20°-25°C).
- Store REQUIP at room temperature out of direct sunlight.
- Keep REQUIP in a tightly closed container.
- Keep REQUIP out of the reach of children.

Other Information about REQUIP

- Do not share REQUIP with other people, even if they have the same symptoms you have.
- Studies of people with Parkinson's disease show that they may be at an increased risk of developing melanoma, a form of skin cancer, when compared to people without Parkinson's disease. It is not known if this problem is associated with Parkinson's disease or the medicines used to treat Parkinson's disease. REQUIP is one of the medicines used to treat Parkinson's disease; therefore, patients being treated with REQUIP should have periodic skin examinations.

This patient information leaflet summarizes important information about REQUIP for Restless Legs Syndrome. Medicines are sometimes prescribed for purposes other than those listed in this leaflet. Do not take REQUIP for a condition for which it was not prescribed. For more information, talk with your healthcare provider or pharmacist. They can give you information about REQUIP that is written for healthcare professionals. For more information call 1-888-825-5249 (toll-free) or visit www.requip.com.

What are the ingredients in REQUIP?

The following ingredients are in REQUIP:

Active ingredient: ropinirole (as ropinirole hydrochloride)

Inactive ingredients: croscarmellose sodium, hydrous lactose, magnesium stearate, microcrystalline cellulose, and one or more of the following: carmine, FD&C Blue No. 2 aluminum lake, FD&C Yellow No. 6 aluminum lake, hypromellose, iron oxides, polyethylene glycol, polysorbate 80, titanium dioxide.

GlaxoSmithKline

Research Triangle Park, NC 27709

RXL:3PIL

December 2012

ROTARIX ℞
[*rōt' ə-rix*]
(Rotavirus Vaccine, Live, Oral)
Oral Suspension

HIGHLIGHTS OF PRESCRIBING INFORMATION
These highlights do not include all the information needed to use ROTARIX safely and effectively. See full prescribing information for ROTARIX.
ROTARIX (Rotavirus Vaccine, Live, Oral)
Initial U.S. Approval: 2008

RECENT MAJOR CHANGES

Warnings and Precautions, Shedding and Transmission (5.4)	06/2012
Warnings and Precautions, Intussusception (5.5)	09/2012

INDICATIONS AND USAGE

ROTARIX is a vaccine indicated for the prevention of rotavirus gastroenteritis caused by G1 and non-G1 types (G3, G4, and G9). ROTARIX is approved for use in infants 6 weeks to 24 weeks of age. (1)

DOSAGE AND ADMINISTRATION

FOR ORAL USE ONLY. (2.1)
- Each dose is 1-mL administered orally. (2.2)
- Administer first dose to infants beginning at 6 weeks of age. (2.2)
- Administer second dose after an interval of at least 4 weeks and prior to 24 weeks of age. (2.2)

DOSAGE FORMS AND STRENGTHS

- Vial of lyophilized vaccine to be reconstituted with a liquid diluent in a prefilled oral applicator. (3)
- Each 1-mL dose contains a suspension of at least $10^{6.0}$ median Cell Culture Infective Dose ($CCID_{50}$) of live, attenuated human G1P[8] rotavirus after reconstitution. (3)

CONTRAINDICATIONS

- A demonstrated history of hypersensitivity to the vaccine or any component of the vaccine. (4.1, 11)
- History of uncorrected congenital malformation of the gastrointestinal tract that would predispose the infant to intussusception. (4.2)
- History of intussusception. (4.3)
- History of Severe Combined Immunodeficiency Disease (SCID). (4.4, 6.2)

WARNINGS AND PRECAUTIONS

- The tip caps of the prefilled oral applicators of diluent may contain natural rubber latex which may cause allergic reactions in latex-sensitive individuals. (5.1)
- Administration of ROTARIX in infants suffering from acute diarrhea or vomiting should be delayed. Safety and effectiveness of ROTARIX in infants with chronic gastrointestinal disorders have not been evaluated. (5.2)
- Safety and effectiveness of ROTARIX in infants with known primary or secondary immunodeficiencies have not been established. (5.3)
- In a postmarketing study, cases of intussusception were observed in temporal association within 31 days following the first dose of ROTARIX, with a clustering of cases in the first 7 days. (5.5, 6.2)

ADVERSE REACTIONS

Common (≥5%) solicited adverse events included fussiness/irritability, cough/runny nose, fever, loss of appetite, and vomiting. (6.1)

To report SUSPECTED ADVERSE REACTIONS, contact GlaxoSmithKline at 1-888-825-5249 or VAERS at 1-800-822-7967 or www.vaers.hhs.gov.

See 17 for PATIENT COUNSELING INFORMATION and FDA-approved patient labeling

Revised: 09/2012

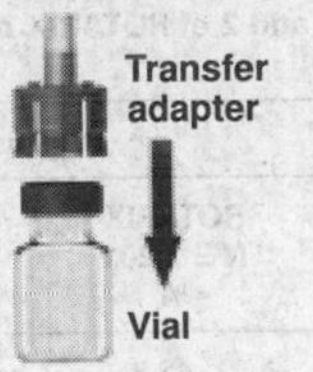

Remove vial cap and push transfer adapter onto vial (lyophilized vaccine).

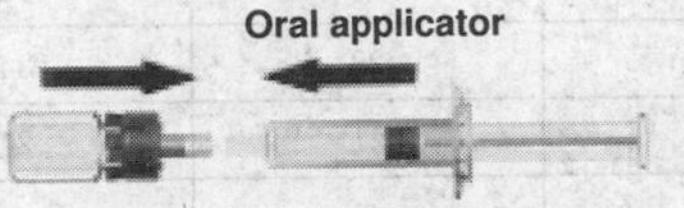

Shake diluent in oral applicator (white, turbid suspension). Connect oral applicator to transfer adapter.

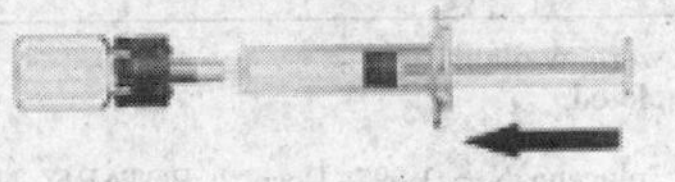

Push plunger of oral applicator to transfer diluent into vial. Suspension will appear white and turbid.

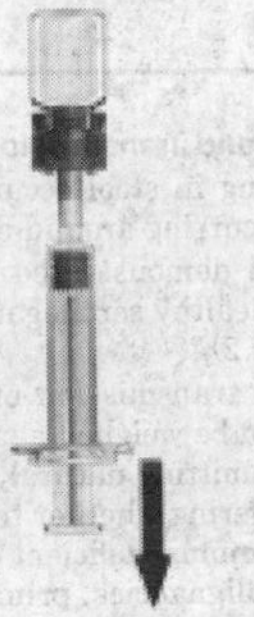

Withdraw vaccine into oral applicator.

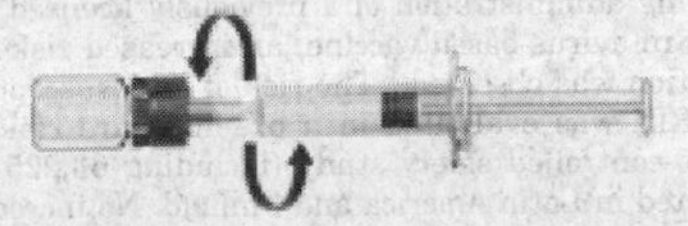

Twist and remove the oral applicator.

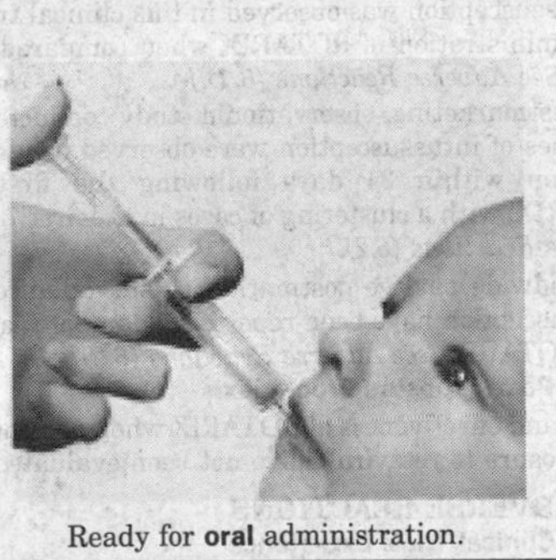

Ready for **oral** administration.

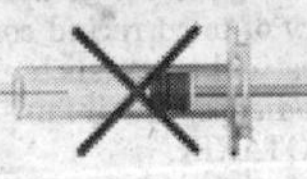

Do not use a needle with ROTARIX. Not for injection.

FULL PRESCRIBING INFORMATION: CONTENTS*

* Sections or subsections omitted from the full prescribing information are not listed

FULL PRESCRIBING INFORMATION

1 INDICATIONS AND USAGE

ROTARIX® is indicated for the prevention of rotavirus gastroenteritis caused by G1 and non-G1 types (G3, G4, and G9) when administered as a 2-dose series *[see Clinical Studies (14.3)]*. ROTARIX is approved for use in infants 6 weeks to 24 weeks of age.

2 DOSAGE AND ADMINISTRATION

2.1 Reconstitution Instructions for Oral Administration

For oral use only. Not for injection.

Reconstitute only with accompanying diluent. Do not mix ROTARIX with other vaccines or solutions.

[See table above]

2.2 Recommended Dose and Schedule

The vaccination series consists of two 1-mL doses administered **orally**. The first dose should be administered to infants beginning at 6 weeks of age. There should be an interval of at least 4 weeks between the first and second dose. The 2-dose series should be completed by 24 weeks of age. Safety and effectiveness have not been evaluated if ROTARIX were administered for the first dose and another rotavirus vaccine were administered for the second dose or vice versa.

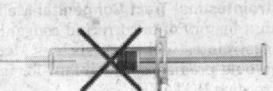

Table 1. Solicited Adverse Events Within 8 Days Following Doses 1 and 2 of ROTARIX or Placebo (Total Vaccinated Cohort)

	Dose 1		Dose 2	
	ROTARIX N = 3,284 %	Placebo N = 2,013 %	ROTARIX N = 3,201 %	Placebo N = 1,973 %
Fussiness/irritability[a]	52	52	42	42
Cough/runny nose[b]	28	30	31	33
Fever[c]	25	33	28	34
Loss of appetite[d]	25	25	21	21
Vomiting	13	11	8	8
Diarrhea	4	3	3	3

Total vaccinated cohort = all vaccinated infants for whom safety data were available.
N = number of infants for whom at least one symptom sheet was completed.
[a]Defined as crying more than usual.
[b]Data not collected in 1 of 7 studies; Dose 1: ROTARIX N = 2,583; placebo N = 1,897; Dose 2: ROTARIX N = 2,522; placebo N = 1,863.
[c]Defined as temperature ≥100.4°F (≥38.0°C) rectally or ≥99.5°F (≥37.5°C) orally.
[d]Defined as eating less than usual.

In the event that the infant spits out or regurgitates most of the vaccine dose, a single replacement dose may be considered at the same vaccination visit.

2.3 Infant Feeding

Breast-feeding was permitted in clinical studies. There was no evidence to suggest that breast-feeding reduced the protection against rotavirus gastroenteritis afforded by ROTARIX. There are no restrictions on the infant's liquid consumption, including breast-milk, either before or after vaccination with ROTARIX.

3 DOSAGE FORMS AND STRENGTHS

ROTARIX is available as a vial of lyophilized vaccine to be reconstituted with a liquid diluent in a prefilled oral applicator.

Each 1-mL dose contains a suspension of at least $10^{6.0}$ median Cell Culture Infective Dose ($CCID_{50}$) of live, attenuated human G1P[8] rotavirus after reconstitution.

4 CONTRAINDICATIONS

4.1 Hypersensitivity

A demonstrated history of hypersensitivity to any component of the vaccine.

Infants who develop symptoms suggestive of hypersensitivity after receiving a dose of ROTARIX should not receive further doses of ROTARIX.

4.2 Gastrointestinal Tract Congenital Malformation

Infants with a history of uncorrected congenital malformation of the gastrointestinal tract (such as Meckel's diverticulum) that would predispose the infant for intussusception should not receive ROTARIX.

4.3 History of Intussusception

Infants with a history of intussusception should not receive ROTARIX *[see Warnings and Precautions (5.5)]*. In postmarketing experience, intussusception resulting in death following a second dose has been reported following a history of intussusception after the first dose *[see Adverse Reactions (6.2)]*.

4.4 Severe Combined Immunodeficiency Disease

Infants with Severe Combined Immunodeficiency Disease (SCID) should not receive ROTARIX. Postmarketing reports of gastroenteritis, including severe diarrhea and prolonged shedding of vaccine virus, have been reported in infants who were administered live, oral rotavirus vaccines and later identified as having SCID *[see Adverse Reactions (6.2)]*.

5 WARNINGS AND PRECAUTIONS

5.1 Latex

The tip caps of the prefilled oral applicators of diluent may contain natural rubber latex which may cause allergic reactions in latex-sensitive individuals. The vial stopper does not contain latex. *[See Description (11).]*

5.2 Gastrointestinal Disorders

Administration of ROTARIX should be delayed in infants suffering from acute diarrhea or vomiting.

Safety and effectiveness of ROTARIX in infants with chronic gastrointestinal disorders have not been evaluated. *[See Contraindications (4.2).]*

5.3 Altered Immunocompetence

Safety and effectiveness of ROTARIX in infants with known primary or secondary immunodeficiencies, including infants with human immunodeficiency virus (HIV), infants on immunosuppressive therapy, or infants with malignant neoplasms affecting the bone marrow or lymphatic system have not been established.

5.4 Shedding and Transmission

Rotavirus shedding in stool occurs after vaccination with peak excretion occurring around day 7 after dose 1.

One clinical trial demonstrated that vaccinees transmit vaccine virus to healthy seronegative contacts *[see Clinical Pharmacology (12.2)]*.

The potential for transmission of vaccine virus following vaccination should be weighed against the possibility of acquiring and transmitting natural rotavirus. Caution is advised when considering whether to administer ROTARIX to individuals with immunodeficient close contacts, such as individuals with malignancies, primary immunodeficiency or receiving immunosuppressive therapy.

5.5 Intussusception

Following administration of a previously licensed oral live rhesus rotavirus-based vaccine, an increased risk of intussusception was observed.[1] The risk of intussusception with ROTARIX was evaluated in a pre-licensure randomized, placebo-controlled safety study (including 63,225 infants) conducted in Latin America and Finland. No increased risk of intussusception was observed in this clinical trial following administration of ROTARIX when compared with placebo. *[See Adverse Reactions (6.1).]*

In a postmarketing, observational study conducted in Mexico, cases of intussusception were observed in temporal association within 31 days following the first dose of ROTARIX, with a clustering of cases in the first 7 days. *[See Adverse Reactions (6.2).]*

In worldwide passive postmarketing surveillance, cases of intussusception have been reported in temporal association with ROTARIX *[see Adverse Reactions (6.2)]*.

5.6 Post-Exposure Prophylaxis

Safety and effectiveness of ROTARIX when administered after exposure to rotavirus have not been evaluated.

6 ADVERSE REACTIONS

6.1 Clinical Trials Experience

Because clinical trials are conducted under widely varying conditions, adverse reaction rates observed in the clinical trials of a vaccine cannot be directly compared to rates in the clinical trials of another vaccine, and may not reflect the rates observed in practice. As with any vaccine, there is the possibility that broad use of ROTARIX could reveal adverse reactions not observed in clinical trials.

Solicited and unsolicited adverse events, serious adverse events and cases of intussusception were collected in 7 clinical studies. Cases of intussusception and serious adverse events were collected in an additional large safety study. These 8 clinical studies evaluated a total of 71,209 infants who received ROTARIX (N = 36,755) or placebo (N = 34,454). The racial distribution for these studies was as follows: Hispanic 73.4%, white 16.2%, black 1.0%, and other 9.4%; 51% were male.

Solicited Adverse Events: In 7 clinical studies, detailed safety information was collected by parents/guardians for 8 consecutive days following vaccination with ROTARIX (i.e., day of vaccination and the next 7 days). A diary card was completed to record fussiness/irritability, cough/runny nose, the infant's temperature, loss of appetite, vomiting, or diarrhea on a daily basis during the first week following each dose of ROTARIX or placebo. Adverse events among recipients of ROTARIX and placebo occurred at similar rates (Table 1).

[See table 1 above]

Unsolicited Adverse Events: Infants were monitored for unsolicited serious and non-serious adverse events that occurred in the 31-day period following vaccination in 7 clinical studies. The following adverse events occurred at a statistically higher incidence (95% Confidence Interval [CI] of Relative Risk excluding 1) among recipients of ROTARIX (N = 5,082) as compared with placebo recipients (N = 2,902): irritability (ROTARIX 11.4%, placebo 8.7%) and flatulence (ROTARIX 2.2%, placebo 1.3%).

Serious Adverse Events (SAEs): Infants were monitored for serious adverse events that occurred in the 31-day period following vaccination in 8 clinical studies. Serious adverse events occurred in 1.7% of recipients of ROTARIX (N = 36,755) as compared with 1.9% of placebo recipients (N = 34,454). Among placebo recipients, diarrhea (placebo 0.07%, ROTARIX 0.02%), dehydration (placebo 0.06%, ROTARIX 0.02%), and gastroenteritis (placebo 0.3%, ROTARIX 0.2%) occurred at a statistically higher incidence (95% CI of Relative Risk excluding 1) as compared with recipients of ROTARIX.

Deaths: During the entire course of 8 clinical studies, there were 68 (0.19%) deaths following administration of ROTARIX (N = 36,755) and 50 (0.15%) deaths following placebo administration (N = 34,454). The most commonly reported cause of death following vaccination was pneumonia, which was observed in 19 (0.05%) recipients of ROTARIX and 10 (0.03%) placebo recipients (Relative Risk: 1.74, 95% CI: 0.76, 4.23).

Intussusception: In a controlled safety study conducted in Latin America and Finland, the risk of intussusception was evaluated in 63,225 infants (31,673 received ROTARIX and 31,552 received placebo). Infants were monitored by active surveillance including independent, complementary methods (prospective hospital surveillance and parent reporting at scheduled study visits) to identify potential cases of intussusception within 31 days after vaccination and, in a subset of 20,169 infants (10,159 received ROTARIX and 10,010 received placebo), up to one year after the first dose. No increased risk of intussusception following administration of ROTARIX was observed within a 31-day period following any dose, and rates were comparable to the placebo group after a median of 100 days (Table 2). In a subset of 20,169 infants (10,159 received ROTARIX and 10,010 received placebo) followed up to one year after dose 1, there were 4 cases of intussusception with ROTARIX compared with 14 cases of intussusception with placebo [Relative Risk: 0.28 (95% CI: 0.10, 0.81)]. All of the infants who developed intussusception recovered without sequelae.

Table 2. Intussusception and Relative Risk With ROTARIX Compared With Placebo

Confirmed Cases of Intussusception	ROTARIX N = 31,673	Placebo N = 31,552
Within 31 days following diagnosis after any dose	6	7
Relative Risk (95% CI)	0.85 (0.30, 2.42)	
Within 100 days following dose 1[a]	9	16
Relative Risk (95% CI)	0.56 (0.25, 1.24)	

CI = Confidence Interval.
[a]Median duration after dose 1 (follow-up visit at 30 to 90 days after dose 2).

Among vaccine recipients, there were no confirmed cases of intussusception within the 0- to 14-day period after the first dose (Table 3), which was the period of highest risk for the previously licensed oral live rhesus rotavirus-based vaccine.[1]

[See table 3 at top of next page]

Kawasaki Disease: Kawasaki disease has been reported in 18 (0.035%) recipients of ROTARIX and 9 (0.021%) placebo recipients from 16 completed or ongoing clinical trials. Of the 27 cases, 5 occurred following ROTARIX in clinical trials that were either not placebo-controlled or 1:1 randomized. In placebo-controlled trials, Kawasaki disease was reported in 17 recipients of ROTARIX and 9 placebo recipients [Relative Risk: 1.71 (95% CI: 0.71, 4.38)]. Three of the 27 cases were reported within 30 days post-vaccination: 2 cases (ROTARIX = 1, placebo = 1) were from placebo-controlled trials [Relative Risk: 1.00 (95% CI: 0.01, 78.35)] and one case following ROTARIX was from a non-placebo-controlled trial. Among recipients of ROTARIX, the time of onset after study dose ranged 3 days to 19 months.

6.2 Postmarketing Experience

The temporal association between vaccination with ROTARIX and intussusception was evaluated in a hospital-based active surveillance study that identified infants with intussusception at participating hospitals in Mexico. Using a self-controlled case series method,[2] the incidence of intussusception during the first 7 days after receipt of ROTARIX and during the 31-day period after receipt of ROTARIX was compared to a control period. The control period was from birth to one year, excluding the pre-defined risk period (first 7 days or first 31 days post-vaccination, respectively).

Over a 2-year period, the participating hospitals provided health services to approximately 1 million infants under 1 year of age. Among 750 infants with intussusception, the relative incidence of intussusception in the 31–day period after the first dose of ROTARIX compared to the control period was 1.96 (95.5% CI: 1.46, 2.63)]; the relative incidence of intussusception in the first 7 days after the first dose of ROTARIX compared to the control period was 6.07 (95.5% CI: 4.20, 8.63).

The Mexico study did not take into account all medical conditions that may predispose infants to intussusception. The results may not be generalizable to US infants who have a lower background rate of intussusception than Mexican infants. However, if a temporal increase in the risk for intussusception following ROTARIX similar in magnitude to that observed in the Mexico study does exist in US infants, it is estimated that approximately 1 to 3 additional cases of intussusception hospitalizations would occur per 100,000 vaccinated infants in the US within 7 days following the first dose of ROTARIX. In the first year of life, the background rate of intussusception hospitalizations in the US has been estimated to be approximately 34 per 100,000 infants.[3]

Worldwide passive postmarketing surveillance data also suggest that most cases of intussusception reported following ROTARIX occur in the 7-day period after the first dose.

The following adverse events have been reported since market introduction of ROTARIX. Because these events are reported voluntarily from a population of uncertain size, it is not always possible to reliably estimate their frequency or establish a causal relationship to vaccination with ROTARIX.

Gastrointestinal Disorders: Intussusception (including death), recurrent intussusception (including death), hematochezia, gastroenteritis with vaccine viral shedding in infants with Severe Combined Immunodeficiency Disease (SCID).

Blood and Lymphatic System Disorders: Idiopathic thrombocytopenic purpura.

Vascular Disorders: Kawasaki disease.

General Disorders and Administration Site Conditions: Maladministration.

7 DRUG INTERACTIONS

7.1 Concomitant Vaccine Administration

In clinical trials, ROTARIX was administered concomitantly with US-licensed and non-US-licensed vaccines. In a US coadministration study in 484 infants, there was no evidence of interference in the immune responses to any of the antigens when PEDIARIX® [Diphtheria and Tetanus Toxoids and Acellular Pertussis Adsorbed, Hepatitis B (Recombinant) and Inactivated Poliovirus Vaccine], a US-licensed 7-valent pneumococcal conjugate vaccine (Wyeth Pharmaceuticals Inc.), and a US-licensed Hib conjugate vaccine (Sanofi Pasteur SA) were coadministered with ROTARIX as compared with separate administration of ROTARIX.

7.2 Immunosuppressive Therapies

Immunosuppressive therapies, including irradiation, antimetabolites, alkylating agents, cytotoxic drugs, and corticosteroids (used in greater than physiologic doses), may reduce the immune response to ROTARIX. *[See Warnings and Precautions (5.3).]*

8 USE IN SPECIFIC POPULATIONS

8.1 Pregnancy

Pregnancy Category C

Animal reproduction studies have not been conducted with ROTARIX. It is also not known whether ROTARIX can cause fetal harm when administered to a pregnant woman or can affect reproduction capacity.

8.4 Pediatric Use

Safety and effectiveness of ROTARIX in infants younger than 6 weeks or older than 24 weeks of age have not been evaluated.

The effectiveness of ROTARIX in pre-term infants has not been established. Safety data are available in pre-term infants (ROTARIX = 134, placebo = 120) with a reported gestational age ≤36 weeks. These pre-term infants were followed for serious adverse events up to 30 to 90 days after dose 2. Serious adverse events were observed in 5.2% of recipients of ROTARIX as compared with 5.0% of placebo recipients. No deaths or cases of intussusception were reported in this population.

11 DESCRIPTION

ROTARIX (Rotavirus Vaccine, Live, Oral), for oral administration, is a live, attenuated rotavirus vaccine derived from the human 89-12 strain which belongs to G1P[8] type. The rotavirus strain is propagated on Vero cells. After reconstitution, the final formulation (1 mL) contains at least $10^{6.0}$ median Cell Culture Infective Dose ($CCID_{50}$) of live, attenuated rotavirus.

Table 3. Intussusception Cases by Day Range in Relation to Dose

Day Range	Dose 1		Dose 2		Any Dose	
	ROTARIX N = 31,673	Placebo N = 31,552	ROTARIX N = 29,616	Placebo N = 29,465	ROTARIX N = 31,673	Placebo N = 31,552
0-7	0	0	2	0	2	0
8-14	0	0	0	2	0	2
15-21	1	1	2	1	3	2
22-30	0	1	1	2	1	3
Total (0-30)	1	2	5	5	6	7

The lyophilized vaccine contains amino acids, dextran, Dulbecco's Modified Eagle Medium (DMEM), sorbitol, and sucrose. DMEM contains the following ingredients: sodium chloride, potassium chloride, magnesium sulfate, ferric (III) nitrate, sodium phosphate, sodium pyruvate, D-glucose, concentrated vitamin solution, L-cystine, L-tyrosine, amino acids solution, L-glutamine, calcium chloride, sodium hydrogenocarbonate, and phenol red.

In the manufacturing process, porcine-derived materials are used. Porcine circovirus type 1 (PCV-1) is present in ROTARIX. PCV-1 is not known to cause disease in humans.

The liquid diluent contains calcium carbonate, sterile water, and xanthan. The diluent includes an antacid component (calcium carbonate) to protect the vaccine during passage through the stomach and prevent its inactivation due to the acidic environment of the stomach.

ROTARIX is available with a vial of lyophilized vaccine and a prefilled oral applicator of liquid diluent. The tip caps of the prefilled oral applicators may contain natural rubber latex. The vial stopper does not contain latex.

ROTARIX contains no preservatives.

12 CLINICAL PHARMACOLOGY

12.1 Mechanism of Action

Prior to rotavirus vaccination programs, rotavirus infected nearly all children by the time they were 5 years of age. Severe, dehydrating rotavirus gastroenteritis occurs primarily among children aged 3 to 35 months.[4] Among children up to 3 years of age, approximately 16% of cases before 6 months of age result in hospitalization.[5]

The exact immunologic mechanism by which ROTARIX protects against rotavirus gastroenteritis is unknown *[see Clinical Pharmacology (12.2)]*. ROTARIX contains a live, attenuated human rotavirus that replicates in the small intestine and induces immunity.

12.2 Pharmacodynamics

Immunogenicity: A relationship between antibody responses to rotavirus vaccination and protection against rotavirus gastroenteritis has not been established. Seroconversion was defined as the appearance of anti-rotavirus IgA antibodies (concentration ≥20 U/mL) post-vaccination in the serum of infants previously negative for rotavirus. In 2 safety and efficacy studies, one to two months after a 2-dose series, 86.5% of 787 recipients of ROTARIX seroconverted compared with 6.7% of 420 placebo recipients and 76.8% of 393 recipients of ROTARIX seroconverted compared with 9.7% of 341 placebo recipients, respectively.

Shedding and Transmission: A prospective, randomized, double-blind, placebo-controlled study was performed in the Dominican Republic in twins within the same household to assess whether transmission of vaccine virus occurs from a vaccinated infant to a non-vaccinated infant. One hundred pairs of healthy twins 6 to 14 weeks of age (gestational age ≥32 weeks) were randomized with one twin to receive ROTARIX (N = 100) and the other twin to receive placebo (N = 100). Twenty subjects in each arm were excluded for reasons such as having rotavirus antibody at baseline. Stool samples were collected on the day of or 1 day prior to each dose, as well as 3 times weekly for 6 consecutive weeks after each dose of ROTARIX or placebo. Transmission was defined as presence of the vaccine virus strain in any stool sample from a twin receiving placebo.

Transmitted vaccine virus was identified in 15 of 80 twins receiving placebo (18.8% [95% CI: 10.9, 29.0]). Median duration of the rotavirus shedding was 10 days in twins who received ROTARIX as compared to 4 days in twins who received placebo in whom the vaccine virus was transmitted. In the 15 twins who received placebo, no gastrointestinal symptoms related to transmitted vaccine virus were observed.

13 NONCLINICAL TOXICOLOGY

13.1 Carcinogenesis, Mutagenesis, Impairment of Fertility

ROTARIX has not been evaluated for carcinogenic or mutagenic potential, or for impairment of fertility.

14 CLINICAL STUDIES

14.1 Efficacy Studies

The data demonstrating the efficacy of ROTARIX in preventing rotavirus gastroenteritis come from 24,163 infants randomized in two placebo-controlled studies conducted in 17 countries in Europe and Latin America. In these studies, oral polio vaccine (OPV) was not coadministered; however, other routine childhood vaccines could be concomitantly administered. Breast-feeding was permitted in both studies.

A randomized, double-blind, placebo-controlled study was conducted in 6 European countries. A total of 3,994 infants were enrolled to receive ROTARIX (n = 2,646) or placebo (n = 1,348). Vaccine or placebo was given to healthy infants as a 2-dose series with the first dose administered orally from 6 through 14 weeks of age followed by one additional dose administered at least 4 weeks after the first dose. The 2-dose series was completed by 24 weeks of age. For both vaccination groups, 98.3% of infants were white and 53% were male.

The clinical case definition of rotavirus gastroenteritis was an episode of diarrhea (passage of 3 or more loose or watery stools within a day), with or without vomiting, where rotavirus was identified in a stool sample. Severity of gastroenteritis was determined by a clinical scoring system, the Vesikari scale, assessing the duration and intensity of diarrhea and vomiting, the intensity of fever, use of rehydration therapy or hospitalization for each episode. Scores range from 0 to 20, where higher scores indicate greater severity. An episode of gastroenteritis with a score of 11 or greater was considered severe.[6]

The primary efficacy endpoint was prevention of any grade of severity of rotavirus gastroenteritis caused by naturally occurring rotavirus from 2 weeks after the second dose through one rotavirus season (according to protocol, ATP). Other efficacy evaluations included prevention of severe rotavirus gastroenteritis, as defined by the Vesikari scale, and reductions in hospitalizations due to rotavirus gastroenteritis and all cause gastroenteritis regardless of presumed etiology. Analyses were also done to evaluate the efficacy of ROTARIX against rotavirus gastroenteritis among infants who received at least one vaccination (total vaccinated cohort, TVC).

Efficacy of ROTARIX against any grade of severity of rotavirus gastroenteritis through one rotavirus season was 87.1% (95% CI: 79.6, 92.1); TVC efficacy was 87.3% (95% CI: 80.3, 92.0). Efficacy against severe rotavirus gastroenteritis through one rotavirus season was 95.8% (95% CI: 89.6, 98.7); TVC efficacy was 96.0% (95% CI: 90.2, 98.8) (Table 4). The protective effect of ROTARIX against any grade of severity of rotavirus gastroenteritis observed immediately following dose 1 administration and prior to dose 2 was 89.8% (95% CI: 8.9, 99.8).

Efficacy of ROTARIX in reducing hospitalizations for rotavirus gastroenteritis through one rotavirus season was 100% (95% CI: 81.8, 100); TVC efficacy was 100% (95% CI: 81.7, 100) (Table 4). ROTARIX reduced hospitalizations for all cause gastroenteritis regardless of presumed etiology by 74.7% (95% CI: 45.5, 88.9).

[See table 4 at top of next page]

A randomized, double-blind, placebo-controlled study was conducted in 11 countries in Latin America and Finland. A total of 63,225 infants received ROTARIX (n = 31,673) or placebo (n = 31,552). An efficacy subset of these infants consisting of 20,169 infants from Latin America received ROTARIX (n = 10,159) or placebo (n = 10,010). Vaccine or placebo was given to healthy infants as a 2-dose series with the first dose administered orally from 6 through 13 weeks of age followed by one additional dose administered at least 4 weeks after the first dose. The 2-dose series was completed by the age of 24 weeks of age. For both vaccination groups, the racial distribution of the efficacy subset was as follows: Hispanic 85.8%, white 7.9%, black 1.1%, and other 5.2%; 51% were male.

The clinical case definition of severe rotavirus gastroenteritis was an episode of diarrhea (passage of 3 or more loose or watery stools within a day), with or without vomiting,

Table 4. Efficacy Evaluation of ROTARIX Through One Rotavirus Season

	According to Protocol [a]		Total Vaccinated Cohort [b]	
Infants in Cohort	**ROTARIX N = 2,572**	**Placebo N = 1,302**	**ROTARIX N = 2,646**	**Placebo N = 1,348**
Gastroenteritis cases				
Any severity	24	94	26	104
Severe[c]	5	60	5	64
Efficacy estimate against RV GE				
Any severity	87.1%[d]		87.3%[d]	
(95% CI)	(79.6, 92.1)		(80.3, 92.0)	
Severe[c]	95.8%[d]		96.0%[d]	
(95% CI)	(89.6, 98.7)		(90.2, 98.8)	
Cases of hospitalization due to RV GE	0	12	0	12
Efficacy in reducing hospitalizations due to RV GE	100%[d]		100%[d]	
(95% CI)	(81.8, 100)		(81.7, 100)	

RV GE = rotavirus gastroenteritis; CI = Confidence Interval.
[a]ATP analysis includes all infants in the efficacy cohort who received two doses of vaccine according to randomization.
[b]TVC analysis includes all infants in the efficacy cohort who received at least one dose of vaccine or placebo.
[c]Severe gastroenteritis defined as ≥11 on the Vesikari scale.
[d]Statistically significant vs. placebo (P <0.001).

Table 5. Efficacy Evaluation of ROTARIX Through One Year

	According to Protocol [a]		Total Vaccinated Cohort [b]	
Infants in Cohort	**ROTARIX N = 9,009**	**Placebo N = 8,858**	**ROTARIX N = 10,159**	**Placebo N = 10,010**
Gastroenteritis cases				
Severe	12	77	18	94
Efficacy estimate against RV GE				
Severe	84.7%[c]		81.1%[c]	
(95% CI)	(71.7, 92.4)		(68.5, 89.3)	
Cases of hospitalization due to RV GE	9	59	14	72
Efficacy in reducing hospitalizations due to RV GE	85.0%[c]		80.8%[c]	
(95% CI)	(69.6, 93.5)		(65.7, 90.0)	

RV GE = rotavirus gastroenteritis; CI = Confidence Interval.
[a]ATP analysis includes all infants in the efficacy cohort who received two doses of vaccine according to randomization.
[b]TVC analysis includes all infants in the efficacy cohort who received at least one dose of vaccine or placebo.
[c]Statistically significant vs. placebo (P <0.001).

where rotavirus was identified in a stool sample, requiring hospitalization and/or rehydration therapy equivalent to World Health Organization (WHO) plan B (oral rehydration therapy) or plan C (intravenous rehydration therapy) in a medical facility.

The primary efficacy endpoint was prevention of severe rotavirus gastroenteritis caused by naturally occurring rotavirus from 2 weeks after the second dose through one year (ATP). Analyses were done to evaluate the efficacy of ROTARIX against severe rotavirus gastroenteritis among infants who received at least one vaccination (TVC). Reduction in hospitalizations due to rotavirus gastroenteritis was also evaluated (ATP).

Efficacy of ROTARIX against severe rotavirus gastroenteritis through one year was 84.7% (95% CI: 71.7, 92.4); TVC efficacy was 81.1% (95% CI: 68.5, 89.3) (Table 5).

Efficacy of ROTARIX in reducing hospitalizations for rotavirus gastroenteritis through one year was 85.0% (95% CI: 69.6, 93.5); TVC efficacy was 80.8% (95% CI: 65.7, 90.0) (Table 5).

[See table 5 above]

14.2 Efficacy Through Two Rotavirus Seasons

The efficacy of ROTARIX persisting through two rotavirus seasons was evaluated in two studies.

In the European study, the efficacy of ROTARIX against any grade of severity of rotavirus gastroenteritis through two rotavirus seasons was 78.9% (95% CI: 72.7, 83.8). Efficacy in preventing any grade of severity of rotavirus gastroenteritis cases occurring only during the second season post-vaccination was 71.9% (95% CI: 61.2, 79.8). The efficacy of ROTARIX against severe rotavirus gastroenteritis through two rotavirus seasons was 90.4% (95% CI: 85.1, 94.1). Efficacy in preventing severe rotavirus gastroenteritis cases occurring only during the second season post-vaccination was 85.6% (95% CI: 75.8, 91.9).

The efficacy of ROTARIX in reducing hospitalizations for rotavirus gastroenteritis through two rotavirus seasons was 96.0% (95% CI: 83.8, 99.5).

In the Latin American study, the efficacy of ROTARIX against severe rotavirus gastroenteritis through two years was 80.5% (95% CI: 71.3, 87.1). Efficacy in preventing severe rotavirus gastroenteritis cases occurring only during the second year post-vaccination was 79.0% (95% CI: 66.4, 87.4). The efficacy of ROTARIX in reducing hospitalizations for rotavirus gastroenteritis through two years was 83.0% (95% CI: 73.1, 89.7).

The efficacy of ROTARIX beyond the second season post-vaccination was not evaluated.

14.3 Efficacy Against Specific Rotavirus Types

The type-specific efficacy against any grade of severity and severe rotavirus gastroenteritis caused by G1P[8], G3P[8], G4P[8], G9P[8], and combined non-G1 (G2, G3, G4, G9) types was statistically significant through one year. Additionally, type-specific efficacy against any grade of severity and severe rotavirus gastroenteritis caused by G1P[8], G2P[4], G3P[8], G4P[8], G9P[8], and combined non-G1 (G2, G3, G4, G9) types was statistically significant through two years (Table 6).

[See table 6 at top of next page]

15 REFERENCES

1. Murphy TV, Gargiullo PM, Massoudi MS, et al. Intussusception among infants given an oral rotavirus vaccine. *N Engl J Med* 2001;344:564–572.
2. Farrington CP, Whitaker HJ, Hocine MN, et al. Case series analysis for censored, perturbed, or curtailed post-event exposures. *Biostatistics* 2009;10(1):3–16.
3. Tate JE, Simonsen L, Viboud C, et al. Trends in intussusception hospitalizations among US infants, 1993–2004: implications for monitoring the safety of the new rotavirus vaccination program. *Pediatrics* 2008;121:e1125-e1132.
4. Centers for Disease Control and Prevention. Prevention of rotavirus gastroenteritis among infants and children. Recommendations of the Advisory Committee on Immunization Practices (ACIP). *MMWR* 2006;55(No. RR-12):1-13.
5. Parashar UD, Holman RC, Clarke MJ, et al. Hospitalizations associated with rotavirus diarrhea in the United States, 1993 through 1995: surveillance based on the new ICD-9-CM rotavirus-specific diagnostic code. *J Infect Dis* 1998;177:13-17.
6. Ruuska T, Vesikari T. Rotavirus disease in Finnish children: use of numerical scores for severity of diarrheal episodes. *Scand J Infect Dis* 1990;22:259-267.

16 HOW SUPPLIED/STORAGE AND HANDLING

ROTARIX is available as a vial of lyophilized vaccine, a prefilled oral applicator of liquid diluent (1 mL) with a plunger stopper, and a transfer adapter for reconstitution.

Supplied as:

NDC 58160-851-01 Vial (contains no latex) and NDC 58160-853-02 Applicator (tip cap may contain latex) in Package of 10: NDC 58160-854-52

16.1 Storage Before Reconstitution

- Vials: Store the vials of lyophilized ROTARIX refrigerated at 2° to 8°C (36° to 46°F). **Protect vials from light.**
- Diluent: The diluent may be stored at a controlled room temperature 20° to 25°C (68° to 77°F). **Do not freeze. Discard if the diluent has been frozen.**

16.2 Storage After Reconstitution

ROTARIX should be administered within 24 hours of reconstitution. It may be stored refrigerated at 2° to 8°C (36° to 46°F) or at room temperature up to 25°C (77°F), after reconstitution. Discard the reconstituted vaccine if not used within 24 hours in biological waste container. **Do not freeze. Discard if the vaccine has been frozen.**

17 PATIENT COUNSELING INFORMATION

See FDA-approved patient labeling. Patient labeling is provided as a tear-off leaflet at the end of this full prescribing information.

17.1 Patient Advice

- Parents or guardians should be informed by the healthcare provider of the potential benefits and risks of immunization with ROTARIX, and of the importance of completing the immunization series.
- The healthcare provider should inform the parents or guardians about the potential for adverse reactions that have been temporally associated with administration of ROTARIX or other vaccines containing similar components.
- The parent or guardian should immediately report any signs and/or symptoms of intussusception.
- The parent or guardian accompanying the recipient should be instructed to report any adverse events to their healthcare provider.
- The parent or guardian should be given the Vaccine Information Statements, which are required by the National Childhood Vaccine Injury Act of 1986 to be given prior to immunization. These materials are available free of charge at the Centers for Disease Control and Prevention (CDC) website (www.cdc.gov/vaccines).

ROTARIX and PEDIARIX are registered trademarks of GlaxoSmithKline.

Manufactured by **GlaxoSmithKline Biologicals**
Rixensart, Belgium, US License 1617
Distributed by **GlaxoSmithKline**
Research Triangle Park, NC 27709

RTX:12PI

PATIENT INFORMATION

ROTARIX® (ROW-tah-rix)

Rotavirus Vaccine, Live, Oral

Read this Patient Information carefully before your baby gets ROTARIX and before your baby receives the next dose of ROTARIX. This leaflet is a summary of information about ROTARIX and does not take the place of talking with your baby's doctor.

What is ROTARIX?

ROTARIX is a vaccine that protects your baby from a kind of virus (called a rotavirus) that can cause bad diarrhea and vomiting. Rotavirus can cause diarrhea and vomiting that is so bad that your baby can lose too much body fluid and need to go to the hospital.

Rotavirus vaccine is a liquid that is given to your baby by mouth. It is not a shot.

Who should not take ROTARIX?

Your baby should not get ROTARIX if:

- He or she has had an allergic reaction after getting a dose of ROTARIX.
- He or she is allergic to any of the ingredients of this vaccine. A list of ingredients can be found at the end of this leaflet.
- A doctor has told you that your baby's digestive system has a defect (is not normal).
- He or she has a history of a serious problem called intussusception that happens when a part of the intestine gets blocked or twisted.

Table 6. Type-Specific Efficacy of ROTARIX Against Any Grade of Severity and Severe Rotavirus Gastroenteritis (According to Protocol)

	Through One Rotavirus Season			Through Two Rotavirus Seasons		
	Number of Cases			Number of Cases		
Type Identified[a]	ROTARIX N = 2,572	Placebo N = 1,302	% Efficacy (95% CI)	ROTARIX N = 2,572	Placebo N = 1,302	% Efficacy (95% CI)
ANY GRADE OF SEVERITY						
G1P[8]	4	46	95.6%[b] (87.9, 98.8)	18	89[c,d]	89.8%[b] (82.9, 94.2)
G2P[4]	3	4[c]	NS	14	17[c]	58.3%[b] (10.1, 81.0)
G3P[8]	1	5	89.9%[b] (9.5, 99.8)	3	10	84.8%[b] (41.0, 97.3)
G4P[8]	3	13	88.3%[b] (57.5, 97.9)	6	18	83.1%[b] (55.6, 94.5)
G9P[8]	13	27	75.6%[b] (51.1, 88.5)	38	71[d]	72.9%[b] (59.3, 82.2)
Combined non-G1 (G2, G3, G4, G9, G12) types[e]	20	49	79.3%[b] (64.6, 88.4)	62	116	72.9%[b] (62.9, 80.5)
SEVERE						
G1P[8]	2	28	96.4%[b] (85.7, 99.6)	4	57	96.4%[b] (90.4, 99.1)
G2P[4]	1	2[c]	NS	2	7[c]	85.5%[b] (24.0, 98.5)
G3P[8]	0	5	100%[b] (44.8, 100)	1	8	93.7%[b] (52.8, 99.9)
G4P[8]	0	7	100%[b] (64.9, 100)	1	11	95.4%[b] (68.3, 99.9)
G9P[8]	2	19	94.7%[b] (77.9, 99.4)	13	44[d]	85.0%[b] (71.7, 92.6)
Combined non-G1 (G2, G3, G4, G9, G12) types[e]	3	33	95.4%[b] (85.3, 99.1)	17	70	87.7%[b] (78.9, 93.2)

CI = Confidence Interval; NS = Not significant.
[a]Statistical analyses done by G type; if more than one rotavirus type was detected from a rotavirus gastroenteritis episode, the episode was counted in each of the detected rotavirus type categories.
[b]Statistically significant vs. placebo (P <0.05).
[c]The P genotype was not typeable for one episode.
[d]P[8] genotype was not detected in one episode.
[e]Two cases of G12P[8] were isolated in the second season (one in each group).

- He or she has Severe Combined Immunodeficiency Disease (SCID), a severe problem with his/her immune system.

Tell your doctor if your baby:

- Is allergic to latex.
- Has problems with his/her immune system.
- Has cancer.
- Will be in close contact with someone who has problems with his/her immune system or is getting treated for cancer as the spread of vaccine virus to non-vaccinated contacts could occur. Hand washing is recommended after diaper changes to help prevent the spread of vaccine virus.

If your baby has been having diarrhea and vomiting, your doctor may want to wait before giving your baby a dose of ROTARIX.

What are possible side effects of ROTARIX?

The most common side effects of ROTARIX are:

- Crying
- Fussiness
- Cough
- Runny nose
- Fever
- Loss of appetite
- Vomiting.

Call your doctor right away or go to the emergency department if your baby has any of these problems after getting ROTARIX, especially if symptoms occur in the first 7 days after the first dose, but even if it has been several weeks since the last vaccine dose because these may be signs of a serious problem called intussusception:

- Bad vomiting
- Bad diarrhea
- Bloody bowel movement
- High fever
- Severe stomach pain (if your baby brings his/her knees to his/her chest while crying or screaming).

A study in Mexico showed an increased risk of intussusception after the first dose, in the first month, but especially in the first 7 days.

Since FDA approval, reports of infants with intussusception have been received by Vaccine Adverse Event Reporting System (VAERS). Intussusception occurred days and sometimes weeks after vaccination. Some infants needed hospitalization, surgery on their intestines, or a special enema to treat this problem. Death due to intussusception has occurred.

Other reported side effects include: Kawasaki disease (a serious condition that can affect the heart; symptoms may include fever, rash, red eyes, red mouth, swollen glands, swollen hands, and feet and, if not treated, death can occur).

Talk to your baby's doctor if your baby has any problems that concern you.

How is ROTARIX given?

ROTARIX is a liquid that is dropped into your baby's mouth and swallowed.

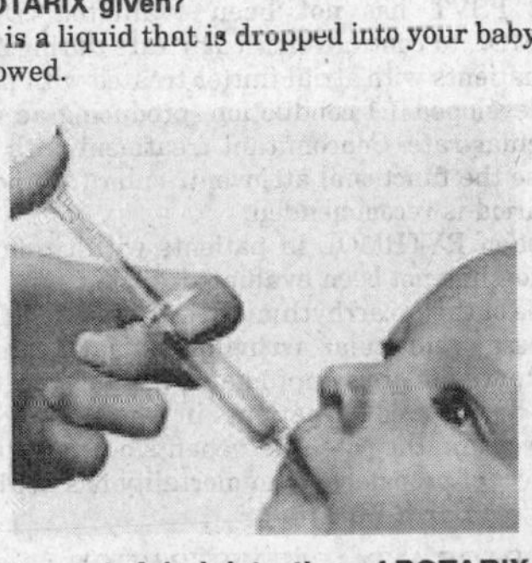

Figure 1. Administration of ROTARIX

Your baby will get the first dose at around 6 weeks old.

The second dose will be at least 4 weeks after the first dose (before 6 months old).

Be sure to plan the time for your baby's second dose with the doctor because it is important that your baby gets both doses of ROTARIX before your baby is 6 months old.

The doctor may decide to give your baby shots at the same time as ROTARIX.

Your baby can be fed normally after getting ROTARIX.

What are the ingredients in ROTARIX?

ROTARIX contains weakened human rotavirus.

ROTARIX also contains dextran, sorbitol, xanthan, and Dulbecco's Modified Eagle Medium (DMEM). The ingredients of DMEM are as follows: sodium chloride, potassium chloride, magnesium sulphate, ferric (III) nitrate, sodium phosphate, sodium pyruvate, D-glucose, concentrated vitamin solution, L-cystine, L-tyrosine, amino acids solution, L-glutamine, calcium chloride, sodium hydrogenocarbonate, and phenol red.

Porcine circovirus type 1 (PCV-1), a virus found in pigs, is present in ROTARIX. PCV-1 is not known to cause disease in humans.

ROTARIX contains no preservatives.

The dropper used to give your baby ROTARIX may contain latex.

ROTARIX is a registered trademark of GlaxoSmithKline.

Manufactured by **GlaxoSmithKline Biologicals**
Rixensart, Belgium, US License 1617
Distributed by **GlaxoSmithKline**
Research Triangle Park, NC 27709

September 2012
RTX:9PIL

RYTHMOL

℞

[*rith'-mol*]
(propafenone hydrochloride)
Tablets for oral use

HIGHLIGHTS OF PRESCRIBING INFORMATION

These highlights do not include all the information needed to use RYTHMOL safely and effectively. See full prescribing information for RYTHMOL.

RYTHMOL (propafenone hydrochloride) Tablets for oral use
Initial U.S. Approval: 1989

WARNING: MORTALITY

See full prescribing information for complete boxed warning.

- **An increased rate of death or reversed cardiac arrest rate was seen in patients treated with encainide or flecainide (Class IC antiarrhythmics) compared with that seen in patients assigned to placebo. At present it is prudent to consider any IC antiarrhythmic to have a significant risk of provoking proarrhythmic events in patients with structural heart disease.**
- **Given the lack of any evidence that these drugs improve survival, antiarrhythmic agents should generally be avoided in patients with non-life-threatening ventricular arrhythmias, even if the patients are experiencing unpleasant, but not life-threatening, symptoms or signs.**

RECENT MAJOR CHANGES

Contraindications (4) 03/2013
Warnings and Precautions, Unmasking Brugada Syndrome (5.2) 03/2013

INDICATIONS AND USAGE

RYTHMOL is an antiarrhythmic indicated to:

- prolong the time to recurrence of symptomatic atrial fibrillation (AF) in patients with episodic (most likely paroxysmal or persistent) AF who do not have structural heart disease. (1)
- prolong the time to recurrence of paroxysmal supraventricular tachycardia (PSVT) associated with disabling symptoms in patients who do not have structural heart disease. (1)
- treat documented life-threatening ventricular arrhythmias. (1)

Usage Considerations:

- Use in patients with permanent atrial fibrillation or with atrial flutter or PSVT has not been evaluated. Do not use to control ventricular rate during atrial fibrillation. (1)
- In patients with atrial fibrillation and atrial flutter, use RYTHMOL with drugs that increase the atrioventricular nodal refractory period. (1)
- Because of proarrhythmic effects, use with lesser ventricular arrhythmias is not recommended, even if patients are symptomatic. (1)

- The effect of propafenone on mortality has not been determined. (1)

DOSAGE AND ADMINISTRATION

- Initiate therapy with 150 mg given every 8 hours. (2)
- As needed, uptitrate in 3-4 days to 225-300 mg every 8 hours. (2)
- Consider reducing the dose in patients with hepatic impairment, significant widening of the QRS complex, or second or third degree AV block. (2)

DOSAGE FORMS AND STRENGTHS

Tablets: 150 mg, 225 mg. (3)

CONTRAINDICATIONS

- Heart failure, cardiogenic shock, or marked hypotension (4)
- Sinoatrial, atrioventricular, and intraventricular disorders of impulse generation or conduction in the absence of pacemaker (4)
- Known Brugada Syndrome (4)
- Bradycardia (4)
- Bronchospastic disorders and severe obstructive pulmonary disease (4)
- Marked electrolyte imbalance (4)

WARNINGS AND PRECAUTIONS

- May cause new or worsened arrhythmias. Evaluate patients via ECG prior to and during therapy. (5.1)
- RYTHMOL may unmask Brugada or Brugada-like Syndrome. (4, 5.2)
- Avoid use with other drugs that prolong the QT interval. (5.3)
- Avoid simultaneous use of propafenone with both a cytochrome P450 2D6 inhibitor and a 3A4 inhibitor. (5.4)
- May provoke overt heart failure. (5.5)
- May cause dose-related first degree AV block or other conduction disturbances. Only use in patients with conduction disorders who have pacemakers. (5.6)
- May affect artificial pacemakers.Monitor pacemaker function. (5.7)
- Agranulocytosis: Patients should report signs of infection. (5.8)
- May exacerbate myasthenia gravis. (5.11)

ADVERSE REACTIONS

The most commonly reported adverse events with propafenone (>5%) included: unusual taste, nausea and/or vomiting, dizziness, constipation, headache, fatigue, first degree AV block, and intraventricular conduction delay. (6.1)

To report SUSPECTED ADVERSE REACTIONS, contact GlaxoSmithKline at 1-888-825-5249 or FDA at 1-800-FDA-1088 or www.fda.gov/medwatch.

DRUG INTERACTIONS

- Inhibitors of CYP2D6, 1A2, and 3A4 increase propafenone exposure. (7.1)
- Propafenone may increase digoxin or warfarin levels. (7.2, 7.3)
- Orlistat may reduce propafenone exposure. Taper orlistat withdrawal. (7.4)
- Lidocaine may increase central nervous system side effects. (7.6)

See 17 for PATIENT COUNSELING INFORMATION and FDA-approved patient labeling

Revised: 06/2013

FULL PRESCRIBING INFORMATION: CONTENTS*

*** Sections or subsections omitted from the full prescribing information are not listed**

FULL PRESCRIBING INFORMATION

WARNING: MORTALITY

- **In the National Heart, Lung and Blood Institute's Cardiac Arrhythmia Suppression Trial (CAST), a long-term, multi-center, randomized, double-blind study in patients with asymptomatic non-life-threatening ventricular arrhythmias who had a myocardial infarction more than 6 days but less than 2 years previously, an increased rate of death or reversed cardiac arrest rate (7.7%; 56/730) was seen in patients treated with encainide or flecainide (Class IC antiarrhythmics) compared with that seen in patients assigned to placebo (3.0%; 22/725). The average duration of treatment with encainide or flecainide in this study was 10 months.**
- **The applicability of the CAST results to other populations (e.g., those without recent myocardial infarction) or other antiarrhythmic drugs is uncertain, but at present, it is prudent to consider any IC antiarrhythmic to have a significant proarrhythmic risk in patients with structural heart disease. Given the lack of any evidence that these drugs improve survival, antiarrhythmic agents should generally be avoided in patients with non-life-threatening ventricular arrhythmias, even if the patients are experiencing unpleasant, but not life-threatening, symptoms or signs.**

1 INDICATIONS AND USAGE

RYTHMOL is indicated to:

- prolong the time to recurrence of paroxysmal atrial fibrillation/flutter (PAF) associated with disabling symptoms in patients without structural heart disease.
- prolong the time to recurrence of paroxysmal supraventricular tachycardia (PSVT) associated with disabling symptoms in patients without structural heart disease.
- treat documented ventricular arrhythmias, such as sustained ventricular tachycardia that, in the judgment of the physician, are life-threatening. Initiate treatment in the hospital.

Usage Considerations:

- The use of RYTHMOL in patients with permanent atrial fibrillation (AF) or in patients exclusively with atrial flutter or PSVT has not been evaluated. Do not use RYTHMOL to control ventricular rate during AF.
- Some patients with atrial flutter treated with propafenone have developed 1:1 conduction, producing an increase in ventricular rate. Concomitant treatment with drugs that increase the functional atrioventricular (AV) nodal refractory period is recommended.
- The use of RYTHMOL in patients with chronic atrial fibrillation has not been evaluated.
- Because of the proarrhythmic effects of RYTHMOL, its use with lesser ventricular arrhythmias is not recommended, even if patients are symptomatic, and any use of the drug should be reserved for patients in whom, in the opinion of the physician, the potential benefits outweigh the risks.
- The effect of propafenone on mortality has not been determined *[see Boxed Warning]*.

2 DOSAGE AND ADMINISTRATION

The dose of RYTHMOL must be individually titrated on the basis of response and tolerance. Initiate therapy with RYTHMOL 150 mg given every eight hours (450 mg/day). Dosage may be increased at a minimum of 3 to 4 day intervals to 225 mg every 8 hours (675 mg/day). If additional therapeutic effect is needed, the dose of RYTHMOL may be increased to 300 mg every 8 hours (900 mg/day). The usefulness and safety of dosages exceeding 900 mg per day have not been established.

In patients with hepatic impairment or those with significant widening of the QRS complex or second or third degree AV block, consider reducing the dose.

As with other antiarrhythmic agents, in the elderly or in ventricular arrhythmia patients with marked previous myocardial damage, the dose of RYTHMOL should be increased more gradually during the initial phase of treatment.

The combination of CYP3A4 inhibition and either CYP2D6 deficiency or CYP2D6 inhibition with the simultaneous administration of propafenone may significantly increase the concentration of propafenone and thereby increase the risk of proarrhythmia and other adverse events. Therefore, avoid simultaneous use of RYTHMOL with both a CYP2D6 inhibitor and a CYP3A4 inhibitor *[see Warnings and Precautions (5.4) and Drug Interactions (7.1)]*.

3 DOSAGE FORMS AND STRENGTHS

150 mg and 225 mg scored, round, film-coated tablets.

4 CONTRAINDICATIONS

RYTHMOL is contraindicated in the following circumstances:

- Heart failure
- Cardiogenic shock
- Sinoatrial, atrioventricular and intraventricular disorders of impulse generation or conduction (e.g., sick sinus node syndrome, AV block) in the absence of an artificial pacemaker
- Known Brugada Syndrome
- Bradycardia
- Marked hypotension
- Bronchospastic disorders or severe obstructive pulmonary disease
- Marked electrolyte imbalance

5 WARNINGS AND PRECAUTIONS

5.1 Proarrhythmic Effects

Propafenone has caused new or worsened arrhythmias. Such proarrhythmic effects include sudden death and life-threatening ventricular arrhythmias such as ventricular fibrillation, ventricular tachycardia, asystole and torsade de pointes. It may also worsen premature ventricular contractions or supraventricular arrhythmias, and it may prolong the QT interval. It is therefore essential that each patient given RYTHMOL be evaluated electrocardiographically prior to and during therapy to determine whether the response to RYTHMOL supports continued treatment. Because propafenone prolongs the QRS interval in the electrocardiogram, changes in the QT interval are difficult to interpret *[see Clinical Pharmacology (12.2)]*.

In a U.S. uncontrolled, open label, multicenter trial in patients with symptomatic supraventricular tachycardia (SVT), 1.9% (9/474) of these patients experienced ventricular tachycardia (VT) or ventricular fibrillation (VF) during the study. However, in 4 of the 9 patients, the ventricular tachycardia was of atrial origin. Six of the nine patients that developed ventricular arrhythmias did so within 14 days of onset of therapy. About 2.3% (11/474) of all patients had a recurrence of SVT during the study which could have been a change in the patients' arrhythmia behavior or could represent a proarrhythmic event. Case reports in patients treated with propafenone for atrial fibrillation/flutter have included increased premature ventricular contractions (PVCs), VT, VF, torsade de pointes, asystole, and death.

Overall in clinical trials with RYTHMOL (which included patients treated for ventricular arrhythmias, atrial fibrillation/flutter, and PSVT), 4.7% of all patients had new or worsened ventricular arrhythmia possibly representing a proarrhythmic event (0.7% was an increase in PVCs; 4.0% a worsening, or new appearance, of VT or VF). Of the patients who had worsening of VT (4%), 92% had a history of VT and/or VT/VF, 71% had coronary artery disease, and 68% had a prior myocardial infarction. The incidence of proarrhythmia in patients with less serious or benign arrhythmias, which include patients with an increase in frequency of PVCs, was 1.6%. Although most proarrhythmic events occurred during the first week of therapy, late events also were seen and the CAST study *[see Boxed Warning: Mortality]* suggests that an increased risk of proarrythmia is present throughout treatment.

In a study of sustained-release propafenone (RYTHMOL SR®), there were too few deaths to assess the long term risk to patients. There were 5 deaths, 3 in the pooled RYTHMOL SR group (0.8%) and 2 in the placebo group (1.6%). In the overall RYTHMOL SR and RYTHMOL immediate-release database of 8 studies, the mortality rate was 2.5% per year on propafenone and 4.0% per year on placebo. Concurrent use of propafenone with other antiarrhythmic agents has not been well studied.

5.2 Unmasking Brugada Syndrome

Brugada Syndrome may be unmasked after exposure to RYTHMOL. Perform an ECG after initiation of RYTHMOL, and discontinue the drug if changes are suggestive of Brugada Syndrome *[see Contraindications (4)]*.

5.3 Use with Drugs that Prolong the QT Interval and Antiarrhythmic Agents

The use of RYTHMOL in conjunction with other drugs that prolong the QT interval has not been extensively studied. Such drugs may include many antiarrhythmics, some phenothiazines, tricyclic antidepressants, and oral macrolides. Withhold Class IA and III antiarrhythmic agents for at least 5 half-lives prior to dosing with RYTHMOL. Avoid the use of propafenone with Class IA and III antiarrhythmic agents (including quinidine and amiodarone). There is only limited experience with the concomitant use of Class IB or IC antiarrhythmics.

5.4 Drug Interactions: Simultaneous Use with Inhibitors of Cytochrome P450 Isoenzymes 2D6 and 3A4

Propafenone is metabolized by CYP2D6, CYP3A4, and CYP1A2 isoenzymes. Approximately 6% of Caucasians in the U.S. population are naturally deficient in CYP2D6 activity and to a somewhat lesser extent in other demographic groups. Drugs that inhibit these CYP pathways (such as desipramine, paroxetine, ritonavir, sertraline for CYP2D6; ketoconazole, erythromycin, saquinavir, and grapefruit juice for CYP3A4; and amiodarone and tobacco smoke for CYP1A2) can be expected to cause increased plasma levels of propafenone.

Increased exposure to propafenone may lead to cardiac arrhythmias and exaggerated beta-adrenergic blocking activity. Because of its metabolism, the combination of CYP3A4 inhibition and either CYP2D6 deficiency or CYP2D6 inhibition in users of propafenone is potentially hazardous. Therefore, avoid simultaneous use of RYTHMOL with both a CYP2D6 inhibitor and a CYP3A4 inhibitor.

5.5 Use in Patients with a History of Heart Failure

Propafenone exerts a negative inotropic activity on the myocardium as well as beta blockade effects and may provoke overt heart failure.

In clinical trial experience with RYTHMOL, new or worsened congestive heart failure (CHF) has been reported in 3.7% of patients with ventricular arrhythmia; of those 0.9% were considered probably or definitely related to propafenone HCl. Of the patients with CHF probably related to propafenone, 80% had preexisting heart failure and 85% had coronary artery disease. CHF attributable to propafenone HCl developed rarely (< 0.2%) in ventricular arrhythmia patients who had no previous history of CHF. CHF occurred in 1.9% of patients studied with PAF or PSVT.

In a U.S. trial of RYTHMOL SR in patients with symptomatic AF, heart failure was reported in 4 (1.0%) patients receiving RYTHMOL SR (all doses), compared to 1 (0.8%) patient receiving placebo.

5.6 Conduction Disturbances

Propafenone slows atrioventricular conduction and may also cause dose-related first degree AV block. Average PR interval prolongation and increases in QRS duration are also dose-related. Do not give propafenone to patients with atrioventricular and intraventricular conduction defects in the absence of a pacemaker *[see Contraindications (4) and Clinical Pharmacology (12.2)]*.

The incidence of first degree, second degree, and third degree AV block observed in 2,127 ventricular arrhythmia patients was 2.5%, 0.6%, and 0.2%, respectively. Development of second or third degree AV block requires a reduction in dosage or discontinuation of propafenone HCl. Bundle branch block (1.2%) and intraventricular conduction delay (1.1%) have been reported in patients receiving propafenone. Bradycardia has also been reported (1.5%). Experience in patients with sick sinus node syndrome is limited and these patients should not be treated with propafenone.

In a U.S. trial in 523 patients with a history of symptomatic AF treated with RYTHMOL SR, sinus bradycardia (rate <50 beats/min) was reported with the same frequency with RYTHMOL SR and placebo.

5.7 Effects on Pacemaker Threshold

Propafenone may alter both pacing and sensing thresholds of implanted pacemakers and defibrillators. During and after therapy, monitor and re-program these devices accordingly.

5.8 Agranulocytosis

Agranulocytosis has been reported in patients receiving propafenone. Generally, the agranulocytosis occurred within the first 2 months of propafenone therapy and upon discontinuation of therapy, the white count usually normalized by 14 days. Unexplained fever or decrease in white cell count, particularly during the initial 3 months of therapy, warrant consideration of possible agranulocytosis or granulocytopenia. Instruct patients to report promptly any signs of infection such as fever, sore throat, or chills.

5.9 Use in Patients with Hepatic Dysfunction

Propafenone is highly metabolized by the liver. Severe liver dysfunction increases the bioavailability of propafenone to approximately 70% compared to 3 to 40% in patients with normal liver function. In 8 patients with moderate to severe liver disease, the mean half-life was approximately 9 hours. Increased bioavailability of propafenone in these patients may result in excessive accumulation. Carefully monitor patients with impaired hepatic function for excessive pharmacological effects *[see Overdosage (10)]*.

5.10 Use in Patients with Renal Dysfunction

Approximately 50% of propafenone metabolites are excreted in the urine following administration of RYTHMOL.

In patients with impaired renal function, monitor for signs of overdosage *[see Overdosage (10)]*.

5.11 Use in Patients with Myasthenia Gravis

Exacerbation of myasthenia gravis has been reported during propafenone therapy.

5.12 Elevated ANA Titers

Positive ANA titers have been reported in patients receiving propafenone. They have been reversible upon cessation of treatment and may disappear even in the face of continued propafenone therapy. These laboratory findings were usually not associated with clinical symptoms, but there is one published case of drug-induced lupus erythematosis (positive rechallenge); it resolved completely upon discontinuation of therapy. Carefully evaluate patients who develop an abnormal ANA test and, if persistent or worsening elevation of ANA titers is detected, consider discontinuing therapy.

5.13 Impaired Spermatogenesis

Reversible disorders of spermatogenesis have been demonstrated in monkeys, dogs and rabbits after high dose intravenous administration of propafenone. Evaluation of the effects of short-term RYTHMOL administration on spermatogenesis in 11 normal subjects suggested that propafenone produced a reversible, short-term drop (within normal range) in sperm count.

6 ADVERSE REACTIONS

6.1 Clinical Trials Experience

Because clinical trials are conducted under widely varying conditions, adverse reaction rates observed in the clinical trials of a drug cannot be directly compared to rates in the clinical trials of another drug and may not reflect the rates observed in practice.

Adverse reactions associated with RYTHMOL occur most frequently in the gastrointestinal, cardiovascular, and central nervous systems. About 20% of patients treated with RYTHMOL have discontinued treatment because of adverse reactions.

Adverse reactions reported for > 1.5% of 474 SVT patients who received RYTHMOL in U.S. clinical trials are presented in Table 1 by incidence and percent discontinuation, reported to the nearest percent.

Table 1: Adverse Reactions Reported for > 1.5% of SVT Patients

	Incidence (N = 480)	% of Pts. Who Discontinued
Unusual Taste	14%	1.3%
Nausea and/or Vomiting	11%	2.9%
Dizziness	9%	1.7%
Constipation	8%	0.2%
Headache	6%	0.8%
Fatigue	6%	1.5%
Blurred Vision	3%	0.6%
Weakness	3%	1.3%
Dyspnea	2%	1.0%
Wide Complex Tachycardia	2%	1.9%
CHF	2%	0.6%
Bradycardia	2%	0.2%
Palpitations	2%	0.2%
Tremor	2%	0.4%
Anorexia	2%	0.2%
Diarrhea	2%	0.4%
Ataxia	2%	0.0%

In controlled trials in patients with ventricular arrhythmia, the most common reactions reported for RYTHMOL and more frequent than on placebo were unusual taste, dizziness, first degree AV block, intraventricular conduction delay, nausea and/or vomiting, and constipation. Headache was relatively common also, but was not increased compared to placebo. Other reactions reported more frequently than on placebo or comparator and not already reported elsewhere included anxiety, angina, second degree AV block, bundle branch block, loss of balance, congestive heart failure, and dyspepsia.

Adverse reactions reported for ≥ 1% of 2,127 ventricular arrhythmia patients who received propafenone in U.S. clinical trials were evaluated by daily dose. The most common adverse reactions appeared dose-related (but note that most patients spent more time at the larger doses), especially dizziness, nausea and/or vomiting, unusual taste, constipation, and blurred vision. Some less common reactions may also have been dose-related such as first degree AV block, congestive heart failure, dyspepsia, and weakness. Other adverse reactions included rash, syncope, chest pain, abdominal pain, ataxia, and hypotension.

In addition, the following adverse reactions were reported less frequently than 1% either in clinical trials or in marketing experience. Causality and relationship to propafenone therapy cannot necessarily be judged from these events.

Cardiovascular System: Atrial flutter, AV dissociation, cardiac arrest, flushing, hot flashes, sick sinus syndrome, sinus pause or arrest, supraventricular tachycardia.

Nervous System: Abnormal dreams, abnormal speech, abnormal vision, confusion, depression, memory loss, numbness, paresthesias, psychosis/mania, seizures (0.3%), tinnitus, unusual smell sensation, vertigo.

Gastrointestinal: Cholestasis , elevated liver enzymes (alkaline phosphatase, serum transaminases) , gastroenteritis, hepatitis .

Hematologic: Agranulocytosis, anemia, bruising, granulocytopenia, leukopenia, purpura, thrombocytopenia.

Other: Alopecia, eye irritation, impotence, increased glucose, positive ANA (0.7%), muscle cramps, muscle weakness, nephrotic syndrome, pain, pruritus.

6.2 Postmarketing Experience

The following adverse reactions have been identified during post-approval use of RYTHMOL. Because these reactions are reported voluntarily from a population of uncertain size, it is not always possible to reliably estimate their frequency or establish a causal relationship to drug exposure.

Gastrointestinal: A number of patients with liver abnormalities associated with propafenone therapy have been reported in post-marketing experience. Some appeared due to hepatocellular injury, some were cholestatic and some showed a mixed picture. Some of these reports were simply discovered through clinical chemistries, others because of clinical symptoms including fulminant hepatitis and death. One case was rechallenged with a positive outcome.

Blood and Lymphatic System: Increased bleeding time

Immune System: Lupus erythematosis

Nervous System: Apnea, coma

Renal and Urinary: Hyponatremia/inappropriate ADH secretion, kidney failure

7 DRUG INTERACTIONS

7.1 CYP2D6 and CYP3A4 Inhibitors

Drugs that inhibit CYP2D6 (such as desipramine, paroxetine, ritonavir, or sertraline) and CYP3A4 (such as ketoconazole, ritonavir, saquinavir, erythromycin, or grapefruit juice) can be expected to cause increased plasma levels of propafenone. The combination of CYP3A4 inhibition and either CYP2D6 deficiency or CYP2D6 inhibition with administration of propafenone may increase the risk of adverse reactions, including proarrhythmia. Therefore, simultaneous use of RYTHMOL with both a CYP2D6 inhibitor and a CYP3A4 inhibitor should be avoided *[see Warnings and Precautions (5.4) and Dosage and Administration (2)]*.

Amiodarone: Concomitant administration of propafenone and amiodarone can affect conduction and repolarization and is not recommended.

Cimetidine: Concomitant administration of propafenone immediate release tablets and cimetidine in 12 healthy subjects resulted in a 20% increase in steady-state plasma concentrations of propafenone.

Fluoxetine: Concomitant administration of propafenone and fluoxetine in extensive metabolizers increased the S-propafenone C_{max} and AUC by 39% and 50% and the R propafenone C_{max} and AUC by 71% and 50%.

Quinidine: Small doses of quinidine completely inhibit the CYP2D6 hydroxylation metabolic pathway, making all patients, in effect, slow metabolizers *[see Clinical Pharmacology (12)]*. Concomitant administration of quinidine (50 mg three times daily) with 150 mg immediate release propafenone three times daily decreased the clearance of propafenone by 60% in extensive metabolizers, making them slow metabolizers. Steady-state plasma concentra-

Table 2: Mean Changes in Electrocardiogram Intervals [a]

	Total Daily Dose (mg)							
	337.5 mg		450 mg		675 mg		900 mg	
Interval	msec	%	msec	%	msec	%	msec	%
RR	-14.5	-1.8	30.6	3.8	31.5	3.9	41.7	5.1
PR	3.6	2.1	19.1	11.6	28.9	17.8	35.6	21.9
QRS	5.6	6.4	5.5	6.1	7.7	8.4	15.6	17.3
QTc	2.7	0.7	-7.5	-1.8	5.0	1.2	14.7	3.7

[a] Change and percent change based on mean baseline values for each treatment group.

tions more than doubled for propafenone, and decreased 50% for 5-OH-propafenone. A 100 mg dose of quinidine tripled steady state concentrations of propafenone. Avoid concomitant use of propafenone and quinidine.

Rifampin: Concomitant administration of rifampin and propafenone in extensive metabolizers decreased the plasma concentrations of propafenone by 67% with a corresponding decrease of 5-OH-propafenone by 65%. The concentrations of norpropafenone increased by 30%. In slow metabolizers, there was a 50% decrease in propafenone plasma concentrations and increased the AUC and C_{max} of norpropafenone by 74% and 20%, respectively. Urinary excretion of propafenone and its metabolites decreased significantly. Similar results were noted in elderly patients: Both the AUC and C_{max} propafenone decreased by 84%, with a corresponding decrease in AUC and C_{max} of 5-OH–propafenone by 69% and 57%.

7.2 Digoxin

Concomitant use of propafenone and digoxin increased steady-state serum digoxin exposure (AUC) in patients by 60% to 270%, and decreased the clearance of digoxin by 31% to 67%. Monitor plasma digoxin levels of patients receiving propafenone and adjust digoxin dosage as needed.

7.3 Warfarin

The concomitant administration of propafenone and warfarin increased warfarin plasma concentrations at steady state by 39% in healthy volunteers and prolonged the prothrombin time (PT) in patients taking warfarin. Adjust the warfarin dose as needed by monitoring INR (international normalized ratio).

7.4 Orlistat

Orlistat may limit the fraction of propafenone available for absorption. In post marketing reports, abrupt cessation of orlistat in patients stabilized on propafenone has resulted in severe adverse events including convulsions, atrioventricular block and acute circulatory failure.

7.5 Beta-Antagonists

Concomitant use of propafenone and propranolol in healthy subjects increased propranolol plasma concentrations at steady state by 113%. In 4 patients, administration of metoprolol with propafenone increased the metoprolol plasma concentrations at steady state by 100% to 400%. The pharmacokinetics of propafenone was not affected by the coadministration of either propranolol or metoprolol. In clinical trials using propafenone immediate release tablets, patients who were receiving beta-blockers concurrently did not experience an increased incidence of side effects.

7.6 Lidocaine

No significant effects on the pharmacokinetics of propafenone or lidocaine have been seen following their concomitant use in patients. However, concomitant use of propafenone and lidocaine has been reported to increase the risks of central nervous system side effects of lidocaine.

8 USE IN SPECIFIC POPULATIONS

8.1 Pregnancy

Pregnancy Category C. There are no adequate and well-controlled studies in pregnant women. RYTHMOL should be used during pregnancy only if the potential benefit justifies the potential risk to the fetus.

Animal Data: *Teratogenic Effects:* Propafenone has been shown to be embryotoxic (decreased survival) in rabbits and rats when given in oral maternally toxic doses of 150 mg/kg day (about 3 times the maximum recommended human dose [MRHD] on a mg/m^2 basis) and 600 mg/kg/day (about 6 times the MRHD on a mg/m^2 basis), respectively. Although maternally tolerated doses (up to 270 mg/kg/day, about 3 times the MRHD on a mg/m^2 basis) produced no evidence of embryotoxicity in rats, post-implantation loss was elevated in all rabbit treatment groups (doses as low as 15 mg/kg/day, about 1/3 the MRHD on a mg/m^2 basis).

Non-teratogenic Effects: In a study in which female rats received daily oral doses of propafenone from mid-gestation through weaning of their offspring, doses as low as 90 mg/kg/day (equivalent to the MRHD on a mg/m^2 basis) produced increases in maternal deaths. Doses of 360 or more mg/kg/day (4 or more times the MRHD on a mg/m^2 basis) resulted in reductions in neonatal survival, body weight gain and physiological development.

8.2 Labor and Delivery

It is not known whether the use of propafenone during labor or delivery has immediate or delayed adverse effects on the fetus, or whether it prolongs the duration of labor or increases the need for forceps delivery or other obstetrical intervention.

8.3 Nursing Mothers

Propafenone is excreted in human milk. Because of the potential for serious adverse reactions in nursing infants from propafenone, decide whether to discontinue nursing or to discontinue the drug, taking into account the importance of the drug to the mother.

8.4 Pediatric Use

The safety and effectiveness of propafenone in pediatric patients have not been established.

8.5 Geriatric Use

Clinical studies of RYTHMOL did not include sufficient numbers of subjects aged 65 and over to determine whether they respond differently from younger subjects. Other reported clinical experience has not identified differences in responses between the elderly and younger patients. In general, dose selection for an elderly patient should be cautious, usually starting at the low end of the dosing range, reflecting the greater frequency of decreased hepatic, renal, or cardiac function, and of concomitant disease or other drug therapy.

10 OVERDOSAGE

The symptoms of overdosage may include hypotension, somnolence, bradycardia, intra-atrial and intraventricular conduction disturbances, and rarely convulsions and high grade ventricular arrhythmias. Defibrillation as well as infusion of dopamine and isoproterenol have been effective in controlling abnormal rhythm and blood pressure. Convulsions have been alleviated with intravenous diazepam. General supportive measures such as mechanical respiratory assistance and external cardiac massage may be necessary. The hemodialysis of propafenone in patients with an overdose is expected to be of limited value in the removal of propafenone as a result of both its high protein binding (>95%) and large volume of distribution.

11 DESCRIPTION

RYTHMOL(propafenone hydrochloride) is an antiarrhythmic drug supplied in scored, film-coated tablets of 150 and 225 mg for oral administration. Propafenone has some structural similarities to beta-blocking agents.

Chemically, propafenone hydrochloride (HCl) is 2′-[2-Hydroxy-3-(propylamino)-propoxy]-3-phenylpropiophenone hydrochloride, with a molecular weight of 377.92. The molecular formula is $C_{21}H_{27}NO_3 \bullet HCl$.The structural formula of propafenone HCl is given below:

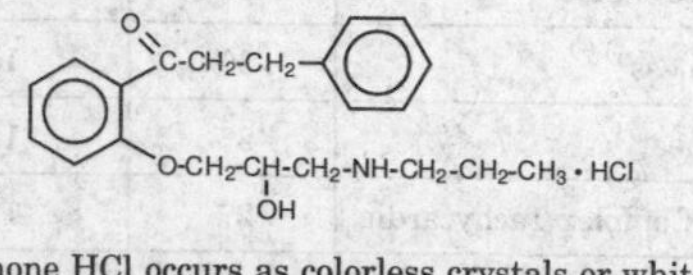

Propafenone HCl occurs as colorless crystals or white crystalline powder with a very bitter taste. It is slightly soluble in water (20°C), chloroform and ethanol. The following inactive ingredients are contained in the tablet: corn starch, hypromellose, magnesium stearate, polyethylene glycol, polysorbate, povidone, propylene glycol, sodium starch glycolate, and titanium dioxide.

12 CLINICAL PHARMACOLOGY

12.1 Mechanism of Action

Propafenone is a Class 1C antiarrhythmic drug with local anesthetic effects, and a direct stabilizing action on myocardial membranes. The electrophysiological effect of propafenone manifests itself in a reduction of upstroke velocity (Phase 0) of the monophasic action potential. In Purkinje fibers, and to a lesser extent myocardial fibers, propafenone reduces the fast inward current carried by sodium ions. Diastolic excitability threshold is increased and effective refractory period prolonged. Propafenone reduces spontaneous automaticity and depresses triggered activity. Studies in anesthetized dogs and isolated organ preparations show that propafenone has beta-sympatholytic activity at about 1/50 the potency of propranolol. Clinical studies employing isoproterenol challenge and exercise testing after single doses of propafenone indicate a beta-adrenergic blocking potency (per mg) about 1/40 that of propranolol in man. In clinical trials, resting heart rate decreases of about 8% were noted at the higher end of the therapeutic plasma concentration range. At very high concentrations in vitro, propafenone can inhibit the slow inward current carried by calcium, but this calcium antagonist effect probably does not contribute to antiarrhythmic efficacy. Moreover, propafenone inhibits a variety of cardiac potassium currents in in vitro studies (i.e. the transient outward, the delayed rectifier, and the inward rectifier current). Propafenone has local anesthetic activity approximately equal to procaine. Compared to propafenone, the main metabolite, 5-hydroxypropafenone, has similar sodium and calcium channel activity, but about 10 times less beta-blocking activity (N-depropylpropafenone has weaker sodium channel activity but equivalent affinity for beta-receptors).

12.2 Pharmacodynamics

Electrophysiology: Electrophysiology studies in patients with ventricular tachycardia have shown that propafenone prolongs atrioventricular conduction while having little or no effect on sinus node function. Both atrioventricular nodal conduction time (AH interval) and His-Purkinje conduction time (HV interval) are prolonged. Propafenone has little or no effect on the atrial functional refractory period, but AV nodal functional and effective refractory periods are prolonged. In patients with Wolff-Parkinson-White syndrome, RYTHMOL reduces conduction and increases the effective refractory period of the accessory pathway in both directions.

Electrocardiograms: Propafenone slows prolongs the PR and QRS intervals. Prolongation of the QRS interval makes it difficult to interpret the effect of propafenone on the QT interval.

[See table 2 above]

In any individual patient, the above ECG changes cannot be readily used to predict either efficacy or plasma concentration.

RYTHMOL causes a dose-related and concentration-related decrease in the rate of single and multiple premature ventricular contractions (PVCs) and can suppress recurrence of ventricular tachycardia. Based on the percent of patients attaining substantial (80% to 90%) suppression of ventricular ectopic activity, it appears that trough plasma levels of 0.2 to 1.5 μg/mL can provide good suppression, with higher concentrations giving a greater rate of good response.

When 600 mg/day propafenone was administered to patients with paroxysmal atrial tachyarrhythmias, mean heart rate during arrhythmia decreased 14 beats/min and 37 beats/min for paroxysmal atrial fibrillation/flutter (PAF) patients and paroxysmal supraventricular tachycardia (PSVT) patients, respectively.

Hemodynamics: Studies in humans have shown that propafenone HCl exerts a negative inotropic effect on the myocardium. Cardiac catheterization studies in patients with moderately impaired ventricular function (mean C.I. = 2.61 L/min/m^2) utilizing intravenous propafenone infusions (loading dose of 2 mg/kg over 10 min followed by 2 mg/min for 30 min) that gave mean plasma concentrations of 3.0 μg/mL (a dose that produces plasma levels of propafenone greater than does recommended oral dosing) showed significant increases in pulmonary capillary wedge pressure, systemic and pulmonary vascular resistances and depression of cardiac output and cardiac index.

12.3 Pharmacokinetics

Absorption/Bioavailability: Propafenone HCl is nearly completely absorbed after oral administration with peak plasma levels occurring approximately 3.5 hours after administration in most individuals. Propafenone exhibits extensive saturable presystemic biotransformation (first pass effect) resulting in a dose dependent and dosage form dependent absolute bioavailability; e.g., a 150 mg tablet had absolute bioavailability of 3.4%, while a 300 mg tablet had absolute bioavailability of 10.6%. A 300 mg solution which was rapidly absorbed had absolute bioavailability of 21.4%. At still larger doses, above those recommended, bioavailability increases still further.

Propafenone HCl follows a nonlinear pharmacokinetic disposition presumably because of saturation of first pass hepatic metabolism as the liver is exposed to higher concentrations of propafenone and shows a very high degree of interindividual variability. For example, for an increase in daily dose from 300 to 900 mg/day there is a 10-fold increase in steady-state plasma concentration. The top 25% of patients given 337.5 mg/day, however, had a mean concentration of propafenone larger than the bottom 25%, and about equal to the second 25%, of patients given a dose of 900 mg. Although food increased peak blood level and bioavailability in a single dose study, during multiple dose administration of propafenone to healthy volunteers food did not change bioavailability significantly.

Distribution: Following intravenous administration of propafenone, plasma levels decline in a bi-phasic manner consistent with a 2 compartment pharmacokinetic model. The average distribution half-life corresponding to the first phase was about 5 minutes. The volume of the central compartment was about 88 liters (1.1 L/kg) and the total volume of distribution about 252 liters.

In serum, propafenone is greater than 95% bound to proteins within the concentration range of 0.5 to 2 µg/mL.

Metabolism: There are two genetically determined patterns of propafenone metabolism. In over 90% of patients, the drug is rapidly and extensively metabolized with an elimination half-life from 2 to 10 hours. These patients metabolize propafenone into two active metabolites: 5-hydroxypropafenone which is formed by CYP2D6 and N-depropylpropafenone (norpropafenone) which is formed by both CYP3A4 and CYP1A2.

In less than 10% of patients, metabolism of propafenone is slower because the 5-hydroxy metabolite is not formed or is minimally formed. In these patients, the estimated propafenone elimination half-life ranges from 10 to 32 hours. Decreased ability to form the 5-hydroxy metabolite of propafenone is associated with a diminished ability to metabolize debrisoquine and a variety of other drugs (such as encainide, metoprolol, and dextromethorphan) whose metabolism is mediated by the CYP2D6 isozyme. In these patients, the N-depropylpropafenone metabolite occurs in quantities comparable to the levels occurring in extensive metabolizers.

There are significant differences in plasma concentrations of propafenone in slow and extensive metabolizers, the former achieving concentrations 1.5 to 2.0 times those of the extensive metabolizers at daily doses of 675 to 900 mg/day. At low doses the differences are greater, with slow metabolizers attaining concentrations more than five times that of extensive metabolizers. Because the difference decreases at high doses and is mitigated by the lack of the active 5-hydroxy metabolite in the slow metabolizers, and because steady state conditions are achieved after 4 to 5 days of dosing in all patients, the recommended dosing regimen is the same for all patients. The greater variability in blood levels require that the drug be titrated carefully in patients with close attention paid to clinical and ECG evidence of toxicity *[see Dosage and Administration (2)]*.

Stereochemistry: RYTHMOL is a racemic mixture. The R- and S-enantiomers of propafenone display stereoselective disposition characteristics. In vitro and in vivo studies have shown that the R-isomer of propafenone is cleared faster than the S-isomer via the 5-hydroxylation pathway (CYP2D6). This results in a higher ratio of S-propafenone to R-propafenone at steady state. Both enantiomers have equivalent potency to block sodium channels; however, the S-enantiomer is a more potent β-antagonist than the R-enantiomer. Following administration of RYTHMOL immediate-release tablets, the S/R ratio for the area under the plasma concentration-time curve was about 1.7. In addition, no difference in the average values of the S/R ratios is evident between genotypes or over time.

Special Populations: *Hepatic Impairment:* Decreased liver function increases the bioavailability of propafenone. Absolute bioavailability of RYTHMOL immediate-release tablets is inversely related to indocyanine green clearance, reaching 60-70% at clearances of 7 mL/min and below. Protein binding decreases to about 88% in patients with severe hepatic dysfunction. The clearance of propafenone is reduced and the elimination half-life increased in patients with significant hepatic dysfunction *[see Warnings and Precautions (5.9)]*.

13 NONCLINICAL TOXICOLOGY

13.1 Carcinogenesis, Mutagenesis, Impairment of Fertility

Lifetime maximally tolerated oral dose studies in mice (up to 360 mg/kg/day, about twice the maximum recommended human oral daily dose [MRHD] on a mg/m^2 basis) and rats (up to 270 mg/kg/day, about 3 times the MRHD on a mg/m^2 basis) provided no evidence of a carcinogenic potential for propafenone HCl.

Propafenone HCl tested negative for mutagenicity in the Ames (salmonella) test and in the in vivo mouse dominant lethal test. It tested negative for clastogenicity in the human lymphocyte chromosome aberration assay in vitro and in rat and Chinese hamster micronucleus tests, and other in vivo tests for chromosomal aberrations in rat bone marrow and Chinese hamster bone marrow and spermatogonia.

Propafenone HCl, administered intravenously to rabbits, dogs, and monkeys, has been shown to decrease spermatogenesis. These effects were reversible, were not found following oral dosing of propafenone HCl, were seen at lethal or near lethal dose levels and were not seen in rats treated either orally or intravenously *[see Warnings and Precautions (5.13)]*. Treatment of male rabbits for 10 weeks prior to mating at an oral dose of 120 mg/kg/day (about 2.4 times the MRHD on a mg/m^2 basis) or an intravenous dose of 3.5 mg/kg/day (a spermatogenesis-impairing dose) did not result in evidence of impaired fertility. Nor was there evidence of impaired fertility when propafenone HCl was administered orally to male and female rats at dose levels up to 270 mg/kg/day (about 3 times the MRHD on a mg/m^2 basis).

13.2 Animal Toxicology and/or Pharmacology

Renal changes have been observed in the rat following 6 months of oral administration of propafenone HCl at doses of 180 and 360 mg/kg/day (about 2 and 4 times, respectively, the MRHD on a mg/m^2 basis). Both inflammatory and non-inflammatory changes in the renal tubules, with accompanying interstitial nephritis, were observed. These changes were reversible, as they were not found in rats allowed to recover for 6 weeks. Fatty degenerative changes of the liver were found in rats following longer durations of administration of propafenone HCl at a dose of 270 mg/kg/day (about 3 times the MRHD on a mg/m^2 basis). There were no renal or hepatic changes at 90 mg/kg/day (equivalent to the MRHD on a mg/m^2 basis).

14 CLINICAL STUDIES

In two randomized, crossover, placebo-controlled, double-blind trials of 60 to 90 days duration in patients with paroxysmal supraventricular arrhythmias [paroxysmal atrial fibrillation/flutter (PAF), or paroxysmal supraventricular tachycardia (PSVT)], propafenone reduced the rate of both arrhythmias, as shown in Table 3.

[See table 3 above]

Table 3: Reduction of Arrythmias in Patients with PAF or PSVT

	Study 1		Study 2	
	Propafenone	Placebo	Propafenone	Placebo
PAF	n = 30	n = 30	n = 9	n = 9
Percent attack free	53%	13%	67%	22%
Median time to first recurrence	> 98 days	8 days	62 days	5 days
PSVT	n = 45	n = 45	n = 15	n = 15
Percent attack free	47%	16%	38%	7%
Median time to first recurrence	> 98 days	12 days	31 days	8 days

The patient population in the above trials was 50% male with a mean age of 57.3 years. Fifty percent of the patients had a diagnosis of PAF and 50% had PSVT. Eighty percent of the patients received 600 mg/day propafenone. No patient died in the above 2 studies.

In U.S. long-term safety trials, 474 patients (mean age: 57.4 ± 14.5 years) with supraventricular arrhythmias [195 with PAF, 274 with PSVT and 5 with both PAF and PSVT] were treated up to 5 years (mean: 14.4 months) with propafenone. Fourteen of the patients died. When this mortality rate was compared to the rate in a similar patient population (n = 194 patients; mean age: 43.0 ± 16.8 years) studied in an arrhythmia clinic, there was no age-adjusted difference in mortality. This comparison was not, however, a randomized trial and the 95% confidence interval around the comparison was large, such that neither a significant adverse or favorable effect could be ruled out.

16 HOW SUPPLIED/STORAGE AND HANDLING

RYTHMOL tablets are supplied as white, biconvex, scored, round, film-coated tablets containing either 150 mg or 225 mg of propafenone hydrochloride and embossed (on the same side) with GS and TF5 for the 150 mg tablet, and GS and F1X for the 225 mg tablet, in the following package sizes:

150 mg bottles of 100: NDC 0173-0792-20
225 mg bottles of 100: NDC 0173-0794-20

Storage: Store at 25°C (77°F); excursions permitted to 15° to 30°C (59° to 86°F). Dispense in a tight, light-resistant container.

17 PATIENT COUNSELING INFORMATION

See FDA-approved patient labeling (Patient Information).

17.1 Information for Patients

- Patients should be instructed to notify their health care providers of any change in over-the-counter, prescription and supplement use. The health care provider should assess the patients' medication history including all over-the-counter, prescription and herbal/natural preparations for those that may affect the pharmacodynamics or kinetics of RYTHMOL *[see Warnings and Precautions (5.4)]*.
- Patients should also check with their health care providers prior to taking a new over-the-counter medicine.
- If patients experience symptoms that may be associated with altered electrolyte balance, such as excessive or prolonged diarrhea, sweating, vomiting, or loss of appetite or thirst, these conditions should be immediately reported to their health care provider.
- Patients should be instructed NOT to double the next dose if a dose is missed. The next dose should be taken at the usual time.

RYTHMOL is a registered trademark of G. Petrik used under license by Abbott Laboratories.

Manufactured for:
GlaxoSmithKline
Research Triangle Park, NC 27709

RML:5PI

PHARMACIST–DETACH HERE AND GIVE INSTRUCTIONS TO PATIENT

PATIENT INFORMATION
RYTHMOL® (RITH-Mall)
(propafenone hydrochloride) Tablets

What is RYTHMOL?

RYTHMOL is a prescription medicine that is used:

- in certain people who have ventricular heart rhythm disorders
- to increase the amount of time between having symptoms of heart rhythm disorders called atrial fibrillation (AF) or paroxysmal supraventricular tachycardia (PSVT)

It is not known if RYTHMOL is safe and effective in children.

Who should not take RYTHMOL?

Do not take RYTHMOL if you have:

- heart failure (weak heart)
- had a recent heart attack
- a heart rate that is too slow, and you do not have a pacemaker
- a heart condition called Brugada Syndrome
- very low blood pressure
- certain breathing problems that make you short of breath or wheeze
- certain abnormal body salt (electrolyte) levels in your blood

Talk to your doctor before taking RYTHMOL if you think you have any of the conditions listed above.

What should I tell my doctor before taking RYTHMOL?

Before you take RYTHMOL, tell your doctor if you:

- have liver or kidney problems
- have breathing problems
- have symptoms including diarrhea, sweating, vomiting, or loss of appetite or thirst that are severe. These symptoms may be a sign of abnormal electrolyte levels in your blood.
- have myasthenia gravis
- have lupus erythematosis
- have been told you have or had an abnormal blood test called Antinuclear Antibody Test or ANA Test
- have any other medical conditions
- are pregnant or plan to become pregnant. It is not known if RYTHMOL will harm your unborn baby.
- are breastfeeding or plan to breastfeed. RYTHMOL can pass into your milk and may harm your baby. You and your doctor should decide if you will breastfeed or take RYTHMOL. You should not do both.

Tell your doctor about all the medicines you take, including prescription and over-the-counter medicines, vitamins, and herbal supplements. RYTHMOL and certain other medicines can affect (interact with) each other and cause serious side effects. You can ask your pharmacist for a list of medicines that interact with RYTHMOL.

Know the medicines you take. Keep a list of them to show your doctor and pharmacist when you get a new medicine.

How should I take RYTHMOL?

- Take RYTHMOL exactly as prescribed. Your doctor will tell you how many tablets to take and how often to take them.
- To help reduce the chance of certain side effects, your doctor may start you with a low dose of RYTHMOL, and then slowly increase the dose.
- You should not drink grapefruit juice during treatment with RYTHMOL.
- If you miss a dose of RYTHMOL, take your next dose at the usual time. Do not take 2 doses at the same time.

• If you take too much RYTHMOL, call your doctor or go to the nearest hospital emergency room right away.
• Call your doctor if your heart problems get worse.

What are possible side effects of RYTHMOL?

RYTHMOL can cause serious side effects including:

- **New or worsened abnormal heart beats, that can cause sudden death or be life-threatening.** Your doctor may do an electrocardiogram (ECG or EKG) before and during treatment to check your heart for these problems.
- **New or worsened heart failure. Tell your doctor about any changes in your heart symptoms, including:**
  - any new or increased swelling in your arms or legs
  - trouble breathing
  - sudden weight gain
- **Effects on pacemaker function.** RYTHMOL may affect how an implanted pacemaker or defibrillator works. Your doctor should check how your pacemaker or defibrillator is working during and after treatment with RYTHMOL. They may need to be re-programmed.
- **Very low white blood cell levels in your blood (agranulocytosis).** Your bone marrow may not produce enough of a certain type of white blood cells called neutrophils. If this happens, you are more likely to get infections. Tell your doctor right away if you have any of these symptoms, especially during the first 3 months of treatment:
  - fever
  - sore throat
  - chills
- **Worsening of myasthenia gravis in people who already have this condition.** Tell your doctor about any change in your symptoms.
- **RYTHMOL may cause lower sperm counts in men.** This could affect the ability to father a child. Talk to your doctor if this is a concern for you.

Common side effects of RYTHMOL include:
1. unusual taste
2. nausea
3. vomiting
4. dizziness
5. constipation
6. headache
7. tiredness
8. irregular heart beats

Tell your doctor if you have any side effect that bothers you or that does not go away.

These are not all the possible side effects of RYTHMOL. For more information, ask your doctor or pharmacist.

Call your doctor for medical advice about side effects. You may report side effects to FDA at 1-800-FDA-1088.

How should I store RYTHMOL?

• Store RYTHMOL at room temperature between 68°F to 77°F (20°C to 25°C).
• Keep the bottle tightly closed.

Keep RYTHMOL and all medicines out of the reach of children.

General information about RYTHMOL

Medicines are sometimes prescribed for purposes other than those listed in a Patient Information Leaflet. Do not use RYTHMOL for a condition for which it was not prescribed. Do not give RYTHMOL to other people, even if they have the same symptoms you have. It may harm them.

If you would like more information, talk with your doctor. You can ask your doctor or pharmacist for information about RYTHMOL that is written for health professionals. For more information about RYTHMOL, call 1-888-825-5249.

What are the ingredients in RYTHMOL?

Active ingredient: propafenone hydrochloride

Inactive ingredients: corn starch, hypromellose, magnesium stearate, polyethylene glycol, polysorbate, povidone, propylene glycol, sodium starch glycolate, and titanium dioxide.

This Patient Information has been approved by the U.S. Food and Drug Administration.

RYTHMOL is a registered trademark of G. Petrik used under license by Abbott Laboratories.

Manufactured for:
GlaxoSmithKline
Research Triangle Park, NC 27709

June 2013
RML:2PIL

RYTHMOL SR ℞

[RITH-Mall]
(propafenone hydrochloride)
Extended-Release Capsules for oral use

HIGHLIGHTS OF PRESCRIBING INFORMATION

These highlights do not include all the information needed to use RYTHMOL SR safely and effectively. See full prescribing information for RYTHMOL SR.

RYTHMOL SR (propafenone hydrochloride) Extended-Release Capsules for oral use
Initial U.S. Approval: 1989

WARNING: MORTALITY
See full prescribing information for complete boxed warning
- **An increased rate of death or reversed cardiac arrest rate was seen in patients treated with encainide or flecainide (Class IC antiarrhythmics) compared with that seen in patients assigned to placebo. At present it is prudent to consider any IC antiarrhythmic to have a significant risk of provoking proarrhythmic events in patients with structural heart disease.**
- **Given the lack of any evidence that these drugs improve survival, antiarrhythmic agents should generally be avoided in patients with non-life-threatening ventricular arrhythmias, even if the patients are experiencing unpleasant, but not life-threatening, symptoms or signs.**

RECENT MAJOR CHANGES

Contraindications (4) 02/2013
Warnings and Precautions, Unmasking Brugada Syndrome (5.2) 02/2013

INDICATIONS AND USAGE

RYTHMOL SR is an antiarrhythmic indicated to prolong the time to recurrence of symptomatic atrial fibrillation (AF) in patients with episodic (most likely paroxysmal or persistent) AF who do not have structural heart disease. (1)

Usage Considerations:
- Use in patients with permanent atrial fibrillation or with atrial flutter or PSVT has not been evaluated. Do not use to control ventricular rate during atrial fibrillation. (1)
- In patients with atrial fibrillation and atrial flutter, use RYTHMOL SR with drugs that increase the atrioventricular nodal refractory period. (1)
- The effect of propafenone on mortality has not been determined. (1)

DOSAGE AND ADMINISTRATION

- Initiate therapy with 225 mg given every 12 hours. (2)
- Dosage may be increased at a minimum of 5 day intervals to 325 mg every 12 hours and, if necessary, to 425 mg every 12 hours. (2)
- Dose reduction should be considered in patients with hepatic impairment, significant widening of the QRS complex, or second or third degree AV block. (2)

DOSAGE FORMS AND STRENGTHS

Capsules: 225 mg, 325 mg, 425 mg. (3)

CONTRAINDICATIONS

- Heart failure (4)
- Cardiogenic shock (4)
- Sinoatrial, atrioventricular, and intraventricular disorders of impulse generation and/or conduction in the absence of pacemaker (4)
- Known Brugada Syndrome (4)
- Bradycardia (4)
- Marked hypotension (4)
- Bronchospastic disorders and severe obstructive pulmonary disease (4)
- Marked electrolyte imbalance (4)

WARNINGS AND PRECAUTIONS

- May cause new or worsened arrhythmias. Evaluate patients via ECG prior to and during therapy. (5.1)
- RYTHMOL SR may unmask Brugada or Brugada-like Syndrome. Evaluate patients via ECG after initiation of therapy. (4, 5.2)
- Avoid use with other antiarrhythmic agents or drugs that prolong the QT interval. (5.3)
- Avoid simultaneous use of propafenone with both a cytochrome P450 2D6 inhibitor and a 3A4 inhibitor. (5.4)
- May provoke overt heart failure. (5.5)
- May cause dose-related first degree AV block or other conduction disturbances. Should not be given to patients with conduction defects in absence of a pacemaker. (5.6)
- May affect artificial pacemakers. Pacemakers should be monitored during therapy. (5.7)
- Agranulocytosis: Patients should report signs of infection. (5.8)
- Administer cautiously to patients with impaired hepatic and renal function. (5.9, 5.10)
- Exacerbation of myasthenia gravis has been reported. (5.11)

ADVERSE REACTIONS

The most commonly reported adverse events with propafenone (>5% and greater than placebo) excluding those not reasonably associated with the use of the drug included the following: dizziness, palpitations, chest pain, dyspnea, taste disturbance, nausea, fatigue, anxiety, constipation, upper respiratory tract infection, edema, and influenza. (6.1)

To report SUSPECTED ADVERSE REACTIONS, contact GlaxoSmithKline at 1-888-825-5249 or FDA at 1-800-FDA-1088 or www.fda.gov/medwatch.

DRUG INTERACTIONS

- Inhibitors of CYP2D6, 1A2, and 3A4 may increase propafenone levels which may lead to cardiac arrhythmias. Simultaneous use with both a CYP3A4 and CYP2D6 inhibitor (or in patients with CYP2D6 deficiency) should be avoided. (7.1)
- Propafenone may increase digoxin or warfarin levels. (7.2, 7.3)
- Orlistat may reduce propafenone concentrations. Abrupt cessation of orlistat in patients stable on RYTHMOL SR has resulted in convulsions, atrioventricular block, and circulatory failure. (7.4)
- Concomitant use of lidocaine may increase central nervous system side effects. (7.6)

See 17 for PATIENT COUNSELING INFORMATION and FDA-approved patient labeling

Revised: 06/2013

FULL PRESCRIBING INFORMATION: CONTENTS*

*** Sections or subsections omitted from the full prescribing information are not listed**

FULL PRESCRIBING INFORMATION

WARNING: MORTALITY
- **In the National Heart, Lung and Blood Institute's Cardiac Arrhythmia Suppression Trial (CAST), a long-term, multi-center, randomized, double-blind study in patients with asymptomatic non-life-threatening ventricular arrhythmias who had a myocardial infarction more than 6 days but less than 2 years previously, an increased rate of death or reversed cardiac arrest rate (7.7%; 56/730) was seen in patients treated with encainide or flecainide (Class IC antiarrhythmics) compared with that seen in patients assigned to placebo (3.0%; 22/725). The average duration of treatment with encainide or flecainide in this study was 10 months.**

- **The applicability of the CAST results to other populations (e.g., those without recent myocardial infarction) or other antiarrhythmic drugs is uncertain, but at present, it is prudent to consider any IC antiarrhythmic to have a significant proarrhythmic risk in patients with structural heart disease. Given the lack of any evidence that these drugs improve survival, antiarrhythmic agents should generally be avoided in patients with non-life-threatening ventricular arrhythmias, even if the patients are experiencing unpleasant, but not life-threatening, symptoms or signs.**

1 INDICATIONS AND USAGE

RYTHMOL SR® is indicated to prolong the time to recurrence of symptomatic atrial fibrillation (AF) in patients with episodic (most likely paroxysmal or persistent) AF who do not have structural heart disease.

Usage Considerations:

- The use of RYTHMOL SR in patients with permanent AF or in patients exclusively with atrial flutter or paroxysmal supraventricular tachycardia (PSVT) has not been evaluated. Do not use RYTHMOL SR to control ventricular rate during AF.
- Some patients with atrial flutter treated with propafenone have developed 1:1 conduction, producing an increase in ventricular rate. Concomitant treatment with drugs that increase the functional atrioventricular (AV) nodal refractory period is recommended.
- The effect of propafenone on mortality has not been determined *[see Boxed Warning]*.

2 DOSAGE AND ADMINISTRATION

RYTHMOL SR can be taken with or without food. Do not crush or further divide the contents of the capsule.

The dose of RYTHMOL SR must be individually titrated on the basis of response and tolerance. Initiate therapy with RYTHMOL SR 225 mg given every 12 hours. Dosage may be increased at a minimum of 5 day interval to 325 mg given every 12 hours. If additional therapeutic effect is needed, the dose of RYTHMOL SR may be increased to 425 mg given every 12 hours.

In patients with hepatic impairment or those with significant widening of the QRS complex or second or third degree AV block, consider reducing the dose.

The combination of CYP3A4 inhibition and either CYP2D6 deficiency or CYP2D6 inhibition with the simultaneous administration of propafenone may significantly increase the concentration of propafenone and thereby increase the risk of proarrhythmia and other adverse events. Therefore, avoid simultaneous use of RYTHMOL SR with both a CYP2D6 inhibitor and a CYP3A4 inhibitor *[see Warnings and Precautions (5.4) and Drug Interactions (7.1)]*.

3 DOSAGE FORMS AND STRENGTHS

RYTHMOL SR (propafenone HCl) capsules are supplied as white, opaque, hard gelatin capsules containing either 225 mg, 325 mg, or 425 mg of propafenone HCl. The 225 mg strength is imprinted in red with GS EUG followed by 225. The 325 mg strength is imprinted in red with GS F1Y followed by 325, and also has a single red band around ¾ of the circumference of the body. The 425 mg strength is imprinted in red with GS UY2 followed by 425, and also has three red bands around ¾ of the circumference of the body.

4 CONTRAINDICATIONS

RYTHMOL SR is contraindicated in the following circumstances:

- Heart failure
- Cardiogenic shock
- Sinoatrial, atrioventricular and intraventricular disorders of impulse generation or conduction (e.g., sick sinus node syndrome, AV block) in the absence of an artificial pacemaker
- Known Brugada Syndrome
- Bradycardia
- Marked hypotension
- Bronchospastic disorders or severe obstructive pulmonary disease
- Marked electrolyte imbalance

5 WARNINGS AND PRECAUTIONS

5.1 Proarrhythmic Effects

Propafenone has caused new or worsened arrhythmias. Such proarrhythmic effects include sudden death and life-threatening ventricular arrhythmias such as ventricular fibrillation, ventricular tachycardia, asystole and torsade de pointes. It may also worsen premature ventricular contractions or supraventricular arrhythmias, and it may prolong the QT interval. It is therefore essential that each patient given RYTHMOL SR be evaluated electrocardiographically prior to and during therapy, to determine whether the response to RYTHMOL SR supports continued treatment. Because propafenone prolongs the QRS interval in the electrocardiogram, changes in the QT interval are difficult to interpret *[see Clinical Pharmacology (12.2)]*.

In the RAFT study *[see Clinical Studies (14)]*, there were too few deaths to assess the long term risk to patients. There were 5 deaths, 3 in the pooled RYTHMOL SR group (0.8%) and 2 in the placebo group (1.6%). In the overall RYTHMOL SR and RYTHMOL immediate-release database of 8 studies, the mortality rate was 2.5% per year on propafenone and 4.0% per year on placebo. Concurrent use of propafenone with other antiarrhythmic agents has not been well studied.

In a U.S. uncontrolled, open label multicenter trial using the immediate-release formulation in patients with symptomatic supraventricular tachycardia (SVT), 1.9% (9/474) of these patients experienced ventricular tachycardia (VT) or ventricular fibrillation (VF) during the study. However, in 4 of the 9 patients, the ventricular tachycardia was of atrial origin. Six of the 9 patients that developed ventricular arrhythmias did so within 14 days of onset of therapy. About 2.3% (11/474) of all patients had recurrence of SVT during the study which could have been a change in the patients' arrhythmia behavior or could represent a proarrhythmic event. Case reports in patients treated with propafenone for atrial fibrillation/flutter have included increased premature ventricular contractions (PVCs), VT, VF, torsades de pointes, asystole, and death.

Overall in clinical trials with RYTHMOL immediate-release (which included patients treated for ventricular arrhythmias, atrial fibrillation/flutter, and PSVT), 4.7% of all patients had new or worsened ventricular arrhythmia possibly representing a proarrhythmic event (0.7% was an increase in PVCs; 4.0% a worsening, or new appearance, of VT or VF). Of the patients who had worsening of VT (4%), 92% had a history of VT and/or VT/VF, 71% had coronary artery disease, and 68% had a prior myocardial infarction. The incidence of proarrhythmia in patients with less serious or benign arrhythmias, which include patients with an increase in frequency of PVCs, was 1.6%. Although most proarrhythmic events occurred during the first week of therapy, late events also were seen and the CAST study *[see Boxed Warning: Mortality]* suggests that an increased risk of proarrythmia is present throughout treatment.

5.2 Unmasking Brugada Syndrome

Brugada Syndrome may be unmasked after exposure to RYTHMOL SR. Perform an ECG after initiation of RYTHMOL SR and discontinue the drug if changes are suggestive of Brugada Syndrome *[see Contraindications (4)]*.

5.3 Use with Drugs that Prolong the QT Interval and Antiarrhythmic Agents

The use of RYTHMOL SR in conjunction with other drugs that prolong the QT interval has not been extensively studied. Such drugs may include many antiarrhythmics, some phenothiazines, tricyclic antidepressants, and oral macrolides. Withhold Class IA and III antiarrhythmic agents for at least 5 half-lives prior to dosing with RYTHMOL SR. Avoid the use of propafenone with Class IA and III antiarrhythmic agents (including quinidine and amiodarone). There is only limited experience with the concomitant use of Class IB or IC antiarrhythmics.

5.4 Drug Interactions: Simultaneous Use with Inhibitors of Cytochrome P450 Isoenzymes 2D6 and 3A4

Propafenone is metabolized by CYP2D6, CYP3A4, and CYP1A2 isoenzymes. Approximately 6% of Caucasians in the U.S. population are naturally deficient in CYP2D6 activity and to a somewhat lesser extent in other demographic groups. Drugs that inhibit these CYP pathways (such as desipramine, paroxetine, ritonavir, sertraline for CYP2D6; ketoconazole, erythromycin, saquinavir, and grapefruit juice for CYP3A4; and amiodarone and tobacco smoke for CYP1A2) can be expected to cause increased plasma levels of propafenone.

Increased exposure to propafenone may lead to cardiac arrhythmias and exaggerated beta-adrenergic blocking activity. Because of its metabolism, the combination of CYP3A4 inhibition and either CYP2D6 deficiency or CYP2D6 inhibition in users of propafenone is potentially hazardous. Therefore, avoid simultaneous use of RYTHMOL SR with both a CYP2D6 inhibitor and a CYP3A4 inhibitor.

5.5 Use in Patients with a History of Heart Failure

Propafenone exerts a negative inotropic activity on the myocardium as well as beta blockade effects and may provoke overt heart failure. In the U.S. trial (RAFT) in patients with symptomatic AF, heart failure was reported in 4 (1.0%) patients receiving RYTHMOL SR (all doses), compared to 1 (0.8%) patient receiving placebo. Proarrhythmic effects more likely occur when propafenone is administered to patients with heart failure (NYHA III and IV) or severe myocardial ischemia *[see Contraindications (4)]*.

In clinical trial experience with RYTHMOL immediate-release, new or worsened heart failure has been reported in 3.7% of patients with ventricular arrhythmia. These events were more likely in subjects with preexisting heart failure and coronary artery disease. New onset of heart failure attributable to propafenone developed in <0.2% of patients with ventricular arrhythmia and in 1.9% of patients with paroxysmal AF or PSVT.

5.6 Conduction Disturbances

Propafenone slows atrioventricular conduction and may also cause dose-related first degree AV block. Average PR interval prolongation and increases in QRS duration are also dose-related. Do not give propafenone to patients with atrioventricular and intraventricular conduction defects in the absence of a pacemaker *[see Contraindications (4) and Clinical Pharmacology (12.2)]*.

In a U.S. trial (RAFT) in 523 patients with a history of symptomatic AF treated with RYTHMOL SR, sinus bradycardia (rate <50 beats/min) was reported with the same frequency with RYTHMOL SR and placebo.

5.7 Effects on Pacemaker Threshold

Propafenone may alter both pacing and sensing thresholds of implanted pacemakers and defibrillators. During and after therapy, monitor and re-program these devices accordingly.

5.8 Agranulocytosis

Agranulocytosis has been reported in patients receiving propafenone. Generally, the agranulocytosis occurred within the first 2 months of propafenone therapy and upon discontinuation of therapy, the white count usually normalized by 14 days. Unexplained fever or decrease in white cell count, particularly during the initial 3 months of therapy, warrant consideration of possible agranulocytosis or granulocytopenia. Instruct patients to report promptly any signs of infection such as fever, sore throat, or chills.

5.9 Use in Patients with Hepatic Dysfunction

Propafenone is highly metabolized by the liver. Severe liver dysfunction increases the bioavailability of propafenone to approximately 70% compared to 3 to 40% in patients with normal liver function when given RYTHMOL immediate-release tablets. In 8 patients with moderate to severe liver disease administered RYTHMOL immediate-release tablets, the mean half-life was approximately 9 hours. No studies have compared bioavailability of propafenone from RYTHMOL SR in patients with normal and impaired hepatic function. Increased bioavailability of propafenone in these patients may result in excessive accumulation. Carefully monitor patients with impaired hepatic function for excessive pharmacological effects *[see Overdosage (10)]*.

5.10 Use in Patients with Renal Dysfunction

Approximately 50% of propafenone metabolites are excreted in the urine following administration of RYTHMOL immediate-release tablets. No studies have been performed to assess the percentage of metabolites eliminated in the urine following the administration of RYTHMOL SR capsules.

In patients with impaired renal function monitor for signs of overdosage *[see Overdosage (10)]*.

5.11 Use in Patients with Myasthenia Gravis

Exacerbation of myasthenia gravis has been reported during propafenone therapy.

5.12 Elevated ANA Titers

Positive ANA titers have been reported in patients receiving propafenone. They have been reversible upon cessation of treatment and may disappear even in the face of continued propafenone therapy. These laboratory findings were usually not associated with clinical symptoms, but there is one published case of drug-induced lupus erythematosis (positive rechallenge); it resolved completely upon discontinuation of therapy. Carefully evaluate patients who develop an abnormal ANA test and if persistent or worsening elevation of ANA titers is detected, consider discontinuing therapy.

5.13 Impaired Spermatogenesis

Reversible disorders of spermatogenesis have been demonstrated in monkeys, dogs and rabbits after high dose intravenous administration of propafenone. Evaluation of the effects of short-term RYTHMOL administration on spermatogenesis in 11 normal subjects suggested that propafenone produced a reversible, short-term drop (within normal range) in sperm count.

6 ADVERSE REACTIONS

6.1 Clinical Trials Experience

Because clinical trials are conducted under widely varying conditions, adverse reaction rates observed in the clinical trials of a drug cannot be directly compared to rates in the clinical trials of another drug and may not reflect the rates observed in practice.

The data described below reflect exposure to RYTHMOL SR 225 mg twice daily in 126 patients, to RYTHMOL SR 325 mg twice daily in 135 patients, to RYTHMOL SR 425 mg twice daily in 136 patients, and to placebo in 126 patients for up to 39 weeks (mean 20 weeks) in a placebo-controlled trial (RAFT) conducted in the US. The most commonly reported adverse events with propafenone (>5% and greater than placebo) excluding those not reasonably associated with the use of the drug or because they were associated with the condition being treated, were dizziness, palpitations, chest pain, dyspnea, taste disturbance, nausea, fatigue, anxiety, constipation, upper respiratory tract infection, edema, and influenza. The frequency of discontinuation due to adverse events was 17%, and the rate was highest during the first 14 days of treatment.

Cardiac-related adverse events occurring in ≥ 2% of the patients in any of the RAFT propafenone SR treatment groups and more common with propafenone than with placebo, excluding those that are common in the population and those not plausibly related to drug therapy, included the following: angina pectoris, atrial flutter, AV block first degree, bradycardia, congestive cardiac failure, cardiac murmur, edema, dyspnea, rales, wheezing, and cardioactive drug level above therapeutic.

Propafenone prolongs the PR and QRS intervals in patients with atrial and ventricular arrhythmias. Prolongation of the QRS interval makes it difficult to interpret the effect of propafenone on the QT interval *[see Clinical Pharmacology (12.2)]*.

Non-cardiac related adverse events occurring in ≥ 2% of the patients in any of the RAFT propafenone SR treatment groups and more common with propafenone than with placebo, excluding those that are common in the population and those not plausibly related to drug therapy, included the following: blurred vision, constipation, diarrhea, dry mouth, flatulence, nausea, vomiting, fatigue, weakness, upper respiratory tract infection, blood alkaline phosphatase increased, hematuria, muscle weakness, dizziness (excluding vertigo), headache, taste disturbance, tremor, somnolence, anxiety, depression, ecchymosis.

No clinically important differences in incidence of adverse reactions were noted by age or gender. Too few non-Caucasian patients were enrolled to assess adverse events according to race.

Adverse events occurring in 2% or more of the patients in any of the ERAFT *[see Clinical Studies (14)]* propafenone SR treatment groups and not listed above include the following: bundle branch block left, bundle branch block right, conduction disorders, sinus bradycardia, and hypotension.

Other adverse events reported with propafenone clinical trials not already listed elsewhere in the prescribing information include the following adverse events by body and preferred term.

Blood and Lymphatic System Disorders

Anemia, lymphadenopathy, spleen disorder, thrombocytopenia.

Cardiac Disorders

Unstable angina, atrial hypertrophy, cardiac arrest, coronary artery disease, extrasystoles, myocardial infarction, nodal arrhythmia, palpitations, pericarditis, sinoatrial block, sinus arrest, sinus arrhythmia, supraventricular extrasystoles, ventricular extrasystoles, ventricular hypertrophy.

Ear and Labyrinth Disorders

Hearing impaired, tinnitus, vertigo.

Eye Disorders

Eye hemorrhage, eye inflammation, eyelid ptosis, miosis, retinal disorder, visual acuity reduced.

Gastrointestinal Disorders

Abdominal distension, abdominal pain, duodenitis, dyspepsia, dysphagia, eructation, gastritis, gastroesophageal reflux disease, gingival bleeding, glossitis, glossodynia, gum pain, halitosis, intestinal obstruction, melena, mouth ulceration, pancreatitis, peptic ulcer, rectal bleeding, sore throat.

General Disorders and Administration Site Conditions

Chest pain, feeling hot, hemorrhage, malaise, pain, pyrexia.

Hepatobiliary Disorders

Hepatomegaly.

Investigations

Abnormal heart sounds, abnormal pulse, carotid bruit, decreased blood chloride, decreased blood pressure, decreased blood sodium, decreased hemoglobin, decreased neutrophil count, decreased platelet count, decreased prothrombin level, decreased red blood cell count, decreased weight, glycosuria present, increased alanine aminotransferase, increased aspartate aminotransferase, increased blood bilirubin, increased blood cholesterol, increased blood creatinine, increased blood glucose, increased blood lactate dehydrogenase, increased blood pressure, increased blood prolactin, increased blood triglycerides, increased blood urea, increased blood uric acid, increased eosinophil count, increased gamma-glutamyltransferase, increased monocyte count, increased prostatic specific antigen, increased prothrombin level, increased weight, increased white blood cell count, ketonuria present, proteinuria present.

Metabolism and Nutrition Disorders

Anorexia, dehydration, diabetes mellitus, gout, hypercholesterolemia, hyperglycemia, hyperlipidemia, hypokalemia.

Musculoskeletal, Connective Tissue and Bone Disorders

Arthritis, bursitis, collagen-vascular disease, costochondritis, joint disorder, muscle cramps, muscle spasms, myalgia, neck pain, pain in jaw, sciatica, tendonitis.

Nervous System Disorders

Amnesia, ataxia, balance impaired, brain damage, cerebrovascular accident, dementia, gait abnormal, hypertonia, hypothesia, insomnia, paralysis, paresthesia, peripheral neuropathy, speech disorder, syncope, tongue hypoesthesia.

Psychiatric Disorders

Decreased libido, emotional disturbance, mental disorder, neurosis, nightmare, sleep disorder.

Renal and Urinary Disorders

Dysuria, nocturia, oliguria, pyuria, renal failure, urinary casts, urinary frequency, urinary incontinence, urinary retention, urine abnormal.

Reproductive System and Breast Disorders

Breast pain, impotence, prostatism.

Respiratory, Thoracic and Mediastinal Disorders

Atelectasis, breath sounds decreased, chronic obstructive airways disease, cough, epistaxis, hemoptysis, lung disorder, pleural effusion, pulmonary congestion, rales, respiratory failure, rhinitis, throat tightness.

Skin and Subcutaneous Tissue Disorders

Alopecia, dermatitis, dry skin, erythema, nail abnormality, petechiae, pruritus, sweating increased, urticaria.

Vascular Disorders

Arterial embolism limb, deep limb venous thrombosis, flushing, hematoma, hypertension, hypertensive crisis, hypotension, labile blood pressure, pallor, peripheral coldness, peripheral vascular disease, thrombosis.

7 DRUG INTERACTIONS

7.1 CYP2D6 and CYP3A4 Inhibitors

Drugs that inhibit CYP2D6 (such as desipramine, paroxetine, ritonavir, sertraline) and CYP3A4 (such as ketoconazole, ritonavir, saquinavir, erythromycin, and grapefruit juice) can be expected to cause increased plasma levels of propafenone. The combination of CYP3A4 inhibition and either CYP2D6 deficiency or CYP2D6 inhibition with administration of propafenone may increase the risk of adverse reactions, including proarrhythmia. Therefore, simultaneous use of RYTHMOL SR with both a CYP2D6 inhibitor and a CYP3A4 inhibitor should be avoided *[see Warnings and Precautions (5.4) and Dosage and Administration (2)]*.

Amiodarone

Concomitant administration of propafenone and amiodarone can affect conduction and repolarization and is not recommended.

Cimetidine

Concomitant administration of propafenone immediate-release tablets and cimetidine in 12 healthy subjects resulted in a 20% increase in steady-state plasma concentrations of propafenone.

Fluoxetine

Concomitant administration of propafenone and fluoxetine in extensive metabolizers increased the S propafenone C_{max} and AUC by 39 and 50% and the R propafenone C_{max} and AUC by 71 and 50%.

Quinidine

Small doses of quinidine completely inhibit the CYP2D6 hydroxylation metabolic pathway, making all patients, in effect, slow metabolizers *[see Clinical Pharmacology (12)]*. Concomitant administration of quinidine (50 mg three times daily) with 150 mg immediate-release propafenone three times daily decreased the clearance of propafenone by 60% in extensive metabolizers, making them poor metabolizers. Steady-state plasma concentrations increased by more than 2-fold for propafenone, and decreased 50% for 5-OH-propafenone. A 100 mg dose of quinidine increased steady state concentrations of propafenone 3-fold. Avoid concomitant use of propafenone and quinidine.

Rifampin

Concomitant administration of rifampin and propafenone in extensive metabolizers decreased the plasma concentrations of propafenone by 67% with a corresponding decrease of 5-OH-propafenone by 65%. The concentrations of norpropafenone increased by 30%. In poor metabolizers, there was a 50% decrease in propafenone plasma concentrations and increased the AUC and C_{max} of norpropafenone by 74 and 20%, respectively. Urinary excretion of propafenone and its metabolites decreased significantly. Similar results were noted in elderly patients: Both the AUC and C_{max} propafenone decreased by 84%, with a corresponding decrease in AUC and C_{max} of 5-OH-propafenone by 69 and 57%.

7.2 Digoxin

Concomitant use of propafenone and digoxin increased steady-state serum digoxin exposure (AUC) in patients by 60 to 270%, and decreased the clearance of digoxin by 31 to 67%. Monitor plasma digoxin levels of patients receiving propafenone and adjust digoxin dosage as needed.

7.3 Warfarin

The concomitant administration of propafenone and warfarin increased warfarin plasma concentrations at steady state by 39% in healthy volunteers and prolonged the prothrombin time (PT) in patients taking warfarin. Adjust the warfarin dose as needed by monitoring INR (international normalized ratio).

7.4 Orlistat

Orlistat may limit the fraction of propafenone available for absorption. In post marketing reports, abrupt cessation of orlistat in patients stabilized on propafenone has resulted in severe adverse events including convulsions, atrioventricular block and acute circulatory failure.

7.5 Beta-Antagonists

Concomitant use of propafenone and propranolol in healthy subjects increased propranolol plasma concentrations at steady state by 113%. In 4 patients, administration of metoprolol with propafenone increased the metoprolol plasma concentrations at steady state by 100 to 400%. The pharmacokinetics of propafenone was not affected by the coadministration of either propranolol or metoprolol. In clinical trials using propafenone immediate-release tablets, patients who were receiving beta-blockers concurrently did not experience an increased incidence of side effects.

7.6 Lidocaine

No significant effects on the pharmacokinetics of propafenone or lidocaine have been seen following their concomitant use in patients. However, concomitant use of propafenone and lidocaine has been reported to increase the risks of central nervous system side effects of lidocaine.

8 USE IN SPECIFIC POPULATIONS

8.1 Pregnancy

Pregnancy Category C. There are no adequate and well-controlled studies in pregnant women. RYTHMOL SR should be used during pregnancy only if the potential benefit justifies the potential risk to the fetus.

Animal Data

Teratogenic Effects

Propafenone has been shown to be embryotoxic (decreased survival) in rabbits and rats when given in oral maternally toxic doses of 150 mg/kg/day (about 3 times the maximum recommended human dose [MRHD] on a mg/m^2 basis) and 600 mg/kg/day (about 6 times the MRHD on a mg/m^2 basis), respectively. Although maternally tolerated doses (up to 270 mg/kg/day, about 3 times the MRHD on a mg/m^2 basis) produced no evidence of embryotoxicity in rats, post-implantation loss was elevated in all rabbit treatment groups (doses as low as 15 mg/kg/day, about 1/3 the MRHD on a mg/m^2 basis).

Non-teratogenic Effects

In a study in which female rats received daily oral doses of propafenone from mid-gestation through weaning of their offspring, doses as low as 90 mg/kg/day (equivalent to the MRHD on a mg/m^2 basis) produced increases in maternal deaths. Doses of 360 or more mg/kg/day (4 or more times the MRHD on a mg/m^2 basis) resulted in reductions in neonatal survival, body weight gain and physiological development.

8.2 Labor and Delivery

It is not known whether the use of propafenone during labor or delivery has immediate or delayed adverse effects on the fetus, or whether it prolongs the duration of labor or increases the need for forceps delivery or other obstetrical intervention.

8.3 Nursing Mothers

Propafenone is excreted in human milk. Because of the potential for serious adverse reactions in nursing infants from propafenone, decide whether to discontinue nursing or to discontinue the drug, taking into account the importance of the drug to the mother.

8.4 Pediatric Use

The safety and effectiveness of propafenone in pediatric patients have not been established.

8.5 Geriatric Use

Of the total number of subjects in Phase 3 clinical studies of RYTHMOL SR (propafenone hydrochloride) 46% were 65 and over, while 16% were 75 and over. No overall differences in safety or effectiveness were observed between these subjects and younger subjects, but greater sensitivity of some older individuals at higher doses cannot be ruled out. The effect of age on the pharmacokinetics and pharmacodynamics of propafenone has not been studied.

10 OVERDOSAGE

The symptoms of overdosage may include hypotension, somnolence, bradycardia, intra-atrial and intraventricular conduction disturbances, and rarely convulsions and high grade ventricular arrhythmias. Defibrillation as well as infusion of dopamine and isoproterenol have been effective in controlling abnormal rhythm and blood pressure. Convulsions have been alleviated with intravenous diazepam. General supportive measures such as mechanical respiratory assistance and external cardiac massage may be necessary. The hemodialysis of propafenone in patients with an overdose is expected to be of limited value in the removal of propafenone as a result of both its high protein binding (>95%) and large volume of distribution.

11 DESCRIPTION

RYTHMOL SR (propafenone hydrochloride) is an antiarrhythmic drug supplied in extended-release capsules of 225, 325 and 425 mg for oral administration.

Chemically, propafenone hydrochloride is 2′-[2-Hydroxy-3-(propylamino)-propoxy]-3-phenylpropiophenone hydrochloride, with a molecular weight of 377.92. The molecular formula is $C_{21}H_{27}NO_3$•HCl.

Propafenone HCl has some structural similarities to beta-blocking agents. The structural formula of propafenone HCl is given below:

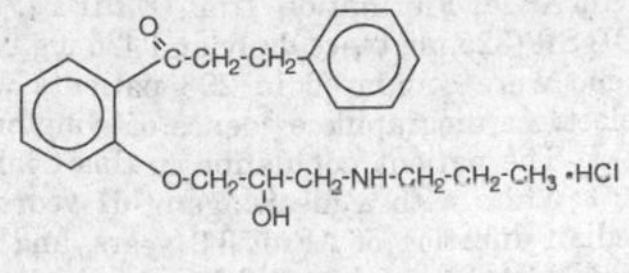

Propafenone HCl occurs as colorless crystals or white crystalline powder with a very bitter taste. It is slightly soluble in water (20°C), chloroform and ethanol. RYTHMOL SR capsules are filled with cylindrical-shaped 2 × 2 mm microtablets containing propafenone and the following inactive ingredients: antifoam, gelatin, hypromellose, magnesium stearate, red iron oxide, shellac, sodium dodecyl sulfate, sodium lauryl sulfate, soy lecithin and titanium dioxide.

12 CLINICAL PHARMACOLOGY

12.1 Mechanism of Action

Propafenone is a Class 1C antiarrhythmic drug with local anesthetic effects, and a direct stabilizing action on myocardial membranes. The electrophysiological effect of propafenone manifests itself in a reduction of upstroke velocity (Phase 0) of the monophasic action potential. In Purkinje fibers, and to a lesser extent myocardial fibers, propafenone reduces the fast inward current carried by sodium ions. Diastolic excitability threshold is increased and effective refractory period prolonged. Propafenone reduces spontaneous automaticity and depresses triggered activity. Studies in anesthetized dogs and isolated organ preparations show that propafenone has beta-sympatholytic activity at about 1/50 the potency of propranolol. Clinical studies employing isoproterenol challenge and exercise testing after single doses of propafenone indicate a beta-adrenergic blocking potency (per mg) about 1/40 that of propranolol in man. In clinical trials with the immediate-release formulation, resting heart rate decreases of about 8% were noted at the higher end of the therapeutic plasma concentration range. At very high concentrations in vitro, propafenone can inhibit the slow inward current carried by calcium, but this calcium antagonist effect probably does not contribute to antiarrhythmic efficacy. Moreover, propafenone inhibits a variety of cardiac potassium currents in in vitro studies (i.e. the transient outward, the delayed rectifier, and the inward rectifier current). Propafenone has local anesthetic activity approximately equal to procaine. Compared to propafenone, the main metabolite, 5-hydroxypropafenone, has similar sodium and calcium channel activity, but about 10 times less beta-blocking activity (N-depropylpropafenone has weaker sodium channel activity but equivalent affinity for beta-receptors).

12.2 Pharmacodynamics

Electrophysiology

Electrophysiology studies in patients with ventricular tachycardia have shown that propafenone prolongs atrioventricular conduction while having little or no effect on sinus node function. Both atrioventricular nodal conduction time (AH interval) and His-Purkinje conduction time (HV interval) are prolonged. Propafenone has little or no effect on the atrial functional refractory period, but AV nodal functional and effective refractory periods are prolonged. In patients with Wolff-Parkinson-White syndrome, RYTHMOL immediate-release tablets reduce conduction and increase the effective refractory period of the accessory pathway in both directions.

Electrocardiograms

Propafenone prolongs the PR and QRS intervals. Prolongation of the QRS interval makes it difficult to interpret the effect of propafenone on the QT interval.

[See table 1 above]

Table 1. Mean Change ± SD in 12-Lead Electrocardiogram Results (RAFT)

	RYTHMOL SR Twice Daily Dosing			Placebo
	225 mg	325 mg	425 mg	
	n = 126	n = 135	n = 136	n = 126
PR (ms)	9 ± 22	12 ± 23	21 ± 24	1 ± 16
QRS (ms)	4 ± 14	6 ± 15	6 ± 15	-2 ± 12
Heart rate	5 ± 24	7 ± 23	2 ± 22	8 ± 27
QTc[a] (ms)	2 ± 30	5 ± 36	6 ± 37	5 ± 35

[a] Calculated using Bazett's correction factor

In RAFT *[see Clinical Studies (14)]*, the distribution of the maximum changes in QTc compared to baseline over the study in each patient was similar in the RYTHMOL SR 225 mg twice daily, 325 mg twice daily, and 425 mg twice daily and placebo dose groups. Similar results were seen in the ERAFT study.

[See table 2 above]

Table 2. Number of Patients According to the Range of Maximum QTc Change Compared to Baseline Over the Study in Each Dose Group (RAFT Study).

Range maximum QTc change	RYTHMOL SR			Placebo
	225 mg twice daily	325 mg twice daily	425 mg twice daily	
	N = 119	N = 129	N = 123	N = 100
	n (%)	n (%)	n (%)	n (%)
>20%	1 (1)	6 (5)	3 (2)	5 (4)
10-20%	19 (16)	28 (22)	32 (26)	24 (20)
0 ≤10%	99 (83)	95 (74)	88 (72)	91 (76)

Hemodynamics

Studies in humans have shown that propafenone exerts a negative inotropic effect on the myocardium. Cardiac catheterization studies in patients with moderately impaired ventricular function (mean C.I. = 2.61 L/min/m^2), utilizing intravenous propafenone infusions (loading dose of 2 mg/kg over 10 min+ followed by 2 mg/min for 30 min) that gave mean plasma concentrations of 3.0 µg/mL (a dose that produces plasma levels of propafenone greater than does recommended oral dosing), showed significant increases in pulmonary capillary wedge pressure, systemic and pulmonary vascular resistances and depression of cardiac output and cardiac index.

12.3 Pharmacokinetics

Absorption/Bioavailability

Maximal plasma levels of propafenone are reached between 3 to 8 hours following the administration of RYTHMOL SR. Propafenone is known to undergo extensive and saturable presystemic biotransformation which results in a dose and dosage form dependent absolute bioavailability; e.g., a 150 mg immediate-release tablet had an absolute bioavailability of 3.4%, while a 300 mg immediate-release tablet had an absolute bioavailability of 10.6%. Absorption from a 300 mg solution dose was rapid, with an absolute bioavailability of 21.4%. At still larger doses, above those recommended, bioavailability of propafenone from immediate-release tablets increased still further.

Relative bioavailability assessments have been performed between RYTHMOL SR capsules and RYTHMOL immediate-release tablets. In extensive metabolizers, the bioavailability of propafenone from the SR formulation was less than that of the immediate-release formulation as the more gradual release of propafenone from the prolonged-release preparations resulted in an increase of overall first pass metabolism *[see Metabolism]*. As a result of the increased first pass effect, higher daily doses of propafenone were required from the SR formulation relative to the immediate-release formulation, to obtain similar exposure to propafenone. The relative bioavailability of propafenone from the 325 twice daily regimens of RYTHMOL SR approximates that of RYTHMOL immediate-release 150 mg three times daily regimen. Mean exposure to 5-hydroxypropafenone was about 20 to 25% higher after SR capsule administration than after immediate-release tablet administration.

Food increased the exposure to propafenone 4-fold after single dose administration of 425 mg of RYTHMOL SR. However, in the multiple dose study (425 mg dose twice daily), the difference between the fed and fasted state was not significant.

Distribution

Following intravenous administration of propafenone, plasma levels decline in a bi-phasic manner consistent with a 2 compartment pharmacokinetic model. The average distribution half-life corresponding to the first phase was about 5 minutes. The volume of the central compartment was about 88 liters (1.1 L/kg) and the total volume of distribution about 252 liters.

In serum, propafenone is greater than 95% bound to proteins within the concentration range of 0.5 to 2 µg/mL.

Metabolism

There are two genetically determined patterns of propafenone metabolism. In over 90% of patients, the drug is rapidly and extensively metabolized with an elimination half-life from 2 to 10 hours. These patients metabolize propafenone into two active metabolites: 5-hydroxypropafenone which is formed by CYP2D6 and N-depropylpropafenone (norpropafenone) which is formed by both CYP3A4 and CYP1A2. In less than 10% of patients, metabolism of propafenone is slower because the 5-hydroxy metabolite is not formed or is minimally formed. In these patients, the estimated propafenone elimination half-life ranges from 10 to 32 hours. Decreased ability to form the 5-hydroxy metabolite of propafenone is associated with a diminished ability to metabolize debrisoquine and a variety of other drugs such as encainide, metoprolol, and dextromethorphan whose metabolism is mediated by the CYP2D6 isozyme. In these patients, the N-depropylpropafenone metabolite occurs in quantities comparable to the levels occurring in extensive metabolizers.

As a consequence of the observed differences in metabolism, administration of RYTHMOL SR to slow and extensive metabolizers results in significant differences in plasma concentrations of propafenone, with slow metabolizers achieving concentrations about twice those of the extensive metabolizers at daily doses of 850 mg/day. At low doses the differences are greater, with slow metabolizers attaining concentrations about 3 to 4 times higher than extensive metabolizers. In extensive metabolizers, saturation of the hydroxylation pathway (CYP2D6) results in greater-than-linear increases in plasma levels following administration of RYTHMOL SR capsules. In slow metabolizers, propafenone pharmacokinetics is linear. Because the difference decreases at high doses and is mitigated by the lack of the active 5-hydroxymetabolite in the slow metabolizers, and because steady-state conditions are achieved after 4 to 5 days of dosing in all patients, the recommended dosing regimen of RYTHMOL SR is the same for all patients. The larger inter-subject variability in blood levels require that the dose of the drug be titrated carefully in patients with close attention paid to clinical and ECG evidence of toxicity *[see Dosage and Administration (2)]*.

The 5-hydroxypropafenone and norpropafenone metabolites have electrophysiologic properties similar to propafenone in vitro. In man after administration of RYTHMOL SR, the 5-hydroxypropafenone metabolite is usually present in concentrations less than 40% of propafenone. The norpropafenone metabolite is usually present in concentrations less than 10% of propafenone.

Inter-Subject Variability

With propafenone, there is a considerable degree of inter-subject variability in pharmacokinetics which is due in large part to the first pass hepatic effect and non-linear pharmacokinetics in extensive metabolizers. A higher degree of inter-subject variability in pharmacokinetic parameters of propafenone was observed following both single and multiple dose administration of RYTHMOL SR capsules. Inter-subject variability appears to be substantially less in the poor metabolizer group than in the extensive metabolizer group, suggesting that a large portion of the variability is intrinsic to CYP2D6 polymorphism rather than to the formulation.

Stereochemistry

RYTHMOL is a racemic mixture. The R- and S-enantiomers of propafenone display stereoselective disposition characteristics. In vitro and in vivo studies have shown that the R-isomer of propafenone is cleared faster than the S-isomer

Table 3. Analysis of Tachycardia-Free Period (Days) from Day 1 of Randomization

Parameter	RYTHMOL SR Dose 225 mg twice daily (N = 126) n (%)	325 mg twice daily (N = 135) n (%)	425 mg twice daily (N = 136) n (%)	Placebo (N = 126) n (%)
Patients completing with terminating event[a]	66 (52)	56 (41)	41 (30)	87 (69)
Comparison of tachycardia-free periods				
Kaplan-Meier Media	112	291	NA[b]	41
Range	0 - 285	0 - 293	0 - 300	0 – 289
p-Value (Log-rank test)	0.014	<0.0001	<0.0001	--
Hazard Ratio compared to placebo	0.67	0.43	0.35	--
95% CI for Hazard Ratio	(0.49, 0.93)	(0.31, 0.61)	(0.24, 0.51)	--

[a] Terminating events comprised 91% AF, 5% atrial flutter, and 4% PSVT.
[b] Not Applicable: Fewer than 50% of the patients had events. The median time is not calculable.

via the 5-hydroxylation pathway (CYP2D6). This results in a higher ratio of S-propafenone to R-propafenone at steady state. Both enantiomers have equivalent potency to block sodium channels; however, the S-enantiomer is a more potent β-antagonist than the R-enantiomer. Following administration of RYTHMOL immediate-release tablets or RYTHMOL SR capsules, the S/R ratio for the area under the plasma concentration-time curve was about 1.7. The S/R ratios of propafenone obtained after administration of 225, 325 and 425 mg RYTHMOL SR are independent of dose. In addition, no difference in the average values of the S/R ratios is evident between genotypes or over time.

Special Populations

Hepatic Impairment

Decreased liver function increases the bioavailability of propafenone. Absolute bioavailability assessments have not been determined for the RYTHMOL SR capsule formulation. Absolute bioavailability of RYTHMOL immediate-release tablets is inversely related to indocyanine green clearance, reaching 60-70% at clearances of 7 mL/min and below. Protein binding decreases to about 88% in patients with severe hepatic dysfunction. The clearance of propafenone is reduced and the elimination half-life increased in patients with significant hepatic dysfunction *[see Warnings and Precautions (5.9)]*.

13 NONCLINICAL TOXICOLOGY

13.1 Carcinogenesis, Mutagenesis, Impairment of Fertility

Lifetime maximally tolerated oral dose studies in mice (up to 360 mg/kg/day, about twice the maximum recommended human oral daily dose [MRHD] on a mg/m^2 basis) and rats (up to 270 mg/kg/day, about 3 times the MRHD on a mg/m^2 basis) provided no evidence of a carcinogenic potential for propafenone HCl.

Propafenone HCl tested negative for mutagenicity in the Ames (salmonella) test and in the in vivo mouse dominant lethal test. It tested negative for clastogenicity in the human lymphocyte chromosome aberration assay in vitro and in rat and Chinese hamster micronucleus tests, and other in vivo tests for chromosomal aberrations in rat bone marrow and Chinese hamster bone marrow and spermatogonia.

Propafenone HCl, administered intravenously to rabbits, dogs, and monkeys, has been shown to decrease spermatogenesis. These effects were reversible, were not found following oral dosing of propafenone HCl, were seen at lethal or near lethal dose levels and were not seen in rats treated either orally or intravenously *[see Warnings and Precautions (5.13)]*. Treatment of male rabbits for 10 weeks prior to mating at an oral dose of 120 mg/kg/day (about 2.4 times the MRHD on a mg/m^2 basis) or an intravenous dose of 3.5 mg/kg/day (a spermatogenesis-impairing dose) did not result in evidence of impaired fertility. Nor was there evidence of impaired fertility when propafenone HCl was administered orally to male and female rats at dose levels up to 270 mg/kg/day (about 3 times the MRHD on a mg/m^2 basis).

13.2 Animal Toxicology and/or Pharmacology

Renal and Hepatic Toxicity in Animals

Renal changes have been observed in the rat following 6 months of oral administration of propafenone HCl at doses of 180 and 360 mg/kg/day (about 2 and 4 times, respectively, the MRHD on a mg/m^2 basis). Both inflammatory and noninflammatory changes in the renal tubules, with accompanying interstitial nephritis, were observed. These changes were reversible, as they were not found in rats allowed to recover for 6 weeks. Fatty degenerative changes of the liver were found in rats following longer durations of administration of propafenone HCl at a dose of 270 mg/kg/day (about 3 times the MRHD on a mg/m^2 basis). There were no renal or hepatic changes at 90 mg/kg/day equivalent to the MRHD on a mg/m^2 basis).

14 CLINICAL STUDIES

RYTHMOL SR has been evaluated in patients with a history of electrocardiographically documented recurrent episodes of symptomatic AF in 2 randomized, double-blind, placebo controlled trials.

RAFT: In one US multicenter study (Rythmol SR Atrial Fibrillation Trial, RAFT), 3 doses of RYTHMOL SR (225 mg twice daily, 325 mg twice daily and 425 mg twice daily) and placebo were compared in 523 patients with symptomatic, episodic AF. The patient population in this trial was 59% male with a mean age of 63 years, 91% White and 6% Black. The patients had a median history of AF of 13 months, and documented symptomatic AF within 12 months of study entry. Over 90% were NYHA Class I, and 21% had a prior electrical cardioversion. At baseline, 24% were treated with calcium channel blockers, 37% with beta blockers, and 38% with digoxin. Symptomatic arrhythmias after randomization were documented by transtelephonic electrocardiogram and centrally read and adjudicated by a blinded adverse event committee. RYTHMOL SR administered for up to 39 weeks was shown to prolong significantly the time to the first recurrence of symptomatic atrial arrhythmia, predominantly AF, from Day 1 of randomization (primary efficacy variable) compared to placebo, as shown in Table 3.

[See table 3 above]

There was a dose response for RYTHMOL SR for the tachycardia free period as shown in the proportional hazard analysis and the Kaplan-Meier curves presented in Figure 1.

Figure 1. RAFT Kaplan-Meier Analysis for the Tachycardia-Free Period From Day 1 of Randomization:

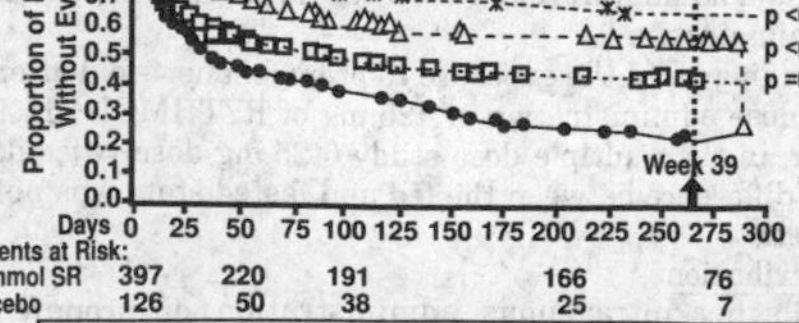

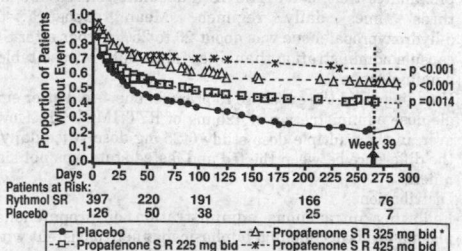

* Patient closeout started on Day 273 (week 39) and lasted until 300 days. On day 291, of the 2 patients that were left on 325 mg, 1 had an event, causing a 50% decline in the Kaplan-Meier curves

In additional analyses, RYTHMOL SR (225 mg twice daily, 325 mg twice daily, and 425 mg twice daily) was also shown to prolong time to the first recurrence of symptomatic AF from Day 5 (steady-state pharmacokinetics were attained). The antiarrhythmic effect of RYTHMOL SR was not influenced by age, gender, history of cardioversion, duration of AF, frequency of AF or use of medication that lowers heart rate. Similarly, the antiarrhythmic effect of RYTHMOL SR was not influenced by the individual use of calcium channel blockers, beta-blockers or digoxin. Too few non-White patients were enrolled to assess the influence of race on effects of RYTHMOL SR (propafenone hydrochloride).

No difference in the average heart rate during the first recurrence of symptomatic arrhythmia between RYTHMOL SR and placebo was observed.

ERAFT: In a European multicenter trial [European Rythmonorm SR Atrial Fibrillation Trial (ERAFT)], 2 doses of RYTHMOL SR (325 mg twice daily and 425 mg twice daily) and placebo were compared in 293 patients with documented electrocardiographic evidence of symptomatic paroxysmal AF. The patient population in this trial was 61% male, 100% White with a mean age of 61 years. Patients had a median duration of AF of 3.3 years, and 61% were taking medications that lowered heart rate. At baseline, 15% of the patients were treated with calcium channel blockers (verapamil and diltiazem), 42% with beta-blockers and 8% with digoxin. During a qualifying period of up to 28 days, patients had to have 1 ECG-documented incident of symptomatic AF. The double-blind treatment phase consisted of a 4 day loading period followed by a 91-day efficacy period. Symptomatic arrhythmias were documented by electrocardiogram monitoring.

In ERAFT, RYTHMOL SR was shown to prolong the time to the first recurrence of symptomatic atrial arrhythmia from Day 5 of randomization (primary efficacy analysis). The proportional hazard analysis revealed that both RYTHMOL SR doses were superior to placebo. The antiarrhythmic effect of propafenone SR was not influenced by age, gender, duration of AF, frequency of AF or use of medication that lowers heart rate. It was also not influenced by the individual use of calcium channel blockers, beta-blockers or digoxin. Too few non-White patients were enrolled to assess the influence of race on the effects of RYTHMOL SR. There was a slight increase in the incidence of centrally diagnosed asymptomatic AF or atrial flutter in each of the 2 RYTHMOL SR treatment groups compared to placebo.

16 HOW SUPPLIED/STORAGE AND HANDLING

RYTHMOL SR (propafenone HCl) capsules are supplied as white, opaque, hard gelatin capsules containing either 225 mg, 325 mg, or 425 mg of propafenone HCl. The 225 mg strength is imprinted in red with GS EUG followed by 225. The 325 mg strength is imprinted in red with GS F1Y followed by 325, and also has a single red band around ¾ of the circumference of the body. The 425 mg strength is imprinted in red with GS UY2 followed by 425, and also has three red bands around ¾ of the circumference of the body.

Capsule Strength	60 count bottle NDC
225 mg	0173-0823-18
325 mg	0173-0824-18
425 mg	0173-0826-18

Storage: Store at 25°C (77°F); excursions permitted to 15° to 30°C (59° to 86°F). Dispense in a tight container.

17 PATIENT COUNSELING INFORMATION

See FDA-approved patient labeling (Patient Information).

17.1 Information for Patients

- Patients should be instructed to notify their health care providers of any change in over-the-counter, prescription and supplement use. The health care provider should assess the patients' medication history including all over-the-counter, prescription and herbal/natural preparations for those that may affect the pharmacodynamics or kinetics of RYTHMOL SR *[see Warnings and Precautions (5.4)]*.
- Patients should also check with their health care providers prior to taking a new over-the-counter medicine.
- If patients experience symptoms that may be associated with altered electrolyte balance, such as excessive or prolonged diarrhea, sweating, vomiting, or loss of appetite or thirst, these conditions should be immediately reported to their health care provider.
- Patients should be instructed NOT to double the next dose if a dose is missed. The next dose should be taken at the usual time.

RYTHMOL SR is a registered trademark of G. Petrik used under license by Abbott Laboratories.

Manufactured for:
GlaxoSmithKline
Research Triangle Park, NC 27709

RMS:8PI

PHARMACIST-DETACH HERE AND GIVE INSTRUCTIONS TO PATIENT

PATIENT INFORMATION

RYTHMOL SR® (RITH-Mall)

(propafenone hydrochloride) Extended-Release Capsules

Read this Patient Information Leaflet before you start taking RYTHMOL SR and each time you get a refill. There may be new information. This information does not take the place of talking with your doctor about your medical condition or your treatment.

What is RYTHMOL SR?
RYTHMOL SR is a prescription medicine that is used:
- in certain people who have a heart rhythm disorder called atrial fibrillation (AF)
- to increase the amount of time between having symptoms of AF

It is not known if RYTHMOL SR is safe and effective in children.

Who should not take RYTHMOL SR?
Do not take RYTHMOL SR if you have:
- heart failure (weak heart)
- had a recent heart attack
- have a heart condition called Brugada Syndrome
- a heart rate that is too slow, and you do not have a pacemaker
- very low blood pressure
- certain breathing problems that make you short of breath or wheeze
- certain abnormal body salt (electrolyte) levels in your blood

Talk to your doctor before taking RYTHMOL SR if you think you have any of the conditions listed above.

What should I tell my doctor before taking RYTHMOL SR?
Before you take RYTHMOL SR, tell your doctor if you:
- have liver or kidney problems
- have breathing problems
- have symptoms including diarrhea, sweating, vomiting, or loss of appetite or thirst that are severe. These symptoms may be a sign of abnormal electrolyte levels in your blood.
- have myasthenia gravis
- have lupus erythematosis
- have been told you have or had an abnormal blood test called Antinuclear Antibody Test or ANA Test
- are pregnant or plan to become pregnant. It is not known if RYTHMOL SR will harm your unborn baby.
- are breastfeeding or plan to breastfeed. RYTHMOL SR can pass into your milk and may harm your baby. You and your doctor should decide if you will breastfeed or take RYTHMOL SR. You should not do both.
- have any other medical conditions

Tell your doctor about all the medicines you take, including prescription and non-prescription medicines, vitamins, and herbal supplements. RYTHMOL SR and certain other medicines can affect each other and cause serious side effects. RYTHMOL SR may affect the way other medicines work, and other medicines may affect how RYTHMOL SR works.

Especially tell your doctor if you take:
- amiodarone or other medicines for your abnormal heart beats
- an antidepressant medicine
- a medicine to treat anxiety
- ritonavir (for example, KALETRA®, NORVIR®) or saquinavir (for example, INVIRASE®)
- an antibiotic medicine
- ketoconazole (for example, NIZORAL®)
- digoxin (LANOXIN®)
- warfarin sodium (for example, COUMADIN®, JANTOVEN®)

Know the medicines you take. Keep a list of them to show your doctor and pharmacist when you get a new medicine.

How should I take RYTHMOL SR?
- Take RYTHMOL SR exactly as prescribed. Your doctor will tell you how many capsules to take and how often to take them.
- To help reduce the chance of certain side effects, your doctor may start you with a low dose of RYTHMOL SR, and then slowly increase the dose.
- Do not open or crush the capsule.
- You may take RYTHMOL SR with or without food.
- You should not drink grapefruit juice during treatment with RYTHMOL SR.
- If you miss a dose of RYTHMOL SR, take your next dose at the usual time. Do not take 2 doses at the same time.
- If you take too much RYTHMOL SR, call your doctor or go to the nearest hospital emergency room right away.
- Call your doctor if your heart problems get worse.

What are possible side effects of RYTHMOL SR?
RYTHMOL SR can cause serious side effects including:
- **New or worsened abnormal heart beats, that can cause sudden death or be life-threatening.** Your doctor may do an electrocardiogram (ECG or EKG) before and during treatment to check your heart for these problems.
- **New or worsened heart failure. Tell your doctor about any changes in your heart symptoms, including:**
  - any new or increased swelling in your arms or legs
  - trouble breathing
  - sudden weight gain
- **Effects on pacemaker function.** RYTHMOL SR may affect how an implanted pacemaker or defibrillator works. Your doctor should check how your pacemaker or defibrillator is working during and after treatment with RYTHMOL SR. They may need to be re-programmed.
- **Very low white blood cell levels in your blood (agranulocytosis).** Your bone marrow may not produce enough of a certain type of white blood cells called neutrophils. If this happens, you are more likely to get infections. Tell your doctor right away if you have any of these symptoms, especially during the first 3 months of treatment:
  - fever
  - sore throat
  - chills
- **Worsening of myasthenia gravis in people who already have this condition.** Tell your doctor about any change in your symptoms.
- **RYTHMOL SR may cause lower sperm counts in men.** This could affect the ability to father a child. Talk to your doctor if this is a concern for you.

Common side effects of RYTHMOL SR include:
- dizziness
- fast or irregular heart beats
- chest pain
- trouble breathing
- taste changes
- nausea
- tiredness
- feeling anxious
- constipation
- upper respiratory infection or flu
- swelling

Tell your doctor if you have any side effect that bothers you or that does not go away.
These are not all the possible side effects of RYTHMOL SR. For more information, ask your doctor or pharmacist.
Call your doctor for medical advice about side effects. You may report side effects to FDA at 1-800-FDA-1088.

How should I store RYTHMOL SR?
- Store RYTHMOL SR at room temperature between 59°F to 86°F (15°C to 30°C).
- Keep the bottle tightly closed.

Keep RYTHMOL SR and all medicines out of the reach of children.

General information about RYTHMOL SR
Medicines are sometimes prescribed for conditions other than those described in patient information leaflets. Do not use RYTHMOL SR for a condition for which it was not prescribed by your doctor. Do not give RYTHMOL SR to other people, even if they have the same symptoms you have. It may harm them.
This leaflet summarizes the most important information about RYTHMOL SR. If you would like more information, talk with your doctor. You can ask your doctor or pharmacist for information about RYTHMOL SR that is written for healthcare professionals. For more information about RYTHMOL SR, call 1-888-825-5249.

What are the ingredients in RYTHMOL SR?
Active Ingredient: Propafenone hydrochloride
Inactive Ingredients: Antifoam, gelatin, hypromellose, magnesium stearate, red iron oxide, shellac, sodium dodecyl sulfate, sodium lauryl sulfate, soy lecithin and titanium dioxide.

RYTHMOL is a registered trademark of G. Petrik used under license by Abbott Laboratories. The other brands listed are trademarks of their respective owners and are not trademarks of GlaxoSmithKline. The makers of these brands are not affiliated with and do not endorse GlaxoSmithKline or its products.
Manufactured for:
GlaxoSmithKline
Research Triangle Park, NC 27709

June 2013
RMS:3PIL

SEREVENT DISKUS ℞

[ser′ ə-vent dĭsk′ us]
(salmeterol xinafoate inhalation powder)
FOR ORAL INHALATION

HIGHLIGHTS OF PRESCRIBING INFORMATION
These highlights do not include all the information needed to use SEREVENT DISKUS safely and effectively. See full prescribing information for SEREVENT DISKUS.
SEREVENT DISKUS
(salmeterol xinafoate inhalation powder)
FOR ORAL INHALATION
Initial U.S. Approval: 1994

WARNING: ASTHMA-RELATED DEATH
See full prescribing information for complete boxed warning
- **Long-acting $beta_2$-adrenergic agonists (LABA), such as salmeterol, the active ingredient in SEREVENT DISKUS, increase the risk of asthma-related death. A US study showed an increase in asthma-related deaths in patients receiving salmeterol (13 deaths out of 13,176 patients treated for 28 weeks on salmeterol versus 3 out of 13,179 patients on placebo). Currently available data are inadequate to determine whether concurrent use of inhaled corticosteroids or other long-term asthma control drugs mitigates the increased risk of asthma-related death from LABA. (5.1)**
- **Prescribe SEREVENT DISKUS only as additional therapy for patients with asthma who are currently taking but are inadequately controlled on a long-term asthma control medication, such as an inhaled corticosteroid. Once asthma control is achieved and maintained, assess the patient at regular intervals and step down therapy (e.g., discontinue SEREVENT DISKUS) if possible without loss of asthma control and maintain the patient on a long-term asthma control medication, such as an inhaled corticosteroid. Do not use SEREVENT DISKUS for patients whose asthma is adequately controlled on low- or medium-dose inhaled corticosteroids. (1.1, 5.1)**
- **Available data from controlled clinical trials suggest that LABA increase the risk of asthma-related hospitalization in pediatric and adolescent patients. (5.1)**

INDICATIONS AND USAGE

SEREVENT DISKUS is a LABA indicated for:
- Treatment of asthma in patients aged 4 years and older. (1.1)
- Prevention of exercise-induced bronchospasm (EIB) in patients aged 4 years and older. (1.2)
- Maintenance treatment of bronchospasm associated with chronic obstructive pulmonary disease (COPD). (1.3)

Important limitation:
- Not indicated for the relief of acute bronchospasm. (1.1, 1.3)

DOSAGE AND ADMINISTRATION

For oral inhalation only.
- Treatment of asthma in patients ≥4 years: 1 inhalation twice daily in addition to concomitant treatment with an inhaled corticosteroid. (2.1)
- EIB: One inhalation at least 30 minutes before exercise. (2.2)
- Maintenance treatment of bronchospasm associated with COPD: 1 inhalation twice daily. (2.3)

DOSAGE FORMS AND STRENGTHS

DISKUS device containing salmeterol (50 mcg) as an oral inhalation powder. (3)

CONTRAINDICATIONS

- Asthma: Without concomitant use of a long-term asthma control medication such as an inhaled corticosteroid. (4)
- Primary treatment of status asthmaticus or acute episodes of asthma or COPD requiring intensive measures. (4)
- Severe hypersensitivity to milk proteins. (4)

WARNINGS AND PRECAUTIONS

- Asthma-related death and asthma-related hospitalizations: Long-acting $beta_2$-adrenergic agonists increase the risk. Prescribe for asthma only as concomitant therapy with an inhaled corticosteroid. (5.1)
- Deterioration of disease and acute episodes: Do not initiate during rapidly deteriorating asthma. Do not use to treat acute symptoms. (5.2)
- Corticosteroids: Not a substitute for corticosteroids. Patients with asthma must take a concomitant inhaled corticosteroid. (5.3)
- Use with additional long-acting $beta_2$-agonist: Do not use in combination because of risk of overdose. (5.4)
- Paradoxical bronchospasm: Discontinue SEREVENT DISKUS and institute alternative therapy if paradoxical bronchospasm occurs. (5.5)
- Patients with cardiovascular or central nervous system disorders: Use with caution because of beta-adrenergic stimulation. (5.6)
- Strong cytochrome P450 3A4 inhibitors (e.g., ketoconazole): Risk of cardiovascular effects. Use not recommended with SEREVENT DISKUS. (5.8)
- Coexisting conditions: Use with caution in patients with convulsive disorders, thyrotoxicosis, diabetes mellitus, and ketoacidosis. (5.9)
- Metabolic effects: Be alert to hypokalemia and hyperglycemia. (5.10)

ADVERSE REACTIONS

The most common adverse reactions (incidence ≥5%) are:
- Asthma: Headache, influenza, nasal/sinus congestion, pharyngitis, rhinitis tracheitis/bronchitis. (6.1)
- COPD: Cough, headache, musculoskeletal pain, throat irritation, viral respiratory infection. (6.2)

To report SUSPECTED ADVERSE REACTIONS, contact GlaxoSmithKline at 1-888-825-5249 or FDA at 1-800-FDA-1088 or www.fda.gov/medwatch

DRUG INTERACTIONS

- Strong cytochrome P450 3A4 inhibitors (e.g., ritonavir): Use not recommended. May increase risk of cardiovascular effects. (7.1)
- Monoamine oxidase inhibitors and tricyclic antidepressants: Use with extreme caution. May potentiate effect of salmeterol on vascular system. (7.2)
- Beta-blockers: Use with caution. May block bronchodilatory effects of beta-agonists and produce severe bronchospasm. (7.3)
- Diuretics: Use with caution. Electrocardiographic changes and/or hypokalemia associated with nonpotassium-sparing diuretics may worsen with concomitant beta-agonists. (7.4)

USE IN SPECIFIC POPULATIONS

Hepatic impairment: Monitor patients for signs of increased drug exposure. (8.6)

See 17 for PATIENT COUNSELING INFORMATION and Medication Guide

Revised: 01/2012

FULL PRESCRIBING INFORMATION: CONTENTS*

*** Sections or subsections omitted from the full prescribing information are not listed**

FULL PRESCRIBING INFORMATION

WARNING: ASTHMA-RELATED DEATH

Long-acting beta$_2$-adrenergic agonists (LABA), such as salmeterol, the active ingredient in SEREVENT® DISKUS®, increase the risk of asthma-related death. Data from a large placebo-controlled US study that compared the safety of salmeterol (SEREVENT® Inhalation Aerosol) or placebo added to usual asthma therapy showed an increase in asthma-related deaths in patients receiving salmeterol (13 deaths out of 13,176 patients treated for 28 weeks on salmeterol versus 3 deaths out of 13,179 patients on placebo). Currently available data are inadequate to determine whether concurrent use of inhaled corticosteroids or other long-term asthma control drugs mitigates the increased risk of asthma-related death from LABA.

Because of this risk, use of SEREVENT DISKUS for the treatment of asthma without a concomitant long-term asthma control medication, such as an inhaled corticosteroid, is contraindicated. Use SEREVENT DISKUS only as additional therapy for patients with asthma who are currently taking but are inadequately controlled on a long-term asthma control medication, such as an inhaled corticosteroid. Once asthma control is achieved and maintained, assess the patient at regular intervals and step down therapy (e.g., discontinue SEREVENT DISKUS) if possible without loss of asthma control and maintain the patient on a long-term asthma control medication, such as an inhaled corticosteroid. Do not use SEREVENT DISKUS for patients whose asthma is adequately controlled on low- or medium-dose inhaled corticosteroids.

Pediatric and Adolescent Patients: Available data from controlled clinical trials suggest that LABA increase the risk of asthma-related hospitalization in pediatric and adolescent patients. For pediatric and adolescent patients with asthma who require addition of a LABA to an inhaled corticosteroid, a fixed-dose combination product containing both an inhaled corticosteroid and a LABA should ordinarily be used to ensure adherence with both drugs. In cases where use of a separate long-term asthma control medication (e.g., inhaled corticosteroid) and a LABA is clinically indicated, appropriate steps must be taken to ensure adherence with both treatment components. If adherence cannot be assured, a fixed-dose combination product containing both an inhaled corticosteroid and a LABA is recommended.

1 INDICATIONS AND USAGE

1.1 Treatment of Asthma

SEREVENT DISKUS is indicated for the treatment of asthma and in the prevention of bronchospasm only as concomitant therapy with a long-term asthma control medication, such as an inhaled corticosteroid, in patients aged 4 years and older with reversible obstructive airway disease, including patients with symptoms of nocturnal asthma. LABA, such as salmeterol, the active ingredient in SEREVENT DISKUS, increase the risk of asthma-related death *[see Warnings and Precautions (5.1)]*. Use of SEREVENT DISKUS for the treatment of asthma without concomitant use of a long-term asthma control medication, such as an inhaled corticosteroid, is contraindicated *[see Contraindications (4)]*. Use SEREVENT DISKUS only as additional therapy for patients with asthma who are currently taking but are inadequately controlled on a long-term asthma control medication, such as an inhaled corticosteroid. Once asthma control is achieved and maintained, assess the patient at regular intervals and step down therapy (e.g., discontinue SEREVENT DISKUS) if possible without loss of asthma control and maintain the patient on a long-term asthma control medication, such as an inhaled corticosteroid. Do not use SEREVENT DISKUS for patients whose asthma is adequately controlled on low- or medium-dose inhaled corticosteroids.

Pediatric and Adolescent Patients: Available data from controlled clinical trials suggest that LABA increase the risk of asthma-related hospitalization in pediatric and adolescent patients. For pediatric and adolescent patients with asthma who require addition of a LABA to an inhaled corticosteroid, a fixed-dose combination product containing both an inhaled corticosteroid and a LABA should ordinarily be used to ensure adherence with both drugs. In cases where use of a separate long-term asthma control medication (e.g., inhaled corticosteroid) and a LABA is clinically indicated, appropriate steps must be taken to ensure adherence with both treatment components. If adherence cannot be assured, a fixed-dose combination product containing both an inhaled corticosteroid and a LABA is recommended.

Important Limitation of Use: SEREVENT DISKUS is NOT indicated for the relief of acute bronchospasm.

1.2 Prevention of Exercise-Induced Bronchospasm

SEREVENT DISKUS is also indicated for prevention of exercise-induced bronchospasm (EIB) in patients aged 4 years and older. Use of SEREVENT DISKUS as a single agent for the prevention of EIB may be clinically indicated in patients who do not have persistent asthma. In patients with persistent asthma, use of SEREVENT DISKUS for the prevention of EIB may be clinically indicated, but the treatment of asthma should include a long-term asthma control medication, such as an inhaled corticosteroid.

1.3 Maintenance Treatment of Chronic Obstructive Pulmonary Disease

SEREVENT DISKUS is indicated for the long-term twice-daily (morning and evening) administration in the maintenance treatment of bronchospasm associated with chronic obstructive pulmonary disease (COPD) (including emphysema and chronic bronchitis).

Important Limitation of Use: SEREVENT DISKUS is NOT indicated for the relief of acute bronchospasm.

2 DOSAGE AND ADMINISTRATION

SEREVENT DISKUS should be administered by the orally inhaled route only.

For both asthma and COPD, adverse effects are more likely to occur with higher doses of salmeterol, and more frequent administration or administration of a larger number of inhalations (more than 1 inhalation twice daily) is not recommended. Patients using SEREVENT DISKUS should not use additional LABA for any reason. *[See Warnings and Precautions (5.4, 5.6).]*

2.1 Asthma

LABA, such as salmeterol, the active ingredient in SEREVENT DISKUS, increase the risk of asthma-related death *[see Warnings and Precautions (5.1)]*.

Because of this risk, use of SEREVENT DISKUS for the treatment of asthma without concomitant use of a long-term asthma control medication, such as an inhaled corticosteroid is contraindicated. Use SEREVENT DISKUS only as additional therapy for patients with asthma who are currently taking but are inadequately controlled on a long-term asthma control medication, such as an inhaled corticosteroid. Once asthma control is achieved and maintained, assess the patient at regular intervals and step down therapy (e.g., discontinue SEREVENT DISKUS) if possible without loss of asthma control and maintain the patient on a long-term asthma control medication, such as an inhaled corticosteroid. Do not use SEREVENT DISKUS for patients whose asthma is adequately controlled on low- or medium-dose inhaled corticosteroids.

Pediatric and Adolescent Patients: Available data from controlled clinical trials suggest that LABA increase the risk of asthma-related hospitalization in pediatric and adolescent patients. For patients with asthma less than 18 years of age who require addition of a LABA to an inhaled corticosteroid, a fixed-dose combination product containing both an inhaled corticosteroid and a LABA should ordinarily be used to ensure adherence with both drugs. In cases where use of a separate long-term asthma control medication (e.g., inhaled corticosteroid) and a LABA is clinically indicated, appropriate steps must be taken to ensure adherence with both treatment components. If adherence cannot be assured, a fixed-dose combination product containing both an inhaled corticosteroid and a LABA is recommended.

For bronchodilatation and prevention of symptoms of asthma, including the symptoms of nocturnal asthma, the usual dosage for adults and children aged 4 years and older is 1 inhalation (50 mcg) twice daily (morning and evening, approximately 12 hours apart). If a previously effective dosage regimen fails to provide the usual response, medical advice should be sought immediately as this is often a sign of destabilization of asthma. Under these circumstances, the therapeutic regimen should be reevaluated. If symptoms arise in the period between doses, an inhaled, short-acting beta$_2$-agonist should be taken for immediate relief.

2.2 Exercise-Induced Bronchospasm

Use of SEREVENT DISKUS as a single agent for the prevention of EIB may be clinically indicated in patients who do not have persistent asthma. In patients with persistent asthma, use of SEREVENT DISKUS for the prevention of EIB may be clinically indicated, but the treatment of asthma should include a long-term asthma control medication, such as an inhaled corticosteroid. One inhalation of SEREVENT DISKUS at least 30 minutes before exercise has been shown to protect patients against EIB. When used intermittently as needed for prevention of EIB, this protection may last up to 9 hours in adolescents and adults and up to 12 hours in patients aged 4 to 11 years. Additional doses of SEREVENT should not be used for 12 hours after the administration of this drug. Patients who are receiving SEREVENT DISKUS twice daily should not use additional SEREVENT for prevention of EIB.

2.3 Chronic Obstructive Pulmonary Disease
For maintenance treatment of bronchospasm associated with COPD (including chronic bronchitis and emphysema), the dosage for adults is 1 inhalation (50 mcg) twice daily (morning and evening, approximately 12 hours apart).

3 DOSAGE FORMS AND STRENGTHS

Disposable teal green device with 60 blisters containing salmeterol (50 mcg) as an oral inhalation powder formulation. An institutional pack containing 28 blisters is also available.

4 CONTRAINDICATIONS

Because of the risk of asthma-related death and hospitalization, use of SEREVENT DISKUS for the treatment of asthma without concomitant use of a long-term asthma control medication, such as an inhaled corticosteroid, is contraindicated *[see Warnings and Precautions (5.1)]*.
SEREVENT DISKUS is contraindicated as primary treatment of status asthmaticus or other acute episodes of asthma or COPD where intensive measures are required *[see Warnings and Precautions (5.2)]*.
SEREVENT DISKUS is contraindicated in patients with severe hypersensitivity to milk proteins *[see Warnings and Precautions (5.7), Adverse Reactions (6.3), Description (11)]*.

5 WARNINGS AND PRECAUTIONS

5.1 Asthma-Related Death
LABA, such as salmeterol, the active ingredient in SEREVENT DISKUS, increase the risk of asthma-related death. Currently available data are inadequate to determine whether concurrent use of inhaled corticosteroids or other long-term asthma control drugs mitigates the increased risk of asthma-related death from LABA.
Because of this risk, use of SEREVENT DISKUS for the treatment of asthma without concomitant use of a long-term asthma control medication, such as an inhaled corticosteroid, is contraindicated. Use SEREVENT DISKUS only as additional therapy for patients with asthma who are currently taking but are inadequately controlled on a long-term asthma control medication, such as an inhaled corticosteroid. Once asthma control is achieved and maintained, assess the patient at regular intervals and step down therapy (e.g., discontinue SEREVENT DISKUS) if possible without loss of asthma control and maintain the patient on a long-term asthma control medication, such as an inhaled corticosteroid. Do not use SEREVENT DISKUS for patients whose asthma is adequately controlled on low- or medium-dose inhaled corticosteroids.
Pediatric and Adolescent Patients: **Available data from controlled clinical trials suggest that LABA increase the risk of asthma-related hospitalization in pediatric and adolescent patients. For pediatric and adolescent patients with asthma who require addition of a LABA to an inhaled corticosteroid, a fixed-dose combination product containing both an inhaled corticosteroid and a LABA should ordinarily be used to ensure adherence with both drugs. In cases where use of a separate long-term asthma control medication (e.g., inhaled corticosteroid) and a LABA is clinically indicated, appropriate steps must be taken to ensure adherence with both treatment components. If adherence cannot be assured, a fixed-dose combination product containing both an inhaled corticosteroid and a LABA is recommended.**
The Salmeterol Multi-center Asthma Research Trial (SMART) was a large 28-week placebo-controlled US study comparing the safety of salmeterol (SEREVENT Inhalation Aerosol) with placebo, each added to usual asthma therapy, that showed an increase in asthma-related deaths in patients receiving salmeterol *[see Clinical Studies (14.1)]*. Given the similar basic mechanisms of action of beta$_2$-agonists, the findings seen in the SMART study are considered a class effect.
A 16-week clinical study performed in the United Kingdom, the Salmeterol Nationwide Surveillance (SNS) study, showed results similar to the SMART study. In the SNS study, the rate of asthma-related death was numerically, though not statistically significantly, greater in patients with asthma treated with salmeterol (42 mcg twice daily) than those treated with albuterol (180 mcg 4 times daily) added to usual asthma therapy.
The SNS and SMART studies enrolled patients with asthma. No studies have been conducted that were adequate to determine whether the rate of death in patients with COPD is increased by LABA.

5.2 Deterioration of Disease and Acute Episodes
SEREVENT DISKUS should not be initiated in patients during rapidly deteriorating or potentially life-threatening episodes of asthma or COPD. SEREVENT DISKUS has not been studied in patients with acutely deteriorating asthma or COPD. The initiation of SEREVENT DISKUS in this setting is not appropriate.
Serious acute respiratory events, including fatalities, have been reported when salmeterol has been initiated in patients with significantly worsening or acutely deteriorating asthma. In most cases, these have occurred in patients with severe asthma (e.g., patients with a history of corticosteroid dependence, low pulmonary function, intubation, mechanical ventilation, frequent hospitalizations, previous life-threatening acute asthma exacerbations) and in some patients with acutely deteriorating asthma (e.g., patients with significantly increasing symptoms; increasing need for inhaled, short-acting beta$_2$-agonists; decreasing response to usual medications; increasing need for systemic corticosteroids; recent emergency room visits; deteriorating lung function). However, these events have occurred in a few patients with less severe asthma as well. It was not possible from these reports to determine whether salmeterol contributed to these events.
Increasing use of inhaled, short-acting beta$_2$-agonists is a marker of deteriorating asthma. In this situation, the patient requires immediate reevaluation with reassessment of the treatment regimen, giving special consideration to the possible need for adding additional inhaled corticosteroid or initiating systemic corticosteroids. Patients should not use more than 1 inhalation twice daily (morning and evening) of SEREVENT DISKUS.
SEREVENT DISKUS should not be used for the relief of acute symptoms, i.e., as rescue therapy for the treatment of acute episodes of bronchospasm. An inhaled, short-acting beta$_2$-agonist, not SEREVENT DISKUS, should be used to relieve acute symptoms such as shortness of breath. When prescribing SEREVENT DISKUS, the physician must also provide the patient with an inhaled, short-acting beta$_2$-agonist (e.g., albuterol) for treatment of acute symptoms.
When beginning treatment with SEREVENT DISKUS, patients who have been taking oral or inhaled, short-acting beta$_2$-agonists on a regular basis (e.g., 4 times a day) should be instructed to discontinue the regular use of these drugs.

5.3 SEREVENT DISKUS is Not a Substitute for Corticosteroids
There are no data demonstrating that SEREVENT DISKUS has a clinical anti-inflammatory effect such as that associated with corticosteroids. When initiating and throughout treatment with SEREVENT DISKUS in patients receiving oral or inhaled corticosteroids for treatment of asthma, patients must continue taking a suitable dosage of corticosteroids to maintain clinical stability even if they feel better as a result of initiating SEREVENT DISKUS. Any change in corticosteroid dosage should be made ONLY after clinical evaluation.

5.4 Excessive Use of SEREVENT DISKUS and Use With Other Long-Acting Beta$_2$-Agonists
As with other inhaled beta$_2$-adrenergic drugs, SEREVENT DISKUS should not be used more often or at higher doses than recommended, or in conjunction with other medications containing LABA, as an overdose may result. Clinically significant cardiovascular effects and fatalities have been reported in association with excessive use of inhaled sympathomimetic drugs. Patients using SEREVENT DISKUS should not use an additional LABA (e.g., formoterol fumarate, arformoterol tartrate) for any reason.

5.5 Paradoxical Bronchospasm and Upper Airway Symptoms
As with other inhaled medications, SEREVENT DISKUS can produce paradoxical bronchospasm, which may be life threatening. If paradoxical bronchospasm occurs following dosing with SEREVENT DISKUS, it should be treated immediately with an inhaled, short-acting bronchodilator; SEREVENT DISKUS should be discontinued immediately; and alternative therapy should be instituted. Upper airway symptoms of laryngeal spasm, irritation, or swelling, such as stridor and choking, have been reported in patients receiving SEREVENT DISKUS.

5.6 Cardiovascular and Central Nervous System Effects
Excessive beta-adrenergic stimulation has been associated with seizures, angina, hypertension or hypotension, tachycardia with rates up to 200 beats/min, arrhythmias, nervousness, headache, tremor, palpitation, nausea, dizziness, fatigue, malaise, and insomnia *[see Overdosage (10)]*. Therefore, SEREVENT DISKUS, like all products containing sympathomimetic amines, should be used with caution in patients with cardiovascular disorders, especially coronary insufficiency, cardiac arrhythmias, and hypertension.
Salmeterol can produce a clinically significant cardiovascular effect in some patients as measured by pulse rate, blood pressure, and/or symptoms. Although such effects are uncommon after administration of salmeterol at recommended doses, if they occur, the drug may need to be discontinued. In addition, beta-agonists have been reported to produce ECG changes, such as flattening of the T wave, prolongation of the QTc interval, and ST segment depression. The clinical significance of these findings is unknown. Large doses of inhaled or oral salmeterol (12 to 20 times the recommended dose) have been associated with clinically significant prolongation of the QTc interval, which has the potential for producing ventricular arrhythmias. Fatalities have been reported in association with excessive use of inhaled sympathomimetic drugs.

5.7 Immediate Hypersensitivity Reactions
Immediate hypersensitivity reactions may occur after administration of SEREVENT DISKUS, as demonstrated by cases of urticaria, angioedema, rash, and bronchospasm. There have been reports of anaphylactic reactions in patients with severe milk protein allergy; therefore, patients with severe milk protein allergy should not take SEREVENT DISKUS *[see Contraindications (4)]*.

5.8 Drug Interactions With Strong Cytochrome P450 3A4 Inhibitors
Because of the potential for drug interactions and the potential for increased risk of cardiovascular adverse events, the concomitant use of SEREVENT DISKUS with strong cytochrome P450 3A4 (CYP3A4) inhibitors (e.g., ketoconazole, ritonavir, atazanavir, clarithromycin, indinavir, itraconazole, nefazodone, nelfinavir, saquinavir, telithromycin) is not recommended *[see Drug Interactions (7.1)]*.

5.9 Coexisting Conditions
SEREVENT DISKUS, like all medications containing sympathomimetic amines, should be used with caution in patients with convulsive disorders or thyrotoxicosis and in those who are unusually responsive to sympathomimetic amines. Doses of the related beta$_2$-adrenoceptor agonist albuterol, when administered intravenously, have been reported to aggravate preexisting diabetes mellitus and ketoacidosis.

5.10 Hypokalemia and Hyperglycemia
Beta-adrenergic agonist medications may produce significant hypokalemia in some patients, possibly through intracellular shunting, which has the potential to produce adverse cardiovascular effects *[see Clinical Pharmacology (12.2)]*. The decrease in serum potassium is usually transient, not requiring supplementation. Clinically significant and dose-related changes in blood glucose and/or serum potassium were seen infrequently during clinical studies with SEREVENT DISKUS at recommended doses.

6 ADVERSE REACTIONS

LABA, including salmeterol, the active ingredient in SEREVENT DISKUS, increase the risk of asthma-related death. Data from a large 28-week placebo-controlled US study that compared the safety of salmeterol (SEREVENT Inhalation Aerosol) or placebo added to usual asthma therapy showed an increase in asthma-related deaths in patients receiving salmeterol. Available data from controlled clinical trials suggest that LABA increase the risk of asthma-related hospitalization in pediatric and adolescent patients *[see Warnings and Precautions (5.1), Clinical Studies (14.1)]*.
Because clinical trials are conducted under widely varying conditions, adverse reaction rates observed in the clinical trials of a drug cannot be directly compared with rates in the clinical trials of another drug and may not reflect the rates observed in practice.

6.1 Clinical Trials Experience in Asthma
Adult and Adolescent Patients Aged 12 Years and Older: Two multicenter, 12-week, controlled studies evaluated twice-daily doses of SEREVENT DISKUS in patients aged 12 years and older with asthma. Table 1 reports the incidence of adverse reactions in these 2 studies.
[See table 1 at top of next page]
Table 1 includes all events (whether considered drug-related or nondrug-related by the investigator) that occurred at a rate of 3% or greater in the group receiving SEREVENT DISKUS and were more common than in the placebo group.
Pharyngitis, sinusitis, upper respiratory tract infection, and cough occurred at ≥3% but were more common in the placebo group. However, throat irritation has been described at rates exceeding that of placebo in other controlled clinical trials.
Additional Adverse Reactions: Other adverse reactions not previously listed, whether considered drug-related or not by the investigators, that were reported more frequently by patients with asthma treated with SEREVENT DISKUS compared with patients treated with placebo include the following: contact dermatitis, eczema, localized aches and pains, nausea, oral mucosal abnormality, pain in joint, paresthesia, pyrexia of unknown origin, sinus headache, and sleep disturbance.
Pediatric Patients Aged 4 to 11 Years: Two multicenter, 12-week, controlled studies have evaluated twice-daily doses of SEREVENT DISKUS in patients aged 4 to 11 years with asthma. Table 2 includes all events (whether considered drug-related or nondrug-related by the investigator) that occurred at a rate of 3% or greater in the group receiving SEREVENT DISKUS and were more common than in the placebo group.
[See table 2 at top of next page]
The following events were reported at an incidence of >1% in the salmeterol group and with a higher incidence than in

the albuterol and placebo groups: gastrointestinal signs and symptoms, lower respiratory signs and symptoms, photodermatitis, and arthralgia and articular rheumatism.

In clinical trials evaluating concurrent therapy of salmeterol with inhaled corticosteroids, adverse events were consistent with those previously reported for salmeterol, or with events that would be expected with the use of inhaled corticosteroids.

Laboratory Test Abnormalities: Elevation of hepatic enzymes was reported in ≥1% of patients in clinical trials. The elevations were transient and did not lead to discontinuation from the studies. In addition, there were no clinically relevant changes noted in glucose or potassium.

6.2 Clinical Trials Experience in Chronic Obstructive Pulmonary Disease

Two multicenter, 24-week, controlled studies have evaluated twice-daily doses of SEREVENT DISKUS in patients with COPD. For presentation (Table 3), the placebo data from a third trial, identical in design, patient entrance criteria, and overall conduct but comparing fluticasone propionate with placebo, were integrated with the placebo data from these 2 studies (total N = 341 for salmeterol and 576 for placebo).

Table 3. Adverse Reactions With ≥3% Incidence in US Controlled Clinical Trials With SEREVENT DISKUS in Patients With Chronic Obstructive Pulmonary Disease[a]

Adverse Event	Percent of Patients: Placebo (N = 576)	SEREVENT DISKUS 50 mcg Twice Daily (N = 341)
Cardiovascular		
Hypertension	2	4
Ear, nose, and throat		
Throat irritation	6	7
Nasal congestion/blockage	3	4
Sinusitis	2	4
Ear signs and symptoms	1	3
Gastrointestinal		
Nausea and vomiting	3	3
Lower respiratory		
Cough	4	5
Rhinitis	2	4
Viral respiratory infection	4	5
Musculoskeletal		
Musculoskeletal pain	10	12
Muscle cramps and spasms	1	3
Neurological		
Headache	11	14
Dizziness	2	4
Average duration of exposure (days)	128.9	138.5

[a]Table 3 includes all events (whether considered drug-related or nondrug-related by the investigator) that occurred at a rate of 3% or greater in the group receiving SEREVENT DISKUS and were more common in the group receiving SEREVENT DISKUS than in the placebo group.

Additional Adverse Reactions: Other events occurring in the group receiving SEREVENT DISKUS that occurred at a frequency of ≥1% and were more common than in the placebo group were as follows: anxiety; arthralgia and articular rheumatism; bone and skeletal pain; candidiasis mouth/throat; dental discomfort and pain; dyspeptic symptoms; edema and swelling; gastrointestinal infections; hyperglycemia; hyposalivation; keratitis and conjunctivitis; lower respiratory signs and symptoms; migraines; muscle pain; muscle stiffness, tightness, and rigidity; musculoskeletal inflammation; pain; and skin rashes.

Adverse reactions to salmeterol are similar in nature to those seen with other selective beta$_2$-adrenoceptor agonists,

Table 1. Adverse Reaction Incidence in Two 12-Week Clinical Trials in Adult and Adolescent Patients With Asthma

Adverse Event	Percent of Patients: Placebo (N = 152)	SEREVENT DISKUS 50 mcg Twice Daily (N = 149)	Albuterol Inhalation Aerosol 180 mcg 4 Times Daily (N = 150)
Ear, nose, and throat			
Nasal/sinus congestion, pallor	6	9	8
Rhinitis	4	5	4
Neurological			
Headache	9	13	12
Respiratory			
Asthma	1	3	<1
Tracheitis/bronchitis	4	7	3
Influenza	2	5	5

Table 2. Adverse Reaction Incidence in Two 12-Week Pediatric Clinical Trials in Patients With Asthma

Adverse Event	Percent of Patients: Placebo (N = 215)	SEREVENT DISKUS 50 mcg Twice Daily (N = 211)	Albuterol Inhalation Aerosol 200 mcg 4 Times Daily (N = 115)
Ear, nose, and throat			
Ear signs and symptoms	3	4	9
Pharyngitis	3	6	3
Neurological			
Headache	14	17	20
Respiratory			
Asthma	2	4	<1
Skin			
Skin rashes	3	4	2
Urticaria	0	3	2

e.g., tachycardia; palpitations; immediate hypersensitivity reactions, including urticaria, angioedema, rash, bronchospasm; headache; tremor; nervousness; and paradoxical bronchospasm.

Laboratory Abnormalities: There were no clinically relevant changes in these trials. Specifically, no changes in potassium were noted.

6.3 Postmarketing Experience

In addition to adverse reactions reported from clinical trials, the following adverse reactions have been identified during postapproval use of salmeterol. Because these reactions are reported voluntarily from a population of uncertain size, it is not always possible to reliably estimate their frequency or establish a causal relationship to drug exposure. These events have been chosen for inclusion due to either their seriousness, frequency of reporting, or causal connection to salmeterol or a combination of these factors.

In extensive US and worldwide postmarketing experience with salmeterol, serious exacerbations of asthma, including some that have been fatal, have been reported. In most cases, these have occurred in patients with severe asthma and/or in some patients in whom asthma has been acutely deteriorating *[see Warnings and Precautions (5.2)]*, but they have also occurred in a few patients with less severe asthma. It was not possible from these reports to determine whether salmeterol contributed to these events.

Cardiovascular: Arrhythmias (including atrial fibrillation, supraventricular tachycardia, extrasystoles) and anaphylaxis.

Non-Site Specific: Very rare anaphylactic reaction in patients with severe milk protein allergy.

Respiratory: Reports of upper airway symptoms of laryngeal spasm, irritation, or swelling such as stridor or choking; oropharyngeal irritation.

7 DRUG INTERACTIONS

7.1 Inhibitors of Cytochrome P450 3A4

In a drug interaction study in 20 healthy subjects, coadministration of salmeterol (50 mcg twice daily) and ketoconazole (400 mg once daily) for 7 days resulted in greater systemic exposure to salmeterol (AUC increased 16-fold and C_{max} increased 1.4-fold). Three (3) subjects were withdrawn due to beta$_2$-agonist side effects (2 with prolonged QTc and 1 with palpitations and sinus tachycardia). Although there was no statistical effect on the mean QTc, coadministration of salmeterol and ketoconazole was associated with more frequent increases in QTc duration compared with salmeterol and placebo administration. Due to the potential increased risk of cardiovascular adverse events, the concomitant use of salmeterol with strong CYP3A4 inhibitors (e.g., ketoconazole, ritonavir, atazanavir, clarithromycin, indinavir, itraconazole, nefazodone, nelfinavir, saquinavir, telithromycin) is not recommended.

7.2 Monoamine Oxidase Inhibitors and Tricyclic Antidepressants

SEREVENT DISKUS should be administered with extreme caution to patients being treated with monoamine oxidase inhibitors or tricyclic antidepressants, or within 2 weeks of discontinuation of such agents, because the action of salmeterol on the vascular system may be potentiated by these agents.

7.3 Beta-Adrenergic Receptor Blocking Agents

Beta-blockers not only block the pulmonary effect of beta-agonists, such as SEREVENT DISKUS, but may also produce severe bronchospasm in patients with asthma or COPD. Therefore, patients with asthma or COPD should not normally be treated with beta-blockers. However, under certain circumstances, there may be no acceptable alternatives to the use of beta-adrenergic blocking agents for these patients; cardioselective beta-blockers could be considered, although they should be administered with caution.

7.4 Diuretics

The ECG changes and/or hypokalemia that may result from the administration of nonpotassium-sparing diuretics (such as loop or thiazide diuretics) can be acutely worsened by beta-agonists, especially when the recommended dose of the beta-agonist is exceeded. Although the clinical relevance of these effects is not known, caution is advised in the coadministration of SEREVENT DISKUS with nonpotassium-sparing diuretics.

8 USE IN SPECIFIC POPULATIONS

8.1 Pregnancy

Teratogenic Effects: Pregnancy Category C. There are no adequate and well-controlled studies with SEREVENT DISKUS in pregnant women. SEREVENT DISKUS should be used during pregnancy only if the potential benefit justifies the potential risk to the fetus.

No teratogenic effects occurred in rats at oral doses approximately 160 times the maximum recommended daily inhalation dose (MRHD) on an mg/m^2 basis. In pregnant Dutch rabbits administered oral doses approximately 50 times the MRHD based on comparison of the AUCs, salmeterol exhibited fetal toxic effects characteristically resulting from beta-adrenoceptor stimulation. These included precocious eyelid openings, cleft palate, sternebral fusion, limb and paw flexures, and delayed ossification of the frontal cranial bones. No such effects occurred at an oral dose approximately 20 times the MRHD based on comparison of the AUCs.

New Zealand White rabbits were less sensitive since only delayed ossification of the frontal cranial bones was seen at an oral dose approximately 1,600 times the MRHD on an mg/m^2 basis. Extensive use of other beta-agonists has provided no evidence that these class effects in animals are relevant to their use in humans.

8.2 Labor and Delivery

There are no well-controlled human studies that have investigated effects of salmeterol on preterm labor or labor at term. Because of the potential for beta-agonist interference with uterine contractility, use of SEREVENT DISKUS during labor should be restricted to those patients in whom the benefits clearly outweigh the risks.

8.3 Nursing Mothers

Plasma levels of salmeterol, a component of SEREVENT DISKUS, after inhaled therapeutic doses are very low. In rats, salmeterol xinafoate is excreted in the milk. Since there are no data from controlled trials on the use of salmeterol by nursing mothers, a decision should be made whether to discontinue nursing or to discontinue SEREVENT DISKUS, taking into account the importance of SEREVENT DISKUS to the mother. Caution should be exercised when SEREVENT DISKUS is administered to a nursing woman.

8.4 Pediatric Use

Available data from controlled clinical trials suggest that LABA increase the risk of asthma-related hospitalization in pediatric and adolescent patients. For pediatric and adolescent patients with asthma who require addition of a LABA to an inhaled corticosteroid, a fixed-dose combination product containing both an inhaled corticosteroid and a LABA should ordinarily be used to ensure adherence with both drugs *[see Indications and Usage (1.1), Warnings and Precautions (5.1)]*.

The safety and efficacy of SEREVENT DISKUS in adolescents (aged 12 years and older) has been established based on adequate and well-controlled trials conducted in adults and adolescents *[see Clinical Studies (14.1)]*. A large 28-week placebo-controlled US study comparing salmeterol (SEREVENT Inhalation Aerosol) and placebo, each added to usual asthma therapy, showed an increase in asthma-related deaths in patients receiving salmeterol *[see Clinical Studies (14.1)]*. Post-hoc analyses in pediatric patients aged 12 to 18 years were also performed. Pediatric patients accounted for approximately 12% of patients in each treatment arm. Respiratory-related death or life-threatening experience occurred at a similar rate in the salmeterol group (0.12% [2/1,653]) and the placebo group (0.12% [2/1,622]; relative risk: 1.0 [95% CI: 0.1, 7.2]). All-cause hospitalization, however, was increased in the salmeterol group (2% [35/1,653]) versus the placebo group (<1% [16/1,622]; relative risk: 2.1 [95% CI: 1.1, 3.7]).

The safety and efficacy of SEREVENT DISKUS have been evaluated in over 2,500 patients aged 4 to 11 years with asthma, 346 of whom were administered SEREVENT DISKUS for 1 year. Based on available data, no adjustment of dosage of SEREVENT DISKUS in pediatric patients is warranted for either asthma or EIB.

In 2 randomized, double-blind, controlled clinical trials of 12 weeks' duration, SEREVENT DISKUS 50 mcg was administered to 211 pediatric patients with asthma who did and who did not receive concurrent inhaled corticosteroids. The efficacy of SEREVENT DISKUS was demonstrated over the 12-week treatment period with respect to peak expiratory flow (PEF) and forced expiratory volume in 1 second (FEV_1). SEREVENT DISKUS was effective in demographic subgroups (gender and age) of the population.

In 2 randomized studies in children aged 4 to 11 years with asthma and EIB, a single 50-mcg dose of SEREVENT DISKUS prevented EIB when dosed 30 minutes prior to exercise, with protection lasting up to 11.5 hours in repeat testing following this single dose in many patients.

8.5 Geriatric Use

Of the total number of adolescent and adult patients with asthma who received SEREVENT DISKUS in chronic dosing clinical trials, 209 were aged 65 years or older. Of the total number of patients with COPD who received SEREVENT DISKUS in chronic dosing clinical trials, 167 were aged 65 years or older and 45 were aged 75 years or older. No apparent differences in the safety of SEREVENT DISKUS were observed when geriatric patients were compared with younger patients in clinical trials. As with other beta$_2$-agonists, however, special caution should be observed when using SEREVENT DISKUS in geriatric patients who have concomitant cardiovascular disease that could be adversely affected by this class of drug. Data from the trials in patients with COPD suggested a greater effect on FEV_1 of SEREVENT DISKUS in the <65 years age-group, as compared with the ≥65 years age-group. However, based on available data, no adjustment of dosage of SEREVENT DISKUS in geriatric patients is warranted.

8.6 Hepatic Impairment

The pharmacokinetics of salmeterol base has not been studied in patients with hepatic impairment. Since salmeterol is predominantly cleared by hepatic metabolism, liver function impairment may lead to accumulation of salmeterol in plasma. Therefore, patients with hepatic disease should be closely monitored.

10 OVERDOSAGE

The expected signs and symptoms with overdosage of SEREVENT DISKUS are those of excessive beta-adrenergic stimulation and/or occurrence or exaggeration of any of the following: seizures, angina, hypertension or hypotension, tachycardia with rates up to 200 beats/min, arrhythmias, nervousness, headache, tremor, muscle cramps, dry mouth, palpitation, nausea, dizziness, fatigue, malaise, insomnia. Overdosage with SEREVENT DISKUS can lead to clinically significant prolongation of the QTc interval, which can produce ventricular arrhythmias. Other signs of overdosage may include hypokalemia and hyperglycemia.

As with all sympathomimetic medications, cardiac arrest and even death may be associated with abuse of SEREVENT DISKUS.

Treatment consists of discontinuation of SEREVENT DISKUS together with appropriate symptomatic therapy. The judicious use of a cardioselective beta-receptor blocker may be considered, bearing in mind that such medication can produce bronchospasm. There is insufficient evidence to determine if dialysis is beneficial for overdosage of SEREVENT DISKUS. Cardiac monitoring is recommended in cases of overdosage.

No deaths were seen in rats given salmeterol at an inhalation dose of 2.9 mg/kg (approximately 240 and 110 times the MRHD for adults and children, respectively, on an mg/m^2 basis) and in dogs at an inhalation dose of 0.7 mg/kg (approximately 190 and 90 times the MRHD for adults and children, respectively, on an mg/m^2 basis). By the oral route, no deaths occurred in mice at 150 mg/kg (approximately 6,100 and 2,900 times the MRHD for adults and children, respectively, on an mg/m^2 basis) and in rats at 1,000 mg/kg (approximately 81,000 and 38,000 times the MRHD for adults and children, respectively, on an mg/m^2 basis).

11 DESCRIPTION

SEREVENT DISKUS contains salmeterol xinafoate as the racemic form of the 1-hydroxy-2-naphthoic acid salt of salmeterol. The active component of the formulation is salmeterol base, a selective beta$_2$-adrenergic bronchodilator. The chemical name of salmeterol xinafoate is 4-hydroxy-α^1-[[[6-(4-phenylbutoxy)hexyl]amino]methyl]-1,3-benzenedimethanol, 1-hydroxy-2-naphthalenecarboxylate. Salmeterol xinafoate has the following chemical structure:

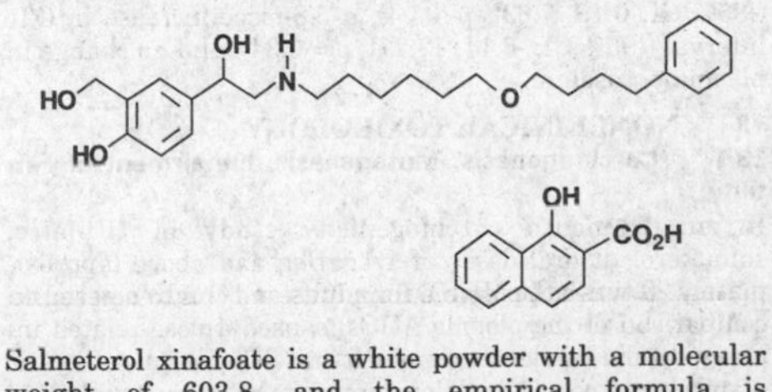

Salmeterol xinafoate is a white powder with a molecular weight of 603.8, and the empirical formula is $C_{25}H_{37}NO_4 \bullet C_{11}H_8O_3$. It is freely soluble in methanol; slightly soluble in ethanol, chloroform, and isopropanol; and sparingly soluble in water.

SEREVENT DISKUS is a specially designed plastic device containing a double-foil blister strip of a powder formulation of salmeterol xinafoate intended for oral inhalation only. Each blister on the double-foil strip within the device contains 50 mcg of salmeterol base administered as the salmeterol xinafoate salt in 12.5 mg of formulation containing lactose (which contains milk proteins). After a blister containing medication is opened by activating the device, the medication is dispersed into the airstream created by the patient inhaling through the mouthpiece.

Under standardized in vitro test conditions, SEREVENT DISKUS delivers 47 mcg when tested at a flow rate of 60 L/min for 2 seconds. In adult patients with obstructive lung disease and severely compromised lung function (mean FEV_1 20% to 30% of predicted), mean peak inspiratory flow (PIF) through a DISKUS® inhalation device was 82.4 L/min (range: 46.1 to 115.3 L/min).

The actual amount of drug delivered to the lung will depend on patient factors, such as inspiratory flow profile.

12 CLINICAL PHARMACOLOGY

12.1 Mechanism of Action

Salmeterol is a selective LABA. In vitro studies show salmeterol to be at least 50 times more selective for beta$_2$-adrenoceptors than albuterol. Although beta$_2$-adrenoceptors are the predominant adrenergic receptors in bronchial smooth muscle and beta$_1$-adrenoceptors are the predominant receptors in the heart, there are also beta$_2$-adrenoceptors in the human heart comprising 10% to 50% of the total beta-adrenoceptors. The precise function of these receptors has not been established, but their presence raises the possibility that even highly selective beta$_2$-agonists may have cardiac effects.

The pharmacologic effects of beta$_2$-adrenoceptor agonist drugs, including salmeterol, are at least in part attributable to stimulation of intracellular adenyl cyclase, the enzyme that catalyzes the conversion of adenosine triphosphate (ATP) to cyclic-3′,5′-adenosine monophosphate (cyclic AMP). Increased cyclic AMP levels cause relaxation of bronchial smooth muscle and inhibition of release of mediators of immediate hypersensitivity from cells, especially from mast cells.

In vitro tests show that salmeterol is a potent and long-lasting inhibitor of the release of mast cell mediators, such as histamine, leukotrienes, and prostaglandin D_2, from human lung. Salmeterol inhibits histamine-induced plasma protein extravasation and inhibits platelet-activating factor–induced eosinophil accumulation in the lungs of guinea pigs when administered by the inhaled route. In humans, single doses of salmeterol administered via inhalation aerosol attenuate allergen-induced bronchial hyper-responsiveness.

12.2 Pharmacodynamics

Inhaled salmeterol, like other beta-adrenergic agonist drugs, can in some patients produce dose-related cardiovascular effects and effects on blood glucose and/or serum potassium *[see Warnings and Precautions (5.6, 5.10)]*. The cardiovascular effects (heart rate, blood pressure) associated with salmeterol inhalation aerosol occur with similar frequency, and are of similar type and severity, as those noted following albuterol administration.

The effects of rising doses of salmeterol and standard inhaled doses of albuterol were studied in volunteers and in patients with asthma. Salmeterol doses up to 84 mcg administered as inhalation aerosol resulted in heart rate increases of 3 to 16 beats/min, about the same as albuterol dosed at 180 mcg by inhalation aerosol (4 to 10 beats/min). Adolescent and adult patients receiving 50-mcg doses of salmeterol inhalation powder (N = 60) underwent continuous electrocardiographic monitoring during two 12-hour periods after the first dose and after 1 month of therapy, and no clinically significant dysrhythmias were noted. Also, pediatric patients receiving 50-mcg doses of salmeterol inhalation powder (N = 67) underwent continuous electrocardiographic monitoring during two 12-hour periods after the first dose and after 3 months of therapy, and no clinically significant dysrhythmias were noted.

In 24-week clinical studies in patients with COPD, the incidence of clinically significant abnormalities on the predose electrocardiograms (ECGs) at Weeks 12 and 24 in patients who received salmeterol 50 mcg was not different compared with placebo.

No effect of treatment with salmeterol 50 mcg was observed on pulse rate and systolic and diastolic blood pressure in a subset of patients with COPD who underwent 12-hour serial vital sign measurements after the first dose (N = 91) and after 12 weeks of therapy (N = 74). Median changes from baseline in pulse rate and systolic and diastolic blood pressure were similar for patients receiving either salmeterol or placebo *[see Adverse Reactions (6.1)]*.

Concomitant Use of SEREVENT DISKUS With Other Respiratory Medications: *Short-Acting Beta$_2$-Agonists:* In two 12-week repetitive-dose adolescent and adult clinical trials in patients with asthma (N = 149), the mean daily need for additional beta$_2$-agonist in patients using SEREVENT DISKUS was approximately 1½ inhalations/day. Twenty-six percent (26%) of the patients in these trials

Table 4. Daily Efficacy Measurements in Two 12-Week Clinical Trials (Combined Data)

Parameter	Time	Placebo	SEREVENT DISKUS	Albuterol Inhalation Aerosol
No. of randomized subjects		152	149	148
Mean AM peak expiratory flow (L/min)	Baseline	394	395	394
	12 weeks	396	427[a]	394
Mean % days with no asthma symptoms	Baseline	14	13	12
	12 weeks	20	33	21
Mean % nights with no awakenings	Baseline	70	63	68
	12 weeks	73	85[a]	71
Rescue medications (mean no. of inhalations per day)	Baseline	4.2	4.3	4.3
	12 weeks	3.3	1.6[b]	2.2
Asthma exacerbations (%)		14	15	16

[a]Statistically superior to placebo and albuterol (p<0.001).
[b]Statistically superior to placebo (p<0.001).

used between 8 and 24 inhalations of short-acting beta-agonist per day on 1 or more occasions. Nine percent (9%) of the patients in these trials averaged over 4 inhalations/day over the course of the 12-week trials. No increase in frequency of cardiovascular events was observed among the 3 patients who averaged 8 to 11 inhalations/day; however, the safety of concomitant use of more than 8 inhalations/day of short-acting $beta_2$-agonist with SEREVENT DISKUS has not been established. In 29 patients who experienced worsening of asthma while receiving SEREVENT DISKUS during these trials, albuterol therapy administered via either nebulizer or inhalation aerosol (1 dose in most cases) led to improvement in FEV_1 and no increase in occurrence of cardiovascular adverse events.

In 2 clinical trials in patients with COPD, the mean daily need for additional $beta_2$-agonist for patients using SEREVENT DISKUS was approximately 4 inhalations/day. Twenty-four percent (24%) of the patients using SEREVENT DISKUS in these trials averaged 6 or more inhalations of albuterol per day over the course of the 24-week trials. No increase in frequency of cardiovascular adverse reactions was observed among patients who averaged 6 or more inhalations per day.

Methylxanthines: The concurrent use of intravenously or orally administered methylxanthines (e.g., aminophylline, theophylline) by patients receiving salmeterol has not been completely evaluated. In 1 clinical asthma trial, 87 patients receiving SEREVENT Inhalation Aerosol 42 mcg twice daily concurrently with a theophylline product had adverse event rates similar to those in 71 patients receiving SEREVENT Inhalation Aerosol without theophylline. Resting heart rates were slightly higher in the patients on theophylline but were little affected by therapy with SEREVENT Inhalation Aerosol.

In 2 clinical trials in patients with COPD, 39 patients receiving SEREVENT DISKUS concurrently with a theophylline product had adverse event rates similar to those in 302 patients receiving SEREVENT DISKUS without theophylline. Based on the available data, the concomitant administration of methylxanthines with SEREVENT DISKUS did not alter the observed adverse event profile.

Cromoglycate: In clinical trials, inhaled cromolyn sodium did not alter the safety profile of salmeterol when administered concurrently.

12.3 Pharmacokinetics

Salmeterol xinafoate, an ionic salt, dissociates in solution so that the salmeterol and 1-hydroxy-2-naphthoic acid (xinafoate) moieties are absorbed, distributed, metabolized, and eliminated independently. Salmeterol acts locally in the lung; therefore, plasma levels do not predict therapeutic effect.

Absorption: Because of the small therapeutic dose, systemic levels of salmeterol are low or undetectable after inhalation of recommended doses (50 mcg of salmeterol inhalation powder twice daily). Following chronic administration of an inhaled dose of 50 mcg of salmeterol inhalation powder twice daily, salmeterol was detected in plasma within 5 to 45 minutes in 7 patients with asthma; plasma concentrations were very low, with mean peak concentrations of 167 pg/mL at 20 minutes and no accumulation with repeated doses.

Distribution: The percentage of salmeterol bound to human plasma proteins averages 96% in vitro over the concentration range of 8 to 7,722 ng of salmeterol base per milliliter, much higher concentrations than those achieved following therapeutic doses of salmeterol.

Metabolism: Salmeterol base is extensively metabolized by hydroxylation, with subsequent elimination predominantly in the feces. No significant amount of unchanged salmeterol base was detected in either urine or feces.

An in vitro study using human liver microsomes showed that salmeterol is extensively metabolized to α-hydroxysalmeterol (aliphatic oxidation) by CYP3A4. Ketoconazole, a strong inhibitor of CYP3A4, essentially completely inhibited the formation of α-hydroxysalmeterol in vitro.

Elimination: In 2 healthy adult subjects who received 1 mg of radiolabeled salmeterol (as salmeterol xinafoate) orally, approximately 25% and 60% of the radiolabeled salmeterol was eliminated in urine and feces, respectively, over a period of 7 days. The terminal elimination half-life was about 5.5 hours (1 volunteer only).

The xinafoate moiety has no apparent pharmacologic activity. The xinafoate moiety is highly protein bound (>99%) and has a long elimination half-life of 11 days.

Drug Interactions: *Inhibitors of Cytochrome P450 3A4: Ketoconazole:* In a placebo-controlled crossover drug interaction study in 20 healthy male and female subjects, coadministration of salmeterol (50 mcg twice daily) and the strong CYP3A4 inhibitor ketoconazole (400 mg once daily) for 7 days resulted in a significant increase in plasma salmeterol exposure as determined by a 16-fold increase in AUC (ratio with and without ketoconazole 15.76 [90% CI: 10.66, 23.31]) mainly due to increased bioavailability of the swallowed portion of the dose. Peak plasma salmeterol concentrations were increased by 1.4-fold (90% CI: 1.23, 1.68). Three (3) out of 20 subjects (15%) were withdrawn from salmeterol and ketoconazole coadministration due to beta-agonist–mediated systemic effects (2 with QTc prolongation and 1 with palpitations and sinus tachycardia). Coadministration of salmeterol and ketoconazole did not result in a clinically significant effect on mean heart rate, mean blood potassium, or mean blood glucose. Although there was no statistical effect on the mean QTc, coadministration of salmeterol and ketoconazole was associated with more frequent increases in QTc duration compared with salmeterol and placebo administration.

Erythromycin: In a repeat-dose study in 13 healthy subjects, concomitant administration of erythromycin (a moderate CYP3A4 inhibitor) and salmeterol inhalation aerosol resulted in a 40% increase in salmeterol C_{max} at steady state (ratio with and without erythromycin 1.4 [90% CI: 0.96, 2.03], p = 0.12), a 3.6-beat/min increase in heart rate ([95% CI: 0.19, 7.03], p<0.04), a 5.8-msec increase in QTc interval ([95% CI: -6.14, 17.77], p = 0.34), and no change in plasma potassium.

13 NONCLINICAL TOXICOLOGY

13.1 Carcinogenesis, Mutagenesis, Impairment of Fertility

In an 18-month carcinogenicity study in CD-mice, salmeterol at oral doses of 1.4 mg/kg and above (approximately 20 times the MRHD for adults and children based on comparison of the plasma AUCs) caused a dose-related increase in the incidence of smooth muscle hyperplasia, cystic glandular hyperplasia, leiomyomas of the uterus, and ovarian cysts. No tumors were seen at 0.2 mg/kg (approximately 3 times the MRHD for adults and children based on comparison of the AUCs).

In a 24-month oral and inhalation carcinogenicity study in Sprague Dawley rats, salmeterol caused a dose-related increase in the incidence of mesovarian leiomyomas and ovarian cysts at doses of 0.68 mg/kg and above (approximately 55 and 25 times the MRHD for adults and children, respectively, on an mg/m^2 basis). No tumors were seen at 0.21 mg/kg (approximately 15 and 8 times the MRHD for adults and children, respectively, on an mg/m^2 basis). These findings in rodents are similar to those reported previously for other beta-adrenergic agonist drugs. The relevance of these findings to human use is unknown.

Salmeterol produced no detectable or reproducible increases in microbial and mammalian gene mutation in vitro. No clastogenic activity occurred in vitro in human lymphocytes or in vivo in a rat micronucleus test. No effects on fertility were identified in rats treated with salmeterol at oral doses up to 2 mg/kg (approximately 160 times the MRHD for adults on an mg/m^2 basis).

13.2 Animal Toxicology and/or Pharmacology

Preclinical: Studies in laboratory animals (minipigs, rodents, and dogs) have demonstrated the occurrence of cardiac arrhythmias and sudden death (with histologic evidence of myocardial necrosis) when beta-agonists and methylxanthines are administered concurrently. The clinical relevance of these findings is unknown.

Reproductive Toxicology Studies: No teratogenic effects occurred in rats at oral doses up to 2 mg/kg (approximately 160 times the MRHD on an mg/m^2 basis).

In Dutch rabbits administered oral doses of 1 mg/kg and above (approximately 50 times and above the MRHD based on comparison of the AUCs), salmeterol exhibited fetal toxic effects characteristically resulting from beta-adrenoceptor stimulation. These included precocious eyelid openings, cleft palate, sternebral fusion, limb and paw flexures, and delayed ossification of the frontal cranial bones. No such effects occurred at an oral dose of 0.6 mg/kg (approximately 20 times the MRHD based on comparison of the AUCs). New Zealand White rabbits were less sensitive since only delayed ossification of the frontal bones was seen at an oral dose of 10 mg/kg (approximately 1,600 times the MRHD on an mg/m^2 basis).

Salmeterol crossed the placenta following oral administration to mice and rats.

14 CLINICAL STUDIES

14.1 Asthma

The initial studies supporting the approval of SEREVENT DISKUS for the treatment of asthma did not require the regular use of inhaled corticosteroids. However, for the treatment of asthma, SEREVENT DISKUS is currently indicated only as concomitant therapy with an inhaled corticosteroid *[see Indications and Usage (1.1)]*.

Adult and Adolescent Patients Aged 12 Years and Older: In 2 randomized double-blind studies, SEREVENT DISKUS was compared with albuterol inhalation aerosol and placebo in adolescent and adult patients with mild-to-moderate asthma (protocol defined as 50% to 80% predicted FEV_1, actual mean of 67.7% at baseline), including patients who did and who did not receive concurrent inhaled corticosteroids. The efficacy of SEREVENT DISKUS was demonstrated over the 12-week period with no change in effectiveness over this time period (see Figure 1). There were no gender- or age-related differences in safety or efficacy. No development of tachyphylaxis to the bronchodilator effect was noted in these studies. FEV_1 measurements (mean change from baseline) from these two 12-week studies are shown in Figure 1 for both the first and last treatment days.

[See figure 1 at top of next column]

Table 4 shows the treatment effects seen during daily treatment with SEREVENT DISKUS for 12 weeks in adolescent and adult patients with mild-to-moderate asthma.

[See table 4 above]

Maintenance of efficacy for periods up to 1 year has been documented.

SEREVENT DISKUS and SEREVENT Inhalation Aerosol were compared with placebo in 2 additional randomized double-blind clinical trials in adolescent and adult patients with mild-to-moderate asthma. SEREVENT DISKUS 50 mcg and SEREVENT Inhalation Aerosol 42 mcg, both administered twice daily, produced significant improvements in pulmonary function compared with placebo over the 12-week period. While no statistically significant differences were observed between the active treatments for any of the efficacy assessments or safety evaluations performed, there were some efficacy measures on which the metered-dose inhaler appeared to provide better results. Similar findings were noted in 2 randomized, single-dose, crossover comparisons of SEREVENT DISKUS and SEREVENT Inhalation Aerosol for the prevention of EIB. Therefore, while SEREVENT DISKUS was comparable to SEREVENT Inhalation Aerosol in clinical trials in mild-to-moderate patients with asthma, it should not be assumed that they will produce clinically equivalent outcomes in all patients.

Patients on Concomitant Inhaled Corticosteroids: In 4 clinical trials in adult and adolescent patients with asthma (N = 1,922), the effect of adding SEREVENT Inhalation Aerosol to inhaled corticosteroid therapy was evaluated over a

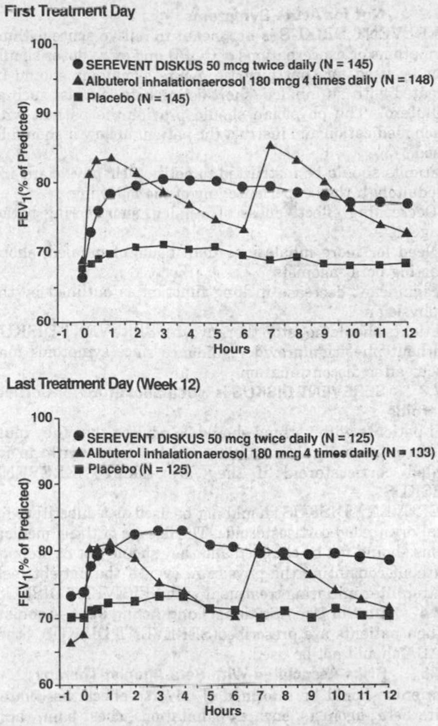

Figure 1. Serial 12-Hour FEV_1 From Two 12-Week Clinical Trials in Patients With Asthma

24-week treatment period. The studies compared the addition of salmeterol therapy to an increase (at least doubling) of the inhaled corticosteroid dose.

Two randomized, double-blind, controlled, parallel-group clinical trials (N = 997) enrolled patients (aged 18 to 82 years) with persistent asthma who were previously maintained but not adequately controlled on inhaled corticosteroid therapy. During the 2-week run-in period, all patients were switched to beclomethasone dipropionate (BDP) 168 mcg twice daily. Patients still not adequately controlled were randomized to either the addition of SEREVENT Inhalation Aerosol 42 mcg twice daily or an increase of BDP to 336 mcg twice daily. As compared with the doubled dose of BDP, the addition of SEREVENT Inhalation Aerosol resulted in statistically significantly greater improvements in pulmonary function and asthma symptoms, and statistically significantly greater reduction in supplemental albuterol use. The percent of patients who experienced asthma exacerbations overall was not different between groups (i.e., 16.2% in the group receiving SEREVENT Inhalation Aerosol versus 17.9% in the higher-dose beclomethasone dipropionate group).

Two randomized, double-blind, controlled, parallel-group clinical trials (N = 925) enrolled patients (aged 12 to 78 years) with persistent asthma who were previously maintained but not adequately controlled on prior asthma therapy. During the 2- to 4-week run-in period, all patients were switched to fluticasone propionate 88 mcg twice daily. Patients still not adequately controlled were randomized to either the addition of SEREVENT Inhalation Aerosol 42 mcg twice daily or an increase of fluticasone propionate to 220 mcg twice daily. As compared with the increased (2.5 times) dose of fluticasone propionate, the addition of SEREVENT Inhalation Aerosol resulted in statistically significantly greater improvements in pulmonary function and asthma symptoms, and statistically significantly greater reductions in supplemental albuterol use. Fewer patients receiving SEREVENT Inhalation Aerosol experienced asthma exacerbations than those receiving the higher dose of fluticasone propionate (8.8% versus 13.8%).

Table 5 shows the treatment effects seen during daily treatment with SEREVENT Inhalation Aerosol for 24 weeks in adolescent and adult patients with mild-to-moderate asthma.

Onset of Action: During the initial treatment day in several multiple-dose clinical trials with SEREVENT DISKUS in patients with asthma, the median time to onset of clinically significant bronchodilatation (≥15% improvement in FEV_1) ranged from 30 to 48 minutes after a 50-mcg dose.

One hour after a single dose of 50 mcg of SEREVENT DISKUS, the majority of patients had ≥15% improvement in FEV_1. Maximum improvement in FEV_1 generally occurred within 180 minutes, and clinically significant improvement continued for 12 hours in most patients.

Table 5: Asthma-Related Deaths in the 28-Week Salmeterol Multi-center Asthma Research Trial (SMART)

	Salmeterol n (%[a])	Placebo n (%[a])	Relative Risk[b] (95% Confidence Interval)	Excess Deaths Expressed per 10,000 Patients[c] (95% Confidence Interval)
Total Population[d]				
Salmeterol: N = 13,176	13 (0.10%)		4.37 (1.25, 15.34)	8 (3, 13)
Placebo: N = 13,179		3 (0.02%)		
Caucasian				
Salmeterol: N = 9,281	6 (0.07%)		5.82 (0.70, 48.37)	6 (1, 10)
Placebo: N = 9,361		1 (0.01%)		
African American				
Salmeterol: N = 2,366	7 (0.31%)		7.26 (0.89, 58.94)	27 (8, 46)
Placebo: N = 2,319		1 (0.04%)		

[a]Life-table 28-week estimate, adjusted according to the patients' actual lengths of exposure to study treatment to account for early withdrawal of patients from the study.
[b]Relative risk is the ratio of the rate of asthma-related death in the salmeterol group and the rate in the placebo group. The relative risk indicates how many more times likely an asthma-related death occurred in the salmeterol group than in the placebo group in a 28-week treatment period.
[c] Estimate of the number of additional asthma-related deaths in patients treated with salmeterol in SMART, assuming 10,000 patients received salmeterol for a 28-week treatment period. Estimate calculated as the difference between the salmeterol and placebo groups in the rates of asthma-related death multiplied by 10,000.
[d]The Total Population includes the following ethnic origins listed on the case report form: Caucasian, African American, Hispanic, Asian, and "Other." In addition, the Total Population includes those patients whose ethnic origin was not reported. The results for Caucasian and African American subpopulations are shown above. No asthma-related deaths occurred in the Hispanic (salmeterol n = 996, placebo n = 999), Asian (salmeterol n = 173, placebo n = 149), or "Other" (salmeterol n = 230, placebo n = 224) subpopulations. One asthma-related death occurred in the placebo group in the subpopulation whose ethnic origin was not reported (salmeterol n = 130, placebo n = 127).

Pediatric Patients: In a randomized, double-blind, controlled study (N = 449), 50 mcg of SEREVENT DISKUS was administered twice daily to pediatric patients with asthma who did and who did not receive concurrent inhaled corticosteroids. The efficacy of salmeterol inhalation powder was demonstrated over the 12-week treatment period with respect to periodic serial PEF (36% to 39% postdose increase from baseline) and FEV_1 (32% to 33% postdose increase from baseline). Salmeterol was effective in demographic subgroup analyses (gender and age) and was effective when coadministered with other inhaled asthma medications such as short-acting bronchodilators and inhaled corticosteroids. A second randomized, double-blind, placebo-controlled study (N = 207) with 50 mcg of salmeterol inhalation powder via an alternate device supported the findings of the trial with the DISKUS.

Salmeterol Multi-center Asthma Research Trial: The SMART study was a randomized double-blind study that enrolled LABA-naive patients with asthma (average age of 39 years; 71% Caucasian, 18% African American, 8% Hispanic) to assess the safety of salmeterol (SEREVENT Inhalation Aerosol) 42 mcg twice daily over 28 weeks compared with placebo when added to usual asthma therapy.

A planned interim analysis was conducted when approximately half of the intended number of patients had been enrolled (N = 26,355), which led to premature termination of the study. The results of the interim analysis showed that patients receiving salmeterol were at increased risk for fatal asthma events (see Table 5 and Figure 2). In the total population, a higher rate of asthma-related death occurred in patients treated with salmeterol than those treated with placebo (0.10% versus 0.02%, relative risk: 4.37 [95% CI: 1.25, 15.34]).

Post-hoc subpopulation analyses were performed. In Caucasians, asthma-related death occurred at a higher rate in patients treated with salmeterol than in patients treated with placebo (0.07% versus 0.01%, relative risk: 5.82 [95% CI: 0.70, 48.37]). In African Americans also, asthma-related death occurred at a higher rate in patients treated with salmeterol than those treated with placebo (0.31% versus 0.04%, relative risk: 7.26 [95% CI: 0.89, 58.94]). Although the relative risks of asthma-related death were similar in Caucasians and African Americans, the estimate of excess deaths in patients treated with salmeterol was greater in African Americans because there was a higher overall rate of asthma-related death in African American patients (see Table 5).

Post-hoc analyses in pediatric patients aged 12 to 18 years were also performed. Pediatric patients accounted for approximately 12% of patients in each treatment arm. Respiratory-related death or life-threatening experience occurred at a similar rate in the salmeterol group (0.12% [2/1,653]) and the placebo group (0.12% [2/1,622]; relative risk: 1.0 [95% CI: 0.1, 7.2]). All-cause hospitalization, however, was increased in the salmeterol group (2% [35/1,653]) versus the placebo group (<1% [16/1,622]; relative risk: 2.1 [95% CI: 1.1, 3.7]).

The data from the SMART study are not adequate to determine whether concurrent use of inhaled corticosteroids or other long-term asthma control therapy mitigates the risk of asthma-related death.

[See table 5 above]

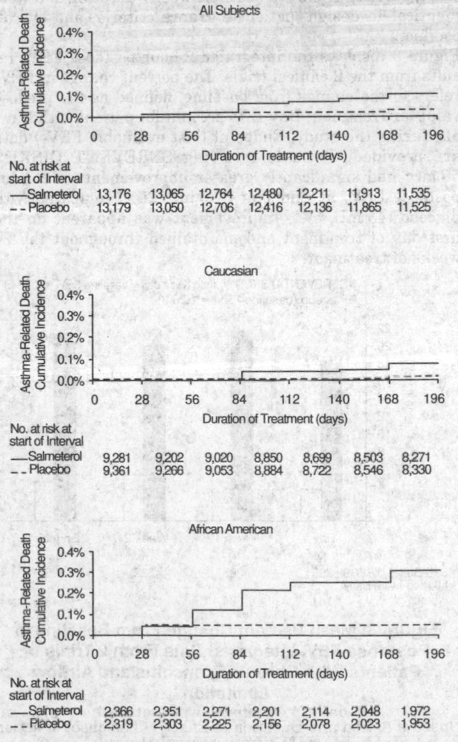

Figure 2. Cumulative Incidence of Asthma-Related Deaths in the 28-Week Salmeterol Multi-center Asthma Research Trial (SMART), by Duration of Treatment

14.2 Exercise-Induced Bronchospasm

In 2 randomized, single-dose, crossover studies in adolescents and adults with EIB (N = 52), 50 mcg of SEREVENT

Table 6. Results of 2 Exercise-Induced Bronchospasm Studies in Adolescents and Adults

		Placebo (N = 52)		SEREVENT DISKUS (N = 52)	
		n	% Total	n	% Total
0.5-Hour postdose exercise challenge	% Fall in FEV_1				
	<10%	15	29	31	60
	≥10%, <20%	3	6	11	21
	≥20%	34	65	10	19
Mean maximal % fall in FEV_1 (SE)		-25% (1.8)		-11% (1.9)	
8.5-Hour postdose exercise challenge	% Fall in FEV_1				
	<10%	12	23	26	50
	≥10%, <20%	7	13	12	23
	≥20%	33	63	14	27
Mean maximal % fall in FEV_1 (SE)		-27% (1.5)		-16% (2.0)	

DISKUS prevented EIB when dosed 30 minutes prior to exercise. For some patients, this protective effect against EIB was still apparent up to 8.5 hours following a single dose (see Table 6).

[See table 6 above]

In 2 randomized studies in children aged 4 to 11 years with asthma and EIB (N = 50), a single 50-mcg dose of SEREVENT DISKUS prevented EIB when dosed 30 minutes prior to exercise, with protection lasting up to 11.5 hours in repeat testing following this single dose in many patients.

14.3 Chronic Obstructive Pulmonary Disease

In 2 clinical trials evaluating twice-daily treatment with SEREVENT DISKUS 50 mcg (N = 336) compared with placebo (N = 366) in patients with chronic bronchitis with airflow limitation, with or without emphysema, improvements in pulmonary function endpoints were greater with salmeterol 50 mcg than with placebo. Treatment with SEREVENT DISKUS did not result in significant improvements in secondary endpoints assessing COPD symptoms in either clinical trial. Both trials were randomized, double-blind, parallel-group studies of 24 weeks' duration and were identical in design, patient entrance criteria, and overall conduct.

Figure 3 displays the integrated 2-hour postdose FEV_1 results from the 2 clinical trials. The percent change in FEV_1 refers to the change from baseline, defined as the predose value on Treatment Day 1. To account for patient withdrawals during the study, Endpoint (last evaluable FEV_1) data are provided. Patients receiving SEREVENT DISKUS 50 mcg had significantly greater improvements in 2-hour postdose FEV_1 at Endpoint (216 mL, 20%) compared with placebo (43 mL, 5%). Improvement was apparent on the first day of treatment and maintained throughout the 24 weeks of treatment.

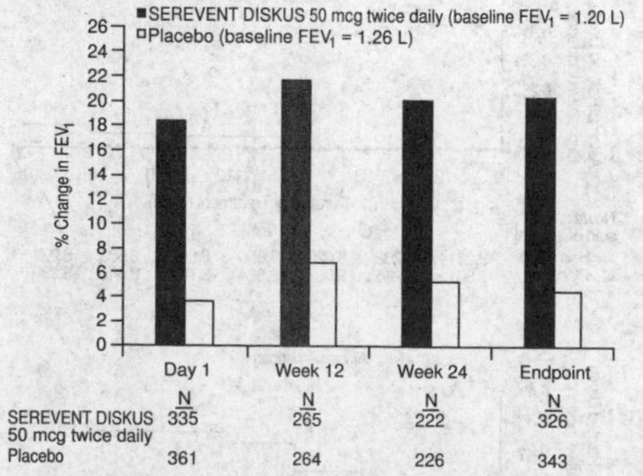

Figure 3. Mean Percent Change From Baseline in Postdose FEV_1 Integrated Data From 2 Trials of Patients With Chronic Bronchitis and Airflow Limitation

Onset of Action and Duration of Effect: The onset of action and duration of effect of SEREVENT DISKUS were evaluated in a subset of patients (n = 87) from 1 of the 2 clinical trials discussed above. Following the first 50-mcg dose, significant improvement in pulmonary function (mean FEV_1 increase of 12% or more and at least 200 mL) occurred at 2 hours. The mean time to peak bronchodilator effect was 4.75 hours. As seen in Figure 4, evidence of bronchodilatation was seen throughout the 12-hour period. Figure 4 also demonstrates that the bronchodilating effect after 12 weeks of treatment was similar to that observed after the first dose. The mean time to peak bronchodilator effect after 12 weeks of treatment was 3.27 hours.

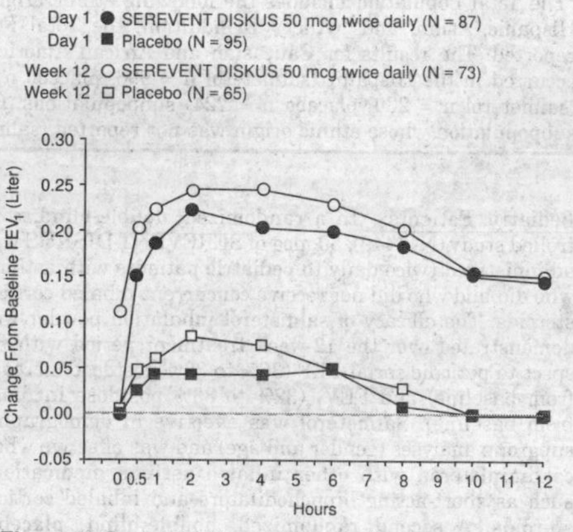

Figure 4. Serial 12-Hour FEV_1 on the First Day and at Week 12 of Treatment

16 HOW SUPPLIED/STORAGE AND HANDLING

SEREVENT DISKUS is supplied as a disposable teal green device containing 60 blisters. The DISKUS inhalation device is packaged within a plastic-coated, moisture-protective foil pouch (NDC 0173-0521-00).

SEREVENT DISKUS is also supplied in an institutional pack of 1 disposable teal green unit containing 28 blisters. The drug product is packaged within a plastic-coated, moisture-protective foil pouch (NDC 0173-0520-00).

Store at controlled room temperature (see USP), 20° to 25°C (68° to 77°F) in a dry place away from direct heat or sunlight. Keep out of reach of children. The DISKUS inhalation device is not reusable. The device should be discarded 6 weeks after removal from the moisture-protective foil pouch or after all blisters have been used (when the dose indicator reads "0"), whichever comes first. Do not attempt to take the DISKUS apart.

17 PATIENT COUNSELING INFORMATION

See FDA-approved patient labeling (Medication Guide and Instructions for Use).

17.1 Asthma-Related Death

Patients should be informed that salmeterol increases the risk of asthma-related death and may increase the risk of asthma-related hospitalization in pediatric and adolescent patients. Patients should be informed that SEREVENT DISKUS should not be the only therapy for the treatment of asthma and must only be used as additional therapy when long-term asthma control medications (e.g., inhaled corticosteroids) do not adequately control asthma symptoms. They should also be informed that currently available data are inadequate to determine whether concurrent use of inhaled corticosteroids or other long-term asthma control drugs mitigates the increased risk of asthma-related death from LABA.Patients should be informed that when SEREVENT DISKUS is added to their treatment regimen they must continue to use their long-term asthma control medication.

17.2 Not for Acute Symptoms

SEREVENT DISKUS is not meant to relieve acute asthma symptoms or exacerbations of COPD and extra doses should not be used for that purpose. Acute symptoms should be treated with an inhaled, short-acting $beta_2$-agonist such as albuterol. The physician should provide the patient with such medication and instruct the patient in how it should be used.

Patients should be instructed to notify their physicians immediately if they experience any of the following:

- Decreasing effectiveness of inhaled, short-acting $beta_2$-agonists
- Need for more inhalations than usual of inhaled, short-acting $beta_2$-agonists
- Significant decrease in lung function as outlined by the physician

Patients should not stop therapy with SEREVENT DISKUS without physician/provider guidance since symptoms may recur after discontinuation.

17.3 SEREVENT DISKUS is Not a Substitute for Corticosteroids

All patients with asthma should be advised that they must also continue regular maintenance treatment with an inhaled corticosteroid if they are taking SEREVENT DISKUS.

SEREVENT DISKUS should not be used as a substitute for oral or inhaled corticosteroids. The dosage of these medications should not be changed and they should not be stopped without consulting the physician, even if the patient feels better after initiating treatment with SEREVENT DISKUS.

17.4 Do Not Use Additional Long-Acting $Beta_2$-Agonists

When patients are prescribed SEREVENT DISKUS, other LABA should not be used.

17.5 Risks Associated With Beta-Agonist Therapy

Patients should be informed of adverse effects associated with $beta_2$-agonists, such as palpitations, chest pain, rapid heart rate, tremor, or nervousness.

17.6 Treatment of Exercise-Induced Bronchospasm

When used for the treatment of EIB, additional doses of SEREVENT should not be used for 12 hours. Patients who are receiving SEREVENT DISKUS twice daily should not use additional SEREVENT for prevention of EIB.

SEREVENT and DISKUS are registered trademarks of GlaxoSmithKline.

GlaxoSmithKline
Research Triangle Park, NC 27709

January 2012
SRD:9PI

MEDICATION GUIDE

SEREVENT® [*ser' uh-vent*] DISKUS®

(salmeterol xinafoate inhalation powder)

Read the Medication Guide that comes with SEREVENT DISKUS before you start using it and each time you get a refill. There may be new information. This Medication Guide does not take the place of talking to your healthcare provider about your medical condition or treatment.

What is the most important information I should know about SEREVENT DISKUS?

SEREVENT DISKUS can cause serious side effects, including:

1. **People with asthma who take long-acting $beta_2$-adrenergic agonist (LABA) medicines such as salmeterol (SEREVENT DISKUS), have an increased risk of death from asthma problems.**
   - Call your healthcare provider if breathing problems worsen over time while using SEREVENT DISKUS. You may need a different treatment.
   - Get emergency medical care if:
     - breathing problems worsen quickly, and
     - you use your rescue inhaler medicine, but it does not relieve your breathing problems.
2. **Do not use SEREVENT DISKUS as your only asthma medicine. SEREVENT DISKUS must only be used with a long-term asthma-control medicine, such as an inhaled corticosteroid.**
3. When your asthma is well controlled, your healthcare provider may tell you to stop taking SEREVENT DISKUS. Your healthcare provider will decide if you can stop SEREVENT DISKUS without loss of asthma control. You will continue taking your long-term asthma-control medicine, such as an inhaled corticosteroid.
4. Children and adolescents who take LABA medicines may have an increased risk of being hospitalized for asthma problems.

What is SEREVENT DISKUS?

- SEREVENT DISKUS is a LABA medicine. LABA medicines help the muscles around the airways in your lungs stay relaxed to prevent symptoms, such as wheezing and shortness of breath. These symptoms can happen when the muscles around the airways tighten. This makes it hard to breathe. In severe cases, wheezing can stop your breathing and cause death if not treated right away.

- SEREVENT DISKUS is used for asthma, exercise-induced bronchospasm (EIB), and chronic obstructive pulmonary disease (COPD) as follows:

Asthma:

SEREVENT DISKUS is used in adults and children aged 4 years and older, with a long-term asthma control medicine, such as an inhaled corticosteroid:

- to control symptoms of asthma, and
- to prevent symptoms such as wheezing.

LABA medicines, such as SEREVENT DISKUS, increase the risk of death from asthma problems. SEREVENT DISKUS is not for adults and children with asthma who are well controlled with a long-term asthma-control medicine, such as a low to medium dose of an inhaled corticosteroid medicine.

Exercise-Induced Bronchospasm:

SEREVENT DISKUS is used to prevent wheezing caused by exercise in adults and children aged 4 years and older.

- If you have EIB only, your healthcare provider may prescribe only SEREVENT DISKUS for your condition.
- If you have EIB and asthma, your healthcare provider should also prescribe an asthma control medicine, such as an inhaled corticosteroid.

Chronic Obstructive Pulmonary Disease:

SEREVENT DISKUS is used long term, 2 times each day (morning and evening) to control symptoms of COPD and prevent wheezing in adults with COPD.

Who should not use SEREVENT DISKUS?

Do not take SEREVENT DISKUS:

- to treat your asthma without an asthma medicine known as an inhaled corticosteroid
- if you are allergic to salmeterol or any of the ingredients in SEREVENT DISKUS. Ask your healthcare provider if you are not sure. See the end of this Medication Guide for a complete list of ingredients in SEREVENT DISKUS.

What should I tell my healthcare provider before using SEREVENT DISKUS?

Tell your healthcare provider about all of your health conditions, including if you:

- have heart problems
- have high blood pressure
- have seizures
- have thyroid problems
- have diabetes
- have liver problems
- are pregnant or planning to become pregnant. It is not known if SEREVENT DISKUS may harm your unborn baby.
- are breastfeeding. It is not known if SEREVENT DISKUS passes into your milk and if it can harm your baby.
- are allergic to SEREVENT DISKUS, any other medicines, or food products. See the end of this Medication Guide for a complete list of ingredients in SEREVENT DISKUS.

Tell your healthcare provider about all the medicines you take including prescription and non-prescription medicines, vitamins, and herbal supplements. SEREVENT DISKUS and certain other medicines, especially those used to treat infections, may interact with each other. This may cause serious side effects.

Know the medicines you take. Keep a list and show it to your healthcare provider and pharmacist each time you get a new medicine.

How do I use SEREVENT DISKUS?

See the step-by-step instructions for using the SEREVENT DISKUS at the end of this Medication Guide. Do not use SEREVENT DISKUS unless your healthcare provider has taught you and you understand everything. Ask your healthcare provider or pharmacist if you have any questions.

- Children should use SEREVENT DISKUS with an adult's help, as instructed by the child's healthcare provider.
- Use SEREVENT DISKUS exactly as prescribed. Do not use SEREVENT DISKUS more often than prescribed.
- For asthma and COPD, the usual dose is 1 inhalation 2 times each day (morning and evening). The 2 doses should be about 12 hours apart.
- For preventing exercise-induced bronchospasm, take 1 inhalation at least 30 minutes before exercise. Do not use SEREVENT DISKUS more often than every 12 hours. Do not use extra SEREVENT DISKUS before exercise if you already use it 2 times each day.
- If you miss a dose of SEREVENT DISKUS, just skip that dose. Take your next dose at your usual time. Do not take 2 doses at one time.
- Do not use a spacer device with SEREVENT DISKUS.
- Do not breathe into SEREVENT DISKUS.
- While you are using SEREVENT DISKUS 2 times each day, do not use other medicines that contain a long-acting beta$_2$-agonist or LABA for any reason. Ask your healthcare provider or pharmacist for a list of these medicines.
- Do not stop using SEREVENT DISKUS or any of your asthma medicines unless told to do so by your healthcare provider because your symptoms might get worse. Your healthcare provider will change your medicines as needed.
- SEREVENT DISKUS does not relieve sudden symptoms. Always have a rescue inhaler medicine with you to treat sudden symptoms. If you do not have an inhaled, short-acting bronchodilator, contact your healthcare provider to have one prescribed for you.
- Call your healthcare provider or get medical care right away if:
  - your breathing problems worsen with SEREVENT DISKUS
  - you need to use your rescue inhaler medicine more often than usual
  - your rescue inhaler medicine does not work as well for you at relieving symptoms
  - you need to use 4 or more inhalations of your rescue inhaler medicine for 2 or more days in a row
  - you use 1 whole canister of your rescue inhaler medicine in 8 weeks' time
  - your peak flow meter results decrease. Your healthcare provider will tell you the numbers that are right for you.
  - you have asthma and your symptoms do not improve after using SEREVENT DISKUS regularly for 1 week.
  - after a change in your asthma medicines you have any worsening of your asthma symptoms or an increase in the need for your rescue inhaler medicine.

What are the possible side effects with SEREVENT DISKUS?

SEREVENT DISKUS can cause serious side effects, including:

- **See "What is the most important information I should know about SEREVENT DISKUS?"**
- **serious allergic reactions.** Call your healthcare provider or get emergency medical care if you get any of the following symptoms of a serious allergic reaction:
  - rash
  - hives
  - swelling of the face, mouth, and tongue
  - breathing problems.
- **sudden breathing problems immediately after inhaling your medicine**
- **effects on heart**
  - increased blood pressure
  - a fast and irregular heartbeat
  - chest pain
- **effects on nervous system**
  - tremor
  - nervousness
- **changes in blood (sugar, potassium)**

Common side effects of SEREVENT DISKUS include:

Asthma in adults and children:

- headache
- nasal congestion
- bronchitis
- throat irritation
- runny nose
- flu

Chronic obstructive pulmonary disease:

- headache
- musculoskeletal pain
- throat irritation
- cough
- respiratory infection

Tell your healthcare provider about any side effect that bothers you or that does not go away.

These are not all the side effects with SEREVENT DISKUS. Ask your healthcare provider or pharmacist for more information.

Call your doctor for medical advice about side effects. You may report side effects to FDA at 1-800-FDA-1088.

How do I store SEREVENT DISKUS?

- Store SEREVENT DISKUS at room temperature between 68°F to 77°F (20°C to 25°C). Keep in a dry place away from heat and sunlight.
- Safely discard SEREVENT DISKUS 6 weeks after you remove it from the foil pouch, or after the dose indicator reads "0", whichever comes first.
- Keep SEREVENT DISKUS and all medicines out of the reach of children.

General Information about SEREVENT DISKUS

Medicines are sometimes prescribed for purposes not mentioned in a Medication Guide. Do not use SEREVENT DISKUS for a condition for which it was not prescribed. Do not give your SEREVENT DISKUS to other people, even if they have the same condition that you have. It may harm them.

This Medication Guide summarizes the most important information about SEREVENT DISKUS. If you would like more information, talk with your healthcare provider or pharmacist. You can ask your healthcare provider or pharmacist for information about SEREVENT DISKUS that was written for healthcare professionals. You can also contact the company that makes SEREVENT DISKUS (toll free) at 1-888-825-5249 or at www.serevent.com.

What are the ingredients in SEREVENT DISKUS?

Active ingredient: salmeterol xinafoate

Inactive ingredient: lactose (contains milk proteins)

Instructions for Using SEREVENT DISKUS

Follow the instructions below for using your SEREVENT DISKUS. **You will breathe in (inhale) the medicine from the DISKUS.** If you have any questions, ask your healthcare provider or pharmacist.

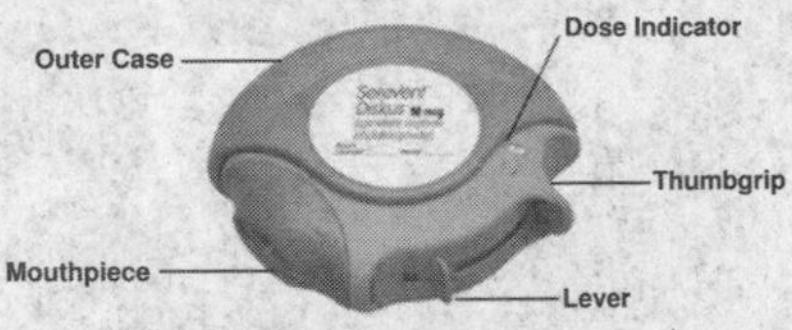

Take the SEREVENT DISKUS out of the box and foil pouch. Write the **"Pouch opened"** and **"Use by"** dates on the label on top of the DISKUS. **The "Use by" date is 6 weeks from date of opening the pouch.**

- The DISKUS will be in the closed position when the pouch is opened.
- The **dose indicator** on the top of the DISKUS tells you how many doses are left. The dose indicator number will decrease each time you use the DISKUS. After you have used 55 doses from the DISKUS, the numbers 5 to 0 will appear in **red** to warn you that there are only a few doses left *(see Figure 1).*

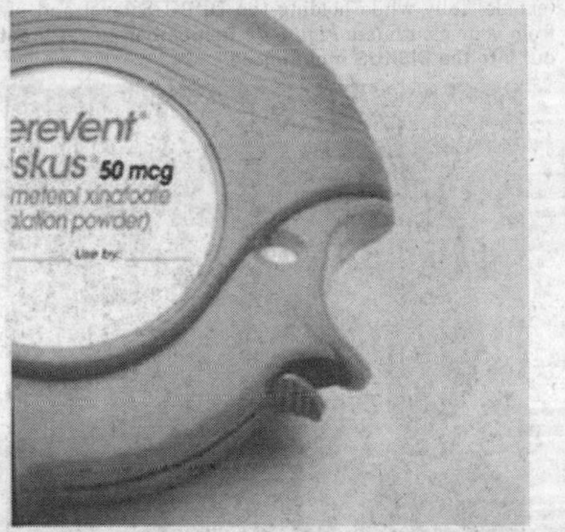

Figure 1

Taking a dose from the DISKUS requires the following 3 simple steps: Open, Click, Inhale.

1. OPEN

Hold the DISKUS in one hand and put the thumb of your other hand on the **thumbgrip**. Push your thumb away from you as far as it will go until the mouthpiece appears and snaps into position *(see Figure 2).*

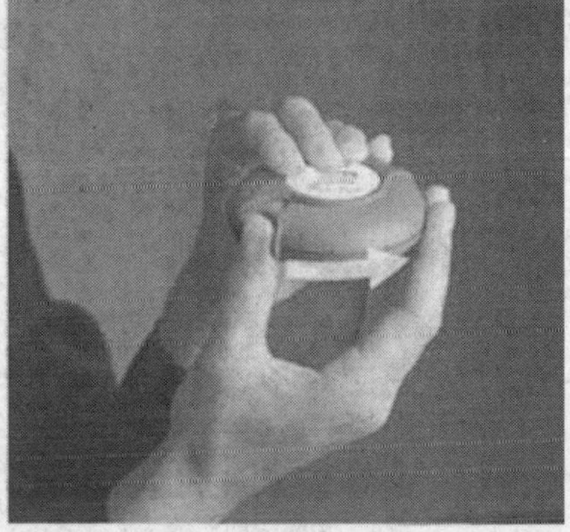

Figure 2

2. CLICK

Hold the DISKUS in a level, flat position with the mouthpiece towards you. Slide the **lever** away from you as far as it will go until it **clicks** *(see Figure 3).* The DISKUS is now ready to use.

[See figure 3 at top of next column]

Every time the **lever** is pushed back, a dose is ready to be inhaled. This is shown by a decrease in numbers on the dose counter. **To avoid releasing or wasting doses once the DISKUS is ready:**

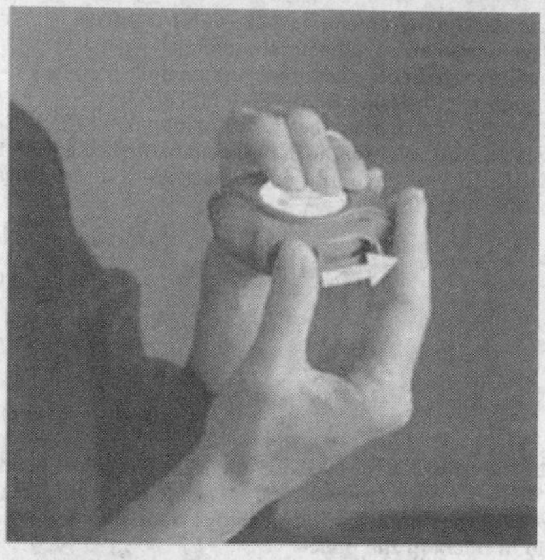

Figure 3

- **Do not close the DISKUS.**
- **Do not tilt the DISKUS.**
- **Do not play with the lever.**
- **Do not move the lever more than once.**

3. INHALE

Before inhaling your dose from the DISKUS, breathe out (exhale) fully while holding the DISKUS level and away from your mouth *(see Figure 4)*. **Remember, never breathe out into the DISKUS mouthpiece.**

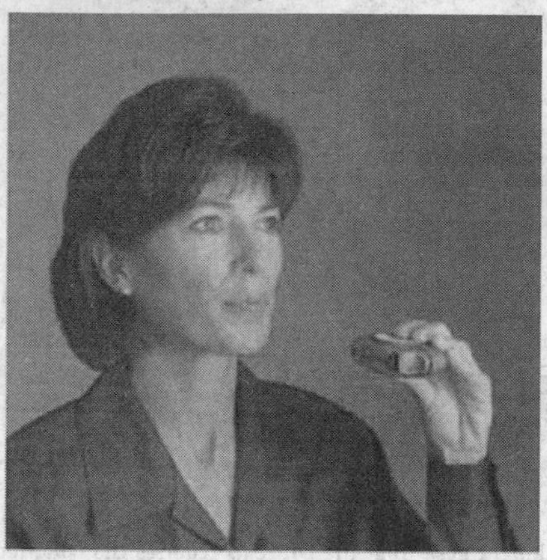

Figure 4

Put the mouthpiece to your lips *(see Figure 5)*. Breathe in quickly and deeply through the DISKUS. Do not breathe in through your nose.

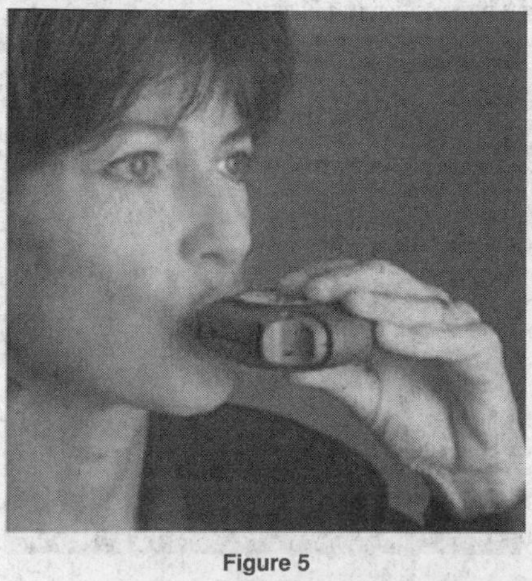

Figure 5

Remove the DISKUS from your mouth. Hold your breath for about 10 seconds, or for as long as is comfortable. Breathe out slowly.

The DISKUS delivers your dose of medicine as a very fine powder. Most patients can taste or feel the powder. Do not use another dose from the DISKUS if you do not feel or taste the medicine.

4. Close the DISKUS when you are finished taking a dose so that the DISKUS will be ready for you to take your next dose. Put your thumb on the thumbgrip and slide the thumbgrip back towards you as far as it will go *(see Figure 6)*. The DISKUS will click shut. The lever will automatically return to its original position. The DISKUS is now ready for you to take your next scheduled dose, due in about 12 hours. (Repeat steps 1 to 4.)

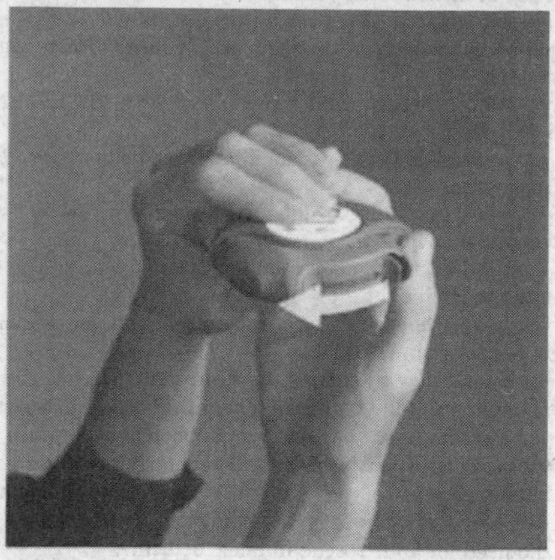

Figure 6

Remember:
- Never breathe into the DISKUS.
- Never take the DISKUS apart.
- Always ready and use the DISKUS in a level, flat position.
- Do not use the DISKUS with a spacer device.
- Never wash the mouthpiece or any part of the DISKUS. **Keep it dry.**
- Always keep the DISKUS in a dry place.
- Never take an extra dose, even if you did not taste or feel the medicine.

This Medication Guide has been approved by the U.S. Food and Drug Administration.

SEREVENT and DISKUS are registered trademarks of GlaxoSmithKline.

GlaxoSmithKline
Research Triangle Park, NC 27709

December 2010
SRD:4MG

TAFINLAR ℞
(dabrafenib)
capsules for oral use

HIGHLIGHTS OF PRESCRIBING INFORMATION
These highlights do not include all the information needed to use TAFINLAR safely and effectively. See full prescribing information for TAFINLAR.
TAFINLAR(dabrafenib) capsules for oral use
Initial U.S. Approval: 2013

INDICATIONS AND USAGE

TAFINLAR is a kinase inhibitor indicated for the treatment of patients with unresectable or metastatic melanoma with BRAF V600E mutation as detected by an FDA-approved test. (1, 2.1)

Limitation of use: TAFINLAR is not indicated for treatment of patients with wild-type BRAF melanoma. (1, 5.2)

DOSAGE AND ADMINISTRATION

- Confirm the presence of BRAF V600E mutation in tumor specimens prior to initiation of treatment with TAFINLAR. (2.1)
- The recommended dose is 150 mg orally twice daily taken at least 1 hour before or at least 2 hours after a meal. (2.2)

DOSAGE FORMS AND STRENGTHS

Capsules: 50 mg, 75 mg. (3)

CONTRAINDICATIONS

- None. (4)

WARNINGS AND PRECAUTIONS

- New Primary Cutaneous Malignancies: Perform dermatologic evaluations prior to initiation of therapy, every 2 months while on therapy, and for up to 6 months following discontinuation of TAFINLAR. (5.1)
- Tumor Promotion in BRAF Wild-Type Melanoma: Increased cell proliferation can occur with BRAF inhibitors. (5.2)
- Serious Febrile Drug Reactions: Withhold TAFINLAR if fever ≥101.3°F or complicated fever occurs. (5.3)
- Hyperglycemia: Monitor serum glucose levels in patients with pre-existing diabetes or hyperglycemia. (5.4)
- Uveitis and Iritis: Monitor patients routinely for visual symptoms. (5.5)
- Glucose-6-Phosphate Dehydrogenase Deficiency: Closely monitor for hemolytic anemia. (5.6)
- Embryofetal Toxicity: Can cause fetal harm. Advise females of reproductive potential of potential risk to a fetus. TAFINLAR may render hormonal contraceptives less effective and an alternative method of contraception should be used. (5.7, 8.1)

ADVERSE REACTIONS

Most common adverse reactions (≥20%) for TAFINLAR are hyperkeratosis, headache, pyrexia, arthralgia, papilloma, alopecia, and palmar-plantar erythrodysesthesia syndrome. (6.1)

To report SUSPECTED ADVERSE REACTIONS, contact GlaxoSmithKline at 1-888-825-5249 or FDA at 1-800-FDA-1088 or www.fda.gov/medwatch.

DRUG INTERACTIONS

- Concurrent administration of strong inhibitors of CYP3A4 or CYP2C8 is not recommended. (7.1)
- Concurrent administration of strong inducers of CYP3A4 or CYP2C8 is not recommended. (7.1)
- Drugs that increase gastric pH may decrease dabrafenib concentrations. (7.1)
- Concomitant use with agents that are sensitive substrates of CYP3A4, CYP2C8, CYP2C9, CYP2C19, or CYP2B6 may result in loss of efficacy of these agents. (7.2)

USE IN SPECIFIC POPULATIONS

- Nursing Mothers: Discontinue drug or nursing. (8.3)
- Females and Males of Reproductive Potential: Advise female patients to use highly effective contraception during treatment and for 4 weeks following discontinuation of treatment. Advise male patients of potential risk for impaired spermatogenesis. (8.6)

See 17 for PATIENT COUNSELING INFORMATION and Medication Guide

Revised: 05/2013

FULL PRESCRIBING INFORMATION: CONTENTS*

*** Sections or subsections omitted from the full prescribing information are not listed**

FULL PRESCRIBING INFORMATION

1 INDICATIONS AND USAGE

TAFINLAR® is indicated for the treatment of patients with unresectable or metastatic melanoma with BRAF V600E mutation as detected by an FDA-approved test.

Limitation of use: TAFINLAR is not indicated for treatment of patients with wild-type BRAF melanoma *[see Warnings and Precautions (5.2)]*.

2 DOSAGE AND ADMINISTRATION

2.1 Patient Selection

Confirm the presence of BRAF V600E mutation in tumor specimens prior to initiation of treatment with TAFINLAR *[see Warnings and Precautions (5.2)]*. Information on FDA-approved tests for the detection of BRAF V600 mutations in melanoma is available at http://www.fda.gov/CompanionDiagnostics.

2.2 Recommended Dosing

The recommended dose for TAFINLAR is 150 mg orally taken twice daily, approximately 12 hours apart, until disease progression or unacceptable toxicity occurs. Take either at least 1 hour before or at least 2 hours after a meal *[see Clinical Pharmacology (12.3)]*.

A missed dose can be taken up to 6 hours prior to the next dose. Do not open, crush, or break TAFINLAR capsule.

2.3 Dose Modifications

For New Primary Cutaneous Malignancies: No dose modifications are recommended.

[See table 1 above]

Table 1. Recommended Dose Modifications for TAFINLAR

Target Organ	Adverse Reactions[a]	Dose Modification
Febrile Drug Reaction	• Fever of 101.3°F to 104°F	Withhold TAFINLAR until adverse reaction resolves. Then resume TAFINLAR at same dose or at a reduced dose level (see Table 2).
	• Fever higher than 104°F • Fever complicated by rigors, hypotension, dehydration, or renal failure	Either • Permanently discontinue TAFINLAR Or • Withhold TAFINLAR until adverse reaction resolves. Then resume TAFINLAR at a reduced dose level (see Table 2).
Other	• Intolerable Grade 2 Adverse Reactions • Any Grade 3 Adverse Reactions	Withhold TAFINLAR until adverse reaction resolves to Grade 1 or less. Then resume TAFINLAR at a reduced dose level (see Table 2).
	• First occurrence of Any Grade 4 Adverse Reaction	Either • Permanently discontinue TAFINLAR Or • Withhold TAFINLAR until adverse reaction resolves to Grade 1 or less. Then resume TAFINLAR at a reduced dose level (see Table 2).
	• Recurrent Grade 4 Adverse Reaction • Intolerable Grade 2 or Any Grade 3 or 4 Adverse Reaction on TAFINLAR 50 mg twice daily	Permanently discontinue TAFINLAR.

[a] Common Terminology Criteria for Adverse Events (CTCAE) version 4.0.

Table 2. Recommended TAFINLAR Dose Reductions

Dose Reductions	Dose and Schedule
First dose reduction	100 mg orally twice daily
Second dose reduction	75 mg orally twice daily
Third dose reduction	50 mg orally twice daily
If unable to tolerate 50 mg twice daily	Discontinue TAFINLAR

3 DOSAGE FORMS AND STRENGTHS

50 mg Capsules: Dark red capsule imprinted with 'GS TEW' and '50 mg'.

75 mg Capsules: Dark pink capsule imprinted with 'GS LHF' and '75 mg'.

4 CONTRAINDICATIONS

None.

5 WARNINGS AND PRECAUTIONS

5.1 New Primary Cutaneous Malignancies

TAFINLAR results in an increased incidence of cutaneous squamous cell carcinoma, keratoacanthoma, and melanoma. In Trial 1, cutaneous squamous cell carcinomas and keratoacanthomas (cuSCC) occurred in 7% (14/187) of patients treated with TAFINLAR and in none of the patients treated with dacarbazine. Across clinical trials of TAFINLAR (n = 586), the incidence of cuSCC was 11%. The median time to first cuSCC was 9 weeks (range: 1 to 53 weeks). Of those patients who developed a cuSCC, approximately 33% developed one or more cuSCC with continued TAFINLAR. The median time between diagnosis of the first cuSCC and the second cuSCC was 6 weeks.

In Trial 1, the incidence of new primary malignant melanomas was 2% (3/187) for patients receiving TAFINLAR while no chemotherapy-treated patient was diagnosed with new primary malignant melanoma.

Perform dermatologic evaluations prior to initiation of TAFINLAR, every 2 months while on therapy, and for up to 6 months following discontinuation of TAFINLAR.

5.2 Tumor Promotion in BRAF Wild-Type Melanoma

In vitro experiments have demonstrated paradoxical activation of MAP-kinase signaling and increased cell proliferation in BRAF wild-type cells which are exposed to BRAF inhibitors. Confirm evidence of BRAF V600E mutation status prior to initiation of TAFINLAR *[see Indications and Usage (1) and Dosage and Administration (2.1)]*.

5.3 Serious Febrile Drug Reactions

In Trial 1, serious febrile drug reactions, defined as serious cases of fever or fever of any severity accompanied by hypotension, rigors or chills, dehydration, or renal failure in the absence of another identifiable cause (e.g., infection) occurred in 3.7% (7/187) of patients treated with TAFINLAR and in none of the patients treated with dacarbazine. The incidence of fever (serious and non-serious) was 28% in patients treated with TAFINLAR and 10% in patients treated with dacarbazine. In patients treated with TAFINLAR, the median time to initial onset of fever (any severity) was 11 days (range: 1 to 202 days) and the median duration of fever was 3 days (range: 1 to 129 days).

Withhold TAFINLAR for fever of 101.3°F or greater or for any serious febrile drug reaction and evaluate for signs and symptoms of infection. Refer to Table 1 for recommended dose modifications for adverse reactions *[see Dosage and Administration (2.3)]*. Prophylaxis with antipyretics may be required when resuming TAFINLAR.

5.4 Hyperglycemia

Hyperglycemia requiring an increase in the dose of, or initiation of insulin or oral hypoglycemic agent therapy can occur with TAFINLAR. In Trial 1, five of 12 patients with a history of diabetes required more intensive hypoglycemic therapy while taking TAFINLAR. The incidence of Grade 3 hyperglycemia based on laboratory values was 6% (12/187) in patients treated with TAFINLAR compared to none of the dacarbazine-treated patients.

Monitor serum glucose levels as clinically appropriate during treatment with TAFINLAR in patients with pre-existing diabetes or hyperglycemia. Advise patients to report symptoms of severe hyperglycemia such as excessive thirst or any increase in the volume or frequency of urination.

5.5 Uveitis and Iritis

Uveitis (including iritis) occurred in 1% (6/586) of patients treated with TAFINLAR across clinical trials. Symptomatic treatment employed in clinical trials included steroid and mydriatic ophthalmic drops. Monitor patients for visual signs and symptoms of uveitis (e.g., change in vision, photophobia, and eye pain).

5.6 Glucose-6-Phosphate Dehydrogenase Deficiency

TAFINLAR, which contains a sulfonamide moiety, confers a potential risk of hemolytic anemia in patients with glucose-6-phosphate dehydrogenase (G6PD) deficiency. Closely observe patients with G6PD deficiency for signs of hemolytic anemia.

5.7 Embryofetal Toxicity

Based on its mechanism of action, TAFINLAR can cause fetal harm when administered to a pregnant woman. Dabrafenib was teratogenic and embryotoxic in rats at doses three times greater than the human exposure at the recommended clinical dose. If this drug is used during pregnancy or if the patient becomes pregnant while taking this drug, the patient should be apprised of the potential hazard to a fetus *[see Use in Specific Populations (8.1)]*.

Advise female patients of reproductive potential to use a highly effective non-hormonal method of contraception during treatment and for 4 weeks after treatment since TAFINLAR can render hormonal contraceptives ineffective. Advise patients to contact their healthcare provider if they become pregnant, or if pregnancy is suspected, while taking TAFINLAR *[see Drug Interactions (7.2), Use in Specific Populations (8.6)]*.

6 ADVERSE REACTIONS

The following adverse reactions are discussed in greater detail in another section of the label.

- New Primary Cutaneous Malignancies *[see Warnings and Precautions (5.1)]*
- Tumor Promotion in BRAF Wild-Type Melanoma *[see Warnings and Precautions (5.2)]*
- Serious Febrile Drug Reactions *[see Warnings and Precautions (5.3)]*
- Hyperglycemia *[see Warnings and Precautions (5.4)]*
- Uveitis and Iritis *[see Warnings and Precautions (5.5)]*

6.1 Clinical Trials Experience

Because clinical trials are conducted under widely varying conditions, adverse reaction rates observed in the clinical trials of a drug cannot be directly compared to rates in the clinical trials of another drug and may not reflect the rates observed in practice.

The safety of TAFINLAR was evaluated in 586 patients with BRAF V600 mutation-positive unresectable or metastatic melanoma, previously treated or untreated, who received TAFINLAR 150 mg orally twice daily as monotherapy until disease progression or unacceptable toxicity, including 181 patients treated for at least 6 months and 86 additional patients treated for more than 12 months. TAFINLAR was studied in open-label, single-arm trials and in an open-label, randomized, active-controlled trial. The median daily dose of TAFINLAR was 300 mg (range: 118 to 300 mg).

Table 3 and Table 4 present adverse drug reactions and laboratory abnormalities identified from analyses of Trial 1 *[see Clinical Studies (14)]*. Trial 1, a multi-center, international, open-label, randomized (3:1), controlled trial allocated 250 patients with unresectable or metastatic BRAF V600E mutation-positive melanoma to receive TAFINLAR 150 mg orally twice daily (n = 187) or dacarbazine 1,000 mg/m^2 intravenously every 3 weeks (n = 63). The trial excluded patients with abnormal left ventricular ejection fraction or cardiac valve morphology (≥Grade 2), corrected QT interval ≥480 milliseconds on electrocardiogram, or a known history of glucose-6-phosphate dehydrogenase deficiency. The median duration on treatment was 4.9 months for patients treated with TAFINLAR and 2.8 months for dacarbazine-treated patients. The population exposed to TAFINLAR was 60% male, 99% white, and had a median age of 53 years.

The most commonly occurring adverse reactions (≥20%) in patients treated with TAFINLAR were, in order of decreasing frequency: hyperkeratosis, headache, pyrexia, arthralgia, papilloma, alopecia, and palmar-plantar erythrodysesthesia syndrome (PPES).

The incidence of adverse events resulting in permanent discontinuation of study medication in Trial 1 was 3% for patients treated with TAFINLAR and 3% for patients treated with dacarbazine. The most frequent (≥2%) adverse reactions leading to dose reduction of TAFINLAR were pyrexia (9%), PPES (3%), chills (3%), fatigue (2%), and headache (2%).

[See table 3 at top of next page]
[See table 4 at top of next page]

Other clinically important adverse reactions observed in <10% of patients (N = 586) treated with TAFINLAR were:

Gastrointestinal Disorders: Pancreatitis.

Immune System Disorders: Hypersensitivity manifesting as bullous rash.

Renal and Urinary Disorders: Interstitial nephritis.

7 DRUG INTERACTIONS

7.1 Effects of Other Drugs on Dabrafenib

Drugs that Inhibit or Induce Drug-Metabolizing Enzymes: Dabrafenib is primarily metabolized by CYP2C8 and CYP3A4. Strong inhibitors or inducers of CYP3A4 or CYP2C8 may increase or decrease, respectively, concentrations of dabrafenib *[see Clinical Pharmacology (12.3)]*. Substitution of strong inhibitors or strong inducers of CYP3A4 or CYP2C8 is recommended during treatment with TAFINLAR. If concomitant use of strong inhibitors (e.g., ke-

Table 3. Selected Common Adverse Reactions Occurring in ≥10% (All Grades) or ≥2% (Grades 3 or 4) of Patients Treated with TAFINLAR[a]

	TAFINLAR N = 187		Dacarbazine N = 59	
Primary System Organ Class Preferred Term	**All Grades (%)**	**Grades 3 and 4[b] (%)**	**All Grades (%)**	**Grades 3 and 4 (%)**
Skin and subcutaneous tissue disorders				
Hyperkeratosis	37	1	0	0
Alopecia	22	NA[f]	2	NA[f]
Palmar-plantar erythrodysesthesia syndrome	20	2	2	0
Rash	17	0	0	0
Nervous system disorders				
Headache	32	0	8	0
General disorders and administration site conditions				
Pyrexia	28	3	10	0
Musculoskeletal and connective tissue disorders				
Arthralgia	27	1	2	0
Back pain	12	3	7	0
Myalgia	11	0	0	0
Neoplasms benign, malignant and unspecified (including cysts and polyps)				
Papilloma[c]	27	0	2	0
cuSCC[d, e]	7	4	0	0
Gastrointestinal disorders				
Constipation	11	2	14	0
Respiratory, thoracic, and mediastinal disorders				
Cough	12	0	5	0
Infections and infestations				
Nasopharyngitis	10	0	3	0

[a] Adverse drug reactions, reported using MedDRA and graded using CTCAE version 4.0 for assessment of toxicity.
[b] Grade 4 adverse reactions limited to hyperkeratosis (n = 1) and constipation (n = 1).
[c] Includes skin papilloma and papilloma.
[d] Includes squamous cell carcinoma of the skin and keratoacanthoma.
[e] Cases of cutaneous squamous cell carcinoma were required to be reported as Grade 3 per protocol.
[f] NA = not applicable

Table 4. Incidence of Laboratory Abnormalities Increased from Baseline Occurring at a Higher Incidence in Patients Treated with TAFINLAR in Trial 1 [Between Arm Difference of ≥5% (All Grades) or ≥2% (Grades 3 or 4)]

	Dabrafenib N = 187		DTIC N = 59	
	All Grades (%)	**Grades 3 and 4 (%)**	**All Grades (%)**	**Grades 3 and 4 (%)**
Hyperglycemia	50	6	43	0
Hypophosphatemia	37	6[a]	14	2
Increased Alkaline phosphatase	19	0	14	2
Hyponatremia	8	2	3	0

[a] Grade 4 laboratory abnormality limited to hypophosphatemia (n = 1).

toconazole, nefazodone, clarithromycin, gemfibrozil) or strong inducers (e.g., rifampin, phenytoin, carbamazepine, phenobarbital, St John's wort) of CYP3A4 or CYP2C8 is unavoidable, monitor patients closely for adverse reactions when taking strong inhibitors or loss of efficacy when taking strong inducers.

Drugs that Affect Gastric pH: Drugs that alter the pH of the upper GI tract (e.g., proton pump inhibitors, H_2-receptor antagonists, antacids) may alter the solubility of dabrafenib and reduce its bioavailability. However, no formal clinical trial has been conducted to evaluate the effect of gastric pH-altering agents on the systemic exposure of dabrafenib. When TAFINLAR is coadministered with a proton pump inhibitor, H_2-receptor antagonist, or antacid, systemic exposure of dabrafenib may be decreased and the effect on efficacy of TAFINLAR is unknown.

7.2 Effects of Dabrafenib on Other Drugs

Dabrafenib induces CYP3A4 and may induce other enzymes including CYP2B6, CYP2C8, CYP2C9, CYP2C19, and UDP glucuronosyltransferases (UGT) and may induce transporters. Dabrafenib decreased the maximum concentration (C_{max}) and area under the curve (AUC) of midazolam (a substrate of CYP3A4) by 61% and 74%, respectively *[see Clinical Pharmacology (12.3)]*. Coadministration of TAFINLAR with other substrates of these enzymes, including warfarin, dexamethasone, or hormonal contraceptives, can result in decreased concentrations and loss of efficacy *[see Use in Specific Populations (8.1, 8.6)]*. Substitute for these medications or monitor patients for loss of efficacy if use of these medications is unavoidable.

8 USE IN SPECIFIC POPULATIONS

8.1 Pregnancy

Pregnancy Category D

Risk Summary: Based on its mechanism of action, TAFINLAR can cause fetal harm when administered to a pregnant woman. Dabrafenib was teratogenic and embryotoxic in rats at doses 3 times greater than the human exposure at the recommended clinical dose of 150 mg twice daily based on AUC. If this drug is used during pregnancy or if the patient becomes pregnant while taking this drug, the patient should be apprised of the potential hazard to a fetus *[see Warnings and Precautions (5.7)]*.

Animal Data: In a combined female fertility and embryo-fetal development study in rats, developmental toxicity consisted of embryo-lethality, ventricular septal defects, and variation in thymic shape at a dabrafenib dose of 300 mg/kg/day (approximately 3 times the human exposure at the recommended dose based on AUC). At doses of 20 mg/kg/day or greater (equivalent to the human exposure at the recommended dose based on AUC), rats demonstrated delays in skeletal development and reduced fetal body weight.

8.3 Nursing Mothers

It is not known whether this drug is present in human milk. Because many drugs are present in human milk and because of the potential for serious adverse reactions from TAFINLAR in nursing infants, a decision should be made whether to discontinue nursing or discontinue the drug, taking into account the importance of the drug to the mother.

8.4 Pediatric Use

The safety and effectiveness of TAFINLAR have not been established in pediatric patients.

8.5 Geriatric Use

One hundred and twenty-six (22%) of 586 patients in clinical trials of TAFINLAR and 40 (21%) of the 187 patients receiving TAFINLAR in Trial 1 were ≥65 years of age. No overall differences in the effectiveness or safety of TAFINLAR were observed in the elderly in Trial 1.

8.6 Females and Males of Reproductive Potential

Contraception:

Females

Advise female patients of reproductive potential to use highly effective contraception during treatment and for 4 weeks after treatment. Counsel patients to use a non-hormonal method of contraception since TAFINLAR can render hormonal contraceptives ineffective. Advise patients to contact their healthcare provider if they become pregnant, or if pregnancy is suspected, while taking TAFINLAR *[see Warnings and Precautions (5.7), Drug Interactions (7.1), Use in Specific Populations (8.1)]*.

Infertility:

Males

Effects on spermatogenesis have been observed in animals. Advise male patients of the potential risk for impaired spermatogenesis, and to seek counseling on fertility and family planning options prior to starting treatment with TAFINLAR *[see Nonclinical Toxicology (13.1)]*.

8.7 Hepatic Impairment

No formal pharmacokinetic trial in patients with hepatic impairment has been conducted. Dose adjustment is not recommended for patients with mild hepatic impairment based on the results of the population pharmacokinetic analysis. As hepatic metabolism and biliary secretion are the primary routes of elimination of dabrafenib and its metabolites, patients with moderate to severe hepatic impairment may have increased exposure. An appropriate dose has not been established for patients with moderate to severe hepatic impairment *[see Clinical Pharmacology (12.3)]*.

8.8 Renal Impairment

No formal pharmacokinetic trial in patients with renal impairment has been conducted. Dose adjustment is not recommended for patients with mild or moderate renal impairment based on the results of the population pharmacokinetic analysis. An appropriate dose has not been established for patients with severe renal impairment *[see Clinical Pharmacology (12.3)]*.

10 OVERDOSAGE

There is no information on overdosage of TAFINLAR.

11 DESCRIPTION

Dabrafenib mesylate is a kinase inhibitor. The chemical name for dabrafenib mesylate is N-{3-[5-(2-Amino-4-pyrimidinyl)-2-(1,1-dimethylethyl)-1,3-thiazol-4-yl]-2-fluorophenyl}-2,6-difluorobenzene sulfonamide, methanesulfonate salt. It has the molecular formula $C_{23}H_{20}F_3N_5O_2S_2 \cdot CH_4O_3S$ and a molecular weight of 615.68. Dabrafenib mesylate has the following chemical structure.

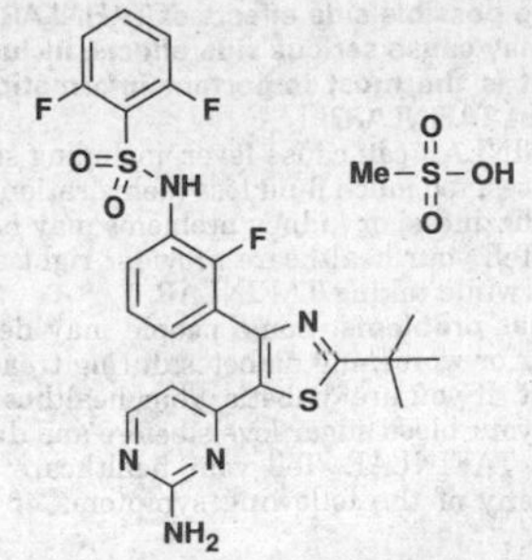

Dabrafenib mesylate is a white to slightly colored solid with three pK_as: 6.6, 2.2, and -1.5. It is very slightly soluble at pH 1 and practically insoluble above pH 4 in aqueous media.

TAFINLAR (dabrafenib) capsules are supplied as 50 mg and 75 mg capsules for oral administration. Each 50 mg capsule contains 59.25 mg dabrafenib mesylate equivalent to 50 mg of dabrafenib free base. Each 75 mg capsule contains 88.88 mg dabrafenib mesylate equivalent to 75 mg of dabrafenib free base.

The inactive ingredients of TAFINLAR are colloidal silicon dioxide, magnesium stearate, and microcrystalline cellulose. Capsule shells contain hypromellose, red iron oxide (E172), and titanium dioxide (E171).

12 CLINICAL PHARMACOLOGY

12.1 Mechanism of Action

Dabrafenib is an inhibitor of some mutated forms of BRAF kinases with in vitro IC_{50} values of 0.65, 0.5, and 1.84 nM for BRAF V600E, BRAF V600K, and BRAF V600D enzymes, respectively. Dabrafenib also inhibits wild-type BRAF and CRAF kinases with IC_{50} values of 3.2 and 5.0 nM, respectively, and other kinases such as SIK1, NEK11, and LIMK1 at higher concentrations. Some mutations in the BRAF gene, including those that result in BRAF V600E, can result in constitutively activated BRAF kinases that may stimulate tumor cell growth *[see Indications and Usage (1)]*. Dabrafenib inhibits BRAF V600 mutation-positive melanoma cell growth in vitro and in vivo.

12.3 Pharmacokinetics

Absorption: After oral administration, median time to achieve peak plasma concentration (T_{max}) is 2 hours. Mean absolute bioavailability of oral dabrafenib is 95%. Following a single dose, dabrafenib exposure (C_{max} and AUC) increased in a dose-proportional manner across the dose range of 12 to 300 mg, but the increase was less than dose-proportional after repeat twice daily dosing. After repeat twice daily dosing of 150 mg, the mean accumulation ratio was 0.73 and the inter-subject variability (CV%) of AUC at steady-state was 38%.

Administration of dabrafenib with a high-fat meal decreased C_{max} by 51%, decreased AUC by 31%, and delayed median T_{max} by 3.6 hours as compared to the fasted state *[see Dosage and Administration (2.2)]*.

Distribution: Dabrafenib is 99.7% bound to human plasma proteins. The apparent volume of distribution (V_c/F) is 70.3 L.

Metabolism: The metabolism of dabrafenib is primarily mediated by CYP2C8 and CYP3A4 to form hydroxy-dabrafenib. Hydroxy-dabrafenib is further oxidized via CYP3A4 to form carboxy-dabrafenib and subsequently excreted in bile and urine. Carboxy-dabrafenib is decarboxylated to form desmethyl-dabrafenib; desmethyl-dabrafenib may be reabsorbed from the gut. Desmethyl-dabrafenib is further metabolized by CYP3A4 to oxidative metabolites. Hydroxy-dabrafenib terminal half-life (10 hours) parallels that of dabrafenib while the carboxy- and desmethyl-dabrafenib metabolites exhibited longer half-lives (21 to 22 hours). Mean metabolite-to-parent AUC ratios following repeat-dose administration are 0.9, 11, and 0.7 for hydroxy-, carboxy-, and desmethyl-dabrafenib, respectively. Based on systemic exposure, relative potency, and pharmacokinetic properties, both hydroxy- and desmethyl-dabrafenib are likely to contribute to the clinical activity of dabrafenib.

Elimination: The mean terminal half-life of dabrafenib is 8 hours after oral administration. The apparent clearance of dabrafenib is 17.0 L/h after single dosing and 34.4 L/h after 2 weeks of twice daily dosing.

Fecal excretion is the major route of elimination accounting for 71% of radioactive dose while urinary excretion accounted for 23% of total radioactivity as metabolites only.

Specific Populations:

Age, Body Weight and Gender: Based on the population pharmacokinetics analysis, age has no effect on dabrafenib pharmacokinetics. Pharmacokinetic differences based on gender and on weight are not clinically relevant.

Pediatric: Pharmacokinetics of dabrafenib have not been studied in pediatric patients.

Renal: No formal pharmacokinetic trial in patients with renal impairment has been conducted. The pharmacokinetics of dabrafenib were evaluated using a population analysis in 233 patients with mild renal impairment (GFR 60 to 89 mL/min/1.73 m^2) and 30 patients with moderate renal impairment (GFR 30 to 59 mL/min/1.73 m^2) enrolled in clinical trials. Mild or moderate renal impairment has no effect on systemic exposure to dabrafenib and its metabolites. No data are available in patients with severe renal impairment.

Hepatic: No formal pharmacokinetic trial in patients with hepatic impairment has been conducted. The pharmacokinetics of dabrafenib were evaluated using a population analysis in 65 patients with mild hepatic impairment enrolled in clinical trials. Mild hepatic impairment has no effect on systemic exposure to dabrafenib and its metabolites. No data are available in patients with moderate to severe hepatic impairment.

Drug Interactions:

Human liver microsome studies show that dabrafenib is a substrate of CYP3A4 and CYP2C8 while hydroxy-dabrafenib and desmethyl-dabrafenib are CYP3A4 substrates. Dabrafenib is a substrate of human P-glycoprotein (Pgp) and breast cancer resistance protein (BCRP) in vitro. In human hepatocytes, dabrafenib produced dose-dependent increases in CYP2B6 and CYP3A4 mRNA levels up to 32 times the control levels and is a moderate inducer of CYP3A4 in vivo. In a clinical trial in 12 subjects following coadministration of repeat doses of dabrafenib and a single dose of midazolam (a CYP3A4 substrate), midazolam C_{max} and $AUC_{(0-\infty)}$ were decreased 61% and 74%, respectively. Dabrafenib is a moderate inducer of CYP3A4 and may induce other enzymes such as CYP2B6, CYP2C8, CYP2C9, CYP2C19, and UDP glucuronosyltransferases (UGT) and may induce transporters.

Dabrafenib and its metabolites, hydroxy-dabrafenib, carboxy-dabrafenib, and desmethyl-dabrafenib, were inhibitors of human organic anion transporting polypeptide OATP1B1, OATP1B3, organic anion transporter OAT1 and OAT3 in vitro. Dabrafenib and desmethyl-dabrafenib are moderate inhibitors of BCRP in vitro.

13 NONCLINICAL TOXICOLOGY

13.1 Carcinogenesis, Mutagenesis, Impairment of Fertility

Carcinogenicity studies with dabrafenib have not been conducted. TAFINLAR increased the risk of cutaneous squamous cell carcinomas in patients in clinical trials.

Dabrafenib was not mutagenic in vitro in the bacterial reverse mutation assay (Ames test) or the mouse lymphoma assay, and was not clastogenic in an in vivo rat bone marrow micronucleus test.

In a combined female fertility and embryofetal development study in rats, a reduction in fertility was noted at doses greater than or equal to 20 mg/kg/day (equivalent to the human exposure at the recommended dose based on AUC). A reduction in the number of ovarian corpora lutea was noted in pregnant females at 300 mg/kg/day (which is approximately three times the human exposure at the recommended dose based on AUC).

Male fertility studies with dabrafenib have not been conducted; however, in repeat-dose studies, testicular degeneration/depletion was seen in rats and dogs at doses equivalent to and three times the human exposure at the recommended dose based on AUC, respectively.

13.2 Animal Toxicology and/or Pharmacology

Adverse cardiovascular effects were noted in dogs at dabrafenib doses of 50 mg/kg/day (approximately five times the human exposure at the recommended dose based on AUC) or greater, when administered for up to 4 weeks. Adverse effects consisted of coronary arterial degeneration/necrosis and hemorrhage, as well as cardiac atrioventricular valve hypertrophy/hemorrhage.

14 CLINICAL STUDIES

In Trial 1, the safety and efficacy of TAFINLAR were demonstrated in an international, multi-center, randomized (3:1), open-label, active-controlled trial conducted in 250 patients with previously untreated BRAF V600E mutation-positive, unresectable or metastatic melanoma. Patients with any prior use of BRAF inhibitors or MEK inhibitors were excluded. Patients were randomized to receive TAFINLAR 150 mg by mouth twice daily (n = 187) or dacarbazine 1,000 mg/m^2 intravenously every 3 weeks (n = 63). Randomization was stratified by disease stage at baseline [unresectable stage III (regional nodal or in-transit metastases), M1a (distant skin, subcutaneous, or nodal metastases), or M1b (lung metastases) vs. M1c melanoma (all other visceral metastases or elevated serum LDH)]. The main efficacy outcome measure was progression-free survival (PFS) as assessed by the investigator. In addition, an independent radiology review committee (IRRC) assessed the following efficacy outcome measures in pre-specified supportive analyses: PFS, confirmed objective response rate (ORR), and duration of response.

The median age of patients in Trial 1 was 52 years. The majority of the trial population was male (60%), white (99%), had an ECOG performance status of 0 (67%), M1c disease (66%), and normal LDH (62%). All patients had tumor tissue with mutations in BRAF V600E as determined by a clinical trial assay at a centralized testing site. Tumor samples from 243 patients (97%) were tested retrospectively, using an FDA-approved companion diagnostic test, THxID™-BRAF assay.

The median duration of follow-up prior to initiation of alternative treatment in the TAFINLAR arm was 5.1 months and in the dacarbazine arm was 3.5 months. Twenty-eight (44%) patients crossed over from the dacarbazine arm at the time of disease progression to receive TAFINLAR.

Trial 1 demonstrated a statistically significant increase in progression-free survival in the patients treated with TAFINLAR. Table 5 and Figure 1 summarize the PFS results.

Table 5. Investigator-Assessed Progression-Free Survival and Confirmed Objective Response Results

	TAFINLAR N = 187	Dacarbazine N = 63
Progression-free Survival		
Number of Events (%)	78 (42%)	41 (65%)
Progressive Disease	76	41
Death	2	0
Median, months (95% CI)	5.1 (4.9, 6.9)	2.7 (1.5, 3.2)
HR[a] (95% CI)	0.33 (0.20, 0.54)	
P value[b]	*P* <0.0001	
Confirmed Tumor Responses		
Objective Response Rate	52%	17%
(95% CI)	(44, 59)	(9, 29)
CR, n (%)	6 (3%)	0
PR, n (%)	91 (48%)	11 (17%)
Duration of Response		
Median, months (95% CI)	5.6 (5.4, NR)	NR (5.0, NR)

[a] Pike estimator, stratified by disease state.
[b] Stratified log rank test.
CI = Confidence interval; CR = complete response; HR = hazard ratio; NR = not reached; PR = partial response

Figure 1. Kaplan-Meier Curves of Investigator-Assessed Progression-Free Survival

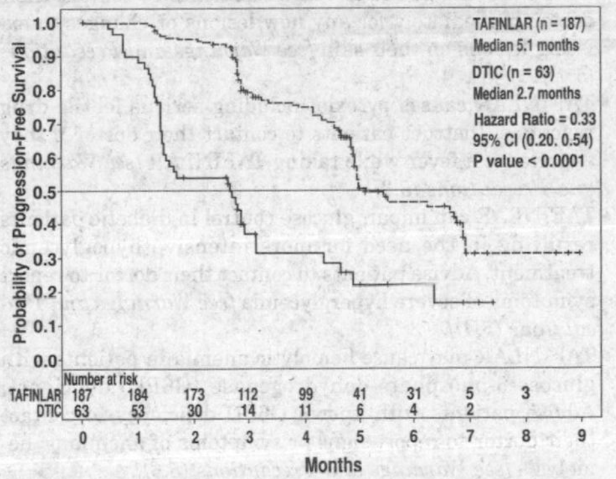

In supportive analyses based on IRRC assessment and in an exploratory subgroup analysis of patients with retrospectively confirmed V600E mutation-positive melanoma with the THxID™-BRAF assay, the PFS results were consistent with those of the primary efficacy analysis.

The activity of TAFINLAR for the treatment of BRAF V600E mutation-positive melanoma, metastatic to the brain was evaluated in a single arm, open-label, two-cohort, multi-center trial (Trial 2). All patients received TAFINLAR 150 mg twice daily. Patients in Cohort A (n = 74) had received no prior local therapy for brain metastases, while patients in Cohort B (n = 65) had received at least one local therapy for brain metastases, including, but not limited to, surgical resection, whole brain radiotherapy, or stereotactic radiosurgery such as gamma knife, linear-accelerated-based radiosurgery, charged particles, or CyberKnife. In addition, patients in Cohort B were required to have evidence of disease progression in a previously treated lesion or an untreated lesion. Additional eligibility criteria were at least one measurable lesion of 0.5 cm or greater in largest diameter on contrast-enhanced MRI, stable or decreasing corticosteroid dose, and no more than two prior systemic regimens for treatment of metastatic disease. The primary outcome measure was estimation of the overall intracranial response rate (OIRR) in each cohort.

The median age of patients in Cohort A was 50 years, 72% were male, 100% were white, 59% had a pre-treatment ECOG performance status of 0, and 57% had an elevated LDH value at baseline. The median age of patients in Cohort B was 51 years, 63% were male, 98% were white, 66% had a pre-treatment ECOG performance status of 0, and 54% had an elevated LDH value at baseline. Efficacy results as determined by an independent radiology review committee, masked to investigator response assessments, are provided in Table 6.

Table 6. Efficacy Results in Patients with BRAF V600E Melanoma Brain Metastases (Trial 2)

	IRRC Assessed Response	
Endpoint	**Cohort A N = 74**	**Cohort B N = 65**
Overall Intracranial Response Rate (OIRR)		
% (95% CI)	18 (9.7, 28.2)	18 (9.9, 30.0)
Duration of OIRR	(N = 13)	(N = 12)
Median, months (95% CI)	4.6 (2.8, NR)	4.6 (1.9, 4.6)

IRRC = Independent radiology review committee; CI = Confidence interval; NR = not reached

16 HOW SUPPLIED/STORAGE AND HANDLING

50 mg Capsules: Dark red capsule imprinted with 'GS TEW' and '50 mg' available in bottles of 120 (NDC 0173-0846-08). Each bottle contains a silica gel desiccant.

75 mg Capsules: Dark pink capsule imprinted with 'GS LHF' and '75 mg' available in bottles of 120 (NDC 0173-0847-08). Each bottle contains a silica gel desiccant.

Store at 25°C (77°F); excursions permitted to 15° to 30°C (59° to 86°F) [see USP Controlled Room Temperature].

17 PATIENT COUNSELING INFORMATION

See FDA-approved patient labeling (Medication Guide).

Inform patients of the following:

- Evidence of BRAF V600E mutation in the tumor specimen is necessary to identify patients for whom treatment with TAFINLAR is indicated *[see Dosage and Administration (2.1)]*.
- TAFINLAR increases the risk of developing new primary cutaneous malignancies. Advise patients to contact their doctor immediately for any new lesions or changes to existing lesions on their skin *[see Warnings and Precautions (5.1)]*.
- TAFINLAR causes pyrexia including serious febrile drug reactions. Instruct patients to contact their doctor if they experience a fever while taking TAFINLAR *[see Warnings and Precautions (5.3)]*.
- TAFINLAR can impair glucose control in diabetic patients resulting in the need for more intensive hypoglycemic treatment. Advise patients to contact their doctor to report symptoms of severe hyperglycemia *[see Warnings and Precautions (5.4)]*.
- TAFINLAR may cause hemolytic anemia in patients with glucose-6-phosphate dehydrogenase (G6PD) deficiency. Advise patients with known G6PD deficiency to contact their doctor to report signs or symptoms of anemia or hemolysis *[see Warnings and Precautions (5.6)]*.
- TAFINLAR can cause fetal harm if taken during pregnancy. Instruct female patients to use non-hormonal, highly effective contraception during treatment and for 4 weeks after treatment. Advise patients to contact their doctor if they become pregnant, or if pregnancy is suspected, while taking TAFINLAR *[see Use in Specific Populations (8.1)]*.
- Nursing infants may experience serious adverse reactions if the mother is taking TAFINLAR during breastfeeding. Advise breastfeeding mothers to discontinue nursing while taking TAFINLAR *[see Use in Specific Populations (8.3)]*.
- Male patients are at an increased risk for impaired spermatogenesis *[see Use in Specific Populations (8.6)]*.
- TAFINLAR should be taken either at least 1 hour before or at least 2 hours after a meal *[see Dosage and Administration (2.1)]*.

TAFINLAR is a registered trademark of GlaxoSmithKline.
THxID is a trademark of bioMérieux.

GlaxoSmithKline
Research Triangle Park, NC 27709

TFR:1PI

MEDICATION GUIDE
TAFINLAR® (TAFF-in-lar)
(dabrafenib)
capsules

What is the most important information I should know about TAFINLAR?

TAFINLAR may cause serious side effects, including:

Risk of new cancers. TAFINLAR may cause new cancers, including cutaneous squamous cell carcinoma (cuSCC) that can spread to other parts of the body. Talk with your healthcare provider about your risk for developing skin cancers.

Check your skin and tell your healthcare provider right away about any skin changes including a:

- new wart
- skin sore or reddish bump that bleeds or does not heal
- change in size or color of a mole

Your healthcare provider should check your skin before you start taking TAFINLAR, and every two months while taking TAFINLAR to look for any new skin cancers. Your healthcare provider may continue to check your skin for six months after you stop taking TAFINLAR.

See "What are the possible side effects of TAFINLAR?" for more information about side effects.

What is TAFINLAR?

TAFINLAR is a prescription medicine used to treat a type of skin cancer called melanoma:

- that has spread to other parts of the body or cannot be removed by surgery, and
- that has a certain type of abnormal "BRAF" gene.

Your healthcare provider will perform a test to make sure that TAFINLAR is right for you.

TAFINLAR is not used to treat people with a type of skin cancer called wild-type BRAF melanoma.

It is not known if TAFINLAR is safe and effective in children.

What should I tell my healthcare provider before taking TAFINLAR?

Before you start taking TAFINLAR, tell your healthcare provider if you:

- have liver or kidney problems
- have diabetes
- plan to have surgery, dental, or other medical procedures
- have a deficiency of the glucose-6-phosphate dehydrogenase (G6PD) enzyme
- have any other medical conditions
- are pregnant or plan to become pregnant. TAFINLAR can harm your unborn baby.
  - Females who are able to become pregnant should use birth control during treatment and for 4 weeks after stopping TAFINLAR.
  - Birth control using hormones (such as birth control pills, injections, or patches) may not work as well while you are taking TAFINLAR. You should use another effective method of birth control while taking TAFINLAR. Talk to your healthcare provider about birth control methods that may be right for you.
  - Tell your healthcare provider right away if you become pregnant during treatment with TAFINLAR.
- are breastfeeding or plan to breastfeed. It is not known if TAFINLAR passes into your breast milk. You and your healthcare provider should decide if you will take TAFINLAR or breastfeed. You should not do both.

TAFINLAR may cause lower sperm counts in men. This could affect the ability to father a child. Talk to your healthcare provider if this is a concern for you. Talk to your healthcare provider about family planning options that might be right for you.

Tell your healthcare provider about all the medicines you take including prescription and over-the-counter medicines, vitamins, and herbal supplements. TAFINLAR and certain other medicines can affect each other, causing side effects. TAFINLAR may affect the way other medicines work, and other medicines may affect how TAFINLAR works. You can ask your pharmacist for a list of medicines that may interact with TAFINLAR.

Know the medicines you take. Keep a list of them to show your healthcare provider and pharmacist when you get a new medicine.

How should I take TAFINLAR?

- Take TAFINLAR exactly as your healthcare provider tells you. Do not change your dose or stop TAFINLAR unless your healthcare provider tells you.
- Take TAFINLAR 2 times a day, about 12 hours apart.
- Take TAFINLAR at least 1 hour before or 2 hours after a meal.
- Do not open, crush, or break TAFINLAR capsules.
- If you miss a dose, take it as soon as you remember. If it is within 6 hours of your next scheduled dose, just take your next dose at your regular time. Do not make up for the missed dose. If you take too much TAFINLAR, call your healthcare provider or go to the nearest hospital emergency room right away.

What are the possible side effects of TAFINLAR?

TAFINLAR may cause serious side effects, including:

- **See "What is the most important information I should know about TAFINLAR?"**
- **Fever.** TAFINLAR can cause fever, including severe fever. In some cases, too much fluid loss (dehydration), low blood pressure, dizziness, or kidney problems may happen with the fever. Tell your healthcare provider right away if you get a fever while taking TAFINLAR.
- **Blood sugar problems.** Some people may develop high blood sugar or worsening diabetes during treatment with TAFINLAR. If you are diabetic, your healthcare provider will check your blood sugar levels before and during treatment with TAFINLAR. Tell your healthcare provider if you have any of the following symptoms of high blood sugar:
  - increased thirst
  - urinating more often than normal
  - your breath smells like fruit
- **Eye problems.** You should have your eyes examined before and while you are taking TAFINLAR. Tell your healthcare provider right away if you get these symptoms during treatment with TAFINLAR:
  - eye pain, swelling, or redness
  - blurred vision or other vision changes during treatment with TAFINLAR

The most common side effects of TAFINLAR include:

- thickening of the outer layers of the skin
- headache
- joint aches
- warts
- hair loss
- redness, swelling, peeling, or tenderness of hands or feet

Tell your healthcare provider if you have any side effect that bothers you or that does not go away.

These are not all of the possible side effects of TAFINLAR. For more information about side effects, ask your healthcare provider or pharmacist.

Call your doctor for medical advice about side effects. You may report side effects to FDA at 1-800-FDA-1088. You may also report side effects to GSK at 1-888-825-5249.

How should I store TAFINLAR?

- Store TAFINLAR at room temperature, between 68°F to 77°F (20°C to 25°C).
- Ask your healthcare provider or pharmacist how to safely throw away TAFINLAR that is out of date or no longer needed.

Keep TAFINLAR and all medicine out of the reach of children.

General information about TAFINLAR

Medicines are sometimes prescribed for purposes other than those listed in a Medication Guide. Do not use TAFINLAR for a condition for which it was not prescribed. Do not give TAFINLAR to other people, even if they have the same symptoms that you have. It may harm them.

If you would like more information, talk with your healthcare provider. You can ask your healthcare provider or pharmacist for information about TAFINLAR that is written for health professionals.

For more information, call GlaxoSmithKline at 1-888-825-5249 or go to www.TAFINLAR.com.

What are the ingredients in TAFINLAR?

Active ingredient: dabrafenib

Inactive ingredients: colloidal silicon dioxide, magnesium stearate, microcrystalline cellulose

Capsule shells contain: hypromellose, red iron oxide (E172), titanium dioxide (E171).

This Medication Guide has been approved by the U.S. Food and Drug Administration.

TAFINLAR is a registered trademark of GlaxoSmithKline.

GlaxoSmithKline
Research Triangle Park, NC 27709

Issued: May 2013
TFR:1MG

TIMENTIN ℞

(ticarcillin disodium and clavulanate potassium) for Injection

TIMENTIN

(ticarcillin disodium and clavulanate potassium) for Injection: Pharmacy Bulk Package

TIMENTIN

(ticarcillin disodium and clavulanate potassium) Injection: GALAXY

HIGHLIGHTS OF PRESCRIBING INFORMATION

These highlights do not include all the information needed to use TIMENTIN safely and effectively. See full prescribing information for TIMENTIN.

TIMENTIN (ticarcillin disodium and clavulanate potassium) for Injection

TIMENTIN (ticarcillin disodium and clavulanate potassium) for Injection: Pharmacy Bulk Package

TIMENTIN (ticarcillin disodium and clavulanate potassium) Injection: GALAXY

Initial U.S. Approval: 1985

To reduce the development of drug-resistant bacteria and maintain the effectiveness of TIMENTIN and other antibacterial drugs, TIMENTIN should be used only to treat infections that are proven or strongly suspected to be caused by bacteria.

INDICATIONS AND USAGE

TIMENTIN is a combination of a β–lactam antibacterial and a β–lactamase inhibitor indicated for the treatment of the following infections due to designated susceptible bacteria:

- Septicemia (1.1)
- Lower respiratory infections (1.2)
- Bone and joint infections (1.3)
- Skin and skin structure infections (1.4)
- Urinary tract infections (1.5)
- Gynecologic infections (1.6)
- Intra–abdominal infections (1.7)

DOSAGE AND ADMINISTRATION

Administer TIMENTIN by intravenous infusion (30 minutes). (2)

Adults:

- Systemic and urinary tract infections: 3.1 g every 4 to 6 hours. (2.1)
- Gynecologic infections: 200 to 300 mg/kg/day in divided doses every 4 to 6 hours depending on severity of infection. (2.1)

Pediatric Patients:

- <60 kg: 200 to 300 mg/kg/day in divided doses every 4 to 6 hours depending on severity of infection. (2.2)
- 60 kg: 3.1 grams every 4 to 6 hours depending on severity of infection. (2.2)

DOSAGE FORMS AND STRENGTHS

- 3.1 gram vial of TIMENTIN for Injection containing ticarcillin disodium equivalent to 3 grams ticarcillin and clavulanate potassium equivalent to 0.1 gram clavulanic acid. (3)
- 31-gram Pharmacy Bulk Package of TIMENTIN for Injection containing ticarcillin disodium equivalent to 30 grams ticarcillin and clavulanate potassium equivalent to 1 gram clavulanic acid. (3)
- 100–mL single-dose GALAXY (PL 2040) Plastic bag of TIMENTIN for Injection containing ticarcillin disodium equivalent to 3.0 grams ticarcillin and clavulanate potassium equivalent to 0.1 gram clavulanic acid as a frozen solution. (3)

CONTRAINDICATIONS

History of a serious hypersensitivity reaction (anaphylaxis or Stevens-Johnson syndrome) to TIMENTIN or to other β–lactams (e.g., penicillins and cephalosporins). (4)

WARNINGS AND PRECAUTIONS

- Serious hypersensitivity (anaphylactic) reactions have been reported in patients on penicillin therapy. Discontinue TIMENTIN and institute appropriate therapy. (5.1)
- *Clostridium difficile* associated diarrhea (CDAD) has been reported with nearly all systemic antibacterial agents: If diarrhea occurs, evaluate patients for CDAD. (5.2)
- Convulsions: Patients may experience convulsions when the dose of TIMENTIN exceeds the recommended dose, especially in the presence of impaired renal function. (5.3)

ADVERSE REACTIONS

Most common adverse reactions (1%) are rash, nausea, diarrhea, and phlebitis at injection site. (6.1)

To report SUSPECTED ADVERSE REACTIONS, contact GlaxoSmithKline at 1-888-825-5249 or FDA at 1-800-FDA-1088 or www.fda.gov/medwatch

DRUG INTERACTIONS

- Aminoglycosides: Mixing with TIMENTIN for parenteral administration can inactivate the aminoglycoside. (7.1)
- Probenecid: Interferes with renal tubular secretion of ticarcillin, therefore increases exposure to ticarcillin. (7.2)
- Oral Contraceptives: Effects on gut flora may lower estrogen reabsorption and reduce efficacy of oral contraceptives. (7.3)

USE IN SPECIFIC POPULATIONS

Renal Impairment: Adjust dose based on creatinine clearance and type of dialysis. (2.3, 8.6)

See 17 for PATIENT COUNSELING INFORMATION

Revised: 12/2012

FULL PRESCRIBING INFORMATION: CONTENTS*

*** Sections or subsections omitted from the full prescribing information are not listed**

FULL PRESCRIBING INFORMATION

1 INDICATIONS AND USAGE

TIMENTIN® is indicated in the treatment of infections caused by susceptible isolates of the designated bacteria in the conditions listed below:

1.1 Septicemia

Septicemia (including bacteremia) caused by β–lactamase–producing isolates of *Klebsiella* spp.*, *Escherichia coli**, *Staphylococcus aureus**, or *Pseudomonas aeruginosa** (or other *Pseudomonas* species*)

1.2 Lower Respiratory Infections

Lower respiratory infections caused by β–lactamase–producing isolates of *S. aureus*, *Haemophilus influenzae**, or *Klebsiella* spp.*

1.3 Bone and Joint Infections

Bone and joint infections caused by β–lactamase–producing isolates of *S. aureus*

1.4 Skin and Skin Structure Infections

Skin and skin structure infections caused by β–lactamase–producing isolates of *S. aureus*, *Klebsiella* spp.*, or *E. coli**

1.5 Urinary Tract Infections

Urinary tract infections (complicated and uncomplicated) caused by β–lactamase–producing isolates of *E. coli*, *Klebsiella* spp., *P. aeruginosa** (or other *Pseudomonas* spp.*), *Citrobacter* spp.*, *Enterobacter cloacae**, *Serratia marcescens**, or *S. aureus**

1.6 Gynecologic Infections

Endometritis caused by β–lactamase–producing isolates of *Prevotella melaninogenicus**, *Enterobacter* spp. (including *E. cloacae**), *E. coli*, *Klebsiella pneumoniae**, *S. aureus*, or *Staphylococcus epidermidis*

1.7 Intra-abdominal Infections

Peritonitis caused by β–lactamase–producing isolates of *E. coli*, *K. pneumoniae*, or *Bacteroides fragilis** group

*Efficacy for this organism in this organ system was studied in fewer than 10 infections.

To reduce the development of drug–resistant bacteria and maintain the effectiveness of TIMENTIN and other antibacterial drugs, TIMENTIN should be used only to treat infections that are proven or strongly suspected to be caused by susceptible bacteria. When culture and susceptibility information are available, they should be considered in selecting or modifying antibacterial therapy. In the absence of such data, local epidemiology and susceptibility patterns may contribute to the empiric selection of therapy.

2 DOSAGE AND ADMINISTRATION

2.1 Adults

The usual recommended dosage for systemic and urinary tract infections for adults is 3.1 grams of TIMENTIN (3 grams ticarcillin and 100 mg clavulanic acid) given every 4 to 6 hours. For gynecologic infections, TIMENTIN should be administered as follows (based on ticarcillin content): Moderate infections, 200 mg/kg/day in divided doses every 6 hours; Severe infections, 300 mg/kg/day in divided doses every 4 hours. For patients weighing less than 60 kg, the recommended dosage is 200 to 300 mg/kg/day given in divided doses every 4 to 6 hours.

The duration of therapy depends upon the severity of infection. The usual duration is 10 to 14 days; however, in difficult and complicated infections, more prolonged therapy may be required.

2.2 Pediatric Patients (≥3 Months)

Patients <60 kg: Mild to moderate infections, 200 mg/kg/day based on ticarcillin content in divided doses every 6 hours; Severe infections, 300 mg/kg/day in divided doses every 4 hours.

Patients ≥60 kg: Mild to moderate infections, 3.1 grams every 6 hours; Severe infections, 3.1 grams every 4 hours.

2.3 Renal Impairment

For patients with renal insufficiency, an initial loading dose of 3.1 grams should be followed by doses based on creatinine clearance and type of dialysis as indicated in Table 1.

Table 1. Dosage Adjustments for Renal Impairment

Creatinine Clearance (mL/minute)[a]	Dosage[b]
Over 60	3 grams every 4 hours
30 to 60	2 grams every 4 hours
10 to 30	2 grams every 8 hours
Less than 10	2 grams every 12 hours
Less than 10 with hepatic dysfunction	2 grams every 24 hours
Patients on peritoneal dialysis	3 grams every 12 hours
Patients on hemodialysis	2 grams every 12 hours supplemented with 3 grams after each dialysis

[a] To calculate creatinine clearance[1] from a serum creatinine value use the following formula:
$C_{cr} = \underline{(140\text{–Age})\ (\text{weight in kg})}/72 \times S_{cr}$ (mg/100 mL)
This is the calculated creatinine clearance for adult males; for females it is 15% less.

[b] Based on ticarcillin content.

2.4 Administration and Directions for Use

TIMENTIN should be administered by intravenous infusion over a 30-minute period.

Directions for Reconstitution and Further Dilution:

3.1–gram Glass Vials: The 3.1–gram vial should be reconstituted by adding approximately 13 mL of Sterile Water for Injection, USP, or Sodium Chloride Injection, USP, and shaking well. When dissolved, the concentration of ticarcillin will be approximately 200 mg/mL with a corresponding concentration of 6.7 mg/mL for clavulanic acid. The color of reconstituted solutions of TIMENTIN normally ranges from light to dark yellow, depending on concentration, duration, and temperature of storage.

The dissolved drug should be further diluted to desired volume using the recommended solution listed under Stability below *[see Dosage and Administration (2.5)]* to a concentration between 10 mg/mL to 100 mg/mL.

Pharmacy Bulk Package: The container closure may be penetrated only one time utilizing a suitable sterile transfer device or dispensing set that allows measured distribution of the contents. A sterile substance that must be reconstituted prior to use may require a separate closure entry.

Restrict use of Pharmacy Bulk Packages to an aseptic area such as a laminar flow hood.

Reconstituted contents of the vial should be withdrawn immediately. However, if this is not possible, aliquoting operations must be completed within 4 hours of reconstitution. Discard the reconstituted stock solution 4 hours after initial entry.

Add 76 mL of Sterile Water for Injection, USP, or Sodium Chloride Injection, USP, to the 31–gram Pharmacy Bulk Package and shake well. For ease of reconstitution, the diluent may be added in 2 portions. Each 1 mL of the resulting concentrated stock solution contains approximately 300 mg of ticarcillin and 10 mg of clavulanic acid.

The desired dosage should be withdrawn from the stock solution and further diluted to desired volume using the recommended solution listed under Stability below *[see Dosage and Administration (2.5)]* to a concentration between 10 mg/mL to 100 mg/mL.

Directions for Intravenous Infusion: After reconstitution and further dilution and prior to administration, TIMENTIN should be inspected visually for particulate matter. If particulate matter is present, the solution should be discarded.

The solution of reconstituted drug may be administered over a 30-minute period by direct infusion or through a Y–type intravenous infusion set. If this method of administration is used, it is advisable to temporarily discontinue the administration of any other solutions during the infusion of TIMENTIN.

When TIMENTIN is given in combination with another antimicrobial, such as an aminoglycoside, each drug should be given separately in accordance with the recommended dosage and routes of administration for each drug. *[See Drug Interactions (7.1)]*

GALAXY Container: Prior to administration, TIMENTIN should be inspected visually for particulate matter. If particulate matter is present, the solution should be discarded.

Caution: Do not use plastic containers in series connections. Such use could result in an embolism due to residual air being drawn from the primary container before administration of the fluid from the secondary container is completed.

Preparation for Administration: See How Supplied/Storage and Handling (16) for thawing and handling instructions:

- Suspend the container from eyelet support.
- Remove protector from outlet port at bottom of container.
- Attach administration set. Refer to complete directions accompanying set.

2.5 Stability

NOTE: TIMENTIN is incompatible with Sodium Bicarbonate.

3.1–gram Glass Vials: The concentrated stock solution at 200 mg/mL is stable for up to 6 hours at room temperature 21° to 24°C (70° to 75°F) or up to 72 hours under refrigeration 4°C (40°F).

If the concentrated stock solution (200 mg/mL) is held for up to 6 hours at room temperature 21° to 24°C (70° to 75°F) or up to 72 hours under refrigeration 4°C (40°F) and further diluted to a concentration between 10 mg/mL and 100 mg/mL with any of the diluents listed below, then the following stability periods apply.

STABILITY PERIOD

(3.1–gram Vials)

Intravenous Solution (ticarcillin concentrations of 10 mg/mL to 100 mg/mL)	Room Temperature 21° to 24°C (70° to 75°F)	Refrigerated 4°C (40°F)
Dextrose Injection 5%, USP	24 hours	3 days
Sodium Chloride Injection, USP	24 hours	7 days
Lactated Ringer's Injection, USP	24 hours	7 days

If the concentrated stock solution (200 mg/mL) is stored for up to 6 hours at room temperature and then further diluted to a concentration between 10 mg/mL and 100 mg/mL, solutions of Sodium Chloride Injection, USP, and Lactated Ringer's Injection, USP, may be stored frozen –18°C (0°F) for up to 30 days. Solutions prepared with Dextrose Injection 5%, USP, may be stored frozen –18°C (0°F) for up to 7 days. All thawed solutions should be used within 8 hours or discarded. Once thawed, solutions should not be refrozen.

Unused solutions must be discarded after the time periods listed above.

Pharmacy Bulk Package: Aliquots of the reconstituted stock solution at 300 mg/mL are stable for up to 6 hours between 21° and 24°C (70° and 75°F) or up to 72 hours under refrigeration 4°C (40°F). The reconstituted stock solution should be held under refrigeration 4°C (40°F).

If the aliquots of the reconstituted stock solution (300 mg/mL) are held up to 6 hours between 21° and 24°C (70° and 75°F) or up to 72 hours under refrigeration 4°C (40°F) and further diluted to a concentration between 10 mg/mL and 100 mg/mL with any of the diluents listed below, then the following stability periods apply.

STABILITY PERIOD

(31–gram Pharmacy Bulk Package)

Intravenous Solution (ticarcillin concentrations of 10 mg/mL to 100 mg/mL)	Room Temperature 21° to 24°C (70° to 75°F)	Refrigerated 4°C (40°F)
Dextrose Injection 5%, USP	24 hours	3 days
Sodium Chloride Injection 0.9%, USP	24 hours	4 days
Lactated Ringer's Injection, USP	24 hours	4 days
Sterile Water for Injection, USP	24 hours	4 days

If an aliquot of concentrated stock solution (300 mg/mL) is stored for up to 6 hours between 21° and 24°C (70° and 75°F) and then further diluted to a concentration between 10 mg/mL and 100 mg/mL, solutions of Sodium Chloride Injection, USP, Lactated Ringer's Injection, USP, and Sterile Water for Injection, USP, may be stored frozen –18°C (0°F) for up to 30 days. Solutions prepared with Dextrose Injection 5%, USP, may be stored frozen –18°C (0°F) for up to 7 days. All thawed solutions should be used within 8 hours or discarded. Once thawed, solutions should not be refrozen.

Unused solutions must be discarded after the time periods listed above.

GALAXY containers: Do not add supplementary medication to the bag. The thawed solution is stable for 24 hours at room temperature 22°C (72°F) or for 7 days under refrigeration at 4°C (39°F).

3 DOSAGE FORMS AND STRENGTHS

The 3.1–gram glass vial of TIMENTIN for Injection is a white to pale yellow sterile powder for reconstitution containing ticarcillin disodium equivalent to 3 grams ticarcillin and clavulanate potassium equivalent to 0.1 gram clavulanic acid.

The 31–gram Pharmacy Bulk Package of TIMENTIN for Injection is a white to pale yellow sterile powder for reconstitution containing ticarcillin disodium equivalent to 30 grams ticarcillin and clavulanate potassium equivalent to 1 gram clavulanic acid.

The 100-mL single-dose GALAXY® Plastic Container of TIMENTIN is a frozen solution containing ticarcillin disodium equivalent to 3.0 grams ticarcillin and clavulanate potassium equivalent to 0.1 gram clavulanic acid.

4 CONTRAINDICATIONS

TIMENTIN is contraindicated in patients who have a history of hypersensitivity reaction (e.g., anaphylaxis or erythema multiforme) to TIMENTIN or to other β–lactam antibacterials (e.g., penicillins and cephalosporins).

5 WARNINGS AND PRECAUTIONS

5.1 Anaphylactic Reactions

Serious and occasionally fatal hypersensitivity (anaphylactic) reactions have been reported in patients on penicillin therapy. These reactions are more likely to occur in individuals with a history of penicillin hypersensitivity and/or a history of sensitivity to multiple allergens. There have been reports of individuals with a history of penicillin hypersensitivity who have experienced severe reactions when treated with cephalosporins. Before initiating therapy with TIMENTIN, careful inquiry should be made regarding previous hypersensitivity reactions to penicillins, cephalosporins, or other allergens. If an allergic reaction occurs, TIMENTIN should be discontinued and the appropriate therapy instituted. Serious anaphylactic reactions require immediate emergency treatment with epinephrine. Oxygen, intravenous steroids, and airway management, including intubation, should also be provided as indicated.

5.2 *Clostridium difficile* Associated Diarrhea

Clostridium difficile associated diarrhea (CDAD) has been reported with use of nearly all antibacterial agents, including TIMENTIN, and may range in severity from mild diarrhea to fatal colitis. Treatment with antibacterial agents alters the normal flora of the colon leading to overgrowth of *C. difficile.*

C. difficile produces toxins A and B, which contribute to the development of CDAD. Hypertoxin producing strains of *C. difficile* cause increased morbidity and mortality, as these infections can be refractory to antimicrobial therapy and may require colectomy. CDAD must be considered in all patients who present with diarrhea following antibacterial use. Careful medical history is necessary since CDAD has been reported to occur over two months after the administration of antibacterial agents.

If CDAD is suspected or confirmed, ongoing antibacterial use not directed against *C. difficile* may need to be discontinued. Appropriate fluid and electrolyte management, protein supplementation, antibacterial treatment of *C. difficile*, and surgical evaluation should be instituted as clinically indicated.

5.3 Convulsions

Patients may experience convulsions when the dose of TIMENTIN exceeds the recommended dose, especially in the presence of impaired renal function *[see Adverse Reactions (6.2) and Overdosage (10)].*

5.4 Risk of Bleeding

Some patients receiving β-lactam antibacterials have experienced bleeding associated with abnormalities in coagulation tests. These adverse reactions are more likely to occur in patients with renal impairment. If bleeding manifestations appear, treatment with TIMENTIN should be discontinued and appropriate therapy instituted.

5.5 Potential for Microbial Overgrowth or Bacterial Resistance

The possibility of superinfections with fungal or bacterial pathogens should be considered during therapy. If superinfections occur, appropriate measures should be taken.

Prescribing TIMENTIN either in the absence of a proven or strongly suspected bacterial infection is unlikely to provide benefit to the patient and increases the risk of the development of drug–resistant bacteria.

5.6 Interference with Laboratory Tests

High urine concentrations of ticarcillin may produce false-positive protein reactions (pseudoproteinuria) *[see Drug Interactions (7.4)].*

Clavulanic acid may cause a nonspecific binding of IgG and albumin by red cell membranes, leading to a false-positive Coombs test *[see Drug Interactions (7.4)].*

5.7 Electrolyte Imbalance

Hypokalemia has been reported during treatment with TIMENTIN. Serum potassium should be monitored in patients with fluid and electrolyte imbalance and in patients receiving prolonged therapy. The theoretical sodium content is 4.51 mEq (103.6 mg) per gram of TIMENTIN. This should be considered when treating patients requiring restricted salt intake.

6 ADVERSE REACTIONS

The following are discussed in more detail in other sections of the labeling:

- Anaphylactic Reactions *[see Warnings and Precautions (5.1)]*
- *Clostridium difficile* Associated Diarrhea *[see Warnings and Precautions (5.2)]*

6.1 Clinical Trials Experience

Because clinical trials are conducted under widely varying conditions, adverse reaction rates observed in the clinical trials of a drug cannot be directly compared to rates in the clinical trials of another drug and may not reflect the rates observed in practice.

Adverse reactions occurring in ≥1% of 867 patients receiving TIMENTIN 3.1 grams in clinical studies included rash, nausea, diarrhea, and phlebitis at the injection site. The most common laboratory abnormalities (≥3%) were elevations in eosinophils, serum aspartate aminotransferase (AST), and serum alanine aminotransferase (ALT).

Available safety data for pediatric patients treated with TIMENTIN demonstrate a similar adverse event profile to that observed in adult patients.

6.2 Postmarketing Experience

In addition to adverse reactions reported from clinical trials, the following adverse reactions have been identified during post–marketing use of TIMENTIN. Because they are reported voluntarily from a population of unknown size, estimates of frequency cannot be made. These adverse reactions have been chosen for inclusion due to a combination of their seriousness, frequency of reporting, or potential causal connection to TIMENTIN.

Hypersensitivity Reactions: Skin rash, pruritus, urticaria, arthralgia, myalgia, drug fever, chills, chest discomfort, anaphylactic reactions, and bullous reactions (including erythema multiforme, toxic epidermal necrolysis, and Stevens–Johnson syndrome).

Central Nervous System: Headache, giddiness, neuromuscular hyperirritability, or convulsive seizures.

Gastrointestinal Disturbances: Disturbances of taste and smell, stomatitis, flatulence, nausea, vomiting and diarrhea, epigastric pain, and pseudomembranous colitis have been reported. Onset of pseudomembranous colitis symptoms may occur during or after antibacterial treatment *[see Warnings and Precautions (5.2)].*

Hemic and Lymphatic Systems: Thrombocytopenia, leukopenia, neutropenia, eosinophilia, reduction of hemoglobin or hematocrit, and prolongation of prothrombin time and bleeding time.
Abnormalities of Hepatic Function Tests: Elevation of AST, ALT, serum alkaline phosphatase, serum LDH, and serum bilirubin. There have been reports of transient hepatitis and cholestatic jaundice, as with some other penicillins and some cephalosporins.
Renal and Urinary Effects: Hemorrhagic cystitis, elevation of serum creatinine and/or BUN, hypernatremia, reduction in serum potassium, and uric acid.
Local Reactions: Pain, burning, swelling, and induration at the injection site and thrombophlebitis with intravenous administration.

7 DRUG INTERACTIONS

7.1 Aminoglycosides

The mixing of TIMENTIN with an aminoglycoside in solutions for parenteral administration can result in substantial inactivation of the aminoglycoside.

7.2 Probenecid

Probenecid interferes with the renal tubular secretion of ticarcillin, thereby increasing serum concentrations and prolonging serum half–life of ticarcillin. Probenecid does not affect the serum levels of clavulanic acid.

7.3 Oral Contraceptives

Ticarcillin disodium/clavulanate potassium may affect the gut flora, leading to lower estrogen reabsorption and reduced efficacy of combined oral estrogen/progesterone contraceptives.

7.4 Effects on Laboratory Tests

High urine concentrations of ticarcillin may produce false–positive protein reactions (pseudoproteinuria) with certain methods. The bromphenol blue reagent strip test has been reported to be a reliable method for testing protein reactions *[see Warnings and Precautions (5.6)]*.
Clavulanic acid in TIMENTIN may cause a nonspecific binding of IgG and albumin by red cell membranes, leading to a false–positive Coombs test. A positive Coombs test should be interpreted with caution during TIMENTIN treatment *[see Warnings and Precautions (5.6)]*.

8 USE IN SPECIFIC POPULATIONS

8.1 Pregnancy

Teratogenic Effects: Pregnancy Category B: Reproduction studies have been performed in rats given doses up to 1,050 mg/kg/day (approximately half of the recommended human dose on a body surface area basis) and have revealed no evidence of impaired fertility or harm to the fetus due to TIMENTIN. There are, however, no adequate and well–controlled studies in pregnant women. Because animal reproduction studies are not always predictive of human response, this drug should be used during pregnancy only if clearly needed.

8.3 Nursing Mothers

It is not known whether ticarcillin or clavulanic acid is excreted in human milk. Because many drugs are excreted in human milk, caution should be exercised when TIMENTIN is administered to a nursing woman.

8.4 Pediatric Use

The safety and effectiveness of TIMENTIN have been established in the age group of 3 months to 16 years. Use of TIMENTIN in these age groups is supported by evidence from adequate and well–controlled studies of TIMENTIN in adults with additional efficacy, safety, and pharmacokinetic data from both comparative and non–comparative studies in pediatric patients. There are insufficient data to support the use of TIMENTIN in pediatric patients under 3 months of age.
If meningitis is suspected or documented, an alternative agent with demonstrated clinical efficacy in this setting should be used.

8.5 Geriatric Use

An analysis of clinical studies of TIMENTIN was conducted to determine whether subjects aged 65 and over respond differently from younger subjects. Of the 1,078 subjects treated with at least one dose of TIMENTIN, 67.5% were <65 years old, and 32.5% were ≥65 years old. No overall differences in safety or efficacy were observed between older and younger subjects, and other reported clinical experience have not identified differences in responses between the elderly and younger patients, but a greater sensitivity of some older individuals cannot be ruled out.
This drug is known to be substantially excreted by the kidney, and the risk of toxic reactions to this drug may be greater in patients with impaired renal function. Because elderly patients are more likely to have decreased renal function, care should be taken in dose selection, and it may be useful to monitor renal function *[see Dosage and Administration (2.3)]*.
TIMENTIN contains 103.6 mg (4.51 mEq) of sodium per gram of TIMENTIN. At the usual recommended doses, patients would receive between 1,285 and 1,927 mg/day (56 and 84 mEq) of sodium. The geriatric population may respond with a blunted natriuresis to salt loading. This may be clinically important with regard to such diseases as congestive heart failure.

8.6 Renal Impairment

Ticarcillin is predominantly excreted by the kidney *[see Clinical Pharmacology (12.3)]*.Dosage adjustments should be made for patients with renal impairment *[see Dosage and Administration (2.3)]*.

10 OVERDOSAGE

In case of overdosage, discontinue TIMENTIN, treat symptomatically, and institute supportive measures as required. Ticarcillin and clavulanic acid may be removed from circulation by hemodialysis.

11 DESCRIPTION

TIMENTIN (ticarcillin disodium and clavulanate potassium) for Injection, 3.1–gram glass vial, 31–gram Pharmacy Bulk Package, and TIMENTIN (ticarcillin disodium and clavulanate potassium) Injection in the GALAXY bag are a combination of ticarcillin disodium and the β–lactamase inhibitor clavulanate potassium (the potassium salt of clavulanic acid) for intravenous administration. Ticarcillin is derived from the basic penicillin nucleus, 6–amino–penicillanic acid.
Chemically, ticarcillin disodium is *N*-(2-Carboxy-3,3-dimethyl-7-oxo-4-thia-1-azabicyclo[3.2.0]hept-6-yl)-3-thiophenemalonamic acid disodium salt and may be represented as:

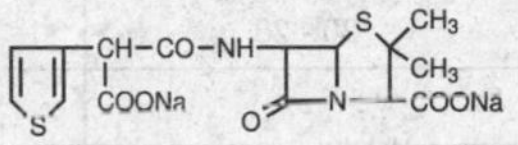

Clavulanic acid is produced by the fermentation of *Streptomyces clavuligerus*. It is a β–lactam structurally related to the penicillins and possesses the ability to inactivate a wide variety of β–lactamases by blocking the active sites of these enzymes. Clavulanic acid is particularly active against the clinically important plasmid–mediated β–lactamases frequently responsible for transferred drug resistance to penicillins and cephalosporins.
Chemically, clavulanate potassium is potassium (*Z*)-(2*R*,5*R*)-3-(2-hydroxyethylidene)-7-oxo-4-oxa-1-azabicyclo [3.2.0]heptane-2-carboxylate and may be represented structurally as:

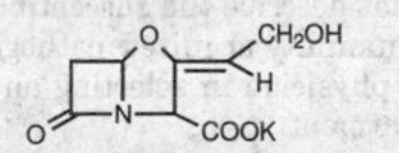

TIMENTIN (ticarcillin disodium and clavulanate potassium) for Injection, the 3.1–gram glass vial or the 31–gram Pharmacy Bulk Package, are white to pale yellow sterile powders to be reconstituted and diluted for intravenous infusion. The reconstituted solution is clear, colorless or pale yellow, with a pH of 5.5 to 7.5. The 3.1–gram glass vial of TIMENTIN for Injection contains ticarcillin disodium equivalent to 3 grams ticarcillin and clavulanate potassium equivalent to 0.1 gram clavulanic acid. The 31–gram TIMENTIN for Injection Pharmacy Bulk Package contains ticarcillin disodium equivalent to 30 grams ticarcillin and clavulanate potassium equivalent to 1 gram clavulanic acid.
TIMENTIN (ticarcillin disodium and clavulanate potassium) Injection in GALAXY bag is an iso–osmotic, sterile, nonpyrogenic, frozen solution containing 3.0 grams ticarcillin as ticarcillin disodium and 0.1 gram clavulanic acid as clavulanate potassium and approximately 0.3 gram sodium citrate hydrous as a buffer. The solution is intended for intravenous use after thawing to room temperature. The pH of thawed solution ranges from 5.5 to 7.5.
For the 3.1-gram dosage of TIMENTIN, the theoretical sodium content is 4.51 mEq (103.6 mg) per gram of TIMENTIN. The theoretical potassium content is 0.15 mEq (6 mg) per gram of TIMENTIN.

12 CLINICAL PHARMACOLOGY

12.1 Mechanism of Action

TIMENTIN is an antibacterial drug *[see Microbiology (12.4)]*.

12.3 Pharmacokinetics

Absorption: After an intravenous infusion (30 minutes) of 3.1 grams of TIMENTIN, peak serum concentrations of both ticarcillin and clavulanic acid were attained immediately after completion of the infusion. Ticarcillin serum levels were similar to those produced by the administration of equivalent amounts of ticarcillin alone with a mean peak serum level of 324 mcg/mL. The corresponding mean peak serum level for clavulanic acid was 8 mcg/mL. (See Table 2.)

Table 2. Mean Peak Serum Levels (mcg/mL) in Adults After a 30 Minute IV Infusion of 3.1 gram of TIMENTIN

Time	Ticarcillin Peak (Range)	Clavulanic Acid Peak (Range)
0	324 (293 388)	8.0 (5.3–10.3)
15 minutes	223 (184–293)	4.6 (3.0–7.6)
30 minutes	176 (135–235)	2.6 (1.8–3.4)
1 hour	131 (102–195)	1.8 (1.6–2.2)
1.5 hours	90 (65–119)	1.2 (0.8–1.6)
3.5 hours	27 (19–37)	0.3 (0.2–0.3)
5.5 hours	6 (5–7)	0

The mean area under the serum concentration curve was 485 mcg•hr/mL for ticarcillin and 8.2 mcg•hr/mL for clavulanic acid.
Distribution: Ticarcillin has been found to be approximately 45% bound to human serum protein and clavulanic acid approximately 25% bound. Ticarcillin can be detected in tissues and interstitial fluid following parenteral administration.
Distribution of ticarcillin into bile and pleural fluid has been demonstrated. The results of experiments involving the administration of clavulanic acid to animals suggest that this compound, like ticarcillin, is well distributed in body tissues.
Elimination: Approximately 60% to 70% of ticarcillin and approximately 35% to 45% of clavulanic acid are excreted unchanged in urine during the first 6 hours after administration of a single dose of TIMENTIN to normal volunteers with normal renal function. Two hours after an intravenous injection of 3.1 grams of TIMENTIN, concentrations of ticarcillin in urine generally exceed 1,500 mcg/mL. The corresponding concentrations of clavulanic acid in urine generally exceed 40 mcg/mL. By 4 to 6 hours after injection, the urine concentrations of ticarcillin and clavulanic acid usually decline to approximately 190 mcg/mL and 2 mcg/mL, respectively.
The mean serum half–life of both ticarcillin and clavulanic acid in healthy volunteers was 1.1 hours.
Pediatrics: In pediatric patients receiving approximately 50 mg/kg of TIMENTIN (30:1 ratio ticarcillin to clavulanate), mean ticarcillin serum half–lives were 4.4 hours in neonates (n = 18) and 1.0 hour in infants and children (n = 41). The corresponding clavulanate serum half–lives averaged 1.9 hours in neonates (n = 14) and 0.9 hour in infants and children (n = 40). Area under the serum concentration time curves averaged 339 mcg•hr/mL in infants and children (n = 41), whereas the corresponding mean clavulanate area under the serum concentration time curves was approximately 7 mcg•hr/mL in the same population (n = 40).
Renal Impairment: An inverse relationship exists between the serum half–life of ticarcillin and creatinine clearance. The half–life of ticarcillin in patients with renal failure is approximately 13 hours. The dosage of TIMENTIN need only be adjusted in cases of severe renal impairment *[see Dosage and Administration (2.3)]*.
Ticarcillin may be removed from patients undergoing dialysis; the actual amount removed depends on the duration and type of dialysis.

12.4 Microbiology

Mechanism of Action: Ticarcillin disrupts bacterial cell wall development by inhibiting peptidoglycan synthesis and/or by interacting with penicillin–binding proteins.
Ticarcillin is susceptible to degradation by β–lactamases, so the spectrum of activity does not normally include organisms which produce these enzymes.
Clavulanic acid is a β–lactam, structurally related to the penicillins, which inactivates some β–lactamase enzymes commonly found in bacteria resistant to penicillins and cephalosporins. In particular, it has good activity against the clinically important plasmid–mediated β–lactamases frequently responsible for transferred drug resistance.
The formulation of ticarcillin with clavulanic acid in TIMENTIN protects ticarcillin from degradation by β–lactamase enzymes, effectively extending the antibacterial spectrum of ticarcillin to include many bacteria normally resistant to ticarcillin and other β–lactam antibacterials.
Interaction with other Antimicrobials: In vitro synergism between TIMENTIN and gentamicin, tobramycin, or amikacin against multi-resistant isolates of *Pseudomonas aeruginosa* has been demonstrated.
Ticarcillin/clavulanic acid has been shown to be active against most isolates of the following bacteria, both in vitro and in clinical infections *[see Indications and Usage (1)]*.

Table 3. Susceptibility Test Interpretive Criteria for Ticarcillin/Clavulanic Acid

Microorganism	Minimum Inhibitory Concentration (mcg/mL)			Disc Diffusion Zone Diameter (mm)		
	S	I	R	S	I	R
Anaerobes	≤32/2	64/2	≥128/2	-	-	-
Enterobacteriaceae	≤16/2	32/2 – 64/2	≥128/2	≥20	15 - 19	≤14
Pseudomonas aeruginosa	≤16/2	32/2-64/2	≥128/2	≥24	16-23	≤15
Staphylococci	≤8/2	-	≥16/2	≥23	-	≤22

Table 4. Acceptable Quality Control Ranges for Ticarcillin/Clavulanic Acid

QC Strain	Broth MIC (mcg/mL)	Zone Diameter (mm)	Agar Dilution MIC (mcg/mL)
Bacteroides thetaiotaomicron ATCC 29741	0.5/2 – 2/2		0.5/2 – 2/2
Escherichia coli ATCC 25922	4/2 – 16/2	24 - 30	-
Escherichia coli ATCC 35218	8/2 – 32/2	21 - 25	-
Eubacteriumlentum ATCC 43055	8/2 – 32/2	-	16/2 -64/2
Pseudomonas aeruginosa ATCC 27853	8/2 – 32/2	20 - 28	-
Staphylococcus aureus ATCC 29213	0.5/2 – 2/2	-	-
Staphylococcus aureus ATCC 25923	-	29 – 37	-

ATCC = American Type Culture Collection

Gram-positive bacteria
Staphylococcus aureus (methicillin-susceptible isolates only)
Staphylococcus epidermidis (methicillin-susceptible isolates only)
Gram-negative bacteria
Citrobacter species
Enterobacter species
E. cloacae
Escherichia coli
Haemophilus influenzae[a]
Klebsiella species
K. pneumoniae
Pseudomonas species
P. aeruginosa
Serratia marcescens
Anaerobic bacteria
Bacteroides fragilis group
Prevotella melaninogenicus

[a] β-lactamase-negative, ampicillin-resistant (BLNAR) isolates of *H. influenzae* must be considered resistant to ticarcillin/clavulanic acid.

The following in vitro data are available, but their clinical significance is unknown. At least 90 percent of the following bacteria exhibit an in vitro minimum inhibitory concentration (MIC) less than or equal to the susceptible breakpoint for ticarcillin/clavulanic acid. However, the efficacy of ticarcillin/clavulanic acid in treating clinical infections due to these bacteria have not been established in adequate and well-controlled clinical trials.

Gram positive bacteria
Staphylococcus saprophyticus
Streptococcus agalactiae (Group B)
Streptococcus bovis
Streptococcus pneumonia (penicillin-susceptible isolates only)
Streptococcus pyogenes
Viridans group streptococci
Gram negative bacteria
Moraxella catarrhalis
Morganella morganii
Neisseria gonorrhoeae
Pasteurell amultocida
Proteus mirabilis
Proteus penneri
Proteus vulgaris
Providencia rettgeri
Providencia stuartii
Anaerobic bacteria
Clostridium species
C. perfringens
C. difficile
C. sporogenes
C. ramosum
C. bifermentans
Eubacterium species
Fusobacterium species
F. nucleatum
F. necrophorum
Peptostreptococcus species
Veillonella species

Susceptibility Testing: When available, the clinical microbiology laboratory should provide the results of in vitro susceptibility test results for antimicrobial drug products used in local hospitals and practice areas to the physician as periodic reports that describe the susceptibility profile of nosocomial and community-acquired pathogens. These reports should aid the physician in selecting an antibacterial drug product for treatment.

Dilution Techniques: Quantitative methods are used to determine antimicrobial MICs. These MICs provide estimates of the susceptibility of bacteria to antimicrobial compounds. The MICs should be determined using a standardized test method[2,4] (broth and/or agar). The MIC values should be interpreted according to criteria provided in Table 3.

Diffusion Techniques: Quantitative methods that require measurement of zone diameters can also provide reproducible estimates of the susceptibility of bacteria to antimicrobial compounds. The zone size provides an estimate of the susceptibility of bacteria to antimicrobial compounds. The zone size should be determined using a standardized test method.[3,4] These procedures use paper disks impregnated with 85 mcg of ticarcillin/clavulanate potassium (75 mcg ticarcillin plus 10 mcg clavulanate potassium) to test the susceptibility of bacteria to ticarcillin/clavulanic acid. The disc diffusion interpretive criteria are provided in Table 3.

Anaerobic Techniques: For anaerobic bacteria, susceptibility to ticarcillin/clavulanic acid can be determined by standardized test methods[4,5]. The MIC values obtained should be interpreted according to the criteria in Table 3.
[See table 3 above]

A report of "Susceptible" indicates the antimicrobial is likely to inhibit growth of the pathogen if the antimicrobial compound reaches the concentrations at the infection site necessary to inhibit growth of the pathogen. A report of "Intermediate" indicates that the result should be considered equivocal, and, if the bacterium is not fully susceptible to alternative, clinically feasible drugs, the test should be repeated. This category implies possible clinical applicability in body sites where the drug product is physiologically concentrated or in situations where a high dosage of the drug product can be used. This category also provides a buffer zone that prevents small uncontrolled technical factors from causing major discrepancies in interpretation. A report of "Resistant" indicates that the antimicrobial is not likely to inhibit growth of the pathogen if the antimicrobial compound reaches the concentrations usually achievable at the infection site; other therapy should be selected.

Quality Control: Standardized susceptibility test procedures require the use of laboratory controls to monitor and ensure the accuracy and precision of supplies and reagents used in the assay, and the techniques of the individual performing the tests.[2,3,4,5] Standard ticarcillin/clavulanic acid powder should provide the following range of MIC values noted in Table 4. For the diffusion technique using the 85 mcg of ticarcillin/clavulanate potassium (75 mcg ticarcillin plus 10 mcg clavulanate potassium), the criteria in Table 4 should be achieved.
[See table 4 above]

13 NONCLINICAL TOXICOLOGY

13.1 Carcinogenesis, Mutagenesis, Impairment of Fertility

Long–term studies in animals have not been performed to evaluate carcinogenic potential. Results from in vitro assays in bacteria (Ames tests), yeast, and human lymphocytes, and in vivo in mouse bone marrow (micronucleus test) indicate TIMENTIN is without genotoxic potential.

14 CLINICAL STUDIES

TIMENTIN has been studied in 296 pediatric patients (excluding neonates and infants less than 3 months) in 6 controlled clinical trials. The majority of patients studied had intra–abdominal infections, and the primary comparator was clindamycin and gentamicin with or without ampicillin. At the end–of–therapy visit, comparable efficacy was reported in the trial arms using TIMENTIN and an appropriate comparator.

TIMENTIN was also evaluated in an additional 408 pediatric patients (excluding neonates and infants less than 3 months) in 3 uncontrolled US clinical trials. Patients had a broad range of presenting diagnoses including: Infections in bone and joint, skin and skin structure, lower respiratory tract, urinary tract, as well as intra–abdominal and gynecologic infections. Patients received TIMENTIN, either 300 mg/kg/day (based on the ticarcillin component) divided every 4 hours for severe infection or 200 mg/kg/day (based on the ticarcillin component) divided every 6 hours for mild to moderate infections. Efficacy rates were comparable to those obtained in controlled trials.

The adverse event profile in these 704 pediatric patients treated with TIMENTIN was comparable to that seen in adult patients.

15 REFERENCES

1. Cockcroft, DW, et al. Prediction of Creatinine clearance from Serum Creatinine. *Nephron* 16:31-41, 1976.
2. Clinical and Laboratory Standards Institute (CLSI). Methods for Dilution Antimicrobial Susceptibility Tests for Bacteria that Grow Aerobically; Approved Standard – 9th ed. CLSI Document M07-A9. CLSI, 950 West Valley Rd., Suite 2500, Wayne, PA 19087, 2012.
3. CLSI. Performance Standards for Antimicrobial Disk Susceptibility Tests; Approved Standard – 11th ed. CLSI Document M02-A11. CLSI, 2012.
4. CLSI. Performance Standards for Antimicrobial Susceptibility Testing; 22nd Informational Supplement. CLSI document M100-S22. CLSI, 2012.
5. CLSI. Methods for Antimicrobial Susceptibility Testing of Anaerobic Bacteria; Approved Standard – 8th ed. CLSI Document M11-A8. CLSI, 2012.

16 HOW SUPPLIED/STORAGE AND HANDLING

Each 3.1–gram vial of TIMENTIN for Injection contains sterile ticarcillin disodium equivalent to 3 grams ticarcillin and sterile clavulanate potassium equivalent to 0.1 gram clavulanic acid.

NDC 0029-6571-26 3.1–gram Vial

Each 31–gram Pharmacy Bulk Package of TIMENTIN for Injection contains sterile ticarcillin disodium equivalent to 30 grams ticarcillin and sterile clavulanate potassium equivalent to 1 gram clavulanic acid.

NDC 0029-6579-21 31–gram Pharmacy Bulk Package

Each 100–mL single-dose GALAXY (PL 2040) Plastic bag of TIMENTIN Injection in contains ticarcillin disodium equivalent to 3.0 grams ticarcillin and clavulanate potassium equivalent to 0.1 gram clavulanic acid.

NDC 0029-6575-31 100 mL GALAXY (PL 2040) Plastic Bag

3.1-gram Vials and 31-gram Pharmacy Bulk Packages of TIMENTIN for Injection should be stored at or below 24°C (75°F).

GALAXY (PL 2040) Plastic bags of TIMENTIN Injection should be stored at or below -20°C (-4°F). Avoid unnecessary handling of bags.

Thawing of Plastic Bags: Thaw frozen bag at room temperature 22°C (72°F) or in a refrigerator 4°C (39°F). [Do not force thaw by immersion in water baths or by microwave irradiation.] Check for minute leaks by squeezing bag firmly. If leaks are detected discard solution as sterility may be impaired. Do not add supplementary medication.

The bag should be visually inspected. Thawed solutions should not be used unless clear; solutions will be light to dark yellow in color. Components of the solution may precipitate in the frozen state and will dissolve upon reaching room temperature with little or no agitation. If, after visual inspection, the solution remains cloudy or if an insoluble precipitate is noted or if any seals or outlet ports are not intact, the bag should be discarded.

The thawed solution is stable for 24 hours at room temperature 22°C (72°F) or for 7 days under refrigeration 4°C (39°F).

Do not refreeze.

17 PATIENT COUNSELING INFORMATION

17.1 Information for Patients

- Patients should be counseled that antibacterial drugs, including TIMENTIN, should only be used to treat bacterial infections. They do not treat viral infections (e.g., the common cold). When TIMENTIN is prescribed to treat a bacterial infection, patients should be told that although it is common to feel better early in the course of therapy, the medication should be taken exactly as directed. Skipping doses or not completing the full course of therapy may: (1) decrease the effectiveness of the immediate treatment, and (2) increase the likelihood that bacteria will develop resistance and will not be treatable by TIMENTIN or other antibacterial drugs in the future.
- Patients should be counseled that diarrhea is a common problem caused by antibacterials, and it usually ends when the antibacterial is discontinued. Sometimes after starting treatment with antibacterials, patients can develop watery and bloody stools (with or without stomach cramps and fever) even as late as 2 or more months after having taken their last dose of the antibacterial. If this occurs, patients should contact their physician as soon as possible.
- Patients should be aware that TIMENTIN contains a penicillin that can cause allergic reactions in some individuals.

TIMENTIN is a registered trademark of GlaxoSmithKline.
GALAXY is a registered trademark of Baxter International, Inc.

GlaxoSmithKline
Research Triangle Park, NC 27709

TMN:22PI

TREXIMET® ℞

[*trĕx' ə-mĕt*]
(sumatriptan and naproxen sodium)
Tablets

WARNINGS

Cardiovascular Risk: TREXIMET may cause an increased risk of serious cardiovascular thrombotic events, myocardial infarction, and stroke, which can be fatal. This risk may increase with duration of use. Patients with cardiovascular disease or risk factors for cardiovascular disease may be at greater risk (see WARNINGS: Cardiovascular Effects).

Gastrointestinal Risk: TREXIMET contains a nonsteroidal anti-inflammatory drug (NSAID). NSAID-containing products cause an increased risk of serious gastrointestinal adverse events including bleeding, ulceration, and perforation of the stomach or intestines, which can be fatal. These events can occur at any time during use and without warning symptoms. Elderly patients are at greater risk for serious gastrointestinal events (see WARNINGS: Risk of Gastrointestinal Ulceration, Bleeding, and Perforation With Nonsteroidal Anti-inflammatory Drug Therapy).

DESCRIPTION

TREXIMET contains sumatriptan (as the succinate), a selective 5-hydroxytryptamine$_1$ (5-HT$_1$) receptor subtype agonist, and naproxen sodium, a member of the arylacetic acid group of nonsteroidal anti-inflammatory drugs (NSAIDs).

Sumatriptan succinate is chemically designated as 3-[2-(dimethylamino)ethyl]-N-methyl-indole-5-methanesulfonamide succinate (1:1), and it has the following structure:

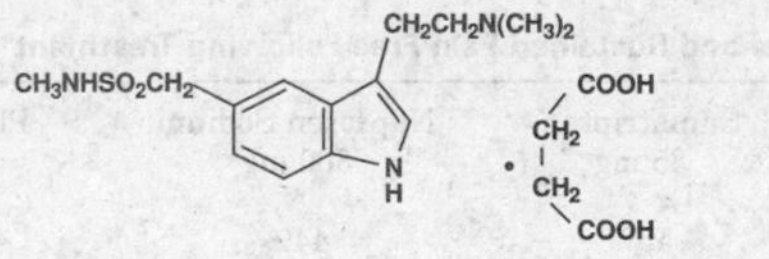

The empirical formula is $C_{14}H_{21}N_3O_2S \bullet C_4H_6O_4$, representing a molecular weight of 413.5. Sumatriptan succinate is a white to off-white powder that is readily soluble in water and in saline.

Naproxen sodium is chemically designated as (S)-6-methoxy-α-methyl-2-naphthaleneacetic acid, sodium salt, and it has the following structure:

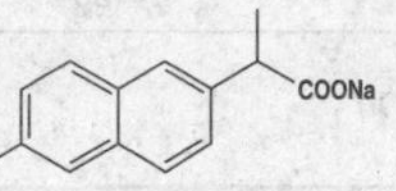

The empirical formula is $C_{14}H_{13}NaO_3$, representing a molecular weight of 252.23. Naproxen sodium is a white-to-creamy white crystalline solid, freely soluble in water at neutral pH.

Each TREXIMET Tablet for oral administration contains 119 mg of sumatriptan succinate equivalent to 85 mg of sumatriptan and 500 mg of naproxen sodium. Each tablet also contains the inactive ingredients croscarmellose sodium, dextrose monohydrate, dibasic calcium phosphate, FD&C Blue No. 2, lecithin, magnesium stearate, maltodextrin, microcrystalline cellulose, povidone, sodium bicarbonate, sodium carboxymethylcellulose, talc, and titanium dioxide.

CLINICAL PHARMACOLOGY

Mechanism of Action

TREXIMET contains sumatriptan, a 5-HT$_1$ receptor agonist that mediates vasoconstriction of the human basilar artery and vasculature of human dura mater, which correlates with the relief of migraine headache. It also contains naproxen, an NSAID that inhibits the synthesis of inflammatory mediators. Therefore, sumatriptan and naproxen contribute to the relief of migraine through pharmacologically different mechanisms of action.

Sumatriptan is a 5-HT$_1$ receptor agonist that binds with high affinity to 5-HT$_{1B}$ and 5-HT$_{1D}$ receptors. Sumatriptan has only a weak affinity for 5-HT$_{1A}$, 5-HT$_{5A}$, and 5-HT$_7$ receptors and no significant affinity (as measured using standard radioligand binding assays) or pharmacological activity at 5-HT$_2$, 5-HT$_3$, or 5-HT$_4$ receptor subtypes or at alpha$_1$-, alpha$_2$-, or beta-adrenergic; dopamine$_1$; dopamine$_2$; muscarinic; or benzodiazepine receptors. In addition to causing vasoconstriction, experimental data from animal studies show that sumatriptan also activates 5-HT$_1$ receptors on peripheral terminals of the trigeminal nerve innervating cranial blood vessels. Such an action may contribute to the antimigrainous effect of sumatriptan in humans. In the anesthetized dog, sumatriptan selectively reduces carotid arterial blood flow with little or no effect on arterial blood pressure or total peripheral resistance.

Naproxen sodium is an NSAID with analgesic and antipyretic properties. The sodium salt of naproxen has been developed as a more rapidly absorbed formulation of naproxen for use as an analgesic. The mechanism of action of the naproxen anion, like that of other NSAIDs, is not completely understood but may be related to prostaglandin synthetase inhibition.

Pharmacokinetics

TREXIMET is a formulation of 85 mg of sumatriptan (as sumatriptan succinate) and 500 mg of naproxen sodium with a distinct pharmacokinetic profile. C_{max} (median, range) for sumatriptan following administration of TREXIMET occurs at approximately 1 hour (0.3 to 4.0 hours). C_{max} (median, range) for naproxen following administration of TREXIMET occurs at approximately 5 hours (0.3 to 12 hours). The sumatriptan half-life is approximately 2 hours (15% to 43% CV) and the naproxen half-life is approximately 19 hours (13% to 15% CV). The mean C_{max} for sumatriptan when given as TREXIMET is similar to that of sumatriptan when given as IMITREX® (sumatriptan succinate) Tablets 100 mg alone. The median sumatriptan T_{max} is only slightly different (1 hour for TREXIMET and 1.5 hours for IMITREX). The C_{max} for naproxen is approximately 36% lower, and the T_{max} occurs approximately 4 hours later from TREXIMET than from ANAPROX® DS (naproxen sodium tablets) 550 mg. AUC values for sumatriptan and for naproxen are similar for TREXIMET compared to IMITREX or ANAPROX DS, respectively. In a crossover study in 16 patients, the pharmacokinetics of both components administered as TREXIMET were similar during a migraine attack and during a migraine-free period.

Absorption and Bioavailability: Bioavailability of sumatriptan is approximately 15%, primarily due to presystemic (first-pass) metabolism and partly due to incomplete absorption.

Naproxen is rapidly and completely absorbed from the gastrointestinal tract with an in vivo bioavailability of 95%.

Food Effects: Food had no significant effect on the bioavailability of sumatriptan or naproxen administered as TREXIMET, but slightly delayed the T_{max} of sumatriptan by about 0.6 hour. These data indicate that TREXIMET may be administered without regard to food.

Distribution: The volume of distribution of sumatriptan is 2.4 L/kg. Plasma protein binding is 14% to 21%. The effect of sumatriptan on the protein binding of other drugs has not been evaluated, but would be expected to be minor, given the low protein binding.

The volume of distribution of naproxen is 0.16 L/kg. At therapeutic levels naproxen is greater than 99% albumin bound. At doses of naproxen greater than 500 mg/day, there is a less than proportional increase in plasma levels due to an increase in clearance caused by saturation of plasma protein binding at higher doses (average trough C_{ss} = 36.5, 49.2, and 56.4 mg/L with 500, 1,000, and 1,500 mg daily doses of naproxen, respectively). However, the concentration of unbound naproxen continues to increase proportionally to dose.

Metabolism: Most of a radiolabeled dose of sumatriptan excreted in the urine is the major metabolite indole acetic acid (IAA) or the IAA glucuronide, both of which are inactive. Three percent of the dose can be recovered as unchanged sumatriptan. In vitro studies with human microsomes suggest that sumatriptan is metabolized by monoamine oxidase (MAO), predominantly the A isoenzyme, and inhibitors of that enzyme may alter sumatriptan pharmacokinetics to increase systemic exposure (see CONTRAINDICATIONS and PRECAUTIONS: Drug Interactions: *Monoamine Oxidase-A Inhibitors*). No significant effect was seen with an MAO-B inhibitor.

Naproxen is extensively metabolized to 6-0-desmethyl naproxen, and both parent and metabolites do not induce metabolizing enzymes.

Elimination: Radiolabeled ^{14}C-sumatriptan administered orally is largely renally excreted (about 60%), with about 40% found in the feces. The elimination half-life of sumatriptan is approximately 2 hours.

The clearance of naproxen is 0.13 mL/min/kg. Approximately 95% of the naproxen from any dose is excreted in the urine, primarily as naproxen (less than 1%), 6-0-desmethyl naproxen (less than 1%), or their conjugates (66% to 92%). The plasma half-life of the naproxen anion in humans is approximately 19 hours. The corresponding half-lives of both metabolites and conjugates of naproxen are shorter than 12 hours, and their rates of excretion have been found to coincide closely with the rate of naproxen disappearance from the plasma. In patients with renal failure, metabolites may accumulate (see PRECAUTIONS: Renal Effects).

Special Populations

Renal Impairment: TREXIMET is not recommended for use in patients with creatinine clearance less than 30 mL/min (see PRECAUTIONS: Renal Effects). The effect of renal impairment on the pharmacokinetics of TREXIMET has not been studied.

Minimal change in clinical effect would be expected with regard to sumatriptan as it is largely metabolized to an inactive substance.

Since naproxen and its metabolites and conjugates are primarily excreted by the kidney, the potential exists for naproxen metabolites to accumulate in the presence of renal insufficiency. Elimination of naproxen is decreased in patients with severe renal impairment.

Hepatic Impairment: Because TREXIMET is a fixed-dose combination that cannot be adjusted for this patient population, it is contraindicated in patients with hepatic impairment (see CONTRAINDICATIONS and PRECAUTIONS: Hepatic Effects). The effect of hepatic impairment on the pharmacokinetics of TREXIMET has not been studied. Sumatriptan is contraindicated in patients with severe hepatic impairment and the dose is limited to 50 mg in patients with liver disease.

Age: The effect of age (elderly or pediatric patients) on the pharmacokinetics of TREXIMET has not been studied. Elderly patients are more likely to have decreased hepatic function and decreased renal function (see PRECAUTIONS: Geriatric Use).

The pharmacokinetics of oral sumatriptan in the elderly (mean age: 72 years, 2 males and 4 females) and in patients with migraine (mean age: 38 years, 25 males and 155 females) were similar to that in healthy male subjects (mean age: 30 years).

Gender: In a pooled analysis of 5 pharmacokinetic studies, there was no effect of gender on the systemic exposure of TREXIMET. In a study comparing the pharmacokinetics of sumatriptan in females and males, no differences were observed between genders for AUC, C_{max}, T_{max}, and T½.

Race: The effect of race on the pharmacokinetics of TREXIMET has not been studied. The systemic clearance and C_{max} of sumatriptan were similar in black (n = 34) and Caucasian (n = 38) healthy male subjects.

Drug Interactions

No formal drug interaction studies have been conducted with TREXIMET.

Table 1. Percentage of Patients With 2-Hour Pain Relief and Sustained Pain Free Following Treatment[a]

	TREXIMET	Sumatriptan 85 mg	Naproxen Sodium 500 mg	Placebo
2-Hour Pain Relief				
Study 1 (all patients)	65%[b]	55%	44%	28%
	n = 364	n = 361	n = 356	n = 360
Study 2 (all patients)	57%[b]	50%	43%	29%
	n = 362	n = 362	n = 364	n = 382
Sustained Pain Free (2-24 Hours)				
Study 1	25%[c]	16%	10%	8%
	n = 364	n = 361	n = 356	n = 360
Study 2	23%[c]	14%	10%	7%
	n = 362	n = 362	n = 364	n = 382

[a]*P* values provided only for prespecified comparisons.
[b]*P*<0.05 versus placebo and sumatriptan.
[c]*P*<0.01 versus placebo, sumatriptan, and naproxen sodium.

Monoamine Oxidase Inhibitors: TREXIMET is contraindicated in patients taking MAO-A inhibitors (see CONTRAINDICATIONS and PRECAUTIONS: Drug Interactions). Treatment with MAO-A inhibitors generally leads to an increase of sumatriptan plasma levels. This interaction has not been seen with an MAO-B inhibitor.

Alcohol: The effect of alcohol consumption on the pharmacokinetics of TREXIMET has not been studied. Alcohol consumed 30 minutes prior to sumatriptan ingestion had no effect on the pharmacokinetics of sumatriptan.

CLINICAL TRIALS

The efficacy of TREXIMET in providing relief from migraine was demonstrated in 2 randomized, double-blind, multicenter, parallel-group trials utilizing placebo and each individual active component of TREXIMET (sumatriptan and naproxen sodium) as comparison treatments. Patients enrolled in these 2 trials were predominately female (87%) and Caucasian (88%), with a mean age of 40 years (range 18 to 65 years). Patients were instructed to treat a migraine of moderate to severe pain with 1 tablet. No rescue medication was allowed within 2 hours postdose. Patients evaluated their headache pain 2 hours after taking 1 dose of study medication; headache relief was defined as a reduction in headache severity from moderate or severe pain to mild or no pain. Associated symptoms of nausea, photophobia, and phonophobia were also evaluated. Sustained pain free was defined as a reduction in headache severity from moderate or severe pain to no pain at 2 hours postdose without a return of mild, moderate, or severe pain and no use of rescue medication for 24 hours postdose. The results from the 2 controlled clinical trials are summarized in Table 1. In both trials, the percentage of patients achieving headache pain relief 2 hours after treatment was significantly greater among patients receiving TREXIMET (65% and 57%) compared with those who received placebo (28% and 29%).

Further, the percentage of patients who remained pain free without use of other medications through 24 hours postdose was significantly greater among patients receiving a single dose of TREXIMET (25% and 23%) compared with those who received placebo (8% and 7%) or either sumatriptan (16% and 14%) or naproxen sodium (10%) alone.

[See table 1 above]

Note that comparisons of the performance of different drugs based upon results obtained in different clinical trials are never reliable. Because studies are generally conducted at different times, with different samples of patients, by different investigators, employing different criteria and/or different interpretations of the same criteria, under different conditions (dose, dosing regimen, etc.), quantitative estimates of treatment response and the timing of response may be expected to vary considerably from study to study.

The percentage of patients achieving initial headache pain relief within 2 hours following treatment with TREXIMET is shown in Figure 1.

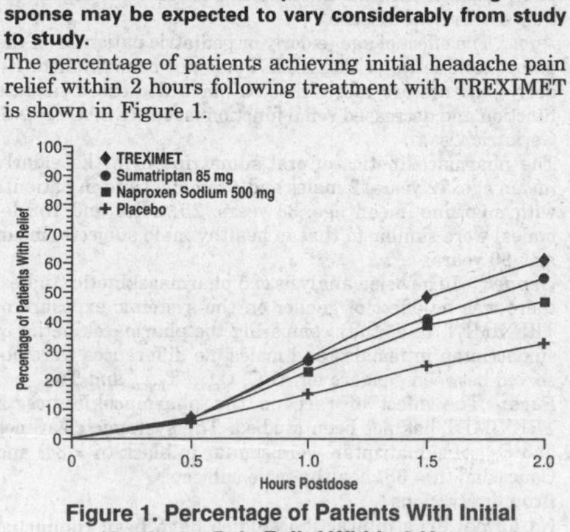

Figure 1. Percentage of Patients With Initial Headache Pain Relief Within 2 Hours

Compared with placebo, there was a decreased incidence of photophobia, phonophobia, and nausea 2 hours after the administration of TREXIMET. The estimated probability of taking a rescue medication over the first 24 hours is shown in Figure 2.

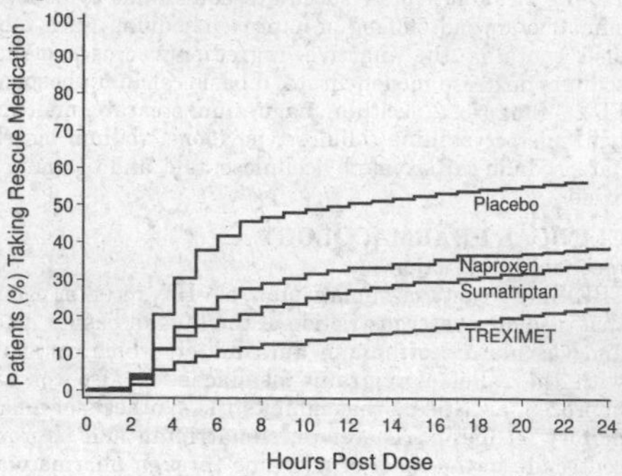

Figure 2. Estimated Probability of Taking a Rescue Medication Over the 24 Hours Following the First Dose[a]

[a]Kaplan-Meier plot based on data obtained in the 2 clinical controlled trials providing evidence of efficacy with patients not using additional treatments censored to 24 hours. Plot also includes patients who had no response to the initial dose. No rescue medication was allowed within 2 hours postdose.

TREXIMET was more effective than placebo regardless of the presence of aura; duration of headache prior to treatment; gender, age, or weight of the patient; or concomitant use of oral contraceptives or common migraine prophylactic drugs (e.g., beta-blockers, anti-epileptic drugs, tricyclic antidepressants).

INDICATIONS AND USAGE

TREXIMET is indicated for the acute treatment of migraine attacks with or without aura in adults. Carefully consider the potential benefits and risks of TREXIMET and other treatment options when deciding to use TREXIMET.

TREXIMET is not intended for the prophylactic therapy of migraine or for use in the management of hemiplegic or basilar migraine (see CONTRAINDICATIONS). Safety and effectiveness of TREXIMET have not been established for cluster headache.

CONTRAINDICATIONS

Cardiac, Cerebrovascular, or Peripheral Vascular Disease

TREXIMET should not be given to patients with history, symptoms, or signs of ischemic cardiac, cerebrovascular, or peripheral vascular syndromes. In addition, patients with other significant underlying cardiovascular diseases should not receive TREXIMET, nor should patients who have had coronary artery bypass graft (CABG) surgery. Ischemic cardiac syndromes include, but are not limited to, angina pectoris of any type (e.g., stable angina of effort and vasospastic forms of angina, such as the Prinzmetal variant), all forms of myocardial infarction, and silent myocardial ischemia. Cerebrovascular syndromes include, but are not limited to, strokes of any type as well as transient ischemic attacks. Peripheral vascular disease includes, but is not limited to, ischemic bowel disease (see WARNINGS: Cardiovascular Effects).

Uncontrolled Hypertension

TREXIMET should not be given to patients with uncontrolled hypertension because the components have been shown to increase blood pressure.

Monoamine Oxidase-A Inhibitors

Concurrent administration of MAO-A inhibitors or use of TREXIMET within 2 weeks of discontinuation of MAO-A inhibitor therapy is contraindicated (see CLINICAL PHARMACOLOGY: Drug Interactions and PRECAUTIONS: Drug Interactions).

Ergotamine-Containing or Ergot-Type Medications

TREXIMET and any ergotamine-containing or ergot-type medication (like dihydroergotamine or methysergide) should not be used within 24 hours of each other (see PRECAUTIONS: Drug Interactions).

Other 5-HT$_1$ Agonists

Since TREXIMET contains sumatriptan, it should not be administered within 24 hours of another 5-HT$_1$ agonist.

Hemiplegic or Basilar Migraine

TREXIMET should not be administered to patients with hemiplegic or basilar migraine.

Hepatic Impairment

TREXIMET is contraindicated in patients with hepatic impairment (see CLINICAL PHARMACOLOGY: Special Populations, PRECAUTIONS: Hepatic Effects, and PRECAUTIONS: Geriatric Use).

Allergy to Naproxen/Asthma, Nasal Polyps, Urticaria, and Hypotension Associated With Nonsteroidal Anti-inflammatory Drugs

TREXIMET is contraindicated in patients who have had allergic reactions to prescription as well as to over-the-counter products containing naproxen. It is also contraindicated in patients in whom aspirin or other nonsteroidal anti-inflammatory/analgesic drugs induce the syndrome of asthma, rhinitis, and nasal polyps. Anaphylactic/anaphylactoid reactions to naproxen, whether of the true allergic type or the pharmacologic idiosyncratic type (e.g., aspirin hypersensitivity syndrome), usually but not always occur in patients with a known history of such reactions. Both types of reactions have the potential of being fatal. Therefore, careful questioning of patients for medical conditions such as asthma, nasal polyps, urticaria, and hypotension associated with NSAIDs before starting therapy is important. In addition, if such symptoms occur during therapy, treatment should be discontinued (see WARNINGS: Anaphylactic/Anaphylactoid Reactions and PRECAUTIONS: Preexisting Asthma).

Hypersensitivity to Sumatriptan or Naproxen

TREXIMET is contraindicated in patients with hypersensitivity to sumatriptan, naproxen, or any other component of the product.

WARNINGS

TREXIMET should only be used where a clear diagnosis of migraine headache has been established.

Cardiovascular Effects

Risk of Myocardial Ischemia and/or Infarction and Other Adverse Cardiac Events: **TREXIMET should not be given to patients with documented ischemic or vasospastic coronary artery disease (CAD) or to patients with a history of CABG surgery (see CONTRAINDICATIONS). It is strongly recommended that sumatriptan-containing products not be given to patients in whom unrecognized CAD is predicted by the presence of risk factors (e.g., hypertension, hypercholesterolemia, smoker, obesity, diabetes, strong family history of CAD, female with surgical or physiological menopause, male over 40 years of age) unless a cardiovascular evaluation provides satisfactory clinical evidence that the patient is reasonably free of CAD and ischemic myocardial disease or other significant underlying cardiovascular disease. The sensitivity of cardiac diagnostic procedures to detect cardiovascular disease or predisposition to coronary artery vasospasm is modest, at best. If, during the cardiovascular evaluation, the patient's medical history or electrocardiographic investigations reveal findings indicative of, or consistent with, coronary artery vasospasm or myocardial ischemia, TREXIMET should not be administered (see CONTRAINDICATIONS).**

For patients with risk factors predictive of CAD who are determined to have a satisfactory cardiovascular evaluation, it is strongly recommended that administration of the first dose of TREXIMET take place in the setting of a physician's office or similar medically staffed and equipped facility unless the patient has previously received sumatriptan. Because cardiac ischemia can occur in the absence of clinical symptoms, consideration should be given to obtaining an electrocardiogram (ECG) immediately following first-time use of TREXIMET in patients with risk factors.

It is recommended that patients who are intermittent long-term users of TREXIMET and who have or acquire risk factors predictive of CAD as described above undergo periodic cardiovascular evaluation as they continue to use TREXIMET.

The systematic approach described above is intended to reduce the likelihood that patients with unrecognized cardiovascular disease will be inadvertently exposed to sumatriptan-containing products.

Cardiac Events and Fatalities Associated With 5-HT$_1$ Agonists: Serious adverse cardiac events, including acute myocardial infarction, life-threatening disturbances of cardiac rhythm, and death have been reported within a few hours following the administration of sumatriptan. Considering the extent of use of 5-HT$_1$ agonists in patients with migraine, the incidence of these events is extremely low.

The fact that sumatriptan can cause coronary vasospasm, that some of these events have occurred in patients with no prior cardiac disease history and with documented absence of CAD, and the close proximity of the events to sumatriptan use support the conclusion that some of these cases were caused by the drug. In cases, however, where there has been known underlying coronary artery disease, the relationship is uncertain.

Cardiovascular Thrombotic Events and Fatalities Associated With Nonsteroidal Anti-inflammatory Drugs: Clinical trials of several COX-2 selective and nonselective NSAIDs of up to 3 years' duration have shown an increased risk of serious cardiovascular thrombotic events, myocardial infarction, and stroke, which can be fatal. All NSAIDs, both COX-2 selective and nonselective, may have a similar risk. Patients with known cardiovascular disease or risk factors for cardiovascular disease may be at greater risk. To minimize the potential risk for an adverse cardiovascular event in patients treated with an NSAID, the lowest effective dose should be used for the shortest duration possible. Physicians and patients should remain alert for the development of such events, even in the absence of previous cardiovascular symptoms. Patients should be informed about the signs and/or symptoms of serious cardiovascular events and the steps to take if they occur.

There is no consistent evidence that concurrent use of aspirin mitigates the increased risk of serious cardiovascular thrombotic events associated with NSAID use. The concurrent use of aspirin and an NSAID does increase the risk of serious gastrointestinal events (see WARNINGS: Risk of Gastrointestinal Ulceration, Bleeding, and Perforation With Nonsteroidal Anti-inflammatory Drug Therapy).

Premarketing Experience With TREXIMET: Among 3,302 patients with migraine who received TREXIMET in premarketing controlled and uncontrolled clinical trials, a 47-year-old female with cardiac risk factors in an open-label 12-month safety study experienced signs and symptoms of acute coronary syndrome approximately 2 hours after receiving TREXIMET.

Drug-Associated Cerebrovascular Events and Fatalities: Cerebral hemorrhage, subarachnoid hemorrhage, stroke, and other cerebrovascular events have been reported in patients treated with oral or subcutaneous sumatriptan, and some have resulted in fatalities. The relationship of sumatriptan to these events is uncertain. In a number of cases, it appears possible that the cerebrovascular events were primary, sumatriptan having been administered in the incorrect belief that the symptoms experienced were a consequence of migraine when they were not. As with other acute migraine therapies, before treating headaches in patients not previously diagnosed as migraineurs, and in migraineurs who present with atypical symptoms, care should be taken to exclude other potentially serious neurological conditions. It should also be noted that patients with migraine may be at increased risk of certain cerebrovascular events (e.g., cerebrovascular accident, transient ischemic attack).

Other Vasospasm-Related Events: Sumatriptan may cause vasospastic reactions other than coronary artery vasospasm. Both peripheral vascular ischemia and colonic ischemia with abdominal pain and bloody diarrhea have been reported. Transient and permanent blindness and significant partial vision loss have been reported with the use of sumatriptan. Visual disorders may also be part of a migraine attack.

Increase in Blood Pressure: TREXIMET is contraindicated in patients with uncontrolled hypertension (see CONTRAINDICATIONS). TREXIMET should be used with caution in patients with controlled hypertension.

Significant elevation in blood pressure, including hypertensive crisis, has been reported in patients with and without a history of hypertension receiving sumatriptan. Sumatriptan-containing products should be administered with caution to patients with controlled hypertension as transient increases in blood pressure and peripheral vascular resistance have been observed.

NSAID-containing products can lead to onset of new hypertension or worsening of preexisting hypertension, either of which may contribute to the increased incidence of cardiovascular events. Patients taking thiazides or loop diuretics may have impaired response to these therapies when taking NSAIDs. The potential effect on blood pressure associated with long-term use of TREXIMET has not been studied. Blood pressure should be monitored closely during the initiation of NSAID treatment and throughout the course of therapy.

Congestive Heart Failure and Edema: TREXIMET should be used with caution in patients with fluid retention or heart failure. Fluid retention and edema have been observed in some patients taking NSAIDs. Since each TREXIMET tablet contains 61.2 mg of sodium (about 2.7 mEq/500 mg of naproxen sodium), this should be considered in patients whose overall intake of sodium must be severely restricted.

Serotonin Syndrome

The development of a potentially life-threatening serotonin syndrome may occur with triptans, including treatment with TREXIMET, particularly during combined use with selective serotonin reuptake inhibitors (SSRIs) or serotonin norepinephrine reuptake inhibitors (SNRIs). If concomitant treatment with TREXIMET and an SSRI (e.g., fluoxetine, paroxetine, sertraline, fluvoxamine, citalopram, escitalopram) or SNRI (e.g., venlafaxine, duloxetine) is clinically warranted, careful observation of the patient is advised, particularly during treatment initiation and dose increases. Serotonin syndrome symptoms may include mental status changes (e.g., agitation, hallucinations, coma), autonomic instability (e.g., tachycardia, labile blood pressure, hyperthermia), neuromuscular aberrations (e.g., hyperreflexia, incoordination), and/or gastrointestinal symptoms (e.g., nausea, vomiting, diarrhea) (see PRECAUTIONS: Drug Interactions).

Risk of Gastrointestinal Ulceration, Bleeding, and Perforation With Nonsteroidal Anti-inflammatory Drug Therapy

TREXIMET contains an NSAID. NSAID-containing products can cause serious gastrointestinal adverse events including inflammation, bleeding, ulceration, and perforation of the stomach, small intestine, or large intestine, which can be fatal.

These serious adverse events can occur at any time, with or without warning symptoms, in patients treated with NSAIDs. Only 1 in 5 patients who develop a serious upper gastrointestinal adverse event on NSAID therapy is symptomatic. Upper gastrointestinal ulcers, gross bleeding, or perforation caused by NSAIDs appear to occur in approximately 1% of patients treated daily for 3 to 6 months and in about 2% to 4% of patients treated for 1 year. These trends continue with longer duration of use, increasing the likelihood of developing a serious gastrointestinal event at some time during the course of therapy. However, even short-term therapy is not without risk. Among 3,302 patients with migraine who received TREXIMET in premarketing controlled and uncontrolled clinical trials, 1 patient experienced a recurrence of gastric ulcer after taking 8 doses over 3 weeks, and 1 patient developed a gastric ulcer after treating an average of 8 attacks per month over 7 months.

NSAID-containing products, including TREXIMET, should be prescribed with extreme caution in those with a prior history of ulcer disease or gastrointestinal bleeding. Patients with a prior history of peptic ulcer disease and/or gastrointestinal bleeding who use NSAIDs have a greater than 10-fold increased risk for developing gastrointestinal bleeding compared to patients with neither of these risk factors. Other factors that increase the risk for gastrointestinal bleeding in patients treated with NSAIDs include concomitant use of oral corticosteroids or anticoagulants, longer duration of NSAID therapy, smoking, use of alcohol, older age, and poor general health status. Most spontaneous reports of fatal gastrointestinal events are in elderly or debilitated patients, and therefore special care should be taken in treating this population.

To minimize the potential risk for an adverse gastrointestinal event in patients treated with an NSAID-containing product, the lowest effective dose should be used for the shortest possible duration. Patients and physicians should remain alert for signs and symptoms of gastrointestinal ulceration and bleeding during NSAID therapy and promptly initiate additional evaluation and treatment if a serious gastrointestinal adverse event is suspected. This should include discontinuation of the NSAID until a serious gastrointestinal adverse event is ruled out. For high-risk patients, alternate therapies that do not involve NSAIDs should be considered.

NSAIDs should be given with care to patients with a history of inflammatory bowel disease (ulcerative colitis, Crohn's disease) as their condition may be exacerbated.

Renal Effects

Long-term administration of NSAIDs has resulted in renal papillary necrosis and other renal injury. Renal toxicity has also been seen in patients in whom renal prostaglandins have a compensatory role in the maintenance of renal perfusion. In these patients administration of an NSAID may cause a dose-dependent reduction in prostaglandin formation and, secondarily, in renal blood flow, which may precipitate overt renal decompensation. Patients at greatest risk of this reaction are those with impaired renal function, heart failure, liver dysfunction, those taking diuretics and angiotensin-converting enzyme (ACE) inhibitors, and the elderly. Discontinuation of NSAID therapy is usually followed by recovery to the pretreatment state.

Advanced Renal Disease: Treatment with TREXIMET is not recommended in patients with advanced renal disease. If therapy with TREXIMET must be initiated, close monitoring of the patient's renal function is advisable (see CLINICAL PHARMACOLOGY: Pharmacokinetics and PRECAUTIONS: Renal Effects). No information is available from controlled clinical studies regarding the use of TREXIMET in patients with advanced renal disease.

Anaphylactic/Anaphylactoid Reactions

As with other NSAID-containing products, anaphylactic/anaphylactoid reactions may occur in patients without known prior exposure to naproxen. TREXIMET should not be given to patients with the aspirin triad. This symptom complex typically occurs in patients with asthma who experience rhinitis with or without nasal polyps, or who exhibit severe, potentially fatal bronchospasm after taking aspirin or other NSAIDs (see CONTRAINDICATIONS, PRECAUTIONS: Preexisting Asthma, and PRECAUTIONS: Drug Interactions).

Anaphylactic/anaphylactoid reactions have occurred in patients receiving sumatriptan. Such reactions can be life-threatening or fatal. In general, anaphylactic reactions to drugs are more likely to occur in individuals with a history of sensitivity to multiple allergens (see CONTRAINDICATIONS). Emergency help should be sought in cases where an anaphylactoid reaction occurs. Anaphylactoid reactions, like anaphylaxis, may have a fatal outcome.

Skin Reactions

NSAID-containing products, including TREXIMET, can cause serious adverse events such as exfoliative dermatitis, Stevens-Johnson syndrome, and toxic epidermal necrolysis, which can be fatal. These serious events may occur without warning. Patients should be informed about the signs and symptoms of serious skin manifestations and use of the drug should be discontinued at the first appearance of skin rash or any other sign of hypersensitivity.

Pregnancy

TREXIMET should not be used in late pregnancy because NSAID-containing products have been shown to cause premature closure of the ductus arteriosus. TREXIMET should not be used during early pregnancy unless the potential benefit justifies the potential risk to the fetus (see PRECAUTIONS: Pregnancy).

PRECAUTIONS

Naproxen-Containing Products

TREXIMET and other naproxen-containing products should not be used concomitantly since they all circulate in the plasma as the naproxen anion.

Chest, Jaw, or Neck Pain/Discomfort

Chest discomfort and jaw or neck tightness have been reported following use of sumatriptan. Only rarely have these symptoms been associated with ischemic ECG changes. However, because sumatriptan may cause coronary artery vasospasm, patients who experience signs or symptoms suggestive of angina following TREXIMET should be evaluated for the presence of CAD or a predisposition to Prinzmetal variant angina before receiving additional doses of TREXIMET and should be monitored electrocardiographically if dosing is resumed and similar symptoms recur. Similarly, patients who experience other symptoms or signs suggestive of decreased arterial flow, such as ischemic bowel syndrome or Raynaud syndrome, following TREXIMET should be evaluated for atherosclerosis or predisposition to vasospasm (see WARNINGS: Cardiovascular Effects).

Diseases That May Alter the Absorption, Metabolism, or Excretion of Drugs

TREXIMET should also be administered with caution to patients with diseases that may alter the absorption, metabolism, or excretion of drugs, such as impaired renal function.

Seizures

TREXIMET should be used with caution in patients with a history of epilepsy or conditions associated with a lowered seizure threshold. There have been reports of seizure following administration of sumatriptan.

Other Potentially Serious Neurologic Conditions

Care should be taken to exclude other potentially serious neurologic conditions before treating headache in patients not previously diagnosed with migraine headache or who experience a headache that is atypical for them. There have been reports where patients received sumatriptan for severe headaches that were subsequently shown to have been secondary to an evolving neurologic lesion (see WARNINGS: Drug-Associated Cerebrovascular Events and Fatalities). For a given attack, if a patient does not respond to the first dose of TREXIMET, the diagnosis of migraine should be reconsidered before administration of a second dose.

Hepatic Effects

TREXIMET is contraindicated in patients with hepatic impairment (see CONTRAINDICATIONS and CLINICAL PHARMACOLOGY). A patient with symptoms and/or signs suggesting liver dysfunction or in whom an abnormal liver test has occurred should be evaluated for evidence of the development of a more severe hepatic reaction while on therapy with TREXIMET. Borderline elevations of 1 or more liver tests may occur in up to 15% of patients who take NSAID-containing products. These abnormalities may progress, may remain essentially unchanged, or may be transient with continued therapy. Notable (3 times the upper limit of normal) elevations of SGPT (ALT) or SGOT (AST) have been reported in approximately 1% of patients in clinical trials with NSAIDs. In addition, cases of severe hepatic reactions, including jaundice and fatal fulminant hepatitis, liver necrosis, and hepatic failure, some of them with fatal outcomes, have been reported with NSAIDs. A patient with symptoms and/or signs suggesting liver dysfunction, or in whom an abnormal liver test has occurred, should be evaluated for evidence of the development of a more severe hepatic reaction while on therapy with TREXIMET. If clinical signs and symptoms consistent with liver disease develop, or if systemic manifestations occur (e.g., eosinophilia, rash), TREXIMET should be discontinued.

Overuse

Overuse of acute migraine drugs (e.g., ergotamine, triptans, opioids, or a combination of drugs for 10 or more days per month) may lead to exacerbation of headache (medication overuse headache). Medication overuse headache may present as migraine-like daily headaches, or as a marked increase in frequency of migraine attacks. Detoxification of patients, including withdrawal of the overused drugs, and treatment of withdrawal symptoms (which often includes a transient worsening of headache) may be necessary. Migraine patients should be informed about the risks of medication overuse, and encouraged to record headache frequency and drug use.

Binding to Melanin-Containing Tissues

In rats treated with a single subcutaneous dose (0.5 mg/kg) or oral dose (2 mg/kg) of radiolabeled sumatriptan, the elimination half-life of radioactivity from the eye was 15 and 23 days, respectively, suggesting that sumatriptan and/or its metabolites bind to the melanin of the eye. Because there could be an accumulation in melanin-rich tissues over time, sumatriptan could possibly cause toxicity in these tissues after extended use. However, no effects on the retina related to treatment with sumatriptan were noted in any of the oral or subcutaneous toxicity studies. Although no systematic monitoring of ophthalmologic function was undertaken in clinical trials and no specific recommendations for ophthalmologic monitoring are offered, prescribers should be aware of the possibility of long-term ophthalmologic effects.

Corneal Opacities

Sumatriptan causes corneal opacities and defects in the corneal epithelium in dogs (see ANIMAL TOXICOLOGY). Adverse eye findings have also been observed in animal studies with some NSAIDs. Patients were not systematically evaluated for these changes in clinical trials. However, since the animal findings raise the possibility that adverse effects on the eye may occur in humans, it is recommended that ophthalmic studies be carried out if any change or disturbance in vision occurs.

Renal Effects

Caution is recommended in patients with preexisting kidney disease or dehydration (see WARNINGS: Renal Effects). Naproxen and its metabolites are eliminated primarily by the kidneys; therefore, TREXIMET should be used with caution in patients with significantly impaired renal function, and monitoring of serum creatinine and/or creatinine clearance is advised in these patients. TREXIMET is not recommended for use in patients with creatinine clearance less than 30 mL/min (see CLINICAL PHARMACOLOGY: Special Populations).

Hematological Effects

Patients on long-term treatment with NSAIDs, including TREXIMET, should have their hemoglobin or hematocrit checked if they exhibit any signs or symptoms of anemia. Anemia is sometimes seen in patients receiving NSAIDs. This may be due to fluid retention, occult or gross gastrointestinal blood loss, or an incompletely described effect upon erythropoiesis. Patients receiving TREXIMET who may be adversely affected by alterations in platelet function, such as those with coagulation disorders or patients receiving anticoagulants, should be carefully monitored. NSAID-containing products inhibit platelet aggregation and have been shown to prolong bleeding time in some patients. Unlike aspirin, their effect on platelet function is quantitatively less, of shorter duration, and reversible.

Preexisting Asthma

Patients with asthma may have aspirin-sensitive asthma. The use of aspirin in patients with aspirin-sensitive asthma has been associated with severe bronchospasm that can be fatal. Since cross reactivity, including bronchospasm, between aspirin and other NSAIDs has been reported in such aspirin-sensitive patients, TREXIMET should not be administered to patients with this form of aspirin sensitivity and should be used with caution in patients with preexisting asthma.

Information for Patients

Patients should be informed of the following information before initiating therapy with TREXIMET and periodically during the course of ongoing therapy. Patients should also be encouraged to read the Medication Guide that accompanies each prescription dispensed.

1. TREXIMET may cause serious cardiovascular side effects such as myocardial infarction or stroke, which may result in hospitalization and even death. Although serious cardiovascular events can occur without warning symptoms, patients should be alert for the signs and symptoms of chest pain, shortness of breath, weakness, slurring of speech, and should ask for medical advice when observing any indicative sign or symptoms. Patients should be apprised of the importance of this follow-up (see WARNINGS: Cardiovascular Effects).
2. TREXIMET, like other NSAID-containing products, may cause gastrointestinal discomfort and, rarely, serious gastrointestinal side effects such as ulcers and bleeding, which may result in hospitalization and even death. Although serious gastrointestinal tract ulcerations and bleeding can occur without warning symptoms, patients should be alert for the signs and symptoms of ulcerations and bleeding and should ask for medical advice when observing any indicative sign or symptoms, including epigastric pain, dyspepsia, melena, and hematemesis. Patients should be apprised of the importance of this follow-up (see WARNINGS: Risk of Gastrointestinal Ulceration, Bleeding, and Perforation With Nonsteroidal Anti-inflammatory Drug Therapy).
3. TREXIMET, like other NSAID-containing products, may increase the risk of serious skin side effects such as exfoliative dermatitis, Stevens-Johnson syndrome, and toxic epidermal necrolysis, which may result in hospitalizations and even death. Although serious skin reactions may occur without warning, patients should be alert for the signs and symptoms of skin rash and blisters, fever, or other signs of hypersensitivity such as itching and should ask for medical advice when observing any indicative signs or symptoms. Patients should be advised to stop the drug immediately if they develop any type of rash and contact their physicians as soon as possible.
4. Patients should promptly report signs or symptoms of unexplained weight gain or edema to their physicians.
5. Patients should be informed of the warning signs and symptoms of hepatotoxicity (e.g., nausea, fatigue, lethargy, pruritus, jaundice, right upper quadrant tenderness, flu-like symptoms). If these occur, patients should be instructed to stop therapy and seek immediate medical therapy.
6. Patients should be informed of the signs of an anaphylactic/anaphylactoid reaction (e.g., difficulty breathing, swelling of the face or throat). If these occur, patients should be instructed to seek immediate emergency help (see WARNINGS: Anaphylactic/Anaphylactoid Reactions).
7. TREXIMET should not be used in late pregnancy because NSAID-containing products have been shown to cause premature closure of the ductus arteriosus. TREXIMET should not be used during early pregnancy unless the potential benefit justifies the potential risk to the fetus.
8. Patients should be cautioned about the risk of serotonin syndrome, particularly during concomitant use with SSRIs or SNRIs.
9. Caution should be exercised by patients whose activities require alertness if they experience drowsiness, dizziness, vertigo, or depression during therapy with TREXIMET.

Laboratory Tests

Because serious gastrointestinal tract ulcerations and bleeding can occur without warning symptoms, physicians should monitor for signs or symptoms of gastrointestinal bleeding. If clinical signs and symptoms consistent with liver or renal disease develop, systemic manifestations occur (e.g., eosinophilia, rash), or abnormal liver tests persist or worsen, TREXIMET should be discontinued.

Drug Interactions

Monoamine Oxidase-A Inhibitors: The use of TREXIMET in patients receiving MAO-A inhibitors is contraindicated (see CLINICAL PHARMACOLOGY: Drug Interactions and CONTRAINDICATIONS). MAO-A inhibitors reduce sumatriptan clearance, significantly increasing systemic exposure. In patients taking MAO-A inhibitors, sumatriptan plasma levels attained after treatment with recommended doses are 7-fold higher following oral administration than those obtained under other conditions.

Ergot-Containing Drugs: Ergot-containing drugs have been reported to cause prolonged vasospastic reactions. Because there is a theoretical basis that these effects may be additive, use of ergotamine-containing or ergot-type medications (e.g., dihydroergotamine, methysergide) and TREXIMET within 24 hours of each other should be avoided (see CONTRAINDICATIONS).

Methotrexate: Caution should be used if TREXIMET is administered concomitantly with methotrexate. Naproxen sodium and other NSAIDs have been reported to reduce the tubular secretion of methotrexate in an animal model, possibly increasing the toxicity of methotrexate. Concomitant administration of some NSAIDs with high-dose methotrexate therapy has been reported to elevate and prolong serum methotrexate levels, resulting in deaths from severe hematologic and gastrointestinal toxicity.

Aspirin: When naproxen is administered with aspirin, its protein binding is reduced, although the clearance of free naproxen is not altered. The clinical significance of this interaction is not known; however, as with other NSAID-containing products, concomitant administration of TREXIMET and aspirin is not generally recommended because of the potential of increased adverse effects.

Selective Serotonin Reuptake Inhibitors/Serotonin Norepinephrine Reuptake Inhibitors and Serotonin Syndrome: Cases of life-threatening serotonin syndrome have been reported during combined use of SSRIs or SNRIs and triptans (see WARNINGS: Serotonin Syndrome).

Angiotensin-Converting Enzyme Inhibitors: Reports suggest that NSAIDs may diminish the antihypertensive effect of ACE inhibitors. The use of TREXIMET in patients who are receiving ACE inhibitors may potentiate renal disease states (see WARNINGS: Renal Effects).

Furosemide: Clinical studies, as well as postmarketing observations, have shown that NSAIDs can reduce the natriuretic effect of furosemide and thiazides in some patients. This response has been attributed to inhibition of renal prostaglandin synthesis. During concomitant therapy with NSAIDs, the patient should be observed closely for signs of renal failure (see WARNINGS: Renal Effects), as well as to assure diuretic efficacy.

Lithium: NSAIDs have produced an elevation of plasma lithium levels and a reduction in renal lithium clearance. The mean minimum lithium concentration increased 15%, and the renal clearance was decreased by approximately 20%. These effects have been attributed to inhibition of renal prostaglandin synthesis by the NSAID. Thus, when TREXIMET and lithium are administered concurrently, patients should be observed carefully for signs of lithium toxicity.

Probenecid: Probenecid given concurrently increases naproxen anion plasma levels and extends its plasma half-life significantly.

Propranolol and Other Beta-Blockers: Propranolol 80 mg given twice daily had no significant effect on sumatriptan pharmacokinetics. Naproxen and other NSAIDs can reduce the antihypertensive effect of propranolol and other beta-blockers.

Warfarin: The effects of warfarin and NSAIDs on gastrointestinal bleeding are synergistic, such that patients taking both drugs have a higher risk of serious gastrointestinal bleeding than patients taking either drug alone.

Drug/Laboratory Test Interactions

The ability of TREXIMET to interfere with commonly employed clinical laboratory tests has not been investigated. Sumatriptan is not known to interfere with commonly employed clinical laboratory tests. Naproxen may decrease platelet aggregation and prolong bleeding time. This effect should be kept in mind when bleeding times are determined.

The administration of naproxen sodium may result in increased urinary values for 17-ketogenic steroids because of an interaction between the drug and/or its metabolites with m-di-nitrobenzene used in this assay. Although 17-hydroxy-corticosteroid measurements (Porter-Silber test) do not appear to be artifactually altered, it is suggested that therapy with naproxen be temporarily discontinued 72 hours before adrenal function tests are performed if the Porter-Silber test is to be used.

Naproxen may interfere with some urinary assays of 5-hydroxy indoleacetic acid (5HIAA).

Carcinogenesis, Mutagenesis, Impairment of Fertility

Carcinogenesis: The carcinogenic potential of TREXIMET has not been studied.

The carcinogenic potential of sumatriptan was evaluated in oral carcinogenicity studies in mice (78 weeks) and rats (104 weeks). The highest dose administered to mice and rats (160 mg/kg/day) is approximately 9 and 18 times, respectively, the recommended human oral daily dose of 85 mg sumatriptan on a mg/m^2 basis. There was no evidence of an increase in tumors in either species related to sumatriptan administration.

The carcinogenic potential of naproxen sodium was evaluated in a 2-year oral carcinogenicity study in rats at doses of 8, 16, and 24 mg/kg/day and in another 2-year oral carcinogenicity study in rats at a dose of 8 mg/kg/day. No evidence of tumorigenicity was found in either study, at doses up to approximately 0.5 times the recommended human oral daily dose of 500 mg/day naproxen sodium on a mg/m^2 basis.

Mutagenesis: Sumatriptan and naproxen sodium tested alone and in combination were negative in an in vitro bacterial reverse mutation assay, and in an in vivo micronucleus assay in mice.

The combination of sumatriptan and naproxen sodium was negative in an in vitro mouse lymphoma tk assay in the presence and absence of metabolic activation. However, in separate in vitro mouse lymphoma tk assays, naproxen sodium alone was reproducibly positive in the presence of metabolic activation.

Naproxen sodium alone and in combination with sumatriptan was positive in an in vitro clastogenicity assay in mammalian cells in the presence and absence of metabolic activation. The clastogenic effect for the combination was reproducible within this assay and was greater than observed with naproxen sodium alone. Sumatriptan alone was negative in these assays.

Chromosomal aberrations were not induced in peripheral blood lymphocytes following 7 days of twice-daily dosing with TREXIMET in human volunteers.

In previous studies, sumatriptan alone was not mutagenic in 2 gene mutation assays (the Ames test and the in vitro Chinese Hamster V79/HGPRT assay) and was not clastogenic in 2 cytogenetics assays (the in vitro human lymphocyte assay and the in vivo rat micronucleus assay).

Impairment of Fertility: The effect of TREXIMET on fertility in animals has not been studied.

In a study in which male and female rats were dosed daily with oral sumatriptan prior to and throughout the mating period, there was a treatment-related decrease in fertility secondary to a decrease in mating in animals treated with 50 and 500 mg/kg/day. The highest no-effect dose for this finding was 5 mg/kg/day, or approximately 0.5 times the recommended human oral daily dose of 85 mg sumatriptan on a mg/m^2 basis. It is not clear whether the problem is associated with treatment of the males or females or both combined. In a similar study of sumatriptan by the subcutaneous route there was no evidence of impaired fertility at doses up to 60 mg/kg/day.

Pregnancy

Pregnancy Category C. In developmental toxicity studies in rabbits, oral treatment with sumatriptan combined with naproxen sodium (5/9, 25/45, or 50/90 mg/kg/day sumatriptan/naproxen sodium) or each drug alone (50/0 or 0/90 mg/kg/day sumatriptan/naproxen sodium) resulted in decreased fetal body weight in all treated groups and in increased embryofetal death at the highest dose of naproxen, alone and in combination with sumatriptan. Naproxen sodium, alone and in combination with sumatriptan, increased the total incidences of fetal abnormalities at all doses and increased the incidences of specific malformations (cardiac interventricular septal defect in the 50/90-mg/kg/day group, fused caudal vertebrae in the 50/0- and 0/90-mg/kg/day groups) and variations (absent intermediate lobe of the lung, irregular ossification of the skull, incompletely ossified sternal centra) in the 50/0- and 0/90-mg/kg/day groups. A no-effect dose for development toxicity in rabbits was not established. The lowest effect dose was 5/9 mg/kg/day sumatriptan/naproxen sodium, which was associated with plasma exposures (AUC) to sumatriptan and naproxen that were 1.4 and 0.14 times, respectively, those attained at the maximum recommended human oral daily dose of 85 mg sumatriptan and 500 mg naproxen sodium.

In previous developmental toxicity studies in rats and rabbits, oral treatment with sumatriptan was associated with embryolethality, fetal abnormalities, and pup mortality. Oral treatment of pregnant rats with sumatriptan during the period of organogenesis resulted in an increased incidence of fetal blood vessel (cervicothoracic and umbilical) abnormalities and decreased pup survival at doses of 250 mg/kg/day or higher. The highest no-effect dose was approximately 60 mg/kg/day, which is approximately 7 times the recommended human oral daily dose of 85 mg sumatriptan on a mg/m^2 basis. Oral treatment of pregnant rabbits with sumatriptan during the period of organogenesis resulted in an increased incidence of cervicothoracic vascular and skeletal abnormalities at a dose of 50 mg/kg/day and embryolethality at 100 mg/kg/day. The highest no-effect dose for embryotoxicity in rabbits was 15 mg/kg/day, or approximately 3 times the recommended human oral daily dose of 85 mg sumatriptan on a mg/m^2 basis.

Inhibitors of prostaglandin synthesis (including naproxen) are known to delay parturition. Because of this and the known effects of drugs of this class on the human fetal cardiovascular system (closure of the ductus arteriosus), use during third trimester should be avoided.

There are no adequate and well-controlled studies in pregnant women.

TREXIMET should not be used during pregnancy unless the potential benefit justifies the potential risk to the fetus.

Labor and Delivery

In rat studies with NSAIDs, as with other drugs known to inhibit prostaglandin synthesis, an increased incidence of dystocia, delayed parturition, and decreased pup survival occurred. Naproxen-containing products are not recommended in labor and delivery because, through its prostaglandin synthesis inhibitory effect, naproxen may adversely affect fetal circulation and inhibit uterine contractions, thus increasing the risk of uterine hemorrhage.

Nursing Mothers

Both active components of TREXIMET, sumatriptan and naproxen sodium, have been reported to be excreted in human breast milk. Because of the possible adverse effects of these drugs on neonates, use of TREXIMET in nursing mothers should be avoided.

Table 2. Treatment-Emergent Adverse Events Reported by at Least 2% of Patients in 2 Controlled Migraine Trials[a]

Adverse Event	Percent of Patients Reporting			
	TREXIMET (n = 737)	Placebo (n = 752)	Sumatriptan 85 mg (n = 735)	Naproxen Sodium 500 mg (n = 732)
Nervous system disorders				
Dizziness	4	2	2	2
Somnolence	3	2	2	2
Paresthesia	2	<1	2	<1
Gastrointestinal disorders				
Nausea	3	1	3	<1
Dyspepsia	2	1	2	1
Dry mouth	2	1	2	<1
Pain and other pressure sensations				
Chest discomfort/chest pain	3	<1	2	1
Neck/throat/jaw pain/tightness/pressure	3	1	3	1

[a]Events that occurred at a frequency of 2% or more in the group treated with TREXIMET and that occurred more frequently in the group treated with TREXIMET than in the placebo group.

Pediatric Use

Safety and effectiveness of TREXIMET in pediatric patients have not been established.

Geriatric Use

TREXIMET is contraindicated for use in elderly patients who have abnormal hepatic function, and is not recommended for use in elderly patients who have decreased renal function, higher risk for unrecognized CAD, and increases in blood pressure that may be more pronounced in the elderly (see CONTRAINDICATIONS: Hepatic Impairment, WARNINGS: Cardiovascular Effects, and CLINICAL PHARMACOLOGY: Pharmacokinetics).

ADVERSE REACTIONS

The adverse reactions reported below are specific to the clinical trials with TREXIMET. See also the full prescribing information for naproxen and sumatriptan products.

Incidence in Controlled Clinical Trials

Table 2 lists adverse events that occurred in 2 placebo-controlled clinical trials evaluating patients who took at least 1 dose of study drug. Only events that occurred at a frequency of 2% or more with TREXIMET and were more frequent than in the placebo group are included in Table 2. The events cited reflect experience gained under closely monitored conditions of clinical trials in a highly selected patient population. In actual clinical practice or in other clinical trials, these frequency estimates may not apply, as the conditions of use, reporting behavior, and the kinds of patients treated may differ.

[See table 2 above]

Other events that occurred in more than 1% of patients receiving TREXIMET and occurred at a frequency greater than the placebo group included asthenia, feeling hot, muscle tightness, and palpitations.

TREXIMET was generally well tolerated. Most adverse reactions were mild and transient. The incidence of adverse events in controlled clinical trials was not affected by gender or age of the patients. There were insufficient data to assess the impact of race on the incidence of adverse events.

Other Events Observed in Migraine Clinical Trials Associated With the Administration of TREXIMET

The occurrence of less commonly reported adverse clinical events is presented in this section. Because the reports include events observed in an open-label, long-term safety study in which TREXIMET was used as needed for up to 12 months, the role of TREXIMET cannot be reliably determined. Furthermore, variability associated with adverse event reporting, the terminology used to describe adverse events, etc., limit the value of quantitative frequency estimates provided. Event frequencies are calculated as the number of patients who used TREXIMET and reported an event divided by the total number of patients (N = 3,302) exposed to TREXIMET. Events listed in the previous table and text are not included below. Those events described too generally to be informative or those unlikely to be associated with the use of TREXIMET are excluded. Events are further classified within body system categories and enumerated in order of decreasing frequency using the following definitions: frequent adverse events are those occurring in at least 1/100 patients, infrequent adverse events are those occurring in 1/100 to 1/1,000 patients, and rare adverse events are those occurring in fewer than 1/1,000 patients.

Blood and Lymphatic Disorders: Infrequent was lymphadenopathy. Rare were anemia, ecchymosis, leukopenia.

Cardiac Disorders: Infrequent was tachycardia. Rare were acute coronary syndrome, cardiac flutter, congestive cardiac failure, right ventricular failure, ventricular extrasystoles.

Ear and Labyrinth Disorders: Infrequent were ear pain, tinnitus. Rare were motion sickness, vertigo.

Endocrine, Metabolic, and Nutrition Disorders: Rare were diabetes mellitus, goiter, hypoglycemia, hypothyroidism.

Eye Disorders: Infrequent was conjunctivitis. Rare were cataract, conjunctival hemorrhage, visual disturbance.

Gastrointestinal Disorders: Frequent was abdominal pain. Infrequent were abdominal distention, constipation, diarrhea, dysgeusia, dysphagia, flatulence, gastritis, gastroesophageal reflux disease, vomiting. Rare were colitis, diverticulitis, gastric ulcer, irritable bowel syndrome, oral mucosal blistering, swollen tongue.

General Disorders: Frequent was fatigue. Infrequent were feeling jittery, lethargy, malaise, peripheral edema, pyrexia, temperature intolerance, thirst. Rare was difficulty in walking.

Hepatobiliary Disorders: Rare was biliary colic.

Infections and Infestations: Rare were kidney infection, pneumonia, sepsis, staphylococcal infection, viral myocarditis.

Musculoskeletal and Connective Tissue: Infrequent were arthralgia, back pain, muscular weakness, myalgia, sensation of heaviness.

Nervous System Disorders: Infrequent were burning sensation, disturbance of attention, insomnia, mental impairment, tremor. Rare were aphasia, facial palsy, impairment of psychomotor skills, sedation.

Psychiatric Disorders: Infrequent were anxiety, depression, irritability, nervousness. Rare were disorientation, panic attack.

Renal and Urinary Disorders: Infrequent was nephrolithiasis. Rare was renal insufficiency.

Respiratory, Thoracic, and Mediastinal: Infrequent were asthma, cough, dyspnea, oropharyngeal swelling. Rare was pleurisy.

Skin and Subcutaneous Disorders: Infrequent were facial swelling, hyperhydrosis, pruritus, rash, urticaria. Rare was systemic lupus erythematosus.

Vascular Disorders: Infrequent were flushing, hot flush, hypertension. Rare were epistaxis, peripheral coldness.

DRUG ABUSE AND DEPENDENCE

The potential for abuse with TREXIMET has not been studied.

One clinical study with sumatriptan succinate injection enrolling 12 patients with a history of substance abuse failed to induce subjective behavior and/or physiologic response ordinarily associated with drugs that have an established potential for abuse.

OVERDOSAGE

Because strategies for the management of overdose are continually evolving, it is advisable to contact a Poison Control Center to determine the latest recommendations for the management of an overdose of any drug.

There have been no reports of overdosage with TREXIMET. Since sumatriptan and naproxen have pharmacologically different actions, it is difficult to predict how an individual will respond to an overdosage with TREXIMET.

Patients (N = 670) have received single oral doses of 140 to 300 mg of sumatriptan without significant adverse effects. Volunteers (N = 174) have received single oral doses of 140 to 400 mg without serious adverse events. Overdose of sumatriptan in animals has been fatal and has been heralded by convulsions, tremor, paralysis, inactivity, ptosis, erythema of the extremities, abnormal respiration, cyanosis, ataxia, mydriasis, salivation, and lacrimation.

Significant naproxen overdosage may be characterized by lethargy, dizziness, drowsiness, epigastric pain, abdominal discomfort, heartburn, indigestion, nausea, transient alterations in liver function, hypoprothrombinemia, renal dysfunction, metabolic acidosis, apnea, disorientation, or vomiting. Gastrointestinal bleeding can occur. Hypertension, acute renal failure, respiratory depression, and coma may occur, but are rare. Anaphylactoid reactions have been reported with therapeutic ingestion of NSAIDs, and may occur following an overdose. Because naproxen sodium may be rapidly absorbed, high and early blood levels should be anticipated. A few patients have experienced seizures, but it is not clear whether or not these were drug related. It is not known what dose of the drug would be life threatening.

In animals 0.5 g/kg of activated charcoal was effective in reducing plasma levels of naproxen. Patients should be managed by symptomatic and supportive care. There are no specific antidotes. Hemodialysis does not decrease the plasma concentration of naproxen because of the high degree of its protein binding. It is unknown what effect hemodialysis or peritoneal dialysis has on the serum concentrations of sumatriptan. Emesis and/or activated charcoal (60 to 100 g in adults, 1 to 2 g/kg in children) and/or osmotic cathartic may be indicated in patients seen within 4 hours of ingestion with symptoms or following a large overdose. Forced diuresis, alkalinization of urine, or hemoperfusion may not be useful due to high protein binding.

DOSAGE AND ADMINISTRATION

TREXIMET is a fixed combination containing doses of sumatriptan (85 mg) and naproxen sodium (500 mg) within the approved dosage ranges of the individual components (25 to 100 mg of sumatriptan and 220 to 825 mg of naproxen sodium). TREXIMET contains a dose of sumatriptan higher than the lowest effective dose. Individuals may vary in response to doses of sumatriptan. The choice of the dose of sumatriptan, and of the use of a fixed combination such as in TREXIMET should therefore be made on an individual basis, weighing the possible benefit of a higher dose of sumatriptan with the potential for a greater risk of adverse events. Carefully consider the potential benefits and risks of TREXIMET and other treatment options when deciding to use TREXIMET.

The recommended dose is 1 tablet. In controlled clinical trials, single doses of TREXIMET were effective for the acute treatment of migraine in adults (see CLINICAL TRIALS). The efficacy of taking a second dose has not been established. Do not take more than 2 TREXIMET tablets in 24 hours. Dosing of tablets should be at least 2 hours apart. The safety of treating an average of more than 5 migraine headaches in a 30-day period has not been established.

TREXIMET may be administered with or without food. Tablets should not be split, crushed, or chewed.

The combined use of TREXIMET with MAO-A inhibitors or use of TREXIMET within 2 weeks of discontinuation of MAO-A inhibitor therapy is contraindicated (see CONTRAINDICATIONS, CLINICAL PHARMACOLOGY: Drug Interactions, PRECAUTIONS: Drug Interactions).

TREXIMET and any ergotamine-containing or ergot-type medication (like dihydroergotamine or methysergide) should not be used within 24 hours of each other. TREXIMET and other 5-HT_1 agonists should not be administered within 24 hours of each other (see CONTRAINDICATIONS and PRECAUTIONS: Drug Interactions).

TREXIMET is contraindicated in patients with hepatic impairment (see CONTRAINDICATIONS and CLINICAL PHARMACOLOGY: Special Populations).

TREXIMET is not recommended for use in patients with creatinine clearance less than 30 mL/min (see CLINICAL PHARMACOLOGY: Special Populations and PRECAUTIONS: Renal Effects).

HOW SUPPLIED

TREXIMET contains 119 mg of sumatriptan succinate equivalent to 85 mg of sumatriptan and 500 mg of naproxen sodium and is supplied as blue film-coated tablets debossed on one side with *TREXIMET* in bottles of 9 tablets with desiccant (NDC 0173-0750-49).

Store at 25°C (77°F); excursions permitted to 15°-30°C (59°-86°F) [see USP Controlled Room Temperature]. Do not repackage; dispense and store in original container with desiccant.

ANIMAL TOXICOLOGY

Corneal Opacities

Dogs receiving oral sumatriptan developed corneal opacities and defects in the corneal epithelium. Corneal opacities were seen at the lowest dosage tested, 2 mg/kg/day, and were present after 1 month of treatment. Defects in the corneal epithelium were noted in a 60-week study. Earlier examinations for these toxicities were not conducted and no-effect doses were not established; the lowest dose tested is approximately 0.8 times the recommended human oral daily dose of 85 mg sumatriptan on a mg/m^2 basis. There was evidence of alterations in corneal appearance on the first day of intranasal dosing to dogs at all doses tested.

TREXIMET and IMITREX are registered trademarks of GlaxoSmithKline.

ANAPROX is a registered trademark of F. Hoffmann-La Roche Ltd.

GlaxoSmithKline
Research Triangle Park, NC 27709

October 2012
TRX:10PI

MEDICATION GUIDE

TREXIMET®*[trex' i-met]* Tablets
(sumatriptan and naproxen sodium)

What is the most important information I should know about TREXIMET?

1. TREXIMET may increase your chance of a heart attack or stroke that can lead to death. TREXIMET contains 2 medicines: sumatriptan and naproxen sodium (a nonsteroidal anti-inflammatory drug [NSAID]).

Your chance of a heart attack or stroke increases:
- with longer use of NSAID medicines
- if you have heart disease.

2. TREXIMET should never be used right before or after a heart surgery called a coronary artery bypass graft (CABG).

3. TREXIMET can cause ulcers and bleeding in the stomach and intestines at any time during your treatment.

Ulcers and bleeding:
- can happen without warning symptoms
- may cause death.

Your chance of getting an ulcer or bleeding increases with:
- the use of medicines called steroid hormones (corticosteroids) and blood thinners (anticoagulants)
- longer use
- more frequent use
- smoking
- drinking alcohol
- older age
- having poor health.

4. TREXIMET is not recommended for people with risk factors for heart disease unless a heart exam is done and shows no problems.

Risk factors for heart disease include:
- high blood pressure
- high cholesterol levels
- smoking
- obesity
- diabetes
- family history of heart disease
- female who has gone through menopause
- male over age 40.

5. "Serotonin syndrome" is a serious and life-threatening problem that may occur with TREXIMET, especially if used with antidepressant medicines called selective serotonin reuptake inhibitors (SSRIs) or selective norepinephrine reuptake inhibitors (SNRIs).

Commonly used SSRIs are:
- CELEXA® (citalopram HBr)
- LEXAPRO® (escitalopram oxalate)
- PAXIL® (paroxetine)
- PROZAC®/SARAFEM® (fluoxetine)
- SYMBYAX® (olanzapine/fluoxetine)
- ZOLOFT® (sertraline)
- LUVOX® (fluvoxamine).

Commonly used SNRIs are:
- CYMBALTA® (duloxetine)
- EFFEXOR® (venlafaxine).

Call your healthcare provider if you have symptoms of serotonin syndrome, which include:
- mental changes (hallucinations, agitation, coma)
- fast heartbeat
- changes in blood pressure
- high body temperature or sweating
- tight muscles
- trouble walking
- nausea, vomiting, diarrhea.

6. TREXIMET should only be used:
- exactly as prescribed
- at the lowest dose possible for your treatment
- for the shortest time needed.

7. TREXIMET already contains an NSAID (naproxen). Do not use TREXIMET with other medicines to lessen pain or fever without talking to your healthcare provider first, because they may contain an NSAID also.

What is TREXIMET?

TREXIMET is a prescription medicine used to treat migraine attacks in adults. It does not prevent or lessen the number of migraines you have, and it is not for other types of headaches. TREXIMET contains 2 medicines: sumatriptan and naproxen sodium (an NSAID). This Medication Guide provides important information you need to know before taking TREXIMET. It does not take the place of talking with your healthcare provider about your medical condition or your treatment.

How should I take TREXIMET?
- Take 1 TREXIMET tablet to treat your migraine headache. Do not take more than 2 TREXIMET tablets in 24 hours. Doses should be separated by at least 2 hours.
- TREXIMET can be taken with or without food.
- Do not split, crush, or chew TREXIMET tablets.
- If you take too much TREXIMET, call the Poison Control Center at 1-800-222-1222.

Who should not take TREXIMET?

Do not take TREXIMET right before or after heart bypass surgery. Do not take TREXIMET if you have or have had:
- uncontrolled high blood pressure
- hemiplegic or basilar migraine. (Ask your doctor if you are not sure what type of migraine you have.)
- liver problems
- an asthma attack, hives, or other allergic reaction with aspirin or any other NSAID medicine
- a heart attack or a history or symptoms of heart disease (such as chest pain or angina)
- a stroke, mini-stroke (transient ischemic attack or TIA), or other stroke-like syndrome
- problems with blood circulation to parts of your body, such as less blood flow to your intestines (ischemic bowel disease)
- allergic reactions to sumatriptan, naproxen, or other ingredients in TREXIMET.

Do not take TREXIMET if you take or have taken an antidepressant medicine called a monoamine oxidase (MAO) inhibitor within the last 2 weeks. Common MAO inhibitors are isocarboxazid (MARPLAN®), phenelzine (NARDIL®), tranylcypromine (PARNATE®), and selegiline (ELDEPRYL®, EMSAM®). Ask your healthcare provider if you are not sure if your medicine is an MAO inhibitor.

Do not take TREXIMET if you have taken other migraine medicines in the last 24 hours such as:
- ergotamine-containing medicine or
- another triptan medicine.

Before starting TREXIMET, tell your healthcare provider about:
- all of your medical conditions including kidney or liver problems
- all allergies to any medicines
- chest pain, shortness of breath, irregular heartbeats
- medicines you may take for migraines, depression, or other health problems such as MAO inhibitors, SSRIs, or SNRIs
- all the prescription and non-prescription medicines you take, including vitamins and herbal supplements. Some medicines can interact with TREXIMET and cause serious side effects.

Keep a list of your medicines to show to your healthcare provider. Before starting TREXIMET, tell your healthcare provider if you:
- are pregnant, think you might be pregnant, or are trying to become pregnant. **TREXIMET should not be used by pregnant women late in their pregnancy.**
- are breastfeeding
- have a headache that is different from your usual migraine
- have or have had epilepsy or seizures.

What are the possible side effects of TREXIMET?

Serious side effects include:	Other side effects include:
• heart attack • heartbeat problems • stroke • high blood pressure • heart failure from body swelling (fluid retention) • kidney problems including kidney failure • bleeding and ulcers in the stomach and intestine • low red blood cells (anemia) • life-threatening skin reactions • life-threatening allergic reactions • liver problems including liver failure • asthma attacks in people who have asthma • loss of blood circulation to areas of your body • serotonin syndrome (See list of symptoms in "What is the most important information I should know about TREXIMET?")	• pain, tightness, or pressure in the chest, neck, and throat • stomach pain • constipation • diarrhea • gas • heartburn • nausea • vomiting • dizziness • drowsiness • tiredness • weakness • tingling and numbness • unusual body sensations • redness of face (flushed)

Get emergency help right away if you have any of the following symptoms:
- shortness of breath or trouble breathing
- chest pain
- swelling of the face or throat

• weakness in one part or on one side of your body
• slurred speech.

Stop TREXIMET and call your healthcare provider right away if you have any of the following symptoms:

• nausea that seems out of proportion to your migraine
• stomach pain
• sudden/severe pain in your belly
• vomit blood
• blood in your bowel movement or it is black and sticky like tar
• itching
• skin rash or blisters with fever
• yellow skin or eyes
• swelling of the arms and legs, hands, feet, face, lips, or tongue
• unusual weight gain
• more tired or weaker than usual
• flu-like symptoms
• serotonin syndrome. See list of symptoms in "What is the most important information I should know about TREXIMET?"

Tell your healthcare provider if you have any side effects that bother you or do not go away. These are not all of the side effects of TREXIMET. For more information ask your healthcare provider.

Call your healthcare provider for medical advice about side effects. You may report side effects to FDA at 1-800-FDA-1088.

How should I store TREXIMET?

• Store TREXIMET at room temperature, 59° to 86°F (15° to 30°C).
• Keep TREXIMET and all medicines out of the reach of children.

General information about TREXIMET

• Medicines are sometimes prescribed for purposes other than those listed in a Medication Guide. Do not use TREXIMET for a condition for which it was not prescribed.
• Do not give TREXIMET to other people, even if they have the same problem you have. It may harm them.
• This Medication Guide contains the most important information about TREXIMET. If you would like more information, talk with your healthcare provider.
• You can ask your healthcare provider for information written for healthcare professionals.
• For more information call 1-888-825-5249 (toll-free), or visit www.TREXIMET.com.

What are the ingredients in TREXIMET?

Active ingredients: sumatriptan succinate and naproxen sodium

Inactive ingredients: croscarmellose sodium, dextrose monohydrate, dibasic calcium phosphate, FD&C Blue No. 2, lecithin, magnesium stearate, maltodextrin, microcrystalline cellulose, povidone, sodium bicarbonate, sodium carboxymethylcellulose, talc, and titanium dioxide.

This Medication Guide has been approved by the U.S. Food and Drug Administration.

TREXIMET, PARNATE, and PAXIL are registered trademarks of GlaxoSmithKline.

The other brands listed are trademarks of their respective owners and are not trademarks of GlaxoSmithKline. The makers of these brands are not affiliated with and do not endorse GlaxoSmithKline or its products.

GlaxoSmithKline
Research Triangle Park, NC 27709

March 2012
TRX:4MG

TWINRIX ℞

[twin'rix]

[Hepatitis A & Hepatitis B (Recombinant) Vaccine]
Suspension for Intramuscular Injection

HIGHLIGHTS OF PRESCRIBING INFORMATION

These highlights do not include all the information needed to use TWINRIX safely and effectively. See full prescribing information for TWINRIX.

TWINRIX [Hepatitis A & Hepatitis B (Recombinant) Vaccine]
Suspension for Intramuscular Injection
Initial U.S. Approval: 2001

RECENT MAJOR CHANGES

Warnings and Precautions, Syncope (5.2) 03/2012

INDICATIONS AND USAGE

TWINRIX is a vaccine indicated for active immunization against disease caused by hepatitis A virus and infection by all known subtypes of hepatitis B virus. TWINRIX is approved for use in persons 18 years of age or older. (1)

DOSAGE AND ADMINISTRATION

• TWINRIX is administered by intramuscular injection. (2.2)
• Standard Dosing: A series of 3 doses (1 mL each) given on a 0-, 1-, and 6-month schedule. (2.3)
• Accelerated Dosing: A series of 4 doses (1 mL each) given on days 0, 7, and 21 to 30 followed by a booster dose at month 12. (2.3)

DOSAGE FORMS AND STRENGTHS

Suspension for injection available in 1-mL single-dose vials and prefilled syringes. (3, 11, 16)

CONTRAINDICATIONS

Severe allergic reaction (e.g., anaphylaxis) after a previous dose of any hepatitis A-containing or hepatitis B-containing vaccine, or to any component of TWINRIX, including yeast and neomycin. (4)

WARNINGS AND PRECAUTIONS

• TWINRIX is available in vials and 2 types of prefilled syringes. One type of prefilled syringe has a tip cap which may contain natural rubber latex. The other type has a tip cap and a rubber plunger which contain dry natural latex rubber. Use of these syringes may cause allergic reactions in latex-sensitive individuals. (5.1, 16)
• Syncope (fainting) can occur in association with administration of injectable vaccines, including TWINRIX. Procedures should be in place to avoid falling injury and to restore cerebral perfusion following syncope. (5.2)

ADVERSE REACTIONS

Following any dose of TWINRIX, the most common (≥10%) solicited injection site reactions were injection site soreness (35% to 41%) and redness (8% to 11%); the most common solicited systemic adverse events were headache (13% to 22%) and fatigue (11% to 14%). (6.1)

To report SUSPECTED ADVERSE REACTIONS, contact GlaxoSmithKline at 1-888-825-5249 or VAERS at 1-800-822-7967 or www.vaers.hhs.gov

DRUG INTERACTIONS

Do not mix TWINRIX with any other vaccine or product in the same syringe or vial. (7)

USE IN SPECIFIC POPULATIONS

• Safety and effectiveness of TWINRIX have not been established in pregnant women, nursing mothers, and pediatric patients. (8.1, 8.3, 8.4)
• Register women who receive TWINRIX while pregnant in the pregnancy registry by calling 1-888-452-9622. (8.1)

See 17 for PATIENT COUNSELING INFORMATION

Revised: 08/2012

FULL PRESCRIBING INFORMATION: CONTENTS*

*** Sections or subsections omitted from the full prescribing information are not listed**

FULL PRESCRIBING INFORMATION

1 INDICATIONS AND USAGE

TWINRIX® is indicated for active immunization against disease caused by hepatitis A virus and infection by all known subtypes of hepatitis B virus. TWINRIX is approved for use in persons 18 years of age or older.

2 DOSAGE AND ADMINISTRATION

2.1 Preparation for Administration

Shake well before use. With thorough agitation, TWINRIX is a slightly turbid white suspension. Do not administer if it appears otherwise. Parenteral drug products should be inspected visually for particulate matter and discoloration prior to administration, whenever solution and container permit. If either of these conditions exists, the vaccine should not be administered.

For the prefilled syringes, attach a sterile needle and administer intramuscularly.

For the vials, use a sterile needle and sterile syringe to withdraw the 1-mL dose and administer intramuscularly. Changing needles between drawing vaccine from a vial and injecting it into a recipient is not necessary unless the needle has been damaged or contaminated. Use a separate sterile needle and syringe for each individual.

2.2 Administration

TWINRIX should be administered by intramuscular injection only as a 1-mL dose. Administer in the deltoid region. Do not administer in the gluteal region; such injections may result in a suboptimal response.

Do not administer this product intravenously, intradermally, or subcutaneously.

2.3 Recommended Dose and Schedule

Standard dosing schedule consists of 3 doses (1 mL each), given intramuscularly at 0, 1, and 6 months. Alternatively, an accelerated schedule of 4 doses (1 mL each), given intramuscularly on days 0, 7, and 21 to 30 followed by a booster dose at month 12 may be used.

3 DOSAGE FORMS AND STRENGTHS

Suspension for injection available in 1-mL single-dose vials and prefilled TIP-LOK® syringes *[see Description (11) and How Supplied/Storage and Handling (16)]*.

4 CONTRAINDICATIONS

Severe allergic reaction (e.g., anaphylaxis) after a previous dose of any hepatitis A-containing or hepatitis B-containing vaccine, or to any component of TWINRIX, including yeast and neomycin, is a contraindication to administration of TWINRIX *[see Description (11)]*.

5 WARNINGS AND PRECAUTIONS

5.1 Latex

TWINRIX is available in vials and 2 types of prefilled syringes. One type of prefilled syringe has a tip cap which may contain natural rubber latex. The other type has a tip cap and a rubber plunger which contain dry natural latex rubber. Use of these syringes may cause allergic reactions in latex-sensitive individuals. The vial stopper does not contain latex. *[See How Supplied/Storage and Handling (16).]*

5.2 Syncope

Syncope (fainting) can occur in association with administration of injectable vaccines, including TWINRIX. Syncope can be accompanied by transient neurological signs such as visual disturbance, paresthesia, and tonic-clonic limb movements. Procedures should be in place to avoid falling injury and to restore cerebral perfusion following syncope.

5.3 Preventing and Managing Allergic Vaccine Reactions

Prior to immunization, the healthcare provider should review the immunization history for possible vaccine sensitivity and previous vaccination-related adverse reactions to allow an assessment of benefits and risks. Appropriate medical treatment and supervision must be available to manage possible anaphylactic reactions following administration of the vaccine. *[See Contraindications (4).]*

5.4 Moderate or Severe Acute Illness

To avoid diagnostic confusion between manifestations of an acute illness and possible vaccine adverse effects, vaccination with TWINRIX should be postponed in persons with moderate or severe acute febrile illness unless they are at immediate risk of hepatitis A or hepatitis B infection.

5.5 Altered Immunocompetence

Immunocompromised persons, including individuals receiving immunosuppressive therapy, may have a diminished immune response to TWINRIX.

Table 1. Rates of Local Adverse Reactions and Systemic Adverse Events Within 4 Days of Vaccination[a] With TWINRIX[b] or ENGERIX-B and HAVRIX[c]

	TWINRIX			ENGERIX-B			HAVRIX	
	Dose 1	Dose 2	Dose 3	Dose 1	Dose 2	Dose 3	Dose 1	Dose 2
Local	(N = 385) %	(N = 382) %	(N = 374) %	(N = 382) %	(N = 376) %	(N = 369) %	(N = 382) %	(N = 369) %
Soreness	37	35	41	41	25	30	53	47
Redness	8	9	11	6	7	9	7	9
Swelling	4	4	6	3	5	5	5	5

	TWINRIX			ENGERIX-B and HAVRIX		
	Dose 1	Dose 2	Dose 3	Dose 1[d]	Dose 2[e]	Dose 3[d]
Systemic	(N = 385) %	(N = 382) %	(N = 374) %	(N = 382) %	(N = 376) %	(N = 369) %
Headache	22	15	13	19	12	14
Fatigue	14	13	11	14	9	10
Diarrhea	5	4	6	5	3	3
Nausea	4	3	2	7	3	5
Fever	4	3	2	4	2	4
Vomiting	1	1	0	1	1	1

[a] Within 4 days of vaccination defined as day of vaccination and the next 3 days.
[b] 389 subjects received at least 1 dose of TWINRIX.
[c] 384 subjects received at least 1 dose each of ENGERIX-B and HAVRIX.
[d] Doses 1 and 3 included ENGERIX-B and HAVRIX in the control group receiving separate vaccinations.
[e] Dose 2 included only ENGERIX-B in the control group receiving separate vaccinations.

5.6 Multiple Sclerosis

Results from 2 clinical studies indicate that there is no association between hepatitis B vaccination and the development of multiple sclerosis,[1] and that vaccination with hepatitis B vaccine does not appear to increase the short-term risk of relapse in multiple sclerosis.[2]

5.7 Limitations of Vaccine Effectiveness

Hepatitis A and hepatitis B have relatively long incubation periods. The vaccine may not prevent hepatitis A or hepatitis B infection in individuals who have an unrecognized hepatitis A or hepatitis B infection at the time of vaccination. Additionally, vaccination with TWINRIX may not protect all individuals.

6 ADVERSE REACTIONS

6.1 Clinical Trials Experience

Because clinical trials are conducted under widely varying conditions, adverse reaction rates observed in the clinical trials of a vaccine cannot be directly compared to rates in the clinical trials of another vaccine and may not reflect the rates observed in practice. As with any vaccine, there is the possibility that broad use of TWINRIX could reveal adverse events not observed in clinical trials.

Following any dose of TWINRIX, the most common (≥10%) solicited injection site reactions were injection site soreness (35% to 41%) and redness (8% to 11%); the most common solicited systemic adverse events were headache (13% to 22%) and fatigue (11% to 14%).

The safety of TWINRIX has been evaluated in clinical trials involving the administration of approximately 7,500 doses to more than 2,500 individuals.

In a US study, 773 subjects (18 to 70 years of age) were randomized 1:1 to receive TWINRIX (0-, 1-, and 6-month schedule) or concurrent administration of ENGERIX-B (0-, 1-, and 6-month schedule) and HAVRIX (0- and 6-month schedule). Solicited local adverse reactions and systemic adverse events were recorded by parents/guardians on diary cards for 4 days (days 0 to 3) after vaccination. Unsolicited adverse events were recorded for 31 days after vaccination. Solicited events reported following the administration of TWINRIX or ENGERIX-B and HAVRIX are presented in Table 1.

[See table 1 above]

Most solicited local adverse reactions and systemic adverse events seen with TWINRIX were considered by the subjects as mild and self-limiting and did not last more than 48 hours.

In a clinical trial in which TWINRIX was given on a 0-, 7-, and 21- to 30-day schedule followed by a booster dose at 12 months, solicited local adverse reactions or systemic adverse events were comparable to those seen in other clinical trials of TWINRIX given on a 0-, 1-, and 6-month schedule.

Among 2,299 subjects in 14 clinical trials, the following adverse events were reported to occur within 30 days following vaccination:

Incidence 1% to 10% of Injections, Seen in Clinical Trials With TWINRIX:

Infections and Infestations: Upper respiratory tract infections.

General Disorders and Administration Site Conditions: Injection site induration.

Incidence <1% of Injections, Seen in Clinical Trials With TWINRIX:

Infections and Infestations: Respiratory tract illnesses.
Metabolism and Nutrition Disorders: Anorexia.
Psychiatric Disorders: Agitation, insomnia.
Nervous System Disorders: Dizziness, migraine, paresthesia, somnolence, syncope.
Ear and Labyrinth Disorders: Vertigo.
Vascular Disorders: Flushing.
Gastrointestinal Disorders: Abdominal pain, vomiting.
Skin and Subcutaneous Tissue Disorders: Erythema, petechiae, rash, sweating, urticaria.
Musculoskeletal and Connective Tissue Disorders: Arthralgia, back pain, myalgia.
General Disorders and Administration Site Conditions: Injection site ecchymosis, injection site pruritus, influenza-like symptoms, irritability, weakness.

Incidence <1% of Injections, Seen in Clinical Trials With HAVRIX and/or ENGERIX-B:

Blood and Lymphatic System Disorders: Lymphadenopathy.[1]
Nervous System Disorders: Dysgeusia,[2] hypertonia,[2] tingling.[3]
Eye Disorders: Photophobia.[2]
Vascular Disorders: Hypotension.[3]
Gastrointestinal Disorders: Constipation.[3]
Investigations: Creatine phosphokinase increased.

Adverse events within 30 days of vaccination in the US clinical trial of TWINRIX given on a 0-, 7-, and 21- to 30-day schedule followed by a booster dose at 12 months were comparable to those reported in other clinical trials.

[1]Following either HAVRIX or ENGERIX-B.
[2]Following HAVRIX.
[3]Following ENGERIX-B.

6.2 Postmarketing Experience

The following adverse events have been identified during postapproval use of TWINRIX, HAVRIX, or ENGERIX-B. Because these events are reported voluntarily from a population of uncertain size, it is not possible to reliably estimate their frequency or establish a causal relationship to product exposure.

Postmarketing Experience with TWINRIX: The following list includes serious events or events which have suspected causal connection to components of TWINRIX.

Infections and Infestations: Herpes zoster, meningitis.
Blood and Lymphatic System Disorders: Thrombocytopenia, thrombocytopenic purpura.
Immune System Disorders: Allergic reaction, anaphylactoid reaction, anaphylaxis, serum sickness–like syndrome days to weeks after vaccination (including arthralgia/arthritis, usually transient, fever, urticaria, erythema multiforme, ecchymoses, and erythema nodosum).
Nervous System Disorders: Bell's palsy, convulsions, encephalitis, encephalopathy, Guillain-Barré syndrome, hypoesthesia, myelitis, multiple sclerosis, neuritis, neuropathy, optic neuritis, paralysis, paresis, transverse myelitis.
Eye Disorders: Conjunctivitis, visual disturbances.
Ear and Labyrinth Disorders: Earache, tinnitus.
Cardiac Disorders: Palpitations, tachycardia.
Vascular Disorders: Vasculitis.
Respiratory, Thoracic and Mediastinal Disorders: Bronchospasm including asthma-like symptoms, dyspnea.
Gastrointestinal Disorders: Dyspepsia.
Hepatobiliary Disorders: Hepatitis, jaundice.
Skin and Subcutaneous Tissue Disorders: Alopecia, angioedema, eczema, erythema multiforme, erythema nodosum, hyperhydrosis, lichen planus.
Musculoskeletal and Connective Tissue Disorders: Arthritis, muscular weakness.
General Disorders and Administration Site Conditions: Chills, immediate injection site pain, stinging, and burning sensation, injection site reaction, malaise.
Investigations: Abnormal liver function tests.

Postmarketing Experience With HAVRIX and/or ENGERIX-B: The following list includes serious events or events which have suspected causal connection to components of HAVRIX and/or ENGERIX-B, not already reported above for TWINRIX.

Eye Disorders: Keratitis.[4]
Skin and Subcutaneous Tissue Disorders: Stevens-Johnson syndrome.[4]
Congenital, Familial and Genetic Disorders: Congenital abnormality.[5]

[4]Following ENGERIX-B.
[5]Following HAVRIX.

7 DRUG INTERACTIONS

7.1 Concomitant Administration With Vaccines and Immune Globulin

Do not mix TWINRIX with any other vaccine or product in the same syringe or vial.

When concomitant administration of immunoglobulin is required, it should be given with a different syringe and at a different injection site.

There are no data to assess the concomitant use of TWINRIX with other vaccines.

7.2 Immunosuppressive Therapies

Immunosuppressive therapies, including irradiation, antimetabolites, alkylating agents, cytotoxic drugs, and corticosteroids (used in greater than physiologic doses), may reduce the immune response to TWINRIX.

8 USE IN SPECIFIC POPULATIONS

8.1 Pregnancy

Pregnancy Category C

Animal reproduction studies have not been conducted with TWINRIX. It is also not known whether TWINRIX can cause fetal harm when administered to a pregnant woman or can affect reproduction capacity. TWINRIX should be given to a pregnant woman only if clearly needed.

Pregnancy Registry: GlaxoSmithKline maintains a surveillance registry to collect data on pregnancy outcomes and newborn health status outcomes following vaccination with TWINRIX during pregnancy. Women who receive TWINRIX during pregnancy should be encouraged to contact GlaxoSmithKline directly or their healthcare provider should contact GlaxoSmithKline by calling 1-888-452-9622.

8.3 Nursing Mothers

It is not known whether TWINRIX is excreted in human milk. Because many drugs are excreted in human milk, caution should be exercised when TWINRIX is administered to a nursing woman.

8.4 Pediatric Use

Safety and effectiveness in pediatric patients below the age of 18 years have not been established.

8.5 Geriatric Use

Clinical studies of TWINRIX did not include sufficient numbers of subjects aged 65 years and older to determine whether they respond differently from younger subjects *[see Clinical Studies (14.1, 14.3)]*.

11 DESCRIPTION

TWINRIX [Hepatitis A & Hepatitis B (Recombinant) Vaccine] is a bivalent vaccine containing the antigenic components used in producing HAVRIX® (Hepatitis A Vaccine) and ENGERIX-B® [Hepatitis B Vaccine (Recombinant)]. TWINRIX is a sterile suspension for intramuscular administration that contains inactivated hepatitis A virus (strain HM175) and noninfectious hepatitis B virus surface antigen (HBsAg). The hepatitis A virus is propagated in MRC-5 human diploid cells and inactivated with formalin. The purified HBsAg is obtained by culturing genetically engineered *Saccharomyces cerevisiae* yeast cells, which carry the surface antigen gene of the hepatitis B virus. Bulk preparations of each antigen are adsorbed separately onto aluminum salts and then pooled during formulation.

A 1-mL dose of vaccine contains 720 ELISA Units of inactivated hepatitis A virus and 20 mcg of recombinant HBsAg protein. One dose of vaccine also contains 0.45 mg of aluminum in the form of aluminum phosphate and aluminum hydroxide as adjuvants, amino acids, sodium chloride, phosphate buffer, polysorbate 20, and Water for Injection. From the manufacturing process each 1-mL dose of

TWINRIX also contains residual formalin (not more than 0.1 mg), MRC-5 cellular proteins (not more than 2.5 mcg), neomycin sulfate (an aminoglycoside antibiotic included in the cell growth media; not more than 20 ng) and yeast protein (no more than 5%).

TWINRIX is available in vials and 2 types of prefilled syringes. One type of prefilled syringe has a tip cap which may contain natural rubber latex. The other type has a tip cap and a rubber plunger which contain dry natural latex rubber. The vial stopper does not contain latex. *[See How Supplied/Storage and Handling (16).]*

TWINRIX is formulated without preservatives.

12 CLINICAL PHARMACOLOGY

12.1 Mechanism of Action

Hepatitis A: The course of infection with hepatitis A virus (HAV) is extremely variable, ranging from asymptomatic infection to fulminant hepatitis.[3]

The presence of antibodies to HAV (anti-HAV) confers protection against hepatitis A disease. However, the lowest titer needed to confer protection has not been determined. Natural infection provides lifelong immunity even when antibodies to hepatitis A are undetectable. Seroconversion is defined as antibody titers equal to or greater than the assay cut-off (cut-off values vary depending on the assay used) in those previously seronegative.

Hepatitis B: Infection with hepatitis B virus (HBV) can have serious consequences including acute massive hepatic necrosis and chronic active hepatitis. Chronically infected persons are at increased risk for cirrhosis and hepatocellular carcinoma.

Antibody concentrations ≥10 mIU/mL against HBsAg are recognized as conferring protection against hepatitis B virus infection.[4]

13 NONCLINICAL TOXICOLOGY

13.1 Carcinogenesis, Mutagenesis, Impairment of Fertility

TWINRIX has not been evaluated for its carcinogenic or mutagenic potential, or for impairment of fertility.

14 CLINICAL STUDIES

14.1 Immunogenicity: Standard 0-, 1-, and 6-Month Dosing Schedule

In 11 clinical trials, sera from 1,551 healthy adults 17 to 70 years of age, including 555 male subjects and 996 female subjects, were analyzed following administration of 3 doses of TWINRIX on a 0-, 1-, and 6-month schedule. Seroconversion (defined as equal to or greater than assay cut-off depending on assay used) for antibodies against HAV was elicited in 99.9% of vaccinees, and protective antibodies (defined as ≥10 mIU/mL) against HBV surface antigen were detected in 98.5% of vaccinees, 1 month after completion of the 3-dose series (Table 2).

Table 2. Seroconversion and Seroprotection Rates in Worldwide Clinical Trials

TWINRIX Dose	N	% Seroconversion for Hepatitis A[a]	% Seroprotection for Hepatitis B[b]
1	1,587	93.8	30.8
2	1,571	98.8	78.2
3	1,551	99.9	98.5

[a] Anti-HAV titer ≥assay cut-off: 20 mIU/mL (HAVAB Test) or 33 mIU/mL (ENZYMUN-TEST®).
[b] Anti-HBsAg titer ≥10 mIU/mL (AUSAB® Test).

One of the 11 trials was a comparative trial conducted in a US population given either TWINRIX (on a 0-, 1-, and 6-month schedule) or HAVRIX (0- and 6-month schedule) and ENGERIX-B (0-, 1-, and 6-month schedule). The monovalent vaccines were given concurrently in opposite arms. Of the 773 adults (18 to 70 years of age) enrolled in this trial, an immunogenicity analysis was performed in 533 subjects who completed the study according to protocol. Of these, 264 subjects received TWINRIX and 269 subjects received HAVRIX and ENGERIX-B. Seroconversion rates against HAV and seroprotection rates against HBV are presented in Table 3; GMTs are presented in Table 4. The absolute difference in anti-HAV seropositivity rates between groups was 0.36% (90% CI: -1.8, 3.1). Non-inferiority in terms of anti-HAV response was demonstrated (lower limit of the 90% CI was higher than the pre-specified non-inferiority criterion of -4.3%). The absolute difference in anti-HBsAg seroprotection rates between groups was 2.8% (90% CI: -1.3, 7.7). Non-inferiority in terms of anti-HBV response was demonstrated (lower limit of the 90% CI was higher than the pre-specified non-inferiority criterion of -9.4%).

[See table 3 above]

[See table 4 above]

Table 3. Seroconversion and Seroprotection Rates in a US Clinical Trial

Vaccine	N	Timepoint	% Seroconversion for Hepatitis A[a] (95% CI)	% Seroprotection for Hepatitis B[b] (95% CI)
TWINRIX	264	Month 1	91.6	17.9
		Month 2	97.7	61.2
		Month 7	99.6 (97.9, 100.0)	95.1 (91.7, 97.4)
HAVRIX and ENGERIX-B	269	Month 1	98.1	7.5
		Month 2	98.9	50.4
		Month 7	99.3 (97.3, 99.9)	92.2 (88.3, 95.1)

CI = Confidence Interval
[a] Anti-HAV titer ≥assay cut-off: 33 mIU/mL (ENZYMUN-TEST).
[b] Anti-HBsAg titer ≥10 mIU/mL (AUSAB Test).

Table 4. Geometric Mean Titers in a US Clinical Trial

Vaccine	N	Timepoint	GMT to Hepatitis A (95% CI)	GMT to Hepatitis B (95% CI)
TWINRIX	263	Month 1	335	8
	259	Month 2	636	23
	264	Month 7	4756 (4152, 5448)	2099 (1663, 2649)
HAVRIX and ENGERIX-B	268	Month 1	444	6
	269	Month 2	257	18
	269	Month 7	2948 (2638, 3294)	1871 (1428, 2450)

GMT = Geometric mean titer; CI = Confidence Interval

Table 5. Seroconversion and Seroprotection Rates up to One Month After the Last Dose of Vaccines (According To Protocol Cohort)

	Timepoint	TWINRIX[a] (N = 194-204)	HAVRIX and ENGERIX-B[b] (N = 197-207)
% Seroconversion for Hepatitis A[c] (95% CI)	Day 37	98.5 (95.8, 99.7)	98.6 (95.8, 99.7)
	Day 90	100 (98.2, 100)	95.6 (91.9, 98.0)
	Month 12	96.9 (93.4, 98.9)	86.9 (81.4, 91.2)
	Month 13	100 (98.1, 100)	100 (98.1, 100)
% Seroprotection for Hepatitis B[d] (95% CI)	Day 37	63.2 (56.2, 69.9)	43.5 (36.6, 50.5)
	Day 90	83.2 (77.3, 88.1)	76.7 (70.3, 82.3)
	Month 12	82.1 (75.9, 87.2)	77.8 (71.3, 83.4)
	Month 13	96.4 (92.7, 98.5)	93.4 (89.0, 96.4)

CI = Confidence Interval
[a] TWINRIX given on a 0-, 7-, and 21- to 30-day schedule followed by a booster at month 12.
[b] HAVRIX 1440 EL.U./1 mL given on a 0- and 12-month schedule and ENGERIX-B 20 mcg/1 mL given on a 0-, 1-, 2-, and 12-month schedule.
[c] Anti-HAV titer ≥assay cut-off: 15 mIU/mL (anti-HAV Behring Test).
[d] Anti-HBsAg titer ≥10 mIU/mL (AUSAB Test).

Since the immune responses to hepatitis A and hepatitis B induced by TWINRIX were non-inferior to the monovalent vaccines, efficacy is expected to be similar to the efficacy for each of the monovalent vaccines.

The antibody titers achieved 1 month after the final dose of TWINRIX were higher than titers achieved 1 month after the final dose of HAVRIX in this clinical trial. This may have been due to a difference in the recommended dosage regimens for these 2 vaccines, whereby TWINRIX vaccinees received 3 doses of 720 EL.U. of hepatitis A antigen at 0, 1, and 6 months, whereas HAVRIX vaccinees received 2 doses of 1440 EL.U. of the same antigen (at 0 and 6 months). However, these differences in peak titer have not been shown to be clinically significant.

14.2 Immunogenicity: Accelerated Dosing Schedule (Day 0-, 7-, and 21-30, Month 12)

In 496 healthy adults, the safety and immunogenicity of TWINRIX given on a 0-, 7-, and 21- to 30-day schedule followed by a booster dose at 12 months (N = 250), was compared to separate vaccinations with monovalent hepatitis A vaccine (HAVRIX at 0 and 12 months) and hepatitis B vaccine (ENGERIX-B at 0, 1, 2, and 12 months) as a control group (N = 246).

Following a booster dose at month 12, seroprotection rates for hepatitis B and seroconversion rates for hepatitis A at month 13 following TWINRIX were non-inferior to the control group. The absolute difference in anti-HBs seroprotection rates between groups (HAVRIX + ENGERIX-B minus TWINRIX) was -2.99 (95% CI: -7.80, 1.49). Non-inferiority was demonstrated as the upper limit of the 95% CI was lower than the pre-defined limit of 7%. The absolute difference in anti-HAV seroprotection rates between groups (HAVRIX + ENGERIX-B minus TWINRIX) was 0 (95% CI: -1.91, 1.94). Non-inferiority was demonstrated as the upper limit of the 95% CI was lower than the pre-defined limit of 7%. The immune responses are presented in Table 5.

[See table 5 above]

14.3 Immunogenicity in Adults Older Than 40 Years of Age

The effect of age on immune response to TWINRIX was studied in 2 trials. The first trial evaluated subjects 41 to 63 years of age (N = 72; mean age = 50). All subjects were seropositive for anti-HAV antibodies following the third dose of TWINRIX. For the hepatitis B response, 94% of subjects were seroprotected after the third dose of TWINRIX.

The second trial included subjects 19 years of age and older with a comparison between those older than 40 years of age (N = 183, 41 to 70 years of age; mean age = 48) with those 40 years of age or younger (N = 191; 19 to 40 years of age; mean age 33). Over 99% of subjects in both age groups achieved a seropositive response for anti-HAV antibodies and GMTs were comparable between the age groups. In the older subjects who received TWINRIX, 92.9% (95% CI: 88.2, 96.2) achieved seroprotection against hepatitis B compared to 96.9% (95% CI: 93.3, 98.8) of the younger subjects. The GMT was 1,890 mIU/mL in the older subjects compared to 2,285 mIU/mL in the younger subjects.

14.4 Duration of Immunity

Two clinical trials involving a total of 129 subjects demonstrated that antibodies to both HAV and HBV surface antigen persisted for at least 4 years after the first vaccine dose in a 3-dose series of TWINRIX, given on a 0-, 1-, and 6-month schedule. For comparison, after the recommended immunization regimens for HAVRIX and ENGERIX-B, respectively, similar studies involving a total of 114 subjects have shown that seropositivity to HAV and HBV also persists for at least 4 years.

15 REFERENCES

1. Ascherio A, Zhang SM, Hernán MA, et al. Hepatitis B vaccination and the risk of multiple sclerosis. *N Engl J Med.* 2001;344(5):327-332.

2. Confavreux C, Suissa S, Saddier P, et al. Vaccination and the risk of relapse in multiple sclerosis. *N Engl J Med.* 2001;344(5):319-326.
3. Lemon SM. Type A viral hepatitis: new developments in an old disease. *N Engl J Med.* 1985;313(17):1059-1067.
4. Frisch-Niggemeyer W, Ambrosch F, Hofmann H. The assessment of immunity against hepatitis B after vaccination. *J Bio Stand.* 1986;14(3):255-258.

16 HOW SUPPLIED/STORAGE AND HANDLING

TWINRIX is available in 1-mL single-dose vials and 1-mL single-dose prefilled disposable TIP-LOK syringes (packaged without needles) (Preservative Free Formulation):
NDC 58160-815-01 Vial (contains no latex) in Package of 10: NDC 58160-815-11
NDC 58160-815-05 Syringe (tip cap may contain latex) in Package of 1: NDC 58160-815-34
NDC 58160-815-34 Syringe (tip cap may contain latex) in Package of 1: NDC 58160-815-34
NDC 58160-815-43 Syringe (tip cap may contain latex) in Package of 5: NDC 58160-815-48
NDC 58160-815-43 Syringe (tip cap may contain latex) in Package of 10: NDC 58160-815-52
NDC 58160-815-41 Syringe (tip cap and plunger contain latex) in Package of 5: NDC 58160-815-46
Store refrigerated between 2° and 8°C (36° and 46°F). Do not freeze; discard if product has been frozen.

17 PATIENT COUNSELING INFORMATION

- Inform vaccine recipients of the potential benefits and risks of immunization with TWINRIX.
- Emphasize, when educating vaccine recipients regarding potential side effects, that components of TWINRIX cannot cause hepatitis A or hepatitis B infection.
- Instruct vaccine recipients to report any adverse events to their healthcare provider.
- Inform that safety and efficacy have not been established in pregnant women. Register women who receive TWINRIX while pregnant in the pregnancy registry by calling 1-888-452-9622.
- Give vaccine recipients the Vaccine Information Statements, which are required by the National Childhood Vaccine Injury Act of 1986 to be given prior to immunization. These materials are available free of charge at the Centers for Disease Control and Prevention (CDC) website (www.cdc.gov/vaccines).

TWINRIX, HAVRIX, ENGERIX-B, and TIP-LOK are registered trademarks of GlaxoSmithKline. ENZYMUN-TEST is a registered trademark of Boehringer Mannheim Immunodiagnostics. AUSAB is a registered trademark of Abbott Laboratories.
Manufactured by **GlaxoSmithKline Biologicals**
Rixensart, Belgium, US License No. 1617
Distributed by **GlaxoSmithKline**
Research Triangle Park, NC 27709

TWR:21PI

TYKERB ℞

[*tī'kerb*]
(lapatinib)
tablets

HIGHLIGHTS OF PRESCRIBING INFORMATION
These highlights do not include all the information needed to use TYKERB safely and effectively. See full prescribing information for TYKERB.
TYKERB (lapatinib) tablets
Initial U.S. Approval: 2007

> **WARNING: HEPATOTOXICITY**
> ***See full prescribing information for complete boxed warning.***
> **Hepatotoxicity has been observed in clinical trials and postmarketing experience. The hepatotoxicity may be severe and deaths have been reported. Causality of the deaths is uncertain. *[See Warnings and Precautions (5.2).]***

RECENT MAJOR CHANGES

Dosage and Administration, Dose Modification Guidelines (2.2)	12/2012
Warnings and Precautions, Diarrhea (5.4)	06/2013

INDICATIONS AND USAGE

TYKERB, a kinase inhibitor, is indicated in combination with: (1)
- capecitabine, for the treatment of patients with advanced or metastatic breast cancer whose tumors overexpress HER2 and who have received prior therapy including an anthracycline, a taxane, and trastuzumab.
- letrozole for the treatment of postmenopausal women with hormone receptor positive metastatic breast cancer that overexpresses the HER2 receptor for whom hormonal therapy is indicated.

TYKERB in combination with an aromatase inhibitor has not been compared to a trastuzumab-containing chemotherapy regimen for the treatment of metastatic breast cancer.

DOSAGE AND ADMINISTRATION

The recommended dosage of TYKERB for advanced or metastatic breast cancer is 1,250 mg (5 tablets) given orally once daily on Days 1-21 continuously in combination with capecitabine 2,000 mg/m^2/day (administered orally in 2 doses approximately 12 hours apart) on Days 1-14 in a repeating 21 day cycle. (2.1)
The recommended dose of TYKERB for hormone receptor positive, HER2 positive metastatic breast cancer is 1500 mg (6 tablets) given orally once daily continuously in combination with letrozole. When TYKERB is coadministered with letrozole, the recommended dose of letrozole is 2.5 mg once daily. (2.1)
- TYKERB should be taken at least one hour before or one hour after a meal. However, capecitabine should be taken with food or within 30 minutes after food. (2.1)
- TYKERB should be taken once daily. Do not divide daily doses of TYKERB. (2.1, 12.3)
- Modify dose for cardiac and other toxicities, severe hepatic impairment, diarrhea, and CYP3A4 drug interactions. (2.2)

DOSAGE FORMS AND STRENGTHS

250 mg tablets (3)

CONTRAINDICATIONS

Known severe hypersensitivity (e.g., anaphylaxis) to this product or any of its components. (4)

WARNINGS AND PRECAUTIONS

- Decreases in left ventricular ejection fraction have been reported. Confirm normal LVEF before starting TYKERB and continue evaluations during treatment. (5.1)
- Lapatinib has been associated with hepatotoxicity. Monitor liver function tests before initiation of treatment, every 4 to 6 weeks during treatment, and as clinically indicated. Discontinue and do not restart TYKERB if patients experience severe changes in liver function tests. (5.2)
- Dose reduction in patients with severe hepatic impairment should be considered. (2.2, 5.3, 8.7)
- Diarrhea, including severe diarrhea, has been reported during treatment. Manage with anti-diarrheal agents, and replace fluids and electrolytes if severe. (5.4)
- Lapatinib has been associated with interstitial lung disease and pneumonitis. Discontinue TYKERB if patients experience severe pulmonary symptoms. (5.5)
- Lapatinib may prolong the QT interval in some patients. Consider ECG and electrolyte monitoring. (5.6, 12.4)
- Fetal harm can occur when administered to a pregnant woman. Women should be advised not to become pregnant when taking TYKERB. (5.7)

ADVERSE REACTIONS

The most common (>20%) adverse reactions during treatment with TYKERB plus capecitabine were diarrhea, palmar-plantar erythrodysesthesia, nausea, rash, vomiting, and fatigue. The most common (≥20%) adverse reactions during treatment with TYKERB plus letrozole were diarrhea, rash, nausea, and fatigue. (6.1)
To report SUSPECTED ADVERSE REACTIONS, contact GlaxoSmithKline at 1-888-825-5249 or FDA at 1-800-FDA-1088 or www.fda.gov/medwatch.

DRUG INTERACTIONS

- TYKERB is likely to increase exposure to concomitantly administered drugs which are substrates of CYP3A4, CYP2C8, or P-glycoprotein (ABCB1). (7.1)
- Avoid strong CYP3A4 inhibitors. If unavoidable, consider dose reduction of TYKERB in patients coadministered a strong CYP3A4 inhibitor. (2.2, 7.2)
- Avoid strong CYP3A4 inducers. If unavoidable, consider gradual dose increase of TYKERB in patients coadministered a strong CYP3A4 inducer. (2.2, 7.2)

See 17 for PATIENT COUNSELING INFORMATION and FDA-approved patient labeling

Revised: 06/2013

FULL PRESCRIBING INFORMATION: CONTENTS*

*** Sections or subsections omitted from the full prescribing information are not listed**

FULL PRESCRIBING INFORMATION

> **WARNING: HEPATOTOXICITY**
> **Hepatotoxicity has been observed in clinical trials and postmarketing experience. The hepatotoxicity may be severe and deaths have been reported. Causality of the deaths is uncertain. *[See Warnings and Precautions (5.2).]***

1 INDICATIONS AND USAGE

TYKERB® is indicated in combination with:
- capecitabine for the treatment of patients with advanced or metastatic breast cancer whose tumors overexpress HER2 and who have received prior therapy including an anthracycline, a taxane, and trastuzumab.
- letrozole for the treatment of postmenopausal women with hormone receptor positive metastatic breast cancer that overexpresses the HER2 receptor for whom hormonal therapy is indicated.

TYKERB in combination with an aromatase inhibitor has not been compared to a trastuzumab-containing chemotherapy regimen for the treatment of metastatic breast cancer.

2 DOSAGE AND ADMINISTRATION

2.1 Recommended Dosing

HER2 Positive Metastatic Breast Cancer: The recommended dose of TYKERB is 1,250 mg given orally once daily on Days 1-21 continuously in combination with capecitabine 2,000 mg/m^2/day (administered orally in 2 doses approximately 12 hours apart) on Days 1-14 in a repeating 21 day cycle. TYKERB should be taken at least one hour before or one hour after a meal. The dose of TYKERB should be once daily (5 tablets administered all at once); dividing the daily dose is not recommended *[see Clinical Pharmacology (12.3)]*. Capecitabine should be taken with food or within 30 minutes after food. If a day's dose is missed, the patient should not double the dose the next day. Treatment should be continued until disease progression or unacceptable toxicity occurs.

Hormone Receptor Positive, HER2 Positive Metastatic Breast Cancer: The recommended dose of TYKERB is 1,500 mg given orally once daily continuously in combination with letrozole. When coadministered with TYKERB, the recommended dose of letrozole is 2.5 mg once daily. TYKERB should be taken at least one hour before or one hour after a meal. The dose of TYKERB should be once daily (6 tablets administered all at once); dividing the daily dose is not recommended *[see Clinical Pharmacology (12.3)]*.

2.2 Dose Modification Guidelines

Cardiac Events: TYKERB should be discontinued in patients with a decreased left ventricular ejection fraction (LVEF) that is Grade 2 or greater by National Cancer Institute Common Terminology Criteria for Adverse Events (NCI CTCAE v3) and in patients with an LVEF that drops below the institution's lower limit of normal *[see Warnings and Precautions (5.1) and Adverse Reactions (6.1)]*. TYKERB in combination with capecitabine may be restarted at a reduced dose (1,000 mg/day) and in combination with letrozole may be restarted at a reduced dose of 1,250 mg/day after a minimum of 2 weeks if the LVEF recovers to normal and the patient is asymptomatic.

Hepatic Impairment: Patients with severe hepatic impairment (Child-Pugh Class C) should have their dose of TYKERB reduced. A dose reduction from 1,250 mg/day to 750 mg/day (HER2 positive metastatic breast cancer indication) or from 1,500 mg/day to 1,000 mg/day (hormone receptor positive, HER2 positive breast cancer indication) in patients with severe hepatic impairment is predicted to adjust the area under the curve (AUC) to the normal range and should be considered. However, there are no clinical data with this dose adjustment in patients with severe hepatic impairment.

Diarrhea: TYKERB should be interrupted in patients with diarrhea which is NCI CTCAE Grade 3 or Grade 1 or 2 with complicating features (moderate to severe abdominal cramping, nausea or vomiting ≥NCI CTCAE Grade 2, decreased performance status, fever, sepsis, neutropenia, frank bleeding, or dehydration). TYKERB may be reintroduced at a lower dose (reduced from 1,250 mg/day to 1,000 mg/day or from 1,500 mg/day to 1,250 mg/day) when diarrhea resolves to Grade 1 or less. TYKERB should be permanently discontinued in patients with diarrhea which is NCI CTCAE Grade 4 *[see Warnings and Precautions (5.4) and Adverse Reactions (6.1)]*.

Concomitant Strong CYP3A4 Inhibitors: The concomitant use of strong CYP3A4 inhibitors should be avoided (e.g., ketoconazole, itraconazole, clarithromycin, atazanavir, indinavir, nefazodone, nelfinavir, ritonavir, saquinavir, telithromycin, voriconazole). Grapefruit may also increase plasma concentrations of lapatinib and should be avoided. If patients must be coadministered a strong CYP3A4 inhibitor, based on pharmacokinetic studies, a dose reduction to 500 mg/day of lapatinib is predicted to adjust the lapatinib AUC to the range observed without inhibitors and should be considered. However, there are no clinical data with this dose adjustment in patients receiving strong CYP3A4 inhibitors. If the strong inhibitor is discontinued, a washout period of approximately 1 week should be allowed before the lapatinib dose is adjusted upward to the indicated dose. *[See Drug Interactions (7.2).]*

Concomitant Strong CYP3A4 Inducers: The concomitant use of strong CYP3A4 inducers should be avoided (e.g., dexamethasone, phenytoin, carbamazepine, rifampin, rifabutin, rifapentin, phenobarbital, St. John's Wort). If patients must be coadministered a strong CYP3A4 inducer, based on pharmacokinetic studies, the dose of lapatinib should be titrated gradually from 1,250 mg/day up to 4,500 mg/day (HER2 positive metastatic breast cancer indication) or from 1,500 mg/day up to 5,500 mg/day (hormone receptor positive, HER2 positive breast cancer indication) based on tolerability. This dose of lapatinib is predicted to adjust the lapatinib AUC to the range observed without inducers and should be considered. However, there are no clinical data with this dose adjustment in patients receiving strong CYP3A4 inducers. If the strong inducer is discontinued the lapatinib dose should be reduced to the indicated dose. *[See Drug Interactions (7.2).]*

Other Toxicities: Discontinuation or interruption of dosing with TYKERB may be considered when patients develop ≥Grade 2 NCI CTCAE toxicity and can be restarted at 1,250 mg/day when the toxicity improves to Grade 1 or less. If the toxicity recurs, then TYKERB in combination with capecitabine should be restarted at a lower dose (1,000 mg/day) and in combination with letrozole should be restarted at a lower dose of 1,250 mg/day.

See manufacturer's prescribing information for the coadministered product dosage adjustment guidelines in the event of toxicity and other relevant safety information or contraindications.

3 DOSAGE FORMS AND STRENGTHS

250 mg tablets — oval, biconvex, orange, film-coated with GS XJG debossed on one side.

4 CONTRAINDICATIONS

TYKERB is contraindicated in patients with known severe hypersensitivity (e.g., anaphylaxis) to this product or any of its components.

5 WARNINGS AND PRECAUTIONS

5.1 Decreased Left Ventricular Ejection Fraction

TYKERB has been reported to decrease LVEF *[see Adverse Reactions (6.1)]*. In clinical trials, the majority (>57%) of LVEF decreases occurred within the first 12 weeks of treatment; however, data on long-term exposure are limited. Caution should be taken if TYKERB is to be administered to patients with conditions that could impair left ventricular function. LVEF should be evaluated in all patients prior to initiation of treatment with TYKERB to ensure that the patient has a baseline LVEF that is within the institution's normal limits. LVEF should continue to be evaluated during treatment with TYKERB to ensure that LVEF does not decline below the institution's normal limits *[see Dosage and Administration (2.2)]*.

Table 1. Adverse Reactions Occurring in ≥10% of Patients

	TYKERB 1,250 mg/day + Capecitabine 2,000 mg/m²/day (N = 198)			Capecitabine 2,500 mg/m²/day (N = 191)		
	All Grades[a]	Grade 3	Grade 4	All Grades[a]	Grade 3	Grade 4
Reactions	**%**	**%**	**%**	**%**	**%**	**%**
Gastrointestinal disorders						
Diarrhea	65	13	1	40	10	0
Nausea	44	2	0	43	2	0
Vomiting	26	2	0	21	2	0
Stomatitis	14	0	0	11	<1	0
Dyspepsia	11	<1	0	3	0	0
Skin and subcutaneous tissue disorders						
Palmar-plantar erythrodysesthesia	53	12	0	51	14	0
Rash[b]	28	2	0	14	1	0
Dry skin	10	0	0	6	0	0
General disorders and administrative site conditions						
Mucosal inflammation	15	0	0	12	2	0
Musculoskeletal and connective tissue disorders						
Pain in extremity	12	1	0	7	<1	0
Back pain	11	1	0	6	<1	0
Respiratory, thoracic, and mediastinal disorders						
Dyspnea	12	3	0	8	2	0
Psychiatric disorders						
Insomnia	10	<1	0	6	0	0

[a] National Cancer Institute Common Terminology Criteria for Adverse Events, version 3.
[b] Grade 3 dermatitis acneiform was reported in <1% of patients in TYKERB plus capecitabine group.

5.2 Hepatotoxicity

Hepatotoxicity (ALT or AST >3 times the upper limit of normal and total bilirubin >2 times the upper limit of normal) has been observed in clinical trials (<1% of patients) and postmarketing experience. The hepatotoxicity may be severe and deaths have been reported. Causality of the deaths is uncertain. The hepatotoxicity may occur days to several months after initiation of treatment. Liver function tests (transaminases, bilirubin, and alkaline phosphatase) should be monitored before initiation of treatment, every 4 to 6 weeks during treatment, and as clinically indicated. If changes in liver function are severe, therapy with TYKERB should be discontinued and patients should not be retreated with TYKERB *[see Adverse Reactions (6.1)]*.

5.3 Patients with Severe Hepatic Impairment

If TYKERB is to be administered to patients with severe pre-existing hepatic impairment, dose reduction should be considered *[see Dosage and Administration (2.2) and Use in Specific Populations (8.7)]*. In patients who develop severe hepatotoxicity while on therapy, TYKERB should be discontinued and patients should not be retreated with TYKERB *[see Warnings and Precautions (5.2)]*.

5.4 Diarrhea

Diarrhea has been reported during treatment with TYKERB *[see Adverse Reactions (6.1)]*. The diarrhea may be severe, and deaths have been reported. Diarrhea generally occurs early during treatment with TYKERB, with almost half of those patients with diarrhea first experiencing it within 6 days. This usually lasts 4 to 5 days. Lapatinib-induced diarrhea is usually low-grade, with severe diarrhea of NCI CTCAE Grades 3 and 4 occurring in <10% and <1% of patients, respectively. Early identification and intervention is critical for the optimal management of diarrhea. Patients should be instructed to report any change in bowel patterns immediately. Prompt treatment of diarrhea with anti-diarrheal agents (such as loperamide) after the first unformed stool is recommended. Severe cases of diarrhea may require administration of oral or intravenous electrolytes and fluids, use of antibiotics such as fluoroquinolones (especially if diarrhea is persistent beyond 24 hours, there is fever, or Grade 3 or 4 neutropenia), and interruption or discontinuation of therapy with TYKERB *[(see Dosage and Administration (2.2)]*.

5.5 Interstitial Lung Disease/Pneumonitis

Lapatinib has been associated with interstitial lung disease and pneumonitis in monotherapy or in combination with other chemotherapies *[see Adverse Reactions (6.1)]*. Patients should be monitored for pulmonary symptoms indicative of interstitial lung disease or pneumonitis. TYKERB should be discontinued in patients who experience pulmonary symptoms indicative of interstitial lung disease/pneumonitis which are ≥Grade 3 (NCI CTCAE).

5.6 QT Prolongation

QT prolongation was observed in an uncontrolled, open-label dose escalation study of lapatinib in advanced cancer patients *[see Clinical Pharmacology (12.4)]*. Lapatinib should be administered with caution to patients who have or may develop prolongation of QTc. These conditions include patients with hypokalemia or hypomagnesemia, with congenital long QT syndrome, patients taking anti-arrhythmic medicines or other medicinal products that lead to QT prolongation, and cumulative high-dose anthracycline therapy. Hypokalemia or hypomagnesemia should be corrected prior to lapatinib administration.

5.7 Use in Pregnancy

TYKERB can cause fetal harm when administered to a pregnant woman. Based on findings in animals, TYKERB is

Table 2. Selected Laboratory Abnormalities

	TYKERB 1,250 mg/day + Capecitabine 2,000 mg/m²/day			Capecitabine 2,500 mg/m²/day		
	All Grades[a]	Grade 3	Grade 4	All Grades[a]	Grade 3	Grade 4
Parameters	%	%	%	%	%	%
Hematologic						
Hemoglobin	56	<1	0	53	1	0
Platelets	18	<1	0	17	<1	<1
Neutrophils	22	3	<1	31	2	1
Hepatic						
Total Bilirubin	45	4	0	30	3	0
AST	49	2	<1	43	2	0
ALT	37	2	0	33	1	0

[a] National Cancer Institute Common Terminology Criteria for Adverse Events, version 3.

Table 3. Adverse Reactions Occurring in ≥10% of Patients

	TYKERB 1,500 mg/day + Letrozole 2.5 mg/day (N = 654)			Letrozole 2.5 mg/day (N = 624)		
	All Grades[a]	Grade 3	Grade 4	All Grades[a]	Grade 3	Grade 4
Reactions	%	%	%	%	%	%
Gastrointestinal disorders						
Diarrhea	64	9	<1	20	<1	0
Nausea	31	<1	0	21	<1	0
Vomiting	17	1	<1	11	<1	<1
Anorexia	11	<1	0	9	<1	0
Skin and subcutaneous tissue disorders						
Rash[b]	44	1	0	13	0	0
Dry skin	13	<1	0	4	0	0
Alopecia	13	<1	0	7	0	0
Pruritus	12	<1	0	9	<1	0
Nail Disorder	11	<1	0	<1	0	0
General disorders and administrative site conditions						
Fatigue	20	2	0	17	<1	0
Asthenia	12	<1	0	11	<1	0
Nervous system disorders						
Headache	14	<1	0	13	<1	0
Respiratory, thoracic, and mediastinal disorders						
Epistaxis	11	<1	0	2	<1	0

[a] National Cancer Institute Common Terminology Criteria for Adverse Events, version 3.
[b] In addition to the rash reported under "Skin and subcutaneous tissue disorders", 3 additional subjects in each treatment arm had rash under "Infections and infestations"; none were Grade 3 or 4.

expected to result in adverse reproductive effects. Lapatinib administered to rats during organogenesis and through lactation led to death of offspring within the first 4 days after birth *[see Use in Specific Populations (8.1)]*.

There are no adequate and well-controlled studies with TYKERB in pregnant women. Women should be advised not to become pregnant when taking TYKERB. If this drug is used during pregnancy, or if the patient becomes pregnant while taking this drug, the patient should be apprised of the potential hazard to the fetus.

6 ADVERSE REACTIONS

6.1 Clinical Trials Experience

Because clinical trials are conducted under widely varying conditions, adverse reaction rates observed in the clinical trials of a drug cannot be directly compared to rates in the clinical trials of another drug and may not reflect the rates observed in practice.

HER2 Positive Metastatic Breast Cancer: The safety of TYKERB has been evaluated in more than 12,000 patients in clinical trials. The efficacy and safety of TYKERB in combination with capecitabine in breast cancer was evaluated in 198 patients in a randomized, Phase 3 trial. *[See Clinical Studies (14.1).]* Adverse reactions which occurred in at least 10% of patients in either treatment arm and were higher in the combination arm are shown in Table 1.

The most common adverse reactions (>20%) during therapy with TYKERB plus capecitabine were gastrointestinal (diarrhea, nausea, and vomiting), dermatologic (palmar-plantar erythrodysesthesia and rash), and fatigue. Diarrhea was the most common adverse reaction resulting in discontinuation of study medication.

The most common Grade 3 and 4 adverse reactions (NCI CTCAE v3) were diarrhea and palmar-plantar erythrodysesthesia. Selected laboratory abnormalities are shown in Table 2.

[See table 1 at top of previous page]
[See table 2 above]

Hormone Receptor Positive, Metastatic Breast Cancer: In a randomized clinical trial of patients (N = 1,286) with hormone receptor positive, metastatic breast cancer, who had not received chemotherapy for their metastatic disease, patients received letrozole with or without TYKERB. In this trial, the safety profile of TYKERB was consistent with previously reported results from trials of TYKERB in the advanced or metastatic breast cancer population. Adverse reactions which occurred in at least 10% of patients in either treatment arm and were higher in the combination arm are shown in Table 3. Selected laboratory abnormalities are shown in Table 4.

[See table 3 above]
[See table 4 at top of next page]

Decreases in Left Ventricular Ejection Fraction: Due to potential cardiac toxicity with HER2 (ErbB2) inhibitors, LVEF was monitored in clinical trials at approximately 8-week intervals. LVEF decreases were defined as signs or symptoms of deterioration in left ventricular cardiac function that are ≥Grade 3 (NCI CTCAE), or a ≥20% decrease in left ventricular cardiac ejection fraction relative to baseline which is below the institution's lower limit of normal. Among 198 patients who received TYKERB/capecitabine combination treatment, 3 experienced Grade 2 and one had Grade 3 LVEF adverse reactions (NCI CTCAE v3). *[See Warnings and Precautions (5.1).]* Among 654 patients who received TYKERB/letrozole combination treatment, 26 patients experienced Grade 1 or 2 and 6 patients had Grade 3 or 4 LVEF adverse reactions.

Hepatotoxicity: TYKERB has been associated with hepatotoxicity *[see Boxed Warning and Warnings and Precautions (5.2)]*.

Interstitial Lung Disease/Pneumonitis: TYKERB has been associated with interstitial lung disease and pneumonitis in monotherapy or in combination with other chemotherapies *[see Warnings and Precautions (5.5)]*.

6.2 Postmarketing Experience

The following adverse reactions have been identified during post-approval use of TYKERB. Because these reactions are reported voluntarily from a population of uncertain size, it is not always possible to reliably estimate their frequency or establish a causal relationship to drug exposure.

Immune System Disorders: Hypersensitivity reactions including anaphylaxis *[see Contraindications (4)]*.

Skin and Subcutaneous Tissue Disorders: Nail disorders including paronychia.

7 DRUG INTERACTIONS

7.1 Effects of Lapatinib on Drug Metabolizing Enzymes and Drug Transport Systems

Lapatinib inhibits CYP3A4, CYP2C8, and P-glycoprotein (P-gp, ABCB1) in vitro at clinically relevant concentrations and is a weak inhibitor of CYP3A4 in vivo. Caution should be exercised and dose reduction of the concomitant substrate drug should be considered when dosing TYKERB concurrently with medications with narrow therapeutic windows that are substrates of CYP3A4, CYP2C8, or P-gp. Lapatinib did not significantly inhibit the following enzymes in human liver microsomes: CYP1A2, CYP2C9, CYP2C19, and CYP2D6 or UGT enzymes in vitro, however, the clinical significance is unknown.

Midazolam: Following coadministration of TYKERB and midazolam (CYP3A4 substrate), 24-hour systemic exposure (AUC) of orally administered midazolam increased 45%, while 24-hour AUC of intravenously administered midazolam increased 22%.

Paclitaxel: In cancer patients receiving TYKERB and paclitaxel (CYP2C8 and P-gp substrate), 24-hour systemic exposure (AUC) of paclitaxel was increased 23%. This increase in paclitaxel exposure may have been underestimated from the in vivo evaluation due to study design limitations.

Digoxin: Following coadministration of TYKERB and digoxin (P-gp substrate), systemic AUC of an oral digoxin dose increased approximately 2.8-fold. Serum digoxin concentrations should be monitored prior to initiation of TYKERB and throughout coadministration. If digoxin serum concentration is >1.2 ng/mL, the digoxin dose should be reduced by half.

7.2 Drugs that Inhibit or Induce Cytochrome P450 3A4 Enzymes

Lapatinib undergoes extensive metabolism by CYP3A4, and concomitant administration of strong inhibitors or inducers of CYP3A4 alter lapatinib concentrations significantly *(see Ketoconazole and Carbamazepine sections, below)*. Dose adjustment of lapatinib should be considered for patients who must receive concomitant strong inhibitors or concomitant strong inducers of CYP3A4 enzymes *[see Dosage and Administration (2.2)]*.

Ketoconazole: In healthy subjects receiving ketoconazole, a CYP3A4 inhibitor, at 200 mg twice daily for 7 days, systemic exposure (AUC) to lapatinib was increased to approximately 3.6-fold of control and half-life increased to 1.7-fold of control.

Carbamazepine: In healthy subjects receiving the CYP3A4 inducer, carbamazepine, at 100 mg twice daily for 3 days and 200 mg twice daily for 17 days, systemic exposure (AUC) to lapatinib was decreased approximately 72%.

7.3 Drugs that Inhibit Drug Transport Systems

Lapatinib is a substrate of the efflux transporter P-glycoprotein (P-gp, ABCB1). If TYKERB is administered with drugs that inhibit P-gp, increased concentrations of lapatinib are likely, and caution should be exercised.

7.4 Acid Reducing Agents

The aqueous solubility of lapatinib is pH dependent, with higher pH resulting in lower solubility. However, esomeprazole, a proton pump inhibitor, administered at a dose of 40 mg once daily for 7 days, did not result in a clinically meaningful reduction in lapatinib steady-state exposure.

8 USE IN SPECIFIC POPULATIONS

8.1 Pregnancy

Pregnancy Category D *[see Warnings and Precautions (5.7)]*.

Based on findings in animals, TYKERB can cause fetal harm when administered to a pregnant woman. Lapatinib administered to rats during organogenesis and through lactation led to death of offspring within the first 4 days after birth. When administered to pregnant animals during the period of organogenesis, lapatinib caused fetal anomalies (rats) or abortions (rabbits) at maternally toxic doses. There are no adequate and well-controlled studies with TYKERB in pregnant women. Women should be advised not to become pregnant when taking TYKERB. If this drug is used during pregnancy, or if the patient becomes pregnant while taking this drug, the patient should be apprised of the potential hazard to the fetus.

In a study where pregnant rats were dosed with lapatinib during organogenesis and through lactation, at a dose of 120 mg/kg/day (approximately 6.4 times the human clinical exposure based on AUC following 1,250 mg dose of lapatinib plus capecitabine), 91% of the pups had died by the fourth day after birth, while 34% of the 60 mg/kg/day pups were dead. The highest no-effect dose for this study was 20 mg/kg/day (approximately equal to the human clinical exposure based on AUC).

Lapatinib was studied for effects on embryo-fetal development in pregnant rats and rabbits given oral doses of 30, 60, and 120 mg/kg/day. There were no teratogenic effects; however, minor anomalies (left-sided umbilical artery, cervical rib, and precocious ossification) occurred in rats at the maternally toxic dose of 120 mg/kg/day (approximately 6.4 times the human clinical exposure based on AUC following 1,250 mg dose of lapatinib plus capecitabine). In rabbits, lapatinib was associated with maternal toxicity at 60 and 120 mg/kg/day (approximately 0.07 and 0.2 times the human clinical exposure, respectively, based on AUC following 1,250 mg dose of lapatinib plus capecitabine) and abortions at 120 mg/kg/day. Maternal toxicity was associated with decreased fetal body weights and minor skeletal variations.

8.3 Nursing Mothers

It is not known whether lapatinib is excreted in human milk. Because many drugs are excreted in human milk and because of the potential for serious adverse reactions in nursing infants from TYKERB, a decision should be made whether to discontinue nursing or to discontinue the drug, taking into account the importance of the drug to the mother.

8.4 Pediatric Use

The safety and effectiveness of TYKERB in pediatric patients have not been established.

8.5 Geriatric Use

Of the total number of metastatic breast cancer patients in clinical studies of TYKERB in combination with capecitabine (N = 198), 17% were 65 years of age and older, and 1% were 75 years of age and older. Of the total number of hormone receptor positive, HER2 positive metastatic breast cancer patients in clinical studies of TYKERB in combination with letrozole (N = 642), 44% were 65 years of age and older, and 12% were 75 years of age and older. No overall differences in safety or effectiveness were observed between elderly subjects and younger subjects, and other reported clinical experience has not identified differences in responses between the elderly and younger patients, but greater sensitivity of some older individuals cannot be ruled out.

8.6 Renal Impairment

Lapatinib pharmacokinetics have not been specifically studied in patients with renal impairment or in patients undergoing hemodialysis. There is no experience with TYKERB in patients with severe renal impairment. However, renal impairment is unlikely to affect the pharmacokinetics of lapatinib given that less than 2% (lapatinib and metabolites) of an administered dose is eliminated by the kidneys.

Table 4. Selected Laboratory Abnormalities

	TYKERB 1,500 mg/day + Letrozole 2.5 mg/day			Letrozole 2.5 mg/day		
	All Grades[a]	Grade 3	Grade 4	All Grades[a]	Grade 3	Grade 4
Hepatic Parameters	%	%	%	%	%	%
AST	53	6	0	36	2	<1
ALT	46	5	<1	35	1	0
Total Bilirubin	22	<1	<1	11	1	<1

[a] National Cancer Institute Common Terminology Criteria for Adverse Events, version 3.

8.7 Hepatic Impairment

The pharmacokinetics of lapatinib were examined in subjects with pre-existing moderate (n = 8) or severe (n = 4) hepatic impairment (Child-Pugh Class B/C, respectively) and in 8 healthy control subjects. Systemic exposure (AUC) to lapatinib after a single oral 100-mg dose increased approximately 14% and 63% in subjects with moderate and severe pre-existing hepatic impairment, respectively. Administration of TYKERB in patients with severe hepatic impairment should be undertaken with caution due to increased exposure to the drug. A dose reduction should be considered for patients with severe pre-existing hepatic impairment *[see Dosage and Administration (2.2)]*. In patients who develop severe hepatotoxicity while on therapy, TYKERB should be discontinued and patients should not be retreated with TYKERB *[see Warnings and Precautions (5.2)]*.

10 OVERDOSAGE

There is no known antidote for overdoses of TYKERB. The maximum oral doses of lapatinib that have been administered in clinical trials are 1,800 mg once daily. More frequent ingestion of TYKERB could result in serum concentrations exceeding those observed in clinical trials and could result in increased toxicity. Therefore, missed doses should not be replaced and dosing should resume with the next scheduled daily dose.

Asymptomatic and symptomatic cases of overdose have been reported. The doses ranged from 2,500 to 9,000 mg daily and where reported, the duration varied between 1 and 17 days. Symptoms observed include lapatinib-associated events *[see Adverse Reactions (6.1)]* and in some cases sore scalp, sinus tachycardia (with otherwise normal ECG) and/or mucosal inflammation.

Because lapatinib is not significantly renally excreted and is highly bound to plasma proteins, hemodialysis would not be expected to be an effective method to enhance the elimination of lapatinib.

Treatment of overdose with TYKERB should consist of general supportive measures.

11 DESCRIPTION

Lapatinib is a small molecule and a member of the 4-anilinoquinazoline class of kinase inhibitors. It is present as the monohydrate of the ditosylate salt, with chemical name *N*-(3-chloro-4-{[(3-fluorophenyl)methyl]oxy}phenyl)-6-[5-({[2-(methylsulfonyl)ethyl]amino}methyl)-2-furanyl]-4-quinazolinamine bis(4-methylbenzenesulfonate) monohydrate. It has the molecular formula $C_{29}H_{26}ClFN_4O_4S$ $(C_7H_8O_3S)_2$ H_2O and a molecular weight of 943.5. Lapatinib ditosylate monohydrate has the following chemical structure:

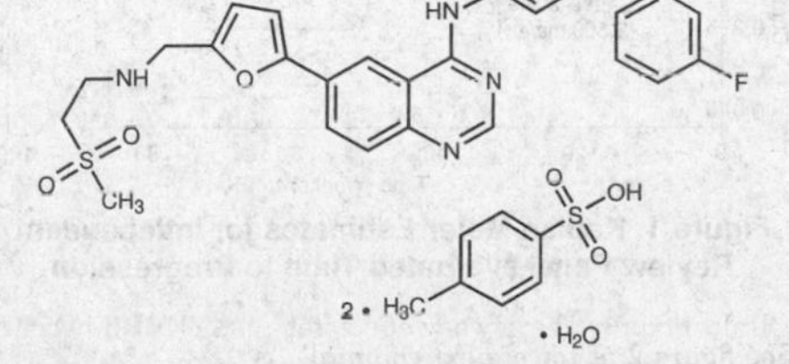

Lapatinib is a yellow solid, and its solubility in water is 0.007 mg/mL and in 0.1N HCl is 0.001 mg/mL at 25°C.

Each 250 mg tablet of TYKERB contains 405 mg of lapatinib ditosylate monohydrate, equivalent to 398 mg of lapatinib ditosylate or 250 mg lapatinib free base.

The inactive ingredients of TYKERB are: **Tablet Core:** Magnesium stearate, microcrystalline cellulose, povidone, sodium starch glycolate. **Coating:** Orange film-coat: FD&C yellow No. 6/sunset yellow FCF aluminum lake, hypromellose, macrogol/PEG 400, polysorbate 80, titanium dioxide.

12 CLINICAL PHARMACOLOGY

12.1 Mechanism of Action

Lapatinib is a 4-anilinoquinazoline kinase inhibitor of the intracellular tyrosine kinase domains of both Epidermal Growth Factor Receptor (EGFR [ErbB1]) and of Human Epidermal Receptor Type 2 (HER2 [ErbB2]) receptors (estimated K_i^{app}values of 3nM and 13nM, respectively) with a dissociation half-life of ≥300 minutes. Lapatinib inhibits ErbB-driven tumor cell growth in vitro and in various animal models.

An additive effect was demonstrated in an in vitro study when lapatinib and 5-FU (the active metabolite of capecitabine) were used in combination in the 4 tumor cell lines tested. The growth inhibitory effects of lapatinib were evaluated in trastuzumab-conditioned cell lines. Lapatinib retained significant activity against breast cancer cell lines selected for long-term growth in trastuzumab-containing medium in vitro. These in vitro findings suggest non-cross-resistance between these two agents.

Hormone receptor positive breast cancer cells (with ER [Estrogen Receptor] and/or PgR [Progesterone Receptor]) that coexpress the HER2 tend to be resistant to established endocrine therapies. Similarly, hormone receptor positive breast cancer cells that initially lack EGFR or HER2 upregulate these receptor proteins as the tumor becomes resistant to endocrine therapy.

12.3 Pharmacokinetics

Absorption: Absorption following oral administration of TYKERB is incomplete and variable. Serum concentrations appear after a median lag time of 0.25 hours (range 0 to 1.5 hour). Peak plasma concentrations (C_{max}) of lapatinib are achieved approximately 4 hours after administration. Daily dosing of TYKERB results in achievement of steady state within 6 to 7 days, indicating an effective half-life of 24 hours.

At the dose of 1,250 mg daily, steady state geometric mean (95% confidence interval) values of C_{max} were 2.43 mcg/mL (1.57 to 3.77 mcg/mL) and AUC were 36.2 mcg.hr/mL (23.4 to 56 mcg.hr/mL).

Divided daily doses of TYKERB resulted in approximately 2-fold higher exposure at steady state (steady state AUC) compared to the same total dose administered once daily.

Systemic exposure to lapatinib is increased when administered with food. Lapatinib AUC values were approximately 3- and 4-fold higher (C_{max} approximately 2.5- and 3-fold higher) when administered with a low fat (5% fat-500 calories) or with a high fat (50% fat-1,000 calories) meal, respectively.

Distribution: Lapatinib is highly bound (>99%) to albumin and alpha-1 acid glycoprotein. In vitro studies indicate that lapatinib is a substrate for the transporters breast cancer resistance protein (BCRP, ABCG2) and P-glycoprotein (P-gp, ABCB1). Lapatinib has also been shown to inhibit P-gp, BCRP, and the hepatic uptake transporter OATP 1B1, in vitro at clinically relevant concentrations.

Metabolism: Lapatinib undergoes extensive metabolism, primarily by CYP3A4 and CYP3A5, with minor contributions from CYP2C19 and CYP2C8 to a variety of oxidated metabolites, none of which accounts for more than 14% of the dose recovered in the feces or 10% of lapatinib concentration in plasma.

Elimination: At clinical doses, the terminal phase half-life following a single dose was 14.2 hours; accumulation with repeated dosing indicates an effective half-life of 24 hours. Elimination of lapatinib is predominantly through metabolism by CYP3A4/5 with negligible (<2%) renal excretion. Recovery of parent lapatinib in feces accounts for a median of 27% (range 3 to 67%) of an oral dose.

Effects of Age, Gender, or Race: Studies of the effects of age, gender, or race on the pharmacokinetics of lapatinib have not been performed.

12.4 QT Prolongation

The QT prolongation potential of lapatinib was assessed as part of an uncontrolled, open-label dose escalation study in

Table 5. Efficacy Results

	Independent Assessment[a]		Investigator Assessment	
	TYKERB 1,250 mg/day + Capecitabine 2,000 mg/m²/day	Capecitabine 2,500 mg/m²/day	TYKERB 1,250 mg/day + Capecitabine 2,000 mg/m²/day	Capecitabine 2,500 mg/m²/day
	(N = 198)	(N = 201)	(N = 198)	(N = 201)
Number of TTP events	82	102	121	126
Median TTP, weeks (25th, 75th, Percentile), weeks	27.1 (17.4, 49.4)	18.6 (9.1, 36.9)	23.9 (12.0, 44.0)	18.3 (6.9, 35.7)
Hazard Ratio (95% CI) *P* value	0.57 (0.43, 0.77) 0.00013		0.72 (0.56, 0.92) 0.00762	
Response Rate (%) (95% CI)	23.7 (18.0, 30.3)	13.9 (9.5, 19.5)	31.8 (25.4, 38.8)	17.4 (12.4, 23.4)

TTP = Time to progression.
[a] The time from last tumor assessment to the data cut-off date was >100 days in approximately 30% of patients in the independent assessment. The pre-specified assessment interval was 42 or 84 days.

Table 7. Efficacy Results

	HER2(+) Population		HER2(-) Population	
	TYKERB 1500 mg/day + Letrozole 2.5 mg/day	Letrozole 2.5 mg/day	TYKERB 1500 mg/day + Letrozole 2.5 mg/day	Letrozole 2.5 mg/day
	(N = 111)	(N = 108)	(N = 478)	(N = 474)
Median PFS[a], weeks (95% CI)	35.4 (24.1, 39.4)	13.0 (12.0, 23.7)	59.7 (48.6, 69.7)	58.3 (47.9, 62.0)
Hazard Ratio (95% CI) ***P* value**	0.71 (0.53, 0.96) 0.019		0.90 (0.77, 1.05) 0.188	
Response Rate (%) (95% CI)	27.9 (19.8, 37.2)	14.8 (8.7, 22.9)	32.6 (28.4, 37.0)	31.6 (27.5, 36.0)

PFS = progression-free survival; CI = confidence interval.
[a] Kaplan-Meier estimate.

advanced cancer patients. Eighty-one patients received daily doses of lapatinib ranging from 175 mg/day to 1,800 mg/day. Serial ECGs were collected on Day 1 and Day 14 to evaluate the effect of lapatinib on QT intervals. Analysis of the data suggested a consistent concentration-dependent increase in QTc interval.

13 NONCLINICAL TOXICOLOGY

13.1 Carcinogenesis, Mutagenesis, Impairment of Fertility

Two-year carcinogenicity studies with lapatinib are ongoing.

Lapatinib was not clastogenic or mutagenic in the Chinese hamster ovary chromosome aberration assay, microbial mutagenesis (Ames) assay, human lymphocyte chromosome aberration assay or the in vivo rat bone marrow chromosome aberration assay at single doses up to 2,000 mg/kg. However, an impurity in the drug product (up to 4 ppm or 8 mcg/day) was genotoxic when tested alone in both in vitro and in vivo assays.

There were no effects on male or female rat mating or fertility at doses up to 120 mg/kg/day in females and 180 mg/kg/day in males (approximately 6.4 times and 2.6 times the expected human clinical exposure based on AUC following 1,250 mg dose of lapatinib plus capecitabine, respectively). The effect of lapatinib on human fertility is unknown. However, when female rats were given oral doses of lapatinib during breeding and through the first 6 days of gestation, a significant decrease in the number of live fetuses was seen at 120 mg/kg/day and in the fetal body weights at ≥60 mg/kg/day (approximately 6.4 times and 3.3 times the expected human clinical exposure based on AUC following 1,250 mg dose of lapatinib plus capecitabine, respectively).

14 CLINICAL STUDIES

14.1 HER2 Positive Metastatic Breast Cancer

The efficacy and safety of TYKERB in combination with capecitabine in breast cancer were evaluated in a randomized, Phase 3 trial. Patients eligible for enrollment had HER2 (ErbB2) overexpressing (IHC 3+ or IHC 2+ confirmed by FISH), locally advanced or metastatic breast cancer, progressing after prior treatment that included anthracyclines, taxanes, and trastuzumab.

Patients were randomized to receive either TYKERB 1,250 mg once daily (continuously) plus capecitabine 2,000 mg/m²/day on Days 1-14 every 21 days, or to receive capecitabine alone at a dose of 2,500 mg/m²/day on Days 1-14 every 21 days. The endpoint was time to progression (TTP). TTP was defined as time from randomization to tumor progression or death related to breast cancer. Based on the results of a pre-specified interim analysis, further enrollment was discontinued. Three hundred and ninety-nine (399) patients were enrolled in this study. The median age was 53 years and 14% were older than 65 years. Ninety-one percent (91%) were Caucasian. Ninety-seven percent (97%) had stage IV breast cancer, 48% were estrogen receptor+ (ER+) or progesterone receptor+ (PR+), and 95% were ErbB2 IHC 3+ or IHC 2+ with FISH confirmation. Approximately 95% of patients had prior treatment with anthracyclines, taxanes, and trastuzumab.

Efficacy analyses 4 months after the interim analysis are presented in Table 5, Figure 1, and Figure 2.

[See table 5 above]

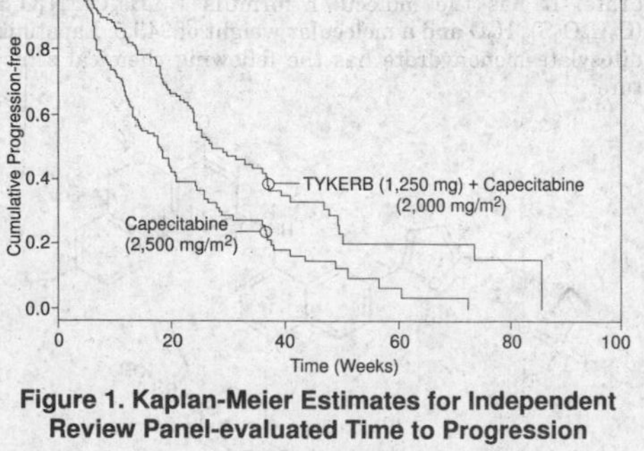

Figure 1. Kaplan-Meier Estimates for Independent Review Panel-evaluated Time to Progression

[See figure 2 at top of next column]

At the time of above efficacy analysis, the overall survival data were not mature (32% events). However, based on the TTP results, the study was unblinded and patients receiving capecitabine alone were allowed to cross over to TYKERB plus capecitabine treatment. The survival data were followed for an additional 2 years to be mature and the analysis is summarized in Table 6.

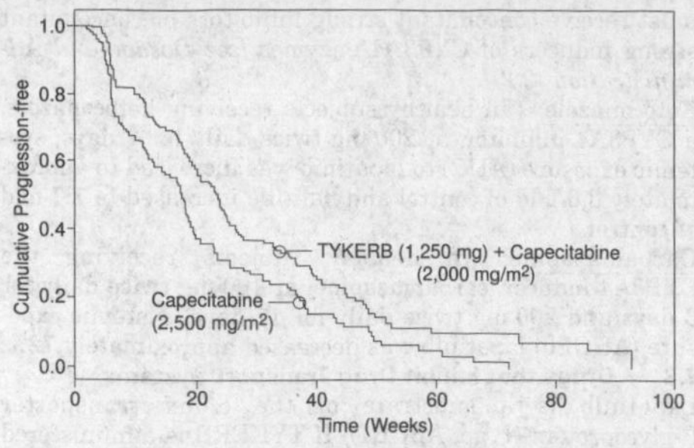

Figure 2. Kaplan-Meier Estimates for Investigator Assessment Time to Progression

Table 6: Overall Survival Data

	TYKERB 1,250 mg/day + Capecitabine 2,000 mg/m²/day (N = 207)	Capecitabine 2,500 mg/m²/day (N = 201)
Overall Survival		
Died	76%	82%
Median Overall Survival (weeks)	75.0	65.9
Hazard ratio, 95% CI (*P* value)	0.89 (0.71, 1.10) 0.276	

CI = confidence interval

14.2 Hormone Receptor Positive, HER2 Positive Metastatic Breast Cancer

The efficacy and safety of TYKERB in combination with letrozole were evaluated in a double-blind, placebo-controlled, multi-center study. A total of 1,286 postmenopausal women with hormone receptor positive (ER positive and/or PgR positive) metastatic breast cancer, who had not received prior therapy for metastatic disease, were randomly assigned to receive either TYKERB (1,500 mg once daily) plus letrozole (2.5 mg once daily) (n = 642) or letrozole (2.5 mg once daily) alone (n = 644). Of all patients randomized to treatment, 219 (17%) patients had tumors overexpressing the HER2 receptor, defined as fluorescence in situ hybridization (FISH) (≥2 or 3+ immunohistochemistry (IHC). There were 952 (74%) patients who were HER2 negative and 115 (9%) patients did not have their HER2 receptor status confirmed. The primary objective was to evaluate and compare progression-free survival (PFS) in the HER2 positive population. Progression-free survival was defined as the interval of time between date of randomization and the earlier date of first documented sign of disease progression or death due to any cause.

The baseline demographic and disease characteristics were balanced between the two treatment arms. The median age was 63 years and 45% were 65 years of age or older. Eighty-four percent (84%) of the patients were White. Approximately 50% of the HER2 positive population had prior adjuvant/neo-adjuvant chemotherapy and 56% had prior hormonal therapy. Only 2 patients had prior trastuzumab. In the HER2 positive subgroup (n = 219), the addition of TYKERB to letrozole resulted in an improvement in PFS. In the HER2 negative subgroup, there was no improvement in PFS of the TYKERB plus letrozole combination compared to the letrozole plus placebo. Overall response rate (ORR) was also improved with the TYKERB plus letrozole combination therapy. The overall survival (OS) data were not mature. Efficacy analyses for the hormone receptor positive, HER2 positive and HER2 negative subgroups are presented in Table 7 and Figure 3.

[See table 7 above]

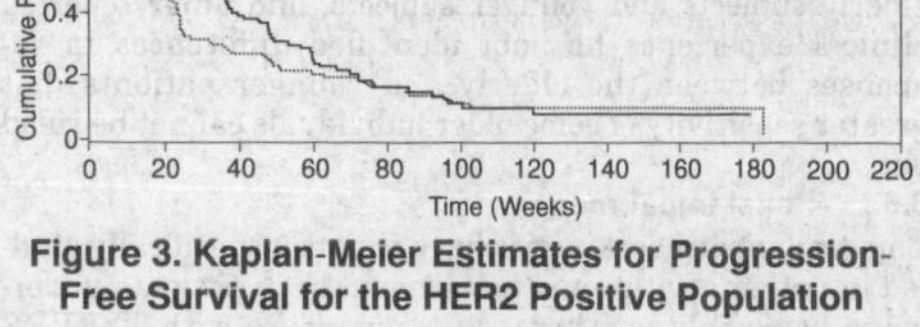

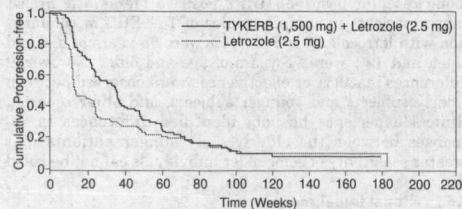

Figure 3. Kaplan-Meier Estimates for Progression-Free Survival for the HER2 Positive Population

16 HOW SUPPLIED/STORAGE AND HANDLING

The 250 mg tablets of TYKERB are oval, biconvex, orange, and film-coated with GS XJG debossed on one side and are available in:

Bottles of 150 tablets: NDC 0173-0752-00

Store at 25°C (77°F); excursions permitted to 15° to 30°C (59° to 86°F) [see USP Controlled Room Temperature].

17 PATIENT COUNSELING INFORMATION

See FDA-approved patient labeling (17.2).

17.1 Information for Patients

Patients should be informed of the following:

- TYKERB has been reported to decrease left ventricular ejection fraction which may result in shortness of breath, palpitations, and/or fatigue. Patients should inform their physician if they develop these symptoms while taking TYKERB.
- TYKERB often causes diarrhea which may be severe in some cases. Patients should be told how to manage and/or prevent diarrhea and to inform their physician immediately if there is any change in bowel patterns or severe diarrhea occurs during treatment with TYKERB.
- TYKERB may interact with many drugs; therefore, patients should be advised to report to their healthcare provider the use of any other prescription or nonprescription medication or herbal products.
- TYKERB may interact with grapefruit. Patients should not take TYKERB with grapefruit products.
- TYKERB should be taken at least one hour before or one hour after a meal, in contrast to capecitabine which should be taken with food or within 30 minutes after food.
- The dose of TYKERB should be taken once daily. Dividing the daily dose is not recommended.

17.2 FDA-Approved Patient Labeling

Patient labeling is provided as a tear-off leaflet at the end of this full prescribing information.

TYKERB is a registered trademark of GlaxoSmithKline.

GlaxoSmithKline
Research Triangle Park, NC 27709

TKB:12PI

PHARMACIST - DETACH HERE AND GIVE INSTRUCTIONS TO PATIENT

PATIENT INFORMATION

TYKERB (TIE-curb)
(lapatinib) tablets

Read this leaflet before you start taking TYKERB® and each time you get a refill. There may be new information. This information does not take the place of talking with your doctor about your medical condition or treatment.

What is TYKERB?

TYKERB is used with the medicine capecitabine for the treatment of patients with advanced or metastatic breast cancer that is HER2 positive (tumors that produce large amounts of a protein called human epidermal growth factor receptor-2), and who have already had certain other breast cancer treatments.

TYKERB is also used with a type of medicine called letrozole for the treatment of postmenopausal women with hormone receptor positive, HER2 positive metastatic breast cancer for whom hormonal therapy is indicated. TYKERB in combination with an aromatase inhibitor has not been compared to a trastuzumab-containing chemotherapy regimen for the treatment of metastatic breast cancer.

Who should not take TYKERB?

Do not take TYKERB if you are allergic to any of its ingredients. See the end of this leaflet for a list of ingredients in TYKERB.

Before you start taking TYKERB, tell your doctor about all of your medical conditions, including if you:

- ever had a severe allergic (hypersensitivity) reaction to TYKERB. Check with your doctor if you think this applies to you. Don't take TYKERB.
- have heart problems.
- have liver problems. You may need a lower dose of TYKERB.
- are pregnant or may become pregnant. TYKERB may harm an unborn baby. If you become pregnant during treatment with TYKERB, tell your doctor as soon as possible.
- are breast-feeding. It is not known if TYKERB passes into your breast milk or if it can harm your baby. If you are a woman who has or will have a baby, talk with your doctor about the best way to feed your baby.

Tell your doctor about all the medicines you take, including prescription and nonprescription medicines, vitamins, and herbal and dietary supplements. TYKERB and many other medicines may interact with each other. Your doctor needs to know what medicines you take so he or she can choose the right dose of TYKERB for you.

Especially tell your doctor if you take:

- antibiotics and anti-fungals (drugs used to treat infections)
- HIV (AIDS) treatments
- anticonvulsant drugs (drugs used to treat seizures)
- calcium channel blockers (drugs used to treat certain heart disorders or high blood pressure)
- antidepressants
- drugs that decrease stomach acidity
- St. John's Wort or other herbal supplements

Know the medicines you take. Keep a list of your medicines with you to show your doctor. Do not take other medicines during treatment with TYKERB without first checking with your doctor.

Because TYKERB is given with other drugs called capecitabine or letrozole, you should also discuss with your doctor or pharmacist any medicines that should be avoided during treatment.

How should I take TYKERB?

- Take TYKERB exactly as your doctor tells you to take it. Your doctor may change your dose of TYKERB if needed.
  - For patients with advanced or metastatic breast cancer, TYKERB and capecitabine are taken in 21 day cycles. The usual dose of TYKERB is 1,250 mg (5 tablets) taken by mouth all at once, **one time a day on days 1 to 21**. Your doctor will tell you the dose of capecitabine you should take and when you should take it.
  - For patients with hormone receptor positive, HER2 positive breast cancer, TYKERB and letrozole are taken daily. The usual dose of TYKERB is 1,500 mg (6 tablets) taken by mouth all at once, **one time a day**. Your doctor will tell you the dose of letrozole you should take and when you should take it.
- TYKERB should be taken at least one hour before, or at least one hour after food.
- Do not eat or drink grapefruit products while taking TYKERB.
- If you forget to take your dose of TYKERB, do not take two doses at one time. Take your next dose at your scheduled time.
- If you take too much TYKERB, call your doctor or poison control center, or go to the nearest hospital emergency room right away. Take TYKERB tablets with you when possible.

What are the possible side effects of TYKERB?

Serious side effects include:

- **heart problems** including, decreased pumping of blood from the heart and an abnormal heartbeat. Signs and symptoms of an abnormal heartbeat include:
  - feeling like your heart is pounding or racing
  - dizziness
  - tiredness
  - feeling lightheaded
  - shortness of breath
  - ■ Your doctor should check your heart function before you start taking TYKERB and during treatment.
- **liver problems.** Signs and symptoms of liver problems include:
  - itching
  - yellow eyes or skin
  - dark urine
  - pain or discomfort in the right upper stomach area
  - death
  - ■ Your doctor should do blood tests to check your liver before you start taking TYKERB and during treatment.
- **diarrhea**, which may cause you to become dehydrated. Follow your doctors instructions for what to do to help prevent or treat diarrhea. Call your doctor immediately at the first sign of diarrhea, as it is important that this is treated right away.
- **lung problems.** Symptoms of a lung problem with TYKERB include a cough that will not go away or shortness of breath.

Call your doctor right away if you have any of the signs or symptoms of the serious side effects listed above.

Common side effects of TYKERB in combination with capecitabine or letrozole include:

- diarrhea
- red, painful hands and feet
- nausea
- rash
- vomiting
- tiredness or weakness
- mouth sores
- loss of appetite
- indigestion
- unusual hair loss or thinning
- nose bleeds
- headache
- dry skin
- itching
- nail disorders such as nail bed changes, nail pain, infection and swelling of the cuticles.

Tell your doctor about any side effect that gets serious or that does not go away.

These are not all the side effects with TYKERB. Ask your doctor or pharmacist for more information.

Call your doctor for medical advice about side effects. You may report side effects to FDA at 1-800-FDA-1088.

You may also get side effects from the other drugs taken with TYKERB. Talk to your doctor about possible side effects you may get during treatment.

How should I store TYKERB tablets?

- Store TYKERB tablets at room temperature at 59° to 86°F (15° to 30°C). Keep the container closed tightly.
- Do not keep medicine that is out of date or that you no longer need. Be sure that if you throw any medicine away, it is out of the reach of children.
- **Keep TYKERB and all medicines out of the reach of children.**

General information about TYKERB

Medicines are sometimes prescribed for conditions that are not mentioned in patient information leaflets. Do not use TYKERB for any other condition for which it was not prescribed. Do not give TYKERB to other people, even if they have the same condition that you have. It may harm them.

This leaflet summarizes the most important information about TYKERB. If you would like more information, talk with your doctor. You can ask your doctor or pharmacist for information about TYKERB that is written for health professionals. For more information, you can call toll-free 1-888-825-5249 or by visiting the website www.tykerb.com.

What are the ingredients in TYKERB?

Active Ingredient: Lapatinib.

Inactive Ingredients: Tablet Core: Magnesium stearate, microcrystalline cellulose, povidone, sodium starch glycolate. **Coating:** Orange film-coat: FD&C yellow #6/sunset yellow FCF aluminum lake, hypromellose, macrogol/PEG 400, polysorbate 80, titanium dioxide.

TYKERB tablets are oval, biconvex, orange, film-coated with GS XJG printed on one side.

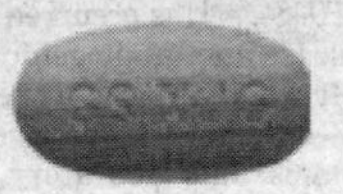

TYKERB is a registered trademark of GlaxoSmithKline.

GlaxoSmithKline
Research Triangle Park, NC 27709

Revised: June 2013

TKB:10PIL

VALTREX ℞

[*val'trĕx*]

(valacyclovir hydrochloride)
Caplets

HIGHLIGHTS OF PRESCRIBING INFORMATION

These highlights do not include all the information needed to use VALTREX safely and effectively. See full prescribing information for VALTREX.

VALTREX (valacyclovir hydrochloride) Caplets
Initial U.S. Approval: 1995

INDICATIONS AND USAGE

VALTREX is a nucleoside analogue DNA polymerase inhibitor indicated for:

Adult Patients (1.1)

- Cold Sores (Herpes Labialis)
- Genital Herpes
  - Treatment in immunocompetent patients (initial or recurrent episode)
  - Suppression in immunocompetent or HIV-1 infected patients
  - Reduction of transmission
- Herpes Zoster

Pediatric Patients (1.2)

- Cold Sores (Herpes Labialis)
- Chickenpox

Limitations of Use (1.3)

- The efficacy and safety of VALTREX have not been established in immunocompromised patients other than for the suppression of genital herpes in HIV-1 infected patients.

DOSAGE AND ADMINISTRATION

Adult Dosage (2.1)

Cold Sores	2 grams every 12 hours for 1 day
Genital Herpes	
Initial episode	1 gram twice daily for 10 days
Recurrent episodes	500 mg twice daily for 3 days

Suppressive therapy Immunocompetent patients	1 gram once daily
Alternate dose in patients with less than or equal to 9 recurrences/year	500 mg once daily
HIV-1 infected patients	500 mg twice daily
Reduction of transmission	500 mg once daily
Herpes Zoster	1 gram 3 times daily for 7 days
Pediatric Dosage (2.2)	
Cold Sores (aged greater than or equal to 12 years)	2 grams every 12 hours for 1 day
Chickenpox (aged 2 to less than 18 years)	20 mg/kg 3 times daily for 5 days; not to exceed 1 gram 3 times daily

Valacyclovir oral suspension (25 mg/mL or 50 mg/mL) can be prepared from the 500 mg VALTREX Caplets. (2.3).

DOSAGE FORMS AND STRENGTHS

Caplets: 500 mg (unscored), 1 gram (partially scored) (3)

CONTRAINDICATIONS

Hypersensitivity to valacyclovir (e.g., anaphylaxis), acyclovir, or any component of the formulation. (4)

WARNINGS AND PRECAUTIONS

- Thrombotic thrombocytopenic purpura/hemolytic uremic syndrome (TTP/HUS): Has occurred in patients with advanced HIV-1 disease and in allogenic bone marrow transplant and renal transplant patients receiving 8 grams per day of VALTREX in clinical trials. Discontinue treatment if clinical symptoms and laboratory findings consistent with TTP/HUS occur. (5.1)
- Acute renal failure: May occur in elderly patients (with or without reduced renal function), patients with underlying renal disease who receive higher than recommended doses of VALTREX for their level of renal function, patients who receive concomitant nephrotoxic drugs, or inadequately hydrated patients. Use with caution in elderly patients and reduce dosage in patients with renal impairment. (2.4, 5.2)
- Central nervous system adverse reactions (e.g., agitation, hallucinations, confusion, and encephalopathy): May occur in both adult and pediatric patients (with or without reduced renal function) and in patients with underlying renal disease who receive higher than recommended doses of VALTREX for their level of renal function. Elderly patients are more likely to have central nervous system adverse reactions. Use with caution in elderly patients and reduce dosage in patients with renal impairment. (2.4, 5.3)

ADVERSE REACTIONS

- **The most common adverse reactions reported in at least one indication by greater than 10% of adult subjects treated with VALTREX and more commonly than in subjects treated with placebo are headache, nausea, and abdominal pain. (6.1)**
- **The only adverse reaction occurring in greater than 10% of pediatric subjects less than 18 years of age was headache. (6.2)**

To report SUSPECTED ADVERSE REACTIONS, contact GlaxoSmithKline at 1-888-825-5249 or FDA at 1-800-FDA-1088 or www.fda.gov/medwatch.

See 17 for PATIENT COUNSELING INFORMATION and FDA-approved patient labeling

Revised: 01/2013

FULL PRESCRIBING INFORMATION: CONTENTS*

*** Sections or subsections omitted from the full prescribing information are not listed**

FULL PRESCRIBING INFORMATION

1 INDICATIONS AND USAGE

1.1 Adult Patients

Cold Sores (Herpes Labialis): VALTREX® (valacyclovir hydrochloride) Caplets are indicated for treatment of cold sores (herpes labialis). The efficacy of VALTREX initiated after the development of clinical signs of a cold sore (e.g., papule, vesicle, or ulcer) has not been established.

Genital Herpes: *Initial Episode:* VALTREX is indicated for treatment of the initial episode of genital herpes in immunocompetent adults. The efficacy of treatment with VALTREX when initiated more than 72 hours after the onset of signs and symptoms has not been established.

Recurrent Episodes: VALTREX is indicated for treatment of recurrent episodes of genital herpes in immunocompetent adults. The efficacy of treatment with VALTREX when initiated more than 24 hours after the onset of signs and symptoms has not been established.

Suppressive Therapy: VALTREX is indicated for chronic suppressive therapy of recurrent episodes of genital herpes in immunocompetent and in HIV-1 infected adults. The efficacy and safety of VALTREX for the suppression of genital herpes beyond 1 year in immunocompetent patients and beyond 6 months in HIV-1 infected patients have not been established.

Reduction of Transmission: VALTREX is indicated for the reduction of transmission of genital herpes in immunocompetent adults. The efficacy of VALTREX for the reduction of transmission of genital herpes beyond 8 months in discordant couples has not been established. The efficacy of VALTREX for the reduction of transmission of genital herpes in individuals with multiple partners and non-heterosexual couples has not been established. Safer sex practices should be used with suppressive therapy (see current Centers for Disease Control and Prevention [CDC] *Sexually Transmitted Diseases Treatment Guidelines*).

Herpes Zoster: VALTREX is indicated for the treatment of herpes zoster (shingles) in immunocompetent adults. The efficacy of VALTREX when initiated more than 72 hours after the onset of rash and the efficacy and safety of VALTREX for treatment of disseminated herpes zoster have not been established.

1.2 Pediatric Patients

Cold Sores (Herpes Labialis): VALTREX is indicated for the treatment of cold sores (herpes labialis) in pediatric patients aged greater than or equal to 12 years. The efficacy of VALTREX initiated after the development of clinical signs of a cold sore (e.g., papule, vesicle, or ulcer) has not been established.

Chickenpox: VALTREX is indicated for the treatment of chickenpox in immunocompetent pediatric patients aged 2 to less than 18 years. Based on efficacy data from clinical trials with oral acyclovir, treatment with VALTREX should be initiated within 24 hours after the onset of rash *[see Clinical Studies (14.4)]*.

1.3 Limitations of Use

The efficacy and safety of VALTREX have not been established in:

- Immunocompromised patients other than for the suppression of genital herpes in HIV-1 infected patients with a CD4+ cell count greater than or equal to 100 cells/mm^3.
- Patients aged less than 12 years with cold sores (herpes labialis).
- Patients aged less than 2 years or greater than or equal to 18 years with chickenpox.
- Patients aged less than 18 years with genital herpes.
- Patients aged less than 18 years with herpes zoster.
- Neonates and infants as suppressive therapy following neonatal herpes simplex virus (HSV) infection.

2 DOSAGE AND ADMINISTRATION

- VALTREX may be given without regard to meals.
- Valacyclovir oral suspension (25 mg/mL or 50 mg/mL) may be prepared extemporaneously from 500-mg VALTREX Caplets for use in pediatric patients for whom a solid dosage form is not appropriate *[see Dosage and Administration (2.3)]*.

2.1 Adult Dosing Recommendations

Cold Sores (Herpes Labialis): The recommended dosage of VALTREX for treatment of cold sores is 2 grams twice daily for 1 day taken 12 hours apart. Therapy should be initiated at the earliest symptom of a cold sore (e.g., tingling, itching, or burning).

Genital Herpes: *Initial Episode:* The recommended dosage of VALTREX for treatment of initial genital herpes is 1 gram twice daily for 10 days. Therapy was most effective when administered within 48 hours of the onset of signs and symptoms.

Recurrent Episodes: The recommended dosage of VALTREX for treatment of recurrent genital herpes is 500 mg twice daily for 3 days. Initiate treatment at the first sign or symptom of an episode.

Suppressive Therapy: The recommended dosage of VALTREX for chronic suppressive therapy of recurrent genital herpes is 1 gram once daily in patients with normal immune function. In patients with a history of 9 or fewer recurrences per year, an alternative dose is 500 mg once daily. In HIV-1 infected patients with a CD4+ cell count greater than or equal to 100 cells/mm^3, the recommended dosage of VALTREX for chronic suppressive therapy of recurrent genital herpes is 500 mg twice daily.

Reduction of Transmission: The recommended dosage of VALTREX for reduction of transmission of genital herpes in patients with a history of 9 or fewer recurrences per year is 500 mg once daily for the source partner.

Herpes Zoster: The recommended dosage of VALTREX for treatment of herpes zoster is 1 gram 3 times daily for 7 days. Therapy should be initiated at the earliest sign or symptom of herpes zoster and is most effective when started within 48 hours of the onset of rash.

2.2 Pediatric Dosing Recommendations

Cold Sores (Herpes Labialis): The recommended dosage of VALTREX for the treatment of cold sores in pediatric patients aged greater than or equal to 12 years is 2 grams twice daily for 1 day taken 12 hours apart. Therapy should be initiated at the earliest symptom of a cold sore (e.g., tingling, itching, or burning).

Chickenpox: The recommended dosage of VALTREX for treatment of chickenpox in immunocompetent pediatric patients aged 2 to less than 18 years is 20 mg/kg administered 3 times daily for 5 days. The total dose should not exceed 1 gram 3 times daily. Therapy should be initiated at the earliest sign or symptom *[see Use in Specific Populations (8.4), Clinical Pharmacology (12.3), Clinical Studies (14.4)]*.

2.3 Extemporaneous Preparation of Oral Suspension

Ingredients and Preparation per USP-NF: VALTREX Caplets 500 mg, cherry flavor, and Suspension Structured Vehicle USP-NF (SSV). Valacyclovir oral suspension (25 mg/mL or 50 mg/mL) should be prepared in lots of 100 mL.

Prepare Suspension at Time of Dispensing as Follows:

- Prepare SSV according to the USP-NF.
- Using a pestle and mortar, grind the required number of VALTREX 500 mg Caplets until a fine powder is produced (5 VALTREX Caplets for 25 mg/mL suspension; 10 VALTREX Caplets for 50 mg/mL suspension).
- Gradually add approximately 5-mL aliquots of SSV to the mortar and triturate the powder until a paste has been produced. Ensure that the powder has been adequately wetted.
- Continue to add approximately 5-mL aliquots of SSV to the mortar, mixing thoroughly between additions, until a concentrated suspension is produced, to a minimum total quantity of 20 mL SSV and a maximum total quantity of 40 mL SSV for both the 25-mg/mL and 50-mg/mL suspensions.
- Transfer the mixture to a suitable 100-mL measuring flask.
- Transfer the cherry flavor* to the mortar and dissolve in approximately 5 mL of SSV. Once dissolved, add to the measuring flask.
- Rinse the mortar at least 3 times with approximately 5-mL aliquots of SSV, transferring the rinsing to the measuring flask between additions.

- Make the suspension to volume (100 mL) with SSV and shake thoroughly to mix.
- Transfer the suspension to an amber glass medicine bottle with a child-resistant closure.
- The prepared suspension should be labeled with the following information "Shake well before using. Store suspension between 2° to 8°C (36° to 46°F) in a refrigerator. Discard after 28 days."

*The amount of cherry flavor added is as instructed by the suppliers of the cherry flavor.

2.4 Patients With Renal Impairment

Dosage recommendations for adult patients with reduced renal function are provided in Table 1 *[see Use in Specific Populations (8.5, 8.6), Clinical Pharmacology (12.3)]*. Data are not available for the use of VALTREX in pediatric patients with a creatinine clearance less than 50 mL/min/1.73 m^2.

[See table 1 above]

Table 1. VALTREX Dosage Recommendations for Adults With Renal Impairment

Indications	Normal Dosage Regimen (Creatinine Clearance ≥50 mL/min)	Creatinine Clearance (mL/min)		
		30-49	10-29	<10
Cold sores (Herpes labialis) **Do not exceed 1 day of treatment.**	Two 2 gram doses taken 12 hours apart	Two 1 gram doses taken 12 hours apart	Two 500 mg doses taken 12 hours apart	500 mg single dose
Genital herpes: Initial episode	1 gram every 12 hours	no reduction	1 gram every 24 hours	500 mg every 24 hours
Genital herpes: Recurrent episode	500 mg every 12 hours	no reduction	500 mg every 24 hours	500 mg every 24 hours
Genital herpes: Suppressive therapy				
Immunocompetent patients	1 gram every 24 hours	no reduction	500 mg every 24 hours	500 mg every 24 hours
Alternate dose for immunocompetent patients with less than or equal to 9 recurrences/year	500 mg every 24 hours	no reduction	500 mg every 48 hours	500 mg every 48 hours
HIV-1 infected patients	500 mg every 12 hours	no reduction	500 mg every 24 hours	500 mg every 24 hours
Herpes zoster	1 gram every 8 hours	1 gram every 12 hours	1 gram every 24 hours	500 mg every 24 hours

Hemodialysis: Patients requiring hemodialysis should receive the recommended dose of VALTREX after hemodialysis. During hemodialysis, the half-life of acyclovir after administration of VALTREX is approximately 4 hours. About one-third of acyclovir in the body is removed by dialysis during a 4-hour hemodialysis session.

Peritoneal Dialysis: There is no information specific to administration of VALTREX in patients receiving peritoneal dialysis. The effect of chronic ambulatory peritoneal dialysis (CAPD) and continuous arteriovenous hemofiltration/dialysis (CAVHD) on acyclovir pharmacokinetics has been studied. The removal of acyclovir after CAPD and CAVHD is less pronounced than with hemodialysis, and the pharmacokinetic parameters closely resemble those observed in patients with end-stage renal disease (ESRD) not receiving hemodialysis. Therefore, supplemental doses of VALTREX should not be required following CAPD or CAVHD.

3 DOSAGE FORMS AND STRENGTHS

Caplets:
- 500-mg: blue, film-coated, capsule-shaped tablets printed with "VALTREX 500 mg."
- 1-gram: blue, film-coated, capsule-shaped tablets, with a partial scorebar on both sides, printed with "VALTREX 1 gram."

4 CONTRAINDICATIONS

VALTREX is contraindicated in patients who have had a demonstrated clinically significant hypersensitivity reaction (e.g., anaphylaxis) to valacyclovir, acyclovir, or any component of the formulation *[see Adverse Reactions (6.3)]*.

5 WARNINGS AND PRECAUTIONS

5.1 Thrombotic Thrombocytopenic Purpura/Hemolytic Uremic Syndrome (TTP/HUS)

TTP/HUS, in some cases resulting in death, has occurred in patients with advanced HIV-1 disease and also in allogeneic bone marrow transplant and renal transplant recipients participating in clinical trials of VALTREX at doses of 8 grams per day. Treatment with VALTREX should be stopped immediately if clinical signs, symptoms, and laboratory abnormalities consistent with TTP/HUS occur.

5.2 Acute Renal Failure

Cases of acute renal failure have been reported in:
- Elderly patients with or without reduced renal function. Caution should be exercised when administering VALTREX to geriatric patients, and dosage reduction is recommended for those with impaired renal function *[see Dosage and Administration (2.4), Use in Specific Populations (8.5)]*.
- Patients with underlying renal disease who received higher-than-recommended doses of VALTREX for their level of renal function. Dosage reduction is recommended when administering VALTREX to patients with renal impairment *[see Dosage and Administration (2.4), Use in Specific Populations (8.6)]*.
- Patients receiving other nephrotoxic drugs. Caution should be exercised when administering VALTREX to patients receiving potentially nephrotoxic drugs.
- Patients without adequate hydration. Precipitation of acyclovir in renal tubules may occur when the solubility (2.5 mg/mL) is exceeded in the intratubular fluid. Adequate hydration should be maintained for all patients.

In the event of acute renal failure and anuria, the patient may benefit from hemodialysis until renal function is restored *[see Dosage and Administration (2.4), Adverse Reactions (6.3)]*.

5.3 Central Nervous System Effects

Central nervous system adverse reactions, including agitation, hallucinations, confusion, delirium, seizures, and encephalopathy, have been reported in both adult and pediatric patients with or without reduced renal function and in patients with underlying renal disease who received higher-than-recommended doses of VALTREX for their level of renal function. Elderly patients are more likely to have central nervous system adverse reactions. VALTREX should be discontinued if central nervous system adverse reactions occur *[see Adverse Reactions (6.3), Use in Specific Populations (8.5, 8.6)]*.

6 ADVERSE REACTIONS

The following serious adverse reactions are discussed in greater detail in other sections of the labeling:
- Thrombotic Thrombocytopenic Purpura/Hemolytic Uremic Syndrome *[see Warnings and Precautions (5.1)]*.
- Acute Renal Failure *[see Warnings and Precautions (5.2)]*.
- Central Nervous System Effects *[see Warnings and Precautions (5.3)]*.

The most common adverse reactions reported in at least 1 indication by greater than 10% of adult subjects treated with VALTREX and observed more frequently with VALTREX compared to placebo are headache, nausea, and abdominal pain. The only adverse reaction reported in greater than 10% of pediatric subjects aged less than 18 years was headache.

6.1 Clinical Trials Experience in Adult Subjects

Because clinical trials are conducted under widely varying conditions, adverse reaction rates observed in the clinical trials of a drug cannot be directly compared with rates in the clinical trials of another drug and may not reflect the rates observed in practice.

Cold Sores (Herpes Labialis): In clinical trials for the treatment of cold sores, the adverse reactions reported by subjects receiving VALTREX 2 grams twice daily (n = 609) or placebo (n = 609) for 1 day, respectively, included headache (14%, 10%) and dizziness (2%, 1%). The frequencies of abnormal ALT (greater than 2 × ULN) were 1.8% for subjects receiving VALTREX compared with 0.8% for placebo. Other laboratory abnormalities (hemoglobin, white blood cells, alkaline phosphatase, and serum creatinine) occurred with similar frequencies in the 2 groups.

Genital Herpes: *Initial Episode:* In a clinical trial for the treatment of initial episodes of genital herpes, the adverse reactions reported by greater than or equal to 5% of subjects receiving VALTREX 1 gram twice daily for 10 days (n = 318) or oral acyclovir 200 mg 5 times daily for 10 days (n = 318), respectively, included headache (13%, 10%) and nausea (6%, 6%). For the incidence of laboratory abnormalities see Table 2.

Recurrent Episodes: In 3 clinical trials for the episodic treatment of recurrent genital herpes, the adverse reactions reported by greater than or equal to 5% of subjects receiving VALTREX 500 mg twice daily for 3 days (n = 402), VALTREX 500 mg twice daily for 5 days (n = 1,136) or placebo (n = 259), respectively, included headache (16%, 11%, 14%) and nausea (5%, 4%, 5%). For the incidence of laboratory abnormalities see Table 2.

Suppressive Therapy: Suppression of Recurrent Genital Herpes in Immunocompetent Adults: In a clinical trial for the suppression of recurrent genital herpes infections, the adverse reactions reported by subjects receiving VALTREX 1 gram once daily (n = 269), VALTREX 500 mg once daily (n = 266), or placebo (n = 134), respectively, included headache (35%, 38%, 34%), nausea (11%, 11%, 8%), abdominal pain (11%, 9%, 6%), dysmenorrhea (8%, 5%, 4%), depression (7%, 5%, 5%), arthralgia (6%, 5%, 4%), vomiting (3%, 3%, 2%), and dizziness (4%, 2%, 1%). For the incidence of laboratory abnormalities see Table 2.

Suppression of Recurrent Genital Herpes in HIV-1 Infected Subjects: In HIV-1 infected subjects, frequently reported adverse reactions for VALTREX (500 mg twice daily; n = 194, median days on therapy = 172) and placebo (n = 99, median days on therapy = 59), respectively, included headache (13%, 8%), fatigue (8%, 5%), and rash (8%, 1%). Post-randomization laboratory abnormalities that were reported more frequently in valacyclovir subjects versus placebo included elevated alkaline phosphatase (4%, 2%), elevated ALT (14%, 10%), elevated AST (16%, 11%), decreased neutrophil counts (18%, 10%), and decreased platelet counts (3%, 0%), respectively.

Reduction of Transmission: In a clinical trial for the reduction of transmission of genital herpes, the adverse reactions reported by subjects receiving VALTREX 500 mg once daily (n = 743) or placebo once daily (n = 741), respectively, included headache (29%, 26%), nasopharyngitis (16%, 15%), and upper respiratory tract infection (9%, 10%).

Herpes Zoster: In 2 clinical trials for the treatment of herpes zoster, the adverse reactions reported by subjects receiving VALTREX 1 gram 3 times daily for 7 to 14 days (n = 967) or placebo (n = 195), respectively, included nausea (15%, 8%), headache (14%, 12%), vomiting (6%, 3%), dizziness (3%, 2%), and abdominal pain (3%, 2%). For the incidence of laboratory abnormalities see Table 2.

[See table 2 at top of next page]

6.2 Clinical Trials Experience in Pediatric Subjects

The safety profile of VALTREX has been studied in 177 pediatric subjects aged 1 month to less than 18 years. Sixty-five of these pediatric subjects, aged 12 to less than 18 years, received oral caplets for 1 to 2 days for treatment of cold sores. The remaining 112 pediatric subjects, aged 1 month to less than 12 years, participated in 3 pharmacokinetic and safety trials and received valacyclovir oral suspension. Fifty-one of these 112 pediatric subjects received oral suspension for 3 to 6 days. The frequency, intensity, and nature of clinical adverse reactions and laboratory abnormalities were similar to those seen in adults.

Pediatric Subjects Aged 12 to Less Than 18 Years (Cold Sores): In clinical trials for the treatment of cold sores, the adverse reactions reported by adolescent subjects receiving VALTREX 2 grams twice daily for 1 day, or VALTREX 2 grams twice daily for 1 day followed by 1 gram twice daily for 1 day (n = 65, across both dosing groups), or placebo (n = 30), respectively, included headache (17%, 3%) and nausea (8%, 0%).

Pediatric Subjects Aged 1 Month to Less Than 12 Years: Adverse events reported in more than 1 subject across the 3 pharmacokinetic and safety trials in children aged 1 month to less than 12 years were diarrhea (5%), pyrexia (4%), dehydration (2%), herpes simplex (2%), and rhinorrhea (2%). No clinically meaningful changes in laboratory values were observed.

6.3 Postmarketing Experience

In addition to adverse events reported from clinical trials, the following events have been identified during postmarketing use of VALTREX. Because they are reported voluntarily from a population of unknown size, estimates of frequency cannot be made. These events have been chosen for inclusion due to a combination of their seriousness, frequency of reporting, or potential causal connection to VALTREX.

General: Facial edema, hypertension, tachycardia.

Allergic: Acute hypersensitivity reactions including anaphylaxis, angioedema, dyspnea, pruritus, rash, and urticaria *[see Contraindications (4)]*.

Table 2. Incidence (%) of Laboratory Abnormalities in Herpes Zoster and Genital Herpes Trial Populations

Laboratory Abnormality	Herpes Zoster		Genital Herpes Treatment			Genital Herpes Suppression		
	VALTREX 1 gram 3 times daily (n = 967)	Placebo (n = 195)	VALTREX 1 gram twice daily (n = 1,194)	VALTREX 500 mg twice daily (n = 1,159)	Placebo (n = 439)	VALTREX 1 gram once daily (n = 269)	VALTREX 500 mg once daily (n = 266)	Placebo (n = 134)
Hemoglobin (<0.8 × LLN)	0.8%	0%	0.3%	0.2%	0%	0%	0.8%	0.8%
White blood cells (<0.75 × LLN)	1.3%	0.6%	0.7%	0.6%	0.2%	0.7%	0.8%	1.5%
Platelet count (<100,000/mm^3)	1.0%	1.2%	0.3%	0.1%	0.7%	0.4%	1.1%	1.5%
AST (SGOT) (>2 × ULN)	1.0%	0%	1.0%	[a]	0.5%	4.1%	3.8%	3.0%
Serum creatinine (>1.5 × ULN)	0.2%	0%	0.7%	0%	0%	0%	0%	0%

[a] Data were not collected prospectively.
LLN = Lower limit of normal.
ULN = Upper limit of normal.

CNS Symptoms: Aggressive behavior; agitation; ataxia; coma; confusion; decreased consciousness; dysarthria; encephalopathy; mania; and psychosis, including auditory and visual hallucinations, seizures, tremors *[see Warnings and Precautions (5.3), Use in Specific Populations (8.5), (8.6)]*.
Eye: Visual abnormalities.
Gastrointestinal: Diarrhea.
Hepatobiliary Tract and Pancreas: Liver enzyme abnormalities, hepatitis.
Renal: Renal failure, renal pain (may be associated with renal failure) *[see Warnings and Precautions (5.2), Use in Specific Populations (8.5), (8.6)]*.
Hematologic: Thrombocytopenia, aplastic anemia, leukocytoclastic vasculitis, TTP/HUS *[see Warnings and Precautions (5.1)]*.
Skin: Erythema multiforme, rashes including photosensitivity, alopecia.

7 DRUG INTERACTIONS

No clinically significant drug-drug or drug-food interactions with VALTREX are known *[see Clinical Pharmacology (12.3)]*.

8 USE IN SPECIFIC POPULATIONS

8.1 Pregnancy

Pregnancy Category B. There are no adequate and well-controlled trials of VALTREX or acyclovir in pregnant women. Based on prospective pregnancy registry data on 749 pregnancies, the overall rate of birth defects in infants exposed to acyclovir in-utero appears similar to the rate for infants in the general population. VALTREX should be used during pregnancy only if the potential benefit justifies the potential risk to the fetus.

A prospective epidemiologic registry of acyclovir use during pregnancy was established in 1984 and completed in April 1999. There were 749 pregnancies followed in women exposed to systemic acyclovir during the first trimester of pregnancy resulting in 756 outcomes. The occurrence rate of birth defects approximates that found in the general population. However, the small size of the registry is insufficient to evaluate the risk for less common defects or to permit reliable or definitive conclusions regarding the safety of acyclovir in pregnant women and their developing fetuses.

Animal reproduction studies performed at oral doses that provided up to 10 and 7 times the human plasma levels during the period of major organogenesis in rats and rabbits, respectively, revealed no evidence of teratogenicity.

8.3 Nursing Mothers

Following oral administration of a 500 mg dose of VALTREX to 5 nursing mothers, peak acyclovir concentrations (C_{max}) in breast milk ranged from 0.5 to 2.3 times (median 1.4) the corresponding maternal acyclovir serum concentrations. The acyclovir breast milk AUC ranged from 1.4 to 2.6 times (median 2.2) maternal serum AUC. A 500 mg maternal dosage of VALTREX twice daily would provide a nursing infant with an oral acyclovir dosage of approximately 0.6 mg/kg/day. This would result in less than 2% of the exposure obtained after administration of a standard neonatal dose of 30 mg/kg/day of intravenous acyclovir to the nursing infant. Unchanged valacyclovir was not detected in maternal serum, breast milk, or infant urine. Caution should be exercised when VALTREX is administered to a nursing woman.

8.4 Pediatric Use

VALTREX is indicated for treatment of cold sores in pediatric patients aged greater than or equal to 12 years and for treatment of chickenpox in pediatric patients aged 2 to less than 18 years *[see Indications and Usage (1.2), Dosage and Administration (2.2)]*.

The use of VALTREX for treatment of cold sores is based on 2 double-blind, placebo-controlled clinical trials in healthy adults and adolescents (aged greater than or equal to 12 years) with a history of recurrent cold sores *[see Clinical Studies (14.1)]*.

The use of VALTREX for treatment of chickenpox in pediatric patients aged 2 to less than 18 years is based on single-dose pharmacokinetic and multiple-dose safety data from an open-label trial with valacyclovir and supported by efficacy and safety data from 3 randomized, double-blind, placebo-controlled trials evaluating oral acyclovir in pediatric subjects with chickenpox *[see Dosage and Administration (2.2), Adverse Reactions (6.2), Clinical Pharmacology (12.3), Clinical Studies (14.4)]*.

The efficacy and safety of valacyclovir have not been established in pediatric patients:
- aged less than 12 years with cold sores
- aged less than 18 years with genital herpes
- aged less than 18 years with herpes zoster
- aged less than 2 years with chickenpox
- for suppressive therapy following neonatal HSV infection.

The pharmacokinetic profile and safety of valacyclovir oral suspension in children aged less than 12 years were studied in 3 open–label trials. No efficacy evaluations were conducted in any of the 3 trials.

Trial 1 was a single–dose pharmacokinetic, multiple–dose safety trial in 27 pediatric subjects aged 1 to less than 12 years with clinically suspected varicella-zoster virus (VZV) infection *[see Dosage and Administration (2.2), Adverse Reactions (6.2), Clinical Pharmacology (12.3), Clinical Studies (14.4)]*.

Trial 2 was a single–dose pharmacokinetic and safety trial in pediatric subjects aged 1 month to less than 6 years who had an active herpes virus infection or who were at risk for herpes virus infection. Fifty-seven subjects were enrolled and received a single dose of 25 mg/kg valacyclovir oral suspension. In infants and children aged 3 months to less than 6 years, this dose provided comparable systemic acyclovir exposures to that from a 1-gram dose of valacyclovir in adults (historical data). In infants aged 1 month to less than 3 months, mean acyclovir exposures resulting from a 25-mg/kg dose were higher (C_{max}: ↑30%, AUC: ↑60%) than acyclovir exposures following a 1-gram dose of valacyclovir in adults. Acyclovir is not approved for suppressive therapy in infants and children following neonatal HSV infections; therefore valacyclovir is not recommended for this indication because efficacy cannot be extrapolated from acyclovir.

Trial 3 was a single–dose pharmacokinetic, multiple–dose safety trial in 28 pediatric subjects aged 1 to less than 12 years with clinically suspected HSV infection. None of the subjects enrolled in this trial had genital herpes. Each subject was dosed with valacyclovir oral suspension, 10 mg/kg twice daily for 3 to 5 days. Acyclovir systemic exposures in pediatric subjects following valacyclovir oral suspension were compared with historical acyclovir systemic exposures in immunocompetent adults receiving the solid oral dosage form of valacyclovir or acyclovir for the treatment of recurrent genital herpes. The mean projected daily acyclovir systemic exposures in pediatric subjects across all age–groups (1 to less than 12 years) were lower (C_{max}: ↓20%, AUC: ↓33%) compared with the acyclovir systemic exposures in adults receiving valacyclovir 500 mg twice daily, but were higher (daily AUC: ↑16%) than systemic exposures in adults receiving acyclovir 200 mg 5 times daily. Insufficient data are available to support valacyclovir for the treatment of recurrent genital herpes in this age–group because clinical information on recurrent genital herpes in young children is limited; therefore, extrapolating efficacy data from adults to this population is not possible. Moreover, valacyclovir has not been studied in children aged 1 to less than 12 years with recurrent genital herpes.

8.5 Geriatric Use

[Of the total number of subjects in clinical trials of VALTREX, 906 were 65 and over, and 352 were 75 and over. In a clinical trial of herpes zoster, the duration of pain after healing (post-herpetic neuralgia) was longer in subjects 65 and older compared with younger adults. Elderly patients are more likely to have reduced renal function and require dose reduction. Elderly patients are also more likely to have renal or CNS adverse events *[see Dosage and Administration (2.4), Warnings and Precautions (5.2, 5.3), Clinical Pharmacology (12.3)]*.

8.6 Renal Impairment

Dosage reduction is recommended when administering VALTREX to patients with renal impairment *[see Dosage and Administration (2.4), Warnings and Precautions (5.2, 5.3)]*.

10 OVERDOSAGE

Caution should be exercised to prevent inadvertent overdose *[see Use in Specific Populations (8.5), (8.6)]*. Precipitation of acyclovir in renal tubules may occur when the solubility (2.5 mg/mL) is exceeded in the intratubular fluid. In the event of acute renal failure and anuria, the patient may benefit from hemodialysis until renal function is restored *[see Dosage and Administration (2.4)]*.

11 DESCRIPTION

VALTREX (valacyclovir hydrochloride) is the hydrochloride salt of the *L*-valyl ester of the antiviral drug acyclovir.

VALTREX Caplets are for oral administration. Each caplet contains valacyclovir hydrochloride equivalent to 500 mg or 1 gram valacyclovir and the inactive ingredients carnauba wax, colloidal silicon dioxide, crospovidone, FD&C Blue No. 2 Lake, hypromellose, magnesium stearate, microcrystalline cellulose, polyethylene glycol, polysorbate 80, povidone, and titanium dioxide. The blue, film-coated caplets are printed with edible white ink.

The chemical name of valacyclovir hydrochloride is *L*-valine, 2-[(2-amino-1,6-dihydro-6-oxo-9*H*-purin-9-yl)methoxy]ethyl ester, monohydrochloride. It has the following structural formula:

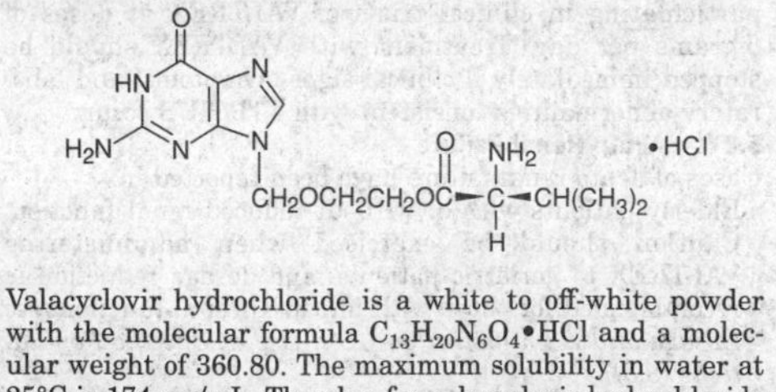

Valacyclovir hydrochloride is a white to off-white powder with the molecular formula $C_{13}H_{20}N_6O_4$•HCl and a molecular weight of 360.80. The maximum solubility in water at 25°C is 174 mg/mL. The pk_as for valacyclovir hydrochloride are 1.90, 7.47, and 9.43.

12 CLINICAL PHARMACOLOGY

12.1 Mechanism of Action

Valacyclovir is an antiviral drug *[see Clinical Pharmacology (12.4)]*.

12.3 Pharmacokinetics

The pharmacokinetics of valacyclovir and acyclovir after oral administration of VALTREX have been investigated in 14 volunteer trials involving 283 adults and in 3 trials involving 112 pediatric subjects aged 1 month to less than 12 years.

Pharmacokinetics in Adults: *Absorption and Bioavailability:* After oral administration, valacyclovir hydrochloride is rapidly absorbed from the gastrointestinal tract and nearly completely converted to acyclovir and *L*-valine by first-pass intestinal and/or hepatic metabolism.

The absolute bioavailability of acyclovir after administration of VALTREX is 54.5% ± 9.1% as determined following a 1-gram oral dose of VALTREX and a 350-mg intravenous acyclovir dose to 12 healthy volunteers. Acyclovir bioavailability from the administration of VALTREX is not altered by administration with food (30 minutes after an 873 Kcal breakfast, which included 51 grams of fat).

Acyclovir pharmacokinetic parameter estimates following administration of VALTREX to healthy adult volunteers are presented in Table 3. There was a less than dose-proportional increase in acyclovir maximum concentration (C_{max}) and area under the acyclovir concentration-time curve (AUC) after single-dose and multiple-dose administration (4 times daily) of VALTREX from doses between 250 mg to 1 gram.

There is no accumulation of acyclovir after the administration of valacyclovir at the recommended dosage regimens in adults with normal renal function.

[See table 3 above]

Distribution: The binding of valacyclovir to human plasma proteins ranges from 13.5% to 17.9%. The binding of acyclovir to human plasma proteins ranges from 9% to 33%.

Metabolism: Valacyclovir is converted to acyclovir and L-valine by first-pass intestinal and/or hepatic metabolism. Acyclovir is converted to a small extent to inactive metabolites by aldehyde oxidase and by alcohol and aldehyde dehydrogenase. Neither valacyclovir nor acyclovir is metabolized by cytochrome P450 enzymes. Plasma concentrations of unconverted valacyclovir are low and transient, generally becoming non-quantifiable by 3 hours after administration. Peak plasma valacyclovir concentrations are generally less than 0.5 mcg/mL at all doses. After single-dose administration of 1 gram of VALTREX, average plasma valacyclovir concentrations observed were 0.5, 0.4, and 0.8 mcg/mL in subjects with hepatic dysfunction, renal insufficiency, and in healthy subjects who received concomitant cimetidine and probenecid, respectively.

Elimination: The pharmacokinetic disposition of acyclovir delivered by valacyclovir is consistent with previous experience from intravenous and oral acyclovir. Following the oral administration of a single 1 gram dose of radiolabeled valacyclovir to 4 healthy subjects, 46% and 47% of administered radioactivity was recovered in urine and feces, respectively, over 96 hours. Acyclovir accounted for 89% of the radioactivity excreted in the urine. Renal clearance of acyclovir following the administration of a single 1-gram dose of VALTREX to 12 healthy subjects was approximately 255 ± 86 mL/min which represents 42% of total acyclovir apparent plasma clearance.

The plasma elimination half–life of acyclovir typically averaged 2.5 to 3.3 hours in all trials of VALTREX in subjects with normal renal function.

Specific Populations: *Renal Impairment:* Reduction in dosage is recommended in patients with renal impairment *[see Dosage and Administration (2.4), Use in Specific Populations (8.5), (8.6)].*

Following administration of VALTREX to subjects with ESRD, the average acyclovir half–life is approximately 14 hours. During hemodialysis, the acyclovir half–life is approximately 4 hours. Approximately one–third of acyclovir in the body is removed by dialysis during a 4–hour hemodialysis session. Apparent plasma clearance of acyclovir in subjects on dialysis was 86.3 ± 21.3 mL/min/1.73 m^2 compared with 679.16 ± 162.76 mL/min/1.73 m^2 in healthy subjects.

Hepatic Impairment: Administration of VALTREX to subjects with moderate (biopsy-proven cirrhosis) or severe (with and without ascites and biopsy-proven cirrhosis) liver disease indicated that the rate but not the extent of conversion of valacyclovir to acyclovir is reduced, and the acyclovir half-life is not affected. Dosage modification is not recommended for patients with cirrhosis.

HIV-1 Disease: In 9 subjects with HIV-1 disease and CD4+ cell counts less than 150 cells/mm^3 who received VALTREX at a dosage of 1 gram 4 times daily for 30 days, the pharmacokinetics of valacyclovir and acyclovir were not different from that observed in healthy subjects.

Geriatrics: After single-dose administration of 1 gram of VALTREX in healthy geriatric subjects, the half-life of acyclovir was 3.11 ± 0.51 hours, compared with 2.91 ± 0.63 hours in healthy younger adult subjects. The pharmacokinetics of acyclovir following single- and multiple–dose oral administration of VALTREX in geriatric subjects varied with renal function. Dose reduction may be required in geriatric patients, depending on the underlying renal status of the patient *[see Dosage and Administration (2.4), Use in Specific Populations (8.5), (8.6)].*

Pediatrics: Acyclovir pharmacokinetics have been evaluated in a total of 98 pediatric subjects (aged 1 month to less than 12 years) following administration of the first dose of an extemporaneous oral suspension of valacyclovir *[see Adverse Reactions (6.2), Use in Specific Populations (8.4)].* Acyclovir pharmacokinetic parameter estimates following a 20-mg/kg dose are provided in Table 4.

[See table 4 above]

Drug Interactions: When VALTREX is coadministered with antacids, cimetidine and/or probenicid, digoxin, or thiazide diuretics in patients with normal renal function, the effects are not considered to be of clinical significance (see below). Therefore, when VALTREX is coadministered with these drugs in patients with normal renal function, no dosage adjustment is recommended.

Antacids: The pharmacokinetics of acyclovir after a single dose of VALTREX (1 gram) were unchanged by coadministration of a single dose of antacids (Al^{3+} or Mg^{++}).

Table 3. Mean (±SD) Plasma Acyclovir Pharmacokinetic Parameters Following Administration of VALTREX to Healthy Adult Volunteers

Dose	Single-Dose Administration (N = 8)		Multiple-Dose Administration[a] (N = 24, 8 per treatment arm)	
	C_{max} (±SD) (mcg/mL)	AUC (±SD) (hr•mcg/mL)	C_{max} (±SD) (mcg/mL)	AUC (±SD) (hr•mcg/mL)
100 mg	0.83 (±0.14)	2.28 (±0.40)	ND	ND
250 mg	2.15 (±0.50)	5.76 (±0.60)	2.11 (±0.33)	5.66 (±1.09)
500 mg	3.28 (±0.83)	11.59 (±1.79)	3.69 (±0.87)	9.88 (±2.01)
750 mg	4.17 (±1.14)	14.11 (±3.54)	ND	ND
1,000 mg	5.65 (±2.37)	19.52 (±6.04)	4.96 (±0.64)	15.70 (±2.27)

[a] Administered 4 times daily for 11 days.
ND = not done.

Table 4. Mean (±SD) Plasma Acyclovir Pharmacokinetic Parameter Estimates Following First-Dose Administration of 20 mg/kg Valacyclovir Oral Suspension to Pediatric Subjects vs. 1-Gram Single Dose of VALTREX to Adults

Parameter	Pediatric Subjects (20 mg/kg Oral Suspension)			Adults 1-gram Solid Dose of VALTREX[a] (N = 15)
	1 - <2 yr (N = 6)	2 - <6 yr (N = 12)	6 - <12 yr (N = 8)	
AUC (mcg•hr/mL)	14.4 (±6.26)	10.1 (±3.35)	13.1 (±3.43)	17.2 (±3.10)
C_{max} (mcg/mL)	4.03 (±1.37)	3.75 (±1.14)	4.71 (±1.20)	4.72 (±1.37)

[a] Historical estimates using pediatric pharmacokinetic sampling schedule.

Cimetidine: Acyclovir C_{max} and AUC following a single dose of VALTREX (1 gram) increased by 8% and 32%, respectively, after a single dose of cimetidine (800 mg).

Cimetidine Plus Probenecid: Acyclovir C_{max} and AUC following a single dose of VALTREX (1 gram) increased by 30% and 78%, respectively, after a combination of cimetidine and probenecid, primarily due to a reduction in renal clearance of acyclovir.

Digoxin: The pharmacokinetics of digoxin were not affected by coadministration of VALTREX 1 gram 3 times daily, and the pharmacokinetics of acyclovir after a single dose of VALTREX (1 gram) was unchanged by coadministration of digoxin (2 doses of 0.75 mg).

Probenecid: Acyclovir C_{max} and AUC following a single dose of VALTREX (1 gram) increased by 22% and 49%, respectively, after probenecid (1 gram).

Thiazide Diuretics: The pharmacokinetics of acyclovir after a single dose of VALTREX (1 gram) were unchanged by coadministration of multiple doses of thiazide diuretics.

12.4 Microbiology

Mechanism of Action: Valacyclovir is a nucleoside analogue DNA polymerase inhibitor. Valacyclovir hydrochloride is rapidly converted to acyclovir which has demonstrated antiviral activity against HSV types 1 (HSV-1) and 2 (HSV-2) and VZV both in cell culture and in vivo.

The inhibitory activity of acyclovir is highly selective due to its affinity for the enzyme thymidine kinase (TK) encoded by HSV and VZV. This viral enzyme converts acyclovir into acyclovir monophosphate, a nucleotide analogue. The monophosphate is further converted into diphosphate by cellular guanylate kinase and into triphosphate by a number of cellular enzymes. In biochemical assays, acyclovir triphosphate inhibits replication of herpes viral DNA. This is accomplished in 3 ways: 1) competitive inhibition of viral DNA polymerase, 2) incorporation and termination of the growing viral DNA chain, and 3) inactivation of the viral DNA polymerase. The greater antiviral activity of acyclovir against HSV compared with VZV is due to its more efficient phosphorylation by the viral TK.

Antiviral Activities: The quantitative relationship between the cell culture susceptibility of herpesviruses to antivirals and the clinical response to therapy has not been established in humans, and virus sensitivity testing has not been standardized. Sensitivity testing results, expressed as the concentration of drug required to inhibit by 50% the growth of virus in cell culture (EC_{50}), vary greatly depending upon a number of factors. Using plaque-reduction assays, the EC_{50} values against herpes simplex virus isolates range from 0.09 to 60 µM (0.02 to 13.5 mcg/mL) for HSV-1 and from 0.04 to 44 µM (0.01 to 9.9 mcg/mL) for HSV-2. The EC_{50} values for acyclovir against most laboratory strains and clinical isolates of VZV range from 0.53 to 48 µM (0.12 to 10.8 mcg/mL). Acyclovir also demonstrates activity against the Oka vaccine strain of VZV with a mean EC_{50} of 6 µM (1.35 mcg/mL).

Resistance: Resistance of HSV and VZV to acyclovir can result from qualitative and quantitative changes in the viral TK and/or DNA polymerase. Clinical isolates of VZV with reduced susceptibility to acyclovir have been recovered from patients with AIDS. In these cases, TK-deficient mutants of VZV have been recovered.

Resistance of HSV and VZV to acyclovir occurs by the same mechanisms. While most of the acyclovir-resistant mutants isolated thus far from immunocompromised patients have been found to be TK-deficient mutants, other mutants involving the viral TK gene (TK partial and TK altered) and DNA polymerase have also been isolated. TK-negative mutants may cause severe disease in immunocompromised patients. The possibility of viral resistance to valacyclovir (and therefore, to acyclovir) should be considered in patients who show poor clinical response during therapy.

13 NONCLINICAL TOXICOLOGY

13.1 Carcinogenesis, Mutagenesis, Impairment of Fertility

The data presented below include references to the steady-state acyclovir AUC observed in humans treated with 1 gram VALTREX given orally 3 times a day to treat herpes zoster. Plasma drug concentrations in animal studies are expressed as multiples of human exposure to acyclovir *[see Clinical Pharmacology (12.3)].*

Valacyclovir was noncarcinogenic in lifetime carcinogenicity bioassays at single daily doses (gavage) of valacyclovir giving plasma acyclovir concentrations equivalent to human levels in the mouse bioassay and 1.4 to 2.3 times human levels in the rat bioassay. There was no significant difference in the incidence of tumors between treated and control animals, nor did valacyclovir shorten the latency of tumors.

Valacyclovir was tested in 5 genetic toxicity assays. An Ames assay was negative in the absence or presence of metabolic activation. Also negative were an in vitro cytogenetic study with human lymphocytes and a rat cytogenetic study. In the mouse lymphoma assay, valacyclovir was not mutagenic in the absence of metabolic activation. In the presence of metabolic activation (76% to 88% conversion to acyclovir), valacyclovir was mutagenic.

Valacyclovir was mutagenic in a mouse micronucleus assay.

Valacyclovir did not impair fertility or reproduction in rats at 6 times human plasma levels.

14 CLINICAL STUDIES

14.1 Cold Sores (Herpes Labialis)

Two double–blind, placebo–controlled clinical trials were conducted in 1,856 healthy adults and adolescents (aged greater than or equal to 12 years) with a history of recurrent cold sores. Subjects self–initiated therapy at the earliest symptoms and prior to any signs of a cold sore. The majority of subjects initiated treatment within 2 hours of onset of symptoms. Subjects were randomized to VALTREX 2 grams twice daily on Day 1 followed by placebo on Day 2, VALTREX 2 grams twice daily on Day 1 followed by 1 gram twice daily on Day 2, or placebo on Days 1 and 2.

The mean duration of cold sore episodes was about 1 day shorter in treated subjects as compared with placebo. The

Table 5. Recurrence Rates in Immunocompetent Adults at 6 and 12 Months

Outcome	6 Months			12 Months		
	VALTREX 1 gram once daily (n = 269)	Oral acyclovir 400 mg twice daily (n = 267)	Placebo (n = 134)	VALTREX 1 gram once daily (n = 269)	Oral acyclovir 400 mg twice daily (n = 267)	Placebo (n = 134)
Recurrence free	55%	54%	7%	34%	34%	4%
Recurrences	35%	36%	83%	46%	46%	85%
Unknown[a]	10%	10%	10%	19%	19%	10%

[a] Includes lost to follow-up, discontinuations due to adverse events, and consent withdrawn.

2-day regimen did not offer additional benefit over the 1-day regimen.

No significant difference was observed between subjects receiving VALTREX or placebo in the prevention of progression of cold sore lesions beyond the papular stage.

14.2 Genital Herpes Infections

Initial Episode: Six hundred forty-three immunocompetent adults with first-episode genital herpes who presented within 72 hours of symptom onset were randomized in a double-blind trial to receive 10 days of VALTREX 1 gram twice daily (n = 323) or oral acyclovir 200 mg 5 times a day (n = 320). For both treatment groups the median time to lesion healing was 9 days, the median time to cessation of pain was 5 days, and the median time to cessation of viral shedding was 3 days.

Recurrent Episodes: Three double-blind trials (2 of them placebo-controlled) in immunocompetent adults with recurrent genital herpes were conducted. Subjects self-initiated therapy within 24 hours of the first sign or symptom of a recurrent genital herpes episode.

In 1 trial, subjects were randomized to receive 5 days of treatment with either VALTREX 500 mg twice daily (n = 360) or placebo (n = 259). The median time to lesion healing was 4 days in the group receiving VALTREX 500 mg versus 6 days in the placebo group, and the median time to cessation of viral shedding in subjects with at least 1 positive culture (42% of the overall trial population) was 2 days in the group receiving VALTREX 500 mg versus 4 days in the placebo group. The median time to cessation of pain was 3 days in the group receiving VALTREX 500 mg versus 4 days in the placebo group. Results supporting efficacy were replicated in a second trial.

In a third trial, subjects were randomized to receive VALTREX 500 mg twice daily for 5 days (n = 398) or VALTREX 500 mg twice daily for 3 days (and matching placebo twice daily for 2 additional days) (n = 402). The median time to lesion healing was about 4½ days in both treatment groups. The median time to cessation of pain was about 3 days in both treatment groups.

Suppressive Therapy: Two clinical trials were conducted, one in immunocompetent adults and one in HIV-1-infected adults.

A double–blind, 12–month, placebo– and active–controlled trial enrolled immunocompetent adults with a history of 6 or more recurrences per year. Outcomes for the overall trial population are shown in Table 5.

[See table 5 above]

Subjects with 9 or fewer recurrences per year showed comparable results with VALTREX 500 mg once daily.

In a second trial, 293 HIV–1-infected adults on stable antiretroviral therapy with a history of 4 or more recurrences of ano–genital herpes per year were randomized to receive either VALTREX 500 mg twice daily (n = 194) or matching placebo (n = 99) for 6 months. The median duration of recurrent genital herpes in enrolled subjects was 8 years, and the median number of recurrences in the year prior to enrollment was 5. Overall, the median pretrial HIV–1 RNA was 2.6 $\log_{10}$ copies/mL. Among subjects who received VALTREX, the pretrial median CD4+ cell count was 336 cells/mm^3; 11% had less than 100 cells/mm^3, 16% had 100 to 199 cells/mm^3, 42% had 200 to 499 cells/mm^3, and 31% had greater than or equal to 500 cells/mm^3. Outcomes for the overall trial population are shown in Table 6.

Table 6. Recurrence Rates in HIV-1-Infected Adults at 6 Months

Outcome	VALTREX 500 mg twice daily (n = 194)	Placebo (n = 99)
Recurrence free	65%	26%
Recurrences	17%	57%
Unknown[a]	18%	17%

[a] Includes lost to follow-up, discontinuations due to adverse events, and consent withdrawn.

Reduction of Transmission of Genital Herpes: A double-blind, placebo-controlled trial to assess transmission of genital herpes was conducted in 1,484 monogamous, heterosexual, immunocompetent adult couples. The couples were discordant for HSV-2 infection. The source partner had a history of 9 or fewer genital herpes episodes per year. Both partners were counseled on safer sex practices and were advised to use condoms throughout the trial period. Source partners were randomized to treatment with either VALTREX 500 mg once daily or placebo once daily for 8 months. The primary efficacy endpoint was symptomatic acquisition of HSV-2 in susceptible partners. Overall HSV-2 acquisition was defined as symptomatic HSV-2 acquisition and/or HSV-2 seroconversion in susceptible partners. The efficacy results are summarized in Table 7.

Table 7. Percentage of Susceptible Partners Who Acquired HSV-2 Defined by the Primary and Selected Secondary Endpoints

Endpoint	VALTREX[a] (n = 743)	Placebo (n = 741)
Symptomatic HSV-2 acquisition	4 (0.5%)	16 (2.2%)
HSV-2 seroconversion	12 (1.6%)	24 (3.2%)
Overall HSV-2 acquisition	14 (1.9%)	27 (3.6%)

[a] Results show reductions in risk of 75% (symptomatic HSV-2 acquisition), 50% (HSV-2 seroconversion), and 48% (overall HSV-2 acquisition) with VALTREX versus placebo. Individual results may vary based on consistency of safer sex practices.

14.3 Herpes Zoster

Two randomized double–blind clinical trials in immunocompetent adults with localized herpes zoster were conducted. VALTREX was compared with placebo in subjects aged less than 50 years, and with oral acyclovir in subjects aged greater than 50 years. All subjects were treated within 72 hours of appearance of zoster rash. In subjects aged less than 50 years, the median time to cessation of new lesion formation was 2 days for those treated with VALTREX compared with 3 days for those treated with placebo. In subjects aged greater than 50 years, the median time to cessation of new lesions was 3 days in subjects treated with either VALTREX or oral acyclovir. In subjects aged less than 50 years, no difference was found with respect to the duration of pain after healing (post–herpetic neuralgia) between the recipients of VALTREX and placebo. In subjects aged greater than 50 years, among the 83% who reported pain after healing (post–herpetic neuralgia), the median duration of pain after healing [95% confidence interval] in days was: 40 [31, 51], 43 [36, 55], and 59 [41, 77] for 7–day VALTREX, 14–day VALTREX, and 7–day oral acyclovir, respectively.

14.4 Chickenpox

The use of VALTREX for treatment of chickenpox in pediatric subjects aged 2 to less than 18 years is based on single–dose pharmacokinetic and multiple–dose safety data from an open–label trial with valacyclovir and supported by safety and extrapolated efficacy data from 3 randomized, double–blind, placebo–controlled trials evaluating oral acyclovir in pediatric subjects.

The single–dose pharmacokinetic and multiple–dose safety trial enrolled 27 pediatric subjects aged 1 to less than 12 years with clinically suspected VZV infection. Each subject was dosed with valacyclovir oral suspension, 20 mg/kg 3 times daily for 5 days. Acyclovir systemic exposures in pediatric subjects following valacyclovir oral suspension were compared with historical acyclovir systemic exposures in immunocompetent adults receiving the solid oral dosage form of valacyclovir or acyclovir for the treatment of herpes zoster. The mean projected daily acyclovir exposures in pediatric subjects across all age–groups (1 to less than 12 years) were lower (C_{max}: ↓13%, AUC: ↓30%) than the mean daily historical exposures in adults receiving valacyclovir 1 gram 3 times daily, but were higher (daily AUC: ↑50%) than the mean daily historical exposures in adults receiving acyclovir 800 mg 5 times daily. The projected daily exposures in pediatric subjects were greater (daily AUC approximately 100% greater) than the exposures seen in immunocompetent pediatric subjects receiving acyclovir 20 mg/kg 4 times daily for the treatment of chickenpox. Based on the pharmacokinetic and safety data from this trial and the safety and extrapolated efficacy data from the acyclovir trials, oral valacyclovir 20 mg/kg 3 times a day for 5 days (not to exceed 1 gram 3 times daily) is recommended for the treatment of chickenpox in pediatric patients aged 2 to less than 18 years. Because the efficacy and safety of acyclovir for the treatment of chickenpox in children aged less than 2 years have not been established, efficacy data cannot be extrapolated to support valacyclovir treatment in children aged less than 2 years with chickenpox. Valacyclovir is also not recommended for the treatment of herpes zoster in children because safety data up to 7 days' duration are not available *[see Use in Specific Populations (8.4)]*.

16 HOW SUPPLIED/STORAGE AND HANDLING

VALTREX Caplets (blue, film-coated, capsule-shaped tablets) containing valacyclovir hydrochloride equivalent to 500 mg valacyclovir and printed with "VALTREX 500 mg."

Bottle of 30 (NDC 0173-0933-08).

Bottle of 90 (NDC 0173-0933-10).

Unit dose pack of 100 (NDC 0173-0933-56).

VALTREX Caplets (blue, film-coated, capsule-shaped tablets, with a partial scorebar on both sides) containing valacyclovir hydrochloride equivalent to 1 gram valacyclovir and printed with "VALTREX 1 gram."

Bottle of 30 (NDC 0173-0565-04).

Bottle of 90 (NDC 0173-0565-10).

Storage:

Store at 15° to 25°C (59° to 77°F). Dispense in a well-closed container as defined in the USP.

17 PATIENT COUNSELING INFORMATION

See FDA-Approved Patient Labeling

17.1 Importance of Adequate Hydration

Patients should be advised to maintain adequate hydration.

17.2 Cold Sores (Herpes Labialis)

Patients should be advised to initiate treatment at the earliest symptom of a cold sore (e.g., tingling, itching, or burning). There are no data on the effectiveness of treatment initiated after the development of clinical signs of a cold sore (e.g., papule, vesicle, or ulcer). Patients should be instructed that treatment for cold sores should not exceed 1 day (2 doses) and that their doses should be taken about 12 hours apart. Patients should be informed that VALTREX is not a cure for cold sores.

17.3 Genital Herpes

Patients should be informed that VALTREX is not a cure for genital herpes. Because genital herpes is a sexually transmitted disease, patients should avoid contact with lesions or intercourse when lesions and/or symptoms are present to avoid infecting partners. Genital herpes is frequently transmitted in the absence of symptoms through asymptomatic viral shedding. Therefore, patients should be counseled to use safer sex practices in combination with suppressive therapy with VALTREX. Sex partners of infected persons should be advised that they might be infected even if they have no symptoms. Type-specific serologic testing of asymptomatic partners of persons with genital herpes can determine whether risk for HSV-2 acquisition exists.

VALTREX has not been shown to reduce transmission of sexually transmitted infections other than HSV-2.

If medical management of a genital herpes recurrence is indicated, patients should be advised to initiate therapy at the first sign or symptom of an episode.

There are no data on the effectiveness of treatment initiated more than 72 hours after the onset of signs and symptoms of a first episode of genital herpes or more than 24 hours after the onset of signs and symptoms of a recurrent episode.

There are no data on the safety or effectiveness of chronic suppressive therapy of more than 1 year's duration in otherwise healthy patients. There are no data on the safety or effectiveness of chronic suppressive therapy of more than 6 months' duration in HIV-1 infected patients.

17.4 Herpes Zoster

There are no data on treatment initiated more than 72 hours after onset of the zoster rash. Patients should be advised to initiate treatment as soon as possible after a diagnosis of herpes zoster.

17.5 Chickenpox

Patients should be advised to initiate treatment at the earliest sign or symptom of chickenpox.

Distributed by:
GlaxoSmithKline
Research Triangle Park, NC 27709

Manufactured by:
GlaxoSmithKline
Research Triangle Park, NC 27709
or
DSM Pharmaceuticals, Inc.
Greenville, NC 27834

VTX:5PI

PHARMACIST-DETACH HERE AND GIVE INSTRUCTIONS TO PATIENT

Patient Information

VALTREX® (VAL-trex)

(valacyclovir hydrochloride) Caplets

Read the Patient Information that comes with VALTREX before you start using it and each time you get a refill. There may be new information. This information does not take the place of talking to your healthcare provider about your medical condition or treatment. Ask your healthcare provider or pharmacist if you have questions.

What is VALTREX?

VALTREX is a prescription antiviral medicine. VALTREX lowers the ability of herpes viruses to multiply in your body.

VALTREX is used in adults:

- to treat cold sores (also called fever blisters or herpes labialis)
- to treat shingles (also called herpes zoster)
- to treat or control genital herpes outbreaks in adults with normal immune systems
- to control genital herpes outbreaks in adults infected with the human immunodeficiency virus (HIV-1) with CD4+ cell count greater than 100 cells/mm^3
- with safer sex practices to lower the chances of spreading genital herpes to others. Even with safer sex practices, it is still possible to spread genital herpes.

VALTREX used daily with the following safer sex practices can lower the chances of passing genital herpes to your partner.

- **Do not have sexual contact with your partner when you have any symptom or outbreak of genital herpes.**
- **Use a condom** made of latex or polyurethane whenever you have sexual contact.

VALTREX is used in children:

- to treat cold sores (for children aged greater than or equal to 12 years)
- to treat chickenpox (for children aged 2 to less than 18 years).

VALTREX does not cure herpes infections (cold sores, chickenpox, shingles, or genital herpes).

The efficacy of VALTREX has not been studied in children who have not reached puberty.

What are cold sores, chickenpox, shingles, and genital herpes?

Cold sores are caused by a herpes virus that may be spread by kissing or other physical contact with the infected area of the skin. They are small, painful ulcers that you get in or around your mouth. It is not known if VALTREX can stop the spread of cold sores to others.

Chickenpox is caused by a herpes virus. It causes an itchy rash of multiple small, red bumps that look like pimples or insect bites usually appearing first on the abdomen or back and face. It can spread to almost everywhere else on the body and may be accompanied by flu-like symptoms.

Shingles is caused by the same herpes virus that causes chickenpox. It causes small, painful blisters that happen on your skin. Shingles occurs in people who have already had chickenpox. Shingles can be spread to people who have not had chickenpox or the chickenpox vaccine by contact with the infected areas of the skin. It is not known if VALTREX can stop the spread of shingles to others.

Genital herpes is a sexually transmitted disease. It causes small, painful blisters on your genital area. You can spread genital herpes to others, even when you have no symptoms. If you are sexually active, you can still pass herpes to your partner, even if you are taking VALTREX. VALTREX, taken every day as prescribed and used with the following **safer sex practices**, can lower the chances of passing genital herpes to your partner.

- Do not have sexual contact with your partner when you have any symptom or outbreak of genital herpes.
- Use a condom made of latex or polyurethane whenever you have sexual contact.

Ask your healthcare provider for more information about safer sex practices.

Who should not take VALTREX?

Do not take VALTREX if you are allergic to any of its ingredients or to acyclovir. The active ingredient is valacyclovir. See the end of this leaflet for a complete list of ingredients in VALTREX.

Before taking VALTREX, tell your healthcare provider:

About all of your medical conditions, including:

- **if you have had a bone marrow transplant or kidney transplant, or if you have advanced HIV-1 disease or "AIDS".** Patients with these conditions may have a higher chance for getting a blood disorder called thrombotic thrombocytopenic purpura/hemolytic uremic syndrome (TTP/HUS). TTP/HUS can result in death.
- **if you have kidney problems.** Patients with kidney problems may have a higher chance for getting side effects or more kidney problems with VALTREX. Your healthcare provider may give you a lower dose of VALTREX.
- **if you are aged 65 years or older.** Elderly patients have a higher chance of certain side effects. Also, elderly patients are more likely to have kidney problems. Your healthcare provider may give you a lower dose of VALTREX.
- **if you are pregnant or planning to become pregnant.** Talk with your healthcare provider about the risks and benefits of taking prescription drugs (including VALTREX) during pregnancy.
- **if you are breastfeeding.** VALTREX may pass into your milk and it may harm your baby. Talk with your healthcare provider about the best way to feed your baby if you are taking VALTREX.
- **about all the medicines you take,** including prescription and non-prescription medicines, vitamins, and herbal supplements. VALTREX may affect other medicines, and other medicines may affect VALTREX. It is a good idea to keep a complete list of all the medicines you take. Show this list to your healthcare provider and pharmacist any time you get a new medicine.

How should I take VALTREX?

Take VALTREX exactly as prescribed by your healthcare provider. Your dose of VALTREX and length of treatment will depend on the type of herpes infection that you have and any other medical problems that you have.

- Do not stop VALTREX or change your treatment without talking to your healthcare provider.
- VALTREX can be taken with or without food.
- If you are taking VALTREX to treat cold sores, chickenpox, shingles, or genital herpes, you should start treatment as soon as possible after your symptoms start. VALTREX may not help you if you start treatment too late.
- If you miss a dose of VALTREX, take it as soon as you remember and then take your next dose at its regular time. However, if it is almost time for your next dose, do not take the missed dose. Wait and take the next dose at the regular time.
- Do not take more than the prescribed number of VALTREX Caplets each day. Call your healthcare provider right away if you take too much VALTREX.

What are the possible side effects of VALTREX?

Kidney failure and nervous system problems are not common, but can be serious in some patients taking VALTREX. Nervous system problems include aggressive behavior, unsteady movement, shaky movements, confusion, speech problems, hallucinations (seeing or hearing things that are really not there), seizures, and coma. Kidney failure and nervous system problems have happened in patients who already have kidney disease and in elderly patients whose kidneys do not work well due to age. **Always tell your healthcare provider if you have kidney problems before taking VALTREX. Call your doctor right away if you get a nervous system problem while you are taking VALTREX.**

Common side effects of VALTREX in adults include headache, nausea, stomach pain, vomiting, and dizziness. Side effects in HIV-1-infected adults include headache, tiredness, and rash. These side effects usually are mild and do not cause patients to stop taking VALTREX.

Other less common side effects in adults include painful periods in women, joint pain, depression, low blood cell counts, and changes in tests that measure how well the liver and kidneys work.

The most common side effect seen in children aged less than 18 years was headache.

Talk to your healthcare provider if you develop any side effects that concern you.

These are not all the side effects of VALTREX. For more information ask your healthcare provider or pharmacist.

How should I store VALTREX?

- Store VALTREX Caplets at room temperature, 59° to 77°F (15° to 25°C).
- Store VALTREX suspension between 2° to 8°C (36° to 46°F) in a refrigerator. Discard after 28 days.
- Keep VALTREX in a tightly closed container.
- Do not keep medicine that is out of date or that you no longer need.
- Keep VALTREX and all medicines out of the reach of children.

General information about VALTREX

Medicines are sometimes prescribed for conditions that are not mentioned in patient information leaflets. Do not use VALTREX for a condition for which it was not prescribed. Do not give VALTREX to other people, even if they have the same symptoms you have. It may harm them.

This leaflet summarizes the most important information about VALTREX. If you would like more information, talk with your healthcare provider. You can ask your healthcare provider or pharmacist for information about VALTREX that is written for health professionals. More information is available at www.VALTREX.com.

What are the ingredients in VALTREX?

Active Ingredient: valacyclovir hydrochloride

Inactive Ingredients: carnauba wax, colloidal silicon dioxide, crospovidone, FD&C Blue No. 2 Lake, hypromellose, magnesium stearate, microcrystalline cellulose, polyethylene glycol, polysorbate 80, povidone, and titanium dioxide.

Distributed by:
GlaxoSmithKline
Research Triangle Park, NC 27709
Manufactured by:
GlaxoSmithKline
Research Triangle Park, NC 27709
or
DSM Pharmaceuticals, Inc.
Greenville, NC 27834

January 2013
VTX:4PIL

VENTOLIN HFA ℞

[vent'ō-lin]

(albuterol sulfate)

Inhalation Aerosol

HIGHLIGHTS OF PRESCRIBING INFORMATION

These highlights do not include all the information needed to use VENTOLIN HFA safely and effectively. See full prescribing information for VENTOLIN HFA.

VENTOLIN HFA (albuterol sulfate) Inhalation Aerosol

Initial U.S. Approval: 1981

INDICATIONS AND USAGE

VENTOLIN HFA is a beta$_2$-adrenergic agonist indicated for:

- Treatment or prevention of bronchospasm in patients 4 years of age and older with reversible obstructive airway disease. (1.1)
- Prevention of exercise-induced bronchospasm in patients 4 years of age and older. (1.2)

DOSAGE AND ADMINISTRATION

FOR ORAL INHALATION ONLY.

- Treatment or prevention of bronchospasm in adults and children 4 years of age and older: 2 inhalations every 4 to 6 hours. For some patients, 1 inhalation every 4 hours may be sufficient. (2.1)
- Prevention of exercise-induced bronchospasm in adults and children 4 years of age and older: 2 inhalations 15 to 30 minutes before exercise. (2.2)
- Priming information: Prime VENTOLIN HFA before using for the first time, when the inhaler has not been used for more than 2 weeks, or when the inhaler has been dropped. To prime VENTOLIN HFA, release 4 sprays into the air away from the face, shaking well before each spray. (2.3)
- Cleaning information: At least once a week, wash the actuator with warm water and let it air-dry completely. (2.3)

DOSAGE FORMS AND STRENGTHS

Inhalation aerosol: 108 mcg albuterol sulfate (90 mcg albuterol base) from mouthpiece per actuation. Supplied in 18-g canister containing 200 actuations and 8-g canister containing 60 actuations. (3)

CONTRAINDICATIONS

Hypersensitivity to albuterol sulfate or any of the ingredients of VENTOLIN HFA. (4)

WARNINGS AND PRECAUTIONS

- Paradoxical bronchospasm may occur and should be treated immediately with alternative therapy. (5.1)
- Need for more doses of VENTOLIN HFA than usual may be a sign of deterioration of asthma and requires reevaluation of treatment. (5.2)
- Cardiovascular effects may occur with beta-adrenergic agonists use. Consider discontinuation of VENTOLIN HFA if these effects occur. Use with caution in patients with underlying cardiovascular disorders. (5.4)
- Immediate hypersensitivity reactions may occur. Discontinue VENTOLIN HFA if immediate hypersensitivity reactions occur. (5.6)

ADVERSE REACTIONS

Most common adverse reactions (incidence ≥3%) are throat irritation, viral respiratory infections, upper respiratory inflammation, cough, and musculoskeletal pain. (6)

To report SUSPECTED ADVERSE REACTIONS, contact GlaxoSmithKline at 1-888-825-5249 or FDA at 1-800-FDA-1088 or www.fda.gov/medwatch.

DRUG INTERACTIONS

- Beta-blockers: May block bronchodilatory effects of beta-agonists and produce severe bronchospasm. Patients with asthma should not normally be treated with beta-blockers. (7.1)
- Diuretics: Electrocardiographic changes and/or hypokalemia associated with diuretics may worsen with concomitant beta-agonists. Consider monitoring potassium levels. (7.2)
- Monoamine oxidase inhibitors (MAOs) or tricyclic antidepressants: May potentiate effect of albuterol on the vascular system. Consider alternative therapy in patients taking MAOs or tricyclic antidepressants. (7.4)

See 17 for PATIENT COUNSELING INFORMATION and FDA-approved patient labeling

Revised: 10/2012

FULL PRESCRIBING INFORMATION: CONTENTS*

*** Sections or subsections omitted from the full prescribing information are not listed**

FULL PRESCRIBING INFORMATION

1 INDICATIONS AND USAGE

1.1 Bronchospasm

VENTOLIN® HFA is indicated for the treatment or prevention of bronchospasm in patients 4 years of age and older with reversible obstructive airway disease.

1.2 Exercise-Induced Bronchospasm

VENTOLIN HFA is indicated for the prevention of exercise-induced bronchospasm in patients 4 years of age and older.

2 DOSAGE AND ADMINISTRATION

Administer VENTOLIN HFA by oral inhalation only. Shake VENTOLIN HFA well before each spray.

2.1 Bronchospasm

For treatment of acute episodes of bronchospasm or prevention of symptoms associated with bronchospasm, the usual dosage for adults and children is 2 inhalations repeated every 4 to 6 hours; in some patients, 1 inhalation every 4 hours may be sufficient. More frequent administration or a larger number of inhalations is not recommended.

2.2 Exercise-Induced Bronchospasm

The usual dosage for adults and children 4 years of age and older is 2 inhalations 15 to 30 minutes before exercise.

2.3 Administration Information

Priming: Priming VENTOLIN HFA is essential to ensure appropriate albuterol content in each actuation. Prime VENTOLIN HFA before using for the first time, when the inhaler has not been used for more than 2 weeks, or when the inhaler has been dropped. To prime VENTOLIN HFA, release 4 sprays into the air away from the face, shaking well before each spray.

Cleaning: To ensure proper dosing and to prevent actuator orifice blockage, wash the actuator with warm water and let it air-dry completely at least once a week.

Dose Counter: VENTOLIN HFA has a dose counter attached to the canister that starts at 204 or 64 and counts down each time a spray is released *[see Dosage Forms and Strengths (3)]*. When the counter reads 020, the patient should contact the pharmacist for a refill of medication or consult the physician to determine whether a prescription refill is needed.

VENTOLIN HFA comes in a moisture-protective foil pouch, which should be removed prior to use. Discard VENTOLIN HFA when the counter reads 000 or 12 months after removal from the moisture-protective foil pouch, whichever comes first *[see Dosage Forms and Strengths (3)]*.

See Patient Information tear-off leaflet for instructions on how to prime and clean the inhaler to ensure proper dosing and to prevent actuator orifice blockage.

3 DOSAGE FORMS AND STRENGTHS

VENTOLIN HFA is an inhalation aerosol. Each actuation contains 108 mcg albuterol sulfate (90 mcg albuterol base) from the mouthpiece. VENTOLIN HFA is supplied as an 18-g pressurized aluminum canister with dose counter fitted with a blue plastic actuator and a blue strapcap; this canister contains 200 actuations. VENTOLIN HFA is also supplied as an 8-g pressurized aluminum canister with dose counter fitted with a blue plastic actuator and a blue strapcap; this canister contains 60 actuations.

4 CONTRAINDICATIONS

VENTOLIN HFA is contraindicated in patients with a history of hypersensitivity to albuterol or any other components of VENTOLIN HFA. Rare cases of hypersensitivity reactions, including urticaria, angioedema, and rash have been reported after the use of albuterol sulfate.

5 WARNINGS AND PRECAUTIONS

5.1 Paradoxical Bronchospasm

Inhaled albuterol sulfate can produce paradoxical bronchospasm, which may be life threatening. If paradoxical bronchospasm occurs, VENTOLIN HFA should be discontinued immediately and alternative therapy instituted. It should be recognized that paradoxical bronchospasm, when associated with inhaled formulations, frequently occurs with the first use of a new canister.

5.2 Deterioration of Asthma

Asthma may deteriorate acutely over a period of hours or chronically over several days or longer. If the patient needs more doses of VENTOLIN HFA than usual, this may be a marker of destabilization of asthma and requires reevaluation of the patient and treatment regimen, giving special consideration to the possible need for anti-inflammatory treatment, e.g., corticosteroids.

5.3 Use of Anti-Inflammatory Agents

The use of beta-adrenergic agonist bronchodilators alone may not be adequate to control asthma in many patients. Early consideration should be given to adding anti-inflammatory agents, e.g., corticosteroids, to the therapeutic regimen.

5.4 Cardiovascular Effects

VENTOLIN HFA, like all other beta$_2$-adrenergic agonists, can produce clinically significant cardiovascular effects in some patients such as changes in pulse rate or blood pressure. If such effects occur, VENTOLIN HFA may need to be discontinued. In addition, beta-agonists have been reported to produce electrocardiogram (ECG) changes, such as flattening of the T wave, prolongation of the QTc interval, and ST segment depression. The clinical relevance of these findings is unknown. Therefore, VENTOLIN HFA, like all other sympathomimetic amines, should be used with caution in patients with underlying cardiovascular disorders, especially coronary insufficiency, cardiac arrhythmias, and hypertension.

5.5 Do Not Exceed Recommended Dose

Fatalities have been reported in association with excessive use of inhaled sympathomimetic drugs in patients with asthma. The exact cause of death is unknown, but cardiac arrest following an unexpected development of a severe acute asthmatic crisis and subsequent hypoxia is suspected.

5.6 Immediate Hypersensitivity Reactions

Immediate hypersensitivity reactions may occur after administration of albuterol sulfate inhalation aerosol, as demonstrated by cases of urticaria, angioedema, rash, bronchospasm, anaphylaxis, and oropharyngeal edema. Discontinue VENTOLIN HFA if immediate hypersensitivity reactions occur.

5.7 Coexisting Conditions

VENTOLIN HFA, like other sympathomimetic amines, should be used with caution in patients with convulsive disorders, hyperthyroidism, or diabetes mellitus and in patients who are unusually responsive to sympathomimetic amines. Large doses of intravenous albuterol have been reported to aggravate preexisting diabetes mellitus and ketoacidosis.

5.8 Hypokalemia

As with other beta-agonists, albuterol may produce significant hypokalemia in some patients, possibly through intracellular shunting, which has the potential to produce adverse cardiovascular effects. The decrease is usually transient, not requiring supplementation.

6 ADVERSE REACTIONS

Use of VENTOLIN HFA may be associated with the following:

- Paradoxical bronchospasm *[see Warnings and Precautions (5.1)]*
- Cardiovascular effects *[see Warnings and Precautions (5.4)]*
- Immediate hypersensitivity reactions *[see Warnings and Precautions (5.6)]*
- Hypokalemia *[see Warnings and Precautions (5.8)]*

6.1 Clinical Trials Experience

The safety data described below reflects exposure to VENTOLIN HFA in 248 patients treated with VENTOLIN HFA in 3 placebo-controlled clinical trials of 2 to 12 weeks' duration. The data from adults and adolescents is based upon 2 clinical trials in which 202 patients with asthma 12 years of age and older were treated with VENTOLIN HFA 2 inhalations 4 times daily for 12 weeks' duration. The adult/adolescent population was 92 female, 110 male and 163 white, 19 black, 18 Hispanic, 2 other. The data from pediatric patients are based upon 1 clinical trial in which 46 patients with asthma 4 to 11 years of age were treated with VENTOLIN HFA 2 inhalations 4 times daily for 2 weeks' duration. The population was 21 female, 25 male and 25 white, 17 black, 3 Hispanic, 1 other.

Because clinical trials are conducted under widely varying conditions, adverse reaction rates observed in the clinical trials of a drug cannot be directly compared to rates in the clinical trials of another drug and may not reflect the rates observed in practice.

Adults and Adolescents 12 Years of Age and Older: The two 12-week, randomized, double-blind studies in 610 adolescent and adult patients with asthma that compared VENTOLIN HFA, a CFC 11/12-propelled albuterol inhaler, and an HFA-134a placebo inhaler. Overall, the incidence and nature of the adverse reactions reported for VENTOLIN HFA and a CFC 11/12-propelled albuterol inhaler were comparable. Table 1 lists the incidence of all adverse reactions (whether considered by the investigator to be related or unrelated to drug) from these studies that occurred at a rate of 3% or greater in the group treated with VENTOLIN HFA and more frequently in the group treated with VENTOLIN HFA than in the HFA-134a placebo inhaler group.

[See table 1 at top of next page]

Adverse reactions reported by less than 3% of the adolescent and adult patients receiving VENTOLIN HFA and by a greater proportion of patients receiving VENTOLIN HFA than receiving HFA-134a placebo inhaler and that have the potential to be related to VENTOLIN HFA include diarrhea, laryngitis, oropharyngeal edema, cough, lung disorders, tachycardia, and extrasystoles. Palpitation and dizziness have also been observed with VENTOLIN HFA.

Pediatric Patients: Results from the 2-week pediatric clinical study in patients with asthma 4 to 11 years of age showed that this pediatric population had an adverse reaction profile similar to that of the adolescent and adult populations.

Three studies have been conducted to evaluate the safety and efficacy of VENTOLIN HFA in patients between birth and 4 years of age. The results of these studies did not establish the efficacy of VENTOLIN HFA in this age-group *[see Pediatric Use (8.4)]*. Since the efficacy of VENTOLIN HFA has not been demonstrated in children between birth and 48 months of age, the safety of VENTOLIN HFA in this age-group cannot be established. However, the safety profile observed in the pediatric population under 4 years of age was comparable to that observed in the older pediatric patients and in adolescents and adults. Where adverse reaction incidence rates were greater in patients under 4 years of age compared with older patients, the higher incidence rates were noted in all treatment arms, including placebo. These adverse reactions included upper respiratory tract infection, nasopharyngitis, pyrexia, and tachycardia.

6.2 Postmarketing Experience

In addition to the adverse reactions listed in section 6.1, the following adverse reactions have been identified during postapproval use of VENTOLIN HFA. Because these reactions are reported voluntarily from a population of uncertain size, it is not always possible to reliably estimate their frequency or establish a causal relationship to drug exposure.

Cases of paradoxical bronchospasm, hoarseness, arrhythmias (including atrial fibrillation, supraventricular tachycardia), and hypersensitivity reactions (including urticaria, angioedema, rash) have been reported after the use of VENTOLIN HFA.

In addition, albuterol, like other sympathomimetic agents, can cause adverse reactions such as hypokalemia, hypertension, peripheral vasodilatation, angina, tremor, central nervous system stimulation, hyperactivity, sleeplessness, headache, muscle cramps, drying or irritation of the oropharynx, and metabolic acidosis.

7 DRUG INTERACTIONS

Other short-acting sympathomimetic aerosol bronchodilators should not be used concomitantly with albuterol. If additional adrenergic drugs are to be administered by any route, they should be used with caution to avoid deleterious cardiovascular effects.

7.1 Beta-Blockers

Beta-adrenergic receptor blocking agents not only block the pulmonary effect of beta-agonists, such as VENTOLIN HFA, but may produce severe bronchospasm in patients with asthma. Therefore, patients with asthma should not normally be treated with beta-blockers. However, under certain circumstances, e.g., as prophylaxis after myocardial infarction, there may be no acceptable alternatives to the use of beta-adrenergic blocking agents in patients with asthma. In this setting, cardioselective beta-blockers should be considered, although they should be administered with caution.

7.2 Diuretics

The ECG changes and/or hypokalemia that may result from the administration of nonpotassium-sparing diuretics (such as loop or thiazide diuretics) can be acutely worsened by beta-agonists, especially when the recommended dose of the beta-agonist is exceeded. Although the clinical relevance of these effects is not known, caution is advised in the coadministration of beta-agonists with nonpotassium-sparing diuretics. Consider monitoring potassium levels.

7.3 Digoxin

Mean decreases of 16% to 22% in serum digoxin levels were demonstrated after single-dose intravenous and oral administration of albuterol, respectively, to normal volunteers who had received digoxin for 10 days. The clinical relevance of these findings for patients with obstructive airway disease who are receiving inhaled albuterol and digoxin on a chronic basis is unclear. Nevertheless, it would be prudent to carefully evaluate the serum digoxin levels in patients who are currently receiving digoxin and albuterol.

7.4 Monoamine Oxidase Inhibitors or Tricyclic Antidepressants

VENTOLIN HFA should be administered with extreme caution to patients being treated with monoamine oxidase inhibitors or tricyclic antidepressants, or within 2 weeks of discontinuation of such agents, because the action of albuterol on the vascular system may be potentiated. Consider alternative therapy in patients taking MAOs or tricyclic antidepressants.

Table 1. Overall Adverse Reactions With ≥3% Incidence in 2 Large 12-Week Clinical Trials in Adolescents and Adults[a]

Adverse Reaction	Percent of Patients		
	VENTOLIN HFA (n = 202) %	CFC 11/12-Propelled Albuterol Inhaler (n = 207) %	Placebo HFA-134a (n = 201) %
Ear, nose, and throat			
Throat irritation	10	6	7
Upper respiratory inflammation	5	5	2
Lower respiratory			
Viral respiratory infections	7	4	4
Cough	5	2	2
Musculoskeletal			
Musculoskeletal pain	5	5	4

[a]This table includes all adverse reactions (whether considered by the investigator to be drug-related or unrelated to drug) that occurred at an incidence rate of at least 3.0% in the group treated with VENTOLIN HFA and more frequently in the group treated with VENTOLIN HFA than in the HFA-134a placebo inhaler group.

Table 2. In Vitro Medication Delivery Through AeroChamber Plus® Valved Holding Chamber With a Facemask

Age	Facemask	Flow Rate (L/min)	Holding Time (seconds)	Mean Medication Delivery Through AeroChamber Plus (mcg/actuation)	Body Weight 50th Percentile (kg)[a]	Medication Delivered per Actuation (mcg/kg)[b]
6 to 12 Months	Small	4.9	0	18.2	7.5-9.9	1.8-2.4
			2	19.8		2.0-2.6
			5	13.8		1.4-1.8
			10	15.4		1.6-2.1
2 to 5 Years	Small	8.0	0	17.8	12.3-18.0	1.0-1.4
			2	16.0		0.9-1.3
			5	16.3		0.9-1.3
			10	18.3		1.0-1.5
2 to 5 Years	Medium	8.0	0	21.1	12.3-18.0	1.2-1.7
			2	15.3		0.8-1.2
			5	18.3		1.0-1.5
			10	18.2		1.0-1.5
>5 Years	Medium	12.0	0	26.8	18.0	1.5
			2	20.9		1.2
			5	19.6		1.1
			10	20.3		1.1

[a]Centers for Disease Control growth charts, developed by the National Center for Health Statistics in collaboration with the National Center for Chronic Disease Prevention and Health Promotion (2000). Ranges correspond to the average of the 50th percentile weight for boys and girls at the ages indicated.

[b]A single inhalation of VENTOLIN HFA in a 70-kg adult without use of a valved holding chamber and facemask delivers approximately 90 mcg, or 1.3 mcg/kg.

8 USE IN SPECIFIC POPULATIONS

8.1 Pregnancy

Teratogenic Effects: Pregnancy Category C.

There are no adequate and well-controlled studies of VENTOLIN HFA or albuterol sulfate in pregnant women. During worldwide marketing experience, various congenital anomalies, including cleft palate and limb defects, have been reported in the offspring of patients being treated with albuterol. Some of the mothers were taking multiple medications during their pregnancies. No consistent pattern of defects can be discerned, and a relationship between albuterol use and congenital anomalies has not been established. Animal reproduction studies in mice and rabbits revealed evidence of teratogenicity. VENTOLIN HFA should be used during pregnancy only if the potential benefit justifies the potential risk to the fetus.

In a mouse reproduction study, subcutaneously administered albuterol sulfate produced cleft palate formation in 5 of 111 (4.5%) fetuses at exposures approximately equal to the maximum recommended human dose (MRHD) for adults on a mg/m^2 basis and in 10 of 108 (9.3%) fetuses at approximately 8 times the MRHD. Similar effects were not observed at approximately one eleventh of the MRHD. Cleft palate also occurred in 22 of 72 (30.5%) fetuses from females treated subcutaneously with isoproterenol (positive control).

In a rabbit reproduction study, orally administered albuterol sulfate produced cranioschisis in 7 of 19 fetuses (37%) at approximately 680 times the MRHD.

In another rabbit study, an albuterol sulfate/HFA-134a formulation administered by inhalation produced enlargement of the frontal portion of the fetal fontanelles at approximately one third of the MRHD *[see Animal Toxicology and/or Pharmacology (13.2)]*.

8.2 Labor and Delivery

Because of the potential for beta-agonist interference with uterine contractility, use of VENTOLIN HFA for relief of bronchospasm during labor should be restricted to those patients in whom the benefits clearly outweigh the risk.

8.3 Nursing Mothers

Plasma levels of albuterol sulfate and HFA-134a after inhaled therapeutic doses are very low in humans, but it is not known whether the components of VENTOLIN HFA are excreted in human milk. Because of the potential for tumorigenicity shown for albuterol in animal studies and lack of experience with the use of VENTOLIN HFA by nursing mothers, a decision should be made whether to discontinue nursing or to discontinue the drug, taking into account the importance of the drug to the mother. Caution should be exercised when VENTOLIN HFA is administered to a nursing woman.

8.4 Pediatric Use

The safety and effectiveness of VENTOLIN HFA in children 4 years of age and older has been established based upon two 12-week clinical trials in patients 12 years of age and older with asthma and one 2-week clinical trial in patients 4 to 11 years of age with asthma *[see Clinical Studies (14.1), Adverse Reactions (6.1)]*. The safety and effectiveness of VENTOLIN HFA in children under 4 years of age has not been established. Three studies have been conducted to evaluate the safety and efficacy of VENTOLIN HFA in patients under 4 years of age and the findings are described below.

Two 4-week randomized, double-blind, placebo-controlled studies were conducted in 163 pediatric patients from birth to 48 months of age with symptoms of bronchospasm associated with obstructive airway disease (presenting symptoms included: wheeze, cough, dyspnea, or chest tightness). VENTOLIN HFA or placebo HFA was delivered with either an AeroChamber Plus® Valved Holding Chamber or an Optichamber® Valved Holding Chamber with mask 3 times daily. In one study, VENTOLIN HFA 90 mcg (N = 26), VENTOLIN HFA 180 mcg (N = 25), and placebo HFA (N = 26) were administered to children between 24 and 48 months of age. In the second study, VENTOLIN HFA 90 mcg (N = 29), VENTOLIN HFA 180 mcg (N = 29), and placebo HFA (N = 28) were administered to children between birth and 24 months of age. Over the 4-week treatment period, there were no treatment differences in asthma symptom scores between the groups receiving VENTOLIN HFA 90 mcg, VENTOLIN HFA 180 mcg, and placebo in either study.

In a third study, VENTOLIN HFA was evaluated in 87 pediatric patients younger than 24 months of age for the treatment of acute wheezing. VENTOLIN HFA was delivered with an AeroChamber Plus Valved Holding Chamber in this study. There were no significant differences in asthma symptom scores and mean change from baseline in an asthma symptom score between VENTOLIN HFA 180 mcg and VENTOLIN HFA 360 mcg.

In vitro dose characterization studies were performed to evaluate the delivery of VENTOLIN HFA via holding chambers with facemasks. The studies were conducted with 2 different holding chambers with facemasks (small and medium size). The in vitro study data when simulated to patients suggest that the dose of VENTOLIN HFA presented for inhalation via a valved holding chamber with facemask will be comparable to the dose delivered in adults without a spacer and facemask per kilogram of body weight (Table 2). However, clinical studies in children under 4 years of age described above suggest that either the optimal dose of VENTOLIN HFA has not been defined in this age-group or VENTOLIN HFA is not effective in this age-group. The safety and effectiveness of VENTOLIN HFA administered with or without a spacer device in children under 4 years of age has not been demonstrated.

[See table 2 above]

8.5 Geriatric Use

Clinical studies of VENTOLIN HFA did not include sufficient numbers of subjects aged 65 and over to determine whether they respond differently from younger subjects. Other reported clinical experience has not identified differences in responses between the elderly and younger patients. In general, dose selection for an elderly patient should be cautious, usually starting at the low end of the dosing range, reflecting the greater frequency of decreased hepatic, renal, or cardiac function, and of concomitant disease or other drug therapy.

10 OVERDOSAGE

The expected symptoms with overdosage are those of excessive beta-adrenergic stimulation and/or occurrence or exaggeration of any of the symptoms listed under ADVERSE REACTIONS, e.g., seizures, angina, hypertension or hypotension, tachycardia with rates up to 200 beats/min, arrhythmias, nervousness, headache, tremor, dry mouth, palpitation, nausea, dizziness, fatigue, malaise, sleeplessness. Hypokalemia and metabolic acidosis may also occur.

As with all sympathomimetic aerosol medications, cardiac arrest and even death may be associated with abuse of VENTOLIN HFA. Treatment consists of discontinuation of VENTOLIN HFA together with appropriate symptomatic therapy. The judicious use of a cardioselective beta-receptor blocker may be considered, bearing in mind that such medication can produce bronchospasm. There is insufficient evidence to determine if dialysis is beneficial for overdosage of VENTOLIN HFA.

The oral median lethal dose of albuterol sulfate in mice is greater than 2,000 mg/kg (approximately 6,800 times the maximum recommended daily inhalation dose for adults on a mg/m^2 basis and approximately 3,200 times the maximum recommended daily inhalation dose for children on a mg/m^2 basis). In mature rats, the subcutaneous median lethal dose of albuterol sulfate is approximately 450 mg/kg (approximately 3,000 times the maximum recommended daily inhalation dose for adults on a mg/m^2 basis and approximately 1,400 times the maximum recommended daily inhalation dose for children on a mg/m^2 basis). In young rats, the subcutaneous median lethal dose is approximately 2,000 mg/kg (approximately 14,000 times the maximum recommended daily inhalation dose for adults on a mg/m^2 basis and approximately 6,400 times the maximum recommended daily inhalation dose for children on a mg/m^2 basis). The inhalation median lethal dose has not been determined in animals.

11 DESCRIPTION

The active component of VENTOLIN HFA is albuterol sulfate, USP, the racemic form of albuterol and a relatively selective beta$_2$-adrenergic bronchodilator. Albuterol sulfate has the chemical name α^1-[(*tert*-butylamino)methyl]-4-hydroxy-*m*-xylene-α, α'-diol sulfate (2:1)(salt) and the following chemical structure:

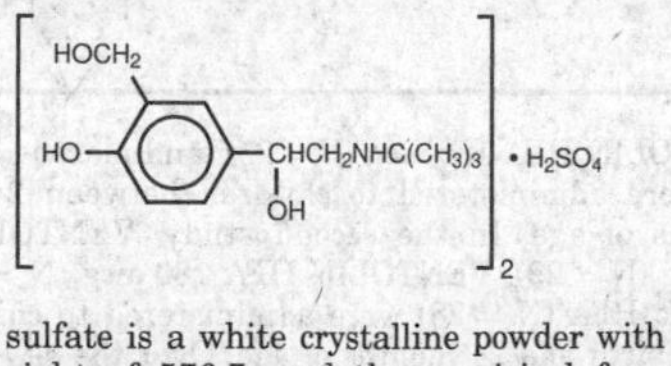

Albuterol sulfate is a white crystalline powder with a molecular weight of 576.7, and the empirical formula is $(C_{13}H_{21}NO_3)_2 \bullet H_2SO_4$. It is soluble in water and slightly soluble in ethanol.

The World Health Organization recommended name for albuterol base is salbutamol.

VENTOLIN HFA is a pressurized metered-dose aerosol unit fitted with a counter. VENTOLIN HFA is intended for oral inhalation only. Each unit contains a microcrystalline suspension of albuterol sulfate in propellant HFA-134a (1,1,1,2-tetrafluoroethane). It contains no other excipients.

Priming VENTOLIN HFA is essential to ensure appropriate albuterol content in each actuation. To prime the inhaler, release 4 sprays into the air away from the face, shaking well before each spray. The inhaler should be primed before using it for the first time, when it has not been used for more than 2 weeks, or when it has been dropped.

After priming, each actuation of the inhaler delivers 120 mcg of albuterol sulfate, USP in 75 mg of suspension from the valve and 108 mcg of albuterol sulfate, USP from the mouthpiece (equivalent to 90 mcg of albuterol base from the mouthpiece).

Each 18-g canister provides 200 inhalations. Each 8-g canister provides 60 inhalations.

This product does not contain chlorofluorocarbons (CFCs) as the propellant.

12 CLINICAL PHARMACOLOGY

12.1 Mechanism of Action

In vitro studies and in vivo pharmacologic studies have demonstrated that albuterol has a preferential effect on beta$_2$-adrenergic receptors compared with isoproterenol. While it is recognized that beta$_2$-adrenergic receptors are the predominant receptors in bronchial smooth muscle, data indicate that there is a population of beta$_2$-receptors in the human heart existing in a concentration between 10% and 50% of cardiac beta-adrenergic receptors. The precise function of these receptors has not been established *[see Warnings and Precautions (5.4)]*.

Activation of beta$_2$-adrenergic receptors on airway smooth muscle leads to the activation of adenylcyclase and to an increase in the intracellular concentration of cyclic-3′,5′-adenosine monophosphate (cyclic AMP). This increase of cyclic AMP leads to the activation of protein kinase A, which inhibits the phosphorylation of myosin and lowers intracellular ionic calcium concentrations, resulting in relaxation. Albuterol relaxes the smooth muscles of all airways, from the trachea to the terminal bronchioles. Albuterol acts as a functional antagonist to relax the airway irrespective of the spasmogen involved, thus protecting against all bronchoconstrictor challenges. Increased cyclic AMP concentrations are also associated with the inhibition of release of mediators from mast cells in the airway.

Albuterol has been shown in most controlled clinical trials to have more effect on the respiratory tract, in the form of bronchial smooth muscle relaxation, than isoproterenol at comparable doses while producing fewer cardiovascular effects. Controlled clinical studies and other clinical experience have shown that inhaled albuterol, like other beta-adrenergic agonist drugs, can produce a significant cardiovascular effect in some patients, as measured by pulse rate, blood pressure, symptoms, and/or electrocardiographic changes *[see Warnings and Precautions (5.4)]*.

12.2 Pharmacokinetics

The systemic levels of albuterol are low after inhalation of recommended doses. A study conducted in 12 healthy male and female subjects using a higher dose (1,080 mcg of albuterol base) showed that mean peak plasma concentrations of approximately 3 ng/mL occurred after dosing when albuterol was delivered using propellant HFA-134a. The mean time to peak concentrations (T_{max}) was delayed after administration of VENTOLIN HFA (T_{max} = 0.42 hours) as compared to CFC-propelled albuterol inhaler (T_{max} = 0.17 hours). Apparent terminal plasma half-life of albuterol is approximately 4.6 hours. No further pharmacokinetic studies for VENTOLIN HFA were conducted in neonates, children, or elderly subjects.

13 NONCLINICAL TOXICOLOGY

13.1 Carcinogenesis, Mutagenesis, Impairment of Fertility

In a 2-year study in Sprague-Dawley rats, albuterol sulfate caused a dose-related increase in the incidence of benign leiomyomas of the mesovarium at and above dietary doses of 2.0 mg/kg (approximately 14 times the maximum recommended daily inhalation dose for adults on a mg/m^2 basis and approximately 6 times the maximum recommended daily inhalation dose for children on a mg/m^2 basis). In another study this effect was blocked by the coadministration of propranolol, a non-selective beta-adrenergic antagonist.

In an 18-month study in CD-1 mice, albuterol sulfate showed no evidence of tumorigenicity at dietary doses of up to 500 mg/kg (approximately 1,700 times the maximum recommended daily inhalation dose for adults on a mg/m^2 basis and approximately 800 times the maximum recommended daily inhalation dose for children on a mg/m^2 basis). In a 22-month study in Golden hamsters, albuterol sulfate showed no evidence of tumorigenicity at dietary doses of up to 50 mg/kg (approximately 225 times the maximum recommended daily inhalation dose for adults on a mg/m^2 basis and approximately 110 times the maximum recommended daily inhalation dose for children on a mg/m^2 basis).

Albuterol sulfate was not mutagenic in the Ames test or a mutation test in yeast. Albuterol sulfate was not clastogenic in a human peripheral lymphocyte assay or in an AH1 strain mouse micronucleus assay.

Reproduction studies in rats demonstrated no evidence of impaired fertility at oral doses of albuterol sulfate up to 50 mg/kg (approximately 340 times the maximum recommended daily inhalation dose for adults on a mg/m^2 basis).

13.2 Animal Toxicology and/or Pharmacology

Preclinical: Intravenous studies in rats with albuterol sulfate have demonstrated that albuterol crosses the blood-brain barrier and reaches brain concentrations amounting to approximately 5.0% of the plasma concentrations. In structures outside the blood-brain barrier (pineal and pituitary glands), albuterol concentrations were found to be 100 times those in the whole brain.

Studies in laboratory animals (minipigs, rodents, and dogs) have demonstrated the occurrence of cardiac arrhythmias and sudden death (with histologic evidence of myocardial necrosis) when beta-agonists and methylxanthines are administered concurrently. The clinical relevance of these findings is unknown.

Propellant HFA-134a is devoid of pharmacological activity except at very high doses in animals (380 to 1,300 times the maximum human exposure based on comparisons of AUC values), primarily producing ataxia, tremors, dyspnea, or salivation. These are similar to effects produced by the structurally related CFCs, which have been used extensively in metered-dose inhalers.

In animals and humans, propellant HFA-134a was found to be rapidly absorbed and rapidly eliminated, with an elimination half-life of 3 to 27 minutes in animals and 5 to 7 minutes in humans. Time to maximum plasma concentration (T_{max}) and mean residence time are both extremely short, leading to a transient appearance of HFA-134a in the blood with no evidence of accumulation.

Reproductive Toxicology Studies: A study in CD-1 mice given albuterol sulfate subcutaneously showed cleft palate formation in 5 of 111 (4.5%) fetuses at 0.25 mg/kg (less than the maximum recommended daily inhalation dose for adults on a mg/m^2 basis) and in 10 of 108 (9.3%) fetuses at 2.5 mg/kg (approximately 8 times the maximum recommended daily inhalation dose for adults on a mg/m^2 basis). The drug did not induce cleft palate formation at a dose of 0.025 mg/kg (less than the maximum recommended daily inhalation dose for adults on a mg/m^2 basis). Cleft palate also occurred in 22 of 72 (30.5%) fetuses from females treated subcutaneously with 2.5 mg/kg of isoproterenol (positive control).

A reproduction study in Stride Dutch rabbits revealed cranioschisis in 7 of 19 fetuses (37%) when albuterol sulfate was administered orally at a 50 mg/kg dose (approximately 680 times the maximum recommended daily inhalation dose for adults on a mg/m^2 basis).

In an inhalation reproduction study in New Zealand white rabbits, albuterol sulfate/HFA-134a formulation exhibited enlargement of the frontal portion of the fetal fontanelles at and above inhalation doses of 0.0193 mg/kg (less than the maximum recommended daily inhalation dose for adults on a mg/m^2 basis).

A study in which pregnant rats were dosed with radiolabeled albuterol sulfate demonstrated that drug-related material is transferred from the maternal circulation to the fetus.

14 CLINICAL STUDIES

14.1 Bronchospasm Associated With Asthma

Adult and Adolescent Patients 12 Years of Age and Older: The efficacy of VENTOLIN HFA was evaluated in two 12-week, randomized, double-blind, placebo controlled trials in patients 12 years of age and older with mild to moderate asthma. These trials included a total of 610 patients (323 males, 287 females). In each trial, patients received 2 inhalations of VENTOLIN HFA, CFC 11/12-propelled albuterol, or HFA-134a placebo 4 times daily for 12 weeks' duration. Patients taking the HFA-134a placebo inhaler also took VENTOLIN HFA for asthma symptom relief on an as-needed basis. Some patients who participated in these clinical trials were using concomitant inhaled steroid therapy. Efficacy was assessed by serial forced expiratory volume in 1 second (FEV_1). In each of these trials, 2 inhalations of VENTOLIN HFA produced significantly greater improvement in FEV_1 over the pretreatment value than placebo. Results from the 2 clinical trials are described below.

In a 12-week, randomized, double-blind study, VENTOLIN HFA (101 patients) was compared to CFC 11/12-propelled albuterol (99 patients) and an HFA-134a placebo inhaler (97 patients) in adolescent and adult patients 12 to 76 years of age with mild to moderate asthma. Serial FEV_1 measurements [shown below as percent change from test-day baseline at Day 1 (n = 297) and at Week 12 (n = 249)] demonstrated that 2 inhalations of VENTOLIN HFA produced significantly greater improvement in FEV_1 over the pretreatment value than placebo.

[See first figure at top of next column]
[See second figure at top of next column]

In the responder population (≥15% increase in FEV_1 within 30 minutes postdose) treated with VENTOLIN HFA, the mean time to onset of a 15% increase in FEV_1 over the pretreatment value was 5.4 minutes, and the mean time to peak effect was 56 minutes. The mean duration of effect as measured by a 15% increase in FEV_1 over the pretreatment value was approximately 4 hours. In some patients, duration of effect was as long as 6 hours.

The second 12-week randomized, double-blind study was conducted to evaluate the efficacy and safety of switching patients from CFC 11/12-propelled albuterol to VENTOLIN HFA. During the 3-week run-in phase of the study, all patients received CFC 11/12-propelled albuterol. During the double-blind treatment phase, VENTOLIN HFA (91 patients) was compared to CFC 11/12-propelled albuterol (100 patients) and an HFA-134a placebo inhaler (95 patients) in adolescent and adult patients with mild to moderate asthma. Serial FEV_1 measurements demonstrated that 2 inhalations of VENTOLIN HFA produced significantly greater improvement in pulmonary function than placebo. The switching from CFC 11/12-propelled albuterol inhaler to VENTOLIN HFA did not reveal any clinically significant changes in the efficacy profile.

FEV_1 as Percent Change From Predose in a Large, 12-Week Clinical Trial

Day 1

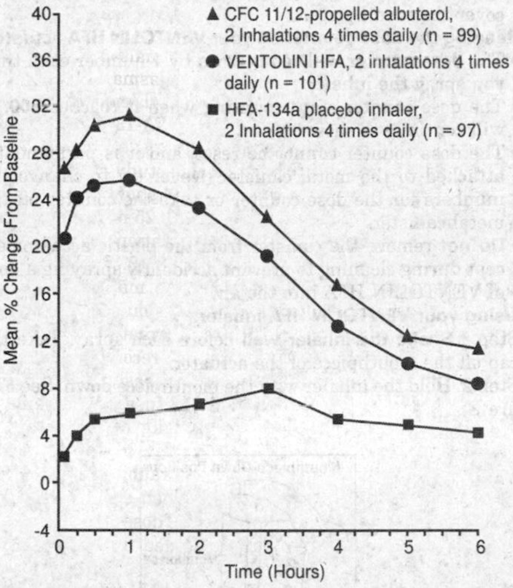

Week 12

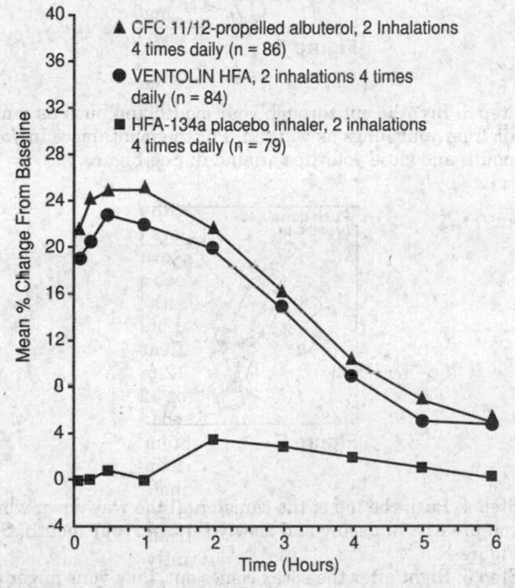

In the 2 adult studies, the efficacy results from VENTOLIN HFA were significantly greater than placebo and were clinically comparable to those achieved with CFC 11/12-propelled albuterol, although small numerical differences in mean FEV_1 response and other measures were observed. Physicians should recognize that individual responses to beta-adrenergic agonists administered via different propellants may vary and that equivalent responses in individual patients should not be assumed.

Pediatric Patients 4 Years of Age: The efficacy of VENTOLIN HFA was evaluated in one 2-week, randomized, double-blind, placebo-controlled trial in 135 pediatric patients 4 to 11 years of age with mild to moderate asthma. In this trial, patients received VENTOLIN HFA, CFC 11/12-propelled albuterol, or HFA-134a placebo. Serial pulmonary function measurements demonstrated that 2 inhalations of VENTOLIN HFA produced significantly greater improvement in pulmonary function than placebo and that there were no significant differences between the groups treated with VENTOLIN HFA and CFC 11/12-propelled albuterol. In the responder population treated with VENTOLIN HFA, the mean time to onset of a 15% increase in peak expiratory flow rate (PEFR) over the pretreatment value was 7.8 minutes, and the mean time to peak effect was approximately 90 minutes. The mean duration of effect as measured by a 15% increase in PEFR over the pretreatment value was greater than 3 hours. In some patients, duration of effect was as long as 6 hours.

14.2 Exercise-Induced Bronchospasm

One controlled clinical study in adult patients with asthma (N = 24) demonstrated that 2 inhalations of VENTOLIN HFA taken approximately 30 minutes prior to exercise significantly prevented exercise-induced bronchospasm (as measured by maximum percentage fall in FEV_1 following exercise) compared to an HFA-134a placebo inhaler. In addition, VENTOLIN HFA was shown to be clinically comparable to a CFC 11/12-propelled albuterol inhaler for this indication.

16 HOW SUPPLIED/STORAGE AND HANDLING

VENTOLIN HFA (albuterol sulfate) Inhalation Aerosol is supplied in the following packs as a pressurized aluminum canister fitted with a counter with a blue plastic actuator and a blue strapcap packaged within a moisture-protective foil pouch that also contains a desiccant:

NDC 0173-0682-20 18-g canister containing 200 actuations
NDC 0173-0682-21 8-g canister containing 60 actuations
NDC 0173-0682-24 8-g institutional pack canister containing 60 actuations

Before using, VENTOLIN HFA should be removed from the moisture-protective foil pouch. The pouch and desiccant should be discarded. VENTOLIN HFA should be discarded 12 months after removal from the pouch.

Priming VENTOLIN HFA is essential to ensure appropriate albuterol content in each actuation. To prime the inhaler, release 4 sprays into the air away from the face, shaking well before each spray. The inhaler should be primed before using it for the first time, when the inhaler has not been used for more than 2 weeks, or when it has been dropped. After priming, each actuation delivers 120 mcg of albuterol sulfate, USP in 75 mg of suspension from the valve and 108 mcg of albuterol sulfate, USP from the mouthpiece (equivalent to 90 mcg of albuterol base from the mouthpiece).

To ensure proper dosing and to prevent actuator orifice blockage, wash the actuator with warm water and let it air-dry completely at least once a week [see the Patient Information tear-off leaflet].

The blue actuator supplied with VENTOLIN HFA should not be used with any other product canisters, and actuators from other products should not be used with a VENTOLIN HFA canister.

VENTOLIN HFA has a counter attached to the canister. The counter starts at 204 or 64 and counts down each time a spray is released. The correct amount of medication in each inhalation cannot be assured after the counter reads 000, even though the canister is not completely empty and will continue to operate. VENTOLIN HFA should be discarded when the counter reads 000 or 12 months after removal from the moisture-protective foil pouch, whichever comes first. Never immerse the canister in water to determine the amount of drug remaining in the canister.

Keep out of reach of children. Avoid spraying in eyes.

Contents Under Pressure: Do not puncture. Do not use or store near heat or open flame. Exposure to temperatures above 120°F may cause bursting. Never throw container into fire or incinerator.

Store between 15° and 25°C (59° and 77°F). Store the inhaler with the mouthpiece down. For best results, the inhaler should be at room temperature before use. SHAKE WELL BEFORE EACH SPRAY.

VENTOLIN HFA does not contain chlorofluorocarbons (CFCs) as the propellant.

17 PATIENT COUNSELING INFORMATION

See FDA-approved patient labeling (Patient Information and Instructions for Use).

17.1 Frequency of Use

The action of VENTOLIN HFA should last up to 4 to 6 hours. VENTOLIN HFA should not be used more frequently than recommended. Do not increase the dose or frequency of doses of VENTOLIN HFA without consulting the physician. If patients find that treatment with VENTOLIN HFA becomes less effective for symptomatic relief, symptoms become worse, and/or they need to use the product more frequently than usual, they should seek medical attention immediately.

17.2 Priming and Cleaning

Priming: Patients should be instructed that priming VENTOLIN HFA is essential to ensure appropriate albuterol content in each actuation. Patients should prime VENTOLIN HFA before using for the first time, when the inhaler has not been used for more than 2 weeks, or when the inhaler has been dropped. To prime VENTOLIN HFA, patients should release 4 sprays into the air away from the face, shaking well before each spray.

Cleaning: To ensure proper dosing and to prevent actuator orifice blockage, patients should be instructed to wash the actuator and dry thoroughly at least once a week. Patients should be informed that detailed cleaning instructions are included in the Patient Information leaflet.

17.3 Dose Counter

Patients should be informed that VENTOLIN HFA has a dose counter that starts at 204 or 64 and counts down each time a spray is released. Patients should be informed to discard VENTOLIN HFA when the counter reads 000 or 12 months after removal from the moisture-protective foil pouch, whichever comes first. When the counter reads 020, the patient should contact the pharmacist for a refill of medication or consult the physician to determine whether a prescription refill is needed. Patients should never try to alter the numbers or remove the counter from the metal canister. Patients should never immerse the canister in water to determine the amount of drug remaining in the canister.

17.4 Paradoxical Bronchospasm

Patients should be informed that VENTOLIN HFA can produce paradoxical bronchospasm. If paradoxical bronchospasm occurs, patients should discontinue VENTOLIN HFA.

17.5 Concomitant Drug Use

While patients are using VENTOLIN HFA, other inhaled drugs and asthma medications should be taken only as directed by the physician.

17.6 Common Adverse Effects

Common adverse effects of treatment with inhaled albuterol include palpitations, chest pain, rapid heart rate, tremor, and nervousness.

17.7 Pregnancy

Patients who are pregnant or nursing should contact their physicians about the use of VENTOLIN HFA.

VENTOLIN is a registered trademark of GlaxoSmithKline.
AeroChamber Plus is a registered trademark of Monaghan Medical Inc.
OptiChamber is a registered trademark of Respironics Inc.

GlaxoSmithKline
Research Triangle Park, NC 27709

VNT:8PI

PHARMACIST—DETACH HERE AND GIVE LEAFLET TO PATIENT

Patient Information

VENTOLIN® HFA *(vent' o-lin)*
(albuterol sulfate)
Inhalation Aerosol

Read this Patient Information before you start using VENTOLIN HFA and each time you get a refill. There may be new information. This information does not take the place of talking to your healthcare provider about your medical condition or your treatment.

What is VENTOLIN HFA?

VENTOLIN HFA is a prescription medicine used in people 4 years of age and older to:

- treat or prevent bronchospasm in people who have reversible obstructive airway disease
- prevent exercise-induced bronchospasm

It is not known if VENTOLIN HFA is safe and effective in children under 4 years of age.

Who should not use VENTOLIN HFA?

Do not use VENTOLIN HFA if you are allergic to albuterol sulfate or any of the ingredients in VENTOLIN HFA. See the end of this Patient Information leaflet for a complete list of ingredients in VENTOLIN HFA.

What should I tell my healthcare provider before I use VENTOLIN HFA?

Before you use VENTOLIN HFA, tell your healthcare provider if you:

- have heart problems
- have high blood pressure (hypertension)
- have convulsions (seizures)
- have thyroid problems
- have diabetes
- have low potassium levels in your blood
- are pregnant or plan to become pregnant. It is not known if VENTOLIN HFA will harm your unborn baby. Talk to your healthcare provider if you are pregnant or plan to become pregnant.
- are breastfeeding or plan to breastfeed. It is not known if VENTOLIN HFA passes into your breast milk. Talk to your healthcare provider about the best way to feed your baby if you are using VENTOLIN HFA.

Tell your healthcare provider about all the medicines you take, including prescription and nonprescription medicines, vitamins, and herbal supplements.

VENTOLIN HFA and other medicines may affect each other and cause side effects. VENTOLIN HFA may affect the way other medicines work, and other medicines may affect the way VENTOLIN HFA works.

Especially tell your healthcare provider if you take:

- other inhaled medicines or asthma medicines
- beta-blocker medicines
- diuretics
- digoxin
- monoamine oxidase inhibitors
- tricyclic antidepressants

Ask your healthcare provider or pharmacist for a list of these medicines if you are not sure.

Know the medicines you take. Keep a list of them to show your healthcare provider and pharmacist when you get a new medicine.

How should I use VENTOLIN HFA?

- For detailed instructions, see **"Instructions for Use"** at the end of this Patient Information.

- Use VENTOLIN HFA exactly as your healthcare provider tells you to use it.
- **Do not** increase your dose or take extra doses of VENTOLIN HFA without first talking to your healthcare provider.
- If your child needs to use VENTOLIN HFA, watch your child closely to make sure your child uses the inhaler correctly. Your healthcare provider will show you how your child should use VENTOLIN HFA.
- Each dose of VENTOLIN HFA should last up to 4 hours to 6 hours.
- Get medical help right away if VENTOLIN HFA no longer helps your symptoms.
- Get medical help right away if your symptoms get worse or if you need to use your inhaler more often.
- While you are using VENTOLIN HFA, use other inhaled medicines and asthma medicines only as directed by your healthcare provider.
- Call your healthcare provider if your asthma symptoms like wheezing and trouble breathing become worse over a few hours or days. Your healthcare provider may need to give you another medicine to treat your symptoms.

What are the possible side effects of VENTOLIN HFA?

VENTOLIN HFA may cause serious side effects, including:

- **worsening trouble breathing, coughing, and wheezing (paradoxical bronchospasm).** If this happens, stop using VENTOLIN HFA and call your healthcare provider or get emergency help right away. Paradoxical bronchospasm is more likely to happen with your first use of a new canister of medicine.
- **heart problems, including faster heart rate and higher blood pressure**
- **possible death in people with asthma who use too much VENTOLIN HFA**
- **allergic reactions.** Call your healthcare provider right away if you have any of the following symptoms of an allergic reaction:
  - itchy skin
  - swelling beneath your skin or in your throat
  - rash
  - worsening trouble breathing
- **low potassium levels in your blood**
- **worsening of other medical problems in people who also use VENTOLIN HFA, including increases in blood sugar**

Common side effects of VENTOLIN HFA include:

- your heart feels like it is pounding or racing (palpitations)
- chest pain
- fast heart rate
- shakiness
- nervousness
- headache
- pain
- dizziness
- sore throat
- runny nose

Tell your healthcare provider if you have any side effect that bothers you or that does not go away.

These are not all the possible side effects of VENTOLIN HFA. For more information, ask your healthcare provider or pharmacist.

Call your doctor for medical advice about side effects. You may report side effects to FDA at 1-800-FDA-1088.

How should I store VENTOLIN HFA?

- Store VENTOLIN HFA at room temperature between 59°F and 77°F (15°C and 25°C) with the mouthpiece down.
- Avoid exposure to extreme heat and cold.
- Shake the VENTOLIN HFA canister well before use.
- **Do not** puncture the VENTOLIN HFA canister.
- **Do not** store the VENTOLIN HFA canister near heat or a flame. Temperatures above 120°F may cause the canister to burst.
- **Do not** throw the VENTOLIN HFA canister into a fire or an incinerator.
- Avoid spraying VENTOLIN HFA in your eyes.

Keep VENTOLIN HFA and all medicines out of the reach of children.

General information about the safe and effective use of VENTOLIN HFA

Medicines are sometimes prescribed for purposes other than those listed in a Patient Information leaflet. Do not use VENTOLIN HFA for a condition for which it was not prescribed. Do not give VENTOLIN HFA to other people, even if they have the same symptoms that you have. It may harm them.

This Patient Information leaflet summarizes the most important information about VENTOLIN HFA. If you would like more information, talk with your healthcare provider. You can ask your pharmacist or healthcare provider for information about VENTOLIN HFA that is written for healthcare professionals.

For more information, go to www.ventolin.com or call 1-888-825-5249.

What are the ingredients in VENTOLIN HFA?

Active ingredient: albuterol sulfate

Inactive ingredient: propellant HFA-134a

Instructions for Use

VENTOLIN® HFA *(vent' o-lin)*

(albuterol sulfate)

Inhalation Aerosol

Read this Instructions for Use before you start using VENTOLIN HFA and each time you get a refill. There may be new information. This information does not take the place of talking to your healthcare provider about your medical condition or your treatment.

The parts of your VENTOLIN HFA inhaler:

There are 2 main parts of your VENTOLIN HFA inhaler:

- the blue plastic actuator that sprays the medicine into your mouth. See Figure A.
- the metal canister that holds the medicine. See Figure A.

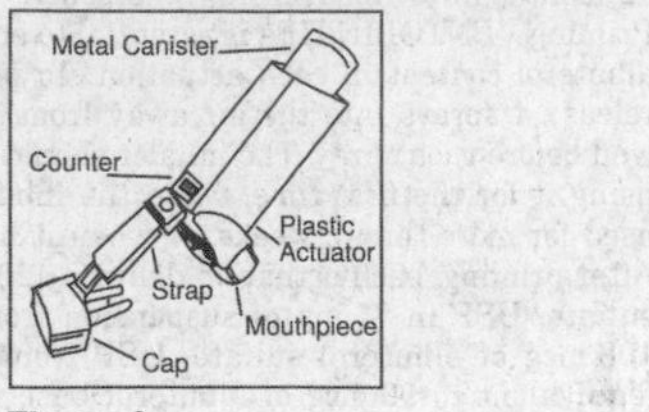

Figure A

The actuator has a protective cap that covers the mouthpiece. The strap on the cap will stay attached to the actuator.

Do not use this actuator with a canister of medicine from any other inhaler.

Do not use this canister of medicine with an actuator from any other inhaler.

The canister has a counter that shows you how many sprays of medicine you have left. The number shows through a window in the back of the actuator. The counter starts at either 204 or 64, depending on which size inhaler you have. See Figure B.

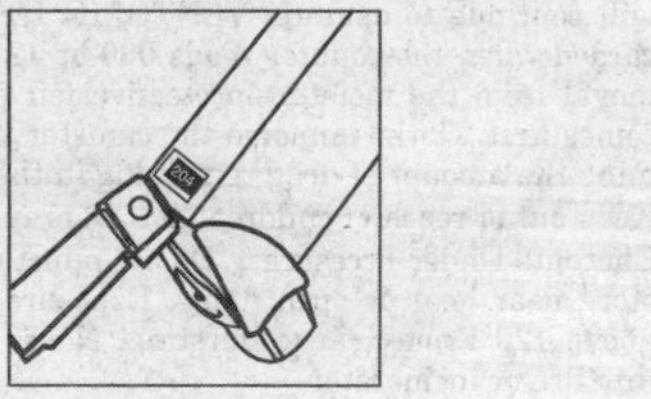

Figure B

Priming your VENTOLIN HFA inhaler:

Your VENTOLIN HFA inhaler must be primed before you use it for the first time, when it has not been used for more than 14 days in a row, or if it has been dropped. Do not prime your VENTOLIN HFA every day.

- Remove your VENTOLIN HFA inhaler from its packaging.
- Throw away the pouch and the drying packet that comes inside the pouch.
- Remove the protective cap from the mouthpiece.
- Shake the inhaler well, and spray it into the air away from your face. See Figure C.

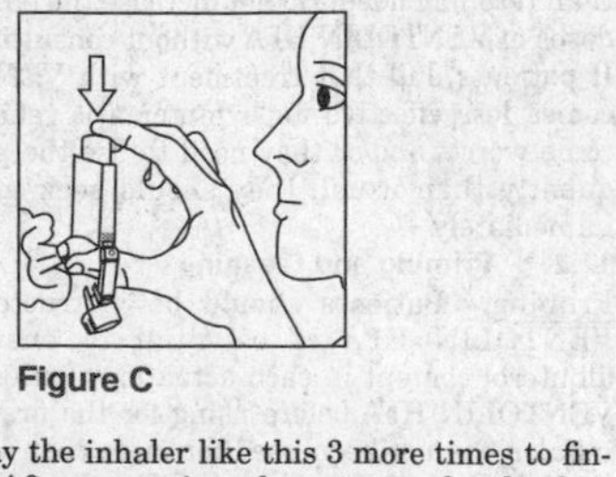

Figure C

- Shake and spray the inhaler like this 3 more times to finish priming it. After you prime the actuator for the first time, the dose counter in the window on the back of the actuator should show the number 200 or 60, depending on which size inhaler you have. See Figure D.

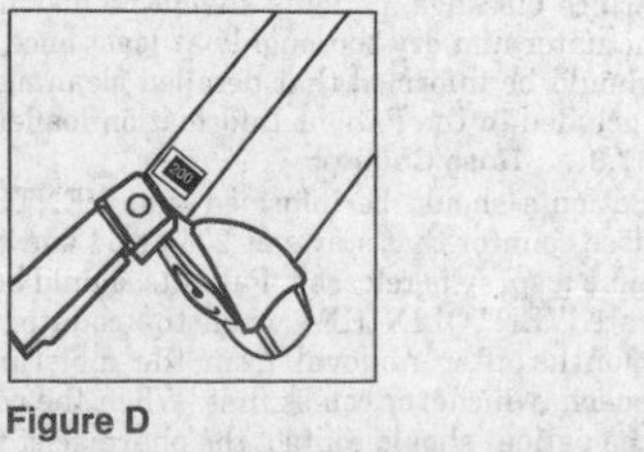

Figure D

Each time you use your VENTOLIN HFA inhaler:

- Make sure the canister fits firmly in the plastic actuator.
- Look into the mouthpiece to make sure there are no foreign objects there, especially if the strap is no longer attached to the actuator or the cap has not been used to cover the mouthpiece.

Reading the dose counter on your VENTOLIN HFA actuator:

- The dose counter will count down by 1 number each time you spray the inhaler.
- The dose counter stops counting when it reaches **000.** It will continue to show **000.**
- The dose counter cannot be reset, and it is permanently attached to the metal canister. **Never** try to change the numbers for the dose counter or take the counter off the metal canister.
- **Do not** remove the canister from the plastic actuator except during cleaning to prevent accidently spraying a dose of VENTOLIN HFA into the air.

Using your VENTOLIN HFA inhaler:

Step 1.**Shake the inhaler well** before each spray. Take the cap off the mouthpiece of the actuator.

Step 2. Hold the inhaler with the mouthpiece down. See Figure E.

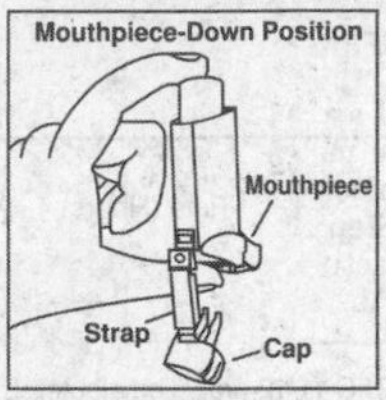

Figure E

Step 3. Breathe out through your mouth and push as much air from your lungs as you can. Put the mouthpiece in your mouth and close your lips around it. See Figure F.

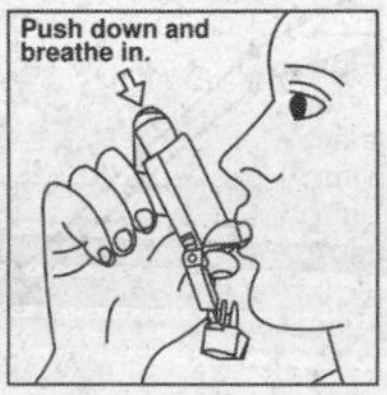

Figure F

Step 4. Push the top of the canister all the way down while you breathe in deeply and slowly through your mouth. See Figure F.

Step 5. Right after the spray comes out, take your finger off the canister. After you have breathed in all the way, take the inhaler out of your mouth and close your mouth.

Step 6.**Hold your breath as long as you can**, up to 10 seconds, then breathe normally.

If your healthcare provider has told you to use more sprays, wait 1 minute and shake the inhaler again. Repeat Steps 2 through Step 6.

Step 7. Put the cap back on the mouthpiece after every time you use the inhaler. Make sure the cap snaps firmly into place.

Cleaning your VENTOLIN HFA actuator:

It is very important to keep the plastic actuator clean so the medicine will not build-up and block the spray. See Figure G.

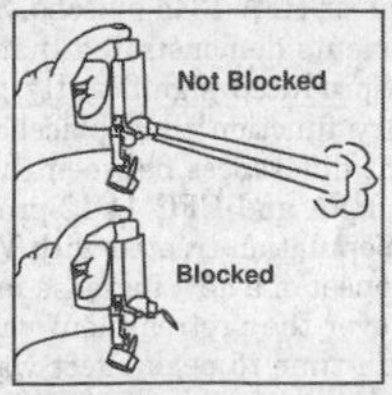

Figure G

- **Do not try to clean the metal canister or let it get wet.** The inhaler may stop spraying if it is not cleaned correctly.
- **Wash the actuator** at least once a week as follows:

Step 8. Take the canister out of the actuator, and take the cap off the mouthpiece. The strap on the cap will stay attached to the actuator.

Step 9. Hold the actuator under the faucet and run warm water through it for about 30 seconds. See Figure H.

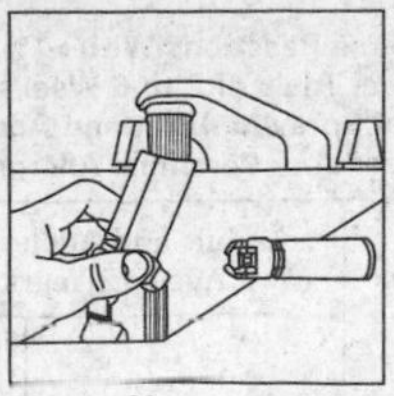

Figure H

Step 10. Turn the actuator upside down and run warm water through the mouthpiece for about 30 seconds. See Figure I.

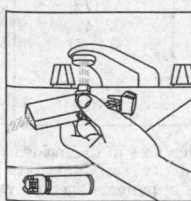

Figure I

Step 11. Shake off as much water from the actuator as you can. Look into the mouthpiece to make sure any medicine build-up has been completely washed away. If there is any build-up, repeat Steps 9 and 10.

Step 12. Let the actuator air-dry completely, such as overnight. See Figure J.

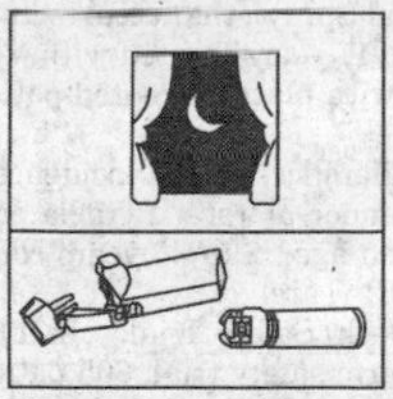

Figure J

Step 13. When the actuator is dry, put the canister in the actuator and make sure it fits firmly. Shake the inhaler well and spray it once into the air away from your face. (The counter will count down by 1 number.) Put the cap back on the mouthpiece.

If you need to use your inhaler before the actuator is completely dry:

- Shake as much water off the actuator as you can.
- Put the canister in the actuator and make sure it fits firmly.
- Shake the inhaler well and spray it once into the air away from your face.
- Take your VENTOLIN HFA dose as prescribed.
- Follow cleaning Steps 8 through 13 above.

Replacing your VENTOLIN HFA inhaler:

- **When the dose counter on the actuator shows the number 020,** you need to refill your prescription or ask your doctor for another prescription for VENTOLIN HFA.
- **Throw the VENTOLIN HFA inhaler away** as soon as the dose counter shows **000**, after the expiration date on the VENTOLIN HFA packaging, or 12 months after you open the foil pouch, whichever comes first. You should not keep using the inhaler after the dose counter shows **000** even though the canister may not be completely empty. You cannot be sure you will receive the right amount of medicine.

VENTOLIN is a registered trademark of GlaxoSmithKline.

This Patient Information and Instructions for Use has been approved by the U.S. Food and Drug Administration.

GlaxoSmithKline
Research Triangle Park, NC 27709

October 2012
VNT:8PIL

VERAMYST ℞

[ver'ə-mist]
(fluticasone furoate)
Nasal Spray

HIGHLIGHTS OF PRESCRIBING INFORMATION

These highlights do not include all the information needed to use VERAMYST safely and effectively. See full prescribing information for VERAMYST.

VERAMYST (fluticasone furoate) Nasal Spray
Initial U.S. Approval: 2007

RECENT MAJOR CHANGES

Use in Specific Populations, Pediatric Use (8.4) — August 2012

INDICATIONS AND USAGE

VERAMYST Nasal Spray is a corticosteroid indicated for treatment of symptoms of seasonal and perennial allergic rhinitis in adults and children ≥2 years. (1.1)

DOSAGE AND ADMINISTRATION

For intranasal use only. Usual starting dosages:

- Adults and adolescents ≥12 years: 110 mcg (2 sprays per nostril) once daily. (2.1)
- Children 2-11 years: 55 mcg (1 spray per nostril) once daily. (2.2)
- Priming information: Prime VERAMYST Nasal Spray before using for the first time, when not used for more than 30 days, or if the cap has been left off the bottle for 5 days or longer. (2)

DOSAGE FORMS AND STRENGTHS

Nasal spray: 27.5 mcg of fluticasone furoate in each 50-microliter spray. (3)

Supplied in 10-g bottle containing 120 sprays. (16)

CONTRAINDICATIONS

Hypersensitivity to ingredients. (4)

WARNINGS AND PRECAUTIONS

- Epistaxis, nasal ulceration, *Candida albicans* infection, nasal septal perforation, impaired wound healing. Monitor patients periodically for signs of adverse effects on the nasal mucosa. Avoid use in patients with recent nasal ulcers, nasal surgery, or nasal trauma. (5.1)
- Development of glaucoma or posterior subcapsular cataracts. Monitor patients closely with a change in vision or with a history of increased intraocular pressure, glaucoma, and/or cataracts. (5.2)
- Hypersensitivity reactions, including anaphylaxis, angioedema, rash, and urticaria, may occur after administration of VERAMYST Nasal Spray. (5.3)
- Potential worsening of existing tuberculosis; fungal, bacterial, viral, or parasitic infections; or ocular herpes simplex. More serious or even fatal course of chickenpox or measles in susceptible patients. Use caution in patients with the above because of the potential for worsening of these infections. (5.4)
- Hypercorticism and adrenal suppression with very high dosages or at the regular dosage in susceptible individuals. If such changes occur, discontinue VERAMYST Nasal Spray slowly. (5.5)
- Potential reduction in growth velocity in children. Monitor growth routinely in pediatric patients receiving VERAMYST Nasal Spray. (5.7, 8.4)

ADVERSE REACTIONS

The most common adverse reactions (>1% incidence) included headache, epistaxis, pharyngolaryngeal pain, nasal ulceration, back pain, pyrexia, and cough. (6.1)

To report SUSPECTED ADVERSE REACTIONS, contact GlaxoSmithKline at 1-888-825-5249 or FDA at 1-800-FDA-1088 or www.fda.gov/medwatch.

DRUG INTERACTIONS

Potent inhibitors of cytochrome P450 3A4 (CYP3A4) may increase exposure to fluticasone furoate.

- Coadministration of ritonavir is not recommended. (5.6, 7)
- Use caution with coadministration of other potent CYP3A4 inhibitors, such as ketoconazole. (5.6, 7)

USE IN SPECIFIC POPULATIONS

Hepatic impairment may increase exposure to fluticasone furoate. Use with caution in patients with severe hepatic impairment. (8.6)

See 17 for PATIENT COUNSELING INFORMATION and FDA-approved patient labeling

Revised: 08/2012

FULL PRESCRIBING INFORMATION: CONTENTS*

*** Sections or subsections omitted from the full prescribing information are not listed**

FULL PRESCRIBING INFORMATION

1 INDICATIONS AND USAGE

1.1 Treatment of Allergic Rhinitis

VERAMYST® (fluticasone furoate) Nasal Spray is indicated for the treatment of the symptoms of seasonal and perennial allergic rhinitis in patients aged 2 years and older.

2 DOSAGE AND ADMINISTRATION

Administer VERAMYST Nasal Spray by the intranasal route only. Prime VERAMYST Nasal Spray before using for the first time by shaking the contents well and releasing 6 sprays into the air away from the face. When VERAMYST Nasal Spray has not been used for more than 30 days or if the cap has been left off the bottle for 5 days or longer, prime the pump again until a fine mist appears. Shake VERAMYST Nasal Spray well before each use.

Titrate an individual patient to the minimum effective dosage to reduce the possibility of side effects.

2.1 Adults and Adolescents Aged 12 Years and Older

The recommended starting dosage is 110 mcg once daily administered as 2 sprays (27.5 mcg/spray) in each nostril. When the maximum benefit has been achieved and symptoms have been controlled, reducing the dosage to 55 mcg (1 spray in each nostril) once daily may be effective in maintaining control of allergic rhinitis symptoms.

2.2 Children Aged 2 to 11 Years

The recommended starting dosage in children is 55 mcg once daily administered as 1 spray (27.5 mcg/spray) in each nostril. Children not adequately responding to 55 mcg may use 110 mcg (2 sprays in each nostril) once daily. Once symptoms have been controlled, dosage reduction to 55 mcg once daily is recommended.

3 DOSAGE FORMS AND STRENGTHS

VERAMYST Nasal Spray is a nasal spray suspension. Each spray (50 microliters) delivers 27.5 mcg of fluticasone furoate.

4 CONTRAINDICATIONS

VERAMYST Nasal Spray is contraindicated in patients with hypersensitivity to any of its ingredients *[see Warnings and Precautions (5.3)]*.

5 WARNINGS AND PRECAUTIONS

5.1 Local Nasal Effects

Epistaxis and Nasal Ulceration: In clinical studies of 2 to 52 weeks' duration, epistaxis and nasal ulcerations were observed more frequently and some epistaxis events were more severe in patients treated with VERAMYST Nasal Spray than those who received placebo *[see Adverse Reactions (6.1)]*.

Candida Infection: Evidence of localized infections of the nose with *Candida albicans* was seen on nasal exams in 7 of 2,745 patients treated with VERAMYST Nasal Spray during clinical trials and was reported as an adverse event in 3 patients. When such an infection develops, it may require treatment with appropriate local therapy and discontinuation of VERAMYST Nasal Spray. Therefore, patients using VERAMYST Nasal Spray over several months or longer should be examined periodically for evidence of *Candida* infection or other signs of adverse effects on the nasal mucosa.

Table 2. Adverse Reactions With >3% Incidence in Controlled Clinical Trials of 2 to 12 Weeks' Duration With VERAMYST Nasal Spray in Pediatric Patients With Seasonal or Perennial Allergic Rhinitis

Adverse Event	Pediatric Patients Aged 2 to <12 Years		
	Vehicle Placebo (n = 429)	VERAMYST Nasal Spray 55 mcg Once Daily (n = 369)	VERAMYST Nasal Spray 110 mcg Once Daily (n = 426)
Headache	31 (7%)	28 (8%)	33 (8%)
Nasopharyngitis	21 (5%)	20 (5%)	21 (5%)
Epistaxis	19 (4%)	17 (5%)	17 (4%)
Pyrexia	7 (2%)	17 (5%)	19 (4%)
Pharyngolaryngeal pain	14 (3%)	16 (4%)	12 (3%)
Cough	12 (3%)	12 (3%)	16 (4%)

Nasal Septal Perforation: Postmarketing cases of nasal septal perforation have been reported in patients following the intranasal application of VERAMYST Nasal Spray *[see Adverse Reactions (6.2)]*.

Impaired Wound Healing: Because of the inhibitory effect of corticosteroids on wound healing, patients who have experienced recent nasal ulcers, nasal surgery, or nasal trauma should not use VERAMYST Nasal Spray until healing has occurred.

5.2 Glaucoma and Cataracts

Nasal and inhaled corticosteroids may result in the development of glaucoma and/or cataracts. Therefore, close monitoring is warranted in patients with a change in vision or with a history of increased intraocular pressure (IOP), glaucoma, and/or cataracts.

Glaucoma and cataract formation was evaluated with intraocular pressure measurements and slit lamp examinations in 1 controlled 12-month study in 806 adolescent and adult patients aged 12 years and older and in 1 controlled 12-week study in 558 children aged 2 to 11 years. The patients had perennial allergic rhinitis and were treated with either VERAMYST Nasal Spray (110 mcg once daily in adult and adolescent patients and 55 or 110 mcg once daily in pediatric patients) or placebo. Intraocular pressure remained within the normal range (<21 mmHg) in ≥98% of the patients in any treatment group in both studies. However, in the 12-month study in adolescents and adults, 12 patients, all treated with VERAMYST Nasal Spray 110 mcg once daily, had intraocular pressure measurements that increased above normal levels (≥21 mmHg). In the same study, 7 patients (6 treated with VERAMYST Nasal Spray 110 mcg once daily and 1 patient treated with placebo) had cataracts identified during the study that were not present at baseline.

5.3 Hypersensitivity Reactions, Including Anaphylaxis

Hypersensitivity reactions, including anaphylaxis, angioedema, rash, and urticaria, may occur after administration of VERAMYST Nasal Spray. Discontinue VERAMYST Nasal Spray if such reactions occur *[see Contraindications (4)]*.

5.4 Immunosuppression

Persons who are using drugs that suppress the immune system are more susceptible to infections than healthy individuals. Chickenpox and measles, for example, can have a more serious or even fatal course in susceptible children or adults using corticosteroids. In children or adults who have not had these diseases or have not been properly immunized, particular care should be taken to avoid exposure. How the dose, route, and duration of corticosteroid administration affect the risk of developing a disseminated infection is not known. The contribution of the underlying disease and/or prior corticosteroid treatment to the risk is also not known. If a patient is exposed to chickenpox, prophylaxis with varicella zoster immune globulin (VZIG) may be indicated. If a patient is exposed to measles, prophylaxis with pooled intramuscular immunoglobulin (IG) may be indicated. (See the respective package inserts for complete VZIG and IG prescribing information.) If chickenpox or measles develops, treatment with antiviral agents may be considered.

Corticosteroids should be used with caution, if at all, in patients with active or quiescent tuberculous infections of the respiratory tract, untreated local or systemic fungal or bacterial infections, systemic viral or parasitic infections, or ocular herpes simplex because of the potential for worsening of these infections.

5.5 Hypothalamic-Pituitary-Adrenal Axis Effects

Hypercorticism and Adrenal Suppression: When intranasal steroids are used at higher than recommended dosages or in susceptible individuals at recommended dosages, systemic corticosteroid effects such as hypercorticism and adrenal suppression may appear. If such changes occur, the dosage of VERAMYST Nasal Spray should be discontinued slowly, consistent with accepted procedures for discontinuing oral corticosteroid therapy.

The replacement of a systemic corticosteroid with a topical corticosteroid can be accompanied by signs of adrenal insufficiency. In addition, some patients may experience symptoms of corticosteroid withdrawal, e.g., joint and/or muscular pain, lassitude, depression. Patients previously treated for prolonged periods with systemic corticosteroids and transferred to topical corticosteroids should be carefully monitored for acute adrenal insufficiency in response to stress. In those patients who have asthma or other clinical conditions requiring long-term systemic corticosteroid treatment, rapid decreases in systemic corticosteroid dosages may cause a severe exacerbation of their symptoms.

5.6 Use of Cytochrome P450 3A4 Inhibitors

Coadministration with ritonavir is not recommended because of the risk of systemic effects secondary to increased exposure to fluticasone furoate. Use caution with the coadministration of VERAMYST Nasal Spray and other potent cytochrome P450 3A4(CYP3A4) inhibitors, such as ketoconazole *[see Drug Interactions (7)]*.

5.7 Effect on Growth

Corticosteroids may cause a reduction in growth velocity when administered to pediatric patients. Monitor the growth routinely of pediatric patients receiving VERAMYST Nasal Spray. To minimize the systemic effects of intranasal corticosteroids, including VERAMYST Nasal Spray, titrate each patient's dose to the lowest dosage that effectively controls his/her symptoms *[see Use in Specific Populations (8.4)]*.

6 ADVERSE REACTIONS

Systemic and local corticosteroid use may result in the following:

- Epistaxis, ulcerations, *Candida albicans* infection, impaired wound healing, and nasal septal perforation *[see Warnings and Precautions (5.1)]*
- Cataracts and glaucoma *[see Warnings and Precautions (5.2)]*
- Immunosuppression *[see Warnings and Precautions (5.4)]*
- Hypothalamic-pituitary-adrenal (HPA) axis effects, including growth reduction *[see Warnings and Precautions (5.5), Use in Specific Populations (8.4)]*

6.1 Clinical Trials Experience

The safety data described below reflect exposure to VERAMYST Nasal Spray in 1,563 patients with seasonal or perennial allergic rhinitis in 9 controlled clinical trials of 2 to 12 weeks' duration. The data from adults and adolescents are based upon 6 clinical trials in which 768 patients with seasonal or perennial allergic rhinitis (473 females and 295 males aged 12 years and older) were treated with VERAMYST Nasal Spray 110 mcg once daily for 2 to 6 weeks. The racial distribution of adult and adolescent patients receiving VERAMYST Nasal Spray was 82% white, 5% black, and 13% other. The data from pediatric patients are based upon 3 clinical trials in which 795 children with seasonal or perennial rhinitis (352 females and 443 males aged 2 to 11 years) were treated with VERAMYST Nasal Spray 55 or 110 mcg once daily for 2 to 12 weeks. The racial distribution of pediatric patients receiving VERAMYST Nasal Spray was 75% white, 11% black, and 14% other.

Because clinical trials are conducted under widely varying conditions, adverse reaction rates observed in the clinical trials of a drug cannot be directly compared with rates in the clinical trials of another drug and may not reflect the rates observed in practice.

Adults and Adolescents Aged 12 Years and Older: Overall adverse reactions were reported with approximately the same frequency by patients treated with VERAMYST Nasal Spray and those receiving placebo. Less than 3% of patients in clinical trials discontinued treatment because of adverse reactions. The rate of withdrawal among patients receiving VERAMYST Nasal Spray was similar or lower than the rate among patients receiving placebo.

Table 1 displays the common adverse reactions (>1% in any patient group receiving VERAMYST Nasal Spray) that occurred more frequently in patients aged 12 years and older treated with VERAMYST Nasal Spray compared with placebo-treated patients.

Table 1. Adverse Reactions With >1% Incidence in Controlled Clinical Trials of 2 to 6 Weeks' Duration With VERAMYST Nasal Spray in Adult and Adolescent Patients With Seasonal or Perennial Allergic Rhinitis

Adverse Event	Adult and Adolescent Patients Aged 12 Years and Older	
	Vehicle Placebo (n = 774)	VERAMYST Nasal Spray 110 mcg Once Daily (n = 768)
Headache	54 (7%)	72 (9%)
Epistaxis	32 (4%)	45 (6%)
Pharyngolaryngeal pain	8 (1%)	15 (2%)
Nasal ulceration	3 (<1%)	11 (1%)
Back pain	7 (<1%)	9 (1%)

There were no differences in the incidence of adverse reactions based on gender or race. Clinical trials did not include sufficient numbers of patients aged 65 years and older to determine whether they respond differently from younger subjects.

Pediatric Patients Aged 2 to 11 Years: In the 3 clinical trials in pediatric patients aged 2 to <12 years, overall adverse reactions were reported with approximately the same frequency by patients treated with VERAMYST Nasal Spray and those receiving placebo. Table 2 displays the common adverse reactions (>3% in any patient group receiving VERAMYST Nasal Spray), that occurred more frequently in patients aged 2 to 11 years treated with VERAMYST Nasal Spray compared with placebo-treated patients.

[See table 2 above]

There were no differences in the incidence of adverse reactions based on gender or race. Pyrexia occurred more frequently in children aged 2 to <6 years compared with children aged 6 to <12 years.

Long-Term (52-Week) Safety Trial: In a 52-week, placebo-controlled, long-term safety trial, 605 patients (307 females and 298 males aged 12 years and older) with perennial allergic rhinitis were treated with VERAMYST Nasal Spray 110 mcg once daily for 12 months and 201 were treated with placebo nasal spray. While most adverse reactions were similar in type and rate between the treatment groups, epistaxis occurred more frequently in patients who received VERAMYST Nasal Spray (123/605, 20%) than in patients who received placebo (17/201, 8%). Epistaxis tended to be more severe in patients treated with VERAMYST Nasal Spray. All 17 reports of epistaxis that occurred in patients who received placebo were of mild intensity, while 83, 39, and 1 of the total 123 epistaxis events in patients treated with VERAMYST Nasal Spray were of mild, moderate, and severe intensity, respectively. No patient experienced a nasal septal perforation during this trial.

6.2 Postmarketing Experience

In addition to adverse reactions reported from clinical trials, the following adverse reactions have been identified during postmarketing use of VERAMYST Nasal Spray. Because these reactions are reported voluntarily from a population of uncertain size, it is not always possible to reliably estimate their frequency or establish a causal relationship to drug exposure. These events have been chosen for inclusion due to either their seriousness, frequency of reporting, or causal connection to fluticasone furoate or a combination of these factors.

Immune System Disorders: Hypersensitivity reactions, including anaphylaxis, angioedema, rash, and urticaria.

Respiratory, Thoracic, and Mediastinal Disorders: Rhinalgia, nasal discomfort (including nasal burning, nasal irritation, and nasal soreness), nasal dryness, and nasal septal perforation.

7 DRUG INTERACTIONS

Fluticasone furoate is cleared by extensive first-pass metabolism mediated by CYP3A4. In a drug interaction study of intranasal fluticasone furoate and the CYP3A4 inhibitor ketoconazole given as a 200-mg once-daily dose for 7 days, 6 of 20 subjects receiving fluticasone furoate and ketoconazole had measurable but low levels of fluticasone furoate compared with 1 of 20 receiving fluticasone furoate and placebo. Based on this study and the low systemic exposure, there was a 5% reduction in 24-hour serum cortisol levels with ketoconazole compared with placebo. The data from this study should be carefully interpreted because the study was conducted with ketoconazole 200 mg once daily rather than 400 mg, which is the maximum recommended dosage. Therefore, caution is required with the coadministration of VERAMYST Nasal Spray and ketoconazole or other potent CYP3A4 inhibitors.

Based on data with another glucocorticoid, fluticasone propionate, metabolized by CYP3A4, coadministration of

VERAMYST Nasal Spray with the potent CYP3A4 inhibitor ritonavir is not recommended because of the risk of systemic effects secondary to increased exposure to fluticasone furoate. High exposure to corticosteroids increases the potential for systemic side effects, such as cortisol suppression.

Enzyme induction and inhibition data suggest that fluticasone furoate is unlikely to significantly alter the cytochrome P450-mediated metabolism of other compounds at clinically relevant intranasal dosages.

8 USE IN SPECIFIC POPULATIONS

8.1 Pregnancy

Teratogenic Effects: Pregnancy Category C. Corticosteroids have been shown to be teratogenic in laboratory animals when administered systemically at relatively low dosage levels.

There were no teratogenic effects in rats and rabbits at inhaled fluticasone furoate dosages of up to 91 and 8 mcg/kg/day, respectively (approximately 7 and 1 times, respectively, the maximum recommended daily intranasal dose in adults on a mcg/m^2 basis). There was also no effect on pre- or postnatal development in rats treated with up to 27 mcg/kg/day by inhalation during gestation and lactation (approximately 2 times the maximum recommended daily intranasal dose in adults on a mcg/m^2 basis).

There are no adequate and well-controlled studies in pregnant women. VERAMYST Nasal Spray should be used during pregnancy only if the potential benefit justifies the potential risk to the fetus.

Nonteratogenic Effects: Hypoadrenalism may occur in infants born of mothers receiving corticosteroids during pregnancy. Such infants should be carefully monitored.

8.3 Nursing Mothers

It is not known whether fluticasone furoate is excreted in human breast milk. However, other corticosteroids have been detected in human milk. Since there are no data from controlled trials on the use of intranasal fluticasone furoate by nursing mothers, caution should be exercised when VERAMYST Nasal Spray is administered to a nursing woman.

8.4 Pediatric Use

Controlled clinical trials with VERAMYST Nasal Spray included 1,224 patients aged 2 to 11 years and 344 adolescent patients aged 12 to 17 years *[see Clinical Studies (14)]*. The safety and effectiveness of VERAMYST Nasal Spray in children younger than 2 years have not been established.

Controlled clinical studies have shown that intranasal corticosteroids may cause a reduction in growth velocity in pediatric patients. This effect has been observed in the absence of laboratory evidence of HPA axis suppression, suggesting that growth velocity is a more sensitive indicator of systemic corticosteroid exposure in pediatric patients than some commonly used tests of HPA axis function. The long-term effects of reduction in growth velocity associated with intranasal corticosteroids, including the impact on final adult height, are unknown. The potential for "catch-up" growth following discontinuation of treatment with intranasal corticosteroids has not been adequately studied. The growth of pediatric patients receiving intranasal corticosteroids, including VERAMYST Nasal Spray, should be monitored routinely (e.g., via stadiometry). The potential growth effects of prolonged treatment should be weighed against the clinical benefits obtained and the risks/benefits of treatment alternatives. To minimize the systemic effects of intranasal corticosteroids, including VERAMYST Nasal Spray, each patient's dose should be titrated to the lowest dosage that effectively controls his/her symptoms.

A randomized, double-blind, parallel-group, multicenter, 1-year placebo-controlled clinical growth study evaluated the effect of 110 mcg of VERAMYST Nasal Spray once daily on growth velocity in 474 prepubescent children (girls aged 5 to 7.5 years and boys aged 5 to 8.5 years) with stadiometry. Mean growth velocity over the 52-week treatment period was lower in the patients receiving VERAMYST Nasal Spray (5.19 cm/year compared with placebo (5.46 cm/year). The mean treatment difference was -0.27 cm/year [95% CI: -0.48 to -0.06] *[see Warnings and Precautions (5.7)]*.

8.5 Geriatric Use

Clinical studies of VERAMYST Nasal Spray did not include sufficient numbers of subjects aged 65 years and older to determine whether they respond differently from younger subjects. Other reported clinical experience has not identified differences in responses between the elderly and younger patients. In general, dose selection for an elderly patient should be cautious, usually starting at the low end of the dosing range, reflecting the greater frequency of decreased hepatic, renal, or cardiac function, and of concomitant disease or other drug therapy.

8.6 Hepatic Impairment

Use VERAMYST Nasal Spray with caution in patients with severe hepatic impairment *[see Clinical Pharmacology (12.3)]*.

8.7 Renal Impairment

No dosage adjustment is required in patients with renal impairment *[see Clinical Pharmacology (12.3)]*.

10 OVERDOSAGE

Chronic overdosage may result in signs/symptoms of hypercorticism *[see Warnings and Precautions (5.5)]*. There are no data on the effects of acute or chronic overdosage with VERAMYST Nasal Spray. Because of low systemic bioavailability and an absence of acute drug-related systemic findings in clinical studies (with dosages of up to 440 mcg/day for 2 weeks [4 times the maximum recommended daily dose]), overdose is unlikely to require any therapy other than observation.

Intranasal administration of up to 2,640 mcg/day (24 times the recommended adult dose) of fluticasone furoate was administered to healthy human volunteers for 3 days. Single- and repeat-dose studies with orally inhaled fluticasone furoate doses of 50 to 4,000 mcg have shown decreased mean serum cortisol at doses of 500 mcg or higher. The oral median lethal dose in mice and rats was >2,000 mg/kg (approximately 74,000 and 147,000 times, respectively, the maximum recommended daily intranasal dose in adults and 52,000 and 105,000 times, respectively, the maximum recommended daily intranasal dose in children, on a mcg/m^2 basis).

Acute overdosage with the intranasal dosage form is unlikely since 1 bottle of VERAMYST Nasal Spray contains approximately 3 mg of fluticasone furoate, and the bioavailability of fluticasone furoate is <1% for 2.64 mg/day given intranasally and 1% for 2 mg/day given as an oral solution.

11 DESCRIPTION

Fluticasone furoate, the active component of VERAMYST Nasal Spray, is a synthetic fluorinated corticosteroid having the chemical name (6α,11β,16α,17α)-6,9-difluoro-17-{[(fluoro-methyl)thio]carbonyl}-11-hydroxy-16-methyl-3-oxoandrosta-1,4-dien-17-yl 2-furancarboxylate and the following chemical structure:

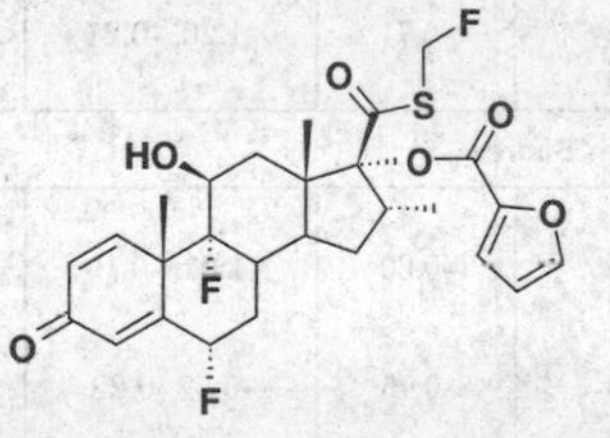

Fluticasone furoate is a white powder with a molecular weight of 538.6, and the empirical formula is $C_{27}H_{29}F_3O_6S$. It is practically insoluble in water.

VERAMYST Nasal Spray is an aqueous suspension of micronized fluticasone furoate for topical administration to the nasal mucosa by means of a metering (50 microliters), atomizing spray pump. After initial priming *[see Dosage and Administration (2)]*, each actuation delivers 27.5 mcg of fluticasone furoate in a volume of 50 microliters of nasal spray suspension. VERAMYST Nasal Spray also contains 0.015% w/w benzalkonium chloride, dextrose anhydrous, edetate disodium, microcrystalline cellulose and carboxymethylcellulose sodium, polysorbate 80, and purified water. It has a pH of approximately 6.

12 CLINICAL PHARMACOLOGY

12.1 Mechanism of Action

Fluticasone furoate is a synthetic trifluorinated corticosteroid with potent anti-inflammatory activity. The precise mechanism through which fluticasone furoate affects rhinitis symptoms is not known. Corticosteroids have been shown to have a wide range of actions on multiple cell types (e.g., mast cells, eosinophils, neutrophils, macrophages, lymphocytes) and mediators (e.g., histamine, eicosanoids, leukotrienes, cytokines) involved in inflammation. Specific effects of fluticasone furoate demonstrated in in vitro and in vivo models included activation of the glucocorticoid response element, inhibition of pro-inflammatory transcription factors such as NFkB, and inhibition of antigen-induced lung eosinophilia in sensitized rats.

Fluticasone furoate has been shown in vitro to exhibit a binding affinity for the human glucocorticoid receptor that is approximately 29.9 times that of dexamethasone and 1.7 times that of fluticasone propionate. The clinical relevance of these findings is unknown.

12.2 Pharmacodynamics

Adrenal Function: The effects of VERAMYST Nasal Spray on adrenal function have been evaluated in 4 controlled clinical trials in patients with perennial allergic rhinitis. Two 6-week clinical trials were designed specifically to assess the effect of VERAMYST Nasal Spray on the HPA axis with assessments of both 24-hour urinary cortisol excretion and serum cortisol levels in domiciled patients. In addition, one 52-week safety study and one 12-week safety and efficacy study included assessments of 24-hour urinary cortisol excretion. Details of the studies and results are described below. In all 4 studies, since serum fluticasone determinations were generally below the limit of quantification, compliance was assured by efficacy assessments.

Clinical Trials Specifically Designed to Assess Hypothalamic-Pituitary-Adrenal Axis Effect: In a 6-week randomized, double-blind, parallel-group study in adult and adolescent patients aged 12 years and older with perennial allergic rhinitis, VERAMYST Nasal Spray 110 mcg was compared with both placebo nasal spray and prednisone as a positive-control group that received prednisone 10 mg orally once daily for the final 7 days of the treatment period. Adrenal function was assessed by 24-hour urinary cortisol excretion before and after 6 weeks of treatment and by serial serum cortisol levels. Patients were domiciled for collection of 24-hour urinary cortisol. After 6 weeks of treatment, there was a change from baseline in the mean 24-hour urinary cortisol excretion in the group treated with VERAMYST Nasal Spray (n = 43) of -1.16 mcg/day compared with -3.48 mcg/day in the placebo group (n = 42). The difference from placebo in the group treated with VERAMYST Nasal Spray was 2.32 mcg/day (95% CI: -6.76, 11.39). Urinary cortisol data were not available for the positive-control (prednisone) treatment group. For serum cortisol levels, after 6 weeks of treatment there was a change from baseline in the mean (0-24 hours) of -0.38 and 0.08 mcg/dL for the group treated with VERAMYST Nasal Spray (n = 43) and the placebo group (n = 44), respectively, with a difference between the group treated with VERAMYST Nasal Spray and the placebo group of -0.47 mcg/dL (95% CI: -1.31, 0.37). For comparison, in the positive-control (prednisone, n = 12) treatment group, there was a change in mean serum cortisol (0-24 hours) from baseline of -4.49 mcg/dL with a difference between the prednisone and placebo group of -4.57 mcg/dL (95% CI: -5.83, -3.31).

The second 6-week study conducted in children aged 2 to 11 years was of similar design to the adult study, including adrenal function assessments, but did not include a prednisone positive-control arm. Patients were treated once daily with VERAMYST Nasal Spray 110 mcg or placebo nasal spray. After 6 weeks of treatment, there was a change in the mean 24-hour urinary cortisol excretion in the group treated with VERAMYST Nasal Spray (n = 43) of 0.49 mcg/day compared with 1.92 mcg/day in the placebo group (n = 41), with a difference between the group treated with VERAMYST Nasal Spray and the placebo group of -1.43 mcg/day (95% CI: -5.21, 2.35). For serum cortisol levels, after 6 weeks, there was a change from baseline in mean (0-24 hours) of -0.34 and -0.23 mcg/dL for the group treated with VERAMYST Nasal Spray (n = 48) and for the placebo group (n = 47), respectively, with a difference between the group treated with VERAMYST Nasal Spray and the placebo group of -0.11 mcg/dL (95% CI: -0.88, 0.66).

Additional Hypothalamic-Pituitary-Adrenal Axis Assessments: In the 52-week safety trial in adolescents and adults aged 12 years and older with perennial allergic rhinitis, VERAMYST Nasal Spray 110 mcg (n = 605) was compared with placebo nasal spray (n = 201). Adrenal function was assessed by 24-hour urinary cortisol excretion in a subset of patients who received VERAMYST Nasal Spray (n = 370) or placebo (n = 120) before and after 52 weeks of treatment. After 52 weeks of treatment, the mean change from baseline 24-hour urinary cortisol excretion was 5.84 mcg/day in the group treated with VERAMYST Nasal Spray and 3.34 mcg/day in the placebo group. The difference from placebo in mean change from baseline 24-hour urinary cortisol excretion was 2.50 mcg/day (95% CI: -5.49, 10.49).

In the 12-week safety and efficacy trial in children aged 2 to 11 years with perennial allergic rhinitis, VERAMYST Nasal Spray 55 mcg (n = 185) and VERAMYST Nasal Spray 110 mcg (n = 185) were compared with placebo nasal spray (n = 188). Adrenal function was assessed by measurement of 24-hour urinary free cortisol in a subset of patients who were aged 6 to 11 years (103 to 109 patients per group) before and after 12 weeks of treatment. After 12 weeks of treatment, there was a decrease in mean 24-hour urinary cortisol excretion from baseline in the group treated with VERAMYST Nasal Spray 55 mcg (n = 109) of -2.93 mcg/day and in the group treated with VERAMYST Nasal Spray 110 mcg (n = 103) of -2.07 mcg/day compared with an increase in the placebo group (n = 107) of 0.08 mcg/day. The difference from placebo in mean change from baseline in 24-hour urinary cortisol excretion for the group treated with VERAMYST Nasal Spray 55 mcg was -3.01 mcg/day (95% CI: -6.16, 0.13) and -2.14 mcg/day (95% CI: -5.33, 1.04) for the group treated with VERAMYST Nasal Spray 110 mcg. When the results of the HPA axis assessments described above are taken as a whole, an effect of intranasal fluticasone furoate on adrenal function cannot be ruled out, especially in pediatric patients.

Cardiac Effects: A QT/QTc study did not demonstrate an effect of fluticasone furoate administration on the QTc interval. The effect of a single dose of 4,000 mcg of orally inhaled fluticasone furoate on the QTc interval was evaluated over

Table 3. Mean Change From Baseline in Reflective Total Nasal Symptom Score Over 2 Weeks in Patients With Seasonal Allergic Rhinitis

Treatment	n	Baseline (AM + PM)	Change From Baseline	Difference From Placebo		
				LS Mean	95% CI	P Value
Fluticasone furoate 440 mcg	130	9.6	-4.02	-2.19	-2.75, -1.62	<0.001
Fluticasone furoate 220 mcg	129	9.5	-3.19	-1.36	-1.93, -0.79	<0.001
Fluticasone furoate 110 mcg	127	9.5	-3.84	-2.01	-2.58, -1.44	<0.001
Fluticasone furoate 55 mcg	125	9.6	-3.50	-1.68	-2.25, -1.10	<0.001
Placebo	128	9.6	-1.83			

Table 4. Mean Changes in Efficacy Variables in Adult and Adolescent Patients With Seasonal or Perennial Allergic Rhinitis

Treatment	n	Baseline	Change From Baseline – LS Mean	Difference From Placebo		
				LS Mean	95% CI	P Value
Reflective Total Nasal Symptom Scores						
Seasonal allergic rhinitis trial						
Fluticasone furoate 110 mcg	151	9.6	-3.55	-1.47	-2.01, -0.94	<0.001
Placebo	147	9.9	-2.07			
Perennial allergic rhinitis trial						
Fluticasone furoate 110 mcg	149	8.6	-2.78	-0.71	-1.20, -0.21	0.005
Placebo	153	8.7	-2.08			
Instantaneous Total Nasal Symptom Scores						
Seasonal allergic rhinitis trial						
Fluticasone furoate 110 mcg	151	9.4	-2.90	-1.38	-1.90, -0.85	<0.001
Placebo	147	9.3	-1.53			
Perennial allergic rhinitis trial						
Fluticasone furoate 110 mcg	149	8.2	-2.45	-0.71	-1.20, -0.21	0.006
Placebo	153	8.3	-1.75			
Reflective Total Ocular Symptom Scores						
Seasonal allergic rhinitis trial						
Fluticasone furoate 110 mcg	151	6.6	-2.23	-0.60	-1.01, -0.19	0.004
Placebo	147	6.5	-1.63			
Perennial allergic rhinitis trial						
Fluticasone furoate 110 mcg	149	4.8	-1.39	-0.15	-0.52, 0.22	0.428
Placebo	153	5.0	-1.24			
Rhinoconjunctivitis Quality of Life Questionnaire						
Seasonal allergic rhinitis trial						
Fluticasone furoate 110 mcg	144	3.9	-1.77	-0.60	-0.93, -0.28	<0.001
Placebo	144	3.9	-1.16			
Perennial allergic rhinitis trial						
Fluticasone furoate 110 mcg	143	3.5	-1.41	-0.23	-0.59, 0.13	0.214
Placebo	151	3.4	-1.18			

24 hours in 40 healthy male and female subjects in a placebo and positive (a single dose of 400 mg oral moxifloxacin) controlled cross-over study. The QTcF maximal mean change from baseline following fluticasone furoate was similar to that observed with placebo with a treatment difference of 0.788 msec (90% CI: -1.802, 3.378). In contrast, moxifloxacin given as a 400-mg tablet resulted in prolongation of the QTcF maximal mean change from baseline compared with placebo with a treatment difference of 9.929 msec (90% CI: 7.339, 12.520). While a single dose of fluticasone furoate had no effect on the QTc interval, the effects of fluticasone furoate may not be at steady state following single dose. The effect of fluticasone furoate on the QTc interval following multiple dose administration is unknown.

12.3 Pharmacokinetics

Absorption: Following intranasal administration of fluticasone furoate, most of the dose is eventually swallowed and undergoes incomplete absorption and extensive first-pass metabolism in the liver and gut, resulting in negligible systemic exposure. At the highest recommended intranasal dosage of 110 mcg once daily for up to 12 months in adults and up to 12 weeks in children, plasma concentrations of fluticasone furoate are typically not quantifiable despite the use of a sensitive HPLC-MS/MS assay with a lower limit of quantification (LOQ) of 10 pg/mL. However, in a few isolated cases (<0.3%) fluticasone furoate was detected in high concentrations above 500 pg/mL, and in a single case the concentration was as high as 1,430 pg/mL in the 52-week study. There was no relationship between these concentrations and cortisol levels in these subjects. The reasons for these high concentrations are unknown.

Absolute bioavailability was evaluated in 16 male and female subjects following supratherapeutic dosages of fluticasone furoate (880 mcg given intranasally at 8-hour intervals for 10 doses, or 2,640 mcg/day). The average absolute bioavailability was 0.50% (90% CI: 0.34%, 0.74%).

Due to the low bioavailability by the intranasal route, the majority of the pharmacokinetic data was obtained via other routes of administration. Studies using oral solution and intravenous dosing of radiolabeled drug have demonstrated that at least 30% of fluticasone furoate is absorbed and then rapidly cleared from plasma. Oral bioavailability is on average 1.26%, and the majority of the circulating radioactivity is due to inactive metabolites.

Distribution: Following intravenous administration, the mean volume of distribution at steady state is 608 L.

Binding of fluticasone furoate to human plasma proteins is greater than 99%.

Metabolism: In vivo studies have revealed no evidence of cleavage of the furoate moiety to form fluticasone. Fluticasone furoate is cleared (total plasma clearance of 58.7 L/h) from systemic circulation principally by hepatic metabolism via CYP3A4. The principal route of metabolism is hydrolysis of the S-fluoromethyl carbothioate function to form the inactive 17β-carboxylic acid metabolite.

Elimination: Fluticasone furoate and its metabolites are eliminated primarily in the feces, accounting for approximately 101% and 90% of the orally and intravenously administered dose, respectively. Urinary excretion accounted for approximately 1% and 2% of the orally and intravenously administered dose, respectively. The elimination phase half-life averaged 15.1 hours following intravenous administration.

Population Pharmacokinetics: Fluticasone furoate is typically not quantifiable in plasma following intranasal dosing of 110 mcg once daily with the exception of isolated cases of very high plasma levels (see Absorption). Overall, quantifiable levels (>10 pg/mL) were observed in <31% of patients aged 12 years and older and in <16% of children (aged 2 to 11 years) following intranasal dosing of 110 mcg once daily and in <7% of children following intranasal dosing of 55 mcg once daily. There was no evidence to suggest that the presence or absence of detectable levels of fluticasone furoate was related to gender, age, or race.

Hepatic Impairment: Reduced liver function may affect the elimination of corticosteroids. Since fluticasone furoate undergoes extensive first-pass metabolism by the hepatic CYP3A4, the pharmacokinetics of fluticasone furoate may be altered in patients with hepatic impairment. A study of a single 400-mcg dose of orally inhaled fluticasone furoate in patients with moderate hepatic impairment (Child-Pugh Class B) resulted in increased C_{max} (42%) and $AUC_{(0-\infty)}$ (172%), resulting in an approximately 20% reduction in serum cortisol level in patients with hepatic impairment compared with healthy subjects. The systemic exposure would be expected to be higher than that observed had the study been conducted after multiple doses and/or in patients with severe hepatic impairment. Therefore, use VERAMYST Nasal Spray with caution in patients with severe hepatic impairment.

Renal Impairment: Fluticasone furoate is not detectable in urine from healthy subjects following intranasal dosing. Less than 1% of dose-related material is excreted in urine. No dosage adjustment is required in patients with renal impairment.

13 NONCLINICAL TOXICOLOGY

13.1 Carcinogenesis, Mutagenesis, Impairment of Fertility

Fluticasone furoate produced no treatment-related increases in the incidence of tumors in 2-year inhalation studies in rats and mice at doses of up to 9 and 19 mcg/kg/day, respectively (less than the maximum recommended daily intranasal dose in adults and children on a mcg/m^2 basis).

Fluticasone furoate did not induce gene mutation in bacteria or chromosomal damage in a mammalian cell mutation test in mouse lymphoma L5178Y cells in vitro. There was also no evidence of genotoxicity in the in vivo micronucleus test in rats.

No evidence of impairment of fertility was observed in reproductive studies conducted in male and female rats at inhaled fluticasone furoate doses of up to 24 and 91 mcg/kg/day, respectively (approximately 2 and 7 times, respectively, the maximum recommended daily intranasal dose in adults on a mcg/m^2 basis).

14 CLINICAL STUDIES

14.1 Seasonal and Perennial Allergic Rhinitis

Adult and Adolescent Patients Aged 12 Years and Older: The efficacy and safety of VERAMYST Nasal Spray was evaluated in 5 randomized, double-blind, parallel-group, multicenter, placebo-controlled clinical trials of 2 to 4 weeks' duration in adult and adolescent patients aged 12 years and older with symptoms of seasonal or perennial allergic rhinitis. The 5 clinical trials included one 2-week dose-ranging trial in patients with seasonal allergic rhinitis, three 2-week confirmatory efficacy trials in patients with seasonal allergic rhinitis, and one 4-week efficacy trial in patients with perennial allergic rhinitis. These trials included 1,829 patients (697 males and 1,132 females). About 75% of patients were Caucasian, and the mean age was 36 years. Of these patients, 722 received VERAMYST Nasal Spray 110 mcg once daily administered as 2 sprays in each nostril.

Assessment of efficacy was based on total nasal symptom score (TNSS). TNSS is calculated as the sum of the patients' scoring of the 4 individual nasal symptoms (rhinorrhea, nasal congestion, sneezing, and nasal itching) on a 0 to 3 categorical severity scale (0 = absent, 1 = mild, 2 = moderate, 3 = severe) as reflective(rTNSS) or instantaneous (iTNSS). rTNSS required the patients to record symptom severity over the previous 12 hours; iTNSS required patients to record symptom severity at the time immediately prior to the next dose. Morning and evening rTNSS scores were averaged over the treatment period and the difference from placebo in the change from baseline rTNSS was the primary efficacy endpoint. The morning iTNSS (AM iTNSS) reflects the TNSS at the end of the 24-hour dosing interval and is an indication of whether the effect was maintained over the 24-hour dosing interval.

Additional secondary efficacy variables were assessed, including the total ocular symptom score (TOSS) and the Rhinoconjunctivitis Quality of Life Questionnaire (RQLQ). TOSS is calculated as the sum of the patients' scoring of the 3 individual ocular symptoms (itching/burning, tearing/watering, and redness) on a 0 to 3 categorical severity scale (0 = absent, 1 = mild, 2 = moderate, 3 = severe) as reflective (rTOSS) or instantaneous scores (iTOSS). To assess efficacy, rTOSS and AM iTOSS were evaluated as described above for the TNSS. Patients' perceptions of disease-specific quality of life were evaluated through use of the RQLQ, which assesses the impact of allergic rhinitis treatment through 28 items in 7 domains (activities, sleep, non-nose/eye symptoms, practical problems, nasal symptoms, eye symptoms, and emotional) on a 7-point scale where 0 = no impairment and 6 = maximum impairment. An overall RQLQ score is calculated from the mean of all items in the instrument. An absolute difference of ≥0.5 in mean change from baseline over placebo is considered the minimally important difference (MID) for the RQLQ.

Dose-Ranging Trial: The dose-ranging trial was a 2-week trial that evaluated the efficacy of 4 dosages of fluticasone furoate nasal spray (440, 220, 110, and 55 mcg) in patients with seasonal allergic rhinitis. In this trial, each of the 4 dosages of fluticasone furoate nasal spray demonstrated greater decreases in the rTNSS than placebo, and the difference was statistically significant (Table 3).

[See table 3 at top of previous page]

Each of the 4 dosages of fluticasone furoate nasal spray also demonstrated greater decreases in the AM iTNSS than placebo, and the difference between each of the 4 fluticasone furoate treatment groups and placebo was statistically significant, indicating that the effect was maintained over the 24-hour dosing interval.

Seasonal Allergic Rhinitis Trials: Three clinical trials were designed to evaluate the efficacy of VERAMYST Nasal Spray 110 mcg once daily compared with placebo in patients with seasonal allergic rhinitis over a 2-week treatment period. In all 3 trials, VERAMYST Nasal Spray 110 mcg demonstrated a greater decrease from baseline in the rTNSS and AM iTNSS than placebo, and the difference from placebo was statistically significant. In terms of ocular symptoms, in all 3 seasonal allergic rhinitis trials, VERAMYST Nasal Spray 110 mcg demonstrated a greater decrease from baseline in the rTOSS than placebo and the difference from placebo was statistically significant. For the RQLQ in all 3 seasonal allergic rhinitis trials, VERAMYST Nasal Spray 110 mcg demonstrated greater decrease from baseline in the overall RQLQ than placebo, and the difference from placebo was statistically significant. The difference in the overall RQLQ score mean change from baseline between the groups treated with VERAMYST Nasal Spray and placebo ranged from -0.60 to -0.70 in the 3 trials, meeting the minimally important difference criterion. Table 4 displays the efficacy results from a representative trial in patients with seasonal allergic rhinitis.

Perennial Allergic Rhinitis Trials: One clinical trial was designed to evaluate the efficacy of VERAMYST Nasal Spray 110 mcg once daily compared with placebo in patients with perennial allergic rhinitis over a 4-week treatment period. VERAMYST Nasal Spray 110 mcg demonstrated a greater decrease from baseline in the rTNSS and AM iTNSS than placebo, and the difference from placebo was statistically significant. Similar to patients with seasonal allergic rhinitis, the improvement of nasal symptoms with VERAMYST Nasal Spray in patients with perennial allergic rhinitis persisted for a full 24 hours, as evaluated by AM iTNSS immediately prior to the next dose. However, unlike the trials in patients with seasonal allergic rhinitis, patients with perennial allergic rhinitis who were treated with VERAMYST Nasal Spray 110 mcg did not demonstrate statistically significant improvement from baseline in rTOSS or in disease-specific quality of life as measured by the RQLQ compared with placebo. In addition, the overall RQLQ score mean change from baseline difference between the group treated with VERAMYST Nasal Spray and the placebo group was -0.23, which did not meet the minimally important difference of ≥0.5. Table 4 displays the efficacy results from the clinical trial in patients with perennial allergic rhinitis.

[See table 4 at top of previous page]

Onset of action was evaluated by frequent instantaneous TNSS assessments after the first dose in the clinical trials in patients with seasonal allergic rhinitis and perennial allergic rhinitis. Onset of action was generally observed within 24 hours in patients with seasonal allergic rhinitis. In patients with perennial rhinitis, onset of action was observed after 4 days of treatment. Continued improvement in symptoms was observed over approximately 1 and 3 weeks in patients with seasonal or perennial allergic rhinitis, respectively.

Pediatric Patients Aged 2 to 11 Years: The efficacy and safety of VERAMYST Nasal Spray were evaluated in 1,112 children (633 boys and 479 girls), mean age of 8 years with seasonal or perennial allergic rhinitis in 2 controlled clinical trials. The pediatric patients were treated with VERAMYST Nasal Spray 55 or 110 mcg once daily for 2 to 12 weeks (n = 369 for each dose). The trials were similar in design to the trials conducted in adolescents and adults; however, the efficacy determination was made from patient- or parent/guardian-reported TNSS for children aged 6 to <12 years. Children treated with VERAMYST Nasal Spray generally exhibited greater decreases in nasal symptoms than placebo-treated patients. In seasonal allergic rhinitis, the difference in rTNSS was statistically significant only for the 110-mcg dose. In perennial allergic rhinitis, the difference in rTNSS was statistically significant only for the 55-mcg dose. Changes in rTOSS in the seasonal allergic rhinitis trial were not statistically significant compared with placebo for either dose. rTOSS was not assessed in the perennial allergic rhinitis trial. Table 5 displays the efficacy results from the clinical trials in patients with perennial allergic rhinitis and seasonal allergic rhinitis in children aged 6 to <12 years. Efficacy in children aged 2 to <6 years was supported by a numerical decrease in the rTNSS.

[See table 5 above]

Table 5. Mean Changes in Efficacy Variables in Pediatric Patients Aged 6 to <12 Years With Seasonal or Perennial Allergic Rhinitis

Treatment	n	Baseline	Change From Baseline – LS Mean	Difference From Placebo		
				LS Mean	95% CI	*P* Value
Reflective Total Nasal Symptom Scores						
Seasonal allergic rhinitis trial						
Fluticasone furoate 55 mcg	151	8.6	-2.71	-0.16	-0.69, 0.37	0.553
Fluticasone furoate 110 mcg	146	8.5	-3.16	-0.62	-1.15, -0.08	0.025
Placebo	149	8.4	-2.54			
Perennial allergic rhinitis trial						
Fluticasone furoate 55 mcg	144	8.5	-4.16	-0.75	-1.24, -0.27	0.003
Fluticasone furoate 110 mcg	140	8.6	-3.86	-0.45	-0.95, 0.04	0.073
Placebo	147	8.5	-3.41			
Instantaneous Total Nasal Symptom Scores						
Seasonal allergic rhinitis trial						
Fluticasone furoate 55 mcg	151	8.4	-2.37	-0.23	-0.77, 0.30	0.389
Fluticasone furoate 110 mcg	146	8.3	-2.80	-0.67	-1.21, -0.13	0.015
Placebo	149	8.4	-2.13			
Perennial allergic rhinitis trial						
Fluticasone furoate 55 mcg	144	8.3	-3.62	-0.75	-1.24, -0.27	0.002
Fluticasone furoate 110 mcg	140	8.3	-3.52	-0.65	-1.14, -0.16	0.009
Placebo	147	8.3	-2.87			
Reflective Total Ocular Symptom Scores						
Seasonal allergic rhinitis trial						
Fluticasone furoate 55 mcg	151	4.4	-1.26	0.04	-0.33, 0.41	0.826
Fluticasone furoate 110 mcg	146	4.1	-1.45	-0.15	-0.52, 0.22	0.426
Placebo	149	3.8	-1.30			

16 HOW SUPPLIED/STORAGE AND HANDLING

VERAMYST Nasal Spray, 27.5 mcg per spray, is supplied in a brown glass bottle enclosed in a nasal device with a nozzle and a mist-release button to actuate the spray in a box of 1 (NDC 0173-0753-00) with FDA-Approved Patient Labeling (see Patient Instructions for Use for proper actuation of the device). Each bottle contains a net fill weight of 10 g of white, liquid suspension and will provide 120 metered sprays. After priming *[see Dosage and Administration (2)]*, each spray delivers a fine mist containing 27.5 mcg of fluticasone furoate in 50 microliters of formulation through the nozzle. The contents of the bottle can be viewed through an indicator window. Shake the contents well before each use. The correct amount of medication in each spray cannot be assured before the initial priming and after 120 sprays have been used, even though the bottle is not completely empty. The nasal device should be discarded after 120 sprays have been used.

Store the device in the upright position with the cap in place between 15° and 30°C (59° and 86°F). Do not freeze or refrigerate.

17 PATIENT COUNSELING INFORMATION

See FDA-approved patient labeling (Patient Information and Instructions for Use).

17.1 Local Nasal Effects

Patients should be informed that treatment with VERAMYST Nasal Spray may lead to adverse reactions, which include epistaxis and nasal ulceration. *Candida* infection may also occur with treatment with VERAMYST Nasal Spray. In addition, nasal corticosteroids are associated with nasal septal perforation and impaired wound healing. Patients who have experienced recent nasal ulcers, nasal surgery, or nasal trauma should not use VERAMYST Nasal Spray until healing has occurred *[see Warnings and Precautions (5.1)]*.

17.2 Cataracts and Glaucoma

Patients should be informed that glaucoma and cataracts are associated with nasal and inhaled corticosteroid use. Patients should inform his/her health care provider if a change in vision is noted while using VERAMYST Nasal Spray *[see Warnings and Precautions (5.2)]*.

17.3 Hypersensitivity Reactions, Including Anaphylaxis

Patients should be aware that hypersensitivity reactions, including anaphylaxis, angioedema, rash, and urticaria, may occur after administration of VERAMYST Nasal Spray. If such reactions occur, patients should discontinue use of VERAMYST Nasal Spray *[see Warnings and Precautions (5.3)]*.

17.4 Immunosuppression

Patients who are on immunosuppressant doses of corticosteroids should be warned to avoid exposure to chickenpox or measles and, if exposed, to consult their physician without delay. Patients should be informed of potential worsening of existing tuberculosis, fungal, bacterial, viral or parasitic infections, or ocular herpes simplex *[see Warnings and Precautions (5.4)]*.

17.5 Effect on Growth

Parents should be advised that VERAMYST Nasal Spray may slow growth in children. A child taking VERAMYST Nasal Spray should have his/her growth checked regularly *[see Warnings and Precautions (5.7) and Pediatric Use (8.4)]*.

17.6 Use Daily for Best Effect

Patients should use VERAMYST Nasal Spray on a regular once-daily basis for optimal effect. VERAMYST Nasal Spray, like other corticosteroids, does not have an immediate effect on rhinitis symptoms. Although significant improvement is usually achieved within 24 hours in patients with seasonal allergic rhinitis and 4 days in patients with perennial allergic rhinitis, maximum benefit may not be reached for several days. The patient should not increase the prescribed dosage but should contact the physician if symptoms do not improve or if the condition worsens.

17.7 Keep Spray Out of Eyes

Patients should be informed to avoid spraying VERAMYST Nasal Spray in their eyes.

17.8 Potential Drug Interactions

Patients should be advised that coadministration of VERAMYST Nasal Spray and ritonavir is not recommended and to be cautious if coadministrating with ketoconazole.

GlaxoSmithKline
Research Triangle Park, NC 27709

VRM:9PI

Patient Information
VERAMYST®*[VAIR-uh-mist]*
(fluticasonefuroate)
Nasal Spray
For Intranasal Use Only

Read the Patient Information that comes with VERAMYST Nasal Spray carefully before you start using it and each time you get a refill. There may be new information. Keep the leaflet for reference because it gives you a summary of important information about VERAMYST Nasal Spray. This leaflet does not take the place of talking to your healthcare provider about your medical condition or your treatment.

What is VERAMYST Nasal Spray?

VERAMYST Nasal Spray is a medicine that treats seasonal and year-round allergy symptoms in adults and children 2 years old and older.

VERAMYST Nasal Spray contains fluticasone furoate, which is a man-made (synthetic) corticosteroid. When you spray VERAMYST Nasal Spray into your nose, it helps reduce the nasal symptoms of allergic rhinitis (inflammation of the lining of the nose), such as stuffy nose, runny nose, nasal itching, and sneezing. VERAMYST Nasal Spray may also help red, itchy, and watery eyes in adults and teenagers with seasonal allergic rhinitis.

Your healthcare provider has prescribed VERAMYST Nasal Spray to treat your symptoms of allergic rhinitis.

It is not known if VERAMYST Nasal Spray is safe and effective in children under 2 years of age.

Who should not use VERAMYST Nasal Spray?

Do not use VERAMYST Nasal Spray if you are allergic to fluticasone furoate or any of the ingredients in VERAMYST Nasal Spray. See the end of this Patient Information leaflet for a complete list of ingredients in VERAMYST Nasal Spray.

What should I tell my healthcare provider before taking VERAMYST Nasal Spray?

Tell your healthcare provider about all of your medical conditions, including if you:

- have had recent nasal sores, nasal surgery, or nasal injury
- have eye or vision problems, such as cataracts or glaucoma (increased pressure in your eye)
- have tuberculosis or any untreated fungal, bacterial, viral infections, or eye infections caused by herpes
- are exposed to chickenpox or measles.
- are feeling unwell or have any symptoms that you do not understand.
- are pregnant or plan to become pregnant. It is not known if VERAMYST Nasal Spray will harm your unborn baby. Talk to your healthcare provider if you are pregnant or plan to become pregnant.
- are breastfeeding or plan to breastfeed. It is not known if VERAMYST Nasal Spray can pass into your breast milk. Talk to your healthcare provider about the best way to feed your baby if you take VERAMYST Nasal Spray.

Tell your healthcare provider about all the medicines you take, including prescription and non-prescription medicines, vitamins, and herbal products. VERAMYST Nasal Spray and other medicines may affect each other, causing side effects. **Be certain to tell your healthcare provider if you are taking a medicine that contains ritonavir (commonly used to treat HIV infection or AIDS).**

How should I use VERAMYST Nasal Spray?

- This medicine is for use in the nose only. Do not spray it in your eyes or mouth.
- An adult should help a young child use this medicine.
- This medicine has been prescribed for you by your healthcare provider. Do not give this medicine to anyone else.
- Use VERAMYST Nasal Spray exactly as your healthcare provider tells you to. Do not take more of your medicine or take it more often than your healthcare provider tells you. The prescription label will usually tell you how many sprays to take and how often. If it does not or if you are not sure, ask your healthcare provider or pharmacist.
- **For people aged 12 years and older,** the usual starting dosage is **2 sprays in each nostril, 1 time a day.** After you begin to feel better, your healthcare provider may tell you that 1 spray in each nostril 1 time a day may be enough for you.
- **For children aged 2 to 11 years,** the usual starting dosage is **1 spray in each nostril, 1 time a day.** Your healthcare provider may tell you to take 2 sprays in each nostril 1 time a day. After you begin to feel better, your healthcare provider may change the dosage to 1 spray in each nostril 1 time a day. An adult should help a young child use this medicine.
- Do not use VERAMYST Nasal Spray after 120 sprays (plus the initial priming sprays) have been used or after the expiration date, whichever comes first. (The sample bottle contains 30 sprays.) The bottle may not be completely empty. The expiration date is printed as "EXP" on the product label and box. Before you throw away VERAMYST Nasal Spray, talk to your healthcare provider to see if you need a refill of your prescription. If your healthcare provider tells you to continue using VERAMYST Nasal Spray, throw away the empty or expired bottle and use a new bottle of VERAMYST Nasal Spray. Follow the **Instructions for Use** below.
- Do not take extra doses or stop taking VERAMYST Nasal Spray without telling your healthcare provider.
- VERAMYST Nasal Spray may begin to work within 24 hours after you take your first dose. It may take several days before it has its greatest effect. If your symptoms do not improve or get worse, call your healthcare provider.
- You will get the best results if you keep using VERAMYST Nasal Spray regularly each day without missing a dose. If you miss a dose by several hours, just take your next dose at the usual time. Do not take an extra dose.

What are the possible side effects of VERAMYST Nasal Spray?

VERAMYST Nasal Spray may cause serious side effects, including:

- **thrush (candidiasis), a fungal infection in your mouth and throat.** Tell your healthcare provider if you have any redness or white colored patches in your mouth or throat.
- **hole in the cartilage in the nose (nasal septal perforation).** Symptoms of nasal septal perforation may include:
  - crusting in the nose
  - nosebleeds
  - runny nose
  - whistling sound when you breathe
- **slow wound healing.** You should not use VERAMYST Nasal Spray until your nose has healed if you have a sore in your nose, have had surgery on your nose, or if your nose has been injured.
- **eye problems such as glaucoma and cataracts.** If you have a history of glaucoma or cataracts or have a family history of these eye problems, you should have regular eye exams while you use VERAMYST Nasal Spray.
- **serious allergic reactions.** Serious allergic reactions can happen with VERAMYST Nasal Spray. **Stop using VERAMYST Nasal Spray and call your healthcare provider right away if you have any of the following signs of a serious allergic reaction:**
  - shortness of breath or trouble breathing
  - skin rash, redness, or swelling
  - severe itching
  - swelling of the lips, tongue, or face
- **immune system problems that may increase your risk of infections.** You are more likely to get infections if you take medicines that may weaken your body's ability to fight infections. Avoid contact with people who have contagious diseases such as chicken pox or measles while you use VERAMYST Nasal Spray. Symptoms of an infection may include:
  - fever
  - pain
  - aches
  - chills
  - feeling tired
  - nausea
  - vomiting
- **adrenal insufficiency.** Adrenal insufficiency is a condition in which the adrenal glands do not make enough steroid hormones. Symptoms of adrenal insufficiency may include:
  - tiredness
  - weakness
  - dizziness
  - nausea
  - vomiting
- **slowed or delayed growth in children.** A child's growth should be checked regularly while using VERAMYST Nasal Spray.

The most common side effects of VERAMYST Nasal Spray include:

- **adults and adolescents 12 years of age and older**
  - headaches
  - nose bleeds
  - sore throat
  - nose sores
  - back pain
- **children 2 to 12 years of age**
  - headaches
  - sore throat
  - nose bleeds
  - fever
  - cough

Tell your healthcare provider if you have any side effect that bothers you or does not go away.

These are not all of the possible side effects of VERAMYST Nasal Spray. For more information, ask your healthcare provider or pharmacist.

Call your doctor for medical advice about side effects. You may report side effects to FDA at 1-800-FDA-1088.

What should I know about allergic rhinitis?

"Rhinitis" means inflammation of the lining of the nose. It is sometimes called "hay fever." Allergic rhinitis can be caused by allergies to pollen, animal dander, house dust mite, and mold spores. If you have allergic rhinitis, your nose becomes stuffy, runny, and itchy. You may also sneeze a lot. You may also have red, itchy, watery eyes; itchy throat; or blocked, itchy ears.

What are the ingredients in VERAMYST Nasal Spray?

Active ingredient: fluticasone furoate

Inactive ingredients: 0.015% w/w benzalkonium chloride, dextrose anhydrous, edetate disodium, microcrystalline cellulose, carboxymethylcellulose sodium, polysorbate 80, and purified water

Instructions for Use

Read this leaflet carefully before you start to use VERAMYST Nasal Spray. If you have any questions, ask your healthcare provider or pharmacist.

The parts of the VERAMYST Nasal Spray

VERAMYST Nasal Spray comes in a brown glass bottle inside a nasal device. It contains 120 sprays (or 30 sprays if it is a sample) plus the first priming sprays. Be careful not to drop it. If you accidentally drop the device, check it for damage. If the device is damaged, return it to your pharmacist.

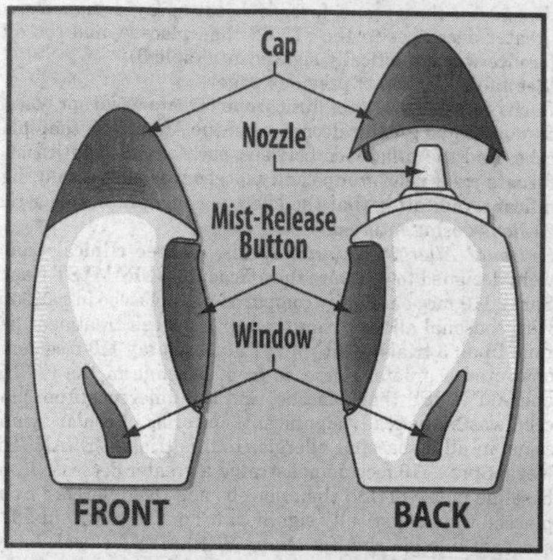

The **Cap** has a tab that keeps the **Mist-Release Button** from being pressed accidentally. It also helps keep the nozzle clean. Do not throw the cap away. Always keep the cap on the device when you are not using it.

The **Nozzle** is small and short, so it will fit inside your nose. The medicine comes out of the nozzle.

Pressing the **Mist-Release Button** sprays a measured amount of medicine from the nozzle as a gentle, fine mist. Because the button is on the side of the device, you can keep the nozzle in the right place in your nose while you press the button.

The **Window** lets you see if there is medicine left in the bottle when you hold it in front of a bright light. (You may not be able to see the medicine in a full bottle because the liquid level is above the window.)

How to prime your VERAMYST Nasal Spray

Priming helps to make sure you always get the same full dose of medicine. You need to prime VERAMYST Nasal Spray:

- before you use a new bottle for the first time.
- if you have not used your VERAMYST Nasal Spray for 30 days or longer.
- if the cap has been left off the bottle for 5 days or longer.
- if the device does not seem to be working right.

To prime VERAMYST Nasal Spray:

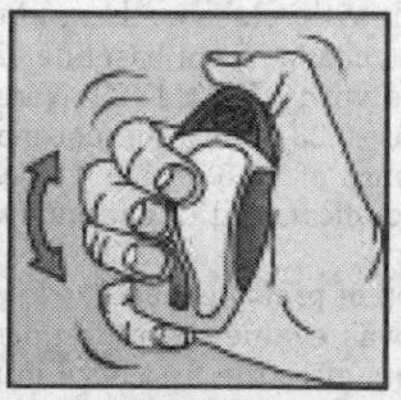

Figure 1

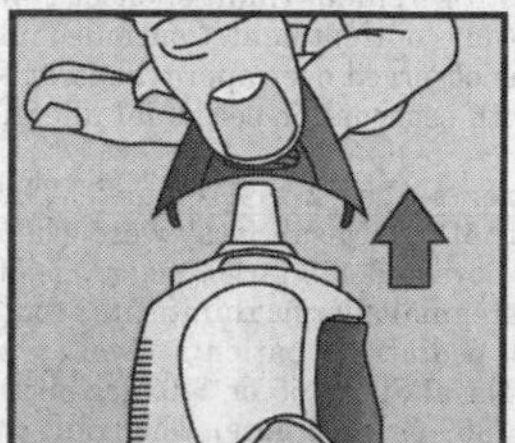

Figure 2

[See figure 3 at top of next column]

1. With the cap on, shake the device well (Figure 1). This is important to make the medicine a liquid that will spray.
2. Take the cap off by **squeezing** the finger grips and pulling it straight off (Figure 2).

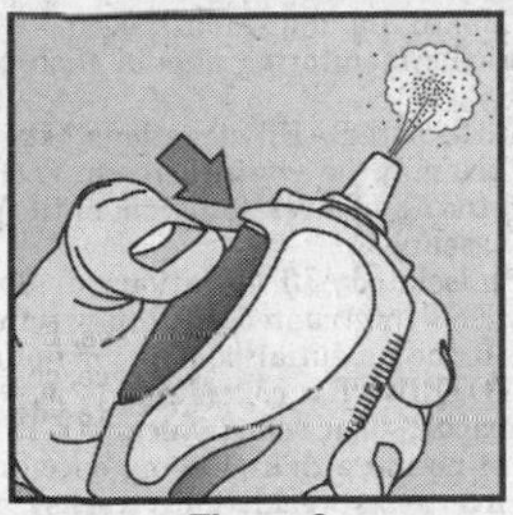

Figure 3

3. Hold the device with the nozzle pointing up and away from you. Place your thumb or fingers on the button. Press the button all the way in 6 times or until a fine mist sprays from the nozzle (Figure 3). Your VERAMYST Nasal Spray is now ready to use.

How to use your VERAMYST Nasal Spray

Follow the instructions below. If you have any questions, ask your healthcare provider or pharmacist.

Before taking a dose of VERAMYST Nasal Spray, gently blow your nose to clear your nostrils. Shake the bottle well. Then do these 3 simple steps: **Place, Press, Repeat.**

Figure 4

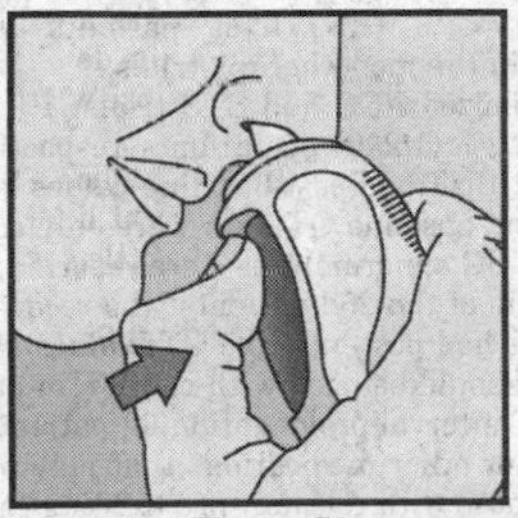

Figure 5

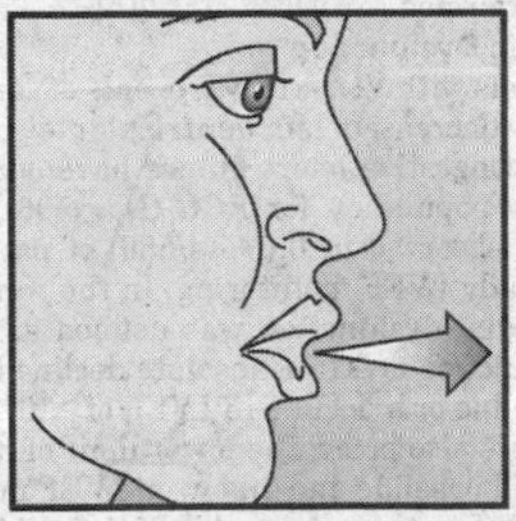

Figure 6

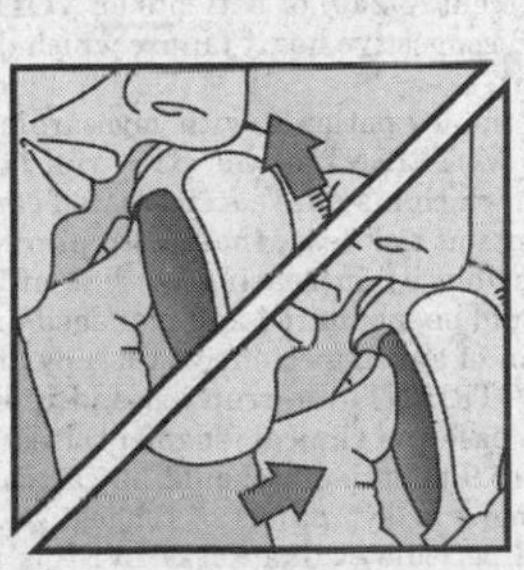

Figure 7

1. PLACE

Tilt your head forward a little bit. Hold the device upright. **PLACE** the nozzle in one of your nostrils (Figure 4). Point the end of the nozzle toward the side of your nose, away from the center of your nose (septum). This helps get the medicine to the right part of your nose.

2. PRESS

PRESS the button all the way in 1 time to spray the medicine in your nose while you are breathing in (Figure 5).

Do not get any spray in your eyes. If you do, rinse your eyes well with water.

Take the nozzle out of your nose. Breathe out through your mouth (Figure 6).

3. REPEAT

To deliver the medicine to the other nostril, **REPEAT** Steps 1 and 2 in the other nostril (Figure 7).

If your healthcare provider has told you to take 2 sprays in each nostril, do Steps 1-3 again.

Put the cap back on the device after you have finished taking your dose.

How to clean your VERAMYST Nasal Spray

After each use: wipe the nozzle with a clean, dry tissue (Figure 8). **Never try to clean the nozzle with a pin or anything sharp because this will damage the nozzle.** Do not use water to clean the nozzle.

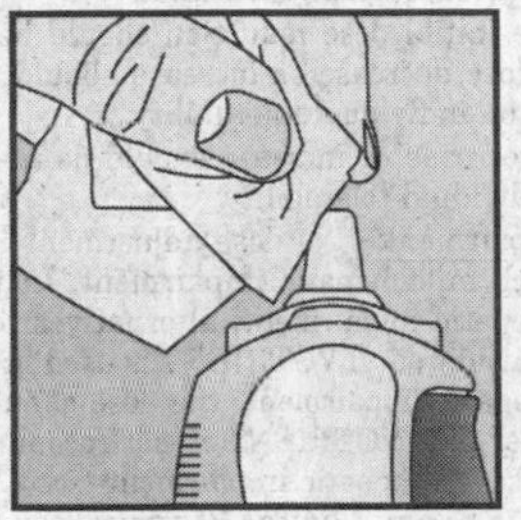

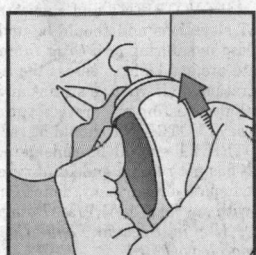

Figure 8

Once a week: clean the inside of the cap with a clean, dry tissue (Figure 9). This will help keep the nozzle from getting blocked.

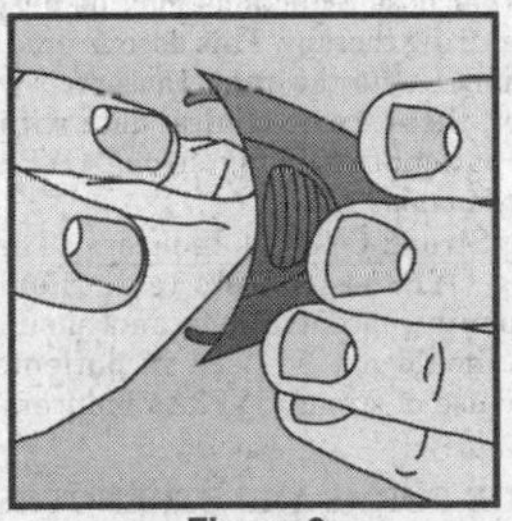

Figure 9

How to store your VERAMYST Nasal Spray

- Keep your VERAMYST Nasal Spray and all medicines out of the reach of children.
- Store between 59°F and 86°F (15°C and 30°C). Do not refrigerate or freeze.
- Store with the cap on.
- Store in an upright position.

This Patient Information has been approved by the U.S. Food and Drug Administration.

GlaxoSmithKline
Research Triangle Park, NC 27709

August 2012
VRM:9PIL

VOTRIENT ℞

[vo' trē-ent]
(pazopanib)
tablets

HIGHLIGHTS OF PRESCRIBING INFORMATION

These highlights do not include all the information needed to use VOTRIENT safely and effectively. See full prescribing information for VOTRIENT.

VOTRIENT (pazopanib) tablets
Initial U.S. Approval: 2009

> **WARNING: HEPATOTOXICITY**
> ***See full prescribing information for complete boxed warning.***
> **Severe and fatal hepatotoxicity has been observed in clinical trials. Monitor hepatic function and interrupt, reduce, or discontinue dosing as recommended *[see Warnings and Precautions (5.1)]*.**

RECENT MAJOR CHANGES

Indications and Usage (1)	04/2012
Dosage and Administration (2.2)	04/2012
Warnings and Precautions (5.1)	02/2013
Warnings and Precautions (5.1-5.9, 5.11-5.14)	04/2012
Warnings and Precautions (5.15)	11/2012

INDICATIONS AND USAGE

VOTRIENT is a kinase inhibitor indicated for the treatment of patients with:

- advanced renal cell carcinoma. (1)
- advanced soft tissue sarcoma who have received prior chemotherapy. (1)

Limitation of Use:

The efficacy of VOTRIENT for the treatment of patients with adipocytic soft tissue sarcoma or gastrointestinal stromal tumors has not been demonstrated.

DOSAGE AND ADMINISTRATION

- 800 mg orally once daily without food (at least 1 hour before or 2 hours after a meal). (2.1)
- Baseline moderate hepatic impairment – 200 mg orally once daily. Not recommended in patients with severe hepatic impairment. (2.2)

DOSAGE FORMS AND STRENGTHS

200 mg tablets (3)

CONTRAINDICATIONS

None (4)

WARNINGS AND PRECAUTIONS

- Increases in serum transaminase levels and bilirubin were observed. Severe and fatal hepatotoxicity has occurred. Measure liver chemistries before the initiation of treatment and regularly during treatment. (5.1)
- Prolonged QT intervals and torsades de pointes have been observed. Use with caution in patients at higher risk of developing QT interval prolongation. Monitoring electrocardiograms and electrolytes should be considered. (5.2)
- Cardiac dysfunction such as congestive heart failure and decreased left ventricular ejection fraction have occurred. Monitor blood pressure and manage hypertension promptly. Baseline and periodic evaluation of LVEF is recommended in patients at risk of cardiac dysfunction. (5.3)
- Fatal hemorrhagic events have been reported. VOTRIENT has not been studied in patients who have a history of hemoptysis, cerebral, or clinically significant gastrointestinal hemorrhage in the past 6 months and should not be used in those patients. (5.4)
- Arterial thrombotic events have been observed and can be fatal. Use with caution in patients who are at increased risk for these events. (5.5)
- Venous thrombotic events (VTE) have been observed, including fatal pulmonary emboli (PE). Monitor for signs and symptoms of VTE and PE. (5.6)
- Gastrointestinal perforation or fistula has occurred. Fatal perforation events have occurred. Use with caution in patients at risk for gastrointestinal perforation or fistula. (5.7)
- Reversible Posterior Leukoencephalopathy Syndrome (RPLS) has been observed. Permanently discontinue VOTRIENT if signs or symptoms of RPLS occur. (5.8)
- Hypertension including hypertensive crisis has been observed. Blood pressure should be well-controlled prior to initiating VOTRIENT. Monitor blood pressure within one week after starting VOTRIENT and frequently thereafter. (5.9)
- Interruption of therapy with VOTRIENT is recommended in patients undergoing surgical procedures. (5.10)
- Hypothyroidism may occur. Monitoring of thyroid function tests is recommended. (5.11)
- Proteinuria: Monitor urine protein. Interrupt treatment for 24-hour urine protein ≥3 grams and discontinue for repeat episodes despite dose reductions. (5.12)
- Infection: Serious infections (with or without neutropenia), some with fatal outcome, have been reported. Monitor for signs and symptoms and treat active infection promptly. Consider discontinuation of VOTRIENT. (5.13)
- Animal studies have demonstrated VOTRIENT can severely affect organ growth and maturation during early post-natal development. The safety and effectiveness in pediatric patients have not been established. (5.15)
- VOTRIENT can cause fetal harm when administered to a pregnant woman. Women of childbearing potential should be advised of the potential hazard to the fetus and to avoid becoming pregnant while taking VOTRIENT. (5.16, 8.1)

ADVERSE REACTIONS

The most common adverse reactions in patients with advanced renal cell carcinoma (≥20%) are diarrhea, hypertension, hair color changes (depigmentation), nausea, anorexia, and vomiting. (6.1)

The most common adverse reactions in patients with advanced soft tissue sarcoma (≥20%) are fatigue, diarrhea, nausea, decreased weight, hypertension, decreased appetite, vomiting, tumor pain, hair color changes, musculoskeletal pain, headache, dysgeusia, dyspnea and skin hypopigmentation. (6.1)

To report SUSPECTED ADVERSE REACTIONS, contact GlaxoSmithKline at 1-888-825-5249 or FDA at 1-800-FDA-1088 or www.fda.gov/medwatch

DRUG INTERACTIONS

- CYP3A4 Inhibitors: Avoid use of strong inhibitors. Reduce the dose of VOTRIENT when administered with strong CYP3A4 inhibitors. (7.1)
- CYP3A4 Inducers: Consider an alternate concomitant medication with no or minimal enzyme induction potential or avoid VOTRIENT. (7.1)
- CYP Substrates: Concomitant use of VOTRIENT with agents with narrow therapeutic windows that are metabolized by CYP3A4, CYP2D6, or CYP2C8 is not recommended. (7.2)
- Concomitant use of VOTRIENT and simvastatin increases the risk of ALT elevations and should be undertaken with caution and close monitoring. (7.3)

See 17 for PATIENT COUNSELING INFORMATION and Medication Guide

Revised: 02/2013

FULL PRESCRIBING INFORMATION: CONTENTS*

*** Sections or subsections omitted from the full prescribing information are not listed**

FULL PRESCRIBING INFORMATION

WARNING: HEPATOTOXICITY

Severe and fatal hepatotoxicity has been observed in clinical trials. Monitor hepatic function and interrupt, reduce, or discontinue dosing as recommended *[see Warnings and Precautions (5.1)]*.

1 INDICATIONS AND USAGE

VOTRIENT® is indicated for the treatment of patients with advanced renal cell carcinoma (RCC).

VOTRIENT is indicated for the treatment of patients with advanced soft tissue sarcoma (STS) who have received prior chemotherapy.

Limitation of Use:

The efficacy of VOTRIENT for the treatment of patients with adipocytic STS or gastrointestinal stromal tumors has not been demonstrated.

2 DOSAGE AND ADMINISTRATION

2.1 Recommended Dosing

The recommended starting dose of VOTRIENT is 800 mg orally once daily without food (at least 1 hour before or 2 hours after a meal) *[see Clinical Pharmacology (12.3)]*. The dose of VOTRIENT should not exceed 800 mg.

Do not crush tablets due to the potential for increased rate of absorption which may affect systemic exposure *[see Clinical Pharmacology (12.3)]*.

If a dose is missed, it should not be taken if it is less than 12 hours until the next dose.

2.2 Dose Modification Guidelines

In RCC, the initial dose reduction should be 400 mg, and additional dose decrease or increase should be in 200 mg steps based on individual tolerability.

In STS, a decrease or increase should be in 200 mg steps based on individual tolerability.

Hepatic Impairment: No dose adjustment is required in patients with mild hepatic impairment. In patients with moderate hepatic impairment, alternatives to VOTRIENT should be considered. If VOTRIENT is used in patients with moderate hepatic impairment, the dose should be reduced to 200 mg per day. VOTRIENT is not recommended in patients with severe hepatic impairment *[see Use in Specific Populations (8.6) and Clinical Pharmacology (12.3)]*.

Concomitant Strong CYP3A4 Inhibitors: The concomitant use of strong CYP3A4 inhibitors (e.g., ketoconazole, ritonavir, clarithromycin) increases pazopanib concentrations and should be avoided. If coadministration of a strong CYP3A4 inhibitor is warranted, reduce the dose of VOTRIENT to 400 mg. Further dose reductions may be needed if adverse effects occur during therapy. This dose is predicted to adjust the pazopanib AUC to the range observed without inhibitors. However, there are no clinical data with this dose adjustment in patients receiving strong CYP3A4 inhibitors *[see Drug Interactions (7.1)]*.

Concomitant Strong CYP3A4 Inducer: The concomitant use of strong CYP3A4 inducers (e.g., rifampin) may decrease pazopanib concentrations and should be avoided. VOTRIENT should not be used in patients who cannot avoid chronic use of strong CYP3A4 inducers *[see Drug Interactions (7.1)]*.

3 DOSAGE FORMS AND STRENGTHS

200 mg tablets of VOTRIENT — modified capsule-shaped, gray, film-coated with GS JT debossed on one side. Each tablet contains 216.7 mg of pazopanib hydrochloride equivalent to 200 mg of pazopanib.

4 CONTRAINDICATIONS

None.

5 WARNINGS AND PRECAUTIONS

5.1 Hepatic Toxicity and Hepatic Impairment

In clinical trials with VOTRIENT, hepatotoxicity, manifested as increases in serum transaminases (ALT, AST) and bilirubin, was observed. This hepatotoxicity can be severe and fatal. Transaminase elevations occur early in the course of treatment (92.5% of all transaminase elevations of any grade occurred in the first 18 weeks) *[see Dosage and Administration (2.2)]*.

In the randomized RCC trial, ALT >3 × ULN was reported in 18% and 3% of the VOTRIENT and placebo groups, respectively. ALT >10 × ULN was reported in 4% of patients who received VOTRIENT and in <1% of patients who received placebo. Concurrent elevation in ALT >3 × ULN and bilirubin >2 × ULN in the absence of significant alkaline phosphatase >3 × ULN occurred in 2% (5/290) of patients on VOTRIENT and 1% (2/145) on placebo.

In the randomized STS trial, ALT >3 × ULN was reported in 18% and 5% of the VOTRIENT and placebo groups, respectively. ALT >8 × ULN was reported in 5% and 2% of the VOTRIENT and placebo groups, respectively. Concurrent elevation in ALT >3 × ULN and bilirubin >2 × ULN in the absence of significant alkaline phosphatase >3 × ULN occurred in 2% (4/240) of patients on VOTRIENT and <1% (1/123) on placebo.

Two-tenths percent of the patients (2/977) from trials that supported the RCC indication died with disease progression and hepatic failure and 0.4% of patients (1/240) in the randomized STS trial died of hepatic failure.

- Monitor serum liver tests before initiation of treatment with VOTRIENT and at Weeks 3, 5, 7, and 9. Thereafter, monitor at Month 3 and at Month 4, and as clinically indicated. Periodic monitoring should then continue after Month 4.
- Patients with isolated ALT elevations between 3 × ULN and 8 × ULN may be continued on VOTRIENT with weekly monitoring of liver function until ALT return to Grade 1 or baseline.
- Patients with isolated ALT elevations of >8 × ULN should have VOTRIENT interrupted until they return to Grade 1 or baseline. If the potential benefit for reinitiating treatment with VOTRIENT is considered to outweigh the risk for hepatotoxicity, then reintroduce VOTRIENT at a reduced dose of no more than 400 mg once daily and measure serum liver tests weekly for 8 weeks *[see Dosage and Administration (2.2)]*. Following reintroduction of VOTRIENT, if ALT elevations >3 × ULN recur, then VOTRIENT should be permanently discontinued.
- If ALT elevations >3 × ULN occur concurrently with bilirubin elevations >2 × ULN, VOTRIENT should be permanently discontinued. Patients should be monitored until resolution. VOTRIENT is a UGT1A1 inhibitor. Mild, indirect (unconjugated) hyperbilirubinemia may occur in patients with Gilbert's syndrome *[see Clinical Pharmacology (12.5)]*. Patients with only a mild indirect hyperbilirubinemia, known Gilbert's syndrome, and elevation in ALT >3 × ULN should be managed as per the recommendations outlined for isolated ALT elevations.

Concomitant use of VOTRIENT and simvastatin increases the risk of ALT elevations and should be undertaken with caution and close monitoring *[see Drug Interactions (7.3)]*. Insufficient data are available to assess the risk of concomitant administration of alternative statins and VOTRIENT.

In patients with pre-existing moderate hepatic impairment, the starting dose of VOTRIENT should be reduced or alternatives to VOTRIENT should be considered. Treatment with VOTRIENT is not recommended in patients with pre-existing severe hepatic impairment, defined as total bilirubin >3 × ULN with any level of ALT *[see Dosage and Administration (2.2), Use in Specific Populations (8.6), and Clinical Pharmacology (12.3)]*.

5.2 QT Prolongation and Torsades de Pointes

In the RCC trials of VOTRIENT, QT prolongation (≥500 msec) was identified on routine electrocardiogram monitoring in 2% (11/558) of patients. Torsades de pointes occurred in <1% (2/977) of patients who received VOTRIENT in the monotherapy trials.

In the randomized RCC and STS trials, 1% (3/290) of patients and 0.2% (1/240) of patients respectively, who received VOTRIENT had post-baseline values between 500 to 549 msec. Post-baseline QT data were only collected in the STS trial if ECG abnormalities were reported as an adverse reaction. None of the 268 patients who received placebo on the two trials had post-baseline QTc values ≥500 msec.

VOTRIENT should be used with caution in patients with a history of QT interval prolongation, in patients taking antiarrhythmics or other medications that may prolong QT interval, and those with relevant pre-existing cardiac disease. When using VOTRIENT, baseline and periodic monitoring of electrocardiograms and maintenance of electrolytes (e.g., calcium, magnesium, potassium) within the normal range should be performed.

5.3 Cardiac Dysfunction

In clinical trials with VOTRIENT, events of cardiac dysfunction such as decreased left ventricular ejection fraction (LVEF) and congestive heart failure have occurred. In the overall safety population for RCC (N = 586), cardiac dysfunction was observed in 0.6% (4/586) of patients without routine on-study LVEF monitoring. In the randomized STS trial, myocardial dysfunction was defined as symptoms of cardiac dysfunction or ≥15% absolute decline in LVEF compared to baseline or a decline in LVEF of ≥10% compared to baseline that is also below the lower limit of normal. In patients who had baseline and follow up LVEF measurements, myocardial dysfunction occurred in 11% (16/142) of patients on VOTRIENT compared to 5% (2/40) of patients on placebo. One percent (3/240) of patients on VOTRIENT in the STS trial had congestive heart failure which did not resolve in one patient.

Fourteen of the 16 patients with myocardial dysfunction treated with VOTRIENT in the STS trial had concurrent hypertension which may have exacerbated cardiac dysfunction in patients at risk (e.g., those with prior anthracycline therapy) possibly by increasing cardiac afterload. Blood pressure should be monitored and managed promptly using a combination of anti-hypertensive therapy and dose modification of VOTRIENT (interruption and re-initiation at a reduced dose based on clinical judgment) [see Warnings and Precautions (5.9)]. Patients should be carefully monitored for clinical signs or symptoms of congestive heart failure. Baseline and periodic evaluation of LVEF is recommended in patients at risk of cardiac dysfunction including previous anthracycline exposure.

5.4 Hemorrhagic Events

Fatal hemorrhage occurred in 0.9% (5/586) in the RCC trials; there were no reports of fatal hemorrhage in the STS trials. In the randomized RCC trial, 13% (37/290) of patients treated with VOTRIENT and 5% (7/145) of patients on placebo experienced at least 1 hemorrhagic event. The most common hemorrhagic events in the patients treated with VOTRIENT were hematuria (4%), epistaxis (2%), hemoptysis (2%), and rectal hemorrhage (1%). Nine of 37 patients treated with VOTRIENT who had hemorrhagic events experienced serious events including pulmonary, gastrointestinal, and genitourinary hemorrhage. One percent (4/290) of patients treated with VOTRIENT died from hemorrhage compared with no (0/145) patients on placebo. In the overall safety population in RCC (N = 586), cerebral/intracranial hemorrhage was observed in <1% (2/586) of patients treated with VOTRIENT.

In the randomized STS trial, 22% (53/240) of patients treated with VOTRIENT compared to 8% (10/123) treated with placebo experienced at least 1 hemorrhagic event. The most common hemorrhagic events were epistaxis (8%), mouth hemorrhage (3%), and anal hemorrhage (2%). Grade 4 hemorrhagic events in the STS population occurred in 1% (3/240) patients and included intracranial hemorrhage, subarachnoid hemorrhage, and peritoneal hemorrhage.

VOTRIENT has not been studied in patients who have a history of hemoptysis, cerebral, or clinically significant gastrointestinal hemorrhage in the past 6 months and should not be used in those patients.

5.5 Arterial Thrombotic Events

Fatal arterial thromboembolic events were observed in 0.3% (2/586) of patients in the RCC trials and in no patients in the STS trials. In the randomized RCC trial, 2% (5/290) of patients receiving VOTRIENT experienced myocardial infarction or ischemia, 0.3% (1/290) had a cerebrovascular accident and 1% (4/290) had an event of transient ischemic attack. In the randomized STS trial, 2% (4/240) of patients receiving VOTRIENT experienced a myocardial infarction or ischemia, 0.4% (1/240) had a cerebrovascular accident and there were no incidents of transient ischemic attack. No arterial thrombotic events were reported in patients who received placebo in either trial. VOTRIENT should be used with caution in patients who are at increased risk for these events or who have had a history of these events. VOTRIENT has not been studied in patients who have had an arterial thrombotic event within the previous 6 months and should not be used in those patients.

5.6 Venous Thromboembolic Events

In RCC and STS trials of VOTRIENT, venous thromboembolic events including venous thrombosis and fatal pulmonary embolus have occurred. In the randomized STS trial, venous thromboembolic events were reported in 5% of patients treated with VOTRIENT compared to 2% with placebo. In the randomized RCC trial, the rate was 1% in both arms. Fatal pulmonary embolus occurred in 1% (2/240) of STS patients receiving VOTRIENT and in no patients receiving placebo. There were no fatal pulmonary emboli in the RCC trial. Monitor for signs and symptoms of VTE and PE.

5.7 Gastrointestinal Perforation and Fistula

In the RCC and STS trials, gastrointestinal perforation or fistula occurred in 0.9% (5/586) of patients and 1% (4/382) of patients receiving VOTRIENT, respectively. Fatal perforations occurred in 0.3% (2/586) of these patients in the RCC trials and in 0.3% (1/382) of these patients in the STS trials. Monitor for signs and symptoms of gastrointestinal perforation or fistula.

5.8 Reversible Posterior Leukoencephalopathy Syndrome

Reversible Posterior Leukoencephalopathy Syndrome (RPLS) has been reported in patients receiving VOTRIENT and may be fatal.

RPLS is a neurological disorder which can present with headache, seizure, lethargy, confusion, blindness, and other visual and neurologic disturbances. Mild to severe hypertension may be present. The diagnosis of RPLS is optimally confirmed by magnetic resonance imaging. Discontinue VOTRIENT in patients developing RPLS.

5.9 Hypertension

Hypertension (systolic blood pressure ≥150 or diastolic blood pressure ≥100 mm Hg) and hypertensive crisis were observed in patients treated with VOTRIENT. Blood pressure should be well-controlled prior to initiating VOTRIENT. Hypertension occurs early in the course of treatment (40% of cases occurred by Day 9 and 90% of cases occurred in the first 18 weeks). Blood pressure should be monitored early after starting treatment (no longer than one week) and frequently thereafter to ensure blood pressure control. Approximately 40% of patients who received VOTRIENT experienced hypertension. Grade 3 hypertension was reported in 4% to 7% of patients receiving VOTRIENT *[see Adverse Reactions (6.1)]*.

Increased blood pressure should be treated promptly with standard anti-hypertensive therapy and dose reduction or interruption of VOTRIENT as clinically warranted. VOTRIENT should be discontinued if there is evidence of hypertensive crisis or if hypertension is severe and persistent despite anti-hypertensive therapy and dose reduction. Approximately 1% of patients required permanent discontinuation of VOTRIENT because of hypertension *[see Dosage and Administration (2.2)]*.

5.10 Wound Healing

No formal trials on the effect of VOTRIENT on wound healing have been conducted. Since vascular endothelial growth factor receptor (VEGFR) inhibitors such as pazopanib may impair wound healing, treatment with VOTRIENT should be stopped at least 7 days prior to scheduled surgery. The decision to resume VOTRIENT after surgery should be based on clinical judgment of adequate wound healing. VOTRIENT should be discontinued in patients with wound dehiscence.

5.11 Hypothyroidism

Hypothyroidism, confirmed based on a simultaneous rise of TSH and decline of T4, was reported in 7% (19/290) of patients treated with VOTRIENT in the randomized RCC trial and in 5% (11/240) of patients treated with VOTRIENT in the randomized STS trial. No patients on the placebo arm of either trial had hypothyroidism. In RCC and STS trials of VOTRIENT, hypothyroidism was reported as an adverse reaction in 4% (26/586) and 5% (20/382) of patients, respectively. Proactive monitoring of thyroid function tests is recommended.

5.12 Proteinuria

In the randomized RCC trial, proteinuria was reported as an adverse reaction in 9% (27/290) of patients receiving VOTRIENT and in no patients receiving placebo. In 2 patients, proteinuria led to discontinuation of treatment with VOTRIENT. In the randomized STS trial, proteinuria was reported as an adverse reaction in 1% (2/240) of patients, and nephrotic syndrome was reported in 1 patient, treated with VOTRIENT compared to none in patients receiving placebo. Treatment was withdrawn in the patient with nephrotic syndrome.

Baseline and periodic urinalysis during treatment is recommended with follow up measurement of 24-hour urine protein as clinically indicated. Interrupt VOTRIENT and dose reduce for 24-hour urine protein ≥3 grams; discontinue VOTRIENT for repeat episodes despite dose reductions [see Dosage and Administration (2.2)].

5.13 Infection

Serious infections (with or without neutropenia), including some with fatal outcome, have been reported. Monitor patients for signs and symptoms of infection. Institute appropriate anti-infective therapy promptly and consider interruption or discontinuation of VOTRIENT for serious infections.

5.14 Increased Toxicity with Other Cancer Therapy

VOTRIENT is not indicated for use in combination with other agents. Clinical trials of VOTRIENT in combination with pemetrexed and lapatinib were terminated early due to concerns over increased toxicity and mortality. The fatal toxicities observed included pulmonary hemorrhage, gastrointestinal hemorrhage, and sudden death. A safe and effective combination dose has not been established with these regimens.

5.15 Increased Toxicity in Developing Organs

The safety and effectiveness of VOTRIENT in pediatric patients have not been established. VOTRIENT is not indicated for use in pediatric patients. Based on its mechanism of action, pazopanib may have severe effects on organ growth and maturation during early post-natal development. Administration of pazopanib to juvenile rats less than 21 days old resulted in toxicity to the lungs, liver, heart, and kidney and in death at doses significantly lower than the clinically recommended dose or doses tolerated in older animals. VOTRIENT may potentially cause serious adverse effects on organ development in pediatric patients, particularly in patients younger than 2 years of age *[see Use in Specific Populations (8.4)]*.

5.16 Pregnancy

VOTRIENT can cause fetal harm when administered to a pregnant woman. Based on its mechanism of action, VOTRIENT is expected to result in adverse reproductive effects. In pre-clinical studies in rats and rabbits, pazopanib was teratogenic, embryotoxic, fetotoxic, and abortifacient. There are no adequate and well-controlled studies of VOTRIENT in pregnant women. If this drug is used during pregnancy, or if the patient becomes pregnant while taking this drug, the patient should be apprised of the potential hazard to the fetus. Women of childbearing potential should be advised to avoid becoming pregnant while taking VOTRIENT *[see Use in Specific Populations (8.1)]*.

6 ADVERSE REACTIONS

6.1 Clinical Trials Experience

Because clinical trials are conducted under widely varying conditions, adverse reaction rates observed in the clinical trials of a drug cannot be directly compared to rates in the clinical trials of another drug and may not reflect the rates observed in practice.

Potentially serious adverse reactions with VOTRIENT included:

- Hepatotoxicity *[see Warnings and Precautions (5.1)]*
- QT prolongation and torsades de pointes *[see Warnings and Precautions (5.2)]*
- Cardiac dysfunction *[see Warnings and Precautions (5.3)]*
- Hemorrhagic events *[see Warnings and Precautions (5.4)]*
- Arterial and venous thrombotic events *[see Warnings and Precautions (5.5 and 5.6)]*
- Gastrointestinal perforation and fistula *[see Warnings and Precautions (5.7)]*
- Reversible Posterior Leukoencephalopathy Syndrome (RPLS) *[see Warnings and Precautions (5.8)]*
- Hypertension *[see Warnings and Precautions (5.9)]*
- Infection *[see Warnings and Precautions (5.13)]*
- Increased toxicity with other cancer therapies *[see Warnings and Precautions (5.14)]*

Renal Cell Carcinoma: The safety of VOTRIENT has been evaluated in 977 patients in the monotherapy trials which included 586 patients with RCC at the time of NDA submission. With a median duration of treatment of 7.4 months (range 0.1 to 27.6), the most commonly observed adverse reactions (≥20%) in the 586 patients were diarrhea, hypertension, hair color change, nausea, fatigue, anorexia, and vomiting.

The data described below reflect the safety profile of VOTRIENT in 290 RCC patients who participated in a randomized, double-blind, placebo-controlled trial *[see Clinical Studies (14.1)]*. The median duration of treatment was 7.4 months (range 0 to 23) for patients who received VOTRIENT and 3.8 months (range 0 to 22) for the placebo

Table 1. Adverse Reactions Occurring in ≥10% of Patients with RCC who Received VOTRIENT

	VOTRIENT (N = 290)			Placebo (N = 145)		
	All Grades[a]	Grade 3	Grade 4	All Grades[a]	Grade 3	Grade 4
Adverse Reactions	%	%	%	%	%	%
Diarrhea	52	3	<1	9	<1	0
Hypertension	40	4	0	10	<1	0
Hair color changes	38	<1	0	3	0	0
Nausea	26	<1	0	9	0	0
Anorexia	22	2	0	10	<1	0
Vomiting	21	2	<1	8	2	0
Fatigue	19	2	0	8	1	1
Asthenia	14	3	0	8	0	0
Abdominal pain	11	2	0	1	0	0
Headache	10	0	0	5	0	0

[a] National Cancer Institute Common Terminology Criteria for Adverse Events, version 3.

Table 2. Selected Laboratory Abnormalities Occurring in >10% of Patients with RCC who Received VOTRIENT and More Commonly (≥5%) in Patients who Received VOTRIENT Versus Placebo

	VOTRIENT (N = 290)			Placebo (N = 145)		
	All Grades[a]	Grade 3	Grade 4	All Grades[a]	Grade 3	Grade 4
Parameters	%	%	%	%	%	%
Hematologic						
Leukopenia	37	0	0	6	0	0
Neutropenia	34	1	<1	6	0	0
Thrombocytopenia	32	<1	<1	5	0	<1
Lymphocytopenia	31	4	<1	24	1	0
Chemistry						
ALT increased	53	10	2	22	1	0
AST increased	53	7	<1	19	<1	0
Glucose increased	41	<1	0	33	1	0
Total bilirubin increased	36	3	<1	10	1	<1
Phosphorus decreased	34	4	0	11	0	0
Sodium decreased	31	4	1	24	4	0
Magnesium decreased	26	<1	1	14	0	0
Glucose decreased	17	0	<1	3	0	0

[a] National Cancer Institute Common Terminology Criteria for Adverse Events, version 3.

arm. Forty-two percent of patients on VOTRIENT required a dose interruption. Thirty-six percent of patients on VOTRIENT were dose reduced. Table 1 presents the most common adverse reactions occurring in ≥10% of patients who received VOTRIENT.

[See table 1 at top of previous page]

Other adverse reactions observed more commonly in patients treated with VOTRIENT than placebo and that occurred in <10% (any grade) were alopecia (8% versus <1%), chest pain (5% versus 1%), dysgeusia (altered taste) (8% versus <1%), dyspepsia (5% versus <1%), dysphonia (4% versus <1%), facial edema (1% versus 0%), palmar-plantar erythrodysesthesia (hand-foot syndrome) (6% versus <1%), proteinuria (9% versus 0%), rash (8% versus 3%), skin depigmentation (3% versus 0%), and weight decreased (9% versus 3%).

Table 2 presents the most common laboratory abnormalities occurring in >10% of patients who received VOTRIENT and more commonly (≥5%) in patients who received VOTRIENT versus placebo.

[See table 2 above]

Soft Tissue Sarcoma: The safety of VOTRIENT has been evaluated in 382 patients with advanced soft tissue sarcoma, with a median duration of treatment of 3.6 months (range 0 to 53). The most commonly observed adverse reactions (≥20%) in the 382 patients were fatigue, diarrhea, nausea, decreased weight, hypertension, decreased appetite, vomiting, tumor pain, hair color changes, musculoskeletal pain, headache, dysgeusia, dyspnea, and skin hypopigmentation.

The data described below reflect the safety profile of VOTRIENT in 240 patients who participated in a randomized, double-blind, placebo-controlled trial *[see Clinical Studies (14.2)]*. The median duration of treatment was 4.5 months (range 0 to 24) for patients who received VOTRIENT and 1.9 months (range 0 to 24) for the placebo arm. Fifty-eight percent of patients on VOTRIENT required a dose interruption. Thirty-eight percent of patients on VOTRIENT had their dose reduced. Fourteen percent of patients who received VOTRIENT discontinued therapy due to adverse reactions. Table 3 presents the most common adverse reactions occurring in ≥10% of patients who received VOTRIENT.

[See table 3 at top of next page]

Other adverse reactions observed more commonly in patients treated with VOTRIENT that occurred in ≥5% of patients and at an incidence of more than 2% difference from placebo included insomnia (9% versus 6%), hypothyroidism (8% versus 0), dysphonia (8% versus 2%), epistaxis (8% versus 2%), left ventricular dysfunction (8% versus 4%), dyspepsia (7% versus 2%), dry skin (6% versus <1%), chills (5% versus 1%), vision blurred (5% versus 2%), and nail disorder (5% versus 0%).

Table 4 presents the most common laboratory abnormalities occurring in >10% of patients who received VOTRIENT and more commonly (≥5%) in patients who received VOTRIENT versus placebo.

[See table 4 at top of page 1288]

Diarrhea: Diarrhea occurred frequently and was predominantly mild to moderate in severity in both the RCC and STS clinical trials. Patients should be advised how to manage mild diarrhea and to notify their healthcare provider if moderate to severe diarrhea occurs so appropriate management can be implemented to minimize its impact.

Lipase Elevations: In a single-arm RCC trial, increases in lipase values were observed for 27% (48/181) of patients. Elevations in lipase as an adverse reaction were reported for 4% (10/225) of patients and were Grade 3 for 6 patients and Grade 4 for 1 patient. In the RCC trials of VOTRIENT, clinical pancreatitis was observed in <1% (4/586) of patients.

Pneumothorax: Two of 290 patients treated with VOTRIENT and no patient on the placebo arm in the randomized RCC trial developed a pneumothorax. In the randomized trial of VOTRIENT for the treatment of STS, pneumothorax occurred in 3% (8/240) of patients treated with VOTRIENT and in no patients on the placebo arm.

6.2 Postmarketing Experience

The following adverse reactions have been identified during post approval use of VOTRIENT. Because these reactions are reported voluntarily from a population of uncertain size it is not always possible to reliably estimate the frequency or establish a causal relationship to drug exposure.

Reversible Posterior Leukoencephalopathy Syndrome *[see Warnings and Precautions (5.8)]*

7 DRUG INTERACTIONS

7.1 Drugs That Inhibit or Induce Cytochrome P450 3A4 Enzymes

In vitro studies suggested that the oxidative metabolism of pazopanib in human liver microsomes is mediated primarily by CYP3A4, with minor contributions from CYP1A2 and CYP2C8. Therefore, inhibitors and inducers of CYP3A4 may alter the metabolism of pazopanib.

CYP3A4 Inhibitors: Coadministration of pazopanib with strong inhibitors of CYP3A4 (e.g., ketoconazole, ritonavir, clarithromycin) increases pazopanib concentrations and should be avoided. Reduce the dose of VOTRIENT when it must be coadministered with strong CYP3A4 inhibitors *[see Dosage and Administration (2.2)]*. Grapefruit juice should be avoided as it inhibits CYP3A4 activity and may also increase plasma concentrations of pazopanib.

CYP3A4 Inducers: CYP3A4 inducers such as rifampin may decrease plasma pazopanib concentrations. VOTRIENT should not be used if chronic use of strong CYP3A4 inducers cannot be avoided *[see Dosage and Administration (2.2)]*.

7.2 Effects of Pazopanib on CYP Substrates

Results from drug-drug interaction trials conducted in cancer patients suggest that pazopanib is a weak inhibitor of CYP3A4, CYP2C8, and CYP2D6 in vivo, but had no effect on CYP1A2, CYP2C9, or CYP2C19 *[see Clinical Pharmacology (12.3)]*.

Concomitant use of VOTRIENT with agents with narrow therapeutic windows that are metabolized by CYP3A4, CYP2D6, or CYP2C8 is not recommended. Coadministration may result in inhibition of the metabolism of these products and create the potential for serious adverse events *[see Clinical Pharmacology (12.3)]*.

7.3 Effect of Concomitant use of VOTRIENT and Simvastatin

Concomitant use of VOTRIENT and simvastatin increases the incidence of ALT elevations. Across monotherapy studies with VOTRIENT, ALT >3 × ULN was reported in 126/895 (14%) of patients who did not use statins, compared with 11/41 (27%) of patients who had concomitant use of simvastatin. If a patient receiving concomitant simvastatin develops ALT elevations, follow dosing guidelines for VOTRIENT or consider alternatives to VOTRIENT *[see Warnings and Precautions (5.1)]*. Alternatively, consider discontinuing simvastatin *[see Warnings and Precautions (5.1)]*. Insufficient data are available to assess the risk of concomitant administration of alternative statins and VOTRIENT.

8 USE IN SPECIFIC POPULATIONS

8.1 Pregnancy

Pregnancy Category D *[see Warnings and Precautions (5.16)]*.

VOTRIENT can cause fetal harm when administered to a pregnant woman. There are no adequate and well-controlled studies of VOTRIENT in pregnant women.

In pre-clinical studies in rats and rabbits, pazopanib was teratogenic, embryotoxic, fetotoxic, and abortifacient. Administration of pazopanib to pregnant rats during organogenesis at a dose level of ≥3 mg/kg/day (approximately 0.1 times the human clinical exposure based on AUC) resulted in teratogenic effects including cardiovascular malformations (retroesophageal subclavian artery, missing innominate artery, changes in the aortic arch) and incomplete or absent ossification. In addition, there was reduced fetal body weight, and pre- and post-implantation embryolethality in rats administered pazopanib at doses ≥3 mg/kg/day. In rabbits, maternal toxicity (reduced food consumption, increased post-implantation loss, and abortion) was observed at doses ≥30 mg/kg/day (approximately 0.007 times the human clinical exposure). In addition, severe maternal body weight loss and 100% litter loss were observed at doses ≥100 mg/kg/day (0.02 times the human clinical exposure), while fetal weight was reduced at doses ≥3 mg/kg/day (AUC not calculated).

If this drug is used during pregnancy, or if the patient becomes pregnant while taking this drug, the patient should be apprised of the potential hazard to the fetus. Women of childbearing potential should be advised to avoid becoming pregnant while taking VOTRIENT.

8.3 Nursing Mothers

It is not known whether this drug is excreted in human milk. Because many drugs are excreted in human milk and because of the potential for serious adverse reactions in nursing infants from VOTRIENT, a decision should be made whether to discontinue nursing or to discontinue the drug, taking into account the importance of the drug to the mother.

8.4 Pediatric Use

The safety and effectiveness of VOTRIENT in pediatric patients have not been established.

In rats, weaning occurs at day 21 postpartum which approximately equates to a human pediatric age of 2 years. In a juvenile animal toxicology study performed in rats, when animals were dosed from day 9 through day 14 postpartum (pre-weaning), pazopanib caused abnormal organ growth/maturation in the kidney, lung, liver, and heart at approximately 0.1 times the clinical exposure, based on AUC in adult patients receiving VOTRIENT. At approximately 0.4 times the clinical exposure (based on the AUC in adult patients), pazopanib administration resulted in mortality.

In repeat-dose toxicology studies in rats including 4-week, 13-week, and 26-week administration, toxicities in bone, teeth, and nail beds were observed at doses ≥3 mg/kg/day (approximately 0.07 times the human clinical exposure based on AUC). Doses of 300 mg/kg/day (approximately 0.8 times the human clinical exposure based on AUC) were not tolerated in 13- and 26-week studies and animals required dose reductions due to body weight loss and morbidity. Hypertrophy of epiphyseal growth plates, nail abnormalities (including broken, overgrown, or absent nails) and tooth abnormalities in growing incisor teeth (including excessively long, brittle, broken and missing teeth, and dentine and enamel degeneration and thinning) were observed in rats at doses ≥30 mg/kg/day (approximately 0.35 times the human clinical exposure based on AUC) at 26 weeks, with the onset of tooth and nail bed alterations noted clinically after 4 to 6 weeks. Similar findings were noted in repeat-dose studies in juvenile rats dosed with pazopanib beginning day 21 post-partum (post-weaning). In the post-weaning animals, the occurrence of changes in teeth and bones occurred earlier and with greater severity than in older animals. There was evidence of tooth degeneration and decreased bone growth at doses ≥30 mg/kg (approximately 0.1 to 0.2 times the AUC in human adults at the clinically recommended dose). Pazopanib exposure in juvenile rats was lower than that seen at the same dose levels in adult animals, based on comparative AUC values. At pazopanib doses approximately 0.5 to 0.7 times the exposure in adult patients at the clinically recommended dose, decreased bone growth in juvenile rats persisted even after the end of the dosing period. Finally, despite lower pazopanib exposures than those reported in adult animals or adult humans, juvenile animals administered 300 mg/kg/dose pazopanib required dose reduction within 4 weeks of dosing initiation due to significant toxicity, although adult animals could tolerate this same dose for at least 3 times as long *[see Warnings and Precautions (5.15)]*.

8.5 Geriatric Use

In clinical trials with VOTRIENT for the treatment of RCC, 33% (196/582) of patients were aged ≥65 years. No overall differences in safety or effectiveness of VOTRIENT were observed between these patients and younger patients. However, patients >60 years of age may be at greater risk for an ALT >3 × ULN. In the STS trials, 24% (93/382) of patients were age ≥65 years. Patients ≥ 65 years had increased Grade 3 or 4 fatigue (19% versus 12% for <65), hypertension (10% versus 6%), decreased appetite (11% versus 2%) and ALT (3% versus 2 %) or AST elevations (4% versus 1%). Other reported clinical experience has not identified differences in responses between elderly and younger patients, but greater sensitivity of some older individuals cannot be ruled out.

8.6 Hepatic Impairment

In clinical studies for VOTRIENT, patients with total bilirubin ≤1.5 × ULN and AST and ALT ≤2 × ULN were included *[see Warnings and Precautions (5.1)]*.

An analysis of data from a pharmacokinetic study of pazopanib in patients with varying degrees of hepatic dysfunction suggested that no dose adjustment is required in patients with mild hepatic impairment [either total bilirubin within normal limit (WNL) with ALT >ULN or bilirubin >1 × to 1.5 × ULN regardless of the ALT value]. The maximum tolerated dose in patients with moderate hepatic impairment (total bilirubin >1.5 × to 3 × ULN regardless of the ALT value) was 200 mg per day (N = 11). The median steady-state C_{max} and $AUC_{(0-24)}$ achieved at this dose was approximately 40% and 29%, respectively of that seen in patients with normal hepatic function at the recommended daily dose of 800 mg. The maximum dose explored in patients with severe hepatic impairment (total bilirubin >3 × ULN regardless of the ALT value) was 200 mg per day (N = 14). This dose was not well tolerated. Median exposures achieved at this dose were approximately 18% and 15% of those seen in patients with normal liver function at the recommended daily dose of 800 mg. Therefore, VOTRIENT is not recommended in these patients *[see Clinical Pharmacology (12.3)]*.

8.7 Renal Impairment

Patients with renal cell cancer and mild/moderate renal impairment (creatinine clearance ≥30 mL/min) were included in clinical trials for VOTRIENT.

There are no clinical or pharmacokinetic data in patients with severe renal impairment or in patients undergoing peritoneal dialysis or hemodialysis. However, renal impairment is unlikely to significantly affect the pharmacokinetics of pazopanib since <4% of a radiolabeled oral dose was recovered in the urine. In a population pharmacokinetic analysis using 408 patients with various cancers, creatinine clearance (30-150 mL/min) did not influence clearance of pazopanib. Therefore, renal impairment is not expected to influence pazopanib exposure, and dose adjustment is not necessary.

10 OVERDOSAGE

Pazopanib doses up to 2,000 mg have been evaluated in clinical trials. Dose-limiting toxicity (Grade 3 fatigue) and Grade 3 hypertension were each observed in 1 of 3 patients dosed at 2,000 mg daily and 1,000 mg daily, respectively.

Treatment of overdose with VOTRIENT should consist of general supportive measures. There is no specific antidote for overdosage of VOTRIENT.

Hemodialysis is not expected to enhance the elimination of VOTRIENT because pazopanib is not significantly renally excreted and is highly bound to plasma proteins.

11 DESCRIPTION

VOTRIENT (pazopanib) is a tyrosine kinase inhibitor (TKI). Pazopanib is presented as the hydrochloride salt, with the

Table 3. Adverse Reactions Occurring in ≥10% of Patients with STS who Received VOTRIENT

	VOTRIENT (N = 240)			Placebo (N = 123)		
	All Grades[a]	Grade 3	Grade 4	All Grades[a]	Grade 3	Grade 4
Adverse Reactions	%	%	%	%	%	%
Fatigue	65	13	1	48	4	1
Diarrhea	59	5	0	15	1	0
Nausea	56	3	0	22	2	0
Weight decreased	48	4	0	15	0	0
Hypertension	42	7	0	6	0	0
Appetite decreased	40	6	0	19	0	0
Hair color changes	39	0	0	2	0	0
Vomiting	33	3	0	11	1	0
Tumor pain	29	8	0	21	7	2
Dysgeusia	28	0	0	3	0	0
Headache	23	1	0	8	0	0
Musculoskeletal pain	23	2	0	20	2	0
Myalgia	23	2	0	9	0	0
Gastrointestinal pain	23	3	0	9	4	0
Dyspnea	20	5	<1	17	5	1
Exfoliative rash	18	<1	0	9	0	0
Cough	17	<1	0	12	<1	0
Peripheral edema	14	2	0	9	2	0
Mucositis	12	2	0	2	0	0
Alopecia	12	0	0	1	0	0
Dizziness	11	1	0	4	0	0
Skin disorder[b]	11	2	0	1	0	0
Skin hypopigmentation	11	0	0	0	0	0
Stomatitis	11	<1	0	3	0	0
Chest pain	10	2	0	6	0	0

[a] National Cancer Institute Common Terminology Criteria for Adverse Events, version 3.
[b] 27 of the 28 cases of skin disorder were palmar-plantar erythrodysesthesia.

chemical name 5-[[4-[(2,3-dimethyl-2H-indazol-6-yl)methyl-amino]-2-pyrimidinyl]amino]-2-methylbenzenesulfonamide monohydrochloride. It has the molecular formula $C_{21}H_{23}N_7O_2S \bullet HCl$ and a molecular weight of 473.99. Pazopanib hydrochloride has the following chemical structure:

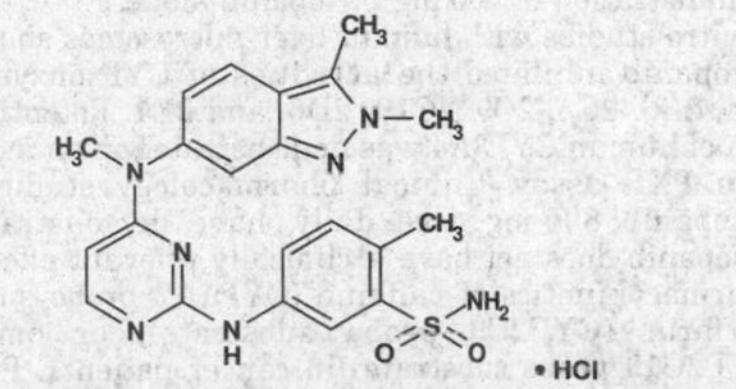

Pazopanib hydrochloride is a white to slightly yellow solid. It is very slightly soluble at pH 1 and practically insoluble above pH 4 in aqueous media.

Tablets of VOTRIENT are for oral administration. Each 200 mg tablet of VOTRIENT contains 216.7 mg of pazopanib hydrochloride, equivalent to 200 mg of pazopanib free base.

The inactive ingredients of VOTRIENT are: **Tablet Core:** Magnesium stearate, microcrystalline cellulose, povidone, sodium starch glycolate. **Coating:** Gray film-coat: Hypromellose, iron oxide black, macrogol/polyethylene glycol 400 (PEG 400), polysorbate 80, titanium dioxide.

12 CLINICAL PHARMACOLOGY

12.1 Mechanism of Action

Pazopanib is a multi-tyrosine kinase inhibitor of vascular endothelial growth factor receptor (VEGFR)-1, VEGFR-2, VEGFR-3, platelet-derived growth factor receptor (PDGFR)-α and -β, fibroblast growth factor receptor (FGFR) -1 and -3, cytokine receptor (Kit), interleukin-2 receptor inducible T-cell kinase (Itk), leukocyte-specific protein tyrosine kinase (Lck), and transmembrane glycoprotein receptor tyrosine kinase (c-Fms). In vitro, pazopanib inhibited ligand-induced autophosphorylation of VEGFR-2, Kit and PDGFR-β receptors. In vivo, pazopanib inhibited VEGF-induced VEGFR-2 phosphorylation in mouse lungs, angiogenesis in a mouse model, and the growth of some human tumor xenografts in mice.

12.2 Pharmacodynamics

Increases in blood pressure have been observed and are related to steady-state trough plasma pazopanib concentrations.

The QT prolongation potential of pazopanib was assessed in a randomized, blinded, parallel trial (N = 96) using moxifloxacin as a positive control. Pazopanib 800 mg was dosed under fasting conditions on Days 2 to 8 and 1,600 mg was dosed on Day 9 after a meal in order to increase exposure to pazopanib and its metabolites. No large changes (i.e., >20 msec) in QTc interval following the treatment of pazopanib were detected in this QT trial. The trial was not able to exclude small changes (<10 msec) in QTc interval, because assay sensitivity below this threshold (<10 msec) was not established in this trial *[see Warnings and Precautions (5.2)]*.

Table 4. Selected Laboratory Abnormalities Occurring in >10% of Patients with STS who Received VOTRIENT and More Commonly (≥5%) in Patients who Received VOTRIENT Versus Placebo

	VOTRIENT (N = 240)			Placebo (N = 123)		
	All Grades[a]	Grade 3	Grade 4	All Grades[a]	Grade 3	Grade 4
Parameters	%	%	%	%	%	%
Hematologic						
Leukopenia	44	1	0	15	0	0
Lymphocytopenia	43	10	0	36	9	2
Thrombocytopenia	36	3	1	6	0	0
Neutropenia	33	4	0	7	0	0
Chemistry						
AST increased	51	5	3	22	2	0
ALT increased	46	8	2	18	2	1
Glucose increased	45	<1	0	35	2	0
Albumin decreased	34	1	0	21	0	0
Alkaline phosphatase increased	32	3	0	23	1	0
Sodium decreased	31	4	0	20	3	0
Total bilirubin increased	29	1	0	7	2	0
Potassium increased	16	1	0	11	0	0

[a]National Cancer Institute Common Terminology Criteria for Adverse Events, version 3.

12.3 Pharmacokinetics

Absorption: Pazopanib is absorbed orally with median time to achieve peak concentrations of 2 to 4 hours after the dose. Daily dosing at 800 mg results in geometric mean AUC and C_{max} of 1,037 hr•µg/mL and 58.1 µg/mL (equivalent to 132 µM), respectively. There was no consistent increase in AUC or C_{max} at pazopanib doses above 800 mg.

Administration of a single pazopanib 400 mg crushed tablet increased $AUC_{(0-72)}$ by 46% and C_{max} by approximately 2 fold and decreased t_{max} by approximately 2 hours compared to administration of the whole tablet. These results indicate that the bioavailability and the rate of pazopanib oral absorption are increased after administration of the crushed tablet relative to administration of the whole tablet. Therefore, due to this potential for increased exposure, tablets of VOTRIENT should not be crushed.

Systemic exposure to pazopanib is increased when administered with food. Administration of pazopanib with a high-fat or low-fat meal results in an approximately 2 fold increase in AUC and C_{max}. Therefore, pazopanib should be administered at least 1 hour before or 2 hours after a meal *[see Dosage and Administration (2.1)]*.

Distribution: Binding of pazopanib to human plasma protein in vivo was greater than 99% with no concentration dependence over the range of 10 to 100 µg/mL. In vitro studies suggest that pazopanib is a substrate for P-glycoprotein (Pgp) and breast cancer resistant protein (BCRP).

Metabolism: In vitro studies demonstrated that pazopanib is metabolized by CYP3A4 with a minor contribution from CYP1A2 and CYP2C8.

Elimination: Pazopanib has a mean half-life of 30.9 hours after administration of the recommended dose of 800 mg. Elimination is primarily via feces with renal elimination accounting for <4% of the administered dose.

Hepatic Impairment: Mild hepatic impairment was defined as either total bilirubin WNL with ALT >ULN or bilirubin >1 × to 1.5 × ULN regardless of the ALT value. The median steady-state pazopanib C_{max} and $AUC_{(0-24)}$ after a once daily dose of 800 mg/day in patients (N = 12) with mild impairment were 34 µg/ml (range 11 to 104) and 774 µg•hr/ml (range 215 to 2,034), respectively. These were in a similar range as the median steady-state pazopanib C_{max} and $AUC_{(0-24)}$ in patients (N = 18) with no hepatic impairment (52 µg/ml, range 17 to 86 and 888 µg•hr/ml, range 346 to 1,482, respectively) *[see Dosage and Administration (2.2)]*.

Moderate hepatic impairment was defined as total bilirubin >1.5 × to 3 × ULN regardless of the ALT value. The maximum tolerated pazopanib dose in patients with moderate impairment was 200 mg once daily. The median (N = 11) steady-state C_{max} with that regimen was 22 µg/ml (range 4.2 to 33), and the median $AUC_{(0-24)}$ was 257 µg•hr/ml (range 66 to 488). These values were approximately 43% and 29% those of the corresponding median values after administration of 800 mg once daily in patients with normal hepatic function (N = 18) *[see Dosage and Administration (2.2)]*.

Severe hepatic impairment was defined as total bilirubin >3 × ULN regardless of the ALT value. Median exposures in patients with severe hepatic impairment receiving 200 mg once daily (N = 14) were unexpectedly lower than those observed in patients with moderate hepatic impairment receiving 200 mg once daily. The median steady-state C_{max} was 9.4 µg/ml (range 2.4 to 24), and the median $AUC_{(0-24)}$ was 131 µg•hr/ml (range 47 to 473). These values were approximately 18% and 15% that of the corresponding median values after administration of 800 mg once daily in patients with normal hepatic function. Despite the observed concentrations, the dose of 200 mg was not well tolerated in patients with severe hepatic impairment. Use of VOTRIENT is not recommended in patients with severe hepatic impairment *[see Use in Specific Populations (8.6)]*.

Drug Interactions: Coadministration of multiple doses of oral pazopanib 400 mg with multiple doses of oral ketoconazole 400 mg (strong CYP3A4/P-gp inhibitor) resulted in a 1.7 fold increase in the $AUC_{(0-24)}$ and a 1.5 fold increase in the C_{max} of pazopanib compared to when pazopanib was administered alone. Concurrent administration of a single dose of pazopanib eye drops with ketoconazole in healthy volunteers resulted in a 2 fold and 1.5 fold increase in mean $AUC_{(0-t)}$ and C_{max} values, respectively *[see Dosage and Administration (2.2) and Drug Interactions (7.1)]*.

Administration of 1,500 mg lapatinib, a substrate and weak inhibitor of CYP3A4, Pgp, and BCRP, with 800 mg pazopanib resulted in an approximately 50% to 60% increase in mean pazopanib $AUC_{(0-24)}$ and C_{max} compared to administration of 800 mg pazopanib alone.

In vitro studies with human liver microsomes showed that pazopanib inhibited the activities of CYP enzymes 1A2, 3A4, 2B6, 2C8, 2C9, 2C19, 2D6, and 2E1. Potential induction of human CYP3A4 was demonstrated in an in vitro human PXR assay. Clinical pharmacology studies, using pazopanib 800 mg once daily, have demonstrated that pazopanib does not have a clinically relevant effect on the pharmacokinetics of caffeine (CYP1A2 probe substrate), warfarin (CYP2C9 probe substrate), or omeprazole (CYP2C19 probe substrate) in cancer patients. Pazopanib resulted in an increase of approximately 30% in the mean AUC and C_{max} of midazolam (CYP3A4 probe substrate) and increases of 33% to 64% in the ratio of dextromethorphan to dextrorphan concentrations in the urine after oral administration of dextromethorphan (CYP2D6 probe substrate). Coadministration of pazopanib 800 mg once daily and paclitaxel 80 mg/m^2 (CYP3A4 and CYP2C8 substrate) once weekly resulted in a mean increase of 26% and 31% in paclitaxel AUC and C_{max}, respectively *[see Drug Interactions (7.2)]*.

In vitro studies also showed that pazopanib inhibits UGT1A1 and OATP1B1 with IC50s of 1.2 and 0.79 µM, respectively. Pazopanib may increase concentrations of drugs eliminated by UGT1A1 and OATP1B1.

12.5 Pharmacogenomics

Pazopanib can increase serum total bilirubin levels *[see Warnings and Precautions (5.1)]*. In vitro studies showed that pazopanib inhibits UGT1A1, which glucuronidates bilirubin for elimination. A pooled pharmacogenetic analysis of 236 Caucasian patients evaluated the TA repeat polymorphism of UGT1A1 and its potential association with hyperbilirubinemia during pazopanib treatment. In this analysis, the (TA)7/(TA)7 genotype (UGT1A1*28/*28) (underlying genetic susceptibility to Gilbert's syndrome) was associated with a statistically significant increase in the incidence of hyperbilirubinemia relative to the (TA)6/(TA)6 and (TA)6/(TA)7 genotypes.

13 NONCLINICAL TOXICOLOGY

13.1 Carcinogenesis, Mutagenesis, Impairment of Fertility

Carcinogenicity studies with pazopanib have not been conducted. However, in a 13-week study in mice, proliferative lesions in the liver including eosinophilic foci in 2 females and a single case of adenoma in another female was observed at doses of 1,000 mg/kg/day (approximately 2.5 times the human clinical exposure based on AUC).

Pazopanib did not induce mutations in the microbial mutagenesis (Ames) assay and was not clastogenic in both the in vitro cytogenetic assay using primary human lymphocytes and in the in vivo rat micronucleus assay.

Pazopanib may impair fertility in humans. In female rats, reduced fertility including increased pre-implantation loss and early resorptions were noted at dosages ≥30 mg/kg/day (approximately 0.4 times the human clinical exposure based on AUC). Total litter resorption was seen at 300 mg/kg/day (approximately 0.8 times the human clinical exposure based on AUC). Post-implantation loss, embryolethality, and decreased fetal body weight were noted in females administered doses ≥10 mg/kg/day (approximately 0.3 times the human clinical exposure based on AUC). Decreased corpora lutea and increased cysts were noted in mice given ≥100 mg/kg/day for 13 weeks and ovarian atrophy was noted in rats given ≥300 mg/kg/day for 26 weeks (approximately 1.3 and 0.85 times the human clinical exposure based on AUC, respectively). Decreased corpora lutea was also noted in monkeys given 500 mg/kg/day for up to 34 weeks (approximately 0.4 times the human clinical exposure based on AUC).

Pazopanib did not affect mating or fertility in male rats. However, there were reductions in sperm production rates and testicular sperm concentrations at doses ≥3 mg/kg/day, epididymal sperm concentrations at doses ≥30 mg/kg/day, and sperm motility at ≥100 mg/kg/day following 15 weeks of dosing. Following 15 and 26 weeks of dosing, there were decreased testicular and epididymal weights at doses of ≥30 mg/kg/day (approximately 0.35 times the human clinical exposure based on AUC); atrophy and degeneration of the testes with aspermia, hypospermia and cribiform change in the epididymis was also observed at this dose in the 6-month toxicity studies in male rats.

14 CLINICAL STUDIES

14.1 Renal Cell Carcinoma

The safety and efficacy of VOTRIENT in renal cell carcinoma (RCC) were evaluated in a randomized, double-blind, placebo-controlled, multicenter, Phase 3 trial. Patients (N = 435) with locally advanced and/or metastatic RCC who had received either no prior therapy or one prior cytokine-based systemic therapy were randomized (2:1) to receive VOTRIENT 800 mg once daily or placebo once daily. The primary objective of the trial was to evaluate and compare the 2 treatment arms for progression-free survival (PFS); the secondary endpoints included overall survival (OS), overall response rate (RR), and duration of response.

Of the total of 435 patients enrolled in this trial, 233 patients had no prior systemic therapy (treatment-naïve subgroup) and 202 patients received one prior IL-2 or INFα-based therapy (cytokine-pretreated subgroup). The baseline demographic and disease characteristics were balanced between the VOTRIENT and placebo arms. The majority of patients were male (71%) with a median age of 59 years. Eighty-six percent of patients were Caucasian, 14% were Asian, and less than 1% were other. Forty-two percent were ECOG performance status 0 and 58% were ECOG performance status 1. All patients had clear cell histology (90%) or predominantly clear cell histology (10%). Approximately 50% of all patients had 3 or more organs involved with metastatic disease. The most common metastatic sites at baseline were lung (74%), lymph nodes (56%), bone (27%), and liver (25%).

A similar proportion of patients in each arm were treatment-naïve and cytokine-pretreated (see Table 5). In the cytokine-pretreated subgroup, the majority (75%) had received interferon-based treatment. Similar proportions of patients in each arm had prior nephrectomy (89% and 88% for VOTRIENT and placebo, respectively).

The analysis of the primary endpoint PFS was based on disease assessment by independent radiological review in the entire trial population. Efficacy results are presented in Table 5 and Figure 1.

[See table 5 above]

Figure 1. Kaplan-Meier Curve for Progression-Free Survival in RCC by Independent Assessment for the Overall Population (Treatment-Naïve and Cytokine Pre-Treated Populations)

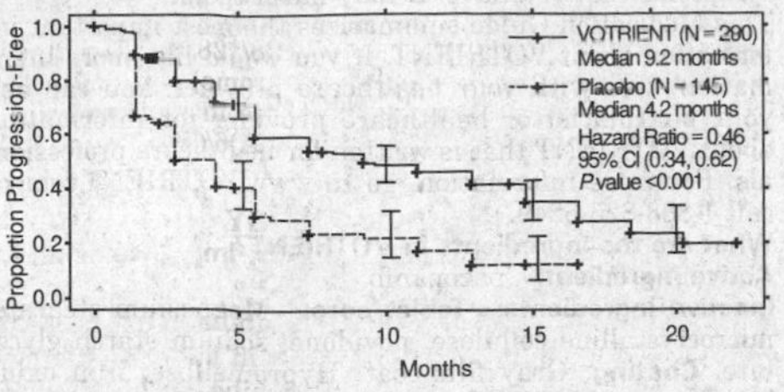

At the protocol-specified final analysis of OS, the median OS was 22.9 months for patients randomized to VOTRIENT and 20.5 months for the placebo arm [HR = 0.91 (95% CI: 0.71, 1.16)]. The median OS for the placebo arm includes 79 patients (54%) who discontinued placebo treatment because of disease progression and crossed over to treatment with VOTRIENT. In the placebo arm, 95 (66%) patients received at least one systemic anti-cancer treatment after progression compared to 88 (30%) patients randomized to VOTRIENT.

14.2 Soft Tissue Sarcoma

The safety and efficacy of VOTRIENT in patients with STS were evaluated in a randomized, double-blind, placebo-controlled, multicenter trial. Patients (N = 369) with metastatic STS who had received prior chemotherapy, including anthracycline treatment, or were unsuited for such therapy, were randomized (2:1) to receive VOTRIENT 800 mg once daily or placebo. Patients with gastrointestinal stromal tumors (GIST) or adipocytic sarcoma were excluded from the trial. Randomization was stratified by the factors of WHO performance status (WHO PS) 0 or 1 at baseline and the number of lines of prior systemic therapy for advanced disease (0 or 1 versus 2+). Progression-free survival (PFS) was assessed by independent radiological review. Other efficacy endpoints included overall survival (OS), overall response rate, and duration of response.

The majority of patients were female (59%) with a median age of 55 years. Seventy-two percent of patients were Caucasian, 22% were Asian, and 6% were Other. Forty-three percent of patients had leiomyosarcoma, 10% had synovial sarcoma, and 47% had other soft tissue sarcomas. Fifty-six percent of patients had received 2 or more lines of prior systemic therapy and 44% had received 0 or 1 lines of prior systemic therapy. The median duration of treatment was 4.5 months for patients on the pazopanib arm and 1.9 months for patients on the placebo arm.

Efficacy results are presented in Table 6 and Figure 2.

[See table 6 above]

Table 5. Efficacy Results in RCC Patients by Independent Assessment

Endpoint/Trial Population	VOTRIENT	Placebo	HR (95% CI)
PFS			
Overall ITT	N = 290	N = 145	
Median (months)	9.2	4.2	0.46[a] (0.34, 0.62)
Treatment-naïve subgroup	N = 155 (53%)	N = 78 (54%)	
Median (months)	11.1	2.8	0.40 (0.27, 0.60)
Cytokine pre-treated subgroup	N = 135 (47%)	N = 67 (46%)	
Median (months)	7.4	4.2	0.54 (0.35, 0.84)
Response Rate (CR + PR)	N = 290	N = 145	
% (95% CI)	30 (25.1, 35.6)	3 (0.5, 6.4)	–
Duration of response			
Median (weeks) (95% CI)	58.7 (52.1, 68.1)	–[b]	

HR = Hazard Ratio; ITT = Intent to Treat; PFS = Progression-free Survival; CR = Complete Response; PR = Partial Response

[a]P value <0.001

[b]There were only 5 objective responses.

Table 6. Efficacy Results in STS Patients by Independent Assessment

Endpoint/Trial Population	VOTRIENT	Placebo	HR (95% CI)
PFS			
Overall ITT	N = 246	N = 123	0.35[a]
Median (months)	4.6	1.6	(0.26, 0.48)
Leiomyosarcoma subgroup	N = 109	N = 49	0.37
Median (months)	4.6	1.9	(0.23, 0.60)
Synovial sarcoma subgroup	N = 25	N = 13	0.43
Median (months)	4.1	0.9	(0.19, 0.98)
'Other soft tissue sarcoma' subgroup	N = 112	N = 61	0.39
Median (months)	4.6	1.0	(0.25, 0.60)
Response Rate (CR + PR)			
% (95% CI)	4 (2.3, 7.9)[b]	0 (0.0, 3.0)	–
Duration of response			
Median (months) (95% CI)	9.0 (3.9, 9.2)		

HR = Hazard Ratio; ITT = Intent to Treat; PFS = Progression-free Survival; CR = Complete Response; PR = Partial Response

[a]P value <0.001

[b]There were 11 partial responses and 0 complete responses.

Figure 2. Kaplan-Meier Curve for Progression-Free Survival in STS by Independent Assessment for the Overall Population

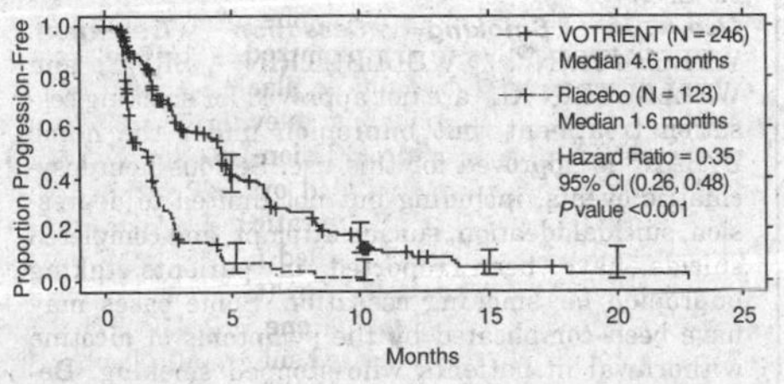

At the protocol-specified final analysis of OS, the median OS was 12.6 months for patients randomized to VOTRIENT and 10.7 months for the placebo arm [HR = 0.87 (95% CI: 0.67, 1.12)].

16 HOW SUPPLIED/STORAGE AND HANDLING

The 200 mg tablets of VOTRIENT are modified capsule-shaped, gray, film-coated with GS JT debossed on one side and are available in:

Bottles of 120 tablets: NDC NDC 0173-0804-09

Store at room temperature between 20°C and 25°C (68°F to 77°F); excursions permitted to 15°C to 30°C (59°F to 86°F) [See USP Controlled Room Temperature].

17 PATIENT COUNSELING INFORMATION

See Medication Guide. The Medication Guide is contained in a separate leaflet that accompanies the product. However, inform patients of the following:

- Therapy with VOTRIENT may result in hepatobiliary laboratory abnormalities. Monitor serum liver tests (ALT, AST, and bilirubin) prior to initiation of VOTRIENT and at Weeks 3, 5, 7, and 9. Thereafter, monitor at Month 3 and at Month 4, and as clinically indicated. Inform patients that they should report signs and symptoms of liver dysfunction to their healthcare provider right away.
- Prolonged QT intervals and torsades de pointes have been observed. Patients should be advised that ECG monitoring may be performed. Patients should be advised to inform their physicians of concomitant medications.
- Cardiac dysfunction (such as CHF and LVEF decrease) has been observed in patients at risk (e.g., prior anthracycline therapy) particularly in association with development or worsening of hypertension. Patients should be advised to report hypertension or signs and symptoms of congestive heart failure.
- Serious hemorrhagic events have been reported. Patients should be advised to report unusual bleeding.
- Arterial thrombotic events have been reported. Patients should be advised to report signs or symptoms of an arterial thrombosis.
- Reports of pneumothorax and venous thromboembolic events including pulmonary embolus have been reported. Patients should be advised to report if new onset of dyspnea, chest pain, or localized limb edema occurs.
- Advise patients to inform their doctor if they have worsening of neurological function consistent with RPLS (headache, seizure, lethargy, confusion, blindness, and other visual and neurologic disturbances).
- Hypertension and hypertensive crisis have been reported. Patients should be advised to monitor blood pressure early in the course of therapy and frequently thereafter and report increases of blood pressure or symptoms such as blurred vision, confusion, severe headache, or nausea and vomiting.
- GI perforation or fistula has occurred. Advise patients to report signs and symptoms of a GI perforation or fistula.
- VEGFR inhibitors such as VOTRIENT may impair wound healing. Advise patients to stop VOTRIENT at least 7 days prior to a scheduled surgery.
- Hypothyroidism and proteinuria have been reported. Advise patients that thyroid function testing and urinalysis will be performed during treatment.
- Serious infections including some with fatal outcomes have been reported. Advise patients to promptly report any signs or symptoms of infection.
- Women of childbearing potential should be advised of the potential hazard to the fetus and to avoid becoming pregnant.
- Gastrointestinal adverse reactions such as diarrhea, nausea, and vomiting have been reported with VOTRIENT. Patients should be advised how to manage diarrhea and to notify their healthcare provider if moderate to severe diarrhea occurs.
- Patients should be advised to inform their healthcare providers of all concomitant medications, vitamins, or dietary and herbal supplements.
- Patients should be advised that depigmentation of the hair or skin may occur during treatment with VOTRIENT.
- Patients should be advised to take VOTRIENT without food (at least 1 hour before or 2 hours after a meal).

VOTRIENT is a registered trademark of GlaxoSmithKline.

GlaxoSmithKline
Research Triangle Park, NC 27709

VTR:9PI

MEDICATION GUIDE
VOTRIENT® (VO-tree-ent)
(pazopanib)
tablets

Read the Medication Guide that comes with VOTRIENT before you start taking it and each time you get a refill. There may be new information. This Medication Guide does not take the place of talking with your healthcare provider about your medical condition or treatment.

What is the most important information I should know about VOTRIENT?

- **VOTRIENT can cause serious liver problems including death.** Your healthcare provider will do blood tests to check your liver before you start and while you take VOTRIENT.

Tell your healthcare provider right away if you get any of these signs of liver problems during treatment with VOTRIENT:

- yellowing of your skin or the whites of your eyes (jaundice)
- dark urine
- tiredness
- nausea or vomiting
- loss of appetite

- pain on the right side of your stomach area (abdomen)
- bruise easily

Your healthcare provider may need to prescribe a lower dose of VOTRIENT for you or tell you to stop taking VOTRIENT if you develop liver problems during treatment.

What is VOTRIENT?

VOTRIENT is a prescription medicine used to treat people with:

- advanced renal cell cancer (RCC)
- advanced soft tissue sarcoma (STS) who have received chemotherapy in the past

It is not known if VOTRIENT is effective in treating certain soft tissue sarcomas or certain gastrointestinal tumors.

It is not known if VOTRIENT is safe and effective in children under 18 years of age.

What should I tell my healthcare provider before taking VOTRIENT?

Before you take VOTRIENT, tell your healthcare provider if you:

- have or had liver problems. You may need a lower dose of VOTRIENT or your healthcare provider may prescribe a different medicine to treat your advanced renal cell cancer or advanced soft tissue sarcoma.
- have high blood pressure
- have heart problems or an irregular heartbeat including QT prolongation
- have a history of a stroke
- have headaches, seizures, or vision problems
- have coughed up blood in the last 6 months
- had bleeding of your stomach or intestines in the last 6 months
- have a history of a tear (perforation) in your stomach or intestine, or an abnormal connection between two parts of your gastrointestinal tract (fistula)
- have had blood clots in a vein or in the lung
- have thyroid problems
- had recent surgery (within the last 7 days) or are going to have surgery
- have any other medical conditions
- are pregnant or plan to become pregnant. VOTRIENT can harm your unborn baby. You should not become pregnant while you are taking VOTRIENT.
- are breastfeeding or plan to breastfeed. It is not known if VOTRIENT passes into your breast milk. You and your healthcare provider should decide if you will take VOTRIENT or breastfeed. You should not do both.

Tell your healthcare provider about all the medicines you take including prescription and non-prescription medicines, vitamins, and herbal supplements. VOTRIENT may affect the way other medicines work and other medicines may affect how VOTRIENT works.

Especially, tell your healthcare provider if you:

- take medicines that can affect how your liver enzymes work such as:
  - certain antibiotics (used to treat infections)
  - certain medicines used to treat HIV
  - certain medicines used to treat depression
  - medicines used to treat irregular heart beats
- take a medicine that contains simvastatin to treat high cholesterol levels
- drink grapefruit juice

Ask your healthcare provider if you are not sure if your medicine is one that is listed above.

Know the medicines you take. Keep a list of them and show it to your healthcare provider and pharmacist when you get a new medicine.

How should I take VOTRIENT?

- Take VOTRIENT exactly as your healthcare provider tells you. Your healthcare provider will tell you how much VOTRIENT to take.
- Your healthcare provider may change your dose.
- Take VOTRIENT on an empty stomach, at least 1 hour before or 2 hours after food.
- Do not crush VOTRIENT tablets.
- Do not eat grapefruit or drink grapefruit juice during treatment with VOTRIENT. Grapefruit products may increase the amount of VOTRIENT in your body.
- If you miss a dose, take it as soon as you remember. Do not take it if it is close (within 12 hours) to your next dose. Just take the next dose at your regular time. Do not take more than 1 dose of VOTRIENT at a time.
- Your healthcare provider will test your urine, blood, and heart before you start and while you take VOTRIENT.
- Tell your healthcare provider if you plan to have surgery while taking VOTRIENT. You will need to stop taking VOTRIENT at least 7 days before surgery because VOTRIENT may affect healing after surgery.

What are the possible side effects of VOTRIENT?

VOTRIENT may cause serious side effects including:

- See **"What is the most important information I should know about VOTRIENT?"**
- **irregular or fast heartbeat or fainting**
- **heart failure.** This is a condition where your heart does not pump as well as it should and may cause you to have shortness of breath.
- **heart attack or stroke.** Heart attack and stroke can happen with VOTRIENT and may cause death.
  Symptoms may include: chest pain or pressure, pain in your arms, back, neck or jaw, shortness of breath, numbness or weakness on one side of your body, trouble talking, headache, or dizziness.
- **blood clots.** Blood clots may form in a vein, especially in your legs (deep vein thrombosis or DVT). Pieces of a blood clot may travel to your lungs (pulmonary embolism). This may be life-threatening and cause death.
  Symptoms may include: new chest pain, trouble breathing or shortness of breath that starts suddenly, leg pain, and swelling of the arms and hands, or legs and feet, a cool or pale arm or leg.
- **bleeding problems.** These bleeding problems may be severe and cause death.
  Symptoms may include: unusual bleeding, bruising, or wounds that do not heal.
- **tear in your stomach or intestinal wall (perforation) or an abnormal connection between two parts of your gastrointestinal tract (fistula).**
  Symptoms may include: pain, swelling in your stomach-area, vomiting blood, and black sticky stools.
- **Reversible Posterior Leukoencephalopathy (RPLS).** RPLS is a condition that can happen while taking VOTRIENT that may cause death.
  Symptoms may include: headaches, seizures, lack of energy, confusion, high blood pressure, blindness or changes in vision, and problems thinking.
- **high blood pressure. High blood pressure can happen with VOTRIENT, including a sudden and severe rise in blood pressure which may be life-threatening.** These blood pressure increases usually happen in the first several months of treatment. Your blood pressure should be well controlled before you start taking VOTRIENT. Your healthcare provider should begin checking your blood pressure within 1 week of you starting VOTRIENT and often during treatment to make sure that your blood pressure is well controlled.
  Have someone call your healthcare provider or get medical help right away for you, if you get symptoms of a severe increase in blood pressure, including: severe chest pain, severe headache, blurred vision, confusion, nausea and vomiting, severe anxiety, shortness of breath, seizures, or you pass out (become unconscious).
- **thyroid problems.** Your healthcare provider should check you for this during treatment with VOTRIENT.
- **protein in your urine.** Your healthcare provider will check you for this problem. If there is too much protein in your urine, your healthcare provider may tell you to stop taking VOTRIENT.
- **serious infections. Serious infections can happen with VOTRIENT and can cause death.**
  Symptoms of an infection may include: fever, cold symptoms, such as runny nose or sore throat that do not go away, flu symptoms, such as cough, tiredness, and body aches, pain when urinating, cuts, scrapes or wounds that are red, warm, swollen or painful.
- **collapsed lung (pneumothorax).** A collapsed lung can happen with VOTRIENT. Air may get trapped in the space between your lung and chest wall. This may cause you to have shortness of breath.

Call your healthcare provider right away, if you have any of the symptoms listed above.

The most common side effects in people who take VOTRIENT include:

- diarrhea
- change in hair color
- nausea or vomiting
- loss of appetite

Other common side effects in people with advanced soft tissue sarcoma who take VOTRIENT include:

- feeling tired
- decreased weight
- tumor pain
- muscle or bone pain
- headache
- taste changes
- trouble breathing
- change in skin color

Tell your healthcare provider if you have any side effect that bothers you or that does not go away.

These are not all the possible side effects of VOTRIENT. For more information, ask your healthcare provider or pharmacist.

Call your doctor for medical advice about side effects. You may report side effects to FDA at 1-800-FDA-1088.

How should I store VOTRIENT tablets?

Store VOTRIENT at room temperature between 68°F and 77°F (20°C to 25°C).

Keep VOTRIENT and all medicines out of the reach of children.

General information about the safe and effective use of VOTRIENT.

Medicines are sometimes prescribed for purposes other than those listed in a Medication Guide. Do not use VOTRIENT for a condition for which it was not prescribed. Do not give VOTRIENT to other people even if they have the same symptoms that you have. It may harm them.

This Medication Guide summarizes the most important information about VOTRIENT. If you would like more information, talk with your healthcare provider. You can ask your pharmacist or healthcare provider for information about VOTRIENT that is written for healthcare professionals. For more information, go to www.VOTRIENT.com or call 1-888-825-5249.

What are the ingredients in VOTRIENT?

Active ingredient: pazopanib.

Inactive ingredients: Tablet core: Magnesium stearate, microcrystalline cellulose, povidone, sodium starch glycolate. **Coating:** Gray film-coat: Hypromellose, iron oxide black, macrogol/polyethylene glycol 400 (PEG 400), polysorbate 80, titanium dioxide.

This Medication Guide has been approved by the U.S. Food and Drug Administration.

GlaxoSmithKline
Research Triangle Park, NC 27709
Revised: April 2012

VTR:6MG

WELLBUTRIN® ℞
(bupropion hydrochloride)
Tablets

WARNING

Suicidality and Antidepressant Drugs

Use in Treating Psychiatric Disorders: Antidepressants increased the risk compared to placebo of suicidal thinking and behavior (suicidality) in children, adolescents, and young adults in short-term studies of major depressive disorder (MDD) and other psychiatric disorders. Anyone considering the use of WELLBUTRIN or any other antidepressant in a child, adolescent, or young adult must balance this risk with the clinical need. Short-term studies did not show an increase in the risk of suicidality with antidepressants compared to placebo in adults beyond age 24; there was a reduction in risk with antidepressants compared to placebo in adults aged 65 and older. Depression and certain other psychiatric disorders are themselves associated with increases in the risk of suicide. Patients of all ages who are started on antidepressant therapy should be monitored appropriately and observed closely for clinical worsening, suicidality, or unusual changes in behavior. Families and caregivers should be advised of the need for close observation and communication with the prescriber. WELLBUTRIN is not approved for use in pediatric patients. (See WARNINGS: Clinical Worsening and Suicide Risk in Treating Psychiatric Disorders, PRECAUTIONS: Information for Patients, and PRECAUTIONS: Pediatric Use.)

Use in Smoking Cessation Treatment: WELLBUTRIN®, WELLBUTRIN SR®, and WELLBUTRIN XL® are not approved for smoking cessation treatment, but bupropion under the name ZYBAN® is approved for this use. Serious neuropsychiatric events, including but not limited to depression, suicidal ideation, suicide attempt, and completed suicide have been reported in patients taking bupropion for smoking cessation. Some cases may have been complicated by the symptoms of nicotine withdrawal in patients who stopped smoking. Depressed mood may be a symptom of nicotine withdrawal. Depression, rarely including suicidal ideation, has been reported in smokers undergoing a smoking cessation attempt without medication. However, some of these symptoms have occurred in patients taking bupropion who continued to smoke.

All patients being treated with bupropion for smoking cessation treatment should be observed for neuropsychiatric symptoms including changes in behavior, hostility, agitation, depressed mood, and suicide-related events, including ideation, behavior, and attempted suicide. These symptoms, as well as worsening of pre-existing psychiatric illness and completed suicide have been reported in some patients attempting to quit smoking while taking ZYBAN in the postmarketing experience. When symptoms were reported, most were during treatment with ZYBAN, but some were following discontinuation of treatment with ZYBAN. These events have occurred in patients with and without pre-existing psychiatric disease; some have experienced worsening of their psychiatric illnesses. Patients with serious psychiatric illness such as schizophrenia, bipolar disorder, and major depressive disorder did not participate in the premarketing studies of ZYBAN.

Advise patients and caregivers that the patient using bupropion for smoking cessation should stop taking bupropion and contact a healthcare provider immediately if agitation, hostility, depressed mood, or changes in thinking or behavior that are not typical for the patient are observed, or if the patient develops suicidal ideation or suicidal behavior. In many postmarketing cases, resolution of symptoms after discontinuation of ZYBAN was reported, although in some cases the symptoms persisted; therefore, ongoing monitoring and supportive care should be provided until symptoms resolve.

The risks of using bupropion for smoking cessation should be weighed against the benefits of its use. ZYBAN has been demonstrated to increase the likelihood of abstinence from smoking for as long as 6 months compared to treatment with placebo. The health benefits of quitting smoking are immediate and substantial. (See WARNINGS: Neuropsychiatric Symptoms and Suicide Risk in Smoking Cessation Treatment and PRECAUTIONS: Information for Patients.)

DESCRIPTION

WELLBUTRIN (bupropion hydrochloride), an antidepressant of the aminoketone class, is chemically unrelated to tricyclic, tetracyclic, selective serotonin re-uptake inhibitor, or other known antidepressant agents. Its structure closely resembles that of diethylpropion; it is related to phenylethylamines. It is designated as (±)-1-(3-chlorophenyl)-2-[(1,1 dimethylethyl)amino]-1-propanone hydrochloride. The molecular weight is 276.2. The empirical formula is $C_{13}H_{18}ClNO \cdot HCl$. Bupropion hydrochloride powder is white, crystalline, and highly soluble in water. It has a bitter taste and produces the sensation of local anesthesia on the oral mucosa. The structural formula is:

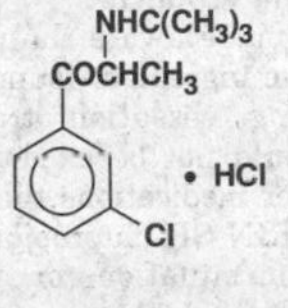

WELLBUTRIN is supplied for oral administration as 75-mg (yellow-gold) and 100-mg (red) film-coated tablets. Each tablet contains the labeled amount of bupropion hydrochloride and the inactive ingredients: 75-mg tablet – D&C Yellow No. 10 Lake, FD&C Yellow No. 6 Lake, hydroxypropyl cellulose, hypromellose, microcrystalline cellulose, polyethylene glycol, talc, and titanium dioxide; 100-mg tablet – FD&C Red No. 40 Lake, FD&C Yellow No. 6 Lake, hydroxypropyl cellulose, hypromellose, microcrystalline cellulose, polyethylene glycol, talc, and titanium dioxide.

CLINICAL PHARMACOLOGY

Pharmacodynamics

The neurochemical mechanism of the antidepressant effect of bupropion is not known. Bupropion is a relatively weak inhibitor of the neuronal uptake of norepinephrine and dopamine, and does not inhibit monoamine oxidase or the re-uptake of serotonin.

Bupropion produces dose-related central nervous system (CNS) stimulant effects in animals, as evidenced by increased locomotor activity, increased rates of responding in various schedule-controlled operant behavior tasks, and, at high doses, induction of mild stereotyped behavior.

Bupropion causes convulsions in rodents and dogs at doses approximately tenfold the dose recommended as the human antidepressant dose.

Pharmacokinetics

Bupropion is a racemic mixture. The pharmacological activity and pharmacokinetics of the individual enantiomers have not been studied. In humans, following oral administration of WELLBUTRIN, peak plasma bupropion concentrations are usually achieved within 2 hours, followed by a biphasic decline. The terminal phase has a mean half-life of 14 hours, with a range of 8 to 24 hours. The distribution phase has a mean half-life of 3 to 4 hours. The mean elimination half-life (±SD) of bupropion after chronic dosing is 21 (±9) hours, and steady-state plasma concentrations of bupropion are reached within 8 days. Plasma bupropion concentrations are dose-proportional following single doses of 100 to 250 mg; however, it is not known if the proportionality between dose and plasma level is maintained in chronic use.

Absorption: The absolute bioavailability of WELLBUTRIN in humans has not been determined because an intravenous formulation for human use is not available. However, it appears likely that only a small proportion of any orally administered dose reaches the systemic circulation intact.

Distribution: In vitro tests show that bupropion is 84% bound to human plasma protein at concentrations up to 200 mcg/mL. The extent of protein binding of the hydroxybupropion metabolite is similar to that for bupropion, whereas the extent of protein binding of the threohydrobupropion metabolite is about half that seen with bupropion.

Metabolism: Bupropion is extensively metabolized in humans. Three metabolites have been shown to be active: hydroxybupropion, which is formed via hydroxylation of the *tert*-butyl group of bupropion, and the amino-alcohol isomers threohydrobupropion and erythrohydrobupropion, which are formed via reduction of the carbonyl group. In vitro findings suggest that cytochrome P450IIB6 (CYP2B6) is the principal isoenzyme involved in the formation of hydroxybupropion, while cytochrome P450 isoenzymes are not involved in the formation of threohydrobupropion. Oxidation of the bupropion side chain results in the formation of a glycine conjugate of meta-chlorobenzoic acid, which is then excreted as the major urinary metabolite. The potency and toxicity of the metabolites relative to bupropion have not been fully characterized. However, it has been demonstrated in an antidepressant screening test in mice that hydroxybupropion is one-half as potent as bupropion, while threohydrobupropion and erythrohydrobupropion are 5-fold less potent than bupropion. This may be of clinical importance because their plasma concentrations are as high as or higher than those of bupropion.

Because bupropion is extensively metabolized, there is the potential for drug-drug interactions, particularly with those agents that are metabolized by or which inhibit/induce the cytochrome P450IIB6 (CYP2B6) isoenzyme, such as ritonavir or efavirenz. In a healthy volunteer study, ritonavir at a dose of 100 mg twice daily reduced the AUC and C_{max} of bupropion by 22% and 21%, respectively. The exposure of the hydroxybupropion metabolite was decreased by 23%, the threohydrobupropion decreased by 38%, and the erythrohydrobupropion decreased by 48%.

In a second healthy volunteer study, ritonavir at a dose of 600 mg twice daily decreased the AUC and the C_{max} of bupropion by 66% and 62%, respectively. The exposure of the hydroxybupropion metabolite was decreased by 78%, the threohydrobupropion decreased by 50%, and the erythrohydrobupropion decreased by 68%.

In another healthy volunteer study, KALETRA® (lopinavir 400 mg/ritonavir 100 mg twice daily) decreased bupropion AUC and C_{max} by 57%. The AUC and C_{max} of hydroxybupropion were decreased by 50% and 31%, respectively (see PRECAUTIONS: Drug Interactions).

In a study in healthy volunteers, efavirenz 600 mg once daily for 2 weeks reduced the AUC and C_{max} of bupropion by approximately 55% and 34%, respectively. The AUC of hydroxybupropion was unchanged, whereas C_{max} of hydroxybupropion was increased by 50%.

Although bupropion is not metabolized by cytochrome P450IID6 (CYP2D6), there is the potential for drug-drug interactions when bupropion is coadministered with drugs metabolized by this isoenzyme (see PRECAUTIONS: Drug Interactions).

Following a single dose in humans, peak plasma concentrations of hydroxybupropion occur approximately 3 hours after administration of WELLBUTRIN. Peak plasma concentrations of hydroxybupropion are approximately 10 times the peak level of the parent drug at steady state. The elimination half-life of hydroxybupropion is approximately 20 (±5) hours and its AUC at steady state is about 17 times that of bupropion. The times to peak concentrations for the erythrohydrobupropion and threohydrobupropion metabolites are similar to that of the hydroxybupropion metabolite. However, their elimination half-lives are longer, 33 (±10) and 37 (±13) hours, respectively, and steady-state AUCs are 1.5 and 7 times that of bupropion, respectively.

Bupropion and its metabolites exhibit linear kinetics following chronic administration of 300 to 450 mg/day.

Elimination: Following oral administration of 200 mg of ^{14}C-bupropion in humans, 87% and 10% of the radioactive dose were recovered in the urine and feces, respectively. However, the fraction of the oral dose of WELLBUTRIN excreted unchanged was only 0.5%, a finding consistent with the extensive metabolism of bupropion.

Populations Subgroups: Factors or conditions altering metabolic capacity (e.g., liver disease, congestive heart failure [CHF], age, concomitant medications, etc.) or elimination may be expected to influence the degree and extent of accumulation of the active metabolites of bupropion. The elimination of the major metabolites of bupropion may be affected by reduced renal or hepatic function because they are moderately polar compounds and are likely to undergo further metabolism or conjugation in the liver prior to urinary excretion.

Hepatic: The effect of hepatic impairment on the pharmacokinetics of bupropion was characterized in 2 single-dose studies, one in patients with alcoholic liver disease and one in patients with mild-to-severe cirrhosis. The first study showed that the half-life of hydroxybupropion was significantly longer in 8 patients with alcoholic liver disease than in 8 healthy volunteers (32 ± 14 hours versus 21 ± 5 hours, respectively). Although not statistically significant, the AUCs for bupropion and hydroxybupropion were more variable and tended to be greater (by 53% to 57%) in volunteers with alcoholic liver disease. The differences in half-life for bupropion and the other metabolites in the 2 patient groups were minimal.

The second study showed that there were no statistically significant differences in the pharmacokinetics of bupropion and its active metabolites in 9 patients with mild-to-moderate hepatic cirrhosis compared to 8 healthy volunteers. However, more variability was observed in some of the pharmacokinetic parameters for bupropion (AUC, C_{max}, and T_{max}) and its active metabolites ($t_{½}$) in patients with mild-to-moderate hepatic cirrhosis. In addition, in patients with severe hepatic cirrhosis, the bupropion C_{max} and AUC were substantially increased (mean difference: by approximately 70% and 3-fold, respectively) and more variable when compared to values in healthy volunteers; the mean bupropion half-life was also longer (29 hours in patients with severe hepatic cirrhosis vs. 19 hours in healthy subjects). For the metabolite hydroxybupropion, the mean C_{max} was approximately 69% lower. For the combined amino-alcohol isomers threohydrobupropion and erythrohydrobupropion, the mean C_{max} was approximately 31% lower. The mean AUC increased by about 1½-fold for hydroxybupropion and about 2½-fold for threo/erythrohydrobupropion. The median T_{max} was observed 19 hours later for hydroxybupropion and 31 hours later for threo/erythrohydrobupropion. The mean half-lives for hydroxybupropion and threo/erythrohydrobupropion were increased 5- and 2-fold, respectively, in patients with severe hepatic cirrhosis compared to healthy volunteers (see WARNINGS, PRECAUTIONS, and DOSAGE AND ADMINISTRATION).

Renal: There is limited information on the pharmacokinetics of bupropion in patients with renal impairment. An inter-study comparison between normal subjects and patients with end-stage renal failure demonstrated that the parent drug C_{max} and AUC values were comparable in the 2 groups, whereas the hydroxybupropion and threohydrobupropion metabolites had a 2.3– and 2.8–fold increase, respectively, in AUC for patients with end-stage renal failure. A second study, comparing normal subjects and patients with moderate-to-severe renal impairment (GFR 30.9 ± 10.8 mL/min) showed that exposure to a single 150-mg dose of sustained-release bupropion was approximately 2-fold higher in patients with impaired renal function while levels of the hydroxybupropion and threo/erythrohydrobupropion (combined) metabolites were similar in the 2 groups. The elimination of bupropion and/or the major metabolites of bupropion may be reduced by impaired renal function (see PRECAUTIONS: Renal Impairment).

Left Ventricular Dysfunction: During a chronic dosing study in 14 depressed patients with left ventricular dysfunction (history of CHF or an enlarged heart on x-ray), no apparent effect on the pharmacokinetics of bupropion or its metabolites was revealed, compared to healthy volunteers.

Age: The effects of age on the pharmacokinetics of bupropion and its metabolites have not been fully characterized, but an exploration of steady-state bupropion concentrations from several depression efficacy studies involving patients dosed in a range of 300 to 750 mg/day, on a 3 times daily schedule, revealed no relationship between age (18 to 83 years) and plasma concentration of bupropion. A single-dose pharmacokinetic study demonstrated that the disposition of bupropion and its metabolites in elderly subjects was similar to that of younger subjects. These data suggest there is no prominent effect of age on bupropion concentration; however, another pharmacokinetic study, single and multiple dose, has suggested that the elderly are at increased risk for accumulation of bupropion and its metabolites (see PRECAUTIONS: Geriatric Use).

Gender: A single-dose study involving 12 healthy male and 12 healthy female volunteers revealed no sex-related differences in the pharmacokinetic parameters of bupropion.

Smokers: The effects of cigarette smoking on the pharmacokinetics of bupropion were studied in 34 healthy male and female volunteers; 17 were chronic cigarette smokers and 17 were nonsmokers. Following oral administration of a single 150-mg dose of bupropion, there were no statistically significant differences in C_{max}, half-life, T_{max}, AUC or clearance of bupropion or its active metabolites between smokers and nonsmokers.

INDICATIONS AND USAGE

WELLBUTRIN is indicated for the treatment of major depressive disorder. A physician considering WELLBUTRIN for the management of a patient's first episode of depression should be aware that the drug may cause generalized seizures in a dose-dependent manner with an approximate incidence of 0.4% (4/1,000). This incidence of seizures may exceed that of other marketed antidepressants by as much as 4-fold. This relative risk is only an approximate estimate because no direct comparative studies have been conducted (see WARNINGS).

The efficacy of WELLBUTRIN has been established in 3 placebo-controlled trials, including 2 of approximately 3 weeks' duration in depressed inpatients and one of approximately 6 weeks' duration in depressed outpatients. The depressive disorder of the patients studied corresponds most closely to the Major Depression category of the APA Diagnostic and Statistical Manual III.

Major Depression implies a prominent and relatively persistent depressed or dysphoric mood that usually interferes with daily functioning (nearly every day for at least 2 weeks); it should include at least 4 of the following 8 symptoms: change in appetite, change in sleep, psychomotor agitation or retardation, loss of interest in usual activities or decrease in sexual drive, increased fatigability, feelings of guilt or worthlessness, slowed thinking or impaired concentration, and suicidal ideation or attempts.

Effectiveness of WELLBUTRIN in long-term use, that is, for more than 6 weeks, has not been systematically evaluated in controlled trials. Therefore, the physician who elects to use WELLBUTRIN for extended periods should periodically reevaluate the long-term usefulness of the drug for the individual patient.

CONTRAINDICATIONS

WELLBUTRIN is contraindicated in patients with a seizure disorder.

WELLBUTRIN is contraindicated in patients treated with ZYBAN® (bupropion hydrochloride) Sustained-Release Tablets; WELLBUTRIN SR® (bupropion hydrochloride), the sustained-release formulation; WELLBUTRIN XL® (bupropion hydrochloride), the extended-release formulation; or any other medications that contain bupropion because the incidence of seizure is dose dependent.

WELLBUTRIN is contraindicated in patients with a current or prior diagnosis of bulimia or anorexia nervosa because of a higher incidence of seizures noted in such patients treated with WELLBUTRIN.

WELLBUTRIN is contraindicated in patients undergoing abrupt discontinuation of alcohol or sedatives (including benzodiazepines).

The use of monoamine oxidase inhibitors or MAOIs (intended to treat psychiatric disorders) concomitantly with WELLBUTRIN or within 14 days of stopping treatment with WELLBUTRIN is contraindicated. There is an increased risk of hypertensive reactions when bupropion is used concomitantly with other drugs that inhibit the reuptake of dopamine or norepinephrine or inhibit their metabolism (e.g., MAOIs). The use of WELLBUTRIN within 14 days of stopping treatment with an MAOI is also contraindicated. Starting WELLBUTRIN in a patient treated with reversible MAOIs such as linezolid or intravenous methylene blue is contraindicated (see DOSAGE AND ADMINISTRATION and DRUG INTERACTIONS).

WELLBUTRIN is contraindicated in patients who have shown an allergic response to bupropion or the other ingredients that make up WELLBUTRIN.

WARNINGS

Clinical Worsening and Suicide Risk in Treating Psychiatric Disorders

Patients with major depressive disorder (MDD), both adult and pediatric, may experience worsening of their depression and/or the emergence of suicidal ideation and behavior (suicidality) or unusual changes in behavior, whether or not they are taking antidepressant medications, and this risk may persist until significant remission occurs. Suicide is a known risk of depression and certain other psychiatric disorders, and these disorders themselves are the strongest predictors of suicide. There has been a long-standing concern, however, that antidepressants may have a role in inducing worsening of depression and the emergence of suicidality in certain patients during the early phases of treatment. Pooled analyses of short-term placebo-controlled trials of antidepressant drugs (SSRIs and others) showed that these drugs increase the risk of suicidal thinking and behavior (suicidality) in children, adolescents, and young adults (ages 18-24) with major depressive disorder (MDD) and other psychiatric disorders. Short-term studies did not show an increase in the risk of suicidality with antidepressants compared to placebo in adults beyond age 24; there was a reduction with antidepressants compared to placebo in adults aged 65 and older.

The pooled analyses of placebo-controlled trials in children and adolescents with MDD, obsessive compulsive disorder (OCD), or other psychiatric disorders included a total of 24 short-term trials of 9 antidepressant drugs in over 4,400 patients. The pooled analyses of placebo-controlled trials in adults with MDD or other psychiatric disorders included a total of 295 short-term trials (median duration of 2 months) of 11 antidepressant drugs in over 77,000 patients. There was considerable variation in risk of suicidality among drugs, but a tendency toward an increase in the younger patients for almost all drugs studied. There were differences in absolute risk of suicidality across the different indications, with the highest incidence in MDD. The risk differences (drug vs. placebo), however, were relatively stable within age strata and across indications. These risk differences (drug-placebo difference in the number of cases of suicidality per 1,000 patients treated) are provided in Table 1.

Table 1

Age Range	Drug-Placebo Difference in Number of Cases of Suicidality per 1,000 Patients Treated
Increases Compared to Placebo	
<18	14 additional cases
18-24	5 additional cases
Decreases Compared to Placebo	
25-64	1 fewer case
≥65	6 fewer cases

No suicides occurred in any of the pediatric trials. There were suicides in the adult trials, but the number was not sufficient to reach any conclusion about drug effect on suicide.

It is unknown whether the suicidality risk extends to longer-term use, i.e., beyond several months. However, there is substantial evidence from placebo-controlled maintenance trials in adults with depression that the use of antidepressants can delay the recurrence of depression.

All patients being treated with antidepressants for any indication should be monitored appropriately and observed closely for clinical worsening, suicidality, and unusual changes in behavior, especially during the initial few months of a course of drug therapy, or at times of dose changes, either increases or decreases.

The following symptoms, anxiety, agitation, panic attacks, insomnia, irritability, hostility, aggressiveness, impulsivity, akathisia (psychomotor restlessness), hypomania, and mania, have been reported in adult and pediatric patients being treated with antidepressants for major depressive disorder as well as for other indications, both psychiatric and nonpsychiatric. Although a causal link between the emergence of such symptoms and either the worsening of depression and/or the emergence of suicidal impulses has not been established, there is concern that such symptoms may represent precursors to emerging suicidality.

Consideration should be given to changing the therapeutic regimen, including possibly discontinuing the medication, in patients whose depression is persistently worse, or who are experiencing emergent suicidality or symptoms that might be precursors to worsening depression or suicidality, especially if these symptoms are severe, abrupt in onset, or were not part of the patient's presenting symptoms.

Families and caregivers of patients being treated with antidepressants for major depressive disorder or other indications, both psychiatric and nonpsychiatric, should be alerted about the need to monitor patients for the emergence of agitation, irritability, unusual changes in behavior, and the other symptoms described above, as well as the emergence of suicidality, and to report such symptoms immediately to healthcare providers. Such monitoring should include daily observation by families and caregivers. Prescriptions for WELLBUTRIN should be written for the smallest quantity of tablets consistent with good patient management, in order to reduce the risk of overdose.

Neuropsychiatric Symptoms and Suicide Risk in Smoking Cessation Treatment: WELLBUTRIN, WELLBUTRIN SR, and WELLBUTRIN XL are not approved for smoking cessation treatment, but bupropion under the name ZYBAN is approved for this use. Serious neuropsychiatric symptoms have been reported in patients taking bupropion for smoking cessation **(see BOXED WARNING, ADVERSE REACTIONS). These have included changes in mood (including depression and mania), psychosis, hallucinations, paranoia, delusions, homicidal ideation, hostility, agitation, aggression, anxiety, and panic, as well as suicidal ideation, suicide attempt, and completed suicide.** Some reported cases may have been complicated by the symptoms of nicotine withdrawal in patients who stopped smoking. Depressed mood may be a symptom of nicotine withdrawal. Depression, rarely including suicidal ideation, has been reported in smokers undergoing a smoking cessation attempt without medication. However, some of these symptoms have occurred in patients taking bupropion who continued to smoke. When symptoms were reported, most were during bupropion treatment, but some were following discontinuation of bupropion therapy.

These events have occurred in patients with and without pre-existing psychiatric disease; some have experienced worsening of their psychiatric illnesses. All patients being treated with bupropion as part of smoking cessation treatment should be observed for neuropsychiatric symptoms or worsening of pre-existing psychiatric illness.

Patients with serious psychiatric illness such as schizophrenia, bipolar disorder, and major depressive disorder did not participate in the pre-marketing studies of ZYBAN.

Advise patients and caregivers that the patient using bupropion for smoking cessation should stop taking bupropion and contact a healthcare provider immediately if agitation, depressed mood, or changes in behavior or thinking that are not typical for the patient are observed, or if the patient develops suicidal ideation or suicidal behavior. In many postmarketing cases, resolution of symptoms after discontinuation of ZYBAN was reported, although in some cases the symptoms persisted, therefore, ongoing monitoring and supportive care should be provided until symptoms resolve.

The risks of using bupropion for smoking cessation should be weighed against the benefits of its use. ZYBAN has been demonstrated to increase the likelihood of abstinence from smoking for as long as six months compared to treatment with placebo. The health benefits of quitting smoking are immediate and substantial.

Screening Patients for Bipolar Disorder

A major depressive episode may be the initial presentation of bipolar disorder. It is generally believed (though not established in controlled trials) that treating such an episode with an antidepressant alone may increase the likelihood of precipitation of a mixed/manic episode in patients at risk for bipolar disorder. Whether any of the symptoms described above represent such a conversion is unknown. However, prior to initiating treatment with an antidepressant, patients with depressive symptoms should be adequately screened to determine if they are at risk for bipolar disorder; such screening should include a detailed psychiatric history, including a family history of suicide, bipolar disorder, and depression. It should be noted that WELLBUTRIN is not approved for use in treating bipolar depression.

Bupropion-Containing Products

Patients should be made aware that WELLBUTRIN contains the same active ingredient found in ZYBAN, used as an aid to smoking cessation treatment, and that WELLBUTRIN should not be used in combination with ZYBAN, or any other medications that contain bupropion, such as WELLBUTRIN SR (bupropion hydrochloride), the sustained-release formulation or WELLBUTRIN XL (bupropion hydrochloride), the extended-release formulation.

Seizures

Bupropion is associated with seizures in approximately 0.4% (4/1,000) of patients treated at doses up to 450 mg/day. This incidence of seizures may exceed that of other marketed antidepressants by as much as 4-fold. This relative risk is only an approximate estimate because no direct comparative studies have been conducted. The estimated seizure incidence for WELLBUTRIN increases almost tenfold between 450 and 600 mg/day, which is twice the usually required daily dose (300 mg) and one and one-third the maximum recommended daily dose (450 mg). Given the wide variability among individuals and their capacity to metabolize and eliminate drugs this disproportionate increase in seizure incidence with dose incrementation calls for caution in dosing.

During the initial development, 25 among approximately 2,400 patients treated with WELLBUTRIN experienced seizures. At the time of seizure, 7 patients were receiving daily doses of 450 mg or below for an incidence of 0.33% (3/1,000) within the recommended dose range. Twelve patients experienced seizures at 600 mg/day (2.3% incidence); 6 additional patients had seizures at daily doses between 600 and 900 mg (2.8% incidence).

A separate, prospective study was conducted to determine the incidence of seizure during an 8-week treatment exposure in approximately 3,200 additional patients who received daily doses of up to 450 mg. Patients were permitted to continue treatment beyond 8 weeks if clinically indicated. Eight seizures occurred during the initial 8-week treatment period and 5 seizures were reported in patients continuing treatment beyond 8 weeks, resulting in a total seizure incidence of 0.4%.

The risk of seizure appears to be strongly associated with dose. Sudden and large increments in dose may contribute to increased risk. While many seizures occurred early in the course of treatment, some seizures did occur after several weeks at fixed dose. WELLBUTRIN should be discontinued and not restarted in patients who experience a seizure while on treatment.

The risk of seizure is also related to patient factors, clinical situations, and concomitant medications, which must be considered in selection of patients for therapy with WELLBUTRIN.

• Patient factors: Predisposing factors that may increase the risk of seizure with bupropion use include history of head trauma or prior seizure, central nervous system (CNS) tumor, the presence of severe hepatic cirrhosis, and concomitant medications that lower seizure threshold.
• Clinical situations: Circumstances associated with an increased seizure risk include, among others, excessive use of alcohol or sedatives (including benzodiazepines); addiction to opiates, cocaine, or stimulants; use of over-the-counter stimulants and anorectics; and diabetes treated with oral hypoglycemics or insulin.
• Concomitant medications: Many medications (e.g., antipsychotics, antidepressants, theophylline, systemic steroids) are known to lower seizure threshold.

Recommendations for Reducing the Risk of Seizure: **Retrospective analysis of clinical experience gained during the development of WELLBUTRIN suggests that the risk of seizure may be minimized if**
• the total daily dose of WELLBUTRIN does *not* exceed 450 mg,
• the daily dose is administered 3 times daily, with each single dose *not* to exceed 150 mg to avoid high peak concentrations of bupropion and/or its metabolites, and
• the rate of incrementation of dose is very gradual.

WELLBUTRIN should be administered with extreme caution to patients with a history of seizure, cranial trauma, or other predisposition(s) toward seizure, or patients treated with other agents (e.g., antipsychotics, other antidepressants, theophylline, systemic steroids, etc.) that lower seizure threshold.

Hepatic Impairment

WELLBUTRIN should be used with extreme caution in patients with severe hepatic cirrhosis. In these patients a reduced dose and/or frequency is required, as peak bupropion, as well as AUC, levels are substantially increased and accumulation is likely to occur in such patients to a greater extent than usual. The dose should not exceed 75 mg once a day in these patients (see CLINICAL PHARMACOLOGY, PRECAUTIONS, and DOSAGE AND ADMINISTRATION).

Potential for Hepatotoxicity

In rats receiving large doses of bupropion chronically, there was an increase in incidence of hepatic hyperplastic nodules and hepatocellular hypertrophy. In dogs receiving large doses of bupropion chronically, various histologic changes were seen in the liver, and laboratory tests suggesting mild hepatocellular injury were noted.

PRECAUTIONS

General: ***Agitation and Insomnia:*** A substantial proportion of patients treated with WELLBUTRIN experience some degree of increased restlessness, agitation, anxiety, and insomnia, especially shortly after initiation of treatment. In clinical studies, these symptoms were sometimes of sufficient magnitude to require treatment with sedative/hypnotic drugs. In approximately 2% of patients, symptoms were sufficiently severe to require discontinuation of treatment with WELLBUTRIN.

Psychosis, Confusion, and Other Neuropsychiatric Phenomena: Depressed patients treated with WELLBUTRIN have been reported to show a variety of neuropsychiatric signs and symptoms including delusions, hallucinations, psychosis, concentration disturbance, paranoia, and confusion. Because of the uncontrolled nature of many studies, it is impossible to provide a precise estimate of the extent of risk imposed by treatment with WELLBUTRIN. In several cases, neuropsychiatric phenomena abated upon dose reduction and/or withdrawal of treatment.

Activation of Psychosis and/or Mania: Antidepressants can precipitate manic episodes in bipolar disorder patients during the depressed phase of their illness and may activate latent psychosis in other susceptible patients. WELLBUTRIN is expected to pose similar risks.

Altered Appetite and Weight: A weight loss of greater than 5 lbs occurred in 28% of patients receiving WELLBUTRIN. This incidence is approximately double that seen in comparable patients treated with tricyclics or placebo. Furthermore, while 35% of patients receiving tricyclic antidepressants gained weight, only 9.4% of patients treated with WELLBUTRIN did. Consequently, if weight loss is a major presenting sign of a patient's depressive illness, the anorectic and/or weight reducing potential of WELLBUTRIN should be considered.

Allergic Reactions: Anaphylactoid/anaphylactic reactions characterized by symptoms such as pruritus, urticaria, angioedema, and dyspnea requiring medical treatment have been reported in clinical trials with bupropion. In addition, there have been rare spontaneous postmarketing reports of erythema multiforme, Stevens-Johnson syndrome, and anaphylactic shock associated with bupropion. A patient should stop taking WELLBUTRIN and consult a doctor if experiencing allergic or anaphylactoid/anaphylactic reactions (e.g., skin rash, pruritus, hives, chest pain, edema, and shortness of breath) during treatment.

Arthralgia, myalgia, and fever with rash and other symptoms suggestive of delayed hypersensitivity have been reported in association with bupropion. These symptoms may resemble serum sickness.

Cardiovascular Effects: In clinical practice, hypertension, in some cases severe, requiring acute treatment, has been reported in patients receiving bupropion alone and in combination with nicotine replacement therapy. These events have been observed in both patients with and without evidence of preexisting hypertension.

Data from a comparative study of the sustained-release formulation of bupropion (ZYBAN® Sustained-Release Tablets), nicotine transdermal system (NTS), the combination of sustained-release bupropion plus NTS, and placebo as an aid to smoking cessation suggest a higher incidence of treatment-emergent hypertension in patients treated with the combination of sustained-release bupropion and NTS. In this study, 6.1% of patients treated with the combination of sustained-release bupropion and NTS had treatment-emergent hypertension compared to 2.5%, 1.6%, and 3.1% of patients treated with sustained-release bupropion, NTS, and placebo, respectively. The majority of these patients had evidence of preexisting hypertension. Three patients (1.2%) treated with the combination of ZYBAN and NTS and 1 patient (0.4%) treated with NTS had study medication discontinued due to hypertension compared to none of the patients treated with ZYBAN or placebo. Monitoring of blood pressure is recommended in patients who receive the combination of bupropion and nicotine replacement.

There is no clinical experience establishing the safety of WELLBUTRIN in patients with a recent history of myocardial infarction or unstable heart disease. Therefore, care should be exercised if it is used in these groups. Bupropion was well tolerated in depressed patients who had previously developed orthostatic hypotension while receiving tricyclic antidepressants and was also generally well tolerated in a group of 36 depressed inpatients with stable congestive heart failure (CHF). However, bupropion was associated with a rise in supine blood pressure in the study of patients with CHF, resulting in discontinuation of treatment in 2 patients for exacerbation of baseline hypertension.

Hepatic Impairment: WELLBUTRIN should be used with extreme caution in patients with severe hepatic cirrhosis. In these patients, a reduced dose and frequency is required. WELLBUTRIN should be used with caution in patients with hepatic impairment (including mild-to-moderate hepatic cirrhosis) and a reduced frequency and/or dose should be considered in patients with mild-to-moderate hepatic cirrhosis.

All patients with hepatic impairment should be closely monitored for possible adverse effects that could indicate high drug and metabolite levels (see CLINICAL PHARMACOLOGY, WARNINGS, and DOSAGE AND ADMINISTRATION).

Renal Impairment: There is limited information on the pharmacokinetics of bupropion in patients with renal impairment. An inter-study comparison between normal subjects and patients with end-stage renal failure demonstrated that the parent drug C_{max} and AUC values were comparable in the 2 groups, whereas the hydroxybupropion and threohydrobupropion metabolites had a 2.3– and 2.8–fold increase, respectively, in AUC for patients with end-stage renal failure. A second study, comparing normal subjects and patients with moderate-to-severe renal impairment (GFR 30.9 ± 10.8 mL/min) showed that exposure to a single 150-mg dose of sustained-release bupropion was approximately 2-fold higher in patients with impaired renal function while levels of the hydroxybupropion and threo/erythrohydrobupropion (combined) metabolites were similar in the 2 groups. Bupropion is extensively metabolized in the liver to active metabolites, which are further metabolized and subsequently excreted by the kidneys. WELLBUTRIN should be used with caution in patients with renal impairment and a reduced frequency and/or dose should be considered as bupropion and the metabolites of bupropion may accumulate in such patients to a greater extent than usual. The patient should be closely monitored for possible adverse effects that could indicate high drug or metabolite levels.

Information for Patients

Prescribers or other health professionals should inform patients, their families, and their caregivers about the benefits and risks associated with treatment with WELLBUTRIN and should counsel them in its appropriate use. A patient Medication Guide about "Antidepressant Medicines, Depression and Other Serious Mental Illnesses, and Suicidal Thoughts or Actions," "Quitting Smoking, Quit-Smoking Medication, Changes in Thinking and Behavior, Depression, and Suicidal Thoughts or Actions,"and "What Other Important Information Should I Know About WELLBUTRIN?" is available for WELLBUTRIN. The prescriber or health professional should instruct patients, their families, and their caregivers to read the Medication Guide and should assist them in understanding its contents. Patients should be given the opportunity to discuss the contents of the Medication Guide and to obtain answers to any questions they may have. The complete text of the Medication Guide is reprinted at the end of this document.

Patients should be advised of the following issues and asked to alert their prescriber if these occur while taking WELLBUTRIN.

Clinical Worsening and Suicide Risk in Treating Psychiatric Disorders: Patients, their families, and their caregivers should be encouraged to be alert to the emergence of anxiety, agitation, panic attacks, insomnia, irritability, hostility, aggressiveness, impulsivity, akathisia (psychomotor restlessness), hypomania, mania, other unusual changes in behavior, worsening of depression, and suicidal ideation, especially early during antidepressant treatment and when the dose is adjusted up or down. Families and caregivers of patients should be advised to look for the emergence of such symptoms on a day-to-day basis, since changes may be abrupt. Such symptoms should be reported to the patient's prescriber or health professional, especially if they are severe, abrupt in onset, or were not part of the patient's presenting symptoms. Symptoms such as these may be associated with an increased risk for suicidal thinking and behavior and indicate a need for very close monitoring and possibly changes in the medication.

Neuropsychiatric Symptoms and Suicide Risk in Smoking Cessation Treatment: Although WELLBUTRIN is not indicated for smoking cessation treatment, it contains the same active ingredient as ZYBAN which is approved for this use. Patients should be informed that quitting smoking, with or without ZYBAN, may be associated with nicotine withdrawal symptoms (including depression or agitation), or exacerbation of pre-existing psychiatric illness. Furthermore, some patients have experienced changes in mood (including depression and mania), psychosis, hallucinations, paranoia, delusions, homicidal ideation aggression, anxiety, and panic, as well as suicidal ideation, suicide attempt, and completed suicide when attempting to quit smoking while taking ZYBAN. If patients develop agitation, hostility, depressed mood, or changes in thinking or behavior that are not typical for them, or if patients develop suicidal ideation or behavior, they should be urged to report these symptoms to their healthcare provider immediately.

Bupropion-Containing Products: Patients should be made aware that WELLBUTRIN contains the same active ingredient found in ZYBAN, used as an aid to smoking cessation, and that WELLBUTRIN should not be used in combination with ZYBAN or any other medications that contain bupropion hydrochloride (such as WELLBUTRIN SR, the sustained-release formulation and WELLBUTRIN XL, the extended-release formulation).

Patients should be instructed to take WELLBUTRIN in equally divided doses 3 or 4 times a day to minimize the risk of seizure.

Patients should be told that WELLBUTRIN should be discontinued and not restarted if they experience a seizure while on treatment.

Patients should be told that any CNS-active drug like WELLBUTRIN may impair their ability to perform tasks requiring judgment or motor and cognitive skills. Consequently, until they are reasonably certain that WELLBUTRIN does not adversely affect their performance, they should refrain from driving an automobile or operating complex, hazardous machinery.

Patients should be told that the excessive use or abrupt discontinuation of alcohol or sedatives (including benzodiazepines) may alter the seizure threshold. Some patients have reported lower alcohol tolerance during treatment with WELLBUTRIN. Patients should be advised that the consumption of alcohol should be minimized or avoided.

Patients should be advised to inform their physicians if they are taking or plan to take any prescription or over-the-counter drugs. Concern is warranted because WELLBUTRIN and other drugs may affect each other's metabolism.

Patients should be advised to notify their physicians if they become pregnant or intend to become pregnant during therapy.

Laboratory Tests

There are no specific laboratory tests recommended.

Drug Interactions

Because bupropion is extensively metabolized, the coadministration of other drugs may affect its clinical activity. In vitro studies indicate that bupropion is primarily metabolized to hydroxybupropion by the CYP2B6 isoenzyme. Therefore, the potential exists for a drug interaction between WELLBUTRIN and drugs that are substrates of or inhibitors/inducers of the CYP2B6 isoenzyme (e.g., orphenadrine, thiotepa, cyclophosphamide, ticlopidine, and clopidogrel). In addition, in vitro studies suggest that paroxetine, sertraline, norfluoxetine, and fluvoxamine as well as nelfinavir inhibit the hydroxylation of bupropion. No clinical studies have been performed to evaluate this finding. The threohydrobupropion metabolite of bupropion does not appear to be produced by the cytochrome P450 isoenzymes. The effects of concomitant administration of cimetidine on the pharmacokinetics of bupropion and its active metabolites were studied in 24 healthy young male volunteers. Following oral administration of two 150-mg sustained-release tablets with and without 800 mg of cimetidine, the pharmacokinetics of bupropion and hydroxybupropion were unaffected. However, there were 16% and 32% increases in the AUC and C_{max}, respectively, of the combined moieties of threohydrobupropion and erythrohydrobupropion.

In a series of studies in healthy volunteers, ritonavir (100 mg twice daily or 600 mg twice daily) or ritonavir 100 mg plus lopinavir 400 mg (KALETRA) twice daily reduced the exposure of bupropion and its major metabolites in a dose dependent manner by approximately 20% to 80%. Similarly, efavirenz 600 mg once daily for 2 weeks reduced the exposure of bupropion by approximately 55%. This effect of ritonavir, KALETRA, and efavirenz is thought to be due to the induction of bupropion metabolism. Patients receiving any of these drugs with bupropion may need increased doses of bupropion, but the maximum recommended dose of bupropion should not be exceeded (see CLINICAL PHARMACOLOGY: Metabolism).

While not systematically studied, certain drugs may induce the metabolism of bupropion (e.g., carbamazepine, phenobarbital, phenytoin).

Multiple oral doses of bupropion had no statistically significant effects on the single dose pharmacokinetics of lamotrigine in 12 healthy volunteers.

Animal data indicated that bupropion may be an inducer of drug-metabolizing enzymes in humans. In one study, following chronic administration of bupropion, 100 mg 3 times daily to 8 healthy male volunteers for 14 days, there was no evidence of induction of its own metabolism. Nevertheless, there may be the potential for clinically important alterations of blood levels of coadministered drugs.

Drugs Metabolized by Cytochrome P450IID6 (CYP2D6): Many drugs, including most antidepressants (SSRIs, many tricyclics), beta-blockers, antiarrhythmics, and antipsychotics are metabolized by the CYP2D6 isoenzyme. Although bupropion is not metabolized by this isoenzyme, bupropion and hydroxybupropion are inhibitors of the CYP2D6 isoenzyme in vitro. In a study of 15 male subjects (ages 19 to 35 years) who were extensive metabolizers of the CYP2D6 isoenzyme, daily doses of bupropion given as 150 mg twice daily followed by a single dose of 50 mg desipramine increased the C_{max}, AUC, and $t_{1/2}$ of desipramine by an average of approximately 2-, 5- and 2-fold, respectively. The effect was present for at least 7 days after the last dose of bupropion. Concomitant use of bupropion with other drugs metabolized by CYP2D6 has not been formally studied.

Therefore, coadministration of bupropion with drugs that are metabolized by CYP2D6 isoenzyme including certain antidepressants (e.g., nortriptyline, imipramine, desipramine, paroxetine, fluoxetine, sertraline), antipsychotics (e.g., haloperidol, risperidone, thioridazine), beta-blockers (e.g., metoprolol), and Type 1C antiarrhythmics (e.g., propafenone, flecainide), should be approached with caution and should be initiated at the lower end of the dose range of the concomitant medication. If bupropion is added to the treatment regimen of a patient already receiving a drug metabolized by CYP2D6, the need to decrease the dose of the original medication should be considered, particularly for those concomitant medications with a narrow therapeutic index.

Drugs which require metabolic activation by CYP2D6 in order to be effective (e.g., tamoxifen) theoretically could have reduced efficacy when administered concomitantly with inhibitors of CYP2D6 such as bupropion.

Although citalopram is not primarily metabolized by CYP2D6, in one study bupropion increased the C_{max} and AUC of citalopram by 30% and 40%, respectively. Citalopram did not affect the pharmacokinetics of bupropion and its 3 metabolites.

MAO Inhibitors: Concomitant use of MAOIs and bupropion is contraindicated. Bupropion inhibits the reuptake of dopamine and norepinephrine and can increase risk of hypertensive reactions when used concomitantly with drugs that also inhibit the reuptake of dopamine or norepinephrine, including MAOIs. In addition, MAOIs decrease the metabolism of dopamine and norepinephrine. These effects can increase dopaminergic and noradrenergic activity. Studies in animals demonstrate that the acute toxicity of bupropion is enhanced by the MAO inhibitor phenelzine (see CONTRAINDICATIONS and DOSAGE AND ADMINISTRATION).

Levodopa and Amantadine: Limited clinical data suggest a higher incidence of adverse experiences in patients receiving bupropion concurrently with either levodopa or amantadine. Administration of WELLBUTRIN to patients receiving either levodopa or amantadine concurrently should be undertaken with caution, using small initial doses and small gradual dose increases.

Drugs that Lower Seizure Threshold: Concurrent administration of WELLBUTRIN and agents (e.g., antipsychotics, other antidepressants, theophylline, systemic steroids, etc.) that lower seizure threshold should be undertaken only with extreme caution (see WARNINGS). Low initial dosing and small gradual dose increases should be employed.

Nicotine Transdermal System: (see PRECAUTIONS: Cardiovascular Effects).

Alcohol: In postmarketing experience, there have been rare reports of adverse neuropsychiatric events or reduced alcohol tolerance in patients who were drinking alcohol during treatment with WELLBUTRIN. The consumption of alcohol during treatment with WELLBUTRIN should be minimized or avoided (also see CONTRAINDICATIONS).

Drug-Laboratory Test Interactions: False-positive urine immunoassay screening tests for amphetamines have been reported in patients taking bupropion. This is due to lack of specificity of some screening tests. False-positive test results may result even following discontinuation of bupropion therapy. Confirmatory tests, such as gas chromatography/mass spectrometry, will distinguish bupropion from amphetamines.

Carcinogenesis, Mutagenesis, Impairment of Fertility

Lifetime carcinogenicity studies were performed in rats and mice at doses up to 300 and 150 mg/kg/day, respectively. In the rat study there was an increase in nodular proliferative lesions of the liver at doses of 100 to 300 mg/kg/day; lower doses were not tested. The question of whether or not such lesions may be precursors of neoplasms of the liver is currently unresolved. Similar liver lesions were not seen in the mouse study, and no increase in malignant tumors of the liver and other organs was seen in either study.

Bupropion produced a borderline positive response (2 to 3 times control mutation rate) in some strains in the Ames bacterial mutagenicity test, and a high oral dose (300 mg/kg, but not 100 or 200 mg/kg) produced a low incidence of chromosomal aberrations in rats. The relevance of these results in estimating the risk of human exposure to therapeutic doses is unknown.

A fertility study was performed in rats; no evidence of impairment of fertility was encountered at oral doses up to 300 mg/kg/day.

Pregnancy

Teratogenic Effects: Pregnancy Category C. In studies conducted in rats and rabbits, bupropion was administered orally at doses up to 450 and 150 mg/kg/day, respectively (approximately 11 and 7 times the MRHD, respectively, on a mg/m^2 basis), during the period of organogenesis. No clear evidence of teratogenic activity was found in either species; however, in rabbits, slightly increased incidences of fetal malformations and skeletal variations were observed at the lowest dose tested (25 mg/kg/day, approximately equal to the MRHD on a mg/m^2 basis) and greater. Decreased fetal weights were seen at 50 mg/kg and greater.

When rats were administered bupropion at oral doses of up to 300 mg/kg/day (approximately 7 times the MRHD on a mg/m^2 basis) prior to mating and throughout pregnancy and lactation, there were no apparent adverse effects on offspring development.

One study has been conducted in pregnant women. This retrospective, managed-care database study assessed the risk of congenital malformations overall and cardiovascular malformations specifically, following exposure to bupropion in the first trimester compared to the risk of these malformations following exposure to other antidepressants in the first trimester and bupropion outside of the first trimester. This study included 7,005 infants with antidepressant exposure during pregnancy, 1,213 of whom were exposed to bupropion in the first trimester. The study showed no greater risk for congenital malformations overall or cardiovascular malformations specifically, following first trimester bupropion exposure compared to exposure to all other antidepressants in the first trimester, or bupropion outside of the first trimester. The results of this study have not been corroborated. WELLBUTRIN should be used during pregnancy only if the potential benefit justifies the potential risk to the fetus.

Labor and Delivery

The effect of WELLBUTRIN on labor and delivery in humans is unknown.

Nursing Mothers

Like many other drugs, bupropion and its metabolites are secreted in human milk. Because of the potential for serious adverse reactions in nursing infants from WELLBUTRIN, a decision should be made whether to discontinue nursing or to discontinue the drug, taking into account the importance of the drug to the mother.

Pediatric Use

Safety and effectiveness in the pediatric population have not been established (see BOX WARNING and WARNINGS: Clinical Worsening and Suicide Risk in Treating Psychiatric Disorders). Anyone considering the use of WELLBUTRIN in a child or adolescent must balance the potential risks with the clinical need.

Geriatric Use

Of the approximately 6,000 patients who participated in clinical trials with bupropion sustained-release tablets (depression and smoking cessation studies), 275 were 65 and over and 47 were 75 and over. In addition, several hundred patients 65 and over participated in clinical trials using the immediate-release formulation of bupropion (depression studies). No overall differences in safety or effectiveness were observed between these subjects and younger subjects, and other reported clinical experience has not identified differences in responses between the elderly and younger patients, but greater sensitivity of some older individuals cannot be ruled out.

A single-dose pharmacokinetic study demonstrated that the disposition of bupropion and its metabolites in elderly subjects was similar to that of younger subjects; however, another pharmacokinetic study, single and multiple dose, has suggested that the elderly are at increased risk for accumulation of bupropion and its metabolites (see CLINICAL PHARMACOLOGY).

Bupropion is extensively metabolized in the liver to active metabolites, which are further metabolized and excreted by the kidneys. The risk of toxic reaction to this drug may be greater in patients with impaired renal function. Because elderly patients are more likely to have decreased renal function, care should be taken in dose selection, and it may be useful to monitor renal function (see PRECAUTIONS: Renal Impairment and DOSAGE AND ADMINISTRATION).

ADVERSE REACTIONS

(See also WARNINGS and PRECAUTIONS.)

Adverse events commonly encountered in patients treated with WELLBUTRIN are agitation, dry mouth, insomnia, headache/migraine, nausea/vomiting, constipation, and tremor.

Adverse events were sufficiently troublesome to cause discontinuation of treatment with WELLBUTRIN in approximately 10% of the 2,400 patients and volunteers who participated in clinical trials during the product's initial development. The more common events causing discontinuation include neuropsychiatric disturbances (3.0%), primarily agitation and abnormalities in mental status; gastrointestinal disturbances (2.1%), primarily nausea and vomiting; neurological disturbances (1.7%), primarily seizures, headaches, and sleep disturbances; and dermatologic problems (1.4%), primarily rashes. It is important to note, however, that many of these events occurred at doses that exceed the recommended daily dose.

Accurate estimates of the incidence of adverse events associated with the use of any drug are difficult to obtain. Estimates are influenced by drug dose, detection technique, setting, physician judgments, etc. Consequently, Table 2 is presented solely to indicate the relative frequency of adverse events reported in representative controlled clinical studies conducted to evaluate the safety and efficacy of WELLBUTRIN under relatively similar conditions of daily dosage (300 to 600 mg), setting, and duration (3 to 4 weeks). The figures cited cannot be used to predict precisely the incidence of untoward events in the course of usual medical practice where patient characteristics and other factors must differ from those which prevailed in the clinical trials. These incidence figures also cannot be compared with those obtained from other clinical studies involving related drug products as each group of drug trials is conducted under a different set of conditions.

Finally, it is important to emphasize that the tabulation does not reflect the relative severity and/or clinical importance of the events. A better perspective on the serious adverse events associated with the use of WELLBUTRIN is provided in WARNINGS and PRECAUTIONS.

Table 2. Treatment-Emergent Adverse Experience Incidence in Placebo-Controlled Clinical Trials[a] (Percent of Patients Reporting)

Adverse Experience	WELLBUTRIN Patients (n = 323)	Placebo Patients (n = 185)
Cardiovascular		
Cardiac arrhythmias	5.3	4.3
Dizziness	22.3	16.2
Hypertension	4.3	1.6
Hypotension	2.5	2.2
Palpitations	3.7	2.2
Syncope	1.2	0.5
Tachycardia	10.8	8.6
Dermatologic		
Pruritus	2.2	0.0
Rash	8.0	6.5

Gastrointestinal		
Anorexia	18.3	18.4
Appetite increase	3.7	2.2
Constipation	26.0	17.3
Diarrhea	6.8	8.6
Dyspepsia	3.1	2.2
Nausea/vomiting	22.9	18.9
Weight gain	13.6	22.7
Weight loss	23.2	23.2
Genitourinary		
Impotence	3.4	3.1
Menstrual complaints	4.7	1.1
Urinary frequency	2.5	2.2
Urinary retention	1.9	2.2
Musculoskeletal		
Arthritis	3.1	2.7
Neurological		
Akathisia	1.5	1.1
Akinesia/bradykinesia	8.0	8.6
Cutaneous temperature disturbance	1.9	1.6
Dry mouth	27.6	18.4
Excessive sweating	22.3	14.6
Headache/migraine	25.7	22.2
Impaired sleep quality	4.0	1.6
Increased salivary flow	3.4	3.8
Insomnia	18.6	15.7
Muscle spasms	1.9	3.2
Pseudoparkinsonism	1.5	1.6
Sedation	19.8	19.5
Sensory disturbance	4.0	3.2
Tremor	21.1	7.6
Neuropsychiatric		
Agitation	31.9	22.2
Anxiety	3.1	1.1
Confusion	8.4	4.9
Decreased libido	3.1	1.6
Delusions	1.2	1.1
Disturbed concentration	3.1	3.8
Euphoria	1.2	0.5
Hostility	5.6	3.8
Nonspecific		
Fatigue	5.0	8.6
Fever/chills	1.2	0.5
Respiratory		
Upper respiratory complaints	5.0	11.4
Special Senses		
Auditory disturbance	5.3	3.2
Blurred vision	14.6	10.3
Gustatory disturbance	3.1	1.1

[a]Events reported by at least 1% of patients receiving WELLBUTRIN are included.

Other Events Observed During the Development of WELLBUTRIN

The conditions and duration of exposure to WELLBUTRIN varied greatly, and a substantial proportion of the experience was gained in open and uncontrolled clinical settings. During this experience, numerous adverse events were reported; however, without appropriate controls, it is impossible to determine with certainty which events were or were not caused by WELLBUTRIN. The following enumeration is organized by organ system and describes events in terms of their relative frequency of reporting in the data base. Events of major clinical importance are also described in WARNINGS and PRECAUTIONS.

The following definitions of frequency are used: Frequent adverse events are defined as those occurring in at least 1/100 patients. Infrequent adverse events are those occurring in 1/100 to 1/1,000 patients, while rare events are those occurring in less than 1/1,000 patients.

Cardiovascular: Frequent was edema; infrequent were chest pain, electrocardiogram (ECG) abnormalities (premature beats and nonspecific ST-T changes), and shortness of breath/dyspnea; rare were flushing, pallor, phlebitis, and myocardial infarction.

Dermatologic: Frequent were nonspecific rashes; infrequent were alopecia and dry skin; rare were change in hair color, hirsutism, and acne.

Endocrine: Infrequent was gynecomastia; rare were glycosuria and hormone level change.

Gastrointestinal: Infrequent were dysphagia, thirst disturbance, and liver damage/jaundice; rare were rectal complaints, colitis, gastrointestinal bleeding, intestinal perforation, and stomach ulcer.

Genitourinary: Frequent was nocturia; infrequent were vaginal irritation, testicular swelling, urinary tract infection, painful erection, and retarded ejaculation; rare were dysuria, enuresis, urinary incontinence, menopause, ovarian disorder, pelvic infection, cystitis, dyspareunia, and painful ejaculation.

Hematologic/Oncologic: Rare were lymphadenopathy, anemia, and pancytopenia.

Musculoskeletal: Rare was musculoskeletal chest pain.

Neurological: (see WARNINGS) Frequent were ataxia/incoordination, seizure, myoclonus, dyskinesia, and dystonia; infrequent were mydriasis, vertigo, and dysarthria; rare were electroencephalogram (EEG) abnormality, abnormal neurological exam, impaired attention, sciatica, and aphasia.

Neuropsychiatric: (see PRECAUTIONS) Frequent were mania/hypomania, increased libido, hallucinations, decrease in sexual function, and depression; infrequent were memory impairment, depersonalization, psychosis, dysphoria, mood instability, paranoia, formal thought disorder, and frigidity; rare was suicidal ideation.

Oral Complaints: Frequent was stomatitis; infrequent were toothache, bruxism, gum irritation, and oral edema; rare was glossitis.

Respiratory: Infrequent were bronchitis and shortness of breath/dyspnea; rare were epistaxis, rate or rhythm disorder, pneumonia, and pulmonary embolism.

Special Senses: Infrequent was visual disturbance; rare was diplopia.

Nonspecific: Frequent were flu-like symptoms; infrequent was nonspecific pain; rare were body odor, surgically related pain, infection, medication reaction, and overdose.

Postintroduction Reports

Voluntary reports of adverse events temporally associated with bupropion that have been received since market introduction and which may have no causal relationship with the drug include the following:

Body (General): arthralgia, myalgia, and fever with rash and other symptoms suggestive of delayed hypersensitivity. These symptoms may resemble serum sickness (see PRECAUTIONS).

Cardiovascular: hypertension (in some cases severe, see PRECAUTIONS), orthostatic hypotension, third degree heart block

Endocrine: syndrome of inappropriate antidiuretic hormone secretion, hyperglycemia, hypoglycemia

Gastrointestinal: esophagitis, hepatitis, liver damage

Hemic and Lymphatic: ecchymosis, leukocytosis, leukopenia, thrombocytopenia. Altered PT and/or INR, infrequently associated with hemorrhagic or thrombotic complications, were observed when bupropion was coadministered with warfarin.

Musculoskeletal: arthralgia, myalgia, muscle rigidity/fever/rhabdomyolysis, muscle weakness

Nervous: aggression, coma, completed suicide, delirium, dream abnormalities, paranoid ideation, paresthesia, restlessness, suicide attempt, unmasking of tardive dyskinesia

Skin and Appendages: Stevens-Johnson syndrome, angioedema, exfoliative dermatitis, urticaria

Special Senses: tinnitus, increased intraocular pressure

DRUG ABUSE AND DEPENDENCE

Humans

Controlled clinical studies conducted in normal volunteers, in subjects with a history of multiple drug abuse, and in depressed patients showed some increase in motor activity and agitation/excitement.

In a population of individuals experienced with drugs of abuse, a single dose of 400 mg of WELLBUTRIN produced mild amphetamine-like activity as compared to placebo on the Morphine-Benzedrine Subscale of the Addiction Research Center Inventories (ARCI) and a score intermediate between placebo and amphetamine on the Liking Scale of the ARCI. These scales measure general feelings of euphoria and drug desirability.

Findings in clinical trials, however, are not known to predict the abuse potential of drugs reliably. Nonetheless, evidence from single-dose studies does suggest that the recommended daily dosage of bupropion when administered in divided doses is not likely to be especially reinforcing to amphetamine or stimulant abusers. However, higher doses that could not be tested because of the risk of seizure might be modestly attractive to those who abuse stimulant drugs.

Animals

Studies in rodents have shown that bupropion exhibits some pharmacologic actions common to psychostimulants including increases in locomotor activity and the production of a mild stereotyped behavior and increases in rates of responding in several schedule-controlled behavior paradigms. Drug discrimination studies in rats showed stimulus generalization between bupropion and amphetamine and other psychostimulants. Rhesus monkeys have been shown to self-administer bupropion intravenously.

OVERDOSAGE

Human Overdose Experience

Overdoses of up to 30 g or more of bupropion have been reported. Seizure was reported in approximately one-third of all cases. Other serious reactions reported with overdoses of bupropion alone included hallucinations, loss of consciousness, sinus tachycardia, and ECG changes such as conduction disturbances (including QRS prolongation) or arrhythmias. Fever, muscle rigidity, rhabdomyolysis, hypotension, stupor, coma, and respiratory failure have been reported mainly when bupropion was part of multiple drug overdoses.

Although most patients recovered without sequelae, deaths associated with overdoses of bupropion alone have been reported in patients ingesting large doses of the drug. Multiple uncontrolled seizures, bradycardia, cardiac failure, and cardiac arrest prior to death were reported in these patients.

Overdosage Management

Ensure an adequate airway, oxygenation, and ventilation. Monitor cardiac rhythm and vital signs. EEG monitoring is also recommended for the first 48 hours post-ingestion. General supportive and symptomatic measures are also recommended. Induction of emesis is not recommended.

Activated charcoal should be administered. There is no experience with the use of forced diuresis, dialysis, hemoperfusion, or exchange transfusion in the management of bupropion overdoses. No specific antidotes for bupropion are known.

Due to the dose-related risk of seizures with WELLBUTRIN, hospitalization following suspected overdose should be considered. Based on studies in animals, it is recommended that seizures be treated with intravenous benzodiazepine administration and other supportive measures, as appropriate.

In managing overdosage, consider the possibility of multiple drug involvement. The physician should consider contacting a poison control center for additional information on the treatment of any overdose. Telephone numbers for certified poison control centers are listed in the *Physicians' Desk Reference* (PDR).

DOSAGE AND ADMINISTRATION

General Dosing Considerations

It is particularly important to administer WELLBUTRIN in a manner most likely to minimize the risk of seizure (see WARNINGS). Increases in dose should not exceed 100 mg/day in a 3-day period. Gradual escalation in dosage is also important if agitation, motor restlessness, and insomnia, often seen during the initial days of treatment, are to be minimized. If necessary, these effects may be managed by temporary reduction of dose or the short-term administration of an intermediate to long-acting sedative hypnotic. A sedative hypnotic usually is not required beyond the first week of treatment. Insomnia may also be minimized by avoiding bedtime doses. If distressing, untoward effects supervene, dose escalation should be stopped.

No single dose of WELLBUTRIN should exceed 150 mg. WELLBUTRIN should be administered 3 times daily, preferably with at least 6 hours between successive doses.

Usual Dosage for Adults

The usual adult dose is 300 mg/day, given 3 times daily. Dosing should begin at 200 mg/day, given as 100 mg twice daily. Based on clinical response, this dose may be increased to 300 mg/day, given as 100 mg 3 times daily, no sooner than 3 days after beginning therapy (see Table 3).

[See table 3 above]

Table 3. Dosing Regimen

Treatment Day	Total Daily Dose	Tablet Strength	Number of Tablets		
			Morning	Midday	Evening
1	200 mg	100 mg	1	0	1
4	300 mg	100 mg	1	1	1

Increasing the Dosage Above 300 mg/Day

As with other antidepressants, the full antidepressant effect of WELLBUTRIN may not be evident until 4 weeks of treatment or longer. An increase in dosage, up to a maximum of 450 mg/day, given in divided doses of not more than 150 mg each, may be considered for patients in whom no clinical improvement is noted after several weeks of treatment at 300 mg/day. Dosing above 300 mg/day may be accomplished using the 75- or 100-mg tablets. The 100-mg tablet must be administered 4 times daily with at least 4 hours between successive doses, in order not to exceed the limit of 150 mg in a single dose. WELLBUTRIN should be discontinued in patients who do not demonstrate an adequate response after an appropriate period of treatment at 450 mg/day.

Maintenance Treatment

The lowest dose that maintains remission is recommended. Although it is not known how long the patient should remain on WELLBUTRIN, it is generally recognized that acute episodes of depression require several months or longer of antidepressant drug treatment.

Dosage Adjustment for Patients With Impaired Hepatic Function

WELLBUTRIN should be used with extreme caution in patients with severe hepatic cirrhosis. The dose should not exceed 75 mg once a day in these patients. WELLBUTRIN should be used with caution in patients with hepatic impairment (including mild-to-moderate hepatic cirrhosis) and a reduced frequency and/or dose should be considered in patients with mild-to-moderate hepatic cirrhosis (see CLINICAL PHARMACOLOGY, WARNINGS, and PRECAUTIONS).

Dosage Adjustment for Patients With Impaired Renal Function

WELLBUTRIN should be used with caution in patients with renal impairment and a reduced frequency and/or dose should be considered (see CLINICAL PHARMACOLOGY and PRECAUTIONS).

Switching a Patient To or From a Monoamine Oxidase Inhibitor (MAOI) Antidepressant

At least 14 days should elapse between discontinuation of an MAOI intended to treat depression and initiation of therapy with WELLBUTRIN. Conversely, at least 14 days should be allowed after stopping WELLBUTRIN before starting an MAOI antidepressant (see CONTRAINDICATIONS and DRUG INTERACTIONS).

Use of WELLBUTRIN With Reversible MAOIs Such as Linezolid or Methylene Blue

Do not start WELLBUTRIN in a patient who is being treated with a reversible MAOI such as linezolid or intravenous methylene blue. Drug interactions can increase the risk of hypertensive reactions. In a patient who requires more urgent treatment of a psychiatric condition, non-pharmacological interventions, including hospitalization, should be considered (see CONTRAINDICATIONS and DRUG INTERACTIONS).

In some cases, a patient already receiving therapy with WELLBUTRIN may require urgent treatment with linezolid or intravenous methylene blue. If acceptable alternatives to linezolid or intravenous methylene blue treatment are not available and the potential benefits of linezolid or intravenous methylene blue treatment are judged to outweigh the risks of hypertensive reactions in a particular patient, WELLBUTRIN should be stopped promptly, and linezolid or intravenous methylene blue can be administered. The patient should be monitored for 2 weeks or until 24 hours after the last dose of linezolid or intravenous methylene blue, whichever comes first. Therapy with WELLBUTRIN may be resumed 24 hours after the last dose of linezolid or intravenous methylene blue.

The risk of administering methylene blue by non-intravenous routes (such as oral tablets or by local injection) or in intravenous doses much lower than 1 mg/kg with WELLBUTRIN is unclear. The clinician should, nevertheless, be aware of the possibility of a drug interaction with such use (see CONTRAINDICATIONS and DRUG INTERACTIONS).

HOW SUPPLIED

WELLBUTRIN Tablets, 75 mg of bupropion hydrochloride, are yellow-gold, round, biconvex tablets printed with "WELLBUTRIN 75" in bottles of 100 (NDC 0173-0177-55).

WELLBUTRIN Tablets, 100 mg of bupropion hydrochloride, are red, round, biconvex tablets printed with "WELLBUTRIN 100" in bottles of 100 (NDC 0173-0178-55).

Store at 15° to 25°C (59° to 77°F). Protect from light and moisture.

WELLBUTRIN, WELLBUTRIN SR, WELLBUTRIN XL, and ZYBAN are registered trademarks of GlaxoSmithKline. KALETRA is a registered trademark of Abbott Laboratories.

Distributed by:
GlaxoSmithKline
Research Triangle Park, NC 27709
Manufactured by:
DSM Pharmaceuticals, Inc.
Greenville, NC 27834 for
GlaxoSmithKline
Research Triangle Park, NC 27709

March 2013
WLT:9PI

MEDICATION GUIDE

WELLBUTRIN® (WELL byu-trin)
(bupropion hydrochloride) Tablets

Read this Medication Guide carefully before you start using WELLBUTRIN and each time you get a refill. There may be new information. This information does not take the place of talking with your doctor about your medical condition or your treatment. If you have any questions about WELLBUTRIN, ask your doctor or pharmacist.

IMPORTANT: Be sure to read the three sections of this Medication Guide. The first section is about the risk of suicidal thoughts and actions with antidepressant medicines; the second section is about the risk of changes in thinking and behavior, depression and suicidal thoughts or actions with medicines used to quit smoking; and the third section is entitled "What Other Important Information Should I Know About WELLBUTRIN?"

Antidepressant Medicines, Depression and Other Serious Mental Illnesses, and Suicidal Thoughts or Actions

This section of the Medication Guide is only about the risk of suicidal thoughts and actions with antidepressant medicines. **Talk to your, or your family member's, healthcare provider about:**

- all risks and benefits of treatment with antidepressant medicines
- all treatment choices for depression or other serious mental illness

What is the most important information I should know about antidepressant medicines, depression and other serious mental illnesses, and suicidal thoughts or actions?

1. **Antidepressant medicines may increase suicidal thoughts or actions in some children, teenagers, and young adults within the first few months of treatment.**
2. **Depression and other serious mental illnesses are the most important causes of suicidal thoughts and actions. Some people may have a particularly high risk of having suicidal thoughts or actions.** These include people who have (or have a family history of) bipolar illness (also called manic-depressive illness) or suicidal thoughts or actions.
3. **How can I watch for and try to prevent suicidal thoughts and actions in myself or a family member?**
   - Pay close attention to any changes, especially sudden changes, in mood, behaviors, thoughts, or feelings. This is very important when an antidepressant medicine is started or when the dose is changed.
   - Call the healthcare provider right away to report new or sudden changes in mood, behavior, thoughts, or feelings.
   - Keep all follow-up visits with the healthcare provider as scheduled. Call the healthcare provider between visits as needed, especially if you have concerns about symptoms.

Call a healthcare provider right away if you or your family member has any of the following symptoms, especially if they are new, worse, or worry you:

• thoughts about suicide or dying	• trouble sleeping (insomnia)
• attempts to commit suicide	• new or worse irritability
• new or worse depression	• acting aggressive, being angry, or violent
• new or worse anxiety	• acting on dangerous impulses
• feeling very agitated or restless	• an extreme increase in activity and talking (mania)
• panic attacks	• other unusual changes in behavior or mood

What else do I need to know about antidepressant medicines?

- **Never stop an antidepressant medicine without first talking to a healthcare provider.** Stopping an antidepressant medicine suddenly can cause other symptoms.
- **Antidepressants are medicines used to treat depression and other illnesses.** It is important to discuss all the risks of treating depression and also the risks of not treating it. Patients and their families or other caregivers should discuss all treatment choices with the healthcare provider, not just the use of antidepressants.
- **Antidepressant medicines have other side effects.** Talk to the healthcare provider about the side effects of the medicine prescribed for you or your family member.
- **Antidepressant medicines can interact with other medicines.** Know all of the medicines that you or your family member takes. Keep a list of all medicines to show the healthcare provider. Do not start new medicines without first checking with your healthcare provider.
- **Not all antidepressant medicines prescribed for children are FDA approved for use in children.** Talk to your child's healthcare provider for more information.

WELLBUTRIN has not been studied in children under the age of 18 and is not approved for use in children and teenagers.

Quitting Smoking, Quit-Smoking Medications, Changes in Thinking and Behavior, Depression, and Suicidal Thoughts or Actions

This section of the Medication Guide is only about the risk of changes in thinking and behavior, depression and suicidal thoughts or actions with drugs used to quit smoking. Although WELLBUTRIN is not a treatment for quitting smoking, it contains the same active ingredient (bupropion hydrochloride) as ZYBAN® which is used to help patients quit smoking.

Some people have had changes in behavior, hostility, agitation, depression, suicidal thoughts or actions while taking bupropion to help them quit smoking. These symptoms can develop during treatment with bupropion or after stopping treatment with bupropion.

If you, your family member, or your caregiver notice agitation, hostility, depression, or changes in thinking or behavior that are not typical for you, or you have any of the following symptoms, stop taking bupropion and call your healthcare provider right away:

• thoughts about suicide or dying	• an extreme increase in activity and talking (mania)
• attempts to commit suicide	• abnormal thoughts or sensations
• new or worse depression	• seeing or hearing things that are not there (hallucinations)
• new or worse anxiety	• feeling people are against you (paranoia)
• panic attacks	• feeling confused
• feeling very agitated or restless	• other unusual changes in behavior or mood
• acting aggressive, being angry, or violent	
• acting on dangerous impulses	

When you try to quit smoking, with or without bupropion, you may have symptoms that may be due to nicotine withdrawal, including urge to smoke, depressed mood, trouble sleeping, irritability, frustration, anger, feeling anxious, difficulty concentrating, restlessness, decreased heart rate, and increased appetite or weight gain. Some people have even experienced suicidal thoughts when trying to quit smoking without medication. Sometimes quitting smoking can lead to worsening of mental health problems that you already have, such as depression.

Before taking bupropion, tell your healthcare provider if you have ever had depression or other mental illnesses. You should also tell your doctor about any symptoms you had during other times you tried to quit smoking, with or without bupropion.

What Other Important Information Should I Know About WELLBUTRIN?

- **Seizures: There is a chance of having a seizure (convulsion, fit) with WELLBUTRIN, especially in people:**
   - with certain medical problems.
   - who take certain medicines.

The chance of having seizures increases with higher doses of WELLBUTRIN. For more information, see the sections "Who should not take WELLBUTRIN?" and "What should I tell my doctor before using WELLBUTRIN?" Tell your doctor about all of your medical conditions and all the medicines you take. **Do not take any other medicines while you are using WELLBUTRIN unless your doctor has said it is okay to take them.**

If you have a seizure while taking WELLBUTRIN, stop taking the tablets and call your doctor right away. Do not take WELLBUTRIN again if you have a seizure.

- **High blood pressure (hypertension).Some people get high blood pressure, that can be severe, while taking WELLBUTRIN.** The chance of high blood pressure may be higher if you also use nicotine replacement therapy (such as a nicotine patch) to help you stop smoking.
- **Severe allergic reactions. Some people have severe allergic reaction to WELLBUTRIN. Stop taking WELLBUTRIN and call your doctor right away** if you get a rash, itching, hives, fever, swollen lymph glands, painful sores in the mouth or around the eyes, swelling of the lips or tongue, chest pain, or have trouble breathing. These could be signs of a serious allergic reaction.
- **Unusual thoughts or behaviors.** Some patients have unusual thoughts or behaviors while taking WELLBUTRIN, including delusions (believe you are someone else), hallucinations (seeing or hearing things that are not there), paranoia (feeling that people are against you), or feeling confused. If this happens to you, call your doctor.

What is WELLBUTRIN?

WELLBUTRIN is a prescription medicine used to treat adults with a certain type of depression called major depressive disorder.

Who should not take WELLBUTRIN?

Do not take WELLBUTRIN if you:

- have or had a seizure disorder or epilepsy.
- **are taking ZYBAN (used to help people stop smoking) or any other medicines that contain bupropion hydrochloride, such as WELLBUTRIN SR Sustained-Release Tablets or WELLBUTRIN XL Extended-Release Tablets.** Bupropion is the same active ingredient that is in WELLBUTRIN.
- drink a lot of alcohol and abruptly stop drinking, or use medicines called sedatives (these make you sleepy) or benzodiazepines and you stop using them all of a sudden.
- take a monoamine oxidase inhibitor (MAOI). Ask your healthcare provider or pharmacist if you are not sure if you take an MAOI, including the antibiotic linezolid.
  - do not take an MAOI within 2 weeks of stopping WELLBUTRIN unless directed to do so by your physician.
  - do not start WELLBUTRIN if you stopped taking an MAOI in the last 2 weeks unless directed to do so by your physician.
- have or had an eating disorder such as anorexia nervosa or bulimia.
- are allergic to the active ingredient in WELLBUTRIN, bupropion, or to any of the inactive ingredients. See the end of this leaflet for a complete list of ingredients in WELLBUTRIN.

What should I tell my doctor before using WELLBUTRIN?

Tell your doctor if you have ever had depression, suicidal thoughts or actions, or other mental health problems. See "Antidepressant Medicines, Depression and Other Serious Mental Illnesses, and Suicidal Thoughts or Actions."

- **Tell your doctor about your other medical conditions including if you:**
  - **are pregnant or plan to become pregnant.** It is not known if WELLBUTRIN can harm your unborn baby.
  - **are breastfeeding.** WELLBUTRIN passes through your milk. It is not known if WELLBUTRIN can harm your baby.
  - **have liver problems**, especially cirrhosis of the liver.
  - have kidney problems.
  - have an eating disorder, such as anorexia nervosa or bulimia.
  - have had a head injury.
  - have had a seizure (convulsion, fit).
  - have a tumor in your nervous system (brain or spine).
  - have had a heart attack, heart problems, or high blood pressure.
  - are a diabetic taking insulin or other medicines to control your blood sugar.
  - drink a lot of alcohol.
  - abuse prescription medicines or street drugs.
- **Tell your doctor about all the medicines you take,** including prescription and non-prescription medicines, vitamins, and herbal supplements. Many medicines increase your chances of having seizures or other serious side effects if you take them while you are using WELLBUTRIN.

How should I take WELLBUTRIN?

- Take WELLBUTRIN exactly as prescribed by your doctor.
- Take WELLBUTRIN at the same time each day.
- Take your doses of WELLBUTRIN at least 6 hours apart.
- You may take WELLBUTRIN with or without food.
- If you miss a dose, do not take an extra tablet to make up for the dose you forgot. Wait and take your next tablet at the regular time. **This is very important.** Too much WELLBUTRIN can increase your chance of having a seizure.
- If you take too much WELLBUTRIN, or overdose, call your local emergency room or poison control center right away.
- **Do not take any other medicines while using WELLBUTRIN unless your doctor has told you it is okay.**
- It may take several weeks for you to feel that WELLBUTRIN is working. Once you feel better, it is important to keep taking WELLBUTRIN exactly as directed by your doctor. Call your doctor if you do not feel WELLBUTRIN is working for you.
- Do not change your dose or stop taking WELLBUTRIN without talking with your doctor first.

What should I avoid while taking WELLBUTRIN?

- Do not drink a lot of alcohol while taking WELLBUTRIN. If you usually drink a lot of alcohol, talk with your doctor before suddenly stopping. If you suddenly stop drinking alcohol, you may increase your risk of having seizures.
- Do not drive a car or use heavy machinery until you know how WELLBUTRIN affects you. WELLBUTRIN can impair your ability to perform these tasks.

What are possible side effects of WELLBUTRIN?

WELLBUTRIN can cause serious side effects. Read this entire Medication Guide for more information about these serious side effects.

The most common side effects of WELLBUTRIN are nervousness, constipation, trouble sleeping, dry mouth, headache, nausea, vomiting, and shakiness (tremor).

If you have nausea, take your medicine with food. If you have trouble sleeping, do not take your medicine too close to bedtime.

These are not all the side effects of WELLBUTRIN. For a complete list, ask your doctor or pharmacist.

Call your doctor for medical advice about side effects. You may report side effects to FDA at 1-800-FDA-1088.

How should I store WELLBUTRIN?

- Store WELLBUTRIN at room temperature. Store out of direct sunlight. Keep WELLBUTRIN in its tightly closed bottle.

General Information about WELLBUTRIN.

Medicines are sometimes prescribed for purposes other than those listed in a Medication Guide. Do not use WELLBUTRIN for a condition for which it was not prescribed. Do not give WELLBUTRIN to other people, even if they have the same symptoms you have. It may harm them.

Keep WELLBUTRIN out of the reach of children.

If you take a urine drug screening test, WELLBUTRIN may make the test result positive for amphetamines. If you tell the person giving you the drug screening test that you are taking WELLBUTRIN, they can do a more specific drug screening test that should not have this problem.

This Medication Guide summarizes important information about WELLBUTRIN. For more information, talk to your doctor. You can ask your doctor or pharmacist for information about WELLBUTRIN that is written for health professionals.

What are the ingredients in WELLBUTRIN?

Active ingredient: bupropion hydrochloride.

Inactive ingredients: 75-mg tablet – D&C Yellow No. 10 Lake, FD&C Yellow No. 6 Lake, hydroxypropyl cellulose, hypromellose, microcrystalline cellulose, polyethylene glycol, talc, and titanium dioxide; 100-mg tablet – FD&C Red No. 40 Lake, FD&C Yellow No. 6 Lake, hydroxypropyl cellulose, hypromellose, microcrystalline cellulose, polyethylene glycol, talc, and titanium dioxide.

This Medication Guide has been approved by the U.S. Food and Drug Administration.

WELLBUTRIN, WELLBUTRIN SR, WELLBUTRIN XL, and ZYBAN are registered trademarks of GlaxoSmithKline.

Distributed by:
GlaxoSmithKline
Research Triangle Park, NC 27709

Manufactured by:
DSM Pharmaceuticals, Inc.
Greenville, NC 27834 for
GlaxoSmithKline
Research Triangle Park, NC 27709

March 2013
WLT:8MG

WELLBUTRIN SR® ℞

[wel'byü-trin]

(bupropion hydrochloride)
Sustained-Release Tablets

WARNING

Suicidality and Antidepressant Drugs

Use in Treating Psychiatric Disorders: **Antidepressants increased the risk compared to placebo of suicidal thinking and behavior (suicidality) in children, adolescents, and young adults in short-term studies of major depressive disorder (MDD) and other psychiatric disorders. Anyone considering the use of WELLBUTRIN SR or any other antidepressant in a child, adolescent, or young adult must balance this risk with the clinical need. Short-term studies did not show an increase in the risk of suicidality with antidepressants compared to placebo in adults beyond age 24; there was a reduction in risk with antidepressants compared to placebo in adults aged 65 and older. Depression and certain other psychiatric disorders are themselves associated with increases in the risk of suicide. Patients of all ages who are started on antidepressant therapy should be monitored appropriately and observed closely for clinical worsening, suicidality, or unusual changes in behavior. Families and caregivers should be advised of the need for close observation and communication with the prescriber. WELLBUTRIN SR is not approved for use in pediatric patients. (See WARNINGS: Clinical Worsening and Suicide Risk in Treating Psychiatric Disorders, PRECAUTIONS: Information for Patients, and PRECAUTIONS: Pediatric Use.)**

Use in Smoking Cessation Treatment: **WELLBUTRIN®, WELLBUTRIN SR®, and WELLBUTRIN XL® are not approved for smoking cessation treatment, but bupropion under the name ZYBAN® is approved for this use. Serious neuropsychiatric events, including but not limited to depression, suicidal ideation, suicide attempt, and completed suicide have been reported in patients taking bupropion for smoking cessation. Some cases may have been complicated by the symptoms of nicotine withdrawal in patients who stopped smoking. Depressed mood may be a symptom of nicotine withdrawal. Depression, rarely including suicidal ideation, has been reported in smokers undergoing a smoking cessation attempt without medication. However, some of these symptoms have occurred in patients taking bupropion who continued to smoke.**

All patients being treated with bupropion for smoking cessation treatment should be observed for neuropsychiatric symptoms including changes in behavior, hostility, agitation, depressed mood, and suicide-related events, including ideation, behavior, and attempted suicide. These symptoms, as well as worsening of pre-existing psychiatric illness and completed suicide have been reported in some patients attempting to quit smoking while taking ZYBAN in the postmarketing experience. When symptoms were reported, most were during treatment with ZYBAN, but some were following discontinuation of treatment with ZYBAN. These events have occurred in patients with and without pre-existing psychiatric disease; some have experienced worsening of their psychiatric illnesses. Patients with serious psychiatric illness such as schizophrenia, bipolar disorder, and major depressive disorder did not participate in the premarketing studies of ZYBAN.

Advise patients and caregivers that the patient using bupropion for smoking cessation should stop taking bupropion and contact a healthcare provider immediately if agitation, hostility, depressed mood, or changes in thinking or behavior that are not typical for the patient are observed, or if the patient develops suicidal ideation or suicidal behavior. In many postmarketing cases, resolution of symptoms after discontinuation of ZYBAN was reported, although in some cases the symptoms persisted; therefore, ongoing monitoring and supportive care should be provided until symptoms resolve.

The risks of using bupropion for smoking cessation should be weighed against the benefits of its use. ZYBAN has been demonstrated to increase the likelihood of abstinence from smoking for as long as 6 months compared to treatment with placebo. The health benefits of quitting smoking are immediate and substantial. (See WARNINGS: Neuropsychiatric Symptoms and Suicide Risk in Smoking Cessation Treatment and PRECAUTIONS: Information for Patients.)

DESCRIPTION

WELLBUTRIN SR (bupropion hydrochloride), an antidepressant of the aminoketone class, is chemically unrelated to tricyclic, tetracyclic, selective serotonin re-uptake inhibitor, or other known antidepressant agents. Its structure closely resembles that of diethylpropion; it is related to phenylethylamines. It is designated as (±)-1-(3-chlorophenyl)-2-[(1,1-dimethylethyl)amino]-1-propanone hydrochloride. The molecular weight is 276.2. The molecular formula is $C_{13}H_{18}ClNO \bullet HCl$. Bupropion hydrochloride powder is white, crystalline, and highly soluble in water. It has a bitter taste and produces the sensation of local anesthesia on the oral mucosa. The structural formula is:

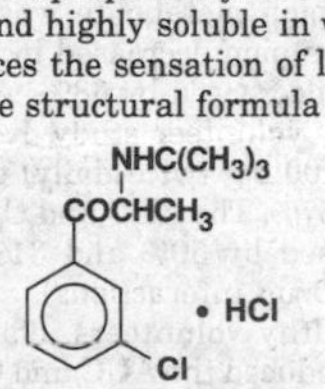

WELLBUTRIN SR is supplied for oral administration as 100-mg (blue), 150-mg (purple), and 200-mg (light pink), film-coated, sustained-release tablets. Each tablet contains the labeled amount of bupropion hydrochloride and the inactive ingredients: carnauba wax, cysteine hydrochloride, hypromellose, magnesium stearate, microcrystalline cellulose, polyethylene glycol, polysorbate 80, and titanium dioxide and is printed with edible black ink. In addition, the 100-mg tablet contains FD&C Blue No. 1 Lake, the 150-mg tablet contains FD&C Blue No. 2 Lake and FD&C Red No. 40 Lake, and the 200-mg tablet contains FD&C Red No. 40 Lake.

CLINICAL PHARMACOLOGY

Pharmacodynamics

Bupropion is a relatively weak inhibitor of the neuronal uptake of norepinephrine and dopamine, and does not inhibit monoamine oxidase or the re-uptake of serotonin. While the mechanism of action of bupropion, as with other antidepressants, is unknown, it is presumed that this action is mediated by noradrenergic and/or dopaminergic mechanisms.

Pharmacokinetics

Bupropion is a racemic mixture. The pharmacologic activity and pharmacokinetics of the individual enantiomers have not been studied. The mean elimination half-life (±SD) of bupropion after chronic dosing is 21 (±9) hours, and steady-state plasma concentrations of bupropion are reached within 8 days. In a study comparing chronic dosing with WELLBUTRIN SR 150 mg twice daily to the immediate-release formulation of bupropion at 100 mg 3 times daily, peak plasma concentrations of bupropion at steady state for WELLBUTRIN SR were approximately 85% of those achieved with the immediate-release formulation. There was equivalence for bupropion AUCs, as well as equivalence for both peak plasma concentration and AUCs for all 3 of the detectable bupropion metabolites. Thus, at steady state, WELLBUTRIN SR, given twice daily, and the immediate-release formulation of bupropion, given 3 times daily, are essentially bioequivalent for both bupropion and the 3 quantitatively important metabolites.

Absorption: Exposure to bupropion may be increased when WELLBUTRIN SR tablets are taken with food. Three studies in healthy volunteers demonstrated peak plasma concentrations (C_{max}) of bupropion increased by 11% to 35% when administered with food, while overall exposure (AUC) to bupropion increased by 16% to 19%. The food effect is not considered clinically significant and WELLBUTRIN SR can be taken with or without food.

Distribution: In vitro tests show that bupropion is 84% bound to human plasma proteins at concentrations up to 200 mcg/mL. The extent of protein binding of the hydroxybupropion metabolite is similar to that for bupropion, whereas the extent of protein binding of the threohydrobupropion metabolite is about half that seen with bupropion.

Metabolism: Bupropion is extensively metabolized in humans. Three metabolites have been shown to be active: hydroxybupropion, which is formed via hydroxylation of the *tert*-butyl group of bupropion, and the amino-alcohol isomers threohydrobupropion and erythrohydrobupropion, which are formed via reduction of the carbonyl group. In vitro findings suggest that cytochrome P450IIB6 (CYP2B6) is the principal isoenzyme involved in the formation of hydroxybupropion, while cytochrome P450 isoenzymes are not involved in the formation of threohydrobupropion. Oxidation of the bupropion side chain results in the formation of a glycine conjugate of meta-chlorobenzoic acid, which is then excreted as the major urinary metabolite. The potency and toxicity of the metabolites relative to bupropion have not been fully characterized. However, it has been demonstrated in an antidepressant screening test in mice that hydroxybupropion is one-half as potent as bupropion, while threohydrobupropion and erythrohydrobupropion are 5-fold less potent than bupropion. This may be of clinical importance because the plasma concentrations of the metabolites are as high as or higher than those of bupropion.

Because bupropion is extensively metabolized, there is the potential for drug-drug interactions, particularly with those agents that are metabolized by or which inhibit/induce the cytochrome P450IIB6 (CYP2B6) isoenzyme, such as ritonavir or efavirenz. In a healthy volunteer study, ritonavir at a dose of 100 mg twice daily reduced the AUC and C_{max} of bupropion by 22% and 21%, respectively. The exposure of the hydroxybupropion metabolite was decreased by 23%, the threohydrobupropion decreased by 38%, and the erythrohydrobupropion decreased by 48%.

In a second healthy volunteer study, ritonavir at a dose of 600 mg twice daily decreased the AUC and the C_{max} of bupropion by 66% and 62%, respectively. The exposure of the hydroxybupropion metabolite was decreased by 78%, the threohydrobupropion decreased by 50%, and the erythrohydrobupropion decreased by 68%.

In another healthy volunteer study, KALETRA® (lopinavir 400 mg/ritonavir 100 mg twice daily) decreased bupropion AUC and C_{max} by 57%. The AUC and C_{max} of hydroxybupropion were decreased by 50% and 31%, respectively (see PRECAUTIONS: Drug Interactions).

In a study in healthy volunteers, efavirenz 600 mg once daily for 2 weeks reduced the AUC and C_{max} of bupropion by approximately 55% and 34%, respectively. The AUC of hydroxybupropion was unchanged, whereas C_{max} of hydroxybupropion was increased by 50%.

Although bupropion is not metabolized by cytochrome P450IID6 (CYP2D6), there is the potential for drug-drug interactions when bupropion is coadministered with drugs metabolized by this isoenzyme (see PRECAUTIONS: Drug Interactions).

Following a single dose in humans, peak plasma concentrations of hydroxybupropion occur approximately 6 hours after administration of WELLBUTRIN SR. Peak plasma concentrations of hydroxybupropion are approximately 10 times the peak level of the parent drug at steady state. The elimination half-life of hydroxybupropion is approximately 20 (±5) hours and its AUC at steady state is about 17 times that of bupropion. The times to peak concentrations for the erythrohydrobupropion and threohydrobupropion metabolites are similar to that of the hydroxybupropion metabolite. However, their elimination half-lives are longer, 33 (±10) and 37 (±13) hours, respectively, and steady-state AUCs are 1.5 and 7 times that of bupropion, respectively.

Bupropion and its metabolites exhibit linear kinetics following chronic administration of 300 to 450 mg/day.

Elimination: Following oral administration of 200 mg of ^{14}C-bupropion in humans, 87% and 10% of the radioactive dose were recovered in the urine and feces, respectively. However, the fraction of the oral dose of bupropion excreted unchanged was only 0.5%, a finding consistent with the extensive metabolism of bupropion.

Population Subgroups: Factors or conditions altering metabolic capacity (e.g., liver disease, congestive heart failure [CHF], age, concomitant medications, etc.) or elimination may be expected to influence the degree and extent of accumulation of the active metabolites of bupropion. The elimination of the major metabolites of bupropion may be affected by reduced renal or hepatic function because they are moderately polar compounds and are likely to undergo further metabolism or conjugation in the liver prior to urinary excretion

Hepatic: The effect of hepatic impairment on the pharmacokinetics of bupropion was characterized in 2 single-dose studies, one in patients with alcoholic liver disease and one in patients with mild-to-severe cirrhosis. The first study showed that the half-life of hydroxybupropion was significantly longer in 8 patients with alcoholic liver disease than in 8 healthy volunteers (32 ± 14 hours versus 21 ± 5 hours, respectively). Although not statistically significant, the AUCs for bupropion and hydroxybupropion were more variable and tended to be greater (by 53% to 57%) in patients with alcoholic liver disease. The differences in half-life for bupropion and the other metabolites in the 2 patient groups were minimal.

The second study showed no statistically significant differences in the pharmacokinetics of bupropion and its active metabolites in 9 patients with mild-to-moderate hepatic cirrhosis compared to 8 healthy volunteers. However, more variability was observed in some of the pharmacokinetic parameters for bupropion (AUC, C_{max}, and T_{max}) and its active metabolites ($t_{1/2}$) in patients with mild-to-moderate hepatic cirrhosis. In addition, in patients with severe hepatic cirrhosis, the bupropion C_{max} and AUC were substantially increased (mean difference: by approximately 70% and 3-fold, respectively) and more variable when compared to values in healthy volunteers; the mean bupropion half-life was also longer (29 hours in patients with severe hepatic cirrhosis vs. 19 hours in healthy subjects). For the metabolite hydroxybupropion, the mean C_{max} was approximately 69% lower. For the combined amino-alcohol isomers threohydrobupropion and erythrohydrobupropion, the mean C_{max} was approximately 31% lower. The mean AUC increased by about 1½-fold for hydroxybupropion and about 2½-fold for threo/erythrohydrobupropion. The median T_{max} was observed 19 hours later for hydroxybupropion and 31 hours later for threo/erythrohydrobupropion. The mean half-lives for hydroxybupropion and threo/erythrohydrobupropion were increased 5- and 2-fold, respectively, in patients with severe hepatic cirrhosis compared to healthy volunteers (see WARNINGS, PRECAUTIONS, and DOSAGE AND ADMINISTRATION).

Renal: There is limited information on the pharmacokinetics of bupropion in patients with renal impairment. An inter-study comparison between normal subjects and patients with end-stage renal failure demonstrated that the parent drug C_{max} and AUC values were comparable in the 2 groups, whereas the hydroxybupropion and threohydrobupropion metabolites had a 2.3- and 2.8-fold increase, respectively, in AUC for patients with end-stage renal failure. A second study, comparing normal subjects and patients with moderate-to-severe renal impairment (GFR 30.9 ± 10.8 mL/min) showed that exposure to a single 150-mg dose of sustained-release bupropion was approximately 2-fold higher in patients with impaired renal function while levels of the hydroxybupropion and threo/erythrohydrobupropion (combined) metabolites were similar in the 2 groups. The elimination of bupropion and/or the major metabolites of bupropion may be reduced by impaired renal function (see PRECAUTIONS: Renal Impairment).

Left Ventricular Dysfunction: During a chronic dosing study with bupropion in 14 depressed patients with left ventricular dysfunction (history of CHF or an enlarged heart on x-ray), no apparent effect on the pharmacokinetics of bupropion or its metabolites was revealed, compared to healthy volunteers.

Age: The effects of age on the pharmacokinetics of bupropion and its metabolites have not been fully characterized, but an exploration of steady-state bupropion concentrations from several depression efficacy studies involving patients dosed in a range of 300 to 750 mg/day, on a 3 times daily schedule, revealed no relationship between age (18 to 83 years) and plasma concentration of bupropion. A single-dose pharmacokinetic study demonstrated that the disposition of bupropion and its metabolites in elderly subjects was similar to that of younger subjects. These data suggest there is no prominent effect of age on bupropion concentration; however, another pharmacokinetic study, single and multiple dose, has suggested that the elderly are at increased risk for accumulation of bupropion and its metabolites (see PRECAUTIONS: Geriatric Use).

Gender: A single-dose study involving 12 healthy male and 12 healthy female volunteers revealed no sex-related differences in the pharmacokinetic parameters of bupropion.

Smokers: The effects of cigarette smoking on the pharmacokinetics of bupropion were studied in 34 healthy male and female volunteers; 17 were chronic cigarette smokers and 17 were nonsmokers. Following oral administration of a single 150-mg dose of bupropion, there was no statistically significant difference in C_{max}, half-life, T_{max}, AUC, or clearance of bupropion or its active metabolites between smokers and nonsmokers.

CLINICAL TRIALS

The efficacy of the immediate-release formulation of bupropion as a treatment for depression was established in two 4-week, placebo-controlled trials in adult inpatients with depression and in one 6-week, placebo-controlled trial in adult outpatients with depression. In the first study, patients were titrated in a bupropion dose range of 300 to 600 mg/day on a 3 times daily schedule; 78% of patients received maximum doses of 450 mg/day or less. This trial demonstrated the effectiveness of the immediate-release formulation of bupropion on the Hamilton Depression Rating Scale (HDRS) total score, the depressed mood item (item 1) from that scale, and the Clinical Global Impressions (CGI) severity score. A second study included 2 fixed doses of the immediate-release formulation of bupropion (300 and 450 mg/day) and placebo. This trial demonstrated the effectiveness of the immediate-release formulation of bupropion, but only at the 450-mg/day dose; the results were positive for the HDRS total score and the CGI severity score, but not for HDRS item 1. In the third study, outpatients received 300 mg/day of the immediate-release formulation of bupropion. This study demonstrated the effectiveness of the immediate-release formulation of bupropion on the HDRS total score, HDRS item 1, the Montgomery-Asberg Depression Rating Scale, the CGI severity score, and the CGI improvement score.

Although there are not as yet independent trials demonstrating the antidepressant effectiveness of the sustained-release formulation of bupropion, studies have demonstrated the bioequivalence of the immediate-release and sustained-release forms of bupropion under steady-state conditions, i.e., bupropion sustained-release 150 mg twice daily was shown to be bioequivalent to 100 mg 3 times daily of the immediate-release formulation of bupropion, with regard to both rate and extent of absorption, for parent drug and metabolites.

In a longer-term study, outpatients meeting DSM-IV criteria for major depressive disorder, recurrent type, who had responded during an 8-week open trial on WELLBUTRIN SR (150 mg twice daily) were randomized to continuation of their same dose of WELLBUTRIN SR or placebo, for up to 44 weeks of observation for relapse. Response during the open phase was defined as CGI Improvement score of 1 (very much improved) or 2 (much improved) for each of the final 3 weeks. Relapse during the double-blind phase was defined as the investigator's judgment that drug treatment was needed for worsening depressive symptoms. Patients receiving continued treatment with WELLBUTRIN SR experienced significantly lower relapse rates over the subsequent 44 weeks compared to those receiving placebo.

INDICATIONS AND USAGE

WELLBUTRIN SR is indicated for the treatment of major depressive disorder.

The efficacy of bupropion in the treatment of a major depressive episode was established in two 4-week controlled trials of depressed inpatients and in one 6-week controlled trial of depressed outpatients whose diagnoses corresponded most closely to the Major Depression category of the APA Diagnostic and Statistical Manual (DSM) (see CLINICAL PHARMACOLOGY).

A major depressive episode (DSM-IV) implies the presence of 1) depressed mood or 2) loss of interest or pleasure; in addition, at least 5 of the following symptoms have been present during the same 2-week period and represent a change from previous functioning: depressed mood, markedly diminished interest or pleasure in usual activities, significant change in weight and/or appetite, insomnia or hypersomnia, psychomotor agitation or retardation, increased fatigue, feelings of guilt or worthlessness, slowed thinking or impaired concentration, a suicide attempt or suicidal ideation.

The efficacy of WELLBUTRIN SR in maintaining an antidepressant response for up to 44 weeks following 8 weeks of acute treatment was demonstrated in a placebo-controlled trial (see CLINICAL PHARMACOLOGY). Nevertheless, the physician who elects to use WELLBUTRIN SR for extended periods should periodically reevaluate the long-term usefulness of the drug for the individual patient.

CONTRAINDICATIONS

WELLBUTRIN SR is contraindicated in patients with a seizure disorder.

WELLBUTRIN SR is contraindicated in patients treated with ZYBAN (bupropion hydrochloride) Sustained-Release Tablets; WELLBUTRIN (bupropion hydrochloride), the immediate-release formulation; WELLBUTRIN XL (bupropion hydrochloride), the extended-release formulation; or any other medications that contain bupropion because the incidence of seizure is dose dependent.

WELLBUTRIN SR is contraindicated in patients with a current or prior diagnosis of bulimia or anorexia nervosa because of a higher incidence of seizures noted in patients treated for bulimia with the immediate-release formulation of bupropion.

WELLBUTRIN SR is contraindicated in patients undergoing abrupt discontinuation of alcohol or sedatives (including benzodiazepines).

The use of monoamine oxidase inhibitors or MAOIs (intended to treat psychiatric disorders) concomitantly with WELLBUTRIN SR or within 14 days of stopping treatment with WELLBUTRIN SR is contraindicated. There is an increased risk of hypertensive reactions when bupropion is used concomitantly with other drugs that inhibit the reuptake of dopamine or norepinephrine or inhibit their metabolism (e.g., MAOIs). The use of WELLBUTRIN SR within 14 days of stopping treatment with an MAOI is also contraindicated. Starting WELLBUTRIN SR in a patient treated with reversible MAOIs such as linezolid or intravenous methylene blue is contraindicated (see DOSAGE AND ADMINISTRATION and DRUG INTERACTIONS).

WELLBUTRIN SR is contraindicated in patients who have shown an allergic response to bupropion or the other ingredients that make up WELLBUTRIN SR.

WARNINGS

Clinical Worsening and Suicide Risk in Treating Psychiatric Disorders

Patients with major depressive disorder (MDD), both adult and pediatric, may experience worsening of their depression and/or the emergence of suicidal ideation and behavior (suicidality) or unusual changes in behavior, whether or not they are taking antidepressant medications, and this risk may persist until significant remission occurs. Suicide is a known risk of depression and certain other psychiatric disorders, and these disorders themselves are the strongest predictors of suicide. There has been a long-standing concern, however, that antidepressants may have a role in inducing worsening of depression and the emergence of suicidality in certain patients during the early phases of treatment. Pooled analyses of short-term placebo-controlled trials of antidepressant drugs (SSRIs and others) showed that these drugs increase the risk of suicidal thinking and behavior (suicidality) in children, adolescents, and young adults (ages 18-24) with major depressive disorder (MDD) and other psychiatric disorders. Short-term studies did not show an increase in the risk of suicidality with antidepressants compared to placebo in adults beyond age 24; there was a reduction with antidepressants compared to placebo in adults aged 65 and older.

The pooled analyses of placebo-controlled trials in children and adolescents with MDD, obsessive compulsive disorder (OCD), or other psychiatric disorders included a total of 24 short-term trials of 9 antidepressant drugs in over 4,400 patients. The pooled analyses of placebo-controlled trials in adults with MDD or other psychiatric disorders included a total of 295 short-term trials (median duration of 2 months) of 11 antidepressant drugs in over 77,000 patients. There was considerable variation in risk of suicidality among drugs, but a tendency toward an increase in the younger patients for almost all drugs studied. There were differences in absolute risk of suicidality across the different indications, with the highest incidence in MDD. The risk differences (drug vs. placebo), however, were relatively stable within age strata and across indications. These risk differences (drug-placebo difference in the number of cases of suicidality per 1,000 patients treated) are provided in Table 1.

Table 1

Age Range	Drug-Placebo Difference in Number of Cases of Suicidality per 1,000 Patients Treated
	Increases Compared to Placebo
<18	14 additional cases
18-24	5 additional cases
	Decreases Compared to Placebo
25-64	1 fewer case
≥65	6 fewer cases

No suicides occurred in any of the pediatric trials. There were suicides in the adult trials, but the number was not sufficient to reach any conclusion about drug effect on suicide.

It is unknown whether the suicidality risk extends to longer-term use, i.e., beyond several months. However, there is substantial evidence from placebo-controlled maintenance trials in adults with depression that the use of antidepressants can delay the recurrence of depression.

All patients being treated with antidepressants for any indication should be monitored appropriately and observed closely for clinical worsening, suicidality, and unusual changes in behavior, especially during the initial few months of a course of drug therapy, or at times of dose changes, either increases or decreases.

The following symptoms, anxiety, agitation, panic attacks, insomnia, irritability, hostility, aggressiveness, impulsivity, akathisia (psychomotor restlessness), hypomania, and mania, have been reported in adult and pediatric patients being treated with antidepressants for major depressive disorder as well as for other indications, both psychiatric and nonpsychiatric. Although a causal link between the emergence of such symptoms and either the worsening of depression and/or the emergence of suicidal impulses has not been established, there is concern that such symptoms may represent precursors to emerging suicidality.

Consideration should be given to changing the therapeutic regimen, including possibly discontinuing the medication, in patients whose depression is persistently worse, or who are experiencing emergent suicidality or symptoms that might be precursors to worsening depression or suicidality, especially if these symptoms are severe, abrupt in onset, or were not part of the patient's presenting symptoms.

Families and caregivers of patients being treated with antidepressants for major depressive disorder or other indications, both psychiatric and nonpsychiatric, should be alerted about the need to monitor patients for the emergence of agitation, irritability, unusual changes in behavior, and the other symptoms described above, as well as the emergence of suicidality, and to report such symptoms immediately to healthcare providers.Such monitoring should include daily observation by families and caregivers. Prescriptions for WELLBUTRIN SR should be written for the smallest quantity of tablets consistent with good patient management, in order to reduce the risk of overdose.

Neuropsychiatric Symptoms and Suicide Risk in Smoking Cessation Treatment

WELLBUTRIN, WELLBUTRIN SR, and WELLBUTRIN XL are not approved for smoking cessation treatment, but bupropion under the name ZYBAN is approved for this use. Serious neuropsychiatric symptoms have been reported in patients taking bupropion for smoking cessation **(see BOXED WARNING, ADVERSE REACTIONS). These have included changes in mood (including depression and mania), psychosis, hallucinations, paranoia, delusions, homicidal ideation, hostility, agitation, aggression, anxiety, and panic, as well as suicidal ideation, suicide attempt, and completed suicide.** Some reported cases may have been complicated by the symptoms of nicotine withdrawal in patients who stopped smoking. Depressed mood may be a symptom of nicotine withdrawal. Depression, rarely including suicidal ideation, has been reported in smokers undergoing a smoking cessation attempt without medication. However, some of these symptoms have occurred in patients taking bupropion who continued to smoke. When symptoms were reported, most were during bupropion treatment, but some were following discontinuation of bupropion therapy. These events have occurred in patients with and without pre-existing psychiatric disease; some have experienced worsening of their psychiatric illnesses. All patients being treated with bupropion as part of smoking cessation treatment should be observed for neuropsychiatric symptoms or worsening of pre-existing psychiatric illness.

Patients with serious psychiatric illness such as schizophrenia, bipolar disorder, and major depressive disorder did not participate in the pre-marketing studies of ZYBAN.

Advise patients and caregivers that the patient using bupropion for smoking cessation should stop taking bupropion and contact a healthcare provider immediately if agitation, depressed mood, or changes in behavior or thinking that are not typical for the patient are observed, or if the patient develops suicidal ideation or suicidal behavior. In many postmarketing cases, resolution of symptoms after discontinuation of ZYBAN was reported, although in some cases the symptoms persisted, therefore, ongoing monitoring and supportive care should be provided until symptoms resolve.

The risks of using bupropion for smoking cessation should be weighed against the benefits of its use. ZYBAN has been demonstrated to increase the likelihood of abstinence from smoking for as long as six months compared to treatment with placebo. The health benefits of quitting smoking are immediate and substantial.

Screening Patients for Bipolar Disorder

A major depressive episode may be the initial presentation of bipolar disorder. It is generally believed (though not established in controlled trials) that treating such an episode with an antidepressant alone may increase the likelihood of precipitation of a mixed/manic episode in patients at risk for bipolar disorder. Whether any of the symptoms described above represent such a conversion is unknown. However, prior to initiating treatment with an antidepressant, patients with depressive symptoms should be adequately screened to determine if they are at risk for bipolar disorder; such screening should include a detailed psychiatric history, including a family history of suicide, bipolar disorder, and depression. It should be noted that WELLBUTRIN SR is not approved for use in treating bipolar depression.

Bupropion-Containing Products

Patients should be made aware that WELLBUTRIN SR contains the same active ingredient found in ZYBAN, used as an aid to smoking cessation treatment, and that WELLBUTRIN SR should not be used in combination with ZYBAN, or any other medications that contain bupropion, such as WELLBUTRIN (bupropion hydrochloride), the immediate-release formulation or WELLBUTRIN XL (bupropion hydrochloride), the extended-release formulation.

Seizures

Bupropion is associated with a dose-related risk of seizures. The risk of seizures is also related to patient factors, clinical situations, and concomitant medications, which must be considered in selection of patients for therapy with WELLBUTRIN SR. WELLBUTRIN SR should be discontinued and not restarted in patients who experience a seizure while on treatment.

- **Dose: At doses of WELLBUTRIN SR up to a dose of 300 mg/day, the incidence of seizure is approximately 0.1% (1/1,000) and increases to approximately 0.4% (4/1,000) at the maximum recommended dose of 400 mg/day.**

Data for the immediate-release formulation of bupropion revealed a seizure incidence of approximately 0.4% (i.e., 13 of 3,200 patients followed prospectively) in patients treated at doses in a range of 300 to 450 mg/day. The 450-mg/day upper limit of this dose range is close to the currently recommended maximum dose of 400 mg/day for WELLBUTRIN SR. This seizure incidence (0.4%) may exceed that of other marketed antidepressants and WELLBUTRIN SR up to 300 mg/day by as much as 4-fold. This relative risk is only an approximate estimate because no direct comparative studies have been conducted.

Additional data accumulated for the immediate-release formulation of bupropion suggested that the estimated seizure incidence increases almost tenfold between 450 and 600 mg/day, which is twice the usual adult dose and one and one-half the maximum recommended daily dose (400 mg) of WELLBUTRIN SR. This disproportionate increase in seizure incidence with dose incrementation calls for caution in dosing.

Data for WELLBUTRIN SR revealed a seizure incidence of approximately 0.1% (i.e., 3 of 3,100 patients followed prospectively) in patients treated at doses in a range of 100 to 300 mg/day. It is not possible to know if the lower seizure incidence observed in this study involving the sustained-release formulation of bupropion resulted from the different formulation or the lower dose used. However, as noted above, the immediate-release and sustained-release formulations are bioequivalent with regard to both rate and extent of absorption during steady state (the most pertinent condition to estimating seizure incidence), since most observed seizures occur under steady-state conditions.

- **Patient factors: Predisposing factors that may increase the risk of seizure with bupropion use include history of head trauma or prior seizure, central nervous system (CNS) tumor, the presence of severe hepatic cirrhosis, and concomitant medications that lower seizure threshold.**
- **Clinical situations: Circumstances associated with an increased seizure risk include, among others, excessive use of alcohol or sedatives (including benzodiazepines); addiction to opiates, cocaine, or stimulants; use of over-the-counter stimulants and anorectics; and diabetes treated with oral hypoglycemics or insulin.**
- **Concomitant medications: Many medications (e.g., antipsychotics, antidepressants, theophylline, systemic steroids) are known to lower seizure threshold.**

***Recommendations for Reducing the Risk of Seizure:* Retrospective analysis of clinical experience gained during the development of bupropion suggests that the risk of seizure may be minimized if**

- **the total daily dose of WELLBUTRIN SR does *not* exceed 400 mg,**
- **the daily dose is administered twice daily, and**
- **the rate of incrementation of dose is gradual.**
- **No single dose should exceed 200 mg to avoid high peak concentrations of bupropion and/or its metabolites.**

WELLBUTRIN SR should be administered with extreme caution to patients with a history of seizure, cranial trauma, or other predisposition(s) toward seizure, or patients treated with other agents (e.g., antipsychotics, other antidepressants, theophylline, systemic steroids, etc.) that lower seizure threshold.

Hepatic Impairment

WELLBUTRIN SR should be used with extreme caution in patients with severe hepatic cirrhosis. In these patients a

reduced frequency and/or dose is required, as peak bupropion, as well as AUC, levels are substantially increased and accumulation is likely to occur in such patients to a greater extent than usual. The dose should not exceed 100 mg every day or 150 mg every other day in these patients (see CLINICAL PHARMACOLOGY, PRECAUTIONS, and DOSAGE AND ADMINISTRATION).

Potential for Hepatotoxicity

In rats receiving large doses of bupropion chronically, there was an increase in incidence of hepatic hyperplastic nodules and hepatocellular hypertrophy. In dogs receiving large doses of bupropion chronically, various histologic changes were seen in the liver, and laboratory tests suggesting mild hepatocellular injury were noted.

PRECAUTIONS

General

Agitation and Insomnia: Patients in placebo-controlled trials with WELLBUTRIN SR experienced agitation, anxiety, and insomnia as shown in Table 2.

Table 2. Incidence of Agitation, Anxiety, and Insomnia in Placebo-Controlled Trials

Adverse Event Term	WELLBUTRIN SR 300 mg/day (n = 376)	WELLBUTRIN SR 400 mg/day (n = 114)	Placebo (n = 385)
Agitation	3%	9%	2%
Anxiety	5%	6%	3%
Insomnia	11%	16%	6%

In clinical studies, these symptoms were sometimes of sufficient magnitude to require treatment with sedative/hypnotic drugs.

Symptoms were sufficiently severe to require discontinuation of treatment in 1% and 2.6% of patients treated with 300 and 400 mg/day, respectively, of WELLBUTRIN SR and 0.8% of patients treated with placebo.

Psychosis, Confusion, and Other Neuropsychiatric Phenomena: Depressed patients treated with an immediate-release formulation of bupropion or with WELLBUTRIN SR have been reported to show a variety of neuropsychiatric signs and symptoms, including delusions, hallucinations, psychosis, concentration disturbance, paranoia, and confusion. In some cases, these symptoms abated upon dose reduction and/or withdrawal of treatment.

Activation of Psychosis and/or Mania: Antidepressants can precipitate manic episodes in bipolar disorder patients during the depressed phase of their illness and may activate latent psychosis in other susceptible patients. WELLBUTRIN SR is expected to pose similar risks.

Altered Appetite and Weight: In placebo-controlled studies, patients experienced weight gain or weight loss as shown in Table 3.

Table 3. Incidence of Weight Gain and Weight Loss in Placebo-Controlled Trials

Weight Change	WELLBUTRIN SR 300 mg/day (n = 339)	WELLBUTRIN SR 400 mg/day (n = 112)	Placebo (n = 347)
Gained >5 lbs	3%	2%	4%
Lost >5 lbs	14%	19%	6%

In studies conducted with the immediate-release formulation of bupropion, 35% of patients receiving tricyclic antidepressants gained weight, compared to 9% of patients treated with the immediate-release formulation of bupropion. If weight loss is a major presenting sign of a patient's depressive illness, the anorectic and/or weight-reducing potential of WELLBUTRIN SR should be considered.

Allergic Reactions: Anaphylactoid/anaphylactic reactions characterized by symptoms such as pruritus, urticaria, angioedema, and dyspnea requiring medical treatment have been reported in clinical trials with bupropion. In addition, there have been rare spontaneous postmarketing reports of erythema multiforme, Stevens-Johnson syndrome, and anaphylactic shock associated with bupropion. A patient should stop taking WELLBUTRIN SR and consult a doctor if experiencing allergic or anaphylactoid/anaphylactic reactions (e.g., skin rash, pruritus, hives, chest pain, edema, and shortness of breath) during treatment.

Arthralgia, myalgia, and fever with rash and other symptoms suggestive of delayed hypersensitivity have been reported in association with bupropion. These symptoms may resemble serum sickness.

Cardiovascular Effects: In clinical practice, hypertension, in some cases severe, requiring acute treatment, has been reported in patients receiving bupropion alone and in combination with nicotine replacement therapy. These events have been observed in both patients with and without evidence of preexisting hypertension.

Data from a comparative study of the sustained-release formulation of bupropion (ZYBAN® Sustained-Release Tablets), nicotine transdermal system (NTS), the combination of sustained-release bupropion plus NTS, and placebo as an aid to smoking cessation suggest a higher incidence of treatment-emergent hypertension in patients treated with the combination of sustained-release bupropion and NTS. In this study, 6.1% of patients treated with the combination of sustained-release bupropion and NTS had treatment-emergent hypertension compared to 2.5%, 1.6%, and 3.1% of patients treated with sustained-release bupropion, NTS, and placebo, respectively. The majority of these patients had evidence of preexisting hypertension. Three patients (1.2%) treated with the combination of ZYBAN and NTS and 1 patient (0.4%) treated with NTS had study medication discontinued due to hypertension compared to none of the patients treated with ZYBAN or placebo. Monitoring of blood pressure is recommended in patients who receive the combination of bupropion and nicotine replacement.

There is no clinical experience establishing the safety of WELLBUTRIN SR Tablets in patients with a recent history of myocardial infarction or unstable heart disease. Therefore, care should be exercised if it is used in these groups. Bupropion was well tolerated in depressed patients who had previously developed orthostatic hypotension while receiving tricyclic antidepressants, and was also generally well tolerated in a group of 36 depressed inpatients with stable congestive heart failure (CHF). However, bupropion was associated with a rise in supine blood pressure in the study of patients with CHF, resulting in discontinuation of treatment in 2 patients for exacerbation of baseline hypertension.

Hepatic Impairment: WELLBUTRIN SR should be used with extreme caution in patients with severe hepatic cirrhosis. In these patients, a reduced frequency and/or dose is required. WELLBUTRIN SR should be used with caution in patients with hepatic impairment (including mild-to-moderate hepatic cirrhosis) and reduced frequency and/or dose should be considered in patients with mild-to-moderate hepatic cirrhosis.

All patients with hepatic impairment should be closely monitored for possible adverse effects that could indicate high drug and metabolite levels (see CLINICAL PHARMACOLOGY, WARNINGS, and DOSAGE AND ADMINISTRATION).

Renal Impairment: There is limited information on the pharmacokinetics of bupropion in patients with renal impairment. An inter-study comparison between normal subjects and patients with end-stage renal failure demonstrated that the parent drug C_{max} and AUC values were comparable in the 2 groups, whereas the hydroxybupropion and threohydrobupropion metabolites had a 2.3- and 2.8-fold increase, respectively, in AUC for patients with end-stage renal failure. A second study, comparing normal subjects and patients with moderate-to-severe renal impairment (GFR 30.9 ± 10.8 mL/min) showed that exposure to a single 150-mg dose of sustained-release bupropion was approximately 2-fold higher in patients with impaired renal function while levels of the hydroxybupropion and threo/erythrohydrobupropion (combined) metabolites were similar in the 2 groups. Bupropion is extensively metabolized in the liver to active metabolites, which are further metabolized and subsequently excreted by the kidneys. WELLBUTRIN SR should be used with caution in patients with renal impairment and a reduced frequency and/or dose should be considered as bupropion and the metabolites of bupropion may accumulate in such patients to a greater extent than usual. The patient should be closely monitored for possible adverse effects that could indicate high drug or metabolite levels.

Information for Patients

Prescribers or other health professionals should inform patients, their families, and their caregivers about the benefits and risks associated with treatment with WELLBUTRIN SR and should counsel them in its appropriate use. A patient Medication Guide about "Antidepressant Medicines, Depression and Other Serious Mental Illnesses, and Suicidal Thoughts or Actions," "Quitting Smoking, Quit-Smoking Medication, Changes in Thinking and Behavior, Depression, and Suicidal Thoughts or Actions," and "What Other Important Information Should I Know About WELLBUTRIN SR?" is available for WELLBUTRIN SR. The prescriber or health professional should instruct patients, their families, and their caregivers to read the Medication Guide and should assist them in understanding its contents. Patients should be given the opportunity to discuss the contents of the Medication Guide and to obtain answers to any questions they may have. The complete text of the Medication Guide is reprinted at the end of this document.

Patients should be advised of the following issues and asked to alert their prescriber if these occur while taking WELLBUTRIN SR.

Clinical Worsening and Suicide Risk in Treating Psychiatric Disorders

Patients, their families, and their caregivers should be encouraged to be alert to the emergence of anxiety, agitation, panic attacks, insomnia, irritability, hostility, aggressiveness, impulsivity, akathisia (psychomotor restlessness), hypomania, mania, other unusual changes in behavior, worsening of depression, and suicidal ideation, especially early during antidepressant treatment and when the dose is adjusted up or down. Families and caregivers of patients should be advised to look for the emergence of such symptoms on a day-to-day basis, since changes may be abrupt. Such symptoms should be reported to the patient's prescriber or health professional, especially if they are severe, abrupt in onset, or were not part of the patient's presenting symptoms. Symptoms such as these may be associated with an increased risk for suicidal thinking and behavior and indicate a need for very close monitoring and possibly changes in the medication.

Neuropsychiatric Symptoms and Suicide Risk in Smoking Cessation Treatment

Although WELLBUTRIN SR is not indicated for smoking cessation treatment, it contains the same active ingredient as ZYBAN which is approved for this use. Patients should be informed that quitting smoking, with or without ZYBAN, may be associated with nicotine withdrawal symptoms (including depression or agitation), or exacerbation of preexisting psychiatric illness. Furthermore, some patients have experienced changes in mood (including depression and mania), psychosis, hallucinations, paranoia, delusions, homicidal ideation, aggression, anxiety, and panic, as well as suicidal ideation, suicide attempt, and completed suicide when attempting to quit smoking while taking ZYBAN. If patients develop agitation, hostility, depressed mood, or changes in thinking or behavior that are not typical for them, or if patients develop suicidal ideation or behavior, they should be urged to report these symptoms to their healthcare provider immediately.

Bupropion-Containing Products

Patients should be made aware that WELLBUTRIN SR contains the same active ingredient found in ZYBAN, used as an aid to smoking cessation treatment, and that WELLBUTRIN SR should not be used in combination with ZYBAN or any other medications that contain bupropion hydrochloride (such as WELLBUTRIN, the immediate-release formulation and WELLBUTRIN XL, the extended-release formulation).

As dose is increased during initial titration to doses above 150 mg/day, patients should be instructed to take WELLBUTRIN SR in 2 divided doses, preferably with at least 8 hours between successive doses, to minimize the risk of seizures.

Patients should be told that WELLBUTRIN SR should be discontinued and not restarted if they experience a seizure while on treatment.

Patients should be told that any CNS-active drug like WELLBUTRIN SR may impair their ability to perform tasks requiring judgment or motor and cognitive skills. Consequently, until they are reasonably certain that WELLBUTRIN SR does not adversely affect their performance, they should refrain from driving an automobile or operating complex, hazardous machinery.

Patients should be told that the excessive use or abrupt discontinuation of alcohol or sedatives (including benzodiazepines) may alter the seizure threshold. Some patients have reported lower alcohol tolerance during treatment with WELLBUTRIN SR. Patients should be advised that the consumption of alcohol should be minimized or avoided.

Patients should be advised to inform their physicians if they are taking or plan to take any prescription or over-the-counter drugs. Concern is warranted because WELLBUTRIN SR and other drugs may affect each other's metabolism.

Patients should be advised to notify their physicians if they become pregnant or intend to become pregnant during therapy.

Patients should be advised to swallow WELLBUTRIN SR tablets whole so that the release rate is not altered. Do not chew, divide, or crush tablets, as this may lead to an increased risk of adverse effects, including seizures.

Laboratory Tests

There are no specific laboratory tests recommended.

Drug Interactions

Because bupropion is extensively metabolized, the coadministration of other drugs may affect its clinical activity. In vitro studies indicate that bupropion is primarily metabolized to hydroxybupropion by the CYP2B6 isoenzyme. Therefore, the potential exists for a drug interaction between WELLBUTRIN SR and drugs that are substrates of or inhibitors/inducers of the CYP2B6 isoenzyme (e.g., orphenadrine, thiotepa, cyclophosphamide, ticlopidine, and clopidogrel). In addition, in vitro studies suggest that paroxetine, sertraline, norfluoxetine, and fluvoxamine as well as nelfinavir inhibit the hydroxylation of bupropion. No clinical studies have been performed to evaluate this finding. The threohydrobupropion metabolite of bupropion does not appear to be produced by the cytochrome P450 isoenzymes. The effects of concomitant administration of cimetidine on the pharmacokinetics of bupropion and its active metabolites were studied in 24 healthy young male volunteers. Following oral administration of two 150-mg WELLBUTRIN SR tablets with and without 800 mg of cimetidine, the pharmacokinetics of bupropion and hydroxybupropion were unaffected. However, there were 16% and 32% increases in the AUC and C_{max}, respectively, of the combined moieties of threohydrobupropion and erythrohydrobupropion.

In a series of studies in healthy volunteers, ritonavir (100 mg twice daily or 600 mg twice daily) or ritonavir 100 mg plus lopinavir 400 mg (KALETRA) twice daily reduced the exposure of bupropion and its major metabolites in a dose dependent manner by approximately 20% to 80%. Similarly, efavirenz 600 mg once daily for 2 weeks reduced the exposure of bupropion by approximately 55%. This effect of ritonavir, KALETRA, and efavirenz is thought to be due to the induction of bupropion metabolism. Patients receiving any of these drugs with bupropion may need increased doses of bupropion, but the maximum recommended dose of bupropion should not be exceeded (see CLINICAL PHARMACOLOGY: Metabolism).

While not systematically studied, certain drugs may induce the metabolism of bupropion (e.g., carbamazepine, phenobarbital, phenytoin).

Multiple oral doses of bupropion had no statistically significant effects on the single-dose pharmacokinetics of lamotrigine in 12 healthy volunteers.

Animal data indicated that bupropion may be an inducer of drug-metabolizing enzymes in humans. In one study, following chronic administration of bupropion, 100 mg 3 times daily to 8 healthy male volunteers for 14 days, there was no evidence of induction of its own metabolism. Nevertheless, there may be the potential for clinically important alterations of blood levels of coadministered drugs.

Drugs Metabolized By Cytochrome P450IID6 (CYP2D6): Many drugs, including most antidepressants (SSRIs, many tricyclics), beta-blockers, antiarrhythmics, and antipsychotics are metabolized by the CYP2D6 isoenzyme. Although bupropion is not metabolized by this isoenzyme, bupropion and hydroxybupropion are inhibitors of CYP2D6 isoenzyme in vitro. In a study of 15 male subjects (aged 19 to 35 years) who were extensive metabolizers of the CYP2D6 isoenzyme, daily doses of bupropion given as 150 mg twice daily followed by a single dose of 50 mg desipramine increased the C_{max}, AUC, and $t_{1/2}$ of desipramine by an average of approximately 2-, 5-, and 2-fold, respectively. The effect was present for at least 7 days after the last dose of bupropion. Concomitant use of bupropion with other drugs metabolized by CYP2D6 has not been formally studied.

Therefore, coadministration of bupropion with drugs that are metabolized by CYP2D6 isoenzyme including certain antidepressants (e.g., nortriptyline, imipramine, desipramine, paroxetine, fluoxetine, sertraline), antipsychotics (e.g., haloperidol, risperidone, thioridazine), beta-blockers (e.g., metoprolol), and Type 1C antiarrhythmics (e.g., propafenone, flecainide), should be approached with caution and should be initiated at the lower end of the dose range of the concomitant medication. If bupropion is added to the treatment regimen of a patient already receiving a drug metabolized by CYP2D6, the need to decrease the dose of the original medication should be considered, particularly for those concomitant medications with a narrow therapeutic index.

Drugs which require metabolic activation by CYP2D6 in order to be effective (e.g., tamoxifen) theoretically could have reduced efficacy when administered concomitantly with inhibitors of CYP2D6 such as bupropion.

Although citalopram is not primarily metabolized by CYP2D6, in one study bupropion increased the C_{max} and AUC of citalopram by 30% and 40%, respectively. Citalopram did not affect the pharmacokinetics of bupropion and its 3 metabolites.

MAO Inhibitors: Concomitant use of MAOIs and bupropion is contraindicated. Bupropion inhibits the reuptake of dopamine and norepinephrine and can increase risk of hypertensive reactions when used concomitantly with drugs that also inhibit the reuptake of dopamine or norepinephrine, including MAOIs. In addition, MAOIs decrease the metabolism of dopamine and norepinephrine. These effects can increase dopaminergic and noradrenergic activity. Studies in animals demonstrate that the acute toxicity of bupropion is enhanced by the MAO inhibitor phenelzine (see CONTRAINDICATIONS and DOSAGE AND ADMINISTRATION).

Levodopa and Amantadine: Limited clinical data suggest a higher incidence of adverse experiences in patients receiving bupropion concurrently with either levodopa or amantadine. Administration of WELLBUTRIN SR to patients receiving either levodopa or amantadine concurrently should be undertaken with caution, using small initial doses and gradual dose increases.

Drugs That Lower Seizure Threshold: Concurrent administration of WELLBUTRIN SR and agents (e.g., antipsychotics, other antidepressants, theophylline, systemic steroids, etc.) that lower seizure threshold should be undertaken only with extreme caution (see WARNINGS). Low initial dosing and gradual dose increases should be employed.

Nicotine Transdermal System: (see PRECAUTIONS: Cardiovascular Effects).

Alcohol: In postmarketing experience, there have been rare reports of adverse neuropsychiatric events or reduced alcohol tolerance in patients who were drinking alcohol during treatment with WELLBUTRIN SR. The consumption of alcohol during treatment with WELLBUTRIN SR should be minimized or avoided (also see CONTRAINDICATIONS).

Drug-Laboratory Test Interactions

False-positive urine immunoassay screening tests for amphetamines have been reported in patients taking bupropion. This is due to lack of specificity of some screening tests. False-positive test results may result even following discontinuation of bupropion therapy. Confirmatory tests, such as gas chromatography/mass spectrometry, will distinguish bupropion from amphetamines.

Carcinogenesis, Mutagenesis, Impairment of Fertility

Lifetime carcinogenicity studies were performed in rats and mice at doses up to 300 and 150 mg/kg/day, respectively. These doses are approximately 7 and 2 times the maximum recommended human dose (MRHD), respectively, on a mg/m^2 basis. In the rat study there was an increase in nodular proliferative lesions of the liver at doses of 100 to 300 mg/kg/day (approximately 2 to 7 times the MRHD on a mg/m^2 basis); lower doses were not tested. The question of whether or not such lesions may be precursors of neoplasms of the liver is currently unresolved. Similar liver lesions were not seen in the mouse study, and no increase in malignant tumors of the liver and other organs was seen in either study.

Bupropion produced a positive response (2 to 3 times control mutation rate) in 2 of 5 strains in the Ames bacterial mutagenicity test and an increase in chromosomal aberrations in 1 of 3 in vivo rat bone marrow cytogenetic studies.

A fertility study in rats at doses up to 300 mg/kg/day revealed no evidence of impaired fertility.

Pregnancy

Teratogenic Effects: Pregnancy Category C. In studies conducted in rats and rabbits, bupropion was administered orally at doses up to 450 and 150 mg/kg/day, respectively (approximately 11 and 7 times the MRHD, respectively, on a mg/m^2 basis), during the period of organogenesis. No clear evidence of teratogenic activity was found in either species; however, in rabbits, slightly increased incidences of fetal malformations and skeletal variations were observed at the lowest dose tested (25 mg/kg/day, approximately equal to the MRHD on a mg/m^2 basis) and greater. Decreased fetal weights were seen at 50 mg/kg and greater.

When rats were administered bupropion at oral doses of up to 300 mg/kg/day (approximately 7 times the MRHD on a mg/m^2 basis) prior to mating and throughout pregnancy and lactation, there were no apparent adverse effects on offspring development.

One study has been conducted in pregnant women. This retrospective, managed-care database study assessed the risk of congenital malformations overall and cardiovascular malformations specifically, following exposure to bupropion in the first trimester compared to the risk of these malformations following exposure to other antidepressants in the first trimester and bupropion outside of the first trimester. This study included 7,005 infants with antidepressant exposure during pregnancy, 1,213 of whom were exposed to bupropion in the first trimester. The study showed no greater risk for congenital malformations overall or cardiovascular malformations specifically, following first trimester bupropion exposure compared to exposure to all other antidepressants in the first trimester, or bupropion outside of the first trimester. The results of this study have not been corroborated. WELLBUTRIN SR should be used during pregnancy only if the potential benefit justifies the potential risk to the fetus.

Labor and Delivery

The effect of WELLBUTRIN SR on labor and delivery in humans is unknown.

Nursing Mothers

Like many other drugs, bupropion and its metabolites are secreted in human milk. Because of the potential for serious adverse reactions in nursing infants from WELLBUTRIN SR, a decision should be made whether to discontinue nursing or to discontinue the drug, taking into account the importance of the drug to the mother.

Pediatric Use

Safety and effectiveness in the pediatric population have not been established (see BOX WARNING and WARNINGS: Clinical Worsening and Suicide Risk in Treating Psychiatric Disorders). Anyone considering the use of WELLBUTRIN SR in a child or adolescent must balance the potential risks with the clinical need.

Geriatric Use

Of the approximately 6,000 patients who participated in clinical trials with bupropion sustained-release tablets (depression and smoking cessation studies), 275 were 65 and over and 47 were 75 and over. In addition, several hundred patients 65 and over participated in clinical trials using the immediate-release formulation of bupropion (depression studies). No overall differences in safety or effectiveness were observed between these subjects and younger subjects, and other reported clinical experience has not identified differences in responses between the elderly and younger patients, but greater sensitivity of some older individuals cannot be ruled out.

A single-dose pharmacokinetic study demonstrated that the disposition of bupropion and its metabolites in elderly subjects was similar to that of younger subjects; however, another pharmacokinetic study, single and multiple dose, has suggested that the elderly are at increased risk for accumulation of bupropion and its metabolites (see CLINICAL PHARMACOLOGY).

Bupropion is extensively metabolized in the liver to active metabolites, which are further metabolized and excreted by the kidneys. The risk of toxic reaction to this drug may be greater in patients with impaired renal function. Because elderly patients are more likely to have decreased renal function, care should be taken in dose selection, and it may be useful to monitor renal function (see PRECAUTIONS: Renal Impairment and DOSAGE AND ADMINISTRATION).

ADVERSE REACTIONS

(See also WARNINGS and PRECAUTIONS.)

The information included under the Incidence in Controlled Trials subsection of ADVERSE REACTIONS is based primarily on data from controlled clinical trials with WELLBUTRIN SR. Information on additional adverse events associated with the sustained-release formulation of bupropion in smoking cessation trials, as well as the immediate-release formulation of bupropion, is included in a separate section (see Other Events Observed During the Clinical Development and Postmarketing Experience of Bupropion).

Incidence in Controlled Trials With WELLBUTRIN SR

Adverse Events Associated With Discontinuation of Treatment Among Patients Treated With WELLBUTRIN SR: In placebo-controlled clinical trials, 9% and 11% of patients treated with 300 and 400 mg/day, respectively, of WELLBUTRIN SR and 4% of patients treated with placebo discontinued treatment due to adverse events. The specific adverse events in these trials that led to discontinuation in at least 1% of patients treated with either 300 or 400 mg/day of WELLBUTRIN SR and at a rate at least twice the placebo rate are listed in Table 4.

Table 4. Treatment Discontinuations Due to Adverse Events in Placebo-Controlled Trials

Adverse Event Term	WELLBUTRIN SR 300 mg/day (n = 376)	WELLBUTRIN SR 400 mg/day (n = 114)	Placebo (n = 385)
Rash	2.4%	0.9%	0.0%
Nausea	0.8%	1.8%	0.3%
Agitation	0.3%	1.8%	0.3%
Migraine	0.0%	1.8%	0.3%

Adverse Events Occurring at an Incidence of 1% or More Among Patients Treated With WELLBUTRIN SR: Table 5 enumerates treatment-emergent adverse events that occurred among patients treated with 300 and 400 mg/day of WELLBUTRIN SR and with placebo in placebo-controlled trials. Events that occurred in either the 300- or 400-mg/day group at an incidence of 1% or more and were more frequent than in the placebo group are included. Reported adverse events were classified using a COSTART-based Dictionary.

Accurate estimates of the incidence of adverse events associated with the use of any drug are difficult to obtain. Estimates are influenced by drug dose, detection technique, setting, physician judgments, etc. The figures cited cannot be used to predict precisely the incidence of untoward events in the course of usual medical practice where patient characteristics and other factors differ from those that prevailed in the clinical trials. These incidence figures also cannot be compared with those obtained from other clinical studies involving related drug products as each group of drug trials is conducted under a different set of conditions.

Finally, it is important to emphasize that the tabulation does not reflect the relative severity and/or clinical importance of the events. A better perspective on the serious adverse events associated with the use of WELLBUTRIN SR is provided in the WARNINGS and PRECAUTIONS sections.

[See table 5 at top of next page]

Table 5. Treatment-Emergent Adverse Events in Placebo-Controlled Trials[a]

Body System/ Adverse Event	WELLBUTRIN SR 300 mg/day (n = 376)	WELLBUTRIN SR 400 mg/day (n = 114)	Placebo (n = 385)
Body (General)			
Headache	26%	25%	23%
Infection	8%	9%	6%
Abdominal pain	3%	9%	2%
Asthenia	2%	4%	2%
Chest pain	3%	4%	1%
Pain	2%	3%	2%
Fever	1%	2%	—
Cardiovascular			
Palpitation	2%	6%	2%
Flushing	1%	4%	—
Migraine	1%	4%	1%
Hot flashes	1%	3%	1%
Digestive			
Dry mouth	17%	24%	7%
Nausea	13%	18%	8%
Constipation	10%	5%	7%
Diarrhea	5%	7%	6%
Anorexia	5%	3%	2%
Vomiting	4%	2%	2%
Dysphagia	0%	2%	0%
Musculoskeletal			
Myalgia	2%	6%	3%
Arthralgia	1%	4%	1%
Arthritis	0%	2%	0%
Twitch	1%	2%	—
Nervous system			
Insomnia	11%	16%	6%
Dizziness	7%	11%	5%
Agitation	3%	9%	2%
Anxiety	5%	6%	3%
Tremor	6%	3%	1%
Nervousness	5%	3%	3%
Somnolence	2%	3%	2%
Irritability	3%	2%	2%
Memory decreased	—	3%	1%
Paresthesia	1%	2%	1%
Central nervous system stimulation	2%	1%	1%
Respiratory			
Pharyngitis	3%	11%	2%
Sinusitis	3%	1%	2%
Increased cough	1%	2%	1%
Skin			
Sweating	6%	5%	2%
Rash	5%	4%	1%
Pruritus	2%	4%	2%
Urticaria	2%	1%	0%
Special senses			
Tinnitus	6%	6%	2%
Taste perversion	2%	4%	—
Blurred vision or diplopia	3%	2%	2%
Urogenital			
Urinary frequency	2%	5%	2%
Urinary urgency	—	2%	0%
Vaginal hemorrhage[b]	0%	2%	—
Urinary tract infection	1%	0%	—

[a] Adverse events that occurred in at least 1% of patients treated with either 300 or 400 mg/day of WELLBUTRIN SR, but equally or more frequently in the placebo group, were: abnormal dreams, accidental injury, acne, appetite increased, back pain, bronchitis, dysmenorrhea, dyspepsia, flatulence, flu syndrome, hypertension, neck pain, respiratory disorder, rhinitis, and tooth disorder.

[b]Incidence based on the number of female patients.

— Hyphen denotes adverse events occurring in greater than 0 but less than 0.5% of patients.

Incidence of Commonly Observed Adverse Events in Controlled Clinical Trials: Adverse events from Table 5 occurring in at least 5% of patients treated with WELLBUTRIN SR and at a rate at least twice the placebo rate are listed below for the 300- and 400-mg/day dose groups.

WELLBUTRIN SR 300 mg/day: Anorexia, dry mouth, rash, sweating, tinnitus, and tremor.

WELLBUTRIN SR 400 mg/day: Abdominal pain, agitation, anxiety, dizziness, dry mouth, insomnia, myalgia, nausea, palpitation, pharyngitis, sweating, tinnitus, and urinary frequency.

Other Events Observed During the Clinical Development and Postmarketing Experience of Bupropion

In addition to the adverse events noted above, the following events have been reported in clinical trials and postmarketing experience with the sustained-release formulation of bupropion in depressed patients and in nondepressed smokers, as well as in clinical trials and postmarketing clinical experience with the immediate-release formulation of bupropion.

Adverse events for which frequencies are provided below occurred in clinical trials with the sustained-release formulation of bupropion. The frequencies represent the proportion of patients who experienced a treatment-emergent adverse event on at least one occasion in placebo-controlled studies for depression (n = 987) or smoking cessation (n = 1,013), or patients who experienced an adverse event requiring discontinuation of treatment in an open-label surveillance study with WELLBUTRIN SR (n = 3,100). All treatment-emergent adverse events are included except those listed in Tables 2 through 5, those events listed in other safety-related sections, those adverse events subsumed under COSTART terms that are either overly general or excessively specific so as to be uninformative, those events not reasonably associated with the use of the drug, and those events that were not serious and occurred in fewer than 2 patients. Events of major clinical importance are described in the WARNINGS and PRECAUTIONS sections of the labeling.

Events are further categorized by body system and listed in order of decreasing frequency according to the following definitions of frequency: Frequent adverse events are defined as those occurring in at least 1/100 patients. Infrequent adverse events are those occurring in 1/100 to 1/1,000 patients, while rare events are those occurring in less than 1/1,000 patients.

Adverse events for which frequencies are not provided occurred in clinical trials or postmarketing experience with bupropion. Only those adverse events not previously listed for sustained-release bupropion are included. The extent to which these events may be associated with WELLBUTRIN SR is unknown.

Body (General): Infrequent were chills, facial edema, musculoskeletal chest pain, and photosensitivity. Rare was malaise. Also observed were arthralgia, myalgia, and fever with rash and other symptoms suggestive of delayed hypersensitivity. These symptoms may resemble serum sickness (see PRECAUTIONS).

Cardiovascular: Infrequent were postural hypotension, stroke, tachycardia, and vasodilation. Rare was syncope. Also observed were complete atrioventricular block, extrasystoles, hypotension, hypertension (in some cases severe, see PRECAUTIONS), myocardial infarction, phlebitis, and pulmonary embolism.

Digestive: Infrequent were abnormal liver function, bruxism, gastric reflux, gingivitis, glossitis, increased salivation, jaundice, mouth ulcers, stomatitis, and thirst. Rare was edema of tongue. Also observed were colitis, esophagitis, gastrointestinal hemorrhage, gum hemorrhage, hepatitis, intestinal perforation, liver damage, pancreatitis, and stomach ulcer.

Endocrine: Also observed were hyperglycemia, hypoglycemia, and syndrome of inappropriate antidiuretic hormone.

Hemic and Lymphatic: Infrequent was ecchymosis. Also observed were anemia, leukocytosis, leukopenia, lymphadenopathy, pancytopenia, and thrombocytopenia. Altered PT and/or INR, infrequently associated with hemorrhagic or thrombotic complications, were observed when bupropion was coadministered with warfarin.

Metabolic and Nutritional: Infrequent were edema and peripheral edema. Also observed was glycosuria.

Musculoskeletal: Infrequent were leg cramps. Also observed were muscle rigidity/fever/rhabdomyolysis and muscle weakness.

Nervous System: Infrequent were abnormal coordination, decreased libido, depersonalization, dysphoria, emotional lability, hostility, hyperkinesia, hypertonia, hypesthesia, suicidal ideation, and vertigo. Rare were amnesia, ataxia, derealization, and hypomania. Also observed were abnormal electroencephalogram (EEG), akinesia, aggression, aphasia, coma, completed suicide, delirium, delusions, dysarthria, dyskinesia, dystonia, euphoria, extrapyramidal syndrome, hallucinations, hypokinesia, increased libido, manic reaction, neuralgia, neuropathy, paranoid ideation, restlessness, suicide attempt, and unmasking tardive dyskinesia.

Respiratory: Rare was bronchospasm. Also observed was pneumonia.

Skin: Rare was maculopapular rash. Also observed were alopecia, angioedema, exfoliative dermatitis, and hirsutism.

Special Senses: Infrequent were accommodation abnormality and dry eye. Also observed were deafness, diplopia, increased intraocular pressure, and mydriasis.

Urogenital: Infrequent were impotence, polyuria, and prostate disorder. Also observed were abnormal ejaculation, cystitis, dyspareunia, dysuria, gynecomastia, menopause, painful erection, salpingitis, urinary incontinence, urinary retention, and vaginitis.

DRUG ABUSE AND DEPENDENCE

Controlled Substance Class

Bupropion is not a controlled substance.

Humans

Controlled clinical studies of bupropion (immediate-release formulation) conducted in normal volunteers, in subjects with a history of multiple drug abuse, and in depressed patients showed some increase in motor activity and agitation/excitement.

In a population of individuals experienced with drugs of abuse, a single dose of 400 mg of bupropion produced mild amphetamine-like activity as compared to placebo on the Morphine-Benzedrine Subscale of the Addiction Research Center Inventories (ARCI), and a score intermediate between placebo and amphetamine on the Liking Scale of the ARCI. These scales measure general feelings of euphoria and drug desirability.

Findings in clinical trials, however, are not known to reliably predict the abuse potential of drugs. Nonetheless, evidence from single-dose studies does suggest that the recommended daily dosage of bupropion when administered in divided doses is not likely to be especially reinforcing to amphetamine or stimulant abusers. However, higher doses that could not be tested because of the risk of seizure might be modestly attractive to those who abuse stimulant drugs.

Animals

Studies in rodents and primates have shown that bupropion exhibits some pharmacologic actions common to psychostimulants. In rodents, it has been shown to increase locomotor activity, elicit a mild stereotyped behavioral response, and increase rates of responding in several schedule-controlled behavior paradigms. In primate models to assess the positive reinforcing effects of psychoactive drugs, bupropion was self-administered intravenously. In rats, bupropion produced amphetamine-like and cocaine-like discriminative stimulus effects in drug discrimination paradigms used to characterize the subjective effects of psychoactive drugs.

OVERDOSAGE

Human Overdose Experience

Overdoses of up to 30 g or more of bupropion have been reported. Seizure was reported in approximately one-third of all cases. Other serious reactions reported with overdoses of bupropion alone included hallucinations, loss of consciousness, sinus tachycardia, and ECG changes such as conduction disturbances (including QRS prolongation) or arrhythmias. Fever, muscle rigidity, rhabdomyolysis, hypotension, stupor, coma, and respiratory failure have been reported mainly when bupropion was part of multiple drug overdoses.

Although most patients recovered without sequelae, deaths associated with overdoses of bupropion alone have been reported in patients ingesting large doses of the drug. Multiple uncontrolled seizures, bradycardia, cardiac failure, and cardiac arrest prior to death were reported in these patients.

Overdosage Management

Ensure an adequate airway, oxygenation, and ventilation. Monitor cardiac rhythm and vital signs. EEG monitoring is also recommended for the first 48 hours post-ingestion. General supportive and symptomatic measures are also recommended. Induction of emesis is not recommended.

Activated charcoal should be administered. There is no experience with the use of forced diuresis, dialysis, hemoperfusion, or exchange transfusion in the management of bupropion overdoses. No specific antidotes for bupropion are known.

Due to the dose-related risk of seizures with WELLBUTRIN SR, hospitalization following suspected overdose should be considered. Based on studies in animals, it is recommended that seizures be treated with intravenous benzodiazepine administration and other supportive measures, as appropriate.

In managing overdosage, consider the possibility of multiple drug involvement. The physician should consider contacting a poison control center for additional information on the treatment of any overdose. Telephone numbers for certified poison control centers are listed in the *Physicians' Desk Reference* (PDR).

DOSAGE AND ADMINISTRATION

General Dosing Considerations

It is particularly important to administer WELLBUTRIN SR in a manner most likely to minimize the risk of seizure (see WARNINGS). Gradual escalation in dosage is also important if agitation, motor restlessness, and insomnia, often seen during the initial days of treatment, are to be minimized. If necessary, these effects may be managed by temporary reduction of dose or the short-term administration of an intermediate to long-acting sedative hypnotic. A sedative hypnotic usually is not required beyond the first week of treatment. Insomnia may also be minimized by avoiding bedtime doses. If distressing, untoward effects supervene, dose escalation should be stopped. WELLBUTRIN SR should be swallowed whole and not crushed, divided, or chewed, as this may lead to an increased risk of adverse effects including seizures.

Initial Treatment

The usual adult target dose for WELLBUTRIN SR is 300 mg/day, given as 150 mg twice daily. Dosing with WELLBUTRIN SR should begin at 150 mg/day given as a single daily dose in the morning. If the 150-mg initial dose is adequately tolerated, an increase to the 300-mg/day target dose, given as 150 mg twice daily, may be made as early as day 4 of dosing. There should be an interval of at least 8 hours between successive doses.

Increasing the Dosage Above 300 mg/day

As with other antidepressants, the full antidepressant effect of WELLBUTRIN SR may not be evident until 4 weeks of treatment or longer. An increase in dosage to the maximum of 400 mg/day, given as 200 mg twice daily, may be considered for patients in whom no clinical improvement is noted after several weeks of treatment at 300 mg/day.

Maintenance Treatment

It is generally agreed that acute episodes of depression require several months or longer of sustained pharmacological therapy beyond response to the acute episode. In a study in which patients with major depressive disorder, recurrent type, who had responded during 8 weeks of acute treatment with WELLBUTRIN SR were assigned randomly to placebo or to the same dose of WELLBUTRIN SR (150 mg twice daily) during 44 weeks of maintenance treatment as they had received during the acute stabilization phase, longer-term efficacy was demonstrated (see CLINICAL TRIALS under CLINICAL PHARMACOLOGY). Based on these limited data, it is unknown whether or not the dose of WELLBUTRIN SR needed for maintenance treatment is identical to the dose needed to achieve an initial response. Patients should be periodically reassessed to determine the need for maintenance treatment and the appropriate dose for such treatment.

Dosage Adjustment for Patients With Impaired Hepatic Function

WELLBUTRIN SR should be used with extreme caution in patients with severe hepatic cirrhosis. The dose should not exceed 100 mg every day or 150 mg every other day in these patients. WELLBUTRIN SR should be used with caution in patients with hepatic impairment (including mild-to-moderate hepatic cirrhosis) and a reduced frequency and/or dose should be considered in patients with mild-to-moderate hepatic cirrhosis (see CLINICAL PHARMACOLOGY, WARNINGS, and PRECAUTIONS).

Dosage Adjustment for Patients With Impaired Renal Function

WELLBUTRIN SR should be used with caution in patients with renal impairment and a reduced frequency and/or dose should be considered (see CLINICAL PHARMACOLOGY and PRECAUTIONS).

Switching a Patient To or From a Monoamine Oxidase Inhibitor (MAOI) Antidepressant

At least 14 days should elapse between discontinuation of an MAOI intended to treat depression and initiation of therapy with WELLBUTRIN SR. Conversely, at least 14 days should be allowed after stopping WELLBUTRIN SR before starting an MAOI antidepressant (see CONTRAINDICATIONS and DRUG INTERACTIONS).

Use of WELLBUTRIN SR With Reversible MAOIs Such as Linezolid or Methylene Blue

Do not start WELLBUTRIN SR in a patient who is being treated with a reversible MAOI such as linezolid or intravenous methylene blue. Drug interactions can increase the risk of hypertensive reactions. In a patient who requires more urgent treatment of a psychiatric condition, non-pharmacological interventions, including hospitalization, should be considered (see CONTRAINDICATIONS and DRUG INTERACTIONS).

In some cases, a patient already receiving therapy with WELLBUTRIN SR may require urgent treatment with linezolid or intravenous methylene blue. If acceptable alternatives to linezolid or intravenous methylene blue treatment are not available and the potential benefits of linezolid or intravenous methylene blue treatment are judged to outweigh the risks of hypertensive reactions in a particular patient, WELLBUTRIN SR should be stopped promptly, and linezolid or intravenous methylene blue can be administered. The patient should be monitored for 2 weeks or until 24 hours after the last dose of linezolid or intravenous methylene blue, whichever comes first. Therapy with WELLBUTRIN SR may be resumed 24 hours after the last dose of linezolid or intravenous methylene blue.

The risk of administering methylene blue by non-intravenous routes (such as oral tablets or by local injection) or in intravenous doses much lower than 1 mg/kg with WELLBUTRIN SR is unclear. The clinician should, nevertheless, be aware of the possibility of a drug interaction with such use (see CONTRAINDICATIONS and DRUG INTERACTIONS).

HOW SUPPLIED

WELLBUTRIN SR Sustained-Release Tablets, 100 mg of bupropion hydrochloride, are blue, round, biconvex, film-coated tablets printed with "WELLBUTRIN SR 100" in bottles of 60 (NDC 0173-0947-55) tablets.

WELLBUTRIN SR Sustained-Release Tablets, 150 mg of bupropion hydrochloride, are purple, round, biconvex, film-coated tablets printed with "WELLBUTRIN SR 150" in bottles of 60 (NDC 0173-0135-55) tablets.

WELLBUTRIN SR Sustained-Release Tablets, 200 mg of bupropion hydrochloride, are light pink, round, biconvex, film-coated tablets printed with "WELLBUTRIN SR 200" in bottles of 60 (NDC 0173-0722-00) tablets.

Store at controlled room temperature, 20° to 25°C (68° to 77°F) [see USP]. Dispense in a tight, light-resistant container as defined in the USP.

WELLBUTRIN, WELLBUTRIN SR, WELLBUTRIN XL, and ZYBAN are registered trademarks of GlaxoSmithKline. KALETRA is a registered trademark of Abbott Laboratories.

Distributed by:
GlaxoSmithKline
Research Triangle Park, NC 27709

Manufactured by:
GlaxoSmithKline
Research Triangle Park, NC 27709
or DSM Pharmaceuticals, Inc.
Greenville, NC 27834

March 2013
WLS:9PI

MEDICATION GUIDE

WELLBUTRIN SR® (WELL byu-trin)

(bupropion hydrochloride) Sustained-Release Tablets

Read this Medication Guide carefully before you start using WELLBUTRIN SR and each time you get a refill. There may be new information. This information does not take the place of talking with your doctor about your medical condition or your treatment. If you have any questions about WELLBUTRIN SR, ask your doctor or pharmacist.

IMPORTANT: Be sure to read the three sections of this Medication Guide. The first section is about the risk of suicidal thoughts and actions with antidepressant medicines; the second section is about the risk of changes in thinking and behavior, depression and suicidal thoughts or actions with medicines used to quit smoking; and the third section is entitled "What Other Important Information Should I Know About WELLBUTRIN SR?"

Antidepressant Medicines, Depression and Other Serious Mental Illnesses, and Suicidal Thoughts or Actions

This section of the Medication Guide is only about the risk of suicidal thoughts and actions with antidepressant medicines. **Talk to your, or your family member's, healthcare provider about:**

- all risks and benefits of treatment with antidepressant medicines
- all treatment choices for depression or other serious mental illness

What is the most important information I should know about antidepressant medicines, depression and other serious mental illnesses, and suicidal thoughts or actions?

1. **Antidepressant medicines may increase suicidal thoughts or actions in some children, teenagers, and young adults within the first few months of treatment.**
2. **Depression and other serious mental illnesses are the most important causes of suicidal thoughts and actions. Some people may have a particularly high risk of having suicidal thoughts or actions.** These include people who have (or have a family history of) bipolar illness (also called manic-depressive illness) or suicidal thoughts or actions.
3. **How can I watch for and try to prevent suicidal thoughts and actions in myself or a family member?**
   - Pay close attention to any changes, especially sudden changes, in mood, behaviors, thoughts, or feelings. This is very important when an antidepressant medicine is started or when the dose is changed.
   - Call the healthcare provider right away to report new or sudden changes in mood, behavior, thoughts, or feelings.
   - Keep all follow-up visits with the healthcare provider as scheduled. Call the healthcare provider between visits as needed, especially if you have concerns about symptoms.

Call a healthcare provider right away if you or your family member has any of the following symptoms, especially if they are new, worse, or worry you:

• thoughts about suicide or dying	• trouble sleeping (insomnia)
• attempts to commit suicide	• new or worse irritability
• new or worse depression	• acting aggressive, being angry, or violent
• new or worse anxiety	• acting on dangerous impulses
• feeling very agitated or restless	• an extreme increase in activity and talking (mania)
• panic attacks	• other unusual changes in behavior or mood

What else do I need to know about antidepressant medicines?

- **Never stop an antidepressant medicine without first talking to a healthcare provider.** Stopping an antidepressant medicine suddenly can cause other symptoms.
- **Antidepressants are medicines used to treat depression and other illnesses.** It is important to discuss all the risks of treating depression and also the risks of not treating it.

Patients and their families or other caregivers should discuss all treatment choices with the healthcare provider, not just the use of antidepressants.

- **Antidepressant medicines have other side effects.** Talk to the healthcare provider about the side effects of the medicine prescribed for you or your family member.
- **Antidepressant medicines can interact with other medicines.** Know all of the medicines that you or your family member takes. Keep a list of all medicines to show the healthcare provider. Do not start new medicines without first checking with your healthcare provider.
- **Not all antidepressant medicines prescribed for children are FDA approved for use in children.** Talk to your child's healthcare provider for more information.

WELLBUTRIN SR has not been studied in children under the age of 18 and is not approved for use in children and teenagers.

Quitting Smoking, Quit-Smoking Medications, Changes in Thinking and Behavior, Depression, and Suicidal Thoughts or Actions

This section of the Medication Guide is only about the risk of changes in thinking and behavior, depression and suicidal thoughts or actions with drugs used to quit smoking.

Although WELLBUTRIN SR is not a treatment for quitting smoking, it contains the same active ingredient (bupropion hydrochloride) as ZYBAN® which is used to help patients quit smoking.

Some people have had changes in behavior, hostility, agitation, depression, suicidal thoughts or actions while taking bupropion to help them quit smoking. These symptoms can develop during treatment with bupropion or after stopping treatment with bupropion.

If you, your family member, or your caregiver notice agitation, hostility, depression, or changes in thinking or behavior that are not typical for you, or you have any of the following symptoms, stop taking bupropion and call your healthcare provider right away:

• thoughts about suicide or dying	• an extreme increase in activity and talking (mania)
• attempts to commit suicide	• abnormal thoughts or sensations
• new or worse depression	• seeing or hearing things that are not there (hallucinations)
• new or worse anxiety	• feeling people are against you (paranoia)
• panic attacks	• feeling confused
• feeling very agitated or restless	• other unusual changes in behavior or mood
• acting aggressive, being angry, or violent	
• acting on dangerous impulses	

When you try to quit smoking, with or without bupropion, you may have symptoms that may be due to nicotine withdrawal, including urge to smoke, depressed mood, trouble sleeping, irritability, frustration, anger, feeling anxious, difficulty concentrating, restlessness, decreased heart rate, and increased appetite or weight gain. Some people have even experienced suicidal thoughts when trying to quit smoking without medication. Sometimes quitting smoking can lead to worsening of mental health problems that you already have, such as depression.

Before taking bupropion, tell your healthcare provider if you have ever had depression or other mental illnesses. You should also tell your doctor about any symptoms you had during other times you tried to quit smoking, with or without bupropion.

What Other Important Information Should I Know About WELLBUTRIN SR?

- **Seizures: There is a chance of having a seizure (convulsion, fit) with WELLBUTRIN SR, especially in people:**
  - with certain medical problems.
  - who take certain medicines.

The chance of having seizures increases with higher doses of WELLBUTRIN SR. For more information, see the sections "Who should not take WELLBUTRIN SR?" and "What should I tell my doctor before using WELLBUTRIN SR?" Tell your doctor about all of your medical conditions and all the medicines you take. **Do not take any other medicines while you are using WELLBUTRIN SR unless your doctor has said it is okay to take them.**

If you have a seizure while taking WELLBUTRIN SR, stop taking the tablets and call your doctor right away. Do not take WELLBUTRIN SR again if you have a seizure.

- **High blood pressure (hypertension).Some people get high blood pressure, that can be severe, while taking WELLBUTRIN SR.** The chance of high blood pressure may be higher if you also use nicotine replacement therapy (such as a nicotine patch) to help you stop smoking.
- **Severe allergic reactions. Some people have severe allergic reaction to WELLBUTRIN SR. Stop taking WELLBUTRIN SR and call your doctor right away** if you get a rash, itching, hives, fever, swollen lymph glands, painful sores in the mouth or around the eyes, swelling of the lips or tongue, chest pain, or have trouble breathing. These could be signs of a serious allergic reaction.
- **Unusual thoughts or behaviors.** Some patients have unusual thoughts or behaviors while taking WELLBUTRIN SR, including delusions (believe you are someone else), hallucinations (seeing or hearing things that are not there), paranoia (feeling that people are against you), or feeling confused. If this happens to you, call your doctor.

What is WELLBUTRIN SR?

WELLBUTRIN SR is a prescription medicine used to treat adults with a certain type of depression called major depressive disorder.

Who should not take WELLBUTRIN SR?

Do not take WELLBUTRIN SR if you:

- have or had a seizure disorder or epilepsy.
- **are taking ZYBAN® (used to help people stop smoking) or any other medicines that contain bupropion hydrochloride, such as WELLBUTRIN® Tablets or WELLBUTRIN XL® Extended-Release Tablets.** Bupropion is the same active ingredient that is in WELLBUTRIN SR.
- drink a lot of alcohol and abruptly stop drinking, or use medicines called sedatives (these make you sleepy) or benzodiazepines and you stop using them all of a sudden.
- take a monoamine oxidase inhibitor (MAOI). Ask your healthcare provider or pharmacist if you are not sure if you take an MAOI, including the antibiotic linezolid.
  - do not take an MAOI within 2 weeks of stopping WELLBUTRIN SR unless directed to do so by your physician.
  - do not start WELLBUTRIN SR if you stopped taking an MAOI in the last 2 weeks unless directed to do so by your physician.
- have or had an eating disorder such as anorexia nervosa or bulimia.
- are allergic to the active ingredient in WELLBUTRIN SR, bupropion, or to any of the inactive ingredients. See the end of this leaflet for a complete list of ingredients in WELLBUTRIN SR.

What should I tell my doctor before using WELLBUTRIN SR?

Tell your doctor if you have ever had depression, suicidal thoughts or actions, or other mental health problems. See "Antidepressant Medicines, Depression and Other Serious Mental Illnesses, and Suicidal Thoughts or Actions."

- Tell your doctor about your other medical conditions including if you:
  - **are pregnant or plan to become pregnant.** It is not known if WELLBUTRIN SR can harm your unborn baby.
  - **are breastfeeding.** WELLBUTRIN SR passes through your milk. It is not known if WELLBUTRIN SR can harm your baby.
  - **have liver problems,** especially cirrhosis of the liver.
  - have kidney problems.
  - have an eating disorder such as anorexia nervosa or bulimia.
  - have had a head injury.
  - have had a seizure (convulsion, fit).
  - have a tumor in your nervous system (brain or spine).
  - have had a heart attack, heart problems, or high blood pressure.
  - are a diabetic taking insulin or other medicines to control your blood sugar.
  - drink a lot of alcohol.
  - abuse prescription medicines or street drugs.
- **Tell your doctor about all the medicines you take,** including prescription and non-prescription medicines, vitamins, and herbal supplements. Many medicines increase your chances of having seizures or other serious side effects if you take them while you are using WELLBUTRIN SR.

How should I take WELLBUTRIN SR?

- Take WELLBUTRIN SR exactly as prescribed by your doctor.
- **Do not chew, cut, or crush WELLBUTRIN SR tablets.** If you do, the medicine will be released into your body too quickly. If this happens you may be more likely to get side effects including seizures. You must swallow the tablets whole. **Tell your doctor if you cannot swallow medicine tablets.**
- Take WELLBUTRIN SR at the same time each day.
- Take your doses of WELLBUTRIN SR at least 8 hours apart.
- You may take WELLBUTRIN SR with or without food.
- If you miss a dose, do not take an extra tablet to make up for the dose you forgot. Wait and take your next tablet at the regular time. **This is very important.** Too much WELLBUTRIN SR can increase your chance of having a seizure.
- If you take too much WELLBUTRIN SR, or overdose, call your local emergency room or poison control center right away.
- **Do not take any other medicines while using WELLBUTRIN SR unless your doctor has told you it is okay.**
- It may take several weeks for you to feel that WELLBUTRIN SR is working. Once you feel better, it is important to keep taking WELLBUTRIN SR exactly as directed by your doctor. Call your doctor if you do not feel WELLBUTRIN SR is working for you.
- Do not change your dose or stop taking WELLBUTRIN SR without talking with your doctor first.

What should I avoid while taking WELLBUTRIN SR?

- Do not drink a lot of alcohol while taking WELLBUTRIN SR. If you usually drink a lot of alcohol, talk with your doctor before suddenly stopping. If you suddenly stop drinking alcohol, you may increase your chance of having seizures.
- Do not drive a car or use heavy machinery until you know how WELLBUTRIN SR affects you. WELLBUTRIN SR can impair your ability to perform these tasks.

What are possible side effects of WELLBUTRIN SR?

WELLBUTRIN SR can cause serious side effects. Read this entire Medication Guide for more information about these serious side effects.

The most common side effects of WELLBUTRIN SR are loss of appetite, dry mouth, skin rash, sweating, ringing in the ears, shakiness, stomach pain, agitation, anxiety, dizziness, trouble sleeping, muscle pain, nausea, fast heartbeat, sore throat, and urinating more often.

If you have nausea, take your medicine with food. If you have trouble sleeping, do not take your medicine too close to bedtime.

These are not all the side effects of WELLBUTRIN SR. For a complete list, ask your doctor or pharmacist.

Call your doctor for medical advice about side effects. You may report side effects to FDA at 1-800-FDA-1088.

How should I store WELLBUTRIN SR?

- Store WELLBUTRIN SR at room temperature. Store out of direct sunlight. Keep WELLBUTRIN SR in its tightly closed bottle.
- WELLBUTRIN SR tablets may have an odor.

General Information about WELLBUTRIN SR.

Medicines are sometimes prescribed for purposes other than those listed in a Medication Guide. Do not use WELLBUTRIN SR for a condition for which it was not prescribed. Do not give WELLBUTRIN SR to other people, even if they have the same symptoms you have. It may harm them. Keep WELLBUTRIN SR out of the reach of children.

If you take a urine drug screening test, WELLBUTRIN SR may make the test result positive for amphetamines. If you tell the person giving you the drug screening test that you are taking WELLBUTRIN SR, they can do a more specific drug screening test that should not have this problem.

This Medication Guide summarizes important information about WELLBUTRIN SR. For more information, talk with your doctor. You can ask your doctor or pharmacist for information about WELLBUTRIN SR that is written for health professionals.

What are the ingredients in WELLBUTRIN SR?

Active ingredient: bupropion hydrochloride.

Inactive ingredients: carnauba wax, cysteine hydrochloride, hypromellose, magnesium stearate, microcrystalline cellulose, polyethylene glycol, polysorbate 80, and titanium dioxide. In addition, the 100-mg tablet contains FD&C Blue No. 1 Lake, the 150-mg tablet contains FD&C Blue No. 2 Lake and FD&C Red No. 40 Lake, and the 200-mg tablet contains FD&C Red No. 40 Lake. The tablets are printed with edible black ink.

This Medication Guide has been approved by the U.S. Food and Drug Administration.

WELLBUTRIN, WELLBUTRIN SR, WELLBUTRIN XL and ZYBAN are registered trademarks of GlaxoSmithKline.

Distributed by:
GlaxoSmithKline
Research Triangle Park, NC 27709

Manufactured by:
GlaxoSmithKline
Research Triangle Park, NC 27709
or DSM Pharmaceuticals, Inc.
Greenville, NC 27834

March 2013
WLS:8MG

ZANTAC® 150 ℞
(ranitidine hydrochloride)
Tablets, USP

ZANTAC® 300 ℞
(ranitidine hydrochloride)
Tablets, USP

ZANTAC® ℞
(ranitidine hydrochloride)
Syrup, USP

DESCRIPTION

The active ingredient in ZANTAC 150 Tablets, ZANTAC 300 Tablets, and ZANTAC Syrup is ranitidine hydrochloride

(HCl), USP, a histamine H_2-receptor antagonist. Chemically it is N[2-[[[5-[(dimethylamino)methyl]-2-furanyl]methyl]thio]ethyl]-N′-methyl-2-nitro-1,1-ethenediamine, HCl. It has the following structure:

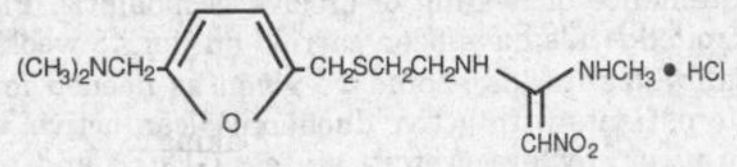

The empirical formula is $C_{13}H_{22}N_4O_3S \cdot HCl$, representing a molecular weight of 350.87.
Ranitidine HCl is a white to pale yellow, granular substance that is soluble in water. It has a slightly bitter taste and sulfur-like odor.
Each ZANTAC 150 Tablet for oral administration contains 168 mg of ranitidine HCl equivalent to 150 mg of ranitidine. Each tablet also contains the inactive ingredients FD&C Yellow No. 6 Aluminum Lake, hypromellose, magnesium stearate, microcrystalline cellulose, titanium dioxide, triacetin, and yellow iron oxide.
Each ZANTAC 300 Tablet for oral administration contains 336 mg of ranitidine HCl equivalent to 300 mg of ranitidine. Each tablet also contains the inactive ingredients croscarmellose sodium, D&C Yellow No. 10 Aluminum Lake, hypromellose, magnesium stearate, microcrystalline cellulose, titanium dioxide, and triacetin.
Each 1 mL of ZANTAC Syrup contains 16.8 mg of ranitidine HCl equivalent to 15 mg of ranitidine. ZANTAC Syrup also contains the inactive ingredients alcohol (7.5%), butylparaben, dibasic sodium phosphate, hypromellose, peppermint flavor, monobasic potassium phosphate, propylparaben, purified water, saccharin sodium, sodium chloride, and sorbitol.

CLINICAL PHARMACOLOGY

ZANTAC is a competitive, reversible inhibitor of the action of histamine at the histamine H_2-receptors, including receptors on the gastric cells. ZANTAC does not lower serum Ca++ in hypercalcemic states. ZANTAC is not an anticholinergic agent.

Pharmacokinetics

Absorption: ZANTAC is 50% absorbed after oral administration, compared to an intravenous (IV) injection with mean peak levels of 440 to 545 ng/mL occurring 2 to 3 hours after a 150-mg dose. The syrup is bioequivalent to the tablets. Absorption is not significantly impaired by the administration of food or antacids. Propantheline slightly delays and increases peak blood levels of ranitidine, probably by delaying gastric emptying and transit time. In one study, simultaneous administration of high-potency antacid (150 mmol) in fasting subjects has been reported to decrease the absorption of ZANTAC.

Distribution: The volume of distribution is about 1.4 L/kg. Serum protein binding averages 15%.

Metabolism: In humans, the N-oxide is the principal metabolite in the urine; however, this amounts to <4% of the dose. Other metabolites are the S-oxide (1%) and the desmethyl ranitidine (1%). The remainder of the administered dose is found in the stool. Studies in patients with hepatic dysfunction (compensated cirrhosis) indicate that there are minor, but clinically insignificant, alterations in ranitidine half-life, distribution, clearance, and bioavailability.

Excretion: The principal route of excretion is the urine, with approximately 30% of the orally administered dose collected in the urine as unchanged drug in 24 hours. Renal clearance is about 410 mL/min, indicating active tubular excretion. The elimination half-life is 2.5 to 3 hours. Four patients with clinically significant renal function impairment (creatinine clearance 25 to 35 mL/min) administered 50 mg of ranitidine intravenously had an average plasma half-life of 4.8 hours, a ranitidine clearance of 29 mL/min, and a volume of distribution of 1.76 L/kg. In general, these parameters appear to be altered in proportion to creatinine clearance (see DOSAGE AND ADMINISTRATION).

Geriatrics: The plasma half-life is prolonged and total clearance is reduced in the elderly population due to a decrease in renal function. The elimination half-life is 3 to 4 hours. Peak levels average 526 ng/mL following a 150-mg twice-daily dose and occur in about 3 hours (see PRECAUTIONS: Geriatric Use and DOSAGE AND ADMINISTRATION: Dosage Adjustment for Patients With Impaired Renal Function).

Pediatrics: There are no significant differences in the pharmacokinetic parameter values for ranitidine in pediatric patients (from 1 month up to 16 years of age) and healthy adults when correction is made for body weight. The average bioavailability of ranitidine given orally to pediatric patients is 48%, which is comparable to the bioavailability of ranitidine in the adult population. All other pharmacokinetic parameter values ($t_{1/2}$, Vd, and CL) are similar to those observed with intravenous ranitidine use in pediatric patients. Estimates of C_{max} and T_{max} are displayed in Table 1.
[See table 1 above]

Table 1. Ranitidine Pharmacokinetics in Pediatric Patients Following Oral Dosing

Population (age)	n	Dosage Form (dose)	C_{max} (ng/mL)	T_{max} (hours)
Gastric or duodenal ulcer (3.5 to 16 years)	12	Tablets (1 to 2 mg/kg)	54 to 492	2.0
Otherwise healthy requiring ZANTAC (0.7 to 14 years, Single dose)	10	Syrup (2 mg/kg)	244	1.61
Otherwise healthy requiring ZANTAC (0.7 to 14 years, Multiple dose)	10	Syrup (2 mg/kg)	320	1.66

Table 2. Effect of Oral ZANTAC on Gastric Acid Secretion

	Time After Dose, hours	% Inhibition of Gastric Acid Output by Dose, mg			
		75-80	100	150	200
Basal	Up to 4		99	95	
Nocturnal	Up to 13	95	96	92	
Betazole	Up to 3		97	99	
Pentagastrin	Up to 5	58	72	72	80
Meal	Up to 3		73	79	95

Table 3. Duodenal Ulcer Patient Healing Rates

	ZANTAC[a]		Placebo[a]	
	Number Entered	Healed/ Evaluable	Number Entered	Healed/ Evaluable
Outpatients Week 2	195	69/182 (38%)[b]	188	31/164 (19%)
Week 4		137/187 (73%)[b]		76/168 (45%)

[a]All patients were permitted antacids as needed for relief of pain.
[b]$P<0.0001$.

Plasma clearance measured in 2 neonatal patients (younger than 1 month of age) was considerably lower (3 mL/min/kg) than children or adults and is likely due to reduced renal function observed in this population (see PRECAUTIONS: Pediatric Use and DOSAGE AND ADMINISTRATION: Pediatric Use).

Pharmacodynamics

Serum concentrations necessary to inhibit 50% of stimulated gastric acid secretion are estimated to be 36 to 94 ng/mL. Following a single oral dose of 150 mg, serum concentrations of ranitidine are in this range up to 12 hours. However, blood levels bear no consistent relationship to dose or degree of acid inhibition.

Antisecretory Activity: 1. Effects on Acid Secretion: ZANTAC inhibits both daytime and nocturnal basal gastric acid secretions as well as gastric acid secretion stimulated by food, betazole, and pentagastrin, as shown in Table 2.
[See table 2 above]
It appears that basal-, nocturnal-, and betazole-stimulated secretions are most sensitive to inhibition by ZANTAC, responding almost completely to doses of 100 mg or less, while pentagastrin- and food-stimulated secretions are more difficult to suppress.

2. Effects on Other Gastrointestinal Secretions:

Pepsin: Oral ZANTAC does not affect pepsin secretion. Total pepsin output is reduced in proportion to the decrease in volume of gastric juice.

Intrinsic Factor: Oral ZANTAC has no significant effect on pentagastrin-stimulated intrinsic factor secretion.

Serum Gastrin: ZANTAC has little or no effect on fasting or postprandial serum gastrin.

Other Pharmacologic Actions:

1. Gastric bacterial flora—increase in nitrate-reducing organisms, significance not known.
2. Prolactin levels—no effect in recommended oral or IV dosage, but small, transient, dose-related increases in serum prolactin have been reported after IV bolus injections of 100 mg or more.
3. Other pituitary hormones—no effect on serum gonadotropins, TSH, or GH. Possible impairment of vasopressin release.
4. No change in cortisol, aldosterone, androgen, or estrogen levels.
5. No antiandrogenic action.
6. No effect on count, motility, or morphology of sperm.

Pediatrics: Oral doses of 6 to 10 mg/kg/day in 2 or 3 divided doses maintain gastric pH >4 throughout most of the dosing interval.

Clinical Trials

Active Duodenal Ulcer: In a multicenter, double-blind, controlled, US study of endoscopically diagnosed duodenal ulcers, earlier healing was seen in the patients treated with ZANTAC as shown in Table 3.
[See table 3 above]
In these studies, patients treated with ZANTAC reported a reduction in both daytime and nocturnal pain, and they also consumed less antacid than the placebo-treated patients.

Table 4. Mean Daily Doses of Antacid

	Ulcer Healed	Ulcer Not Healed
ZANTAC	0.06	0.71
Placebo	0.71	1.43

Foreign studies have shown that patients heal equally well with 150 mg twice daily and 300 mg at bedtime (85% versus 84%, respectively) during a usual 4-week course of therapy. If patients require extended therapy of 8 weeks, the healing rate may be higher for 150 mg twice daily as compared to 300 mg at bedtime (92% versus 87%, respectively).
Studies have been limited to short-term treatment of acute duodenal ulcer. Patients whose ulcers healed during therapy had recurrences of ulcers at the usual rates.

Maintenance Therapy in Duodenal Ulcer: Ranitidine has been found to be effective as maintenance therapy for patients following healing of acute duodenal ulcers. In 2 independent, double-blind, multicenter, controlled trials, the number of duodenal ulcers observed was significantly less in patients treated with ZANTAC (150 mg at bedtime) than in patients treated with placebo over a 12-month period.
[See table 5 at top of next page]
As with other H_2-antagonists, the factors responsible for the significant reduction in the prevalence of duodenal ulcers include prevention of recurrence of ulcers, more rapid healing of ulcers that may occur during maintenance therapy, or both.

Table 5. Duodenal Ulcer Prevalence

Double-Blind, Multicenter, Placebo-Controlled Trials					
Multicenter Trial	Drug	Duodenal Ulcer Prevalence			No. of Patients
		0-4 Months	0-8 Months	0-12 Months	
USA	RAN	20%[a]	24%	35%[a]	138
	PLC	44%	54%	59%	139
Foreign	RAN	12%[a]	21%[a]	28%[a]	174
	PLC	56%	64%	68%	165

% = Life table estimate.
[a] = $P<0.05$ (ZANTAC versus comparator).
RAN = ranitidine (ZANTAC).
PLC = placebo.

Table 6. Gastric Ulcer Patient Healing Rates

	ZANTAC[a]		Placebo[a]	
	Number Entered	Healed/ Evaluable	Number Entered	Healed/ Evaluable
Outpatients Week 2	92	16/83 (19%)	94	10/83 (12%)
Week 6		50/73 (68%)[b]		35/69 (51%)

[a]All patients were permitted antacids as needed for relief of pain.
[b]$P= 0.009$.

Gastric Ulcer: In a multicenter, double-blind, controlled, US study of endoscopically diagnosed gastric ulcers, earlier healing was seen in the patients treated with ZANTAC as shown in Table 6.

[See table 6 above]

In this multicenter trial, significantly more patients treated with ZANTAC became pain free during therapy.

Maintenance of Healing of Gastric Ulcers: In 2 multicenter, double-blind, randomized, placebo-controlled, 12-month trials conducted in patients whose gastric ulcers had been previously healed, ZANTAC 150 mg at bedtime was significantly more effective than placebo in maintaining healing of gastric ulcers.

Pathological Hypersecretory Conditions (such as Zollinger-Ellison syndrome): ZANTAC inhibits gastric acid secretion and reduces occurrence of diarrhea, anorexia, and pain in patients with pathological hypersecretion associated with Zollinger-Ellison syndrome, systemic mastocytosis, and other pathological hypersecretory conditions (e.g., postoperative, "short-gut" syndrome, idiopathic). Use of ZANTAC was followed by healing of ulcers in 8 of 19 (42%) patients who were intractable to previous therapy.

Gastroesophageal Reflux Disease (GERD): In 2 multicenter, double-blind, placebo-controlled, 6-week trials performed in the United States and Europe, ZANTAC 150 mg twice daily was more effective than placebo for the relief of heartburn and other symptoms associated with GERD. Ranitidine-treated patients consumed significantly less antacid than did placebo-treated patients.

The US trial indicated that ZANTAC 150 mg twice daily significantly reduced the frequency of heartburn attacks and severity of heartburn pain within 1 to 2 weeks after starting therapy. The improvement was maintained throughout the 6-week trial period. Moreover, patient response rates demonstrated that the effect on heartburn extends through both the day and night time periods.

In 2 additional US multicenter, double-blind, placebo-controlled, 2-week trials, ZANTAC 150 mg twice daily was shown to provide relief of heartburn pain within 24 hours of initiating therapy and a reduction in the frequency of severity of heartburn.

Erosive Esophagitis: In 2 multicenter, double-blind, randomized, placebo-controlled, 12-week trials performed in the United States, ZANTAC 150 mg 4 times daily was significantly more effective than placebo in healing endoscopically diagnosed erosive esophagitis and in relieving associated heartburn. The erosive esophagitis healing rates were as follows:

Table 7. Erosive Esophagitis Patient Healing Rates

	Healed/Evaluable	
	Placebo[a] n = 229	ZANTAC 150 mg 4 times daily[a] n = 215
Week 4	43/198 (22%)	96/206 (47%)[b]
Week 8	63/176 (36%)	142/200 (71%)[b]
Week 12	92/159 (58%)	162/192 (84%)[b]

[a]All patients were permitted antacids as needed for relief of pain.
[b]$P<0.001$ versus placebo.

No additional benefit in healing of esophagitis or in relief of heartburn was seen with a ranitidine dose of 300 mg 4 times daily.

Maintenance of Healing of Erosive Esophagitis: In 2 multicenter, double-blind, randomized, placebo-controlled, 48-week trials conducted in patients whose erosive esophagitis had been previously healed, ZANTAC 150 mg twice daily was significantly more effective than placebo in maintaining healing of erosive esophagitis.

INDICATIONS AND USAGE

ZANTAC is indicated in:

1. Short-term treatment of active duodenal ulcer. Most patients heal within 4 weeks. Studies available to date have not assessed the safety of ranitidine in uncomplicated duodenal ulcer for periods of more than 8 weeks.
2. Maintenance therapy for duodenal ulcer patients at reduced dosage after healing of acute ulcers. No placebo-controlled comparative studies have been carried out for periods of longer than 1 year.
3. The treatment of pathological hypersecretory conditions (e.g., Zollinger-Ellison syndrome and systemic mastocytosis).
4. Short-term treatment of active, benign gastric ulcer. Most patients heal within 6 weeks and the usefulness of further treatment has not been demonstrated. Studies available to date have not assessed the safety of ranitidine in uncomplicated, benign gastric ulcer for periods of more than 6 weeks.
5. Maintenance therapy for gastric ulcer patients at reduced dosage after healing of acute ulcers. Placebo-controlled studies have been carried out for 1 year.
6. Treatment of GERD. Symptomatic relief commonly occurs within 24 hours after starting therapy with ZANTAC 150 mg twice daily.
7. Treatment of endoscopically diagnosed erosive esophagitis. Symptomatic relief of heartburn commonly occurs within 24 hours of therapy initiation with ZANTAC 150 mg 4 times daily.
8. Maintenance of healing of erosive esophagitis. Placebo-controlled trials have been carried out for 48 weeks.

Concomitant antacids should be given as needed for pain relief to patients with active duodenal ulcer; active, benign gastric ulcer; hypersecretory states; GERD; and erosive esophagitis.

CONTRAINDICATIONS

ZANTAC is contraindicated for patients known to have hypersensitivity to the drug or any of the ingredients (see PRECAUTIONS).

PRECAUTIONS

General:

1. Symptomatic response to therapy with ZANTAC does not preclude the presence of gastric malignancy.
2. Since ZANTAC is excreted primarily by the kidney, dosage should be adjusted in patients with impaired renal function (see DOSAGE AND ADMINISTRATION). Caution should be observed in patients with hepatic dysfunction since ZANTAC is metabolized in the liver.
3. Rare reports suggest that ZANTAC may precipitate acute porphyric attacks in patients with acute porphyria. ZANTAC should therefore be avoided in patients with a history of acute porphyria.

Laboratory Tests

False-positive tests for urine protein with MULTISTIX® may occur during therapy with ZANTAC, and therefore testing with sulfosalicylic acid is recommended.

Drug Interactions

Ranitidine has been reported to affect the bioavailability of other drugs through several different mechanisms such as competition for renal tubular secretion, alteration of gastric pH, and inhibition of cytochrome P450 enzymes.

Procainamide: Ranitidine, a substrate of the renal organic cation transport system, may affect the clearance of other drugs eliminated by this route. High doses of ranitidine (e.g., such as those used in the treatment of Zollinger-Ellison syndrome) have been shown to reduce the renal excretion of procainamide and N-acetylprocainamide resulting in increased plasma levels of these drugs. Although this interaction is unlikely to be clinically relevant at usual ranitidine doses, it may be prudent to monitor for procainamide toxicity when administered with oral ranitidine at a dose exceeding 300 mg per day.

Warfarin: There have been reports of altered prothrombin time among patients on concomitant warfarin and ranitidine therapy. Due to the narrow therapeutic index, close monitoring of increased or decreased prothrombin time is recommended during concurrent treatment with ranitidine.

Ranitidine may alter the absorption of drugs in which gastric pH is an important determinant of bioavailability. This can result in either an increase in absorption (e.g., triazolam, midazolam, glipizide) or a decrease in absorption (e.g., ketoconazole, atazanavir, delavirdine, gefitinib). Appropriate clinical monitoring is recommended.

Atazanavir: Atazanavir absorption may be impaired based on known interactions with other agents that increase gastric pH. Use with caution. See atazanavir label for specific recommendations.

Delavirdine: Delavirdine absorption may be impaired based on known interactions with other agents that increase gastric pH. Chronic use of H_2-receptor antagonists with delavirdine is not recommended.

Gefitinib: Gefitinib exposure was reduced by 44% with the coadministration of ranitidine and sodium bicarbonate (dosed to maintain gastric pH above 5.0). Use with caution.

Glipizide: In diabetic patients, glipizide exposure was increased by 34% following a single 150-mg dose of oral ranitidine. Use appropriate clinical monitoring when initiating or discontinuing ranitidine.

Ketoconazole: Oral ketoconazole exposure was reduced by up to 95% when oral ranitidine was coadministered in a regimen to maintain a gastric pH of 6 or above. The degree of interaction with usual dose of ranitidine (150 mg twice daily) is unknown.

Midazolam: Oral midazolam exposure in 5 healthy volunteers was increased by up to 65% when administered with oral ranitidine at a dose of 150 mg twice daily. However, in another interaction study in 8 volunteers receiving IV midazolam, a 300 mg oral dose of ranitidine increased midazolam exposure by about 9%. Monitor patients for excessive or prolonged sedation when ranitidine is coadministered with oral midazolam.

Triazolam: Triazolam exposure in healthy volunteers was increased by approximately 30% when administered with oral ranitidine at a dose of 150 mg twice daily. Monitor patients for excessive or prolonged sedation.

Carcinogenesis, Mutagenesis, Impairment of Fertility
There was no indication of tumorigenic or carcinogenic effects in life-span studies in mice and rats at dosages up to 2,000 mg/kg/day.
Ranitidine was not mutagenic in standard bacterial tests (*Salmonella, Escherichia coli*) for mutagenicity at concentrations up to the maximum recommended for these assays.
In a dominant lethal assay, a single oral dose of 1,000 mg/kg to male rats was without effect on the outcome of 2 matings per week for the next 9 weeks.
Pregnancy
Teratogenic Effects: Pregnancy Category B. Reproduction studies have been performed in rats and rabbits at doses up to 160 times the human dose and have revealed no evidence of impaired fertility or harm to the fetus due to ZANTAC. There are, however, no adequate and well-controlled studies in pregnant women. Because animal reproduction studies are not always predictive of human response, this drug should be used during pregnancy only if clearly needed.
Nursing Mothers
Ranitidine is secreted in human milk. Caution should be exercised when ZANTAC is administered to a nursing mother.
Pediatric Use
The safety and effectiveness of ZANTAC have been established in the age-group of 1 month to 16 years for the treatment of duodenal and gastric ulcers, gastroesophageal reflux disease and erosive esophagitis, and the maintenance of healed duodenal and gastric ulcer. Use of ZANTAC in this age-group is supported by adequate and well-controlled studies in adults, as well as additional pharmacokinetic data in pediatric patients and an analysis of the published literature (see CLINICAL PHARMACOLOGY: Pediatrics and DOSAGE AND ADMINISTRATION: Pediatric Use).
Safety and effectiveness in pediatric patients for the treatment of pathological hypersecretory conditions or the maintenance of healing of erosive esophagitis have not been established.
Safety and effectiveness in neonates (younger than 1 month of age) have not been established (see CLINICAL PHARMACOLOGY: Pediatrics).
Geriatric Use
Of the total number of subjects enrolled in US and foreign controlled clinical trials of oral formulations of ZANTAC, for which there were subgroup analyses, 4,197 were aged 65 and older, while 899 were aged 75 and older. No overall differences in safety or effectiveness were observed between these subjects and younger subjects, and other reported clinical experience has not identified differences in responses between the elderly and younger patients, but greater sensitivity of some older individuals cannot be ruled out.
This drug is known to be substantially excreted by the kidney and the risk of toxic reactions to this drug may be greater in patients with impaired renal function. Because elderly patients are more likely to have decreased renal function, caution should be exercised in dose selection, and it may be useful to monitor renal function (see CLINICAL PHARMACOLOGY: Pharmacokinetics: Geriatrics and DOSAGE AND ADMINISTRATION: Dosage Adjustment for Patients With Impaired Renal Function).

ADVERSE REACTIONS

The following have been reported as events in clinical trials or in the routine management of patients treated with ZANTAC. The relationship to therapy with ZANTAC has been unclear in many cases. Headache, sometimes severe, seems to be related to administration of ZANTAC.
Central Nervous System
Rarely, malaise, dizziness, somnolence, insomnia, and vertigo. Rare cases of reversible mental confusion, agitation, depression, and hallucinations have been reported, predominantly in severely ill elderly patients. Rare cases of reversible blurred vision suggestive of a change in accommodation have been reported. Rare reports of reversible involuntary motor disturbances have been received.
Cardiovascular
As with other H_2-blockers, rare reports of arrhythmias such as tachycardia, bradycardia, atrioventricular block, and premature ventricular beats.
Gastrointestinal
Constipation, diarrhea, nausea/vomiting, abdominal discomfort/pain, and rare reports of pancreatitis.
Hepatic
There have been occasional reports of hepatocellular, cholestatic, or mixed hepatitis, with or without jaundice. In such circumstances, ranitidine should be immediately discontinued. These events are usually reversible, but in rare circumstances death has occurred. Rare cases of hepatic failure have also been reported. In normal volunteers, SGPT values were increased to at least twice the pretreatment levels in 6 of 12 subjects receiving 100 mg intravenously 4 times daily for 7 days, and in 4 of 24 subjects receiving 50 mg intravenously 4 times daily for 5 days.
Musculoskeletal
Rare reports of arthralgias and myalgias.
Hematologic
Blood count changes (leukopenia, granulocytopenia, and thrombocytopenia) have occurred in a few patients. These were usually reversible. Rare cases of agranulocytosis, pancytopenia, sometimes with marrow hypoplasia, and aplastic anemia and exceedingly rare cases of acquired immune hemolytic anemia have been reported.
Endocrine
Controlled studies in animals and man have shown no stimulation of any pituitary hormone by ZANTAC and no antiandrogenic activity, and cimetidine-induced gynecomastia and impotence in hypersecretory patients have resolved when ZANTAC has been substituted. However, occasional cases of impotence and loss of libido have been reported in male patients receiving ZANTAC, but the incidence did not differ from that in the general population. Rare cases of breast symptoms and conditions, including galactorrhea and gynecomastia, have been reported in both males and females.
Integumentary
Rash, including rare cases of erythema multiforme. Rare cases of alopecia and vasculitis.
Respiratory
A large epidemiological study suggested an increased risk of developing pneumonia in current users of histamine-2-receptor antagonists (H_2RAs) compared to patients who had stopped H_2RA treatment, with an observed adjusted relative risk of 1.63 (95% CI, 1.07–2.48). However, a causal relationship between use of H_2RAs and pneumonia has not been established.
Other
Rare cases of hypersensitivity reactions (e.g., bronchospasm, fever, rash, eosinophilia), anaphylaxis, angioneurotic edema, acute interstitial nephritis, and small increases in serum creatinine.

OVERDOSAGE

There has been limited experience with overdosage. Reported acute ingestions of up to 18 g orally have been associated with transient adverse effects similar to those encountered in normal clinical experience (see ADVERSE REACTIONS). In addition, abnormalities of gait and hypotension have been reported.
When overdosage occurs, the usual measures to remove unabsorbed material from the gastrointestinal tract, clinical monitoring, and supportive therapy should be employed.
Studies in dogs receiving dosages of ZANTAC in excess of 225 mg/kg/day have shown muscular tremors, vomiting, and rapid respiration. Single oral doses of 1,000 mg/kg in mice and rats were not lethal. Intravenous LD_{50} values in mice and rats were 77 and 83 mg/kg, respectively.

DOSAGE AND ADMINISTRATION

Active Duodenal Ulcer
The current recommended adult oral dosage of ZANTAC for duodenal ulcer is 150 mg or 10 mL of syrup (2 teaspoonfuls of syrup equivalent to 150 mg of ranitidine) twice daily. An alternative dosage of 300 mg or 20 mL of syrup (4 teaspoonfuls of syrup equivalent to 300 mg of ranitidine) once daily after the evening meal or at bedtime can be used for patients in whom dosing convenience is important. The advantages of one treatment regimen compared to the other in a particular patient population have yet to be demonstrated (see Clinical Trials: Active Duodenal Ulcer). Smaller doses have been shown to be equally effective in inhibiting gastric acid secretion in US studies, and several foreign trials have shown that 100 mg twice daily is as effective as the 150-mg dose.
Antacid should be given as needed for relief of pain (see CLINICAL PHARMACOLOGY: Pharmacokinetics).
Maintenance of Healing of Duodenal Ulcers
The current recommended adult oral dosage is 150 mg or 10 mL of syrup (2 teaspoonfuls of syrup equivalent to 150 mg of ranitidine) at bedtime.
Pathological Hypersecretory Conditions (such as Zollinger-Ellison syndrome)
The current recommended adult oral dosage is 150 mg or 10 mL of syrup (2 teaspoonfuls of syrup equivalent to 150 mg of ranitidine) twice daily. In some patients it may be necessary to administer ZANTAC 150-mg doses more frequently. Dosages should be adjusted to individual patient needs, and should continue as long as clinically indicated. Dosages up to 6 g/day have been employed in patients with severe disease.
Benign Gastric Ulcer
The current recommended adult oral dosage is 150 mg or 10 mL of syrup (2 teaspoonfuls of syrup equivalent to 150 mg of ranitidine) twice daily.
Maintenance of Healing of Gastric Ulcers
The current recommended adult oral dosage is 150 mg or 10 mL of syrup (2 teaspoonfuls of syrup equivalent to 150 mg of ranitidine) at bedtime.
GERD
The current recommended adult oral dosage is 150 mg or 10 mL of syrup (2 teaspoonfuls of syrup equivalent to 150 mg of ranitidine) twice daily.
Erosive Esophagitis
The current recommended adult oral dosage is 150 mg or 10 mL of syrup (2 teaspoonfuls of syrup equivalent to 150 mg of ranitidine) 4 times daily.
Maintenance of Healing of Erosive Esophagitis
The current recommended adult oral dosage is 150 mg or 10 mL of syrup (2 teaspoonfuls of syrup equivalent to 150 mg of ranitidine) twice daily.
Pediatric Use
The safety and effectiveness of ZANTAC have been established in the age-group of 1 month to 16 years. There is insufficient information about the pharmacokinetics of ZANTAC in neonatal patients (younger than 1 month of age) to make dosing recommendations.
The following 3 subsections provide dosing information for each of the pediatric indications.
Treatment of Duodenal and Gastric Ulcers: The recommended oral dose for the treatment of active duodenal and gastric ulcers is 2 to 4 mg/kg twice daily to a maximum of 300 mg/day. This recommendation is derived from adult clinical studies and pharmacokinetic data in pediatric patients.
Maintenance of Healing of Duodenal and Gastric Ulcers: The recommended oral dose for the maintenance of healing of duodenal and gastric ulcers is 2 to 4 mg/kg once daily to a maximum of 150 mg/day. This recommendation is derived from adult clinical studies and pharmacokinetic data in pediatric patients.
Treatment of GERD and Erosive Esophagitis: Although limited data exist for these conditions in pediatric patients, published literature supports a dosage of 5 to 10 mg/kg/day, usually given as 2 divided doses.
Dosage Adjustment for Patients With Impaired Renal Function
On the basis of experience with a group of subjects with severely impaired renal function treated with ZANTAC, the recommended dosage in patients with a creatinine clearance <50 mL/min is 150 mg or 10 mL of syrup (2 teaspoonfuls of syrup equivalent to 150 mg of ranitidine) every 24 hours. Should the patient's condition require, the frequency of dosing may be increased to every 12 hours or even further with caution. Hemodialysis reduces the level of circulating ranitidine. Ideally, the dosing schedule should be adjusted so that the timing of a scheduled dose coincides with the end of hemodialysis.
Elderly patients are more likely to have decreased renal function, therefore caution should be exercised in dose selection, and it may be useful to monitor renal function (see CLINICAL PHARMACOLOGY: Pharmacokinetics: Geriatrics and PRECAUTIONS: Geriatric Use).

HOW SUPPLIED

ZANTAC 150 Tablets (ranitidine HCl equivalent to 150 mg of ranitidine) are peach, film-coated, 5-sided tablets embossed with "ZANTAC 150" on one side and "Glaxo" on the other. They are available in bottles of 60 (NDC 0173-0344-42) and 500 (NDC 0173-0344-14) tablets.
ZANTAC 300 Tablets (ranitidine HCl equivalent to 300 mg of ranitidine) are yellow, film-coated, capsule-shaped tablets embossed with "ZANTAC 300" on one side and "Glaxo" on the other. They are available in bottles of 30 (NDC 0173-0393-40) tablets.
Store between 15°and 30°C (59° and 86°F) in a dry place. Protect from light. Replace cap securely after each opening.
ZANTAC Syrup, a clear, pale yellow, peppermint-flavored liquid, contains 16.8 mg of ranitidine HCl equivalent to 15 mg of ranitidine per 1 mL (75 mg/5 mL) in bottles of 16 fluid ounces (1 pint) (NDC 0173-0383-54).
Store between 4° and 25°C (39° and 77°F). Dispense in tight, light-resistant containers as defined in the USP/NF.
GlaxoSmithKline
Research Triangle Park, NC 27709
ZANTAC is a registered trademarks of Warner-Lambert Company, used under license.
MULTISTIX is a registered trademark of Bayer Healthcare LLC.

July 2013
ZNT:7PI

ZOFRAN® ℞
[*zō' fran*]
(ondansetron hydrochloride)
injection for intravenous use

HIGHLIGHTS OF PRESCRIBING INFORMATION
These highlights do not include all the information needed to use ZOFRAN safely and effectively. See full prescribing information for ZOFRAN.

ZOFRAN® (ondansetron hydrochloride) injection for intravenous use
Initial U.S. Approval: 1991

RECENT MAJOR CHANGES

Dosage and Administration, Prevention of Nausea and Vomiting Associated with Initial and Repeat Courses of Emetogenic Chemotherapy – Removal of 32 mg single intravenous dose (2.1) 11/2012
Warnings and Precautions, QT Prolongation (5.2) 11/2012

INDICATIONS AND USAGE

ZOFRAN Injection is a 5-HT_3 receptor antagonist indicated:
- Prevention of nausea and vomiting associated with initial and repeat courses of emetogenic cancer chemotherapy. (1.1)
- Prevention of postoperative nausea and/or vomiting. (1.2)

DOSAGE AND ADMINISTRATION

Prevention of nausea and vomiting associated with initial and repeat courses of emetogenic cancer chemotherapy (2.1):
- Adults and Pediatric patients (6 months to 18 years): Three 0.15 mg/kg doses, up to a maximum of 16 mg per dose, infused intravenously over 15 minutes. The first dose should be administered 30 minutes before the start of chemotherapy. Subsequent doses are administered 4 and 8 hours after the first dose.

Prevention of postoperative nausea and/or vomiting (2.2):

Population	Age	ZOFRAN Injection Dosage	Intravenous Infusion Rate
Adults	> 12 yrs	4 mg × 1	over 2 - 5 min
Pediatrics (> 40 kg)	1 mo. – 12 yrs	4 mg × 1	over 2 - 5 min
Pediatrics (≤ 40 kg)	1 mo. – 12 yrs	0.1 mg/kg × 1	over 2 - 5 min

- In patients with severe hepatic impairment, a total daily dose of 8 mg should not be exceeded. (2.4)

DOSAGE FORMS AND STRENGTHS

ZOFRAN Injection (2 mg/mL): 20 mL multidose vials. (3)

CONTRAINDICATIONS

- Patients known to have hypersensitivity (e.g., anaphylaxis) to this product or any of its components. (4)
- Concomitant use of apomorphine. (4)

WARNINGS AND PRECAUTIONS

- Hypersensitivity reactions including anaphylaxis and bronchospasm, have been reported in patients who have exhibited hypersensitivity to other selective 5-HT_3 receptor antagonists. (5.1)
- QT prolongation occurs in a dose-dependent manner. Cases of Torsade de Pointes have been reported. Avoid ZOFRAN in patients with congenital long QT syndrome. (5.2)
- Use in patients following abdominal surgery or in patients with chemotherapy-induced nausea and vomiting may mask a progressive ileus and/or gastric distention. (5.3)(5.4)

ADVERSE REACTIONS

Chemotherapy-Induced Nausea and Vomiting –
- The most common adverse reactions (≥ 7%) in adults are diarrhea, headache, and fever. (6.1)

Postoperative Nausea and Vomiting –
- The most common adverse reaction (≥ 10%) which occurs at a higher frequency compared to placebo in adults is headache. (6.1)
- The most common adverse reaction (≥ 2%) which occurs at a higher frequency compared to placebo in pediatric patients 1 to 24 months of age is diarrhea. (6.1)

To report SUSPECTED ADVERSE REACTIONS, contact GlaxoSmithKline at 1-888-825-5249 or FDA at 1-800-FDA-1088 or www.fda.gov/medwatch

DRUG INTERACTIONS

- Apomorphine – profound hypotension and loss of consciousness. Concomitant use with ondansetron is contraindicated. (7.2)

See 17 for PATIENT COUNSELING INFORMATION
Revised: 05/2013

FULL PRESCRIBING INFORMATION: CONTENTS*

*** Sections or subsections omitted from the full prescribing information are not listed**

FULL PRESCRIBING INFORMATION

1 INDICATIONS AND USAGE

1.1 Prevention of Nausea and Vomiting Associated with Initial and Repeat Courses of Emetogenic Cancer Chemotherapy

ZOFRAN Injection is indicated for the prevention of nausea and vomiting associated with initial and repeat courses of emetogenic cancer chemotherapy, including high-dose cisplatin *[see Clinical Studies (14.1)]*.
ZOFRAN is approved for patients aged 6 months and older.

1.2 Prevention of Postoperative Nausea and/or Vomiting

ZOFRAN Injection is indicated for the prevention of postoperative nausea and/or vomiting. As with other antiemetics, routine prophylaxis is not recommended for patients in whom there is little expectation that nausea and/or vomiting will occur postoperatively. In patients in whom nausea and/or vomiting must be avoided postoperatively, ZOFRAN Injection is recommended even when the incidence of postoperative nausea and/or vomiting is low. For patients who do not receive prophylactic ZOFRAN Injection and experience nausea and/or vomiting postoperatively, ZOFRAN Injection may be given to prevent further episodes *[see Clinical Studies (14.3)]*.
ZOFRAN is approved for patients aged 1 month and older.

2 DOSAGE AND ADMINISTRATION

2.1 Prevention of Nausea and Vomiting Associated with Initial and Repeat Courses of Emetogenic Chemotherapy

ZOFRAN Injection should be diluted in 50 mL of 5% Dextrose Injection or 0.9% Sodium Chloride Injection before administration.

Adults

The recommended adult intravenous dosage of ZOFRAN is three 0.15-mg/kg doses up to a maximum of 16 mg per dose *[see Clinical Pharmacology (12.2)]*. The first dose is infused over 15 minutes beginning 30 minutes before the start of emetogenic chemotherapy. Subsequent doses (0.15 mg/kg up to a maximum of 16 mg per dose) are administered 4 and 8 hours after the first dose of ZOFRAN.

Pediatrics

For pediatric patients 6 months through 18 years of age, the intravenous dosage of ZOFRAN is three 0.15-mg/kg doses up to a maximum of 16 mg per dose *[see Clinical Studies (14.1) and Clinical Pharmacology (12.2 and 12.3)]*. The first dose is to be administered 30 minutes before the start of moderately to highly emetogenic chemotherapy. Subsequent doses (0.15 mg/kg up to a maximum of 16 mg per dose) are administered 4 and 8 hours after the first dose of ZOFRAN. The drug should be infused intravenously over 15 minutes.

2.2 Prevention of Postoperative Nausea and Vomiting

ZOFRAN Injection should not be mixed with solutions for which physical and chemical compatibility have not been established. In particular, this applies to alkaline solutions as a precipitate may form.

Adults

The recommended adult intravenous dosage of ZOFRAN is 4 mg *undiluted* administered intravenously in not less than 30 seconds, preferably over 2 to 5 minutes, immediately before induction of anesthesia, or postoperatively if the patient did not receive prophylactic antiemetics and experiences nausea and/or vomiting occurring within 2 hours after surgery. Alternatively, 4 mg *undiluted* may be administered intramuscularly as a single injection for adults. While recommended as a fixed dose for patients weighing more than 40 kg, few patients above 80 kg have been studied. In patients who do not achieve adequate control of postoperative nausea and vomiting following a single, prophylactic, preinduction, intravenous dose of ondansetron 4 mg, administration of a second intravenous dose of 4 mg ondansetron postoperatively does not provide additional control of nausea and vomiting.

Pediatrics

For pediatric patients 1 month through 12 years of age, the dosage is a single 0.1-mg/kg dose for patients weighing 40 kg or less, or a single 4-mg dose for patients weighing more than 40 kg. The rate of administration should not be less than 30 seconds, preferably over 2 to 5 minutes immediately prior to or following anesthesia induction, or postoperatively if the patient did not receive prophylactic antiemetics and experiences nausea and/or vomiting occurring shortly after surgery. Prevention of further nausea and vomiting was only studied in patients who had not received prophylactic ZOFRAN.

2.3 Stability and Handling

After dilution, do not use beyond 24 hours. Although ZOFRAN Injection is chemically and physically stable when diluted as recommended, sterile precautions should be observed because diluents generally do not contain preservative.

ZOFRAN Injection is stable at room temperature under normal lighting conditions for 48 hours after dilution with the following intravenous fluids: 0.9% Sodium Chloride Injection, 5% Dextrose Injection, 5% Dextrose and 0.9% Sodium Chloride Injection, 5% Dextrose and 0.45% Sodium Chloride Injection, and 3% Sodium Chloride Injection.

Note: Parenteral drug products should be inspected visually for particulate matter and discoloration before administration whenever solution and container permit.

Precaution: Occasionally, ondansetron precipitates at the stopper/vial interface in vials stored upright. Potency and safety are not affected. If a precipitate is observed, resolubilize by shaking the vial vigorously.

2.4 Dosage Adjustment for Patients with Impaired Hepatic Function

In patients with severe hepatic impairment (Child-Pugh score of 10 or greater), a single maximal daily dose of 8 mg infused over 15 minutes beginning 30 minutes before the start of the emetogenic chemotherapy is recommended. There is no experience beyond first-day administration of ondansetron in these patients *[see Clinical Pharmacology (12.3)]*.

3 DOSAGE FORMS AND STRENGTHS

ZOFRAN Injection, 2 mg/mL is a clear, colorless, nonpyrogenic, sterile solution available as a 20 mL multidose vial.

4 CONTRAINDICATIONS

ZOFRAN Injection is contraindicated for patients known to have hypersensitivity (e.g., anaphylaxis) to this product or any of its components. Anaphylactic reactions have been reported in patients taking ondansetron. *[See Adverse Reactions (6.2)].*

The concomitant use of apomorphine with ondansetron is contraindicated based on reports of profound hypotension and loss of consciousness when apomorphine was administered with ondansetron.

5 WARNINGS AND PRECAUTIONS

5.1 Hypersensitivity Reactions

Hypersensitivity reactions, including anaphylaxis and bronchospasm, have been reported in patients who have exhibited hypersensitivity to other selective 5-HT_3 receptor antagonists.

5.2 QT Prolongation

Ondansetron prolongs the QT interval in a dose-dependent manner *[see Clinical Pharmacology (12.2)].* In addition, post-marketing cases of Torsade de Pointes have been reported in patients using ondansetron. Avoid ZOFRAN in patients with congenital long QT syndrome. ECG monitoring is recommended in patients with electrolyte abnormalities (e.g., hypokalemia or hypomagnesemia), congestive heart failure, bradyarrhythmias, or patients taking other medicinal products that lead to QT prolongation.

5.3 Masking of Progressive Ileus and Gastric Distension

The use of ZOFRAN in patients following abdominal surgery or in patients with chemotherapy-induced nausea and vomiting may mask a progressive ileus and gastric distension.

5.4 Effect on Peristalsis

ZOFRAN is not a drug that stimulates gastric or intestinal peristalsis. It should not be used instead of nasogastric suction.

6 ADVERSE REACTIONS

6.1 Clinical Trials Experience

Because clinical trials are conducted under widely varying conditions, adverse reaction rates observed in the clinical trials of a drug cannot be directly compared to rates in the clinical trials of another drug and may not reflect the rates observed in clinical practice.

The following adverse reactions have been reported in clinical trials of adult patients treated with ondansetron, the active ingredient of intravenous ZOFRAN across a range of dosages. A causal relationship to therapy with ZOFRAN (ondansetron) was unclear in many cases.

Chemotherapy-Induced Nausea and Vomiting

Table 1. Adverse Reactions Reported in > 5% of Adult Patients Who Received Ondansetron at a Dosage of Three 0.15-mg/kg Doses

	Number of Adult Patients With Reaction		
Adverse Reaction	ZOFRAN Injection 0.15 mg/kg × 3 n = 419	Metoclopramide n = 156	Placebo n = 34
Diarrhea	16%	44%	18%
Headache	17%	7%	15%
Fever	8%	5%	3%

Cardiovascular

Rare cases of angina (chest pain), electrocardiographic alterations, hypotension, and tachycardia have been reported.

Gastrointestinal

Constipation has been reported in 11% of chemotherapy patients receiving multiday ondansetron.

Hepatic

In comparative trials in cisplatin chemotherapy patients with normal baseline values of aspartate transaminase (AST) and alanine transaminase (ALT), these enzymes have been reported to exceed twice the upper limit of normal in approximately 5% of patients. The increases were transient and did not appear to be related to dose or duration of therapy. On repeat exposure, similar transient elevations in transaminase values occurred in some courses, but symptomatic hepatic disease did not occur.

Integumentary

Rash has occurred in approximately 1% of patients receiving ondansetron.

Neurological

There have been rare reports consistent with, but not diagnostic of, extrapyramidal reactions in patients receiving ZOFRAN Injection, and rare cases of grand mal seizure.

Other

Rare cases of hypokalemia have been reported.

Postoperative Nausea and Vomiting

The adverse reactions in Table 2 have been reported in ≥ 2% of adults receiving ondansetron at a dosage of 4 mg intravenous over 2 to 5 minutes in clinical trials.

Table 2. Adverse Reactions Reported in ≥ 2% (and With Greater Frequency than the Placebo Group) of Adult Patients Receiving Ondansetron at a Dosage of 4 mg Intravenous over 2 to 5 Minutes

Adverse Reaction[a,b]	ZOFRAN Injection 4 mg Intravenous n = 547 patients	Placebo n = 547 patients
Headache	92 (17%)	77 (14%)
Drowsiness/sedation	44 (8%)	37 (7%)
Injection site reaction	21 (4%)	18 (3%)
Fever	10 (2%)	6 (1%)
Cold sensation	9 (2%)	8 (1%)
Pruritus	9 (2%)	3 (< 1%)
Paresthesia	9 (2%)	2 (< 1%)

[a] Adverse Reactions: Rates of these reactions were not significantly different in the ondansetron and placebo groups

[b] Patients were receiving multiple concomitant perioperative and postoperative medications

Pediatric Use

Rates of adverse reactions were similar in both the ondansetron and placebo groups in pediatric patients receiving ondansetron (a single 0.1 mg/kg dose for pediatric patients weighing 40 kg or less, or 4 mg for pediatric patients weighing more than 40 kg) administered intravenously over at least 30 seconds. Diarrhea was seen more frequently in patients taking ZOFRAN (2%) compared to placebo (<1%) in the 1 month to 24 month age group. These patients were receiving multiple concomitant perioperative and postoperative medications.

6.2 Postmarketing Experience

The following adverse reactions have been identified during post-approval use of ondansetron. Because these reactions are reported voluntarily from a population of uncertain size, it is not always possible to reliably estimate their frequency or establish a causal relationship to drug exposure. The reactions have been chosen for inclusion due to a combination of their seriousness, frequency of reporting, or potential causal connection to ondansetron.

Cardiovascular

Arrhythmias (including ventricular and supraventricular tachycardia, premature ventricular contractions, and atrial fibrillation), bradycardia, electrocardiographic alterations (including second-degree heart block, QT/QTc interval prolongation, and ST segment depression), palpitations, and syncope. Rarely and predominantly with intravenous ondansetron, transient ECG changes including QT/QTc interval prolongation have been reported *[see Warnings and Precautions (5.2)].*

General

Flushing. Rare cases of hypersensitivity reactions, sometimes severe (e.g., anaphylactic reactions, angioedema, bronchospasm, cardiopulmonary arrest, hypotension, laryngeal edema, laryngospasm, shock, shortness of breath, stridor) have also been reported. A positive lymphocyte transformation test to ondansetron has been reported, which suggests immunologic sensitivity to ondansetron.

Hepatobiliary

Liver enzyme abnormalities have been reported. Liver failure and death have been reported in patients with cancer receiving concurrent medications including potentially hepatotoxic cytotoxic chemotherapy and antibiotics.

Local Reactions

Pain, redness, and burning at site of injection.

Lower Respiratory

Hiccups

Neurological

Oculogyric crisis, appearing alone, as well as with other dystonic reactions. Transient dizziness during or shortly after intravenous infusion.

Skin

Urticaria, toxic skin eruption, including toxic epidermal necrolysis.

Eye Disorders

Cases of transient blindness, predominantly during intravenous administration, have been reported. These cases of transient blindness were reported to resolve within a few minutes up to 48 hours. Transient blurred vision, in some cases associated with abnormalities of accommodation, have also been reported.

7 DRUG INTERACTIONS

7.1 Drugs Affecting Cytochrome P-450 Enzymes

Ondansetron does not appear to induce or inhibit the cytochrome P-450 drug-metabolizing enzyme system of the liver. Because ondansetron is metabolized by hepatic cytochrome P-450 drug-metabolizing enzymes (CYP3A4, CYP2D6, CYP1A2), inducers or inhibitors of these enzymes may change the clearance and, hence, the half-life of ondansetron *[see Clinical Pharmacology (12.3)].* On the basis of limited available data, no dosage adjustment is recommended for patients on these drugs.

7.2 Apomorphine

Based on reports of profound hypotension and loss of consciousness when apomorphine was administered with ondansetron, the concomitant use of apomorphine with ondansetron is contraindicated *[see Contraindications (4)].*

7.3 Phenytoin, Carbamazepine, and Rifampin

In patients treated with potent inducers of CYP3A4 (i.e., phenytoin, carbamazepine, and rifampin), the clearance of ondansetron was significantly increased and ondansetron blood concentrations were decreased. However, on the basis of available data, no dosage adjustment for ondansetron is recommended for patients on these drugs *[see Clinical Pharmacology (12.3)].*

7.4 Tramadol

Although there are no data on pharmacokinetic drug interactions between ondansetron and tramadol, data from two small studies indicate that concomitant use of ondansetron may result in reduced analgesic activity of tramadol. Patients on concomitant ondansetron self administered tramadol more frequently in these studies, leading to an increased cumulative dose in patient controlled administration (PCA) of tramadol.

7.5 Chemotherapy

In humans, carmustine, etoposide, and cisplatin do not affect the pharmacokinetics of ondansetron.

In a crossover study in 76 pediatric patients, intravenous ondansetron did not increase blood levels of high-dose methotrexate.

7.6 Temazepam

The coadministration of ondansetron had no effect on the pharmacokinetics and pharmacodynamics of temazepam.

7.7 Alfentanil and Atracurium

Ondansetron does not alter the respiratory depressant effects produced by alfentanil or the degree of neuromuscular blockade produced by atracurium. Interactions with general or local anesthetics have not been studied.

8 USE IN SPECIFIC POPULATIONS

8.1 Pregnancy

Pregnancy Category B. Reproduction studies have been performed in pregnant rats and rabbits at intravenous doses up to 4 mg/kg per day (approximately 1.4 and 2.9 times the recommended human intravenous dose of 0.15 mg/kg given three times a day, respectively, based on body surface area) and have revealed no evidence of impaired fertility or harm to the fetus due to ondansetron. There are, however, no adequate and well-controlled studies in pregnant women. Because animal reproduction studies are not always predictive of human response, this drug should be used during pregnancy only if clearly needed.

8.3 Nursing Mothers

Ondansetron is excreted in the breast milk of rats. It is not known whether ondansetron is excreted in human milk. Because many drugs are excreted in human milk, caution should be exercised when ondansetron is administered to a nursing woman.

8.4 Pediatric Use

Little information is available about the use of ondansetron in pediatric surgical patients younger than 1 month of age. *[See Clinical Studies (14.2)].* Little information is available about the use of ondansetron in pediatric cancer patients younger than 6 months of age. *[See Clinical Studies (14.1) and Dosage and Administration (2)].*

The clearance of ondansetron in pediatric patients 1 month to 4 months of age is slower and the half-life is ~2.5 fold longer than patients who are > 4 to 24 months of age. As a precaution, it is recommended that patients less than 4 months of age receiving this drug be closely monitored. *[See Clinical Pharmacology (12.3)].*

8.5 Geriatric Use

Of the total number of subjects enrolled in cancer chemotherapy-induced and postoperative nausea and vomiting in US- and foreign-controlled clinical trials, 862 were 65 years of age and over. No overall differences in safety or effectiveness were observed between these subjects and younger subjects, and other reported clinical experience has not identified differences in responses between the elderly and younger patients, but greater sensitivity of some older individuals cannot be ruled out. Dosage adjustment is not needed in patients over the age of 65 *[see Clinical Pharmacology (12.3)].*

Table 3. Pharmacokinetics in Normal Adult Volunteers

Age-group (years)	n	Peak Plasma Concentration (ng/mL)	Mean Elimination Half-life (h)	Plasma Clearance (L/h/kg)
19-40	11	102	3.5	0.381
61-74	12	106	4.7	0.319
≥ 75	11	170	5.5	0.262

8.6 Hepatic Impairment

In patients with severe hepatic impairment (Child-Pugh score of 10 or greater), clearance is reduced and apparent volume of distribution is increased with a resultant increase in plasma half-life *[see Clinical Pharmacology (12.3)]*. In such patients, a total daily dose of 8 mg should not be exceeded *[see Dosage and Administration (2.3)]*.

8.7 Renal Impairment

Although plasma clearance is reduced in patients with severe renal impairment (creatinine clearance < 30 mL/min), no dosage adjustment is recommended *[see Clinical Pharmacology (12.3)]*.

9 DRUG ABUSE AND DEPENDENCE

Animal studies have shown that ondansetron is not discriminated as a benzodiazepine nor does it substitute for benzodiazepines in direct addiction studies.

10 OVERDOSAGE

There is no specific antidote for ondansetron overdose. Patients should be managed with appropriate supportive therapy. Individual intravenous doses as large as 150 mg and total daily intravenous doses as large as 252 mg have been inadvertently administered without significant adverse events. These doses are more than 10 times the recommended daily dose.

In addition to the adverse reactions listed above, the following events have been described in the setting of ondansetron overdose: "Sudden blindness" (amaurosis) of 2 to 3 minutes' duration plus severe constipation occurred in one patient that was administered 72 mg of ondansetron intravenously as a single dose. Hypotension (and faintness) occurred in another patient that took 48 mg of ondansetron hydrochloride tablets. Following infusion of 32 mg over only a 4-minute period, a vasovagal episode with transient second-degree heart block was observed. In all instances, the events resolved completely.

11 DESCRIPTION

The active ingredient of ZOFRAN Injection is ondansetron hydrochloride, a selective blocking agent of the serotonin 5-HT_3 receptor type. Its chemical name is (±) 1, 2, 3, 9-tetrahydro-9-methyl-3-[(2-methyl-1H-imidazol-1-yl)methyl]-4H-carbazol-4-one, monohydrochloride, dihydrate. It has the following structural formula:

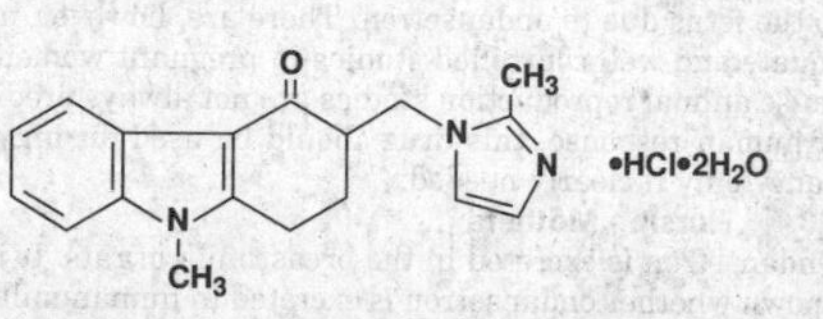

The empirical formula is $C_{18}H_{19}N_3O \cdot HCl \cdot 2H_2O$, representing a molecular weight of 365.9.

Ondansetron HCl is a white to off-white powder that is soluble in water and normal saline.

Each 1 mL of aqueous solution in the 20 mL multidose vial contains 2 mg of ondansetron as the hydrochloride dihydrate; 8.3 mg of sodium chloride, USP; 0.5 mg of citric acid monohydrate, USP and 0.25 mg of sodium citrate dihydrate, USP as buffers; and 1.2 mg of methylparaben, NF and 0.15 mg of propylparaben, NF as preservatives in Water for Injection, USP.

ZOFRAN Injection is a clear, colorless, nonpyrogenic, sterile solution for intravenous use. The pH of the injection solution is 3.3 to 4.0.

12 CLINICAL PHARMACOLOGY

12.1 Mechanism of Action

Ondansetron is a selective 5-HT_3 receptor antagonist. While ondansetron's mechanism of action has not been fully characterized, it is not a dopamine-receptor antagonist.

12.2 Pharmacodynamics

QTc interval prolongation was studied in a double blind, single intravenous dose, placebo- and positive-controlled, crossover study in 58 healthy subjects. The maximum mean (95% upper confidence bound) difference in QTcF from placebo after baseline-correction was 19.5 (21.8) ms and 5.6 (7.4) ms after 15 minute intravenous infusions of 32mg and 8 mg ZOFRAN, respectively. A significant exposure-reponse relationship was identified between ondansetron concentration and ΔΔQTcF. Using the established exposure-response relationship, 24 mg infused intravenously over 15 min had a mean predicted (95% upper prediction interval) ΔΔQTcF of 14.0 (16.3) ms. In contrast, 16 mg infused intravenously over 15 min using the same model had a mean predicted (95% upper prediction interval) ΔΔQTcF of 9.1 (11.2) ms.

In normal volunteers, single intravenous doses of 0.15 mg/kg of ondansetron had no effect on esophageal motility, gastric motility, lower esophageal sphincter pressure, or small intestinal transit time. In another study in six normal male volunteers, a 16-mg dose infused over 5 minutes showed no effect of the drug on cardiac output, heart rate, stroke volume, blood pressure, or electrocardiogram (ECG). Multiday administration of ondansetron has been shown to slow colonic transit in normal volunteers. Ondansetron has no effect on plasma prolactin concentrations. In a gender-balanced pharmacodynamic study (n = 56), ondansetron 4 mg administered intravenously or intramuscularly was dynamically similar in the prevention of nausea and vomiting using the ipecacuanha model of emesis.

12.3 Pharmacokinetics

In normal adult volunteers, the following mean pharmacokinetic data have been determined following a single 0.15-mg/kg intravenous dose.

[See table 3 above]

Absorption

A study was performed in normal volunteers (n = 56) to evaluate the pharmacokinetics of a single 4-mg dose administered as a 5-minute infusion compared to a single intramuscular injection. Systemic exposure as measured by mean AUC were equivalent, with values of 156 [95% CI 136, 180] and 161 [95% CI 137, 190] ng•h/mL for intravenous and intramuscular groups, respectively. Mean peak plasma concentrations were 42.9 [95% CI 33.8, 54.4] ng/mL at 10 minutes after intravenous infusion and 31.9 [95% CI 26.3, 38.6] ng/mL at 41 minutes after intramuscular injection.

Distribution

Plasma protein binding of ondansetron as measured in vitro was 70% to 76%, over the pharmacologic concentration range of 10 to 500 ng/mL. Circulating drug also distributes into erythrocytes.

Metabolism

Ondansetron is extensively metabolized in humans, with approximately 5% of a radiolabeled dose recovered as the parent compound from the urine. The primary metabolic pathway is hydroxylation on the indole ring followed by subsequent glucuronide or sulfate conjugation.

Although some nonconjugated metabolites have pharmacologic activity, these are not found in plasma at concentrations likely to significantly contribute to the biological activity of ondansetron. The metabolites are observed in the urine.

In vitro metabolism studies have shown that ondansetron is a substrate for multiple human hepatic cytochrome P-450 enzymes, including CYP1A2, CYP2D6, and CYP3A4. In terms of overall ondansetron turnover, CYP3A4 plays a predominant role while formation of the major in vivo metabolites is apparently mediated by CYP1A2. The role of CYP2D6 in ondansetron in vivo metabolism is relatively minor.

The pharmacokinetics of intravenous ondansetron did not differ between subjects who were poor metabolisers of CYP2D6 and those who were extensive metabolisers of CYP2D6, further supporting the limited role of CYP2D6 in ondansetron disposition in vivo.

Elimination

In adult cancer patients, the mean ondansetron elimination half-life was 4.0 hours, and there was no difference in the multidose pharmacokinetics over a 4-day period. In a dose proportionality study, systemic exposure to 32 mg of ondansetron was not proportional to dose as measured by comparing dose-normalized AUC values to an 8-mg dose. This is consistent with a small decrease in systemic clearance with increasing plasma concentrations.

Geriatrics

A reduction in clearance and increase in elimination half-life are seen in patients over 75 years of age. In clinical trials with cancer patients, safety and efficacy were similar in patients over 65 years of age and those under 65 years of age; there was an insufficient number of patients over 75 years of age to permit conclusions in that age-group. No dosage adjustment is recommended in the elderly.

Pediatrics

Pharmacokinetic samples were collected from 74 cancer patients 6 to 48 months of age, who received a dose of 0.15 mg/kg of intravenous ondansetron every 4 hours for 3 doses during a safety and efficacy trial. These data were combined with sequential pharmacokinetics data from 41 surgery patients 1 month to 24 months of age, who received a single dose of 0.1 mg/kg of ondansetron prior to surgery with general anesthesia, and a population pharmacokinetic analysis was performed on the combined data set. The results of this analysis are included in Table 4 and are compared to the pharmacokinetic results in cancer patients 4 to 18 years of age.

Table 4. Pharmacokinetics in Pediatric Cancer Patients 1 Month to 18 Years of Age

Subjects and Age Group	N	CL (L/h/kg)	Vd_{ss} (L/kg)	$T_{1/2}$ (h)
		Geometric Mean		Mean
Pediatric Cancer Patients 4 to 18 years of age	N = 21	0.599	1.9	2.8
Population PK Patients[a] 1 month to 48 months of age	N = 115	0.582	3.65	4.9

[a] Population PK (Pharmacokinetic) Patients: 64% cancer patients and 36% surgery patients.

Based on the population pharmacokinetic analysis, cancer patients 6 to 48 months of age who receive a dose of 0.15 mg/kg of intravenous ondansetron every 4 hours for 3 doses would be expected to achieve a systemic exposure (AUC) consistent with the exposure achieved in previous pediatric studies in cancer patients (4 to 18 years of age) at similar doses.

In a study of 21 pediatric patients (3 to 12 years of age) who were undergoing surgery requiring anesthesia for a duration of 45 minutes to 2 hours, a single intravenous dose of ondansetron, 2 mg (3 to 7 years) or 4 mg (8 to 12 years), was administered immediately prior to anesthesia induction. Mean weight-normalized clearance and volume of distribution values in these pediatric surgical patients were similar to those previously reported for young adults. Mean terminal half-life was slightly reduced in pediatric patients (range, 2.5 to 3 hours) in comparison with adults (range, 3 to 3.5 hours).

In a study of 51 pediatric patients (1 month to 24 months of age) who were undergoing surgery requiring general anesthesia, a single intravenous dose of ondansetron, 0.1 or 0.2 mg/kg, was administered prior to surgery. As shown in Table 5, the 41 patients with pharmacokinetic data were divided into 2 groups, patients 1 month to 4 months of age and patients 5 to 24 months of age, and are compared to pediatric patients 3 to 12 years of age.

Table 5. Pharmacokinetics in Pediatric Surgery Patients 1 Month to 12 Years of Age

Subjects and Age Group	N	CL (L/h/kg)	Vd_{ss} (L/kg)	$T_{1/2}$ (h)
		Geometric Mean		Mean
Pediatric Surgery Patients 3 to 12 years of age	N = 21	0.439	1.65	2.9
Pediatric Surgery Patients 5 to 24 months of age	N = 22	0.581	2.3	2.9
Pediatric Surgery Patients 1 month to 4 months of age	N = 19	0.401	3.5	6.7

In general, surgical and cancer pediatric patients younger than 18 years tend to have a higher ondansetron clearance compared to adults leading to a shorter half-life in most pediatric patients. In patients 1 month to 4 months of age, a longer half-life was observed due to the higher volume of distribution in this age group.

In a study of 21 pediatric cancer patients (4 to 18 years of age) who received three intravenous doses of 0.15 mg/kg of ondansetron at 4-hour intervals, patients older than 15 years of age exhibited ondansetron pharmacokinetic parameters similar to those of adults.

Renal Impairment

Due to the very small contribution (5%) of renal clearance to the overall clearance, renal impairment was not expected to significantly influence the total clearance of ondansetron. However, ondansetron mean plasma clearance was reduced by about 41% in patients with severe renal impairment (creatinine clearance < 30 mL/min). This reduction in clearance is variable and was not consistent with an increase in half-life. No reduction in dose or dosing frequency in these patients is warranted.

Hepatic Impairment

In patients with mild-to-moderate hepatic impairment, clearance is reduced 2-fold and mean half-life is increased to 11.6 hours compared to 5.7 hours in those without hepatic impairment. In patients with severe hepatic impairment (Child-Pugh score of 10 or greater), clearance is reduced 2-fold to 3-fold and apparent volume of distribution is increased with a resultant increase in half-life to 20 hours. In patients with severe hepatic impairment, a total daily dose of 8 mg should not be exceeded.

13 NONCLINICAL TOXICOLOGY

13.1 Carcinogenesis, Mutagenesis, Impairment of Fertility

Carcinogenic effects were not seen in 2-year studies in rats and mice with oral ondansetron doses up to 10 and 30 mg/kg per day, respectively (approximately 3.6 and 5.4 times the recommended human intravenous dose of 0.15 mg/kg given three times a day, based on body surface area). Ondansetron was not mutagenic in standard tests for mutagenicity.

Oral administration of ondansetron up to 15 mg/kg per day (approximately 3.8 times the recommended human intravenous dose, based on body surface area) did not affect fertility or general reproductive performance of male and female rats.

14 CLINICAL STUDIES

The clinical efficacy of ondansetron hydrochloride, the active ingredient of ZOFRAN, was assessed in clinical trials as described below.

14.1 Chemotherapy-Induced Nausea and Vomiting

Adults

In a double-blind study of three different dosing regimens of ZOFRAN Injection, 0.015 mg/kg, 0.15 mg/kg, and 0.30 mg/kg, each given three times during the course of cancer chemotherapy, the 0.15-mg/kg dosing regimen was more effective than the 0.015-mg/kg dosing regimen. The 0.30-mg/kg dosing regimen was not shown to be more effective than the 0.15-mg/kg dosing regimen.

Cisplatin-Based Chemotherapy

In a double-blind study in 28 patients, ZOFRAN Injection (three 0.15-mg/kg doses) was significantly more effective than placebo in preventing nausea and vomiting induced by cisplatin-based chemotherapy. Therapeutic response was as shown in Table 6.

[See table 6 above]

Table 6. Therapeutic Response in Prevention of Chemotherapy-Induced Nausea and Vomiting in Single-Day Cisplatin Therapy[a] in Adults

	Zofran Injection (0.15 mg/kg × 3)	Placebo	*P* Value[b]
Number of patients	14	14	
Treatment response			
0 Emetic episodes	2 (14%)	0 (0%)	
1-2 Emetic episodes	8 (57%)	0 (0%)	
3-5 Emetic episodes	2 (14%)	1 (7%)	
More than 5 emetic episodes/rescued	2 (14%)	13 (93%)	0.001
Median number of emetic episodes	1.5	Undefined[c]	
Median time to first emetic episode (h)	11.6	2.8	0.001
Median nausea scores (0-100)[d]	3	59	0.034
Global satisfaction with control of nausea and vomiting (0-100)[e]	96	10.5	0.009

[a] Chemotherapy was high dose (100 and 120 mg/m^2; ZOFRAN Injection n = 6, placebo n = 5) or moderate dose (50 and 80 mg/m^2; ZOFRAN Injection n = 8, placebo n = 9). Other chemotherapeutic agents included fluorouracil, doxorubicin, and cyclophosphamide. There was no difference between treatments in the types of chemotherapy that would account for differences in response.

[b] Efficacy based on "all patients treated" analysis.

[c] Median undefined since at least 50% of the patients were rescued or had more than five emetic episodes.

[d] Visual analog scale assessment of nausea: 0 = no nausea, 100 = nausea as bad as it can be.

[e] Visual analog scale assessment of satisfaction: 0 = not at all satisfied, 100 = totally satisfied.

Ondansetron injection (0.15-mg/kg × 3 doses) was compared with metoclopramide (2 mg/kg × 6 doses) in a single-blind trial in 307 patients receiving cisplatin ≥ 100 mg/m^2 with or without other chemotherapeutic agents. Patients received the first dose of ondansetron or metoclopramide 30 minutes before cisplatin. Two additional ondansetron doses were administered 4 and 8 hours later, or five additional metoclopramide doses were administered 2, 4, 7, 10, and 13 hours later. Cisplatin was administered over a period of 3 hours or less. Episodes of vomiting and retching were tabulated over the period of 24 hours after cisplatin. The results of this study are summarized in Table 7.

[See table 7 above]

Table 7. Therapeutic Response in Prevention of Vomiting Induced by Cisplatin (≥ 100 mg/m^2) Single-Day Therapy[a] in Adults

	Zofran Injection	Metoclopramide	*P* Value
Dose	0.15 mg/kg × 3	2 mg/kg × 6	
Number of patients in efficacy population	136	138	
Treatment response			
0 Emetic episodes	54 (40%)	41 (30%)	
1-2 Emetic episodes	34 (25%)	30 (22%)	
3-5 Emetic episodes	19 (14%)	18 (13%)	
More than 5 emetic episodes/rescued	29 (21%)	49 (36%)	
Comparison of treatments with respect to			
0 Emetic episodes	54/136	41/138	0.083
More than 5 emetic episodes/rescued	29/136	49/138	0.009
Median number of emetic episodes	1	2	0.005
Median time to first emetic episode (h)	20.5	4.3	< 0.001
Global satisfaction with control of nausea and vomiting (0-100)[b]	85	63	0.001
Acute dystonic reactions	0	8	0.005
Akathisia	0	10	0.002

[a] In addition to cisplatin, 68% of patients received other chemotherapeutic agents, including cyclophosphamide, etoposide, and fluorouracil. There was no difference between treatments in the types of chemotherapy that would account for differences in response.

[b] Visual analog scale assessment: 0 = not at all satisfied, 100 = totally satisfied.

Cyclophosphamide-Based Chemotherapy

In a double-blind, placebo-controlled study of ZOFRAN Injection (three 0.15-mg/kg doses) in 20 patients receiving cyclophosphamide (500 to 600 mg/m^2) chemotherapy, ZOFRAN Injection was significantly more effective than placebo in preventing nausea and vomiting. The results are summarized in Table 8.

[See table 8 above and on next page]

Table 8. Therapeutic Response in Prevention of Chemotherapy-Induced Nausea and Vomiting in Single-Day Cyclophosphamide Therapy[a] in Adults

	Zofran Injection (0.15 mg/kg × 3)	Placebo	*P* Value[b]
Number of patients	10	10	
Treatment response			
0 Emetic episodes	7 (70%)	0 (0%)	0.001
1-2 Emetic episodes	0 (0%)	2 (20%)	
3-5 Emetic episodes	2 (20%)	4 (40%)	
More than 5 emetic episodes/rescued	1 (10%)	4 (40%)	0.131
Median number of emetic episodes	0	4	0.008
Median time to first emetic episode (h)	Undefined[c]	8.79	

(Table continued on next page)

Re-treatment

In uncontrolled trials, 127 patients receiving cisplatin (median dose, 100 mg/m^2) and ondansetron who had two or fewer emetic episodes were re-treated with ondansetron and chemotherapy, mainly cisplatin, for a total of 269 re-treatment courses (median, 2; range, 1 to 10). No emetic episodes occurred in 160 (59%), and two or fewer emetic episodes occurred in 217 (81%) re-treatment courses.

Pediatrics

Four open-label, noncomparative (one US, three foreign) trials have been performed with 209 pediatric cancer patients 4 to 18 years of age given a variety of cisplatin or noncisplatin-regimens. In the three foreign trials, the initial ZOFRAN Injection dose ranged from 0.04 to 0.87 mg/kg for a total dose of 2.16 to 12 mg. This was followed by the oral administration of ondansetron ranging from 4 to 24 mg daily for 3 days. In the US trial, ZOFRAN was administered intravenously (only) in three doses of 0.15 mg/kg each for a total daily dose of 7.2 to 39 mg. In these studies, 58% of the 196 evaluable patients had a complete response (no emetic episodes) on day 1. Thus, prevention of vomiting in these pediatric patients was essentially the same as for patients older than 18 years of age.

An open-label, multicenter, noncomparative trial has been performed in 75 pediatric cancer patients 6 to 48 months of age receiving at least one moderately or highly emetogenic chemotherapeutic agent. Fifty-seven percent (57%) were fe-

Table 8 *(cont.)*. Therapeutic Response in Prevention of Chemotherapy-Induced Nausea and Vomiting in Single-Day Cyclophosphamide Therapy[a] in Adults

	Zofran Injection (0.15 mg/kg × 3)	Placebo	*P* Value[b]
Median nausea scores (0-100)[d]	0	60	0.001
Global satisfaction with control of nausea and vomiting (0-100)[e]	100	52	0.008

[a] Chemotherapy consisted of cyclophosphamide in all patients, plus other agents, including fluorouracil, doxorubicin, methotrexate, and vincristine. There was no difference between treatments in the type of chemotherapy that would account for differences in response.
[b] Efficacy based on "all patients treated" analysis.
[c] Median undefined since at least 50% of patients did not have any emetic episodes.
[d] Visual analog scale assessment of nausea: 0 = no nausea, 100 = nausea as bad as it can be.
[e] Visual analog scale assessment of satisfaction: 0 = not at all satisfied, 100 = totally satisfied.

Table 9. Therapeutic Response in Prevention of Postoperative Nausea and Vomiting in Adult Patients

	Ondansetron 4 mg Intravenous	Placebo	*P* Value
Study 1			
Emetic episodes:			
Number of patients	136	139	
Treatment response over 24-h postoperative period			
0 Emetic episodes	103 (76%)	64 (46%)	< 0.001
1 Emetic episode	13 (10%)	17 (12%)	
More than 1 emetic episode/rescued	20 (15%)	58 (42%)	
Nausea assessments:			
Number of patients	134	136	
No nausea over 24-h postoperative period	56 (42%)	39 (29%)	
Study 2			
Emetic episodes:			
Number of patients	136	143	
Treatment response over 24-h postoperative period			
0 Emetic episodes	85 (63%)	63 (44%)	0.002
1 Emetic episode	16 (12%)	29 (20%)	
More than 1 emetic episode/rescued	35 (26%)	51 (36%)	
Nausea assessments:			
Number of patients	125	133	
No nausea over 24-h postoperative period	48 (38%)	42 (32%)	

Table 11. Therapeutic Response in Prevention of Further Postoperative Nausea and Vomiting in Adult Patients

	Ondansetron 4 mg Intravenous	Placebo	*P* Value
Study 1			
Emetic episodes:			
Number of patients	104	117	
Treatment response 24 h after study drug			
0 Emetic episodes	49 (47%)	19 (16%)	< 0.001
1 Emetic episode	12 (12%)	9 (8%)	
More than 1 emetic episode/rescued	43 (41%)	89 (76%)	
Median time to first emetic episode (min)[a]	55.0	43.0	
Nausea assessments:			
Number of patients	98	102	
Mean nausea score over 24-h postoperative period[b]	1.7	3.1	
Study 2			
Emetic episodes:			
Number of patients	112	108	
Treatment response 24 h after study drug			
0 Emetic episodes	49 (44%)	28 (26%)	0.006
1 Emetic episode	14 (13%)	3 (3%)	
More than 1 emetic episode/rescued	49 (44%)	77 (71%)	
Median time to first emetic episode (min)[a]	60.5	34.0	
Nausea assessments:			
Number of patients	105	85	
Mean nausea score over 24-h postoperative period[b]	1.9	2.9	

[a] After administration of study drug.
[b] Nausea measured on a scale of 0-10 with 0 = no nausea, 10 = nausea as bad as it can be.

males; 67% were white, 18% were American Hispanic, and 15% were black patients. ZOFRAN was administered intravenously over 15 minutes in three doses of 0.15 mg/kg. The first dose was administered 30 minutes before the start of chemotherapy, the second and third doses were administered 4 and 8 hours after the first dose, respectively. Eighteen patients (25%) received routine prophylactic dexamethasone (i.e., not given as rescue). Of the 75 evaluable patients, 56% had a complete response (no emetic episodes) on day 1. Thus, prevention of vomiting in these pediatric patients was comparable to the prevention of vomiting in patients 4 years of age and older.

14.2 Prevention of Postoperative Nausea and/or Vomiting

Adults

Adult surgical patients who received ondansetron immediately before the induction of general balanced anesthesia (barbiturate: thiopental, methohexital, or thiamylal; opioid: alfentanil or fentanyl; nitrous oxide; neuromuscular blockade: succinylcholine/curare and/or vecuronium or atracurium; and supplemental isoflurane) were evaluated in two double-blind US studies involving 554 patients. ZOFRAN Injection (4 mg) intravenous given over 2 to 5 minutes was significantly more effective than placebo. The results of these studies are summarized in Table 9.

[See table 9 above]

The study populations in Table 9 consisted mainly of females undergoing laparoscopic procedures.

In a placebo-controlled study conducted in 468 males undergoing outpatient procedures, a single 4-mg intravenous ondansetron dose prevented postoperative vomiting over a 24-hour study period in 79% of males receiving drug compared to 63% of males receiving placebo ($P < 0.001$).

Two other placebo-controlled studies were conducted in 2,792 patients undergoing major abdominal or gynecological surgeries to evaluate a single 4-mg or 8-mg intravenous ondansetron dose for prevention of postoperative nausea and vomiting over a 24-hour study period. At the 4-mg dosage, 59% of patients receiving ondansetron versus 45% receiving placebo in the first study ($P < 0.001$) and 41% of patients receiving ondansetron versus 30% receiving placebo in the second study ($P = 0.001$) experienced no emetic episodes. No additional benefit was observed in patients who received intravenous ondansetron 8 mg compared to patients who received intravenous ondansetron 4 mg.

Pediatrics

Three double-blind, placebo-controlled studies have been performed (one US, two foreign) in 1,049 male and female patients (2 to 12 years of age) undergoing general anesthesia with nitrous oxide. The surgical procedures included tonsillectomy with or without adenoidectomy, strabismus surgery, herniorrhaphy, and orchidopexy. Patients were randomized to either single intravenous doses of ondansetron (0.1 mg/kg for pediatric patients weighing 40 kg or less, 4 mg for pediatric patients weighing more than 40 kg) or placebo. Study drug was administered over at least 30 seconds, immediately prior to or following anesthesia induction. Ondansetron was significantly more effective than placebo in preventing nausea and vomiting. The results of these studies are summarized in Table 10.

Table 10. Therapeutic Response in Prevention of Postoperative Nausea and Vomiting in Pediatric Patients 2 to 12 Years of Age

Treatment Response Over 24 Hours	Ondansetron n (%)	Placebo n (%)	*P* Value
Study 1			
Number of patients	205	210	
0 Emetic episodes	140 (68%)	82 (39%)	0.001
Failure[a]	65 (32%)	128 (61%)	
Study 2			
Number of patients	112	110	
0 Emetic episodes	68 (61%)	38 (35%)	0.001
Failure[a]	44 (39%)	72 (65%)	
Study 3			
Number of patients	206	206	
0 Emetic episodes	123 (60%)	96 (47%)	0.01
Failure[a]	83 (40%)	110 (53%)	
Nausea assessments[b]:			
Number of patients	185	191	
None	119 (64%)	99 (52%)	0.01

[a] Failure was one or more emetic episodes, rescued, or withdrawn.
[b] Nausea measured as none, mild, or severe.

A double-blind, multicenter, placebo-controlled study was conducted in 670 pediatric patients 1 month to 24 months of age who were undergoing routine surgery under general anesthesia. Seventy-five percent (75%) were males; 64% were white, 15% were black, 13% were American Hispanic, 2% were Asian, and 6% were "other race" patients. A single 0.1-mg/kg intravenous dose of ondansetron administered within 5 minutes following induction of anesthesia was statistically significantly more effective than placebo in preventing vomiting. In the placebo group, 28% of patients experienced vomiting compared to 11% of subjects who received ondansetron ($P \leq 0.01$). Overall, 32 (10%) of placebo patients and 18 (5%) of patients who received ondansetron received antiemetic rescue medication(s) or prematurely withdrew from the study.

14.3 Prevention of Further Postoperative Nausea and Vomiting

Adults

Adult surgical patients receiving general balanced anesthesia (barbiturate: thiopental, methohexital, or thiamylal; opioid: alfentanil or fentanyl; nitrous oxide; neuromuscular blockade: succinylcholine/curare and/or vecuronium or atracurium; and supplemental isoflurane) who received no prophylactic antiemetics and who experienced nausea and/or vomiting within 2 hours postoperatively were evaluated in two double-blind US studies involving 441 patients. Patients who experienced an episode of postoperative nausea and/or vomiting were given ZOFRAN Injection (4 mg) intravenous over 2 to 5 minutes, and this was significantly more effective than placebo. The results of these studies are summarized in Table 11.

[See table 11 at top of previous page]

The study populations in Table 11 consisted mainly of women undergoing laparoscopic procedures.

Repeat Dosing in Adults

In patients who do not achieve adequate control of postoperative nausea and vomiting following a single, prophylactic, preinduction, intravenous dose of ondansetron 4 mg, administration of a second intravenous dose of ondansetron 4 mg postoperatively does not provide additional control of nausea and vomiting.

Pediatrics

One double-blind, placebo-controlled, US study was performed in 351 male and female outpatients (2 to 12 years of age) who received general anesthesia with nitrous oxide and no prophylactic antiemetics. Surgical procedures were unrestricted. Patients who experienced two or more emetic episodes within 2 hours following discontinuation of nitrous oxide were randomized to either single intravenous doses of ondansetron (0.1 mg/kg for pediatric patients weighing 40 kg or less, 4 mg for pediatric patients weighing more than 40 kg) or placebo administered over at least 30 seconds. Ondansetron was significantly more effective than placebo in preventing further episodes of nausea and vomiting. The results of the study are summarized in Table 12.

Table 12. Therapeutic Response in Prevention of Further Postoperative Nausea and Vomiting in Pediatric Patients 2 to 12 Years of Age

Treatment Response Over 24 Hours	Ondansetron n (%)	Placebo n (%)	*P* Value
Number of patients	180	171	
0 Emetic episodes	96 (53%)	29 (17%)	0.001
Failure[a]	84 (47%)	142 (83%)	

[a] Failure was one or more emetic episodes, rescued, or withdrawn.

16 HOW SUPPLIED/STORAGE AND HANDLING

ZOFRAN Injection, 2 mg/mL, is supplied as follows:
NDC 0173-0442-00 20-mL multidose vials (Singles)

Storage: Store vials between 2° and 30°C (36° and 86°F). Protect from light.

17 PATIENT COUNSELING INFORMATION

- Patients should be informed that ZOFRAN may cause serious cardiac arrhythmias such as QT prolongation. Patients should be instructed to tell their healthcare provider right away if they perceive a change in their heart rate, if they feel lightheaded, or if they have a syncopal episode.
- Patients should be informed that the chances of developing severe cardiac arrhythmias such as QT prolongation and Torsade de Pointes are higher in the following people:
  - Patients with a personal or family history of abnormal heart rhythms, such as congenital long QT syndrome;
  - Patients who take medications, such as diuretics, which may cause electrolyte abnormalities
  - Patients with hypokalemia or hypomagnesemia

  ZOFRAN should be avoided in these patients, since they may be more at risk for cardiac arrhythmias such as QT prolongation and Torsade de Pointes.
- Inform patients that ZOFRAN may cause hypersensitivity reactions, some as severe as anaphylaxis and bronchospasm. The patient should report any signs and symptoms of hypersensitivity reactions, including fever, chills, rash, or breathing problems.
- The patient should report the use of all medications, especially apomorphine, to their healthcare provider. Concomitant use of apomorphine and ZOFRAN may cause a significant drop in blood pressure and loss of consciousness.
- Inform patients that ZOFRAN may cause headache, drowsiness/sedation, constipation, fever and diarrhea.

GlaxoSmithKline
Research Triangle Park, NC 27709

ZFJ:7PI

ZOFRAN®
(ondansetron hydrochloride)
Tablets
ZOFRAN ODT®
(ondansetron)
Orally Disintegrating Tablets
ZOFRAN®
(ondansetron hydrochloride)
Oral Solution

DESCRIPTION

The active ingredient in ZOFRAN Tablets and ZOFRAN Oral Solution is ondansetron hydrochloride (HCl) as the dihydrate, the racemic form of ondansetron and a selective blocking agent of the serotonin 5-HT_3 receptor type. Chemically it is (±) 1, 2, 3, 9-tetrahydro-9-methyl-3-[(2-methyl-1H-imidazol-1-yl)methyl]-4H-carbazol-4-one, monohydrochloride, dihydrate. It has the following structural formula:

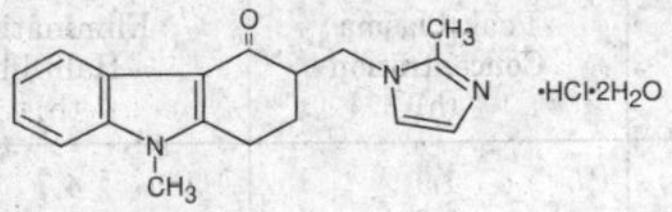

The empirical formula is $C_{18}H_{19}N_3O \bullet HCl \bullet 2H_2O$, representing a molecular weight of 365.9.

Ondansetron HCl dihydrate is a white to off-white powder that is soluble in water and normal saline.

The active ingredient in ZOFRAN ODT Orally Disintegrating Tablets is ondansetron base, the racemic form of ondansetron, and a selective blocking agent of the serotonin 5-HT_3 receptor type. Chemically it is (±) 1, 2, 3, 9-tetrahydro-9-methyl-3-[(2-methyl-1H-imidazol-1-yl)methyl]-4H-carbazol-4-one. It has the following structural formula:

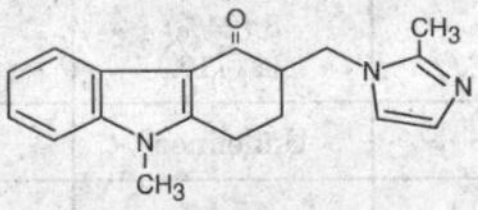

The empirical formula is $C_{18}H_{19}N_3O$ representing a molecular weight of 293.4.

Each 4-mg ZOFRAN Tablet for oral administration contains ondansetron HCl dihydrate equivalent to 4 mg of ondansetron. Each 8-mg ZOFRAN Tablet for oral administration contains ondansetron HCl dihydrate equivalent to 8 mg of ondansetron. Each tablet also contains the inactive ingredients lactose, microcrystalline cellulose, pregelatinized starch, hypromellose, magnesium stearate, titanium dioxide, triacetin, and iron oxide yellow (8-mg tablet only).

Each 4-mg ZOFRAN ODT Orally Disintegrating Tablet for oral administration contains 4 mg ondansetron base. Each 8-mg ZOFRAN ODT Orally Disintegrating Tablet for oral administration contains 8 mg ondansetron base. Each ZOFRAN ODT Tablet also contains the inactive ingredients aspartame, gelatin, mannitol, methylparaben sodium, propylparaben sodium, and strawberry flavor. ZOFRAN ODT Tablets are a freeze-dried, orally administered formulation of ondansetron which rapidly disintegrates on the tongue and does not require water to aid dissolution or swallowing.

Each 5 mL of ZOFRAN Oral Solution contains 5 mg of ondansetron HCl dihydrate equivalent to 4 mg of ondansetron. ZOFRAN Oral Solution contains the inactive ingredients citric acid anhydrous, purified water, sodium benzoate, sodium citrate, sorbitol, and strawberry flavor.

CLINICAL PHARMACOLOGY

Pharmacodynamics

Ondansetron is a selective 5-HT_3 receptor antagonist. While its mechanism of action has not been fully characterized, ondansetron is not a dopamine-receptor antagonist. Serotonin receptors of the 5-HT_3 type are present both peripherally on vagal nerve terminals and centrally in the chemoreceptor trigger zone of the area postrema. It is not certain whether ondansetron's antiemetic action is mediated centrally, peripherally, or in both sites. However, cytotoxic chemotherapy appears to be associated with release of serotonin from the enterochromaffin cells of the small intestine. In humans, urinary 5-HIAA (5-hydroxyindoleacetic acid) excretion increases after cisplatin administration in parallel with the onset of emesis. The released serotonin may stimulate the vagal afferents through the 5-HT_3 receptors and initiate the vomiting reflex.

In animals, the emetic response to cisplatin can be prevented by pretreatment with an inhibitor of serotonin synthesis, bilateral abdominal vagotomy and greater splanchnic nerve section, or pretreatment with a serotonin 5-HT_3 receptor antagonist.

In normal volunteers, single intravenous doses of 0.15 mg/kg of ondansetron had no effect on esophageal motility, gastric motility, lower esophageal sphincter pressure, or small intestinal transit time. Multiday administration of ondansetron has been shown to slow colonic transit in normal volunteers. Ondansetron has no effect on plasma prolactin concentrations.

Ondansetron does not alter the respiratory depressant effects produced by alfentanil or the degree of neuromuscular blockade produced by atracurium. Interactions with general or local anesthetics have not been studied.

Pharmacokinetics

Ondansetron is well absorbed from the gastrointestinal tract and undergoes some first-pass metabolism. Mean bioavailability in healthy subjects, following administration of a single 8-mg tablet, is approximately 56%.

Ondansetron systemic exposure does not increase proportionately to dose. AUC from a 16-mg tablet was 24% greater than predicted from an 8-mg tablet dose. This may reflect some reduction of first-pass metabolism at higher oral doses. Bioavailability is also slightly enhanced by the presence of food but unaffected by antacids.

Ondansetron is extensively metabolized in humans, with approximately 5% of a radiolabeled dose recovered as the parent compound from the urine. The primary metabolic pathway is hydroxylation on the indole ring followed by subsequent glucuronide or sulfate conjugation. Although some nonconjugated metabolites have pharmacologic activity, these are not found in plasma at concentrations likely to significantly contribute to the biological activity of ondansetron.

In vitro metabolism studies have shown that ondansetron is a substrate for human hepatic cytochrome P-450 enzymes, including CYP1A2, CYP2D6, and CYP3A4. In terms of overall ondansetron turnover, CYP3A4 played the predominant role. Because of the multiplicity of metabolic enzymes capable of metabolizing ondansetron, it is likely that inhibition or loss of one enzyme (e.g., CYP2D6 genetic deficiency) will be compensated by others and may result in little change in overall rates of ondansetron elimination. Ondansetron elimination may be affected by cytochrome P-450 inducers. In a pharmacokinetic study of 16 epileptic patients maintained chronically on CYP3A4 inducers, carbamazepine, or phenytoin, reduction in AUC, C_{max}, and T½ of ondansetron was observed.[1] This resulted in a significant increase in clearance. However, on the basis of available data, no dosage adjustment for ondansetron is recommended (see PRECAUTIONS: Drug Interactions).

In humans, carmustine, etoposide, and cisplatin do not affect the pharmacokinetics of ondansetron.

Gender differences were shown in the disposition of ondansetron given as a single dose. The extent and rate of ondansetron's absorption is greater in women than men. Slower clearance in women, a smaller apparent volume of distribution (adjusted for weight), and higher absolute bioavailability resulted in higher plasma ondansetron levels. These higher plasma levels may in part be explained by differences in body weight between men and women. It is not known whether these gender-related differences were clinically important. More detailed pharmacokinetic information is contained in Tables 1 and 2 taken from 2 studies.

[See table 1 at top of next page]
[See table 2 at top of next page]

A reduction in clearance and increase in elimination half-life are seen in patients over 75 years of age. In clinical trials with cancer patients, safety and efficacy were similar in patients over 65 years of age and those under 65 years of age; there was an insufficient number of patients over 75 years of age to permit conclusions in that age-group. No dosage adjustment is recommended in the elderly.

In patients with mild-to-moderate hepatic impairment, clearance is reduced 2-fold and mean half-life is increased to 11.6 hours compared to 5.7 hours in normals. In patients with severe hepatic impairment (Child-Pugh[2] score of 10 or greater), clearance is reduced 2-fold to 3-fold and apparent volume of distribution is increased with a resultant increase in half-life to 20 hours. In patients with severe hepatic impairment, a total daily dose of 8 mg should not be exceeded.

Due to the very small contribution (5%) of renal clearance to the overall clearance, renal impairment was not expected to significantly influence the total clearance of ondansetron. However, ondansetron oral mean plasma clearance was reduced by about 50% in patients with severe renal impairment (creatinine clearance < 30 mL/min). This reduction in clearance is variable and was not consistent with an increase in half-life. No reduction in dose or dosing frequency in these patients is warranted.

Plasma protein binding of ondansetron as measured in vitro was 70% to 76% over the concentration range of 10 to 500 ng/mL. Circulating drug also distributes into erythrocytes.

Four- and 8-mg doses of either ZOFRAN Oral Solution or ZOFRAN ODT Orally Disintegrating Tablets are bioequiva-

Table 1. Pharmacokinetics in Normal Volunteers: Single 8-mg ZOFRAN Tablet Dose

Age-group (years)	Mean Weight (kg)	n	Peak Plasma Concentration (ng/mL)	Time of Peak Plasma Concentration (h)	Mean Elimination Half-life (h)	Systemic Plasma Clearance L/h/kg	Absolute Bioavailability
18-40 M	69.0	6	26.2	2.0	3.1	0.403	0.483
F	62.7	5	42.7	1.7	3.5	0.354	0.663
61-74 M	77.5	6	24.1	2.1	4.1	0.384	0.585
F	60.2	6	52.4	1.9	4.9	0.255	0.643
≥ 75 M	78.0	5	37.0	2.2	4.5	0.277	0.619
F	67.6	6	46.1	2.1	6.2	0.249	0.747

Table 2. Pharmacokinetics in Normal Volunteers: Single 24-mg ZOFRAN Tablet Dose

Age-group (years)	Mean Weight (kg)	n	Peak Plasma Concentration (ng/mL)	Time of Peak Plasma Concentration (h)	Mean Elimination Half-life (h)
18-43 M	84.1	8	125.8	1.9	4.7
F	71.8	8	194.4	1.6	5.8

Table 3. Emetic Episodes: Treatment Response

	Ondansetron 8-mg b.i.d. ZOFRAN Tablets[a]	Placebo	*P* Value
Number of patients	33	34	
Treatment response			
0 Emetic episodes	20 (61%)	2 (6%)	< 0.001
1-2 Emetic episodes	6 (18%)	8 (24%)	< 0.001
More than 2 emetic episodes/withdrawn	7 (21%)	24 (71%)	
Median number of emetic episodes	0.0	Undefined[b]	
Median time to first emetic episode (h)	Undefined[c]	6.5	

[a] The first dose was administered 30 minutes before the start of emetogenic chemotherapy, with a subsequent dose 8 hours after the first dose. An 8-mg ZOFRAN Tablet was administered twice a day for 2 days after completion of chemotherapy.
[b] Median undefined since at least 50% of the patients were withdrawn or had more than 2 emetic episodes.
[c] Median undefined since at least 50% of patients did not have any emetic episodes.

Table 4. Emetic Episodes: Treatment Response

	Ondansetron 8-mg b.i.d. ZOFRAN Tablets[a]	Ondansetron 8-mg t.i.d. ZOFRAN Tablets[b]
Number of patients	165	171
Treatment response		
0 Emetic episodes	101 (61%)	99 (58%)
1-2 Emetic episodes	16 (10%)	17 (10%)
More than 2 emetic episodes/withdrawn	48 (29%)	55 (32%)
Median number of emetic episodes	0.0	0.0
Median time to first emetic episode (h)	Undefined[c]	Undefined[c]
Median nausea scores (0-100)[d]	6	6

[a] The first dose was administered 30 minutes before the start of emetogenic chemotherapy, with a subsequent dose 8 hours after the first dose. An 8-mg ZOFRAN Tablet was administered twice a day for 2 days after completion of chemotherapy.
[b] The first dose was administered 30 minutes before the start of emetogenic chemotherapy, with subsequent doses 4 and 8 hours after the first dose. An 8-mg ZOFRAN Tablet was administered 3 times a day for 2 days after completion of chemotherapy.
[c] Median undefined since at least 50% of patients did not have any emetic episodes.
[d] Visual analog scale assessment: 0 = no nausea, 100 = nausea as bad as it can be.

lent to corresponding doses of ZOFRAN Tablets and may be used interchangeably. One 24-mg ZOFRAN Tablet is bioequivalent to and interchangeable with three 8-mg ZOFRAN Tablets.

CLINICAL TRIALS

Chemotherapy-Induced Nausea and Vomiting

Highly Emetogenic Chemotherapy

In 2 randomized, double-blind, monotherapy trials, a single 24-mg ZOFRAN Tablet was superior to a relevant historical placebo control in the prevention of nausea and vomiting associated with highly emetogenic cancer chemotherapy, including cisplatin ≥ 50 mg/m^2. Steroid administration was excluded from these clinical trials. More than 90% of patients receiving a cisplatin dose ≥ 50 mg/m^2 in the historical placebo comparator experienced vomiting in the absence of antiemetic therapy.

The first trial compared oral doses of ondansetron 24 mg once a day, 8 mg twice a day, and 32 mg once a day in 357 adult cancer patients receiving chemotherapy regimens containing cisplatin ≥ 50 mg/m^2. A total of 66% of patients in the ondansetron 24-mg once-a-day group, 55% in the ondansetron 8-mg twice-a-day group, and 55% in the ondansetron 32-mg once-a-day group completed the 24-hour study period with 0 emetic episodes and no rescue antiemetic medications, the primary endpoint of efficacy. Each of the 3 treatment groups was shown to be statistically significantly superior to a historical placebo control.

In the same trial, 56% of patients receiving oral ondansetron 24 mg once a day experienced no nausea during the 24-hour study period, compared with 36% of patients in the oral ondansetron 8-mg twice-a-day group (P = 0.001) and 50% in the oral ondansetron 32-mg once-a-day group.

In a second trial, efficacy of the oral ondansetron 24-mg once-a-day regimen in the prevention of nausea and vomiting associated with highly emetogenic cancer chemotherapy, including cisplatin ≥ 50 mg/m^2, was confirmed.

Moderately Emetogenic Chemotherapy

In 1 double-blind US study in 67 patients, ZOFRAN Tablets 8 mg administered twice a day were significantly more effective than placebo in preventing vomiting induced by cyclophosphamide-based chemotherapy containing doxorubicin. Treatment response is based on the total number of emetic episodes over the 3-day study period. The results of this study are summarized in Table 3:

[See table 3 above]

In 1 double-blind US study in 336 patients, ZOFRAN Tablets 8 mg administered twice a day were as effective as ZOFRAN Tablets 8 mg administered 3 times a day in preventing nausea and vomiting induced by cyclophosphamide-based chemotherapy containing either methotrexate or doxorubicin. Treatment response is based on the total number of emetic episodes over the 3-day study period. The results of this study are summarized in Table 4:

[See table 4 above]

Re-treatment

In uncontrolled trials, 148 patients receiving cyclophosphamide-based chemotherapy were re-treated with ZOFRAN Tablets 8 mg 3 times daily during subsequent chemotherapy for a total of 396 re-treatment courses. No emetic episodes occurred in 314 (79%) of the re-treatment courses, and only 1 to 2 emetic episodes occurred in 43 (11%) of the re-treatment courses.

Pediatric Studies

Three open-label, uncontrolled, foreign trials have been performed with 182 pediatric patients 4 to 18 years old with cancer who were given a variety of cisplatin or noncisplatin regimens. In these foreign trials, the initial dose of ZOFRAN® (ondansetron HCl) Injection ranged from 0.04 to 0.87 mg/kg for a total dose of 2.16 to 12 mg. This was followed by the administration of ZOFRAN Tablets ranging from 4 to 24 mg daily for 3 days. In these studies, 58% of the 170 evaluable patients had a complete response (no emetic episodes) on day 1. Two studies showed the response rates for patients less than 12 years of age who received ZOFRAN Tablets 4 mg 3 times a day to be similar to those in patients 12 to 18 years of age who received ZOFRAN Tablets 8 mg 3 times daily. Thus, prevention of emesis in these pediatric patients was essentially the same as for patients older than 18 years of age. Overall, ZOFRAN Tablets were well tolerated in these pediatric patients.

Radiation-Induced Nausea and Vomiting

Total Body Irradiation

In a randomized, double-blind study in 20 patients, ZOFRAN Tablets (8 mg given 1.5 hours before each fraction of radiotherapy for 4 days) were significantly more effective than placebo in preventing vomiting induced by total body irradiation. Total body irradiation consisted of 11 fractions (120 cGy per fraction) over 4 days for a total of 1,320 cGy. Patients received 3 fractions for 3 days, then 2 fractions on day 4.

Single High-Dose Fraction Radiotherapy

Ondansetron was significantly more effective than metoclopramide with respect to complete control of emesis (0 emetic episodes) in a double-blind trial in 105 patients receiving single high-dose radiotherapy (800 to 1,000 cGy) over an anterior or posterior field size of ≥ 80 cm^2 to the abdomen. Patients received the first dose of ZOFRAN Tablets (8 mg) or metoclopramide (10 mg) 1 to 2 hours before radiotherapy. If radiotherapy was given in the morning, 2 additional doses of study treatment were given (1 tablet late afternoon and 1 tablet before bedtime). If radiotherapy was given in the afternoon, patients took only 1 further tablet that day before bedtime. Patients continued the oral medication on a 3 times a day basis for 3 days.

Daily Fractionated Radiotherapy

Ondansetron was significantly more effective than prochlorperazine with respect to complete control of emesis (0 emetic episodes) in a double-blind trial in 135 patients receiving a 1- to 4-week course of fractionated radiotherapy (180 cGy doses) over a field size of ≥ 100 cm^2 to the abdomen. Patients received the first dose of ZOFRAN Tablets (8 mg) or prochlorperazine (10 mg) 1 to 2 hours before the patient received the first daily radiotherapy fraction, with 2 subsequent doses on a 3 times a day basis. Patients continued the oral medication on a 3 times a day basis on each day of radiotherapy.

Postoperative Nausea and Vomiting

Surgical patients who received ondansetron 1 hour before the induction of general balanced anesthesia (barbiturate:

thiopental, methohexital, or thiamylal; opioid: alfentanil, sufentanil, morphine, or fentanyl; nitrous oxide; neuromuscular blockade: succinylcholine/curare or gallamine and/or vecuronium, pancuronium, or atracurium; and supplemental isoflurane or enflurane) were evaluated in 2 double-blind studies (1 US study, 1 foreign) involving 865 patients. ZOFRAN Tablets (16 mg) were significantly more effective than placebo in preventing postoperative nausea and vomiting.

The study populations in all trials thus far consisted of women undergoing inpatient surgical procedures. No studies have been performed in males. No controlled clinical study comparing ZOFRAN Tablets to ZOFRAN Injection has been performed.

INDICATIONS AND USAGE

1. Prevention of nausea and vomiting associated with highly emetogenic cancer chemotherapy, including cisplatin ≥ 50 mg/m².
2. Prevention of nausea and vomiting associated with initial and repeat courses of moderately emetogenic cancer chemotherapy.
3. Prevention of nausea and vomiting associated with radiotherapy in patients receiving either total body irradiation, single high-dose fraction to the abdomen, or daily fractions to the abdomen.
4. Prevention of postoperative nausea and/or vomiting. As with other antiemetics, routine prophylaxis is not recommended for patients in whom there is little expectation that nausea and/or vomiting will occur postoperatively. In patients where nausea and/or vomiting must be avoided postoperatively, ZOFRAN Tablets, ZOFRAN ODT Orally Disintegrating Tablets, and ZOFRAN Oral Solution are recommended even where the incidence of postoperative nausea and/or vomiting is low.

CONTRAINDICATIONS

The concomitant use of apomorphine with ondansetron is contraindicated based on reports of profound hypotension and loss of consciousness when apomorphine was administered with ondansetron.

ZOFRAN Tablets, ZOFRAN ODT Orally Disintegrating Tablets, and ZOFRAN Oral Solution are contraindicated for patients known to have hypersensitivity to the drug.

WARNINGS

Hypersensitivity reactions have been reported in patients who have exhibited hypersensitivity to other selective 5-HT$_3$ receptor antagonists.

ECG changes including QT interval prolongation has been seen in patients receiving ondansetron. In addition, postmarketing cases of Torsade de Pointes have been reported in patients using ondansetron. Avoid ZOFRAN in patients with congenital long QT syndrome. ECG monitoring is recommended in patients with electrolyte abnormalities (e.g., hypokalemia or hypomagnesemia), congestive heart failure, bradyarrhythmias or patients taking other medicinal products that lead to QT prolongation.

PRECAUTIONS

General

Ondansetron is not a drug that stimulates gastric or intestinal peristalsis. It should not be used instead of nasogastric suction. The use of ondansetron in patients following abdominal surgery or in patients with chemotherapy-induced nausea and vomiting may mask a progressive ileus and/or gastric distension.

Information for Patients

Phenylketonurics

Phenylketonuric patients should be informed that ZOFRAN ODT Orally Disintegrating Tablets contain phenylalanine (a component of aspartame). Each 4-mg and 8-mg orally disintegrating tablet contains < 0.03 mg phenylalanine.

Patients should be instructed not to remove ZOFRAN ODT Tablets from the blister until just prior to dosing. The tablet should not be pushed through the foil. With dry hands, the blister backing should be peeled completely off the blister. The tablet should be gently removed and immediately placed on the tongue to dissolve and be swallowed with the saliva. Peelable illustrated stickers are affixed to the product carton that can be provided with the prescription to ensure proper use and handling of the product.

Drug Interactions

Ondansetron does not itself appear to induce or inhibit the cytochrome P-450 drug-metabolizing enzyme system of the liver (see CLINICAL PHARMACOLOGY, Pharmacokinetics). Because ondansetron is metabolized by hepatic cytochrome P-450 drug-metabolizing enzymes (CYP3A4, CYP2D6, CYP1A2), inducers or inhibitors of these enzymes may change the clearance and, hence, the half-life of ondansetron. On the basis of available data, no dosage adjustment is recommended for patients on these drugs.

Apomorphine

Based on reports of profound hypotension and loss of consciousness when apomorphine was administered with ondansetron, concomitant use of apomorphine with ondansetron is contraindicated (see CONTRAINDICATIONS).

Phenytoin, Carbamazepine, and Rifampicin

In patients treated with potent inducers of CYP3A4 (i.e., phenytoin, carbamazepine, and rifampicin), the clearance of ondansetron was significantly increased and ondansetron blood concentrations were decreased. However, on the basis of available data, no dosage adjustment for ondansetron is recommended for patients on these drugs.[1,3]

Tramadol

Although no pharmacokinetic drug interaction between ondansetron and tramadol has been observed, data from 2 small studies indicate that ondansetron may be associated with an increase in patient controlled administration of tramadol.[4,5]

Chemotherapy

Tumor response to chemotherapy in the P-388 mouse leukemia model is not affected by ondansetron. In humans, carmustine, etoposide, and cisplatin do not affect the pharmacokinetics of ondansetron.

In a crossover study in 76 pediatric patients, I.V. ondansetron did not increase blood levels of high-dose methotrexate.

Use in Surgical Patients

The coadministration of ondansetron had no effect on the pharmacokinetics and pharmacodynamics of temazepam.

Carcinogenesis, Mutagenesis, Impairment of Fertility

Carcinogenic effects were not seen in 2-year studies in rats and mice with oral ondansetron doses up to 10 and 30 mg/kg/day, respectively. Ondansetron was not mutagenic in standard tests for mutagenicity. Oral administration of ondansetron up to 15 mg/kg/day did not affect fertility or general reproductive performance of male and female rats.

Pregnancy

Teratogenic Effects

Pregnancy Category B. Reproduction studies have been performed in pregnant rats and rabbits at daily oral doses up to 15 and 30 mg/kg/day, respectively, and have revealed no evidence of impaired fertility or harm to the fetus due to ondansetron. There are, however, no adequate and well-controlled studies in pregnant women. Because animal reproduction studies are not always predictive of human response, this drug should be used during pregnancy only if clearly needed.

Nursing Mothers

Ondansetron is excreted in the breast milk of rats. It is not known whether ondansetron is excreted in human milk. Because many drugs are excreted in human milk, caution should be exercised when ondansetron is administered to a nursing woman.

Pediatric Use

Little information is available about dosage in pediatric patients 4 years of age or younger (see CLINICAL PHARMACOLOGY and DOSAGE AND ADMINISTRATION sections for use in pediatric patients 4 to 18 years of age).

Geriatric Use

Of the total number of subjects enrolled in cancer chemotherapy-induced and postoperative nausea and vomiting in US- and foreign-controlled clinical trials, for which there were subgroup analyses, 938 were 65 years of age and over. No overall differences in safety or effectiveness were observed between these subjects and younger subjects, and other reported clinical experience has not identified differences in responses between the elderly and younger patients, but greater sensitivity of some older individuals cannot be ruled out. Dosage adjustment is not needed in patients over the age of 65 (see CLINICAL PHARMACOLOGY).

ADVERSE REACTIONS

The following have been reported as adverse events in clinical trials of patients treated with ondansetron, the active ingredient of ZOFRAN. A causal relationship to therapy with ZOFRAN has been unclear in many cases.

Chemotherapy-Induced Nausea and Vomiting

The adverse events in Table 5 have been reported in ≥ 5% of adult patients receiving a single 24-mg ZOFRAN Tablet in 2 trials. These patients were receiving concurrent highly emetogenic cisplatin-based chemotherapy regimens (cisplatin dose ≥ 50 mg/m²).

Table 5. Principal Adverse Events in US Trials: Single Day Therapy With 24-mg ZOFRAN Tablets (Highly Emetogenic Chemotherapy)

Event	Ondansetron 24 mg q.d. n = 300	Ondansetron 8 mg b.i.d. n = 124	Ondansetron 32 mg q.d. n = 117
Headache	33 (11%)	16 (13%)	17 (15%)
Diarrhea	13 (4%)	9 (7%)	3 (3%)

The adverse events in Table 6 have been reported in ≥ 5% of adults receiving either 8 mg of ZOFRAN Tablets 2 or 3 times a day for 3 days or placebo in 4 trials. These patients were receiving concurrent moderately emetogenic chemotherapy, primarily cyclophosphamide-based regimens.

Table 6. Principal Adverse Events in US Trials: 3 Days of Therapy With 8-mg ZOFRAN Tablets (Moderately Emetogenic Chemotherapy)

Event	Ondansetron 8 mg b.i.d. n = 242	Ondansetron 8 mg t.i.d. n = 415	Placebo n = 262
Headache	58 (24%)	113 (27%)	34 (13%)
Malaise/fatigue	32 (13%)	37 (9%)	6 (2%)
Constipation	22 (9%)	26 (6%)	1 (<1%)
Diarrhea	15 (6%)	16 (4%)	10 (4%)
Dizziness	13 (5%)	18 (4%)	12 (5%)

Central Nervous System

There have been rare reports consistent with, but not diagnostic of, extrapyramidal reactions in patients receiving ondansetron.

Hepatic

In 723 patients receiving cyclophosphamide-based chemotherapy in US clinical trials, AST and/or ALT values have been reported to exceed twice the upper limit of normal in approximately 1% to 2% of patients receiving ZOFRAN Tablets. The increases were transient and did not appear to be related to dose or duration of therapy. On repeat exposure, similar transient elevations in transaminase values occurred in some courses, but symptomatic hepatic disease did not occur. The role of cancer chemotherapy in these biochemical changes cannot be clearly determined.

There have been reports of liver failure and death in patients with cancer receiving concurrent medications including potentially hepatotoxic cytotoxic chemotherapy and antibiotics. The etiology of the liver failure is unclear.

Integumentary

Rash has occurred in approximately 1% of patients receiving ondansetron.

Other

Rare cases of anaphylaxis, bronchospasm, tachycardia, angina (chest pain), hypokalemia, electrocardiographic alterations, vascular occlusive events, and grand mal seizures have been reported. Except for bronchospasm and anaphylaxis, the relationship to ZOFRAN was unclear.

Radiation-Induced Nausea and Vomiting

The adverse events reported in patients receiving ZOFRAN Tablets and concurrent radiotherapy were similar to those reported in patients receiving ZOFRAN Tablets and concurrent chemotherapy. The most frequently reported adverse events were headache, constipation, and diarrhea.

Postoperative Nausea and Vomiting

The adverse events in Table 7 have been reported in ≥ 5% of patients receiving ZOFRAN Tablets at a dosage of 16 mg orally in clinical trials. With the exception of headache, rates of these events were not significantly different in the ondansetron and placebo groups. These patients were receiving multiple concomitant perioperative and postoperative medications.

Table 7. Frequency of Adverse Events From Controlled Studies With ZOFRAN Tablets (Postoperative Nausea and Vomiting)

Adverse Event	Ondansetron 16 mg (n = 550)	Placebo (n = 531)
Wound problem	152 (28%)	162 (31%)
Drowsiness/sedation	112 (20%)	122 (23%)
Headache	49 (9%)	27 (5%)
Hypoxia	49 (9%)	35 (7%)
Pyrexia	45 (8%)	34 (6%)
Dizziness	36 (7%)	34 (6%)
Gynecological disorder	36 (7%)	33 (6%)
Anxiety/agitation	33 (6%)	29 (5%)
Bradycardia	32 (6%)	30 (6%)
Shiver(s)	28 (5%)	30 (6%)

Urinary retention	28 (5%)	18 (3%)
Hypotension	27 (5%)	32 (6%)
Pruritus	27 (5%)	20 (4%)

Preliminary observations in a small number of subjects suggest a higher incidence of headache when ZOFRAN ODT Orally Disintegrating Tablets are taken with water, when compared to without water.

Observed During Clinical Practice

In addition to adverse events reported from clinical trials, the following events have been identified during post-approval use of oral formulations of ZOFRAN. Because they are reported voluntarily from a population of unknown size, estimates of frequency cannot be made. The events have been chosen for inclusion due to a combination of their seriousness, frequency of reporting, or potential causal connection to ZOFRAN.

Cardiovascular

Rarely and predominantly with intravenous ondansetron, transient ECG changes including QT interval prolongation have been reported.

General

Flushing. Rare cases of hypersensitivity reactions, sometimes severe (e.g., anaphylaxis/anaphylactoid reactions, angioedema, bronchospasm, shortness of breath, hypotension, laryngeal edema, stridor) have also been reported. Laryngospasm, shock, and cardiopulmonary arrest have occurred during allergic reactions in patients receiving injectable ondansetron.

Hepatobiliary

Liver enzyme abnormalities

Lower Respiratory

Hiccups

Neurology:

Oculogyric crisis, appearing alone, as well as with other dystonic reactions

Skin

Urticaria, toxic skin eruption, including toxic epidermal necrolysis

Special Senses

Eye Disorders

Cases of transient blindness, predominantly during intravenous administration, have been reported. These cases of transient blindness were reported to resolve within a few minutes up to 48 hours.

DRUG ABUSE AND DEPENDENCE

Animal studies have shown that ondansetron is not discriminated as a benzodiazepine nor does it substitute for benzodiazepines in direct addiction studies.

OVERDOSAGE

There is no specific antidote for ondansetron overdose. Patients should be managed with appropriate supportive therapy. Individual intravenous doses as large as 150 mg and total daily intravenous doses as large as 252 mg have been inadvertently administered without significant adverse events. These doses are more than 10 times the recommended daily dose.

In addition to the adverse events listed above, the following events have been described in the setting of ondansetron overdose: "Sudden blindness" (amaurosis) of 2 to 3 minutes' duration plus severe constipation occurred in 1 patient that was administered 72 mg of ondansetron intravenously as a single dose. Hypotension (and faintness) occurred in a patient that took 48 mg of ZOFRAN Tablets. Following infusion of 32 mg over only a 4-minute period, a vasovagal episode with transient second-degree heart block was observed. In all instances, the events resolved completely.

DOSAGE AND ADMINISTRATION

Instructions for Use/Handling ZOFRAN ODT Orally Disintegrating Tablets

Do not attempt to push ZOFRAN ODT Tablets through the foil backing. With dry hands, PEEL BACK the foil backing of 1 blister and GENTLY remove the tablet. IMMEDIATELY place the ZOFRAN ODT Tablet on top of the tongue where it will dissolve in seconds, then swallow with saliva. Administration with liquid is not necessary.

Prevention of Nausea and Vomiting Associated With Highly Emetogenic Cancer Chemotherapy

The recommended adult oral dosage of ZOFRAN is 24 mg given as three 8-mg tablets administered 30 minutes before the start of single-day highly emetogenic chemotherapy, including cisplatin ≥ 50 mg/m^2. Multiday, single-dose administration of a 24 mg dosage has not been studied.

Pediatric Use

There is no experience with the use of a 24 mg dosage in pediatric patients.

Geriatric Use

The dosage recommendation is the same as for the general population.

Prevention of Nausea and Vomiting Associated With Moderately Emetogenic Cancer Chemotherapy

The recommended adult oral dosage is one 8-mg ZOFRAN Tablet or one 8-mg ZOFRAN ODT Tablet or 10 mL (2 teaspoonfuls equivalent to 8 mg of ondansetron) of ZOFRAN Oral Solution given twice a day. The first dose should be administered 30 minutes before the start of emetogenic chemotherapy, with a subsequent dose 8 hours after the first dose. One 8-mg ZOFRAN Tablet or one 8-mg ZOFRAN ODT Tablet or 10 mL (2 teaspoonfuls equivalent to 8 mg of ondansetron) of ZOFRAN Oral Solution should be administered twice a day (every 12 hours) for 1 to 2 days after completion of chemotherapy.

Pediatric Use

For pediatric patients 12 years of age and older, the dosage is the same as for adults. For pediatric patients 4 through 11 years of age, the dosage is one 4-mg ZOFRAN Tablet or one 4-mg ZOFRAN ODT Tablet or 5 mL (1 teaspoonful equivalent to 4 mg of ondansetron) of ZOFRAN Oral Solution given 3 times a day. The first dose should be administered 30 minutes before the start of emetogenic chemotherapy, with subsequent doses 4 and 8 hours after the first dose. One 4-mg ZOFRAN Tablet or one 4-mg ZOFRAN ODT Tablet or 5 mL (1 teaspoonful equivalent to 4 mg of ondansetron) of ZOFRAN Oral Solution should be administered 3 times a day (every 8 hours) for 1 to 2 days after completion of chemotherapy.

Geriatric Use

The dosage is the same as for the general population.

Prevention of Nausea and Vomiting Associated With Radiotherapy, Either Total Body Irradiation, or Single High-Dose Fraction or Daily Fractions to the Abdomen

The recommended oral dosage is one 8-mg ZOFRAN Tablet or one 8-mg ZOFRAN ODT Tablet or 10 mL (2 teaspoonfuls equivalent to 8 mg of ondansetron) of ZOFRAN Oral Solution given 3 times a day.

For total body irradiation, one 8-mg ZOFRAN Tablet or one 8-mg ZOFRAN ODT Tablet or 10 mL (2 teaspoonfuls equivalent to 8 mg of ondansetron) of ZOFRAN Oral Solution should be administered 1 to 2 hours before each fraction of radiotherapy administered each day.

For single high-dose fraction radiotherapy to the abdomen, one 8-mg ZOFRAN Tablet or one 8-mg ZOFRAN ODT Tablet or 10 mL (2 teaspoonfuls equivalent to 8 mg of ondansetron) of ZOFRAN Oral Solution should be administered 1 to 2 hours before radiotherapy, with subsequent doses every 8 hours after the first dose for 1 to 2 days after completion of radiotherapy.

For daily fractionated radiotherapy to the abdomen, one 8-mg ZOFRAN Tablet or one 8-mg ZOFRAN ODT Tablet or 10 mL (2 teaspoonfuls equivalent to 8 mg of ondansetron) of ZOFRAN Oral Solution should be administered 1 to 2 hours before radiotherapy, with subsequent doses every 8 hours after the first dose for each day radiotherapy is given.

Pediatric Use

There is no experience with the use of ZOFRAN Tablets, ZOFRAN ODT Tablets, or ZOFRAN Oral Solution in the prevention of radiation-induced nausea and vomiting in pediatric patients.

Geriatric Use

The dosage recommendation is the same as for the general population.

Postoperative Nausea and Vomiting

The recommended dosage is 16 mg given as two 8-mg ZOFRAN Tablets or two 8-mg ZOFRAN ODT Tablets or 20 mL (4 teaspoonfuls equivalent to 16 mg of ondansetron) of ZOFRAN Oral Solution 1 hour before induction of anesthesia.

Pediatric Use

There is no experience with the use of ZOFRAN Tablets, ZOFRAN ODT Tablets, or ZOFRAN Oral Solution in the prevention of postoperative nausea and vomiting in pediatric patients.

Geriatric Use

The dosage is the same as for the general population.

Dosage Adjustment for Patients With Impaired Renal Function

The dosage recommendation is the same as for the general population. There is no experience beyond first-day administration of ondansetron.

Dosage Adjustment for Patients With Impaired Hepatic Function

In patients with severe hepatic impairment (Child-Pugh[2] score of 10 or greater), clearance is reduced and apparent volume of distribution is increased with a resultant increase in plasma half-life. In such patients, a total daily dose of 8 mg should not be exceeded.

HOW SUPPLIED

ZOFRAN Tablets, 4 mg (ondansetron HCl dihydrate equivalent to 4 mg of ondansetron), are white, oval, film-coated tablets engraved with "Zofran" on one side and "4" on the other in bottles of 30 tablets (NDC 0173-0446-00).

Bottles: Store between 2° and 30°C (36° and 86°F). Protect from light. Dispense in tight, light-resistant container as defined in the USP.

Unit Dose Packs: Store between 2° and 30°C (36° and 86°F). Protect from light. Store blisters in cartons.

ZOFRAN Tablets, 8 mg (ondansetron HCl dihydrate equivalent to 8 mg of ondansetron), are yellow, oval, film-coated tablets engraved with "Zofran" on one side and "8" on the other in daily unit dose packs of 3 tablets (NDC 0173-0447-04), and bottles of 30 tablets (NDC 0173-0447-00).

Bottles: Store between 2° and 30°C (36° and 86°F). Dispense in tight container as defined in the USP.

Unit Dose Packs: Store between 2° and 30°C (36° and 86°F).

ZOFRAN ODT Orally Disintegrating Tablets, 4 mg (as 4 mg ondansetron base) are white, round and plano-convex tablets debossed with a "Z4" on one side in unit dose packs of 30 tablets (NDC 0173-0569-00).

ZOFRAN ODT Orally Disintegrating Tablets, 8 mg (as 8 mg ondansetron base) are white, round and plano-convex tablets debossed with a "Z8" on one side in unit dose packs of 30 tablets (NDC 0173-0570-00).

Store between 2° and 30°C (36° and 86°F).

ZOFRAN Oral Solution, a clear, colorless to light yellow liquid with a characteristic strawberry odor, contains 5 mg of ondansetron HCl dihydrate equivalent to 4 mg of ondansetron per 5 mL in amber glass bottles of 50 mL with child-resistant closures (NDC 0173-0489-00).

Store upright between 15° and 30°C (59° and 86°F). Protect from light. Store bottles upright in cartons.

REFERENCES

1. Britto MR, Hussey EK, Mydlow P, et al. Effect of enzyme inducers on ondansetron (OND) metabolism in humans. *Clin Pharmacol Ther*. 1997;61:228.
2. Pugh RNH, Murray-Lyon IM, Dawson JL, Pietroni MC, Williams R. Transection of the oesophagus for bleeding oesophageal varices. *Brit J Surg*. 1973;60:646-649.
3. Villikka K, Kivisto KT, Neuvonen PJ. The effect of rifampin on the pharmacokinetics of oral and intravenous ondansetron. *Clin Pharmacol Ther*. 1999;65:377-381.
4. De Witte JL, Schoenmaekers B, Sessler DI, et al. *Anesth Analg*. 2001;92:1319-1321.
5. Arcioni R, della Rocca M, Romanò R, et al. *Anesth Analg*. 2002;94:1553-1557.

GlaxoSmithKline
Research Triangle Park, NC 27709
ZOFRAN Tablets and Oral Solution:
GlaxoSmithKline
Research Triangle Park, NC 27709
ZOFRAN ODT Orally Disintegrating Tablets:
Manufactured for GlaxoSmithKline
Research Triangle Park, NC 27709
by Catalent UK Swindon Zydis Ltd.
Blagrove, Swindon, Wiltshire, UK SN5 8RU

May 2013
ZFT:4PI

ZYBAN® ℞

[*zī′ban*]

(bupropion hydrochloride)

Sustained-Release Tablets

> **WARNING**
>
> Serious neuropsychiatric events, including but not limited to depression, suicidal ideation, suicide attempt, and completed suicide have been reported in patients taking ZYBAN for smoking cessation. Some cases may have been complicated by the symptoms of nicotine withdrawal in patients who stopped smoking. Depressed mood may be a symptom of nicotine withdrawal. Depression, rarely including suicidal ideation, has been reported in smokers undergoing a smoking cessation attempt without medication. However, some of these symptoms have occurred in patients taking ZYBAN who continued to smoke.
>
> All patients being treated with ZYBAN should be observed for neuropsychiatric symptoms including changes in behavior, hostility, agitation, depressed mood, and suicide-related events, including ideation, behavior, and attempted suicide. These symptoms, as well as worsening of pre-existing psychiatric illness and completed suicide have been reported in some patients attempting to quit smoking while taking ZYBAN in the postmarketing experience. When symptoms were reported, most were during treatment with ZYBAN, but some were following discontinuation of treatment with ZYBAN. These events have occurred in patients with and without pre-existing psychiatric disease; some have experienced worsening of their psychiatric illnesses. Patients with serious psychiatric

illness such as schizophrenia, bipolar disorder, and major depressive disorder did not participate in the premarketing studies of ZYBAN.

Advise patients and caregivers that the patient should stop taking ZYBAN and contact a healthcare provider immediately if agitation, hostility, depressed mood, or changes in thinking or behavior that are not typical for the patient are observed, or if the patient develops suicidal ideation or suicidal behavior. In many postmarketing cases, resolution of symptoms after discontinuation of ZYBAN was reported, although in some cases the symptoms persisted; therefore, ongoing monitoring and supportive care should be provided until symptoms resolve.

The risks of ZYBAN should be weighed against the benefits of its use. ZYBAN has been demonstrated to increase the likelihood of abstinence from smoking for as long as 6 months compared to treatment with placebo. The health benefits of quitting smoking are immediate and substantial. (See WARNINGS: Neuropsychiatric Symptoms and Suicide Risk in Smoking Cessation Treatment and PRECAUTIONS: Information for Patients.)

Use in Treating Psychiatric Disorders

Although ZYBAN is not indicated for treatment of depression, it contains the same active ingredient as the antidepressant medications WELLBUTRIN®, WELLBUTRIN SR ®, and WELLBUTRIN XL®. Antidepressants increased the risk compared to placebo of suicidal thinking and behavior (suicidality) in children, adolescents, and young adults in short-term studies of major depressive disorder (MDD) and other psychiatric disorders. Anyone considering the use of ZYBAN or any other antidepressant in a child, adolescent, or young adult must balance this risk with the clinical need. Short-term studies did not show an increase in the risk of suicidality with antidepressants compared to placebo in adults beyond age 24; there was a reduction in risk with antidepressants compared to placebo in adults aged 65 and older. Depression and certain other psychiatric disorders are themselves associated with increases in the risk of suicide. Patients of all ages who are started on antidepressant therapy should be monitored appropriately and observed closely for clinical worsening, suicidality, or unusual changes in behavior. Families and caregivers should be advised of the need for close observation and communication with the prescriber. ZYBAN is not approved for use in pediatric patients. (See WARNINGS: Clinical Worsening and Suicide Risk in Treating Psychiatric Disorders, PRECAUTIONS: Information for Patients, and PRECAUTIONS: Pediatric Use.)

DESCRIPTION

ZYBAN (bupropion hydrochloride) Sustained-Release Tablets are a non-nicotine aid to smoking cessation. ZYBAN is chemically unrelated to nicotine or other agents currently used in the treatment of nicotine addiction. Initially developed and marketed as an antidepressant (WELLBUTRIN [bupropion hydrochloride] Tablets and WELLBUTRIN SR [bupropion hydrochloride] Sustained-Release Tablets), ZYBAN is also chemically unrelated to tricyclic, tetracyclic, selective serotonin re-uptake inhibitor, or other known antidepressant agents. Its structure closely resembles that of diethylpropion; it is related to phenylethylamines. It is (±)-1-(3-chlorophenyl)-2-[(1,1-dimethylethyl)amino]-1-propanone hydrochloride. The molecular weight is 276.2. The molecular formula is $C_{13}H_{18}ClNO \bullet HCl$. Bupropion hydrochloride powder is white, crystalline, and highly soluble in water. It has a bitter taste and produces the sensation of local anesthesia on the oral mucosa. The structural formula is:

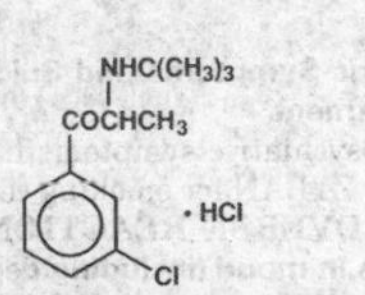

ZYBAN is supplied for oral administration as 150-mg (purple), film-coated, sustained-release tablets. Each tablet contains the labeled amount of bupropion hydrochloride and the inactive ingredients carnauba wax, cysteine hydrochloride, hypromellose, magnesium stearate, microcrystalline cellulose, polyethylene glycol, polysorbate 80 and titanium dioxide and is printed with edible black ink. In addition, the 150-mg tablet contains FD&C Blue No. 2 Lake and FD&C Red No. 40 Lake.

CLINICAL PHARMACOLOGY

Pharmacodynamics

Bupropion is a relatively weak inhibitor of the neuronal uptake of norepinephrine and dopamine, and does not inhibit monoamine oxidase or the re-uptake of serotonin. The mechanism by which ZYBAN enhances the ability of patients to abstain from smoking is unknown. However, it is presumed that this action is mediated by noradrenergic and/or dopaminergic mechanisms.

Pharmacokinetics

Bupropion is a racemic mixture. The pharmacologic activity and pharmacokinetics of the individual enantiomers have not been studied. Bupropion follows biphasic pharmacokinetics best described by a 2-compartment model. The terminal phase has a mean half-life (±% CV) of about 21 hours (±20%), while the distribution phase has a mean half-life of 3 to 4 hours.

Absorption: Bupropion has not been administered intravenously to humans; therefore, the absolute bioavailability of ZYBAN in humans has not been determined. In rat and dog studies, the bioavailability of bupropion ranged from 5% to 20%.

Following oral administration of ZYBAN to healthy volunteers, peak plasma concentrations of bupropion are achieved within 3 hours. The mean peak concentration (C_{max}) values were 91 and 143 ng/mL from 2 single-dose (150-mg) studies. At steady state, the mean C_{max} following a 150-mg dose every 12 hours is 136 ng/mL.

Exposure to bupropion may be increased when ZYBAN tablets are taken with food. Three studies in healthy volunteers demonstrated peak plasma concentrations (C_{max}) of bupropion increased by 11% to 35% when administered with food, while overall exposure (AUC) to bupropion increased by 16% to 19%. The food effect is not considered clinically significant and ZYBAN can be taken with or without food.

Distribution: In vitro tests show that bupropion is 84% bound to human plasma proteins at concentrations up to 200 mcg/mL. The extent of protein binding of the hydroxybupropion metabolite is similar to that for bupropion, whereas the extent of protein binding of the threohydrobupropion metabolite is about half that seen with bupropion. The volume of distribution (V_{ss}/F) estimated from a single 150-mg dose given to 17 subjects is 1,950 L (20% CV).

Metabolism: Bupropion is extensively metabolized in humans. Three metabolites have been shown to be active: hydroxybupropion, which is formed via hydroxylation of the *tert*-butyl group of bupropion, and the amino-alcohol isomers threohydrobupropion and erythrohydrobupropion, which are formed via reduction of the carbonyl group. In vitro findings suggest that cytochrome P450IIB6 (CYP2B6) is the principal isoenzyme involved in the formation of hydroxybupropion, while cytochrome P450 isoenzymes are not involved in the formation of threohydrobupropion. Oxidation of the bupropion side chain results in the formation of a glycine conjugate of meta-chlorobenzoic acid, which is then excreted as the major urinary metabolite. The potency and toxicity of the metabolites relative to bupropion have not been fully characterized. However, it has been demonstrated in an antidepressant screening test in mice that hydroxybupropion is one-half as potent as bupropion, while threohydrobupropion and erythrohydrobupropion are 5-fold less potent than bupropion. This may be of clinical importance because the plasma concentrations of the metabolites are as high or higher than those of bupropion.

Because bupropion is extensively metabolized, there is the potential for drug-drug interactions, particularly with those agents that are metabolized by or which inhibit/induce the cytochrome P450IIB6 (CYP2B6) isoenzyme, such as ritonavir or efavirenz. In a healthy volunteer study, ritonavir at a dose of 100 mg twice daily reduced the AUC and C_{max} of bupropion by 22% and 21%, respectively. The exposure of the hydroxybupropion metabolite was decreased by 23%, the threohydrobupropion decreased by 38%, and the erythrohydrobupropion decreased by 48%.

In a second healthy volunteer study, ritonavir at a dose of 600 mg twice daily decreased the AUC and the C_{max} of bupropion by 66% and 62%, respectively. The exposure of the hydroxybupropion metabolite was decreased by 78%, the threohydrobupropion decreased by 50%, and the erythrohydrobupropion decreased by 68%.

In another healthy volunteer study, KALETRA® (lopinavir 400 mg/ritonavir 100 mg twice daily) decreased bupropion AUC and C_{max} by 57%. The AUC and C_{max} of hydroxybupropion were decreased by 50% and 31%, respectively (see PRECAUTIONS: Drug Interactions).

In a study in healthy volunteers, efavirenz 600 mg once daily for 2 weeks reduced the AUC and C_{max} of bupropion by approximately 55% and 34%, respectively. The AUC of hydroxybupropion was unchanged, whereas C_{max} of hydroxybupropion was increased by 50%.

Although bupropion is not metabolized by cytochrome P450IID6 (CYP2D6), there is the potential for drug-drug interactions when bupropion is coadministered with drugs metabolized by this isoenzyme (see PRECAUTIONS: Drug Interactions).

Following a single dose in humans, peak plasma concentrations of hydroxybupropion occur approximately 6 hours after administration of ZYBAN. Peak plasma concentrations of hydroxybupropion are approximately 10 times the peak level of the parent drug at steady state. The elimination half-life of hydroxybupropion is approximately 20 (±5) hours and its AUC at steady state is about 17 times that of bupropion. The times to peak concentrations for the erythrohydrobupropion and threohydrobupropion metabolites are similar to that of the hydroxybupropion metabolite; however, their elimination half-lives are longer, 33 (±10) and 37 (±13) hours, respectively, and steady-state AUCs are 1.5 and 7 times that of bupropion, respectively.

Bupropion and its metabolites exhibit linear kinetics following chronic administration of 300 to 450 mg/day.

Elimination: The mean (±% CV) apparent clearance (Cl/F) estimated from 2 single-dose (150-mg) studies are 135 (±20%) and 209 L/hr (±21%). Following chronic dosing of 150 mg of ZYBAN every 12 hours for 14 days (n = 34), the mean Cl/F at steady state was 160 L/hr (±23%). The mean elimination half-life of bupropion estimated from a series of studies is approximately 21 hours. Estimates of the half-lives of the metabolites determined from a multiple-dose study were 20 hours (±25%) for hydroxybupropion, 37 hours (±35%) for threohydrobupropion, and 33 hours (±30%) for erythrohydrobupropion. Steady-state plasma concentrations of bupropion and metabolites are reached within 5 and 8 days, respectively.

Following oral administration of 200 mg of ^{14}C-bupropion in humans, 87% and 10% of the radioactive dose were recovered in the urine and feces, respectively. The fraction of the oral dose of bupropion excreted unchanged was only 0.5%.

The effects of cigarette smoking on the pharmacokinetics of bupropion were studied in 34 healthy male and female volunteers; 17 were chronic cigarette smokers and 17 were nonsmokers. Following oral administration of a single 150-mg dose of ZYBAN, there was no statistically significant difference in C_{max}, half-life, T_{max}, AUC, or clearance of bupropion or its major metabolites between smokers and nonsmokers.

In a study comparing the treatment combination of ZYBAN and nicotine transdermal system (NTS) versus ZYBAN alone, no statistically significant differences were observed between the 2 treatment groups of combination ZYBAN and NTS (n = 197) and ZYBAN alone (n = 193) in the plasma concentrations of bupropion or its active metabolites at weeks 3 and 6.

Population Subgroups

Factors or conditions altering metabolic capacity (e.g., liver disease, congestive heart failure [CHF], age, concomitant medications, etc.) or elimination may be expected to influence the degree and extent of accumulation of the active metabolites of bupropion. The elimination of the major metabolites of bupropion may be affected by reduced renal or hepatic function because they are moderately polar compounds and are likely to undergo further metabolism or conjugation in the liver prior to urinary excretion.

Hepatic: The effect of hepatic impairment on the pharmacokinetics of bupropion was characterized in 2 single-dose studies, one in patients with alcoholic liver disease and one in patients with mild-to-severe cirrhosis. The first study showed that the half-life of hydroxybupropion was significantly longer in 8 patients with alcoholic liver disease than in 8 healthy volunteers (32 ± 14 hours versus 21 ± 5 hours, respectively). Although not statistically significant, the AUCs for bupropion and hydroxybupropion were more variable and tended to be greater (by 53% to 57%) in patients with alcoholic liver disease. The differences in half-life for bupropion and the other metabolites in the 2 patient groups were minimal.

The second study showed that there were no statistically significant differences in the pharmacokinetics of bupropion and its active metabolites in 9 patients with mild-to-moderate hepatic cirrhosis compared to 8 healthy volunteers. However, more variability was observed in some of the pharmacokinetic parameters for bupropion (AUC, C_{max}, and T_{max}) and its active metabolites ($t_{½}$) in patients with mild-to-moderate hepatic cirrhosis. In addition, in patients with severe hepatic cirrhosis, the bupropion C_{max} and AUC were substantially increased (mean difference: by approximately 70% and 3-fold, respectively) and more variable when compared to values in healthy volunteers; the mean bupropion half-life was also longer (29 hours in patients with severe hepatic cirrhosis vs. 19 hours in healthy subjects). For the metabolite hydroxybupropion, the mean C_{max} was approximately 69% lower. For the combined amino-alcohol isomers threohydrobupropion and erythrohydrobupropion, the mean C_{max} was approximately 31% lower. The mean AUC increased by 28% for hydroxybupropion and 50% for threo/erythrohydrobupropion. The median T_{max} was observed 19 hours later for hydroxybupropion and 21 hours later for threo/erythrohydrobupropion. The mean half-lives for hydroxybupropion and threo/erythrohydrobupropion were increased 2- and 4-fold, respectively, in patients with severe hepatic cirrhosis compared to healthy volunteers (see WARNINGS, PRECAUTIONS, and DOSAGE AND ADMINISTRATION).

Renal: There is limited information on the pharmacokinetics of bupropion in patients with renal impairment. An inter-study comparison between normal subjects and patients with end-stage renal failure demonstrated that the parent drug C_{max} and AUC values were comparable in the 2 groups, whereas the hydroxybupropion and threohydrobupropion metabolites had a 2.3– and 2.8–fold increase, respectively, in AUC for patients with end-stage renal failure. A second study, comparing normal subjects and patients with moderate-to-severe renal impairment (GFR 30.9 ± 10.8 mL/min) showed that exposure to a single 150-mg dose

Table 1. Dose-Response Trial: Quit Rates by Treatment Group

Abstinence From Week 4 Through Specified Week	Treatment Groups			
	Placebo (n = 151) % (95% CI)	ZYBAN 100 mg/day (n = 153) % (95% CI)	ZYBAN 150 mg/day (n = 153) % (95% CI)	ZYBAN 300 mg/day (n = 156) % (95% CI)
Week 7 (4-week quit)	17% (11-23)	22% (15-28)	27%[a] (20-35)	36%[a] (28-43)
Week 12	14% (8-19)	20% (13-26)	20% (14-27)	25%[a] (18-32)
Week 26	11% (6-16)	16% (11-22)	18% (12-24)	19%[a] (13-25)

[a] Significantly different from placebo ($P \leq 0.05$).

Table 2. Comparative Trial: Quit Rates by Treatment Group

Abstinence From Week 4 Through Specified Week	Treatment Groups			
	Placebo (n = 160) % (95% CI)	Nicotine Transdermal System (NTS) 21 mg/day (n = 244) % (95% CI)	ZYBAN 300 mg/day (n = 244) % (95% CI)	ZYBAN 300 mg/day and NTS 21 mg/day (n = 245) % (95% CI)
Week 7 (4-week quit)	23% (17-30)	36% (30-42)	49% (43-56)	58% (51-64)
Week 10	20% (14-26)	32% (26-37)	46% (39-52)	51% (45-58)

of sustained-release bupropion was approximately 2-fold higher in patients with impaired renal function while levels of the hydroxybupropion and threo/erythrohydrobupropion (combined) metabolites were similar in the 2 groups. The elimination of bupropion and/or the major metabolites of bupropion may be reduced by impaired renal function (see PRECAUTIONS: Renal Impairment).

Left Ventricular Dysfunction: During a chronic dosing study with bupropion in 14 depressed patients with left ventricular dysfunction (history of CHF or an enlarged heart on x-ray), no apparent effect on the pharmacokinetics of bupropion or its metabolites, compared to healthy normal volunteers, was revealed.

Age: The effects of age on the pharmacokinetics of bupropion and its metabolites have not been fully characterized, but an exploration of steady-state bupropion concentrations from several depression efficacy studies involving patients dosed in a range of 300 to 750 mg/day, on a 3-times-a-day schedule, revealed no relationship between age (18 to 83 years) and plasma concentration of bupropion. A single-dose pharmacokinetic study demonstrated that the disposition of bupropion and its metabolites in elderly subjects was similar to that of younger subjects. These data suggest there is no prominent effect of age on bupropion concentration; however, another pharmacokinetic study, single and multiple dose, has suggested that the elderly are at increased risk for accumulation of bupropion and its metabolites (see PRECAUTIONS: Geriatric Use).

Gender: A single-dose study involving 12 healthy male and 12 healthy female volunteers revealed no sex-related differences in the pharmacokinetic parameters of bupropion.

CLINICAL TRIALS

The efficacy of ZYBAN as an aid to smoking cessation was demonstrated in 3 placebo-controlled, double-blind trials in nondepressed chronic cigarette smokers (n = 1,940, ≥15 cigarettes per day). In these studies, ZYBAN was used in conjunction with individual smoking cessation counseling.

The first study was a dose-response trial conducted at 3 clinical centers. Patients in this study were treated for 7 weeks with 1 of 3 doses of ZYBAN (100, 150, or 300 mg/day) or placebo; quitting was defined as total abstinence during the last 4 weeks of treatment (weeks 4 through 7). Abstinence was determined by patient daily diaries and verified by carbon monoxide levels in expired air.

Results of this dose-response trial with ZYBAN demonstrated a dose-dependent increase in the percentage of patients able to achieve 4-week abstinence (weeks 4 through 7). Treatment with ZYBAN at both 150 and 300 mg/day was significantly more effective than placebo in this study.

Table 1 presents quit rates over time in the multicenter trial by treatment group. The quit rates are the proportions of all persons initially enrolled (i.e., intent-to-treat analysis) who abstained from week 4 of the study through the specified week. Treatment with ZYBAN (150 or 300 mg/day) was more effective than placebo in helping patients achieve 4-week abstinence. In addition, treatment with ZYBAN (7 weeks at 300 mg/day) was more effective than placebo in helping patients maintain continuous abstinence through week 26 (6 months) of the study.

[See table 1 above]

The second study was a comparative trial conducted at 4 clinical centers. Four treatments were evaluated: ZYBAN 300 mg/day, nicotine transdermal system (NTS) 21 mg/day, combination of ZYBAN 300 mg/day plus NTS 21 mg/day, and placebo. Patients were treated for 9 weeks. Treatment with ZYBAN was initiated at 150 mg/day while the patient was still smoking and was increased after 3 days to 300 mg/day given as 150 mg twice daily. NTS 21 mg/day was added to treatment with ZYBAN after approximately 1 week when the patient reached the target quit date. During weeks 8 and 9 of the study, NTS was tapered to 14 and 7 mg/day, respectively. Quitting, defined as total abstinence during weeks 4 through 7, was determined by patient daily diaries and verified by expired air carbon monoxide levels. In this study, patients treated with any of the 3 treatments achieved greater 4-week abstinence rates than patients treated with placebo.

Table 2 presents quit rates over time by treatment group for the comparative trial.

[See table 2 above]

When patients in this study were followed out to one year, the superiority of ZYBAN and the combination of ZYBAN and NTS over placebo in helping patients to achieve abstinence from smoking was maintained. The continuous abstinence rate was 30% (95% CI 24-35) in the patients treated with ZYBAN, and 33% (95% CI 27-39) for patients treated with the combination at 26 weeks compared with 13% (95% CI 7-18) in the placebo group. At 52 weeks, the continuous abstinence rate was 23% (95% CI 18-28) in the patients treated with ZYBAN , and 28% (95% CI 23-34) for patients treated with the combination, compared with 8% (95% CI 3-12) in the placebo group. Although the treatment combination of ZYBAN and NTS displayed the highest rates of continuous abstinence throughout the study, the quit rates for the combination were not significantly higher ($P>0.05$) than for ZYBAN alone.

The comparisons between ZYBAN, NTS, and combination treatment in this study have not been replicated, and, therefore should not be interpreted as demonstrating the superiority of any of the active treatment arms over any other.

The third study was a long-term maintenance trial conducted at 5 clinical centers. Patients in this study received open-label ZYBAN 300 mg/day for 7 weeks. Patients who quit smoking while receiving ZYBAN (n = 432) were then randomized to ZYBAN 300 mg/day or placebo for a total study duration of 1 year. Abstinence from smoking was determined by patient self-report and verified by expired air carbon monoxide levels. This trial demonstrated that at 6 months, continuous abstinence rates were significantly higher for patients continuing to receive ZYBAN than for those switched to placebo ($P<0.05$; 55% versus 44%).

Quit rates in clinical trials are influenced by the population selected. Quit rates in an unselected population may be lower than the above rates. Quit rates for ZYBAN were similar in patients with and without prior quit attempts using nicotine replacement therapy.

Treatment with ZYBAN reduced withdrawal symptoms compared to placebo. Reductions on the following withdrawal symptoms were most pronounced: irritability, frustration, or anger; anxiety; difficulty concentrating; restlessness; and depressed mood or negative affect. Depending on the study and the measure used, treatment with ZYBAN showed evidence of reduction in craving for cigarettes or urge to smoke compared to placebo.

Use In Patients With Chronic Obstructive Pulmonary Disease (COPD)

ZYBAN was evaluated in a randomized, double-blind, comparative study of 404 patients with mild-to-moderate COPD, defined as $FEV_1 \geq 35\%$, $FEV_1/FVC \leq 70\%$ and a diagnosis of chronic bronchitis, emphysema and/or small airways disease. Patients aged 36 to 76 years were randomized to ZYBAN 300 mg/day (n = 204) or placebo (n = 200) and treated for 12 weeks. Treatment with ZYBAN was initiated at 150 mg/day for 3 days while the patient was still smoking and increased to 150 mg twice daily for the remaining treatment period. Abstinence from smoking was determined by patient daily diaries and verified by carbon monoxide levels in expired air. Quitters are defined as subjects who were abstinent during the last 4 weeks of treatment. Table 3 shows quit rates in the COPD Trial.

Table 3. COPD Trial: Quit Rates by Treatment Group

4-Week Abstinence Period	Treatment Groups	
	Placebo (n = 200) % (95% CI)	ZYBAN 300 mg/day (n = 204) % (95% CI)
Weeks 9 through 12	12% (8-16)	22%[a] (17-27)

[a]Significantly different from placebo ($P<0.05$).

INDICATIONS AND USAGE

ZYBAN is indicated as an aid to smoking cessation treatment.

CONTRAINDICATIONS

ZYBAN is contraindicated in patients with a seizure disorder.

ZYBAN is contraindicated in patients treated with WELLBUTRIN (bupropion hydrochloride), the immediate-release formulation; WELLBUTRIN SR (bupropion hydrochloride), the sustained-release formulation; WELLBUTRIN XL (bupropion hydrochloride), the extended-release formulation; or any other medications that contain bupropion because the incidence of seizure is dose dependent.

ZYBAN is contraindicated in patients with a current or prior diagnosis of bulimia or anorexia nervosa because of a higher incidence of seizures noted in patients treated for bulimia with the immediate-release formulation of bupropion.

ZYBAN is contraindicated in patients undergoing abrupt discontinuation of alcohol or sedatives (including benzodiazepines).

The concurrent administration of ZYBAN and a monoamine oxidase (MAO) inhibitor is contraindicated. At least 14 days should elapse between discontinuation of an MAO inhibitor and initiation of treatment with ZYBAN.

ZYBAN is contraindicated in patients who have shown an allergic response to bupropion or the other ingredients that make up ZYBAN.

WARNINGS

Neuropsychiatric Symptoms and Suicide Risk in Smoking Cessation Treatment

Serious neuropsychiatric symptoms have been reported in patients taking ZYBAN for smoking cessation **(see BOXED WARNING, ADVERSE REACTIONS). These have included changes in mood (including depression and mania), psychosis, hallucinations, paranoia, delusions, homicidal ideation, hostility, agitation, aggression, anxiety, and panic, as well as suicidal ideation, suicide attempt, and completed suicide.** Some reported cases may have been complicated by the symptoms of nicotine withdrawal in patients who stopped smoking. Depressed mood may be a symptom of nicotine withdrawal. Depression, rarely including suicidal ideation, has been reported in smokers undergoing a smoking cessation attempt without medication. However, some of these symptoms have occurred in patients taking ZYBAN who continued to smoke. When symptoms were reported, most were during treatment with ZYBAN, but some were following discontinuation of treatment with ZYBAN.

These events have occurred in patients with and without pre-existing psychiatric disease; some patients have experienced worsening of their psychiatric illnesses. All patients being treated with ZYBAN should be observed for neuropsychiatric symptoms or worsening of pre-existing psychiatric illness.

Patients with serious psychiatric illness such as schizophrenia, bipolar disorder, and major depressive disorder did not participate in the premarketing studies of ZYBAN.

Advise patients and caregivers that the patient should stop taking ZYBAN and contact a healthcare provider immediately if agitation, depressed mood, or changes in behavior or thinking that are not typical for the patient are observed, or if the patient develops suicidal ideation or suicidal behavior. In many postmarketing cases, resolution of symptoms after discontinuation of ZYBAN was reported, although in some cases the symptoms persisted, therefore, ongoing monitoring and supportive care should be provided until symptoms resolve.

The risks of ZYBAN should be weighed against the benefits of its use. ZYBAN has been demonstrated to increase the likelihood of abstinence from smoking for as long as six months compared to treatment with placebo. The health benefits of quitting smoking are immediate and substantial.

Clinical Worsening and Suicide Risk in Treating Psychiatric Disorders

Patients with major depressive disorder (MDD), both adult and pediatric, may experience worsening of their depression and/or the emergence of suicidal ideation and behavior (suicidality) or unusual changes in behavior, whether or not they are taking antidepressant medications, and this risk may persist until significant remission occurs. Suicide is a known risk of depression and certain other psychiatric disorders, and these disorders themselves are the strongest predictors of suicide. There has been a long-standing concern, however, that antidepressants may have a role in inducing worsening of depression and the emergence of suicidality in certain patients during the early phases of treatment. Pooled analyses of short-term placebo-controlled trials of antidepressant drugs (SSRIs and others) showed that these drugs increase the risk of suicidal thinking and behavior (suicidality) in children, adolescents, and young adults (ages 18-24) with major depressive disorder (MDD) and other psychiatric disorders. Short-term studies did not show an increase in the risk of suicidality with antidepressants compared to placebo in adults beyond age 24; there was a reduction with antidepressants compared to placebo in adults aged 65 and older.

The pooled analyses of placebo-controlled trials in children and adolescents with MDD, obsessive compulsive disorder (OCD), or other psychiatric disorders included a total of 24 short-term trials of 9 antidepressant drugs in over 4,400 patients. The pooled analyses of placebo-controlled trials in adults with MDD or other psychiatric disorders included a total of 295 short-term trials (median duration of 2 months) of 11 antidepressant drugs in over 77,000 patients. There was considerable variation in risk of suicidality among drugs, but a tendency toward an increase in the younger patients for almost all drugs studied. There were differences in absolute risk of suicidality across the different indications, with the highest incidence in MDD. The risk differences (drug vs. placebo), however, were relatively stable within age strata and across indications. These risk differences (drug-placebo difference in the number of cases of suicidality per 1,000 patients treated) are provided in Table 4.

Table 4.

Age Range	Drug-Placebo Difference in Number of Cases of Suicidality per 1,000 Patients Treated
	Increases Compared to Placebo
<18	14 additional cases
18-24	5 additional cases
	Decreases Compared to Placebo
25-64	1 fewer case
≥65	6 fewer cases

No suicides occurred in any of the pediatric trials. There were suicides in the adult trials, but the number was not sufficient to reach any conclusion about drug effect on suicide.

It is unknown whether the suicidality risk extends to longer-term use, i.e., beyond several months. However, there is substantial evidence from placebo-controlled maintenance trials in adults with depression that the use of antidepressants can delay the recurrence of depression.

All patients being treated with antidepressants for any indication should be monitored appropriately and observed closely for clinical worsening, suicidality, and unusual changes in behavior, especially during the initial few months of a course of drug therapy, or at times of dose changes, either increases or decreases.

The following symptoms, anxiety, agitation, panic attacks, insomnia, irritability, hostility, aggressiveness, impulsivity, akathisia (psychomotor restlessness), hypomania, and mania, have been reported in adult and pediatric patients being treated with antidepressants for major depressive disorder as well as for other indications, both psychiatric and nonpsychiatric. Although a causal link between the emergence of such symptoms and either the worsening of depression and/or the emergence of suicidal impulses has not been established, there is concern that such symptoms may represent precursors to emerging suicidality.

Consideration should be given to changing the therapeutic regimen, including possibly discontinuing the medication, in patients whose depression is persistently worse, or who are experiencing emergent suicidality or symptoms that might be precursors to worsening depression or suicidality, especially if these symptoms are severe, abrupt in onset, or were not part of the patient's presenting symptoms.

Families and caregivers of patients being treated with antidepressants for major depressive disorder or other indications, both psychiatric and nonpsychiatric, should be alerted about the need to monitor patients for the emergence of agitation, irritability, unusual changes in behavior, and the other symptoms described above, as well as the emergence of suicidality, and to report such symptoms immediately to healthcare providers. Such monitoring should include daily observation by families and caregivers. Prescriptions for ZYBAN should be written for the smallest quantity of tablets consistent with good patient management, in order to reduce the risk of overdose.

Screening Patients for Bipolar Disorder

A major depressive episode may be the initial presentation of bipolar disorder. It is generally believed (though not established in controlled trials) that treating such an episode with an antidepressant alone may increase the likelihood of precipitation of a mixed/manic episode in patients at risk for bipolar disorder. Whether any of the symptoms described above represent such a conversion is unknown. However, prior to initiating treatment with an antidepressant, patients with depressive symptoms should be adequately screened to determine if they are at risk for bipolar disorder; such screening should include a detailed psychiatric history, including a family history of suicide, bipolar disorder, and depression. It should be noted that ZYBAN is not approved for use in treating bipolar depression.

Bupropion-Containing Products

Patients should be made aware that ZYBAN contains the same active ingredient found in WELLBUTRIN, WELLBUTRIN SR, and WELLBUTRIN XL used to treat depression, and that ZYBAN should not be used in combination with WELLBUTRIN (bupropion hydrochloride), the immediate-release formulation; WELLBUTRIN SR (bupropion hydrochloride), the sustained-release formulation; WELLBUTRIN XL (bupropion hydrochloride), the extended-release formulation; or any other medications that contain bupropion.

Seizures

Because the use of bupropion is associated with a dose-dependent risk of seizures, *clinicians should not prescribe doses over 300 mg/day for smoking cessation.* The risk of seizures is also related to patient factors, clinical situation, and concomitant medications, which must be considered in selection of patients for therapy with ZYBAN. ZYBAN should be discontinued and not restarted in patients who experience a seizure while on treatment.

- **Dose: *For smoking cessation, doses above 300 mg/day should not be used.* The seizure rate associated with doses of sustained-release bupropion up to 300 mg/day is approximately 0.1% (1/1,000). This incidence was prospectively determined during an 8-week treatment exposure in approximately 3,100 depressed patients.**

Data for the immediate-release formulation of bupropion revealed a seizure incidence of approximately 0.4% (4/1,000) in depressed patients treated at doses in a range of 300 to 450 mg/day. In addition, the estimated seizure incidence increases almost tenfold between 450 and 600 mg/day.

- **Patient factors: Predisposing factors that may increase the risk of seizure with bupropion use include history of head trauma or prior seizure, central nervous system (CNS) tumor, the presence of severe hepatic cirrhosis, and concomitant medications that lower seizure threshold.**
- **Clinical situations: Circumstances associated with an increased seizure risk include, among others, excessive use of alcohol or sedatives (including benzodiazepines); addiction to opiates, cocaine, or stimulants; use of over-the-counter stimulants and anorectics; and diabetes treated with oral hypoglycemics or insulin.**
- **Concomitant medications: Many medications (e.g., antipsychotics, antidepressants, theophylline, systemic steroids) are known to lower seizure threshold.**

Recommendations for Reducing the Risk of Seizure: **Retrospective analysis of clinical experience gained during the development of bupropion suggests that the risk of seizure may be minimized if**

- **the total daily dose of ZYBAN does *not* exceed 300 mg (the maximum recommended dose for smoking cessation), and**
- **the recommended daily dose for most patients (300 mg/day) is administered in divided doses (150 mg twice daily).**
- **No single dose should exceed 150 mg to avoid high peak concentrations of bupropion and/or its metabolites.**

ZYBAN should be administered with extreme caution to patients with a history of seizure, cranial trauma, or other predisposition(s) toward seizure, or patients treated with other agents (e.g., antipsychotics, antidepressants, theophylline, systemic steroids, etc.) that lower seizure threshold.

Hepatic Impairment

ZYBAN should be used with extreme caution in patients with severe hepatic cirrhosis. In these patients a reduced frequency of dosing is required, as peak bupropion levels are substantially increased and accumulation is likely to occur in such patients to a greater extent than usual. The dose should not exceed 150 mg every other day in these patients (see CLINICAL PHARMACOLOGY, PRECAUTIONS, and DOSAGE AND ADMINISTRATION).

Potential for Hepatotoxicity

In rats receiving large doses of bupropion chronically, there was an increase in incidence of hepatic hyperplastic nodules and hepatocellular hypertrophy. In dogs receiving large doses of bupropion chronically, various histologic changes were seen in the liver, and laboratory tests suggesting mild hepatocellular injury were noted.

PRECAUTIONS

General

Allergic Reactions: Anaphylactoid/anaphylactic reactions characterized by symptoms such as pruritus, urticaria, angioedema, and dyspnea requiring medical treatment have been reported at a rate of about 1 to 3 per thousand in clinical trials of ZYBAN. In addition, there have been rare spontaneous postmarketing reports of erythema multiforme, Stevens-Johnson syndrome, and anaphylactic shock associated with bupropion. A patient should stop taking ZYBAN and consult a doctor if experiencing allergic or anaphylactoid/anaphylactic reactions (e.g., skin rash, pruritus, hives, chest pain, edema, and shortness of breath) during treatment.

Arthralgia, myalgia, and fever with rash and other symptoms suggestive of delayed hypersensitivity have been reported in association with bupropion. These symptoms may resemble serum sickness.

Insomnia: In the dose-response smoking cessation trial, 29% of patients treated with 150 mg/day of ZYBAN and 35% of patients treated with 300 mg/day of ZYBAN experienced insomnia, compared to 21% of placebo-treated patients. Symptoms were sufficiently severe to require discontinuation of treatment in 0.6% of patients treated with ZYBAN and none of the patients treated with placebo.

In the comparative trial, 40% of the patients treated with 300 mg/day of ZYBAN, 28% of the patients treated with 21 mg/day of NTS, and 45% of the patients treated with the combination of ZYBAN and NTS experienced insomnia compared to 18% of placebo-treated patients. Symptoms were sufficiently severe to require discontinuation of treatment in 0.8% of patients treated with ZYBAN and none of the patients in the other 3 treatment groups.

Insomnia may be minimized by avoiding bedtime doses and, if necessary, reduction in dose.

Psychosis, Confusion, and Other Neuropsychiatric Phenomena: Depressed patients treated with bupropion in depression trials have been reported to show a variety of neuropsychiatric signs and symptoms including delusions, hallucinations, psychosis, concentration disturbance, paranoia, and confusion. In some cases, these symptoms abated upon dose reduction and/or withdrawal of treatment. In clinical trials with ZYBAN conducted in nondepressed smokers, the incidence of neuropsychiatric side effects was generally comparable to placebo. However, in the postmarketing experience, patients taking ZYBAN to quit smoking have reported similar types of neuropsychiatric symptoms to those reported by patients in the clinical trials of bupropion for depression.

Activation of Psychosis and/or Mania: Antidepressants can precipitate manic episodes in bipolar disorder patients during the depressed phase of their illness and may activate latent psychosis in other susceptible individuals. The sustained-release formulation of bupropion is expected to pose similar risks. There were no reports of activation of psychosis or mania in clinical trials with ZYBAN conducted in nondepressed smokers.

Cardiovascular Effects: In clinical practice, hypertension, in some cases severe, requiring acute treatment, has been reported in patients receiving bupropion alone and in combination with nicotine replacement therapy. These events have been observed in both patients with and without evidence of preexisting hypertension.

Data from a comparative study of ZYBAN, nicotine transdermal system (NTS), the combination of sustained-release bupropion plus NTS, and placebo as an aid to smoking cessation suggest a higher incidence of treatment-emergent hypertension in patients treated with the combination of ZYBAN and NTS. In this study, 6.1% of patients treated with the combination of ZYBAN and NTS had treatment-emergent hypertension compared to 2.5%, 1.6%, and 3.1% of patients treated with ZYBAN, NTS, and placebo, respectively. The majority of these patients had evidence of preexisting hypertension. Three patients (1.2%) treated with the combination of ZYBAN and NTS and 1 patient (0.4%) treated with NTS had study medication discontinued due to hypertension compared to none of the patients treated with ZYBAN or placebo. Monitoring of blood pressure is recommended in patients who receive the combination of bupropion and nicotine replacement.

There is no clinical experience establishing the safety of ZYBAN in patients with a recent history of myocardial infarction or unstable heart disease. Therefore, care should be exercised if it is used in these groups. Bupropion was well tolerated in depressed patients who had previously developed orthostatic hypotension while receiving tricyclic antidepressants, and was also generally well tolerated in a group of 36 depressed inpatients with stable congestive heart failure (CHF). However, bupropion was associated with a rise in supine blood pressure in the study of patients with CHF, resulting in discontinuation of treatment in 2 patients for exacerbation of baseline hypertension.

Hepatic Impairment: ZYBAN should be used with extreme caution in patients with severe hepatic cirrhosis. In these patients, a reduced frequency of dosing is required. ZYBAN should be used with caution in patients with hepatic impairment (including mild-to-moderate hepatic cirrhosis) and reduced frequency of dosing should be considered in patients with mild-to-moderate hepatic cirrhosis.

All patients with hepatic impairment should be closely monitored for possible adverse effects that could indicate high drug and metabolite levels (see CLINICAL PHARMACOLOGY, WARNINGS, and DOSAGE AND ADMINISTRATION).

Renal Impairment: There is limited information on the pharmacokinetics of bupropion in patients with renal impairment. An inter-study comparison between normal subjects and patients with end-stage renal failure demonstrated that the parent drug C_{max} and AUC values were comparable in the 2 groups, whereas the hydroxybupropion and threohydrobupropion metabolites had a 2.3– and 2.8–fold increase, respectively, in AUC for patients with end-stage renal failure. A second study, comparing normal subjects and patients with moderate-to-severe renal impairment (GFR 30.9 ± 10.8 mL/min) showed that exposure to a single 150-mg dose of sustained-release bupropion was approximately 2-fold higher in patients with impaired renal function while levels of the hydroxybupropion and threo/erythrohydrobupropion (combined) metabolites were similar in the 2 groups. Bupropion is extensively metabolized in the liver to active metabolites, which are further metabolized and subsequently excreted by the kidneys. ZYBAN should be used with caution in patients with renal impairment and a reduced frequency of dosing should be considered as bupropion and the metabolites of bupropion may accumulate in such patients to a greater extent than usual. The patient should be closely monitored for possible adverse effects that could indicate high drug or metabolite levels.

Information for Patients

Although ZYBAN is not indicated for treatment of depression, it contains the same active ingredient as the antidepressant medications WELLBUTRIN, WELLBUTRIN SR, and WELLBUTRIN XL. Prescribers or other health professionals should inform patients, their families, and their caregivers about the benefits and risks associated with treatment with ZYBAN and should counsel them in its appropriate use. A patient Medication Guide about "Quitting Smoking, Quit-Smoking Medication, Changes in Thinking and Behavior, Depression, and Suicidal Thoughts or Actions," "Antidepressant Medicines, Depression and Other Serious Mental Illnesses, and Suicidal Thoughts or Actions," and "What Other Important Information Should I Know About ZYBAN?" is available for ZYBAN. The prescriber or health professional should instruct patients, their families, and their caregivers to read the Medication Guide and should assist them in understanding its contents. Patients should be given the opportunity to discuss the contents of the Medication Guide and to obtain answers to any questions they may have. The complete text of the Medication Guide is reprinted at the end of this document.

Patients should be advised of the following issues and asked to alert their prescriber if these occur while taking ZYBAN.

Neuropsychiatric Symptoms and Suicide Risk in Smoking Cessation Treatment: Patients should be informed that quitting smoking, with or without ZYBAN, may be associated with nicotine withdrawal symptoms (including depression or agitation), or exacerbation of pre-existing psychiatric illness. Furthermore, some patients have experienced changes in mood (including depression and mania), psychosis, hallucinations, paranoia, delusions, homicidal ideation, aggression, anxiety, and panic, as well as suicidal ideation, suicide attempt, and completed suicide when attempting to quit smoking while taking ZYBAN. If patients develop agitation, hostility, depressed mood, or changes in thinking or behavior that are not typical for them, or if patients develop suicidal ideation or behavior, they should be urged to report these symptoms to their healthcare provider immediately.

Clinical Worsening and Suicide Risk in Treating Psychiatric Disorders: Patients, their families, and their caregivers should be encouraged to be alert to the emergence of anxiety, agitation, panic attacks, insomnia, irritability, hostility, aggressiveness, impulsivity, akathisia (psychomotor restlessness), hypomania, mania, other unusual changes in behavior, worsening of depression, and suicidal ideation, especially early during antidepressant treatment and when the dose is adjusted up or down. Families and caregivers of patients should be advised to look for the emergence of such symptoms on a day-to-day basis, since changes may be abrupt. Such symptoms should be reported to the patient's prescriber or health professional, especially if they are severe, abrupt in onset, or were not part of the patient's presenting symptoms. Symptoms such as these may be associated with an increased risk for suicidal thinking and behavior and indicate a need for very close monitoring and possibly changes in the medication.

Bupropion-Containing Products: Patients should be made aware that ZYBAN contains the same active ingredient found in WELLBUTRIN, WELLBUTRIN SR, and WELLBUTRIN XL used to treat depression and that ZYBAN should not be used in conjunction with WELLBUTRIN, the immediate-release formulation; WELLBUTRIN SR, the sustained-release formulation; WELLBUTRIN XL, the extended-release formulation; or any other medications that contain bupropion hydrochloride.

Laboratory Tests

There are no specific laboratory tests recommended.

Drug Interactions

In vitro studies indicate that bupropion is primarily metabolized to hydroxybupropion by the CYP2B6 isoenzyme. Therefore, the potential exists for a drug interaction between ZYBAN and drugs that are substrates of or inhibitors/inducers of the CYP2B6 isoenzyme (e.g., orphenadrine, thiotepa, cyclophosphamide, ticlopidine, and clopidogrel). In addition, in vitro studies suggest that paroxetine, sertraline, norfluoxetine, and fluvoxamine as well as nelfinavir inhibit the hydroxylation of bupropion. No clinical studies have been performed to evaluate this finding. The threohydrobupropion metabolite of bupropion does not appear to be produced by the cytochrome P450 isoenzymes.

In a series of studies in healthy volunteers, ritonavir (100 mg twice daily or 600 mg twice daily) or ritonavir 100 mg plus lopinavir 400 mg (KALETRA) twice daily reduced the exposure of bupropion and its major metabolites in a dose dependent manner by approximately 20% to 80%. Similarly, efavirenz 600 mg once daily for 2 weeks reduced the exposure of bupropion by approximately 55%. This effect of ritonavir, KALETRA, and efavirenz is thought to be due to the induction of bupropion metabolism. Patients receiving of these drugs with bupropion may need increased doses of bupropion, but the maximum recommended dose of bupropion should not be exceeded (see CLINICAL PHARMACOLOGY: Metabolism).

Multiple oral doses of bupropion had no statistically significant effects on the single dose pharmacokinetics of lamotrigine in 12 healthy volunteers.

Animal data indicated that bupropion may be an inducer of drug-metabolizing enzymes in humans. However, following chronic administration of bupropion, 100 mg three times daily to 8 healthy male volunteers for 14 days, there was no evidence of induction of its own metabolism. Because bupropion is extensively metabolized, the coadministration of other drugs may affect its clinical activity. In particular, certain drugs may induce the metabolism of bupropion (e.g., carbamazepine, phenobarbital, phenytoin), while other drugs may inhibit the metabolism of bupropion (e.g., cimetidine). The effects of concomitant administration of cimetidine on the pharmacokinetics of bupropion and its active metabolites were studied in 24 healthy young male volunteers. Following oral administration of two 150-mg ZYBAN tablets with and without 800 mg of cimetidine, the pharmacokinetics of bupropion and its hydroxy metabolite were unaffected. However, there were 16% and 32% increases, respectively, in the AUC and C_{max} of the combined moieties of threohydro- and erythrohydro- bupropion.

Drugs Metabolized by Cytochrome P450IID6 (CYP2D6): Many drugs, including most antidepressants (SSRIs, many tricyclics), beta-blockers, antiarrhythmics, and antipsychotics are metabolized by the CYP2D6 isoenzyme. Although bupropion is not metabolized by this isoenzyme, bupropion and hydroxybupropion are inhibitors of the CYP2D6 isoenzyme in vitro. In a study of 15 male subjects (aged 19 to 35 years) who were extensive metabolizers of the CYP2D6 isoenzyme, daily doses of bupropion given as 150 mg twice daily followed by a single dose of 50 mg desipramine increased the C_{max}, AUC, and $t_{1/2}$ of desipramine by an average of approximately 2-, 5- and 2-fold, respectively. The effect was present for at least 7 days after the last dose of bupropion. Concomitant use of bupropion with other drugs metabolized by CYP2D6 has not been formally studied.

Therefore, coadministration of bupropion with drugs that are metabolized by CYP2D6 isoenzyme including certain antidepressants (e.g., nortriptyline, imipramine, desipramine, paroxetine, fluoxetine, sertraline), antipsychotics (e.g., haloperidol, risperidone, thioridazine), beta-blockers (e.g., metoprolol), and Type 1C antiarrhythmics (e.g., propafenone, flecainide), should be approached with caution and should be initiated at the lower end of the dose range of the concomitant medication. If bupropion is added to the treatment regimen of a patient already receiving a drug metabolized by CYP2D6, the need to decrease the dose of the original medication should be considered, particularly for those concomitant medications with a narrow therapeutic index.

Drugs which require metabolic activation by CYP2D6 in order to be effective (e.g., tamoxifen) theoretically could have reduced efficacy when administered concomitantly with inhibitors of CYP2D6 such as bupropion.

Although citalopram is not primarily metabolized by CYP2D6, in one study bupropion increased the C_{max} and AUC of citalopram by 30% and 40%, respectively. Citalopram did not affect the pharmacokinetics of bupropion and its three metabolites.

MAO Inhibitors: Studies in animals demonstrate that the acute toxicity of bupropion is enhanced by the MAO inhibitor phenelzine (see CONTRAINDICATIONS).

Levodopa and Amantadine: Limited clinical data suggest a higher incidence of adverse experiences in patients receiving bupropion concurrently with either levodopa or amantadine. Administration of ZYBAN to patients receiving either levodopa or amantadine concurrently should be undertaken with caution, using small initial doses and gradual dose increases.

Drugs that Lower Seizure Threshold: Concurrent administration of ZYBAN and agents (e.g., antipsychotics, antidepressants, theophylline, systemic steroids, etc.) that lower seizure threshold should be undertaken only with extreme caution (see WARNINGS).

Nicotine Transdermal System: (see PRECAUTIONS: Cardiovascular Effects).

Smoking Cessation: Physiological changes resulting from smoking cessation itself, with or without treatment with ZYBAN, may alter the pharmacokinetics of some concomitant medications, which may require dosage adjustment. Blood concentrations of concomitant medications that are extensively metabolized, such as theophylline and warfarin, may be expected to increase following smoking cessation due to de-induction of hepatic enzymes.

Alcohol: In postmarketing experience, there have been rare reports of adverse neuropsychiatric events or reduced alcohol tolerance in patients who were drinking alcohol during treatment with ZYBAN. The consumption of alcohol during treatment with ZYBAN should be minimized or avoided (also see CONTRAINDICATIONS).

Drug-Laboratory Test Interactions: False-positive urine immunoassay screening tests for amphetamines have been reported in patients taking bupropion. This is due to lack of specificity of some screening tests. False-positive test results may result even following discontinuation of bupropion therapy. Confirmatory tests, such as gas chromatography/mass spectrometry, will distinguish bupropion from amphetamines.

Carcinogenesis, Mutagenesis, Impairment of Fertility

Lifetime carcinogenicity studies were performed in rats and mice at doses up to 300 and 150 mg/kg/day, respectively. These doses are approximately 10 and 2 times the maximum recommended human dose (MRHD), respectively, on a mg/m^2 basis. In the rat study, there was an increase in nodular proliferative lesions of the liver at doses of 100 to 300 mg/kg/day (approximately 3 to 10 times the MRHD on a mg/m^2 basis); lower doses were not tested. The question of whether or not such lesions may be precursors of neoplasms of the liver is currently unresolved. Similar liver lesions were not seen in the mouse study, and no increase in malignant tumors of the liver and other organs was seen in either study.

Bupropion produced a positive response (2 to 3 times control mutation rate) in 2 of 5 strains in the Ames bacterial mutagenicity test and an increase in chromosomal aberrations in 1 of 3 in vivo rat bone marrow cytogenic studies.

A fertility study in rats at doses up to 300 mg/kg revealed no evidence of impaired fertility.

Pregnancy

Teratogenic Effects: Pregnancy Category C, In studies conducted in rats and rabbits, bupropion was administered orally at doses up to 450 and 150 mg/kg/day, respectively (approximately 14 and 10 times the MRHD, respectively, on a mg/m^2 basis), during the period of organogenesis. No clear evidence of teratogenic activity was found in either species; however, in rabbits, slightly increased incidences of fetal malformations and skeletal variations were observed at the lowest dose tested (25 mg/kg/day, approximately 2 times the MRHD on a mg/m^2 basis) and greater. Decreased fetal weights were seen at 50 mg/kg and greater.

When rats were administered bupropion at oral doses of up to 300 mg/kg/day (approximately 10 times the MRHD on a mg/m^2 basis) prior to mating and throughout pregnancy and lactation, there were no apparent adverse effects on offspring development.

One study has been conducted in pregnant women. This retrospective, managed-care database study assessed the risk of congenital malformations overall and cardiovascular malformations specifically, following exposure to bupropion in the first trimester compared to the risk of these malformations following exposure to other antidepressants in the first trimester and bupropion outside of the first trimester. This study included 7,005 infants with antidepressant exposure during pregnancy, 1,213 of whom were exposed to bupropion in the first trimester. The study showed no greater risk for congenital malformations overall or cardiovascular malformations specifically, following first trimester bupropion exposure compared to exposure to all other antidepressants in the first trimester, or bupropion outside of the first trimester. The results of this study have not been corroborated. ZYBAN should be used during pregnancy only if the potential benefit justifies the potential risk to the fetus. Pregnant smokers should be encouraged to attempt cessation using educational and behavioral interventions before pharmacological approaches are used.

Labor and Delivery

The effect of ZYBAN on labor and delivery in humans is unknown.

Nursing Mothers

Bupropion and its metabolites are secreted in human milk. Because of the potential for serious adverse reactions in nursing infants from ZYBAN, a decision should be made whether to discontinue nursing or to discontinue the drug, taking into account the importance of the drug to the mother.

Pediatric Use

Safety and effectiveness in the pediatric population have not been established (see BOX WARNING and WARNINGS: Clinical Worsening and Suicide Risk in Treating Psychiatric Disorders). Anyone considering the use of ZYBAN in a child or adolescent must balance the potential risks with the clinical need.

Geriatric Use

Of the approximately 6,000 patients who participated in clinical trials with bupropion sustained-release tablets (depression and smoking cessation studies), 275 were 65 and over and 47 were 75 and over. In addition, several hundred patients 65 and over participated in clinical trials using the immediate-release formulation of bupropion (depression studies). No overall differences in safety or effectiveness were observed between these subjects and younger subjects, and other reported clinical experience has not identified differences in responses between the elderly and younger patients, but greater sensitivity of some older individuals cannot be ruled out.

A single-dose pharmacokinetic study demonstrated that the disposition of bupropion and its metabolites in elderly subjects was similar to that of younger subjects; however, another pharmacokinetic study, single and multiple dose, has suggested that the elderly are at increased risk for accumulation of bupropion and its metabolites (see CLINICAL PHARMACOLOGY).

Bupropion is extensively metabolized in the liver to active metabolites, which are further metabolized and excreted by the kidneys. The risk of toxic reaction to this drug may be greater in patients with impaired renal function. Because elderly patients are more likely to have decreased renal function, care should be taken in dose selection, and it may be useful to monitor renal function (see PRECAUTIONS: Renal Impairment and DOSAGE AND ADMINISTRATION).

ADVERSE REACTIONS

(See also WARNINGS and PRECAUTIONS.)

The information included under ADVERSE REACTIONS is based primarily on data from the dose-response trial and the comparative trial that evaluated ZYBAN for smoking cessation (see CLINICAL TRIALS). Information on additional adverse events associated with the sustained-release formulation of bupropion in depression trials, as well as the immediate-release formulation of bupropion, is included in a separate section (see Other Events Observed During the Clinical Development and Postmarketing Experience of Bupropion).

Adverse Events Associated With the Discontinuation of Treatment

Adverse events were sufficiently troublesome to cause discontinuation of treatment in 8% of the 706 patients treated with ZYBAN and 5% of the 313 patients treated with placebo. The more common events leading to discontinuation of treatment with ZYBAN included nervous system disturbances (3.4%), primarily tremors, and skin disorders (2.4%), primarily rashes.

Incidence of Commonly Observed Adverse Events

The most commonly observed adverse events consistently associated with the use of ZYBAN were dry mouth and insomnia. The most commonly observed adverse events were defined as those that consistently occurred at a rate of 5 percentage points greater than that for placebo across clinical studies.

Dose Dependency of Adverse Events

The incidence of dry mouth and insomnia may be related to the dose of ZYBAN. The occurrence of these adverse events may be minimized by reducing the dose of ZYBAN. In addition, insomnia may be minimized by avoiding bedtime doses.

Adverse Events Occurring at an Incidence of 1% or More Among Patients Treated With ZYBAN

Table 5 enumerates selected treatment-emergent adverse events from the dose-response trial that occurred at an incidence of 1% or more and were more common in patients treated with ZYBAN compared to those treated with placebo. Table 6 enumerates selected treatment-emergent adverse events from the comparative trial that occurred at an incidence of 1% or more and were more common in patients treated with ZYBAN, NTS, or the combination of ZYBAN and NTS compared to those treated with placebo. Reported adverse events were classified using a COSTART-based dictionary.

Table 5. Treatment-Emergent Adverse Event Incidence in the Dose-Response Trial[a]

Body System/ Adverse Experience	ZYBAN 100 to 300 mg/day (n = 461) %	Placebo (n = 150) %
Body (General)		
Neck pain	2	<1
Allergic reaction	1	0
Cardiovascular		
Hot flashes	1	0
Hypertension	1	<1
Digestive		
Dry mouth	11	5
Increased appetite	2	<1
Anorexia	1	<1
Musculoskeletal		
Arthralgia	4	3
Myalgia	2	1
Nervous system		
Insomnia	31	21
Dizziness	8	7
Tremor	2	1
Somnolence	2	1
Thinking abnormality	1	0
Respiratory		
Bronchitis	2	0
Skin		
Pruritus	3	<1
Rash	3	<1
Dry skin	2	0
Urticaria	1	0
Special senses		
Taste perversion	2	<1

[a]Selected adverse events with an incidence of at least 1% of patients treated with ZYBAN and more frequent than in the placebo group.

[See table 6 at top of next page]

ZYBAN was well tolerated in the long-term maintenance trial that evaluated chronic administration of ZYBAN for up to 1 year and in the COPD trial that evaluated patients with mild-to-moderate COPD for a 12-week period. Adverse events in both studies were quantitatively and qualitatively similar to those observed in the dose-response and comparative trials.

Other Events Observed During the Clinical Development and Postmarketing Experience of Bupropion

In addition to the adverse events noted above, the following events have been reported in clinical trials and postmarketing experience with the sustained-release formulation of bupropion in depressed patients and in nondepressed smokers, as well as in clinical trials and postmarketing clinical experience with the immediate-release formulation of bupropion.

Adverse events for which frequencies are provided below occurred in clinical trials with the sustained-release formulation of bupropion . The frequencies represent the proportion of patients who experienced a treatment-emergent adverse event on at least one occasion in placebo-controlled studies for depression (n = 987) or smoking cessation (n = 1,013), or patients who experienced an adverse event requiring discontinuation of treatment in an open-label surveillance study with bupropion sustained-release tablets (n = 3,100). All treatment-emergent adverse events are included except those listed in Tables 5 and 6, those events listed in other safety-related sections of the insert, those adverse events subsumed under COSTART terms that are either overly general or excessively specified so as to be uninformative, those events not reasonably associated with the use of the drug, and those events that were not serious and occurred in fewer than 2 patients.

Events are further categorized by body system and listed in order of decreasing frequency according to the following definitions of frequency: Frequent adverse events are defined as those occurring in at least 1/100 patients. Infrequent adverse events are those occurring in 1/100 to 1/1,000 patients, while rare events are those occurring in less than 1/1,000 patients.

Adverse events for which frequencies are not provided occurred in clinical trials or postmarketing experience with bupropion. Only those adverse events not previously listed for sustained-release bupropion are included. The extent to which these events may be associated with ZYBAN is unknown.

Body (General): Frequent were asthenia, fever, and headache. Infrequent were back pain, chills, inguinal hernia, musculoskeletal chest pain, pain, and photosensitivity. Rare was malaise. Also observed were arthralgia, myalgia, and fever with rash and other symptoms suggestive of delayed hypersensitivity. These symptoms may resemble serum sickness (see PRECAUTIONS).

Cardiovascular: Infrequent were flushing, migraine, postural hypotension, stroke, tachycardia, and vasodilation. Rare was syncope. Also observed were cardiovascular disorder, complete AV block, extrasystoles, hypotension, hypertension (in some cases severe, see PRECAUTIONS), myocardial infarction, phlebitis, and pulmonary embolism.

Digestive: Frequent were dyspepsia, flatulence, and vomiting. Infrequent were abnormal liver function, bruxism, dysphagia, gastric reflux, gingivitis, glossitis, jaundice, and stomatitis. Rare was edema of tongue. Also observed were colitis, esophagitis, gastrointestinal hemorrhage, gum hemorrhage, hepatitis, increased salivation, intestinal perforation, liver damage, pancreatitis, stomach ulcer, and stool abnormality.

Endocrine: Also observed were hyperglycemia, hypoglycemia, and syndrome of inappropriate antidiuretic hormone.

Hemic and Lymphatic: Infrequent was ecchymosis. Also observed were anemia, leukocytosis, leukopenia, lymphadenopathy, pancytopenia, and thrombocytopenia. Altered PT and/or INR, infrequently associated with hemorrhagic or thrombotic complications, were observed when bupropion was coadministered with warfarin.

Metabolic and Nutritional: Infrequent were edema, increased weight, and peripheral edema. Also observed was glycosuria.

Musculoskeletal: Infrequent were leg cramps and twitching. Also observed were arthritis and muscle rigidity/fever/rhabdomyolysis, and muscle weakness.

Nervous System: Frequent were agitation, depression, and irritability. Infrequent were abnormal coordination, CNS stimulation, confusion, decreased libido, decreased memory, depersonalization, emotional lability, hostility, hyperkinesia, hypertonia, hypesthesia, paresthesia, suicidal ideation, and vertigo. Rare were amnesia, ataxia, derealization, and hypomania. Also observed were abnormal electroencephalogram (EEG), aggression, akinesia, aphasia, coma, completed suicide, delirium, delusions, dysarthria, dyskinesia, dystonia, euphoria, extrapyramidal syndrome, hallucinations, hypokinesia, increased libido, manic reaction, neuralgia, neuropathy, paranoid ideation, restlessness, suicide attempt, and unmasking tardive dyskinesia.

Respiratory: Rare was bronchospasm. Also observed was pneumonia.

Skin: Frequent was sweating. Infrequent was acne and dry skin. Rare was maculopapular rash. Also observed were alopecia, angioedema, exfoliative dermatitis, and hirsutism.

Special Senses: Frequent was blurred vision or diplopia. Infrequent were accommodation abnormality and dry eye. Also observed were deafness, increased intraocular pressure, and mydriasis.

Urogenital: Frequent was urinary frequency. Infrequent were impotence, polyuria, and urinary urgency. Also observed were abnormal ejaculation, cystitis, dyspareunia, dysuria, gynecomastia, menopause, painful erection, prostate disorder, salpingitis, urinary incontinence, urinary retention, urinary tract disorder, and vaginitis.

DRUG ABUSE AND DEPENDENCE

ZYBAN is likely to have a low abuse potential.

Humans

There have been few reported cases of drug dependence and withdrawal symptoms associated with the immediate-release formulation of bupropion. In human studies of abuse

Table 6. Treatment-Emergent Adverse Event Incidence in the Comparative Trial[a]

Adverse Experience (COSTART Term)	ZYBAN 300 mg/day (n = 243) %	Nicotine Transdermal System (NTS) 21 mg/day (n = 243) %	ZYBAN and NTS (n = 244) %	Placebo (n = 159) %
Body				
Abdominal pain	3	4	1	1
Accidental injury	2	2	1	1
Chest pain	<1	1	3	1
Neck pain	2	1	<1	0
Facial edema	<1	0	1	0
Cardiovascular				
Hypertension	1	<1	2	0
Palpitations	2	0	1	0
Digestive				
Nausea	9	7	11	4
Dry mouth	10	4	9	4
Constipation	8	4	9	3
Diarrhea	4	4	3	1
Anorexia	3	1	5	1
Mouth ulcer	2	1	1	0
Thirst	<1	<1	2	0
Musculoskeletal				
Myalgia	4	3	5	3
Arthralgia	5	3	3	2
Nervous system				
Insomnia	40	28	45	18
Dream abnormality	5	18	13	3
Anxiety	8	6	9	6
Disturbed concentration	9	3	9	4
Dizziness	10	2	8	6
Nervousness	4	<1	2	2
Tremor	1	<1	2	0
Dysphoria	<1	1	2	1
Respiratory				
Rhinitis	12	11	9	8
Increased cough	3	5	<1	1
Pharyngitis	3	2	3	0
Sinusitis	2	2	2	1
Dyspnea	1	0	2	1
Epistaxis	2	1	1	0
Skin				
Application site reaction[b]	11	17	15	7
Rash	4	3	3	2
Pruritus	3	1	5	1
Urticaria	2	0	2	0
Special Senses				
Taste perversion	3	1	3	2
Tinnitus	1	0	<1	0

[a]Selected adverse events with an incidence of at least 1% of patients treated with either ZYBAN, NTS, or the combination of ZYBAN and NTS and more frequent than in the placebo group.
[b]Patients randomized to ZYBAN or placebo received placebo patches.

liability, individuals experienced with drugs of abuse reported that bupropion produced a feeling of euphoria and desirability. In these subjects, a single dose of 400 mg (1.33 times the recommended daily dose) of bupropion produced mild amphetamine-like effects compared to placebo on the Morphine-Benzedrine Subscale of the Addiction Research Center Inventories (ARCI), which is indicative of euphorigenic properties and a score intermediate between placebo and amphetamine on the Liking Scale of the ARCI.

Animals

Studies in rodents and primates have shown that bupropion exhibits some pharmacologic actions common to psychostimulants. In rodents, it has been shown to increase locomotor activity, elicit a mild stereotyped behavioral response, and increase rates of responding in several schedule-controlled behavior paradigms. In primate models to assess the positive reinforcing effects of psychoactive drugs, bupropion was self-administered intravenously. In rats, bupropion produced amphetamine- and cocaine-like discriminative stimulus effects in drug discrimination paradigms used to characterize the subjective effects of psychoactive drugs.

The possibility that bupropion may induce dependence should be kept in mind when evaluating the desirability of including the drug in smoking cessation programs of individual patients.

OVERDOSAGE

Human Overdose Experience

Overdoses of up to 30 g or more of bupropion have been reported. Seizure was reported in approximately one-third of all cases. Other serious reactions reported with overdoses of bupropion alone included hallucinations, loss of consciousness, sinus tachycardia, and ECG changes such as conduction disturbances (including QRS prolongation) or arrhythmias. Fever, muscle rigidity, rhabdomyolysis, hypotension, stupor, coma, and respiratory failure have been reported mainly when bupropion was part of multiple drug overdoses.

Although most patients recovered without sequelae, deaths associated with overdoses of bupropion alone have been reported in patients ingesting large doses of the drug. Multiple uncontrolled seizures, bradycardia, cardiac failure, and cardiac arrest prior to death were reported in these patients.

Overdosage Management

Ensure an adequate airway, oxygenation, and ventilation. Monitor cardiac rhythm and vital signs. EEG monitoring is also recommended for the first 48 hours post-ingestion. General supportive and symptomatic measures are also recommended. Induction of emesis is not recommended.

Activated charcoal should be administered. There is no experience with the use of forced diuresis, dialysis, hemoperfusion, or exchange transfusion in the management of bupropion overdoses. No specific antidotes for bupropion are known.

Due to the dose-related risk of seizures with ZYBAN, hospitalization following suspected overdose should be considered. Based on studies in animals, it is recommended that seizures be treated with intravenous benzodiazepine administration and other supportive measures, as appropriate.

In managing overdosage, consider the possibility of multiple drug involvement. The physician should consider contacting a poison control center for additional information on the treatment of any overdose. Telephone numbers for certified poison control centers are listed in the *Physicians' Desk Reference* (PDR).

DOSAGE AND ADMINISTRATION

Usual Dosage for Adults

The recommended and maximum dose of ZYBAN is 300 mg/day, given as 150 mg twice daily. Dosing should begin at 150 mg/day given every day for the first 3 days, followed by a dose increase for most patients to the recommended usual dose of 300 mg/day. There should be an interval of at least 8 hours between successive doses. Doses above 300 mg/day should not be used (see WARNINGS). ZYBAN should be swallowed whole and not crushed, divided, or chewed, as this may lead to an increased risk of adverse effects including seizures. Treatment with ZYBAN should be initiated **while the patient is still smoking,** since approximately 1 week of treatment is required to achieve steady-state blood levels of bupropion. Patients should set a "target quit date" within the first 2 weeks of treatment with ZYBAN, generally in the second week. Treatment with ZYBAN should be continued for 7 to 12 weeks; longer treatment should be guided by the relative benefits and risks for individual patients. If a patient has not made significant progress towards abstinence by the seventh week of therapy with ZYBAN, it is unlikely that he or she will quit during that attempt, and treatment should probably be discontinued. Conversely, a patient who successfully quits after 7 to 12 weeks of treatment should be considered for ongoing therapy with ZYBAN. Dose tapering of ZYBAN is not required when discontinuing treatment. It is important that patients continue to receive counseling and support throughout treatment with ZYBAN, and for a period of time thereafter.

Individualization of Therapy

Patients are more likely to quit smoking and remain abstinent if they are seen frequently and receive support from their physicians or other healthcare professionals. It is important to ensure that patients read the instructions provided to them and have their questions answered. Physicians should review the patient's overall smoking cessation program that includes treatment with ZYBAN. Patients should be advised of the importance of participating in the behavioral interventions, counseling, and/or support services to be used in conjunction with ZYBAN. See Medication Guide at the end of the prescribing information.

The goal of therapy with ZYBAN is complete abstinence. If a patient has not made significant progress towards abstinence by the seventh week of therapy with ZYBAN, it is unlikely that he or she will quit during that attempt, and treatment should probably be discontinued.

Patients who fail to quit smoking during an attempt may benefit from interventions to improve their chances for success on subsequent attempts. Patients who are unsuccessful should be evaluated to determine why they failed. A new quit attempt should be encouraged when factors that contributed to failure can be eliminated or reduced, and conditions are more favorable.

Maintenance: Nicotine dependence is a chronic condition. Some patients may need continuous treatment. Systematic evaluation of ZYBAN 300 mg/day for maintenance therapy demonstrated that treatment for up to 6 months was efficacious. Whether to continue treatment with ZYBAN for periods longer than 12 weeks for smoking cessation must be determined for individual patients.

Combination Treatment With ZYBAN and a Nicotine Transdermal System (NTS)

Combination treatment with ZYBAN and NTS may be prescribed for smoking cessation. The prescriber should review the complete prescribing information for both ZYBAN and NTS before using combination treatment. See also CLINICAL TRIALS for methods and dosing used in the ZYBAN and NTS combination trial. Monitoring for treatment-emergent hypertension in patients treated with the combination of ZYBAN and NTS is recommended.

Dosage Adjustment for Patients with Impaired Hepatic Function

ZYBAN should be used with extreme caution in patients with severe hepatic cirrhosis. The dose should not exceed 150 mg every other day in these patients. ZYBAN should be used with caution in patients with hepatic impairment (including mild-to-moderate hepatic cirrhosis) and a reduced frequency of dosing should be considered in patients with mild-to-moderate hepatic cirrhosis (see CLINICAL PHARMACOLOGY, WARNINGS, and PRECAUTIONS).

Dosage Adjustment for Patients with Impaired Renal Function

ZYBAN should be used with caution in patients with renal impairment and a reduced frequency of dosing should be considered (see CLINICAL PHARMACOLOGY and PRECAUTIONS).

HOW SUPPLIED

ZYBAN Sustained-Release Tablets, 150 mg of bupropion hydrochloride, are purple, round, biconvex, film-coated tablets printed with "ZYBAN 150" in bottles of 60 (NDC 0173-0556-02) tablets and the ZYBAN Advantage Pack® containing 1 bottle of 60 (NDC 0173-0556-01) tablets.

Store at controlled room temperature, 20° to 25°C (68° to 77°F) (see USP). Dispense in tight, light-resistant containers as defined in the USP.

ZYBAN, WELLBUTRIN, WELLBUTRIN SR, WELLBUTRIN XL are registered trademarks of GlaxoSmithKline.KALETRA is a registered trademark of Abbott Laboratories.

Distributed by:
GlaxoSmithKline
Research Triangle Park, NC 27709
Manufactured by:
GlaxoSmithKline
Research Triangle Park
or DSM Pharmaceuticals, Inc.
Greenville, NC 27834

January 2012
ZYB:7PI

MEDICATION GUIDE

ZYBAN® (zi ban)

(bupropion hydrochloride) Sustained-Release Tablets

Read this Medication Guide carefully before you start using ZYBAN and each time you get a refill. There may be new information. This information does not take the place of talking with your doctor about your medical condition or your treatment. If you have any questions about ZYBAN, ask your doctor or pharmacist.

IMPORTANT: Be sure to read the three sections of this Medication Guide. The first section is about the risk of changes in thinking and behavior, depression and suicidal thoughts or actions with medicines used to quit smoking; the second section is about the risk of suicidal thoughts and actions with antidepressant medicines; and the third section is entitled "What Other Important Information Should I Know About ZYBAN?"

Quitting Smoking, Quit-Smoking Medications, Changes in Thinking and Behavior, Depression, and Suicidal Thoughts or Actions

This section of the Medication Guide is only about the risk of changes in thinking and behavior depression and suicidal thoughts or actions with drugs used to quit smoking.

Some people have had changes in behavior, hostility, agitation, depression, suicidal thoughts or actions while taking ZYBAN to help them quit smoking. These symptoms can develop during treatment with ZYBAN or after stopping treatment with ZYBAN.

If you, your family member, or your caregiver notice agitation, hostility, depression, or changes in thinking or behavior that are not typical for you, or you have any of the following symptoms, stop taking ZYBAN and call your healthcare provider right away:

- thoughts about suicide or dying
- attempts to commit suicide
- new or worse depression
- new or worse anxiety
- panic attacks
- feeling very agitated or restless
- acting aggressive, being angry, or violent
- acting on dangerous impulses
- an extreme increase in activity and talking (mania)
- abnormal thoughts or sensations
- seeing or hearing things that are not there (hallucinations)
- feeling people are against you (paranoia)
- feeling confused
- other unusual changes in behavior or mood

When you try to quit smoking, with or without ZYBAN, you may have symptoms that may be due to nicotine withdrawal, including urge to smoke, depressed mood, trouble sleeping, irritability, frustration, anger, feeling anxious, difficulty concentrating, restlessness, decreased heart rate, and increased appetite or weight gain. Some people have even experienced suicidal thoughts when trying to quit smoking without medication. Sometimes quitting smoking can lead to worsening of mental health problems that you already have, such as depression.

Before taking ZYBAN, tell your healthcare provider if you have ever had depression or other mental health problems. You should also tell your doctor about any symptoms you had during other times you tried to quit smoking, with or without ZYBAN.

Antidepressant Medicines, Depression and Other Serious Mental Illnesses, and Suicidal Thoughts or Actions

Although ZYBAN is not a treatment for depression, it contains bupropion, the same active ingredient as the antidepressant medications WELLBUTRIN®, WELLBUTRIN SR®, and WELLBUTRIN XL®.

This section of the Medication Guide is only about the risk of suicidal thoughts and actions with antidepressant medicines. **Talk to your doctor, or your family member's healthcare provider about:**

- all risks and benefits of treatment with antidepressant medicines
- all treatment choices for depression or other serious mental illness

What is the most important information I should know about antidepressant medicines, depression and other serious mental illnesses, and suicidal thoughts or actions?

1. **Antidepressant medicines may increase suicidal thoughts or actions in some children, teenagers, and young adults within the first few months of treatment.**
2. **Depression and other serious mental illnesses are the most important causes of suicidal thoughts and actions. Some people may have a particularly high risk of having suicidal thoughts or actions.** These include people who have (or have a family history of) bipolar illness (also called manic-depressive illness) or suicidal thoughts or actions.
3. **How can I watch for and try to prevent suicidal thoughts and actions in myself or a family member?**
   - Pay close attention to any changes, especially sudden changes, in mood, behaviors, thoughts, or feelings. This is very important when an antidepressant medicine is started or when the dose is changed.
   - Call the healthcare provider right away to report new or sudden changes in mood, behavior, thoughts, or feelings.
   - Keep all follow-up visits with the healthcare provider as scheduled. Call the healthcare provider between visits as needed, especially if you have concerns about symptoms.

Call a healthcare provider right away if you or your family member has any of the following symptoms, especially if they are new, worse, or worry you:

- thoughts about suicide or dying
- attempts to commit suicide
- new or worse depression
- new or worse anxiety
- feeling very agitated or restless
- panic attacks
- trouble sleeping (insomnia)
- new or worse irritability
- acting aggressive, being angry, or violent
- acting on dangerous impulses
- an extreme increase in activity and talking (mania)
- other unusual changes in behavior or mood

What else do I need to know about antidepressant medicines?

- **Never stop an antidepressant medicine without first talking to a healthcare provider.** Stopping an antidepressant medicine suddenly can cause other symptoms.
- **Antidepressants are medicines used to treat depression and other illnesses.** It is important to discuss all the risks of treating depression and also the risks of not treating it. Patients and their families or other caregivers should discuss all treatment choices with the healthcare provider, not just the use of antidepressants.
- **Antidepressant medicines have other side effects.** Talk to the healthcare provider about the side effects of the medicine prescribed for you or your family member.
- **Antidepressant medicines can interact with other medicines.** Know all of the medicines that you or your family member takes. Keep a list of all medicines to show the healthcare provider. Do not start new medicines without first checking with your healthcare provider.
- **Not all antidepressant medicines prescribed for children are FDA approved for use in children.** Talk to your child's healthcare provider for more information.

ZYBAN has not been studied in children under the age of 18 and is not approved for use in children and teenagers.

What Other Important Information Should I Know About ZYBAN?

- **Seizures: There is a chance of having a seizure (convulsion, fit) with ZYBAN, especially in people:**
  - with certain medical problems.
  - who take certain medicines.

The chance of having seizures increases with higher doses of ZYBAN. For more information, see the sections "Who should not take ZYBAN?" and "What should I tell my doctor before using ZYBAN?" Tell your doctor about all of your medical conditions and all the medicines you take. **Do not take any other medicines while you are using ZYBAN unless your doctor has said it is okay to take them.**

If you have a seizure while taking ZYBAN, stop taking the tablets and call your doctor right away. Do not take ZYBAN again if you have a seizure.

- **High blood pressure (hypertension): Some people get high blood pressure that can be severe, while taking ZYBAN.** The chance of high blood pressure may be higher if you also use nicotine replacement therapy (such as a nicotine patch) to help you stop smoking (see "Can ZYBAN be used at the same time as nicotine patches?").
- **Severe allergic reactions: Some people have severe allergic reactions to ZYBAN. Stop taking ZYBAN and call your doctor right away** if you get a rash, itching, hives, fever, swollen lymph glands, painful sores in your mouth or around your eyes, swelling of your lips or tongue, chest pain, or have trouble breathing. These could be signs of a serious allergic reaction.

What is ZYBAN?

ZYBAN is a prescription medicine to help people quit smoking. Studies have shown that more than one third of people quit smoking for at least 1 month while taking ZYBAN and participating in a patient support program. For many patients, ZYBAN reduces withdrawal symptoms and the urge to smoke. ZYBAN should be used with a patient support program. It is important to participate in the behavioral program, counseling, or other support program your healthcare professional recommends.

Who should not take ZYBAN?

Do not take ZYBAN if you:

- have or had a seizure disorder or epilepsy.
- **are taking WELLBUTRIN, WELLBUTRIN SR, WELLBUTRIN XL, or any other medicines that contain bupropion hydrochloride.** Bupropion is the same active ingredient that is in ZYBAN.
- drink a lot of alcohol and abruptly stop drinking, or use medicines called sedatives (these make you sleepy) or benzodiazepines and you stop using them all of a sudden.
- have taken within the last 14 days medicine for depression called a monoamine oxidase inhibitor (MAOI), such as NARDIL® (phenelzine sulfate), PARNATE®(tranylcypromine sulfate), or MARPLAN® (isocarboxazid).
- have or had an eating disorder such as anorexia nervosa or bulimia.
- are allergic to the active ingredient in ZYBAN, bupropion, or to any of the inactive ingredients. See the end of this leaflet for a complete list of ingredients in ZYBAN.

What should I tell my doctor before using ZYBAN?

Tell your doctor if you have ever had depression, suicidal thoughts or actions, or other mental health problems. You should also tell your doctor about any symptoms you had during other times you tried to quit smoking, with or without ZYBAN. See "Quitting Smoking, Quit-Smoking Medications, Changes in Thinking and Behavior, Depression, and Suicidal Thoughts or Actions."

- **Tell your doctor about your other medical conditions, including if you:**
- **are pregnant or plan to become pregnant.** It is not known if ZYBAN can harm your unborn baby.
- **are breastfeeding.** ZYBAN passes through your milk. It is not known if ZYBAN can harm your baby.
- **have liver problems,** especially cirrhosis of the liver.
- have kidney problems.
- have an eating disorder such as anorexia nervosa or bulimia.
- have had a head injury.
- have had a seizure (convulsion, fit).
- have a tumor in your nervous system (brain or spine).
- have had a heart attack, heart problems, or high blood pressure.
- are a diabetic taking insulin or other medicines to control your blood sugar.
- drink a lot of alcohol.
- abuse prescription medicines or street drugs.
- **Tell your doctor about all the medicines you take,** including prescription and non-prescription medicines, vitamins, and herbal supplements. Many medicines increase your chances of getting seizures or other serious side effects if you take them while you are using ZYBAN.

How should I take ZYBAN?

- Take ZYBAN exactly as prescribed by your doctor.
- **Do not chew, cut, or crush ZYBAN tablets.** If you do, the medicine will be released into your body too quickly. If this happens you may be more likely to get side effects including seizures. You must swallow the tablets whole. **Tell your doctor if you cannot swallow medicine tablets.**
- Take ZYBAN at the same time each day.
- Take your doses of ZYBAN at least 8 hours apart.
- If you miss a dose, do not take an extra tablet to make up for the dose you forgot. Wait and take your next tablet at the regular time. **This is very important.** Too much ZYBAN can increase your chance of having a seizure.
- If you take too much ZYBAN, or overdose, call your local emergency room or poison control center right away.
- **Do not take any other medicines while using ZYBAN unless your doctor has told you it is okay.**
- Do not change your dose or stop taking ZYBAN without talking with your doctor first.

How long should I take ZYBAN?

Most people should take ZYBAN for at least 7 to 12 weeks. Some people may need to take ZYBAN for a longer period of time to assist in their smoking cessation efforts. Follow your doctor's instructions.

When should I stop smoking?
It takes about 1 week for ZYBAN to start working. For your best chance of quitting, you should not stop smoking until you have been taking ZYBAN for 1 week. You should set a date to stop smoking during the second week you're taking ZYBAN.

Can I smoke while taking ZYBAN?
It is not physically dangerous to smoke and use ZYBAN at the same time. But you will seriously lower your chance of breaking your smoking habit if you smoke after the date you set to stop smoking.

Can ZYBAN be used at the same time as nicotine patches?
Yes, ZYBAN and nicotine patches can be used at the same time but should only be used together under the supervision of your doctor. Using ZYBAN and nicotine patches together may raise your blood pressure, sometimes severely. Tell your doctor if you are planning to use nicotine replacement therapy because your doctor should check your blood pressure regularly.

Do not smoke at any time if you are using a nicotine patch or any other nicotine product along with ZYBAN. It is possible to get too much nicotine and have serious side effects.

What should I avoid while taking ZYBAN?
- Do not drink a lot of alcohol while taking ZYBAN. If you usually drink a lot of alcohol, talk with your doctor before suddenly stopping. If you suddenly stop drinking alcohol, you may increase your chance of having seizures.
- Do not drive a car or use heavy machinery until you know how ZYBAN affects you. ZYBAN can affect your ability to do these things safely.

What are possible side effects of ZYBAN?
ZYBAN can cause serious side effects. Read this entire Medication Guide for more information about these serious side effects.

The most common side effects of ZYBAN are dry mouth and trouble sleeping. These side effects are generally mild and often disappear after a few weeks. If you have trouble sleeping, do not take ZYBAN too close to bedtime.

These are not all the side effects of ZYBAN. For a complete list, ask your doctor or pharmacist.

Call your doctor for medical advice about side effects. You may report side effects to FDA at 1-800-FDA-1088.

How should I store ZYBAN?
- Store ZYBAN at room temperature.
- Store out of direct sunlight.
- Keep ZYBAN in its tightly closed bottle.
- ZYBAN may have an odor.

General Information about ZYBAN.
Medicines are sometimes prescribed for purposes other than those listed in a Medication Guide. Do not use ZYBAN for a condition for which it was not prescribed. Do not give ZYBAN to other people, even if they have the same symptoms you have. It may harm them. Keep ZYBAN out of the reach of children.

If you take a urine drug screening test, ZYBAN may make the test result positive for amphetamines. If you tell the person giving you the drug screening test that you are taking ZYBAN, they can do a more specific drug screening test that should not have this problem.

This Medication Guide summarizes important information about ZYBAN. For more information, talk with your doctor. You can ask your doctor or pharmacist for information about ZYBAN that is written for health professionals.

What are the ingredients in ZYBAN?
Active ingredient: bupropion hydrochloride.
Inactive ingredients: carnauba wax, cysteine hydrochloride, hypromellose, magnesium stearate, microcrystalline cellulose, polyethylene glycol, polysorbate 80 and titanium dioxide. The tablets are printed with edible black ink. In addition, the 150-mg tablet contains FD&C Blue No. 2 Lake and FD&C Red No. 40 Lake.

This Medication Guide has been approved by the U.S. Food and Drug Administration.

ZYBAN, WELLBUTRIN, WELLBUTRIN SR, WELLBUTRIN XL, and PARNATE are registered trademarks of GlaxoSmithKline.

The following are registered trademarks of their respective manufacturers: NARDIL®/Warner Lambert Company; MARPLAN®/Oxford Pharmaceutical Services, Inc.

Distributed by:
GlaxoSmithKline
Research Triangle Park, NC 27709
Manufactured by:
GlaxoSmithKline
Research Triangle Park
or DSM Pharmaceuticals, Inc.
Greenville, NC 27834

January 2012
ZYB:7MG

Glenwood

111 CEDAR LANE
ENGLEWOOD, NJ 07631

Direct Inquiries to:
Professional Services Department
201 569-0050
800 542-0772
For Medical Information Contact:
In Emergencies:
Professional Services Department
201 569-0050
800 542-0772

POTABA® ℞

Aminobenzoate Potassium, USP
Systemic ANTIFIBROSIS THERAPY

FORMULA: POTABA® is chemically pure potassium p-aminobenzoate.

DESCRIPTION
POTABA® (Aminobenzoate Potassium, USP) is available in Capsules. Each Capsule contains the following inactive ingredients: Colloidal Silicon Dioxide, Stearic Acid. Capsule Shell contains: Gelatin and Titanium Dioxide. The imprinting ink contains Titanium Dioxide.

INDICATIONS
Based on a review of this drug by the National Academy of Sciences-National Research Council and/or other information, FDA has classified the indications as follows:
"Possibly" effective: Potassium aminobenzoate is possibly effective in the treatment of scleroderma, dermatomyositis, morphea, linear scleroderma, pemphigus, and Peyronie's disease.
Final classification of the less-than-effective indications requires further investigation.

ADVANTAGES: POTABA® offers a means of treatment of serious and often chronic entities involving fibrosis and nonsuppurative inflammation.

PHARMACOLOGY
p-Aminobenzoate is considered a member of the vitamin B complex. Small amounts are found in cereal, eggs, milk and meats. Detectable amounts are normally present in human blood, spinal fluid, urine, and sweat. PABA is a component of several biologically important systems, and it participates in a number of fundamental biological processes.
It has been suggested that the antifibrosis action of POTABA® is due to its mediation of increased oxygen uptake at the tissue level. Fibrosis is believed to occur from either too much serotonin or too little monoamine oxidase (MAO) activity over a period of time. Monoamine oxidase requires an adequate supply of oxygen to function properly. By increasing oxygen supply at the tissue level POTABA® may enhance MAO activity and prevent or bring about regression of fibrosis.[3]

CLINICAL USES
PEYRONIE'S DISEASE: 21 patients with Peyronie's disease were placed on POTABA® therapy for periods ranging from 3 months to 2 years. Pain disappeared from 16 of 16 cases in which it had been present. There was objective improvement in penile deformity in 10 of 17 patients, and decrease in plaque size in 16 of 21. The authors suggest that this medication offers no hazard of further local injury as may result from other therapy. There were no significant untoward effects encountered on long-term POTABA® therapy.[5,10]
SCLERODERMA: Of 135 patients with diffuse systemic sclerosis treated with POTABA® every patient but one has shown softening of the involved skin if treatment has been continued for 3 months or longer. The responses have been reported in a number of publications.[9] The treatment program consists of systemic antifibrosis therapy with POTABA®, physical therapy, including deep breathing exercises and dynamic traction splints where indicated, and bethanechol chloride for relief of dysphagia as well as small doses of reserpine for amelioration of Raynaud's phenomena.[1,3]
DERMATOMYOSITIS: Five patients with scleroderma and 2 with dermatomyositis were treated with POTABA®. There was striking clinical improvement in each patient. Doses of 15-20 grams per day were well tolerated, and patients were easily able to take these doses.[6]
MORPHEA and LINEAR SCLERODERMA: All 14 patients with localized forms of scleroderma placed on long-term POTABA® treatment showed softening of the sclerotic component of their disorder. Treatment is particularly indicated in patients where persistent compressive sclerosis may contribute even greater disfigurement or functional embarrassment from secondary pressure atrophy.[8,9]

DOSAGE & ADMINISTRATION
The average adult daily dose of POTABA® is 12 grams, usually given in four to six divided doses. Capsules 0.5 gram are given at the rate of 4 capsules 6 times daily, or 6 given four times daily, usually with meals, and at bedtime with a snack.
Children are given 1 gram of POTABA® daily in divided doses for each 10 lbs. of body weight.
SIDE EFFECTS: Anorexia, nausea, fever and rash have occurred infrequently and subside with omission of the drug. Desensitization can be accomplished and treatment resumed.
USAGE IN PREGNANCY: Safety for use in pregnancy or during lactation has not been established.

PRECAUTIONS
Should anorexia or nausea occur, therapy is interrupted until the patient is eating normally again. This permits prompt subsidence of symptoms and also avoids the possible development of hypoglycemia. Give cautiously to patients with renal disease. If hypersensitivity reaction should occur, POTABA® should be stopped.

CONTRAINDICATIONS
POTABA® should not be administered to patients taking sulfonamides.

HOW SUPPLIED
POTABA® (Aminobenzoate Potassium, USP) Capsules 0.5 grams are supplied as No. 0 White/White Opaque Hard Gelatin Capsule Printed "POTABA 51" in black ink.
NDC-0516-0051-10 bottle of 1000
Rx only.

REFERENCES
1. From: Inflammation and Diseases of Connective Tissue, Edited by Drs. Lewis C. Mills and John H. Moyer, Published by W. B. Saunders Company, Phila. 1961.
3. Zarafonetis, Chris J. D.: Treatment of Scleroderma, Annals of Int. Med. 50:343-365 (1959).
5. Zarafonetis, C. J. D., and Horrax, T.M.: Treatment of Peyronie's Disease with POTABA, Journ. of Urology 81:770-772 (June 1959).
6. Grace. William J., Kennedy, Richard J., Formato, Anthony: Therapy of Scleroderma and Dermatomyositis, N.Y. State J. of Med. 63:140-144, 1963.
8. Zarafonetis, C. J. D.: Treatment of Localized Forms of Scleroderma, Am. J. Med. Sci. 243:147-158. 1962.
9. Zarafonetis, Chris J. D.: Antifibrotic Therapy With POTABA, Amer. Jrnl. of Med. Sci. 248: No. 5/551-561 (Nov. 1964).
10. Horrax, Trudeau M.: Peyronie's Disease, Scientific Exhibit, Amer. Urological Assn. Annl. Meet., New Orleans, May 1965.

GLENWOOD, LLC
111 Cedar Lane
Englewood, NJ 07631
REV. 11/10

Shown in Product Identification Guide, page 307

Gordon Laboratories

6801 LUDLOW STREET
UPPER DARBY, PA 19082

Direct inquiries to:
Customer Service
(610) 734-2011
Fax (610) 734-2049
Website: http://www.gordonlabs.net
E-mail: gordonlabs@att.net
For medical emergencies contact:
David Dercher (610) 734-2011
Fax (610) 734-2049

FORMADON ℞

INDICATIONS
Used as a drying agent for pre and postsurgical removal of warts; and as an antiperspirant in the treatment of severe conditions of hyperhidrosis and bromidrosis.
ACTIVE INGREDIENT: Formaldehyde (10% of U.S.P. strength).

DESCRIPTION

Formadon provides a preferable vehicle for the topical application of formalin solution (10% U.S.P. strength formaldehyde). It is formulated with an aqueous perfumed base which helps minimize the characteristic pungent odor.

PHARMACOLOGY

Formalin, a solution of formaldehyde, has been extensively used as a drying agent as well as a disinfectant. Direct topical application of formalin solution has been an extremely useful way of dealing with odor-causing bacteria on the surface of the skin. The elimination of hyperhidrosis is of paramount importance in reducing bacteria associated with odor and wetness. Formalin, in drying the skin surface, reduces bacteria flora which can thrive in moisture.

CONTRAINDICATIONS/WARNINGS

Avoid frequent use. Avoid contact with eyes or mucous membranes. Do not apply to open wounds. Should signs of irritation develop, medication should be discontinued. Irritates eyes, nose, and throat. Avoid breathing vapors. Use with adequate ventilation. In the event of eye contact, flush copiously with water and get medical attention. **Keep out of reach of children. For external use only.** Harmful if swallowed. Contact a local Poison Control Center immediately. **Do not Induce vomiting.** If conscious, give eight ounces (240 mL) of milk, water or water with activated charcoal. Keep well closed in a cool place. **Federal law prohibits dispensing without a prescription.**

DIRECTIONS

Apply to feet twice weekly or as prescribed by a Physician.

HOW SUPPLIED

2 oz. sponge tip bottle NDC 10481-1050-05
4 oz. plastic bottle NDC 10481-1050-2
Shown in Product Identification Guide, page 307

GORDOCHOM™ Solution OTC

[*gŏrdō'kōm*]

DESCRIPTION

Gordochom is an antifungal solution for topical use containing 25% Undecylenic Acid and Chloroxylenol as its active ingredients in a penetrating oil base. Undecylenic Acid is chemically 10 hendecenoic acid having the empirical formula $C_{11}H_{20}O_2$ and the chemical bond structure CH_2=CH $(CH_2)8\ CO_2H$.
Undecylenic Acid is a colorless to pale yellow liquid. It is insoluble in water and soluble in alcohol, chloroform and ether.
Chloroxylenol is chemically 2-chloro-5-hydroxy-1,3-dimethylbenzene having the empirical formula C_8H_9ClO.

CLINICAL PHARMACOLOGY

Undecylenic Acid is a fungistatic agent employed in the treatment of tinea pedis, ringworm and dermatophytosis.
Chloroxylenol is a topical antiseptic, germicide and antifungal agent effective against a wide variety of causative fungi and yeast organisms. Among those affected by Chloroxylenol are candida albicans, aspergillus niger, aspergillus flavus, trichophyton rubrum, trichophyton mentagrophytes, penicillum luteum and epidermophyton floccosum.
The penetrating oil base vehicle serves as a delivery system, enhancing the impregnation of Undecylenic Acid and Chloroxylenol as antimicrobial agents.

INDICATIONS

Cures athlete's foot (tinea pedis), and ringworm (tinea corporis).

CONTRAINDICATIONS

Gordochom is contraindicated in patients who are sensitive to Undecylenic Acid or Chloroxylenol.

WARNINGS

For external use only. Not for opthalmic or optic use. Avoid inhaling and contact with eyes or other mucous membranes. Not to be applied over blistered, raw or oozing areas of skin or over deep puncture wounds.

PRECAUTIONS

If a reaction suggesting sensitivity or chemical irritation should occur with the use of Gordochom, treatment should be discontinued. Use of Gordochom in pregnancy has not been established. **Keep out of reach of children.**

ADVERSE REACTIONS

No significant adverse reactions have been reported. However, attention should be paid to localized hypersensitivity.

DOSAGE AND ADMINISTRATION

Cleanse and dry affected areas. Apply a thin application twice a day (morning and night) to the affected area, or as recommended by your physician. For athlete's foot, pay special attention to the spaces between the toes; wear well-fitting, ventilated shoes, and change shoes and socks at least once daily. For athlete's foot and ringworm, use daily for 4 weeks. If condition persists longer, consult a physician. This product has not been proven effective on the scalp or nails.

HOW SUPPLIED

Gordochom is available in 1 oz. bottles with special brush applicator. (NDC 10481-8010-2)
Store at controlled room temperatures (59°–86°F).
Shown in Product Identification Guide, page 307

Halozyme Therapeutics, Inc.

11388 SORRENTO VALLEY ROAD
SAN DIEGO, CA 92121

Direct Inquires to:
858-704-8288

HYLENEX RECOMBINANT ℞

(hyaluronidase human injection)

HIGHLIGHTS OF PRESCRIBING INFORMATION

These highlights do not include all the information needed to use HYLENEX recombinant safely and effectively. See full prescribing information for HYLENEX recombinant.
HYLENEX recombinant (hyaluronidase human injection)
Initial U.S. Approval: 2005

INDICATIONS AND USAGE

HYLENEX recombinant is a tissue permeability modifier indicated as an adjuvant

- in subcutaneous fluid administration for achieving hydration (1.1)
- to increase the dispersion and absorption of other injected drugs (1.2)
- in subcutaneous urography for improving resorption of radiopaque agents (1.3)

DOSAGE AND ADMINISTRATION

- Subcutaneous fluid administration:
  Inject 150 U HYLENEX recombinant prior to subcutaneous fluid administration. It will facilitate absorption of 1,000 mL or more of solution. The dosage of subcutaneous fluids administered is dependent upon the age, weight, and clinical condition of the patient as well as laboratory determinations. The rate and volume of subcutaneous fluid administration should not exceed those employed for intravenous infusion. (2.1)
- Increasing dispersion and absorption of injected or subcutaneously infused drugs:
  Inject 50-300 U (most typically 150 U) HYLENEX recombinant prior to drug administration. Alternatively, add 50-300 U (most typically 150 U) HYLENEX recombinant to the injection solution. (2.2)
- Subcutaneous Urography:
  Inject 75 U HYLENEX recombinant subcutaneously over each scapula, followed by injection of the contrast medium at the same sites. (2.3)

DOSAGE FORMS AND STRENGTHS

- 150 USP units/mL single dose vials (3)

CONTRAINDICATIONS

- Hypersensitivity (4)

WARNINGS AND PRECAUTIONS

- Spread of Localized Infection (5.1)
- Ocular Damage (5.2)
- Enzyme Inactivation with Intravenous Administration (5.3)
- Products Containing Plasma-derived Albumin (5.4)

ADVERSE REACTIONS

- Allergic and anaphylactic-like reactions have been reported, rarely. (6)

To report SUSPECTED ADVERSE REACTIONS, contact Halozyme Therapeutics, Inc. at 1-877-877-1679 or FDA at 1-800-FDA-1088 or *www.fda.gov/medwatch.*

DRUG INTERACTIONS

- Furosemide, the benzodiazepines and phenytoin are incompatible with hyaluronidase. (7.1)
- Hyaluronidase should not be used to enhance the dispersion and absorption of dopamine and/or alpha agonist drugs. (7.2)
- Local anesthetics: Hyaluronidase hastens onset and shortens duration of effect, increases incidence of systemic reactions. (7.3)
- Large doses of salicylates, cortisone, ACTH, estrogens or antihistamines may require larger amounts of hyaluronidase for equivalent dispersing effect. (7.4)

USE IN SPECIFIC POPULATIONS

- Pediatric Use: The dosage of subcutaneous fluids administered is dependent upon the age, weight, and clinical condition of the patient. For premature infants or during the neonatal period, the daily dosage should not exceed 25 mL/kg of body weight, and the rate of administration should not be greater than 2 mL per minute. Special care must be taken in pediatric patients to avoid over hydration by controlling the rate and total volume of the infusion. (2.1, 8.4, 14)

See 17 for PATIENT COUNSELING INFORMATION

Revised: 09/2012

FULL PRESCRIBING INFORMATION: CONTENTS*

*** Sections or subsections omitted from the full prescribing information are not listed**

FULL PRESCRIBING INFORMATION

1 INDICATIONS AND USAGE

1.1 Subcutaneous Fluid Administration

HYLENEX recombinant is indicated as an adjuvant in subcutaneous fluid administration for achieving hydration.

1.2 Dispersion and Absorption of Injected Drugs

HYLENEX recombinant is indicated as an adjuvant to increase the dispersion and absorption of other injected drugs.

1.3 Subcutaneous Urography

HYLENEX recombinant is indicated as an adjunct in subcutaneous urography for improving resorption of radiopaque agents.

2 DOSAGE AND ADMINISTRATION

Parenteral drug products should be inspected visually for particulate matter and discoloration prior to administration whenever solution and container permit.
Always use aseptic precautions. Lightly pinch the skin up into a small mound and insert the needle/catheter into the subcutaneous space. Inject HYLENEX recombinant through the catheter hub or injection port closest to the needle/catheter. Begin administration of solution. Solution should start in readily.

2.1 Subcutaneous Fluid Administration

150 U of HYLENEX recombinant injected prior to start of subcutaneous fluid administration will facilitate absorption

of 1,000 mL or more of solution. As with all parenteral fluid therapy, observe effect closely, with the same precautions for restoring fluid and electrolyte balance as in intravenous injections. The dose, the rate of injection, and the type of solution (saline, glucose, Ringer's, etc.) must be adjusted carefully to the individual patient. When solutions devoid of inorganic electrolytes are administered subcutaneously, hypovolemia may occur. This may be prevented by using solutions containing adequate amounts of inorganic electrolytes and/or controlling the volume and speed of administration.

HYLENEX recombinant may be added to small volumes of solution, such as fluid replacement solutions or solutions of drugs for subcutaneous injection. Subcutaneous fluids should be administered as directed by a physician. The dosage of subcutaneous fluids administered is dependent upon the age, weight, and clinical condition of the patient as well as laboratory determinations. The rate and volume of subcutaneous fluid administration should not exceed those employed for intravenous infusion. For premature infants or during the neonatal period, the daily dosage should not exceed 25 mL/kg of body weight, and the rate of administration should not be greater than 2 mL per minute.

2.2 Dispersion and Absorption of Injected Drugs

Dispersion and absorption of other injected or subcutaneously infused drugs may be enhanced by pre-administration of HYLENEX recombinant or by adding 50-300 U, most typically 150 U hyaluronidase, to the injection solution.

2.3 Subcutaneous Urography

The subcutaneous route of administration of urographic contrast media is indicated when intravenous administration cannot be successfully accomplished, particularly in infants and small children. With the patient prone, 75 U of HYLENEX recombinant is injected subcutaneously over each scapula, followed by injection of the contrast medium at the same sites.

3 DOSAGE FORMS AND STRENGTHS

150 USP units/mL single dose vials

4 CONTRAINDICATIONS

HYLENEX recombinant is contraindicated in patients with known hypersensitivity to hyaluronidase or any of the excipients in HYLENEX recombinant. A preliminary skin test for hypersensitivity to HYLENEX recombinant can be performed. The skin test is made by an intradermal injection of approximately 0.02 mL (3 Units) of a 150 Unit/mL solution. A positive reaction consists of a wheal with pseudopods appearing within 5 minutes and persisting for 20 to 30 minutes and accompanied by localized itching. Transient vasodilation at the site of the test, i.e., erythema, is not a positive reaction. Discontinue HYLENEX recombinant if sensitization occurs.

5 WARNINGS AND PRECAUTIONS

5.1 Spread of Localized Infection

Hyaluronidase should not be injected into or around an infected or acutely inflamed area because of the danger of spreading a localized infection.

Hyaluronidase should not be used to reduce the swelling of bites or stings.

5.2 Ocular Damage

Hyaluronidase should not be applied directly to the cornea. It is not for topical use.

5.3 Enzyme Inactivation with Intravenous Administration

HYLENEX recombinant should not be administered intravenously. Its effects relative to dispersion and absorption of other drugs are not produced when it is administered intravenously because the enzyme is rapidly inactivated.

5.4 Products Containing Plasma-derived Albumin

This product contains albumin, a derivative of human blood. Based on effective donor screening and product manufacturing processes, it carries an extremely remote risk for transmission of viral diseases and variant Creutzfeldt-Jakob disease (vCJD). There is a theoretical risk for transmission of Creutzfeldt-Jakob disease (CJD), but if that risk actually exists, the risk of transmission would also be considered extremely remote. No cases of transmission of viral diseases, CJD, or vCJD have ever been identified for licensed albumin or albumin contained in other licensed products.

6 ADVERSE REACTIONS

The following adverse reactions have been identified during post-approval use of hyaluronidase products. Because these reactions are reported voluntarily from a population of uncertain size, it is not always possible to reliably estimate their frequency or establish a causal relationship to drug exposure.

The most frequently reported adverse reactions have been mild local injection site reactions such as erythema and pain. Hyaluronidase has been reported to enhance the adverse reactions associated with co-administered drug products. Edema has been reported most frequently in association with subcutaneous fluid administration. Allergic reactions (urticaria or angioedema) have been reported in less than 0.1% of patients receiving hyaluronidase. Anaphylactic-like reactions following retrobulbar block or intravenous injections have occurred, rarely.

7 DRUG INTERACTIONS

It is recommended that appropriate references be consulted regarding physical or chemical incompatibilities before adding HYLENEX recombinant to a solution containing another drug.

7.1 Incompatibilities

Furosemide, the benzodiazepines and phenytoin have been found to be incompatible with hyaluronidase.

7.2 Drug-Specific Precautions

Hyaluronidase should not be used to enhance the dispersion and absorption of dopamine and/or alpha agonist drugs.

When considering the administration of any other drug with hyaluronidase, it is recommended that appropriate references first be consulted to determine the usual precautions for the use of the other drug.

7.3 Local Anesthetics

When hyaluronidase is added to a local anesthetic agent, it hastens the onset of analgesia and tends to reduce the swelling caused by local infiltration, but the wider spread of the local anesthetic solution increases its absorption; this shortens its duration of action and tends to increase the incidence of systemic reaction.

7.4 Salicylates, Cortisone, ACTH, Estrogens and Antihistamines

Patients receiving large doses of salicylates, cortisone, ACTH, estrogens or antihistamines may require larger amounts of hyaluronidase for equivalent dispersing effect, since these drugs apparently render tissues partly resistant to the action of hyaluronidase.

8 USE IN SPECIFIC POPULATIONS

8.1 Pregnancy

Pregnancy Category C. In an embryo-fetal study, mice have been dosed daily by subcutaneous injection with recombinant human hyaluronidase at dose levels up to 2,200,000 U/kg. The study found no evidence of teratogenicity. Reduced fetal weight and increased numbers of fetal resorptions were observed, with no effects found at a daily dose of 360,000 U/kg, which represents several orders of magnitude over the suggested human dose range of 50-300 U of HYLENEX recombinant (0.8-5 U/kg in a 60 kg subject).

In a pre- and postnatal development study, mice have been dosed daily by subcutaneous injection with recombinant human hyaluronidase at dose levels up to 1,100,000 U/kg. The study found no adverse effects on sexual maturation, learning and memory of offspring, or their ability to produce another generation of offspring.

It is also not known whether HYLENEX recombinant can cause fetal harm when administered to a pregnant woman. HYLENEX recombinant should be given to a pregnant woman only if clearly needed.

8.2 Labor and Delivery

Administration of hyaluronidase during labor was reported to cause no complications: no increase in blood loss or differences in cervical trauma were observed.

8.3 Nursing Mothers

It is not known whether hyaluronidase is excreted in human milk. Because many drugs are excreted in human milk, caution should be exercised when hyaluronidase is administered to a nursing woman.

8.4 Pediatric Use

Clinical hydration requirements for children can be achieved through administration of subcutaneous fluids facilitated with HYLENEX recombinant.

The dosage of subcutaneous fluids administered is dependent upon the age, weight, and clinical condition of the patient as well as laboratory determinations. The potential for chemical or physical incompatibilities should be kept in mind *[see Drug Interactions (7)]*.

The rate and volume of subcutaneous fluid administration should not exceed those employed for intravenous infusion. For premature infants or during the neonatal period, the daily dosage should not exceed 25 mL/kg of body weight, and the rate of administration should not be greater than 2 mL per minute.

During subcutaneous fluid administration, special care must be taken in pediatric patients to avoid over hydration by controlling the rate and total volume of the infusion *[see Dosage and Administration (2.1)]*.

8.5 Geriatric Use

No overall differences in safety or effectiveness have been observed between elderly and younger adult patients.

11 DESCRIPTION

HYLENEX recombinant is a purified preparation of the enzyme recombinant human hyaluronidase. HYLENEX recombinant is produced by genetically engineered Chinese Hamster Ovary (CHO) cells containing a DNA plasmid encoding for a soluble fragment of human hyaluronidase (PH20). The purified hyaluronidase glycoprotein contains 447 amino acids with an approximate molecular weight of 61,000 Daltons.

HYLENEX recombinant is supplied as a sterile, clear, colorless, nonpreserved, ready for use solution. Each mL contains 150 USP units of recombinant human hyaluronidase with 8.5 mg sodium chloride, 1.4 mg dibasic sodium phosphate, 1 mg albumin human, 0.9 mg edetate disodium, 0.3 mg calcium chloride, and sodium hydroxide added for pH adjustment.

HYLENEX recombinant has an approximate pH of 7.0 and an osmolality of 290 to 350 mOsm.

12 CLINICAL PHARMACOLOGY

12.1 Mechanism of Action

Hyaluronidase is a dispersion agent, which modifies the permeability of connective tissue through the hydrolysis of hyaluronic acid, a polysaccharide found in the intercellular ground substance of connective tissue, and of certain specialized tissues, such as the umbilical cord and vitreous humor. Hyaluronic acid is also present in the capsules of type A and C hemolytic streptococci. Hyaluronidase hydrolyzes hyaluronic acid by splitting the glucosaminidic bond between C1 of an N-acetylglucosamine moiety and C4 of a glucuronic acid moiety. This temporarily decreases the viscosity of the cellular cement and promotes dispersion of injected fluids or of localized transudates or exudates, thus facilitating their absorption.

Hyaluronidase cleaves glycosidic bonds of hyaluronic acid and, to a variable degree, some other acid mucopolysaccharides of the connective tissue. The activity is measured in vitro by monitoring the decrease in the amount of an insoluble serum albumin-hyaluronic acid complex as the enzyme cleaves the hyaluronic acid component.

12.2 Pharmacodynamics

In the absence of hyaluronidase, material injected subcutaneously disperses very slowly. Hyaluronidase facilitates dispersion, provided local interstitial pressure is adequate to furnish the necessary mechanical impulse. Such an impulse is normally initiated by injected solutions. The rate and extent of dispersion and absorption is proportionate to the amount of hyaluronidase and the volume of solution.

The reconstitution of the dermal barrier removed by intradermal injection of hyaluronidase (20, 2, 0.2, 0.02, and 0.002 U/mL) to adult humans indicated that at 24 hours the restoration of the barrier is incomplete and inversely related to the dosage of hyaluronidase; at 48 hours, the barrier is completely restored in all treated areas.

Results from an experimental study, in humans, on the influence of hyaluronidase in bone repair support the conclusion that hyaluronidase alone, in the usual clinical dosage, does not deter bone healing.

12.3 Pharmacokinetics

Knowledge of the mechanisms involved in the disappearance of injected hyaluronidase is limited. It is known, however, that the components in blood of a number of mammalian species bring about the inactivation of hyaluronidase. Studies have demonstrated that hyaluronidase is antigenic; repeated injections of relatively large amounts of hyaluronidase preparations may result in the formation of neutralizing antibodies.

13 NONCLINICAL TOXICOLOGY

13.1 Carcinogenesis, Mutagenesis, Impairment of Fertility

Hyaluronidase is found in most tissues of the body. Long-term animal studies have not been performed to assess the carcinogenic or mutagenic potential of hyaluronidase.

Human studies on the effect of intravaginal hyaluronidase in sterility due to oligospermia indicated that hyaluronidase may have aided conception. Thus, it appears that hyaluronidase may not adversely affect fertility in females. In addition, when recombinant human hyaluronidase was administered to cynomolgus monkeys for 39 weeks at dose levels up to 220,000 U/kg, no evidence of toxicity to the male or female reproductive system was found through periodic monitoring of in-life parameters, e.g., semen analyses, hormone levels, menstrual cycles, and also from gross pathology, histopathology and organ weight data.

14 CLINICAL STUDIES

HYLENEX recombinant facilitated the administration of subcutaneous fluids in pediatric patients with mild to moderate dehydration in an open-label, multicenter, single arm study in fifty-one (51) patients. A subcutaneous injection of 1 mL (150 U) of HYLENEX recombinant was immediately followed by subcutaneous infusion of isotonic fluids in either the mid-anterior thigh or the inter-scapular area of the upper back.

The safety and flow rate of subcutaneously administered Lactated Ringer's (LR) solution with and without HYLENEX recombinant was evaluated in a prospective, randomized, double-blinded, placebo-controlled, within-subject, single-center study in fifty-four (54) healthy volunteers. The mean HYLENEX recombinant facilitated infusion rate was 464 mL/hr versus 118 mL/hr for the saline control ($p < 0.001$, paired t-test).

16 HOW SUPPLIED/STORAGE AND HANDLING

HYLENEX recombinant is supplied sterile as 150 USP units of nonpreserved recombinant human hyaluronidase per mL in a single-use glass vial.
HYLENEX recombinant is supplied in the following packaging:
1 mL Single Dose Vial (NDC 18657-102-01) available in boxes of 4 (NDC 18657-102-04)
Store unopened in a refrigerator at 2° to 8°C (36° to 46° F).
DO NOT FREEZE.

17 PATIENT COUNSELING INFORMATION

17.1 Important Precautions Regarding HYLENEX recombinant

Instruct patient that HYLENEX recombinant is being used to increase the dispersion and absorption of fluids or other injected drugs, as appropriate to the intended use.
Instruct patient that there may be mild local injection site signs and symptoms, such as redness, swelling, itching, or pain localized to the site of injection.

17.2 What Patients Should Know About Adverse Reactions

Patients should be advised that the most frequently reported adverse reactions have been mild local injection site reactions such as redness, swelling, itching, or pain.
Anaphylactic-like reactions, and allergic reactions, such as hives, have been reported rarely in patients receiving hyaluronidases.

17.3 Patients Should Inform Their Doctors If Taking Other Medications

Instruct patients that they may not receive furosemide, the benzodiazepines, phenytoin, dopamine and/or alpha agonists with HYLENEX recombinant. These medications have been found to be incompatible with hyaluronidase.
Patients should be advised that if they are taking salicylates (e.g., aspirin), steroids (e.g., cortisone or estrogens), or antihistamines, they may need to be prescribed larger amounts of hyaluronidase for equivalent dispersing effect.
Halozyme and Hylenex are registered trademarks of Halozyme, Inc.
U.S. Patent No. 7,767,429
Manufactured for and Marketed by: Halozyme Therapeutics, Inc.
San Diego, CA 92121
For Product Inquiry: 1-855-495 3639
Rev. September 2012
LBL293-04

Shown in Product Identification Guide, page 307

High Chemical Company

3901 NEBRASKA AVENUE, SUITE A
LEVITTOWN, PA 19056 - 3333

Phone: 800-447-8792, 215-788-3113
Email: sarapin@gmail.com

SARAPIN ℞

DESCRIPTION

A sterile aqueous solution of soluble salts of the volatile bases from Sarraceniaceae (Pitcher Plant). Benzyl Alcohol 0.75%.

ACTIONS

The painful syndromes most commonly encountered in general practice which are relieved by SARAPIN® treatment are as follows:
Sciatic Pain
Intercostal Neuralgia
Occipital Neuritis
Brachial Plexus Neuralgia
Meralgia Paresthetica
Lumbar Neuralgia
Trigeminal Neuralgia

ADMINISTRATION

These and allied conditions may be treated with success in a majority of cases by nerve block or local infiltration:
Paravertebral—Careful localization of the zone of tenderness permits a determination of the corresponding trunk levels to be injected.
Perineural—In some instances, as in sciatica, the affected nerve can be injected at a site distant from its origin.
Local Infiltration—Multiple injections throughout an area of tenderness provide for diffusion into all the affected parts.

DOSAGE AND ADMINISTRATION

Paravertebral Injections

Cervical	2–3 ml
Thoracic	5–10 ml
Lumbar	5–10 ml
Sacral	3–5 ml
Sciatic Nerve	10 ml
Local Infiltration	5–10 ml

WARNINGS

Withdraw plunger of syringe to make sure the needle point is not in a blood vessel.

PRECAUTIONS

Procedure should be gentle and unhurried.
SARAPIN® is intended only for professional use. Its successful employment depends upon a thorough knowledge of the anatomy involved.

ADVERSE REACTIONS

Patients should be maintained in a recumbent position for 10 to 15 minutes following injection. A local sensation is to be expected, limited to the distribution of the nerve injected, and usually appearing as a temporary feeling of heaviness, although some cases will feel heat or a transitory aggravation of symptoms.

CONTRAINDICATIONS

SARAPIN® is non-toxic, has no side effects other than above and is contraindicated only in areas of infection.

HOW SUPPLIED

50 ml Multiple Dose Vial.
NDC-10541-0012-2
CAUTION: Federal law prohibits dispensing without prescription.
HIGH CHEMICAL COMPANY
3901 Nebraska Avenue, Suite A
Levittown, PA 19056 - 3333
800-447-8792, 215-788-3113
www.sarapin.com
sarapin@gmail.com

Shown in Product Identification Guide, page 307

Ironwood Pharmaceuticals, Inc.

301 BINNEY STREET, 2ND FLOOR
CAMBRIDGE, MA 02142

LINZESS ℞
(linaclotide)
capsules, for oral use

HIGHLIGHTS OF PRESCRIBING INFORMATION
These highlights do not include all the information needed to use LINZESS safely and effectively. See full prescribing information for LINZESS.
LINZESS (linaclotide) capsules, for oral use
Initial U.S. Approval: 2012

> **WARNING: PEDIATRIC RISK**
> ***See full prescribing information for complete boxed warning.***
> **LINZESS is contraindicated in pediatric patients up to 6 years of age. Avoid use of LINZESS in pediatric patients 6 through 17 years of age. Linaclotide caused deaths in young juvenile mice (4, 5.1, 8.4, 13.2).**

INDICATIONS AND USAGE

LINZESS is a guanylate cyclase-C agonist indicated in adults for treatment of:
- Irritable bowel syndrome with constipation (IBS-C) (1.1)
- Chronic idiopathic constipation (CIC) (1.2)

DOSAGE AND ADMINISTRATION

- IBS-C: Take 290 mcg orally once daily (2.1)
- CIC: Take 145 mcg orally once daily (2.2)
- Take on empty stomach at least 30 minutes prior to first meal of the day (2.1, 2.2)

DOSAGE FORMS AND STRENGTHS

Capsules: 145 mcg and 290 mcg (3)

CONTRAINDICATIONS

- Pediatric patients up to 6 years of age (4)
- Patients with known or suspected mechanical gastrointestinal obstruction (4)

WARNINGS AND PRECAUTIONS

- *Diarrhea:* Patients may experience severe diarrhea. Hold or stop LINZESS (5.2)

ADVERSE REACTIONS

Most common adverse reactions (incidence of at least 2%) reported in IBS-C or CIC patients are diarrhea, abdominal pain, flatulence and abdominal distension. (6.1)
To report SUSPECTED ADVERSE REACTIONS, contact Forest Pharmaceuticals, Inc., at 1- 800- 678-1605 or FDA at 1-800-FDA-1088 or www.fda.gov/medwatch.
See 17 for PATIENT COUNSELING INFORMATION and Medication Guide

Revised: 08/2013

FULL PRESCRIBING INFORMATION: CONTENTS*

*** Sections or subsections omitted from the full prescribing information are not listed**

FULL PRESCRIBING INFORMATION

> **WARNING: PEDIATRIC RISK**
> **LINZESS is contraindicated in pediatric patients up to 6 years of age. Avoid use in pediatric patients 6 through 17 years of age. In nonclinical studies, administration of a single, clinically relevant adult oral dose of linaclotide caused deaths in young juvenile mice *[see Contraindications (4), Warnings and Precautions (5.1), Use in Specific Populations (8.4) and Nonclinical Toxicology (13.2)].***

1 INDICATIONS AND USAGE

1.1 Irritable Bowel Syndrome with Constipation (IBS-C)

LINZESS (linaclotide) is indicated in adults for the treatment of irritable bowel syndrome with constipation (IBS-C).

1.2 Chronic Idiopathic Constipation (CIC)

LINZESS is indicated in adults for the treatment of chronic idiopathic constipation (CIC).

2 DOSAGE AND ADMINISTRATION

2.1 Irritable Bowel Syndrome with Constipation (IBS-C)

The recommended dose of LINZESS is 290 mcg taken orally once daily on an empty stomach, at least 30 minutes prior to the first meal of the day.

2.2 Chronic Idiopathic Constipation (CIC)

The recommended dose of LINZESS is 145 mcg taken orally once daily on an empty stomach, at least 30 minutes prior to the first meal of the day.

2.3 Important Administration Instructions

Swallow capsules whole; do not break apart or chew.

3 DOSAGE FORMS AND STRENGTHS

- 145 mcg capsules are white to off-white opaque with gray imprint "FL 145"
- 290 mcg capsules are white to off-white opaque with gray imprint "FL 290"

4 CONTRAINDICATIONS

LINZESS is contraindicated in:
- Pediatric patients up to 6 years of age *[see Warnings and Precautions (5.1), Use in Specific Populations (8.4) and Nonclinical Toxicology (13.2)]*
- Patients with known or suspected mechanical gastrointestinal obstruction

5 WARNINGS AND PRECAUTIONS

5.1 Pediatric Risk

LINZESS is contraindicated in pediatric patients up to 6 years of age. In nonclinical studies, deaths occurred within 24 hours in young juvenile mice (1 to 3 week-old mice; approximately equivalent to human pediatric patients less than 2 years of age) following administration of one or two daily oral doses of linaclotide *[see Contraindications (4), Use in Specific Populations (8.4) and Nonclinical Toxicology (13.2)]*.

Avoid the use of LINZESS in pediatric patients 6 through 17 years of age. Linaclotide did not cause deaths in older juvenile mice (approximately equivalent to humans ages 12 to 17 years). Although there were no deaths in older juvenile mice, given the deaths in young juvenile mice and the lack of clinical safety and efficacy data in pediatric patients, avoid the use of LINZESS in pediatric patients 6 through 17 years of age *[see Use in Specific Populations (8.4) and Nonclinical Toxicology (13.2)]*.

5.2 Diarrhea

Diarrhea was the most common adverse reaction of LINZESS-treated patients in the pooled IBS-C and CIC double-blind placebo-controlled trials. Severe diarrhea was reported in 2% of the LINZESS-treated patients. The incidence of diarrhea was similar between the IBS-C and CIC populations *[see Adverse Reactions (6.1)]*.

Instruct patients to stop LINZESS if severe diarrhea occurs and to contact their healthcare provider, who should consider dose suspension *[see Patient Counseling Information (17)]*.

6 ADVERSE REACTIONS

6.1 Clinical Trials Experience

Because clinical trials are conducted under widely varying conditions, adverse reaction rates observed in the clinical trials of a drug cannot be directly compared with rates in the clinical trials of another drug and may not reflect the rates observed in practice.

During clinical development, approximately 2570, 2040, and 1220 patients with either IBS-C or CIC were treated with LINZESS for 6 months or longer, 1 year or longer, and 18 months or longer, respectively (not mutually exclusive).

Irritable Bowel Syndrome with Constipation (IBS-C)

Most Common Adverse Reactions

The data described below reflect exposure to LINZESS in the two placebo-controlled clinical trials involving 1605 adult patients with IBS-C (Trials 1 and 2). Patients were randomized to receive placebo or 290 mcg LINZESS once daily on an empty stomach for up to 26 weeks. Demographic characteristics were comparable between treatment groups *[see Clinical Studies (14.1)]*. **Table 1** provides the incidence of adverse reactions reported in at least 2% of IBS-C patients in the LINZESS treatment group and at an incidence that was greater than in the placebo group.

Table 1: Adverse Reactions Reported in at least 2% of LINZESS-treated Patients and at an Incidence Greater than in Placebo Group Patients in the Two Phase 3 Placebo-controlled Trials (1 and 2) in IBS-C

Adverse Reactions	LINZESS 290 mcg [N=807] %	Placebo [N=798] %
Gastrointestinal		
Diarrhea	20	3
Abdominal pain[a]	7	5
Flatulence	4	2
Abdominal distension	2	1
Infections and Infestations		
Viral Gastroenteritis	3	1
Nervous System Disorders		
Headache	4	3

a: "Abdominal pain" term includes abdominal pain, upper abdominal pain, and lower abdominal pain.

Diarrhea

Diarrhea was the most commonly reported adverse reaction of the LINZESS-treated patients in the pooled IBS-C pivotal placebo-controlled trials. In these trials, 20% of LINZESS-treated patients reported diarrhea compared to 3% of placebo-treated patients. Severe diarrhea was reported in 2% of the LINZESS-treated patients versus less than 1% of the placebo-treated patients, and 5% of LINZESS-treated patients discontinued due to diarrhea vs less than 1% of placebo-treated patients. The majority of reported cases of diarrhea started within the first 2 weeks of LINZESS treatment. Fecal incontinence and dehydration were each reported in less than or equal to 1% of patients in the LINZESS treatment group *[see Warnings and Precautions (5.2)]*.

Adverse Reactions Leading to Discontinuation

In placebo-controlled trials in patients with IBS-C, 9% of patients treated with LINZESS and 3% of patients treated with placebo discontinued prematurely due to adverse reactions. In the LINZESS treatment group, the most common reasons for discontinuation due to adverse reactions were diarrhea (5%) and abdominal pain (1%). In comparison, less than 1% of patients in the placebo group withdrew due to diarrhea or abdominal pain.

Adverse Reactions Leading to Dose Reductions

In the open-label, long-term trials, 2147 patients with IBS-C received 290 mcg of LINZESS daily for up to 18 months. In these trials, 29% of patients had their dose reduced or suspended secondary to adverse reactions, the majority of which were diarrhea or other GI adverse reactions.

Other Adverse Reactions

Adverse reactions that were reported in at least 1% and less than 2% of IBS-C patients in the LINZESS treatment group and at an incidence greater than in the placebo treatment group are listed below by body system:

Gastrointestinal Disorders: gastroesophageal reflux disease, vomiting

General Disorders and Administration Site Conditions: fatigue

Other Adverse Events

In placebo-controlled trials in patients with IBS-C, less than 1% LINZESS-treated patients and no placebo-treated patients reported hematochezia; no patient in either treatment group reported melena. Less than 1% of LINZESS-treated and placebo-treated patients reported allergic reactions, urticaria, or hives as adverse events.

Chronic Idiopathic Constipation (CIC)

Most Common Adverse Reactions

The data described below reflect exposure to LINZESS in the two double-blind placebo-controlled clinical trials of 1275 adult patients with CIC (Trials 3 and 4). Patients were randomized to receive placebo or 145 mcg LINZESS or 290 mcg LINZESS once daily on an empty stomach, for at least 12 weeks. Demographic characteristics were comparable between both LINZESS treatment groups and placebo *[see Clinical Studies (14.2)]*. Only data for the recommended LINZESS 145 mcg dose and placebo are presented. **Table 2** provides the incidence of adverse reactions reported in at least 2% of CIC patients in the 145 mcg LINZESS treatment group and at an incidence that was greater than in the placebo treatment group.

Table 2: Adverse Reactions Reported in at least 2% of 145 mcg LINZESS-treated Patients and at an Incidence Greater than in Placebo Group Patients in the Two Phase 3 Placebo-controlled Trials (3 and 4) in CIC

Adverse Reactions	LINZESS 145 mcg [N=430] %	Placebo [N=423] %
Gastrointestinal		
Diarrhea	16	5
Abdominal pain[a]	7	6
Flatulence	6	5
Abdominal distension	3	2
Infections and Infestations		
Upper respiratory tract infection	5	4
Sinusitis	3	2

a: "Abdominal pain" term includes abdominal pain, upper abdominal pain, and lower abdominal pain.

Diarrhea

Diarrhea was the most commonly reported adverse reaction of the LINZESS-treated patients in the pooled CIC placebo-controlled trials. In these trials, 16% of LINZESS-treated patients reported diarrhea compared to 5% of placebo-treated patients. Severe diarrhea was reported in 2% of the 145 mcg LINZESS-treated patients versus less than 1% of the placebo-treated patients, and 5% of LINZESS-treated patients discontinued due to diarrhea vs less than 1% of placebo-treated patients. The majority of reported cases of diarrhea started within the first 2 weeks of LINZESS treatment. Fecal incontinence was reported in 1% of patients in the LINZESS treatment group, compared with less than 1% in the placebo group. Dehydration was reported in less than 1% of patients in the LINZESS treatment group *[see Warnings and Precautions (5.2)]*.

Adverse Reactions Leading to Discontinuation

In placebo-controlled trials in patients with CIC, 8% of patients treated with LINZESS and 4% of patients treated with placebo discontinued prematurely due to adverse reactions. In the 145 mcg LINZESS treatment group, the most common reasons for discontinuation due to adverse reactions were diarrhea (5%) and abdominal pain (1%). In comparison, less than 1% of patients in the placebo group withdrew due to diarrhea or abdominal pain.

Adverse Reactions Leading to Dose Reductions

In the open-label, long-term trials, 1129 patients with CIC received 290 mcg of LINZESS daily for up to 18 months. In these trials, 27% of patients had their dose reduced or suspended secondary to adverse reactions, the majority of which were diarrhea or other GI adverse reactions.

Other Adverse Reactions

Adverse reactions that were reported in at least 1% of and less than 2% of CIC patients in the 145 mcg LINZESS treatment group and at an incidence greater than in the placebo treatment group are listed below by body system:

Gastrointestinal Disorders: dyspepsia, fecal incontinence

Infections and Infestations: viral gastroenteritis

Other Adverse Events

In placebo-controlled trials in patients with CIC, less than 1% of both LINZESS-treated and placebo-treated patients reported rectal hemorrhage, hematochezia or melena. Less than 1% of LINZESS-treated and placebo-treated patients reported allergic reactions, urticaria, or hives as adverse events.

7 DRUG INTERACTIONS

No drug-drug interaction studies have been conducted with LINZESS. Linaclotide and its active metabolite are not measurable in plasma following administration of the recommended clinical doses; hence, no systemic drug-drug interactions or drug interactions mediated by plasma protein binding of linaclotide or its metabolite are anticipated *[see Clinical Pharmacology (12.3)]*.

Linaclotide does not interact with the cytochrome P450 enzyme system based on the results of *in vitro* studies. In addition, linaclotide is neither a substrate nor an inhibitor of the efflux transporter P-glycoprotein (P-gp).

8 USE IN SPECIFIC POPULATIONS

8.1 Pregnancy

Pregnancy Category C

Risk Summary

There are no adequate and well-controlled studies with LINZESS in pregnant women. In animal developmental studies, adverse fetal effects were observed only with maternal toxicity and at doses of linaclotide much higher than the maximum recommended human dose. LINZESS should be used during pregnancy only if the potential benefit justifies the potential risk to the fetus.

Animal Data

The potential for linaclotide to cause teratogenic effects was studied in rats, rabbits and mice. Oral administration of up to 100,000 mcg/kg/day in rats and 40,000 mcg/kg/day in rabbits produced no maternal toxicity and no effects on embryo-fetal development. In mice, oral dose levels of at least 40,000 mcg/kg/day produced severe maternal toxicity including death, reduction of gravid uterine and fetal weights, and effects on fetal morphology. Oral doses of 5000 mcg/kg/day did not produce maternal toxicity or any adverse effects on embryo-fetal development in mice.

The maximum recommended human dose is approximately 5 mcg/kg/day, based on a 60-kg body weight. Limited systemic exposure to linaclotide was achieved at the tested dose levels in animals (AUC = 40, 640, and 25 ng•hr/mL in rats, rabbits, and mice, respectively, at the highest dose levels), whereas no detectable exposure occurred in humans. Therefore, animal and human doses should not be compared directly for evaluating relative exposure.

8.3 Nursing Mothers

It is not known whether linaclotide is excreted in human milk; however, linaclotide and its active metabolite are not measurable in plasma following administration of the recommended clinical doses *[see Clinical Pharmacology (12.3)]*. Caution should be exercised when LINZESS is administered to nursing women *[see Contraindications (4), Warnings and Precautions (5.1) and Use in Specific Populations (8.4)]*.

8.4 Pediatric Use

Safety and effectiveness in pediatric patients have not been established.

LINZESS is contraindicated in pediatric patients up to 6 years of age. In nonclinical studies, deaths occurred within 24 hours in young juvenile mice (1 to 3 week-old-mice; approximately equivalent to human pediatric patients less than 2 years of age) following administration of one or two daily oral doses of linaclotide *[see Contraindications (4), Warnings and Precautions (5.1) and Nonclinical Toxicology (13.2)]*.

Avoid the use of LINZESS in pediatric patients 6 through 17 years of age. Linaclotide did not cause deaths in older juvenile mice (approximately equivalent to humans age 12 to 17 years). Although there were no deaths in older juvenile mice, given the deaths in young juvenile mice and the lack of clinical safety and efficacy data in pediatric patients, avoid the use of LINZESS in pediatric patients 6 through 17 years of age *[see Warnings and Precautions (5.1) and Nonclinical Toxicology (13.2)]*.

8.5 Geriatric Use

Irritable Bowel Syndrome with Constipation (IBS-C)

Of 1605 IBS-C patients in the placebo-controlled clinical studies of LINZESS, 85 (5%) were at least 65 years of age, while 20 (1%) were at least 75 years old. Clinical studies of LINZESS did not include sufficient numbers of subjects aged 65 and over to determine whether they respond differently from younger subjects.

Chronic Idiopathic Constipation (CIC)

Of 1275 CIC patients in the placebo-controlled clinical studies of LINZESS, 155 (12%) were at least 65 years of age, while 30 (2%) were at least 75 years old. Clinical trials of LINZESS did not include sufficient numbers of subjects aged 65 and over to determine whether they respond differently from younger subjects.

8.6 Hepatic or Renal Impairment

No dose adjustment is necessary based on hepatic or renal function *[see Clinical Pharmacology (12.3)]*.

10 OVERDOSAGE

There is limited experience with overdose of LINZESS. During the clinical development program of LINZESS, single doses of 2897 mcg were administered to 22 healthy volunteers; the safety profile in these subjects was consistent with that in the overall LINZESS-treated population, with diarrhea being the most commonly reported adverse reaction.

11 DESCRIPTION

LINZESS (linaclotide) is a guanylate cyclase-C agonist. Linaclotide is a 14-amino acid peptide with the following chemical name: L-cysteinyl L cysteinyl-L-glutamyl-L-tyrosyl-L-cysteinyl-L-cysteinyl-L-asparaginyl-L-prolyl-L-alanyl-L-cysteinyl-L-threonyl-glycyl-L-cysteinyl-L-tyrosine, cyclic (1-6), (2-10), (5-13)-tris (disulfide).

The molecular formula of linaclotide is $C_{59}H_{79}N_{15}O_{21}S_6$ and its molecular weight is 1526.8. The amino acid sequence for linaclotide is shown below:

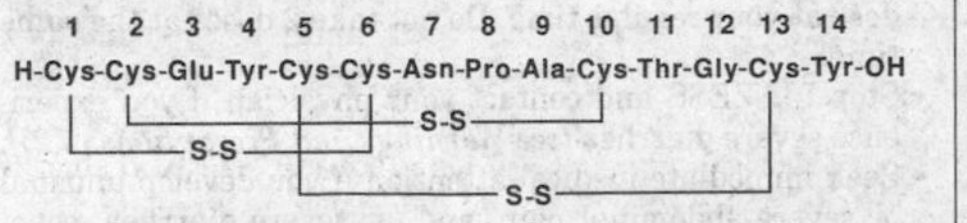

Linaclotide is an amorphous, white to off-white powder. It is slightly soluble in water and aqueous sodium chloride (0.9%). LINZESS contains linaclotide-coated beads in hard gelatin capsules. LINZESS is available as 145 mcg and 290 mcg capsules for oral administration.

The inactive ingredients of LINZESS capsules include: calcium chloride dihydrate, L-leucine, hypromellose, microcrystalline cellulose, gelatin, and titanium dioxide.

12 CLINICAL PHARMACOLOGY

12.1 Mechanism of Action

Linaclotide is a guanylate cyclase-C (GC-C) agonist. Both linaclotide and its active metabolite bind to GC-C and act locally on the luminal surface of the intestinal epithelium. Activation of GC-C results in an increase in both intracellular and extracellular concentrations of cyclic guanosine monophosphate (cGMP). Elevation in intracellular cGMP stimulates secretion of chloride and bicarbonate into the intestinal lumen, mainly through activation of the cystic fibrosis transmembrane conductance regulator (CFTR) ion channel, resulting in increased intestinal fluid and accelerated transit. In animal models, linaclotide has been shown to both accelerate GI transit and reduce intestinal pain. The linaclotide-induced reduction in visceral pain in animals is thought to be mediated by increased extracellular cGMP, which was shown to decrease the activity of pain-sensing nerves.

12.2 Pharmacodynamics

Although the pharmacologic effects of LINZESS in humans have not been fully evaluated, in clinical studies, LINZESS has been shown to change stool consistency as measured by the Bristol Stool Form Scale (BSFS) and increase stool frequency.

12.3 Pharmacokinetics

Absorption

LINZESS is minimally absorbed with low systemic availability following oral administration. Concentrations of linaclotide and its active metabolite in plasma are below the limit of quantitation after oral doses of 145 mcg or 290 mcg were administered. Therefore, standard pharmacokinetic parameters such as area under the curve (AUC), maximum concentration (C_{max}), and half-life ($t_{1/2}$) cannot be calculated.

Distribution

Given that linaclotide plasma concentrations following therapeutic oral doses are not measurable, linaclotide is expected to be minimally distributed to tissues.

Metabolism

Linaclotide is metabolized within the gastrointestinal tract to its principal, active metabolite by loss of the terminal tyrosine moiety. Both linaclotide and the metabolite are proteolytically degraded within the intestinal lumen to smaller peptides and naturally occurring amino acids.

Elimination

Active peptide recovery in the stool samples of fed and fasted subjects following the daily administration of 290 mcg of LINZESS for seven days averaged about 5% (fasted) and about 3% (fed) and virtually all as the active metabolite.

Food Effect

In a cross-over study, 18 healthy subjects were given LINZESS 290 mcg for 7 days both in the non-fed and fed state. Neither linaclotide nor its active metabolite was detected in the plasma. Taking LINZESS immediately after the high fat breakfast resulted in looser stools and a higher stool frequency compared with taking it in the fasted state *[see Dosage and Administration (2.1, 2.2)]*. In clinical trials, LINZESS was administered on an empty stomach, at least 30 minutes before breakfast.

Specific Populations

Age and Gender

Clinical studies to determine the impact of age and gender on the pharmacokinetics of LINZESS have not been conducted. See *Use in Specific Populations (8.5)* for information regarding patients aged 65 years and older.

Hepatic Impairment

LINZESS has not been specifically studied in patients who have hepatic impairment. Hepatic impairment is not expected to affect the metabolism or clearance of the parent drug or its metabolite because linaclotide is metabolized within the gastrointestinal tract *[see Use in Specific Populations (8.6)]*.

Renal Impairment

LINZESS has not been specifically studied in patients who have renal impairment. Renal impairment is not expected to affect clearance of the parent drug or its metabolite because linaclotide has low systemic availability following oral administration and is metabolized within the gastrointestinal tract *[see Use in Specific Populations (8.6)]*.

13 NONCLINICAL TOXICOLOGY

13.1 Carcinogenesis, Mutagenesis, Impairment of Fertility

Carcinogenesis

In 2-year carcinogenicity studies, linaclotide was not tumorigenic in rats at doses up to 3500 mcg/kg/day or in mice at doses up to 6000 mcg/kg/day. The maximum recommended human dose is approximately 5 mcg/kg/day based on a 60-kg bodyweight. Limited systemic exposure to linaclotide was achieved at the tested dose levels in animals, whereas no detectable exposure occurred in humans. Therefore, animal and human doses should not be compared directly for evaluating relative exposure.

Mutagenesis

Linaclotide was not genotoxic in an *in vitro* bacterial reverse mutation (Ames) assay or in the *in vitro* chromosomal aberration assay in cultured human peripheral blood lymphocytes.

Impairment of Fertility

Linaclotide had no effect on fertility or reproductive function in male and female rats at oral doses of up to 100,000 mcg/kg/day.

13.2 Animal Toxicology and/or Pharmacology

Linaclotide caused deaths in two separate toxicology studies in juvenile mice. The mechanism for these deaths is unknown *[see Contraindications (4) and Warnings and Precautions (5.1)]*.

Linaclotide caused deaths at 10 mcg/kg/day in neonatal mice after oral administration of 1 or 2 daily doses, starting on post partum day 7. Deaths were also observed in juvenile mice after a single oral administration on post partum day 14 (100 mcg/kg) and post partum day 21 (600 mcg/kg). The deaths were identified in mice with ages approximately equivalent to human infants and children less than 2 years of age. There were no deaths in the control groups. There are currently no data for mice between ages of 21 days and 6 weeks. Linaclotide did not cause death in a study in older juvenile mice age 6 weeks (approximately equivalent to humans age 12 to 17 years) at a dose of 20,000 mcg/kg/day for 28 days. Linaclotide did not cause death in adult mice, rats, rabbits and monkeys at dose levels up to 5,000 mcg/kg/day. The maximum recommended dose in adults is approximately 5 mcg/kg/day, based on a 60-kg body weight. Animal and human doses of linaclotide should not be compared directly for evaluating relative exposure *[see Nonclinical Toxicology (13.1)]*.

14 CLINICAL STUDIES

14.1 Irritable Bowel Syndrome with Constipation (IBS-C)

The efficacy of LINZESS for the management of symptoms of IBS-C was established in two double-blind, placebo-controlled, randomized, multicenter trials in adult patients (Trials 1 and 2). A total of 800 patients in Trial 1 and 804 patients in Trial 2 [overall mean age of 44 years (range 18 - 87 years with 5% at least 65 years of age), 90% female, 77% white, 19% black, and 12% Hispanic] received treatment with LINZESS 290 mcg or placebo once daily and were evaluated for efficacy. All patients met Rome II criteria for IBS and were required, during the 2-week baseline period, to meet the following criteria:

- a mean abdominal pain score of at least 3 on a 0-to-10-point numeric rating scale
- less than 3 complete spontaneous bowel movements (CSBMs) per week [a CSBM is a spontaneous bowel movement (SBM) that is associated with a sense of complete evacuation; a SBM is a bowel movement occurring in the absence of laxative use], and
- less than or equal to 5 SBMs per week.

The trial designs were identical through the first 12 weeks, and thereafter differed only in that Trial 1 included a 4-week randomized withdrawal (RW) period, and Trial 2 continued for 14 additional weeks (total of 26 weeks) of double-blind treatment. During the trials, patients were allowed to continue stable doses of bulk laxatives or stool softeners but were not allowed to take laxatives, bismuth, prokinetic agents, or other drugs to treat IBS-C or chronic constipation.

Efficacy of LINZESS was assessed using overall responder analyses and change-from-baseline endpoints. Results for endpoints were based on information provided daily by patients in diaries.

The 4 primary efficacy responder endpoints were based on a patient being a weekly responder for either at least 9 out of the first 12 weeks of treatment or at least 6 out of the first 12 weeks of treatment. For the 9 out of 12 weeks combined primary responder endpoint, a patient had to have at least a

Table 3: Efficacy Responder Rates in the Two Placebo-controlled IBS-C Trials: at Least 9 Out of 12 Weeks

	Trial 1			Trial 2		
	LINZESS 290 mcg (N=405)	Placebo (N=395)	Treatment Difference [95% CI]	LINZESS 290 mcg (N=401)	Placebo (N=403)	Treatment Difference [95% CI]
Combined Responder* (Abdominal Pain and CSBM Responder)	12.1%	5.1%	7.0% [3.2%, 10.9%]	12.7%	3.0%	9.7% [6.1%, 13.4%]
Abdominal Pain Responder* (≥ 30% Abdominal Pain Reduction)	34.3%	27.1%	7.2% [0.9%, 13.6%]	38.9%	19.6%	19.3% [13.2%, 25.4%]
CSBM Responder* (≥ 3 CSBMs and Increase ≥1 CSBM from Baseline)	19.5%	6.3%	13.2% [8.6%, 17.7%]	18.0%	5.0%	13.0% [8.7%, 17.3%]

* Primary Endpoints
Note: Analyses based on first 12 weeks of treatment for both Trials 1 and 2
CI =Confidence Interval

Table 4: Efficacy Responder Rates in the Two Placebo-controlled IBS-C Trials: at Least 6 Out of 12 Weeks

	Trial 1			Trial 2		
	LINZESS 290 mcg (N=405)	**Placebo (N=395)**	**Treatment Difference [95% CI]**	**LINZESS 290 mcg (N=401)**	**Placebo (N=403)**	**Treatment Difference [95% CI]**
Combined Responder* (Abdominal Pain and CSBM Responder)	33.6%	21.0%	12.6% [6.5%, 18.7%]	33.7%	13.9%	19.8% [14.0%, 25.5%]
Abdominal Pain Responder** (≥ 30% Abdominal Pain Reduction)	50.1%	37.5%	12.7% [5.8%, 19.5%]	48.9%	34.5%	14.4% [7.6%, 21.1%]
CSBM Responder** (Increase ≥ 1 CSBM from Baseline)	48.6%	29.6%	19.0% [12.4%, 25.7%]	47.6%	22.6%	25.1% [18.7%, 31.4%]

* Primary Endpoint, ** Secondary Endpoints
Note: Analyses based on first 12 weeks of treatment for both Trials 1 and 2
CI =Confidence Interval

Table 5: Efficacy Responder Rates in the Two Placebo-controlled CIC Trials: at Least 9 Out of 12 Weeks

	Trial 3			Trial 4		
	LINZESS 145 mcg (N=217)	**Placebo (N=209)**	**Treatment Difference [95% CI]**	**LINZESS 145 mcg (N=213)**	**Placebo (N=215)**	**Treatment Difference [95% CI]**
CSBM Overall Responder* (≥ 3 CSBMs and Increase ≥ 1 CSBM from Baseline)	20.3%	3.3%	16.9% [11.0%, 22.8%]	15.5%	5.6%	9.9% [4.2%, 15.7%]

*Primary Endpoint
CI=Confidence Interval

30% reduction from baseline in mean abdominal pain, at least 3 CSBMs and an increase of at least 1 CSBM from baseline, all in the same week, for at least 9 out of the first 12 weeks of treatment. Each of the 2 components of the 9 out of 12 weeks combined responder endpoint, abdominal pain and CSBMs, was also a primary endpoint.

For the 6 out of 12 weeks combined primary responder endpoint, a patient had to have at least a 30% reduction from baseline in mean abdominal pain and an increase of at least 1 CSBM from baseline, all in the same week, for at least 6 out of the first 12 weeks of treatment. To be considered a responder for this analysis, patients did not have to have at least 3 CSBMs per week.

The efficacy results for the 9 out of 12 weeks and the 6 out of 12 weeks responder endpoints are shown in **Tables 3 and 4**, respectively. In both trials, the proportion of patients who were responders to LINZESS 290 mcg was statistically significantly higher than with placebo.

[See table 3 at top of previous page]
[See table 4 above]

In each trial, improvement from baseline in abdominal pain and CSBM frequency was seen over the first 12-weeks of the treatment periods. For change from baseline in the 11-point abdominal pain scale, LINZESS 290 mcg began to separate from placebo in the first week. Maximum effects were seen at weeks 6 - 9 and were maintained until the end of the study. The mean treatment difference from placebo at week 12 was a decrease in pain score of approximately 1.0 point in both trials (using an 11-point scale). Maximum effect on CSBM frequency occurred within the first week, and for change from baseline in CSBM frequency at week 12, the difference between placebo and LINZESS was approximately 1.5 CSBMs per week in both trials.

During the 4-week randomized withdrawal period in Trial 1, patients who received LINZESS during the 12-week treatment period were re-randomized to receive placebo or continue treatment on LINZESS 290 mcg. In LINZESS-treated patients re-randomized to placebo, CSBM frequency and abdominal-pain severity returned toward baseline within 1 week and did not result in worsening compared to baseline. Patients who continued on LINZESS maintained their response to therapy over the additional 4 weeks. Patients on placebo who were allocated to LINZESS had an increase in CSBM frequency and a decrease in abdominal pain levels that were similar to the levels observed in patients taking LINZESS during the treatment period.

14.2 Chronic Idiopathic Constipation (CIC)

The efficacy of LINZESS for the management of symptoms of CIC was established in two double-blind, placebo-controlled, randomized, multicenter clinical trials in adult patients (Trials 3 and 4). A total of 642 patients in Trial 3 and 630 patients in Trial 4 [overall mean age of 48 years (range 18 - 85 years with 12% at least 65 years of age), 89% female, 76% white, 22% black, 10% Hispanic] received treatment with LINZESS 145 mcg, 290 mcg, or placebo once daily and were evaluated for efficacy. All patients met modified Rome II criteria for functional constipation. Modified Rome II criteria were less than 3 Spontaneous Bowel Movements (SBMs) per week and 1 of the following symptoms for at least 12 weeks, which need not be consecutive, in the preceding 12 months:

- Straining during greater than 25% of bowel movements
- Lumpy or hard stools during greater than 25% of bowel movements
- Sensation of incomplete evacuation during greater than 25% of bowel movements

Patients were also required to have less than 3 CSBMs per week and less than or equal to 6 SBMs per week during a 2-week baseline period. Patients were excluded if they met criteria for IBS-C or had fecal impaction that required emergency room treatment.

The trial designs were identical through the first 12 weeks. Trial 3 also included an additional 4-week randomized withdrawal (RW) period. During the trials, patients were allowed to continue stable doses of bulk laxatives or stool softeners but were not allowed to take laxatives, bismuth, prokinetic agents, or other drugs to treat chronic constipation.

Efficacy of LINZESS was assessed using overall responder analysis and change-from-baseline endpoints. Results for endpoints were based on information provided daily by patients in diaries.

A CSBM overall responder in the CIC trials was defined as a patient who had at least 3 CSBMs and an increase of at least 1 CSBM from baseline in a given week for at least 9 weeks out of the 12-week treatment period. The CSBM responder rates are shown in **Table 5**. During the individual double-blind placebo-controlled trials, LINZESS 290 mcg did not consistently offer additional clinically meaningful treatment benefit over placebo than that observed with the LINZESS 145 mcg dose. Therefore, the 145 mcg dose is the recommended dose. Only the data for the approved 145 mcg dose of LINZESS are presented in **Table 5**.

In Trials 3 and 4, the proportion of patients who were CSBM responders was statistically significantly greater with the LINZESS 145 mcg dose than with placebo.

[See table 5 above]

CSBM frequency reached maximum level during week 1 and was also demonstrated over the remainder of the 12-week treatment period in Trial 3 and Trial 4. For the mean change from baseline in CSBM frequency at week 12, the difference between placebo and LINZESS was approximately 1.5 CSBMs.

On average, patients who received LINZESS across the 2 trials had significantly greater improvements compared with patients receiving placebo in stool frequency (CSBMs/week and SBMs/week), and stool consistency (as measured by the BSFS).

During the 4-week randomized withdrawal period in Trial 3, patients who received LINZESS during the 12-week treatment period were re-randomized to receive placebo or continue treatment on the same dose of LINZESS taken during the treatment period. In LINZESS-treated patients re-randomized to placebo, CSBM and SBM frequency returned toward baseline within 1 week and did not result in worsening compared to baseline. Patients who continued on LINZESS maintained their response to therapy over the additional 4 weeks. Patients on placebo who were allocated to LINZESS had an increase in CSBM and SBM frequency similar to the levels observed in patients taking LINZESS during the treatment period.

16 HOW SUPPLIED/STORAGE AND HANDLING

How Supplied

- **145 mcg Capsules**: White to off-white opaque hard gelatin capsules with grey imprint "FL 145"
  Bottle of 30: NDC 0456-1201-30
- **290 mcg Capsules**: White to off-white opaque hard gelatin capsules with grey imprint "FL 290"
  Bottle of 30: NDC 0456-1202-30

Storage

Store at 25°C (77°F); excursions permitted between 15°C and 30°C (59°F and 86°F) [see USP Controlled Room Temperature].

Keep LINZESS in the original container. Do not subdivide or repackage. Protect from moisture. Do not remove desiccant from the container. Keep bottles tightly closed in a dry place.

17 PATIENT COUNSELING INFORMATION

See FDA-approved patient labeling (Medication Guide).

Patients should be instructed as follows:

- **Do not give LINZESS to children who are under 6 years of age. You should not give LINZESS to children 6 to 17 years of age. It may harm them** *[see Contraindications (4), Warnings and Precautions (5.1), Use in Specific Populations (8.4) and Nonclinical Toxicology (13.2)].*
- Keep LINZESS in the original container. Do not subdivide or repackage. Protect from moisture. Do not remove desiccant from the container. Keep bottles closed tightly in a dry place *[see How Supplied/Storage and Handling (16)].*
- Take LINZESS once daily on an empty stomach as prescribed. Swallow the capsule whole and do not break apart or chew *[see Dosage and Administration (2.1 and 2.2)].*
- If you miss a dose, skip the missed dose. Just take the next dose at your regular time. Do not take 2 doses at the same time.
- Stop LINZESS and contact your physician if you experience severe diarrhea *[see Warnings and Precautions (5.2)].*
- Seek immediate medical attention if you develop unusual or severe abdominal pain, and /or severe diarrhea, especially if in combination with hematochezia or melena *[see Adverse Reactions (6.1)].*

LINZESS® is a registered trademark of Ironwood Pharmaceuticals, Inc.

Distributed by:
Forest Pharmaceuticals, Inc.
Subsidiary of Forest Laboratories, Inc.
St. Louis, Missouri, 63045

Marketed by:
Forest Pharmaceuticals, Inc.
Subsidiary of Forest Laboratories, Inc.
St. Louis, Missouri, 63045
Ironwood Pharmaceuticals, Inc.
Cambridge, MA, 02142

MEDICATION GUIDE
LINZESS® (lin-ZESS)
(linaclotide)
capsules

Read this Medication Guide before you start taking LINZESS and each time you get a refill. There may be new information. This information does not take the place of talking to your doctor about your medical condition or your treatment.

What is the most important information I should know about LINZESS?

- **Do not give LINZESS to children who are under 6 years of age. It may harm them.**
- **You should not give LINZESS to children 6 to 17 years of age. It may harm them.**

See the section **"What are the possible side effects of LINZESS?"** for more information about side effects.

What is LINZESS?

LINZESS is a prescription medication used in adults to treat

- irritable bowel syndrome with constipation (IBS-C)

- a type of constipation called chronic idiopathic constipation (CIC). "Idiopathic" means the cause of the constipation is unknown.

It is not known if LINZESS is safe and effective in children.

Who should not take LINZESS?

- **Do not give LINZESS to children who are under 6 years of age.**
- Do not take LINZESS if a doctor has told you that you have a bowel blockage (intestinal obstruction).

What should I tell my doctor before taking LINZESS?

Before you take LINZESS, tell your doctor if you:

- have any other medical conditions
- are pregnant or plan to become pregnant. It is not known if LINZESS will harm your unborn baby.
- are breastfeeding or plan to breastfeed. It is not known if LINZESS passes into your breast milk. Talk with your doctor about the best way to feed your baby, if you take LINZESS.

Tell your doctor about all the medicines you take, including prescription and non-prescription medicines, vitamins and herbal supplements.

How should I take LINZESS?

- Take LINZESS exactly as your doctor tells you to take it.
- Take LINZESS one time each day on an empty stomach, at least 30 minutes before your first meal of the day.
- Swallow LINZESS capsules whole. Do not break or chew the capsules.
- If you miss a dose, skip the missed dose. Just take the next dose at your regular time. Do not take 2 doses at the same time.

What are the possible side effects of LINZESS?

LINZESS can cause serious side effects, including:

- **See "What is the most important information I should know about LINZESS?"**
- **Diarrhea is the most common side effect of LINZESS, and it can sometimes be severe.**
  - Diarrhea often begins within the first 2 weeks of LINZESS treatment.
  - **Stop taking LINZESS and call your doctor right away if you get severe diarrhea during treatment with LINZESS.**

Other common side effects of LINZESS include:

- gas
- stomach-area (abdomen) pain
- swelling, or a feeling of fullness or pressure in your abdomen (distention)

Tell your doctor if you have any side effect that bothers you or that does not go away.

These are not all the possible side effects of LINZESS. For more information, ask your doctor or pharmacist.

In addition, call your doctor or go to the nearest hospital emergency room right away, if you develop unusual or severe stomach-area (abdomen) pain, especially if you also have bright red, bloody stools or black stools that look like tar.

Call your doctor for medical advice about side effects. You may report side effects to FDA at 1-800-FDA-1088.

How should I store LINZESS?

- Store LINZESS at room temperature between 68°F to 77°F (20°C to 25°C).
- Keep LINZESS in the bottle that it comes in.
- The LINZESS bottle contains a desiccant packet to help keep your medicine dry (protect it from moisture). Do not remove the desiccant packet from the bottle.
- Keep the container of LINZESS tightly closed and in a dry place.

Keep LINZESS and all medicines out of the reach of children.

General information about LINZESS

Medicines are sometimes prescribed for purposes other than those listed in a Medication Guide. Do not use LINZESS for a condition for which it was not prescribed. Do not give LINZESS to other people, even if they have the same symptoms that you have. It may harm them.

This Medication Guide summarizes the most important information about LINZESS. If you would like more information, talk with your doctor. You can ask your doctor or pharmacist for information about LINZESS that is written for health professionals. For more information, go to www.LINZESS.com or call 1-800-678-1605.

What are the ingredients in LINZESS?

Active ingredient: linaclotide

Inactive ingredients: calcium chloride dihydrate, L-leucine, hypromellose, microcrystalline cellulose, gelatin, and titanium dioxide.

This Medication Guide has been approved by the U.S. Food and Drug Administration.

Revised: August 2013

LINZESS® is a registered trademark of Ironwood Pharmaceuticals, Inc.

Distributed by:
Forest Pharmaceuticals, Inc.
Subsidiary of Forest Laboratories, Inc.
St. Louis, Missouri, 63045

Marketed by:
Forest Pharmaceuticals, Inc.
Subsidiary of Forest Laboratories, Inc.
St. Louis, Missouri, 63045
Ironwood Pharmaceuticals, Inc.
Cambridge, MA, 02142

Jacobus Pharmaceutical Co., Inc.

37 CLEVELAND LANE
P.O. BOX 5290
PRINCETON, NJ 08540

Direct All Inquiries to:
(609) 921-7447
FAX: (609) 799-1176

DAPSONE ℞

[*dap 'sōne*]
Tablets, USP
25 mg & 100 mg

DESCRIPTION

Dapsone-USP, 4,4′-diaminodiphenylsulfone (DDS), is a primary treatment for Dermatitis herpetiformis. It is an antibacterial drug for susceptible cases of leprosy. It is a white, odorless crystalline powder, practically insoluble in water and insoluble in fixed and vegetable oils.

Dapsone is issued on prescription in tablets of 25 and 100 mg for oral use.

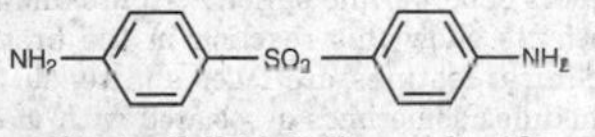

Inactive Ingredients: Colloidal silicone dioxide, magnesium stearate, microcrystalline cellulose and corn starch.

CLINICAL PHARMACOLOGY

Actions: The mechanism of action in Dermatitis herpetiformis has not been established. By the kinetic method in mice, Dapsone is bactericidal as well as bacteriostatic against *Mycobacterium leprae.*

Absorption and Excretion: Dapsone, when given orally, is rapidly and almost completely absorbed. About 85 percent of the daily intake is recoverable from the urine mainly in the form of water-soluble metabolites. Excretion of the drug is slow and a constant blood level can be maintained with the usual dosage.

Blood Levels: Detected a few minutes after ingestion, the drug reaches peak concentration in 4-8 hours. Daily administration for at least eight days is necessary to achieve a plateau level. With doses of 200 mg daily, this level averaged 2.3 µg/ml with a range of 0.1-7.0 µg/ml. The half-life in the plasma in different individuals varies from ten hours to fifty hours and averages twenty-eight hours. Repeat tests in the same individual are constant. Daily administration (50-100 mg) in leprosy patients will provide blood levels in excess of the usual minimum inhibitory concentration even for patients with a short Dapsone half-life.

INDICATIONS AND USAGE

Dermatitis herpetiformis: (D.H.)

Leprosy: All forms of leprosy except for cases of proven Dapsone resistance.

CONTRAINDICATION

Hypersensitivity to Dapsone and/or its derivatives.

WARNINGS

The patient should be warned to respond to the presence of clinical signs such as sore throat, fever, pallor, purpura or jaundice. Deaths associated with the administration of Dapsone have been reported from agranulocytosis, aplastic anemia and other blood dyscrasias. Complete blood counts should be done frequently in patients receiving Dapsone. The FDA Dermatology Advisory Committee recommended that, when feasible, counts should be done weekly for the first month, monthly for six months and semi-annually thereafter. If a significant reduction in leucocytes, platelets or hemopoiesis is noted, Dapsone should be discontinued and the patient followed intensively. Folic acid antagonists have similar effects and may increase the incidence of hematologic reactions; if co-administered with Dapsone the patient should be monitored more frequently. Patients on weekly pyrimethamine and Dapsone have developed agranulocytosis during the second and third month of therapy.

Severe anemia should be treated prior to initiation of therapy and hemoglobin monitored. Hemolysis and methemoglobin may be poorly tolerated by patients with severe cardiopulmonary disease.

Cutaneous reactions, especially bullous, include exfoliative dermatitis and are probably one of the most serious, though rare, complications of sulfone therapy. They are directly due to drug sensitization. Such reactions include toxic erythema, erythema multiforme, toxic epidermal necrolysis, morbilliform and scarlatiniform reactions, urticaria and erythema nodosum. If new or toxic dermatologic reactions occur, sulfone therapy must be promptly discontinued and appropriate therapy instituted. Leprosy reactional states, including cutaneous, are not hypersensitivity reactions to Dapsone and do not require discontinuation. See special section.

PRECAUTIONS

General: Hemolysis and Heinz body formation may be exaggerated in individuals with a glucose-6-phosphate dehydrogenase (G6PD) deficiency, or methemoglobin reductase deficiency, or hemoglobin M. This reaction is frequently dose-related. Dapsone should be given with caution to these patients or if the patient is exposed to other agents or conditions such as infection or diabetic ketosis capable of producing hemolysis. Drugs or chemicals which have produced significant hemolysis in G6PD or methemoglobin reductase deficient patients include Dapsone, sulfanilamide, nitrite, aniline, phenylhydrazine, napthalene, niridazole, nitrofurantoin and 8-amino-antimalarials such as primaquine.

Toxic hepatitis and cholestatic jaundice have been reported early in therapy. Hyperbilirubinemia may occur more often in G6PD deficient patients. When feasible, baseline and subsequent monitoring of liver function is recommended; if abnormal, Dapsone should be discontinued until the source of the abnormality is established.

Drug Interactions: Rifampin lowers Dapsone levels 7 to 10-fold by accelerating plasma clearance; in leprosy this reduction has not required a change in dosage. Folic acid antagonists such as pyrimethamine may increase the likelihood of hematologic reactions.

A modest interaction has been reported for patients receiving 100 mg Dapsone daily in combination with trimethoprim 5 mg/kg q6h. On Day 7, the serum Dapsone levels averaged 2.1 ± 1.0 µg/mL in comparison to 1.5 ± 0.5 µg/mL for Dapsone alone. On Day 7, trimethoprim levels averaged 18.4 ± 5.2 µg/mL in comparison to 12.4 ± 4.5 µg/mL for patients not receiving Dapsone. Thus, there is a mutual interaction between Dapsone and trimethoprim in which each raises the level of the other about 1.5 times.

A crossover study[1] designed to assess the potential of a drug interaction between Dapsone, 100 mg/day and trimethoprim, 200 mg every 12 hours, in eight asymptomatic HIV positive volunteers (average CD4 count 524 cells/mm^3) demonstrated that there was not a significant drug intreraction between Dapsone and trimethoprim. However, an earlier report[2] also by Lee et al, in 78 HIV infected patients with acute *Pneumocystis carinii* pneumonia, receiving Dapsone, 100 mg/day and higher trimethoprim dose, 20 mg/kg/day, demonstrated that the serum levels of Dapsone were increased by 40% and trimethoprim levels were increased by 48% when the drugs were administered concurrently.

Carcinogenesis, mutagenesis: Dapsone has been found carcinogenic (sarcomagenic) for male rats and female mice causing mesenchymal tumors in the spleen and peritoneum, and thyroid carcinoma in female rats. Dapsone is not mutagenic with or without microsomal activation in *S. typhimurium* tester strains 1535, 1537, 1538, 98, or 100.

Pregnancy: Teratogenic Effects. Pregnancy Category C: Animal reproduction studies have not been conducted with Dapsone. Extensive, but uncontrolled experience and two published surveys on the use of Dapsone in pregnant women have not shown that Dapsone increases the risk of fetal abnormalities if administered during all trimesters of pregnancy or can affect reproduction capacity. Because of the lack of animal studies or controlled human experience, Dapsone should be given to a pregnant woman only if clearly needed. In general, for leprosy, USPHS at Carville recommends maintenance of Dapsone. Dapsone has been important for the management of some pregnant D.H. patients.

Nursing Mothers: Dapsone is excreted in breast milk in substantial amounts. Hemolytic reactions can occur in neonates. See section on hemolysis. Because of the potential for tumorgenicity shown for Dapsone in animal studies a decision should be made whether to discontinue nursing or discontinue the drug taking into account the importance of drug to the mother.

Pediatric Use: Pediatric patients are treated on the same schedule as adults but with correspondingly smaller doses. Dapsone is generally not considered to have an effect on the later growth, development and functional development of the pediatric patient.

ADVERSE REACTIONS

In addition to the warnings listed above, the following syndromes and serious reactions have been reported in patients on Dapsone.

Hematologic Effects: Dose-related hemolysis is the most common adverse effect and is seen in patients with or without G6PD deficiency. Almost all patients demonstrate the inter-related changes of a loss of 1-2g of hemoglobin, an increase in the reticulocytes (2-12%), a shortened red cell life span and a rise in methemoglobin. G6PD deficient patients have greater responses.

Nervous System Effects: Peripheral neuropathy is a definite but unusual complication of Dapsone therapy in non-leprosy patients. Motor loss is predominant. If muscle weakness appears, Dapsone should be withdrawn. Recovery on withdrawal is usually substantially complete. The mechanism of recovery is reported by axonal regeneration. Some recovered patients have tolerated retreatment at reduced dosage. In leprosy this complication may be difficult to distinguish from a leprosy reactional state.

Body As A Whole: In addition to the warnings and adverse effects reported above, additional adverse reactions include: nausea, vomiting, abdominal pains, pancreatitis, vertigo, blurred vision, tinnitus, insomnia, fever, headache, psychosis, phototoxicity, pulmonary eosinophilia, tachycardia, albuminuria, the nephrotic syndrome, hypoalbuminemia without proteinuria, renal papillary necrosis, male infertility, drug-induced Lupus erythematosus and an infectious mononucleosis-like syndrome. In general, with the exception of the complications of severe anoxia from overdosage (retinal and optic nerve damage, etc.) these adverse reactions have regressed off drug.

OVERDOSAGE

Nausea, vomiting, hyperexcitability can appear a few minutes up to 24 hours after ingestion of an overdosage. Methemoglobin induced depression, convulsions or severe cyanosis requires prompt treatment. In normal and methemoglobin reductase deficient patients, methylene blue, 1-2 mg/kg of body weight, given slowly intravenously, is the treatment of choice. The effect is complete in 30 minutes, but may have to be repeated if methemoglobin reaccumulates. For non-emergencies, if treatment is needed, methylene blue may be given orally in doses of 3-5 mg/kg every 4-6 hours. Methylene blue reduction depends on G6PD and should not be given to fully expressed G6PD deficient patients.

DOSAGE AND ADMINISTRATION

Dermatitis herpetiformis: The dosage should be individually titrated starting in adults with 50 mg daily and correspondingly smaller doses in children. If full control is not achieved within the range of 50-300 mg daily, higher doses may be tried. Dosage should be reduced to a minimum maintenance level as soon as possible. In responsive patients there is a prompt reduction in pruritus followed by clearance of skin lesions. There is no effect on the gastrointestinal component of the disease. Dapsone levels are influenced by acetylation rates. Patients with high acetylation rates, or who are receiving treatment affecting acetylation may require an adjustment in dosage.

A strict gluten free diet is an option for the patient to elect, permitting many to reduce or eliminate the need for Dapsone; the average time for dosage reduction is 8 months with a range of 4 months to 2 1/2 years and for dosage elimination 29 months with a range of 6 months to 9 years.

Leprosy: In order to reduce secondary Dapsone resistance, the WHO Expert Committee on Leprosy and the USPHS at Carville, LA, recommended that Dapsone should be commenced in combination with one or more anti-leprosy drugs. In the multidrug program Dapsone should be maintained at the full dosage of 100 mg daily without interruption (with corresponding smaller doses for children) and provided to all patients who have sensitive organisms with new or recrudescent disease or who have not yet completed a two year course of Dapsone monotherapy. For advice and other drugs, the USPHS at Carville, LA (1-800-642-2477) should be contacted. Before using other drugs consult appropriate product labeling.

In bacteriologically negative tuberculoid and indeterminate disease, the recommendation is the coadministration of Dapsone 100 mg daily with six months of Rifampin 600 mg daily. Under WHO, daily Rifampin may be replaced by 600 mg Rifampin monthly, if supervised. The Dapsone is continued until all signs of clinical activity are controlled - usually after an additional six months. Then Dapsone should be continued for an additional three years for tuberculoid and indeterminate patients and for five years for borderline tuberculoid patients.

In lepromatous and borderline lepromatous patients, the recommendation is the co-administration of Dapsone 100 mg daily with two years of Rifampin 600 mg daily. Under WHO daily Rifampin may be replaced by 600 mg Rifampin monthly, if supervised. One may elect the concurrent administration of a third anti-leprosy drug, usually either Clofazamine 50-100 mg daily or Ethionamide 250-500 mg daily. Dapsone 100 mg daily is continued 3-10 years until all signs of clinical activity are controlled with skin scrapings and biopsies negative for one year. Dapsone should then be continued for an additional 10 years for borderline patients and for life for lepromatous patients.

Secondary Dapsone resistance should be suspected whenever a lepromatous or borderline lepromatous patient receiving Dapsone treatment relapses clinically and bacteriologically, solid staining bacilli being found in the smears taken from the new active lesions. If such cases show no response to regular and supervised Dapsone therapy within three to six months or good compliance for the past 3-6 months can be assured, Dapsone resistance should be considered confirmed clinically. Determination of drug sensitivity using the mouse footpad method is recommended and, after prior arrangement, is available without charge from the USPHS, Carville, LA. Patients with proven Dapsone resistance should be treated with other drugs.

LEPROSY REACTIONAL STATES

Abrupt changes in clinical activity occur in leprosy with any effective treatment and are known as reactional states. The majority can be classified into two groups. The "Reversal" reaction (Type 1) may occur in borderline or tuberculoid leprosy patients often soon after chemotherapy is started. The mechanism is presumed to result from a reduction in the antigenic load: the patient is able to mount an enhanced delayed hypersensitivity response to residual infection leading to swelling ("Reversal") of existing skin and nerve lesions. If severe, or if neuritis is present, large doses of steroids should always be used. If severe, the patient should be hospitalized. In general anti-leprosy treatment is continued and therapy to suppress the reaction is indicated such as analgesics, steroids, or surgical decompression of swollen nerve trunks. USPHS at Carville, LA should be contacted for advice in management.

Erythema nodosum leprosum (ENL) (lepromatous reaction) (Type 2 reaction) occurs mainly in lepromatous patients and small numbers of borderline patients. Approximately 50% of treated patients show this reaction in the first year. The principal clinical features are fever and tender erythematous skin nodules sometimes associated with malaise, neuritis, orchitis, albuminuria, joint swelling, iritis, epistaxis or depression. Skin lesions can become pustular and/or ulcerate. Histologically there is a vasculitis with an intense polymorphonuclear infiltrate. Elevated circulating immune complexes are considered to be the mechanism of reaction. If severe, patients should be hospitalized. In general, anti-leprosy treatment is continued. Analgesics, steroids, and other agents available from USPHS, Carville, LA, are used to suppress the reaction.

HOW SUPPLIED

Dapsone Tablets USP, 25 mg are available as round white scored tablets, debossed "25" above and "102" below the score and on the obverse "JACOBUS" in a Unit of Use carton of 30 tablets (2 × 15). The blisters are light and child-resistant. NDC 49938-102-30.

Dapsone Tablets USP, 100 mg are available as round white scored tablets, debossed "100" above and "101" below the score and on the obverse "JACOBUS" in a Unit of Use carton of 30 tablets (2 × 15). The blisters are light and child-resistant. NDC 49938-101-30.

Dapsone Tablets USP, 25 mg are available as round white scored tablets, debossed "25" above and "102" below the score and on the obverse "JACOBUS" in a Unit of Use carton of 28 tablets (2 × 14). The blisters are light and child-resistant. NDC 49938-102-28.

Dapsone Tablets USP, 100 mg are available as round white scored tablets, debossed "100" above and "101" below the score and on the obverse "JACOBUS" in a Unit of Use carton of 28 tablets (2 × 14). The blisters are light and child-resistant. NDC 49938-101-28.

REFERENCES

1. Lee, B., et al., Zidovudine, Trimethoprim, and Dapsone Pharmacokinetic Interactions in Patients with HIV Infection. *Antimicrobial Agents and Chemotherapy*, May 1996; 1231-1236.
2. Lee, B., et al., Dapsone, Trimethoprim, and Sulfamethoxazole Plasma Levels During Treatment of Pneumocystis Carinii Pneumonia in Patients with AIDS, *Annals of Internal Medicine*, 1989; 110:606-611.

Store at 20°-25° C (68°-77°F). [see USP Controlled Room Temperature]. Protect from light.

Rx only. Keep this and all medication out of the reach of children.

JACOBUS PHARMACEUTICAL CO., INC.
P.O. Box 5290
Princeton, NJ 08540
Revised August 2009
0826A09

PASER® GRANULES ℞

[*Pa - ser*]

(4 grams aminosalicylic acid delayed-release granules)

DESCRIPTION

PASER granules are a delayed release granule preparation of aminosalicylic acid (p-aminosalicylic acid; 4-aminosalicylic acid) for use with other anti-tuberculosis drugs for the treatment of all forms of active tuberculosis due to susceptible strains of tubercle bacilli. The granules are designed for gradual release to avoid high peak levels not useful (and perhaps toxic) with bacteriostatic drugs. Aminosalicylic acid is rapidly degraded in acid media; the protective acid-resistant outer coating is rapidly dissolved in neutral media so a mildly acidic food such as orange, apple or tomato juice, yogurt or apple sauce should be used.

Aminosalicylic acid (p-aminosalicylic acid) is 4-Amino-2-hydroxybenzoic acid. PASER granules are the free base of aminosalicylic acid and do NOT contain sodium or a sugar. The molecular formula is $C_7H_7NO_3$ with a molecular weight of 153.14. With heat p-aminosalicylic acid is decarboxylated to produce CO_2 and m-aminophenol. If the airtight packets are swollen, storage has been improper. DO NOT USE if packets are swollen or the granules have lost their tan color and are dark brown or purple.

The structural formula is:

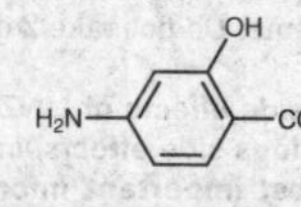

PASER granules are supplied as off-white tan colored granules with an average diameter of 1.5 mm and an average content of 60% aminosalicylic acid by weight. The acid resistant outer coating will be completely removed by a few minutes at a neutral pH. The inert ingredients are:

- colloidal silicon dioxide
- dibutyl sebacate
- hydroxypropyl methyl cellulose
- methacrylic acid copolymer
- microcrystalline cellulose
- talc

The packets contain 4 grams of aminosalicylic acid for oral administration three times a day by sprinkling on apple sauce or yogurt to be eaten without chewing. Suspension in an acidic fruit drink such as orange juice or tomato juice will protect the coating for at least 2 hours. Swirling the juice in the glass will help resuspend the granules if they sink.

CLINICAL PHARMACOLOGY

Mechanism of Action: Aminosalicylic acid is bacteriostatic against Mycobacterium tuberculosis. It inhibits the onset of bacterial resistance to streptomycin and isoniazid. The mechanism of action has been postulated to be inhibition of folic acid synthesis (but without potentiation with antifolic compounds) and/or inhibition of synthesis of the cell wall component, mycobactin, thus reducing iron uptake by M. tuberculosis.

Characteristics: The two major considerations in the clinical pharmacology of aminosalicylic acid are the prompt production of a toxic inactive metabolite under acid conditions and the short serum half life of one hour for the free drug. Both are discussed below.

After two hours in simulated gastric fluid, 10% of unprotected aminosalicylic acid is decarboxylated to form meta-aminophenol, a known hepatotoxin. The acid-resistant coating of the PASER granules protects against degradation in the stomach. The small granules are designed to escape the usual restriction on gastric emptying of large particles. Under neutral conditions such as are found in the small intestine or in neutral foods, the acid-resistant coating is dissolved within one minute. Care must be taken in the administration of these granules to protect the acid-resistant coating by maintaining the granules in an acidic food during dosage administration. Patients who have neutralized gastric acid with antacids will not need to protect the acid resistant coating with an acidic food since no acid is present to spoil the drug. Antacids may influence the absorption of other medications and are not necessary for PASER consumed with an acidic food.

Because PASER granules are protected by an enteric coating absorption does not commence until they leave the stomach; the soft skeletons of the granules remain and may be seen in the stool.

Absorption and excretion: In a single 4 gram pharmacokinetic study with food in normal volunteers the initial time to a 2μg/mL serum level of aminosalicylic acid was 2 hours with a range of 45 minutes to 24 hours; the median time to peak was 6 hours with a range of 1.5 to 24 hours; the mean peak level was 20 μg/mL with a range of 9 to 35 μg/mL; a level of 2 μg/mL was maintained for an average of 7.9 hours

with a range of 5 to 9; a level of 1 µg/mL was maintained for an average of 8.8 hours with a range of 6 to 11.5 hours. The recommended schedule is 4 grams every 8 hours.
80% of aminosalicylic acid is excreted in the urine, with 50% or more of the dosage excreted in acetylated form. The acetylation process is not genetically determined as is the case for isoniazid. Aminosalicylic acid is excreted by glomerular filtration, although previously reported otherwise, probenecid, a tubular blocking agent, does not enhance plasma concentration. In a 1954 study thyroxine synthesis but not iodide uptake was reported reduced about 40% when the sodium salt (not PASER granules) of aminosalicylic acid was administered one hour before radio-iodine; the sodium salt typically produces a serum level over 120 µg/mL at one hour lasting one hour. Occasional goiter development can be prevented by the administration of thyroxine but not iodide. Penetration into the cerebrospinal fluid occurs only if the meminges are inflamed.
Approximately 50-60% of aminosalicylic acid is protein bound; binding is reported to be reduced 50% in kwashiorkor.
Microbiology: The aminosalicylic acid MIC for M. tuberculosis in 7H11 agar was less than 1.0 µg/mL for nine strains including three multidrug resistant strains, but 4 and 8 µg/mL for two other multidrug resistant strains. The 90% inhibition in 7H12 broth (Bactec) showed little dose response but was interpreted as being less than or equal to 0.12-0.25 µg/mL for eight strains of which three were multiresistant, 0.50 µg/mL for one resistant strain, questionable for four non-resistant strains and greater than 1µg/mL for one non-resistant and three resistant strains. Aminosalicylic acid is not active in vitro against M. avium.

INDICATIONS AND USAGE

PASER is indicated for the treatment of tuberculosis in combination with other active agents. It is most commonly used in patients with Multi-drug Resistant TB (MDR-TB) or in situations when therapy with isoniazid and rifampin is not possible due to a combination of resistance and/or intolerance. When PASER is added to the treatment regimen in patients proven or suspected drug resistance, it should be accompanied by at least one and preferably two other new agents to which the patient's organism is known or expected to be susceptible.

CONTRAINDICATIONS

Hypersensitivity to any component of this medication.
Severe renal disease.
Patients with severe renal disease will accumulate aminosalicylic acid and its acetyl metabolite but will continue to acetylate, thus leading exclusively to the inactive acetylated form; deacetylation, if any, is not significant.
The half life of free aminosalicylic acid in renal disease is 30.8 minutes in comparison to 26.4 minutes in normal volunteers. but the half life of the inactive metabolite is 309 minutes in uremic patients in comparison to 51 minutes in normal volunteers. Although aminosalicylic acid passes dialysis membranes, the frequency of dialysis usually is not comparable to the half-life of 50 minutes for the free acid. Patients with end stage renal disease should not receive aminosalicylic acid.

WARNINGS

Liver Function

In one retrospective study of 7492 patients on rapidly absorbed aminosalicylic acid preparations, drug-induced hepatitis occurred in 38 patients (0.5%); in these 38 the first symptom usually appeared within three months of the start of therapy with a rash as the most common event followed by fever and much less frequently by GI disturbances of anorexia, nausea or diarrhea. Only one patient was diagnosed on routine biochemistry.
Premonitory symptoms in 90% of these 38 patients preceded jaundice by a few days to several weeks with the mean time of onset 33 days with a range of 7-90 days. Half of the adverse reactions occurred during the third, fourth or fifth weeks. When aminosalicylic acid-induced hepatitis was diagnosed, hepatomegaly was invariably present with lymphadenopathy in 46%, leucocytosis in 79%, and eosinophilia in 55%. Prompt recognition with discontinuation led to the recovery of all 38 patients. If recognized in the premonitory stage, the reaction is reported to "settle" in 24 hours and no jaundice ensues. From other reported studies failure to recognize the reaction can result in a mortality of up to 21%. The patient must be monitored carefully during the first three months of therapy and treatment must be discontinued immediately at the first sign of a rash, fever or other premonitory signs of intolerance.

PRECAUTIONS

(1) General:

All drugs should be stopped at the first sign suggesting a hypersensitivity reaction. They may be restarted one at a time in very small but gradually increasing doses to determine whether the manifestations are drug-induced and, if so, which drug is responsible.
Desensitization has been accomplished successfully in 15 of 17 patients starting with 10 mg aminosalicylic acid given as a single dose. The dosage is doubled every 2 days until reaching a total of 1 gram after which the dosage is divided to follow the regular schedule of administration. If a mild temperature rise or skin reaction develops, the increment is to be dropped back one level or the progression held for one cycle. Reactions are rare after a total dosage of 1.5 grams.
Patients with hepatic disease may not tolerate aminosalicylic acid as well as normal patients, even though the metabolism in patients with hepatic disease has been reported to be comparable to that in normal volunteers.

(2) Information for Patients:

The patient should be advised that the first signs of hypersensitivity include a rash, often followed by fever, and much less frequently, GI disturbances of anorexia, nausea or diarrhea. If such symptoms develop, the patient should immediately cease taking the medication and arrange for a prompt clinical visit.
Patients should be advised that poor compliance in taking anti-TB medication often leads to treatment failure, and, not infrequently, to the development of resistance of the organisms in the individual patient.
Patients should be advised that the skeleton of the granules may be seen in the stool.
The coating to protect the PASER granules dissolves promptly under neutral conditions; the granules therefore should be administered by sprinkling on acidic foods such as apple sauce or yogurt or by suspension in a fruit drink which will protect the coating, but the granules sink and will have to be swirled. The coating will last at least 2 hours in either system. All juices tested to date have been satisfactory; tested are: tomato, orange, grapefruit, grape, cranberry, apple, "fruit punch".
Patients should be advised to store PASER in a refrigerator or freezer. PASER packets may be stored at room temperature for short periods of time.
Patients should be advised NOT to use if the packets are swollen or the granules have lost their tan color and are dark brown or purple. The patient should inform the pharmacist or physician immediately and return the medication.

(3) Laboratory Tests:

Aminosalicylic acid has been reported to interfere technically with the serum determinations of albumin by dye-binding, SGOT by the azoene dye method and with qualitative urine tests for ketones, bilirubin, urobilinogen or porphobilinogen.

(4) Drug Interactions:

Aminosalicylic acid at a dosage of 12 grams in a rapidly available form has been reported to produce a 20 percent reduction in the acetylation of isoniazid, especially in patients who are rapid acetylators; INH serum levels, half lives and excretions in fast acetylators still remain half of the levels seen in slow acetylators with or without p-aminosalicylic acid. The effect is dose related and, while it has not been studied with the current delayed release preparation, the lower serum levels with this preparation will result in a reduced effect on the acetylation of INH.
Aminosalicylic acid has previously been reported to block the absorption of rifampin. A subsequent report has shown that this blockade was due to an excipient not included in PASER granules. Oral administration of a solution containing both aminosalicylic acid and rifampin showed full absorption of each product.
As a result of competition, Vitamin B_{12} absorption has been reduced 55% by 5 grams of aminosalicylic acid with clinically significant erythrocyte abnormalities developing after depletion; patients on therapy of more than one month should be considered for maintenance B_{12}.
A malabsorption syndrome can develop in patients on aminosalicylic acid but is usually not complete. The complete syndrome includes steatorrhea, an abnormal small bowel pattern on x-ray, villus atrophy, depressed cholesterol, reduced D-xylose and iron absorption. Triglyceride absorption always is normal.
In one literature report 8 hours after the last dosage of aminosalicylic acid at 2 gm qid serum digoxin levels were reduced 40% in two of ten patients but not changed in the remaining eight.

(5) Carcinogenesis, mutagenesis, impairment of fertility:

Sodium aminosalicylate produced an occipital bone defect, probably with a dose response, when administered to ten pregnant Wistar rats at five doses from 3.85 to 385 mg/kg from days 6 to 14. There were no significant changes from controls in any group in corpora lutea, early resorptions, total resorptions, fetal death, litter size, or hematomas. For all except the 77 mg/kg group, fetal weights were significantly greater than controls. Chinchilla rabbits on 5 mg/kg from days 7 to 14 did not show any significant differences as compared to controls for the same parameters studied.
Sodium aminosalicylic acid was not mutagenic in Ames tester strain TA 100. In human lymphocyte cultures in-vitro clastogenic effects of achromatic, chromatid, isochromatic breaks or chromatid translocations were not seen at 153 or 600 µg/mL. At 1500 and 3000 µg/mL there was a dose related increase in chromatid aberrations.
Patients on isoniazid and aminosalicylic acid have been reported to have an increased number of chromosomal aberrations as compared to controls.

(6) Pregnancy: Pregnancy Category C:

Aminosalicylic acid has been reported to produce occipital malformations in rats when given at doses within the human dose range. Although there probably is a dose response, the frequency of abnormalities was comparable to controls at the highest level tested (two times the human dosage). When administered to rabbits at 5 mg/kg, throughout all three trimesters, no teratologic or embryocidal effects were seen. Literature reports on aminosalicylic acid in pregnant women always report coadministration of other medications. Because there are no adequate and well controlled studies of aminosalicylic acid in humans, PASER granules should be given to a pregnant woman only if clearly needed.

(8) Nursing mothers:

After administration of a different preparation of aminosalicylic acid to one patient, the maximum concentration in the milk was 1 µg/mL at 3 hours with a half-life of 2.5 hours; the maximum maternal plasma concentration was 70 µg/mL at two hours.

ADVERSE EFFECTS

The most common side effect is gastrointestinal intolerance manifested by nausea, vomiting, diarrhea, and abdominal pain.
Hypersensitivity reactions: Fever, skin eruptions of various types, including exfoliative dermatitis, infectious mononucleosis-like, or lymphoma-like syndrome, leucopenia, agranulocytosis, thrombocytopenia, Coombs' positive hemolytic anemia, jaundice, hepatitis, pericarditis, hypoglycemia, optic neuritis, encephalopathy, Leoffler's syndrome, vasculitis and a reduction in prothrombin.
Crystalluria may be prevented by the maintenance of urine at a neutral or an alkaline pH.

OVERDOSAGE

Overdosage has not been reported.

DOSAGE AND ADMINISTRATION

PASER granules should be administered with other drugs to which the organism is known or expected to be susceptible. It is most commonly administered to patients with Multi-drug Resistant TB (MDR-TB) or in other situations in which therapy with isoniazid or rifampin is not possible due to a combination of resistance and/or intolerance. The adult dosage of four grams (one packet) three times per day or correspondingly smaller doses in children should be given by sprinkling on apple sauce or yogurt or by swirling in the glass to suspend the granules in an acidic drink such as tomato or orange juice.
DO NOT USE if packet is swollen or the granules have lost their tan color, turning dark brown or purple.

HOW SUPPLIED

Carton of 30 PASER packets (NDC 49938-107-04).
Each packet contains four grams aminosalicylic acid.
PASER granules are supplied in packets containing 4 grams of aminosalicylic acid for administration three times a day by suspension in an acidic drink or food with a pH less than 5. Examples include apple sauce, yogurt, tomato or orange juice.
Distributors and Pharmacists: Store below 59°F (15°C) (in a refrigerator or freezer).
Patients are urged to store PASER in a refrigerator or freezer. PASER packets may be stored at room temperature for short periods of time.
AVOID EXCESSIVE HEAT. DO NOT USE if packet is swollen or the granules have lost their tan color, turning dark brown or purple.
JACOBUS PHARMACEUTICAL CO. INC.
P.O. Box 5290
Princeton, NJ 08540
2A JULY, 1996

Janssen Pharmaceuticals, Inc.
1000 ROUTE 202 S
RARITAN, NJ 08869-0602
and
1125 TRENTON-HARBOURTON ROAD
TITUSVILLE, NJ 08560-0200
http://www.janssenpharmaceuticalsinc.com

Direct General Inquiries to:
(800) 526-7736
Medical Emergency Contact:
Ph: (800) 457-6399 or 908-218-7325
For Medical Information/Adverse Experience Reporting Contact:
Ph: (800) 457-6399

DURAGESIC® CII

[*dər 'ă-jēsĭk*]
(Fentanyl Transdermal System)
for transdermal administration

HIGHLIGHTS OF PRESCRIBING INFORMATION
These highlights do not include all the information needed to use DURAGESIC® safely and effectively. See full prescribing information for DURAGESIC.
DURAGESIC (Fentanyl Transdermal System) for transdermal administration, CII
Initial U.S. Approval: 1968

WARNING: ABUSE POTENTIAL, RESPIRATORY DEPRESSION and DEATH, ACCIDENTAL EXPOSURE, CYTOCHROME P450 3A4 INTERACTION, AND EXPOSURE TO HEAT

See full prescribing information for complete boxed warning.

- **Contains a high concentration of fentanyl, a Schedule II controlled substance, which is subject to misuse, abuse, addiction, and criminal diversion. (9)**
- **Fatal respiratory depression could occur in patients who are not opioid-tolerant and in patients that are opioid-tolerant even if DURAGESIC is not misused or abused. (5)**
- **Accidental exposure of DURAGESIC, especially in children, can result in a fatal overdose of fentanyl. (5)**
- **CYP 3A4 inhibitors can result in a fatal overdose of fentanyl from DURAGESIC. (5)**
- **Avoid exposing the DURAGESIC application site and surrounding area to direct external heat sources. Temperature dependent increases in fentanyl release from the system may result in overdose and death. (5)**

RECENT MAJOR CHANGES

Boxed Warning	7/2012
Indications and Usage (1)	7/2012
Dosage and Administration (2)	7/2012
Contraindications (4)	7/2012
Warnings and Precautions (5)	7/2012

INDICATIONS AND USAGE

- DURAGESIC contains fentanyl, a full opioid agonist.
- DURAGESIC is indicated for the management of persistent, moderate to severe chronic pain in **opioid-tolerant** patients 2 years of age and older when a continuous, around-the-clock opioid analgesic is needed for an extended period of time. (1)
- DURAGESIC is NOT intended for use as an as-needed analgesic. (1)

DOSAGE AND ADMINISTRATION

- Individualize treatment in every case as part of a pain management plan. (2)
- Initial dose selection: carefully select initial dose based on the status of each patient, consult conversion instructions. (2.1)
- Each transdermal system is intended to be worn for 72 hours. (2.2)
- Individually titrate to a tolerable dose that provides adequate analgesia. (2.2)
- Adhere to instructions concerning administration and disposal of DURAGESIC. (2.3)
- When DURAGESIC is no longer needed by the patient, taper the dose as part of a pain management plan. (2.4)
- Use with caution in the hepatic, and renally impaired patients. (2.2)

DOSAGE FORMS AND STRENGTHS

- **Transdermal system:** 12 mcg/h, 25 mcg/h, 50 mcg/h, 75 mcg/h, 100 mcg/h. (3)

CONTRAINDICATIONS

- Opioid non-tolerant patients. (4)
- Impaired pulmonary function. (4)
- Paralytic ileus. (4)
- Known hypersensitivity to fentanyl or any of the components of the transdermal system. (4)

WARNINGS AND PRECAUTIONS

- DURAGESIC can be abused. Use caution when prescribing if there is an increased risk of misuse, abuse, or diversion. (5.1)
- Fatal respiratory depression can occur with DURAGESIC. Monitor patients accordingly. Use with extreme caution in patients at risk of respiratory depression. (5.2)
- Accidental exposure of DURAGESIC, especially in children, can result in a fatal overdose of fentanyl. (5.3)
- Use DURAGESIC with extreme caution in patients susceptible to intracranial effects of CO_2 retention. (5.6)
- DURAGESIC may have additive effects when used in conjunction with other CNS depressants, alcohol, and drugs of abuse. (5.7)
- Use of DURAGESIC with a CYP3A4 inhibitor may result in an increase in fentanyl plasma concentrations. Monitor patients accordingly and adjust dosage if necessary. (5.8)
- DURAGESIC may produce bradycardia. Administer with caution to patients with bradyarrhythmias. (5.11)
- Use DURAGESIC with caution in patients with pancreatic/biliary disease. (5.14)

ADVERSE REACTIONS

The most common adverse reactions (≥5%) in a double-blind, randomized, placebo-controlled clinical trial in patients with severe pain were nausea, vomiting, somnolence, dizziness, insomnia, constipation, hyperhidrosis, fatigue, feeling cold, and anorexia. Other common adverse reactions (≥5%) reported in clinical trials in patients with chronic malignant or nonmalignant pain were headache and diarrhea. (6.0)

To report SUSPECTED ADVERSE REACTIONS, call 1-800-526-7736 or FDA at 1-800-FDA-1088 or *www.fda.gov/medwatch.*

DRUG INTERACTIONS

- Monitor patients receiving DURAGESIC and any CYP3A4 inhibitor for an extended period of time and adjust dosage, if necessary. (7.1)
- Use CNS Depressants with caution and in reduced dosage in patients who are receiving DURAGESIC. (7.2)
- Avoid DURAGESIC in patients taking a monoamine oxidase (MAO) inhibitor or within 14 days of stopping such treatment. (7.3)

USE IN SPECIFIC POPULATIONS

- Pregnancy: Based on animal data, may cause fetal harm. (8.1)
- Nursing Mothers: Breast-feeding is not advised in mothers treated with DURAGESIC. (8.3)
- Pediatric Use: Safety and efficacy in pediatric patients below the age of 2 years have not been established. To guard against accidental ingestion by children, use caution when choosing the application site for DURAGESIC. (8.4)
- Geriatric Use: Administer DURAGESIC with caution, and in reduced dosages in elderly patients. (8.5)
- Hepatic or Renal Impairment: Administer DURAGESIC with caution. Monitor for signs of fentanyl toxicity and reduce dosage, if necessary. (8.6, 8.7)

See 17 for PATIENT COUNSELING INFORMATION and Medication Guide

Revised: 07/2012

FULL PRESCRIBING INFORMATION: CONTENTS*

*** Sections or subsections omitted from the full prescribing information are not listed**

FULL PRESCRIBING INFORMATION

WARNING: ABUSE POTENTIAL , RESPIRATORY DEPRESSION and DEATH, ACCIDENTAL EXPOSURE, CYTOCHROME P450 3A4 INTERACTION, AND EXPOSURE TO HEAT

Abuse Potential

DURAGESIC contains fentanyl, an opioid agonist and a Schedule II controlled substance with an abuse liability similar to other opioid analgesics. DURAGESIC can be abused in a manner similar to other opioid agonists, legal or illicit. Persons at increased risk for opioid abuse include those with a personal or family history of substance abuse (including drug or alcohol abuse or addiction) or mental illness (e.g., major depression). Assess patients for their clinical risks for opioid abuse or addiction prior to prescribing DURAGESIC and then routinely monitor all patients for signs of misuse, abuse and addiction during treatment *[see Warnings and Precautions (5.1) and Drug Abuse and Dependence (9)]*.

Respiratory Depression and Death

Respiratory depression and death may occur with use of DURAGESIC, even when DURAGESIC has been used as recommended and not misused or abused. Proper dosing and titration are essential and DURAGESIC should only be prescribed by healthcare professionals who are knowledgeable in the use of potent opioids for the management of chronic pain. DURAGESIC is contraindicated for use in conditions in which the risk of life-threatening respiratory depression is significantly increased, including use as an as-needed analgesic, use in non-opioid tolerant patients, acute pain, and postoperative pain. Monitor for respiratory depression, especially during the first two applications following initiation of dosing, or following an increase in dosage *[see Contraindications (4) and Warnings and Precautions (5.2)]*.

Accidental Exposure

Death and other serious medical problems have occurred when children and adults were accidentally

exposed to DURAGESIC. Advise patients about strict adherence to the recommended handling and disposal instructions in order to prevent accidental exposure *[see Dosage and Administration (2.3) (2.4) and Warnings and Precautions (5.3)]*.

Cytochrome P450 3A4 Interaction

The concomitant use of DURAGESIC with all cytochrome P450 3A4 inhibitors may result in an increase in fentanyl plasma concentrations, which could increase or prolong adverse drug effects and may cause potentially fatal respiratory depression. Monitor patients receiving DURAGESIC and any CYP3A4 inhibitor *[see Warnings and Precautions (5.8), and Clinical Pharmacology (12.3)]*.

Exposure To Heat

The DURAGESIC application site and surrounding area must not be exposed to direct external heat sources, such as heating pads or electric blankets, heat or tanning lamps, sunbathing, hot baths, saunas, hot tubs, and heated water beds. Exposure to heat may increase fentanyl absorption and there have been reports of overdose and death as a result of exposure to heat *(5.9)*. Patients wearing DURAGESIC systems who develop fever or increased core body temperature due to strenuous exertion are also at risk for increased fentanyl exposure and may require an adjustment in the dose of DURAGESIC to avoid overdose and death *(5.10)*.

1 INDICATIONS AND USAGE

DURAGESIC is a transdermal formulation of fentanyl indicated for the management of persistent, moderate to severe chronic pain in opioid-tolerant patients 2 years of age and older when a continuous, around-the-clock opioid analgesic is required for an extended period of time, and the patient cannot be managed by other means such as non-steroidal analgesics, opioid combination products, or immediate-release opioids.

Patients considered opioid-tolerant are those who are taking at least 60 mg of morphine daily, or at least 30 mg of oral oxycodone daily, or at least 8 mg of oral hydromorphone daily, or an equianalgesic dose of another opioid for a week or longer.

2 DOSAGE AND ADMINISTRATION

2.1 Proper Patient Selection

Abuse Potential

Assess patients for their clinical risks for opioid abuse or addiction prior to being prescribing DURAGESIC *[see Warnings and Precautions (5.1)]*.

Opioid Tolerance

Opioid tolerance to an opioid of comparable potency must be established before prescribing DURAGESIC *[see Warnings and Precautions (5.2)]*.

Patients considered opioid-tolerant are those who are taking at least 60 mg of morphine daily, or at least 30 mg of oral oxycodone daily, or at least 8 mg of oral hydromorphone daily or an equianalgesic dose of another opioid for a week or longer.

2.2 Dosing

Conversion to DURAGESIC in Opioid-Tolerant Patients

The recommended starting dose when converting from other opioids to DURAGESIC is intended to minimize the potential for overdosing patients with the first dose. Monitor patients closely for respiratory depression, especially within the first 24–72 hours of initiating therapy with DURAGESIC *[see Warnings and Precautions (5.2)]*.

In selecting an initial DURAGESIC dose, take the following factors into account:

1. the daily dose, potency, and characteristics of the opioid the patient has been taking previously (e.g., whether it is a pure agonist or mixed agonist-antagonist);
2. the reliability of the relative potency estimates used to calculate the DURAGESIC dose needed (potency estimates may vary with the route of administration);
3. the degree of opioid tolerance;
4. the general condition and medical status of the patient.

To convert adult and pediatric patients from oral or parenteral opioids to DURAGESIC, use Table 1. **Do not use Table 1 to convert from DURAGESIC to other therapies because this conversion to DURAGESIC is conservative and will overestimate the dose of the new agent.**

[See table 1 above]

TABLE 1*: DOSE CONVERSION GUIDELINES

Current Analgesic	Daily Dosage (mg/day)			
Oral morphine	60–134	135–224	225–314	315–404
Intramuscular or Intravenous morphine	10–22	23–37	38–52	53–67
Oral oxycodone	30–67	67.5–112	112.5–157	157.5–202
Oral codeine	150–447			
Oral hydromorphone	8–17	17.1–28	28.1–39	39.1–51
Intravenous hydromorphone	1.5–3.4	3.5–5.6	5.7–7.9	8–10
Intramuscular meperidine	75–165	166–278	279–390	391–503
Oral methadone	20–44	45–74	75–104	105–134
	⇓	⇓	⇓	⇓
Recommended DURAGESIC Dose	25 mcg/hour	50 mcg/hour	75 mcg/hour	100 mcg/hour

Alternatively, for adult and pediatric patients taking opioids or doses not listed in Table 1, use the conversion methodology outlined above with Table 2.

* Table 1 should not be used to convert from DURAGESIC to other therapies because this conversion to DURAGESIC is conservative. Use of Table 1 for conversion to other analgesic therapies can overestimate the dose of the new agent. Overdosage of the new analgesic agent is possible *[see Dosage and Administration (2.3)]*.

Alternatively, for adult and pediatric patients taking opioids or doses not listed in Table 1, use the following methodology:

1. Calculate the previous 24-hour analgesic requirement.
2. Convert this amount to the equianalgesic oral morphine dose using a reliable reference.
   Refer to Table 2 for the range of 24-hour oral morphine doses that are recommended for conversion to each DURAGESIC dose. Use this table to find the calculated 24-hour morphine dose and the corresponding DURAGESIC dose. Initiate DURAGESIC treatment using the recommended dose and titrate patients upwards (no more frequently than 3 days after the initial dose and every 6 days thereafter) until analgesic efficacy is attained.
3. **Do not use Table 2 to convert from DURAGESIC to other therapies** because this conversion to DURAGESIC is conservative and will overestimate the dose of the new agent.

TABLE 2*: RECOMMENDED INITIAL DURAGESIC DOSE BASED UPON DAILY ORAL MORPHINE DOSE

Oral 24-hour Morphine (mg/day)	DURAGESIC Dose (mcg/hour)
60–134	25
135–224	50
225–314	75
315–404	100
405–494	125
495–584	150
585–674	175
675–764	200
765–854	225
855–944	250
945–1034	275
1035–1124	300

NOTE: In clinical trials, these ranges of daily oral morphine doses were used as a basis for conversion to DURAGESIC.

* Table 2 should not be used to convert from DURAGESIC to other therapies because this conversion to DURAGESIC is conservative. Use of Table 2 for conversion to other analgesic therapies can overestimate the dose of the new agent. Overdosage of the new analgesic agent is possible *[see Dosage and Administration (2.3)]*.

For delivery rates in excess of 100 mcg/hour, multiple systems may be used.

Hepatic Impairment

Avoid the use of DURAGESIC in patients with severe hepatic impairment. In patients with mild to moderate hepatic impairment, start with one half of the usual dosage of DURAGESIC. Closely monitor for signs of sedation and respiratory depression, including at each dosage increase *[see Warnings and Precautions (5.12), Use in Specific Populations (8.6) and Clinical Pharmacology (12.3)]*.

Renal Impairment

Avoid the use of DURAGESIC in patients with severe renal impairment. In patients with mild to moderate renal impairment, start with one half of the usual dosage of DURAGESIC. Closely monitor for signs of sedation and respiratory depression, including at each dosage increase *[see Warnings and Precautions (5.13), Use in Specific Populations (8.7) and Clinical Pharmacology (12.3)]*.

2.3 Titration and Maintenance of Therapy

Once therapy is initiated, assess pain intensity and opioid adverse reactions frequently, especially respiratory depression *[see Warnings and Precautions (5.2)]*. Routinely monitor all patients for signs of misuse, abuse and addiction *[see Warnings and Precautions (5.1)]*.

The initial DURAGESIC dose may be increased after 3 days based on the daily dose of supplemental opioid analgesics required by the patient on the second or third day of the initial application.

It may take up to 6 days for fentanyl levels to reach equilibrium on a new dose *[see Clinical Pharmacology (12.3)]*. Therefore, evaluate patients for further titration after no less than two 3-day applications before any further increase in dosage is made.

Base dosage increments on the daily dosage of supplementary opioids, using the ratio of 45 mg/24 hours of oral morphine to a 12 mcg/hour increase in DURAGESIC dose.

The majority of patients are adequately maintained with DURAGESIC administered every 72 hours. Some patients may not achieve adequate analgesia using this dosing interval and may require systems to be applied at 48 hours rather than at 72 hours, only if adequate pain control cannot be achieved using a 72-hour regimen. An increase in the DURAGESIC dose should be evaluated before changing dosing intervals in order to maintain patients on a 72-hour regimen. Dosing intervals less than every 72 hours were not studied in children and adolescents and are not recommended.

Discontinuation of DURAGESIC

To convert patients to another opioid, remove DURAGESIC and titrate the dose of the new analgesic based upon the patient's report of pain until adequate analgesia has been attained. Upon system removal, 17 hours or more are required for a 50% decrease in serum fentanyl concentrations. Withdrawal symptoms are possible in some patients after conversion or dose adjustment *[see Warnings and Precautions (5.15)]*.

Do not use Tables 1 and 2 to convert from DURAGESIC to other therapies to avoid overestimating the dose of the new agent potentially resulting in overdose of the new analgesic and death.

When discontinuing DURAGESIC and not converting to another opioid, use a gradual downward titration, such as halving the dose every 6 days, in order to reduce the possibility of withdrawal symptoms *[see Warnings and Precautions (5.15)]*. It is not known at what dose level DURAGESIC may be discontinued without producing the signs and symptoms of opioid withdrawal.

2.4 Administration of DURAGESIC

DURAGESIC patches are for transdermal use, only.

Proper handling of DURAGESIC is advised in order to prevent adverse reactions, including death, associated with accidental secondary exposure to DURAGESIC *[see Warnings and Precautions (5.3)]*.

Application and Handling Instructions

- Patients should apply DURAGESIC to intact, non-irritated, and non-irradiated skin on a flat surface such as the chest, back, flank, or upper arm. In young children and persons with cognitive impairment, adhesion should be monitored and the upper back is the preferred location to minimize the potential of inappropriate patch removal. Hair at the application site may be clipped (not shaved) prior to system application. If the site of DURAGESIC application must be cleansed prior to application of the patch, do so with clear water. Do not use soaps, oils, lotions, alcohol, or any other agents that might irritate the skin or alter its characteristics. Allow the skin to dry completely prior to patch application.
- Patients should apply DURAGESIC immediately upon removal from the sealed package. The patch must not be altered (e.g., cut) in any way prior to application. DURAGESIC should not be used if the pouch seal is broken or if the patch is cut or damaged.
- The transdermal system is pressed firmly in place with the palm of the hand for 30 seconds, making sure the contact is complete, especially around the edges.
- Each DURAGESIC patch may be worn continuously for 72 hours. The next patch is applied to a different skin site after removal of the previous transdermal system.
- If problems with adhesion of the DURAGESIC patch occur, the edges of the patch may be taped with first aid tape. If problems with adhesion persist, the patch may be overlayed with a transparent adhesive film dressing.

- If the patch falls off before 72 hours, dispose of it by folding in half and flushing down the toilet. A new patch may be applied to a different skin site.
- Patients (or caregivers who apply DURAGESIC) should wash their hands immediately with soap and water after applying DURAGESIC.
- Contact with unwashed or unclothed application sites can result in secondary exposure to DURAGESIC and should be avoided. Examples of accidental exposure include transfer of a DURAGESIC patch from an adult's body to a child while hugging, sharing the same bed as the patient, accidental sitting on a patch and possible accidental exposure of a caregiver's skin to the medication in the patch while applying or removing the patch.
- Instruct patients, family members, and caregivers to keep patches in a secure location out of the reach of children and of others for whom DURAGESIC was not prescribed.

Avoidance of Heat

Instruct patients to avoid exposing the DURAGESIC application site and surrounding area to direct external heat sources, such as heating pads or electric blankets, heat or tanning lamps, sunbathing, hot baths, saunas, hot tubs, and heated water beds, while wearing the system *[see Warnings and Precautions (5.9)]*.

2.5 Disposal Instructions

Proper disposal of DURAGESIC is advised in order to prevent adverse reactions, including death, associated with accidental secondary exposure to DURAGESIC *[see Warnings and Precautions (5.3)]*.

Patients should dispose of used patches by folding the adhesive side of the patch to itself, then flush the patch down the toilet immediately upon removal.

Patients should dispose of any patches remaining from a prescription as soon as they are no longer needed. Unused patches should be removed from their pouches, fold so that the adhesive side of the patch adheres to itself, and flush down the toilet.

3 DOSAGE FORMS AND STRENGTHS

DURAGESIC is available as:

- DURAGESIC 12 mcg/hour[1] Transdermal System (system size 5.25 cm^2) is orange in color.
- DURAGESIC 25 mcg/hour Transdermal System (system size 10.5 cm^2) is pink in color.
- DURAGESIC 50 mcg/hour Transdermal System (system size 21 cm^2) is green in color.
- DURAGESIC 75 mcg/hour Transdermal System (system size 31.5 cm^2) is blue in color.
- DURAGESIC 100 mcg/hour Transdermal System (system size 42 cm^2) is gray in color.

[1]This lowest dosage is designated as 12 mcg/hour (however, the actual dosage is 12.5 mcg/hour) to distinguish it from a 125 mcg/h dosage that could be prescribed by multiple patches.

4 CONTRAINDICATIONS

DURAGESIC is contraindicated in the following patients and situations due to the risk of fatal respiratory depression:

- in patients who are not opioid-tolerant *[see Warnings and Precautions (5.2)]*.
- in the management of acute or intermittent pain, or in patients who require opioid analgesia for a short period of time *[see Warnings and Precautions (5.2)]*.
- in the management of post-operative pain, including use after out-patient or day surgeries, (e.g., tonsillectomies) *[see Warnings and Precautions (5.2)]*.
- in the management of mild pain [see Warnings and Precautions (5.2)].
- in patients with significant respiratory compromise, especially if adequate monitoring and resuscitative equipment are not readily available [see Warnings and Precautions (5.2)].
- in patients who have acute or severe bronchial asthma [see Warnings and Precautions (5.2)].

DURAGESIC is also contraindicated:

- in patients who have or are suspected of having paralytic ileus
- in patients with known hypersensitivity to fentanyl or any components of the transdermal system. Severe hypersensitivity reactions, including anaphylaxis have been observed with DURAGESIC *[see Adverse Reactions (6.2]*.

5 WARNINGS AND PRECAUTIONS

5.1 Abuse Potential

DURAGESIC contains fentanyl, an opioid agonist and a Schedule II controlled substance with an abuse liability similar to other opioid analgesics. Schedule II opioid substances which include hydromorphone, morphine, oxycodone, fentanyl, oxymorphone and methadone have the highest potential for abuse and risk of fatal overdose due to respiratory depression. DURAGESIC can be abused in a manner similar to other opioid agonists, legal or illicit. These risks should be considered when administering, prescribing, or dispensing DURAGESIC in situations where the healthcare professional is concerned about increased risk of misuse, abuse, or diversion *[see Drug Abuse and Dependence (9)]*.

Assess patients for their clinical risks for opioid abuse or addiction prior to being prescribed opioids. Routinely monitor all patients receiving opioids for signs of misuse, abuse and addiction since use of opioid analgesic products carries the risk of addiction even under appropriate medical use. Persons at increased risk for opioid abuse include those with a personal or family history of substance abuse (including drug or alcohol abuse or addiction) or mental illness (e.g., major depression). Patients at increased risk may still be appropriately treated with modified-release opioid formulations; however these patients will require intensive monitoring for signs of misuse, abuse, or addiction. Concerns about abuse, addiction, and diversion should not prevent the proper management of pain.

Contact local state professional licensing board or state controlled substances authority for information on how to prevent and detect abuse or diversion of this product.

5.2 Respiratory Depression and Death

Respiratory depression is the chief hazard of DURAGESIC. Respiratory depression, if not immediately recognized and treated, may lead to respiratory arrest and death.

DURAGESIC has a narrow indication and should be prescribed only by healthcare professionals who are knowledgeable in the administration of potent opioids and management of chronic pain *[see Indications and Usage (1)]*.

DURAGESIC is contraindicated for use in conditions in which the risk of life-threatening respiratory depression is significantly increased, including use as an as-needed analgesic, use in non-opioid tolerant patients, acute pain, and postoperative pain *[see Contraindications (4)]*. Proper dosing and titration of DURAGESIC are essential *[see Dosage and Administration (2.3)]*. Overestimating the DURAGESIC dose when converting patients from another opioid medication, can result in fatal overdose with the first dose. However, respiratory depression has also been reported with use of DURAGESIC in patients who are opioid-tolerant, even when DURAGESIC has been used as recommended and not misused or abused.

The mean half-life of fentanyl when delivered by DURAGESIC is approximately 20–27 hours. Serum fentanyl concentrations continue to rise for the first two system applications. In addition, significant amounts of fentanyl continue to be absorbed from the skin for 24 hours or more after the patch is removed *[see Clinical Pharmacology (12.3)]*.

Respiratory depression from opioids is manifested by a reduced urge to breathe and a decreased rate of respiration, often associated with a "sighing" pattern of breathing (deep breaths separated by abnormally long pauses). Carbon dioxide retention from opioid-induced respiratory depression can exacerbate the sedating effects of opioids.

While serious, life-threatening or fatal respiratory depression can occur at any time during the use of DURAGESIC, the potential for serious, life threatening, or fatal respiratory depression is greatest during the first two applications following initiation of dosing, or following an increase in dosage. Closely monitor patients for respiratory depression when initiating therapy with DURAGESIC, especially within the initial 24–72 hours when serum concentrations from the initial patch will peak, and following increases in dosage. Because significant amounts of fentanyl continue to be absorbed from the skin for 24 hours or more after the patch is removed, respiratory depression may persist beyond the removal of DURAGESIC. Monitor patients for respiratory depression after patch removal to ensure that the patient's respiration has stabilized for at least 24 to 72 hours or longer as clinical symptoms dictate.

Management of respiratory depression may include close observation, supportive measures, and use of opioid antagonists, depending on the patient's clinical status *[see Overdose (10.2)]*.

5.3 Accidental Exposure

A considerable amount of active fentanyl remains in DURAGESIC even after use as directed. Death and other serious medical problems have occurred when children and adults were accidentally exposed to DURAGESIC. Accidental or deliberate application or ingestion by a child or adolescent will cause respiratory depression that could result in death. Placing DURAGESIC in the mouth, chewing it, swallowing it, or using it in ways other than indicated may cause choking or overdose that could result in death.

Advise patients about strict adherence to the recommended handling and disposal instructions in order to prevent accidental exposure to DURAGESIC *(see Dosage and Administration (2.4) (2.5)]*.

5.4 Elderly, Cachectic, and Debilitated Patients

Respiratory depression is more likely to occur in elderly, cachectic, or debilitated patients as they may have altered pharmacokinetics due to poor fat stores, muscle wasting, or altered clearance. Therefore, monitor these patients closely, particularly when initiating therapy with DURAGESIC and when given in conjunction with other drugs that depress respiration *[see Warnings and Precautions (5.2) and Use in Specific Populations (8.5)]*.

5.5 Chronic Pulmonary Disease

Monitor patients with significant chronic obstructive pulmonary disease or cor pulmonale, and patients having a substantially decreased respiratory reserve, hypoxia, hypercapnia, or pre-existing respiratory depression for respiratory depression, particularly when initiating therapy with DURAGESIC, as in these patients, even usual therapeutic doses of DURAGESIC may decrease respiratory drive to the point of apnea *[see Warnings and Precautions (5.2)]*. Consider the use of alternative non-opioid analgesics in these patients if possible.

5.6 Head Injuries and Increased Intracranial Pressure

Avoid use of DURAGESIC in patients who may be particularly susceptible to the intracranial effects of CO_2 retention such as those with evidence of increased intracranial pressure, impaired consciousness, or coma *[see Warnings and Precautions (5.2)]*. In addition, opioids may obscure the clinical course of patients with head injury. Monitor patients with brain tumors who may be susceptible to the intracranial effects of CO_2 retention for signs of sedation and respiratory depression, particularly when initiating therapy with DURAGESIC, as DURAGESIC may reduce respiratory drive and CO_2 retention can further increase intracranial pressure.

5.7 Interactions with Other CNS Depressants, Alcohol, and Drugs of Abuse

The concomitant use of DURAGESIC with other central nervous system depressants, including, but not limited to, other opioids, sedatives, hypnotics, tranquilizers (e.g., benzodiazepines), general anesthetics, phenothiazines, skeletal muscle relaxants, and alcohol, may cause respiratory depression, hypotension, and profound sedation or coma. Monitor patients prescribed concomitant CNS active drugs for signs of sedation and respiratory depression, particularly when initiating therapy with DURAGESIC, and reduce the dose of one or both agents *[see Warnings and Precautions (5.2)]*.

5.8 Interactions with CYP3A4 Inhibitors

The concomitant use of DURAGESIC with a CYP3A4 inhibitors (such as ritonavir, ketoconazole, itraconazole, troleandomycin, clarithromycin, nelfinavir, nefazadone, amiodarone, amprenavir, aprepitant, diltiazem, erythromycin, fluconazole, fosamprenavir, verapamil) may result in an increase in fentanyl plasma concentrations, which could increase or prolong adverse drug effects and may cause potentially fatal respiratory depression. Carefully monitor patients receiving DURAGESIC and any CYP3A4 inhibitor for signs of sedation and respiratory depression for an extended period of time, and make dosage adjustments if warranted *[see Warnings and Precautions (5.2), Drug Interactions (7.1) and Clinical Pharmacology (12.3)]*.

5.9 Application of External Heat

Exposure to heat may increase fentanyl absorption and there have been reports of overdose and death as a result of exposure to heat. A clinical pharmacology study conducted in healthy adult subjects has shown that the application of heat over the DURAGESIC system increased fentanyl exposure *[see Clinical Pharmacology (12.3)]*.

Warn patients to avoid exposing the DURAGESIC application site and surrounding area to direct external heat sources *[see Dosage and Administration (2.4)]*.

5.10 Patients with Fever

Based on a pharmacokinetic model, serum fentanyl concentrations could theoretically increase by approximately one-third for patients with a body temperature of 40°C (104°F) due to temperature-dependent increases in fentanyl released from the system and increased skin permeability. Monitor patients wearing DURAGESIC systems who develop fever closely for opioid side effects and reduce the DURAGESIC dose if necessary. Warn patients to avoid strenuous exertion that leads to increased core body temperature while wearing DURAGESIC to avoid the risk of potential overdose and death.

5.11 Cardiac Disease

DURAGESIC may produce bradycardia. Monitor patients with bradyarrhythmias closely for changes in heart rate, particularly when initiating therapy with DURAGESIC.

5.12 Hepatic Impairment

A clinical pharmacology study with DURAGESIC in patients with cirrhosis has shown that systemic fentanyl exposure increased in these patients. Because of the long half-life of fentanyl when administered as DURAGESIC and hepatic metabolism of fentanyl, avoid use of DURAGESIC in patients with severe hepatic impairment. Insufficient information exists to make precise dosing recommendations regarding the use of DURAGESIC in patients with impaired hepatic function. Therefore, to avoid starting patients with mild to moderate hepatic impairment on too high of a dose, start with one half of the usual dosage of DURAGESIC. Closely monitor for signs of sedation and respiratory depression, including at each dosage increase. *[see Dosing and Administration (2.2),Use in Specific Populations (8.6) and Clinical Pharmacology (12.3)].*

5.13 Renal Impairment

A clinical pharmacology study with intravenous fentanyl in patients undergoing kidney transplantation has shown that patients with high blood urea nitrogen level had low fentanyl clearance. Because of the long half-life of fentanyl when administered as DURAGESIC, avoid the use of DURAGESIC in patients with severe renal impairment. Insufficient information exists to make precise dosing recommendations regarding the use of DURAGESIC in patients with impaired renal function. Therefore, to avoid starting patients with mild to moderate renal impairment on too high of a dose, start with one half of the usual dosage of DURAGESIC. Closely monitor for signs of sedation and respiratory depression, including at each dosage increase *[see Dosing and Administration (2.2), Use in Specific Populations (8.7) and Clinical Pharmacology (12.3)].*

5.14 Use in Pancreatic/Biliary Tract Disease

DURAGESIC may cause spasm of the sphincter of Oddi. Monitor patients with biliary tract disease, including acute pancreatitis for worsened symptoms. DURAGESIC may cause increases in the serum amylase concentration.

5.15 Avoidance of Withdrawal

Opioid withdrawal symptoms (such as nausea, vomiting, diarrhea, anxiety, and shivering) are possible in some patients after conversion to another opioid or when decreasing or discontinuing DURAGESIC. Gradual reduction of the dose of DURAGESIC is recommended *[see Dosage and Administration (2.3) and Drug Abuse and Dependence (9)].*

5.16 Driving and Operating Machinery

Strong opioid analgesics impair the mental or physical abilities required for the performance of potentially dangerous tasks, such as driving a car or operating machinery. Warn patients not to drive or operate dangerous machinery unless they are tolerant to the effects of the DURAGESIC.

6 ADVERSE REACTIONS

The following serious adverse reactions are discussed elsewhere in the labeling:

- Abuse Potential *[see Warnings and Precautions (5.1)]*
- Respiratory Depression *[see Warnings and Precautions (5.2)]*
- Accidental Exposure *[see Warnings and Precautions (5.3)]*
- Elderly, Cachetic, and Debilitated Patients *[see Warnings and Precautions (5.4)]*
- Chronic Pulmonary Disease *[see Warnings and Precautions (5.5)]*
- Head Injuries and Increased Intracranial Pressure *[see Warnings and Precautions (5.6)]*
- Interactions with Other CNS Depressants, Alcohol, and Drugs of Abuse *[see Warnings and Precautions (5.7)]*
- Interactions with CYP3A4 Inhibitors *[see Warnings and Precautions (5.8)]*
- Application of External Heat *[see Warnings and Precautions (5.9)]*
- Patients with Fever *[see Warnings and Precautions (5.10)]*
- Cardiac Disease *[see Warnings and Precautions (5.11)]*
- Hepatic Impairment *[see Warnings and Precautions (5.12)]*
- Renal Impairment *[see Warnings and Precautions (5.13)]*
- Use in Pancreatic/Biliary Tract Disease *[see Warnings and Precautions (5.14)]*
- Avoidance of Withdrawal *[see Warnings and Precautions (5.15)]*
- Driving and Operating Machinery *[see Warnings and Precautions (5.16)]*

Because clinical trials are conducted under widely varying conditions, adverse reaction rates observed in the clinical trials of a drug cannot be directly compared to rates in the clinical trials of another drug and may not reflect the rates observed in clinical practice.

6.1 Clinical Trial Experience

The safety of DURAGESIC was evaluated in 216 patients who took at least one dose of DURAGESIC in a multicenter, double-blind, randomized, placebo-controlled clinical trial of DURAGESIC. This trial examined patients over 40 years of age with severe pain induced by osteoarthritis of the hip or knee and who were in need of and waiting for joint replacement.

The most common adverse reactions (≥5%) in a double-blind, randomized, placebo controlled clinical trial in patients with severe pain were nausea, vomiting, somnolence, dizziness, insomnia, constipation, hyperhidrosis, fatigue, feeling cold, and anorexia. Other common adverse reactions (≥5%) reported in clinical trials in patients with chronic malignant or nonmalignant pain were headache and diarrhea. Adverse reactions reported for ≥1% of DURAGESIC-treated patients and with an incidence greater than placebo-treated patients are shown in Table 3.

The most common adverse reactions that were associated with discontinuation in patients with pain (causing discontinuation in ≥1% of patients) were depression, dizziness, somnolence, headache, nausea, vomiting, constipation, hyperhidrosis, and fatigue.

Table 3. Adverse Reactions Reported by ≥1% of DURAGESIC-treated Patients and With an Incidence Greater Than Placebo-treated Patients in 1 Double-Blind, Placebo-Controlled Clinical Trial of DURAGESIC

System/Organ Class Adverse Reaction	DURAGESIC % (N=216)	Placebo % (N=200)
Cardiac disorders		
Palpitations	4	1
Ear and labyrinth disorders		
Vertigo	2	1
Gastrointestinal disorders		
Nausea	41	17
Vomiting	26	3
Constipation	9	1
Abdominal pain upper	3	2
Dry mouth	2	0
General disorders and administration site conditions		
Fatigue	6	3
Feeling cold	6	2
Malaise	4	1
Asthenia	2	0
Edema peripheral	1	1
Metabolism and nutrition disorders		
Anorexia	5	0
Musculoskeletal and connective tissue disorders		
Muscle spasms	4	2
Nervous system disorders		
Somnolence	19	3
Dizziness	10	4
Psychiatric disorders		
Insomnia	10	7
Depression	1	0
Skin and subcutaneous tissue disorders		
Hyperhidrosis	6	1
Pruritus	3	2
Rash	2	1

Adverse reactions not reported in Table 1 that were reported by ≥1% of DURAGESIC-treated adult and pediatric patients (N=1854) in 11 controlled and uncontrolled clinical trials of DURAGESIC used for the treatment of chronic malignant or nonmalignant pain are shown in Table 4.

Table 4. Adverse Reactions Reported by ≥1% of DURAGESIC-treated Patients in 11 Clinical Trials of DURAGESIC

System/Organ Class Adverse Reaction	DURAGESIC % (N=1854)
Gastrointestinal disorders	
Diarrhea	10
Abdominal pain	3
Immune system disorders	
Hypersensitivity	1
Nervous system disorders	
Headache	12
Tremor	3
Paresthesia	2
Psychiatric disorders	
Anxiety	3
Confusional state	2
Hallucination	1
Renal and urinary disorders	
Urinary retention	1
Skin and subcutaneous tissue disorders	
Erythema	1

The following adverse reactions occurred in adult and pediatric patients with an overall frequency of <1% and are listed in descending frequency within each System/Organ Class:

Cardiac disorders: cyanosis

Eye disorders: miosis

Gastrointestinal disorders: subileus

General disorders and administration site conditions: application site reaction, influenza-like illness, application site hypersensitivity, drug withdrawal syndrome, application site dermatitis

Musculoskeletal and connective tissue disorders: muscle twitching

Nervous system disorders: hypoesthesia

Psychiatric disorders: disorientation, euphoric mood

Reproductive system and breast disorders: erectile dysfunction, sexual dysfunction

Respiratory, thoracic and mediastinal disorders: respiratory depression

Skin and subcutaneous tissue disorders: eczema, dermatitis allergic, dermatitis contact

Pediatrics

The safety of DURAGESIC was evaluated in three open-label trials in 289 pediatric patients with chronic pain, 2 years of age through 18 years of age. Adverse reactions reported by ≥1% of DURAGESIC-treated pediatric patients are shown in Table 5.

Table 5. Adverse Reactions Reported by ≥1% of DURAGESIC-treated Pediatric Patients in 3 Clinical Trials of DURAGESIC

System/Organ Class Adverse Reaction	DURAGESIC % (N=289)
Gastrointestinal disorders	
Vomiting	34
Nausea	24
Constipation	13
Diarrhea	13
Abdominal pain	9
Abdominal pain upper	4
Dry mouth	2
General disorders and administration site conditions	
Edema peripheral	5
Fatigue	2
Application site reaction	1
Asthenia	1
Immune system disorders	
Hypersensitivity	3
Metabolism and nutrition disorders	
Anorexia	4
Musculoskeletal and connective tissue disorders	
Muscle spasms	2
Nervous system disorders	
Headache	16
Somnolence	5
Dizziness	2
Tremor	2
Hypoesthesia	1
Psychiatric disorders	
Insomnia	6
Anxiety	4
Depression	2
Hallucination	2
Renal and urinary disorders	
Urinary retention	3
Respiratory, thoracic and mediastinal disorders	
Respiratory depression	1
Skin and subcutaneous tissue disorders	
Pruritus	13
Rash	6
Hyperhidrosis	3
Erythema	3

6.2 Post-Marketing Experience

The following adverse reactions have been identified during post-approval use of DURAGESIC. Because these reactions are reported voluntarily from a population of uncertain size, it is not always possible to reliably estimate their frequency.

Cardiac Disorders: Tachycardia, Bradycardia

Eye Disorders: Vision blurred

Gastrointestinal Disorders: Ileus, Dyspepsia

General Disorders and Administration Site Conditions: Feeling of body temperature change

Immune System Disorders: Anaphylactic shock, Anaphylactic reaction, Anaphylactoid reaction

Investigations: Weight decreased

Nervous System Disorders: Convulsions (including Clonic convulsions and Grand mal convulsion), Amnesia

Psychiatric Disorders: Agitation

Respiratory, Thoracic, and Mediastinal Disorders: Respiratory distress, Apnea, Bradypnea, Hypoventilation, Dyspnea

Vascular Disorders: Hypotension, Hypertension

7 DRUG INTERACTIONS

7.1 Agents Affecting Cytochrome P450 3A4 Isoenzyme System

Fentanyl is metabolized mainly via the human cytochrome P450 3A4 isoenzyme system (CYP3A4). Coadministration with agents that induce CYP3A4 activity may reduce the efficacy of DURAGESIC. The concomitant use of DURAGESIC with a CYP3A4 inhibitor (such as ritonavir, ketoconazole, itraconazole, troleandomycin, clarithromycin, nelfanivir, nefazadone, amiodarone, amprenavir, aprepitant, diltiazem, erythromycin, fluconazole, fosamprenavir, verapamil, or grapefruit juice) may result in an increase in fentanyl plasma concentrations, which could increase or prolong adverse drug effects and may cause fatal respiratory depression. Closely monitor patients receiving DURAGESIC and any CYP3A4 inhibitor and reduce the dosage of DURAGESIC if warranted *[see Clinical Pharmacology (12.3)]*.

7.2 Central Nervous System Depressants

The concomitant use of DURAGESIC with other central nervous system depressants, including but not limited to other opioids, sedatives, hypnotics, tranquilizers (e.g., benzodiazepines), general anesthetics, phenothiazines, skeletal muscle relaxants, and alcohol, may cause respiratory depression, hypotension, and profound sedation, or potentially result in coma or death. Monitor patients closely when central nervous system depressants are used concomitantly with DURAGESIC and reduce the dose of one or both agents.

7.3 MAO Inhibitors

Avoid use of DURAGESIC in the patient who would require the concomitant administration of a monoamine oxidase (MAO) inhibitor, or within 14 days of stopping such treatment because severe and unpredictable potentiation by MAO inhibitors has been reported with opioid analgesics.

8 USE IN SPECIFIC POPULATIONS

8.1 Pregnancy

Teratogenic Effects

Pregnancy C: There are no adequate and well-controlled studies in pregnant women. DURAGESIC should be used during pregnancy only if the potential benefit justifies the potential risk to the fetus.

The potential effects of fentanyl on embryo-fetal development were studied in the rat, mouse, and rabbit models. Published literature reports that administration of fentanyl (0, 10, 100, or 500 μg/kg/day) to pregnant female Sprague-Dawley rats from day 7 to 21 via implanted microosmotic minipumps did not produce any evidence of teratogenicity (the high dose is approximately 2 times the daily human dose administered by a 100 mcg/hr patch on a mg/m^2 basis). In contrast, the intravenous administration of fentanyl (0, 0.01, or 0.03 mg/kg) to bred female rats from gestation day 6 to 18 suggested evidence of embryotoxicity and a slight increase in mean delivery time in the 0.03 mg/kg/day group. There was no clear evidence of teratogenicity noted.

Pregnant female New Zealand White rabbits were treated with fentanyl (0, 0.025, 0.1, 0.4 mg/kg) via intravenous infusion from day 6 to day 18 of pregnancy. Fentanyl produced a slight decrease in the body weight of the live fetuses at the high dose, which may be attributed to maternal toxicity. Under the conditions of the assay, there was no evidence for fentanyl induced adverse effects on embryo-fetal development at doses up to 0.4 mg/kg (approximately 3 times the daily human dose administered by a 100 mcg/hr patch on a mg/m^2 basis).

Nonteratogenic Effects

Chronic maternal treatment with fentanyl during pregnancy has been associated with transient respiratory depression, behavioral changes, or seizures characteristic of neonatal abstinence syndrome in newborn infants. Symptoms of neonatal respiratory or neurological depression were no more frequent than expected in most studies of infants born to women treated acutely during labor with intravenous or epidural fentanyl. Transient neonatal muscular rigidity has been observed in infants whose mothers were treated with intravenous fentanyl.

The potential effects of fentanyl on prenatal and postnatal development were examined in the rat model. Female Wistar rats were treated with 0, 0.025, 0.1, or 0.4 mg/kg/day fentanyl via intravenous infusion from day 6 of pregnancy through 3 weeks of lactation. Fentanyl treatment (0.4 mg/kg/day) significantly decreased body weight in male and female pups and also decreased survival in pups at day 4. Both the mid-dose and high-dose of fentanyl animals demonstrated alterations in some physical landmarks of development (delayed incisor eruption and eye opening) and transient behavioral development (decreased locomotor activity at day 28 which recovered by day 50). The mid-dose and the high-dose are 0.4 and 1.6 times the daily human dose administered by a 100 mcg/hr patch on a mg/m^2 basis.

8.2 Labor and Delivery

Fentanyl readily passes across the placenta to the fetus; therefore, DURAGESIC is not recommended for analgesia during labor and delivery.

8.3 Nursing Mothers

Fentanyl is excreted in human milk; therefore, DURAGESIC is not recommended for use in nursing women because of the possibility of effects in their infants.

8.4 Pediatric Use

The safety of DURAGESIC was evaluated in three open-label trials in 289 pediatric patients with chronic pain, 2 years of age through 18 years of age. Starting doses of 25 mcg/h and higher were used by 181 patients who had been on prior daily opioid doses of at least 45 mg/day of oral morphine or an equianalgesic dose of another opioid. Initiation of DURAGESIC therapy in pediatric patients taking less than 60 mg/day of oral morphine or an equianalgesic dose of another opioid has not been evaluated in controlled clinical trials.

The safety and effectiveness of DURAGESIC in children under 2 years of age have not been established.

To guard against excessive exposure to DURAGESIC by young children, advise caregivers to strictly adhere to recommended DURAGESIC application and disposal instructions *[see Dosage and Administration (2.4)(2.5) and Warnings and Precautions (5.3)]*.

8.5 Geriatric Use

Clinical studies of DURAGESIC did not include sufficient numbers of subjects aged 65 and over to determine whether they respond differently from younger subjects. Other reported clinical experience has not identified differences in responses between the elderly and younger patients. In general, dose selection for an elderly patient should be cautious, usually starting at the low end of the dosing range, reflecting the greater frequency of decreased hepatic, renal, or cardiac function, and of concomitant disease or other drug therapy.

Data from intravenous studies with fentanyl suggest that the elderly patients may have reduced clearance and a prolonged half-life. Moreover, elderly patients may be more sensitive to the active substance than younger patients. A study conducted with the DURAGESIC patch in elderly patients demonstrated that fentanyl pharmacokinetics did not differ significantly from young adult subjects, although peak serum concentrations tended to be lower and mean half-life values were prolonged to approximately 34 hours *[see Clinical Pharmacology (12.3)]*.

Monitor geriatric patients closely for signs of sedation and respiratory depression, particularly when initiating therapy with DURAGESIC and when given in conjunction with other drugs that depress respiration *[see Warnings and Precautions (5.2)(5.4)]*.

8.6 Hepatic Impairment

The effect of hepatic impairment on the pharmacokinetics of DURAGESIC has not been fully evaluated. A clinical pharmacology study with DURAGESIC in patients with cirrhosis has shown that systemic fentanyl exposure increased in these patients. Because there is *in-vitro* and *in-vivo* evidence of extensive hepatic contribution to the elimination of DURAGESIC, hepatic impairment would be expected to have significant effects on the pharmacokinetics of DURAGESIC. Avoid use of DURAGESIC in patients with severe hepatic impairment *[see Dosing and Administration (2.2), Warnings and Precautions (5.12) and Clinical Pharmacology 12.3)]*.

8.7 Renal Impairment

The effect of renal impairment on the pharmacokinetics of DURAGESIC has not been fully evaluated. A clinical pharmacology study with intravenous fentanyl in patients undergoing kidney transplantation has shown that patients with high blood urea nitrogen level had low fentanyl clearance. Because there is *in-vivo* evidence of renal contribution to the elimination of DURAGESIC, renal impairment would be expected to have significant effects on the pharmacokinetics of DURAGESIC. Avoid the use of DURAGESIC in patients with severe renal impairment *[see Dosing and Administration (2.2), Warnings and Precautions (5.13) and Clinical Pharmacology (12.3)]*.

8.8 Neonatal Opioid Withdrawal Syndrome

Chronic maternal use of fentanyl can affect the neonate with subsequent withdrawal signs. Neonatal withdrawal syndrome presents as irritability, hyperactivity, and abnormal sleep pattern, high pitched cry, tremor, vomiting, diarrhea, and failure to gain weight. The onset, duration and severity of neonatal withdrawal syndrome vary based on the drug used, duration of use, the dosage of last maternal use, and rate of elimination of the drug by the newborn. Neonatal opioid withdrawal syndrome, unlike opioid withdrawal syndrome in adults, may be life-threatening and should be treated according to protocols developed by neonatology experts.

9 DRUG ABUSE AND DEPENDENCE

9.1 Controlled Substance

DURAGESIC contains fentanyl, a potent Schedule II opioid agonist. Schedule II opioid substances, which include hydromorphone, methadone, morphine, oxycodone, and oxymorphone, have the highest potential for abuse and risk of fatal overdose due to respiratory depression. DURAGESIC can be abused and is subject to criminal diversion *[see Warnings and Precautions (5.1)]*.

9.2 Abuse

Addiction is a primary, chronic, neurobiologic disease, with genetic, psychosocial, and environmental factors influencing its development and manifestations. It is characterized by behaviors that include one or more of the following: impaired control over drug use, compulsive use, continued use despite harm, and craving. Drug addiction is a treatable disease, utilizing a multidisciplinary approach, but relapse is common.

"Drug seeking" behavior is very common in addicts and drug abusers. Drug-seeking tactics include emergency calls or visits near the end of office hours, refusal to undergo appropriate examination, testing or referral, repeated "loss" of prescriptions, tampering with prescriptions and reluctance to provide prior medical records or contact information for other treating physician(s). "Doctor shopping" to obtain additional prescriptions is common among drug abusers and people suffering from untreated addiction.

Abuse and addiction are separate and distinct from physical dependence and tolerance. Physicians should be aware that addiction may be accompanied by concurrent tolerance and symptoms of physical dependence. In addition, abuse of opioids can occur in the absence of true addiction and is characterized by misuse for non-medical purposes, often in combination with other psychoactive substances. Since DURAGESIC may be diverted for non-medical use, careful recordkeeping of prescribing information, including quantity, frequency, and renewal requests is strongly advised.

Proper assessment of the patient, proper prescribing practices, periodic reevaluation of therapy, and proper dispensing and storage are appropriate measures that help to limit abuse of opioid drugs.

9.3 Dependence

Tolerance is a state of adaptation in which exposure to a drug induces changes that result in a diminution of one or more of the drug's effects over time. Tolerance may occur to both the desired and undesired effects of drugs, and may develop at different rates for different effects.

Physical dependence is a state of adaptation that is manifested by an opioid specific withdrawal syndrome that can be produced by abrupt cessation, rapid dose reduction, decreasing blood concentration of the drug, and/or administration of an antagonist. The opioid abstinence or withdrawal syndrome is characterized by some or all of the following: restlessness, lacrimation, rhinorrhea, yawning, perspiration, chills, piloerection, myalgia, mydriasis, irritability, anxiety, backache, joint pain, weakness, abdominal cramps, insomnia, nausea, anorexia, vomiting, diarrhea, or increased blood pressure, respiratory rate, or heart rate. In general, opioids should not be abruptly discontinued *[see Dosage and Administration (2.3)]*.

10 OVERDOSAGE

10.1 Clinical Presentation

Acute overdosage with opioids can be manifested by respiratory depression, somnolence progressing to stupor or coma, skeletal muscle flaccidity, cold and clammy skin, constricted pupils, and sometimes bradycardia, hypotension and death. The pharmacokinetic characteristics of DURAGESIC must also be taken into account when treating the overdose. Even in the face of improvement, continued medical monitoring is required because of the possibility of extended effects. Deaths due to overdose have been reported with abuse and misuse of DURAGESIC.

10.2 Treatment

Give primary attention to the reestablishment of a patent airway and institution of assisted or controlled ventilation. Employ supportive measures (including oxygen and vasopressors) in the management of circulatory shock and pulmonary edema accompanying overdose as indicated. Cardiac arrest or arrhythmias will require advanced life support techniques. Remove all DURAGESIC systems.

The pure opioid antagonists, such as naloxone, are specific antidotes to respiratory depression from opioid overdose. Since the duration of reversal is expected to be less than the duration of action of fentanyl, carefully monitor the patient until spontaneous respiration is reliably reestablished. After DURAGESIC system removal, serum fentanyl concentrations decline gradually, falling about 50% in approximately 20–27 hours. Therefore, management of an overdose must be monitored accordingly, at least 72 to 96 hours beyond the overdose.

Only administer opioid antagonists in the presence of clinically significant respiratory or circulatory depression secondary to hydromorphone overdose. In patients who are physically dependent on any opioid agonist including DURAGESIC, an abrupt or complete reversal of opioid effects may precipitate an acute abstinence syndrome. The severity of the withdrawal syndrome produced will depend on the degree of physical dependence and the dose of the antagonist administered. Please see the prescribing information for the specific opioid antagonist for details of their proper use.

11 DESCRIPTION

DURAGESIC (fentanyl transdermal system) is a transdermal system containing fentanyl. The chemical name is N-Phenyl-N-(1-(2-phenylethyl)-4-piperidinyl) propanamide. The structural formula is:

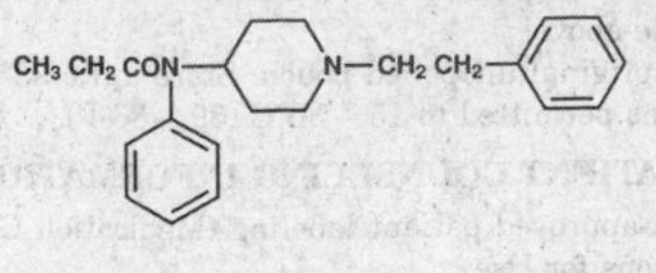

The molecular weight of fentanyl base is 336.5, and the empirical formula is $C_{22}H_{28}N_2O$. The n-octanol: water partition coefficient is 860:1. The pKa is 8.4.

System Components and Structure

The amount of fentanyl released from each system per hour is proportional to the surface area (25 mcg/h per 10.5 cm^2). The composition per unit area of all system sizes is identical.

Dose* (mcg/h)	Size (cm^2)	Fentanyl Content (mg)	Color of Printing on Back of Patch
12†	5.25	2.1	Orange
25	10.5	4.2	Pink
50	21	8.4	Green
75	31.5	12.6	Blue
100	42	16.8	Gray

* Nominal delivery rate per hour
† Nominal delivery rate is 12.5 mcg/hr

DURAGESIC is a rectangular transparent unit comprising a protective liner and two functional layers. Proceeding from the outer surface toward the surface adhering to skin, these layers are:
1) a backing layer of polyester/ethyl vinyl acetate film; 2) a drug-in-adhesive layer. Before use, a protective liner covering the adhesive layer is removed and discarded.

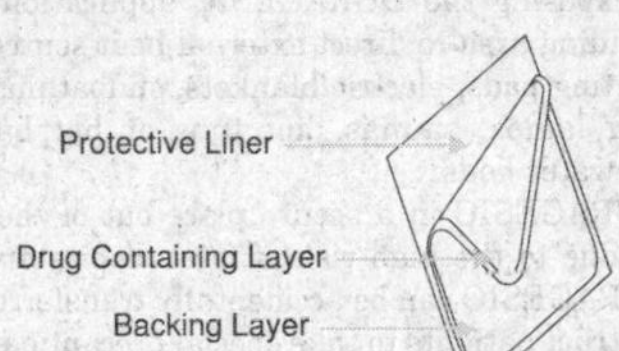

12 CLINICAL PHARMACOLOGY

12.1 Mechanism of Action

Fentanyl is an opioid analgesic. Fentanyl interacts predominately with the opioid mu-receptor. These mu-binding sites are distributed in the human brain, spinal cord, and other tissues.

12.2 Pharmacodynamics

Central Nervous System Effects

Fentanyl exerts its principal pharmacologic effects on the central nervous system. Central nervous system effects increase with increasing serum fentanyl concentrations.

In addition to analgesia, alterations in mood, euphoria, dysphoria, and drowsiness commonly occur. Fentanyl depresses the respiratory centers, depresses the cough reflex, and constricts the pupils. Analgesic blood concentrations of fentanyl may cause nausea and vomiting directly by stimulating the chemoreceptor trigger zone, but nausea and vomiting are significantly more common in ambulatory than in recumbent patients, as is postural syncope.

Ventilatory Effects

In clinical trials of 357 non-opioid tolerant subjects treated with DURAGESIC, 13 subjects experienced hypoventilation. Hypoventilation was manifested by respiratory rates of less than 8 breaths/minute or a pCO_2 greater than 55 mm Hg. In these studies, the incidence of hypoventilation was higher in nontolerant women (10) than in men (3) and in subjects weighing less than 63 kg (9 of 13). Although subjects with prior impaired respiration were not common in the trials, they had higher rates of hypoventilation. In addition, post-marketing reports have been received that describe opioid-naive post-operative patients who have experienced clinically significant hypoventilation and death with DURAGESIC.

Hypoventilation can occur throughout the therapeutic range of fentanyl serum concentrations, especially for patients who have an underlying pulmonary condition or who receive concomitant opioids or other CNS drugs associated with hypoventilation. The use of DURAGESIC is contraindicated in patients who are not tolerant to opioid therapy.

Gastrointestinal Tract and Other Smooth Muscle

Opioids increase the tone and decrease the propulsive contractions of the smooth muscle of the gastrointestinal tract. The resultant prolongation in gastrointestinal transit time may be responsible for the constipating effect of fentanyl.

TABLE 6: FENTANYL PHARMACOKINETIC PARAMETERS FOLLOWING FIRST 72-HOUR APPLICATION OF DURAGESIC

	Mean (SD) Time to Maximal Concentration Tmax (h)	Mean (SD) Maximal Concentration Cmax (ng/mL)
DURAGESIC 12 mcg/h	28.8 (13.7)	0.38 (0.13)*
DURAGESIC 25 mcg/h	31.7 (16.5)	0.85 (0.26)†
DURAGESIC 50 mcg/h	32.8 (15.6)	1.72 (0.53)†
DURAGESIC 75 mcg/h	35.8 (14.1)	2.32 (0.86)†
DURAGESIC 100 mcg/h	29.9 (13.3)	3.36 (1.28)†

NOTE: After system removal there is continued systemic absorption from residual fentanyl in the skin so that serum concentrations fall 50%, on average, in approximately 20–27 hours.
* Cmax values dose normalized from 4 × 12.5 mcg/h: Study 2003-038 in healthy volunteers
† Cmax values: Study C-2002-048 dose proportionality study in healthy volunteers

TABLE 7: RANGE OF PHARMACOKINETIC PARAMETERS OF INTRAVENOUS FENTANYL IN PATIENTS

	Clearance (L/h) Range [70 kg]	Volume of Distribution V_{SS} (L/kg) Range	Half-Life $t_{1/2}$ (h) Range
Surgical Patients	27 – 75	3 – 8	3 – 12
Hepatically Impaired Patients	3 – 80*	0.8 – 8*	4 – 12*
Renally Impaired Patients	30 – 78	–	–

NOTE: Information on volume of distribution and half-life not available for renally impaired patients.
* Estimated

Because opioids may increase biliary tract pressure, some patients with biliary colic may experience worsening rather than relief of pain.

While opioids generally increase the tone of urinary tract smooth muscle, the net effect tends to be variable, in some cases producing urinary urgency, in others, difficulty in urination.

Cardiovascular Effects

Fentanyl may cause orthostatic hypotension and fainting. Fentanyl may infrequently produce bradycardia. The incidence of bradycardia in clinical trials with DURAGESIC was less than 1%.

Histamine assays and skin wheal testing in clinical studies indicate that clinically significant histamine release rarely occurs with fentanyl administration. Clinical assays show no clinically significant histamine release in dosages up to 50 mcg/kg.

12.3 Pharmacokinetics

Absorption

DURAGESIC is a drug-in-adhesive matrix designed formulation. Fentanyl is released from the matrix at a nearly constant amount per unit time. The concentration gradient existing between the matrix and the lower concentration in the skin drives drug release. Fentanyl moves in the direction of the lower concentration at a rate determined by the matrix and the diffusion of fentanyl through the skin layers. While the actual rate of fentanyl delivery to the skin varies over the 72-hour application period, each system is labeled with a nominal flux which represents the average amount of drug delivered to the systemic circulation per hour across average skin.

While there is variation in dose delivered among patients, the nominal flux of the systems (12.5, 25, 50, 75, and 100 mcg of fentanyl per hour) is sufficiently accurate as to allow individual titration of dosage for a given patient.

Following DURAGESIC application, the skin under the system absorbs fentanyl, and a depot of fentanyl concentrates in the upper skin layers. Fentanyl then becomes available to the systemic circulation. Serum fentanyl concentrations increase gradually following initial DURAGESIC application, generally leveling off between 12 and 24 hours and remaining relatively constant, with some fluctuation, for the remainder of the 72-hour application period. Peak serum concentrations of fentanyl generally occurred between 20 and 72 hours after initial application (see Table 6). Serum fentanyl concentrations achieved are proportional to the DURAGESIC delivery rate. With continuous use, serum fentanyl concentrations continue to rise for the first two system applications. By the end of the second 72-hour application, a steady-state serum concentration is reached and is maintained during subsequent applications of a patch of the same size (see Figure 1). Patients reach and maintain a steady-state serum concentration that is determined by individual variation in skin permeability and body clearance of fentanyl.

After system removal, serum fentanyl concentrations decline gradually, falling about 50% in approximately 20–27 hours. Continued absorption of fentanyl from the skin accounts for a slower disappearance of the drug from the serum than is seen after an IV infusion, where the apparent half-life is approximately 7 (range 3–12) hours.

A clinical pharmacology study conducted in healthy adult subjects has shown that the application of heat over the DURAGESIC system increased mean overall fentanyl exposure by 120% and average maximum fentanyl level by 61%. [See table 6 above]

Figure 1 Serum Fentanyl Concentrations Following Single and Multiple Applications of DURAGESIC 100 mcg/h

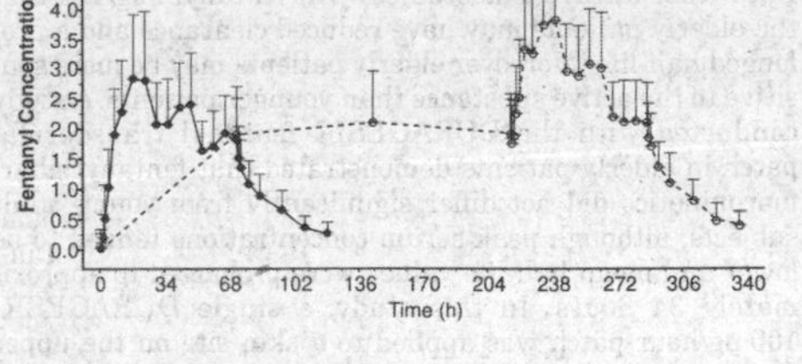

[See table 7 above]

Distribution

Fentanyl plasma protein binding capacity decreases with increasing ionization of the drug. Alterations in pH may affect its distribution between plasma and the central nervous system. Fentanyl accumulates in the skeletal muscle and fat and is released slowly into the blood. The average volume of distribution for fentanyl is 6 L/kg (range 3–8; N=8).

Metabolism

Fentanyl is metabolized primarily via human cytochrome P450 3A4 isoenzyme system. In humans, the drug appears to be metabolized primarily by oxidative N-dealkylation to norfentanyl and other inactive metabolites that do not contribute materially to the observed activity of the drug.

Excretion

Within 72 hours of IV fentanyl administration, approximately 75% of the dose is excreted in urine, mostly as metabolites with less than 10% representing unchanged drug. Approximately 9% of the dose is recovered in the feces, primarily as metabolites. Mean values for unbound fractions of fentanyl in plasma are estimated to be between 13 and 21%. Skin does not appear to metabolize fentanyl delivered transdermally. This was determined in a human keratinocyte cell assay and in clinical studies in which 92% of the dose delivered from the system was accounted for as unchanged fentanyl that appeared in the systemic circulation.

DURAGESIC Dose (mcg/h)	System Size (cm^2)	Fentanyl Content (mg)	Color of Printing on Back of Patch	NDC Number
DURAGESIC-12*	5.25	2.1	Orange	50458-090-05
DURAGESIC-25	10.5	4.2	Pink	50458-091-05
DURAGESIC-50	21	8.4	Green	50458-092-05
DURAGESIC-75	31.5	12.6	Blue	50458-093-05
DURAGESIC-100	42	16.8	Gray	50458-094-05

* This lowest dosage is designated as 12 mcg/h (however, the actual dosage is 12.5 mcg/h) to distinguish it from a 125 mcg/h dosage that could be prescribed by using multiple patches.

Hepatic Impairment

Information on the effect of hepatic impairment on the pharmacokinetics of DURAGESIC is limited. The pharmacokinetics of DURAGESIC delivering 50 µg/hour of fentanyl for 72 hours was evaluated in patients hospitalized for surgery. Compared to the controlled patients (n=8), Cmax and AUC in the patients with cirrhosis (n=9) increased 35% and 73%, respectively.

Because there is *in-vitro* and *in-vivo* evidence of extensive hepatic contribution to the elimination of DURAGESIC, hepatic impairment would be expected to have significant effects on the pharmacokinetics of DURAGESIC. Avoid use of DURAGESIC in patients with severe hepatic impairment *[see Dosing and Administration (2.2), Warnings and Precautions (5.12) and Use in Specific Populations (8.6)].*

Renal Impairment

Information on the effect of renal impairment on the pharmacokinetics of DURAGESIC is limited. The pharmacokinetics of intravenous injection of 25 µg/kg fentanyl was evaluated in patients (n=8) undergoing kidney transplantation. An inverse relationship between blood urea nitrogen level and fentanyl clearance was found.

Because there is *in-vivo* evidence of renal contribution to the elimination of DURAGESIC, renal impairment would be expected to have significant effects on the pharmacokinetics of DURAGESIC. Avoid the use of DURAGESIC in patients with severe renal impairment *[see Dosing and Administration (2.2), Warnings and Precautions (5.13) and Use in Specific Populations (8.7)].*

Pediatric Use

In 1.5 to 5 year old, non-opioid-tolerant pediatric patients, the fentanyl plasma concentrations were approximately twice as high as that of adult patients. In older pediatric patients, the pharmacokinetic parameters were similar to that of adults. However, these findings have been taken into consideration in determining the dosing recommendations for opioid-tolerant pediatric patients (2 years of age and older). For pediatric dosing information, refer to *[see Dosing and Administration (2.2)].*

Geriatric Use

Data from intravenous studies with fentanyl suggest that the elderly patients may have reduced clearance and a prolonged half-life. Moreover elderly patients may be more sensitive to the active substance than younger patients. A study conducted with the DURAGESIC fentanyl transdermal patch in elderly patients demonstrated that fentanyl pharmacokinetics did not differ significantly from young adult subjects, although peak serum concentrations tended to be lower and mean half-life values were prolonged to approximately 34 hours. In this study, a single DURAGESIC 100 µg/hour patch was applied to a skin site on the upper outer arm in a group of healthy elderly Caucasians ≥65 years old (n=21, mean age 71 years) and worn for 72 hours. The mean Cmax and AUC∞ values were approximately 8% lower and 7% higher, respectively, in the elderly subjects as compared with subjects 18 to 45 years old. Inter-subject variability in AUC∞ was higher in elderly subjects than in healthy adult subjects 18 to 45 years (58% and 37%, respectively). The mean half-life value was longer in subjects ≥65 years old than in subjects 18 to 45 years old (34.4 hours versus 23.5 hours) *[see Warnings and Precautions (5.4) and Use in Specific Populations (8.5)].*

Drug Interactions

The interaction between ritonavir, a CPY3A4 inhibitor, and fentanyl was investigated in eleven healthy volunteers in a randomized crossover study. Subjects received oral ritonavir or placebo for 3 days. The ritonavir dose was 200 mg tid on Day 1 and 300 mg tid on Day 2 followed by one morning dose of 300 mg on Day 3. On Day 2, fentanyl was given as a single IV dose at 5 mcg/kg two hours after the afternoon dose of oral ritonavir or placebo. Naloxone was administered to counteract the side effects of fentanyl. The results suggested that ritonavir might decrease the clearance of fentanyl by 67%, resulting in a 174% (range 52%–420%) increase in fentanyl $AUC_{0-\infty}$. Coadministration of ritonavir in patients receiving DURAGESIC has not been studied; however, an increase in fentanyl AUC is expected *[see Box Warning and Warnings and Precautions (5.7) and Drug Interactions (7.1)].*

Fentanyl is metabolized mainly via the human cytochrome P450 3A4 isoenzyme system (CYP3A4), therefore, potential interactions may occur when DURAGESIC is given concurrently with agents that affect CYP3A4 activity. Coadministration with agents that induce CYP3A4 activity may reduce the efficacy of DURAGESIC. The concomitant use of transdermal fentanyl with all CYP3A4 inhibitors (such as ritonavir, ketoconazole, itraconazole, troleandomycin, clarithromycin, nelfinavir, nefazadone, amiodarone, amprenavir, aprepitant, diltiazem, erythromycin, fluconazole, fosamprenavir, verapamil, or grapefruit juice) may result in an increase in fentanyl plasma concentrations, which could increase or prolong adverse drug effects and may cause potentially fatal respiratory depression. Carefully monitor patients receiving DURAGESIC and any CYP3A4 inhibitor for signs of respiratory depression for an extended period of time and adjust the dosage if warranted *[see Box Warning and Warnings and Precautions (5.7)].*

13 NON-CLINICAL TOXICOLOGY

13.1 Carcinogenesis, Mutagenesis, and Impairment of Fertility

Carcinogenesis

In a two-year carcinogenicity study conducted in rats, fentanyl was not associated with an increased incidence of tumors at subcutaneous doses up to 33 µg/kg/day in males or 100 µg/kg/day in females (0.16 and 0.39 times the human daily exposure obtained via the 100 mcg/h patch based on AUC_{0-24h} comparison).

Mutagenesis

There was no evidence of mutagenicity in the Ames Salmonella mutagenicity assay, the primary rat hepatocyte unscheduled DNA synthesis assay, the BALB/c 3T3 transformation test, and the human lymphocyte and CHO chromosomal aberration in-vitro assays.

Impairment of Fertility

The potential effects of fentanyl on male and female fertility were examined in the rat model via two separate experiments. In the male fertility study, male rats were treated with fentanyl (0, 0.025, 0.1 or 0.4 mg/kg/day) via continuous intravenous infusion for 28 days prior to mating; female rats were not treated. In the female fertility study, female rats were treated with fentanyl (0, 0.025, 0.1 or 0.4 mg/kg/day) via continuous intravenous infusion for 14 days prior to mating until day 16 of pregnancy; male rats were not treated. Analysis of fertility parameters in both studies indicated that an intravenous dose of fentanyl up to 0.4 mg/kg/day to either the male or the female alone produced no effects on fertility (this dose is approximately 1.6 times the daily human dose administered by a 100 mcg/hr patch on a mg/m^2 basis). In a separate study, a single daily bolus dose of fentanyl was shown to impair fertility in rats when given in intravenous doses of 0.3 times the human dose for a period of 12 days.

14 CLINICAL STUDIES

DURAGESIC as therapy for pain due to cancer has been studied in 153 patients. In this patient population, DURAGESIC has been administered in doses of 25 µg/h to 600 µg/h. Individual patients have used DURAGESIC continuously for up to 866 days. At one month after initiation of DURAGESIC therapy, patients generally reported lower pain intensity scores as compared to a prestudy analgesic regimen of oral morphine.

The duration of DURAGESIC use varied in cancer patients; 56% of patients used DURAGESIC for over 30 days, 28% continued treatment for more than 4 months, and 10% used DURAGESIC for more than 1 year.

In the pediatric population, the safety of DURAGESIC has been evaluated in 289 patients with chronic pain 2–18 years of age. The duration of DURAGESIC use varied; 20% of pediatric patients were treated for ≤ 15 days; 46% for 16–30 days; 16% for 31–60 days; and 17% for at least 61 days. Twenty-five patients were treated with DURAGESIC for at least 4 months and 9 patients for more than 9 months.

16 HOW SUPPLIED/STORAGE AND HANDLING

DURAGESIC (fentanyl transdermal system) is supplied in cartons containing 5 individually packaged systems. See chart for information regarding individual systems.

[See table above]

Store in original unopened pouch. Store up to 25°C (77°F); excursions permitted to 15 – 30°C (59 – 86°F).

17 PATIENT COUNSELING INFORMATION

See FDA-approved patient labeling (Medication Guide and Instructions for Use)

Provide patients receiving DURAGESIC patches the following information:

- DURAGESIC patches contain fentanyl, an opioid pain medicine that can cause serious breathing problems and death, especially if used in the wrong way and therefore should be taken only as directed. Instruct patients to call their doctor immediately or seek emergency medical help if they experience breathing problems while taking DURAGESIC.
- DURAGESIC contains fentanyl which has a high potential for abuse. Instruct patients, family members, and caregivers to protect DURAGESIC from theft or misuse in the work or home environment.
- Instruct patients to never give DURAGESIC to anyone other than the individual for whom it was prescribed because of the risk of death or other serious medical problems to that person for whom it was not intended.
- Advise patients never to change the dose of DURAGESIC or the number of patches applied to the skin unless instructed to do so by the prescribing healthcare professional.
- Warn patients of the potential for temperature-dependent increases in fentanyl release from the patch that could result in an overdose of fentanyl. Instruct patients to contact their healthcare provider if they develop a high fever. Instruct patients to:
  - avoid strenuous exertion that can increase body temperature while wearing the patch
  - avoid exposing the DURAGESIC application site and surrounding area to direct external heat sources including heating pads, electric blankets, sunbathing, heat or tanning lamps, saunas, hot tubs or hot baths, and heated water beds.
- Keep DURAGESIC in a secure place out of the reach of children due to the high risk of **fatal respiratory depression**. DURAGESIC can be accidentally transferred to children. Instruct patients to take special precautions to avoid accidental contact when holding or caring for children.
- If the patch dislodges and accidentally sticks to the skin of another person, to immediately take the patch off, wash the exposed area with water and seek medical attention for the accidentally exposed individual as accidental exposure may lead to death or other serious medical problems.
- To properly disposal of used and unneeded, unused DURAGESIC, remove them from their pouches, fold them so that the adhesive side of the patch adheres to itself, and flush them down the toilet.
- DURAGESIC may impair mental and/or physical ability required for the performance of potentially hazardous tasks (e.g., driving, operating machinery). Instruct patients to refrain from any potentially dangerous activity when starting on DURAGESIC or when their dose is being adjusted, until it is established that they have not been adversely affected.
- Advise women of childbearing potential who become, or are planning to become pregnant, to consult a healthcare provider prior to initiating or continuing therapy with DURAGESIC.
- Instruct patients not to use alcohol or other CNS depressants (e.g. sleep medications, tranquilizers) while using DURAGESIC because dangerous additive effects may occur, resulting in serious injury or death.
- Advise patients of the potential for severe constipation.
- When no longer needed, DURAGESIC should not be stopped abruptly to avoid the risk of precipitating withdrawal symptoms.

Medication Guide

DURAGESIC® (Dur-ah-GEE-zik)

(fentanyl) Transdermal System, CII

DURAGESIC® is:

- A strong prescription pain medicine that contains an opioid (narcotic) that is used to treat moderate to severe around-the-clock pain, in people who are already regularly using opioid pain medicine.

Important information about DURAGESIC®:

- Get emergency help right away if you use too much DURAGESIC® (overdose). DURAGESIC® overdose can cause life threatening breathing problems that can lead to death.
- Never give anyone else your DURAGESIC®. They could die from using it. Store DURAGESIC® away from children and in a safe place to prevent stealing or abuse. Selling or giving away DURAGESIC® is against the law.

Do not use DURAGESIC® if you have:
- severe asthma, trouble breathing, or other lung problems.
- a bowel blockage or have narrowing of the stomach or intestines.

Before applying DURAGESIC®, tell your healthcare provider if you have a history of:
- head injury, seizures
- liver, kidney, thyroid problems
- problems urinating
- pancreas or gallbladder problems
- abuse of street or prescription drugs, alcohol addiction, or mental health problems.

Tell your healthcare provider if you:
- have a fever
- **are pregnant or planning to become pregnant.** DURAGESIC® may harm your unborn baby.
- **are breastfeeding.** DURAGESIC® passes into breast milk and may harm your baby.
- are taking prescription or over-the-counter medicines, vitamins, or herbal supplements.

When using DURAGESIC®:
- Do not change your dose. Apply DURAGESIC® exactly as prescribed by your healthcare provider.
- See the detailed Instructions for Use for information about how to apply and dispose of the DURAGESIC® patch.
- Do not wear more than 1 patch at the same time unless your healthcare provider tells you to.
- **Call your healthcare provider if the dose you are using does not control your pain.**
- **Do not stop using DURAGESIC® without talking to your healthcare provider.**

While using DURAGESIC® Do Not:
- Take hot baths or sunbathe, use hot tubs, saunas, heating pads, electric blankets, heated waterbeds, or tanning lamps, or engage in exercise that increases your body temperature. These can cause an overdose that can lead to death.
- Drive or operate heavy machinery, until you know how DURAGESIC® affects you. DURAGESIC® can make you sleepy, dizzy, or lightheaded.
- Drink alcohol or use prescription or over-the-counter medicines that contain alcohol.

The possible side effects of DURAGESIC® are:
- constipation, nausea, sleepiness, vomiting, tiredness, headache, dizziness, abdominal pain, itching, redness, or rash where the patch is applied. Call your healthcare provider if you have any of these symptoms and they are severe.

Get emergency medical help if you have:
- trouble breathing, shortness of breath, fast heartbeat, chest pain, swelling of your face, tongue or throat, extreme drowsiness, or you are feeling faint.

These are not all the possible side effects of DURAGESIC®. Call your doctor for medical advice about side effects. You may report side effects to FDA at 1-800-FDA-1088. **For more information go to dailymed.nlm.nih.gov**

Manufactured by: Alza Corporation, Vacaville, CA 95688; Manufactured for: Janssen Pharmaceuticals, Inc. Titusville, NJ 08560, www.Duragesic.com or call 1-800-526-7736

This Medication Guide has been approved by the U.S. FDA.

Issue: July 2012

DURAGESIC® (Dur-ah-GEE-zik)
(Fentanyl Transdermal System) CII

Instructions for Applying a DURAGESIC® patch

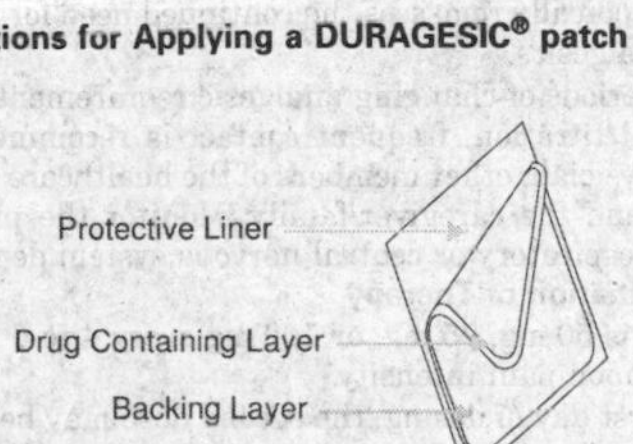

Before Applying DURAGESIC®
- **Each DURAGESIC® patch is sealed in its own protective pouch. Do not remove a DURAGESIC® patch from the pouch until you are ready to use it.**
- **Do not use a DURAGESIC® patch if the pouch seal is broken or the patch is cut, damaged or changed in any way.**
- **DURAGESIC® patches are available in 5 different doses and patch sizes. Make sure you have the right dose patch or patches that have been prescribed for you.**

Applying a DURAGESIC® Patch

1. Skin Areas Where the DURAGESIC® Patch May Be Applied:

For adults:
- Put the patch on the chest, back, flank (sides of the waist), or upper arm in a place where there is no hair (see Figures 1-4).

Figure 1

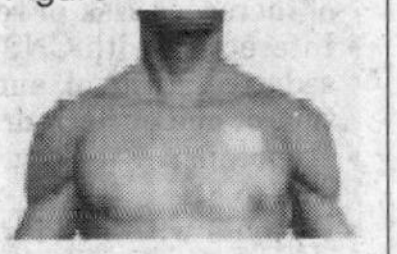

Figure 2

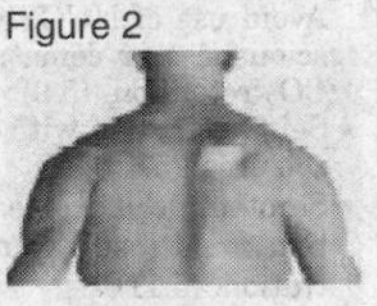

For children (and adults with mental impairment):
- **Put the patch on the upper back (see Figure 2).** This will lower the chances that the child will remove the patch and put it in their mouth.

Figure 3

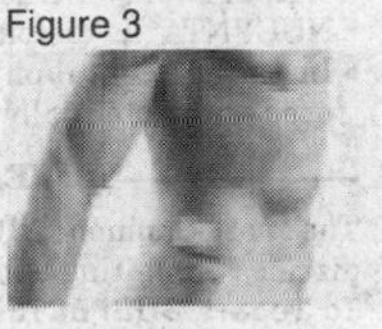

For adults and children
- Do not put a DURAGESIC® patch on skin that is very oily, burned, broken out, cut, irritated, or damaged in any way.
- Avoid sensitive areas or those that move around a lot. If there is hair, **do not shave (shaving irritates the skin).** Instead, clip hair as close to the skin as possible (see Figure 5).
- **Talk to your doctor if you have questions about skin application sites.**

Figure 4

Figure 5

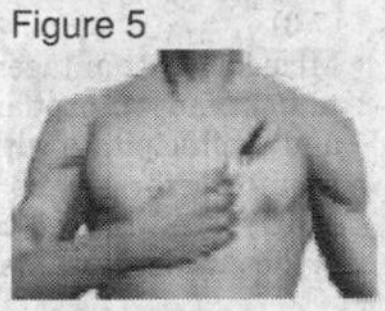

2. Prepare to Apply a DURAGESIC® Patch:
- Choose the time of day that is best for you to apply DURAGESIC®. Change it at about the same time of day (3 days or 72 hours after you apply the patch) or as directed by your doctor.
- Do not wear more than one DURAGESIC® patch at a time unless your doctor tells you to do so. Before putting on a new DURAGESIC® patch, remove the patch you have been wearing.
- Clean the skin area with clear water **only. Pat skin completely dry.** Do not use anything on the skin such as soaps, lotions, oils, or alcohol before the patch is applied.

3. Open the Pouch: Fold and tear at slit, or cut at slit taking care so as not to cut the patch, and remove the DURAGESIC® patch. Each DURAGESIC® patch is sealed in its own protective pouch. Do not remove the DURAGESIC® patch from the pouch until you are ready to use it (see Figure 6).

Figure 6

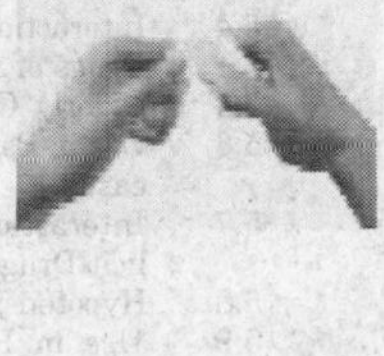

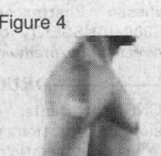

4. Peel: Peel off both parts of the protective liner from the patch. Each DURAGESIC® patch has a clear plastic backing that can be peeled off in two pieces. This covers the sticky side of the patch. Carefully peel this backing off. Throw the clear plastic backing away. **Touch the sticky side of the DURAGESIC® patch as little as possible** (see Figure 7).

Figure 7

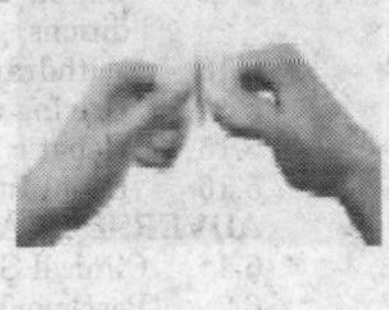

5. Press: Press the patch onto the chosen skin site **with the palm of your hand and hold there for at least 30 seconds** (see Figure 8). Make sure it sticks well, especially at the edges.

Figure 8

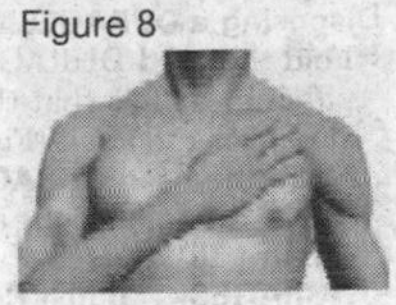

- DURAGESIC® may not stick to all patients. You need to check the patches often to make sure that they are sticking well to the skin.
- If the patch falls off right away after applying, throw it away and put a new one on at a different skin site (see Disposing a DURAGESIC® Patch).
- If you have a problem with the patch not sticking
  - Apply first aid tape only to the edges of the patch.
  - If you continue to have problems with the patch sticking, you may cover the patch with Bioclusive™ or Tegaderm™. These are special see-through adhesive dressings. **Never cover a DURAGESIC® patch with any other bandage or tape.** Remove the backing from the Bioclusive™ or Tegaderm™ dressing and place it carefully over the DURAGESIC® patch, smoothing it over the patch and your skin.
- **If your patch falls off later, but before 3 days (72 hours) of use, discard it properly (see Disposing a DURAGESIC® patch) and put a new one on at a different skin site. Be sure to let your doctor know that this has happened, and do not replace the new patch until 3 days (72 hours) after you put it on (or as directed by your doctor).**

6. Wash your hands when you have finished applying a DURAGESIC® patch.

7. Remove a DURAGESIC® patch after wearing it for 3 days (72 hours) (see "Disposing a DURAGESIC® Patch"). Choose a **different** place on the skin to apply a new DURAGESIC® patch and repeat Steps 2 through 6.
Do not apply the new patch to the same place as the last one.

Water and DURAGESIC®
- You can bathe, swim or shower while you are wearing a DURAGESIC® patch. If the patch falls off before 3 days (72 hours) after application, discard it properly (see Disposing a DURAGESIC® Patch) and put a new one on at a different skin site. Be sure to let your doctor know that this has happened, and do not replace the new patch until 3 days (72 hours) after you put it on (or as directed by your doctor).

Disposing a DURAGESIC® Patch

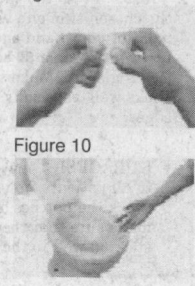

- Fold the used DURAGESIC® patch in half so that the sticky side sticks to itself (Figure 9). **Flush the used DURAGESIC® down the toilet right away** (Figure 10). **A used DURAGESIC® patch CAN be VERY dangerous for or even lead to death in babies, children, pets, and adults who have not been prescribed DURAGESIC®.**
- Throw away any DURAGESIC® patches that are left over from your prescription as soon as they are no longer needed. Remove the leftover patches from their protective pouch and remove the protective liner. **Fold the patches in half with the sticky sides together, and flush the patches down the toilet.** Do not flush the pouch or the protective liner down the toilet. These items can be thrown away in a trashcan.

Figure 9

Figure 10

Bioclusive™ is a trademark of Ethicon, Inc.
Tegaderm™ is a trademark of 3M
Rx Only
Manufactured by:
ALZA Corporation
Vacaville, CA 95688
Manufactured for:
Janssen Pharmaceuticals, Inc.
Titusville, NJ 08560
©Janssen Pharmaceuticals, Inc. 2009
October 2011

Shown in Product Identification Guide, page 307

NUCYNTA® Ⓒℐℐ

[new-sinn'-tah]
(tapentadol)
immediate-release oral tablets C-II

HIGHLIGHTS OF PRESCRIBING INFORMATION
These highlights do not include all the information needed to use NUCYNTA® safely and effectively. See full prescribing information for NUCYNTA®.
NUCYNTA® (tapentadol) immediate-release oral tablets C-II
Initial U.S. Approval: 2008

RECENT MAJOR CHANGES

Contraindications (4)	07/2013
Warnings and Precautions (5)	07/2013

INDICATIONS AND USAGE

NUCYNTA® is an opioid analgesic indicated for the management of moderate to severe acute pain in adults. (1)

DOSAGE AND ADMINISTRATION

- Individualize dosing according to the severity of pain being treated, the previous experience with similar drugs and the ability to monitor the patient. (2.1)
- Initiate NUCYNTA® with or without food at a dose of 50 mg, 75 mg, or 100 mg every 4 to 6 hours depending upon pain intensity. On the first day of dosing, the second dose may be administered as soon as one hour after the first dose, if adequate pain relief is not attained with the first dose. Subsequent dosing is 50 mg, 75 mg, or 100 mg every 4 to 6 hours and should be adjusted to maintain adequate analgesia with acceptable tolerability. Daily doses greater than 700 mg on the first day of therapy and 600 mg on subsequent days have not been studied and are, therefore, not recommended. (2.2)

DOSAGE FORMS AND STRENGTHS

Tablets: 50 mg, 75 mg, 100 mg (3)

CONTRAINDICATIONS

- Significant respiratory depression (4)
- Acute or severe bronchial asthma, hypercarbia (4)
- Known or suspected paralytic ileus (4)
- Hypersensitivity to tapentadol or to any other ingredients of the product (4)
- Concurrent use of monoamine oxidase (MAO) inhibitors or use within the last 14 days. (4)

WARNINGS AND PRECAUTIONS

- Misuse, Abuse and Diversion: NUCYNTA® is a Schedule II controlled substance with abuse liability similar to other opioids: monitor patients closely for signs of misuse, abuse and addiction. (5.1)
- Elderly, cachectic, and debilitated patients and patients with chronic pulmonary disease: Monitor closely because of increased risk of respiratory depression. (5.5)
- Interaction with CNS depressants including other opioids, sedatives, alcohol, and illicit drugs: Consider dose reduction of one or both drugs because of additive effects. (5.7)
- Hypotensive effect: Monitor for signs of hypotension.(5.8)
- Patients with head injury or increased intracranial pressure: Monitor for sedation and respiratory depression. Avoid use of NUCYNTA® in patients with impaired consciousness or coma susceptible to intracranial effects of CO_2 retention. (5.9)
- Seizures: Use with caution in patients with a history of seizures. (5.10)
- Serotonin Syndrome: Potentially life-threatening condition could result from concomitant serotonergic administration. (5.11)
- Withdrawal: Withdrawal symptoms may occur if NUCYNTA® is discontinued abruptly. (5.13)
- Impaired mental/physical abilities: Caution must be used with potentially hazardous activities. (5.14)

ADVERSE REACTIONS

The most common (≥10%) adverse reactions were nausea, dizziness, vomiting and somnolence. (6)
To report SUSPECTED ADVERSE REACTIONS, contact Janssen Pharmaceuticals, Inc. at 1-800-526-7736 (1-800-JANSSEN) or FDA at 1-800-FDA-1088 or *www.fda.gov/medwatch*

DRUG INTERACTIONS

- CNS depressants: Increased risk of respiratory depression, hypotension, profound sedation, coma or death. When combined therapy with CNS depressant is contemplated, the dose of one or both agents should be reduced. (7.3)
- Mixed agonist/antagonist opioids (i.e., pentazocine, nalbuphine, and butorphanol): May reduce analgesic effect and/or precipitate withdrawal symptoms. (7.5)
- Monitor for signs of serotonin syndrome when NUCYNTA® is used concurrently with SSRIs, SNRIs, tricyclic antidepressants, or triptans. (7.4)

USE IN SPECIFIC POPULATIONS

- Pregnancy: Based on animal data, may cause fetal harm. (8.1)
- Nursing mothers: Closely monitor infants of nursing women receiving NUCYNTA®. (8.3)
- Renal or hepatic impairment: not recommended in patients with severe renal or hepatic impairment. Reduce dose in patients with moderate hepatic impairment. (8.7, 8.8)

See 17 for PATIENT COUNSELING INFORMATION
Revised: 07/2013

FULL PRESCRIBING INFORMATION: CONTENTS*

*** Sections or subsections omitted from the full prescribing information are not listed**

FULL PRESCRIBING INFORMATION

1 INDICATIONS AND USAGE

NUCYNTA® (tapentadol) is indicated for the management of moderate to severe acute pain in adults.

2 DOSAGE AND ADMINISTRATION

2.1 Individualization of Dosage

As with any opioid drug product, adjust the dosing regimen for each patient individually, taking into account the patient's prior analgesic treatment experience. In the selection of the initial dose of tapentadol, give attention to the following:

- the total daily dose, potency and specific characteristics of the opioid the patient has been taking previously;
- the reliability of the relative potency estimate used to calculate the equivalent morphine sulfate dose needed;
- the patient's degree of opioid tolerance;
- the general condition and medical status of the patient;
- concurrent medications;
- the type and severity of the patient's pain;
- risk factors for abuse, addiction or diversion, including a prior history of abuse, addiction or diversion.

The following dosing recommendations, therefore, can only be considered suggested approaches to what is actually a series of clinical decisions over time in the management of the pain of each individual patient.

Continual re-evaluation of the patient receiving tapentadol is important, with special attention to the maintenance of pain control and the relative incidence of side effects associated with therapy.

During chronic therapy, especially for non-cancer-related pain, periodically re-assess the continued need for the use of opioid analgesics.

During periods of changing analgesic requirements, including initial titration, frequent contact is recommended between physician, other members of the healthcare team, the patient, and the caregiver/family. Monitor the patient for signs of respiratory or central nervous system depression.

2.2 Initiation of Therapy

The dose is 50 mg, 75 mg, or 100 mg every 4 to 6 hours depending upon pain intensity.

On the first day of dosing, the second dose may be administered as soon as one hour after the first dose, if adequate pain relief is not attained with the first dose. Subsequent dosing is 50 mg, 75 mg, or 100 mg every 4 to 6 hours and should be adjusted to maintain adequate analgesia with acceptable tolerability.

Daily doses greater than 700 mg on the first day of therapy and 600 mg on subsequent days have not been studied and are not recommended.

NUCYNTA® may be given with or without food *[see Clinical Pharmacology (12.3)]*.

2.3 Renal Impairment

Use of NUCYNTA® in patients with severe renal impairment is not recommended *[see Warnings and Precautions (5.16) and Clinical Pharmacology (12.3)]*.

No dosage adjustment is recommended in patients with mild or moderate renal impairment.

2.4 Hepatic Impairment

The safety and efficacy of NUCYNTA® has not been studied in patients with severe hepatic impairment (Child-Pugh Score 10–15) and use in this population is not recommended *[see Warnings and Precautions (5.15)]*.

Initiate treatment of patients with moderate hepatic impairment (Child-Pugh Score 7 to 9) with 50 mg no more frequently than once every 8 hours (maximum of three doses in 24 hours). Further treatment should reflect maintenance of analgesia with acceptable tolerability, to be achieved by either shortening or lengthening the dosing interval *[see Clinical Pharmacology (12.3)]*.

No dosage adjustment is recommended in patients with mild hepatic impairment (Child-Pugh Score 5 to 6) *[see Clinical Pharmacology (12.3)]*.

2.5 Elderly Patients

In general, recommended dosing for elderly patients with normal renal and hepatic function is the same as for younger adult patients with normal renal and hepatic function. Because elderly patients are more likely to have decreased renal and hepatic function, consideration should be given to starting elderly patients with the lower range of recommended doses.

2.6 Cessation of Therapy

When the patient no longer requires therapy with tapentadol, gradually taper the dose to prevent signs and symptoms of withdrawal in the physically dependent patient *[see Warnings and Precautions (5.13)]*.

3 DOSAGE FORMS AND STRENGTHS

NUCYNTA® Tablets are round, biconvex and film-coated and are available in the following strengths, colors, and debossings: 50 mg of tapentadol (yellow with "O-M" on one side and "50" on the other side), 75 mg of tapentadol (yellow-orange with "O-M" on one side and "75" on the other side), and 100 mg of tapentadol (orange with "O-M" on one side and "100" on the other side) *[see Description (11) and How Supplied/Storage and Handling (16)]*.

4 CONTRAINDICATIONS

NUCYNTA® is contraindicated in:

- Patients with significant respiratory depression
- Patients with acute or severe bronchial asthma or hypercarbia in an unmonitored setting or in the absence of resuscitative equipment
- Patients with known or suspected paralytic ileus
- Patients with hypersensitivity (e.g. anaphylaxis, angioedema) to tapentadol or to any other ingredients of the product *[see Adverse Reactions (6.2)]*.
- Patients who are receiving monoamine oxidase (MAO) inhibitors or who have taken them within the last 14 days due to potential additive effects on norepinephrine levels which may result in adverse cardiovascular events *[see Drug Interactions (7.2)]*.

5 WARNINGS AND PRECAUTIONS

5.1 Abuse Potential

NUCYNTA® contains tapentadol, an opioid agonist and a Schedule II controlled substance. Tapentadol can be abused in a manner similar to other opioid agonists legal or illicit. Opioid agonists are sought by drug abusers and people with addiction disorders and are subject to criminal diversion. Consider these risks when prescribing or dispensing NUCYNTA® in situations where there is concern about increased risks of misuse, abuse, or diversion. Concerns about abuse, addiction, and diversion should not, however, prevent the proper management of pain.

Assess each patient's risk for opioid abuse or addiction prior to prescribing NUCYNTA®. The risk for opioid abuse is increased in patients with a personal or family history of substance abuse (including drug or alcohol abuse or addiction) or mental illness (e.g., major depression). Patients at increased risk may still be appropriately treated with opioids; however these patients will require intensive monitoring for signs of misuse, abuse, or addiction. Routinely monitor all patients receiving opioids for signs of misuse, abuse, and addiction because these drugs carry a risk for addiction even under appropriate medical use.

Misuse or abuse of NUCYNTA® by crushing, chewing, snorting or injecting will pose a significant risk that could result in overdose and death *[see Overdosage (10)]*.

Contact local state professional licensing board or state controlled substances authority for information on how to prevent and detect abuse or diversion of this product *[see Drug Abuse and Dependence (9)]*.

5.2 Life Threatening Respiratory Depression

Respiratory depression is the chief hazard of opioid agonists, including NUCYNTA®. Respiratory depression, if not immediately recognized and treated, may lead to respiratory arrest and death. Respiratory depression from opioids is manifested by a reduced urge to breathe and a decreased rate of respiration, often associated with a "sighing" pattern of breathing (deep breaths separated by abnormally long pauses). Carbon dioxide (CO_2) retention from opioid-induced respiratory depression can exacerbate the sedating effects of opioids. Management of respiratory depression may include close observation, supportive measures, and use of opioid antagonists, depending on the patient's clinical status *[see Overdosage (10)]*.

Instruct patients against use by individuals other than the patient for whom NUCYNTA® was prescribed and to keep NUCYNTA® out of the reach of children, as such inappropriate use may result in fatal respiratory depression.

Patients with conditions accompanied by hypoxia, hypercarbia or decreased respiratory reserve such as: asthma, chronic obstructive pulmonary disease or cor pulmonale, central nervous system (CNS) depression, or coma may be at increased risk for increased airway resistance and decreased respiratory drive to the point of apnea even with usual therapeutic doses of NUCYNTA®. Consider the use of alternative non-mu-opioid agonist analgesics and use NUCYNTA® only under careful medical supervision at the lowest effective dose in such patients. If respiratory depression occurs, treat the patient for mu-opioid agonist-induced respiratory depression *[see Overdosage (10.2)]*. To reduce the risk of respiratory depression, proper dosing of NUCYNTA® is essential *[see Dosage and Administration (2)]*.

5.3 Accidental Exposure

Accidental ingestion of NUCYNTA®, especially in children, can result in a fatal overdose of tapentadol.

5.4 Interactions with Alcohol, Other Opioids, and Drugs of Abuse

Due to its mu-opioid agonist activity, NUCYNTA® may be expected to have additive effects when used in conjunction with alcohol, other opioids, or illicit drugs that cause central nervous system depression, respiratory depression, hypotension, and profound sedation, coma or death *[see Drug Interactions (7.3)]*. Instruct patients not to consume alcoholic beverages or use prescription or non-prescription products containing alcohol, other opioids, or drugs of abuse while on NUCYNTA® therapy *[see Drug Interactions (7.1)]*.

5.5 Elderly, Cachectic, and Debilitated Patients

Respiratory depression is more likely to occur in elderly, cachectic, or debilitated patients as they may have altered pharmacokinetics or altered clearance compared to younger, healthier patients. Therefore, closely monitor such patients, particularly when NUCYNTA® is given concomitantly with other drugs that depress respiration *[see Warnings and Precautions (5.2)]*.

5.6 Use in Patients with Chronic Pulmonary Disease

Monitor for respiratory depression those patients with significant chronic obstructive pulmonary disease or cor pulmonale, and patients having a substantially decreased respiratory reserve, hypoxia, hypercarbia, or pre-existing respiratory depression, as in these patients, even usual therapeutic doses of NUCYNTA® may decrease respiratory drive to the point of apnea *[see Warnings and Precautions (5.2)]*. Consider the use of alternative non-opioid analgesics in these patients if possible.

5.7 Interactions with CNS Depressants and Illicit Drugs

Hypotension, and profound sedation, coma or respiratory depression may result if NUCYNTA® is used concomitantly with other CNS depressants (e.g., sedatives, anxiolytics, hypnotics, neuroleptics, muscle relaxants, other opioids and illicit drugs). When considering the use of NUCYNTA® in a patient taking a CNS depressant, assess the duration of use of the CNS depressant and the patient's response, including the degree of tolerance that has developed to CNS depression. Additionally, consider the patient's use, if any, of alcohol and/or illicit drugs that can cause CNS depression. If NUCYNTA® therapy is to be initiated in a patient taking a CNS depressant, start with a lower NUCYNTA® dose than usual and monitor patients for signs of sedation and respiratory depression and consider using a lower dose of the concomitant CNS depressant *[see Drug Interactions (7.3)]*.

5.8 Hypotensive Effect

NUCYNTA® may cause severe hypotension. There is an increased risk in patients whose ability to maintain blood pressure has already been compromised by a reduced blood volume or concurrent administration of certain CNS depressant drugs (e.g., phenothiazines or general anesthetics) *[see Drug Interactions (7.3)]*. Monitor these patients for signs of hypotension after the dose of NUCYNTA®. In patients with circulatory shock, NUCYNTA® may cause vasodilation that can further reduce cardiac output and blood pressure. Avoid the use of NUCYNTA® in patients with circulatory shock.

5.9 Use in Patients with Head Injury or Increased Intracranial Pressure

Monitor patients taking NUCYNTA® who may be susceptible to the intracranial effects of CO_2 retention (e.g., those with evidence of increased intracranial pressure or brain tumors) for signs of sedation and respiratory depression. NUCYNTA® may reduce respiratory drive, and the resultant CO_2 retention can further increase intracranial pressure. Opioids may also obscure the clinical course in a patient with a head injury.

Avoid the use of NUCYNTA® in patients with impaired consciousness or coma.

5.10 Seizures

NUCYNTA® has not been evaluated in patients with a predisposition to a seizure disorder, and such patients were excluded from clinical studies. The active ingredient tapentadol in NUCYNTA® may aggravate convulsions in patients with convulsive disorders, and may induce or aggravate seizures in some clinical settings. Monitor patients with a history of seizure disorders for worsened seizure control during NUCYNTA® therapy.

5.11 Serotonin Syndrome Risk

Cases of life-threatening serotonin syndrome have been reported with the concurrent use of tapentadol and serotonergic drugs. Serotonergic drugs comprise Selective Serotonin Reuptake Inhibitors (SSRIs), Serotonin and Norepinephrine Reuptake Inhibitors (SNRIs), tricyclic antidepressants (TCAs), triptans, drugs that affect the serotonergic neurotransmitter system (e.g. mirtazapine, trazodone, and tramadol), and drugs that impair metabolism of serotonin (including MAOIs). This may occur within the recommended dose. Serotonin syndrome may include mental-status changes (e.g., agitation, hallucinations, coma), autonomic instability (e.g., tachycardia, labile blood pressure, hyperthermia), neuromuscular aberrations (e.g., hyperreflexia, incoordination) and/or gastrointestinal symptoms (e.g., nausea, vomiting, diarrhea) and can be fatal *[see Drug Interactions (7.4)]*.

5.12 Use in Patients with Gastrointestinal Conditions

NUCYNTA® is contraindicated in patients with GI obstruction, including paralytic ileus. The tapentadol in NUCYNTA® may cause spasm of the sphincter of Oddi. Monitor patients with biliary tract disease, including acute pancreatitis, for worsening symptoms.

5.13 Withdrawal

Withdrawal symptoms may occur if NUCYNTA® is discontinued abruptly. These symptoms may include: anxiety, sweating, insomnia, rigors, pain, nausea, tremors, diarrhea, upper respiratory symptoms, piloerection, and rarely, hallucinations. Withdrawal symptoms may be reduced by tapering NUCYNTA® *[see Drug Abuse and Dependence (9.3)]*.

5.14 Driving and Operating Heavy Machinery

NUCYNTA® may impair the mental or physical abilities needed to perform potentially hazardous activities such as driving a car or operating machinery. Warn patients not to drive or operate dangerous machinery unless they are tolerant to the effects of NUCYNTA® and know how they will react to the medication.

5.15 Hepatic Impairment

A study with NUCYNTA® in subjects with hepatic impairment showed higher serum concentrations of tapentadol than in those with normal hepatic function. Avoid use of NUCYNTA® in patients with severe hepatic impairment. Reduce the dose of NUCYNTA® in patients with moderate hepatic impairment *[see Dosage and Administration (2.4) and Clinical Pharmacology (12.3)]*. Closely monitor patients with moderate hepatic impairment for respiratory and central nervous system depression when receiving NUCYNTA®.

5.16 Renal Impairment

Use of NUCYNTA® in patients with severe renal impairment is not recommended due to accumulation of a metabolite formed by glucuronidation of tapentadol. The clinical relevance of the elevated metabolite is not known *[see Clinical Pharmacology (12.3)]*.

6 ADVERSE REACTIONS

The following adverse reactions are discussed in more detail in other sections of the labeling:

- Respiratory Depression *[see Warnings and Precautions (5.2)]*
- Interaction with Alcohol *[see Warnings and Precautions (5.4)]*
- Chronic Pulmonary Disease *[see Warnings and Precautions (5.6)]*
- Hypotensive Effects *[see Warnings and Precautions (5.8)]*
- Interactions with Other CNS Depressants *[see Warnings and Precautions (5.7)]*
- Drug abuse, addiction, and dependence *[see Drug Abuse and Dependence (9.2, 9.3)]*
- Gastrointestinal Effects *[see Warnings and Precautions (5.12)]*
- Seizures *[see Warnings and Precautions (5.10)]*
- Serotonin Syndrome *[see Warnings and Precautions (5.11)]*

6.1 Clinical Studies Experience

Because clinical trials are conducted under widely varying conditions, adverse reaction rates observed in the clinical trials of a drug cannot be directly compared to rates in the clinical trials of another drug and may not reflect the rates observed in clinical practice.

Based on data from nine Phase 2/3 studies that administered multiple doses (seven placebo- and/or active-controlled, one noncontrolled and one Phase 3 active-controlled safety study) the most common adverse reactions (reported by ≥10% in any NUCYNTA® dose group) were: nausea, dizziness, vomiting and somnolence.

The most common reasons for discontinuation due to adverse reactions in the studies described above (reported by ≥1% in any NUCYNTA® dose group) were dizziness (2.6% vs. 0.5%), nausea (2.3% vs. 0.6%), vomiting (1.4% vs. 0.2%), somnolence (1.3% vs. 0.2%) and headache (0.9% vs. 0.2%) for NUCYNTA®- and placebo-treated patients, respectively. Seventy-six percent of NUCYNTA®-treated patients from the nine studies experienced adverse events.

NUCYNTA® was studied in multiple-dose, active- or placebo-controlled studies, or noncontrolled studies (n = 2178), in single-dose studies (n = 870), in open-label study extension (n = 483) and in Phase 1 studies (n = 597). Of these, 2034 patients were treated with doses of 50 mg to 100 mg of NUCYNTA® dosed every 4 to 6 hours.

The data described below reflect exposure to NUCYNTA® in 3161 patients, including 449 exposed for 45 days. NUCYNTA® was studied primarily in placebo- and active-controlled studies (n = 2266, and n = 2944, respectively). The population was 18 to 85 years old (mean age 46 years), 68% were female, 75% white and 67% were postoperative. Most patients received NUCYNTA® doses of 50 mg, 75 mg, or 100 mg every 4 to 6 hours.

Table 1 Adverse Reactions Reported by ≥1% of NUCYNTA®-Treated Patients In Seven Phase 2/3 Placebo- and/or Oxycodone-Controlled, One Non-controlled, and One Phase 3 Oxycodone-Controlled Safety, Multiple-Dose Clinical Studies

System/Organ Class MedDRA Preferred Term	NUCYNTA® 21 mg – 120 mg (n=2178) %	Placebo (n=619) %
Gastrointestinal disorders		
Nausea	30	13
Vomiting	18	4
Constipation	8	3
Dry mouth	4	<1
Dyspepsia	2	<1
General disorders and administration site conditions		
Fatigue	3	<1
Feeling hot	1	<1
Infections and infestations		
Nasopharyngitis	1	<1
Upper respiratory tract infection	1	<1
Urinary tract infection	1	<1
Metabolism and nutrition disorders		
Decreased appetite	2	0
Nervous system disorders		
Dizziness	24	8
Somnolence	15	3
Tremor	1	<1
Lethargy	1	<1
Psychiatric disorders		
Insomnia	2	<1
Confusional state	1	0
Abnormal dreams	1	<1
Anxiety	1	<1
Skin and subcutaneous tissue disorders		
Pruritus	5	1
Hyperhidrosis	3	<1
Pruritus generalized	3	<1
Rash	1	<1
Vascular disorders		
Hot flush	1	<1

The following adverse drug reactions occurred in less than 1% of NUCYNTA®-treated patients in the pooled safety data from nine Phase 2/3 clinical studies:

Cardiac disorders: heart rate increased, heart rate decreased

Eye disorders: visual disturbance

Gastrointestinal disorders: abdominal discomfort, impaired gastric emptying

General disorders and administration site conditions: irritability, edema, drug withdrawal syndrome, feeling drunk

Immune system disorders: hypersensitivity

Investigations: gamma-glutamyltransferase increased, alanine aminotransferase increased, aspartate aminotransferase increased

Musculoskeletal and connective tissue disorders: involuntary muscle contractions, sensation of heaviness

Nervous system disorders: hypoesthesia, paresthesia, disturbance in attention, sedation, dysarthria, depressed level of consciousness, memory impairment, ataxia, presyncope, syncope, coordination abnormal, seizure

Psychiatric disorders: euphoric mood, disorientation, restlessness, agitation, nervousness, thinking abnormal

Renal and urinary disorders: urinary hesitation, pollakiuria

Respiratory, thoracic and mediastinal disorders: oxygen saturation decreased, cough, dyspnea, respiratory depression

Skin and subcutaneous tissue disorders: urticaria

Vascular disorders: blood pressure decreased

In the pooled safety data, the overall incidence of adverse reactions increased with increased dose of NUCYNTA®, as did the percentage of patients with adverse reactions of nausea, dizziness, vomiting, somnolence, and pruritus.

6.2 Post-marketing Experience

The following additional adverse reactions have been identified during post-approval use of NUCYNTA®. Because these reactions are reported voluntarily from a population of uncertain size, it is not always possible to estimate their frequency reliably.

Gastrointestinal disorders: diarrhea

Nervous system disorders: headache

Psychiatric disorders: hallucination, suicidal ideation

Cardiac disorders: palpitations

Anaphylaxis, angioedema, and anaphylactic shock have been reported very rarely with ingredients contained in NUCYNTA®. Advise patients how to recognize such reactions and when to seek medical attention.

7 DRUG INTERACTIONS

NUCYNTA® is mainly metabolized by glucuronidation. The following substances have been included in a set of interaction studies without any clinically significant finding: acetaminophen, acetylsalicylic acid, naproxen and probenecid *[see Clinical Pharmacology (12.3)]*.

The pharmacokinetics of tapentadol were not affected when gastric pH or gastrointestinal motility were increased by omeprazole and metoclopramide, respectively *[see Clinical Pharmacology (12.3)]*.

7.1 Alcohol, Other Opioids, and Drugs of Abuse

Due to its mu-opioid agonist activity, NUCYNTA® may be expected to have additive effects when used in conjunction with alcohol, other opioids, or illicit drugs that cause central nervous system depression, respiratory depression, hypotension, and profound sedation, coma or death. Instruct patients not to consume alcoholic beverages or use prescription or non-prescription products containing alcohol, other opioids, or drugs of abuse while on NUCYNTA® therapy *[see Warnings and Precautions (5.4)]*.

7.2 Monoamine Oxidase Inhibitors

NUCYNTA® is contraindicated in patients who are receiving monoamine oxidase (MAO) inhibitors or who have taken them within the last 14 days due to potential additive effects on norepinephrine levels which may result in adverse cardiovascular events *[see Contraindications (4)]*.

7.3 CNS Depressants

Concurrent use of NUCYNTA® and other central nervous system (CNS) depressants including sedatives or hypnotics, general anesthetics, phenothiazines, tranquilizers, and alcohol can increase the risk of respiratory depression, hypotension, profound sedation or coma. Monitor patients receiving CNS depressants and NUCYNTA® for signs of respiratory depression and hypotension. When such combined therapy is contemplated, start NUCYNTA® at ⅓ to ½ of the usual dosage and consider using a lower dose of the concomitant CNS depressant *[see Warnings and Precautions (5.7)]*.

7.4 Serotonergic Drugs

There have been post-marketing reports of serotonin syndrome with the concomitant use of tapentadol and serotonergic drugs (e.g., SSRIs and SNRIs). Caution is advised when NUCYNTA® is co-administered with other drugs that may affect serotonergic neurotransmitter systems such as SSRIs, SNRIs, MAOIs, and triptans. If concomitant treatment of NUCYNTA® with a drug affecting the serotonergic neurotransmitter system is clinically warranted, careful observation of the patient is advised *[see Warning and Precautions (5.11)]*.

7.5 Mixed Agonist/Antagonist Opioid Analgesics

The concomitant use of NUCYNTA® with mixed agonist/antagonists (e.g., butorphanol, nalbuphine, and pentazocine) and partial agonists (e.g., buprenorphine) may precipitate withdrawal symptoms. Avoid the use of agonist/antagonists and partial agonists with NUCYNTA®.

7.6 Anticholinergics

The use of NUCYNTA® with anticholinergic products may increase the risk of urinary retention and/or severe constipation, which may lead to paralytic ileus.

8 USE IN SPECIFIC POPULATIONS

8.1 Pregnancy

Pregnancy Category C: There are no adequate and well-controlled studies of NUCYNTA® in pregnant women. NUCYNTA® should be used during pregnancy only if the potential benefit justifies the potential risk to the fetus.

Tapentadol HCl was evaluated for teratogenic effects in pregnant rats and rabbits following intravenous and subcutaneous exposure during the period of embryofetal organogenesis. When tapentadol was administered twice daily by the subcutaneous route in rats at dose levels of 10, 20, or 40 mg/kg/day [producing up to 1 times the plasma exposure at the maximum recommended human dose (MRHD) of 700 mg/day based on an area under the time-curve (AUC) comparison], no teratogenic effects were observed. Evidence of embryofetal toxicity included transient delays in skeletal maturation (i.e. reduced ossification) at the 40 mg/kg/day dose which was associated with significant maternal toxicity. Administration of tapentadol HCl in rabbits at doses of 4, 10, or 24 mg/kg/day by subcutaneous injection [producing 0.2, 0.6, and 1.85 times the plasma exposure at the MRHD based on an AUC comparison] revealed embryofetal toxicity at doses ≥10 mg/kg/day. Findings included reduced fetal viability, skeletal delays and other variations. In addition, there were multiple malformations including gastroschisis/thoracogastroschisis, amelia/phocomelia, and cleft palate at doses ≥10 mg/kg/day and above, and ablepharia, encephalopathy, and spina bifida at the high dose of 24 mg/kg/day. Embryofetal toxicity, including malformations, may be secondary to the significant maternal toxicity observed in the study.

In a study of pre- and postnatal development in rats, oral administration of tapentadol at doses of 20, 50, 150, or 300 mg/kg/day to pregnant and lactating rats during the late gestation and early postnatal period [resulting in up to 1.7 times the plasma exposure at the MRHD on an AUC basis] did not influence physical or reflex development, the outcome of neurobehavioral tests or reproductive parameters. Treatment-related developmental delay was observed, including incomplete ossification, and significant reductions in pup body weights and body weight gains at doses associated with maternal toxicity (150 mg/kg/day and above). At maternal tapentadol doses ≥150 mg/kg/day, a dose-related increase in pup mortality was observed through postnatal Day 4.

8.2 Labor and Delivery

NUCYNTA® is not for use in women during and immediately prior to labor. Occasionally, opioid analgesics may prolong labor by temporarily reducing the strength, duration, and frequency of uterine contractions. However, these effects are not consistent and may be offset by an increased rate of cervical dilatation which tends to shorten labor.

Opioids cross the placenta and may produce respiratory depression and psychophysiologic effects in neonates. Closely observe neonates whose mothers received opioid analgesics during labor for signs of respiratory depression. An opioid antagonist, such as naloxone, should be available for reversal of opioid-induced respiratory depression in the neonate in such situations.

8.3 Nursing Mothers

There is insufficient/limited information on the excretion of tapentadol in human or animal breast milk. Physicochemical and available pharmacodynamic/toxicological data on tapentadol point to excretion in breast milk and risk to the breastfeeding child cannot be excluded.

Because of the potential for adverse reactions in nursing infants from NUCYNTA®, a decision should be made whether to discontinue nursing or discontinue the drug, taking into account the importance of the drug to the mother.

Withdrawal symptoms can occur in breast-feeding infants when maternal administration of NUCYNTA® is stopped.

8.4 Pediatric Use

The safety and effectiveness of NUCYNTA® in pediatric patients less than 18 years of age have not been established.

8.5 Geriatric Use

Of the total number of patients in Phase 2/3 double-blind, multiple-dose clinical studies of NUCYNTA®, 19% were 65 and over, while 5% were 75 and over. No overall differences in effectiveness were observed between these patients and younger patients. The rate of constipation was higher in subjects greater than or equal to 65 years than those less than 65 years (12% vs. 7%).

In general, recommended dosing for elderly patients with normal renal and hepatic function is the same as for younger adult patients with normal renal and hepatic function. Because elderly patients are more likely to have decreased renal and hepatic function, consideration should be given to starting elderly patients with the lower range of recommended doses *[see Clinical Pharmacology (12.3)]*.

8.6 Neonatal Withdrawal Syndrome

Chronic maternal use of NUCYNTA® during pregnancy can affect the neonate with subsequent withdrawal signs. Neonatal withdrawal syndrome presents as irritability, hyperactivity and abnormal sleep pattern, high pitched cry, tremor, vomiting, diarrhea and failure to gain weight. The onset, duration and severity of neonatal withdrawal syndrome vary based on the drug used, duration of use, the dose of last maternal use, and rate of elimination drug by the newborn. Neonatal opioid withdrawal syndrome may be life-threatening and should be treated according to protocols developed by neonatology experts.

8.7 Renal Impairment

The safety and effectiveness of NUCYNTA® has not been established in patients with severe renal impairment (CLCR <30 mL/min). Use of NUCYNTA® in patients with severe renal impairment is not recommended due to accumulation of a metabolite formed by glucuronidation of tapentadol. The clinical relevance of the elevated metabolite is not known *[see Clinical Pharmacology (12.3)]*.

8.8 Hepatic Impairment

Administration of tapentadol resulted in higher exposures and serum levels of tapentadol in subjects with impaired hepatic function compared to subjects with normal hepatic function *[see Clinical Pharmacology (12.3)]*. The dose of NUCYNTA® should be reduced in patients with moderate hepatic impairment (Child-Pugh Score 7 to 9) *[see Dosage and Administration (2.2)]*.

Use of NUCYNTA® is not recommended in patients with severe hepatic impairment (Child-Pugh Score 10 to 15) *[see Warnings and Precautions (5.15)]*.

9 DRUG ABUSE AND DEPENDENCE

9.1 Controlled Substance

NUCYNTA® contains tapentadol, a Schedule II controlled substance with a high potential for abuse similar to fentanyl, methadone, morphine, oxycodone, and oxymorphone. NUCYNTA® is subject to misuse, abuse, addiction, and criminal diversion *[see Warnings and Precautions (5.1)]*.

9.2 Abuse

All patients treated with opioids require careful monitoring for signs of abuse and addiction, because use of opioid analgesic products carries the risk of addiction even under appropriate medical use.

Drug abuse is the intentional non-therapeutic use of an over-the-counter or prescription drug, even once, for its rewarding psychological or physiological effects. Drug abuse includes, but is not limited to the following examples: the use of a prescription or over-the-counter drug to get "high", or the use of steroids for performance enhancement and muscle build up.

Drug addiction is a cluster of behavioral, cognitive, and physiological phenomena that develop after repeated substance use and include: a strong desire to take the drug, difficulties in controlling its use, persisting in its use despite harmful consequences, a higher priority given to drug use than to other activities and obligations, increased tolerance, and sometimes a physical withdrawal.

"Drug seeking" behavior is very common in addicts, and drug abusers. Drug-seeking tactics include emergency calls or visits near the end of office hours, refusal to undergo appropriate examination, testing or referral, repeated claims of loss of prescriptions, tampering with prescriptions and reluctance to provide prior medical records or contact information for other treating physician(s). "Healthcare professional shopping" (visiting multiple prescribers) to obtain additional prescriptions is common among drug abusers, people suffering from untreated addiction and criminals seeking drugs to sell.

Abuse and addiction are separate and distinct from physical dependence and tolerance. Physicians should be aware that addiction may not be accompanied by concurrent tolerance and symptoms of physical dependence in all addicts. In addition, abuse of opioids can occur in the absence of true addiction and is characterized by misuse for non-medical purposes, often in combination with other psychoactive substances.

NUCYNTA® can be diverted for non-medical use into illicit channels of distribution. Careful record-keeping of prescribing information, including quantity, frequency, and renewal requests, as required by law, is strongly advised.

Proper assessment of the patient, proper prescribing practices, periodic re-evaluation of therapy, and proper dispensing and storage are appropriate measures that help to limit abuse of opioid drugs.

9.3 Dependence

Both tolerance and physical dependence can develop during chronic opioid therapy. Tolerance is the need for increasing doses of opioids to maintain a defined effect such as analgesia (in the absence of disease progression or other external factors). Tolerance may occur to both the desired and undesired effects of drugs, and may develop at different rates for different effects.

Physical dependence results in withdrawal symptoms after abrupt discontinuation or a significant dose reduction of a drug. Withdrawal also may be precipitated through the administration of drugs with opioid antagonist activity, e.g., naloxone, nalmefene, or mixed agonist/antagonist analgesics (pentazocine, butorphanol, buprenorphine, nalbuphine). Physical dependence may not occur to a clinically significant degree until after several days to weeks of continued opioid usage. Some or all of the following can characterize this syndrome: restlessness, lacrimation, rhinorrhea, yawning, perspiration, chills, piloerection, myalgia, mydriasis, irritability, anxiety, backache, joint pain, weakness, abdominal cramps, insomnia, nausea, anorexia, vomiting, diarrhea, increased blood pressure, respiratory rate, or heart rate. Withdrawal symptoms may be reduced by tapering NUCYNTA®.

Infants born to mothers physically dependent on opioids will also be physically dependent and may exhibit respiratory difficulties and withdrawal symptoms *[see Use in Specific Populations (8.1, 8.2)]*.

10 OVERDOSAGE

10.1 Clinical Presentation

Acute overdosage with opioids can be manifested by respiratory depression, somnolence progressing to stupor or coma, skeletal muscle flaccidity, cold and clammy skin, constricted pupils, and sometimes pulmonary edema, bradycardia, hypotension and death. Marked mydriasis rather than miosis may be seen due to severe hypoxia in overdose situations.

10.2 Management

In case of overdose, priorities are the re-establishment of a patent and protected airway and institution of assisted or controlled ventilation if needed. Employ other supportive measures (including oxygen, vasopressors) in the management of circulatory shock and pulmonary edema as indicated. Cardiac arrest or arrhythmias will require advanced life support techniques.

The opioid antagonists, naloxone or nalmefene, are specific antidotes to respiratory depression resulting from opioid overdose. Opioid antagonists should not be administered in the absence of clinically significant respiratory or circulatory depression secondary to tapentadol overdose. Such agents should be administered cautiously to patients who are known, or suspected to be, physically dependent on NUCYNTA®. In such cases, an abrupt or complete reversal of opioid effects may precipitate an acute withdrawal syndrome.

Because the duration of reversal would be expected to be less than the duration of action of tapentadol in NUCYNTA®, carefully monitor the patient until spontaneous respiration is reliably re-established. If the response to opioid antagonists is suboptimal or not sustained, additional antagonist should be given as directed in the product's prescribing information.

In an individual physically dependent on opioids, administration of an opioid receptor antagonist may precipitate an acute withdrawal. The severity of the withdrawal produced will depend on the degree of physical dependence and the dose of the antagonist administered. If a decision is made to treat serious respiratory depression in the physically dependent patient, administration of the antagonist should be begun with care and by titration with smaller than usual doses of the antagonist.

11 DESCRIPTION

NUCYNTA® (tapentadol) is a mu-opioid receptor agonist, supplied in immediate-release film-coated tablets for oral administration, containing 58.24, 87.36 and 116.48 mg of tapentadol hydrochloride in each tablet strength, corresponding to 50, 75, and 100 mg of tapentadol free-base, respectively. The chemical name is 3-[(1*R*,2*R*)-3-(dimethylamino)-1-ethyl-2-methylpropyl]phenol monohydrochloride. The structural formula is:

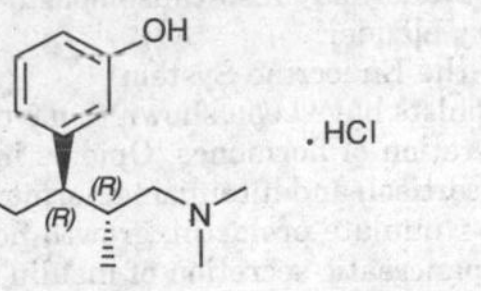

The molecular weight of tapentadol HCl is 257.80, and the molecular formula is $C_{14}H_{23}NO \bullet HCl$. The n-octanol:water partition coefficient log P value is 2.87. The pKa values are 9.34 and 10.45.

In addition to the active ingredient tapentadol HCl, NUCYNTA® tablets also contain the following inactive ingredients: croscarmellose sodium, lactose monohydrate, magnesium stearate, microcrystalline cellulose, povidone. The film coatings for all tablet strengths contain polyvinyl alcohol, titanium dioxide, polyethylene glycol, talc, and the colorant FD&C Yellow #6 aluminum lake; the film coatings for the 50 mg and 75 mg tablets also contain the additional colorant D&C Yellow #10 aluminum lake.

12 CLINICAL PHARMACOLOGY

12.1 Mechanism of Action

Tapentadol is a centrally-acting synthetic analgesic. The exact mechanism of action is unknown. Although the clinical relevance is unclear, preclinical studies have shown that tapentadol is a mu-opioid receptor (MOR) agonist and a norepinephrine reuptake inhibitor (NRI). Analgesia in animal models is derived from both of these properties.

12.2 Pharmacodynamics

Tapentadol is 18 times less potent than morphine in binding to the human mu-opioid receptor and is 2–3 times less potent in producing analgesia in animal models. Tapentadol has been shown to inhibit norepinephrine reuptake in the brains of rats resulting in increased norepinephrine concentrations. In preclinical models, the analgesic activity due to the mu-opioid receptor agonist activity of tapentadol can be antagonized by selective mu-opioid antagonists (e.g., naloxone), whereas the norepinephrine reuptake inhibition is sensitive to norepinephrine modulators. Tapentadol exerts its analgesic effects without a pharmacologically active metabolite.

Concentration-Efficacy Relationships

The minimum effective plasma concentration of tapentadol for analgesia varies widely among patients, especially among patients who have been previously treated with agonist opioids.

Concentration-Adverse Experience Relationships

There is a general relationship between increasing opioid plasma concentration and increasing frequency of adverse experiences such as nausea, vomiting, CNS effects, and respiratory depression.

Effects on the Cardiovascular System

There was no effect of therapeutic and supratherapeutic doses of tapentadol on the QT interval. In a randomized, double-blind, placebo- and positive-controlled crossover study, healthy subjects were administered five consecutive doses of NUCYNTA® 100 mg every 6 hours, NUCYNTA® 150 mg every 6 hours, placebo and a single oral dose of moxifloxacin. Similarly, NUCYNTA® had no relevant effect on other ECG parameters (heart rate, PR interval, QRS duration, T-wave or U-wave morphology).

Tapentadol produces peripheral vasodilation which may result in orthostatic hypotension.

Effects on the Central Nervous System (CNS)

The principal therapeutic action of tapentadol is analgesia. Tapentadol causes respiratory depression, in part by a direct effect on the brainstem respiratory centers. The respiratory depression involves a reduction in the responsiveness of the brain stem respiratory centers to both increases in carbon dioxide tension and electrical stimulation. Tapentadol depresses the cough reflex by direct effect on the cough center in the medulla.

Tapentadol causes miosis, even in total darkness. Pinpoint pupils are a sign of opioid overdose but are not pathognomonic (e.g., pontine lesions of hemorrhagic or ischemic origin may produce similar findings). Marked mydriasis rather than miosis may be seen with hypoxia in overdose situations *[see Overdosage (10)]*. Other effects of tapentadol include anxiolysis, euphoria, and feeling of relaxation, drowsiness and changes in mood.

Effects on the Gastrointestinal Tract and on Other Smooth Muscle

Gastric, biliary and pancreatic secretions are decreased by tapentadol. Tapentadol causes a reduction in motility and is associated with an increase in tone in the antrum of the stomach and duodenum. Digestion of food in the small intestine is delayed and propulsive contractions are decreased. Propulsive peristaltic waves in the colon are decreased, while tone is increased to the point of spasm. The end result is constipation. Tapentadol can cause a marked increase in biliary tract pressure as a result of spasm of the sphincter of Oddi, and transient elevations in serum amylase. Tapentadol may also cause spasm of the sphincter of the urinary bladder.

Effects on the Endocrine System

Opioid agonists have been shown to have a variety of effects on the secretion of hormones. Opioids inhibit the secretion of ACTH, cortisol, and luteinizing hormone (LH) in humans. They also stimulate prolactin, growth hormone (GH) secretion, and pancreatic secretion of insulin and glucagon.

Effects on the Immune System

Opioids have been shown to have a variety of effects on components of the immune system in *in vitro* and animal models. The clinical significance of these findings is unknown.

CNS Depressant/Alcohol Interaction

Additive pharmacodynamic effects may be expected when NUCYNTA® is used in conjunction with alcohol, other opioids, or illicit drugs that cause central nervous system depression.

12.3 Pharmacokinetics

Absorption

The mean absolute bioavailability after single-dose administration (fasting) of NUCYNTA® is approximately 32% due to extensive first-pass metabolism. Maximum serum concentrations of tapentadol are typically observed at around 1.25 hours after dosing.

Dose-proportional increases in the C_{max} and AUC values of tapentadol have been observed over the 50 to 150 mg dose range.

A multiple (every 6 hour) dose study with doses ranging from 75 to 175 mg tapentadol showed a mean accumulation factor of 1.6 for the parent drug and 1.8 for the major metabolite tapentadol-O-glucuronide, which are primarily determined by the dosing interval and apparent half-life of tapentadol and its metabolite.

Food Effect

The AUC and C_{max} increased by 25% and 16%, respectively, when NUCYNTA® was administered after a high-fat, high-calorie breakfast. NUCYNTA® may be given with or without food.

Distribution

Tapentadol is widely distributed throughout the body. Following intravenous administration, the volume of distribution (Vz) for tapentadol is 540 +/- 98 L. The plasma protein binding is low and amounts to approximately 20%.

Metabolism and Elimination

In humans, about 97% of the parent compound is metabolized. Tapentadol is mainly metabolized via Phase 2 pathways, and only a small amount is metabolized by Phase 1 oxidative pathways. The major pathway of tapentadol metabolism is conjugation with glucuronic acid to produce glucuronides. After oral administration approximately 70% (55% O-glucuronide and 15% sulfate of tapentadol) of the dose is excreted in urine in the conjugated form. A total of 3% of drug was excreted in urine as unchanged drug. Tapentadol is additionally metabolized to N-desmethyl tapentadol (13%) by CYP2C9 and CYP2C19 and to hydroxy tapentadol (2%) by CYP2D6, which are further metabolized by conjugation. Therefore, drug metabolism mediated by cytochrome P450 system is of less importance than phase 2 conjugation.

None of the metabolites contribute to the analgesic activity. Tapentadol and its metabolites are excreted almost exclusively (99%) via the kidneys. The terminal half-life is on average 4 hours after oral administration. The total clearance is 1530 +/- 177 mL/min.

Special Populations

Geriatric Patients

The mean exposure (AUC) to tapentadol was similar in elderly subjects compared to young adults, with a 16% lower mean C_{max} observed in the elderly subject group compared to young adult subjects.

Renal Impairment

AUC and C_{max} of tapentadol were comparable in subjects with varying degrees of renal function (from normal to severely impaired). In contrast, increasing exposure (AUC) to tapentadol-O-glucuronide was observed with increasing degree of renal impairment. In subjects with mild (CL_{CR} = 50 to <80 mL/min), moderate (CL_{CR} = 30 to <50 mL/min), and severe (CL_{CR} = <30 mL/min) renal impairment, the AUC of tapentadol-O-glucuronide was 1.5-, 2.5-, and 5.5-fold higher compared with normal renal function, respectively.

Hepatic Impairment

Administration of NUCYNTA® resulted in higher exposures and serum levels to tapentadol in subjects with impaired hepatic function compared to subjects with normal hepatic function. The ratio of tapentadol pharmacokinetic parameters for the mild hepatic impairment group (Child-Pugh Score 5 to 6) and moderate hepatic impairment group (Child-Pugh Score 7 to 9) in comparison to the normal hepatic function group were 1.7 and 4.2, respectively, for AUC; 1.4 and 2.5, respectively, for C_{max}; and 1.2 and 1.4, respectively, for $t_{1/2}$. The rate of formation of tapentadol-O-glucuronide was lower in subjects with increased liver impairment.

Pharmacokinetic Drug Interactions

Tapentadol is mainly metabolized by Phase 2 glucuronidation, a high capacity/low affinity system; therefore, clinically relevant interactions caused by Phase 2 metabolism are unlikely to occur. Naproxen and probenecid increased the AUC of tapentadol by 17% and 57%, respectively. These changes are not considered clinically relevant and no change in dose is required.

No changes in the pharmacokinetic parameters of tapentadol were observed when acetaminophen and acetylsalicylic acid were given concomitantly.

In vitro studies did not reveal any potential of tapentadol to either inhibit or induce cytochrome P450 enzymes. Furthermore, a minor amount of NUCYNTA® is metabolized via the oxidative pathway. Thus, clinically relevant interactions mediated by the cytochrome P450 system are unlikely to occur.

The pharmacokinetics of tapentadol were not affected when gastric pH or gastrointestinal motility were increased by omeprazole and metoclopramide, respectively.

Plasma protein binding of tapentadol is low (approximately 20%). Therefore, the likelihood of pharmacokinetic drug-drug interactions by displacement from the protein binding site is low.

13 NON-CLINICAL TOXICOLOGY

13.1 Carcinogenesis, Mutagenesis, Impairment of Fertility

Carcinogenesis

Tapentadol was administered to rats (diet) and mice (oral gavage) for two years.

In mice, tapentadol HCl was administered by oral gavage at dosages of 50, 100 and 200 mg/kg/day for 2 years (up to 0.2 times the plasma exposure at the maximum recommended human dose [MRHD] on an area under the time-curve [AUC] basis). No increase in tumor incidence was observed at any dose level.

In rats, tapentadol HCl was administered in diet at dosages of 10, 50, 125 and 250 mg/kg/day for two years (up to 0.2 times in the male rats and 0.6 times in the female rats the MRHD on an AUC basis). No increase in tumor incidence was observed at any dose level.

Mutagenesis

Tapentadol did not induce gene mutations in bacteria, but was clastogenic with metabolic activation in a chromosomal aberration test in V79 cells. The test was repeated and was negative in the presence and absence of metabolic activation. The one positive result for tapentadol was not confirmed *in vivo* in rats, using the two endpoints of chromosomal aberration and unscheduled DNA synthesis, when tested up to the maximum tolerated dose.

Impairment of Fertility

Tapentadol HCl was administered intravenously to male or female rats at dosages of 3, 6, or 12 mg/kg/day (representing exposures of up to approximately 0.4 times the exposure at the MRHD on an AUC basis, based on extrapolation from toxicokinetic analyses in a separate 4-week intravenous study in rats). Tapentadol did not alter fertility at any dose level. Maternal toxicity and adverse effects on embryonic development, including decreased number of implantations, decreased numbers of live conceptuses, and increased pre- and post-implantation losses occurred at dosages ≥6 mg/kg/day.

13.2 Animal Toxicology and/or Pharmacology

In toxicological studies with tapentadol, the most common systemic effects of tapentadol were related to the mu-opioid receptor agonist and norepinephrine reuptake inhibition pharmacodynamic properties of the compound. Transient, dose-dependent and predominantly CNS-related findings were observed, including impaired respiratory function and convulsions, the latter occurring in the dog at plasma levels (C_{max}) which are in the range associated with the maximum recommended human dose (MRHD).

14 CLINICAL STUDIES

The efficacy and safety of NUCYNTA® in the treatment of moderate to severe acute pain has been established in two randomized, double-blind, placebo- and active-controlled studies of moderate to severe pain from first metatarsal bunionectomy and end-stage degenerative joint disease.

14.1 Orthopedic Surgery – Bunionectomy

A randomized, double-blind, parallel-group, active- and placebo-controlled, multiple-dose study demonstrated the efficacy of 50 mg, 75 mg, and 100 mg NUCYNTA® given every 4 to 6 hours for 72 hours in patients aged 18 to 80 years experiencing moderate to severe pain following unilateral, first metatarsal bunionectomy surgery. Patients who qualified for the study with a baseline pain score of ≥4 on an 11-point rating scale ranging from 0 to 10 were randomized to 1 of 5 treatments. Patients were allowed to take a second dose of study medication as soon as 1 hour after the first dose on study Day 1, with subsequent dosing every 4 to 6 hours. If rescue analgesics were required, the patients were discontinued for lack of efficacy. Efficacy was evaluated by comparing the sum of pain intensity difference over the first 48 hours (SPID48) versus placebo. NUCYNTA® at each dose provided a greater reduction in pain compared to placebo based on SPID48 values.

For various degrees of improvement from baseline to the 48-hour endpoint, Figure 1 shows the fraction of patients achieving that level of improvement. The figures are cumulative, such that every patient that achieves a 50% reduction in pain from baseline is included in every level of improvement below 50%. Patients who did not complete the 48-hour observation period in the study were assigned 0% improvement.

Figure 1: Percentage of Patients Achieving Various Levels of Pain Relief as Measured by Pain Severity at 48 Hours Compared to Baseline- Post Operative Bunionectomy

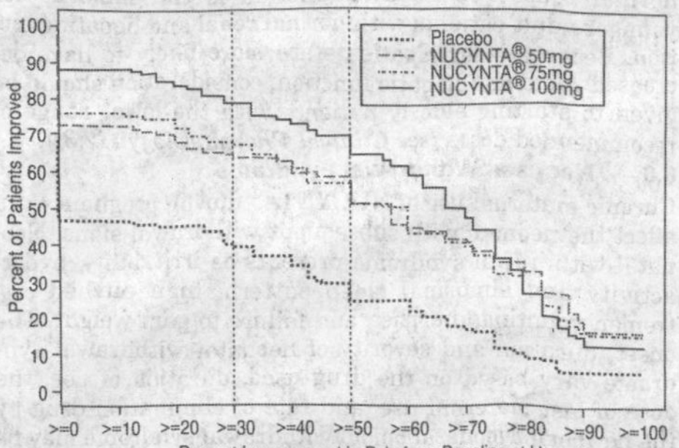

The proportions of patients who showed reduction in pain intensity at 48 hours of 30% or greater, or 50% or greater were significantly higher in patients treated with NUCYNTA® at each dose versus placebo.

14.2 End-Stage Degenerative Joint Disease

A randomized, double-blind, parallel-group, active- and placebo-controlled, multiple-dose study evaluated the efficacy and safety of 50 mg and 75 mg NUCYNTA® given every 4 to 6 hours during waking hours for 10 days in patients aged 18 to 80 years, experiencing moderate to severe pain from end stage degenerative joint disease of the hip or knee, defined as a 3-day mean pain score of ≥5 on an 11-point pain intensity scale, ranging from 0 to 10. Pain scores were assessed twice daily and assessed the pain the patient had experienced over the previous 12 hours. Patients were allowed to continue non-opioid analgesic therapy for which they had been on a stable regimen before screening throughout the study. Eighty-three percent (83%) of patients in the tapentadol treatment groups and the placebo group took such analgesia during the study. The 75 mg treatment group was dosed at 50 mg for the first day of the study, followed by 75 mg for the remaining nine days. Patients requiring rescue analgesics other than study medication were discontinued for lack of efficacy. Efficacy was evaluated by comparing the sum of pain intensity difference (SPID) versus placebo over the first five days of treatment. NUCYNTA® 50 mg and 75 mg provided improvement in pain compared with placebo based on the 5-Day SPID.

For various degrees of improvement from baseline to the Day 5 endpoint, Figure 2 shows the fraction of patients achieving that level of improvement. The figures are cumulative, such that every patient that achieves a 50% reduction in pain from baseline is included in every level of improvement below 50%. Patients who did not complete the 5-day observation period in the study were assigned 0% improvement.

Figure 2: Percentage of Patients Achieving Various Levels of Pain Relief as Measured by Average Pain Severity for the Previous 12 hours, Measured on Study Day 5 Compared to Baseline — End Stage Degenerative Joint Disease

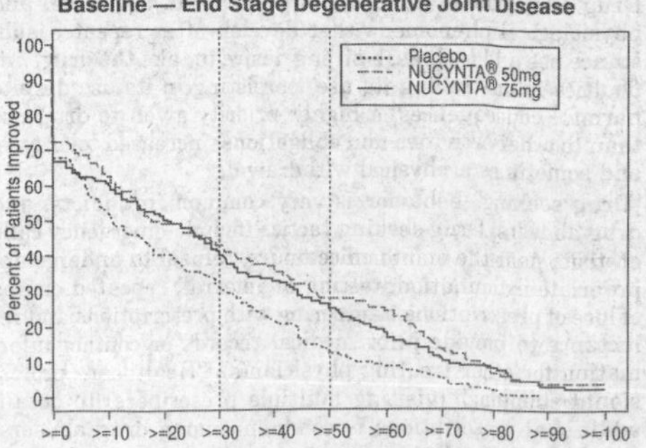

The proportions of patients who showed reduction in pain intensity at 5 days of 30% or greater, or 50% or greater were significantly higher in patients treated with NUCYNTA® at each dose versus placebo.

16 HOW SUPPLIED/STORAGE AND HANDLING

NUCYNTA® Tablets are available in the following strengths and packages. All tablets are round and biconvex-shaped.

50 mg tablets are yellow and debossed with "O-M" on one side and "50" on the other side, and are available in bottles of 100 (NDC 50458-820-04) and hospital unit dose blister packs of 10 (NDC 50458-820-02).

75 mg tablets are yellow-orange and debossed with "O-M" on one side and "75" on the other side, and are available in bottles of 100 (NDC 50458-830-04) and hospital unit dose blister packs of 10 (NDC 50458-830-02).

100 mg tablets are orange and debossed with "O-M" on one side and "100" on the other side, and are available in bottles of 100 (NDC 50458-840-04) and hospital unit dose blister packs of 10 (NDC 50458-840-02).

Storage and Handling

Store up to 25°C (77°F); excursions permitted to 15° – 30°C (59° – 86°F) [see USP Controlled Room Temperature]. Protect from moisture.

Keep NUCYNTA® in a secure place out of reach of children. NUCYNTA® tablets that are no longer needed should be destroyed by flushing down the toilet.

17 PATIENT COUNSELING INFORMATION

Instruct patients to take NUCYNTA® only as prescribed.

Abuse Potential

Inform patients that NUCYNTA® contains tapentadol, a Schedule II controlled substance that is subject to abuse. Instruct patients not to share NUCYNTA® with others and to take steps to protect NUCYNTA® from theft or misuse.

Life-threatening Respiratory Depression

Discuss the risk of respiratory depression with patients, explaining that the risk is greatest when starting NUCYNTA® or when the dose is increased. Advise patients how to recognize respiratory depression and to seek medical attention if they are experiencing breathing difficulties.

Accidental Exposure

Instruct patients to take steps to store NUCYNTA® securely. Accidental exposure, especially in children, may results in serious harm or death. Advise patients to dispose of unused NUCYNTA® by flushing the tablets down the toilet.

Important Administration Instructions

Instruct patients how to properly take NUCYNTA®, including the following:

- Using NUCYNTA® exactly as prescribed to reduce the risk of life-threatening adverse reactions (e.g., respiratory depression).
- Not discontinuing NUCYNTA® without first discussing the need for a tapering regimen with the prescriber.

Risks from Concomitant Use of Alcohol and other CNS Depressants

Inform patients that the concomitant use of alcohol with NUCYNTA® can increase the risk of life-threatening respiratory depression. Instruct patients not to consume alcoholic beverages, as well as prescription and over-the-counter drug products that contain alcohol, during treatment with NUCYNTA®.

Inform patients that potentially serious additive effects may occur if NUCYNTA® is used with other CNS depressants, and not to use such drugs unless supervised by a health care provider.

Concurrent use of MAOI

Inform patients not to take NUCYNTA® while using any drugs that inhibit monoamine oxidase. Patients should not start any new medications while taking NUCYNTA®.

Seizures

Inform patients that NUCYNTA® could cause seizures if they are at risk for seizures or have epilepsy. Patients should be advised to stop taking NUCYNTA® if they have a seizure while taking NUCYNTA® and call their healthcare provider right away.

Serotonin Syndrome

Inform patients that NUCYNTA® could cause a rare but potentially life-threatening condition resulting from concomitant administration of serotonergic drugs (including Serotonin Reuptake Inhibitors, Serotonin and Norepinephrine Reuptake Inhibitors and tricyclic antidepressants). Warn patients of the symptoms of serotonin syndrome and to seek medical attention right away if symptoms develop.

Instruct patients to inform their physicians if they are taking or plan to take additional medications, including CNS Depressants, MAO inhibitors, mixed agonists/antagonist opioid analgesics, anticholinergics, SSRIs, SNRIs, or tricyclic antidepressants.

Hypotension

Inform patients that NUCYNTA® may cause orthostatic hypotension and syncope. Instruct patients how to recognize symptoms of low blood pressure and how to reduce the risk of serious consequences should hypotension occur (e.g., sit or lie down, carefully rise from a sitting or lying position).

Driving or Operating Heavy Machinery

Inform patients that NUCYNTA® may impair the ability to perform potentially hazardous activities such as driving a car or operating heavy machinery. Advise patients not to perform such tasks until they know how they will react to the medication.

Constipation

Advise patients of the potential for severe constipation, including management instructions and when to seek medical attention.

Anaphylaxis

Inform patients that anaphylaxis has been reported with ingredients contained in NUCYNTA®. Advise patients how to recognize such a reaction and when to seek medical attention.

Pregnancy

Advise female patients that NUCYNTA® can cause fetal harm and to inform the prescriber if they are pregnant or plan to become pregnant.

Manufactured by:
Janssen Ortho, LLC
Gurabo, PR 00778
Manufactured for:
Janssen Pharmaceuticals, Inc.
Titusville, NJ 08560
Revised: July 2013

Shown in Product Identification Guide, page 307

NUCYNTA® ER CII

[new-SINN-tah E-R]
(tapentadol)
extended-release oral tablets

HIGHLIGHTS OF PRESCRIBING INFORMATION

These highlights do not include all the information needed to use NUCYNTA® ER safely and effectively. See full prescribing information for NUCYNTA® ER.

NUCYNTA® ER (tapentadol) extended-release oral tablets C-II

Initial U.S. Approval: 2008

WARNING: ABUSE POTENTIAL, LIFE-THREATENING RESPIRATORY DEPRESSION, ACCIDENTAL EXPOSURE, and INTERACTION WITH ALCOHOL

See full prescribing information for complete boxed warning.

- **NUCYNTA® ER contains tapentadol, a Schedule II controlled substance. Monitor for signs of misuse, abuse, and addiction during NUCYNTA® ER therapy. (5.1)**
- **Fatal respiratory depression may occur, with highest risk at initiation and with dose increases. Instruct patients on proper administration of NUCYNTA® ER tablets to reduce the risk. (5.2)**
- **Accidental ingestion of NUCYNTA® ER can result in fatal overdose of tapentadol, especially in children. (5.3)**
- **Instruct patients not to consume alcoholic beverages or use prescription or non-prescription products containing alcohol while taking NUCYNTA® ER because of the risk of increased and potentially fatal plasma tapentadol levels. (5.4)**

RECENT MAJOR CHANGES

Indications and Usage, Neuropathic pain associated with diabetic peripheral neuropathy (1) 8/2012
Dosage and Administration (2) 8/2012

INDICATIONS AND USAGE

NUCYNTA® ER is an opioid agonist indicated for the management of:

- moderate to severe chronic pain in adults (1)
- neuropathic pain associated with diabetic peripheral neuropathy (DPN) in adults (1)

when a continuous, around-the-clock opioid analgesic is needed for an extended period of time.

Limitations of Use

- NUCYNTA® ER is not for use:
  - As an as-needed (prn) analgesic (1)
  - For pain that is mild or not expected to persist for an extended period of time (1)
  - For acute pain (1)
  - For postoperative pain, unless the patient is already receiving chronic opioid therapy prior to surgery, or if the postoperative pain is expected to be moderate to severe and persist for an extended period of time. (1)

DOSAGE AND ADMINISTRATION

Continuous line is replaced with dotted line before and after the headings

- Individualize dosing based on patient's prior analgesic treatment experience, and titrate as needed to provide adequate analgesia and minimize adverse reactions. (2.1, 2.2)
- The initial dose in patients not currently taking opioid analgesics is 50 mg twice a day. (2.1).
- Instruct patients to swallow NUCYNTA® ER tablets whole. (2.7)
- Use a gradual downward titration when NUCYNTA® ER is discontinued in a physically dependent patient. (2.3, 5.13)
- Reduce the dose of NUCYNTA® ER in patients with moderate hepatic impairment. (2.4)
- NUCYNTA® ER use in patients with severe renal impairment is not recommended. (2.5)
- Conservative initial dosing of NUCYNTA® ER in elderly patients is recommended due to possible decreased renal and hepatic function. (2.6)

DOSAGE FORMS AND STRENGTHS

- Extended-Release Tablets: 50 mg, 100 mg, 150 mg, 200 mg, 250 mg (3)

CONTRAINDICATIONS

- Significant respiratory depression (4)
- Acute or severe bronchial asthma, hypercarbia (4)
- Known or suspected paralytic ileus (4)
- Hypersensitivity to tapentadol or to any other ingredients of the product (4)
- Concurrent use of monoamine oxidase inhibitors (MAOI) or use within the last 14 days. (4)

WARNINGS AND PRECAUTIONS

See Boxed WARNINGS

- Elderly, cachectic, and debilitated patients and patients with chronic pulmonary disease: Monitor closely because of increased risk of respiratory depression. (5.5)
- Interaction with CNS depressants: Consider dose reduction of one or both drugs because of additive effects. (5.7, 7.3)
- Hypotensive effect: Monitor during dose initiation and titration. (5.8)
- Patients with head injury or increased intracranial pressure: Monitor for sedation and respiratory depression. Avoid use of NUCYNTA® ER in patients with impaired consciousness or coma susceptible to intracranial effects of CO_2 retention. (5.9)
- Seizures: Use with caution in patients with a history of seizures. (5.10)
- Serotonin Syndrome: Potentially life-threatening condition could result from concomitant administration of drugs with serotonergic activity. (5.11)

ADVERSE REACTIONS

The most common (≥10%) adverse reactions were nausea, constipation, dizziness, headache, and somnolence. (6)

To report SUSPECTED ADVERSE REACTIONS, contact Janssen Pharmaceuticals, Inc. at 1–800–526–7736 (1-800-JANSSEN) or FDA at 1-800-FDA-1088 or *www.fda.gov/medwatch.*

DRUG INTERACTIONS

- CNS depressants: Increased risk of respiratory depression, hypotension, profound sedation, coma or death. When combined therapy with CNS depressant is contemplated, the dose of one or both agents should be reduced. (7.3)
- Mixed agonist/antagonist opioids (i.e., pentazocine, nalbuphine, and butorphanol): May reduce analgesic effect and/or precipitate withdrawal symptoms. (7.5)
- Monitor for signs of serotonin syndrome when NUCYNTA® ER is used concurrently with SSRIs, SNRIs, tricyclic antidepressants, or triptans. (7.4)

USE IN SPECIFIC POPULATIONS

- Pregnancy: Based on animal data, may cause fetal harm. (8.1)
- Nursing mothers: Closely monitor infants of nursing women receiving. NUCYNTA® ER. (8.3)
- Renal or hepatic impairment: not recommended in patients with severe renal or hepatic impairment. Reduce dose in patients with moderate hepatic impairment. (8.7, 8.8)

See 17 for PATIENT COUNSELING INFORMATION and Medication Guide

Revised: 07/2013

FULL PRESCRIBING INFORMATION: CONTENTS*

*** Sections or subsections omitted from the full prescribing information are not listed**

FULL PRESCRIBING INFORMATION

WARNING: ABUSE POTENTIAL, LIFE-THREATENING RESPIRATORY DEPRESSION, ACCIDENTAL EXPOSURE, and INTERACTION WITH ALCOHOL

Abuse Potential

NUCYNTA® ER contains tapentadol, an opioid agonist and Schedule II controlled substance with an abuse liability similar to other opioid agonists, legal or illicit *[see Warnings and Precautions (5.1)]*. Assess each patient's risk for opioid abuse or addiction prior to prescribing NUCYNTA® ER. The risk for opioid abuse is increased in patients with a personal or family history of substance abuse (including drug or alcohol abuse or addiction) or mental illness (e.g., major depressive disorder). Routinely monitor all patients receiving NUCYNTA® ER for signs of misuse, abuse, and addiction during treatment *[see Drug Abuse and Dependence (9)]*.

Life-threatening Respiratory Depression

Respiratory depression, including fatal cases, may occur with use of NUCYNTA® ER, even when the drug has been used as recommended and not misused or abused *[see Warnings and Precautions (5.2)]*. Proper dosing and titration are essential and NUCYNTA® ER should only be prescribed by health-care professionals who are knowledgeable in the use of potent opioids for the management of chronic pain. Monitor for respiratory depression, especially during initiation of NUCYNTA® ER or following a dose increase. Instruct patients to swallow NUCYNTA® ER tablets whole. Crushing, dissolving, or chewing NUCYNTA® ER can cause rapid release and absorption of a potentially fatal dose of tapentadol.

Accidental Exposure

Accidental ingestion of NUCYNTA® ER, especially in children, can result in a fatal overdose of tapentadol *[see Warnings and Precautions (5.3)]*.

Interaction with Alcohol

The co-ingestion of alcohol with NUCYNTA® ER may result in an increase of plasma levels and potentially fatal overdose of tapentadol *[see Warnings and Precautions (5.4)]*. Instruct patients not to consume alcoholic beverages or use prescription or non-prescription products that contain alcohol while on NUCYNTA® ER.

1 INDICATIONS AND USAGE

NUCYNTA® ER (tapentadol) is indicated for the management of:

- moderate to severe chronic pain in adults
- neuropathic pain associated with diabetic peripheral neuropathy (DPN) in adults

when a continuous, around-the-clock opioid analgesic is needed for an extended period of time *[see Clinical Studies (14.1, 14.2)]*.

Limitations of Usage

NUCYNTA® ER is not intended for use:

- As an as-needed (prn) analgesic
- For pain that is mild or not expected to persist for an extended period of time
- For acute pain
- For postoperative pain unless the patient is already receiving chronic opioid therapy prior to surgery or if the postoperative pain is expected to be moderate to severe and persist for an extended period of time.

2 DOSAGE AND ADMINISTRATION

2.1 Initial Dosing

Initiate the dosing regimen for each patient individually, taking into account the patient's prior analgesic treatment experience. Monitor patients closely for respiratory depression, especially within the first 72 hours of initiating therapy with NUCYNTA® ER *[see Warnings and Precautions (5.2)]*.

Consider the following factors when selecting an initial dose of NUCYNTA® ER:

- Total daily dose, potency, and kind of any prior analgesic the patient has been taking previously;
- Reliability of the relative potency estimate used to calculate the equivalent dose of tapentadol needed (Note: potency estimates may vary with the route of administration);
- Patient's degree of opioid experience and opioid tolerance;
- General condition and medical status of the patient;
- Concurrent medication;
- Type and severity of the patient's pain.

NUCYNTA® ER tablets must be taken whole, one tablet at a time, with enough water to ensure complete swallowing immediately after placing in the mouth *[see Patient Counseling Information (17)]*.

NUCYNTA® ER is administered at a frequency of twice daily (every 12 hours).

Discontinue all other tapentadol and tramadol products when beginning and while taking NUCYNTA® ER *[see Warnings and Precautions (5.11)]*. Although the maximum approved total daily dose of NUCYNTA® immediate-release formulation is 600 mg per day, the maximum total daily dose of NUCYNTA® ER is 500 mg. Do not exceed a total daily dose of NUCYNTA® ER of 500 mg.

Use of NUCYNTA® ER as the First Opioid Analgesic

Initiate NUCYNTA® ER therapy with the 50 mg tablet twice daily (at 12 hour intervals).

Conversion from NUCYNTA® to NUCYNTA® ER

Patients can be converted from NUCYNTA® to NUCYNTA® ER using the equivalent total daily dose of NUCYNTA® and dividing it into two equal doses of NUCYNTA® ER separated by approximately 12-hour intervals. As an example, a patient receiving 50 mg of NUCYNTA® four times per day (200 mg/day) may be converted to 100 mg NUCYNTA® ER twice a day.

Conversion from other Opioids to NUCYNTA® ER

While there are useful tables of oral and parenteral equivalents, there is substantial inter-patient variation in the relative potency of different opioid drugs and formulations. Specific recommendations are not available because of a lack of systematic evidence for these types of analgesic substitutions. As such, it is safer to underestimate a patient's 24-hour NUCYNTA® ER requirement and provide rescue medication (e.g., immediate-release opioid or non-opioid) than to overestimate and manage an adverse reaction. In general, begin with half of the estimated daily tapentadol requirement as the initial dose, managing inadequate analgesia by supplementation with immediate-release rescue medication.

Published relative potency/equianalgesia data are available and may be referred to in clinical practice guidelines such as those published by authorities in the field of pain medicine, but such ratios are approximations. Consider contacting your specific state medical or pharmacy professional societies for further information on how to safely convert patients from one opioid to another.

2.2 Titration and Maintenance of Therapy

Individually titrate NUCYNTA® ER to a dose that provides adequate analgesia and minimizes adverse reactions. Continually reevaluate patients receiving NUCYNTA® ER to assess the maintenance of pain control and the relative incidence of adverse reactions. During chronic therapy, especially for non-cancer-related pain (or pain associated with other terminal illnesses), periodically reassess the continued need for the use of opioid analgesics.

Titrate patients to adequate analgesia with dose increases of 50 mg no more than twice daily every three days. In clinical studies, efficacy with NUCYNTA® ER was demonstrated relative to placebo in the dosage range of 100 mg to 250 mg twice daily *[see Clinical Studies (14)]*.

If the level of pain increases, attempt to identify the source of increased pain, while adjusting the NUCYNTA® ER dose to decrease the level of pain.

Patients who experience breakthrough pain may require dosage adjustment or rescue medication with an appropriate dose of an immediate-release opioid or non-opioid medication.

If signs of excessive opioid-related adverse reactions are observed, the next dose may be reduced. Adjust the dose to obtain an appropriate balance between management of pain and opioid-related adverse reactions.

During chronic, around-the-clock opioid therapy, especially for non-cancer pain syndromes, reassess the continued need for around-the-clock opioid therapy regularly (e.g., every 6 to 12 months) as appropriate.

2.3 Discontinuation of NUCYNTA® ER

When the patient no longer requires therapy with NUCYNTA® ER tablets, use a gradual downward titration of the dose to prevent signs and symptoms of withdrawal in the physically-dependent patient.

2.4 Patients with Hepatic Impairment

The use of NUCYNTA® ER in patients with severe hepatic impairment (Child-Pugh Score 10–15) is not recommended.

In patients with moderate hepatic impairment (Child-Pugh Score 7 to 9), initiate treatment using 50 mg NUCYNTA® ER and administer no more frequently than once every 24 hours. The maximum recommended dose for patients with moderate hepatic impairment is 100 mg of NUCYNTA® ER once daily *[see Clinical Pharmacology (12.3)]*.

No dosage adjustment is recommended in patients with mild hepatic impairment (Child-Pugh Score 5 to 6) *[see Warnings and Precautions (5.15)* and *Clinical Pharmacology (12.3)]*.

2.5 Patients with Renal Impairment

No dosage adjustment is recommended in patients with mild or moderate renal impairment. Use of NUCYNTA® ER in patients with severe renal impairment is not recommended *[see Warnings and Precautions (5.16)* and *Clinical Pharmacology (12.3)]*.

2.6 Elderly Patients

In general, recommended dosing for elderly patients with normal renal and hepatic function is the same as for younger adult patients with normal renal and hepatic function. Because elderly patients are more likely to have decreased renal and hepatic function, consideration should be given to starting elderly patients with the lower range of recommended doses *[see Clinical Pharmacology (12.3)]*.

2.7 Administration of NUCYNTA® ER

Instruct patients to swallow NUCYNTA® ER tablets whole. The tablets are not to be cut, crushed, dissolved, or chewed due to the risk of rapid release and absorption of a potentially fatal dose of tapentadol *[see Warnings and Precautions (5.1, 5.2)]*.

Instruct patients to take NUCYNTA® ER one tablet at a time and with enough water to ensure complete swallowing immediately after placing in the mouth *[see Warnings and Precautions (5.2),* and *Patient Counseling Information (17)]*.

3 DOSAGE FORMS AND STRENGTHS

NUCYNTA® ER 50 mg, 100 mg, 150 mg, 200 mg and 250 mg extended-release tablets are available in the following colors and prints:

- 50 mg extended-release tablets are white oblong-shaped with a black print "OMJ 50" on one side
- 100 mg extended-release tablets are light-blue oblong-shaped with a black print "OMJ 100" on one side
- 150 mg extended-release tablets are blue-green oblong-shaped with a black print "OMJ 150" on one side
- 200 mg extended-release tablets are blue oblong-shaped with a depression in the middle running lengthwise on each side and a black print "OMJ 200" on one side
- 250 mg extended-release tablets are dark blue oblong-shaped with a depression in the middle running lengthwise on each side and a white print "OMJ 250" on one side.

4 CONTRAINDICATIONS

NUCYNTA® ER is contraindicated in:

- Patients with significant respiratory depression
- Patients with acute or severe bronchial asthma or hypercarbia in an unmonitored setting or in the absence of resuscitative equipment
- Patients with known or suspected paralytic ileus
- Patients with hypersensitivity (e.g. anaphylaxis, angioedema) to tapentadol or to any other ingredients of the product *[see Adverse Reactions (6.2)]*.
- Patients who are receiving monoamine oxidase inhibitors (MAOI) or who have taken them within the last 14 days due to potential additive effects on norepinephrine levels which may result in adverse cardiovascular events *[see Drug Interactions(7.2)]*.

5 WARNINGS AND PRECAUTIONS

5.1 Abuse Potential

NUCYNTA® ER contains tapentadol, an opioid agonist and a Schedule II controlled substance. Tapentadol can be abused in a manner similar to other opioid agonists legal or illicit. Opioid agonists are sought by drug abusers and people with addiction disorders and are subject to criminal diversion. Consider these risks when prescribing or dispensing NUCYNTA® ER in situations where there is concern about increased risks of misuse, abuse, or diversion. Concerns about abuse, addiction, and diversion should not, however, prevent the proper management of pain.

Assess each patient's risk for opioid abuse or addiction prior to prescribing NUCYNTA® ER. The risk for opioid abuse is increased in patients with a personal or family history of substance abuse (including drug or alcohol abuse or addiction) or mental illness (e.g., major depression). Patients at increased risk may still be appropriately treated with modified-release opioid formulations; however these patients will require intensive monitoring for signs of misuse, abuse, or addiction. Routinely monitor all patients receiving opioids for signs of misuse, abuse, and addiction because these drugs carry a risk for addiction even under appropriate medical use.

Misuse or abuse of NUCYNTA® ER by crushing, chewing, snorting, or injecting the dissolved product will result in the uncontrolled delivery of the opioid and pose a significant risk that could result in overdose and death *[see Overdosage (10)]*.

Contact local state professional licensing board or state controlled substances authority for information on how to prevent and detect abuse or diversion of this product *[see Drug Abuse and Dependence (9)]*.

5.2 Life Threatening Respiratory Depression

Respiratory depression is the chief hazard of opioid agonists, including NUCYNTA® ER. Respiratory depression, if not immediately recognized and treated, may lead to respiratory arrest and death. Respiratory depression from opioids is manifested by a reduced urge to breathe and a decreased rate of respiration, often associated with a "sighing" pattern of breathing (deep breaths separated by abnormally long pauses). Carbon dioxide (CO_2) retention from opioid-induced respiratory depression can exacerbate the sedating effects of opioids. Management of respiratory depression may include close observation, supportive measures, and use of opioid antagonists, depending on the patient's clinical status *[see Overdosage (10)]*.

While serious, life-threatening, or fatal respiratory depression can occur at any time during the use of NUCYNTA® ER, the risk is greatest during the initiation of therapy or following a dose increase. Closely monitor patients for respiratory depression when initiating therapy with NUCYNTA® ER and following dose increases. Instruct patients against use by individuals other than the patient for whom NUCYNTA® ER was prescribed and to keep NUCYNTA® ER out of the reach of children, as such inappropriate use may result in fatal respiratory depression.

To reduce the risk of respiratory depression, proper dosing and titration of NUCYNTA® ER are essential *[see Dosage and Administration (2)]*. Overestimating the NUCYNTA® ER dose when converting patients from another opioid product can result in fatal overdose with the first dose. Respiratory depression has also been reported with use of modified-release opioids when used as recommended and not misused or abused.

To further reduce the risk of respiratory depression, consider the following:

- Proper dosing and titration are essential and NUCYNTA® ER should only be prescribed by healthcare professionals who are knowledgeable in the use of potent opioids for the management of chronic pain.
- Instruct patients to swallow NUCYNTA® ER tablets whole. The tablets are not to be cut, crushed, dissolved, or chewed. The resulting tapentadol dose may be fatal, particularly in opioid-naïve individuals.
- NUCYNTA® ER is contraindicated in patients with respiratory depression and in patients with conditions that increase the risk of life-threatening respiratory depression *[see Contraindications (4)]*.

5.3 Accidental Exposure

Accidental ingestion of NUCYNTA® ER, especially in children, can result in a fatal overdose of tapentadol.

5.4 Interaction with Alcohol

The co-ingestion of alcohol with NUCYNTA® ER can result in an increase of tapentadol plasma levels and potentially fatal overdose of tapentadol. Instruct patients not to consume alcoholic beverages or use prescription or non-prescription products containing alcohol while on NUCYNTA® ER therapy *[see Drug Interactions (7.1)* and *Clinical Pharmacology (12.3)]*.

5.5 Elderly, Cachectic, and Debilitated Patients

Respiratory depression is more likely to occur in elderly, cachectic, or debilitated patients as they may have altered pharmacokinetics or altered clearance compared to younger, healthier patients. Therefore, closely monitor such patients, particularly when initiating and titrating NUCYNTA® ER and when NUCYNTA® ER is given concomitantly with other drugs that depress respiration *[see Warnings and Precautions (5.2)]*.

5.6 Use in Patients with Chronic Pulmonary Disease

Monitor for respiratory depression those patients with significant chronic obstructive pulmonary disease or cor pulmonale, and patients having a substantially decreased respiratory reserve, hypoxia, hypercarbia, or pre-existing respiratory depression, particularly when initiating therapy and titrating with NUCYNTA® ER, as in these patients, even usual therapeutic doses of NUCYNTA® ER may decrease respiratory drive to the point of apnea *[see Warnings and Precautions (5.2)]*. Consider the use of alternative non-opioid analgesics in these patients if possible.

5.7 Interactions with CNS Depressants and Illicit Drugs

Hypotension, and profound sedation, coma or respiratory depression may result if NUCYNTA® ER is used concomitantly with other CNS depressants (e.g., sedatives, anxiolytics, hypnotics, neuroleptics, muscle relaxants, other opioids and illicit drugs). When considering the use of NUCYNTA® ER in a patient taking a CNS depressant, assess the duration of use of the CNS depressant and the patient's response, including the degree of tolerance that has developed to CNS depression. Additionally, consider the patient's use, if any, of alcohol and/or illicit drugs that can cause CNS depression. If NUCYNTA® ER therapy is to be initiated in a patient taking a CNS depressant, start with a lower NUCYNTA® ER dose than usual and monitor patients for signs of sedation and respiratory depression and consider using a lower dose of the concomitant CNS depressant *[see Drug Interactions (7.3)]*.

5.8 Hypotensive Effect

NUCYNTA® ER may cause severe hypotension. There is an increased risk in patients whose ability to maintain blood pressure has already been compromised by a reduced blood volume or concurrent administration of certain CNS depressant drugs (e.g., phenothiazines or general anesthetics) *[see Drug Interactions (7.3)]*. Monitor these patients for signs of hypotension after initiating or titrating the dose of NUCYNTA® ER. In patients with circulatory shock, NUCYNTA® ER may cause vasodilation that can further reduce cardiac output and blood pressure. Avoid the use of NUCYNTA® ER in patients with circulatory shock.

5.9 Use in Patients with Head Injury or Increased Intracranial Pressure

Monitor patients taking NUCYNTA® ER who may be susceptible to the intracranial effects of CO_2 retention (e.g., those with evidence of increased intracranial pressure or brain tumors) for signs of sedation and respiratory depression, particularly when initiating therapy with NUCYNTA® ER. NUCYNTA® ER may reduce respiratory drive, and the resultant CO_2 retention can further increase intracranial pressure. Opioids may also obscure the clinical course in a patient with a head injury.

Avoid the use of NUCYNTA® ER in patients with impaired consciousness or coma.

5.10 Seizures

NUCYNTA® ER has not been evaluated in patients with a predisposition to a seizure disorder, and such patients were excluded from clinical studies. The active ingredient tapentadol in NUCYNTA® ER may aggravate convulsions in patients with convulsive disorders, and may induce or aggravate seizures in some clinical settings. Monitor patients with a history of seizure disorders for worsened seizure control during NUCYNTA® ER therapy.

5.11 Serotonin Syndrome Risk

Cases of life-threatening serotonin syndrome have been reported with the concurrent use of tapentadol and serotonergic drugs. Serotonergic drugs comprise Selective Serotonin Reuptake Inhibitors (SSRIs), Serotonin and Norepinephrine Reuptake Inhibitors (SNRIs), tricyclic antidepressants (TCAs), triptans, drugs that affect the serotonergic neurotransmitter system (e.g. mirtazapine, trazodone, and tramadol), and drugs that impair metabolism of serotonin (including MAOIs). This may occur within the recommended dose. Serotonin syndrome may include mental-status changes (e.g., agitation, hallucinations, coma), autonomic instability (e.g., tachycardia, labile blood pressure, hyperthermia), neuromuscular aberrations (e.g., hyperreflexia, incoordination) and/or gastrointestinal symptoms (e.g., nausea, vomiting, diarrhea) and can be fatal *[see Drug Interactions (7.4)]*.

5.12 Use in Patients with Gastrointestinal Conditions

NUCYNTA® ER is contraindicated in patients with GI obstruction, including paralytic ileus. The tapentadol in NUCYNTA® ER may cause spasm of the sphincter of Oddi. Monitor patients with biliary tract disease, including acute pancreatitis, for worsening symptoms.

5.13 Avoidance of Withdrawal

Avoid the use of mixed agonist/antagonist analgesics (i.e., pentazocine, nalbuphine, and butorphanol) in patients who have received or are receiving a course of therapy with a full opioid agonist analgesic, including NUCYNTA® ER. In these patients, mixed agonists/antagonists analgesics may reduce the analgesic effect and/or may precipitate withdrawal symptoms.

When discontinuing NUCYNTA® ER, gradually taper the dose *[see Dosage and Administration (2.3)]*.

5.14 Driving and Operating Heavy Machinery

NUCYNTA® ER may impair the mental or physical abilities needed to perform potentially hazardous activities such as driving a car or operating machinery. Warn patients not to drive or operate dangerous machinery unless they are tolerant to the effects of NUCYNTA® ER and know how they will react to the medication.

5.15 Hepatic Impairment

A study with an immediate-release formulation of tapentadol in subjects with hepatic impairment showed higher serum concentrations of tapentadol than in those with normal hepatic function. Avoid use of NUCYNTA® ER in patients with severe hepatic impairment. Reduce the dose of NUCYNTA® ER in patients with moderate hepatic impairment *[see Dosage and Administration (2.4) and Clinical Pharmacology (12.3)]*. Closely monitor patients with moderate hepatic impairment for respiratory and central nervous system depression when initiating and titrating NUCYNTA® ER.

5.16 Renal Impairment

Use of NUCYNTA® ER in patients with severe renal impairment is not recommended due to accumulation of a metabolite formed by glucuronidation of tapentadol. The clinical relevance of the elevated metabolite is not known *[see Clinical Pharmacology (12.3)]*.

6 ADVERSE REACTIONS

The following adverse reactions are discussed in more detail in other sections of the labeling:

- Respiratory Depression *[see Warnings and Precautions (5.2)]*
- Interaction with Alcohol *[see Warnings and Precautions (5.4)]*
- Chronic Pulmonary Disease *[see Warnings and Precautions (5.6)]*
- Hypotensive Effects *[see Warnings and Precautions (5.8)]*
- Interactions with Other CNS Depressants *[see Warnings and Precautions (5.7)]*
- Drug abuse, addiction, and dependence *[see Drug Abuse and Dependence (9.2, 9.3)]*
- Gastrointestinal Effects *[see Warnings and Precautions (5.12)]*
- Seizures *[see Warnings and Precautions (5.10)]*
- Serotonin Syndrome *[see Warnings and Precautions (5.11)]*

6.1 Clinical Studies Experience

Because clinical trials are conducted under widely varying conditions, adverse reaction rates observed in the clinical trials of a drug cannot be directly compared to rates in the clinical trials of another drug and may not reflect the rates observed in clinical practice.

Commonly-Observed Adverse Reactions in Clinical Studies with NUCYNTA® ER in Patients with Chronic Pain due to Low Back Pain or Osteoarthritis

The safety data described in Table 1 below are based on three pooled, randomized, double-blind, placebo-controlled, parallel group, 15-week studies of NUCYNTA® ER (dosed 100 to 250 mg BID after a 50 mg BID starting dose) in patients with chronic pain due to low back pain (LBP) and osteoarthritis (OA). These trials included 980 NUCYNTA® ER-treated patients and 993 placebo-treated patients. The mean age was 57 years old; 63% were female and 37% were male; 83% were White, 10% were Black, and 5% were Hispanic.

The most common adverse reactions (reported by ≥10% in any NUCYNTA® ER dose group) were: nausea, constipation, dizziness, headache, and somnolence.

The most common reasons for discontinuation due to adverse reactions in eight Phase 2/3 pooled studies reported by ≥1% in any NUCYNTA® ER dose group for NUCYNTA® ER- and placebo-treated patients were nausea (4% vs. 1%), dizziness (3% vs. <1%), vomiting (3% vs. <1%), somnolence (2% vs. <1%), constipation (1% vs. <1%), headache (1% vs. <1%), and fatigue (1% vs. <1%), respectively.

Table 1: Adverse Drug Reactions Reported by ≥ 1% of NUCYNTA® ER-Treated Patients and Greater than Placebo-treated Patients in Pooled Parallel-Group Trials*

	NUCYNTA® ER 50 to 250 mg BID† (n=980)	Placebo (n=993)
Nausea	21%	7%
Constipation	17%	7%
Dizziness	17%	6%
Headache	15%	13%
Somnolence	12%	4%
Fatigue	9%	4%
Vomiting	8%	3%
Dry mouth	7%	2%
Hyperhidrosis	5%	<1%
Pruritus	5%	2%
Insomnia	4%	2%
Dyspepsia	3%	2%
Lethargy	2%	<1%
Asthenia	2%	<1%
Anxiety	2%	1%
Decreased appetite	2%	<1%
Vertigo	2%	<1%
Hot flush	2%	<1%
Disturbance in attention	1%	<1%
Tremor	1%	<1%
Chills	1%	0%
Abnormal dreams	1%	<1%
Depression	1%	<1%
Vision blurred	1%	<1%
Erectile dysfunction	1%	<1%

* MedDRA preferred terms. The trials included forced titration during the first week of dosing.

† NUCYNTA® ER dosed between 100 and 250 mg BID after a starting dose of 50 mg BID

Commonly-Observed Adverse Reactions in Clinical Studies with NUCYNTA® ER in Patients with Neuropathic Pain Associated with Diabetic Peripheral Neuropathy

The types of adverse reactions seen in the studies of patients with painful diabetic peripheral neuropathy (DPN) were similar to what was seen in the low back pain and osteoarthritis trials. The safety data described in Table 2 below are based on two pooled, randomized withdrawal, double-blind, placebo-controlled, 12-week studies of NUCYNTA® ER (dosed 100 to 250 mg BID) in patients with neuropathic pain associated with diabetic peripheral neuropathy. These trials included 1040 NUCYNTA® ER-treated patients and 343 placebo-treated patients. The mean age was 60 years old; 40% were female and 60% were male; 76% were White, 12% were Black, and 12% were "Other". The most commonly reported ADRs (incidence ≥ 10% in NUCYNTA® ER-treated subjects) were: nausea, constipation, vomiting, dizziness, somnolence, and headache.

Table 2 lists the common adverse reactions reported in 1% or more of NUCYNTA® ER-treated patients and greater than placebo-treated patients with neuropathic pain associated with diabetic peripheral neuropathy in the two pooled studies.

Table 2: Adverse Drug Reactions Reported by ≥ 1% of NUCYNTA® ER-Treated Patients and Greater than Placebo-Treated Patients in Pooled Trials (Studies DPN-1 and DPN-2) *

	NUCYNTA® ER 50 to 250 mg BID† (n=1040)	Placebo‡ (n=343)
Nausea	27%	8%
Dizziness	18%	2%
Somnolence	14%	<1%
Constipation	13%	<1%
Vomiting	12%	3%
Headache	10%	5%
Fatigue	9%	<1%
Pruritus	8%	0%
Dry mouth	7%	<1%
Diarrhea	7%	5%
Decreased appetite	6%	<1%
Anxiety	5%	4%
Insomnia	4%	3%
Hyperhidrosis	3%	2%
Hot flush	3%	2%
Tremor§	3%	3%
Abnormal dreams	2%	0%
Lethargy	2%	0%
Asthenia	2%	<1%
Irritability	2%	1%
Dyspnea	1%	0%
Nervousness	1%	0%
Sedation	1%	0%
Vision blurred	1%	0%
Pruritus generalized	1%	0%
Vertigo	1%	<1%
Abdominal discomfort	1%	<1%
Hypotension	1%	<1%
Dyspepsia	1%	<1%
Hypoesthesia	1%	<1%
Depression	1%	<1%
Rash	1%	<1%
Chills§	1%	1%
Feeling cold§	1%	1%
Drug withdrawal syndrome	1%	<1%

* MedDRA preferred terms.

† NUCYNTA® ER dosed between 100 and 250 mg BID after a starting dose of 50 mg BID. It includes ADR reported in the open-label titration period for all subjects and in the double-blind maintenance period for the subjects who were randomized to NUCYNTA® ER.

‡ It includes ADR reported in the double-blind maintenance period for the subjects who were randomized to placebo after receiving NUCYNTA® ER during the open-label titration period.

§ Tremor was observed in 3.4% of NUCYNTA® ER-treated subjects vs. 3.2% in placebo group, chills- in 1.3% vs.1.2% in placebo, and feeling cold- in 1.3% vs.1.2% in placebo.

Other Adverse Reactions Observed During the Premarketing Evaluation of NUCYNTA® ER

The following additional adverse drug reactions occurred in less than 1% of NUCYNTA® ER-treated patients in ten Phase 2/3 clinical studies:

Nervous System Disorders: paresthesia, balance disorder, syncope, memory impairment, mental impairment, depressed level of consciousness, dysarthria, presyncope, coordination abnormal

Gastrointestinal disorders: impaired gastric emptying

General disorders and administration site conditions: feeling abnormal, feeling drunk

Psychiatric disorders: perception disturbances, disorientation, confusional state, agitation, euphoric mood, drug dependence, thinking abnormal, nightmare

Skin and subcutaneous tissue disorders: urticaria

Metabolism and nutrition disorders: weight decreased

Cardiac disorders: heart rate increased, palpitations, heart rate decreased, left bundle branch block

Vascular Disorder: blood pressure decreased

Respiratory, thoracic and mediastinal disorders: respiratory depression

Renal and urinary disorders: urinary hesitation, pollakiuria

Reproductive system and breast disorders: sexual dysfunction

Eye disorders: visual disturbance

Immune system disorders: drug hypersensitivity

6.2 Postmarketing Experience

The following adverse reactions, not noted in Section 6.1 above, have been identified during post approval use of tapentadol. Because these reactions are reported voluntarily from a population of uncertain size, it is not always possible to reliably estimate their frequency or establish a causal relationship to drug exposure.

Psychiatric disorders: hallucination, suicidal ideation

Anaphylaxis, angioedema, and anaphylactic shock have been reported very rarely with ingredients contained in NUCYNTA® ER. Advise patients how to recognize such reactions and when to seek medical attention.

7 DRUG INTERACTIONS

7.1 Alcohol

Concomitant use of alcohol with NUCYNTA® ER can result in an increase of tapentadol plasma levels and potentially fatal overdose of tapentadol. Instruct patients not to consume alcoholic beverages or use prescription or non-prescription products containing alcohol while on NUCYNTA® ER therapy *[see Clinical Pharmacology (12.3)]*.

7.2 Monoamine Oxidase Inhibitors

NUCYNTA® ER is contraindicated in patients who are receiving monoamine oxidase inhibitors (MAOI) or who have taken them within the last 14 days due to potential additive effects on norepinephrine levels, which may result in adverse cardiovascular events *[see Contraindications (4)]*.

7.3 CNS Depressants

Concurrent use of NUCYNTA® ER and other central nervous system (CNS) depressants including sedatives or hypnotics, general anesthetics, phenothiazines, tranquilizers, and alcohol can increase the risk of respiratory depression, hypotension, profound sedation or coma. Monitor patients receiving CNS depressants and NUCYNTA® ER for signs of respiratory depression and hypotension. When such combined therapy is contemplated, start NUCYNTA® ER at ⅓ to ½ of the usual dosage and consider using a lower dose of the concomitant CNS depressant *[see Warnings and Precautions (5.7)]*.

7.4 Serotonergic Drugs

There have been post-marketing reports of serotonin syndrome with the concomitant use of tapentadol and serotonergic drugs (e.g., SSRIs and SNRIs). Caution is advised when NUCYNTA® ER is co-administered with other drugs that may affect serotonergic neurotransmitter systems such as SSRIs, SNRIs, MAOIs, and triptans. If concomitant treatment of NUCYNTA® ER with a drug affecting the serotonergic neurotransmitter system is clinically warranted, careful observation of the patient is advised, particularly during treatment initiation and dose increases *[see Warning and Precautions (5.11)]*.

7.5 Mixed Agonist/Antagonist Opioid Analgesics

The concomitant use of NUCYNTA® ER with mixed agonist/antagonists (e.g., butorphanol, nalbuphine, and pentazocine) and partial agonists (e.g., buprenorphine) may precipitate withdrawal symptoms. Avoid the use of agonist/antagonists and partial agonists with NUCYNTA® ER.

7.6 Anticholinergics

The use of NUCYNTA® ER with anticholinergic products may increase the risk of urinary retention and/or severe constipation, which may lead to paralytic ileus.

8 USE IN SPECIFIC POPULATIONS

8.1 Pregnancy

Pregnancy Category C: There are no adequate and well-controlled studies of NUCYNTA® ER in pregnant women. NUCYNTA® ER should be used during pregnancy only if the potential benefit justifies the potential risk to the fetus.

Tapentadol HCl was evaluated for teratogenic effects in pregnant rats and rabbits following intravenous and subcutaneous exposure during the period of embryofetal organogenesis. When tapentadol was administered twice daily by the subcutaneous route in rats at dose levels of 10, 20, or 40 mg/kg/day [producing up to 1.36 times the plasma exposure at the maximum recommended human dose (MRHD) of 500 mg/day for NUCYNTA® ER based on an area under the time-curve (AUC) comparison], no teratogenic effects were observed. Evidence of embryofetal toxicity included transient delays in skeletal maturation (i.e., reduced ossification) at the 40 mg/kg/day dose which was associated with significant maternal toxicity. Administration of tapentadol HCl in rabbits at doses of 4, 10, or 24 mg/kg/day by subcutaneous injection [producing 0.3, 0.8, and 2.5 times the plasma exposure at the MRHD based on an AUC comparison, respectively] revealed embryofetal toxicity at doses ≥10 mg/kg/day. Findings included reduced fetal viability, skeletal delays and other variations. In addition, there were multiple malformations including gastroschisis/thoracogastroschisis, amelia/phocomelia, and cleft palate at doses ≥10 mg/kg/day and above, and ablepharia, encephalopathy, and spina bifida at the high dose of 24 mg/kg/day. Embryofetal toxicity, including malformations, may be secondary to the significant maternal toxicity observed in the study.

In a study of pre- and postnatal development in rats, oral administration of tapentadol at doses of 20, 50, 150, or 300 mg/kg/day to pregnant and lactating rats during the late gestation and early postnatal period [resulting in up to 2.28 times the plasma exposure at the MRHD on an AUC basis] did not influence physical or reflex development, the outcome of neurobehavioral tests or reproductive parameters. At maternal tapentadol doses ≥150 mg/kg/day, a dose-related increase in pup mortality was observed to postnatal Day 4. Treatment-related developmental delay was observed in the dead pups, including incomplete ossification. In addition, significant reductions in pup body weights and body weight gains at doses associated with maternal toxicity (150 mg/kg/day and above) was seen throughout lactation.

8.2 Labor and Delivery

NUCYNTA® ER is not for use in women during and immediately prior to labor, where shorter acting analgesics or other analgesic techniques are more appropriate. Occasionally, opioid analgesics may prolong labor by temporarily reducing the strength, duration, and frequency of uterine contractions. However, these effects are not consistent and may be offset by an increased rate of cervical dilatation which tends to shorten labor.

Opioids cross the placenta and may produce respiratory depression and psychophysiologic effects in neonates. Closely observe neonates whose mothers received opioid analgesics during labor for signs of respiratory depression. An opioid antagonist, such as naloxone, should be available for reversal of opioid-induced respiratory depression in the neonate in such situations.

8.3 Nursing Mothers

There is insufficient/limited information on the excretion of tapentadol in human or animal breast milk. Physicochemical and available pharmacodynamic/toxicological data on tapentadol point to excretion in breast milk and risk to the breastfeeding child cannot be excluded.

Because of the potential for adverse reactions in nursing infants from NUCYNTA® ER, a decision should be made whether to discontinue nursing or discontinue the drug, taking into account the importance of the drug to the mother.

Withdrawal symptoms can occur in breast-feeding infants when maternal administration of NUCYNTA® ER is stopped.

8.4 Pediatric Use

The safety and efficacy of NUCYNTA® ER in pediatric patients less than 18 years of age have not been established.

8.5 Geriatric Use

Of the total number of patients in Phase 2/3 double-blind, multiple-dose clinical studies of NUCYNTA® ER, 28% (1023/3613) were 65 years and over, while 7% (245/3613) were 75 years and over. No overall differences in effectiveness or tolerability were observed between these patients and younger patients.

In general, recommended dosing for elderly patients with normal renal and hepatic function is the same as for younger adult patients with normal renal and hepatic function. Because elderly patients are more likely to have decreased renal and hepatic function, consideration should be given to starting elderly patients with the lower range of recommended doses *[see Clinical Pharmacology (12.3)]*.

8.6 Neonatal Withdrawal Syndrome

Chronic maternal use of NUCYNTA® ER during pregnancy can affect the neonate with subsequent withdrawal signs. Neonatal withdrawal syndrome presents as irritability, hyperactivity and abnormal sleep pattern, high pitched cry, tremor, vomiting, diarrhea and failure to gain weight. The onset, duration and severity of neonatal withdrawal syndrome vary based on the drug used, duration of use, the dose of last maternal use, and rate of elimination drug by the newborn. Neonatal opioid withdrawal syndrome may be life-threatening and should be treated according to protocols developed by neonatology experts.

8.7 Renal Impairment

The safety and effectiveness of NUCYNTA® ER has not been established in patients with severe renal impairment (CL_{CR} <30 mL/min). Use of NUCYNTA® ER in patients with severe renal impairment is not recommended due to accumulation of a metabolite formed by glucuronidation of tapentadol. The clinical relevance of the elevated metabolite is not known *[see Clinical Pharmacology (12.3)]*.

8.8 Hepatic Impairment

Administration of tapentadol resulted in higher exposures and serum levels of tapentadol in subjects with impaired hepatic function compared to subjects with normal hepatic function *[see Clinical Pharmacology (12.3)]*. The dose of NUCYNTA® ER should be reduced in patients with moderate hepatic impairment (Child-Pugh Score 7 to 9) *[see Dosage and Administration (2.4)]*.

Use of NUCYNTA® ER is not recommended in severe hepatic impairment (Child-Pugh Score 10 to 15) *[see Warnings and Precautions (5.15)]*.

9 DRUG ABUSE AND DEPENDENCE

9.1 Controlled Substance

NUCYNTA® ER contains tapentadol, a Schedule II controlled substance with a high potential for abuse similar to fentanyl, methadone, morphine, oxycodone, and oxymorphone. NUCYNTA® ER is subject to misuse, abuse, addiction, and criminal diversion *[see Warnings and Precautions (5.1)]*. The high drug content in the extended release formulation adds to the risk of adverse outcomes from abuse and misuse.

9.2 Abuse

All patients treated with opioids require careful monitoring for signs of abuse and addiction, because use of opioid analgesic products carries the risk of addiction even under appropriate medical use.

Drug abuse is the intentional non-therapeutic use of an over-the-counter or prescription drug, even once, for its rewarding psychological or physiological effects. Drug abuse includes, but is not limited to the following examples: the use of a prescription or over-the-counter drug to get "high", or the use of steroids for performance enhancement and muscle build up.

Drug addiction is a cluster of behavioral, cognitive, and physiological phenomena that develop after repeated substance use and include: a strong desire to take the drug, difficulties in controlling its use, persisting in its use despite harmful consequences, a higher priority given to drug use than to other activities and obligations, increased tolerance, and sometimes a physical withdrawal.

"Drug-seeking" behavior is very common to addicts and drug abusers. Drug-seeking tactics include emergency calls or visits near the end of office hours, refusal to undergo appropriate examination, testing or referral, repeated claims of loss of prescriptions, tampering with prescriptions and reluctance to provide prior medical records or contact information for other treating physician(s). "Healthcare professional shopping" (visiting multiple prescribers) to obtain additional prescriptions is common among drug abusers, people suffering from untreated addiction and criminals seeking drugs to sell.

Abuse and addiction are separate and distinct from physical dependence and tolerance. Physicians should be aware that addiction may not be accompanied by concurrent tolerance and symptoms of physical dependence in all addicts. In addition, abuse of opioids can occur in the absence of true addiction and is characterized by misuse for non-medical purposes, often in combination with other psychoactive substances.

NUCYNTA® ER can be diverted for non-medical use into illicit channels of distribution. Careful record-keeping of prescribing information, including quantity, frequency, and renewal requests, as required by law, is strongly advised.

Proper assessment of the patient, proper prescribing practices, periodic re-evaluation of therapy, and proper dispensing and storage are appropriate measures that help to limit abuse of opioid drugs.

9.3 Dependence

Both tolerance and physical dependence can develop during chronic opioid therapy. Tolerance is the need for increasing doses of opioids to maintain a defined effect such as analgesia (in the absence of disease progression or other external factors). Tolerance may occur to both the desired and undesired effects of drugs, and may develop at different rates for different effects.

Physical dependence results in withdrawal symptoms after abrupt discontinuation or a significant dose reduction of a drug. Withdrawal also may be precipitated through the administration of drugs with opioid antagonist activity, e.g., naloxone, nalmefene, or mixed agonist/antagonist analgesics (pentazocine, butorphanol, buprenorphine, nalbuphine). Physical dependence may not occur to a clinically significant degree until after several days to weeks of continued opioid usage.

NUCYNTA® ER should be discontinued by a gradual downward titration *[see Dosage and Administration (2.3)]*. If NUCYNTA® ER is abruptly discontinued in a physically-dependent patient, an abstinence syndrome may occur. Some or all of the following can characterize this syndrome: restlessness, lacrimation, rhinorrhea, yawning, perspiration, chills, piloerection, myalgia, mydriasis, irritability, anxiety, backache, joint pain, weakness, abdominal cramps, insomnia, nausea, anorexia, vomiting, diarrhea, increased blood pressure, respiratory rate, or heart rate.

Infants born to mothers physically dependent on opioids will also be physically dependent and may exhibit respiratory difficulties and withdrawal symptoms *[see Use in Specific Populations (8.1, 8.2, 8.6)]*.

10 OVERDOSAGE

10.1 Clinical Presentation

Acute overdosage with opioids can be manifested by respiratory depression, somnolence progressing to stupor or coma, skeletal muscle flaccidity, cold and clammy skin, constricted pupils, and sometimes pulmonary edema, bradycardia, hypotension and death. Marked mydriasis rather than miosis may be seen due to severe hypoxia in overdose situations.

10.2 Management

In case of overdose, priorities are the re-establishment of a patent and protected airway and institution of assisted or controlled ventilation if needed. Employ other supportive measures (including oxygen, vasopressors) in the management of circulatory shock and pulmonary edema as indicated. Cardiac arrest or arrhythmias will require advanced life support techniques.

The opioid antagonists, naloxone or nalmefene, are specific antidotes to respiratory depression resulting from opioid overdose. Opioid antagonists should not be administered in the absence of clinically significant respiratory or circulatory depression secondary to tapentadol overdose. Such agents should be administered cautiously to patients who are known, or suspected to be, physically dependent on NUCYNTA® ER. In such cases, an abrupt or complete reversal of opioid effects may precipitate an acute withdrawal syndrome.

Because the duration of reversal would be expected to be less than the duration of action of tapentadol in NUCYNTA® ER, carefully monitor the patient until spontaneous respiration is reliably re-established. NUCYNTA® ER will continue to release tapentadol adding to the tapentadol load for up to 24 hours after administration necessitating prolonged monitoring. If the response to opioid antagonists is suboptimal or not sustained, additional antagonist should be given as directed in the product's prescribing information.

In an individual physically dependent on opioids, administration of an opioid receptor antagonist may precipitate an acute withdrawal. The severity of the withdrawal produced will depend on the degree of physical dependence and the dose of the antagonist administered. If a decision is made to treat serious respiratory depression in the physically dependent patient, administration of the antagonist should be begun with care and by titration with smaller than usual doses of the antagonist.

11 DESCRIPTION

NUCYNTA® ER (tapentadol) is a mu-opioid receptor agonist, supplied in extended-release film-coated tablets for oral administration, containing 58.24, 116.48, 174.72, 232.96, and 291.20 mg of tapentadol hydrochloride in each tablet strength, corresponding to 50, 100, 150, 200, and 250 mg of tapentadol free-base, respectively. The chemical name is 3-[(1*R*,2*R*)-3-(dimethylamino)-1-ethyl-2-methylpropyl]phenol monohydrochloride. The structural formula is:

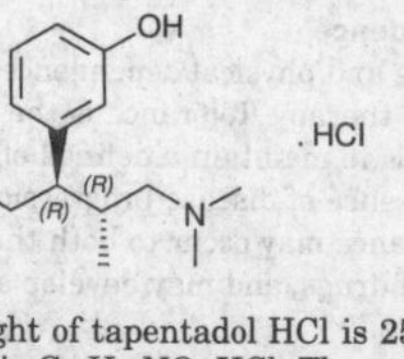

The molecular weight of tapentadol HCl is 257.80, and the molecular formula is $C_{14}H_{23}NO \bullet HCl$. The n-octanol: water partition coefficient log P value is 2.89. The pKa values are 9.36 and 10.45. In addition to the active ingredient tapentadol HCl, tablets also contain the following inactive ingredients: alpha-tocopherol (vitamin E), hypromellose, polyethylene glycol, and polyethylene oxide. The film coating is comprised of polyvinyl alcohol, polyethylene glycol, talc, titanium dioxide, and the colorant FD&C Blue #2 aluminum lake is used for 100, 150, 200, and 250 mg strengths; and additionally, yellow iron oxide is used in 150 mg tablets. Printing inks contain shellac glaze and propylene glycol for all strengths, and black iron oxide (50, 100, 150 and 200 mg tablets) or titanium dioxide (250 mg tablets).

12 CLINICAL PHARMACOLOGY

12.1 Mechanism of Action

Tapentadol is a centrally-acting synthetic analgesic. The exact mechanism of action is unknown. Although the clinical relevance is unclear, preclinical studies have shown that tapentadol is a mu-opioid receptor (MOR) agonist and a norepinephrine reuptake inhibitor (NRI). Analgesia in animal models is derived from both of these properties.

12.2 Pharmacodynamics

Tapentadol is 18 times less potent than morphine in binding to the human mu-opioid receptor and is 2–3 times less potent in producing analgesia in animal models. Tapentadol has been shown to inhibit norepinephrine reuptake in the brains of rats resulting in increased norepinephrine concentrations. In preclinical models, the analgesic activity due to the mu-opioid receptor agonist activity of tapentadol can be antagonized by selective mu-opioid antagonists (e.g., naloxone), whereas the norepinephrine reuptake inhibition is sensitive to norepinephrine modulators. Tapentadol exerts its analgesic effects without a pharmacologically active metabolite.

Concentration-Efficacy Relationships

The minimum effective plasma concentration of tapentadol for analgesia varies widely among patients, especially among patients who have been previously treated with agonist opioids. As a result, individually titrate patients to achieve a balance between therapeutic and adverse effects. The minimum effective analgesic concentration of tapentadol for any individual patient may increase over time due to an increase in pain, progression of disease, development of a new pain syndrome and/or potential development of analgesic tolerance.

Concentration-Adverse Experience Relationships

There is a general relationship between increasing opioid plasma concentration and increasing frequency of adverse experiences such as nausea, vomiting, CNS effects, and respiratory depression.

Effects on the Cardiovascular System

There was no effect of therapeutic and supratherapeutic doses of tapentadol on the QT interval. In a randomized, double-blind, placebo- and positive-controlled crossover study, healthy subjects were administered five consecutive immediate-release formulation doses of tapentadol 100 mg every 6 hours, tapentadol 150 mg every 6 hours, placebo and a single oral dose of moxifloxacin. Similarly, the immediate-release formulation tapentadol had no relevant effect on other ECG parameters (heart rate, PR interval, QRS duration, T-wave or U-wave morphology).

Tapentadol produces peripheral vasodilation which may result in orthostatic hypotension.

Effects on the Central Nervous System (CNS)

The principal therapeutic action of tapentadol is analgesia. Tapentadol causes respiratory depression, in part by a direct effect on the brainstem respiratory centers. The respiratory depression involves a reduction in the responsiveness of the brain stem respiratory centers to both increases in carbon dioxide tension and electrical stimulation. Tapentadol depresses the cough reflex by direct effect on the cough center in the medulla.

Tapentadol causes miosis, even in total darkness. Pinpoint pupils are a sign of opioid overdose but are not pathognomonic (e.g., pontine lesions of hemorrhagic or ischemic origin may produce similar findings). Marked mydriasis rather than miosis may be seen with hypoxia in overdose situations *[see Overdosage (10)]*. Other effects of tapentadol include anxiolysis, euphoria, and feeling of relaxation, drowsiness and changes in mood.

Effects on the Gastrointestinal Tract and on Other Smooth Muscle

Gastric, biliary and pancreatic secretions are decreased by tapentadol. Tapentadol causes a reduction in motility and is associated with an increase in tone in the antrum of the stomach and duodenum. Digestion of food in the small intestine is delayed and propulsive contractions are decreased. Propulsive peristaltic waves in the colon are decreased, while tone is increased to the point of spasm. The end result is constipation. Tapentadol can cause a marked increase in biliary tract pressure as a result of spasm of the sphincter of Oddi, and transient elevations in serum amylase. Tapentadol may also cause spasm of the sphincter of the urinary bladder.

Effects on the Endocrine System

Opioid agonists have been shown to have a variety of effects on the secretion of hormones. Opioids inhibit the secretion of ACTH, cortisol, and luteinizing hormone (LH) in humans. They also stimulate prolactin, growth hormone (GH) secretion, and pancreatic secretion of insulin and glucagon.

Effects on the Immune System

Opioids have been shown to have a variety of effects on components of the immune system in *in vitro* and animal models. The clinical significance of these findings is unknown.

CNS Depressant/Alcohol Interaction

Additive pharmacodynamic effects may be expected when NUCYNTA® ER is used in conjunction with alcohol, other opioids, or illicit drugs that cause central nervous system depression.

12.3 Pharmacokinetics

Absorption

The mean absolute bioavailability after single-dose administration (fasting) of NUCYNTA® ER is approximately 32% due to extensive first-pass metabolism. Maximum serum concentrations of tapentadol are observed between 3 and 6 hours after administration of NUCYNTA® ER. Dose proportional increases for AUC have been observed after administration of NUCYNTA® ER over the therapeutic dose range. Steady-state exposure of tapentadol is attained after the third dose (i.e., 24 hours after first twice daily multiple dose administration). Following dosing with 250 mg every 12 hours, minimal accumulation was observed.

Food Effect

The AUC and C_{max} increased by 6% and 17%, respectively, when NUCYNTA® ER tablet was administered after a high-fat, high-calorie breakfast. NUCYNTA® ER may be given with or without food.

Distribution

Tapentadol is widely distributed throughout the body. Following intravenous administration, the volume of distribution (Vz) for tapentadol is 540 +/- 98 L. The plasma protein binding is low and amounts to approximately 20%.

Metabolism

In humans, about 97% of the parent compound is metabolized. Tapentadol is mainly metabolized via Phase 2 pathways, and only a small amount is metabolized by Phase 1 oxidative pathways. The major pathway of tapentadol metabolism is conjugation with glucuronic acid to produce glucuronides. After oral administration approximately 70% (55% O-glucuronide and 15% sulfate of tapentadol) of the dose is excreted in urine in the conjugated form. A total of 3% of drug was excreted in urine as unchanged drug. Tapentadol is additionally metabolized to N-desmethyl tapentadol (13%) by CYP2C9 and CYP2C19 and to hydroxy tapentadol (2%) by CYP2D6, which are further metabolized by conjugation. Therefore, drug metabolism mediated by cytochrome P450 system is of less importance than phase 2 conjugation.

None of the metabolites contribute to the analgesic activity.

Excretion

Tapentadol and its metabolites are excreted almost exclusively (99%) via the kidneys. The terminal half-life is on average 5 hours after oral administration. The total clearance of tapentadol is 1603 +/-227 mL/min.

Special Populations

Geriatric Patients

The mean exposure (AUC) to tapentadol was similar in elderly subjects compared to young adults, with a 16% lower mean C_{max} observed in the elderly subject group compared to young adult subjects.

Renal Impairment

AUC and C_{max} of tapentadol were comparable in subjects with varying degrees of renal function (from normal to severely impaired). In contrast, increasing exposure (AUC) to tapentadol-O-glucuronide was observed with increasing degree of renal impairment. In subjects with mild (CL_{CR}= 50 to <80 mL/min), moderate (CL_{CR}= 30 to <50 mL/min), and severe (CL_{CR}= <30 mL/min) renal impairment, the AUC of tapentadol-O-glucuronide was 1.5-, 2.5-, and 5.5-fold higher compared with normal renal function, respectively.

Hepatic Impairment

Administration of tapentadol resulted in higher exposures and serum levels to tapentadol in subjects with impaired hepatic function compared to subjects with normal hepatic function. The ratio of tapentadol pharmacokinetic parameters for the mild hepatic impairment group (Child-Pugh Score 5 to 6) and moderate hepatic impairment group (Child-Pugh Score 7 to 9) in comparison to the normal hepatic function group were 1.7 and 4.2, respectively, for AUC; 1.4 and 2.5, respectively, for C_{max}; and 1.2 and 1.4, respectively, for $t_{1/2}$. The rate of formation of tapentadol-O-glucuronide was lower in subjects with increased liver impairment.

Pharmacokinetic Drug Interactions

Tapentadol is mainly metabolized by Phase 2 glucuronidation, a high capacity/low affinity system; therefore, clinically relevant interactions caused by Phase 2 metabolism are unlikely to occur. Naproxen and probenecid increased the AUC of tapentadol by 17% and 57%, respectively. These changes are not considered clinically relevant and no change in dose is required.

No changes in the pharmacokinetic parameters of tapentadol were observed when acetaminophen and acetylsalicylic acid were given concomitantly.

In vitro studies did not reveal any potential of tapentadol to either inhibit or induce cytochrome P450 enzymes. Furthermore, a minor amount of tapentadol is metabolized via the oxidative pathway. Thus, clinically relevant interactions mediated by the cytochrome P450 system are unlikely to occur.

The pharmacokinetics of tapentadol were not affected when gastric pH or gastrointestinal motility were increased by omeprazole and metoclopramide, respectively.

Plasma protein binding of tapentadol is low (approximately 20%). Therefore, the likelihood of pharmacokinetic drug-drug interactions by displacement from the protein binding site is low.

Drug Interaction / Alcohol Interaction

NUCYNTA® ER may be expected to have additive effects when used in conjunction with alcohol, other opioids, or illicit drugs that cause central nervous system depression, because respiratory depression, hypotension, hypertension, and profound sedation, coma or death may result *[see Warnings and Precautions (5.4)]*.

An *in vivo* study examined the effect of alcohol (240 mL of 40%) on the bioavailability of a single dose of 100 mg and 250 mg of NUCYNTA® ER tablet in healthy, fasted volunteers. After co-administration of a 100 mg NUCYNTA® ER tablet and alcohol, the mean C_{max} value increased by 48% compared to control with a range of 0.99-fold to 4.38-fold. The mean tapentadol AUC_{last} and AUC_{inf} were increased by 17%; the T_{max} and $t_{1/2}$ were unchanged. After co-administration of a 250 mg NUCYNTA® ER tablet and alcohol, the mean C_{max} value increased by 28% compared to control with a range of 0.90-fold to 2.67-fold. The mean tapentadol AUC_{last} and AUC_{inf} were increased by 16%; the T_{max} and $t_{1/2}$ were unchanged.

13 NONCLINICAL TOXICOLOGY

13.1 Carcinogenesis, Mutagenesis, Impairment of Fertility

Carcinogenesis

Tapentadol was administered to rats (diet) and mice (oral gavage) for two years.

In mice, tapentadol HCl was administered by oral gavage at dosages of 50, 100 and 200 mg/kg/day for 2 years (up to 0.34 times in the male mice and 0.25 times in the female mice the plasma exposure at the maximum recommended human dose [MRHD] for NUCYNTA® ER on an area under the time-curve [AUC] basis). No increase in tumor incidence was observed at any dose level.

In rats, tapentadol HCl was administered in diet at dosages of 10, 50, 125 and 250 mg/kg/day for two years (up to 0.20 times in the male rats and 0.75 times in the female rats the MRHD on an AUC basis). No increase in tumor incidence was observed at any dose level.

Mutagenesis

Tapentadol did not induce gene mutations in bacteria, but was clastogenic with metabolic activation in a chromosomal aberration test in V79 cells. The test was repeated and was negative in the presence and absence of metabolic activation. The one positive result for tapentadol was not confirmed *in vivo* in rats, using the two endpoints of chromosomal aberration and unscheduled DNA synthesis, when tested up to the maximum tolerated dose.

Impairment of Fertility

Tapentadol HCl was administered intravenously to male or female rats at dosages of 3, 6, or 12 mg/kg/day (representing exposures of up to approximately 0.56 times in the male rats and 0.50 times in the female rats the exposure at the MRHD on an AUC basis, based on extrapolation from toxicokinetic analyses in a separate 4-week intravenous study in rats). Tapentadol did not alter fertility at any dose level. Maternal toxicity and adverse effects on embryonic development, including decreased number of implantations, decreased numbers of live conceptuses, and increased pre- and post-implantation losses occurred at dosages ≥6 mg/kg/day.

13.2 Animal Toxicology and/or Pharmacology

In toxicological studies with tapentadol, the most common systemic effects of tapentadol were related to the mu-opioid receptor agonist and norepinephrine reuptake inhibition pharmacodynamic properties of the compound. Transient, dose-dependent and predominantly CNS-related findings were observed, including impaired respiratory function and convulsions, the latter occurring in the dog at plasma levels (C_{max}), which are in the range associated with the maximum recommended human dose (MRHD).

14 CLINICAL STUDIES

The efficacy of NUCYNTA® ER was studied in five studies in patients with moderate to severe chronic pain and DPN. Efficacy was demonstrated in one randomized, double-blind, placebo- and active-controlled study in patients with chronic low back pain (LBP), and two randomized, double-blind, placebo-controlled studies in patients with pain related to diabetic peripheral neuropathy (DPN-1 and DPN-2).

14.1 Moderate to Severe Chronic Low Back Pain

In the LBP study, patients 18 years of age or older with chronic low back pain and a baseline pain score of ≥5 on an 11-point numerical rating scale (NRS), ranging from 0 to 10 were enrolled and randomized to 1 of 3 treatments: NUCYNTA® ER, active-control (an extended-release Schedule II opioid analgesic), or placebo.

Patients randomized to NUCYNTA® ER initiated therapy with a dose of 50 mg twice daily for three days. After three days, the dose was increased to 100 mg twice daily. Subsequent titration was allowed over a 3-week titration period to a dose up to 250 mg twice daily, followed by a 12-week maintenance period. There were 981 patients randomized. The mean age of the study population was 50 (range 18 to 89) years; the mean baseline pain intensity score was 8 (SD 1). Approximately half of the patients were opioid-naïve (had not taken opioids during the three months prior to the screening visit).

The number of patients completing the study was 51% in the placebo group, 54% in the NUCYNTA® ER group and 43% in the active-control group. Lack of efficacy was the most common reason for discontinuation among placebo-treated patients (21%), whereas adverse events were the most common reason for discontinuation among the active treatment groups (17% and 32% for NUCYNTA® ER and active-control, respectively).

After 15 weeks of treatment, patients taking NUCYNTA® ER had a significantly greater pain reduction compared to placebo. The proportion of patients with various degrees of improvement is shown in Figure 1. The figure is cumulative, such that patients, whose change from baseline is, for example 50%, are also included at every level of improvement below 50%. Patients who did not complete the study were assigned 0% improvement.

Figure 1: Percentage of Patients Achieving Various Levels of Improvement in Pain Intensity - Study LBP*

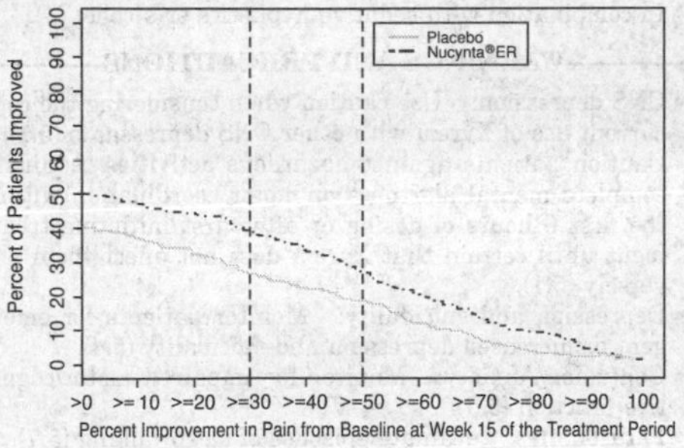

* The last week of Study LBP was Week 15.

14.2 Neuropathic Pain Associated with Diabetic Peripheral Neuropathy

In the two DPN studies, patients 18 years of age or older with pain due to diabetic peripheral neuropathy and a pain score of ≥5 on an 11-point numerical rating scale (NRS) ranging from 0 (no pain) to 10 (worst possible pain) were enrolled. Following an open-label treatment period in which NUCYNTA® ER was administered to all patients for three weeks and titrated to an individually stable dose, patients who had tolerated the drug and demonstrated at least a 1-point improvement in pain intensity on the NRS at the end of the open-label titration period were randomized to either continue the NUCYNTA® ER dose (100 mg to 250 mg twice a day) reached during the open-label titration period, or receive placebo for 12 weeks of maintenance treatment. During the first 4 days of the double-blind maintenance period patients were permitted to take tapentadol ER 25 mg up to two times a day as additional medication. After the first 4 days, patients were allowed to take tapentadol ER 25 mg once daily as needed for pain, in addition to the patient's assigned study drug. Patients recorded their pain in a diary twice daily.

Study DPN-1: A total of 591 patients entered open-label treatment and 389 patients met the criteria for randomization into the double-blind treatment period. The mean age of the randomized population was 60 (range 29 to 87) years; approximately two-thirds of the patients were opioid-naïve (had not taken opioids during the three months prior to the screening visit).

During the titration period, 34% of patients discontinued open-label NUCYNTA® ER. The most common reasons for discontinuation in the double blind treatment period were lack of efficacy in the placebo group (14%) and adverse events in the NUCYNTA® ER group (15%).

After 12 weeks of treatment, NUCYNTA® ER provided a significantly greater reduction in pain intensity from baseline to the end of the 12-week double-blind period compared to placebo. Figure 2 displays the proportion of randomized patients achieving various degrees of improvement in pain intensity from the start of the open-label titration period to the last week of the randomized withdrawal period. The figure is cumulative, such that patients, whose change from baseline is, for example 50%, are also included at every level of improvement below 50%. Patients who did not complete the study were assigned 0% improvement.

Figure 2: Percentage of Patients Achieving Various Levels of Improvement in Pain Intensity - DPN-1

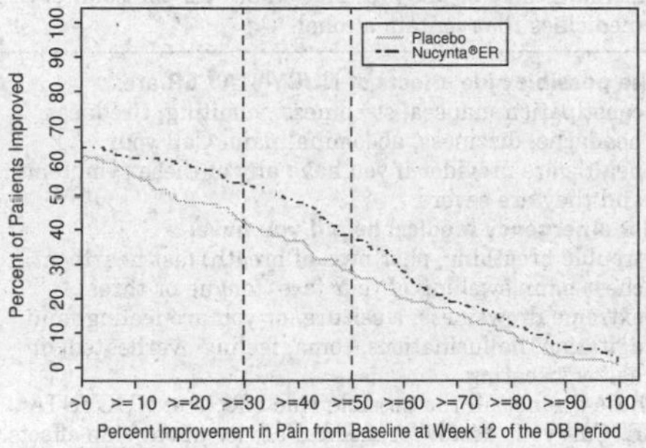

Study DPN-2: A total of 459 patients entered open-label treatment and 320 patients met the criteria for randomization into the double-blind treatment period. The mean age of the randomized population was 59 (range 28 to 83) years; approximately two-thirds of the patients were opioid-naïve (had not taken opioids during the three months prior to the screening visit).

During the titration period, 22% of patients discontinued open-label NUCYNTA® ER and 6% of patients were not subsequently randomized because they failed to have at least 1-point improvement in pain intensity. The most common reason for discontinuation in the double-blind treatment period was adverse events in both the placebo group (9%) and the NUCYNTA® ER group (14%).

After 12 weeks of treatment, NUCYNTA® ER provided a significantly greater reduction in pain intensity from baseline to the end of the 12-week double-blind period compared to placebo. Figure 3 displays the proportion of randomized patients achieving various degrees of improvement in pain intensity from the start of the open-label titration period to the last week of the randomized withdrawal period. The figure is cumulative, such that patients, whose change from baseline is, for example 50%, are also included at every level of improvement below 50%. Patients who did not complete the study were assigned 0% improvement.

Figure 3: Percentage of Patients Achieving Various Levels of Improvement in Pain Intensity-DPN-2

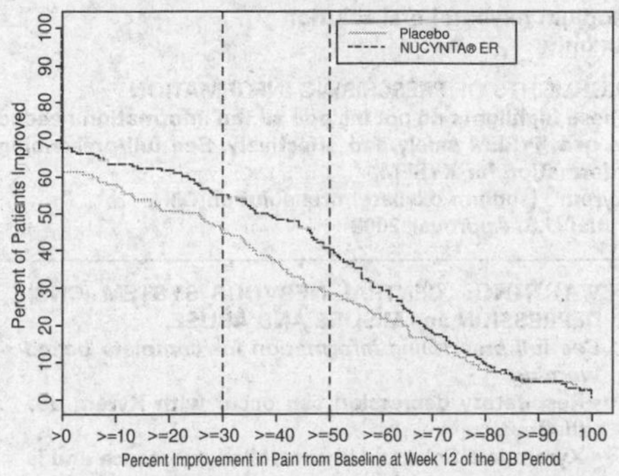

16 HOW SUPPLIED/STORAGE AND HANDLING

NUCYNTA® ER tablets are available in the following strengths and packages:

50 mg extended-release tablets are white oblong-shaped with a black print "OMJ 50" on one side and are available in bottles of 60 with child-resistant closure (NDC 50458-860-01) and unit dose blister packs of 100 (10 blister strips of 10 tablets each), for hospital use only (NDC 50458-860-02).

100 mg extended-release tablets are light-blue oblong-shaped with a black print "OMJ 100" on one side and are available in bottles of 60 with child-resistant closure (NDC 50458-861-01) and unit dose blister packs of 100 (10 blister strips of 10 tablets each), for hospital use only (NDC 50458-861-02).

150 mg extended-release tablets are blue-green oblong-shaped with a black print "OMJ 150" on one side and are available in bottles of 60 with child-resistant closure (NDC 50458-862-01) and unit dose blister packs of 100 (10 blister strips of 10 tablets each), for hospital use only (NDC 50458-862-02).

200 mg extended-release tablets are blue oblong-shaped with a depression in the middle running lengthwise on each side and with a black print "OMJ 200" on one side, and are available in bottles of 60 with child-resistant closure (NDC 50458-863-01) and unit dose blister packs of 100 (10 blister strips of 10 tablets each), for hospital use only (NDC 50458-863-02).

250 mg extended-release tablets are dark blue oblong-shaped with a depression in the middle running lengthwise on each side and with a white print "OMJ 250" on one side, and are available in bottles of 60 with child-resistant closure (NDC 50458-864-01) and unit dose blister packs of 100 (10 blister strips of 10 tablets each), for hospital use only (NDC 50458-864-02).

Storage and Handling

Store up to 25°C (77°F); excursions permitted to 15° – 30°C (59° – 86°F) [see USP Controlled Room Temperature].

Protect from moisture.

Keep NUCYNTA® ER in a secure place out of reach of children.

NUCYNTA® ER tablets that are no longer needed should be destroyed by flushing down the toilet.

17 PATIENT COUNSELING INFORMATION

See *FDA-approved patient labeling (Medication Guide)*

Abuse Potential

Inform patients that NUCYNTA® ER contains tapentadol, a Schedule II controlled substance that is subject to abuse. Instruct patients not to share NUCYNTA® ER with others and to take steps to protect NUCYNTA® ER from theft or misuse.

Life-threatening Respiratory Depression

Discuss the risk of respiratory depression with patients, explaining that the risk is greatest when starting NUCYNTA® ER or when the dose is increased. Advise patients how to recognize respiratory depression and to seek medical attention if they are experiencing breathing difficulties.

Accidental Exposure

Instruct patients to take steps to store NUCYNTA® ER securely. Accidental exposure, especially in children, may results in serious harm or death. Advise patients to dispose of unused NUCYNTA® ER by flushing the tablets down the toilet.

Risks from Concomitant Use of Alcohol and other CNS Depressants

Inform patients that the concomitant use of alcohol with NUCYNTA® ER can increase the risk of life-threatening respiratory depression. Instruct patients not to consume alcoholic beverages, as well as prescription and over-the-counter drug products that contain alcohol, during treatment with NUCYNTA® ER.

Inform patients that potentially serious additive effects may occur if NUCYNTA® ER is used with other CNS depressants, and not to use such drugs unless supervised by a health care provider.

Concurrent use of MAOI

Inform patients not to take NUCYNTA® ER while using any drugs that inhibit monoamine oxidase. Patients should not start MAOIs while taking NUCYNTA® ER.

Seizures

Inform patients that NUCYNTA® ER could cause seizures if they are at risk for seizures or have epilepsy. Patients should be advised to stop taking NUCYNTA® ER if they have a seizure while taking NUCYNTA® ER and call their healthcare provider right away.

Serotonin Syndrome

Inform patients that NUCYNTA® ER could cause a rare but potentially life-threatening condition resulting from concomitant administration of serotonergic drugs (including Serotonin Reuptake Inhibitors, Serotonin and Norepinephrine Reuptake Inhibitors and tricyclic antidepressants. Warn patients of the symptoms of serotonin syndrome and to seek medical attention right away if symptoms develop. Instruct patients to inform their physicians if they are taking, or plan to take additional medications including CNS

Depressants, MAO inhibitors, mixed agonists/antagonist opioid analgesics, anticholinergics, SSRIs, SNRIs, or tricyclic antidepressants.

Important Administration Instructions

Instruct patients how to properly take NUCYNTA® ER, including the following:

- Swallowing NUCYNTA® ER tablets whole
- Not cutting, crushing, chewing, or dissolving the tablets
- Using NUCYNTA® ER exactly as prescribed to reduce the risk of life-threatening adverse reactions (e.g., respiratory depression)
- Not discontinuing NUCYNTA® ER without first discussing the need for a tapering regimen with the prescriber
- To take each tablet with enough water to ensure complete swallowing immediately after placing in mouth.

Hypotension

Inform patients that NUCYNTA® ER may cause orthostatic hypotension and syncope. Instruct patients how to recognize symptoms of low blood pressure and how to reduce the risk of serious consequences should hypotension occur (e.g., sit or lie down, carefully rise from a sitting or lying position).

Driving or Operating Heavy Machinery

Inform patients that NUCYNTA® ER may impair the ability to perform potentially hazardous activities such as driving a car or operating heavy machinery. Advise patients not to perform such tasks until they know how they will react to the medication.

Constipation

Advise patients of the potential for severe constipation, including management instructions and when to seek medical attention.

Anaphylaxis

Inform patients that anaphylaxis has been reported with ingredients contained in NUCYNTA® ER. Advise patients how to recognize such a reaction and when to seek medical attention.

Pregnancy

Advise female patients that NUCYNTA® ER can cause fetal harm and to inform the prescriber if they are pregnant or plan to become pregnant.

Manufactured by:
Janssen Ortho, LLC
Gurabo, PR 00778
Manufactured for:
Janssen Pharmaceuticals, Inc.
Titusville, NJ 08560

Revised: July 2013

Medication Guide
NUCYNTA® ER (new-SINN-tah E-R)
(tapentadol) extended-release oral tablets, CII

NUCYNTA® ER is:

- A strong prescription pain medicine that contains an opioid (narcotic) that is used to treat moderate to severe around-the-clock pain and pain from damaged nerves (neuropathic pain) that happens with diabetes.

Important information about NUCYNTA® ER:

- Get emergency help right away if you take too much NUCYNTA® ER (overdose). NUCYNTA® ER overdose can cause life threatening breathing problems that can lead to death.
- Never give anyone else your NUCYNTA® ER. They could die from taking it. Store NUCYNTA® ER away from children and in a safe place to prevent stealing or abuse. Selling or giving away NUCYNTA® ER is against the law.

Do not take NUCYNTA® ER if you have:

- severe asthma, trouble breathing, or other lung problems.
- a bowel blockage or have narrowing of the stomach or intestines.
- taken a monoamine oxidase inhibitor (MAOI) medicine or have taken a MAOI medicine within the last 14 days.

Before taking NUCYNTA® ER, tell your healthcare provider if you have a history of:

- head injury, seizures • liver, kidney, thyroid problems
- problems urinating • pancreas or gallbladder problems
- abuse of street or prescription drugs, alcohol addiction, or mental health problems.

Tell your healthcare provider if you are:

- **pregnant or planning to become pregnant.** NUCYNTA® ER may harm your unborn baby.
- **breastfeeding.** NUCYNTA® ER passes into breast milk and may harm your baby.
- taking prescription or over-the-counter medicines, vitamins, or herbal supplements.

When taking NUCYNTA® ER:

- Do not change your dose. Take NUCYNTA® ER exactly as prescribed by your healthcare provider.
- Take your prescribed dose every 12 hours at the same time every day. Do not take more than your prescribed dose in 24 hours. If you miss a dose take the missed dose as soon as possible. If it is almost time for your next dose, skip the missed dose and go back to your regular dosing schedule.
- Swallow NUCYNTA® ER whole with enough water to make sure that you completely swallow the tablet right away. Do not cut, break, chew, crush, dissolve, or inject NUCYNTA® ER.
- **Call your healthcare provider if the dose you are taking does not control your pain.**
- **Do not stop taking NUCYNTA® ER without talking to your healthcare provider.**
- After you stop taking NUCYNTA® ER flush any unused tablets down the toilet.

While taking NUCYNTA® ER Do Not:

- Drive or operate heavy machinery, until you know how NUCYNTA® ER affects you. NUCYNTA® ER can make you sleepy, dizzy, or lightheaded.
- Drink alcohol or use prescription or over-the-counter medicines that contain alcohol.

The possible side effects of NUCYNTA® ER are:

- constipation, nausea, sleepiness, vomiting, tiredness, headache, dizziness, abdominal pain. Call your healthcare provider if you have any of these symptoms and they are severe.

Get emergency medical help if you have:

- trouble breathing, shortness of breath, fast heartbeat, chest pain, swelling of your face, tongue or throat, extreme drowsiness, a seizure, or you are feeling faint.
- agitation, hallucinations, coma, feeling overheated, or heavy sweating.

These are not all the possible side effects of NUCYNTA® ER. Call your doctor for medical advice about side effects. You may report side effects to FDA at 1-800-FDA-1088.
For more information go to *dailymed.nlm.nih.gov*
Manufactured by: Janssen Ortho LLC, Gurabo, PR 00778; Manufactured for: Janssen Pharmaceuticals, Inc. Titusville, NJ 08560, *www.Nucynta.com* or call 1-800-526-7736

This Medication Guide has been approved by the U.S. FDA
Revised: 8/2012

Shown in Product Identification Guide, page 307

Jazz Pharmaceuticals, Inc.
3180 PORTER DRIVE
PALO ALTO, CA 94304

Direct Inquiries to:
Phone: (650) 496-3777
Fax: (650) 496-3781
E-mail: customercare@jazzpharma.com
For medical information:
E-mail: jazzpharma@medcomsol.com
For media information:
E-mail: mediainfo@jazzpharma.com

XYREM® Ⓒ III
(sodium oxybate) oral solution
Rx only

HIGHLIGHTS OF PRESCRIBING INFORMATION
These highlights do not include all the information needed to use XYREM safely and effectively. See full prescribing information for XYREM.
Xyrem® (sodium oxybate) oral solution CIII
Initial U.S. Approval: 2002

WARNING: CENTRAL NERVOUS SYSTEM (CNS) DEPRESSION and MISUSE AND ABUSE.
See full prescribing information for complete boxed warning.

- **Respiratory depression can occur with Xyrem use (5.4)**
- **Xyrem is a Schedule III controlled substance and is the sodium salt of gamma hydroxybutyrate (GHB), a Schedule I controlled substance. Abuse or misuse of illicit GHB is associated with CNS adverse reactions, including seizure, respiratory depression, decreased consciousness, coma and death (5.2, 9.2)**
- **Because of the risks of CNS depression, abuse, and misuse, Xyrem is available only through a restricted distribution program called the Xyrem Success Program® using a centralized pharmacy. Prescribers and patients must enroll in the program. (5.3)**

RECENT MAJOR CHANGES

Contraindications, concomitant use with alcohol (4) 12/2012

INDICATIONS AND USAGE

Xyrem is a central nervous system depressant indicated for the treatment of:

- Cataplexy in narcolepsy (1.1).
- Excessive daytime sleepiness (EDS) in narcolepsy (1.2).

Xyrem may only be dispensed to patients enrolled in the Xyrem Success Program (1).

DOSAGE AND ADMINISTRATION

- Initiate dose at 4.5 grams (g) per night administered orally in two equal, divided doses: 2.25 g at bedtime and 2.25 g taken 2.5 to 4 hours later (2.1)
- Titrate to effect in increments of 1.5 g per night at weekly intervals (0.75 g at bedtime and 0.75 g taken 2.5 to 4 hours later) (2.1).
- Recommended dose range: 6 g to 9 g per night orally (2.1).

Total Nightly Dose	Take at Bedtime	Take 2.5 to 4 Hours Later
4.5 g per night	2.25 g	2.25 g
6 g per night	3 g	3 g
7.5 g per night	3.75 g	3.75 g
9 g per night	4.5 g	4.5 g

- Take each dose while in bed and lie down after dosing (2.2).
- Allow 2 hours after eating before dosing (2.2).
- Prepare both doses prior to bedtime; dilute each dose with approximately ¼ cup of water in pharmacy-provided vials (2.2).
- Patients with Hepatic Impairment: starting dose is 2.25 g per night administered orally in two equal, divided doses of approximately 1.13 g at bedtime and approximately 1.13 g taken 2.5 to 4 hours later (2.3).

DOSAGE FORMS AND STRENGTHS

Oral solution, 0.5 g per mL (3)

CONTRAINDICATIONS

- Succinic semialdehyde dehydrogenase deficiency (4).
- In combination with sedative hypnotics or alcohol (4).

WARNINGS AND PRECAUTIONS

- CNS depression: Use caution when considering the concurrent use of Xyrem with other CNS depressants (5.1).
- Caution patients against hazardous activities requiring complete mental alertness or motor coordination within the first 6 hours of dosing or after first initiating treatment until certain that Xyrem does not affect them adversely (5.1).
- Depression and suicidality: Monitor patients for emergent or increased depression and suicidality (5.4).
- Confusion/Anxiety: Monitor for impaired motor/cognitive function (5.5).
- Parasomnias: evaluate episodes of sleepwalking (5.7).
- High sodium content in Xyrem: Monitor patients with heart failure, hypertension, or impaired renal function (5.7).

ADVERSE REACTIONS

Most common adverse reactions (≥ 5% and at least twice the incidence with placebo) were nausea, dizziness, vomiting, somnolence, enuresis, and tremor (6.1).
To report SUSPECTED ADVERSE REACTIONS, contact Jazz Pharmaceuticals at 1-800-520-5568, or FDA at 1-800-FDA-1088 or www.fda.gov/Medwatch.

USE IN SPECIFIC POPULATIONS

- Pregnancy: Based on animal data, may cause fetal harm (8.1).
- Geriatric patients: Monitor for impaired motor and/or cognitive function when taking Xyrem (8.5).

See 17 for PATIENT COUNSELING INFORMATION and Medication Guide

Revised: 12/2012

FULL PRESCRIBING INFORMATION: CONTENTS*

*** Sections or subsections omitted from the full prescribing information are not listed**

FULL PRESCRIBING INFORMATION

WARNING: CENTRAL NERVOUS SYSTEM DEPRESSION and MISUSE AND ABUSE.

Xyrem (sodium oxybate) is a CNS depressant. In clinical trials at recommended doses obtundation and clinically significant respiratory depression occurred in Xyrem-treated patients. Almost all of the patients who received Xyrem during clinical trials in narcolepsy were receiving central nervous system stimulants[*see Warnings and Precautions (5.1)*].

Xyrem® (sodium oxybate) is the sodium salt of gamma hydroxybutyrate (GHB). Abuse of GHB, either alone or in combination with other CNS depressants, is associated with CNS adverse reactions, including seizure, respiratory depression, decreases in the level of consciousness, coma, and death [*see Warnings and Precautions (5.2)*].

Because of the risks of CNS depression, abuse, and misuse, Xyrem is available only through a restricted distribution program called the Xyrem Success Program®, using a centralized pharmacy. Prescribers and patients must enroll in the program. For further information go to www.XYREM.com or call 1-866-XYREM88® (1-866-997-3688).[*see Warnings and Precautions (5.3)*].

1 INDICATIONS AND USAGE

Limitations of Use

Xyrem may only be dispensed to patients enrolled in the Xyrem Success Program *[see Warnings and Precautions (5.3)]*.

1.1 Cataplexy in Narcolepsy

Xyrem (sodium oxybate) oral solution is indicated for the treatment of cataplexy in narcolepsy *[see Clinical Studies (14.1)]*.

1.2 Excessive Daytime Sleepiness in Narcolepsy

Xyrem (sodium oxybate) oral solution is indicated for the treatment of excessive daytime sleepiness (EDS) in narcolepsy *[see Clinical Studies (14.2)]*.

2 DOSAGE AND ADMINISTRATION

Healthcare professionals who prescribe Xyrem must enroll in the Xyrem Success Program and must comply with the requirements to ensure safe use of Xyrem *[see Warnings and Precautions (5.3)]*.

2.1 Dosing Information

The recommended starting dose is 4.5 grams (g) per night administered orally in two equal, divided doses: 2.25 g at bedtime and 2.25 g taken 2.5 to 4 hours later (see Table 1). Increase the dose by 1.5 g per night at weekly intervals (additional 0.75 g at bedtime and 0.75 g taken 2.5 to 4 hours later) to the effective dose range of 6 g to 9 g per night orally. Doses higher than 9 g per night have not been studied and should not ordinarily be administered.

Table 1: Xyrem Dose Regimen (g = grams)

If A Patient's Total Nightly Dose is:	Take at Bedtime:	Take 2.5 to 4 Hours Later:
4.5 g per night	2.25 g	2.25 g
6 g per night	3 g	3 g
7.5 g per night	3.75 g	3.75 g
9 g per night	4.5 g	4.5 g

2.2 Important Administration Instructions

Take the first dose of Xyrem at least 2 hours after eating because food significantly reduces the bioavailability of sodium oxybate.

Prepare both doses of Xyrem prior to bedtime. Prior to ingestion, each dose of Xyrem should be diluted with approximately ¼ cup (approximately 60 mL) of water in the empty pharmacy vials provided. Patients should take Xyrem while in bed and lie down immediately after dosing as Xyrem may cause them to fall asleep abruptly without first feeling drowsy. Patients will often fall asleep within 5 minutes of taking Xyrem, and will usually fall asleep within 15 minutes, though the time it takes any individual patient to fall asleep may vary from night to night. Rarely, patients may take up to 2 hours to fall asleep. Therefore, patients should remain in bed following ingestion of the first dose, and should not take the second dose until 2.5 to 4 hours later. Patients may need to set an alarm to awaken for the second dose.

2.3 Dose Modification in Patients with Hepatic Impairment

The recommended starting dose in patients with hepatic impairment is 2.25 g per night administered orally in two equal, divided doses: approximately 1.13 g at bedtime and approximately 1.13 g taken 2.5 to 4 hours later *[see Use in Specific Populations (8.6); Clinical Pharmacology (12.3)]*.

3 DOSAGE FORMS AND STRENGTHS

Xyrem is a clear to slightly opalescent oral solution, in a concentration of 0.5 g per mL.

4 CONTRAINDICATIONS

Xyrem is contraindicated in patients being treated with sedative hypnotic agents.

Patients should not drink alcohol when using Xyrem.

Xyrem is contraindicated in patients with succinic semialdehyde dehydrogenase deficiency. This is a rare disorder of inborn error of metabolism variably characterized by mental retardation, hypotonia, and ataxia.

5 WARNINGS AND PRECAUTIONS

5.1 Central Nervous System Depression

Xyrem is a central nervous system (CNS) depressant. Alcohol and sedative hypnotics are contraindicated in patients who are using Xyrem. The concurrent use of Xyrem with other CNS depressants, including but not limited to opioid analgesics, benzodiazepines, sedating antidepressants or antipsychotics, general anesthetics, muscle relaxants, and/or illicit CNS depressants, may increase the risk of respiratory depression, hypotension, profound sedation, syncope, and death. If use of these CNS depressants in combination with Xyrem is required, dose reduction or discontinuation of one or more CNS depressants (including Xyrem) should be considered. In addition, if short-term use of an opioid (e.g. post- or perioperative) is required, interruption of treatment with Xyrem should be considered.

Healthcare providers should caution patients about operating hazardous machinery, including automobiles or airplanes, until they are reasonably certain that Xyrem does not affect them adversely (e.g., impair judgment, thinking, or motor skills). Patients should not engage in hazardous occupations or activities requiring complete mental alertness or motor coordination, such as operating machinery or a motor vehicle or flying an airplane, for at least 6 hours after taking the second nightly dose of Xyrem. Patients should be queried about CNS depression–related events upon initiation of Xyrem therapy and periodically thereafter [See Warnings and Precautions (5.3)].

5.2 Abuse and Misuse

Xyrem is a Schedule III controlled substance. The active ingredient of Xyrem, sodium oxybate or gamma-hydroxybutyrate (GHB), is a Schedule I controlled substance. Abuse of illicit GHB, either alone or in combination with other CNS depressants, is associated with CNS adverse reactions, including seizure, respiratory depression, decreases in the level of consciousness, coma, and death. The rapid onset of sedation, coupled with the amnestic features of Xyrem, particularly when combined with alcohol, has proven to be dangerous for the voluntary and involuntary user (e.g., assault victim). Because illicit use and abuse of GHB have been reported, physicians should carefully evaluate patients for a history of drug abuse and follow such patients closely, observing them for signs of misuse or abuse of GHB (e.g. increase in size or frequency of dosing, drug-seeking behavior, feigned cataplexy) [see Warnings and Precautions (5.3); Drug Abuse and Dependence (9.2)].

5.3 Xyrem Success Program

Because of the risks of central nervous system depression and abuse/misuse, Xyrem is available only through a restricted distribution program called the Xyrem Success Program.

Required components of the Xyrem Success Program are:

- Use of a centralized pharmacy
- Healthcare Providers who prescribe Xyrem must complete the enrollment forms and comply with the requirements.
- To receive Xyrem, patients must understand the risks and benefits of Xyrem.

Further information is available at www.XYREM.com or 1-866-XYREM88® (1-866-997-3688).

5.4 Respiratory Depression and Sleep-Disordered Breathing

Xyrem may impair respiratory drive, especially in patients with compromised respiratory function. In overdoses, life-threatening respiratory depression has been reported [see Overdosage (10)].

In a study assessing the respiratory-depressant effects of Xyrem at doses up to 9 g per night in 21 patients with narcolepsy, no dose-related changes in oxygen saturation were demonstrated in the group as a whole. One of the four patients with preexisting, moderate-to-severe sleep apnea had significant worsening of the apnea/hypopnea index during treatment.

In a study assessing the effects of Xyrem 9 g per night in 50 patients with obstructive sleep apnea, Xyrem did not increase the severity of sleep-disordered breathing and did not adversely affect the average duration and severity of oxygen desaturation overall. However, there was a significant increase in the number of central apneas in patients taking Xyrem, and clinically significant oxygen desaturation (< 55%) was measured in three patients (6%) after Xyrem administration, with one patient withdrawing from the study and two continuing after single brief instances of desaturation. Prescribers should be aware that increased central apneas and clinically relevant desaturation events have been observed with Xyrem administration.

In clinical trials in 128 patients with narcolepsy, two subjects had profound CNS depression, which resolved after supportive respiratory intervention. Two other patients discontinued sodium oxybate because of severe difficulty breathing and an increase in obstructive sleep apnea. In two controlled trials assessing polysomnographic (PSG) measures in patients with narcolepsy, 40 of 477 patients were included with a baseline apnea/hypopnea index of 16 to 67 events per hour, indicative of mild to severe sleep-disordered breathing. None of the 40 patients had a clinically significant worsening of respiratory function as measured by apnea/hypopnea index and pulse oximetry at doses of 4.5 g to 9 g per night.

Prescribers should be aware that sleep-related breathing disorders tend to be more prevalent in obese patients and in postmenopausal women not on hormone replacement therapy as well as among patients with narcolepsy.

5.5 Depression and Suicidality

In clinical trials in patients with narcolepsy (n=781), there were two suicides and two attempted suicides in Xyrem-treated patients, including three patients with a previous history of depressive psychiatric disorder. Of the two suicides, one patient used Xyrem in conjunction with other drugs. Xyrem was not involved in the second suicide. Adverse reactions of depression were reported by 7% of 781 Xyrem-treated patients, with four patients (< 1%) discontinuing because of depression. In most cases, no change in Xyrem treatment was required.

In a controlled trial, with patients randomized to fixed doses of 3 g, 6 g, or 9 g per night Xyrem or placebo, there was a single event of depression at the 3 g per night dose. In another controlled trial, with patients titrated from an initial

4.5 g per night starting dose, the incidences of depression were 1 (1.7%), 1 (1.5%), 2 (3.2%), and 2 (3.6%) for the placebo, 4.5 g, 6 g, and 9 g per night doses, respectively.

The emergence of depression in patients treated with Xyrem requires careful and immediate evaluation. Patients with a previous history of a depressive illness and/or suicide attempt should be monitored carefully for the emergence of depressive symptoms while taking Xyrem.

5.6 Other Behavioral or Psychiatic Adverse Reactions

During clinical trials in narcolepsy, 3% of 781 patients treated with Xyrem experienced confusion, with incidence generally increasing with dose.

Less than 1% of patients discontinued the drug because of confusion. Confusion was reported at all recommended doses from 6 g to 9 g per night. In a controlled trial where patients were randomized to fixed total daily doses of 3 g, 6 g, or 9 g per night or placebo, a dose-response relationship for confusion was demonstrated, with 17% of patients at 9 g per night experiencing confusion. In all cases in that controlled trial, the confusion resolved soon after termination of treatment. In Trial 3 where sodium oxybate was titrated from an initial 4.5 g per night dose, there was a single event of confusion in one patient at the 9 g per night dose. In the majority of cases in all clinical trials in narcolepsy, confusion resolved either soon after termination of dosing or with continued treatment. However, patients treated with Xyrem who become confused should be evaluated fully, and appropriate intervention considered on an individual basis.

Anxiety occurred in 5.8% of the 874 patients receiving Xyrem in clinical trials in another population. The emergence of or increase in anxiety in patients taking Xyrem should be carefully monitored.

Other neuropsychiatric reactions reported in Xyrem clinical trials included hallucinations, paranoia, psychosis, and agitation. The emergence of thought disorders and/or behavior abnormalities requires careful and immediate evaluation.

5.7 Parasomnias

Sleepwalking, defined as confused behavior occurring at night and at times associated with wandering, was reported in 6% of 781 patients with narcolepsy treated with Xyrem in controlled and long-term open-label studies, with < 1% of patients discontinuing due to sleepwalking. Rates of sleepwalking were similar for patients taking placebo and patients taking Xyrem in controlled trials It is unclear if some or all of the reported sleepwalking episodes correspond to true somnambulism, which is a parasomnia occurring during non-REM sleep, or to any other specific medical disorder. Five instances of significant injury or potential injury were associated with sleepwalking during a clinical trial of Xyrem in patients with narcolepsy.

Parasomnias including sleepwalking have been reported in postmarketing experience with Xyrem. Therefore, episodes of sleepwalking should be fully evaluated and appropriate interventions considered.

5.8 Use in Patients Sensitive to High Sodium Intake

Xyrem has a high salt content. In patients sensitive to salt intake (e.g., those with heart failure, hypertension, or renal impairment) consider the amount of daily sodium intake in each dose of Xyrem. Table 2 provides the approximate sodium content per Xyrem dose.

Table 2

Approximate Sodium Content per Total Nightly Dose of Xyrem (g = grams)

Xyrem Dose	Sodium Content/Total Nightly Exposure
3 g per night	550 mg
4.5 g per night	820 mg
6 g per night	1100 mg
7.5 g per night	1400 mg
9 g per night	1640 mg

6 ADVERSE REACTIONS

The following adverse reactions appear in other sections of the labeling:

- CNS depression [*see Warnings and Precautions (5.1)*]
- Abuse and Misuse [*see Warnings and Precautions (5.2)*]
- Respiratory Depression and Sleep-disordered Breathing [*see Warnings and Precautions (5.4)*]
- Depression and Suicidality [*see Warnings and Precautions (5.5)*]
- Other Behavioral or Psychiatic Adverse Reactions [*see Warnings and Precautions (5.6)*]
- Parasomnias [*see Warnings and Precautions (5.7)*]
- Use in Patients Sensitive to High Sodium Intake [*see Warnings and Precautions (5.8)*]

Table 3

Adverse Reactions Occurring in ≥2% of Patients and More Frequently with Xyrem than Placebo in Three Controlled Trials (N1, N3, N4) by Body System and Dose at Onset

System Organ Class /MedDRA Preferred Term	Placebo (n=213) %	Xyrem 4.5g (n=185) %	Xyrem 6g (n=258)%	Xyrem 9g (n=178) %
ANY ADVERSE REACTION	62	45	55	70
GASTROINTESTINAL DISORDERS				
Nausea	3	8	13	20
Vomiting	1	2	4	11
Diarrhea	2	4	3	4
Abdominal pain upper	2	3	1	2
Dry mouth	2	1	2	1
GENERAL DISORDERS AND ADMINISTRATIVE SITE CONDITIONS				
Pain	1	1	<1	3
Feeling drunk	1	0	<1	3
Edema peripheral	1	3	0	0
MUSCULOSKELETAL AND CONNECTIVE TISSUE DISORDERS				
Pain in extremity	1	3	1	1
Cataplexy	1	1	1	2
Muscle spasms	2	2	<1	2
NERVOUS SYSTEM DISORDERS				
Dizziness	4	9	11	15
Somnolence	4	1	3	8
Tremor	0	0	2	5
Paresthesia	1	2	1	3
Disturbance in attention	0	1	0	4
Sleep paralysis	1	0	1	3
PSYCHIATRIC DISORDERS				
Disorientation	1	1	2	3
Anxiety	1	1	1	2
Irritability	1	0	<1	3
Sleep walking	0	0	0	3
RENAL AND URINARY DISORDERS				
Enuresis	1	3	3	7
SKIN AND SUBCUTANEOUS TISSUE DISORDERS				
Hyperhidrosis	0	1	1	3

6.1 Clinical Trial Experience

Because clinical trials are conducted under widely varying conditions, adverse reaction rates observed in the clinical trials of a drug cannot be directly compared to rates in the clinical trials of another drug and may not reflect the rates observed in clinical practice.

Xyrem was studied in three placebo-controlled clinical trials (Trials N1, N3, and N4, described in Sections 14.1 and 14.2) in 611 patients with narcolepsy (398 subjects treated with Xyrem, and 213 with placebo).A total of 781 patients with narcolepsy were treated with Xyrem in controlled and uncontrolled clinical trials.

Section 6.1 and Table 3 presents adverse reactions from three pooled, controlled trials (N1, N3, N4,) in patients with narcolepsy.

Adverse Reactions Leading to Treatment Discontinuation

Of the 398 Xyrem-treated patients with narcolepsy, 10.3% of patients discontinued because of adverse reactions compared with 2.8% of patients receiving placebo. The most common adverse reaction leading to discontinuation was nausea (2.8%). The majority of adverse reactions leading to discontinuation began during the first few weeks of treatment.

Commonly Observed Adverse Reactions in Controlled Clinical Trials:

The most common adverse reactions (incidence ≥ 5% and twice the rate seen with placebo) in Xyrem-treated patients were nausea, dizziness, vomiting, somnolence, enuresis, and tremor.

Adverse Reactions Occurring at an Incidence of 2% or greater:

Table 3 lists adverse reactions that occurred at a frequency of 2% or more in any treatment group for three controlled trials and were more frequent in any Xyrem treatment group than with placebo. Adverse reactions are summarized by dose at onset. Nearly all patients in these studies initiated treatment at 4.5 g per night. In patients who remained on treatment, adverse reactions tended to occur early and to diminish over time.

[See table 3 above]

Dose-Response Information

In clinical trials in narcolepsy, a dose-response relationship was observed for nausea, vomiting, paresthesia, disorientation, irritability, disturbance in attention, feeling drunk, sleepwalking, and enuresis. The incidence of all these reactions was notably higher at 9 g per night.

In controlled trials in narcolepsy, discontinuations of treatment due to adverse reactions were greater at higher doses of Xyrem.

6.2 Postmarketing Experience

The following additional adverse reactions that have a likely causal relationship to Xyrem exposure have been identified during postmarketing use of Xyrem. These adverse reactions include: arthralgia, decreased appetite, fall, fluid retention, hangover, headache, hypersensitivity, hypertension, memory impairment, panic attack, vision blurred, and weight decreased. Because these reactions are reported voluntarily, it is not always possible to reliably estimate their frequency.

7 DRUG INTERACTIONS

Xyrem should not be used in combination with alcohol or sedative hypnotics. Use of other CNS depressants may potentiate the CNS-depressant effects of Xyrem.

8 USE IN SPECIFIC POPULATIONS

8.1 Pregnancy

Pregnancy Category C

There are no adequate and well-controlled studies in pregnant women. Xyrem should be used during pregnancy only if the potential benefit justifies the potential risk to the fetus. Oral administration of sodium oxybate to pregnant rats (150, 350, or 1,000 mg/kg/day) or rabbits (300, 600, or 1,200 mg/kg/day) throughout organogenesis produced no clear evidence of developmental toxicity. The highest doses tested in rats and rabbits were approximately 1 and 3 times, respectively, the maximum recommended human dose (MRHD) of 9 g per night on a body surface area (mg/m^2) basis.

Oral administration of sodium oxybate (150, 350, or 1,000 mg/kg/day) to rats throughout pregnancy and lactation resulted in increased stillbirths and decreased offspring postnatal viability and body weight gain at the highest dose tested. The no-effect dose for pre- and post-natal developmental toxicity in rats is less than the MRHD on a mg/m^2 basis.

8.2 Labor and Delivery

Xyrem has not been studied in labor or delivery. In obstetric anesthesia using an injectable formulation of sodium oxybate, newborns had stable cardiovascular and respiratory measures but were very sleepy, causing a slight decrease in Apgar scores. There was a fall in the rate of uterine contractions 20 minutes after injection. Placental transfer is rapid, but umbilical vein levels of sodium oxybate were no more than 25% of the maternal concentration. No sodium oxybate was detected in the infant's blood 30 minutes after delivery. Elimination curves of sodium oxybate between a 2-day-old infant and a 15-year-old patient were similar. Subsequent effects of sodium oxybate on later growth, development, and maturation in humans are unknown.

8.3 Nursing Mothers

It is not known whether sodium oxybate is excreted in human milk. Because many drugs are excreted in human milk, caution should be exercised when Xyrem is administered to a nursing woman.

8.4 Pediatric Use

Safety and effectiveness in pediatric patients have not been established.

8.5 Geriatric Use

Clinical studies of Xyrem in patients with narcolepsy did not include sufficient numbers of subjects age 65 years and older to determine whether they respond differently from younger subjects. In controlled trials in another population, 39 (5%) of 874 patients were 65 years or older. Discontinuations of treatment due to adverse reactions were increased in the elderly compared to younger adults (20.5% v. 18.9%). Frequency of headaches was markedly increased in the elderly (38.5% v. 18.9%). The most common adverse reactions were similar in both age categories. In general, dose selection for an elderly patient should be cautious, usually starting at the low end of the dosing range, reflecting the greater frequency of decreased hepatic, renal, or cardiac function, and of concomitant disease or other drug therapy.

8.6 Hepatic Impairment

The starting dose of Xyrem should be reduced by one half in patients with liver impairment *[see Dosage and Administration (2.3), Clinical Pharmacology (12.3)]*.

9 DRUG ABUSE AND DEPENDENCE

9.1 Controlled Substance

Xyrem is a Schedule III controlled substance under the Federal Controlled Substances Act. Non-medical use of Xyrem could lead to penalties assessed under the higher Schedule I controls.

9.2 Abuse

Xyrem (sodium oxybate), the sodium salt of GHB, produces dose-dependent central nervous system effects, including hypnotic and positive subjective reinforcing effects. The onset of effect is rapid, enhancing its potential for abuse or misuse.

The rapid onset of sedation, coupled with the amnestic features of Xyrem, particularly when combined with alcohol, has proven to be dangerous for the voluntary and involuntary user (e.g., assault victim).

Illicit GHB is abused in social settings primarily by young adults. Some of the doses estimated to be abused are in a similar dosage range to that used for treatment of patients with cataplexy. GHB has some commonalties with ethanol over a limited dose range, and some cross tolerance with ethanol has been reported as well. Cases of severe dependence and craving for GHB have been reported when the drug is taken around the clock. Patterns of abuse indicative of dependence include: 1) the use of increasingly large doses, 2) increased frequency of use, and 3) continued use despite adverse consequences.

Because illicit use and abuse of GHB have been reported, physicians should carefully evaluate patients for a history of drug abuse and follow such patients closely, observing them for signs of misuse or abuse of GHB (e.g. increase in size or frequency of dosing, drug-seeking behavior, feigned cataplexy). Dispose of Xyrem according to state and federal regulations. It is safe to dispose of Xyrem down the sanitary sewer.

9.3 Dependence

There have been case reports of withdrawal, ranging from mild to severe, following discontinuation of illicit use of GHB at frequent repeated doses (18 g to 250 g per day) in excess of the therapeutic dose range. Signs and symptoms of GHB withdrawal following abrupt discontinuation included insomnia, restlessness, anxiety, psychosis, lethargy, nausea, tremor, sweating, muscle cramps, tachycardia, headache, dizziness, rebound fatigue and sleepiness, confusion, and, particularly in the case of severe withdrawal, visual hallucinations, agitation, and delirium. These symptoms generally abated in 3 to 14 days. In cases of severe withdrawal, hospitalization may be required. The discontinuation effects of Xyrem have not been systematically evaluated in controlled clinical trials. In the clinical trial experience with Xyrem in narcolepsy/cataplexy patients at therapeutic doses, two patients reported anxiety and one reported insomnia following abrupt discontinuation at the termination of the clinical trial; in the two patients with anxiety, the frequency of cataplexy had increased markedly at the same time.

Tolerance

Tolerance to Xyrem has not been systematically studied in controlled clinical trials. There have been some case reports of symptoms of tolerance developing after illicit use at dosages far in excess of the recommended Xyrem dosage regimen. Clinical studies of sodium oxybate in the treatment of alcohol withdrawal suggest a potential cross-tolerance with alcohol. The safety and effectiveness of Xyrem in the treatment of alcohol withdrawal have not been established.

10 OVERDOSAGE

10.1 Human Experience

Information regarding overdose with Xyrem is derived largely from reports in the medical literature that describe symptoms and signs in individuals who have ingested GHB illicitly. In these circumstances the co-ingestion of other drugs and alcohol was common, and may have influenced the presentation and severity of clinical manifestations of overdose.

In clinical trials two cases of overdose with Xyrem were reported. In the first case, an estimated dose of 150 g, more than 15 times the maximum recommended dose, caused a patient to be unresponsive with brief periods of apnea and to be incontinent of urine and feces. This individual recovered without sequelae. In the second case, death was reported following a multiple drug overdose consisting of Xyrem and numerous other drugs.

10.2 Signs and Symptoms

Information about signs and symptoms associated with overdosage with Xyrem derives from reports of its illicit use. Patient presentation following overdose is influenced by the dose ingested, the time since ingestion, the co-ingestion of other drugs and alcohol, and the fed or fasted state. Patients have exhibited varying degrees of depressed consciousness that may fluctuate rapidly between a confusional, agitated combative state with ataxia and coma. Emesis (even when obtunded), diaphoresis, headache, and impaired psychomotor skills have been observed. No typical pupillary changes have been described to assist in diagnosis; pupillary reactivity to light is maintained. Blurred vision has been reported. An increasing depth of coma has been observed at higher doses. Myoclonus and tonic-clonic seizures have been reported. Respiration may be unaffected or compromised in rate and depth. Cheyne-Stokes respiration and apnea have been observed. Bradycardia and hypothermia may accompany unconsciousness, as well as muscular hypotonia, but tendon reflexes remain intact.

10.3 Recommended Treatment of Overdose

General symptomatic and supportive care should be instituted immediately, and gastric decontamination may be considered if co-ingestants are suspected. Because emesis may occur in the presence of obtundation, appropriate posture (left lateral recumbent position) and protection of the airway by intubation may be warranted. Although the gag reflex may be absent in deeply comatose patients, even unconscious patients may become combative to intubation, and rapid-sequence induction (without the use of sedative) should be considered. Vital signs and consciousness should be closely monitored. The bradycardia reported with GHB overdose has been responsive to atropine intravenous administration. No reversal of the central depressant effects of Xyrem can be expected from naloxone or flumazenil administration. The use of hemodialysis and other forms of extracorporeal drug removal have not been studied in GHB overdose. However, due to the rapid metabolism of sodium oxybate, these measures are not warranted.

10.4 Poison Control Center

As with the management of all cases of drug overdosage, the possibility of multiple drug ingestion should be considered. The healthcare provider is encouraged to collect urine and blood samples for routine toxicologic screening, and to consult with a regional poison control center (1-800-222-1222) for current treatment recommendations.

11 DESCRIPTION

Sodium oxybate, a CNS depressant, is the active ingredient in Xyrem. The chemical name for sodium oxybate is sodium 4 hydroxybutyrate. The molecular formula is C4H7NaO3, and the molecular weight is 126.09 g/mole. The chemical structure is:

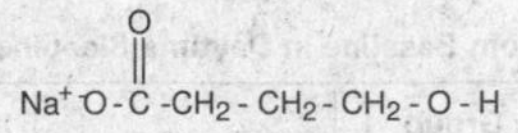

Sodium oxybate is a white to off-white, crystalline powder that is very soluble in aqueous solutions. Each mL of Xyrem contains 0.5 g of sodium oxybate in USP Purified Water, neutralized to pH 7.5 with malic acid.

12 CLINICAL PHARMACOLOGY

12.1 Mechanism of Action

Xyrem is a CNS depressant. The mechanism of action of Xyrem in the treatment of narcolepsy is unknown. Sodium oxybate is the sodium salt of gamma hydroxybutyrate, an endogenous compound and metabolite of the neurotransmitter GABA. It is hypothesized that the therapeutic effects of Xyrem on cataplexy and excessive daytime sleepiness are mediated through $GABA_B$ actions at noradrenergic and dopaminergic neurons, as well as at thalamocortical neurons.

12.3 Pharmacokinetics

Pharmacokinetics of sodium oxybate are nonlinear and are similar following single or repeat dosing.

Absorption

Following oral administration, sodium oxybate is absorbed rapidly across the clinical dose range, with an absolute bioavailability of about 88%. The average peak plasma concentrations (C_{max}) following administration of each of the two 2.25 g doses given under fasting conditions 4 hours apart were similar. The average time to peak plasma concentration (T_{max}) ranged from 0.5 to 1.25 hours. Following oral administration, the plasma levels of sodium oxybate increased more than dose-proportionally, with blood levels increasing 3.7–fold as total daily dose is doubled from 4.5 g to 9 g. Single doses greater than 4.5 g have not been studied. Administration of Xyrem immediately after a high-fat meal resulted in delayed absorption (average T_{max} increased from 0.75 hr to 2 hr) and a reduction in C_{max} by a mean of 59% and of systemic exposure (AUC) by 37%.

Distribution

Sodium oxybate is a hydrophilic compound with an apparent volume of distribution averaging 190 mL/kg to 384 mL/kg. At sodium oxybate concentrations ranging from 3 mcg/mL to 300 mcg/mL, less than 1% is bound to plasma proteins.

Metabolism

Animal studies indicate that metabolism is the major elimination pathway for sodium oxybate, producing carbon dioxide and water via the tricarboxylic acid (Krebs) cycle and secondarily by beta-oxidation. The primary pathway involves a cytosolic $NADP^+$-linked enzyme, GHB dehydrogenase, that catalyzes the conversion of sodium oxybate to succinic semialdehyde, which is then biotransformed to succinic acid by the enzyme succinic semialdehyde dehydrogenase. Succinic acid enters the Krebs cycle where it is metabolized to carbon dioxide and water. A second mitochondrial oxidoreductase enzyme, a transhydrogenase, also catalyzes the conversion to succinic semialdehyde in the presence of α-ketoglutarate. An alternate pathway of biotransformation involves β-oxidation via 3,4–dihydroxybutyrate to carbon dioxide and water. No active metabolites have been identified.

Elimination

The clearance of sodium oxybate is almost entirely by biotransformation to carbon dioxide, which is then eliminated by expiration. On average, less than 5% of unchanged drug appears in human urine within 6 to 8 hours after dosing. Fecal excretion is negligible. Sodium oxybate has an elimination half-life of 0.5 to 1 hour.

Table 4
Median Number of Cataplexy Attacks in Trials N1 and N2

Trial/Dosage Group	Baseline	Median Change from Baseline	Comparison to Placebo (p-value)
Trial N1 (Prospective, Randomized, Parallel Group Trial)			
		(median attacks/week)	
Placebo (n=33)	20.5	-4	–
Xyrem 6 g per night (n=31)	23.0	-10	0.0451
Xyrem 9 g per night (n=33)	23.5	-16	0.0016
Trial N2 (Randomized Withdrawal Trial)			
		(median attacks/2 weeks)	
Placebo (n=29)	4.0	21	–
Xyrem (n=26)	1.9	0	< 0.001

Table 5
Change from Baseline in Daytime Sleepiness Score (Epworth Sleepiness Scale) at Week 8 in Trial N3 (Range 0-24)

Treatment Group	Baseline	Week 8	Median Change from Baseline at Week 8	p-value
Placebo (n=59)	17.5	17.0	-0.5	-
Xyrem 6 g per night (n=58)	19.0	16.0	-2.0	< 0.001
Xyrem 9 g per night (n=47)	19.0	12.0	-5.0	< 0.001

Specific Populations

Geriatric

There is limited experience with Xyrem in the elderly. Results from a pharmacokinetic study (n=20) in another studied population indicate that the pharmacokinetic characteristics of sodium oxybate are consistent among younger (age 48 to 64 years) and older (age 65 to 75 years) adults.

Pediatric

The pharmacokinetics of sodium oxybate in patients younger than 18 years of age have not been studied.

Gender

In a study of 18 female and 18 male healthy adult volunteers, no gender differences were detected in the pharmacokinetics of sodium oxybate oral solution following a single oral dose of 4.5 g.

Race

There are insufficient data to evaluate any pharmacokinetic differences among races.

Renal Impairment

No pharmacokinetic study in patients with renal impairment has been conducted.

Hepatic Impairment

The pharmacokinetics of Xyrem in 16 cirrhotic patients, half without ascites (Child's Class A) and half with ascites (Child's Class C), were compared to the kinetics in 8 subjects with normal hepatic function after a single oral dose of 25 mg/kg. AUC values were double in the cirrhotic patients, with apparent oral clearance reduced from 9.1 mL/min/kg in healthy adults to 4.5 and 4.1 mL/min/kg in Class A and Class C patients, respectively. Elimination half-life was significantly longer in Class C and Class A patients than in control patients (mean $t_{1/2}$ of 59 and 32 minutes, respectively, versus 22 minutes). The starting dose of Xyrem should be reduced by one-half in patients with liver impairment *[see Dosage and Administration (2.3); Use in Specific Populations (8.6)]*.

Drug Interactions Studies

Studies *in vitro* with pooled human liver microsomes indicate that sodium oxybate does not significantly inhibit the activities of the human isoenzymes CYP1A2, CYP2C9, CYP2C19, CYP2D6, CYP2E1, or CYP3A up to the concentration of 3 mM (378 mcg/mL), a level considerably higher than levels achieved with therapeutic doses.

Drug interaction studies in healthy adults demonstrated no pharmacokinetic interactions between sodium oxybate and protriptyline hydrochloride, zolpidem tartrate, and modafinil. Also, there were no pharmacokinetic interactions with the alcohol dehydrogenase inhibitor fomepizole. However, pharmacodynamic interactions with these drugs cannot be ruled out. Alteration of gastric pH with omeprazole produced no significant change in the oxybate kinetics *[see Drug Interactions (7)]*. In addition, drug interaction studies in healthy adults demonstrated no pharmacokinetic or clinically significant pharmacodynamic interactions between sodium oxybate and the SNRI duloxetine HCl.

13 NONCLINICAL TOXICOLOGY

13.1 Carcinogenesis, Mutagenesis, Impairment of Fertility

Carcinogenesis

Administration of sodium oxybate to rats at oral doses of up to 1,000 mg/kg/day for 83 (males) or 104 (females) weeks resulted in no increase in tumors. Plasma exposure (AUC) at the highest dose tested was 2 times that in humans at the maximum recommend human dose (MRHD) of 9 g per night.

The results of 2-year carcinogenicity studies in mouse and rat with gamma-butyrolactone, a compound that is metabolized to sodium oxybate in vivo, showed no clear evidence of carcinogenic activity. The plasma AUCs of sodium oxybate achieved at the highest doses tested in these studies were less than that in humans at the MRHD.

Mutagenesis

Sodium oxybate was negative in the in vitro bacterial gene mutation assay, an in vitro chromosomal aberration assay in mammalian cells, and in an in vivo rat micronucleus assay.

Impairment of Fertility

Oral administration of sodium oxybate (150, 350, or 1,000 mg/kg/day) to male and female rats prior to and throughout mating and continuing in females through early gestation resulted in no adverse effects on fertility. The highest dose tested is approximately equal to the MRHD on a mg/m2 basis.

14 CLINICAL STUDIES

14.1 Cataplexy in Narcolepsy

The effectiveness of Xyrem in the treatment of cataplexy was established in two randomized, double-blind, placebo-controlled, multicenter, parallel-group trials (Trials N1 and N2) in patients with narcolepsy (see Table 4). In Trials N1 and N2, 85% and 80% of patients, respectively, were also being treated with CNS stimulants. The high percentages of concomitant stimulant use make it impossible to assess the efficacy and safety of Xyrem independent of stimulant use. In each trial, the treatment period was 4 weeks and the total nightly Xyrem doses ranged from 3 g to 9 g, with the total nightly dose administered as two equal doses. The first dose each night was taken at bedtime and the second dose was taken 2.5 to 4 hours later. There were no restrictions on the time between food consumption and dosing.

Trial N1 enrolled 136 narcoleptic patients with moderate to severe cataplexy (median of 21 cataplexy attacks per week) at baseline. Prior to randomization, medications with possible effects on cataplexy were withdrawn, but stimulants were continued at stable doses. Patients were randomized to receive placebo, Xyrem 3 g per night, Xyrem 6 g per night, or Xyrem 9 g per night.

Trial N2 was a randomized withdrawal trial with 55 narcoleptic patients who had been taking open-label Xyrem for 7 to 44 months prior to study entry. To be included, patients were required to have a history of at least 5 cataplexy attacks per week prior to any treatment for cataplexy. Patients were randomized to continued treatment with Xyrem at their stable dose (ranging from 3 g to 9 g per night) or to placebo for 4 weeks. Trial N2 was designed specifically to evaluate the continued efficacy of sodium oxybate after long-term use

The primary efficacy measure in Trials N1 and N2 was the frequency of cataplexy attacks.

[See table 4 above]

In Trial N1, both the 6 g and 9 g per night Xyrem doses resulted in statistically significant reductions in the frequency of cataplexy attacks. The 3 g per night dose had little effect. In Trial N2, patients randomized to placebo after discontinuing long-term open-label Xyrem therapy experienced a significant increase in cataplexy attacks ($p < 0.001$), providing evidence of long-term efficacy of Xyrem. In Trial N2, the response was numerically similar for patients treated with doses of 6 g to 9 g per night, but there was no effect seen in patients treated with doses less than 6 g per night, suggesting little effect at these doses.

14.2 Excessive Daytime Sleepiness in Narcolepsy

The effectiveness of Xyrem in the treatment of excessive daytime sleepiness in patients with narcolepsy was established in two randomized, double-blind, placebo-controlled trials (Trials N3 and N4) (see Tables 7 to 9). Seventy-eight percent of patients in Trial N3 were also being treated with CNS stimulants.

Trial N3 was a multicenter randomized, double-blind, placebo-controlled, parallel-group trial that evaluated 228 patients with moderate to severe symptoms at entry into the study including a median Epworth Sleepiness Scale (see below) score of 18, and a Maintenance of Wakefulness Test (see below) score of 8.3 minutes. Patients were randomized to one of 4 treatment groups: placebo, Xyrem 4.5 g per night, Xyrem 6 g per night, or Xyrem 9 g per night. The period of double-blind treatment in this trial was 8 weeks. Antidepressants were withdrawn prior to randomization; stimulants were continued at stable doses.

The primary efficacy measures in Trial N3 were the Epworth Sleepiness Scale and the Clinical Global Impression of Change. The Epworth Sleepiness Scale is intended to evaluate the extent of sleepiness in everyday situations by asking the patient a series of questions. In these questions, patients were asked to rate their chances of dozing during each of 8 activities on a scale from 0-3 (0=never; 1=slight; 2=moderate; 3=high). Higher total scores indicate a greater tendency to sleepiness. The Clinical Global Impression of Change is evaluated on a 7-point scale, centered at *No Change*, and ranging from *Very Much Worse* to *Very Much Improved*. In Trial N3, patients were rated by evaluators who based their assessments on the severity of narcolepsy at baseline.

In Trial N3, statistically significant improvements were seen on the Epworth Sleepiness Scale score at Week 8 and on the Clinical Global Impression of Change score at Week 8 with the 6 g and 9 g per night doses of Xyrem compared to the placebo group.

[See table 5 above]

Table 6
Proportion of patients with a very much or much improved Clinical Global Impression of Change in Daytime and Nighttime Symptoms in Trial N3

Treatment Group	Percentages of Responders (Very Much Improved or Much Improved)	Change from Baseline Significance Compared to Placebo (p-value)
Placebo (59)	22%	-
Xyrem 6 g per night (n=58)	52%	< 0.001
Xyrem 9 g per night (n=47)	64%	< 0.001

Trial N4 was a multicenter randomized, double-blind, placebo-controlled, parallel-group trial that evaluated 222 patients with moderate to severe symptoms at entry into the study including a median Epworth Sleepiness Scale score of 15, and a Maintenance of Wakefulness Test (see below) score of 10.3 minutes. At entry, patients had to be taking modafinil at stable doses of 200 mg, 400 mg, or 600 mg daily for at least 1 month prior to randomization. The patients enrolled in the study were randomized to one of 4 treatment groups: placebo, Xyrem, modafinil, or Xyrem plus modafinil. Xyrem was administered in a dose of 6 g per night for 4 weeks, followed by 9 g per night for 4 weeks. Modafinil was continued in the modafinil alone and the Xyrem plus modafinil treatment groups at the patient's prior dose. Trial N4 was not designed to compare the effects of Xyrem to modafinil because patients receiving modafinil were not titrated to a maximal dose. Patients randomized to placebo or to Xyrem treatment were withdrawn from their stable dose of modafinil. Patients taking antidepressants could continue these medications at stable doses.

The primary efficacy measure in Trial N4 was the Maintenance of Wakefulness Test. The Maintenance of Wakefulness Test measures latency to sleep onset (in minutes) averaged over 4 sessions at 2-hour intervals following nocturnal polysomnography. For each test session, the subject was asked to remain awake without using extraordinary measures. Each test session is terminated after 20 minutes if no sleep occurs, or after 10 minutes, if sleep occurs. The overall score is the mean sleep latency for the 4 sessions.

In Trial N4, a statistically significant improvement in the change in the Maintenance of Wakefulness Test score from baseline at Week 8 was seen in the Xyrem and Xyrem plus modafinil groups compared to the placebo group.

This trial was not designed to compare the effects of Xyrem to modafinil, because patients receiving modafinil were not titrated to a maximally effective dose.

[See table 7 above]

Table 7
Change in Baseline in the Maintenance of Wakefulness Test Score (in minutes) at Week 8 in Trial N4

Treatment Group	Baseline	Week 8	Mean Change from Baseline at Week 8	p-value
Placebo (modafinil withdrawn) (n=55)	9.7	6.9	-2.7	-
Xyrem (modafinil withdrawn) (n=50)	11.3	12.0	0.6	<0.001
Xyrem plus modafinil (n=54)	10.4	13.2	2.7	<0.001

16 HOW SUPPLIED/STORAGE AND HANDLING

16.1 How Supplied

Xyrem is a clear to slightly opalescent oral solution. Each prescription includes a carton containing one bottle of Xyrem, a press-in-bottle-adaptor, an oral measuring device (plastic syringe), and a Medication Guide. The pharmacy provides two empty vials with child-resistant caps with each Xyrem shipment.

Each amber bottle contains Xyrem oral solution at a concentration of 0.5 g per mL and has a child-resistant cap.

Carton containing one 180 mL bottle NDC 68727-100-01

16.2 Storage

Keep out of reach of children.

Xyrem should be stored at 25°C (77°F); excursions permitted to 15° to 30°C (59° to 86°F) (see USP Controlled Room Temperature).

Dispense in tight containers.

16.3 Handling and Disposal

Xyrem is a Schedule III drug under the Controlled Substances Act. Xyrem should be handled according to state and federal regulations. It is safe to dispose of Xyrem down the sanitary sewer.

17 PATIENT COUNSELING INFORMATION

See FDA-approved patient labeling (Medication Guide).

Xyrem Success Program

- Inform patients that Xyrem is available only through a restricted distribution program called the Xyrem Success Program.
- The contents of the Xyrem Medication Guide and educational materials are reviewed with every patient before initiating treatment with Xyrem.
- Patients must read and understand the materials in the Xyrem Success Program prior to initiating treatment. Inform the patient that they should be seen by the prescriber frequently to review dose titration, symptom response, and adverse reactions; a follow-up of every three months is recommended.
- Discuss safe and proper use of Xyrem and dosing information with patients prior to the initiation of treatment. Instruct patients to store Xyrem bottles and Xyrem doses in a secure place, out of the reach of children and pets.

Alcohol or Sedative Hypnotics

Advise patients not to drink alcohol or take other sedative hypnotics if they are taking Xyrem.

Sedation

Inform patients that after taking Xyrem they are likely to fall asleep quickly (often within 5 and usually within 15 minutes), but the time it takes to fall asleep can vary from night to night. The sudden onset of sleep, including in a standing position or while rising from bed, has led to falls complicated by injuries, in some cases requiring hospitalization. Instruct patients to remain in bed following ingestion of their first dose, and not to take their second dose until 2.5 to 4 hours later.

Food Effects on Xyrem

Inform patients to take the first dose at least 2 hours after eating.

Respiratory Depression

Inform patients that Xyrem can be associated with respiratory depression.

Operating Hazardous Machinery

Inform patients that until they are reasonably certain that Xyrem does not affect them adversely (e.g., impair judgment, thinking, or motor skills) they should not operate hazardous machinery, including automobiles or airplanes.

Suicidality

Instruct patients or families to contact a healthcare provider immediately if the patient develops depressed mood, markedly diminished interest or pleasure in usual activities, significant change in weight and/or appetite, psychomotor agitation or retardation, increased fatigue, feelings of guilt or worthlessness, slowed thinking or impaired concentration, or suicidal ideation.

Sleepwalking

Instruct patients and their families that Xyrem has been associated with sleepwalking and to contact their healthcare provider if this occurs.

Sodium Intake

Instruct patients who are sensitive to salt intake (e.g., those with heart failure, hypertension, or renal impairment) that Xyrem contains a significant amount of sodium and they should limit their sodium intake.

MEDICATION GUIDE

Xyrem® (ZIE-rem)
(sodiumoxybate)
oral solution C III

Read this Medication Guide carefully before you start taking Xyrem and each time you get a refill. There may be new information. This information does not take the place of talking to your doctor about your medical condition or your treatment.

What is the most important information I should know about Xyrem?

Xyrem can cause serious side effects including slow breathing or changes in your alertness. Do not drink alcohol or take medicines intended to make you fall asleep while you are taking Xyrem because they can make these side effects worse. Call your doctor right away if you have any of these serious side effects.

- The active ingredient of Xyrem is a form of gamma-hydroxybutyrate (GHB). GHB is a chemical that has been abused and misused. Abuse and misuse of Xyrem can cause serious medical problems, including:
  - seizures
  - trouble breathing
  - changes in alertness
  - coma
  - death
- Do not drive a car, use heavy machinery, fly an airplane, or do anything that is dangerous or that requires you to be fully awake for at least 6 hours after you take Xyrem. You should not do those activities until you know how Xyrem affects you.
- Xyrem is available only by prescription and filled through the central pharmacy in the Xyrem Success Program. Before you receive Xyrem, your doctor or pharmacist will make sure that you understand how to use Xyrem safely and effectively. If you have any questions about Xyrem, ask your doctor or call the Xyrem Success Program® at 1-866-997-3688.

What is Xyrem?

Xyrem is a prescription medicine used to treat the following symptoms in people who fall asleep frequently during the day, often at unexpected times (narcolepsy):

- suddenly weak or paralyzed muscles when they feel strong emotions (cataplexy)
- excessive daytime sleepiness (EDS) in people who have narcolepsy

It is not known if Xyrem is safe and effective in children. Xyrem is a controlled substance (CIII) because it contains sodium oxybate that can be a target for people who abuse prescription medicines or street drugs. Keep your Xyrem in a safe place to protect it from theft. Never give your Xyrem to anyone else because it may cause death or harm them. Selling or giving away this medicine is against the law.

Who should not take Xyrem?

Do not take Xyrem if you:

- take other sleep medicines or sedatives (medicines that cause sleepiness)
- drink alcohol
- have a rare problem called succinic semialdehyde dehydrogenase deficiency

Before you take Xyrem, tell your doctor if you:

- have short periods of not breathing while you sleep (sleep apnea)
- snore, have trouble breathing, or have lung problems. You may have a higher chance of having serious breathing problems when you take Xyrem.
- have or had depression or have tried to harm yourself. You should be watched carefully for new symptoms of depression.
- have liver problems
- are on a salt-restricted diet. Xyrem contains a lot of sodium (salt) and may not be right for you.
- have high blood pressure
- have heartfailure
- have kidney problems
- are pregnant or plan to become pregnant. It is not known if Xyrem can harm your unborn baby.
- are breastfeeding or plan to breastfeed. It is not known if Xyrem passes into your breast milk. You and your doctor should decide if you will take Xyrem or breastfeed.

Tell your doctor about all the medicines you take, including prescription and non-prescription medicines, vitamins, and herbal supplements.

Especially, tell your doctor if you take other medicines to help you sleep (sedatives). Do not take medicines that make you sleepy with Xyrem.

Know the medicines you take. Keep a list of them to show your doctor and pharmacist when you get a new medicine.

How should I take Xyrem?

- Read the **Instructions for Use** at the end of this Medication Guide for detailed instructions on how to take Xyrem.
- Take Xyrem exactly as your doctor tells you to take it.
- Never change your Xyrem dose without talking to your doctor.
- Xyrem can cause sleep very quickly. You should fall asleep soon. Some patients fall asleep within 5 minutes and most fall asleep within 15 minutes. Some patients take less time to fall asleep and some take more time. The time it takes you to fall asleep might be different from night to night.
- Take your first Xyrem dose at bedtime while you are in bed. Take your second Xyrem dose 2 ½ to 4 hours after you take your first Xyrem dose. You may want to set an alarm clock to make sure you wake up to take your second Xyrem dose.
- If you miss your second Xyrem dose, skip that dose and do not take Xyrem again until the next night. Never take 2 Xyrem doses at 1 time.
- Wait at least 2 hours after eating before you take Xyrem.
- You should see your doctor every 3 months for a check-up while taking Xyrem. Your doctor should check to see if Xyrem is helping to lessen your symptoms and if you feel any side effects while you take Xyrem.
- If you take too much Xyrem, call your doctor or go to the nearest hospital emergency room right away.

What are the possible side effects of Xyrem?

Xyrem can cause serious side effects, including:

- See **"What is the most important information I should know about Xyrem?"**
- **Breathing problems, including:**
  - slower breathing
  - trouble breathing
  - short periods of not breathing while sleeping (sleep apnea). People who already have breathing or lung problems have a higher chance of having breathing problems when they use Xyrem.
- **Mental health problems, including:**
  - confusion
  - seeing or hearing things that are not real (hallucinations)

- ○ unusual or disturbing thoughts (abnormal thinking)
- ○ feeling anxious or upset
- ○ depression
- ○ thoughts of killing yourself or trying to kill yourself

Call your doctor right away if you have symptoms of mental health problems.

- **Sleepwalking.** Sleepwalking can cause injuries. Call your doctor if you start sleepwalking.Your doctor should check you.

The most common side effects of Xyrem include:

- ○ nausea
- ○ dizziness
- ○ vomiting
- ○ bedwetting
- ○ diarrhea

Your side effects may increase when you take higher doses of Xyrem.

Xyrem can cause physical dependence and craving for the medicine when it is not taken as directed.

These are not all the possible side effects of Xyrem. For more information, ask your doctor or pharmacist.

Call your doctor for medical advice about side effects. You may report side effects to FDA at 1-800-FDA-1088.

How should I store Xyrem?

- **Always store Xyrem in the original bottle or in pharmacy containers with child-resistant caps provided by the pharmacy.**
- **Keep Xyrem in a safe place out of the reach of children and pets.**
- **Get emergency medical help right away if a child drinks your Xyrem.**
- Store Xyrem between 68°F to 77°F (20°C to 24°C). When you have finished using a Xyrem bottle:
- ○ empty any unused Xyrem down the sink drain
- ○ cross out the label on the Xyrem bottle with a marker
- ○ place the empty Xyrem bottle in the trash

General information about the safe and effective use of Xyrem

Medicines are sometimes prescribed for purposes other than those listed in a Medication Guide. Do not use Xyrem for a condition for which it was not prescribed. Do not give Xyrem to other people, even if they have the same symptoms that you have. It may harm them.

This Medication Guide summarizes the most important information about Xyrem. If you would like more information, talk with your doctor. You can ask your pharmacist or doctor for information about Xyrem that is written for health professionals.

For more information, go to www.XYREM.com or call the Xyrem Success Program at 1-866-997-3688.

What are the ingredients in Xyrem?

Active Ingredients: sodium oxybate

Inactive Ingredients: purified water and malic acid

This Medication Guide has been approved by the U. S. Food and Drug Administration.

Distributed By:

Jazz Pharmaceuticals, Inc.

Palo Alto, CA 94304

Instructions for Use

Xyrem®(ZIE-rem)

(sodiumoxybate)

oral solution C III

Read these Instructions for Use carefully before you start taking Xyrem and each time you get a refill. There may be new information. This information does not take the place of talking to your doctor about your medical condition or your treatment.

Note:

- **You will need to split your prescribed Xyrem dose into 2 separate pharmacy containers for mixing.**
- **You will need to mix Xyrem with water before you take your dose.**

Supplies you will need for mixing and taking Xyrem: See Figure A.

- bottle of your Xyrem medicine
  - press-in bottle adaptor with straw attached
- syringe for drawing up your Xyrem dose
- a measuring cup containing about ¼ cup of water (not provided with your Xyrem prescription)
- 2 **empty** pharmacy containers with child-resistant caps
- alarm clock by your bedside (alarm clock may be included in your first shipment of Xyrem)

[See figure A at top of next column]

Step 1. Take the Xyrem bottle, press-in-bottle adaptor, and syringe out of the box.

Step 2. Remove the bottle cap from the Xyrem bottle by pushing down while turning the cap counterclockwise (to the left). See Figure B.

[See figure B at top of next column]

Step 3.

- The press-in-bottle adaptor may already be put in place by the pharmacy. If it is not already in place, you will have to do it yourself. After removing the cap from the Xyrem bottle, set the bottle upright on a tabletop.

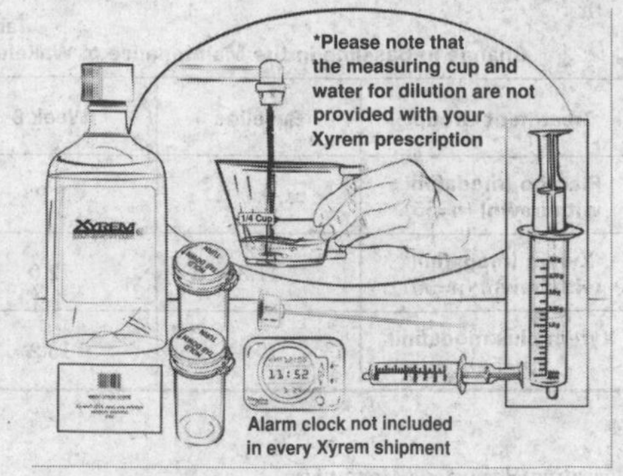
*Please note that the measuring cup and water for dilution are not provided with your Xyrem prescription
Alarm clock not included in every Xyrem shipment

Figure A

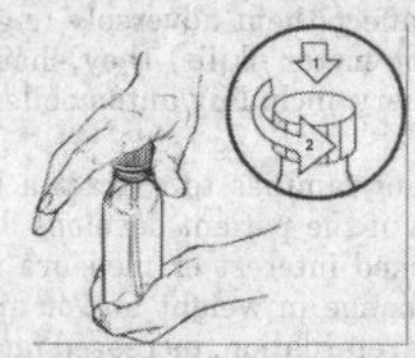

Figure B

- While holding the Xyrem bottle in its upright position, insert the press-in-bottle-adaptor into the neck of the Xyrem bottle. See Figure C.

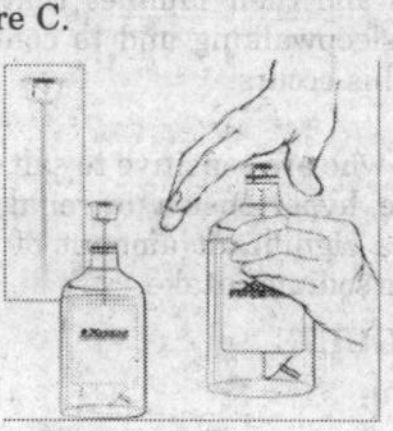

Figure C

- Tilt the straw toward the edge of the bottom of the bottle to be sure you can draw out your dose of the medicine. You only need to do this the first time you open the bottle. See Figure D.

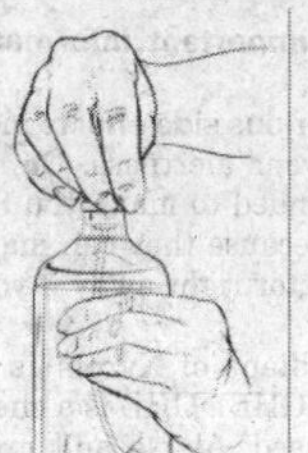

Figure D

- After you draw out your dose of the medicine, leave the adaptor in the bottle for all your future uses. See Figure E.

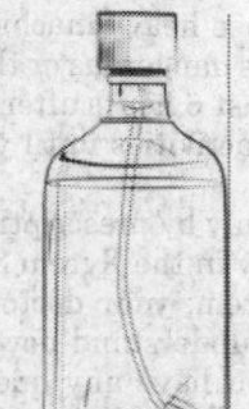

Figure E

Step 4.

- Take the syringe out of the plastic wrapper. Use only the syringe provided with your Xyrem prescription.
- While holding the Xyrem bottle upright on the tabletop, insert the tip of the syringe into the opening on top of the Xyrem bottle and press down firmly. See Figure F.

[See figure F at top of next column]

Step 5.

- Hold the bottle and syringe down with one hand, and draw up one-half (1/2) of your total prescribed nightly dose with the other hand by pulling up on the plunger. For example, if your total nightly dose of Xyrem is 4.5 grams a night, you will need to draw up 2 separate doses of 2.25 grams each, one for each pharmacy container. See Figure G.

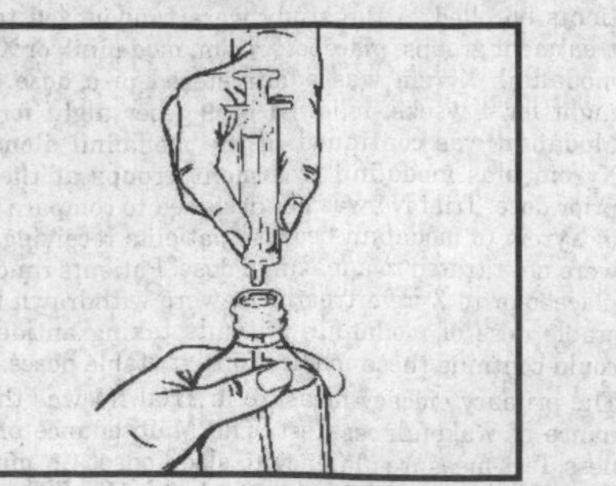

Figure F

Note: The Xyrem medicine will not flow into the syringe unless you keep the bottle upright.

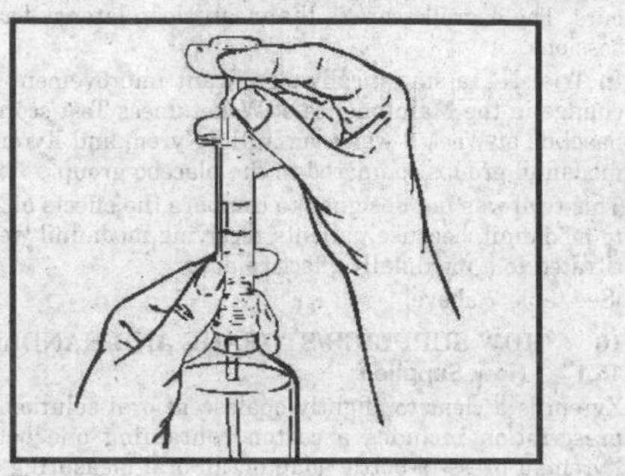

Figure G

Step 6.

- After you draw up each separate Xyrem dose, remove the syringe from the opening of the Xyrem bottle. Put the tip into 1 of the **empty** containers with child-resistant caps provided by the pharmacy.
- **Make sure the pharmacy container is empty and does not contain any medicine from your previous night's dose.**
  - ○ Empty each separate Xyrem dose into 1 of the **empty** pharmacy containers by pushing down on the plunger. (See Figure H).
- Using a measuring cup, pour about ¼ cup of water into each container. **Be careful to add only water to each container and not more Xyrem. All shipped bottles of Xyrem contain the concentrated medicine. Water for mixing the medicine is not provided in the shipment.**

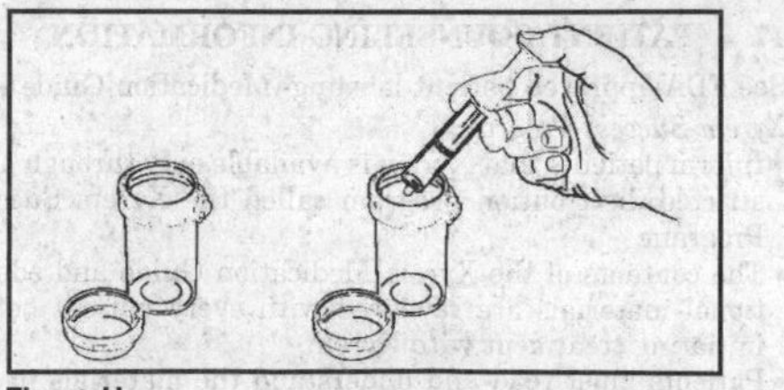

Figure H

Step 7.

- Place the child-resistant caps provided on the filled pharmacy containers and turn each cap clockwise (to the right) until it clicks and locks into its child-resistant position. See Figure I.

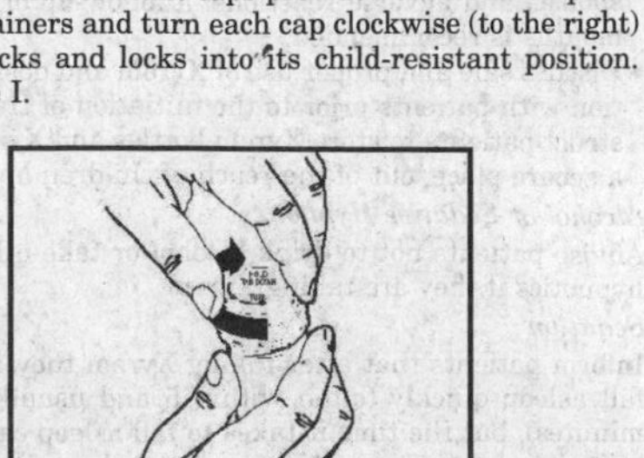

Figure I

- Put the cap back on the Xyrem bottle and store it in a safe and secure place. Store in a locked place if needed. Keep Xyrem out of the reach of children and pets.
- Rinse the syringe out with water and squirt the liquid into the sink drain.

Step 8.

- At bedtime, and before you take your first Xyrem dose, put your second Xyrem dose in a safe place near your bed.

- You may want to set an alarm clock to make sure you wake up to take the second dose.
- When it is time to take your first Xyrem dose, remove the cap from the container by pressing down on the child-resistant locking tab and turning the cap counterclockwise (to the left).
- Drink all of your first Xyrem dose at bedtime. Put the cap back on the first container before lying down to sleep.
- You should fall asleep soon. Some patients fall asleep within 5 minutes and most fall asleep within 15 minutes. Some patients take less time to fall asleep, and some take more time. The time it takes you to fall asleep might be different from night to night.

Step 9.

- When you wake up 2½ to 4 hours later, take the cap off the second pharmacy container.
- If you wake up before the alarm and it has been at least 2½ hours since your first Xyrem dose, turn off your alarm and take your second Xyrem dose.
- While sitting in bed, drink all of the second Xyrem dose and put the cap back on the second pharmacy container before lying down to continue sleeping.

Distributed By:
Jazz Pharmaceuticals, Inc.
Palo Alto, CA 94304
These Instructions for Use have been approved by the U.S. Food and Drug Administration.
Revised December 2012

Lupin Pharmaceuticals, Inc.
HARBOR PLACE TOWER
111 SOUTH CALVERT STREET, 21ST FLOOR
BALTIMORE, MD 21202

Direct Inquiries to:
Phone (410) 576-2000

SUPRAX ℞

[sū-praks]
(cefixime)
Tablets USP, 400 mg
SUPRAX
(cefixime)
Capsules USP, 400 mg
SUPRAX
(cefixime)
Chewable Tablets, 100 mg, 150 mg and 200 mg
SUPRAX
(cefixime)
for Oral Suspension USP, 100 mg/5 mL
SUPRAX
(cefixime)
for Oral Suspension USP, 200 mg/5 mL
SUPRAX
(cefixime)
for Oral Suspension USP, 500 mg/5 mL
For oral administration

HIGHLIGHTS OF PRESCRIBING INFORMATION
These highlights do not include all the information needed to use SUPRAX safely and effectively. See full prescribing information for SUPRAX.
Suprax (cefixime) Tablets USP, 400 mg
Suprax (cefixime) Capsules, 400 mg
Suprax (cefixime) Chewable Tablets, 100 mg, 150 mg and 200 mg
Suprax (cefixime) for Oral Suspension USP, 100 mg/5 mL
Suprax (cefixime) for Oral Suspension USP, 200 mg/5 mL
Suprax (cefixime) for Oral Suspension USP, 500 mg/5 mL
For oral administration
Initial U.S. Approval:1986
To reduce the development of drug-resistant bacteria and maintain the effectiveness of Suprax and other antibacterial drugs, Suprax should be used only to treat infections that are proven or strongly suspected to be caused by bacteria.

INDICATIONS AND USAGE

Suprax (cefixime) is a cephalosporin antibacterial drug indicated for

- Uncomplicated Urinary Tract Infections (1.1)
- Otitis Media (1.2)
- Pharyngitis and Tonsillitis (1.3)
- Acute Exacerbations of Chronic Bronchitis (1.4)
- Uncomplicated Gonorrhea (cervical/urethral) (1.5)

DOSAGE AND ADMINISTRATION

- Adults: 400 mg daily (2.1)
- Children: 8 mg/kg/day (2.2)

Table 1. Suggested doses for pediatric patients

PEDIATRIC DOSAGE CHART
Doses are suggested for each weight range and rounded for ease of administration

		Suprax (cefixime) for Oral Suspension			Suprax (cefixime) Chewable Tablet
		100 mg/5 mL	200 mg/5 mL	500 mg/5 mL	
Patient Weight (kg)	Dose/Day (mg)	Dose/Day (mL)	Dose/Day (mL)	Dose/Day (mL)	Dose
5 to 7.5*	50	2.5	--	--	--
7.6 to 10*	80	4	2	--	--
10.1 to 12.5	100	5	2.5	1	1 tablet of 100 mg
12.6 to 20.5	150	7.5	4	1.5	1 tablet of 150 mg
20.6 to 28	200	10	5	2	1 tablet of 200 mg
28.1 to 33	250	12.5	6	2.5	1 tablet of 100 mg and 1 tablet of 150 mg
33.1 to 40	300	15	7.5	3	2 tablets of 150 mg
40.1to 45	350	17.5	9	3.5	1 tablet of 150 mg and 1 tablet of 200 mg
45.1 or greater	400	20	10	4	2 tablets of 200 mg

* The preferred concentrations of oral suspension to use are 100 mg/5 mL or 200 mg/5 mL for pediatric patients in these weight ranges.

DOSAGE FORMS AND STRENGTHS

- Film-coated, scored Tablets: 400 mg (3)
- Capsules: 400 mg (3)
- Chewable Tablets: 100 mg, 150 mg and 200 mg (3)
- Oral Suspension: 100 mg/5 mL, 200 mg/5 mL and 500 mg/5 mL (3)

CONTRAINDICATIONS

- Contraindicated in patients with known allergy to cefixime or other cephalosporins. (4)

WARNINGS AND PRECAUTIONS

- Hypersensitivity reactions including shock and fatalities have been reported with cefixime. Discontinue use if a reaction occurs. (5.1)
- *Clostridium difficile* associated diarrhea: Evaluate if diarrhea occurs. (5.2)

ADVERSE REACTIONS

Most common adverse reactions are gastrointestinal such as diarrhea (16%), nausea (7%), loose stools (6%), abdominal pain (3%), dyspepsia (3%), and vomiting. (6)
To report SUSPECTED ADVERSE REACTIONS, contact Lupin Pharma at 1-800-399-2561 or FDA at 1-800-FDA-1088 or *www.fda.gov/medwatch.*

DRUG INTERACTIONS

- Elevated carbamazepine levels have been reported in postmarketing experience when cefixime is administered concomitantly. (7.1)
- Increased prothrombin time, with or without clinical bleeding, has been reported when cefixime is administered concomitantly with warfarin and anticoagulants. (7.2)

USE IN SPECIFIC POPULATIONS

- Pregnancy: Cefixime should be used during pregnancy only if clearly needed. (8.1)
- Nursing Mothers: Consideration should be given to discontinuing nursing temporarily during treatment with cefixime. (8.3)
- Children: Efficacy and safety in infants aged less than six months have not been established. (8.4)
- Geriatric Use: Clinical studies did not include sufficient numbers of subjects aged 65 and older to determine whether they respond differently than younger subjects. Other reported clinical experience has not identified differences in responses between the elderly and younger patients. (8.5)
- Renal Impairment: Cefixime may be administered in the presence of impaired renal function. Dose adjustment is required in patients whose creatinine clearance is less than 60 mL/min. (8.6)

See 17 for PATIENT COUNSELING INFORMATION
Revised: 03/2013

FULL PRESCRIBING INFORMATION: CONTENTS*

*** Sections or subsections omitted from the full prescribing information are not listed**

FULL PRESCRIBING INFORMATION

1. INDICATIONS AND USAGE

To reduce the development of drug resistant bacteria and maintain the effectiveness of Suprax (cefixime) and other antibacterial drugs, Suprax should be used only to treat infections that are proven or strongly suspected to be caused by susceptible bacteria. When culture and susceptibility information are available, they should be considered in selecting or modifying antimicrobial therapy. In the absence of such data, local epidemiology and susceptibility patterns may contribute to the empiric selection of therapy.

Table 2. Doses for Adults with Renal Impairment

Renal Dysfunction	Suprax (cefixime) for Oral Suspension			Tablet	Chewable Tablet
Creatinine Clearance (mL/min)	**100 mg/5 mL**	**200 mg/5 mL**	**500 mg/5 mL**	**400 mg**	**200 mg**
	Dose/Day (mL)	Dose/Day (mL)	Dose/Day (mL)	Dose/Day	Dose/Day
60 or greater	Normal dose	Normal dose	Normal dose	Normal dose	Normal dose
21 to 59* OR renal hemodialysis*	13	6.5	2.6	Not Appropriate	Not Appropriate
20 or less OR continuous peritoneal dialysis	8.6	4.4	1.8	0.5 tablet	1 tablet

* The preferred concentrations of oral suspension to use are 200 mg/5 mL or 500 mg/5 mL for patients with this renal dysfunction

Strength	Bottle Size	Reconstitution Directions
100 mg/5 mL and 200 mg/5 mL	100 mL	To reconstitute, suspend with **68 mL water.** Method: Tap the bottle several times to loosen powder contents prior to reconstitution. Add approximately half the total amount of water for reconstitution and shake well. Add the remainder of water and shake well.
100 mg/5 mL and 200 mg/5 mL	75 mL	To reconstitute, suspend with **51 mL water.** Method: Tap the bottle several times to loosen powder contents prior to reconstitution. Add approximately half the total amount of water for reconstitution and shake well. Add the remainder of water and shake well.
100 mg/5 mL and 200 mg/5 mL	50 mL	To reconstitute, suspend with **34 mL water.** Method: Tap the bottle several times to loosen powder contents prior to reconstitution. Add approximately half the total amount of water for reconstitution and shake well. Add the remainder of water and shake well.
200 mg/5 mL	37.5 mL	To reconstitute, suspend with **26 mL water.** Method: Tap the bottle several times to loosen powder contents prior to reconstitution. Add approximately half the total amount of water for reconstitution and shake well. Add the remainder of water and shake well.
200 mg/5 mL	25 mL	To reconstitute, suspend with **17 mL water.** Method: Tap the bottle several times to loosen powder contents prior to reconstitution. Add approximately half the total amount of water for reconstitution and shake well. Add the remainder of water and shake well.
500 mg/5 mL	20 mL	To reconstitute, suspend with **14 mL water.** Method: Tap the bottle several times to loosen powder contents prior to reconstitution. Add approximately half the total amount of water for reconstitution and shake well. Add the remainder of water and shake well.
500 mg/5 mL	10 mL	To reconstitute, suspend with **8 mL water.** Method: Tap the bottle several times to loosen powder contents prior to reconstitution. Add approximately half the total amount of water for reconstitution and shake well. Add the remainder of water and shake well.

Suprax (cefixime) is a cephalosporin antibacterial drug indicated in the treatment of adults and pediatric patients six months of age or older with the following infections when caused by susceptible isolates of the designated bacteria:

1.1 Uncomplicated Urinary Tract Infections

Uncomplicated Urinary Tract Infections caused by *Escherichia coli* and *Proteus mirabilis.*

1.2 Otitis Media

Otitis Media caused by *Haemophilus influenzae, Moraxella catarrhalis,* and *Streptococcus pyogenes.* (Efficacy for *Streptococcus pyogenes* in this organ system was studied in fewer than 10 infections.)

Note: For patients with otitis media caused by *Streptococcus pneumoniae,* overall response was approximately 10% lower for cefixime than for the comparator. [See **CLINICAL STUDIES (14)**].

1.3 Pharyngitis and Tonsillitis

Pharyngitis and Tonsillitis caused by *Streptococcus pyogenes.* (Note: Penicillin is the usual drug of choice in the treatment of *Streptococcus pyogenes* infections. Suprax is generally effective in the eradication of *Streptococcus pyogenes* from the nasopharynx; however, data establishing the efficacy of Suprax in the subsequent prevention of rheumatic fever is not available.)

1.4 Acute Exacerbations of Chronic Bronchitis

Acute Exacerbations of Chronic Bronchitis caused by *Streptococcus pneumoniae* and *Haemophilus influenzae.*

1.5 Uncomplicated Gonorrhea (cervical/urethral)

Uncomplicated Gonorrhea (cervical/urethral) caused by *Neisseria gonorrhoeae* (penicillinase-and non-penicillinase-producing isolates).

2. DOSAGE AND ADMINISTRATION

2.1 Adults

The recommended dose of cefixime is 400 mg daily. This may be given as a 400 mg tablet or capsule daily or the 400 mg tablet may be split and given as one half tablet every 12 hours. For the treatment of uncomplicated cervical/urethral gonococcal infections, a single oral dose of 400 mg is recommended. The capsule and tablet may be administered without regard to food.

In the treatment of infections due to *Streptococcus pyogenes,* a therapeutic dosage of cefixime should be administered for at least 10 days.

2.2 Pediatric Patients (6 months or older)

The recommended dose is 8 mg/kg/day of the suspension. This may be administered as a single daily dose or may be given in two divided doses, as 4 mg/kg every 12 hours.

Note: A suggested dose has been determined for each pediatric weight range. Refer to Table 1. Ensure all orders that specify a dose in milliliters include a concentration, because Suprax for oral suspension is available in three different concentrations (100 mg/5 mL, 200 mg/5 mL, and 500 mg/5 mL).

[See table 1 at top of previous page]

Children weighing more than 45 kg or older than 12 years should be treated with the recommended adult dose. Suprax (cefixime) Chewable Tablets must be chewed or crushed before swallowing.

Otitis media should be treated with the chewable tablets or suspension. Clinical trials of otitis media were conducted with the chewable tablets or suspension, and the chewable tablets or suspension results in higher peak blood levels than the tablet when administered at the same dose.

Therefore, the tablet or capsule should not be substituted for the chewable tablets or suspension in the treatment of otitis media. [See **CLINICAL PHARMACOLOGY (12.3)**]

In the treatment of infections due to *Streptococcus pyogenes,* a therapeutic dosage of cefixime should be administered for at least 10 days.

2.3 Renal Impairment

Suprax may be administered in the presence of impaired renal function. Normal dose and schedule may be employed in patients with creatinine clearances of 60 mL/min or greater. Refer to Table 2 for dose adjustments for adults with renal impairment. Neither hemodialysis nor peritoneal dialysis removes significant amounts of drug from the body.

[See table 2 above]

2.4 Reconstitution Directions for Oral Suspension

[See second table above]

After reconstitution, the suspension may be kept for 14 days either at room temperature, or under refrigeration, without significant loss of potency. Keep tightly closed. Shake well before using. Discard unused portion after 14 days.

3. DOSAGE FORMS AND STRENGTHS

Suprax is available for oral administration in the following dosage forms and strengths:

- Film-coated tablets provide 400 mg of cefixime as trihydrate. These are white to off-white, film-coated, capsule shaped tablets with beveled edges and a divided score line on each side. The tablet is debossed with "SUPRAX" across one side and "LUPIN" across the other side.
- Capsules provide 400 mg of cefixime as trihydrate. These are size "00EL" capsules with pink opaque cap and pink opaque body with "LU" on the cap and "U43" on the body in black ink. Capsules contain white to yellowish white granular powder.
- Chewable tablets provide either 100 mg or 150 mg or 200 mg of cefixime as trihydrate. The 100 mg tablet is pink, round tablet, debossed with "SUPRAX 100" on one side and "LUPIN" on other side. The 150 mg tablet is pink, round tablet, debossed with "SUPRAX 150" on one side and "LUPIN" on other side. The 200 mg tablet is pink, round tablet, debossed with "SUPRAX 200" on one side and "LUPIN" on other side.
- Powder for oral suspension, when reconstituted, provides either 100 mg/5 mL or 200 mg/5 mL or 500 mg/5 mL of cefixime as trihydrate. For 100 mg/5 mL and 200 mg/5 mL, the powder has an off white to pale yellow color and is strawberry flavored. For 500 mg/5 mL, the powder has an off white to cream color and is strawberry flavored.

4. CONTRAINDICATIONS

Suprax (cefixime) is contraindicated in patients with known allergy to cefixime or other cephalosporins.

5. WARNINGS AND PRECAUTIONS

5.1 Hypersensitivity Reactions

Anaphylactic/anaphylactoid reactions (including shock and fatalities) have been reported with the use of cefixime.

Before therapy with Suprax is instituted, careful inquiry should be made to determine whether the patient has had previous hypersensitivity reactions to cephalosporins, penicillins, or other drugs. If this product is to be given to penicillin-sensitive patients, caution should be exercised because cross hypersensitivity among beta-lactam antibiotics has been clearly documented and may occur in up to 10% of patients with a history of penicillin allergy. If an allergic reaction to Suprax occurs, discontinue the drug.

5.2 Clostridium difficile-Associated Diarrhea

Clostridium difficile associated diarrhea (CDAD) has been reported with use of nearly all antibacterial agents, including Suprax, and may range in severity from mild diarrhea to fatal colitis. Treatment with antibacterial agents alters the normal flora of the colon leading to overgrowth of *C. difficile.*

C. difficile produces toxins A and B which contribute to the development of CDAD. Hypertoxin producing isolates of *C. difficile* cause increased morbidity and mortality, as these infections can be refractory to antimicrobial therapy and may require colectomy. CDAD must be considered in all patients who present with diarrhea following antibiotic use. Careful medical history is necessary since CDAD has been reported to occur over two months after the administration of antibacterial agents.

If CDAD is suspected or confirmed, ongoing antibiotic use not directed against *C. difficile* may need to be discontinued. Appropriate fluid and electrolyte management, protein supplementation, antibiotic treatment of *C. difficile,* and surgical evaluation should be instituted as clinically indicated.

5.3 Dose Adjustment in Renal Impairment

The dose of Suprax should be adjusted in patients with renal impairment as well as those undergoing continuous ambulatory peritoneal dialysis (CAPD) and hemodialysis (HD). Patients on dialysis should be monitored carefully [See **DOSAGE AND ADMINISTRATION (2)**].

5.4 Coagulation Effects

Cephalosporins, including Suprax, may be associated with a fall in prothrombin activity. Those at risk include patients with renal or hepatic impairment, or poor nutritional state, as well as patients receiving a protracted course of antimicrobial therapy, and patients previously stabilized on anticoagulant therapy. Prothrombin time should be monitored in patients at risk and exogenous vitamin K administered as indicated.

5.5 Development of Drug-Resistant Bacteria

Prescribing Suprax (cefixime) in the absence of a proven or strongly suspected bacterial infection is unlikely to provide benefit to the patient and increases the risk of the development of drug-resistant bacteria.

6. ADVERSE REACTIONS

6.1 Clinical Trials Experience

Because clinical trials are conducted under widely varying conditions, adverse reaction rates observed in the clinical trials of a drug cannot be directly compared to rates in the clinical trials of another drug and may not reflect the rates observed in practice.

The most commonly seen adverse reactions in U.S. trials of the tablet formulation were gastrointestinal events, which were reported in 30% of adult patients on either the twice daily or the once daily regimen. Five percent (5%) of patients in the U.S. clinical trials discontinued therapy because of drug-related adverse reactions. Individual adverse reactions included diarrhea 16%, loose or frequent stools 6%, abdominal pain 3%, nausea 7%, dyspepsia 3%, and flatulence 4%. The incidence of gastrointestinal adverse reactions, including diarrhea and loose stools, in pediatric patients receiving the suspension was comparable to the incidence seen in adult patients receiving tablets.

6.2 Post-marketing Experience

The following adverse reactions have been reported following the use of cefixime. Incidence rates were less than 1 in 50 (less than 2%).

Gastrointestinal

Several cases of documented pseudomembranous colitis were identified in clinical trials. The onset of pseudomembranous colitis symptoms may occur during or after therapy.

Hypersensitivity Reactions

Anaphylactic/anaphylactoid reactions (including shock and fatalities), skin rashes, urticaria, drug fever, pruritus, angioedema, and facial edema. Erythema multiforme, Stevens-Johnson syndrome, and serum sickness-like reactions have been reported.

Hepatic

Transient elevations in SGPT, SGOT, alkaline phosphatase, hepatitis, jaundice.

Renal

Transient elevations in BUN or creatinine, acute renal failure.

Central Nervous System

Headaches, dizziness, seizures.

Hemic and Lymphatic System

Transient thrombocytopenia, leukopenia, neutropenia, prolongation in prothrombin time, elevated LDH, pancytopenia, agranulocytosis, and eosinophilia.

Abnormal Laboratory Tests

Hyperbilirubinemia.

Other Adverse Reactions

Genital pruritus, vaginitis, candidiasis, toxic epidermal necrolysis.

Adverse Reactions Reported for Cephalosporin-class Drugs

Allergic reactions, superinfection, renal dysfunction, toxic nephropathy, hepatic dysfunction including cholestasis, aplastic anemia, hemolytic anemia, hemorrhage, and colitis.

Several cephalosporins have been implicated in triggering seizures, particularly in patients with renal impairment when the dosage was not reduced. [See **DOSAGE AND ADMINISTRATION (2)** and **OVERDOSAGE (10)**]. If seizures associated with drug therapy occur, the drug should be discontinued. Anticonvulsant therapy can be given if clinically indicated.

7. DRUG INTERACTIONS

7.1 Carbamazepine

Elevated carbamazepine levels have been reported in postmarketing experience when cefixime is administered concomitantly. Drug monitoring may be of assistance in detecting alterations in carbamazepine plasma concentrations.

7.2 Warfarin and Anticoagulants

Increased prothrombin time, with or without clinical bleeding, has been reported when cefixime is administered concomitantly.

7.3 Drug/Laboratory Test Interactions

A false-positive reaction for ketones in the urine may occur with tests using nitroprusside but not with those using nitroferricyanide.

The administration of cefixime may result in a false-positive reaction for glucose in the urine using Clinitest®[1], Benedict's solution, or Fehling's solution. It is recommended that glucose tests based on enzymatic glucose oxidase reactions (such as Clinistix®[1] or TesTape®[1]) be used. A false-positive direct Coombs test has been reported during treatment with other cephalosporins; therefore, it should be recognized that a positive Coombs test may be due to the drug.

[1]Clinitest® and Clinistix® are registered trademarks of Ames Division, Miles Laboratories, Inc. Tes-Tape® is a registered trademark of Eli Lilly and Company.

Table 3: Susceptibility interpretive criteria for cefixime

Pathogen	Minimum Inhibitory Concentrations (mcg/mL)			Disk Diffusion Zone Diameter (mm)		
	S	I	R	S	I	R
Neisseria gonorrhoeae	≤ 0.25	-*	-	≥ 31	-	-
H. influenzae	≤1	-	-	≥21	-	-
E. coli and *P. mirabilis*	≤ 1	2	≥ 4	≥ 19	16 - 18	≤ 15

* Insufficient information is available to determine Intermediate or Resistant interpretive criteria

Bacteriological Outcome of Otitis Media at Two to Four Weeks Post-Therapy Based on Repeat Middle Ear Fluid Culture or Extrapolation from Clinical Outcome

Organism	Cefixime(a) 4 mg/kg BID	Cefixime(a) 8 mg/kg QD	Control(a) drugs
Streptococcus pneumoniae	48/70 (69%)	18/22 (82%)	82/100 (82%)
Haemophilus influenzae beta-lactamase negative	24/34 (71%)	13/17 (76%)	23/34 (68%)
Haemophilus influenzae beta-lactamase positive	17/22 (77%)	9/12 (75%)	1/1 (b)
Moraxella catarrhalis	26/31 (84%)	5/5	18/24 (75%)
S. pyogenes	5/5	3/3	6/7
All Isolates	120/162 (74%)	48/59 (81%)	130/166 (78%)

(a)Number eradicated/number isolated.

(b)An additional 20 beta-lactamase positive isolates of *Haemophilus influenzae* were isolated, but were excluded from this analysis because they were resistant to the control antibiotic. In nineteen of these, the clinical course could be assessed and a favorable outcome occurred in 10. When these cases are included in the overall bacteriological evaluation of therapy with the control drugs, 140/185 (76%) of pathogens were considered to be eradicated.

8. USE IN SPECIFIC POPULATIONS

8.1 Pregnancy

Pregnancy Category B. Reproduction studies have been performed in mice and rats at doses up to 40 times the human dose and have revealed no evidence of harm to the fetus due to cefixime. There are no adequate and well-controlled studies in pregnant women. Because animal reproduction studies are not always predictive of human response, this drug should be used during pregnancy only if clearly needed.

8.2 Labor And Delivery

Cefixime has not been studied for use during labor and delivery. Treatment should only be given if clearly needed.

8.3 Nursing Mothers

It is not known whether cefixime is excreted in human milk. Consideration should be given to discontinuing nursing temporarily during treatment with this drug.

8.4 Pediatric Use

Safety and effectiveness of cefixime in children aged less than six months old have not been established. The incidence of gastrointestinal adverse reactions, including diarrhea and loose stools, in the pediatric patients receiving the suspension, was comparable to the incidence seen in adult patients receiving tablets.

8.5 Geriatric Use

Clinical studies did not include sufficient numbers of subjects aged 65 and older to determine whether they respond differently than younger subjects. Other reported clinical experience has not identified differences in responses between the elderly and younger patients. A pharmacokinetic study in the elderly detected differences in pharmacokinetic parameters [See **CLINICAL PHARMACOLOGY (12.3)**]. These differences were small and do not indicate a need for dosage adjustment of the drug in the elderly.

8.6 Renal Impairment

The dose of cefixime should be adjusted in patients with renal impairment as well as those undergoing continuous ambulatory peritoneal dialysis (CAPD) and hemodialysis (HD). Patients on dialysis should be monitored carefully [See **DOSAGE AND ADMINISTRATION (2.3)**].

10. OVERDOSAGE

Gastric lavage may be indicated; otherwise, no specific antidote exists. Cefixime is not removed in significant quantities from the circulation by hemodialysis or peritoneal dialysis. Adverse reactions in small numbers of healthy adult volunteers receiving single doses up to 2 g of cefixime did not differ from the profile seen in patients treated at the recommended doses.

11. DESCRIPTION

Cefixime is a semisynthetic, cephalosporin antibacterial for oral administration. Chemically, it is *(6R,7R)*-7-[2-(2-Amino-4-thiazolyl)glyoxylamido]-8-oxo-3-vinyl-5-thia-1-azabicyclo [4.2.0] oct-2-ene-2-carboxylic acid, 7^2-*(Z)*-[*O*-(carboxy methyl) oxime] trihydrate.

Molecular weight = 507.50 as the trihydrate. Chemical Formula is $C_{16}H_{15}N_5O_7S_2.3H_2O$

The structural formula for cefixime is:

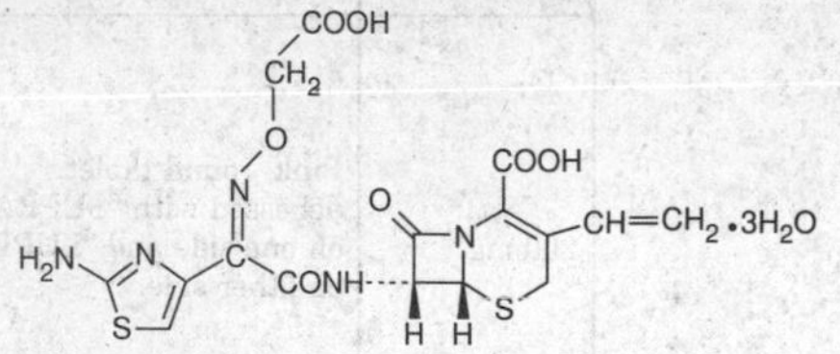

- Inactive ingredients contained in Suprax® (cefixime) 400 mg tablets are: dibasic calcium phosphate, hypromellose, lactose monohydrate, magnesium stearate, microcrystalline cellulose, polyethylene glycol, pregelatinized starch, titanium dioxide, and triacetin.
- Inactive ingredients contained in Suprax® (cefixime) 400 mg capsules are: colloidal silicon dioxide, crospovidone, low substituted hydroxy propyl cellulose, magnesium stearate, and mannitol. The capsule shell contains the following inactive ingredients: ferric oxide black, ferric oxide red, gelatin, potassium hydroxide, propylene glycol, shellac, sodium lauryl sulfate, and titanium dioxide.
- Inactive ingredients contained in Suprax® (cefixime) 100 mg or 150 mg or 200 mg chewable tablets are: aspartame, colloidal silicon dioxide, crospovidone, FD&C Red # 40 Aluminium Lake, low substituted hydroxypropyl cellulose, magnesium stearate, mannitol, fantasy flavor permaseal, and tutti frutti flavor.
- Inactive ingredients contained in Suprax® (cefixime) powder for oral suspension are: colloidal silicon dioxide, sodium benzoate, strawberry flavor, sucralose (only in 500 mg/5 mL strength), sucrose, and xanthan gum.

12. CLINICAL PHARMACOLOGY

12.1 Mechanism of Action

Cefixime is a semisynthetic cephalosporin antibacterial drug [see **Microbiology (12.4)**].

12.3 Pharmacokinetics

Suprax chewable tablets are bioequivalent to oral suspension.

Dosage Form	Strength	Description	Package Size	NDC Code	Storage
Suprax® (cefixime) Tablets USP	400 mg	White to off-white, film-coated, capsule shaped tablets with beveled edges and a divided score line on each side, debossed with "SUPRAX" across one side and "LUPIN" across other side, containing 400 mg of cefixime as the trihydrate.	Bottles of 10 tablets	27437-201-10	Store at 20 to 25°C (68 to 77°F) [See USP Controlled Room Temperature].
			Bottle of 50 tablets	27437-201-08	
			Bottle of 100 tablets	27437-201-01	
Suprax® (cefixime) Capsules	400 mg	Size "00EL" capsules with pink opaque cap and pink opaque body, imprinted with "LU" on cap and "U43" on body in black ink, containing white to yellowish white granular powder containing 400 mg of cefixime as the trihydrate.	Bottle of 50 capsules	27437-208-08	Store at 20 to 25°C (68 to 77°F) [See USP Controlled Room Temperature].
			Unit Dose Package of 10 (1 blister of 10 capsules)	27437-208-11	
Suprax® (cefixime) Chewable Tablets	100 mg	Pink, round tablet, debossed with "SUPRAX 100" on one side and "LUPIN" on other side.	Bottles of 10 tablets	27437-203-10	
			Bottle of 50 tablets	27437-203-08	
			Unit Dose Package of 10 (1 blister of 10 tablets)	27437-203-11	
	150 mg	Pink, round tablet, debossed with "SUPRAX 150" on one side and "LUPIN" on other side.	Bottles of 10 tablets	27437-204-10	
			Bottle of 50 tablets	27437-204-08	Store at 20 to 25°C (68 to 77°F) [See USP Controlled Room Temperature].
			Unit Dose Package of 10 (1 blister of 10 tablets)	27437-204-11	
	200 mg	Pink, round tablet, debossed with "SUPRAX 200" on one side and "LUPIN" on other side.	Bottles of 10 tablets	27437-205-10	
			Bottle of 50 tablets	27437-205-08	
			Unit Dose Package of 10 (1 blister of 10 tablets)	27437-205-11	

(Table continued on next page)

Suprax tablets and suspension, given orally, are about 40% to 50% absorbed whether administered with or without food; however, time to maximal absorption is increased approximately 0.8 hours when administered with food. A single 200 mg tablet of cefixime produces an average peak serum concentration of approximately 2 mcg/mL (range 1 to 4 mcg/mL); a single 400 mg tablet produces an average peak concentration of approximately 3.7 mcg/mL (range 1.3 to 7.7 mcg/mL). The oral suspension produces average peak concentrations approximately 25% to 50% higher than the tablets, when tested in normal *adult* volunteers. Two hundred and 400 mg doses of oral suspension produce average peak concentrations of 3 mcg/mL (range 1 to 4.5 mcg/mL) and 4.6 mcg/mL (range 1.9 to 7.7 mcg/mL), respectively, when tested in normal *adult* volunteers. The area under the time versus concentration curve (AUC) is greater by approximately 10% to 25% with the oral suspension than with the tablet after doses of 100 to 400 mg, when tested in normal *adult* volunteers. This increased absorption should be taken into consideration if the oral suspension is to be substituted for the tablet. Because of the lack of bioequivalence, tablets should not be substituted for oral suspension in the treatment of otitis media [See **DOSAGE AND ADMINISTRATION (2)**]. Cross-over studies of tablet versus suspension have not been performed in children.

The 400 mg capsule is bioequivalent to the 400 mg tablet under fasting conditions. However, food reduces the absorption following administration of the capsule by approximately 15% based on AUC and 25% based on C_{max}.

Peak serum concentrations occur between 2 and 6 hours following oral administration of a single 200 mg tablet, a single 400 mg tablet or 400 mg of cefixime suspension. Peak serum concentrations occur between 2 and 5 hours following a single administration of 200 mg of suspension. Peak serum concentrations occur between 3 and 8 hours following oral administration of a single 400 mg capsule.

Distribution

Serum protein binding is concentration independent with a bound fraction of approximately 65%. In a multiple dose study conducted with a research formulation which is less bioavailable than the tablet or suspension, there was little accumulation of drug in serum or urine after dosing for 14 days. Adequate data on CSF levels of cefixime are not available.

Metabolism and Excretion

There is no evidence of metabolism of cefixime *in vivo*. Approximately 50% of the absorbed dose is excreted unchanged in the urine in 24 hours. In animal studies, it was noted that cefixime is also excreted in the bile in excess of 10% of the administered dose. The serum half-life of cefixime in healthy subjects is independent of dosage form and averages 3 to 4 hours but may range up to 9 hours in some normal volunteers.

Special Populations

Geriatrics: Average AUCs at steady state in elderly patients are approximately 40% higher than average AUCs in other healthy adults. Differences in the pharmacokinetic parameters between 12 young and 12 elderly subjects who received 400 mg of cefixime once daily for 5 days are summarized as follows:

Pharmacokinetic Parameters (mean ± SD) for Cefixime in Both Young & Elderly Subjects

Pharmacokinetic parameter	Young	Elderly
C_{max} (mg/L)	4.74 ± 1.43	5.68 ± 1.83
T_{max} (h)*	3.9 ± 0.3	4.3 ± 0.6
AUC (mg.h/L)*	34.9 ± 12.2	49.5 ± 19.1
$T_{1/2}$ (h)*	3.5 ± 0.6	4.2 ± 0.4
C_{ave} (mg/L)*	1.42 ±0.50	1.99 ± 0.75

* Difference between age groups was significant. ($p<0.05$)

However, these increases were not clinically significant [See **DOSAGE AND ADMINISTRATION (2)**].

Renal Impairment: In subjects with moderate impairment of renal function (20 to 40 mL/min creatinine clearance), the average serum half-life of cefixime is prolonged to 6.4 hours. In severe renal impairment (5 to 20 mL/min creatinine clearance), the half-life increased to an average of 11.5 hours. The drug is not cleared significantly from the blood by hemodialysis or peritoneal dialysis. However, a study indicated that with doses of 400 mg, patients undergoing hemodialysis have similar blood profiles as subjects with creatinine clearances of 21 to 60 mL/min.

12.4 Microbiology

Mechanism of Action

Bactericidal action of cefixime results from inhibition of cell-wall synthesis.

Cefixime has been shown to be active against most isolates of the following bacteria both *in vitro* and in clinical infections [see **INDICATIONS AND USAGE (1)**]:

Gram-positive bacteria
Streptococcus pneumoniae
Streptococcus pyogenes
Gram-negative bacteria
Haemophilus influenzae
Moraxella catarrhalis
Escherichia coli
Proteus mirabilis
Neisseria gonorrhoeae

The following *in vitro* data are available, but their clinical significance is unknown. Suprax exhibits *in vitro* MICs of 1 mcg/mL or less against most (≥ 90%) isolates of the following bacteria; however, the safety and effectiveness of Suprax in treating clinical infections due to these bacteria have not been established in adequate and well-controlled clinical trials.

Gram-positive bacteria
Streptococcus agalactiae
Gram-negative bacteria
Haemophilus parainfluenzae
Proteus vulgaris
Klebsiella pneumoniae
Klebsiella oxytoca
Pasteurella multocida
Providencia species
Salmonella species
Shigella species
Citrobacter amalonaticus
Citrobacter diversus
Serratia marcescens

Susceptibility Tests Methods

When available, the clinical microbiology laboratory should provide the results of *in vitro* susceptibility test results for antimicrobial drugs used in resident hospitals to the physician as periodic reports that describe the susceptibility profile of nosocomial and community-acquired pathogens. These reports should aid the physician in selecting an antibacterial drug product for treatment.

Dilution Techniques: Quantitative methods are used to determine the minimum inhibitory concentrations (MICs). These MICs provide estimates of the susceptibility of bacteria to antimicrobial compounds. The MICs should be determined using standardized test methods [1,2] (broth, and/or agar). The MIC values should be interpreted according to the criteria in Table 3.

Diffusion Techniques: Quantitative methods that require measurement of zone diameters can also provide reproducible estimates of the susceptibility of bacteria to antimicrobial compounds. The zone size provides an estimate of the susceptibility of bacteria to antimicrobial compounds. The zone size should be determined using standardized method.[2,3] This procedure uses paper disks impregnated with 5 mcg of cefixime to test the susceptibility of bacteria to cefixime. The disk diffusion interpretive criteria are provided in Table 3.

[See table 3 at top of page 1363]

A report of "Susceptible" indicates that the antimicrobial is likely to inhibit growth of the pathogen if the antimicrobial compound reaches the concentration at the infection site necessary to inhibit growth of the pathogen. A report of "Intermediate" indicates that the result should be considered equivocal, and if the microorganism is not fully susceptible to alternative clinically feasible drugs, the test should be repeated. This category implies possible clinical applicability in body sites where the drug is physiologically concentrated. This category also provides a buffer zone that prevents small uncontrolled technical factors from causing major discrepancies in interpretation. A report of "Resistant" indicates that the antimicrobial is not likely to inhibit growth of the pathogen if the antimicrobial compound reaches the concentrations usually achievable at the infection site; other therapy should be selected.

Quality Control

Standardized susceptibility test procedures require the use of laboratory controls to monitor and ensure the accuracy and precision of supplies and reagents used in the assay, and the techniques of the individuals performing the test.[1, 2, 3] The standard cefixime powder should provide the following range of MIC values provided in Table 4. For the diffusion technique using the 5-mcg cefixime disk the criteria provided in Table 4 should be achieved.

Table 4: Acceptable Quality Control Ranges for Susceptibility Testing

Quality Control Organisms	Minimum Inhibitory Concentrations (mcg/mL)	Disk Diffusion (zone diameters in mm)
E. coli ATCC 25922	0.25 - 1	23 - 27
S. aureus ATCC 29213	8 - 32	--
H. influenzae ATCC 49247	0.12-1	25-33
N. gonorrhoeae ATCC 49226	0.004 - 0.03	37 - 45

13. NONCLINICAL TOXICOLOGY

13.1 Carcinogenesis, Mutagenesis, Impairment Of Fertility

Lifetime studies in animals to evaluate carcinogenic potential have not been conducted. Cefixime did not cause point mutations in bacteria or mammalian cells, DNA damage, or chromosome damage *in vitro* and did not exhibit clastogenic potential *in vivo* in the mouse micronucleus test. In rats, fertility and reproductive performance were not affected by cefixime at doses up to 25 times the adult therapeutic dose.

14. CLINICAL STUDIES

Comparative clinical trials of otitis media were conducted in nearly 400 children between the ages of 6 months to 10 years. *Streptococcus pneumoniae* was isolated from 47% of the patients, *Haemophilus influenzae* from 34%, *Moraxella catarrhalis* from 15% and *S. pyogenes* from 4%.

The overall response rate of *Streptococcus pneumoniae* to cefixime was approximately 10% lower and that of *Haemophilus influenzae* or *Moraxella catarrhalis* approximately 7% higher (12% when beta-lactamase positive isolates of *H. influenzae* are included) than the response rates of these organisms to the active control drugs.

In these studies, patients were randomized and treated with either cefixime at dose regimens of 4 mg/kg twice a day or 8 mg/kg once a day, or with a comparator. Sixty-nine to 70% of the patients in each group had resolution of signs and symptoms of otitis media when evaluated 2 to 4 weeks post-treatment, but persistent effusion was found in 15% of the patients. When evaluated at the completion of therapy, 17% of patients receiving cefixime and 14% of patients receiving effective comparative drugs (18% including those patients who had *Haemophilus influenzae* resistant to the control drug and who received the control antibiotic) were considered to be treatment failures. By the 2 to 4 week follow-up, a total of 30%-31% of patients had evidence of either treatment failure or recurrent disease.

[See table at top of page 1363]

15. REFERENCES

1. Clinical and Laboratory Standards Institute (CLSI) Methods for Dilution Antimicrobial Susceptibility Tests for Bacteria that Grow Aerobically: Approved Standard-9th Edition. CLSI Document M07-A9. CLSI, 950 West Valley Rd., Suite 2500, Wayne, PA 19087, 2012.
2. Clinical and Laboratory Standards Institute (CLSI). Performance Standards for Antimicrobial Susceptibility Testing 21st Informational Supplement, CLSI document M100-S22,CLSI, 2012.
3. CLSI. Performance Standards for Antimicrobial Disk Diffusion Susceptibility Tests. Approved Standard-11th Edition, CLSI document M02-A11, 2012.
4. Faulkner RD, Bohayachuk W, Lanc RA, et al.: Pharmacokinetics of cefixime in the young and elderly. *J Antimicrob Chemother* 1988; 21(6): 787-794.

16. HOW SUPPLIED/STORAGE AND HANDLING

Suprax® is available for oral administration in following dosage forms, strengths and packages listed in the table below:

continued

Dosage Form	Strength	Description	Package Size	NDC Code	Storage
Suprax® (cefixime) for Oral Suspension USP	100 mg/5 mL	Off-white to pale yellow colored powder. After reconstituted as directed, each 5 mL of reconstituted suspension contains 100 mg of cefixime as the trihydrate.	Bottle of 50 mL	68180-202-03	Prior to reconstitution: Store drug powder at 20 to 25°C (68 to 77°F) [See USP Controlled Room Temperature]. After reconstitution: Store at room temperature or under refrigeration. Keep tightly closed.
			Bottle of 75 mL	68180-202-02	
			Bottle of 100 mL	68180-202-01	
	200 mg/5 mL	Off-white to pale yellow colored powder. After reconstituted as directed, each 5 mL of reconstituted suspension contains 200 mg of cefixime as the trihydrate.	Bottle of 25 mL	27437-206-05	
			Bottle of 37.5 mL	27437-206-06	
			Bottle of 50 mL	27437-206-03	
			Bottle of 75 mL	27437-206-02	
			Bottle of 100 mL	27437-206-01	
	500 mg/5 mL	Off white to cream colored powder forming off-white to pale yellow suspension with characteristic fruity odor on constitution. After reconstituted as directed, each mL of reconstituted suspension contains 100 mg of cefixime as the trihydrate.	Bottle of 10 mL	27437-207-02	
			Bottle of 20 mL	27437-207-03	

Products	Manufactured for:	Manufactured by:
Suprax® (cefixime) Tablets USP, 400 mg	**Lupin Pharma** Baltimore, Maryland 21202 United States.	**Lupin Limited** Mandideep 462 046 India.
Suprax® (cefixime) Capsules, 400 mg		
Suprax® (cefixime) Chewable Tablets, 100 mg, 150 mg and 200 mg		
Suprax® (cefixime) for Oral Suspension USP, 200 mg/5 mL		
Suprax® (cefixime) for Oral Suspension USP, 500 mg/5 mL		
Suprax® (cefixime) for Oral Suspension USP, 100 mg/5 mL	**Lupin Pharmaceuticals, Inc.** Baltimore, Maryland 21202 United States.	

[See table on previous page and above]

17. PATIENT COUNSELING INFORMATION

17.1 Information for Patients

Patients should be counseled that antibacterial drugs, including cefixime, should only be used to treat bacterial infections. They do not treat viral infections (e.g., the common cold). When cefixime is prescribed to treat a bacterial infection, patients should be told that although it is common to feel better early in the course of therapy, the medication should be taken exactly as directed. Skipping doses or not completing the full course of therapy may: (1) decrease the effectiveness of the immediate treatment and (2) increase the likelihood that bacteria will develop resistance and will not be treatable by cefixime for oral suspension or cefixime chewable tablets or other antibacterial drugs in the future.

Phenylketonurics: Suprax (cefixime) Chewable Tablets contains 3.3 mg, 5 mg and 6.7 mg of phenylalanine per 100 mg, 150 mg and 200 mg strength, respectively.

Diarrhea is a common problem caused by antibiotics which usually ends when the antibiotic is discontinued. Sometimes after starting treatment with antibiotics, patients can develop watery and bloody stools (with or without stomach cramps and fever) even as late as two or more months after having taken the last dose of the antibiotic. If this occurs, patients should contact their physician as soon as possible.

[See second table above]

Revised: March 15th, 2013

ID#: 231653

McNeil Consumer Healthcare
Division of McNEIL-PPC, Inc.
7050 CAMP HILL ROAD
FORT WASHINGTON, PA 19034

Direct Inquiries to:
Consumer Care Center
(800) 962-5357
www.mcneil-consumer.com

BENADRYL® ALLERGY OTC
Ultratab Tablets and Liqui-Gels

Active ingredient (in each tablet/capsule)	*Purpose*
Diphenhydramine HCl 25 mg	Antihistamine

Uses

- temporarily relieves these symptoms due to hay fever or other upper respiratory allergies:
  - runny nose • sneezing • itchy, watery eyes • itching of the nose or throat
- temporarily relieves these symptoms due to the common cold:
  - runny nose • sneezing

Warnings

Do not use
- to make a child sleepy
- with any other product containing diphenhydramine, even one used on skin

Ask a doctor before use if you have
- a breathing problem such as emphysema or chronic bronchitis
- glaucoma
- trouble urinating due to an enlarged prostate gland

Ask a doctor or pharmacist before use if you are taking sedatives or tranquilizers

When using this product
- marked drowsiness may occur
- avoid alcoholic drinks
- alcohol, sedatives, and tranquilizers may increase drowsiness
- be careful when driving a motor vehicle or operating machinery
- excitability may occur, especially in children

If pregnant or breast-feeding, ask a health professional before use.

Keep out of reach of children. In case of overdose, get medical help or contact a Poison Control Center right away. (1-800-222-1222)

Directions

- take every 4 to 6 hours, or as directed by a doctor
- do not take more than 6 times in 24 hours

adults and children 12 years and over	1 to 2 tablets or capsules
children 6 to under 12 years	1 tablet or capsule
children under 6 years	do not use

Other information

Benadryl Allergy Ultratab
- each tablet contains: calcium 20mg
- store between 20–25°C (68–77°F). Avoid high humidity. Protect from light.

Benadryl Allergy Liqui-Gels
- Store at 59°–77°F in a dry place. Protect from heat, humidity, and light.

Benadryl Allergy Ultratab

Inactive ingredients carnauba wax, croscarmellose sodium, D&C red no. 27 aluminum lake, dibasic calcium phosphate, hypromellose, magnesium stearate, microcrystalline cellulose, polyethylene glycol, polysorbate 80, titanium dioxide

Benadryl Allergy Liqui-gels

Inactive ingredients gelatin, glycerin, polyethylene glycol, purified water, sorbitol. Capsules are imprinted with edible dye-free ink.

For information or questions, visit our website www.benadryl.com

CHILDREN'S BENADRYL® ALLERGY CHERRY FLAVORED LIQUID OTC

CHILDREN'S BENADRYL® DYE-FREE ALLERGY BUBBLE GUM FLAVORED LIQUID

Active ingredient (in each 5 mL = 1 teaspoonful)	*Purpose*
Diphenhydramine HCl 12.5 mg	Antihistamine

Uses

- temporarily relieves these symptoms due to hay fever or other upper respiratory allergies:
  - runny nose • sneezing • itchy, watery eyes • itching of the nose or throat

Warnings

Do not use
- to make a child sleepy
- with any other product containing diphenhydramine, even one used on skin

Ask a doctor before use if the child has
- a breathing problem such as chronic bronchitis
- glaucoma
- a sodium-restricted diet (CHILDREN'S BENADRYL ALLERGY CHERRY FLAVORED LIQUID only)

Ask a doctor or pharmacist before use if the child is taking sedatives or tranquilizers

When using this product
- marked drowsiness may occur
- sedatives and tranquilizers may increase drowsiness
- excitability may occur, especially in children

Keep out of reach of children. In case of overdose, get medical help or contact a Poison Control Center right away. (1-800-222-1222)

Directions

- find right dose on chart
- mL = milliliter; tsp = teaspoonful
- take every 4 to 6 hours, or as directed by a doctor
- do not take more than 6 doses in 24 hours

Age (yr)	Dose (mL or tsp)
children under 2 years	do not use
children 2 to 5 years	do not use unless directed by a doctor
children 6 to 11 years	5 mL (1 tsp) to 10 mL (2 tsp)

Attention: use only enclosed dosing cup specifically designed for use with this product. Do not use any other dosing device.

Other information

- **each 5 mL (1 tsp) contains:** sodium 14 mg (CHILDREN'S BENADRYL® ALLERGY CHERRY FLAVORED LIQUID only)
- **each 5 mL (1 tsp) contains:** sodium 11 mg (CHILDREN'S BENADRYL® DYE-FREE ALLERGY BUBBLE GUM FLAVORED LIQUID only)
- store between 20–25°C (68–77°F). Protect from light. Store in outer carton until contents used. (CHILDREN'S BENADRYL® ALLERGY CHERRY FLAVORED LIQUID only)
- store at 59–77°F (CHILDREN'S BENADRYL® DYE-FREE ALLERGY BUBBLE GUM FLAVORED LIQUID)

Inactive ingredients CHILDREN'S BENADRYL® ALLERGY CHERRY FLAVORED LIQUID anhydrous citric acid, D&C red no. 33, FD&C red no. 40, flavors, glycerin, monoammonium glycyrrhizinate, poloxamer 407, purified water, sodium benzoate, sodium chloride, sodium citrate, sucrose

CHILDREN'S BENADRYL® DYE-FREE ALLERGY BUBBLE GUM FLAVORED LIQUID

anhydrous citric acid, carboxymethylcellulose sodium, flavors, glycerin, purified water, saccharin sodium, sodium benzoate, sodium citrate, sorbitol solution.

For information or questions, visit our website www.benadryl.com

CHILDREN'S BENADRYL-D® ALLERGY & SINUS OTC
Grape Flavored Liquid

Active ingredients (in each 5 mL = 1 teaspoonful)	*Purpose*
Diphenhydramine HCl 12.5 mg	Antihistamine
Phenylephrine HCl 5 mg	Nasal decongestant

Uses

- temporarily relieves these symptoms due to hay fever or other upper respiratory allergies:
  - runny nose ■ sneezing ■ itchy, watery eyes
  - itching of the nose or throat ■ nasal congestion ■ stuffy nose
- temporarily relieves these symptoms due to the common cold:
  - runny nose ■ sneezing ■ nasal congestion ■ stuffy nose
- temporarily relieves sinus congestion and pressure

Warnings

Do not use
- to make a child sleepy
- with any other product containing diphenhydramine, even one used on skin
- if you are now taking a prescription monoamine oxidase inhibitor (MAOI) (certain drugs for depression, psychiatric or emotional conditions, or Parkinson's disease), or for 2 weeks after stopping the MAOI drug. If you do not know if your prescription drug contains an MAOI, ask a doctor or pharmacist before taking this product.

Ask a doctor before use if you have
- heart disease ■ high blood pressure ■ thyroid disease
- diabetes
- trouble urinating due to an enlarged prostate gland
- a breathing problem such as emphysema or chronic bronchitis
- glaucoma

Ask a doctor or pharmacist before use if you are taking sedatives or tranquilizers

When using this product
- **do not exceed recommended dose**
- marked drowsiness may occur
- avoid alcoholic drinks
- alcohol, sedatives, and tranquilizers may increase drowsiness
- be careful when driving a motor vehicle or operating machinery
- excitability may occur, especially in children

Stop use and ask a doctor if
- nervousness, dizziness, or sleeplessness occur
- symptoms do not improve within 7 days or occur with a fever

If pregnant or breast-feeding, ask a health professional before use.

Keep out of reach of children. In case of overdose, get medical help or contact a Poison Control Center right away. (1-800-222-1222)

Directions

- find right dose on chart below
- mL = milliliter; tsp = teaspoonful
- take every 4 hours
- do not take more than 6 doses in 24 hours

Age (yr)	Dose (mL or tsp)
children under 4 years	do not use
children 4 to 5 years	do not use unless directed by a doctor
children 6 to 11 years	5 mL (1 tsp)
adults and children 12 years and over	10 mL (2 tsp)

Attention: use only enclosed dosing cup specifically designed for use with this product. Do not use any other dosing device.

Other information

- **each 5 mL (1 tsp) contains:** sodium 10 mg
- store between 20-25°C (68–77°F). Protect from light. Store in outer carton until contents are used.

Inactive ingredients anhydrous citric acid, carboxymethylcellulose sodium, edetate disodium, FD&C blue no. 1, FD&C red no. 40, flavors, glycerin, purified water, sodium benzoate, sodium citrate, sorbitol solution, sucralose

For information or questions, visit our website www.benadryl.com

IMODIUM® A-D OTC
Liquid, Caplets, and EZ Chews (loperamide hydrochloride)

Active ingredient	*Purpose*
IMODIUM® A-D Liquid (in each 7.5mL = 1½ teaspoonful) Loperamide HCl 1mg	Anti-diarrheal

IMODIUM® A-D Caplet
(in each caplet)
Loperamide HCl 2mg Anti-diarrheal
IMODIUM® A-D EZ Chew
(in each tablet)
Loperamide HCl 2mg Anti-diarrheal

Use controls symptoms of diarrhea, including Travelers' Diarrhea

Warnings

Allergy alert: Do not use if you have ever had a rash or other allergic reaction to loperamide HCl

Do not use if you have bloody or black stool

Ask a doctor before use if you have
• fever • mucus in the stool • a history of liver disease

Ask a doctor or pharmacist before use if you are taking antibiotics

When using this product tiredness, drowsiness or dizziness may occur. Be careful when driving or operating machinery.

Stop use and ask a doctor if
• symptoms get worse • diarrhea lasts for more than 2 days
• you get abdominal swelling or bulging. These may be signs of a serious condition.

If pregnant or breast-feeding, ask a health professional before use.

Keep out of reach of children. In case of overdose, get medical help or contact a Poison Control Center right away. (1-800-222-1222)

Directions

Imodium A-D Caplets and EZ Chews
• **drink plenty of clear fluids to help prevent dehydration caused by diarrhea**
• take only on an empty stomach (1 hour before or 2 hours after a meal) (EZ Chews only)
• find right dose on chart. If possible, use weight to dose; otherwise, use age.

adults and children 12 years and over	2 caplets or chew 2 tablets after the first loose stool; 1 caplet or chew 1 tablet after each subsequent loose stool; but no more than 4 caplets or tablets in 24 hours
children 9–11 years (60–95 lbs)	1 caplet or chew 1 tablet after the first loose stool; ½ caplet or chew ½ tablet after each subsequent loose stool; but no more than 3 caplets or tablets in 24 hours
children 6–8 years (48–59 lbs)	1 caplet or chew 1 tablet after the first loose stool; ½ caplet or chew ½ tablet after each subsequent loose stool; but no more than 2 caplets or tablets in 24 hours
children under 6 years (up to 47 lbs)	ask a doctor

Imodium A-D Liquid
• **drink plenty of clear fluids to help prevent dehydration caused by diarrhea**
• find right dose on chart. If possible, use weight to dose; otherwise use age.
• shake well before using
• only use attached measuring cup to dose product

adults and children 12 years and over	30 mL (6 tsp) after the first loose stool; 15 mL (3 tsp) after each subsequent loose stool; but no more than 60 mL (12 tsp) in 24 hours
children 9–11 years (60–95 lbs)	15 mL (3 tsp) after first loose stool; 7.5 mL (1½ tsp) after each subsequent loose stool; but no more than 45 mL (9 tsp) in 24 hours
children 6–8 years (48–59 lbs)	15 mL (3 tsp) after first loose stool; 7.5 mL (1½ tsp) after each subsequent loose stool; but no more than 30 mL (6 tsp) in 24 hours
children under 6 years (up to 47 lbs)	ask a doctor

Imodium A-D Liquid Professional Dosage Schedule for children 2–5 years old (24–47 lbs): 1½ teaspoonful after first loose bowel movement, followed by 1½ teaspoonful after each subsequent loose bowel movement. Do not exceed 4½ teaspoonful a day.

Other information:

Liquid:
• **each 30 mL (6 tsp) contains:** sodium 16 mg
• store between 20–25°C (68–77°F)

Caplets:
• **each caplet contains:** calcium 10 mg
• store between 20–25°C (68–77°F)

EZ Chews:
• **contains milk**
• store between 20–25°C (68–77°F)

Professional Information:
Overdosage information

For emergency information, contact your local Poison Control Center (1-800-222-1222)

Overdosage of loperamide HCl may include in constipation, CNS depression, respiratory depression, and nausea. A slurry of activated charcoal administered promptly after ingestion of loperamide hydrochloride can reduce the amount of drug that is absorbed. If vomiting occurs spontaneously upon ingestion, a slurry of activated charcoal can be administered orally as soon as fluids can be retained. In the event of overdosage, patients should be monitored for signs of CNS depression or respiratory depression for at least 24 hours. Children may be more sensitive to CNS effects than adults. Naloxone may be administered if CNS depression or respiratory depression is observed.

Inactive ingredients:

Liquid: anhydrous citric acid, caramel color, D&C yellow no. 10, FD&C blue no. 1, flavor, glycerin, microcrystalline cellulose and carboxymethylcellulose sodium, propylene glycol, purified water, simethicone emulsion, sodium benzoate, sucralose, titanium dioxide, xanthan gum.

Caplets: colloidal silicon dioxide, dibasic calcium phosphate, D&C yellow no. 10 aluminum lake, FD&C blue no. 1 aluminum lake, magnesium stearate, microcrystalline cellulose

EZ Chews: acesulfame potassium, basic polymethacrylate, cellulose acetate, confectioner's sugar, crospovidone, D&C yellow #10 aluminum lake, dextrose excipient, FD&C blue #1 aluminum lake, flavors, magnesium stearate, microcrystalline cellulose, milk powder, sucralose

For information or questions, visit our website www.imodium.com

IMODIUM® MULTI-SYMPTOM RELIEF OTC
Caplets & Chewable Tablets

Active Ingredients (in each caplet/tablet) ***Purpose***
Loperamide HCl 2mg Anti-diarrheal
Simethicone 125 mg Anti-gas

Uses relieves symptoms of diarrhea plus bloating, pressure, and cramps, commonly referred to as gas

Warnings

Allergy alert: Do not use if you have ever had a rash or other allergic reaction to loperamide HCl

Do not use if you have bloody or black stool

Ask a doctor before use if you have
• fever • mucus in the stool • a history of liver disease

Ask a doctor or pharmacist before use if you are taking antibiotics

When using this product tiredness, drowsiness or dizziness may occur. Be careful when driving or operating machinery.

Stop use and ask a doctor if
• symptoms get worse • diarrhea lasts for more than 2 days
• you get abdominal swelling or bulging. These may be signs of a serious condition.

If pregnant or breast-feeding, ask a health professional before use.

Keep out of reach of children. In case of overdose, get medical help or contact a Poison Control Center right away. (1-800-222-1222)

Directions
• **drink plenty of clear fluids to help prevent dehydration caused by diarrhea**
• take only on an empty stomach (1 hour before or 2 hours after a meal) (caplets only)
• find right dose on chart. If possible, use weight to dose; otherwise, use age.

adults and children 12 years and over	2 caplets or chew 2 tablets and take with water (for chewables) after the first loose stool; 1 caplet or chew 1 tablet and take with water (for chewables) after each subsequent loose stool; but no more than 4 caplets or chewable tablets in 24 hours
children 9–11 years (60–95 lbs)	1 caplet or chew 1 tablet and take with water (for chewables) after the first loose stool; ½ caplet or chew ½ tablet and take with water (for chewables) after each subsequent loose stool; but no more than 3 caplets/tablets in 24 hours
children 6–8 years (48–59 lbs)	1 caplet or chew 1 tablet and take with water (for chewables) after the first loose stool; ½ caplet or chew ½ tablet and take with water (for chewables) after each subsequent loose stool; but no more than 2 caplets/tablets in 24 hours
children under 6 years (up to 47 lbs)	ask a doctor

Other information:

Caplets:
• each caplet contains: **calcium 165 mg, sodium 4 mg**
• store between 20–25°C (68–77°F). Protect from light.

Chewable Tablets:
• each tablet contains: **calcium 50 mg**
• **contains milk**
• store between 20–25°C (68–77°F)

Professional Information:
Overdosage information

For emergency information, contact your local Poison Control Center (1-800-222-1222).

Overdosage of loperamide HCl may include in constipation, CNS depression, respiratory depression, and nausea. A slurry of activated charcoal administered promptly after ingestion of loperamide hydrochloride can reduce the amount of drug that is absorbed. If vomiting occurs spontaneously upon ingestion, a slurry of activated charcoal can be administered orally as soon as fluids can be retained. In the event of overdosage, patients should be monitored for signs of CNS depression or respiratory depression for at least 24 hours. Children may be more sensitive to central nervous system effects than adults. Naloxone may be administered if CNS depression or respiratory depression is observed. No treatment is necessary for the simethicone ingestion in this circumstance.

Inactive ingredients:

Caplets: acesulfame potassium, croscarmellose sodium, dibasic calcium phosphate, flavor, microcrystalline cellulose, stearic acid

Chewable Tablets: cellulose acetate, confectioner's sugar, D&C yellow # 10 aluminum lake, dextrates, FD&C blue # 1 aluminum lake, flavors, microcrystalline cellulose, milk powder, polymethacrylates, saccharin sodium, sorbitol, stearic acid, tribasic calcium phosphate

For information or questions, visit our website www.imodium.com

INFANTS' MOTRIN® and CHILDREN'S MOTRIN® Dosing Chart

Find the right dose on the chart below. If possible, use weight to dose; otherwise use age.

[See table at top of next page]

• **this product does not contain directions or complete warnings for adult use**
• **do not give more than directed**
• shake well before using
• find right dose on chart. If possible, use weight to dose; otherwise use age.
• if needed, repeat dose every **6-8 hours**
• do not use more than **4 times a day**
• Children's MOTRIN® Suspension:
 ◦ use only enclosed measuring cup
 ◦ replace original bottle cap to maintain child resistance

		Weight and Age**							
Product	Concentration*	6-11 lbs (0-5 mos)	12-17 lbs (6-11 mos)	18-23 lbs (12-23 mos)	24-35 lbs (2-3 yrs)	36-47 lbs (4-5 yrs)	48-59 lbs (6-8 yrs)	60-71 lbs (9-10 yrs)	72-95 lbs (11 yrs)
Concentrated Motrin® Infants' Drops	Ibuprofen 50 mg per 1.25 mL	ask a doctor	1.25 mL	1.875 mL	-	-	-	-	-
Children's MOTRIN® Suspension	Ibuprofen 100 mg per 5 mL	ask a doctor	ask a doctor	ask a doctor	5 mL (1 tsp)	7.5 mL (1 ½ tsp)	10 mL (2 tsp)	12.5 mL (2 ½ tsp)	15 mL (3 tsp)

mL = milliliter; tsp = teaspoonful
5 mL = 1 teaspoon
*Concentrated Motrin® Infants' Drops are more concentrated than Children's Motrin® Suspension. The Concentrated Motrin® Infants' Drops have been specifically designed for use only with enclosed dosing device. Do not use any other dosing device with this product.
** Under 6 mos, ask a doctor.

• Concentrated Motrin® Infants' Drops
  ◦ measure with the dosing device provided. Do not use with any other device.
  ◦ dispense liquid slowly into the child's mouth, toward the inner cheek

MOTRIN® IB (Ibuprofen) Caplets — OTC

Active ingredient (in each caplet) — ***Purpose***
Ibuprofen 200 mg (NSAID)* — Pain reliever/fever reducer
*nonsteroidal anti-inflammatory drug

Uses
• temporarily relieves minor aches and pains due to:
  • headache • muscular aches • minor pain of arthritis
  • toothache • backache • the common cold • menstrual cramps
• temporarily reduces fever

Warnings
Allergy alert: Ibuprofen may cause a severe allergic reaction, especially in people allergic to aspirin. Symptoms may include:
• hives • facial swelling • asthma (wheezing) • shock • skin reddening • rash • blisters
If an allergic reaction occurs, stop use and seek medical help right away.
Stomach bleeding warning: This product contains an NSAID, which may cause severe stomach bleeding. The chance is higher if you:
• are age 60 or older
• have had stomach ulcers or bleeding problems
• take a blood thinning (anticoagulant) or steroid drug
• take other drugs containing prescription or nonprescription NSAIDs (aspirin, ibuprofen, naproxen, or others)
• have 3 or more alcoholic drinks every day while using this product
• take more or for a longer time than directed

Do not use
• if you have ever had an allergic reaction to any other pain reliever/fever reducer
• right before or after heart surgery

Ask a doctor before use if
• you have problems or serious side effects from taking pain relievers or fever reducers
• the stomach bleeding warning applies to you
• you have a history of stomach problems, such as heartburn
• you have high blood pressure, heart disease, liver cirrhosis, or kidney disease
• you have asthma
• you are taking a diuretic

Ask a doctor or pharmacist before use if you are
• taking aspirin for heart attack or stroke, because ibuprofen may decrease this benefit of aspirin
• under a doctor's care for any serious condition
• taking any other drug

When using this product
• take with food or milk if stomach upset occurs
• the risk of heart attack or stroke may increase if you use more than directed or for longer than directed

Stop use and ask a doctor if
• you experience any of the following signs of stomach bleeding
  • feel faint
  • vomit blood
  • have bloody or black stools
  • have stomach pain that does not get better
• pain gets worse or lasts more than 10 days
• fever gets worse or lasts more than 3 days
• redness or swelling is present in the painful area
• any new symptoms appear

If pregnant or breast-feeding, ask a health professional before use. It is especially important not to use ibuprofen during the last 3 months of pregnancy unless definitely directed to do so by a doctor because it may cause problems in the unborn child or complications during delivery.

Keep out of reach of children. In case of overdose, get medical help or contact a Poison Control Center right away. (1-800-222-1222)

Directions
• **do not take more than directed**
• **the smallest effective dose should be used**

adults and children 12 years and older	• take 1 caplet every 4 to 6 hours while symptoms persist • if pain or fever does not respond to 1 caplet, 2 caplets may be used • do not exceed 6 caplets in 24 hours, unless directed by a doctor
children under 12 years	• ask a doctor

Other information
• store between 20–25°C (68–77°F)

Inactive ingredients:
carnauba wax, colloidal silicon dioxide, corn starch, FD&C yellow no. 6, hypromellose, iron oxide, magnesium stearate, polydextrose, polyethylene glycol, pregelatinized starch, propylene glycol, shellac, stearic acid, titanium dioxide

Professional Information:
Overdosage information FOR ADULT MOTRIN®

For emergency information, contact your local Poison Control Center (1-800-222-1222).

IBUPROFEN

The *toxicity of ibuprofen* overdose is dependent upon the amount of drug ingested and the time elapsed since ingestion, though individual response may vary, which makes it necessary to evaluate each case individually. Although uncommon, serious toxicity and death have been reported in the medical literature with ibuprofen overdosage. The most frequently reported symptoms of ibuprofen overdose include abdominal pain, nausea, vomiting, lethargy and drowsiness. Other central nervous system symptoms include headache, tinnitus, CNS depression and seizures. Metabolic acidosis, coma, acute renal failure and apnea (primarily in very young children) may rarely occur. Cardiovascular toxicity, including hypotension, bradycardia, tachycardia and atrial fibrillation, also have been reported. The *treatment of acute ibuprofen overdose* is primarily supportive. Management of hypotension, acidosis and gastrointestinal bleeding may be necessary. Orally administered activated charcoal may help in reducing the absorption and reabsorption of ibuprofen. In children, the estimated amount of ibuprofen ingested per body weight may be helpful to predict the potential for development of toxicity although each case must be evaluated. Ingestion of less than 100 mg/kg is unlikely to produce toxicity. Activated Charcoal bonds ibuprofen and can be administered after overdoses of more than 200 mg/kg. Children ingesting greater than 400 mg/kg require immediate medical referral, careful observation and appropriate supportive therapy. Ipecac-induced emesis is not recommended in overdoses greater than 400 mg/kg because of the risk of convulsions and the potential for aspiration of gastric contents. In adult patients the history of the dose reportedly ingested does not appear to be predictive of toxicity. The need for referral and follow-up must be judged by the circumstances at the time of the overdose ingestion. Symptomatic adults should be admitted to a health care facility for observation.

For information or questions, visit our website www.motrin.com

INFANTS' MOTRIN® ibuprofen Concentrated Drops — OTC
CHILDREN'S MOTRIN® ibuprofen Oral Suspension

Product information for all dosages of Children's MOTRIN have been combined under this heading

INFANTS' MOTRIN® Concentrated Drops
Active ingredient (in each 1.25 mL) — ***Purpose***
Ibuprofen 50 mg (NSAID)* — Pain Reliever/fever reducer

CHILDREN'S MOTRIN® Oral Suspension
Active ingredient (in each 5 mL = 1 teaspoon) — ***Purpose***
Ibuprofen 100 mg (NSAID)* — Pain Reliever/fever reducer
*nonsteroidal anti-inflammatory drug

Uses temporarily:
• reduces fever
• relieves minor aches and pains due to the common cold, flu, sore throat, headaches and toothaches

Directions See Children's Motrin Dosing Chart above

Warnings
Allergy alert: Ibuprofen may cause a severe allergic reaction, especially in people allergic to aspirin. Symptoms may include:
• hives • facial swelling • asthma (wheezing) • shock • skin reddening • rash • blisters
If an allergic reaction occurs, stop use and seek medical help right away.
Stomach bleeding warning: This product contains an NSAID, which may cause severe stomach bleeding. The chance is higher if your child:
• has had stomach ulcers or bleeding problems
• takes a blood thinning (anticoagulant) or steroid drug
• takes other drugs containing prescription or nonprescription NSAIDs (aspirin, ibuprofen, naproxen, or others)
• takes more or for a longer time than directed
Sore throat warning: Severe or persistent sore throat or sore throat accompanied by high fever, headache, nausea, and vomiting may be serious. Consult doctor promptly. Do not use more than 2 days or administer to children under 3 years of age unless directed by doctor.

Do not use
• if the child has ever had an allergic reaction to any other pain reliever/fever reducer
• right before or after heart surgery

Ask a doctor before use if
• stomach bleeding warnings applies to your child
• child has a history of stomach problems, such as heartburn
• child has problems or serious side effects from taking pain relievers or fever reducers
• child has not been drinking fluids
• child has lost a lot of fluid due to vomiting or diarrhea
• child has high blood pressure, heart disease, liver cirrhosis, or kidney disease
• child has asthma
• child is taking a diuretic

Ask a doctor or pharmacist before use if the child is
• under a doctor's care for any serious condition
• taking any other drug

When using this product
• take with food or milk if stomach upset occurs
• the risk of heart attack or stroke may increase if you use more than directed or for longer than directed

Stop use and ask a doctor if
• child experiences any of the following signs of stomach bleeding
  • feels faint • vomits blood • has bloody or black stools
  • has stomach pain that does not get better
• the child does not get any relief within first day (24 hours) of treatment
• fever or pain gets worse or lasts more than 3 days
• redness or swelling is present in the painful area
• any new symptoms appear

Keep out of reach of children. In case of overdose, get medical help or contact a Poison Control Center right away (1-800-222-1222).

Other information
Infants' and Children's MOTRIN® products:
• store between 20–25°C *(68–77°F)*
Children's MOTRIN® Suspension Liquid:
• **each teaspoon contains:** sodium 2 mg

Inactive ingredients

Concentrated MOTRIN® Infants' Drops: **Berry-Flavored:** anhydrous citric acid, caramel, FD&C red no. 40, flavors, glycerin, polysorbate 80, pregelatinized starch, purified water, sodium benzoate, sorbitol solution, sucrose, xanthan gum. **Dye-Free Berry-Flavored:** anhydrous citric acid, caramel, flavors, glycerin, polysorbate 80, pregelatinized starch, purified water, sodium benzoate, sorbitol solution, sucrose, xanthan gum.

Children's MOTRIN® Oral Suspension: **Berry-Flavored:** acesulfame potassium, anhydrous citric acid, D&C yellow no. 10, FD&C red no. 40, flavors, glycerin, polysorbate 80, pregelatinized starch, purified water, sodium benzoate, sucrose, xanthan gum. **Dye-Free Berry-Flavored:** acesulfame potassium, anhydrous citric acid, flavors, glycerin, polysorbate 80, pregelatinized starch, purified water, sodium benzoate, sucrose, xanthan gum.

Professional Information:

Overdosage information for all infants' & children's MOTRIN® products

For emergency information, contact your local Poison Control Center (1-800-222-1222).

Ibuprofen: The *toxicity of ibuprofen* overdose is dependent upon the amount of drug ingested and the time elapsed since ingestion, though individual response may vary, which makes it necessary to evaluate each case individually. Although uncommon, serious toxicity and death have been reported in the medical literature with ibuprofen overdosage. The most frequently reported symptoms of ibuprofen overdose include abdominal pain, nausea, vomiting, lethargy and drowsiness. Other central nervous system symptoms include headache, tinnitus, CNS depression and seizures. Metabolic acidosis, coma, acute renal failure and apnea (primarily in very young children) may rarely occur. Cardiovascular toxicity, including hypotension, bradycardia, tachycardia and atrial fibrillation, also have been reported.

The *treatment of acute ibuprofen overdose* is primarily supportive. Management of hypotension, acidosis and gastrointestinal bleeding may be necessary. Orally administered activated charcoal may help in reducing the absorption and reabsorption of ibuprofen. In children, the estimated amount of ibuprofen ingested per body weight may be helpful to predict the potential for development of toxicity although each case must be evaluated. Ingestion of less than 100 mg/kg is unlikely to produce toxicity. Activated charcoal binds ibuprofen and can be administered after overdoses of more than 200 mg/kg. Children ingesting greater than 400 mg/kg require immediate medical referral, careful observation and appropriate supportive therapy. Ipecac-induced emesis is not recommended in overdoses greater than 400 mg/kg because of the risk of convulsions and the potential for aspiration of gastric contents.

In adult patients the history of the dose reportedly ingested does not appear to be predictive of toxicity. The need for referral and follow-up must be judged by the circumstances at the time of the overdose ingestion. Symptomatic adults should be admitted to a health care facility for observation.

For information or questions, visit our website www.motrin.com

---

MOTRIN® PM Caplets — OTC

Active ingredients (in each caplet)	*Purposes*
Diphenhydramine citrate 38 mg	Nighttime sleep-aid
Ibuprofen 200 mg (NSAID)*	Pain reliever

*nonsteroidal anti-inflammatory drug

Uses

- for relief of occasional sleeplessness when associated with minor aches and pains
- helps you fall asleep and stay asleep

Warnings

Allergy alert: Ibuprofen may cause a severe allergic reaction, especially in people allergic to aspirin. Symptoms may include:

- hives • facial swelling • asthma (wheezing) • shock • skin reddening • rash • blisters

If an allergic reaction occurs, stop use and seek medical help right away.

Stomach bleeding warning: This product contains an NSAID, which may cause severe stomach bleeding. The chance is higher if you:

- are age 60 or older
- have had stomach ulcers or bleeding problems
- take a blood thinning (anticoagulant) or steroid drug
- take other drugs containing prescription or nonprescription NSAIDs (aspirin, ibuprofen, naproxen, or others)
- have 3 or more alcoholic drinks every day while using this product
- take more or for a longer time than directed

Do not use

- if you have ever had an allergic reaction to any other pain reliever/fever reducer
- unless you have time for a full night's sleep
- in children under 12 years of age
- right before or after heart surgery
- with any other product containing diphenhydramine, even one used on skin
- if you have sleeplessness without pain

Ask a doctor before use if

- the stomach bleeding warning applies to you
- you have problems or serious side effects from taking pain relievers or fever reducers
- you have a history of stomach problems, such as heartburn
- you have high blood pressure, heart disease, liver cirrhosis, kidney disease, or asthma
- you are taking a diuretic
- you have a breathing problem such as emphysema or chronic bronchitis
- you have glaucoma
- you have trouble urinating due to an enlarged prostate gland

Ask a doctor or pharmacist before use if you are

- taking sedatives or tranquilizers, or any other sleep-aid
- under a doctor's care for any continuing medical illness
- taking any other antihistamines
- taking aspirin for heart attack or stroke, because ibuprofen may decrease this benefit of aspirin
- taking any other drug

When using this product

- drowsiness will occur
- avoid alcoholic drinks
- do not drive a motor vehicle or operate machinery
- take with food or milk if stomach upset occurs
- the risk of heart attack or stroke may increase if you use more than directed or for longer than directed

Stop use and ask a doctor if

- you experience any of the following signs of stomach bleeding:
  - feel faint • vomit blood • have bloody or black stools
  - have stomach pain that does not get better
- pain gets worse or lasts more than 10 days
- sleeplessness persists continuously for more than 2 weeks. Insomnia may be a symptom of a serious underlying medical illness.
- redness or swelling is present in the painful area
- any new symptoms appear

If pregnant or breast-feeding, ask a health professional before use. It is especially important not to use ibuprofen during the last 3 months of pregnancy unless definitely directed to do so by a doctor because it may cause problems in the unborn child or complications during delivery.

Keep out of reach of children. In case of overdose, get medical help or contact a Poison Control Center right away. (1-800-222-1222)

Directions

- **do not take more than directed**
- adults and children 12 years and over: take 2 caplets at bedtime
- do not take more than 2 caplets in 24 hours

Other information

- read all warnings and directions before use. Keep carton.
- store at 20°-25°C (68°-77°F)
- avoid excessive heat above 40°C (104°F)

Inactive ingredients colloidal silicon dioxide, croscarmellose sodium, glyceryl behenate, hydroxypropyl cellulose, lactose monohydrate, magnesium stearate, microcrystalline cellulose, polyethylene glycol, polyvinyl alcohol, pregelatinized starch, talc, titanium dioxide

For information or questions, visit our website www.motrin.com

---

SIMPLY SLEEP® Caplet — OTC

Drug Facts

Active ingredient (in each caplet)	*Purpose*
Diphenhydramine HCl 25 mg	Nighttime sleep aid

Use for relief of occasional sleeplessness

Warnings

Do not use

- in children under 12 years of age
- with any other product containing diphenhydramine, even one used on skin

Ask a doctor before use if you have

- a breathing problem such as emphysema or chronic bronchitis
- glaucoma
- trouble urinating due to an enlarged prostate gland

Ask a doctor or pharmacist before use if you are taking sedatives or tranquilizers

When using this product

- avoid alcoholic drinks
- drowsiness will occur
- do not drive a motor vehicle or operate machinery

Stop use and ask a doctor if

- sleeplessness persists continuously for more than 2 weeks. Insomnia may be a symptom of serious underlying medical illness.

If pregnant or breast-feeding, ask a health professional before use.

Keep out of reach of children.

Overdose warning: In case of overdose, get medical help or contact a Poison Control Center right away. (1-800-222-1222)

Directions

adults and children 12 years and over	take 2 caplets at bedtime if needed, or as directed by a doctor
children under 12 years	do not use

Other information

- **each caplet contains:** calcium 14 mg
- store between 20-25°C (68-77°F). Avoid high humidity. Protect from light.

Inactive ingredients carnauba wax, croscarmellose sodium, dibasic calcium phosphate, FD&C blue no. 1 aluminum lake, hypromellose, magnesium stearate, microcrystalline cellulose, polyethylene glycol, polysorbate 80, titanium dioxide

---

SUDAFED® 12 HOUR PRESSURE AND PAIN — OTC
Non-Drowsy Caplets

Drug Facts

Active ingredients (in each caplet)	*Purposes*
Naproxen sodium 220 mg (naproxen 200 mg) (NSAID)*	Pain reliever/fever reducer
Pseudoephedrine HCl 120 mg, extended-release	Nasal decongestant

*nonsteroidal anti-inflammatory drug

Uses

temporarily relieves these cold, sinus, and flu symptoms:

- sinus pressure ■ minor body aches and pains
- headache ■ nasal and sinus congestion (promotes sinus drainage and restores freer breathing through the nose)
- fever

Warnings

Allergy alert: Naproxen sodium may cause a severe allergic reaction, especially in people allergic to aspirin. Symptoms may include:

- hives ■ facial swelling ■ asthma (wheezing)
- shock ■ skin reddening ■ rash
- blisters

If an allergic reaction occurs, stop use and seek medical help right away.

Stomach bleeding warning: This product contains an NSAID, which may cause severe stomach bleeding. The chance is higher if you:

- are age 60 or older
- have had stomach ulcers or bleeding problems
- take a blood thinning (anticoagulant) or steroid drug
- take other drugs containing prescription or nonprescription NSAIDs (aspirin, ibuprofen, naproxen, or others)
- have 3 or more alcoholic drinks every day while using this product
- take more or for a longer time than directed

Do not use

- if you have ever had an allergic reaction to any other pain reliever/fever reducer
- right before or after heart surgery
- if you are now taking a prescription monoamine oxidase inhibitor (MAOI) (certain drugs for depression, psychiatric, or emotional conditions, or Parkinson's disease), or for 2 weeks after stopping the MAOI drug. If you do not know if your prescription drug contains an MAOI, ask a doctor or pharmacist before taking this product.
- in children under 12 years of age

Ask a doctor before use if

- the stomach bleeding warning applies to you
- you have a history of stomach problems, such as heartburn

- you have high blood pressure, heart disease, liver cirrhosis, or kidney disease
- you are taking a diuretic
- you have problems or serious side effects from taking pain relievers or fever reducers
- you have
  - asthma ■ diabetes ■ thyroid disease
  - trouble urinating due to an enlarged prostate gland

Ask a doctor or pharmacist before use if you are
- under a doctor's care for any serious condition
- taking any other drug

When using this product
- take with food or milk if stomach upset occurs
- the risk of heart attack or stroke may increase if you use more than directed or for longer than directed

Stop use and ask a doctor if
- you experience any of the following signs of stomach bleeding:
  - feel faint ■ vomit blood ■ have bloody or black stools
  - have stomach pain that does not get better
- redness or swelling is present in the painful area
- any new symptoms appear
- fever gets worse or lasts more than 3 days
- you have difficulty swallowing or the caplet feels stuck in your throat
- you get nervous, dizzy, or sleepless
- nasal congestion lasts more than 7 days

If pregnant or breast-feeding, ask a health professional before use. It is especially important not to use naproxen sodium during the last 3 months of pregnancy unless definitely directed to do so by a doctor because it may cause problems in the unborn child or complications during delivery.

Keep out of reach of children. In case of overdose, get medical help or contact a Poison Control Center right away. (1-800-222-1222)

Directions
- **do not take more than directed**
- **the smallest effective dose should be used**
- **swallow whole;** do not crush or chew
- **drink a full glass of water with each dose**

adults and children 12 years and older	■ **1 caplet every 12 hours** ■ do not take more than 2 caplets in 24 hours
children under 12 years	■ do not use

Other information
- **each caplet contains:** sodium 22 mg
- **Do not use if carton is opened or if blister unit is broken**
- store at 20-25°C (68-77°F)
- store in a dry place

Inactive ingredients colloidal silicon dioxide, hypromellose, lactose monohydrate, magnesium stearate, microcrystalline cellulose, polyethylene glycol, polysorbate 80, povidone, talc, titanium dioxide

For information or questions, visit our website www.sudafed.com

CHILDREN'S SUDAFED® NON-DROWSY NASAL DECONGESTANT LIQUID OTC

Drug Facts

Active ingredient: (in each 5 mL = 1 teaspoonful) ***Purpose***
Pseudoephedrine HCl 15 mg Nasal decongestant

Uses
- temporarily relieves nasal congestion due to the common cold, hay fever or other upper respiratory allergies
- temporarily relieves sinus congestion and pressure
- promotes nasal and/or sinus drainage

Warnings
Do not use in a child who is taking a prescription monoamine oxidase inhibitor (MAOI) (certain drugs for depression, psychiatric or emotional conditions, or Parkinson's disease), or for 2 weeks after stopping the MAOI drug. If you do not know if your child's prescription drug contains an MAOI, ask a doctor or pharmacist before giving this product.

Ask a doctor before use if the child has
- heart disease
- high blood pressure
- thyroid disease
- diabetes

When using this product do not exceed recommended dose

Stop use and ask a doctor if
- nervousness, dizziness, or sleeplessness occur
- symptoms do not improve within 7 days or occur with a fever

Keep out of reach of children. In case of overdose, get medical help or contact a Poison Control Center right away. (1-800-222-1222)

Directions
- find right dose on chart
- mL = milliliter; tsp = teaspoonful
- repeat dose every 4 to 6 hours
- do not use more than 4 times in 24 hours

Age (yr)	Dose (mL or tsp)
under 4 years	do not use
4 to 5 years	5 mL (1 tsp)
6 to 11 years	10 mL (2 tsp)

Attention: use only enclosed dosing cup designed for use with this product. Do not use any other dosing device.

Other information
- **each 5 mL (1 tsp) contains:** sodium 5 mg
- store between 20–25°C (68–77°F)

Inactive ingredients anhydrous citric acid, edetate disodium, FD&C blue no. 1, FD&C red no. 40, flavor, glycerin, menthol, poloxamer 407, polyethylene glycol, povidone K-90, purified water, saccharin sodium, sodium benzoate, sodium citrate, sorbitol solution

For information or questions, visit our website www.sudafed.com

CHILDREN'S SUDAFED PE® COLD & COUGH (Grape) OTC

Drug Facts

Active ingredients (in each 5 mL = 1 teaspoonful) ***Purpose***
Dextromethorphan HBr 5 mg Cough suppressant
Phenylephrine HCl 2.5 mg Nasal decongestant

Use
- temporarily relieves these symptoms due to the common cold, hay fever, or other upper respiratory allergies:
  - cough ■ nasal congestion

Warnings
Do not use in a child who is taking a prescription monoamine oxidase inhibitor (MAOI) (certain drugs for depression, psychiatric or emotional conditions, or Parkinson's disease), or for 2 weeks after stopping the MAOI drug. If you do not know if your child's prescription drug contains an MAOI, ask a doctor or pharmacist before giving this product.

Ask a doctor before use if the child has
- heart disease ■ high blood pressure ■ thyroid disease
- diabetes
- persistent or chronic cough such as occurs with asthma
- cough that occurs with too much phlegm (mucus)
- a sodium-restricted diet

When using this product do not exceed recommended dose

Stop use and ask a doctor if
- nervousness, dizziness, or sleeplessness occur
- symptoms do not improve within 7 days or occur with a fever
- cough gets worse or lasts for more than 7 days
- cough tends to come back or occurs with fever, rash or headache that lasts

These could be signs of a serious condition.

Keep out of reach of children. In case of overdose, get medical help or contact a Poison Control Center right away. (1-800-222-1222)

Directions
- find right dose on chart (*use if appropriate*)
- mL = milliliter; tsp = teaspoonful
- repeat dose every 4 hours
- do not give more than 6 times in 24 hours

Age (yr)	Dose (mL or tsp)
Under 4 years	do not use
4 to 5 years	5 mL (1 tsp)
6 to 11 years	10 mL (2 tsp)

Attention: use only enclosed dosing cup specifically designed for use with this product. Do not use any other dosing device.

Other information
- **each 5 mL (1 tsp) contains:** sodium 15 mg
- store between 20-25°C (68-77°F). Protect from light.

Inactive ingredients anhydrous citric acid, carboxymethylcellulose sodium, edetate disodium, FD&C blue #1, FD&C red #40, flavors, glycerin, purified water, sodium benzoate, sodium citrate, sorbitol solution, sucralose

For information or questions, visit our website www.benadryl.com

CHILDREN'S SUDAFED PE® NASAL DECONGESTANT LIQUID OTC

Active ingredient (in each 5 mL = 1 teaspoonful) ***Purpose***
Phenylephrine HCl 2.5 mg Nasal decongestant

Use temporarily relieves nasal congestion due to the common cold, hay fever or other upper respiratory allergies

Warnings
Do not use in a child who is taking a prescription monoamine oxidase inhibitor (MAOI) (certain drugs for depression, psychiatric, or emotional conditions, or Parkinson's disease), or for 2 weeks after stopping the MAOI drug. If you do not know if your child's prescription drug contains an MAOI, ask a doctor or pharmacist before giving this product.

Ask a doctor before use if the child has
- heart disease
- high blood pressure
- thyroid disease
- diabetes
- a sodium-restricted diet

When using this product do not exceed recommended dose

Stop use and ask a doctor if
- nervousness, dizziness, or sleeplessness occur
- symptoms do not improve within 7 days or occur with a fever

Keep out of reach of children. In case of overdose, get medical help or contact a Poison Control Center right away. (1-800-222-1222)

Directions
- find right dose on chart
- mL = milliliter; tsp = teaspoonful
- repeat dose every 4 hours
- do not use more than 6 times in 24 hours

Age (yr)	Dose (mL or tsp)
under 4 years	do not use
4 to 5 years	5 mL (1 tsp)
6 to 11 years	10 mL (2 tsp)

Attention: use only enclosed dosing cup designed for use with this product. Do not use any other dosing device.

Other information
- **each 5 mL (1 tsp) contains:** sodium 14 mg
- store between 20°-25°C (68°-77°F). Protect from light. Store in outer carton until contents are used.

Inactive ingredients: anhydrous citric acid, carboxymethylcellulose sodium, edetate disodium, FD&C red # 40, flavors, glycerin, purified water, sodium benzoate, sodium citrate, sorbitol solution, sucralose

For information or questions, visit our website www.sudafed.com

SUDAFED® OTC

Active ingredient (in each tablet/caplet) ***Purpose***
SUDAFED® 12 Hour Caplets
Pseudoephedrine HCl 120 mg Nasal decongestant
SUDAFED® 24 Hour Tablets
Pseudoephedrine HCl 240 mg Nasal decongestant

Uses
SUDAFED® 12 Hour Caplets
SUDAFED® 24 Hour Tablets
- temporarily relieves nasal congestion due to the common cold, hay fever or other upper respiratory allergies
- temporarily relieves sinus congestion and pressure (SUDAFED® 12 Hour Caplets)
- reduces swelling of nasal passages (SUDAFED® 24 Hour Caplets)
- relieves sinus pressure (SUDAFED® 24 Hour Caplets)

Warnings
Do not use if you are now taking a prescription monoamine oxidase inhibitor (MAOI) (certain drugs for depression, psychiatric or emotional conditions, or Parkinson's disease), or for 2 weeks after stopping the MAOI drug. If you do not know if your prescription drug contains an MAOI, ask a doctor or pharmacist before taking this product.

Ask a doctor before use if you have
- heart disease
- high blood pressure
- thyroid disease
- diabetes
- trouble urinating due to an enlarged prostate gland

SUDAFED® 24 HOUR Tablets
- had obstruction or narrowing of the bowel.
  Rarely tablets of this kind may cause bowel obstruction (blockage), usually in people with severe narrowing of the bowel (esophagus, stomach or intestine)

When using this product do not exceed recommended dose

Stop use and ask a doctor if
- nervousness, dizziness, or sleeplessness occur
- symptoms do not improve within 7 days or occur with a fever

SUDAFED® 24 HOUR Tablets
- you experience persistent abdominal pain or vomiting

If pregnant or breast-feeding, ask a health professional before use.

Keep out of reach of children. In case of overdose, get medical help or contact a Poison Control Center right away. (1-800-222-1222)

Directions

SUDAFED® 12 HOUR Caplets

adults and children 12 years and over	• take 1 tablet every 12 hours • do not take more than 2 tablets in 24 hours
children under 12 years	• do not use this product in children under 12 years of age

SUDAFED® 24 HOUR Tablets

adults and children 12 years and over	• **swallow one** whole tablet with water every 24 hours • **do not exceed one tablet in 24 hours** • **do not divide, crush, chew or dissolve the tablet** • the tablet does not completely dissolve and may be seen in the stool (this is normal)
children under 12 years	• do not use the product in children under 12 years of age

Other information

SUDAFED® 12 HOUR Caplets
- store at 59° to 77°F in a dry place. Protect from light.

SUDAFED® 24 HOUR Tablets
- **each tablet contains:** sodium 10 mg
- store at 15° to 25°C (59° to 77°F) in a dry place.

SUDAFED® 12 HOUR Caplets

Inactive ingredients candelilla wax, FD&C blue no. 1 aluminum lake, hypromellose, magnesium stearate, microcrystalline cellulose, polyethylene glycol, povidone, propylene glycol, shellac, talc, titanium dioxide

SUDAFED® 24 HOUR Tablets

Inactive ingredients cellulose triacetate, hydroxypropylcellulose, hypromellose, iron oxide, magnesium stearate, microcrystalline cellulose, polyethylene glycol, polysorbate 80, povidine, propylene glycol, shellac, sodium chloride, and titanium dioxide

For information or questions, visit our website www.sudafed.com

SUDAFED PE® Congestion Tablets — OTC

Active ingredient (in each tablet) — ***Purpose***

Phenylephrine HCl 10 mg — Nasal decongestant

Uses
- temporarily relieves sinus congestion and pressure
- temporarily relieves nasal congestion due to the common cold, hay fever or other upper respiratory allergies

Warnings

Do not use if you are now taking a prescription monoamine oxidase inhibitor (MAOI) (certain drugs for depression, psychiatric or emotional conditions, or Parkinson's disease), or for 2 weeks after stopping the MAOI drug. If you do not know if your prescription drug contains an MAOI, ask a doctor or pharmacist before taking this product.

Ask a doctor before use if you have
- heart disease
- high blood pressure
- thyroid disease
- diabetes
- trouble urinating due to an enlarged prostate gland

When using this product do not exceed recommended dose

Stop use and ask a doctor if
- nervousness, dizziness, or sleeplessness occur
- symptoms do not improve within 7 days or occur with a fever

If pregnant or breast-feeding, ask a health professional before use.

Keep out of reach of children. In case of overdose, get medical help or contact a Poison Control Center right away. (1-800-222-1222)

Directions

adults and children 12 years and over	• take 1 tablet every 4 hours • do not take more than 6 tablets in 24 hours
children under 12 years	• ask a doctor

Other information
- store between 20-25° C (68-77° F)

Inactive ingredients carnauba wax, corn starch, D&C yellow no. 10 alumium lake, FD&C red no. 40 aluminum lake, FD&C yellow no. 6 aluminum lake, magnesium stearate, microcrystalline cellulose, polyethylene glycol, polyvinyl alcohol, powdered cellulose, pregelatinized starch, sodium starch glycolate, talc, titanium dioxide.

For information or questions, visit our website www.sudafed.com

SUDAFED PE® PRESSURE + PAIN CAPLETS (Daytime) — OTC

Drug Facts

Active ingredients (in each caplet) — ***Purpose***

Acetaminophen 325 mg — Pain reliever/fever reducer
Phenylephrine HCl 5 mg — Nasal decongestant

Uses
- temporarily relieves these symptoms associated with hay fever or other respiratory allergies, and the common cold:
  - sinus congestion and pressure
  - headache
  - minor aches and pains
  - nasal congestion
- promotes sinus drainage
- temporarily reduces fever

Warnings

Liver warning: This product contains acetaminophen. The maximum daily dose of this product is 10 caplets (3,250 mg acetaminophen) in 24 hours. Severe liver damage may occur if you take
- more than 4,000 mg of acetaminophen in 24 hours
- with other drugs containing acetaminophen
- 3 or more alcoholic drinks every day while using this product

Do not use
- with any other drug containing acetaminophen (prescription or nonprescription). If you are not sure whether a drug contains acetaminophen, ask a doctor or pharmacist.
- if you are now taking a prescription monoamine oxidase inhibitor (MAOI) (certain drugs for depression, psychiatric or emotional conditions, or Parkinson's disease), or for 2 weeks after stopping the MAOI drug. If you do not know if your prescription drug contains an MAOI, ask a doctor or pharmacist before taking this product.
- if you have ever had an allergic reaction to this product or any of its ingredients

Ask a doctor before use if you have
- liver disease
- heart disease
- high blood pressure
- thyroid disease
- diabetes
- trouble urinating due to an enlarged prostate gland

Ask a doctor or pharmacist before use if you are taking the blood thinning drug warfarin

When using this product do not exceed recommended dose

Stop use and ask a doctor if
- nervousness, dizziness, or sleeplessness occur
- pain or nasal congestion gets worse or lasts more than 7 days
- fever gets worse or lasts more than 3 days
- redness or swelling is present
- new symptoms occur

These could be signs of a serious condition.

If pregnant or breast-feeding, ask a health professional before use.

Keep out of reach of children.

Overdose warning: In case of overdose, get medical help or contact a Poison Control Center right away. (1-800-222-1222) Quick medical attention is critical for adults as well as for children even if you do not notice any signs or symptoms.

Directions
- **do not use more than directed (see overdose warning)**

adults and children 12 years and over	■ take 2 caplets every 4 hours ■ do not take more than 10 caplets in 24 hours
children under 12 years	ask a doctor

Other information
- store between 20-25°C (68-77°F)

Inactive ingredients carnauba wax, corn starch, FD&C yellow no. 6 aluminum lake, hypromellose, magnesium stearate, microcrystalline cellulose, polyethylene glycol, polysorbate 80, powdered cellulose, pregelatinized starch, sodium starch glycolate, titanium dioxide

For information or questions, visit our website www.sudafed.com

SUDAFED PE® PRESSURE + PAIN + Cough Caplets — OTC

SUDAFED PE® PRESSURE + PAIN + Cold Caplets

SUDAFED PE® PRESSURE + PAIN + Mucus Caplets

Drug Facts

Active ingredients (in each caplet) — **Purpose**

SUDAFED PE ® PRESSURE + PAIN + COUGH Caplets
Acetaminophen 325 mg — Pain reliever/fever reducer
Dextromethorphan HBr 10 mg — Cough suppressant
Phenylephrine HCl 5 mg — Nasal decongestant

SUDAFED PE ® PRESSURE + PAIN + COLD Caplets
Acetaminophen 325 mg — Pain reliever/fever reducer
Dextromethorphan HBr 10 mg — Cough suppressant
Guaifenesin 100 mg — Expectorant
Phenylephrine HCl 5 mg — Nasal decongestant

SUDAFED PE ® PRESSURE + PAIN + MUCUS Caplets
Acetaminophen 325 mg — Pain reliever/fever reducer
Guaifenesin 200 mg — Expectorant
Phenylephrine HCl 5 mg — Nasal decongestant

Uses

SUDAFED PE ® PRESSURE + PAIN + COUGH Caplets
- temporarily relieves these common cold/flu symptoms:
  - sinus congestion and pressure
  - nasal congestion
  - cough
  - sore throat
  - minor aches and pains
  - headache
  - promotes nasal and sinus drainage
- temporarily reduces fever

SUDAFED PE ® PRESSURE + PAIN + COLD Caplets
- temporarily relieves these symptoms due to the common cold:
  - nasal congestion
  - headache
  - minor aches and pains
  - cough
  - sore throat
- helps loosen phlegm (mucus) and thin bronchial secretions to drain bronchial tubes and make coughs more productive
- temporarily reduces fever

SUDAFED PE ® PRESSURE + PAIN + MUCUS Caplets
- temporarily relieves these symptoms associated with hay fever or other respiratory allergies, and the common cold:
  - sinus congestion and pressure
  - headache
  - minor aches and pains
  - nasal congestion
- helps loosen phlegm (mucus) and thin bronchial secretions to rid the bronchial passageways of bothersome mucus and make coughs more productive
- temporarily reduces fever

Warnings

Liver warning: This product contains acetaminophen. The maximum daily dose of this product is 10 caplets (3,250 mg acetaminophen) in 24 hours. Severe liver damage may occur if you take

- more than 4,000 mg of acetaminophen in 24 hours
- with other drugs containing acetaminophen
- 3 or more alcoholic drinks every day while using this product

Sore throat warning: If sore throat is severe, persists for more than 2 days, is accompanied or followed by fever, headache, rash, nausea, or vomiting, consult a doctor promptly.

(SUDAFED PE ® PRESSURE + PAIN + COUGH and SUDAFED PE ® PRESSURE + PAIN + COLD only)

Do not use

- with any other drug containing acetaminophen (prescription or nonprescription). If you are not sure whether a drug contains acetaminophen, ask a doctor or pharmacist.
- if you are now taking a prescription monoamine oxidase inhibitor (MAOI) (certain drugs for depression, psychiatric or emotional conditions, or Parkinson's disease), or for 2 weeks after stopping the MAOI drug. If you do not know if your prescription drug contains an MAOI, ask a doctor or pharmacist before taking this product.
- if you have ever had an allergic reaction to this product or any of its ingredients

Ask a doctor before use if you have

- liver disease
- heart disease
- high blood pressure
- thyroid disease
- diabetes
- trouble urinating due to an enlarged prostate gland
- persistent or chronic cough such as occurs with smoking, chronic bronchitis, asthma or emphysema (SUDAFED PE® Pressure + Pain + Cold Caplets and SUDAFED PE® Pressure + Pain + Mucus Caplets only)
- persistent or chronic cough such as occurs with smoking, asthma, or emphysema (SUDAFED PE® Pressure + Pain + Cough Caplets only)
- cough that occurs with too much phlegm (mucus)

Ask a doctor or pharmacist before use if you are taking the blood thinning drug warfarin

When using this product do not exceed recommended dose

Stop use and ask a doctor if

- nervousness, dizziness, or sleeplessness occur
- pain, nasal congestion or cough gets worse or lasts more than 7 days
- fever gets worse or lasts more than 3 days
- redness or swelling is present
- new symptoms occur
- cough comes back or occurs with rash or headache that lasts

These could be signs of a serious condition.

If pregnant or breast-feeding, ask a health professional before use.

Keep out of reach of children.

Overdose warning: In case of overdose, get medical help or contact a Poison Control Center right away. (1-800-222-1222) Quick medical attention is critical for adults as well as for children even if you do not notice any signs or symptoms.

Directions

- **do not take more than directed (see overdose warning)**

adults and children 12 years and over	■ take 2 caplets every 4 hours ■ do not take more than 10 caplets in 24 hours
children under 12 years	ask a doctor

Other information

- store between 20-25°C (68-77°F)
- each caplet contains: sodium 3 mg (SUDAFED PE® PRESSURE + PAIN + COLD AND SUDAFED PE ® PRESSURE + PAIN + MUCUS only)
- contains FD&C yellow no. 5 aluminum lake (tartrazine) as a color additive (SUDAFED PE® PRESSURE + PAIN + COLD only)

Inactive ingredients

SUDAFED PE ® PRESSURE + PAIN + COUGH Caplets
carnauba wax, corn starch, hypromellose, magnesium stearate, microcrystalline cellulose, powdered cellulose, pregelatinized starch, sodium starch glycolate

SUDAFED PE ® PRESSURE + PAIN + COLD Caplets
carnauba wax, croscarmellose sodium, FD&C yellow no. 5 aluminum lake (tartrazine), FD&C yellow no. 6 aluminum lake, hydroxypropyl cellulose, hypromellose, magnesium stearate, microcrystalline cellulose, polyethylene glycol, polysorbate 80, pregelatinized starch, titanium dioxide

SUDAFED PE ® PRESSURE + PAIN + MUCUS Caplets
carnauba wax, croscarmellose sodium, hydroxypropyl cellulose, hypromellose, magnesium stearate, microcrystalline cellulose, pregelatinized starch, titanium dioxide, triacetin

For information or questions, visit our website www.sudafed.com

INFANTS' TYLENOL® OTC
acetaminophen Oral Suspension

CHILDREN'S TYLENOL®
acetaminophen Oral Suspension

Product information for all dosages of CHILDREN'S TYLENOL® have been combined under this heading

Description

Infants' TYLENOL® Oral Suspension Liquid in each 5 mL contains 160 mg acetaminophen. *Children's TYLENOL® Oral Suspension Liquid* in each 5 mL (1 teaspoonful) contains 160 mg acetaminophen. *Infants' TYLENOL Oral Suspension Liquid* includes SimpleMeasure™ dosing system with a protective opening and push-in syringe designed to: 1) provide accurate dosing and easy administration to infants; 2) allow for better control when dispensing with fewer spills; and 3) further reduce the risk of children getting to the medicine in the bottle. *Children's TYLENOL Oral Suspension Liquid* includes a protective opening and dosing cup.

Actions

Acetaminophen is a clinically proven analgesic/antipyretic. Acetaminophen is thought to produce analgesia by elevation of the pain threshold and antipyresis through action on the hypothalamic heat-regulating center. Acetaminophen is equal to aspirin in analgesic and antipyretic effectiveness and it is unlikely to produce many of the side effects associated with aspirin and aspirin-containing products.

Uses

Infants' TYLENOL® Oral Suspension Liquid:
temporarily:

- reduces fever
- relieves minor aches and pains due to:
  - the common cold
  - flu
  - headache
  - sore throat
  - toothache

Children's TYLENOL® Oral Suspension Liquid
temporarily:

- reduces fever
- relieves minor aches and pains due to
  - the common cold
  - flu
  - headache
  - sore throat
  - toothache

Directions

Refer to Infants' and Children's TYLENOL Dosing chart for Important Instructions/Directions for Proper Use

Infants' TYLENOL® Oral Suspension

- **this product does not contain directions or complete warnings for adult use.**
- **do not give more than directed (see overdose warning)**
- **shake well before using**
- mL = milliliter
- find right dose on chart. If possible, use weight to dose; otherwise, use age.
- push air out of syringe. Insert syringe tip into bottle opening
- flip bottle upside down. Pull yellow part of syringe to the correct dose
- dispense liquid slowly into child's mouth, toward inner cheek
- repeat dose every 4 hours while symptoms last
- do not give more than 5 times in 24 hours
- replace cap tightly to maintain child resistance

Children's TYLENOL® Oral Suspension

- **this product does not contain directions or complete warnings for adult use.**
- **do not give more than directed (see overdose warning)**
- **shake well before using**
- mL = milliliter; tsp = teaspoonful
- find right dose on chart. If possible, use weight to dose; otherwise, use age.
- remove the child protective cap and squeeze your child's dose in to the dosing cup
- repeat dose every 4 hours while symptoms last
- do not give more than 5 times in 24 hours

Warnings

Liver warning: This product contains acetaminophen. Severe liver damage may occur if your child takes

- more than 5 doses in 24 hours, which is the maximum daily amount
- with other drugs containing acetaminophen

Sore throat warning: if sore throat is severe, persists for more than 2 days, is accompanied or followed by fever, headache, rash, nausea, or vomiting, consult a doctor promptly.

Do not use

- with any other drug containing acetaminophen (prescription or nonprescription). If you are not sure whether a drug contains acetaminophen, ask a doctor or pharmacist.
- if your child is allergic to acetaminophen or any of the inactive ingredients in this product.

Ask a doctor before use if your child has liver disease

Ask a doctor or pharmacist before use if you child is taking the blood thinning drug warfarin

When using this product do not exceed recommended dose (see overdose warning)

Stop use and ask a doctor if

- pain gets worse or lasts more than 5 days
- fever gets worse or lasts more than 3 days
- new symptoms occur
- redness or swelling is present

These could be signs of a serious condition

Keep out of reach of children.

Overdose warning: In case of overdose, get medical help or contact a Poison Control Center right away. (1-800-222-1222) Quick medical attention is critical for adults as well as for children even if you do not notice any signs or symptoms.

Other information

Infants' TYLENOL® Oral Suspension Liquid:

- store between 20-25°C (68-77°F)

Children's TYLENOL® Oral Suspension Liquid:

- **each 5 mL (1 tsp) contains:** sodium 2 mg
- store between 20-25°C (68-77°F)

Inactive Ingredients

Infants' TYLENOL® Oral Suspension Liquids: Cherry: anhydrous citric acid, butylparaben, FD&C red no. 40, flavors, glycerin, high fructose corn syrup, microcrystalline cellulose and carboxymethylcellulose sodium, propylene glycol, purified water, sodium benzoate, sorbitol solution, sucralose, xanthan gum **Grape:** anhydrous citric acid, butylparaben, D&C red no. 33, FD&C blue no. 1, flavors, glycerin, high fructose corn syrup, microcrystalline cellulose and carboxymethylcellulose sodium, propylene glycol, purified water, sodium benzoate, sorbitol solution, sucralose, xanthan gum

Children's TYLENOL® Oral Suspension Liquids: Cherry Blast: anhydrous citric acid, butylparaben, FD&C red no. 40, flavors, glycerin, high fructose corn syrup, microcrystalline cellulose and carboxymethylcellulose sodium, propylene glycol, purified water, sodium benzoate, sorbitol solution, sucralose, xanthan gum **Grape Splash:** anhydrous citric acid, butylparaben, D&C red no. 33, FD&C blue no. 1, flavors, glycerin, high fructose corn syrup, microcrystalline cellulose and carboxymethylcellulose sodium, propylene glycol, purified water, sodium benzoate, sorbitol solution, sucralose, xanthan gum

Dye-Free Cherry: anhydrous citric acid, butylparaben, flavors, glycerin, microcrystalline cellulose and carboxymethylcellulose sodium, propylene glycol, propylparaben, purified water, sorbitol solution, sucralose, sucrose, xanthan gum.

PROFESSIONAL INFORMATION: OVERDOSAGE INFORMATION for all Infants', Children's & Jr. TYLENOL® Products

For emergency information, contact your local Poison Control Center (1-800-222-1222) or call the Rocky Mountain Poison Center toll-free, (1-800-526-6155).

Acetaminophen:

Acetaminophen in massive overdosage may cause hepatic toxicity in some patients. In adults and adolescents (≥ 12 years of age), hepatic toxicity may occur following ingestion of greater than 7.5 to 10 grams over a period of 8 hours or less. Fatalities are infrequent (less than 3–4% of untreated cases) and have rarely been reported with overdoses of less than 15 grams. In children (<12 years of age), an acute overdosage of less than 150 mg/kg has not been associated with hepatic toxicity. Early symptoms following a potentially hepatotoxic overdose may include: nausea, vomiting, diaphoresis and general malaise. Clinical and laboratory evidence of hepatic toxicity may not be apparent until 48 to 72 hours postingestion. In adults and adolescents, any individual presenting with an unknown amount of acetaminophen ingested or with a questionable or unreliable history about the time of ingestion should have a plasma acetaminophen level drawn and be treated with *N*-acetylcysteine. For full prescribing information, refer to the *N*-acetylcysteine package insert. Do not await results of assays for plasma acetaminophen levels before initiating treatment with *N*-acetylcysteine. The following additional procedures are recommended: Promptly initiate gastric decontamination of the stomach. A plasma acetaminophen assay should be obtained as early as possible, but no sooner than four hours following ingestion. If an acetaminophen *extended-release* product is involved, it may be appropriate to obtain an ad-

INFANTS' TYLENOL® and CHILDREN'S TYLENOL® Dosing Chart

Product	Concentration	Weight and Age							
		6-11 lbs (0-3 mos)	12-17 lbs (4-11 mos)	18-23 lbs (12-23 mos)	24-35 lbs (2-3 yrs)	36-47 lbs (4-5 yrs)	48-59 lbs (6-8 yrs)	60-71 lbs (9-10 yrs)	72-95 lbs (11 yrs)
Infants' TYLENOL® Oral Suspension	Acetaminophen 160 mg (in each 5 mL)	1.25 mL	2.5 mL	3.75 mL	5 mL	–	–	–	–
Children's TYLENOL® Oral Suspension	Acetaminophen 160 mg (in each 5 mL = 1 tsp)	–	–	–	5 mL (1 tsp)	7.5 mL (1 ½ tsp)	10 mL (2 tsp)	12.5 mL (2 ½ tsp)	15 mL (3 tsp)

mL = milliliter; tsp = teaspoonful
Attention: use only the enclosed dosing device specifically designed for use with the product. Do not use any other dosing device.

ditional plasma acetaminophen level 4–6 hours following the initial acetaminophen level. If either acetaminophen level plots above the treatment line on the acetaminophen overdose nomogram, *N*-acetylcysteine treatment should be continued for a full course of therapy. Liver function studies should be obtained initially and repeated at 24-hour intervals. Serious toxicity or fatalities have been extremely infrequent following an acute acetaminophen overdose in young children, possibly because of differences in the way they metabolize acetaminophen. In children, the maximum potential amount ingested can be more easily estimated. If more than 150 mg/kg or an unknown amount was ingested, obtain a plasma acetaminophen level as soon as possible, but no sooner than 4 hours following ingestion. If an acetaminophen *extended-release* product is involved, it may be appropriate to obtain an additional plasma acetaminophen level 4–6 hours following the initial acetaminophen level. If either acetaminophen level plots above the treatment line on the acetaminophen overdose nomogram, *N*-acetylcysteine treatment should be initiated and continued for a full course of therapy. If an assay cannot be obtained and the estimated acetaminophen ingestion exceeds 150 mg/kg, dosing with *N*-acetylcysteine should be initiated and continued for a full course of therapy.

For information or questions, visit our website www.tylenol.com

INFANTS' TYLENOL® and CHILDREN'S TYLENOL® Dosing Chart Chart — OTC

[Note:] If possible, use weight to dose, otherwise use age. To arrive at the correct dose, weigh your child before giving TYLENOL®.
[A healthcare professional should be consulted for dosing in children under the age of two years.]
[See table above]

Important Instructions for Proper Use
- Read and follow the label instructions on all TYLENOL® products
- Do NOT use with any other product containing acetaminophen
- Do NOT administer adult medicines to children
- Find the right dose on the chart above. If possible, use weight to dose; otherwise use age.
- Repeat dose every 4 hours while symptoms last.
- Do not give more than 5 times in 24 hours.
- If you have any questions, contact your healthcare professional or call 1-877-895-3665

TYLENOL® Cold Extra Strength Sore Throat Liquid — OTC
(Cool Burst)

Drug Facts

Active ingredient (in each 15 mL = 1 tablespoon) — ***Purpose***
Acetaminophen 500 mg — Pain reliever/fever reducer

Uses
- temporarily relieves minor aches and pains due to:
  - the common cold
  - headache
  - sore throat
- temporarily reduces fever

Warnings
Liver warning: This product contains acetaminophen. Severe liver damage may occur if you take
- more than 4,000 mg of acetaminophen in 24 hours
- with other drugs containing acetaminophen
- 3 or more alcoholic drinks every day while using this product

Sore throat warning: If sore throat is severe, persists for more than 2 days, is accompanied or followed by fever, headache, rash, nausea, or vomiting, consult a doctor promptly.
Do not use
- with any other drug containing acetaminophen (prescription or nonprescription). If you are not sure whether a drug contains acetaminophen, ask a doctor or pharmacist.
- if you are allergic to acetaminophen or any of the inactive ingredients in this product

Ask a doctor before use if you have liver disease
Ask a doctor or pharmacist before use if you are taking the blood thinning drug warfarin
Stop use and ask a doctor if
- pain gets worse or lasts more than 10 days
- fever gets worse or lasts more than 3 days
- new symptoms occur
- redness or swelling is present

These could be signs of a serious condition.
If pregnant or breast-feeding, ask a health professional before use.
Keep out of reach of children.
Overdose warning: In case of overdose, get medical help or contact a Poison Control Center right away. (1-800-222-1222) Quick medical attention is critical for adults as well as for children even if you do not notice any signs or symptoms.

Directions
- **do not take more than directed (see overdose warning)**
- mL = milliliter; TBSP = tablespoon; FL OZ = fluid ounce
- use only enclosed dosing cup designed for use with this product. Do not use any other dosing device.

adults and children 12 years and over	■ take 30 mL (2 TBSP) (1 FL OZ) in the dosing cup provided every 6 hours while symptoms last ■ do not take more than 90 mL (6 TBSP) (3 FL OZ) in 24 hours, unless directed by a doctor ■ do not use for more than 10 days unless directed by a doctor
children under 12 years	ask a doctor

Other Information
- **each 15 mL (1 TBSP) (½ FL OZ) contains:** sodium 11 mg
- store between 20-25°C (68-77°F)

Inactive ingredients anhydrous citric acid, carboxymethylcellulose sodium, FD&C blue no. 1, flavors, polyethylene glycol, propylene glycol, purified water, sodium benzoate, sorbitol solution, sucralose, sucrose
Questions or comments? call **1-877-895-3665** (toll-free) or **215-273-8755** (collect)

TYLENOL® COLD HEAD CONGESTION SEVERE — OTC
Caplets
TYLENOL® COLD & FLU SEVERE
Caplets
TYLENOL® COLD & FLU SEVERE
Warming Liquid

TYLENOL®
Active ingredients — ***Purpose***

TYLENOL® Cold Head Congestion Severe Caplet (in each caplet)
Acetaminophen 325 mg — Pain reliever/fever reducer
Guaifenesin 200 mg — Expectorant
Phenylephrine HCl 5 mg — Nasal decongestant

TYLENOL® Cold & Flu Severe Caplet (in each caplet)
Acetaminophen 325 mg — Pain reliever/fever reducer
Dextromethorphan HBr 10 mg — Cough suppressant
Guaifenesin 200 mg — Expectorant
Phenylephrine HCl 5 mg — Nasal decongestant

TYLENOL® Cold & Flu Severe Warming Liquid (in each 15 mL=1 tablespoon)
Acetaminophen 325 mg — Pain reliever/fever reducer
Dextromethorphan HBr 10 mg — Cough suppressant
Guaifenesin 200 mg — Expectorant
Phenylephrine HCl 5 mg — Nasal decongestant

Uses
TYLENOL® Cold & Flu Severe Caplets and TYLENOL® Cold & Flu Severe Warming Liquid
- for the temporary relief of the following cold/flu symptoms:
  - minor aches and pains
  - headache
  - sore throat
  - nasal congestion
  - cough
- helps loosen phlegm (mucus) and thin bronchial secretions to make coughs more productive
- temporarily reduces fever

TYLENOL® Cold Head Congestion Severe Caplets
- for the temporary relief of the following cold symptoms:
  - minor aches and pains
  - headache
  - sore throat
  - nasal congestion
  - sinus congestion and pressure
- helps loosen phlegm (mucus) and thin bronchial secretions to make coughs more productive
- temporarily reduces fever

Warnings
TYLENOL® Cold & Flu Severe Warming Liquid
Liver warning: This product contains acetaminophen. Severe liver damage may occur if you take
- more than 4,000 mg of acetaminophen in 24 hours
- with other drugs containing acetaminophen
- 3 or more alcoholic drinks every day while using this product

TYLENOL® Cold and Flu Severe Caplets and *TYLENOL® Cold Head Congestion Severe Caplets*
Liver warning: This product contains acetaminophen. The maximum daily dose of this product is 10 caplets (3,250 mg acetaminophen) in 24 hours. Severe liver damage may occur if you take
- more than 4,000 mg of acetaminophen in 24 hours
- with other drugs containing acetaminophen
- 3 or more alcoholic drinks every day while using this product

Follow for all products: TYLENOL® Cold Head Congestion Severe Caplets, TYLENOL® Cold & Flu Severe Caplets, and TYLENOL® Cold & Flu Severe Warming Liquid:
Sore throat warning: If sore throat is severe, persists for more than 2 days, is accompanied or followed by fever, headache, rash, nausea or vomiting, consult a doctor promptly.
Do not use
- with any other drug containing acetaminophen (prescription or nonprescription). If you are not sure whether a drug contains acetaminophen, ask a doctor or pharmacist.
- if you are now taking a prescription monoamine oxidase inhibitor (MAOI) (certain drugs for depression, psychiatric or emotional conditions, or Parkinson's disease), or for 2 weeks after stopping the MAOI drug. If you do not know if your prescription drug contains an MAOI, ask a doctor or pharmacist before taking this product.
- if you have ever had an allergic reaction to this product or any of its ingredients

Ask a doctor before use if you have
- liver disease
- heart disease

- high blood pressure
- thyroid disease
- diabetes
- trouble urinating due to an enlarged prostate gland
- persistent or chronic cough such as occurs with smoking, asthma, chronic bronchitis or emphysema
- cough that occurs with too much phlegm (mucus)

Ask a doctor or pharmacist before use if you are taking the blood thinning drug warfarin

When using this product do not exceed recommended dose

Stop use and ask a doctor if

- nervousness, dizziness, or sleeplessness occur
- pain, nasal congestion or cough gets worse or lasts more than 7 days
- fever gets worse or lasts more than 3 days
- redness or swelling is present
- new symptoms occur
- cough comes back or occurs with rash or headache that lasts

These could be signs of a serious condition.

If pregnant or breastfeeding, ask a health professional before use.

Keep out of reach of children.

Overdose warning: In case of overdose, get medical help or contact a Poison Control Center right away. (1-800-222-1222) Quick medical attention is critical for adults as well as for children even if you do not notice any signs or symptoms.

Directions

TYLENOL® Cold Head Congestion Severe Caplets

- **do not take more than directed (see overdose warning)**

adults and children 12 years and over	■ take 2 caplets every 4 hours ■ swallow whole; do not crush, chew or dissolve ■ do not take more than 10 caplets in 24 hours
children under 12 years	ask a doctor

TYLENOL® Cold and Flu Severe Caplets

- **do not take more than directed (see overdose warning)**

adults and children 12 years and over	■ take 2 caplets every 4 hours ■ swallow whole; do not crush, chew or dissolve ■ do not take more than 10 caplets in 24 hours
children under 12 years	ask a doctor

TYLENOL® Cold & Flu Severe Warming Liquid

- **do not take more than directed (see overdose warning)**
- mL=milliliter; TBSP=tablespoon; FL OZ=fluid ounce
- use only enclosed dosing cup designed for use with this product. Do not use any other dosing device.

adults and children 12 years and over	■ take 30 mL (2 TBSP) (1 FL OZ) in the dosing cup provided every 4 hours while symptoms last ■ do not take more than 150 mL (10 TBSP) (5 FL OZ) in 24 hours, unless directed by a doctor
children under 12 years	ask a doctor

Other information

- **each 15 mL (1 TBSP) (½ FL OZ) contains:** sodium 5 mg (*TYLENOL® Cold & Flu Severe Warming Liquid*)
- store between 20-25°C (68-77°F). Do not refrigerate (*TYLENOL® Cold & Flu Severe Warming Liquid*)
- each caplet contains: sodium 3 mg (*TYLENOL® Cold & Flu Severe Caplets* and *TYLENOL® Cold Head Congestion Severe Caplets*)
- store between 20-25°C (68-77°F) (TYLENOL® COLD & FLU SEVERE Caplets and TYLENOL® COLD Head Congestion Severe Caplets)

Inactive Ingredients:

TYLENOL® Cold Head Congestion Severe Caplets: carnauba wax, croscarmellose sodium, flavor, hydroxypropyl cellulose, hypromellose, magnesium stearate, microcrystalline cellulose, pregelatinized starch, sucralose, titanium dioxide, triacetin

TYLENOL® Cold & Flu Severe Caplets: carnauba wax, croscarmellose sodium, D&C yellow no. 10 aluminum lake, flavor, hydroxypropyl cellulose, hypromellose, magnesium stearate, microcrystalline cellulose, polyethylene glycol, pregelatinized starch, sucralose, titanium dioxide

TYLENOL® Cold & Flu Severe Warming Liquid: anhydrous citric acid, FD&C blue no. 1, FD&C red no. 40, FD&C yellow no. 6, flavor, glycerin, propylene glycol, purified water, sodium benzoate, sorbitol solution, sucralose

For information or questions, visit our website www.tylenol.com.

TYLENOL® COLD MULTI-SYMPTOM OTC
Daytime Caplets

TYLENOL® COLD MULTI-SYMPTOM
Daytime Liquid with Citrus Burst

TYLENOL® COLD MULTI-SYMPTOM NIGHTTIME
Liquid with CoolBurst™

TYLENOL® COLD MULTI-SYMPTOM SEVERE
Liquid with CoolBurst™

Product information for all forms of TYLENOL® Cold Multi-SYMPTOM products listed above have been combined under this heading.

Active Ingredients	Purpose
TYLENOL® Cold Multi-Symptom Daytime Caplet (in each caplet)	
Acetaminophen 325 mg	Pain reliever/fever reducer
Dextromethorphan HBr 10 mg	Cough suppressant
Phenylephrine HCl 5 mg	Nasal decongestant
TYLENOL® Cold Multi-Symptom Daytime Liquid with Citrus Burst™ (in each 15 ml = 1 tablespoon)	
Acetaminophen 325 mg	Pain reliever/fever reducer
Dextromethorphan HBr 10 mg	Cough suppressant
Phenylephrine HCl 5 mg	Nasal decongestant
TYLENOL® Cold Multi-Symptom Nighttime Liquid with Cool Burst™ (in each 15 ml = 1 tablespoon)	
Acetaminophen 325 mg	Pain reliever/fever reducer
Dextromethorphan HBr 10 mg	Cough suppressant
Doxylamine succinate 6.25 mg	Antihistamine
Phenylephrine HCl 5 mg	Nasal decongestant
TYLENOL® Cold Multi-Symptom Severe Liquid with Cool Burst™ (in each 15 ml = 1 tablespoon)	
Acetaminophen 325 mg	Pain reliever/fever reducer
Dextromethorphan HBr 10 mg	Cough suppressant
Guaifenesin 200 mg	Expectorant
Phenylephrine HCl 5 mg	Nasal decongestant

Uses

TYLENOL® Cold Mult-Symptom Daytime Caplets and TYLENOL® Cold Multi-Symptom Daytime Liquid with Citrus Burst™

- temporarily relieves these common cold/flu symptoms:
  - minor aches and pains
  - headache
  - sore throat
  - nasal congestion
  - cough
  - sinus congestion and pressure
- helps clear nasal passages
- promotes nasal and sinus drainage
- temporarily reduces fever

TYLENOL® Cold Multi-Symptom Nighttime Liquid with Cool Burst™

- temporarily relieves these common cold/flu symptoms:
  - minor aches and pains
  - headache
  - sore throat
  - nasal congestion
  - runny nose and sneezing
  - cough
  - sinus congestion and pressure
- helps clear nasal passages
- relieves cough to help you sleep
- temporarily reduces fever

TYLENOL ® Cold Multi-Symptom Severe Liquid with Cool Burst™

- for the temporary relief of the following cold/flu symptoms:
  - minor aches and pains
  - headache
  - sore throat
  - nasal congestion
  - cough
- helps loosen phlegm (mucus) and thin bronchial secretions to make coughs more productive
- temporarily reduces fever

Warnings

TYLENOL® Cold Multi-Symptom Daytime Liquid with Citrus Burst™, TYLENOL ® *Cold Multi-Symptom Nighttime Liquid with Cool Burst™*, and TYLENOL ® *Cold Multi-Symptom Severe Liquid with Cool Burst™*

Liver warning: This product contains acetaminophen. Severe liver damage may occur if you take

- more than 4,000 mg of acetaminophen in 24 hours
- with other drugs containing acetaminophen
- 3 or more alcoholic drinks every day while using this product

TYLENOL® *Cold Multi-Symptom Daytime Caplets*:

Liver warning: This product contains acetaminophen. The maximum daily dose of this product is 10 caplets (3,250 mg acetaminophen) in 24 hours. Severe liver damage may occur if you take

- more than 4,000 mg of acetaminophen in 24 hours
- with other drugs containing acetaminophen
- 3 or more alcoholic drinks every day while using this product

Sore throat warning: If sore throat is severe, persists for more than 2 days, is accompanied or followed by fever, headache, rash, nausea, or vomiting, consult a doctor promptly.

Do not use

- with any other drug containing acetaminophen (prescription or nonprescription). If you are not sure whether a drug contains acetaminophen, ask a doctor or pharmacist.
- if you are now taking a prescription monoamine oxidase inhibitor (MAOI) (certain drugs for depression, psychiatric or emotional conditions, or Parkinson's disease), or for 2 weeks after stopping the MAOI drug. If you do not know if your prescription drug contains an MAOI, ask a doctor or pharmacist before taking this product.
- if you have ever had an allergic reaction to this product or any of its ingredients

Ask a doctor before use if you have

- liver disease
- heart disease
- high blood pressure
- thyroid disease
- diabetes
- trouble urinating due to an enlarged prostate gland
- persistent or chronic cough such as occurs with smoking, asthma or emphysema
- cough that occurs with too much phlegm (mucus)
- a breathing problem such as emphysema or chronic bronchitis (applies to TYLENOL® *Cold Multi-Symptom Nighttime Liquid with Cool Burst™* only).
- glaucoma (applies to TYLENOL® *Cold Multi-Symptom Nighttime Liquid with Cool Burst™* only).

Ask a doctor or pharmacist before use if you are

- taking the blood thinning drug warfarin
- taking sedatives or tranquilizers (applies to TYLENOL® *Cold Multi-Symptom Nighttime Liquid with Cool Burst™* only).

When using this product

TYLENOL® *Cold Multi-Symptom Daytime Liquid with Citrus Burst™*, TYLENOL ® *Cold Multi-Symptom Severe Liquid with Cool Burst™* and TYLENOL® *Cold Multi-Symptom Daytime Caplets*:

- **do not exceed recommended dosage**

TYLENOL® *Cold Multi-Symptom Nighttime Liquid with Cool Burst™*

- **do not exceed recommended dosage**
- excitability may occur, especially in children
- marked drowsiness may occur
- alcohol, sedatives and tranquilizers may increase drowsiness
- avoid alcoholic drinks
- be careful when driving a motor vehicle or operating machinery

Stop use and ask a doctor if

- nervousness, dizziness, or sleeplessness occur
- pain, nasal congestion or cough gets worse or lasts more than 7 days
- fever gets worse or lasts more than 3 days
- redness or swelling is present
- new symptoms occur
- cough comes back or occurs with rash or headache that lasts

These could be signs of a serious condition.

If pregnant or breastfeeding, ask a health care professional before use

Keep out of reach of children.

Overdose warning: In case of overdose, get medical help or contact a Poison Control Center right away. (1-800-222-1222) Quick medical attention is critical for adults as well as for children even if you do not notice any signs or symptoms.

Directions

TYLENOL® *Cold Multi-Symptom Daytime Caplets*

■ **do not take more than directed (see overdose warning)**

adults and children 12 years and older	■ take 2 caplets every 4 hours ■ swallow whole; do not crush, chew or dissolve ■ do not take more than 10 caplets in 24 hours
children under 12 years	Ask a doctor

TYLENOL® *Cold Multi-Symptom Daytime Liquid with Citrus Burst™*, TYLENOL ® *Cold Multi-Symptom Nighttime Liquid with Cool Burst™*, and TYLENOL ® *Cold Multi-Symptom Severe Liquid with Cool Burst™*

■ **do not take more than directed (see overdose warning)**

■ mL = milliliter; TBSP = tablespoon; FL OZ = fluid ounce

■ use only enclosed dosing cup designed for use with this product. Do not use any other dosing device

adults and children 12 years and older	■ take 30 mL (2 TBSP) (1 FL OZ) in the dosing cup provided every 4 hours while symptoms last ■ do not take more than 150 mL (10 TBSP) (5 FL OZ) in 24 hours, unless directed by a doctor
children under 12 years	Ask a doctor

Other information

TYLENOL® *Cold Multi-Symptom Daytime Caplets*

■ store between 20-25° C (68-77°F).

TYLENOL® *Cold Multi-Symptom Nighttime Liquid with Cool Burst™*, TYLENOL® *Cold Multi-Symptom Daytime Liquid with Citrus Burst™*, and TYLENOL® *Cold Multi-Symptom Severe Liquid with Cool Burst™*

■ **each 15 mL (1 TBSP) (1/2 FL OZ) contains:** sodium 5 mg

■ store between 20-25° C (68-77°F). Do not refrigerate

Inactive Ingredients

TYLENOL® Cold *Multi-Symptom Daytime Liquid with Citrus Burst™*: alcohol, anhydrous citric acid, FD&C yellow no. 6, flavors, glycerin, propylene glycol, purified water, sodium benzoate, sorbitol solution, sucralose

TYLENOL® *Cold Multi-Symptom Daytime Caplets*: anhydrous citric acid, carnauba wax, corn starch, flavors, hypromellose, magnesium stearate, microcrystalline cellulose, potassium sorbate, powdered cellulose, pregelatinized starch, sodium benzoate, sodium citrate, sodium starch glycolate, sucralose.

TYLENOL® *Cold Multi-Symptom Nighttime Liquid with Cool Burst™*: alcohol, anhydrous citric acid, FD&C blue no. 1, flavor, glycerin, propylene glycol, purified water, sodium benzoate, sorbitol solution, sucralose

TYLENOL® *Cold Multi-Symptom Nighttime Liquid with Cool Burst™*: alcohol, anhydrous citric acid, FD&C blue no. 1, flavor, glycerin, propylene glycol, purified water, sodium benzoate, sorbitol solution, sucralose

For information or questions, visit our website www.tylenol.com

TYLENOL® PM EXTRA STRENGTH CAPLET OTC

Acetaminophen, Diphenhydramine HCl
Pain Reliever Nighttime Sleep Aid
Caplets

Drug Facts

Active ingredients (in each caplet)	***Purpose***
Acetaminophen 500 mg	Pain reliever
Diphenhydramine HCl 25 mg	Nighttime sleep aid

Uses temporary relief of occasional headaches and minor aches and pains with accompanying sleeplessness

Warnings

Liver warning: This product contains acetaminophen. Severe liver damage may occur if you take
- more than 4,000 mg of acetaminophen in 24 hours
- with other drugs containing acetaminophen
- 3 or more alcoholic drinks every day while using this product

Do not use
- with any other drug containing acetaminophen (prescription or nonprescription). If you are not sure whether a drug contains acetaminophen, ask a doctor or pharmacist.
- with any other product containing diphenhydramine, even one used on skin
- in children under 12 years of age
- if you have ever had an allergic reaction to this product or any of its ingredients

Ask a doctor before use if you have
- liver disease
- a breathing problem such as emphysema or chronic bronchitis
- trouble urinating due to an enlarged prostate gland
- glaucoma

Ask a doctor or pharmacist before use if you are
- taking the blood thinning drug warfarin
- taking sedatives or tranquilizers

When using this product
- drowsiness will occur
- avoid alcoholic drinks
- do not drive a motor vehicle or operate machinery

Stop use and ask a doctor if
- sleeplessness persists continuously for more than 2 weeks. Insomnia may be a symptom of serious underlying medical illness.
- pain gets worse or lasts more than 10 days
- fever gets worse or lasts more than 3 days
- redness or swelling is present
- new symptoms occur

These could be signs of a serious condition.

If pregnant or breast-feeding, ask a health professional before use.

Keep out of reach of children.

Overdose warning: In case of overdose, get medical help or contact a Poison Control Center right away. (1-800-222-1222) Quick medical attention is critical for adults as well as for children even if you do not notice any signs or symptoms.

Directions

- **do not take more than directed (see overdose warning)**

adults and children 12 years and over	• take 2 caplets at bedtime • do not take more than 2 caplets of this product in 24 hours
children under 12 years	do not use

Other information
- store between 20-25°C (68-77°F)

Inactive ingredients

carnauba wax, FD&C blue no. 1 aluminum lake, FD&C blue no. 2 aluminum lake, hypromellose, magnesium stearate, polyethylene glycol, polysorbate 80, powdered cellulose, pregelatinized starch, propylene glycol, shellac, sodium citrate, sodium starch glycolate, titanium dioxide

For information or questions, visit our website www.tylenol.com

REGULAR STRENGTH TYLENOL® OTC
acetaminophen Tablets
EXTRA STRENGTH TYLENOL®
acetaminophen Caplets
EXTRA STRENGTH TYLENOL®
acetaminophen Rapid Release Gels
EXTRA STRENGTH TYLENOL®
acetaminophen Adult Rapid Blast Liquid
TYLENOL® ARTHRITIS PAIN
acetaminophen extended-release tablets

Product information for all dosage forms of Adult TYLENOL® acetaminophen has been combined under this heading.

Description

Each Regular Strength TYLENOL® Tablet contains acetaminophen 325 mg. Each Extra Strength TYLENOL® Caplet or Rapid Release Gel contains acetaminophen 500 mg. Extra Strength TYLENOL® Adult Rapid Blast Liquid is alcohol-free and each 15 mL (1 tablespoonful) contains 500 mg acetaminophen. Each TYLENOL® Arthritis Pain extended-release tablet contains acetaminophen 650 mg.

Actions

Acetaminophen is a clinically proven analgesic/antipyretic. Acetaminophen is thought to produce analgesia by elevation of the pain threshold and antipyresis through action on the hypothalamic heat-regulating center. Acetaminophen is equal to aspirin in analgesic and antipyretic effectiveness and it is unlikely to produce many of the side effects associated with aspirin and aspirin-containing products. TYLENOL® Arthritis Pain extended-release tablets are a bilayer caplet. The first layer dissolves quickly while the second layer is time released to provide up to 8 hours of relief.

Uses

Regular Strength TYLENOL® Tablets; Extra Strength TYLENOL® Caplets, Rapid Release Gels, and TYLENOL® Adult Liquid:
- temporarily relieve minor aches and pains due to:
  - headache
  - muscular aches
  - backache
  - minor pain of arthritis
  - the common cold
  - toothache
  - premenstrual and menstrual cramps
- temporarily reduces fever

TYLENOL® Arthritis Pain extended-release tablets:
- temporarily relieve minor aches and pains due to:
  - minor pain of arthritis
  - muscular aches
  - backache
  - premenstrual and menstrual cramps
  - the common cold
  - headache
  - toothache
- temporarily reduces fever

Directions

Regular Strength TYLENOL® Tablets:
- **do not take more than directed (see overdose warning)**

adults and children 12 years and over	• take 2 tablets every 4 to 6 hours while symptoms last • do not take more than 10 tablets in 24 hours • do not use for more than 10 days unless directed by a doctor
children 6–11 years	• take 1 tablet every 4 to 6 hours while symptoms last • do not take more than 5 tablets in 24 hours • do not use for more than 5 days unless directed by a doctor
children under 6 years	ask a doctor

Extra Strength TYLENOL® Caplets or Rapid Release Gels:
- **do not take more than directed (see overdose warning)**

adults and children 12 years and over	• take 2 caplets or gelcaps every 6 hours while symptoms last • do not take more than 6 caplets or gelcaps in 24 hours, unless directed by a doctor • do not use for more than 10 days unless directed by a doctor
children under 12 years	ask a doctor

Extra Strength TYLENOL® Adult Rapid Blast Liquid:
- **do not take more than directed (see overdose warning)**
- mL = milliliter; TBSP = tablespoon; FL OZ = fluid ounce
- use only enclosed dosing cup designed for use with this product. Do not use any other dosing device.

adults and children 12 years and over	• take 30 mL (2 TBSP) (1 FL OZ) in the dosing cup provided every 6 hours while symptoms last • do not take more than 90 mL (6 TBSP) (3 FL OZ) in 24 hours, unless directed by a doctor • do not use for more than 10 days unless directed by a doctor
children under 12 years	ask a doctor

TYLENOL® Arthritis Pain extended-release tablets
• do not take more than directed (see overdose warning)

adults	• take 2 caplets every 8 hours with water • swallow whole; do not crush, chew, split or dissolve • do not take more than 6 caplets in 24 hours • do not use for more than 10 days unless directed by a doctor
under 18 years of age	• ask a doctor

Warnings
Regular Strength TYLENOL® Tablets
Liver warning: This product contains acetaminophen. The maximum daily dose of this product is 10 tablets (3,250 mg) in 24 hours for adults or 5 tablets (1,625 mg) in 24 hours for children. Severe liver damage may occur if
- adult takes more than 4,000 mg of acetaminophen in 24 hours
- child takes more than 5 doses in 24 hours, which is the maximum daily amount
- taken with other drugs containing acetaminophen
- adult has 3 or more alcoholic drinks every day while using this product

Do not use
- with any other drug containing acetaminophen (prescription or nonprescription). If you are not sure whether a drug contains acetaminophen, ask a doctor or pharmacist.
- if you are allergic to acetaminophen or any of the inactive ingredients in this product

Ask a doctor before use if the user has liver disease
Ask a doctor or pharmacist before use if the user is taking the blood thinning drug warfarin
Stop use and ask a doctor if
- pain gets worse or lasts more than 10 days in adults
- pain gets worse or lasts more than 5 days in children under 12 years
- fever gets worse or lasts more than 3 days
- new symptoms occur
- redness or swelling is present

These could be signs of a serious condition.
If pregnant or breast-feeding, ask a health professional before use.
Keep out of reach of children.
Overdose warning: In case of overdose, get medical help or contact a Poison Control Center right away. (1-800-222-1222) Quick medical attention is critical for adults as well as for children even if you do not notice any signs or symptoms.
Extra Strength TYLENOL® Caplets, Rapid Release Gels or Adult Rapid Blast Liquid
Liver warning: This product contains acetaminophen. Severe liver damage may occur if you take
- more than 4,000 mg of acetaminophen in 24 hours
- with other drugs containing acetaminophen
- 3 or more alcoholic drinks every day while using this product

Do not use
- with any other drug containing acetaminophen (prescription or nonprescription). If you are not sure whether a drug contains acetaminophen, ask a doctor or pharmacist.
- if you are allergic to acetaminophen or any of the inactive ingredients in this product

Ask a doctor before use if you have liver disease
Ask a doctor or pharmacist before use if you are taking the blood thinning drug warfarin
Stop use and ask a doctor if
- pain gets worse or lasts more than 10 days
- fever gets worse or lasts more than 3 days
- new symptoms occur
- redness or swelling is present

These could be signs of a serious condition.
If pregnant or breast-feeding, ask a health professional before use.
Keep out of reach of children.
Overdose warning: In case of overdose, get medical help or contact a Poison Control Center right away. (1-800-222-1222) Quick medical attention is critical for adults as well as for children even if you do not notice any signs or symptoms.
TYLENOL® Arthritis Pain extended-release tablet
Liver warning: This product contains acetaminophen. Severe liver damage may occur if you take
- more than 6 caplets in 24 hours, which is the maximum daily amount
- with other drugs containing acetaminophen
- 3 or more alcoholic drinks every day while using this product

Do not use
- with any other drug containing acetaminophen (prescription or nonprescription). If you are not sure whether a drug contains acetaminophen, ask a doctor or pharmacist.
- if you are allergic to acetaminophen or any of the inactive ingredients in this product

Ask a doctor before use if you have liver disease
Ask a doctor or pharmacist before use if you are taking the blood thinning drug warfarin
Stop use and ask a doctor if
- pain gets worse or lasts more than 10 days
- fever gets worse or lasts more than 3 days
- new symptoms occur
- redness or swelling is present

These could be signs of a serious condition.
If pregnant or breast-feeding, ask a health professional before use.
Keep out of reach of children.
Overdose warning: In case of overdose, get medical help or contact a Poison Control Center right away. (1-800-222-1222) Quick medical attention is critical for adults as well as for children even if you do not notice any signs or symptoms.
Other information
Regular Strength TYLENOL® Tablets
- store between 20–25°C (68–77°F)

Extra Strength TYLENOL® Caplets or Rapid Release Gels
- store between 20–25°C (68–77°F) *(Caplet)*
- store between 20–25°C (68–77°F). Avoid high humidity. *(Rapid Release Gel)*

Extra Strength TYLENOL® Adult Rapid Blast Liquid
- **each 15 mL (1 TBSP) (½ FL OZ) contains:** sodium 9 mg
- store between 20–25°C (68–77°F)

TYLENOL® Arthritis Pain extended-release tablets
- store between 20–25°C (68–77°F). Avoid excessive heat 40°C (104°F).

Inactive ingredients
Regular Strength TYLENOL® Tablets: corn starch, magnesium stearate, powdered cellulose, pregelatinized starch, sodium starch glycolate
Extra Strength TYLENOL® **Caplets:** carnauba wax*, castor oil*, corn starch, FD&C red no. 40 aluminum lake, hypromellose, magnesium stearate, polyethylene glycol*, powdered cellulose, pregelatinized starch, propylene glycol, shellac, sodium starch glycolate, titanium dioxide.
*contains one or more of these ingredients. **Rapid Release Gels:** benzyl alcohol, butylparaben, carboxymethylcellulose sodium, corn starch, D&C yellow no. 10, edetate calcium disodium, FD&C blue no. 1, FD&C red no. 40, gelatin, hypromellose, iron oxide, magnesium stearate, methylparaben, polyethylene glycol, polysorbate 80, powdered cellulose, pregelatinized starch, propylene glycol, propylparaben, red iron oxide, sodium lauryl sulfate, sodium propionate, sodium starch glycolate, titanium dioxide, yellow iron oxide
Extra Strength TYLENOL® Adult Rapid Blast Liquid: anhydrous citric acid, D&C red no. 33, FD&C red no. 40, flavor, high fructose corn syrup, polyethylene glycol, propylene glycol, purified water, saccharin sodium, sodium benzoate, sorbitol solution
TYLENOL® Arthritis Pain extended-release Tablets: carnauba wax, corn starch, hydroxyethyl cellulose, hypromellose, magnesium stearate, microcrystalline cellulose, povidone, powdered cellulose, pregelatinized starch, sodium starch glycolate, titanium dioxide, triacetin

Professional Information:
Overdosage information for all adult TYLENOL® products
For emergency information, contact your local Poison Control Center (1-800-222-1222) or call the Rocky Mountain Poison Center toll-free, (1-800-526-6155).
Acetaminophen: Acetaminophen in massive overdosage may cause hepatic toxicity in some patients. In adults and adolescents (≥ 12 years of age), hepatic toxicity may occur following ingestion of greater than 7.5 to 10 grams over a period of 8 hours or less. Fatalities are infrequent (less than 3–4% of untreated cases) and have rarely been reported with overdoses of less than 15 grams. In children (<12 years of age), an acute overdosage of less than 150 mg/kg has not been associated with hepatic toxicity. Early symptoms following a potentially hepatotoxic overdose may include: nausea, vomiting, diaphoresis and general malaise. Clinical and laboratory evidence of hepatic toxicity may not be apparent until 48 to 72 hours postingestion. In adults and adolescents, any individual presenting with an unknown amount of acetaminophen ingested or with a questionable or unreliable history about the time of ingestion should have a plasma acetaminophen level drawn and be treated with *N*-acetylcysteine. For full prescribing information, refer to the *N*-acetylcysteine package insert. Do not await results of assays for plasma acetaminophen levels before initiating treatment with *N*-acetylcysteine. The following additional procedures are recommended: Promptly initiate gastric decontamination of the stomach. A plasma acetaminophen assay should be obtained as early as possible, but no sooner than four hours following ingestion. If an acetaminophen extended-release product is involved, it may be appropriate to obtain an additional plasma acetaminophen level 4–6 hours following the initial acetaminophen level. If either acetaminophen level plots above the treatment line on the acetaminophen overdose nomogram, *N*-acetylcysteine treatment should be continued for a full course of therapy. Liver function studies should be obtained initially and repeated at 24-hour intervals. Serious toxicity or fatalities have been extremely infrequent following an acute acetaminophen overdose in young children, possibly because of differences in the way they metabolize acetaminophen. In children, the maximum potential amount ingested can be more easily estimated. If more than 150 mg/kg or an unknown amount was ingested, obtain a plasma acetaminophen level as soon as possible, but no sooner than 4 hours following ingestion. If an acetaminophen extended-release product is involved, it may be appropriate to obtain an additional plasma acetaminophen level 4–6 hours following the initial acetaminophen level. If either acetaminophen level plots above the treatment line on the acetaminophen overdose nomogram, *N*-acetylcysteine treatment should be initiated and continued for a full course of therapy. If an assay cannot be obtained and the estimated acetaminophen ingestion exceeds 150 mg/kg, dosing with *N*-acetylcysteine should be initiated and continued for a full course of therapy. For additional emergency information, call your regional poison center or call the Rocky Mountain Poison Center toll-free, (1-800-525-6115).
Our adult TYLENOL® combination products contain active ingredients in addition to acetaminophen. The following is basic overdose information regarding those ingredients.
Chlorpheniramine: Chlorpheniramine toxicity should be treated as you would an anthihistamine/anticholinergic overdose and is likely to be present within a few hours after acute ingestion.
Dextromethorphan: Acute dextromethorphan overdose usually does not result in serious signs and symptoms unless massive amounts have been ingested. Signs and symptoms of a substantial overdose may include nausea and vomiting, visual disturbances, CNS disturbances and urinary retention.
Diphenhydramine: Diphenhydramine toxicity should be treated as you would an antihistamine/anticholinergic overdose and is likely to be present within a few hours after acute ingestion.
Doxylamine: Doxylamine toxicity should be treated as you would an antihistamine/anticholinergic overdose and is likely to be present within a few hours after acute ingestion.
Guaifenesin: Guaifenesin should be treated as a nontoxic ingestion.
Phenylephrine: Symptoms from phenylephrine overdose most often consist of hypertension, anxiety, nervousness, restlessness, tachycardia, bradycardia, headache, dizziness, and/or palpitations. Symptoms usually are transient and typically require no treatment.
Pseudoephedrine: Symptoms from pseudoephedrine overdose consist most often of mild anxiety, tachycardia and/or mild hypertension. Symptoms usually appear within 4 to 8 hours of ingestion and are transient, usually requiring no treatment.
Alcohol Information: Chronic heavy alcohol abusers may be at increased risk of liver toxicity from excessive acetaminophen use, although reports of this event are rare. Reports usually involve cases of severe chronic alcoholics and the dosages of acetaminophen most often exceed recommended doses and often involve substantial overdose. Healthcare professionals should alert their patients who regularly consume large amounts of alcohol not to exceed recommended doses of acetaminophen.

For information or questions, visit our website www.tylenol.com

---

TYLENOL® SINUS CONGESTION & PAIN OTC
Caplets (Daytime)

TYLENOL® SINUS CONGESTION & PAIN SEVERE
Caplets

Drug Facts
Active ingredients
TYLENOL® Sinus Congestion & Pain Caplets (Daytime) (in each caplet) ***Purpose***
Acetaminophen 325 mg Pain reliever/fever reducer
Phenylephrine HCl 5 mg Nasal decongestant

TYLENOL® Sinus Congestion & Pain Severe Caplets
(in each caplet) ***Purpose***

Acetaminophen 325 mg	Pain reliever/fever reducer
Guaifenesin 200 mg	Expectorant
Phenylephrine HCl 5 mg	Nasal decongestant

Uses
- temporarily relieves these symptoms associated with hay fever or other respiratory allergies, and the common cold:
- headache
- sinus congestion and pressure
- nasal congestion
- minor aches and pains
- temporarily reduces fever
- helps decongest sinus openings and passages (TYLENOL® Sinus Congestion & Pain only)
- promotes sinus drainage (TYLENOL® Sinus Congestion & Pain only)
- helps clear nasal passages (TYLENOL® Sinus Congestion & Pain only)
- helps loosen phlegm (mucus) and thin bronchial secretions to make coughs more productive (TYLENOL® Sinus Congestion & Pain Severe only)

Warnings

Liver warning: This product contains acetaminophen. The maximum daily dose of this product is 10 caplets (3,250 mg acetaminophen) in 24 hours Severe liver damage may occur if you take
- more than 4,000 mg of acetaminophen in 24 hours
- with other drugs containing acetaminophen
- 3 or more alcoholic drinks every day while using this product

Do not use
- with any other drug containing acetaminophen (prescription or nonprescription). If you are not sure whether a drug contains acetaminophen, ask a doctor or pharmacist.
- if you are now taking a prescription monoamine oxidase inhibitor (MAOI) (certain drugs for depression, psychiatric or emotional conditions, or Parkinson's disease), or for 2 weeks after stopping the MAOI drug. If you do not know if your prescription drug contains an MAOI, ask a doctor or pharmacist before taking this product.
- if you have ever had an allergic reaction to this product or any of its ingredients

Ask a doctor before use if you have
- liver disease
- heart disease
- high blood pressure
- thyroid disease
- diabetes
- trouble urinating due to an enlarged prostate gland
- persistent or chronic cough such as occurs with smoking, asthma, chronic bronchitis, or emphysema (TYLENOL® Sinus Congestion & Pain Severe only)
- cough that occurs with too much phlegm (mucus) (TYLENOL® Sinus Congestion & Pain Severe only)

Ask a doctor or pharmacist before use if you are taking the blood thinning drug warfarin

When using this product do not exceed recommended dose

Stop use and ask a doctor if
- nervousness, dizziness, or sleeplessness occur
- pain, nasal congestion or cough gets worse or lasts more than 7 days
- fever gets worse or lasts more than 3 days
- redness or swelling is present
- new symptoms occur
- cough comes back or occurs with rash or headache that lasts (TYLENOL® Sinus Congestion & Pain Severe only)

These could be signs of a serious condition.

If pregnant or breast-feeding, ask a health professional before use.

Keep out of reach of children.

Overdose warning: In case of overdose, get medical help or contact a Poison Control Center right away. (1-800-222-1222) Quick medical attention is critical for adults as well as for children even if you do not notice any signs or symptoms.

Directions
- **do not take more than directed (see overdose warning)**

adults and children 12 years and over	■ take 2 caplets every 4 hours ■ swallow whole; do not crush, chew or dissolve ■ do not take more than 10 caplets in 24 hours
children under 12 years	ask a doctor

Other information
- store between 20-25°C (68-77°F)
- **each caplet contains:** sodium 3 mg (TYLENOL® Sinus Congestion & Pain Severe only)

Inactive ingredients

TYLENOL® Sinus Congestion & Pain
anhydrous citric acid, carnauba wax, corn starch, D&C yellow no. 10 aluminum lake, FD&C blue no. 1 aluminum lake, FD&C red no. 40 aluminum lake, flavors, hypromellose, magnesium stearate, microcrystalline cellulose, polyethylene glycol, polysorbate 80, potassium sorbate, powdered cellulose, pregelatinized starch, sodium benzoate, sodium citrate, sodium starch glycolate, sucralose, titanium dioxide

TYLENOL® Sinus Congestion & Pain Severe
carnauba wax, croscarmellose sodium, flavor, hydroxypropyl cellulose, hypromellose, magnesium stearate, microcrystalline cellulose, pregelatinized starch, sucralose, titanium dioxide, triacetin

For information or questions, visit our website www.tylenol.com

ZYRTEC® ALLERGY — OTC
Tablets, Liquid Gels, and Orally Disintegrating Tablets

Active ingredient (in each tablet/capsule) ***Purpose***
Cetirizine HCl 10 mg — Antihistamine

Uses
temporarily relieves these symptoms due to hay fever or other upper respiratory allergies:
- runny nose • sneezing • itchy, watery eyes
- itching of the nose or throat

Warnings

Do not use if you have ever had an allergic reaction to this product or any of its ingredients or to an antihistamine containing hydroxyzine.

Ask a doctor before use if you have liver or kidney disease. Your doctor should determine if you need a different dose.

Ask a doctor or pharmacist before use if you are taking tranquilizers or sedatives.

When using this product
- drowsiness may occur
- avoid alcoholic drinks
- alcohol, sedatives, and tranquilizers may increase drowsiness
- be careful when driving a motor vehicle or operating machinery

Stop use and ask a doctor if an allergic reaction to this product occurs. Seek medical help right away.

If pregnant or breast-feeding:
- if breast-feeding: not recommended
- if pregnant: ask a health professional before use.

Keep out of reach of children. In case of overdose, get medical help or contact a Poison Control Center right away. (1-800-222-1222)

Directions
Tablet melts in mouth. Can be taken with or without water. (Orally Disintegrating Tablets only)

adults and children 6 years and over	one 10 mg tablet/capsule once daily; do not take more than one 10 mg tablet/capsule in 24 hours. A 5 mg product may be appropriate for less severe symptoms.
adults 65 years and over	ask a doctor
children under 6 years of age	ask a doctor
consumers with liver or kidney disease	ask a doctor

Other information
- store between 20° to 25°C (68° to 77°F)
- Avoid high humidity (Orally Disintegrating Tablets only)
- avoid high humidity and excessive heat above 40°C (104°F) [Liquid gels only]
- protect from light (Liquid gels only).
- meets USP Dissolution Test 2 (Tablets only)

ZYRTEC® Tablet Inactive ingredients colloidal silicon dioxide, croscarmellose sodium, hypromellose, lactose monohydrate, magnesium stearate, microcrystalline cellulose, polyethylene glycol, titanium dioxide

ZYRTEC® Liquid Gel Inactive ingredients gelatin, glycerin, mannitol, pharmaceutical ink, polyethylene glycol 400, purified water, sodium hydroxide, sorbitan, sorbitol

ZYRTEC® Orally Disintegrating Tablets Inactive ingredients amino methacrylate copolymer, anhydrous citric acid, colloidal silicon dioxide, crospovidone, flavors, hydroxypropyl cellulose, magnesium stearate, mannitol, microcrystalline cellulose, sodium bicarbonate, sodium starch glycolate, sucralose

For information or questions, visit our website www.zyrtec.com

ZYRTEC-D® Allergy & Congestion — OTC
Extended Release Tablets

Active ingredients (in each extended release tablet) ***Purpose***

Cetirizine HCl 5 mg	Antihistamine
Pseudoephedrine HCl 120 mg	Nasal decongestant

Uses
- temporarily relieves these symptoms due to hay fever or other upper respiratory allergies:
  - runny nose ■ sneezing
  - itchy, watery eyes ■ itching of the nose or throat
  - nasal congestion
- reduces swelling of nasal passages
- temporarily relieves sinus congestion and pressure
- temporarily restores freer breathing through the nose

Warnings

Do not use
- if you have ever had an allergic reaction to this product or any of its ingredients or to an antihistamine containing hydroxyzine.
- if you are now taking a prescription monoamine oxidase inhibitor (MAOI) (certain drugs for depression, psychiatric, or emotional conditions, or Parkinson's disease), or for 2 weeks after stopping the MAOI drug. If you do not know if your prescription drug contains an MAOI, ask a doctor or pharmacist before taking this product.

Ask a doctor before use if you have
- heart disease
- thyroid disease
- diabetes
- glaucoma
- high blood pressure
- trouble urinating due to an enlarged prostate gland
- liver or kidney disease. Your doctor should determine if you need a different dose.

Ask a doctor or pharmacist before use if you are taking tranquilizers or sedatives.

When using this product
- **do not use more than directed**
- drowsiness may occur
- avoid alcoholic drinks
- alcohol, sedatives, and tranquilizers may increase drowsiness
- be careful when driving a motor vehicle or operating machinery

Stop use and ask a doctor if
- an allergic reaction to this product occurs. Seek medical help right away.
- you get nervous, dizzy, or sleepless
- symptoms do not improve within 7 days or are accompanied by fever

If pregnant or breast-feeding:
- if breast-feeding: not recommended
- if pregnant: ask a health professional before use.

Keep out of reach of children. In case of overdose, get medical help or contact a Poison Control Center right away. (1-800-222-1222)

Directions
- do not break or chew tablet; swallow tablet whole

adults and children 12 years and over	take 1 tablet every 12 hours; do not take more than 2 tablets in 24 hours.
adults 65 years and over	ask a doctor
children under 12 years of age	ask a doctor
consumers with liver or kidney disease	ask a doctor

Other information
- store between 20° to 25°C (68° to 77°F)

Inactive ingredients
colloidal silicon dioxide, croscarmellose sodium, hypromellose, lactose monohydrate, magnesium stearate, microcrystalline cellulose, polyethylene glycol, titanium dioxide

For information or questions, visit our website www.zyrtec.com

McNeil Consumer Pharmaceuticals Co.
7050 CAMP HILL ROAD
FORT WASHINGTON, PA 19034

Direct Inquiries to:
Consumer Care Center
(800) 962-5357
www.mcneil-consumer.com

PEPCID® AC® OTC

Original Strength PEPCID® AC® Tablets
Maximum Strength PEPCID® AC® Tablets

Active ingredient (in each tablet)	Purpose
Original Strength PEPCID® AC® tablets	
Famotidine 10 mg	Acid reducer
Maximum Strength PEPCID® AC® tablets	
Famotidine 20 mg	Acid reducer

Uses
- relieves heartburn associated with acid indigestion and sour stomach
- prevents heartburn associated with acid indigestion and sour stomach brought on by eating or drinking certain food and beverages.

Warnings
Allergy alert: Do not use if you are allergic to famotidine or other acid reducers
Do not use
- if you have trouble or pain swallowing food, vomiting with blood, or bloody or black stools. These may be signs of a serious condition. See your doctor.
- if you have kidney disease, except under the advice and supervision of a doctor (Maximum Strength PEPCID® AC®).
- with other acid reducers

Ask a doctor before use if you have
- had heartburn over 3 months. This may be a sign of a more serious condition.
- heartburn with **lightheadedness, sweating, or dizziness**
- chest pain or shoulder pain with shortness of breath; sweating; pain spreading to arms, neck or shoulder; or lightheadedness
- frequent **chest pain**
- frequent wheezing, particularly with heartburn
- unexplained weight loss
- nausea or vomiting
- stomach pain

Stop use and ask a doctor if
- your heartburn continues or worsens
- you need to take this product for more than 14 days

If pregnant or breast-feeding, ask a health professional before use.
Keep out of reach of children. In case of overdose, get medical help or contact a Poison Control Center right away. (1-800-222-1222)

Directions
Original Strength PEPCID® AC®:
- adults and children 12 years and over:
  - to **relieve** symptoms, swallow 1 tablet with a glass of water. Do not chew.
  - to **prevent** symptoms, swallow 1 tablet with a glass of water at any time from **15 to 60 minutes before** eating food or drinking beverages that cause heartburn
  - do not use more than 2 tablets in 24 hours
- children under 12 years: ask a doctor

Maximum Strength PEPCID® AC®:
- adults and children 12 years and over:
  - to **relieve** symptoms, swallow 1 tablet with a glass of water. Do not chew.
  - to **prevent** symptoms, swallow 1 tablet with a glass of water at any time from **10 to 60 minutes before** eating food or drinking beverages that cause heartburn
  - do not use more than 2 tablets in 24 hours
- children under 12 years: ask a doctor

Other information
- read the directions and warnings before use
- keep the carton. It contains important information.
- store at 20°–25°C (68°–77°F)
- protect from moisture

Inactive ingredients (Orig. Strength PEPCID® AC®)
carnauba wax, hydroxypropyl cellulose, hypromellose, magnesium stearate, microcrystalline cellulose, pregelatinized starch, red iron oxide, talc, titanium dioxide

Inactive ingredients (Max. Strength PEPCID® AC®)
carnauba wax, hydroxypropyl cellulose, hypromellose, magnesium stearate, microcrystalline cellulose, pregelatinized starch, talc, titanium dioxide
For information or questions, visit our website www.pepcid.com

PEPCID® COMPLETE® OTC

Acid Reducer + Antacid Chewable Tablets

Active Ingredients (in each chewable tablet):	***Purpose:***
Famotidine 10 mg	Acid Reducer
Calcium carbonate 800 mg	Antacid
Magnesium hydroxide 165 mg	Antacid

Use relieves heartburn associated with acid indigestion and sour stomach

Warnings
Allergy alert: Do not use if you are allergic to famotidine or other acid reducers
Do not use
- if you have trouble or pain swallowing food, vomiting with blood, or bloody or black stools. These may be signs of a serious condition. See your doctor.
- with other acid reducers

Ask a doctor before use if you have
- had heartburn over 3 months. This may be a sign of a more serious condition.
- heartburn with **lightheadedness, sweating, or dizziness**
- chest pain or shoulder pain with shortness of breath; sweating; pain spreading to arms, neck or shoulders; or lightheadedness
- frequent **chest pain**
- frequent wheezing, particularly with heartburn
- unexplained weight loss
- nausea or vomiting
- stomach pain

Ask a doctor or pharmacist before use if you are presently taking a prescription drug. Antacids may interact with certain prescription drugs.
Stop use and ask a doctor if
- your heartburn continues or worsens
- you need to take this product for more than 14 days
- **If pregnant or breast-feeding,** ask a health professional before use.
- **Keep out of reach of children.** In case of overdose, get medical help or contact a Poison Control Center right away. (1-800-222-1222)

Directions
- adults and children 12 years and over:
  - **do not swallow tablet whole: chew completely**
  - to relieve symptoms, **chew** 1 tablet before swallowing
  - do not use more than 2 chewable tablets in 24 hours
- children under 12 years: ask a doctor

Other information
- **each tablet contains:** calcium 320 mg; magnesium 70 mg.
- contains FD&C yellow no. 5 (tartrazine) as a color additive (Tropical Fruit flavor only)
- read the directions and warnings before use
- keep the carton. It contains important information.
- store at 20°–25°C (68°–77°F).
- protect from moisture

Inactive Ingredients:
Mint flavor: Cellulose acetate, corn starch, crospovidone, D&C yellow no. 10 aluminum lake, dextrose excipient, FD&C blue no. 1 aluminum lake, flavors, gum arabic, hydroxypropyl cellulose, hypromellose, lactose monohydrate, magnesium stearate, maltodextrin, mineral oil, sucralose.
Berry flavor: Cellulose acetate, corn starch, crospovidone, D&C red no. 7 calcium lake, dextrose excipient, FD&C blue no. 1 aluminum lake, FD&C red no. 40 aluminum lake, flavors, gum arabic, hydroxypropyl cellulose, hypromellose, lactose monohydrate, magnesium stearate, maltodextrin, mineral oil, sucralose
Tropical Fruit flavor: Cellulose acetate, corn starch, corn syrup solids, crospovidone, dextrose excipient, FD&C yellow no. 5 aluminum lake (tartrazine), FD&C yellow no. 6 aluminum lake, flavors, gum arabic, hydroxypropyl cellulose, hypromellose, lactose monohydrate, magnesium stearate, maltodextrin, mineral oil, sucralose, triacetin

Tips for Managing Heartburn
Do not lie flat or bend over after eating ■ Do not wear tight-fitting clothing around the stomach ■ Do not eat before bedtime ■ Raise the head of your bed ■ Avoid heartburn-causing foods such as rich, spicy, fatty or fried foods, chocolate, caffeine, alcohol, and certain fruits and vegetables ■ Eat slowly and avoid big meals ■ If overweight, lose weight ■ Quit smoking
For information or questions, visit our website www.pepcid.com

Merck
ONE MERCK DRIVE
P.O. BOX 100
WHITEHOUSE STATION, NJ 08889-0100 USA

For updates to the product information listed below, please check the Merck Web site, http://www.merck.com.

U.S. Healthcare Professionals
To speak with a Merck health care professional about Merck products or to report an adverse experience with a specific Merck product, please call the Merck National Service Center at (800) 444-2080. The Merck National Service Center is pleased to assist you Monday through Friday from 8 AM to 7 PM ET.

Adverse experiences and product-related emergencies can be reported at any time by dialing (800) 444-2080.

Merck U.S. operating companies include: Merck, Sharp & Dohme Corp.

AFLURIA ℞

Influenza Virus Vaccine
Suspension for Intramuscular Injection

HIGHLIGHTS OF PRESCRIBING INFORMATION
These highlights do not include all the information needed to use AFLURIA safely and effectively. See full prescribing information for AFLURIA.
AFLURIA, Influenza Virus Vaccine
Suspension for Intramuscular Injection
2012-2013 Formula
Initial U.S. Approval: 2007

RECENT MAJOR CHANGES

Indications and Usage (1)	11/2011
Dosage and Administration (2)	11/2011
Warnings and Precautions (5)	11/2011

INDICATIONS AND USAGE
- AFLURIA is an inactivated influenza virus vaccine indicated for active immunization against influenza disease caused by influenza virus subtypes A and type B present in the vaccine. (1)
- AFLURIA is approved for use in persons 5 years of age and older. (1)

DOSAGE AND ADMINISTRATION
For intramuscular (IM) injection only (0.5 mL). (2.2)
Children
- **5 years through 8 years of age**
  Previously unvaccinated children, or vaccinated for the first time last season with only one dose: two 0.5 mL doses, one on Day 1 followed by another approximately 4 weeks later. (2.1)
  Children vaccinated with two doses last season or with at least one dose two or more years ago: one 0.5 mL dose. (2.1)
- **9 years of age and older**
  A single 0.5 mL dose. (2.1)

Adults
A single 0.5 mL dose. (2.1)

DOSAGE FORMS AND STRENGTHS
AFLURIA is a suspension for injection supplied in two presentations:
- 0.5 mL pre-filled syringe (single dose) (3, 11)
- 5 mL multi-dose vial (ten 0.5 mL doses) (3, 11)

CONTRAINDICATIONS
- Severe allergic reaction (e.g., anaphylaxis) to any component of the vaccine including egg protein, or to a previous dose of any influenza vaccine. (4, 11)

WARNINGS AND PRECAUTIONS
- Administration of CSL's 2010 Southern Hemisphere influenza vaccine was associated with increased rates of fever and febrile seizures in children predominantly below the age of 5 years as compared to previous years. Febrile events were also observed in children 5 to less than 9 years of age. (5.1)
- If Guillain-Barré Syndrome (GBS) has occurred within 6 weeks of previous influenza vaccination, the decision to give AFLURIA should be based on careful consideration of the potential benefits and risks. (5.2)
- Appropriate medical treatment and supervision must be available to manage possible anaphylactic reactions following administration of the vaccine. (5.3)

• Immunocompromised persons may have a diminished immune response to AFLURIA. (5.4)

ADVERSE REACTIONS

• In children 5 through 17 years of age, the most common injection-site adverse reactions were pain (≥60%), redness (≥20%) and swelling (≥10%). The most common systemic adverse reactions were headache, myalgia (≥20%), malaise and fever (≥10%). (6.1)
• In adults 18 through 64 years of age, the most common injection-site adverse reactions were tenderness (≥60%) and pain (≥40%). The most common systemic adverse reactions were headache, malaise, and muscle aches (≥20%). (6.1)
• In adults 65 years of age and older, the most common injection-site adverse reactions were tenderness (≥30%) and pain (≥10%). (6.1)

To report SUSPECTED ADVERSE REACTIONS, contact Merck Sharp & Dohme Corp., a subsidiary of Merck & Co., Inc. at 1-877-888-4231 or VAERS at 1-800-822-7967 or www.vaers.hhs.gov.

USE IN SPECIFIC POPULATIONS

• Safety and effectiveness of AFLURIA have not been established in pregnant women or nursing mothers. (8.1, 8.3)
• Antibody responses were lower in geriatric subjects than in younger subjects. (8.5)
• AFLURIA is not approved for use in children less than 5 years of age because of increased rates of fever and febrile seizures. One comparator-controlled trial demonstrated higher rates of fever in recipients of AFLURIA as compared to a trivalent inactivated influenza vaccine control. (8.4)

See 17 for PATIENT COUNSELING INFORMATION

Revised: 07/2012

FULL PRESCRIBING INFORMATION: CONTENTS*

*** Sections or subsections omitted from the full prescribing information are not listed**

FULL PRESCRIBING INFORMATION

1 INDICATIONS AND USAGE

AFLURIA® is an inactivated influenza virus vaccine indicated for active immunization against influenza disease caused by influenza virus subtypes A and type B present in the vaccine. AFLURIA is approved for use in persons 5 years of age and older.

Table 1: Proportion of Subjects 5 through 17 Years of Age with Solicited Local or Systemic Adverse Events within 7 Days after Administration of First or Second Dose of AFLURIA, Irrespective of Causality (Study 1)

Solicited Adverse Event	Age Group			
	Subjects ≥ 5 to < 9 years		Subjects ≥ 9 to < 18 years	
	AFLURIA N=161	Comparator N=166	AFLURIA N=254	Comparator N=250
After the First Dose				
Local				
Pain	63%	60%	66%	60%
Redness	23%	27%	17%	17%
Induration	17%	17%	15%	16%
Systemic				
Myalgia	34%	30%	40%	37%
Malaise	24%	13%	22%	20%
Headache	21%	20%	27%	26%
Any Fever Fever ≥102.2°F	16% 5%	8% 1%	6% 3%	4% 1%
Nausea/vomiting	12%	8%	9%	10%
Diarrhea	7%	7%	8%	10%
	AFLURIA N=39	Comparator N=53		
After the Second Dose				
Local				
Pain	36%	38%	-	-
Redness	10%	19%	-	-
Induration	8%	17%	-	-
Systemic				
Diarrhea	13%	6%	-	-
Headache	13%	13%	-	-
Myalgia	13%	17%	-	-
Malaise	5%	8%	-	-
Nausea/vomiting	3%	8%	-	-
Any Fever Fever ≥102.2°F	0% 0%	2% 0%	- -	- -

2 DOSAGE AND ADMINISTRATION

For intramuscular (IM) injection only (0.5 mL).

2.1 Dose and Schedule

Children

Children 5 years through 8 years of age not previously vaccinated with an influenza vaccine, or vaccinated for the first time last season with only one dose: Administer two 0.5 mL doses, one on Day 1 and another approximately 4 weeks later.

Children 5 years through 8 years of age given two doses last season, or at least one dose two or more years ago: Administer a single 0.5 mL dose.

Children 9 years of age and older: Administer a single 0.5 mL dose.

Adults

Administer a single 0.5 mL dose.

2.2 Administration

Shake thoroughly and inspect visually before use. Parenteral drug products should be inspected visually for particulate matter and discoloration prior to administration, whenever suspension and container permit. If either of these conditions exists, the vaccine should not be administered.

When using a single-dose syringe, shake the syringe thoroughly and administer the dose immediately.

When using the multi-dose vial, shake the vial thoroughly before withdrawing each dose, and administer the dose immediately. Draw up the exact dose using a separate sterile needle and syringe for each individual patient. It is recommended that small syringes (0.5 mL or 1 mL) be used to minimize any product loss.

Between uses, return the multi-dose vial to the recommended storage conditions between 2–8°C (36–46°F). **Do not freeze.** Discard if the vaccine has been frozen.

For intramuscular injection. The preferred site for intramuscular injection is the deltoid muscle of the upper arm.

3 DOSAGE FORMS AND STRENGTHS

AFLURIA is a sterile suspension for intramuscular injection (*see Description [11]*).

AFLURIA is supplied in two presentations:
• 0.5 mL pre-filled syringe (single dose).
• 5 mL multi-dose vial (ten 0.5 mL doses).

4 CONTRAINDICATIONS

AFLURIA is contraindicated in individuals with known severe allergic reactions (e.g., anaphylaxis), to any component of the vaccine including egg protein, or to a previous dose of any influenza vaccine (*see Description [11]*).

5 WARNINGS AND PRECAUTIONS

5.1 Fever and Febrile Seizures

Administration of CSL's 2010 Southern Hemisphere influenza vaccine was associated with postmarketing reports of increased rates of fever and febrile seizures in children predominantly below the age of 5 years as compared to previous years; these increased rates were confirmed by postmarketing studies. Febrile events were also observed in children 5 to less than 9 years of age.

5.2 Guillain-Barré Syndrome

Guillain-Barré Syndrome (GBS) has occurred following vaccination with AFLURIA. If GBS has occurred within 6 weeks of previous influenza vaccination, the decision to give AFLURIA should be based on careful consideration of the potential benefits and risks.

Table 2: Proportion of Subjects 5 through 17 Years of Age with Solicited Local or Systemic Adverse Events Within 7 Days after Administration of AFLURIA, Irrespective of Causality (Studies 2 and 3)

Solicited Adverse Event	Studies 2 and 3 Subjects ≥ 5 to < 9 years		Study 2 Subjects ≥ 9 to < 18 years
	Dose 1 N=595	Dose 2 N=430	Dose 1 N=398
Local			
Pain	61%	55%	68%
Erythema	24%	23%	17%
Swelling	18%	17%	13%
Systemic			
Headache	17%	10%	27%
Malaise or feeling generally unwell*	16%	8%	17%
Any Fever Fever ≥ 102.2°F	13% 2%	6% 2%	5% 1%
General Muscle Ache (Myalgia)	12%	8%	20%
Nausea/vomiting*	7%	3%	5%
Vomiting/Diarrhea†	5%	6%	-
Diarrhea*	4%	2%	5%
Irritability	3%	3%	-
Loss of appetite	1%	1%	-

* These preferred terms were used to describe Solicited Adverse Events in Study 2.
† These preferred terms were used to describe Solicited Adverse Events in Study 3.

Table 3: Proportion of Subjects 18 Years of Age and Older with Solicited Local or Systemic Adverse Events within 5 Days after Administration of AFLURIA or Placebo, Irrespective of Causality (Studies 4, 5 and 6)

Solicited Adverse Event	Study 4 Subjects ≥ 18 to < 65 years		Study 5 Subjects ≥ 18 to < 65 years		Study 6 Subjects ≥ 65 years	
	AFLURIA N = 1089	Placebo N = 268	AFLURIA N=10,015	Placebo N=5005	AFLURIA N=630	Comparator N=636
Local						
Tenderness (Pain on touching)	60%	18%	69%	17%	36%	31%
Pain (without touching)	40%	9%	48%	11%	15%	14%
Redness	16%	8%	4%	<1%	3%	1%
Swelling	9%	1%	4%	<1%	7%	8%
Bruising	5%	1%	1%	<1%	1%	1%
Systemic						
Headache	26%	26%	25%	23%	9%	10%
Malaise	20%	19%	29%	26%	7%	6%
Muscle aches	13%	9%	21%	12%	9%	8%
Nausea	6%	9%	7%	6%	2%	1%
Chills/Shivering	3%	2%	5%	4%	2%	2%
Fever	1%	1%	3%	2%	0%	0%

5.3 Preventing and Managing Allergic Reactions
Appropriate medical treatment and supervision must be available to manage possible anaphylactic reactions following administration of the vaccine.

5.4 Altered Immunocompetence
If AFLURIA is administered to immunocompromised persons, including those receiving immunosuppressive therapy, the immune response may be diminished.

5.5 Limitations of Vaccine Effectiveness
Vaccination with AFLURIA may not protect all individuals.

6 ADVERSE REACTIONS

In children 5 through 17 years of age, the most common injection-site reactions observed in clinical studies with AFLURIA were pain (≥60%), redness (≥20%) and swelling (≥10%). The most common systemic adverse events were headache, myalgia (≥20%), malaise and fever (≥10%).

In adults 18 through 64 years of age, the most common injection-site adverse reactions observed in clinical studies with AFLURIA were tenderness (≥60%) and pain (≥40%). The most common systemic adverse events observed were headache, malaise, and muscle aches (≥20%).

In adults 65 years of age and older, the most common injection-site adverse reactions observed in clinical studies with AFLURIA were tenderness (≥30%) and pain (≥10%).

6.1 Clinical Trials Experience
Because clinical studies are conducted under widely varying conditions, adverse reaction rates observed in the clinical studies of a vaccine cannot be directly compared to rates in the clinical studies of another vaccine and may not reflect the rates observed in clinical practice.

Children
In clinical studies, AFLURIA has been administered to, and safety information collected for, 3,009 children ages 6 months to less than 18 years. Clinical safety data for AFLURIA in children is presented from three clinical studies (Studies 1, 2 and 3). Data from a comparator-controlled trial (Study 1) are presented, followed by pooled data from two open label studies (Studies 2 and 3). Subjects 6 months through 8 years of age received one or two vaccinations as determined by previous vaccination history (for further details on clinical study design, dosing and demographics *see Clinical Studies [14]*).

Study 1 included 1,468 subjects for safety analysis, ages 6 months to less than 18 years, randomized to receive AFLURIA (735 subjects) or another U.S.-licensed trivalent inactivated influenza vaccine (manufactured by Sanofi Pasteur, Inc.) (733 subjects).

Study 2 included 1,976 subjects for safety analysis, ages 6 months to less than 18 years. All subjects received AFLURIA.

Study 3 included 298 subjects for safety analysis, ages 6 months to less than 9 years. All subjects received AFLURIA.

The safety assessment was similar for the three pediatric studies. Local (injection site) and systemic adverse events were solicited for 7 days post-vaccination (Tables 1 and 2). Unsolicited adverse events were collected for 30 days post-vaccination. All adverse events are presented regardless of any treatment causality assigned by study investigators.

Among the pediatric studies, there were no vaccine-related deaths or vaccine-related serious adverse events reported in children 5 years of age and older.

In the comparator-controlled trial (Study 1), the rate of fever after the first dose of AFLURIA in subjects aged 5 to less than 9 years was 16% as compared to 8% in subjects who received the comparator. The rate of fever in subjects aged 9 to less than 18 years following a single dose of AFLURIA was 6% as compared to 4% in subjects who received the comparator. In all three pediatric studies, the rates of fever in subjects aged 5 to less than 9 years who received AFLURIA were lower after dose 2 than dose 1.

Data in Tables 1 and 2 are presented for children 5 years and older.

[See table 1 at top of previous page]

[See table 2 above]

In Study 1, unsolicited adverse events that occurred in ≥ 5% of subjects who received AFLURIA in ages 5 years to less than 9 years following the first or second dose included cough (15%) and pyrexia (9%). Unsolicited adverse events that occurred in ≥ 5% of subjects who received AFLURIA in ages 9 years to less than 18 years following the first dose included cough (7%), oropharyngeal pain (7%), headache (7%) and nasal congestion (6%).

In Studies 2 and 3, unsolicited adverse events that occurred in ≥ 5% subjects ages 5 years to less than 9 years after the first or second dose included the following: upper respiratory tract infection (13%), cough (10%), rhinorrhoea (7%), headache (5%), nasopharyngitis (5%) and pyrexia (5%). Unsolicited adverse events that occurred in ≥ 5% of subjects who received AFLURIA in ages 9 years to less than 18 years following the first dose included upper respiratory tract infection (9%) and headache (8%).

Adults
In clinical studies, a single dose of AFLURIA was administered to, and safety information collected for, 11,104 subjects ages 18 to less than 65 years and 836 subjects ages 65 years and older. Clinical safety data for AFLURIA in adults are presented from three clinical studies (Studies 4 through 6). In all adult studies, there were no vaccine-related deaths or vaccine-related serious adverse events reported.

Study 4 included 1,357 subjects for safety analysis, ages 18 to less than 65 years, randomized to receive AFLURIA (1,089 subjects) or placebo (268 subjects) (*see Clinical Studies [14]*).

Study 5 included 15,020 subjects for safety analysis, ages 18 to less than 65 years, randomized to receive AFLURIA (10,015 subjects) or placebo (5,005 subjects) (*see Clinical Studies [14]*).

Study 6 included 1,266 subjects for safety analysis, ages 65 years and older, randomized to receive AFLURIA (630 subjects) or another U.S.-licensed trivalent inactivated influenza vaccine (manufactured by Sanofi Pasteur SA) as an active control (636 subjects) (*see Clinical Studies [14]*).

The safety assessment was identical for the three adult studies. Local (injection-site) and systemic adverse events were solicited for 5 days post-vaccination (Table 3). Unsolicited adverse events were collected for 21 days post-vaccination. All adverse events are presented regardless of any treatment causality assigned by study investigators.

[See table 3 above]

In Study 4, headache was the only unsolicited adverse event that occurred in ≥ 5% of subjects who received AFLURIA or placebo (8% versus 6%, respectively).

In Study 5, headache was the only unsolicited adverse event that occurred in ≥ 5% of subjects who received AFLURIA or placebo (12% versus 11%, respectively).

In Study 6, unsolicited adverse events that occurred in ≥ 5% of subjects who received AFLURIA included headache (8%), nasal congestion (7%), cough (5%), rhinorrea (5%), and pharyngolaryngeal pain (5%).

6.2 Postmarketing Experience

Because postmarketing reporting of adverse reactions is voluntary and from a population of uncertain size, it is not always possible to reliably estimate their frequency or establish a causal relationship to vaccine exposure. The adverse reactions described have been included in this section because they: 1) represent reactions that are known to occur following immunizations generally or influenza immunizations specifically; 2) are potentially serious; or 3) have been reported frequently. These adverse reactions reflect experience in both children and adults and include those identified during post-approval use of AFLURIA outside the US since 1985.

Blood and lymphatic system disorders

Transient thrombocytopenia

Immune system disorders

Allergic reactions including anaphylactic shock and serum sickness

Nervous system disorders

Neuralgia, paresthesia, convulsions (including febrile seizures), encephalopathy, neuritis or neuropathy, transverse myelitis, and GBS

Vascular disorders

Vasculitis with transient renal involvement

Skin and subcutaneous tissue disorders

Pruritus, urticaria, and rash

6.3 Adverse Reactions Associated With Influenza Vaccination

Anaphylaxis has been reported after administration of AFLURIA. Egg protein can induce immediate hypersensitivity reactions among persons who have severe egg allergy. Allergic reactions include hives, angioedema, asthma, and systemic anaphylaxis *(see Contraindications [4])*.

The 1976 swine influenza vaccine was associated with an increased frequency of GBS. Evidence for a causal relation of GBS with subsequent vaccines prepared from other influenza viruses is unclear. If influenza vaccine does pose a risk, it is probably slightly more than one additional case per 1 million persons vaccinated.

Neurological disorders temporally associated with influenza vaccination, such as encephalopathy, optic neuritis/neuropathy, partial facial paralysis, and brachial plexus neuropathy, have been reported.

Microscopic polyangiitis (vasculitis) has been reported temporally associated with influenza vaccination.

7 DRUG INTERACTIONS

7.1 Concurrent Use With Other Vaccines

There are no data to assess the concomitant administration of AFLURIA with other vaccines. If AFLURIA is to be given at the same time as another injectable vaccine(s), the vaccine(s) should be administered at different injection sites.

AFLURIA should not be mixed with any other vaccine in the same syringe or vial.

7.2 Concurrent Use With Immunosuppressive Therapies

The immunological response to AFLURIA may be diminished in individuals receiving corticosteroid or immunosuppressive therapies.

8 USE IN SPECIFIC POPULATIONS

8.1 Pregnancy

Pregnancy Category B: A reproductive and developmental toxicity study has been performed in female rats at a dose approximately 265 times the human dose (on a mg/kg basis) and revealed no evidence of impaired female fertility or harm to the fetus due to AFLURIA. There are, however, no adequate and well-controlled studies in pregnant women. Because animal reproduction studies are not always predictive of human response, AFLURIA should be given to a pregnant woman only if clearly needed.

In the reproductive and developmental toxicity study, the effect of AFLURIA on embryo-fetal and pre-weaning development was evaluated in pregnant rats. Animals were administered AFLURIA by intramuscular injection twice prior to gestation, once during the period of organogenesis (gestation day 6), and once later in pregnancy (gestation day 20), 0.5 mL/rat/occasion (approximately a 265-fold excess relative to the projected human dose on a body weight basis). No adverse effects on mating, female fertility, pregnancy, parturition, lactation parameters, and embryo-fetal or pre-weaning development were observed. There were no vaccine-related fetal malformations or other evidence of teratogenesis.

8.3 Nursing Mothers

AFLURIA has not been evaluated in nursing mothers. It is not known whether AFLURIA is excreted in human milk. Because many drugs are excreted in human milk, caution should be exercised when AFLURIA is administered to a nursing woman.

Table 4: Laboratory-confirmed Influenza Infection Rate and Vaccine Efficacy in Adults 18 to less than 65 Years of Age (Study 5)

	Subjects*	Laboratory-confirmed Influenza Cases	Influenza Infection Rate	Vaccine Efficacy†	
	N	n	n/N %	%	Lower Limit of the 95% CI
Vaccine-matched Strains					
AFLURIA	9889	58	0.59	60	41
Placebo	4960	73	1.47		
Any Influenza Virus Strain					
AFLURIA	9889	222	2.24	42	28
Placebo	4960	192	3.87		

Abbreviations: CI, confidence interval

* The Per Protocol Population was identical to the Evaluable Population in this study.

† Vaccine efficacy = 1 minus the ratio of AFLURIA/placebo infection rates. The objective of the study was to demonstrate that the lower limit of the CI for vaccine efficacy was greater than 40%.

8.4 Pediatric Use

AFLURIA is not approved for use in children less than 5 years of age. In a clinical study in which children received AFLURIA or a US-licensed comparator vaccine (Study 1, *see Clinical Trials Experience, [6.1]*), the incidence of fever in children 6 months to less than 3 years of age following the first and second doses of AFLURIA were 37% and 15%, respectively, as compared to 14% following each dose in the comparator group. Among children 3 years to less than 5 years of age, the incidence of fever following the first and second doses of AFLURIA were 32% and 14%, respectively, as compared to 11% and 16% in the comparator. In an open-label study (Study 2), fever, irritability, loss of appetite, and vomiting/diarrhea occurred more frequently in children 6 months to less than 3 years of age as compared to older children. Across three pediatric studies of AFLURIA (Studies 1, 2, and 3), 1.2% of eligible children (n=1,764) were discontinued from the second vaccination because of severe fever (>104°F) within 48 hours of the first vaccination. Across the three pediatric studies, two children, a 7-month old and a 3-year old, experienced vaccine-related febrile seizures (rate of 0.07% across studies), one of which was serious.

Administration of CSL's 2010 Southern Hemisphere influenza vaccine was associated with increased rates of fever and febrile seizures, predominantly in children below the age of 5 years as compared to previous years, in postmarketing reports confirmed by postmarketing studies *(see Warnings and Precautions [5.1])*.

8.5 Geriatric Use

In clinical studies, AFLURIA has been administered to, and safety information collected for, 836 subjects ages 65 years and older *(see Clinical Trials Experience [6.1])*. After administration of AFLURIA, hemagglutination-inhibiting antibody responses in persons 65 years of age and older were lower as compared to younger adult subjects *(see Clinical Studies [14])*.

11 DESCRIPTION

AFLURIA, Influenza Virus Vaccine for intramuscular injection, is a sterile, clear, colorless to slightly opalescent suspension with some sediment that resuspends upon shaking to form a homogeneous suspension. AFLURIA is prepared from influenza virus propagated in the allantoic fluid of embryonated chicken eggs. Following harvest, the virus is purified in a sucrose density gradient using continuous flow zonal centrifugation. The purified virus is inactivated with beta-propiolactone, and the virus particles are disrupted using sodium taurodeoxycholate to produce a "split virion". The disrupted virus is further purified and suspended in a phosphate buffered isotonic solution.

AFLURIA is standardized according to USPHS requirements for the 2012-2013 influenza season and is formulated to contain 45 mcg hemagglutinin (HA) per 0.5 mL dose in the recommended ratio of 15 mcg HA for each of the three influenza strains recommended for the 2012-2013 Northern Hemisphere influenza season: A/California/7/2009 (H1N1), NYMC X-181, A/Victoria/361/2011 (H3N2), IVR-165, and B/Hubei-Wujiagang/158/2009, NYMC BX-39 (a B/Wisconsin/1/2010-like strain).

Thimerosal, a mercury derivative, is not used in the manufacturing process for the single dose presentations; therefore these products contain no preservative. The multi-dose presentation contains thimerosal, added as a preservative; each 0.5 mL dose contains 24.5 mcg of mercury.

A single 0.5 mL dose of AFLURIA contains sodium chloride (4.1 mg), monobasic sodium phosphate (80 mcg), dibasic sodium phosphate (300 mcg), monobasic potassium phosphate (20 mcg), potassium chloride (20 mcg), and calcium chloride (1.5 mcg). From the manufacturing process, each 0.5 mL dose may also contain residual amounts of sodium taurodeoxycholate (≤ 10 ppm), ovalbumin (≤ 1 mcg), neomycin sulfate (≤ 3 nanograms [ng]), polymyxin B (≤ 0.5 ng), and beta-propiolactone (≤ 2 ng).

The rubber tip cap and plunger used for the preservative-free, single-dose syringes and the rubber stoppers used for the multi-dose vial contain no latex.

12 CLINICAL PHARMACOLOGY

12.1 Mechanism of Action

Influenza illness and its complications follow infection with influenza viruses. Global surveillance of influenza identifies yearly antigenic variants. For example, since 1977 antigenic variants of influenza A (H1N1 and H3N2) and influenza B viruses have been in global circulation. Specific levels of hemagglutination inhibition (HI) antibody titers post-vaccination with inactivated influenza virus vaccine have not been correlated with protection from influenza virus. In some human studies, antibody titers of 1:40 or greater have been associated with protection from influenza illness in up to 50% of subjects.[2,3]

Antibody against one influenza virus type or subtype confers limited or no protection against another. Furthermore, antibody to one antigenic variant of influenza virus might not protect against a new antigenic variant of the same type or subtype. Frequent development of antigenic variants through antigenic drift is the virologic basis for seasonal epidemics and the reason for the usual change to one or more new strains in each year's influenza vaccine. Therefore, inactivated influenza vaccines are standardized to contain the HA of three strains (i.e., typically two type A and one type B) representing the influenza viruses likely to be circulating in the US during the upcoming winter.

Annual revaccination with the current vaccine is recommended because immunity declines during the year after vaccination and circulating strains of influenza virus change from year to year.[1]

13 NONCLINICAL TOXICOLOGY

13.1 Carcinogenesis, Mutagenesis, Impairment of Fertility

AFLURIA has not been evaluated for carcinogenic or mutagenic potential.

14 CLINICAL STUDIES

14.1 Efficacy Against Laboratory-Confirmed Influenza

In Study 5, the efficacy of AFLURIA was demonstrated in a randomized, observer-blind, placebo-controlled study conducted in 15,044 subjects. Healthy subjects 18 to less than 65 years of age were randomized in a 2:1 ratio to receive a single dose of AFLURIA (enrolled subjects: 10,033; evaluable subjects: 9,889) or placebo (enrolled subjects: 5,011; evaluable subjects: 4,960). The mean age of all randomized subjects was 35.5 years. 54.4% were female and 90.2% were White. Laboratory-confirmed influenza was assessed by active and passive surveillance of influenza-like illness (ILI) beginning 2 weeks post-vaccination until the end of the influenza season, approximately 6 months post-vaccination. ILI was defined as at least one respiratory symptom (e.g., cough, sore throat, nasal congestion) and at least one systemic symptom (e.g., oral temperature of 100.0°F or higher, feverishness, chills, body aches). Nasal and throat swabs were collected from subjects who presented with an ILI for laboratory confirmation by viral culture and real-time reverse transcription polymerase chain reaction. Influenza virus strain was further characterized using gene sequencing and pyrosequencing.

Attack rates and vaccine efficacy, defined as the relative reduction in the influenza infection rate for AFLURIA com-

Table 5: Post-Vaccination HI Antibody GMTs, Seroconversion Rates, and Analyses of Non-Inferiority of AFLURIA to a U.S. Licensed Comparator, Subjects 5 to less than 18 Years of Age (Study 1)

Strain	Post-vaccination GMT		GMT Ratio*	Seroconversion %†		Difference	Met both pre-defined non-inferiority criteria? ‡
	Comparator N=381	AFLURIA N=380	Comparator over AFLURIA (95% CI)	Comparator N=381	AFLURIA N=380	Comparator minus AFLURIA (95% CI)	
A(H1N1)	526.2	507.4	1.03 (0.88, 1.21)	62.7	62.6	0.1 (-6.8, 7.0)	Yes
A(H3N2)	1060.0	961.3	1.07 (0.94, 1.23)	72.2	69.7	2.4 (-4.0, 8.9)	Yes
B	123.3	110.1	1.10 (0.94, 1.29)	75.1	70.0	5.1 (-1.3, 11.4)	No

Abbreviations: CI, confidence interval; GMT, geometric mean titer.
* GMT ratios are adjusted for baseline HI titers
† Seroconversion rate is defined as a 4-fold increase in post-vaccination HI antibody titer from pre-vaccination titer ≥ 1:10 or an increase in titer from < 1:10 to ≥ 1:40.
‡ Note that the study was powered to assess the pre-specified non-inferiority criteria based on 1400 evaluable subjects.

Table 7: Post-Vaccination HI Antibody GMTs, Seroconversion Rates, and Analyses of Non-Inferiority of AFLURIA to a U.S. Licensed Comparator, Adults 65 Years of Age and Older (Study 6)

Strain	Post-vaccination GMT		GMT Ratio*	Seroconversion %†		Difference	Met both pre-defined non-inferiority criteria?
	Comparator N=610	AFLURIA N=605	Comparator over AFLURIA (95% CI)	Comparator N=610	AFLURIA N=605	Comparator minus AFLURIA (95% CI)	
A (H1N1)	59.2	59.4	1.04 (0.92, 1.18)	43.0	38.8	4.1 (-1.4, 9.6)	Yes
A (H3N2)	337.7	376.8	0.95 (0.83, 1.08)	68.7	69.4	-0.7 (-5.9, 4.5)	Yes
B	33.4	30.4	1.12 (1.01, 1.25)	34.4	29.3	5.2 (-0.1, 10.4)	No

Abbreviations: CI, confidence interval; GMT, geometric mean titer.
* Post-vaccination GMTs were adjusted for baseline HI titers.
† Seroconversion rate is defined as a 4-fold increase in post-vaccination HI antibody titer from pre-vaccination titer ≥ 1:10 or an increase in titer from < 1:10 to ≥ 1:40.

pared to placebo, were calculated using the per protocol population. Vaccine efficacy against laboratory-confirmed influenza infection due to influenza A or B virus strains contained in the vaccine was 60% with a lower limit of the 95% CI of 41% (Table 4).
[See table 4 at top of previous page]

14.2 Immunogenicity in Children

Study 1 was a randomized, observer-blind, comparator-controlled study to evaluate the immunological non-inferiority of AFLURIA to a U.S.-licensed trivalent inactivated influenza vaccine (manufactured by Sanofi Pasteur, Inc.) in subjects 6 months to less than 18 years of age. Results are presented for children 5 to less than 18 years of age (Table 5). A total of 832 subjects (aged 5 to less than 18 years) were enrolled. Subjects were randomized in a 1:1 ratio to receive AFLURIA (enrolled subjects: 417; evaluable subjects: 383) or the comparator vaccine (enrolled subjects: 415; evaluable subjects: 383).

Children 6 months to less than 9 years of age with no history of influenza vaccination received 2 doses approximately 28 days apart. Children 6 months to less than 9 years of age with a history of influenza vaccination and children 9 years of age and older received 1 dose. Children 6 months to less than 3 years of age received 0.25 mL of AFLURIA or comparator influenza vaccine, and children 3 years of age and older received 0.5 mL of AFLURIA or comparator influenza vaccine. Nearly equal proportions of subjects were male (49.9%) and female (50.1%), and the majority were White (85.0%) or Black (10.3%).

Immunogenicity assessments were performed prior to vaccination and at 21 days after vaccination. The co-primary endpoints were HI Geometric Mean Titer (GMT) ratios (adjusted for baseline HI titers) and the difference in seroconversion rates for each vaccine strain 21 days after the final vaccination. Pre-specified non-inferiority criteria required that the upper bound of the 2-sided 95% CI of the GMT ratio (Comparator/AFLURIA) did not exceed 1.5 and the upper bound of the 2-sided 95% CI of the seroconversion rate difference (Comparator minus AFLURIA) did not exceed 10.0% for each strain. As shown in Table 5, non-inferiority of AFLURIA to the comparator vaccine was demonstrated in the per protocol population for influenza A subtypes A(H1N1) and A(H3N2), but not for influenza type B. For influenza type B, non-inferiority was demonstrated for HI GMTs, but not for seroconversion rates. Note that the study was powered to assess the pre-specified non-inferiority criteria based on 1400 evaluable subjects. Analysis of the 761 subjects aged 5 to less than 18 years reduced the power of the study and widened the confidence intervals. In the pre-specified analysis, AFLURIA was not inferior to the comparator vaccine for all three virus strains. Post hoc analyses of immunogenicity by gender did not demonstrate significant differences between males and females. The study was not sufficiently diverse to assess differences between races or ethnicities.
[See table 5 above]

14.3 Immunogenicity in Adults and Older Adults

Two randomized, controlled clinical studies of AFLURIA evaluated the immune responses by measuring HI antibody titers to each virus strain in the vaccine in adults. In these studies, post-vaccination immunogenicity was evaluated on sera obtained 21 days after administration of a single dose of AFLURIA.

Study 4 was a randomized, double-blinded, placebo-controlled, multicenter study in healthy subjects ages 18 to less than 65 years. A total of 1,357 subjects were vaccinated (1,089 subjects with AFLURIA and 268 with a placebo). Subjects who received AFLURIA were vaccinated using either the preservative-free or thimerosal-containing presentation. The evaluable population consisted of 1,341 subjects (1,077 in the AFLURIA group and 264 in the placebo group). The mean age of the entire evaluable population receiving AFLURIA was 38 years. 62.5% of subjects were female, 81.3% were White, 12.1% were Black, and 6.2% were Asian. Serum HI antibody responses to AFLURIA met the pre-specified co-primary endpoint criteria for all three virus strains (Table 6). Similar responses were observed between genders. The study was not sufficiently diverse to assess immunogenicity by race or ethnicity.

Table 6: Serum Antibody Responses in Subjects 18 through 64 Years of Age Receiving AFLURIA (Study 4)

Strain Variable	AFLURIA N=1077 value (95% CI)	Placebo N=264 value (95% CI)
A (H1N1)		
HI Titer ≥ 1:40*	97.8% (96.7, 98.6)	74.6% (68.9, 79.8)
Seroconversion Rate (%)†	48.7% (45.6, 51.7)	2.3% (0.8, 4.9)
A (H3N2)		
HI Titer ≥ 1:40*	99.9% (99.5, 100.0)	72.0% (66.1, 77.3)
Seroconversion Rate (%)†	71.5% (68.7, 74.2)	0.0% (N/A)
B		
HI Titer ≥ 1:40*	94.2% (92.7, 95.6)	47.0% (40.8, 53.2)
Seroconversion Rate (%)†	69.7% (66.9, 72.5)	0.4% (< 0.1, 2.1)

* HI titer ≥ 1:40 is defined as the proportion of subjects with a minimum post-vaccination HI antibody titer of 1:40. Lower bound of 95% CI for HI antibody titer ≥ 1:40 should be > 70% for the study population.
† Seroconversion rate is defined as a 4-fold increase in post-vaccination HI antibody titer from pre-vaccination titer ≥ 1:10 or an increase in titer from < 1:10 to ≥ 1:40. Lower bound of 95% CI for seroconversion should be > 40% for the study population.

Study 6 was a randomized, observer-blind, comparator-controlled study that enrolled 1,268 subjects 65 years of age and older (Table 7). This study compared the immune response following administration of AFLURIA to that following a US-licensed trivalent inactivated influenza vaccine (manufactured by Sanofi Pasteur SA). Subjects were randomized in a 1:1 ratio to receive a single vaccination of AFLURIA (enrolled subjects: 631; evaluable subjects: 605) or the comparator vaccine (enrolled subjects: 637; evaluable subjects: 610). Immunogenicity assessments were performed prior to vaccination and at 21 days after vaccination. Most of the subjects in the per-protocol immunogenicity population were female (56.7%) and White (97.4%). 2.0% were Black and less than 1.0% were of other races or ethnicities.

The co-primary endpoints were HI GMT ratios (adjusted for baseline HI titers) and the difference in seroconversion rates for each vaccine strain 21 days after vaccination. Pre-specified non-inferiority criteria required that the upper bound of the 2-sided 95% CI of the GMT ratio (Comparator/AFLURIA) did not exceed 1.5 and the upper bound of the 2-sided 95% CI of the seroconversion rate difference (Comparator minus AFLURIA) did not exceed 10.0% for each strain. As shown in Table 7, non-inferiority of AFLURIA to the comparator vaccine was demonstrated in the per protocol population for influenza A subtypes A(H1N1) and A(H3N2), but not for influenza type B. For the B strain, non-inferiority was demonstrated for HI GMTs, but not for seroconversion rates. Post hoc analyses of immunogenicity by gender did not demonstrate significant differences between males and females. The study was not sufficiently diverse to assess differences between races or ethnicities.
[See table 7 above]

15 REFERENCES

1. Centers for Disease Control and Prevention. Prevention and Control of Influenza: Recommendations of the Advisory Committee on Immunization Practices (ACIP). *MMWR Recomm Rep* 2010;59 (RR-8):1-62.
2. Hannoun C, Megas F, Piercy J. Immunogenicity and Protective Efficacy of Influenza Vaccination. *Virus Res* 2004;103:133-138.
3. Hobson D, Curry RL, Beare AS, et al. The Role of Serum Hemagglutination-Inhibiting Antibody in Protection against Challenge Infection with Influenza A2 and B Viruses. *J Hyg Camb* 1972;70:767-777.

16 HOW SUPPLIED/STORAGE AND HANDLING

16.1 How Supplied

Each product presentation includes a package insert and the following components:

Presentation	Carton NDC Number	Components
Pre-Filled Syringe	33332-012-01	• Ten 0.5 mL single-dose syringes without needles [NDC 33332-012-02]
Multi-Dose Vial	33332-112-10	• One 5 mL vial, which contains ten 0.5 mL doses [NDC 33332-112-11]

16.2 Storage and Handling

- Store refrigerated at 2–8°C (36–46°F).
- Do not freeze. Discard if product has been frozen.
- Protect from light.
- Do not use AFLURIA beyond the expiration date printed on the label.
- Once the stopper of the multi-dose vial has been pierced, the vial must be discarded within 28 days.

17 PATIENT COUNSELING INFORMATION

The vaccine recipient or guardian should be:
- informed of the potential benefits and risks of immunization with AFLURIA.

- informed that AFLURIA is an inactivated vaccine that cannot cause influenza but stimulates the immune system to produce antibodies that protect against influenza, and that the full effect of the vaccine is generally achieved approximately 3 weeks after vaccination.
- instructed to report any severe or unusual adverse reactions to their healthcare provider.
- provided with Vaccine Information Statements which are required by the National Childhood Vaccine Injury Act of 1986 to be given prior to immunization. These materials are available free of charge at the Centers for Disease Control and Prevention (CDC) website (www.cdc.gov/vaccines).
- instructed that annual revaccination is recommended.

Manufactured by:
CSL Limited
Parkville, Victoria, 3052, Australia
US License No. 1764
Distributed by:
Merck Sharp & Dohme Corp., a subsidiary of
MERCK & CO., INC., Whitehouse Station, NJ 08889, USA
AFLURIA is a registered trademark of CSL Limited.
CSL Biotherapies is a division of CSL Limited.

AMINOHIPPURATE SODIUM "PAH" ℞

[*am-ino-hip-pur-ate*]
Injection

DESCRIPTION

Aminohippurate sodium[1] is an agent to measure effective renal plasma flow (ERPF). It is the sodium salt of para-aminohippuric acid, commonly abbreviated "PAH". It is water soluble, lipid-insoluble, and has a pKa of 3.83. The empirical formula of the anhydrous salt is $C_9H_9N_2NaO_3$ and its structural formula is:

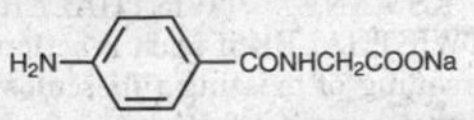

It is provided as a sterile, non-preserved 20 percent aqueous solution for injection, with a pH of 6.7 to 7.6. Each 10 mL contains: Aminohippurate sodium 2 g. Inactive ingredients: Sodium hydroxide to adjust pH, water for injection, q.s.

[1] Formerly referred to as Sodium para-Aminohippurate.

CLINICAL PHARMACOLOGY

PAH is filtered by the glomeruli and is actively secreted by the proximal tubules. At low plasma concentrations (1.0 to 2.0 mg/100 mL), an average of 90 percent of PAH is cleared by the kidneys from the renal blood stream in a single circulation. It is ideally suited for measurement of ERPF since it has a high clearance, is essentially nontoxic at the plasma concentrations reached with recommended doses, and its analytical determination is relatively simple and accurate.
PAH is also used to measure the functional capacity of the renal tubular secretory mechanism or transport maximum (Tm_{PAH}). This is accomplished by elevating the plasma concentration to levels (40-60 mg/100 mL) sufficient to saturate the maximal capacity of the tubular cells to secrete PAH.
Inulin clearance is generally measured during Tm_{PAH} determinations since glomerular filtration rate (GFR) must be known before calculations of secretory Tm measurements can be done (see DOSAGE AND ADMINISTRATION, Calculations).

INDICATIONS AND USAGE

Estimation of effective renal plasma flow.
Measurement of the functional capacity of the renal tubular secretory mechanism.

CONTRAINDICATIONS

Hypersensitivity to this product or to its components.

PRECAUTIONS

General
Intravenous solutions must be given with caution to patients with low cardiac reserve, since a rapid increase in plasma volume can precipitate congestive heart failure.
For measurement of ERPF, small doses of PAH are used. However, in research procedures to measure Tm_{PAH}, high plasma levels are required to saturate the capacity of the tubular cells. During these procedures, the intravenous administration of PAH solutions should be carried out slowly and with caution. The patient should be continuously observed for any adverse reactions.
Use caution when injecting this product into latex-sensitive individuals, since the vial stopper contains dry natural latex rubber that may cause allergic reactions.
Drug Interactions
Renal clearance measurements of PAH cannot be made with any significant accuracy in patients receiving sulfonamides, procaine, or thiazolesulfone. These compounds interfere with chemical color development essential to the analytical procedures.
Probenecid depresses tubular secretion of certain weak acids such as PAH. Therefore, patients receiving probenecid will have erroneously low ERPF and Tm_{PAH} values.
Carcinogenesis, Mutagenesis, Impairment of Fertility
Long-term studies in animals have not been done to evaluate any effects upon fertility or carcinogenic potential of PAH.
Pregnancy
Pregnancy Category C
Animal reproduction studies have not been done with PAH. It is also not known whether PAH can cause fetal harm when given to a pregnant woman or can affect reproduction capacity. PAH should be given to a pregnant woman only if clearly needed.
Nursing Mothers
It is not known whether this drug is excreted in human milk. Because many drugs are excreted in human milk, caution should be exercised when PAH is administered to a nursing woman.
Pediatric Use
Safety and effectiveness in pediatric patients have not been established.
Geriatric Use
Clinical studies of PAH did not include sufficient numbers of subjects aged 65 and over to determine whether they respond differently from younger subjects. Other reported clinical experience has not identified differences in responses between the elderly and younger patients.

ADVERSE REACTIONS

Hypersensitivity reactions including anaphylaxis, angioedema, urticaria, vasomotor disturbances, flushing, tingling, nausea, vomiting, and cramps may occur.
Patients may have a sensation of warmth or the desire to defecate or urinate during or shortly following initiation of infusion.

OVERDOSE

The intravenous LD_{50} in female mice is 7.22 g/kg.

DOSAGE AND ADMINISTRATION

For intravenous use only
Clearance measurements using single injection techniques are generally inaccurate, particularly in the measurement of ERPF. For this reason, intravenous infusions at fixed rates are used to sustain the plasma PAH concentration at the desired level.
To measure ERPF, the concentration of PAH in the plasma should be maintained at 2 mg per 100 mL, which can be achieved with a priming dose of 6 to 10 mg/kg and an infusion dose of 10 to 24 mg/min.
As a research procedure for the measurement of Tm_{PAH}, the plasma level of PAH must be sufficient to saturate the capacity of the tubular secretory cells. Concentrations from 40 to 60 mg per 100 mL are usually necessary.
Technical details of these tests may be found in Smith {1}; Wesson {2}; Bauer {3}; Pitts{4}; and Schnurr {5}.
Parenteral drug products should be inspected visually for particulate matter and discoloration prior to use, whenever solution and container permit. NOTE: The normal color range for this product is a colorless to yellow/brown solution. The efficacy is not affected by color changes within this range.
Calculations
Effective Renal Plasma Flow (ERPF)
The clearance of PAH, which is extracted almost completely from the plasma during its passage through the renal circulation, constitutes a measure of ERPF. Hence:
$ERPF = U_{PAH}V/P_{PAH}$
Where U_{PAH} = concentration of PAH (mg/mL) in the urine
V = rate of urine excretion (mL/min), and
P_{PAH} = plasma concentration of PAH (mg/mL).
Example:
$U_{PAH} = 8.0$ mg/mL
V = 1.5 mL/min
$P_{PAH} = 0.02$ mg/mL
$ERPF = 8.0 \times 1.5/0.02 = 600$ mL/min
Based on PAH clearance studies, the normal values for ERPF are:
men 675 ± 150 mL/min
women 595 ± 125 mL/min
Maximum Tubular Secretory
(Tm_{PAH}) Mechanism
The quantity of PAH secreted by the tubules (Tm_{PAH}) is given by the difference between the total rate of excretion ($U_{PAH}V$) and the quantity filtered by the glomeruli (GFR × P_{PAH}). Hence:
$Tm_{PAH} = U_{PAH}V - (GFR \times P_{PAH} \times 0.83)$
The factor, 0.83, corrects for that portion of PAH which is bound to plasma protein and hence is unfilterable.
Example:
$U_{PAH} = 9.55$ mg/mL
V = 16.68 mL/min
GFR = 120 mL/min
$P_{PAH} = 0.60$ mg/mL
Then $Tm_{PAH} = 9.55 \times 16.68 - (120 \times 0.60 \times 0.83) = 100$ mg/min.
Average normal values of Tm_{PAH} are 80-90 mg/min.
The value of the expression $U_{PAH}V$, used in calculations of ERPF and Tm_{PAH}, may be found by determining the amount of PAH in a measured volume of urine excreted within a specific period of time.
These calculations are based on a body surface area of 1.73 m^2. Corrections for variations in surface area are made by multiplying the values obtained for ERPF and Tm_{PAH} by 1.73/A, where A is the subject surface area.

HOW SUPPLIED

No. 95 — Aminohippurate Sodium, 20 percent sterile solution for intravenous injection, is supplied as follows:
NDC 0006-3395-11 in 10 mL vials.
Storage
Store at 25°C (77°F); excursions permitted to 15-30°C (59-86°F) [see USP Controlled Room Temperature].

REFERENCES

1. Smith, H.W.: Lectures on the kidney, University Extension Division, University of Kansas, Lawrence, Kansas, 1943.
2. Wesson, L.G., Jr.: "Physiology of the Human Kidney," New York, Grune & Stratton, 1969, pp. 632-655.
3. Bauer, J.D.; Ackermann, P.G.; Toro, G.: "Brays Clinical Laboratory Methods," ed. 7, St. Louis, Mosby, 1968.
4. Pitts, R.F.: "Physiology of the Kidney and Body Fluids," ed. 2, Chicago, Year Book Medical Publishers, 1968.
5. Schnurr, E.; Lahme, W.; Kuppers, H.: Measurement of renal clearance of inulin and PAH in the steady state without urine collection; Clinical Nephrology, *13*(1): (26-29), 1980.

Merck Sharp & Dohme Corp., a subsidiary of
MERCK & CO., INC., Whitehouse Station, NJ 08889, USA
Issued January 2011
Printed in USA
9051026

ANTIVENIN ℞

[*an-tiv-en-in*]
(Latrodectus mactans)
(Black Widow Spider Antivenin)
Equine Origin

DESCRIPTION

Antivenin (Latrodectus mactans), is a sterile, non-pyrogenic preparation derived by drying a frozen solution of specific venom-neutralizing globulins obtained from the blood serum of healthy horses immunized against venom of black widow spiders (Latrodectus mactans). It is standardized by biological assay on mice, in terms of one dose of Antivenin neutralizing the venom in not less than 6000 mouse LD_{50} of Latrodectus mactans. Thimerosal (mercury derivative) 1:10,000 is added as a preservative. When constituted as specified, it is opalescent, ranging in color from light (straw) to very dark (iced tea), and contains not more than 20.0 percent of solids.
Each vial contains not less than 6000 Antivenin units. One unit of Antivenin will neutralize one average mouse lethal dose of black widow spider venom when the Antivenin and the venom are injected simultaneously in mice under suitable conditions.

CLINICAL PHARMACOLOGY

The pharmacological mode of action is unknown and metabolic and pharmacokinetic data in humans are unavailable.

INDICATIONS AND USAGE

Antivenin (Latrodectus mactans), is used to treat patients with symptoms due to bites by the black widow spider (Latrodectus mactans). Early use of the Antivenin is emphasized for prompt relief.
Local muscular cramps begin from 15 minutes to several hours after the bite which usually produces a sharp pain similar to that caused by puncture with a needle. The exact sequence of symptoms depends somewhat on the location of the bite. The venom acts on the myoneural junctions or on the nerve endings, causing an ascending motor paralysis or destruction of the peripheral nerve endings. The groups of muscles most frequently affected at first are those of the thigh, shoulder, and back. After a varying length of time, the pain becomes more severe, spreading to the abdomen, and weakness and tremor usually develop. The abdominal muscles assume a boardlike rigidity, but tenderness is slight. Respiration is thoracic. The patient is restless and anxious. Feeble pulse, cold, clammy skin, labored breathing and speech, light stupor, and delirium may occur. Convulsions also may occur, particularly in small children. The temperature may be normal or slightly elevated. Urinary

retention, shock, cyanosis, nausea and vomiting, insomnia, and cold sweats also have been reported. The syndrome following the bite of the black widow spider may be confused easily with any medical or surgical condition with acute abdominal symptoms.

The symptoms of black widow spider bite increase in severity for several hours, perhaps a day, and then very slowly become less severe, gradually passing off in the course of two or three days except in fatal cases. Residual symptoms such as general weakness, tingling, nervousness, and transient muscle spasm may persist for weeks or months after recovery from the acute stage.

If possible, the patient should be hospitalized. Other additional measures giving greatest relief are prolonged warm baths and intravenous injection of 10 mL of 10 percent solution of calcium gluconate repeated as necessary to control muscle pain. Morphine also may be required to control pain. Barbiturates may be used for extreme restlessness. However, as the venom is a neurotoxin, it can cause respiratory paralysis. This must be borne in mind when considering use of morphine or a barbiturate. Adrenocorticosteroids have been used with varying degrees of success. Supportive therapy is indicated by the condition of the patient. Local treatment of the site of the bite is of no value. Nothing is gained by applying a tourniquet or by attempting to remove venom from the site of the bite by incision and suction.

In otherwise healthy individuals between the ages of 16 and 60, the use of Antivenin may be deferred and treatment with muscle relaxants may be considered.

WARNINGS

Prior to treatment with any product prepared from horse serum, a careful review of the patient's history should be taken emphasizing prior exposure to horse serum or any allergies. Serum sickness and even death could result from the use of horse serum in a sensitive patient. A skin or conjunctival test should be performed prior to administration of Antivenin. However, an anaphylactic reaction to Antivenin may occur even following a negative skin or conjunctival test (see ADVERSE REACTIONS).

Skin test: Inject into (not under) the skin not more than 0.02 mL of the test material (1:10 dilution of normal horse serum in physiologic saline). Evaluate result in 10 minutes. A positive reaction is an urticarial wheal surrounded by a zone of erythema. A control test using Sodium Chloride Injection facilitates interpretation of the results.

Conjunctival test: For adults instill into the conjunctival sac one drop of a 1:10 dilution of horse serum and for children one drop of 1:100 dilution. Itching of the eye and reddening of the conjunctiva indicate a positive reaction, usually within 10 minutes.

Patients should be observed for serum sickness for an average of 8 to 12 days following administration of Antivenin.

Desensitization should be attempted only when the administration of Antivenin is considered necessary to save life. Epinephrine must be available in case of untoward reaction.

Desensitization: If the history is positive or the results of the sensitivity tests are mildly or questionably positive, Antivenin should be administered as follows to reduce the risk of an immediate severe allergic reaction:

1. In separate sterile vials or syringes prepare 1:10 or 1:100 dilutions of Antivenin in Sodium Chloride for Injection.
2. Allow at least 15 but preferably 30 minutes between injections and only proceed with the next dose if no reactions occurred following the previous dose.
3. Using a tuberculin syringe, inject subcutaneously 0.1, 0.2 and 0.5 mL of the 1:100 dilution at 15 or 30 minute intervals; repeat with the 1:10 dilution, and finally the undiluted Antivenin.
4. If there is a reaction after any of the injections, place a tourniquet proximal to the sites of injection and administer epinephrine, 1:1000 (0.3 to 1.0 mL subcutaneously, 0.05 to 0.1 mL intravenously), proximal to the tourniquet or into another extremity. Wait at least 30 minutes before giving another injection of Antivenin, the amount of which should be the same as the last one not evoking a reaction.
5. If no reaction has occurred after 0.5 mL of undiluted Antivenin has been given, it is probably safe to continue the dose at 15 minute intervals until the entire dose has been injected.

PRECAUTIONS

Patients with Asthma

Anaphylactic reactions and death have been reported in patients with a medical history of asthma.

Carcinogenesis, Mutagenesis, Impairment of Fertility

No long term studies in animals have been performed to evaluate the potential for carcinogenesis, mutagenesis, or impairment of fertility.

Pregnancy

Pregnancy Category C. Animal reproduction studies have not been conducted with Black Widow Spider Antivenin. It is also not known whether Black Widow Spider Antivenin can cause fetal harm when administered to a pregnant woman or can affect reproduction capacity. Black Widow Spider Antivenin should be given to a pregnant woman only if clearly needed.

Nursing Mothers

It is not known whether this drug is excreted in human milk. Because many drugs are excreted in human milk, caution should be exercised when Black Widow Spider Antivenin is administered to a nursing woman.

Pediatric Use

Controlled clinical studies for safety and effectiveness in children have not been conducted.

Geriatric Use

Reported clinical experience has not identified differences in responses between the elderly and younger patients. Because of the increased risk of complications from envenomation in elderly patients, the standard of care described in the literature suggests that patients older than 60 years of age should be given Antivenin as a preferred initial therapy (see INDICATIONS AND USAGE).

ADVERSE REACTIONS

The following adverse reactions have been reported following the use of Antivenin: Hypersensitivity reactions including anaphylaxis and serum sickness. Muscle cramps have also been reported.

DOSAGE AND ADMINISTRATION

Using a sterile syringe, remove from the accompanying vial 2.5 mL of Sterile Diluent for Antivenin and inject into the vial of Antivenin. With the needle still in the rubber stopper, shake the vial to dissolve the contents completely.

Parenteral drug products should be inspected visually for particulate matter prior to administration, whenever solution and container permit (see DESCRIPTION).

The dose for adults and children is the entire contents of a restored vial (2.5 mL) of Antivenin. It may be given intramuscularly, preferably in the region of the anterolateral thigh so that a tourniquet may be applied in the event of a systemic reaction. Symptoms usually subside in 1 to 3 hours. Although one dose of Antivenin usually is adequate, a second dose may be necessary in some cases.

Antivenin also may be given intravenously in 10 to 50 mL of saline solution over a 15 minute period. It is the preferred route in severe cases, or when the patient is under 12, or in shock. One restored vial usually is enough.

HOW SUPPLIED

No. 4084 — Antivenin (Latrodectus mactans), equine origin is a white to gray crystalline powder, each vial containing not less than 6000 Antivenin units. Thimerosal (mercury derivative) 1:10,000 is added as preservative, **NDC** 0006-4084-00. A 2.5 mL vial of Sterile Diluent for Antivenin is included. Also supplied is a 1 mL vial of normal horse serum (1:10 dilution) for sensitivity testing. Thimerosal (mercury derivative) 1:10,000 is added as preservative.

Storage

Antivenin must be stored and shipped at 2-8°C (36-46°F). When reconstituted as directed, the color of Antivenin ranges from light (straw) to very dark (iced tea), but the color has no effect on potency. *Do not freeze.*

REFERENCES

Barron, W. E.: Spider Bites, J. Med. Ass. Georgia *49:* 511-512, Oct. 1960.

Micks, D. W.: Insects and Other Arthropods of Medical Importance in Texas, Tex. Rep. Biol. & Med. *18:* 624-635, Winter 1960.

Prince, G. E.: Arachnidism in Children, J. Pediat. *49:* 101-108, July 1956.

Russell, F. E.: Injuries by Venomous Animals in the United States, J. Amer. Med. Ass. *177:* 903-907, Sept. 30, 1961.

Russell, F. E.: Muscle Relaxants in Black Widow Spider (Latrodectus mactans) Poisoning, Amer. J. Med. Sci. *243:* 159-162, Feb. 1962.

Russell, F. E.: Venom Poisoning, Rational Drug Therap. *5:* 5-6, Aug. 1971.

Merck Sharp & Dohme Corp., a subsidiary of
MERCK & CO., INC., Whitehouse Station, NJ 08889, USA
Revised: 05/2013
USPI-I-90011305R019

ASMANEX TWISTHALER ℞

[ăs-măn-ĕcks]
110 mcg, 220 mcg
(mometasone furoate inhalation powder)

HIGHLIGHTS OF PRESCRIBING INFORMATION
These highlights do not include all the information needed to use ASMANEX TWISTHALER safely and effectively. See full prescribing information for ASMANEX TWISTHALER.
ASMANEX TWISTHALER 110 mcg, 220 mcg (mometasone furoate inhalation powder)
Initial U.S. Approval: 1987

INDICATIONS AND USAGE

ASMANEX TWISTHALER is a corticosteroid indicated for:
- Maintenance treatment of asthma as prophylactic therapy in patients 4 years of age and older. (1.1)

ASMANEX TWISTHALER is NOT indicated for the relief of acute bronchospasm (1.1, 5.2) or in children less than 4 years of age (1.1, 8.4).

DOSAGE AND ADMINISTRATION

- FOR ORAL INHALATION ONLY. (2)
- Instruct patients to inhale rapidly and deeply and to rinse mouth after inhalation. (2)

[See table at top of next page]

DOSAGE FORMS AND STRENGTHS

- 220 mcg TWISTHALER: delivers 200 mcg mometasone furoate per actuation. (3)
- 110 mcg TWISTHALER: delivers 100 mcg mometasone furoate per actuation. (3)

CONTRAINDICATIONS

- Patients with status asthmaticus or other acute episodes of asthma where intensive measures are required. (4.1)
- Patients with a *known* hypersensitivity to milk proteins or any ingredients of ASMANEX TWISTHALER. (4.2)

WARNINGS AND PRECAUTIONS

- *Candida albicans* infection of the mouth and pharynx. Monitor patients periodically for signs of adverse effects in the mouth and pharynx.
  Advise patients to rinse mouth after inhalation. (5.1)
- Deterioration of asthma or acute episodes: ASMANEX TWISTHALER should not be used for relief of acute symptoms. Patients require immediate re-evaluation during rapidly deteriorating asthma. (5.2)
- Hypersensitivity reactions including anaphylaxis, angioedema, pruritus, and rash have been reported with the use of ASMANEX TWISTHALER. Discontinue ASMANEX TWISTHALER if such reactions occur. (5.3)
- Potential worsening of existing tuberculosis; fungal, bacterial, viral, or parasitic infection; or ocular herpes simplex. More serious or even fatal course of chickenpox or measles in susceptible patients. Use caution in patients with the above because of the potential for worsening of these infections. (5.4)
- Risk of impaired adrenal function when transferring from oral steroids to inhaled corticosteroids. Taper patients slowly from systemic corticosteroids if transferring to ASMANEX TWISTHALER. (5.5)
- Hypercorticism, suppression of hypothalamic-pituitary-adrenal (HPA) function, with very high dosages or at the regular dosage in susceptible individuals. If such changes occur discontinue ASMANEX TWISTHALER slowly. (5.6)
- Reduction in bone mineral density with long-term administration. Monitor patients with major risk factors for decreased bone mineral content. (5.7)
- Suppression of growth in children. Monitor growth routinely in pediatric patients receiving ASMANEX TWISTHALER. (5.8)
- Development of glaucoma, increased intraocular pressure, and posterior subcapsular cataracts. Monitor patients with a change in vision or with a history of increased intraocular pressure, glaucoma, and/or cataracts closely. (5.9)
- Paradoxical bronchospasm may occur with ASMANEX TWISTHALER. Treat bronchospasm immediately with a fast-acting inhaled bronchodilator and discontinue use of ASMANEX TWISTHALER. (5.10)

ADVERSE REACTIONS

The most common adverse reactions (incidence ≥5%) are headache, allergic rhinitis, pharyngitis, upper respiratory tract infection, sinusitis, oral candidiasis, dysmenorrhea, musculoskeletal pain, back pain, and dyspepsia. (6.1)

To report SUSPECTED ADVERSE REACTIONS, contact Merck Sharp & Dohme Corp., a subsidiary of Merck & Co., Inc., at 1-877-888-4231 or FDA at 1-800-FDA-1088 or www.fda.gov/medwatch.

See 17 for PATIENT COUNSELING INFORMATION and FDA-approved patient labeling

Revised: 01/2013

FULL PRESCRIBING INFORMATION: CONTENTS*

*** Sections or subsections omitted from the full prescribing information are not listed**

Recommended Dosages for ASMANEX TWISTHALER Treatment

Previous Therapy	Recommended Starting Dose	Highest Recommended Daily Dose
Patients ≥12 years who received bronchodilators alone	220 mcg once daily in the evening*	440 mcg†
Patients ≥12 years who received inhaled corticosteroids	220 mcg once daily in the evening*	440 mcg†
Patients ≥12 years who received oral corticosteroids‡	440 mcg twice daily	880 mcg
Children 4-11 years of age§	110 mcg once daily in the evening*	110 mcg*

*,†,‡,§Please refer to section 2.1 for full dosage recommendations and details.

Table 1: Recommended Dosages for ASMANEX TWISTHALER Treatment

Previous Therapy	Recommended Starting Dose	Highest Recommended Daily Dose
Patients ≥12 years who received bronchodilators alone	220 mcg once daily in the evening*	440 mcg†
Patients ≥12 years who received inhaled corticosteroids	220 mcg once daily in the evening*	440 mcg†
Patients ≥12 years who received oral corticosteroids‡	440 mcg twice daily	880 mcg
Children 4-11 years of age§	110 mcg once daily in the evening*	110 mcg*

* When administered once daily, ASMANEX TWISTHALER should be taken only in the evening.
† The 440 mcg daily dose may be administered in divided doses of 220 mcg twice daily or as 440 mcg once daily.
‡ **For Patients Currently Receiving Chronic Oral Corticosteroid Therapy:** Prednisone should be reduced no faster than 2.5 mg/day on a weekly basis, beginning after at least 1 week of ASMANEX TWISTHALER therapy. Monitor patients carefully for signs of asthma instability, including serial objective measures of airflow, and for signs of adrenal insufficiency during steroid taper and following discontinuation of oral corticosteroid therapy *[see Warnings and Precautions (5.5)]*.
§ Recommended pediatric dosage is 110 mcg once daily in the evening regardless of prior therapy.

FULL PRESCRIBING INFORMATION

1 INDICATIONS AND USAGE

1.1 Treatment of Asthma

ASMANEX® TWISTHALER® is indicated for the maintenance treatment of asthma as prophylactic therapy in patients 4 years of age and older.

Important Limitations of Use

ASMANEX TWISTHALER is NOT indicated for the relief of acute bronchospasm.

ASMANEX TWISTHALER is NOT indicated in children less than 4 years of age.

2 DOSAGE AND ADMINISTRATION

Administer ASMANEX TWISTHALER by the orally inhaled route only. Instruct patients to inhale rapidly and deeply. Advise patients to rinse the mouth after inhalation. Individual patients will experience a variable time to onset and degree of symptom relief. Maximum benefit may not be achieved for 1 to 2 weeks or longer after initiation of treatment. After asthma stability has been achieved, it is desirable to titrate to the lowest effective dosage to reduce the possibility of side effects. For patients ≥12 years of age who do not respond adequately to the starting dose after 2 weeks of therapy, higher doses may provide additional asthma control. The safety and efficacy of ASMANEX TWISTHALER when administered in excess of recommended doses have not been established.

2.1 Recommended Dosages in Patients 4 Years of Age and Older

The recommended starting doses and highest recommended daily dose for ASMANEX TWISTHALER treatment based on prior asthma therapy are provided in **Table 1**.

[See table 1 above]

3 DOSAGE FORMS AND STRENGTHS

ASMANEX TWISTHALER is a dry powder for inhalation that is available in 2 strengths.

ASMANEX TWISTHALER 220 mcg delivers 200 mcg mometasone furoate per actuation from the mouthpiece.

ASMANEX TWISTHALER 110 mcg delivers 100 mcg mometasone furoate per actuation from the mouthpiece.

4 CONTRAINDICATIONS

4.1 Status Asthmaticus

ASMANEX TWISTHALER therapy is contraindicated in the primary treatment of status asthmaticus or other acute episodes of asthma where intensive measures are required.

4.2 Hypersensitivity

ASMANEX TWISTHALER is contraindicated in patients with *known* hypersensitivity to milk proteins or any ingredients of ASMANEX TWISTHALER *[see Warnings and Precautions (5.3) and Description (11)]*.

5 WARNINGS AND PRECAUTIONS

5.1 Local Effects

In clinical trials, the development of localized infections of the mouth and pharynx with *Candida albicans* occurred in 195 of 3007 patients treated with ASMANEX TWISTHALER. If oropharyngeal candidiasis develops, it should be treated with appropriate local or systemic (i.e., oral) antifungal therapy while remaining on treatment with ASMANEX TWISTHALER therapy, but at times therapy with the ASMANEX TWISTHALER may need to be interrupted. Advise patients to rinse the mouth after inhalation of ASMANEX TWISTHALER.

5.2 Acute Asthma Episodes

ASMANEX TWISTHALER is not a bronchodilator and is not indicated for rapid relief of bronchospasm or other acute episodes of asthma. Instruct patients to contact their physician immediately if episodes of asthma that are not responsive to bronchodilators occur during the course of treatment with ASMANEX TWISTHALER. During such episodes, patients may require therapy with oral corticosteroids.

5.3 Hypersensitivity Reactions Including Anaphylaxis

Hypersensitivity reactions including rash, pruritus, angioedema, and anaphylactic reaction have been reported with use of ASMANEX TWISTHALER. Discontinue ASMANEX TWISTHALER if such reactions occur *[see Contraindications (4.2) and Postmarketing Experience (6.2)]*.

ASMANEX TWISTHALER contains small amounts of lactose, which contains trace levels of milk proteins. In postmarketing experience with ASMANEX TWISTHALER, anaphylactic reactions in patients with milk protein allergy have been reported *[see Contraindications (4.2) and Postmarketing Experience (6.2)]*.

5.4 Immunosuppression

Persons who are using drugs that suppress the immune system are more susceptible to infections than healthy individuals. Chickenpox and measles, for example, can have a more serious or even fatal course in susceptible children or adults using corticosteroids. In such children or adults who have not had these diseases or who are not properly immunized, particular care should be taken to avoid exposure. How the dose, route, and duration of corticosteroid administration affect the risk of developing a disseminated infection is not known. The contribution of the underlying disease and/or prior corticosteroid treatment to the risk is also not known. If exposed to chickenpox, prophylaxis with varicella zoster immune globulin (VZIG) may be indicated. If exposed to measles, prophylaxis with pooled intramuscular immunoglobulin (IG) may be indicated. (See the respective package inserts for complete VZIG and IG prescribing information.) If chickenpox develops, treatment with antiviral agents may be considered.

Inhaled corticosteroids should be used with caution, if at all, in patients with active or quiescent tuberculosis infection of the respiratory tract; untreated systemic fungal, bacterial, viral, or parasitic infections; or ocular herpes simplex.

5.5 Transferring Patients from Systemic Corticosteroid Therapy

Particular care is needed for patients who are transferred from systemically active corticosteroids to ASMANEX TWISTHALER because deaths due to adrenal insufficiency have occurred in asthmatic patients during and after transfer from systemic corticosteroids to less systemically available inhaled corticosteroids. After withdrawal from systemic corticosteroids, a number of months are required for recovery of hypothalamic-pituitary-adrenal (HPA) function.

Patients who have been previously maintained on 20 mg or more per day of prednisone (or its equivalent) may be most susceptible, particularly when their systemic corticosteroids have been almost completely withdrawn. During this period of HPA suppression, patients may exhibit signs and symptoms of adrenal insufficiency when exposed to trauma, surgery, or infection (particularly gastroenteritis) or other conditions associated with severe electrolyte loss. Although ASMANEX TWISTHALER may improve control of asthma symptoms during these episodes, in recommended doses it supplies less than normal physiological amounts of corticosteroid systemically and does NOT provide the mineralocorticoid activity necessary for coping with these emergencies.

During periods of stress or severe asthma attack, patients who have been withdrawn from systemic corticosteroids should be instructed to resume oral corticosteroids (in large doses) immediately and to contact their physicians for further instruction. These patients should also be instructed to carry a medical identification card indicating that they may need supplementary systemic corticosteroids during periods of stress or severe asthma attack.

Patients requiring oral corticosteroids should be weaned slowly from systemic corticosteroid use after transferring to ASMANEX TWISTHALER. Prednisone reduction can be accomplished by reducing the daily prednisone dose by 2.5 mg on a weekly basis during treatment with ASMANEX TWISTHALER *[see Dosage and Administration (2.1)]*. Lung function (FEV_1 or PEFR), beta-agonist use, and asthma

Table 2: Adverse Reactions with ≥3% Incidence in 10 Controlled Clinical Trials with ASMANEX TWISTHALER in Patients 12 Years of Age and Older Previously on Bronchodilators and/or Inhaled Corticosteroids

	(%) of Patients			
	ASMANEX TWISTHALER			
Adverse Reaction	220 mcg twice daily (n=433)	440 mcg once daily (n=497)	220 mcg once daily in the evening (n=232)	Placebo (n=720)
Headache	22	17	20	20
Allergic Rhinitis	15	11	14	13
Pharyngitis	11	8	13	7
Upper Respiratory Infection	10	8	15	7
Sinusitis	6	6	5	5
Candidiasis, oral	6	4	4	2
Dysmenorrhea*	9	4	4	4
Musculoskeletal Pain	8	4	4	5
Back Pain	6	3	3	4
Dyspepsia	5	3	3	3
Myalgia	3	2	3	2
Abdominal Pain	3	2	3	2
Nausea	3	1	3	2
Average Duration of Exposure (Days)	81	70	80	62

* Percentages are based on the number of female patients.

symptoms should be carefully monitored during withdrawal of oral corticosteroids. In addition to monitoring asthma signs and symptoms, patients should be observed for signs and symptoms of adrenal insufficiency such as fatigue, lassitude, weakness, nausea and vomiting, and hypotension.

Transfer of patients from systemic corticosteroid therapy to ASMANEX TWISTHALER may unmask allergic conditions previously suppressed by the systemic corticosteroid therapy, e.g., rhinitis, conjunctivitis, eczema, arthritis, and eosinophilic conditions.

During withdrawal from oral corticosteroids, some patients may experience symptoms of systemically active corticosteroid withdrawal, e.g., joint and/or muscular pain, lassitude, and depression, despite maintenance or even improvement of respiratory function.

5.6 Hypercorticism and Adrenal Suppression

ASMANEX TWISTHALER will often help control asthma symptoms with less suppression of HPA function than therapeutically similar oral doses of prednisone. Since individual sensitivity to effects on cortisol production exists, physicians should consider this information when prescribing ASMANEX TWISTHALER. Particular care should be taken in observing patients postoperatively or during periods of stress for evidence of inadequate adrenal response. It is possible that systemic corticosteroid effects such as hypercorticism and adrenal suppression may appear in a small number of patients, particularly when ASMANEX TWISTHALER is administered at higher than recommended doses over prolonged periods of time. If such effects occur, the dosage of ASMANEX TWISTHALER should be reduced slowly, consistent with accepted procedures for reducing systemic corticosteroids and for management of asthma.

5.7 Reduction in Bone Mineral Density

Decreases in bone mineral density (BMD) have been observed with long-term administration of products containing inhaled corticosteroids, including mometasone furoate. The clinical significance of small changes in BMD with regard to long-term outcomes is unknown. Patients with major risk factors for decreased bone mineral content, such as prolonged immobilization, family history of osteoporosis, or chronic use of drugs that can reduce bone mass (e.g., anticonvulsants and corticosteroids) should be monitored and treated with established standards of care.

In a 2-year double-blind study in 103 male and female asthma patients 18 to 50 years of age previously maintained on bronchodilator therapy (baseline FEV_1 85%–88% predicted), treatment with ASMANEX TWISTHALER 220 mcg twice daily resulted in significant reductions in lumbar spine (LS) BMD at the end of the treatment period compared to placebo. The mean change from baseline to endpoint in the lumbar spine BMD was -0.015 (-1.43%) for the ASMANEX TWISTHALER group compared to 0.002 (0.25%) for the placebo group. In another 2-year double-blind study in 87 male and female asthma patients 18 to 50 years of age previously maintained on bronchodilator therapy (baseline FEV_1 82%–83% predicted), treatment with ASMANEX TWISTHALER 440 mcg twice daily demonstrated no statistically significant changes in lumbar spine BMD at the end of the treatment period compared to placebo. The mean change from baseline to endpoint in the lumbar spine BMD was -0.018 (-1.57%) for the ASMANEX TWISTHALER group compared to -0.006 (-0.43%) for the placebo group.

5.8 Effect on Growth

Orally inhaled corticosteroids, including ASMANEX TWISTHALER, may cause a reduction in growth velocity when administered to pediatric patients. Monitor the growth of pediatric patients receiving ASMANEX TWISTHALER routinely (e.g., via stadiometry). To minimize the systemic effects of orally inhaled corticosteroids, including ASMANEX TWISTHALER, titrate each patient's dose to the lowest dosage that effectively controls his/her symptoms *[see Use in Specific Populations (8.4)]*.

5.9 Glaucoma and Cataracts

In clinical trials, glaucoma, increased intraocular pressure, and cataracts have been reported in 8 of 3007 patients following the administration of ASMANEX TWISTHALER. Close monitoring is warranted in patients with a change in vision or with a history of increased intraocular pressure, glaucoma, and/or cataracts.

5.10 Paradoxical Bronchospasm

As with other inhaled asthma medications, bronchospasm may occur with an immediate increase in wheezing after dosing. If bronchospasm occurs following dosing with ASMANEX TWISTHALER, it should be treated immediately with a fast-acting inhaled bronchodilator.

Treatment with ASMANEX TWISTHALER should be discontinued and alternative therapy instituted.

6 ADVERSE REACTIONS

Systemic and local corticosteroid use may result in the following:

- *Candida albicans* infection *[see Warnings and Precautions (5.1)]*
- Immunosuppression *[see Warnings and Precautions (5.4)]*
- Hypercorticism and adrenal suppression *[see Warnings and Precautions (5.6)]*
- Growth effects *[see Warnings and Precautions (5.8) and Use in Specific Populations (8.4)]*
- Glaucoma and cataracts *[see Warnings and Precautions (5.9)]*

6.1 Clinical Studies Experience

The safety data described below reflect exposure to ASMANEX TWISTHALER in 2380 patients with asthma exposed for 8 to 12 weeks and 627 patients with asthma exposed for 1 year in a total of 17 clinical trials.

In adult and adolescent patients 12 years of age and older, ASMANEX TWISTHALER was studied in 10 placebo-controlled clinical trials of 8 to 12 weeks duration with a total of 1750 patients receiving ASMANEX TWISTHALER. There were also 3 trials with a total of 475 patients receiving ASMANEX TWISTHALER for 1 year. In the 8- to 12-week clinical trials, the population was 12 to 83 years of age; 38% males and 62% females; and 83% Caucasian, 8% black, 6% Hispanic, and 3% other race/ethnicity. Patients received ASMANEX TWISTHALER 110 mcg twice daily (n=133), 220 mcg once daily in the morning (n=209), 220 mcg once daily in the evening (n=232), 220 mcg twice daily (n=433), 440 mcg once daily in the morning (n=419), 440 mcg once daily in the evening (n=250), or 440 mcg twice daily (n=74). In 3 long-term safety trials (two 9-month extensions of efficacy trials and one 52-week active-controlled safety trial), 475 patients with asthma (12-83 years of age, 44% males, 56% females, 87% Caucasian, 8% black, 4% Hispanic, and 1% other race/ethnicity) received various doses of ASMANEX TWISTHALER for 1 year.

In pediatric patients 4 to 11 years of age, ASMANEX TWISTHALER was studied in 3 placebo-controlled clinical trials of 12 weeks duration with a total of 630 patients receiving ASMANEX TWISTHALER and a 52-week, active-controlled safety trial with a total of 152 patients receiving ASMANEX TWISTHALER. In the 12-week clinical trials, the population was 4 to 11 years of age; 63% males and 37% females; and 67% Caucasian, 13% black, 17% Hispanic, and 3% other race/ethnicity. Patients received ASMANEX TWISTHALER 110 mcg once daily in the evening (n=98), 110 mcg once daily in the morning (n=181), 110 mcg twice daily (n=179), or 220 mcg once daily in the morning (n=172). In the long-term active-controlled safety trial (n=152), patients with asthma (4 to 11 years of age, 60% males and 40% females, 84% Caucasian, 11% Black, and 5% Hispanic) received ASMANEX TWISTHALER 110 mcg twice daily or 220 mcg once daily in the morning for 52 weeks.

Because clinical trials are conducted under widely varying conditions, adverse reaction rates observed in the clinical trials of a drug cannot be directly compared to rates in the clinical trials of another drug and may not reflect the rates observed in practice.

Adults and Adolescents 12 Years of Age and Older: The safety results of the 10 trials that were 8 to 12 weeks in duration were pooled because patients with asthma in these studies were previously maintained on bronchodilators and/or inhaled corticosteroids. The safety results of the one 12-week clinical trial in patients with asthma previously treated with oral corticosteroids are presented separately.

In the pooled 8- to 12-week clinical trials, adverse reactions were reported in 70% of patients treated with ASMANEX TWISTHALER (n=1750) compared to 65% of patients taking placebo (n=720). **Table 2** displays the common adverse reactions (≥3% in any patient group receiving ASMANEX TWISTHALER) that occurred more frequently in patients treated with ASMANEX TWISTHALER compared to patients treated with placebo.

[See table 2 above]

The following other adverse reactions occurred in these clinical trials with an incidence of at least 1% but less than 3% and were more common on ASMANEX TWISTHALER therapy than on placebo:

Body as a Whole: fatigue, flu-like symptoms, pain
Gastrointestinal: gastroenteritis, vomiting, anorexia
Hearing, Vestibular: earache
Resistance Mechanism: infection
Respiratory: dysphonia, epistaxis, nasal irritation, respiratory disorder, throat dry

In the 12-week trial in adult asthmatics who previously required oral corticosteroids, the effects of ASMANEX TWISTHALER therapy administered as two 220-mcg inhalations twice daily (n=46) were compared with those of placebo (n=43). Adverse reactions, whether considered drug-related or not by the investigators, reported in more than 3 patients in the ASMANEX TWISTHALER treatment group, and which occurred more frequently than in placebo were (ASMANEX TWISTHALER % vs. placebo %): musculoskeletal pain (22% vs. 14%), oral candidiasis (22% vs. 9%), sinusitis (22% vs. 19%), allergic rhinitis (20% vs. 5%), upper respiratory infection (15% vs. 14%), arthralgia (13% vs. 7%), fatigue (13% vs. 2%), depression (11% vs. 0%), and sinus congestion (9% vs. 0%). In considering these data, an increased duration of exposure for patients on ASMANEX TWISTHALER treatment (77 days vs. 58 days on placebo) should be taken into account.

Long-Term Clinical Trials Experience - 12 Years of Age and Older: In 3 long-term safety trials, 475 patients with asthma 12 years of age and older were treated with ASMANEX TWISTHALER 220 mcg twice daily (n=60), 220 mcg once daily in the morning (n=41), 220 mcg once daily in the evening (n=40), 440 mcg once daily in the morning (n=44), 440 mcg once daily in the evening (n=41), 440 mcg twice daily (n=62), 880 mcg once daily (n=59), or at variable doses (n=128) for 52 weeks. The safety profile of

ASMANEX TWISTHALER in the 52-week trials was similar to the findings in the 8- to 12-week clinical trials. In patients previously on inhaled corticosteroids, cataracts were reported in 3 patients (0.9%) treated with ASMANEX TWISTHALER, compared to 1 patient (1.7%) treated with the active comparator medication. Increased ocular pressure at the end of the study was observed in 2 patients, both on ASMANEX TWISTHALER 880 mcg once daily in the morning. Oral candidiasis, dysphonia, and dysmenorrhea were seen at a higher frequency with long-term administration than in the 8- to 12-week trials.

Pediatric Patients 4 to 11 Years of Age: In the three 12-week clinical trials in pediatric patients 4 to 11 years of age, patients with asthma were previously maintained on bronchodilators and/or inhaled corticosteroids. The safety results from 1 trial are described in **Table 3** for ASMANEX TWISTHALER 110 mcg once daily in the evening. The safety results from the other 2 trials showed similar findings.

Overall adverse reactions were reported with approximately the same frequency by patients treated with ASMANEX TWISTHALER and those receiving placebo. **Table 3** displays the common adverse reactions (≥2% in any patient group receiving ASMANEX TWISTHALER) that occurred more frequently in patients 4 to 11 years of age treated with ASMANEX TWISTHALER compared with placebo-treated patients.

Table 3: Adverse Reactions with ≥2% Incidence in a 12-Week Study with ASMANEX TWISTHALER in Patients 4 to 11 Years of Age Previously on Bronchodilators and/or Inhaled Corticosteroids

	(%) of Patients	
	ASMANEX TWISTHALER	
Adverse Reaction	110 mcg once daily in the evening (n=98)	Placebo (n=99)
Fever	7	5
Allergic Rhinitis	4	3
Abdominal Pain	6	2
Vomiting	3	2
Urinary Tract Infection	2	1
Bruise	2	0
Average Duration of Exposure (Days)	72	68

Long-Term Clinical Trials Experience in Children 4 to 11 Years of Age: In a 52-week, active-controlled, long-term safety trial, 152 patients with asthma 4 to 11 years of age were treated with ASMANEX TWISTHALER 110 mcg twice daily (n=74) or 220 mcg once daily (n=78). The safety profile for ASMANEX TWISTHALER in the 52-week trial was similar to the findings in the 12-week clinical trials.

6.2 Postmarketing Experience

The following adverse reactions have been reported during post-approval use of ASMANEX TWISTHALER. Because they are reported voluntarily from a population of uncertain size, it is not always possible to reliably estimate their frequency or establish a causal relationship to drug exposure.

Immune System Disorders: Immediate and delayed hypersensitivity reactions including rash, pruritus, angioedema and anaphylactic reaction *[see Warnings and Precautions (5.3) and Contraindications (4.2)]*.

Respiratory, Thoracic and Mediastinal Disorders: Asthma aggravation, which may include cough, dyspnea, wheezing and bronchospasm.

7 DRUG INTERACTIONS

In clinical studies, the concurrent administration of ASMANEX TWISTHALER and other drugs commonly used in the treatment of asthma was not associated with any unusual adverse reactions.

7.1 Inhibitors of Cytochrome P450 3A4

Ketoconazole, a strong inhibitor of cytochrome P450 3A4, may increase plasma levels of mometasone furoate during concomitant dosing *[see Clinical Pharmacology (12.3)]*.

8 USE IN SPECIFIC POPULATIONS

8.1 Pregnancy

Pregnancy Category C:

There are no adequate and well-controlled studies of ASMANEX TWISTHALER use in pregnant women. Animal reproduction studies in mice, rats, and rabbits revealed evidence of teratogenicity. Asthma is a serious and potentially life-threatening condition. Poorly controlled asthma during pregnancy is associated with adverse outcomes for mother and fetus. ASMANEX TWISTHALER should be used during pregnancy only if the potential benefit justifies the potential risk to the fetus.

There is a natural increase in corticosteroid production during pregnancy; therefore, most women require a lower exogenous corticosteroid dose and may not need corticosteroid treatment during pregnancy. Infants born to mothers taking substantial oral corticosteroid doses during pregnancy should be monitored for signs of hypoadrenalism.

When administered to pregnant mice, rats, and rabbits, mometasone furoate increased fetal malformations and decreased fetal growth (measured by lower fetal weights and/or delayed ossification). Dystocia and related complications were also observed when mometasone furoate was administered to rats late in gestation. However, experience with oral corticosteroids suggests that rodents are more prone to teratogenic effects from corticosteroid exposure than humans.

In a mouse reproduction study, subcutaneous mometasone furoate produced cleft palate at approximately one-third of the maximum recommended daily human dose (MRHD) for adults on an mcg/m^2 basis and decreased fetal survival at approximately 1 times the MRHD. No toxicity was observed at approximately one-tenth of the MRHD.

In a rat reproduction study, mometasone furoate produced umbilical hernia at topical dermal doses approximately 6 times the MRHD and delays in ossification at approximately 3 times the MRHD.

In another study, rats received subcutaneous doses of mometasone throughout pregnancy or late in gestation. Treated animals had prolonged and difficult labor, fewer live births, lower birth weight, and reduced early pup survival at a dose that was approximately 6 times the MRHD for adults on an area under the curve (AUC) basis. Similar effects were not observed at approximately 3 times the MRHD.

In rabbits, mometasone furoate caused multiple malformations (e.g., flexed front paws, gallbladder agenesis, umbilical hernia, hydrocephaly) at topical dermal doses approximately 3 times the maximum recommended daily inhalation dose in adults on an mcg/m^2 basis. In an oral study, mometasone furoate increased resorptions and caused cleft palate and/or head malformations (hydrocephaly and domed head) at a dose less than the MRHD for adults based on AUC. At a dose approximately 2 times the MRHD in adults based on AUC, most litters were aborted or resorbed *[see Nonclinical Toxicology (13.2)]*.

8.3 Nursing Mothers

Systemic absorption of a single inhaled 400 mcg mometasone dose was less than 1%. It is not known if mometasone furoate is excreted in human milk. Because other corticosteroids are excreted in human milk, caution should be used when ASMANEX TWISTHALER is administered to nursing women.

8.4 Pediatric Use

The safety and effectiveness of ASMANEX TWISTHALER have been established in children 4 years of age and older. Use of ASMANEX TWISTHALER in children 12 years of age and older is supported by evidence from adequate and well-controlled clinical trials in this patient population *[see Clinical Studies (14.1) and Adverse Reactions (6.1)]*.

Use of ASMANEX TWISTHALER in pediatric patients 4 to 11 years of age is supported by evidence from adequate and well-controlled clinical trials of 12 weeks duration in 630 patients 4 to 11 years of age receiving ASMANEX TWISTHALER and one 52-week safety trial in 152 patients *[see Clinical Studies (14.1) and Adverse Reactions (6.1)]*.

Controlled clinical studies have shown that inhaled corticosteroids may cause a reduction in growth in pediatric patients. In these studies, the mean reduction in growth velocity was approximately 1 cm per year (range: 0.3–1.8 per year) and appears to depend upon dose and duration of exposure. This effect was observed in the absence of laboratory evidence of HPA axis suppression, suggesting that growth velocity is a more sensitive indicator of systemic corticosteroid exposure in pediatric patients than some commonly used tests of HPA axis function. The long-term effects of this reduction in growth velocity associated with orally inhaled corticosteroids, including the impact on final adult height, are unknown. The potential for "catch-up" growth following discontinuation of treatment with orally inhaled corticosteroids has not been adequately studied. The growth of children and adolescents (4 years of age and older) receiving orally inhaled corticosteroids, including ASMANEX TWISTHALER, should be monitored routinely (e.g., via stadiometry).

A 52-week, placebo-controlled, parallel-group study was conducted to assess the potential growth effects of ASMANEX TWISTHALER in 187 prepubescent children (131 males and 56 females) 4 to 9 years of age with asthma who were previously maintained on an inhaled beta-agonist. Treatment groups included ASMANEX TWISTHALER 110 mcg twice daily (n=44), 220 mcg once daily in the morning (n=50), 110 mcg once daily in the morning (n=48), and placebo (n=45). For each patient, an average growth rate was determined using an individual regression approach. The mean growth rates, expressed as least-squares mean in cm per year, for ASMANEX TWISTHALER 110 mcg twice daily, 220 mcg once daily in the morning, 110 mcg once daily in the morning, and placebo were 5.34, 5.93, 6.15, and 6.44, respectively. The differences from placebo and the corresponding 2-sided 95% CI of growth rates for ASMANEX TWISTHALER 110 mcg twice daily, 220 mcg once daily in the morning, and 110 mcg once daily in the morning were -1.11 (95% CI: -2.34, 0.12), -0.51 (95% CI: -1.69, 0.67), and -0.30 (95% CI: -1.48, 0.89), respectively.

The potential growth effects of prolonged treatment with orally inhaled corticosteroids should be weighed against clinical benefits obtained and the availability of safe and effective noncorticosteroid treatment alternatives. To minimize the systemic effects of orally inhaled corticosteroids, including ASMANEX TWISTHALER, each patient should be titrated to his/her lowest effective dose.

8.5 Geriatric Use

A total of 175 patients 65 years of age and over (23 of whom were 75 years of age and older) have been treated with ASMANEX TWISTHALER in controlled clinical trials. No overall differences in safety or effectiveness were observed between these and younger patients, and other reported clinical experience has not identified differences in responses between the elderly and younger patients, but greater sensitivity of some older individuals cannot be ruled out.

8.6 Hepatic Impairment

Concentrations of mometasone furoate appear to increase with severity of hepatic impairment *[see Clinical Pharmacology (12.3)]*.

10 OVERDOSAGE

Chronic overdosage may result in signs/symptoms of hypercorticism *[see Warnings and Precautions (5.6)]*. Because of low systemic bioavailability and an absence of acute drug-related systemic findings in clinical studies, acute overdose is unlikely to require any treatment other than observation. Single daily doses as high as 1200 mcg per day for 28 days were well tolerated and did not cause a significant reduction in plasma cortisol AUC (94% of placebo AUC). Single oral doses up to 8000 mcg have been studied on human volunteers with no adverse reactions reported.

11 DESCRIPTION

Mometasone furoate, the active component of the ASMANEX TWISTHALER product, is a corticosteroid with the chemical name 9,21-dichloro-11(Beta),17-dihydroxy-16(alpha)-methylpregna-1,4-diene-3,20-dione 17-(2-furoate) and the following chemical structure:

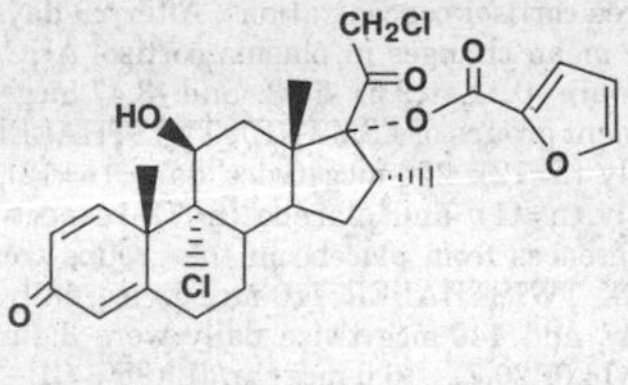

Mometasone furoate is a white powder with an empirical formula of $C_{27}H_{30}Cl_2O_6$, and molecular weight of 521.44 Daltons.

The ASMANEX TWISTHALER 110 mcg and 220 mcg products are cap-activated, inhalation-driven, multidose dry powder inhalers containing mometasone furoate and anhydrous lactose (which contains trace amounts of milk proteins).

Each actuation of the ASMANEX TWISTHALER 110 mcg or 220 mcg inhaler provides a measured dose of approximately 0.75 or 1.5 mg mometasone furoate inhalation powder, containing 110 or 220 mcg of mometasone furoate, respectively. This results in delivery of 100 or 200 mcg mometasone furoate from the mouthpiece, respectively, based on *in vitro* testing at flow rates of 30 L/min and 60 L/min with constant volume of 2 L. The amount of mometasone furoate emitted from the inhaler *in vitro* does not differ significantly for flow rates ranging from 28.3 L/min to 70 L/min at a constant volume of 2 L. However, the amount of drug delivered to the lung will depend on patient factors such as inspiratory flow and peak inspiratory flow through the device. In adult and adolescent patients (aged ≥12 years) with varied asthma severity, mean peak inspiratory flow rate through the device was 69 L/min (range: 54–77 L/min). In pediatric patients (aged 5-12 years) diagnosed with asthma, mean peak inspiratory flow rate in the 5- to 8-year-old subgroup was >50 L/min (minimum of 46 L/min) and for the 9- to 12-year-old subgroup was >60 L/min (minimum of 48 L/min).

12 CLINICAL PHARMACOLOGY

12.1 Mechanism of Action

Mometasone furoate is a corticosteroid demonstrating potent anti-inflammatory activity. The precise mechanism of corticosteroid action on asthma is not known. Inflammation is an important component in the pathogenesis of asthma. Corticosteroids have been shown to have a wide range of inhibitory effects on multiple cell types (e.g., mast cells, eosinophils, neutrophils, macrophages, and lymphocytes) and mediators (e.g., histamine, eicosanoids, leukotrienes, and cytokines) involved in inflammation and in the asthmatic response. These anti-inflammatory actions of corticosteroids may contribute to their efficacy in asthma.

Mometasone furoate has been shown *in vitro* to exhibit a binding affinity for the human glucocorticoid receptor, which is approximately 12 times that of dexamethasone, 7 times that of triamcinolone acetonide, 5 times that of budesonide, and 1.5 times that of fluticasone. The clinical significance of these findings is unknown.

Though effective for the treatment of asthma, corticosteroids do not affect asthma symptoms immediately. Maximum improvement in symptoms following inhaled administration of mometasone furoate may not be achieved for 1 to 2 weeks or longer after starting treatment. When corticosteroids are discontinued, asthma stability may persist for several days or longer.

12.2 Pharmacodynamics

Adrenal Function: The effects of ASMANEX TWISTHALER on adrenal function have been evaluated in 2 clinical studies: 1 in adults 18 years of age and older and 1 in pediatric patients 6 to 11 years of age. Both clinical studies were specifically designed to assess the effect of ASMANEX TWISTHALER on adrenal function.

In a 29-day, randomized, double-blind, placebo-controlled study in 64 adult and adolescent patients 18 years of age and older with asthma, ASMANEX TWISTHALER 440 mcg twice daily and 880 mcg twice daily (twice the highest recommended daily dose) were compared to both placebo and prednisone 10 mg once daily as a positive control. The 30-minute post-Cosyntropin stimulation serum cortisol concentration on Day 29 was 23.2 mcg/dL for the ASMANEX 440 mcg twice daily group (n=16) and 20.8 mcg/dL for the ASMANEX 880 mcg twice daily group (n=16), compared to 14.5 mcg/dL for the oral prednisone 10-mg group (n=16) and 25 mcg/dL for the placebo group (n=16). The difference between ASMANEX 880 mcg twice daily (twice the maximum recommended dose) and placebo was statistically significant.

In a 29-day, randomized, double-blind, placebo-controlled, parallel-group clinical trial in 50 pediatric patients 6 to 11 years of age with asthma, ASMANEX TWISTHALER 110 mcg twice daily, 220 mcg twice daily, and 440 mcg twice daily (2-8 times the highest pediatric daily recommended daily dose) were compared to placebo. HPA-axis function was assessed by 12-hour plasma cortisol AUC and 24-hour urinary-free cortisol concentrations. After 29 days of treatment, the mean changes in plasma cortisol AUC_{0-12h} from baseline were -0.11, -19.5, -21.3, and -3.47 mcg•hr/dL for the treatment groups of ASMANEX TWISTHALER 110 mcg twice daily (n=12), 220 mcg twice daily (n=12), 440 mcg twice daily (n=11), and placebo (n=7), respectively. The mean differences from placebo in the groups treated with ASMANEX TWISTHALER 110 mcg twice daily, 220 mcg twice daily, and 440 mcg twice daily were 3.4 mcg•hr/dL (95% CI: -14.0, 20.7), -16.0 mcg•hr/dL (95% CI: -33.9, 1.9), and -17.9 mcg•hr/dL (95% CI: -35.8, 0.0), respectively. For 24-hour urinary-free cortisol, after 29 days of treatment, the mean changes from baseline were -1.53, -1.33, -6.70, and -4.68 mcg/day for the groups treated with ASMANEX TWISTHALER 110 mcg twice daily (n=12), 220 mcg twice daily (n=12), 440 mcg twice daily (n=12), and placebo (n=10), respectively. The mean differences in urinary-free cortisol changes from baseline compared to placebo were 3.1 mcg/day (95% CI: -3.3, 9.6), 3.3 mcg/day (95% CI: -3.0, 9.7), and -2.0 mcg/day (95% CI: -8.6, 4.6) for the groups treated with 110 mcg twice daily, 220 mcg twice daily, and 440 mcg twice daily, respectively.

12.3 Pharmacokinetics

Absorption: Following a 1000 mcg inhaled dose of tritiated mometasone furoate inhalation powder to 6 healthy human subjects, plasma concentrations of unchanged mometasone furoate were shown to be very low compared to the total radioactivity in plasma. Following an inhaled single 400 mcg dose of ASMANEX TWISTHALER treatment to 24 healthy subjects, plasma concentrations for most subjects were near or below the lower limit of quantitation for the assay (50 pcg/mL). The mean absolute systemic bioavailability of the above single inhaled 400 mcg dose, compared to an intravenous 400 mcg dose of mometasone furoate, was determined to be less than 1%. Following administration of the recommended highest inhaled dose (400 mcg twice daily) to 64 patients for 28 days, concentration-time profiles were discernible, but with large intersubject variability. The coefficient of variation for C_{max} and AUC ranged from approximately 50% to 100%. The mean peak plasma concentrations at steady state ranged from approximately 94 to 114 pcg/mL and the mean time to peak levels ranged from approximately 1.0 to 2.5 hours.

Distribution: Based on the study employing a 1000 mcg inhaled dose of tritiated mometasone furoate inhalation powder in humans, no appreciable accumulation of mometasone furoate in the red blood cells was found. Following an intravenous 400 mcg dose of mometasone furoate, the plasma concentrations showed a biphasic decline, with a mean terminal half-life of about 5 hours and the mean steady-state volume of distribution of 152 L. The *in vitro* protein binding for mometasone furoate was reported to be 98% to 99% (in a concentration range of 5–500 ng/mL).

Metabolism: Studies have shown that mometasone furoate is primarily and extensively metabolized in the liver of all species investigated and undergoes extensive metabolism to multiple metabolites. *In vitro* studies have confirmed the primary role of CYP 3A4 in the metabolism of this compound; however, no major metabolites were identified.

Excretion: Following an intravenous dosing, the terminal half-life was reported to be about 5 hours. Following the inhaled dose of tritiated 1000 mcg mometasone furoate, the radioactivity is excreted mainly in the feces (a mean of 74%), and to a small extent in the urine (a mean of 8%) up to 7 days. No radioactivity was associated with unchanged mometasone furoate in the urine.

Special Populations:

Hepatic Impairment: Administration of a single inhaled dose of 400 mcg mometasone furoate to subjects with mild (n=4), moderate (n=4), and severe (n=4) hepatic impairment resulted in only 1 or 2 subjects in each group having detectable peak plasma concentrations of mometasone furoate (ranging from 50–105 pcg/mL). The observed peak plasma concentrations appear to increase with severity of hepatic impairment; however, the numbers of detectable levels were few.

Renal Impairment: The effects of renal impairment on mometasone furoate pharmacokinetics have not been adequately investigated.

Pediatric: Mometasone furoate pharmacokinetics have not been investigated in the pediatric population *[see Use in Specific Populations (8.4)]*.

Gender: The effects of gender on mometasone furoate pharmacokinetics have not been adequately investigated.

Race: The effects of race on mometasone furoate pharmacokinetics have not been adequately investigated.

Drug-Drug Interaction: *Inhibitors of Cytochrome P450 3A4:* In a drug interaction study, an inhaled dose of mometasone furoate 400 mcg was given to 24 healthy subjects twice daily for 9 days and ketoconazole 200 mg (as well as placebo) were given twice daily concomitantly on Days 4 to 9. Mometasone furoate plasma concentrations were <150 pcg/mL on Day 3 prior to coadministration of ketoconazole or placebo. Following concomitant administration of ketoconazole, 4 out of 12 subjects in the ketoconazole treatment group (n=12) had peak plasma concentrations of mometasone furoate >200 pcg/mL on Day 9 (211–324 pcg/mL).

13 NONCLINICAL TOXICOLOGY

13.1 Carcinogenesis, Mutagenesis, Impairment of Fertility

In a 2-year carcinogenicity study in Sprague Dawley® rats, mometasone furoate demonstrated no statistically significant increase in the incidence of tumors at inhalation doses up to 67 mcg/kg (approximately 8 times the maximum recommended daily inhalation dose in adults on an AUC basis and 2 times the maximum recommended daily inhalation dose in pediatric patients based on an mcg/m^2 basis). In a 19-month carcinogenicity study in Swiss CD-1 mice, mometasone furoate demonstrated no statistically significant increase in the incidence of tumors at inhalation doses up to 160 mcg/kg (approximately 10 times the maximum recommended daily inhalation dose in adults on an AUC basis and 2 times the maximum recommended daily inhalation dose in pediatric patients based on an mcg/m^2 basis).

Mometasone furoate increased chromosomal aberrations in an *in vitro* Chinese hamster ovary cell assay, but did not have this effect in an *in vitro* Chinese hamster lung cell assay. Mometasone furoate was not mutagenic in the Ames test or mouse lymphoma assay, and was not clastogenic in an *in vivo* mouse micronucleus assay, a rat bone marrow chromosomal aberration assay, or a mouse male germ-cell chromosomal aberration assay. Mometasone furoate also did not induce unscheduled DNA synthesis *in vivo* in rat hepatocytes.

In reproductive studies in rats, impairment of fertility was not produced by subcutaneous doses up to 15 mcg/kg (approximately 6 times the maximum recommended daily inhalation dose in adults on an AUC basis).

13.2 Animal Toxicology and/or Pharmacology

Reproductive Toxicology Studies: In mice, mometasone furoate caused cleft palate at subcutaneous doses of 60 mcg/kg and above (less than the maximum recommended daily inhalation dose in adults on an mcg/m^2 basis). Fetal survival was reduced at 180 mcg/kg (approximately equal to the maximum recommended daily inhalation dose in adults on an mcg/m^2 basis). No toxicity was observed at 20 mcg/kg (less than the maximum recommended daily inhalation dose in adults on an mcg/m^2 basis).

In rats, mometasone furoate produced umbilical hernia at topical dermal doses of 600 mcg/kg and above (approximately 6 times the maximum recommended daily inhalation dose in adults on an mcg/m^2 basis). A dose of 300 mcg/kg (approximately 3 times the maximum recommended daily inhalation dose in adults on an mcg/m^2 basis) produced delays in ossification but no malformations.

When rats received subcutaneous doses of mometasone furoate throughout pregnancy or during the later stages of pregnancy, 15 mcg/kg (approximately 6 times the maximum recommended daily inhalation dose in adults on an AUC basis) caused prolonged and difficult labor and reduced the number of live births, birth weight, and early pup survival. Similar effects were not observed at 7.5 mcg/kg (approximately 3 times the maximum recommended daily inhalation dose in adults on an AUC basis).

In rabbits, mometasone furoate caused multiple malformations (e.g., flexed front paws, gallbladder agenesis, umbilical hernia, hydrocephaly) at topical dermal doses of 150 mcg/kg and above (approximately 3 times the maximum recommended daily inhalation dose in adults on an mcg/m^2 basis). In an oral study, mometasone furoate increased resorptions and caused cleft palate and/or head malformations (hydrocephaly and domed head) at 700 mcg/kg (less than the maximum recommended daily inhalation dose in adults on an area under the curve [AUC] basis). At 2800 mcg/kg (approximately 2 times the maximum recommended daily inhalation dose in adults on an AUC basis) most litters were aborted or resorbed. No toxicity was observed at 140 mcg/kg (less than the maximum recommended daily inhalation dose in adults on an AUC basis).

14 CLINICAL STUDIES

14.1 Asthma

Adults and Adolescents 12 Years of Age and Older: The efficacy of ASMANEX TWISTHALER in patients with asthma 12 years and older was evaluated in ten 8- to 12-week, randomized, double-blind, placebo-controlled, parallel-group clinical trials. These trials included 1750 patients ranging from 12 to 83 years of age; 38% male and 62% female; and 83% Caucasian, 8% black, 6% Hispanic, and 3% other race/ethnicity. Patients received ASMANEX TWISTHALER 110 mcg twice daily (n=133), 220 mcg once daily in the morning (n=209), 220 mcg once daily in the evening (n=232), 220 mcg twice daily (n=433), 440 mcg once daily in the morning (n=419), 440 mcg once daily in the evening (n=250), or 440 mcg twice daily (n=74). The results of the clinical trials are presented based upon previous asthma therapy.

Patients ≥12 Years of Age Previously Maintained on Bronchodilators Alone: ASMANEX TWISTHALER was studied in three 12-week, double-blind trials in 737 patients with mild to moderate asthma (mean baseline FEV_1=2.6 L, 72% of predicted normal) who were maintained on short-acting $beta_2$-agonists alone. The first 2 trials evaluated doses of 440 mcg administered as 2 inhalations once daily in the morning and 1 of these studies also evaluated 220 mcg twice daily. In both trials, AM predose FEV_1 was significantly improved at endpoint (last observation) following treatment with 440 mcg ASMANEX TWISTHALER once daily in the morning as compared to placebo (14% vs. 2.5%, respectively, in 1 trial and 16% vs. 5.5% in the other). There was also a significant improvement in AM predose FEV_1 at endpoint following treatment with ASMANEX TWISTHALER 220 mcg twice daily. Other measures of lung function (AM and PM PEFR) also showed improvement compared to placebo. Patients receiving ASMANEX TWISTHALER treatment had reduced frequency of $beta_2$-agonist rescue medication use compared to those on placebo (mean reductions at endpoint 2.2 and 0.5 puffs per day, respectively, from a baseline of 4.1 puffs/day). Additionally, fewer patients receiving ASMANEX TWISTHALER 440 mcg once daily experienced asthma worsening than did patients receiving placebo.

In the third trial, 195 asthmatic patients were treated with ASMANEX TWISTHALER 220 mcg once daily in the evening or placebo. The AM FEV_1 at endpoint was significantly improved compared to placebo (mean change at endpoint 0.43 L or 16.8% vs. 0.16 L or 6%, respectively, see **Figure 1**). Evening PEF increased 24.96 L/min (7%) from baseline in the ASMANEX TWISTHALER group compared to 8.67 L/min (4%) in placebo.

FIGURE 1: A 12-Week Trial in Patients Previously Maintained on Inhaled Beta$_2$-agonists

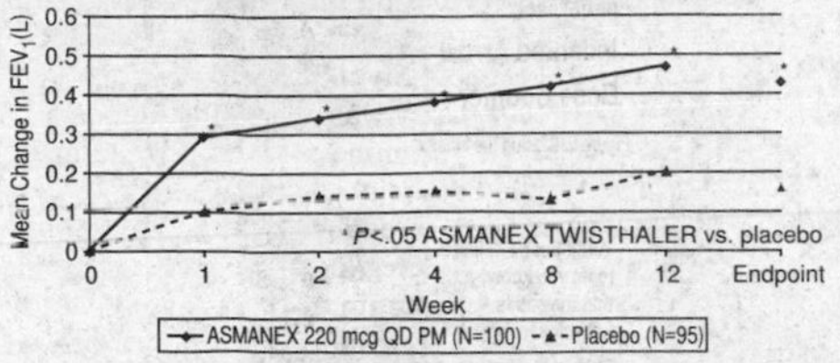

Patients ≥12 Years of Age Previously Maintained on Inhaled Corticosteroids: The efficacy and safety of ASMANEX TWISTHALER in doses ranging from 110 mcg twice daily to 440 mcg twice daily was evaluated in 3 trials in 1072 patients previously maintained on inhaled corticosteroids. In the first 2 trials, asthmatic patients (mean baseline FEV_1 ~2.6 L, 76% predicted) were previously on either beclomethasone dipropionate [84–1200 mcg/day], flunisolide [100–2000 mcg/day], fluticasone propionate [110–880 mcg/day], or triamcinolone acetonide [300–2400 mcg/day]. The first trial included 307 patients who were treated in an open-label fashion with ASMANEX TWISTHALER 220 mcg (110 mcg × 2 inhalations) twice daily for 2 weeks followed by 12 weeks of double-blind treatment with ASMANEX TWISTHALER 440 mcg once daily in the morning or placebo. The second trial involved 365 patients who continued on their previous dose of inhaled corticosteroids during a 2-week screening period before being switched to ASMANEX TWISTHALER 440 mcg twice daily, 220 mcg twice daily, 110 mcg twice daily, beclomethasone dipropionate 168 mcg twice daily, or placebo for 12 weeks.

In the first trial, AM predose FEV_1 was effectively maintained (-1.4% change from baseline to endpoint) over the 12 weeks in the patients who were randomized to ASMANEX TWISTHALER 440 mcg once daily in the morning, while decreasing 10% at endpoint in those switched to placebo. In addition, fewer patients treated with ASMANEX TWISTHALER experienced worsening of asthma compared to placebo.

In the second trial, AM predose FEV_1 was significantly increased at endpoint when patients were switched to ASMANEX TWISTHALER 220 mcg twice daily (7% increase) or 440 mcg twice daily (6.2% increase) as compared to a decrease of 7% when switched to placebo. Additionally, beta$_2$-agonist rescue medication use was decreased for patients who received ASMANEX TWISTHALER treatment relative to those on placebo (mean reduction from baseline to endpoint 1.1 puffs/day vs. increase of 0.7 puffs/day). Fewer patients receiving ASMANEX TWISTHALER treatment experienced asthma worsening than did patients receiving placebo.

The third trial evaluated the efficacy and safety of ASMANEX TWISTHALER compared to placebo in 400 asthmatic patients (mean FEV_1 67% predicted at baseline) previously maintained on beclomethasone dipropionate (hydrofluoroalkane [HFA] or chlorofluorocarbon [CFC]) 168–600 mcg/day, budesonide 200–1200 mcg/day, flunisolide 500–2000 mcg/day, fluticasone propionate 88–880 mcg/day, or triamcinolone acetonide 400–1600 mcg/day. Following a 28-day inhaled corticosteroid dose-reduction phase, patients were randomized to ASMANEX TWISTHALER 440 mcg once daily in the evening, 220 mcg once daily in the evening, 220 mcg twice daily, or placebo. At endpoint, patients who received ASMANEX TWISTHALER 220 mcg once daily in the evening, 440 mcg once daily in the evening, or 220 mcg twice daily had a significant improvement in AM FEV_1 [0.41 L (19%), 0.49 L (22%), and 0.51 L (24%) in the 220 mcg once daily in the evening, 440 mcg once daily in the evening, and 220 mcg twice daily treatment group, respectively] compared to placebo [0.16 L (8%)] (see **Figure 2**). Evening PEF increased 15.65 L/min (4.1%) with the 220 mcg once daily in the evening dose, 39.26 L/min (10.7%) with the 440 mcg once daily in the evening dose, and 36.7 L/min (10.8%) with the 220 mcg twice daily dose, respectively, compared to a 1.4 L/min (1%) increase with placebo. Patients receiving all doses of ASMANEX TWISTHALER treatment had reduced frequency of beta-agonist rescue medication use compared to those on placebo (mean reductions at endpoint of 1.4–1.8 puffs/day from a baseline of more than 3 puffs/day compared to an increase in use by 0.5 puffs/day for placebo). In addition, fewer patients receiving ASMANEX TWISTHALER experienced asthma worsening than did those on placebo.

FIGURE 2: A 12-Week Trial in Patients Previously Maintained on Inhaled Corticosteroids

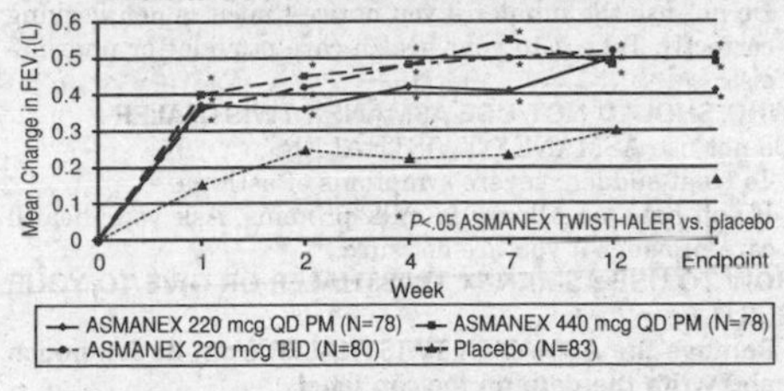

Patients ≥12 Years of Age Previously Maintained on Oral Corticosteroids: The efficacy of ASMANEX TWISTHALER 440 mcg and 880 mcg twice daily was evaluated in one 12-week, double-blind trial in patients previously maintained on oral corticosteroids. A total of 132 patients requiring oral prednisone (baseline mean daily oral prednisone requirement approximately 12 mg; baseline FEV_1 of 1.8 L, 59% of predicted normal), most of whom were also on inhaled corticosteroids (baseline inhaled steroid: beclomethasone dipropionate [168–840 mcg/day], budesonide [800–1600 mcg/day], flunisolide [1000–2000 mcg/day], fluticasone propionate [440–1760 mcg/day], or triamcinolone acetonide [400–2400 mcg/day]) were studied. Patients who received ASMANEX TWISTHALER 440 mcg twice daily had a significant reduction in their oral prednisone (46%) as compared to placebo (164% increase in oral prednisone dose). Additionally, 40% of patients on ASMANEX TWISTHALER 440 mcg twice daily were able to completely discontinue their use of prednisone, whereas 60% of patients on placebo had an increase in daily prednisone use. Patients on ASMANEX TWISTHALER had significant improvement in lung function (14% increase) compared to a 12% decrease in FEV_1 in the placebo group. Additionally, mean rescue beta$_2$-agonist use was reduced to approximately 3 puffs/day from a baseline of 4–5 puffs/day with ASMANEX TWISTHALER treatment, compared to an increase of 0.3 puffs/day on placebo. Patients who received ASMANEX TWISTHALER 880 mcg twice daily experienced no additional benefit beyond that seen with 440 mcg twice daily.

Pediatric Patients 4 to 11 Years of Age: The efficacy of ASMANEX TWISTHALER in patients with asthma 4 to 11 years of age was evaluated in three 12-week, randomized, double-blind, placebo-controlled, parallel-group clinical trials. These trials included 630 patients receiving ASMANEX TWISTHALER, ranging from 4 to 11 years of age; 63% male and 37% female; and 67% Caucasian, 13% black, 17% Hispanic, and 3% other race/ethnicity. Patients received ASMANEX TWISTHALER 110 mcg once daily in the evening (n=98), 110 mcg once daily in the morning (n=181), 110 mcg twice daily (n=179), or 220 mcg once daily in the morning (n=172). The results for 1 clinical trial are described below. The other 2 clinical trials support the efficacy of ASMANEX TWISTHALER.

A 12-week, placebo-controlled trial of 296 patients 4 to 11 years of age with asthma of at least 6 months duration (mean % predicted FEV_1 at baseline ranging from 77.3%–79.7%) was conducted to demonstrate the efficacy of the ASMANEX TWISTHALER in the treatment of asthma. Patients were treated with ASMANEX TWISTHALER 110 mcg once daily in the evening (n=98) or placebo (n=99) for 12 weeks. Assessment of efficacy was based upon morning predose FEV_1. The primary endpoint was the mean change from baseline to endpoint in percent-predicted FEV_1. For the primary endpoint, improvement in the ASMANEX TWISTHALER 110 mcg once daily in the evening treatment group (4.73) was statistically significant compared to placebo (-1.77). **Figure 3** displays the results for % predicted FEV_1 change from baseline at endpoint.

In this study, secondary endpoints of morning and evening peak expiratory flow and rescue medication use were supportive of efficacy of ASMANEX TWISTHALER.

FIGURE 3: A 12-Week Trial in Children 4 to 11 Years of Age: % Predicted FEV_1 Change from Baseline Over Time and at Endpoint by Treatment Group

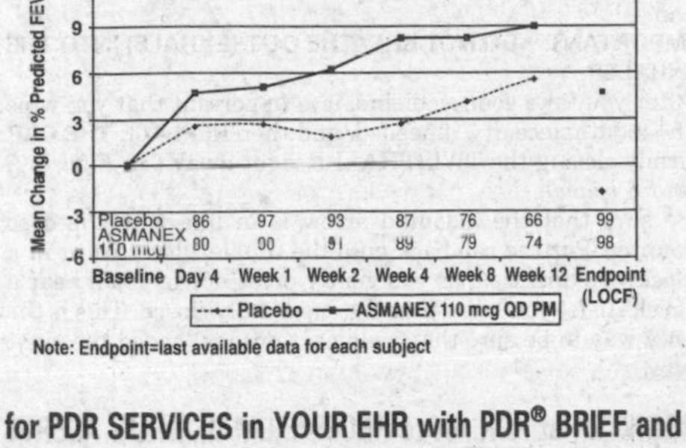

Note: Endpoint=last available data for each subject

16 HOW SUPPLIED/STORAGE AND HANDLING

The ASMANEX TWISTHALER 220 mcg product is comprised of an assembled plastic cap–activated dosing mechanism with dose counter, drug-product storage unit, drug-product formulation (135 mg for the 14 and 30 inhalation units and 240 mg for the 60 and 120 inhalation units), and mouthpiece, covered by a white screw cap that bears the product label. The body of the inhaler is white and the turning grip is pink with a clear plastic window indicating the number of doses remaining. The inhaler will not deliver subsequent doses once the counter reaches zero ("00").

The ASMANEX TWISTHALER 110 mcg product is comprised of an assembled plastic cap–activated dosing mechanism with dose counter, drug-product storage unit, drug-product formulation (135 mg), and mouthpiece, covered by a white screw cap that bears the product label. The body of the inhaler is white and the turning grip is gray with a clear plastic window indicating the number of doses remaining. The inhaler will not deliver subsequent doses once the counter reaches zero ("00").

The ASMANEX TWISTHALER product is available as:

ASMANEX TWISTHALER 220 mcg, which delivers 200 mcg mometasone furoate from the mouthpiece: 14 inhalation units (Institutional Use Only; NDC# 0085-1341-04 and NDC# 0085-1341-06); 30 inhalation units (NDC# 0085-1341-03 and NDC# 0085-1341-07); 60 inhalation units (for more than 1 inhalation daily; NDC# 0085-1341-02); or 120 inhalation units (for more than 2 inhalations daily; NDC# 0085-1341-01).

ASMANEX TWISTHALER 110 mcg, which delivers 100 mcg mometasone furoate from the mouthpiece: 7 inhalation units (Institutional Use Only; NDC# 0085-1461-07); 30 inhalation units (NDC# 0085-1461-02).

Each inhaler is supplied in a protective foil pouch with Patient's Instructions for Use.

Store in a dry place at 25°C (77°F); excursions permitted to 15–30°C (59–86°F) [see USP Controlled Room Temperature].

Discard the inhaler 45 days after opening the foil pouch or when dose counter reads "00", whichever comes first.

17 PATIENT COUNSELING INFORMATION

See FDA-Approved Patient Labeling (Patient Information).

17.1 Oral Candidiasis

Patients should be advised that localized infections with *Candida albicans* occurred in the mouth and pharynx in some patients. If oropharyngeal candidiasis develops, it should be treated with appropriate local or systemic (i.e., oral) antifungal therapy while still continuing with ASMANEX TWISTHALER therapy, but at times therapy with ASMANEX TWISTHALER may need to be temporarily interrupted under close medical supervision. Rinsing the mouth after inhalation is advised *[see Warnings and Precautions (5.1)]*.

17.2 Acute Asthma Episodes

Patients should be advised that ASMANEX TWISTHALER is not a bronchodilator and should not be used to treat status asthmaticus or to relieve acute asthma symptoms. Acute asthma symptoms should be treated with an inhaled, short-acting beta$_2$-agonist such as albuterol *[see Warnings and Precautions (5.2)]*.

17.3 Hypersensitivity Reactions Including Anaphylaxis

Hypersensitivity reactions including rash, pruritus, angioedema and anaphylactic reaction have been reported with use of ASMANEX TWISTHALER. Discontinue ASMANEX TWISTHALER if such reactions occur *[see Contraindications (4.2), Warnings and Precautions 5.3, and Postmarketing Experience (6.2)]*.

ASMANEX TWISTHALER contains small amounts of lactose, which contains trace levels of milk proteins. In postmarketing experience with ASMANEX TWISTHALER, anaphylactic reactions in patients with milk protein allergy have been reported *[see Contraindications (4.2) and Postmarketing Experience (6.2)]*.

17.4 Immunosuppression

Patients who are on immunosuppressant doses of corticosteroids should be warned to avoid exposure to chickenpox or measles and, if exposed, to consult their physician without delay. Patients should be informed of potential worsening of existing tuberculosis; fungal, bacterial, viral, or parasitic infections; or ocular herpes simplex *[see Warnings and Precautions (5.4)]*.

17.5 Hypercorticism and Adrenal Suppression

Patients should be advised that ASMANEX TWISTHALER may cause systemic corticosteroid effects of hypercorticism and adrenal suppression. Additionally, patients should be instructed that deaths due to adrenal insufficiency have occurred during and after transfer from systemic corticosteroids. Patients should taper slowly from systemic corticosteroids if transferring to ASMANEX TWISTHALER *[see Warnings and Precautions (5.6)]*.

17.6 Reduction in Bone Mineral Density

Patients who are at an increased risk for decreased BMD should be advised that the use of corticosteroids may pose an additional risk and should be monitored and, where appropriate, be treated for this condition *[see Warnings and Precautions (5.7)]*.

17.7 Reduced Growth Velocity

Patients should be informed that orally inhaled corticosteroids, including mometasone furoate inhalation powder, may cause a reduction in growth velocity when administered to pediatric patients. Physicians should closely follow the growth of children and adolescents taking corticosteroids by any route *[see Warnings and Precautions (5.8)]*.

17.8 Use Daily for Best Effect

Patients should be advised to use ASMANEX TWISTHALER at regular intervals, since its effectiveness depends on regular use. Maximum benefit may not be achieved for 1 to 2 weeks or longer after starting treatment. If symptoms do not improve in that time frame or if the condition worsens, patients should be instructed to contact their physician.

17.9 Instructions for Use

Patients should be instructed to record the date of pouch opening on the cap label and discard the inhaler 45 days after opening the foil pouch or when the dose counter reads "00" and the final dose has been inhaled, whichever comes first. The inhaler should be held upright while removing the cap. The medication should be taken as directed, breathing rapidly and deeply, and patients should not breathe out through the inhaler. The mouthpiece should be wiped dry and the cap replaced immediately following each inhalation and rotated fully until the click is heard. Rinsing of mouth after inhalation is advised. Patients should store the unit as instructed. The dose counter displays the doses remaining. When the dose counter indicates zero, the cap will lock and the unit must be discarded. Patients should be advised that if the dose counter is not working correctly, the unit should not be used and it should be brought to their physician or pharmacist.

Manufactured for: Merck Sharp & Dohme Corp., a subsidiary of
MERCK & CO., INC., Whitehouse Station, NJ 08889, USA
Manufactured by:
MSD International GmbH (Singapore Branch)
Singapore 638030, Singapore
Or
Merck Sharp & Dohme Corp., a subsidiary of
Merck & Co., Inc., Whitehouse Station, NJ 08889, USA
U.S. Patent Nos. 5,687,710; 5,829,434; 6,240,918; and 6,503,537.

Revised: 01/2013
032088-AS-PwIH-USPI.14

Patient Information

ASMANEX® TWISTHALER® 220 mcg (mometasone furoate inhalation powder)

ASMANEX® TWISTHALER® 110 mcg (mometasone furoate inhalation powder)

FOR ORAL INHALATION ONLY

Please read this leaflet carefully before taking ASMANEX® TWISTHALER®.

This leaflet does not contain the complete information about this medication. If you have any questions about ASMANEX TWISTHALER, ask your health care provider or pharmacist.

IMPORTANT POINTS TO REMEMBER ABOUT ASMANEX TWISTHALER

- Your health care provider has prescribed ASMANEX TWISTHALER for you or your child. It contains a medicine called mometasone furoate, which is a man-made corticosteroid. This medicine is used as maintenance treatment that helps prevent and control asthma symptoms.
- ASMANEX TWISTHALER is not a bronchodilator and should not be used for sudden symptoms of shortness of breath. Use an inhaled short-acting bronchodilator such as albuterol to relieve sudden symptoms of shortness of breath.
- Your health care provider may prescribe bronchodilators such as albuterol for emergency relief if an acute asthma attack occurs.
- Use your ASMANEX TWISTHALER regularly and at the same time each day, as prescribed by your health care provider. You or your child may not get the most benefit for 1 to 2 weeks or longer after starting ASMANEX. If you or your child's symptoms do not improve in that time frame or if your condition gets worse, contact your health care provider.
- The cap is needed to use the ASMANEX TWISTHALER. Do not twist the mouthpiece with your hand. When the cap is removed from the TWISTHALER, the dose counter will count down by one, and show the number of doses available after this use.
- The inhaler delivers your medicine as a very fine powder that **you or your child may not taste, smell, or feel.** Do not take or give extra doses unless your health care provider has told you to.
- It is important to replace the cap after each inhalation to protect the inhaler from moisture.
- Do not use the inhaler if you notice that it is not working correctly. Take it to your health care provider or pharmacist.

WHO SHOULD NOT USE ASMANEX TWISTHALER

Do not use ASMANEX TWISTHALER:
- To treat sudden, severe symptoms of asthma.
- If you have an allergy to milk proteins. Ask your health care provider if you are not sure.

HOW TO USE ASMANEX TWISTHALER OR GIVE TO YOUR CHILD

- **Remove the ASMANEX TWISTHALER from its foil pouch and write the date on the cap label.**
- **Throw away the inhaler 45 days after this date or when the dose counter reads "00", indicating the final dose has been inhaled, whichever comes first.**
- **Follow steps 1 and 2 below each time you inhale a dose from your ASMANEX TWISTHALER.**

Inhaler Parts:

See Figures 1 and 2 below to become familiar with the inhaler parts.

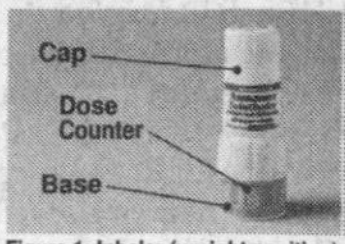

Figure 1: Inhaler (upright position)

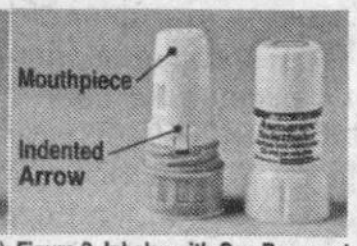

Figure 2: Inhaler with Cap Removed

Step 1: Open inhaler

Hold the inhaler straight up (upright position) with the colored portion (the base) on the bottom *(see Figure 3 below)*. It is important that you remove the cap of the TWISTHALER while it is in this upright position to make sure that you get the right amount of medicine with each dose.

Holding the colored base, twist the cap in a counterclockwise direction to remove it *(see Figure 3 below)*. As you lift off the cap, the dose counter on the base will count down by one. Removing the cap loads the TWISTHALER with the medicine that you are now ready to inhale.

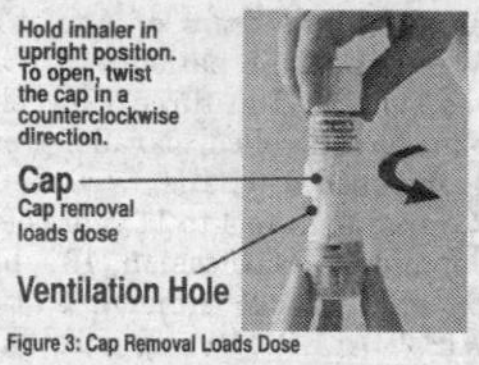

Figure 3: Cap Removal Loads Dose

IT IS IMPORTANT TO NOTE that the indented arrow (located on the white portion of the TWISTHALER, directly above the colored base) is pointing to the dose counter *(see Figure 2)*.

Step 2: Inhale dose

Breathe out fully. Then bring the TWISTHALER up to your mouth or your child's mouth with the mouthpiece facing toward you or your child. Place the mouthpiece in your mouth or your child's mouth, holding it in a horizontal (on its side) position as shown below *(see Figure 4)*. Firmly close your lips around the mouthpiece and take in a fast, deep breath. Since the medicine is a very fine powder, you may not be able to taste, smell, or feel it after inhalation. Do not cover the ventilation holes while inhaling the dose.

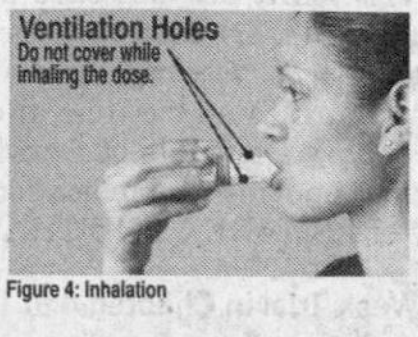

Figure 4: Inhalation

Remove the TWISTHALER from your mouth and hold your breath for about 10 seconds, or as long as you comfortably can.

IMPORTANT: DO NOT BREATHE OUT (EXHALE) INTO THE INHALER.

After you take your medicine, it is important that you wipe the mouthpiece dry, if needed, and then **REPLACE THE CAP,** firmly closing the TWISTHALER right away *(see Figures 5 and 6 below)*.

Be sure that the indented arrow is in line with the dose counter. Put the cap back onto the inhaler and turn it in a clockwise direction, as you gently press down. You'll hear a "click" to let you know that the cap is fully closed. This is the only way to be sure that your next dose is loaded the right way.

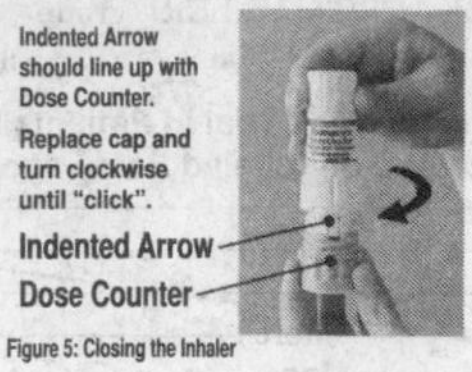

Indented Arrow should line up with Dose Counter.
Replace cap and turn clockwise until "click".
Indented Arrow
Dose Counter

Figure 5: Closing the Inhaler

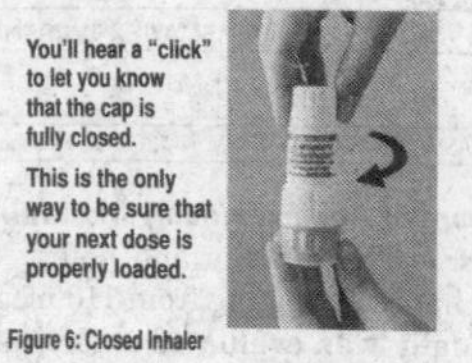

Figure 6: Closed Inhaler

IT IS IMPORTANT TO REPEAT STEPS 1 AND 2 EACH TIME YOU INHALE.

Rinse your mouth after using.

STORING YOUR INHALER

- Keep your inhaler clean and dry at all times. If the mouthpiece needs cleaning, gently wipe the mouthpiece with a dry cloth or tissue as needed. Do not wash the inhaler. Avoid contact with any liquids.
- **Store in a dry place at 25°C (77°F) [may range between 15–30°C (59–86°F)].**
- Keep your inhaler out of the reach of children.

HOW TO KNOW WHEN YOUR INHALER IS EMPTY

The inhaler has a dose counter on the colored base, which shows the number of doses left to use. As you lift off the cap to take your dose, the dose counter on the base will count down by one (if you began with the dose counter reading "30" this will cause the dose counter to now read "29"). Read the numbers from top to bottom.

When the unit reads "01" this indicates the last remaining dose. After dose "01" the counter will read "00". When you replace the cap, the unit will lock and then must be thrown away. Start using a new ASMANEX TWISTHALER as instructed by your health care provider.

POSSIBLE SIDE EFFECTS WITH ASMANEX TWISTHALER

Serious Side Effects may include:

- **Fungal infections in the mouth and throat.** Patients who use inhaled steroid medicines for asthma may develop a fungal infection of the mouth. Rinse your mouth after using ASMANEX TWISTHALER.
- Worsening asthma or sudden asthma attacks
- **Serious allergic reactions.** Call your health care provider or get emergency medical care if you get any symptoms of a serious allergic reaction, including:
  - Rash
  - Swelling of the face, mouth and tongue
  - Breathing problems
- **Possible increased risk of infection due to a weakened immune system with using steroid medicines.** Tell your health care provider if you or your child have or had TB, are exposed to anyone with chickenpox or measles, or about any other infections you or your child had before or while using ASMANEX TWISTHALER.
- **Adrenal insufficiency (your adrenal gland cannot produce enough steroids since you were on oral steroid medicine).** If you or your child took steroids by mouth and are having them decreased (tapered) or you are being switched to ASMANEX TWISTHALER, you should be followed closely by your health care professional.
  Death can occur. Tell your health care professional right away about any symptoms such as feeling tired or exhausted, weakness, nausea, vomiting, or symptoms of low blood pressure (such as dizziness or faintness). If you or your child is under stress, such as with surgery, after surgery or trauma, you may need steroids by mouth again.
- **Decreased bone mass (bone mineral density).** Patients who use inhaled steroid medicines for a long time may have an increased risk of decreased bone mass, which can affect bone strength. Talk with your health care provider about any questions about bone health.

The most common side effects with ASMANEX TWISTHALER include: headache, nasal allergy symptoms, sore throat, upper respiratory tract infection, sinus infection, fungal infections in the mouth, painful menstrual periods, muscle and bone pain, back pain, and upset stomach. Tell your health care professional about any side effects that bother you or do not go away. These are not all of the possible side effects with ASMANEX TWISTHALER. For more information, ask your health care professional.

Manufactured for: Merck Sharp & Dohme Corp., a subsidiary of
MERCK & CO., INC., Whitehouse Station, NJ 08889, USA

Manufactured by:
MSD International GmbH (Singapore Branch)
Singapore 638030, Singapore
Or
Merck Sharp & Dohme Corp., a subsidiary of
Merck & Co., Inc., Whitehouse Station, NJ 08889, USA
U.S. Patent Nos. 5,687,710; 5,829,434; 6,240,918; and 6,503,537.

Revised: 01/2013
032088-AS-PwIH-PPI.9

AVELOX ℞
[ă'vĕ-lŏks]
(moxifloxacin hydrochloride)
Tablet, film-coated
AVELOX
(moxifloxacin hydrochloride)
Injection, solution for IV use

HIGHLIGHTS OF PRESCRIBING INFORMATION
These highlights do not include all the information needed to use AVELOX safely and effectively. See full prescribing information for AVELOX.
AVELOX (moxifloxacin) hydrochloride Tablet, film-coated
AVELOX (moxifloxacin) hydrochloride Injection, solution for IV use
Initial U.S. Approval: 1999

WARNING:
Fluoroquinolones, including AVELOX®, are associated with an increased risk of tendinitis and tendon rupture in all ages. This risk is further increased in older patients usually over 60 years of age, in patients taking corticosteroid drugs, and in patients with kidney, heart or lung transplants *[see Warnings and Precautions (5.1)]*.
Fluoroquinolones, including AVELOX, may exacerbate muscle weakness in persons with myasthenia gravis. Avoid AVELOX in patients with known history of myasthenia gravis *[see Warnings and Precautions (5.2).]*

To reduce the development of drug-resistant bacteria and maintain the effectiveness of AVELOX and other antibacterial drugs, AVELOX should be used only to treat or prevent infections that are proven or strongly suspected to be caused by susceptible bacteria. (1)

RECENT MAJOR CHANGES

Warnings and Precautions, Peripheral Neuropathy (5.8) 8/13

INDICATIONS AND USAGE

AVELOX is a fluoroquinolone antibacterial indicated for treating infections in adults ≥ 18 years of age caused by designated, susceptible bacteria. (1, 12.4)
- Acute Bacterial Sinusitis (1.1)
- Acute Bacterial Exacerbation of Chronic Bronchitis (1.2)
- Community Acquired Pneumonia (1.3)
- Skin and Skin Structure Infections: Uncomplicated (1.4) and Complicated (1.5)
- Complicated Intra-Abdominal Infections (1.6)

DOSAGE AND ADMINISTRATION

Type of Infection	Dose Every 24 hours	Duration (days)
Acute Bacterial Sinusitis (1.1)	400 mg	10
Acute Bacterial Exacerbation of Chronic Bronchitis (1.2)	400 mg	5
Community Acquired Pneumonia (1.3)	400 mg	7-14
Uncomplicated Skin and Skin Structure Infections (SSSI) (1.4)	400 mg	7
Complicated SSSI (1.5)	400 mg	7-21
Complicated Intra-Abdominal Infections (1.6)	400 mg	5-14

- No dosage adjustment in patients with renal or hepatic impairment. (8.6, 8.7)
- AVELOX Tablets: Administer 4 hours before or 8 hours after antacids, sucralfate, multivitamins and other products with multivalent cations. (2.2)
- AVELOX IV: Slow IV infusion over 60 minutes. Avoid rapid or bolus IV. (2.3)
- Do not mix with other medications in IV bag or in IV line (2.3)

DOSAGE FORMS AND STRENGTHS

- AVELOX Tablets 400 mg moxifloxacin hydrochloride
- AVELOX IV 250 mL flexibag containing 400 mg moxifloxacin hydrochloride in sodium chloride injection (3.2)

CONTRAINDICATIONS

Known hypersensitivity to AVELOX or other quinolones (4, 5.4)

WARNINGS AND PRECAUTIONS

- Increased risk of tendinitis and tendon rupture. This risk is further increased in older patients usually over 60 years of age, in patients taking corticosteroids, and in patients with kidney, heart or lung transplants. Discontinue if pain or inflammation in a tendon occurs. (5.1, 8.5)
- Prolongation of the QT interval and isolated cases of torsade de pointes has been reported. Avoid use in patients with known prolongation, hypokalemia, and with drugs that prolong the QT interval. (5.3, 7.4, 8.5). Use caution in patients with proarrhythmic conditions such as clinically significant bradycardia or acute myocardial ischemia. (5.3)
- Serious and sometimes fatal hypersensitivity reactions, including anaphylactic reactions, may occur after first or subsequent doses. Discontinue drug use at first sign of skin rash, jaundice or any other sign of hypersensitivity. (5.4, 5.5)
- Central nervous system (CNS) events including dizziness, confusion, hallucination, depression, and rarely suicidal thoughts or acts may occur after first dose. Use caution in patients with known or suspected CNS disorders that may predispose to seizures or lower the seizure threshold. (5.6)
- Clostridium difficile-associated diarrhea: Evaluate if diarrhea occurs. (5.7)
- Peripheral neuropathy: Discontinue if symptoms occur. (5.8)

ADVERSE REACTIONS

Most common reactions (≥3%) were nausea, diarrhea, headache, and dizziness (6.2)

To report SUSPECTED ADVERSE REACTIONS, contact Bayer HealthCare Pharmaceuticals Inc. at 1-888-842-2937 or FDA at 1-800-FDA-1088 or www.fda.gov/medwatch

DRUG INTERACTIONS

Interacting Drug	Interaction
Antacids, sucralfate, multivitamins, and other products containing multivalent cations	Moxifloxacin absorption is decreased. Administer AVELOX Tablet at least 4 hours before or 8 hours after these products. (2.2, 7.1, 12.3, 17.2)
Warfarin	Anticoagulant effect of warfarin may be enhanced. Monitor prothrombin time/INR, watch for bleeding. (6.4, 7.2, 12.3)
Class IA and Class III antiarrhythmics:	Proarrhythmic effect may be enhanced. Avoid concomitant use. (5.3, 7.4)

USE IN SPECIFIC POPULATIONS

- **Pregnancy:** Based on animal data may cause fetal harm (8.1)
- **Geriatrics:** Increased risk for severe tendon disorders further increased by concomitant corticosteroid therapy and increased risk of prolongation of the QT interval. (5.1, 5.3, 8.5)

See 17 for PATIENT COUNSELING INFORMATION and FDA-approved patient labeling

Revised: 08/2013

FULL PRESCRIBING INFORMATION: CONTENTS*

*** Sections or subsections omitted from the full prescribing information are not listed**

FULL PRESCRIBING INFORMATION

WARNING:
Fluoroquinolones, including AVELOX®, are associated with an increased risk of tendinitis and tendon rupture in all ages. This risk is further increased in older patients usually over 60 years of age, in patients taking corticosteroid drugs, and in patients with kidney, heart or lung transplants. *[see Warnings and Precautions (5.1)]*.
Fluoroquinolones, including AVELOX, may exacerbate muscle weakness in persons with myasthenia gravis. Avoid AVELOX in patients with known history of myasthenia gravis *[see Warnings and Precautions (5.2)]*.

1 INDICATIONS AND USAGE

To reduce the development of drug-resistant bacteria and maintain the effectiveness of AVELOX® and other antibacterial drugs, AVELOX should be used only to treat or prevent infections that are proven or strongly suspected to be caused by susceptible bacteria. When culture and susceptibility information are available, they should be considered in selecting or modifying antibacterial therapy. In the absence of such data, local epidemiology and susceptibility patterns may contribute to the empiric selection of therapy.

AVELOX® Tablets and IV are indicated for the treatment of adults (≥ 18 years of age) with infections caused by susceptible isolates of the designated microorganisms in the conditions listed below *[see Dosage and Administration (2) and Use In Specific Populations (8.5)].*

Culture and Susceptibility Testing

Appropriate culture and susceptibility tests should be performed before treatment in order to isolate and identify organisms causing infection and to determine their susceptibility to moxifloxacin *[see Clinical Pharmacology (12.4)].* Therapy with AVELOX may be initiated before results of these tests are known; once results become available, appropriate therapy should be continued.

1.1 Acute Bacterial Sinusitis

AVELOX is indicated for the treatment of Acute Bacterial Sinusitis caused by *Streptococcus pneumoniae, Haemophilus influenzae,* or *Moraxella catarrhalis [see Clinical Studies (14.4)].*

1.2 Acute Bacterial Exacerbation of Chronic Bronchitis

AVELOX is indicated for the treatment of Acute Bacterial Exacerbation of Chronic Bronchitis caused by *Streptococcus pneumoniae, Haemophilus influenzae, Haemophilus parainfluenzae, Klebsiella pneumoniae,* methicillin-susceptible *Staphylococcus aureus,* or *Moraxella catarrhalis [see Clinical Studies (14.1)].*

1.3 Community Acquired Pneumonia

AVELOX is indicated for the treatment of Community Acquired Pneumonia caused by *Streptococcus pneumoniae* (including multi-drug resistant isolates*), *Haemophilus influenzae, Moraxella catarrhalis,* methicillin-susceptible *Staphylococcus aureus, Klebsiella pneumoniae, Mycoplasma pneumoniae, or Chlamydophila pneumoniae.*

* MDRSP, Multi-drug resistant *Streptococcus pneumoniae* includes isolates previously known as PRSP (Penicillin-resistant *S. pneumoniae*), and are isolates resistant to two or more of the following antibiotics: penicillin (minimum inhibitory concentrations [MIC] ≥ 2 mcg/mL), 2nd generation cephalosporins (for example, cefuroxime), macrolides, tetracyclines, and trimethoprim/sulfamethoxazole *[see Clinical Studies (14.2)].*

1.4 Uncomplicated Skin and Skin Structure Infections

AVELOX is indicated for the treatment of Uncomplicated Skin and Skin Structure Infections caused by methicillin-susceptible *Staphylococcus aureus* or *Streptococcus pyogenes [see Clinical Studies (14.5)].*

1.5 Complicated Skin and Skin Structure Infections

AVELOX is indicated for the treatment of Complicated Skin and Skin Structure Infections caused by methicillin-susceptible *Staphylococcus aureus, Escherichia coli, Klebsiella pneumoniae,* or *Enterobacter cloacae [see Clinical Studies (14.6)].*

1.6 Complicated Intra-Abdominal Infections

AVELOX is indicated for the treatment of Complicated Intra-Abdominal Infections including polymicrobial infections such as abscess caused by *Escherichia coli, Bacteroides fragilis, Streptococcus anginosus, Streptococcus constellatus, Enterococcus faecalis, Proteus mirabilis, Clostridium perfringens, Bacteroides thetaiotaomicron, or Peptostreptococcus*species *[see Clinical Studies (14.7)].*

2 DOSAGE AND ADMINISTRATION

2.1 Dosage in Adult Patients

The dose of AVELOX is 400 mg (orally or as an intravenous infusion) once every 24 hours. The duration of therapy depends on the type of infection as described in **Table 1**.

Table 1 Dosage and Duration of Therapy in Adult Patients

Type of Infection*	Dose Every 24 hours	Duration (days)
Acute Bacterial Sinusitis (1.1)	400 mg	10
Acute Bacterial Exacerbation of Chronic Bronchitis (1.2)	400 mg	5
Community Acquired Pneumonia	400 mg	7–14
Uncomplicated Skin and Skin Structure Infections (SSSI) (1.4)	400 mg	7
Complicated SSSI (1.5)	400 mg	7–21
Complicated Intra-Abdominal Infections (1.6)	400 mg	5–14

* Due to the designated pathogens *[see Indications and Usage (1), for IV use, see Use in Specific Populations (8.5)].*

Intravenous formulation is indicated when it offers a route of administration advantageous to the patient (for example, patient cannot tolerate an oral dosage form). When switching from intravenous to oral formulation, no dosage adjustment is necessary. Patients whose therapy is started with AVELOX IV may be switched to AVELOX Tablets when clinically indicated at the discretion of the physician.

2.2 Drug Interactions with Multivalent Cations

Oral doses of AVELOX should be administered at least 4 hours before or 8 hours after products containing magnesium, aluminum, iron or zinc, including antacids, sucralfate, multivitamins and VIDEX® (didanosine) chewable/buffered tablets or the pediatric powder for oral solution *[see Drug Interactions (7.1) and Clinical Pharmacology (12.3)].*

2.3 Administration Instructions

AVELOX Film-Coated Tablets

AVELOX Tablets can be taken with or without food, drink fluids liberally.

AVELOX IV Solution for Infusion

Parenteral drug products should be inspected visually for particulate matter and discoloration prior to administration, whenever solution and container permit.

AVELOX IV should be administered by INTRAVENOUS infusion only. It is not intended for intra-arterial, intramuscular, intrathecal, intraperitoneal, or subcutaneous administration.

AVELOX IV should be administered by intravenous infusion over a period of 60 minutes by direct infusion or through a Y-type intravenous infusion set which may already be in place. Caution: rapid or bolus intravenous infusion must be avoided.

Because only limited data are available on the compatibility of AVELOX intravenous injection with other intravenous substances, additives or other medications should not be added to AVELOX IV or infused simultaneously through the same intravenous line. If the same intravenous line or a Y-type line is used for sequential infusion of other drugs, or if the "piggyback" method of administration is used, the line should be flushed before and after infusion of AVELOX IV with an infusion solution compatible with AVELOX IV as well as with other drug(s) administered via this common line.

AVELOX IV is compatible with the following intravenous solutions at ratios from 1:10 to 10:1

0.9% Sodium Chloride Injection, USP	Sterile Water for Injection, USP
1M Sodium Chloride Injection	10% Dextrose for Injection, USP
5% Dextrose Injection, USP	Lactated Ringer's for Injection

2.4 Preparation for Administration of AVELOX IV

To prepare AVELOX IV injection premix in flexible containers:

1. Close flow control clamp of administration set.
2. Remove cover from port at bottom of container.
3. Insert piercing pin from an appropriate transfer set (for example, one that does not require excessive force, such as ISO compatible administration set) into port with a gentle twisting motion until pin is firmly seated.

NOTE: Refer to complete directions that have been provided with the administration set.

3 DOSAGE FORMS AND STRENGTHS

3.1 AVELOX Tablets

- Containing moxifloxacin hydrochloride (equivalent to 400 mg moxifloxacin)
- Oblong, dull red film-coated tablets
- Imprinted with BAYER on one side and M400 on the other

3.2 AVELOX IV

- Containing 400 mg moxifloxacin in 0.8% saline (moxifloxacin hydrochloride in sodium chloride injection) with pH ranging from 4.1 to 4.6.
- Ready-to-use 250 mL latex-free flexibags. No further dilution is necessary
- Sterile, preservative free, 0.8% sodium chloride aqueous solution of moxifloxacin hydrochloride

4 CONTRAINDICATIONS

AVELOX is contraindicated in persons with a history of hypersensitivity to moxifloxacin or any member of the quinolone class of antimicrobial agents.

5 WARNINGS AND PRECAUTIONS

5.1 Tendinopathy and Tendon Rupture

Fluoroquinolones, including AVELOX, are associated with an increased risk of tendinitis and tendon rupture in all ages. This adverse reaction most frequently involves the Achilles tendon, and rupture of the Achilles tendon may require surgical repair. Tendinitis and tendon rupture in the rotator cuff (the shoulder), the hand, the biceps, the thumb, and other tendon sites have also been reported. The risk of developing fluoroquinolone-associated tendinitis and tendon rupture is further increased in older patients usually over 60 years of age, in patients taking corticosteroid drugs, and in patients with kidney, heart or lung transplants. Factors, in addition to age and corticosteroid use, that may independently increase the risk of tendon rupture include strenuous physical activity, renal failure, and previous tendon disorders such as rheumatoid arthritis. Tendinitis and tendon rupture have also occurred in patients taking fluoroquinolones who do not have the above risk factors. Tendon rupture can occur during or after completion of therapy; cases occurring up to several months after completion of therapy have been reported. AVELOX should be discontinued if the patient experiences pain, swelling, inflammation or rupture of a tendon. Patients should be advised to rest at the first sign of tendinitis or tendon rupture, and to contact their healthcare provider regarding changing to a non-quinolone antimicrobial drug. *[see Adverse Reactions (6.4) and Patient Counseling Information (17.3).]*

5.2 Exacerbation of Myasthenia Gravis

Fluoroquinolones, including AVELOX, have neuromuscular blocking activity and may exacerbate muscle weakness in persons with myasthenia gravis. Postmarketing serious adverse events, including deaths and requirement for ventilatory support, have been associated with fluoroquinolone use in persons with myasthenia gravis. Avoid AVELOX in patients with known history of myasthenia gravis *[see Patient Counseling Information (17.3)].*

5.3 QT Prolongation

AVELOX has been shown to prolong the QT interval of the electrocardiogram in some patients. Following oral dosing with 400 mg of AVELOX the mean (± SD) change in QTc from the pre-dose value at the time of maximum drug concentration was 6 msec (± 26) (n = 787). Following a course of daily intravenous dosing (400 mg; 1 hour infusion each day) the mean change in QTc from the Day 1 pre-dose value was 10 msec (±22) on Day 1 (n=667) and 7 msec (± 24) on Day 3 (n = 667).

The drug should be avoided in patients with known prolongation of the QT interval, patients with uncorrected hypokalemia and patients receiving Class IA (for example, quinidine, procainamide) or Class III (for example, amiodarone, sotalol) antiarrhythmic agents, due to the lack of clinical experience with the drug in these patient populations.

Pharmacokinetic studies between AVELOX and other drugs that prolong the QT interval such as cisapride, erythromycin, antipsychotics, and tricyclic antidepressants have not been performed. An additive effect of AVELOX and these drugs cannot be excluded; therefore caution should be exercised when AVELOX is given concurrently with these drugs.

In premarketing clinical trials, the rate of cardiovascular adverse events was similar in 798 AVELOX and 702 comparator treated patients who received concomitant therapy with drugs known to prolong the QTc interval.

AVELOX should be used with caution in patients with ongoing proarrhythmic conditions, such as clinically significant bradycardia, acute myocardial ischemia. The magnitude of QT prolongation may increase with increasing concentrations of the drug or increasing rates of infusion of the intravenous formulation. Therefore the recommended dose or infusion rate should not be exceeded. QT prolongation may lead to an increased risk for ventricular arrhythmias including torsade de pointes. No excess in cardiovascular morbidity or mortality attributable to QTc prolongation occurred with AVELOX treatment in over 15,500 patients in controlled clinical studies, including 759 patients who were hypokalemic at the start of treatment, and there was no increase in mortality in over 18,000 AVELOX tablet treated patients in a postmarketing observational study in which ECGs were not performed. Elderly patients using IV AVELOX may be more susceptible to drug-associated QT prolongation. *[see Use In Specific Populations, (8.5).]* In addition, AVELOX should be used with caution in patients with mild, moderate, or severe liver cirrhosis. *[See Clinical Pharmacology (12.3) and Patient Counseling Information (17.3).]*

5.4 Hypersensitivity Reactions

Serious anaphylactic reactions, some following the first dose, have been reported in patients receiving quinolone therapy, including AVELOX. Some reactions were accompanied by cardiovascular collapse, loss of consciousness, tingling, pharyngeal or facial edema, dyspnea, urticaria, and itching. Serious anaphylactic reactions require immediate emergency treatment with epinephrine. AVELOX should be discontinued at the first appearance of a skin rash or any other sign of hypersensitivity. Oxygen, intravenous steroids, and airway management, including intubation, may be administered as indicated. *[see Adverse Reactions (6) and Patient Counseling Information (17.3).]*

5.5 Other Serious and Sometimes Fatal Reactions

Other serious and sometimes fatal events, some due to hypersensitivity, and some due to uncertain etiology, have been reported rarely in patients receiving therapy with quinolones, including AVELOX . These events may be severe and generally occur following the administration of multiple doses. Clinical manifestations may include one or more of the following:

- Fever, rash, or severe dermatologic reactions (for example, toxic epidermal necrolysis, Stevens-Johnson syndrome)
- Vasculitis; arthralgia; myalgia; serum sickness
- Allergic pneumonitis
- Interstitial nephritis; acute renal insufficiency or failure
- Hepatitis; jaundice; acute hepatic necrosis or failure
- Anemia, including hemolytic and aplastic; thrombocytopenia, including thrombotic thrombocytopenic purpura; leukopenia; agranulocytosis; pancytopenia; and/or other hematologic abnormalities

The drug should be discontinued immediately at the first appearance of a skin rash, jaundice, or any other sign of hypersensitivity and supportive measures instituted *[see Patient Counseling Information (17.3) and Adverse Reactions (6.4)*.

5.6 Central Nervous System Effects

Fluoroquinolones, including AVELOX, may cause central nervous system (CNS) events, including: nervousness, agitation, insomnia, anxiety, nightmares or paranoia *[see Adverse Reactions (6.2, 6.4)]*.

Convulsions and increased intracranial pressure (including pseudotumor cerebri) have been reported in patients receiving fluoroquinolones. Fluoroquinolones may also cause central nervous system (CNS) events including: dizziness, confusion, tremors, hallucinations, depression, and, rarely, suicidal thoughts or acts. These reactions may occur following the first dose. If these reactions occur in patients receiving AVELOX, the drug should be discontinued and appropriate measures instituted. As with all fluoroquinolones, AVELOX should be used with caution in patients with known or suspected CNS disorders (for example, severe cerebral arteriosclerosis, epilepsy) or in the presence of other risk factors that may predispose to seizures or lower the seizure threshold. *[See Drug Interactions (7.4) Adverse Reactions (6.2, 6.4) and Patient Counseling Information (17.3).]*

5.7 *Clostridium Difficile*-Associated Diarrhea

Clostridium difficile-associated diarrhea (CDAD) has been reported with use of nearly all antibacterial agents, including AVELOX, and may range in severity from mild diarrhea to fatal colitis. Treatment with antibacterial agents alters the normal flora of the colon leading to overgrowth of *C. difficile*.

C. difficile produces toxins A and B which contribute to the development of CDAD. Hypertoxin producing strains of *C. difficile* cause increased morbidity and mortality, as these infections can be refractory to antimicrobial therapy and may require colectomy. CDAD must be considered in all patients who present with diarrhea following antibiotic use. Careful medical history is necessary since CDAD has been reported to occur over two months after the administration of antibacterial agents.

If CDAD is suspected or confirmed, ongoing antibiotic use not directed against *C. difficile* may need to be discontinued. Appropriate fluid and electrolyte management, protein supplementation, antibiotic treatment of *C. difficile*, and surgical evaluation should be instituted as clinically indicated *[see Adverse Reactions (6.2) and Patient Counseling Information (17.3)]*.

5.8 Peripheral Neuropathy

Cases of sensory or sensorimotor axonal polyneuropathy affecting small and/or large axons resulting in paresthesias, hypoesthesias, dysesthesias and weakness have been reported in patients receiving fluoroquinolones including AVELOX. Symptoms may occur soon after initiation of AVELOX and may be irreversible. AVELOX should be discontinued immediately if the patient experiences symptoms of peripheral neuropathy including pain, burning, tingling, numbness, and/or weakness or other alterations of sensation including light touch, pain, temperature, position sense, and vibratory sensation *[see Adverse Reactions (6.2, 6.4) and Patient Counseling Information (17.3)]*.

5.9 Arthropathic Effects in Animals

The oral administration of AVELOX caused lameness in immature dogs. Histopathological examination of the weight-bearing joints of these dogs revealed permanent lesions of the cartilage. Related quinolone-class drugs also produce erosions of cartilage of weight-bearing joints and other signs of arthropathy in immature animals of various species. *[See Animal Toxicology and/or Pharmacology (13.2).]*

5.10 Photosensitivity/Phototoxicity

Moderate to severe photosensitivity/phototoxicity reactions, the latter of which may manifest as exaggerated sunburn reactions (for example, burning, erythema, exudation, vesicles, blistering, edema) involving areas exposed to light (typically the face, "V" area of the neck, extensor surfaces of the forearms, dorsa of the hands), can be associated with the use of quinolone antibiotics after sun or UV light exposure. Therefore, excessive exposure to these sources of light should be avoided. Drug therapy should be discontinued if phototoxicity occurs. *[see Adverse Reactions (6.4) and Pharmacokinetics (12.3).]*

5.11 Development of Drug Resistant Bacteria

Prescribing AVELOX in the absence of a proven or strongly suspected bacterial infection or a prophylactic indication is unlikely to provide benefit to the patient and increases the risk of the development of drug-resistant bacteria *[see Patient Counseling Information (17.1)]*.

6 ADVERSE REACTIONS

6.1 Serious and Otherwise Important Adverse Reactions

The following serious and otherwise important adverse reactions are discussed in greater detail in the warnings and precautions section of the label:

- Tendinopathy and Tendon Rupture *[see Warnings and Precautions (5.1)]*
- QT Prolongation *[see Warnings and Precautions (5.3)]*
- Hypersensitivity Reactions *[see Warnings and Precautions (5.4)]*
- Other Serious and Sometimes Fatal Reactions *[see Warnings and Precautions (5.5)]*
- Central Nervous System Effects *[see Warnings and Precautions (5.6)]*
- Clostridium difficile-Associated Diarrhea *[see Warnings and Precautions (5.7)]*
- Peripheral Neuropathy that may be irreversible *[see Warnings and Precautions (5.8)]*
- Photosensitivity/Phototoxicity *[see Warnings and Precautions (5.10)]*
- Development of Drug Resistant Bacteria *[see Warnings and Precautions (5.11)]*

6.2 Clinical Trial Experience

Because clinical trials are conducted under widely varying conditions, adverse reaction rates observed in the clinical trials of a drug cannot be directly compared to rates in the clinical trials of another drug and may not reflect the rates observed in practice.

The data described below reflect exposure to AVELOX in 14981 patients in 71 active controlled Phase II- IV clinical trials in different indications *[see Indications and Usage (1)]*. The population studied had a mean age of 50 years (approximately 73% of the population was <65 years of age), 50% were male, 63% were Caucasian, 12% were Asian and 9% were Black. Patients received AVELOX 400 mg once daily PO, IV, or sequentially (IV followed by PO). Treatment duration was usually 6-10 days, and the mean number of days on therapy was 9 days.

Discontinuation of AVELOX due to adverse events occurred in 5.0% of patients overall, 4.1% of patients treated with 400 mg PO, 3.9% with 400 mg IV and 8.2% with sequential therapy 400 mg PO/IV. The most common adverse events leading to discontinuation with the 400 mg PO doses were nausea (0.8%), diarrhea (0.5%), dizziness (0.5%), and vomiting (0.4%). The most common adverse event leading to discontinuation with the 400 mg IV dose was rash (0.5%). The most common adverse events leading to discontinuation with the 400 mg IV/PO sequential dose were diarrhea (0.5%), pyrexia (0.4%).

Adverse reactions occurring in ≥1% of AVELOX-treated patients and less common adverse reactions, occurring in 0.1 to <1% of AVELOX-treated patients, are shown in **Tables 2** and **Table 3**, respectively. The most common adverse drug reactions (≥3%) are nausea, diarrhea, headache, and dizziness.

Table 2 Common (≥ 1.0%) Adverse Reactions Reported in Active-Controlled Clinical Trials with AVELOX

System Organ Class	Adverse Reactions*	% (N=14,981)
Blood and Lymphatic System Disorders	Anemia	1.1
Gastrointestinal Disorders	Nausea	6.9
	Diarrhea	6.0
	Vomiting	2.4
	Constipation	1.9
	Abdominal pain	1.5
	Abdominal pain upper	1.1
	Dyspepsia	1.0
General Disorders and Administration Site Conditions	Pyrexia	1.1
Investigations	Alanine aminotransferase increased	1.1
Metabolism and Nutritional Disorder	Hypokalemia	1
Nervous System Disorders	Headache	4.2
	Dizziness	3.0
Psychiatric Disorders	Insomnia	1.9

* MedDRA Version 12.0

Table 3 Less Common (0.1 to <1.0%) Adverse Reactions Reported in Active-Controlled Clinical Trials with AVELOX (N=14,981)

System Organ Class	Adverse Reactions[a]
Blood and Lymphatic System Disorders	Thrombocythemia Eosinophilia Neutropenia Thrombocytopenia Leukopenia Leukocytosis
Cardiac Disorders	Atrial fibrillation Palpitations Tachycardia Cardiac failure congestive Angina pectoris Cardiac failure Cardiac arrest Bradycardia
Ear and Labyrinth Disorders	Vertigo Tinnitus
Eye Disorders	Vision blurred
Gastrointestinal Disorders	Dry mouth Abdominal discomfort Flatulence Abdominal distention Gastritis Gastroesophageal reflux disease
General Disorders and Administration Site Conditions	Fatigue Chest pain Asthenia Edema peripheral Pain Malaise Infusion site extravasation Edema Chills Chest discomfort Facial pain
Hepatobiliary disorders	Hepatic function abnormal
Infections and Infestations	Vulvovaginal candidiasis Oral candidiasis Vulvovaginal mycotic infection Candidiasis Vaginal infection Oral fungal infection Fungal infection Gastroenteritis
Investigations	Aspartate aminotransferase increased Gamma-glutamyltransferase increased Blood alkaline phosphatase increased Hepatic enzyme increased Electrocardiogram QT prolonged Blood lactate dehydrogenase increased Platelet count increased Blood amylase increased Blood glucose increased Lipase increased Hemoglobin decreased Blood creatinine increased Transaminases increased White blood cell count increased Blood urea increased

	Liver function test abnormal Hematocrit decreased Prothrombin time prolonged Eosinophil count increased Activated partial thromboplastin time prolonged Blood bilirubin increased Blood triglycerides increased Blood uric acid increased Blood pressure increased
Metabolism and Nutrition Disorders	Hyperglycemia Anorexia Hypoglycemia Hyperlipidemia Decreased appetite Dehydration
Musculoskeletal and Connective Tissue Disorders	Back pain Pain in extremity Arthralgia Myalgia Muscle spasms Musculoskeletal chest pain Musculoskeletal pain
Nervous System Disorders	Dysgeusia Somnolence Tremor Lethargy Paresthesia Tension headache Hypoesthesia Syncope
Psychiatric Disorders	Anxiety Confusional state Agitation Depression Nervousness Restlessness Hallucination Disorientation
Renal and Urinary Disorders	Renal failure Dysuria Renal failure acute
Reproductive System and Breast Disorders	Vulvovaginal pruritus
Respiratory, Thoracic, and Mediastinal Disorders	Dyspnea Asthma Wheezing Bronchospasm
Skin and Subcutaneous Tissue Disorders	Rash Pruritus Hyperhidrosis Erythema Urticaria Dermatitis allergic Night sweats
Vascular Disorders	Hypertension Hypotension Phlebitis

[a]MedDRA Version 12.0

6.3 Laboratory Changes

Changes in laboratory parameters, without regard to drug relationship, which are not listed above and which occurred in ≥ 2% of patients and at an incidence greater than in controls included: increases in MCH, neutrophils, WBCs, PT ratio, ionized calcium, chloride, albumin, globulin, bilirubin; decreases in hemoglobin, RBCs, neutrophils, eosinophils, basophils, PT ratio, glucose, pO_2, bilirubin, and amylase. It cannot be determined if any of the above laboratory abnormalities were caused by the drug or the underlying condition being treated.

6.4 Postmarketing Experience

Table 4 lists adverse reactions that have been identified during post-approval use of AVELOX. Because these events are reported voluntarily from a population of uncertain size, it is not always possible to reliably estimate their frequency or establish a causal relationship to drug exposure.

Table 4 Postmarketing Reports of Adverse Drug Reactions

System/Organ Class	Adverse Reaction
Blood and Lymphatic System Disorders	Agranulocytosis Pancytopenia *[see Warnings and Precautions (5.5)]*
Cardiac Disorders	Ventricular tachyarrhythmias (including in very rare cases cardiac arrest and torsade de pointes, and usually in patients with concurrent severe underlying proarrhythmic conditions)
Ear and Labyrinth Disorders	Hearing impairment, including deafness (reversible in majority of cases)
Eye Disorders	Vision loss (especially in the course of CNS reactions, transient in majority of cases)
Hepatobiliary Disorders	Hepatitis (predominantly cholestatic) Hepatic failure (including fatal cases) Jaundice Acute hepatic necrosis *[see Warnings and Precautions (5.5)]*
Immune System Disorders	Anaphylactic reaction Anaphylactic shock Angioedema (including laryngeal edema) *[see Warnings and Precautions (5.4, 5.5)]*
Musculoskeletal and Connective Tissue Disorders	Tendon rupture *[see Warnings and Precautions (5.1)]*
Nervous System Disorders	Altered coordination Abnormal gait *[see Warnings and Precautions (5.8)]* Myasthenia gravis (exacerbation of) *[see Warnings and Precautions (5.2)]* Muscle weakness Peripheral neuropathy, (that may be irreversible), polyneuropathy *[see Warnings and Precautions (5.8)]*
Psychiatric Disorders	Psychotic reaction (very rarely culminating in self-injurious behavior, such as suicidal ideation/thoughts or suicide attempts *[see Warnings and Precautions (5.6)]*
Renal and Urinary Disorders	Renal dysfunction Interstitial nephritis *[see Warnings and Precautions (5.5)]*
Respiratory, Thoracic and Mediastinal Disorders	Allergic pneumonitis *[see Warnings and Precautions (5.5)]*
Skin and Subcutaneous Tissue Disorders	Photosensitivity/phototoxicity reaction *[see Warnings and Precautions (5.10)]* Stevens-Johnson syndrome Toxic epidermal necrolysis *[see Warnings and Precautions (5.5)]*

7 DRUG INTERACTIONS

7.1 Antacids, Sucralfate, Multivitamins and other products containing Multivalent Cations

Quinolones form chelates with alkaline earth and transition metal cations. Oral administration of quinolones with antacids containing aluminum or magnesium, with sucralfate, with metal cations such as iron, or with multivitamins containing iron or zinc, or with formulations containing divalent and trivalent cations such as VIDEX® (didanosine) chewable/buffered tablets or the pediatric powder for oral solution, may substantially interfere with the absorption of quinolones, resulting in systemic concentrations considerably lower than desired. Therefore, AVELOX should be taken at least 4 hours before or 8 hours after these agents. *[see Dosage and Administration (2.2), Pharmacokinetics (12.3), and Patient Counseling Information (17.2).]*

7.2 Warfarin

Quinolones, including AVELOX, have been reported to enhance the anticoagulant effects of warfarin or its derivatives in the patient population. In addition, infectious disease and its accompanying inflammatory process, age, and general status of the patient are risk factors for increased anticoagulant activity. Therefore the prothrombin time, International Normalized Ratio (INR), or other suitable anticoagulation tests should be closely monitored if a quinolone is administered concomitantly with warfarin or its derivatives. *[see Adverse Reactions (6.2, 6.3), Pharmacokinetics (12.3), and Patient Counseling Information (17.3).]*

7.3 Nonsteroidal Anti-Inflammatory Drugs (NSAIDs)

Although not observed with AVELOX in preclinical and clinical trials, the concomitant administration of a nonsteroidal anti-inflammatory drug with a quinolone may increase the risks of CNS stimulation and convulsions *[see Warnings and Precautions (5.6), and Patient Counseling Information (17.3)].*

7.4 Drugs that Prolong QT

There is limited information available on the potential for a pharmacodynamic interaction in humans between AVELOX and other drugs that prolong the QTc interval of the electrocardiogram. Sotalol, a Class III antiarrhythmic, has been shown to further increase the QTc interval when combined with high doses of intravenous (IV) AVELOX in dogs. Therefore, AVELOX should be avoided with Class IA and Class III antiarrhythmics. *[see Warnings and Precautions, (5.3), Nonclinical Toxicology (13.2), and Patient Counseling Information (17.3).]*

8 USE IN SPECIFIC POPULATIONS

8.1 Pregnancy

Pregnancy Category C.

Because no adequate or well-controlled studies have been conducted in pregnant women, AVELOX should be used during pregnancy only if the potential benefit justifies the potential risk to the fetus.

Moxifloxacin was not teratogenic when administered to pregnant rats during organogenesis at oral doses as high as 500 mg/kg/day or 0.24 times the maximum recommended human dose based on systemic exposure (AUC), but decreased fetal body weights and slightly delayed fetal skeletal development (indicative of fetotoxicity) were observed. Intravenous administration of 80 mg/kg/day (approximately 2 times the maximum recommended human dose based on body surface area (mg/m^2) to pregnant rats resulted in maternal toxicity and a marginal effect on fetal and placental weights and the appearance of the placenta. There was no evidence of teratogenicity at intravenous doses as high as 80 mg/kg/day. Intravenous administration of 20 mg/kg/day (approximately equal to the maximum recommended human oral dose based upon systemic exposure) to pregnant rabbits during organogenesis resulted in decreased fetal body weights and delayed fetal skeletal ossification. When rib and vertebral malformations were combined, there was an increased fetal and litter incidence of these effects. Signs of maternal toxicity in rabbits at this dose included mortality, abortions, marked reduction of food consumption, decreased water intake, body weight loss and hypoactivity. There was no evidence of teratogenicity when pregnant cynomolgus monkeys were given oral doses as high as 100 mg/kg/day (2.5 times the maximum recommended human dose based upon systemic exposure). An increased incidence of smaller fetuses was observed at 100 mg/kg/day. In an oral pre- and postnatal development study conducted in rats, effects observed at 500 mg/kg/day included slight increases in duration of pregnancy and prenatal loss, reduced pup birth weight and decreased neonatal survival. Treatment-related maternal mortality occurred during gestation at 500 mg/kg/day in this study.

8.3 Nursing Mothers

Moxifloxacin is excreted in the breast milk of rats. Moxifloxacin may also be excreted in human milk. Because of the potential for serious adverse reactions in infants who are nursing from mothers taking AVELOX, a decision should be made whether to discontinue nursing or to discontinue the drug, taking into account the importance of the drug to the mother.

8.4 Pediatric Use

Safety and effectiveness in pediatric patients and adolescents less than 18 years of age have not been established. AVELOX causes arthropathy in juvenile animals *[see Boxed Warning, Warnings and Precautions (5.9), and Clinical Pharmacology (12.3)]*.

8.5 Geriatric Use

Geriatric patients are at increased risk for developing severe tendon disorders including tendon rupture when being treated with a fluoroquinolone such as AVELOX. This risk is further increased in patients receiving concomitant corticosteroid therapy. Tendinitis or tendon rupture can involve the Achilles, hand, shoulder, or other tendon sites and can occur during or after completion of therapy; cases occurring up to several months after fluoroquinolone treatment have been reported. Caution should be used when prescribing AVELOX to elderly patients especially those on corticosteroids. Patients should be informed of this potential side effect and advised to discontinue AVELOX and contact their healthcare provider if any symptoms of tendinitis or tendon rupture occur. *[see Boxed Warning, Warnings and Precautions (5.1), and Adverse Reactions (6.2).]*

In controlled multiple-dose clinical trials, 23% of patients receiving oral AVELOX were greater than or equal to 65 years of age and 9% were greater than or equal to 75 years of age. The clinical trial data demonstrate that there is no difference in the safety and efficacy of oral AVELOX in patients aged 65 or older compared to younger adults.

In trials of intravenous use, 42% of AVELOX patients were greater than or equal to 65 years of age, and 23% were greater than or equal to 75 years of age. The clinical trial data demonstrate that the safety of intravenous AVELOX in patients aged 65 or older was similar to that of comparator-treated patients. In general, elderly patients may be more susceptible to drug-associated effects of the QT interval. Therefore, AVELOX should be avoided in patients taking drugs that can result in prolongation of the QT interval (for example, class IA or class III antiarrhythmics) or in patients with risk factors for torsade de pointes (for example, known QT prolongation, uncorrected hypokalemia). *[see Warnings and Precautions (5.3), Drug Interactions (7.4), and Clinical Pharmacology (12.3).]*

8.6 Renal Impairment

The pharmacokinetic parameters of moxifloxacin are not significantly altered in mild, moderate, severe, or end-stage renal disease. No dosage adjustment is necessary in patients with renal impairment, including those patients requiring hemodialysis (HD) or continuous ambulatory peritoneal dialysis (CAPD) *[see Dosage and Administration (2), and Clinical Pharmacology (12.3).]*

8.7 Hepatic Impairment

No dosage adjustment is recommended for mild, moderate, or severe hepatic insufficiency (Child-Pugh Classes A, B, or C). However, due to metabolic disturbances associated with hepatic insufficiency, which may lead to QT prolongation, AVELOX should be used with caution in these patients *[see Warnings and Precaution (5.3), and Clinical Pharmacology, (12.3)]*.

10 OVERDOSAGE

Single oral overdoses up to 2.8 g were not associated with any serious adverse events. In the event of acute overdose, the stomach should be emptied and adequate hydration maintained. ECG monitoring is recommended due to the possibility of QT interval prolongation. The patient should be carefully observed and given supportive treatment. The administration of activated charcoal as soon as possible after oral overdose may prevent excessive increase of systemic moxifloxacin exposure. About 3% and 9% of the dose of moxifloxacin, as well as about 2% and 4.5% of its glucuronide metabolite are removed by continuous ambulatory peritoneal dialysis and hemodialysis, respectively.

Single oral AVELOX doses of 2000, 500, and 1500 mg/kg were lethal to rats, mice, and cynomolgus monkeys, respectively. The minimum lethal intravenous dose in mice and rats was 100 mg/kg. Adverse clinical signs included CNS and gastrointestinal effects such as decreased activity, somnolence, tremor, convulsions, vomiting and diarrhea.

11 DESCRIPTION

AVELOX (moxifloxacin) hydrochloride is a synthetic broad spectrum antibacterial agent for oral and intravenous administration. Moxifloxacin, a fluoroquinolone, is available as the monohydrochloride salt of 1-cyclopropyl-7-[(S,S)-2,8-diazabicyclo[4.3.0]non-8-yl]-6-fluoro-8-methoxy-1,4-dihydro-4-oxo-3 quinoline carboxylic acid. It is a slightly yellow to yellow crystalline substance with a molecular weight of 437.9. Its empirical formula is $C_{21}H_{24}FN_3O_4$*HCl and its chemical structure is as follows:

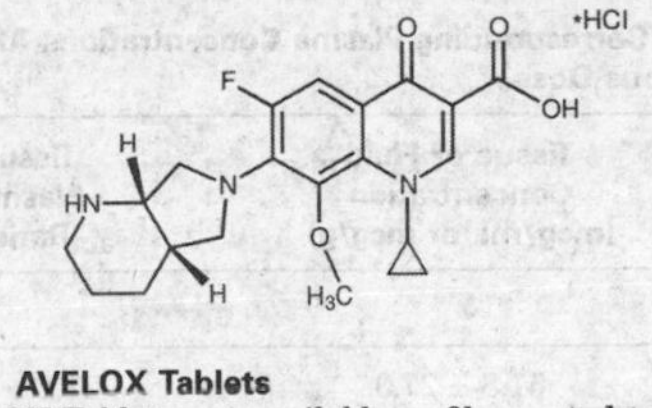

11.1 AVELOX Tablets

- AVELOX Tablets are available as film-coated tablets containing moxifloxacin hydrochloride (equivalent to 400 mg moxifloxacin).
- The inactive ingredients are microcrystalline cellulose, lactose monohydrate, croscarmellose sodium, magnesium stearate, hypromellose, titanium dioxide, polyethylene glycol and ferric oxide.

11.2 AVELOX IV

- AVELOX IV is available in ready-to-use 250 mL latex-free flexibags as a sterile, preservative free, 0.8% sodium chloride aqueous solution of moxifloxacin hydrochloride (containing 400 mg moxifloxacin) with pH ranging from 4.1 to 4.6.
- The appearance of the intravenous solution is yellow. The color does not affect, nor is it indicative of, product stability.
- The inactive ingredients are sodium chloride, USP, Water for Injection, USP, and may include hydrochloric acid and/or sodium hydroxide for pH adjustment.
- AVELOX IV contains approximately 34.2 mEq (787 mg) of sodium in 250 mL.

12 CLINICAL PHARMACOLOGY

12.1 Mechanism of Action

AVELOX is a member of the fluoroquinolone class of antibacterial agents *[see Microbiology (12.4)]*.

12.3 Pharmacokinetics

Absorption

Moxifloxacin, given as an oral tablet, is well absorbed from the gastrointestinal tract. The absolute bioavailability of moxifloxacin is approximately 90 percent. Coadministration with a high fat meal (that is, 500 calories from fat) does not affect the absorption of moxifloxacin.

Consumption of 1 cup of yogurt with moxifloxacin does not significantly affect the extent or rate of systemic absorption (AUC).

Table 5 Mean (± SD) C_{max} and AUC values following single and multiple doses of 400 mg moxifloxacin given orally

	C_{max} (mg/L)	AUC (mg•h/L)	Half-life (hr)
Single Dose Oral			
Healthy (n = 372)	3.1 ± 1	36.1 ± 9.1	11.5–15.6*
Multiple Dose Oral			
Healthy young male/female (n = 15)	4.5 ± 0.5	48 ± 2.7	12.7 ± 1.9
Healthy elderly male (n = 8)	3.8 ± 0.3	51.8 ± 6.7	
Healthy elderly female (n = 8)	4.6 ± 0.6	54.6 ± 6.7	
Healthy young male (n = 8)	3.6 ± 0.5	48.2 ± 9	
Healthy young female (n = 9)	4.2 ± 0.5	49.3 ± 9.5	

* Range of means from different studies

Table 6 Mean (± SD) C_{max} and AUC values following single and multiple doses of 400 mg moxifloxacin given by 1 hour IV infusion

	C_{max} (mg/L)	AUC (mg•h/L)	Half-life (hr)
Single Dose IV			
Healthy young male/female (n = 56)	3.9 ± 0.9	39.3 ± 8.6	8.2 - 15.4*
Patients (n = 118)			
Male (n = 64)	4.4 ± 3.7		
Female (n = 54)	4.5 ± 2		
< 65 years (n = 58)	4.6 ± 4.2		
≥ 65 years (n = 60)	4.3 ± 1.3		
Multiple Dose IV			
Healthy young male (n = 8)	4.2 ± 0.8	38 ± 4.7	14.8 ± 2.2
Healthy elderly (n =12; 8 male, 4 female)	6.1 ± 1.3	48.2 ± 0.9	10.1 ± 1.6
Patients† (n = 107)			
Male (n = 58)	4.2 ± 2.6		
Female (n = 49)	4.6 ± 1.5		
<65 years (n = 52)	4.1 ± 1.4		
≥65 years (n = 55)	4.7 ± 2.7		

* Range of means from different studies

† Expected C_{max} (concentration obtained around the time of the end of the infusion)

Plasma concentrations increase proportionately with dose up to the highest dose tested (1200 mg single oral dose). The mean (± SD) elimination half-life from plasma is 12 ± 1.3 hours; steady-state is achieved after at least three days with a 400 mg once daily regimen.

Figure 1 Mean Steady-State Plasma Concentrations of Moxifloxacin Obtained With Once Daily Dosing of 400 mg Either Orally (n=10) or by IV Infusion (n=12)

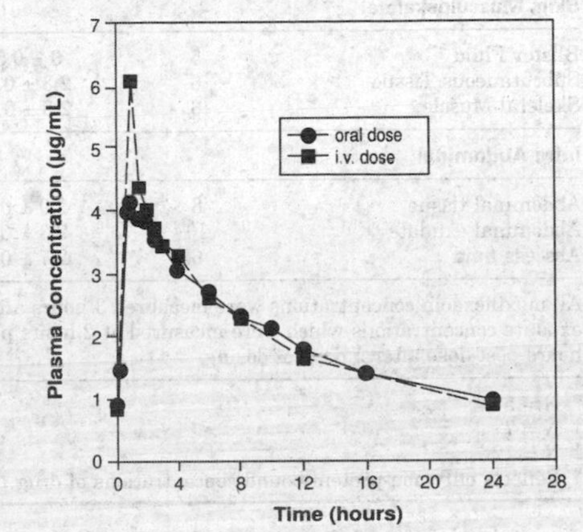

Distribution

Moxifloxacin is approximately 30-50% bound to serum proteins, independent of drug concentration. The volume of distribution of moxifloxacin ranges from 1.7 to 2.7 L/kg. Moxifloxacin is widely distributed throughout the body, with tissue concentrations often exceeding plasma concentrations. Moxifloxacin has been detected in the saliva, nasal and bronchial secretions, mucosa of the sinuses, skin blister fluid, subcutaneous tissue, skeletal muscle, and abdominal tissues and fluids following oral or intravenous administration of 400 mg. Moxifloxacin concentrations measured post-dose in various tissues and fluids following a 400 mg oral or IV dose are summarized in **Table 7**. The rates of elimination of moxifloxacin from tissues generally parallel the elimination from plasma.

[See table 7 at top of next page]

Metabolism

Approximately 52% of an oral or intravenous dose of moxifloxacin is metabolized via glucuronide and sulfate conjugation. The cytochrome P450 system is not involved in moxifloxacin metabolism, and is not affected by moxifloxacin. The sulfate conjugate (M1) accounts for approximately 38% of the dose, and is eliminated primarily in the feces. Approximately 14% of an oral or intravenous dose is converted to a glucuronide conjugate (M2), which is excreted exclusively in the urine. Peak plasma concentrations of M2 are approximately 40% those of the parent drug, while plasma concentrations of M1 are generally less than 10% those of moxifloxacin.

In vitro studies with cytochrome (CYP) P450 enzymes indicate that moxifloxacin does not inhibit CYP3A4, CYP2D6, CYP2C9, CYP2C19, or CYP1A2, suggesting that moxifloxacin is unlikely to alter the pharmacokinetics of drugs metabolized by these enzymes.

Excretion

Approximately 45% of an oral or intravenous dose of moxifloxacin is excreted as unchanged drug (~20% in urine and ~25% in feces). A total of 96% ± 4% of an oral dose is excreted as either unchanged drug or known metabolites. The mean (± SD) apparent total body clearance and renal clearance are 12 ± 2 L/hr and 2.6 ± 0.5 L/hr, respectively.

Pharmacokinetics in Specific Populations

Geriatric

Following oral administration of 400 mg moxifloxacin for 10 days in 16 elderly (8 male; 8 female) and 17 young (8 male; 9 female) healthy volunteers, there were no age-related changes in moxifloxacin pharmacokinetics. In 16 healthy male volunteers (8 young; 8 elderly) given a single 200 mg dose of oral moxifloxacin, the extent of systemic exposure (AUC and C_{max}) was not statistically different between young and elderly males and elimination half-life was unchanged. No dosage adjustment is necessary based on age. In large phase III studies, the concentrations around the

Table 7 Moxifloxacin Concentrations (mean ± SD) in Tissues and the Corresponding Plasma Concentrations After a Single 400 mg Oral or Intravenous Dose

Tissue or Fluid	N	Plasma Concentration (mcg/mL)	Tissue or Fluid Concentration (mcg/mL or mcg/g)	Tissue Plasma Ratio
Respiratory				
Alveolar Macrophages	5	3.3 ± 0.7	61.8 ± 27.3	21.2 ± 10
Bronchial Mucosa	8	3.3 ± 0.7	5.5 ± 1.3	1.7 ± 0.3
Epithelial Lining Fluid	5	3.3 ± 0.7	24.4 ± 14.7	8.7 ± 6.1
Sinus				
Maxillary Sinus Mucosa	4	3.7 ± 1.1*	7.6 ± 1.7	2 ± 0.3
Anterior Ethmoid Mucosa	3	3.7 ± 1.1*	8.8 ± 4.3	2.2 ± 0.6
Nasal Polyps	4	3.7 ± 1.1*	9.8 ± 4.5	2.6 ± 0.6
Skin, Musculoskeletal				
Blister Fluid	5	3 ± 0.5†	2.6 ± 0.9	0.9 ± 0.2
Subcutaneous Tissue	6	2.3 ± 0.4‡	0.9 ± 0.3§	0.4 ± 0.6
Skeletal Muscle	6	2.3 ± 0.4‡	0.9 ± 0.2§	0.4 ± 0.1
Intra-Abdominal				
Abdominal tissue	8	2.9 ± 0.5	7.6 ± 2	2.7 ± 0.8
Abdominal exudate	10	2.3 ± 0.5	3.5 ±1.2	1.6 ± 0.7
Abscess fluid	6	2.7 ± 0.7	2.3 ±1.5	0.8±0.4

All moxifloxacin concentrations were measured 3 hours after a single 400 mg dose, except the abdominal tissue and exudate concentrations which were measured at 2 hours post-dose and the sinus concentrations which were measured 3 hours post-dose after 5 days of dosing.

* N = 5
† N = 7
‡ N = 12
§ Reflects only non-protein bound concentrations of drug.

time of the end of the infusion in elderly patients following intravenous infusion of 400 mg were similar to those observed in young patients. *[see Use In Specific Populations (8.5).]*

Pediatric

The pharmacokinetics of moxifloxacin in pediatric subjects has not been studied *[see Use In Specific Populations (8.4)]*.

Gender

Following oral administration of 400 mg moxifloxacin daily for 10 days to 23 healthy males (19-75 years) and 24 healthy females (19-70 years), the mean AUC and C_{max} were 8% and 16% higher, respectively, in females compared to males. There are no significant differences in moxifloxacin pharmacokinetics between male and female subjects when differences in body weight are taken into consideration.

A 400 mg single dose study was conducted in 18 young males and females. The comparison of moxifloxacin pharmacokinetics in this study (9 young females and 9 young males) showed no differences in AUC or C_{max} due to gender. Dosage adjustments based on gender are not necessary.

Race

Steady-state moxifloxacin pharmacokinetics in male Japanese subjects were similar to those determined in Caucasians, with a mean C_{max} of 4.1 mcg/mL, an AUC_{24} of 47 mcg•h/mL, and an elimination half-life of 14 hours, following 400 mg p.o. daily.

Renal Insufficiency

The pharmacokinetic parameters of moxifloxacin are not significantly altered in mild, moderate, severe, or end-stage renal disease. No dosage adjustment is necessary in patients with renal impairment, including those patients requiring hemodialysis (HD) or continuous ambulatory peritoneal dialysis (CAPD).

In a single oral dose study of 24 patients with varying degrees of renal function from normal to severely impaired, the mean peak concentrations (C_{max}) of moxifloxacin were reduced by 21% and 28% in the patients with moderate ($CL_{CR} \geq 30$ and ≤ 60 mL/min) and severe ($CL_{CR} < 30$ mL/min) renal impairment, respectively. The mean systemic exposure (AUC) in these patients was increased by 13%. In the moderate and severe renally impaired patients, the mean AUC for the sulfate conjugate (M1) increased by 1.7-fold (ranging up to 2.8-fold) and mean AUC and C_{max} for the glucuronide conjugate (M2) increased by 2.8-fold (ranging up to 4.8-fold) and 1.4-fold (ranging up to 2.5-fold), respectively. *[see Use in Specific Populations (8.6).]*

The pharmacokinetics of single dose and multiple dose moxifloxacin were studied in patients with $CL_{CR} < 20$ mL/min on either hemodialysis or continuous ambulatory peritoneal dialysis (8 HD, 8 CAPD). Following a single 400 mg oral dose, the AUC of moxifloxacin in these HD and CAPD patients did not vary significantly from the AUC generally found in healthy volunteers. C_{max} values of moxifloxacin were reduced by about 45% and 33% in HD and CAPD patients, respectively, compared to healthy, historical controls. The exposure (AUC) to the sulfate conjugate (M1) increased by 1.4- to 1.5-fold in these patients. The mean AUC of the glucuronide conjugate (M2) increased by a factor of 7.5, whereas the mean C_{max} values of the glucuronide conjugate (M2) increased by a factor of 2.5 to 3, compared to healthy subjects. The sulfate and the glucuronide conjugates of moxifloxacin are not microbiologically active, and the clinical implication of increased exposure to these metabolites in patients with renal disease including those undergoing HD and CAPD has not been studied.

Oral administration of 400 mg QD AVELOX for 7 days to patients on HD or CAPD produced mean systemic exposure (AUC_{ss}) to moxifloxacin similar to that generally seen in healthy volunteers. Steady-state C_{max} values were about 22% lower in HD patients but were comparable between CAPD patients and healthy volunteers. Both HD and CAPD removed only small amounts of moxifloxacin from the body (approximately 9% by HD, and 3% by CAPD). HD and CAPD also removed about 4% and 2% of the glucuronide metabolite (M2), respectively.

Hepatic Insufficiency

No dosage adjustment is recommended for mild, moderate, or severe hepatic insufficiency (Child-Pugh Classes A, B, or C). However, due to metabolic disturbances associated with hepatic insufficiency, which may lead to QT prolongation, AVELOX should be used with caution in these patients *[see Warnings and Precautions (5.3), Use in Specific Populations (8.7)]*.

In 400 mg single oral dose studies in 6 patients with mild (Child-Pugh Class A) and 10 patients with moderate (Child-Pugh Class B) hepatic insufficiency, moxifloxacin mean systemic exposure (AUC) was 78% and 102%, respectively, of 18 healthy controls and mean peak concentration (C_{max}) was 79% and 84% of controls.

The mean AUC of the sulfate conjugate of moxifloxacin (M1) increased by 3.9-fold (ranging up to 5.9-fold) and 5.7-fold (ranging up to 8-fold) in the mild and moderate groups, respectively. The mean C_{max} of M1 increased by approximately 3-fold in both groups (ranging up to 4.7- and 3.9-fold). The mean AUC of the glucuronide conjugate of moxifloxacin (M2) increased by 1.5-fold (ranging up to 2.5-fold) in both groups. The mean C_{max} of M2 increased by 1.6- and 1.3-fold (ranging up to 2.7- and 2.1-fold), respectively. The clinical significance of increased exposure to the sulfate and glucuronide conjugates has not been studied. In a subset of patients participating in a clinical trial, the plasma concentrations of moxifloxacin and metabolites determined approximately at the moxifloxacin T_{max} following the first intravenous or oral AVELOX dose in the Child-Pugh Class C patients (n=10) were similar to those in the Child-Pugh Class A/B patients (n=5), and also similar to those observed in healthy volunteer studies.

Photosensitivity Potential

A study of the skin response to ultraviolet (UVA and UVB) and visible radiation conducted in 32 healthy volunteers (8 per group) demonstrated that AVELOX does not show phototoxicity in comparison to placebo. The minimum erythematous dose (MED) was measured before and after treatment with AVELOX (200 mg or 400 mg once daily), lomefloxacin (400 mg once daily), or placebo. In this study, the MED measured for both doses of AVELOX were not significantly different from placebo, while lomefloxacin significantly lowered the MED.

It is difficult to ascribe relative photosensitivity/phototoxicity among various fluoroquinolones during actual patient use because other factors play a role in determining a subject's susceptibility to this adverse event such as: a patient's skin pigmentation, frequency and duration of sun and artificial ultraviolet light (UV) exposure, wearing of sunscreen and protective clothing, the use of other concomitant drugs and the dosage and duration of fluoroquinolone therapy *[see Warnings and Precautions (5.10), Adverse Reactions (6.3), and Patient Counseling Information (17.3)]*.

Drug-Drug Interactions

The following drug interactions were studied in healthy volunteers or patients.

Antacids and iron significantly reduced bioavailability of moxifloxacin, as observed with other quinolones *[see Drug Interactions (7.1)]*.

Calcium, digoxin, itraconazole, morphine, probenecid, ranitidine, theophylline, and warfarin did not significantly affect the pharmacokinetics of moxifloxacin. These results and the data from *in vitro* studies suggest that moxifloxacin is unlikely to significantly alter the metabolic clearance of drugs metabolized by CYP3A4, CYP2D6, CYP2C9, CYP2C19, or CYP1A2 enzymes.

Moxifloxacin had no clinically significant effect on the pharmacokinetics of atenolol, digoxin, glyburide, itraconazole, oral contraceptives, theophylline, and warfarin *[see Drug Interactions (7.2)]*.

Antacids

When moxifloxacin (single 400 mg tablet dose) was administered two hours before, concomitantly, or 4 hours after an aluminum/magnesium-containing antacid (900 mg aluminum hydroxide and 600 mg magnesium hydroxide as a single oral dose) to 12 healthy volunteers there was a 26%, 60% and 23% reduction in the mean AUC of moxifloxacin, respectively. Moxifloxacin should be taken at least 4 hours before or 8 hours after antacids containing magnesium or aluminum, as well as sucralfate, metal cations such as iron, and multivitamin preparations with zinc, or VIDEX® (didanosine) chewable/ buffered tablets or the pediatric powder for oral solution. *[see Dosage and Administration (2.2), Drug Interactions (7.1)]*.

Atenolol

In a crossover study involving 24 healthy volunteers (12 male; 12 female), the mean atenolol AUC following a single oral dose of 50 mg atenolol with placebo was similar to that observed when atenolol was given concomitantly with a single 400 mg oral dose of moxifloxacin. The mean C_{max} of single dose atenolol decreased by about 10% following coadministration with a single dose of moxifloxacin.

Calcium

Twelve healthy volunteers were administered concomitant moxifloxacin (single 400 mg dose) and calcium (single dose of 500 mg Ca^{++} dietary supplement) followed by an additional two doses of calcium 12 and 24 hours after moxifloxacin administration. Calcium had no significant effect on the mean AUC of moxifloxacin. The mean C_{max} was slightly reduced and the time to maximum plasma concentration was prolonged when moxifloxacin was given with calcium compared to when moxifloxacin was given alone (2.5 hours versus 0.9 hours). These differences are not considered to be clinically significant.

Digoxin

No significant effect of moxifloxacin (400 mg once daily for two days) on digoxin (0.6 mg as a single dose) AUC was detected in a study involving 12 healthy volunteers. The mean digoxin C_{max} increased by about 50% during the distribution phase of digoxin. This transient increase in digoxin C_{max} is not viewed to be clinically significant. Moxifloxacin pharmacokinetics were similar in the presence or absence of digoxin. No dosage adjustment for moxifloxacin or digoxin is required when these drugs are administered concomitantly.

Glyburide

In diabetics, glyburide (2.5 mg once daily for two weeks pretreatment and for five days concurrently) mean AUC and C_{max} were 12% and 21% lower, respectively, when taken with moxifloxacin (400 mg once daily for five days) in comparison to placebo. Nonetheless, blood glucose levels were decreased slightly in patients taking glyburide and moxifloxacin in comparison to those taking glyburide alone, suggesting no interference by moxifloxacin on the activity of glyburide. These interaction results are not viewed as clinically significant.

Iron

When moxifloxacin tablets were administered concomitantly with iron (ferrous sulfate 100 mg once daily for two days), the mean AUC and C_{max} of moxifloxacin was reduced by 39% and 59%, respectively. Moxifloxacin should only be taken more than 4 hours before or 8 hours after iron products. *[see Dosage and Administration (2.2), Drug Interactions (7.1)].*

Itraconazole

In a study involving 11 healthy volunteers, there was no significant effect of itraconazole (200 mg once daily for 9 days), a potent inhibitor of cytochrome P4503A4, on the pharmacokinetics of moxifloxacin (a single 400 mg dose given on the 7th day of itraconazole dosing). In addition, moxifloxacin was shown not to affect the pharmacokinetics of itraconazole.

Morphine

No significant effect of morphine sulfate (a single 10 mg intramuscular dose) on the mean AUC and C_{max} of moxifloxacin (400 mg single dose) was observed in a study of 20 healthy male and female volunteers.

Oral Contraceptives

A placebo-controlled study in 29 healthy female subjects showed that moxifloxacin 400 mg daily for 7 days did not interfere with the hormonal suppression of oral contraception with 0.15 mg levonorgestrel/0.03 mg ethinylestradiol (as measured by serum progesterone, FSH, estradiol, and LH), or with the pharmacokinetics of the administered contraceptive agents.

Probenecid

Probenecid (500 mg twice daily for two days) did not alter the renal clearance and total amount of moxifloxacin (400 mg single dose) excreted renally in a study of 12 healthy volunteers.

Ranitidine

No significant effect of ranitidine (150 mg twice daily for three days as pretreatment) on the pharmacokinetics of moxifloxacin (400 mg single dose) was detected in a study involving 10 healthy volunteers.

Theophylline

No significant effect of moxifloxacin (200 mg every twelve hours for 3 days) on the pharmacokinetics of theophylline (400 mg every twelve hours for 3 days) was detected in a study involving 12 healthy volunteers. In addition, theophylline was not shown to affect the pharmacokinetics of moxifloxacin. The effect of co-administration of a 400 mg dose of moxifloxacin with theophylline has not been studied, but it is not expected to be clinically significant based on *in vitro* metabolic data showing that moxifloxacin does not inhibit the CYP1A2 isoenzyme.

Warfarin

No significant effect of moxifloxacin (400 mg once daily for eight days) on the pharmacokinetics of R- and S-warfarin (25 mg single dose of warfarin sodium on the fifth day) was detected in a study involving 24 healthy volunteers. No significant change in prothrombin time was observed. *[see Adverse Reactions (6.2), Drug Interactions (7.2)].*

12.4 Microbiology

Mechanism of Action

The bactericidal action of moxifloxacin results from inhibition of the topoisomerase II (DNA gyrase) and topoisomerase IV required for bacterial DNA replication, transcription, repair, and recombination. It appears that the C8-methoxy moiety contributes to enhanced activity and lower selection of resistant mutants of Gram-positive bacteria compared to the C8-H moiety. The presence of the bulky bicycloamine substituent at the C-7 position prevents active efflux, associated with the *NorA* or *pmrA* genes seen in certain Gram-positive bacteria.

Mechanism of Resistance

The mechanism of action for fluoroquinolones, including moxifloxacin, is different from that of macrolides, beta-lactams, aminoglycosides, or tetracyclines; therefore, microorganisms resistant to these classes of drugs may be susceptible to moxifloxacin. Resistance to fluoroquinolones occurs primarily by a mutation in topoisomerase II (DNA gyrase) or topoisomerase IV genes, decreased outer membrane permeability or drug efflux. *In vitro* resistance to moxifloxacin develops slowly via multiple-step mutations. Resistance to moxifloxacin occurs *in vitro* at a general frequency of between 1.8×10^{-9} to $< 1 \times 10^{-11}$ for Gram-positive bacteria.

Cross Resistance

Cross-resistance has been observed between moxifloxacin and other fluoroquinolones against Gram-negative bacteria. Gram-positive bacteria resistant to other fluoroquinolones may, however, still be susceptible to moxifloxacin. There is no known cross-resistance between moxifloxacin and other classes of antimicrobials.

Moxifloxacin has been shown to be active against most isolates of the following bacteria, both *in vitro* and in clinical infections. *[see Indications and Usage (1)].*

Gram-positive bacteria

- *Enterococcus faecalis*
- *Staphylococcus aureus*
- *Streptococcus anginosus*

Table 8 Susceptibility Test Interpretive Criteria for Moxifloxacin

	MIC (mcg/mL)			Zone Diameter (mm)		
Species	**S**	**I**	**R**	**S**	**I**	**R**
Enterobacteriaceae	≤2	4	≥8	≥19	16–18	≤15
Enterococcus faecalis	≤1	2	≥4	≥18	15 17	≤14
Staphylococcus aureus	≤2	4	≥8	≥19	16–18	≤15
Haemophilus influenzae	≤1	-*	-*	≥18	-*	-*
Haemophilus parainfluenzae	≤1	-*	-*	≥18	-*	-*
Streptococcus pneumoniae	≤1	2	≥4	≥18	15–17	≤14†
Streptococcus species	≤1	2	≥4	≥18	15–17	≤14†
Anaerobic bacteria	≤2	4	≥8	-	-	-

S=susceptible, I=Intermediate, and R=resistant.

* The current absence of data on moxifloxacin-resistant isolates precludes defining any results other than "Susceptible".
† Isolates yielding test results (MIC or zone diameter) other than susceptible, should be submitted to a reference laboratory for additional testing.

- *Streptococcus constellatus*
- *Streptococcus pneumoniae* (including multi-drug resistant isolates [MDRSP]**)
- *Streptococcus pyogenes*

**MDRSP, Multi-drug resistant *Streptococcus pneumoniae* includes isolates previously known as PRSP (Penicillin-resistant *S. pneumoniae*), and are isolates resistant to two or more of the following antibiotics: penicillin (MIC) ≥2 mcg/mL), 2nd generation cephalosporins (for example, cefuroxime), macrolides, tetracyclines, and trimethoprim/sulfamethoxazole.

Gram-negative bacteria

- *Enterobacter cloacae*
- *Escherichia coli*
- *Haemophilus influenzae*
- *Haemophilus parainfluenzae*
- *Klebsiella pneumoniae*
- *Moraxella catarrhalis*
- *Proteus mirabilis*

Anaerobic bacteria

- *Bacteroides fragilis*
- *Bacteroides thetaiotaomicron*
- *Clostridium perfringens*
- *Peptostreptococcus species*

Other microorganisms

- *Chlamydophila pneumoniae*
- *Mycoplasma pneumoniae*

The following *in vitro* data are available, **but their clinical significance is unknown.** At least 90 percent of the following bacteria exhibit an *in vitro* minimum inhibitory concentration (MIC) less than or equal to the susceptible breakpoint for moxifloxacin. However, the efficacy of AVELOX in treating clinical infections due to these bacteria **has not been** established in adequate and well controlled clinical trials.

Gram-positive bacteria

- *Staphylococcus epidermidis*
- *Streptococcus agalactiae*
- *Streptococcus viridans group*

Gram-negative bacteria

- *Citrobacter freundii*
- *Klebsiellao xytoca*
- *Legionella pneumophila*

Anaerobic bacteria

- *Fusobacterium species*
- *Prevotella species*

Susceptibility Tests Methods

When available, the clinical microbiology laboratory should provide the results of *in vitro* susceptibility test results for antimicrobial drug products used in resident hospitals to the physician as periodic reports that describe the susceptibility profile of nosocomial and community acquired pathogens. These reports should aid the physician in selecting an antibacterial drug product for treatment.

• Dilution Techniques

Quantitative methods are used to determine antimicrobial minimum inhibitory concentrations (MICs). These MICs provide estimates of the susceptibility of bacteria to antimicrobial compounds. The MICs should be determined using a standardized procedure. Standardized procedures are based on a dilution method (broth and/or agar). [1] The MIC values should be interpreted according to the criteria in Table 8.

• Diffusion Techniques

Quantitative methods that require measurement of zone diameters can also provide reproducible estimates of the susceptibility of bacteria to antimicrobial compounds. The zone size provides an estimate of the susceptibility of bacteria to antimicrobial compounds. The zone size prove should be determined using a standardized test method.[2,3] This procedure uses paper disks impregnated with 5 mcg moxifloxacin to test the susceptibility of bacteria to moxifloxacin. The disc diffusion interpretive criteria are provided in Table 8.

• Anaerobic Techniques

For anaerobic bacteria, the susceptibility to moxifloxacin can be determined by a standardized test method.[4] The MIC values obtained should be interpreted according to the criteria provided in Table 8.

[See table 8 above]

A report of "Susceptible" indicates that the antimicrobial is likely to inhibit growth of the pathogen if the antimicrobial compound reaches the concentrations at the infection site necessary to inhibit growth of the pathogen. A report of "Intermediate" indicates that the result should be considered equivocal, and, if the microorganism is not fully susceptible to alternative, clinically feasible drugs, the test should be repeated. This category implies possible clinical applicability in body sites where the drug is physiologically concentrated or in situations where a high dosage of the drug product can be used. This category also provides a buffer zone that prevents small uncontrolled technical factors from causing major discrepancies in interpretation. A report of "Resistant" indicates that the antimicrobial is not likely to inhibit growth of the pathogen if the antimicrobial compound reaches the concentrations usually achievable at the infection site; other therapy should be selected.

• Quality Control

Standardized susceptibility test procedures require the use of laboratory controls to monitor and ensure the accuracy and precision of supplies and reagents used in the assay and the techniques of the individuals performing the test.[1,2,3,4] Standard moxifloxacin powder should provide the following range of MIC values noted in Table 9. For the diffusion technique using the 5 mcg moxifloxacin disk, the criteria in Table 9 should be achieved.

Table 9 Acceptable Quality Control Ranges for Moxifloxacin

Strains	MIC range (mcg/mL)	Zone Diameter (mm)
Enterococcus faecalis ATCC 29212	0.06–0.5	-
Escherichia coli ATCC 25922	0.008–0.06	28–35
Haemophilus influenzae ATCC 49247	0.008–0.03	31–39
Staphylococcus aureus ATCC29213	0.015–0.06	-
Staphylococcus aureus ATCC25923	-	28–35
Streptococcus pneumoniae ATCC 49619	0.06–0.25	25–31
Bacteroides fragilis ATCC 25285	0.125–0.5	-
Bacteroides thetaiotaomicron ATCC 29741	1–4	-

Table 12 Clinical and Bacteriological Success Rates for AVELOX-Treated MDRSP CAP Patients (Population: Valid for Efficacy)

Screening Susceptibility	Clinical Success		Bacteriological Success	
	n/N*	%	n/N†	%
Penicillin-resistant	21/21	100%‡	21/21	100%‡
2nd generation cephalosporin-resistant	25/26	96%‡	25/26	96%‡
Macrolide-resistant§	22/23	96%	22/23	96%
Trimethoprim/sulfamethoxazole-resistant	28/30	93%	28/30	93%
Tetracycline-resistant	17/18	94%	17/18	94%

* n = number of patients successfully treated; N = number of patients with MDRSP (from a total of 37 patients)
† n = number of patients successfully treated (presumed eradication or eradication); N = number of patients with MDRSP (from a total of 37 patients)
‡ One patient had a respiratory isolate that was resistant to penicillin and cefuroxime but a blood isolate that was intermediate to penicillin and cefuroxime. The patient is included in the database based on the respiratory isolate.
§ Azithromycin, clarithromycin, and erythromycin were the macrolide antimicrobials tested.

Eubacterium lentum ATCC 43055	0.125–0.5	-

13 NONCLINICAL TOXICOLOGY

13.1 Carcinogenesis, Mutagenesis, Impairment of Fertility

Long term studies in animals to determine the carcinogenic potential of moxifloxacin have not been performed.

Moxifloxacin was not mutagenic in 4 bacterial strains (TA 98, TA 100, TA 1535, TA 1537) used in the Ames *Salmonella* reversion assay. As with other quinolones, the positive response observed with moxifloxacin in strain TA 102 using the same assay may be due to the inhibition of DNA gyrase. Moxifloxacin was not mutagenic in the CHO/HGPRT mammalian cell gene mutation assay. An equivocal result was obtained in the same assay when v79 cells were used. Moxifloxacin was clastogenic in the v79 chromosome aberration assay, but it did not induce unscheduled DNA synthesis in cultured rat hepatocytes. There was no evidence of genotoxicity *in vivo* in a micronucleus test or a dominant lethal test in mice.

Moxifloxacin had no effect on fertility in male and female rats at oral doses as high as 500 mg/kg/day, approximately 12 times the maximum recommended human dose based on body surface area (mg/m^2), or at intravenous doses as high as 45 mg/kg/day, approximately equal to the maximum recommended human dose based on body surface area (mg/m^2). At 500 mg/kg orally there were slight effects on sperm morphology (head-tail separation) in male rats and on the estrous cycle in female rats.

13.2 Animal Toxicology and/or Pharmacology

Quinolones have been shown to cause arthropathy in immature animals. In studies in juvenile dogs oral doses of moxifloxacin ≥ 30 mg/kg/day (approximately 1.5 times the maximum recommended human dose based upon systemic exposure) for 28 days resulted in arthropathy. There was no evidence of arthropathy in mature monkeys and rats at oral doses up to 135 and 500 mg/kg/day, respectively.

Moxifloxacin at an oral dose of 300 mg/kg did not show an increase in acute toxicity or potential for CNS toxicity (for example, seizures) in mice when used in combination with NSAIDs such as diclofenac, ibuprofen, or fenbufen. Some quinolones have been reported to have proconvulsant activity that is exacerbated with concomitant use of non-steroidal anti-inflammatory drugs (NSAIDs).

A QT-prolonging effect of moxifloxacin was found in dog studies, at plasma concentrations about five times the human therapeutic level. The combined infusion of sotalol, a Class III antiarrhythmic agent, with moxifloxacin induced a higher degree of QTc prolongation in dogs than that induced by the same dose (30 mg/kg) of moxifloxacin alone. Electrophysiological *in vitro* studies suggested an inhibition of the rapid activating component of the delayed rectifier potassium current (I_{Kr}) as an underlying mechanism.

No signs of local intolerability were observed in dogs when moxifloxacin was administered intravenously. After intraarterial injection, inflammatory changes involving the periarterial soft tissue were observed suggesting that intraarterial administration of AVELOX should be avoided.

14 CLINICAL STUDIES

14.1 Acute Bacterial Exacerbation of Chronic Bronchitis

AVELOX Tablets (400 mg once daily for five days) were evaluated for the treatment of acute bacterial exacerbation of chronic bronchitis in a randomized, double-blind, controlled clinical trial conducted in the US. This study compared AVELOX with clarithromycin (500 mg twice daily for 10 days) and enrolled 629 patients. Clinical success was assessed at 7-17 days post-therapy. The clinical success for AVELOX was 89% (222/250) compared to 89% (224/251) for clarithromycin.

Table 10 Clinical Success Rates at Follow-Up Visit for Clinically Evaluable Patients by Pathogen (Acute Bacterial Exacerbation of Chronic Bronchitis)

PATHOGEN	AVELOX	Clarithromycin
Streptococcus pneumoniae	16/16 (100%)	20/23 (87%)
Haemophilus influenzae	33/37 (89%)	36/41 (88%)
Haemophilus parainfluenzae	16/16 (100%)	14/14 (100%)
Moraxella catarrhalis	29/34 (85%)	24/24 (100%)
Staphylococcus aureus	15/16 (94%)	6/8 (75%)
Klebsiella pneumoniae	18/20 (90%)	10/11 (91%)

The microbiological eradication rates (eradication plus presumed eradication) in AVELOX treated patients were *Streptococcus pneumoniae* 100%, *Haemophilus influenzae* 89%, *Haemophilus parainfluenzae* 100%, *Moraxella catarrhalis* 85%, *Staphylococcus aureus* 94%, and *Klebsiella pneumonia* 85%.

14.2 Community Acquired Pneumonia

A randomized, double-blind, controlled clinical trial was conducted in the US to compare the efficacy of AVELOX Tablets (400 mg once daily) to that of high-dose clarithromycin (500 mg twice daily) in the treatment of patients with clinically and radiologically documented community acquired pneumonia. This study enrolled 474 patients (382 of whom were valid for the efficacy analysis conducted at the 14 - 35 day follow-up visit). Clinical success for clinically evaluable patients was 95% (184/194) for AVELOX and 95% (178/188) for high dose clarithromycin.

A randomized, double-blind, controlled trial was conducted in the US and Canada to compare the efficacy of sequential IV/PO AVELOX 400 mg QD for 7-14 days to an IV/PO fluoroquinolone control (trovafloxacin or levofloxacin) in the treatment of patients with clinically and radiologically documented community acquired pneumonia. This study enrolled 516 patients, 362 of whom were valid for the efficacy analysis conducted at the 7-30 day post-therapy visit. The clinical success rate was 86% (157/182) for AVELOX therapy and 89% (161/180) for the fluoroquinolone comparators.

An open-label ex-US study that enrolled 628 patients compared AVELOX to sequential IV/PO amoxicillin/clavulanate (1.2 g IV q8h/625 mg PO q8h) with or without high-dose IV/PO clarithromycin (500 mg BID). The intravenous formulations of the comparators are not FDA approved. The clinical success rate at Day 5-7 for AVELOX therapy was 93% (241/258) and demonstrated superiority to amoxicillin/clavulanate ± clarithromycin (85%, 239/280) [95% C.I. of difference in success rates between moxifloxacin and comparator (2.9%, 13.2%)]. The clinical success rate at the 21-28 days post-therapy visit for AVELOX was 84% (216/258), which also demonstrated superiority to the comparators (74%, 208/280) [95% C.I. of difference in success rates between moxifloxacin and comparator (2.6%, 16.3%)].

The clinical success rates by pathogen across four CAP studies are presented in **Table 11**.

Table 11 Clinical Success Rates By Pathogen (Pooled CAP Studies)

PATHOGEN	AVELOX	
Streptococcus pneumoniae	80/85	(94%)
Staphylococcus aureus	17/20	(85%)
Klebsiella pneumoniae	11/12	(92%)
Haemophilus influenzae	56/61	(92%)
Chlamydophila pneumoniae	119/128	(93%)
Mycoplasma pneumoniae	73/76	(96%)
Moraxella catarrhalis	11/12	(92%)

14.3 Community Acquired Pneumonia caused by Multi-Drug Resistant *Streptococcus pneumoniae* (MDRSP)*

AVELOX was effective in the treatment of community acquired pneumonia (CAP) caused by multi-drug resistant *Streptococcus pneumoniae* MDRSP* isolates. Of 37 microbiologically evaluable patients with MDRSP isolates, 35 patients (95%) achieved clinical and bacteriological success post-therapy. The clinical and bacteriological success rates based on the number of patients treated are shown in **Table 12**.

* MDRSP, Multi-drug resistant *Streptococcus pneumoniae* includes isolates previously known as PRSP (Penicillin-resistant *S. pneumoniae*), and are isolates resistant to two or more of the following antibiotics: penicillin (MIC ≥ 2 mcg/mL), 2nd generation cephalosporins (for example, cefuroxime), macrolides, tetracyclines, and trimethoprim/sulfamethoxazole.

[See table 12 above]

Not all isolates were resistant to all antimicrobial classes tested. Success and eradication rates are summarized in Table 13.

Table 13 Clinical Success Rates and Microbiological Eradication Rates for Resistant Streptococcus pneumoniae (Community Acquired Pneumonia)

S. pneumoniae with MDRSP	Clinical Success	Bacteriological Eradication Rate
Resistant to 2 antimicrobials	12/13 (92.3 %)	12/13 (92.3 %)
Resistant to 3 antimicrobials	10/11 (90.9 %)*	10/11 (90.9 %)*
Resistant to 4 antimicrobials	6/6 (100%)	6/6 (100%)
Resistant to 5 antimicrobials	7/7 (100%)*	7/7 (100%)*
Bacteremia with MDRSP	9/9 (100%)	9/9 (100%)

* One patient had a respiratory isolate resistant to 5 antimicrobials and a blood isolate resistant to 3 antimicrobials. The patient was included in the category resistant to 5 antimicrobials.

14.4 Acute Bacterial Sinusitis

In a controlled double-blind study conducted in the US, AVELOX Tablets (400 mg once daily for ten days) were compared with cefuroxime axetil (250 mg twice daily for ten days) for the treatment of acute bacterial sinusitis. The trial included 457 patients valid for the efficacy analysis. Clinical success (cure plus improvement) at the 7 to 21 day post-therapy test of cure visit was 90% for AVELOX and 89% for cefuroxime.

An additional non-comparative study was conducted to gather bacteriological data and to evaluate microbiological eradication in adult patients treated with AVELOX 400 mg once daily for seven days. All patients (n = 336) underwent antral puncture in this study. Clinical success rates and eradication/presumed eradication rates at the 21 to 37 day follow-up visit were 97% (29 out of 30) for *Streptococcus pneumoniae*, 83% (15 out of 18) for *Moraxella catarrhalis*, and 80% (24 out of 30) for *Haemophilusinfluenzae*.

14.5 Uncomplicated Skin and Skin Structure Infections

A randomized, double-blind, controlled clinical trial conducted in the US compared the efficacy of AVELOX 400 mg once daily for seven days with cephalexin HCl 500 mg three times daily for seven days. The percentage of patients treated for uncomplicated abscesses was 30%, furuncles 8%, cellulitis 16%, impetigo 20%, and other skin infections 26%. Adjunctive procedures (incision and drainage or debridement) were performed on 17% of the AVELOX treated patients and 14% of the comparator treated patients. Clinical success rates in evaluable patients were 89% (108/122) for AVELOX and 91% (110/121) for cephalexin HCl.

14.6 Complicated Skin and Skin Structure Infections

Two randomized, active controlled trials of cSSSI were performed. A double-blind trial was conducted primarily in North America to compare the efficacy of sequential IV/PO AVELOX 400 mg QD for 7-14 days to an IV/PO beta-lactam/beta-lactamase inhibitor control in the treatment of patients with cSSSI. This study enrolled 617 patients, 335 of which were valid for the efficacy analysis. A second open-label International study compared AVELOX 400 mg QD for 7-21 days to sequential IV/PO beta-lactam/beta-lactamase inhibitor control in the treatment of patients with cSSSI. This study enrolled 804 patients, 632 of which were valid for the efficacy analysis. Surgical incision and drainage or debridement was performed on 55% of the AVELOX treated and 53% of the comparator treated patients in these studies and formed an integral part of therapy for this indication. Success rates varied with the type of diagnosis ranging from 61% in patients with infected ulcers to 90% in patients with complicated erysipelas. These rates were similar to those seen with comparator drugs. The overall success rates in the evaluable patients and the clinical success by pathogen are shown in **Tables 14 and 15.**

Table 14 Overall Clinical Success Rates in Patients with Complicated Skin and Skin Structure Infections

Study	AVELOX n/ N (%)	Comparator n/N (%)	95% Confidence Interval*
North America	125/162 (77.2%)	141/173 (81.5%)	(-14.4%, 2%)
International	254/315 (80.6%)	268/317 (84.5%)	(-9.4%, 2.2%)

* of difference in success rates between Moxifloxacin and comparator (Moxifloxacin – comparator)

Table 15 Clinical Success Rates by Pathogen in Patients with Complicated Skin and Skin Structure Infections

Pathogen	AVELOX n/ N (%)	Comparator n/N (%)
Staphylococcus aureus (methicillin-susceptible isolates)*	106/129 (82.2%)	120/137 (87.6%)
Escherichia coli	31/38 (81.6 %)	28/33 (84.8 %)
Klebsiella pneumoniae	11/12 (91.7 %)	7/10 (70%)
Enterobacter cloacae	9/11 (81.8%)	4/7 (57.1%)

* methicillin susceptibility was only determined in the North American Study

14.7 Complicated Intra-Abdominal Infections

Two randomized, active controlled trials of cIAI were performed. A double-blind trial was conducted primarily in North America to compare the efficacy of sequential IV/PO AVELOX 400 mg QD for 5-14 days to IV/ piperacillin/tazobactam followed by PO amoxicillin/clavulanic acid in the treatment of patients with cIAI, including peritonitis, abscesses, appendicitis with perforation, and bowel perforation. This study enrolled 681 patients, 379 of which were considered clinically evaluable. A second open-label international study compared AVELOX 400 mg QD for 5-14 days to IV ceftriaxone plus IV metronidazole followed by PO amoxicillin/clavulanic acid in the treatment of patients with cIAI. This study enrolled 595 patients, 511 of which were considered clinically evaluable. The clinically evaluable population consisted of subjects with a surgically confirmed complicated infection, at least 5 days of treatment and a 25-50 day follow-up assessment for patients at the Test of Cure visit. The overall clinical success rates in the clinically evaluable patients are shown in **Table 16.**

Table 16 Clinical Success Rates in Patients with Complicated Intra-Abdominal Infections

Study	AVELOX n/ N (%)	Comparator n/N (%)	95% Confidence Interval*
North America (overall)	146/183 (79.8 %)	153/196 (78.1 %)	(-7.4%, 9.3%)
Abscess	40/57 (70.2 %)	49/63 (77.8 %)†	NA‡
Non-abscess	106/126 (84.1 %)	104/133 (78.2 %)	NA‡
International (overall)	199/246 (80.9 %)	218/265 (82.3 %)	(-8.9 %, 4.2%)
Abscess	73/93 (78.5 %)	86/99 (86.9 %)	NA
Non-abscess	126/153 (82.4 %)	132/166 (79.5 %)	NA

* of difference in success rates between AVELOX and comparator (AVELOX – comparator)
† Excludes 2 patients who required additional surgery within the first 48 hours.
‡ NA - not applicable

15 REFERENCES

1. Clinical and Laboratory Standards Institute (CLSI), Methods for Dilution Antimicrobial Susceptibility Tests for Bacteria That Grow Aerobically 9th edition. Approved Standard CLSI Document M7-A9, CLSI, 950 West Valley Rd., Suite 2500, Wayne, PA 19087, 2012.
2. CLSI , Performance Standards for Antimicrobial Susceptibility Testing 22 Informational Supplement. CLSI Document M100-S22, 2012.
3. CLSI , Performance Standards for Antimicrobial Disk Susceptibility Tests 11th edition. Approved Standard CLSI Document M2-A11, 2012.
4. CLSI , Methods for Antimicrobial Susceptibility Testing of Anaerobic Bacteria 8th edition; Approved Standard CLSI Document M11-A8, 2012

16 HOW SUPPLIED/STORAGE AND HANDLING

16.1 AVELOX Tablets

AVELOX (moxifloxacin) hydrochloride tablets are available as oblong, dull red film-coated tablets containing 400 mg moxifloxacin.

The tablet is coded with the word "BAYER" on one side and "M400" on the reverse side.

Package	NDC Code
Bottles of 30:	0085-1733-01
Unit Dose Pack of 50:	0085-1733-02
ABC Pack of 5:	0085-1733-03

Store at 25°C (77°F); excursions permitted to 15–30°C (59–86°F) *[see USP Controlled Room Temperature]*. Avoid high humidity.

16.2 AVELOX Intravenous Solution – Premix Bags

AVELOX IV (moxifloxacin) hydrochloride in sodium chloride injection) is available in ready-to-use 250 mL latex-free flexible bags containing 400 mg of moxifloxacin in 0.8% saline. NO FURTHER DILUTION OF THIS PREPARATION IS NECESSARY.

Package	NDC Code
250 mL flexible container	0085-1737-01

Parenteral drug products should be inspected visually for particulate matter prior to administration. Samples containing visible particulates should not be used.

Because the premix flexible containers are for single-use only, any unused portion should be discarded.

Store at 25°C (77°F); excursions permitted to 15–30°C (59–86°F) *[see USP Controlled Room Temperature]*.

DO NOT REFRIGERATE – PRODUCT PRECIPITATES UPON REFRIGERATION.

17 PATIENT COUNSELING INFORMATION

See FDA-Approved Medication Guide

17.1 Antibacterial Resistance

Antibacterial drugs including AVELOX should only be used to treat bacterial infections. They do not treat viral infections (for example, the common cold). When AVELOX is prescribed to treat a bacterial infection, patients should be told that although it is common to feel better early in the course of therapy, the medication should be taken exactly as directed. Skipping doses or not completing the full course of therapy may (1) decrease the effectiveness of the immediate treatment and (2) increase the likelihood that bacteria will develop resistance and will not be treatable by AVELOX or other antibacterial drugs in the future.

17.2 Administration With Food, Fluids, and Drug Products Containing Multivalent Cations

Patients should be informed that AVELOX tablets may be taken with or without food. Patients should be advised to drink fluids liberally.

AVELOX tablets should be taken at least 4 hours before or 8 hours after multivitamins (containing iron or zinc), antacids (containing magnesium or aluminum), sucralfate, or VIDEX® (didanosine) chewable/buffered tablets or the pediatric powder for oral solution.

17.3 Serious and Potentially Serious Adverse Reactions

To assure safe and effective use of AVELOX, patients should be informed of the following serious adverse reactions that have been associated with AVELOX and other fluoroquinolone use:

- **Tendon Disorders:** Patients should contact their healthcare provider if they experience pain, swelling, or inflammation of a tendon, or weakness or inability to use one of their joints; rest and refrain from exercise; and discontinue AVELOX treatment. The risk of severe tendon disorder with fluoroquinolones is higher in older patients usually over 60 years of age, in patients taking corticosteroid drugs, and in patients with kidney, heart or lung transplants.
- **Exacerbation of Myasthenia Gravis:** fluoroquinolones like AVELOX may cause worsening of myasthenia gravis symptoms, including muscle weakness and breathing problems. Patients should call their healthcare provider right away if they have any worsening muscle weakness or breathing problems.
- **Prolongation of the QT interval:** AVELOX may produce changes in the electrocardiogram (QTc interval prolongation). AVELOX should be avoided in patients receiving Class IA (for example quinidine, procainamide) or Class III (for example amiodarone, sotalol) antiarrhythmic agents. AVELOX may add to the QTc prolonging effects of other drugs such as cisapride, erythromycin, antipsychotics, and tricyclic antidepressants. The patients should inform their physician of any personal or family history of QTc prolongation or proarrhythmic conditions such as recent hypokalemia, significant bradycardia, and acute myocardial ischemia. Patients should contact their physician if they experience palpitations or fainting spells while taking AVELOX.
- **Hypersensitivity Reactions:** Patients should be advised that AVELOX may be associated with hypersensitivity reactions, including anaphylactic reactions, even following a single dose. Patients should discontinue AVELOX at the first sign of a skin rash or other signs of an allergic reaction.
- **Convulsions:** Convulsions have been reported in patients receiving quinolones, and they should notify their physician before taking AVELOX if there is a history of this condition. Patients should also inform their physician if they are taking NSAIDs concurrently with AVELOX.
- **Neurologic Adverse Effects (for example, dizziness, lightheadedness):** AVELOX may cause dizziness, lightheadedness and vision disorders; therefore, patients should know how they react to this drug before they operate an automobile or machinery or engage in activities requiring mental alertness or coordination.
- **Psychotic Reaction:** Psychotic reactions sometimes resulting in self-injurious behavior have been reported in patients receiving quinolones. Patients should notify their physician if they have a history of psychiatric illness before taking AVELOX.
- **Peripheral Neuropathies:** Patients should be informed that peripheral neuropathy has been associated with AVELOX use. Symptoms may occur soon after initiation of therapy and may be irreversible. If symptoms of peripheral neuropathy including pain, burning, tingling, numbness, and/or weakness develop, patients should immediately discontinue AVELOX and contact their physician.
- **Photosensitivity/Phototoxicity:** Patients should be informed that photosensitivity/phototoxicity has been reported in patients receiving quinolones. Patients should minimize or avoid exposure to natural or artificial sunlight (tanning beds or UVA/B treatment) while taking quinolones. If patients need to be outdoors while using quinolones, they should wear loose-fitting clothes that protect skin from sun exposure and discuss other sun protection measures with their physician. If a sunburn-like reaction or skin eruption occurs, patients should contact their physician.
- **Diarrhea:** Diarrhea is a common problem caused by antibiotics which usually ends when the antibiotic is discontinued. Sometimes after starting treatment with antibiotics, patients can develop watery and bloody stools (with or without stomach cramps and fever) even as late as two or more months after having taken the last dose of the antibiotic. If this occurs, patients should contact their physician as soon as possible.

FDA-Approved Medication Guide

MEDICATION GUIDE
AVELOX® (AV-eh-locks)
(moxifloxacin hydrochloride)
Tablets
AVELOX® IV (*AV-eh-locks*)
(moxifloxacin hydrochloride)
Injection Solution for IV use

Read the Medication Guide that comes with AVELOX® before you start taking it and each time you get a refill. There may be new information. This Medication Guide does not take the place of talking to your healthcare provider about your medical condition or your treatment.

What is the most important information I should know about AVELOX?

AVELOX belongs to a class of antibiotics called fluoroquinolones. AVELOX can cause side effects that may be serious or even cause death. If you get any of the following serious side effects, get medical help right away. Talk with your healthcare provider about whether you should continue to take AVELOX.

1. Tendon rupture or swelling of the tendon (tendinitis).

- **Tendon problems can happen in people of all ages who take AVELOX.** Tendons are tough cords of tissue that connect muscles to bones. Symptoms of tendon problems may include:
  - Pain, swelling, tears and inflammation of tendons including the back of the ankle (Achilles), shoulder, hand, or other tendon sites.
- **The risk of getting tendon problems while you take AVELOX is higher if you:**
  - Are over 60 years of age
  - Are taking steroids (corticosteroids)
  - Have had a kidney, heart or lung transplant

Tendon problems can happen in people who do not have the above risk factors when they take AVELOX.

- **Other reasons that can increase your risk of tendon problems can include:**
  - Physical activity or exercise
  - Kidney failure
  - Tendon problems in the past, such as in people with rheumatoid arthritis (RA)
- **Call your healthcare provider right away at the first sign of tendon pain, swelling or inflammation.** Stop taking AVELOX until tendinitis or tendon rupture has been ruled out by your healthcare provider. Avoid exercise and using the affected area. The most common area of pain and swelling is in the Achilles tendon at the back of your ankle. This can also happen with other tendons.
- **Talk to your healthcare provider about the risk of tendon rupture with continued use of AVELOX.** You may need a different antibiotic that is not a fluoroquinolone to treat your infection.
- **Tendon rupture can happen while you are taking or after you have finished taking AVELOX.** Tendon ruptures have happened up to several months after patients have finished taking their fluoroquinolone.
- **Get medical help right away if you get any of the following signs or symptoms of a tendon rupture:**
  - Hear or feel a snap or pop in a tendon area
  - Bruising right after an injury in a tendon area
  - Unable to move the affected area or bear weight

2. Worsening of myasthenia gravis (a disease which causes muscle weakness). Fluoroquinolones like AVELOX may cause worsening of myasthenia gravis symptoms, including muscle weakness and breathing problems. Call your healthcare provider right away if you have any worsening muscle weakness or breathing problems.

See the section **"What are the possible side effects of AVELOX?"** for more information about side effects.

What is AVELOX?

AVELOX is a fluoroquinolone antibiotic medicine used to treat certain types of infections caused by certain germs called bacteria in adults 18 years or older. It is not known if AVELOX is safe and works in people under 18 years of age. Children have a higher chance of getting bone, joint, and tendon (musculoskeletal) problems while taking fluoroquinolone antibiotic medicines.

Sometimes infections are caused by viruses rather than by bacteria. Examples include viral infections in the sinuses and lungs, such as the common cold or flu. Antibiotics, including AVELOX, do not kill viruses.

Call your healthcare provider if you think your condition is not getting better while you are taking AVELOX.

Who should not take AVELOX?

Do not take AVELOX if you have ever had a severe allergic reaction to an antibiotic known as a fluoroquinolone, or if you are allergic to any of the ingredients in AVELOX. Ask your healthcare provider if you are not sure. See the list of ingredients in AVELOX at the end of this Medication Guide.

What should I tell my healthcare provider before taking AVELOX?

See **"What is the most important information I should know about AVELOX?"**

Tell your healthcare provider about all your medical conditions, including if you:

- Have tendon problems
- Have a disease that causes muscle weakness (myasthenia gravis)
- Have central nervous system problems (such as epilepsy)
- Have nerve problems
- Have or anyone in your family has an irregular heartbeat, especially a condition called "QT prolongation"
- Have low blood potassium (hypokalemia)
- Have a slow heartbeat (bradycardia)
- Have a history of seizures
- Have kidney problems
- Have rheumatoid arthritis (RA) or other history of joint problems
- Are pregnant or planning to become pregnant. It is not known if AVELOX will harm your unborn child.
- Are breast-feeding or planning to breast-feed. It is not known if AVELOX passes into breast milk. You and your healthcare provider should decide whether you will take AVELOX or breast-feed.

Tell your healthcare provider about all the medicines you take, including prescription and non-prescription medicines, vitamins and herbal and dietary supplements. AVELOX and other medicines can affect each other causing side effects. Especially tell your healthcare provider if you take:

- An NSAID (Non-Steroidal Anti-Inflammatory Drug). Many common medicines for pain relief are NSAIDs. Taking an NSAID while you take AVELOX or other fluoroquinolones may increase your risk of central nervous system effects and seizures. See **"What are the possible side effects of AVELOX?"**
- A blood thinner (warfarin, Coumadin, Jantoven).
- A medicine to control your heart rate or rhythm (antiarrhythmic) See **"What are the possible side effects of AVELOX?"**
- An anti-psychotic medicine.
- A tricyclic antidepressant.
- Erythromycin.
- A water pill (diuretic).
- A steroid medicine. Corticosteroids taken by mouth or by injection may increase the chance of tendon injury. See **"What is the most important information I should know about AVELOX?"**
- Certain medicines may keep AVELOX from working correctly. Take AVELOX either 4 hours before or 8 hours after taking these products:
  - An antacid, multivitamin, or other product that has magnesium, aluminum, iron, or zinc
  - Sucralfate (Carafate)
  - Didanosine (Videx®, Videx EC®)

Ask your healthcare provider if you are not sure if any of your medicines are listed above.

Know the medicines you take. Keep a list of your medicines and show it to your healthcare provider and pharmacist when you get a new medicine.

How should I take AVELOX?

- **Take AVELOX once a day exactly as prescribed by your healthcare provider.**
- **Take AVELOX at about the same time each day.**
- **AVELOX Tablets should be swallowed.**
- **AVELOX can be taken with or without food.**
- **Drink plenty of fluids while taking AVELOX.**
- **AVELOX IV is given to you by intravenous (IV) infusion into your vein slowly, over 60 minutes, as prescribed by your healthcare provider.**
- **Do not skip any doses, or stop taking AVELOX even if you begin to feel better, until you finish your prescribed treatment, unless:**
  - You have tendon effects (see **"What is the most important information I should know about AVELOX?"**).
  - You have a serious allergic reaction (see **"What are the possible side effects of AVELOX?"**), or your healthcare provider tells you to stop.
- This will help make sure that all of the bacteria are killed and lower the chance that the bacteria will become resistant to AVELOX. If this happens, AVELOX and other antibiotic medicines may not work in the future.
- **If you miss a dose of AVELOX, take it as soon as you remember. Do not take more than 1 dose of AVELOX in one day.**
- **If you take too much, call your healthcare provider or get medical help immediately.**

What should I avoid while taking AVELOX?

- AVELOX can make you feel dizzy and lightheaded. Do not drive, operate machinery, or do other activities that require mental alertness or coordination until you know how AVELOX affects you.
- Avoid sunlamps, tanning beds, and try to limit your time in the sun. AVELOX can make your skin sensitive to the sun (photosensitivity) and the light from sunlamps and tanning beds. You could get severe sunburn, blisters or swelling of your skin. If you get any of these symptoms while taking AVELOX, call your healthcare provider right away. You should use a sunscreen and wear a hat and clothes that cover your skin if you have to be in sunlight.

What are the possible side effects of AVELOX?

AVELOX can cause side effects that may be serious or even cause death. See **"What is the most important information I should know about AVELOX?"**

Other serious side effects of AVELOX include:

- **Central Nervous System effects**

Seizures have been reported in people who take fluoroquinolone antibiotics including AVELOX. Tell your healthcare provider if you have a history of seizures. Ask your healthcare provider whether taking AVELOX will change your risk of having a seizure.

Central Nervous System (CNS) side effects may happen as soon as after taking the first dose of AVELOX. Talk to your healthcare provider right away if you have any of these side effects, or other changes in mood or behavior:

- Feeling dizzy
- Seizures
- Hear voices, see things, or sense things that are not there (hallucinations)
- Feel restless
- Tremors
- Feel anxious or nervous
- Confusion
- Depression
- Trouble sleeping
- Feel more suspicious (paranoia)
- Suicidal thoughts or acts
- Nightmares
- Vision Loss
- **Serious allergic reactions**

Allergic reactions can happen in people taking fluoroquinolones, including AVELOX, even after only one dose. Stop taking AVELOX and get emergency medical help right away if you get any of the following symptoms of a severe allergic reaction:

- Hives
- Trouble breathing or swallowing
- Swelling of the lips, tongue, face
- Throat tightness, hoarseness
- Rapid heartbeat
- Faint
- Yellowing of the skin or eyes. Stop taking AVELOX and tell your healthcare provider right away if you get yellowing of your skin or white part of your eyes, or if you have dark urine. These can be signs of a serious reaction to AVELOX (a liver problem).
- **Skin rash**

Skin rash may happen in people taking AVELOX even after only one dose. Stop taking AVELOX at the first sign of a skin rash and call your healthcare provider. Skin rash may be a sign of a more serious reaction to AVELOX.

- **Serious heart rhythm changes** (QT prolongation and torsade de pointes)

Tell your healthcare provider right away if you have a change in your heart beat (a fast or irregular heartbeat), or if you faint. AVELOX may cause a rare heart problem known as prolongation of the QT interval. This condition can cause an abnormal heartbeat and can be very dangerous. The chances of this event are higher in people:

- Who are elderly
- With a family history of prolonged QT interval
- With low blood potassium (hypokalemia)
- Who take certain medicines to control heart rhythm (antiarrhythmics)
- **Intestine infection** (Pseudomembranous colitis)

Pseudomembranous colitis can happen with most antibiotics, including AVELOX. Call your healthcare provider right away if you get watery diarrhea, diarrhea that does not go away, or bloody stools. You may have stomach cramps and a fever. Pseudomembranous colitis can happen 2 or more months after you have finished your antibiotic.

- **Changes in sensation and nerve damage (Peripheral Neuropathy)**

Damage to the nerves in arms, hands, legs, or feet can happen in people taking fluoroquinolones, including AVELOX. Stop AVELOX and talk with your healthcare provider right away if you get any of the following symptoms of peripheral neuropathy in your arms, hands, legs, or feet:

- Pain
- Burning
- Tingling
- Numbness
- Weakness

The nerve damage may be permanent.

- **Sensitivity to sunlight** (photosensitivity)

See **"What should I avoid while taking AVELOX?"**

The most common side effects of AVELOX include nausea and diarrhea.

These are not all the possible side effects of AVELOX. Tell your healthcare provider about any side effect that bothers you or that does not go away.

Call your doctor for medical advice about side effects. You may report side effects to FDA at 1-800-FDA-1088.

How should I store AVELOX?

AVELOX Tablets

- Store AVELOX 59–86°F (15–30°C)
- Keep AVELOX away from moisture (humidity)

Keep AVELOX and all medicines out of the reach of children.

General Information about AVELOX

Medicines are sometimes prescribed for purposes other than those listed in a Medication Guide. Do not use AVELOX for a condition for which it is not prescribed. Do not give AVELOX to other people, even if they have the same symptoms that you have. It may harm them.

This Medication Guide summarizes the most important information about AVELOX. If you would like more information about AVELOX, talk with your healthcare provider. You can ask your healthcare provider or pharmacist for information about AVELOX that is written for healthcare professionals. For more information go to www.AVELOX.com or call 1-800-526-4099.

What are the ingredients in AVELOX?

- **AVELOX Tablets:**
  - Active ingredient: moxifloxacin hydrochloride
  - Inactive ingredients: microcrystalline cellulose, lactose monohydrate, croscarmellose sodium, magnesium stearate, hypromellose, titanium dioxide, polyethylene glycol, and ferric oxide
- **AVELOX IV:**
  - Active ingredient: moxifloxacin hydrochloride
  - Inactive ingredients: sodium chloride, USP, water for injection, USP, and may include hydrochloric acid and/or sodium hydroxide for pH adjustment

Revised August 2013

This Medication Guide has been approved by the U.S. Food and Drug Administration.

Manufactured for:
Bayer HealthCare Pharmaceuticals Inc.
Wayne, NJ 07470

AVELOX Tablets manufactured in Germany
AVELOX IV manufactured in Germany
or
AVELOX IV manufactured in Norway by
Fresenius Kabi Norge AS
NO-1753 Halden, Norway

Distributed by:
Merck Sharp & Dohme Corp., a subsidiary of
Merck & Co, Inc.
Whitehouse Station, NJ 08889, USA

AVELOX® is a registered trademark of Bayer Aktiengesellschaft and is used under license by Merck Sharp & Dohme Corp., a subsidiary of **Merck & Co.**, Inc.

Rx Only

83680831, R.4

Shown in Product Identification Guide, page 307

AZASITE® ℞

(azithromycin ophthalmic solution) 1%
Sterile topical ophthalmic drops

HIGHLIGHTS OF PRESCRIBING INFORMATION

These highlights do not include all the information needed to use AzaSite safely and effectively. See full prescribing information for AzaSite.

AzaSite® (azithromycin ophthalmic solution) 1%
Sterile topical ophthalmic drops
Initial U.S. Approval: 2007

RECENT MAJOR CHANGES

Contraindications (4) 07/2012

INDICATIONS AND USAGE

AzaSite is a macrolide antibiotic indicated for the treatment of bacterial conjunctivitis caused by susceptible isolates of the following microorganisms: CDC coryneform group G, *Haemophilus influenzae, Staphylococcus aureus, Streptococcus mitis* group, and *Streptococcus pneumoniae.* (1)

DOSAGE AND ADMINISTRATION

Instill 1 drop in the affected eye(s) twice daily, eight to twelve hours apart for the first two days and then instill 1 drop in the affected eye(s) once daily for the next five days. (2)

DOSAGE FORMS AND STRENGTHS

2.5 mL of 1% sterile topical ophthalmic solution. (3)

CONTRAINDICATIONS

Hypersensitivity (4)

WARNINGS AND PRECAUTIONS

- For topical ophthalmic use only. (5.1)
- Anaphylaxis and hypersensitivity have been reported with systemic use of azithromycin. (5.2)
- Growth of resistant organisms may occur with prolonged use. (5.3)
- Patients should not wear contact lenses if they have signs or symptoms of bacterial conjunctivitis. (5.4)

ADVERSE REACTIONS

Most common adverse reaction reported in patients was eye irritation (1-2% of patients). (6)

To report SUSPECTED ADVERSE REACTIONS, contact Inspire Pharmaceuticals, Inc., a subsidiary of Merck & Co., Inc., at 1-800-672-6372 or FDA at 1-800-FDA-1088 or www.fda.gov/medwatch.

See 17 for PATIENT COUNSELING INFORMATION and FDA-approved patient labeling

Revised: 10/2012

FULL PRESCRIBING INFORMATION: CONTENTS*

*** Sections or subsections omitted from the full prescribing information are not listed**

FULL PRESCRIBING INFORMATION

1 INDICATIONS AND USAGE

AzaSite® is indicated for the treatment of bacterial conjunctivitis caused by susceptible isolates of the following microorganisms:

CDC coryneform group G[1]
Haemophilus influenzae
Staphylococcus aureus
Streptococcus mitis group
Streptococcus pneumoniae

[1] *Efficacy for this organism was studied in fewer than 10 infections.*

2 DOSAGE AND ADMINISTRATION

The recommended dosage regimen for the treatment of bacterial conjunctivitis is:

Instill 1 drop in the affected eye(s) twice daily, eight to twelve hours apart for the first two days and then instill 1 drop in the affected eye(s) once daily for the next five days.

3 DOSAGE FORMS AND STRENGTHS

2.5 mL of a 1% sterile topical ophthalmic solution.

4 CONTRAINDICATIONS

Hypersensitivity to any component of this product.

5 WARNINGS AND PRECAUTIONS

5.1 Topical Ophthalmic Use Only

NOT FOR INJECTION. AzaSite is indicated for topical ophthalmic use only, and should not be administered systemically, injected subconjunctivally, or introduced directly into the anterior chamber of the eye.

5.2 Anaphylaxis and Hypersensitivity with Systemic Use of Azithromycin

In patients receiving systemically administered azithromycin, serious allergic reactions, including angioedema, anaphylaxis, and dermatologic reactions including Stevens-Johnson syndrome and toxic epidermal necrolysis have been reported rarely in patients on azithromycin therapy. Although rare, fatalities have been reported. The potential for anaphylaxis or other hypersensitivity reactions should be considered based on known hypersensitivity to azithromycin when administered systemically.

5.3 Growth of Resistant Organisms with Prolonged Use

As with other anti-infectives, prolonged use may result in overgrowth of non-susceptible organisms, including fungi. If super-infection occurs, discontinue use and institute alternative therapy. Whenever clinical judgment dictates, the patient should be examined with the aid of magnification, such as slit-lamp biomicroscopy, and where appropriate, fluorescein staining.

5.4 Avoidance of Contact Lenses

Patients should be advised not to wear contact lenses if they have signs or symptoms of bacterial conjunctivitis.

6 ADVERSE REACTIONS

Because clinical trials are conducted under widely varying conditions, adverse reaction rates observed in one clinical trial of a drug cannot be directly compared with the rates in the clinical trials of the same or another drug and may not reflect the rates observed in practice.

The data described below reflect exposure to AzaSite in 698 patients. The population was between 1 and 87 years old with clinical signs and symptoms of bacterial conjunctivitis. The most frequently reported ocular adverse reaction reported in patients receiving AzaSite was eye irritation. This reaction occurred in approximately 1-2% of patients. Other adverse reactions associated with the use of AzaSite were reported in less than 1% of patients and included ocular reactions (blurred vision, burning, stinging and irritation upon instillation, contact dermatitis, corneal erosion, dry eye, eye pain, itching, ocular discharge, punctate keratitis, visual acuity reduction) and non-ocular reactions (dysgeusia, facial swelling, hives, nasal congestion, periocular swelling, rash, sinusitis, urticaria).

8 USE IN SPECIFIC POPULATIONS

8.1 Pregnancy

Pregnancy Category B. Reproduction studies have been performed in rats and mice at doses up to 200 mg/kg/day. The highest dose was associated with moderate maternal toxicity. These doses are estimated to be approximately 5,000 times the maximum human ocular daily dose of 2 mg. In the animal studies, no evidence of harm to the fetus due to azithromycin was found. There are, however, no adequate and well-controlled studies in pregnant women. Because animal reproduction studies are not always predictive of human response, azithromycin should be used during pregnancy only if clearly needed.

8.3 Nursing Mothers

It is not known whether azithromycin is excreted in human milk. Because many drugs are excreted in human milk, caution should be exercised when azithromycin is administered to a nursing woman.

8.4 Pediatric Use

The safety and effectiveness of AzaSite solution in pediatric patients below 1 year of age have not been established. The efficacy of AzaSite in treating bacterial conjunctivitis in pediatric patients one year or older has been demonstrated in controlled clinical trials *[see Clinical Studies (14)]*.

8.5 Geriatric Use

No overall differences in safety or effectiveness have been observed between elderly and younger patients.

11 DESCRIPTION

AzaSite (azithromycin ophthalmic solution) is a 1% sterile aqueous topical ophthalmic solution of azithromycin formulated in DuraSite® (polycarbophil, edetate disodium, sodium chloride). AzaSite is an off-white, viscous liquid with an osmolality of approximately 290 mOsm/kg.

Preservative: 0.003% benzalkonium chloride. **Inactives:** mannitol, citric acid, sodium citrate, poloxamer 407, polycarbophil, edetate disodium (EDTA), sodium chloride, water for injection, and sodium hydroxide to adjust pH to 6.3.

Azithromycin is a macrolide antibiotic with a 15-membered ring. Its chemical name is (2R,3S,4R,5R,8R,10R,11R,12S,13S,14R)-13-[(2,6-dideoxy-3-C-methyl-3-O-methyl-α-L-ribo-hexopyranosyl)oxy]-2-ethyl-3,4,10-trihydroxy-3,5,6,8,10,12,14-heptamethyl-11-[[3,4,6-trideoxy-3-(dimethylamino)-β-D-xylo-hexopyranosyl]oxy]-1-oxa-6-aza-cyclopentadecan-15-one, and the structural formula is:

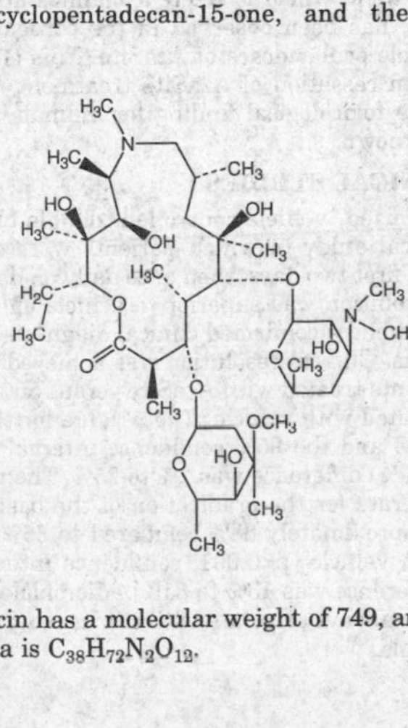

Azithromycin has a molecular weight of 749, and its empirical formula is $C_{38}H_{72}N_2O_{12}$.

12 CLINICAL PHARMACOLOGY

12.1 Mechanism of Action

Azithromycin is a macrolide antibiotic *[see Clinical Pharmacology (12.4)]*.

12.3 Pharmacokinetics

The plasma concentration of azithromycin following ocular administration of AzaSite (azithromycin ophthalmic solution) in humans is unknown. Based on the proposed dose of one drop to each eye (total dose of 100 mcL or 1 mg) and exposure information from systemic administration, the systemic concentration of azithromycin following ocular administration is estimated to be below quantifiable limits (≤10 ng/mL) at steady-state in humans, assuming 100% systemic availability.

12.4 Microbiology

Azithromycin acts by binding to the 50S ribosomal subunit of susceptible microorganisms and interfering with microbial protein synthesis.

Azithromycin has been shown to be active against most isolates of the following microorganisms, both *in vitro* and clinically in conjunctival infections *[see Indications and Usage (1)]*.

CDC coryneform group G[2]
Haemophilus influenzae
Staphylococcus aureus
Streptococcus mitis group
Streptococcus pneumoniae

The following *in vitro* data are also available, **but their clinical significance in ophthalmic infections is unknown.** The safety and effectiveness of AzaSite in treating ophthalmological infections due to these microorganisms have not been established.

The following microorganisms are considered susceptible when evaluated using systemic breakpoints. However, a correlation between the *in vitro* systemic breakpoint and ophthalmological efficacy has not been established. This list of microorganisms is provided as an aid only in assessing the potential treatment of conjunctival infections. Azithromycin exhibits *in vitro* minimal inhibitory concentrations (MICs) of equal or less (systemic susceptible breakpoint) against most (≥90%) of isolates of the following ocular pathogens:

Chlamydia pneumoniae
Chlamydia trachomatis
Legionella pneumophila
Moraxella catarrhalis
Mycoplasma hominis
Mycoplasma pneumoniae
Neisseria gonorrhoeae
Peptostreptococcus species
Streptococci (Groups C, F, G)
Streptococcus pyogenes
Streptococcus agalactiae
Ureaplasma urealyticum
Viridans group streptococci

[2] *Efficacy for this organism was studied in fewer than 10 infections.*

13 NONCLINICAL TOXICOLOGY

13.1 Carcinogenesis, Mutagenesis, Impairment of Fertility

Long-term studies in animals have not been performed to evaluate carcinogenic potential. Azithromycin has shown no mutagenic potential in standard laboratory tests: mouse lymphoma assay, human lymphocyte clastogenic assay, and mouse bone marrow clastogenic assay. No evidence of impaired fertility due to azithromycin was found in mice or rats that received oral doses of up to 200 mg/kg/day.

13.2 Animal Toxicology and/or Pharmacology

Phospholipidosis (intracellular phospholipid accumulation) has been observed in some tissues of mice, rats, and dogs given multiple systemic doses of azithromycin. Cytoplasmic microvacuolation, which is likely a manifestation of phospholipidosis, has been observed in the corneas of rabbits given multiple ocular doses of AzaSite. This effect was reversible upon cessation of AzaSite treatment. The significance of this toxicological finding for animals and for humans is unknown.

14 CLINICAL STUDIES

In a randomized, vehicle-controlled, double-blind, multicenter clinical study in which patients were dosed twice daily for the first two days, then once daily on days 3, 4, and 5, AzaSite solution was superior to vehicle on days 6-7 in patients who had a confirmed clinical diagnosis of bacterial conjunctivitis. Clinical resolution was achieved in 63% (82/130) of patients treated with AzaSite versus 50% (74/149) of patients treated with vehicle. The p-value for the comparison was 0.03 and the 95% confidence interval around the 13% (63%-50%) difference was 2% to 25%. The microbiological success rate for the eradication of the baseline pathogens was approximately 88% compared to 66% of patients treated with vehicle (p<0.001, confidence interval around the 22% difference was 13% to 31%). Microbiologic eradication does not always correlate with clinical outcome in anti-infective trials.

16 HOW SUPPLIED/STORAGE AND HANDLING

AzaSite is a sterile aqueous topical ophthalmic formulation of 1% azithromycin.

NDC 31357-040-25: 2.5 mL in 5 mL bottle containing a total of 25 mg of azithromycin in a white, round, low-density polyethylene (LDPE) bottle, with a clear LDPE dropper tip, and a tan colored high density polyethylene (HDPE) eyedropper cap. A white tamper evident over-cap is provided.

NDC 31357-040-03: 2.5 mL in 4 mL bottle containing a total of 25 mg of azithromycin in a white, round, low-density polyethylene (LDPE) bottle, with a clear LDPE dropper tip, and a tan colored high density polyethylene (HDPE) eyedropper cap. A white tamper evident over-cap is provided.

Storage and Handling:

Store unopened bottle under refrigeration at 2°C to 8°C (36°F to 46°F). Once the bottle is opened, store at 2°C to 25°C (36°F to 77°F) for up to 14 days. Discard after the 14 days.

17 PATIENT COUNSELING INFORMATION

See FDA-Approved Patient Labeling (Patient Information).

Patients should be advised to avoid contaminating the applicator tip by allowing it to touch the eye, fingers or other sources.

Patients should be directed to discontinue use and contact a physician if any signs of an allergic reaction occur.

Patients should be told that although it is common to feel better early in the course of the therapy, the medication should be taken exactly as directed. Skipping doses or not completing the full course of therapy may (1) decrease the effectiveness of the immediate treatment and (2) increase the likelihood that bacteria will develop resistance and will not be treatable by AzaSite (azithromycin ophthalmic solution) or other antibacterial drugs in the future.

Patients should be advised not to wear contact lenses if they have signs or symptoms of bacterial conjunctivitis.

Patients should be advised to thoroughly wash hands prior to using AzaSite.

Patients should be advised to invert the closed bottle (upside down) and shake once before each use. Remove cap with bottle still in the inverted position. Tilt head back, and with bottle inverted, gently squeeze bottle to instill one drop into the affected eye(s).

Manufactured for: Inspire Pharmaceuticals, Inc., a subsidiary of
MERCK & CO., INC., Whitehouse Station, NJ 08889, USA
Manufactured by:
Catalent Pharma Solutions, LLC
Woodstock, IL 60098
U.S. Patent Nos.: 6,159,458; 6,239,113; 6,569,443; 6,861,411; 7,056,893; and Patents Pending
AzaSite is a registered trademark of InSite Vision Inc.

Revised: 10/2012
USPI-OS-82431210R002

PATIENT INFORMATION

AzaSite® (A-zuh-site)
(azithromycin ophthalmic solution) 1%

Read this Patient Information before you start using AzaSite® and each time you get a refill. There may be new information. This information does not take the place of talking to your doctor about your medical condition or treatment.

What is AzaSite?

AzaSite is a prescription sterile eye drop solution. AzaSite is used to treat bacterial conjunctivitis which is an infection of the eye caused by certain bacteria.

It is not known if AzaSite is safe and effective in children less than 1 year of age.

Information about bacterial conjunctivitis.

Bacterial conjunctivitis is a bacterial infection of the mucous membranes which line the inside of the eyelids. Symptoms may include redness of the eye and discharge. The infection can be spread to other people and to both eyes.

Who should not use AzaSite?

Do not use AzaSite if you are allergic to azithromycin or any of the ingredients in AzaSite. See the end of this Patient Information leaflet for a complete list of the ingredients in AzaSite.

What should I tell my doctor before using AzaSite?

Before you use AzaSite, tell your doctor if you:

- wear contact lenses. Do not wear contact lenses if you have signs or symptoms of bacterial conjunctivitis.
- are pregnant or plan to become pregnant. It is not known if AzaSite will harm your unborn baby. Talk to your doctor if you are pregnant or plan to become pregnant.
- are breast-feeding or plan to breast-feed. It is not known if AzaSite passes into your breast milk. Talk to your doctor about the best way to feed your baby if you are using AzaSite.

Tell your doctor about all the medicines you take, including prescription and non-prescription medicines, vitamins, and herbal supplements.

Know the medicines you take. Keep a list of them to show your doctors and pharmacist when you get a new medicine.

How should I use AzaSite?

- **Read the Instructions for Use at the end of this Patient Information** leaflet for the right way to use AzaSite.
- Use AzaSite exactly as your doctor tells you to use it.
- For the first 2 days place 1 drop of AzaSite in your eye (or eyes) each morning and 1 drop in your eye (or eyes) each evening. Wait 8 to 12 hours after placing your morning drops before you place evening drops in your eye (or eyes).
- For the next 5 days place 1 drop of AzaSite in your eye (or eyes) 1 time each day.
- Make sure you continue to use AzaSite as directed by your doctor even if you feel better after you start using it. Skipping drops can increase the chances that:
  - your medicine will not work well
  - Bacteria can develop resistance, which means in the future your bacterial conjunctivitis may not improve from AzaSite or other drugs that treat infections from bacteria.

What should I be aware of while using AzaSite?

Do not wear contact lenses if you have signs or symptoms of bacterial conjunctivitis and until you have finished your prescribed course of treatment. The symptoms of bacterial conjunctivitis may include:

- discharge coming from the eye
- eye redness
- eye irritation

Only your doctor can tell you if you have bacterial conjunctivitis.

Severe allergic reactions have been reported rarely when azithromycin has been taken by mouth.

- Serious rash or serious allergic reactions may occur. Azithromycin, the active ingredient in AzaSite, may cause a serious rash or a serious allergic reaction. Both of these reactions may need to be treated in a hospital and may be life-threatening.
- Stop taking AzaSite and call your doctor right away or get emergency help if you have any of these symptoms:
  - skin rash, hives, sores in your mouth, or your skin blisters and peels
  - swelling of your face, eyes, lips, tongue, or throat
  - trouble swallowing or breathing

Increased risk of other infections caused by bacteria or fungi.

- Using AzaSite for a long time may cause other bacteria or fungi to grow. If this happens you may get a new infection. Tell your doctor right away if your symptoms do not get better.

What are the possible side effects of AzaSite?

The most common side effect of AzaSite is eye irritation.

Other side effects seen with AzaSite include:

- eye burning, stinging and irritation when the drop hits your eye
- irritation on your eyelid and the skin around your eye
- a feeling of discomfort and irritation or that something is in your eye
- dry eye
- eye pain
- eye itching
- discharge coming from your eye
- changes to the surface of your eye
- blurred vision
- changes in your taste
- hives and rash on your skin
- stuffy nose and sinus infection
- swelling around your eye or of your face

Tell your doctor about any side effect that bothers you or that does not go away.

These are not all of the possible side effects of AzaSite. For more information, ask your doctor or pharmacist.

Call your doctor for medical advice about side effects. You may report side effects to FDA at 1-800-FDA-1088.

How should I store AzaSite?

- Before you open your AzaSite, store it in the refrigerator between 36°F to 46°F (2°C to 8°C).
- After you open your AzaSite, store it at room temperature or the refrigerator between 36°F to 77°F (2°C to 25°C).
- **AzaSite should not be stored for more than 14 days after opening. After 14 days, throw the AzaSite bottle away.**
- Safely throw away medicine that is out of date or no longer needed.

Keep AzaSite and all medicines out of reach of children.

General information about the safe and effective use of AzaSite

Medicines are sometimes prescribed for purposes other than those listed in a Patient Information leaflet. Do not use AzaSite for a condition for which it was not prescribed. Do not give AzaSite to other people, even if they have the same symptoms that you have. It may harm them.

☐ ☐	Day 1: ______	1 drop in the morning and 1 drop in the evening
☐ ☐	Day 2: ______	1 drop in the morning and 1 drop in the evening
☐	Day 3: ______	1 drop anytime during the day
☐	Day 4: ______	1 drop anytime during the day
☐	Day 5: ______	1 drop anytime during the day
☐	Day 6: ______	1 drop anytime during the day
☐	Day 7: ______	1 drop anytime during the day

This Patient Information summarizes the most important information about AzaSite. If you would like more information, talk with your doctor. You can ask your pharmacist or doctor for information about AzaSite that is written for health professionals.

For more information, go to www.azasite.com or call 1-800-622-4477.

What are the ingredients in AzaSite?

Active ingredient: azithromycin

Inactive ingredients: 0.003% benzalkonium chloride, mannitol, citric acid, sodium citrate, poloxamer 407, polycarbophil, edetate disodium (EDTA), sodium chloride, water, and sodium hydroxide.

Instructions for Use

AzaSite® (A-zuh-site)

(azithromycin ophthalmic solution) 1%

Read this Instructions for Use for AzaSite before you start using it and each time you get a refill. There may be new information. This leaflet does not take the place of talking to your doctor about your medical condition or treatment.

Important:

- **AzaSite is for use as an eye drop only.**

The checklist below tells you when to use your medicine for each eye that has bacterial conjunctivitis:

[See table above]

This is a total of 9 drops of AzaSite for each infected eye.

- Avoid letting the applicator tip touch your eye, your fingers, or other objects.
- If a drop misses your eye, try again.
- Follow the steps below to use AzaSite correctly.

Before using a new bottle of AzaSite:

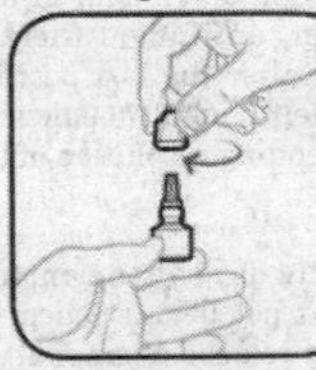

Figure A

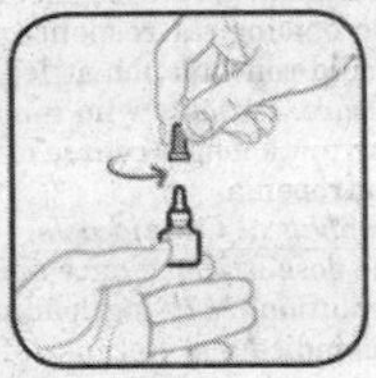

Figure B

- Turn the white cap clockwise until it comes off. Throw away the white cap. **See Figure A**
- Hold the bottle straight, turn the tan cap counterclockwise until it comes off. Put the tan cap back on the bottle and close tightly. (This lets out the air.) **See Figure B**

Wash your hands each time you use AzaSite.

To use AzaSite:

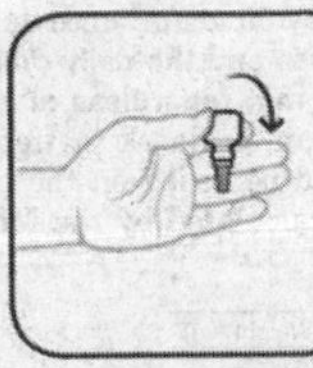

Figure C

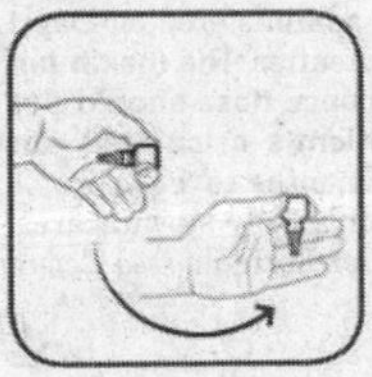

Figure D

Step 1. Turn the closed bottle upside down. **See Figure C**

Step 2. Shake your hand firmly. This helps move the medicine into the tip of the bottle. **See Figure D**

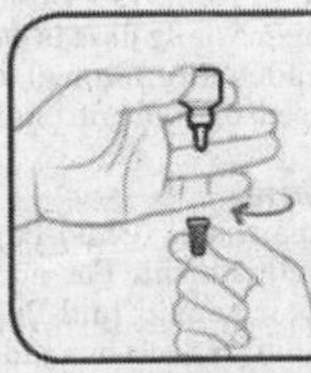

Figure E

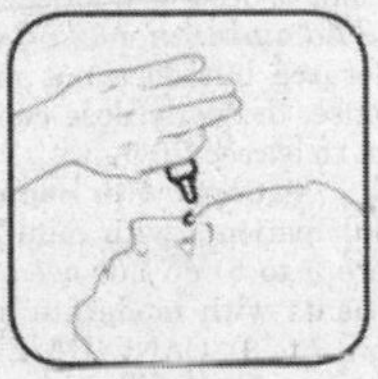

Figure F

Step 3. Hold the bottle upside down and take off the tan cap. **See Figure E**

Step 4. Tilt your head back. Hold the bottle over your eye and gently squeeze the bottle to let 1 drop into each eye that has bacterial conjunctivitis. Put the tan cap back on the bottle and close tightly. **See Figure F**

If a drop does not come out of the bottle, repeat steps one to four.

This Patient Information and Instructions for Use have been approved by the U.S. Food and Drug Administration.

Manufactured for: Inspire Pharmaceuticals, Inc., a subsidiary of

MERCK & CO., INC., Whitehouse Station, NJ 08889, USA

Manufactured by:

Catalent Pharma Solutions, LLC

Woodstock, IL 60098

U.S. Patent Nos.: 6,159,458; 6,239,113; 6,569,443; 6,861,411; 7,056,893; and Patents Pending

AzaSite is a registered trademark of InSite Vision Inc.

Revised: 10/2012

USPPI-OS-82431210R002

Shown in Product Identification Guide, page 307

CANCIDAS® ℞

[*kan-si-das*]

(caspofungin acetate)

for injection, for intravenous use

HIGHLIGHTS OF PRESCRIBING INFORMATION

These highlights do not include all the information needed to use CANCIDAS safely and effectively. See full prescribing information for CANCIDAS.

CANCIDAS® (caspofungin acetate) for injection, for intravenous use

Initial U.S. Approval: 2001

RECENT MAJOR CHANGES

Warnings and Precautions, Hypersensitivity (5.1) 01/2013

INDICATIONS AND USAGE

CANCIDAS is an echinocandin antifungal drug indicated in adults and pediatric patients (3 months and older) for:

- Empirical therapy for presumed fungal infections in febrile, neutropenic patients. (1)
- Treatment of candidemia and the following *Candida* infections: intra-abdominal abscesses, peritonitis and pleural space infections. (1)
- Treatment of esophageal candidiasis. (1)
- Treatment of invasive aspergillosis in patients who are refractory to or intolerant of other therapies (e.g., amphotericin B, lipid formulations of amphotericin B, itraconazole). (1)

DOSAGE AND ADMINISTRATION

For All Patients (2.1):

- Administer by slow intravenous (IV) infusion over approximately 1 hour. Not for IV bolus administration.
- Do not mix or co-infuse CANCIDAS with other medications. Do not use diluents containing dextrose (α-D-glucose).

Adults [≥18 years of age] (2.2):

- Administer a single 70-mg loading dose on Day 1, followed by 50 mg once daily for all indications except esophageal candidiasis.
- For esophageal candidiasis, use 50 mg once daily with no loading dose.

Pediatric Patients [3 months to 17 years of age] (2.3):

- Dosing should be based on the patient's body surface area.
- For all indications, administer a single 70-mg/m^2 loading dose on Day 1, followed by 50 mg/m^2 once daily thereafter.
- **Maximum loading dose and daily maintenance dose should not exceed 70 mg, regardless of the patient's calculated dose.**

Dosing With Rifampin and Other Inducers of Drug Clearance (2.5):

- Use 70-mg once daily dose for adult patients on rifampin.
- Consider dose increase to 70 mg once daily for adult patients on nevirapine, efavirenz, carbamazepine, dexamethasone, or phenytoin.
- Pediatric patients receiving these same concomitant medications may also require an increase in dose to 70 mg/m^2 once daily (maximum daily dose not to exceed 70 mg).

DOSAGE FORMS AND STRENGTHS

- Vials: 50 or 70 mg lyophilized powder (plus allowance for overfill). (3)

CONTRAINDICATIONS

- CANCIDAS is contraindicated in patients with hypersensitivity to any component of this product. (4)

WARNINGS AND PRECAUTIONS

- Hypersensitivity: Anaphylaxis has been reported. If this occurs, CANCIDAS should be discontinued and appropriate treatment administered. Possible histamine-mediated adverse reactions, including rash, facial swelling, angioedema, pruritus, sensation of warmth or bronchospasm have been reported and may require discontinuation and/or administration of appropriate treatment. (5.1)
- Use with cyclosporine: Limit use to patients for whom potential benefit outweighs potential risk. Monitor patients who develop abnormal liver function tests (LFTs) during concomitant therapy and evaluate risk/benefit of continuing CANCIDAS. (5.2)
- Hepatic effects: Can cause abnormalities in LFTs and isolated cases of clinically significant hepatic dysfunction, hepatitis, or hepatic failure. Monitor patients who develop abnormal LFTs for evidence of worsening hepatic function, and evaluate risk/benefit of continuing CANCIDAS. (5.3)

ADVERSE REACTIONS

- *Adults:* Most common adverse reactions (incidence ≥10%) are diarrhea, pyrexia, ALT/AST increased, blood alkaline phosphatase increased, and blood potassium decreased. (6.1)
- *Pediatric patients:* Most common adverse reactions (incidence ≥10%) are pyrexia, diarrhea, rash, ALT/AST increased, blood potassium decreased, hypotension, and chills. (6.2)

To report SUSPECTED ADVERSE REACTIONS, contact Merck Sharp & Dohme Corp., a subsidiary of Merck & Co., Inc., at 1-877-888-4231 or FDA at 1-800-FDA-1088 or www.fda.gov/medwatch.

USE IN SPECIFIC POPULATIONS

- Pregnancy: Based on animal data, may cause fetal harm. (8.1)
- Pediatric use: Safety and efficacy in neonates and infants less than 3 months old have not been established. (8.4)
- Hepatic impairment: Reduce dose for adult patients with moderate hepatic impairment (35 mg once daily, with a 70-mg loading dose on Day 1 where appropriate). No data are available in adults with severe impairment or in pediatric patients with any degree of impairment. (8.6, 12.3)

See 17 for PATIENT COUNSELING INFORMATION

Revised: 01/2013

FULL PRESCRIBING INFORMATION: CONTENTS*

Table 2: Adverse Reactions Among Patients with Persistent Fever and Neutropenia* Incidence ≥7.5% for at Least One Treatment Group by System Organ Class or Preferred Term

Adverse Reaction (MedDRA v10.1 System Organ Class and Preferred Term)	CANCIDAS† N=564 (percent)	AmBisome‡ N=547 (percent)
All Systems, Any Adverse Reaction	**95**	**97**
Investigations	**58**	**63**
Alanine Aminotransferase Increased	18	20
Blood Alkaline Phosphatase Increased	15	23
Blood Potassium Decreased	15	23
Aspartate Aminotransferase Increased	14	17
Blood Bilirubin Increased	10	14
Blood Albumin Decreased	7	8
Blood Magnesium Decreased	7	9
Blood Glucose Increased	6	9
Bilirubin Conjugated Increased	5	9
Blood Urea Increased	4	8
Blood Creatinine Increased	3	11
General Disorders and Administration Site Conditions	**57**	**63**
Pyrexia	27	29
Chills	23	31
Edema Peripheral	11	12
Mucosal Inflammation	6	8
Gastrointestinal Disorders	**50**	**55**
Diarrhea	20	16
Nausea	11	20
Abdominal Pain	9	11
Vomiting	9	17
Respiratory, Thoracic and Mediastinal Disorders	**47**	**49**
Cough	11	10
Dyspnea	9	10
Rales	7	8
Infections and Infestations	**45**	**42**
Pneumonia	11	10
Skin and Subcutaneous Tissue Disorders	**42**	**37**
Rash	16	14
Nervous System Disorders	**25**	**27**
Headache	11	12
Metabolism and Nutrition Disorders	**21**	**24**
Hypokalemia	6	8
Vascular Disorders	**20**	**23**
Hypotension	6	10
Cardiac Disorders	**16**	**19**
Tachycardia	7	9

Within any system organ class, individuals may experience more than 1 adverse reaction.
* Regardless of causality
† 70 mg on Day 1, then 50 mg once daily for the remainder of treatment; daily dose was increased to 70 mg for 73 patients.
‡ 3 mg/kg/day; daily dose was increased to 5 mg/kg for 74 patients.

*** Sections or subsections omitted from the full prescribing information are not listed**

FULL PRESCRIBING INFORMATION

1 INDICATIONS AND USAGE

CANCIDAS® is indicated in adults and pediatric patients (3 months and older) for:

- Empirical therapy for presumed fungal infections in febrile, neutropenic patients
- Treatment of candidemia and the following *Candida* infections: intra-abdominal abscesses, peritonitis and pleural space infections. CANCIDAS has not been studied in endocarditis, osteomyelitis, and meningitis due to *Candida*.
- Treatment of esophageal candidiasis *[see Clinical Studies (14.3)]*
- Treatment of invasive aspergillosis in patients who are refractory to or intolerant of other therapies (e.g., amphotericin B, lipid formulations of amphotericin B, itraconazole). CANCIDAS has not been studied as initial therapy for invasive aspergillosis.

2 DOSAGE AND ADMINISTRATION

2.1 Instructions for Use in All Patients

CANCIDAS should be administered by slow intravenous (IV) infusion over approximately 1 hour. CANCIDAS should not be administered by IV bolus administration.

Do not mix or co-infuse CANCIDAS with other medications, as there are no data available on the compatibility of CANCIDAS with other intravenous substances, additives, or medications. DO NOT USE DILUENTS CONTAINING DEXTROSE (α-D-GLUCOSE), as CANCIDAS is not stable in diluents containing dextrose.

2.2 Recommended Dosing in Adult Patients [≥18 years of age]

The usual dose is 50 mg once daily (following a 70-mg loading dose for most indications). The safety and efficacy of a dose of 150 mg daily (range: 1 to 51 days; median: 14 days) have been studied in 100 adult patients with candidemia and other *Candida* infections. The efficacy of CANCIDAS at this higher dose was not significantly better than the efficacy of the 50-mg daily dose of CANCIDAS. The efficacy of doses higher than 50 mg daily in the other adult patients for whom CANCIDAS is indicated is not known *[see Clinical Studies (14.2)]*.

Empirical Therapy

A single 70-mg loading dose should be administered on Day 1, followed by 50 mg once daily thereafter. Duration of treatment should be based on the patient's clinical response. Empirical therapy should be continued until resolution of neutropenia. Patients found to have a fungal infection should be treated for a minimum of 14 days; treatment should continue for at least 7 days after both neutropenia and clinical symptoms are resolved. If the 50-mg dose is well tolerated but does not provide an adequate clinical response, the daily dose can be increased to 70 mg.

Candidemia and Other Candida Infections [see Clinical Studies (14.2)]

A single 70-mg loading dose should be administered on Day 1, followed by 50 mg once daily thereafter. Duration of treatment should be dictated by the patient's clinical and microbiological response. In general, antifungal therapy should continue for at least 14 days after the last positive culture. Patients who remain persistently neutropenic may warrant a longer course of therapy pending resolution of the neutropenia.

Esophageal Candidiasis

The dose is 50 mg once daily for 7 to 14 days after symptom resolution. A 70-mg loading dose has not been studied for this indication. Because of the risk of relapse of oropharyngeal candidiasis in patients with HIV infections, suppressive oral therapy could be considered *[see Clinical Studies (14.3)]*.

Invasive Aspergillosis

A single 70-mg loading dose should be administered on Day 1, followed by 50 mg once daily thereafter. Duration of treatment should be based upon the severity of the patient's underlying disease, recovery from immunosuppression, and clinical response.

2.3 Recommended Dosing in Pediatric Patients [3 months to 17 years of age]

For all indications, a single 70-mg/m² loading dose should be administered on Day 1, followed by 50 mg/m² once daily thereafter. **The maximum loading dose and the daily maintenance dose should not exceed 70 mg, regardless of the patient's calculated dose.** Dosing in pediatric patients (3 months to 17 years of age) should be based on the patient's body surface area (BSA) as calculated by the Mosteller Formula *[see References (15)]*:

$$\text{BSA (m}^2) = \sqrt{\frac{\text{Height (cm) X Weight (kg)}}{3600}}$$

Following calculation of the patient's BSA, the loading dose in milligrams should be calculated as BSA (m^2) × 70 mg/m^2. The maintenance dose in milligrams should be calculated as BSA (m^2) × 50 mg/m^2.

Duration of treatment should be individualized to the indication, as described for each indication in adults *[see Dosage and Administration (2.2)]*. If the 50-mg/m² daily dose is well tolerated but does not provide an adequate clinical response, the daily dose can be increased to 70 mg/m² daily (not to exceed 70 mg).

2.4 Patients with Hepatic Impairment

Adult patients with mild hepatic impairment (Child-Pugh score 5 to 6) do not need a dosage adjustment. For adult patients with moderate hepatic impairment (Child-Pugh score 7 to 9), CANCIDAS 35 mg once daily is recommended based upon pharmacokinetic data *[see Clinical Pharmacology (12.3)]*. However, where recommended, a 70-mg loading dose should still be administered on Day 1. There is no clinical experience in adult patients with severe hepatic impairment (Child-Pugh score >9) and in pediatric patients with any degree of hepatic impairment.

2.5 Patients Receiving Concomitant Inducers of Drug Clearance

Adult patients on rifampin should receive 70 mg of CANCIDAS once daily. Adult patients on nevirapine, efavirenz, carbamazepine, dexamethasone, or phenytoin may require an increase in dose to 70 mg of CANCIDAS once daily *[see Drug Interactions (7)]*.

When CANCIDAS is co-administered to pediatric patients with inducers of drug clearance, such as rifampin, efavirenz, nevirapine, phenytoin, dexamethasone, or carbamazepine, a CANCIDAS dose of 70 mg/m^2 once daily (not to exceed 70 mg) should be considered *[see Drug Interactions (7)]*.

2.6 Preparation and Reconstitution for Administration

Do not mix or co-infuse CANCIDAS with other medications, as there are no data available on the compatibility of CANCIDAS with other intravenous substances, additives, or medications. DO NOT USE DILUENTS CONTAINING DEXTROSE (α-D-GLUCOSE), as CANCIDAS is not stable in diluents containing dextrose.

Preparation of CANCIDAS for Infusion

A. Equilibrate the refrigerated vial of CANCIDAS to room temperature.

B. Aseptically add 10.8 mL of 0.9% Sodium Chloride Injection, Sterile Water for Injection, Bacteriostatic Water for Injection with methylparaben and propylparaben, or Bacteriostatic Water for Injection with 0.9% benzyl alcohol to the vial.

Each vial of CANCIDAS contains an intentional overfill of CANCIDAS. Thus, the drug concentration of the resulting solution is listed in Table 1 below.

Table 1: Information for Preparation of CANCIDAS

CANCIDAS vial	Total Drug Content (including overfill)	Reconstitution Volume to be added	Resulting Concentration following Reconstitution
50 mg	54.6 mg	10.8 mL	5 mg/mL
70 mg	75.6 mg	10.8 mL	7 mg/mL

The white to off-white cake will dissolve completely. Mix gently until a clear solution is obtained. Visually inspect the reconstituted solution for particulate matter or discoloration during reconstitution and prior to infusion. Do not use if the solution is cloudy or has precipitated.

The reconstituted solution may be stored for up to one hour at ≤25°C (≤77°F).

CANCIDAS vials are for single use only; the remaining solution should be discarded.

C. Aseptically transfer the appropriate volume (mL) of reconstituted CANCIDAS to an IV bag (or bottle) containing 250 mL of 0.9%, 0.45%, or 0.225% Sodium Chloride Injection or Lactated Ringers Injection. Alternatively, the volume (mL) of reconstituted CANCIDAS can be added to a reduced volume of 0.9%, 0.45%, or 0.225% Sodium Chloride Injection or Lactated Ringers Injection, not to exceed a final concentration of 0.5 mg/mL.

This infusion solution must be used within 24 hours if stored at ≤25°C (≤77°F) or within 48 hours if stored refrigerated at 2 to 8°C (36 to 46°F).

Special Considerations for Pediatric Patients >3 Months of Age

Follow the reconstitution procedures described above using either the 70-mg or 50-mg vial to create the reconstituted solution *[see Dosage and Administration (2.3)]*. From the reconstituted solution in the vial, remove the volume of drug equal to the calculated loading dose or calculated maintenance dose based on a concentration of 7 mg/mL (if reconstituted from the 70-mg vial) or a concentration of 5 mg/mL (if reconstituted from the 50-mg vial).

The choice of vial should be based on total milligram dose of drug to be administered to the pediatric patient. To help ensure accurate dosing, it is recommended for pediatric doses less than 50 mg that 50-mg vials (with a concentration of 5 mg/mL) be used if available. The 70-mg vial should be reserved for pediatric patients requiring doses greater than 50 mg.

The maximum loading dose and the daily maintenance dose should not exceed 70 mg, regardless of the patient's calculated dose.

3 DOSAGE FORMS AND STRENGTHS

CANCIDAS 50 mg is a white to off-white powder/cake for infusion in a vial with a red aluminum band and a plastic cap. CANCIDAS 50-mg vial contains 54.6 mg of caspofungin.

CANCIDAS 70 mg is a white to off-white powder/cake for infusion in a vial with a yellow/orange aluminum band and a plastic cap. CANCIDAS 70-mg vial contains 75.6 mg of caspofungin.

Table 3: Adverse Reactions Among Patients with Candidemia or other Candida Infections*, † Incidence ≥10% for at Least One Treatment Group by System Organ Class or Preferred Term

Adverse Reaction (MedDRA v10.1 System Organ Class and Preferred Term)	CANCIDAS 50 mg‡ N=114 (percent)	Amphotericin B N=125 (percent)
All Systems, Any Adverse Reaction	**96**	**99**
Investigations	**67**	**82**
Blood Potassium Decreased	23	32
Blood Alkaline Phosphatase Increased	21	32
Hemoglobin Decreased	18	23
Alanine Aminotransferase Increased	16	15
Aspartate Aminotransferase Increased	16	14
Blood Bilirubin Increased	13	17
Hematocrit Decreased	13	18
Blood Creatinine Increased	11	28
Red Blood Cells Urine Positive	10	10
Blood Urea Increased	9	23
Bilirubin Conjugated Increased	8	14
Gastrointestinal Disorders	**49**	**53**
Vomiting	17	16
Diarrhea	14	10
Nausea	9	17
Infections and Infestations	**48**	**54**
Septic Shock	11	9
Pneumonia	4	10
General Disorders and Administration Site Conditions	**47**	**63**
Pyrexia	13	33
Edema Peripheral	11	12
Chills	9	30
Respiratory, Thoracic and Mediastinal Disorders	**40**	**54**
Respiratory Failure	11	12
Pleural Effusion	9	14
Tachypnea	1	11
Cardiac Disorders	**26**	**34**
Tachycardia	8	12
Skin and Subcutaneous Tissue Disorders	**25**	**28**
Rash	4	10
Vascular Disorders	**25**	**38**
Hypotension	10	16
Blood and Lymphatic System Disorders	**15**	**13**
Anemia	11	9

Within any system organ class, individuals may experience more than 1 adverse reaction.
* Intra-abdominal abscesses, peritonitis and pleural space infections.
† Regardless of causality
‡ Patients received CANCIDAS 70 mg on Day 1, then 50 mg once daily for the remainder of their treatment.

4 CONTRAINDICATIONS

CANCIDAS is contraindicated in patients with hypersensitivity (e.g., anaphylaxis) to any component of this product *[see Adverse Reactions (6)]*.

5 WARNINGS AND PRECAUTIONS

5.1 Hypersensitivity

Anaphylaxis has been reported during administration of CANCIDAS. If this occurs, CANCIDAS should be discontinued and appropriate treatment administered.

Possible histamine-mediated adverse reactions, including rash, facial swelling, angioedema, pruritus, sensation of warmth or bronchospasm have been reported and may require discontinuation and/or administration of appropriate treatment.

5.2 Concomitant Use with Cyclosporine

Concomitant use of CANCIDAS with cyclosporine should be limited to patients for whom the potential benefit outweighs the potential risk. In one clinical study, 3 of 4 healthy adult subjects who received CANCIDAS 70 mg on Days 1 through 10, and also received two 3 mg/kg doses of cyclosporine 12 hours apart on Day 10, developed transient elevations of alanine transaminase (ALT) on Day 11 that were 2 to 3 times the upper limit of normal (ULN). In a separate panel of adult subjects in the same study, 2 of 8 who received CANCIDAS 35 mg daily for 3 days and cyclosporine (two 3 mg/kg doses administered 12 hours apart) on Day 1 had small increases in ALT (slightly above the ULN) on Day 2. In both groups, elevations in aspartate transaminase (AST) paralleled ALT elevations, but were of lesser magnitude. In another clinical study, 2 of 8 healthy men developed transient ALT elevations of less than 2× ULN. In this study, cyclosporine (4 mg/kg) was administered on Days 1 and 12, and CANCIDAS was administered (70 mg) daily on Days 3 through 13. In one subject, the ALT elevation occurred on Days 7 and 9 and, in the other subject, the ALT elevation occurred on Day 19. These elevations returned to normal by Day 27. In all groups, elevations in AST paralleled ALT elevations but were of lesser magnitude. In these clinical studies, cyclosporine (one 4 mg/kg dose or two 3 mg/kg doses) increased the AUC of caspofungin by approximately 35%.

In a retrospective postmarketing study, 40 immunocompromised patients, including 37 transplant recipients, were treated with CANCIDAS and cyclosporine for 1 to 290 days (median 17.5 days). Fourteen patients (35%) developed transaminase elevations >5× upper limit of normal or >3× baseline during concomitant therapy or the 14-day follow-up period; five were considered possibly related to concomitant therapy. One patient had elevated bilirubin considered possibly related to concomitant therapy. No patient developed clinical evidence of hepatotoxicity or serious hepatic events. Discontinuations due to laboratory abnormalities in hepatic enzymes from any cause occurred in four patients. Of these, 2 were considered possibly related to therapy with CANCIDAS and/or cyclosporine as well as to other possible causes.

Table 4: Adverse Reactions Among Patients with Candidemia or other Candida Infections*, † Incidence ≥5% for at Least One Treatment Group by System Organ Class or Preferred Term

Adverse Reaction (MedDRA v11.0 System Organ Class and Preferred Term)	CANCIDAS 50 mg‡ N=104 (percent)	CANCIDAS 150 mg N=100 (percent)
All Systems, Any Adverse Reaction	**83**	**83**
Infections and Infestations	**44**	**43**
Septic Shock	13	14
Pneumonia	5	7
Sepsis	5	7
General Disorders and Administration Site Conditions	**33**	**27**
Pyrexia	6	6
Gastrointestinal Disorders	**30**	**33**
Vomiting	11	6
Diarrhea	6	7
Nausea	5	7
Investigations	**28**	**35**
Alkaline Phosphatase Increased	12	9
Aspartate Aminotransferase Increased	6	9
Blood potassium decreased	6	8
Alanine Aminotransferase Increased	4	7
Respiratory, Thoracic and Mediastinal Disorders	**23**	**26**
Respiratory Failure	6	2
Vascular Disorders	**19**	**18**
Hypotension	7	3
Hypertension	5	6
Skin and Subcutaneous Tissue Disorders	**15**	**15**
Decubitus Ulcer	3	5

Within any system organ class, individuals may experience more than 1 adverse event
* Intra-abdominal abscesses, peritonitis and pleural space infections.
† Regardless of causality
‡ Patients received CANCIDAS 70 mg on Day 1, then 50 mg once daily for the remainder of their treatment.

In the prospective invasive aspergillosis and compassionate use studies, there were 4 adult patients treated with CANCIDAS (50 mg/day) and cyclosporine for 2 to 56 days. None of these patients experienced increases in hepatic enzymes.

Given the limitations of these data, CANCIDAS and cyclosporine should only be used concomitantly in those patients for whom the potential benefit outweighs the potential risk. Patients who develop abnormal liver function tests during concomitant therapy should be monitored and the risk/benefit of continuing therapy should be evaluated.

5.3 Hepatic Effects

Laboratory abnormalities in liver function tests have been seen in healthy volunteers and in adult and pediatric patients treated with CANCIDAS. In some adult and pediatric patients with serious underlying conditions who were receiving multiple concomitant medications with CANCIDAS, isolated cases of clinically significant hepatic dysfunction, hepatitis, and hepatic failure have been reported; a causal relationship to CANCIDAS has not been established. Patients who develop abnormal liver function tests during CANCIDAS therapy should be monitored for evidence of worsening hepatic function and evaluated for risk/benefit of continuing CANCIDAS therapy.

6 ADVERSE REACTIONS

The following serious adverse reactions are discussed in detail in another section of the labeling:

- Hepatic effects *[see Warnings and Precautions (5.3)]*
- Hypersensitivity *[see Warnings and Precautions (5.1)]*

Because clinical trials are conducted under widely varying conditions, adverse reaction rates observed in clinical trials of CANCIDAS cannot be directly compared to rates in clinical trials of another drug and may not reflect the rates observed in practice. The adverse reaction information from clinical trials does provide a basis for identifying adverse reactions that appear to be related to drug use and for approximating rates.

6.1 Clinical Trials Experience in Adults

The overall safety of CANCIDAS was assessed in 1865 adult individuals who received single or multiple doses of CANCIDAS: 564 febrile, neutropenic patients (empirical therapy study); 382 patients with candidemia and/or intra-abdominal abscesses, peritonitis, or pleural space infections (including 4 patients with chronic disseminated candidiasis); 297 patients with esophageal and/or oropharyngeal candidiasis; 228 patients with invasive aspergillosis; and 394 individuals in phase I studies. In the empirical therapy study patients had undergone hematopoietic stem-cell transplantation or chemotherapy. In the studies involving patients with documented *Candida* infections, the majority of the patients had serious underlying medical conditions (e.g., hematologic or other malignancy, recent major surgery, HIV) requiring multiple concomitant medications. Patients in the noncomparative *Aspergillus* studies often had serious predisposing medical conditions (e.g., bone marrow or peripheral stem cell transplants, hematologic malignancy, solid tumors or organ transplants) requiring multiple concomitant medications.

Empirical Therapy

In the randomized, double-blinded empirical therapy study, patients received either CANCIDAS 50 mg/day (following a 70-mg loading dose) or AmBisome® (amphotericin B liposome for injection, 3 mg/kg/day). In this study clinical or laboratory hepatic adverse reactions were reported in 39% and 45% of patients in the CANCIDAS and AmBisome groups, respectively. Also reported was an isolated, serious adverse reaction of hyperbilirubinemia considered possibly related to CANCIDAS. Adverse reactions occurring in ≥7.5% of the patients in either treatment group are presented in Table 2.

[See table 2 at top of page 1404]

The proportion of patients who experienced an infusion-related adverse reaction (defined as a systemic event, such as pyrexia, chills, flushing, hypotension, hypertension, tachycardia, dyspnea, tachypnea, rash, or anaphylaxis, that developed during the study therapy infusion and one hour following infusion) was significantly lower in the group treated with CANCIDAS (35%) than in the group treated with AmBisome (52%).

To evaluate the effect of CANCIDAS and AmBisome on renal function, nephrotoxicity was defined as doubling of serum creatinine relative to baseline or an increase of ≥1 mg/dL in serum creatinine if baseline serum creatinine was above the upper limit of the normal range. Among patients whose baseline creatinine clearance was >30 mL/min, the incidence of nephrotoxicity was significantly lower in the group treated with CANCIDAS (3%) than in the group treated with AmBisome (12%). Clinical renal events, regardless of causality, were similar between CANCIDAS (75/564, 13%) and AmBisome (85/547, 16%).

Candidemia and Other Candida Infections

In the randomized, double-blinded invasive candidiasis study, patients received either CANCIDAS 50 mg/day (following a 70-mg loading dose) or amphotericin B 0.6 to 1 mg/kg/day. Adverse reactions occurring in ≥10% of the patients in either treatment group are presented in Table 3.

[See table 3 at top of previous page]

The proportion of patients who experienced an infusion-related adverse reaction (defined as a systemic event, such as pyrexia, chills, flushing, hypotension, hypertension, tachycardia, dyspnea, tachypnea, rash, or anaphylaxis, that developed during the study therapy infusion and one hour following infusion) was significantly lower in the group treated with CANCIDAS (20%) than in the group treated with amphotericin B (49%).

To evaluate the effect of CANCIDAS and amphotericin B on renal function, nephrotoxicity was defined as doubling of serum creatinine relative to baseline or an increase of ≥1 mg/dL in serum creatinine if baseline serum creatinine was above the upper limit of the normal range. In a subgroup of patients whose baseline creatinine clearance was >30 mL/min, the incidence of nephrotoxicity was significantly lower in the group treated with CANCIDAS than in the group treated with amphotericin B.

In a second randomized, double-blinded invasive candidiasis study, patients received either CANCIDAS 50 mg/day (following a 70-mg loading dose) or CANCIDAS 150 mg/day. The proportion of patients who experienced any adverse reaction was similar in the 2 treatment groups; however, this study was not large enough to detect differences in rare or unexpected adverse events. Adverse reactions occurring in ≥5% of the patients in either treatment group are presented in Table 4.

[See table 4 above]

Esophageal Candidiasis and Oropharyngeal Candidiasis

Adverse reactions occurring in ≥10% of patients with esophageal and/or oropharyngeal candidiasis are presented in Table 5.

[See table 5 at top of next page]

Invasive Aspergillosis

In an open-label, noncomparative aspergillosis study, in which 69 patients received CANCIDAS (70-mg loading dose on Day 1 followed by 50 mg daily), the following treatment-emergent adverse reactions were observed with an incidence of ≥12.5%: blood alkaline phosphatase increased (22%), hypotension (20%), respiratory failure (20%), pyrexia (17%), diarrhea (15%), nausea (15%), headache (15%), rash (13%), aspergillosis (13%), alanine aminotransferase increased (13%), aspartate aminotransferase increased (13%), blood bilirubin increased (13%), and blood potassium decreased (13%). Also reported infrequently in this patient population were pulmonary edema, ARDS (adult respiratory distress syndrome), and radiographic infiltrates.

6.2 Clinical Trials Experience in Pediatric Patients (3 months to 17 years of age)

The overall safety of CANCIDAS was assessed in 171 pediatric patients who received single or multiple doses of CANCIDAS. The distribution among the 153 pediatric patients who were over the age of 3 months was as follows: 104 febrile, neutropenic patients; 38 patients with candidemia and/or intra-abdominal abscesses, peritonitis, or pleural space infections; 1 patient with esophageal candidiasis; and 10 patients with invasive aspergillosis. The overall safety profile of CANCIDAS in pediatric patients is comparable to that in adult patients. Table 6 shows the incidence of adverse reactions reported in ≥7.5% of pediatric patients in clinical studies.

One patient (0.6%) receiving CANCIDAS, and three patients (12%) receiving AmBisome developed a serious drug-related adverse reaction. Two patients (1%) were discontinued from CANCIDAS and three patients (12%) were discontinued from AmBisome due to a drug-related adverse reaction. The proportion of patients who experienced an infusion-related adverse reaction (defined as a systemic event, such as pyrexia, chills, flushing, hypotension, hypertension, tachycardia, dyspnea, tachypnea, rash, or anaphylaxis, that developed during the study therapy infusion and one hour following infusion) was 22% in the group treated with CANCIDAS and 35% in the group treated with AmBisome.

[See table 6 at top of page 1408]

6.3 Overall Safety Experience of CANCIDAS in Clinical Trials

The overall safety of CANCIDAS was assessed in 2036 individuals (including 1642 adult or pediatric patients and 394 volunteers) from 34 clinical studies. These individuals received single or multiple (once daily) doses of CANCIDAS, ranging from 5 mg to 210 mg. Full safety data is available from 1951 individuals, as the safety data from 85 patients enrolled in 2 compassionate use studies was limited solely to serious adverse reactions. Treatment emergent adverse reactions, regardless of causality, which occurred in ≥5% of all individuals who received CANCIDAS in these trials, are shown in Table 7.

Overall, 1665 of the 1951 (85%) patients/volunteers who received CANCIDAS experienced an adverse reaction.

Table 7: Treatment-Emergent* Adverse Reactions in Patients Who Received CANCIDAS in Clinical Trials† Incidence ≥5% for at Least One Treatment Group by System Organ Class or Preferred Term

Adverse Reaction‡ (MedDRA v10 System Organ Class and Preferred Term)	CANCIDAS (N = 1951) n	(%)
All Systems, Any Adverse Reaction	**1665**	**(85)**
Investigations	**901**	**(46)**
Alanine Aminotransferase Increased	258	(13)
Aspartate Aminotransferase Increased	233	(12)
Blood Alkaline Phosphatase Increased	232	(12)
Blood Potassium Decreased	220	(11)
Blood Bilirubin Increased	117	(6)
General Disorders and Administration Site Conditions	**843**	**(43)**
Pyrexia	381	(20)
Chills	192	(10)
Edema Peripheral	110	(6)
Gastrointestinal Disorders	**754**	**(39)**
Diarrhea	273	(14)
Nausea	166	(9)
Vomiting	146	(8)
Abdominal Pain	112	(6)
Infections and Infestations	**730**	**(37)**
Pneumonia	115	(6)
Respiratory, Thoracic, and Mediastinal Disorders	**613**	**(31)**
Cough	111	(6)
Skin and Subcutaneous Tissue Disorders	**520**	**(27)**
Rash	159	(8)
Erythema	98	(5)
Nervous System Disorders	**412**	**(21)**
Headache	193	(10)
Vascular Disorders	**344**	**(18)**
Hypotension	118	(6)

* Defined as an adverse reaction, regardless of causality, while on CANCIDAS or during the 14-day post-CANCIDAS follow-up period.
† Incidence for each preferred term is ≥5% among individuals who received at least 1 dose of CANCIDAS.
‡ Within any system organ class, individuals may experience more than 1 adverse event.

Clinically significant adverse reactions, regardless of causality or incidence which occurred in less than 5% of patients are listed below.

- ***Blood and lymphatic system disorders:*** anemia, coagulopathy, febrile neutropenia, neutropenia, thrombocytopenia
- ***Cardiac disorders:*** arrhythmia, atrial fibrillation, bradycardia, cardiac arrest, myocardial infarction, tachycardia
- ***Gastrointestinal disorders:*** abdominal distension, abdominal pain upper, constipation, dyspepsia
- ***General disorders and administration site conditions:*** asthenia, fatigue, infusion site pain/pruritus/swelling, mucosal inflammation, edema
- ***Hepatobiliary disorders:*** hepatic failure, hepatomegaly, hepatotoxicity, hyperbilirubinemia, jaundice
- ***Infections and infestations:*** bacteremia, sepsis, urinary tract infection
- ***Metabolic and nutrition disorders:*** anorexia, decreased appetite, fluid overload, hypomagnesemia, hypercalcemia, hyperglycemia, hypokalemia
- ***Musculoskeletal, connective tissue, and bone disorders:*** arthralgia, back pain, pain in extremity
- ***Nervous system disorders:*** convulsion, dizziness, somnolence, tremor

Table 5: Adverse Reactions Among Patients with Esophageal and/or Oropharyngeal Candidiasis* Incidence ≥10% for at Least One Treatment Group by System Organ Class or Preferred Term

Adverse Reaction (MedDRA v10.1 System Organ Class and Preferred Term)	CANCIDAS 50 mg† N=83 (percent)	Fluconazole IV 200 mg† N=94 (percent)
All Systems, Any Adverse Reaction	**90**	**93**
Gastrointestinal Disorders	**58**	**50**
Diarrhea	27	18
Nausea	15	15
Investigations	**53**	**61**
Hemoglobin Decreased	21	16
Hematocrit Decreased	18	16
Aspartate Aminotransferase Increased	13	19
Blood Alkaline Phosphatase Increased	13	17
Alanine Aminotransferase Increased	12	17
White Blood Cell Count Decreased	12	19
General Disorders and Administration Site Conditions	**31**	**36**
Pyrexia	21	21
Vascular Disorders	**19**	**15**
Phlebitis	18	11
Nervous System Disorders	**18**	**17**
Headache	15	9

Within any system organ class, individuals may experience more than 1 adverse reaction.
* Regardless of causality
† Derived from a comparator-controlled clinical study.

- ***Psychiatric disorders:*** anxiety, confusional state, depression, insomnia
- ***Renal and urinary disorders:*** hematuria, renal failure
- ***Respiratory, thoracic, and mediastinal disorders:*** dyspnea, epistaxis, hypoxia, tachypnea
- ***Skin and subcutaneous tissue disorders:*** erythema, petechiae, skin lesion, urticaria
- ***Vascular disorders:*** flushing, hypertension, phlebitis

6.4 Postmarketing Experience

The following additional adverse reactions have been identified during the post-approval use of CANCIDAS. Because these reactions are reported voluntarily from a population of uncertain size, it is not always possible to reliably estimate their frequency or establish a causal relationship to drug exposure.

- *Gastrointestinal disorders:* pancreatitis
- *Hepatobiliary disorders:* hepatic necrosis
- *Skin and subcutaneous tissue disorders:* erythema multiforme, Stevens-Johnson, skin exfoliation
- *Renal and urinary disorders:* clinically significant renal dysfunction
- *General disorders and administration site conditions:* swelling and peripheral edema

7 DRUG INTERACTIONS

[See Clinical Pharmacology (12.3).]

In clinical studies, caspofungin did not induce the CYP3A4 metabolism of other drugs. Caspofungin is not a substrate for P-glycoprotein and is a poor substrate for cytochrome P450 enzymes.

Clinical studies in adult healthy volunteers show that the pharmacokinetics of CANCIDAS are not altered by itraconazole, amphotericin B, mycophenolate, nelfinavir, or tacrolimus. CANCIDAS has no effect on the pharmacokinetics of itraconazole, amphotericin B, or the active metabolite of mycophenolate.

Cyclosporine: In two adult clinical studies, cyclosporine (one 4 mg/kg dose or two 3 mg/kg doses) increased the AUC of caspofungin by approximately 35%. CANCIDAS did not increase the plasma levels of cyclosporine. There were transient increases in liver ALT and AST when CANCIDAS and cyclosporine were co-administered *[see Warnings and Precautions (5.2)]*.

Tacrolimus: For patients receiving CANCIDAS and tacrolimus, standard monitoring of tacrolimus blood concentrations and appropriate tacrolimus dosage adjustments are recommended.

Rifampin: Adult patients on rifampin should receive 70 mg of CANCIDAS daily.

Other inducers of drug clearance:

Adults: When CANCIDAS is co-administered to adult patients with inducers of drug clearance, such as efavirenz, nevirapine, phenytoin, dexamethasone, or carbamazepine, use of a daily dose of 70 mg of CANCIDAS should be considered.

Pediatric Patients: When CANCIDAS is co-administered to pediatric patients with inducers of drug clearance, such as rifampin, efavirenz, nevirapine, phenytoin, dexamethasone, or carbamazepine, a CANCIDAS dose of 70 mg/m^2 daily (not to exceed an actual daily dose of 70 mg) should be considered.

8 USE IN SPECIFIC POPULATIONS

8.1 Pregnancy

Pregnancy Category C

There are no adequate and well-controlled studies with the use of CANCIDAS in pregnant women. In animal studies, caspofungin caused embryofetal toxicity, including increased resorptions, increased peri-implantation loss, and incomplete ossification at multiple fetal sites. CANCIDAS should be used during pregnancy only if the potential benefit justifies the potential risk to the fetus.

In offspring born to pregnant rats treated with caspofungin at doses comparable to the human dose based on body surface area comparisons, there was incomplete ossification of the skull and torso and increased incidences of cervical rib. There was also an increase in resorptions and peri-implantation losses. In pregnant rabbits treated with caspofungin at doses comparable to 2 times the human dose based on body surface area comparisons, there was an increased incidence of incomplete ossification of the talus/calcaneus in offspring and increases in fetal resorptions. Caspofungin crossed the placenta in rats and rabbits and was detectable in fetal plasma.

8.3 Nursing Mothers

It is not known whether caspofungin is present in human milk. Caspofungin was found in the milk of lactating, drug-treated rats. Because many drugs are excreted in human milk, caution should be exercised when caspofungin is administered to a nursing woman.

8.4 Pediatric Use

The safety and effectiveness of CANCIDAS in pediatric patients 3 months to 17 years of age are supported by evidence from adequate and well-controlled studies in adults, pharmacokinetic data in pediatric patients, and additional data from prospective studies in pediatric patients 3 months to 17 years of age for the following indications *[see Indications and Usage (1)]*:

- Empirical therapy for presumed fungal infections in febrile, neutropenic patients.
- Treatment of candidemia and the following *Candida* infections: intra-abdominal abscesses, peritonitis, and pleural space infections.
- Treatment of esophageal candidiasis.
- Treatment of invasive aspergillosis in patients who are refractory to or intolerant of other therapies (e.g., amphotericin B, lipid formulations of amphotericin B, itraconazole).

Table 6: Adverse Reactions Among Pediatric Patients (0 months to 17 years of age)* Incidence ≥7.5% for at Least One Treatment Group by System Organ Class or Preferred Term

Adverse Reaction (MedDRA v10.0 System Organ Class and Preferred Term)	Noncomparative Clinical Studies	Comparator-Controlled Clinical Study of Empirical Therapy	
	CANCIDAS Any Dose N=115 (percent)	CANCIDAS 50 mg/m²† N=56 (percent)	AmBisome 3 mg/kg N=26 (percent)
All Systems, Any Adverse Reaction	**95**	**96**	**89**
Investigations	**55**	**41**	**50**
Blood Potassium Decreased	18	9	27
Aspartate Aminotransferase Increased	17	2	12
Alanine Aminotransferase Increased	14	5	12
Blood Potassium Increased	3	0	8
Protein Total Decreased	0	0	8
General Disorders and Administration Site Conditions	**47**	**59**	**42**
Pyrexia	29	30	23
Chills	10	13	8
Mucosal Inflammation	10	4	4
Edema	3	4	8
Respiratory, Thoracic and Mediastinal Disorders	**43**	**32**	**27**
Respiratory Distress	8	0	4
Cough	6	9	8
Gastrointestinal Disorders	**42**	**41**	**35**
Diarrhea	17	7	15
Vomiting	8	11	12
Abdominal Pain	7	4	12
Nausea	4	4	8
Infections and Infestations	**40**	**30**	**35**
Central Line Infection	1	9	0
Skin and Subcutaneous Tissue Disorders	**33**	**41**	**39**
Pruritus	7	6	8
Rash	6	23	8
Erythema	4	9	0
Vascular Disorders	**24**	**21**	**19**
Hypotension	12	9	8
Hypertension	10	9	4
Metabolism and Nutrition Disorders	**22**	**11**	**23**
Hypokalemia	8	5	4
Cardiac Disorders	**17**	**13**	**19**
Tachycardia	4	11	19
Nervous System Disorders	**13**	**16**	**8**
Headache	5	9	4
Musculoskeletal and Connective Tissue Disorders	**11**	**14**	**12**
Back Pain	4	0	8
Blood and Lymphatic System Disorders	**10**	**2**	**15**
Anemia	2	0	8
Immune System Disorders	**7**	**7**	**12**
Graft Versus Host Disease	1	4	8

Within any system organ class, individuals may experience more than 1 adverse reaction.
* Regardless of causality
† 70 mg/m² on Day 1, then 50 mg/m² once daily for the remainder of the treatment.

The efficacy and safety of CANCIDAS has not been adequately studied in prospective clinical trials involving neonates and infants under 3 months of age. Although limited pharmacokinetic data were collected in neonates and infants below 3 months of age, these data are insufficient to establish a safe and effective dose of caspofungin in the treatment of neonatal candidiasis. Invasive candidiasis in neonates has a higher rate of CNS and multi-organ involvement than in older patients; the ability of CANCIDAS to penetrate the blood-brain barrier and to treat patients with meningitis and endocarditis is unknown.

CANCIDAS has not been studied in pediatric patients with endocarditis, osteomyelitis, and meningitis due to *Candida*. CANCIDAS has also not been studied as initial therapy for invasive aspergillosis in pediatric patients.

In clinical trials, 171 pediatric patients (0 months to 17 years of age), including 18 patients who were less than 3 months of age, were given intravenous CANCIDAS. Pharmacokinetic studies enrolled a total of 66 pediatric patients, and an additional 105 pediatric patients received CANCIDAS in safety and efficacy studies *[see Clinical Pharmacology (12.3) and Clinical Studies (14.5)]*. The majority of the pediatric patients received CANCIDAS at a once-daily maintenance dose of 50 mg/m² for a mean duration of 12 days (median 9, range 1-87 days). In all studies, safety was assessed by the investigator throughout study therapy and for 14 days following cessation of study therapy. The most common adverse reactions in pediatric patients treated with CANCIDAS were pyrexia (29%), blood potassium decreased (15%), diarrhea (14%), increased aspartate aminotransferase (12%), rash (12%), increased alanine aminotransferase (11%), hypotension (11%), and chills (11%) *[see Adverse Reactions (6.2)]*.

Postmarketing hepatobiliary adverse reactions have been reported in pediatric patients with serious underlying medical conditions *[see Warnings and Precautions (5.3)]*.

8.5 Geriatric Use

Clinical studies of CANCIDAS did not include sufficient numbers of patients aged 65 and over to determine whether they respond differently from younger patients. Although the number of elderly patients was not large enough for a statistical analysis, no overall differences in safety or efficacy were observed between these and younger patients. Plasma concentrations of caspofungin in healthy older men and women (≥65 years of age) were increased slightly (approximately 28% in AUC) compared to young healthy men. A similar effect of age on pharmacokinetics was seen in patients with candidemia or other *Candida* infections (intra-abdominal abscesses, peritonitis, or pleural space infections). No dose adjustment is recommended for the elderly; however, greater sensitivity of some older individuals cannot be ruled out.

8.6 Patients with Hepatic Impairment

Adult patients with mild hepatic impairment (Child-Pugh score 5 to 6) do not need a dosage adjustment. For adult patients with moderate hepatic impairment (Child-Pugh score 7 to 9), CANCIDAS 35 mg once daily is recommended based upon pharmacokinetic data *[see Clinical Pharmacology (12.3)]*. However, where recommended, a 70-mg loading dose should still be administered on Day 1 *[see Dosage and Administration (2.4) and Clinical Pharmacology (12.3)]*. There is no clinical experience in adult patients with severe hepatic impairment (Child-Pugh score >9) and in pediatric patients 3 months to 17 years of age with any degree of hepatic impairment.

8.7 Patients with Renal Impairment

No dosage adjustment is necessary for patients with renal impairment. Caspofungin is not dialyzable; thus, supplementary dosing is not required following hemodialysis *[see Clinical Pharmacology (12.3)]*.

10 OVERDOSAGE

In 6 healthy subjects who received a single 210-mg dose, no significant adverse reactions were reported. Multiple doses above 150 mg daily have not been studied. Caspofungin is not dialyzable. The minimum lethal dose of caspofungin in rats was 50 mg/kg, a dose which is equivalent to 10 times the recommended daily dose based on relative body surface area comparison.

In clinical trials, one pediatric patient (16 years of age) unintentionally received a single dose of caspofungin of 113 mg (on Day 1), followed by 80 mg daily for an additional 7 days. No clinically significant adverse reactions were reported.

11 DESCRIPTION

CANCIDAS is a sterile, lyophilized product for intravenous (IV) infusion that contains a semisynthetic lipopeptide (echinocandin) compound synthesized from a fermentation product of *Glarea lozoyensis*. CANCIDAS is an echinocandin that inhibits the synthesis of β (1,3)-D-glucan, an integral component of the fungal cell wall.

CANCIDAS (caspofungin acetate) is 1-[(4*R*,5*S*)-5-[(2-aminoethyl)amino]-N^2-(10,12-dimethyl-1-oxotetradecyl)-4-hydroxy-L-ornithine]-5-[(3*R*)-3-hydroxy-L-ornithine] pneumocandin B_0 diacetate (salt). CANCIDAS 50 mg also contains: 39 mg sucrose, 26 mg mannitol, glacial acetic acid, and sodium hydroxide. CANCIDAS 70 mg also contains 54 mg sucrose, 36 mg mannitol, glacial acetic acid, and sodium hydroxide. Caspofungin acetate is a hygroscopic, white to off-white powder. It is freely soluble in water and methanol, and slightly soluble in ethanol. The pH of a saturated aqueous solution of caspofungin acetate is approximately 6.6. The empirical formula is $C_{52}H_{88}N_{10}O_{15}\bullet 2C_2H_4O_2$ and the formula weight is 1213.42. The structural formula is:

[See chemical structure at top of next column]

12 CLINICAL PHARMACOLOGY

12.1 Mechanism of Action

Caspofungin is an antifungal drug *[see Clinical Pharmacology (12.4)]*.

12.3 Pharmacokinetics

Adult and pediatric pharmacokinetic parameters are presented in Table 8.

Distribution

Plasma concentrations of caspofungin decline in a polyphasic manner following single 1-hour IV infusions. A short α-phase occurs immediately postinfusion, followed by a

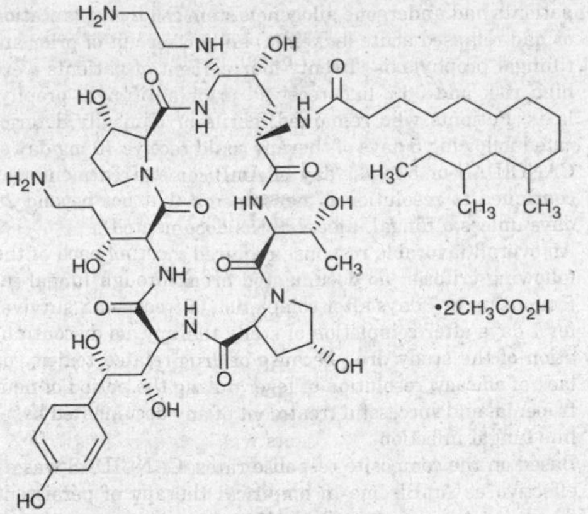

β-phase (half-life of 9 to 11 hours) that characterizes much of the profile and exhibits clear log-linear behavior from 6 to 48 hours postdose during which the plasma concentration decreases 10-fold. An additional, longer half-life phase, γ-phase, (half-life of 40-50 hours), also occurs. Distribution, rather than excretion or biotransformation, is the dominant mechanism influencing plasma clearance. Caspofungin is extensively bound to albumin (~97%), and distribution into red blood cells is minimal. Mass balance results showed that approximately 92% of the administered radioactivity was distributed to tissues by 36 to 48 hours after a single 70-mg dose of [^{3}H] caspofungin acetate. There is little excretion or biotransformation of caspofungin during the first 30 hours after administration.

Metabolism

Caspofungin is slowly metabolized by hydrolysis and N-acetylation. Caspofungin also undergoes spontaneous chemical degradation to an open-ring peptide compound, L-747969. At later time points (≥5 days postdose), there is a low level (≤7 picomoles/mg protein, or ≤1.3% of administered dose) of covalent binding of radiolabel in plasma following single-dose administration of [^{3}H] caspofungin acetate, which may be due to two reactive intermediates formed during the chemical degradation of caspofungin to L-747969. Additional metabolism involves hydrolysis into constitutive amino acids and their degradates, including dihydroxyhomotyrosine and N-acetyl-dihydroxyhomotyrosine. These two tyrosine derivatives are found only in urine, suggesting rapid clearance of these derivatives by the kidneys.

Excretion

Two single-dose radiolabeled pharmacokinetic studies were conducted. In one study, plasma, urine, and feces were collected over 27 days, and in the second study plasma was collected over 6 months. Plasma concentrations of radioactivity and of caspofungin were similar during the first 24 to 48 hours postdose; thereafter drug levels fell more rapidly. In plasma, caspofungin concentrations fell below the limit of quantitation after 6 to 8 days postdose, while radiolabel fell below the limit of quantitation at 22.3 weeks postdose. After single intravenous administration of [^{3}H] caspofungin acetate, excretion of caspofungin and its metabolites in humans was 35% of dose in feces and 41% of dose in urine. A small amount of caspofungin is excreted unchanged in urine (~1.4% of dose). Renal clearance of parent drug is low (~0.15 mL/min) and total clearance of caspofungin is 12 mL/min.

Special Populations

Renal Impairment

In a clinical study of single 70-mg doses, caspofungin pharmacokinetics were similar in healthy adult volunteers with mild renal impairment (creatinine clearance 50 to 80 mL/min) and control subjects. Moderate (creatinine clearance 31 to 49 mL/min), severe (creatinine clearance 5 to 30 mL/min), and end-stage (creatinine clearance <10 mL/min and dialysis dependent) renal impairment moderately increased caspofungin plasma concentrations after single-dose administration (range: 30 to 49% for AUC). However, in adult patients with invasive aspergillosis, candidemia, or other *Candida* infections (intra-abdominal abscesses, peritonitis, or pleural space infections) who received multiple daily doses of CANCIDAS 50 mg, there was no significant effect of mild to end-stage renal impairment on caspofungin concentrations. No dosage adjustment is necessary for patients with renal impairment. Caspofungin is not dialyzable, thus supplementary dosing is not required following hemodialysis.

Hepatic Impairment

Plasma concentrations of caspofungin after a single 70-mg dose in adult patients with mild hepatic impairment (Child-Pugh score 5 to 6) were increased by approximately 55% in AUC compared to healthy control subjects. In a 14-day multiple-dose study (70 mg on Day 1 followed by 50 mg daily thereafter), plasma concentrations in adult patients with mild hepatic impairment were increased modestly (19 to 25% in AUC) on Days 7 and 14 relative to healthy control subjects. No dosage adjustment is recommended for patients with mild hepatic impairment.

Adult patients with moderate hepatic impairment (Child-Pugh score 7 to 9) who received a single 70-mg dose of CANCIDAS had an average plasma caspofungin increase of 76% in AUC compared to control subjects. A dosage reduction is recommended for adult patients with moderate hepatic impairment based upon these pharmacokinetic data *[see Dosage and Administration (2.4)]*.

There is no clinical experience in adult patients with severe hepatic impairment (Child-Pugh score >9) or in pediatric patients with any degree of hepatic impairment.

Gender

Plasma concentrations of caspofungin in healthy adult men and women were similar following a single 70-mg dose. After 13 daily 50-mg doses, caspofungin plasma concentrations in women were elevated slightly (approximately 22% in area under the curve [AUC]) relative to men. No dosage adjustment is necessary based on gender.

Race

Regression analyses of patient pharmacokinetic data indicated that no clinically significant differences in the pharmacokinetics of caspofungin were seen among Caucasians, Blacks, and Hispanics. No dosage adjustment is necessary on the basis of race.

Geriatric Patients

Plasma concentrations of caspofungin in healthy older men and women (≥65 years of age) were increased slightly (approximately 28% AUC) compared to young healthy men after a single 70-mg dose of caspofungin. In patients who were treated empirically or who had candidemia or other *Candida* infections (intra-abdominal abscesses, peritonitis, or pleural space infections), a similar modest effect of age was seen in older patients relative to younger patients. No dosage adjustment is necessary for the elderly *[see Use in Specific Populations (8.5)]*.

Pediatric Patients

CANCIDAS has been studied in five prospective studies involving pediatric patients under 18 years of age, including three pediatric pharmacokinetic studies [initial study in adolescents (12-17 years of age) and children (2-11 years of age) followed by a study in younger patients (3-23 months of age) and then followed by a study in neonates and infants (<3 months)] *[see Use in Specific Populations (8.4)]*.

Pharmacokinetic parameters following multiple doses of CANCIDAS in pediatric and adult patients are presented in Table 8.

[See table 8 above]

Table 8: Pharmacokinetic Parameters Following Multiple Doses of CANCIDAS in Pediatric (3 months to 17 years) and Adult Patients

			Pharmacokinetic Parameters (Mean ± Standard Deviation)				
Population	N	Daily Dose	AUC_{0-24hr} (μg·hr/mL)	C_{1hr} (μg/mL)	C_{24hr} (μg/mL)	$t_{1/2}$ (hr)*	Cl (mL/min)
PEDIATRIC PATIENTS							
Adolescents, Aged 12-17 years	8	50 mg/m^2	124.9 ± 50.4	14.0 ± 6.9	2.4 ± 1.0	11.2 ± 1.7	12.6 ± 5.5
Children, Aged 2-11 years	9	50 mg/m^2	120.0 ± 33.4	16.1 ± 4.2	1.7 ± 0.8	8.2 ± 2.4	6.4 ± 2.6
Young Children, Aged 3-23 months	8	50 mg/m^2	131.2 ± 17.7	17.6 ± 3.9	1.7 ± 0.7	8.8 ± 2.1	3.2 ± 0.4
ADULT PATIENTS							
Adults with Esophageal Candidiasis	6†	50 mg	87.3 ± 30.0	8.7 ± 2.1	1.7 ± 0.7	13.0 ± 1.9	10.6 ± 3.8
Adults receiving Empirical Therapy	119‡	50 mg§	--	8.0 ± 3.4	1.6 ± 0.7	--	--

* Harmonic Mean ± jackknife standard deviation
† N=5 for C_{1hr} and AUC_{0-24hr}; N=6 for C_{24hr}
‡ N=117 for C_{24hr}; N=119 for C_{1hr}
§ Following an initial 70-mg loading dose on day 1

Drug Interactions [see Drug Interactions (7)]

Studies in *vitro* show that caspofungin acetate is not an inhibitor of any enzyme in the cytochrome P450 (CYP) system. In clinical studies, caspofungin did not induce the CYP3A4 metabolism of other drugs. Caspofungin is not a substrate for P-glycoprotein and is a poor substrate for cytochrome P450 enzymes.

Clinical studies in adult healthy volunteers show that the pharmacokinetics of CANCIDAS are not altered by itraconazole, amphotericin B, mycophenolate, nelfinavir, or tacrolimus. CANCIDAS has no effect on the pharmacokinetics of itraconazole, amphotericin B, or the active metabolite of mycophenolate.

Cyclosporine: In two adult clinical studies, cyclosporine (one 4 mg/kg dose or two 3 mg/kg doses) increased the AUC of caspofungin by approximately 35%. CANCIDAS did not increase the plasma levels of cyclosporine. There were transient increases in liver ALT and AST when CANCIDAS and cyclosporine were co-administered *[see Warnings and Precautions (5.2)]*.

Tacrolimus: CANCIDAS reduced the blood AUC_{0-12} of tacrolimus (FK-506, Prograf®) by approximately 20%, peak blood concentration (C_{max}) by 16%, and 12-hour blood concentration (C_{12hr}) by 26% in healthy adult subjects when tacrolimus (2 doses of 0.1 mg/kg 12 hours apart) was administered on the 10th day of CANCIDAS 70 mg daily, as compared to results from a control period in which tacrolimus was administered alone. For patients receiving both therapies, standard monitoring of tacrolimus blood concentrations and appropriate tacrolimus dosage adjustments are recommended.

Rifampin: A drug-drug interaction study with rifampin in adult healthy volunteers has shown a 30% decrease in caspofungin trough concentrations. Adult patients on rifampin should receive 70 mg of CANCIDAS daily.

Other inducers of drug clearance

Adults: In addition, results from regression analyses of adult patient pharmacokinetic data suggest that co-administration of other inducers of drug clearance (efavirenz, nevirapine, phenytoin, dexamethasone, or carbamazepine) with CANCIDAS may result in clinically meaningful reductions in caspofungin concentrations. It is not known which drug clearance mechanism involved in caspofungin disposition may be inducible. When CANCIDAS is co-administered to adult patients with inducers of drug clearance, such as efavirenz, nevirapine, phenytoin, dexamethasone, or carbamazepine, use of a daily dose of 70 mg of CANCIDAS should be considered.

Pediatric patients: In pediatric patients, results from regression analyses of pharmacokinetic data suggest that co-administration of dexamethasone with CANCIDAS may result in clinically meaningful reductions in caspofungin trough concentrations. This finding may indicate that pediatric patients will have similar reductions with inducers as seen in adults. When CANCIDAS is co-administered to pediatric patients with inducers of drug clearance, such as rifampin, efavirenz, nevirapine, phenytoin, dexamethasone, or carbamazepine, a CANCIDAS dose of 70 mg/m^2 daily (not to exceed an actual daily dose of 70 mg) should be considered.

12.4 Microbiology

Mechanism of Action

Caspofungin, an echinocandin, inhibits the synthesis of β (1,3)-D-glucan, an essential component of the cell wall of susceptible *Aspergillus* species and *Candida* species. β (1,3)-D-glucan is not present in mammalian cells. Caspofungin has shown activity against *Candida* species and in regions of active cell growth of the hyphae of *Aspergillus fumigatus*.

Activity in vitro

Caspofungin has been shown to be active **both *in vitro* and in clinical infections** against most strains of the following microorganisms:

Aspergillus fumigatus
Aspergillus flavus
Aspergillus terreus
Candida albicans
Candida glabrata
Candida guilliermondii

Table 11: Favorable Response of Patients with Persistent Fever and Neutropenia

	CANCIDAS*	AmBisome*	% Difference (Confidence Interval)†
Number of Patients‡	556	539	
Overall Favorable Response	190 (33.9%)	181 (33.7%)	0.2 (-5.6, 6.0)
No documented breakthrough fungal infection	527 (94.8%)	515 (95.5%)	-0.8
Survival 7 days after end of treatment	515 (92.6%)	481 (89.2%)	3.4
No discontinuation due to toxicity or lack of efficacy	499 (89.7%)	461 (85.5%)	4.2
Resolution of fever during neutropenia	229 (41.2%)	223 (41.4%)	-0.2

* CANCIDAS: 70 mg on Day 1, then 50 mg once daily for the remainder of treatment (daily dose increased to 70 mg for 73 patients); AmBisome: 3 mg/kg/day (daily dose increased to 5 mg/kg for 74 patients).
† Overall Response: estimated % difference adjusted for strata and expressed as CANCIDAS – AmBisome (95.2% CI); Individual criteria presented above are not mutually exclusive. The percent difference calculated as CANCIDAS – AmBisome.
‡ Analysis population excluded subjects who did not have fever or neutropenia at study entry.

Candida krusei
Candida parapsilosis
Candida tropicalis
Susceptibility Testing Methods [see References (15)]
Aspergillus Species and Other Filamentous fungi
No interpretive criteria have been established for *Aspergillus* species and other filamentous fungi.
Candida Species
The interpretive standards for caspofungin against *Candida* species are applicable only to tests performed using Clinical Laboratory and Standards Institute (CLSI) microbroth dilution reference method M27A for MIC (partial inhibition endpoint) read at 24 hours.
Broth Microdilution Techniques: Quantitative methods are used to determine antifungal minimum inhibitory concentrations (MICs). These MICs provide estimates of the susceptibility of *Candida* spp. to antifungal agents. MICs should be determined using a standardized procedure at 24 hours *[see References (15)]*. Standardized procedures are based on a microdilution method (broth) with standardized inoculum concentrations and standardized concentrations of caspofungin powder. The MIC values should be interpreted according to the criteria provided in Table 9.

Table 9: Susceptibility Interpretive Criteria for Caspofungin

Pathogen	Broth Microdilution MIC* (µg/mL) at 24 hours		
	S	I	R
Candida species	≤2	(†)	(†)

* A report of "Susceptible" indicates that the pathogen is likely to be inhibited if the antimicrobial compound in the blood reaches the concentrations usually achievable.
† The current absence of data on caspofungin-resistant isolates precludes defining any categories other than "Susceptible." Isolates yielding test results suggestive of a "Non-Susceptible" category should be retested, and if the result is confirmed, the isolate should be submitted to a reference laboratory for further testing.

Quality Control
Standardized susceptibility test procedures require the use of quality control organisms to control the technical aspects of the test procedures. Standard caspofungin powder should provide the following range of values noted in Table 10.
NOTE: Quality control microorganisms are specific strains of organisms with intrinsic biological properties relating to resistance mechanisms and their genetic expression within fungi; the specific strains used for microbiological control are not clinically significant.

Table 10: Acceptable Quality Control Ranges* for Caspofungin to be used in Validation of Susceptibility Test Results

QC strain	Broth microdilution (MIC in µg/mL) at 24-hour
Candida parapsilosis ATCC† 22019	0.25 – 1.0
Candida krusei ATCC 6258	0.12 – 1.0

* Quality control ranges have not been established for this strain/antifungal agent combination due to their extensive interlaboratory variation during initial quality control studies.
† ATCC is a registered trademark of the American Type Culture Collection.

Activity in vivo
Caspofungin was active when parenterally administered to immunocompetent and immunosuppressed mice as long as 24 hours after disseminated infections with *C. albicans*, in which the endpoints were prolonged survival of infected mice and reduction of *C. albicans* from target organs. Caspofungin, administered parenterally to immunocompetent and immunosuppressed rodents, as long as 24 hours after disseminated or pulmonary infection with *Aspergillus fumigatus*, has shown prolonged survival, which has not been consistently associated with a reduction in mycological burden.
Drug Resistance
A caspofungin MIC of ≤2 µg/mL (Susceptible) indicates that the *Candida* isolate is likely to be inhibited if caspofungin therapeutic concentrations are achieved; there is insufficient treatment outcome information on isolates with reduced caspofungin susceptibility to define categories other than susceptible. Breakthrough infections with *Candida* isolates requiring caspofungin concentrations >2 µg/mL for growth inhibition have developed in a mouse model of *C. albicans* infection and in some patients with *Candida* infections. Some of these isolates had mutations in the FKS1 gene. The incidence of drug resistance by various clinical isolates of *Candida* and *Aspergillus* species is unknown.
Drug Interactions
Studies *in vitro* and *in vivo* of caspofungin, in combination with amphotericin B, suggest no antagonism of antifungal activity against either *A. fumigatus* or *C. albicans*. The clinical significance of these results is unknown.

13 NONCLINICAL TOXICOLOGY

13.1 Carcinogenesis, Mutagenesis, Impairment of Fertility

No long-term studies in animals have been performed to evaluate the carcinogenic potential of caspofungin.
Caspofungin did not show evidence of mutagenic or genotoxic potential when evaluated in the following *in vitro* assays: bacterial (Ames) and mammalian cell (V79 Chinese hamster lung fibroblasts) mutagenesis assays, the alkaline elution/rat hepatocyte DNA strand break test, and the chromosome aberration assay in Chinese hamster ovary cells. Caspofungin was not genotoxic when assessed in the mouse bone marrow chromosomal test at doses up to 12.5 mg/kg (equivalent to a human dose of 1 mg/kg based on body surface area comparisons), administered intravenously.
Fertility and reproductive performance were not affected by the intravenous administration of caspofungin to rats at doses up to 5 mg/kg. At 5 mg/kg exposures were similar to those seen in patients treated with the 70-mg dose.

13.2 Animal Toxicology and/or Pharmacology

In one 5-week study in monkeys at doses which produced exposures approximately 4 to 6 times those seen in adult patients treated with a 70-mg dose, scattered small foci of subcapsular necrosis were observed microscopically in the livers of some animals (2/8 monkeys at 5 mg/kg and 4/8 monkeys at 8 mg/kg); however, this histopathological finding was not seen in another study of 27 weeks duration at similar doses.
No treatment-related findings were seen in a 5-week study in infant monkeys at doses which produced exposures approximately 3 times those achieved in pediatric patients receiving a maintenance dose of 50 mg/m^2 daily.

14 CLINICAL STUDIES

The results of the adult clinical studies are presented by indications in Section 14.1 to 14.4. Results of pediatric clinical trials are in Section 14.5.

14.1 Empirical Therapy in Febrile, Neutropenic Patients

A double-blind study enrolled 1111 febrile, neutropenic (<500 cells/mm^3) patients who were randomized to treatment with daily doses of CANCIDAS (50 mg/day following a 70-mg loading dose on Day 1) or AmBisome (3 mg/kg/day). Patients were stratified based on risk category (high-risk patients had undergone allogeneic stem cell transplantation or had relapsed acute leukemia) and on receipt of prior antifungal prophylaxis. Twenty-four percent of patients were high risk and 56% had received prior antifungal prophylaxis. Patients who remained febrile or clinically deteriorated following 5 days of therapy could receive 70 mg/day of CANCIDAS or 5 mg/kg/day of AmBisome. Treatment was continued to resolution of neutropenia (but not beyond 28 days unless a fungal infection was documented).
An overall favorable response required meeting each of the following criteria: no documented breakthrough fungal infections up to 7 days after completion of treatment, survival for 7 days after completion of study therapy, no discontinuation of the study drug because of drug-related toxicity or lack of efficacy, resolution of fever during the period of neutropenia, and successful treatment of any documented baseline fungal infection.
Based on the composite response rates, CANCIDAS was as effective as AmBisome in empirical therapy of persistent febrile neutropenia (see Table 11).
[See table 11 above]
The rate of successful treatment of documented baseline infections, a component of the primary endpoint, was not statistically different between treatment groups.
The response rates did not differ between treatment groups based on either of the stratification variables: risk category or prior antifungal prophylaxis.

14.2 Candidemia and the Following other *Candida* Infections: Intra-Abdominal Abscesses, Peritonitis and Pleural Space Infections

In a randomized, double-blind study, patients with a proven diagnosis of invasive candidiasis received daily doses of CANCIDAS (50 mg/day following a 70-mg loading dose on Day 1) or amphotericin B deoxycholate (0.6 to 0.7 mg/kg/day for non-neutropenic patients and 0.7 to 1 mg/kg/day for neutropenic patients). Patients were stratified by both neutropenic status and APACHE II score. Patients with *Candida* endocarditis, meningitis, or osteomyelitis were excluded from this study.
Patients who met the entry criteria and received one or more doses of IV study therapy were included in the modified intention-to-treat [MITT] analysis of response at the end of IV study therapy. A favorable response at this time point required both symptom/sign resolution/improvement and microbiological clearance of the *Candida* infection.
Two hundred thirty-nine patients were enrolled. Patient disposition is shown in Table 12.
[See table 12 at top of next page]
Of the 239 patients enrolled, 224 met the criteria for inclusion in the MITT population (109 treated with CANCIDAS and 115 treated with amphotericin B). Of these 224 patients, 186 patients had candidemia (92 treated with CANCIDAS and 94 treated with amphotericin B). The majority of the patients with candidemia were non-neutropenic (87%) and had an APACHE II score less than or equal to 20 (77%) in both arms. Most candidemia infections were caused by *C. albicans* (39%), followed by *C. parapsilosis* (20%), *C. tropicalis* (17%), *C. glabrata* (8%), and *C. krusei* (3%).
At the end of IV study therapy, CANCIDAS was comparable to amphotericin B in the treatment of candidemia in the MITT population. For the other efficacy time points (Day 10 of IV study therapy, end of all antifungal therapy, 2-week post-therapy follow-up, and 6- to 8-week post-therapy follow-up), CANCIDAS was as effective as amphotericin B.
Outcome, relapse and mortality data are shown in Table 13.
[See table 13 at top of next page]
In this study, the efficacy of CANCIDAS in patients with intra-abdominal abscesses, peritonitis and pleural space *Candida* infections was evaluated in 19 non-neutropenic patients. Two of these patients had concurrent candidemia. *Candida* was part of a polymicrobial infection that required adjunctive surgical drainage in 11 of these 19 patients. A favorable response was seen in 9 of 9 patients with peritonitis, 3 of 4 with abscesses (liver, parasplenic, and urinary bladder abscesses), 2 of 2 with pleural space infections, 1 of 2 with mixed peritoneal and pleural infection, 1 of 1 with mixed abdominal abscess and peritonitis, and 0 of 1 with *Candida* pneumonia.
Overall, across all sites of infection included in the study, the efficacy of CANCIDAS was comparable to that of amphotericin B for the primary endpoint.
In this study, the efficacy data for CANCIDAS in neutropenic patients with candidemia were limited. In a separate compassionate use study, 4 patients with hepatosplenic candidiasis received prolonged therapy with CANCIDAS following other long-term antifungal therapy; three of these patients had a favorable response.
In a second randomized, double-blind study, 197 patients with proven invasive candidiasis received CANCIDAS 50 mg/day (following a 70-mg loading dose on Day 1) or

CANCIDAS 150 mg/day. The diagnostic criteria, evaluation time points, and efficacy endpoints were similar to those employed in the prior study. Patients with *Candida* endocarditis, meningitis, or osteomyelitis were excluded. Although this study was designed to compare the safety of the two doses, it was not large enough to detect differences in rare or unexpected adverse events *[see Adverse Reactions (6.1)]*. A significant improvement in efficacy with the 150-mg daily dose was not seen when compared to the 50-mg dose.

14.3 Esophageal Candidiasis (and information on oropharyngeal candidiasis)

The safety and efficacy of CANCIDAS in the treatment of esophageal candidiasis was evaluated in one large, controlled, noninferiority, clinical trial and two smaller dose-response studies.

In all 3 studies, patients were required to have symptoms and microbiological documentation of esophageal candidiasis; most patients had advanced AIDS (with CD4 counts <50/mm^3).

Of the 166 patients in the large study who had culture-confirmed esophageal candidiasis at baseline, 120 had *Candida albicans* and 2 had *Candida tropicalis* as the sole baseline pathogen whereas 44 had mixed baseline cultures containing *C. albicans* and one or more additional *Candida* species.

In the large, randomized, double-blind study comparing CANCIDAS 50 mg/day versus intravenous fluconazole 200 mg/day for the treatment of esophageal candidiasis, patients were treated for an average of 9 days (range 7-21 days). Favorable overall response at 5 to 7 days following discontinuation of study therapy required both complete resolution of symptoms and significant endoscopic improvement. The definition of endoscopic response was based on severity of disease at baseline using a 4-grade scale and required at least a two-grade reduction from baseline endoscopic score or reduction to grade 0 for patients with a baseline score of 2 or less.

The proportion of patients with a favorable overall response was comparable for CANCIDAS and fluconazole as shown in Table 14.

[See table 14 below]

The proportion of patients with a favorable symptom response was also comparable (90.1% and 89.4% for CANCIDAS and fluconazole, respectively). In addition, the proportion of patients with a favorable endoscopic response was comparable (85.2% and 86.2% for CANCIDAS and fluconazole, respectively).

As shown in Table 15, the esophageal candidiasis relapse rates at the Day 14 post-treatment visit were similar for the two groups. At the Day 28 post-treatment visit, the group treated with CANCIDAS had a numerically higher incidence of relapse; however, the difference was not statistically significant.

[See table 15 at top of next page]

In this trial, which was designed to establish noninferiority of CANCIDAS to fluconazole for the treatment of esophageal candidiasis, 122 (70%) patients also had oropharyngeal candidiasis. A favorable response was defined as complete resolution of all symptoms of oropharyngeal disease and all visible oropharyngeal lesions. The proportion of patients with a favorable oropharyngeal response at the 5- to 7-day post-treatment visit was numerically lower for CANCIDAS; however, the difference was not statistically significant. Oropharyngeal candidiasis relapse rates at Day 14 and Day 28 post-treatment visits were statistically significantly higher for CANCIDAS than for fluconazole. The results are shown in Table 16.

[See table 16 at top of next page]

The results from the two smaller dose-ranging studies corroborate the efficacy of CANCIDAS for esophageal candidiasis that was demonstrated in the larger study.

CANCIDAS was associated with favorable outcomes in 7 of 10 esophageal *C. albicans* infections refractory to at least 200 mg of fluconazole given for 7 days, although the *in vitro* susceptibility of the infecting isolates to fluconazole was not known.

14.4 Invasive Aspergillosis

Sixty-nine patients between the ages of 18 and 80 with invasive aspergillosis were enrolled in an open-label, noncomparative study to evaluate the safety, tolerability, and efficacy of CANCIDAS. Enrolled patients had previously been refractory to or intolerant of other antifungal therapy(ies). Refractory patients were classified as those who had disease progression or failed to improve despite therapy for at least 7 days with amphotericin B, lipid formulations of amphotericin B, itraconazole, or an investigational azole with reported activity against *Aspergillus*. Intolerance to previous therapy was defined as a doubling of creatinine (or creatinine ≥2.5 mg/dL while on therapy), other acute reactions, or infusion-related toxicity. To be included in the study, patients with pulmonary disease must have had definite (positive tissue histopathology or positive culture from tissue obtained by an invasive procedure) or probable (positive radiographic or computed tomography evidence with supporting culture from bronchoalveolar lavage or sputum, galactomannan enzyme-linked immunosorbent assay, and/or polymerase chain reaction) invasive aspergillosis. Patients with extrapulmonary disease had to have definite invasive aspergillosis. The definitions were modeled after the Mycoses Study Group Criteria *[see References (15)]*. Patients were administered a single 70-mg loading dose of CANCIDAS and subsequently dosed with 50 mg daily. The mean duration of therapy was 33.7 days, with a range of 1 to 162 days.

An independent expert panel evaluated patient data, including diagnosis of invasive aspergillosis, response and tolerability to previous antifungal therapy, treatment course on CANCIDAS, and clinical outcome.

A favorable response was defined as either complete resolution (complete response) or clinically meaningful improvement (partial response) of all signs and symptoms and attributable radiographic findings. Stable, nonprogressive disease was considered to be an unfavorable response.

Among the 69 patients enrolled in the study, 63 met entry diagnostic criteria and had outcome data; and of these, 52 patients received treatment for >7 days. Fifty-three (84%) were refractory to previous antifungal therapy and 10 (16%) were intolerant. Forty-five patients had pulmonary disease and 18 had extrapulmonary disease. Underlying conditions were hematologic malignancy (N=24), allogeneic bone marrow transplant or stem cell transplant (N=18), organ transplant (N=8), solid tumor (N=3), or other conditions (N=10).

Table 12: Disposition in Candidemia and Other Candida Infections (Intra-abdominal abscesses, peritonitis, and pleural space infections)

	CANCIDAS*	Amphotericin B
Randomized patients	114	125
Patients completing study†	63 (55.3%)	69 (55.2%)
DISCONTINUATIONS OF STUDY†		
All Study Discontinuations	51 (44.7%)	56 (44.8%)
Study Discontinuations due to clinical adverse events	39 (34.2%)	43 (34.4%)
Study Discontinuations due to laboratory adverse events	0 (0%)	1 (0.8%)
DISCONTINUATIONS OF STUDY THERAPY		
All Study Therapy Discontinuations	48 (42.1%)	58 (46.4%)
Study Therapy Discontinuations due to clinical adverse events	30 (26.3%)	37 (29.6%)
Study Therapy Discontinuations due to laboratory adverse events	1 (0.9%)	7 (5.6%)
Study Therapy Discontinuations due to all drug-related‡ adverse events	3 (2.6%)	29 (23.2%)

* Patients received CANCIDAS 70 mg on Day 1, then 50 mg once daily for the remainder of their treatment.
† Study defined as study treatment period and 6-8 week follow-up period.
‡ Determined by the investigator to be possibly, probably, or definitely drug-related.

Table 13: Outcomes, Relapse, & Mortality in Candidemia and Other Candida Infections (Intra-abdominal abscesses, peritonitis, and pleural space infections)

	CANCIDAS*	Amphotericin B	% Difference† after adjusting for strata (Confidence Interval)‡
Number of MITT§ patients	109	115	
FAVORABLE OUTCOMES (MITT) AT THE END OF IV STUDY THERAPY			
All MITT patients	81/109 (74.3%)	78/115 (67.8%)	7.5 (-5.4, 20.3)
Candidemia	67/92 (72.8%)	63/94 (67.0%)	7.0 (-7.0, 21.1)
Neutropenic	6/14 (43%)	5/10 (50%)	
Non-neutropenic	61/78 (78%)	58/84 (69%)	
Endophthalmitis	0/1	2/3	
Multiple Sites	4/5	4/4	
Blood / Pleural	1/1	1/1	
Blood / Peritoneal	1/1	1/1	
Blood / Urine	-	1/1	
Peritoneal / Pleural	1/2	-	
Abdominal / Peritoneal	-	1/1	
Subphrenic / Peritoneal	1/1	-	
DISSEMINATED INFECTIONS, RELAPSES AND MORTALITY			
Disseminated Infections in neutropenic patients	4/14 (28.6%)	3/10 (30.0%)	
All relapses¶	7/81 (8.6%)	8/78 (10.3%)	
Culture-confirmed relapse	5/81 (6%)	2/78 (3%)	
Overall study# mortality in MITT	36/109 (33.0%)	35/115 (30.4%)	
Mortality during study therapy	18/109 (17%)	13/115 (11%)	
Mortality attributed to *Candida*	4/109 (4%)	7/115 (6%)	

* Patients received CANCIDAS 70 mg on Day 1, then 50 mg once daily for the remainder of their treatment.
† Calculated as CANCIDAS – amphotericin B
‡ 95% CI for candidemia, 95.6% for all patients
§ Modified intention-to-treat
¶ Includes all patients who either developed a culture-confirmed recurrence of *Candida* infection or required antifungal therapy for the treatment of a proven or suspected *Candida* infection in the follow-up period.
\# Study defined as study treatment period and 6-8 week follow-up period.

Table 14: Favorable Response Rates for Patients with Esophageal Candidiasis*

	CANCIDAS	Fluconazole	% Difference† (95% CI)
Day 5-7 post-treatment	66/81 (81.5%)	80/94 (85.1%)	-3.6 (-14.7, 7.5)

* Analysis excluded patients without documented esophageal candidiasis or patients not receiving at least 1 day of study therapy.
† Calculated as CANCIDAS – fluconazole

Table 15: Relapse Rates at 14 and 28 Days Post-Therapy in Patients with Esophageal Candidiasis at Baseline

	CANCIDAS	Fluconazole	% Difference* (95% CI)
Day 14 post-treatment	7/66 (10.6%)	6/76 (7.9%)	2.7 (-6.9, 12.3)
Day 28 post-treatment	18/64 (28.1%)	12/72 (16.7%)	11.5 (-2.5, 25.4)

* Calculated as CANCIDAS – fluconazole

Table 16: Oropharyngeal Candidiasis Response Rates at 5 to 7 Days Post-Therapy and Relapse Rates at 14 and 28 Days Post-Therapy in Patients with Oropharyngeal and Esophageal Candidiasis at Baseline

	CANCIDAS	Fluconazole	% Difference* (95% CI)
Response Rate Day 5-7 post-treatment	40/56 (71.4%)	55/66 (83.3%)	-11.9 (-26.8, 3.0)
Relapse Rate Day 14 post-treatment	17/40 (42.5%)	7/53 (13.2%)	29.3 (11.5, 47.1)
Relpase Rate Day 28 post-treatment	23/39 (59.0%)	18/51 (35.3%)	23.7 (3.4, 43.9)

* Calculated as CANCIDAS – fluconazole

All patients in the study received concomitant therapies for their other underlying conditions. Eighteen patients received tacrolimus and CANCIDAS concomitantly, of whom 8 also received mycophenolate mofetil.

Overall, the expert panel determined that 41% (26/63) of patients receiving at least one dose of CANCIDAS had a favorable response. For those patients who received >7 days of therapy with CANCIDAS, 50% (26/52) had a favorable response. The favorable response rates for patients who were either refractory to or intolerant of previous therapies were 36% (19/53) and 70% (7/10), respectively. The response rates among patients with pulmonary disease and extrapulmonary disease were 47% (21/45) and 28% (5/18), respectively. Among patients with extrapulmonary disease, 2 of 8 patients who also had definite, probable, or possible CNS involvement had a favorable response. Two of these 8 patients had progression of disease and manifested CNS involvement while on therapy.

CANCIDAS is effective for the treatment of invasive aspergillosis in patients who are refractory to or intolerant of itraconazole, amphotericin B, and/or lipid formulations of amphotericin B. However, the efficacy of CANCIDAS for initial treatment of invasive aspergillosis has not been evaluated in comparator-controlled clinical studies.

14.5 Pediatric Patients

The safety and efficacy of CANCIDAS were evaluated in pediatric patients 3 months to 17 years of age in two prospective, multicenter clinical trials.

The first study, which enrolled 82 patients between 2 to 17 years of age, was a randomized, double-blind study comparing CANCIDAS (50 mg/m^2 IV once daily following a 70-mg/m^2 loading dose on Day 1 [not to exceed 70 mg daily]) to AmBisome (3 mg/kg IV daily) in a 2:1 treatment fashion (56 on caspofungin, 26 on AmBisome) as empirical therapy in pediatric patients with persistent fever and neutropenia. The study design and criteria for efficacy assessment were similar to the study in adult patients *[see Clinical Studies (14.1)]*. Patients were stratified based on risk category (high-risk patients had undergone allogeneic stem cell transplantation or had relapsed acute leukemia). Twenty-seven percent of patients in both treatment groups were high risk. Favorable overall response rates of pediatric patients with persistent fever and neutropenia are presented in Table 17.

Table 17: Favorable Overall Response Rates of Pediatric Patients with Persistent Fever and Neutropenia

	CANCIDAS	AmBisome*
Number of Patients	56	25
Overall Favorable Response	26/56 (46.4%)	8/25 (32.0%)
High risk	9/15 (60.0%)	0/7 (0.0%)
Low risk	17/41 (41.5%)	8/18 (44.4%)

* One patient excluded from analysis due to no fever at study entry.

The second study was a prospective, open-label, non-comparative study estimating the safety and efficacy of caspofungin in pediatric patients (ages 3 months to 17 years) with candidemia and other *Candida* infections, esophageal candidiasis, and invasive aspergillosis (as salvage therapy). The study employed diagnostic criteria which were based on established EORTC/MSG criteria of proven or probable infection; these criteria were similar to those criteria employed in the adult studies for these various indications. Similarly, the efficacy time points and endpoints used in this study were similar to those employed in the corresponding adult studies *[see Clinical Studies (14.2, 14.3, and 14.4)]*. All patients received CANCIDAS at 50 mg/m^2 IV once daily following a 70-mg/m^2 loading dose on Day 1 (not to exceed 70 mg daily). Among the 49 enrolled patients who received CANCIDAS, 48 were included in the efficacy analysis (one patient excluded due to not having a baseline *Aspergillus* or *Candida* infection). Of these 48 patients, 37 had candidemia or other *Candida* infections, 10 had invasive aspergillosis, and 1 patient had esophageal candidiasis. Most candidemia and other *Candida* infections were caused by *C. albicans* (35%), followed by *C. parapsilosis* (22%), *C. tropicalis* (14%), and *C. glabrata* (11%). The favorable response rate, by indication, at the end of caspofungin therapy was as follows: 30/37 (81%) in candidemia or other *Candida* infections, 5/10 (50%) in invasive aspergillosis, and 1/1 in esophageal candidiasis.

15 REFERENCES

1. Mosteller RD: Simplified Calculation of Body Surface Area. N Engl J Med 1987 Oct 22;317(17): 1098 (letter).
2. Reference Method for Broth Dilution Antifungal Susceptibility Testing of Filamentous Fungi; Approved Standard M38-A2 Clinical and Laboratory Standards Institute, Wayne, PA, USA.
3. Reference Method for Broth Dilution Antifungal Susceptibility Testing of Yeasts; Approved Standard M27-A3 Clinical and Laboratory Standards Institute, Wayne, PA, USA.
4. Denning DW, Lee JY, Hostetler JS, et al. NIAID Mycoses Study Group multicenter trial of oral itraconazole therapy for invasive aspergillosis. Am J Med 1994; 97:135-144.

16 HOW SUPPLIED/STORAGE AND HANDLING

How Supplied

CANCIDAS 50 mg is a white to off-white powder/cake for infusion in a vial with a red aluminum band and a plastic cap.

NDC 0006-3822-10 supplied as one single-use vial.

CANCIDAS 70 mg is a white to off-white powder/cake for infusion in a vial with a yellow/orange aluminum band and a plastic cap.

NDC 0006-3823-10 supplied as one single-use vial.

Storage and Handling

Vials

The lyophilized vials should be stored refrigerated at 2° to 8°C (36° to 46°F).

Reconstituted Concentrate

Reconstituted CANCIDAS in the vial may be stored at ≤25°C (≤77°F) for one hour prior to the preparation of the patient infusion solution.

Diluted Product

The final patient infusion solution in the IV bag or bottle can be stored at ≤25°C (≤77°F) for 24 hours or at 2 to 8°C (36 to 46°F) for 48 hours.

17 PATIENT COUNSELING INFORMATION

17.1 Hypersensitivity

Inform patients that anaphylactic reactions have been reported during administration of CANCIDAS. CANCIDAS can cause hypersensitivity reactions, including rash, facial swelling, angioedema, pruritus, sensation of warmth, or bronchospasm. Inform patients to report these signs or symptoms to their healthcare providers.

17.2 Hepatic Effects

Inform patients that there have been isolated reports of serious hepatic effects from CANCIDAS therapy. Physicians will assess the risk/benefit of continuing CANCIDAS therapy if abnormal liver function tests occur during treatment.

Distributed by: Merck Sharp & Dohme Corp., a subsidiary of
MERCK & CO., INC., Whitehouse Station, NJ 08889, USA

Revised: 01/2013
USPI-I-09910113R002

Shown in Product Identification Guide, page 307

CELESTONE® SOLUSPAN®¹ ℞

brand of betamethasone sodium phosphate and betamethasone acetate
Injectable Suspension USP
6 mg per mL

DESCRIPTION

CELESTONE® SOLUSPAN®[1] Injectable Suspension is a sterile aqueous suspension containing 3 mg per milliliter betamethasone, as betamethasone sodium phosphate, and 3 mg per milliliter betamethasone acetate. Inactive ingredients per mL: 7.1 mg dibasic sodium phosphate; 3.4 mg monobasic sodium phosphate; 0.1 mg edetate disodium; and 0.2 mg benzalkonium chloride as preservative. The pH is adjusted to between 6.8 and 7.2.

The formula for betamethasone sodium phosphate is $C_{22}H_{28}FNa_2O_8P$ and it has a molecular weight of 516.40. Chemically, it is 9-Fluoro-11β,17,21-trihydroxy-16β-methylpregna-1,4-diene-3,20-dione 21-(disodium phosphate).

The formula for betamethasone acetate is $C_{24}H_{31}FO_6$ and it has a molecular weight of 434.50. Chemically, it is 9-Fluoro-11β,17,21-trihydroxy-16β-methylpregna-1,4-diene-3,20-dione 21-acetate.

The chemical structures for betamethasone sodium phosphate and betamethasone acetate are as follows:

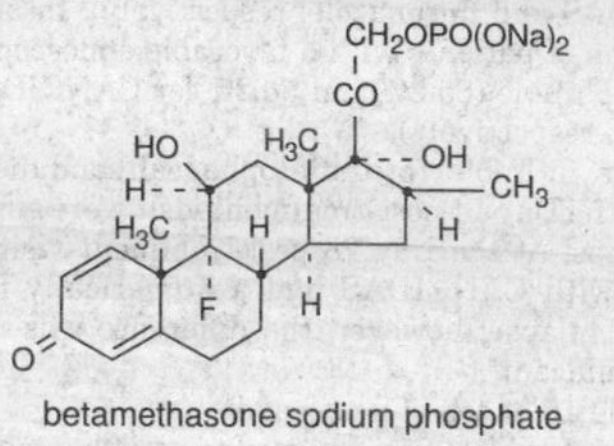

betamethasone sodium phosphate

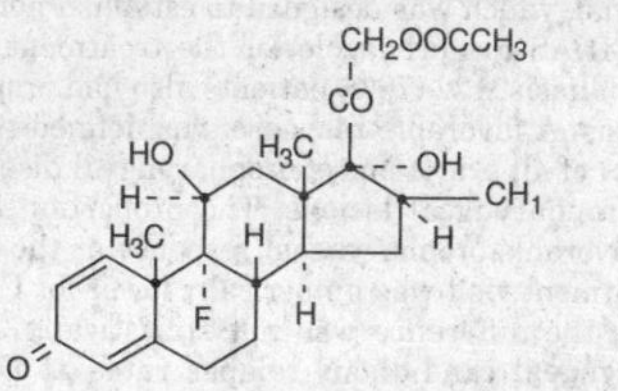

betamethasone acetate

Betamethasone sodium phosphate is a white to practically white, odorless powder, and is hygroscopic. It is freely soluble in water and in methanol, but is practically insoluble in acetone and in chloroform.

Betamethasone acetate is a white to creamy white, odorless powder that sinters and resolidifies at about 165°C, and remelts at about 200°C-220°C with decomposition. It is practically insoluble in water, but freely soluble in acetone, and is soluble in alcohol and in chloroform.

[1]brand of rapid and repository injectable

CLINICAL PHARMACOLOGY

Glucocorticoids, naturally occurring and synthetic, are adrenocortical steroids that are readily absorbed from the gastrointestinal tract.

Naturally occurring glucocorticoids (hydrocortisone and cortisone), which also have salt-retaining properties, are used as replacement therapy in adrenocortical deficiency states. Their synthetic analogs are primarily used for their anti-inflammatory effects in disorders of many organ systems. A derivative of prednisolone, betamethasone has a 16ß-methyl group that enhances the anti-inflammatory action of the molecule and reduces the sodium- and water-retaining properties of the fluorine atom bound at carbon 9.

Betamethasone sodium phosphate, a soluble ester, provides prompt activity, while betamethasone acetate is only slightly soluble and affords sustained activity.

INDICATIONS AND USAGE

When oral therapy is not feasible, the **intramuscular use** of CELESTONE® SOLUSPAN®[1] Injectable Suspension is indicated as follows:

Allergic States

Control of severe or incapacitating allergic conditions intractable to adequate trials of conventional treatment in asthma, atopic dermatitis, contact dermatitis, drug hypersensitivity reactions, perennial or seasonal allergic rhinitis, serum sickness, transfusion reactions.

Dermatologic Diseases

Bullous dermatitis herpetiformis, exfoliative erythroderma, mycosis fungoides, pemphigus, severe erythema multiforme (Stevens-Johnson syndrome).

Endocrine Disorders

Congenital adrenal hyperplasia, hypercalcemia associated with cancer, nonsuppurative thyroiditis.

Hydrocortisone or cortisone is the drug of choice in primary or secondary adrenocortical insufficiency. Synthetic analogs may be used in conjunction with mineralocorticoids where applicable; in infancy mineralocorticoid supplementation is of particular importance.

Gastrointestinal Diseases

To tide the patient over a critical period of the disease in regional enteritis and ulcerative colitis.

Hematologic Disorders

Acquired (autoimmune) hemolytic anemia, Diamond-Blackfan anemia, pure red cell aplasia, selected cases of secondary thrombocytopenia.

Miscellaneous

Trichinosis with neurologic or myocardial involvement, tuberculous meningitis with subarachnoid block or impending block when used with appropriate antituberculous chemotherapy.

Neoplastic Diseases

For palliative management of leukemias and lymphomas.

Nervous System

Acute exacerbations of multiple sclerosis; cerebral edema associated with primary or metastatic brain tumor or craniotomy.

Ophthalmic Diseases

Sympathetic ophthalmia, temporal arteritis, uveitis and ocular inflammatory conditions unresponsive to topical corticosteroids.

Renal Diseases

To induce diuresis or remission of proteinuria in idiopathic nephrotic syndrome or that due to lupus erythematosus.

Respiratory Diseases

Berylliosis, fulminating or disseminated pulmonary tuberculosis when used concurrently with appropriate antituberculous chemotherapy, idiopathic eosinophilic pneumonias, symptomatic sarcoidosis.

Rheumatic Disorders As adjunctive therapy for short-term administration (to tide the patient over an acute episode or exacerbation) in acute gouty arthritis; acute rheumatic carditis; ankylosing spondylitis; psoriatic arthritis; rheumatoid arthritis, including juvenile rheumatoid arthritis (selected cases may require low-dose maintenance therapy). For the treatment of dermatomyositis, polymyositis, and systemic lupus erythematosus.

The **intra-articular or soft tissue administration** of CELESTONE SOLUSPAN Injectable Suspension is indicated as adjunctive therapy for short-term administration (to tide the patient over an acute episode or exacerbation) in acute gouty arthritis, acute and subacute bursitis, acute nonspecific tenosynovitis, epicondylitis, rheumatoid arthritis, synovitis of osteoarthritis.

The **intralesional administration** of CELESTONE SOLUSPAN Injectable Suspension is indicated for alopecia areata; discoid lupus erythematosus; keloids; localized hypertrophic, infiltrated, inflammatory lesions of granuloma annulare, lichen planus, lichen simplex chronicus (neurodermatitis), and psoriatic plaques; necrobiosis lipoidica diabeticorum.

CELESTONE SOLUSPAN Injectable Suspension may also be useful in cystic tumors of an aponeurosis or tendon (ganglia).

CONTRAINDICATIONS

CELESTONE® SOLUSPAN®[1] Injectable Suspension is contraindicated in patients who are hypersensitive to any components of this product.

Intramuscular corticosteroid preparations are contraindicated for idiopathic thrombocytopenic purpura.

WARNINGS

General

CELESTONE® SOLUSPAN®[1] Injectable Suspension should not be administered intravenously.

Rare instances of anaphylactoid reactions have occurred in patients receiving corticosteroid therapy (see **ADVERSE REACTIONS**).

In patients on corticosteroid therapy subjected to any unusual stress, hydrocortisone or cortisone is the drug of choice as a supplement during and after the event.

Cardio-renal

Average and large doses of corticosteroids can cause elevation of blood pressure, salt and water retention, and increased excretion of potassium. These effects are less likely to occur with the synthetic derivatives except when used in large doses. Dietary salt restriction and potassium supplementation may be necessary. All corticosteroids increase calcium excretion.

Literature reports suggest an apparent association between use of corticosteroids and left ventricular free wall rupture after a recent myocardial infarction; therefore, therapy with corticosteroids should be used with great caution in these patients.

Endocrine

Corticosteroids can produce reversible hypothalamic pituitary adrenal (HPA) axis suppression with the potential for glucocorticosteroid insufficiency after withdrawal of treatment.

Metabolic clearance of corticosteroids is decreased in hypothyroid patients and increased in hyperthyroid patients. Changes in thyroid status of the patient may necessitate adjustment in dosage.

Infections

General

Patients who are on corticosteroids are more susceptible to infections than are healthy individuals. There may be decreased resistance and inability to localize infection when corticosteroids are used. Infection with any pathogen (viral, bacterial, fungal, protozoan, or helminthic) in any location of the body may be associated with the use of corticosteroids alone or in combination with other immunosuppressive agents. These infections may be mild to severe. With increasing doses of corticosteroids, the rate of occurrence of infectious complications increases. Corticosteroids may also mask some signs of current infection.

Fungal Infections

Corticosteroids may exacerbate systemic fungal infections and therefore should not be used in the presence of such infections unless they are needed to control drug reactions. There have been cases reported in which concomitant use of amphotericin B and hydrocortisone was followed by cardiac enlargement and congestive heart failure (see **PRECAUTIONS, Drug Interactions, Amphotericin B Injection and Potassium-Depleting Agents** section).

Special Pathogens

Latent disease may be activated or there may be an exacerbation of intercurrent infections due to pathogens, including those caused by *Amoeba, Candida, Cryptococcus, Mycobacterium, Nocardia, Pneumocystis,* and *Toxoplasma*.

It is recommended that latent amebiasis or active amebiasis be ruled out before initiating corticosteroid therapy in any patient who has spent time in the tropics or in any patient with unexplained diarrhea.

Similarly, corticosteroids should be used with great care in patients with known or suspected Strongyloides (threadworm) infestation. In such patients, corticosteroid-induced immunosuppression may lead to Strongyloides hyperinfection and dissemination with widespread larval migration, often accompanied by severe enterocolitis and potentially fatal gram-negative septicemia.

Corticosteroids should not be used in cerebral malaria.

Tuberculosis

The use of corticosteroids in active tuberculosis should be restricted to those cases of fulminating or disseminated tuberculosis in which the corticosteroid is used for the management of the disease in conjunction with an appropriate antituberculous regimen.

If corticosteroids are indicated in patients with latent tuberculosis or tuberculin reactivity, close observation is necessary as reactivation of the disease may occur. During prolonged corticosteroid therapy, these patients should receive chemoprophylaxis.

Vaccination

Administration of live or live, attenuated vaccines is contraindicated in patients receiving immunosuppressive doses of corticosteroids. Killed or inactivated vaccines may be administered. However, the response to such vaccines cannot be predicted. Immunization procedures may be undertaken in patients who are receiving corticosteroids as replacement therapy, eg, for Addison's disease.

Viral Infections

Chickenpox and measles can have a more serious or even fatal course in pediatric and adult patients on corticosteroids. In pediatric and adult patients who have not had these diseases, particular care should be taken to avoid exposure. The contribution of the underlying disease and/or prior corticosteroid treatment to the risk is also not known. If exposed to chickenpox, prophylaxis with varicella zoster immune globulin (VZIG) may be indicated. If exposed to measles, prophylaxis with immunoglobulin (IG) may be indicated. (See the respective package inserts for complete VZIG and IG prescribing information.) If chickenpox develops, treatment with antiviral agents should be considered.

Neurologic

Reports of severe medical events have been associated with the intrathecal route of administration (see **ADVERSE REACTIONS, Gastrointestinal** and **Neurologic/Psychiatric** sections).

Results from one multicenter, randomized, placebo-controlled study with methylprednisolone hemisuccinate, an IV corticosteroid, showed an increase in early mortality (at 2 weeks) and late mortality (at 6 months) in patients with cranial trauma who were determined not to have other clear indications for corticosteroid treatment. High doses of corticosteroids, including CELESTONE SOLUSPAN, should not be used for the treatment of traumatic brain injury.

Ophthalmic

Use of corticosteroids may produce posterior subcapsular cataracts, glaucoma with possible damage to the optic nerves, and may enhance the establishment of secondary ocular infections due to bacteria, fungi, or viruses. The use of oral corticosteroids is not recommended in the treatment of optic neuritis and may lead to an increase in the risk of new episodes. Corticosteroids should not be used in active ocular herpes simplex.

PRECAUTIONS

General

This product, like many other steroid formulations, is sensitive to heat. Therefore, it should not be autoclaved when it is desirable to sterilize the exterior of the vial.

The lowest possible dose of corticosteroid should be used to control the condition under treatment. When reduction in dosage is possible, the reduction should be gradual.

Since complications of treatment with glucocorticoids are dependent on the size of the dose and the duration of treatment, a risk/benefit decision must be made in each individual case as to dose and duration of treatment and as to whether daily or intermittent therapy should be used.

Kaposi's sarcoma has been reported to occur in patients receiving corticosteroid therapy, most often for chronic conditions. Discontinuation of corticosteroids may result in clinical improvement.

Cardio-renal

As sodium retention with resultant edema and potassium loss may occur in patients receiving corticosteroids, these agents should be used with caution in patients with congestive heart failure, hypertension, or renal insufficiency.

Endocrine

Drug-induced secondary adrenocortical insufficiency may be minimized by gradual reduction of dosage. This type of relative insufficiency may persist for months after discontinuation of therapy. Therefore, in any situation of stress occurring during that period, naturally occurring glucocorticoids (hydrocortisone cortisone), which also have salt-retaining properties, rather than betamethasone, are the appropriate choices as replacement therapy in adrenocortical deficiency states.

Gastrointestinal

Steroids should be used with caution in active or latent peptic ulcers, diverticulitis, fresh intestinal anastomoses, and nonspecific ulcerative colitis, since they may increase the risk of a perforation.

Signs of peritoneal irritation following gastrointestinal perforation in patients receiving corticosteroids may be minimal or absent.

There is an enhanced effect of corticosteroids in patients with cirrhosis.

Intra-Articular and Soft Tissue Administration

Intra-articular injected corticosteroids may be systemically absorbed.

Appropriate examination of any joint fluid present is necessary to exclude a septic process.

A marked increase in pain accompanied by local swelling, further restriction of joint motion, fever, and malaise are suggestive of septic arthritis. If this complication occurs and the diagnosis of sepsis is confirmed, appropriate antimicrobial therapy should be instituted.

Injection of a steroid into an infected site is to be avoided.

Local injection of a steroid into a previously injected joint is not usually recommended.

Corticosteroid injection into unstable joints is generally not recommended.

Intra-articular injection may result in damage to joint tissues (see **ADVERSE REACTIONS, Musculoskeletal** section).

Musculoskeletal

Corticosteroids decrease bone formation and increase bone resorption both through their effect on calcium regulation (ie, decreasing absorption and increasing excretion) and inhibition of osteoblast function. This, together with a decrease in the protein matrix of the bone secondary to an increase in protein catabolism, and reduced sex hormone production, may lead to inhibition of bone growth in pediatric patients and the development of osteoporosis at any age. Special consideration should be given to patients at increased risk of osteoporosis (ie, postmenopausal women) before initiating corticosteroid therapy.

Neuro-psychiatric

Although controlled clinical trials have shown corticosteroids to be effective in speeding the resolution of acute exacerbations of multiple sclerosis, they do not show that they affect the ultimate outcome or natural history of the disease. The studies do show that relatively high doses of corticosteroids are necessary to demonstrate a significant effect (see **DOSAGE AND ADMINISTRATION**).

An acute myopathy has been observed with the use of high doses of corticosteroids, most often occurring in patients with disorders of neuromuscular transmission (eg, myasthenia gravis), or in patients receiving concomitant therapy with neuromuscular blocking drugs (eg, pancuronium). This acute myopathy is generalized, may involve ocular and respiratory muscles, and may result in quadriparesis. Elevation of creatinine kinase may occur. Clinical improvement or recovery after stopping corticosteroids may require weeks to years.

Psychic derangements may appear when corticosteroids are used, ranging from euphoria, insomnia, mood swings, personality changes, and severe depression to frank psychotic manifestations. Also, existing emotional instability or psychotic tendencies may be aggravated by corticosteroids.

Ophthalmic

Intraocular pressure may become elevated in some individuals. If steroid therapy is continued for more than 6 weeks, intraocular pressure should be monitored.

Information for Patients

Patients should be warned not to discontinue the use of corticosteroids abruptly or without medical supervision, to advise any medical attendants that they are taking corticosteroids and to seek medical advice at once should they develop fever or other signs of infection.

Persons who are on corticosteroids should be warned to avoid exposure to chickenpox or measles. Patients should also be advised that if they are exposed, medical advice should be sought without delay.

Drug Interactions

Aminoglutethimide

Aminoglutethimide may lead to a loss of corticosteroid-induced adrenal suppression.

Amphotericin B Injection and Potassium-Depleting Agents

When corticosteroids are administered concomitantly with potassium-depleting agents (ie, amphotericin B, diuretics), patients should be observed closely for development of hypokalemia. There have been cases reported in which concomitant use of amphotericin B and hydrocortisone was followed by cardiac enlargement and congestive heart failure.

Antibiotics

Macrolide antibiotics have been reported to cause a significant decrease in corticosteroid clearance.

Anticholinesterases

Concomitant use of anticholinesterase agents and corticosteroids may produce severe weakness in patients with myasthenia gravis. If possible, anticholinesterase agents should be withdrawn at least 24 hours before initiating corticosteroid therapy.

Anticoagulants, Oral

Coadministration of corticosteroids and warfarin usually results in inhibition of response to warfarin, although there have been some conflicting reports. Therefore, coagulation indices should be monitored frequently to maintain the desired anticoagulant effect.

Antidiabetics

Because corticosteroids may increase blood glucose concentrations, dosage adjustments of antidiabetic agents may be required.

Antitubercular Drugs

Serum concentrations of isoniazid may be decreased.

Cholestyramine

Cholestyramine may increase the clearance of corticosteroids.

Cyclosporine

Increased activity of both cyclosporine and corticosteroids may occur when the two are used concurrently. Convulsions have been reported with this concurrent use.

Digitalis Glycosides

Patients on digitalis glycosides may be at increased risk of arrhythmias due to hypokalemia.

Estrogens, Including Oral Contraceptives

Estrogens may decrease the hepatic metabolism of certain corticosteroids, thereby increasing their effect.

Hepatic Enzyme Inducers (eg, barbiturates, phenytoin, carbamazepine, rifampin)

Drugs which induce hepatic microsomal drug-metabolizing enzyme activity may enhance the metabolism of corticosteroids and require that the dosage of the corticosteroid be increased.

Ketoconazole

Ketoconazole has been reported to decrease the metabolism of certain corticosteroids by up to 60%, leading to an increased risk of corticosteroid side effects.

Nonsteroidal Anti-inflammatory Agents (NSAIDS)

Concomitant use of aspirin (or other nonsteroidal anti-inflammatory agents) and corticosteroids increases the risk of gastrointestinal side effects. Aspirin should be used cautiously in conjunction with corticosteroids in hypoprothrombinemia. The clearance of salicylates may be increased with concurrent use of corticosteroids.

Skin Tests

Corticosteroids may suppress reactions to skin tests.

Vaccines

Patients on prolonged corticosteroid therapy may exhibit a diminished response to toxoids and live or inactivated vaccines due to inhibition of antibody response. Corticosteroids may also potentiate the replication of some organisms contained in live attenuated vaccines. Route administration of vaccines or toxoids should be deferred until corticosteroid therapy is discontinued if possible (see **WARNINGS, Infections, Vaccination** section).

Carcinogenesis, Mutagenesis, Impairment of Fertility

No adequate studies have been conducted in animals to determine whether corticosteroids have a potential for carcinogenesis or mutagenesis.

Steroids may increase or decrease motility and number of spermatozoa in some patients.

Pregnancy

Teratogenic Effects

Pregnancy Category C

Corticosteroids have been shown to be teratogenic in many species when given in doses equivalent to the human dose. Animal studies in which corticosteroids have been given to pregnant mice, rats, and rabbits have yielded an increased incidence of cleft palate in the offspring. There are no adequate and well-controlled studies in pregnant women. Corticosteroids should be used during pregnancy only if the potential benefit justifies the potential risk to the fetus. Infants born to mothers who have received corticosteroids during pregnancy should be carefully observed for signs of hypoadrenalism.

Nursing Mothers

Systemically administered corticosteroids appear in human milk and could suppress growth, interfere with endogenous corticosteroid production, or cause other untoward effects. Caution should be exercised when corticosteroids are administered to a nursing woman.

Pediatric Use

The efficacy and safety of corticosteroids in the pediatric population are based on the well-established course of effect of corticosteroids, which is similar in pediatric and adult populations. Published studies provide evidence of efficacy and safety in pediatric patients for the treatment of nephrotic syndrome (>2 years of age), and aggressive lymphomas and leukemias (>1 month of age). Other indications for pediatric use of corticosteroids, eg, severe asthma and wheezing, are based on adequate and well-controlled trials conducted in adults, on the premises that the course of the diseases and their pathophysiology are considered to be substantially similar in both populations.

The adverse effects of corticosteroids in pediatric patients are similar to those in adults (see **ADVERSE REACTIONS**). Like adults, pediatric patients should be carefully observed with frequent measurements of blood pressure, weight, height, intraocular pressure, and clinical evaluation for the presence of infection, psychosocial disturbances, thromboembolism, peptic ulcers, cataracts, and osteoporosis. Pediatric patients who are treated with corticosteroids by any route, including systemically administered corticosteroids, may experience a decrease in their growth velocity. This negative impact of corticosteroids on growth has been observed at low systemic doses and in the absence of laboratory evidence of HPA axis suppression (ie, cosyntropin stimulation and basal cortisol plasma levels). Growth velocity may therefore be a more sensitive indicator of systemic corticosteroid exposure in pediatric patients than some commonly used tests of HPA axis function. The linear growth of pediatric patients treated with corticosteroids should be monitored, and the potential growth effects of prolonged treatment should be weighed against clinical benefits obtained and the availability of treatment alternatives. In order to minimize the potential growth effects of corticosteroids, pediatric patients should be titrated to the lowest effective dose.

Geriatric Use

No overall differences in safety or effectiveness were observed between elderly subjects and younger subjects, and other reported clinical experience has not identified differences in responses between the elderly and young patients, but greater sensitivity of some older individuals cannot be ruled out.

ADVERSE REACTIONS (listed alphabetically, under each subsection)

Allergic Reactions

Anaphylactoid reaction, anaphylaxis, angioedema.

Cardiovascular

Bradycardia, cardiac arrest, cardiac arrhythmias, cardiac enlargement, circulatory collapse, congestive heart failure, fat embolism, hypertension, hypertrophic cardiomyopathy in premature infants, myocardial rupture following recent myocardial infarction (see **WARNINGS**), pulmonary edema, syncope, tachycardia, thromboembolism, thrombophlebitis, vasculitis.

Dermatologic

Acne, allergic dermatitis, cutaneous and subcutaneous atrophy, dry scaly skin, ecchymoses and petechiae, edema, erythema, hyperpigmentation, hypopigmentation, impaired wound healing, increased sweating, rash, sterile abscess, striae, suppressed reactions to skin tests, thin fragile skin, thinning scalp hair, urticaria.

Endocrine

Decreased carbohydrate and glucose tolerance, development of cushingoid state, glucosuria, hirsutism, hypertrichosis, increased requirements for insulin or oral hypoglycemic agents, adrenocortical and pituitary unresponsiveness (particularly in times of stress, as in trauma, surgery, or illness), suppression of growth in pediatric patients.

Fluid and Electrolyte Disturbances

Congestive heart failure in susceptible patients, fluid retention, hypokalemic alkalosis, potassium loss, sodium retention.

Gastrointestinal

Abdominal distention, bowel/bladder dysfunction (after intrathecal administration), elevation in serum liver enzyme levels (usually reversible upon discontinuation), hepatomegaly, increased appetite, nausea, pancreatitis, peptic ulcer with possible perforation and hemorrhage, perforation of the small and large intestine (particularly in patients with inflammatory bowel disease), ulcerative esophagitis.

Metabolic

Negative nitrogen balance due to protein catabolism.

Musculoskeletal

Aseptic necrosis of femoral and humeral heads, calcinosis (following intra-articular or intralesional use), Charcot-like arthropathy, loss of muscle mass, muscle weakness, osteoporosis, pathologic fracture of long bones, postinjection flare (following intra-articular use), steroid myopathy, tendon rupture, vertebral compression fractures.

Neurologic/Psychiatric

Convulsions, depression, emotional instability, euphoria, headache, increased intracranial pressure with papilledema (pseudotumor cerebri) usually following discontinuation of treatment, insomnia, mood swings, neuritis, neuropathy, paresthesia, personality changes, psychic disorders, vertigo. Arachnoiditis, meningitis, paraparesis/paraplegia, and sensory disturbances have occurred after intrathecal administration (see **WARNINGS, Neurologic** section).

Ophthalmic

Exophthalmos, glaucoma, increased intraocular pressure, posterior subcapsular cataracts, rare instances of blindness associated with periocular injections.

Other

Abnormal fat deposits, decreased resistance to infection, hiccups, increased or decreased motility and number of spermatozoa, malaise, moon face, weight gain.

OVERDOSAGE

Treatment of acute overdose is by supportive and symptomatic therapy. For chronic overdosage in the face of severe disease requiring continuous steroid therapy, the dosage of the corticosteroid may be reduced only temporarily, or alternate day treatment may be introduced.

DOSAGE AND ADMINISTRATION

Benzyl alcohol as a preservative has been associated with a fatal "Gasping Syndrome" in premature infants and infants of low birth weight. Solutions used for further dilution of this product should be preservative-free when used in the neonate, especially the premature infant. The initial dosage of parenterally administered CELESTONE® SOLUSPAN®[1] Injectable Suspension may vary from 0.25 to 9.0 mg per day depending on the specific disease entity being treated. However, in certain overwhelming, acute, life-threatening situations, administrations in dosages exceeding the usual dosages may be justified and may be in multiples of the oral dosages.

It Should Be Emphasized That Dosage Requirements Are Variable and Must Be Individualized on the Basis of the Disease Under Treatment and the Response of the Patient. After a favorable response is noted, the proper maintenance dosage should be determined by decreasing the initial drug dosage in small decrements at appropriate time intervals until the lowest dosage which will maintain an adequate clinical response is reached. Situations which may make dosage adjustments necessary are changes in clinical status secondary to remissions or exacerbations in the disease process, the patient's individual drug responsiveness, and the effect of patient exposure to stressful situations not directly related to the disease entity under treatment. In this latter

situation it may be necessary to increase the dosage of the corticosteroid for a period of time consistent with the patient's condition. If after long-term therapy the drug is to be stopped, it is recommended that it be withdrawn gradually rather than abruptly.
In the treatment of acute exacerbations of multiple sclerosis, daily doses of 30 mg of betamethasone for a week followed by 12 mg every other day for 1 month are recommended (see **PRECAUTIONS, Neuro-psychiatric** section).
In pediatric patients, the initial dose of betamethasone may vary depending on the specific disease entity being treated. The range of initial doses is 0.02 to 0.3 mg/kg/day in three or four divided doses (0.6 to 9 mg/m²bsa/day).
For the purpose of comparison, the following is the equivalent milligram dosage of the various glucocorticoids:

Cortisone, 25	Triamcinolone, 4
Hydrocortisone, 20	Paramethasone, 2
Prednisolone, 5	Betamethasone, 0.75
Prednisone, 5	Dexamethasone, 0.75
Methylprednisolone, 4	

These dose relationships apply only to oral or intravenous administration of these compounds. When these substances or their derivatives are injected intramuscularly or into joint spaces, their relative properties may be greatly altered.
If coadministration of a local anesthetic is desired, CELESTONE SOLUSPAN Injectable Suspension may be mixed with 1% or 2% lidocaine hydrochloride, using the formulations which do not contain parabens. Similar local anesthetics may also be used. Diluents containing methylparaben, propylparaben, phenol, etc., should be avoided, since these compounds may cause flocculation of the steroid. The required dose of CELESTONE SOLUSPAN Injectable Suspension is first withdrawn from the vial into the syringe. The local anesthetic is then drawn in, and the syringe shaken briefly. **Do not inject local anesthetics into the vial of CELESTONE SOLUSPAN Injectable Suspension.**

Bursitis, Tenosynovitis, Peritendinitis
In acute subdeltoid, subacromial, olecranon, and prepatellar bursitis, one intrabursal injection of 1.0 mL CELESTONE SOLUSPAN Injectable Suspension can relieve pain and restore full range of movement. Several intrabursal injections of corticosteroids are usually required in recurrent acute bursitis and in acute exacerbations of chronic bursitis. Partial relief of pain and some increase in mobility can be expected in both conditions after one or two injections. Chronic bursitis may be treated with reduced dosage once the acute condition is controlled. In tenosynovitis and tendinitis, three or four local injections at intervals of 1 to 2 weeks between injections are given in most cases. Injections should be made into the affected tendon sheaths rather than into the tendons themselves. In ganglions of joint capsules and tendon sheaths, injection of 0.5 mL directly into the ganglion cysts has produced marked reduction in the size of the lesions.

Rheumatoid Arthritis and Osteoarthritis
Following intra-articular administration of 0.5 to 2.0 mL of CELESTONE SOLUSPAN Injectable Suspension, relief of pain, soreness, and stiffness may be experienced. Duration of relief varies widely in both diseases. Intra-articular Injection of CELESTONE SOLUSPAN Injectable Suspension is well tolerated in joints and periarticular tissues. There is virtually no pain on injection, and the "secondary flare" that sometimes occurs a few hours after intra-articular injection of corticosteroids has not been reported with CELESTONE SOLUSPAN Injectable Suspension. Using sterile technique, a 20- to 24-gauge needle on an empty syringe is inserted into the synovial cavity and a few drops of synovial fluid are withdrawn to confirm that the needle is in the joint. The aspirating syringe is replaced by a syringe containing CELESTONE SOLUSPAN Injectable Suspension and injection is then made into the joint.

Recommended Doses for Intra-articular Injection

Size of joint	Location	Dose (mL)
Very large	Hip	1.0-2.0
Large	Knee, ankle, shoulder	1.0
Medium	Elbow, wrist	0.5-1.0
Small (metacarpophalangeal, interphalangeal) (sternoclavicular)	Hand, chest	0.25-0.5

A portion of the administered dose of CELESTONE SOLUSPAN Injectable Suspension is absorbed systemically following intra-articular injection. In patients being treated concomitantly with oral or parenteral corticosteroids, especially those receiving large doses, the systemic absorption of the drug should be considered in determining intra-articular dosage.

Dermatologic Conditions
In intralesional treatment, 0.2 mL/cm² of CELESTONE SOLUSPAN Injectable Suspension is injected intradermally (not subcutaneously) using a tuberculin syringe with a 25-gauge, ½-inch needle. Care should be taken to deposit a uniform depot of medication intradermally. A total of no more than 1.0 mL at weekly intervals is recommended.

Disorders of the Foot
A tuberculin syringe with a 25-gauge, ¾-inch needle is suitable for most injections into the foot. The following doses are recommended at intervals of 3 days to a week.

Diagnosis	CELESTONE SOLUSPAN Injectable Suspension Dose (mL)
Bursitis under heloma durum or heloma molle	0.25-0.5
under calcaneal spur	0.5
over hallux rigidus or digiti quinti varus	0.5
Tenosynovitis, periostitis of cuboid	0.5
Acute gouty arthritis	0.5-1.0

HOW SUPPLIED
CELESTONE® SOLUSPAN®1 Injectable Suspension, 5-mL multiple-dose vial; box of one (NDC 0085-0566-05).
SHAKE WELL BEFORE USING.
Store at 25°C (77°F); excursions permitted to 15°-30°C (59°-86°F) [see USP Controlled Room Temperature].
Protect from light.
Rx only
Manufactured for: Merck Sharp & Dohme Corp., a subsidiary of
MERCK & CO., INC., Whitehouse Station, NJ 08889, USA
Manufactured by: Patheon UK Limited, Covingham, Swindon, Wiltshire, SN3 5BZ, United Kingdom

Revised: 05/2012
31550327T

CLARINEX® ℞
[klā-rĭ-nĕcks]
(desloratadine)
Tablets and Oral Solution
for oral use

HIGHLIGHTS OF PRESCRIBING INFORMATION
These highlights do not include all the information needed to use CLARINEX safely and effectively. See full prescribing information for CLARINEX.
CLARINEX® (desloratadine) Tablets and Oral Solution for oral use
Initial U.S. Approval: 2001

INDICATIONS AND USAGE

CLARINEX is indicated for:
- **Seasonal Allergic Rhinitis:** relief of nasal and non-nasal symptoms in patients 2 years of age and older. (1.1)
- **Perennial Allergic Rhinitis:** relief of nasal and non-nasal symptoms in patients 6 months of age and older. (1.2)
- **Chronic Idiopathic Urticaria:** symptomatic relief of pruritus, reduction in the number of hives, and size of hives in patients 6 months of age and older. (1.3)

DOSAGE AND ADMINISTRATION

Dosage (by age):
Adults and Adolescents 12 Years of Age and Over:
- CLARINEX Tablets - one 5 mg tablet once daily **or**
- CLARINEX Oral Solution - 2 teaspoonfuls (5 mg in 10 mL) once daily (2)

Children 6 to 11 Years of Age:
- CLARINEX Oral Solution - 1 teaspoonful (2.5 mg in 5 mL) once daily (2)

Children 12 Months to 5 Years of Age:
- CLARINEX Oral Solution - 1/2 teaspoonful (1.25 mg in 2.5 mL) once daily (2)

Children 6 to 11 Months of Age:
- CLARINEX Oral Solution - 2 mL (1 mg) once daily (2)

DOSAGE FORMS AND STRENGTHS

- CLARINEX Tablets - 5 mg (3)
- CLARINEX Oral Solution - 0.5 mg/1 mL (3)

CONTRAINDICATIONS

- Hypersensitivity (4, 6.2)

WARNINGS AND PRECAUTIONS

- Hypersensitivity reactions including rash, pruritus, urticaria, edema, dyspnea, and anaphylaxis have been reported. In such cases, stop CLARINEX at once and consider alternative treatments. (5.1)

ADVERSE REACTIONS

- The most common adverse reactions (reported in ≥2% of adult and adolescent patients with allergic rhinitis and greater than placebo) were pharyngitis, dry mouth, myalgia, fatigue, somnolence, dysmenorrhea. (6.1)

To report SUSPECTED ADVERSE REACTIONS, contact Merck Sharp & Dohme Corp., a subsidiary of Merck & Co., Inc., at 1-877-888-4231 or FDA at 1-800-FDA-1088 or www.fda.gov/medwatch.

USE IN SPECIFIC POPULATIONS

- Renal impairment: dosage adjustment is recommended (2.5, 8.6, 12.3)
- Hepatic impairment: dosage adjustment is recommended (2.5, 8.7, 12.3)

See 17 for PATIENT COUNSELING INFORMATION and FDA-approved patient labeling
Revised: 06/2013

FULL PRESCRIBING INFORMATION: CONTENTS*

*** Sections or subsections omitted from the full prescribing information are not listed**

FULL PRESCRIBING INFORMATION

1 INDICATIONS AND USAGE

1.1 Seasonal Allergic Rhinitis

CLARINEX® is indicated for the relief of the nasal and nonnasal symptoms of seasonal allergic rhinitis in patients 2 years of age and older.

1.2 Perennial Allergic Rhinitis

CLARINEX is indicated for the relief of the nasal and nonnasal symptoms of perennial allergic rhinitis in patients 6 months of age and older.

1.3 Chronic Idiopathic Urticaria

CLARINEX is indicated for the symptomatic relief of pruritus, reduction in the number of hives, and size of hives, in patients with chronic idiopathic urticaria 6 months of age and older.

2 DOSAGE AND ADMINISTRATION

CLARINEX Tablets or Oral Solution may be taken without regard to meals.

The age-appropriate dose of CLARINEX Oral Solution should be administered with a commercially available measuring dropper or syringe that is calibrated to deliver 2 mL and 2.5 mL (½ teaspoon).

2.1 Adults and Adolescents 12 Years of Age and Over

The recommended dose of CLARINEX Tablets is one 5-mg tablet once daily. The recommended dose of CLARINEX Oral Solution is 2 teaspoonfuls (5 mg in 10 mL) once daily.

2.2 Children 6 to 11 Years of Age

The recommended dose of CLARINEX Oral Solution is 1 teaspoonful (2.5 mg in 5 mL) once daily.

2.3 Children 12 Months to 5 Years of Age

The recommended dose of CLARINEX Oral Solution is ½ teaspoonful (1.25 mg in 2.5 mL) once daily.

2.4 Children 6 to 11 Months of Age

The recommended dose of CLARINEX Oral Solution is 2 mL (1 mg) once daily.

2.5 Adults with Hepatic or Renal Impairment

In adult patients with liver or renal impairment, a starting dose of one 5-mg tablet every other day is recommended based on pharmacokinetic data. Dosing recommendation for children with liver or renal impairment cannot be made due to lack of data *[see Clinical Pharmacology (12.3)]*.

3 DOSAGE FORMS AND STRENGTHS

CLARINEX Tablets are light blue, film-coated tablets embossed with "C5" containing 5 mg desloratadine.

CLARINEX Oral Solution is a clear orange-colored liquid containing 0.5 mg desloratadine/1 mL.

4 CONTRAINDICATIONS

CLARINEX Tablets and Oral Solution are contraindicated in patients who are hypersensitive to this medication or to any of its ingredients or to loratadine *[see Warnings and Precautions (5.1) and Adverse Reactions (6.2)]*.

5 WARNINGS AND PRECAUTIONS

5.1 Hypersensitivity Reactions

Hypersensitivity reactions including rash, pruritus, urticaria, edema, dyspnea, and anaphylaxis have been reported after administration of desloratadine. If such a reaction occurs, therapy with CLARINEX should be stopped and alternative treatment should be considered. *[See Adverse Reactions (6.2).]*

6 ADVERSE REACTIONS

The following adverse reactions are discussed in greater detail in other sections of the label:

- Hypersensitivity reactions. *[See Warnings and Precautions (5.1).]*

6.1 Clinical Trials Experience

Because clinical trials are conducted under widely varying conditions, adverse reaction rates observed in the clinical trials of a drug cannot be directly compared to rates in the clinical trials of another drug and may not reflect the rates observed in clinical practice.

Adults and Adolescents

Allergic Rhinitis: In multiple-dose placebo-controlled trials, 2834 patients ages 12 years or older received CLARINEX Tablets at doses of 2.5 mg to 20 mg daily, of whom 1655 patients received the recommended daily dose of 5 mg. In patients receiving 5 mg daily, the rate of adverse events was similar between CLARINEX and placebo-treated patients. The percent of patients who withdrew prematurely due to adverse events was 2.4% in the CLARINEX group and 2.6% in the placebo group. There were no serious adverse events in these trials in patients receiving desloratadine. All adverse events that were reported by greater than or equal to 2% of patients who received the recommended daily dose of CLARINEX Tablets (5 mg once daily), and that were more common with CLARINEX Tablets than placebo, are listed in Table 1.

Table 1: Incidence of Adverse Events Reported by ≥2% of Adult and Adolescent Allergic Rhinitis Patients Receiving CLARINEX Tablets

Adverse Event	CLARINEX Tablets 5 mg (n=1655)	Placebo (n=1652)
Infections and Infestations		
Pharyngitis	4.1%	2.0%
Nervous System Disorders		
Somnolence	2.1%	1.8%
Gastrointestinal Disorders		
Dry Mouth	3.0%	1.9%
Musculoskeletal and Connective Tissue Disorders		
Myalgia	2.1%	1.8%
Reproductive System and Breast Disorders		
Dysmenorrhea	2.1%	1.6%
General Disorders and Administration Site Conditions		
Fatigue	2.1%	1.2%

The frequency and magnitude of laboratory and electrocardiographic abnormalities were similar in CLARINEX and placebo-treated patients.

There were no differences in adverse events for subgroups of patients as defined by gender, age, or race.

Chronic Idiopathic Urticaria: In multiple-dose, placebo-controlled trials of chronic idiopathic urticaria, 211 patients ages 12 years or older received CLARINEX Tablets and 205 received placebo. Adverse events that were reported by greater than or equal to 2% of patients who received CLARINEX Tablets and that were more common with CLARINEX than placebo were (rates for CLARINEX and placebo, respectively): headache (14%, 13%), nausea (5%, 2%), fatigue (5%, 1%), dizziness (4%, 3%), pharyngitis (3%, 2%), dyspepsia (3%, 1%), and myalgia (3%, 1%).

Pediatrics

Two hundred and forty-six pediatric subjects 6 months to 11 years of age received CLARINEX Oral Solution for 15 days in three placebo-controlled clinical trials. Pediatric subjects aged 6 to 11 years received 2.5 mg once a day, subjects aged 1 to 5 years received 1.25 mg once a day, and subjects 6 to 11 months of age received 1.0 mg once a day.

In subjects 6 to 11 years of age, no individual adverse event was reported by 2 percent or more of the subjects.

In subjects 2 to 5 years of age, adverse events reported for CLARINEX and placebo in at least 2 percent of subjects receiving CLARINEX Oral Solution and at a frequency greater than placebo were fever (5.5%, 5.4%), urinary tract infection (3.6%, 0%) and varicella (3.6%, 0%).

In subjects 12 months to 23 months of age, adverse events reported for the CLARINEX product and placebo in at least 2 percent of subjects receiving CLARINEX Oral Solution and at a frequency greater than placebo were fever (16.9%, 12.9%), diarrhea (15.4%, 11.3%), upper respiratory tract infections (10.8%, 9.7%), coughing (10.8%, 6.5%), appetite increased (3.1%, 1.6%), emotional lability (3.1%, 0%), epistaxis (3.1%, 0%), parasitic infection (3.1%, 0%), pharyngitis (3.1%, 0%), rash maculopapular (3.1%, 0%).

In subjects 6 months to 11 months of age, adverse events reported for CLARINEX and placebo in at least 2 percent of subjects receiving CLARINEX Oral Solution and at a frequency greater than placebo were upper respiratory tract infections (21.2%, 12.9%), diarrhea (19.7%, 8.1%), fever (12.1%, 1.6%), irritability (12.1%, 11.3%), coughing (10.6%, 9.7%), somnolence (9.1%, 8.1%), bronchitis (6.1%, 0%), otitis media (6.1%, 1.6%), vomiting (6.1%, 3.2%), anorexia (4.5%, 1.6%), pharyngitis (4.5%, 1.6%), insomnia (4.5%, 0%), rhinorrhea (4.5%, 3.2%), erythema (3.0%, 1.6%), and nausea (3.0%, 0%).

There were no clinically meaningful changes in any electrocardiographic parameter, including the QTc interval. Only one of the 246 pediatric subjects receiving CLARINEX Oral Solution in the clinical trials discontinued treatment because of an adverse event.

6.2 Post-Marketing Experience

Because adverse events are reported voluntarily from a population of uncertain size, it is not always possible to reliably estimate their frequency or establish a causal relationship to drug exposure. The following spontaneous adverse events have been reported during the marketing of desloratadine: tachycardia, palpitations, rare cases of hypersensitivity reactions (such as rash, pruritus, urticaria, edema, dyspnea, and anaphylaxis), psychomotor hyperactivity, seizures, and elevated liver enzymes including bilirubin, and very rarely, hepatitis.

7 DRUG INTERACTIONS

7.1 Inhibitors of Cytochrome P450 3A4

In controlled clinical studies co-administration of desloratadine with ketoconazole, erythromycin, or azithromycin resulted in increased plasma concentrations of desloratadine and 3 hydroxydesloratadine, but there were no clinically relevant changes in the safety profile of desloratadine. *[See Clinical Pharmacology (12.3).]*

7.2 Fluoxetine

In controlled clinical studies co-administration of desloratadine with fluoxetine, a selective serotonin reuptake inhibitor (SSRI), resulted in increased plasma concentrations of desloratadine and 3 hydroxydesloratadine, but there were no clinically relevant changes in the safety profile of desloratadine. *[See Clinical Pharmacology (12.3).]*

7.3 Cimetidine

In controlled clinical studies co-administration of desloratadine with cimetidine, a histamine H2-receptor antagonist, resulted in increased plasma concentrations of desloratadine and 3 hydroxydesloratadine, but there were no clinically relevant changes in the safety profile of desloratadine. *[See Clinical Pharmacology (12.3).]*

8 USE IN SPECIFIC POPULATIONS

8.1 Pregnancy

Pregnancy Category C: There are no adequate and well-controlled studies in pregnant women. Because animal reproduction studies are not always predictive of human response, desloratadine should be used during pregnancy only if clearly needed.

Desloratadine was not teratogenic in rats or rabbits at approximately 210 and 230 times, respectively, the area under the concentration-time curve (AUC) in humans at the recommended daily oral dose. An increase in pre-implantation loss and a decreased number of implantations and fetuses were noted, however, in a separate study in female rats at approximately 120 times the AUC in humans at the recommended daily oral dose. Reduced body weight and slow righting reflex were reported in pups at approximately 50 times or greater than the AUC in humans at the recommended daily oral dose. Desloratadine had no effect on pup development at approximately 7 times the AUC in humans at the recommended daily oral dose. The AUCs in comparison referred to the desloratadine exposure in rabbits and the sum of desloratadine and its metabolites exposures in rats, respectively. *[See Nonclinical Toxicology (13.2).]*

8.3 Nursing Mothers

Desloratadine passes into breast milk; therefore, a decision should be made whether to discontinue nursing or to discontinue desloratadine, taking into account the benefit of the drug to the nursing mother and the possible risk to the child.

8.4 Pediatric Use

The recommended dose of CLARINEX Oral Solution in the pediatric population is based on cross-study comparison of the plasma concentration of CLARINEX in adults and pediatric subjects. The safety of CLARINEX Oral Solution has been established in 246 pediatric subjects aged 6 months to 11 years in three placebo-controlled clinical studies. Since the course of seasonal and perennial allergic rhinitis and chronic idiopathic urticaria and the effects of CLARINEX are sufficiently similar in the pediatric and adult populations, it allows extrapolation from the adult efficacy data to pediatric patients. The effectiveness of CLARINEX Oral Solution in these age groups is supported by evidence from adequate and well-controlled studies of CLARINEX Tablets in adults. The safety and effectiveness of CLARINEX Tablets or CLARINEX Oral Solution have not been demonstrated in pediatric patients less than 6 months of age. *[See Clinical Pharmacology (12.3).]*

8.5 Geriatric Use

Clinical studies of desloratadine did not include sufficient numbers of subjects aged 65 and over to determine whether they respond differently from younger subjects. Other reported clinical experience has not identified differences between the elderly and younger patients. In general, dose selection for an elderly patient should be cautious, reflecting the greater frequency of decreased hepatic, renal, or cardiac function, and of concomitant disease or other drug therapy. *[See Clinical Pharmacology (12.3).]*

8.6 Renal Impairment

Dosage adjustment for patients with renal impairment is recommended *[see Dosage and Administration (2.5) and Clinical Pharmacology (12.3)]*.

8.7 Hepatic Impairment

Dosage adjustment for patients with hepatic impairment is recommended *[see Dosage and Administration (2.5) and Clinical Pharmacology (12.3)]*.

9 DRUG ABUSE AND DEPENDENCE

There is no information to indicate that abuse or dependency occurs with CLARINEX Tablets.

10 OVERDOSAGE

In the event of overdose, consider standard measures to remove any unabsorbed drug. Symptomatic and supportive treatment is recommended. Desloratadine and 3-hydroxydesloratadine are not eliminated by hemodialysis. Information regarding acute overdosage is limited to experience from post-marketing adverse event reports and from clinical trials conducted during the development of the CLARINEX product. In a dose-ranging trial, at doses of 10 mg and 20 mg/day somnolence was reported.

In another study, no clinically relevant adverse events were reported in normal male and female volunteers who were given single daily doses of CLARINEX 45 mg for 10 days *[see Clinical Pharmacology (12.2)]*.

Lethality occurred in rats at oral doses of 250 mg/kg or greater (estimated desloratadine and desloratadine metabolite exposures were approximately 120 times the AUC in humans at the recommended daily oral dose). The oral median lethal dose in mice was 353 mg/kg (estimated desloratadine exposures were approximately 290 times the human daily oral dose on a mg/m^2 basis). No deaths occurred at oral doses up to 250 mg/kg in monkeys (estimated desloratadine exposures were approximately 810 times the human daily oral dose on a mg/m^2 basis).

11 DESCRIPTION

CLARINEX (desloratadine) Tablets are light blue, round, film-coated tablets containing 5 mg desloratadine, an antihistamine, to be administered orally. CLARINEX Tablets also contain the following excipients: dibasic calcium phosphate dihydrate USP, microcrystalline cellulose NF, corn starch NF, talc USP, carnauba wax NF, white wax NF, coating material consisting of lactose monohydrate, hypromellose, titanium dioxide, polyethylene glycol, and FD&C Blue #2 Aluminum Lake.

CLARINEX Oral Solution is a clear orange-colored liquid containing 0.5 mg/1 mL desloratadine. The Oral Solution contains the following inactive ingredients: propylene glycol USP, sorbitol solution USP, citric acid (anhydrous) USP, sodium citrate dihydrate USP, sodium benzoate NF, disodium edetate USP, purified water USP. It also contains granulated sugar, natural and artificial flavor for bubble gum, and FDC Yellow #6 dye.

Desloratadine is a white to off-white powder that is slightly soluble in water, but very soluble in ethanol and propylene glycol. It has an empirical formula: $C_{19}H_{19}ClN_2$ and a molecular weight of 310.8. The chemical name is 8-chloro-6,11-dihydro-11-(4-piperdinylidene)-5*H*-benzo[5,6]cyclohepta-[1,2-*b*]pyridine and has the following structure:

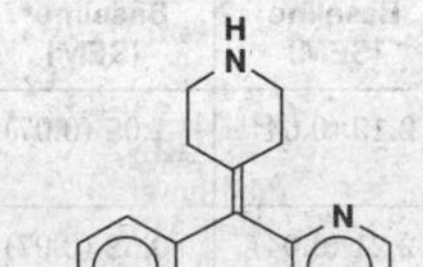

12 CLINICAL PHARMACOLOGY

12.1 Mechanism of Action

Desloratadine is a long-acting tricyclic histamine antagonist with selective H_1-receptor histamine antagonist activity. Receptor binding data indicates that at a concentration of 2–3 ng/mL (7 nanomolar), desloratadine shows significant interaction with the human histamine H_1-receptor. Desloratadine inhibited histamine release from human mast cells *in vitro*. Results of a radiolabeled tissue distribution study in rats and a radioligand H_1-receptor binding study in guinea pigs showed that desloratadine did not readily cross the blood brain barrier. The clinical significance of this finding is unknown.

12.2 Pharmacodynamics

Wheal and Flare: Human histamine skin wheal studies following single and repeated 5-mg doses of desloratadine have shown that the drug exhibits an antihistaminic effect by 1 hour; this activity may persist for as long as 24 hours. There was no evidence of histamine-induced skin wheal tachyphylaxis within the desloratadine 5-mg group over the 28-day treatment period. The clinical relevance of histamine wheal skin testing is unknown.

Effects on QT_c: Single daily doses of 45 mg were given to normal male and female volunteers for 10 days. All ECGs obtained in this study were manually read in a blinded fashion by a cardiologist. In CLARINEX-treated subjects, there was an increase in mean heart rate of 9.2 bpm relative to placebo. The QT interval was corrected for heart rate (QT_c) by both the Bazett and Fridericia methods. Using the QT_c (Bazett) there was a mean increase of 8.1 msec in CLARINEX-treated subjects relative to placebo. Using QT_c (Fridericia) there was a mean increase of 0.4 msec in CLARINEX-treated subjects relative to placebo. No clinically relevant adverse events were reported.

12.3 Pharmacokinetics

Absorption

Following oral administration of a desloratadine 5-mg tablet once daily for 10 days to normal healthy volunteers, the mean time to maximum plasma concentrations (T_{max}) occurred at approximately 3 hours post dose and mean steady state peak plasma concentrations (C_{max}) and AUC of 4 ng/mL and 56.9 ng•hr/mL were observed, respectively. Neither food nor grapefruit juice had an effect on the bioavailability (C_{max} and AUC) of desloratadine.

The pharmacokinetic profile of CLARINEX Oral Solution was evaluated in a three-way crossover study in 30 adult volunteers. A single dose of 10 mL of CLARINEX Oral Solution containing 5 mg of desloratadine was bioequivalent to a single dose of 5-mg CLARINEX Tablet. Food had no effect on the bioavailability (AUC and C_{max}) of CLARINEX Oral Solution.

Distribution

Desloratadine and 3-hydroxydesloratadine are approximately 82% to 87% and 85% to 89% bound to plasma proteins, respectively. Protein binding of desloratadine and 3-hydroxydesloratadine was unaltered in subjects with impaired renal function.

Metabolism

Desloratadine (a major metabolite of loratadine) is extensively metabolized to 3-hydroxydesloratadine, an active metabolite, which is subsequently glucuronidated. The enzyme(s) responsible for the formation of 3-hydroxydesloratadine have not been identified. Data from clinical trials indicate that a subset of the general population has a decreased ability to form 3-hydroxydesloratadine, and are poor metabolizers of desloratadine. In pharmacokinetic studies (n=3748), approximately 6% of subjects were poor metabolizers of desloratadine (defined as a subject with an AUC ratio of 3-hydroxydesloratadine to desloratadine less than 0.1, or a subject with a desloratadine half-life exceeding 50 hours). These pharmacokinetic studies included subjects between the ages of 2 and 70 years, including 977 subjects aged 2 to 5 years, 1575 subjects aged 6 to 11 years, and 1196 subjects aged 12 to 70 years. There was no difference in the prevalence of poor metabolizers across age groups. The frequency of poor metabolizers was higher in Blacks (17%, n=988) as compared to Caucasians (2%, n=1,462) and Hispanics (2%, n=1,063). The median exposure (AUC) to desloratadine in the poor metabolizers was approximately 6-fold greater than in the subjects who are not poor metabolizers. Subjects who are poor metabolizers of desloratadine cannot be prospectively identified and will be exposed to higher levels of desloratadine following dosing with the recommended dose of desloratadine. In multidose clinical safety studies, where metabolizer status was identified, a total of 94 poor metabolizers and 123 normal metabolizers were enrolled and treated with CLARINEX Oral Solution for 15–35 days. In these studies, no overall differences in safety were observed between poor metabolizers and normal metabolizers. Although not seen in these studies, an increased risk of exposure-related adverse events in patients who are poor metabolizers cannot be ruled out.

Elimination

The mean plasma elimination half-life of desloratadine was approximately 27 hours. C_{max} and AUC values increased in a dose proportional manner following single oral doses between 5 and 20 mg. The degree of accumulation after 14 days of dosing was consistent with the half-life and dosing frequency. A human mass balance study documented a recovery of approximately 87% of the ^{14}C-desloratadine dose, which was equally distributed in urine and feces as metabolic products. Analysis of plasma 3-hydroxydesloratadine showed similar T_{max} and half-life values compared to desloratadine.

Special Populations

Geriatric Subjects: In older subjects (≥65 years old; n=17) following multiple-dose administration of CLARINEX Tablets, the mean C_{max} and AUC values for desloratadine were 20% greater than in younger subjects (<65 years old). The oral total body clearance (CL/F) when normalized for body weight was similar between the two age groups. The mean plasma elimination half-life of desloratadine was 33.7 hr in subjects ≥65 years old. The pharmacokinetics for 3-hydroxydesloratadine appeared unchanged in older versus younger subjects. These age-related differences are unlikely to be clinically relevant and no dosage adjustment is recommended in elderly subjects.

Pediatric Subjects: In subjects 6 to 11 years old, a single dose of 5 mL of CLARINEX Oral Solution containing 2.5 mg of desloratadine, resulted in desloratadine plasma concentrations similar to those achieved in adults administered a single 5-mg CLARINEX Tablet. In subjects 2 to 5 years old, a single dose of 2.5 mL of CLARINEX Oral Solution containing 1.25 mg of desloratadine, resulted in desloratadine plasma concentrations similar to those achieved in adults administered a single 5-mg CLARINEX Tablet. However, the C_{max} and AUC of the metabolite (3-hydroxydesloratadine) were 1.27 and 1.61 times higher for the 5-mg dose of Oral Solution administered in adults compared to the C_{max} and AUC obtained in children 2 to 11 years of age receiving 1.25–2.5 mg of CLARINEX Oral Solution.

A single dose of either 2.5 mL or 1.25 mL of CLARINEX Oral Solution containing 1.25 mg or 0.625 mg, respectively, of desloratadine was administered to subjects 6 to 11 months of age and 12 to 23 months of age. The results of a population pharmacokinetic analysis indicated that a dose of 1 mg for subjects aged 6 to 11 months and 1.25 mg for subjects 12 to 23 months of age is required to obtain desloratadine plasma concentrations similar to those achieved in adults administered a single 5-mg dose of CLARINEX Oral Solution.

Renally Impaired: Desloratadine pharmacokinetics following a single dose of 7.5 mg were characterized in patients with mild (n=7; creatinine clearance 51–69 mL/min/1.73 m^2), moderate (n=6; creatinine clearance 34–43 mL/min/1.73 m^2), and severe (n=6; creatinine clearance 5–29 mL/min/1.73 m^2) renal impairment or hemodialysis dependent (n=6) patients. In patients with mild and moderate renal impairment, median C_{max} and AUC values increased by approximately 1.2- and 1.9-fold, respectively, relative to subjects with normal renal function. In patients with severe renal impairment or who were hemodialysis dependent, C_{max} and AUC values increased by approximately 1.7- and 2.5-fold, respectively. Minimal changes in 3-hydroxydesloratadine concentrations were observed. Desloratadine and 3-hydroxydesloratadine were poorly removed by hemodialysis. Plasma protein binding of desloratadine and 3-hydroxydesloratadine was unaltered by renal impairment. Dosage adjustment for patients with renal impairment is recommended *[see Dosage and Administration (2.5)]*.

Hepatically Impaired: Desloratadine pharmacokinetics were characterized following a single oral dose in patients with mild (n=4), moderate (n=4), and severe (n=4) hepatic impairment as defined by the Child-Pugh classification of hepatic function and 8 subjects with normal hepatic function. Patients with hepatic impairment, regardless of severity, had approximately a 2.4-fold increase in AUC as compared with normal subjects. The apparent oral clearance of desloratadine in patients with mild, moderate, and severe hepatic impairment was 37%, 36%, and 28% of that in normal subjects, respectively. An increase in the mean elimination half-life of desloratadine in patients with hepatic impairment was observed. For 3-hydroxydesloratadine, the mean C_{max} and AUC values for patients with hepatic impairment were not statistically significantly different from subjects with normal hepatic function. Dosage adjustment for patients with hepatic impairment is recommended *[see Dosage and Administration (2.5)]*.

Gender: Female subjects treated for 14 days with CLARINEX Tablets had 10% and 3% higher desloratadine C_{max} and AUC values, respectively, compared with male subjects. The 3-hydroxydesloratadine C_{max} and AUC values were also increased by 45% and 48%, respectively, in females compared with males. However, these apparent differences are not likely to be clinically relevant and therefore no dosage adjustment is recommended.

Race: Following 14 days of treatment with CLARINEX Tablets, the C_{max} and AUC values for desloratadine were 18% and 32% higher, respectively, in Blacks compared with Caucasians. For 3-hydroxydesloratadine there was a corresponding 10% reduction in C_{max} and AUC values in Blacks compared to Caucasians. These differences are not likely to be clinically relevant and therefore no dose adjustment is recommended.

Drug Interactions: In two controlled crossover clinical pharmacology studies in healthy male (n=12 in each study) and female (n=12 in each study) volunteers, desloratadine 7.5 mg (1.5 times the daily dose) once daily was coadministered with erythromycin 500 mg every 8 hours or ketoconazole 200 mg every 12 hours for 10 days. In three separate controlled, parallel group clinical pharmacology studies, desloratadine at the clinical dose of 5 mg has been coadministered with azithromycin 500 mg followed by 250 mg once daily for 4 days (n=18) or with fluoxetine 20 mg once daily for 7 days after a 23-day pretreatment period with fluoxetine (n=18) or with cimetidine 600 mg every 12 hours for 14 days (n=18) under steady-state conditions to normal healthy male and female volunteers. Although increased plasma concentrations (C_{max} and $AUC_{0\text{-}24\ hrs}$) of desloratadine and 3-hydroxydesloratadine were observed (see Table 2), there were no clinically relevant changes in the safety profile of desloratadine, as assessed by electrocardiographic parameters (including the corrected QT interval), clinical laboratory tests, vital signs, and adverse events.

[See table 2 at top of next page]

Table 2: Changes in Desloratadine and 3-Hydroxydesloratadine Pharmacokinetics in Healthy Male and Female Volunteers

	Desloratadine		3-Hydroxydesloratadine	
	C_{max}	$AUC_{0\text{-}24\ hrs}$	C_{max}	$AUC_{0\text{-}24\ hrs}$
Erythromycin (500 mg Q8h)	+ 24%	+ 14%	+ 43%	+ 40%
Ketoconazole (200 mg Q12h)	+ 45%	+ 39%	+ 43%	+ 72%
Azithromycin (500 mg day 1, 250 mg QD × 4 days)	+ 15%	+ 5%	+ 15%	+ 4%
Fluoxetine (20 mg QD)	+ 15%	+ 0%	+ 17%	+ 13%
Cimetidine (600 mg Q12h)	+ 12%	+ 19%	- 11%	- 3%

13 NONCLINICAL TOXICOLOGY

13.1 Carcinogenesis, Mutagenesis, Impairment of Fertility

Carcinogenicity Studies

The carcinogenic potential of desloratadine was assessed using a loratadine study in rats and a desloratadine study in mice. In a 2-year study in rats, loratadine was administered in the diet at doses up to 25 mg/kg/day (estimated desloratadine and desloratadine metabolite exposures were approximately 30 times the AUC in humans at the recommended daily oral dose). A significantly higher incidence of hepatocellular tumors (combined adenomas and carcinomas) was observed in males given 10 mg/kg/day of loratadine and in males and females given 25 mg/kg/day of loratadine. The estimated desloratadine and desloratadine metabolite exposures in rats given 10 mg/kg of loratadine were approximately 7 times the AUC in humans at the recommended daily oral dose. The clinical significance of these findings during long-term use of desloratadine is not known.

In a 2-year dietary study in mice, males and females given up to 16 mg/kg/day and 32 mg/kg/day desloratadine, respectively, did not show significant increases in the incidence of any tumors. The estimated desloratadine and desloratadine metabolite exposures in mice at these doses were 12 and 27 times, respectively, the AUC in humans at the recommended daily oral dose.

Genotoxicity Studies

In genotoxicity studies with desloratadine, there was no evidence of genotoxic potential in a reverse mutation assay (*Salmonella/E. coli* mammalian microsome bacterial mutagenicity assay) or in 2 assays for chromosomal aberrations (human peripheral blood lymphocyte clastogenicity assay and mouse bone marrow micronucleus assay).

Impairment of Fertility

There was no effect on female fertility in rats at desloratadine doses up to 24 mg/kg/day (estimated desloratadine and desloratadine metabolite exposures were approximately 130 times the AUC in humans at the recommended daily oral dose). A male specific decrease in fertility, demonstrated by reduced female conception rates, decreased sperm numbers and motility, and histopathologic testicular changes, occurred at an oral desloratadine dose of 12 mg/kg in rats (estimated desloratadine and desloratadine metabolite exposures were approximately 45 times the AUC in humans at the recommended daily oral dose). Desloratadine had no effect on fertility in rats at an oral dose of 3 mg/kg/day (estimated desloratadine and desloratadine metabolite exposures were approximately 8 times the AUC in humans at the recommended daily oral dose).

13.2 Animal Toxicology and/or Pharmacology

Reproductive Toxicology Studies

Desloratadine was not teratogenic in rats at doses up to 48 mg/kg/day (estimated desloratadine and desloratadine metabolite exposures were approximately 210 times the AUC in humans at the recommended daily oral dose) or in rabbits at doses up to 60 mg/kg/day (estimated desloratadine exposures were approximately 230 times the AUC in humans at the recommended daily oral dose). In a separate study, an increase in pre-implantation loss and a decreased number of implantations and fetuses were noted in female rats at 24 mg/kg (estimated desloratadine and desloratadine metabolite exposures were approximately 120 times the AUC in humans at the recommended daily oral dose). Reduced body weight and slow righting reflex were reported in pups at doses of 9 mg/kg/day or greater (estimated desloratadine and desloratadine metabolite exposures were approximately 50 times or greater than the AUC in humans at the recommended daily oral dose). Desloratadine had no effect on pup development at an oral dose of 3 mg/kg/day (estimated desloratadine and desloratadine metabolite exposures were approximately 7 times the AUC in humans at the recommended daily oral dose).

14 CLINICAL STUDIES

14.1 Seasonal Allergic Rhinitis

The clinical efficacy and safety of CLARINEX Tablets were evaluated in over 2300 patients 12 to 75 years of age with seasonal allergic rhinitis. A total of 1838 patients received 2.5 to 20 mg/day of CLARINEX in 4 double-blind, randomized, placebo-controlled clinical trials of 2 to 4 weeks' duration conducted in the United States. The results of these studies demonstrated the efficacy and safety of CLARINEX 5 mg in the treatment of adult and adolescent patients with seasonal allergic rhinitis. In a dose-ranging trial, CLARINEX 2.5 to 20 mg/day was studied. Doses of 5, 7.5, 10, and 20 mg/day were superior to placebo; and no additional benefit was seen at doses above 5.0 mg. In the same study, an increase in the incidence of somnolence was observed at doses of 10 mg/day and 20 mg/day (5.2% and 7.6%, respectively), compared to placebo (2.3%).

In two 4-week studies of 924 patients (aged 15 to 75 years) with seasonal allergic rhinitis and concomitant asthma, CLARINEX Tablets 5 mg once daily improved rhinitis symptoms, with no decrease in pulmonary function. This supports the safety of administering CLARINEX Tablets to adult patients with seasonal allergic rhinitis with mild to moderate asthma.

CLARINEX Tablets 5 mg once daily significantly reduced the Total Symptom Score (the sum of individual scores of nasal and non-nasal symptoms) in patients with seasonal allergic rhinitis. See Table 3.

Table 3: TOTAL SYMPTOM SCORE (TSS) Changes in a 2-Week Clinical Trial in Patients with Seasonal Allergic Rhinitis

Treatment Group (n)	Mean Baseline* (SEM)	Change from Baseline† (SEM)	Placebo Comparison (*P*-value)
CLARINEX 5.0 mg (171)	14.2 (0.3)	-4.3 (0.3)	*P*<0.01
Placebo (173)	13.7 (0.3)	-2.5 (0.3)	

SEM=Standard Error of the Mean

* At baseline, a total nasal symptom score (sum of 4 individual symptoms) of at least 6 and a total non-nasal symptom score (sum of 4 individual symptoms) of at least 5 (each symptom scored 0 to 3 where 0=no symptom and 3=severe symptoms) was required for trial eligibility. TSS ranges from 0=no symptoms to 24=maximal symptoms.

† Mean reduction in TSS averaged over the 2-week treatment period.

There were no significant differences in the effectiveness of CLARINEX Tablets 5 mg across subgroups of patients defined by gender, age, or race.

14.2 Perennial Allergic Rhinitis

The clinical efficacy and safety of CLARINEX Tablets 5 mg were evaluated in over 1300 patients 12 to 80 years of age with perennial allergic rhinitis. A total of 685 patients received 5 mg/day of CLARINEX in two double-blind, randomized, placebo-controlled clinical trials of 4 weeks' duration conducted in the United States and internationally. In one of these studies CLARINEX Tablets 5 mg once daily was shown to significantly reduce the Total Symptom Score in patients with perennial allergic rhinitis (Table 4).

Table 4: TOTAL SYMPTOM SCORE (TSS) Changes in a 4-Week Clinical Trial in Patients with Perennial Allergic Rhinitis

Treatment Group (n)	Mean Baseline* (SEM)	Change from Baseline† (SEM)	Placebo Comparison (*P*-value)
CLARINEX 5.0 mg (337)	12.37 (0.18)	-4.06 (0.21)	*P*=0.01
Placebo (337)	12.30 (0.18)	-3.27 (0.21)	

SEM=Standard Error of the Mean

* At baseline, average of total symptom score (sum of 5 individual nasal symptoms and 3 non-nasal symptoms, each symptom scored 0 to 3 where 0=no symptom and 3=severe symptoms) of at least 10 was required for trial eligibility. TSS ranges from 0=no symptoms to 24=maximal symptoms.

† Mean reduction in TSS averaged over the 4-week treatment period.

14.3 Chronic Idiopathic Urticaria

The efficacy and safety of CLARINEX Tablets 5 mg once daily was studied in 416 chronic idiopathic urticaria patients 12 to 84 years of age, of whom 211 received CLARINEX. In two double-blind, placebo-controlled, randomized clinical trials of six weeks duration, at the prespecified one-week primary time point evaluation, CLARINEX Tablets significantly reduced the severity of pruritus when compared to placebo (Table 5). Secondary endpoints were also evaluated, and during the first week of therapy CLARINEX Tablets 5 mg reduced the secondary endpoints, "Number of Hives" and the "Size of the Largest Hive," when compared to placebo.

Table 5: PRURITUS SYMPTOM SCORE Changes in the First Week of a Clinical Trial in Patients with Chronic Idiopathic Urticaria

Treatment Group (n)	Mean Baseline (SEM)	Change from Baseline* (SEM)	Placebo Comparison (*P*-value)
CLARINEX 5.0 mg (115)	2.19 (0.04)	-1.05 (0.07)	*P*<0.01
Placebo (110)	2.21 (0.04)	-0.52 (0.07)	

Pruritus scored 0 to 3 where 0=no symptom to 3=maximal symptom

SEM=Standard Error of the Mean

* Mean reduction in pruritus averaged over the first week of treatment.

The clinical safety of CLARINEX Oral Solution was documented in three, 15-day, double-blind, placebo-controlled safety studies in pediatric subjects with a documented history of allergic rhinitis, chronic idiopathic urticaria, or subjects who were candidates for antihistamine therapy. In the first study, 2.5 mg of CLARINEX Oral Solution was administered to 60 pediatric subjects 6 to 11 years of age. The second study evaluated 1.25 mg of CLARINEX Oral Solution administered to 55 pediatric subjects 2 to 5 years of age. In the third study, 1.25 mg of CLARINEX Oral Solution was administered to 65 pediatric subjects 12 to 23 months of age and 1.0 mg of CLARINEX Oral Solution was administered to 66 pediatric subjects 6 to 11 months of age. The results of these studies demonstrated the safety of CLARINEX Oral Solution in pediatric subjects 6 months to 11 years of age.

16 HOW SUPPLIED/STORAGE AND HANDLING

CLARINEX Tablets: Embossed "C5", light blue, film-coated tablets that are packaged in high-density polyethylene plastic bottles of 100 (NDC 0085-1264-01) and 500 (NDC 0085-1264-02).

CLARINEX Oral Solution: Clear orange-colored liquid containing 0.5 mg/1 mL desloratadine in a 16-ounce Amber glass bottle (NDC 0085-1334-01) and a 4-ounce Amber glass bottle (NDC 0085-1334-02).

Storage

- **CLARINEX Tablets:** Protect Unit-of-Use packaging and Unit-Dose Hospital Pack from excessive moisture. Store at 25°C (77°F); excursions permitted to 15–30°C (59–86°F) [see USP Controlled Room Temperature]. Heat Sensitive. Avoid exposure at or above 30°C (86°F).
- **CLARINEX Oral Solution:** Store at 25°C (77°F); excursions permitted to 15–30°C (59–86°F) [see USP Controlled Room Temperature]. Protect from light.

17 PATIENT COUNSELING INFORMATION

See FDA-Approved Patient Labeling (Patient Information).

17.1 Information for Patients

- Patients should be instructed to use CLARINEX as directed.
- As there are no food effects on bioavailability, patients can be instructed that CLARINEX Tablets or Oral Solution may be taken without regard to meals.
- Patients should be advised not to increase the dose or dosing frequency as studies have not demonstrated increased effectiveness at higher doses and somnolence may occur.

CLARINEX Tablets and Oral Solution are
Manufactured for: Merck Sharp & Dohme Corp., a subsidiary of
MERCK & CO., INC., Whitehouse Station, NJ 08889, USA
CLARINEX Tablets are
Manufactured by: Merck Sharp & Dohme Corp., a subsidiary of
Merck & Co., Inc., Whitehouse Station, NJ 08889, USA
CLARINEX Oral Solution is
Manufactured by: Schering-Plough Canada, Inc., Pointe Claire, Quebec, Canada
For patent information: www.merck.com/product/patent/home.html

Revised: 06/2013
uspi-mk4117-mtl-1306r005

PATIENT INFORMATION

CLARINEX® (CLA-RI-NEX) (desloratadine) Tablets and Oral Solution

Read the Patient Information that comes with CLARINEX® before you start taking it and each time you get a refill. There may be new information. This leaflet is a summary of the information for patients. Your doctor or pharmacist can give you additional information. This leaflet does not take the place of talking to your doctor about your medical condition or treatment.

What is CLARINEX?

CLARINEX is a prescription medicine that contains the medicine desloratadine (an antihistamine).

CLARINEX is used to help control the symptoms of:

- seasonal allergic rhinitis (sneezing, stuffy nose, runny nose and itching of the nose) in people 2 years of age and older.
- perennial allergic rhinitis (sneezing, stuffy nose, runny nose and itching of the nose) in people 6 months of age and older.
- chronic idiopathic urticaria (long-term itching) and to reduce the number and size of hives in people 6 months of age and older.

CLARINEX is not for children younger than 6 months of age.

Who should not take CLARINEX?

Do not take CLARINEX if you:

- are allergic to desloratadine or any of the ingredients in CLARINEX Tablets or CLARINEX Oral Solution. See the end of this leaflet for a complete list of ingredients.
- are allergic to loratadine (Alavert, Claritin).

Talk to your doctor before taking this medicine if you have any questions about whether or not to take this medicine.

What should I tell my doctor before taking CLARINEX?

Before you take CLARINEX, tell your doctor if you:

- have liver or kidney problems.
- have any other medical conditions.
- are pregnant or plan to become pregnant. It is not known if CLARINEX will harm your unborn baby. Talk to your doctor if you are pregnant or plan to become pregnant.
- are breast-feeding or plan to breast-feed. CLARINEX **can pass into your breast milk.** Talk to your doctor about the best way to feed your baby if you take CLARINEX.

Tell your doctor about all the medicines you take, including prescription and non-prescription medicines, vitamins and herbal supplements. CLARINEX may affect the way other medicines work, and other medicines may affect how CLARINEX works. Especially tell your doctor if you take:

- ketoconazole (Nizoral)
- erythromycin (Ery-tab, Eryc, PCE)
- azithromycin (Zithromax, Zmax)
- antihistamines
- fluoxetine (Prozac)
- cimetidine (Tagamet)

Know the medicines you take. Keep a list of your medicines and show it to your doctor and pharmacist when you get a new medicine.

How should I take CLARINEX?

- Take CLARINEX exactly as your doctor tells you to take it.
- Do not change your dose of CLARINEX or take more often than prescribed.
- CLARINEX can be taken with or without food.
- Take CLARINEX Oral Solution with a measuring dropper or oral syringe that can measure 2 mL or 2.5 mL. Ask your pharmacist for a dropper or syringe if you do not have one.
- If you take too much CLARINEX, call your doctor or get medical attention right away.

What are the possible side effects of CLARINEX Tablets?

CLARINEX may cause serious side effects, including:

- Allergic reactions. Stop taking CLARINEX and call your doctor right away or get emergency help if you have any of these symptoms:
  - rash
  - itching
  - hives
  - swelling of your lips, tongue, face, and throat
  - shortness of breath or trouble breathing

The most common side effects of CLARINEX in adults and children 12 years of age and older with allergic rhinitis include:

- sore throat
- dry mouth
- muscle pain
- tiredness
- sleepiness
- menstrual pain

Increased sleepiness or tiredness can happen if you take more CLARINEX than your doctor prescribed to you.

Tell your doctor if you have any side effect that bothers you or that does not go away.

These are not all of the possible side effects of CLARINEX. For more information, ask your doctor or pharmacist.

Call your doctor for medical advice about side effects. You may report side effects to FDA at 1-800-FDA-1088.

How should I store CLARINEX?

- Store **CLARINEX Tablets** between 59°F to 86°F (15°C to 30°C).
- **CLARINEX Tablets** are sensitive to heat. Do not store above 86°F (30°C).
- Protect **CLARINEX Tablets** from moisture.
- Store **CLARINEX Oral Solution** between 59°F to 86°F (15°C to 30°C). Protect CLARINEX Oral Solution from light.

Keep **CLARINEX Tablets** and **Oral Solution** and all medicines out of the reach of children.

General information about CLARINEX

Medicines are sometimes prescribed for purposes other than those listed in a patient information leaflet. Do not use CLARINEX for a condition for which it was not prescribed. Do not give CLARINEX to other people, even if they have the same condition you have. It may harm them.

This Patient Information leaflet summarizes the most important information about CLARINEX. If you would like more information, talk with your doctor. You can ask your pharmacist or doctor for information about CLARINEX that is written for health professionals.

For more information, go to **www.CLARINEX.com**

What are the ingredients in CLARINEX?

Active ingredient: desloratadine

Inactive ingredients in CLARINEX Tablets: dibasic calcium phosphate dihydrate USP, microcrystalline cellulose NF, corn starch NF, talc USP, carnauba wax NF, white wax NF, coating material consisting of lactose monohydrate, hypromellose, titanium dioxide, polyethylene glycol, and FD&C Blue #2 Aluminum Lake.

Inactive ingredients in CLARINEX Oral Solution: propylene glycol USP, sorbitol solution USP, citric acid (anhydrous) USP, sodium citrate dihydrate USP, sodium benzoate NF, disodium edetate USP, purified water USP. It also contains granulated sugar, natural and artificial flavor for bubble gum and FDC Yellow #6 dye.

CLARINEX Tablets and Oral Solution are
Manufactured for: Merck Sharp & Dohme Corp., a subsidiary of
MERCK & CO., INC., Whitehouse Station, NJ 08889, USA
CLARINEX Tablets are
Manufactured by: Merck Sharp & Dohme Corp., a subsidiary of
Merck & Co., Inc., Whitehouse Station, NJ 08889, USA
CLARINEX Oral Solution is
Manufactured by: Schering-Plough Canada, Inc., Pointe Claire, Quebec, Canada
For patent information: www.merck.com/product/patent/home.html

Revised: 06/2013
usppi-mk4117-mtl-1306r005

Shown in Product Identification Guide, page 307

CLARINEX-D® 12 HOUR ℞

[klă-rĭ-nĕks D]
(desloratadine/pseudoephedrine sulfate)
Extended Release Tablets
for oral use

HIGHLIGHTS OF PRESCRIBING INFORMATION
These highlights do not include all the information needed to use CLARINEX-D 12 HOUR Extended Release Tablets safely and effectively. See full prescribing information for CLARINEX-D 12 HOUR Extended Release Tablets.
CLARINEX-D® 12 HOUR Extended Release Tablets (desloratadine/pseudoephedrine sulfate) for oral use
Initial U.S. Approval: 2005

INDICATIONS AND USAGE

CLARINEX-D 12 HOUR is a combination product containing an H_1-receptor antagonist and a sympathomimetic amine indicated for:

- Relief of nasal and non-nasal symptoms of seasonal allergic rhinitis, including nasal congestion, in adults and adolescents 12 years of age and older. (1)

DOSAGE AND ADMINISTRATION

For oral use only

Adults and adolescents 12 years of age and over: The recommended dose of CLARINEX-D 12 HOUR Extended Release Tablets is one tablet twice a day. (2)

DOSAGE FORMS AND STRENGTHS

Desloratadine 2.5 mg/Pseudoephedrine sulfate 120 mg tablets. (3)

CONTRAINDICATIONS

- Hypersensitivity (4)
- Narrow-Angle Glaucoma (4)
- Urinary Retention (4)
- Patients Receiving MAO Inhibitors or within 14 days of stopping such treatment (4)
- Severe hypertension or severe coronary artery disease. (4)

WARNINGS AND PRECAUTIONS

- Cardiovascular and central nervous system effects: Use with caution in patients with cardiovascular disorders. (5.1)
- Coexisting conditions: Use with caution in patients with increased intraocular pressure, prostatic hypertrophy, diabetes mellitus, or hyperthyroidism. (5.2)

ADVERSE REACTIONS

- The most common adverse reactions (reported in ≥2% of patients) were insomnia, headache, mouth dry, fatigue, somnolence, pharyngitis, dizziness, nausea, and anorexia. (6.1)

To report SUSPECTED ADVERSE REACTIONS, contact Merck Sharp & Dohme Corp., a subsidiary of Merck & Co., Inc., at 1-877-888-4231 or FDA at 1-800-FDA-1088 or *www.fda.gov/medwatch.*

DRUG INTERACTIONS

Monoamine Oxidase (MAO) Inhibitors: Do not use. May potentiate the effect of pseudoephedrine on vascular system. (7.1)

USE IN SPECIFIC POPULATIONS

- Renal impairment: Avoid in patients with renal impairment. (8.6)
- Hepatic impairment: Avoid in patients with hepatic impairment. (8.7)

See 17 for PATIENT COUNSELING INFORMATION and FDA-approved patient labeling

Revised: 10/2012

FULL PRESCRIBING INFORMATION: CONTENTS*

*** Sections or subsections omitted from the full prescribing information are not listed**

FULL PRESCRIBING INFORMATION

1 INDICATIONS AND USAGE

1.1 Seasonal Allergic Rhinitis

CLARINEX-D® 12 HOUR Extended Release Tablets is indicated for the relief of the nasal and non-nasal symptoms of seasonal allergic rhinitis, including nasal congestion, in adults and adolescents 12 years of age and older. CLARINEX-D 12 HOUR Extended Release Tablets should be administered when the antihistaminic properties of desloratadine and the nasal decongestant properties of pseudoephedrine are desired *[see Clinical Pharmacology (12)].*

2 DOSAGE AND ADMINISTRATION

Administer CLARINEX-D 12 HOUR Extended Release Tablet by the oral route only. Do not break, chew, or crush the tablet. Swallow the tablet whole.

2.1 Adults and Adolescents 12 years of Age and Over

The recommended dose of CLARINEX-D 12 HOUR Extended Release Tablets is 1 tablet twice a day, administered approximately 12 hours apart and with or without a meal. Higher doses or increased dosing frequency of CLARINEX-D 12 HOUR Extended Release Tablets have not demonstrated increased effectiveness. Do not exceed the recommended dose as desloratadine and pseudoephedrine, the active components of CLARINEX-D 12 HOUR Extended Release Tablets have been associated with adverse effects at higher doses *[see Overdosage (10.1) and (10.2)].*

3 DOSAGE FORMS AND STRENGTHS

CLARINEX-D 12 HOUR Extended Release Tablets are oval shaped, blue and white bilayer tablets with "D12" embossed in the blue layer. Each tablet contains 2.5 mg desloratadine in the blue immediate-release layer and 120 mg of pseudoephedrine sulfate USP in the white extended-release layer.

4 CONTRAINDICATIONS

CLARINEX-D 12 HOUR Extended Release Tablets are contraindicated in:

- Patients with hypersensitivity to any of its ingredients, or to loratadine *[see Warnings and Precautions (5.4) and Post-Marketing Experience (6.2)]*
- Patients with narrow-angle glaucoma
- Patients with urinary retention
- Patients receiving monoamine oxidase (MAO) inhibitor therapy or within fourteen (14) days of stopping such treatment *[see Drug Interactions (7.1)]*
- Patients with severe hypertension or severe coronary artery disease

5 WARNINGS AND PRECAUTIONS

5.1 Cardiovascular and Central Nervous System Effects

The pseudoephedrine sulfate contained in CLARINEX-D 12 HOUR Extended Release Tablets, like other sympathomimetic amines, can produce cardiovascular and central nervous system (CNS) effects in some patients such as insomnia, dizziness, weakness, tremor, or arrhythmias. In addition, central nervous system stimulation with convulsions or cardiovascular collapse with accompanying hypotension has been reported. Therefore, CLARINEX-D 12 HOUR Extended Release Tablets should be used with caution in patients with cardiovascular disorders, and should not be used in patients with severe hypertension or severe coronary artery disease.

5.2 Coexisting Conditions

CLARINEX-D 12 HOUR Extended Release Tablets contain pseudoephedrine sulfate, a sympathomimetic amine, and therefore should be used with caution in patients with diabetes and hyperthyroidism. Also use with caution in patients with prostatic hypertrophy or increased intraocular pressure, as urinary retention and narrow-angle glaucoma may occur *[see Contraindications (4)].*

5.3 Co-Administration with Monoamine Oxidase (MAO) Inhibitors

CLARINEX-D 12 HOUR Extended Release Tablets should not be used in patients receiving monoamine oxidase (MAO) inhibitor therapy or within fourteen (14) days of stopping such treatment as an increase in blood pressure or hypertensive crisis, may occur *[see Contraindications (4) and Drug Interactions (7.1)].*

5.4 Hypersensitivity Reactions

Hypersensitivity reactions including rash, pruritus, urticaria, edema, dyspnea, and anaphylaxis have been reported after administration of desloratadine a component of CLARINEX-D 12 HOUR Extended Release Tablets. If such a reaction occurs, therapy with CLARINEX-D 12 HOUR Extended Release Tablets should be stopped and alternative treatment should be considered *[see Post-Marketing Experience (6.2)].*

5.5 Renal Impairment

CLARINEX-D 12 HOUR Extended Release Tablets should generally be avoided in patients with renal impairment *[see Clinical Pharmacology (12)].*

5.6 Hepatic Impairment

CLARINEX-D 12 HOUR Extended Release Tablets should generally be avoided in patients with hepatic impairment *[see Clinical Pharmacology (12)].*

6 ADVERSE REACTIONS

The following adverse reactions are discussed in greater detail in other sections of the label:

- Cardiovascular and Central Nervous System effects *[see Warnings and Precautions (5.1)]*
- Increased intraocular pressure *[see Warnings and Precautions (5.2)]*
- Urinary retention in patients with prostatic hypertrophy *[see Warnings and Precautions (5.2)]*
- Hypersensitivity reactions *[see Warnings and Precautions (5.4)]*

6.1 Clinical Trials Experience

Because clinical trials are conducted under widely varying conditions, adverse reaction rates observed in the clinical trials of a drug cannot be directly compared to rates in the clinical trials of another drug and may not reflect the rates observed in clinical practice.

The safety data described below are from 2 clinical trials with CLARINEX-D 12 HOUR Extended Release Tablets that included 1248 patients with seasonal allergic rhinitis, of which 414 patients received CLARINEX-D 12 HOUR Extended Release Tablets twice daily for up to 2 weeks. The majority of patients were between 18 and <65 years of age with a mean age of 35.8 years and were predominantly women (64%). Patient ethnicity was 82% Caucasian, 9% Black, 6% Hispanic and 3% Asian/other ethnicity. The percentage of subjects receiving CLARINEX-D 12 HOUR Extended Release Tablets and who discontinued from the clinical trials because of an adverse event was 3.6%. Adverse reactions that were reported by ≥2% of subjects receiving CLARINEX-D 12 HOUR Extended Release Tablets are shown in **Table 1**.

[See table 1 at left]

Table 1: Incidence of Adverse Reactions Reported by ≥2% of Subjects Receiving CLARINEX-D 12 HOUR Extended Release Tablets

Adverse Reaction	CLARINEX-D 12 HOUR BID (N=414)	Desloratadine 5 mg QD (N=412)	Pseudoephedrine 120 mg BID (N=422)
Gastrointestinal Disorders			
Mouth Dry	8%	2%	8%
Nausea	2%	1%	3%
General Disorders and Administration Site Conditions			
Fatigue	4%	2%	2%
Metabolism and Nutrition Disorders			
Anorexia	2%	0%	2%
Nervous System Disorders			
Headache	8%	8%	9%
Somnolence	3%	4%	2%
Dizziness	3%	2%	2%
Psychiatric Disorders			
Insomnia	10%	3%	13%
Respiratory, Thoracic, and Mediastinal Disorders			
Pharyngitis	3%	3%	3%

There were no relevant differences in adverse reactions for subgroups of patients as defined by gender, age, or race.

6.2 Post-Marketing Experience

In addition to the adverse reactions reported during clinical trials and listed above, adverse events have been identified during post approval use of CLARINEX-D 12 HOUR Extended Release Tablets. Because these events are reported voluntarily from a population of uncertain size, it is not always possible to reliably estimate their frequency or establish a causal relationship to drug exposure. Adverse events identified from post-marketing surveillance on the use of CLARINEX-D 12 HOUR Extended Release Tablets include tachycardia, palpitations, dyspnea, rash and pruritus.

In addition to these events, the following spontaneous adverse events have been reported during the marketing of desloratadine as a single ingredient product: headache, somnolence, dizziness and rarely hypersensitivity reactions (such as urticaria, edema and anaphylaxis), and elevated liver enzymes including bilirubin and, very rarely, hepatitis.

7 DRUG INTERACTIONS

No specific interaction studies have been conducted with CLARINEX-D 12 HOUR Extended Release Tablets.

7.1 Monoamine Oxidase Inhibitors

CLARINEX-D 12 HOUR Extended Release Tablets should not be used in patients receiving monoamine oxidase (MAO) inhibitor therapy or within fourteen (14) days of stopping such treatment because the action of pseudoephedrine a component of CLARINEX-D 12 HOUR Extended Release tablets on the vascular system may be potentiated by these agents *[see Contraindications (4) and Warnings and Precautions (5.3)]*.

7.2 Beta-adrenergic blocking agents

The antihypertensive effects of beta-adrenergic blocking agents, methyldopa, and reserpine, may be reduced by sympathomimetics such as pseudoephedrine. Exercise caution when using CLARINEX-D 12 HOUR Extended Release Tablets with these agents.

7.3 Digitalis

Increased ectopic pacemaker activity can occur when pseudoephedrine is used concomitantly with digitalis. Exercise caution when using CLARINEX-D 12 HOUR Extended Release Tablets with these agents.

7.4 Inhibitors of cytochrome P450 3A4

In controlled clinical studies co-administration of desloratadine with ketoconazole, erythromycin, or azithromycin resulted in increased plasma concentrations of desloratadine and 3-hydroxydesloratadine but there were no clinically relevant changes in the safety profile of desloratadine *[see Clinical Pharmacology (12.3)]*.

7.5 Fluoxetine

In controlled clinical studies co-administration of desloratadine with fluoxetine, a selective serotonin reuptake inhibitor (SSRI), resulted in increased plasma concentrations of desloratadine and 3-hydroxydesloratadine but there were no clinically relevant changes in the safety profile of desloratadine *[see Clinical Pharmacology (12.3)]*.

7.6 Cimetidine

In controlled clinical studies co-administration of desloratadine with cimetidine a histamine H_2-receptor antagonist resulted in increased plasma concentrations of desloratadine and 3-hydroxydesloratadine but there were no clinically relevant changes in the safety profile of desloratadine *[see Clinical Pharmacology (12.3)]*.

8 USE IN SPECIFIC POPULATIONS

8.1 Pregnancy

Pregnancy Category C: There are no adequate and well-controlled studies of desloratadine and pseudoephedrine in combination in pregnant women. Neither are there animal reproduction studies conducted with the combination of desloratadine and pseudoephedrine. Desloratadine was not teratogenic in rats or rabbits but affected implantation in rats. Because animal reproduction studies are not always predictive of human response, CLARINEX-D 12 HOUR Extended Release Tablets should be used during pregnancy only if clearly needed.

Desloratadine was not teratogenic in rats or rabbits at approximately 210 and 230 times, respectively, the AUC in humans at the recommended daily oral dose. An increase in pre-implantation loss and a decreased number of implantations and fetuses were noted, however, in a separate study in female rats at approximately 120 times the AUC in humans at the recommended daily oral dose. Reduced body weight and slow righting reflex were reported in pups at approximately 50 times or greater than the AUC in humans at the recommended daily oral dose. Desloratadine had no effect on pup development at approximately 7 times the AUC in humans at the recommended daily oral dose. The AUCs in comparison referred to the desloratadine exposure in rabbits and the sum of desloratadine and its metabolites exposures in rats, respectively *[see Nonclinical Toxicology (13.2)]*.

8.3 Nursing Mothers

Desloratadine and pseudoephedrine both pass into breast milk; therefore, a decision should be made whether to discontinue nursing or to discontinue CLARINEX-D 12 HOUR Extended Release Tablets, taking into account the benefit of the drug to the nursing mother and the possible risk to the child.

8.4 Pediatric Use

CLARINEX-D 12 HOUR Extended Release Tablets are not indicated for use in pediatric patients under 12 years of age.

8.5 Geriatric Use

The number of subjects (n=10) ≥65 years old treated with CLARINEX-D 12 HOUR Extended Release Tablets was too limited to make any formal statistical comparison regarding the efficacy or safety of this drug product in this age group, or to determine whether they respond differently from younger subjects. Other reported clinical experience has not identified differences between the elderly and younger patients, although the elderly are more likely to have adverse reactions to sympathomimetic amines. In general, dose selection for an elderly patient should be cautious, reflecting the greater frequency of decreased hepatic, renal, or cardiac function, and of concomitant disease or other drug therapy *[see Clinical Pharmacology (12.3)]*.

Pseudoephedrine, desloratadine, and their metabolites are known to be substantially excreted by the kidney, and the risk of adverse reactions may be greater in patients with renal impairment. Because elderly patients are more likely to have decreased renal function, care should be taken in dose selection, and it may be useful to monitor the patient for adverse events *[see Clinical Pharmacology (12.3)]*.

8.6 Renal Impairment

No studies with CLARINEX-D 12 HOUR Extended Release Tablets were conducted in subjects with renal impairment. CLARINEX-D 12 HOUR Extended Release Tablets should generally be avoided in patients with renal impairment *[see Warnings and Precautions (5.5) and Clinical Pharmacology (12.3)]*.

8.7 Hepatic Impairment

No studies with CLARINEX-D 12 HOUR Extended Release Tablets or pseudoephedrine were conducted in subjects with hepatic impairment.

CLARINEX-D 12 HOUR Extended Release Tablets should generally be avoided in patients with hepatic impairment *[see Warnings and Precautions (5.6) and Clinical Pharmacology (12.3)]*.

8.8 Gender

No clinically significant gender-related differences were observed in the pharmacokinetic parameters of desloratadine, 3-hydroxydesloratadine or pseudoephedrine following administration of CLARINEX-D 12 HOUR Extended Release Tablets.

8.9 Race

No studies have been conducted to evaluate the effect of race on the pharmacokinetics of CLARINEX-D 12 HOUR Extended Release Tablets.

9 DRUG ABUSE AND DEPENDENCE

There is no information to indicate that abuse or dependency occurs with CLARINEX or CLARINEX-D 12 HOUR Extended Release Tablets.

10 OVERDOSAGE

In the event of overdose, consider standard measures to remove any unabsorbed drug. Symptomatic and supportive treatment is recommended. Desloratadine and 3-hydroxydesloratadine are not eliminated by hemodialysis.

10.1 Desloratadine

Information regarding acute overdosage with desloratadine is limited to experience from postmarketing adverse event reports and from clinical trials conducted during the development of the CLARINEX product. In the reported cases of overdose, there were no significant adverse events that were attributed to desloratadine. In a dose-ranging trial, at doses of 10 mg and 20 mg/day, somnolence was reported.

In another study, no clinically relevant adverse events were reported in normal male and female volunteers who were given single daily doses of CLARINEX 45 mg for 10 days *[see Clinical Pharmacology (12.2)]*.

Lethality occurred in rats at oral doses of 250 mg/kg or greater (estimated desloratadine and desloratadine metabolite exposures were approximately 120 times the AUC in humans at the recommended daily oral dose). The oral median lethal dose in mice was 353 mg/kg (estimated desloratadine exposure was approximately 290 times the human daily oral dose on an mg/m^2 basis). No deaths occurred at oral doses up to 250 mg/kg in monkeys (estimated desloratadine exposure was approximately 810 times the human daily oral dose on an mg/m^2 basis).

10.2 Sympathomimetics

In large doses, sympathomimetics such as pseudoephedrine may give rise to giddiness, headache, nausea, vomiting, sweating, thirst, tachycardia, precordial pain, palpitations, difficulty in micturition, muscle weakness and tenseness, anxiety, restlessness, and insomnia. Many patients can present a toxic psychosis with delusions and hallucinations. Some may develop cardiac arrhythmias, circulatory collapse, convulsions, coma, and respiratory failure.

11 DESCRIPTION

CLARINEX-D 12 HOUR Extended Release Tablets are oval-shaped blue and white bilayer tablets containing 2.5 mg desloratadine in the blue immediate-release layer and 120 mg of pseudoephedrine sulfate USP in the white extended-release layer which is released slowly, allowing for twice-daily administration.

The inactive ingredients contained in CLARINEX-D 12 HOUR Extended Release Tablets are hypromellose USP, microcrystalline cellulose NF, povidone USP, silicon dioxide NF, magnesium stearate NF, corn starch NF, edetate disodium USP, citric acid anhydrous USP, stearic acid NF, and FD&C Blue No. 2 aluminum lake dye.

Desloratadine, 1 of the 2 active ingredients of CLARINEX-D 12 HOUR Extended Release Tablets, is a white to off-white powder that is slightly soluble in water, but very soluble in ethanol and propylene glycol. It has an empirical formula: $C_{19}H_{19}ClN_2$ and a molecular weight of 310.8. The chemical name is 8-chloro-6,11-dihydro-11-(4-piperdinylidene)-5*H*-benzo[5,6] cyclohepta [1,2-*b*]pyridine and has the following structure:

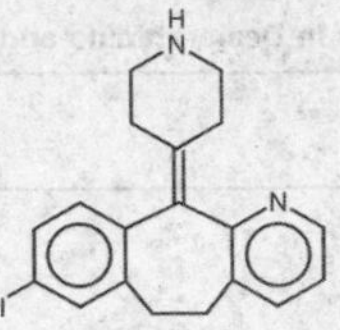

Pseudoephedrine sulfate, the other active ingredient of CLARINEX-D 12 HOUR Extended Release Tablets, is the synthetic salt of one of the naturally occurring dextrorotatory diastereomers of ephedrine and is classified as an indirect sympathomimetic amine. Pseudoephedrine sulfate is a colorless hygroscopic crystal or white, hygroscopic crystalline powder, practically odorless, with a bitter taste. It is very soluble in water, freely soluble in alcohol, and sparingly soluble in ether. The empirical formula for pseudoephedrine sulfate is $(C_{10}H_{15}NO)_2 \bullet H_2SO_4$; the chemical name is benzenemethanol, α-[1-(methylamino) ethyl]-,[*S*-(*R**,*R**)]-, sulfate (2:1)(salt); and the chemical structure is:

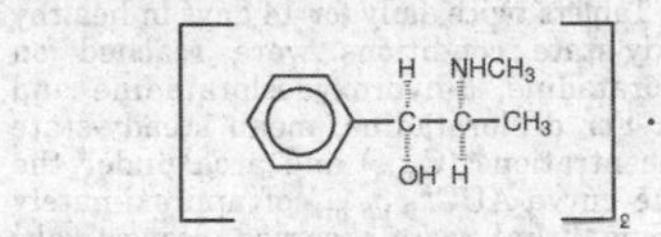

12 CLINICAL PHARMACOLOGY

12.1 Mechanism of Action

Desloratadine is a long acting tricyclic histamine antagonist with selective H_1-receptor histamine antagonist activity. Receptor binding data indicate that at a concentration of 2 to 3 ng/mL (7 nanomolar), desloratadine shows significant interaction with the human histamine H_1 receptor. Desloratadine inhibited histamine release from human mast cells *in vitro*. Results of a radiolabeled tissue distribution study in rats and a radioligand H_1-receptor-binding study in guinea pigs showed that desloratadine does not readily cross the blood brain barrier. The clinical significance of this finding is unknown.

Pseudoephedrine sulfate is an orally active sympathomimetic amine and exerts a decongestant action on the nasal mucosa. Pseudoephedrine sulfate is recognized as an effective agent for the relief of nasal congestion due to allergic rhinitis. Pseudoephedrine produces peripheral effects similar to those of ephedrine and central effects similar to, but less intense than, amphetamines. It has the potential for excitatory side effects.

12.2 Pharmacodynamics

Wheal and Flare: Human histamine skin wheal studies following single and repeated 5 mg doses of desloratadine have shown that the drug exhibits an antihistaminic effect by 1 hour; this activity may persist for as long as 24 hours. There was no evidence of histamine-induced skin wheal tachyphylaxis within the desloratadine 5 mg group over the 28-day treatment period. The clinical relevance of histamine wheal skin testing is unknown.

Effects on QT_c: In clinical trials for CLARINEX-D 12 HOUR Extended Release Tablets, ECGs were recorded at baseline and endpoint within 1 to 3 hours after the last dose. The majority of ECGs were normal at both baseline and endpoint. No clinically meaningful changes were observed following treatment with CLARINEX-D 12 HOUR Extended Release Tablets for any ECG parameter, including the QT_c interval. An increase in the ventricular rate of 7.1 and 6.4 bpm was observed in the CLARINEX-D 12 HOUR Extended Release Tablets and pseudoephedrine groups, respectively, compared to an increase of 3.2 bpm in subjects receiving desloratadine alone. Single daily doses of CLARINEX 45 mg were given to normal male and female volunteers for 10 days.

All ECGs obtained in this study were manually read in a blinded fashion by a cardiologist. In the CLARINEX-treated subjects, there was a mean increase in the maximum heart rate of 9.2 bpm relative to placebo. The QT interval was corrected for heart rate (QT_c) by both Bazett's and Fridericia methods. Using the QT_c (Bazett), there was a mean increase of 8.1 msec in the CLARINEX-treated subjects relative to placebo. Using QT_c (Fridericia) there was a mean increase of 0.4 msec in CLARINEX-treated subjects relative to placebo. No clinically relevant adverse events were reported.

12.3 Pharmacokinetics

Absorption: In a single dose pharmacokinetic study, the mean time to maximum plasma concentrations (T_{max}) for desloratadine occurred at approximately 4 to 5 hours post dose and mean peak plasma concentrations (C_{max}) and area under the concentration-time curve (AUC) of approximately 1.09 ng/mL and 31.6 ng•hr/mL, respectively, were observed. In another pharmacokinetic study, food and grapefruit juice had no effect on the bioavailability (C_{max} and AUC) of desloratadine.

For pseudoephedrine, the mean T_{max} occurred at 6 to 7 hours post dose and mean peak plasma concentrations (C_{max}) and area under the concentration-time curve (AUC)

Table 2: Changes in Desloratadine and 3-hydroxydesloratadine Pharmacokinetics in Healthy Male and Female Subjects

	Desloratadine		3-hydroxydesloratadine	
	C_{max}	AUC $_{0\text{-}24hrs}$	C_{max}	AUC $_{0\text{-}24hrs}$
Erythromycin (500 mg Q8h)	+24%	+14%	+43%	+40%
Ketoconazole (200 mg Q12h)	+45%	+39%	+43%	+72%
Azithromycin (500 mg Day 1, 250 mg QD × 4 days)	+15%	+5%	+15%	+4%
Fluoxetine (20 mg QD)	+15%	+0%	+17%	+13%
Cimetidine (600 mg Q12h)	+12%	+19%	-11%	-3%

of approximately 263 ng/mL and 4588 ng•hr/mL, respectively, were observed. Food had no effect on the bioavailability (C_{max} and AUC) of pseudoephedrine.

Following oral administration of CLARINEX-D 12 HOUR Extended Release Tablets twice daily for 14 days in healthy volunteers, steady-state conditions were reached on Day 10 for desloratadine, 3-hydroxydesloratadine and pseudoephedrine. For desloratadine, mean steady-state peak plasma concentrations (C_{max}) and area under the concentration-time curve AUC $_{0\text{-}12\ hrs}$ of approximately 1.7 ng/mL and 16 ng•hr/mL were observed, respectively. For pseudoephedrine, mean steady-state peak plasma concentrations (C_{max}) and AUC $_{0\text{-}12\ hrs}$ of 459 ng/mL and 4658 ng•hr/mL were observed.

Distribution: Desloratadine and 3-hydroxydesloratadine are approximately 82% to 87% and 85% to 89%, bound to plasma proteins, respectively. Protein binding of desloratadine and 3-hydroxydesloratadine was unaltered in subjects with impaired renal function.

Metabolism: Desloratadine (a major metabolite of loratadine) is extensively metabolized to 3-hydroxydesloratadine, an active metabolite, which is subsequently glucuronidated. The enzyme(s) responsible for the formation of 3-hydroxydesloratadine have not been identified. Data from clinical trials with desloratadine indicate that a subset of the general population has a decreased ability to form 3-hydroxydesloratadine, and are poor metabolizers of desloratadine. In pharmacokinetic studies (n=3748), approximately 6% of subjects were poor metabolizers of desloratadine (defined as a subject with an AUC ratio of 3-hydroxydesloratadine to desloratadine less than 0.1, or a subject with a desloratadine half-life exceeding 50 hours). These pharmacokinetic studies included subjects between the ages of 2 and 70 years, including 977 subjects aged 2 to 5 years, 1575 subjects aged 6 to 11 years, and 1196 subjects aged 12 to 70 years. There was no difference in the prevalence of poor metabolizers across age groups. The frequency of poor metabolizers was higher in Blacks (17%, n=988) as compared to Caucasians (2%, n=1462) and Hispanics (2%, n=1063). The median exposure (AUC) to desloratadine in the poor metabolizers was approximately 6-fold greater than in the subjects who are not poor metabolizers. Subjects who are poor metabolizers of desloratadine cannot be prospectively identified and will be exposed to higher levels of desloratadine following dosing with the recommended dose of desloratadine. In multidose clinical safety studies, where metabolizer status was prospectively identified, a total of 94 poor metabolizers and 123 normal metabolizers were enrolled and treated with CLARINEX Syrup for 15 to 35 days. In these studies, no overall differences in safety were observed between poor metabolizers and normal metabolizers. Although not seen in these studies, an increased risk of exposure-related adverse events in patients who are poor metabolizers cannot be ruled out.

Pseudoephedrine alone is incompletely metabolized (less than 1%) in the liver by N-demethylation to an inactive metabolite. The drug and its metabolite are excreted in the urine. About 55% to 96% of an administered dose of pseudoephedrine hydrochloride is excreted unchanged in the urine.

Elimination: Following single dose administration of CLARINEX-D 12 HOUR Extended Release Tablets, the mean plasma elimination half-life of desloratadine was approximately 27 hours. In another study, following administration of single oral doses of desloratadine 5 mg, C_{max} and AUC values increased in a dose proportional manner following single oral doses between 5 and 20 mg. The degree of accumulation after 14 days of dosing was consistent with the half-life and dosing frequency. A human mass balance study documented a recovery of approximately 87% of the ^{14}C-desloratadine dose, which was equally distributed in urine and feces as metabolic products. Analysis of plasma 3-hydroxydesloratadine showed similar T_{max} and half-life values compared to desloratadine.

The mean elimination half-life of pseudoephedrine is dependent on urinary pH. The elimination half-life is approximately 3 to 6 or 9 to 16 hours when the urinary pH is 5 or 8, respectively.

Geriatric Subjects: Following multiple-dose administration of CLARINEX Tablets, the mean C_{max} and AUC values for desloratadine were 20% greater than in younger subjects (< 65 years old). The oral total body clearance (CL/F) when normalized for body weight was similar between the 2 age groups. The mean plasma elimination half-life of desloratadine was 33.7 hr in subjects ≥65 years old. The pharmacokinetics for 3-hydroxydesloratadine appeared unchanged in older vs. younger subjects. These age-related differences are unlikely to be clinically relevant and no dosage adjustment is recommended in elderly patients.

Pediatric Subjects: CLARINEX-D 12 HOUR Extended Release Tablets are not an appropriate dosage form for use in pediatric patients below 12 years of age.

Renally Impaired: Following a single dose of desloratadine 7.5 mg, pharmacokinetics were characterized in subjects with mild (n=7; creatinine clearance 51–69 mL/min/1.73m^2), moderate (n=6; creatinine clearance 34–43 mL/min/1.73m^2) and severe (n=6; creatinine clearance 5–29 mL/min/1.73m^2) renal impairment or hemodialysis dependent (n=6) subjects. In subjects with mild and moderate renal impairment, median C_{max} and AUC values increased by approximately 1.2- and 1.9-fold, respectively, relative to subjects with normal renal function. In subjects with severe renal impairment or who were hemodialysis dependent, C_{max} and AUC values increased by approximately 1.7- and 2.5-fold, respectively. Minimal changes in 3-hydroxydesloratadine concentrations were observed. Desloratadine and 3-hydroxydesloratadine were poorly removed by hemodialysis. Plasma protein binding of desloratadine and 3-hydroxydesloratadine was unaltered by renal impairment.

Pseudoephedrine is primarily excreted unchanged in the urine as unchanged drug with the remainder apparently being metabolized in the liver. Therefore, pseudoephedrine may accumulate in patients with renal impairment.

Hepatically Impaired: Following a single oral dose of desloratadine, pharmacokinetics were characterized in subjects with mild (n=4), moderate (n=4) and severe (n=4) hepatic impairment as defined by the Child-Pugh classification of hepatic impairment and 8 subjects with normal hepatic function. Subjects with hepatic impairment, regardless of severity, had approximately a 2.4-fold increase in AUC as compared with normal subjects. The apparent oral clearance of desloratadine in subjects with mild, moderate, and severe hepatic impairment was 37%, 36%, and 28% of that in normal subjects, respectively. An increase in the mean elimination half-life of desloratadine in subjects with hepatic impairment was observed. For 3-hydroxydesloratadine, the mean C_{max} and AUC values for subjects with hepatic impairment combined were not statistically significantly different from subjects with normal hepatic function.

Gender: Female subjects treated for 14 days with CLARINEX Tablets had 10% and 3% higher desloratadine C_{max} and AUC values, respectively, compared with male subjects. The 3-hydroxydesloratadine C_{max} and AUC values were also increased by 45% and 48%, respectively, in females compared with males. However, these apparent differences are not considered to be clinically relevant.

Race: Following 14 days of treatment with CLARINEX Tablets, the C_{max} and AUC values for desloratadine were 18% and 32% higher, respectively in Blacks compared with Caucasians. For 3-hydroxydesloratadine there was a corresponding 10% reduction in C_{max} and AUC values in Blacks compared to Caucasians. These differences are not considered to be clinically relevant.

Drug Interaction: In 2 controlled crossover clinical pharmacology studies in healthy male (n=12 in each study) and female (n=12 in each study) subjects, desloratadine 7.5 mg (1.5 times the daily dose) once daily was co-administered with erythromycin 500 mg every 8 hours or ketoconazole 200 mg every 12 hours for 10 days. In 3 separate controlled, parallel group clinical pharmacology studies, desloratadine at the clinical dose of 5 mg has been co-administered with azithromycin 500 mg followed by 250 mg once daily for 4 days (n=18) or with fluoxetine 20 mg once daily for 7 days after a 23-day pretreatment period with fluoxetine (n=18) or with cimetidine 600 mg every 12 hours for 14 days (n=18) under steady state conditions to healthy male and female subjects. Although increased plasma concentrations (C_{max} and AUC $_{0\text{-}24\ hrs}$) of desloratadine and 3-hydroxydesloratadine were observed (see **Table 2**), there were no clinically relevant changes in the safety profile of desloratadine, as assessed by electrocardiographic parameters (including the corrected QT interval), clinical laboratory tests, vital signs and adverse events.

[See table 2 above]

13 NONCLINICAL TOXICOLOGY

13.1 Carcinogenesis, Mutagenesis, Impairment of Fertility

There are no animal or laboratory studies on the combination product of desloratadine and pseudoephedrine sulfate to evaluate carcinogenesis, mutagenesis, or impairment of fertility.

Carcinogenicity Studies: The carcinogenic potential of desloratadine was assessed using a loratadine study in rats and a desloratadine study in mice. In a 2-year study in rats, loratadine was administered in the diet at doses up to 25 mg/kg/day (estimated desloratadine and desloratadine metabolite exposures were approximately 30 times the AUC in humans at the recommended daily oral dose). A significantly higher incidence of hepatocellular tumors (combined adenomas and carcinomas) was observed in males given 10 mg/kg/day of loratadine and in males and females given 25 mg/kg/day of loratadine. The estimated desloratadine and desloratadine metabolite exposures in rats given 10 mg/kg of loratadine were approximately 7 times the AUC in humans at the recommended daily oral dose. The clinical significance of these findings during long-term use of desloratadine is not known.

In a 2-year dietary study in mice, males and females given up to 16 mg/kg/day and 32 mg/kg/day desloratadine, respectively, did not show significant increases in the incidence of any tumors. The estimated desloratadine and desloratadine metabolite exposures in mice at these doses were 12 and 27 times, respectively, the AUC in humans at the recommended daily oral dose.

Genotoxicity Studies: In genotoxicity studies with desloratadine, there was no evidence of genotoxic potential in a reverse mutation assay (*Salmonella*/*E. coli* mammalian microsome bacterial mutagenicity assay) or in 2 assays for chromosomal aberrations (human peripheral blood lymphocyte clastogenicity assay and mouse bone marrow micronucleus assay).

Impairment of Fertility: There was no effect on female fertility in rats at desloratadine doses up to 24 mg/kg/day (estimated desloratadine and desloratadine metabolite exposures were approximately 130 times the AUC in humans at the recommended daily oral dose). A male-specific decrease in fertility, demonstrated by reduced female conception rates, decreased sperm numbers and motility, and histopathologic testicular changes, occurred at an oral desloratadine dose of 12 mg/kg (estimated desloratadine and desloratadine metabolite exposures were approximately 45 times the AUC in humans at the recommended daily oral dose). Desloratadine had no effect on fertility in rats at an oral dose of 3 mg/kg/day (estimated desloratadine and desloratadine metabolite exposures were approximately 8 times the AUC in humans at the recommended daily oral dose).

13.2 Animal Toxicology and/or Pharmacology

Reproductive Toxicology Studies: Desloratadine was not teratogenic in rats at doses up to 48 mg/kg/day (estimated desloratadine and desloratadine metabolite exposures were approximately 210 times the AUC in humans at the recommended daily oral dose) or in rabbits at doses up to 60 mg/kg/day (estimated desloratadine exposures were approximately 230 times the AUC in humans at the recommended daily oral dose). In a separate study, an increase in preimplantation loss and a decreased number of implantations and fetuses were noted in female rats at 24 mg/kg (estimated desloratadine and desloratadine metabolite exposures were approximately 120 times the AUC in humans at the recommended daily oral dose). Reduced body weight and slow righting reflex were reported in pups at doses of 9 mg/kg/day or greater (estimated desloratadine and desloratadine metabolite exposures were approximately 50 times or greater than the AUC in humans at the recommended daily oral dose). Desloratadine had no effect on pup development at an oral dose of 3 mg/kg/day (estimated desloratadine and desloratadine metabolite exposures were approximately 7 times the AUC in humans at the recommended daily oral dose).

14 CLINICAL STUDIES

14.1 Seasonal Allergic Rhinitis

The clinical efficacy and safety of CLARINEX-D 12 HOUR Extended Release Tablets was evaluated in two 2-week multicenter, randomized parallel group clinical trials involving 1248 subjects 12 to 78 years of age with seasonal allergic rhinitis, 414 of whom received CLARINEX-D 12

HOUR Extended Release Tablets. In the 2 trials, subjects were randomized to receive CLARINEX-D 12 HOUR Extended Release Tablets twice daily, CLARINEX Tablets 5 mg once daily, or sustained-release pseudoephedrine tablet 120 mg twice daily for 2 weeks. The majority of patients were between 18 and <65 years of age with a mean age of 35.8 years and were predominantly women (64%). Patient ethnicity was 82% Caucasian, 9% Black, 6% Hispanic and 3% Asian/other ethnicity. Primary efficacy variable was twice-daily reflective patient scoring of 4 nasal symptoms (rhinorrhea, nasal stuffiness/congestion, nasal itching, and sneezing) and four non-nasal symptoms (itching/burning eyes, tearing/watering eyes, redness of eyes, and itching of ears/palate) on a 4 point scale (0=none, 1=mild, 2=moderate, and 3=severe). In both trials, the antihistaminic efficacy of CLARINEX-D 12 HOUR Extended Release Tablets, as measured by total symptom score excluding nasal congestion, was significantly greater than pseudoephedrine alone over the 2-week treatment period; and the decongestant efficacy of CLARINEX-D 12 HOUR Extended Release Tablets, as measured by nasal stuffiness/congestion, was significantly greater than CLARINEX (desloratadine alone) over the 2-week treatment period. Primary efficacy variable results from 1 of 2 trials are shown in **Table 3**.

[See table 3 above]

Table 3: Changes In Symptoms in a 2-Week Clinical Trial in Subjects With Seasonal Allergic Rhinitis

Treatment Group (n)	Mean Baseline* (sem)	Change (% Change) from Baseline† (sem)	CLARINEX-D 12 HOUR Comparison to Components‡ (*P*-value)
Total Symptom Score (Excluding Nasal Congestion)			
CLARINEX-D 12 HOUR Extended Release Tablets BID (199)	14.18 (0.21)	-6.54 (-46.0) (0.30)	-
Pseudoephedrine tablet 120 mg BID (197)	14.06 (0.21)	-5.07 (-35.9) (0.30)	***P*<0.001**
CLARINEX 5 mg Tablets QD (197)	14.82 (0.21)	-5.09 (-33.5) (0.30)	*P*<0.001
Nasal Stuffiness/Congestion			
CLARINEX-D 12 HOUR Extended Release Tablets BID (199)	2.47 (0.027)	-0.93 (-37.4) (0.046)	-
Pseudoephedrine tablet 120 mg BID (197)	2.46 (0.027)	-0.75 (-31.2) (0.046)	*P*=0.006
CLARINEX 5 mg Tablets QD (197)	2.50 (0.027)	-0.66 (-26.7) (0.046)	***P*<0.001**

Sem=Standard Error of the Mean

* To qualify at Baseline, the sum of the twice-daily diary reflective scores for the 3 days prior to Baseline and the morning of the Baseline visit were to total ≥42 for total nasal symptom score (sum of 4 nasal symptoms of rhinorrhea, nasal stuffiness/congestion, nasal itching, and sneezing) and a total of ≥35 for total non-nasal symptoms score (sum of 4 non-nasal symptoms of itching/burning eyes, tearing/watering eyes, redness of eyes, and itching of ears/palate), and a score of ≥14 for each of the individual symptoms of nasal stuffiness/congestion and rhinorrhea. Each symptom was scored on a 4-point severity scale (0=none, 1=mild, 2=moderate, 3=severe).

† Mean reduction in score averaged over the 2-week treatment period.

‡ The comparison of interest is shown bolded.

There were no significant differences in the efficacy of CLARINEX-D 12 HOUR Extended Release Tablets across subgroups of subjects defined by gender, age, or race.

16 HOW SUPPLIED/STORAGE AND HANDLING

CLARINEX-D 12 HOUR Extended Release Tablets are oval-shaped, blue and white bilayer tablets with "D12" embossed in the blue layer, containing 2.5 mg desloratadine in the blue immediate-release layer and 120 mg of pseudoephedrine sulfate USP in the white extended-release layer. CLARINEX-D 12 HOUR Extended Release Tablets are supplied in high-density polyethylene bottles of 100 (NDC 0085-1322-01).

Storage: Store at 25°C (77°F); excursions permitted to 15–30°C (59–86°F) [see USP Controlled Room Temperature]. Avoid exposure at or above 30°C (86°F). Protect from excessive moisture. Protect from light.

17 PATIENT COUNSELING INFORMATION

[see FDA-approved patient labeling]

17.1 Cardiovascular and Central Nervous System Effects

Patients should be informed that pseudoephedrine, one of the active ingredients in CLARINEX-D 12 HOUR Extended Release Tablets may cause cardiovascular or central nervous system effects such as insomnia, dizziness, tremor, or arrhythmia.

17.2 Dosing

Patients should be advised not to increase the dose or dosing frequency of CLARINEX-D 12 HOUR Extended Release Tablets.

17.3 Additional Antihistamines and/or Decongestants

Patients should be advised against the concurrent use of CLARINEX-D 12 HOUR Extended Release Tablets with other antihistamines and/or decongestants.

17.4 Monoamine Oxidase (MAO) Inhibitors

Patients should be informed that due to its pseudoephedrine component, they should not use CLARINEX-D 12 HOUR with a monoamine oxidase (MAO) inhibitor or within 14 days of stopping use of an MAO inhibitor.

17.5 Coexisting Conditions

Patients with severe hypertension or severe coronary artery disease, narrow-angle glaucoma, or urinary retention should be advised not to use CLARINEX-D 12 HOUR Extended Release Tablets.

17.6 Instructions for Use

Patients should be instructed not to break, crush, or chew the tablet; the tablet should be swallowed whole, and can be taken without regard to meals.

Manufactured for: Merck Sharp & Dohme Corp., a subsidiary of
MERCK & CO., INC., Whitehouse Station, NJ 08889, USA
Manufactured by:
Patheon Inc., Whitby, Ontario
L1N 5Z5, Canada
U.S. Patent Nos. 6,100,274; 6,709,676; 7,214,683; 7,618,649.

Revised: 10/2012
000483-DLD12-TB-USPI.3

PATIENT INFORMATION

CLARINEX-D® (CLA-RI-NEX) 12 Hour Extended Release Tablets

(desloratadine and pseudoephedrine sulfate)

Read the Patient Information that comes with CLARINEX-D 12 Hour Extended Release Tablets before you start taking it and each time you get a refill. There may be new information. This leaflet is a summary of the information for patients. Your doctor or pharmacist can give you additional information. This leaflet does not take the place of talking to your doctor about your medical condition or treatment.

What is CLARINEX-D® 12 Hour Extended Release Tablets?

CLARINEX-D 12 Hour Extended Release Tablets is a prescription medicine that contains the medicines desloratadine (an antihistamine) and pseudoephedrine (a nasal decongestant). CLARINEX-D 12 Hour Extended Release Tablets is used to help control the symptoms of seasonal allergic rhinitis (sneezing, stuffy nose, runny nose and itching of the nose) in adults and children 12 years and older.

CLARINEX-D 12 Hour Extended Release Tablets is not for children under 12 years of age.

Who should not take CLARINEX-D® 12 Hour Extended Release Tablets?

Do not take CLARINEX-D 12 Hour Extended Release Tablets if you:

- are allergic to desloratadine or pseudoephedrine sulfate or any of the ingredients in CLARINEX-D 12 Hour Extended Release Tablets. See the end of this leaflet for a complete list of ingredients in CLARINEX-D 12 Hour Extended Release Tablets.
- are allergic to loratadine (Alavert, Claritin)
- have narrow-angle glaucoma
- have problems with urination (urinary retention)
- take a Monoamine Oxidase Inhibitor (MAOI) medicine to treat depression, or if you stopped taking an MAOI medicine within the last 2 weeks. Ask your doctor or pharmacist if you are not sure if you take an MAOI medicine.
- have severe high blood pressure
- have severe heart disease

Talk to your doctor before taking this medicine if you have any of these conditions.

What should I tell my doctor before taking CLARINEX-D® 12 Hour Extended Release Tablets?

Before you take CLARINEX-D 12 Hour Extended Release Tablets, tell your doctor if you:

- have any of the conditions listed in the section "Who should not take CLARINEX-D 12 Hour Extended Release Tablets?"
- diabetes
- hyperthyroidism
- have prostate problems
- have liver or kidney problems
- have any other medical conditions
- are pregnant or plan to become pregnant. It is not known if CLARINEX-D 12 Hour Extended Release Tablets will harm your unborn baby. Talk to your doctor if you are pregnant or plan to become pregnant.
- are breastfeeding or plan to breastfeed. CLARINEX-D 12 Hour Extended Release Tablets **can pass into your breast milk**. Talk to your doctor about the best way to feed your baby if you take CLARINEX-D 12 Hour Extended Release Tablets.

Tell your doctor about all the medicines you take, including prescription and nonprescription medicines, vitamins and herbal supplements. CLARINEX-D® 12 Hour Extended Release Tablets may affect the way other medicines work, and other medicines may affect how CLARINEX-D 12 Hour Extended Release Tablets works. Especially tell your doctor if you take:

- Monoamine Oxidase Inhibitors (MAOIs). You should not use CLARINEX-D 12 Hour Extended Release Tablets if you take an MAOI or within 2 weeks of stopping an MAOI.
- methyldopa
- reserpine (Serpalan)
- digitalis (Digoxin, Lanoxicaps, Lanoxin) ketoconazole (Nizoral)
- erythromycin (Ery-tab, Eryc, PCE)
- azithromycin (Zithromax, Zmax)
- antihistamines
- other decongestant medicines

Know the medicines you take. Keep a list of your medicines and show it to your doctor and pharmacist when you get a new medicine.

How should I take CLARINEX-D® 12 Hour Extended Release Tablets?

Take CLARINEX-D 12 Hour Extended Release Tablets exactly as your doctor tells you to take it.

- CLARINEX-D 12 Hour Extended Release Tablets can be taken with or without food.
- Swallow CLARINEX-D 12 Hour Extended Release Tablets whole. **Do not break, crush, or chew** CLARINEX-D 12 Hour Extended Release Tablets before swallowing. If you cannot swallow CLARINEX-D 12 Hour Extended Release Tablets whole, tell your doctor. You may need a different medicine.
- Take 1 CLARINEX-D 12 Hour Extended Release Tablet 2 times a day (every 12 hours).

What are the possible side effects of CLARINEX-D® 12 Hour Extended Release Tablets?

CLARINEX-D 12 Hour Extended Release Tablets may cause serious side effects, including:

- Cardiovascular and central nervous system effects, such as
  - unable to sleep (insomnia)
  - dizziness
  - weakness
  - tremor
  - irregular heart beat
  - seizure
  - low blood pressure

- Increased sleepiness or tiredness can happen if you take more CLARINEX-D 12 Hour Extended Release Tablets than your doctor prescribed to you.
- Allergic reactions. Stop taking CLARINEX-D 12 Hour Extended Release Tablets and call your doctor right away or get emergency help if you have any of these symptoms:
  - rash
  - itching
  - hives
  - swelling of your lips, tongue, face, and throat
  - shortness of breath or trouble breathing

The most common side effects of CLARINEX-D 12 HOUR Extended Release Tablets include:

- unable to sleep (insomnia)
- sore throat
- headache
- dizziness
- dry mouth
- nausea
- tiredness
- loss of appetite
- sleepiness

Tell your doctor if you have any side effect that bothers you or that does not go away.

These are not all of the possible side effects of CLARINEX-D 12 Hour Extended Release Tablets. For more information, ask your doctor or pharmacist.

Call your doctor for medical advice about side effects. You may report side effects to FDA at 1-800-FDA-1088.

How should I store CLARINEX-D® 12 Hour Extended Release Tablets?

- Store CLARINEX-D 12 Hour Extended Release Tablets at 59°F to 86°F (15°C to 30°C)
- Keep CLARINEX-D 12 Hour Extended Release Tablets dry and out of the light.

Keep CLARINEX-D 12 Hour Extended Release Tablets and all medicines out of the reach of children.

General information about CLARINEX-D® 12 Hour Extended Release Tablets

Medicines are sometimes prescribed for purposes other than those listed in a patient information leaflet. Do not use CLARINEX-D 12 Hour Extended Release Tablets for a condition for which it was not prescribed. Do not give CLARINEX-D 12 Hour Extended Release Tablets to other people, even if they have the same condition you have. It may harm them.

This patient information leaflet summarizes the most important information about CLARINEX-D 12 Hour Extended Release Tablets. If you would like more information, talk with your doctor. You can ask your pharmacist or doctor for information about CLARINEX-D 12 Hour Extended Release Tablets that is written for health professionals.

For more information, go to **www.CLARINEX.com**

What are the ingredients in CLARINEX-D® 12 Hour Extended Release Tablets?

Active ingredients: desloratadine and pseudoephedrine sulfate

Inactive ingredients: hypromellose USP, microcrystalline cellulose NF, povidone USP, silicon dioxide NF, magnesium stearate NF, corn starch NF, edetate disodium USP, citric acid anhydrous USP, stearic acid NF, and FD&C Blue No. 2 aluminum lake dye.

Manufactured for: Merck Sharp & Dohme Corp., a subsidiary of
MERCK & CO., INC., Whitehouse Station, NJ 08889, USA
Manufactured by:
Patheon Inc., Whitby, Ontario
L1N 5Z5, Canada
U.S. Patent Nos. 6,100,274; 6,709,676; 7,214,683; 7,618,649.

Revised: 10/2012
000483-DLD12-TB-PPI.3

Shown in Product Identification Guide, page 307

CLARINEX-D® 24 HOUR ℞

[klă-rĭ-nĕcks]
(desloratadine/pseudoephedrine sulfate)
Extended Release Tablets
for oral use

HIGHLIGHTS OF PRESCRIBING INFORMATION

These highlights do not include all the information needed to use CLARINEX-D® 24 HOUR Extended Release Tablets safely and effectively. See full prescribing information for CLARINEX-D 24 HOUR Extended Release Tablets.
CLARINEX-D 24 HOUR Extended Release Tablets (desloratadine/pseudoephedrine sulfate) for oral use.
Initial U.S. Approval: 2005

INDICATIONS AND USAGE

CLARINEX-D 24 HOUR is a combination product containing an H1-receptor antagonist and a sympathomimetic amine indicated for:

- Relief of nasal and non-nasal symptoms of seasonal allergic rhinitis, including nasal congestion, in adults and adolescents 12 years of age and older. (1)

DOSAGE AND ADMINISTRATION

For oral use only
Adults and adolescents 12 years of age and over: The recommended dose of CLARINEX-D 24 HOUR Extended Release Tablets is one tablet once daily. (2)

DOSAGE FORMS AND STRENGTHS

Desloratadine 5 mg/Pseudoephedrine sulfate 240 mg tablets (3)

CONTRAINDICATIONS

- Hypersensitivity (4)
- Narrow Angle Glaucoma (4)
- Urinary Retention (4)
- Patients Receiving MAO Inhibitors or within 14 days of stopping such treatment (4)
- Severe hypertension or severe coronary artery disease (4)

WARNINGS AND PRECAUTIONS

- Cardiovascular and central nervous system effects: Use with caution in patients with cardiovascular disorders. (5.1).
- Coexisting conditions: Use with caution in patients with increased intraocular pressure, prostatic hypertrophy, diabetes mellitus, or hyperthyroidism (5.2).

ADVERSE REACTIONS

- The most common adverse reactions (reported in ≥2% of patients) were mouth dry, headache, insomnia, fatigue, pharyngitis, somnolence, nausea, dizziness, nervousness, psychomotor hypersensitivity and anorexia. (6.1)

To report SUSPECTED ADVERSE REACTIONS, contact Schering Corporation at 800-526-4099 or FDA at 1-800-FDA-1088 or *www.fda.gov/medwatch*.

DRUG INTERACTIONS

Monoamine Oxidase (MAO) Inhibitors: Do not use. May potentiate the effect of pseudoephedrine on vascular system. (7.1)

USE IN SPECIFIC POPULATIONS

- Renal impairment: Avoid in patients with renal impairment (8.6)
- Hepatic impairment: Avoid in patients with hepatic impairment (8.7)

See 17 for PATIENT COUNSELING INFORMATION and FDA-approved patient labeling

Revised: 12/2009

FULL PRESCRIBING INFORMATION: CONTENTS*

*** Sections or subsections omitted from the full prescribing information are not listed**

FULL PRESCRIBING INFORMATION

1 INDICATIONS AND USAGE

1.1 Seasonal Allergic Rhinitis

CLARINEX-D® 24 HOUR Extended Release Tablets is indicated for the relief of the nasal and non-nasal symptoms of seasonal allergic rhinitis, including nasal congestion, in adults and adolescents 12 years of age and older. CLARINEX-D 24 HOUR Extended Release Tablets should be administered when the antihistaminic properties of desloratadine and the nasal decongestant properties of pseudoephedrine are desired *[see Clinical Pharmacology (12)]*.

2 DOSAGE AND ADMINISTRATION

Administer CLARINEX-D 24 HOUR Extended Release Tablet by the oral route only. Do not break, chew or crush the tablet. Swallow the tablet whole.

2.1 Adults and Adolescents 12 years of Age and Over

The recommended dose of CLARINEX-D 24 HOUR Extended Release Tablets is 1 tablet once daily, administered with or without a meal. Higher doses or increased dosing frequency of CLARINEX-D 24 HOUR Extended Release Tablets have not demonstrated increased effectiveness. Do not exceed the recommended dose as desloratadine and pseudoephedrine, the active components of CLARINEX-D 24 HOUR Extended Release Tablets have been associated with adverse effects at higher doses *[see Overdosage (10.1, 10.2)]*.

3 DOSAGE FORMS AND STRENGTHS

CLARINEX-D 24 HOUR Extended Release Tablets are oval-shaped, light blue coated tablets with "D 24" branded in black on one side. Each tablet contains 5 mg desloratadine in the tablet coating for immediate release and 240 mg pseudoephedrine sulfate, USP in an extended release core.

4 CONTRAINDICATIONS

CLARINEX-D 24 HOUR Extended Release Tablets are contraindicated in:

- Patients with hypersensitivity to any of its ingredients, or to loratadine *[see Warnings and Precautions (5.4) and Post-Marketing Experience (6.2)]*
- Patients with narrow angle glaucoma
- Patients with urinary retention
- Patients receiving monoamine oxidase (MAO) inhibitor therapy or within fourteen (14) days of stopping such treatment *[see Drug Interactions (7.1)]*.
- Patients with severe hypertension or severe coronary artery disease.

5 WARNINGS AND PRECAUTIONS

5.1 Cardiovascular and Central Nervous System Effects

The pseudoephedrine sulfate contained in CLARINEX-D 24 HOUR Extended Release Tablets, like other sympathomimetic amines, can produce cardiovascular and central nervous system (CNS) effects in some patients such as insomnia, dizziness, weakness, tremor, or arrhythmias. In addition, central nervous system stimulation with convulsions or cardiovascular collapse with accompanying hypotension has been reported. Therefore, CLARINEX-D 24 HOUR Extended Release Tablets should be used with caution in patients with cardiovascular disorders, and should not be used in patients with severe hypertension or severe coronary artery disease.

5.2 Coexisting Conditions

CLARINEX-D 24 HOUR Extended Release Tablets contain pseudoephedrine sulfate, a sympathomimetic amine, and therefore should be used with caution in patients with diabetes and hyperthyroidism. Also use with caution in patients with prostatic hypertrophy or increased intraocular pressure, as urinary retention or narrow-angle glaucoma may occur *[see Contraindications (4)]*.

5.3 Co-Administration with Monoamine Oxidase (MAO) Inhibitors

CLARINEX-D 24 HOUR Extended Release Tablets should not be used in patients receiving monoamine oxidase (MAO) inhibitor therapy or within fourteen (14) days of stopping such treatment as an increase in blood pressure or hypertensive crisis, may occur *[see Contraindications (4) and Drug Interactions (7.1)]*.

5.4 Hypersensitivity Reactions

Hypersensitivity reactions including rash, pruritus, urticaria, edema, dyspnea, and anaphylaxis have been reported after administration of desloratadine a component of CLARINEX-D 24 HOUR Extended Release Tablets. If such a reaction occurs, therapy with CLARINEX-D 24 HOUR Extended Release Tablets should be stopped and alternative treatment should be considered *[see Post-marketing (6.2)]*.

5.5 Renal Impairment

CLARINEX-D 24 HOUR Extended Release Tablets should generally be avoided in patients with renal impairment *[see Clinical Pharmacology (12)]*.

5.6 Hepatic Impairment

CLARINEX-D 24 HOUR Extended Release Tablets should generally be avoided in patients with hepatic impairment *[see Clinical Pharmacology (12)]*.

6 ADVERSE REACTIONS

The following adverse reactions are discussed in greater detail in other sections of the label:

- Cardiovascular and Central Nervous System effects *[see Warnings and Precautions (5.1)]*
- Increased Intraocular pressure *[see Warnings and Precautions (5.2)]*
- Urinary retention in patients with prostatic hypertrophy *[see Warnings and Precautions (5.2)]*
- Hypersensitivity reactions *[see Warnings and Precautions (5.4)]*.

6.1 Clinical Trials Experience

Because clinical trials are conducted under widely varying conditions, adverse reaction rates observed in the clinical trials of a drug cannot be directly compared to rates in the clinical trials of another drug and may not reflect the rates observed in clinical practice.

The safety data described below are from 2 clinical trials with CLARINEX-D 24 HOUR Extended Release Tablets that included 2852 patients, of which 708 patients received CLARINEX-D 24 HOUR Extended Release Tablets daily for up to 15 days. The majority of patients were between 18 and <65 years of age with a mean age of 34.3 years and were predominantly women (63%). Patient ethnicity was 79 % Caucasian, 10% Black, 8 % Hispanic and 3% Asian/other ethnicity. The percentage of subjects receiving CLARINEX-D 24 HOUR Extended Release Tablets, and who discontinued from the clinical trials because of an adverse event was 3.4%. Adverse reactions that were reported by ≥ 2% of subjects receiving CLARINEX-D 24 HOUR Extended Release Tablets are shown in Table 1.

[See table 1 above]

TABLE 1: Incidence of Adverse Reactions Reported by ≥2% of Subjects Receiving CLARINEX-D 24 HOUR Extended Release Tablets

Adverse Reaction	CLARINEX-D® 24 HOUR (N =708)	Desloratadine 5 mg (N =712)	Pseudoephedrine 240 mg (N =719)
Gastrointestinal Disorders			
Mouth Dry	8%	2%	11%
Nausea	2%	1%	3%
Anorexia	2%	0%	2%
General Disorders and Administration Site Conditions			
Fatigue	3%	3%	2%
Nervous System Disorders			
Headache	6%	5%	7%
Somnolence	3%	2%	3%
Dizziness	2%	1%	2%
Psychomotor hyperactivity	2%	0%	2%
Psychiatric Disorders			
Insomnia	5%	1%	8%
Nervousness	2%	1%	1%
Respiratory, Thoracic and Mediastinal Disorders			
Pharyngitis	3%	2%	3%

There were no relevant differences in adverse reactions for subgroups of patients as defined by gender, age, or race.

6.2 Post-Marketing Experience

In addition to the adverse reactions reported during clinical trials and listed above, adverse events have been identified during post approval use of CLARINEX-D 24 HOUR Extended Release Tablets. Because these events are reported voluntarily from a population of uncertain size, it is not always possible to reliably estimate their frequency or establish a causal relationship to drug exposure. Adverse events identified from post-marketing surveillance on the use of CLARINEX-D 24 HOUR Extended Release Tablets include palpitations, pruritis and urticaria.

In addition to these events, the following spontaneous adverse events have been reported during the marketing of desloratadine as a single ingredient product: headache, somnolence, dizziness, tachycardia, and rarely hypersensitivity reactions (such as rash, edema, dyspnea, and anaphylaxis), and elevated liver enzymes including bilirubin and very rarely, hepatitis.

7 DRUG INTERACTIONS

No specific interaction studies have been conducted with CLARINEX-D 24 HOUR Extended Release Tablets.

7.1 Monoamine Oxidase Inhibitors

CLARINEX-D 24 HOUR Extended Release Tablets should not be used in patients receiving monoamine oxidase (MAO) inhibitor therapy or within fourteen (14) days of stopping such treatment because the action of pseudoephedrine a component of CLARINEX-D 24 HOUR Extended Release Tablets on the vascular system may be potentiated by these agents. *(See Contraindications (4) and Warnings and Precautions 5.4)*

7.2 Beta-adrenergic blocking agents

The antihypertensive effects of beta-adrenergic blocking agents, methyldopa, and reserpine, may be reduced by sympathomimetics such as pseudoephedrine. Exercise caution when using CLARINEX-D 24 HOUR Extended Release Tablets with these agents.

7.3 Digitalis

Increased ectopic pacemaker activity can occur when pseudoephedrine is used concomitantly with digitalis. Exercise caution when using CLARINEX-D 24 HOUR Extended Release Tablets with these agents.

7.4 Inhibitors of cytochrome P450 3A4

In controlled clinical studies co-administration of desloratadine with ketoconazole, erythromycin, or azithromycin resulted in increased plasma concentrations of desloratadine and 3-hydroxydesloratadine but there were no clinically relevant changes in the safety profile of desloratadine. *[See Clinical Pharmacology (12.3)]*

7.5 Fluoxetine

In controlled clinical studies co-administration of desloratadine with fluoxetine, a selective serotonin reuptake inhibitor (SSRI), resulted in increased plasma concentrations of desloratadine and 3-hydroxydesloratadine but there were no clinically relevant changes in the safety profile of desloratadine *[See Clinical Pharmacology (12.3)]*

7.6 Cimetidine

In controlled clinical studies co-administration of desloratadine with cimetidine a histamine H2-receptor antagonist resulted in increased plasma concentrations of desloratadine and 3-hydroxydesloratadine but there were no clinically relevant changes in the safety profile of desloratadine *[See Clinical Pharmacology (12.3)]*

8 USE IN SPECIFIC POPULATIONS

8.1 Pregnancy

Pregnancy Category C: There are no adequate and well-controlled studies of desloratadine and pseudoephedrine in combination in pregnant women. Neither are there animal reproduction studies conducted with the combination of desloratadine and pseudoephedrine. Desloratadine was not teratogenic in rats or rabbits but affected implantation in rats. Because animal reproduction studies are not always predictive of human response, CLARINEX-D 24 HOUR Extended Release Tablets should be used during pregnancy only if clearly needed.

Desloratadine was not teratogenic in rats or rabbits at approximately 210 and 230 times, respectively, the AUC in humans at the recommended daily oral dose). An increase in pre-implantation loss and a decreased number of implantations and fetuses were noted, however, in a separate study in female rats at approximately 120 times the AUC in humans at the recommended daily oral dose). Reduced body weight and slow righting reflex were reported in pups at approximately 50 times or greater than the AUC in humans at the recommended daily oral dose. Desloratadine had no effect on pup development at approximately 7 times the AUC in humans at the recommended daily oral dose). The AUCs in comparison referred to the desloratadine exposure in rabbits and the sum of desloratadine and its metabolites exposures in rats, respectively *[see Nonclinical Toxicology (13.2)]*.

8.3 Nursing Mothers

Desloratadine and pseudoephedrine both pass into breast milk; therefore, a decision should be made whether to discontinue nursing or to discontinue CLARINEX-D 24 HOUR Extended Release Tablets, taking into account the benefit of the drug to the nursing mother and the possible risk to the child.

8.4 Pediatric Use

CLARINEX-D 24 HOUR Extended Release Tablets are not indicated for use in pediatric patients under 12 years of age.

8.5 Geriatric Use

The number of subjects (n=8) ≥65 years old treated with CLARINEX-D 24 HOUR Extended Release Tablets was too limited to make any formal statistical comparison regarding the efficacy or safety of this drug product in this age group, or to determine whether they respond differently from younger subjects. Other reported clinical experience has not identified differences between the elderly and younger patients, although the elderly are more likely to have adverse reactions to sympathomimetic amines. In general, dose selection for an elderly patient should be cautious, reflecting the greater frequency of decreased hepatic, renal, or cardiac function, and of concomitant disease or other drug therapy *[see Clinical Pharmacology (12)]*.

Pseudoephedrine, desloratadine, and their metabolites are known to be substantially excreted by the kidney, and the risk of adverse reactions may be greater in patients with renal impairment. Because elderly patients are more likely to have decreased renal function, care should be taken in dose selection, and it may be useful to monitor the patient for adverse events *[see Clinical Pharmacology (12.3)]*.

8.6 Renal Impairment

No studies with CLARINEX-D 24 HOUR Extended Release Tablets were conducted in subjects with renal impairment. For CLARINEX-D 24 HOUR Extended Release Tablets should generally be avoided in patients with renal impairment *[see Warnings and Precautions (5.5) and Clinical Pharmacology (12.3)]*.

8.7 Hepatic Impairment

No studies with CLARINEX-D 24 HOUR Extended Release Tablets or pseudoephedrine have been conducted in subjects with hepatic impairment.

CLARINEX-D 24 HOUR Extended Release Tablets should generally be avoided in patients with hepatic impairment. *[see Warnings and Precautions (5.6) and Clinical Pharmacology (12.3)]*.

8.8 Gender

No clinically significant gender-related differences were observed in the pharmacokinetic parameters of desloratadine, 3-hydroxydesloratadine or pseudoephedrine following administration of CLARINEX-D 24 HOUR Extended Release Tablets.

8.9 Race

No studies have been conducted to evaluate the effect of race on the pharmacokinetics of CLARINEX-D 24 HOUR Extended Release Tablets.

9 DRUG ABUSE AND DEPENDENCE

There is no information to indicate that abuse or dependency occurs with CLARINEX or CLARINEX-D 24 HOUR Extended Release Tablets.

10 OVERDOSAGE

In the event of overdose, consider standard measures to remove any unabsorbed drug. Symptomatic and supportive treatment is recommended. Desloratadine and 3-hydroxydesloratadine are not eliminated by hemodialysis.

10.1 Desloratadine

Information regarding acute overdosage with desloratadine is limited to experience from postmarketing adverse event reports and from clinical trials conducted during the development of the CLARINEX product. In the reported cases of overdose, there were no significant adverse events that were attributed to desloratadine. In a dose ranging trial, at doses of 10 mg and 20 mg/day somnolence was reported.

In another study, no clinically relevant adverse events were reported in normal male and female volunteers who were given single daily doses of CLARINEX 45 mg for 10 days *[see Clinical Pharmacology (12.2)]*.

Lethality occurred in rats at oral doses of 250 mg/kg or greater (estimated desloratadine and desloratadine metabolite exposures were approximately 120 times the AUC in humans at the recommended daily oral dose). The oral median lethal dose in mice was 353 mg/kg (estimated desloratadine exposure was approximately 290 times the human daily oral dose on an mg/m^2 basis). No deaths occurred at oral doses up to 250 mg/kg in monkeys (estimated desloratadine exposures were approximately 810 times the human daily oral dose on an mg/m^2 basis).

10.2 Sympathomimetics

In large doses, sympathomimetics such as pseudoephedrine may give rise to giddiness, headache, nausea, vomiting, sweating, thirst, tachycardia, precordial pain, palpitations, difficulty in micturition, muscle weakness and tenseness, anxiety, restlessness, and insomnia. Many patients can present a toxic psychosis with delusions and hallucinations. Some may develop cardiac arrhythmias, circulatory collapse, convulsions, coma and respiratory failure.

11 DESCRIPTION

CLARINEX-D 24 HOUR Extended Release Tablets are light blue oval-shaped tablets containing 5 mg desloratadine in the tablet coating for immediate release and 240 mg pseudoephedrine sulfate USP in the tablet core for extended release.

The inactive ingredients contained in CLARINEX-D 24 HOUR Extended Release Tablets are hypromellose USP, ethylcellulose NF, dibasic calcium phosphate dihydrate USP, magnesium stearate NF, povidone USP, silicone dioxide NF, talc USP, polyacrylate dispersion, polyethylene glycol NF, simethicone USP, Blue Lake Blend 50726 (FD&C Blue No. 2 Lake, titanium dioxide USP and edetate disodium USP), and ink (Opacode® S-1-17746 or Opacode® S-1-4159).

Desloratadine, 1 of the 2 active ingredients of CLARINEX-D 24 HOUR Extended Release Tablets, is a white to off-white powder that is slightly soluble in water, but very soluble in ethanol and propylene glycol. It has an empirical formula: $C_{19}H_{19}ClN_2$ and a molecular weight of 310.8. The chemical name is 8-chloro-6,11-dihydro-11-(4-piperdinylidene)-5*H*-benzo[5,6]cyclohepta[1,2-*b*]pyridine and has the following structure:

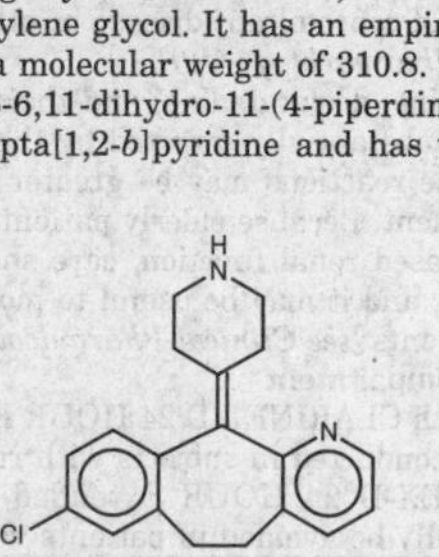

Pseudoephedrine sulfate, the other active ingredient of CLARINEX-D 24 HOUR Extended Release Tablets, is the synthetic salt of one of the naturally occurring dextrorotatory diastereomers of ephedrine and is classified as an indirect sympathomimetic amine. Pseudoephedrine sulfate is a colorless hygroscopic crystal or white, hygroscopic crystalline powder, practically odorless, with a bitter taste. It is very soluble in water, freely soluble in alcohol, and sparingly soluble in ether. The empirical formula for pseudoephedrine sulfate is $(C_{10}H_{15}NO)_2 \bullet H_2SO_4$; the chemical name is benzenemethanol, α-[1-(methylamino) ethyl]-,[*S*-(*R**,*R**)]-, sulfate (2:1)(salt); and the chemical structure is:

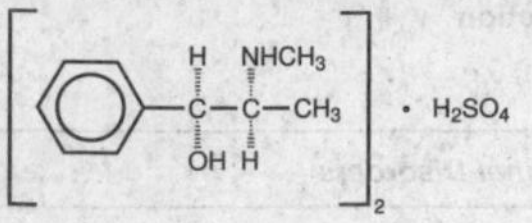

12 CLINICAL PHARMACOLOGY

12.1 Mechanism of Action

Desloratadine is a long-acting tricyclic histamine antagonist with selective H_1-receptor histamine antagonist activity. Receptor binding data indicate that at a concentration of 2 to 3 ng/mL (7 nanomolar), desloratadine shows significant interaction with the human histamine H_1-receptor. Desloratadine inhibited histamine release from human mast cells *in vitro*. Results of a radiolabeled tissue distribution study in rats and a radioligand H_1-receptor binding study in guinea pigs showed that desloratadine does not readily cross the blood brain barrier. The clinical significance of this finding is unknown.

Pseudoephedrine sulfate is an orally active sympathomimetic amine and exerts a decongestant action on the nasal mucosa. Pseudoephedrine sulfate is recognized as an effective agent for the relief of nasal congestion due to allergic rhinitis. Pseudoephedrine produces peripheral effects similar to those of ephedrine and central effects similar to, but less intense than, amphetamines. It has the potential for excitatory side effects.

12.2 Pharmacodynamics

Wheal and Flare: Human histamine skin wheal studies following single and repeated 5 mg doses of desloratadine have shown that the drug exhibits an antihistaminic effect by 1 hour; this activity may persist for as long as 24 hours. There was no evidence of histamine-induced skin wheal tachyphylaxis within the desloratadine 5 mg group over the 28-day treatment period. The clinical relevance of histamine wheal skin testing is unknown.

Effects on QTc: In clinical trials for CLARINEX-D 24 HOUR Extended Release Tablets, ECGs were recorded at baseline and after 2 weeks of treatment within 1 to 3 hours after dosing. No clinically meaningful changes were observed following treatment with CLARINEX-D 24 HOUR Extended Release Tablets for any ECG parameter, including the QTc interval. An increase in the ventricular rate of 6.7 and 5.4 bpm was observed in the CLARINEX-D 24 HOUR Extended Release Tablets and pseudoephedrine groups, respectively, compared to an increase of 2.8 bpm in subjects receiving desloratadine alone. Single daily doses of CLARINEX 45 mg were given to normal male and female volunteers for 10 days. All ECGs obtained in this study were manually read in a blinded fashion by a cardiologist. In the CLARINEX-treated subjects, there was a mean increase in the maximum heart rate of 9.2 bpm relative to placebo. The QT interval was corrected for heart rate (QTc) by both Bazett's and Fridericia methods. Using the QTc (Bazett), there was a mean increase of 8.1 msec in the CLARINEX-treated subjects relative to placebo. Using QTc (Fridericia) there was a mean increase of 0.4 msec in CLARINEX-treated subjects relative to placebo. No clinically relevant adverse events were reported.

12.3 Pharmacokinetics

Absorption:

A bioequivalence study that compared CLARINEX-D 24 HOUR Extended Release Tablets to the monotherapy (desloratadine 5 mg, and pseudoephedrine 240 mg) showed that CLARINEX-D 24 HOUR Extended Release Tablets was not bioequivalent to the monotherapy (desloratadine 5 mg tablet). The systemic exposure to desloratadine and 3-hydroxydesloratadine was 15% to 20% lower from CLARINEX-D 24 HOUR Extended Release Tablets than those from desloratadine 5 mg tablet. Clinical trials were therefore necessary to support efficacy of CLARINEX-D 24 HOUR Extended Release Tablets *[see Clinical Studies (14)]*.

In the above single dose pharmacokinetic study the mean time to maximum plasma concentrations (T_{max}) for desloratadine occurred at approximately 6 to 7 hours post dose and mean peak plasma concentrations (C_{max}) and area under the concentration-time curve (AUC(tf)) of approximately 1.79 ng/mL and 61.1 ng·hr/mL, respectively, were observed. In another pharmacokinetic study, food and grapefruit juice had no effect on the bioavailability (C_{max} and AUC) of desloratadine.

For pseudoephedrine, the mean T_{max} occurred at 8 to 9 hours post dose and mean peak plasma concentrations (C_{max}) and AUC(tf) of 328 ng/mL and 6438 ng·hr/mL, respectively, were observed. The ingestion of food did not affect the absorption of pseudoephedrine from CLARINEX-D 24 HOUR Extended Release Tablets.

Following oral administration of CLARINEX-D 24 HOUR Extended Release Tablets once daily for 14 days in healthy volunteers, steady-state conditions were reached on Day 12 for desloratadine and 3-hydroxydesloratadine, and Day 10 for pseudoephedrine. For desloratadine, mean steady-state C_{max} and AUC (0–24h) of approximately 2.44 ng/mL and 34.8 ng•hr/mL, respectively were observed. For pseudoephedrine, mean steady-state peak plasma concentrations (C_{max}) and AUC (0–24h) of 523 ng/mL and 8795 ng•hr/mL, respectively, were observed.

Distribution:

Desloratadine and 3-hydroxydesloratadine are approximately 82% to 87% and 85% to 89%, bound to plasma proteins, respectively. Protein binding of desloratadine and 3-hydroxydesloratadine was unaltered in subjects with impaired renal function.

Metabolism

Desloratadine (a major metabolite of loratadine) is extensively metabolized to 3-hydroxydesloratadine, an active metabolite, which is subsequently glucuronidated. The enzyme(s) responsible for the formation of 3-hydroxydesloratadine have not been identified. Data from clinical trials with desloratadine indicate that a subset of the general population has a decreased ability to form 3-hydroxydesloratadine, and are poor metabolizers of desloratadine. In pharmacokinetic studies (n=3748), approximately 6% of subjects were poor metabolizers of desloratadine (defined as a subject with an AUC ratio of 3-hydroxydesloratadine to desloratadine less than 0.1, or a subject with a desloratadine half-life exceeding 50 hours). These pharmacokinetic studies included subjects between the ages of 2 and 70 years, including 977 subjects aged 2 to 5 years, 1575 subjects aged 6 to 11 years, and 1196 subjects aged 12 to 70 years. There was no difference in the prevalence of poor metabolizers across age groups. The frequency of poor metabolizers was higher in Blacks (17%, n=988) as compared to Caucasians (2%, n=1462) and Hispanics (2%, n=1063). The median exposure (AUC) to desloratadine in the poor metabolizers was approximately 6-fold greater than in the subjects who are not poor metabolizers. Subjects who are poor metabolizers of desloratadine cannot be prospectively identified and will be exposed to higher levels of desloratadine following dosing with the recommended dose of desloratadine. In multidose clinical safety studies, where metabolizer status was prospectively identified, a total of 94 poor metabolizers and 123 normal metabolizers were enrolled and treated with CLARINEX Syrup for 15 to 35 days. In these studies, no overall differences in safety were observed between poor metabolizers and normal metabolizers. Although not seen in these studies, an increased risk of exposure-related adverse events in patients who are poor metabolizers cannot be ruled out.

Pseudoephedrine alone is incompletely metabolized (less than 1%) in the liver by N-demethylation to an inactive metabolite. The drug and its metabolite are excreted in the urine. About 55% to 96% of an administered dose of pseudoephedrine hydrochloride is excreted unchanged in the urine.

Elimination

Following single dose administration of CLARINEX-D 24 HOUR Extended Release Tablets, the mean plasma elimination half-life of desloratadine was similar to the desloratadine 5 mg tablet, approximately 24 and 27 hours, respectively. In another study, following administration of single oral doses of desloratadine 5 mg, C_{max} and AUC values increased in a dose proportional manner between 5 and 20 mg. The degree of accumulation after 14 days of dosing was consistent with the half-life and dosing frequency. A human mass balance study documented a recovery of approximately 87% of the ^{14}C-desloratadine dose, which was equally distributed in urine and feces as metabolic products. Analysis of plasma 3-hydroxydesloratadine showed similar T_{max} and half-life values compared to desloratadine.

The mean elimination half-life of pseudoephedrine is dependent on urinary pH. The elimination half-life is approximately 3 to 6 or 9 to-16 hours when the urinary pH is 5 or 8, respectively.

Geriatric Subjects: Following multiple-dose administration of CLARINEX Tablets, the mean C_{max} and AUC values for desloratadine were 20% greater than in younger subjects (<65 years old). The oral total body clearance (CL/F) when normalized for body weight was similar between the 2 age groups. The mean plasma elimination half-life of desloratadine was 33.7 hr in subjects ≥ 65 years old. The pharmacokinetics for 3-hydroxydesloratadine appeared unchanged in older vs. younger subjects. These age-related differences are unlikely to be clinically relevant and no dosage adjustment is recommended in elderly patients.

Pediatric Subjects: CLARINEX-D 24 HOUR Extended Release Tablets are not an appropriate dosage form for use in pediatric patients below 12 years of age.

Renally Impaired: Following a single dose of desloratadine 7.5 mg, pharmacokinetics were characterized in subjects with mild (n=7; creatinine clearance 51–69 mL/min/1.73m^2), moderate (n=6; creatinine clearance 34–43 mL/min/1.73 m^2), and severe (n=6; creatinine clearance

5–29 mL/min/1.73m^2) renal impairment or hemodialysis dependent (n=6) subjects. In subjects with mild and moderate renal impairment, median C_{max} and AUC values increased by approximately 1.2- and 1.9-fold, respectively, relative to subjects with normal renal function. In subjects with severe renal impairment or who were hemodialysis dependent, C_{max} and AUC values increased by approximately 1.7- and 2.5-fold, respectively. Minimal changes in 3-hydroxydesloratadine concentrations were observed. Desloratadine and 3-hydroxydesloratadine were poorly removed by hemodialysis. Plasma protein binding of desloratadine and 3-hydroxydesloratadine was unaltered by renal impairment.

Pseudoephedrine is primarily excreted unchanged in the urine as unchanged drug; the remainder is apparently metabolized in the liver. Therefore, pseudoephedrine may accumulate in patients with renal impairment.

Hepatically Impaired: Following a single oral dose of desloratadine, pharmacokinetics were characterized in subjects with mild (n=4), moderate (n=4), and severe (n=4) hepatic impairment as defined by the Child-Pugh classification of hepatic impairment and 8 subjects with normal hepatic function. Subjects with hepatic impairment, regardless of severity, had approximately a 2.4-fold increase in AUC as compared with normal subjects. The apparent oral clearance of desloratadine in subjects with mild, moderate, and severe hepatic impairment was 37%, 36%, and 28% of that in normal subjects, respectively. An increase in the mean elimination half-life of desloratadine in subjects with hepatic impairment was observed. For 3-hydroxydesloratadine, the mean C_{max} and AUC values for subjects with hepatic impairment were not statistically significantly different from subjects with normal hepatic function.

Gender: Female subjects treated for 14 days with CLARINEX Tablets had 10% and 3% higher desloratadine C_{max} and AUC values, respectively, compared with male subjects. The 3-hydroxydesloratadine C_{max} and AUC values were also increased by 45% and 48%, respectively, in females compared with males. However, these apparent differences are not considered to be clinically relevant.

Race: Following 14 days of treatment with CLARINEX Tablets, the C_{max} and AUC values for desloratadine were 18% and 32% higher, respectively, in Blacks compared with Caucasians. For 3-hydroxydesloratadine there was a corresponding 10% reduction in C_{max} and AUC values in Blacks compared to Caucasians. These differences are not considered to be clinically relevant.

Drug interaction: In 2 controlled crossover clinical pharmacology studies in healthy male (n=12 in each study) and female (n=12 in each study) subjects, desloratadine 7.5 mg (1.5 times the daily dose) once daily was co-administered with erythromycin 500 mg every 8 hours or ketoconazole 200 mg every 12 hours for 10 days. In 3 separate controlled, parallel group clinical pharmacology studies, desloratadine at the clinical dose of 5 mg has been co-administered with azithromycin 500 mg followed by 250 mg once daily for 4 days (n=18) or with fluoxetine 20 mg once daily for 7 days after a 23-day pretreatment period with fluoxetine (n=18) or with cimetidine 600 mg every 12 hours for 14 days (n=18) under steady state conditions to healthy male and female subjects. Although increased plasma concentrations (Cmax and AUC 0–24 hrs) of desloratadine and 3-hydroxydesloratadine were observed (see Table 2), there were no clinically relevant changes in the safety profile of desloratadine, as assessed by electrocardiographic parameters (including the corrected QT interval), clinical laboratory tests, vital signs and adverse events.

[See table 2 above]

TABLE 2 Changes in Desloratadine and 3-hydroxydesloratadine Pharmacokinetics in Healthy Male and Female Subjects

	Desloratadine		3-hydroxydesloratadine	
	C_{max}	AUC 0–24 hrs	C_{max}	AUC 0–24 hrs
Erythromycin (500 mg Q8h)	+24%	+14%	+43%	+40%
Ketoconazole (200 mg Q12h)	+45%	+39%	+43%	+72%
Azithromycin (500 mg Day 1, 250 mg QD × 4 days)	+15%	+5%	+15%	+4%
Fluoxetine (20 mg QD)	+15%	+0%	+17%	+13%
Cimetidine (600 mg Q12h)	+12%	+19%	-11%	-3%

TABLE 3 Changes in Symptoms in a 2-Week Clinical Trial in Subjects With Seasonal Allergic Rhinitis

Treatment Group (n)	Mean Baseline* (sem)	Change (% change) from Baseline† (sem)	CLARINEX-D® 24 HOUR Comparison to components‡ (P- value)
Total Symptom Score (Excluding Nasal Congestion)			
CLARINEX-D 24 HOUR Extended Release Tablets (333)	14.84 (0.15)	-5.71 (-37.4) (0.22)	-
Pseudoephedrine tablet 240 mg (337)	15.03 (0.15)	-4.95 (-32.0) (0.22)	**p=0.015**
CLARINEX 5 mg Tablets (337)	15.06 (0.15)	-4.78 (-30.8) (0.22)	p=0.003
Nasal Stuffiness/Congestion			
CLARINEX-D® 24 HOUR Extended Release Tablets (333)	2.56 (0.020)	-0.85 (-32.3) (0.034)	-
Pseudoephedrine tablet 240 mg (337)	2.54 (0.020)	-0.70 (-27.1) (0.034)	p=0.002
CLARINEX 5 mg Tablets (337)	2.57 (0.020)	-0.65 (-24.8) (0.034)	**p<0.001**

Sem=Standard Error of the Mean

*To qualify at Baseline, the sum of the twice-daily diary reflective scores for the 3 days prior to Baseline and the morning of the Baseline visit were to total ≥42 for total nasal symptom score (sum of 4 nasal symptoms of rhinorrhea, nasal stuffiness/congestion, nasal itching, and sneezing) and a total of ≥35 for total non-nasal symptoms score (sum of 4 non-nasal symptoms of itching/burning eyes, tearing/watering eyes, redness of eyes, and itching of ears/palate), and a score of ≥14 for each of the individual symptoms of nasal stuffiness/congestion and rhinorrhea. Each symptom was scored on a 4-point severity scale (0=none, 1=mild, 2=moderate, 3=severe).

†Mean reduction in score averaged over the 2-week treatment period.

‡The comparison of interest is shown bolded.

13 NONCLINICAL TOXICOLOGY

13.1 Carcinogenesis, Mutagenesis, Impairment of Fertility

There are no animal or laboratory studies on the combination product of desloratadine and pseudoephedrine sulfate to evaluate carcinogenesis, mutagenesis, or impairment of fertility.

Carcinogenicity Studies:

The carcinogenic potential of desloratadine was assessed using a loratadine study in rats and a desloratadine study in mice. In a 2-year study in rats, loratadine was administered in the diet at doses up to 25 mg/kg/day (estimated desloratadine and desloratadine metabolite exposures were approximately 30 times the AUC in humans at the recommended daily oral dose). A significantly higher incidence of hepatocellular tumors (combined adenomas and carcinomas) was observed in males given 10 mg/kg/day of loratadine and in males and females given 25 mg/kg/day of loratadine. The estimated desloratadine and desloratadine metabolite exposures in rats given 10 mg/kg of loratadine were approximately 7 times the AUC in humans at the recommended daily oral dose. The clinical significance of these findings during long-term use of desloratadine is not known.

In a 2-year dietary study in mice, males and females given up to 16 mg/kg/day and 32 mg/kg/day desloratadine, respectively, did not show significant increases in the incidence of any tumors. The estimated desloratadine and desloratadine metabolite exposures in mice at these doses were 12 and 27 times, respectively, the AUC in humans at the recommended daily oral dose.

Genotoxicity Studies:

In genotoxicity studies with desloratadine, there was no evidence of genotoxic potential in a reverse mutation assay (*Salmonella*/*E. coli* mammalian microsome bacterial mutagenicity assay) or in 2 assays for chromosomal aberrations (human peripheral blood lymphocyte clastogenicity assay and mouse bone marrow micronucleus assay).

Impairment of Fertility:

There was no effect on female fertility in rats at desloratadine doses up to 24 mg/kg/day (estimated desloratadine and desloratadine metabolite exposures were approximately 130 times the AUC in humans at the recommended daily oral dose). A male specific decrease in fertility, demonstrated by reduced female conception rates, decreased sperm numbers and motility, and histopathologic testicular changes, occurred at an oral desloratadine dose of 12 mg/kg in rats (estimated desloratadine and desloratadine metabolite exposures were approximately 45 times the AUC in humans at the recommended daily oral dose). Desloratadine had no effect on fertility in rats at an oral dose of 3 mg/kg/day (estimated desloratadine and desloratadine metabolite exposures were approximately 8 times the AUC in humans at the recommended daily oral dose).

13.2 Animal Toxicology and/or Pharmacology

Reproductive Toxicology Studies:

Desloratadine was not teratogenic in rats at doses up to 48 mg/kg/day (estimated desloratadine and desloratadine metabolite exposures were approximately 210 times the AUC in humans at the recommended daily oral dose) or in rabbits at doses up to 60 mg/kg/day (estimated desloratadine exposures were approximately 230 times the AUC in humans at the recommended daily oral dose). In a separate study, an increase in pre-implantation loss and a decreased number of implantations and fetuses were noted in female rats at 24 mg/kg (estimated desloratadine and desloratadine metabolite exposures were approximately 120 times the AUC in humans at the recommended daily oral dose). Reduced body weight and slow righting reflex were reported in pups at doses of 9 mg/kg/day or greater (estimated desloratadine and desloratadine metabolite exposures were approximately 50 times or greater than the AUC in humans at the recommended daily oral dose). Desloratadine had no effect on pup development at an oral dose of 3 mg/kg/day (estimated desloratadine and desloratadine metabolite exposures were approximately 7 times the AUC in humans at the recommended daily oral dose).

14 CLINICAL STUDIES

14.1 Seasonal Allergic Rhinitis

The clinical efficacy and safety of CLARINEX-D 24 HOUR Extended Release Tablets was evaluated in two 2-week multicenter, randomized parallel group clinical trials involving 2852 subjects 12 to 78 years of age with seasonal allergic rhinitis, 708 of whom received CLARINEX-D 24 HOUR Extended Release Tablets. In the 2 trials, subjects were randomized to receive CLARINEX-D 24 HOUR Extended Release Tablets once daily, CLARINEX Tablets 5 mg once daily, or sustained-release pseudoephedrine tablet 240 mg once daily for two weeks. The majority of patients were between 18 and <65 years of age with a mean age of 34.3 years and were predominantly women (63%). Patient ethnicity was 79 % Caucasian, 10% Black, 8 % Hispanic and 3% Asian/other ethnicity. Primary efficacy variable was twice-daily reflective patient scoring of 4 nasal symptoms (rhinorrhea, nasal stuffiness/congestion, nasal itching, and sneezing) and 4 non-nasal symptoms (itching/burning eyes, tearing/watering eyes, redness of eyes, and itching of ears/palate) on a four point scale (0=none, 1=mild, 2=moderate, and 3=severe). In both trials, the antihistaminic efficacy of CLARINEX-D 24 HOUR Extended Release Tablets, as measured by total symptom score excluding nasal congestion, was significantly greater than pseudoephedrine alone over the 2-week treatment period; and the decongestant efficacy of CLARINEX-D 24 HOUR Extended Release Tablets, as measured by nasal stuffiness/congestion, was significantly greater than CLARINEX (desloratadine alone) over the 2-week treatment period. Primary efficacy variable results from 1 of 2 trials are shown in Table 3.

[See table 3 at top of previous page]

There were no significant differences in the efficacy of CLARINEX-D 24 HOUR Extended Release Tablets across subgroups of subjects defined by gender, age, or race.

16 HOW SUPPLIED/STORAGE AND HANDLING

CLARINEX-D 24 HOUR Extended Release Tablets are oval-shaped, light blue coated tablets with "D24" branded in black on one side containing 5 mg desloratadine in the tablet coating for immediate release and 240 mg pseudoephedrine sulfate USP in an extended release core. CLARINEX-D 24 HOUR Extended Release Tablets are supplied in high-density polyethylene bottles of 100 (NDC 0085-1317-01).

Storage:

Store at 25°C (77°F), excursions permitted to 15–30°C (59–86°F) [see USP Controlled Room Temperature] Heat Sensitive. Avoid exposure at or above 30°C (86°F). Protect from excessive moisture. Protect from light.

17 PATIENT COUNSELING INFORMATION

[see FDA Approved Patient Labeling]

17.1 Cardiovascular and Central Nervous System Effects

Patients should be informed that pseudoephedrine, on of the active ingredients in CLARINEX-D 24 HOUR Extended Release Tablets may cause cardiovascular or central nervous system effects such as insomnia, dizziness, tremor, or arrhythmia.

17.2 Dosing

Patients should be advised not to increase the dose or dosing frequency of CLARINEX-D 24 HOUR Extended Release Tablets.

17.3 Additional Antihistamines and/or Decongestants

Patients should be advised against the concurrent use of CLARINEX-D 24 HOUR Extended Release Tablets with other antihistamines and/or decongestants.

17.4 Monoamine Oxidase (MAO) Inhibitors

Patients should be informed that due to its pseudoephedrine component, they should not use CLARINEX-D 24 HOUR with a monoamine oxidase (MAO) inhibitor or within 14 days of stopping use of an MAO inhibitor.

17.5 Coexisting Conditions

Patients with severe hypertension or severe coronary artery disease, narrow-angle glaucoma, or urinary retention should be advised not to use CLARINEX-D 24 HOUR Extended Release Tablets.

17.6 Instructions for Use

Patients should be instructed not to break, crush or chew the tablet. The tablet should be swallowed whole, and can be taken without regard to meals.

Manufactured by Schering Corporation, a subsidiary of Schering-Plough Corporation,
Kenilworth, NJ 07033 USA.

U.S. Patent Nos. 4,659,716; 4,863,931; 5,595,997; and 6,100,274

PATIENT INFORMATION

CLARINEX-D (CLA-RI-NEX) 24 Hour Extended Release Tablets

(desloratadine and pseudoephedrine sulfate)

Read the Patient Information that comes with CLARINEX-D 24 Hour Extended Release Tablets before you start taking it and each time you get a refill. There may be new information. This leaflet is a summary of the information for patients. Your doctor or pharmacist can give you additional information. This leaflet does not take the place of talking to your doctor about your medical condition or treatment.

What is CLARINEX-D® 24 Hour Extended Release Tablets?

CLARINEX-D 24 Hour Extended Release Tablets is a prescription medicine that contains the medicines desloratadine (an antihistamine) and pseudoephedrine (a nasal decongestant). CLARINEX-D 24 Hour Extended Release Tablets is used to help control the symptoms of seasonal allergic rhinitis (sneezing, stuffy nose, runny nose and itching of the nose) in adults and children 12 years and older.

CLARINEX-D 24 Hour Extended Release Tablets is not for children under 12 years of age.

Who should not take CLARINEX-D® 24 Hour Extended Release Tablets?

Do not take CLARINEX-D 24 Hour Extended Release Tablets if you:

- are allergic to desloratadine or pseudoephedrine sulfate or any of the ingredients in CLARINEX-D 24 Hour Extended Release Tablets. See the end of this leaflet for a complete list of ingredients in CLARINEX-D 24 Hour Extended Release Tablets.
- are allergic to loratadine (Alavert, Claritin)
- have narrow angle glaucoma
- have problems with urination (urinary retention)
- take a Monoamine Oxidase Inhibitor (MAOI) medicine to treat depression, or if you stopped taking an MAOI medicine within the last 2 weeks. Ask your doctor or pharmacist if you are not sure if you take an MAOI medicine.
- have severe high blood pressure
- have severe heart disease

Talk to your doctor before taking this medicine if you have any of these conditions.

What should I tell my doctor before taking CLARINEX-D® 24 Hour Extended Release Tablets?

Before you take CLARINEX-D 24 Hour Extended Release Tablets, tell your doctor if you:

- have any of the conditions listed in the section "Who should not take CLARINEX-D 24 Hour Extended Release Tablets?"
- diabetes
- hyperthyroidism
- have prostate problems
- have liver or kidney problems
- have any other medical conditions
- are pregnant or plan to become pregnant. It is not known if CLARINEX-D 24 Hour Extended Release Tablets will harm your unborn baby. Talk to your doctor if you are pregnant or plan to become pregnant.
- are breast-feeding or plan to breast-feed. CLARINEX-D 24 Hour Extended Release Tablets **can pass into your breast milk.** Talk to your doctor about the best way to feed your baby if you take CLARINEX-D 24 Hour Extended Release Tablets.

Tell your doctor about all the medicines your take, including prescription and non-prescription medicines, vitamins and herbal supplements. CLARINEX-D 24 Hour Extended Release Tablets may affect the way other medicines work, and other medicines may affect how CLARINEX-D 24 Hour Extended Release Tablets works. Especially tell your doctor if you take:

- Monoamine Oxidase Inhibitors (MAOI). You should not use CLARINEX-D 24 Hour Extended Release Tablets if you take a MAOI or within 2 weeks of stopping an MAOI.
- methyldopa
- reserpine (Serpalan)
- digitalis (Digoxin, Lanoxicaps, Lanoxin)
- ketoconazole (Nizoral)
- erythromycin (Ery-tab, Eryc, PCE)
- azithromycin (Zithromax, Zmax)
- antihistamines
- other decongestant medicines

Know the medicines you take. Keep a list of your medicines and show it to your doctor and pharmacist when you get a new medicine.

How should I take CLARINEX-D 24 Hour Extended Release Tablets?

- Take CLARINEX-D 24 Hour Extended Release Tablets exactly as your doctor tells you to take it.
- CLARINEX-D 24 Hour Extended Release Tablets can be taken with or without food.
- Swallow CLARINEX-D 24 Hour Extended Release Tablets whole. **Do not break, crush, or chew** CLARINEX-D 24 Hour Extended Release Tablets before swallowing. If you can not swallow CLARINEX-D 24 Hour Extended Release Tablets whole, tell your doctor. You may need a different medicine.
- Take 1 CLARINEX-D 24 Hour Extended Release Tablet every day.

What are the possible side effects of CLARINEX-D® 24 Hour Extended Release Tablets?

CLARINEX-D 24 Hour Extended Release Tablets may cause serious side effects, including:

- Cardiovascular and central nervous system effects, such as
  - unable to sleep (insomnia)
  - dizziness
  - weakness
  - tremor
  - irregular heart beat
  - seizure
  - low blood pressure
- Increased sleepiness or tiredness can happen if you take more CLARINEX-D 24 Hour Extended Release Tablets than your doctor prescribed to you.
- Allergic reactions. Stop taking CLARINEX-D 24 Hour Extended Release Tablets and call your doctor right away or get emergency help if you have any of these symptoms:
  - rash
  - itching
  - hives
  - swelling of your lips, tongue, face, and throat
  - shortness of breath or trouble breathing

The most common side effects of CLARINEX-D 24 HOUR Extended Release Tablets include:

- dry mouth
- headache
- unable to sleep (insomnia)
- tiredness
- sore throat
- sleepiness
- nausea
- dizziness
- nervousness
- restlessness
- poor appetite

Tell your doctor if you have any side effect that bothers you or that does not go away.

These are not all of the possible side effects of CLARINEX-D 24 Hour Extended Release Tablets. For more information, ask your doctor or pharmacist.

Call your doctor for medical advice about side effects. You may report side effects to FDA at 1-800-FDA-1088.

How should I store CLARINEX-D® 24 Hour Extended Release Tablets?

- Store CLARINEX-D 24 Hour Extended Release Tablets at 59°F to 86°F (15°C to 30°C)
- Keep CLARINEX-D 24 Hour Extended Release Tablets dry and out of the light.

Keep CLARINEX-D 24 Hour Extended Release Tablets and all medicines out of the reach of children.

General information CLARINEX-D® 24 Hour Extended Release Tablets

Medicines are sometimes prescribed for purposes other than those listed in a patient information leaflet. Do not use CLARINEX-D 24 Hour Extended Release Tablets for a condition for which it was not prescribed. Do not give CLARINEX-D 24 Hour Extended Release Tablets to other people, even if they have the same condition you have. It may harm them.

This patient information leaflet summarizes the most important information about CLARINEX-D 24 Hour Extended Release Tablets. If you would like more information, talk with your doctor. You can ask your pharmacist or doctor for information about CLARINEX-D 24 Hour Extended Release Tablets that is written for health professionals.

For more information, go to **www.CLARINEX.com.**

What are the ingredients in CLARINEX-D® 24 Hour Extended Release Tablets?

Active ingredients: desloratadine and pseudoephedrine sulfate

Inactive ingredients: hypromellose USP, ethylcellulose NF, dibasic calcium phosphate dihydrate USP, magnesium stearate NF, povidone USP, silicone dioxide NF, talc USP, polyacrylate dispersion, polyethylene glycol NF, simethicone USP, Blue Lake Blend 50726 (FD&C Blue No. 2 Lake, titanium dioxide USP and edetate disodium USP), and ink (Opacode® S-1-17746 or Opacode® S-1-4159).

Manufactured by Schering Corporation, a subsidiary of Schering-Plough Corporation,
Kenilworth, NJ 07033 USA.

Rev: Month/Year

U.S. Patent Nos. 4,659,716; 4,863,931; 5,595,997; and 6,100,274

COMVAX® ℞

[com-vax]

[Haemophilus b Conjugate (Meningococcal Protein Conjugate) and Hepatitis B (Recombinant) Vaccine]

DESCRIPTION

COMVAX® [Haemophilus b Conjugate (Meningococcal Protein Conjugate) and Hepatitis B (Recombinant) Vaccine] is a sterile bivalent vaccine made of the antigenic components used in producing PedvaxHIB® [Haemophilus b Conjugate Vaccine (Meningococcal Protein Conjugate)] and RECOMBIVAX HB® [Hepatitis B Vaccine (Recombinant)]. These components are the *Haemophilus influenzae* type b capsular polysaccharide [polyribosylribitol phosphate (PRP)] that is covalently bound to an outer membrane protein complex (OMPC) of *Neisseria meningitidis* and hepatitis B surface antigen (HBsAg) from recombinant yeast cultures.

Haemophilus influenzae type b and *Neisseria meningitidis* serogroup B are grown in complex fermentation media. The primary ingredients of the phenol-inactivated fermentation medium for *Haemophilus influenzae* include an extract of yeast, nicotinamide adenine dinucleotide, hemin chloride, soy peptone, dextrose, and mineral salts and for *Neisseria meningitidis* include an extract of yeast, amino acids and mineral salts. The PRP is purified from the culture broth by purification procedures which include ethanol fractionation, enzyme digestion, phenol extraction and diafiltration. The OMPC from *Neisseria meningitidis* is purified by detergent extraction, ultracentrifugation, diafiltration and sterile filtration.

The PRP-OMPC conjugate is prepared by the chemical coupling of the highly purified PRP (polyribosylribitol phosphate) of *Haemophilus influenzae* type b (Haemophilus b, Ross strain) to an OMPC of the B11 strain of *Neisseria meningitidis* serogroup B. The coupling of the PRP to the OMPC is necessary for enhanced immunogenicity of the PRP. This coupling is confirmed by analysis of the components of the conjugate following chemical treatment which yields a unique amino acid. After conjugation, the aqueous bulk is then adsorbed onto an amorphous aluminum hydroxyphosphate sulfate adjuvant (previously referred to as aluminum hydroxide).

HBsAg is produced in recombinant yeast cells. A portion of the hepatitis B virus gene, coding for HBsAg, is cloned into yeast, and the vaccine for hepatitis B is produced from cultures of this recombinant yeast strain according to methods developed in the Merck Research Laboratories. The antigen is harvested and purified from fermentation cultures of a recombinant strain of the yeast *Saccharomyces cerevisiae* containing the gene for the *adw* subtype of HBsAg. The fermentation process involves growth of *Saccharomyces cerevisiae* on a complex fermentation medium which consists of an extract of yeast, soy peptone, dextrose, amino acids and mineral salts.

The HBsAg protein is released from the yeast cells by mechanical cell disruption and detergent extraction, and purified by a series of physical and chemical methods, which includes ion and hydrophobic chromatography, and diafiltration. The purified protein is treated in phosphate buffer with formaldehyde and then coprecipitated with alum (potassium aluminum sulfate) to form bulk vaccine adjuvanted with amorphous aluminum hydroxyphosphate sulfate. The vaccine contains no detectable yeast DNA, and 1% or less of the protein is of yeast origin.

The individual PRP-OMPC and HBsAg adjuvanted bulks are combined to produce COMVAX. Each 0.5 mL dose of COMVAX is formulated to contain 7.5 mcg PRP conjugated to approximately 125 mcg OMPC, 5 mcg HBsAg, approximately 225 mcg aluminum as amorphous aluminum hydroxyphosphate sulfate, and 35 mcg sodium borate (decahydrate) as a pH stabilizer, in 0.9% sodium chloride. The vaccine contains not more than 0.0004% (w/v) residual formaldehyde.

The potency of the PRP-OMPC component is measured by quantitating the polysaccharide concentration by an HPLC method. The potency of the HBsAg component is measured relative to a standard by an *in vitro* immunoassay.

The product contains no preservative.

COMVAX is a sterile suspension for intramuscular injection.

CLINICAL PHARMACOLOGY

Haemophilus influenzae type b Disease

Prior to the introduction of *Haemophilus b* conjugate vaccines, *Haemophilus influenzae* type b (Hib) was the most frequent cause of bacterial meningitis and a leading cause of serious, systemic bacterial disease in young children worldwide.{1-4}

Hib disease occurred primarily in children under 5 years of age, and in the United States prior to the initiation of a vaccine program was estimated to account for nearly 20,000 cases of invasive infections annually, approximately 12,000 of which were meningitis. The mortality rate from Hib meningitis is about 5%. In addition, up to 35% of survivors develop neurologic sequelae including seizures, deafness, and mental retardation.{5,6} Other invasive diseases caused by this bacterium include cellulitis, epiglottitis, sepsis, pneumonia, septic arthritis, osteomyelitis, and pericarditis.

Prior to the introduction of the vaccine, it was estimated that 17% of all cases of Hib disease occurred in infants less than 6 months of age. The peak incidence of Hib meningitis occurred between 6 to 11 months of age. Forty-seven percent of all cases occurred by one year of age with the remaining 53% of cases occurring over the next four years.{2,20}

Among children under 5 years of age, the risk of invasive Hib disease is increased in certain populations including the following:

- Daycare attendees{7,8,9}
- Lower socio-economic groups{10}
- Blacks{11} (especially those who lack the Km(1) immunoglobulin allotype){12}
- Caucasians who lack the G2m(23) immunoglobulin allotype{13}
- Native Americans{14-16}
- Household contacts of cases{17}
- Individuals with asplenia, sickle cell disease, or antibody deficiency syndromes.{18,19}

Prevention of Hib Disease with Vaccine

An important virulence factor of the Hib bacterium is its polysaccharide capsule (PRP). Antibody to PRP (anti-PRP) has been shown to correlate with protection against Hib disease.{3,21} While the anti-PRP level associated with protection using conjugated vaccines has not yet been determined, the level of anti-PRP associated with protection in studies using bacterial polysaccharide immune globulin or nonconjugated PRP vaccines ranged from ≥0.15 to ≥1.0 mcg/mL.{22-28}

Nonconjugated PRP vaccines are capable of stimulating B-lymphocytes to produce antibody without the help of T-lymphocytes (T-independent). The responses to many other antigens are augmented by helper T-lymphocytes (T-dependent). PedvaxHIB is a PRP-conjugate vaccine in which the PRP is covalently bound to the OMPC carrier{29} producing an antigen which is postulated to convert the T-independent antigen (PRP alone) into a T-dependent antigen resulting in both an enhanced antibody response and immunologic memory.

Clinical Trials with PedvaxHIB

The protective efficacy of the PRP-OMPC component of COMVAX was demonstrated in a randomized, double-blind, placebo-controlled study involving 3486 Native American (Navajo) infants (The Protective Efficacy Study) who completed the primary two-dose regimen for lyophilized PedvaxHIB. This population has a much higher incidence of Hib disease than the United States population as a whole and also has a lower antibody response to Haemophilus b conjugate vaccines, including PedvaxHIB.{14-16,30,31}

Each infant in this study received two doses of either placebo or lyophilized PedvaxHIB (15 mcg Haemophilus b PRP) with the first dose administered at a mean of 8 weeks of age and the second administered approximately two months later; DTP (Diphtheria and Tetanus Toxoids and whole cell Pertussis Vaccine, Adsorbed) and OPV (Poliovirus Vaccine Live Oral Trivalent) were administered concomitantly. In a subset of 416 subjects, lyophilized PedvaxHIB (15 mcg Haemophilus b PRP) induced anti-PRP levels >0.15 mcg/mL in 88% and >1.0 mcg/mL in 52% with a geometric mean titer (GMT) of 0.95 mcg/mL one to three months after the first dose; the corresponding anti-PRP levels one to three months following the second dose were 91% and 60%, respectively, with a GMT of 1.43 mcg/mL. These antibody responses were associated with a high level of protection.

Most subjects were initially followed until 15 to 18 months of age. During this time, 22 cases of invasive Hib disease occurred in the placebo group (8 cases after the first dose and 14 cases after the second dose) and only 1 case in the vaccine group (none after the first dose and 1 after the second dose). Following the primary two-dose regimen, the protective efficacy of lyophilized PedvaxHIB was calculated to be 93% with a 95% confidence interval (C.I.) of 57-98%. In the two months between the first and second doses, the difference in number of cases of disease between placebo and vaccine recipients (8 vs 0 cases, respectively) was statistically significant (p=0.008). At termination of the study, placebo recipients were offered vaccine. All original participants were then followed two years and nine months from termination of the study. During this extended follow-up, invasive Hib disease occurred in an additional 7 of the original placebo recipients prior to receiving vaccine and in 1 of the original vaccine recipients (who had received only 1 dose of vaccine). No cases of invasive Hib disease were observed in placebo recipients after they received at least one dose of vaccine. Efficacy for this follow-up period, estimated from person-days at risk, was 96.6% (95 C.I., 72.2-99.9%) in children under 18 months of age and 100% (95 C.I., 23.5-100%) in children over 18 months of age.{31} Thus, in this study, a protective efficacy of 93% was achieved with an anti-PRP level of >1.0 mcg/mL in 60% of vaccinees and a GMT of 1.43 mcg/mL one to three months after the second dose.

Hepatitis B Disease

Hepatitis B virus is an important cause of viral hepatitis. According to the Centers for Disease Control (CDC), there are an estimated 200,000-300,000 new cases of Hepatitis B infection annually in the United States.{32} There is no specific treatment for this disease. The incubation period for hepatitis B is relatively long; six weeks to six months may elapse between exposure and the onset of clinical symptoms. The prognosis following infection with hepatitis B virus is variable and dependent on at least three factors: (1) Age — infants and younger children usually experience milder initial disease than older persons but are much more likely to remain persistently infected and become at risk of developing serious chronic liver disease; (2) Dose of virus — the higher the dose, the more likely acute icteric hepatitis B will result; and, (3) Severity of associated underlying disease — underlying malignancy or pre-existing hepatic disease predisposes to increased mortality and morbidity.{34}

Hepatitis B infection fails to resolve and progresses to a chronic carrier state in 5 to 10% of older children and adults and in up to 90% of infants; chronic infection also occurs more frequently after initial anicteric hepatitis B than after initial icteric disease.{34} Consequently, carriers of HBsAg frequently give no history of having had recognized acute hepatitis. It has been estimated that more than 285 million people in the world today are persistently infected with hepatitis B virus.{35} The CDC estimates that there are approximately 1 million-1.25 million chronic carriers of hepatitis B virus in the USA.{32} Chronic carriers represent the largest human reservoir of hepatitis B virus.

A serious complication of acute hepatitis B virus infection is massive hepatic necrosis while sequelae of chronic hepatitis B include cirrhosis of the liver, chronic active hepatitis, and hepatocellular carcinoma. Chronic carriers of HBsAg appear to be at increased risk of developing hepatocellular carcinoma. Although a number of etiologic factors are associated with development of hepatocellular carcinoma, the single most important etiologic factor appears to be chronic infection with hepatitis B virus.{36} According to the CDC, hepatitis B vaccine is recognized as the first anti-cancer vaccine because it can prevent primary liver cancer.{67}

The vehicles for transmission of the virus are most often blood and blood products but the viral antigen has also been found in tears, saliva, breast milk, urine, semen, and vaginal secretions. Hepatitis B virus is capable of surviving for days on environmental surfaces exposed to body fluids containing hepatitis B virus. Infection may occur when hepatitis B virus, transmitted by infected body fluids, is implanted via mucous surfaces or percutaneously introduced through accidental or deliberate breaks in the skin. Transmission of hepatitis B virus infection is often associated with close interpersonal contact with an infected individual and with crowded living conditions.{37}

Prevention of Hepatitis B Disease with Vaccine

Hepatitis B infection and disease can be prevented through immunization with vaccines that contain viral surface antigen (HBsAg) and induce formation of protective antibody (anti-HBs).{38-39}

Multiple clinical studies have defined a protective level of anti-HBs as 1) 10 or more sample ratio units (SRU or S/N) as determined by radioimmunoassay or 2) a positive result as determined by enzyme immunoassay.{40-46} Note: 10 SRU is comparable to 10 mIU/mL of antibody.{36} The ACIP and an international group of hepatitis B experts consider an anti-HBs titer ≥10 mIU/mL an adequate response to a complete course of hepatitis B vaccine and protective against clinically significant infection (antigenemia with or without clinical disease).{36,46}

Clinical Trials with RECOMBIVAX HB

In clinical studies, 100% of 92 infants under 1 year of age born of non-carrier mothers developed a protective level of antibody (anti-HBs ≥10 mIU/mL) after receiving three 5-mcg doses of RECOMBIVAX HB at intervals of 0, 1, and 6 months.{31}

In one clinical study of RECOMBIVAX HB (2.5 mcg), which examined a different regimen of RECOMBIVAX HB, protective levels of antibody were achieved in 98% of 52 healthy infants vaccinated at 2, 4, and 12 months of age. Protective anti-HBs levels were achieved in 100% of 50 infants vaccinated at 2, 4, and 15 months of age.{47}

The protective efficacy of three 5-mcg doses of RECOMBIVAX HB, given at birth (with Hepatitis B Immune Globulin), 1, and 6 months of age, has been demonstrated in neonates born of mothers positive for both HBsAg and HBeAg (a core-associated antigenic complex which correlates with high infectivity). In this trial, after nine months of follow-up, chronic infection had not occurred in 96% of 130 infants.{48} The estimated efficacy in prevention of chronic hepatitis B infection was 95% as compared to the infection rate in untreated historical controls.{49}

Immunogenicity of COMVAX

The immunogenicity of COMVAX (7.5 mcg Haemophilus b PRP, 5 mcg HBsAg) was assessed in 1602 infants and children 6 weeks to 15 months of age in 5 clinical studies. In 2 controlled clinical trials (n=684), the immune response of COMVAX was compared with that obtained using the monovalent vaccines, PedvaxHIB (7.5 mcg Haemophilus b PRP) and RECOMBIVAX HB (5 mcg HBsAg) given at separate sites, either concurrently or one month apart. The immunogenicity of COMVAX was further assessed in 2 uncontrolled studies (n=852). In the first, a complete three-dose series of COMVAX was administered concurrently with other routine

Table 1: Antibody Responses to COMVAX, PedvaxHIB, and RECOMBIVAX HB in Infants Not Previously Vaccinated with Hib or Hepatitis B Vaccine

Vaccine	Age (months)	Time	n	Anti-PRP % Subjects with >0.15 mcg/mL	Anti-PRP % Subjects with >1.0 mcg/mL	Anti-PRP GMT (mcg/mL)	n	Anti-HBs % Subjects ≥10 mIU/mL	Anti-HBs GMT (mIU/mL)
COMVAX		Prevaccination	633	34.4	4.7	0.1	603	10.6	0.6
(7.5 mcg PRP,	2	Dose 1*	620	88.9	51.5	1.0	595	34.3	4.2
5 mcg HBsAg)	4	Dose 2*	576	94.8	72.4†	2.5†	571	92.1	113.9
[N=661]	12/15	Dose 3‡	570	99.3	92.6	9.5	571	98.4	4467.5†
PedvaxHIB		Prevaccination	208	33.7	5.8	0.1	196	7.1	0.5
(7.5 mcg PRP)	2	Dose 1*	202	90.1	53.5	1.1	198	41.9	5.3
+	4	Dose 2*	186	95.2	76.3†	2.8†	185	98.4†	255.7
RECOMBIVAX HB	12/15	Dose 3‡	181	98.9	92.3	10.2	179	100.0†	6943.9†
(5 mcg HBsAg)									
[N=221]									

* Postvaccination responses were determined approximately two months after doses 1 and 2.

† C.I.'s of comparisons:

Dose 2 Anti-PRP: 95% C.I. on difference in % >1.0 mcg/mL (-11.2, 3.1); 95% C.I. on ratio of GMT (0.69, 1.17)

Dose 3 Anti-HBs: 95% C.I. on difference in % ≥10 mIU/mL (-2.9, -0.6); 95% C.I. on ratio of GMT (0.49, 0.91)

‡ Postvaccination responses were determined approximately one month after administration of dose 3.

More than three-quarters of the infants in the study received DTP and OPV concomitantly with the first two doses of COMVAX or PedvaxHIB plus RECOMBIVAX HB, and approximately one-third received M-M-R® II (Measles, Mumps, and Rubella Virus Vaccine Live) with the third dose of these vaccines at 12 or 15 months of age.

Table 2: Antibody Responses to COMVAX in Infants Previously Vaccinated with Hepatitis B Vaccine at Birth

Study	Age (months) at Vaccination	Time	n	Anti-PRP % Subjects with >0.15 mcg/mL	Anti-PRP % Subjects with >1.0 mcg/mL	Anti-PRP GMT (mcg/mL)	n	Anti-HBs % Subjects ≥10 mIU/mL	Anti-HBs GMT (mIU/mL)
		Prevaccination	119	24.4	5.9	0.1	71	25.4	2.9
Study 1	2	Dose 1	Not Measured						
[N=126]	4	Dose 2*	111	94.6	81.1	3.3	111	98.2	417.2
	14/15	Dose 3*	88	100	93.2	11.0	87	98.9	3500.7
		Prevaccination	17	58.8	0	0.2	15	6.7	0.7
Study 2	2	Dose 1†	17	88.2	47.1	0.9	16	81.3	35.2
[N=19]	4	Dose 2†	17	100	76.5	2.8	16	100	281.8
	15	Dose 3†	15	100	100	8.5	16	100	3913.4

* Postvaccination responses were determined approximately 2 months after dose 2 and 1 month after dose 3.

† Postvaccination responses were determined approximately 2 months after doses 1, 2, and 3.

Infants in these studies received DTP and OPV or eIPV (enhanced inactivated poliovirus vaccine) concomitantly with the first two doses of COMVAX, while the third dose of COMVAX was given concomitantly with DTaP (diphtheria and tetanus and acellular pertussis), OPV, and M-M-R® II at 14-15 months of age (Study 1) or with just M-M-R® II at 15 months of age (Study 2).

pediatric vaccines. In the second, COMVAX was administered as the third dose of Haemophilus b PRP and HBsAg concurrently with routine pediatric vaccines. COMVAX was also administered as the control arm in the evaluation of an investigational vaccine (n=66).

These studies demonstrate COMVAX to be highly immunogenic. The antibody responses are summarized below.

Antibody Responses to COMVAX in Infants Not Previously Vaccinated with Hib or Hepatitis B Vaccine

In the pivotal, controlled, multicenter, randomized, open-label study, 882 infants approximately 2 months of age, who had not previously received any Hib or hepatitis B vaccine, were assigned to receive a three-dose regimen of either COMVAX or PedvaxHIB plus RECOMBIVAX HB at approximately 2, 4, and 12-15 months of age. The proportions of evaluable vaccinees developing clinically important levels of anti-PRP (percent with >1.0 mcg/mL after the second dose, n=762) and anti-HBs (percent with ≥10 mIU/mL after the third dose, n=750) were similar in children given COMVAX or concurrent PedvaxHIB and RECOMBIVAX HB (Table 1). The anti-PRP response after the second dose among infants given COMVAX in this study was 72.4% (C.I. 68.7, 76.0) >1.0 mcg/mL with a GMT=2.5 mcg/mL (C.I. 2.2, 2.8) and was comparable to that of infants given the PedvaxHIB and RECOMBIVAX HB controls which was 76.3% (C.I. 70.2, 82.5) with a GMT=2.8 mcg/mL (C.I. 2.2, 3.5). These responses exceed the response of Native American (Navajo) infants in a previous study of lyophilized PedvaxHIB (60% >1.0 mcg/mL; GMT=1.43 mcg/mL) that was associated with a 93% reduction in the incidence of invasive Hib disease. The efficacy of COMVAX in the prevention of invasive Hib disease is expected to be similar to that obtained with monovalent lyophilized PedvaxHIB in the Protective Efficacy Trial (see CLINICAL PHARMACOLOGY, Clinical Trials with PedvaxHIB).

The anti-HBs response after the third dose among infants given COMVAX in this study was 98.4% ≥10 mIU/mL (C.I. 97.0, 99.3) with a GMT of 4467.5 (C.I. 3786.3, 5271.3) compared to 100.0% (C.I. 97.9, 100.0) with a GMT of 6943.9 (C.I. 5555.9, 8678.7) among infants given COMVAX or concurrent PedvaxHIB and RECOMBIVAX HB.

Although the difference in anti-HBs GMT is statistically significant (p=0.011), both values are much greater than the level of 10 mIU/mL previously established as marking a protective response to hepatitis B.{42,44-46,51,52} These GMTs are higher than those observed in young infants who received the currently licensed regimen of RECOMBIVAX HB consisting of 5-mcg doses administered on the standard 0, 1, and 6-month schedule (GMT ~ 1359.9 mIU/mL).{53-55} In addition, two studies have shown that infants given 2.5-mcg doses of RECOMBIVAX HB according to the schedule used for COMVAX (2, 4, and 12-15 months of age) developed GMTs of 1245-3424 mIU/mL.{47,64} While a difference in GMT may result in differential retention of ≥10 mIU/mL of anti-HBs after a number of years, this is of no apparent clinical significance because of immunologic memory.{56,57} Because the HBsAg component of COMVAX induces a comparable anti-HBs response to that obtained with RECOMBIVAX HB, the efficacy of COMVAX is expected to be similar (Table 1).

[See table 1 above]

Antibody Responses to COMVAX in Infants Previously Vaccinated with Hepatitis B Vaccine at Birth

Two clinical studies assessed antibody responses to a three-dose series of COMVAX in 128 evaluable infants who were previously given a birth dose of hepatitis B vaccine. Table 2 summarizes the anti-PRP and anti-HBs responses of these infants. The antibody responses were clinically comparable to those observed in the pivotal trial of COMVAX (Table 1).

[See table 2 above]

Interchangeability of COMVAX and Licensed Haemophilus b Conjugate Vaccines or Recombinant Hepatitis B Vaccines

Among 58 children previously given a primary course of PedvaxHIB, 90% (95% C.I. 78.8%, 96.1%) developed an anti-PRP response >1 mcg/mL with a GMT of 9.6 mcg/mL (95% C.I. 6.6, 14.1) in response to a dose of COMVAX at 12-15 months of age. Among 683 children previously given a primary course of another HIB or HIB-containing vaccine, 99% (95% C.I. 97.9%, 99.6%) developed an anti-PRP response >1 mcg/mL with a GMT of 14.9 mcg/mL (95% C.I. 13.7, 16.3) in response to a dose of COMVAX at 12-15 months of age.

In another study, COMVAX was administered either concomitantly or six weeks after vaccination with M-M-R® II and VARIVAX® (Varicella Virus Vaccine Live, Oka/Merck). Among 149 children who previously received 2 doses of monovalent Hepatitis B vaccine, 100% (95% C.I. 97.6%, 100.0%) developed an anti-HBs response ≥10 mIU/mL with a GMT of 2194.6 mIU/mL (95% C.I. 1667.8, 2887.8) in response to a dose of COMVAX at 12-15 months of age.

Antibody Responses to COMVAX and Concurrently Administered Vaccines

Immunogenicity results from open-labeled studies indicate that COMVAX can be administered concomitantly with DTP, DTaP, OPV, IPV (inactivated poliomyelitis vaccine), M-M-R II, and VARIVAX using separate sites and syringes for injectable vaccines.

DTP and DTaP

After a primary series of DTP (2, 4, 6 months of age) given concomitantly with COMVAX (2 and 4 months of age), 98.2% of 57 infants developed a 4-fold rise in antibody to diphtheria, 100% of 57 infants developed a 4-fold rise in antibody to tetanus, and 89.5% to 96.5% of 57 infants developed a 4-fold rise in antibody to pertussis antigens, depending on the assay used and adjusted for maternal antibody. In this trial, after 2 doses of COMVAX, 79.0% of 62 infants developed anti-PRP >1.0 mcg/mL and after 3 doses (2, 4, and 15 months of age), 100% of 59 infants developed ≥10 mIU/mL of anti-HBs.

After a primary series of DTaP and COMVAX given concomitantly at 2, 4, and 6 months of age, 100% of 18 infants had ≥0.01 antitoxin units/mL to diphtheria and tetanus and 94.4% to 100% of 18 infants developed a ≥4-fold rise in antibody to pertussis antigens, depending on the assay used and adjusted for maternal antibody. In this trial, after 2 doses of COMVAX, 85.7% of 63 infants developed anti-PRP >1.0 mcg/mL and after 3 doses administered on the compressed schedule of 2, 4, and 6 months of age, 92.9% of 56 infants developed ≥10 mIU/mL of anti-HBs.

OPV and IPV

After a primary series of OPV (2, 4, 6 months of age) given concomitantly with COMVAX (2 and 4 months of age), 98.3% of 60 infants had neutralizing antibody ≥1:4 to poliovirus type 1, 100% of 57 infants had neutralizing antibody ≥1:4 to poliovirus type 2 and 98.1% of 53 infants had neutralizing antibody ≥1:4 to poliovirus type 3. In this trial, after 2 doses of COMVAX, 79.0% of 62 infants developed anti-PRP >1.0 mcg/mL and after 3 doses, 100% of 59 infants developed ≥10 mIU/mL of anti-HBs.

After a primary series of IPV and COMVAX given concomitantly at 2, 4, and 6 months of age, 100% of 38 infants had neutralizing antibody ≥1:4 to poliovirus types 1, 2, and 3. In this trial, after 2 doses of COMVAX, 85.7% of 63 infants developed anti-PRP >1.0 mcg/mL and after 3 doses administered on the compressed schedule of 2, 4, and 6 months of age, 92.9% of 56 infants developed ≥10 mIU/mL of anti-HBs.

M-M-R II and VARIVAX

After concomitant vaccination of M-M-R II and VARIVAX with COMVAX (12 to 15 months of age), 99.4% of 313 children developed antibody to measles, 99.2% of 354 children developed antibody to mumps, 100% of 358 children developed antibody to rubella and 100% of 276 children developed antibody to varicella. In this trial, infants received the primary series of Hib vaccine and the first two doses of Hepatitis B vaccine in the first year of life. After the dose of COMVAX, 97.8% of 368 infants developed >1.0 mcg/mL of anti-PRP and 99.2% developed ≥10 mIU/mL of anti-HBs.

INDICATIONS AND USAGE

COMVAX is indicated for vaccination against invasive disease caused by *Haemophilus influenzae* type b and against infection caused by all known subtypes of hepatitis B virus in infants 6 weeks to 15 months of age born of HBsAg negative mothers.

Infants born to HBsAg positive mothers should receive Hepatitis B Immune Globulin and Hepatitis B Vaccine (Recombinant) at birth and should complete the hepatitis B vaccination series given according to a particular schedule (see manufacturer's circular for Hepatitis B Vaccine [Recombinant]).

Infants born to mothers of unknown HBsAg status should receive Hepatitis B Vaccine (Recombinant) at birth and should complete the hepatitis B vaccination series given according to a particular schedule (see manufacturer's circular for Hepatitis B Vaccine [Recombinant]).

Vaccination with COMVAX should ideally begin at approximately 2 months of age or as soon thereafter as possible. In order to complete the three-dose regimen of COMVAX, vaccination should be initiated no later than 10 months of age. Infants in whom vaccination with a PRP-OMPC-containing product (i.e., PedvaxHIB, COMVAX) is not initiated until 11 months of age do not require three doses of PRP-OMPC; however, three doses of an HBsAg-containing product are required for complete vaccination against hepatitis B, regardless of age. For infants and children not vaccinated according to the recommended schedule see DOSAGE AND ADMINISTRATION.

COMVAX will not protect against invasive disease caused by *Haemophilus influenzae* other than type b or against invasive disease (such as meningitis or sepsis) caused by other microorganisms. COMVAX will not prevent hepatitis caused by other viruses known to infect the liver. Because of the long incubation period for hepatitis B, it is possible for unrecognized infection to be present at the time the vaccine is given. The vaccine may not prevent hepatitis B in such patients.

As with other vaccines, COMVAX may not induce protective antibody levels immediately following vaccination and may not result in a protective antibody response in all individuals given the vaccine.

Use With Other Vaccines

Immunogenicity results from open-labeled studies indicate that COMVAX can be administered concomitantly with DTP, DTaP, OPV, IPV, M-M-R II, and VARIVAX using separate sites and syringes for injectable vaccines (see CLINICAL PHARMACOLOGY).

CONTRAINDICATIONS

Hypersensitivity to yeast or any component of the vaccine. The decision to administer or delay vaccination because of current or recent febrile illness depends on the severity of symptoms and on the etiology of the disease. The ACIP has recommended that immunization should be delayed during the course of an acute febrile illness.{63} All vaccines can be administered to persons with minor illnesses such as diarrhea, mild upper-respiratory infection with or without low-grade fever, or other low-grade febrile illness. Persons with moderate or severe febrile illness should be vaccinated as soon as they have recovered from the acute phase of the illness.

WARNINGS

Patients who develop symptoms suggestive of hypersensitivity after an injection should not receive further injections of the vaccine (see CONTRAINDICATIONS).

PRECAUTIONS

General

General care is to be taken by the health-care provider for the safe and effective use of this product.

As for any vaccine, adequate treatment provisions, including epinephrine, should be available for immediate use should an anaphylactic or anaphylactoid reaction occur.

Use caution when vaccinating latex-sensitive individuals since the vial stopper contains dry natural latex rubber that may cause allergic reactions.

As reported with Haemophilus b Polysaccharide Vaccine and another Haemophilus b Conjugate Vaccine, cases of Haemophilus b disease may occur in the week after vaccination, prior to the onset of the protective effects of the vaccines.

The packaging stopper of this product contains natural rubber latex which may cause allergic reactions.

Instructions to Health-care Provider

The health-care provider should determine the current health status and previous vaccination history of the vaccinee.

The health-care provider should question the patient, parent or guardian about reactions to a previous dose of COMVAX, PedvaxHIB or other Haemophilus b conjugate vaccines or RECOMBIVAX HB or other hepatitis B vaccines.

Injection of a blood vessel should be avoided.

COMVAX should be given with caution in infants with bleeding disorders such as hemophilia or thrombocytopenia, with steps taken to avoid the risk of hematoma following the injection.

If COMVAX is used in persons with malignancies or those receiving immunosuppressive therapy or who are otherwise immunocompromised, the expected immune response may not be obtained.

COMVAX is not contraindicated in the presence of HIV infection.{68}

Information for Vaccine Recipients and Parents/Guardians

The health-care provider should provide the vaccine information required to be given with each vaccination to the patient, parent or guardian.

The health-care provider should inform the patient, parent or guardian of the benefits and risks associated with vaccination. For risks associated with vaccination, see WARNINGS, PRECAUTIONS, and ADVERSE REACTIONS.

Laboratory Test Interactions

Sensitive tests (e.g., Latex Agglutination Kits) may detect PRP derived from the vaccine in the urine of some vaccinees for at least 30 days following vaccination with lyophilized PedvaxHIB{58}; in clinical studies with lyophilized PedvaxHIB, such children demonstrated a normal immune response to the vaccine. It is not known whether antigenuria will occur after vaccination with COMVAX.

Drug Interaction

Deferral of immunization may be considered in individuals receiving immunosuppressive therapy.

Carcinogenesis, Mutagenesis, Impairment of Fertility

COMVAX has not been evaluated for its carcinogenic or mutagenic potential, or its potential to impair fertility.

Pregnancy

Pregnancy Category C:

Animal reproduction studies have not been conducted with COMVAX. It is also not known whether COMVAX can cause fetal harm when administered to a pregnant woman or can affect reproduction capacity. COMVAX is not recommended for use in women of childbearing age.

Pediatric Use

Safety and effectiveness of COMVAX in infants below the age of 6 weeks and above the age of 15 months have not been established. However, studies have demonstrated that PedvaxHIB is safe and immunogenic when administered to infants and children up to the age of 71 months and RECOMBIVAX HB is safe and immunogenic in persons of all ages.

COMVAX should not be used in infants younger than 6 weeks of age because this will lead to a reduced anti-PRP response and may lead to immune tolerance (impaired ability to respond to subsequent exposure to the PRP antigen).{59-61}

Infants born to HBsAg-positive mothers should not receive COMVAX but instead should receive Hepatitis B Immune Globulin and Hepatitis B Vaccine (Recombinant) at birth and should complete the hepatitis B vaccination series given according to a particular schedule (see manufacturer's circular for Hepatitis B Vaccine [Recombinant]). (See DOSAGE AND ADMINISTRATION.)

Geriatric Use

This vaccine is NOT recommended for use in adult populations.

ADVERSE REACTIONS

In clinical trials involving the administration of 7918 doses of COMVAX to 3561 healthy infants 6 weeks to 15 months of age, COMVAX was generally well tolerated. In these studies, infants received COMVAX with licensed pediatric vaccines (n=1745) or investigational vaccines (n=1816). Serious adverse experience data were available for all 3561 infants and non-serious adverse experience data were available for a subset of 1678 infants.

Pivotal Immunogenicity and Safety Study

In the pivotal, randomized, multicenter study, 882 infants were assigned in a 3:1 ratio to receive either COMVAX or PedvaxHIB plus RECOMBIVAX HB at separate injection sites at 2, 4, and 12-15 months of age. Children may have also received routine pediatric immunizations. The children were monitored daily for five days after each injection for injection-site and systemic adverse experiences. During this time, adverse experiences in infants who received COMVAX were generally similar in type and frequency to those observed in infants who received PedvaxHIB plus RECOMBIVAX HB.

The most frequently cited events were mild, transient signs and symptoms of inflammation at the injection site (i.e., pain/soreness, erythema, and swelling/induration), somnolence, and irritability, all of which were prompted for on report cards filled out by parents of vaccinated children. Table 3 summarizes the frequencies of injection-site and systemic adverse experiences within five days of vaccination that were reported among ≥1.0% of children in this pivotal trial.

[See table 3 above]

Table 3: Local Reactions and Systemic Complaints Within 5 Days After Injection Reported to Occur in ≥1.0%* of Children Given a 3-Dose Course of COMVAX Compared to These Events in Children Given Concomitant Injections of PedvaxHIB and RECOMBIVAX HB

Event	Injection 1† COMVAX (N=660) %	Injection 1† PedvaxHIB and RECOMBIVAX HB‡ (N=221) %	Injection 2† COMVAX (N=645) %	Injection 2† PedvaxHIB and RECOMBIVAX HB‡ (N=213) %	Injection 3 COMVAX (N=593) %	Injection 3 PedvaxHIB and RECOMBIVAX HB‡ (N=193) %
Injection Site Reactions						
Pain/Soreness§	34.5	37.6	24.3	25.8	23.9	21.2
Erythema (>1 in.)§	22.4 (2.7)	25.8 (2.7)	25.7 (1.4)	23.5 (3.3)	27.2 (3.0)	24.4 (1.6)
Swelling/Induration (>1 in.)§	27.6 (3.0)	33.5 (4.1)	30.4 (2.9)	31.0 (3.8)	27.2 (3.2)	29.5 (4.1)
Systemic Complaints						
Irritability§	57.0	46.6	50.7	44.1	32.2	29.0
Somnolence§	49.5	47.1	37.4	31.9	21.1	22.3
Crying—						
unusual, high pitched§	10.6	8.6	6.7	2.3	2.9	3.6
not otherwise specified	2.3	2.3	1.4	2.3	0.7	1.6
prolonged (>4 hrs.)§	2.4	2.3	0.8	1.4	0.2	0
Anorexia	3.9	2.3	2.0	0.9	0.8	0.5
Vomiting	2.1	1.8	2.5	0.9	1.0	1.6
Otitis media	0.5	0	2.0	1.4	2.7	1.6
Fever (°F, rectal equiv.)¶						
101.0-102.9	14.2	11.9	13.8	12.2	10.5	6.4
≥103.0	0.8	0	1.6	1.4	2.7	4.3
Diarrhea	1.7	1.8	0.8	0.9	2.2	0.5
Upper respiratory infection	0.5	0.5	1.1	0.9	1.3	0.5
Rash	0.8	0	0.9	0	0.8	0.5
Rhinorrhea	0.2	0	1.1	0.9	1.3	2.1
Respiratory congestion	0.6	0.5	1.2	0.9	0.3	0.5
Cough	0.2	0	0.9	0.5	0.2	1.0
Candidiasis, oral	0.3	0.5	0.8	0	0.2	0
Rash, diaper	0.5	0.5	0.5	0.9	0.2	0

* Overall frequency of each event listed above is ≥1% even though the frequency after a given dose may be <1%.

† Most children received DTP and OPV concomitantly with the first two doses of COMVAX or PedvaxHIB and RECOMBIVAX HB.

‡ Injection site reactions for PedvaxHIB and RECOMBIVAX HB based on occurrence with either of the monovalent components.

§ Events prompted for on Vaccination Report Card given to parents/guardians of vaccinees.

¶ N for injections 1, 2, and 3 equals 655, 639, and 588, respectively, for COMVAX; N for injections 1, 2, and 3 equals 218, 213, and 187, respectively, for PedvaxHIB and RECOMBIVAX HB.

Infants Previously Vaccinated with Hepatitis B Vaccine

In a group of infants (N=126) given a three-dose course of COMVAX after previously receiving a dose of Hepatitis B Vaccine (Recombinant) at or shortly after birth, the type, frequency, and severity of adverse experiences did not appear to be greater than those observed in infants in the pivotal study who did not receive hepatitis B vaccine at birth.

Infants 6 Weeks to 15 Months of Age

In clinical trials, 3285 doses of COMVAX were administered to 1678 infants who were monitored for injection-site and systemic adverse experiences from Days 0 to 5 after each injection of vaccine. Of these, 855 infants had safety data following vaccination at approximately 2 months of age, 836 infants at approximately 4 months of age and 1573 infants at 12 to 15 months of age. The most frequently reported adverse experiences (≥1% of subjects for at least one injection), without regard to causality are listed in decreasing order of frequency within each body system:

Injection Site Reactions: Pain/tenderness/soreness, swelling/induration, erythema; *Body as a Whole:* Fever; *Digestive System:* Anorexia, diarrhea, vomiting; *Nervous System/Psychiatric:* Irritability, somnolence, crying; *Respiratory System:* Upper respiratory infection, rhinorrhea, cough, rhinitis; *Skin:* Rash; *Special Senses:* Otitis media.

Post-Marketing Experience

As with any vaccine, there is the possibility that broad use of COMVAX could reveal adverse experiences not observed in clinical trials. The following additional adverse reactions have been reported with the use of the marketed vaccine.

Hypersensitivity

Anaphylaxis, angioedema, urticaria, erythema multiforme

Hematologic

Thrombocytopenia

Nervous System

Seizure, febrile seizures

Potential Adverse Effects

In addition, a variety of adverse effects have been reported with marketed use of either PedvaxHIB or RECOMBIVAX HB in infants and children through 71 months of age. These adverse effects are listed below.

PedvaxHIB

Hematologic/Lymphatic

Lymphadenopathy

Skin

Sterile injection-site abscess; pain at the injection site

RECOMBIVAX HB

Hypersensitivity

Symptoms of hypersensitivity including reports of rash, pruritus, edema, arthralgia, dyspnea, hypotension, and ecchymoses

Cardiovascular System

Tachycardia; syncope

Digestive System

Elevation of liver enzymes

Hematologic

Increased erythrocyte sedimentation rate

Musculoskeletal System

Arthritis

Nervous System

Bell's Palsy; Guillain-Barré Syndrome

Psychiatric/Behavioral

Agitation; somnolence; irritability

Skin

Stevens-Johnson Syndrome; alopecia

Special Senses

Conjunctivitis; visual disturbances

Adverse Event Reporting

Patients, parents and guardians should be instructed to report any serious adverse reactions to their health-care provider who in turn should report such events to the U.S. Department of Health and Human Services through the Vaccine Adverse Event Reporting System (VAERS), 1-800-822-7967. The health-care provider should inform the parent or guardian of the National Vaccine Injury Compensation Program (NVICP), 1-800-338-2382.

DOSAGE AND ADMINISTRATION

FOR INTRAMUSCULAR ADMINISTRATION

Do not inject intravenously, intradermally, or subcutaneously.

Recommended Schedule

Infants born to HBsAg negative mothers should be vaccinated with three 0.5 mL doses of COMVAX, ideally at 2, 4, and 12-15 months of age. If the recommended schedule cannot be followed, the interval between the first two doses should be at least six weeks and the interval between the second and third dose should be as close as possible to eight to eleven months.

Infants born to HBsAg-positive mothers should receive Hepatitis B Immune Globulin and Hepatitis B Vaccine (Recombinant) at birth and should complete the hepatitis B vaccination series given according to a particular schedule (see manufacturer's circular for Hepatitis B Vaccine [Recombinant]).

Infants born to mothers of unknown HBsAg status should receive Hepatitis B Vaccine (Recombinant) at birth and should complete the hepatitis B vaccination series given according to a particular schedule (see manufacturer's circular for Hepatitis B Vaccine [Recombinant]).

The subsequent administration of COMVAX for completion of the hepatitis B vaccination series in infants who were born to HBsAg positive mothers and received HBIG or infants born to mothers of unknown status has not been studied.

COMVAX should not be administered to any infant before the age of 6 weeks.

Modified Schedules

Children previously vaccinated with one or more doses of either hepatitis B vaccine or Haemophilus b conjugate vaccine

Children who receive one dose of hepatitis B vaccine at or shortly after birth may be administered COMVAX on the schedule of 2, 4, and 12-15 months of age. There are no data to support the use of a three-dose series of COMVAX in infants who have previously received more than one dose of hepatitis B vaccine. However, COMVAX may be administered to children otherwise scheduled to receive concurrent RECOMBIVAX HB and PedvaxHIB.

Children not vaccinated according to recommended schedule for COMVAX

Vaccination schedules for children not vaccinated according to the recommended schedule should be considered on an individual basis. The number of doses of a PRP-OMPC-containing product (i.e., COMVAX, PedvaxHIB) depends on the age that vaccination is begun. An infant 2 to 10 months of age should receive three doses of a product containing PRP-OMPC. An infant 11 to 14 months of age should receive two doses of a product containing PRP-OMPC. A child 15 to 71 months of age should receive one dose of a product containing PRP-OMPC. Infants and children, regardless of age, should receive three doses of an HBsAg-containing product.

COMVAX is for intramuscular injection. The *anterolateral thigh* is the recommended site for intramuscular injection in infants. Data suggests that injections given in the buttocks frequently are given into fatty tissue instead of into muscle. Such injections have resulted in a lower seroconversion rate (for hepatitis B vaccine) than was expected.

Injection must be accomplished with a needle long enough to ensure intramuscular deposition of the vaccine. The ACIP has recommended that for intramuscular injections, the needle should be of sufficient length to reach the muscle mass itself. In a clinical trial with COMVAX (see CLINICAL PHARMACOLOGY, Antibody Responses to COMVAX in Infants Not Previously Vaccinated with Hib or Hepatitis B Vaccine, Table 1) vaccination was accomplished with a needle length of 5/8 inches in accordance with ACIP recommendations in effect at that time.(62) ACIP currently recommends that needles of longer length (7/8 to 1 inch) be used.(63)

The vaccine should be used as supplied; no reconstitution is necessary.

Shake well before withdrawal and use. Thorough agitation is necessary to maintain suspension of the vaccine.

Parenteral drug products should be inspected visually for extraneous particulate matter and discoloration prior to administration whenever solution and container permit. After thorough agitation, COMVAX is a slightly opaque, white suspension.

It is important to use a separate sterile syringe and needle for each patient to prevent transmission of infectious agents from one person to another.

Interchangeability of COMVAX and Licensed Haemophilus b Conjugate Vaccines or Recombinant Hepatitis B Vaccines

Since 1990, the Advisory Committee on Immunization Practices (ACIP) and the Committee on Infectious Diseases of the American Academy of Pediatrics (AAP) have recommended routine immunization of infants starting at 2 months of age with a polysaccharide-protein conjugate vaccine to prevent invasive Hib disease.(32,33)

Three Hib vaccines are licensed for infant vaccination: 1) oligosaccharide conjugate Hib vaccine (HbOC) (HibTITER®[1]), 2) polyribosylribitol phosphate-tetanus toxoid conjugate (PRP-T) (ActHIB®[1] and OmniHIB®[1]), and 3) Haemophilus b conjugate vaccine (meningococcal protein conjugate) (PRP-OMPC) (PedvaxHIB). According to the ACIP, these products are now considered interchangeable for primary as well as booster vaccination.(66)

Because vaccination recommendations limited to high-risk individuals have failed to substantially lower the overall incidence of hepatitis B infection, both the Advisory Committee on Immunization Practices (ACIP) and the Committee on Infectious Diseases of the American Academy of Pediatrics (AAP) have endorsed universal infant immunization as part of a comprehensive strategy for the control of hepatitis B infection.(32,50)

[1] HibTITER is a registered trademark of Lederle Laboratories, ActHIB is a registered trademark of Aventis Pasteur Inc. and OmniHIB is a registered trademark of GlaxoSmithKline.

HOW SUPPLIED

No. 4898 — COMVAX is supplied as 7.5 mcg PRP polysaccharide conjugated to approximately 125 mcg OMPC and 5 mcg HBsAg in a box of 10 single dose vials.

NDC 0006-4898-00.

Storage

Store vaccine at 2-8°C (36-46°F). Storage above or below the recommended temperature may reduce potency.

DO NOT FREEZE since freezing destroys potency.

REFERENCES

1. Cochi, S.L., et al. JAMA *253:* 521-529, 1985.
2. Schlech, W.F., III, et al. JAMA *253:* 1749-1754, 1985.
3. Peltola, H., et al. N Engl J Med *310:* 1561-1566, 1984.
4. Cardoz, M., et al. Bull WHO *59:* 575-584, 1981.
5. Sell, S.H., et al. Pediatr *49:* 206-217, 1972.
6. Taylor, H.G., et al. Pediatr *74:* 198-205, 1984.
7. Hay, J.W., et al. Pediatr *80*(3): 319-329, 1987.
8. Redmond, S.R., et al. JAMA *252:* 2581-2584, 1984.
9. Istre, G.R., et al. J Pediatr *106:* 190-195, 1985.
10. Fraser, D.W., et al. J Infect Dis *127:* 271-277, 1973.
11. Tarr, P.I., et al. J Pediatr *92:* 884-888, 1978.
12. Granoff, D.M., et al. J Clin Invest *74:* 1708-1714, 1984.
13. Ambrosino, D.M., et al. J Clin Invest *75:* 1935-1942, 1985.
14. Coulehan, J.L., et al. Pub Health Rep *99:* 404-409, 1984.
15. Losonsky, G.A., et al. Pediatr Infect Dis J *3:* 539-547, 1985.
16. Ward, J.I., et al. Lancet *1:* 1281-1285, 1981.
17. Ward, J.I., et al. N Engl J Med *301:* 122-126, 1979.
18. Ward, J.I., et al. J Pediatr *88:* 261-263, 1976.
19. Bartlett, A.V., et al. J Pediatr *102:* 55-58, 1983.
20. Centers for Disease Control. MMWR *34*(15): 201-205, 1985.
21. Santosham, M., et al. N Engl J Med *317:* 923-929, 1987.
22. Siber, G.R., et al. Infect Immun *45:* 248-254, 1984.
23. Smith, D.H., et al. Pediatr *52:* 637-644, 1973.
24. Robbins, J.B., et al. Pediatr Res *7:* 103-110, 1973.
25. Kaythy, H., et al. J Infect Dis *147:* 1100, 1983.
26. Peltola, H., et al. Pediatr *60:* 730-737, 1977.
27. Ward, J.I., et al. Pediatr *81:* 886-893, 1988.
28. Daum, R.S., et al. Pediatr *81:* 893-897, 1988.
29. Marburg, S., et al. J Am Chem Soc *108:* 5282-5287, 1986.
30. Letson, G.W., et al. Pediatr Infect Dis J *7*(111): 747-752, 1988.
31. Data on file at Merck Research Laboratories.
32. Centers for Disease Control. MMWR *40*(RR-1):1-25, 1991.
33. Committee on Infectious Disease. Update Pediatrics *88*(1): 169-172, 1991.
34. Robinson, W.S. "Principles and Practice of Infectious Diseases," G.L. Mandell; R.G. Douglas; J.E. Bennett (eds), vol. 2, New York, John Wiley & Sons, 1985, pp. 1002-1029.
35. Maynard, J. E., et al. "Viral Hepatitis and Liver Disease", A.J. Zuckerman (ed.), Alan R. Liss, Inc., 1988, pp. 967-969.
36. Centers for Disease Control. MMWR *39*(RR-2): 5-26, 1990.
37. Wands, J.R., et al. "Principles of Internal Medicine," G.W. Thorn, R.D. Adams, E. Braunwald, K.J. Isselbacher, R.G. Petersdorf (eds), vol. 2, McGraw-Hill, 1977, pp. 1590-1598.
38. Sitrin, R.D., Wampler, D.E., Ellis, R.W. Survey of licensed hepatitis B vaccines and their production processes. In: Ellis RW, ed. Hepatitis B vaccines in clinical practice. New York: Marcel Dekker, Inc., 1993, pp. 83-101.
39. West, D.J. Scope and design of hepatitis B vaccine clinical trials. In Ellis RW, ed. Hepatitis B vaccines in clinical practice. New York: Marcel Dekker, Inc., 1993, pp. 159-177.
40. Hadler, S.C., et al. NEJM *315*(4): 209-214, 1986.
41. Szmuness, W., et al. NEJM *303:* 833-841, 1980.
42. Francis, D.P., et al. Ann Int Med *97:* 362-366, 1982.
43. Szmuness, W., et al. NEJM *307:* 1481-1486, 1982.
44. Szmuness, W., et al. Hepatology *1:* 377-385, 1981.
45. Coutinho, R.A., et al. BMJ *286:* 1305-1308, 1983.
46. International Group: Immunisation against hepatitis B, Lancet *1*(8590): 875-876, 1988.
47. Keyserling, H.L., et al. J Pediatr *125*(1): 67-69, 1994.
48. Stevens, C.E.; Taylor, P.E.; Tong, M.J., et al. "Viral Hepatitis and Liver Diseases." A.J. Zuckerman (ed.), Alan R. Liss, Inc., 1988, pp. 982-983.
49. Stevens, C.E., et al. Pediatr *90*(1, Part 2): 170-173, 1992.
50. Universal Hepatitis B Immunization, Committee on Infectious Diseases. Pediatr *89*(4): 795-800, 1992.
51. Centers for Disease Control. MMWR *34:* 313-24, 329-35, 1985.
52. Centers for Disease Control. MMWR *36:* 353-60, 366, 1987.
53. West, D.J., et al. Pediatr Clin North Am *37:* 585-601, 1990.
54. Seto, D., et al. Pediatr Res *31*(4 Pt 2): 179A, 1992.
55. Froehlich, H. Pediatr Res *31*(4 Pt 2): 92A, 1992.
56. Jilg, W., et al. Infection *17:* 70-6, 1989.
57. West, D.J., et al. Vaccine *14*: 1019-27, 1996.
58. Goep, J.G., et al. Pediatr Infect Dis J *1*(1): 2-5, 1992.
59. Keyserling, H.L., et al. Program and Abstracts of the 30th ICAAC, 1990. (Abst. 63).
60. Ward, J.I., et al. Program and Abstracts of the 32nd ICAAC, 1992. (Abst. 984).
61. Lieberman, J.M., et al. Infect Dis, 199 (Abst.1028).
62. Centers for Disease Control. MMWR *38*(13): 205-228, 1989.
63. Centers for Disease Control. MMWR *43*(RR-1): 1994.
64. Reisenger, K.S., et al. Pediatr Res (4 pt. 2): 179A, 1993.
65. Centers for Disease Control. MMWR *46*(54): 74, 1998.

66. Centers for Disease Control. MMWR *47*(1): 9, 1998.
67. Centers for Disease Control. Federal Register, *64*(35):9044-9045, February 23, 1999.
68. Centers for Disease Control. MMWR *42*(RR-4): 1-18, April 9, 1993.

Manuf. and Dist. by: Merck Sharp & Dohme Corp., a subsidiary of
MERCK & CO., INC., Whitehouse Station, NJ 08889, USA
Issued December 2010
Printed in USA

9882603

COSOPT® PF ℞

(dorzolamide hydrochloride - timolol maleate ophthalmic solution)
2%/0.5%

HIGHLIGHTS OF PRESCRIBING INFORMATION
These highlights do not include all the information needed to use COSOPT PF safely and effectively. See full prescribing information for COSOPT PF.
COSOPT® PF (dorzolamide hydrochloride-timolol maleate ophthalmic solution) 2%/0.5%
Initial U.S. Approval: 1998

INDICATIONS AND USAGE

- COSOPT PF is a carbonic anhydrase inhibitor with a beta-adrenergic receptor blocking agent indicated for the reduction of elevated intraocular pressure (IOP) in patients with open-angle glaucoma or ocular hypertension who are insufficiently responsive to beta-blockers.
- The IOP-lowering of COSOPT twice daily was slightly less than that seen with the concomitant administration of 0.5% timolol twice daily, and 2% dorzolamide three times daily. (1)

DOSAGE AND ADMINISTRATION

The dose is one drop of COSOPT PF in the affected eye(s) two times daily. (2)

DOSAGE FORMS AND STRENGTHS

Solution containing 20 mg/mL dorzolamide and 5 mg/mL timolol. (3)

CONTRAINDICATIONS

COSOPT PF is contraindicated in patients with:
- Bronchial asthma or a history of bronchial asthma, severe chronic obstructive pulmonary disease. (4.1)
- Sinus bradycardia, second or third degree atrioventricular block, overt cardiac failure, cardiogenic shock. (4.2)
- Hypersensitivity to any component of this product. (4.3, 5.3)

WARNINGS AND PRECAUTIONS

- Potentiation of Respiratory Reactions Including Asthma (5.1)
- Cardiac Failure (5.2)
- Sulfonamide Hypersensitivity (5.3)
- Obstructive Pulmonary Disease (5.4)
- Increased Reactivity to Allergens (5.5)
- Potentiation of Muscle Weakness (5.6)
- Masking of Hypoglycemic Symptoms in Patients with Diabetes Mellitus (5.7)
- Masking of Thyrotoxicosis (5.8)
- Renal and Hepatic Impairment (5.9)
- Impairment of Beta-Adrenergically Mediated Reflexes During Surgery (5.10)

ADVERSE REACTIONS

The most frequently reported adverse reactions were taste perversion (bitter, sour, or unusual taste) or ocular burning and/or stinging in up to 30% of patients. Conjunctival hyperemia, blurred vision, superficial punctate keratitis or eye itching were reported between 5-15% of patients. (6)
To report SUSPECTED ADVERSE REACTIONS, contact Merck Sharp & Dohme Corp., a subsidiary of Merck & Co., Inc., at 1-877-888-4231 or FDA at 1-800-FDA-1088 or www.fda.gov/medwatch.

DRUG INTERACTIONS

- Potential additive effect of oral carbonic anhydrase inhibitor with COSOPT PF. (7.1)
- Potential acid-base and electrolyte disturbances. (7.2)
- Concomitant use with systemic beta-blockers may potentiate systemic beta-blockade. (7.3)
- Oral or intravenous calcium antagonists may cause atrioventricular conduction disturbances, left ventricular failure, and hypotension. (7.4)
- Catecholamine-depleting drugs may have additive effects and produce hypotension and/or marked bradycardia. (7.5)
- Digitalis and calcium antagonists may have additive effects in prolonging atrioventricular conduction time. (7.6)
- CYP2D6 inhibitors may potentiate systemic beta-blockade. (7.7)

See 17 for PATIENT COUNSELING INFORMATION and FDA-approved patient labeling

Revised: 05/2012

FULL PRESCRIBING INFORMATION: CONTENTS*

*** Sections or subsections omitted from the full prescribing information are not listed**

FULL PRESCRIBING INFORMATION

1 INDICATIONS AND USAGE

COSOPT® PF is indicated for the reduction of elevated intraocular pressure (IOP) in patients with open-angle glaucoma or ocular hypertension who are insufficiently responsive to beta-blockers (failed to achieve target IOP determined after multiple measurements over time). The IOP-lowering of COSOPT® administered twice a day was slightly less than that seen with the concomitant administration of 0.5% timolol administered twice a day and 2% dorzolamide administered three times a day *[see Clinical Studies (14.1)]*.

2 DOSAGE AND ADMINISTRATION

The dose is one drop of COSOPT PF in the affected eye(s) two times daily.
If more than one topical ophthalmic drug is being used, the drugs should be administered at least five minutes apart *[see Drug Interactions (7.3)]*.
The solution from one individual unit is to be used immediately after opening for administration to one or both eyes. Since sterility cannot be maintained after the individual unit is opened, the remaining contents should be discarded immediately after administration.

3 DOSAGE FORMS AND STRENGTHS

Solution containing 20 mg/mL dorzolamide (22.26 mg of dorzolamide hydrochloride) and 5 mg/mL timolol (6.83 mg timolol maleate).

4 CONTRAINDICATIONS

4.1 Asthma, COPD

COSOPT PF is contraindicated in patients with bronchial asthma, a history of bronchial asthma, or severe chronic obstructive pulmonary disease *[see Warnings and Precautions (5.1)]*.

4.2 Sinus Bradycardia, AV Block, Cardiac Failure, Cardiogenic Shock

COSOPT PF is contraindicated in patients with sinus bradycardia, second or third degree atrioventricular block, overt cardiac failure, and cardiogenic shock *[see Warnings and Precautions (5.2)]*.

4.3 Hypersensitivity

COSOPT PF is contraindicated in patients who are hypersensitive to any component of this product *[see Warnings and Precautions (5.3)]*.

5 WARNINGS AND PRECAUTIONS

5.1 Potentiation of Respiratory Reactions Including Asthma

COSOPT PF contains timolol maleate, a beta-adrenergic blocking agent; and although administered topically, is absorbed systemically. Therefore, the same types of adverse reactions that are attributable to systemic administration of beta-adrenergic blocking agents may occur with topical administration. For example, severe respiratory reactions, including death due to bronchospasm in patients with asthma, and rarely death in association with cardiac failure, have been reported following systemic or ophthalmic administration of timolol maleate *[see Contraindications (4.1) and Patient Counseling Information (17.1)]*.

5.2 Cardiac Failure

Sympathetic stimulation may be essential for support of the circulation in individuals with diminished myocardial contractility, and its inhibition by beta-adrenergic receptor blockade may precipitate more severe failure.
In patients without a history of cardiac failure continued depression of the myocardium with beta-blocking agents over a period of time can, in some cases, lead to cardiac failure. At the first sign or symptom of cardiac failure, COSOPT PF should be discontinued *[see Contraindications (4.2) and Patient Counseling Information (17.2)]*.

5.3 Sulfonamide Hypersensitivity

COSOPT PF contains dorzolamide, a sulfonamide; and although administered topically, it is absorbed systemically. Therefore, the same types of adverse reactions that are attributable to sulfonamides may occur with topical administration of COSOPT PF. Fatalities have occurred, although rarely, due to severe reactions to sulfonamides including Stevens-Johnson syndrome, toxic epidermal necrolysis, fulminant hepatic necrosis, agranulocytosis, aplastic anemia, and other blood dyscrasias. Sensitization may recur when a sulfonamide is readministered irrespective of the route of administration. If signs of serious reactions or hypersensitivity occur, discontinue the use of this preparation *[see Contraindications (4.3) and Patient Counseling Information (17.3)]*.

5.4 Obstructive Pulmonary Disease

Patients with chronic obstructive pulmonary disease (e.g., chronic bronchitis, emphysema) of mild or moderate severity, bronchospastic disease, or a history of bronchospastic disease (other than bronchial asthma or a history of bronchial asthma, in which COSOPT PF is contraindicated) should, in general, not receive beta-blocking agents, including COSOPT PF *[see Contraindications (4.1) and Patient Counseling Information (17.1)]*.

5.5 Increased Reactivity to Allergens

While taking beta-blockers, patients with a history of atopy or a history of severe anaphylactic reactions to a variety of allergens may be more reactive to repeated accidental, diagnostic, or therapeutic challenge with such allergens. Such patients may be unresponsive to the usual doses of epinephrine used to treat anaphylactic reactions.

5.6 Potentiation of Muscle Weakness

Beta-adrenergic blockade has been reported to potentiate muscle weakness consistent with certain myasthenic symptoms (e.g., diplopia, ptosis, and generalized weakness). Timolol has been reported rarely to increase muscle weakness in some patients with myasthenia gravis or myasthenic symptoms.

5.7 Masking of Hypoglycemic Symptoms in Patients with Diabetes Mellitus

Beta-adrenergic blocking agents should be administered with caution in patients subject to spontaneous hypoglycemia or to diabetic patients (especially those with labile diabetes) who are receiving insulin or oral hypoglycemic agents. Beta-adrenergic receptor blocking agents may mask the signs and symptoms of acute hypoglycemia.

5.8 Masking of Thyrotoxicosis

Beta-adrenergic blocking agents may mask certain clinical signs (e.g., tachycardia) of hyperthyroidism. Patients suspected of developing thyrotoxicosis should be managed carefully to avoid abrupt withdrawal of beta-adrenergic blocking agents that might precipitate a thyroid storm.

5.9 Renal and Hepatic Impairment

Dorzolamide has not been studied in patients with severe renal impairment (CrCl <30 mL/min). Because dorzolamide and its metabolite are excreted predominantly by the kidney, COSOPT PF is not recommended in such patients.

Dorzolamide has not been studied in patients with hepatic impairment and should therefore be used with caution in such patients.

5.10 Impairment of Beta-Adrenergically Mediated Reflexes During Surgery

The necessity or desirability of withdrawal of beta-adrenergic blocking agents prior to major surgery is controversial. Beta-adrenergic receptor blockade impairs the ability of the heart to respond to beta-adrenergically mediated reflex stimuli. This may augment the risk of general anesthesia in surgical procedures. Some patients receiving beta-adrenergic receptor blocking agents have experienced protracted severe hypotension during anesthesia. Difficulty in restarting and maintaining the heartbeat has also been reported. For these reasons, in patients undergoing elective surgery, some authorities recommend gradual withdrawal of beta-adrenergic receptor blocking agents.

If necessary during surgery, the effects of beta-adrenergic blocking agents may be reversed by sufficient doses of adrenergic agonists.

5.11 Corneal Endothelium

Carbonic anhydrase activity has been observed in both the cytoplasm and around the plasma membranes of the corneal endothelium. There is an increased potential for developing corneal edema in patients with low endothelial cell counts. Caution should be used when prescribing COSOPT PF to this group of patients.

6 ADVERSE REACTIONS

6.1 Clinical Studies Experience

Because clinical trials are conducted under widely varying conditions, adverse reaction rates observed in the clinical trials of a drug cannot be directly compared to rates in the clinical trials of another drug and may not reflect the rates observed in practice.

COSOPT and COSOPT PF

COSOPT and COSOPT PF were evaluated in patients with elevated intraocular pressure treated for open-angle glaucoma or ocular hypertension for up to 15 months. Approximately 5% of all patients discontinued therapy because of adverse reactions.

The most frequently reported adverse reactions occurring in up to 30% of patients were taste perversion (bitter, sour, or unusual taste) or ocular burning and/or stinging. The following adverse reactions were reported in 5-15% of patients: conjunctival hyperemia, blurred vision, superficial punctate keratitis or eye itching.

The following adverse reactions were reported in 1-5% of patients: abdominal pain, back pain, blepharitis, bronchitis, cloudy vision, conjunctival discharge, conjunctival edema, conjunctival follicles, conjunctival injection, conjunctivitis, corneal erosion, corneal staining, cortical lens opacity, cough, dizziness, dryness of eyes, dyspepsia, eye debris, eye discharge, eye pain, eye tearing, eyelid edema, eyelid erythema, eyelid exudate/scales, eyelid pain or discomfort, foreign body sensation, glaucomatous cupping, headache, hypertension, influenza, lens nucleus coloration, lens opacity, nausea, nuclear lens opacity, pharyngitis, post-subcapsular cataract, sinusitis, upper respiratory infection, urinary tract infection, visual field defect, vitreous detachment.

Other adverse reactions that have been reported with the individual components are listed below:

Dorzolamide 2%

Angioedema, asthenia/fatigue, bronchospasm, contact dermatitis, epistaxis, eyelid crusting, ocular discomfort, photophobia, signs and symptoms of ocular allergic reaction, transient myopia.

Timolol (ocular administration)

Body as a Whole: Asthenia/fatigue; *Cardiovascular:* Arrhythmia, syncope, cerebral ischemia, worsening of angina pectoris, palpitation, cardiac arrest, pulmonary edema, edema, claudication, Raynaud's phenomenon, and cold hands and feet; *Digestive:* Anorexia; *Immunologic:* Systemic lupus erythematosus; *Nervous System/Psychiatric:* Increase in signs and symptoms of myasthenia gravis, somnolence, insomnia, nightmares, behavioral changes and psychic disturbances including confusion, hallucinations, anxiety, disorientation, nervousness, and memory loss; *Skin:* Alopecia, psoriasiform rash or exacerbation of psoriasis; *Hypersensitivity:* Signs and symptoms of systemic allergic reactions, including anaphylaxis, angioedema, urticaria, and localized and generalized rash; *Respiratory:* Bronchospasm (predominantly in patients with pre-existing bronchospastic disease); *Endocrine:* Masked symptoms of hypoglycemia in diabetic patients; *Special Senses:* Ptosis, decreased corneal sensitivity, cystoid macular edema, visual disturbances including refractive changes and diplopia, pseudopemphigoid, and tinnitus; *Urogenital:* Retroperitoneal fibrosis, decreased libido, impotence, and Peyronie's disease.

6.2 Post-Marketing Experience

The following adverse reactions have been identified during post-approval use of COSOPT or COSOPT PF. Because these reactions are reported voluntarily from a population of uncertain size, it is not always possible to reliably estimate their frequency or establish a causal relationship to drug exposure: bradycardia, cardiac failure, cerebral vascular accident, chest pain, choroidal detachment following filtration surgery, depression, diarrhea, dry mouth, dyspnea, heart block, hypotension, iridocyclitis, myocardial infarction, nasal congestion, Stevens-Johnson syndrome, toxic epidermal necrolysis, paresthesia, photophobia, respiratory failure, skin rashes, urolithiasis, and vomiting.

Timolol (oral administration)

The following additional adverse reactions have been reported in clinical experience with ORAL timolol maleate or other ORAL beta-blocking agents and may be considered potential effects of ophthalmic timolol maleate: *Allergic:* Erythematous rash, fever combined with aching and sore throat, laryngospasm with respiratory distress; *Body as a Whole:* Extremity pain, decreased exercise tolerance, weight loss; *Cardiovascular:* Worsening of arterial insufficiency, vasodilatation; *Digestive:* Gastrointestinal pain, hepatomegaly, mesenteric arterial thrombosis, ischemic colitis; *Hematologic:* Nonthrombocytopenic purpura; thrombocytopenic purpura, agranulocytosis; *Endocrine:* Hyperglycemia, hypoglycemia; *Skin:* Pruritus, skin irritation, increased pigmentation, sweating; *Musculoskeletal:* Arthralgia; *Nervous System/Psychiatric:* Vertigo, local weakness, diminished concentration, reversible mental depression progressing to catatonia, an acute reversible syndrome characterized by disorientation for time and place, emotional lability, slightly clouded sensorium, and decreased performance on neuropsychometrics; *Respiratory:* Rales, bronchial obstruction; *Urogenital:* Urination difficulties.

7 DRUG INTERACTIONS

7.1 Oral Carbonic Anhydrase Inhibitors

There is a potential for an additive effect on the known systemic effects of carbonic anhydrase inhibition in patients receiving an oral carbonic anhydrase inhibitor and COSOPT PF. The concomitant administration of COSOPT PF and oral carbonic anhydrase inhibitors is not recommended.

7.2 High-Dose Salicylate Therapy

Although acid-base and electrolyte disturbances were not reported in the clinical trials with dorzolamide hydrochloride ophthalmic solution, these disturbances have been reported with oral carbonic anhydrase inhibitors and have, in some instances, resulted in drug interactions (e.g., toxicity associated with high-dose salicylate therapy). Therefore, the potential for such drug interactions should be considered in patients receiving COSOPT PF.

7.3 Beta-Adrenergic Blocking Agents

Patients who are receiving a beta-adrenergic blocking agent orally and COSOPT PF should be observed for potential additive effects of beta-blockade, both systemic and on intraocular pressure. The concomitant use of two topical beta-adrenergic blocking agents is not recommended.

7.4 Calcium Antagonists

Caution should be used in the coadministration of beta-adrenergic blocking agents, such as COSOPT PF, and oral or intravenous calcium antagonists because of possible atrioventricular conduction disturbances, left ventricular failure, and hypotension. In patients with impaired cardiac function, coadministration should be avoided.

7.5 Catecholamine-Depleting Drugs

Close observation of the patient is recommended when a beta-blocker is administered to patients receiving catecholamine-depleting drugs such as reserpine, because of possible additive effects and the production of hypotension and/or marked bradycardia, which may result in vertigo, syncope, or postural hypotension.

7.6 Digitalis and Calcium Antagonists

The concomitant use of beta-adrenergic blocking agents with digitalis and calcium antagonists may have additive effects in prolonging atrioventricular conduction time.

7.7 CYP2D6 Inhibitors

Potentiated systemic beta-blockade (e.g., decreased heart rate, depression) has been reported during combined treatment with CYP2D6 inhibitors (e.g., quinidine, SSRIs) and timolol.

7.8 Clonidine

Oral beta-adrenergic blocking agents may exacerbate the rebound hypertension which can follow the withdrawal of clonidine. There have been no reports of exacerbation of rebound hypertension with ophthalmic timolol maleate.

8 USE IN SPECIFIC POPULATIONS

8.1 Pregnancy

Teratogenic Effects. Pregnancy Category C. Developmental toxicity studies with dorzolamide hydrochloride in rabbits at oral doses of ≥2.5 mg/kg/day (31 times the recommended human ophthalmic dose) revealed malformations of the vertebral bodies. These malformations occurred at doses that caused metabolic acidosis with decreased body weight gain in dams and decreased fetal weights. No treatment-related malformations were seen at 1 mg/kg/day (13 times the recommended human ophthalmic dose).

Teratogenicity studies with timolol in mice, rats, and rabbits at oral doses up to 50 mg/kg/day (7,000 times the systemic exposure following the maximum recommended human ophthalmic dose) demonstrated no evidence of fetal malformations. Although delayed fetal ossification was observed at this dose in rats, there were no adverse effects on postnatal development of offspring. Doses of 1000 mg/kg/day (142,000 times the systemic exposure following the maximum recommended human ophthalmic dose) were maternotoxic in mice and resulted in an increased number of fetal resorptions. Increased fetal resorptions were also seen in rabbits at doses of 14,000 times the systemic exposure following the maximum recommended human ophthalmic dose, in this case without apparent maternotoxicity.

There are no adequate and well-controlled studies in pregnant women. COSOPT PF should be used during pregnancy only if the potential benefit justifies the potential risk to the fetus.

8.3 Nursing Mothers

It is not known whether dorzolamide is excreted in human milk. Timolol maleate has been detected in human milk following oral and ophthalmic drug administration. Because of the potential for serious adverse reactions from COSOPT PF in nursing infants, a decision should be made whether to discontinue nursing or to discontinue the drug, taking into account the importance of the drug to the mother.

8.4 Pediatric Use

The safety and effectiveness of dorzolamide hydrochloride ophthalmic solution and timolol maleate ophthalmic solution have been established when administered individually in pediatric patients aged 2 years and older. Use of these drug products in these children is supported by evidence from adequate and well-controlled studies in children and adults. Safety and efficacy in pediatric patients below the age of 2 years have not been established.

8.5 Geriatric Use

No overall differences in safety or effectiveness have been observed between elderly and younger patients.

10 OVERDOSAGE

Symptoms consistent with systemic administration of beta-blockers or carbonic anhydrase inhibitors may occur, including electrolyte imbalance, development of an acidotic state, dizziness, headache, shortness of breath, bradycardia, bronchospasm, cardiac arrest and possible central nervous system effects. Serum electrolyte levels (particularly potassium) and blood pH levels should be monitored. *[See Adverse Reactions (6).]*

A study of patients with renal failure showed that timolol did not dialyze readily.

11 DESCRIPTION

COSOPT PF (dorzolamide hydrochloride-timolol maleate ophthalmic solution) is the combination of a topical carbonic anhydrase inhibitor and a topical beta-adrenergic receptor blocking agent.

Dorzolamide hydrochloride is described chemically as: (4*S*-*trans*)-4-(ethylamino)-5,6-dihydro-6-methyl-4*H*-thieno[2,3-*b*]thiopyran-2-sulfonamide 7,7-dioxide monohydrochloride. Dorzolamide hydrochloride is optically active. The specific rotation is:

[α] $^{25°C}_{405\ nm}$ (C=1, water) = ~ -17°.

Its empirical formula is $C_{10}H_{16}N_2O_4S_3$•HCl and its structural formula is:

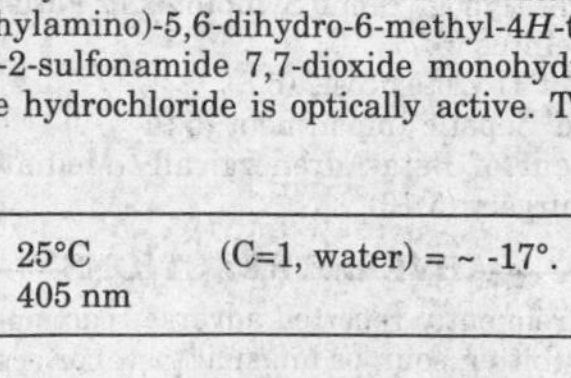

Dorzolamide hydrochloride has a molecular weight of 360.91. It is a white to off-white, crystalline powder, which is soluble in water and slightly soluble in methanol and ethanol.

Timolol maleate is described chemically as: (-)-1-(*tert*-butylamino)-3-[(4-morpholino-1,2,5-thiadiazol-3-yl)oxy]-2-propanol maleate (1:1) (salt). Timolol maleate possesses an asymmetric carbon atom in its structure and is provided as the levo-isomer. The optical rotation of timolol maleate is:

[α]	25°C	in 1N HCl (C = 5) = -12.2° (-11.7° to -12.5°).
	405 nm	

Its molecular formula is $C_{13}H_{24}N_4O_3S \bullet C_4H_4O_4$ and its structural formula is:

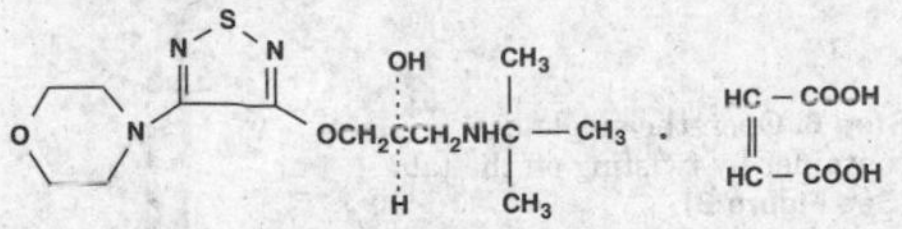

Timolol maleate has a molecular weight of 432.50. It is a white, odorless, crystalline powder which is soluble in water, methanol, and alcohol. Timolol maleate is stable at room temperature.

COSOPT PF is supplied as a sterile, clear, colorless to nearly colorless, isotonic, buffered, slightly viscous, aqueous solution. The pH of the solution is approximately 5.65, and the osmolarity is 242-323 mOsM. Each mL of COSOPT PF contains 20 mg dorzolamide (22.26 mg of dorzolamide hydrochloride) and 5 mg timolol (6.83 mg timolol maleate). Inactive ingredients are sodium citrate, hydroxyethyl cellulose, sodium hydroxide, mannitol, and water for injection. COSOPT PF does not contain a preservative.

12 CLINICAL PHARMACOLOGY

12.1 Mechanism of Action

COSOPT PF is comprised of two components: dorzolamide hydrochloride and timolol maleate. Each of these two components decreases elevated intraocular pressure, whether or not associated with glaucoma, by reducing aqueous humor secretion. Elevated intraocular pressure is a major risk factor in the pathogenesis of optic nerve damage and glaucomatous visual field loss. The higher the level of intraocular pressure, the greater the likelihood of glaucomatous field loss and optic nerve damage.

Dorzolamide hydrochloride is an inhibitor of human carbonic anhydrase II. Inhibition of carbonic anhydrase in the ciliary processes of the eye decreases aqueous humor secretion, presumably by slowing the formation of bicarbonate ions with subsequent reduction in sodium and fluid transport. Timolol maleate is a $beta_1$ and $beta_2$ (non-selective) adrenergic receptor blocking agent that does not have significant intrinsic sympathomimetic, direct myocardial depressant, or local anesthetic (membrane-stabilizing) activity. The combined effect of these two agents administered as COSOPT PF administered twice daily results in additional intraocular pressure reduction compared to either component administered alone, but the reduction is not as much as when dorzolamide administered three times daily and timolol twice daily are administered concomitantly. *[See Clinical Studies (14).]*

12.3 Pharmacokinetics

Dorzolamide Hydrochloride

When topically applied, dorzolamide reaches the systemic circulation. To assess the potential for systemic carbonic anhydrase inhibition following topical administration, drug and metabolite concentrations in RBCs and plasma and carbonic anhydrase inhibition in RBCs were measured. Dorzolamide accumulates in RBCs during chronic dosing as a result of binding to CA-II. The parent drug forms a single N-desethyl metabolite, which inhibits CA-II less potently than the parent drug but also inhibits CA-I. The metabolite also accumulates in RBCs where it binds primarily to CA-I. Plasma concentrations of dorzolamide and metabolite are generally below the assay limit of quantitation (15nM). Dorzolamide binds moderately to plasma proteins (approximately 33%).

Dorzolamide is primarily excreted unchanged in the urine; the metabolite also is excreted in the urine. After dosing is stopped, dorzolamide washes out of RBCs nonlinearly, resulting in a rapid decline of drug concentration initially, followed by a slower elimination phase with a half-life of about four months.

To simulate the systemic exposure after long-term topical ocular administration, dorzolamide was given orally to eight healthy subjects for up to 20 weeks. The oral dose of 2 mg twice daily closely approximates the amount of drug delivered by topical ocular administration of dorzolamide 2% three times daily. Steady state was reached within 8 weeks. The inhibition of CA-II and total carbonic anhydrase activities was below the degree of inhibition anticipated to be necessary for a pharmacological effect on renal function and respiration in healthy individuals.

Timolol Maleate

In a study of plasma drug concentrations in six subjects, the systemic exposure to timolol was determined following twice daily topical administration of timolol maleate ophthalmic solution 0.5%. The mean peak plasma concentration following morning dosing was 0.46 ng/mL.

13 NONCLINICAL TOXICOLOGY

13.1 Carcinogenesis, Mutagenesis, Impairment of Fertility

In a two-year study of dorzolamide hydrochloride administered orally to male and female Sprague-Dawley rats, urinary bladder papillomas were seen in male rats in the highest dosage group of 20 mg/kg/day (250 times the recommended human ophthalmic dose). Papillomas were not seen in rats given oral doses equivalent to approximately 12 times the recommended human ophthalmic dose. No treatment-related tumors were seen in a 21-month study in female and male mice given oral doses up to 75 mg/kg/day (~900 times the recommended human ophthalmic dose).

The increased incidence of urinary bladder papillomas seen in the high-dose male rats is a class-effect of carbonic anhydrase inhibitors in rats. Rats are particularly prone to developing papillomas in response to foreign bodies, compounds causing crystalluria, and diverse sodium salts.

No changes in bladder urothelium were seen in dogs given oral dorzolamide hydrochloride for one year at 2 mg/kg/day (25 times the recommended human ophthalmic dose) or monkeys dosed topically to the eye at 0.4 mg/kg/day (~5 times the recommended human ophthalmic dose) for one year.

In a two-year study of timolol maleate administered orally to rats, there was a statistically significant increase in the incidence of adrenal pheochromocytomas in male rats administered 300 mg/kg/day (approximately 42,000 times the systemic exposure following the maximum recommended human ophthalmic dose). Similar differences were not observed in rats administered oral doses equivalent to approximately 14,000 times the maximum recommended human ophthalmic dose.

In a lifetime oral study of timolol maleate in mice, there were statistically significant increases in the incidence of benign and malignant pulmonary tumors, benign uterine polyps and mammary adenocarcinomas in female mice at 500 mg/kg/day, (approximately 71,000 times the systemic exposure following the maximum recommended human ophthalmic dose), but not at 5 or 50 mg/kg/day (approximately 700 or 7,000, respectively, times the systemic exposure following the maximum recommended human ophthalmic dose). In a subsequent study in female mice, in which post-mortem examinations were limited to the uterus and the lungs, a statistically significant increase in the incidence of pulmonary tumors was again observed at 500 mg/kg/day.

The increased occurrence of mammary adenocarcinomas was associated with elevations in serum prolactin which occurred in female mice administered oral timolol at 500 mg/kg/day, but not at doses of 5 or 50 mg/kg/day. An increased incidence of mammary adenocarcinomas in rodents has been associated with administration of several other therapeutic agents that elevate serum prolactin, but no correlation between serum prolactin levels and mammary tumors has been established in humans. Furthermore, in adult human female subjects who received oral dosages of up to 60 mg of timolol maleate (the maximum recommended human oral dosage), there were no clinically meaningful changes in serum prolactin.

The following tests for mutagenic potential were negative for dorzolamide: (1) *in vivo* (mouse) cytogenetic assay; (2) *in vitro* chromosomal aberration assay; (3) alkaline elution assay; (4) V-79 assay; and (5) Ames test.

Timolol maleate was devoid of mutagenic potential when tested *in vivo* (mouse) in the micronucleus test and cytogenetic assay (doses up to 800 mg/kg) and *in vitro* in a neoplastic cell transformation assay (up to 100 µg/mL). In Ames tests the highest concentrations of timolol employed, 5,000 or 10,000 µg/plate, were associated with statistically significant elevations of revertants observed with tester strain TA100 (in seven replicate assays), but not in the remaining three strains. In the assays with tester strain TA100, no consistent dose response relationship was observed, and the ratio of test to control revertants did not reach 2. A ratio of 2 is usually considered the criterion for a positive Ames test.

Reproduction and fertility studies in rats with either timolol maleate or dorzolamide hydrochloride demonstrated no adverse effect on male or female fertility at doses up to approximately 100 times the systemic exposure following the maximum recommended human ophthalmic dose.

14 CLINICAL STUDIES

14.1 COSOPT Efficacy

Clinical studies of 3 to 15 months duration were conducted to compare the IOP-lowering effect over the course of the day of COSOPT twice daily (dosed morning and bedtime) to individually- and concomitantly-administered 0.5% timolol twice daily and 2.0% dorzolamide twice and three times daily. The IOP-lowering effect of COSOPT twice daily was greater (1-3 mmHg) than that of monotherapy with either 2.0% dorzolamide three times daily or 0.5% timolol twice daily. The IOP-lowering effect of COSOPT twice daily was approximately 1 mmHg less than that of concomitant therapy with 2.0% dorzolamide three times daily and 0.5% timolol twice daily.

Open-label extensions of two studies were conducted for up to 12 months. During this period, the IOP-lowering effect of COSOPT twice daily was consistent during the 12 month follow-up period.

14.2 COSOPT PF Equivalence Study

In an active-treatment controlled, parallel, double-masked study in 261 patients with elevated intraocular pressure ≥22 mmHg in one or both eyes, COSOPT PF had an IOP-lowering effect equivalent to that of COSOPT.

16 HOW SUPPLIED/STORAGE AND HANDLING

COSOPT PF is supplied in a foil pouch containing 15 low density polyethylene 0.2 mL single-use containers.

NDC 0006-3629-60, package of 60 single-use vials.

NDC 0006-3629-62, package of 180 single-use vials.

Store COSOPT PF at 20-25°C (68-77°F). Do not freeze.

Store in the original pouch. After the pouch is opened, store the remaining single-use containers in the foil pouch to protect from light. Write down the date you open the foil pouch in the space provided on the pouch. Discard any unused containers 15 days after first opening the pouch.

17 PATIENT COUNSELING INFORMATION

See FDA-Approved Patient Labeling (Patient Information).

17.1 Potential for Exacerbation of Asthma and COPD

COSOPT PF may cause severe worsening of asthma and COPD symptoms including death due to bronchospasm. Patients with bronchial asthma, a history of bronchial asthma, severe chronic obstructive pulmonary disease should be advised not to take this product. *[See Contraindications (4.1).]*

17.2 Potential of Cardiovascular Effects

COSOPT PF may cause worsening of cardiac symptoms. Patients with sinus bradycardia, second or third degree atrioventricular block, or cardiac failure should be advised not to take this product. *[See Contraindications (4.2).]*

17.3 Sulfonamide Reactions

COSOPT PF contains dorzolamide (which is a sulfonamide) and, although administered topically, is absorbed systemically. Therefore the same types of adverse reactions that are attributable to sulfonamides may occur with topical administration, including severe skin reactions. Patients should be advised that if serious or unusual reactions or signs of hypersensitivity occur, they should discontinue the use of the product and seek their physician's advice. *[See Warnings and Precautions (5.3).]*

17.4 Handling the Single-Use Container

COSOPT PF is a sterile solution that does not contain a preservative. The solution from one individual unit is to be used immediately after opening for administration to one or both eyes. Since sterility cannot be maintained after the individual unit is opened, the remaining contents should be discarded immediately after administration.

17.5 Intercurrent Ocular Conditions

Patients also should be advised that if they have ocular surgery or develop an intercurrent ocular condition (e.g., trauma or infection), they should immediately seek their physician's advice concerning the continued use of this product.

17.6 Concomitant Topical Ocular Therapy

If more than one topical ophthalmic drug is being used, the drugs should be administered at least five minutes apart.

Manuf. for: Merck Sharp & Dohme Corp., a subsidiary of **MERCK & CO., INC.**, Whitehouse Station, NJ 08889, USA

By: Catalent Pharma Solutions, LLC

Woodstock, IL 60098, USA

Revised: 05/2012

6081301

Patient Information

COSOPT® PF (CO-sopt PEA EHF)

(dorzolamide hydrochloride-timolol maleate ophthalmic solution) 2%/0.5%

Read this information before you start using COSOPT PF and each time you get a refill. There may be new information. This information does not take the place of talking to your doctor about your medical condition or your treatment.

What is COSOPT PF?

COSOPT PF is a prescription sterile eye drop solution that contains 2 medicines, dorzolamide hydrochloride (a sulfonamide carbonic anhydrase inhibitor) and timolol maleate (a beta-adrenergic blocker). COSOPT PF is used to lower the pressure in the eye (intraocular pressure) in people with open-angle glaucoma or ocular hypertension, when their eye pressure is too high and beta-adrenergic blocker medicines alone have not adequately lowered the pressure.

It is not known if COSOPT PF is safe and effective in children under 2 years of age.

Who should not use COSOPT PF?
Do not use COSOPT PF if you:
- have or have had asthma
- have or have had severe lung problems (chronic obstructive pulmonary disease)
- have heart problems, including slow or irregular heartbeat or heart failure
- are allergic to dorzolamide hydrochloride, timolol maleate, or any of the ingredients in COSOPT PF. See the end of this leaflet for a complete list of ingredients in COSOPT PF.

Talk to your healthcare provider before taking this medicine if you have any of these conditions.

What should I tell my doctor before using COSOPT PF?
Before you use COSOPT PF, tell your doctor if you:
- have problems with muscle weakness (myasthenia gravis)
- have diabetes or problems with low blood sugar (hypoglycemia)
- have thyroid, kidney, or liver problems
- are planning to have surgery
- are allergic to sulfa drugs
- have or have had eye problems, including any surgery on your eye or eyes, or are using any other eye medicines
- have any other medical problems
- are pregnant or plan to become pregnant. It is not known if COSOPT PF will harm your unborn baby. If you become pregnant while using COSOPT PF talk to your doctor right away.
- are breastfeeding or plan to breastfeed. It is not known whether dorzolamide passes into your breast milk however, timolol has been detected in breast milk. Talk to your doctor about the best way to feed your baby if you use COSOPT PF.

Tell your doctor about all the medicines you take, including prescription and non-prescription medicines, vitamins, and herbal supplements.
COSOPT PF and other medicines may affect each other causing side effects. COSOPT PF may affect the way other medicines work, and other medicines may affect how COSOPT PF works.
Know the medicines you take. Keep a list of them to show your doctor and pharmacist when you get a new medicine.

How should I use COSOPT PF?
Read the Instructions for Use at the end of this Patient Information leaflet for additional instructions about the right way to use COSOPT PF.
- Use COSOPT PF exactly as your doctor tells you.
- **Use 1 drop of COSOPT PF in your eye (or eyes) in the morning and 1 drop in the evening.**
- If you use other medicines in your eye, wait at least 5 minutes between using COSOPT PF and your other eye medicines.
- Use your COSOPT PF right away after opening. Each COSOPT PF single-use container is sterile and is to be used 1 time then thrown away.
- Do not save any COSOPT PF that may be left over after you use a single-use container. Using COSOPT PF that is not sterile may cause other eye problems.

What are the possible side effects of COSOPT PF?
COSOPT PF may cause serious side effects including:
- **severe breathing problems.** These breathing problems can happen in people who have asthma, chronic obstructive pulmonary disease, or heart failure and can cause death. Tell your doctor right away if you have breathing problems while taking COSOPT PF.
- **heart failure.** This can happen in people who already have heart failure and in people who have never had heart failure before. Tell your doctor right away if you get any of these symptoms of heart failure while taking COSOPT PF:
  - shortness of breath
  - irregular heartbeat (palpitations)
  - swelling of your ankles or feet
  - sudden weight gain
- **severe allergic reactions.** These allergic reactions can happen the first time you use COSOPT PF or after you have been using COSOPT PF for a while and may cause death.
  Stop taking COSOPT PF and call your doctor right away or get emergency help if you get any of these symptoms of an allergic reaction:
  - swelling of your face, lips, mouth, or tongue
  - trouble breathing
  - wheezing
  - severe itching
  - skin rash, redness, or swelling
  - dizziness or fainting
  - fast heartbeat or pounding in your chest (tachycardia)
  - sweating
- **worsening muscle weakness.** COSOPT PF can cause muscle weakness to get worse in people who already have problems with muscle weakness (myasthenia gravis).
- **kidney problems.** Your doctor may do tests to check your kidney function while you use COSOPT PF.
- **swelling of your eye (cornea)**

The most common side effects of COSOPT PF include:
- a bitter, sour, or unusual taste in your mouth after using COSOPT PF
- burning, stinging, redness, or itching of the eye
- blurred vision
- painful, red, watery eyes with increased sensitivity (superficial punctate keratitis)

Tell your doctor if you have any new eye problems while using COSOPT PF including:
- an eye injury
- an eye infection
- a sudden loss of vision
- eye surgery
- swelling and redness of and around your eye (conjunctivitis)
- problems with your eyelids

Tell your doctor if you have any other side effects that bother you.
These are not all the possible side effects of COSOPT PF. For more information, ask your doctor or pharmacist.
Call your doctor about medical advice about side effects. You may report side effects to FDA at 1-800-FDA-1088.

What should I do in case of an overdose?
If you swallow the contents of the container, contact your doctor immediately. Among other effects, you may feel lightheaded, have difficulty breathing, or feel your heart rate has slowed.

How should I store COSOPT PF?
- Store COSOPT PF at room temperature between 68°F to 77°F (20°C to 25°C). Do not freeze.
- Keep the COSOPT PF single-use containers in their original foil pouch to protect from light.
- Write down the date you open the foil pouch in the space provided on the pouch.
- Throw away all unused COSOPT PF single-use containers 15 days after first opening the pouch.

Keep COSOPT PF and all medicines out of the reach of children.

General information about the safe and effective use of COSOPT PF.
Medicines are sometimes prescribed for purposes other than those listed in a Patient Information leaflet. Do not use COSOPT PF for a condition for which it was not prescribed. Do not give COSOPT PF to other people, even if they have the same symptoms you have. It may harm them. This Patient Information leaflet summarizes the most important information about COSOPT PF. If you would like more information, talk with your doctor. You can ask your pharmacist or doctor for information about COSOPT PF that is written for health professionals.

What are the ingredients in COSOPT PF?
Active ingredients: dorzolamide hydrochloride and timolol maleate
Inactive ingredients: sodium citrate, hydroxyethyl cellulose, sodium hydroxide, mannitol, and water for injection.

Instructions for Use
Read these instructions before using your COSOPT PF and each time you get a refill. There may be new information. This leaflet does not take the place of talking with your doctor about your medical condition or your treatment.
Important:
- **COSOPT PF is for the eye only. Do not swallow COSOPT PF.**
- COSOPT PF single-use containers are packaged in a foil pouch.
- Write down the date you open the foil pouch in the space provided on the pouch.

Every time you use COSOPT PF:

Step 1. Wash your hands.
Step 2. Take the strip of single-use containers from the pouch.
Step 3. Pull off 1 single-use container from the strip.
Step 4. Put the remaining strip of single-use containers back in the pouch and fold the edge to close the pouch.

Step 5. Hold the single-use container upright. Make sure that the solution is in the bottom part of the single-use container **(See Figure A).**

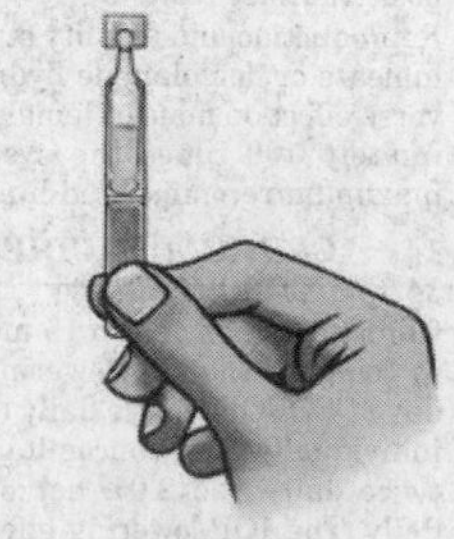

(Figure A)

Step 6. Open the single-use container by twisting off the tab **(See Figure B).**

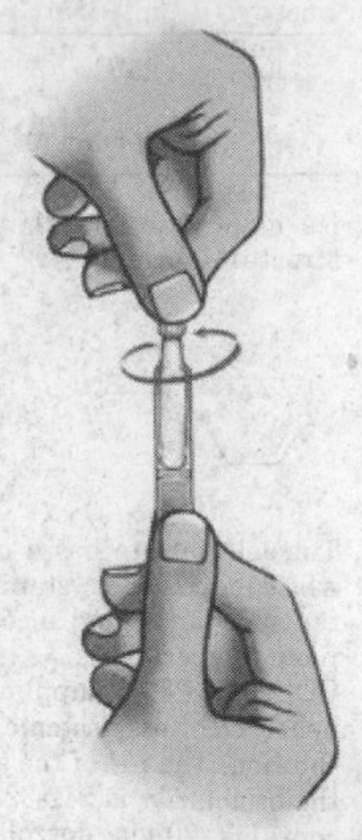

(Figure B)

Step 7. Tilt your head backwards. If you are unable to tilt your head, lie down.
Step 8. Place the tip of the single-use container close to your eye. Be careful not to touch your eye with the tip of the single-use container **(See Figure C).**

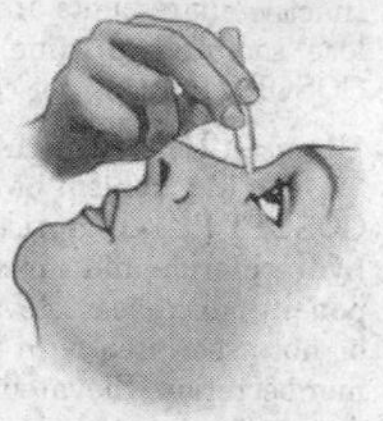

(Figure C)

Step 9. Pull the lower eyelid downwards and look up.
Step 10. Gently squeeze the container and let 1 drop of COSOPT PF fall into the space between your lower eyelid and your eye. If a drop misses your eye, try again **(See Figure D).**

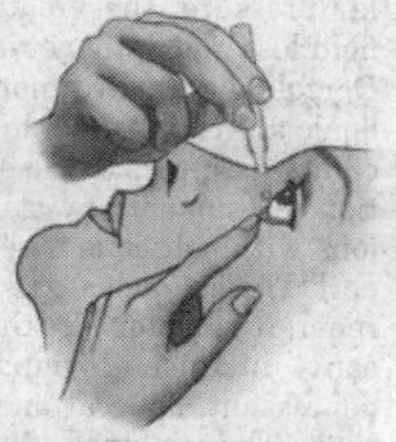

(Figure D)

Step 11. Blot any excess solution from the skin around the eye with a tissue.

- If your doctor has told you to use drops in both eyes, repeat steps 7 to 11 for your other eye.
- There is enough COSOPT PF in 1 single-use container for 1 or both of your eyes.
- **Throw away the opened single-use container with any remaining COSOPT PF right away.**

This Patient Information and Instructions for Use have been approved by the U.S. Food and Drug Administration.
Manuf. for: Merck Sharp & Dohme Corp., a subsidiary of **MERCK & CO., INC.,** Whitehouse Station, NJ 08889, USA
By: Catalent Pharma Solutions, LLC
Woodstock, IL 60098, USA

Issued: May 2012
6081301

Shown in Product Identification Guide, page 307

CRIXIVAN® ℞
(INDINAVIR SULFATE)
CAPSULES

DESCRIPTION
CRIXIVAN® (indinavir sulfate) is an inhibitor of the human immunodeficiency virus (HIV) protease. CRIXIVAN Capsules are formulated as a sulfate salt and are available for oral administration in strengths of 100, 200, and 400 mg of indinavir (corresponding to 125, 250, and 500 mg indinavir sulfate, respectively). Each capsule also contains the inactive ingredients anhydrous lactose and magnesium stearate. The capsule shell has the following inactive ingredients and dyes: gelatin and titanium dioxide.
The chemical name for indinavir sulfate is [1(1*S*,2*R*),5(*S*)]-2,3,5-trideoxy-*N*-(2,3-dihydro-2-hydroxy-1*H*-inden-1-yl)-5-[2-[[(1,1-dimethylethyl)amino]carbonyl]-4-(3-pyridinyl-

methyl)-1-piperazinyl]-2-(phenylmethyl)-D-*erythro*-pentonamide sulfate (1:1) salt. Indinavir sulfate has the following structural formula:

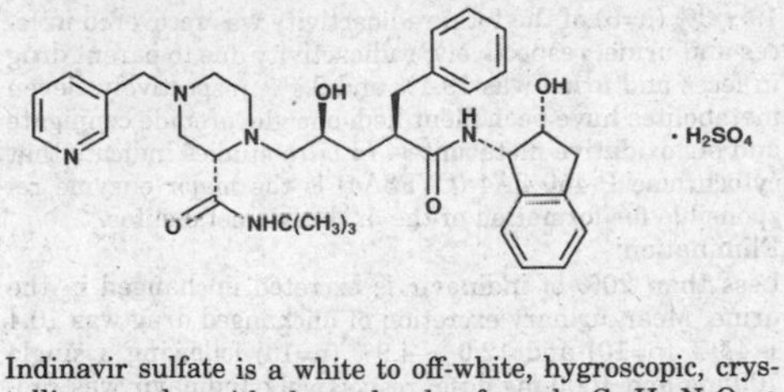

Indinavir sulfate is a white to off-white, hygroscopic, crystalline powder with the molecular formula $C_{36}H_{47}N_5O_4 \bullet H_2SO_4$ and a molecular weight of 711.88. It is very soluble in water and in methanol.

MICROBIOLOGY

Mechanism of Action:

HIV-1 protease is an enzyme required for the proteolytic cleavage of the viral polyprotein precursors into the individual functional proteins found in infectious HIV-1. Indinavir binds to the protease active site and inhibits the activity of the enzyme. This inhibition prevents cleavage of the viral polyproteins resulting in the formation of immature non-infectious viral particles.

Antiretroviral Activity *In Vitro:*

The *in vitro* activity of indinavir was assessed in cell lines of lymphoblastic and monocytic origin and in peripheral blood lymphocytes. HIV-1 variants used to infect the different cell types include laboratory-adapted variants, primary clinical isolates and clinical isolates resistant to nucleoside analogue and nonnucleoside inhibitors of the HIV-1 reverse transcriptase. The IC_{95} (95% inhibitory concentration) of indinavir in these test systems was in the range of 25 to 100 nM. In drug combination studies with the nucleoside analogues zidovudine and didanosine, indinavir showed synergistic activity in cell culture. The relationship between *in vitro* susceptibility of HIV-1 to indinavir and inhibition of HIV-1 replication in humans has not been established.

Drug Resistance:

Isolates of HIV-1 with reduced susceptibility to the drug have been recovered from some patients treated with indinavir. Viral resistance was correlated with the accumulation of mutations that resulted in the expression of amino acid substitutions in the viral protease. Eleven amino acid residue positions, (L10I/V/R, K20I/M/R, L24I, M46I/L, I54A/V, L63P, I64V, A71T/V, V82A/F/T, I84V, and L90M), at which substitutions are associated with resistance, have been identified. Resistance was mediated by the co-expression of multiple and variable substitutions at these positions. No single substitution was either necessary or sufficient for measurable resistance (≥4-fold increase in IC_{95}). In general, higher levels of resistance were associated with the co-expression of greater numbers of substitutions, although their individual effects varied and were not additive. At least 3 amino acid substitutions must be present for phenotypic resistance to indinavir to reach measurable levels. In addition, mutations in the p7/ p1 and p1/ p6 gag cleavage sites were observed in some indinavir resistant HIV-1 isolates.

In vitro phenotypic susceptibilities to indinavir were determined for 38 viral isolates from 13 patients who experienced virologic rebounds during indinavir monotherapy. Pre-treatment isolates from five patients exhibited indinavir IC_{95} values of 50-100 nM. At or following viral RNA rebound (after 12-76 weeks of therapy), IC_{95} values ranged from 25 to >3000 nM, and the viruses carried 2 to 10 mutations in the protease gene relative to baseline.

Cross-Resistance to Other Antiviral Agents:

Varying degrees of HIV-1 cross-resistance have been observed between indinavir and other HIV-1 protease inhibitors. In studies with ritonavir, saquinavir, and amprenavir, the extent and spectrum of cross-resistance varied with the specific mutational patterns observed. In general, the degree of cross-resistance increased with the accumulation of resistance-associated amino acid substitutions. Within a panel of 29 viral isolates from indinavir-treated patients that exhibited measurable (≥4-fold) phenotypic resistance to indinavir, all were resistant to ritonavir. Of the indinavir resistant HIV-1 isolates, 63% showed resistance to saquinavir and 81% to amprenavir.

CLINICAL PHARMACOLOGY

Pharmacokinetics

Absorption:

Indinavir was rapidly absorbed in the fasted state with a time to peak plasma concentration (T_{max}) of 0.8 ± 0.3 hours (mean ± S.D.) (n=11). A greater than dose-proportional increase in indinavir plasma concentrations was observed over the 200-1000 mg dose range. At a dosing regimen of 800 mg every 8 hours, steady-state area under the plasma concentration time curve (AUC) was 30,691 ± 11,407 nM•hour (n=16), peak plasma concentration (C_{max}) was 12,617 ± 4037 nM (n=16), and plasma concentration eight hours post dose (trough) was 251 ± 178 nM (n=16).

Table 1

PK Parameter	% change in PK parameter for females relative to males	90% Confidence Interval
AUC_{0-8h} (nM•hr)	↓13%	(↓32%, ↑12%)
C_{max} (nM)	↓13%	(↓32%, ↑10%)
C_{8h} (nM)	↓22%	(↓47%, ↑15%)

↓Indicates a decrease in the PK parameter; ↑indicates an increase in the PK parameter.

Table 2: Drug Interactions: Pharmacokinetic Parameters for Indinavir in the Presence of the Coadministered Drug (See PRECAUTIONS, Table 9 for Recommended Alterations in Dose or Regimen)

Coadministered drug	Dose of Coadministered drug (mg)	Dose of CRIXIVAN (mg)	n	Ratio (with/without coadministered drug) of Indinavir Pharmacokinetic Parameters (90% CI); No Effect = 1.00		
				C_{max}	AUC	C_{min}
Cimetidine	600 twice daily, 6 days	400 single dose	12	1.07 (0.77, 1.49)	0.98 (0.81, 1.19)	0.82 (0.69, 0.99)
Clarithromycin	500 q12h, 7 days	800 three times daily, 7 days	10	1.08 (0.85, 1.38)	1.19 (1.00, 1.42)	1.57 (1.16, 2.12)
Delavirdine	400 three times daily	400 three times daily, 7 days	28	0.64* (0.48, 0.86)	No significant change*	2.18* (1.16, 4.12)
Delavirdine	400 three times daily	600 three times daily, 7 days	28	No significant change	1.53* (1.07, 2.20)	3.98* (2.04, 7.78)
Efavirenz†	600 once daily, 10 days	1000 three times daily, 10 days	20			
		After morning dose		No significant change*	0.67* (0.61, 0.74)	0.61* (0.49, 0.76)
		After afternoon dose		No significant change*	0.63* (0.54, 0.74)	0.48* (0.43, 0.53)
		After evening dose		0.71* (0.57, 0.89)	0.54* (0.46, 0.63)	0.43* (0.37, 0.50)
Fluconazole†	400 once daily, 8 days	1000 three times daily, 7 days	11	0.87 (0.72, 1.05)	0.76 (0.59, 0.98)	0.90 (0.72, 1.12)
Grapefruit Juice	8 oz.	400 single dose	10	0.65 (0.53, 0.79)	0.73 (0.60, 0.87)	0.90 (0.71, 1.15)
Isoniazid	300 once daily in the morning, 8 days	800 three times daily, 7 days	11	0.95 (0.88, 1.03)	0.99 (0.87, 1.13)	0.89 (0.75, 1.06)
Itraconazole	200 twice daily, 7 days	600 three times daily, 7 days	12	0.78* (0.69, 0.88)	0.99* (0.91, 1.06)	1.49* (1.28, 1.74)
Ketoconazole	400 once daily, 7 days	600 three times daily, 7 days	12	0.69* (0.61, 0.78)	0.80* (0.74, 0.87)	1.29* (1.11, 1.51)
	400 once daily, 7 days	400 three times daily, 7 days	12	0.42* (0.37, 0.47)	0.44* (0.41, 0.48)	0.73* (0.62, 0.85)
Methadone	20-60 once daily in the morning, 8 days	800 three times daily, 8 days	10	See text below for discussion of interaction.		
Quinidine	200 single dose	400 single dose	10	0.96 (0.79, 1.18)	1.07 (0.89, 1.28)	0.93 (0.73, 1.19)
Rifabutin	150 once daily in the morning, 10 days	800 three times daily, 10 days	14	0.80 (0.72, 0.89)	0.68 (0.60, 0.76)	0.60 (0.51, 0.72)
Rifabutin	300 once daily in the morning, 10 days	800 three times daily, 10 days	10	0.75 (0.61, 0.91)	0.66 (0.56, 0.77)	0.61 (0.50, 0.75)
Rifampin	600 once daily in the morning, 8 days	800 three times daily, 7 days	12	0.13 (0.08, 0.22)	0.08 (0.06, 0.11)	Not Done
Ritonavir	100 twice daily, 14 days	800 twice daily, 14 days	10, 16‡	See text below for discussion of interaction.		
Ritonavir	200 twice daily, 14 days	800 twice daily,14 days	9, 16‡	See text below for discussion of interaction.		
Sildenafil	25 single dose	800 three times daily	6	See text below for discussion of interaction.		

(Table continued on next page)

Effect of Food on Oral Absorption:

Administration of indinavir with a meal high in calories, fat, and protein (784 kcal, 48.6 g fat, 31.3 g protein) resulted in a 77% ± 8% reduction in AUC and an 84% ± 7% reduction in C_{max} (n=10). Administration with lighter meals (e.g., a

Table 2 *(cont.)*: Drug Interactions: Pharmacokinetic Parameters for Indinavir in the Presence of the Coadministered Drug (See PRECAUTIONS, Table 9 for Recommended Alterations in Dose or Regimen)

Coadministered drug	Dose of Coadministered drug (mg)	Dose of CRIXIVAN (mg)	n	Ratio (with/without coadministered drug) of Indinavir Pharmacokinetic Parameters (90% CI); No Effect = 1.00		
				C_{max}	AUC	C_{min}
St. John's wort (*Hypericum perforatum*, standardized to 0.3 % hypericin)	300 three times daily with meals, 14 days	800 three times daily	8	Not Available	0.46 (0.34, 0.58)§	0.19 (0.06, 0.33)§
Stavudine (d4T)†	40 twice daily, 7 days	800 three times daily, 7 days	11	0.95 (0.80, 1.11)	0.95 (0.80, 1.12)	1.13 (0.83, 1.53)
Trimethoprim/ Sulfamethoxazole	800 Trimethoprim/ 160 Sulfamethoxazole q12h, 7 days	400 four times daily, 7 days	12	1.12 (0.87, 1.46)	0.98 (0.81, 1.18)	0.83 (0.72, 0.95)
Zidovudine†	200 three times daily, 7 days	1000 three times daily, 7 days	12	1.06 (0.91, 1.25)	1.05 (0.86, 1.28)	1.02 (0.77, 1.35)
Zidovudine/ Lamivudine (3TC)†	200/150 three times daily, 7 days	800 three times daily, 7 days	6, 9¶	1.05 (0.83, 1.33)	1.04 (0.67, 1.61)	0.98 (0.56, 1.73)

All interaction studies conducted in healthy, HIV-negative adult subjects, unless otherwise indicated.
* Relative to indinavir 800 mg three times daily alone.
† Study conducted in HIV-positive subjects.
‡ Comparison to historical data on 16 subjects receiving indinavir alone.
§ 95% CI.
¶ Parallel group design; n for indinavir + coadministered drug, n for indinavir alone.

Table 3: Drug Interactions: Pharmacokinetic Parameters for Coadministered Drug in the Presence of Indinavir (See PRECAUTIONS, Table 9 for Recommended Alterations in Dose or Regimen)

Coadministered drug	Dose of Coadministered drug (mg)	Dose of CRIXIVAN (mg)	n	Ratio (with/without CRIXIVAN) of Coadministered Drug Pharmacokinetic Parameters (90% CI); No Effect = 1.00		
				C_{max}	AUC	C_{min}
Clarithromycin	500 twice daily, 7 days	800 three times daily, 7 days	12	1.19 (1.02, 1.39)	1.47 (1.30, 1.65)	1.97 (1.58, 2.46) n=11
Efavirenz	200 once daily, 14 days	800 three times daily, 14 days	20	No significant change	No significant change	--
Ethinyl Estradiol (ORTHO-NOVUM 1/35)*	35 mcg, 8 days	800 three times daily, 8 days	18	1.02 (0.96, 1.09)	1.22 (1.15, 1.30)	1.37 (1.24, 1.51)
Isoniazid	300 once daily in the morning, 8 days	800 three times daily, 8 days	11	1.34 (1.12, 1.60)	1.12 (1.03, 1.22)	1.00 (0.92, 1.08)
Methadone†	20-60 once daily in the morning, 8 days	800 three times daily, 8 days	12	0.93 (0.84, 1.03)	0.96 (0.86, 1.06)	1.06 (0.94, 1.19)
Norethindrone (ORTHO-NOVUM 1/35)*	1 mcg, 8 days	800 three times daily, 8 days	18	1.05 (0.95, 1.16)	1.26 (1.20, 1.31)	1.44 (1.32, 1.57)
Rifabutin 150 mg once daily in the morning, 11 days + indinavir compared to 300 mg once daily in the morning, 11 days alone	150 once daily in the morning, 10 days 300 once daily in the morning, 10 days	800 three times daily, 10 days 800 three times daily, 10 days	14 10	1.29 (1.05, 1.59) 2.34 (1.64, 3.35)	1.54 (1.33, 1.79) 2.73 (1.99, 3.77)	1.99 (1.71, 2.31) n=13 3.44 (2.65, 4.46) n=9
Ritonavir	100 twice daily, 14 days 200 twice daily, 14 days	800 twice daily, 14 days 800 twice daily, 14 days	10, 4‡ 9, 5‡	1.61 (1.13, 2.29) 1.19 (0.85, 1.66)	1.72 (1.20, 2.48) 1.96 (1.39, 2.76)	1.62 (0.93, 2.85) 4.71 (2.66, 8.33) n=9, 4

(Table continued on next page)

meal of dry toast with jelly, apple juice, and coffee with skim milk and sugar or a meal of corn flakes, skim milk and sugar) resulted in little or no change in AUC, C_{max} or trough concentration.

Distribution:
Indinavir was approximately 60% bound to human plasma proteins over a concentration range of 81 nM to 16,300 nM.
Metabolism:
Following a 400-mg dose of ^{14}C-indinavir, 83 ± 1% (n=4) and 19 ± 3% (n=6) of the total radioactivity was recovered in feces and urine, respectively; radioactivity due to parent drug in feces and urine was 19.1% and 9.4%, respectively. Seven metabolites have been identified, one glucuronide conjugate and six oxidative metabolites. *In vitro* studies indicate that cytochrome P-450 3A4 (CYP3A4) is the major enzyme responsible for formation of the oxidative metabolites.
Elimination:
Less than 20% of indinavir is excreted unchanged in the urine. Mean urinary excretion of unchanged drug was 10.4 ± 4.9% (n=10) and 12.0 ± 4.9% (n=10) following a single 700-mg and 1000-mg dose, respectively. Indinavir was rapidly eliminated with a half-life of 1.8 ± 0.4 hours (n=10). Significant accumulation was not observed after multiple dosing at 800 mg every 8 hours.

Special Populations

Hepatic Insufficiency:
Patients with mild to moderate hepatic insufficiency and clinical evidence of cirrhosis had evidence of decreased metabolism of indinavir resulting in approximately 60% higher mean AUC following a single 400-mg dose (n=12). The half-life of indinavir increased to 2.8 ± 0.5 hours. Indinavir pharmacokinetics have not been studied in patients with severe hepatic insufficiency (see DOSAGE AND ADMINISTRATION, Hepatic Insufficiency).
Renal Insufficiency:
The pharmacokinetics of indinavir have not been studied in patients with renal insufficiency.
Gender:
The effect of gender on the pharmacokinetics of indinavir was evaluated in 10 HIV seropositive women who received CRIXIVAN 800 mg every 8 hours with zidovudine 200 mg every 8 hours and lamivudine 150 mg twice a day for one week. Indinavir pharmacokinetic parameters in these women were compared to those in HIV seropositive men (pooled historical control data). Differences in indinavir exposure, peak concentrations, and trough concentrations between males and females are shown in Table 1 below:
[See table 1 at top of previous page]
The clinical significance of these gender differences in the pharmacokinetics of indinavir is not known.
Race:
Pharmacokinetics of indinavir appear to be comparable in Caucasians and Blacks based on pharmacokinetic studies including 42 Caucasians (26 HIV-positive) and 16 Blacks (4 HIV-positive).
Pediatric:
The optimal dosing regimen for use of indinavir in pediatric patients has not been established. In HIV-infected pediatric patients (age 4-15 years), a dosage regimen of indinavir capsules, 500 mg/m^2 every 8 hours, produced $AUC_{0\text{-}8hr}$ of 38,742 ± 24,098 nM•hour (n=34), C_{max} of 17,181 ± 9809 nM (n=34), and trough concentrations of 134 ± 91 nM (n=28). The pharmacokinetic profiles of indinavir in pediatric patients were not comparable to profiles previously observed in HIV-infected adults receiving the recommended dose of 800 mg every 8 hours. The AUC and C_{max} values were slightly higher and the trough concentrations were considerably lower in pediatric patients. Approximately 50% of the pediatric patients had trough values below 100 nM; whereas, approximately 10% of adult patients had trough levels below 100 nM. The relationship between specific trough values and inhibition of HIV replication has not been established.
Pregnant Patients:
The optimal dosing regimen for use of indinavir in pregnant patients has not been established. A CRIXIVAN dose of 800 mg every 8 hours (with zidovudine 200 mg every 8 hours and lamivudine 150 mg twice a day) has been studied in 16 HIV-infected pregnant patients at 14 to 28 weeks of gestation at enrollment (study PACTG 358). The mean indinavir plasma $AUC_{0\text{-}8hr}$ at weeks 30-32 of gestation (n=11) was 9231 nM•hr, which is 74% (95% CI: 50%, 86%) lower than that observed 6 weeks postpartum. Six of these 11 (55%) patients had mean indinavir plasma concentrations 8 hours post-dose (C_{min}) below assay threshold of reliable quantification. The pharmacokinetics of indinavir in these 11 patients at 6 weeks postpartum were generally similar to those observed in non-pregnant patients in another study (see PRECAUTIONS, Pregnancy).

Drug Interactions:

(also see CONTRAINDICATIONS, WARNINGS, PRECAUTIONS, Drug Interactions)
Indinavir is an inhibitor of the cytochrome P450 isoform CYP3A4. Coadministration of CRIXIVAN and drugs primarily metabolized by CYP3A4 may result in increased plasma concentrations of the other drug, which could increase or prolong its therapeutic and adverse effects (see

Table 3 *(cont.)*: Drug Interactions: Pharmacokinetic Parameters for Coadministered Drug in the Presence of Indinavir (See PRECAUTIONS, Table 9 for Recommended Alterations in Dose or Regimen)

Coadministered drug	Dose of Coadministered drug (mg)	Dose of CRIXIVAN (mg)	n	Ratio (with/without CRIXIVAN) of Coadministered Drug Pharmacokinetic Parameters (90% CI); No Effect = 1.00		
				C_{max}	AUC	C_{min}
Saquinavir						
Hard gel formulation	600 single dose	800 three times daily, 2 days	6	4.7 (2.7, 8.1)	6.0 (4.0, 9.1)	2.9 (1.7, 4.7)§
Soft gel formulation	800 single dose	800 three times daily, 2 days	6	6.5 (4.7, 9.1)	7.2 (4.3, 11.9)	5.5 (2.2, 14.1)§
Soft gel formulation	1200 single dose	800 three times daily, 2 days	6	4.0 (2.7, 5.9)	4.6 (3.2, 6.7)	5.5 (3.7, 8.3)§
Sildenafil	25 single dose	800 three times daily	6	See text below for discussion of interaction.		
Stavudine¶	40 twice daily, 7 days	800 three times daily, 7 days	13	0.86 (0.73, 1.03)	1.21 (1.09, 1.33)	Not Done
Theophylline	250 single dose (on Days 1 and 7)	800 three times daily, 6 days (Days 2 to 7)	12, 4‡	0.88 (0.76, 1.03)	1.14 (1.04, 1.24)	1.13 (0.86, 1.49) n=7, 3
Trimethoprim/ Sulfamethoxazole						
Trimethoprim	800 Trimethoprim/ 160 Sulfamethoxazole q12h, 7 days	400 q6h, 7 days	12	1.18 (1.05, 1.32)	1.18 (1.05, 1.33)	1.18 (1.00, 1.39)
Trimethoprim/ Sulfamethoxazole						
Sulfamethoxazole	800 Trimethoprim/ 160 Sulfamethoxazole q12h, 7 days	400 q6h, 7 days	12	1.01 (0.95, 1.08)	1.05 (1.01, 1.09)	1.05 (0.97, 1.14)
Vardenafil	10 single dose	800 three times daily	18	See text below for discussion of interaction.		
Zidovudine¶	200 three times daily, 7 days	1000 three times daily, 7 days	12	0.89 (0.73, 1.09)	1.17 (1.07, 1.29)	1.51 (0.71, 3.20) n=4
Zidovudine/ Lamivudine¶						
Zidovudine	200/150 three times daily, 7 days	800 three times daily, 7 days	6, 7‡	1.23 (0.74, 2.03)	1.39 (1.02, 1.89)	1.08 (0.77, 1.50) n=5, 5
Zidovudine/ Lamivudine¶						
Lamivudine	200/150 three times daily, 7 days	800 three times daily, 7 days	6, 7‡	0.73 (0.52, 1.02)	0.91 (0.66, 1.26)	0.88 (0.59, 1.33)

All interaction studies conducted in healthy, HIV-negative adult subjects, unless otherwise indicated.
* Registered trademark of Ortho Pharmaceutical Corporation.
† Study conducted in subjects on methadone maintenance.
‡ Parallel group design; n for coadministered drug + indinavir, n for coadministered drug alone.
§ C_{6hr}
¶ Study conducted in HIV-positive subjects.

CONTRAINDICATIONS and WARNINGS). Based on *in vitro* data in human liver microsomes, indinavir does not inhibit CYP1A2, CYP2C9, CYP2E1 and CYP2B6. However, indinavir may be a weak inhibitor of CYP2D6.
Indinavir is metabolized by CYP3A4. Drugs that induce CYP3A4 activity would be expected to increase the clearance of indinavir, resulting in lowered plasma concentrations of indinavir. Coadministration of CRIXIVAN and other drugs that inhibit CYP3A4 may decrease the clearance of indinavir and may result in increased plasma concentrations of indinavir.
Drug interaction studies were performed with CRIXIVAN and other drugs likely to be coadministered and some drugs commonly used as probes for pharmacokinetic interactions. The effects of coadministration of CRIXIVAN on the AUC, C_{max} and C_{min} are summarized in Table 2 (effect of other drugs on indinavir) and Table 3 (effect of indinavir on other drugs). For information regarding clinical recommendations, see Table 9 in PRECAUTIONS.
[See table 2 on pages 1437 and 1438]
[See table 3 on previous page and above]
Delavirdine: Delavirdine inhibits the metabolism of indinavir such that coadministration of 400-mg or 600-mg indinavir three times daily with 400-mg delavirdine three times daily alters indinavir AUC, C_{max} and C_{min} (see Table 2). Indinavir had no effect on delavirdine pharmacokinetics (see DOSAGE AND ADMINISTRATION, Concomitant Therapy, Delavirdine), based on a comparison to historical delavirdine pharmacokinetic data.

Methadone: Administration of indinavir (800 mg every 8 hours) with methadone (20 mg to 60 mg daily) for one week in subjects on methadone maintenance resulted in no change in methadone AUC. Based on a comparison to historical data, there was little or no change in indinavir AUC.
Ritonavir: Compared to historical data in patients who received indinavir 800 mg every 8 hours alone, twice-daily coadministration to volunteers of indinavir 800 mg and ritonavir with food for two weeks resulted in a 2.7-fold increase of indinavir AUC_{24h}, a 1.6-fold increase in indinavir C_{max}, and an 11-fold increase in indinavir C_{min} for a 100-mg ritonavir dose and a 3.6-fold increase of indinavir AUC_{24h}, a 1.8-fold increase in indinavir C_{max}, and a 24-fold increase in indinavir C_{min} for a 200-mg ritonavir dose. In the same study, twice-daily coadministration of indinavir (800 mg) and ritonavir (100 or 200 mg) resulted in ritonavir AUC_{24h} increases versus the same doses of ritonavir alone (see Table 3).
Sildenafil: The results of one published study in HIV-infected men (n=6) indicated that coadministration of indinavir (800 mg every 8 hours chronically) with a single 25-mg dose of sildenafil resulted in an 11% increase in average AUC_{0-8hr} of indinavir and a 48% increase in average indinavir peak concentration (C_{max}) compared to 800 mg every 8 hours alone. Average sildenafil AUC was increased by 340% following coadministration of sildenafil and indinavir compared to historical data following administration of sildenafil alone (see CONTRAINDICATIONS, WARNINGS, Drug Interactions and PRECAUTIONS, Drug Interactions).

Vardenafil: Indinavir (800 mg every 8 hours) coadministered with a single 10-mg dose of vardenafil resulted in a 16-fold increase in vardenafil AUC, a 7-fold increase in vardenafil C_{max}, and a 2-fold increase in vardenafil half-life (see WARNINGS, Drug Interactions and PRECAUTIONS, Drug Interactions).

INDICATIONS AND USAGE

CRIXIVAN in combination with antiretroviral agents is indicated for the treatment of HIV infection.
This indication is based on two clinical trials of approximately 1 year duration that demonstrated: 1) a reduction in the risk of AIDS-defining illnesses or death; 2) a prolonged suppression of HIV RNA.

Description of Studies

In all clinical studies, with the exception of ACTG 320, the AMPLICOR HIV MONITOR assay was used to determine the level of circulating HIV RNA in serum. This is an experimental use of the assay. HIV RNA results should not be directly compared to results from other trials using different HIV RNA assays or using other sample sources.
Study ACTG 320 was a multicenter, randomized, double-blind clinical endpoint trial to compare the effect of CRIXIVAN in combination with zidovudine and lamivudine with that of zidovudine plus lamivudine on the progression to an AIDS-defining illness (ADI) or death. Patients were protease inhibitor and lamivudine naive and zidovudine experienced, with CD4 cell counts of ≤200 cells/mm^3. The study enrolled 1156 HIV-infected patients (17% female, 28% Black, 18% Hispanic, mean age 39 years). The mean baseline CD4 cell count was 87 cells/mm^3. The mean baseline HIV RNA was 4.95 log_{10} copies/mL (89,035 copies/mL). The study was terminated after a planned interim analysis, resulting in a median follow-up of 38 weeks and a maximum follow-up of 52 weeks. Results are shown in Table 4 and Figures 1 & 2.

Table 4: ACTG 320

Endpoint	Number (%) of Patients with AIDS-defining Illness or Death	
	IDV+ZDV+L (n=577)	ZDV+L (n=579)
HIV Progression or Death	35 (6.1)	63 (10.9)
Death*	10 (1.7)	19 (3.3)

IDV = Indinavir, ZDV = Zidovudine, L = Lamivudine
* The number of deaths is inadequate to assess the impact of Indinavir on survival.

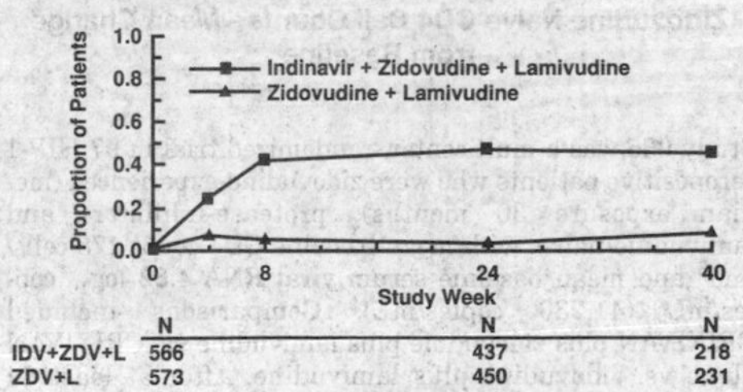

Study ACTG 320: Figure 1 - Indinavir Protocol ACTG 320 Zidovudine Experienced Plasma Viral RNA - Proportions Below 400 copies/mL

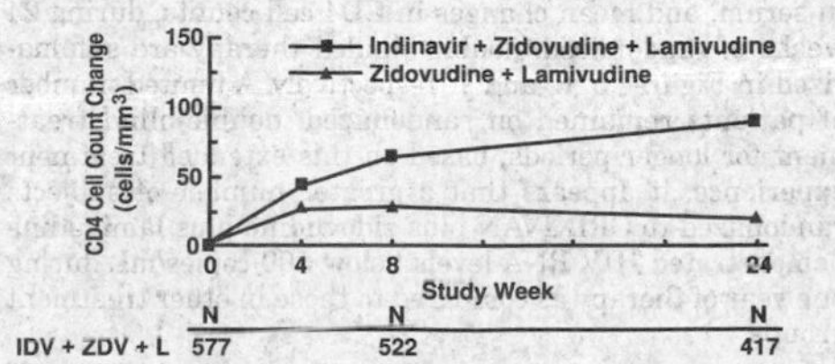

Study ACTG 320: Figure 2 - ACTG 320 Zidovudine Experienced CD4 Cell Counts - Mean Change from Baseline

Study 028, a double-blind, multicenter, randomized, clinical endpoint trial conducted in Brazil, compared the effects of CRIXIVAN plus zidovudine with those of CRIXIVAN alone or zidovudine alone on the progression to an ADI or death, and on surrogate marker responses. All patients were antiretroviral naive with CD4 cell counts of 50 to 250 cells/mm^3. The study enrolled 996 HIV-1 seropositive patients [28% female, 11% Black, 1% Asian/Other, median age 33 years, mean baseline CD4 cell count of 152 cells/mm^3, mean serum viral RNA of 4.44 log_{10} copies/mL (27,824 copies/mL)]. Treatment regimens containing zidovudine were modified in a blinded manner with the optional addition of lamivudine (median time: week 40). The median length of follow-up was 56 weeks with a maximum of 97 weeks. The study was terminated after a planned interim analysis, resulting in a median follow-up of 56 weeks and a maximum follow-up of 97 weeks. Results are shown in Table 5 and Figures 3 and 4.

Table 5: Protocol 028

Endpoint	Number (%) of Patients with AIDS-defining Illness or Death		
	IDV+ZDV (n=332)	IDV (n=332)	ZDV (n=332)
HIV Progression or Death	21 (6.3)	27 (8.1)	62 (18.7)
Death*	8 (2.4)	5 (1.5)	11 (3.3)

* The number of deaths is inadequate to assess the impact of Indinavir on survival.

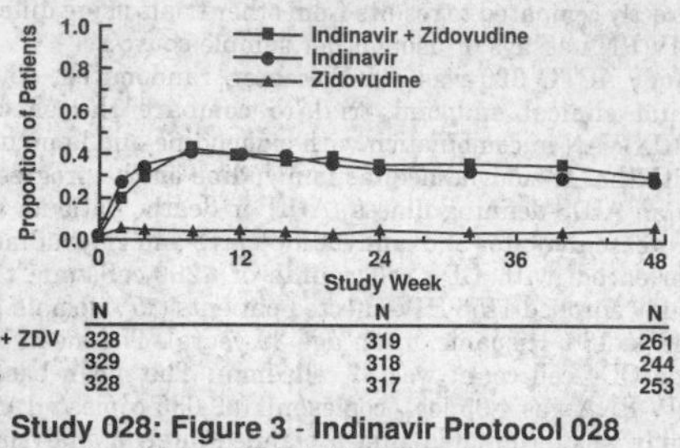

Study 028: Figure 3 - Indinavir Protocol 028 Zidovudine Naive Viral RNA - Proportions Below 500 Copies/mL in Serum

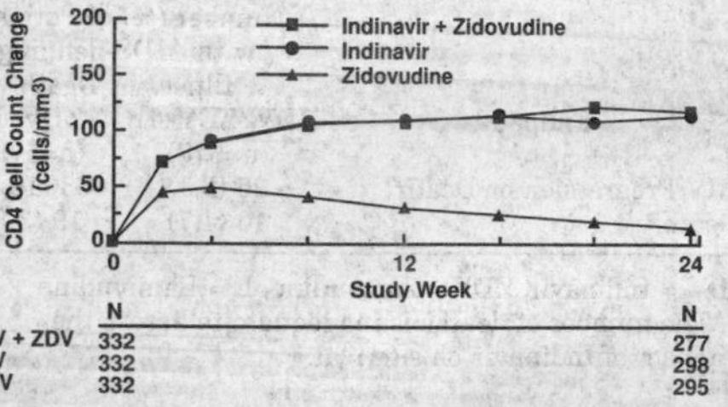

Study 028: Figure 4 - Indinavir Protocol 028 Zidovudine Naive CD4 Cell Counts - Mean Change from Baseline

Study 035 was a multicenter, randomized trial in 97 HIV-1 seropositive patients who were zidovudine-experienced (median exposure 30 months), protease-inhibitor- and lamivudine-naive, with mean baseline CD4 count 175 cells/mm^3 and mean baseline serum viral RNA 4.62 log_{10} copies/mL (41,230 copies/mL). Comparisons included CRIXIVAN plus zidovudine plus lamivudine vs. CRIXIVAN alone vs. zidovudine plus lamivudine. After at least 24 weeks of randomized, double-blind therapy, patients were switched to open-label CRIXIVAN plus lamivudine plus zidovudine. Mean changes in log_{10} viral RNA in serum, the proportions of patients with viral RNA below 500 copies/mL in serum, and mean changes in CD4 cell counts, during 24 weeks of randomized, double-blinded therapy are summarized in Figures 5, 6, and 7, respectively. A limited number of patients remained on randomized, double-blind treatment for longer periods; based on this extended treatment experience, it appears that a greater number of subjects randomized to CRIXIVAN plus zidovudine plus lamivudine demonstrated HIV RNA levels below 500 copies/mL during one year of therapy as compared to those in other treatment groups.

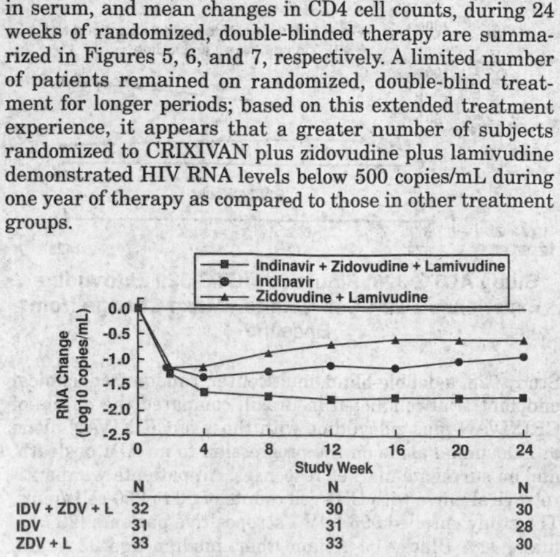

Study 035: Figure 5 - Indinavir Protocol 035 Zidovudine Experienced Viral RNA - Mean Log10 Change from Baseline in Serum

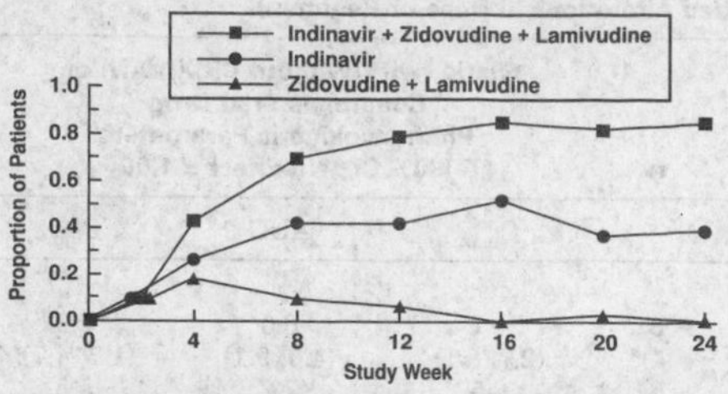

Study 035: Figure 6 - Indinavir Protocol 035 Zidovudine Experienced Viral RNA - Proportions Below 500 Copies/mL in Serum

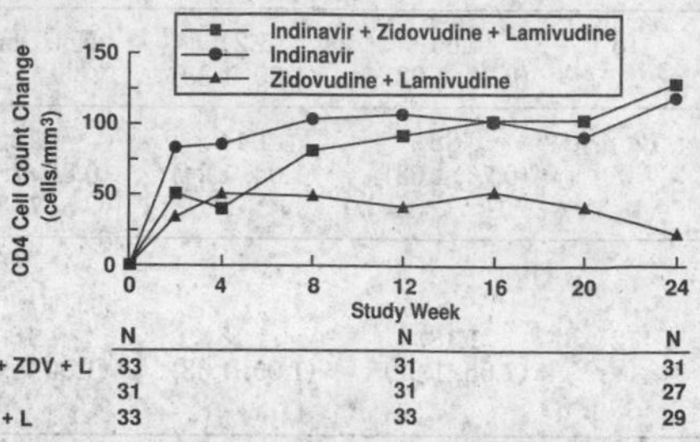

Study 035: Figure 7 - Indinavir Protocol 035 Zidovudine Experienced CD4 Cell Counts - Mean Change from Baseline

Genotypic Resistance in Clinical Studies

Study 006 (10/15/93-10/12/94) was a dose-ranging study in which patients were initially treated with CRIXIVAN at a dose of <2.4 g/day followed by 2.4 g/day. Study 019 (6/23/94-4/10/95) was a randomized comparison of CRIXIVAN 600 mg every 6 hours, CRIXIVAN plus zidovudine, and zidovudine alone. Table 6 shows the incidence of genotypic resistance at 24 weeks in these studies.

Table 6: Genotypic Resistance at 24 Weeks

Treatment Group	Resistance to IDV n/N*	Resistance to ZDV n/N*
IDV	—	—
<2.4 g/day	31/37 (84%)	—
2.4 g/day	9/21 (43%)	1/17 (6%)
IDV/ZDV	4/22 (18%)	1/22 (5%)
ZDV	1/18 (6%)	11/17 (65%)

* N - includes patients with non-amplifiable virus at 24 weeks who had amplifiable virus at week 0.

CONTRAINDICATIONS

CRIXIVAN is contraindicated in patients with clinically significant hypersensitivity to any of its components.

Inhibition of CYP3A4 by CRIXIVAN can result in elevated plasma concentrations of the following drugs, potentially causing serious or life-threatening reactions:

Table 7: Drug Interactions With Crixivan: Contraindicated Drugs

Drug Class	Drugs Within Class That Are Contraindicated With CRIXIVAN
Alpha 1-adrenoreceptor antagonist	alfuzosin
Antiarrhythmics	amiodarone
Ergot derivatives	dihydroergotamine, ergonovine, ergotamine, methylergonovine
GI motility agents	cisapride
HMG-CoA Reductase Inhibitors	lovastatin, simvastatin
Neuroleptics	pimozide
PDE5 Inhibitors	Revatio* (sildenafil) [for treatment of pulmonary arterial hypertension]
Sedative/hypnotics	oral midazolam, triazolam, alprazolam

* Registered trademark of Pfizer, Inc.

WARNINGS

ALERT: Find out about medicines that should NOT be taken with CRIXIVAN. This statement is included on the product's bottle label.

Nephrolithiasis/Urolithiasis

Nephrolithiasis/urolithiasis has occurred with CRIXIVAN therapy. The cumulative frequency of nephrolithiasis is substantially higher in pediatric patients (29%) than in adult patients (12.4%; range across individual trials: 4.7% to 34.4%). The cumulative frequency of nephrolithiasis events increases with increasing exposure to CRIXIVAN; however, the risk over time remains relatively constant. In some cases, nephrolithiasis/urolithiasis has been associated with renal insufficiency or acute renal failure, pyelonephritis with or without bacteremia. If signs or symptoms of nephrolithiasis/urolithiasis occur, (including flank pain, with or without hematuria or microscopic hematuria), temporary interruption (e.g., 1-3 days) or discontinuation of therapy may be considered. **Adequate hydration is recommended in all patients treated with CRIXIVAN. (See ADVERSE REACTIONS and DOSAGE AND ADMINISTRATION, Nephrolithiasis/Urolithiasis.)**

Hemolytic Anemia

Acute hemolytic anemia, including cases resulting in death, has been reported in patients treated with CRIXIVAN. Once a diagnosis is apparent, appropriate measures for the treatment of hemolytic anemia should be instituted, including discontinuation of CRIXIVAN.

Hepatitis

Hepatitis including cases resulting in hepatic failure and death has been reported in patients treated with CRIXIVAN. Because the majority of these patients had confounding medical conditions and/or were receiving concomitant therapy(ies), a causal relationship between CRIXIVAN and these events has not been established.

Hyperglycemia

New onset diabetes mellitus, exacerbation of pre-existing diabetes mellitus and hyperglycemia have been reported during post-marketing surveillance in HIV-infected patients receiving protease inhibitor therapy. Some patients required either initiation or dose adjustments of insulin or oral hypoglycemic agents for treatment of these events. In some cases, diabetic ketoacidosis has occurred. In those patients who discontinued protease inhibitor therapy, hyperglycemia persisted in some cases. Because these events have been reported voluntarily during clinical practice, estimates of frequency cannot be made and a causal relationship between protease inhibitor therapy and these events has not been established.

Drug Interactions

Concomitant use of CRIXIVAN with lovastatin or simvastatin is contraindicated due to an increased risk of myopathy including rhabdomyolysis. Caution should be exercised if CRIXIVAN is used concurrently with atorvastatin or rosuvastatin. Titrate the atorvastatin and rosuvastatin doses carefully and use the lowest necessary dose with CRIXIVAN. (See PRECAUTIONS, Drug Interactions.)

Midazolam is extensively metabolized by CYP3A4. Coadministration with CRIXIVAN with or without ritonavir may cause a large increase in the concentration of this benzodiazepine. No drug interaction study has been performed for the co-administration of CRIXIVAN with benzodiazepines. Based on data from other CYP3A4 inhibitors, plasma concentrations of midazolam are expected to be significantly higher when midazolam is given orally. Therefore CRIXIVAN should not be co-administered with orally administered midazolam (see CONTRAINDICATIONS), whereas caution should be used with co-administration of CRIXIVAN and parenteral midazolam. Data from concomitant use of parenteral midazolam with other protease inhibitors suggest a possible 3-4 fold increase in midazolam plasma levels. If CRIXIVAN with or without ritonavir is coadministered with parenteral midazolam, it should be done in a setting which ensures close clinical monitoring and appropriate medical management in case of respiratory depression and/or prolonged sedation. Dosage reduction for midazolam should be considered, especially if more than a single dose of midazolam is administered.

Particular caution should be used when prescribing sildenafil, tadalafil, or vardenafil in patients receiving indinavir. Coadministration of CRIXIVAN with these medications is expected to substantially increase plasma concentrations of sildenafil, tadalafil, and vardenafil and may result in an increase in adverse events, including hypotension, visual changes, and priapism, which have been associated with sildenafil, tadalafil, and vardenafil (see CONTRAINDICATIONS and PRECAUTIONS, Drug Interactions and Information for Patients, and the manufacturer's complete prescribing information for sildenafil, tadalafil, or vardenafil).

Concomitant use of CRIXIVAN and St. John's wort (*Hypericum perforatum*) or products containing St. John's wort is not recommended. Coadministration of CRIXIVAN and St. John's wort has been shown to substantially decrease indinavir concentrations (see CLINICAL PHARMACOLOGY, Drug Interactions) and may lead to loss of virologic response and possible resistance to CRIXIVAN or to the class of protease inhibitors.

PRECAUTIONS

General

Indirect hyperbilirubinemia has occurred frequently during treatment with CRIXIVAN and has infrequently been associated with increases in serum transaminases (see also ADVERSE REACTIONS, Clinical Trials and Post-Marketing Experience). It is not known whether CRIXIVAN will exacerbate the physiologic hyperbilirubinemia seen in neonates. (See Pregnancy.)

Tubulointerstitial Nephritis

Reports of tubulointerstitial nephritis with medullary calcification and cortical atrophy have been observed in patients with asymptomatic severe leukocyturia (>100 cells/ high power field). Patients with asymptomatic severe leukocyturia should be followed closely and monitored frequently with urinalyses. Further diagnostic evaluation may be warranted, and discontinuation of CRIXIVAN should be considered in all patients with severe leukocyturia.

Immune reconstitution syndrome has been reported in patients treated with combination antiretroviral therapy, including CRIXIVAN. During the initial phase of combination antiretroviral treatment, patients whose immune system responds may develop an inflammatory response to indolent or residual opportunistic infections (such as *Mycobacterium avium* infection, cytomegalovirus, *Pneumocystis jirovecii* pneumonia [PCP], or tuberculosis), which may necessitate further evaluation and treatment.

Autoimmune disorders (such as Graves' disease, polymyositis, and Guillain-Barré syndrome) have also been reported to occur in the setting of immune reconstitution; however, the time to onset is more variable, and can occur many months after initiation of treatment.

Coexisting Conditions

Patients with hemophilia: There have been reports of spontaneous bleeding in patients with hemophilia A and B treated with protease inhibitors. In some patients, additional factor VIII was required. In many of the reported cases, treatment with protease inhibitors was continued or restarted. A causal relationship between protease inhibitor therapy and these episodes has not been established. (See ADVERSE REACTIONS, Post-Marketing Experience.)

Patients with hepatic insufficiency due to cirrhosis: In these patients, the dosage of CRIXIVAN should be lowered because of decreased metabolism of CRIXIVAN (see DOSAGE AND ADMINISTRATION).

Patients with renal insufficiency: Patients with renal insufficiency have not been studied.

Fat Redistribution

Redistribution/accumulation of body fat including central obesity, dorsocervical fat enlargement (buffalo hump), peripheral wasting, facial wasting, breast enlargement, and "cushingoid appearance" have been observed in patients receiving antiretroviral therapy. The mechanism and long-term consequences of these events are currently unknown. A causal relationship has not been established.

Information for Patients

A statement to patients and health care providers is included on the product's bottle label. **ALERT: Find out about medicines that should NOT be taken with CRIXIVAN.** A Patient Package Insert (PPI) for CRIXIVAN is available for patient information.

CRIXIVAN is not a cure for HIV-1 infection and patients may continue to experience illnesses associated with HIV-1 infection, including opportunistic infections. Patients should remain under the care of a physician when using CRIXIVAN.

Patients should be advised to avoid doing things that can spread HIV-1 infection to others.

- **Do not share needles or other injection equipment.**
- **Do not share personal items that can have blood or body fluids on them, like toothbrushes and razor blades.**
- **Do not have any kind of sex without protection.** Always practice safe sex by using a latex or polyurethane condom to lower the chance of sexual contact with semen, vaginal secretions, or blood.
- **Do not breastfeed.** We do not know if CRIXIVAN can be passed to your baby in your breast milk and whether it could harm your baby. Also, mothers with HIV-1 should not breastfeed because HIV-1 can be passed to the baby in the breast milk.

Patients should be advised to remain under the care of a physician when using CRIXIVAN and should not modify or discontinue treatment without first consulting the physician. Therefore, if a dose is missed, patients should take the next dose at the regularly scheduled time and should not double this dose. Therapy with CRIXIVAN should be initiated and maintained at the recommended dosage.

CRIXIVAN may interact with some drugs; therefore, patients should be advised to report to their doctor the use of any other prescription, non-prescription medication or herbal products, particularly St. John's wort.

For optimal absorption, CRIXIVAN should be administered without food but with water 1 hour before or 2 hours after a meal. Alternatively, CRIXIVAN may be administered with other liquids such as skim milk, juice, coffee, or tea, or with a light meal, e.g., dry toast with jelly, juice, and coffee with skim milk and sugar; or corn flakes, skim milk and sugar (see CLINICAL PHARMACOLOGY, Effect of Food on Oral Absorption and DOSAGE AND ADMINISTRATION). Ingestion of CRIXIVAN with a meal high in calories, fat, and protein reduces the absorption of indinavir.

Patients receiving a phosphodiesterase type 5 (PDE5) inhibitor (sildenafil, tadalafil, or vardenafil) should be advised that they may be at an increased risk of PDE5 inhibitor-associated adverse events including hypotension, visual changes, and priapism, and should promptly report any symptoms to their doctors (see CONTRAINDICATIONS and WARNINGS, Drug Interactions).

Patients should be informed that redistribution or accumulation of body fat may occur in patients receiving antiretroviral therapy and that the cause and long-term health effects of these conditions are not known at this time.

CRIXIVAN Capsules are sensitive to moisture. Patients should be informed that CRIXIVAN should be stored and used in the original container and the desiccant should remain in the bottle.

Drug Interactions

Indinavir is an inhibitor of the cytochrome P450 isoform CYP3A4. Coadministration of CRIXIVAN and drugs primarily metabolized by CYP3A4 may result in increased plasma concentrations of the other drug, which could increase or prolong its therapeutic and adverse effects (see CONTRAINDICATIONS and WARNINGS).

Indinavir is metabolized by CYP3A4. Drugs that induce CYP3A4 activity would be expected to increase the clearance of indinavir, resulting in lowered plasma concentrations of indinavir. Coadministration of CRIXIVAN and other drugs that inhibit CYP3A4 may decrease the clearance of indinavir and may result in increased plasma concentrations of indinavir.

Table 8: Drugs That Should Not Be Coadministered with CRIXIVAN

Drug Class: Drug Name	Clinical Comment
Alpha 1-adrenoreceptor antagonist: alfuzosin	Potentially increased alfuzosin concentrations can result in hypotension.
Antiarrhythmics: amiodarone	CONTRAINDICATED due to potential for serious and/or life-threatening reactions such as cardiac arrhythmias.
Antimycobacterial: rifampin	May lead to loss of virologic response and possible resistance to CRIXIVAN or to the class of protease inhibitors or other coadministered antiretroviral agents.
Ergot derivatives: dihydroergotamine, ergonovine, ergotamine, methylergonovine	CONTRAINDICATED due to potential for serious and/or life-threatening reactions such as acute ergot toxicity characterized by peripheral vasospasm and ischemia of the extremities and other tissues.
GI motility agents: cisapride	CONTRAINDICATED due to potential for serious and/or life-threatening reactions such as cardiac arrhythmias.
Herbal products: St. John's wort (*Hypericum perforatum*)	May lead to loss of virologic response and possible resistance to CRIXIVAN or to the class of protease inhibitors.
HMG-CoA Reductase inhibitors: lovastatin, simvastatin	CONTRAINDICATED due to an increased risk for serious reactions such as myopathy including rhabdomyolysis.
Neuroleptic: pimozide	CONTRAINDICATED due to potential for serious and/or life-threatening reactions such as cardiac arrhythmias.
PDE5 inhibitor: Revatio* (sildenafil) [for treatment of pulmonary arterial hypertension]	A safe and effective dose has not been established when used with CRIXIVAN. There is increased potential for sildenafil-associated adverse events (which include visual disturbances, hypotension, prolonged erection, and syncope).
Protease inhibitor: atazanavir	Both CRIXIVAN and atazanavir are associated with indirect (unconjugated) hyperbilirubinemia. Combinations of these drugs have not been studied and coadministration of CRIXIVAN and atazanavir is not recommended.
Sedative/hypnotics: Oral midazolam, triazolam, alprazolam	CONTRAINDICATED due to potential for serious and/or life-threatening reactions such as prolonged or increased sedation or respiratory depression.

* Registered trademark of Pfizer, Inc.

[See table 9 on pages 1442 and 1443]

Carcinogenesis, Mutagenesis, Impairment of Fertility

Carcinogenicity studies were conducted in mice and rats. In mice, no increased incidence of any tumor type was observed. The highest dose tested in rats was 640 mg/kg/day; at this dose a statistically significant increased incidence of thyroid adenomas was seen only in male rats. At that dose, daily systemic exposure in rats was approximately 1.3 times higher than daily systemic exposure in humans. No evidence of mutagenicity or genotoxicity was observed in *in vitro* microbial mutagenesis (Ames) tests, *in vitro* alkaline elution assays for DNA breakage, *in vitro* and *in vivo* chromosomal aberration studies, and *in vitro* mammalian cell mutagenesis assays. No treatment-related effects on mating, fertility, or embryo survival were seen in female rats and no treatment-related effects on mating performance were seen in male rats at doses providing systemic exposure comparable to or slightly higher than that with the clinical dose. In addition, no treatment-related effects were observed in fecundity or fertility of untreated females mated to treated males.

Pregnancy

Pregnancy Category C:

Developmental toxicity studies were performed in rabbits (at doses up to 240 mg/kg/day), dogs (at doses up to 80 mg/kg/day), and rats (at doses up to 640 mg/kg/day). The highest doses in these studies produced systemic exposures in these species comparable to or slightly greater than human exposure. No treatment-related external, visceral, or skeletal changes were observed in rabbits or dogs. No treatment-related external or visceral changes were observed in rats. Treatment-related increases over controls in the incidence of supernumerary ribs (at exposures at or below those in humans) and of cervical ribs (at exposures comparable to or slightly greater than those in humans) were seen in rats. In all three species, no treatment-related effects on embryonic/fetal survival or fetal weights were observed.

In rabbits, at a maternal dose of 240 mg/kg/day, no drug was detected in fetal plasma 1 hour after dosing. Fetal plasma drug levels 2 hours after dosing were approximately 3% of maternal plasma drug levels. In dogs, at a maternal dose of 80 mg/kg/day, fetal plasma drug levels were approximately 50% of maternal plasma drug levels both 1 and 2 hours after dosing. In rats, at maternal doses of 40 and 640 mg/kg/day, fetal plasma drug levels were approximately 10 to 15% and 10 to 20% of maternal plasma drug levels 1 and 2 hours after dosing, respectively.

Indinavir was administered to Rhesus monkeys during the third trimester of pregnancy (at doses up to 160 mg/kg twice daily) and to neonatal Rhesus monkeys (at doses up to 160 mg/kg twice daily). When administered to neonates, indinavir caused an exacerbation of the transient physiologic hyperbilirubinemia seen in this species after birth; serum bilirubin values were approximately fourfold above controls at 160 mg/kg twice daily. A similar exacerbation did not occur in neonates after *in utero* exposure to indinavir during the third trimester of pregnancy. In Rhesus monkeys, fetal plasma drug levels were approximately 1 to 2% of maternal plasma drug levels approximately 1 hour after maternal dosing at 40, 80, or 160 mg/kg twice daily.

Hyperbilirubinemia has occurred during treatment with CRIXIVAN (see PRECAUTIONS and ADVERSE REACTIONS). It is unknown whether CRIXIVAN administered to the mother in the perinatal period will exacerbate physiologic hyperbilirubinemia in neonates.

There are no adequate and well-controlled studies in pregnant patients. CRIXIVAN should be used during pregnancy only if the potential benefit justifies the potential risk to the fetus.

Table 9: Established and Other Potentially Significant Drug Interactions: Alteration in Dose or Regimen May Be Recommended Based on Drug Interaction Studies or Predicted Interaction (See also CLINICAL PHARMACOLOGY for magnitude of interaction, WARNINGS and DOSAGE AND ADMINISTRATION.)

Drug Name	Effect	Clinical Comment
HIV Antiviral Agents		
Delavirdine	↑ indinavir concentration	Dose reduction of CRIXIVAN to 600 mg every 8 hours should be considered when taking delavirdine 400 mg three times a day.
Didanosine		Indinavir and didanosine formulations containing buffer should be administered at least one hour apart on an empty stomach.
Efavirenz	↓ indinavir concentration	The optimal dose of indinavir, when given in combination with efavirenz, is not known. Increasing the indinavir dose to 1000 mg every 8 hours does not compensate for the increased indinavir metabolism due to efavirenz.
Nelfinavir	↑ indinavir concentration	The appropriate doses for this combination, with respect to efficacy and safety, have not been established.
Nevirapine	↓ indinavir concentration	Indinavir concentrations may be decreased in the presence of nevirapine. The appropriate doses for this combination, with respect to efficacy and safety, have not been established.
Ritonavir	↑ indinavir concentration ↑ ritonavir concentration	The appropriate doses for this combination, with respect to efficacy and safety, have not been established. Preliminary clinical data suggest that the incidence of nephrolithiasis is higher in patients receiving indinavir in combination with ritonavir than those receiving CRIXIVAN 800 mg q8h.
Saquinavir	↑ saquinavir concentration	The appropriate doses for this combination, with respect to efficacy and safety, have not been established.
Other Agents		
Antiarrhythmics: bepridil, lidocaine(systemic) and quinidine	↑ antiarrhythmic agents concentration	Caution is warranted and therapeutic concentration monitoring is recommended for antiarrhythmics when coadministered with CRIXIVAN.
Anticonvulsants: carbamazepine, phenobarbital, phenytoin	↓ indinavir concentration	Use with caution. CRIXIVAN may not be effective due to decreased indinavir concentrations in patients taking these agents concomitantly.
Antidepressant: Trazodone	↑ trazodone concentration	Concomitant use of trazodone and CRIXIVAN may increase plasma concentrations of trazodone. Adverse events of nausea, dizziness, hypotension and syncope have been observed following coadministration of trazodone and ritonavir. If trazodone is used with a CYP3A4 inhibitor such as CRIXIVAN, the combination should be used with caution and a lower dose of trazodone should be considered.
Anti-gout: Colchicine	↑ colchicine concentration	Patients with renal or hepatic impairment should not be given colchicine with CRIXIVAN. ***Treatment of gout flares:*** Co-administration of colchicine in patients on CRIXIVAN: 0.6 mg (1 tablet) × 1 dose, followed by 0.3 mg (half tablet) 1 hour later. Dose to be repeated no earlier than 3 days. ***Prophylaxis of gout flares:*** Co-administration of colchicine in patients on CRIXIVAN: If the original colchicine regimen was 0.6 mg twice a day, the regimen should be adjusted to 0.3 mg once a day. If the original colchicine regimen was 0.6 mg once a day, the regimen should be adjusted to 0.3 mg once every other day. ***Treatment of familial Mediterranean fever (FMF):*** Co-administration of colchicine in patients on CRIXIVAN: Maximum daily dose of 0.6 mg (may be given as 0.3 mg twice a day).
Calcium Channel Blockers, Dihydropyridine: e.g., felodipine, nifedipine, nicardipine	↑ dihydropyridine calcium channel blockers concentration	Caution is warranted and clinical monitoring of patients is recommended.
Clarithromycin	↑ clarithromycin concentration ↑ indinavir concentration	The appropriate doses for this combination, with respect to efficacy and safety, have not been established.
Endothelin receptor antagonist: Bosentan	↑ bosentan concentration	Co-administration of bosentan in patients on CRIXIVAN or co-administration of CRIXIVAN in patients on bosentan: Start at or adjust bosentan to 62.5 mg once daily or every other day based upon individual tolerability.

(Table continued on next page)

A CRIXIVAN dose of 800 mg every 8 hours (with zidovudine 200 mg every 8 hours and lamivudine 150 mg twice a day) has been studied in 16 HIV-infected pregnant patients at 14 to 28 weeks of gestation at enrollment (study PACTG 358). Given the substantially lower antepartum exposures observed and the limited data in this patient population, indinavir use is not recommended in HIV-infected pregnant patients (see CLINICAL PHARMACOLOGY, Pregnant Patients).

Antiretroviral Pregnancy Registry

To monitor maternal-fetal outcomes of pregnant patients exposed to CRIXIVAN, an Antiretroviral Pregnancy Registry has been established. Physicians are encouraged to register patients by calling 1-800-258-4263.

Nursing Mothers

Studies in lactating rats have demonstrated that indinavir is excreted in milk. Although it is not known whether CRIXIVAN is excreted in human milk, there exists the potential for adverse effects from indinavir in nursing infants. Mothers should be instructed to discontinue nursing if they are receiving CRIXIVAN. This is consistent with the recommendation by the U.S. Public Health Service Centers for Disease Control and Prevention that HIV-infected mothers not breast-feed their infants to avoid risking postnatal transmission of HIV.

Pediatric Use

The optimal dosing regimen for use of indinavir in pediatric patients has not been established. A dose of 500 mg/m^2 every eight hours has been studied in uncontrolled studies of 70 children, 3 to 18 years of age. The pharmacokinetic profiles of indinavir at this dose were not comparable to profiles previously observed in adults receiving the recommended dose (see CLINICAL PHARMACOLOGY, Pediatric). Although viral suppression was observed in some of the 32 children who were followed on this regimen through 24 weeks, a substantially higher rate of nephrolithiasis was reported when compared to adult historical data (see WARNINGS, Nephrolithiasis/Urolithiasis). Physicians considering the use of indinavir in pediatric patients without other protease inhibitor options should be aware of the limited data available in this population and the increased risk of nephrolithiasis.

Geriatric Use

Clinical studies of CRIXIVAN did not include sufficient numbers of subjects aged 65 and over to determine whether they respond differently from younger subjects. In general, dose selection for an elderly patient should be cautious, reflecting the greater frequency of decreased hepatic, renal or cardiac function and of concomitant disease or other drug therapy.

ADVERSE REACTIONS

Clinical Trials in Adults

Nephrolithiasis/urolithiasis, including flank pain with or without hematuria (including microscopic hematuria), has been reported in approximately 12.4% (301/2429; range across individual trials: 4.7% to 34.4%) of patients receiving CRIXIVAN at the recommended dose in clinical trials with a median follow-up of 47 weeks (range: 1 day to 242 weeks; 2238 patient-years follow-up). The cumulative frequency of nephrolithiasis events increases with duration of exposure to CRIXIVAN; however, the risk over time remains relatively constant. Of the patients treated with CRIXIVAN who developed nephrolithiasis/urolithiasis in clinical trials during the double-blind phase, 2.8% (7/246) were reported to develop hydronephrosis and 4.5% (11/246) underwent stent placement. Following the acute episode, 4.9% (12/246) of patients discontinued therapy. (See WARNINGS and DOSAGE AND ADMINISTRATION, Nephrolithiasis/Urolithiasis.)

Asymptomatic hyperbilirubinemia (total bilirubin ≥2.5 mg/dL), reported predominantly as elevated indirect bilirubin, has occurred in approximately 14% of patients treated with CRIXIVAN. In <1% this was associated with elevations in ALT or AST.

Hyperbilirubinemia and nephrolithiasis/urolithiasis occurred more frequently at doses exceeding 2.4 g/day compared to doses ≤2.4 g/day.

Clinical adverse experiences reported in ≥2% of patients treated with CRIXIVAN alone, CRIXIVAN in combination with zidovudine or zidovudine plus lamivudine, zidovudine alone, or zidovudine plus lamivudine are presented in Table 10.

[See table 10 at top of page 1444]

In Phase I and II controlled trials, the following adverse events were reported significantly more frequently by those randomized to the arms containing CRIXIVAN than by those randomized to nucleoside analogues: rash, upper respiratory infection, dry skin, pharyngitis, taste perversion.

Selected laboratory abnormalities of severe or life-threatening intensity reported in patients treated with CRIXIVAN alone, CRIXIVAN in combination with zidovudine or zidovudine plus lamivudine, zidovudine alone, or zidovudine plus lamivudine are presented in Table 11.

[See table 11 at top of page 1444]

Post-Marketing Experience

Body As A Whole: redistribution/accumulation of body fat (see PRECAUTIONS, Fat Redistribution).

Cardiovascular System: cardiovascular disorders including myocardial infarction and angina pectoris; cerebrovascular disorder.

Digestive System: liver function abnormalities; hepatitis including reports of hepatic failure (see WARNINGS); pancreatitis; jaundice; abdominal distention; dyspepsia.
Hematologic: increased spontaneous bleeding in patients with hemophilia (see PRECAUTIONS); acute hemolytic anemia (see WARNINGS).
Endocrine/Metabolic: new onset diabetes mellitus, exacerbation of pre-existing diabetes mellitus, hyperglycemia (see WARNINGS).
Hypersensitivity: anaphylactoid reactions; urticaria; vasculitis.
Musculoskeletal System: arthralgia.
Nervous System/Psychiatric: oral paresthesia; depression.
Skin and Skin Appendage: rash including erythema multiforme and Stevens-Johnson syndrome; hyperpigmentation; alopecia; ingrown toenails and/or paronychia; pruritus.
Urogenital System: nephrolithiasis/urolithiasis, in some cases resulting in renal insufficiency or acute renal failure, pyelonephritis with or without bacteremia (see WARNINGS); interstitial nephritis sometimes with indinavir crystal deposits; in some patients, the interstitial nephritis did not resolve following discontinuation of CRIXIVAN; renal insufficiency; renal failure; leukocyturia (see PRECAUTIONS), crystalluria; dysuria.

Laboratory Abnormalities

Increased serum triglycerides; increased serum cholesterol.

OVERDOSAGE

There have been more than 60 reports of acute or chronic human overdosage (up to 23 times the recommended total daily dose of 2400 mg) with CRIXIVAN. The most commonly reported symptoms were renal (e.g., nephrolithiasis/urolithiasis, flank pain, hematuria) and gastrointestinal (e.g., nausea, vomiting, diarrhea).

It is not known whether CRIXIVAN is dialyzable by peritoneal or hemodialysis.

DOSAGE AND ADMINISTRATION

The recommended dosage of CRIXIVAN is 800 mg (usually **two** 400-mg capsules) orally every 8 hours.

CRIXIVAN must be taken at intervals of 8 hours. For optimal absorption, CRIXIVAN should be administered without food but with water 1 hour before or 2 hours after a meal. Alternatively, CRIXIVAN may be administered with other liquids such as skim milk, juice, coffee, or tea, or with a light meal, e.g., dry toast with jelly, juice, and coffee with skim milk and sugar; or corn flakes, skim milk and sugar. (See CLINICAL PHARMACOLOGY, Effect of Food on Oral Absorption.)

To ensure adequate hydration, it is recommended that adults drink at least 1.5 liters (approximately 48 ounces) of liquids during the course of 24 hours.

Concomitant Therapy

(See CLINICAL PHARMACOLOGY, Drug Interactions, and/or PRECAUTIONS, Drug Interactions.)

Delavirdine

Dose reduction of CRIXIVAN to 600 mg every 8 hours should be considered when administering delavirdine 400 mg three times a day.

Didanosine

If indinavir and didanosine are administered concomitantly, they should be administered at least one hour apart on an empty stomach (consult the manufacturer's product circular for didanosine).

Itraconazole

Dose reduction of CRIXIVAN to 600 mg every 8 hours is recommended when administering itraconazole 200 mg twice daily concurrently.

Ketoconazole

Dose reduction of CRIXIVAN to 600 mg every 8 hours is recommended when administering ketoconazole concurrently.

Rifabutin

Dose reduction of rifabutin to half the standard dose (consult the manufacturer's product circular for rifabutin) and a dose increase of CRIXIVAN to 1000 mg every 8 hours are recommended when rifabutin and CRIXIVAN are coadministered.

Hepatic Insufficiency

The dosage of CRIXIVAN should be reduced to 600 mg every 8 hours in patients with mild-to-moderate hepatic insufficiency due to cirrhosis.

Nephrolithiasis/Urolithiasis

In addition to adequate hydration, medical management in patients who experience nephrolithiasis/urolithiasis may include temporary interruption (e.g., 1 to 3 days) or discontinuation of therapy.

HOW SUPPLIED

CRIXIVAN Capsules are supplied as follows:

No. 3755 — 100 mg capsules: semi-translucent white capsules coded **"CRIXIVAN™ 100 mg"** in green. Available as:

Table 9 *(cont.)*: Established and Other Potentially Significant Drug Interactions: Alteration in Dose or Regimen May Be Recommended Based on Drug Interaction Studies or Predicted Interaction (See also CLINICAL PHARMACOLOGY for magnitude of interaction, WARNINGS and DOSAGE AND ADMINISTRATION.)

Drug Name	Effect	Clinical Comment
HMG-CoA Reductase Inhibitors: atorvastatin, rosuvastatin	↑ atorvastatin concentration ↑ rosuvastatin concentration	The atorvastatin and rosuvastatin doses should be carefully titrated; use the lowest dose necessary with careful monitoring during treatment with CRIXIVAN.
Immunosuppressants: cyclosporine, tacrolimus, sirolimus	↑ immunosuppressant agents concentration	Plasma concentrations may be increased by CRIXIVAN.
Inhaled beta agonist: Salmeterol	↑ salmeterol	Concurrent administration of salmeterol with CRIXIVAN is not recommended. The combination may result in increased risk of cardiovascular adverse events associated with salmeterol, including QT prolongation, palpitations and sinus tachycardia.
Inhaled/nasal steroid: Fluticasone	↑ fluticasone concentration	Concomitant use of fluticasone propionate and CRIXIVAN may increase plasma concentrations of fluticasone propionate. Use with caution. Consider alternatives to fluticasone propionate, particularly for long-term use. Fluticasone use is not recommended in situations where CRIXIVAN is coadministered with a potent CYP3A4 inhibitor such as ritonavir unless the potential benefit to the patient outweighs the risk of systemic corticosteroid side effects.
Itraconazole	↑ indinavir concentration	Dose reduction of CRIXIVAN to 600 mg every 8 hours is recommended when administering itraconazole concurrently.
Ketoconazole	↑ indinavir concentration	Dose reduction of CRIXIVAN to 600 mg every 8 hours should be considered.
Midazolam (parenteral administration)	↑ midazolam concentration	Concomitant use of parenteral midazolam with CRIXIVAN may increase plasma concentrations of midazolam. Coadministration should be done in a setting which ensures close clinical monitoring and appropriate medical management in case of respiratory depression and/or prolonged sedation. Dosage reduction for midazolam should be considered, especially if more than a single dose of midazolam is administered. Coadministration of oral midazolam with CRIXIVAN is CONTRAINDICATED (see Table 8).
Rifabutin	↓ indinavir concentration ↑ rifabutin concentration	Dose reduction of rifabutin to half the standard dose and a dose increase of CRIXIVAN to 1000 mg every 8 hours are recommended when rifabutin and CRIXIVAN are coadministered.
Sildenafil	↑ sildenafil concentration (only the use of sildenafil at doses used for treatment of erectile dysfunction has been studied with CRIXIVAN)	May result in an increase in PDE5 inhibitor-associated adverse events, including hypotension, syncope, visual disturbances, and priapism. ***Use of sildenafil for pulmonary arterial hypertension (PAH):*** Use of Revatio* (sildenafil) is contraindicated when used for the treatment of pulmonary arterial hypertension (PAH) [see CONTRAINDICATIONS]. ***Use of sildenafil for erectile dysfunction:*** Sildenafil dose should not exceed a maximum of 25 mg in a 48-hour period in patients receiving concomitant CRIXIVAN therapy. Use with increased monitoring for adverse events.
Tadalafil	↑ tadalafil concentration	May result in an increase in PDE5 inhibitor-associated adverse events, including hypotension, visual disturbances, and priapism. ***Use of tadalafil for pulmonary arterial hypertension (PAH):*** The following dose adjustments are recommended for use of Adcirca† (tadalafil) with CRIXIVAN: Co-administration of Adcirca in patients on CRIXIVAN or co-administration of CRIXIVAN in patients on Adcirca: Start at or adjust Adcirca to 20 mg once daily. Increase to 40 mg once daily based upon individual tolerability. ***Use of tadalafil for erectile dysfunction:*** Tadalafil dose should not exceed a maximum of 10 mg in a 72-hour period in patients receiving concomitant CRIXIVAN therapy. Use with increased monitoring for adverse events.
Vardenafil	↑ vardenafil concentration	Vardenafil dose should not exceed a maximum of 2.5 mg in a 24-hour period in patients receiving concomitant indinavir therapy.
Venlafaxine	↓ indinavir concentration	In a study of 9 healthy volunteers, venlafaxine administered under steady-state conditions at 150 mg/day resulted in a 28% decrease in the AUC of a single 800 mg oral dose of indinavir and a 36% decrease in indinavir C_{max}. Indinavir did not affect the pharmacokinetics of venlafaxine and ODV. The clinical significance of this finding is unknown.

Note: ↑ = increase; ↓ = decrease
* Registered trademark of Pfizer, Inc.
† Registered trademark of Eli Lilly and Company.

Table 10: Clinical Adverse Experiences Reported in ≥2% of Patients

	Study 028 Considered Drug-Related and of Moderate or Severe Intensity			Study ACTG 320 of Unknown Drug Relationship and of Severe or Life-threatening Intensity	
Adverse Experience	CRIXIVAN Percent (n=332)	CRIXIVAN plus Zidovudine Percent (n=332)	Zidovudine Percent (n=332)	CRIXIVAN plus Zidovudine plus Lamivudine Percent (n=571)	Zidovudine plus Lamivudine Percent (n=575)
Body as a Whole					
Abdominal pain	16.6	16.0	12.0	1.9	0.7
Asthenia/fatigue	2.1	4.2	3.6	2.4	4.5
Fever	1.5	1.5	2.1	3.8	3.0
Malaise	2.1	2.7	1.8	0	0
Digestive System					
Nausea	11.7	31.9	19.6	2.8	1.4
Diarrhea	3.3	3.0	2.4	0.9	1.2
Vomiting	8.4	17.8	9.0	1.4	1.4
Acid regurgitation	2.7	5.4	1.8	0.4	0
Anorexia	2.7	5.4	3.0	0.5	0.2
Appetite increase	2.1	1.5	1.2	0	0
Dyspepsia	1.5	2.7	0.9	0	0
Jaundice	1.5	2.1	0.3	0	0
Hemic and Lymphatic System					
Anemia	0.6	1.2	2.1	2.4	3.5
Musculoskeletal System					
Back pain	8.4	4.5	1.5	0.9	0.7
Nervous System/Psychiatric					
Headache	5.4	9.6	6.0	2.4	2.8
Dizziness	3.0	3.9	0.9	0.5	0.7
Somnolence	2.4	3.3	3.3	0	0
Skin and Skin Appendage					
Pruritus	4.2	2.4	1.8	0.5	0
Rash	1.2	0.6	2.4	1.1	0.5
Respiratory System					
Cough	1.5	0.3	0.6	1.6	1.0
Difficulty breathing/ dyspnea/ shortness of breath	0	0.6	0.3	1.8	1.0
Urogenital System					
Nephrolithiasis/urolithiasis*	8.7	7.8	2.1	2.6	0.3
Dysuria	1.5	2.4	0.3	0.4	0.2
Special Senses					
Taste perversion	2.7	8.4	1.2	0.2	0

* Including renal colic, and flank pain with and without hematuria

Table 11: Selected Laboratory Abnormalities of Severe or Life-threatening Intensity Reported in Studies 028 and ACTG 320

	Study 028			Study ACTG 320	
	CRIXIVAN Percent (n=329)	CRIXIVAN plus Zidovudine Percent (n=320)	Zidovudine Percent (n=330)	CRIXIVAN plus Zidovudine plus Lamivudine Percent (n=571)	Zidovudine plus Lamivudine Percent (n=575)
Hematology					
Decreased hemoglobin <7.0 g/dL	0.6	0.9	3.3	2.4	3.5
Decreased platelet count <50 THS/mm^3	0.9	0.9	1.8	0.2	0.9
Decreased neutrophils <0.75 THS/mm^3	2.4	2.2	6.7	5.1	14.6
Blood chemistry					
Increased ALT >500% ULN*	4.9	4.1	3.0	2.6	2.6
Increased AST >500% ULN	3.7	2.8	2.7	3.3	2.8
Total serum bilirubin >250% ULN	11.9	9.7	0.6	6.1	1.4
Increased serum amylase >200% ULN	2.1	1.9	1.8	0.9	0.3
Increased glucose >250 mg/dL	0.9	0.9	0.6	1.6	1.9
Increased creatinine >300% ULN	0	0	0.6	0.2	0

* Upper limit of the normal range.

NDC 0006-0570-62 unit-of-use bottles of 180 (with desiccant).

No. 3756 — 200 mg capsules: semi-translucent white capsules coded **"CRIXIVAN™ 200 mg"** in blue. Available as:

NDC 0006-0571-43 unit-of-use bottles of 360 (with desiccant).

No. 3758 — 400 mg capsules: semi-translucent white capsules coded **"CRIXIVAN™ 400 mg"** in green. Available as:

NDC 0006-0573-40 unit-of-use bottles of 120 (with desiccant)

NDC 0006-0573-62 unit-of-use bottles of 180 (with desiccant)

NDC 0006-0573-54 unit-of-use bottles of 90 (with desiccant)

Storage

Bottles: Store in a tightly-closed container at room temperature, 15-30°C (59-86°F). Protect from moisture. CRIXIVAN Capsules are sensitive to moisture. CRIXIVAN should be dispensed and stored in the original container. The desiccant should remain in the original bottle.

Dist. by: Merck Sharp & Dohme Corp., a subsidiary of **MERCK & CO., INC.**, Whitehouse Station, NJ 08889, USA
U.S. Patent Nos.: 6,645,961

Issued April 2012
9640615

CRIXIVAN® (indinavir sulfate) Capsules

Patient Information about

CRIXIVAN (KRIK-sih-van)

for HIV (Human Immunodeficiency Virus) Infection

Generic name: indinavir (in-DIH-nuh-veer) sulfate

ALERT: Find out about medicines that should NOT be taken with CRIXIVAN®. Please also read the section "MEDICINES YOU SHOULD NOT TAKE WITH CRIXIVAN".

Please read this information before you start taking CRIXIVAN. Also, read the leaflet each time you renew your prescription, just in case anything has changed. Remember, this leaflet does not take the place of careful discussions with your doctor. You and your doctor should discuss CRIXIVAN when you start taking your medication and at regular checkups. You should remain under a doctor's care when using CRIXIVAN and should not change or stop treatment without first talking with your doctor.

What is CRIXIVAN?

CRIXIVAN is an oral capsule used for the treatment of HIV (Human Immunodeficiency Virus). HIV is the virus that causes AIDS (acquired immune deficiency syndrome). CRIXIVAN is a type of HIV drug called a protease (PRO-tee-ase) inhibitor.

How does CRIXIVAN work?

CRIXIVAN is a protease inhibitor that fights HIV. CRIXIVAN can help reduce your chances of getting illnesses associated with HIV. CRIXIVAN can also help lower the amount of HIV in your body (called "viral load") and raise your CD4 (T) cell count. CRIXIVAN may not have these effects in all patients.

CRIXIVAN is usually prescribed with other anti-HIV drugs such as ZDV (also called AZT), 3TC, ddI, ddC, or d4T. CRIXIVAN works differently from these other anti-HIV drugs. Talk with your doctor about how you should take CRIXIVAN.

How should I take CRIXIVAN?

There are six important things you must do to help you benefit from CRIXIVAN:

1. **Take CRIXIVAN capsules every day as prescribed by your doctor.** Continue taking CRIXIVAN unless your doctor tells you to stop. Take the exact amount of CRIXIVAN that your doctor tells you to take, right from the very start. To help make sure you will benefit from CRIXIVAN, you must not skip doses or take "drug holidays". If you don't take CRIXIVAN as prescribed, the activity of CRIXIVAN may be reduced (due to resistance).
2. **Take CRIXIVAN capsules every 8 hours around the clock, *every day.*** It may be easier to remember to take CRIXIVAN if you take it at the same time every day. If you have questions about when to take CRIXIVAN, your doctor or health care provider can help you decide what schedule works for you.
3. **If you miss a dose by more than 2 hours, wait and then take the next dose at the regularly scheduled time.** However, if you miss a dose by less than 2 hours, take your missed dose immediately. Then take your next dose at the regularly scheduled time. Do not take more or less than your prescribed dose of CRIXIVAN at any one time.
4. **Take CRIXIVAN with water.** You can also take CRIXIVAN with other beverages such as skim or non-fat milk, juice, coffee, or tea.
5. **Ideally, take each dose of CRIXIVAN without food but with water at least one hour before or two hours after a meal.** Or you can take CRIXIVAN with a light meal. Examples of light meals include:
   dry toast with jelly, juice, and coffee (with skim or non-fat milk and sugar if you want)
   cornflakes with skim or non-fat milk and sugar
   Do not take CRIXIVAN at the same time as any meals that are high in calories, fat, and protein (for example — a bacon and egg breakfast). When taken at the same time as CRIXIVAN, these foods can interfere with CRIXIVAN being absorbed into your bloodstream and may lessen its effect.
6. **It is critical to drink plenty of fluids while taking CRIXIVAN.** Adults should drink at least six 8-ounce glasses of liquids (preferably water) throughout the day, every day. Your health care provider will give you further instructions on the amount of fluid that you should drink. **CRIXIVAN can cause kidney stones.** Having enough fluids in your body should help reduce the chances of forming a kidney stone. Call your doctor or other health care provider if you develop kidney pains (middle to lower stomach or back pain) or blood in the urine.

Does CRIXIVAN cure HIV or AIDS?

CRIXIVAN does not cure HIV infection or AIDS and you may continue to experience illnesses associated with HIV-1 infection, including opportunistic infections. You should remain under the care of a doctor when using CRIXIVAN. Avoid doing things that can spread HIV-1 infection.

- **Do not share needles or other injection equipment.**
- **Do not share personal items that can have blood or body fluids on them, like toothbrushes and razor blades.**
- **Do not have any kind of sex without protection.** Always practice safe sex by using a latex or polyurethane condom to lower the chance of sexual contact with semen, vaginal secretions, or blood.

Who should not take CRIXIVAN?

Do not take CRIXIVAN if you have had a serious allergic reaction to CRIXIVAN or any of its components.

What other medical problems or conditions should I discuss with my doctor?

Talk to your doctor if:

- You are pregnant or if you become pregnant while you are taking CRIXIVAN. We do not yet know how CRIXIVAN affects pregnant women or their developing babies.
- You are breastfeeding. **Do not breastfeed.** We do not know if CRIXIVAN can be passed to your baby in your breast milk and whether it could harm your baby. Also, mothers with HIV-1 should not breastfeed because HIV-1 can be passed to the baby in the breast milk.

Also talk to your doctor if you have:

- Problems with your liver, especially if you have mild or moderate liver disease caused by cirrhosis
- Problems with your kidneys
- Diabetes
- Hemophilia
- High cholesterol and you are taking cholesterol-lowering medicines called "statins"

Tell your doctor about any medicines you are taking or plan to take, including non-prescription medicines, herbal products including St. John's wort (*Hypericum perforatum*), or dietary supplements.

Can CRIXIVAN be taken with other medications?

MEDICINES YOU SHOULD NOT TAKE WITH CRIXIVAN

Oral VERSED® (midazolam)	HALCION® (triazolam)
ORAP® (pimozide)	XANAX® (alprazolam)
PROPULSID® (cisapride)	REVATIO® (sildenafil for the treatment of pulmonary arterial hypertension)
CORDARONE® (amiodarone)	UROXATRAL® (alfuzosin)
HISMANAL® (astemizole)	Ergot medications (e.g., Wigraine®, Cafergot®, D.H.E. 45®, Migranal®, Ergotrate®, and Methergine®)
	ZOCOR® (simvastatin)
	MEVACOR® (lovastatin)

Taking CRIXIVAN with the above medications could result in serious or life-threatening problems (such as irregular heartbeat or excessive sleepiness).

In addition, you should not take CRIXIVAN with the following:

Rifampin, known as RIFADIN®, RIFAMATE®, RIFATER®, or RIMACTANE®.

There is also an increased risk of drug interactions between CRIXIVAN and LIPITOR® (atorvastatin) and CRESTOR® (rosuvastatin); talk to your doctor before you take any of these cholesterol-reducing drugs with CRIXIVAN.

Taking CRIXIVAN with REYATAZ® (atazanavir) is not recommended because they can both sometimes cause increased levels of bilirubin in the blood.

Taking CRIXIVAN with St. John's wort (*Hypericum perforatum*), an herbal product sold as a dietary supplement, or products containing St. John's wort is not recommended. Taking St. John's wort has been shown to decrease CRIXIVAN levels and may lead to increased viral load and possible resistance to CRIXIVAN or cross resistance to other antiretroviral drugs.

Before you take VIAGRA® (sildenafil), CIALIS® (tadalafil), or LEVITRA® (vardenafil) with CRIXIVAN, talk to your doctor about possible drug interactions and side effects. If you take any of these medicines together with CRIXIVAN, you may be at increased risk of side effects such as low blood pressure, visual changes, and penile erection lasting more than 4 hours, which have been associated with sildenafil, tadalafil, and vardenafil. If an erection lasts longer than 4 hours, you should seek immediate medical assistance to avoid permanent damage to your penis. Your doctor can explain these symptoms to you.

MEDICINES YOU CAN TAKE WITH CRIXIVAN

RETROVIR® (zidovudine, ZDV also called AZT)	EPIVIR™ (lamivudine, 3TC)
ZERIT® (stavudine, d4T)	isoniazid (INH)
BACTRIM®/SEPTRA® (trimethoprim/ sulfamethoxazole)	DIFLUCAN® (fluconazole)
BIAXIN® (clarithromycin)	ORTHO-NOVUM 1/35® (oral contraceptive)
TAGAMET® (cimetidine)	Methadone

VIDEX® (didanosine, ddI) — If you take CRIXIVAN with VIDEX, take them at least one hour apart.

MYCOBUTIN® (rifabutin) — If you take CRIXIVAN with MYCOBUTIN, your doctor may adjust both the dose of MYCOBUTIN and the dose of CRIXIVAN.

NIZORAL® (ketoconazole) — If you take CRIXIVAN with NIZORAL, your doctor may adjust the dose of CRIXIVAN.

RESCRIPTOR® (delavirdine) — If you take CRIXIVAN with RESCRIPTOR, your doctor may adjust the dose of CRIXIVAN.

SPORANOX® (itraconazole) — If you take CRIXIVAN with SPORANOX, your doctor may adjust the dose of CRIXIVAN.

SUSTIVA™ (efavirenz) — If you take CRIXIVAN with SUSTIVA, check with your doctor.

Intravenous VERSED® (midazolam) — If you take CRIXIVAN with Intravenous VERSED®, your doctor may adjust the dose of VERSED®.

Talk to your doctor about any medications you are taking.

Calcium Channel Blockers: Tell your doctor if you are taking calcium channel blockers (e.g., amlodipine, felodipine).

Antiarrhythmics: Tell your doctor if you are taking antiarrhythmics (e.g., quinidine).

Anticonvulsants: Tell your doctor if you are taking anticonvulsants (e.g., phenobarbital, phenytoin, or carbamazepine).

Steroids: Tell your doctor if you are taking steroids (e.g., dexamethasone).

What are the possible side effects of CRIXIVAN?

Like all prescription drugs, CRIXIVAN can cause side effects. The following is **not** a complete list of side effects reported with CRIXIVAN when taken either alone or with other anti-HIV drugs. Do not rely on this leaflet alone for information about side effects. Your doctor can discuss with you a more complete list of side effects.

Some patients treated with CRIXIVAN developed kidney stones. In some of these patients this led to more severe kidney problems, including kidney failure or inflammation of the kidneys or kidney infection which sometimes spread to the blood. Drinking at least six 8-ounce glasses of liquids (preferably water) each day should help reduce the chances of forming a kidney stone (see How should I take CRIXIVAN?). Call your doctor or other health care provider if you develop kidney pains (middle to lower stomach or back pain) or blood in the urine.

Some patients treated with CRIXIVAN have had rapid breakdown of red blood cells (hemolytic anemia) which in some cases was severe or resulted in death.

Some patients treated with CRIXIVAN have had liver problems including liver failure and death. Some patients had other illnesses or were taking other drugs. It is uncertain if CRIXIVAN caused these liver problems.

Diabetes and high blood sugar (hyperglycemia) have occurred in patients taking protease inhibitors. In some of these patients, this led to ketoacidosis, a serious condition caused by poorly controlled blood sugar. Some patients had diabetes before starting protease inhibitors, others did not. Some patients required adjustments to their diabetes medication. Others needed new diabetes medication.

In some patients with hemophilia, increased bleeding has been reported.

Severe muscle pain and weakness have occurred in patients taking protease inhibitors, including CRIXIVAN, together with some of the cholesterol-lowering medicines called "statins". Call your doctor if you develop severe muscle pain or weakness.

Changes in body fat have been seen in some patients taking antiretroviral therapy. These changes may include increased amount of fat in the upper back and neck ("buffalo hump"), breast, and around the trunk. Loss of fat from the legs, arms and face may also happen. The cause and long term health effects of these conditions are not known at this time.

In some patients with advanced HIV infection (AIDS), signs and symptoms of inflammation from opportunistic infections may occur when combination antiretroviral treatment is started.

Clinical Studies

Increases in bilirubin (one laboratory test of liver function) have been reported in approximately 14% of patients. Usually, this finding has not been associated with liver problems. However, on rare occasions, a person may develop yellowing of the skin and/or eyes.

Side effects occurring in 2% or more of patients included: abdominal pain, fatigue or weakness, low red blood cell count, flank pain, painful urination, feeling unwell, nausea, upset stomach, diarrhea, vomiting, acid regurgitation, increased or decreased appetite, back pain, headache, dizziness, taste changes, rash, itchy skin, yellowing of the skin and/or eyes, upper respiratory infection, dry skin, and sore throat.

Swollen kidneys due to blocked urine flow occurred rarely.

Marketing Experience

Other side effects reported since CRIXIVAN has been marketed include: allergic reactions; severe skin reactions; yellowing of the skin and/or eyes; heart problems including heart attack; stroke; abdominal swelling; indigestion; inflammation of the kidneys; decreased kidney function; inflammation of the pancreas; joint pain; depression; itching; hives; change in skin color; hair loss; ingrown toenails with or without infection; crystals in the urine; painful urination; numbness of the mouth and increased cholesterol.

Tell your doctor promptly about these or any other unusual symptoms. If the condition persists or worsens, seek medical attention.

How should I store CRIXIVAN capsules?

- Keep CRIXIVAN capsules in the bottle they came in and at room temperature (59°-86°F).
- Keep CRIXIVAN capsules dry by leaving the small desiccant in the bottle. Keep the bottle closed.

This medication was prescribed for your particular condition. Do not use it for any other condition or give it to anybody else. Keep CRIXIVAN and all medicines out of the reach of children. If you suspect that more than the prescribed dose of this medicine has been taken, contact your local poison control center or emergency room immediately.

This leaflet provides a summary of information about CRIXIVAN. If you have any questions or concerns about either CRIXIVAN or HIV, talk to your doctor.

Distributed by:
Merck Sharp & Dohme Corp., a subsidiary of Merck & Co., Inc.
Whitehouse Station, NJ 08889, USA
U.S. Patent Nos.: 6,645,961

Issued April 2012
9640615

Shown in Product Identification Guide, page 307

DIPROLENE® AF ℞

[*dĭp-rō-lēn*]

brand of augmented betamethasone dipropionate[1]
Cream 0.05%
(potency expressed as betamethasone)
[1]Vehicle augments the penetration of the steroid.

For Dermatologic Use Only - Not for Ophthalmic Use

DESCRIPTION

DIPROLENE® AF Cream 0.05% contains betamethasone dipropionate USP, a synthetic adrenocorticosteroid, for dermatologic use in an emollient base. Betamethasone, an analog of prednisolone, has a high degree of corticosteroid activity and a slight degree of mineralocorticoid activity. Betamethasone dipropionate is the 17,21-dipropionate ester of betamethasone.

Chemically, betamethasone dipropionate is 9-fluoro-11β,17,21-trihydroxy-16β-methylpregna-1,4-diene-3,20-dione 17,21-dipropionate, with the empirical formula $C_{28}H_{37}FO_7$, a molecular weight of 504.6, and the following structural formula:

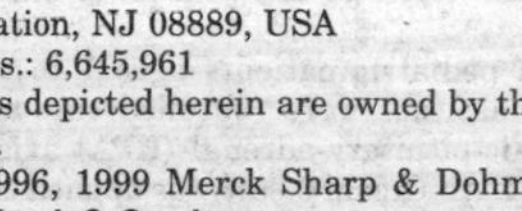

Betamethasone dipropionate is a white to creamy white, odorless crystalline powder, insoluble in water.

Each gram of DIPROLENE AF Cream 0.05% contains: 0.643 mg betamethasone dipropionate USP (equivalent to 0.5 mg betamethasone) in an emollient cream base of purified water; chlorocresol; propylene glycol; white petrolatum; white wax; cyclomethicone; sorbitol solution; glyceryl oleate/propylene glycol; ceteareth-30; carbomer 940; and sodium hydroxide.

CLINICAL PHARMACOLOGY

The corticosteroids are a class of compounds comprising steroid hormones secreted by the adrenal cortex and their synthetic analogs. In pharmacologic doses, corticosteroids are used primarily for their anti-inflammatory and/or immunosuppressive effects.

Topical corticosteroids, such as betamethasone dipropionate, are effective in the treatment of corticosteroid-responsive dermatoses primarily because of their anti-inflammatory, antipruritic, and vasoconstrictive actions. However, while the physiologic, pharmacologic, and clinical effects of the corticosteroids are well known, the exact mechanisms of their actions in each disease are uncertain. Betamethasone dipropionate, a corticosteroid, has been shown to have topical (dermatologic) and systemic pharmacologic and metabolic effects characteristic of this class of drugs.

Pharmacokinetics

The extent of percutaneous absorption of topical corticosteroids is determined by many factors including the vehicle, the integrity of the epidermal barrier, and the use of occlusive dressings (see **DOSAGE AND ADMINISTRATION**).

Topical corticosteroids can be absorbed through normal intact skin. Inflammation and/or other disease processes in the skin may increase percutaneous absorption. Occlusive dressings substantially increase the percutaneous absorption of topical corticosteroids (see **DOSAGE AND ADMINISTRATION**).

Once absorbed through the skin, topical corticosteroids enter pharmacokinetic pathways similar to systemically administered corticosteroids. Corticosteroids are bound to plasma proteins in varying degrees, are metabolized primarily in the liver, and excreted by the kidneys. Some of the topical corticosteroids and their metabolites are also excreted into the bile.

DIPROLENE® AF Cream 0.05% was applied once daily at 7 grams per day for 1 week to diseased skin, in adult patients with psoriasis or atopic dermatitis, to study its effects on the hypothalamic-pituitary-adrenal (HPA) axis. The results suggested that the drug caused a slight lowering of adrenal corticosteroid secretion, although in no case did plasma cortisol levels go below the lower limit of the normal range.

Sixty-seven pediatric patients ages 1 to 12 years, with atopic dermatitis, were enrolled in an open-label, hypothalamic-pituitary-adrenal (HPA) axis safety study. DIPROLENE AF Cream 0.05% was applied twice daily for 2 to 3 weeks over a mean body surface area of 58% (range 35% to 95%). In 19 of 60 (32%) evaluable patients, adrenal suppression was indicated by either a ≤5 mcg/dL prestimulation cortisol, or a cosyntropin post-stimulation cortisol ≤18 mcg/dL and/or an increase of <7 mcg/dL from the baseline cortisol. Studies performed with DIPROLENE AF Cream 0.05% indicate that it is in the high range of potency as compared with other topical corticosteroids.

INDICATIONS AND USAGE

DIPROLENE® AF Cream 0.05% is a high-potency corticosteroid indicated for relief of the inflammatory and pruritic manifestations of corticosteroid-responsive dermatoses in patients 13 years and older.

CONTRAINDICATIONS

DIPROLENE® AF Cream 0.05% is contraindicated in patients who are hypersensitive to betamethasone dipropionate, to other corticosteroids, or to any ingredient in this preparation.

PRECAUTIONS

General

Systemic absorption of topical corticosteroids has produced reversible HPA axis suppression, manifestations of Cushing's syndrome, hyperglycemia, and glucosuria in some patients.

Conditions which augment systemic absorption include the application of the more potent corticosteroids, use over large surface areas, prolonged use, and the addition of occlusive dressings. Use of more than one corticosteroid-containing product at the same time may increase total systemic glucocorticoid exposure (see **DOSAGE AND ADMINISTRATION**).

Therefore, patients receiving a large dose of a potent topical steroid applied to a large surface area should be evaluated periodically for evidence of HPA axis suppression by using the urinary-free cortisol and ACTH stimulation tests. If HPA axis suppression is noted, an attempt should be made to withdraw the drug, to reduce the frequency of application, or to substitute a less potent steroid.

Recovery of HPA axis function is generally prompt and complete upon discontinuation of the drug. In an open-label pediatric study of 60 evaluable patients, of the 19 who showed evidence of suppression, 4 patients were tested 2 weeks after discontinuation of DIPROLENE® AF Cream 0.05%, and 3 of the 4 (75%) had complete recovery of HPA axis function. Infrequently, signs and symptoms of steroid withdrawal may occur, requiring supplemental systemic corticosteroids. Children may absorb proportionally larger amounts of topical corticosteroids and thus be more susceptible to systemic toxicity (see **PRECAUTIONS, Pediatric Use** section).

If irritation develops, topical corticosteroids should be discontinued and appropriate therapy instituted.

In the presence of dermatological infections, the use of an appropriate antifungal or antibacterial agent should be instituted. If a favorable response does not occur promptly, the corticosteroid should be discontinued until the infection has been adequately controlled.

Information for Patients

Patients using topical corticosteroids should receive the following information and instructions. This information is intended to aid in the safe and effective use of this medication. It is not a disclosure of all possible adverse or intended effects.

1. This medication is to be used as directed by the physician and should not be used longer than the prescribed time period. It is for external use only. Avoid contact with the eyes.
2. Patients should be advised not to use this medication for any disorder other than that for which it was prescribed.
3. The treated skin area should not be bandaged or otherwise covered or wrapped as to be occlusive (see **DOSAGE AND ADMINISTRATION**).
4. Patients should report any signs of local adverse reactions.
5. Other corticosteroid-containing products should not be used with DIPROLENE AF Cream 0.05% without first talking to your physician.

Laboratory Tests

The following tests may be helpful in evaluating HPA axis suppression:

Urinary-free cortisol test
ACTH stimulation test

Carcinogenesis, Mutagenesis, and Impairment of Fertility

Long-term animal studies have not been performed to evaluate the carcinogenic potential of betamethasone dipropionate.

Betamethasone was negative in the bacterial mutagenicity assay (*Salmonella typhimurium* and *Escherichia coli*), and in the mammalian cell mutagenicity assay (CHO/HGPRT). It was positive in the *in vitro* human lymphocyte chromosome aberration assay, and equivocal in the *in vivo* mouse bone marrow micronucleus assay. This pattern of response is similar to that of dexamethasone and hydrocortisone.

Reproductive studies with betamethasone dipropionate carried out in rabbits at doses of 1.0 mg/kg by the intramuscular route and in mice up to 33 mg/kg by the intramuscular route indicated no impairment of fertility except for dose-related increases in fetal resorption rates in both species. These doses are approximately 5- and 38-fold the human dose based on a mg/m^2 comparison, respectively.

Pregnancy

Teratogenic Effects
Pregnancy Category C

Corticosteroids are generally teratogenic in laboratory animals when administered systemically at relatively low dosage levels.

Betamethasone dipropionate has been shown to be teratogenic in rabbits when given by the intramuscular route at doses of 0.05 mg/kg. This dose is approximately 0.2-fold the maximum human dose based on a mg/m^2 comparison. The abnormalities observed included umbilical hernias, cephalocele, and cleft palates.

Some corticosteroids have been shown to be teratogenic after dermal application in laboratory animals. There are no adequate and well-controlled studies in pregnant women on teratogenic effects from topically applied corticosteroids. Therefore, topical corticosteroids should be used during pregnancy only if the potential benefit justifies the potential risk to the fetus. Drugs of this class should not be used extensively on pregnant patients, in large amounts, or for prolonged periods of time.

Nursing Mothers

It is not known whether topical administration of corticosteroids can result in sufficient systemic absorption to produce detectable quantities in breast milk. Systemically administered corticosteroids are secreted into breast milk in quantities not likely to have a deleterious effect on the infant. Nevertheless, a decision should be made whether to discontinue nursing or to discontinue the drug, taking into account the importance of the drug to the mother.

Pediatric Use

Use of DIPROLENE AF Cream 0.05% in pediatric patients 12 years of age and younger is not recommended (see **CLINICAL PHARMACOLOGY** and **ADVERSE REACTIONS**). In an open-label study, 19 of 60 (32%) evaluable pediatric patients (aged 3 months-12 years old) using DIPROLENE AF Cream 0.05% for treatment of atopic dermatitis demonstrated HPA axis suppression. The proportion of patients with adrenal suppression in this study was progressively greater, the younger the age group (see **CLINICAL PHARMACOLOGY, Pharmacokinetics** section). Pediatric patients may demonstrate greater susceptibility to topical corticosteroid-induced HPA axis suppression and Cushing's syndrome than mature patients because of a larger skin surface area to body weight ratio. The study described above supports this premise, as adrenal suppression in 9-12 year olds, 6-8 year olds, 2-5 year olds, and 3 months-1 year old was 17%, 32%, 38%, and 50%, respectively.

Hypothalamic-pituitary-adrenal (HPA) axis suppression, Cushing's syndrome, and intracranial hypertension have been reported in children receiving topical corticosteroids. Manifestations of adrenal suppression in children include linear growth retardation, delayed weight gain, low plasma cortisol levels, and absence of response to ACTH stimulation. Manifestations of intracranial hypertension include bulging fontanelles, headaches, and bilateral papilledema. Chronic corticosteroid therapy may interfere with the growth and development of children.

Geriatric Use

Clinical studies of DIPROLENE AF Cream 0.05% included 104 subjects who were 65 years of age and over and 8 subjects who were 75 years of age and over. No overall differences in safety or effectiveness were observed between these subjects and younger subjects, and other reported clinical experience has not identified differences in responses between the elderly and younger patients. However, greater sensitivity of some older individuals cannot be ruled out.

ADVERSE REACTIONS

The only local adverse reaction reported to be possibly or probably related to treatment with DIPROLENE® AF Cream 0.05% during adult-controlled clinical studies was stinging. It occurred in 1 patient, 0.4%, of the 242 patients or subjects involved in the studies.

Adverse reactions reported to be possibly or probably related to treatment with DIPROLENE AF Cream 0.05% during a pediatric clinical study include signs of skin atrophy (telangiectasia, bruising, shininess). Skin atrophy occurred in 7 of 67 (10%) patients, involving all age groups from 3 months – 12 years of age.

The following local adverse reactions are reported infrequently when topical corticosteroids are used as recommended. These reactions are listed in an approximate decreasing order of occurrence: burning, itching, irritation, dryness, folliculitis, hypertrichosis, acneiform eruptions, hypopigmentation, perioral dermatitis, allergic contact dermatitis, maceration of the skin, secondary infection, skin atrophy, striae, miliaria.

Systemic absorption of topical corticosteroids has produced reversible hypothalamic-pituitary-adrenal (HPA) axis suppression, manifestations of Cushing's syndrome, hyperglycemia, and glucosuria in some patients.

OVERDOSAGE

Topically applied corticosteroids can be absorbed in sufficient amounts to produce systemic effects (see **PRECAUTIONS**).

DOSAGE AND ADMINISTRATION

Apply a thin film of DIPROLENE® AF Cream 0.05% to the affected skin areas once or twice daily. Treatment with DIPROLENE AF Cream 0.05% should be limited to 50 g per week.

DIPROLENE AF Cream 0.05% is not to be used with occlusive dressings.

HOW SUPPLIED

DIPROLENE® AF Cream 0.05% is supplied in 15-g (NDC 0085-0517-01) and 50-g (NDC 0085-0517-04) tubes; boxes of one.

Store at 25°C (77°F); excursions permitted to 15-30°C (59-86°F) [see USP Controlled Room Temperature].

Manufactured for: Merck Sharp & Dohme Corp., a subsidiary of
MERCK & CO., INC., Whitehouse Station, NJ 08889, USA
Manufactured by: Schering Plough Canada, Inc.
Pointe Claire, Quebec, Canada

Rev. 05/12
011460-DPL-CR-USPI.2

DIPROLENE® LOTION 0.05% ℞

[*dĭp-rō-lēn*]

brand of augmented betamethasone dipropionate[1]
Lotion 0.05% (potency expressed as betamethasone)
[1]Vehicle augments the penetration of the steroid.

For Dermatologic Use Only
Not for Ophthalmic Use

DESCRIPTION

DIPROLENE® (augmented betamethasone dipropionate) Lotion contains betamethasone dipropionate USP, a synthetic adrenocorticosteroid, for dermatologic use. Betamethasone, an analog of prednisolone, has a high degree of corticosteroid activity and a slight degree of mineralocorticoid activity. Betamethasone dipropionate is the 17, 21-dipropionate ester of betamethasone.

Chemically, betamethasone dipropionate is 9-fluoro-11β,17,21-trihydroxy-16β-methylpregna-1,4-diene-3,20-dione 17,21-dipropionate, with the empirical formula $C_{28}H_{37}FO_7$, a molecular weight of 504.6, and the following structural formula:

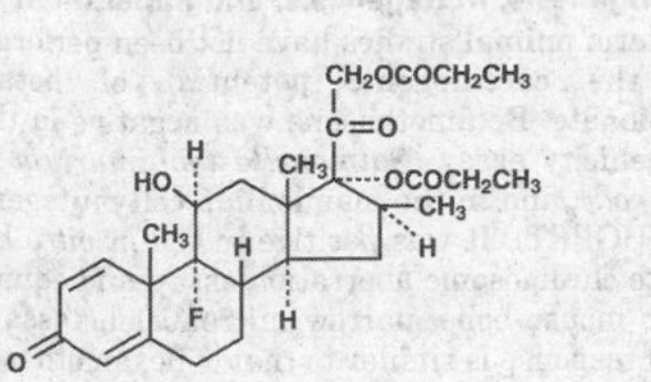

It is a white to creamy-white, odorless powder insoluble in water; freely soluble in acetone and in chloroform; sparingly soluble in alcohol.

Each gram of DIPROLENE Lotion 0.05% contains 0.643 mg betamethasone dipropionate USP (equivalent to 0.5 mg betamethasone), in an augmented lotion base of purified water; isopropyl alcohol (30%); hydroxypropyl cellulose; propylene glycol; sodium phosphate monobasic monohydrate; and phosphoric acid used to adjust the pH.

CLINICAL PHARMACOLOGY

The corticosteroids are a class of compounds comprising steroid hormones secreted by the adrenal cortex and their synthetic analogs. In pharmacologic doses, corticosteroids are used primarily for their anti-inflammatory and/or immunosuppressive effects.

Topical corticosteroids, such as betamethasone dipropionate, are effective in the treatment of corticosteroid-responsive dermatoses primarily because of their anti-inflammatory, antipruritic, and vasoconstrictive actions. However, while the physiologic, pharmacologic, and clinical effects of the corticosteroids are well known, the exact mechanisms of their actions in each disease are uncertain. Betamethasone dipropionate, a corticosteroid, has been shown to have topical (dermatologic) and systemic pharmacologic and metabolic effects characteristic of this class of drugs.

Pharmacokinetics

The extent of percutaneous absorption of topical corticosteroids is determined by many factors including the vehicle, the integrity of the epidermal barrier, and the use of occlusive dressings (see **DOSAGE AND ADMINISTRATION**).

Topical corticosteroids can be absorbed through normal intact skin. Inflammation and/or other disease processes in the skin may increase percutaneous absorption. Occlusive dressings substantially increase the percutaneous absorption of topical corticosteroids (see **DOSAGE AND ADMINISTRATION**).

Once absorbed through the skin, topical corticosteroids enter pharmacokinetic pathways similar to systemically administered corticosteroids. Corticosteroids are bound to plasma proteins in varying degrees, are metabolized primarily in the liver, and excreted by the kidneys. Some of the topical corticosteroids and their metabolites are also excreted into the bile.

Studies performed with DIPROLENE® Lotion indicate that it is in the super-high range of potency as compared with other topical corticosteroids.

INDICATIONS AND USAGE

DIPROLENE® Lotion is a super-high potency corticosteroid indicated for the relief of the inflammatory and pruritic manifestations of corticosteroid-responsive dermatoses in patients 13 years of age and older. The total dose should not exceed 50 mL per week because of the potential for the drug to suppress the hypothalamic-pituitary-adrenal (HPA) axis.

CONTRAINDICATIONS

DIPROLENE® Lotion is contraindicated in patients who are hypersensitive to betamethasone dipropionate, to other corticosteroids, or to any ingredient in this preparation.

PRECAUTIONS

General

Systemic absorption of topical corticosteroids has produced reversible HPA axis suppression, manifestations of Cushing's syndrome, hyperglycemia, and glucosuria in some patients.

Conditions which augment systemic absorption include the application of the more potent corticosteroids, use over large surface areas, prolonged use, and the addition of occlusive dressings. Use of more than one corticosteroid-containing product at the same time may increase total systemic glucocorticoid exposure (see **DOSAGE AND ADMINISTRATION**).

Therefore, patients receiving a large dose of a potent topical steroid applied to a large surface area should be evaluated periodically for evidence of HPA axis suppression by using the urinary-free cortisol and ACTH stimulation tests. If HPA axis suppression is noted, an attempt should be made to withdraw the drug, to reduce the frequency of application, or to substitute a less potent steroid.

Recovery of HPA axis function is generally prompt and complete upon discontinuation of the drug. Patients should not be treated with amounts of DIPROLENE® Lotion greater than 50 mL per week because of the potential for the drug to suppress HPA axis. Patients receiving super-potent corticosteroids should not be treated for more than 2 weeks at a time and only small areas should be treated at any one time due to the increased risk of HPA axis suppression.

DIPROLENE Lotion was applied once daily at 7 mL per day for 21 days to diseased scalp and body skin in patients with scalp psoriasis to study its effects on the HPA axis. In 2 out of 11 patients, the drug lowered plasma cortisol levels below normal limits. HPA axis suppression in these patients was transient and returned to normal within a week. In one of these patients, plasma cortisol levels returned to normal while treatment continued.

Infrequently, signs and symptoms of steroid withdrawal may occur, requiring supplemental systemic corticosteroids.

Pediatric patients may absorb proportionally larger amounts of topical corticosteroids and thus be more susceptible to systemic toxicity (see **PRECAUTIONS, Pediatric Use** section).

If irritation develops, topical corticosteroids should be discontinued and appropriate therapy instituted.

In the presence of dermatological infections, the use of an appropriate antifungal or antibacterial agent should be instituted. If a favorable response does not occur promptly, the corticosteroid should be discontinued until the infection has been adequately controlled.

DIPROLENE Lotion should not be used in the treatment of rosacea or perioral dermatitis, and it should not be used on the face, groin, or in the axillae.

Information for Patients

Patients using topical corticosteroids should receive the following information and instructions. This information is intended to aid in the safe and effective use of this medication. It is not a disclosure of all possible adverse or intended effects.

1. This medication is to be used as directed by the physician and should not be used longer than the prescribed time period. It is for external use only. Avoid contact with the eyes.
2. This medication should not be used for any disorder other than that for which it was prescribed.
3. The treated skin area should not be bandaged, or otherwise covered or wrapped, so as to be occlusive (see **DOSAGE AND ADMINISTRATION**).
4. Patients should report to their physician any signs of local adverse reactions.
5. Patients should be advised not to use DIPROLENE® Lotion in the treatment of diaper dermatitis. DIPROLENE Lotion should not be applied in the diaper areas as diapers or plastic pants may constitute occlusive dressing (see **DOSAGE AND ADMINISTRATION**).
6. This medication should not be used on the face, underarms, or groin areas unless directed by the physician.
7. As with other corticosteroids, therapy should be discontinued when control is achieved. If no improvement is seen within 2 weeks, contact the physician.
8. Other corticosteroid-containing products should not be used with DIPROLENE Lotion.

Laboratory Tests

The following tests may be helpful in evaluating patients for HPA axis suppression:

ACTH stimulation test

Urinary-free cortisol test

Carcinogenesis, Mutagenesis, and Impairment of Fertility

Long-term animal studies have not been performed to evaluate the carcinogenic potential of betamethasone dipropionate. Betamethasone was negative in the bacterial mutagenicity assay (*Salmonella typhimurium* and *Escherichia coli*), and in the mammalian cell mutagenicity assay (CHO/HGPRT). It was positive in the *in vitro* human lymphocyte chromosome aberration assay, and equivocal in the *in vivo* mouse bone marrow micronucleus assay. This pattern of response is similar to that of dexamethasone and hydrocortisone. Studies in rabbits, mice, and rats using intramuscular doses up to 1, 33, and 2 mg/kg, respectively, resulted in dose-related increases in fetal resorptions in rabbits and mice.

Pregnancy

Teratogenic Effects

Pregnancy Category C

Corticosteroids have been shown to be teratogenic in laboratory animals when administered systemically at relatively low dosage levels. Some corticosteroids have been shown to be teratogenic after dermal application in laboratory animals. Betamethasone dipropionate has been shown to be teratogenic in rabbits when given by the intramuscular route at doses of 0.05 mg/kg. This dose is approximately 0.2 times the human topical dose of DIPROLENE Lotion in mg/m^2 of body surface area, assuming 100% absorption and the use in a 60 kg person of 7 g per day. The abnormalities observed included umbilical hernias, cephalocele, and cleft palate. There are no adequate and well-controlled studies in pregnant women on teratogenic effects from topically applied corticosteroids. DIPROLENE Lotion should be used during pregnancy only if the potential benefit justifies the potential risk to the fetus.

Nursing Mothers

Systemically administered corticosteroids appear in human milk and could suppress growth, interfere with endogenous corticosteroid production, or cause other untoward effects. It is not known whether topical administration of corticosteroids could result in sufficient systemic absorption to produce detectable quantities in human milk. Because many drugs are excreted in human milk, caution should be exercised when DIPROLENE Lotion is administered to a nursing woman.

Pediatric Use

Use of DIPROLENE Lotion, 0.05%, in pediatric patients 12 years of age and younger is not recommended (see **CLINICAL PHARMACOLOGY** and **ADVERSE REACTIONS**).

Pediatric patients may demonstrate greater susceptibility to topical corticosteroid-induced HPA axis suppression and Cushing's syndrome than mature patients because of a larger skin surface area to body weight ratio.

Hypothalamic-pituitary-adrenal (HPA) axis suppression, Cushing's syndrome, and intracranial hypertension have been reported in children receiving topical corticosteroids. Manifestations of adrenal suppression in children include linear growth retardation, delayed weight gain, low plasma cortisol levels, and absence of response to ACTH stimulation. Manifestations of intracranial hypertension include bulging fontanelles, headaches, and bilateral papilledema. Chronic corticosteroid therapy may interfere with the growth and development of children.

Geriatric Use

Seven clinical studies of DIPROLENE Lotion evaluated 407 subjects of which 56 subjects were 65 years of age and over and 9 subjects were 75 years of age and over. No overall differences in safety or effectiveness were observed in these clinical studies between geriatric subjects and younger subjects. There was a numerical difference for application site reactions (most frequently reported events were burning and stinging) which occurred in 15% (10/65) of geriatric subjects and 11% (38/342) of subjects less than 65 years of age. Other reported clinical experience has not identified differences in responses between the elderly and younger patients. However, greater sensitivity of some older individuals cannot be ruled out.

ADVERSE REACTIONS

The local adverse reactions which were reported with DIPROLENE® Lotion during controlled clinical trials were as follows: erythema, folliculitis, pruritus, and vesiculation each occurring in less than 1% of patients.

The following additional local adverse reactions have been reported with topical corticosteroids, and they may occur more frequently with the use of occlusive dressings and higher potency corticosteroids. These reactions are listed in an approximately decreasing order of occurrence: burning, itching, irritation, dryness, folliculitis, hypertrichosis, acneiform eruptions, hypopigmentation, perioral dermatitis, allergic contact dermatitis, secondary infection, skin atrophy, striae, and miliaria.

Systemic absorption of topical corticosteroids has produced reversible hypothalamic-pituitary-adrenal (HPA) axis suppression, manifestations of Cushing's syndrome, hyperglycemia, and glucosuria in some patients.

OVERDOSAGE

Topically applied DIPROLENE® Lotion can be absorbed in sufficient amounts to produce systemic effects (see **PRECAUTIONS**).

DOSAGE AND ADMINISTRATION

Apply a few drops of DIPROLENE® Lotion to the affected skin once or twice daily and massage lightly until the lotion disappears.

DIPROLENE Lotion is a super-high potency topical corticosteroid. **Treatment with DIPROLENE Lotion should be limited to two weeks, and amounts greater than 50 mL per week should not be used.**

As with other highly active corticosteroids, therapy should be discontinued when control is achieved. If no improvement is seen within 2 weeks, reassessment of diagnosis may be necessary.

DIPROLENE Lotion should not be used with occlusive dressings. DIPROLENE Lotion should not be applied to the diaper area if the patient requires diapers or plastic pants as these garments may constitute occlusive dressing.

HOW SUPPLIED

DIPROLENE® Lotion 0.05% is supplied in 30-mL (29 g) (NDC 0085-0962-01) and 60-mL (58 g) (NDC 0085-0962-02) plastic squeeze bottles; boxes of one.

Store at 25°C (77°F); excursions permitted to 15–30°C (59–86°F) [see USP Controlled Room Temperature].

Manufactured for: Merck Sharp & Dohme Corp., a subsidiary of

MERCK & CO., INC., Whitehouse Station, NJ 08889, USA

Manufactured by: Schering Plough Canada, Inc., Pointe Claire, Quebec H9R 1B4, Canada

Revised: 10/2012
011460-DPL-LT-USPI.2

DIPROLENE® ℞

[*dīp-rō-lēn*]

brand of augmented betamethasone dipropionate[1]
Ointment 0.05%
(potency expressed as betamethasone)

[1]Vehicle augments the penetration of the steroid.

For Dermatologic Use Only - Not for Ophthalmic Use

DESCRIPTION

DIPROLENE® (augmented betamethasone dipropionate) Ointment contains betamethasone dipropionate USP, a synthetic adrenocorticosteroid, for dermatologic use. Betamethasone, an analog of prednisolone, has a high degree of corticosteroid activity and a slight degree of mineralocorticoid activity. Betamethasone dipropionate is the 17, 21-dipropionate ester of betamethasone.

Chemically, betamethasone dipropionate is 9-fluoro-11β, 17,21-trihydroxy-16β-methylpregna-1,4-diene-3,20-dione 17,21-dipropionate, with the empirical formula $C_{28}H_{37}FO_7$, a molecular weight of 504.6 and the following structural formula:

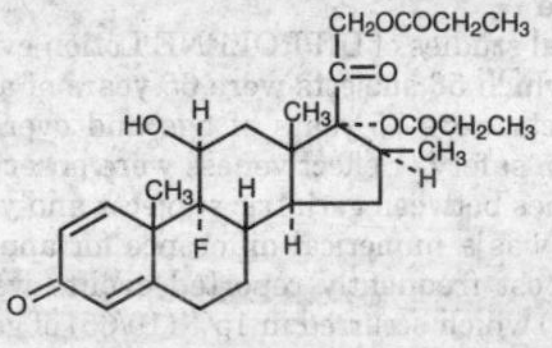

It is a white to creamy-white, odorless powder insoluble in water; freely soluble in acetone and in chloroform; sparingly soluble in alcohol.

Each gram of DIPROLENE Ointment 0.05% contains 0.643 mg betamethasone dipropionate USP (equivalent to 0.5 mg betamethasone), in a vehicle of propylene glycol; propylene glycol stearate; white wax; and white petrolatum.

CLINICAL PHARMACOLOGY

The corticosteroids are a class of compounds comprising steroid hormones secreted by the adrenal cortex and their synthetic analogs. In pharmacologic doses, corticosteroids are used primarily for their anti-inflammatory and/or immunosuppressive effects. Topical corticosteroids, such as betamethasone dipropionate, are effective in the treatment of corticosteroid-responsive dermatoses primarily because of their anti-inflammatory, antipruritic, and vasoconstrictive actions. However, while the physiologic, pharmacologic, and clinical effects of the corticosteroids are well known, the exact mechanisms of their actions in each disease are uncertain. Betamethasone dipropionate, a corticosteroid, has been shown to have topical (dermatologic) and systemic pharmacologic and metabolic effects characteristic of this class of drugs.

Pharmacokinetics

The extent of percutaneous absorption of topical corticosteroids is determined by many factors including the vehicle, the integrity of the epidermal barrier, and the use of occlusive dressings (see **DOSAGE AND ADMINISTRATION**). Topical corticosteroids can be absorbed through normal intact skin. Inflammation and/or other disease processes in the skin may increase percutaneous absorption. Occlusive dressings substantially increase the percutaneous absorption of topical corticosteroids (see **DOSAGE AND ADMINISTRATION**).

Once absorbed through the skin, topical corticosteroids enter pharmacokinetic pathways similar to systemically administered corticosteroids. Corticosteroids are bound to plasma proteins in varying degrees, are metabolized primarily in the liver, and excreted by the kidneys. Some of the topical corticosteroids and their metabolites are also excreted into the bile.

Studies performed with DIPROLENE® Ointment indicate that it is in the super-high range of potency as compared with other topical corticosteroids.

INDICATIONS AND USAGE

DIPROLENE® Ointment is a super-high potency corticosteroid indicated for the relief of the inflammatory and pruritic manifestations of corticosteroid-responsive dermatoses in patients 13 years of age and older. The total dose should not exceed 50 g per week because of the potential for the drug to suppress the hypothalamic-pituitary-adrenal (HPA) axis.

CONTRAINDICATIONS

DIPROLENE® Ointment is contraindicated in patients who are hypersensitive to betamethasone dipropionate, to other corticosteroids, or to any ingredient in this preparation.

PRECAUTIONS

General

Systemic absorption of topical corticosteroids has produced reversible HPA axis suppression, manifestations of Cushing's syndrome, hyperglycemia, and glucosuria in some patients. Conditions which augment systemic absorption include the application of the more potent corticosteroids, use over large surface areas, prolonged use, and the addition of occlusive dressings. Use of more than one corticosteroid-containing product at the same time may increase total systemic glucocorticoid exposure (see **DOSAGE AND ADMINISTRATION**).

Therefore, patients receiving a large dose of a potent topical steroid applied to a large surface area should be evaluated periodically for evidence of HPA axis suppression by using the urinary-free cortisol and ACTH stimulation tests. If HPA axis suppression is noted, an attempt should be made to withdraw the drug, to reduce the frequency of application, or to substitute a less potent steroid.

Recovery of HPA axis function is generally prompt and complete upon discontinuation of the drug. Patients should not be treated with amounts of DIPROLENE® Ointment greater than 50 g per week because of the potential for the drug to suppress HPA axis. Patients receiving super-potent corticosteroids should not be treated for more than 2 weeks at a time and only small areas should be treated at any one time due to the increased risk of HPA suppression.

At 14 g per day DIPROLENE Ointment was shown to depress the plasma levels of adrenal cortical hormones following repeated application to diseased skin in patients with psoriasis. These effects were reversible upon discontinuation of treatment. At 7 g per day DIPROLENE Ointment was shown to cause minimal inhibition of the HPA axis when applied 2 times daily for 2 to 3 weeks in healthy patients and in patients with psoriasis and eczematous disorders.

With 6 to 7 g of DIPROLENE Ointment applied once daily for 3 weeks, no significant inhibition of the HPA axis was observed in patients with psoriasis and atopic dermatitis, as measured by plasma cortisol and 24-hour urinary 17-hydroxy-corticosteroid levels. Infrequently, signs and symptoms of steroid withdrawal may occur, requiring supplemental systemic corticosteroids.

Pediatric patients may absorb proportionally larger amounts of topical corticosteroids and thus be more susceptible to systemic toxicity (see **PRECAUTIONS, Pediatric Use** section).

If irritation develops, topical corticosteroids should be discontinued and appropriate therapy instituted.

In the presence of dermatological infections, the use of an appropriate antifungal or antibacterial agent should be instituted. If a favorable response does not occur promptly, the corticosteroid should be discontinued until the infection has been adequately controlled. DIPROLENE Ointment should not be used in the treatment of rosacea or perioral dermatitis, and it should not be used on the face, groin, or in the axillae.

Information for Patients

Patients using topical corticosteroids should receive the following information and instructions. This information is intended to aid in the safe and effective use of this medication. It is not a disclosure of all possible adverse or intended effects.

1. This medication is to be used as directed by the physician and should not be used longer than the prescribed time period. It is for external use only. Avoid contact with the eyes.
2. This medication should not be used for any disorder other than that for which it was prescribed.
3. The treated skin area should not be bandaged, otherwise covered or wrapped, so as to be occlusive (see **DOSAGE AND ADMINISTRATION**).
4. Patients should report to their physician any signs of local adverse reactions.
5. Patients should be advised not to use DIPROLENE Ointment in the treatment of diaper dermatitis. DIPROLENE Ointment should not be applied in the diaper areas as diapers or plastic pants may constitute occlusive dressing (see **DOSAGE AND ADMINISTRATION**).
6. This medication should not be used on the face, underarms, or groin areas unless directed by the physician.
7. As with other corticosteroids, therapy should be discontinued when control is achieved. If no improvement is seen within 2 weeks, contact the physician.
8. Other corticosteroid-containing products should not be used with DIPROLENE Ointment.

Laboratory Tests

The following tests may be helpful in evaluating patients for HPA axis suppression:
ACTH stimulation test
Urinary-free cortisol test

Carcinogenesis, Mutagenesis, and Impairment of Fertility

Long-term animal studies have not been performed to evaluate the carcinogenic potential of betamethasone dipropionate. Betamethasone was negative in the bacterial mutagenicity assay (*Salmonella typhimurium* and *Escherichia coli*), and in the mammalian cell mutagenicity assay (CHO/HGPRT). It was positive in the *in vitro* human lymphocyte chromosome aberration assay, and equivocal in the *in vivo* mouse bone marrow micronucleus assay. This pattern of response is similar to that of dexamethasone and hydrocortisone. Studies in rabbits, mice, and rats using intramuscular doses up to 1, 33, and 2 mg/kg, respectively, resulted in dose-related increases in fetal resorptions in rabbits and mice.

Pregnancy

Teratogenic Effects

Pregnancy Category C

Corticosteroids have been shown to be teratogenic in laboratory animals when administered systemically at relatively low dosage levels. Some corticosteroids have been shown to be teratogenic after dermal application in laboratory animals. Betamethasone dipropionate has been shown to be teratogenic in rabbits when given by the intramuscular route at doses of 0.05 mg/kg. This dose is approximately 0.2 times the human topical dose of DIPROLENE Ointment in mg/m^2 of body surface area, assuming 100% absorption and the use in a 60 kg person of 7 g per day. The abnormalities observed included umbilical hernias, cephalocele, and cleft palate. There are no adequate and well-controlled studies in pregnant women on teratogenic effects from topically applied corticosteroids. DIPROLENE Ointment should be used during pregnancy only if the potential benefit justifies the potential risk to the fetus.

Nursing Mothers

Systemically administered corticosteroids appear in human milk and could suppress growth, interfere with endogenous corticosteroid production, or cause other untoward effects. It is not known whether topical administration of corticosteroids could result in sufficient systemic absorption to produce detectable quantities in human milk. Because many drugs are excreted in human milk, caution should be exercised when DIPROLENE Ointment is administered to a nursing woman.

Pediatric Use

Use of DIPROLENE Ointment, 0.05%, in pediatric patients 12 years of age and younger is not recommended (see **CLINICAL PHARMACOLOGY** and **ADVERSE REACTIONS**).

Pediatric patients may demonstrate greater susceptibility to topical corticosteroid-induced HPA axis suppression and Cushing's syndrome than mature patients because of a larger skin surface area to body weight ratio.

Hypothalamic-pituitary-adrenal (HPA) axis suppression, Cushing's syndrome, and intracranial hypertension have been reported in children receiving topical corticosteroids. Manifestations of adrenal suppression in children include linear growth retardation, delayed weight gain, low plasma cortisol levels, and an absence of response to ACTH stimulation. Manifestations of intracranial hypertension include bulging fontanelles, headaches, and bilateral papilledema. Chronic corticosteroid therapy may interfere with the growth and development of children.

Geriatric Use

Clinical studies of DIPROLENE Ointment included 225 subjects who were 65 years of age and over and 46 subjects who were 75 years of age and over. No overall differences in safety or effectiveness were observed between these subjects and younger subjects, and other reported clinical experience has not identified differences in responses between the elderly and younger patients. However, greater sensitivity of some older individuals cannot be ruled out.

ADVERSE REACTIONS

The local adverse reactions which were reported with DIPROLENE® Ointment during controlled clinical trials were as follows: erythema, folliculitis, pruritus, and vesiculation each occurring in less than 1% of patients.

The following additional local adverse reactions have been reported with topical corticosteroids, and they may occur more frequently with the use of occlusive dressings and higher potency corticosteroids. These reactions are listed in an approximately decreasing order of occurrence: burning, itching, irritation, dryness, folliculitis, hypertrichosis, acneiform eruptions, hypopigmentation, perioral dermatitis, allergic contact dermatitis, secondary infection, skin atrophy, striae, and miliaria.

Systemic absorption of topical corticosteroids has produced reversible hypothalamic-pituitary-adrenal (HPA) axis suppression, manifestations of Cushing's syndrome, hyperglycemia, and glucosuria in some patients.

OVERDOSAGE

Topically applied DIPROLENE® Ointment can be absorbed in sufficient amounts to produce systemic effects (see **PRECAUTIONS**).

DOSAGE AND ADMINISTRATION

Apply a thin film of DIPROLENE® Ointment to the affected skin once or twice daily. DIPROLENE Ointment is a super-high potency topical corticosteroid. **Treatment with DIPROLENE Ointment should be limited to 50 g per week.** As with other corticosteroids, therapy should be discontinued when control is achieved. If no improvement is seen within 2 weeks, reassessment of diagnosis may be necessary.

DIPROLENE Ointment should not be used with occlusive dressings. DIPROLENE Ointment should not be applied to the diaper area if the patient requires diapers or plastic pants as these garments may constitute occlusive dressing.

HOW SUPPLIED

DIPROLENE® Ointment 0.05% is supplied in 15-g (NDC 0085-0575-02) and 50-g (NDC 0085-0575-05) tubes; boxes of one.

Store at 25°C (77°F); excursions permitted to 15-30°C (59-86°F) [see USP Controlled Room Temperature].

Manufactured for: Merck Sharp & Dohme Corp., a subsidiary of

MERCK & CO., INC., Whitehouse Station, NJ 08889, USA

Manufactured by: Schering Plough Canada, Inc.

Pointe Claire, Quebec, Canada

Rev. 05/12

011460-DPL-OT-USPI.2

DULERA® 100 mcg/5 mcg ℞

[dew-LAIR-ah]

(mometasone furoate 100 mcg and formoterol fumarate dihydrate 5 mcg)

Inhalation Aerosol

DULERA® 200 mcg/5 mcg

(mometasone furoate 200 mcg and formoterol fumarate dihydrate 5 mcg)

Inhalation Aerosol

FOR ORAL INHALATION

HIGHLIGHTS OF PRESCRIBING INFORMATION

These highlights do not include all the information needed to use DULERA safely and effectively. See full prescribing information for DULERA.

DULERA® 100 mcg/5 mcg (mometasone furoate 100 mcg and formoterol fumarate dihydrate 5 mcg) Inhalation Aerosol

DULERA® 200 mcg/5 mcg (mometasone furoate 200 mcg and formoterol fumarate dihydrate 5 mcg) Inhalation Aerosol

FOR ORAL INHALATION

Initial U.S. Approval: 2010

WARNING: ASTHMA-RELATED DEATH

See full prescribing information for complete boxed warning.

- **Long-acting beta$_2$-adrenergic agonists (LABA), such as formoterol, one of the active ingredients in DULERA, increase the risk of asthma-related death. Data from a large placebo-controlled U.S. study that compared the safety of another LABA (salmeterol) or placebo added to usual asthma therapy showed an increase in asthma-related deaths in patients receiving salmeterol. This finding with salmeterol is considered a class effect of the LABA, including formoterol. Currently available data are inadequate to determine whether concurrent use of inhaled corticosteroids or other long-term asthma control drugs mitigates the increased risk of asthma-related death from LABA. Available data from controlled clinical trials suggest that LABA increase the risk of asthma-related hospitalization in pediatric and adolescent patients.**
- **When treating patients with asthma, prescribe DULERA only for patients with asthma not adequately controlled on a long-term asthma control medication, such as an inhaled corticosteroid or whose disease severity clearly warrants initiation of treatment with both an inhaled corticosteroid and LABA. Once asthma control is achieved and maintained, assess the patient at regular intervals and step down therapy (e.g., discontinue DULERA) if possible without loss of asthma control, and maintain the patient on a long-term asthma control medication, such as an inhaled corticosteroid. Do not use DULERA for patients whose asthma is adequately controlled on low or medium dose inhaled corticosteroids. (1.1, 5.1)**

RECENT MAJOR CHANGES

Warnings and Precautions, Coexisting Conditions (5.15) 07/2013

INDICATIONS AND USAGE

DULERA is a combination product containing a corticosteroid and a long-acting beta$_2$-adrenergic agonist indicated for:

- Treatment of asthma in patients 12 years of age and older. (1.1)

Important limitations:

- Not indicated for the relief of acute bronchospasm. (1.1)

DOSAGE AND ADMINISTRATION

For oral inhalation only.

Treatment of asthma in patients ≥12 years: 2 inhalations twice daily of DULERA 100 mcg/5 mcg or 200 mcg/5 mcg. Starting dosage is based on prior asthma therapy. (2.2)

DOSAGE FORMS AND STRENGTHS

Inhalation aerosol containing a combination of mometasone furoate (100 or 200 mcg) and formoterol fumarate dihydrate (5 mcg) per actuation. (3)

CONTRAINDICATIONS

- Primary treatment of status asthmaticus or acute episodes of asthma requiring intensive measures. (4.1)
- Hypersensitivity to any of the ingredients of DULERA. (4.2)

WARNINGS AND PRECAUTIONS

- Asthma-related death: Long-acting beta$_2$-adrenergic agonists increase the risk. Prescribe only for recommended patient populations. (5.1)
- Deterioration of disease and acute episodes: Do not initiate in acutely deteriorating asthma or to treat acute symptoms. (5.2)
- Use with additional long-acting beta$_2$-agonist: Do not use in combination because of risk of overdose. (5.3)
- Localized infections: *Candida albicans* infection of the mouth and throat may occur. Monitor patients periodically for signs of adverse effects on the oral cavity. Advise patients to rinse the mouth following inhalation. (5.4)
- Immunosuppression: Potential worsening of existing tuberculosis, fungal, bacterial, viral, or parasitic infection; or ocular herpes simplex infections. More serious or even fatal course of chickenpox or measles can occur in susceptible patients. Use with caution in patients with these infections because of the potential for worsening of these infections. (5.5)
- Transferring patients from systemic corticosteroids: Risk of impaired adrenal function when transferring from oral steroids. Taper patients slowly from systemic corticosteroids if transferring to DULERA. (5.6)
- Hypercorticism and adrenal suppression: May occur with very high dosages or at the regular dosage in susceptible individuals. If such changes occur, discontinue DULERA slowly. (5.7)
- Strong cytochrome P450 3A4 inhibitors (e.g., ritonavir): Risk of increased systemic corticosteroid effects. Exercise caution when used with DULERA. (5.8)
- Paradoxical bronchospasm: Discontinue DULERA and institute alternative therapy if paradoxical bronchospasm occurs. (5.9)
- Patients with cardiovascular disorders: Use with caution because of beta-adrenergic stimulation. (5.11)
- Decreases in bone mineral density: Monitor patients with major risk factors for decreased bone mineral content. (5.12)
- Effects on growth: Monitor growth of pediatric patients. (5.13)
- Glaucoma and cataracts: Monitor patients with change in vision or with a history of increased intraocular pressure, glaucoma, and/or cataracts closely. (5.14)
- Coexisting conditions: Use with caution in patients with aneurysm, pheochromocytoma, convulsive disorders, thyrotoxicosis, diabetes mellitus, and ketoacidosis. (5.15)
- Hypokalemia and hyperglycemia: Be alert to hypokalemia and hyperglycemia. (5.16)

ADVERSE REACTIONS

Most common adverse reactions (reported in ≥3% of patients) included:

- Nasopharyngitis, sinusitis and headache. (6.1)

To report SUSPECTED ADVERSE REACTIONS, contact Merck Sharp & Dohme Corp., a subsidiary of Merck & Co., Inc., at 1-877-888-4231 or FDA at 1-800-FDA-1088 or *www.fda.gov/medwatch.*

DRUG INTERACTIONS

- Strong cytochrome P450 3A4 inhibitors (e.g., ritonavir): Use with caution. May cause increased systemic corticosteroid effects. (7.1)
- Adrenergic agents: Use with caution. Additional adrenergic drugs may potentiate sympathetic effects. (7.2)
- Xanthine derivatives and diuretics: Use with caution. May potentiate ECG changes and/or hypokalemia. (7.3, 7.4)
- MAO inhibitors, tricyclic antidepressants, macrolides, and drugs that prolong QTc interval: Use with extreme caution. May potentiate effect on the cardiovascular system. (7.5)
- Beta-blockers: Use with caution and only when medically necessary. May decrease effectiveness and produce severe bronchospasm. (7.6)
- Halogenated hydrocarbons: There is an elevated risk of arrhythmias in patients receiving concomitant anesthesia with halogenated hydrocarbons. (7.7)

USE IN SPECIFIC POPULATIONS

- Hepatic impairment: Monitor patients for signs of increased drug exposure. (8.6)

See 17 for PATIENT COUNSELING INFORMATION and Medication Guide

Revised: 07/2013

FULL PRESCRIBING INFORMATION: CONTENTS*

*** Sections or subsections omitted from the full prescribing information are not listed**

FULL PRESCRIBING INFORMATION

WARNING: ASTHMA-RELATED DEATH

Long-acting beta$_2$-adrenergic agonists (LABA), such as formoterol, one of the active ingredients in DULERA, increase the risk of asthma-related death. Data from a large placebo-controlled U.S. study that compared the safety of another long-acting beta$_2$-adrenergic agonist (salmeterol) or placebo added to usual asthma therapy showed an increase in asthma-related deaths in patients receiving salmeterol. This finding with salmeterol is considered a class effect of the LABA, including formoterol. Currently available data are inadequate to determine whether concurrent use of inhaled corticosteroids or other long-term asthma control drugs mitigates the increased risk of asthma-related death from LABA. Available data from controlled clinical trials suggest that LABA increase the risk of asthma-related hospitalization in pediatric and adolescent patients. Therefore, when treating patients with asthma, DULERA should only be used for patients not adequately controlled on a long-term asthma control medication, such as an inhaled corticosteroid or whose disease severity clearly warrants initiation of treatment with both an inhaled corticosteroid and LABA. Once asthma control is achieved and maintained, assess the patient at regular intervals and step down therapy (e.g., discontinue DULERA) if possible without loss of asthma control, and maintain the patient on a long-term asthma control medication, such as an inhaled corticosteroid. Do not use DULERA for patients whose asthma is adequately controlled on low or medium dose inhaled corticosteroids. *[See Warnings and Precautions (5.1).]*

1 INDICATIONS AND USAGE

1.1 Treatment of Asthma

DULERA is indicated for the treatment of asthma in patients 12 years of age and older.

Long-acting beta$_2$-adrenergic agonists, such as formoterol, one of the active ingredients in DULERA, increase the risk of asthma-related death. Available data from controlled clinical trials suggest that LABA increase the risk of asthma-related hospitalization in pediatric and adolescent patients *[see Warnings and Precautions (5.1)]*. Therefore, when treating patients with asthma, DULERA should only be used for patients not adequately controlled on a long-term asthma control medication, such as an inhaled corticosteroid or whose disease severity clearly warrants initiation of treatment with both an inhaled corticosteroid and LABA. Once asthma control is achieved and maintained, assess the patient at regular intervals and step down therapy (e.g., discontinue DULERA) if possible without loss of asthma control, and maintain the patient on a long-term asthma control medication, such as an inhaled corticosteroid. Do not use DULERA for patients whose asthma is adequately controlled on low or medium dose inhaled corticosteroids.

Important Limitation of Use

- DULERA is NOT indicated for the relief of acute bronchospasm.

2 DOSAGE AND ADMINISTRATION

2.1 General

DULERA should be administered only by the orally inhaled route (see Instructions for Using DULERA in the Medication Guide). After each dose, the patient should be advised to rinse his/her mouth with water without swallowing.

The cap from the mouthpiece of the actuator should be removed before using DULERA.

DULERA should be primed before using for the first time by releasing 4 test sprays into the air, away from the face, shaking well before each spray. In cases where the inhaler has not been used for more than 5 days, prime the inhaler again by releasing 4 test sprays into the air, away from the face, shaking well before each spray.

The DULERA canister should only be used with the DULERA actuator. The DULERA actuator should not be used with any other inhalation drug product. Actuators from other products should not be used with the DULERA canister.

2.2 Dosing

DULERA should be administered as two inhalations twice daily every day (morning and evening) by the orally inhaled route.

Shake well prior to each inhalation.

The recommended starting dosages for DULERA treatment are based on prior asthma therapy.

Table 1: Recommended Dosages for DULERA

Previous Therapy	Recommended Dose	Maximum Recommended Daily Dose
Inhaled medium dose corticosteroids	DULERA 100 mcg/5 mcg, 2 inhalations twice daily	400 mcg/20 mcg
Inhaled high dose corticosteroids	DULERA 200 mcg/5 mcg, 2 inhalations twice daily	800 mcg/20 mcg

The maximum daily recommended dose is two inhalations of DULERA 200 mcg/5 mcg twice daily. Do not use more than two inhalations twice daily of the prescribed strength of DULERA as some patients are more likely to experience adverse effects with higher doses of formoterol. If symptoms arise between doses, an inhaled short-acting beta$_2$-agonist should be taken for immediate relief.

If a previously effective dosage regimen of DULERA fails to provide adequate control of asthma, the therapeutic regimen should be re-evaluated and additional therapeutic options, e.g., replacing the current strength of DULERA with a higher strength, adding additional inhaled corticosteroid, or initiating oral corticosteroids, should be considered.

The maximum benefit may not be achieved for 1 week or longer after beginning treatment. Individual patients may experience a variable time to onset and degree of symptom relief. For patients ≥12 years of age who do not respond adequately after 2 weeks of therapy, higher strength may provide additional asthma control.

3 DOSAGE FORMS AND STRENGTHS

DULERA is a pressurized metered dose inhaler that is available in 2 strengths.

DULERA 100 mcg/5 mcg delivers 100 mcg of mometasone furoate and 5 mcg of formoterol fumarate dihydrate per actuation.

DULERA 200 mcg/5 mcg delivers 200 mcg of mometasone furoate and 5 mcg of formoterol fumarate dihydrate per actuation.

4 CONTRAINDICATIONS

4.1 Status Asthmaticus

DULERA is contraindicated in the primary treatment of status asthmaticus or other acute episodes of asthma where intensive measures are required.

4.2 Hypersensitivity

DULERA is contraindicated in patients with known hypersensitivity to mometasone furoate, formoterol fumarate, or any of the ingredients in DULERA *[see Warnings and Precautions (5.10)]*.

5 WARNINGS AND PRECAUTIONS

5.1 Asthma-Related Death

Long-acting beta$_2$-adrenergic agonists, such as formoterol, one of the active ingredients in DULERA, increase the risk of asthma-related death. Currently available data are inadequate to determine whether concurrent use of inhaled corticosteroids or other long-term asthma control drugs mitigates the increased risk of asthma-related death from LABA. Available data from controlled clinical trials suggest that LABA increase the risk of asthma-related hospitalization in pediatric and adolescent patients. Therefore, when treating patients with asthma, physicians should only prescribe DULERA for patients with asthma not adequately controlled on a long-term asthma control medication, such as an inhaled corticosteroid or whose disease severity clearly warrants initiation of treatment with both an inhaled corticosteroid and LABA. Once asthma control is achieved and maintained, assess the patient at regular intervals and step down therapy (e.g., discontinue DULERA) if possible without loss of asthma control, and maintain the patient on a long-term asthma control medication, such as an inhaled corticosteroid. Do not use DULERA for patients whose asthma is adequately controlled on low or medium dose inhaled corticosteroids.

A 28-week, placebo-controlled US study comparing the safety of salmeterol with placebo, each added to usual asthma therapy, showed an increase in asthma-related deaths in patients receiving salmeterol (13/13,176 in patients treated with salmeterol vs. 3/13,179 in patients treated with placebo; RR 4.37, 95% CI 1.25, 15.34). This finding with salmeterol is considered a class effect of the LABAs, including formoterol, one of the active ingredients in DULERA. No study adequate to determine whether the rate of asthma-related death is increased with DULERA has been conducted.

Clinical studies with formoterol suggested a higher incidence of serious asthma exacerbations in patients who received formoterol fumarate than in those who received placebo. The sizes of these studies were not adequate to precisely quantify the differences in serious asthma exacerbation rates between treatment groups.

5.2 Deterioration of Disease and Acute Episodes

DULERA should not be initiated in patients during rapidly deteriorating or potentially life-threatening episodes of asthma. DULERA has not been studied in patients with acutely deteriorating asthma. The initiation of DULERA in this setting is not appropriate.

Increasing use of inhaled, short-acting beta$_2$-agonists is a marker of deteriorating asthma. In this situation, the patient requires immediate re-evaluation with reassessment of the treatment regimen, giving special consideration to the possible need for replacing the current strength of DULERA with a higher strength, adding additional inhaled corticosteroid, or initiating systemic corticosteroids. Patients should not use more than 2 inhalations twice daily (morning and evening) of DULERA.

DULERA is not indicated for the relief of acute symptoms, i.e., as rescue therapy for the treatment of acute episodes of bronchospasm. An inhaled, short-acting beta$_2$-agonist, not DULERA, should be used to relieve acute symptoms such as shortness of breath. When prescribing DULERA, the physician must also provide the patient with an inhaled, short-acting beta$_2$-agonist (e.g., albuterol) for treatment of acute symptoms, despite regular twice-daily (morning and evening) use of DULERA.

When beginning treatment with DULERA, patients who have been taking oral or inhaled, short-acting beta$_2$-agonists on a regular basis (e.g., 4 times a day) should be instructed to discontinue the regular use of these drugs.

5.3 Excessive Use of DULERA and Use with Other Long-Acting Beta$_2$-Agonists

As with other inhaled drugs containing beta$_2$-adrenergic agents, DULERA should not be used more often than recommended, at higher doses than recommended, or in conjunction with other medications containing long-acting beta$_2$-agonists, as an overdose may result. Clinically significant cardiovascular effects and fatalities have been reported in association with excessive use of inhaled sympathomimetic drugs. Patients using DULERA should not use an additional long-acting beta$_2$-agonist (e.g., salmeterol, formoterol fumarate, arformoterol tartrate) for any reason, including prevention of exercise-induced bronchospasm (EIB) or the treatment of asthma.

5.4 Local Effects

In clinical trials, the development of localized infections of the mouth and pharynx with *Candida albicans* have occurred in patients treated with DULERA. If oropharyngeal candidiasis develops, it should be treated with appropriate local or systemic (i.e., oral) antifungal therapy while remaining on treatment with DULERA therapy, but at times therapy with DULERA may need to be interrupted. Advise patients to rinse the mouth after inhalation of DULERA.

5.5 Immunosuppression

Persons who are using drugs that suppress the immune system are more susceptible to infections than healthy individuals.

Chickenpox and measles, for example, can have a more serious or even fatal course in susceptible children or adults using corticosteroids. In such children or adults who have not had these diseases or who are not properly immunized, particular care should be taken to avoid exposure. How the dose, route, and duration of corticosteroid administration affect the risk of developing a disseminated infection is not known. The contribution of the underlying disease and/or prior corticosteroid treatment to the risk is also not known. If exposed to chickenpox, prophylaxis with varicella zoster immune globulin (VZIG) or pooled intravenous immunoglobulin (IVIG) may be indicated. If exposed to measles, prophylaxis with pooled intramuscular immunoglobulin (IG) may be indicated. (See the respective package inserts for complete VZIG and IG prescribing information.) If chickenpox develops, treatment with antiviral agents may be considered.

DULERA should be used with caution, if at all, in patients with active or quiescent tuberculosis infection of the respiratory tract, untreated systemic fungal, bacterial, viral, or parasitic infections; or ocular herpes simplex.

5.6 Transferring Patients from Systemic Corticosteroid Therapy

Particular care is needed for patients who are transferred from systemically active corticosteroids to DULERA because deaths due to adrenal insufficiency have occurred in asthmatic patients during and after transfer from systemic corticosteroids to less systemically available inhaled corticosteroids. After withdrawal from systemic corticosteroids, a number of months are required for recovery of hypothalamic-pituitary-adrenal (HPA) function.

Patients who have been previously maintained on 20 mg or more per day of prednisone (or its equivalent) may be most susceptible, particularly when their systemic corticosteroids have been almost completely withdrawn. During this period of HPA suppression, patients may exhibit signs and symptoms of adrenal insufficiency when exposed to trauma, surgery, or infection (particularly gastroenteritis) or other conditions associated with severe electrolyte loss. Although DULERA may improve control of asthma symptoms during these episodes, in recommended doses it supplies less than normal physiological amounts of corticosteroid systemically and does NOT provide the mineralocorticoid activity necessary for coping with these emergencies.

During periods of stress or severe asthma attack, patients who have been withdrawn from systemic corticosteroids should be instructed to resume oral corticosteroids (in large doses) immediately and to contact their physicians for further instruction. These patients should also be instructed to carry a medical identification card indicating that they may need supplementary systemic corticosteroids during periods of stress or severe asthma attack.

Patients requiring systemic corticosteroids should be weaned slowly from systemic corticosteroid use after transferring to DULERA. Lung function (FEV_1 or PEF), beta-agonist use, and asthma symptoms should be carefully monitored during withdrawal of systemic corticosteroids. In addition to monitoring asthma signs and symptoms, patients should be observed for signs and symptoms of adrenal insufficiency such as fatigue, lassitude, weakness, nausea and vomiting, and hypotension.

Transfer of patients from systemic corticosteroid therapy to DULERA may unmask allergic conditions previously suppressed by the systemic corticosteroid therapy, e.g., rhinitis, conjunctivitis, eczema, arthritis, and eosinophilic conditions.

During withdrawal from oral corticosteroids, some patients may experience symptoms of systemically active corticosteroid withdrawal, e.g., joint and/or muscular pain, lassitude, and depression, despite maintenance or even improvement of respiratory function.

5.7 Hypercorticism and Adrenal Suppression

Mometasone furoate, a component of DULERA, will often help control asthma symptoms with less suppression of HPA function than therapeutically equivalent oral doses of prednisone. Since mometasone furoate is absorbed into the circulation and can be systemically active at higher doses, the beneficial effects of DULERA in minimizing HPA dysfunction may be expected only when recommended dosages are not exceeded and individual patients are titrated to the lowest effective dose.

Because of the possibility of systemic absorption of inhaled corticosteroids, patients treated with DULERA should be observed carefully for any evidence of systemic corticosteroid effects. Particular care should be taken in observing patients postoperatively or during periods of stress for evidence of inadequate adrenal response.

It is possible that systemic corticosteroid effects such as hypercorticism and adrenal suppression (including adrenal crisis) may appear in a small number of patients, particularly when mometasone furoate is administered at higher than recommended doses over prolonged periods of time. If such effects occur, the dosage of DULERA should be reduced slowly, consistent with accepted procedures for reducing systemic corticosteroids and for management of asthma symptoms.

5.8 Drug Interactions with Strong Cytochrome P450 3A4 Inhibitors

Caution should be exercised when considering the coadministration of DULERA with ketoconazole, and other known strong CYP3A4 inhibitors (e.g., ritonavir, atazanavir, clarithromycin, indinavir, itraconazole, nefazodone, nelfinavir, saquinavir, telithromycin) because adverse effects related to increased systemic exposure to mometasone furoate may occur *[see Drug Interactions (7.1) and Clinical Pharmacology (12.3)]*.

5.9 Paradoxical Bronchospasm and Upper Airway Symptoms

DULERA may produce inhalation induced bronchospasm with an immediate increase in wheezing after dosing that may be life-threatening. If inhalation induced bronchospasm occurs, it should be treated immediately with an inhaled, short-acting bronchodilator. DULERA should be discontinued immediately and alternative therapy instituted.

5.10 Immediate Hypersensitivity Reactions

Immediate hypersensitivity reactions may occur after administration of DULERA, as demonstrated by cases of urticaria, flushing, allergic dermatitis, and bronchospasm.

Table 2: Treatment-Emergent Adverse Reactions in DULERA Groups Occurring at an Incidence of ≥3% and More Commonly than Placebo

Adverse Reactions	DULERA*		Mometasone Furoate*		Formoterol*	Placebo*
	100 mcg/5 mcg n=424 n (%)	200 mcg/5 mcg n=255 n (%)	100 mcg n=192 n (%)	200 mcg n=240 n (%)	5 mcg n=202 n (%)	n=196 n (%)
Nasopharyngitis	20 (4.7)	12 (4.7)	15 (7.8)	13 (5.4)	13 (6.4)	7 (3.6)
Sinusitis	14 (3.3)	5 (2.0)	6 (3.1)	4 (1.7)	7 (3.5)	2 (1.0)
Headache	19 (4.5)	5 (2.0)	10 (5.2)	8 (3.3)	6 (3.0)	7 (3.6)
Average Duration of Exposure (days)	116	81	165	79	131	138

* All treatments were administered as two inhalations twice daily.

5.11 Cardiovascular and Central Nervous System Effects

Excessive beta-adrenergic stimulation has been associated with seizures, angina, hypertension or hypotension, tachycardia with rates up to 200 beats/min, arrhythmias, nervousness, headache, tremor, palpitation, nausea, dizziness, fatigue, malaise, and insomnia. Therefore, DULERA should be used with caution in patients with cardiovascular disorders, especially coronary insufficiency, cardiac arrhythmias, and hypertension.

Formoterol fumarate, a component of DULERA, can produce a clinically significant cardiovascular effect in some patients as measured by pulse rate, blood pressure, and/or symptoms. Although such effects are uncommon after administration of DULERA at recommended doses, if they occur, the drug may need to be discontinued. In addition, beta-agonists have been reported to produce ECG changes, such as flattening of the T wave, prolongation of the QTc interval, and ST segment depression. The clinical significance of these findings is unknown. Fatalities have been reported in association with excessive use of inhaled sympathomimetic drugs.

5.12 Reduction in Bone Mineral Density

Decreases in bone mineral density (BMD) have been observed with long-term administration of products containing inhaled corticosteroids, including mometasone furoate, one of the components of DULERA. The clinical significance of small changes in BMD with regard to long-term outcomes, such as fracture, is unknown. Patients with major risk factors for decreased bone mineral content, such as prolonged immobilization, family history of osteoporosis, or chronic use of drugs that can reduce bone mass (e.g., anticonvulsants and corticosteroids) should be monitored and treated with established standards of care.

In a 2-year double-blind study in 103 male and female asthma patients 18 to 50 years of age previously maintained on bronchodilator therapy (Baseline FEV_1 85%–88% predicted), treatment with mometasone furoate dry powder inhaler 200 mcg twice daily resulted in significant reductions in lumbar spine (LS) BMD at the end of the treatment period compared to placebo. The mean change from Baseline to Endpoint in the lumbar spine BMD was -0.015 (-1.43%) for the mometasone furoate group compared to 0.002 (0.25%) for the placebo group. In another 2-year double-blind study in 87 male and female asthma patients 18 to 50 years of age previously maintained on bronchodilator therapy (Baseline FEV_1 82%–83% predicted), treatment with mometasone furoate 400 mcg twice daily demonstrated no statistically significant changes in lumbar spine BMD at the end of the treatment period compared to placebo. The mean change from Baseline to Endpoint in the lumbar spine BMD was -0.018 (-1.57%) for the mometasone furoate group compared to -0.006 (-0.43%) for the placebo group.

5.13 Effect on Growth

Orally inhaled corticosteroids, including DULERA, may cause a reduction in growth velocity when administered to pediatric patients. Monitor the growth of pediatric patients receiving DULERA routinely (e.g., via stadiometry). To minimize the systemic effects of orally inhaled corticosteroids, including DULERA, titrate each patient's dose to the lowest dosage that effectively controls his/her symptoms *[see Use in Specific Populations (8.4)]*.

5.14 Glaucoma and Cataracts

Glaucoma, increased intraocular pressure, and cataracts have been reported following the use of long-term administration of inhaled corticosteroids, including mometasone furoate, a component of DULERA. Therefore, close monitoring is warranted in patients with a change in vision or with a history of increased intraocular pressure, glaucoma, and/or cataracts *[see Adverse Reactions (6)]*.

5.15 Coexisting Conditions

DULERA, like other medications containing sympathomimetic amines, should be used with caution in patients with aneurysm, pheochromocytoma, convulsive disorders, or thyrotoxicosis; and in patients who are unusually responsive to sympathomimetic amines. Doses of the related $beta_2$-agonist albuterol, when administered intravenously, have been reported to aggravate preexisting diabetes mellitus and ketoacidosis.

5.16 Hypokalemia and Hyperglycemia

$Beta_2$-agonist medications may produce significant hypokalemia in some patients, possibly through intracellular shunting, which has the potential to produce adverse cardiovascular effects. The decrease in serum potassium is usually transient, not requiring supplementation. Clinically significant changes in blood glucose and/or serum potassium were seen infrequently during clinical studies with DULERA at recommended doses.

6 ADVERSE REACTIONS

Long-acting $beta_2$-adrenergic agonists, such as formoterol, one of the active ingredients in DULERA, increase the risk of asthma-related death. Currently available data are inadequate to determine whether concurrent use of inhaled corticosteroids or other long-term asthma control drugs mitigates the increased risk of asthma-related death from LABA. Available data from controlled clinical trials suggest that LABA increase the risk of asthma-related hospitalization in pediatric and adolescent patients. Data from a large placebo-controlled US trial that compared the safety of another long-acting $beta_2$-adrenergic agonist (salmeterol) or placebo added to usual asthma therapy showed an increase in asthma-related deaths in patients receiving salmeterol *[see Warnings and Precautions (5.1)]*.

Systemic and local corticosteroid use may result in the following:

- *Candida albicans* infection *[see Warnings and Precautions (5.4)]*
- Immunosuppression *[see Warnings and Precautions (5.5)]*
- Hypercorticism and adrenal suppression *[see Warnings and Precautions (5.7)]*
- Growth effects in pediatrics *[see Warnings and Precautions (5.13)]*
- Glaucoma and cataracts *[see Warnings and Precautions (5.14)]*

Because clinical trials are conducted under widely varying conditions, adverse reaction rates observed in the clinical trials of a drug cannot be directly compared to rates in the clinical trials of another drug and may not reflect the rates observed in practice.

6.1 Clinical Trials Experience

The safety data described below is based on 3 clinical trials which randomized 1913 patients 12 years of age and older with asthma, including 679 patients exposed to DULERA for 12 to 26 weeks and 271 patients exposed for 1 year. DULERA was studied in two placebo- and active-controlled trials (n=781 and n=728, respectively) and in a long-term 52-week safety trial (n=404). In the 12 to 26-week clinical trials, the population was 12 to 84 years of age, 41% male and 59% female, 73% Caucasians, 27% non-Caucasians. Patients received two inhalations twice daily of DULERA (100 mcg/5 mcg or 200 mcg/5 mcg), mometasone furoate MDI (100 mcg or 200 mcg), formoterol MDI (5 mcg) or placebo. In the long-term 52-week active-comparator safety trial, the population was 12 years to 75 years of age with asthma, 37% male and 63% female, 47% Caucasians, 53% non-Caucasians and received two inhalations twice daily of DULERA 100 mcg/5 mcg or 200 mcg/5 mcg, or an active comparator.

The incidence of treatment emergent adverse reactions associated with DULERA in Table 2 below is based upon pooled data from 2 clinical trials 12 to 26 weeks in duration in patients 12 years and older treated with two inhalations twice daily of DULERA (100 mcg/5 mcg or 200 mcg/5 mcg), mometasone furoate MDI (100 mcg or 200 mcg), formoterol MDI (5mcg) or placebo.

[See table 2 above]

Oral candidiasis has been reported in clinical trials at an incidence of 0.7% in patients using DULERA 100 mcg/5 mcg, 0.8 % in patients using DULERA 200 mcg/5 mcg and 0.5 % in the placebo group.

Long-Term Clinical Trial Experience

In a long-term safety trial in patients 12 years and older treated for 52 weeks with DULERA 100 mcg/5 mcg (n=141), DULERA 200 mcg/5 mcg (n=130) or an active comparator (n=133), safety outcomes in general were similar to those observed in the shorter 12 to 26 week controlled trials. No asthma-related deaths were observed. Dysphonia was observed at a higher frequency in the longer term treatment trial at a reported incidence of 7/141 (5%) patients receiving DULERA 100 mcg/5 mcg and 5/130 (3.8%) patients receiving DULERA 200 mcg/5 mcg. No clinically significant changes in blood chemistry, hematology, or ECG were observed.

6.2 Postmarketing Experience

The following adverse reactions have been reported during post-approval use of DULERA or post-approval use with inhaled mometasone furoate or inhaled formoterol fumarate. Because these reactions are reported voluntarily from a population of uncertain size, it is not always possible to reliably estimate their frequency or establish a causal relationship to drug exposure.

Cardiac disorders: angina pectoris, cardiac arrhythmias, e.g., atrial fibrillation, ventricular extrasystoles, tachyarrhythmia

Immune system disorders: immediate and delayed hypersensitivity reactions including anaphylactic reaction, angioedema, severe hypotension, rash, pruritus

Investigations: electrocardiogram QT prolonged, blood pressure increased (including hypertension)

Metabolism and nutrition disorders: hypokalemia, hyperglycemia

Respiratory, thoracic and mediastinal disorders: asthma aggravation, which may include cough, dyspnea, wheezing and bronchospasm

7 DRUG INTERACTIONS

In clinical trials, concurrent administration of DULERA and other drugs, such as short-acting beta$_2$-agonist and intranasal corticosteroids have not resulted in an increased frequency of adverse drug reactions. No formal drug interaction studies have been performed with DULERA. The drug interactions of the combination are expected to reflect those of the individual components.

7.1 Inhibitors of Cytochrome P450 3A4

The main route of metabolism of corticosteroids, including mometasone furoate, a component of DULERA, is via cytochrome P450 (CYP) isoenzyme 3A4 (CYP3A4). After oral administration of ketoconazole, a strong inhibitor of CYP3A4, the mean plasma concentration of orally inhaled mometasone furoate increased. Concomitant administration of CYP3A4 inhibitors may inhibit the metabolism of, and increase the systemic exposure to, mometasone furoate. Caution should be exercised when considering the coadministration of DULERA with long-term ketoconazole and other known strong CYP3A4 inhibitors (e.g., ritonavir, atazanavir, clarithromycin, indinavir, itraconazole, nefazodone, nelfinavir, saquinavir, telithromycin) *[see Warnings and Precautions (5.8) and Clinical Pharmacology (12.3)]*.

7.2 Adrenergic agents

If additional adrenergic drugs are to be administered by any route, they should be used with caution because the pharmacologically predictable sympathetic effects of formoterol, a component of DULERA, may be potentiated.

7.3 Xanthine derivatives

Concomitant treatment with xanthine derivatives may potentiate any hypokalemic effect of formoterol, a component of DULERA.

7.4 Diuretics

Concomitant treatment with diuretics may potentiate the possible hypokalemic effect of adrenergic agonists. The ECG changes and/or hypokalemia that may result from the administration of non-potassium-sparing diuretics (such as loop or thiazide diuretics) can be acutely worsened by beta-agonists, especially when the recommended dose of the beta-agonist is exceeded. Although the clinical significance of these effects is not known, caution is advised in the coadministration of DULERA with non-potassium-sparing diuretics.

7.5 Monoamine oxidase inhibitors, tricyclic antidepressants, and drugs known to prolong the QTc interval

DULERA should be administered with caution to patients being treated with monoamine oxidase inhibitors, tricyclic antidepressants, macrolides, or drugs known to prolong the QTc interval or within 2 weeks of discontinuation of such agents, because the action of formoterol, a component of DULERA, on the cardiovascular system may be potentiated by these agents. Drugs that are known to prolong the QTc interval have an increased risk of ventricular arrhythmias.

7.6 Beta-adrenergic receptor antagonists

Beta-adrenergic receptor antagonists (beta-blockers) and formoterol may inhibit the effect of each other when administered concurrently. Beta-blockers not only block the therapeutic effects of beta$_2$-agonists, such as formoterol, a component of DULERA, but may produce severe bronchospasm in patients with asthma. Therefore, patients with asthma should not normally be treated with beta-blockers. However, under certain circumstances, e.g., as prophylaxis after myocardial infarction, there may be no acceptable alternatives to the use of beta-blockers in patients with asthma. In this setting, cardioselective beta-blockers could be considered, although they should be administered with caution.

7.7 Halogenated Hydrocarbons

There is an elevated risk of arrhythmias in patients receiving concomitant anesthesia with halogenated hydrocarbons.

8 USE IN SPECIFIC POPULATIONS

8.1 Pregnancy

DULERA: Teratogenic Effects: Pregnancy Category C

There are no adequate and well-controlled studies of DULERA, mometasone furoate only or formoterol fumarate only in pregnant women. Animal reproduction studies of mometasone furoate and formoterol in mice, rats, and/or rabbits revealed evidence of teratogenicity as well as other developmental toxic effects. Because animal reproduction studies are not always predictive of human response, DULERA should be used during pregnancy only if the potential benefit justifies the potential risk to the fetus.

Mometasone Furoate: Teratogenic Effects

When administered to pregnant mice, rats, and rabbits, mometasone furoate increased fetal malformations and decreased fetal growth (measured by lower fetal weights and/or delayed ossification). Dystocia and related complications were also observed when mometasone furoate was administered to rats late in gestation. However, experience with oral corticosteroids suggests that rodents are more prone to teratogenic effects from corticosteroid exposure than humans.

In a mouse reproduction study, subcutaneous mometasone furoate produced cleft palate at approximately one-third of the maximum recommended daily human dose (MRHD) on a mcg/m^2 basis and decreased fetal survival at approximately 1 time the MRHD. No toxicity was observed at approximately one-tenth of the MRHD on a mcg/m^2 basis.

In a rat reproduction study, mometasone furoate produced umbilical hernia at topical dermal doses approximately 6 times the MRHD on a mcg/m^2 basis and delays in ossification at approximately 3 times the MRHD on a mcg/m^2 basis.

In another study, rats received subcutaneous doses of mometasone furoate throughout pregnancy or late in gestation. Treated animals had prolonged and difficult labor, fewer live births, lower birth weight, and reduced early pup survival at a dose that was approximately 8 times the MRHD on an area under the curve (AUC) basis. Similar effects were not observed at approximately 4 times MRHD on an AUC basis.

In rabbits, mometasone furoate caused multiple malformations (e.g., flexed front paws, gallbladder agenesis, umbilical hernia, hydrocephaly) at topical dermal doses approximately 3 times the MRHD on a mcg/m^2 basis. In an oral study, mometasone furoate increased resorptions and caused cleft palate and/or head malformations (hydrocephaly and domed head) at a dose less than the MRHD based on AUC. At a dose approximately 2 times the MRHD based on AUC, most litters were aborted or resorbed *[see Nonclinical Toxicology (13.2)]*.

Nonteratogenic Effects:

Hypoadrenalism may occur in infants born to women receiving corticosteroids during pregnancy. Infants born to mothers taking substantial corticosteroid doses during pregnancy should be monitored for signs of hypoadrenalism.

Formoterol Fumarate: Teratogenic Effects

Formoterol fumarate administered throughout organogenesis did not cause malformations in rats or rabbits following oral administration. When given to rats throughout organogenesis, oral doses of approximately 80 times the MRHD on a mcg/m^2 basis and above delayed ossification of the fetus, and doses of approximately 2400 times the MRHD on a mcg/m^2 basis and above decreased fetal weight. Formoterol fumarate has been shown to cause stillbirth and neonatal mortality at oral doses of approximately 2400 times the MRHD on a mcg/m^2 basis and above in rats receiving the drug during the late stage of pregnancy. These effects, however, were not produced at a dose of approximately 80 times the MRHD on a mcg/m^2 basis.

In another testing laboratory, formoterol was shown to be teratogenic in rats and rabbits. Umbilical hernia, a malformation, was observed in rat fetuses at oral doses approximately 1200 times and greater than the MRHD on a mcg/m^2 basis. Brachygnathia, a skeletal malformation, was observed in rat fetuses at an oral dose approximately 6100 times the MRHD on a mcg/m^2 basis. In another study in rats, no teratogenic effects were seen at inhalation doses up to approximately 500 times the MRHD on a mcg/m^2 basis. Subcapsular cysts on the liver were observed in rabbit fetuses at an oral dose approximately 49,000 times the MRHD on a mcg/m^2 basis. No teratogenic effects were observed at oral doses up to approximately 3000 times the MRHD on a mcg/m^2 basis *[see Nonclinical Toxicology (13.2)]*.

8.2 Labor and Delivery

There are no adequate and well-controlled human studies that have studied the effects of DULERA during labor and delivery.

Because beta-agonists may potentially interfere with uterine contractility, DULERA should be used during labor only if the potential benefit justifies the potential risk *[see Nonclinical Toxicology (13.2)]*.

8.3 Nursing Mothers

DULERA: It is not known whether DULERA is excreted in human milk. Because many drugs are excreted in human milk, caution should be exercised when DULERA is administered to a nursing woman.

Since there are no data from well-controlled human studies on the use of DULERA on nursing mothers, based on data for the individual components, a decision should be made whether to discontinue nursing or to discontinue DULERA, taking into account the importance of DULERA to the mother.

Mometasone Furoate: It is not known if mometasone furoate is excreted in human milk. However, other corticosteroids are excreted in human milk.

Formoterol Fumarate: In reproductive studies in rats, formoterol was excreted in the milk. It is not known whether formoterol is excreted in human milk.

8.4 Pediatric Use

The safety and effectiveness of DULERA have been established in patients 12 years of age and older in 3 clinical trials up to 52 weeks in duration. In the 3 clinical trials, 101 patients 12 to 17 years of age were treated with DULERA. Patients in this age-group demonstrated efficacy results similar to those observed in patients 18 years of age and older. There were no obvious differences in the type or frequency of adverse drug reactions reported in this age group compared to patients 18 years of age and older. Similar efficacy and safety results were observed in an additional 22 patients 12 to 17 years of age who were treated with DULERA in another clinical trial. The safety and efficacy of DULERA have not been established in children less than 12 years of age.

Controlled clinical studies have shown that inhaled corticosteroids may cause a reduction in growth velocity in pediatric patients. In these studies, the mean reduction in growth velocity was approximately 1 cm per year (range 0.3 to 1.8 per year) and appears to depend upon dose and duration of exposure. This effect was observed in the absence of laboratory evidence of hypothalamic-pituitary-adrenal (HPA) axis suppression, suggesting that growth velocity is a more sensitive indicator of systemic corticosteroid exposure in pediatric patients than some commonly used tests of HPA axis function. The long-term effects of this reduction in growth velocity associated with orally inhaled corticosteroids, including the impact on final adult height, are unknown. The potential for "catch up" growth following discontinuation of treatment with orally inhaled corticosteroids has not been adequately studied.

The growth of children and adolescents receiving orally inhaled corticosteroids, including DULERA, should be monitored routinely (e.g., via stadiometry). If a child or adolescent on any corticosteroid appears to have growth suppression, the possibility that he/she is particularly sensitive to this effect should be considered. The potential growth effects of prolonged treatment should be weighed against clinical benefits obtained and the risks associated with alternative therapies. To minimize the systemic effects of orally inhaled corticosteroids, including DULERA, each patient should be titrated to his/her lowest effective dose *[see Dosage and Administration (2.2)]*.

8.5 Geriatric Use

A total of 77 patients 65 years of age and older (11 of whom were 75 years and older) have been treated with DULERA in 3 clinical trials up to 52 weeks in duration. Similar efficacy and safety results were observed in an additional 28 patients 65 years of age and older who were treated with DULERA in another clinical trial. No overall differences in safety or effectiveness were observed between these patients and younger patients, but greater sensitivity of some older individuals cannot be ruled out. As with other products containing beta$_2$-agonists, special caution should be observed when using DULERA in geriatric patients who have concomitant cardiovascular disease that could be adversely affected by beta$_2$-agonists. Based on available data for DULERA or its active components, no adjustment of dosage of DULERA in geriatric patients is warranted.

8.6 Hepatic Impairment

Concentrations of mometasone furoate appear to increase with severity of hepatic impairment *[see Clinical Pharmacology (12.3)]*.

10 OVERDOSAGE

10.1 Signs and Symptoms

DULERA: DULERA contains both mometasone furoate and formoterol fumarate; therefore, the risks associated with overdosage for the individual components described below apply to DULERA.

Mometasone Furoate: Chronic overdosage may result in signs/symptoms of hypercorticism *[see Warnings and Precautions (5.7)]*. Single oral doses up to 8000 mcg of mometasone furoate have been studied on human volunteers with no adverse reactions reported.

Formoterol Fumarate: The expected signs and symptoms with overdosage of formoterol are those of excessive beta-adrenergic stimulation and/or occurrence or exaggeration of any of the following signs and symptoms: angina, hypertension or hypotension, tachycardia, with rates up to 200 beats/min., arrhythmias, nervousness, headache, tremor, seizures, muscle cramps, dry mouth, palpitation, nausea, dizziness, fatigue, malaise, hypokalemia, hyperglycemia, and insomnia. Metabolic acidosis may also occur. Cardiac arrest and even death may be associated with an overdose of formoterol.

The minimum acute lethal inhalation dose of formoterol fumarate in rats is 156 mg/kg (approximately 63,000 times the MRHD on a mcg/m^2 basis). The median lethal oral doses in Chinese hamsters, rats, and mice provide even higher multiples of the MRHD.

10.2 Treatment

DULERA: Treatment of overdosage consists of discontinuation of DULERA together with institution of appropriate symptomatic and/or supportive therapy. The judicious use of a cardioselective beta-receptor blocker may be considered, bearing in mind that such medication can produce bronchospasm. There is insufficient evidence to determine if dialysis is beneficial for overdosage of DULERA. Cardiac monitoring is recommended in cases of overdosage.

11 DESCRIPTION

DULERA 100 mcg/5 mcg and DULERA 200 mcg/5 mcg are combinations of mometasone furoate and formoterol fumarate dihydrate for oral inhalation only.

One active component of DULERA is mometasone furoate, a corticosteroid having the chemical name 9,21-dichloro-11(Beta),17-dihydroxy-16 (alpha)-methylpregna-1,4-diene-3,20-dione 17-(2-furoate) with the following chemical structure:

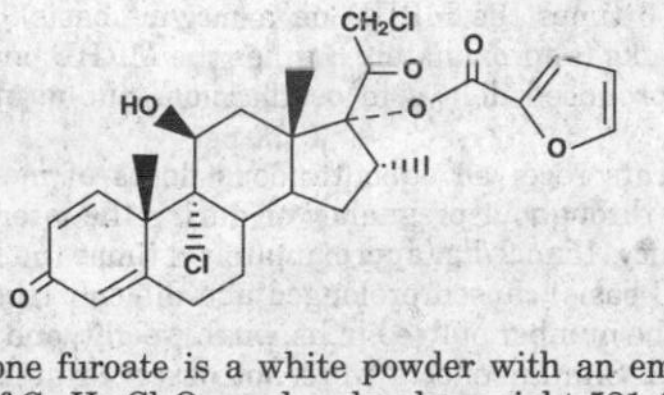

Mometasone furoate is a white powder with an empirical formula of $C_{27}H_{30}Cl_2O_6$, and molecular weight 521.44. It is practically insoluble in water; slightly soluble in methanol, ethanol, and isopropanol; soluble in acetone.

One active component of DULERA is formoterol fumarate dihydrate, a racemate. Formoterol fumarate dihydrate is a selective beta$_2$-adrenergic bronchodilator having the chemical name of (±)-2-hydroxy-5-[(1RS)-1-hydroxy-2-[[(1RS)-2-(4-methoxyphenyl)-1-methylethyl]-amino]ethyl]formanilide fumarate dihydrate with the following chemical structure:

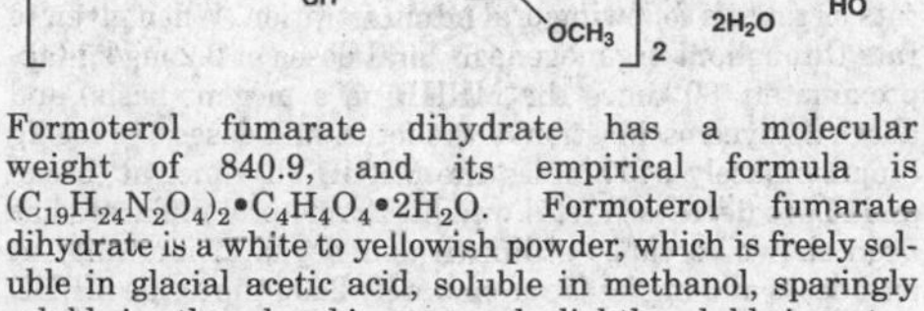

Formoterol fumarate dihydrate has a molecular weight of 840.9, and its empirical formula is $(C_{19}H_{24}N_2O_4)_2 \bullet C_4H_4O_4 \bullet 2H_2O$. Formoterol fumarate dihydrate is a white to yellowish powder, which is freely soluble in glacial acetic acid, soluble in methanol, sparingly soluble in ethanol and isopropanol, slightly soluble in water, and practically insoluble in acetone, ethyl acetate, and diethyl ether.

Each DULERA 100 mcg/5 mcg and 200 mcg/5 mcg is a hydrofluoroalkane (HFA-227) propelled pressurized metered dose inhaler containing sufficient amount of drug for 60 or 120 inhalations *[see How Supplied/Storage and Handling (16)]*. After priming, each actuation of the inhaler delivers 115 or 225 mcg of mometasone furoate and 5.5 mcg of formoterol fumarate dihydrate in 69.6 mg of suspension from the valve and delivers 100 or 200 mcg of mometasone furoate and 5 mcg of formoterol fumarate dihydrate from the actuator. The actual amount of drug delivered to the lung may depend on patient factors, such as the coordination between actuation of the device and inspiration through the delivery system. DULERA also contains anhydrous alcohol as a cosolvent and oleic acid as a surfactant. DULERA should be primed before using for the first time by releasing 4 test sprays into the air, away from the face, shaking well before each spray. In cases where the inhaler has not been used for more than 5 days, prime the inhaler again by releasing 4 test sprays into the air, away from the face, shaking well before each spray.

12 CLINICAL PHARMACOLOGY

12.1 Mechanism of Action

DULERA: DULERA contains both mometasone furoate and formoterol fumarate; therefore, the mechanisms of actions described below for the individual components apply to DULERA. These drugs represent two different classes of medications (a synthetic corticosteroid and a selective long-acting beta$_2$-adrenergic receptor agonist) that have different effects on clinical, physiological, and inflammatory indices of asthma.

Mometasone furoate: Mometasone furoate is a corticosteroid demonstrating potent anti-inflammatory activity. The precise mechanism of corticosteroid action on asthma is not known. Inflammation is an important component in the pathogenesis of asthma. Corticosteroids have been shown to have a wide range of inhibitory effects on multiple cell types (e.g., mast cells, eosinophils, neutrophils, macrophages, and lymphocytes) and mediators (e.g., histamine, eicosanoids, leukotrienes, and cytokines) involved in inflammation and in the asthmatic response. These anti-inflammatory actions of corticosteroids may contribute to their efficacy in asthma. Mometasone furoate has been shown *in vitro* to exhibit a binding affinity for the human glucocorticoid receptor, which is approximately 12 times that of dexamethasone, 7 times that of triamcinolone acetonide, 5 times that of budesonide, and 1.5 times that of fluticasone. The clinical significance of these findings is unknown.

Formoterol fumarate: Formoterol fumarate is a long-acting selective beta$_2$-adrenergic receptor agonist (beta$_2$-agonist). Inhaled formoterol fumarate acts locally in the lung as a bronchodilator. *In vitro* studies have shown that formoterol has more than 200-fold greater agonist activity at beta$_2$-receptors than at beta$_1$-receptors. Although beta$_2$-receptors are the predominant adrenergic receptors in bronchial smooth muscle and beta$_1$-receptors are the predominant receptors in the heart, there are also beta$_2$-receptors in the human heart comprising 10% to 50% of the total beta-adrenergic receptors. The precise function of these receptors has not been established, but they raise the possibility that even highly selective beta$_2$-agonists may have cardiac effects.

The pharmacologic effects of beta$_2$-adrenoceptor agonist drugs, including formoterol, are at least in part attributable to stimulation of intracellular adenyl cyclase, the enzyme that catalyzes the conversion of adenosine triphosphate (ATP) to cyclic-3′, 5′-adenosine monophosphate (cyclic AMP). Increased cyclic AMP levels cause relaxation of bronchial smooth muscle and inhibition of release of mediators of immediate hypersensitivity from cells, especially from mast cells.

In vitro tests show that formoterol is an inhibitor of the release of mast cell mediators, such as histamine and leukotrienes, from the human lung. Formoterol also inhibits histamine-induced plasma albumin extravasation in anesthetized guinea pigs and inhibits allergen-induced eosinophil influx in dogs with airway hyper-responsiveness. The relevance of these *in vitro* and animal findings to humans is unknown.

12.2 Pharmacodynamics

Cardiovascular Effects:

DULERA:

In a single-dose, double-blind placebo-controlled crossover trial in 25 patients with asthma, single-dose treatment of 10 mcg formoterol fumarate in combination with 400 mcg of mometasone furoate delivered via DULERA 200 mcg/5 mcg were compared to formoterol fumarate 10 mcg MDI, formoterol fumarate 12 mcg dry powder inhaler (DPI; nominal dose of formoterol fumarate delivered 10 mcg), or placebo. The degree of bronchodilation at 12 hours after dosing with DULERA was similar to formoterol fumarate delivered alone via MDI or DPI.

ECGs and blood samples for glucose and potassium were obtained prior to dosing and post dose. No downward trend in serum potassium was observed and values were within the normal range and appeared to be similar across all treatments over the 12 hour period. Mean blood glucose appeared similar across all groups for each time point. There was no evidence of significant hypokalemia or hyperglycemia in response to formoterol treatment.

No relevant changes in heart rate or changes in ECG data were observed with DULERA in the trial. No patients had a QTcB (QTc corrected by Bazett's formula) ≥500 msec during treatment.

In a single-dose crossover trial involving 24 healthy subjects, single dose of formoterol fumarate 10, 20, or 40 mcg in combination with 400 mcg of mometasone furoate delivered via DULERA were evaluated for safety (ECG, blood potassium and glucose changes). ECGs and blood samples for glucose and potassium were obtained at baseline and post dose. Decrease in mean serum potassium was similar across all three treatment groups (approximately 0.3 mmol/L) and values were within the normal range. No clinically significant increases in mean blood glucose values or heart rate were observed. No subjects had a QTcB >500 msec during treatment.

Three active- and placebo-controlled trials (study duration ranging from 12, 26, and 52 weeks) evaluated 1913 patients 12 years of age and older with asthma. No clinically meaningful changes were observed in potassium and glucose values, vital signs, or ECG parameters in patients receiving DULERA.

HPA Axis Effects:

The effects of inhaled mometasone furoate administered via DULERA on adrenal function were evaluated in two clinical trials in patients with asthma. HPA-axis function was assessed by 24-hour plasma cortisol AUC. Although both these trials have open-label design and contain small number of subjects per treatment arm, results from these trials taken together demonstrated suppression of 24-hour plasma cortisol AUC for DULERA 200 mcg/5 mcg compared to placebo consistent with the known systemic effects of inhaled corticosteroid.

In a 42-day, open-label, placebo and active-controlled study 60 patients with asthma 18 years of age and older were randomized to receive two inhalations twice daily of 1 of the following treatments: DULERA 100 mcg/5 mcg, DULERA 200 mcg/5 mcg, fluticasone propionate/salmeterol xinafoate 230 mcg/21 mcg, or placebo. At Day 42, the mean change from baseline plasma cortisol AUC$_{(0\text{-}24\ hr)}$ was 8%, 22% and 34% lower compared to placebo for the DULERA 100 mcg/5 mcg (n=13), DULERA 200 mcg/5 mcg (n=15) and fluticasone propionate/salmeterol xinafoate 230 mcg/21 mcg (n=16) treatment groups, respectively.

In a 52-week, open-label safety study, primary analysis of the plasma cortisol 24-hour AUC was performed on 57 patients with asthma who received 2 inhalations twice daily of DULERA 100 mcg/5 mcg, DULERA 200 mcg/5 mcg, fluticasone propionate/salmeterol xinafoate 125/25 mcg, or fluticasone propionate/salmeterol xinafoate 250/25 mcg. At Week 52, the mean plasma cortisol AUC$_{(0\text{-}24\ hr)}$ was 2.2%, 29.6%, 16.7%, and 32.2% lower from baseline for the DULERA 100 mcg/5 mcg (n=18), DULERA 200 mcg/5 mcg (n=20), fluticasone propionate/salmeterol xinafoate 125/25 mcg (n=8), and fluticasone propionate/salmeterol xinafoate 250/25 mcg (n=11) treatment groups, respectively.

Other Mometasone Products

HPA Axis Effects:

The potential effect of mometasone furoate via a dry powder inhaler (DPI) on the HPA axis was assessed in a 29-day study. A total of 64 adult patients with mild to moderate asthma were randomized to one of 4 treatment groups: mometasone furoate DPI 440 mcg twice daily, mometasone furoate DPI 880 mcg twice daily, oral prednisone 10 mg once daily, or placebo. The 30-minute post-Cosyntropin stimulation serum cortisol concentration on Day 29 was 23.2 mcg/dl for the mometasone furoate DPI 440 mcg twice daily group and 20.8 mcg/dl for the mometasone furoate DPI 880 mcg twice daily group, compared to 14.5 mcg/dl for the oral prednisone 10 mg group and 25 mcg/dl for the placebo group. The difference between mometasone furoate DPI 880 mcg twice daily (twice the maximum recommended dose) and placebo was statistically significant.

12.3 Pharmacokinetics

Absorption

Mometasone furoate:

Healthy Subjects: The systemic exposures to mometasone furoate from DULERA versus mometasone furoate delivered via DPI were compared. Following oral inhalation of single and multiple doses of the DULERA, mometasone furoate was absorbed in healthy subjects with median T_{max} values ranging from 0.50 to 4 hours. Following single-dose administration of higher than recommended dose of DULERA (4 inhalations of DULERA 200 mcg/5 mcg) in healthy subjects, the arithmetic mean (CV%) C_{max} and AUC$_{(0\text{-}12\ hr)}$ values for MF were 67.8 (49) pg/mL and 650 (51) pg•hr/mL, respectively while the corresponding estimates following 5 days of BID dosing of DULERA 800 mcg/20 mcg were 241 (36) pg/mL and 2200 (35) pg•hr/mL. Exposure to mometasone furoate increased with increasing inhaled dose of DULERA 100 mcg/5 mcg to 200 mcg/5 mcg. Studies using oral dosing of labeled and unlabeled drug have demonstrated that the oral systemic bioavailability of mometasone furoate is negligible (<1%).

The above study demonstrated that the systemic exposure to mometasone furoate (based on AUC) was approximately 52% and 25% lower on Day 1 and Day 5, respectively, following DULERA administration compared to mometasone furoate via a DPI.

Asthma Patients: Following oral inhalation of single and multiple doses of the DULERA, mometasone furoate was absorbed in asthma patients with median T_{max} values ranging from 1 to 2 hours. Following single-dose administration of DULERA 400 mcg/10 mcg, the arithmetic mean (CV%) C_{max} and $AUC_{(0\text{-}12\ hr)}$ values for MF were 20 (88) pg/mL and 170 (94) pg•hr/mL, respectively while the corresponding estimates following BID dosing of DULERA 400 mcg/10 mcg at steady-state were 60 (36) pg/mL and 577 (40) pg•hr/mL.

Formoterol fumarate:

Healthy Subjects: When DULERA was administered to healthy subjects, formoterol was absorbed with median T_{max} values ranging from 0.167 to 0.5 hour. In a single-dose study with DULERA 400 mcg/10 mcg in healthy subjects, arithmetic mean (CV%) C_{max} and AUC for formoterol were 15 (50) pmol/L and 81 (51) pmol*h/L, respectively. Over the dose range of 10 to 40 mcg for formoterol from DULERA, the exposure to formoterol was dose proportional.

Asthma Patients: When DULERA was administered to patients with asthma, formoterol was absorbed with median T_{max} values ranging from 0.58 to 1.97 hours. In a single-dose study with DULERA 400 mcg/10 mcg in patients with asthma, arithmetic mean (CV%) C_{max} and $AUC_{(0\text{-}12\ hr)}$ for formoterol were 22 (29) pmol/L and 125 (42) pmol*h/L, respectively. Following multiple-dose administration of DULERA 400 mcg/10 mcg, the steady-state arithmetic mean (CV%) C_{max} and $AUC_{(0\text{-}12\ hr)}$ for formoterol were 41 (59) pmol/L and 226 (54) pmol*hr/L.

Distribution

Mometasone furoate: Based on the study employing a 1000 mcg inhaled dose of tritiated mometasone furoate inhalation powder in humans, no appreciable accumulation of mometasone furoate in the red blood cells was found. Following an intravenous 400 mcg dose of mometasone furoate, the plasma concentrations showed a biphasic decline, with a mean steady-state volume of distribution of 152 liters. The *in vitro* protein binding for mometasone furoate was reported to be 98% to 99% (in a concentration range of 5 to 500 ng/mL).

Formoterol fumarate: The binding of formoterol to human plasma proteins *in vitro* was 61% to 64% at concentrations from 0.1 to 100 ng/mL. Binding to human serum albumin *in vitro* was 31% to 38% over a range of 5 to 500 ng/mL. The concentrations of formoterol used to assess the plasma protein binding were higher than those achieved in plasma following inhalation of a single 120 mcg dose.

Metabolism

Mometasone furoate: Studies have shown that mometasone furoate is primarily and extensively metabolized in the liver of all species investigated and undergoes extensive metabolism to multiple metabolites. *In-vitro* studies have confirmed the primary role of human liver cytochrome P-450 3A4 (CYP3A4) in the metabolism of this compound, however, no major metabolites were identified. Human liver CYP3A4 metabolizes mometasone furoate to 6-beta hydroxy mometasone furoate.

Formoterol fumarate: Formoterol is metabolized primarily by direct glucuronidation at either the phenolic or aliphatic hydroxyl group and O-demethylation followed by glucuronide conjugation at either phenolic hydroxyl groups. Minor pathways involve sulfate conjugation of formoterol and deformylation followed by sulfate conjugation. The most prominent pathway involves direct conjugation at the phenolic hydroxyl group. The second major pathway involves O-demethylation followed by conjugation at the phenolic 2′-hydroxyl group. Four cytochrome P450 isozymes (CYP2D6, CYP2C19, CYP2C9 and CYP2A6) are involved in the O-demethylation of formoterol. Formoterol did not inhibit CYP450 enzymes at therapeutically relevant concentrations. Some patients may be deficient in CYP2D6 or 2C19 or both. Whether a deficiency in one or both of these isozymes results in elevated systemic exposure to formoterol or systemic adverse effects has not been adequately explored.

Excretion

Mometasone furoate: Following an intravenous dosing, the terminal half-life was reported to be about 5 hours. Following the inhaled dose of tritiated 1000 mcg mometasone furoate, the radioactivity is excreted mainly in the feces (a mean of 74%), and to a small extent in the urine (a mean of 8%) up to 7 days. No radioactivity was associated with unchanged mometasone furoate in the urine. Absorbed mometasone furoate is cleared from plasma at a rate of approximately 12.5 mL/min/kg, independent of dose. The effective t½ for mometasone furoate following inhalation with DULERA was 25 hours in healthy subjects and in patients with asthma.

Formoterol fumarate: Following oral administration of 80 mcg of radiolabeled formoterol fumarate to 2 healthy subjects, 59% to 62% of the radioactivity was eliminated in the urine and 32% to 34% in the feces over a period of 104 hours. In an oral inhalation study with DULERA, renal clearance of formoterol from the blood was 217 mL/min. In single-dose studies, the mean t½ values for formoterol in plasma were 9.1 hours and 10.8 hours from the urinary excretion data. The accumulation of formoterol in plasma after multiple dose administration was consistent with the increase expected with a drug having a terminal t½ of 9 to 11 hour.

Following single inhaled doses ranging from 10 to 40 mcg to healthy subjects from the MFF MDI, 6.2% to 6.8% of the formoterol dose was excreted in urine unchanged. The (R,R) and (S,S)-enantiomers accounted, respectively, for 37% and 63% of the formoterol recovered in urine. From urinary excretion rates measured in healthy subjects, the mean terminal elimination half-lives for the (R,R)- and (S,S)-enantiomers were determined to be 13 and 9.5 hours, respectively. The relative proportion of the two enantiomers remained constant over the dose range studied.

Special Populations

Hepatic/Renal Impairment: There are no data regarding the specific use of DULERA in patients with hepatic or renal impairment.

A study evaluating the administration of a single inhaled dose of 400 mcg mometasone furoate by a dry powder inhaler to subjects with mild (n=4), moderate (n=4), and severe (n=4) hepatic impairment resulted in only 1 or 2 subjects in each group having detectable peak plasma concentrations of mometasone furoate (ranging from 50–105 pcg/mL). The observed peak plasma concentrations appear to increase with severity of hepatic impairment; however, the numbers of detectable levels were few.

Gender and Race: Specific studies to examine the effects of gender and race on the pharmacokinetics of DULERA have not been specifically studied.

Geriatrics: The pharmacokinetics of DULERA have not been specifically studied in the elderly population.

Drug-Drug Interactions

A single-dose crossover study was conducted to compare the pharmacokinetics of 4 inhalations of the following: mometasone furoate MDI, formoterol MDI, DULERA (mometasone furoate/formoterol fumarate MDI), and mometasone furoate MDI plus formoterol fumarate MDI administered concurrently. The results of the study indicated that there was no evidence of a pharmacokinetic interaction between the two components of DULERA.

Inhibitors of Cytochrome P450 Enzymes: Ketoconazole: In a drug interaction study, an inhaled dose of mometasone furoate 400 mcg delivered by a dry powder inhaler was given to 24 healthy subjects twice daily for 9 days and ketoconazole 200 mg (as well as placebo) were given twice daily concomitantly on Days 4 to 9. Mometasone furoate plasma concentrations were <150 pcg/mL on Day 3 prior to coadministration of ketoconazole or placebo. Following concomitant administration of ketoconazole, 4 out of 12 subjects in the ketoconazole treatment group (n=12) had peak plasma concentrations of mometasone furoate >200 pcg/mL on Day 9 (211–324 pcg/mL). Mometasone furoate plasma levels appeared to increase and plasma cortisol levels appeared to decrease upon concomitant administration of ketoconazole.

Specific drug-drug interaction studies with formoterol have not been performed.

13 NONCLINICAL TOXICOLOGY

13.1 Carcinogenesis, Mutagenesis, Impairment of Fertility

Mometasone furoate: In a 2-year carcinogenicity study in Sprague Dawley® rats, mometasone furoate demonstrated no statistically significant increase in the incidence of tumors at inhalation doses up to 67 mcg/kg (approximately 14 times the MRHD on an AUC basis). In a 19-month carcinogenicity study in Swiss CD-1 mice, mometasone furoate demonstrated no statistically significant increase in the incidence of tumors at inhalation doses up to 160 mcg/kg (approximately 9 times the MRHD on an AUC basis).

Mometasone furoate increased chromosomal aberrations in an *in vitro* Chinese hamster ovary cell assay, but did not have this effect in an *in vitro* Chinese hamster lung cell assay. Mometasone furoate was not mutagenic in the Ames test or mouse lymphoma assay, and was not clastogenic in an *in vivo* mouse micronucleus assay, a rat bone marrow chromosomal aberration assay, or a mouse male germ-cell chromosomal aberration assay. Mometasone furoate also did not induce unscheduled DNA synthesis *in vivo* in rat hepatocytes.

In reproductive studies in rats, impairment of fertility was not produced by subcutaneous doses up to 15 mcg/kg (approximately 8 times the MRHD on an AUC basis).

Formoterol fumarate: The carcinogenic potential of formoterol fumarate has been evaluated in 2-year drinking water and dietary studies in both rats and mice. In rats, the incidence of ovarian leiomyomas was increased at doses of 15 mg/kg and above in the drinking water study and at 20 mg/kg in the dietary study, but not at dietary doses up to 5 mg/kg (AUC exposure approximately 265 times human exposure at the MRHD). In the dietary study, the incidence of benign ovarian theca-cell tumors was increased at doses of 0.5 mg/kg and above (AUC exposure at the low dose of 0.5 mg/kg was approximately 27 times human exposure at the MRHD). This finding was not observed in the drinking water study, nor was it seen in mice (see below).

In mice, the incidence of adrenal subcapsular adenomas and carcinomas was increased in males at doses of 69 mg/kg and above in the drinking water study, but not at doses up to 50 mg/kg (AUC exposure approximately 350 times human exposure at the MRHD) in the dietary study. The incidence of hepatocarcinomas was increased in the dietary study at doses of 20 and 50 mg/kg in females and 50 mg/kg in males, but not at doses up to 5 mg/kg in either males or females (AUC exposure approximately 35 times human exposure at the MRHD). Also in the dietary study, the incidence of uterine leiomyomas and leiomyosarcomas was increased at doses of 2 mg/kg and above (AUC exposure at the low dose of 2 mg/kg was approximately 14 times human exposure at the MRHD). Increases in leiomyomas of the rodent female genital tract have been similarly demonstrated with other beta-agonist drugs.

Formoterol fumarate was not mutagenic or clastogenic in the following tests: mutagenicity tests in bacterial and mammalian cells, chromosomal analyses in mammalian cells, unscheduled DNA synthesis repair tests in rat hepatocytes and human fibroblasts, transformation assay in mammalian fibroblasts and micronucleus tests in mice and rats.

Reproduction studies in rats revealed no impairment of fertility at oral doses up to 3 mg/kg (approximately 1200 times the MRHD on a mcg/m^2 basis).

13.2 Animal Toxicology and/or Pharmacology

Animal Pharmacology

Formoterol fumarate: Studies in laboratory animals (minipigs, rodents, and dogs) have demonstrated the occurrence of cardiac arrhythmias and sudden death (with histologic evidence of myocardial necrosis) when beta-agonists and methylxanthines are administered concurrently. The clinical significance of these findings is unknown.

Reproductive Toxicology Studies

Mometasone furoate: In mice, mometasone furoate caused cleft palate at subcutaneous doses of 60 mcg/kg and above (approximately 1/3 of the maximum recommended human dose MRHD on a mcg/m^2 basis). Fetal survival was reduced at 180 mcg/kg (approximately equal to the MRHD on a mcg/m^2 basis). No toxicity was observed at 20 mcg/kg (approximately one-tenth of the MRHD on a mcg/m^2 basis).

In rats, mometasone furoate produced umbilical hernia at topical dermal doses of 600 mcg/kg and above (approximately 6 times the MRHD on a mcg/m^2 basis). A dose of 300 mcg/kg (approximately 3 times the MRHD on a mcg/m^2 basis) produced delays in ossification, but no malformations.

When rats received subcutaneous doses of mometasone furoate throughout pregnancy or during the later stages of pregnancy, 15 mcg/kg (approximately 8 times the MRHD on an AUC basis) caused prolonged and difficult labor and reduced the number of live births, birth weight, and early pup survival. Similar effects were not observed at 7.5 mcg/kg (approximately 4 times the MRHD on an AUC basis).

In rabbits, mometasone furoate caused multiple malformations (e.g., flexed front paws, gallbladder agenesis, umbilical hernia, hydrocephaly) at topical dermal doses of 150 mcg/kg and above (approximately 3 times the MRHD on a mcg/m^2 basis). In an oral study, mometasone furoate increased resorptions and caused cleft palate and/or head malformations (hydrocephaly and domed head) at 700 mcg/kg (less than the MRHD on an area under the curve [AUC] basis). At 2800 mcg/kg (approximately 2 times the MRHD on an AUC basis) most litters were aborted or resorbed. No toxicity was observed at 140 mcg/kg (less than the MRHD on an AUC basis).

Formoterol fumarate: Formoterol fumarate administered throughout organogenesis did not cause malformations in rats or rabbits following oral administration. When given to rats throughout organogenesis, oral doses of 0.2 mg/kg (approximately 80 times the MRHD on a mcg/m^2 basis) and above delayed ossification of the fetus, and doses of 6 mg/kg (approximately 2400 times the MRHD on a mcg/m^2 basis) and above decreased fetal weight. Formoterol fumarate has been shown to cause stillbirth and neonatal mortality at oral doses of 6 mg/kg (approximately 2400 times the MRHD on a mcg/m^2 basis) and above in rats receiving the drug during the late stage of pregnancy. These effects, however, were not produced at a dose of 0.2 mg/kg (approximately 80 times the MRHD on a mcg/m^2 basis).

In another testing laboratory, formoterol fumarate was shown to be teratogenic in rats and rabbits. Umbilical hernia, a malformation, was observed in rat fetuses at oral doses of 3 mg/kg/day and above (approximately 1200 times greater than the MRHD on a mcg/m^2 basis). Brachygnathia, a skeletal malformation, was observed for rat fetuses at an oral dose of 15 mg/kg/day (approximately 6100 times the MRHD on a mcg/m^2 basis). In another study in rats, no teratogenic effects were seen at inhalation doses up to 1.2 mg/kg/day (approximately 500 times the MRHD on a mcg/m^2 basis). Subcapsular cysts on the liver were observed for rabbit fetuses at an oral dose of 60 mg/kg (approximately 49,000 times the MRHD on a mcg/m^2 basis). No teratogenic effects were observed at oral doses up to 3.5 mg/kg (approximately 3000 times the MRHD on a mcg/m^2 basis).

14 CLINICAL STUDIES

14.1 Asthma

The safety and efficacy of DULERA were demonstrated in two randomized, double-blind, parallel group, multicenter clinical trials of 12 to 26 weeks in duration involving 1509 patients 12 years of age and older with persistent asthma uncontrolled on medium or high dose inhaled corticosteroids (baseline FEV_1 means of 66% to 73% of predicted normal). These studies included a 2 to 3-week run-in period with mometasone furoate to establish a certain level of asthma control. One clinical trial compared DULERA to placebo and the individual components, mometasone furoate and formoterol (Trial 1) and one clinical trial compared two different strengths of DULERA to mometasone furoate alone (Trial 2).

Trial 1: Clinical Trial with DULERA 100 mcg/5 mcg

This 26-week, placebo-controlled trial evaluated 781 patients 12 years of age and older comparing DULERA 100 mcg/5 mcg (n=191 patients), mometasone furoate 100 mcg (n=192 patients), formoterol fumarate 5 mcg (n=202 patients) and placebo (n=196 patients); each administered as 2 inhalations twice daily by metered dose inhalation aerosols. All other maintenance therapies were discontinued. This study included a 2 to 3-week run-in period with mometasone furoate 100 mcg, 2 inhalations twice daily. This trial included patients ranging from 12 to 76 years of age, 41% male and 59% female, and 72% Caucasian and 28% non-Caucasian. Patients had persistent asthma and were not well controlled on medium dose of inhaled corticosteroids prior to randomization. All treatment groups were balanced with regard to baseline characteristics. Mean FEV_1 and mean percent predicted FEV_1 were similar among all treatment groups (2.33 L, 73%). Eight (4%) patients receiving DULERA 100 mcg/5 mcg, 13 (7%) patients receiving mometasone furoate 100 mcg, 47 (23%) patients receiving formoterol fumarate 5 mcg and 46 (23%) patients receiving placebo discontinued the study early due to treatment failure.

FEV_1 $AUC_{(0\text{-}12\ hr)}$ was assessed as a co-primary efficacy endpoint to evaluate the contribution of the formoterol component to DULERA. Patients receiving DULERA 100 mcg/5 mcg had significantly higher increases from baseline at Week 12 in mean FEV_1 $AUC_{(0\text{-}12\ hr)}$ compared to mometasone furoate 100 mcg (the primary treatment comparison) and vs. placebo (both p<0.001) (Figure 1). These differences were maintained through Week 26. Figure 1 shows the change from baseline post-dose serial FEV_1 evaluations in Trial 1.

Figure 1

Trial 1 - DULERA 100 mcg/5 mcg - FEV_1 Serial Evaluations for Observed Cases at Week 12 Change from Baseline by Treatment

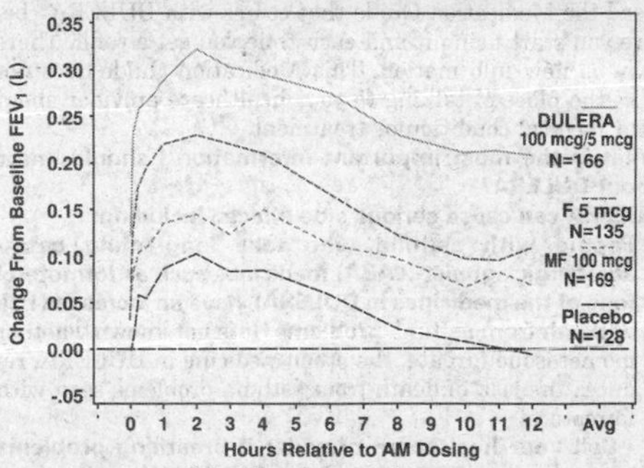

MF = Mometasone furoate
F = Formoterol fumarate
Mean FEV_1 over 12 hours at Week 12 (shown as AVG)

Clinically judged deteriorations in asthma or reductions in lung function were assessed as another primary endpoint to evaluate the contribution of mometasone furoate 100 mcg to DULERA 100 mcg/5 mcg (primary treatment comparison DULERA vs. formoterol). Deteriorations in asthma were defined as any of the following: a 20% decrease in FEV_1; a 30% decrease in PEF on two or more consecutive days; emergency treatment, hospitalization, or treatment with systemic corticosteroids or other asthma medications not allowed per protocol. Fewer patients who received DULERA 100 mcg/5 mcg reported an event compared to patients who received formoterol 5 mcg (p<0.001).
[See table 3 above]

Table 3: Trial 1 - Clinically Judged Deterioration in Asthma or Reduction in Lung Function*

	DULERA 100 mcg/ 5 mcg† (n=191)	Mometasone Furoate 100 mcg† (n=192)	Formoterol 5 mcg† (n=202)	Placebo† (n=196)
Clinically judged deterioration in asthma or reduction in lung function*	58 (30%)	65 (34%)	109 (54%)	109 (56%)
Decrease in FEV_1‡	18 (9%)	19 (10%)	31 (15%)	41 (21%)
Decrease in PEF§	37 (19%)	41 (21%)	62 (31%)	61 (31%)
Emergency treatment	0	1 (<1%)	4 (2%)	1 (<1%)
Hospitalization	1 (<1%)	0	0	0
Treatment with excluded asthma medication¶	2 (1%)	4 (2%)	17 (8%)	8 (4%)

* Includes only the first event day for each patient. Patients could have experienced more than one event criterion.
† Two inhalations, twice daily.
‡ Decrease in absolute FEV_1 below the treatment period stability limit (defined as 80% of the average of the two predose FEV_1 measurements taken 30 minutes and immediately prior to the first dose of randomized trial medication).
§ Decrease in AM or PM peak expiratory flow (PEF) on 2 or more consecutive days below the treatment period stability limit (defined as 70% of the AM or PM PEF obtained over the last 7 days of the run-in period).
¶ Thirty patients received glucocorticosteroids; 1 patient received formoterol via dry powder inhaler in the Formoterol 5 mcg group.

Table 4: Trial 1 – Change in Trough FEV_1 from Baseline to Week 12

Treatment Arm	N	Baseline (L)	Change From Baseline at Week 12 (L)	Treatment Difference from Placebo (L)	P-Value vs. Placebo	P-Value vs. Formoterol
DULERA 100 mcg/5 mcg	167	2.33	0.13	0.18	<0.001	<0.001
Mometasone furoate 100 mcg	175	2.36	0.07	0.12	<0.001	0.058
Formoterol fumarate 5 mcg	141	2.29	0.00	0.05	0.170	
Placebo	145	2.30	-0.05			

LS means and p-values are from Week 12 estimates of a longitudinal analysis model.

Table 6: Trial 2 - Clinically Judged Deterioration in Asthma or Reduction in Lung Function*

	DULERA 100 mcg/ 5 mcg† (n=233)	DULERA 200 mcg/ 5 mcg† (n=255)	Mometasone Furoate 200 mcg† (n=240)
Clinically judged deterioration in asthma or reduction in lung function*	29 (12%)	31 (12%)	44 (18%)
Decrease in FEV_1‡	23 (10%)	17 (7%)	33 (14%)
Decrease in PEF on two consecutive days§	2 (1%)	4 (2%)	3 (1%)
Emergency treatment	2 (1%)	1 (<1%)	1 (<1%)
Hospitalization	0	1 (<1%)	0
Treatment with excluded asthma medication¶	5 (2%)	8 (3%)	12 (5%)

* Includes only the first event day for each patient. Patients could have experienced more than one event criterion.
† Two inhalations, twice daily.
‡ Decrease in absolute FEV_1 below the treatment period stability limit (defined as 80% of the average of the two predose FEV_1 measurements taken 30 minutes and immediately prior to the first dose of randomized trial medication).
§ Decrease in AM or PM peak expiratory flow (PEF) below the treatment period stability limit (defined as 70% of the AM or PM PEF obtained over the last 7 days of the run-in period).
¶ Twenty four patients received glucocorticosteroids; 1 patient received albuterol in the DULERA 200 mcg / 5 mcg group.

The change in mean trough FEV_1 from baseline to Week 12 was assessed as another endpoint to evaluate the contribution of mometasone furoate 100 mcg to DULERA 100 mcg/5 mcg. A significantly greater increase in mean trough FEV_1 was observed for DULERA 100 mcg/5 mcg compared to formoterol 5 mcg (the primary treatment comparison) as well as to placebo (Table 4).
[See table 4 above]

The effect of DULERA 100 mcg/5 mcg, two inhalations twice daily on selected secondary efficacy endpoints, including proportion of nights with nocturnal awakenings (-60% vs. -15%), change in total rescue medication use (-0.6 vs. +1.1 puffs/day), change in morning peak flow (+18.1 vs. -28.4 L/min) and evening peak flow (+10.8 vs. -32.1 L/min) further supports the efficacy of DULERA 100 mcg/5 mcg compared to placebo.

The subjective impact of asthma on patients' health-related quality of life was evaluated by the Asthma Quality of Life Questionnaire (AQLQ(S)) (based on a 7-point scale where 1 = maximum impairment and 7 = no impairment). A change from baseline ≥0.5 points is considered a clinically meaningful improvement. The mean difference in AQLQ between patients receiving DULERA 100 mcg/5 mcg and placebo was 0.5 [95% CI 0.32, 0.68].

Trial 2: Clinical Trial With DULERA 200 mcg/5 mcg

This 12-week double-blind trial evaluated 728 patients 12 years of age and older comparing DULERA 200 mcg/5 mcg (n=255 patients) with DULERA 100 mcg/5 mcg (n=233 patients) and mometasone furoate 200 mcg (n=240 patients), each administered as 2 inhalations twice daily by metered dose inhalation aerosols. All other maintenance therapies were discontinued. This trial included a 2 to 3-week run-in period with mometasone furoate 200 mcg, 2 inhalations twice daily. Patients had persistent asthma and were uncontrolled on high dose inhaled corticosteroids prior to study entry. All treatment groups were balanced with regard to baseline characteristics. This trial included patients ranging from 12 to 84 years of age, 44% male and 56% female, and 89% Caucasian and 11% non-Caucasian. Mean FEV_1 and mean percent predicted FEV_1 values were similar among all treatment groups (2.05 L, 66%). Eleven (5%) patients receiving DULERA 100 mcg/5 mcg, 8 (3%) patients receiving DULERA 200 mcg/5 mcg and 13 (5%) patients receiving mometasone furoate 200 mcg discontinued the trial early due to treatment failure.

The primary efficacy endpoint was the mean change in FEV_1 $AUC_{(0\text{-}12\ hr)}$ from baseline to Week 12. Patients receiving DULERA 100 mcg/5 mcg and DULERA 200 mcg/5 mcg had significantly greater increases from baseline at Day 1 in mean FEV_1 $AUC_{(0\text{-}12\ hr)}$ compared to mometasone furoate 200 mcg. The difference was maintained over 12 weeks of therapy.

Mean change in trough FEV_1 from baseline to Week 12 was also assessed to evaluate the relative contribution of mometasone furoate to DULERA 100 mcg/5 mcg and DULERA 200 mcg/5 mcg (Table 5). A greater numerical increase in the mean trough FEV_1 was observed for DULERA 200 mcg/5 mcg compared to DULERA 100 mcg/5 mcg and mometasone furoate 200 mcg.

Table 5: Trial 2 – Change in Trough FEV_1 from Baseline to Week 12

Treatment Arm	N	Baseline (L)	Change from Baseline at Week 12 (L)
DULERA 100 mcg/5 mcg	232	2.10	0.14
DULERA 200 mcg/5 mcg	255	2.05	0.19
Mometasone furoate 200 mcg	239	2.07	0.10

Clinically judged deterioration in asthma or reduction in lung function was assessed as an additional endpoint. Fewer patients who received DULERA 200 mcg/5 mcg or DULERA 100/5 mcg compared to mometasone furoate 200 mcg alone reported an event, defined as in Trial 1 by any of the following: a 20% decrease in FEV_1; a 30% decrease in PEF on two or more consecutive days; emergency treatment, hospitalization, or treatment with systemic corticosteroids or other asthma medications not allowed per protocol.

[See table 6 at top of previous page]

Other Studies

In addition to Trial 1 and Trial 2, the safety and efficacy of the individual components, mometasone furoate MDI 100 mcg and 200 mcg, in comparison to placebo were demonstrated in three other, 12-week, placebo controlled trials which evaluated the mean change in FEV_1 from baseline as a primary endpoint. The safety and efficacy of formoterol MDI 5 mcg alone in comparison to placebo was replicated in another 26-week trial that evaluated a lower dose of mometasone furoate MDI in combination with formoterol.

16 HOW SUPPLIED/STORAGE AND HANDLING

16.1 How Supplied

DULERA is available in two strengths and supplied in the following package sizes (Table 7):

Table 7

Package	NDC
DULERA 100 mcg/5 mcg 120 inhalations	0085-7206-01
DULERA 100 mcg/5 mcg 60 inhalations (institutional pack)	0085-7206-07
DULERA 200 mcg/5 mcg 120 inhalations	0085-4610-01
DULERA 200 mcg/5 mcg 60 inhalations (institutional pack)	0085-4610-05

Each strength is supplied as a pressurized aluminum canister that has a blue plastic actuator integrated with a dose counter and a blue dust cap. Each 120-inhalation canister has a net fill weight of 13 grams and each 60-inhalation canister has a net fill weight of 8.8 grams. Each canister is placed into a carton. Each carton contains 1 canister and a Medication Guide.

Initially the dose counter will display "64" or "124" actuations. After the initial priming with 4 actuations, the dose counter will read "60" or "120" and the inhaler is now ready for use.

16.2 Storage and Handling

The DULERA canister should only be used with the DULERA actuator. The DULERA actuator should not be used with any other inhalation drug product. Actuators from other products should not be used with the DULERA canister.

The correct amount of medication in each inhalation cannot be ensured after the labeled number of actuations from the canister has been used, even though the inhaler may not feel completely empty and may continue to operate. The inhaler should be discarded when the labeled number of actuations has been used (the dose counter will read "0").

Store at controlled room temperature 20–25°C (68–77°F); excursions permitted to 15–30°C (59–86°F) [see USP Controlled Room Temperature].

The 120-inhalation inhaler does not require specific storage orientation. For the 60-inhalation inhaler, after priming, store the inhaler with the mouthpiece down or in a horizontal position.

For best results, the canister should be at room temperature before use. Shake well and remove the cap from the mouthpiece of the actuator before using. Keep out of reach of children. Avoid spraying in eyes.

Contents Under Pressure: Do not puncture. Do not use or store near heat or open flame. Exposure to temperatures above 120°F may cause bursting. Never throw container into fire or incinerator.

17 PATIENT COUNSELING INFORMATION

See FDA-Approved Patient Labeling (Medication Guide).

17.1 Asthma-Related Death

Patients should be informed that formoterol, one of the active ingredients in DULERA, increases the risk of asthma-related death. In pediatric and adolescent patients, formoterol may increase the risk of asthma-related hospitalization. They should also be informed that data are not adequate to determine whether the concurrent use of inhaled corticosteroids, the other component of DULERA, or other long-term asthma-control therapy mitigates or eliminates this risk *[see Warnings and Precautions (5.1)]*.

17.2 Not for Acute Symptoms

DULERA is not indicated to relieve acute asthma symptoms and extra doses should not be used for that purpose. Acute symptoms should be treated with an inhaled, short-acting, $beta_2$-agonist (the health care provider should prescribe the patient with such medication and instruct the patient in how it should be used).

Patients should be instructed to seek medical attention immediately if they experience any of the following:

- If their symptoms worsen
- Significant decrease in lung function as outlined by the physician
- If they need more inhalations of a short-acting $beta_2$-agonist than usual

Patients should be advised not to increase the dose or frequency of DULERA. The daily dosage of DULERA should not exceed two inhalations twice daily. If they miss a dose, they should be instructed to take their next dose at the same time they normally do. DULERA provides bronchodilation for up to 12 hours.

Patients should not stop or reduce DULERA therapy without physician/provider guidance since symptoms may recur after discontinuation *[see Warnings and Precautions (5.2)]*.

17.3 Do Not Use Additional Long-Acting $Beta_2$-Agonists

When patients are prescribed DULERA, other long-acting $beta_2$-agonists should not be used *[see Warnings and Precautions (5.3)]*.

17.4 Risks Associated With Corticosteroid Therapy

Local Effects: Patients should be advised that localized infections with *Candida albicans* occurred in the mouth and pharynx in some patients. If oropharyngeal candidiasis develops, it should be treated with appropriate local or systemic (i.e., oral) antifungal therapy while still continuing with DULERA therapy, but at times therapy with DULERA may need to be temporarily interrupted under close medical supervision. Rinsing the mouth after inhalation is advised *[see Warnings and Precautions (5.4)]*.

Immunosuppression: Patients who are on immunosuppressant doses of corticosteroids should be warned to avoid exposure to chickenpox or measles and, if exposed, to consult their physician without delay. Patients should be informed of potential worsening of existing tuberculosis, fungal, bacterial, viral, or parasitic infections, or ocular herpes simplex *[see Warnings and Precautions (5.5)]*.

Hypercorticism and Adrenal Suppression: Patients should be advised that DULERA may cause systemic corticosteroid effects of hypercorticism and adrenal suppression. Additionally, patients should be instructed that deaths due to adrenal insufficiency have occurred during and after transfer from systemic corticosteroids. Patients should taper slowly from systemic corticosteroids if transferring to DULERA *[see Warnings and Precautions (5.7)]*.

Reduction in Bone Mineral Density: Patients who are at an increased risk for decreased BMD should be advised that the use of corticosteroids may pose an additional risk and should be monitored and, where appropriate, be treated for this condition *[see Warnings and Precautions (5.12)]*.

Reduced Growth Velocity: Patients should be informed that orally inhaled corticosteroids, a component of DULERA, may cause a reduction in growth velocity when administered to pediatric patients. Physicians should closely follow the growth of pediatric patients taking corticosteroids by any route *[see Warnings and Precautions (5.13)]*.

Glaucoma and Cataracts: Long-term use of inhaled corticosteroids may increase the risk of some eye problems (glaucoma or cataracts); regular eye examinations should be considered *[see Warnings and Precautions (5.14)]*.

17.5 Risks Associated With Beta-Agonist Therapy

Patients should be informed that treatment with $beta_2$-agonists may lead to adverse events which include palpitations, chest pain, rapid heart rate, tremor or nervousness *[see Warnings and Precautions (5.11)]*.

Manufactured for: Merck Sharp & Dohme Corp., a subsidiary of

MERCK & CO., INC., Whitehouse Station, NJ 08889, USA

Manufactured by: 3M Health Care Ltd., Loughborough, United Kingdom.

For patent information: www.merck.com/product/patent/home.html

The trademarks depicted herein are owned by their respective companies.

418131-MFF-AO-USPI.18

Medication Guide

DULERA® [dew-LAIR-ah] 100 mcg/5 mcg

(mometasone furoate 100 mcg and formoterol fumarate dihydrate 5 mcg) Inhalation Aerosol

DULERA® 200 mcg/5 mcg

(mometasone furoate 200 mcg and formoterol fumarate dihydrate 5 mcg) Inhalation Aerosol

Read the Medication Guide that comes with DULERA® before you start using it and each time you get a refill. There may be new information. This Medication Guide does not take the place of talking to your healthcare provider about your medical condition or treatment.

What is the most important information I should know about DULERA?

DULERA can cause serious side effects, including:

1. **People with asthma who take long-acting $beta_2$-adrenergic agonist (LABA) medicines such as formoterol (one of the medicines in DULERA), have an increased risk of death from asthma problems.** It is not known whether mometasone furoate, the other medicine in DULERA, reduces the risk of death from asthma problems seen with formoterol.
   - **Call your healthcare provider if breathing problems worsen over time while using DULERA. You may need different treatment.**
   - **Get emergency medical care if:**
     - breathing problems worsen quickly, and
     - you use your rescue inhaler medicine, but it does not relieve your breathing problems.
2. **DULERA should be used only if your healthcare provider decides that your asthma is not well controlled with a long-term asthma control medicine, such as an inhaled corticosteroid.**
3. When your asthma is well controlled, your healthcare provider may tell you to stop taking DULERA. Your healthcare provider will decide if you can stop DULERA without loss of asthma control. Your healthcare provider may prescribe a different long-term asthma-control medicine for you, such as an inhaled corticosteroid.
4. Children and adolescents who take LABA medicines may have an increased risk of being hospitalized for asthma problems.

What is DULERA?

DULERA combines an inhaled corticosteroid medicine, mometasone furoate (the same medicine found in ASMANEX TWISTHALER), and a long-acting beta$_2$-agonist medicine (LABA), formoterol (the same medicine found in FORADIL® AEROLIZER®).

- Inhaled corticosteroids help to decrease inflammation in the lungs. Inflammation in the lungs can lead to asthma symptoms.
- LABA medicines are used in people with asthma. LABA medicines help the muscles around the airways in your lungs stay relaxed to prevent asthma symptoms, such as wheezing and shortness of breath. These symptoms can happen when the muscles around the airways tighten. This makes it hard to breathe. In severe cases, wheezing can stop your breathing and may lead to death if not treated right away.

DULERA is used to control symptoms of asthma and prevent symptoms such as wheezing in people 12 years of age and older.

DULERA should not be used as a rescue inhaler.

DULERA contains formoterol (the same medicine found in FORADIL AEROLIZER). LABA medicines such as formoterol increase the risk of death from asthma problems.

DULERA is not for children and adults with asthma who:

- are well controlled with an asthma-control medicine, such as a low to medium dose of an inhaled corticosteroid medicine
- only need a rescue inhaler once in awhile

It is not known if DULERA is safe and effective in children less than 12 years of age.

Who should not use DULERA?

Do not use DULERA:

- to treat sudden severe symptoms of asthma
- if you are allergic to any of the ingredients in DULERA. See the end of the Medication Guide for a list of ingredients in DULERA.

What should I tell my healthcare provider before using DULERA?

Tell your healthcare provider about all of your health conditions, including if you:

- **have heart problems**
- **have high blood pressure**
- **have seizures**
- **have thyroid problems**
- **have diabetes**
- **have liver problems**
- **have osteoporosis**
- **have an immune system problem**
- **have eye problems such as increased pressure in the eye, glaucoma, or cataracts**
- **are allergic to any medicines**
- **are exposed to chickenpox or measles**
- **have an aneurysm (swelling of an artery)**
- **have a pheochromocytoma (a tumor of the adrenal gland that can affect your blood pressure)**
- **are scheduled to have surgery**
- **have any other medical problems**
- **are pregnant or planning to become pregnant.** It is not known if DULERA may harm your unborn baby.
- **are breastfeeding.** It is not known if DULERA passes into your milk and if it can harm your baby. You and your healthcare provider should decide if you will take DULERA while breastfeeding.

Tell your healthcare provider about all the medicines you take including prescription and non-prescription medicines, vitamins, and herbal supplements. DULERA and certain other medicines may interact with each other. This may cause serious side effects.

Especially, tell your healthcare provider if you take antifungal medicines, such as ketoconazole, or anti-HIV medicines, such as ritonavir. The anti-HIV medicines NORVIR® (ritonavir capsules) Soft Gelatin, NORVIR® (ritonavir oral solution), and KALETRA® (lopinavir/ritonavir) Tablets contain ritonavir.

Know the medicines you take. Keep a list and show it to your healthcare provider and pharmacist each time you get a new medicine.

How should I use DULERA?

See the step-by-step instructions for using DULERA at the end of this Medication Guide. Do not use DULERA unless your healthcare provider has taught you and you understand everything. Ask your healthcare provider or pharmacist if you have any questions.

- Use DULERA exactly as prescribed. **Do not use DULERA more often than prescribed.** DULERA comes in 2 strengths. Your healthcare provider has prescribed the strength that is best for you. Note the differences between DULERA and your other inhaled medications, including the differences in prescribed use and physical appearance.
- DULERA should be taken every day as 2 puffs in the morning and 2 puffs in the evening.
- If you miss a dose of DULERA, skip your missed dose and take your next dose at your regular time. Do not take DULERA more often or use more puffs than you have been prescribed.
- **While you are using DULERA 2 times each day, do not use other medicines that contain a long-acting beta$_2$-agonist (LABA) for any reason.** Ask your healthcare provider or pharmacist if any of your other medicines are LABA medicines.
- If you take more DULERA than your healthcare provider has prescribed, get medical help right away if you have any unusual symptoms, such as problems breathing, palpitations, chest pain, increased heart rate, nervousness or shakiness.
- Do not change or stop using DULERA or other asthma medicines used to control or treat your breathing problems unless told to do so by your healthcare provider. Your healthcare provider will change your medicines as needed.
- DULERA does not relieve sudden asthma symptoms. Always have a rescue inhaler with you to treat sudden symptoms. Use your rescue inhaler if you have breathing problems between doses of DULERA. If you do not have a rescue inhaler, call your healthcare provider to have one prescribed for you.
- **Remove the cap from the mouthpiece of the actuator before using DULERA.**
- Rinse your mouth with water after each dose (2 puffs) of DULERA. This will help to lessen the chance of getting a yeast infection (thrush) in the mouth and throat.
- Do not spray DULERA in your eyes. If you accidentally get DULERA in your eyes, rinse your eyes with water and if redness or irritation continues, call your healthcare provider.
- **Call your healthcare provider or get medical care right away if:**
  - your breathing problems worsen with DULERA
  - you need to use your rescue inhaler more often than usual
  - your rescue inhaler does not work as well for you at relieving symptoms
  - you need to use 4 or more inhalations of your rescue inhaler for 2 or more days in a row
  - you use 1 whole canister of your rescue inhaler in 8 weeks' time
  - your peak flow meter results decrease. Your healthcare provider will tell you the numbers that are right for you.
  - you have asthma and your symptoms do not improve after using DULERA regularly for 1 to 2 weeks

What are the possible side effects of DULERA?

DULERA can cause serious side effects, including:

- **See "What is the most important information I should know about DULERA?"**
- **Thrush in the mouth and throat.** You may develop a yeast infection (Candida albicans) in your mouth or throat. Rinse your mouth with water after using DULERA to help prevent an infection in your mouth or throat.
- **Immune system effects and a higher chance for infections.**
- Tell your healthcare provider about any signs of infection such as:
  - fever
  - feeling tired
  - pain
  - nausea
  - body aches
  - vomiting
  - chills
- **Adrenal insufficiency.** Adrenal insufficiency is a condition in which the adrenal glands do not make enough steroid hormones. This can happen when you stop taking oral corticosteroid medicines and start inhaled corticosteroid medicines.
- **Increased wheezing right after taking DULERA.** Always have a rescue inhaler with you to treat sudden wheezing.
- **Serious allergic reactions.** Call your healthcare provider or get emergency medical care if you get any of the following symptoms of a serious allergic reaction:
  - rash
  - hives
  - swelling, including swelling of the face, mouth, and tongue
  - breathing problems
- Using too much of a LABA medicine may cause:
  - **chest pain**
  - **increased or decreased blood pressure**
  - **a fast and irregular heartbeat**
  - **headache**
  - **tremor**
  - **nervousness**
  - **dizziness**
  - **weakness**
  - **seizures**
  - **electrocardiogram (ECG) changes**
- **Lower bone mineral density.** This may be a problem for people who already have a higher chance for low bone density (osteoporosis).
- **Slowed growth in children.** A child's growth should be checked often.
- **Eye problems including glaucoma and cataracts.** You should have regular eye exams while using DULERA.
- **Decreases in blood potassium levels (hypokalemia)**
- **Increases in blood sugar levels (hyperglycemia)**

The most common side effects of DULERA include:

- inflammation of the nose and throat (nasopharyngitis)
- inflammation of the sinuses (sinusitis)
- headache

Other side effects:

- Worsening asthma or sudden asthma attacks have been reported with the use of inhaled mometasone furoate (one of the medicines in DULERA).

Tell your healthcare provider about any side effect that bothers you or that does not go away.

These are not all the side effects with DULERA. Ask your healthcare provider or pharmacist for more information.

Call your doctor for medical advice about side effects. You may report side effects to FDA at 1-800-FDA-1088.

You may also report side effects to Merck Sharp & Dohme Corp., a subsidiary of Merck & Co., Inc., at 1-877-888-4231.

How do I store DULERA?

- Store DULERA at room temperature between 59°F to 86°F (15°C to 30°C).
- The 120-actuation inhaler can be stored in any position. For the 60-actuation inhaler, after priming, store the inhaler with the mouthpiece down or sideways.
- The contents of your DULERA are under pressure. Do not puncture. Do not use or store near heat or open flame. Storage above 120°F may cause the canister to burst.
- Do not throw container into fire or incinerator.
- **Keep DULERA and all medicines out of the reach of children.**

General Information about DULERA

Medicines are sometimes prescribed for purposes other than those listed in a Medication Guide. Do not use DULERA for a condition for which it was not prescribed. Do not give your DULERA to other people, even if they have the same condition. It may harm them.

This Medication Guide summarizes the most important information about DULERA. If you would like more information, talk with your healthcare provider. You can ask your healthcare provider or pharmacist for information about DULERA that was written for healthcare professionals. For more information about DULERA, go to www.DULERA.com or call 1-800-622-4477.

What are the ingredients in DULERA?

Active ingredients: mometasone furoate and formoterol fumarate dihydrate

Inactive ingredients: hydrofluoroalkane (HFA-227), anhydrous alcohol and oleic acid

Patient Instructions for Use

DULERA®

DULERA® 100 mcg/5 mcg

(mometasone furoate 100 mcg and formoterol fumarate dihydrate 5 mcg) Inhalation Aerosol

DULERA® 200 mcg/5 mcg

(mometasone furoate 200 mcg and formoterol fumarate dihydrate 5 mcg) Inhalation Aerosol

How to use your DULERA

Before using your DULERA, read the complete instructions and use only as directed.

The parts of your DULERA:

There are 2 main parts to your DULERA inhaler – the metal canister that holds the medicine and the blue plastic actuator that sprays the medicine from the canister. The inhaler also has a cap that covers the mouthpiece of the actuator (see **Figure 1**). The cap from the mouthpiece must be removed before use. The inhaler contains 60 or 120 actuations (puffs).

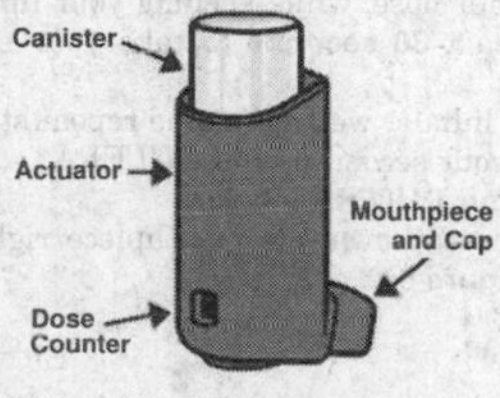

Figure 1

The inhaler comes with dose counter located on the plastic actuator. See **Figure 1.** The counter display will show the number of actuations (puffs) of medicine remaining. The dose counter will initially display "64" or "124" actuations remaining. Each time you press the canister, a puff of medicine is released and the counter will count down by 1. The counter will stop counting at 0.

- You should not remove the canister from the actuator because reinsertion may cause the counter to count down by 1 and discharge a puff.
- Use the DULERA canister only with the actuator supplied with the product. Do not use parts of the DULERA inhaler with parts from any other inhalation medicine.

Before using your DULERA:

REMOVE THE CAP FROM THE MOUTHPIECE OF THE ACTUATOR (see **Figure 2**). Check the mouthpiece for objects before use. Make sure the canister is fully inserted into the actuator.

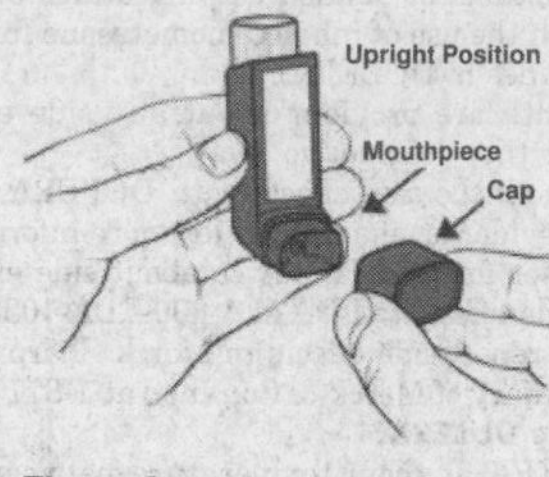

Figure 2

Priming your DULERA Inhaler:

Before you use DULERA for the first time, you must prime the inhaler.

1. To prime the inhaler, hold it in the upright position and release 4 actuations (puffs) into the air, away from your face.
2. Shake the inhaler well before each of the priming actuations. After priming 4 times, the dose counter should read either "60" or "120".
3. **If you do not use your DULERA for more than 5 days, you will need to prime it again before use.**

Using your DULERA

4. **REMOVE THE CAP FROM THE MOUTHPIECE OF THE ACTUATOR** (see **Figure 3**). Check the mouthpiece for objects before use. Make sure the canister is fully inserted into the actuator.
5. Shake the inhaler well before each use.
6. Breathe out as fully as you comfortably can through your mouth. Push out as much air from your lungs as possible. Hold the inhaler in the upright position and place the mouthpiece into your mouth (see **Figure 4**). Close your lips around the mouthpiece.

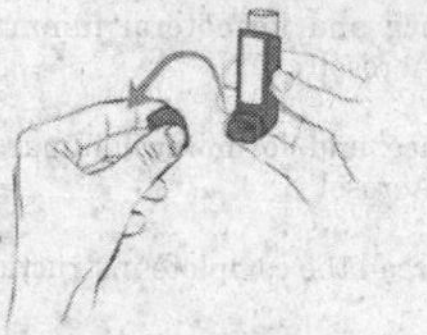

Figure 3 Figure 4

7. Take a deep breath (inhale) in slowly through your mouth. While doing this, press down firmly and fully on the top of the canister until it stops moving in the actuator. Take your finger off the canister.
8. When you have finished breathing in, hold your breath as long as you comfortably can, up to 10 seconds. Then remove the inhaler from your mouth and breathe out through your nose, while keeping your lips closed.
9. Wait at least **30 seconds** to take your second puff of DULERA.
10. Shake the inhaler well again and repeat steps 6 through 8 to take your second puff of DULERA.

After using your DULERA inhaler:

11. Replace the cap over the mouthpiece right away after use (see **Figure 5**).

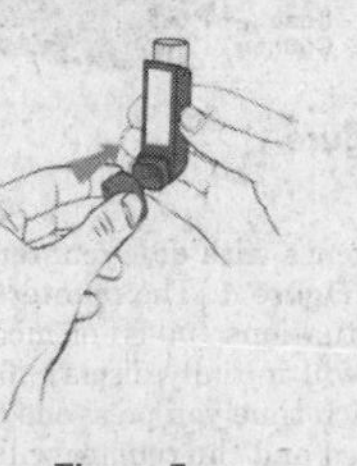

Figure 5

12. After you finish taking DULERA (2 puffs), rinse your mouth with water.

Reading the counter

- The dose counter identifies the number of inhalations (puffs) left in your inhaler.
- The counter will count down each time you release a puff of medicine (either when preparing your DULERA inhaler for use or when taking the medicine).

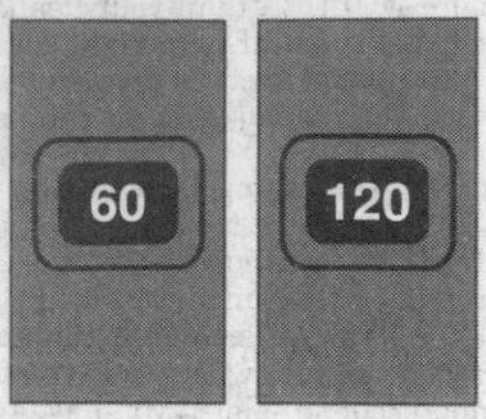

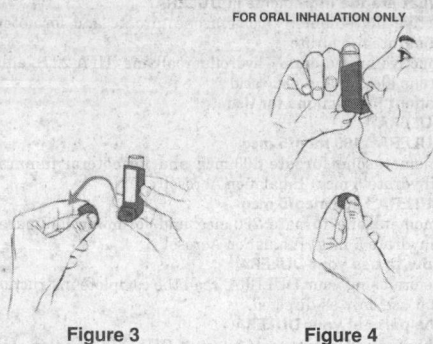

When to replace your DULERA:

- It is important that you pay attention to the number of inhalations (puffs) left in your DULERA inhaler by reading the counter.
- When the counter reads 20, you should refill your prescription or ask your healthcare provider if you need a new prescription for DULERA.
- Throw away DULERA after the counter reaches 0, indicating that you have used the number of actuations on the product label and box. Your inhaler may not feel empty and it may continue to operate, but you will not get the right amount of medicine if you keep using it.
- Never try to change the numbers on the counter or remove the counter from the actuator.
- Do not use the inhaler after the expiration date.

How do I store DULERA?

- Store DULERA at room temperature between 59°F to 86°F (15°C to 30°C).
- The 120-actuation inhaler can be stored in any position. For the 60-actuation inhaler, after priming, store the inhaler with the mouthpiece down or sideways.
- The contents of your DULERA canister are under pressure. Do not puncture or throw the canister into a fire or incinerator. Do not use or store it near heat or open flame. Storage above 120°F (50°C) may cause the canister to burst.
- **Keep DULERA and all medicines out of the reach of children.**

How to clean your DULERA:

The mouthpiece should be cleaned using a dry wipe after every 7 days of use.

Routine cleaning instructions:

- Remove the cap off the mouthpiece. Wipe the inside and outside surfaces of the actuator mouthpiece with a clean, dry, lint-free tissue or cloth. Put the cap back on the mouthpiece after cleaning.
- Do not attempt to unblock the actuator with a sharp object, such as a pin.
- Do not wash or put any parts of your inhaler in water.

Manufactured for: Merck Sharp & Dohme Corp., a subsidiary of

MERCK & CO., INC., Whitehouse Station, NJ 08889, USA

Manufactured by: 3M Health Care Ltd., Loughborough, United Kingdom.

This Medication Guide has been approved by the U.S. Food and Drug Administration.

For patent information: www.merck.com/product/patent/home.html

The trademarks depicted herein are owned by their respective companies.

FORADIL is a registered trademark of Astellas Pharma Inc.

AEROLIZER is a registered trademark of Novartis AG.

NORVIR and KALETRA are registered trademarks of Abbott Laboratories.

Revised: 07/2013

418131-MFF-AO-MG.14

Shown in Product Identification Guide, page 307

ELOCON® ℞

[ĕl'ō-cŏn]

(mometasone furoate)

Cream, 0.1% for topical use

HIGHLIGHTS OF PRESCRIBING INFORMATION

These highlights do not include all the information needed to use ELOCON Cream safely and effectively. See full prescribing information for ELOCON Cream.

ELOCON®(mometasone furoate) Cream, 0.1% for topical use

Initial U.S. Approval: 1987

INDICATIONS AND USAGE

ELOCON Cream is a corticosteroid indicated for the relief of the inflammatory and pruritic manifestations of corticosteroid-responsive dermatoses in patients ≥2 years of age. (1)

DOSAGE AND ADMINISTRATION

- Apply a thin film to the affected skin areas once daily. (2)
- Discontinue therapy when control is achieved. (2)
- If no improvement is seen within 2 weeks, reassess diagnosis. (2)
- The safety and efficacy of ELOCON Cream, 0.1% in pediatric patients for more than 3 weeks of use have not been established. (2)
- Do not use with occlusive dressings unless directed by a physician. (2)

DOSAGE FORMS AND STRENGTHS

- Cream, 0.1%. (3)

CONTRAINDICATIONS

- None. (4)

WARNINGS AND PRECAUTIONS

- Reversible HPA axis suppression with the potential for glucocorticosteroid insufficiency after withdrawal of treatment, Cushing's syndrome, and hyperglycemia may occur due to systemic absorption. Patients applying a topical steroid to a large surface area or to areas under occlusion should be evaluated periodically for evidence of HPA axis suppression. Modify use should HPA axis suppression develop. Pediatric patients may be more susceptible to systemic toxicity. (5.1, 8.4)

ADVERSE REACTIONS

Most common adverse reactions are: burning, pruritus, and skin atrophy. (6)

To report SUSPECTED ADVERSE REACTIONS, contact Merck Sharp & Dohme Corp., a subsidiary of Merck & Co., Inc., at 1-877-888-4231 or FDA at 1-800-FDA-1088 or www.fda.gov/medwatch.

See 17 for PATIENT COUNSELING INFORMATION

Revised: 04/2013

FULL PRESCRIBING INFORMATION: CONTENTS*

*** Sections or subsections omitted from the full prescribing information are not listed**

FULL PRESCRIBING INFORMATION

1 INDICATIONS AND USAGE

ELOCON® Cream is a corticosteroid indicated for the relief of the inflammatory and pruritic manifestations of corticosteroid-responsive dermatoses in patients 2 years of age or older.

2 DOSAGE AND ADMINISTRATION

Apply a thin film of ELOCON Cream to the affected skin areas once daily. ELOCON Cream may be used in pediatric patients 2 years of age or older. Since safety and efficacy of ELOCON Cream have not been established in pediatric patients below 2 years of age; use in this age group is not recommended *[see Warnings and Precautions (5.1) and Use in Specific Populations (8.4)]*.

Therapy should be discontinued when control is achieved. If no improvement is seen within 2 weeks, reassessment of diagnosis may be necessary. Safety and efficacy of ELOCON Cream in pediatric patients for more than 3 weeks of use have not been established.

ELOCON Cream should not be used with occlusive dressings unless directed by a physician. ELOCON Cream should not be applied in the diaper area if the child still requires diapers or plastic pants, as these garments may constitute occlusive dressing.

ELOCON Cream is for topical use only. It is not for oral, ophthalmic, or intravaginal use.

Avoid use on the face, groin, or axillae.

3 DOSAGE FORMS AND STRENGTHS

Cream, 0.1%. Each gram of ELOCON Cream contains 1 mg of mometasone furoate in a white to off-white smooth and homogenous cream base.

4 CONTRAINDICATIONS

None.

5 WARNINGS AND PRECAUTIONS

5.1 Effects on Endocrine System

Systemic absorption of topical corticosteroids can produce reversible hypothalamic-pituitary-adrenal (HPA) axis suppression with the potential for glucocorticosteroid insufficiency. This may occur during treatment or after withdrawal of treatment. Manifestations of Cushing's syndrome, hyperglycemia, and glucosuria can also be produced in some patients by systemic absorption of topical corticosteroids while on treatment. Factors that predispose a patient using a topical corticosteroid to HPA axis suppression include the use of high-potency steroids, large treatment surface areas, prolonged use, use of occlusive dressings, altered skin barrier, liver failure and young age.

Because of the potential for systemic absorption, use of topical corticosteroids may require that patients be periodically evaluated for HPA axis suppression. This may be done by using the adrenocorticotropic hormone (ACTH) stimulation test.

In a study evaluating the effects of mometasone furoate cream on the HPA axis, 15 grams were applied twice daily for 7 days to six adult subjects with psoriasis or atopic dermatitis. The results show that the drug caused a slight lowering of adrenal corticosteroid secretion.

If HPA axis suppression is noted, an attempt should be made to gradually withdraw the drug, to reduce the frequency of application, or to substitute a less potent corticosteroid. Recovery of HPA axis function is generally prompt upon discontinuation of topical corticosteroids. Infrequently, signs and symptoms of glucocorticosteroid insufficiency may occur, requiring supplemental systemic corticosteroids.

Pediatric patients may be more susceptible to systemic toxicity from equivalent doses due to their larger skin surface to body mass ratios *[see Use in Specific Populations (8.4)]*.

5.2 Allergic Contact Dermatitis

If irritation develops, ELOCON Cream should be discontinued and appropriate therapy instituted. Allergic contact dermatitis with corticosteroids is usually diagnosed by observing a failure to heal rather than noting a clinical exacerbation as with most topical products not containing corticosteroids. Such an observation should be corroborated with appropriate diagnostic patch testing.

5.3 Concomitant Skin Infections

If concomitant skin infections are present or develop, an appropriate antifungal or antibacterial agent should be used. If a favorable response does not occur promptly, use of ELOCON Cream should be discontinued until the infection has been adequately controlled.

6 ADVERSE REACTIONS

Because clinical trials are conducted under widely varying conditions, adverse reaction rates observed in the clinical trials of a drug cannot be directly compared to rates in the clinical trials of another drug and may not reflect the rates observed in clinical practice.

In controlled clinical trials involving 319 subjects, the incidence of adverse reactions associated with the use of ELOCON Cream was 1.6%. Reported reactions included burning, pruritus, and skin atrophy. Reports of rosacea associated with the use of ELOCON Cream have also been received. In controlled clinical trials (n=74) involving pediatric subjects 2 to 12 years of age, the incidence of adverse experiences associated with the use of ELOCON Cream was approximately 7%. Reported reactions included stinging, pruritus, and furunculosis.

The following adverse reactions were reported to be possibly or probably related to treatment with ELOCON Cream during clinical trials in 4% of 182 pediatric subjects 6 months to 2 years of age: decreased glucocorticoid levels, 2; paresthesia, 2; folliculitis, 1; moniliasis, 1; bacterial infection, 1; skin depigmentation, 1. The following signs of skin atrophy were also observed among 97 subjects treated with ELOCON Cream in a clinical trial: shininess, 4; telangiectasia, 1; loss of elasticity, 4; loss of normal skin markings, 4; thinness, 1; and bruising, 1.

The following additional local adverse reactions have been reported with topical corticosteroids, but may occur more frequently with the use of occlusive dressings. These reactions are: irritation, dryness, folliculitis, hypertrichosis, acneiform eruptions, hypopigmentation, perioral dermatitis, allergic contact dermatitis, secondary infection, striae, and miliaria.

7 DRUG INTERACTIONS

No drug-drug interaction studies have been conducted with ELOCON Cream.

8 USE IN SPECIFIC POPULATIONS

8.1 Pregnancy

Teratogenic Effects Pregnancy Category C:

There are no adequate and well-controlled studies in pregnant women. Therefore, ELOCON Cream should be used during pregnancy only if the potential benefit justifies the potential risk to the fetus.

Corticosteroids have been shown to be teratogenic in laboratory animals when administered systemically at relatively low dosage levels. Some corticosteroids have been shown to be teratogenic after dermal application in laboratory animals.

When administered to pregnant rats, rabbits, and mice, mometasone furoate increased fetal malformations. The doses that produced malformations also decreased fetal growth, as measured by lower fetal weights and/or delayed ossification. Mometasone furoate also caused dystocia and related complications when administered to rats during the end of pregnancy.

In mice, mometasone furoate caused cleft palate at subcutaneous doses of 60 mcg/kg and above. Fetal survival was reduced at 180 mcg/kg. No toxicity was observed at 20 mcg/kg. (Doses of 20, 60, and 180 mcg/kg in the mouse are approximately 0.01, 0.02, and 0.05 times the estimated maximum clinical topical dose from ELOCON Cream on a mcg/m^2 basis.)

In rats, mometasone furoate produced umbilical hernias at topical doses of 600 mcg/kg and above. A dose of 300 mcg/kg produced delays in ossification, but no malformations. (Doses of 300 and 600 mcg/kg in the rat are approximately 0.2 and 0.4 times the estimated maximum clinical topical dose from ELOCON Cream on a mcg/m^2 basis.)

In rabbits, mometasone furoate caused multiple malformations (e.g., flexed front paws, gallbladder agenesis, umbilical hernia, hydrocephaly) at topical doses of 150 mcg/kg and above (approximately 0.2 times the estimated maximum clinical topical dose from ELOCON Cream on a mcg/m^2 basis). In an oral study, mometasone furoate increased resorptions and caused cleft palate and/or head malformations (hydrocephaly and domed head) at 700 mcg/kg. At 2800 mcg/kg most litters were aborted or resorbed. No toxicity was observed at 140 mcg/kg. (Doses at 140, 700, and 2800 mcg/kg in the rabbit are approximately 0.2, 0.9, and 3.6 times the estimated maximum clinical topical dose from ELOCON Cream on a mcg/m^2 basis.)

When rats received subcutaneous doses of mometasone furoate throughout pregnancy or during the later stages of pregnancy, 15 mcg/kg caused prolonged and difficult labor and reduced the number of live births, birth weight, and early pup survival. Similar effects were not observed at 7.5 mcg/kg. (Doses of 7.5 and 15 mcg/kg in the rat are approximately 0.005 and 0.01 times the estimated maximum clinical topical dose from ELOCON Cream on a mcg/m^2 basis.)

8.3 Nursing Mothers

Systemically administered corticosteroids appear in human milk and could suppress growth, interfere with endogenous corticosteroid production, or cause other untoward effects. It is not known whether topical administration of corticosteroids could result in sufficient systemic absorption to produce detectable quantities in human milk. Because many drugs are excreted in human milk, caution should be exercised when ELOCON Cream is administered to a nursing woman.

8.4 Pediatric Use

ELOCON Cream may be used with caution in pediatric patients 2 years of age or older, although the safety and efficacy of drug use for longer than 3 weeks have not been established. Since safety and efficacy of ELOCON Cream have not been established in pediatric patients below 2 years of age, its use in this age group is not recommended.

In a pediatric trial, 24 atopic dermatitis subjects, of whom 19 subjects were age 2 to 12 years, were treated with ELOCON Cream once daily. The majority of subjects cleared within 3 weeks.

ELOCON Cream caused HPA axis suppression in approximately 16% of pediatric subjects ages 6 to 23 months, who showed normal adrenal function by Cortrosyn test before starting treatment, and were treated for approximately 3 weeks over a mean body surface area of 41% (range 15%-94%). The criteria for suppression were: basal cortisol level of ≤5 mcg/dL, 30-minute post-stimulation level of ≤18 mcg/dL, or an increase of <7 mcg/dL. Follow-up testing 2 to 4 weeks after trial completion, available for 5 of the subjects, demonstrated suppressed HPA axis function in 1 subject, using these same criteria. Long-term use of topical corticosteroids has not been studied in this population *[see Clinical Pharmacology (12.2)]*.

Because of a higher ratio of skin surface area to body mass, pediatric patients are at a greater risk than adults of HPA axis suppression and Cushing's syndrome when they are treated with topical corticosteroids. They are, therefore, also at greater risk of adrenal insufficiency during and/or after withdrawal of treatment. Pediatric patients may be more susceptible than adults to skin atrophy, including striae, when they are treated with topical corticosteroids. Pediatric patients applying topical corticosteroids to greater than 20% of body surface are at higher risk of HPA axis suppression.

HPA axis suppression, Cushing's syndrome, linear growth retardation, delayed weight gain, and intracranial hypertension have been reported in pediatric patients receiving topical corticosteroids. Manifestations of adrenal suppression in children include low plasma cortisol levels and an absence of response to ACTH stimulation. Manifestations of intracranial hypertension include bulging fontanelles, headaches, and bilateral papilledema.

ELOCON Cream should not be used in the treatment of diaper dermatitis.

8.5 Geriatric Use

Clinical studies of ELOCON Cream included 190 subjects who were 65 years of age and over and 39 subjects who were 75 years of age and over. No overall differences in safety or effectiveness were observed between these subjects and younger subjects, and other reported clinical experience has not identified differences in responses between the elderly and younger patients. However, greater sensitivity of some older individuals cannot be ruled out.

10 OVERDOSAGE

Topically applied ELOCON Cream can be absorbed in sufficient amounts to produce systemic effects *[see Warnings and Precautions (5.1)]*.

11 DESCRIPTION

ELOCON (mometasone furoate) Cream, 0.1% contains mometasone furoate for topical use. Mometasone furoate is a synthetic corticosteroid with anti-inflammatory activity. Chemically, mometasone furoate is 9α,21-dichloro-11β,17-dihydroxy-16α-methylpregna-1,4-diene-3,20-dione 17-(2-furoate), with the empirical formula $C_{27}H_{30}Cl_2O_6$, a molecular weight of 521.4 and the following structural formula:

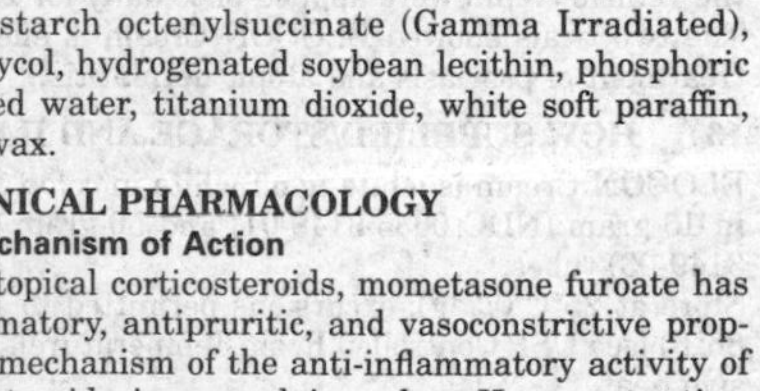

Mometasone furoate is a white to off-white powder practically insoluble in water, slightly soluble in octanol, and moderately soluble in ethyl alcohol.

Each gram of ELOCON Cream, 0.1% contains 1 mg mometasone furoate in a white to off-white cream base of aluminum starch octenylsuccinate (Gamma Irradiated), hexylene glycol, hydrogenated soybean lecithin, phosphoric acid, purified water, titanium dioxide, white soft paraffin, and white wax.

12 CLINICAL PHARMACOLOGY

12.1 Mechanism of Action

Like other topical corticosteroids, mometasone furoate has anti-inflammatory, antipruritic, and vasoconstrictive properties. The mechanism of the anti-inflammatory activity of the topical steroids, in general, is unclear. However, corticosteroids are thought to act by the induction of phospholipase A_2 inhibitory proteins, collectively called lipocortins. It is postulated that these proteins control the biosynthesis of potent mediators of inflammation such as prostaglandins and leukotrienes by inhibiting the release of their common precursor arachidonic acid. Arachidonic acid is released from membrane phospholipids by phospholipase A_2.

12.2 Pharmacodynamics

Studies performed with ELOCON Cream indicate that it is in the medium range of potency as compared with other topical corticosteroids.

In a study evaluating the effects of mometasone furoate cream on the HPA axis, 15 grams were applied twice daily for 7 days to six adult subjects with psoriasis or atopic dermatitis. The cream was applied without occlusion to at least 30% of the body surface. The results showed that the drug caused a slight lowering of adrenal corticosteroid secretion *[see Warnings and Precautions (5.1)]*.

Ninety-seven pediatric subjects ages 6 to 23 months with atopic dermatitis were enrolled in an open-label HPA axis safety study. ELOCON Cream was applied once daily for approximately 3 weeks over a mean body surface area of 41% (range 15%-94%). In approximately 16% of subjects who showed normal adrenal function by Cortrosyn test before starting treatment, adrenal suppression was observed at the end of treatment with ELOCON Cream. The criteria for suppression were: basal cortisol level of ≤5 mcg/dL, 30-minute post-stimulation level of ≤18 mcg/dL, or an increase of <7 mcg/dL. Follow-up testing 2 to 4 weeks after stopping treatment, available for 5 of the subjects, demonstrated suppressed HPA axis function in one subject, using these same criteria *[see Use in Specific Populations (8.4)]*.

12.3 Pharmacokinetics

The extent of percutaneous absorption of topical corticosteroids is determined by many factors including the vehicle and the integrity of the epidermal barrier. Studies in humans indicate that approximately 0.4% of the applied dose of ELOCON Cream enters the circulation after 8 hours of contact on normal skin without occlusion. Inflammation and/or other disease processes in the skin may increase percutaneous absorption.

13 NONCLINICAL TOXICOLOGY

13.1 Carcinogenesis, Mutagenesis, Impairment of Fertility

Long-term animal studies have not been performed to evaluate the carcinogenic potential of ELOCON Cream. Long-term carcinogenicity studies of mometasone furoate were conducted by the inhalation route in rats and mice. In a 2-year carcinogenicity study in Sprague Dawley rats, mometasone furoate demonstrated no statistically significant increase of tumors at inhalation doses up to 67 mcg/kg (approximately 0.04 times the estimated maximum clinical topical dose from ELOCON Cream on a mcg/m^2 basis). In a 19-month carcinogenicity study in Swiss CD-1 mice, mometasone furoate demonstrated no statistically significant increase in the incidence of tumors at inhalation doses up to 160 mcg/kg (approximately 0.05 times the estimated maximum clinical topical dose from ELOCON Cream on a mcg/m^2 basis).

Mometasone furoate increased chromosomal aberrations in an *in vitro* Chinese hamster ovary cell assay, but did not increase chromosomal aberrations in an *in vitro* Chinese hamster lung cell assay. Mometasone furoate was not mutagenic in the Ames test or mouse lymphoma assay, and was not clastogenic in an *in vivo* mouse micronucleus assay, a rat bone marrow chromosomal aberration assay, or a mouse male germ-cell chromosomal aberration assay. Mometasone furoate also did not induce unscheduled DNA synthesis *in vivo* in rat hepatocytes.

In reproductive studies in rats, impairment of fertility was not produced in male or female rats by subcutaneous doses up to 15 mcg/kg (approximately 0.01 times the estimated maximum clinical topical dose from ELOCON Cream on a mcg/m^2 basis).

14 CLINICAL STUDIES

The safety and efficacy of the ELOCON Cream for the treatment of corticosteroid-responsive dermatoses were evaluated in two randomized, double-blind, vehicle-controlled clinical trials, one in psoriasis and one in atopic dermatitis. A total 366 subjects (12-81 years of age), of whom 177 received ELOCON Cream and 181 subjects received vehicle cream, were evaluated in these trials. ELOCON Cream or the vehicle cream were applied once daily for 21 days.

The two trials showed ELOCON Cream is effective in the treatment of psoriasis and atopic dermatitis.

16 HOW SUPPLIED/STORAGE AND HANDLING

ELOCON Cream is white to off-white in color and supplied in 15-gram (NDC 0085-3149-01) and 50-gram (NDC 0085-3149-03) tubes.

Store at 25°C (77°F); excursions permitted to 15-30°C (59-86°F) [see USP Controlled Room Temperature]. Avoid excessive heat.

17 PATIENT COUNSELING INFORMATION

Inform patients of the following:

- Use ELOCON Cream as directed by the physician. It is for external use only.
- Avoid contact with the eyes.
- Do not use ELOCON Cream on the face, underarms, or groin areas unless directed by the physician.
- Do not use ELOCON Cream for any disorder other than that for which it was prescribed.
- The treated skin area should not be bandaged or otherwise covered or wrapped so as to be occlusive, unless directed by the physician.
- Report any signs of local adverse reactions to the physician.
- Advise patients not to use ELOCON Cream in the treatment of diaper dermatitis. Do not apply ELOCON Cream in the diaper area, as diapers or plastic pants may constitute occlusive dressing.
- Discontinue therapy when control is achieved. If no improvement is seen within 2 weeks, contact the physician.
- Do not use other corticosteroid-containing products with ELOCON Cream without first consulting with the physician.

Manufactured for: Merck Sharp & Dohme Corp., a subsidiary of
MERCK & CO., INC., Whitehouse Station, NJ 08889, USA
Manufactured by:
Schering-Plough Labo NV
Heist-op-den-Berg, Belgium

032088-EL-CR-USPI.7

ELOCON® LOTION ℞

[ĕl′ō-cŏn]

mometasone furoate

Lotion, 0.1% for topical use

HIGHLIGHTS OF PRESCRIBING INFORMATION

These highlights do not include all the information needed to use ELOCON Lotion safely and effectively. See full prescribing information for ELOCON Lotion.

ELOCON® (mometasone furoate) Lotion, 0.1% for topical use

Initial U.S. Approval: 1987

INDICATIONS AND USAGE

ELOCON Lotion is a corticosteroid indicated for the relief of the inflammatory and pruritic manifestations of corticosteroid-responsive dermatoses in patients ≥12 years of age. (1)

DOSAGE AND ADMINISTRATION

- Apply a few drops to the affected skin areas once daily and massage lightly until it disappears. (2)
- Discontinue therapy when control is achieved. (2)
- If no improvement is seen within 2 weeks, reassess diagnosis. (2)
- Do not use with occlusive dressings unless directed by a physician. (2)

DOSAGE FORMS AND STRENGTHS

- Lotion, 0.1%. (3)

CONTRAINDICATIONS

- None. (4)

WARNINGS AND PRECAUTIONS

- Reversible HPA axis suppression with the potential for glucocorticosteroid insufficiency after withdrawal of treatment, Cushing's syndrome, and hyperglycemia may occur due to systemic absorption. Patients applying a topical steroid to a large surface area or to areas under occlusion should be evaluated periodically for evidence of HPA axis suppression. Modify use should HPA axis suppression develop. Pediatric patients may be more susceptible to systemic toxicity. (5.1, 8.4)

ADVERSE REACTIONS

Most common adverse reactions included are acneiform reaction, burning, itching and folliculitis. (6)

To report SUSPECTED ADVERSE REACTIONS, contact Merck Sharp & Dohme Corp., a subsidiary of Merck & Co., Inc., at 1-877-888-4231 or FDA at 1-800-FDA-1088 or www.fda.gov/medwatch.

See 17 for PATIENT COUNSELING INFORMATION

Revised: 03/2013

FULL PRESCRIBING INFORMATION: CONTENTS*

*** Sections or subsections omitted from the full prescribing information are not listed**

FULL PRESCRIBING INFORMATION

1 INDICATIONS AND USAGE

ELOCON® Lotion is a corticosteroid indicated for the relief of the inflammatory and pruritic manifestations of corticosteroid-responsive dermatoses in patients 12 years of age or older.

2 DOSAGE AND ADMINISTRATION

Apply a few drops of ELOCON Lotion to the affected skin areas once daily and massage lightly until it disappears.

Therapy should be discontinued when control is achieved. If no improvement is seen within 2 weeks, reassessment of diagnosis may be necessary *[see Warnings and Precautions (5.1) and Use in Specific Populations (8.4)]*.

ELOCON Lotion should not be used with occlusive dressings unless directed by a physician. ELOCON Lotion should not be applied in the diaper area if the patient still requires diapers or plastic pants, as these garments may constitute occlusive dressing.

ELOCON Lotion is for topical use only. It is not for oral, ophthalmic, or intravaginal use.

Avoid use on the face, groin, or axillae.

3 DOSAGE FORMS AND STRENGTHS

Lotion, 0.1%. Each gram of ELOCON Lotion contains 1 mg of mometasone furoate in a colorless, clear to translucent lotion base.

4 CONTRAINDICATIONS

None.

5 WARNINGS AND PRECAUTIONS

5.1 Effects on Endocrine System

Systemic absorption of topical corticosteroids can produce reversible hypothalamic-pituitary-adrenal (HPA) axis suppression with the potential for glucocorticosteroid insufficiency. This may occur during treatment or after withdrawal of treatment. Manifestations of Cushing's syndrome, hyperglycemia, and glucosuria can also be produced in some patients by systemic absorption of topical corticosteroids while on treatment. Factors that predispose a patient using a topical corticosteroid to HPA axis suppression include the use of high potency steroids, large treatment surface areas, prolonged use, use of occlusive dressing, altered skin barrier, liver failure and young age.

Because of the potential for systemic absorption, use of topical corticosteroids may require that patients be periodically evaluated for HPA axis suppression. This may be done by using the adrenocorticotropic hormone (ACTH) stimulation test.

In a study evaluating the effects of mometasone furoate lotion on the HPA axis, 15 mL were applied without occlusion twice daily (30 mL per day) for 7 days to 4 adult subjects with scalp and body psoriasis. At the end of treatment, the plasma cortisol levels for each of the 4 subjects remained within the normal range and changed little from baseline.

If HPA axis suppression is documented, an attempt should be made to gradually withdraw the drug, to reduce the frequency of application, or to substitute a less potent corticosteroid. Recovery of HPA axis function is generally prompt upon discontinuation of topical corticosteroids. Infrequently, signs and symptoms of glucocorticosteroid insufficiency may occur, requiring supplemental systemic corticosteroids.

Pediatric patients may be more susceptible to systemic toxicity from equivalent doses due to their larger skin surface to body mass ratios *[see Use in Specific Populations (8.4)]*.

5.2 Allergic Contact Dermatitis

If irritation develops, ELOCON Lotion should be discontinued and appropriate therapy instituted. Allergic contact dermatitis with corticosteroids is usually diagnosed by observing failure to heal rather than noting a clinical exacerbation. Such an observation should be corroborated with appropriate diagnostic patch testing.

5.3 Concomitant Skin Infections

If concomitant skin infections are present or develop, an appropriate antifungal or antibacterial agent should be used. If a favorable response does not occur promptly, use of ELOCON Lotion should be discontinued until the infection has been adequately controlled.

6 ADVERSE REACTIONS

Because clinical trials are conducted under widely varying conditions, adverse reaction rates observed in the clinical trials of a drug cannot be directly compared to rates in the clinical trials of another drug and may not reflect the rates observed in clinical practice.

In clinical trials involving 209 subjects, the incidence of adverse reactions associated with the use of ELOCON Lotion was 3%. Reported reactions included acneiform reaction, 2; burning, 4; and itching, 1. In an irritation/sensitization study involving 156 normal subjects, the incidence of folliculitis was 3% (4 subjects).

The following adverse reactions were reported to be possibly or probably related to treatment with ELOCON Lotion during a clinical trial in 14% of 65 pediatric subjects 6 months to 2 years of age: decreased glucocorticoid levels, 4; paresthesia, 2; dry mouth,1; an unspecified endocrine disorder, 1; pruritus, 1; and an unspecified skin disorder, 1. The following signs of skin atrophy were also observed among 65 subjects treated with ELOCON Lotion in a clinical trial: shininess, 4; telangiectasia, 2; loss of elasticity, 2; and loss of normal skin markings, 3.

The following additional local adverse reactions have been reported with topical corticosteroids, but may occur more frequently with the use of occlusive dressings. These reactions are: irritation, dryness, hypertrichosis, hypopigmentation, perioral dermatitis, allergic contact dermatitis, secondary infection, skin atrophy, striae, and miliaria.

7 DRUG INTERACTIONS

No drug-drug interaction studies have been conducted with ELOCON Lotion.

8 USE IN SPECIFIC POPULATIONS

8.1 Pregnancy

Teratogenic Effects Pregnancy Category C:

There are no adequate and well-controlled studies in pregnant women. Therefore, ELOCON Lotion should be used during pregnancy only if the potential benefit justifies the potential risk to the fetus.

Corticosteroids have been shown to be teratogenic in laboratory animals when administered systemically at relatively low dosage levels. Some corticosteroids have been shown to be teratogenic after dermal application in laboratory animals.

When administered to pregnant rats, rabbits, and mice, mometasone furoate increased fetal malformations. The doses that produced malformations also decreased fetal growth, as measured by lower fetal weights and/or delayed ossification. Mometasone furoate also caused dystocia and related complications when administered to rats during the end of pregnancy.

In mice, mometasone furoate caused cleft palate at subcutaneous doses of 60 mcg/kg and above. Fetal survival was reduced at 180 mcg/kg. No toxicity was observed at 20 mcg/kg. (Doses of 20, 60, and 180 mcg/kg in the mouse are approximately 0.01, 0.02, and 0.05 times the estimated maximum clinical topical dose from ELOCON Lotion on a mcg/m^2 basis.)

In rats, mometasone furoate produced umbilical hernias at topical doses of 600 mcg/kg and above. A dose of 300 mcg/kg produced delays in ossification, but no malformations. (Doses of 300 and 600 mcg/kg in the rat are approximately 0.2 and 0.4 times the estimated maximum clinical topical dose from ELOCON Lotion on a mcg/m^2 basis.)

In rabbits, mometasone furoate caused multiple malformations (e.g., flexed front paws, gallbladder agenesis, umbilical hernia, hydrocephaly) at topical doses of 150 mcg/kg and above (approximately 0.2 times the estimated maximum clinical topical dose from ELOCON Lotion on a mcg/m^2 basis). In an oral study, mometasone furoate increased resorptions and caused cleft palate and/or head malformations (hydrocephaly and domed head) at 700 mcg/kg. At 2800 mcg/kg most litters were aborted or resorbed. No toxicity was observed at 140 mcg/kg. (Doses at 140, 700, and 2800 mcg/kg in the rabbit are approximately 0.2, 0.9, and 3.6 times the estimated maximum clinical topical dose from ELOCON Lotion on a mcg/m^2 basis.)

When rats received subcutaneous doses of mometasone furoate throughout pregnancy or during the later stages of pregnancy, 15 mcg/kg caused prolonged and difficult labor and reduced the number of live births, birth weight, and early pup survival. Similar effects were not observed at 7.5 mcg/kg. (Doses of 7.5 and 15 mcg/kg in the rat are approximately 0.005 and 0.01 times the estimated maximum clinical topical dose from ELOCON Lotion on a mcg/m^2 basis.)

8.3 Nursing Mothers

Systemically administered corticosteroids appear in human milk and could suppress growth, interfere with endogenous corticosteroid production, or cause other untoward effects. It is not known whether topical administration of corticosteroids could result in sufficient systemic absorption to produce detectable quantities in human milk. Because many drugs are excreted in human milk, caution should be exercised when ELOCON Lotion is administered to a nursing woman.

8.4 Pediatric Use

Since safety and efficacy of ELOCON Lotion have not been established in pediatric patients below 12 years of age, its use in this age group is not recommended.

ELOCON Lotion caused HPA axis suppression in approximately 29% of pediatric subjects ages 6 to 23 months, who showed normal adrenal function by Cortrosyn test before starting treatment, and were treated for approximately 3 weeks over a mean body surface area of 40% (range 16%-90%). The criteria for suppression were: basal cortisol level of ≤5 mcg/dL, 30-minute post-stimulation level of ≤18 mcg/dL, or an increase of <7 mcg/dL. Follow-up testing 2 to 4 weeks after stopping treatment, available for 8 of the subjects, demonstrated suppressed HPA axis function in 1 subject, using these same criteria. Long-term use of topical corticosteroids has not been studied in this population *[see Clinical Pharmacology (12.2)]*.

Because of a higher ratio of skin surface area to body mass, pediatric patients are at a greater risk than adults of HPA axis suppression and Cushing's syndrome when they are treated with topical corticosteroids. They are, therefore, also at greater risk of adrenal insufficiency during and/or after withdrawal of treatment. Pediatric patients may be more susceptible than adults to skin atrophy, including striae, when they are treated with topical corticosteroids. Pediatric patients applying topical corticosteroids to greater than 20% of body surface are at higher risk of HPA axis suppression.

HPA axis suppression, Cushing's syndrome, linear growth retardation, delayed weight gain, and intracranial hypertension have been reported in pediatric patients receiving topical corticosteroids. Manifestations of adrenal suppression in children include low plasma cortisol levels and absence of response to ACTH stimulation. Manifestations of intracranial hypertension include bulging fontanelles, headaches, and bilateral papilledema.

ELOCON Lotion should not be used in the treatment of diaper dermatitis.

8.5 Geriatric Use

Clinical trials of ELOCON Lotion did not include sufficient numbers of subjects aged 65 and over to determine whether they respond differently from younger subjects. Other reported clinical experience has not identified differences in responses between the elderly and younger patients. In general, dose selection for an elderly patient should be cautious usually starting at the low end of the dosing range.

10 OVERDOSAGE

Topically applied ELOCON Lotion can be absorbed in sufficient amounts to produce systemic effects *[see Warnings and Precautions (5.1)]*.

11 DESCRIPTION

ELOCON (mometasone furoate) Lotion, 0.1% contains mometasone furoate for topical use. Mometasone furoate is a synthetic corticosteroid with anti-inflammatory activity. Chemically, mometasone furoate is 9α, 21-dichloro-11β,17-dihydroxy-16α-methylpregna-1,4-diene-3,20-dione 17-(2-furoate), with the empirical formula $C_{27}H_{30}Cl_2O_6$, a molecular weight of 521.4 and the following structural formula:

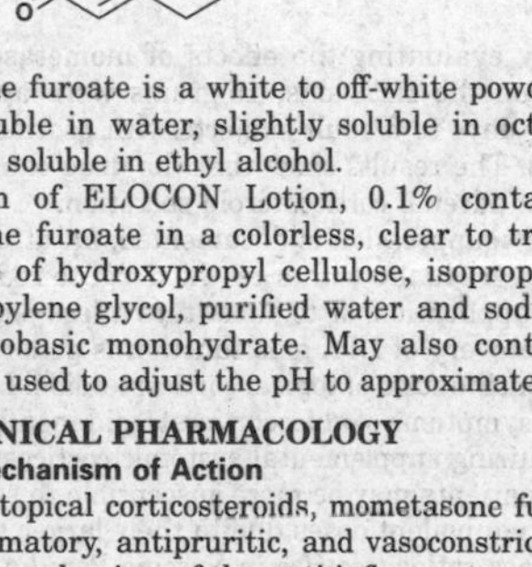

Mometasone furoate is a white to off-white powder practically insoluble in water, slightly soluble in octanol, and moderately soluble in ethyl alcohol.

Each gram of ELOCON Lotion, 0.1% contains 1 mg mometasone furoate in a colorless, clear to translucent lotion base of hydroxypropyl cellulose, isopropyl alcohol (40%), propylene glycol, purified water and sodium phosphate monobasic monohydrate. May also contain phosphoric acid used to adjust the pH to approximately 4.5.

12 CLINICAL PHARMACOLOGY

12.1 Mechanism of Action

Like other topical corticosteroids, mometasone furoate has anti-inflammatory, antipruritic, and vasoconstrictive properties. The mechanism of the anti-inflammatory activity of the topical steroids, in general, is unclear. However, corticosteroids are thought to act by the induction of phospholipase A_2 inhibitory proteins, collectively called lipocortins. It is postulated that these proteins control the biosynthesis of potent mediators of inflammation such as prostaglandins and leukotrienes by inhibiting the release of their common precursor arachidonic acid. Arachidonic acid is released from membrane phospholipids by phospholipase A_2.

12.2 Pharmacodynamics

Studies performed with ELOCON Lotion indicate that it is in the medium range of potency as compared with other topical corticosteroids.

In a study evaluating the effects of mometasone furoate lotion on the HPA axis, 15 mL were applied without occlusion twice daily (30 mL per day) for 7 days to 4 adult subjects with scalp and body psoriasis. At the end of treatment, the plasma cortisol levels for each of the 4 subjects remained within the normal range and changed little from baseline *[see Warnings and Precautions (5.1)]*.

Sixty-five pediatric subjects ages 6 to 23 months, with atopic dermatitis, were enrolled in an open-label, HPA axis safety trial. ELOCON Lotion was applied once daily for approximately 3 weeks over a mean body surface area of 40% (range 16%-90%). In approximately 29% of subjects who showed normal adrenal function by Cortrosyn test before starting treatment, adrenal suppression was observed at the end of treatment with ELOCON Lotion. The criteria for suppression were: basal cortisol level of ≤5 mcg/dL, 30-minute post-stimulation level of ≤18 mcg/dL, or an increase of <7 mcg/dL. Follow-up testing 2 to 4 weeks after stopping treatment, available for 8 of the subjects, demonstrated suppressed HPA axis function in 1 subject, using these same criteria *[see Use in Specific Populations (8.4)]*.

12.3 Pharmacokinetics

The extent of percutaneous absorption of topical corticosteroids is determined by many factors including the vehicle and the integrity of the epidermal barrier. Studies in humans indicate that approximately 0.7% of the applied dose of ELOCON Lotion enters the circulation after 8 hours of contact on normal skin without occlusion. A similar minimal degree of absorption of the corticosteroid from the lotion formulation would be anticipated. Inflammation and/or other disease processes in the skin may increase percutaneous absorption.

13 NONCLINICAL TOXICOLOGY

13.1 Carcinogenesis, Mutagenesis, Impairment of Fertility

Long-term animal studies have not been performed to evaluate the carcinogenic potential of ELOCON Lotion. Long-term carcinogenicity studies of mometasone furoate were conducted by the inhalation route in rats and mice. In a 2-year carcinogenicity study in Sprague Dawley rats, mometasone furoate demonstrated no statistically significant increase of tumors at inhalation doses up to 67 mcg/kg (approximately 0.04 times the estimated maximum clinical topical dose from ELOCON Lotion on a mcg/m^2 basis). In a 19-month carcinogenicity study in Swiss CD-1 mice, mometasone furoate demonstrated no statistically significant increase in the incidence of tumors at inhalation doses up to 160 mcg/kg (approximately 0.05 times the estimated maximum clinical topical dose from ELOCON Lotion on a mcg/m^2 basis).

Mometasone furoate increased chromosomal aberrations in an *in vitro* Chinese hamster ovary cell assay, but did not increase chromosomal aberrations in an *in vitro* Chinese hamster lung cell assay. Mometasone furoate was not mutagenic in the Ames test or mouse lymphoma assay, and was not clastogenic in an *in vivo* mouse micronucleus assay, a rat bone marrow chromosomal aberration assay, or a mouse male germ-cell chromosomal aberration assay. Mometasone furoate also did not induce unscheduled DNA synthesis *in vivo* in rat hepatocytes.

In reproductive studies in rats, impairment of fertility was not produced in male or female rats by subcutaneous doses up to 15 mcg/kg (approximately 0.01 times the estimated maximum clinical topical dose from ELOCON Lotion on a mcg/m^2 basis).

14 CLINICAL STUDIES

The safety and efficacy of ELOCON Lotion, 0.1% for the treatment of corticosteroid-responsive dermatoses was demonstrated in two vehicle-controlled trials, one in scalp psoriasis and one in seborrheic dermatitis. A total of 405 subjects (age range: 12-95 years) received ELOCON Lotion (205 subjects) or the vehicle lotion applied once daily for 21 days.

16 HOW SUPPLIED/STORAGE AND HANDLING

ELOCON Lotion is colorless, clear to translucent and supplied in 30-mL (27.5 gram) (NDC 0085-0854-01) and 60-mL (55 gram) (NDC 0085-0854-02) bottles; boxes of one.

Store ELOCON Lotion, 0.1% at 25°C (77°F); excursions permitted to 15-30°C (59-86°F) [see USP Controlled Room Temperature].

17 PATIENT COUNSELING INFORMATION

Inform patients of the following:

- Use ELOCON Lotion as directed by the physician. It is for external use only.
- Avoid contact with the eyes.
- Do not use ELOCON Lotion on the face, underarms, or groin areas.
- Do not use ELOCON Lotion for any disorder other than that for which it was prescribed.
- The treated skin area should not be bandaged or otherwise covered or wrapped so as to be occlusive, unless directed by the physician.
- Report any signs of local adverse reactions to the physician.
- Advise patients not to use ELOCON Lotion in the treatment of diaper dermatitis. Do not apply ELOCON Lotion in the diaper area, as diapers or plastic pants may constitute occlusive dressing.

- Discontinue therapy when control is achieved. If no improvement is seen within 2 weeks, contact the physician.
- Do not use other corticosteroid-containing products with ELOCON Lotion without first consulting with the physician.

Manufactured for: Merck Sharp & Dohme Corp., a subsidiary of
MERCK & CO., INC., Whitehouse Station, NJ 08889, USA
Manufactured by: Schering Plough Canada, Inc.
Pointe Claire, Quebec, Canada.

032088-EL-LT-USPI.6

ELOCON® ℞

[*el'ō-cŏn*]
(mometasone furoate)
Ointment, 0.1% for topical use

HIGHLIGHTS OF PRESCRIBING INFORMATION
These highlights do not include all the information needed to use ELOCON Ointment safely and effectively. See full prescribing information for ELOCON Ointment.
ELOCON® (mometasone furoate) Ointment, 0.1% for topical use
Initial U.S. Approval: 1987

INDICATIONS AND USAGE

ELOCON Ointment is a corticosteroid indicated for the relief of the inflammatory and pruritic manifestations of corticosteroid-responsive dermatoses in patients ≥2 years of age (1)

DOSAGE AND ADMINISTRATION

- Apply a thin film to the affected skin areas once daily. (2)
- Discontinue therapy when control is achieved. (2)
- If no improvement is seen within 2 weeks, reassess diagnosis. (2)
- The safety and efficacy of ELOCON Ointment in pediatric patients for more than 3 weeks of use have not been established. (2)
- Do not use with occlusive dressings unless directed by a physician. (2)

DOSAGE FORMS AND STRENGTHS

- Ointment, 0.1%. (3)

CONTRAINDICATIONS

- None. (4)

WARNINGS AND PRECAUTIONS

- Reversible HPA axis suppression with the potential for glucocorticosteroid insufficiency after withdrawal of treatment, Cushing's syndrome, and hyperglycemia may occur due to systemic absorption. Patients applying a topical steroid to a large surface area or to areas under occlusion should be evaluated periodically for evidence of HPA axis suppression. Modify use should HPA axis suppression develop. Pediatric patients may be more susceptible to systemic toxicity. (5.1, 8.4)

ADVERSE REACTIONS

Most common adverse reactions are burning, pruritus, skin atrophy, tingling/stinging and furunculosis. (6)
To report SUSPECTED ADVERSE REACTIONS, contact Merck Sharp & Dohme Corp., a subsidiary of Merck & Co., Inc., at 1-877-888-4231 or FDA at 1-800-FDA-1088 or www.fda.gov/medwatch.

See 17 for PATIENT COUNSELING INFORMATION
Revised: 03/2013

FULL PRESCRIBING INFORMATION: CONTENTS*

*** Sections or subsections omitted from the full prescribing information are not listed**

FULL PRESCRIBING INFORMATION

1 INDICATIONS AND USAGE

ELOCON® Ointment is a corticosteroid indicated for the relief of the inflammatory and pruritic manifestations of corticosteroid-responsive dermatoses in patients 2 years of age or older.

2 DOSAGE AND ADMINISTRATION

Apply a thin film of ELOCON Ointment to the affected skin areas once daily.
Therapy should be discontinued when control is achieved. If no improvement is seen within 2 weeks, reassessment of diagnosis may be necessary.
Safety and efficacy of ELOCON Ointment in pediatric patients for more than 3 weeks of use have not been established *[see Warnings and Precautions (5.1) and Use in Specific Populations (8.4)]*.
ELOCON Ointment should not be used with occlusive dressings unless directed by a physician. ELOCON Ointment should not be applied in the diaper area if the child still requires diapers or plastic pants, as these garments may constitute occlusive dressing.
ELOCON Ointment is for topical use only. It is not for oral, ophthalmic, or intravaginal use.
Avoid use on the face, groin, or axillae.

3 DOSAGE FORMS AND STRENGTHS

Ointment, 0.1%. Each gram of ELOCON Ointment contains 1 mg of mometasone furoate in a white to off-white uniform ointment base.

4 CONTRAINDICATIONS

None.

5 WARNINGS AND PRECAUTIONS

5.1 Effects on Endocrine System

Systemic absorption of topical corticosteroids can produce reversible hypothalamic-pituitary-adrenal (HPA) axis suppression with the potential for glucocorticosteroid insufficiency. This may occur during treatment or after withdrawal of treatment. Manifestations of Cushing's syndrome, hyperglycemia, and glucosuria can also be produced in some patients by systemic absorption of topical corticosteroids while on treatment. Factors that predispose a patient using a topical corticosteroid to HPA axis suppression include the use of high-potency steroids, large treatment surface areas, prolonged use, use of occlusive dressings, altered skin barrier, liver failure, and young age.
Because of the potential for systemic absorption, use of topical corticosteroids may require that patients be periodically evaluated for HPA axis suppression. This may be done by using the adrenocorticotropic hormone (ACTH) stimulation test.
In a study evaluating the effects of mometasone furoate ointment on the HPA axis, 15 grams were applied twice daily for 7 days to 6 adult subjects with psoriasis or atopic dermatitis. The results show that the drug caused a slight lowering of adrenal corticosteroid secretion.
If HPA axis suppression is documented, an attempt should be made to gradually withdraw the drug, to reduce the frequency of application, or to substitute a less potent corticosteroid. Recovery of HPA axis function is generally prompt upon discontinuation of topical corticosteroids. Infrequently, signs and symptoms of glucocorticosteroid insufficiency may occur, requiring supplemental systemic corticosteroids.
Pediatric patients may be more susceptible to systemic toxicity from equivalent doses due to their larger skin surface to body mass ratios *[see Use in Specific Populations (8.4)]*.

5.2 Allergic Contact Dermatitis

If irritation develops, ELOCON Ointment should be discontinued and appropriate therapy instituted. Allergic contact dermatitis with corticosteroids is usually diagnosed by observing failure to heal rather than noting a clinical exacerbation. Such an observation should be corroborated with appropriate diagnostic patch testing.

5.3 Concomitant Skin Infections

If concomitant skin infections are present or develop, an appropriate antifungal or antibacterial agent should be used. If a favorable response does not occur promptly, use of ELOCON Ointment should be discontinued until the infection has been adequately controlled.

6 ADVERSE REACTIONS

Because clinical trials are conducted under widely varying conditions, adverse reaction rates observed in the clinical trials of a drug cannot be directly compared to rates in the clinical trials of another drug and may not reflect the rates observed in clinical practice.
In controlled clinical trials involving 812 subjects, the incidence of adverse reactions associated with the use of ELOCON Ointment was 4.8%. Reported reactions included burning, pruritus, skin atrophy, tingling/stinging, and furunculosis. Cases of rosacea associated with the use of ELOCON Ointment have been reported.
The following adverse reactions were reported to be possibly or probably related to treatment with ELOCON Ointment during a clinical study in 5% of 63 pediatric subjects 6 months to 2 years of age: decreased glucocorticoid levels, 1; an unspecified skin disorder, 1; and a bacterial skin infection, 1. The following signs of skin atrophy were also observed among 63 subjects treated with ELOCON Ointment in a clinical trial: shininess, 4; telangiectasia, 1; loss of elasticity, 4; loss of normal skin markings, 4; and thinness, 1.
The following additional local adverse reactions have been reported with topical corticosteroids, but may occur more frequently with the use of occlusive dressings. These reactions are: irritation, dryness, folliculitis, hypertrichosis, acneiform eruptions, hypopigmentation, perioral dermatitis, allergic contact dermatitis, secondary infection, skin atrophy, striae, and miliaria.

7 DRUG INTERACTIONS

No drug-drug interaction studies have been conducted with ELOCON Ointment.

8 USE IN SPECIFIC POPULATIONS

8.1 Pregnancy

Teratogenic Effects Pregnancy Category C:
There are no adequate and well-controlled studies in pregnant women. Therefore, ELOCON Ointment should be used during pregnancy only if the potential benefit justifies the potential risk to the fetus.
Corticosteroids have been shown to be teratogenic in laboratory animals when administered systemically at relatively low dosage levels. Some corticosteroids have been shown to be teratogenic after dermal application in laboratory animals.
When administered to pregnant rats, rabbits, and mice, mometasone furoate increased fetal malformations. The doses that produced malformations also decreased fetal growth, as measured by lower fetal weights and/or delayed ossification. Mometasone furoate also caused dystocia and related complications when administered to rats during the end of pregnancy.
In mice, mometasone furoate caused cleft palate at subcutaneous doses of 60 mcg/kg and above. Fetal survival was reduced at 180 mcg/kg. No toxicity was observed at 20 mcg/kg. (Doses of 20, 60, and 180 mcg/kg in the mouse are approximately 0.01, 0.02, and 0.05 times the estimated maximum clinical topical dose from ELOCON Ointment on a mcg/m^2 basis.)
In rats, mometasone furoate produced umbilical hernias at topical doses of 600 mcg/kg and above. A dose of 300 mcg/kg produced delays in ossification, but no malformations. (Doses of 300 and 600 mcg/kg in the rat are approximately 0.2 and 0.4 times the estimated maximum clinical topical dose from ELOCON Ointment on a mcg/m^2 basis.)
In rabbits, mometasone furoate caused multiple malformations (e.g., flexed front paws, gallbladder agenesis, umbilical hernia, hydrocephaly) at topical doses of 150 mcg/kg and above (approximately 0.2 times the estimated maximum clinical topical dose from ELOCON Ointment on a mcg/m^2 basis). In an oral study, mometasone furoate increased resorptions and caused cleft palate and/or head malformations (hydrocephaly and domed head) at 700 mcg/kg. At 2800 mcg/kg most litters were aborted or resorbed. No toxicity was observed at 140 mcg/kg. (Doses of 140, 700, and 2800 mcg/kg in the rabbit are approximately 0.2, 0.9, and 3.6 times the estimated maximum clinical topical dose from ELOCON Ointment on a mcg/m^2 basis.)
When rats received subcutaneous doses of mometasone furoate throughout pregnancy or during the later stages of pregnancy, 15 mcg/kg caused prolonged and difficult labor and reduced the number of live births, birth weight, and early pup survival. Similar effects were not observed at 7.5 mcg/kg. (Doses of 7.5 and 15 mcg/kg in the rat are approximately 0.005 and 0.01 times the estimated maximum clinical topical dose from ELOCON Ointment on a mcg/m^2 basis.)

8.3 Nursing Mothers

Systemically administered corticosteroids appear in human milk and could suppress growth, interfere with endogenous corticosteroid production, or cause other untoward effects. It is not known whether topical administration of corticosteroids could result in sufficient systemic absorption to produce detectable quantities in human milk. Because many drugs are excreted in human milk, caution should be exercised when ELOCON Ointment is administered to a nursing woman.

8.4 Pediatric Use

ELOCON Ointment may be used with caution in pediatric patients 2 years of age or older, although the safety and efficacy of drug use for longer than 3 weeks have not been established. Since safety and efficacy of ELOCON Ointment have not been established in pediatric patients below 2 years of age, its use in this age group is not recommended.

ELOCON Ointment caused HPA axis suppression in approximately 27% of pediatric subjects ages 6 to 23 months, who showed normal adrenal function by Cortrosyn test before starting treatment, and were treated for approximately 3 weeks over a mean body surface area of 39% (range 15%-99%). The criteria for suppression were: basal cortisol level of ≤5 mcg/dL, 30-minute post-stimulation level of ≤18 mcg/dL, or an increase of <7 mcg/dL. Follow-up testing 2 to 4 weeks after stopping treatment, available for 8 of the subjects, demonstrated suppressed HPA axis function in 3 subjects, using these same criteria. Long-term use of topical corticosteroids has not been studied in this population *[see Clinical Pharmacology (12.2)]*.

Because of a higher ratio of skin surface area to body mass, pediatric patients are at a greater risk than adults of HPA axis suppression and Cushing's syndrome when they are treated with topical corticosteroids. They are, therefore, also at greater risk of glucocorticosteroid insufficiency during and/or after withdrawal of treatment. Pediatric patients may be more susceptible than adults to skin atrophy, including striae, when they are treated with topical corticosteroids. Pediatric patients applying topical corticosteroids to greater than 20% of body surface are at higher risk of HPA axis suppression.

HPA axis suppression, Cushing's syndrome, linear growth retardation, delayed weight gain, and intracranial hypertension have been reported in children receiving topical corticosteroids. Manifestations of adrenal suppression in children include low plasma cortisol levels and absence of response to ACTH stimulation. Manifestations of intracranial hypertension include bulging fontanelles, headaches, and bilateral papilledema.

ELOCON Ointment should not be used in the treatment of diaper dermatitis.

8.5 Geriatric Use

Clinical trials of ELOCON Ointment included 310 subjects who were 65 years of age and over and 57 subjects who were 75 years of age and over. No overall differences in safety or effectiveness were observed between these subjects and younger subjects, and other reported clinical experience has not identified differences in responses between the elderly and younger subjects. However, greater sensitivity of some older individuals cannot be ruled out.

10 OVERDOSAGE

Topically applied ELOCON Ointment can be absorbed in sufficient amounts to produce systemic effects *[see Warnings and Precautions (5.1)]*.

11 DESCRIPTION

ELOCON (mometasone furoate) Ointment, 0.1% contains mometasone furoate for topical use. Mometasone furoate is a synthetic corticosteroid with anti-inflammatory activity.

Chemically, mometasone furoate is 9α,21-dichloro-11β,17-dihydroxy-16α-methylpregna-1,4-diene-3,20-dione 17-(2-furoate), with the empirical formula $C_{27}H_{30}Cl_2O_6$, a molecular weight of 521.4 and the following structural formula:

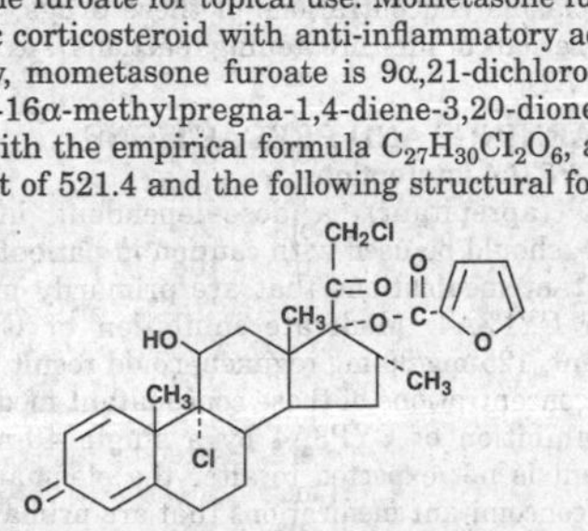

Mometasone furoate is a white to off-white powder practically insoluble in water, slightly soluble in octanol, and moderately soluble in ethyl alcohol.

Each gram of ELOCON Ointment, 0.1% contains 1 mg mometasone furoate in a white to off-white uniform ointment base of hexylene glycol, phosphoric acid, propylene glycol stearate (55% monoester), purified water, white wax, and white petrolatum.

12 CLINICAL PHARMACOLOGY

12.1 Mechanism of Action

Like other topical corticosteroids, mometasone furoate has anti-inflammatory, antipruritic, and vasoconstrictive properties. The mechanism of the anti-inflammatory activity of the topical steroids, in general, is unclear. However, corticosteroids are thought to act by the induction of phospholipase A_2 inhibitory proteins, collectively called lipocortins. It is postulated that these proteins control the biosynthesis of potent mediators of inflammation such as prostaglandins and leukotrienes by inhibiting the release of their common precursor arachidonic acid. Arachidonic acid is released from membrane phospholipids by phospholipase A_2.

12.2 Pharmacodynamics

Studies performed with ELOCON Ointment indicate that it is in the medium range of potency as compared with other topical corticosteroids.

In a study evaluating the effects of mometasone furoate ointment on the HPA axis, 15 grams were applied twice daily for 7 days to 6 adult subjects with psoriasis or atopic dermatitis. The ointment was applied without occlusion to at least 30% of the body surface. The results showed that the drug caused a slight lowering of adrenal corticosteroid secretion *[see Warnings and Precautions (5.1)]*.

Sixty-three pediatric subjects ages 6 to 23 months, with atopic dermatitis, were enrolled in an open-label HPA axis safety study. ELOCON Ointment was applied once daily for approximately 3 weeks over a mean body surface area of 39% (range 15%-99%). In approximately 27% of subjects who showed normal adrenal function by Cortrosyn test before starting treatment, adrenal suppression was observed at the end of treatment with ELOCON Ointment. The criteria for suppression were: basal cortisol level of ≤5 mcg/dL, 30-minute post-stimulation level of ≤18 mcg/dL, or an increase of <7 mcg/dL. Follow-up testing 2 to 4 weeks after stopping treatment, available for 8 of the subjects, demonstrated suppressed HPA axis function in 3 subjects, using these same criteria *[see Use in Specific Populations (8.4)]*.

12.3 Pharmacokinetics

The extent of percutaneous absorption of topical corticosteroids is determined by many factors including the vehicle and the integrity of the epidermal barrier. Studies in humans indicate that approximately 0.7% of the applied dose of ELOCON Ointment enters the circulation after 8 hours of contact on normal skin without occlusion. Inflammation and/or other disease processes in the skin may increase percutaneous absorption.

13 NONCLINICAL TOXICOLOGY

13.1 Carcinogenesis, Mutagenesis, Impairment of Fertility

Long-term animal studies have not been performed to evaluate the carcinogenic potential of ELOCON Ointment. Long-term carcinogenicity studies of mometasone furoate were conducted by the inhalation route in rats and mice. In a 2-year carcinogenicity study in Sprague Dawley rats, mometasone furoate demonstrated no statistically significant increase of tumors at inhalation doses up to 67 mcg/kg (approximately 0.04 times the estimated maximum clinical topical dose from ELOCON Ointment on a mcg/m^2 basis). In a 19-month carcinogenicity study in Swiss CD-1 mice, mometasone furoate demonstrated no statistically significant increase in the incidence of tumors at inhalation doses up to 160 mcg/kg (approximately 0.05 times the estimated maximum clinical topical dose from ELOCON Ointment on a mcg/m^2 basis).

Mometasone furoate increased chromosomal aberrations in an *in vitro* Chinese hamster ovary cell assay, but did not increase chromosomal aberrations in an *in vitro* Chinese hamster lung cell assay. Mometasone furoate was not mutagenic in the Ames test or mouse lymphoma assay, and was not clastogenic in an *in vivo* mouse micronucleus assay, a rat bone marrow chromosomal aberration assay, or a mouse male germ-cell chromosomal aberration assay. Mometasone furoate also did not induce unscheduled DNA synthesis *in vivo* in rat hepatocytes.

In reproductive studies in rats, impairment of fertility was not produced in male or female rats by subcutaneous doses up to 15 mcg/kg (approximately 0.01 times the estimated maximum clinical topical dose from ELOCON Ointment on a mcg/m^2 basis).

14 CLINICAL STUDIES

The safety and efficacy of ELOCON Ointment, 0.1% for the treatment of corticosteroid-responsive dermatoses were demonstrated in two vehicle-controlled trials, one in psoriasis and one in atopic dermatitis. A total of 218 subjects received ELOCON Ointment (109 subjects) or the vehicle ointment applied once daily for 21 days.

16 HOW SUPPLIED/STORAGE AND HANDLING

ELOCON Ointment is a white to off-white uniform ointment and supplied in 15-gram (NDC 0085-0370-01) and 45-gram (NDC 0085-0370-02) tubes; boxes of one.

Store at 25°C (77°F); excursions permitted to 15-30°C (59-86°F) [see USP Controlled Room Temperature].

17 PATIENT COUNSELING INFORMATION

Inform patients of the following:

- Use ELOCON Ointment as directed by the physician. It is for external use only.
- Avoid contact with the eyes.
- Do not use ELOCON Ointment on the face, underarms, or groin areas.
- Do not use ELOCON Ointment for any disorder other than that for which it was prescribed.
- The treated skin area should not be bandaged or otherwise covered or wrapped so as to be occlusive, unless directed by the physician.
- Report any signs of local adverse reactions to the physician.
- Advise patients not to use ELOCON Ointment in the treatment of diaper dermatitis. Do not apply ELOCON Ointment in the diaper area, as diapers or plastic pants may constitute occlusive dressing.
- Discontinue therapy when control is achieved. If no improvement is seen within 2 weeks, contact the physician.
- Do not use other corticosteroid-containing products with ELOCON Ointment without first consulting with the physician.

Manufactured for: Merck Sharp & Dohme Corp., a subsidiary of
MERCK & CO., INC., Whitehouse Station, NJ 08889, USA
Manufactured by: Schering Plough Canada, Inc.
Pointe Claire, Quebec H9R 1B4, Canada

032088-EL-OT-USPI.6

EMEND® ℞
[ē' mĕnd]
(aprepitant)
capsules, for oral use

HIGHLIGHTS OF PRESCRIBING INFORMATION

These highlights do not include all the information needed to use EMEND safely and effectively. See full prescribing information for EMEND.

EMEND (aprepitant) capsules, for oral use
Initial U.S. Approval: 2003

INDICATIONS AND USAGE

EMEND® is a substance P/neurokinin 1 (NK_1) receptor antagonist, indicated:

- in combination with other antiemetic agents for the:
  - prevention of acute and delayed nausea and vomiting associated with initial and repeat courses of highly emetogenic cancer chemotherapy (HEC) including high-dose cisplatin (1.1)
  - prevention of nausea and vomiting associated with initial and repeat courses of moderately emetogenic cancer chemotherapy (MEC) (1.1)
- for the prevention of postoperative nausea and vomiting (PONV) (1.2)

Limitations of Use (1.3)

- Not studied for the treatment of established nausea and vomiting.
- Chronic continuous administration is not recommended.

DOSAGE AND ADMINISTRATION

Prevention of Chemotherapy Induced Nausea and Vomiting (2.1)

- EMEND is given for 3 days as part of the chemotherapy induced nausea and vomiting (CINV) regimen that includes a corticosteroid and a 5-HT_3 antagonist. (2.1)
  - The recommended dose of EMEND is 125 mg orally 1 hour prior to chemotherapy treatment (Day 1) and 80 mg orally once daily in the morning on Days 2 and 3. (2.1)
  - EMEND (fosaprepitant dimeglumine) for Injection may be substituted for oral EMEND (125 mg) on Day 1 only as part of the CINV regimen. (2.1)

Prevention of Postoperative Nausea and Vomiting (2.2)

- The recommended oral dosage of EMEND for the postoperative nausea and vomiting (PONV) indication is 40 mg within 3 hours prior to induction of anesthesia. (2.2)

DOSAGE FORMS AND STRENGTHS

Capsules: 40 mg; 80 mg; 125 mg (3)

CONTRAINDICATIONS

- Hypersensitivity to any component of this medication. (4, 6.2)
- EMEND should not be used concurrently with pimozide, terfenadine, astemizole, or cisapride, since inhibition of CYP3A4 by aprepitant could result in elevated plasma concentrations of these drugs, potentially causing serious or life-threatening reactions. (4)

WARNINGS AND PRECAUTIONS

- Coadministration of aprepitant with warfarin (a CYP2C9 substrate) may result in a clinically significant decrease in International Normalized Ratio (INR) of prothrombin time. (5.2)
- The efficacy of hormonal contraceptives during and for 28 days following the last dose of EMEND may be reduced. Alternative or back-up methods of contraception should be used. (5.3, 7.1)
- EMEND is a dose-dependent inhibitor of CYP3A4, and should be used with caution in patients receiving concomitant medications that are primarily metabolized through CYP3A4. (5.1)
- Caution should be exercised when administered in patients with severe hepatic impairment. (2.5, 5.4, 12.3)

ADVERSE REACTIONS

- Clinical adverse experiences for the CINV regimen in conjunction with highly and moderately emetogenic

	Day 1	Day 2	Day 3	Day 4
EMEND*	125 mg orally	80 mg orally	80 mg orally	none
Dexamethasone†	12 mg orally	8 mg orally	8 mg orally	8 mg orally
5-HT_3 antagonist	See the package insert for the selected 5-HT_3 antagonist for appropriate dosing information.	none	none	none

* EMEND is administered orally 1 hour prior to chemotherapy treatment on Day 1 and in the morning on Days 2 and 3.

† Dexamethasone is administered 30 minutes prior to chemotherapy treatment on Day 1 and in the morning on Days 2 through 4. The dose of dexamethasone accounts for drug interactions.

	Day 1	Day 2	Day 3
EMEND*	125 mg orally	80 mg orally	80 mg orally
Dexamethasone†	12 mg orally	none	none
5-HT_3 antagonist	See the package insert for the selected 5-HT_3 antagonist for appropriate dosing information.	none	none

* EMEND is administered orally 1 hour prior to chemotherapy treatment on Day 1 and in the morning on Days 2 and 3.

† Dexamethasone is administered 30 minutes prior to chemotherapy treatment on Day 1. The dose of dexamethasone accounts for drug interactions.

chemotherapy (incidence >10%) are: alopecia, anorexia, asthenia/fatigue, constipation, diarrhea, headache, hiccups, nausea. (6.1)
- Clinical adverse experiences for the PONV regimen (incidence >5%) are: constipation, hypotension, nausea, pruritus, pyrexia. (6.1)

To report SUSPECTED ADVERSE REACTIONS, contact Merck Sharp & Dohme Corp., a subsidiary of Merck & Co., Inc., at 1-877-888-4231 or FDA at 1-800-FDA-1088 or www.fda.gov/medwatch.

DRUG INTERACTIONS

- Aprepitant is a substrate for CYP3A4; therefore, coadministration of EMEND with drugs that inhibit or induce CYP3A4 activity may result in increased or reduced plasma concentrations of aprepitant, respectively. (5.1, 7.1, 7.2).
- Aprepitant is an inducer of CYP2C9; therefore, coadministration of EMEND with drugs that are metabolized by CYP2C9 (e.g., warfarin, tolbutamide), may result in lower plasma concentrations of these drugs. (5.2, 7.1)

See 17 for PATIENT COUNSELING INFORMATION and FDA-approved patient labeling.

Revised: 12/2012

FULL PRESCRIBING INFORMATION: CONTENTS*

*** Sections or subsections omitted from the full prescribing information are not listed**

FULL PRESCRIBING INFORMATION

1 INDICATIONS AND USAGE

1.1 Prevention of Chemotherapy Induced Nausea and Vomiting (CINV)

EMEND®, in combination with other antiemetic agents, is indicated for the:
- prevention of acute and delayed nausea and vomiting associated with initial and repeat courses of highly emetogenic cancer chemotherapy (HEC) including high-dose cisplatin
- prevention of nausea and vomiting associated with initial and repeat courses of moderately emetogenic cancer chemotherapy (MEC) *[see Dosage and Administration (2.1)]*.

1.2 Prevention of Postoperative Nausea and Vomiting (PONV)

EMEND is indicated for the prevention of postoperative nausea and vomiting *[see Dosage and Administration (2.2)]*.

1.3 Limitations of Use

EMEND has not been studied for the treatment of established nausea and vomiting.

Chronic continuous administration is not recommended *[see Warnings and Precautions (5.5)]*.

2 DOSAGE AND ADMINISTRATION

2.1 Prevention of Chemotherapy Induced Nausea and Vomiting (CINV)

Capsules of EMEND (aprepitant) are given for 3 days as part of a regimen that includes a corticosteroid and a 5-HT_3 antagonist. The recommended dose of EMEND is 125 mg orally 1 hour prior to chemotherapy treatment (Day 1) and 80 mg orally once daily in the morning on Days 2 and 3.

The package insert for the co-administered 5-HT_3 antagonist must be consulted prior to initiation of treatment with EMEND.

EMEND may be taken with or without food.

EMEND (fosaprepitant dimeglumine) for Injection (115 mg) is a prodrug of aprepitant and may be substituted for oral EMEND (125 mg), 30 minutes prior to chemotherapy, on Day 1 only of the CINV regimen as an intravenous infusion administered over 15 minutes.

The following regimen should be used for the prevention of nausea and vomiting associated with highly emetogenic cancer chemotherapy:

[See first table above]

The following regimen should be used for the prevention of nausea and vomiting associated with moderately emetogenic cancer chemotherapy:

[See second table above]

2.2 Prevention of Postoperative Nausea and Vomiting (PONV)

The recommended oral dosage of EMEND is 40 mg within 3 hours prior to induction of anesthesia.

EMEND may be taken with or without food.

2.3 Geriatric Patients

No dosage adjustment is necessary for the elderly.

2.4 Patients with Renal Impairment

No dosage adjustment is necessary for patients with renal impairment or for patients with end stage renal disease (ESRD) undergoing hemodialysis.

2.5 Patients with Hepatic Impairment

No dosage adjustment is necessary for patients with mild to moderate hepatic impairment (Child-Pugh score 5 to 9). There are no clinical data in patients with severe hepatic impairment (Child-Pugh score >9).

2.6 Coadministration with Other Drugs

For additional information on dose adjustment for corticosteroids when coadministered with EMEND, see *Drug Interactions (7.1)*.

Refer to the full prescribing information for coadministered antiemetic agents.

3 DOSAGE FORMS AND STRENGTHS

- Capsules EMEND 40 mg are opaque, hard, gelatin capsules, with white body and mustard yellow cap with "464" and "40 mg" printed radially in black ink on the body.
- Capsules EMEND 80 mg are white, opaque, hard, gelatin capsules, with "461" and "80 mg" printed radially in black ink on the body.
- Capsules EMEND 125 mg are opaque, hard, gelatin capsules, with white body and pink cap with "462" and "125 mg" printed radially in black ink on the body.

4 CONTRAINDICATIONS

EMEND is contraindicated in patients who are hypersensitive to any component of the product.

EMEND is a dose-dependent inhibitor of cytochrome P450 isoenzyme 3A4 (CYP3A4). EMEND should not be used concurrently with pimozide, terfenadine, astemizole, or cisapride. Inhibition of CYP3A4 by aprepitant could result in elevated plasma concentrations of these drugs, potentially causing serious or life-threatening reactions *[see Drug Interactions (7.1)]*.

5 WARNINGS AND PRECAUTIONS

5.1 CYP3A4 Interactions

EMEND (aprepitant), a dose-dependent inhibitor of CYP3A4, should be used with caution in patients receiving concomitant medications that are primarily metabolized through CYP3A4. Moderate inhibition of CYP3A4 by aprepitant, 125-mg/80-mg regimen, could result in elevated plasma concentrations of these concomitant medications.

Weak inhibition of CYP3A4 by a single 40-mg dose of aprepitant is not expected to alter the plasma concentrations of concomitant medications that are primarily metabolized through CYP3A4 to a clinically significant degree.

When aprepitant is used concomitantly with another CYP3A4 inhibitor, aprepitant plasma concentrations could be elevated. When EMEND is used concomitantly with medications that induce CYP3A4 activity, aprepitant plasma concentrations could be reduced and this may result in decreased efficacy of EMEND *[see Drug Interactions (7.1)]*.

Chemotherapy agents that are known to be metabolized by CYP3A4 include docetaxel, paclitaxel, etoposide, irinotecan, ifosfamide, imatinib, vinorelbine, vinblastine and vincristine. In clinical studies, EMEND (125-mg/80-mg regimen) was administered commonly with etoposide, vinorelbine, or paclitaxel. The doses of these agents were not adjusted to account for potential drug interactions.

In separate pharmacokinetic studies, no clinically significant change in docetaxel or vinorelbine pharmacokinetics was observed when EMEND (125-mg/80-mg regimen) was co-administered.

Due to the small number of patients in clinical studies who received the CYP3A4 substrates vinblastine, vincristine, or ifosfamide, particular caution and careful monitoring are advised in patients receiving these agents or other chemotherapy agents metabolized primarily by CYP3A4 that were not studied *[see Drug Interactions (7.1)]*.

5.2 Coadministration with Warfarin (a CYP2C9 substrate)

Coadministration of EMEND with warfarin may result in a clinically significant decrease in International Normalized Ratio (INR) of prothrombin time. In patients on chronic warfarin therapy, the INR should be closely monitored in the 2-week period, particularly at 7 to 10 days, following initiation of the 3-day regimen of EMEND with each chemotherapy cycle, or following administration of a single 40-mg dose of EMEND for the prevention of postoperative nausea and vomiting *[see Drug Interactions (7.1)]*.

5.3 Coadministration with Hormonal Contraceptives

Upon coadministration with EMEND, the efficacy of hormonal contraceptives during and for 28 days following the last dose of EMEND may be reduced. Alternative or back-up methods of contraception should be used during treatment with EMEND and for 1 month following the last dose of EMEND *[see Drug Interactions (7.1)]*.

5.4 Patients with Severe Hepatic Impairment

There are no clinical or pharmacokinetic data in patients with severe hepatic impairment (Child-Pugh score >9). Therefore, caution should be exercised when EMEND is administered in these patients *[see Clinical Pharmacology (12.3) and Dosage and Administration (2.5)]*.

5.5 Chronic Continuous Use

Chronic continuous use of EMEND for prevention of nausea and vomiting is not recommended because it has not been studied; and because the drug interaction profile may change during chronic continuous use.

6 ADVERSE REACTIONS

The overall safety of aprepitant was evaluated in approximately 5300 individuals.

Because clinical trials are conducted under widely varying conditions, adverse reaction rates observed in the clinical trials of a drug cannot be directly compared to rates in the clinical trials of another drug and may not reflect the rates observed in clinical practice.

6.1 Clinical Trials Experience

Chemotherapy Induced Nausea and Vomiting

Highly Emetogenic Chemotherapy

In 2 well-controlled clinical trials in patients receiving highly emetogenic cancer chemotherapy, 544 patients were treated with aprepitant during Cycle 1 of chemotherapy and 413 of these patients continued into the Multiple-Cycle extension for up to 6 cycles of chemotherapy. EMEND was given in combination with ondansetron and dexamethasone.

In Cycle 1, clinical adverse experiences were reported in approximately 69% of patients treated with the aprepitant regimen compared with approximately 68% of patients treated with standard therapy. Table 1 shows the percent of patients with clinical adverse experiences reported at an incidence ≥3%.

Table 1: Percent of Patients Receiving Highly Emetogenic Chemotherapy with Clinical Adverse Experiences (Incidence ≥3%) — Cycle 1

	Aprepitant Regimen (N = 544)	Standard Therapy (N = 550)
Body as a Whole/Site Unspecified		
Asthenia/Fatigue	17.8	11.8
Dizziness	6.6	4.4
Dehydration	5.9	5.1
Abdominal Pain	4.6	3.3
Fever	2.9	3.5
Mucous Membrane Disorder	2.6	3.1
Digestive System		
Nausea	12.7	11.8
Constipation	10.3	12.2
Diarrhea	10.3	7.5
Vomiting	7.5	7.6
Heartburn	5.3	4.9
Gastritis	4.2	3.1
Epigastric Discomfort	4.0	3.1
Eyes, Ears, Nose, and Throat		
Tinnitus	3.7	3.8
Hemic and Lymphatic System		
Neutropenia	3.1	2.9
Metabolism and Nutrition		
Anorexia	10.1	9.5
Nervous System		
Headache	8.5	8.7
Insomnia	2.9	3.1
Respiratory System		
Hiccups	10.8	5.6

In addition, isolated cases of serious adverse experiences, regardless of causality, of bradycardia, disorientation, and perforating duodenal ulcer were reported in highly emetogenic CINV clinical studies.

Moderately Emetogenic Chemotherapy

During Cycle 1 of 2 moderately emetogenic chemotherapy studies, 868 patients were treated with the aprepitant regimen and 686 of these patients continued into extensions for up to 4 cycles of chemotherapy. In the combined analysis of Cycle 1 data for these 2 studies, adverse experiences were reported in approximately 69% of patients treated with the aprepitant regimen compared with approximately 72% of patients treated with standard therapy.

In the combined analysis of Cycle 1 data for these 2 studies, the adverse experience profile in both moderately emetogenic chemotherapy studies was generally comparable to the highly emetogenic chemotherapy studies. Table 2 shows the percent of patients with clinical adverse experiences reported at an incidence ≥3%.

Table 2: Percent of Patients Receiving Moderately Emetogenic Chemotherapy with Clinical Adverse Experiences (Incidence ≥3%) — Cycle 1

	Aprepitant Regimen (N = 868)	Standard Therapy (N = 846)
Blood and Lymphatic System Disorders		
Neutropenia	5.8	5.6
Metabolism and Nutrition Disorders		
Anorexia	6.2	7.2
Psychiatric Disorders		
Insomnia	2.6	3.7
Nervous System Disorders		
Headache	13.2	14.3
Dizziness	2.8	3.4
Gastrointestinal Disorders		
Constipation	10.3	15.5
Diarrhea	7.6	8.7
Dyspepsia	5.8	3.8
Nausea	5.8	5.1
Stomatitis	3.1	2.7
Skin and Subcutaneous Tissue Disorders		
Alopecia	12.4	11.9
General Disorders and General Administration Site Conditions		
Fatigue	15.4	15.6
Asthenia	4.7	4.6

In a combined analysis of these two studies, isolated cases of serious adverse experiences were similar in the two treatment groups.

Highly and Moderately Emetogenic Chemotherapy

The following additional clinical adverse experiences (incidence >0.5% and greater than standard therapy), regardless of causality, were reported in patients treated with aprepitant regimen in either HEC or MEC studies:

Infections and infestations: candidiasis, herpes simplex, lower respiratory infection, oral candidiasis, pharyngitis, septic shock, upper respiratory infection, urinary tract infection.

Neoplasms benign, malignant and unspecified (including cysts and polyps): malignant neoplasm, non-small cell lung carcinoma.

Blood and lymphatic system disorders: anemia, febrile neutropenia, thrombocytopenia.

Metabolism and nutrition disorders: appetite decreased, diabetes mellitus, hypokalemia.

Psychiatric disorders: anxiety disorder, confusion, depression.

Nervous system: peripheral neuropathy, sensory neuropathy, taste disturbance, tremor.

Eye disorders: conjunctivitis.

Cardiac disorders: myocardial infarction, palpitations, tachycardia.

Vascular disorders: deep venous thrombosis, flushing, hot flush, hypertension, hypotension.

Respiratory, thoracic and mediastinal disorders: cough, dyspnea, nasal secretion, pharyngolaryngeal pain, pneumonitis, pulmonary embolism, respiratory insufficiency, vocal disturbance.

Gastrointestinal disorders: abdominal pain upper, acid reflux, deglutition disorder, dry mouth, dysgeusia, dysphagia, eructation, flatulence, obstipation, salivation increased.

Skin and subcutaneous tissue disorders: acne, diaphoresis, pruritus, rash.

Musculoskeletal and connective tissue disorders: arthralgia, back pain, muscular weakness, musculoskeletal pain, myalgia.

Renal and urinary disorders: dysuria, renal insufficiency.

Reproductive system and breast disorders: pelvic pain.

General disorders and administrative site conditions: edema, malaise, pain, rigors.

Investigations: weight loss.

Stevens-Johnson syndrome was reported as a serious adverse experience in a patient receiving aprepitant with cancer chemotherapy in another CINV study.

Laboratory Adverse Experiences

Table 3 shows the percent of patients with laboratory adverse experiences reported at an incidence ≥3% in patients receiving highly emetogenic chemotherapy.

Table 3: Percent of Patients Receiving Highly Emetogenic Chemotherapy with Laboratory Adverse Experiences (Incidence ≥3%) — Cycle 1

	Aprepitant Regimen (N = 544)	Standard Therapy (N = 550)
Proteinuria	6.8	5.3
ALT Increased	6.0	4.3
Blood Urea Nitrogen Increased	4.7	3.5
Serum Creatinine Increased	3.7	4.3
AST Increased	3.0	1.3

The following additional laboratory adverse experiences (incidence >0.5% and greater than standard therapy), regardless of causality, were reported in patients treated with aprepitant regimen: alkaline phosphatase increased, hyperglycemia, hyponatremia, leukocytes increased, erythrocyturia, leukocyturia.

The adverse experience profiles in the Multiple-Cycle extensions of HEC and MEC studies for up to 6 cycles of chemotherapy were generally similar to that observed in Cycle 1.

Postoperative Nausea and Vomiting

In well-controlled clinical studies in patients receiving general anesthesia, 564 patients were administered 40-mg aprepitant orally and 538 patients were administered 4-mg ondansetron IV.

Clinical adverse experiences were reported in approximately 60% of patients treated with 40-mg aprepitant compared with approximately 64% of patients treated with 4-mg ondansetron IV. Table 4 shows the percent of patients with clinical adverse experiences reported at an incidence ≥3% of the combined studies.

Table 4: Percent of Patients Receiving General Anesthesia with Clinical Adverse Experiences (Incidence ≥3%)

	Aprepitant 40 mg (N = 564)	Ondansetron (N = 538)
Infections and Infestations		
Urinary Tract Infection	2.3	3.2
Blood and Lymphatic System Disorders		
Anemia	3.0	4.3
Psychiatric Disorders		
Insomnia	2.1	3.3
Nervous System Disorders		
Headache	5.0	6.5
Cardiac Disorders		
Bradycardia	4.4	3.9

Vascular Disorders		
Hypotension	5.7	4.6
Hypertension	2.1	3.2
Gastrointestinal Disorders		
Nausea	8.5	8.6
Constipation	8.5	7.6
Flatulence	4.1	5.8
Vomiting	2.5	3.9
Skin and Subcutaneous Tissue Disorders		
Pruritus	7.6	8.4
General Disorders and General Administration Site Conditions		
Pyrexia	5.9	10.6

The following additional clinical adverse experiences (incidence >0.5% and greater than ondansetron), regardless of causality, were reported in patients treated with aprepitant:
Infections and infestations: postoperative infection
Metabolism and nutrition disorders: hypokalemia, hypovolemia.
Nervous system disorders: dizziness, hypoesthesia, syncope.
Vascular disorders: hematoma
Respiratory, thoracic and mediastinal disorders: dyspnea, hypoxia, respiratory depression.
Gastrointestinal disorders: abdominal pain, abdominal pain upper, dry mouth, dyspepsia.
Skin and subcutaneous tissue disorders: urticaria
General disorders and administrative site conditions: hypothermia, pain.
Investigations: blood pressure decreased
Injury, poisoning and procedural complications: operative hemorrhage, wound dehiscence.

Other adverse experiences (incidence ≤0.5%) reported in patients treated with aprepitant 40 mg for postoperative nausea and vomiting included:
Nervous system disorders: dysarthria, sensory disturbance.
Eye disorders: miosis, visual acuity reduced.
Respiratory, thoracic and mediastinal disorders: wheezing
Gastrointestinal disorders: bowel sounds abnormal, stomach discomfort.

There were no serious adverse drug-related experiences reported in the postoperative nausea and vomiting clinical studies in patients taking 40-mg aprepitant.

Laboratory Adverse Experiences

One laboratory adverse experience, hemoglobin decreased (40-mg aprepitant 3.8%, ondansetron 4.2%), was reported at an incidence ≥3% in a patient receiving general anesthesia.

The following additional laboratory adverse experiences (incidence >0.5% and greater than ondansetron), regardless of causality, were reported in patients treated with aprepitant 40 mg: blood albumin decreased, blood bilirubin increased, blood glucose increased, blood potassium decreased, glucose urine present.

The adverse experience of ALT increased occurred with similar incidence in patients treated with aprepitant 40 mg (1.1%) as in patients treated with ondansetron 4 mg (1.0%).

Other Studies

In addition, two serious adverse experiences were reported in postoperative nausea and vomiting (PONV) clinical studies in patients taking a higher dose of aprepitant: one case of constipation, and one case of sub-ileus.

Angioedema and urticaria were reported as serious adverse experiences in a patient receiving aprepitant in a non-CINV/non-PONV study.

6.2 Postmarketing Experience

The following adverse reactions have been identified during postmarketing use of aprepitant. Because these reactions are reported voluntarily from a population of uncertain size, it is generally not possible to reliably estimate their frequency or establish a causal relationship to drug exposure.
Skin and subcutaneous tissue disorders: pruritus, rash, urticaria, rarely Stevens-Johnson syndrome/toxic epidermal necrolysis.
Immune system disorders: hypersensitivity reactions including anaphylactic reactions.

7 DRUG INTERACTIONS

Aprepitant is a substrate, a weak-to-moderate (dose-dependent) inhibitor, and an inducer of CYP3A4. Aprepitant is also an inducer of CYP2C9.

7.1 Effect of Aprepitant on the Pharmacokinetics of Other Agents

CYP3A4 substrates:

Weak inhibition of CYP3A4 by a single 40-mg dose of aprepitant is not expected to alter the plasma concentrations of concomitant medications that are primarily metabolized through CYP3A4 to a clinically significant degree. However, higher aprepitant doses or repeated dosing at any aprepitant dose may have a clinically significant effect.

As a moderate inhibitor of CYP3A4 at a dose of 125 mg/80 mg, aprepitant can increase plasma concentrations of concomitantly administered oral medications that are metabolized through CYP3A4 *[see Contraindications (4)]*. The use of fosaprepitant may increase CYP3A4 substrate plasma concentrations to a lesser degree than the use of oral aprepitant (125 mg).

5-HT$_3$ antagonists: In clinical drug interaction studies, aprepitant did not have clinically important effects on the pharmacokinetics of ondansetron, granisetron, or hydrodolasetron (the active metabolite of dolasetron).

Corticosteroids:

Dexamethasone: EMEND, when given as a regimen of 125 mg with dexamethasone coadministered orally as 20 mg on Day 1, and EMEND when given as 80 mg/day with dexamethasone coadministered orally as 8 mg on Days 2 through 5, increased the AUC of dexamethasone, a CYP3A4 substrate, by 2.2-fold on Days 1 and 5. The oral dexamethasone doses should be reduced by approximately 50% when coadministered with EMEND (125-mg/80-mg regimen), to achieve exposures of dexamethasone similar to those obtained when it is given without EMEND. The daily dose of dexamethasone administered in clinical chemotherapy induced nausea and vomiting studies with EMEND reflects an approximate 50% reduction of the dose of dexamethasone *[see Dosage and Administration (2.1)]*. A single dose of EMEND (40 mg) when coadministered with a single oral dose of dexamethasone 20 mg, increased the AUC of dexamethasone by 1.45-fold. Therefore, no dose adjustment is recommended.

Methylprednisolone: EMEND, when given as a regimen of 125 mg on Day 1 and 80 mg/day on Days 2 and 3, increased the AUC of methylprednisolone, a CYP3A4 substrate, by 1.34-fold on Day 1 and by 2.5-fold on Day 3, when methylprednisolone was coadministered intravenously as 125 mg on Day 1 and orally as 40 mg on Days 2 and 3. The IV methylprednisolone dose should be reduced by approximately 25%, and the oral methylprednisolone dose should be reduced by approximately 50% when coadministered with EMEND (125-mg/80-mg regimen) to achieve exposures of methylprednisolone similar to those obtained when it is given without EMEND. Although the concomitant administration of methylprednisolone with the single 40-mg dose of aprepitant has not been studied, a single 40-mg dose of EMEND produces a weak inhibition of CYP3A4 (based on midazolam interaction study) and it is not expected to alter the plasma concentrations of methylprednisolone to a clinically significant degree. Therefore, no dose adjustment is recommended.

Chemotherapeutic agents: *[see Warnings and Precautions (5.1)]*

Docetaxel: In a pharmacokinetic study, EMEND (125-mg/80-mg regimen) did not influence the pharmacokinetics of docetaxel.

Vinorelbine: In a pharmacokinetic study, EMEND (125-mg/80-mg regimen) did not influence the pharmacokinetics of vinorelbine to a clinically significant degree.

CYP2C9 substrates (Warfarin, Tolbutamide):

Aprepitant has been shown to induce the metabolism of S(-) warfarin and tolbutamide, which are metabolized through CYP2C9. Coadministration of EMEND with these drugs or other drugs that are known to be metabolized by CYP2C9, such as phenytoin, may result in lower plasma concentrations of these drugs.

Warfarin: A single 125-mg dose of EMEND was administered on Day 1 and 80 mg/day on Days 2 and 3 to healthy subjects who were stabilized on chronic warfarin therapy. Although there was no effect of EMEND on the plasma AUC of R(+) or S(-) warfarin determined on Day 3, there was a 34% decrease in S(-) warfarin (a CYP2C9 substrate) trough concentration accompanied by a 14% decrease in the prothrombin time (reported as International Normalized Ratio or INR) 5 days after completion of dosing with EMEND. In patients on chronic warfarin therapy, the prothrombin time (INR) should be closely monitored in the 2-week period, particularly at 7 to 10 days, following initiation of the 3-day regimen of EMEND with each chemotherapy cycle, or following administration of a single 40-mg dose of EMEND for the prevention of postoperative nausea and vomiting.

Tolbutamide: EMEND, when given as 125 mg on Day 1 and 80 mg/day on Days 2 and 3, decreased the AUC of tolbutamide (a CYP2C9 substrate) by 23% on Day 4, 28% on Day 8, and 15% on Day 15, when a single dose of tolbutamide 500 mg was administered orally prior to the administration of the 3-day regimen of EMEND and on Days 4, 8, and 15.

EMEND, when given as a 40-mg single oral dose on Day 1, decreased the AUC of tolbutamide (a CYP2C9 substrate) by 8% on Day 2, 16% on Day 4, 15% on Day 8, and 10% on Day 15, when a single dose of tolbutamide 500 mg was administered orally prior to the administration of EMEND 40 mg and on Days 2, 4, 8, and 15. This effect was not considered clinically important.

Oral contraceptives: Aprepitant, when given once daily for 14 days as a 100-mg capsule with an oral contraceptive containing 35 mcg of ethinyl estradiol and 1 mg of norethindrone, decreased the AUC of ethinyl estradiol by 43%, and decreased the AUC of norethindrone by 8%.

In another study, a daily dose of an oral contraceptive containing ethinyl estradiol and norethindrone was administered on Days 1 through 21, and EMEND was given as a 3-day regimen of 125 mg on Day 8 and 80 mg/day on Days 9 and 10 with ondansetron 32 mg IV on Day 8 and oral dexamethasone given as 12 mg on Day 8 and 8 mg/day on Days 9, 10, and 11. In the study, the AUC of ethinyl estradiol decreased by 19% on Day 10 and there was as much as a 64% decrease in ethinyl estradiol trough concentrations during Days 9 through 21. While there was no effect of EMEND on the AUC of norethindrone on Day 10, there was as much as a 60% decrease in norethindrone trough concentrations during Days 9 through 21.

In another study, a daily dose of an oral contraceptive containing ethinyl estradiol and norgestimate (which is converted to norelgestromin) was administered on Days 1 through 21, and EMEND 40 mg was given on Day 8. In the study, the AUC of ethinyl estradiol decreased by 4% and 29% on Day 8 and Day 12, respectively, while the AUC of norelgestromin increased by 18% on Day 8 and decreased by 10% on Day 12. In addition, the trough concentrations of ethinyl estradiol and norelgestromin on Days 8 through 21 were generally lower following coadministration of the oral contraceptive with EMEND 40 mg on Day 8 compared to the trough levels following administration of the oral contraceptive alone.

The coadministration of EMEND may reduce the efficacy of hormonal contraceptives (these can include birth control pills, skin patches, implants, and certain IUDs) during and for 28 days after administration of the last dose of EMEND. Alternative or back-up methods of contraception should be used during treatment with EMEND and for 1 month following the last dose of EMEND.

Midazolam: EMEND increased the AUC of midazolam, a sensitive CYP3A4 substrate, by 2.3-fold on Day 1 and 3.3-fold on Day 5, when a single oral dose of midazolam 2 mg was coadministered on Day 1 and Day 5 of a regimen of EMEND 125 mg on Day 1 and 80 mg/day on Days 2 through 5. The potential effects of increased plasma concentrations of midazolam or other benzodiazepines metabolized via CYP3A4 (alprazolam, triazolam) should be considered when coadministering these agents with EMEND (125 mg/80 mg). A single dose of EMEND (40 mg) increased the AUC of midazolam by 1.2-fold on Day 1, when a single oral dose of midazolam 2 mg was coadministered on Day 1 with EMEND 40 mg; this effect was not considered clinically important.

In another study with intravenous administration of midazolam, EMEND was given as 125 mg on Day 1 and 80 mg/day on Days 2 and 3, and midazolam 2 mg IV was given prior to the administration of the 3-day regimen of EMEND and on Days 4, 8, and 15. EMEND increased the AUC of midazolam by 25% on Day 4 and decreased the AUC of midazolam by 19% on Day 8 relative to the dosing of EMEND on Days 1 through 3. These effects were not considered clinically important. The AUC of midazolam on Day 15 was similar to that observed at baseline.

An additional study was completed with intravenous administration of midazolam and EMEND. Intravenous midazolam 2 mg was given 1 hour after oral administration of a single dose of EMEND 125 mg. The plasma AUC of midazolam was increased by 1.5-fold. Depending on clinical situations (e.g., elderly patients) and degree of monitoring available, dosage adjustment for intravenous midazolam may be necessary when it is coadministered with EMEND for the chemotherapy induced nausea and vomiting indication (125 mg on Day 1 followed by 80 mg on Days 2 and 3).

7.2 Effect of Other Agents on the Pharmacokinetics of Aprepitant

Aprepitant is a substrate for CYP3A4; therefore, coadministration of EMEND with drugs that inhibit CYP3A4 activity may result in increased plasma concentrations of aprepitant. Consequently, concomitant administration of EMEND with strong CYP3A4 inhibitors (e.g., ketoconazole, itraconazole, nefazodone, troleandomycin, clarithromycin, ritonavir, nelfinavir) should be approached with caution. Because moderate CYP3A4 inhibitors (e.g., diltiazem) result in a 2-fold increase in plasma concentrations of aprepitant, concomitant administration should also be approached with caution.

Aprepitant is a substrate for CYP3A4; therefore, coadministration of EMEND with drugs that strongly induce CYP3A4 activity (e.g., rifampin, carbamazepine, phenytoin) may result in reduced plasma concentrations of aprepitant that may result in decreased efficacy of EMEND.

Ketoconazole: When a single 125-mg dose of EMEND was administered on Day 5 of a 10-day regimen of 400 mg/day of ketoconazole, a strong CYP3A4 inhibitor, the AUC of aprepitant increased approximately 5-fold and the mean terminal half-life of aprepitant increased approximately 3-fold. Concomitant administration of EMEND with strong CYP3A4 inhibitors should be approached cautiously.

Rifampin: When a single 375-mg dose of EMEND was administered on Day 9 of a 14-day regimen of 600 mg/day of rifampin, a strong CYP3A4 inducer, the AUC of aprepitant decreased approximately 11-fold and the mean terminal half-life decreased approximately 3-fold.

Coadministration of EMEND with drugs that induce CYP3A4 activity may result in reduced plasma concentrations and decreased efficacy of EMEND.

7.3 Additional Interactions

EMEND is unlikely to interact with drugs that are substrates for the P-glycoprotein transporter, as demonstrated by the lack of interaction of EMEND with digoxin in a clinical drug interaction study.

Diltiazem: In patients with mild to moderate hypertension, administration of aprepitant once daily, as a tablet formulation comparable to 230 mg of the capsule formulation, with diltiazem 120 mg 3 times daily for 5 days, resulted in a 2-fold increase of aprepitant AUC and a simultaneous 1.7-fold increase of diltiazem AUC. These pharmacokinetic effects did not result in clinically meaningful changes in ECG, heart rate or blood pressure beyond those changes induced by diltiazem alone.

Paroxetine: Coadministration of once daily doses of aprepitant, as a tablet formulation comparable to 85 mg or 170 mg of the capsule formulation, with paroxetine 20 mg once daily, resulted in a decrease in AUC by approximately 25% and C_{max} by approximately 20% of both aprepitant and paroxetine.

8 USE IN SPECIFIC POPULATIONS

8.1 Pregnancy

Teratogenic effects

Pregnancy Category B: Reproduction studies have been performed in rats at oral doses up to 1000 mg/kg twice daily (plasma AUC_{0-24hr} of 31.3 mcg•hr/mL, about 1.6 times the human exposure at the recommended dose) and in rabbits at oral doses up to 25 mg/kg/day (plasma AUC_{0-24hr} of 26.9 mcg•hr/mL, about 1.4 times the human exposure at the recommended dose) and have revealed no evidence of impaired fertility or harm to the fetus due to aprepitant. There are, however, no adequate and well-controlled studies in pregnant women. Because animal reproduction studies are not always predictive of human response, this drug should be used during pregnancy only if clearly needed.

8.3 Nursing Mothers

Aprepitant is excreted in the milk of rats. It is not known whether this drug is excreted in human milk. Because many drugs are excreted in human milk and because of the potential for possible serious adverse reactions in nursing infants from aprepitant and because of the potential for tumorigenicity shown for aprepitant in rodent carcinogenicity studies, a decision should be made whether to discontinue nursing or to discontinue the drug, taking into account the importance of the drug to the mother.

8.4 Pediatric Use

Safety and effectiveness of EMEND in pediatric patients have not been established.

8.5 Geriatric Use

In 2 well-controlled chemotherapy-induced nausea and vomiting clinical studies, of the total number of patients (N=544) treated with EMEND, 31% were 65 and over, while 5% were 75 and over. In well-controlled postoperative nausea and vomiting clinical studies, of the total number of patients (N=1120) treated with EMEND, 7% were 65 and over, while 2% were 75 and over. No overall differences in safety or effectiveness were observed between these subjects and younger subjects. Greater sensitivity of some older individuals cannot be ruled out. Dosage adjustment in the elderly is not necessary.

10 OVERDOSAGE

No specific information is available on the treatment of overdosage.

Drowsiness and headache were reported in one patient who ingested 1440 mg of aprepitant.

In the event of overdose, EMEND should be discontinued and general supportive treatment and monitoring should be provided. Because of the antiemetic activity of aprepitant, drug-induced emesis may not be effective.

Aprepitant cannot be removed by hemodialysis.

11 DESCRIPTION

EMEND (aprepitant) is a substance P/neurokinin 1 (NK_1) receptor antagonist, chemically described as 5-[[(2*R*,3*S*)-2-[(1*R*)-1-[3,5-bis(trifluoromethyl)phenyl]ethoxy]-3-(4-fluorophenyl)-4-morpholinyl]methyl]-1,2-dihydro-3*H*-1,2,4-triazol-3-one.

Its empirical formula is $C_{23}H_{21}F_7N_4O_3$, and its structural formula is:

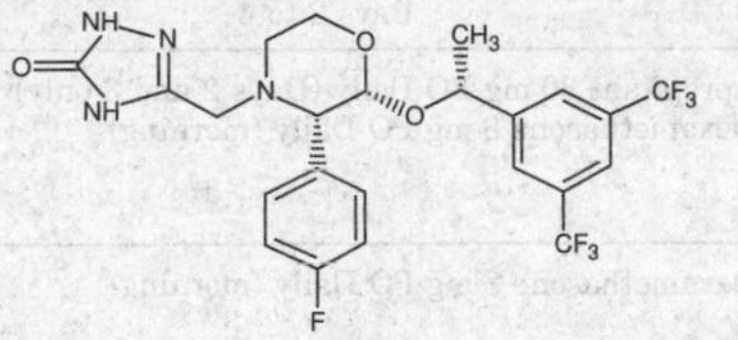

Aprepitant is a white to off-white crystalline solid, with a molecular weight of 534.43. It is practically insoluble in water. Aprepitant is sparingly soluble in ethanol and isopropyl acetate and slightly soluble in acetonitrile.

Each capsule of EMEND for oral administration contains either 40 mg, 80 mg, or 125 mg of aprepitant and the following inactive ingredients: sucrose, microcrystalline cellulose, hydroxypropyl cellulose and sodium lauryl sulfate. The capsule shell excipients are gelatin, titanium dioxide, and may contain sodium lauryl sulfate and silicon dioxide. The 40-mg capsule shell also contains yellow ferric oxide, and the 125-mg capsule also contains red ferric oxide and yellow ferric oxide.

12 CLINICAL PHARMACOLOGY

12.1 Mechanism of Action

Aprepitant is a selective high-affinity antagonist of human substance P/neurokinin 1 (NK_1) receptors. Aprepitant has little or no affinity for serotonin ($5\text{-}HT_3$), dopamine, and corticosteroid receptors, the targets of existing therapies for chemotherapy-induced nausea and vomiting (CINV) and postoperative nausea and vomiting (PONV).

Aprepitant has been shown in animal models to inhibit emesis induced by cytotoxic chemotherapeutic agents, such as cisplatin, via central actions. Animal and human Positron Emission Tomography (PET) studies with aprepitant have shown that it crosses the blood brain barrier and occupies brain NK_1 receptors. Animal and human studies show that aprepitant augments the antiemetic activity of the $5\text{-}HT_3$-receptor antagonist ondansetron and the corticosteroid dexamethasone and inhibits both the acute and delayed phases of cisplatin-induced emesis.

12.2 Pharmacodynamics

NK_1 Receptor Occupancy

In two single-blind, multiple-dose, randomized, and placebo-controlled studies, healthy young men received oral aprepitant doses of 10 mg (N=2), 30 mg (N=3), 100 mg (N=3) or 300 mg (N=5) once daily for 14 days with 2 or 3 subjects on placebo. Both plasma aprepitant concentration and NK_1 receptor occupancy in the corpus striatum by positron emission tomography were evaluated, at predose and 24 hours after the last dose. At aprepitant plasma concentrations of ~10 ng/mL and ~100 ng/mL, the NK_1 receptor occupancies were ~50% and ~90%, respectively. The oral aprepitant regimen for CINV produces mean trough plasma aprepitant concentrations >500 ng/mL, which would be expected to, based on the fitted curve with the Hill equation, result in >95% brain NK_1 receptor occupancy. However, the receptor occupancy for either CINV or PONV dosing regimen has not been determined. In addition, the relationship between NK_1 receptor occupancy and the clinical efficacy of aprepitant has not been established.

Cardiac Electrophysiology

In a randomized, double-blind, positive-controlled, thorough QTc study, a single 200-mg dose of fosaprepitant had no effect on the QTc interval. QT prolongation with the oral dosing regimens for CINV and PONV are not expected.

12.3 Pharmacokinetics

Absorption

Following oral administration of a single 40-mg dose of EMEND in the fasted state, mean area under the plasma concentration-time curve ($AUC_{0-\infty}$) was 7.8 mcg•hr/mL and mean peak plasma concentration (C_{max}) was 0.7 mcg/mL, occurring at approximately 3 hours postdose (T_{max}). The absolute bioavailability at the 40-mg dose has not been determined.

Following oral administration of a single 125-mg dose of EMEND on Day 1 and 80 mg once daily on Days 2 and 3, the AUC_{0-24hr} was approximately 19.6 mcg•hr/mL and 21.2 mcg•hr/mL on Day 1 and Day 3, respectively. The C_{max} of 1.6 mcg/mL and 1.4 mcg/mL were reached in approximately 4 hours (T_{max}) on Day 1 and Day 3, respectively. At the dose range of 80-125 mg, the mean absolute oral bioavailability of aprepitant is approximately 60 to 65%. Oral administration of the capsule with a standard high-fat breakfast had no clinically meaningful effect on the bioavailability of aprepitant.

The pharmacokinetics of aprepitant are non-linear across the clinical dose range. In healthy young adults, the increase in $AUC_{0-\infty}$ was 26% greater than dose proportional between 80-mg and 125-mg single doses administered in the fed state.

Distribution

Aprepitant is greater than 95% bound to plasma proteins. The mean apparent volume of distribution at steady state (Vd_{ss}) is approximately 70 L in humans.

Aprepitant crosses the placenta in rats and rabbits and crosses the blood brain barrier in humans *[see Clinical Pharmacology (12.1)]*.

Metabolism

Aprepitant undergoes extensive metabolism. *In vitro* studies using human liver microsomes indicate that aprepitant is metabolized primarily by CYP3A4 with minor metabolism by CYP1A2 and CYP2C19. Metabolism is largely via oxidation at the morpholine ring and its side chains. No metabolism by CYP2D6, CYP2C9, or CYP2E1 was detected. In healthy young adults, aprepitant accounts for approximately 24% of the radioactivity in plasma over 72 hours following a single oral 300-mg dose of [^{14}C]-aprepitant, indicating a substantial presence of metabolites in the plasma. Seven metabolites of aprepitant, which are only weakly active, have been identified in human plasma.

Excretion

Following administration of a single IV 100-mg dose of [^{14}C]-aprepitant prodrug to healthy subjects, 57% of the radioactivity was recovered in urine and 45% in feces. A study was not conducted with radiolabeled capsule formulation. The results after oral administration may differ.

Aprepitant is eliminated primarily by metabolism; aprepitant is not renally excreted. The apparent plasma clearance of aprepitant ranged from approximately 62 to 90 mL/min. The apparent terminal half-life ranged from approximately 9 to 13 hours.

Specific Populations

Gender

Following oral administration of a single dose of EMEND, the AUC_{0-24hr} and C_{max} are 14% and 22% higher in females as compared with males. The half-life of aprepitant is 25% lower in females as compared with males and T_{max} occurs at approximately the same time. These differences are not considered clinically meaningful. No dosage adjustment is necessary based on gender.

Geriatric

Following oral administration of a single 125-mg dose of EMEND on Day 1 and 80 mg once daily on Days 2 through 5, the AUC_{0-24hr} of aprepitant was 21% higher on Day 1 and 36% higher on Day 5 in elderly (≥65 years) relative to younger adults. The C_{max} was 10% higher on Day 1 and 24% higher on Day 5 in elderly relative to younger adults. These differences are not considered clinically meaningful. No dosage adjustment is necessary in elderly patients.

Race

Following oral administration of a single dose of EMEND, the AUC_{0-24hr} and C_{max} are approximately 42% and 29% higher in Hispanics as compared with Caucasians. The AUC_{0-24hr} and C_{max} are 62% and 41% higher in Asians as compared to Caucasians. There was no difference in AUC_{0-24hr} or C_{max} between Caucasians and Blacks. These differences are not considered clinically meaningful. No dosage adjustment is necessary based on race.

Body Mass Index (BMI)

For every 5 kg/m^2 increase in BMI, AUC_{0-24hr} and C_{max} of aprepitant decrease by 11%. BMI of subjects in the analysis ranged from 18 kg/m^2 to 36 kg/m^2. This change is not considered clinically meaningful. No dosage adjustment is necessary based on BMI.

Hepatic Insufficiency

Following administration of a single 125-mg dose of EMEND on Day 1 and 80 mg once daily on Days 2 and 3 to patients with mild hepatic impairment (Child-Pugh score 5 to 6), the AUC_{0-24hr} of aprepitant was 11% lower on Day 1 and 36% lower on Day 3, as compared with healthy subjects given the same regimen. In patients with moderate hepatic impairment (Child-Pugh score 7 to 9), the AUC_{0-24hr} of aprepitant was 10% higher on Day 1 and 18% higher on Day 3, as compared with healthy subjects given the same regimen. These differences in AUC_{0-24hr} are not considered clinically meaningful; therefore, no dosage adjustment is necessary in patients with mild to moderate hepatic impairment. There are no clinical or pharmacokinetic data in patients with severe hepatic impairment (Child-Pugh score >9) *[see Warnings and Precautions (5.4)]*.

Renal Insufficiency

A single 240-mg dose of EMEND was administered to patients with severe renal impairment (creatinine clearance <30 mL/min/1.73 m^2 as measured by 24-hour urinary creatinine clearance) and to patients with end stage renal disease (ESRD) requiring hemodialysis.

In patients with severe renal impairment, the $AUC_{0-\infty}$ of total aprepitant (unbound and protein bound) decreased by 21% and C_{max} decreased by 32%, relative to healthy subjects (creatinine clearance >80 mL/min estimated by Cockcroft-Gault method). In patients with ESRD undergoing hemodialysis, the $AUC_{0-\infty}$ of total aprepitant decreased by 42% and C_{max} decreased by 32%. Due to modest decreases in protein binding of aprepitant in patients with renal disease, the AUC of pharmacologically active unbound drug was not sig-

Table 5: Treatment Regimens in Highly Emetogenic Chemotherapy Trials

Treatment Regimen	Day 1	Days 2 to 4
Aprepitant	Aprepitant 125 mg PO	Aprepitant 80 mg PO Daily (Days 2 and 3 only) Dexamethasone 8 mg PO Daily (morning)
	Dexamethasone 12 mg PO 5-HT_3 antagonist*	
Standard Therapy	Dexamethasone 20 mg PO	Dexamethasone 8 mg PO Daily (morning)
	5-HT_3 antagonist*	Dexamethasone 8 mg PO Daily (evening)

Aprepitant placebo and dexamethasone placebo were used to maintain blinding.
* Ondansetron 32 mg I.V. was used in the clinical trials of EMEND. Although this dose was used in clinical trials, this is no longer the currently recommended dose. Refer to the ondansetron package insert for the current dosing.

nificantly affected in patients with renal impairment compared with healthy subjects. Hemodialysis conducted 4 or 48 hours after dosing had no significant effect on the pharmacokinetics of aprepitant; less than 0.2% of the dose was recovered in the dialysate.

No dosage adjustment is necessary for patients with renal impairment or for patients with ESRD undergoing hemodialysis.

13 NONCLINICAL TOXICOLOGY

13.1 Carcinogenesis, Mutagenesis, Impairment of Fertility

Carcinogenicity studies were conducted in Sprague-Dawley rats and in CD-1 mice for 2 years. In the rat carcinogenicity studies, animals were treated with oral doses ranging from 0.05 to 1000 mg/kg twice daily. The highest dose produced a systemic exposure to aprepitant (plasma AUC_{0-24hr}) of 0.7 to 1.6 times the human exposure (AUC_{0-24hr} = 19.6 mcg•hr/mL) at the recommended dose of 125 mg/day. Treatment with aprepitant at doses of 5 to 1000 mg/kg twice daily caused an increase in the incidences of thyroid follicular cell adenomas and carcinomas in male rats. In female rats, it produced hepatocellular adenomas at 5 to 1000 mg/kg twice daily and hepatocellular carcinomas and thyroid follicular cell adenomas at 125 to 1000 mg/kg twice daily. In the mouse carcinogenicity studies, the animals were treated with oral doses ranging from 2.5 to 2000 mg/kg/day. The highest dose produced a systemic exposure of about 2.8 to 3.6 times the human exposure at the recommended dose. Treatment with aprepitant produced skin fibrosarcomas at 125 and 500 mg/kg/day doses in male mice.

Aprepitant was not genotoxic in the Ames test, the human lymphoblastoid cell (TK6) mutagenesis test, the rat hepatocyte DNA strand break test, the Chinese hamster ovary (CHO) cell chromosome aberration test and the mouse micronucleus test.

Aprepitant did not affect the fertility or general reproductive performance of male or female rats at doses up to the maximum feasible dose of 1000 mg/kg twice daily (providing exposure in male rats lower than the exposure at the recommended human dose and exposure in female rats at about 1.6 times the human exposure).

14 CLINICAL STUDIES

14.1 Prevention of Chemotherapy Induced Nausea and Vomiting (CINV)

Oral administration of EMEND in combination with ondansetron and dexamethasone (aprepitant regimen) has been shown to prevent acute and delayed nausea and vomiting associated with highly emetogenic chemotherapy including high-dose cisplatin, and nausea and vomiting associated with moderately emetogenic chemotherapy.

Highly Emetogenic Chemotherapy (HEC)

In 2 multicenter, randomized, parallel, double-blind, controlled clinical studies, the aprepitant regimen (see Table 6) was compared with standard therapy in patients receiving a chemotherapy regimen that included cisplatin >50 mg/m^2 (mean cisplatin dose = 80.2 mg/m^2). Of the 550 patients who were randomized to receive the aprepitant regimen, 42% were women, 58% men, 59% White, 3% Asian, 5% Black, 12% Hispanic American, and 21% Multi-Racial. The aprepitant-treated patients in these clinical studies ranged from 14 to 84 years of age, with a mean age of 56 years. 170 patients were 65 years or older, with 29 patients being 75 years or older.

Patients (N = 1105) were randomized to either the aprepitant regimen (N = 550) or standard therapy (N = 555). The treatment regimens are defined in Table 5. [See table 5 above]

During these studies, 95% of the patients in the aprepitant group received a concomitant chemotherapeutic agent in addition to protocol-mandated cisplatin. The most common chemotherapeutic agents and the number of aprepitant patients exposed follows: etoposide (106), fluorouracil (100), gemcitabine (89), vinorelbine (82), paclitaxel (52), cyclophosphamide (50), doxorubicin (38), docetaxel (11).

The antiemetic activity of EMEND was evaluated during the acute phase (0 to 24 hours post-cisplatin treatment), the delayed phase (25 to 120 hours post-cisplatin treatment) and overall (0 to 120 hours post-cisplatin treatment) in Cycle 1. Efficacy was based on evaluation of the following endpoints:

Primary endpoint:
- complete response (defined as no emetic episodes and no use of rescue therapy)

Other prespecified endpoints:
- complete protection (defined as no emetic episodes, no use of rescue therapy, and a maximum nausea visual analogue scale [VAS] score <25 mm on a 0 to 100 mm scale)
- no emesis (defined as no emetic episodes regardless of use of rescue therapy)
- no nausea (maximum VAS <5 mm on a 0 to 100 mm scale)
- no significant nausea (maximum VAS <25 mm on a 0 to 100 mm scale)

A summary of the key study results from each individual study analysis is shown in Table 6 and in Table 7.

Table 6: Percent of Patients Receiving Highly Emetogenic Chemotherapy Responding by Treatment Group and Phase for Study 1 — Cycle 1

ENDPOINTS	Aprepitant Regimen (N = 260)* %	Standard Therapy (N = 261)* %	p-Value
PRIMARY ENDPOINT			
Complete Response			
Overall†	73	52	<0.001
OTHER PRESPECIFIED ENDPOINTS			
Complete Response			
Acute phase‡	89	78	<0.001
Delayed phase§	75	56	<0.001
Complete Protection			
Overall	63	49	0.001
Acute phase	85	75	NS¶
Delayed phase	66	52	<0.001
No Emesis			
Overall	78	55	<0.001
Acute phase	90	79	0.001
Delayed phase	81	59	<0.001
No Nausea			
Overall	48	44	NS#
Delayed phase	51	48	NS#
No Significant Nausea			
Overall	73	66	NS#
Delayed phase	75	69	NS#

Visual analogue scale (VAS) score range: 0 mm = no nausea; 100 mm = nausea as bad as it could be.
* N: Number of patients (older than 18 years of age) who received cisplatin, study drug, and had at least one post-treatment efficacy evaluation.
† Overall: 0 to 120 hours post-cisplatin treatment.
‡ Acute phase: 0 to 24 hours post-cisplatin treatment.
§ Delayed phase: 25 to 120 hours post-cisplatin treatment.
¶ Not statistically significant when adjusted for multiple comparisons.
# Not statistically significant.

Table 7: Percent of Patients Receiving Highly Emetogenic Chemotherapy Responding by Treatment Group and Phase for Study 2 — Cycle 1

ENDPOINTS	Aprepitant Regimen (N = 261)* %	Standard Therapy (N = 263)* %	p-Value
PRIMARY ENDPOINT			
Complete Response			
Overall†	63	43	<0.001
OTHER PRESPECIFIED ENDPOINTS			
Complete Response			
Acute phase‡	83	68	<0.001
Delayed phase§	68	47	<0.001
Complete Protection			
Overall	56	41	<0.001
Acute phase	80	65	<0.001
Delayed phase	61	44	<0.001
No Emesis			
Overall	66	44	<0.001
Acute phase	84	69	<0.001
Delayed phase	72	48	<0.001
No Nausea			
Overall	49	39	NS¶
Delayed phase	53	40	NS¶
No Significant Nausea			
Overall	71	64	NS#
Delayed phase	73	65	NS#

Visual analogue scale (VAS) score range: 0 mm = no nausea; 100 mm = nausea as bad as it could be.
* N: Number of patients (older than 18 years of age) who received cisplatin, study drug, and had at least one post-treatment efficacy evaluation.
† Overall: 0 to 120 hours post-cisplatin treatment.
‡ Acute phase: 0 to 24 hours post-cisplatin treatment.
§ Delayed phase: 25 to 120 hours post-cisplatin treatment.
¶ Not statistically significant when adjusted for multiple comparisons.
# Not statistically significant.

In both studies, a statistically significantly higher proportion of patients receiving the aprepitant regimen in Cycle 1 had a complete response in the overall phase (primary endpoint), compared with patients receiving standard therapy. A statistically significant difference in complete response in favor of the aprepitant regimen was also observed when the acute phase and the delayed phase were analyzed separately.

In both studies, the estimated time to first emesis after initiation of cisplatin treatment was longer with the aprepitant regimen, and the incidence of first emesis was reduced in the aprepitant regimen group compared with standard therapy group as depicted in the Kaplan-Meier curves in Figure 1.

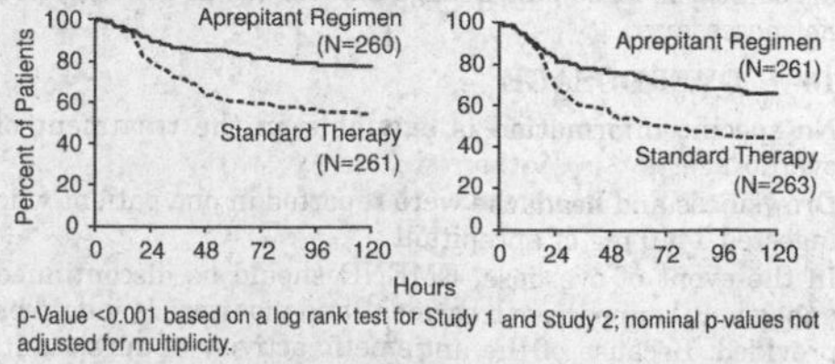

p-Value <0.001 based on a log rank test for Study 1 and Study 2; nominal p-values not adjusted for multiplicity.

Figure 1: Percent of Patients Receiving Highly Emetogenic Chemotherapy Who Remain Emesis Free Over Time — Cycle 1

Patient-Reported Outcomes: The impact of nausea and vomiting on patients' daily lives was assessed in Cycle 1 of both Phase III studies using the Functional Living Index–

Emesis (FLIE), a validated nausea- and vomiting-specific patient-reported outcome measure. Minimal or no impact of nausea and vomiting on patients' daily lives is defined as a FLIE total score >108. In each of the 2 studies, a higher proportion of patients receiving the aprepitant regimen reported minimal or no impact of nausea and vomiting on daily life (Study 1: 74% versus 64%; Study 2: 75% versus 64%).

Multiple-Cycle Extension: In the same 2 clinical studies, patients continued into the Multiple-Cycle extension for up to 5 additional cycles of chemotherapy. The proportion of patients with no emesis and no significant nausea by treatment group at each cycle is depicted in Figure 2. Antiemetic effectiveness for the patients receiving the aprepitant regimen is maintained throughout repeat cycles for those patients continuing in each of the multiple cycles.

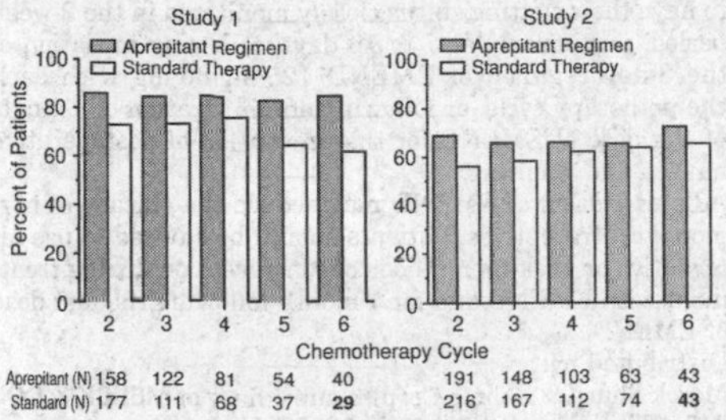

Figure 2: Proportion of Patients Receiving Highly Emetogenic Chemotherapy with No Emesis and No Significant Nausea by Treatment Group and Cycle

Table 8: Treatment Regimens in Moderately Emetogenic Chemotherapy Trials

Treatment Regimen	Day 1	Days 2 to 3
Aprepitant	Aprepitant 125 mg PO* Dexamethasone 12 mg PO† Ondansetron 8 mg PO × 2 doses‡	Aprepitant 80 mg PO Daily
Standard Therapy	Dexamethasone 20 mg PO Ondansetron 8 mg PO × 2 doses	Ondansetron 8 mg PO Daily (every 12 hours)

Aprepitant placebo and dexamethasone placebo were used to maintain blinding.
* 1 hour prior to chemotherapy.
† 30 minutes prior to chemotherapy.
‡ 30 to 60 minutes prior to chemotherapy and 8 hours after first ondansetron dose.

<u>*Moderately Emetogenic Chemotherapy (MEC)*</u>

In a multicenter, randomized, double-blind, parallel-group, clinical study in breast cancer patients, the aprepitant regimen (see Table 9) was compared with a standard of care therapy in patients receiving a moderately emetogenic chemotherapy regimen that included cyclophosphamide 750-1500 mg/m²; or cyclophosphamide 500-1500 mg/m² and doxorubicin (≤60 mg/m²) or epirubicin (≤100 mg/m²).

In this study, the most common combinations were cyclophosphamide + doxorubicin (60.6%); and cyclophosphamide + epirubicin + fluorouracil (21.6%).

Of the 438 patients who were randomized to receive the aprepitant regimen, 99.5% were women. Of these, approximately 80% were White, 8% Black, 8% Asian, 4% Hispanic, and <1% Other. The aprepitant-treated patients in this clinical study ranged from 25 to 78 years of age, with a mean age of 53 years; 70 patients were 65 years or older, with 12 patients being over 74 years.

Patients (N = 866) were randomized to either the aprepitant regimen (N = 438) or standard therapy (N = 428). The treatment regimens are defined in Table 8.

[See table 8 above]

The antiemetic activity of EMEND was evaluated based on the following endpoints:

Primary endpoint:

- complete response (defined as no emetic episodes and no use of rescue therapy) in the overall phase (0 to 120 hours post-chemotherapy)

Other prespecified endpoints:

- no emesis (defined as no emetic episodes regardless of use of rescue therapy)
- no nausea (maximum VAS <5 mm on a 0 to 100 mm scale)
- no significant nausea (maximum VAS <25 mm on a 0 to 100 mm scale)
- complete protection (defined as no emetic episodes, no use of rescue therapy, and a maximum nausea visual analogue scale [VAS] score <25 mm on a 0 to 100 mm scale)
- complete response during the acute and delayed phases.

A summary of the key results from this study is shown in Table 9.

Table 9: Percent of Patients Receiving Moderately Emetogenic Chemotherapy Responding by Treatment Group and Phase — Cycle 1

ENDPOINTS	Aprepitant Regimen (N = 433)* %	Standard Therapy (N = 424)* %	p-Value
PRIMARY ENDPOINT†			
Complete Response	51	42	0.015
OTHER PRESPECIFIED ENDPOINTS†			
No Emesis	76	59	NS‡
No Nausea	33	33	NS
No Significant Nausea	61	56	NS
No Rescue Therapy	59	56	NS
Complete Protection	43	37	NS

* N: Number of patients included in the primary analysis of complete response.
† Overall: 0 to 120 hours post-chemotherapy treatment.
‡ NS when adjusted for prespecified multiple comparisons rule; unadjusted p-value <0.001.

In this study, a statistically significantly (p=0.015) higher proportion of patients receiving the aprepitant regimen (51%) in Cycle 1 had a complete response (primary endpoint) during the overall phase compared with patients receiving standard therapy (42%). The difference between treatment groups was primarily driven by the "No Emesis Endpoint", a principal component of this composite primary endpoint. In addition, a higher proportion of patients receiving the aprepitant regimen in Cycle 1 had a complete response during the acute (0-24 hours) and delayed (25-120 hours) phases compared with patients receiving standard therapy; however, the treatment group differences failed to reach statistical significance, after multiplicity adjustments.

Patient-Reported Outcomes: In a phase III study in patients receiving moderately emetogenic chemotherapy, the impact of nausea and vomiting on patients' daily lives was assessed in Cycle 1 using the FLIE. A higher proportion of patients receiving the aprepitant regimen reported minimal or no impact on daily life (64% versus 56%). This difference between treatment groups was primarily driven by the "No Vomiting Domain" of this composite endpoint.

Multiple-Cycle Extension: Patients receiving moderately emetogenic chemotherapy were permitted to continue into the Multiple-Cycle extension of the study for up to 3 additional cycles of chemotherapy. Antiemetic effect for patients receiving the aprepitant regimen is maintained during all cycles.

Postmarketing Trial: In a postmarketing, multicenter, randomized, double-blind, parallel-group, clinical study in 848 cancer patients, the aprepitant regimen (N=430) was compared with a standard of care therapy (N=418) in patients receiving a moderately emetogenic chemotherapy regimen that included any IV dose of oxaliplatin, carboplatin, epirubicin, idarubicin, ifosfamide, irinotecan, daunorubicin, doxorubicin; cyclophosphamide IV (<1500 mg/m²); or cytarabine IV (>1 g/m²).

Of the 430 patients who were randomized to receive the aprepitant regimen, 76% were women and 24% were men. The distribution by race was 67% White, 6% Black or African American, 11% Asian, and 12% multiracial. Classified by ethnicity, 36% were Hispanic and 64% were non-Hispanic. The aprepitant-treated patients in this clinical study ranged from 22 to 85 years of age, with a mean age of 57 years; approximately 59% of the patients were 55 years or older with 32 patients being over 74 years. Patients receiving the aprepitant regimen were receiving chemotherapy for a variety of tumor types including 50% with breast cancer, 21% with gastrointestinal cancers including colorectal cancer, 13% with lung cancer and 6% with gynecological cancers.

The antiemetic activity of EMEND was evaluated based on no vomiting (with or without rescue therapy) in the overall period (0 to 120 hours post-chemotherapy) and complete response (defined as no vomiting and no use of rescue therapy) in the overall period.

A summary of the key results from this study is shown in Table 10.

Table 10: Percent of Patients Receiving Moderately Emetogenic Chemotherapy Responding by Treatment Group for Study 2 — Cycle 1

ENDPOINTS	Aprepitant Regimen (N = 430)* %	Standard Therapy (N = 418)* %	p-Value
No Vomiting Overall	76	62	<0.0001
Complete Response Overall	69	56	0.0003

* N = Number of patients who received chemotherapy treatment, study drug, and had at least one post-treatment efficacy evaluation.

In this study, a statistically significantly higher proportion of patients receiving the aprepitant regimen (76%) in Cycle 1 had no vomiting during the overall phase compared with patients receiving standard therapy (62%). In addition, a higher proportion of patients receiving the aprepitant regimen (69%) in Cycle 1 had a complete response in the overall phase (0-120 hours) compared with patients receiving standard therapy (56%). In the acute phase (0 to 24 hours following initiation of chemotherapy), a higher proportion of patients receiving aprepitant compared to patients receiving standard therapy were observed to have no vomiting (92% and 84%, respectively) and complete response (89% and 80%, respectively). In the delayed phase (25 to 120 hours following initiation of chemotherapy), a higher proportion of patients receiving aprepitant compared to patients receiving standard therapy were observed to have no vomiting (78% and 67%, respectively) and complete response (71% and 61%, respectively).

In a subgroup analysis by tumor type, a numerically higher proportion of patients receiving aprepitant were observed to have no vomiting and complete response compared to patients receiving standard therapy. For gender, the difference in complete response rates between the aprepitant and standard regimen groups was 14% in females (64.5% and 50.3%, respectively) and 4% in males (82.2% and 78.2%, respectively) during the overall phase. A similar difference for gender was observed for the no vomiting endpoint.

14.2 Prevention of Postoperative Nausea and Vomiting (PONV)

In two multicenter, randomized, double-blind, active comparator-controlled, parallel-group clinical studies (PONV Studies 1 and 2), aprepitant was compared with ondansetron for the prevention of postoperative nausea and vomiting in 1658 patients undergoing open abdominal surgery. Patients were randomized to receive 40-mg aprepitant, 125-mg aprepitant, or 4-mg ondansetron. Aprepitant was given orally with 50 mL of water 1 to 3 hours before anesthesia. Ondansetron was given intravenously immediately before induction of anesthesia. A comparison between the 125-mg dose and the 40-mg dose did not demonstrate any additional clinical benefit. The remainder of this section will focus on the results in the 40-mg aprepitant dose recommended for PONV.

Of the 564 patients who received 40-mg aprepitant, 92% were women and 8% were men; of these, 58% were White, 13% Hispanic American, 7% Multi-Racial, 14% Black, 6% Asian, and 2% Other. The age of patients treated with 40-mg aprepitant ranged from 19 to 84 years, with a mean age of 46.1 years. 46 patients were 65 years or older, with 13 patients being 75 years or older.

The antiemetic activity of EMEND was evaluated during the 0 to 48 hour period following the end of surgery. The two pivotal studies were of similar design; however, they differed in terms of study hypothesis, efficacy analyses and geographic location. PONV Study 1 was a multinational study including the U.S., whereas, PONV Study 2 was conducted entirely in the U.S.

Table 11: PONV Study 1 – Response Rates for Select Efficacy Endpoints (Modified-Intention-to-Treat Population)

Treatment	n/m (%)	Aprepitant vs Ondansetron		
		Δ	Odds ratio*	Analysis
Primary Endpoints				
No Vomiting 0 to 24 hours (Superiority) (no emetic episodes)				
Aprepitant 40 mg	246/293 (84.0)	12.6%	2.1	P<0.001†
Ondansetron	200/280 (71.4)			
Complete Response (Non-inferiority: If LB‡ >0.65) (no emesis and no rescue therapy, 0 to 24 hours)				
Aprepitant 40 mg	187/293 (63.8)	8.8%	1.4	LB=1.02
Ondansetron	154/280 (55.0)			
Complete Response (Superiority: If LB >1.0) (no emesis and no rescue therapy, 0 to 24 hours)				
Aprepitant 40 mg	187/293 (63.8)	8.8%	1.4	LB=1.02§
Ondansetron	154/280 (55.0)			
Secondary Endpoint				
No Vomiting 0 to 48 hours (Superiority) (no emetic episodes)				
Aprepitant 40 mg	238/292 (81.5)	15.2%	2.3	P<0.001†
Ondansetron	185/279 (66.3)			

n/m = Number of responders/number of patients in analysis.
Δ Difference (%): Aprepitant 40 mg minus Ondansetron.
* Estimated odds ratio for Aprepitant versus Ondansetron. A value of >1 favors Aprepitant over Ondansetron.
† P-value of two-sided test <0.05.
‡ LB= lower bound of 1-sided 97.5% confidence interval for the odds ratio.
§ Based on the prespecified fixed sequence multiplicity strategy, Aprepitant 40 mg was not superior to Ondansetron.

Efficacy measures in PONV Study 1 included:
- no emesis (defined as no emetic episodes regardless of use of rescue therapy) in the 0 to 24 hours following the end of surgery (primary)
- complete response (defined as no emetic episodes and no use of rescue therapy) in the 0 to 24 hours following the end of surgery (primary)
- no emesis (defined as no emetic episodes regardless of use of rescue therapy) in the 0 to 48 hours following the end of surgery (secondary)
- time to first use of rescue medication in the 0 to 24 hours following the end of surgery (exploratory)
- time to first emesis in the 0 to 48 hours following the end of surgery (exploratory).

A closed testing procedure was applied to control the type I error for the primary endpoints.
The results of the primary and secondary endpoints for 40-mg aprepitant and 4-mg ondansetron are described in Table 11:
[See table 11 above]
The use of aprepitant did not affect the time to first use of rescue medication when compared to ondansetron. However, compared to the ondansetron group, use of aprepitant delayed the time to first vomiting, as depicted in Figure 3.

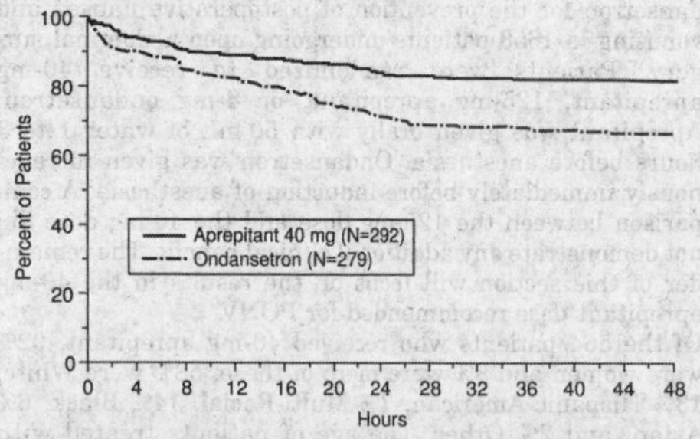

Figure 3: Percent of Patients Who Remain Emesis Free During the 48 Hours Following End of Surgery

Efficacy measures in PONV Study 2 included:
- complete response (defined as no emetic episodes and no use of rescue therapy) in the 0 to 24 hours following the end of surgery (primary)
- no emesis (defined as no emetic episodes regardless of use of rescue therapy) in the 0 to 24 hours following the end of surgery (secondary)
- no use of rescue therapy in the 0 to 24 hours following the end of surgery (secondary)
- no emesis (defined as no emetic episodes regardless of use of rescue therapy) in the 0 to 48 hours following the end of surgery (secondary).

PONV Study 2 failed to satisfy its primary hypothesis that aprepitant is superior to ondansetron in the prevention of PONV as measured by the proportion of patients with complete response in the 24 hours following end of surgery.
The study demonstrated that both dose levels of aprepitant had a clinically meaningful effect with respect to the secondary endpoint "no vomiting" during the first 24 hours after surgery and showed that the use of 40-mg aprepitant was associated with a 16% improvement over ondansetron for the no vomiting endpoint.
[See table 12 at top of next page]

16 HOW SUPPLIED/STORAGE AND HANDLING

No. 3854 — 80-mg capsules: White, opaque, hard gelatin capsule with "461" and "80 mg" printed radially in black ink on the body. They are supplied as follows:
NDC 0006-0461-02 unit-of-use BiPack of 2
NDC 0006-0461-06 unit-dose package of 6.
No. 3855 — 125-mg capsules: Opaque, hard gelatin capsule with white body and pink cap with "462" and "125 mg" printed radially in black ink on the body. They are supplied as follows:
NDC 0006-0462-06 unit-dose package of 6.
No. 3862 — Unit-of-use TriPack containing one 125-mg capsule and two 80-mg capsules.
NDC 0006-3862-03.
No. 6741 — 40-mg capsules: Opaque, hard gelatin capsule with white body and mustard yellow cap with "464" and "40 mg" printed radially in black ink on the body. They are supplied as follows:
NDC 0006-0464-10 unit-of-use package of 1
NDC 0006-0464-05 unit-dose package of 5.

Storage
Store at 20-25°C (68-77°F) [see USP Controlled Room Temperature].

17 PATIENT COUNSELING INFORMATION

"See FDA-Approved Patient Labeling (Patient Information)"
Physicians should instruct their patients to read the patient package insert before starting therapy with EMEND and to reread it each time the prescription is renewed.
Patients should be instructed to take EMEND only as prescribed. For the prevention of chemotherapy induced nausea and vomiting (CINV), patients should be advised to take their first dose (125 mg) of EMEND 1 hour prior to chemotherapy treatment. For the prevention of postoperative nausea and vomiting (PONV), patients should receive their medication (40-mg capsule of EMEND) within 3 hours prior to induction of anesthesia.
Allergic reactions, which may be serious, and may include hives, rash and itching and cause difficulty in breathing or swallowing, have been reported in general use with EMEND. Physicians should instruct their patients to stop taking EMEND and call their doctor right away if they experience an allergic reaction. In addition, severe skin reactions may occur rarely.
EMEND may interact with some drugs including chemotherapy; therefore, patients should be advised to report to their doctor the use of any other prescription, nonprescription medication or herbal products.
Patients on chronic warfarin therapy should be instructed to have their clotting status closely monitored in the 2-week period, particularly at 7 to 10 days, following initiation of the 3-day regimen of EMEND 125 mg/80 mg with each chemotherapy cycle, or following administration of a single 40-mg dose of EMEND for the prevention of postoperative nausea and vomiting.
Administration of EMEND may reduce the efficacy of hormonal contraceptives. Patients should be advised to use alternative or back-up methods of contraception during treatment with EMEND and for 1 month following the last dose of EMEND.

Distributed by:
Merck Sharp & Dohme Corp., a subsidiary of **MERCK & CO., INC.**, Whitehouse Station, NJ 08889, USA
U.S. Patent Nos.: 5,719,147; 6,096,742

USPI-C-08691212R005

Patient Information
EMEND® (EE mend)
(aprepitant)
Capsules

Read the Patient Information that comes with EMEND before you start taking it and each time you refill your prescription. There may be new information. This leaflet does not take the place of talking with your doctor about your medical condition or treatment.

What is EMEND?
EMEND is a prescription medicine used in adults to prevent nausea and vomiting:
- caused by certain anti-cancer (chemotherapy) medicines. When used for this purpose, EMEND is always used with other medicines.
- after surgery.

EMEND is not used to treat nausea and vomiting that you already have.
EMEND should not be used continuously for a long time (chronic use).
It is not known if EMEND is safe and effective in children.

Who should not take EMEND?
Do not take EMEND if you:
- are taking any of the following medicines:
  - ORAP® (pimozide)
  - SELDANE® (terfenadine)
  - HISMANAL® (astemizole)
  - PROPULSID® (cisapride)

  Taking EMEND with any of these medicines could cause serious or life-threatening problems.
- are allergic to any of the ingredients in EMEND. See the end of this leaflet for a list of all the ingredients in EMEND.

What should I tell my doctor before and during treatment with EMEND?
Before you take EMEND, tell your doctor if you:
- have liver problems
- are pregnant or plan to become pregnant. It is not known if EMEND can harm your unborn baby.
  Women who use birth control medicines containing hormones to prevent pregnancy (birth control pills, skin patches, implants, and certain IUDs) should also use a back-up method of birth control during treatment with EMEND and for up to 1 month after using EMEND to prevent pregnancy.
- are breast-feeding. It is not known if EMEND passes into your milk and if it can harm your baby.

Tell your doctor about all the medicines you are taking or plan to take, including prescription and non-prescription medicines, vitamins, and herbal supplements.
EMEND may cause serious life-threatening reactions if used with certain medicines. See the section "Who should not take EMEND?"
EMEND may affect how other medicines work, and other medicines may affect how EMEND works. Ask your doctor or pharmacist before you take any new medicine. They can tell you if it is safe to take the medicine with EMEND.

Table 12: PONV Study 2 (Modified-Intention-to-Treat Population)

Treatment	n/m(%)	Aprepitant vs Ondansetron		
		Δ	Odds ratio*	p-Value
Primary Endpoint				
Complete Response (no emesis and no rescue therapy, 0 to 24 hours)				
Aprepitant 40 mg	111/248 (44.8)	2.5%	1.1	0.61
Ondansetron	104/246 (42.3)			
Secondary Endpoints				
No Vomiting (no emetic episodes, 0 to 24 hours)				
Aprepitant 40 mg	223/248 (89.9)	16.3%	3.2	<0.001†
Ondansetron	181/246 (73.6)			
No Use of Rescue Medication (for established emesis or nausea, 0 to 24 hours)				
Aprepitant 40 mg	112/248 (45.2)	-0.7%	1.0	0.83
Ondansetron	113/246 (45.9)			
No Vomiting 0 to 48 hours (Superiority) (no emetic episodes, 0 to 48 hours)				
Aprepitant 40 mg	209/247 (84.6)	17.7%	2.7	<0.001†
Ondansetron	164/245 (66.9)			

n/m = Number of responders/number of patients in analysis.
Δ Difference (%): Aprepitant 40 mg minus Ondansetron.
* Estimated odds ratio: Aprepitant 40 mg versus Ondansetron.
† Not statistically significant after pre-specified multiplicity adjustment.

Know the medicines you take. Keep a list of them to show your doctor or pharmacist when you get a new medicine.

How should I take EMEND?

- Take EMEND exactly as prescribed.
- If you take too much EMEND, call your doctor, local emergency department or poison control center right away.
- If you are receiving cancer chemotherapy, EMEND is taken as 3 doses over 3 days - starting on the day you have chemotherapy, and the two days after chemotherapy. There are two ways that your doctor may prescribe EMEND for you:

1. Capsules of EMEND by mouth for all 3 doses:
   - You should get a package that has three capsules of EMEND.
   - Day 1 (Day of chemotherapy): Take one 125-mg capsule of EMEND (white and pink) by mouth 1 hour before you start your chemotherapy treatment.
   - Day 2 and Day 3 (the two days after chemotherapy): Take one 80-mg capsule of EMEND (white) by mouth, each morning for the 2 days after your chemotherapy treatment.

   Or
2. Intravenous (IV) injection into a vein the first day, then capsules by mouth on the two days after chemotherapy:
   - Day 1 (Day of chemotherapy): EMEND will be given to you by intravenous (IV) injection in your vein 30 minutes before you start your chemotherapy treatment.
   - You should get a package that has two capsules of EMEND.
   - Day 2 and Day 3 (the two days after chemotherapy): Take one 80-mg capsule of EMEND (white) by mouth, each morning for the 2 days after your chemotherapy treatment.

- If you are receiving chemotherapy, EMEND may be taken with or without food.
- If you are having surgery:
  - Your doctor will prescribe a 40-mg capsule of EMEND for you before surgery. You take EMEND within three hours before surgery.
  - Follow your doctor's instructions about restrictions on eating and drinking before surgery.
- If you take the blood thinner medicine warfarin sodium (COUMADIN®, JANTOVEN®), your doctor may do blood tests after you take EMEND to check your blood clotting.

What are the possible side effects of EMEND?

EMEND may cause serious side effects, including:

- **Serious allergic reactions.** Allergic reactions can happen with EMEND and may be serious. Stop taking EMEND and call your doctor right away if you have any of these signs or symptoms of an allergic reaction:
  - hives
  - rash
  - itching
  - trouble breathing or swallowing.
- Severe skin reactions may occur rarely.

In people taking EMEND to prevent nausea and vomiting caused by chemotherapy, the most common side effects of EMEND include:

- tiredness
- nausea
- hiccups
- constipation
- diarrhea
- loss of appetite
- headache
- hair loss

In people taking EMEND to prevent nausea and vomiting after surgery, the most common side effects are:

- constipation
- nausea
- itch
- fever
- low blood pressure
- headache

Tell your doctor if you have any side effect that bothers you or that does not go away. These are not all of the possible side effects of EMEND. For more information ask your doctor or pharmacist.

Call your doctor for medical advice about side effects. You may report side effects to FDA at 1-800-FDA-1088.

How should I store EMEND?

- Store EMEND at room temperature, between 68°F and 77°F (20°C and 25°C).
- **Keep EMEND and all medicines out of the reach of children.**

General information about EMEND

Medicines are sometimes prescribed for conditions that are not mentioned in patient information leaflets. Do not use EMEND for a condition for which it was not prescribed. Do not give EMEND to other people, even if they have the same symptoms you have. It may harm them.

This Patient Information leaflet summarizes the most important information about EMEND. If you would like to know more information, talk with your doctor. You can ask your doctor or pharmacist for information about EMEND that is written for health professionals. For more information about EMEND call 1-800-622-4477 or go to www.emend.com.

What are the ingredients in EMEND?

Active ingredient: aprepitant

Inactive ingredients: sucrose, microcrystalline cellulose, hydroxypropyl cellulose and sodium lauryl sulfate. The capsule shell excipients are gelatin, titanium dioxide, and may contain sodium lauryl sulfate and silicon dioxide. The 125-mg capsule shell also contains red ferric oxide and yellow ferric oxide. The 40-mg capsule shell also contains yellow ferric oxide.

Distributed by:
Merck Sharp & Dohme Corp., a subsidiary of **MERCK & CO., INC.,** Whitehouse Station, NJ 08889, USA
U.S. Patent Nos.: 5,719,147; 6,096,742

The brands listed in the above sections "Who should not take EMEND?" and "How should I take EMEND?" are the registered trademarks of their respective owners and are not trademarks of Merck Sharp & Dohme Corp., a subsidiary of Merck & Co., Inc.

Revised: 07/2012
USPPI-C-08691207R004

Shown in Product Identification Guide, page 307

EMEND ℞

[ē′mĕnd]

(fosaprepitant dimeglumine)
for Injection, for intravenous use

HIGHLIGHTS OF PRESCRIBING INFORMATION
These highlights do not include all the information needed to use EMEND safely and effectively. See full prescribing information for EMEND.
EMEND (fosaprepitant dimeglumine) for Injection, for intravenous use
Initial U.S. Approval: 2008

INDICATIONS AND USAGE

EMEND® for Injection is a substance P/neurokinin-1 (NK_1) receptor antagonist, in combination with other antiemetic agents, is indicated in adults for the (1):

- prevention of acute and delayed nausea and vomiting associated with initial and repeat courses of highly emetogenic cancer chemotherapy (HEC) including high-dose cisplatin
- prevention of nausea and vomiting associated with initial and repeat courses of moderately emetogenic cancer chemotherapy (MEC)

Limitations of Use (1)

- Chronic continuous administration is not recommended.

DOSAGE AND ADMINISTRATION

- *HEC (Single Dose Regimen):* EMEND for Injection (150 mg) is administered on Day 1 only as an infusion **over 20-30 minutes** initiated approximately 30 minutes prior to chemotherapy. No capsules of EMEND are administered on Days 2 and 3. EMEND for Injection is part of a regimen to prevent nausea and vomiting induced by HEC that includes a corticosteroid and a 5-HT_3 antagonist. (2.1)
- *HEC and MEC (3-Day Dosing Regimen):* EMEND for Injection (115 mg) is administered on Day 1 as an infusion **over 15 minutes** initiated approximately 30 minutes prior to chemotherapy. EMEND capsules (80 mg) are given orally on Days 2 and 3. EMEND for Injection and EMEND capsules are part of a regimen to prevent nausea and vomiting induced by HEC or MEC that includes a corticosteroid and a 5-HT_3 antagonist. (2.1, 2.2)

DOSAGE FORMS AND STRENGTHS

One single dose glass vial supplied as sterile lyophilized powder for intravenous use only after reconstitution and dilution: 150 mg and 115 mg (3)

CONTRAINDICATIONS

- Known hypersensitivity to any component of this drug. (4)
- Do not use concurrently with pimozide or cisapride, since inhibition of CYP3A4 by aprepitant may result in elevated plasma concentrations of these drugs, potentially causing serious or life-threatening reactions. (4)

WARNINGS AND PRECAUTIONS

- Fosaprepitant should be used with caution in patients receiving concomitant medications that are primarily metabolized through CYP3A4. (5.1)
- Immediate hypersensitivity reactions may occur during infusion. Patients have generally responded to discontinuation. It is not recommended to reinitiate the infusion. (5.2)
- Coadministration of fosaprepitant or aprepitant with warfarin (a CYP2C9 substrate) may result in a clinically significant decrease in International Normalized Ratio (INR) of prothrombin time. (5.3)
- The efficacy of hormonal contraceptives during and for 28 days following the last dose of fosaprepitant or aprepitant may be reduced. Alternative or back-up methods of contraception should be used. (5.4)

Table 1: Recommended dosing (Single Dose Regimen of EMEND) for the prevention of nausea and vomiting associated with highly emetogenic cancer chemotherapy

	Day 1	Day 2	Day 3	Day 4
EMEND	150 mg intravenous	none	none	none
Dexamethasone*	12 mg orally	8 mg orally	**8 mg orally twice daily**	**8 mg orally twice daily**
5-HT_3 antagonist	See the package insert for the selected 5-HT_3 antagonist for appropriate dosing information.	none	none	none

* Dexamethasone should be administered 30 minutes prior to chemotherapy treatment on Day 1 and in the morning on Days 2 through 4. The dose of dexamethasone accounts for drug interactions.

Table 2: Recommended dosing (3-Day Dosing Regimen of EMEND) for the prevention of nausea and vomiting associated with highly emetogenic cancer chemotherapy

	Day 1	Day 2	Day 3	Day 4
EMEND	115 mg intravenous	80 mg orally	80 mg orally	none
Dexamethasone*	12 mg orally	8 mg orally	**8 mg orally once daily**	**8 mg orally once daily**
5-HT_3 antagonist	See the package insert for the selected 5-HT_3 antagonist for appropriate dosing information.	none	none	none

* Dexamethasone should be administered 30 minutes prior to chemotherapy treatment on Day 1 and in the morning on Days 2 through 4. The dose of dexamethasone accounts for drug interactions.

ADVERSE REACTIONS

- Adverse reactions for the CINV oral aprepitant regimen in conjunction with highly and moderately emetogenic chemotherapy (incidence ≥1% and greater than standard therapy) are: hiccups, asthenia/fatigue, AST/ALT increased, headache, constipation, anorexia, dyspepsia, diarrhea, eructation. (6.1)
- Adverse reactions reported for EMEND for Injection were generally similar to that seen in prior HEC studies with oral aprepitant. In addition, infusion site reactions (3%) occurred with EMEND for Injection. (6.1)

To report SUSPECTED ADVERSE REACTIONS, contact Merck Sharp & Dohme Corp., a subsidiary of Merck & Co., Inc., at 1-877-888-4231 or FDA at 1-800-FDA-1088 or www.fda.gov/medwatch.

DRUG INTERACTIONS

- Coadministration of fosaprepitant or aprepitant with drugs that inhibit or induce CYP3A4 activity may result in increased or reduced plasma concentrations of aprepitant, respectively. (7.1, 7.2)
- Coadministration of EMEND for Injection with drugs that are metabolized by CYP2C9 (e.g., warfarin, tolbutamide), may result in lower plasma concentrations of these drugs. (7.1)

See 17 for PATIENT COUNSELING INFORMATION and FDA-approved patient labeling

Revised: 12/2012

FULL PRESCRIBING INFORMATION: CONTENTS*

*** Sections or subsections omitted from the full prescribing information are not listed**

FULL PRESCRIBING INFORMATION

1 INDICATIONS AND USAGE

EMEND® for Injection is a substance P/neurokinin-1 (NK_1) receptor antagonist indicated in adults for use in combination with other antiemetic agents for the:

- prevention of acute and delayed nausea and vomiting associated with initial and repeat courses of highly emetogenic cancer chemotherapy (HEC) including high-dose cisplatin *[see Dosage and Administration (2.1)]*
- prevention of nausea and vomiting associated with initial and repeat courses of moderately emetogenic cancer chemotherapy (MEC) *[see Dosage and Administration (2.2)]*.

Limitations of Use

EMEND for Injection has not been studied for the treatment of established nausea and vomiting.

Chronic continuous administration is not recommended *[see Warnings and Precautions (5.5)]*.

2 DOSAGE AND ADMINISTRATION

2.1 Prevention of Nausea and Vomiting Associated with Highly Emetogenic Chemotherapy (HEC)

EMEND for Injection 150 mg (Single Dose Regimen of EMEND):

EMEND for Injection 150 mg is administered intravenously on Day 1 only as an infusion **over 20-30 minutes** initiated approximately 30 minutes prior to chemotherapy. No capsules of EMEND are administered on Days 2 and 3. EMEND for Injection should be administered in conjunction with a corticosteroid and a 5-HT_3 antagonist as specified in Table 1. The recommended dosage of dexamethasone with EMEND for Injection 150 mg differs from the recommended dosage of dexamethasone with EMEND for Injection 115 mg on Days 3 and 4. The package insert for the co-administered 5-HT_3 antagonist must be consulted prior to initiation of treatment with EMEND for Injection.

[See table 1 above]

EMEND for Injection 115 mg (3-Day Dosing Regimen of EMEND):

EMEND for Injection 115 mg is administered on Day 1 only as an infusion **over 15 minutes** initiated 30 minutes prior to chemotherapy. Capsules of EMEND 80 mg should be administered on Days 2 and 3. EMEND for Injection 115 mg should be administered in conjunction with a corticosteroid and a 5-HT_3 antagonist as specified in Table 2. The recommended dosage of dexamethasone with EMEND for Injection 115 mg differs from the recommended dosage of dexamethasone with EMEND for Injection 150 mg on Days 3 and 4. The package insert for the co-administered 5-HT_3 antagonist must be consulted prior to initiation of treatment with EMEND for Injection.

Capsules of EMEND 125 mg may be substituted for EMEND for Injection 115 mg on Day 1.

[See table 2 above]

2.2 Prevention of Nausea and Vomiting Associated with Moderately Emetogenic Chemotherapy (MEC)

EMEND for Injection 115 mg (3-Day Dosing Regimen of EMEND):

EMEND for Injection 115 mg is administered on Day 1 only as an infusion **over 15 minutes** initiated 30 minutes prior to chemotherapy. Capsules of EMEND 80 mg should be administered on Days 2 and 3. EMEND for Injection 115 mg should be administered in conjunction with a corticosteroid and a 5-HT_3 antagonist as specified in Table 3. The recommended dosage of dexamethasone with EMEND for Injection 115 mg differs from the recommended dosage of dexamethasone with EMEND for Injection 150 mg on Days 3 and 4. The package insert for the co-administered 5-HT_3 antagonist must be consulted prior to initiation of treatment with EMEND for Injection.

Capsules of EMEND 125 mg may be substituted for EMEND for Injection 115 mg on Day 1.

Table 3: Recommended dosing (3-Day Dosing Regimen of EMEND) for the prevention of nausea and vomiting associated with moderately emetogenic cancer chemotherapy

	Day 1	Day 2	Day 3
EMEND	115 mg intravenous	80 mg orally	80 mg orally
Dexamethasone*	12 mg orally	none	none
5-HT_3 antagonist	See the package insert for the selected 5-HT_3 antagonist for appropriate dosing information.	none	none

* Dexamethasone should be administered 30 minutes prior to chemotherapy treatment on Day 1. The dose of dexamethasone accounts for drug interactions.

2.3 Preparation of EMEND for Injection

Table 4: Preparation Instructions for EMEND for Injection (115 mg and 150 mg)

	115 mg	***150 mg***
Step 1	Aseptically inject 5 mL 0.9% Sodium Chloride for Injection (normal saline) into the vial. Assure that normal saline is added to the vial along the vial wall in order to prevent foaming. Swirl the vial gently. Avoid shaking and jetting saline into the vial.	Aseptically inject 5 mL 0.9% Sodium Chloride for Injection (normal saline) into the vial. Assure that normal saline is added to the vial along the vial wall in order to prevent foaming. Swirl the vial gently. Avoid shaking and jetting saline into the vial.

Step 2	Aseptically prepare an infusion bag filled with **110 mL** of normal saline.	Aseptically prepare an infusion bag filled with **145 mL** of normal saline.
Step 3	Aseptically withdraw the entire volume from the vial and transfer it into the infusion bag containing **110 mL** of normal saline to yield a total volume of **115 mL** and a final concentration of 1 mg/1 mL.	Aseptically withdraw the entire volume from the vial and transfer it into the infusion bag containing **145 mL** of normal saline to yield a total volume of **150 mL** and a final concentration of 1 mg/1 mL.
Step 4	Gently invert the bag 2-3 times.	Gently invert the bag 2-3 times.
	Note: *The differences in preparation for each dose are displayed as bolded text.*	

The reconstituted final drug solution is stable for 24 hours at ambient room temperature (at or below 25°C).

Parenteral drug products should be inspected visually for particulate matter and discoloration before administration whenever solution and container permit.

Caution: EMEND for Injection should not be mixed or reconstituted with solutions for which physical and chemical compatibility have not been established. EMEND for Injection is incompatible with any solutions containing divalent cations (e.g., Ca^{2+}, Mg^{2+}), including Lactated Ringer's Solution and Hartmann's Solution.

3 DOSAGE FORMS AND STRENGTHS

One 150-mg single dose glass vial: White to off-white lyophilized solid (Sterile lyophilized powder for intravenous use only after reconstitution and dilution).

One 115-mg single dose glass vial: White to off-white lyophilized solid (Sterile lyophilized powder for intravenous use only after reconstitution and dilution).

4 CONTRAINDICATIONS

4.1 Hypersensitivity

EMEND for Injection is contraindicated in patients who are hypersensitive to EMEND for Injection, aprepitant, polysorbate 80 or any other components of the product. Known hypersensitivity reactions include: flushing, erythema, dyspnea, and anaphylactic reactions *[see Adverse Reactions (6.2)]*.

4.2 Concomitant Use with Pimozide or Cisapride

Aprepitant, when administered orally, is a moderate cytochrome P450 isoenzyme 3A4 (CYP3A4) inhibitor following the 3-day antiemetic dosing regimen for CINV. Since fosaprepitant is rapidly converted to aprepitant, do not use fosaprepitant concurrently with pimozide or cisapride. Inhibition of CYP3A4 by aprepitant could result in elevated plasma concentrations of these drugs, potentially causing serious or life-threatening reactions *[see Drug Interactions (7.1)]*.

5 WARNINGS AND PRECAUTIONS

5.1 CYP3A4 Interactions

Fosaprepitant is rapidly converted to aprepitant, which is a moderate inhibitor of CYP3A4 when administered as a 3-day antiemetic dosing regimen for CINV. Fosaprepitant should be used with caution in patients receiving concomitant medications that are primarily metabolized through CYP3A4. Inhibition of CYP3A4 by aprepitant or fosaprepitant could result in elevated plasma concentrations of these concomitant medications. When fosaprepitant is used concomitantly with another CYP3A4 inhibitor, aprepitant plasma concentrations could be elevated. When aprepitant is used concomitantly with medications that induce CYP3A4 activity, aprepitant plasma concentrations could be reduced, and this may result in decreased efficacy of aprepitant *[see Drug Interactions (7.1)]*.

Chemotherapy agents that are known to be metabolized by CYP3A4 include docetaxel, paclitaxel, etoposide, irinotecan, ifosfamide, imatinib, vinorelbine, vinblastine and vincristine. In clinical studies, the oral aprepitant regimen was administered commonly with etoposide, vinorelbine, or paclitaxel. The doses of these agents were not adjusted to account for potential drug interactions.

In separate pharmacokinetic studies, no clinically significant change in docetaxel or vinorelbine pharmacokinetics was observed when the oral aprepitant regimen was coadministered.

Due to the small number of patients in clinical studies who received the CYP3A4 substrates vinblastine, vincristine, or ifosfamide, particular caution and careful monitoring are advised in patients receiving these agents or other chemotherapy agents metabolized primarily by CYP3A4 that were not studied *[see Drug Interactions (7.1)]*.

5.2 Hypersensitivity Reactions

Isolated reports of immediate hypersensitivity reactions including flushing, erythema, dyspnea, and anaphylaxis have occurred during infusion of fosaprepitant. These hypersensitivity reactions have generally responded to discontinuation of the infusion and administration of appropriate therapy. Reinitiation of the infusion is not recommended in patients who experience these symptoms during first-time use.

5.3 Coadministration with Warfarin (a CYP2C9 substrate)

Coadministration of fosaprepitant or aprepitant with warfarin may result in a clinically significant decrease in International Normalized Ratio (INR) of prothrombin time. In patients on chronic warfarin therapy, the INR should be closely monitored in the 2-week period, particularly at 7 to 10 days, following initiation of fosaprepitant with each chemotherapy cycle *[see Drug Interactions (7.1)]*.

5.4 Coadministration with Hormonal Contraceptives

Upon coadministration with fosaprepitant or aprepitant, the efficacy of hormonal contraceptives may be reduced during and for 28 days following the last dose of either fosaprepitant or aprepitant. Alternative or back-up methods of contraception should be used during treatment with and for 1 month following the last dose of fosaprepitant or aprepitant *[see Drug Interactions (7.1)]*.

5.5 Chronic Continuous Use

Chronic continuous use of EMEND for Injection for prevention of nausea and vomiting is not recommended because it has not been studied; and because the drug interaction profile may change during chronic continuous use.

6 ADVERSE REACTIONS

6.1 Clinical Trials Experience

Because clinical trials are conducted under widely varying conditions, adverse reaction rates observed in the clinical trials of a drug cannot be directly compared to rates in the clinical trials of another drug and may not reflect the rates observed in clinical practice.

Since EMEND for Injection is converted to aprepitant, those adverse reactions associated with aprepitant might also be expected to occur with EMEND for Injection.

The overall safety of fosaprepitant was evaluated in approximately 1100 individuals and the overall safety of aprepitant was evaluated in approximately 6500 individuals.

Oral Aprepitant

Highly Emetogenic Chemotherapy (HEC)

In 2 well-controlled clinical trials in patients receiving highly emetogenic cancer chemotherapy, 544 patients were treated with aprepitant during Cycle 1 of chemotherapy and 413 of these patients continued into the Multiple-Cycle extension for up to 6 cycles of chemotherapy. Oral aprepitant was given in combination with ondansetron and dexamethasone.

In Cycle 1, adverse reactions were reported in approximately 17% of patients treated with the aprepitant regimen compared with approximately 13% of patients treated with standard therapy. Treatment was discontinued due to adverse reactions in 0.6% of patients treated with the aprepitant regimen compared with 0.4% of patients treated with standard therapy.

The most common adverse reactions reported in patients treated with the aprepitant regimen with an incidence ≥1% and greater than standard therapy are listed in Table 5.

Table 5: Adverse Reactions (incidence ≥1%) in patients receiving HEC with a greater incidence in the Aprepitant Regimen relative to Standard Therapy

	Aprepitant Regimen (N=544)	Standard Therapy (N=550)
Respiratory System		
hiccups	4.6	2.9
Body as a Whole/ Site Unspecified		
asthenia/fatigue	2.9	1.6
Investigations		
ALT increased	2.8	1.5
AST increased	1.1	0.9
Digestive System		
constipation	2.2	2.0
dyspepsia	1.5	0.7
diarrhea	1.1	0.9
Nervous System		
headache	2.2	1.8
Metabolism and Nutrition		
anorexia	2.0	0.5

A listing of adverse reactions in the aprepitant regimen (incidence <1%) that occurred at a greater incidence than standard therapy are presented in the *Less Common Adverse Reactions* subsection below.

In an additional active-controlled clinical study in 1169 patients receiving aprepitant and highly emetogenic chemotherapy, the adverse experience profile was generally similar to that seen in the other HEC studies with aprepitant.

Moderately Emetogenic Chemotherapy (MEC)

In 2 well-controlled clinical trials in patients receiving moderately emetogenic cancer chemotherapy, 868 patients were treated with the aprepitant regimen during Cycle 1 of chemotherapy and 686 of these patients continued into extensions for up to 4 cycles of chemotherapy. In both studies, oral aprepitant was given in combination with ondansetron and dexamethasone (aprepitant regimen).

In the combined analysis of Cycle 1 data for these 2 studies, adverse reactions were reported in approximately 14% of patients treated with the aprepitant regimen compared with approximately 15% of patients treated with standard therapy. Treatment was discontinued due to adverse reactions in 0.7% of patients treated with the aprepitant regimen compared with 0.2% of patients treated with standard therapy.

The most common adverse reactions reported in patients treated with the aprepitant regimen with an incidence ≥1% and greater than standard therapy are listed in Table 6.

Table 6: Adverse Reactions (incidence ≥1%) in patients receiving MEC with a greater incidence in the Aprepitant Regimen relative to Standard Therapy

	Aprepitant Regimen (N=868)	Standard Therapy (N=846)
Gastrointestinal disorders		
eructation	1.0	0.1
General disorders and administration site conditions		
fatigue	1.4	0.9

A listing of adverse reactions in the aprepitant regimen (incidence <1%) that occurred at a greater incidence than standard therapy are presented in the *Less Common Adverse Reactions* subsection below.

Less Common Adverse Reactions

Adverse reactions reported in either HEC or MEC studies in patients treated with the aprepitant regimen with an incidence <1% and greater than standard therapy are listed in Table 7.

Table 7: Adverse Reactions (incidence <1%) in patients observed in either HEC or MEC Studies with a greater incidence in the Aprepitant Regimen relative to Standard Therapy

Infection and infestations	candidiasis, staphylococcal infection
Blood and the lymphatic system disorders	anemia, febrile neutropenia
Metabolism and nutrition disorders	weight gain, polydipsia
Psychiatric disorders	disorientation, euphoria, anxiety
Nervous system disorders	dizziness, dream abnormality, cognitive disorder, lethargy, somnolence
Eye disorders	conjunctivitis
Ear and labyrinth disorders	tinnitus
Cardiac disorders	bradycardia, cardiovascular disorder, palpitations

Vascular disorders	hot flush, flushing
Respiratory, thoracic and mediastinal disorders	pharyngitis, sneezing, cough, postnasal drip, throat irritation
Gastrointestinal disorders	nausea, acid reflux, dysgeusia, epigastric discomfort, obstipation, gastroesophageal reflux disease, perforating duodenal ulcer, vomiting, abdominal pain, dry mouth, abdominal distension, faeces hard, neutropenic colitis, flatulence, stomatitis
Skin and subcutaneous tissue disorders	rash, acne, photosensitivity, hyperhidrosis, oily skin, pruritus, skin lesion
Musculoskeletal and connective tissue disorders	muscle cramp, myalgia, muscular weakness
Renal and urinary disorders	polyuria, dysuria, pollakiuria
General disorders and administration site condition	edema, chest discomfort, malaise, thirst, chills, gait disturbance
Investigations	alkaline phosphatase increased, hyperglycemia, microscopic hematuria, hyponatremia, weight decreased, neutrophil count decreased

In another chemotherapy induced nausea and vomiting (CINV) study, Stevens-Johnson syndrome was reported as a serious adverse reaction in a patient receiving aprepitant with cancer chemotherapy.

The adverse experience profiles in the Multiple-Cycle extensions of HEC and MEC studies for up to 6 cycles of chemotherapy were similar to that observed in Cycle 1.

Fosaprepitant

In an active-controlled clinical study in patients receiving highly emetogenic chemotherapy, safety was evaluated for 1143 patients receiving the 1-day regimen of EMEND for Injection 150 mg compared to 1169 patients receiving the 3-day regimen of EMEND (aprepitant). The safety profile was generally similar to that seen in prior HEC studies with aprepitant. However, infusion-site reactions occurred at a higher incidence in patients in the fosaprepitant group (3.0%) compared to those in the aprepitant group (0.5%). The reported infusion-site reactions included infusion-site erythema, infusion-site pruritus, infusion-site pain, infusion-site induration, and infusion-site thrombophlebitis.

The following additional adverse reactions occurred with fosaprepitant 150 mg and were not reported with the oral aprepitant regimen in the corresponding section above.

Table 8: Adverse Reactions (incidence >0.1%) in patients receiving Fosaprepitant 150 mg and not reported above for the Oral Aprepitant Regimen

General disorders and administration site conditions	infusion site erythema, infusion site pruritus, infusion site induration, infusion site pain
Investigations	blood pressure increased
Skin and subcutaneous tissue disorders	erythema
Vascular disorders	thrombophlebitis (predominantly, infusion-site thrombophlebitis)

Other Studies with Postoperative Nausea and Vomiting

In well-controlled clinical studies in patients receiving general balanced anesthesia, 564 patients were administered 40-mg aprepitant orally and 538 patients were administered 4-mg ondansetron intravenously.

Adverse reactions were reported in approximately 4% of patients treated with 40-mg aprepitant compared with approximately 6% of patients treated with 4-mg ondansetron intravenously.

In patients treated with aprepitant, increased ALT (1.1%) was seen at a greater incidence than with ondansetron (1.0%). The following additional adverse reactions were observed in patients treated with aprepitant at an incidence <1% and greater than with ondansetron.

Table 9: Adverse Reactions (incidence <1%) in patients receiving Aprepitant 40 mg with a greater incidence in the Aprepitant group relative to ondansetron

Psychiatric disorders	insomnia
Nervous system disorders	dysarthria, hypoesthesia, sensory disturbance
Eye disorders	miosis, visual acuity reduced
Cardiac disorders	bradycardia
Respiratory, thoracic and mediastinal disorders	dyspnea, wheezing
Gastrointestinal disorders	abdominal pain upper, bowel sounds abnormal, dry mouth, nausea, stomach discomfort

In addition, two serious adverse reactions were reported in postoperative nausea and vomiting (PONV) clinical studies in patients taking a higher dose of aprepitant: one case of constipation, and one case of subileus.

Other Studies

Angioedema and urticaria were reported as serious adverse reactions in a patient receiving aprepitant in a non-CINV/non-PONV study.

6.2 Postmarketing Experience

The following adverse reactions have been identified during post approval use of fosaprepitant and aprepitant. Because these reactions are reported voluntarily from a population of uncertain size, it is not always possible to reliably estimate their frequency or establish a causal relationship to drug exposure.

Skin and subcutaneous tissue disorders: pruritus, rash, urticaria, rarely Stevens-Johnson syndrome/toxic epidermal necrolysis.

Immune system disorders: hypersensitivity reactions including anaphylactic reactions.

7 DRUG INTERACTIONS

Drug interactions following administration of fosaprepitant are likely to occur with drugs that interact with oral aprepitant.

Aprepitant is a substrate, a moderate inhibitor, and an inducer of CYP3A4 when administered as a 3-day antiemetic dosing regimen for CINV. Aprepitant is also an inducer of CYP2C9.

Fosaprepitant 150 mg, given as a single dose, is a weak inhibitor of CYP3A4, and does not induce CYP3A4. Fosaprepitant or aprepitant is unlikely to interact with drugs that are substrates for the P-glycoprotein transporter.

The following information was derived from data with oral aprepitant, two studies conducted with fosaprepitant and oral midazolam, and one study conducted with fosaprepitant and dexamethasone.

7.1 Effect of Fosaprepitant/Aprepitant on the Pharmacokinetics of Other Agents

CYP3A4 substrates:

Aprepitant, as a moderate inhibitor of CYP3A4, and fosaprepitant 150 mg, as a weak inhibitor of CYP3A4, can increase plasma concentrations of concomitantly coadministered oral medications that are metabolized through CYP3A4 *[see Contraindications (4)]*.

5-HT_3 antagonists:

In clinical drug interaction studies, aprepitant did not have clinically important effects on the pharmacokinetics of ondansetron, granisetron, or hydrodolasetron (the active metabolite of dolasetron).

Corticosteroids:

Dexamethasone: Fosaprepitant 150 mg administered as a single intravenous dose on Day 1 increased the $AUC_{0\text{-}24hr}$ of dexamethasone, administered as a single 8-mg oral dose on Days 1, 2, and 3, by approximately 2-fold on Days 1 and 2. The oral dexamethasone dose on Days 1 and 2 should be reduced by approximately 50% when coadministered with fosaprepitant 150-mg intravenous on Day 1.

An oral aprepitant regimen of 125 mg on Day 1, and 80 mg/day on Days 2 through 5, coadministered with 20-mg oral dexamethasone on Day 1 and 8-mg oral dexamethasone on Days 2 through 5, increased the AUC of dexamethasone by 2.2-fold on Days 1 and 5. The oral dexamethasone doses should be reduced by approximately 50% when coadministered with a regimen of fosaprepitant 115 mg followed by aprepitant.

Methylprednisolone: An oral aprepitant regimen of 125 mg on Day 1 and 80 mg/day on Days 2 and 3 increased the AUC of methylprednisolone by 1.34-fold on Day 1 and by 2.5-fold on Day 3, when methylprednisolone was coadministered intravenously as 125 mg on Day 1 and orally as 40 mg on Days 2 and 3. The intravenous methylprednisolone dose should be reduced by approximately 25%, and the oral methylprednisolone dose should be reduced by approximately 50% when coadministered with a regimen of fosaprepitant 115 mg followed by aprepitant.

Chemotherapeutic agents:

Docetaxel: In a pharmacokinetic study, oral aprepitant (CINV regimen) did not influence the pharmacokinetics of docetaxel *[see Warnings and Precautions (5.1)]*.

Vinorelbine: In a pharmacokinetic study, oral aprepitant (CINV regimen) did not influence the pharmacokinetics of vinorelbine to a clinically significant degree *[see Warnings and Precautions (5.1)]*.

Oral contraceptives: When oral aprepitant, ondansetron, and dexamethasone were coadministered with an oral contraceptive containing ethinyl estradiol and norethindrone, the trough concentrations of both ethinyl estradiol and norethindrone were reduced by as much as 64% for 3 weeks post-treatment.

The coadministration of fosaprepitant or aprepitant may reduce the efficacy of hormonal contraceptives (these can include birth control pills, skin patches, implants, and certain IUDs) during and for 28 days after administration of the last dose of fosaprepitant or aprepitant. Alternative or back-up methods of contraception should be used during treatment with and for 1 month following the last dose of fosaprepitant or aprepitant.

Midazolam:

Interactions between aprepitant or fosaprepitant and coadministered midazolam are listed in the table below (increase is indicated as "↑", decrease as "↓", no change as "↔").

Table 10: Pharmacokinetic Interaction Data for Fosaprepitant/Aprepitant and Coadministered Midazolam

Dose of fosaprepitant/ aprepitant	Dose of Midazolam	Observed Drug Interactions
fosaprepitant 150 mg on Day 1	oral 2 mg on Days 1 and 4	AUC ↑ 1.8-fold on Day 1 and AUC ↔ on Day 4
fosaprepitant 100 mg on Day 1	oral 2 mg	oral midazolam AUC ↑ 1.6-fold
oral aprepitant 125 mg on Day 1 and 80 mg on Days 2 to 5	oral 2 mg SD on Days 1 and 5	oral midazolam AUC ↑ 2.3-fold on Day 1 and ↑ 3.3-fold on Day 5
oral aprepitant 125 mg on Day 1 and 80 mg on Days 2 and 3	intravenous 2 mg prior to 3-day regimen of aprepitant and on Days 4, 8 and 15	intravenous midazolam AUC ↑ 25% on Day 4, AUC ↓ 19% on Day 8 and AUC ↓ 4% on Day 15
oral aprepitant 125 mg	intravenous 2 mg given 1 hour after aprepitant	intravenous midazolam AUC ↑ 1.5-fold

A difference of less than 2-fold increase of midazolam AUC was not considered clinically important.

The potential effects of increased plasma concentrations of midazolam or other benzodiazepines metabolized via CYP3A4 (alprazolam, triazolam) should be considered when coadministering these agents with fosaprepitant or aprepitant.

CYP2C9 substrates (Warfarin, Tolbutamide):

Warfarin: A single 125-mg dose of oral aprepitant was administered on Day 1 and 80 mg/day on Days 2 and 3 to healthy subjects who were stabilized on chronic warfarin therapy. Although there was no effect of oral aprepitant on the plasma AUC of R(+) or S(-) warfarin determined on Day 3, there was a 34% decrease in S(-) warfarin trough concentration accompanied by a 14% decrease in the prothrombin time (reported as International Normalized Ratio or INR) 5 days after completion of dosing with oral aprepitant. In patients on chronic warfarin therapy, the prothrombin time (INR) should be closely monitored in the 2-week period, particularly at 7 to 10 days, following initiation of fosaprepitant with each chemotherapy cycle.

Tolbutamide: Oral aprepitant, when given as 125 mg on Day 1 and 80 mg/day on Days 2 and 3, decreased the AUC of tolbutamide by 23% on Day 4, 28% on Day 8, and 15% on Day 15, when a single dose of tolbutamide 500 mg was administered orally prior to the administration of the 3-day regimen of oral aprepitant and on Days 4, 8, and 15.

7.2 Effect of Other Agents on the Pharmacokinetics of Aprepitant

Aprepitant is a substrate for CYP3A4; therefore, coadministration of fosaprepitant or aprepitant with drugs that inhibit CYP3A4 activity may result in increased plasma concentrations of aprepitant. Consequently, concomitant administration of fosaprepitant or aprepitant with strong CYP3A4 inhibitors (e.g., ketoconazole, itraconazole, nefazodone, troleandomycin, clarithromycin, ritonavir, nelfinavir) should be approached with caution. Because moderate CYP3A4 inhibitors (e.g., diltiazem) result in a 2-fold increase in plasma concentrations of aprepitant, concomitant administration should also be approached with caution.

Aprepitant is a substrate for CYP3A4; therefore, coadministration of fosaprepitant or aprepitant with drugs that strongly induce CYP3A4 activity (e.g., rifampin, carbamazepine, phenytoin) may result in reduced plasma concentrations and decreased efficacy.

Ketoconazole: When a single 125-mg dose of oral aprepitant was administered on Day 5 of a 10-day regimen of 400 mg/day of ketoconazole, a strong CYP3A4 inhibitor, the AUC of aprepitant increased approximately 5-fold and the mean terminal half-life of aprepitant increased approximately 3-fold. Concomitant administration of fosaprepitant or aprepitant with strong CYP3A4 inhibitors should be approached cautiously.

Rifampin: When a single 375-mg dose of oral aprepitant was administered on Day 9 of a 14-day regimen of 600 mg/day of rifampin, a strong CYP3A4 inducer, the AUC of aprepitant decreased approximately 11-fold and the mean terminal half-life decreased approximately 3-fold.

Coadministration of fosaprepitant or aprepitant with drugs that induce CYP3A4 activity may result in reduced plasma concentrations and decreased efficacy.

7.3 Additional Interactions

Diltiazem: In a study in 10 patients with mild to moderate hypertension, intravenous infusion of 100 mg of fosaprepitant with diltiazem 120 mg 3 times daily, resulted in a 1.5-fold increase of aprepitant AUC and a 1.4-fold increase in diltiazem AUC. It also resulted in a small but clinically meaningful further maximum decrease in diastolic blood pressure [mean (SD) of 24.3 (± 10.2) mm Hg with fosaprepitant versus 15.6 (± 4.1) mm Hg without fosaprepitant] and resulted in a small further maximum decrease in systolic blood pressure [mean (SD) of 29.5 (± 7.9) mm Hg with fosaprepitant versus 23.8 (± 4.8) mm Hg without fosaprepitant], which may be clinically meaningful, but did not result in a clinically meaningful further change in heart rate or PR interval, beyond those changes induced by diltiazem alone.

In the same study, administration of aprepitant once daily, as a tablet formulation comparable to 230 mg of the capsule formulation, with diltiazem 120 mg 3 times daily for 5 days, resulted in a 2-fold increase of aprepitant AUC and a simultaneous 1.7-fold increase of diltiazem AUC. These pharmacokinetic effects did not result in clinically meaningful changes in ECG, heart rate or blood pressure beyond those changes induced by diltiazem alone.

Paroxetine: Coadministration of once daily doses of aprepitant, as a tablet formulation comparable to 85 mg or 170 mg of the capsule formulation, with paroxetine 20 mg once daily, resulted in a decrease in AUC by approximately 25% and C_{max} by approximately 20% of both aprepitant and paroxetine.

8 USE IN SPECIFIC POPULATIONS

8.1 Pregnancy

Teratogenic effects

Pregnancy Category B: In the reproduction studies conducted with fosaprepitant and aprepitant, the highest systemic exposures to aprepitant were obtained following oral administration of aprepitant. Reproduction studies performed in rats at oral doses of aprepitant up to 1000 mg/kg twice daily (plasma $AUC_{0\text{-}24hr}$ of 31.3 mcg•hr/mL, about 1.6 times the human exposure at the recommended dose) and in rabbits at oral doses up to 25 mg/kg/day (plasma $AUC_{0\text{-}24hr}$ of 26.9 mcg•hr/mL, about 1.4 times the human exposure at the recommended dose) revealed no evidence of impaired fertility or harm to the fetus due to aprepitant. There are, however, no adequate and well-controlled studies in pregnant women. Because animal reproduction studies are not always predictive of human response, this drug should be used during pregnancy only if clearly needed.

8.3 Nursing Mothers

Aprepitant is excreted in the milk of rats. It is not known whether this drug is excreted in human milk. Because many drugs are excreted in human milk and because of the potential for possible serious adverse reactions in nursing infants from aprepitant and because of the potential for tumorigenicity shown for aprepitant in rodent carcinogenicity studies, a decision should be made whether to discontinue nursing or to discontinue the drug, taking into account the importance of the drug to the mother.

8.4 Pediatric Use

Safety and effectiveness of EMEND for Injection in pediatric patients have not been established.

8.5 Geriatric Use

In 2 well-controlled chemotherapy-induced nausea and vomiting clinical studies, of the total number of patients (N=544) treated with oral aprepitant, 31% were 65 and over, while 5% were 75 and over. No overall differences in safety or effectiveness were observed between these subjects and younger subjects. Greater sensitivity of some older individuals cannot be ruled out. Dosage adjustment in the elderly is not necessary *[see Clinical Pharmacology (12.3)]*.

8.6 Patients with Severe Hepatic Impairment

There are no clinical or pharmacokinetic data in patients with severe hepatic impairment (Child-Pugh score >9). Therefore, caution should be exercised when fosaprepitant or aprepitant is administered in these patients *[see Clinical Pharmacology (12.3)]*.

10 OVERDOSAGE

There is no specific information on the treatment of overdosage with fosaprepitant or aprepitant.

In the event of overdose, fosaprepitant and/or oral aprepitant should be discontinued and general supportive treatment and monitoring should be provided. Because of the antiemetic activity of aprepitant, drug-induced emesis may not be effective.

Aprepitant cannot be removed by hemodialysis.

Thirteen patients in the randomized controlled trial of EMEND for Injection received both fosaprepitant 150 mg and at least one dose of oral aprepitant, 125 mg or 80 mg. Three patients reported adverse reactions that were similar to those experienced by the total study population.

11 DESCRIPTION

EMEND (fosaprepitant dimeglumine) for Injection is a sterile, lyophilized prodrug of aprepitant, a substance P/neurokinin-1 (NK_1) receptor antagonist, and is chemically described as 1-Deoxy-1-(methylamino)-D-glucitol[3-[[(2*R*, 3*S*)-2-[(1*R*)-1-[3,5-bis(trifluoromethyl)phenyl]ethoxy]-3-(4-fluorophenyl)-4-morpholinyl]methyl]-2,5-dihydro-5-oxo-1*H*-1,2,4-triazol-1-yl]phosphonate (2:1) (salt).

Its empirical formula is $C_{23}H_{22}F_7N_4O_6P \cdot 2(C_7H_{17}NO_5)$ and its structural formula is:

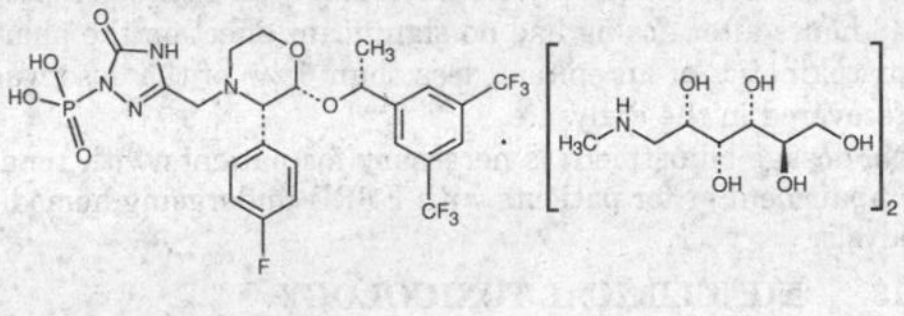

Fosaprepitant dimeglumine is a white to off-white amorphous powder with a molecular weight of 1004.83. It is freely soluble in water.

EMEND for Injection is a lyophilized prodrug of aprepitant containing polysorbate 80 (PS80), to be administered intravenously as an infusion.

Each vial of EMEND for Injection 115 mg for intravenous administration contains 188 mg of fosaprepitant dimeglumine equivalent to 115 mg of fosaprepitant free acid and the following inactive ingredients: edetate disodium (14.4 mg), polysorbate 80 (57.5 mg), lactose anhydrous (287.5 mg), sodium hydroxide and/or hydrochloric acid (for pH adjustment). Each vial of EMEND for Injection 150 mg for intravenous administration contains 245.3 mg of fosaprepitant dimeglumine equivalent to 150 mg of fosaprepitant free acid and the following inactive ingredients: edetate disodium (18.8 mg), polysorbate 80 (75 mg), lactose anhydrous (375 mg), sodium hydroxide and/or hydrochloric acid (for pH adjustment). Fosaprepitant dimeglumine hereafter will be referred to as fosaprepitant.

12 CLINICAL PHARMACOLOGY

Fosaprepitant, a prodrug of aprepitant, when administered intravenously is rapidly converted to aprepitant, a substance P/neurokinin 1 (NK_1) receptor antagonist. Plasma concentrations of fosaprepitant are below the limits of quantification (10 ng/mL) within 30 minutes of the completion of infusion *[see Clinical Pharmacology (12.3)]*. Upon conversion of 188 mg of fosaprepitant dimeglumine (equivalent to 115-mg fosaprepitant free acid) to aprepitant, 18.3 mg of phosphoric acid and 73 mg of meglumine are liberated. Upon conversion of 245.3 mg of fosaprepitant dimeglumine (equivalent to 150-mg fosaprepitant free acid) to aprepitant, 23.9 mg of phosphoric acid and 95.3 mg of meglumine are liberated.

12.1 Mechanism of Action

Fosaprepitant is a prodrug of aprepitant and accordingly, its antiemetic effects are attributable to aprepitant.

Aprepitant is a selective high-affinity antagonist of human substance P/neurokinin 1 (NK_1) receptors. Aprepitant has little or no affinity for serotonin ($5\text{-}HT_3$), dopamine, and corticosteroid receptors, the targets of existing therapies for chemotherapy-induced nausea and vomiting (CINV). Aprepitant has been shown in animal models to inhibit emesis induced by cytotoxic chemotherapeutic agents, such as cisplatin, via central actions. Animal and human Positron Emission Tomography (PET) studies with aprepitant have shown that it crosses the blood brain barrier and occupies brain NK_1 receptors. Animal and human studies show that aprepitant augments the antiemetic activity of the $5\text{-}HT_3$-receptor antagonist ondansetron and the corticosteroid dexamethasone and inhibits both the acute and delayed phases of cisplatin-induced emesis.

12.2 Pharmacodynamics

NK_1 Receptor Occupancy

In two single-blind, multiple-dose, randomized, and placebo control studies, healthy young men received oral aprepitant doses of 10 mg (N=2), 30 mg (N=3), 100 mg (N=3) or 300 mg (N=5) once daily for 14 days with 2 or 3 subjects on placebo. Both plasma aprepitant concentration and NK_1 receptor occupancy in the corpus striatum by positron emission tomography were evaluated, at predose and 24 hours after the last dose. At aprepitant plasma concentrations of ~10 ng/mL and ~100 ng/mL, the NK_1 receptor occupancies were ~50% and ~90%, respectively. The oral aprepitant regimen for CINV produces mean trough plasma aprepitant concentrations >500 ng/mL, which would be expected to, based on the fitted curve with the Hill equation, result in >95% brain NK_1 receptor occupancy. However, the receptor occupancy for either CINV or PONV dosing regimen has not been determined. In addition, the relationship between NK_1 receptor occupancy and the clinical efficacy of aprepitant has not been established.

Cardiac Electrophysiology

In a randomized, double-blind, positive-controlled, thorough QTc study, a single 200-mg dose of fosaprepitant had no effect on the QTc interval.

12.3 Pharmacokinetics

Aprepitant after Fosaprepitant Administration

Following a single intravenous 115-mg dose of fosaprepitant administered as a 15-minute infusion to healthy volunteers the mean $AUC_{0\text{-}\infty}$ of aprepitant was 31.7 (± 14.3) mcg•hr/mL and the mean maximal aprepitant concentration (C_{max}) was 3.27 (± 1.16) mcg/mL. The mean aprepitant plasma concentration at 24 hours postdose was similar between the 125-mg oral aprepitant dose and the 115-mg intravenous fosaprepitant dose. (See Figure 1.)

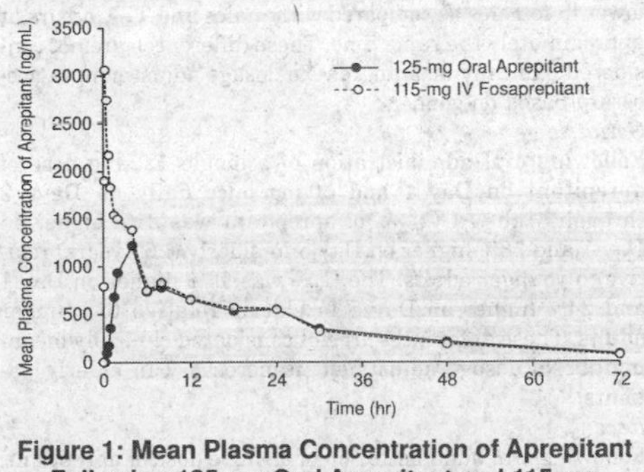

Figure 1: Mean Plasma Concentration of Aprepitant Following 125-mg Oral Aprepitant and 115-mg Intravenous Fosaprepitant

Following a single, intravenous 150-mg dose of fosaprepitant administered as a 20-minute infusion to healthy volunteers, the mean $AUC_{0\text{-}\infty}$ of aprepitant was 37.38 (± 14.75) mcg•hr/mL and the mean maximal aprepitant concentration (C_{max}) was 4.15 (± 1.15) mcg/mL.

Distribution

Fosaprepitant is rapidly converted to aprepitant. Aprepitant is greater than 95% bound to plasma proteins. The mean apparent volume of distribution at steady state (Vd_{ss}) is approximately 70 L in humans.

Aprepitant crosses the placenta in rats and rabbits and crosses the blood brain barrier in humans *[see Clinical Pharmacology (12.1)]*.

Metabolism

Fosaprepitant was rapidly converted to aprepitant in *in vitro* incubations with liver preparations from nonclinical species (rat and dog) and humans. Furthermore, fosaprepitant underwent rapid and nearly complete conversion to aprepitant in S9 preparations from multiple other human tissues including kidney, lung and ileum. Thus, it appears that the conversion of fosaprepitant to aprepitant can occur in multiple extrahepatic tissues in addition to the liver. In humans, fosaprepitant administered intravenously was rapidly converted to aprepitant within 30 minutes following the end of infusion.

Aprepitant undergoes extensive metabolism. *In vitro* studies using human liver microsomes indicate that aprepitant is metabolized primarily by CYP3A4 with minor metabolism by CYP1A2 and CYP2C19. Metabolism is largely via oxidation at the morpholine ring and its side chains. No metabolism by CYP2D6, CYP2C9, or CYP2E1 was detected. In healthy young adults, aprepitant accounts for approximately 24% of the radioactivity in plasma over 72 hours following a single oral 300-mg dose of [^{14}C]-aprepitant, indi-

Table 11: Treatment Regimens — Highly Emetogenic Chemotherapy Trials*

	Day 1	Day 2	Day 3	Day 4
CINV Aprepitant Regimen				
Aprepitant	125 mg orally	80 mg orally	80 mg orally	none
Dexamethasone	12 mg orally	8 mg orally	8 mg orally	8 mg orally
5-HT_3 antagonist†	See package insert	none	none	none
CINV Standard Therapy				
Dexamethasone	20 mg orally	8 mg orally twice daily	8 mg orally twice daily	8 mg orally twice daily
5-HT_3 antagonist†	See package insert	none	none	none

* Aprepitant placebo and dexamethasone placebo were used to maintain blinding.
† Ondansetron 32 mg I.V. was used in the clinical trials of aprepitant. Although this dose was used in clinical trials, this is no longer the currently recommended dose. Refer to the ondansetron package insert for the current dosing.

cating a substantial presence of metabolites in the plasma. Seven metabolites of aprepitant, which are only weakly active, have been identified in human plasma.

Excretion

Following administration of a single intravenous 100-mg dose of [^{14}C]-fosaprepitant to healthy subjects, 57% of the radioactivity was recovered in urine and 45% in feces.

Aprepitant is eliminated primarily by metabolism; aprepitant is not renally excreted. The apparent terminal half-life ranged from approximately 9 to 13 hours.

Specific Populations

Gender

Following oral administration of a single dose of aprepitant, the $AUC_{0\text{-}24hr}$ and C_{max} are 14% and 22% higher in females as compared with males. The half-life of aprepitant is 25% lower in females as compared with males and T_{max} occurs at approximately the same time. These differences are not considered clinically meaningful. No dosage adjustment is necessary based on gender.

Geriatric

Following oral administration of a single 125-mg dose of aprepitant on Day 1 and 80 mg once daily on Days 2 through 5, the $AUC_{0\text{-}24hr}$ of aprepitant was 21% higher on Day 1 and 36% higher on Day 5 in elderly (≥65 years) relative to younger adults. The C_{max} was 10% higher on Day 1 and 24% higher on Day 5 in elderly relative to younger adults. These differences are not considered clinically meaningful. No dosage adjustment is necessary in elderly patients.

Race

Following oral administration of a single dose of aprepitant, the $AUC_{0\text{-}24hr}$ and C_{max} are approximately 42% and 29% higher in Hispanics as compared with Caucasians. The $AUC_{0\text{-}24hr}$ and C_{max} are 62% and 41% higher in Asians as compared to Caucasians. There was no difference in $AUC_{0\text{-}24hr}$ or C_{max} between Caucasians and Blacks. These differences are not considered clinically meaningful. No dosage adjustment is necessary based on race.

Body Mass Index (BMI)

For every 5 kg/m^2 increase in BMI, $AUC_{0\text{-}24hr}$ and C_{max} of aprepitant decrease by 11%. BMI of subjects in the analysis ranged from 18 kg/m^2 to 36 kg/m^2. This change is not considered clinically meaningful. No dosage adjustment is necessary based on BMI.

Hepatic Insufficiency

Fosaprepitant is metabolized in various extrahepatic tissues; therefore hepatic impairment is not expected to alter the conversion of fosaprepitant to aprepitant.

Following administration of a single 125-mg dose of oral aprepitant on Day 1 and 80 mg once daily on Days 2 and 3 to patients with mild hepatic impairment (Child-Pugh score 5 to 6), the $AUC_{0\text{-}24hr}$ of aprepitant was 11% lower on Day 1 and 36% lower on Day 3, as compared with healthy subjects given the same regimen. In patients with moderate hepatic impairment (Child-Pugh score 7 to 9), the $AUC_{0\text{-}24hr}$ of aprepitant was 10% higher on Day 1 and 18% higher on Day 3, as compared with healthy subjects given the same regimen. These differences in $AUC_{0\text{-}24hr}$ are not considered clinically meaningful; therefore, no dosage adjustment is necessary in patients with mild to moderate hepatic impairment. There are no clinical or pharmacokinetic data in patients with severe hepatic impairment (Child-Pugh score >9) *[see Use in Specific Populations (8.6)]*.

Renal Insufficiency

A single 240-mg dose of oral aprepitant was administered to patients with severe renal impairment (creatinine clearance <30 mL/min/1.73 m^2 as measured by 24-hour urinary creatinine clearance) and to patients with end stage renal disease (ESRD) requiring hemodialysis.

In patients with severe renal impairment, the $AUC_{0-\infty}$ of total aprepitant (unbound and protein bound) decreased by 21% and C_{max} decreased by 32%, relative to healthy subjects (creatinine clearance >80 mL/min estimated by Cockcroft-Gault method). In patients with ESRD undergoing hemodialysis, the $AUC_{0-\infty}$ of total aprepitant decreased by 42% and C_{max} decreased by 32%. Due to modest decreases in protein binding of aprepitant in patients with renal disease, the AUC of pharmacologically active unbound drug was not significantly affected in patients with renal impairment compared with healthy subjects. Hemodialysis conducted 4 or 48 hours after dosing had no significant effect on the pharmacokinetics of aprepitant; less than 0.2% of the dose was recovered in the dialysate.

No dosage adjustment is necessary for patients with renal impairment or for patients with ESRD undergoing hemodialysis.

13 NONCLINICAL TOXICOLOGY

13.1 Carcinogenesis, Mutagenesis, Impairment of Fertility

Carcinogenicity studies were conducted in Sprague-Dawley rats and in CD-1 mice for 2 years. In the rat carcinogenicity studies, animals were treated with oral doses ranging from 0.05 to 1000 mg/kg twice daily. The highest dose produced a systemic exposure to aprepitant (plasma $AUC_{0\text{-}24hr}$) of 0.7 to 1.6 times the human exposure ($AUC_{0\text{-}24hr}$ = 19.6 mcg•hr/mL) at the recommended dose of 125 mg/day. Treatment with aprepitant at doses of 5 to 1000 mg/kg twice daily caused an increase in the incidences of thyroid follicular cell adenomas and carcinomas in male rats. In female rats, it produced hepatocellular adenomas at 5 to 1000 mg/kg twice daily and hepatocellular carcinomas and thyroid follicular cell adenomas at 125 to 1000 mg/kg twice daily. In the mouse carcinogenicity studies, the animals were treated with oral doses ranging from 2.5 to 2000 mg/kg/day. The highest dose produced a systemic exposure of about 2.8 to 3.6 times the human exposure at the recommended dose. Treatment with aprepitant produced skin fibrosarcomas at 125 and 500 mg/kg/day doses in male mice. Carcinogenicity studies were not conducted with fosaprepitant.

Aprepitant and fosaprepitant were not genotoxic in the Ames test, the human lymphoblastoid cell (TK6) mutagenesis test, the rat hepatocyte DNA strand break test, the Chinese hamster ovary (CHO) cell chromosome aberration test and the mouse micronucleus test.

Fosaprepitant, when administered intravenously, is rapidly converted to aprepitant. In the fertility studies conducted with fosaprepitant and aprepitant, the highest systemic exposures to aprepitant were obtained following oral administration of aprepitant. Oral aprepitant did not affect the fertility or general reproductive performance of male or female rats at doses up to the maximum feasible dose of 1000 mg/kg twice daily (providing exposure in male rats lower than the exposure at the recommended human dose and exposure in female rats at about 1.6 times the human exposure).

14 CLINICAL STUDIES

Fosaprepitant, a prodrug of aprepitant, when administered intravenously is rapidly converted to aprepitant.

Oral administration of aprepitant in combination with ondansetron and dexamethasone (aprepitant regimen) has been shown to prevent acute and delayed nausea and vomiting associated with highly emetogenic chemotherapy including high-dose cisplatin, and nausea and vomiting associated with moderately emetogenic chemotherapy.

14.1 Highly Emetogenic Chemotherapy (HEC)

EMEND for Injection 115 mg (3-Day Dosing Regimen of EMEND)

Fosaprepitant 115 mg intravenous infused over 15 minutes can be substituted for 125 mg oral aprepitant on Day 1 of a 3-day regimen. Efficacy studies with the 3-day regimen were conducted with oral aprepitant.

In 2 multicenter, randomized, parallel, double-blind, controlled clinical studies, the aprepitant regimen (see Table 11) was compared with standard therapy in patients receiving a chemotherapy regimen that included cisplatin >50 mg/m^2 (mean cisplatin dose = 80.2 mg/m^2). Of the 550 patients who were randomized to receive the aprepitant regimen, 42% were women, 58% men, 59% White, 3% Asian, 5% Black, 12% Hispanic American, and 21% Multi-Racial. The aprepitant-treated patients in these clinical studies ranged from 14 to 84 years of age, with a mean age of 56 years. 170 patients were 65 years or older, with 29 patients being 75 years or older.

Patients (N = 1105) were randomized to either the aprepitant regimen (N = 550) or standard therapy (N = 555). The treatment regimens are defined in Table 11.

[See table 11 above]

During these studies, 95% of the patients in the aprepitant group received a concomitant chemotherapeutic agent in addition to protocol-mandated cisplatin. The most common chemotherapeutic agents and the number of aprepitant patients exposed follow: etoposide (106), fluorouracil (100), gemcitabine (89), vinorelbine (82), paclitaxel (52), cyclophosphamide (50), doxorubicin (38), docetaxel (11).

The antiemetic activity of oral aprepitant was evaluated during the acute phase (0 to 24 hours post-cisplatin treatment), the delayed phase (25 to 120 hours post-cisplatin treatment) and overall (0 to 120 hours post-cisplatin treatment) in Cycle 1. Efficacy was based on evaluation of the following endpoints in which emetic episodes included vomiting, retching, or dry heaves:

Primary endpoint:

- complete response (defined as no emetic episodes and no use of rescue therapy as recorded in patient diaries)

Other prespecified endpoints:

- complete protection (defined as no emetic episodes, no use of rescue therapy, and a maximum nausea visual analogue scale [VAS] score <25 mm on a 0 to 100 mm scale)
- no emesis (defined as no emetic episodes regardless of use of rescue therapy)
- no nausea (maximum VAS <5 mm on a 0 to 100 mm scale)
- no significant nausea (maximum VAS <25 mm on a 0 to 100 mm scale)

A summary of the key study results from each individual study analysis is shown in Table 12 and in Table 13.

Table 12: Percent of Patients Receiving Highly Emetogenic Chemotherapy Responding by Treatment Group and Phase for Study 1 — Cycle 1

ENDPOINTS	Aprepitant Regimen (N = 260)* %	Standard Therapy (N = 261)* %	p-Value
PRIMARY ENDPOINT			
Complete Response			
Overall†	73	52	<0.001
OTHER PRESPECIFIED ENDPOINTS			
Complete Response			
Acute phase‡	89	78	<0.001
Delayed phase§	75	56	<0.001
Complete Protection			
Overall	63	49	0.001
Acute phase	85	75	NS¶
Delayed phase	66	52	<0.001
No Emesis			
Overall	78	55	<0.001
Acute phase	90	79	0.001
Delayed phase	81	59	<0.001
No Nausea			
Overall	48	44	NS#
Delayed phase	51	48	NS#

No Significant Nausea			
Overall	73	66	NS#
Delayed phase	75	69	NS#

Visual analogue scale (VAS) score range: 0 mm = no nausea; 100 mm = nausea as bad as it could be.

* N: Number of patients (older than 18 years of age) who received cisplatin, study drug, and had at least one post-treatment efficacy evaluation.

† Overall: 0 to 120 hours post-cisplatin treatment.

‡ Acute phase: 0 to 24 hours post-cisplatin treatment.

§ Delayed phase: 25 to 120 hours post-cisplatin treatment.

¶ Not statistically significant when adjusted for multiple comparisons.

\# Not statistically significant.

Table 13: Percent of Patients Receiving Highly Emetogenic Chemotherapy Responding by Treatment Group and Phase for Study 2 — Cycle 1

ENDPOINTS	Aprepitant Regimen (N = 261)* %	Standard Therapy (N = 263)* %	p-Value
PRIMARY ENDPOINT			
Complete Response			
Overall†	63	43	<0.001
OTHER PRESPECIFIED ENDPOINTS			
Complete Response			
Acute phase‡	83	68	<0.001
Delayed phase§	68	47	<0.001
Complete Protection			
Overall	56	41	<0.001
Acute phase	80	65	<0.001
Delayed phase	61	44	<0.001
No Emesis			
Overall	66	44	<0.001
Acute phase	84	69	<0.001
Delayed phase	72	48	<0.001
No Nausea			
Overall	49	39	NS¶
Delayed phase	53	40	NS¶
No Significant Nausea			
Overall	71	64	NS#
Delayed phase	73	65	NS#

Visual analogue scale (VAS) score range: 0 mm = no nausea; 100 mm = nausea as bad as it could be.

* N: Number of patients (older than 18 years of age) who received cisplatin, study drug, and had at least one post-treatment efficacy evaluation.

† Overall: 0 to 120 hours post-cisplatin treatment.

‡ Acute phase: 0 to 24 hours post-cisplatin treatment.

§ Delayed phase: 25 to 120 hours post-cisplatin treatment.

¶ Not statistically significant when adjusted for multiple comparisons.

\# Not statistically significant.

In both studies, a statistically significantly higher proportion of patients (both p<0.001) receiving the aprepitant regimen in Cycle 1 had a complete response in the overall phase (primary endpoint), compared with patients receiving standard therapy. A statistically significant difference in complete response in favor of the aprepitant regimen was also observed when the acute phase and the delayed phase were analyzed separately.

In both studies, the estimated time to first emesis after initiation of cisplatin treatment was longer with the aprepitant regimen, and the incidence of first emesis was reduced in the aprepitant regimen group compared with standard therapy group as depicted in the Kaplan-Meier curves in Figure 2.

[See figure 2 at top of next column]

Additional Patient-Reported Outcomes: The impact of nausea and vomiting on patients' daily lives was assessed in Cycle 1 of both phase 3 studies using the Functional Living Index–Emesis (FLIE), a validated nausea- and vomiting-specific patient-reported outcome measure. Minimal or no impact of nausea and vomiting on patients' daily lives is defined as a FLIE total score >108. In each of the 2 studies, a higher proportion of patients receiving the aprepitant regimen reported minimal or no impact of nausea and vomiting on daily life (Study 1: 74% versus 64%; Study 2: 75% versus 64%).

Multiple-Cycle Extension: In the same 2 clinical studies, patients continued into the Multiple-Cycle extension for up to 5 additional cycles of chemotherapy. The proportion of patients with no emesis and no significant nausea by treatment group at each cycle is depicted in Figure 3.

[See figure 3 at top of next column]

Table 14: Treatment Regimens — Highly Emetogenic Chemotherapy Trial*

	Day 1	Day 2	Day 3	Day 4
CINV Fosaprepitant Regimen				
Fosaprepitant	150 mg intravenously	none	none	none
Dexamethasone	12 mg orally	8 mg orally	8 mg orally twice daily	8 mg orally twice daily
5-HT_3 antagonist†	See package insert	none	none	none
CINV Aprepitant Regimen				
Aprepitant	125 mg orally	80 mg orally	80 mg orally	none
Dexamethasone	12 mg orally	8 mg orally	8 mg orally	8 mg orally
5-HT_3 antagonist†	See package insert	none	none	none

* Fosaprepitant placebo, aprepitant placebo and dexamethasone placebo (in the evenings on Days 3 and 4) were used to maintain blinding.

† Ondansetron 32 mg I.V. was used in the clinical trial of EMEND for Injection. Although this dose was used in the clinical trial, this is no longer the currently recommended dose. Refer to the ondansetron package insert for the current dosing.

Table 15: Percent of Patients Receiving Highly Emetogenic Chemotherapy Responding by Treatment Group and Phase — Cycle 1

ENDPOINTS	Fosaprepitant Regimen (N = 1106)* %	Aprepitant Regimen (N = 1134)* %	Difference† (95% CI)
PRIMARY ENDPOINT			
Complete Response‡			
Overall§	71.9	72.3	-0.4 (-4.1, 3.3)
SECONDARY ENDPOINTS			
Complete Response‡			
Delayed phase¶	74.3	74.2	0.1 (-3.5, 3.7)
No Vomiting			
Overall§	72.9	74.6	-1.7 (-5.3, 2.0)

* N: Number of patients included in the primary analysis of complete response.

† Difference and Confidence interval (CI) were calculated using the method proposed by Miettinen and Nurminen and adjusted for Gender.

‡ Complete Response = no vomiting and no use of rescue therapy.

§ Overall = 0 to 120 hours post-initiation of cisplatin chemotherapy.

¶ Delayed phase = 25 to 120 hours post-initiation of cisplatin chemotherapy.

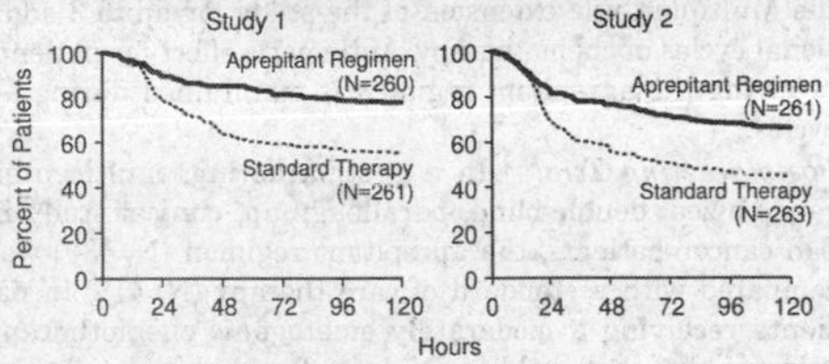

p-Value <0.001 based on a log rank test for Study 1 and Study 2; nominal p-values not adjusted for multiplicity.

Figure 2: Percent of Patients Receiving Highly Emetogenic Chemotherapy Who Remain Emesis Free Over Time — Cycle 1

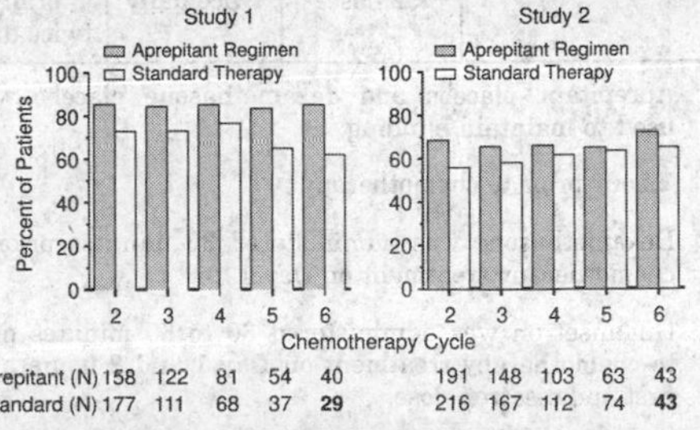

Figure 3: Proportion of Patients Receiving Highly Emetogenic Chemotherapy with No Emesis and No Significant Nausea by Treatment Group and Cycle

EMEND for Injection 150 mg (Single Dose Regimen of EMEND)

EMEND for Injection 150 mg infused over 20-30 minutes is administered on Day 1 only and can be substituted for the 3-day dosing regimen of EMEND for the prevention of nausea and vomiting induced by HEC.

In a randomized, parallel, double-blind, active-controlled study, EMEND for Injection 150 mg (N=1147) was compared with a 3-day oral aprepitant regimen (N=1175) (see Table 14 below) in patients receiving a highly emetogenic chemotherapy regimen that included cisplatin (≥70 mg/m²). Patient demographics were similar between the two treatment groups. Of the total 2322 patients receiving EMEND for Injection or oral aprepitant, 63% were men, 56% White, 26% Asian, 3% American Indian/Alaska Native, 2% Black, 13% Multi-Racial, and 33% Hispanic/Latino ethnicity. Patient ages ranged from 19 to 86 years of age, with a mean age of 56 years. Other concomitant chemotherapy agents were administered similar to those in prior HEC studies described above.

[See table 14 above]

The efficacy of fosaprepitant 150 mg was evaluated based on the primary and secondary endpoints listed in Table 15 below and was shown to be non-inferior to that of the 3-day oral aprepitant regimen with regard to complete response in each of the evaluated phases. The pre-specified non-inferiority margin for complete response in the overall phase was 7%. The pre-specified non-inferiority margin for complete response in the delayed phase was 7.3%. The pre-specified non-inferiority margin for no vomiting in the overall phase was 8.2%.

[See table 15 at top of previous page]

14.2 Moderately Emetogenic Chemotherapy (MEC)

In a multicenter, randomized, double-blind, parallel-group, clinical study in breast cancer patients, the aprepitant regimen (see Table 16) was compared with a standard of care therapy in patients receiving a moderately emetogenic chemotherapy regimen that included cyclophosphamide 750-1500 mg/m^2; or cyclophosphamide 500-1500 mg/m^2 and doxorubicin (≤60 mg/m^2) or epirubicin (≤100 mg/m^2).

In this study, the most common combinations were cyclophosphamide + doxorubicin (60.6%); and cyclophosphamide + epirubicin + fluorouracil (21.6%).

Of the 438 patients who were randomized to receive the aprepitant regimen, 99.5% were women. Of these, approximately 80% were White, 8% Black, 8% Asian, 4% Hispanic, and <1% Other. The aprepitant-treated patients in this clinical study ranged from 25 to 78 years of age, with a mean age of 53 years; 70 patients were 65 years or older, with 12 patients being over 74 years.

Patients (N = 866) were randomized to either the aprepitant regimen (N = 438) or standard therapy (N = 428). The treatment regimens are defined in Table 16.

Table 16: Treatment Regimens — Moderately Emetogenic Chemotherapy Trial*

	Day 1	Day 2	Day 3
CINV Aprepitant Regimen			
Aprepitant	125 mg orally†	80 mg orally	80 mg orally
Dexamethasone	12 mg orally‡	none	none
Ondansetron	8 mg orally × 2 doses§	none	none
CINV Standard Therapy			
Dexamethasone	20 mg orally	none	none
Ondansetron	8 mg orally × 2 doses	8 mg orally twice daily	8 mg orally twice daily

* Aprepitant placebo and dexamethasone placebo were used to maintain blinding.

† 1 hour prior to chemotherapy.

‡ Dexamethasone was administered 30 minutes prior to chemotherapy treatment on Day 1.

§ Ondansetron was administered 30 to 60 minutes prior to chemotherapy treatment on Day 1 and 8 hours after first ondansetron dose.

The antiemetic activity of oral aprepitant was evaluated based on the following endpoints in which emetic episodes included vomiting, retching, or dry heaves:

Primary endpoint:
- complete response (defined as no emetic episodes and no use of rescue therapy as recorded in patient diaries) in the overall phase (0 to 120 hours post-chemotherapy)

Other prespecified endpoints:
- no emesis (defined as no emetic episodes regardless of use of rescue therapy)
- no nausea (maximum VAS <5 mm on a 0 to 100 mm scale)
- no significant nausea (maximum VAS <25 mm on a 0 to 100 mm scale)
- complete protection (defined as no emetic episodes, no use of rescue therapy, and a maximum nausea visual analogue scale [VAS] score <25 mm on a 0 to 100 mm scale)
- complete response during the acute and delayed phases.

A summary of the key results from this study is shown in Table 17.

Table 17: Percent of Patients Receiving Moderately Emetogenic Chemotherapy Responding by Treatment Group and Phase — Cycle 1

ENDPOINTS	Aprepitant Regimen (N = 433)* %	Standard Therapy (N = 424)* %	p-Value
PRIMARY ENDPOINT†			
Complete Response	51	42	0.015
OTHER PRESPECIFIED ENDPOINTS†			
No Emesis	76	59	NS‡
No Nausea	33	33	NS
No Significant Nausea	61	56	NS
No Rescue Therapy	59	56	NS
Complete Protection	43	37	NS

* N: Number of patients included in the primary analysis of complete response.

† Overall: 0 to 120 hours post-chemotherapy treatment.

‡ NS when adjusted for prespecified multiple comparisons rule; unadjusted p-value <0.001.

In this study, a statistically significantly (p=0.015) higher proportion of patients receiving the aprepitant regimen in Cycle 1 had a complete response (primary endpoint) during the overall phase compared with patients receiving standard therapy. The difference between treatment groups was primarily driven by the "No Emesis Endpoint", a principal component of this composite primary endpoint. In addition, a higher proportion of patients receiving the aprepitant regimen in Cycle 1 had a complete response during the acute (0-24 hours) and delayed (25-120 hours) phases compared with patients receiving standard therapy; however, the treatment group differences failed to reach statistical significance, after multiplicity adjustments.

Additional Patient-Reported Outcomes: In a phase 3 study in patients receiving moderately emetogenic chemotherapy, the impact of nausea and vomiting on patients' daily lives was assessed in Cycle 1 using the FLIE. A higher proportion of patients receiving the aprepitant regimen reported minimal or no impact on daily life (64% versus 56%). This difference between treatment groups was primarily driven by the "No Vomiting Domain" of this composite endpoint.

Multiple-Cycle Extension: Patients receiving moderately emetogenic chemotherapy were permitted to continue into the Multiple-Cycle extension of the study for up to 3 additional cycles of chemotherapy. Antiemetic effect for patients receiving the aprepitant regimen is maintained during all cycles.

Postmarketing Trial: In a postmarketing, multicenter, randomized, double-blind, parallel-group, clinical study in 848 cancer patients, the aprepitant regimen (N=430) was compared with a standard of care therapy (N=418) in patients receiving a moderately emetogenic chemotherapy regimen that included any IV dose of oxaliplatin, carboplatin, epirubicin, idarubicin, ifosfamide, irinotecan, daunorubicin, doxorubicin; cyclophosphamide IV (<1500 mg/m^2); or cytarabine IV (>1 g/m^2).

Of the 430 patients who were randomized to receive the aprepitant regimen, 76% were women and 24% were men. The distribution by race was 67% White, 6% Black or African American, 11% Asian, and 12% multiracial. Classified by ethnicity, 36% were Hispanic and 64% were non-Hispanic. The aprepitant-treated patients in this clinical study ranged from 22 to 85 years of age, with a mean age of 57 years; approximately 59% of the patients were 55 years or older with 32 patients being over 74 years. Patients receiving the aprepitant regimen were receiving chemotherapy for a variety of tumor types including 50% with breast cancer, 21% with gastrointestinal cancers including colorectal cancer, 13% with lung cancer and 6% with gynecological cancers.

The antiemetic activity of EMEND was evaluated based on no vomiting (with or without rescue therapy) in the overall period (0 to 120 hours post-chemotherapy) and complete response (defined as no vomiting and no use of rescue therapy) in the overall period.

A summary of the key results from this study is shown in Table 18.

Table 18: Percent of Patients Receiving Moderately Emetogenic Chemotherapy Responding by Treatment Group for Study 2 — Cycle 1

ENDPOINTS	Aprepitant Regimen (N = 430)* %	Standard Therapy (N = 418)* %	p-Value
No Vomiting Overall	76	62	<0.0001
Complete Response Overall	69	56	0.0003

* N = Number of patients who received chemotherapy treatment, study drug, and had at least one post-treatment efficacy evaluation.

In this study, a statistically significantly higher proportion of patients receiving the aprepitant regimen (76%) in Cycle 1 had no vomiting during the overall phase compared with patients receiving standard therapy (62%). In addition, a higher proportion of patients receiving the aprepitant regimen (69%) in Cycle 1 had a complete response in the overall phase (0-120 hours) compared with patients receiving standard therapy (56%). In the acute phase (0 to 24 hours following initiation of chemotherapy), a higher proportion of patients receiving aprepitant compared to patients receiving standard therapy were observed to have no vomiting (92% and 84%, respectively) and complete response (89% and 80%, respectively). In the delayed phase (25 to 120 hours following initiation of chemotherapy), a higher proportion of patients receiving aprepitant compared to patients receiving standard therapy were observed to have no vomiting (78% and 67%, respectively) and complete response (71% and 61%, respectively).

In a subgroup analysis by tumor type, a numerically higher proportion of patients receiving aprepitant were observed to have no vomiting and complete response compared to patients receiving standard therapy. For gender, the difference in complete response rates between the aprepitant and standard regimen groups was 14% in females (64.5% and 50.3%, respectively) and 4% in males (82.2% and 78.2%, respectively) during the overall phase. A similar difference for gender was observed for the no vomiting endpoint.

16 HOW SUPPLIED/STORAGE AND HANDLING

No. 3884 — One 115-mg single dose glass vial: White to off-white lyophilized solid. Supplied as follows:
NDC 0006-3884-32 1 vial per carton.

No. 3941 — One 150-mg single dose glass vial: White to off-white lyophilized solid. Supplied as follows:
NDC 0006-3941-32 1 vial per carton.

Storage

Vials: Store at 2-8°C (36-46°F).

Sterile lyophilized powder for intravenous use only after reconstitution and dilution.

17 PATIENT COUNSELING INFORMATION

"See FDA-Approved Patient Labeling (Patient Information)"

Physicians should instruct their patients to read the patient package insert before starting therapy with EMEND for Injection and to reread it each time the prescription is renewed.

Patients should follow the physician's instructions for the EMEND for Injection regimen.

Allergic reactions, which may be sudden and/or serious, and may include hives, rash, itching, redness of the face/skin and may cause difficulty in breathing or swallowing, have been reported. Physicians should instruct their patients to stop using EMEND and call their doctor right away if they experience an allergic reaction. In addition, severe skin reactions may occur rarely.

Patients who develop an infusion site reaction such as erythema, edema, pain, or thrombophlebitis should be instructed on how to care for the local reaction and when to seek further evaluation.

EMEND for Injection may interact with some drugs including chemotherapy; therefore, patients should be advised to report to their doctor the use of any other prescription, nonprescription medication or herbal products.

Patients on chronic warfarin therapy should be instructed to have their clotting status closely monitored in the 2-week period, particularly at 7 to 10 days, following initiation of fosaprepitant with each chemotherapy cycle.

Administration of EMEND for Injection may reduce the efficacy of hormonal contraceptives. Patients should be advised to use alternative or back-up methods of contraception during treatment with and for 1 month following the last dose of fosaprepitant or aprepitant.

Manufactured for:
Merck Sharp & Dohme Corp., a subsidiary of **MERCK & CO., INC.**, Whitehouse Station, NJ 08889, USA
Manufactured by:
DSM Pharmaceuticals, Inc., 5900 Martin Luther King Jr. Highway, Greenville, NC 27834, USA
U.S. Patent Nos.: 5,512,570; 5,691,336

USPI-IV-05171212R009

Patient Information
EMEND® (EE mend)
(fosaprepitant dimeglumine)
for Injection

Read this Patient Information before you start receiving EMEND for Injection and each time you are scheduled to receive EMEND for Injection. There may be new information. This information does not take the place of talking to your doctor about your medical condition or your treatment.

What is EMEND for Injection?

EMEND for Injection is a prescription medicine used in adults to prevent nausea and vomiting caused by certain anti-cancer (chemotherapy) medicines. EMEND for Injection is always used with other medicines that treat nausea and vomiting.

EMEND for Injection is not used to treat nausea and vomiting that you already have.

EMEND for Injection should not be used continuously for a long time (chronic use).

It is not known if EMEND for Injection is safe and effective in children.

Who should not take EMEND for Injection?

Do not take EMEND for Injection if you:

- are taking any of the following medicines:
  - pimozide (ORAP®)
  - cisapride (PROPULSID®)

Taking EMEND for Injection with any of these medicines could cause serious or life-threatening problems.

- are allergic to any of the ingredients in EMEND for Injection. See the end of this leaflet for a list of all the ingredients in EMEND for Injection.

What should I tell my doctor before receiving EMEND for Injection?

Before you receive EMEND for Injection, tell your doctor if you:

- have liver problems.
- are pregnant or plan to become pregnant. It is not known if EMEND for Injection can harm your unborn baby.
  Women who use birth control medicines containing hormones to prevent pregnancy (birth control pills, skin patches, implants, and certain IUDs) should also use a backup method of birth control during treatment with EMEND for Injection and for up to 1 month after using EMEND for Injection to prevent pregnancy.
- are breastfeeding or plan to breastfeed. It is not known if EMEND for Injection passes into your milk and if it can harm your baby. You and your doctor should decide if you will take EMEND for Injection or breastfeed. You should not do both.

Tell your doctor about all the medicines you take, including prescription and non-prescription medicines, vitamins, and herbal supplements.

EMEND for Injection may cause serious life-threatening reactions if used with certain medicines. See the section "Who should not take EMEND for Injection?".

EMEND for Injection may affect how other medicines work, and other medicines may affect how EMEND for Injection works. Ask your doctor or pharmacist before you take any new medicine. They can tell you if it is safe to take the medicine with EMEND for Injection.

Know the medicines you take. Keep a list of them to show your doctor or pharmacist when you get a new medicine.

How will I receive EMEND for Injection?

You will receive EMEND for Injection in one of two ways:

1. EMEND for Injection 150 mg given on Day 1 only.
- Day 1 (Day of chemotherapy): EMEND for Injection 150 mg will be given to you by infusion in your vein (intravenous) about 30 minutes before you start your chemotherapy treatment.

Or

2. EMEND for Injection 115 mg given along with capsules of EMEND.
- Day 1 (Day of chemotherapy): EMEND for Injection 115 mg will be given to you by infusion in your vein (intravenous) about 30 minutes before you start your chemotherapy treatment.
- You will get a prescription for two capsules of EMEND.
- Day 2 and Day 3 (the two days after chemotherapy): Take one 80-mg capsule of EMEND (white) by mouth, each morning for the 2 days after your chemotherapy treatment.
- If you take the blood thinner medicine warfarin sodium (COUMADIN®, JANTOVEN®), your doctor may do blood tests after you take EMEND to check your blood clotting.

What are the possible side effects of EMEND for Injection?

EMEND for Injection may cause serious side effects, including:

- **Serious allergic reactions.** Allergic reactions can happen suddenly with EMEND for Injection and may be serious. Tell your doctor or nurse right away if you have flushing or redness of your face or skin, or trouble breathing during or soon after you receive EMEND for Injection.
- Severe skin reactions may occur rarely.
  EMEND capsules can also cause allergic reactions. If you receive EMEND for Injection on Day 1, and then take EMEND capsules on Days 2 and 3, stop taking the EMEND capsules and call your doctor right away if you have any of these signs or symptoms of an allergic reaction:
  - hives
  - rash
  - itching
  - redness of the face or skin
  - trouble breathing or swallowing.

The most common side effects of EMEND for Injection include:

- hiccups
- weakness or tiredness
- changes in liver function blood test results. Your doctor will check you for this.
- headache
- constipation
- loss of appetite
- indigestion
- diarrhea
- belching

Infusion-site side effects with EMEND for Injection may include pain, hardening, redness or itching at the site of infusion. Swelling (inflammation) of a vein caused by a blood clot can also happen at the infusion site. Tell your doctor if you get any infusion-site side effects.

Tell your doctor if you have any side effect that bothers you or that does not go away. These are not all of the possible side effects of EMEND for Injection. For more information ask your doctor or pharmacist.

Call your doctor for medical advice about side effects. You may report side effects to FDA at 1-800-FDA-1088.

General information about EMEND for Injection

This Patient Information leaflet summarizes the most important information about EMEND for Injection. If you would like to know more information, talk with your doctor. You can ask your doctor or pharmacist for information about EMEND for Injection that is written for health professionals. For more information about EMEND for Injection call 1-800-622-4477 or go to www.emend.com.

What are the ingredients in EMEND for Injection?

Active ingredient: fosaprepitant dimeglumine

Inactive ingredients: edetate disodium, polysorbate 80, lactose anhydrous, sodium hydroxide and/or hydrochloric acid (for pH adjustment).

Manufactured for:
Merck Sharp & Dohme Corp., a subsidiary of
MERCK & CO., INC., Whitehouse Station, NJ 08889, USA
Manufactured by:
DSM Pharmaceuticals, Inc., 5900 Martin Luther King Jr. Highway, Greenville, NC 27834, USA
U.S. Patent Nos.: 5,512,570; 5,691,336

The brands listed in the above sections "Who should not take EMEND for Injection?" and "How will I receive EMEND for Injection?" are the registered trademarks of their respective owners and are not trademarks of Merck Sharp & Dohme Corp., a subsidiary of Merck & Co., Inc.

Revised: 07/2012
USPPI-IV-05171207R008

FOLLISTIM® AQ CARTRIDGE ℞

[Fol-lis-tim]
(follitropin beta injection)
for subcutaneous use

HIGHLIGHTS OF PRESCRIBING INFORMATION

These highlights do not include all the information needed to use FOLLISTIM® AQ Cartridge safely and effectively. See full prescribing information for FOLLISTIM® AQ Cartridge. FOLLISTIM® AQ Cartridge (follitropin beta injection) for subcutaneous use
Initial U.S. Approval:1997

INDICATIONS AND USAGE

Follistim AQ Cartridge is a gonadotropin indicated:

In Women for:

- Induction of Ovulation and Pregnancy in Anovulatory Infertile Women in Whom the Cause of Infertility is Functional and Not Due to Primary Ovarian Failure (1.1)
- Pregnancy in Normal Ovulatory Women Undergoing Controlled Ovarian Stimulation as Part of an In Vitro Fertilization (IVF) or Intracytoplasmic Sperm Injection (ICSI) Cycle (1.2)

In Men for:

- Induction of Spermatogenesis in Men with Primary and Secondary Hypogonadotropic Hypogonadism (HH) in Whom the Cause of Infertility is Not Due to Primary Testicular Failure (1.3)

DOSAGE AND ADMINISTRATION

See Dose Conversion Table 1 for Follistim AQ Cartridge with Pen Injector (2.1)

In Anovulatory Women Undergoing Ovulation Induction (2.2):

- Starting daily dose of 50 international units of Follistim AQ Cartridge is administered subcutaneously for at least the first 7 days. The dose is increased by 25 or 50 international units at weekly intervals until follicular growth and/or serum estradiol levels indicate an adequate response.
  - When an acceptable pre-ovulatory state is achieved, final oocyte maturation is achieved with 5,000 to 10,000 international units of human chorionic gonadotropin (hCG).
  - The woman and her partner should have intercourse daily, beginning on the day prior to the administration of hCG and until ovulation becomes apparent.

In Normal Ovulatory Women Undergoing Controlled Ovarian Stimulation as Part of an In Vitro Fertilization or Intracytoplasmic Sperm Injection Cycle (2.3):

- Starting dose of 200 international units (actual cartridge doses) of Follistim AQ Cartridge is administered subcutaneously for at least the first 7 days of treatment. Subsequent doses can be adjusted down or up based upon ovarian response as determined by ultrasound evaluation of follicular growth and serum estradiol levels. Dosage reduction in high responders can be considered from the 6th day of treatment onward according to individual response.
  - Final oocyte maturation is induced with a dose of 5,000-10,000 international units of hCG.
  - Oocyte (egg) retrieval is performed 34 to 36 hours later.

Induction of Spermatogenesis in Men (2.4):

- Pretreatment with hCG alone (1,500 international units twice weekly) is required. If serum testosterone levels have not normalized after 8 weeks of hCG treatment, the dose may be increased to 3,000 international units twice a week.
- After normalization of serum testosterone levels, administer 450 international units per week (225 international units twice weekly or 150 international units three times weekly) of Follistim AQ Cartridge subcutaneously with the same pre-treatment hCG dose used to normalize testosterone levels.

DOSAGE FORMS AND STRENGTHS

Injection:	Follistim AQ Cartridge 175 IU per 0.210 mL (3)
Injection:	Follistim AQ Cartridge 350 IU per 0.420 mL (3)
Injection:	Follistim AQ Cartridge 650 IU per 0.780 mL (3)
Injection:	Follistim AQ Cartridge 975 IU per 1.170 mL (3)

CONTRAINDICATIONS

Women and men who exhibit:

- Prior hypersensitivity to recombinant hFSH products (4)
- High levels of FSH indicating primary gonadal failure (4)
- Presence of uncontrolled non-gonadal endocrinopathies (4)
- Hypersensitivity reactions related to streptomycin or neomycin (4)
- Tumors of the ovary, breast, uterus, testis, hypothalamus or pituitary gland (4)

Women who exhibit:

- Pregnancy (4, 8.1)
- Heavy or irregular vaginal bleeding of undetermined origin (4)
- Ovarian cysts or enlargement not due to polycystic ovary syndrome (PCOS) (4)

WARNINGS AND PRECAUTIONS

Treatment with Follistim AQ may result in:

- Abnormal Ovarian Enlargement (5.1)
- Ovarian Hyperstimulation Syndrome (OHSS) (5.2)
- Pulmonary and Vascular Complications (5.3)
- Ovarian Torsion (5.4)
- Multi-fetal Gestation and Birth (5.5)
- Congenital Anomalies (5.6)
- Ectopic Pregnancy (5.7)
- Spontaneous Abortion (5.8)
- Ovarian Neoplasms (5.9)

ADVERSE REACTIONS

The most common adverse reactions (≥2%) in women undergoing ovulation induction are ovarian hyperstimulation syndrome, ovarian cyst, abdominal discomfort, abdominal pain and lower abdominal pain. (6.1)

The most common adverse reactions (≥2%) in women undergoing controlled ovarian stimulation as part of an IVF or ICSI cycle are pelvic discomfort, headache, ovarian hyperstimulation syndrome, pelvic pain, nausea and fatigue. (6.1)
The most common (≥2%) adverse reactions in men undergoing induction of spermatogenesis are headache, acne, injection site reaction, injection site pain, gynecomastia, rash and dermoid cyst. (6.1)

To report SUSPECTED ADVERSE REACTIONS, contact Merck Sharp & Dohme Corp., a subsidiary of Merck & Co., Inc., at 1-877-888-4231 or FDA at 1-800-FDA-1088 or www.fda.gov/medwatch.

USE IN SPECIFIC POPULATIONS

Nursing Mothers: It is not known whether this drug is excreted in human milk. (8.3)

See 17 for PATIENT COUNSELING INFORMATION and FDA-approved patient labeling

Revised: 08/2012

FULL PRESCRIBING INFORMATION: CONTENTS*

*** Sections or subsections omitted from the full prescribing information are not listed**

FULL PRESCRIBING INFORMATION

1 INDICATIONS AND USAGE

Follistim® AQ (follitropin beta injection) Cartridge is indicated:

In Women for:

1.1 Induction of Ovulation and Pregnancy in Anovulatory Infertile Women in Whom the Cause of Infertility is Functional and Not Due to Primary Ovarian Failure

Prior to initiation of treatment with Follistim AQ Cartridge:
- Women should have a complete gynecologic and endocrinologic evaluation.
- Primary ovarian failure should be excluded.
- The possibility of pregnancy should be excluded.
- Tubal patency should be demonstrated.
- The fertility status of the male partner should be evaluated.

1.2 Pregnancy in Normal Ovulatory Women Undergoing Controlled Ovarian Stimulation as Part of an In Vitro Fertilization (IVF) or Intracytoplasmic Sperm Injection (ICSI) Cycle

Prior to initiation of treatment with Follistim AQ Cartridge:
- Women should have a complete gynecologic and endocrinologic evaluation and diagnosis of cause of infertility.
- The possibility of pregnancy should be excluded.
- The fertility status of the male partner should be evaluated.

In Men for:

1.3 Induction of Spermatogenesis in Men with Primary and Secondary Hypogonadotropic Hypogonadism (HH) in Whom the Cause of Infertility is Not Due to Primary Testicular Failure

Prior to initiation of treatment with Follistim AQ Cartridge:
- Men should have a complete medical and endocrinologic evaluation.
- Hypogonadotropic hypogonadism should be confirmed and primary testicular failure should be excluded.
- Serum testosterone levels should be normalized with human chorionic gonadotropin (hCG) treatment.
- The fertility status of the female partner should be evaluated.

2 DOSAGE AND ADMINISTRATION

2.1 General Dosing Information

- Parenteral drug products should be inspected visually for particulate matter and discoloration prior to administration, whenever solution and container permit. If the solution is not clear and colorless or has particles in it, the solution should not be used.
- Do not add any other medicines into the Follistim AQ Cartridge.
- Follistim AQ Cartridge with the pen injector device delivers on average an 18% higher amount of follitropin beta when compared to reconstituted Follistim delivered with a conventional syringe and needle. When administering Follistim AQ Cartridge, a lower starting dose and lower dose adjustments (as compared to reconstituted Follistim) should be considered. For that purpose the following Dose Conversion Table is provided:

Table 1: Follistim AQ Cartridge Administered Subcutaneously With the Follistim Pen Dose Conversion Table*

Lyophilized recombinant FSH dosing with ampules or vials, using conventional syringe	Follistim AQ Cartridge dosing with the Follistim Pen
75 IU	50 IU
150 IU	125 IU
225 IU	175 IU
300 IU	250 IU
375 IU	300 IU
450 IU	375 IU

*** Each value represents an 18% difference rounded to the nearest 25 IU increment.**

2.2 Recommended Dosing in Anovulatory Women Undergoing Ovulation Induction

The dosing scheme is stepwise and is individualized for each woman *[see Clinical Studies (14.1)]*.
- A starting daily dose of 50 international units of Follistim AQ Cartridge is administered *[see Dosage and Administration (2.1)]* subcutaneously daily for at least the first 7 days.
- Subsequent dosage adjustments are made at weekly intervals based upon ovarian response. If an increase in dose is indicated by the ovarian response, the increase should be made by 25 or 50 international units of Follistim AQ Cartridge at weekly intervals until follicular growth and/or serum estradiol levels indicate an adequate ovarian response.

  The following should be considered when planning the woman's individualized dose:
  - Appropriate Follistim AQ Cartridge dose adjustment(s) should be used to prevent multiple follicular growth and cycle cancellation.
  - The maximum, individualized, daily dose of Follistim AQ Cartridge is 250 international units.
- Treatment should continue until ultrasonic visualizations and/or serum estradiol determinations approximate the pre-ovulatory conditions seen in normal individuals.
- When pre-ovulatory conditions are reached, 5,000 to 10,000 international units of hCG are used to induce final oocyte maturation and ovulation.

  The administration of hCG must be withheld in cases where the ovarian monitoring suggests an increased risk of OHSS on the last day of Follistim AQ Cartridge therapy *[see Warnings and Precautions (5.1, 5.2, 5.10)]*.
- The woman and her partner should be encouraged to have intercourse daily, beginning on the day prior to the administration of hCG and until ovulation becomes apparent *[see Warnings and Precautions (5.10)]*.
- During treatment with Follistim AQ Cartridge and during a two-week post-treatment period, the woman should be assessed at least every other day for signs of excessive ovarian stimulation.

It is recommended that Follistim AQ Cartridge administration be stopped if the ovarian monitoring suggests an increased risk of OHSS or abdominal pain occurs. Most OHSS occurs after treatment has been discontinued and reaches its maximum at about seven to ten days post-ovulation.

2.3 Recommended Dosing in Normal Ovulatory Women Undergoing Controlled Ovarian Stimulation as Part of an In Vitro Fertilization (IVF) or Intracytoplasmic Sperm Injection (ICSI) Cycle

The dosing scheme follows a stepwise approach and is individualized for each woman.
- A starting dose of 200 international units (actual cartridge doses) of Follistim AQ Cartridge is administered *[see Dosage and Administration (2.1)]* subcutaneously daily for at least the first 7 days of treatment.
- Subsequent to the first 7 days of treatment, the dose can be adjusted down or up based upon the woman's ovarian response as determined by ultrasound evaluation of follicular growth and serum estradiol levels. Dosage reduction in high responders can be considered from the 6th day of treatment onward according to individual response.

  The following should be considered when planning the woman's individualized dose:
  - For most normal responding women, the daily starting dose can be continued until pre-ovulatory conditions are achieved (seven to twelve days).
  - For low or poor responding women, the daily dose should be increased according to the ovarian response. The maximum, individualized, daily dose of Follistim AQ Cartridge is 500 international units.
  - For high responding women [those at particular risk of abnormal ovarian enlargement and/or ovarian hyperstimulation syndrome (OHSS)], decrease or temporarily stop the daily dose, or discontinue the cycle according to individual response *[see Warnings and Precautions (5.1, 5.2, 5.10)]*.
- When a sufficient number of follicles of adequate size are present, dosing of Follistim AQ Cartridge is stopped and final maturation of the oocytes is induced by administering hCG at a dose of 5,000 to 10,000 international units. The administration of hCG should be withheld in cases where the ovarian monitoring suggests an increased risk of OHSS on the last day of Follistim AQ Cartridge therapy *[see Warnings and Precautions (5.1, 5.2, 5.10)]*.
- Oocyte (egg) retrieval should be performed 34 to 36 hours following the administration of hCG.

2.4 Recommended Dosing for Induction of Spermatogenesis in Men

- Pretreatment with hCG is required prior to concomitant therapy with Follistim AQ Cartridge and hCG. An initial dosage of 1,500 international units of hCG should be administered at twice weekly intervals to normalize serum testosterone levels. If serum testosterone levels have not normalized after 8 weeks of hCG treatment, the hCG dose can be increased to 3,000 international units twice weekly *[see Clinical Studies (14.3)]*.
- After normal serum testosterone levels have been reached, Follistim AQ Cartridge should be administered by subcutaneous injection concomitantly with hCG treatment. Follistim is given at a dosage of 450 international units per week, as either 225 international units twice weekly or 150 international units three times per week, in combination with the same hCG dose used to normalize testosterone levels. Based on delivery of a higher dose of follitropin beta with the Follistim AQ Cartridge and pen injector *[see Dosage and Administration (2.1)]*, a lower

dose of Follistim AQ Cartridge may be considered.

The concomitant therapy should be continued for at least 3 to 4 months before any improvement in spermatogenesis can be expected. If a man has not responded after this period, the combination therapy may be continued. Treatment response has been noted at up to 12 months.

3 DOSAGE FORMS AND STRENGTHS

Injection: Follistim AQ Cartridge 175 international units per 0.210 mL

Injection: Follistim AQ Cartridge 350 international units per 0.420 mL

Injection: Follistim AQ Cartridge 650 international units per 0.780 mL

Injection: Follistim AQ Cartridge 975 international units per 1.170 mL

4 CONTRAINDICATIONS

Follistim AQ Cartridge is contraindicated in women and men who exhibit:

- Prior hypersensitivity to recombinant hFSH products
- High levels of FSH indicating primary gonadal failure
- Presence of uncontrolled non-gonadal endocrinopathies (e.g., thyroid, adrenal, or pituitary disorders) *[see Indications and Usage (1.1, 1.2, 1.3)]*
- Hypersensitivity reactions to streptomycin or neomycin. Follistim AQ may contain traces of these antibiotics
- Tumors of the ovary, breast, uterus, testis, hypothalamus or pituitary gland

Follistim AQ Cartridge is also contraindicated in women who exhibit:

- Pregnancy *[see Use in Specific Populations (8.1)]*
- Heavy or irregular vaginal bleeding of undetermined origin
- Ovarian cysts or enlargement not due to polycystic ovary syndrome (PCOS)

5 WARNINGS AND PRECAUTIONS

Follistim AQ Cartridge should be used only by physicians who are experienced in infertility treatment. Follistim AQ Cartridge contains a potent gonadotropic substance capable of causing Ovarian Hyperstimulation Syndrome (OHSS) *[see Warnings and Precautions (5.2)]* with or without pulmonary or vascular complications *[see Warnings and Precautions (5.3)]* and multiple births *[see Warnings and Precautions (5.5)]*. Gonadotropin therapy requires the availability of appropriate monitoring facilities *[see Warnings and Precautions (5.10)]*.

Careful attention should be given to the diagnosis of infertility and in the selection of candidates for Follistim AQ Cartridge therapy *[see Indications and Usage (1.1, 1.2, 1.3) and Dosage and Administration (2.2, 2.3, 2.4)]*.

Switching to Follistim AQ Cartridge from other brands (manufacturer), types (recombinant, urinary), and/or methods of administration (Follistim Pen, conventional syringe) may necessitate an adjustment of the dose *[see Dosage and Administration (2)]*.

5.1 Abnormal Ovarian Enlargement

In order to minimize the hazards associated with abnormal ovarian enlargement that may occur with Follistim AQ therapy, treatment should be individualized and the lowest effective dose should be used [see *Dosage and Administration (2.2, 2.3)]*. Use of ultrasound monitoring of ovarian response and/or measurement of serum estradiol levels is important to minimize the risk of overstimulation *[see Warnings and Precautions (5.8)]*.

If the ovaries are abnormally enlarged on the last day of Follistim AQ therapy, hCG should not be administered in order to reduce the chances of developing Ovarian Hyperstimulation Syndrome (OHSS). Intercourse should be prohibited in patients with significant ovarian enlargement after ovulation because of the danger of hemoperitoneum resulting from ruptured ovarian cysts *[see Warnings and Precautions (5.3)]*.

5.2 Ovarian Hyperstimulation Syndrome (OHSS)

OHSS is a medical entity distinct from uncomplicated ovarian enlargement and may progress rapidly to become a serious medical condition. OHSS is characterized by a dramatic increase in vascular permeability, which can result in a rapid accumulation of fluid in the peritoneal cavity, thorax, and potentially, the pericardium. The early warning signs of OHSS developing are severe pelvic pain, nausea, vomiting, and weight gain. Abdominal pain, abdominal distension, gastrointestinal symptoms including nausea, vomiting and diarrhea, severe ovarian enlargement, weight gain, dyspnea, and oliguria have been reported with OHSS. Clinical evaluation may reveal hypovolemia, hemoconcentration, electrolyte imbalances, ascites, hemoperitoneum, pleural effusions, hydrothorax, acute pulmonary distress, and thromboembolic reactions *[see Warnings and Precautions (5.3)]*. Transient liver function test abnormalities suggestive of hepatic dysfunction with or without morphologic changes on liver biopsy have also been reported in association with OHSS.

OHSS occurs after gonadotropin treatment has been discontinued, and it can develop rapidly, reaching its maximum about seven to ten days following treatment. Usually, OHSS resolves spontaneously with the onset of menses. If there is a risk for OHSS evident prior to hCG administration *[see Warnings and Precautions (5.1)]*, the hCG must be withheld. Cases of OHSS are more common, more severe, and more protracted if pregnancy occurs; therefore, women should be assessed for the development of OHSS for at least two weeks after hCG administration.

If serious OHSS occurs, gonadotropins, including hCG, should be stopped and consideration should be given as to whether the patient needs to be hospitalized. Treatment is primarily symptomatic and overall should consist of bed rest, fluid and electrolyte management, and analgesics (if needed). Because the use of diuretics can accentuate the diminished intravascular volume, diuretics should be avoided except in the late phase of resolution as described below. The management of OHSS may be divided into three phases as follows:

- *Acute Phase*:
  Management should be directed at preventing hemoconcentration due to loss of intravascular volume to the third space and minimizing the risk of thromboembolic phenomena and kidney damage. Fluid intake and output, weight, hematocrit, serum and urinary electrolytes, urine specific gravity, BUN and creatinine, total proteins with albumin: globulin ratio, coagulation studies, electrocardiogram to monitor for hyperkalemia, and abdominal girth should be thoroughly assessed daily or more often based on the clinical need. Treatment, consisting of limited intravenous fluids, electrolytes, and human serum albumin is intended to normalize electrolytes while maintaining an acceptable but somewhat reduced intravascular volume. Full correction of the intravascular volume deficit may lead to an unacceptable increase in the amount of third space fluid accumulation.
- *Chronic Phase*:
  After the acute phase is successfully managed as above, excessive fluid accumulation in the third space should be limited by instituting severe potassium, sodium, and fluid restriction.
- *Resolution Phase*:
  As third space fluid returns to the intravascular compartment, a fall in hematocrit and increasing urinary output are observed in the absence of any increase in intake. Peripheral and/or pulmonary edema may result if the kidneys are unable to excrete third space fluid as rapidly as it is mobilized. Diuretics may be indicated during the resolution phase, if necessary, to combat pulmonary edema.

OHSS increases the risk of injury to the ovary. The ascitic, pleural, and pericardial fluid should not be removed unless there is the necessity to relieve symptoms such as pulmonary distress or cardiac tamponade. Pelvic examination may cause rupture of an ovarian cyst, which may result in hemoperitoneum, and should therefore be avoided. If bleeding occurs and requires surgical intervention, the clinical objective should be to control the bleeding and retain as much ovarian tissue as possible.

During clinical trials with Follistim or Follistim AQ Cartridge therapy, OHSS occurred in 7.6% of 105 women (OI) and 6.4% of 751 women (IVF or ICSI) treated with Follistim and Follistim AQ Cartridge, respectively.

5.3 Pulmonary and Vascular Complications

Serious pulmonary conditions (e.g., atelectasis, acute respiratory distress syndrome) have been reported in women treated with gonadotropins. In addition, thromboembolic reactions both in association with, and separate from OHSS have been reported following gonadotropin therapy. Intravascular thrombosis, which may originate in venous or arterial vessels, can result in reduced blood flow to vital organs or the extremities. Women with generally recognized risk factors for thrombosis, such as a personal or family history, severe obesity, or thrombophilia, may have an increased risk of venous or arterial thromboembolic events, during or following treatment with gonadotropins. Sequelae of such reactions have included venous thrombophlebitis, pulmonary embolism, pulmonary infarction, cerebral vascular occlusion (stroke), and arterial occlusion resulting in loss of limb and rarely in myocardial infarction. In rare cases, pulmonary complications and/or thromboembolic reactions have resulted in death. In women with recognized risk factors, the benefits of ovulation induction, in vitro fertilization (IVF) or intracytoplasmic sperm injection (ICSI) treatment need to be weighed against the risks. It should be noted, that pregnancy itself also carries an increased risk of thrombosis.

5.4 Ovarian Torsion

Ovarian torsion has been reported after treatment with Follistim AQ Cartridge and after intervention with other gonadotropins. This may be related to OHSS, pregnancy, previous abdominal surgery, past history of ovarian torsion, previous or current ovarian cyst and polycystic ovaries. Damage to the ovary due to reduced blood supply can be limited by early diagnosis and immediate detorsion.

5.5 Multi-fetal Gestation and Birth

Multi-fetal gestation and births have been reported with all gonadotropin treatments including Follistim AQ Cartridge treatment. The woman and her partner should be advised of the potential risk of multi-fetal gestation and births before starting treatment.

5.6 Congenital Anomalies

The incidence of congenital malformations after IVF or ICSI may be slightly higher than after spontaneous conception. This slightly higher incidence is thought to be related to differences in parental characteristics (e.g., maternal age, sperm characteristics) and to the higher incidence of multi-fetal gestations after IVF or ICSI. There are no indications that the use of gonadotropins during IVF or ICSI is associated with an increased risk of congenital malformations.

5.7 Ectopic Pregnancy

Since infertile women undergoing IVF or ICSI often have tubal abnormalities, the incidence of ectopic pregnancies might be increased. Early confirmation of an intrauterine pregnancy should be determined by β-hCG testing and transvaginal ultrasound.

5.8 Spontaneous Abortion

The risk of spontaneous abortions (miscarriage) is increased with gonadotropin products. However, causality has not been established. The increased risk may be a factor of the underlying infertility.

5.9 Ovarian Neoplasms

There have been infrequent reports of ovarian neoplasms, both benign and malignant, in women who have undergone multiple drug regimens for controlled ovarian stimulation; however, a causal relationship has not been established.

5.10 Laboratory Tests

For Women:

In most instances, treatment with Follistim AQ Cartridge will result only in follicular growth and maturation. In order to complete the final phase of follicular maturation and to induce ovulation, hCG must be given following the administration of Follistim AQ Cartridge or when clinical assessment indicates that sufficient follicular maturation has occurred. The degree of follicular maturation and the timing of hCG administration can both be determined with the use of sonographic visualization of the ovaries and endometrial lining in conjunction with measurement of serum estradiol levels. The combination of transvaginal ultrasonography and measurement of serum estradiol levels is also useful for minimizing the risk of OHSS and multi-fetal gestations.

The clinical confirmation of ovulation is obtained by the following direct or indirect indices of progesterone production as well as sonographic evidence of ovulation.

Direct or indirect indices of progesterone production are:

- Urinary or serum luteinizing hormone (LH) rise
- A rise in basal body temperature
- Increase in serum progesterone
- Menstruation following the shift in basal body temperature

The following provide sonographic evidence of ovulation:

- Collapsed follicle
- Fluid in the cul-de-sac
- Features consistent with corpus luteum formation

Sonographic evaluation of the early pregnancy is also important to rule out ectopic pregnancy.

For Men:

Clinical monitoring for spermatogenesis utilizes the following indirect or direct measures:

- Serum testosterone level
- Semen analysis

5.11 Follistim Pen

The Follistim Pen is intended only for use with Follistim AQ Cartridge. The Follistim Pen is not recommended for the blind or visually impaired without the assistance of an individual with good vision who is trained in the proper use of the injection device.

6 ADVERSE REACTIONS

The following serious adverse reactions are discussed elsewhere in the labeling:

- Ovarian Hyperstimulation Syndrome *[see Warnings and Precautions (5.2)]*
- Atelectasis *[see Warnings and Precautions (5.3)]*
- Thromboembolism *[see Warnings and Precautions (5.3)]*
- Ovarian Torsion *[see Warnings and Precautions (5.4)]*
- Multi-fetal Gestation and Birth *[see Warnings and Precautions (5.5)]*
- Congenital Anomalies *[see Warnings and Precautions (5.6)]*
- Ectopic Pregnancy *[see Warnings and Precautions (5.7)]*
- Spontaneous Abortion *[see Warnings and Precautions (5.8)]*

6.1 Clinical Study Experience

Because clinical trials are conducted under widely varying conditions, adverse reactions rates observed in the clinical trials of a drug cannot be directly compared to rates in the clinical trial of another drug and may not reflect the rates observed in practice.

Ovulation Induction

In a single cycle, multi-center, assessor-blind, parallel group, comparative study, a total of 172 chronic anovulatory women who had failed to ovulate and/or conceive with clomiphene citrate therapy, were randomized and treated with Follistim (105) or a urofollitropin comparator. Adverse reactions with an incidence of greater than 2% in either treatment group are listed in Table 2.

Table 2: Common Adverse Reactions Reported at a Frequency of ≥2% in an Assessor-Blind, Comparative Study of Anovulatory Women Receiving Ovulation Induction

System Organ Class/Adverse Reactions	Treatment Number (%) of Women	
	Follistim N=105 n (%)	Comparator N=67 n (%)
Gastrointestinal disorders		
Abdominal discomfort	3 (2.9)	1 (1.5)
Abdominal pain	3 (2.9)	2 (3.0)
Abdominal pain lower	3 (2.9)	1 (1.5)
Reproductive system and breast disorders		
Ovarian cyst	3 (2.9)	2 (3.0)
Ovarian hyperstimulation syndrome	8 (7.6)	3 (4.5)
General disorders and administration site conditions		
Pyrexia	0 (0.0)	2 (3.0)

Adverse reactions reported commonly (greater than or equal to 2% of women treated with Follistim) in other ovulation induction clinical trials were headache, abdominal distension, constipation, diarrhea, nausea, pelvic pain, uterine enlargement, vaginal hemorrhage and injection site reaction.

In Vitro Fertilization/Intracytoplasmic Sperm Injection

In a single cycle, multi-center, double-blind, parallel group, comparative study, a total of 1509 women were randomized to receive controlled ovarian stimulation with either Follistim AQ Cartridge (751 women were treated with Follistim AQ Cartridge) or a comparator and pituitary suppression with a gonadotropin releasing hormone (GnRH) antagonist as part of an in vitro fertilization (IVF) or intracytoplasmic sperm injection (ICSI) cycle. Table 3 lists adverse reactions with an incidence of greater than 2% in the group of women treated with Follistim AQ Cartridge.

Table 3: Common Adverse Reactions Reported At a Frequency of ≥2% in a Randomized, Double-blind, Active-controlled, Comparative Study of Normal Ovulatory Women Undergoing Controlled Ovarian Stimulation as Part of an In Vitro Fertilization or Intracytoplasmic Sperm Injection Cycle

System Organ Class/Adverse Reactions	Follistim AQ Cartridge Treatment N = 751 n* (%)
Nervous System disorders	
Headache	55 (7.3%)
Gastrointestinal disorders	
Nausea	29 (3.9%)
Reproductive system and breast disorders	
Ovarian Hyperstimulation Syndrome	48 (6.4%)
Pelvic discomfort	62 (8.3%)
Pelvic Pain	41 (5.5%)
General disorders and Administration site conditions	
Fatigue	17 (2.3%)

* n = number of women with the adverse reaction

Induction of Spermatogenesis

In an open-label, non-comparative clinical trial, 49 men with hypogonadotropic hypogonadism were enrolled to receive pretreatment with hCG, followed by combination therapy with hCG and Follistim for induction of spermatogenesis. Of the 49 men, 30 received weekly Follistim doses of 450 international units; 24 of these 30 men received a total of 48 weeks of treatment with Follistim. Adverse reactions occurring with an incidence of greater than 2% in the 30 men treated with Follistim are listed in Table 4.

Table 4: Common Adverse Reactions Reported At a Frequency of ≥2% in an Open-Label Clinical Trial in Men with Hypogonadotropic Hypogonadism

System Organ Class/Adverse Reactions	Follistim Treatment N=30 n (%)
Nervous system disorders	
Headache	2 (6.7)
General disorders and administration site disorders	
Injection site reaction	2 (6.7)
Injection site pain	2 (6.7)
Skin and cutaneous tissue disorders	
Acne	2 (6.7)
Rash	1 (3.3)
Reproductive system and breast disorders	
Gynecomastia	1 (3.3)
Neoplasms benign, malignant and unspecified	
Dermoid cyst	1 (3.3)

6.2 Postmarketing Experience

The following adverse reactions have been identified during post approval use of Follistim and/or Follistim AQ Cartridge. Because these reactions are reported voluntarily from a population of uncertain size, it is not always possible to reliably estimate their frequency or establish a causal relationship to drug exposure.

Gastrointestinal disorders

Abdominal distension, abdominal pain, constipation, diarrhea

General disorders and administration site conditions

Injection site reaction

Reproductive system and breast disorders

Breast tenderness, metrorrhagia, ovarian enlargement, vaginal hemorrhage

Skin and subcutaneous tissue disorders

Rash

Vascular disorders

Thromboembolism *[see Warnings and Precautions (5.3)]*

7 DRUG INTERACTIONS

No drug-drug interaction studies have been performed.

8 USE IN SPECIFIC POPULATIONS

8.1 Pregnancy

Pregnancy Category X: Follistim AQ Cartridge should not be used during pregnancy *[see Contraindications (4)]*.

8.3 Nursing Mothers

It is not known whether this drug is excreted in human milk. Because many drugs are excreted in human milk and because of the potential for serious adverse reactions in the nursing infant from Follistim AQ Cartridge, a decision should be made whether to discontinue nursing or to discontinue the drug, taking into account the importance of the drug to the mother.

8.4 Pediatric Use

Safety and effectiveness in pediatric patients have not been established.

8.5 Geriatric Use

Clinical studies of Follistim did not include subjects aged 65 and over.

10 OVERDOSAGE

Aside from the possibility of Ovarian Hyperstimulation Syndrome *[see Warnings and Precautions (5.2, 5.3)]* and multiple gestations *[see Warnings and Precautions (5.5)]*, there is no additional information concerning the consequences of acute overdosage with Follistim AQ Cartridge.

11 DESCRIPTION

Follistim AQ Cartridge contains human follicle-stimulating hormone (hFSH), a glycoprotein hormone which is manufactured by recombinant DNA (rDNA) technology. The active drug substance, follitropin beta, has a dimeric structure containing two glycoprotein subunits (alpha and beta). Both the 92 amino acid alpha-chain and the 111 amino acid beta-chain have complex heterogeneous structures arising from two N-linked oligosaccharide chains. Follitropin beta is synthesized in a Chinese hamster ovary (CHO) cell line that has been transfected with a plasmid containing the two subunit DNA sequences encoding for hFSH. The purification process results in a highly purified preparation with a consistent hFSH isoform profile and high specific activity [as determined by the Ph. Eur. test for FSH *in vivo* bioactivity and on the basis of the molar extinction coefficient at 277 nm (ϵ_s:mg^{-1}cm^{-1}) = 1.066].

The biological activity is determined by measuring the increase in ovary weight in female rats. The intrinsic luteinizing hormone (LH) activity in follitropin beta is less than 1 international unit per 40,000 international units FSH. The compound is considered to contain no LH activity.

The amino acid sequence and tertiary structure of the product are indistinguishable from that of hFSH of urinary source. Also, based on available data derived from physicochemical tests and bioassay, follitropin beta and follitropin alfa, another recombinant follicle-stimulating hormone product, are indistinguishable.

Follistim AQ Cartridge is a ready for use, prefilled with solution, disposable cartridge containing either 175 IU of follitropin beta in 0.210 mL (833 IU/mL), 350 IU in 0.420 mL (833 IU/mL), 650 IU in 0.780 mL (833 IU/mL) or 975 IU in 1.170 mL (833 IU/mL) of aqueous solution for multiple dose use, with a maximal deliverable dose of either 150 IU, 300 IU, 600 IU or 900 IU, respectively. Inactive ingredients in the cartridges include: benzyl alcohol NF 10 mg/mL; L-methionine USP 0.5 mg/mL; polysorbate 20 NF 0.2 mg/mL; sodium citrate (dihydrate) USP 14.7 mg/mL; sucrose NF 50 mg/mL; and water for injection USP. Hydrochloric acid NF and/or sodium hydroxide NF are used to adjust the pH to 7.

Follistim AQ Cartridge is for use only with the Follistim Pen, which features an adjustable dosing system for administering the drug in a microvolume of solution. The Follistim Pen with Follistim AQ Cartridge is intended for SUBCUTANEOUS USE ONLY. The recombinant protein in Follistim AQ Cartridge has been standardized for FSH *in vivo* bioactivity in terms of the WHO International Standard for Follicle Stimulating Hormone (FSH) Recombinant, Human for Bioassay (code 92/642), issued by the World Health Organization Expert Committee on Biological Standardization (1995). Under current storage conditions, Follistim AQ may contain up to 11% of oxidized follitropin beta.

In clinical trials with Follistim, serum antibodies to FSH or anti-CHO cell derived proteins were not detected in any of the treated patients after exposure to Follistim for up to three cycles.

12 CLINICAL PHARMACOLOGY

12.1 Mechanism of Action

<u>*Women:*</u>

Follicle-stimulating hormone (FSH), the active component in Follistim AQ Cartridge, is required for normal follicular growth, maturation, and gonadal steroid production.

In women, the level of FSH is critical for the onset and duration of follicular development, and consequently for the timing and number of follicles reaching maturity. Follistim AQ Cartridge stimulates ovarian follicular growth in women who do not have primary ovarian failure. In order to effect the final phase of follicle maturation, resumption of meiosis and rupture of the follicle in the absence of an endogenous LH surge, human chorionic gonadotropin (hCG) must be given following treatment with Follistim AQ Cartridge when patient monitoring indicates appropriate follicular development parameters have been reached.

<u>*Men:*</u>

Follistim when administered with hCG stimulates spermatogenesis in men with hypogonadotropic hypogonadism. FSH, the active component of Follistim, is the pituitary hormone responsible for spermatogenesis.

12.3 Pharmacokinetics

Pharmacokinetic parameters for Follistim AQ Cartridge were evaluated in an open-label, single-center, randomized study in 20 healthy women. Serum FSH values from a single subcutaneous injection of reconstituted Follistim lyophilized powder administered by conventional syringe were compared to those values following a single subcutaneous injection of Follistim AQ Cartridge administered with the Follistim Pen injector. Administration of follitropin beta with the Follistim Pen resulted an 18% increase in $AUC_{0-\infty}$ and C_{max}. The 18% difference in serum FSH concentrations resulting from administration of the two formulations was due to differences between the anticipated and actual volume delivered with the conventional syringe. The pharmacokinetic parameters for Follistim AQ Cartridge are as follows:

[See table 5 at top of next page]

Absorption:

<u>*Women:*</u>

The bioavailability of Follistim following subcutaneous and intramuscular administration was investigated in healthy, pituitary-suppressed women given a single 300 international units dose. In these women, the area under the curve (AUC), expressed as the mean ± SD, was equivalent between the subcutaneous (455.6 ± 141.4 IU*h/L) and intramuscular (445.7 ± 135.7 IU*h/L) routes of administration. However, equivalence could not be established with respect to the peak serum FSH levels (C_{max}). The C_{max} achieved af-

Table 5: Mean (SD) Pharmacokinetic Parameters of a Single Subcutaneous Injection of 150 IU of Follistim AQ Cartridge (n=20)

	$AUC_{0-\infty}$ (IU/L*h)	C_{max} (IU/L)	t_{max} (h)	$t_{1/2}$ (h)	CL_{app} (L/h/kg)
Follistim AQ Cartridge	215.1 (45.8)	3.4 (0.7)	12.9 (6.2)	33.4 (4.2)	0.01 (0.003)

$AUC_{0-\infty}$ Area under the curve
C_{max} Maximum concentration
t_{max} Time to maximum concentration
$t_{1/2}$ Elimination half-life
CL_{app} Clearance

Table 9: Number of Men Receiving Follistim Who Achieved a Mean Sperm Density of ≥10⁶/mL on Their Last Two Treatment Assessments

	Follistim 150 international units three times a week (n=15)		Follistim 225 international units twice a week (n=15)		Overall (n=30)	
Sperm Density of $\geq 10^6$/mL	n	%	n	%	n	%
Yes	6	40	7	47	13	43
No	9	60	8	53	17	57

ter subcutaneous administration and intramuscular administration was 5.41 ± 0.72 international units/L and 6.86 ± 2.90 international units/L, respectively. After subcutaneous or intramuscular injection the apparent dose absorbed was 77.8% and 76.4%, respectively.

The pharmacokinetics and pharmacodynamics of a single, intramuscular dose (300 international units) of Follistim were also investigated in a group (n=8) of gonadotropin-deficient, but otherwise healthy women. In these women, FSH (mean ± SD) AUC was 339 ± 105 international units*h/L, C_{max} was 4.3 ± 1.7 international units/L. C_{max} occurred at approximately 27 ± 5.4 hours after intramuscular administration.

A multiple dose, dose proportionality, pharmacokinetic study of Follistim was completed in healthy, pituitary-suppressed, female subjects given subcutaneous doses of 75, 150, or 225 international units for 7 days. Steady-state blood concentrations of FSH were reached with all doses after 5 days of treatment based on the trough concentrations of FSH just prior to dosing (C_{trough}). Peak blood concentrations with the 75, 150, and 225 international units dose were 4.30 ± 0.60 international units/L, 8.51 ± 1.16 international units/L and 13.92 ± 1.81 international units/L, respectively.

Men:

No PK studies were conducted using Follistim AQ Cartridge in men. Exposures of follitropin beta from Follistim AQ Cartridge and Follistim are expected to be equivalent after adjusting for the 18% difference in dose *[see Dosage and Administration (2)]*.

Serum levels of FSH were measured in a clinical study that compared the effects of two different dosing schedules of Follistim (150 international units three times a week or 225 international units twice a week) administered by subcutaneous injection concurrently with chorionic gonadotropin for induction of spermatogenesis in hypogonadotropic hypogonadal men. Administration of Follistim was started at Week 17. Mean serum trough concentrations of FSH remained fairly constant over the treatment period. At the end of treatment (Week 64), the mean serum trough concentrations of FSH were 2.09 international units/L in the 150 international units group and 3.22 international units/L in the 225 international units group. Serum trough concentrations of FSH measured prior to the first Follistim injection on the Mondays of active treatment period (Weeks 17 to 64) and one week after the end of treatment period are presented in Figure 1.

[See figure 1 at top of next column]

Distribution:

The volume of distribution of Follistim in healthy, pituitary-suppressed, women following intravenous administration of a 300 international units dose was approximately 8 L.

Metabolism:

The recombinant FSH in Follistim AQ Cartridge is biochemically very similar to urinary FSH and it is therefore anticipated that it is metabolized in the same manner.

Elimination:

The elimination half-life ($t_{1/2}$) following a single subcutaneous injection of 150 IU of Follistim AQ Cartridge in women was 33.4 (4.2) hours. The clearance was 0.01 (0.003) L/h/kg.

Use in Specific Populations:

Body weight: The effect of body weight on the pharmacokinetics of Follistim was evaluated in a group of European

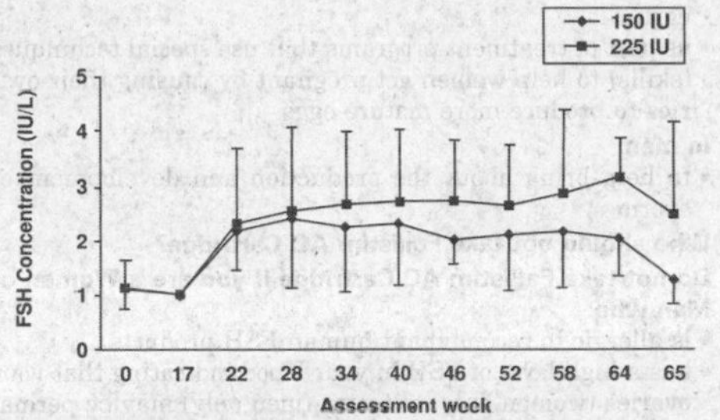

Figure 1: Mean (SD) Serum Trough Concentrations of FSH in Men Following Subcutaneous Administration of Follistim Using Two Different Dosing Schedules (150 International Units Three Times a Week or 225 International Units Twice a Week)

and Japanese women who were significantly different in terms of body weight. The European women had a body weight of (mean ± SD) 67.4 ± 13.5 kg and the Japanese subjects were 46.8 ± 11.6 kg. Following a single intramuscular dose of 300 international units of Follistim, the AUC was significantly smaller in European women (339 ± 105 international units*h/L) than in Japanese women (544 ± 201 international units*h/L). However, clearance per kg of body weight was essentially the same for the respective groups (0.014 and 0.013 L/hr/kg).

Geriatric Use: The pharmacokinetics of Follistim has not been studied in geriatric subjects.

Pediatric Use: The pharmacokinetics of Follistim has not been studied in pediatric subjects.

Renal Impairment: The effect of renal impairment on the pharmacokinetics of Follistim has not been studied.

Hepatic Impairment: The effect of hepatic impairment on the pharmacokinetics of Follistim has not been studied.

13 NONCLINICAL TOXICOLOGY

13.1 Carcinogenesis, Mutagenesis, Impairment of Fertility

Long-term toxicity studies in animals have not been performed with Follistim to evaluate the carcinogenic potential of the drug. Follistim was not mutagenic in the Ames test using *S. typhimurium* and *E. coli* tester strains and did not produce chromosomal aberrations in an in vitro assay using human lymphocytes.

14 CLINICAL STUDIES

14.1 Ovulation Induction

The efficacy of Follistim for ovulation induction was evaluated in a randomized, assessor-blind, parallel-group comparative, multicenter safety and efficacy study of 172 chronic anovulatory women (105 subjects on Follistim) who had previously failed to ovulate and/or conceive during clomiphene citrate treatment. The study results for ovulation rates are summarized in Table 6 and those for pregnancy rates are summarized in Table 7.

Table 6: Cumulative Ovulation Rates

Cycle	Follistim (n=105)
First treatment cycle	72%
Second treatment cycle	82%
Third treatment cycle	85%

Table 7: Cumulative Ongoing*,† Pregnancy Rates

Cycle	Follistim (n=105)
First treatment cycle	14%
Second treatment cycle	19%
Third treatment cycle	23%

* All ongoing pregnancies were confirmed after at least 12 weeks after the hCG injection.
† Study was not powered to demonstrate this outcome.

14.2 Controlled Ovarian Stimulation as Part of an In Vitro Fertilization (IVF) or Intracytoplasmic Sperm Injection (ICSI) Cycle

The efficacy of Follistim AQ Cartridge was evaluated in a randomized, double-blind, active-controlled study of 1,509 healthy normal ovulatory women (mean age, body weight, and body mass index of 32 years, 68 kg and 25 kg/m², respectively) treated for one cycle with controlled ovarian stimulation and pituitary suppression with a GnRH antagonist as part of an in vitro fertilization or intracytoplasmic sperm injection cycle. This 2008 study was conducted in Europe and North America (United States and Canada). Approximately 54% of the subjects were from North America. The overall results, as well as the results from North America only, for clinical pregnancy are summarized in Table 8.

Table 8: Pregnancy Results from Treatment With Follistim AQ Cartridge and a GnRH Antagonist in Normal Ovulatory Women Undergoing Controlled Ovarian Stimulation as Part of an In Vitro Fertilization or Intracytoplasmic Sperm Injection Cycle.* Intent-to-Treat Population (ITT)

Parameter	Follistim AQ Cartridge Overall data (n=750)	Follistim AQ Cartridge North American data (n=403)
Clinical pregnancy rate/ cycle initiation†	41.1%	48.9%

* single treatment cycle results
† Clinical pregnancy was assessed ≥6 weeks after transfer of one or two embryos.

14.3 Induction of Spermatogenesis

The safety and efficacy of Follistim administered by subcutaneous injection concomitantly with chorionic gonadotropin for injection (hCG) has been examined in a multicenter, open-label, non-comparator clinical study for induction of spermatogenesis in hypogonadotropic hypogonadal men. The study compared the effects of two different Follistim dosing schedules on semen parameters and serum levels of follicle stimulating hormone (FSH). The multicenter study involved a 16-week pretreatment phase with hCG at a dosage of 1,500 international units twice a week to normalize serum testosterone levels. If serum testosterone levels did not normalize after 8 weeks of hCG treatment, the hCG dose could have been increased to 3,000 international units twice a week. This phase was followed by a 48-week treatment phase. Men who were still azoospermic after the pretreatment phase were randomized to receive either 225 international units Follistim together with 1,500 international units hCG twice a week or 150 international units Follistim three times a week together with 1,500 international units hCG twice weekly. Men who required 3,000 international units of hCG twice a week in the pretreatment phase were continued on that dosage during the treatment phase. The mean age of patients in both treatment groups was approximately 30 years (range 18 to 47 years). At baseline, mean left and right testis volumes were 4.61 ± 2.94 mL and 4.57 ± 3.00 mL, respectively, in the group receiving three weekly injections of Follistim. For the group receiving two weekly injections of Follistim, the mean left and right testis volumes were 6.54 ± 2.45 mL and 7.21 ± 2.94 mL, respectively, at baseline. The primary efficacy endpoint was the percentage of patients with a mean sperm density of ≥1 × 10⁶/mL on their last two treatment assessments. The outcomes of treatment in the 30 men enrolled in the treatment phase are summarized in Table 9.

[See table 9 at top of previous page]

Overall, the median time to reach a sperm concentration of 10^6 per mL was 165 days (range 25 to 327 days) in patients who demonstrated a sperm concentration of at least 10^6 per mL. The median time to reach a sperm concentration of at least 10^6 per mL was 186 days (range 25 to 327 days) for the 150 international units group and 141 days (range 43 to 204 days) for the 225 international units group. No pregnancy data were collected during the trial.

The local tolerance data were comparable between the two treatment groups. The mean percentage of days without pain calculated for all subjects in the treatment period was 91.3% for patients in the 150 international units (three times a week) and 76.0% for patients in the 225 international units (two times a week) Follistim treatment groups. In the 225 international units (twice per week) group, local symptoms judged as severe by the investigator were: itching in 1 patient (7%), pain in 2 patients (13%), bruising in 2 patients (13%), swelling in 2 patients (13%), and redness in 1 patient (7%). In the 150 international units (three times per week) group, 1 event in 1 patient (bruising, 7%) was judged as severe. No patient discontinued treatment due to injection site reaction or injection site pain.

16 HOW SUPPLIED/STORAGE AND HANDLING

Follistim AQ Cartridge is supplied in a box containing disposable, 29 gauge, ultra-fine, ½-inch, sterile BD Micro-Fine™ Pen Needles (for use with Follistim Pen available separately) and one disposable, blister packed, prefilled 1.5 mL colorless glass cartridge, with grey rubber piston and an aluminum crimp-cap with black rubber inlay and in the following presentations:

NDC 0052-0303-01 Follistim AQ Cartridge 175 international units per 0.210 mL (delivering 150 international units) with orange crimp-caps and 3 BD Micro-Fine Pen Needles

NDC 0052-0313-01 Follistim AQ Cartridge 350 international units per 0.420 mL (delivering 300 international units) with silver crimp-caps and 5 BD Micro-Fine Pen Needles

NDC 0052-0316-01 Follistim AQ Cartridge 650 international units per 0.780 mL (delivering 600 international units) with gold crimp-caps and 7 BD Micro-Fine Pen Needles

NDC 0052-0326-01 Follistim AQ Cartridge 975 international units per 1.170 mL (delivering 900 international units) with blue crimp-caps and 10 BD Micro-Fine Pen Needles

Store refrigerated 2-8°C (36-46°F) until dispensed. Upon dispensing, the product may be stored by the patient at 2-8°C (36-46°F) until the expiration date, or at 25°C (77°F) for 3 months or until expiration date, whichever occurs first. Once the rubber inlay of the Follistim AQ Cartridge has been pierced by a needle, the product can only be stored for a maximum of 28 days at 2-25°C (36-77°F). Protect from light. Do not freeze.

17 PATIENT COUNSELING INFORMATION

"See FDA-Approved Patient Labeling (Patient Information)"

17.1 Dosing and Use of Follistim AQ Cartridge with Pen

Instruct women and men on the correct usage and dosing of Follistim AQ Cartridge in conjunction with the Follistim Pen. Make sure that individuals who have used other gonadotropin products delivered by a syringe are aware of differences arising from use of the pen. Women and men should read and follow all instructions in the Follistim Pen "Instructions for Use" Manual prior to administration of Follistim AQ Cartridge.

Advise women and men of the number of doses which can be extracted from the full unused Follistim AQ Cartridge that you have prescribed.

17.2 Therapy Duration and Necessary Monitoring in Women and Men Undergoing Treatment

Prior to beginning therapy with Follistim AQ Cartridge, inform women and men about the time commitment and monitoring procedures necessary to undergo treatment *[see Dosage and Administration (2), Warnings and Precautions (5.10)]*.

17.3 Instructions on a Missed Dose

Inform women and men that if they miss or forget to take a dose of Follistim AQ Cartridge, the next dose should not be doubled and they should call the healthcare provider for further dosing instructions.

17.4 Ovarian Hyperstimulation Syndrome

Inform women regarding the risks with use of Follistim AQ Cartridge of Ovarian Hyperstimulation Syndrome *[see Warnings and Precautions (5.2)]* and associated symptoms including lung and blood vessel problems *[see Warnings and Precautions (5.3)]* and ovarian torsion *[see Warnings and Precautions (5.4)]*.

17.5 Multi-fetal Gestation and Birth

Inform women regarding the risk of multi-fetal gestations with the use of Follistim AQ Cartridge *[see Warnings and Precautions (5.5)]*.

Manufactured for: Merck Sharp & Dohme Corp., a subsidiary of

MERCK & CO., INC., Whitehouse Station, NJ 08889, USA

Manufactured by: Vetter Pharma-Fertigung GmbH & Co. KG, Ravensburg, Germany

BD, BD Logo and BD Micro-Fine are trademarks of Becton, Dickinson and Company

U.S. Patent Nos. 5,767,251; 5,929,028; 7,446,090 and 7,563,763.

Revised: 08/2012

900328-FTB-SOi-P-USPI.10

PATIENT INFORMATION

Follistim® (Fol'-lis-tim) AQ Cartridge
(follitropin beta injection)

Read the Patient Information that comes with Follistim® AQ Cartridge before you start using it and each time you get a refill. There may be new information. This information does not take the place of talking with your healthcare provider about your medical condition or treatment.

What is Follistim AQ Cartridge?

Follistim AQ is a prescription medicine that contains follicle-stimulating hormone (FSH). The medicine is taken with the Follistim Pen®.

Follistim AQ Cartridge is used:

In women:

- to help healthy ovaries to develop (mature) and release eggs
- as part of treatment programs that use special techniques (skills) to help women get pregnant by causing their ovaries to produce more mature eggs

In men:

- to help bring about the production and development of sperm

Who should not take Follistim AQ Cartridge?

Do not take Follistim AQ Cartridge if you are a Woman or Man who:

- is allergic to recombinant human FSH products
- has a high level of FSH in your blood indicating that your ovaries (women only) or testes (men only) may be permanently damaged and do not work at all
- has uncontrolled thyroid, pituitary, or adrenal gland problems
- is allergic to streptomycin or neomycin (types of antibiotics)
- has a tumor of the hypothalamus, pituitary gland, breast, uterus (women only), ovary (women only), or testis (men only)

Do not take Follistim AQ Cartridge if you are a Woman who:

- is pregnant or think you may be pregnant
- has heavy or irregular vaginal bleeding and the cause is not known
- has ovarian cysts or enlarged ovaries, not due to polycystic ovary syndrome (PCOS)

Talk to your healthcare provider before taking this medicine if you have any of the conditions listed above.

What should I tell my healthcare provider before taking Follistim AQ Cartridge?

Before you take Follistim AQ, tell your healthcare provider if you:

- have an increased risk of blood clots (thrombosis)
- have ever had a blood clot (thrombosis), or anyone in your immediate family has ever had a blood clot (thrombosis)
- had stomach (abdominal) surgery
- had twisting of your ovary (ovarian torsion)
- had or have a cyst in your ovary
- have polycystic ovary disease
- have any other medical conditions
- are breastfeeding or plan to breastfeed. It is not known if the medicine in Follistim AQ Cartridge passes into your breast milk. You and your healthcare provider should decide if you will take Follistim AQ Cartridge or breastfeed. You should not do both.

Tell your healthcare provider about all the medicines you take, including prescription and non-prescription medicines, vitamins, and herbal supplements.

Know the medicines you take. Keep a list of them and show your healthcare provider and pharmacist when you get a new medicine.

How should I use Follistim AQ Cartridge?

- Be sure that you read, understand, and follow the "Patient Instructions for Use" that come with Follistim AQ Cartridge.
- Use Follistim AQ Cartridge exactly as your healthcare provider tells you to.
- Your healthcare provider will tell you how much Follistim AQ Cartridge to use, how to inject it, and how often it should be injected.
- Do not inject Follistim AQ Cartridge at home until your healthcare provider has taught you the right way to put the cartridge and pen device together and to inject yourself.
- Do not mix any other medicines into the cartridge.
- Do not change your dose of Follistim AQ Cartridge unless your healthcare provider tells you to.
- Call your healthcare provider immediately if you use too much Follistim AQ Cartridge.
- If you miss or forget to take a dose, do not double your next dose. Ask your healthcare provider for instructions.
- Use Follistim AQ Cartridge only with the Follistim Pen.
- Do not use the Follistim Pen if you are blind or visually impaired unless you have assistance from an individual with good vision who is trained in the right way to use the pen.
- Do not re-use the BD Micro-Fine™ Pen Needle.
- Your healthcare provider will do blood and urine hormone tests while you are taking Follistim AQ Cartridge. Make sure you follow-up with your healthcare provider to have your blood and urine tested when told to do so.

Women:

- Your healthcare provider may do ultrasound scans of your ovaries. Make sure you follow-up with your healthcare provider to have your ultrasound scans.

Men:

- Your healthcare provider may test your semen while you are taking Follistim AQ Cartridge. Make sure you follow-up with your healthcare provider to give a semen sample for testing.

What are the possible side effects of Follistim AQ Cartridge?

Follistim AQ Cartridge may cause serious side effects.

Serious side effects in women include:

- Ovarian enlargement
- Ovarian hyperstimulation syndrome (OHSS). OHSS is a serious medical problem that can happen when the ovaries are over stimulated. In rare cases it has caused death. OHSS causes fluid to build up suddenly in your stomach and chest areas and can cause blood clots to form. Call your healthcare provider right away if you have:
  - pain in your lower stomach area
  - nausea
  - vomiting
  - weight gain
  - diarrhea
  - decreased urine output
  - trouble breathing
- Lung problems. Follistim AQ Cartridge can cause you to have fluid in your lungs (atelectasis) and trouble breathing (acute respiratory distress syndrome).
- Blood clots. Follistim AQ Cartridge may increase your chance of having blood clots in your blood vessels. Blood clots can cause:
  - blood vessel problems (thrombophlebitis)
  - stroke
  - loss of your arm or leg
  - blood clot in your lungs (pulmonary embolus)
  - heart attack
- Ovarian torsion. Follistim AQ Cartridge may increase the chance of twisting of the ovaries in women with certain conditions such as OHSS, pregnancy and previous abdominal surgery. Twisting of the ovary could cause the blood flow to the ovary to be cut off.
- Pregnancy and birth of multiple babies. Having a pregnancy with more than one baby at a time increases the health risk for you and your babies. Discuss your chances of multiple births with your healthcare provider.
- Birth defects. A woman's age, certain sperm problems, genetic background of both parents and a pregnancy with multiple babies can increase the chance that your baby might have birth defects.
- Ectopic pregnancy (pregnancy outside of the womb). The chance of a pregnancy outside of the womb is increased in women with damaged fallopian tubes.
- Miscarriage. The chance of loss of an early pregnancy may be increased in women who have difficulty with becoming pregnant at all.

The most common side effects of Follistim AQ Cartridge include:

In women:

- headache
- nausea
- stomach pain
- discomfort or pain in the lower stomach area
- cyst (closed sac) in the ovary
- feeling tired

In men:

- headache
- pain at the injection site
- bruising, swelling or redness at the injection site
- breast enlargement
- acne

These are not all the possible side effects of Follistim AQ Cartridge. For more information, ask your healthcare provider or pharmacist.

Call your healthcare provider immediately if you get worsening or strong pain in the lower stomach area (abdomen). Also, call your healthcare provider immediately if this happens some days after the last injection has been given.

Tell your healthcare provider if you have any side effect that bothers you or that does not go away.

Call your doctor for medical advice about side effects. You may report side effects to FDA at 1-800-FDA-1088.

How should I store Follistim AQ Cartridge?

- Store Follistim AQ Cartridge in the refrigerator between 2-8°C (36-46°F) until the expiration date.
- Follistim AQ can be stored at or below 25°C (77°F) for 3 months or until the expiration date, whichever comes first. Once the rubber inlay of the Follistim AQ Cartridge has been pierced by a needle, the product may be stored only for a maximum of 28 days at 2-25°C (36-77°F).
- Keep Follistim AQ Cartridge away from light.
- Do not freeze.

Keep Follistim AQ Cartridge and all medicines out of the reach of children.

General information about Follistim AQ Cartridge

Medicines are sometimes prescribed for purposes other than those listed in the Patient Information leaflet. Do not use Follistim AQ for a condition for which it was not prescribed. Do not give Follistim AQ Cartridge to other people, even if they have the same condition that you have. It may harm them.

This Patient Information leaflet summarizes the most important information about Follistim AQ Cartridge. If you would like more information, talk with your healthcare provider. You can ask your pharmacist or healthcare provider for more information about Follistim AQ Cartridge that is written for healthcare professionals.

For more information, go to **www.follistim.com** or call 1-866-836-5633.

What are the ingredients in Follistim AQ Cartridge?

Active ingredient: follitropin beta

Inactive ingredients: sucrose, sodium citrate, benzyl alcohol NF-10 mg/mL, L-methionine, polysorbate 20, water for injection, hydrochloric acid, and/or sodium hydroxide.

Manufactured for: Merck Sharp & Dohme Corp., a subsidiary of **MERCK & CO., INC.**, Whitehouse Station, NJ 08889, USA

Manufactured by: Vetter Pharma-Fertigung GmbH & Co. KG, Ravensburg, Germany

BD, BD Logo and BD Micro-Fine are trademarks of Becton, Dickinson and Company.

U.S. Patent Nos. 5,767,251; 5,929,028; 7,446,090 and 7,563,763.

Revised: 08/2012

900328-FTB-SOi-P-PPI.10

PATIENT INSTRUCTIONS FOR USE

Follistim® (Fol'-lis-tim) AQ Cartridge

(follitropin beta injection)

Read the Patient Instructions for Use that comes with Follistim® AQ Cartridge before you start using it and each time you get a refill. There may be new information. This information does not take the place of talking with your healthcare provider about your medical condition or treatment.

A. Getting Ready

- Follistim Pen is not recommended for the blind or visually impaired user without the assistance of an individual with good vision, trained in the proper use of the injection device.
- Learn about all of the parts of the Follistim Pen (See Figure 1), Follistim AQ Cartridge (Figure 2) and the BD Micro-Fine™ Pen Needle (Figure 3). You will need to recognize these parts to follow the directions.

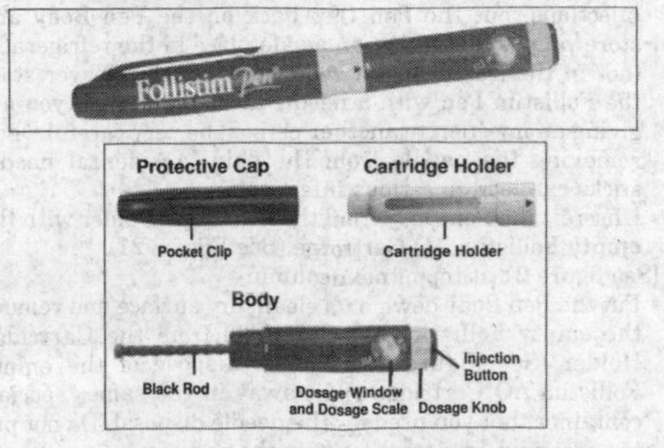

Figure 1. Follistim Pen and its Parts

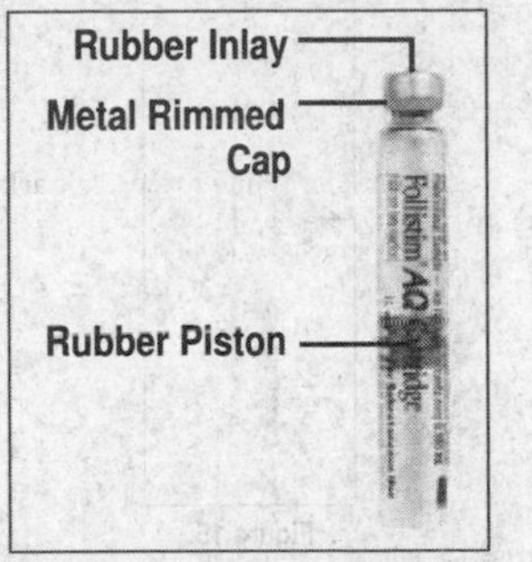

Figure 2. Parts of Follistim AQ Cartridge

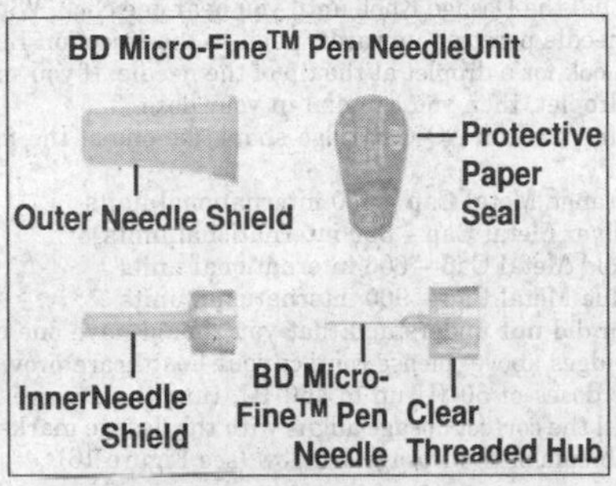

Figure 3. Parts of BD Micro-Fine Pen Needle Unit

- Remove the Cartridge out of the refrigerator.
- Injecting cold drug is likely to cause discomfort. Therefore, it is recommended you allow the drug to reach room temperature before taking the injection.
- Check the liquid in the cartridge. It should appear clear and colorless. If the solution is not clear and colorless or has particles in it, **do not use it.**
- **Gather the supplies you will need for your injection. You will need:**
  - a clean dry surface
  - alcohol
  - cotton balls or alcohol pads
  - sterile gauze
  - a puncture-proof container to throw away the used syringe and needle
- Wash your hands with soap and water and dry them before you use Follistim Pen or when you replace the cartridge.

B. Loading the Follistim Pen with the Follistim AQ Cartridge

- Holding the Pen Body firmly with one hand, pull off the Protective Cap with your other hand (See Figure 4). Put the cap aside on a clean, dry surface.

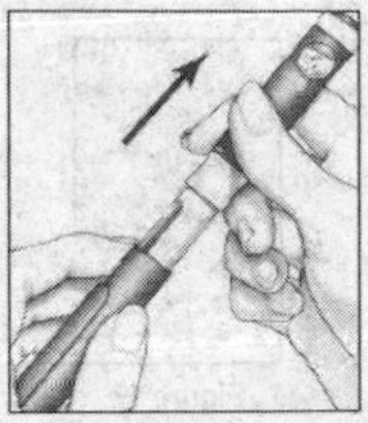

Figure 4

- Unscrew the entire Pen Body from the Cartridge Holder (See Figure 5). Place the Cartridge Holder and the Pen Body aside on a clean, dry surface.

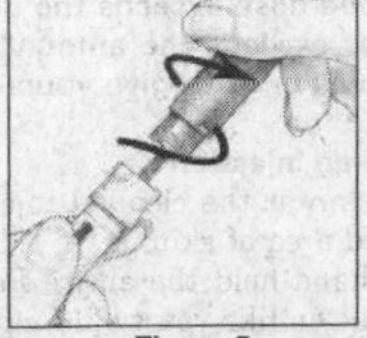

Figure 5

- Take the Follistim AQ Cartridge out of its package. Clean the rubber inlay on the cartridge with an alcohol pad. Pick up the Cartridge Holder. Put the Cartridge into the Cartridge Holder (See Figure 6). The metal rimmed cap goes in first.

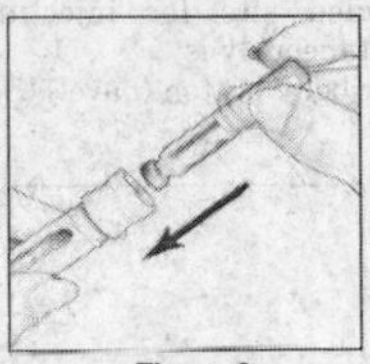

Figure 6

- Pick up the Pen Body and lower it into the Cartridge Holder. The black rod must press against the Rubber Piston on the cartridge. Screw the Pen Body fully onto the Cartridge Holder (See Figure 7). Make sure there is no gap between the Pen Body and the Cartridge Holder. The arrow (▲) on the Cartridge Holder should point to the middle of the yellow alignment mark (■)on the blue Pen Body.

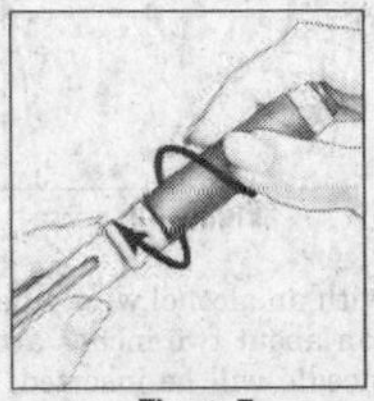

Figure 7

- Clean the open end of the Cartridge Holder with an alcohol pad (See Figure 8).

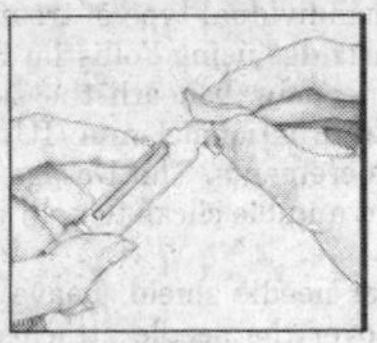

Figure 8

- Pick up a new BD Micro-Fine Pen Needle that is in its Outer Needle Shield. Peel off the protective paper seal (See Figure 9). Do **not** touch the needle. Do not place the open needle on any surface. **Use Only the BD Micro-Fine 0.33 mm × 12.7 mm (29G) Pen Needles as supplied with the Follistim AQ Cartridge.**
- You must use a new BD Micro-Fine Pen Needle with each injection. Never reuse a needle. Attach a new BD Micro-Fine Pen Needle after you make sure there is a Follistim AQ Cartridge in the Cartridge.

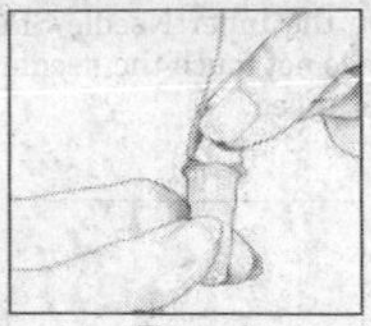

Figure 9

- Hold the Outer Needle Shield firmly in one hand while holding the Cartridge Holder firmly in the other hand. Push the end of the Cartridge Holder into the Outer Needle Shield. Screw them tightly together (See Figure 10). Place your Follistim Pen with the loaded cartridge and attached needle, flat on a clean, dry surface.

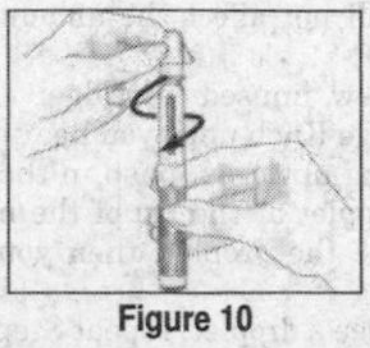

Figure 10

C. Preparing the Injection Site

- Follistim AQ Cartridge can be injected directly into a layer of fat under your skin (subcutaneously).
- When giving a subcutaneous injection, follow your healthcare provider's instructions about changing the site for each injection. This will help lower your chances of having a skin reaction.
- **Do not** inject Follistim AQ Cartridge into an area that is tender, red, bruised, or hard.

- The recommended site for injecting Follistim AQ Cartridge subcutaneously is:
  - ◦ just below your belly button (navel) (See Figure 11)

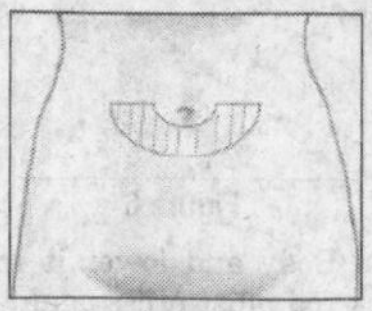

Figure 11

  - ◦ the upper outer area of your thigh (See Figure 12)

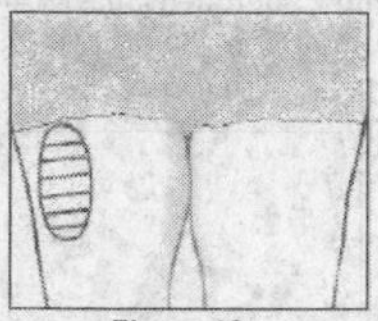

Figure 12

- Clean the skin with an alcohol wipe where the injection is to be made. Clean about two inches around the injection site where the needle will be inserted. Do not touch the cleaned area of skin.

D. Dialing the Dose Before You Give the Injection

- Your healthcare provider will decide on the dose of Follistim AQ Cartridge to be given. This dose may be increased or decreased as your treatment progresses depending on your individual type of treatment.
- Follistim AQ Cartridge using Follistim Pen can be administered subcutaneously (beneath the skin) in prescribed doses from 50 International Units (IU) up to 450 IU, in marked 25 IU increments. The Dosage Scale on the Pen has numbers and audible clicks to help you set the correct dose.
- Pull off the outer needle shield. Leave the Inner Needle Shield in place over the needle attached to the Pen (See Figure 13). Do not throw the Outer Needle Shield away, you will need it later when you throw the needle away.

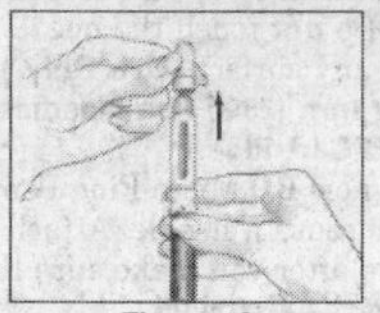

Figure 13

- Carefully remove the Inner Needle Shield and discard it (See Figure 14). Do not touch the needle or let it touch any surface while uncapped.

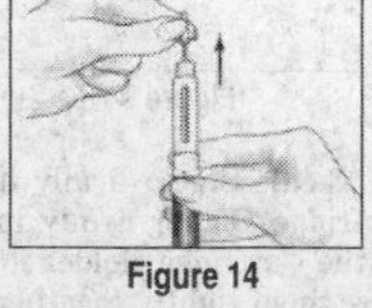

Figure 14

- Hold the Follistim Pen with the needle pointing upwards. Tap the Cartridge Holder gently with your finger to help air bubbles rise to the top of the needle. The small amount of air bubble will not affect the amount of medicine you receive.
- With a loaded new, unused cartridge:
  1. Dial the Dosage Knob until you hear one click. With the needle pointing upwards, push in the Injection Button.
  2. Look for a droplet at the tip of the needle (See Figure 15). If you see the droplet, then you can dial in your dose.
  3. If you do **not** see a droplet, repeat Step 1 (as above) until you see droplet.

     You must **make sure you see a droplet** of medicine (**check the flow of medicine**) or you may **not** inject the correct amount of medicine.

[See figure 15 at top of next column]

- With a partially used cartridge, to give yourself another dose of medicine you will need to attach a new BD Micro-Fine Pen Needle and look for a droplet forming at the tip of the needle (See Figure 15 above). If you see a droplet, then you can dial in your dose.

Figure 15

If **no** droplet:

1. Dial the Dosage Knob until you hear one click. With the needle pointing upwards, push in the Injection Button.
2. Look for a droplet at the tip of the needle. If you see the droplet, then you can dial in your dose.

- Your Follistim AQ Cartridge should be one of the following:
  - ◦ Orange Metal Cap – 150 international units
  - ◦ Silver Metal Cap – 300 international units
  - ◦ Gold Metal Cap – 600 international units
  - ◦ Blue Metal Cap – 900 international units

If you did **not** understand that you should have one of the cartridges above, please contact your healthcare provider.

- For doses of 50 IU up to 450 IU, turn the Dosage Knob until the correct dosage aligns with the dosage markers on each side of the Dosage Window (see Figure 16).

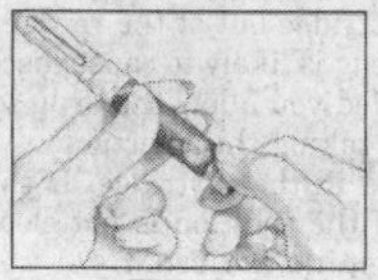

Figure 16

- If by mistake you dial past the correct number, do not try to turn the Dosage Knob backward to fix the mistake. Continue to turn the Dosage Knob in the same direction past the 450 IU mark, as far as it will turn. The Dosage Scale must move freely. Push the Injection Button in all the way. See Figure 17. Start to dial again starting from "0" upwards. By following these directions, you will not lose any medicine from the Follistim AQ Cartridge (See "Checking the Medicine Level Remaining").

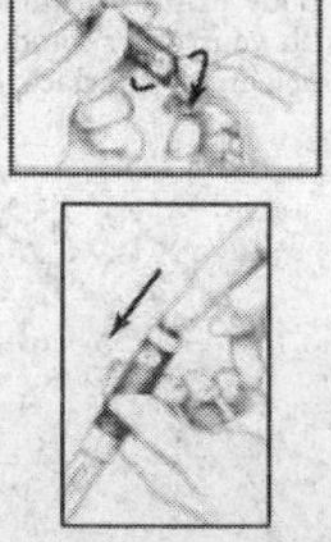

Figure 17

  - ◦ **If you turn the Dosage Knob backward to correct the mistake, it will not damage the Pen, but you will lose some medication from the Follistim AQ Cartridge.**
  - ◦ **Never dial your dose or try to correct a dialing mistake when the needle is still in your skin as this may result in your receiving an incorrect dose.**
  - ◦ **If your prescribed dose exceeds the deliverable dose of Follistim Pen or exceeds the amount remaining in the cartridge, you will need to give yourself more than one injection.**

E. Giving Yourself an Injection

- Pinch a fold of skin at the cleaned injection site. **Do not** touch the cleaned area of skin.
- With the other hand hold the entire Pen with Cartridge loaded and Needle on like you would a pencil. Use a quick "dart-like" motion to insert the needle straight up and down (90-degree angle).
- Press the injection button all the way in to make sure you give yourself a full injection. (See Figure 18). Wait for five seconds before pulling the needle out of the skin. The middle of the Dosage Window should display a dot next to the "0".

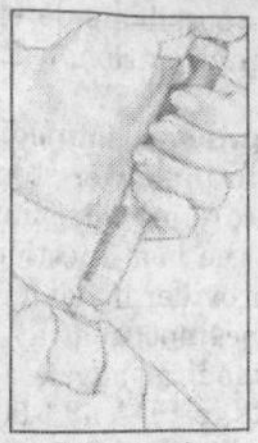

Figure 18

If the injection button does **not** push in all the way, and the number in the Dosage Window does not read "0", it means there is not enough medication left in the cartridge to complete your prescribed dose. The number in the Dosage Window will give you the amount of medicine needed to complete your dose. Write this number down. This will be the number you dial for the completion of your dose. **Start over** with a new Follistim AQ Cartridge and a new needle and follow all the instructions up to this step. Make sure you choose a different injection site to complete your dose of Follistim AQ Cartridge.

- Pull out the BD Micro-Fine Needle and firmly press down on the injection site with an alcohol swab. Use the BD Micro-Fine Pen Needle for one injection only.
- Place the Outer Needle Shield on a flat table surface with the opening pointing up. The opening of the Outer Needle Shield is the wider end with the rim. Without holding on to the Outer Needle Shield, carefully insert the needle (attached to the Follistim Pen) into the opening of the Outer Needle Shield and push down firmly. The Outer Needle Shield should now be attached to the Cartridge Holder and covering the needle (See Figure 19).

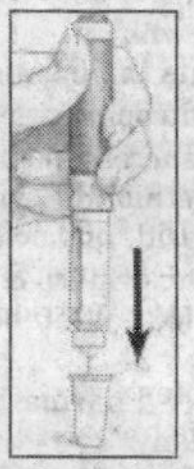

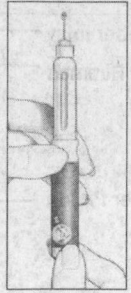

Figure 19

- Grip the Outer Needle Shield and use it to unscrew the needle from the Cartridge Holder (See Figure 20). If there is Follistim AQ Cartridge medicine left for more injections, put the Pen Cap back on the Pen Body and store your Follistim Pen in a safe place in the refrigerator (not in the freezer) or at room temperature. Never store the Follistim Pen with a needle attached to it. If you are giving an injection to another person, be very careful when removing the needle from the skin. Accidental needle sticks can transmit potentially serious or grave infectious diseases.

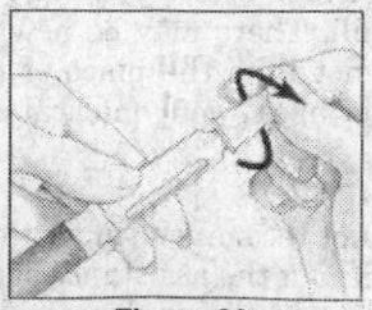

Figure 20

- Throw away the Outer Needle Shield with the used needle right away. Do not throw away in a trash can. Place it in a "special" container. (See " How Do I Throw Away Used Cartridges and Needles?")
- If there is Follistim AQ Cartridge medicine left for more injections, put the Pen Cap back on the Pen Body and store your Follistim Pen in a safe place in the refrigerator (not in the freezer) or at room temperature. Never store the Follistim Pen with a needle attached to it. If you are giving an injection to another person, be very careful when removing the needle from the skin. Accidental needle sticks can lead to serious infections.
- Unscrew the Pen Body from the Cartridge Holder with the **empty** Follistim AQ Cartridge (See Figure 21).

[See figure 21 at top of next column]

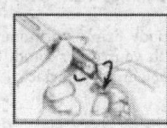

- Put the Pen Body down on a clean, dry surface and remove the empty Follistim AQ Cartridge from the Cartridge Holder (See Figure 22). Safely, dispose of the empty Follistim AQ Cartridge right away in the same "special" container that you used for the needle disposal. Do not put the cartridge in a trash can. At the end of your treatment cycle, your doctor can advise you on how to properly dis-

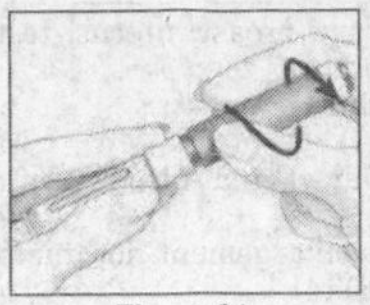

Figure 21

pose of the container. (See "How Do I Throw Away Used Cartridges and Needles?")

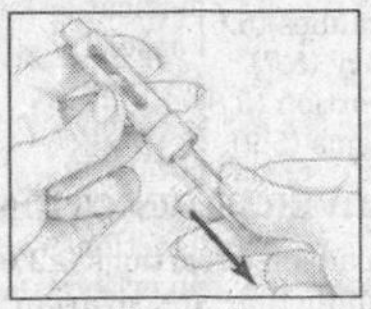

Figure 22

F. Checking the Medicine Level Remaining

For women and men:

Your healthcare provider should advise you of the number of prescribed doses which can be extracted from the full unused Follistim AQ Cartridge.

- **Do not** use the cartridge beyond the advised number of doses. Otherwise, you will run the risk that there will not be enough volume of drug for your prescribed dose.

For women only:

- Keep a Follistim Pen Treatment Diary as follows:
  1. Record the Follistim AQ Cartridge content on Day 1. This will either be 150, 300, 600 or 900 international units depending on what your healthcare provider has prescribed for you.
  2. Record the dose you have been prescribed for your injection.
  3. Subtract your Day 1 dose from the Follistim AQ Cartridge content (150, 300, 600 or 900 international units). (See example – Figure 23.) This will give you the **remaining** Follistim AQ Cartridge content after the Day 1 dose is taken.
  4. Place the number determined as the content after Day 1 (see number 3) in the box as the Follistim AQ Cartridge content **available** for Day 2. (See example – Figure 23.)
  5. Subtract your Day 2 dose from the Follistim AQ Cartridge content you recorded in Step 4. This will give you the **remaining** Follistim AQ Cartridge content after Day 2. Record this number of units. (See example – Figure 23.)
  6. Repeat the steps to determine the Follistim AQ Cartridge content **available** and Follistim AQ Cartridge **remaining** for each day of use.

Day	Date	Dose Prescribed	Follistim AQ Cartridge Content **Available**	Follistim AQ Cartridge Content **Remaining**
1	month/day/year	150	600	450
2	month/day/year	150	450	300
3	month/day/year	150	300	150
4	month/day/year	150	150	0

Figure 23. Example of Treatment Diary Starting with a 600 International Unit Cartridge

If you do not know if there is not enough medicine left in the Follistim AQ Cartridge for your next prescribed dose, see section "If There is Not Enough Follistim AQ in the Cartridge".

G. If There is Not Enough Follistim AQ in the Cartridge

1. If you realize **before** you inject that you do not have enough medicine remaining in your Follistim AQ Cartridge for your complete dose, follow either Option 1 or Option 2, but **not** both.
   - Option 1:
     - Dial your dose and inject the remaining content in the Follistim AQ Cartridge. The Dosage Knob Injection Button will not push in all the way (do not try to force down the button) and the Dosage Window number will not read "0" but will read the number of units you will need to complete your prescribed dose.
     - Write down the number of units needed to complete your dose.
     - Remove the needle and dispose of it properly (see "How Do I Throw Away Used Cartridges and Needles?").
     - Using the Dosage Knob, reset the Dial Window to "0" by turning the Dosage Knob past the 450 IU mark as far as it will turn and push the Injection Button in all the way.
     - Before attempting to replace a Follistim AQ Cartridge, be sure that a BD Micro-Fine Pen Needle is not attached to the Follistim Pen.
     - Insert a new cartridge into the Follistim Pen and attach a new BD Micro-Fine needle.
     - Dial to the number of units you have written down to complete your prescribed dose.
     - Prepare a different injection site and inject the remaining drug to complete your dose (See "Giving Yourself an Injection").
   - Option 2
     - Remove the Follistim AQ Cartridge.
     - **Start over** with a new Follistim AQ Cartridge and Insert into the Follistim Pen.
     - Follow the instructions for "Dialing the Dose" and "Giving Yourself an Injection."

PROBLEM	POSSIBLE CAUSES	WHAT TO DO
The Pen Body will not screw tightly into the Cartridge Holder.	Is something in the way?	Take out the Follistim Cartridge and check the Cartridge Holder to see if anything is in the way. Follow the instructions in this pamphlet to Screw the Pen Body fully onto the Cartridge Holder.
No drug is coming out while checking the flow.	The Cartridge Holder and the Pen Body are not properly screwed together.	Remove the current needle; tighten the Pen Body to the Cartridge Holder ensuring the arrow on the Cartridge Holder is pointing to the middle of the yellow alignment mark on the blue Pen Body. Attach a new needle to the Pen. Recheck the flow as follows: a. Dial the Dosage Knob until you hear one click. With needle pointing upwards, push in the Injection Button. b. Look for a droplet at the tip of the needle.
	Is the Follistim Cartridge empty?	Change to a new cartridge.
	Has the needle been properly attached to the Follistim Pen?	Remove needle and replace with a new one, ensuring that the needle is screwed on tightly to the Pen. Recheck the flow as follows: a. Dial the Dosage Knob until you hear one click. With needle pointing upwards, push in the Injection Button. b. Look for a droplet at the tip of the needle.
You are concerned that you can turn the Dosage Knob to the next number without clicking and the injection button spins freely.	This is not a problem.	The system is in the reset mode. The Injection Button and Dosage Knob must be pushed all the way down to '0' to re-engage the mechanism and the correct dose can now be set. A click will be heard for each setting in the viewing window.
The Dosage Knob does not go back to '0' while you are injecting.	Is the Follistim Cartridge empty?	Change to a new cartridge.
	Is the needle blocked?	a. Remove the needle from the skin and dispose of safely. b. Check the Dosage Window and note how much remaining drug to inject. c. Attach a new needle. Recheck the flow as follows: a. Dial the Dosage Knob until you hear one click. With needle pointing upwards, push in the Injection Button. b. Look for a droplet at the tip of the needle. c. Dial remaining dose.
Some of the drug is dripping out of the needle when you withdraw it from your skin.	Did you take the needle out of your skin before waiting 5 seconds as directed in Step 15?	If this happens you should inform your doctor. To avoid this problem again, you should always wait 5 seconds after you push the Injection Button before you withdraw the needle from your skin.
The needle is left on the Follistim Pen.	Have you missed any of the instructions?	Dispose of the needle in a properly secured container as instructed by your doctor. Change to a new Follistim Cartridge and a new needle.
After your last injection, a remaining volume may be left in the cartridge in addition to the normal quantity of drug dispensed.	The cartridge contains extra volume for checking the drug flow.	This is not a problem.
You cannot get the cartridge out of the Follistim Pen.	Is the needle attached?	Remove the needle from the Follistim Pen and dispose of properly. (Unscrew the Cartridge Holder from the Pen Body and take out the cartridge.)
You are not sure how much drug is left in the cartridge and you do not want to start an injection and then find out that there is not enough drug.	Have you kept good records of your doses?	In case of any doubt, you should load a new, unused Follistim Cartridge into the Follistim Pen. See **"If There is Not Enough Follistim AQ in the Cartridge."** To avoid this problem again, you should record your injections. (Women should use a treatment diary.)

2. If you realize **after** you have inserted the needle at the injection site that you do not have enough medicine remaining in your Follistim AQ Cartridge for your complete dose:
   - Inject the remaining content in the Follistim AQ Cartridge. The Injection Button will not push in all the way and the number in the Dosage Window will not read "0" but will read the number of units you will need to complete your prescribed dose.
   - Wait 5 seconds before withdrawing the needle from your skin and gently apply pressure to the injection site with an alcohol pad.

- Dispose of the used needle (See "How Do I Throw Away Used Cartridges and Needles?").
- Write down the number of units needed to complete your dose.
- Using the Dosage Knob, reset the Dial Window to "0" by turning the Dosage Knob past the 450 IU mark as far as it will turn and push the Injection Button in all the way.
- Insert a new cartridge into the Follistim Pen and attach a new BD Micro-Fine needle.
- Dial to the number you have recorded to complete your prescribed dose.
- Prepare a different injection site and inject the remaining drug to complete your dose (See "Giving Yourself an Injection").

H. How to Solve Problems with Follistim AQ Cartridge and Follistim Pen

If you have problems with using the Follistim AQ Cartridge and the Follistim Pen, see the following chart. If you still have problems after following the chart or if your problem is not on the chart, contact your healthcare provider.

[See table at top of previous page]

Important: If you have a question, always mention the Lot number of your Follistim Pen as printed on the Pen Body. If you have a complaint, please do not discard any product or packaging.

For questions on information contained in this leaflet, call 1-866-836-5633.

www.follistim.com

How Do I Throw Away Used Cartridges and Needles?

Check with your healthcare provider or pharmacist for instructions about the right way to throw away used cartridges and needles. There may be special local or state laws about how to throw away used syringes and needles.

- **Do not** throw away used cartridges and needles in the household trash and do not recycle them.
- Put used and empty cartridges and needles in a closeable, puncture-resistant container. You may use a sharps container (such as a red bio-hazard container), a hard plastic container with a screw-on cap (such as an empty detergent bottle) or in a metal container with a plastic lid, (such as a coffee can).
- When the container is full, tape around the cap or lid to make sure the cap or lid does not come off.
- When your injection is given by another person, this person must also be careful when removing the cartridge and needle and disposing of the cartridge and needle to prevent accidental needle stick injury and passing infection.

How Do I Care for the Follistim Pen?

1. Clean all exposed surfaces of the Follistim Pen with a clean, damp cloth such as a paper towel. Never wash it in water, detergent or strong medical cleaners.
2. Handle the Follistim Pen carefully to avoid causing damage. You could damage the Follistim Pen by dropping it or handling it roughly.
3. Keep the Follistim Pen away from dust and dirt.
4. Never store the Follistim Pen with a needle attached to it. If you store the Follistim Pen with the needle attached, the drug could leak out and there is risk of contamination.
5. If the Follistim Pen breaks or is damaged, do not try to fix it yourself. Contact your healthcare provider.
6. Do not share your Follistim Pen with another person.

How should I store Follistim AQ Cartridge?

- Store Follistim AQ Cartridge in the refrigerator between 2-8°C (36-46°F) until the expiration date.
- Follistim AQ can be stored at or below 25°C (77°F) for 3 months or until the expiration date, whichever comes first. Once the rubber inlay of the Follistim AQ Cartridge has been pierced by a needle, the product may be stored only for a maximum of 28 days at 2-25°C (36-77°F).
- Keep Follistim AQ Cartridge away from light.
- Do not freeze.

Keep Follistim AQ Cartridge, needles, and the disposal container, out of the reach of children.

Manufactured for: Merck Sharp & Dohme Corp., a subsidiary of
MERCK & CO., INC., Whitehouse Station, NJ 08889, USA
Manufactured by: Vetter Pharma-Fertigung GmbH & Co. KG, Ravensburg, Germany

BD, BD Logo and BD Micro-Fine are trademarks of Becton, Dickinson and Company.

U.S. Patent Nos. 5,767,251; 5,929,028; 7,446,090 and 7,563,763.

Revised: 08/2012
900328-FTB-SOi-P-PPI.10

Shown in Product Identification Guide, page 308

FOLLISTIM® AQ ℞
(follitropin beta injection)
for subcutaneous or intramuscular use

HIGHLIGHTS OF PRESCRIBING INFORMATION
These highlights do not include all the information needed to use FOLLISTIM® AQ safely and effectively. See full prescribing information for FOLLISTIM AQ.
FOLLISTIM AQ (follitropin beta injection) for subcutaneous or intramuscular use
Initial U.S. Approval: 1997

RECENT MAJOR CHANGES

Indications and Usage, Induction of Spermatogenesis in Men with Primary and Secondary Hypogonadotropic Hypogonadism (HH) in Whom the Cause of Infertility Is not Due to Primary Testicular Failure (1.3)	6/2010
Dosage and Administration, Recommended Dosing for Induction of Spermatogenesis in Men (2.4)	6/2010
Warnings and Precautions	
• Ovarian Torsion (5.4)	6/2010
• Congenital Anomalies (5.6)	6/2010
• Ectopic Pregnancy (5.7)	6/2010
• Spontaneous Abortion (5.8)	6/2010
• Laboratory Tests For Men (5.10)	6/2010

INDICATIONS AND USAGE

Follistim AQ is a gonadotropin indicated:

In Women for:

- Induction of ovulation and pregnancy in anovulatory infertile women in whom the cause of infertility is functional and not due to primary ovarian failure (1.1)
- Development of multiple follicles in ovulatory women participating in an Assisted Reproductive Technology (ART) program (1.2)

In Men for:

- Induction of spermatogenesis in men with primary and secondary hypogonadotropic hypogonadism (HH) in whom the cause of infertility is not due to primary testicular failure (1.3)

DOSAGE AND ADMINISTRATION

Ovulation Induction in Women (2.2)

- Starting daily dose of 75 international units of Follistim AQ is administered subcutaneously or intramuscularly for at least the first 7 days. The dose is increased by 25 or 50 international units at weekly intervals until follicular growth and/or serum estradiol levels indicate an adequate response
  - ■ When an acceptable pre-ovulatory state is achieved, final oocyte maturation is achieved with 5000 to 10,000 international units of human chorionic gonadotropin (hCG)
  - ■ The woman and her partner should have intercourse daily, beginning on the day prior to the administration of hCG and until ovulation becomes apparent

Assisted Reproductive Technology (ART) in Women (2.3)

- Starting dose of 150 to 225 international units of Follistim AQ is administered subcutaneously or intramuscularly for at least the first 4 days of treatment. Subsequent doses are adjusted based upon ovarian response as determined by ultrasound evaluation of follicular growth and serum estradiol levels
  - ■ Final oocyte maturation is induced with a dose of 5000–10,000 international units of hCG
  - ■ Oocyte (egg) retrieval is performed 34 to 36 hours later

Induction of Spermatogenesis in Men (2.4)

- Pretreatment with hCG alone (1500 international units twice weekly) is required. If serum testosterone levels have not normalized after 8 weeks of hCG treatment, the dose may be increased to 3000 international units twice a week
- After normalization of serum testosterone levels, administer 450 international units per week (225 international units twice weekly or 150 international units three times weekly) of Follistim AQ subcutaneously (only) with the same pre-treatment hCG dose used to normalize testosterone levels

DOSAGE FORMS AND STRENGTHS

Single-Use Vial 75 international units per 0.5 mL (3)
Single-Use Vial 150 international units per 0.5 mL (3)

CONTRAINDICATIONS

Women and men who exhibit:

- Prior hypersensitivity to recombinant hFSH products (4)
- High levels of FSH indicating primary gonadal failure (4)
- Presence of uncontrolled non-gonadal endocrinopathies (4)
- Hypersensitivity reactions related to streptomycin or neomycin (4)
- Tumor of the ovary, breast, uterus, testis, hypothalamus or pituitary gland (4)

Women who exhibit:

- Pregnancy (4, 8.1)
- Heavy or irregular vaginal bleeding of undetermined origin (4)
- Ovarian cysts or enlargement not due to polycystic ovary syndrome (PCOS) (4)

WARNINGS AND PRECAUTIONS

Treatment with Follistim AQ may result in:

- Abnormal Ovarian Enlargement (5.1)
- Ovarian Hyperstimulation Syndrome (OHSS) (5.2)
- Pulmonary and Vascular Complications (5.3)
- Ovarian Torsion (5.4)
- Multi-fetal Gestation and Birth (5.5)
- Congenital Anomalies (5.6)
- Ectopic Pregnancy (5.7)
- Spontaneous Abortion (5.8)
- Ovarian Neoplasms (5.9)

ADVERSE REACTIONS

The most common adverse reactions (≥2%) in women undergoing ovulation induction are: ovarian hyperstimulation syndrome, ovarian cyst, abdominal discomfort, abdominal pain and lower abdominal pain (6.1)

The most common adverse reactions (≥2%) in women receiving ART are ovarian hyperstimulation syndrome and abdominal pain (6.1)

The most common (≥2%) adverse reactions in men undergoing induction of spermatogenesis are headache, acne, injection site reaction, injection site pain, gynecomastia, rash and dermoid cyst (6.1)

To report SUSPECTED ADVERSE REACTIONS, contact Schering Corporation, at 1-800-526-4099 or FDA at 1-800-FDA-1088 or *www.fda.gov/medwatch*.

USE IN SPECIFIC POPULATIONS

- Nursing Mothers: It is not known whether this drug is excreted in human milk (8.1, 8.3)

See 17 for PATIENT COUNSELING INFORMATION and FDA-approved patient labeling

Revised: 06/2010

FULL PRESCRIBING INFORMATION: CONTENTS*

*** Sections or subsections omitted from the full prescribing information are not listed**

FULL PRESCRIBING INFORMATION

1 INDICATIONS AND USAGE

Follistim® AQ (follitropin beta injection) is indicated:

In Women for:

1.1 Induction of ovulation and pregnancy in anovulatory infertile women in whom the cause of infertility is functional and not due to primary ovarian failure.

Prior to initiation of treatment with Follistim AQ:
- Women should have a complete gynecologic and endocrinologic evaluation
- Primary ovarian failure should be excluded
- The possibility of pregnancy should be excluded
- Tubal patency should be demonstrated
- The fertility status of the male partner should be evaluated

1.2 Development of multiple follicles in ovulatory women participating in an Assisted Reproductive Technology (ART) program.

Prior to initiation of treatment with Follistim AQ:
- Women should have a complete gynecologic and endocrinologic evaluation and diagnosis of cause of infertility
- The possibility of pregnancy should be excluded
- The fertility status of the male partner should be evaluated

In Men for:

1.3 Induction of spermatogenesis in men with primary and secondary hypogonadotropic hypogonadism (HH) in whom the cause of infertility is not due to primary testicular failure.

Prior to initiation of treatment with Follistim AQ:
- Men should have a complete medical and endocrinologic evaluation
- Hypogonadotropic hypogonadism should be confirmed and primary testicular failure should be excluded
- Serum testosterone levels should be normalized with human chorionic gonadotropin (hCG) treatment.
- The fertility status of the female partner should be evaluated

2 DOSAGE AND ADMINISTRATION

2.1 General Dosing

- Parenteral drug products should be inspected visually for particulate matter and discoloration prior to administration, whenever solution and container permit. If the solution is not clear and colorless or has particles in it, the solution should not be used
- Do not mix Follistim AQ with any other medicines in the same vial or in the same syringe

2.2 Recommended Dosing for Ovulation Induction

The dosing scheme is stepwise and is individualized for each woman *[see Clinical Studies (14.1)]*.
- A starting daily dose of 75 international units of Follistim AQ is administered for at least the first 7 days
- Subsequent dosage adjustments are made at weekly intervals based upon ovarian response. If an increase in dose is indicated by the ovarian response, the increase should be made by 25 or 50 international units of Follistim AQ at weekly intervals until follicular growth and/or serum estradiol levels indicate an adequate ovarian response

The following should be considered when planning the woman's individualized dose:
- ■ Appropriate Follistim AQ dose adjustment(s) should be used to prevent multiple follicular growth and cycle cancellation
- ■ The maximum, individualized, daily dose of Follistim AQ is 300 international units

- Treatment should continue until ultrasonic visualizations and/or serum estradiol determinations approximate the pre-ovulatory conditions seen in normal individuals.
- When pre-ovulatory conditions are reached, 5000 to 10,000 international units of hCG are used to induce final oocyte maturation and ovulation.
  The administration of hCG must be withheld in cases where the ovarian monitoring suggests an increased risk of OHSS on the last day of Follistim AQ therapy *[see Warnings and Precautions (5.1, 5.2, 5.10)]*.
- The woman and her partner should be encouraged to have intercourse daily, beginning on the day prior to the administration of hCG and until ovulation becomes apparent *[see Warnings and Precautions (5.10)]*.
- During treatment with Follistim AQ and during a two-week post-treatment period, the woman should be assessed at least every other day for signs of excessive ovarian stimulation.
  It is recommended that Follistim AQ administration be stopped if the ovarian monitoring suggests an increased risk of OHSS or abdominal pain occurs. Most OHSS occurs after treatment has been discontinued and reaches its maximum at about seven to ten days post-ovulation.

2.3 Recommended Dosing for ART

The dosing scheme follows a stepwise approach and is individualized for each woman.
- A starting dose of 150 to 225 international units of Follistim AQ is administered subcutaneously or intramuscularly daily for at least the first 4 days of treatment
- Subsequent dosing beyond the first 4 days of treatment is adjusted based upon the woman's ovarian response as determined by ultrasound evaluation of follicular growth and serum estradiol levels

The following should be considered when planning the woman's individualized dose:
- ■ For most normal responding women, the daily starting dose can be continued until pre-ovulatory conditions are achieved (six to twelve days)
- ■ For low or poor responding women, the daily dose should be increased according to the ovarian response. The maximum, individualized, daily dose of Follistim AQ is 600 international units
- ■ For high responding women [those at particular risk of abnormal ovarian enlargement and/or ovarian hyperstimulation syndrome (OHSS)], decrease or temporarily stop the daily dose, or discontinue the cycle according to individual response *[see Warnings and Precautions (5.1, 5.2, 5.10)]*

- When a sufficient number of follicles of adequate size are present, dosing of Follistim AQ is stopped and final maturation of the oocytes is induced by administering hCG at a dose of 5000 to 10,000 international units. The administration of hCG should be withheld in cases where the ovarian monitoring suggests an increased risk of OHSS on the last day of Follistim AQ therapy *[see Warnings and Precautions (5.1, 5.2, 5.10)]*
- Oocyte (egg) retrieval should be performed 34 to 36 hours following the administration of hCG

2.4 Recommended Dosing for Induction of Spermatogenesis in Men

- Pretreatment with hCG is required prior to concomitant therapy with Follistim AQ and hCG. An initial dosage of 1500 international units of hCG should be administered at twice weekly intervals to normalize serum testosterone levels. If serum testosterone levels have not normalized after 8 weeks of hCG treatment, the hCG dose can be increased to 3000 international units twice weekly *[see Clinical Studies (14.3)]*
- After normal serum testosterone levels have been reached, Follistim AQ should be administered by subcutaneous injection concomitantly with hCG treatment. Follistim AQ should be given at a dosage of 450 international units per week, as either 225 international units twice weekly or 150 international units three times per week, in combination with the same hCG dose used to normalize testosterone levels.
  The concomitant therapy should be continued for at least 3 to 4 months before any improvement in spermatogenesis can be expected. If a man has not responded after this period, the combination therapy may be continued. Treatment response has been noted at up to 12 months.

3 DOSAGE FORMS AND STRENGTHS

Follistim AQ Single-Use Vial 75 international units per 0.5 mL

Follistim AQ Single-Use Vial 150 international units per 0.5 mL

4 CONTRAINDICATIONS

Follistim AQ is contraindicated in women and men who exhibit:
- Prior hypersensitivity to recombinant hFSH products
- High levels of FSH indicating primary gonadal failure
- Presence of uncontrolled non-gonadal endocrinopathies (e.g., thyroid, adrenal, or pituitary disorders) *[see Indications and Usage (1.1, 1.2, 1.3)]*
- Hypersensitivity reactions to streptomycin or neomycin. Follistim AQ may contain traces of these antibiotics
- Tumor of the ovary, breast, uterus, testis, hypothalamus or pituitary gland

Follistim AQ is also contraindicated in women who exhibit:
- Pregnancy *[see Use in Specific Populations (8.1)]*
- Heavy or irregular vaginal bleeding of undetermined origin
- Ovarian cysts or enlargement not due to polycystic ovary syndrome (PCOS)

5 WARNINGS AND PRECAUTIONS

Follistim AQ should be used only by physicians who are experienced in infertility treatment. Follistim AQ is a potent gonadotropic substance capable of causing Ovarian Hyperstimulation Syndrome (OHSS) *[see Warnings and Precautions (5.2)]* with or without pulmonary or vascular complications *[see Warnings and Precautions (5.3)]* and multiple births *[see Warnings and Precautions (5.5)]*. Gonadotropin therapy requires the availability of appropriate monitoring facilities *[see Warnings and Precautions (5.10)]*.

Careful attention should be given to the diagnosis of infertility and in the selection of candidates for Follistim AQ therapy *[see Indications and Usage (1.1, 1.2, 1.3) and Dosage and Administration (2.2, 2.3, 2.4)]*.

5.1 Abnormal Ovarian Enlargement

In order to minimize the hazards associated with abnormal ovarian enlargement that may occur with Follistim AQ therapy, treatment should be individualized and the lowest effective dose should be used *[see Dosage and Administration (2.2, 2.3)]*. Use of ultrasound monitoring of ovarian response and/or measurement of serum estradiol levels is important to minimize the risk of overstimulation *[see Warnings and Precautions (5.8)]*.

If the ovaries are abnormally enlarged on the last day of Follistim AQ therapy, hCG should not be administered in order to reduce the chances of developing Ovarian Hyperstimulation Syndrome (OHSS). Intercourse should be prohibited in patients with significant ovarian enlargement after ovulation because of the danger of hemoperitoneum resulting from ruptured ovarian cysts *[see Warnings and Precautions (5.3)]*.

5.2 Ovarian Hyperstimulation Syndrome (OHSS)

OHSS is a medical entity distinct from uncomplicated ovarian enlargement and may progress rapidly to become a serious medical condition. OHSS is characterized by a dramatic increase in vascular permeability, which can result in a rapid accumulation of fluid in the peritoneal cavity, thorax, and potentially, the pericardium. The early warning signs of OHSS developing are severe pelvic pain, nausea, vomiting, and weight gain. Abdominal pain, abdominal distension, gastrointestinal symptoms including nausea, vomiting and diarrhea, severe ovarian enlargement, weight gain, dyspnea, and oliguria have been reported with OHSS. Clinical evaluation may reveal hypovolemia, hemoconcentration, electrolyte imbalances, ascites, hemoperitoneum, pleural effusions, hydrothorax, acute pulmonary distress, and thromboembolic reactions *[see Warnings and Precautions (5.3)]*. Transient liver function test abnormalities suggestive of hepatic dysfunction with or without morphologic changes on liver biopsy have also been reported in association with OHSS.

OHSS occurs after gonadotropin treatment has been discontinued and it can develop rapidly, reaching its maximum about seven to ten days following treatment. Usually, OHSS resolves spontaneously with the onset of menses. If there is evidence that OHSS may be developing prior to hCG administration *[see Warnings and Precautions (5.1)]*, the hCG must be withheld. Cases of OHSS are more common, more severe, and more protracted if pregnancy occurs; therefore, women should be assessed for the development of OHSS for at least two weeks after hCG administration.

If serious OHSS occurs, treatment should be stopped and the patient should be hospitalized. Treatment is primarily symptomatic and overall should consist of bed rest, fluid and electrolyte management, and analgesics (if needed). Because the use of diuretics can accentuate the diminished intravascular volume, diuretics should be avoided except in the late phase of resolution as described below. The management of OHSS may be divided into three phases as follows:
- *Acute Phase:*
  Management should be directed at preventing hemoconcentration due to loss of intravascular volume to the third space and minimizing the risk of thromboembolic phenomena and kidney damage. Fluid intake and output, weight, hematocrit, serum and urinary electrolytes, urine specific gravity, BUN and creatinine, total proteins with albumin: globulin ratio, coagulation studies, electrocardiogram to monitor for hyperkalemia, and abdominal girth should be thoroughly assessed daily or more often based on the clinical need. Treatment, consisting of limited intravenous fluids, electrolytes, human serum albumin, is intended to normalize electrolytes while maintaining an acceptable but somewhat reduced intravascular volume. Full correction of the intravascular volume deficit may lead to an unacceptable increase in the amount of third space fluid accumulation
- *Chronic Phase:*
  After the acute phase is successfully managed as above, excessive fluid accumulation in the third space should be limited by instituting severe potassium, sodium, and fluid restriction
- *Resolution Phase:*
  As third space fluid returns to the intravascular compartment, a fall in hematocrit and increasing urine output are observed in the absence of any increase in take. Peripheral and/or pulmonary edema may

the kidneys are unable to excrete third space fluid as rapidly as it is mobilized. Diuretics may be indicated during the resolution phase, if necessary, to combat pulmonary edema

OHSS increases the risk of injury to the ovary. The ascitic, pleural, and pericardial fluid should not be removed unless there is the necessity to relieve symptoms such as pulmonary distress or cardiac tamponade. Pelvic examination may cause rupture of an ovarian cyst, which may result in hemoperitoneum, and should therefore be avoided. If bleeding occurs and requires surgical intervention, the clinical objective should be to control the bleeding and retain as much ovarian tissue as possible.

During clinical trials with Follistim therapy, OHSS occurred in 7.6% of 105 women (OI) and 5.2% of 591 women (ART) treated with Follistim.

5.3 Pulmonary and Vascular Complications

Serious pulmonary conditions (e.g., atelectasis, acute respiratory distress syndrome) have been reported in women treated with gonadotropins. In addition, thromboembolic reactions both in association with, and separate from, OHSS have been reported following gonadotropin therapy. Intravascular thrombosis, which may originate in venous or arterial vessels, can result in reduced blood flow to vital organs or the extremities. Women with generally recognized risk factors for thrombosis, such as a personal or family history, severe obesity, or thrombophilia, may have an increased risk of venous or arterial thromboembolic events, during or following treatment with gonadotropins. Sequelae of such reactions have included venous thrombophlebitis, pulmonary embolism, pulmonary infarction, cerebral vascular occlusion (stroke), and arterial occlusion resulting in loss of limb and rarely in myocardial infarction. In rare cases, pulmonary complications and/or thromboembolic reactions have resulted in death. In women with recognized risk factors, the benefits of ovulation induction or *in vitro* fertilization (IVF) treatment need to be weighed against the risks. It should be noted that pregnancy itself also carries an increased risk of thrombosis.

5.4 Ovarian Torsion

Ovarian torsion has been reported after treatment with Follistim AQ and after intervention with other gonadotropins. This may be related to OHSS, pregnancy, previous abdominal surgery, past history of ovarian torsion, previous or current ovarian cyst and polycystic ovaries. Damage to the ovary due to reduced blood supply can be limited by early diagnosis and immediate detorsion.

5.5 Multi-fetal Gestation and Birth

Multi-fetal gestation and births have been reported with all gonadotropin treatments including Follistim AQ treatment. The woman and her partner should be advised of the potential risk of multi-fetal gestation and births before starting treatment.

5.6 Congenital Anomalies

The incidence of congenital malformations after ART may be slightly higher than after spontaneous conception. This slightly higher incidence is thought to be related to differences in parental characteristics (e.g., maternal age, sperm characteristics) and to the higher incidence of multi-fetal gestations after ART. There are no indications that the use of gonadotropins during ART is associated with an increased risk of congenital malformations.

5.7 Ectopic Pregnancy

Since infertile women undergoing ART, and particularly IVF, often have tubal abnormalities the incidence of ectopic pregnancies might be increased. Early confirmation of an intrauterine pregnancy should be determined by hCG testing and transvaginal ultrasound.

5.8 Spontaneous Abortion

The risk of spontaneous abortions (miscarriage) is increased with gonadotropin products. However, causality has not been established. The increased risk may be a factor of the underlying infertility.

5.9 Ovarian Neoplasms

There have been infrequent reports of ovarian neoplasms, both benign and malignant, in women who have undergone multiple drug regimens for ovulation induction; however, a causal relationship has not been established.

5.10 Laboratory Tests

For Women:

In most instances, treatment with Follistim AQ will result only in follicular growth and maturation. In order to complete the final phase of follicular maturation and to induce ovulation, hCG must be given following the administration of Follistim AQ or when clinical assessment indicates that sufficient follicular maturation has occurred. The degree of follicular maturation and the timing of hCG administration can both be determined with the use of sonographic visualization of the ovaries and endometrial lining in conjunction with measurement of serum estradiol levels. The combination of transvaginal ultrasonography and measurement of serum estradiol levels is also useful for minimizing the risk f OHSS and multi-fetal gestations.

The clinical confirmation of ovulation is obtained by the following direct or indirect indices of progesterone production as well as sonographic evidence of ovulation.

Direct or indirect indices of progesterone production are:
- Urinary or serum luteinizing hormone (LH) rise
- A rise in basal body temperature
- Increase in serum progesterone
- Menstruation following the shift in basal body temperature

The following provide sonographic evidence of ovulation:
- Collapsed follicle
- Fluid in the cul-de-sac
- Features consistent with corpus luteum formation

Sonographic evaluation of the early pregnancy is also important to rule out ectopic pregnancy.

For Men:

Clinical monitoring for spermatogenesis utilizes the following indirect or direct measures:
- Serum testosterone level
- Semen analysis

6 ADVERSE REACTIONS

The following serious adverse reactions are discussed elsewhere in the labeling:
- Ovarian Hyperstimulation Syndrome *[see Warnings and Precautions(5.2)]*
- Atelectasis *[see Warnings and Precautions (5.3)]*
- Thromboembolism *[see Warnings and Precautions (5.3)]*
- Ovarian Torsion *[see Warnings and Precautions (5.4)]*
- Multi-fetal Gestation *[see Warnings and Precautions (5.5)]*
- Congenital Anomalies *[see Warnings and Precautions (5.6)]*
- Ectopic Pregnancy *[see Warnings and Precautions (5.7)]*
- Spontaneous Abortion *[see Warnings and Precautions (5.8)]*

6.1 Clinical Study Experience

Because clinical trials are conducted under widely varying conditions, adverse reaction rates observed in the clinical trials of a drug cannot be directly compared to rates in the clinical trials of another drug and may not reflect the rates observed in clinical practice.

Ovulation Induction

In a single cycle, multi-center, assessor-blind, parallel group, comparative study, a total of 172 chronic anovulatory women who had failed to ovulate and/or conceive with clomiphene citrate therapy, were randomized and treated with Follistim (105) or a urofollitropin comparator. Adverse reactions with an incidence of greater than 2% in either treatment group are listed in **Table 1**.

TABLE 1: Common Adverse Reactions Reported at a Frequency of ≥2% in an Assessor-Blind, Comparative Study of Women Receiving Ovulation Induction

System Organ Class/Adverse Reactions	Treatment Number (%) of Women: Follistim N=105 n (%)	Comparator N=67 n (%)
Gastrointestinal disorders		
Abdominal discomfort	3 (2.9)	1 (1.5)
Abdominal pain	3 (2.9)	2 (3.0)
Abdominal pain lower	3 (2.9)	1 (1.5)
Reproductive system and breast disorders		
Ovarian cyst	3 (2.9)	2 (3.0)
Ovarian hyperstimulation syndrome	8 (7.6)	3 (4.5)
General disorders and administration site conditions		
Pyrexia	0 (0.0)	2 (3.0)

Adverse reactions reported commonly (greater than or equal to 2% of women treated with Follistim) in other ovulation induction clinical trials were headache, abdominal distension, constipation, diarrhea, nausea, pelvic pain, uterine enlargement, vaginal hemorrhage and injection site reaction.

The following medical events have been reported subsequent to pregnancies resulting from Follistim AQ therapy:
- Ectopic pregnancy *[see Warnings and Precautions (5.7)]*
- Spontaneous abortion *[see Warnings and Precautions (5.8)]*

ART

In a multiple cycle, multi-center, assessor-blind, parallel group, comparative study, after pituitary suppression with a gonadotropin release hormone (GnRH) agonist, a total of 989 women were randomized and treated with Follistim (N=591) or a urofollitropin comparator as part of *in vitro* fertilization therapy (IVF). Adverse reactions with an incidence of greater than 2% in either treatment group are listed in **Table 2**.

TABLE 2: Common Adverse Reactions Reported at a Frequency of ≥2% in an Assessor-Blind, Comparative Study of Women Receiving In Vitro Fertilization (IVF)

System Organ Class/Adverse Reactions	Treatment Number (%) of Women: Follistim N=591 n (%)	Comparator N=398 n (%)
Gastrointestinal disorders		
Abdominal pain	13 (2.2)	4 (1.0)
Reproductive system and breast disorders		
Ovarian hyperstimulation syndrome	31 (5.2)	17 (4.3)

Adverse reactions reported commonly (greater than or equal to 2% of women treated with Follistim) in other IVF clinical trials were headache, abdominal distension, constipation, diarrhea, nausea, pelvic pain, breast tenderness, metrorrhagia, ovarian enlargement, vaginal hemorrhage, injection site reaction and rash.

The following medical events have been reported subsequent to pregnancies resulting from Follistim AQ therapy:
- Ectopic pregnancy *[see Warnings and Precautions (5.7)]*
- Spontaneous abortion *[see Warnings and Precautions (5.8)]*

Induction of Spermatogenesis

In an open-label, non-comparative clinical trial, 49 men with hypogonadotropic hypogonadism were enrolled to receive pretreatment with hCG, followed by combination therapy with hCG and Follistim for induction of spermatogenesis. Of the 49 men, 30 received weekly Follistim doses of 450 international units; 24 of these 30 men received a total of 48 weeks of treatment with Follistim. Adverse reactions occurring with an incidence of greater than 2% in the 30 men treated with Follistim are listed in **Table 3**.

TABLE 3: Common Adverse Reactions Reported at a Frequency of ≥2% in an Open-Label Clinical Trial in Men with Hypogonadotropic Hypogonadism

System Organ Class/Adverse Reactions	Follistim Treatment N=30 n (%)
Nervous system disorders	
Headache	2 (6.7)
General disorders and administration site disorders	
Injection site reaction	2 (6.7)
Injection site pain	2 (6.7)
Skin and subcutaneous tissue disorders	
Acne	2 (6.7)
Rash	1 (3.3)
Reproductive system and breast disorders	
Gynecomastia	1 (3.3)
Neoplasms benign, malignant and unspecified	
Dermoid cyst	1 (3.3)

6.2 Postmarketing Experience

The following adverse reactions have been identified during post approval use of Follistim and/or Follistim AQ. Because these reactions are reported voluntarily from a population of uncertain size, it is not always possible to reliably estimate their frequency or establish a causal relationship to drug exposure.

Vascular disorders:

Thromboembolism *[see Warnings and Precautions (5.3)]*

7 DRUG INTERACTIONS

No drug-drug interaction studies have been performed.

8 USE IN SPECIFIC POPULATIONS

8.1 Pregnancy

Pregnancy Category X: Follistim AQ should not be used during pregnancy *[see Contraindications (4)]*.

8.3 Nursing Mothers

It is not known whether this drug is excreted in human milk. Because many drugs are excreted in human milk and because of the potential for serious adverse reactions in the nursing infant from Follistim AQ, a decision should be made whether to discontinue nursing or to discontinue the drug, taking into account the importance of the drug to the mother.

8.4 Pediatric Use

Safety and effectiveness in pediatric patients have not been established.

8.5 Geriatric Use

Clinical studies of Follistim did not include subjects aged 65 and over.

10 OVERDOSAGE

Aside from the possibility of Ovarian Hyperstimulation Syndrome *[see Warnings and Precautions (5.2, 5.3)]* and multiple gestations *[see Warnings and Precautions (5.5)]*, there is no additional information concerning the consequences of acute overdosage with Follistim AQ.

11 DESCRIPTION

Follistim AQ contains human follicle-stimulating hormone (hFSH), a glycoprotein hormone which is manufactured by recombinant DNA (rDNA) technology. The active drug substance, follitropin beta, has a dimeric structure containing two glycoprotein subunits (alpha and beta). Both the 92 amino acid alpha-chain and the 111 amino acid beta-chain have complex heterogeneous structures arising from two N-linked oligosaccharide chains. Follitropin beta is synthesized in a Chinese hamster ovary (CHO) cell line that has been transfected with a plasmid containing the two subunit DNA sequences encoding for hFSH. The purification process results in a highly purified preparation with a consistent hFSH isoform profile and high specific activity [as determined by the Ph. Eur. test for FSH *in vivo* bioactivity and on the basis of the molar extinction coefficient at 277 nm (ϵ_s:$mg^{-1}cm^{-1}$)=1.066].

The biological activity is determined by measuring the increase in ovary weight in female rats. The intrinsic luteinizing hormone (LH) activity in follitropin beta is less than 1 international unit per 40,000 international units FSH. The compound is considered to contain no LH activity.

The amino acid sequence and tertiary structure of the product are indistinguishable from that of hFSH of urinary source. Also, based on available data derived from physicochemical tests and bioassay, follitropin beta and follitropin alfa, another recombinant follicle-stimulating hormone product, are indistinguishable.

Follistim AQ is presented as a sterile aqueous solution intended for subcutaneous (in men and women) or intramuscular (women only) administration. Each single-use vial of Follistim AQ contains the following per 0.5 mL: 75 international units or 150 international units of FSH activity; 25 mg sucrose NF; 7.35 mg sodium citrate (dihydrate) USP; 0.25 mg L-methionine USP; 0.1 mg polysorbate 20 NF; and water for injection USP. Hydrochloric acid NF and/or sodium hydroxide NF are used to adjust the pH to 7.

The recombinant protein in Follistim AQ has been standardized for FSH *in vivo* bioactivity in terms of the WHO International Standard for Follicle Stimulating Hormone (FSH) Recombinant, Human for Bioassay (code 92/642), issued by the World Health Organization Expert Committee on Biological Standardization (1995). Under current storage conditions, Follistim AQ may contain up to 11% of oxidized follitropin beta.

In clinical trials with Follistim, serum antibodies to FSH or anti-CHO cell derived proteins were not detected in any of the treated patients after exposure to Follistim for up to three cycles.

Therapeutic Class: Infertility.

12 CLINICAL PHARMACOLOGY

12.1 Mechanism of Action

Women:

Follicle-stimulating hormone (FSH), the active component in Follistim AQ, is required for normal follicular growth, maturation, and gonadal steroid production.

In women, the level of FSH is critical for the onset and duration of follicular development, and consequently for the timing and number of follicles reaching maturity. Follistim AQ stimulates ovarian follicular growth in women who do not have primary ovarian failure. In order to effect the final phase of follicle maturation, resumption of meiosis and rupture of the follicle in the absence of an endogenous LH surge, human chorionic gonadotropin (hCG) must be given following treatment with Follistim AQ when patient monitoring indicates appropriate follicular development parameters have been reached.

Men:

Follistim when administered with hCG stimulates spermatogenesis in men with hypogonadotropic hypogonadism. FSH, the active component of Follistim, is the pituitary hormone responsible for spermatogenesis.

12.3 Pharmacokinetics

Exposures of follitropin beta from Follistim AQ and Follistim are expected to be equivalent. The following information is based on studies conducted with Follistim.

Absorption:

Women:

The bioavailability of Follistim following subcutaneous and intramuscular administration was investigated in healthy, pituitary-suppressed, women given a single 300 international units dose. In these women, the area under the curve (AUC), expressed as the mean ± SD, was equivalent between the subcutaneous (455.6 ± 141.4 IU*h/L) and intramuscular (445.7 ± 135.7 IU*h/L) routes of administration. However, equivalence could not be established with respect to the peak serum FSH levels (C_{max}). The C_{max} achieved after subcutaneous administration and intramuscular administration was 5.41 ± 0.72 international units/L and 6.86 ± 2.90 international units/L, respectively. After subcutaneous or intramuscular injection the apparent dose absorbed was 77.8% and 76.4%, respectively.

The pharmacokinetics and pharmacodynamics of a single, intramuscular dose (300 international units) of Follistim were also investigated in a group (n=8) of gonadotropin-deficient, but otherwise healthy women. In these women, FSH (mean ± SD) AUC was 339 ± 105 international units*h/L, Cmax was 4.3 ± 1.7 international units/L. C_{max} occurred at approximately 27 ± 5.4 hours after intramuscular administration.

A multiple dose, dose proportionality, pharmacokinetic study of Follistim was completed in healthy, pituitary-suppressed, women given subcutaneous doses of 75, 150, or 225 international units for 7 days. Steady-state blood concentrations of FSH were reached with all doses after 5 days of treatment based on the trough concentrations of FSH just prior to dosing (C_{trough}). Peak blood concentrations with the 75, 150, and 225 international units dose were 4.30 ± 0.60 international units/L, 8.51 ± 1.16 international units/L and 13.92 ± 1.81 international units/L, respectively.

A multiple dose, dose proportionality, pharmacokinetic study of Follistim was completed in healthy, pituitary-suppressed, women given intramuscular doses of 75, 150, or 225 international units for 7 days. Steady-state blood concentrations of FSH were reached with all doses after 4 days of treatment based on the minimum concentrations of FSH just prior to dosing (C_{min}). Peak blood concentrations with the 75, 150, and 225 international units dose were 4.65 ± 1.49 international units/L, 9.46 ± 2.57 international units/L and 11.30 ± 1.77 international units/L, respectively.

Men:

Serum levels of FSH were measured in a clinical study that compared the effects of two different dosing schedules of Follistim (150 international units three times a week or 225 international units twice a week) administered by subcutaneous injection concurrently with chorionic gonadotropin for injection for induction of spermatogenesis in hypogonadotropic hypogonadal men. Administration of Follistim was started at week 17. Mean serum trough concentrations of FSH remained fairly constant over the treatment period. At the end of treatment (week 64), the mean serum trough concentrations of FSH were 2.09 international units/L in the 150 international units group and 3.22 international units/L in the 225 international units group. Serum trough concentrations of FSH measured prior to the first Follistim injection on the Mondays of active treatment period (weeks 17 to 64) and one week after the end of treatment period are presented in **Figure 1.**

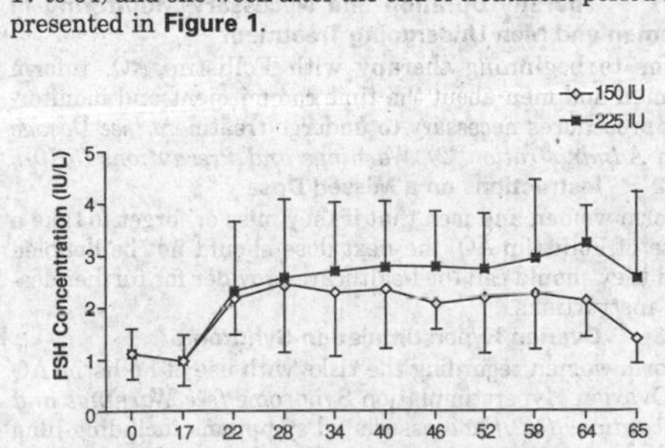

FIGURE 1: Mean (SD) Serum Trough Concentrations of FSH in Men Following Subcutaneous Administration of Follistim Using Two Different Dosing Schedules (150 International Units Three Times a Week or 225 International Units Twice a Week)

Distribution:

The volume of distribution of Follistim in healthy, pituitary-suppressed, women following intravenous administration of a 300 international units dose was approximately 8 L.

Metabolism:

The recombinant FSH in Follistim AQ is biochemically very similar to urinary FSH and it is therefore anticipated that it is metabolized in the same manner.

Elimination:

The elimination half-life ($t_{1/2}$) following a single intramuscular dose (300 international units) of Follistim in women was 43.9 ± 14.1 hours (mean ± SD). The elimination half life following a 7-day intramuscular treatment of women with 75, 150, or 225 international units was 26.9 ± 7.8 hours (mean ± SD), 30.1 ± 6.2 and 28.9 ± 6.5, respectively.

Use in Specific Populations:

Body weight: The effect of body weight on the pharmacokinetics of Follistim was evaluated in a group of European and Japanese women who were significantly different in terms of body weight. The European women had a body weight of (mean ± SD) 67.4 ± 13.5 kg and the Japanese subjects were 46.8 ± 11.6 kg. Following a single intramuscular dose of 300 international units of Follistim, the AUC was significantly smaller in European women (339 ± 105 international units*h/L) than in Japanese women (544 ± 201 international units*h/L). However, clearance per kg of body weight was essentially the same for the respective groups (0.014 and 0.013 L/hr/kg).

Geriatric Use: The pharmacokinetics of Follistim has not been studied in geriatric subjects.

Pediatric Use: The pharmacokinetics of Follistim has not been studied in pediatric subjects.

Renal Impairment: The effect of renal impairment on the pharmacokinetics of Follistim has not been studied.

Hepatic Impairment: The effect of hepatic impairment on the pharmacokinetics of Follistim has not been studied.

13 NONCLINICAL TOXICOLOGY

13.1 Carcinogenesis, Mutagenesis, Impairment of Fertility

Long-term toxicity studies in animals have not been performed with Follistim to evaluate the carcinogenic potential of the drug. Follistim was not mutagenic in the Ames test using *S. typhimurium* and *E. coli* tester strains and did not produce chromosomal aberrations in an *in vitro* assay using human lymphocytes.

14 CLINICAL STUDIES

14.1 Ovulation Induction

The efficacy of Follistim for Ovulation Induction was evaluated in a randomized, assessor-blind, parallel-group comparative, multicenter safety and efficacy study of 172 chronic anovulatory women (105 subjects on Follistim) who had previously failed to ovulate and/or conceive during clomiphene citrate treatment. The study results for ovulation rates are summarized in **Table 4** and those for pregnancy rates are summarized in **Table 5.**

TABLE 4: Cumulative Ovulation Rates

Cycle	Follistim (n=105)
First treatment cycle	72%
Second treatment cycle	82%
Third treatment cycle	85%

TABLE 5: Cumulative Ongoing*, † Pregnancy Rates

Cycle	Follistim (n=105)
First treatment cycle	14%
Second treatment cycle	19%
Third treatment cycle	23%

* All ongoing pregnancies were confirmed after at least 12 weeks after the hCG injection.

† Study was not powered to demonstrate this outcome.

14.2 Assisted Reproductive Technology (ART)

The efficacy of Follistim as part of an Assisted Reproductive Technology (ART) program was established in three studies, two of which are described below.

Follistim was evaluated in a randomized, assessor-blind, parallel-group, comparative, multicenter safety and efficacy study of 981 healthy normal ovulatory infertile women (mean age 32) treated for multiple cycles with *in vitro* fertilization and controlled ovarian stimulation with Follistim (n=585) or urofollitropin (n=396) after pituitary suppression with a GnRH agonist. The first cycle results with Follistim are summarized in **Table 6**.

TABLE 8: Number of Men Receiving Follistim Who Achieved a Mean Sperm Density of ≥10⁶/mL on Their Last Two Treatment Assessments

	Follistim 150 international units three times a week (n=15)		Follistim 225 international units twice a week (n=15)		Overall (n=30)	
Sperm Density of $\geq 10^6$/mL	n	%	n	%	n	%
Yes	6	40	7	47	13	43
No	9	60	8	53	17	57

TABLE 6: Results of First Cycle Treatment of Infertile Women With Follistim and In Vitro Fertilization After Pituitary Suppression With a GnRH Agonist*

Parameter	Follistim (n=585)
Total number of oocytes recovered	10.9
Ongoing† pregnancy rate/attempt‡	22.2%
Ongoing† pregnancy rate/transfer‡,§	26.0%

* All values are means.
† A single vital or multiple vital pregnancy was termed ongoing when a pregnancy, at least 12 weeks after embryo transfer (ET), was confirmed by the investigator.
‡ Study was not powered to demonstrate these secondary endpoints.
§ Transfers were limited to a maximum of three embryos.

Follistim was also evaluated in a randomized, assessor-blind, parallel-group, comparative, single center safety and efficacy study in 89 infertile healthy normal ovulatory women (mean age 32) treated for one cycle with *in vitro* fertilization and controlled ovarian stimulation with Follistim (n=54) or menotropins (n=35) without pituitary suppression with a GnRH agonist. The results with Follistim are summarized in **Table 7**.

TABLE 7: Results of Single Cycle Treatment of Infertile Women Treated With In Vitro Fertilization and Follistim Without Pituitary Suppression*

Parameter	Follistim (n=54)
Total number of oocytes recovered	9.9
Ongoing† pregnancy rate/attempt‡	22.2%
Ongoing† pregnancy rate/transfer‡,§	30.8%

* All values are means.
† A single vital or multiple vital pregnancy was termed ongoing when a pregnancy, at least 12 weeks after embryo transfer (ET), was confirmed by the investigator.
‡ Study was not powered to demonstrate these secondary endpoints.
§ Transfers were limited to a maximum of three embryos.

14.3 Induction of Spermatogenesis

The safety and efficacy of Follistim administered by subcutaneous injection concomitantly chorionic gonadotropin for injection (hCG) has been examined in a multicenter, open-label, non-comparator clinical study for induction of spermatogenesis in hypogonadotropic hypogonadal men. The study compared the effects of two different Follistim dosing schedules on semen parameters and serum levels of follicle stimulating hormone (FSH). The multicenter study involved a 16-week pretreatment phase with hCG at a dosage of 1500 international units twice a week to normalize serum testosterone levels. If serum testosterone levels did not normalize after 8 weeks of hCG treatment, the hCG dose could have been increased to 3000 international units twice a week. This phase was followed by a 48-week treatment phase. Men who were still azoospermic after the pretreatment phase were randomized to receive either 225 international units Follistim together with 1500 international units hCG twice a week or 150 international units Follistim three times a week together with 1500 international units hCG twice weekly. Men who required 3000 international units of hCG twice a week in the pretreatment phase were continued on that dosage during the treatment phase. The mean age of patients in both treatment groups was approximately 30 years (range 18 to 47 years). At baseline, mean left and right testis volumes were 4.61 ± 2.94 mL and 4.57 ± 3.00 mL, respectively, in the group receiving three weekly injections of Follistim. For the group receiving two weekly injections of Follistim, the mean left and right testis volumes were 6.54 ± 2.45 mL and 7.21 ± 2.94 mL, respectively, at baseline. The primary efficacy endpoint was the percentage of patients with a mean sperm density of $\geq 1 \times 10^6$/mL on their last two treatment assessments. The outcomes of treatment in the 30 men enrolled in the treatment phase are summarized in **Table 8.**

[See table 8 above]

Overall, the median time to reach a sperm concentration of 10^6 per mL was 165 days (range 25 to 327 days) in patients who demonstrated a sperm concentration of at least 10^6 per mL. The median time to reach a sperm concentration of at least 10^6 per mL was 186 days (range 25 to 327 days) for the 150 international units group and 141 days (range 43 to 204 days) for the 225 international units group. No pregnancy data were collected during the trial.

The local tolerance data were comparable between the two treatment groups. The mean percentage of days without pain calculated for all subjects in the treatment period was 91.3% for patients in the 150 international units (three times a week) and 76.0% for patients in the 225 international units (two times a week) Follistim treatment groups. In the 225 international units (twice per week) group, local symptoms judged as severe by the investigator were: itching in 1 patient (7%), pain in 2 patients (13%), bruising in 2 patients (13%), swelling in 2 patients (13%), and redness in 1 patient (7%). In the 150 international units (three times per week) group, 1 event in 1 patient (bruising, 7%) was judged as severe. No patient discontinued treatment due to injection site reaction or injection site pain.

16 HOW SUPPLIED/STORAGE AND HANDLING

Follistim AQ (follitropin beta injection) is supplied as a sterile aqueous solution in a 2 mL vial to deliver 0.5 mL of the drug in the following concentrations and packaging:

Follistim AQ Single-Use Vial 75 international units per 0.5 mL

Box of 1 NDC 0052-0308-02

Follistim AQ Single-Use Vial 150 international units per 0.5 mL

Box of 1 NDC 0052-0309-02

Store refrigerated, 2–8°C (36–46°F) until dispensed. Upon dispensing, the product may be stored by the patient at 2–8°C (36–46°F) until the expiration date, or at or below 25°C (77°F) for 3 months or until expiration date, whichever occurs first. Protect from light, keep container in carton. Do not freeze.

17 PATIENT COUNSELING INFORMATION

See FDA-Approved Patient Labeling

17.1 Therapy Duration and Necessary Monitoring in Women and Men Undergoing Treatment

Prior to beginning therapy with Follistim AQ, inform women and men about the time commitment and monitoring procedures necessary to undergo treatment *[see Dosage and Administration (2), Warnings and Precautions (5.10)]*.

17.2 Instructions on a Missed Dose

Inform women and men that if they miss or forget to take a dose of Follistim AQ, the next dose should not be doubled and they should call the healthcare provider for further dosing instructions.

17.3 Ovarian Hyperstimulation Syndrome

Inform women regarding the risks with use of Follistim AQ of Ovarian Hyperstimulation Syndrome *[see Warnings and Precautions (5.2)]* and associated symptoms including lung and blood vessel problems *[see Warnings and Precautions (5.3)]* and ovarian torsion *[see Warnings and Precautions (5.4)]*.

17.4 Multi-fetal Gestation and Birth

Inform women regarding the risk of multi-fetal gestations with the use of Follistim AQ *[see Warnings and Precautions (5.5)]*.

Manufactured for Organon USA Inc.
Roseland, NJ 07068
by Organon (Ireland) Ltd.
Swords, Co. Dublin, Ireland
U.S. Patent Nos. 5,767,251 and 5,929,028.

Rev. 8/10

34306109T
B-33554311
F-33554311 2682
F-33554214 2681

PATIENT INFORMATION

PATIENT INFORMATION LEAFLET

Follistim® *AQ*
(follitropin beta injection)
Single-Use Vial

Read the Patient Information that comes with Follistim® AQ before you start using it and each time you get a refill. There may be new information. This information does not take the place of talking with your healthcare provider about your medical condition or treatment.

What is Follistim AQ?

Follistim AQ is a prescription medicine that contains follicle-stimulating hormone (FSH).

Follistim AQ is used:

In women:
- to help healthy ovaries to develop (mature) and release eggs
- as part of an Assisted Reproductive Technology (ART) program to help the ovaries produce more mature eggs

In men:
- to help bring about the production and development of sperm

Who should not take Follistim AQ?

Do not take Follistim AQ if you are a Woman or Man who:
- is allergic to recombinant human FSH products
- has a high level of FSH in your blood indicating that your ovaries (women only) or testes (men only) may be permanently damaged and do not work at all.
- has uncontrolled thyroid, pituitary, or adrenal gland problems
- is allergic to streptomycin or neomycin (types of antibiotics)
- has a tumor of the hypothalamus, pituitary gland, breast, uterus (women only), ovary (women only), or testis (men only)

Do not take Follistim AQ if you are a Woman who:
- is pregnant or think you may be pregnant
- has heavy or irregular vaginal bleeding and the cause is not known
- has ovarian cysts or enlarged ovaries, not due to polycystic ovary syndrome (PCOS)

Talk to your healthcare provider before taking this medicine if you have any of the conditions listed above.

What should I tell my healthcare provider before taking Follistim AQ?

Before you take Follistim AQ, tell your healthcare provider if you:
- have an increased risk of blood clots (thrombosis)
- have ever had a blood clot (thrombosis), or anyone in your immediate family has ever had a blood clot (thrombosis)
- had stomach (abdominal) surgery
- had twisting of your ovary (ovarian torsion)
- had or have a cyst in your ovary
- have polycystic ovary disease
- have any other medical conditions
- are breastfeeding or plan to breastfeed. It is not known if Follistim AQ passes into your breast milk. You and your healthcare provider should decide if you will take Follistim AQ or breastfeed. You should not do both

Tell your healthcare provider about all the medicines you take, including prescription and nonprescription medicines, vitamins, and herbal supplements.

Know the medicines you take. Keep a list of them and show your healthcare provider and pharmacist when you get a new medicine.

How should I use Follistim AQ?
- Be sure that you read, understand, and follow the "Patient Instructions for Use" that come with Follistim AQ
- Use Follistim AQ exactly as your healthcare provider tells you to
- Your healthcare provider will tell you how much Follistim AQ to use, how to inject it, and how often it should be injected
- Do not inject Follistim AQ at home until your healthcare provider has taught you the right way
- Do not mix Follistim AQ with any other medicines in the same vial or in the same syringe
- Do not change your dose of Follistim AQ unless your healthcare provider tells you to
- **Call your healthcare provider immediately** if you use too much Follistim AQ
- If you miss or forget to take a dose, do not double your next dose. Ask your healthcare provider for instructions
- Your healthcare provider will do blood and urine hormone tests while you are taking Follistim AQ. Make sure you follow-up with your healthcare provider to have your blood and urine tested when told to do so

Women:
- Your healthcare provider may do ultrasound scans of your ovaries. Make sure you follow-up with your healthcare provider to have your ultrasound scans

Men:
- Your healthcare provider may test your semen while you are taking Follistim AQ. Make sure you follow-up with your healthcare provider to give a semen sample for testing

What are the possible side effects of Follistim AQ?
Follistim AQ may cause serious side effects.
Serious side effects in women include:
- **Ovarian enlargement**
- **Ovarian hyperstimulation syndrome (OHSS).** OHSS is a serious medical problem that can happen when the ovaries are over stimulated. In rare cases it has caused death. OHSS causes fluid to build up suddenly in your stomach and chest areas and can cause blood clots to form. Call you healthcare provider right away if you have:
- pain in your lower stomach area
- nausea
- vomiting
- weight gain
- diarrhea
- decreased urine output
- trouble breathing
- **Lung problems.** Follistim AQ can cause you to have fluid in your lungs (atelectasis) and trouble breathing (acute respiratory distress syndrome).
- **Blood clots.** Follistim AQ may increase your chance of having blood clots in your blood vessels. Blood clots can cause:
- blood vessel problems (thrombophlebitis)
- stroke
- loss of your arm or leg
- blood clot in your lungs (pulmonary embolus)
- heart attack
- **Ovarian torsion.** Follistim AQ may increase the chance of twisting of the ovaries in women with certain conditions such as OHSS, pregnancy and previous abdominal surgery. Twisting of the ovary could cause the blood flow to the ovary to be cut off
- **Pregnancy and birth of multiple babies.** Having a pregnancy with more than one baby at a time increases the health risk for you and your babies. Discuss your chances of multiple births with your healthcare provider
- **Birth defects.** A woman's age, certain sperm problems, genetic background of both parents and a pregnancy with multiple babies can increase the chance that your baby might have birth defects
- **Ectopic pregnancy (pregnancy outside of the womb).** The chance of a pregnancy outside of the womb is increased in women with damaged fallopian tubes
- **Miscarriage.** The chance of loss of an early pregnancy may be increased in women who have difficulty with becoming pregnant at all

The most common side effects of Follistim AQ include:
In women:
- Cyst in the ovary
- stomach pain

In Men:
- headache
- pain at the injection site
- bruising, swelling or redness at the injection site
- breast enlargement
- acne

These are not all the possible side effects of Follistim AQ. For more information, ask your healthcare provider or pharmacist.

Call your healthcare provider immediately if you get worsening or strong abdominal pain. Also, call your healthcare provider immediately if this happens some days after the last injection has been given. Tell your healthcare provider if you have any side effect that bothers you or that does not go away

Call your doctor for medical advice about side effects. You may report side effects to FDA at 1-800-FDA-1088.

How should I store Follistim AQ?
- Store Follistim AQ in the refrigerator between 36°F to 46°F (2°C to 8°C) until the expiration date
- Follistim AQ can be stored at or below 77°F (25°C) for 3 months or until the expiration date, whichever comes first
- Keep Follistim AQ away from light
- Do not freeze

Keep Follistim AQ and all medicines out of the reach of children.

General information about Follistim AQ
Medicines are sometimes prescribed for purposes other than those listed in the Patient Information leaflet. Do not use Follistim AQ for a condition for which it was not prescribed. Do not give Follistim AQ to other people, even if they have the same condition that you have. It may harm them.

This Patient Information leaflet summarizes the most important information about Follistim AQ. If you would like more information, talk with your healthcare provider. You can ask your pharmacist or healthcare provider for more information about Follistim AQ that is written for healthcare professionals.

For more information, go to **www.follistim.com** or call 1-866-836-5633.

What are the ingredients in Follistim AQ?
Active ingredient: follitropin beta
Inactive ingredients: sucrose, sodium citrate, L-methionine, polysorbate 20, water for injection, hydrochloric acid, and/or sodium hydroxide.

Manufactured for Organon USA Inc., Roseland, NJ 07068
by Organon (Ireland) Ltd., Swords, Co. Dublin, Ireland
Revised 6/2010

PATIENT INSTRUCTIONS FOR USE
Follistim® (Fol´-lis-tim) AQ
(follitropin beta) for injection
Single-use vial

Read the Patient Instructions for Use that comes with Follistim® AQ before you start using it and each time you get a refill. There may be new information. This information does not take the place of talking with your healthcare provider about your medical condition or treatment.

A. Getting ready
- Remove the vial from the refrigerator
- Check the liquid in the vial. It should appear clear and colorless. If the solution is not clear and colorless or has particles in it, **do not use it**
- **Gather the supplies you will need for your injection. You will need:**
  - a clean dry surface
  - alcohol
  - cotton balls or alcohol pads
  - sterile gauze
  - a puncture-proof container to throw away the used syringe and needle
- Wash your hands and dry them.

B. Preparing your Follistim AQ injection
- Flip off the protective cap on the top of the vial. **Do not** remove the rubber stopper. Wipe the top of the rubber stopper with an alcohol wipe
- Use a syringe and needle that has been recommended by your healthcare provider, attach a needle to the syringe

C. Draw up your dose
- Carefully remove the needle cover (cap) from the needle (See Figure 1)

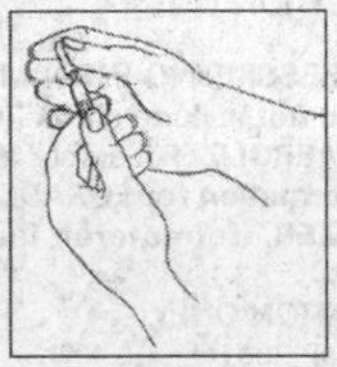

Figure 1

- Pull back on the plunger to draw the amount of air into the syringe equal to the dose needed
- With the vial on a flat work surface, insert the needle straight down through the rubber stopper of the Follistim AQ vial
- Push the plunger of the syringe down to inject the air from the syringe into the vial of Follistim AQ. The air injected into the vial will allow Follistim AQ to be easily withdrawn into the syringe
- Keep the needle inside the vial. Turn the vial and syringe upside down. Be sure that the tip of the Follistim AQ needle is in the liquid. Slowly pull back on the plunger to fill the syringe with Follistim AQ liquid to the number (mL or cc) that matches the dose your healthcare provider prescribed (See Figure 2)

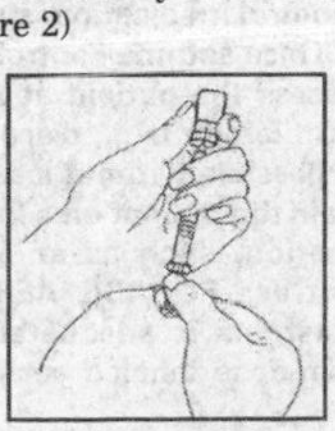

Figure 2

D. Remove the air
- Hold the syringe with the needle pointed up. Check for air bubbles in the syringe. A small amount of air will not hurt you. If you see large air bubbles, gently tap the side of the syringe with your finger until the air bubbles rise to the top of the syringe
- Slowly push the plunger down to force the air bubbles out of the syringe. You will see a drop of liquid on the tip of the needle

[See figure 3 at top of next column]

- Double-check that you have the right dose in the syringe. Lay the syringe down on its side until you have selected and prepared your injection site

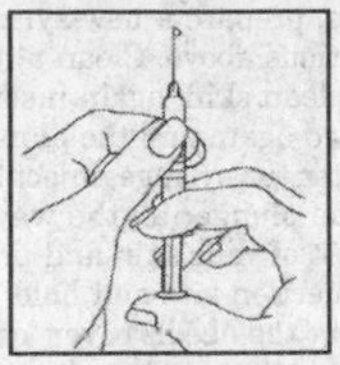

Figure 3

E. Selecting and preparing the injection site
- Follistim AQ can be injected into your body using two different ways (routes) as described below. Follow your healthcare provider's instructions about how you should inject Follistim AQ

1. Subcutaneous Route:
For women and men:
- Follistim AQ can be injected directly into a layer of fat under your skin (subcutaneously)
- When giving a subcutaneous injection, follow your healthcare provider's instructions about changing the site for each injection. This will help lower your chances of having a skin reaction
- **Do not** inject Follistim AQ into an area that is tender, red, bruised, or hard
- Recommended sites for injecting Follistim AQ subcutaneously are:
  - Just below your belly button (navel) (See Figure 4)
  - The upper outer area of your thigh (See Figure 4)

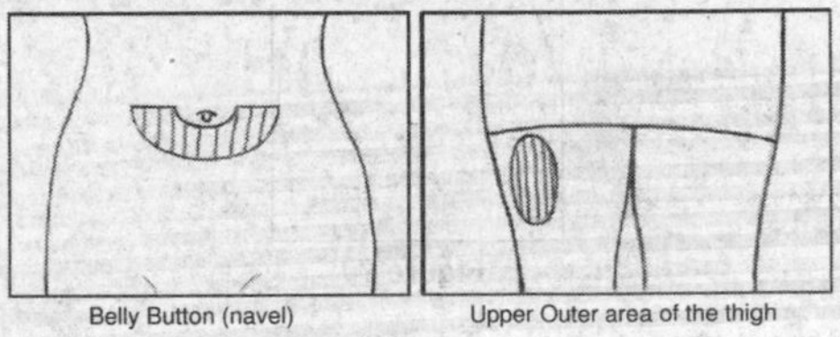

Figure 4

- Clean the skin with an alcohol wipe where the injection is to be made. Be careful not to touch the skin that has been wiped clean
- Pick up the prepared syringe and needle and hold it in the hand that you will use to inject the medicine
- Use the other hand to pinch a fold of skin at the cleaned injection site. **Do not** touch the cleaned area of skin
- Hold the syringe like you would a pencil. Use a quick "dart-like" motion to insert the needle either straight up and down (90-degree angle) or at a slight angle (45-degree angle) (See Figure 5)

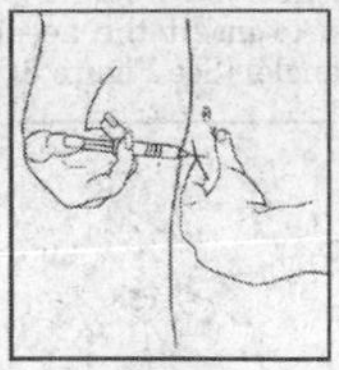

Figure 5

- Let go of the syringe and slowly pull back on the plunger. If blood comes into the syringe, **Do not** inject Follistim AQ because the needle might have entered a blood vessel
- If no blood is seen and the needle is properly placed, push the plunger slowly and steadily to inject the Follistim AQ solution.
- Once you have injected the entire content of the syringe, pull the needle out of your skin and press a cotton ball or gauze over the injection site and hold it there for several seconds (See Figure 6)
- Gently massage the site while still maintaining pressure. This will help disperse the Follistim AQ solution and may relieve any discomfort.
- **Do not** put the needle cover (cap) back on the needle

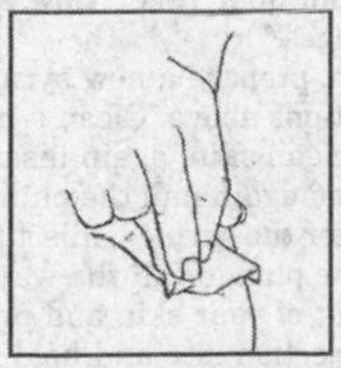

Figure 6

- Throw away the used needle and syringe in your puncture-proof container (See "How should I dispose of needles and syringes?")

- For each injection, prepare a new syringe of Follistim AQ using the instructions above. Clean a new area of skin. In this new area of clean skin, again insert a new needle (as you did before), and again pull the plunger back slightly. If blood does not enter the syringe, inject the Follistim AQ by slowly pushing the plunger all the way down
- Pull the needle out of your skin and press a cotton ball or gauze over the injection site and hold it there for several seconds. Do not put the needle cover (cap) back on the needle
- Throw away the used needle and syringe in your puncture-proof container (See "How should I dispose of needles and syringes?")

2. Intramuscular Route:

For women only:

◦ You will need to ask another person to give you your Follistim AQ injection intramuscularly (IM)

- Follistim AQ can be injected directly into your muscle (intramuscularly)
- When giving an intramuscular injection, follow your healthcare provider's instructions about changing the site for each injection. This will help lower your chances of having a skin reaction
- **Do not** inject Follistim AQ into an area that is tender, red, bruised, or hard
- Recommended site for injecting Follistim AQ intramuscularly is:
  - ◦ The upper outer area of the buttock (See Figure 7).

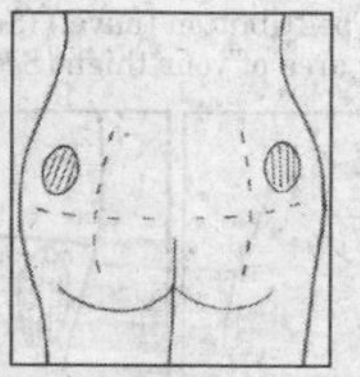

Figure 7

- Relax the muscle first by shifting your weight to the leg opposite of the side that the medicine will be injected into
- Clean the skin with an alcohol wipe where the injection is to be made. Be careful not to touch the skin that has been wiped clean

Instructions for giving an IM injection to the patient:

- Pick up the prepared syringe and needle and hold it in the hand that you will use to inject the medicine
- Use the other hand to stretch a fold of skin at the cleaned injection site. Stretching the skin helps the needle to go in more easily and pushes the tissue beneath the skin out of the way. **Do not** touch the cleaned area of skin (See Figure 8)
- Hold the syringe like you would a pencil. Use a quick "dart-like" motion to insert the needle straight up and down (90-degree angle) (See Figure 8)

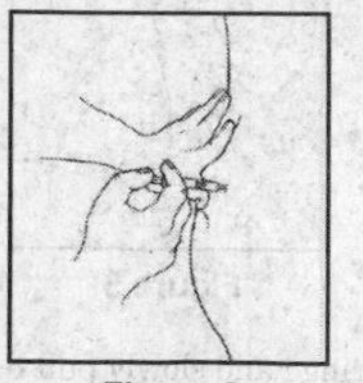

Figure 8

- Let go of the syringe and slowly pull back on the plunger. If blood comes into the syringe, **Do not** inject Follistim AQ because the needle might have entered a blood vessel
- Pull the needle out of your skin and press a cotton ball or gauze over the injection site and hold it there for several seconds. Gently massage the site while still maintaining pressure. This will help disperse the Follistim AQ solution and may relieve any discomfort.
- **Do not** put the needle cover (cap) back on the needle (See Figure 6)
- Throw away the used needle and syringe in your puncture-proof container (See "How should I dispose of needles and syringes?")
- For each injection, prepare a new syringe of Follistim AQ using the instructions above. Clean a new area of skin. In this new area of clean skin, again insert a new needle (as you did before), and again pull the plunger back slightly. If blood does not enter the syringe, inject the Follistim AQ by slowly pushing the plunger all the way down
- Pull the needle out of your skin and press a cotton ball or gauze over the injection site and hold it there for several seconds
- **Do not** put the needle cover (cap) back on the needle
- Throw away the used needle and syringe in your puncture-proof container (See "How should I dispose of needles and syringes?")

How do I throw away used syringes and needles?

Check with your healthcare provider or pharmacist for instructions about the right way to throw away used syringes and needles. There may be special local or state laws about how to throw away used syringes and needles

- **Do not** throw away used syringes and needles in the household trash and do not recycle them
- Put used and empty Follistim AQ syringes, needles, and vials in a closeable, puncture-resistant container. You may use a sharps container (such as a red bio-hazard container), a hard plastic container with a screw-on cap (such as an empty detergent bottle) or in a metal container with a plastic lid, (such as a coffee can)
- When the container is full, tape around the cap or lid to make sure the cap or lid does not come off
- When your injection is given by another person, this person must also be careful when removing the syringe and needle and disposing of the syringe and needle to prevent accidental needle stick injury and passing infection

How should I store Follistim AQ?

- Store Follistim AQ in the refrigerator at 36°F to 46°F (2°C to 8°C) until the expiration date
- Follistim AQ can be stored at or below 77°F (25°C) for 3 months or until the expiration date, whichever comes first
- Keep Follistim AQ away from light
- Do not freeze

Keep Follistim AQ, syringes, needles, and the disposal container out of the reach of children.

Manufactured for Organon USA Inc.
Roseland, NJ 07068
by Organon (Ireland) Ltd.
Swords, Co. Dublin, Ireland
U.S. Patent Nos. 5,767,251 and 5,929,028.
Revised 6/2010

Rev. 9/10
B-33554214
34306206T

FORADIL® AEROLIZER® ℞

[fōr-ă-dil]

(formoterol fumarate inhalation powder)
FOR ORAL INHALATION ONLY

HIGHLIGHTS OF PRESCRIBING INFORMATION

These highlights do not include all the information needed to use FORADIL® AEROLIZER® safely and effectively. See full prescribing information for FORADIL AEROLIZER.

FORADIL AEROLIZER (formoterol fumarate inhalation powder)
FOR ORAL INHALATION ONLY
Initial U.S. Approval: 2001

WARNING: ASTHMA-RELATED DEATH

See full prescribing information for complete boxed warning

- **Long-acting beta$_2$-adrenergic agonists (LABA), such as formoterol the active ingredient in FORADIL, increase the risk of asthma-related death. A large placebo-controlled study with another LABA (salmeterol) showed an increase in asthma-related deaths in patients receiving salmeterol. This finding with salmeterol is considered a class effect of LABA, including formoterol. (5.1)**
- **Prescribe FORADIL AEROLIZER only as additional therapy for patients with asthma who are currently taking but are inadequately controlled on a long-term asthma control medication, such as an inhaled corticosteroid. Once asthma control is achieved and maintained, assess the patient at regular intervals and step down therapy (e.g., discontinue FORADIL AEROLIZER) if possible without loss of asthma control and maintain the patient on a long-term asthma control medication, such as an inhaled corticosteroid. Do not use FORADIL AEROLIZER for patients whose asthma is adequately controlled on low- or medium-dose inhaled corticosteroids. (1.1, 5.1).**
- **Available data from controlled clinical trials suggest that LABA increase the risk of asthma-related hospitalization in pediatric and adolescent patients. (5.1)**

RECENT MAJOR CHANGES

Warnings and Precautions,
Coexisting Conditions (5.8) 09/2012

INDICATIONS AND USAGE

FORADIL AEROLIZER is a LABA indicated for:

- Treatment of asthma in patients ≥5 years as an add-on to a long-term asthma control medication such as an inhaled corticosteroid. (1.1)
- Prevention of exercise-induced bronchospasm (EIB) in patients ≥5 years. (1.2)
- Maintenance treatment of bronchoconstriction in patients with chronic obstructive pulmonary disease (COPD). (1.3)

Important limitations of use:

- NOT indicated for the relief of acute bronchospasm. (1.1, 1.3)

DOSAGE AND ADMINISTRATION

For oral inhalation only. **DO NOT swallow** Foradil capsule. Foradil capsule should be **always** used with Aerolizer inhaler **ONLY**.

- Treatment of asthma in patients ≥5 years: Inhalation of one capsule every 12 hours in addition to concomitant treatment with a long-term control medication such as an inhaled corticosteroid. (2.1)
- EIB: Inhalation of one capsule at least 15 minutes before exercise Additional doses should not be used for 12 hours. (2.2)
- Maintenance treatment of bronchoconstriction in patients with COPD: Inhalation of one capsule every 12 hours. (2.3)

DOSAGE FORMS AND STRENGTHS

Foradil capsules for oral inhalation: 12 mcg formoterol fumarate powder, for use with Aerolizer inhaler. (3)

CONTRAINDICATIONS

- Asthma: Without concomitant use of a long-term asthma control medication such as an inhaled corticosteroid. (4)
- Hypersensitivity to formoterol fumarate or any components of this product. (4)

WARNINGS AND PRECAUTIONS

- Asthma-related deaths and asthma-related hospitalizations: LABA increase the risk. Prescribe for asthma only as concomitant therapy with a long-term control medication such as an inhaled corticosteroid. (5.1)
- Deterioration of asthma and acute episodes: Do not initiate during acutely deteriorating asthma. Do not use to treat acute symptoms. (5.2)
- Corticosteroids: Not a substitute for corticosteroids. Corticosteroids should not be stopped or reduced when FORADIL AEROLIZER is initiated. (5.3)
- Use with additional long-acting beta$_2$-agonist: Do not use in combination because of risk of overdose. (5.4)
- Paradoxical bronchospasm: Discontinue FORADIL AEROLIZER and institute alternative therapy if paradoxical bronchospasm occurs. (5.5)
- Patients with cardiovascular or central nervous system disorders: Use with caution because of beta-adrenergic stimulation. (5.6)
- Coexisting conditions: Use with caution in patients with convulsive disorders, thyrotoxicosis, diabetes mellitus, ketoacidosis, aneurysm, and pheochromocytoma. (5.8)
- Metabolic effects: Be alert to hypokalemia and hyperglycemia. (5.9)

ADVERSE REACTIONS

Most common adverse reactions (incidence ≥1% and more common than placebo) are:

- Asthma: viral infection, bronchitis, chest infection, dyspnea, chest pain, tremor, dizziness, insomnia, tonsillitis, rash, dysphonia, and serious asthma exacerbation. (6.1, 6.3)
- COPD: Upper respiratory tract infection, back pain, pharyngitis, chest pain, sinusitis, fever, leg cramps, muscle cramps, anxiety, pruritus, increased sputum, and dry mouth. (6.2)

To report SUSPECTED ADVERSE REACTIONS, contact Merck Sharp & Dohme Corporation, a subsidiary of Merck & Co., Inc. at 1-877-888-4231 or FDA at 1-800-FDA-1088 or www.fda.gov/medwatch.

DRUG INTERACTIONS

- Adrenergic agents: Use with caution. Additional adrenergic drugs may potentiate sympathetic effects. (7.1)
- Xanthine derivatives, systemic corticosteroids, and non-potassium sparing diuretics: Use with caution. May potentiate hypokalemia or ECG changes. (7.2, 7.3)
- MAO inhibitors, tricyclic antidepressants, macrolides, and drugs that prolong QTc interval: Use with extreme caution. May potentiate effect on cardiovascular system. (7.4)
- Beta-blockers: Use with caution and only when medically necessary. May decrease effectiveness and produce severe bronchospasm. (7.5)
- Halogenated hydrocarbons: There is an elevated risk of arrhythmias in patients receiving concomitant anesthesia with halogenated hydrocarbons. (7.6)

See 17 for PATIENT COUNSELING INFORMATION and Medication Guide

Revised: 11/2012

FULL PRESCRIBING INFORMATION: CONTENTS*

*** Sections or subsections omitted from the full prescribing information are not listed**

FULL PRESCRIBING INFORMATION

WARNING: ASTHMA-RELATED DEATH

Long-acting beta$_2$-adrenergic agonists (LABA), such as formoterol the active ingredient in FORADIL AEROLIZER, increase the risk of asthma-related death. Data from a large placebo controlled US study that compared the safety of another LABA (salmeterol) or placebo added to usual asthma therapy showed an increase in asthma-related deaths in patients receiving salmeterol. This finding with salmeterol is considered a class effect of LABA, including formoterol [*see Warnings and Precautions (5.1)*].

Currently available data are inadequate to determine whether concurrent use of inhaled corticosteroids or other long-term asthma control drugs mitigates the increased risk of asthma-related death from LABA.

Because of this risk, use of FORADIL AEROLIZER for the treatment of asthma without a concomitant long-term asthma control medication, such as an inhaled corticosteroid, is contraindicated. Use FORADIL AEROLIZER only as additional therapy for patients with asthma who are currently taking but are inadequately controlled on a long-term asthma control medication, such as an inhaled corticosteroid. Once asthma control is achieved and maintained, assess the patient at regular intervals and step down therapy (e.g., discontinue FORADIL AEROLIZER) if possible without loss of asthma control, and maintain the patient on a long-term asthma control medication, such as an inhaled corticosteroid. Do not use FORADIL AEROLIZER for patients whose asthma is adequately controlled on low or medium dose inhaled corticosteroids.

Pediatric and Adolescent Patients

Available data from controlled clinical trials suggest that LABA increase the risk of asthma-related hospitalization in pediatric and adolescent patients. For pediatric and adolescent patients with asthma who require addition of a LABA to an inhaled corticosteroid, a fixed-dose combination product containing both an inhaled corticosteroid and LABA should ordinarily be considered to ensure adherence with both drugs. In cases where use of a separate long-term asthma control medication (e.g., inhaled corticosteroid) and LABA is clinically indicated, appropriate steps must be taken to ensure adherence with both treatment components. If adherence cannot be assured, a fixed-dose combination product containing both an inhaled corticosteroid and LABA is recommended.

1 INDICATIONS AND USAGE

1.1 Treatment of Asthma

FORADIL AEROLIZER is indicated for the treatment of asthma and in the prevention of bronchospasm only as concomitant therapy with a long-term asthma control medication, such as an inhaled corticosteroid, in adults and children 5 years of age and older with reversible obstructive airways disease, including patients with symptoms of nocturnal asthma.

Long acting beta$_2$-adrenergic agonists (LABA), such as formoterol, the active ingredient in FORADIL AEROLIZER, increase the risk of asthma-related death. Use of FORADIL AEROLIZER for the treatment of asthma without concomitant use of a long-term asthma control medication, such as an inhaled corticosteroid, is contraindicated. Use FORADIL AEROLIZER only as additional therapy for patients with asthma who are currently taking but are inadequately controlled on a long-term asthma control medication, such as an inhaled corticosteroid. Once asthma control is achieved and maintained, assess the patient at regular intervals and step down therapy (e.g., discontinue FORADIL AEROLIZER) if possible without loss of asthma control, and maintain the patient on a long-term asthma control medication, such as an inhaled corticosteroid. Do not use FORADIL AEROLIZER for patients whose asthma is adequately controlled on low or medium dose inhaled corticosteroids [*see Contraindications (4) and Warnings and Precautions (5.1)*].

Pediatric and Adolescent Patients

Available data from controlled clinical trials suggest that LABA increase the risk of asthma-related hospitalization in pediatric and adolescent patients. For pediatric and adolescent patients with asthma who require addition of a LABA to an inhaled corticosteroid, a fixed-dose combination product containing both an inhaled corticosteroid and LABA should ordinarily be used to ensure adherence with both drugs. In cases where use of a separate long-term asthma control medication (e.g., inhaled corticosteroid) and LABA is clinically indicated, appropriate steps must be taken to ensure adherence with both treatment components. If adherence cannot be assured, a fixed-dose combination product containing both an inhaled corticosteroid and LABA is recommended [*see Warnings and Precautions (5.1)*].

Important Limitation of Use

FORADIL AEROLIZER is NOT indicated for the relief of acute bronchospasm.

1.2 Prevention of Exercise-Induced Bronchospasm

FORADIL AEROLIZER is also indicated for the acute prevention of exercise-induced bronchospasm in adults and children 5 years of age and older, when administered on an occasional, as-needed basis. Use of FORADIL AEROLIZER as a single agent for the prevention of exercise-induced bronchospasm may be clinically indicated in patients who do not have persistent asthma. In patients with persistent asthma, use of FORADIL AEROLIZER for the prevention of exercise-induced bronchospasm may be clinically indicated, but the treatment of asthma should include a long-term asthma control medication, such as an inhaled corticosteroid.

1.3 Maintenance Treatment of Chronic Obstructive Pulmonary Disease

FORADIL AEROLIZER is indicated for the long-term, twice daily (morning and evening) administration in the maintenance treatment of bronchoconstriction in patients with Chronic Obstructive Pulmonary Disease including chronic bronchitis and emphysema.

Important Limitation of Use

FORADIL AEROLIZER is NOT indicated for the relief of acute bronchospasm.

2 DOSAGE AND ADMINISTRATION

FORADIL capsules should be administered only by the oral inhalation route and only using the AEROLIZER Inhaler (see the accompanying Medication Guide). **FORADIL capsules should not be swallowed.** FORADIL capsules should always be stored in the blister, and only removed IMMEDIATELY BEFORE USE.

2.1 Asthma

Long-acting beta$_2$-adrenergic agonists (LABA), such as formoterol, the active ingredient in FORADIL AEROLIZER, increase the risk of asthma-related death [*see Warnings and Precautions (5.1)*]. **Because of this risk, use of FORADIL AEROLIZER for the treatment of asthma without concomitant use of a long-term asthma control medication, such as an inhaled corticosteroid, is contraindicated.** Use FORADIL AEROLIZER only as additional therapy for patients with asthma who are currently taking but are inadequately controlled on a long-term asthma control medication, such as an inhaled corticosteroid. Once asthma control is achieved and maintained, assess the patient at regular intervals and step down therapy (e.g., discontinue FORADIL AEROLIZER) if possible without loss of asthma control, and maintain the patient on a long-term asthma control medication, such as an inhaled corticosteroid. Do not use FORADIL AEROLIZER for patients whose asthma is adequately controlled on low or medium dose inhaled corticosteroids.

Pediatric and Adolescent Patients

For adults and children 5 years of age and older, the usual dosage is the inhalation of the contents of one 12-mcg FORADIL capsule every 12 hours using the AEROLIZER Inhaler. The patient must not exhale into the device. The total daily dose of FORADIL should not exceed one capsule twice daily (24 mcg total daily dose). More frequent administration or administration of a larger number of inhalations is not recommended. If symptoms arise between doses, an inhaled short-acting beta2-agonist should be taken for immediate relief.

Available data from controlled clinical trials suggest that LABA increase the risk of asthma-related hospitalization in pediatric and adolescent patients. For patients with asthma less than 18 years of age who require addition of a LABA to an inhaled corticosteroid, a fixed-dose combination product containing both an inhaled corticosteroid and LABA should ordinarily be used to ensure adherence with both drugs. In cases where use of a separate long-term asthma control medication (e.g., inhaled corticosteroid) and LABA is clinically indicated, appropriate steps must be taken to ensure adherence with both treatment components. If adherence cannot be assured, a fixed-dose combination product containing both an inhaled corticosteroid and LABA is recommended.

2.2 Exercise-Induced Bronchospasm (EIB)

Use of FORADIL AEROLIZER as a single agent for the prevention of exercise induced bronchospasm may be clinically indicated in patients who do not have persistent asthma. In patients with persistent asthma, use of FORADIL AEROLIZER for the prevention of exercise induced bronchospasm may be clinically indicated, but the treatment of asthma should include a long-term asthma control medication, such as an inhaled corticosteroid. For adults and children 5 years of age or older, the usual dosage is the inhalation of the contents of one 12-mcg FORADIL capsule at least 15 minutes before exercise administered on an occasional as needed basis. When used intermittently as needed for prevention, protection may last up to 12 hours. Additional doses of FORADIL AEROLIZER should not be used for 12 hours after the administration of this drug. Regular, twice-daily dosing has not been studied in preventing EIB. Patients who are receiving FORADIL AEROLIZER twice daily for treatment of their asthma should not use additional doses for prevention of EIB and may require a short-acting bronchodilator.

2.3 Chronic Obstructive Pulmonary Disease (COPD)

For maintenance treatment of bronchoconstriction in patients with COPD (including chronic bronchitis and emphysema) the usual dosage is the inhalation of the contents of one 12 mcg FORADIL capsule every 12 hours using the AEROLIZER inhaler.

A total daily dose of greater than 24 mcg is not recommended.

3 DOSAGE FORMS AND STRENGTHS

FORADIL AEROLIZER consists of FORADIL capsules and an AEROLIZER inhaler. FORADIL capsules contain 12 mcg dry powder formulation of formoterol fumarate in a clear, hard gelatin capsule for inhalation use with the AEROLIZER inhaler only.

4 CONTRAINDICATIONS

- **Because of the risk of asthma-related death and hospitalization, use of FORADIL AEROLIZER for the treatment of asthma without concomitant use of a long-term asthma control medication, such as an inhaled corticosteroid, is contraindicated** [*see Warnings and Precautions (5.1)*].
- FORADIL AEROLIZER is contraindicated as primary treatment of status asthmaticus or other acute episodes of asthma or COPD where intensive measures are required [*see Warnings and Precautions (5.2)*].
- FORADIL (formoterol fumarate) is contraindicated in patients with a history of hypersensitivity to formoterol fumarate or to any components of this product [*see Warnings and Precautions (5.7)*].

5 WARNINGS AND PRECAUTIONS

5.1 Asthma-Related Death

Long-acting beta$_2$-adrenergic agonists, such as formoterol, the active ingredient in FORADIL AEROLIZER, increase the risk of asthma-related death. Currently available data are inadequate to determine whether concurrent use of inhaled corticosteroids or other long-term asthma control drugs mitigates the increased risk of asthma-related death from LABA.

Because of this risk, use of FORADIL AEROLIZER for the treatment of asthma without concomitant use of a long-term asthma control medication, such as an inhaled corticosteroid, is contraindicated. Once asthma control is achieved and maintained, assess the patient at regular intervals and step down therapy (e.g., discontinue FORADIL AEROLIZER) if possible without loss of asthma control, and maintain the patient on a long-term asthma control medication, such as an inhaled corticosteroid. Do not use FORADIL AEROLIZER for patients whose asthma is adequately controlled on low or medium dose inhaled corticosteroids.

Pediatric and Adolescent Patients

Available data from controlled clinical trials suggest that LABA increase the risk of asthma-related hospitalization in pediatric and adolescent patients. For pediatric and adolescent patients with asthma who require addition of a LABA to an inhaled corticosteroid, a fixed-dose combination product containing both an inhaled corticosteroid and LABA should ordinarily be considered to ensure adherence with both drugs. In cases where use of a separate long-term asthma control medication (e.g., inhaled corticosteroid) and LABA is clinically indicated, appropriate steps must be taken to ensure adherence with both treatment components. If adherence cannot be assured, a fixed-dose combination product containing both an inhaled corticosteroid and LABA is recommended.

A 28-week, placebo-controlled US study comparing the safety of salmeterol with placebo, each added to usual asthma therapy, showed an increase in asthma-related deaths in patients receiving salmeterol (13/13,176 in patients treated with salmeterol vs. 3/13,179 in patients treated with placebo; RR 4.37, 95% CI 1.25, 15.34). The increased risk of asthma-related death is considered a class effect of the long-acting beta2-adrenergic agonists, including formoterol. No study adequate to determine whether the rate of asthma-related death is increased with FORADIL AEROLIZER has been conducted.

Clinical studies with FORADIL AEROLIZER suggested a higher incidence of serious asthma exacerbations in patients who received FORADIL AEROLIZER than in those who received placebo [*see Adverse Reactions (6.2, 6.3)*]. The sizes of these studies were not adequate to precisely quantify the differences in serious asthma exacerbation rates between treatment groups.

The studies described above enrolled patients with asthma. No studies have been conducted that were adequate to determine whether the rate of death in patients with COPD is increased by long-acting beta$_2$-adrenergic agonists.

5.2 Deterioration of Disease and Acute Episodes

FORADIL AEROLIZER should not be initiated in patients with significantly worsening, acutely deteriorating, or potentially life-threatening episodes of asthma or COPD. The use of FORADIL AEROLIZER in this setting is not appropriate [*see Indications and Usage (1.1, 1.3)*].

Asthma may deteriorate acutely over a period of hours or chronically over several days or longer. It is important to watch for signs of worsening asthma, such as increasing use of inhaled, short-acting beta$_2$-adrenergic agonists or a significant decrease in peak expiratory flow (PEF) or lung function. Such findings require immediate evaluation. Patients should be advised to seek immediate attention should their condition deteriorate. Increasing the daily dosage of FORADIL AEROLIZER beyond the recommended dose in this situation is not appropriate. FORADIL AEROLIZER should not be used more frequently than twice daily (morning and evening) at the recommended dose.

FORADIL AEROLIZER should not be used to treat acute symptoms. FORADIL AEROLIZER has not been studied in the relief of acute symptoms and extra doses should not be used for that purpose. When prescribing FORADIL AEROLIZER, the physician should also provide the patient with an inhaled, short-acting beta$_2$-agonist for treatment of symptoms that occur acutely, despite regular twice-daily (morning and evening) use of FORADIL AEROLIZER. Patients should also be cautioned that increasing inhaled beta$_2$-agonist use is a signal of deteriorating asthma [*see Information for Patients (17) and the accompanying Medication Guide.*]

When beginning treatment with FORADIL AEROLIZER, patients who have been taking inhaled, short-acting beta$_2$-agonists on a regular basis (e.g., four times a day) should be instructed to discontinue the regular use of these drugs and use them only for symptomatic relief of acute symptoms.

5.3 FORADIL AEROLIZER is not a substitute for corticosteroids

There are no data demonstrating that FORADIL has any clinical anti-inflammatory effect and therefore it cannot be expected to take the place of corticosteroids. Corticosteroids should not be stopped or reduced at the time FORADIL AEROLIZER is initiated. Patients who already require oral or inhaled corticosteroids for treatment of asthma should be continued on this type of treatment even if they feel better as a result of initiating FORADIL AEROLIZER. Any change in corticosteroid dosage, in particular a reduction, should be made ONLY after clinical evaluation [*see Patient Counseling Information (17.2)*].

5.4 Excessive Use and Use with Other Long-Acting Beta$_2$-Agonists

FORADIL AEROLIZER should not be used more often or at doses higher than recommended, or in conjunction with other medications containing LABA, as an overdose may result. Patients using FORADIL AEROLIZER should not use an additional LABA (e.g., salmeterol xinafoate, arformoterol tartrate) for any reason. Fatalities have been reported in association with excessive use of inhaled sympathomimetic drugs in patients with asthma. The exact cause of death is unknown, but cardiac arrest following an unexpected development of a severe acute asthmatic crisis and subsequent hypoxia is suspected. In addition, data from clinical trials with FORADIL AEROLIZER suggest that the use of doses higher than recommended is associated with an increased risk of serious asthma exacerbations [*see Adverse Reactions (6.2, 6.3)*].

5.5 Paradoxical Bronchospasm

As with other inhaled beta$_2$-agonists, formoterol can produce paradoxical bronchospasm that may be life-threatening. If paradoxical bronchospasm occurs, FORADIL AEROLIZER should be discontinued immediately and alternative therapy instituted.

5.6 Cardiovascular and Central Nervous System Effects

Excessive beta-adrenergic stimulation has been associated with seizures, angina, hypertension or hypotension, tachycardia with rates up to 200 beats/min, arrhythmias, nervousness, headache, tremor, palpitation, nausea, dizziness, fatigue, malaise, and insomnia. Fatalities have been reported in association with excessive use of inhaled sympathomimetic drugs [*see Overdosage (10)*].

Formoterol fumarate, like other beta$_2$-agonists, can produce a clinically significant cardiovascular effect in some patients as measured by increases in pulse rate, blood pressure, and/or symptoms. Although such effects are uncommon after administration of FORADIL AEROLIZER at recommended doses, if they occur, the drug may need to be discontinued. In addition, beta-agonists have been reported to produce ECG changes, such as flattening of the T wave, prolongation of the QTc interval, and ST segment depression. The clinical significance of these findings is unknown. Therefore, formoterol fumarate, like other sympathomimetic amines, should be used with caution in patients with cardiovascular disorders, especially coronary insufficiency, cardiac arrhythmias, and hypertension.

5.7 Immediate Hypersensitivity Reactions

Immediate hypersensitivity reactions may occur after administration of FORADIL AEROLIZER, as demonstrated by cases of anaphylactic reactions, urticaria, angioedema, rash, and bronchospasm.

FORADIL AEROLIZER contains lactose, which contains trace levels of milk proteins. Allergic reactions to products containing milk proteins may occur in patients with severe milk protein allergy.

5.8 Coexisting Conditions

Formoterol fumarate, like other sympathomimetic amines, should be used with caution in patients with cardiovascular disorders, especially coronary insufficiency, cardiac arrhythmias, hypertension, aneurysm, and pheochromocytoma; in patients with convulsive disorders or thyrotoxicosis; and in patients who are unusually responsive to sympathomimetic amines. Doses of the related beta2-agonist albuterol, when administered intravenously, have been reported to aggravate preexisting diabetes mellitus and ketoacidosis.

5.9 Hypokalemia and Hyperglycemia

Beta-agonist medications may produce significant hypokalemia in some patients, possibly through intracellular shunting, which has the potential to produce adverse cardiovascular effects. The decrease in serum potassium is usually transient, not requiring supplementation.

Clinically significant changes in blood glucose and/or serum potassium were infrequent during clinical studies with long-term administration of FORADIL AEROLIZER at the recommended dose.

5.10 Inappropriate Route of Administration

FORADIL capsules should ONLY be used with the AEROLIZER Inhaler and SHOULD NOT be swallowed.

FORADIL capsules should always be stored in the blister, and only removed IMMEDIATELY before use.

6 ADVERSE REACTIONS

Long-acting beta$_2$-adrenergic agonists (LABA), including formoterol, the active ingredient in FORADIL AEROLIZER, increase the risk of asthma-related death and may increase the risk of asthma-related hospitalizations in pediatric and adolescent patients. Clinical trials with FORADIL AEROLIZER suggested a higher incidence of serious asthma exacerbations in patients who received FORADIL AEROLIZER than in those who received placebo [*see Warnings and Precautions (5.1)*].

Adverse reactions common to LABA drugs include: angina, hypertension or hypotension, tachycardia, arrhythmias, nervousness, headache, tremor, dry mouth, palpitation, muscle cramps, nausea, dizziness, fatigue, malaise, hypokalemia, hyperglycemia, metabolic acidosis, and insomnia.

Because clinical trials are conducted under widely varying conditions, adverse reaction rates observed in the clinical trials of a drug cannot be directly compared to rates in the clinical trials of another drug and may not reflect the rates observed in clinical trials.

6.1 Asthma

Of the 5824 patients in multiple-dose controlled clinical trials, 1985 were treated with FORADIL AEROLIZER at the recommended dose of 12 mcg twice daily. The following table shows treatment-emergent adverse reactions where the frequency was greater than or equal to 1% in the FORADIL twice daily group and where the rates in the FORADIL group exceeded placebo. Three treatment-emergent adverse reactions showed dose ordering among tested doses of 6, 12, and 24 mcg administered twice daily; tremor, dizziness and dysphonia.

Number and Frequency of Treatment-Emergent Adverse Reactions in Patients 5 Years of Age and Older from Multiple-Dose Controlled Clinical Trials

Treatment-Emergent Adverse Reaction	Foradil Aerolizer 12 mcg twice daily n	(%)	Placebo n	(%)
Total Patients	**1985**	**(100)**	**969**	**(100)**
Infection viral	341	(17.2)	166	(17.1)
Bronchitis	92	(4.6)	42	(4.3)
Chest infection	54	(2.7)	4	(0.4)
Dyspnea	42	(2.1)	16	(1.7)
Chest pain	37	(1.9)	13	(1.3)
Tremor	37	(1.9)	4	(0.4)
Dizziness	31	(1.6)	15	(1.5)
Insomnia	29	(1.5)	8	(0.8)
Tonsilitis	23	(1.2)	7	(0.7)
Rash	22	(1.1)	7	(0.7)
Dysphonia	19	(1.0)	9	(0.9)

In patients 5-12 years of age, the numbers and percent of patients who reported treatment-emergent adverse reactions were comparable in the 12 mcg twice daily and placebo groups. In general, the pattern of the treatment-emergent adverse reactions observed in children differed from the usual pattern seen in adults. Treatment-emergent adverse reactions that were more frequent in the formoterol group than in the placebo group reflected infection/inflammation (viral infection, rhinitis, tonsillitis, gastroenteritis) or abdominal complaints (abdominal pain, nausea, dyspepsia).

Serious Asthma Exacerbations in Adolescents and Adults 12 Years of Age and Older

In two 12-week controlled trials with combined enrollment of 1095 patients 12 years of age and older, FORADIL AEROLIZER 12 mcg twice daily was compared to FORADIL AEROLIZER 24 mcg twice daily, albuterol 180 mcg four times daily, and placebo. Serious asthma exacerbations (acute worsening of asthma resulting in hospitalization) occurred more commonly with FORADIL AEROLIZER 24 mcg twice daily than with the recommended dose of FORADIL AEROLIZER 12 mcg twice daily, albuterol, or placebo. The results are shown in the following table.

[See table at top of next page]

In a 16-week, randomized, multi-center, double-blind, parallel-group trial, patients who received either 24 mcg twice daily or 12 mcg twice daily doses of FORADIL AEROLIZER experienced more serious asthma exacerbations than patients who received placebo [*see Clinical Trials (14.1)*]. The results are shown in the following table.

Number and Frequency of Serious Asthma Exacerbations in Patients 12 Years of Age and Older from a 16-Week Trial

	Foradil 12 mcg twice daily	Foradil 24 mcg twice daily	Placebo
Serious asthma exacerbations	3/527 (0.6%)	2/527 (0.4%)	1/514 (0.2%)

Serious Asthma Exacerbations in Children 5-11 Years of Age

The safety of FORADIL AEROLIZER 12 mcg twice daily compared to FORADIL AEROLIZER 24 mcg twice daily and placebo was investigated in one large, multicenter, randomized, double-blind, 52-week clinical trial in 518 children with asthma (ages 5-12 years) in need of daily bronchodilators and anti-inflammatory treatment. More children who received FORADIL AEROLIZER 24 mcg twice daily than children who received FORADIL AEROLIZER 12 mcg twice daily or placebo experienced serious asthma exacerbations, as shown in the next table.

Number and Frequency of Serious Asthma Exacerbations in Patients 5-12 Years of Age from a 52-Week Trial

	Foradil 12 mcg twice daily	Foradil 24 mcg twice daily	Placebo
Serious asthma exacerbations	8/171 (4.7%)	11/171 (6.4%)	0/176 (0)

6.2 COPD

Of the 1634 patients in two pivotal multiple-dose Chronic Obstructive Pulmonary Disease (COPD) controlled trials, 405 were treated with FORADIL AEROLIZER 12 mcg twice daily. Treatment-emergent adverse reactions reported were similar to those seen in asthmatic patients, but with a higher incidence of COPD-related events in both placebo and formoterol treated patients.

The following table shows treatment-emergent adverse reactions where the frequency was greater than or equal to 1% in the FORADIL AEROLIZER group and where the rates in the FORADIL AEROLIZER group exceeded placebo. The two clinical trials included doses of 12 mcg and 24 mcg, administered twice daily. Seven treatment-emergent adverse reactions showed dose ordering among tested doses of 12 and 24 mcg administered twice daily; pharyngitis, fever, muscle cramps, increased sputum, dysphonia, myalgia, and tremor.

Number and Frequency of Treatment-Emergent Adverse Reactions in Adult COPD Patients Treated in Multiple-Dose Controlled Clinical Trials

Treatment-Emergent Adverse Reaction	Foradil Aerolizer 12 mcg twice daily		Placebo	
	n	(%)	n	(%)
Total Patients	**405**	**(100)**	**420**	**(100)**
Upper respiratory tract infection	30	(7.4)	24	(5.7)
Pain back	17	(4.2)	17	(4.0)
Pharyngitis	14	(3.5)	10	(2.4)
Pain chest	13	(3.2)	9	(2.1)
Sinusitis	11	(2.7)	7	(1.7)
Fever	9	(2.2)	6	(1.4)
Cramps leg	7	(1.7)	2	(0.5)
Cramps muscle	7	(1.7)	0	
Anxiety	6	(1.5)	5	(1.2)
Pruritis	6	(1.5)	4	(1.0)
Sputum increased	6	(1.5)	5	(1.2)
Mouth dry	5	(1.2)	4	(1.0)

Overall, the frequency of all cardiovascular treatment-emergent adverse reactions in the two pivotal studies was 6.4% for FORADIL AEROLIZER 12 mcg twice daily, and 6.0% for placebo. There were no frequently-occurring specific cardiovascular treatment-emergent adverse reactions for FORADIL AEROLIZER (frequency greater than or equal to 1% and greater than placebo).

6.3 Postmarketing Experience

The following adverse reactions have been identified during post approval use of FORADIL. Because these reactions are reported voluntarily from a population of uncertain size, it is not always possible to reliably estimate their frequency or establish a causal relationship to drug exposure.

In extensive worldwide marketing experience with FORADIL, serious exacerbations of asthma, including some that have been fatal, have been reported. While most of these cases have been in patients with severe or acutely deteriorating asthma [*see Warnings and Precautions (5.1, 5.2)*], a few have occurred in patients with less severe asthma. It is not possible to determine from these individual case reports whether FORADIL AEROLIZER contributed to the events.

Immune system disorders: rare reports of anaphylactic reactions, including severe hypotension and angioedema
Metabolism and nutrition disorders: Hypokalemia, hyperglycemia
Respiratory, thoracic and mediastinal disorders: Cough
Skin and subcutaneous tissue disorders: Rash
Cardiac disorders: Angina pectoris, cardiac arrhythmias, e.g., atrial fibrillation, ventricular extrasystoles, tachyarrhythmia
Investigations: Electrocardiogram QT prolonged, blood pressure increased (including hypertension)

Number and Frequency of Serious Asthma Exacerbations in Patients 12 Years of Age and Older from Two 12-Week Controlled Clinical Trials

	Foradil 12 mcg twice daily	Foradil 24 mcg twice daily	Albuterol 180 mcg four times daily	Placebo
Trial #1				
Serious asthma exacerbations	0/136 (0)	4/135 (3.0%)[1]	2/134 (1.5%)	0/136 (0)
Trial #2				
Serious asthma exacerbations	1/139 (0.7%)	5/136 (3.7%)[2]	0/138 (0)	2/141 (1.4%)

[1] patient required intubation
[2] patients had respiratory arrest; 1 of the patients died

7 DRUG INTERACTIONS

7.1 Adrenergic Drugs

If additional adrenergic drugs are to be administered by any route, they should be used with caution because the pharmacologically predictable sympathetic effects of formoterol may be potentiated.

7.2 Xanthine Derivatives or Systemic Corticosteroids

Concomitant treatment with xanthine derivatives or systemic corticosteroids may potentiate any hypokalemic effect of adrenergic agonists.

7.3 Diuretics

The ECG changes or hypokalemia that may result from the administration of non-potassium sparing diuretics (such as loop or thiazide diuretics) can be acutely worsened by beta-agonists, especially when the recommended dose of the beta-agonist is exceeded. Although the clinical significance of these effects is not known, caution is advised in the coadministration of beta-agonist with non-potassium sparing diuretics.

7.4 Monoamine Oxidase Inhibitors and Tricyclic Antidepressants, QTc Prolonging Drugs

Formoterol, as with other $beta_2$-agonists, should be administered with extreme caution to patients being treated with monoamine oxidase inhibitors, tricyclic antidepressants, macrolides or drugs known to prolong the QTc interval because the action of adrenergic agonists on the cardiovascular system may be potentiated by these agents. Drugs that are known to prolong the QTc interval have an increased risk of ventricular arrhythmias.

7.5 Beta-blockers

Beta-adrenergic receptor antagonists (beta-blockers) and formoterol may inhibit the effect of each other when administered concurrently. Beta-blockers not only block the therapeutic effects of $beta_2$-agonists, such as formoterol, but may produce severe bronchospasm in asthmatic patients. Therefore, patients with asthma should not normally be treated with beta-blockers. However, under certain circumstances, e.g., as prophylaxis after myocardial infarction, there may be no acceptable alternatives to the use of beta-blockers in patients with asthma. In this setting, cardioselective beta-blockers could be considered, although they should be administered with caution.

7.6 Halogenated Hydrocarbons

There is an elevated risk of arrhythmias in patients receiving concomitant anesthesia with halogenated hydrocarbons.

8 USE IN SPECIFIC POPULATIONS

8.1 Pregnancy

Pregnancy Category C.

Teratogenic Effects: There are no adequate and well-controlled studies of FORADIL AEROLIZER in pregnant women. Animal reproduction studies of formoterol fumarate in rats and rabbits revealed evidence of teratogenicity as well as other developmental toxic effects. Because there are no adequate and well-controlled studies in pregnant women, FORADIL AEROLIZER should be used during pregnancy only if the potential benefit justifies the potential risk to the fetus.

Formoterol fumarate administered throughout organogenesis did not cause malformations in rats or rabbits following oral administration. When given to rats throughout organogenesis, oral doses equal to or greater than 80 times the maximum recommended human dose (MRHD) for adults (on a mcg/m^2 basis for maternal doses of 0.2 mg/kg and above) delayed ossification of the fetus and doses equal to or greater than 2400 times the MRHD for adults (on a mcg/m^2 basis for maternal doses of 6 mg/kg and above) decreased fetal weight. Formoterol fumarate has been shown to cause stillbirth and neonatal mortality at oral doses equal to or greater than 2400 times the MRHD for adults (on a mcg/m^2 basis for maternal doses of 6 mg/kg and above) in rats receiving the drug during the late stage of pregnancy. These effects, however, were not produced at a dose equal to 80 times the MRHD for adults (on a mcg/m^2 basis for a maternal dose of 0.2 mg/kg).

In another testing laboratory, formoterol fumarate was shown to be teratogenic in rats and rabbits. Umbilical hernia, a malformation, was observed in rat fetuses at oral doses equal to or greater than 1200 times the MRHD for adults (on a mcg/m^2 basis for maternal doses of 3 mg/kg/day and above). Brachygnathia, a skeletal malformation, was observed for rat fetuses at an oral dose equal to 6100 times the MRHD for adults (on a mcg/m^2 basis for a maternal dose of 15 mg/kg/day). In another study in rats, no teratogenic effects were seen at inhalation doses up to 500 times the MRHD for adults (on a mcg/m^2 basis for maternal doses up to 1.2 mg/kg/day). Subcapsular cysts on the liver were observed for rabbit fetuses at an oral dose equal to 49000 times the MRHD for adults (on a mcg/m^2 basis for a maternal dose of 60 mg/kg). No teratogenic effects were observed at oral doses up to 3000 times the MRHD for adults (on a mcg/m^2 basis for maternal doses up to 3.5 mg/kg).

8.2 Labor and Delivery

There are no adequate and well-controlled human studies that have investigated the effects of FORADIL AEROLIZER during labor and delivery.

Because beta-agonists may potentially interfere with uterine contractility, FORADIL AEROLIZER should be used during labor only if the potential benefit justifies the potential risk.

Formoterol fumarate has been shown to cause stillbirth and neonatal mortality at oral doses equal to or greater than 2400 times the MRHD for adults (on a mcg/m^2 basis for maternal doses of 6 mg/kg and above) in rats receiving the drug for several days at the end of pregnancy. These effects were not produced at a dose 80 times the MRHD for adults (on a mcg/m^2 basis for a maternal dose of 0.2 mg/kg).

8.3 Nursing Mothers

In reproductive studies in rats, formoterol was excreted in the milk. It is not known whether formoterol is excreted in human milk, but because many drugs are excreted in human milk, caution should be exercised if FORADIL AEROLIZER is administered to nursing women. There are no well-controlled human studies of the use of FORADIL AEROLIZER in nursing mothers.

8.4 Pediatric Use

Asthma

Available data from controlled clinical trials suggest that LABA increase the risk of asthma-related hospitalization in pediatric and adolescent patients. For pediatric and adolescent patients with asthma who require addition of a LABA to an inhaled corticosteroid, a fixed-dose combination product containing both an inhaled corticosteroid and LABA should ordinarily be used to ensure adherence with both drugs [*see Indications and Usage (1.1) and Warnings and Precautions (5.1)*].

A total of 776 children 5 years of age and older with asthma were studied in three multiple-dose controlled clinical trials. Of the 512 children who received formoterol, 508 were 5-12 years of age, and approximately one third were 5-8 years of age [*see Adverse Reactions (6.2, 6.3)*].

Exercise-Induced Bronchospasm

A total of 25 pediatric patients, 4-11 years of age, were studied in two well-controlled single-dose clinical trials.

The safety and effectiveness of FORADIL AEROLIZER in pediatric patients below 5 years of age has not been established [*see Clinical Trials (14.3), and Adverse Reaction (6.2)*].

8.5 Geriatric Use

Of the total number of patients who received FORADIL AEROLIZER in adolescent and adult chronic dosing asthma clinical trials, 318 were 65 years of age or older and 39 were 75 years of age and older. Of the 811 patients who received FORADIL AEROLIZER in two pivotal multiple-dose controlled clinical studies in patients with COPD, 395 (48.7%) were 65 years of age or older while 62 (7.6%) were 75 years of age or older. No overall differences in safety or effectiveness were observed between these subjects and younger subjects. A slightly higher frequency of chest infection was reported in the 39 asthma patients 75 years of age and older, although a causal relationship with FORADIL has not been established. Other reported clinical experience has not identified differences in responses between the elderly and younger adult patients, but greater sensitivity of some older individuals cannot be ruled out.

10 OVERDOSAGE

The expected signs and symptoms with overdosage of FORADIL AEROLIZER are those of excessive beta-adrenergic stimulation and/or occurrence or exaggeration of any of the signs and symptoms listed under ADVERSE REACTIONS, e.g., angina, hypertension or hypotension, tachycardia, with rates up to 200 beats/min., arrhythmias, nervousness, headache, tremor, seizures, muscle cramps, dry mouth, palpitation, nausea, dizziness, fatigue, malaise, hypokalemia, hyperglycemia, and insomnia. Metabolic acidosis may also occur. Cardiac arrest and even death may be associated with an overdose of FORADIL AEROLIZER.

Treatment of overdosage consists of discontinuation of FORADIL AEROLIZER together with institution of appropriate symptomatic and/or supportive therapy. The judicious use of a cardioselective beta-receptor blocker may be considered, bearing in mind that such medication can produce bronchospasm. There is insufficient evidence to determine if dialysis is beneficial for overdosage of FORADIL AEROLIZER. Cardiac monitoring is recommended in cases of overdosage.

11 DESCRIPTION

FORADIL AEROLIZER consists of a dry powder formulation of formoterol fumarate intended for oral inhalation only with the AEROLIZER Inhaler. The inhalation powder is packaged in clear hard gelatin capsules.

Each capsule contains a dry powder blend of 12 mcg of formoterol fumarate and 25 mg of lactose (which contains trace levels of milk proteins) as a carrier.

The active component of FORADIL is formoterol fumarate, a racemate. Formoterol fumarate is a selective beta$_2$-adrenergic agonist. Its chemical name is (±)-2-hydroxy-5-[(1RS)-1-hydroxy-2-[[(1RS)-2-(4-methoxyphenyl)-1-methylethyl]-amino]ethyl]formanilide fumarate dihydrate; its structural formula is:

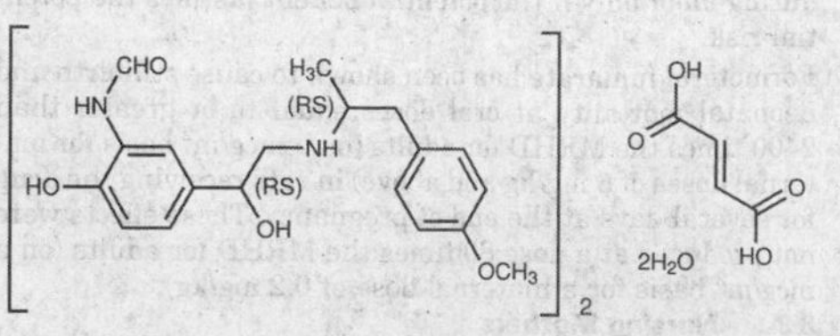

Formoterol fumarate has a molecular weight of 840.9, and its empirical formula is $(C_{19}H_{24}N_2O_4)_2 \bullet C_4H_4O_4 \bullet 2H_2O$. Formoterol fumarate is a white to yellowish crystalline powder, which is freely soluble in glacial acetic acid, soluble in methanol, sparingly soluble in ethanol and isopropanol, slightly soluble in water, and practically insoluble in acetone, ethyl acetate, and diethyl ether.

The AEROLIZER Inhaler is a plastic device used for inhaling FORADIL. The amount of drug delivered to the lung will depend on patient factors, such as inspiratory flow rate and inspiratory time. Under standardized *in vitro* testing at a fixed flow rate of 60 L/min for 2 seconds, the AEROLIZER Inhaler delivered 10 mcg of formoterol fumarate from the mouthpiece. Peak inspiratory flow rates (PIFR) achievable through the AEROLIZER Inhaler were evaluated in 33 adult and adolescent patients and 32 pediatric patients with mild-to-moderate asthma. Mean PIFR was 117.82 L/min (range 34-188 L/min) for adult and adolescent patients, and 99.66 L/min (range 43-187 L/min) for pediatric patients. Approximately ninety percent of each population studied generated a PIFR through the device exceeding 60 L/min.

To use the delivery system, a FORADIL capsule is placed in the well of the AEROLIZER Inhaler, and the capsule is pierced by pressing and releasing the buttons on the side of the device. The formoterol fumarate formulation is dispersed into the air stream when the patient inhales rapidly and deeply through the mouthpiece.

12 CLINICAL PHARMACOLOGY

12.1 Mechanism of Action

Formoterol fumarate is a long-acting beta$_2$-adrenergic receptor agonist (beta$_2$-agonist). Inhaled formoterol fumarate acts locally in the lung as a bronchodilator. *In vitro* studies have shown that formoterol has more than 200-fold greater agonist activity at beta$_2$-receptors than at beta$_1$-receptors. Although beta^2-receptors are the predominant adrenergic receptors in bronchial smooth muscle and beta$_1$-receptors are the predominant receptors in the heart, there are also beta$_2$-receptors in the human heart comprising 10%-50% of the total beta-adrenergic receptors. The precise function of these receptors has not been established, but they raise the possibility that even highly selective beta$_2$-agonists may have cardiac effects.

The pharmacologic effects of beta$_2$-adrenoceptor agonist drugs, including formoterol, are at least in part attributable to stimulation of intracellular adenyl cyclase, the enzyme that catalyzes the conversion of adenosine triphosphate (ATP) to cyclic-3′, 5′-adenosine monophosphate (cyclic AMP). Increased cyclic AMP levels cause relaxation of bronchial smooth muscle and inhibition of release of mediators of immediate hypersensitivity from cells, especially from mast cells.

In vitro tests show that formoterol is an inhibitor of the release of mast cell mediators, such as histamine and leukotrienes, from the human lung. Formoterol also inhibits histamine-induced plasma albumin extravasation in anesthetized guinea pigs and inhibits allergen-induced eosinophil influx in dogs with airway hyper-responsiveness. The relevance of these *in vitro* and animal findings to humans is unknown.

12.2 Pharmacodynamics

Systemic Safety and Pharmacokinetic/Pharmacodynamic Relationships

The major adverse effects of inhaled beta$_2$-agonists occur as a result of excessive activation of the systemic beta-adrenergic receptors. The most common adverse effects in adults and adolescents include skeletal muscle tremor and cramps, insomnia, tachycardia, decreases in plasma potassium, and increases in plasma glucose.

Pharmacokinetic/pharmacodynamic (PK/PD) relationships between heart rate, ECG parameters, and serum potassium levels and the urinary excretion of formoterol were evaluated in 10 healthy male volunteers (25 to 45 years of age) following inhalation of single doses containing 12, 24, 48, or 96 mcg of formoterol fumarate. There was a linear relationship between urinary formoterol excretion and decreases in serum potassium, increases in plasma glucose, and increases in heart rate.

In a second study, PK/PD relationships between plasma formoterol levels and pulse rate, ECG parameters, and plasma potassium levels were evaluated in 12 healthy volunteers following inhalation of a single 120 mcg dose of formoterol fumarate (10 times the recommended clinical dose). Reductions of plasma potassium concentration were observed in all subjects. Maximum reductions from baseline ranged from 0.55 to 1.52 mmol/L with a median maximum reduction of 1.01 mmol/L. The formoterol plasma concentration was highly correlated with the reduction in plasma potassium concentration. Generally, the maximum effect on plasma potassium was noted 1 to 3 hours after peak formoterol plasma concentrations were achieved. A mean maximum increase of pulse rate of 26 bpm was observed 6 hours post dose. The maximum increase of mean corrected QT interval (QTc) was 25 msec when calculated using Bazett's correction and was 8 msec when calculated using Fridericia's correction. The QTc returned to baseline within 12-24 hours post-dose. Formoterol plasma concentrations were weakly correlated with pulse rate and increase of QTc duration. The effects on plasma potassium, pulse rate, and QTc interval are known pharmacological effects of this class of study drug and were not unexpected at the very high formoterol dose (120 mcg single dose, 10 times the recommended single dose) tested in this study. These effects were well-tolerated by the healthy volunteers.

The electrocardiographic and cardiovascular effects of FORADIL AEROLIZER were compared with those of albuterol and placebo in two pivotal 12-week double-blind studies of patients with asthma. A subset of patients underwent continuous electrocardiographic monitoring during three 24-hour periods. No important differences in ventricular or supraventricular ectopy between treatment groups were observed. In these two studies, the total number of patients with asthma exposed to any dose of FORADIL AEROLIZER who had continuous electrocardiographic monitoring was about 200.

Continuous electrocardiographic monitoring was performed in an 8-week, randomized, double-blind, and placebo controlled trial in 204 COPD patients treated with FORADIL AEROLIZER 12 mcg twice daily or placebo. Holter monitoring was used to evaluate predefined proarrhythmic events. Non-sustained ventricular tachycardia occurred in 2 (2.2%) of FORADIL AEROLIZER treated patients compared to none in the placebo group. An increase in ventricular premature beats (VPB) occurred in 3 (3.3 %) of FORADIL AEROLIZER treated patients compared to 2 (1.9%) in the placebo group. There were no events of sustained ventricular tachycardia, ventricular flutter or fibrillation, or symptomatic runs of VPB. One patient in the FORADIL AEROLIZER group had a serious adverse event of atrial flutter.

The electrocardiographic effects of FORADIL AEROLIZER were evaluated versus placebo in a 12-month pivotal double-blind study of patients with COPD. An analysis of ECG intervals was performed for patients who participated at study sites in the United States, including 46 patients treated with FORADIL AEROLIZER 12 mcg twice daily, and 50 patients treated with FORADIL AEROLIZER 24 mcg twice daily. ECGs were performed predose, and at 5-15 minutes and 2 hours post-dose at study baseline and after 3, 6, and 12 months of treatment. The results showed that there was no clinically meaningful acute or chronic effect on ECG intervals, including QTc, resulting from treatment with FORADIL AEROLIZER.

Tachyphylaxis/Tolerance

In a clinical study in 19 adult patients with mild asthma, the bronchoprotective effect of formoterol, as assessed by methacholine challenge, was studied following an initial dose of 24 mcg (twice the recommended dose) and after 2 weeks of 24 mcg twice daily. Tolerance to the bronchoprotective effects of formoterol was observed as evidenced by a diminished bronchoprotective effect on FEV$_1$ after 2 weeks of dosing, with loss of protection at the end of the 12 hour dosing period.

Rebound bronchial hyper-responsiveness after cessation of chronic formoterol therapy has not been observed.

In three large clinical trials in patients with asthma, while efficacy of formoterol versus placebo was maintained, a slightly reduced bronchodilatory response (as measured by 12-hour FEV$_1$ AUC) was observed within the formoterol arms over time, particularly with the 24 mcg twice daily dose (twice the daily recommended dose). A similarly reduced FEV$_1$ AUC over time was also noted in the albuterol treatment arms (180 mcg four times daily by metered-dose inhaler).

12.3 Pharmacokinetics

Information on the pharmacokinetics of formoterol in plasma has been obtained in healthy subjects by oral inhalation of doses higher than the recommended range and in Chronic Obstructive Pulmonary Disease (COPD) patients after oral inhalation of doses at and above the therapeutic dose. Urinary excretion of unchanged formoterol was used as an indirect measure of systemic exposure. Plasma drug disposition data parallel urinary excretion, and the elimination half-lives calculated for urine and plasma are similar.

Absorption

Following inhalation of a single 120 mcg dose of formoterol fumarate by 12 healthy subjects, formoterol was rapidly absorbed into plasma, reaching a maximum drug concentration of 92 pg/mL within 5 minutes of dosing. In COPD patients treated for 12 weeks with formoterol fumarate 12 or 24 mcg twice daily, the mean plasma concentrations of formoterol obtained at 10 min, 2 h, and 6 h post inhalation ranged between 4.0 and 8.8 pg/mL and 8.0 and 17.3 pg/mL, respectively.

Following inhalation of 12 to 96 mcg of formoterol fumarate by 10 healthy males, urinary excretion of both (R,R)- and (S,S)-enantiomers of formoterol increased proportionally to the dose. Thus, absorption of formoterol following inhalation appeared linear over the dose range studied.

In a study in patients with asthma, when formoterol 12 or 24 mcg twice daily was given by oral inhalation for 4 weeks or 12 weeks, the accumulation index, based on the urinary excretion of unchanged formoterol ranged from 1.63 to 2.08 in comparison with the first dose. For COPD patients, when formoterol 12 or 24 mcg twice daily was given by oral inhalation for 12 weeks, the accumulation index, based on the urinary excretion of unchanged formoterol was 1.19 - 1.38. This suggests some accumulation of formoterol in plasma with multiple dosing. The excreted amounts of formoterol at steady-state were close to those predicted based on single-dose kinetics. As with many drug products for oral inhalation, it is likely that the majority of the inhaled formoterol fumarate delivered is swallowed and then absorbed from the gastrointestinal tract.

Distribution
The binding of formoterol to human plasma proteins *in vitro* was 61%-64% at concentrations from 0.1 to 100 ng/mL. Binding to human serum albumin *in vitro* was 31%-38% over a range of 5 to 500 ng/mL. The concentrations of formoterol used to assess the plasma protein binding were higher than those achieved in plasma following inhalation of a single 120 mcg dose.

Metabolism
Formoterol is metabolized primarily by direct glucuronidation at either the phenolic or aliphatic hydroxyl group and O demethylation followed by glucuronide conjugation at either phenolic hydroxyl groups. Minor pathways involve sulfate conjugation of formoterol and deformylation followed by sulfate conjugation. The most prominent pathway involves direct conjugation at the phenolic hydroxyl group. The second major pathway involves O-demethylation followed by conjugation at the phenolic 2′-hydroxyl group. Four cytochrome P450 isozymes (CYP2D6, CYP2C19, CYP2C9, and CYP2A6) are involved in the O-demethylation of formoterol. Formoterol did not inhibit CYP450 enzymes at therapeutically relevant concentrations. Some patients may be deficient in CYP2D6 or 2C19 or both. Whether a deficiency in one or both of these isozymes results in elevated systemic exposure to formoterol or systemic adverse effects has not been adequately explored.

Excretion
Following oral administration of 80 mcg of radiolabeled formoterol fumarate to 2 healthy subjects, 59%-62% of the radioactivity was eliminated in the urine and 32%-34% in the feces over a period of 104 hours. Renal clearance of formoterol from blood in these subjects was about 150 mL/min. Following inhalation of a 12 mcg or 24 mcg dose by 16 patients with asthma, about 10% and 15%-18% of the total dose was excreted in the urine as unchanged formoterol and direct conjugates of formoterol, respectively. Following inhalation of 12 mcg or 24 mcg dose by 18 patients with COPD the corresponding values were 7% and 6-9% of the dose, respectively.

Based on plasma concentrations measured following inhalation of a single 120 mcg dose by 12 healthy subjects, the mean terminal elimination half-life was determined to be 10 hours. From urinary excretion rates measured in these subjects, the mean terminal elimination half-lives for the (R,R)- and (S,S)-enantiomers were determined to be 13.9 and 12.3 hours, respectively. The (R,R)- and (S,S)-enantiomers represented about 40% and 60% of unchanged drug excreted in the urine, respectively, following single inhaled doses between 12 and 120 mcg in healthy volunteers and single and repeated doses of 12 and 24 mcg in patients with asthma. Thus, the relative proportion of the two enantiomers remained constant over the dose range studied and there was no evidence of relative accumulation of one enantiomer over the other after repeated dosing.

Special Populations
Gender: After correction for body weight, formoterol pharmacokinetics did not differ significantly between males and females.

Geriatric and Pediatric: The pharmacokinetics of formoterol have not been studied in the elderly population, and limited data are available in pediatric patients.

In a study of children with asthma who were 5 to 12 years of age, when formoterol fumarate 12 or 24 mcg was given twice daily by oral inhalation for 12 weeks, the accumulation index ranged from 1.18 to 1.84 based on urinary excretion of unchanged formoterol. Hence, the accumulation in children did not exceed that in adults, where the accumulation index ranged from 1.63 to 2.08 (see above). Approximately 6% and 6.5% to 9% of the dose was recovered in the urine of the children as unchanged and conjugated formoterol, respectively.

Hepatic/Renal Impairment
The pharmacokinetics of formoterol have not been studied in subjects with hepatic or renal impairment.

13 NONCLINICAL TOXICOLOGY

13.1 Carcinogenesis, Mutagenesis, Impairment of Fertility

The carcinogenic potential of formoterol fumarate has been evaluated in 2-year drinking water and dietary studies in both rats and mice. In rats, the incidence of ovarian leiomyomas was increased at doses of 15 mg/kg and above in the drinking water study and at 20 mg/kg in the dietary study, but not at dietary doses up to 5 mg/kg (AUC exposure approximately 450 times human exposure at the maximum recommended human dose [MRHD]). In the dietary study, the incidence of benign ovarian theca-cell tumors was increased at doses of 0.5 mg/kg and above (AUC exposure at the low dose of 0.5 mg/kg was approximately 45 times human exposure at the MRHD). This finding was not observed in the drinking water study, nor was it seen in mice (see below).

In mice, the incidence of adrenal subcapsular adenomas and carcinomas was increased in males at doses of 69 mg/kg and above in the drinking water study, but not at doses up to 50 mg/kg (AUC exposure approximately 590 times human exposure at the MRHD) in the dietary study. The incidence of hepatocarcinomas was increased in the dietary study at doses of 20 and 50 mg/kg in females and 50 mg/kg in males, but not at doses up to 5 mg/kg in either males or females (AUC exposure approximately 60 times human exposure at the MRHD). Also in the dietary study, the incidence of uterine leiomyomas and leiomyosarcomas was increased at doses of 2 mg/kg and above (AUC exposure at the low dose of 2 mg/kg was approximately 25 times human exposure at the MRHD). Increases in leiomyomas of the rodent female genital tract have been similarly demonstrated with other beta-agonist drugs.

Formoterol fumarate was not mutagenic or clastogenic in the following tests: mutagenicity tests in bacterial and mammalian cells, chromosomal analyses in mammalian cells, unscheduled DNA synthesis repair tests in rat hepatocytes and human fibroblasts, transformation assay in mammalian fibroblasts and micronucleus tests in mice and rats.

Reproduction studies in rats revealed no impairment of fertility at oral doses up to 3 mg/kg (approximately 1200 times the MRHD on a mcg/m^2 basis).

13.2 Animal Toxicology and/or Pharmacology

Studies in laboratory animals (minipigs, rodents, and dogs) have demonstrated the occurrence of cardiac arrhythmias and sudden death (with histologic evidence of myocardial necrosis) when beta-agonists and methylxanthines are administered concurrently. The clinical significance of these findings is unknown.

14 CLINICAL STUDIES

14.1 Asthma

Adults and Adolescents 12 Years of Age and Older
In a placebo-controlled, single-dose clinical trial, the onset of bronchodilation (defined as a 15% or greater increase from baseline in FEV$_1$) was similar for FORADIL AEROLIZER and albuterol 180 mcg by metered-dose inhaler.

In single-dose and multiple-dose clinical trials, the maximum improvement in FEV$_1$ for FORADIL AEROLIZER 12 mcg generally occurred within 1 to 3 hours, and an increase in FEV$_1$ above baseline was observed for 12 hours in most patients.

FORADIL AEROLIZER 12 mcg twice daily was compared to FORADIL AEROLIZER 24 mcg twice daily, albuterol 180 mcg four times daily by metered-dose inhaler, and placebo in a total of 1095 adult and adolescent patients 12 years of age and above with mild-to-moderate asthma (defined as FEV$_1$ 40%-80% of the patient's predicted normal value) who participated in two pivotal, 12-week, multi-center, randomized, double-blind, parallel group trials.

The results of both clinical trials showed that FORADIL AEROLIZER 12 mcg twice daily resulted in significantly greater post-dose bronchodilation (as measured by serial FEV$_1$ for 12 hours post-dose) throughout the 12-week treatment period. There was no significant difference in post-dose bronchodilation between FORADIL AEROLIZER 12 mcg twice daily and FORADIL AEROLIZER 24 mcg twice daily, but serious asthma exacerbations occurred more commonly in the higher dose group [*see Warnings and Precautions (5.1) and Adverse Reactions (6.2)*]. Mean FEV$_1$ measurements from both studies are shown below for the first and last treatment days (see Figures 1 and 2).

[See figures 1a and 1b at top of next column]
[See figures 2a and 2b at top of next column]

Compared with placebo and albuterol, patients treated with FORADIL AEROLIZER 12 mcg demonstrated improvement in many secondary efficacy endpoints, including improved combined and nocturnal asthma symptom scores, fewer nighttime awakenings, fewer nights in which patients used rescue medication, and higher morning and evening peak flow rates. FORADIL AEROLIZER 24 mcg twice daily did not provide any additional improvements in these secondary endpoints compared to FORADIL AEROLIZER 12 mcg twice daily.

A 16-week, randomized, multi-center, double-blind, parallel-group trial enrolled 1568 patients 12 years of age and older with mild-to-moderate asthma (defined as FEV$_1$ ≥40% of the patient's predicted normal value) in three treatment groups: FORADIL AEROLIZER 12 mcg twice daily, FORADIL AEROLIZER 24 mcg twice daily, and placebo. The trial's primary endpoint was the incidence of serious asthma-related adverse events. Serious asthma exacerbations occurred in 3 (0.6%) patients who received FORADIL AEROLIZER 12 mcg twice daily, 2 (0.4%) patients who received FORADIL AEROLIZER 24 mcg twice daily, and 1 (0.2%) patient who received placebo. The size of this trial was not adequate to precisely quantify the differences in serious asthma exacerbation rates between treatment groups. All serious asthma exacerbations resulted in hospitalizations. While there were no deaths in the trial, the duration and size of this trial were not adequate to quantify the rate of asthma-related death. See [*Warnings and Precautions (5.1)*] for information about a trial that compared another long-acting beta$_2$-adrenergic agonist to placebo.

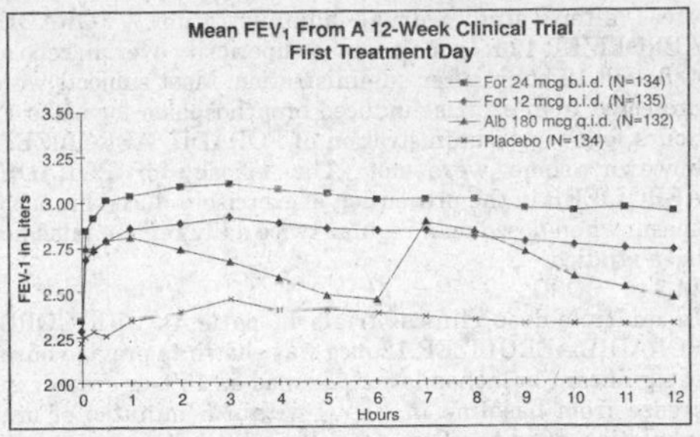

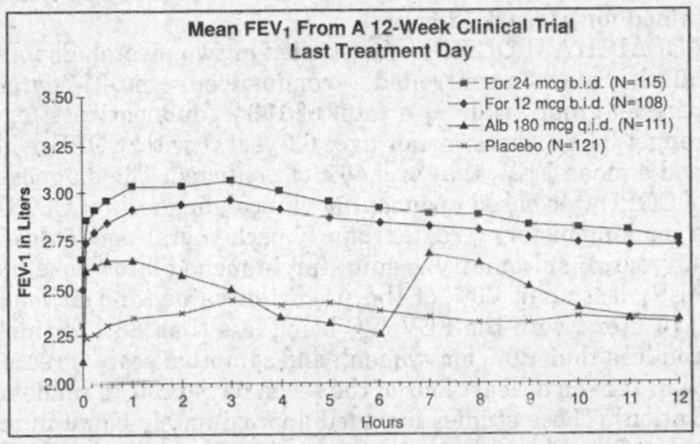

Figures 1a and 1b: Mean FEV$_1$ from Clinical Trial A

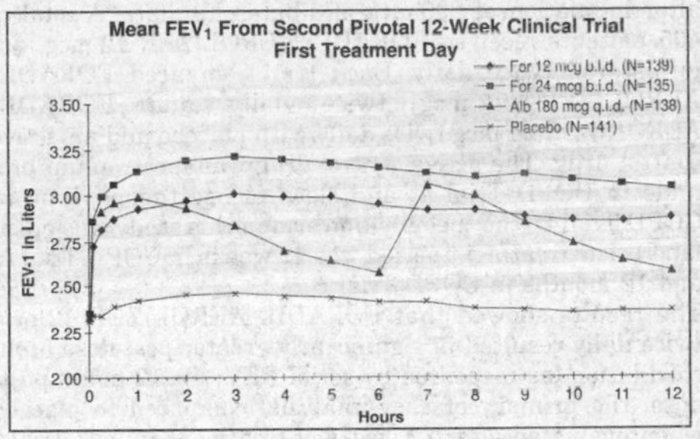

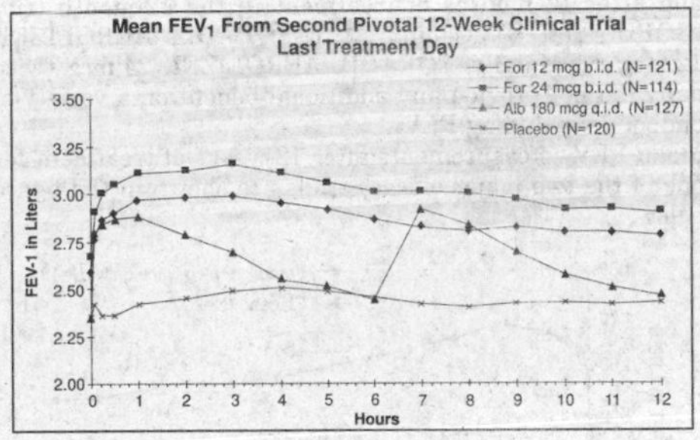

Figures 2a and 2b: Mean FEV$_1$ from Clinical Trial B

Children 5-11 Years of Age
A 12-month, multi-center, randomized, double-blind, parallel-group, trial compared FORADIL AEROLIZER 12 mcg twice daily and FORADIL AEROLIZER 24 mcg twice daily to placebo in a total of 518 children with asthma (ages 5-12 years) who required daily bronchodilators and anti-inflammatory treatment. Efficacy was evaluated on the first day of treatment, at Week 12, and at the end of treatment.

FORADIL AEROLIZER 12 mcg twice daily demonstrated a greater 12-hour FEV$_1$ AUC compared to placebo on the first day of treatment, after twelve weeks of treatment, and after one year of treatment. FORADIL AEROLIZER 24 mcg twice daily did not result in any additional improvement in 12-hour FEV$_1$ AUC compared to FORADIL AEROLIZER 12 mcg twice daily.

14.2 Exercise-Induced Bronchospasm

The effect of FORADIL AEROLIZER on exercise-induced bronchospasm (defined as >20% fall in FEV$_1$) was examined in four randomized, single-dose, double-blind, crossover trials in a total of 77 patients 4 to 41 years of age with exercise-induced bronchospasm. Exercise challenge testing was conducted 15 minutes, and 4, 8, and 12 hours following administration of a single dose of study drug (FORADIL AEROLIZER 12 mcg, albuterol 180 mcg by metered-dose inhaler, or placebo) on separate test days. FORADIL AEROLIZER 12 mcg and albuterol 180 mcg were each superior to placebo for FEV$_1$ measurements obtained 15 minutes after study drug administration. FORADIL AEROLIZER 12 mcg maintained superiority over placebo at 4, 8, and 12 hours after administration. Most subjects were protected from exercise-induced bronchospasm for up to 12 hours following administration of FORADIL AEROLIZER, however, some were not. The efficacy of FORADIL AEROLIZER in the prevention of exercise-induced bronchospasm when dosed on a regular twice daily regimen has not been studied.

14.3 COPD

In multiple-dose clinical trials in patients with COPD, FORADIL AEROLIZER 12 mcg was shown to provide onset of significant bronchodilation (defined as 15% or greater increase from baseline in FEV_1) within 5 minutes of oral inhalation after the first dose. Bronchodilation was maintained for at least 12 hours.

FORADIL AEROLIZER was studied in two pivotal, double-blind, placebo-controlled, randomized, multi-center, parallel-group trials in a total of 1634 adult patients (age range: 34-88 years; mean age: 63 years) with COPD who had a mean FEV_1 that was 46% of predicted. The diagnosis of COPD was based upon a prior clinical diagnosis of COPD, a smoking history (greater than 10 pack-years), age (at least 40 years), spirometry results (prebronchodilator baseline FEV_1 less than 70% of the predicted value, and at least 0.75 liters, with the FEV_1/VC being less than 88% for men and less than 89% for women), and symptom score (greater than zero on at least four of the seven days prior to randomization). These studies included approximately equal numbers of patients with and without baseline bronchodilator reversibility, defined as a 15% or greater increase FEV_1 after inhalation of 200 mcg of albuterol sulfate. A total of 405 patients received FORADIL AEROLIZER 12 mcg, administered twice daily. Each trial compared FORADIL AEROLIZER 12 mcg twice daily and FORADIL AEROLIZER 24 mcg twice daily with placebo and an active control drug. The active control drug was ipratropium bromide in COPD Trial A, and slow-release theophylline in COPD Trial B (the theophylline arm in this study was open-label). The treatment period was 12 weeks in COPD Trial A, and 12 months in COPD Trial B.

The results showed that FORADIL AEROLIZER 12 mcg twice daily resulted in significantly greater post-dose bronchodilation (as measured by serial FEV_1 for 12 hours post-dose; the primary efficacy analysis) compared to placebo when evaluated after 12 weeks of treatment in both trials, and after 12 months of treatment in the 12-month trial (COPD Trial B). Compared to FORADIL AEROLIZER 12 mcg twice daily, FORADIL AEROLIZER 24 mcg twice daily did not provide any additional benefit on a variety of endpoints including FEV_1.

Mean FEV_1 measurements after 12 weeks of treatment for one of the two major efficacy trials are shown in the figure below.

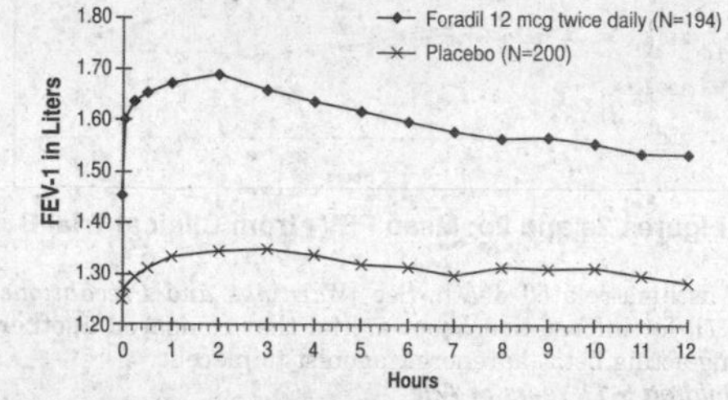

Figure 3 Mean FEV_1 After 12 Weeks of Treatment from COPD Trial A

FORADIL AEROLIZER 12 mcg twice daily was statistically superior to placebo at all post-dose timepoints tested (from 5 minutes to 12 hours post-dose) throughout the 12-week (COPD Trial A) and 12-month (COPD Trial B) treatment periods.

In both pivotal trials compared with placebo, patients treated with FORADIL AEROLIZER 12 mcg demonstrated improved morning premedication peak expiratory flow rates and took fewer puffs of rescue albuterol.

16 HOW SUPPLIED/STORAGE AND HANDLING

16.1 How Supplied

FORADIL AEROLIZER contains: aluminum blister-packaged 12-mcg FORADIL (formoterol fumarate) clear gelatin capsules with "CG" printed on one end and "FXF" printed on the opposite end; one AEROLIZER Inhaler; and Medication Guide.

Unit Dose (blister pack)	
Box of 12 (strips of 6)	NDC 0085-1402-01
Unit Dose (blister pack)	
Box of 60 (strips of 6)	NDC 0085-1401-01

16.2 Storage and Handling

Prior to dispensing: Store in a refrigerator, 2°C to 8°C (36°F to 46°F)

After dispensing to patient: Store at 20°C to 25°C (68°F to 77°F) [*see USP Controlled Room Temperature*]. Protect from heat and moisture. **Capsules should always be stored in the blister and only removed from the blister immediately before use.**

FORADIL capsules should be used with the AEROLIZER Inhaler only. The AEROLIZER Inhaler should not be used with any other capsules.

Always discard the FORADIL capsules and AEROLIZER Inhaler by the "Use by" date and always use the new AEROLIZER Inhaler provided with each new prescription. Keep out of the reach of children.

17 PATIENT COUNSELING INFORMATION

See FDA-approved **patient labeling** (Medication Guide and Instructions for Use)

Patients should be instructed to read the accompanying Medication Guide with each new prescription and refill. The complete text of the Medication Guide is reprinted at the end of this document. Patients should be given the following information:

17.1 Asthma-Related Death

Patients should be informed that long-acting $beta_2$-adrenergic agonists (LABA), including formoterol, the active ingredient in FORADIL AEROLIZER, increase the risk of asthma-related death and may increase the risk of asthma-related hospitalizations in pediatric and adolescent patients. Currently available data are inadequate to determine whether concurrent use of inhaled corticosteroids or other long-term asthma control drugs mitigates the increased risk of asthma- related death from LABA.

Patients should be informed that FORADIL AEROLIZER should not be the only therapy for the treatment of asthma and must only be used as additional therapy when a long-term asthma control medication (e.g., inhaled corticosteroids) do not adequately control asthma symptoms. Patients should be informed that when FORADIL AEROLIZER is added to their treatment regimen they must continue to use their long-term asthma control medication.

17.2 Not for Acute Symptoms

FORADIL AEROLIZER is not indicated to relieve acute asthma symptoms or exacerbations of COPD and extra doses should not be used for that purpose. Acute symptoms should be treated with an inhaled, short-acting, $beta_2$-agonist (the health-care provider should prescribe the patient with such medication and instruct the patient in how it should be used). Patients should be instructed to seek medical attention if their symptoms worsen, if FORADIL AEROLIZER treatment becomes less effective, or if they need more inhalations of a short-acting $beta_2$-agonist than usual. Patients should not inhale more than the contents of one capsule at any one time. The daily dosage of FORADIL AEROLIZER should not exceed one capsule twice daily (24 mcg total daily dose).

17.3 Required Concomitant Therapy

Patients with asthma should be advised that FORADIL AEROLIZER must always be used with a long-term asthma control medication such as an inhaled corticosteroid.

FORADIL AEROLIZER should not be used as a substitute for oral or inhaled corticosteroids. The dosage of these medications should not be changed and they should not be stopped without consulting the physician, even if the patient feels better after initiating treatment with FORADIL AEROLIZER.

17.4 Common Adverse Reactions

Patients should be informed that treatment with $beta_2$-agonists may lead to adverse events which include palpitations, chest pain, rapid heart rate, tremor or nervousness.

17.5 Appropriate Dosing

The active ingredient of FORADIL (formoterol fumarate) is a long-acting, bronchodilator used for the treatment of asthma, including nocturnal asthma, for the prevention of exercise-induced bronchospasm, and for the maintenance treatment of bronchoconstriction in patients with Chronic Obstructive Pulmonary Disease including chronic bronchitis and emphysema. FORADIL AEROLIZER provides bronchodilation for up to 12 hours. Patients should be advised not to increase the dose or frequency of FORADIL AEROLIZER without consulting the prescribing physician. Patients should be warned not to stop or reduce concomitant asthma therapy without medical advice.

For asthma and COPD, the usual dose is one FORADIL capsule inhaled through the AEROLIZER inhaler 2 times each day (morning and evening). The 2 doses should be about 12 hours apart. Patients should be advised not to use other LABA when using FORADIL AEROLIZER.

When FORADIL AEROLIZER is used for the prevention of EIB, the contents of one capsule should be taken at least 15 minutes prior to exercise. Additional doses of FORADIL AEROLIZER should not be used for 12 hours. Prevention of EIB has not been studied in patients who are receiving chronic FORADIL AEROLIZER administration twice daily and these patients should not use additional FORADIL AEROLIZER for prevention of EIB.

17.6 Instructions for Administration

It is important for patients to understand how to correctly administer FORADIL capsules using the AEROLIZER Inhaler and how FORADIL should be used in relation to other asthma medications they are taking (see the accompanying Medication Guide).

Patients should be instructed that FORADIL capsules should only be administered via the AEROLIZER device and the AEROLIZER device should not be used for administering other medications. The contents of FORADIL capsules are for oral inhalation only and must not be swallowed.

Patients should be informed never to use FORADIL AEROLIZER with a spacer and never to exhale into the device.

Patients should avoid exposing the FORADIL capsules to moisture and should handle the capsules with dry hands. The AEROLIZER Inhaler should never be washed and should be kept dry. The patient should always use the new AEROLIZER Inhaler that comes with each refill.

Patients should be told that in rare cases, the gelatin capsule might break into small pieces. These pieces should be retained by the screen built into the AEROLIZER Inhaler. However, it remains possible that rarely, tiny pieces of gelatin might reach the mouth or throat after inhalation. The capsule is less likely to shatter when pierced if: storage conditions are strictly followed, capsules are removed from the blister immediately before use, and the capsules are only pierced once.

Women should be advised to contact their physician if they become pregnant or if they are nursing.

Manufactured for: Merck Sharp & Dohme Corp., a subsidiary of
MERCK & CO., INC., Whitehouse Station, NJ 08889, USA
Manufactured by:
Novartis Pharma AG, Basle, Switzerland

T2012-217
November 2012

MEDICATION GUIDE

Foradil® [FOR-a-dil] **Aerolizer®**

(formoterol fumarate inhalation powder)

> **Important: Do not swallow FORADIL capsules. FORADIL capsules are used only with the Aerolizer inhaler that comes with FORADIL AEROLIZER. Never place a capsule in the mouthpiece of the AEROLIZER Inhaler.**

Read the Medication Guide that comes with FORADIL AEROLIZER before you start using it and each time you get a refill. There may be new information. This Medication Guide does not take the place of talking to your health care provider about your medical condition or treatment.

What is the most important information I should know about FORADIL AEROLIZER?

FORADIL AEROLIZER can cause serious side effects, including:

1. People with asthma who take long-acting $beta_2$-adrenergic agonist (LABA) medicines, such as formoterol fumarate inhalation powder (FORADIL AEROLIZER), have an increased risk of death from asthma problems.

- Call your healthcare provider if breathing problems worsen over time while using FORADIL AEROLIZER. You may need a different treatment.
- Get emergency medical care if:
  - breathing problems worsen quickly, and
  - you use your rescue inhaler medicine, but it does not relieve your breathing problems.

2. Do not use FORADIL AEROLIZER as your only asthma medicine. FORADIL AEROLIZER must only be used with a long-term asthma control medicine, such as an inhaled corticosteroid.

3. When your asthma is well controlled, your healthcare provider may tell you to stop taking FORADIL AEROLIZER. Your healthcare provider will decide if you can stop FORADIL AEROLIZER without loss of asthma control. You will continue taking your long-term asthma control medicine, such as an inhaled corticosteroid.

4. Children and adolescents who take LABA medicines may have an increased risk of being hospitalized for asthma problems.

What is FORADIL AEROLIZER?

FORADIL AEROLIZER is a long-acting $beta_2$-agonist (LABA). LABA medicines help the muscles around the airways in your lungs stay relaxed to prevent asthma symptoms, such as wheezing and shortness of breath. These symptoms can happen when the muscles around the airways tighten. This makes it hard to breathe. In severe cases, wheezing can stop your breathing and cause death if not treated right away.

FORADIL AEROLIZER is used for asthma, exercise-induced bronchospasm (EIB) and chronic obstructive pulmonary disease (COPD) as follows:

Asthma

FORADIL AEROLIZER is used with a long-term asthma control medicine, such as an inhaled corticosteroid, in adults and children ages 5 and older:
- to control symptoms of asthma, and
- to prevent symptoms such as wheezing

LABA medicines, such as FORADIL AEROLIZER, increase the risk of death from asthma problems. FORADIL AEROLIZER is not for adults and children with asthma who are well controlled with long-term asthma control medicine, such as low to medium dose of an inhaled corticosteroid medicine.

Exercise-Induced Bronchospasm (EIB)

FORADIL AEROLIZER is used to prevent wheezing caused by exercise in adults and children 5 years of age and older.
- If you have EIB only, your healthcare provider may prescribe only FORADIL AEROLIZER for your condition
- If you have EIB and asthma, your healthcare provider should also prescribe a long-term asthma control medicine, such as an inhaled corticosteroid

Chronic Obstructive Pulmonary Disease (COPD)

FORADIL AEROLIZER is used long-term, 2 times each day (morning and evening), to control symptoms of COPD and prevent wheezing in adults with COPD.

It is not known if FORADIL AEROLIZER is safe and effective in children under 5 years of age.

Who should not use FORADIL AEROLIZER?

Do not take FORADIL AEROLIZER:
- to treat your asthma without a long-term asthma control medicine, such as an inhaled corticosteroid
- to treat sudden symptoms of asthma or COPD
- if you are allergic to formoterol fumarate or any of the ingredients in FORADIL AEROLIZER. Ask your healthcare provider if you are not sure. See the end of this Medication Guide for a complete list of ingredients in FORADIL AEROLIZER.

What should I tell my healthcare provider before using FORADIL AEROLIZER?

Tell your healthcare provider about all of your health conditions, including if you:
- have heart problems
- have high blood pressure
- have seizures
- have thyroid problems
- have diabetes
- have an aneurysm (swelling of an artery)
- have a pheochromocytoma (a tumor of the adrenal gland that can affect your blood pressure)
- are scheduled to have surgery
- are pregnant or planning to become pregnant. It is not known if FORADIL AEROLIZER may harm your unborn baby.
- are breastfeeding. It is not known if FORADIL AEROLIZER passes into your milk and if it can harm your baby.
- are allergic to FORADIL AEROLIZER, any other medicines, or food products.

FORADIL AEROLIZER contains lactose (milk sugar) and a small amount of milk proteins. It is possible that allergic reactions may happen in patients who have a severe milk protein allergy.

Tell your healthcare provider about all the medicines you take including prescription and non-prescription medicines, vitamins, and herbal supplements. FORADIL AEROLIZER and certain other medicines may interact with each other. This may cause serious side effects.

Know the medicines you take. Keep a list and show it to your healthcare provider and pharmacist each time you get a new medicine.

How do I use FORADIL capsules with the Aerolizer inhaler?

See the step-by-step instructions for using FORADIL Capsules with the Aerolizer inhaler at the end of this Medication Guide.
- Do not use FORADIL unless your healthcare provider has taught you and you understand everything. Ask your healthcare provider or pharmacist if you have any questions.
- Children should use FORADIL AEROLIZER with an adult's help, as instructed by the child's healthcare provider.
- Use FORADIL AEROLIZER exactly as prescribed. **Do not use FORADIL AEROLIZER more often than prescribed.**
- For asthma and COPD, the usual dose is 1 FORADIL capsule inhaled through the AEROLIZER inhaler 2 times each day (morning and evening). The 2 doses should be about 12 hours apart.
- For preventing exercise-induced bronchospasm, the usual dose is 1 FORADIL capsule inhaled through the AEROLIZER inhaler at least 15 minutes before exercise, as needed. Do not use FORADIL AEROLIZER more often than every 12 hours. Do not use extra FORADIL AEROLIZER before exercise if you already use it 2 times each day.
- If you miss a dose of FORADIL AEROLIZER, just skip that dose. Take your next dose at your usual time. Never take 2 doses at one time.
- Do not use a spacer device with FORADIL AEROLIZER.
- Do not breathe into FORADIL AEROLIZER.
- While you are using FORADIL AEROLIZER 2 times each day, do not use other medicines that contain a long-acting $beta_2$-agonist (LABA) for any reason. Ask your healthcare provider or pharmacist for a list of these medicines.
- Do not stop using FORADIL AEROLIZER or any of your asthma medicines unless told to do so by your healthcare provider because your symptoms might get worse. Your healthcare provider will change your medicines as needed.
- FORADIL AEROLIZER does not relieve sudden symptoms. Always have a rescue inhaler medicine with you to treat sudden symptoms. If you do not have an inhaled, short-acting bronchodilator, contact your healthcare provider to have one prescribed for you.

Call your healthcare provider or get medical care right away if:
- your breathing problems worsen with FORADIL AEROLIZER
- you need to use your rescue inhaler medicine more often than usual
- your rescue inhaler medicine does not work as well for you at relieving symptoms
- you need to use 4 or more inhalations of your rescue inhaler medicine for 2 or more days in a row
- you use 1 whole canister of your rescue inhaler medicine in 8 weeks time
- your peak flow meter results decrease. Your healthcare provider will tell you the numbers that are right for you.
- you have asthma and your symptoms do not improve after using FORADIL AEROLIZER regularly for 1 week.

What are the possible side effects with FORADIL AEROLIZER?

FORADIL AEROLIZER may cause serious side effects, including:

See "What is the most important information I should know about FORADIL AEROLIZER?"
- **Sudden breathing problems immediately after inhaling your medicine** (wheezing or coughing and difficulty breathing)
- **Fast or irregular heart beat** (palpitations)
- **Serious allergic reactions including rash, hives, swelling of the face, mouth, and tongue, and breathing problems.** Call your healthcare provider or get emergency medical care if you get any symptoms of a serious allergic reaction.
- **Low blood potassium** (which may cause symptoms of muscle spasm, muscle weakness or abnormal heart rhythm)
- **Increases in blood sugar levels** (hyperglycemia)
- Using too much of a LABA medicine may cause:
  - chest pain
  - increased blood pressure
  - a fast or irregular heart beat
  - headache
  - tremor
  - nervousness
  - dizziness
  - weakness
  - trouble sleeping
  - electrocardiogram (ECG) changes
  - seizures

Common side effects with FORADIL AEROLIZER include:

Asthma in Adults and Adolescents:
- headache
- tremor
- chest infection
- chest pain
- trouble sleeping

Asthma in Children 5-12 Years of Age:
- viral infections
- runny nose
- tonsillitis
- gastroenteritis
- abdominal pain
- nausea
- dyspepsia

COPD:
- respiratory infection
- throat infection
- chest pain
- sinus infection
- fever
- leg cramps
- muscle cramps

Tell your healthcare provider about any side effect that bothers you or that does not go away.

These are not all the side effects with FORADIL AEROLIZER. Ask your healthcare provider or pharmacist for more information.

Call your doctor for medical advice about side effects. You may report side effects to FDA at 1-800-FDA-1088.

How do I store FORADIL AEROLIZER?
- Store FORADIL AEROLIZER at room temperature between 68°F and 77°F (20°C to 25°C).
- Protect FORADIL AEROLIZER from heat and moisture.
- Do not remove FORADIL capsules from their foil blister package until just before use.
- Always discard the old AEROLIZER inhaler by the "Use by" date and use the new one provided with each new prescription.
- Safely discard FORADIL capsules and the Aerolizer inhaler if no longer needed or is out-of-date.

Keep FORADIL AEROLIZER and all medicines out of the reach of children.

General Information about FORADIL AEROLIZER

Medicines are sometimes prescribed for purposes other than those listed in a Medication Guide. Do not use FORADIL AEROLIZER for a condition for which it was not prescribed. Do not give FORADIL AEROLIZER to other people, even if they have the same condition. It may harm them.

This Medication Guide summarizes the most important information about FORADIL AEROLIZER. If you would like more information, talk with your healthcare provider. You can ask your healthcare provider or pharmacist for information about FORADIL AEROLIZER that was written for healthcare professionals. If you have any questions about the use of FORADIL AEROLIZER, call (toll-free) 1-800-622-4477 or go to www.foradil.us.

What are the ingredients in FORADIL AEROLIZER?

Active ingredient: formoterol fumarate

Inactive ingredients: lactose (contains milk proteins), gelatin (capsule shell)

T2012-118

November 2012

INSTRUCTIONS FOR USE

Do not swallow FORADIL capsules.

Follow the instructions below for using your FORADIL AEROLIZER. **You will breathe-in (inhale) the medicine in the FORADIL capsules from the FORADIL AEROLIZER.** If you have any questions, ask your healthcare provider or pharmacist.

FORADIL AEROLIZER
- **FORADIL AEROLIZER consists of FORADIL capsules and a AEROLIZER Inhaler.**
- **FORADIL capsules come on blister cards.**
- **Keep your FORADIL and AEROLIZER Inhaler dry. Handle with DRY hands.**

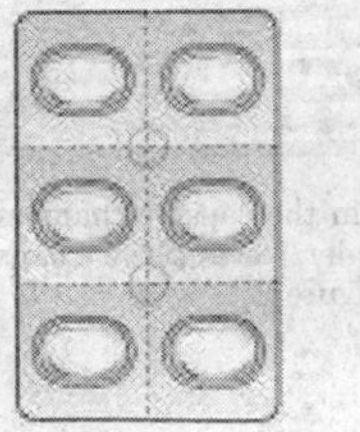

Foil blister card

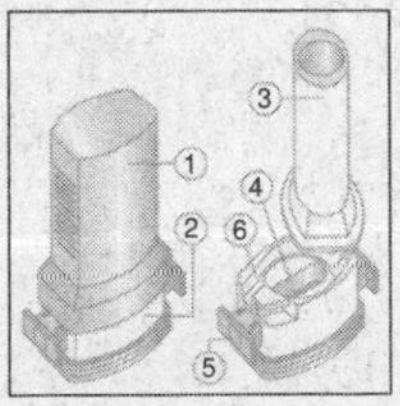

The Aerolizer consists of the following parts:
1. A cap to protect the mouthpiece of the base
2. A base that allows the proper release of medicine from the capsule. The base consists of:
3. A mouth piece
4. A capsule chamber
5. A button with "winglets" (projecting side pieces) and pins on each side
6. An air inlet channel.

With each new prescription of FORADIL AEROLIZER or refill, your pharmacist should have written the "Use by" date on the sticker on the outside of the FORADIL AEROLIZER box. Remove the "Use by" sticker on the box and place it on the AEROLIZER Inhaler cover that comes with FORADIL. If the sticker is blank, count 4 months from the date you got your FORADIL AEROLIZER from the pharmacy and write this date on the sticker. Also, check the expiration date stamped on the box. If this date is less than 4 months from your purchase date, write this date on the sticker.

Do not use FORADIL capsules with any other capsule inhaler, and do not use the AEROLIZER inhaler to take any other capsule medicine.

Taking a dose of FORADIL AEROLIZER requires the following steps:

1. Do not remove a FORADIL capsule from the blister card until you are ready for a dose.

2. Pull off the AEROLIZER Inhaler cover. (Figure A)

Figure A

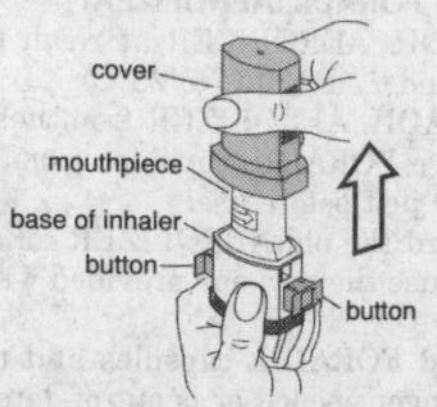

3. Hold the base of the AEROLIZER Inhaler firmly and twist the mouthpiece in the direction of the arrow to open. (Figure B) Push the buttons in on each side to make sure that you can see 4 pins in the capsule well of the AEROLIZER Inhaler.

Figure B

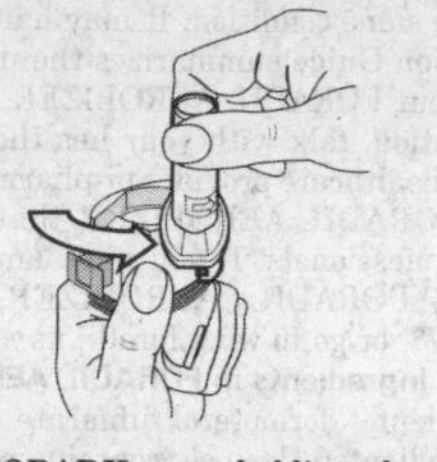

4. Separate one FORADIL capsule blister by tearing at the precut lines. (Figure C)

Figure C

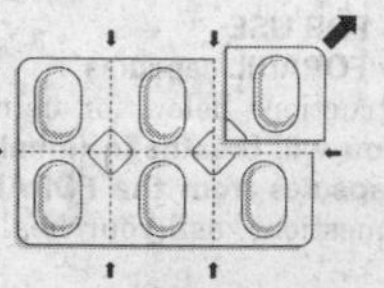

5. Peel the paper backing that covers one FORADIL capsule on the blister card. Push the FORADIL capsule through the foil. (Figure D)

Figure D

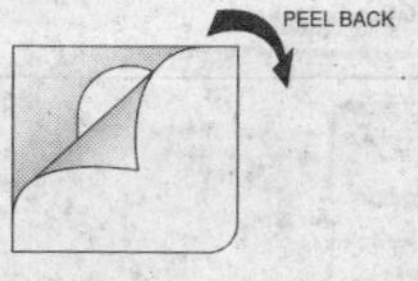

6. Place the FORADIL capsule in the capsule-chamber in the base of the AEROLIZER Inhaler. **Never place a capsule directly into the mouthpiece.** (Figure E)

Figure E

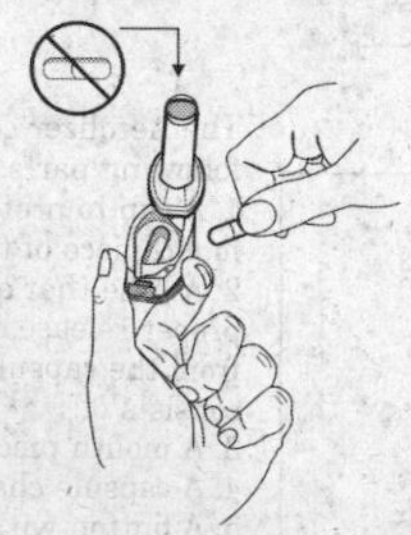

7. Twist the mouthpiece back to the closed position. (Figure F)

Figure F

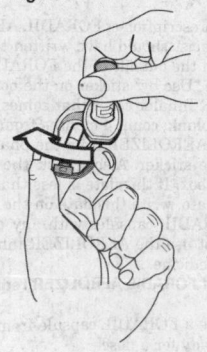

8. Hold the mouthpiece of the AEROLIZER Inhaler upright and press both buttons at the same time. Only press the buttons **ONCE**. You should hear a click as the FORADIL capsule is being pierced. (Figure G)

Figure G

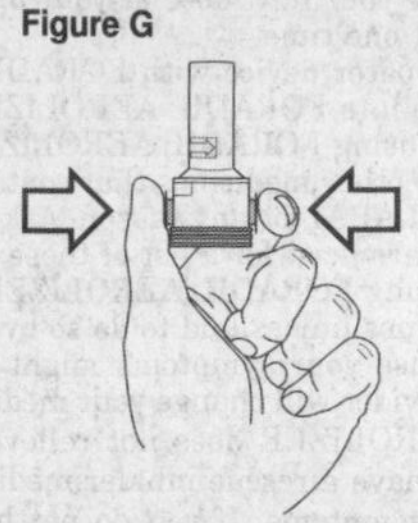

9. Release the buttons. If the buttons stay stuck, grasp the wings on the buttons and pull them out of the stuck position before the next step. Do not push the buttons a second time. This may cause the FORADIL capsule to break into small pieces. There is a screen built into the AEROLIZER Inhaler to hold these small pieces. It is possible that tiny pieces of a FORADIL capsule might reach your mouth or throat when you inhale the medicine. This will not harm you, but to avoid this, only pierce the capsule once. The FORADIL capsules are also less likely to break into small pieces if you store them the right way (See "How do I store FORADIL AEROLIZER?").

10. Breathe out (exhale) fully. **Do not exhale into the AEROLIZER mouthpiece.** (Figure H)

Figure H

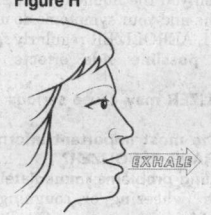

11. Tilt your head back slightly. Keep the AEROLIZER Inhaler level, with the blue buttons to the left and right (**not up and down**). Place the mouthpiece in your mouth and close your lips around the mouthpiece. (Figures I and J)

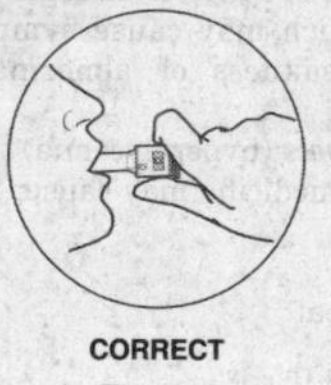

CORRECT

Figure I

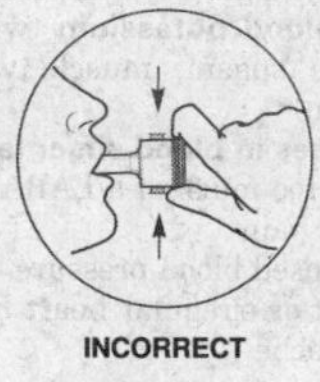

INCORRECT

Figure J

12. Breathe in quickly and deeply (Figure K). This will cause the FORADIL capsule to spin around in the chamber and deliver your dose of medicine. You should hear a whirring noise and experience a sweet taste in your mouth. If you do not hear the whirring noise, the capsule may be stuck. If this occurs, open the AEROLIZER Inhaler and loosen the capsule allowing it to spin freely. **Do not try to loosen the capsule by pressing the buttons again.** (You will have to repeat steps 10 to 12 again to get your dose.)

Figure K

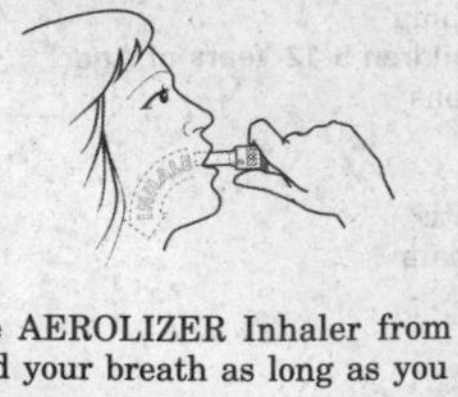

13. Remove the AEROLIZER Inhaler from your mouth. Continue to hold your breath as long as you can and then exhale.

14. Open the AEROLIZER Inhaler to see if any powder is still in the capsule. If any powder remains in the capsule repeat steps 10 to 13. Most people are able to empty the capsule in one or two inhalations.

15. After use, open the AEROLIZER Inhaler, remove and discard the empty capsule. Do not leave a used capsule in the chamber.

16. Close the mouthpiece and replace the cover.

Remember:

- Never breathe into the AEROLIZER Inhaler.
- Never take the AEROLIZER Inhaler apart.
- Never place a FORADIL capsule directly into the mouthpiece of the AEROLIZER Inhaler.
- Never leave a used FORADIL capsule in the AEROLIZER Inhaler chamber.
- Always use the AEROLIZER Inhaler in a level position.
- Never wash the AEROLIZER Inhaler. **Keep it dry.**
- Always keep the AEROLIZER Inhaler and FORADIL capsules in a dry place.
- Always use the new AEROLIZER Inhaler that comes with your refill.

This Medication Guide and Instructions for Use has been approved by the U.S. Food and Drug Administration.

FORADIL® is a registered trademark of Astellas Pharma Inc.

AEROLIZER® is a registered trademark of Novartis AG.

Manufactured for: Merck Sharp & Dohme Corp., a subsidiary of

MERCK & CO., INC., Whitehouse Station, NJ 08889, USA

Manufactured by:

Novartis Pharma AG, Basle, Switzerland

T2012-219

November 2012

FOSAMAX® ℞

[*FOSS-ah-max*]

(alendronate sodium) tablets, for oral use

FOSAMAX® ℞

(alendronate sodium) oral solution

HIGHLIGHTS OF PRESCRIBING INFORMATION

These highlights do not include all the information needed to use FOSAMAX safely and effectively. See full prescribing information for FOSAMAX.

FOSAMAX® (alendronate sodium) tablets, for oral use

FOSAMAX (alendronate sodium) oral solution

Initial U.S. Approval: 1995

RECENT MAJOR CHANGES

Indications and Usage (1.6)	04/2013
Dosage and Administration (2)	06/2012
Warnings and Precautions (5.4)	04/2013

INDICATIONS AND USAGE

FOSAMAX is a bisphosphonate indicated for:

- Treatment and prevention of osteoporosis in postmenopausal women (1.1, 1.2)
- Treatment to increase bone mass in men with osteoporosis (1.3)
- Treatment of glucocorticoid-induced osteoporosis (1.4)
- Treatment of Paget's disease of bone (1.5)

Limitations of use:

Optimal duration of use has not been determined. For patients at low-risk for fracture, consider drug discontinuation after 3 to 5 years of use. (1.6)

DOSAGE AND ADMINISTRATION

- Treatment of osteoporosis in postmenopausal women and in men: 10 mg daily or 70 mg (tablet or oral solution) once weekly. (2.1, 2.3)
- Prevention of osteoporosis in postmenopausal women: 5 mg daily or 35 mg once weekly. (2.2)
- Glucocorticoid-induced osteoporosis: 5 mg daily; or 10 mg daily in postmenopausal women not receiving estrogen. (2.4)
- Paget's disease: 40 mg daily for six months. (2.5)
- Instruct patients to: (2.6)
  - Swallow tablets whole with 6-8 ounces plain water at least 30 minutes before the first food, drink, or medication of the day.
  - Swallow oral solution followed by at least 2 ounces of water.
  - Not lie down for at least 30 minutes after taking FOSAMAX and until after food.

DOSAGE FORMS AND STRENGTHS

Tablets: 70 mg (3)

Oral Solution: 70 mg (3)

CONTRAINDICATIONS

- Abnormalities of the esophagus which delay emptying such as stricture or achalasia (4, 5.1)
- Inability to stand/sit upright for at least 30 minutes (2.6, 4, 5.1)
- Do not administer FOSAMAX oral solution to patients at increased risk of aspiration. (4)
- Hypocalcemia (4, 5.2)
- Hypersensitivity to any component of this product (4, 6.2)

WARNINGS AND PRECAUTIONS

- *Upper Gastrointestinal Adverse Reactions* can occur. Instruct patients to follow dosing instructions. Discontinue if new or worsening symptoms occur. (5.1)
- *Hypocalcemia* can worsen and must be corrected prior to use. (5.2)
- *Severe Bone, Joint, Muscle Pain* may occur. Discontinue use if severe symptoms develop. (5.3)
- *Osteonecrosis of the Jaw* has been reported. (5.4)
- *Atypical Femur Fractures* have been reported. Patients with new thigh or groin pain should be evaluated to rule out an incomplete femoral fracture. (5.5)

ADVERSE REACTIONS

Most common adverse reactions (greater than or equal to 3%) are abdominal pain, acid regurgitation, constipation, diarrhea, dyspepsia, musculoskeletal pain, nausea. (6.1)

To report SUSPECTED ADVERSE REACTIONS, contact Merck Sharp & Dohme Corp., a subsidiary of Merck & Co., Inc., at 1-877-888-4231 or FDA at 1-800-FDA-1088 or www.fda.gov/medwatch.

DRUG INTERACTIONS

- Calcium supplements, antacids, or oral medications containing multivalent cations interfere with absorption of alendronate. (2.6, 7.1)
- Use caution when co-prescribing aspirin/nonsteroidal anti-inflammatory drugs that may worsen gastrointestinal irritation. (7.2, 7.3)

USE IN SPECIFIC POPULATIONS

- FOSAMAX is not indicated for use in pediatric patients. (8.4)
- FOSAMAX is not recommended in patients with renal impairment (creatinine clearance less than 35 mL/min). (5.6, 8.6)

See 17 for PATIENT COUNSELING INFORMATION and Medication Guide

Revised: 04/2013

FULL PRESCRIBING INFORMATION: CONTENTS*

*** Sections or subsections omitted from the full prescribing information are not listed**

FULL PRESCRIBING INFORMATION

1 INDICATIONS AND USAGE

1.1 Treatment of Osteoporosis in Postmenopausal Women

FOSAMAX is indicated for the treatment of osteoporosis in postmenopausal women. In postmenopausal women, FOSAMAX increases bone mass and reduces the incidence of fractures, including those of the hip and spine (vertebral compression fractures). *[See Clinical Studies (14.1).]*

1.2 Prevention of Osteoporosis in Postmenopausal Women

FOSAMAX is indicated for the prevention of postmenopausal osteoporosis *[see Clinical Studies (14.2)]*.

1.3 Treatment to Increase Bone Mass in Men with Osteoporosis

FOSAMAX is indicated for treatment to increase bone mass in men with osteoporosis *[see Clinical Studies (14.3)]*.

1.4 Treatment of Glucocorticoid-Induced Osteoporosis

FOSAMAX is indicated for the treatment of glucocorticoid-induced osteoporosis in men and women receiving glucocorticoids in a daily dosage equivalent to 7.5 mg or greater of prednisone and who have low bone mineral density *[see Clinical Studies (14.4)]*.

1.5 Treatment of Paget's Disease of Bone

FOSAMAX is indicated for the treatment of Paget's disease of bone in men and women. Treatment is indicated in patients with Paget's disease of bone who have alkaline phosphatase at least two times the upper limit of normal, or those who are symptomatic, or those at risk for future complications from their disease. *[See Clinical Studies (14.5).]*

1.6 Important Limitations of Use

The optimal duration of use has not been determined. The safety and effectiveness of FOSAMAX for the treatment of osteoporosis are based on clinical data of four years duration. All patients on bisphosphonate therapy should have the need for continued therapy re-evaluated on a periodic basis. Patients at low-risk for fracture should be considered for drug discontinuation after 3 to 5 years of use. Patients who discontinue therapy should have their risk for fracture re-evaluated periodically.

2 DOSAGE AND ADMINISTRATION

Although alendronate tablets 5 mg, 10 mg, 35 mg, and 40 mg are available in the marketplace, FOSAMAX is no longer marketed in the 5 mg, 10 mg, 35 mg, and 40 mg strengths.

2.1 Treatment of Osteoporosis in Postmenopausal Women

The recommended dosage is:

- one 70 mg tablet once weekly

or

- one bottle of 70 mg oral solution once weekly

or

- one 10 mg tablet once daily

2.2 Prevention of Osteoporosis in Postmenopausal Women

The recommended dosage is:

- one 35 mg tablet once weekly

or

- one 5 mg tablet once daily

2.3 Treatment to Increase Bone Mass in Men with Osteoporosis

The recommended dosage is:

- one 70 mg tablet once weekly

or

- one bottle of 70 mg oral solution once weekly

or

- one 10 mg tablet once daily

2.4 Treatment of Glucocorticoid-Induced Osteoporosis

The recommended dosage is one 5 mg tablet once daily, except for postmenopausal women not receiving estrogen, for whom the recommended dosage is one 10 mg tablet once daily.

2.5 Treatment of Paget's Disease of Bone

The recommended treatment regimen is 40 mg once a day for six months.

Re-treatment of Paget's Disease

Re-treatment with FOSAMAX may be considered, following a six-month post-treatment evaluation period in patients who have relapsed, based on increases in serum alkaline phosphatase, which should be measured periodically. Re-treatment may also be considered in those who failed to normalize their serum alkaline phosphatase.

2.6 Important Administration Instructions

Instruct patients to do the following:

- Take FOSAMAX *at least* one-half hour before the first food, beverage, or medication of the day with plain water only *[see Patient Counseling Information (17.2)]*. Other beverages (including mineral water), food, and some medications are likely to reduce the absorption of FOSAMAX *[see Drug Interactions (7.1)]*. Waiting less than 30 minutes, or taking FOSAMAX with food, beverages (other than plain water) or other medications will lessen the effect of FOSAMAX by decreasing its absorption into the body.
- Take FOSAMAX upon arising for the day. To facilitate delivery to the stomach and thus reduce the potential for esophageal irritation, a FOSAMAX tablet should be swallowed with a full glass of water (6-8 ounces). To facilitate gastric emptying FOSAMAX oral solution should be followed by at least 2 ounces (a quarter of a cup) of water. Patients should not lie down for at least 30 minutes and until after their first food of the day. FOSAMAX should not be taken at bedtime or before arising for the day. Failure to follow these instructions may increase the risk of esophageal adverse experiences *[see Warnings and Precautions (5.1) and Patient Counseling Information (17.2)]*.

2.7 Recommendations for Calcium and Vitamin D Supplementation

Instruct patients to take supplemental calcium if dietary intake is inadequate *[see Warnings and Precautions (5.2)]*. Patients at increased risk for vitamin D insufficiency (e.g., over the age of 70 years, nursing home-bound, or chronically ill) may need vitamin D supplementation. Patients with gastrointestinal malabsorption syndromes may require higher doses of vitamin D supplementation and measurement of 25-hydroxyvitamin D should be considered.

Patients treated with glucocorticoids should receive adequate amounts of calcium and vitamin D.

2.8 Administration Instructions for Missed Doses

If a once-weekly dose of FOSAMAX (tablet or oral solution) is missed, instruct patients to take one dose on the morning after they remember. They should not take two doses on the same day but should return to taking one dose once a week, as originally scheduled on their chosen day.

3 DOSAGE FORMS AND STRENGTHS

- 70 mg tablets are white, oval, uncoated tablets with code 31 on one side and an outline of a bone image on the other.
- 70 mg oral solution is a clear, colorless solution with a raspberry flavor.

4 CONTRAINDICATIONS

FOSAMAX is contraindicated in patients with the following conditions:

- Abnormalities of the esophagus which delay esophageal emptying such as stricture or achalasia *[see Warnings and Precautions (5.1)]*
- Inability to stand or sit upright for at least 30 minutes *[see Dosage and Administration (2.6); Warnings and Precautions (5.1)]*
- Do not administer FOSAMAX oral solution to patients at increased risk of aspiration.
- Hypocalcemia *[see Warnings and Precautions (5.2)]*
- Hypersensitivity to any component of this product. Hypersensitivity reactions including urticaria and angioedema have been reported *[see Adverse Reactions (6.2)]*.

5 WARNINGS AND PRECAUTIONS

5.1 Upper Gastrointestinal Adverse Reactions

FOSAMAX, like other bisphosphonates administered orally, may cause local irritation of the upper gastrointestinal mucosa. Because of these possible irritant effects and a potential for worsening of the underlying disease, caution should be used when FOSAMAX is given to patients with active upper gastrointestinal problems (such as known Barrett's esophagus, dysphagia, other esophageal diseases, gastritis, duodenitis, or ulcers).

Esophageal adverse experiences, such as esophagitis, esophageal ulcers and esophageal erosions, occasionally with bleeding and rarely followed by esophageal stricture or perforation, have been reported in patients receiving treatment with oral bisphosphonates including FOSAMAX. In some cases these have been severe and required hospitalization. Physicians should therefore be alert to any signs or symptoms signaling a possible esophageal reaction and patients should be instructed to discontinue FOSAMAX and seek medical attention if they develop dysphagia, odynophagia, retrosternal pain or new or worsening heartburn.

Table 1: Osteoporosis Treatment Studies in Postmenopausal Women Adverse Reactions Considered Possibly, Probably, or Definitely Drug Related by the Investigators and Reported in Greater Than or Equal to 1% of Patients

	United States/Multinational Studies		Fracture Intervention Trial	
	FOSAMAX* % (n=196)	Placebo % (n=397)	FOSAMAX† % (n=3236)	Placebo % (n=3223)
Gastrointestinal				
abdominal pain	6.6	4.8	1.5	1.5
nausea	3.6	4.0	1.1	1.5
dyspepsia	3.6	3.5	1.1	1.2
constipation	3.1	1.8	0.0	0.2
diarrhea	3.1	1.8	0.6	0.3
flatulence	2.6	0.5	0.2	0.3
acid regurgitation	2.0	4.3	1.1	0.9
esophageal ulcer	1.5	0.0	0.1	0.1
vomiting	1.0	1.5	0.2	0.3
dysphagia	1.0	0.0	0.1	0.1
abdominal distention	1.0	0.8	0.0	0.0
gastritis	0.5	1.3	0.6	0.7
Musculoskeletal				
musculoskeletal (bone, muscle or joint) pain	4.1	2.5	0.4	0.3
muscle cramp	0.0	1.0	0.2	0.1
Nervous System / Psychiatric				
headache	2.6	1.5	0.2	0.2
dizziness	0.0	1.0	0.0	0.1
Special Senses				
taste perversion	0.5	1.0	0.1	0.0

* 10 mg/day for three years
† 5 mg/day for 2 years and 10 mg/day for either 1 or 2 additional years

The risk of severe esophageal adverse experiences appears to be greater in patients who lie down after taking oral bisphosphonates including FOSAMAX and/or who fail to swallow oral bisphosphonates including FOSAMAX with the recommended full glass (6-8 ounces) of water, and/or who continue to take oral bisphosphonates including FOSAMAX after developing symptoms suggestive of esophageal irritation. Therefore, it is very important that the full dosing instructions are provided to, and understood by, the patient *[see Dosage and Administration (2.6)]*. In patients who cannot comply with dosing instructions due to mental disability, therapy with FOSAMAX should be used under appropriate supervision.

There have been post-marketing reports of gastric and duodenal ulcers with oral bisphosphonate use, some severe and with complications, although no increased risk was observed in controlled clinical trials *[see Adverse Reactions (6.2)]*.

5.2 Mineral Metabolism

Hypocalcemia must be corrected before initiating therapy with FOSAMAX *[see Contraindications (4)]*. Other disorders affecting mineral metabolism (such as vitamin D deficiency) should also be effectively treated. In patients with these conditions, serum calcium and symptoms of hypocalcemia should be monitored during therapy with FOSAMAX.

Presumably due to the effects of FOSAMAX on increasing bone mineral, small, asymptomatic decreases in serum calcium and phosphate may occur, especially in patients with Paget's disease, in whom the pretreatment rate of bone turnover may be greatly elevated, and in patients receiving glucocorticoids, in whom calcium absorption may be decreased.

Ensuring adequate calcium and vitamin D intake is especially important in patients with Paget's disease of bone and in patients receiving glucocorticoids.

5.3 Musculoskeletal Pain

In post-marketing experience, severe and occasionally incapacitating bone, joint, and/or muscle pain has been reported in patients taking bisphosphonates that are approved for the prevention and treatment of osteoporosis *[see Adverse Reactions (6.2)]*. This category of drugs includes FOSAMAX (alendronate). Most of the patients were postmenopausal women. The time to onset of symptoms varied from one day to several months after starting the drug. Discontinue use if severe symptoms develop. Most patients had relief of symptoms after stopping. A subset had recurrence of symptoms when rechallenged with the same drug or another bisphosphonate.

In placebo-controlled clinical studies of FOSAMAX, the percentages of patients with these symptoms were similar in the FOSAMAX and placebo groups.

5.4 Osteonecrosis of the Jaw

Osteonecrosis of the jaw (ONJ), which can occur spontaneously, is generally associated with tooth extraction and/or local infection with delayed healing, and has been reported in patients taking bisphosphonates, including FOSAMAX. Known risk factors for osteonecrosis of the jaw include invasive dental procedures (e.g., tooth extraction, dental implants, boney surgery), diagnosis of cancer, concomitant therapies (e.g., chemotherapy, corticosteroids), poor oral hygiene, and co-morbid disorders (e.g., periodontal and/or other pre-existing dental disease, anemia, coagulopathy, infection, ill-fitting dentures). The risk of ONJ may increase with duration of exposure to bisphosphonates.

For patients requiring invasive dental procedures, discontinuation of bisphosphonate treatment may reduce the risk for ONJ. Clinical judgment of the treating physician and/or oral surgeon should guide the management plan of each patient based on individual benefit/risk assessment.

Patients who develop osteonecrosis of the jaw while on bisphosphonate therapy should receive care by an oral surgeon. In these patients, extensive dental surgery to treat ONJ may exacerbate the condition. Discontinuation of bisphosphonate therapy should be considered based on individual benefit/risk assessment.

5.5 Atypical Subtrochanteric and Diaphyseal Femoral Fractures

Atypical, low-energy, or low trauma fractures of the femoral shaft have been reported in bisphosphonate-treated patients. These fractures can occur anywhere in the femoral shaft from just below the lesser trochanter to above the supracondylar flare and are transverse or short oblique in orientation without evidence of comminution. Causality has not been established as these fractures also occur in osteoporotic patients who have not been treated with bisphosphonates.

Atypical femur fractures most commonly occur with minimal or no trauma to the affected area. They may be bilateral and many patients report prodromal pain in the affected area, usually presenting as dull, aching thigh pain, weeks to months before a complete fracture occurs. A number of reports note that patients were also receiving treatment with glucocorticoids (e.g. prednisone) at the time of fracture.

Any patient with a history of bisphosphonate exposure who presents with thigh or groin pain should be suspected of having an atypical fracture and should be evaluated to rule out an incomplete femur fracture. Patients presenting with an atypical fracture should also be assessed for symptoms and signs of fracture in the contralateral limb. Interruption of bisphosphonate therapy should be considered, pending a risk/benefit assessment, on an individual basis.

5.6 Renal Impairment

FOSAMAX is not recommended for patients with creatinine clearance less than 35 mL/min.

5.7 Glucocorticoid-Induced Osteoporosis

The risk versus benefit of FOSAMAX for treatment at daily dosages of glucocorticoids less than 7.5 mg of prednisone or equivalent has not been established *[see Indications and Usage (1.4)]*. Before initiating treatment, the gonadal hormonal status of both men and women should be ascertained and appropriate replacement considered.

A bone mineral density measurement should be made at the initiation of therapy and repeated after 6 to 12 months of combined FOSAMAX and glucocorticoid treatment.

6 ADVERSE REACTIONS

6.1 Clinical Trials Experience

Because clinical trials are conducted under widely varying conditions, adverse reaction rates observed in the clinical trials of a drug cannot be directly compared to rates in the clinical trials of another drug and may not reflect the rates observed in clinical practice.

Treatment of Osteoporosis in Postmenopausal Women

Daily Dosing

The safety of FOSAMAX in the treatment of postmenopausal osteoporosis was assessed in four clinical trials that enrolled 7453 women aged 44-84 years. Study 1 and Study 2 were identically designed, three-year, placebo-controlled, double-blind, multicenter studies (United States and Multinational n=994); Study 3 was the three year vertebral fracture cohort of the Fracture Intervention Trial [FIT] (n=2027) and Study 4 was the four-year clinical fracture cohort of FIT (n=4432). Overall, 3620 patients were exposed to placebo and 3432 patients exposed to FOSAMAX. Patients with pre-existing gastrointestinal disease and concomitant use of non-steroidal anti-inflammatory drugs were included in these clinical trials. In Study 1 and Study 2 all women received 500 mg elemental calcium as carbonate. In Study 3 and Study 4 all women with dietary calcium intake less than 1000 mg per day received 500 mg calcium and 250 international units Vitamin D per day.

Among patients treated with alendronate 10 mg or placebo in Study 1 and Study 2, and all patients in Study 3 and Study 4, the incidence of all-cause mortality was 1.8% in the placebo group and 1.8% in the FOSAMAX group. The incidence of serious adverse event was 30.7% in the placebo group and 30.9% in the FOSAMAX group. The percentage of patients who discontinued the study due to any clinical adverse event was 9.5% in the placebo group and 8.9% in the FOSAMAX group. Adverse reactions from these studies considered by the investigators as possibly, probably, or definitely drug related in greater than or equal to 1% of patients treated with either FOSAMAX or placebo are presented in Table 1.

[See table 1 above]

Rash and erythema have occurred.

Gastrointestinal Adverse Reactions: One patient treated with FOSAMAX (10 mg/day), who had a history of peptic ulcer disease and gastrectomy and who was taking concomitant aspirin, developed an anastomotic ulcer with mild hemorrhage, which was considered drug related. Aspirin and FOSAMAX were discontinued and the patient recovered. In the Study 1 and Study 2 populations, 49-54% had a history of gastrointestinal disorders at baseline and 54-89% used nonsteroidal anti-inflammatory drugs or aspirin at some time during the studies. *[See Warnings and Precautions (5.1).]*

Laboratory Test Findings: In double-blind, multicenter, controlled studies, asymptomatic, mild, and transient decreases in serum calcium and phosphate were observed in approximately 18% and 10%, respectively, of patients taking FOSAMAX versus approximately 12% and 3% of those taking placebo. However, the incidences of decreases in serum calcium to less than 8.0 mg/dL (2.0 mM) and serum phosphate to less than or equal to 2.0 mg/dL (0.65 mM) were similar in both treatment groups.

Weekly Dosing

The safety of FOSAMAX 70 mg once weekly for the treatment of postmenopausal osteoporosis was assessed in a one-year, double-blind, multicenter study comparing FOSAMAX 70 mg once weekly and FOSAMAX 10 mg daily. The overall safety and tolerability profiles of once weekly FOSAMAX 70 mg and FOSAMAX 10 mg daily were similar. The adverse reactions considered by the investigators as possibly, probably, or definitely drug related in greater than or equal to 1% of patients in either treatment group are presented in Table 2.

Table 2: Osteoporosis Treatment Studies in Postmenopausal Women Adverse Reactions Considered Possibly, Probably, or Definitely Drug Related by the Investigators and Reported in Greater Than or Equal to 1% of Patients

	Once Weekly FOSAMAX 70 mg % (n=519)	FOSAMAX 10 mg/day % (n=370)
Gastrointestinal		
abdominal pain	3.7	3.0
dyspepsia	2.7	2.2
acid regurgitation	1.9	2.4
nausea	1.9	2.4
abdominal distention	1.0	1.4
constipation	0.8	1.6
flatulence	0.4	1.6
gastritis	0.2	1.1
gastric ulcer	0.0	1.1
Musculoskeletal		
musculoskeletal (bone, muscle, joint) pain	2.9	3.2
muscle cramp	0.2	1.1

Prevention of Osteoporosis in Postmenopausal Women
Daily Dosing
The safety of FOSAMAX 5 mg/day in postmenopausal women 40-60 years of age has been evaluated in three double-blind, placebo-controlled studies involving over 1,400 patients randomized to receive FOSAMAX for either two or three years. In these studies the overall safety profiles of FOSAMAX 5 mg/day and placebo were similar. Discontinuation of therapy due to any clinical adverse event occurred in 7.5% of 642 patients treated with FOSAMAX 5 mg/day and 5.7% of 648 patients treated with placebo.
Weekly Dosing
The safety of FOSAMAX 35 mg once weekly compared to FOSAMAX 5 mg daily was evaluated in a one-year, double-blind, multicenter study of 723 patients. The overall safety and tolerability profiles of once weekly FOSAMAX 35 mg and FOSAMAX 5 mg daily were similar.
The adverse reactions from these studies considered by the investigators as possibly, probably, or definitely drug related in greater than or equal to 1% of patients treated with either once weekly FOSAMAX 35 mg, FOSAMAX 5 mg/day or placebo are presented in Table 3.
[See table 3 above]

Table 3: Osteoporosis Prevention Studies in Postmenopausal Women Adverse Reactions Considered Possibly, Probably, or Definitely Drug Related by the Investigators and Reported in Greater Than or Equal to 1% of Patients

	Two/Three-Year Studies		One-Year Study	
	FOSAMAX 5 mg/day % (n=642)	Placebo % (n=648)	FOSAMAX 5 mg/day % (n=361)	Once Weekly FOSAMAX 35 mg % (n=362)
Gastrointestinal				
dyspepsia	1.9	1.4	2.2	1.7
abdominal pain	1.7	3.4	4.2	2.2
acid regurgitation	1.4	2.5	4.2	4.7
nausea	1.4	1.4	2.5	1.4
diarrhea	1.1	1.7	1.1	0.6
constipation	0.9	0.5	1.7	0.3
abdominal distention	0.2	0.3	1.4	1.1
Musculoskeletal				
musculoskeletal (bone, muscle or joint) pain	0.8	0.9	1.9	2.2

Concomitant Use with Estrogen/Hormone Replacement Therapy
In two studies (of one and two years' duration) of postmenopausal osteoporotic women (total: n=853), the safety and tolerability profile of combined treatment with FOSAMAX 10 mg once daily and estrogen ± progestin (n=354) was consistent with those of the individual treatments.
Osteoporosis in Men
In two placebo-controlled, double-blind, multicenter studies in men (a two-year study of FOSAMAX 10 mg/day and a one-year study of once weekly FOSAMAX 70 mg) the rates of discontinuation of therapy due to any clinical adverse event were 2.7% for FOSAMAX 10 mg/day vs. 10.5% for placebo, and 6.4% for once weekly FOSAMAX 70 mg vs. 8.6% for placebo. The adverse reactions considered by the investigators as possibly, probably, or definitely drug related in greater than or equal to 2% of patients treated with either FOSAMAX or placebo are presented in Table 4.
[See table 4 above]

Table 4: Osteoporosis Studies in Men Adverse Reactions Considered Possibly, Probably, or Definitely Drug Related by the Investigators and Reported in Greater Than or Equal to 2% of Patients

	Two-year Study		One-year Study	
	FOSAMAX 10 mg/day % (n=146)	Placebo % (n=95)	Once Weekly FOSAMAX 70 mg % (n=109)	Placebo % (n=58)
Gastrointestinal				
acid regurgitation	4.1	3.2	0.0	0.0
flatulence	4.1	1.1	0.0	0.0
gastroesophageal reflux disease	0.7	3.2	2.8	0.0
dyspepsia	3.4	0.0	2.8	1.7
diarrhea	1.4	1.1	2.8	0.0
abdominal pain	2.1	1.1	0.9	3.4
nausea	2.1	0.0	0.0	0.0

Glucocorticoid-Induced Osteoporosis
In two, one-year, placebo-controlled, double-blind, multicenter studies in patients receiving glucocorticoid treatment, the overall safety and tolerability profiles of FOSAMAX 5 and 10 mg/day were generally similar to that of placebo. The adverse reactions considered by the investigators as possibly, probably, or definitely drug related in greater than or equal to 1% of patients treated with either FOSAMAX 5 or 10 mg/day or placebo are presented in Table 5.

Table 5: One-Year Studies in Glucocorticoid-Treated Patients Adverse Reactions Considered Possibly, Probably, or Definitely Drug Related by the Investigators and Reported in Greater Than or Equal to 1% of Patients

	FOSAMAX 10 mg/day % (n=157)	FOSAMAX 5 mg/day % (n=161)	Placebo % (n=159)
Gastrointestinal			
abdominal pain	3.2	1.9	0.0
acid regurgitation	2.5	1.9	1.3
constipation	1.3	0.6	0.0
melena	1.3	0.0	0.0
nausea	0.6	1.2	0.6
diarrhea	0.0	0.0	1.3
Nervous System/ Psychiatric			
headache	0.6	0.0	1.3

The overall safety and tolerability profile in the glucocorticoid-induced osteoporosis population that continued therapy for the second year of the studies (FOSAMAX: n=147) was consistent with that observed in the first year.
Paget's Disease of Bone
In clinical studies (osteoporosis and Paget's disease), adverse events reported in 175 patients taking FOSAMAX 40 mg/day for 3-12 months were similar to those in postmenopausal women treated with FOSAMAX 10 mg/day. However, there was an apparent increased incidence of upper gastrointestinal adverse reactions in patients taking FOSAMAX 40 mg/day (17.7% FOSAMAX vs. 10.2% placebo). One case of esophagitis and two cases of gastritis resulted in discontinuation of treatment.
Additionally, musculoskeletal (bone, muscle or joint) pain, which has been described in patients with Paget's disease treated with other bisphosphonates, was considered by the investigators as possibly, probably, or definitely drug related in approximately 6% of patients treated with FOSAMAX 40 mg/day versus approximately 1% of patients treated with placebo, but rarely resulted in discontinuation of therapy. Discontinuation of therapy due to any clinical adverse events occurred in 6.4% of patients with Paget's disease treated with FOSAMAX 40 mg/day and 2.4% of patients treated with placebo.

6.2 Post-Marketing Experience
The following adverse reactions have been identified during post-approval use of FOSAMAX. Because these reactions are reported voluntarily from a population of uncertain size, it is not always possible to reliably estimate their frequency or establish a causal relationship to drug exposure.
Body as a Whole: hypersensitivity reactions including urticaria and angioedema. Transient symptoms of myalgia, malaise, asthenia and fever have been reported with FOSAMAX, typically in association with initiation of treatment. Symptomatic hypocalcemia has occurred, generally in association with predisposing conditions. Peripheral edema.
Gastrointestinal: esophagitis, esophageal erosions, esophageal ulcers, esophageal stricture or perforation, and oropharyngeal ulceration. Gastric or duodenal ulcers, some severe and with complications, have also been reported *[see Dosage and Administration (2.6); Warnings and Precautions (5.1)]*.
Localized osteonecrosis of the jaw, generally associated with tooth extraction and/or local infection with delayed healing, has been reported *[see Warnings and Precautions (5.4)]*.
Musculoskeletal: bone, joint, and/or muscle pain, occasionally severe, and incapacitating *[see Warnings and Precautions (5.3)]*; joint swelling; low-energy femoral shaft and subtrochanteric fractures *[see Warnings and Precautions (5.5)]*.
Nervous System: dizziness and vertigo.
Pulmonary: acute asthma exacerbations.
Skin: rash (occasionally with photosensitivity), pruritus, alopecia, severe skin reactions, including Stevens-Johnson syndrome and toxic epidermal necrolysis.
Special Senses: uveitis, scleritis or episcleritis.

7 DRUG INTERACTIONS

7.1 Calcium Supplements/Antacids
Co-administration of FOSAMAX and calcium, antacids, or oral medications containing multivalent cations will interfere with absorption of FOSAMAX. Therefore, instruct patients to wait at least one-half hour after taking FOSAMAX before taking any other oral medications.

7.2 Aspirin
In clinical studies, the incidence of upper gastrointestinal adverse events was increased in patients receiving concomitant therapy with daily doses of FOSAMAX greater than 10 mg and aspirin-containing products.

7.3 Nonsteroidal Anti-Inflammatory Drugs
FOSAMAX may be administered to patients taking nonsteroidal anti-inflammatory drugs (NSAIDs). In a 3-year, controlled, clinical study (n=2027) during which a majority of patients received concomitant NSAIDs, the incidence of upper gastrointestinal adverse events was similar in patients taking FOSAMAX 5 or 10 mg/day compared to those taking placebo. However, since NSAID use is associated with gastrointestinal irritation, caution should be used during concomitant use with FOSAMAX.

8 USE IN SPECIFIC POPULATIONS

8.1 Pregnancy
Pregnancy Category C:
There are no studies in pregnant women. FOSAMAX should be used during pregnancy only if the potential benefit justifies the potential risk to the mother and fetus.
Bisphosphonates are incorporated into the bone matrix, from which they are gradually released over a period of years. The amount of bisphosphonate incorporated into adult bone, and hence, the amount available for release back into the systemic circulation, is directly related to the dose and duration of bisphosphonate use. There are no data on fetal risk in humans. However, there is a theoretical risk of fetal harm, predominantly skeletal, if a woman becomes pregnant after completing a course of bisphosphonate therapy. The impact of variables such as time between cessation of bisphosphonate therapy to conception, the particular bisphosphonate used, and the route of administration (intravenous versus oral) on the risk has not been studied.
Reproduction studies in rats showed decreased postimplantation survival and decreased body weight gain in normal pups at doses less than half of the recommended clinical dose. Sites of incomplete fetal ossification were statistically significantly increased in rats beginning at approximately 3 times the clinical dose in vertebral (cervical, thoracic, and lumbar), skull, and sternebral bones. No similar fetal effects were seen when pregnant rabbits were treated with doses approximately 10 times the clinical dose.
Both total and ionized calcium decreased in pregnant rats at approximately 4 times the clinical dose resulting in delays and failures of delivery. Protracted parturition due to maternal hypocalcemia occurred in rats at doses as low as one tenth the clinical dose when rats were treated from before mating through gestation. Maternotoxicity (late pregnancy deaths) also occurred in the female rats treated at approximately 4 times the clinical dose for varying periods of time ranging from treatment only during pre-mating to treatment only during early, middle, or late gestation; these deaths were lessened but not eliminated by cessation of treatment. Calcium supplementation either in the drinking

water or by minipump could not ameliorate the hypocalcemia or prevent maternal and neonatal deaths due to delays in delivery; intravenous calcium supplementation prevented maternal, but not fetal deaths.

Exposure multiples based on surface area, mg/m^2, were calculated using a 40-mg human daily dose. Animal dose ranged between 1 and 15 mg/kg/day in rats and up to 40 mg/kg/day in rabbits.

8.3 Nursing Mothers

It is not known whether alendronate is excreted in human milk. Because many drugs are excreted in human milk, caution should be exercised when FOSAMAX is administered to nursing women.

8.4 Pediatric Use

FOSAMAX is not indicated for use in pediatric patients.

The safety and efficacy of FOSAMAX were examined in a randomized, double-blind, placebo-controlled two-year study of 139 pediatric patients, aged 4-18 years, with severe osteogenesis imperfecta (OI). One-hundred-and-nine patients were randomized to 5 mg FOSAMAX daily (weight less than 40 kg) or 10 mg FOSAMAX daily (weight greater than or equal to 40 kg) and 30 patients to placebo. The mean baseline lumbar spine BMD Z-score of the patients was -4.5. The mean change in lumbar spine BMD Z-score from baseline to Month 24 was 1.3 in the FOSAMAX-treated patients and 0.1 in the placebo-treated patients. Treatment with FOSAMAX did not reduce the risk of fracture. Sixteen percent of the FOSAMAX patients who sustained a radiologically-confirmed fracture by Month 12 of the study had delayed fracture healing (callus remodeling) or fracture non-union when assessed radiographically at Month 24 compared with 9% of the placebo-treated patients. In FOSAMAX-treated patients, bone histomorphometry data obtained at Month 24 demonstrated decreased bone turnover and delayed mineralization time; however, there were no mineralization defects. There were no statistically significant differences between the FOSAMAX and placebo groups in reduction of bone pain. The oral bioavailability in children was similar to that observed in adults.

The overall safety profile of FOSAMAX in osteogenesis imperfecta patients treated for up to 24 months was generally similar to that of adults with osteoporosis treated with FOSAMAX. However, there was an increased occurrence of vomiting in osteogenesis imperfecta patients treated with FOSAMAX compared to placebo. During the 24-month treatment period, vomiting was observed in 32 of 109 (29.4%) patients treated with FOSAMAX and 3 of 30 (10%) patients treated with placebo.

In a pharmacokinetic study, 6 of 24 pediatric osteogenesis imperfecta patients who received a single oral dose of FOSAMAX 35 or 70 mg developed fever, flu-like symptoms, and/or mild lymphocytopenia within 24 to 48 hours after administration. These events, lasting no more than 2 to 3 days and responding to acetaminophen, are consistent with an acute-phase response that has been reported in patients receiving bisphosphonates, including FOSAMAX. *[See Adverse Reactions (6.2).]*

8.5 Geriatric Use

Of the patients receiving FOSAMAX in the Fracture Intervention Trial (FIT), 71% (n=2302) were greater than or equal to 65 years of age and 17% (n=550) were greater than or equal to 75 years of age. Of the patients receiving FOSAMAX in the United States and Multinational osteoporosis treatment studies in women, osteoporosis studies in men, glucocorticoid-induced osteoporosis studies, and Paget's disease studies *[see Clinical Studies (14.1), (14.3), (14.4), (14.5)]*, 45%, 54%, 37%, and 70%, respectively, were 65 years of age or over. No overall differences in efficacy or safety were observed between these patients and younger patients, but greater sensitivity of some older individuals cannot be ruled out.

8.6 Renal Impairment

FOSAMAX is not recommended for patients with creatinine clearance less than 35 mL/min. No dosage adjustment is necessary in patients with creatinine clearance values between 35-60 mL/min *[see Clinical Pharmacology (12.3)]*.

8.7 Hepatic Impairment

As there is evidence that alendronate is not metabolized or excreted in the bile, no studies were conducted in patients with hepatic impairment. No dosage adjustment is necessary *[see Clinical Pharmacology (12.3)]*.

10 OVERDOSAGE

Significant lethality after single oral doses was seen in female rats and mice at 552 mg/kg (3256 mg/m^2) and 966 mg/kg (2898 mg/m^2), respectively. In males, these values were slightly higher, 626 and 1280 mg/kg, respectively. There was no lethality in dogs at oral doses up to 200 mg/kg (4000 mg/m^2).

No specific information is available on the treatment of overdosage with FOSAMAX. Hypocalcemia, hypophosphatemia, and upper gastrointestinal adverse events, such as upset stomach, heartburn, esophagitis, gastritis, or ulcer, may result from oral overdosage. Milk or antacids should be given to bind alendronate. Due to the risk of esophageal irritation, vomiting should not be induced and the patient should remain fully upright.

Dialysis would not be beneficial.

11 DESCRIPTION

FOSAMAX (alendronate sodium) is a bisphosphonate that acts as a specific inhibitor of osteoclast-mediated bone resorption. Bisphosphonates are synthetic analogs of pyrophosphate that bind to the hydroxyapatite found in bone.

Alendronate sodium is chemically described as (4-amino-1-hydroxybutylidene) bisphosphonic acid monosodium salt trihydrate.

The empirical formula of alendronate sodium is $C_4H_{12}NNaO_7P_2 \bullet 3H_2O$ and its formula weight is 325.12. The structural formula is:

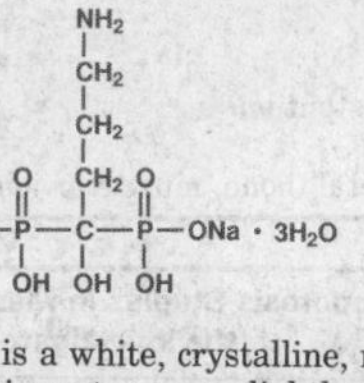

Alendronate sodium is a white, crystalline, nonhygroscopic powder. It is soluble in water, very slightly soluble in alcohol, and practically insoluble in chloroform.

FOSAMAX tablets for oral administration contain 91.37 mg of alendronate monosodium salt trihydrate, which is the molar equivalent of 70 mg of free acid, and the following inactive ingredients: microcrystalline cellulose, anhydrous lactose, croscarmellose sodium, and magnesium stearate.

Each bottle of the oral solution contains 91.35 mg of alendronate monosodium salt trihydrate, which is the molar equivalent to 70 mg of free acid. Each bottle also contains the following inactive ingredients: sodium citrate dihydrate and citric acid anhydrous as buffering agents, sodium saccharin, artificial raspberry flavor, and purified water. Added as preservatives are sodium propylparaben 0.0225% and sodium butylparaben 0.0075%.

12 CLINICAL PHARMACOLOGY

12.1 Mechanism of Action

Animal studies have indicated the following mode of action. At the cellular level, alendronate shows preferential localization to sites of bone resorption, specifically under osteoclasts. The osteoclasts adhere normally to the bone surface but lack the ruffled border that is indicative of active resorption. Alendronate does not interfere with osteoclast recruitment or attachment, but it does inhibit osteoclast activity. Studies in mice on the localization of radioactive [^{3}H]alendronate in bone showed about 10-fold higher uptake on osteoclast surfaces than on osteoblast surfaces. Bones examined 6 and 49 days after [^{3}H]alendronate administration in rats and mice, respectively, showed that normal bone was formed on top of the alendronate, which was incorporated inside the matrix. While incorporated in bone matrix, alendronate is not pharmacologically active. Thus, alendronate must be continuously administered to suppress osteoclasts on newly formed resorption surfaces. Histomorphometry in baboons and rats showed that alendronate treatment reduces bone turnover (i.e., the number of sites at which bone is remodeled). In addition, bone formation exceeds bone resorption at these remodeling sites, leading to progressive gains in bone mass.

12.2 Pharmacodynamics

Alendronate is a bisphosphonate that binds to bone hydroxyapatite and specifically inhibits the activity of osteoclasts, the bone-resorbing cells. Alendronate reduces bone resorption with no direct effect on bone formation, although the latter process is ultimately reduced because bone resorption and formation are coupled during bone turnover.

Osteoporosis in Postmenopausal Women

Osteoporosis is characterized by low bone mass that leads to an increased risk of fracture. The diagnosis can be confirmed by the finding of low bone mass, evidence of fracture on x-ray, a history of osteoporotic fracture, or height loss or kyphosis, indicative of vertebral (spinal) fracture. Osteoporosis occurs in both males and females but is most common among women following the menopause, when bone turnover increases and the rate of bone resorption exceeds that of bone formation. These changes result in progressive bone loss and lead to osteoporosis in a significant proportion of women over age 50. Fractures, usually of the spine, hip, and wrist, are the common consequences. From age 50 to age 90, the risk of hip fracture in white women increases 50-fold and the risk of vertebral fracture 15- to 30-fold. It is estimated that approximately 40% of 50-year-old women will sustain one or more osteoporosis-related fractures of the spine, hip, or wrist during their remaining lifetimes. Hip fractures, in particular, are associated with substantial morbidity, disability, and mortality.

Daily oral doses of alendronate (5, 20, and 40 mg for six weeks) in postmenopausal women produced biochemical changes indicative of dose-dependent inhibition of bone resorption, including decreases in urinary calcium and urinary markers of bone collagen degradation (such as deoxypyridinoline and cross-linked N-telopeptides of type I collagen). These biochemical changes tended to return toward baseline values as early as 3 weeks following the discontinuation of therapy with alendronate and did not differ from placebo after 7 months.

Long-term treatment of osteoporosis with FOSAMAX 10 mg/day (for up to five years) reduced urinary excretion of markers of bone resorption, deoxypyridinoline and cross-linked N-telopeptides of type I collagen, by approximately 50% and 70%, respectively, to reach levels similar to those seen in healthy premenopausal women. Similar decreases were seen in patients in osteoporosis prevention studies who received FOSAMAX 5 mg/day. The decrease in the rate of bone resorption indicated by these markers was evident as early as one month and at three to six months reached a plateau that was maintained for the entire duration of treatment with FOSAMAX. In osteoporosis treatment studies FOSAMAX 10 mg/day decreased the markers of bone formation, osteocalcin and bone specific alkaline phosphatase by approximately 50%, and total serum alkaline phosphatase by approximately 25 to 30% to reach a plateau after 6 to 12 months. In osteoporosis prevention studies FOSAMAX 5 mg/day decreased osteocalcin and total serum alkaline phosphatase by approximately 40% and 15%, respectively. Similar reductions in the rate of bone turnover were observed in postmenopausal women during one-year studies with once weekly FOSAMAX 70 mg for the treatment of osteoporosis and once weekly FOSAMAX 35 mg for the prevention of osteoporosis. These data indicate that the rate of bone turnover reached a new steady-state, despite the progressive increase in the total amount of alendronate deposited within bone.

As a result of inhibition of bone resorption, asymptomatic reductions in serum calcium and phosphate concentrations were also observed following treatment with FOSAMAX. In the long-term studies, reductions from baseline in serum calcium (approximately 2%) and phosphate (approximately 4 to 6%) were evident the first month after the initiation of FOSAMAX 10 mg. No further decreases in serum calcium were observed for the five-year duration of treatment; however, serum phosphate returned toward prestudy levels during years three through five. Similar reductions were observed with FOSAMAX 5 mg/day. In one-year studies with once weekly FOSAMAX 35 and 70 mg, similar reductions were observed at 6 and 12 months. The reduction in serum phosphate may reflect not only the positive bone mineral balance due to FOSAMAX but also a decrease in renal phosphate reabsorption.

Osteoporosis in Men

Treatment of men with osteoporosis with FOSAMAX 10 mg/day for two years reduced urinary excretion of cross-linked N-telopeptides of type I collagen by approximately 60% and bone-specific alkaline phosphatase by approximately 40%. Similar reductions were observed in a one-year study in men with osteoporosis receiving once weekly FOSAMAX 70 mg.

Glucocorticoid-Induced Osteoporosis

Sustained use of glucocorticoids is commonly associated with development of osteoporosis and resulting fractures (especially vertebral, hip, and rib). It occurs both in males and females of all ages. Osteoporosis occurs as a result of inhibited bone formation and increased bone resorption resulting in net bone loss. Alendronate decreases bone resorption without directly inhibiting bone formation.

In clinical studies of up to two years' duration, FOSAMAX 5 and 10 mg/day reduced cross-linked N-telopeptides of type I collagen (a marker of bone resorption) by approximately 60% and reduced bone-specific alkaline phosphatase and total serum alkaline phosphatase (markers of bone formation) by approximately 15 to 30% and 8 to 18%, respectively. As a result of inhibition of bone resorption, FOSAMAX 5 and 10 mg/day induced asymptomatic decreases in serum calcium (approximately 1 to 2%) and serum phosphate (approximately 1 to 8%).

Paget's Disease of Bone

Paget's disease of bone is a chronic, focal skeletal disorder characterized by greatly increased and disorderly bone remodeling. Excessive osteoclastic bone resorption is followed by osteoblastic new bone formation, leading to the replacement of the normal bone architecture by disorganized, enlarged, and weakened bone structure.

Clinical manifestations of Paget's disease range from no symptoms to severe morbidity due to bone pain, bone deformity, pathological fractures, and neurological and other complications. Serum alkaline phosphatase, the most frequently used biochemical index of disease activity, provides an objective measure of disease severity and response to therapy.

FOSAMAX decreases the rate of bone resorption directly, which leads to an indirect decrease in bone formation. In clinical trials, FOSAMAX 40 mg once daily for six months produced significant decreases in serum alkaline phosphatase as well as in urinary markers of bone collagen degradation. As a result of the inhibition of bone resorption, FOSAMAX induced generally mild, transient, and asymptomatic decreases in serum calcium and phosphate.

12.3 Pharmacokinetics

Absorption

Relative to an intravenous reference dose, the mean oral bioavailability of alendronate in women was 0.64% for doses ranging from 5 to 70 mg when administered after an overnight fast and two hours before a standardized breakfast. Oral bioavailability of the 10 mg tablet in men (0.59%) was similar to that in women when administered after an overnight fast and 2 hours before breakfast.

FOSAMAX 70 mg oral solution and FOSAMAX 70 mg tablet are equally bioavailable.

A study examining the effect of timing of a meal on the bioavailability of alendronate was performed in 49 postmenopausal women. Bioavailability was decreased (by approximately 40%) when 10 mg alendronate was administered either 0.5 or 1 hour before a standardized breakfast, when compared to dosing 2 hours before eating. In studies of treatment and prevention of osteoporosis, alendronate was effective when administered at least 30 minutes before breakfast.

Bioavailability was negligible whether alendronate was administered with or up to two hours after a standardized breakfast. Concomitant administration of alendronate with coffee or orange juice reduced bioavailability by approximately 60%.

Distribution

Preclinical studies (in male rats) show that alendronate transiently distributes to soft tissues following 1 mg/kg intravenous administration but is then rapidly redistributed to bone or excreted in the urine. The mean steady-state volume of distribution, exclusive of bone, is at least 28 L in humans. Concentrations of drug in plasma following therapeutic oral doses are too low (less than 5 ng/mL) for analytical detection. Protein binding in human plasma is approximately 78%.

Metabolism

There is no evidence that alendronate is metabolized in animals or humans.

Excretion

Following a single intravenous dose of [^{14}C]alendronate, approximately 50% of the radioactivity was excreted in the urine within 72 hours and little or no radioactivity was recovered in the feces. Following a single 10 mg intravenous dose, the renal clearance of alendronate was 71 mL/min (64, 78; 90% confidence interval [CI]), and systemic clearance did not exceed 200 mL/min. Plasma concentrations fell by more than 95% within 6 hours following intravenous administration. The terminal half-life in humans is estimated to exceed 10 years, probably reflecting release of alendronate from the skeleton. Based on the above, it is estimated that after 10 years of oral treatment with FOSAMAX (10 mg daily) the amount of alendronate released daily from the skeleton is approximately 25% of that absorbed from the gastrointestinal tract.

Specific Populations

Gender: Bioavailability and the fraction of an intravenous dose excreted in urine were similar in men and women.

Geriatric: Bioavailability and disposition (urinary excretion) were similar in elderly and younger patients. No dosage adjustment is necessary in elderly patients.

Race: Pharmacokinetic differences due to race have not been studied.

Renal Impairment: Preclinical studies show that, in rats with kidney failure, increasing amounts of drug are present in plasma, kidney, spleen, and tibia. In healthy controls, drug that is not deposited in bone is rapidly excreted in the urine. No evidence of saturation of bone uptake was found after 3 weeks dosing with cumulative intravenous doses of 35 mg/kg in young male rats. Although no formal renal impairment pharmacokinetic study has been conducted in patients, it is likely that, as in animals, elimination of alendronate via the kidney will be reduced in patients with impaired renal function. Therefore, somewhat greater accumulation of alendronate in bone might be expected in patients with impaired renal function.

No dosage adjustment is necessary for patients with creatinine clearance 35 to 60 mL/min. FOSAMAX is not recommended for patients with creatinine clearance less than 35 mL/min due to lack of experience with alendronate in renal failure.

Hepatic Impairment: As there is evidence that alendronate is not metabolized or excreted in the bile, no studies were conducted in patients with hepatic impairment. No dosage adjustment is necessary.

Drug Interactions

Intravenous ranitidine was shown to double the bioavailability of oral alendronate. The clinical significance of this increased bioavailability and whether similar increases will occur in patients given oral H_2-antagonists is unknown.

Table 6: Effect of FOSAMAX on Fracture Incidence in the Three-Year Study of FIT (patients with vertebral fracture at baseline)

	Percent of Patients			
	FOSAMAX (n=1022)	Placebo (n=1005)	Absolute Reduction in Fracture Incidence	Relative Reduction in Fracture Risk %
Patients with:				
Vertebral fractures (diagnosed by X-ray)*				
≥1 new vertebral fracture	7.9	15.0	7.1	47†
≥2 new vertebral fractures	0.5	4.9	4.4	90†
Clinical (symptomatic) fractures				
Any clinical (symptomatic) fracture	13.8	18.1	4.3	26‡
≥1 clinical (symptomatic) vertebral fracture	2.3	5.0	2.7	54§
Hip fracture	1.1	2.2	1.1	51¶
Wrist (forearm) fracture	2.2	4.1	1.9	48¶

* Number evaluable for vertebral fractures: FOSAMAX, n=984; placebo, n=966
† p<0.001,
‡ p=0.007,
§ p<0.01,
¶ p<0.05

In healthy subjects, oral prednisone (20 mg three times daily for five days) did not produce a clinically meaningful change in the oral bioavailability of alendronate (a mean increase ranging from 20 to 44%).

Products containing calcium and other multivalent cations are likely to interfere with absorption of alendronate.

13 NONCLINICAL TOXICOLOGY

13.1 Carcinogenesis, Mutagenesis, Impairment of Fertility

Harderian gland (a retro-orbital gland not present in humans) adenomas were increased in high-dose female mice (p=0.003) in a 92-week oral carcinogenicity study at doses of alendronate of 1, 3, and 10 mg/kg/day (males) or 1, 2, and 5 mg/kg/day (females). These doses are equivalent to approximately 0.1 to 1 times a maximum recommended daily dose of 40 mg (Paget's disease) based on surface area, mg/m^2. The relevance of this finding to humans is unknown.

Parafollicular cell (thyroid) adenomas were increased in high-dose male rats (p=0.003) in a 2-year oral carcinogenicity study at doses of 1 and 3.75 mg/kg body weight. These doses are equivalent to approximately 0.3 and 1 times a 40 mg human daily dose based on surface area, mg/m^2. The relevance of this finding to humans is unknown.

Alendronate was not genotoxic in the *in vitro* microbial mutagenesis assay with and without metabolic activation, in an *in vitro* mammalian cell mutagenesis assay, in an *in vitro* alkaline elution assay in rat hepatocytes, and in an *in vivo* chromosomal aberration assay in mice. In an *in vitro* chromosomal aberration assay in Chinese hamster ovary cells, however, alendronate gave equivocal results.

Alendronate had no effect on fertility (male or female) in rats at oral doses up to 5 mg/kg/day (approximately 1 times a 40 mg human daily dose based on surface area, mg/m^2).

13.2 Animal Toxicology and/or Pharmacology

The relative inhibitory activities on bone resorption and mineralization of alendronate and etidronate were compared in the Schenk assay, which is based on histological examination of the epiphyses of growing rats. In this assay, the lowest dose of alendronate that interfered with bone mineralization (leading to osteomalacia) was 6000-fold the antiresorptive dose. The corresponding ratio for etidronate was one to one. These data suggest that alendronate administered in therapeutic doses is highly unlikely to induce osteomalacia.

14 CLINICAL STUDIES

14.1 Treatment of Osteoporosis in Postmenopausal Women

Daily Dosing

The efficacy of FOSAMAX 10 mg daily was assessed in four clinical trials. Study 1, a three-year, multicenter double-blind, placebo-controlled, US clinical study enrolled 478 patients with a BMD T-score at or below minus 2.5 with or without a prior vertebral fracture; Study 2, a three-year, multicenter double blind placebo controlled Multinational clinical study enrolled 516 patients with a BMD T-score at or below minus 2.5 with or without a prior vertebral fracture; Study 3, the Three-Year Study of the Fracture Intervention Trial (FIT) a study which enrolled 2027 postmenopausal patients with at least one baseline vertebral fracture; and Study 4, the Four-Year Study of FIT: a study which enrolled 4432 postmenopausal patients with low bone mass but without a baseline vertebral fracture.

Effect on Fracture Incidence

To assess the effects of FOSAMAX on the incidence of vertebral fractures (detected by digitized radiography; approximately one third of these were clinically symptomatic), the U.S. and Multinational studies were combined in an analysis that compared placebo to the pooled dosage groups of FOSAMAX (5 or 10 mg for three years or 20 mg for two years followed by 5 mg for one year). There was a statistically significant reduction in the proportion of patients treated with FOSAMAX experiencing one or more new vertebral fractures relative to those treated with placebo (3.2% vs. 6.2%; a 48% relative risk reduction). A reduction in the total number of new vertebral fractures (4.2 vs. 11.3 per 100 patients) was also observed. In the pooled analysis, patients who received FOSAMAX had a loss in stature that was statistically significantly less than was observed in those who received placebo (-3.0 mm vs. -4.6 mm).

The Fracture Intervention Trial (FIT) consisted of two studies in postmenopausal women: the Three-Year Study of patients who had at least one baseline radiographic vertebral fracture and the Four-Year Study of patients with low bone mass but without a baseline vertebral fracture. In both studies of FIT, 96% of randomized patients completed the studies (i.e., had a closeout visit at the scheduled end of the study); approximately 80% of patients were still taking study medication upon completion.

Fracture Intervention Trial: Three-Year Study (patients with at least one baseline radiographic vertebral fracture)

This randomized, double-blind, placebo-controlled, 2027-patient study (FOSAMAX, n=1022; placebo, n=1005) demonstrated that treatment with FOSAMAX resulted in statistically significant reductions in fracture incidence at three years as shown in Table 6.

[See table 6 above]

Furthermore, in this population of patients with baseline vertebral fracture, treatment with FOSAMAX significantly reduced the incidence of hospitalizations (25.0% vs. 30.7%).

In the Three-Year Study of FIT, fractures of the hip occurred in 22 (2.2%) of 1005 patients on placebo and 11 (1.1%) of 1022 patients on FOSAMAX, p=0.047. Figure 1 displays the cumulative incidence of hip fractures in this study.

Figure 1:

Cumulative Incidence of Hip Fractures in the Three-Year Study of FIT (patients with radiographic vertebral fracture at baseline)

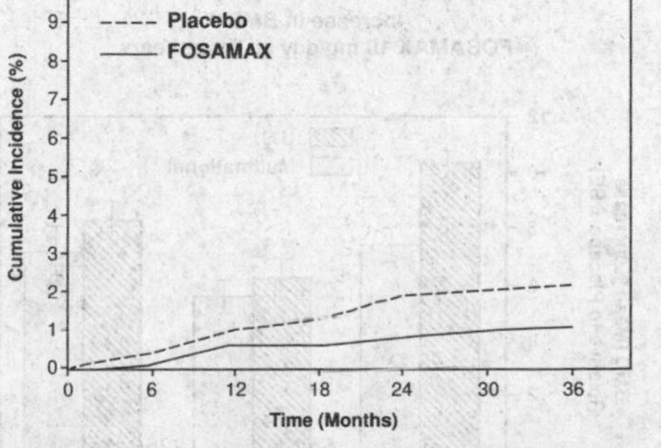

Fracture Intervention Trial: Four-Year Study (patients with low bone mass but without a baseline radiographic vertebral fracture)

This randomized, double-blind, placebo-controlled, 4432-patient study (FOSAMAX, n=2214; placebo, n=2218) further investigated the reduction in fracture incidence due to FOSAMAX. The intent of the study was to recruit women with osteoporosis, defined as a baseline femoral neck BMD at least two standard deviations below the mean for young

Table 7: Effect of FOSAMAX on Fracture Incidence in Osteoporotic* Patients in the Four-Year Study of FIT (patients without vertebral fracture at baseline)

	Percent of Patients			
	FOSAMAX (n=1545)	Placebo (n=1521)	Absolute Reduction in Fracture Incidence	Relative Reduction in Fracture Risk (%)
Patients with:				
Vertebral fractures (diagnosed by X-ray)†				
≥1 new vertebral fracture	2.5	4.8	2.3	48‡
≥2 new vertebral fractures	0.1	0.6	0.5	78§
Clinical (symptomatic) fractures				
Any clinical (symptomatic) fracture	12.9	16.2	3.3	22¶
≥1 clinical (symptomatic) vertebral fracture	1.0	1.6	0.6	41 (NS)#
Hip fracture	1.0	1.4	0.4	29 (NS)#
Wrist (forearm) fracture	3.9	3.8	-0.1	NS#

* Baseline femoral neck BMD at least 2 SD below the mean for young adult women
† Number evaluable for vertebral fractures: FOSAMAX, n=1426; placebo, n=1428
‡ p<0.001,
§ p=0.035,
¶ p=0.01
\# Not significant. This study was not powered to detect differences at these sites.

adult women. However, due to subsequent revisions to the normative values for femoral neck BMD, 31% of patients were found not to meet this entry criterion and thus this study included both osteoporotic and non-osteoporotic women. The results are shown in Table 7 for the patients with osteoporosis.

[See table 7 above]

Fracture Results Across Studies

In the Three-Year Study of FIT, FOSAMAX reduced the percentage of women experiencing at least one new radiographic vertebral fracture from 15.0% to 7.9% (47% relative risk reduction, p<0.001); in the Four-Year Study of FIT, the percentage was reduced from 3.8% to 2.1% (44% relative risk reduction, p=0.001); and in the combined U.S./Multinational studies, from 6.2% to 3.2% (48% relative risk reduction, p=0.034).

FOSAMAX reduced the percentage of women experiencing multiple (two or more) new vertebral fractures from 4.2% to 0.6% (87% relative risk reduction, p<0.001) in the combined U.S./Multinational studies and from 4.9% to 0.5% (90% relative risk reduction, p<0.001) in the Three-Year Study of FIT. In the Four-Year Study of FIT, FOSAMAX reduced the percentage of osteoporotic women experiencing multiple vertebral fractures from 0.6% to 0.1% (78% relative risk reduction, p=0.035).

Thus, FOSAMAX reduced the incidence of radiographic vertebral fractures in osteoporotic women whether or not they had a previous radiographic vertebral fracture.

Effect on Bone Mineral Density

The bone mineral density efficacy of FOSAMAX 10 mg once daily in postmenopausal women, 44 to 84 years of age, with osteoporosis (lumbar spine bone mineral density [BMD] of at least 2 standard deviations below the premenopausal mean) was demonstrated in four double-blind, placebo-controlled clinical studies of two or three years' duration. Figure 2 shows the mean increases in BMD of the lumbar spine, femoral neck, and trochanter in patients receiving FOSAMAX 10 mg/day relative to placebo-treated patients at three years for each of these studies.

Figure 2:

Osteoporosis Treatment Studies in Postmenopausal Women

Increase in BMD
FOSAMAX 10 mg/day at Three Years

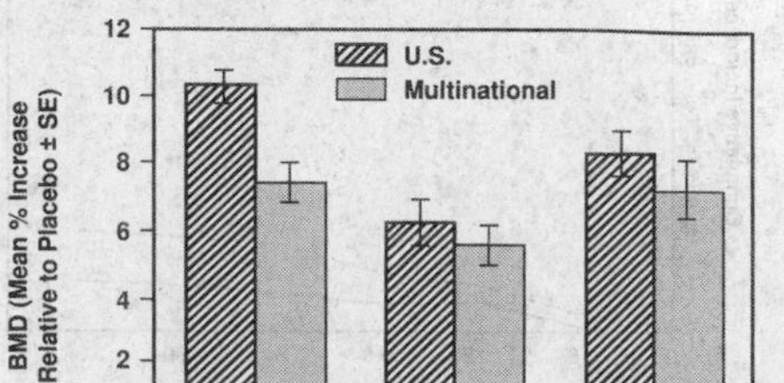

At three years significant increases in BMD, relative both to baseline and placebo, were seen at each measurement site in each study in patients who received FOSAMAX 10 mg/day. Total body BMD also increased significantly in each study, suggesting that the increases in bone mass of the spine and hip did not occur at the expense of other skeletal sites. Increases in BMD were evident as early as three months and continued throughout the three years of treatment. (See Figure 3 for lumbar spine results.) In the two-year extension of these studies, treatment of 147 patients with FOSAMAX 10 mg/day resulted in continued increases in BMD at the lumbar spine and trochanter (absolute additional increases between years 3 and 5: lumbar spine, 0.94%; trochanter, 0.88%). BMD at the femoral neck, forearm and total body were maintained. FOSAMAX was similarly effective regardless of age, race, baseline rate of bone turnover, and baseline BMD in the range studied (at least 2 standard deviations below the premenopausal mean).

Figure 3:

Osteoporosis Treatment Studies in Postmenopausal Women

Time Course of Effect of FOSAMAX 10 mg/day Versus Placebo: Lumbar Spine BMD Percent Change From Baseline

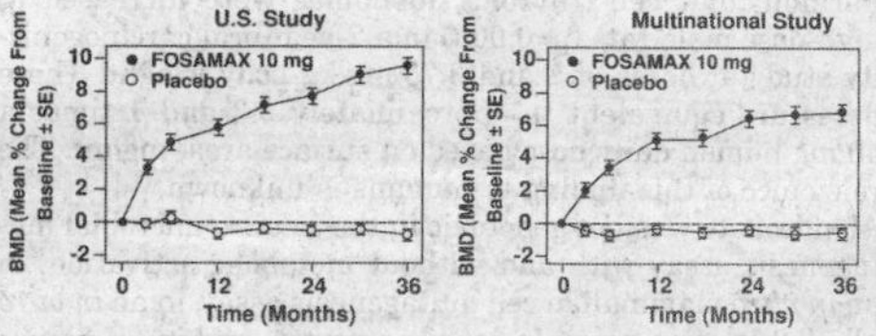

In patients with postmenopausal osteoporosis treated with FOSAMAX 10 mg/day for one or two years, the effects of treatment withdrawal were assessed. Following discontinuation, there were no further increases in bone mass and the rates of bone loss were similar to those of the placebo groups.

Bone Histology

Bone histology in 270 postmenopausal patients with osteoporosis treated with FOSAMAX at doses ranging from 1 to 20 mg/day for one, two, or three years revealed normal mineralization and structure, as well as the expected decrease in bone turnover relative to placebo. These data, together with the normal bone histology and increased bone strength observed in rats and baboons exposed to long-term alendronate treatment, support the conclusion that bone formed during therapy with FOSAMAX is of normal quality.

Effect on Height

FOSAMAX, over a three- or four-year period, was associated with statistically significant reductions in loss of height vs. placebo in patients with and without baseline radiographic vertebral fractures. At the end of the FIT studies the between-treatment group differences were 3.2 mm in the Three-Year Study and 1.3 mm in the Four-Year Study.

Weekly Dosing

The therapeutic equivalence of once weekly FOSAMAX 70 mg (n=519) and FOSAMAX 10 mg daily (n=370) was demonstrated in a one-year, double-blind, multicenter study of postmenopausal women with osteoporosis. In the primary analysis of completers, the mean increases from baseline in lumbar spine BMD at one year were 5.1% (4.8, 5.4%; 95% CI) in the 70-mg once-weekly group (n=440) and 5.4% (5.0, 5.8%; 95% CI) in the 10-mg daily group (n=330). The two treatment groups were also similar with regard to BMD increases at other skeletal sites. The results of the intention-to-treat analysis were consistent with the primary analysis of completers.

Concomitant Use with Estrogen/Hormone Replacement Therapy (HRT)

The effects on BMD of treatment with FOSAMAX 10 mg once daily and conjugated estrogen (0.625 mg/day) either alone or in combination were assessed in a two-year, double-blind, placebo-controlled study of hysterectomized postmenopausal osteoporotic women (n=425). At two years, the increases in lumbar spine BMD from baseline were significantly greater with the combination (8.3%) than with either estrogen or FOSAMAX alone (both 6.0%).

The effects on BMD when FOSAMAX was added to stable doses (for at least one year) of HRT (estrogen ± progestin) were assessed in a one-year, double-blind, placebo-controlled study in postmenopausal osteoporotic women (n=428). The addition of FOSAMAX 10 mg once daily to HRT produced, at one year, significantly greater increases in lumbar spine BMD (3.7%) vs. HRT alone (1.1%).

In these studies, significant increases or favorable trends in BMD for combined therapy compared with HRT alone were seen at the total hip, femoral neck, and trochanter. No significant effect was seen for total body BMD.

Histomorphometric studies of transiliac biopsies in 92 subjects showed normal bone architecture. Compared to placebo there was a 98% suppression of bone turnover (as assessed by mineralizing surface) after 18 months of combined treatment with FOSAMAX and HRT, 94% on FOSAMAX alone, and 78% on HRT alone. The long-term effects of combined FOSAMAX and HRT on fracture occurrence and fracture healing have not been studied.

14.2 Prevention of Osteoporosis in Postmenopausal Women

Daily Dosing

Prevention of bone loss was demonstrated in two double-blind, placebo-controlled studies of postmenopausal women 40-60 years of age. One thousand six hundred nine patients (FOSAMAX 5 mg/day; n=498) who were at least six months postmenopausal were entered into a two-year study without regard to their baseline BMD. In the other study, 447 patients (FOSAMAX 5 mg/day; n=88), who were between six months and three years postmenopause, were treated for up to three years. In the placebo-treated patients BMD losses of approximately 1% per year were seen at the spine, hip (femoral neck and trochanter) and total body. In contrast, FOSAMAX 5 mg/day prevented bone loss in the majority of patients and induced significant increases in mean bone mass at each of these sites (see Figure 4). In addition, FOSAMAX 5 mg/day reduced the rate of bone loss at the forearm by approximately half relative to placebo. FOSAMAX 5 mg/day was similarly effective in this population regardless of age, time since menopause, race and baseline rate of bone turnover.

Figure 4:

Osteoporosis Prevention Studies in Postmenopausal Women

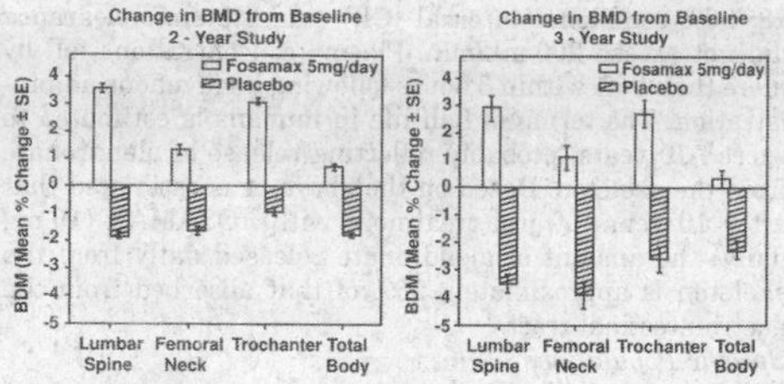

Bone Histology

Bone histology was normal in the 28 patients biopsied at the end of three years who received FOSAMAX at doses of up to 10 mg/day.

Weekly Dosing

The therapeutic equivalence of once weekly FOSAMAX 35 mg (n=362) and FOSAMAX 5 mg daily (n=361) was demonstrated in a one-year, double-blind, multicenter study of postmenopausal women without osteoporosis. In the primary analysis of completers, the mean increases from baseline in lumbar spine BMD at one year were 2.9% (2.6, 3.2%; 95% CI) in the 35-mg once-weekly group (n=307) and 3.2% (2.9, 3.5%; 95% CI) in the 5-mg daily group (n=298). The two treatment groups were also similar with regard to BMD increases at other skeletal sites. The results of the intention-to-treat analysis were consistent with the primary analysis of completers.

14.3 Treatment to Increase Bone Mass in Men with Osteoporosis

The efficacy of FOSAMAX in men with hypogonadal or idiopathic osteoporosis was demonstrated in two clinical studies.

Daily Dosing

A two-year, double-blind, placebo-controlled, multicenter study of FOSAMAX 10 mg once daily enrolled a total of 241 men between the ages of 31 and 87 (mean, 63). All patients in the trial had either a BMD T-score less than or equal to -2 at the femoral neck and less than or equal to -1 at the lumbar spine, or a baseline osteoporotic fracture and a BMD T-score less than or equal to -1 at the femoral neck. At two years, the mean increases relative to placebo in BMD in men receiving FOSAMAX 10 mg/day were significant at the following sites: lumbar spine, 5.3%; femoral neck, 2.6%; trochanter, 3.1%; and total body, 1.6%. Treatment with FOSAMAX also reduced height loss (FOSAMAX, -0.6 mm vs. placebo, -2.4 mm).

Weekly Dosing

A one-year, double-blind, placebo-controlled, multicenter study of once weekly FOSAMAX 70 mg enrolled a total of 167 men between the ages of 38 and 91 (mean, 66). Patients in the study had either a BMD T-score less than or equal to -2 at the femoral neck and less than or equal to -1 at the lumbar spine, or a BMD T-score less than or equal to -2 at the lumbar spine and less than or equal to -1 at the femoral neck, or a baseline osteoporotic fracture and a BMD T-score less than or equal to -1 at the femoral neck. At one year, the mean increases relative to placebo in BMD in men receiving FOSAMAX 70 mg once weekly were significant at the following sites: lumbar spine, 2.8%; femoral neck, 1.9%; trochanter, 2.0%; and total body, 1.2%. These increases in BMD were similar to those seen at one year in the 10 mg once-daily study.

In both studies, BMD responses were similar regardless of age (greater than or equal to 65 years vs. less than 65 years), gonadal function (baseline testosterone less than 9 ng/dL vs. greater than or equal to 9 ng/dL), or baseline BMD (femoral neck and lumbar spine T-score less than or equal to -2.5 vs. greater than -2.5).

14.4 Treatment of Glucocorticoid-Induced Osteoporosis

The efficacy of FOSAMAX 5 and 10 mg once daily in men and women receiving glucocorticoids (at least 7.5 mg/day of prednisone or equivalent) was demonstrated in two, one-year, double-blind, randomized, placebo-controlled, multicenter studies of virtually identical design, one performed in the United States and the other in 15 different countries (Multinational [which also included FOSAMAX 2.5 mg/day]). These studies enrolled 232 and 328 patients, respectively, between the ages of 17 and 83 with a variety of glucocorticoid-requiring diseases. Patients received supplemental calcium and vitamin D. Figure 5 shows the mean increases relative to placebo in BMD of the lumbar spine, femoral neck, and trochanter in patients receiving FOSAMAX 5 mg/day for each study.

Figure 5:

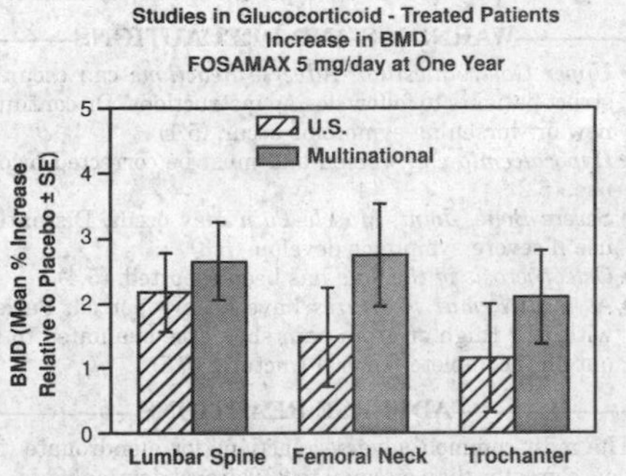

After one year, significant increases relative to placebo in BMD were seen in the combined studies at each of these sites in patients who received FOSAMAX 5 mg/day. In the placebo-treated patients, a significant decrease in BMD occurred at the femoral neck (-1.2%), and smaller decreases were seen at the lumbar spine and trochanter. Total body BMD was maintained with FOSAMAX 5 mg/day. The increases in BMD with FOSAMAX 10 mg/day were similar to those with FOSAMAX 5 mg/day in all patients except for postmenopausal women not receiving estrogen therapy. In these women, the increases (relative to placebo) with FOSAMAX 10 mg/day were greater than those with FOSAMAX 5 mg/day at the lumbar spine (4.1% vs. 1.6%) and trochanter (2.8% vs. 1.7%), but not at other sites. FOSAMAX was effective regardless of dose or duration of glucocorticoid use. In addition, FOSAMAX was similarly effective regardless of age (less than 65 vs. greater than or equal to 65 years), race (Caucasian vs. other races), gender, underlying disease, baseline BMD, baseline bone turnover, and use with a variety of common medications.

Bone histology was normal in the 49 patients biopsied at the end of one year who received FOSAMAX at doses of up to 10 mg/day.

Of the original 560 patients in these studies, 208 patients who remained on at least 7.5 mg/day of prednisone or equivalent continued into a one-year double-blind extension. After two years of treatment, spine BMD increased by 3.7% and 5.0% relative to placebo with FOSAMAX 5 and 10 mg/day, respectively. Significant increases in BMD (relative to placebo) were also observed at the femoral neck, trochanter, and total body.

After one year, 2.3% of patients treated with FOSAMAX 5 or 10 mg/day (pooled) vs. 3.7% of those treated with placebo experienced a new vertebral fracture (not significant). However, in the population studied for two years, treatment with FOSAMAX (pooled dosage groups: 5 or 10 mg for two years or 2.5 mg for one year followed by 10 mg for one year) significantly reduced the incidence of patients with a new vertebral fracture (FOSAMAX 0.7% vs. placebo 6.8%).

14.5 Treatment of Paget's Disease of Bone

The efficacy of FOSAMAX 40 mg once daily for six months was demonstrated in two double-blind clinical studies of male and female patients with moderate to severe Paget's disease (alkaline phosphatase at least twice the upper limit of normal): a placebo-controlled, multinational study and a U.S. comparative study with etidronate disodium 400 mg/day. Figure 6 shows the mean percent changes from baseline in serum alkaline phosphatase for up to six months of randomized treatment.

Figure 6:

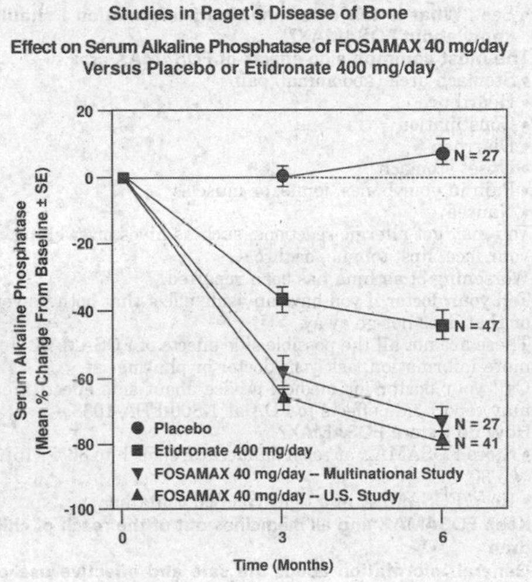

At six months the suppression in alkaline phosphatase in patients treated with FOSAMAX was significantly greater than that achieved with etidronate and contrasted with the complete lack of response in placebo-treated patients. Response (defined as either normalization of serum alkaline phosphatase or decrease from baseline greater than or equal to 60%) occurred in approximately 85% of patients treated with FOSAMAX in the combined studies vs. 30% in the etidronate group and 0% in the placebo group. FOSAMAX was similarly effective regardless of age, gender, race, prior use of other bisphosphonates, or baseline alkaline phosphatase within the range studied (at least twice the upper limit of normal).

Bone histology was evaluated in 33 patients with Paget's disease treated with FOSAMAX 40 mg/day for 6 months. As in patients treated for osteoporosis *[see Clinical Studies (14.1)]*, FOSAMAX did not impair mineralization, and the expected decrease in the rate of bone turnover was observed. Normal lamellar bone was produced during treatment with FOSAMAX, even where preexisting bone was woven and disorganized. Overall, bone histology data support the conclusion that bone formed during treatment with FOSAMAX is of normal quality.

16 HOW SUPPLIED/STORAGE AND HANDLING

How Supplied

No. 3814 — FOSAMAX Tablets, 70 mg, are white, oval, uncoated tablets with code 31 on one side and an outline of a bone image on the other:

- **NDC** 0006-0031-44 unit-of-use blister package of 4.

No. 3833 — FOSAMAX Oral Solution, 70 mg, is a clear, colorless solution with a raspberry flavor:

- **NDC** 0006-3833-34 unit-of-use cartons of 4 single-dose bottles containing 75 mL each.

Storage

FOSAMAX Tablets:

Store in a well-closed container at room temperature, 15-30°C (59-86°F).

FOSAMAX Oral Solution:

Store at 25°C (77°F), excursions permitted to 15-30°C (59-86°F). [See USP Controlled Room Temperature.] Do not freeze.

17 PATIENT COUNSELING INFORMATION

See FDA-approved patient labeling (Medication Guide).

Instruct patients to read the Medication Guide before starting therapy with FOSAMAX and to reread it each time the prescription is renewed.

17.1 Osteoporosis Recommendations, Including Calcium and Vitamin D Supplementation

Instruct patients to take supplemental calcium and vitamin D, if daily dietary intake is inadequate. Weight-bearing exercise should be considered along with the modification of certain behavioral factors, such as cigarette smoking and/or excessive alcohol consumption, if these factors exist.

17.2 Dosing Instructions

Instruct patients that the expected benefits of FOSAMAX may only be obtained when it is taken with plain water the first thing upon arising for the day at least 30 minutes before the first food, beverage, or medication of the day. Even dosing with orange juice or coffee has been shown to markedly reduce the absorption of FOSAMAX *[see Clinical Pharmacology (12.3)]*.

Instruct patients not to chew or suck on the tablet because of a potential for oropharyngeal ulceration.

Instruct patients to swallow each tablet of FOSAMAX with a full glass of water (6-8 ounces) to facilitate delivery to the stomach and thus reduce the potential for esophageal irritation. Instruct patients to drink at least 2 ounces (a quarter of a cup) of water after taking FOSAMAX oral solution to facilitate gastric emptying.

Instruct patients not to lie down for at least 30 minutes and until after their first food of the day.

Instruct patients not to take FOSAMAX at bedtime or before arising for the day. Patients should be informed that failure to follow these instructions may increase their risk of esophageal problems.

Instruct patients that if they develop symptoms of esophageal disease (such as difficulty or pain upon swallowing, retrosternal pain or new or worsening heartburn) they should stop taking FOSAMAX and consult their physician.

If patients miss a dose of once weekly FOSAMAX, instruct patients to take one dose on the morning after they remember. They should not take two doses on the same day but should return to taking one dose once a week, as originally scheduled on their chosen day.

Distributed by:
Merck Sharp & Dohme Corp., a subsidiary of
MERCK & CO., INC., Whitehouse Station, NJ 08889, USA
Manufactured by:
Merck Sharp & Dohme Corp., a subsidiary of **Merck & Co., Inc.**
Whitehouse Station, NJ 08889, USA
FOSAMAX Tablets, 70 mg, are also manufactured by:
Merck Sharp & Dohme (Italia) S.p.A.
Via Emilia, 21, 27100 - Pavia, Italy

Revised: 04/2013
uspi-mf-02171304r016

MEDICATION GUIDE
FOSAMAX® (FOSS-ah-max)
(alendronate sodium)
Tablets and Oral Solution

Read the Medication Guide that comes with FOSAMAX® before you start taking it and each time you get a refill. There may be new information. This Medication Guide does not take the place of talking with your doctor about your medical condition or treatment. Talk to your doctor if you have any questions about FOSAMAX.

What is the most important information I should know about FOSAMAX?

FOSAMAX can cause serious side effects including:

1. Esophagus problems
2. Low calcium levels in your blood (hypocalcemia)
3. Bone, joint, or muscle pain
4. Severe jaw bone problems (osteonecrosis)
5. Unusual thigh bone fractures

1. Esophagus problems.

Some people who take FOSAMAX may develop problems in the esophagus (the tube that connects the mouth and the stomach). These problems include irritation, inflammation, or ulcers of the esophagus which may sometimes bleed.

- **It is important that you take FOSAMAX exactly as prescribed to help lower your chance of getting esophagus problems. (See the section "How should I take FOSAMAX?")**
- **Stop taking FOSAMAX and call your doctor right away if you get chest pain, new or worsening heartburn, or have trouble or pain when you swallow.**

2. Low calcium levels in your blood (hypocalcemia).

FOSAMAX may lower the calcium levels in your blood. If you have low blood calcium before you start taking FOSAMAX, it may get worse during treatment. Your low blood calcium must be treated before you take FOSAMAX. Most people with low blood calcium levels do not have symptoms, but some people may have symptoms. Call your doctor right away if you have symptoms of low blood calcium such as:

- Spasms, twitches, or cramps in your muscles
- Numbness or tingling in your fingers, toes, or around your mouth

Your doctor may prescribe calcium and vitamin D to help prevent low calcium levels in your blood, while you take

FOSAMAX. Take calcium and vitamin D as your doctor tells you to.

3. **Bone, joint, or muscle pain.**
Some people who take FOSAMAX develop severe bone, joint, or muscle pain.
4. **Severe jaw bone problems (osteonecrosis).**
Severe jaw bone problems may happen when you take FOSAMAX. Your doctor should examine your mouth before you start FOSAMAX. Your doctor may tell you to see your dentist before you start FOSAMAX. It is important for you to practice good mouth care during treatment with FOSAMAX.
5. **Unusual thigh bone fractures.**
Some people have developed unusual fractures in their thigh bone. Symptoms of a fracture may include new or unusual pain in your hip, groin, or thigh.

Call your doctor right away if you have any of these side effects.

What is FOSAMAX?

FOSAMAX is a prescription medicine used to:

- Treat or prevent osteoporosis in women after menopause. It helps reduce the chance of having a hip or spinal fracture (break).
- Increase bone mass in men with osteoporosis.
- Treat osteoporosis in either men or women who are taking corticosteroid medicines.
- Treat certain men and women who have Paget's disease of the bone.

It is not known how long FOSAMAX works for the treatment and prevention of osteoporosis. You should see your doctor regularly to determine if FOSAMAX is still right for you.

FOSAMAX is not for use in children.

Who should not take FOSAMAX?

Do not take FOSAMAX if you:

- Have certain problems with your esophagus, the tube that connects your mouth with your stomach
- Cannot stand or sit upright for at least 30 minutes
- Have low levels of calcium in your blood
- Are allergic to FOSAMAX or any of its ingredients. A list of ingredients is at the end of this leaflet.

What should I tell my doctor before taking FOSAMAX?

Before you start FOSAMAX, be sure to talk to your doctor if you:

- Have problems with swallowing
- Have stomach or digestive problems
- Have low blood calcium
- Plan to have dental surgery or teeth removed
- Have kidney problems
- Have been told you have trouble absorbing minerals in your stomach or intestines (malabsorption syndrome)
- Are pregnant, or plan to become pregnant. It is not known if FOSAMAX can harm your unborn baby.
- Are breast-feeding or plan to breast-feed. It is not known if FOSAMAX passes into your milk and may harm your baby.

Especially tell your doctor if you take:

- antacids
- aspirin
- Nonsteroidal Anti-Inflammatory (NSAID) medicines

Tell your doctor about all the medicines you take, including prescription and non-prescription medicines, vitamins, and herbal supplements. Certain medicines may affect how FOSAMAX works.

Know the medicines you take. Keep a list of them and show it to your doctor and pharmacist each time you get a new medicine.

How should I take FOSAMAX?

- Take FOSAMAX exactly as your doctor tells you.
- **FOSAMAX works only if taken on an empty stomach.**
- Take FOSAMAX, **after** you get up for the day and **before** taking your first food, drink, or other medicine.
- Take FOSAMAX while you are sitting or standing.
- **Do not chew or suck on a tablet of FOSAMAX.**
- Swallow FOSAMAX tablet with a full glass (6-8 oz) of plain water only.
- **Do not** take FOSAMAX with mineral water, coffee, tea, soda, or juice.
  - If you take **Alendronate Daily**:
    - Take 1 alendronate tablet one time a day, every day **after** you get up for the day and **before** taking your first food, drink, or other medicine.
  - If you take **Once Weekly FOSAMAX**:
    - Choose the day of the week that best fits your schedule.
    - Take 1 dose of FOSAMAX every week on your chosen day **after** you get up for the day and **before** taking your first food, drink, or other medicine.
  - If you take **FOSAMAX Oral Solution**:
    - Drink your prescribed dose of FOSAMAX Oral Solution every week on your chosen day **after** you get up for the day and **before** taking your first food, drink or other medicine. Drink at least 2 ounces of plain water after you drink FOSAMAX Oral Solution.

After swallowing FOSAMAX tablet or oral solution, wait at least 30 minutes:

- Before you lie down. You may sit, stand or walk, and do normal activities like reading.
- Before you take your first food or drink except for plain water.
- Before you take other medicines, including antacids, calcium, and other supplements and vitamins.

Do not lie down for at least 30 minutes after you take FOSAMAX and after you eat your first food of the day.

If you miss a dose of FOSAMAX, do not take it later in the day. Take your missed dose on the next morning after you remember and then return to your normal schedule. Do not take 2 doses on the same day.

If you take too much FOSAMAX, call your doctor. Do not try to vomit. Do not lie down.

What are the possible side effects of FOSAMAX?

FOSAMAX may cause serious side effects.

- See **"What is the most important information I should know about FOSAMAX?"**

The most common side effects of FOSAMAX are:

- Stomach area (abdominal) pain
- Heartburn
- Constipation
- Diarrhea
- Upset stomach
- Pain in your bones, joints, or muscles
- Nausea

You may get allergic reactions, such as hives or swelling of your face, lips, tongue, or throat.

Worsening of asthma has been reported.

Tell your doctor if you have any side effect that bothers you or that does not go away.

These are not all the possible side effects of FOSAMAX. For more information, ask your doctor or pharmacist.

Call your doctor for medical advice about side effects. You may report side effects to FDA at 1-800-FDA-1088.

How do I store FOSAMAX?

- Store FOSAMAX at room temperature, 59°F to 86°F (15°C to 30°C).
- Keep FOSAMAX in a tightly closed container.

Keep FOSAMAX and all medicines out of the reach of children.

General information about the safe and effective use of FOSAMAX.

Medicines are sometimes prescribed for purposes other than those listed in a Medication Guide. Do not use FOSAMAX for a condition for which it was not prescribed. Do not give FOSAMAX to other people, even if they have the same symptoms you have. It may harm them.

This Medication Guide summarizes the most important information about FOSAMAX. If you would like more information, talk with your doctor. You can ask your doctor or pharmacist for information about FOSAMAX that is written for health professionals. For more information, go to: www.FOSAMAX.com or call 1-800-622-4477 (toll-free).

What are the ingredients in FOSAMAX?

Tablets:

Active ingredient: alendronate sodium

Inactive ingredients: microcrystalline cellulose, anhydrous lactose, croscarmellose sodium, magnesium stearate.

Oral Solution:

Active ingredient: alendronate monosodium salt trihydrate

Inactive ingredients: sodium citrate dihydrate, citric acid anhydrous, sodium saccharin, artificial raspberry flavor, water, sodium propylparaben 0.0225%, sodium butylparaben 0.0075%.

Distributed by:
Merck Sharp & Dohme Corp., a subsidiary of
MERCK & CO., INC., Whitehouse Station, NJ 08889, USA
Manufactured by:
Merck Sharp & Dohme Corp., a subsidiary of **Merck & Co., Inc.**
Whitehouse Station, NJ 08889, USA
FOSAMAX Tablets, 70 mg, are also manufactured by:
Merck Sharp & Dohme (Italia) S.p.A.
Via Emilia, 21, 27100 - Pavia, Italy

Revised: 04/2013
usmg-mf-02171304r016

This Medication Guide has been approved by the U.S. Food and Drug Administration.

Shown in Product Identification Guide, page 308

FOSAMAX® PLUS D ℞

[FOSS-ah-max PLUS D]

(alendronate sodium/cholecalciferol) tablets

HIGHLIGHTS OF PRESCRIBING INFORMATION

These highlights do not include all the information needed to use FOSAMAX PLUS D safely and effectively. See full prescribing information for FOSAMAX PLUS D.

FOSAMAX® PLUS D
(alendronate sodium/cholecalciferol) tablets
Initial U.S. Approval: 2005

RECENT MAJOR CHANGES

Indications and Usage (1.3) 04/2013
Warnings and Precautions (5.4) 04/2013

INDICATIONS AND USAGE

FOSAMAX PLUS D is a combination of a bisphosphonate and vitamin D indicated for:

- Treatment of osteoporosis in postmenopausal women (1.1)
- Treatment to increase bone mass in men with osteoporosis (1.2)

Limitations of use:

- FOSAMAX PLUS D alone should not be used to treat vitamin D deficiency. (1.3)
- Optimal duration of use has not been determined. For patients at low-risk for fracture, consider drug discontinuation after 3 to 5 years of use. (1.3)

DOSAGE AND ADMINISTRATION

- 70 mg alendronate/2800 international units vitamin D_3 or 70 mg alendronate/5600 international units vitamin D_3 tablet once weekly. (2.1, 2.2)
- Instruct patients to: (2.3)
  - Swallow tablets whole with 6-8 ounces plain water at least 30 minutes before the first food, drink, or medication of the day.
  - Not lie down for at least 30 minutes after taking FOSAMAX PLUS D and until after food.

DOSAGE FORMS AND STRENGTHS

Tablets: 70 mg/2800 international units and 70 mg/5600 international units (3)

CONTRAINDICATIONS

- Abnormalities of the esophagus which delay emptying such as stricture or achalasia (4, 5.1)
- Inability to stand/sit upright for at least 30 minutes (4, 5.1)
- Hypocalcemia (4, 5.2)
- Hypersensitivity to any component of this product (4, 6.2)

WARNINGS AND PRECAUTIONS

- *Upper Gastrointestinal Adverse Reactions* can occur. Instruct patients to follow dosing instructions. Discontinue if new or worsening symptoms occur. (5.1)
- *Hypocalcemia* can worsen and must be corrected prior to use. (5.2)
- *Severe Bone, Joint, Muscle Pain* may occur. Discontinue use if severe symptoms develop. (5.3)
- *Osteonecrosis of the Jaw* has been reported. (5.4)
- *Atypical Femur Fractures* have been reported. Patients with new thigh or groin pain should be evaluated to rule out an incomplete femoral fracture. (5.5)

ADVERSE REACTIONS

The most common adverse reactions for alendronate (incidence greater than or equal to 3%) are: abdominal pain, acid regurgitation, constipation, diarrhea, dyspepsia, musculoskeletal pain, nausea. (6.1)

To report SUSPECTED ADVERSE REACTIONS, contact Merck Sharp & Dohme Corp., a subsidiary of Merck & Co., Inc., at 1-877-888-4231 or FDA at 1-800-FDA-1088 or www.fda.gov/medwatch.

DRUG INTERACTIONS

- Calcium supplements/antacids and some medications will likely interfere with absorption of alendronate. (2.3, 7.1)
- Use caution when co-prescribing aspirin/nonsteroidal anti-inflammatory drugs that may worsen gastrointestinal irritation. (7.2, 7.3)
- Some drugs may impair the absorption or increase the catabolism of cholecalciferol (vitamin D_3). Additional vitamin D supplementation should be considered. (7.4, 7.5, 12.3)

USE IN SPECIFIC POPULATIONS

- FOSAMAX PLUS D is not indicated for use in children. (8.4)
- FOSAMAX PLUS D is not recommended in patients with severe renal insufficiency (creatinine clearance less than 35 mL/min). (5.6)

See 17 for PATIENT COUNSELING INFORMATION and Medication Guide

Revised: 04/2013

FULL PRESCRIBING INFORMATION: CONTENTS*

*** Sections or subsections omitted from the full prescribing information are not listed**

FULL PRESCRIBING INFORMATION

1 INDICATIONS AND USAGE

FOSAMAX® PLUS D is indicated for:

1.1 Treatment of Osteoporosis in Postmenopausal Women

For the treatment of osteoporosis, FOSAMAX PLUS D increases bone mass and reduces the incidence of fractures, including those of the hip and spine (vertebral compression fractures).

1.2 Treatment to Increase Bone Mass in Men with Osteoporosis

1.3 Important Limitations of Use

FOSAMAX PLUS D alone should not be used to treat vitamin D deficiency.

The optimal duration of use has not been determined. The safety and effectiveness of FOSAMAX PLUS D for the treatment of osteoporosis are based on clinical data of four years duration. All patients on bisphosphonate therapy should have the need for continued therapy re-evaluated on a periodic basis. Patients at low risk for fracture should be considered for drug discontinuation after 3 to 5 years of use. Patients who discontinue therapy should have their risk for fracture re-evaluated periodically.

2 DOSAGE AND ADMINISTRATION

2.1 Treatment of Osteoporosis in Postmenopausal Women

The recommended dosage is one 70 mg alendronate/2800 international units vitamin D_3 or one 70 mg alendronate/5600 international units vitamin D_3 tablet once weekly. For most osteoporotic women, the appropriate dose is FOSAMAX PLUS D (70 mg alendronate/5600 international units vitamin D_3) once weekly.

2.2 Treatment to Increase Bone Mass in Men with Osteoporosis

The recommended dosage is one 70 mg alendronate/2800 international units vitamin D_3 or one 70 mg alendronate/5600 international units vitamin D_3 tablet once weekly. For most osteoporotic men, the appropriate dose is FOSAMAX PLUS D (70 mg alendronate/5600 international units vitamin D_3) once weekly.

2.3 Important Administration Instructions

Instruct patients to do the following:

- Take FOSAMAX PLUS D *at least* one-half hour before the first food, beverage, or medication of the day with plain water only *[see Medication Guide]*. Other beverages (including mineral water), food, and some medications are likely to reduce the absorption of alendronate *[see Drug Interactions (7.1)]*. Waiting less than 30 minutes, or taking FOSAMAX PLUS D with food, beverages (other than plain water) or other medications will lessen the effect of alendronate by decreasing its absorption into the body.
- Take FOSAMAX PLUS D upon arising for the day. To facilitate delivery to the stomach and thus reduce the potential for esophageal irritation, a FOSAMAX PLUS D tablet should be swallowed with a full glass of water (6-8 ounces). Patients should not lie down for at least 30 minutes and until after their first food of the day. FOSAMAX PLUS D should not be taken at bedtime or before arising for the day. Failure to follow these instructions may increase the risk of esophageal adverse experiences *[see Warnings and Precautions (5.1); Medication Guide]*.

2.4 Recommendations for Calcium and Vitamin D Supplementation

Instruct patients to take supplemental calcium if dietary intake is inadequate *[see Warnings and Precautions (5.2)]*. Patients at increased risk for vitamin D insufficiency (e.g., over the age of 70 years, nursing home bound, or chronically ill) may need additional vitamin D supplementation. Patients with gastrointestinal malabsorption syndromes may require higher doses of vitamin D supplementation and measurement of 25-hydroxyvitamin D should be considered.

The recommended intake of vitamin D is 400-800 international units daily. FOSAMAX PLUS D 70 mg/2800 international units and 70 mg/5600 international units are intended to provide seven days' worth of 400 and 800 international units daily vitamin D in a single, once-weekly dose, respectively.

2.5 Administration Instructions for Missed Doses

If a once-weekly dose of FOSAMAX PLUS D is missed, instruct patients to take one tablet on the morning after they remember. They should not take two tablets on the same day but should return to taking one tablet once a week, as originally scheduled on their chosen day.

3 DOSAGE FORMS AND STRENGTHS

- 70 mg/2800 international units tablets are white to off-white, modified capsule-shaped tablets with code 710 on one side and an outline of a bone image on the other.
- 70 mg/5600 international units tablets are white to off-white, modified rectangle-shaped tablets with code 270 on one side and an outline of a bone image on the other.

4 CONTRAINDICATIONS

FOSAMAX PLUS D is contraindicated in patients with the following conditions:

- Abnormalities of the esophagus which delay esophageal emptying such as stricture or achalasia *[see Warnings and Precautions (5.1)]*
- Inability to stand or sit upright for at least 30 minutes *[see Dosage and Administration (2.3), Warnings and Precautions (5.1)]*
- Hypocalcemia *[see Warnings and Precautions (5.2)]*
- Hypersensitivity to any component of this product. Hypersensitivity reactions including urticaria and angioedema have been reported *[see Adverse Reactions (6.2)]*.

5 WARNINGS AND PRECAUTIONS

5.1 Upper Gastrointestinal Adverse Reactions

FOSAMAX PLUS D, like other bisphosphonates administered orally, may cause local irritation of the upper gastrointestinal mucosa. Because of these possible irritant effects and a potential for worsening of the underlying disease, caution should be used when FOSAMAX PLUS D is given to patients with active upper gastrointestinal problems (such as known Barrett's esophagus, dysphagia, other esophageal diseases, gastritis, duodenitis, or ulcers).

Esophageal adverse experiences, such as esophagitis, esophageal ulcers and esophageal erosions, occasionally with bleeding and rarely followed by esophageal stricture or perforation, have been reported in patients receiving treatment with oral bisphosphonates including FOSAMAX PLUS D. In some cases these have been severe and required hospitalization. Physicians should therefore be alert to any signs or symptoms signaling a possible esophageal reaction and patients should be instructed to discontinue FOSAMAX PLUS D and seek medical attention if they develop dysphagia, odynophagia, retrosternal pain or new or worsening heartburn.

The risk of severe esophageal adverse experiences appears to be greater in patients who lie down after taking oral bisphosphonates including FOSAMAX PLUS D and/or who fail to swallow oral bisphosphonates including FOSAMAX PLUS D with the recommended full glass (6-8 ounces) of water, and/or who continue to take oral bisphosphonates including FOSAMAX PLUS D after developing symptoms suggestive of esophageal irritation. Therefore, it is very important that the full dosing instructions are provided to, and understood by, the patient *[see Dosage and Administration (2.3)]*. In patients who cannot comply with dosing instructions due to mental disability, therapy with FOSAMAX PLUS D should be used under appropriate supervision.

There have been post-marketing reports of gastric and duodenal ulcers with oral bisphosphonate use, some severe and with complications, although no increased risk was observed in controlled clinical trials *[see Adverse Reactions (6.2)]*.

5.2 Mineral Metabolism

Alendronate Sodium

Hypocalcemia must be corrected before initiating therapy with FOSAMAX PLUS D *[see Contraindications (4)]*. Other disorders affecting mineral metabolism (such as vitamin D deficiency) should also be effectively treated. In patients with these conditions, serum calcium and symptoms of hypocalcemia should be monitored during therapy with FOSAMAX PLUS D.

Presumably due to the effects of alendronate on increasing bone mineral, small, asymptomatic decreases in serum calcium and phosphate may occur.

Cholecalciferol

FOSAMAX PLUS D alone should not be used to treat vitamin D deficiency (commonly defined as 25-hydroxyvitamin D level below 9 ng/mL). Patients at increased risk for vitamin D insufficiency may require higher doses of vitamin D supplementation *[see Dosage and Administration (2.4)]*. Patients with gastrointestinal malabsorption syndromes may require higher doses of vitamin D supplementation and measurement of 25-hydroxyvitamin D should be considered.

Vitamin D_3 supplementation may worsen hypercalcemia and/or hypercalciuria when administered to patients with diseases associated with unregulated overproduction of 1,25 dihydroxyvitamin D (e.g., leukemia, lymphoma, sarcoidosis). Urine and serum calcium should be monitored in these patients.

5.3 Musculoskeletal Pain

In post-marketing experience, severe and occasionally incapacitating bone, joint, and/or muscle pain has been reported in patients taking bisphosphonates that are approved for the prevention and treatment of osteoporosis *[see Adverse Reactions (6.2)]*. This category of drugs includes alendronate. Most of the patients were postmenopausal women. The time to onset of symptoms varied from one day to several months after starting the drug. Discontinue use if severe symptoms develop. Most patients had relief of symptoms after stopping. A subset had recurrence of symptoms when rechallenged with the same drug or another bisphosphonate.

In placebo-controlled clinical studies of FOSAMAX, the percentages of patients with these symptoms were similar in the FOSAMAX and placebo groups.

5.4 Osteonecrosis of the Jaw

Osteonecrosis of the jaw (ONJ), which can occur spontaneously, is generally associated with tooth extraction and/or local infection with delayed healing, and has been reported in patients taking bisphosphonates, including FOSAMAX PLUS D. Known risk factors for osteonecrosis of the jaw include invasive dental procedures (e.g., tooth extraction, dental implants, boney surgery), diagnosis of cancer, concomitant therapies (e.g., chemotherapy, corticosteroids), poor oral hygiene, and co-morbid disorders (e.g., periodontal and/or other pre-existing dental disease, anemia, coagulopathy, infection, ill-fitting dentures). The risk of ONJ may increase with duration of exposure to bisphosphonates.

For patients requiring invasive dental procedures, discontinuation of bisphosphonate treatment may reduce the risk for ONJ. Clinical judgment of the treating physician and/or oral surgeon should guide the management plan of each patient based on individual benefit/risk assessment.

Patients who develop osteonecrosis of the jaw while on bisphosphonate therapy should receive care by an oral surgeon. In these patients, extensive dental surgery to treat ONJ may exacerbate the condition. Discontinuation of bisphosphonate therapy should be considered based on individual benefit/risk assessment.

5.5 Atypical Subtrochanteric and Diaphyseal Femoral Fractures

Atypical, low-energy, or low trauma fractures of the femoral shaft have been reported in bisphosphonate-treated patients. These fractures can occur anywhere in the femoral shaft from just below the lesser trochanter to above the supracondylar flare and are transverse or short oblique in orientation without evidence of comminution. Causality has not been established as these fractures also occur in osteoporotic patients who have not been treated with bisphosphonates.

Table 1: Osteoporosis Treatment Studies in Postmenopausal Women: Adverse Experiences Considered Possibly, Probably, or Definitely Drug Related by the Investigators and Reported in Greater Than or Equal to 1% of Patients

	United States/Multinational Studies		Fracture Intervention Trial	
	FOSAMAX* % (n=196)	Placebo % (n=397)	FOSAMAX† % (n=3236)	Placebo % (n=3223)
Gastrointestinal				
abdominal pain	6.6	4.8	1.5	1.5
nausea	3.6	4.0	1.1	1.5
dyspepsia	3.6	3.5	1.1	1.2
constipation	3.1	1.8	0.0	0.2
diarrhea	3.1	1.8	0.6	0.3
flatulence	2.6	0.5	0.2	0.3
acid regurgitation	2.0	4.3	1.1	0.9
esophageal ulcer	1.5	0.0	0.1	0.1
vomiting	1.0	1.5	0.2	0.3
dysphagia	1.0	0.0	0.1	0.1
abdominal distention	1.0	0.8	0.0	0.0
gastritis	0.5	1.3	0.6	0.7
Musculoskeletal				
musculoskeletal (bone, muscle or joint) pain	4.1	2.5	0.4	0.3
muscle cramp	0.0	1.0	0.2	0.1
Nervous System/Psychiatric				
headache	2.6	1.5	0.2	0.2
dizziness	0.0	1.0	0.0	0.1
Special Senses				
taste perversion	0.5	1.0	0.1	0.0

* 10 mg/day for three years
† 5 mg/day for 2 years and 10 mg/day for either 1 or 2 additional years

Table 3: Osteoporosis Studies in Men: Adverse Experiences Considered Possibly, Probably, or Definitely Drug Related by the Investigators and Reported in Greater Than or Equal to 2% of Patients

	Two-year Study		One-year Study	
	FOSAMAX 10 mg/day % (n=146)	Placebo % (n=95)	Once Weekly FOSAMAX 70 mg % (n=109)	Placebo % (n=58)
Gastrointestinal				
acid regurgitation	4.1	3.2	0.0	0.0
flatulence	4.1	1.1	0.0	0.0
gastroesophageal reflux disease	0.7	3.2	2.8	0.0
dyspepsia	3.4	0.0	2.8	1.7
diarrhea	1.4	1.1	2.8	0.0
abdominal pain	2.1	1.1	0.9	3.4
nausea	2.1	0.0	0.0	0.0

Atypical femur fractures most commonly occur with minimal or no trauma to the affected area. They may be bilateral and many patients report prodromal pain in the affected area, usually presenting as dull, aching thigh pain, weeks to months before a complete fracture occurs. A number of reports note that patients were also receiving treatment with glucocorticoids (e.g. prednisone) at the time of fracture.

Any patient with a history of bisphosphonate exposure who presents with thigh or groin pain should be suspected of having an atypical fracture and should be evaluated to rule out an incomplete femur fracture. Patients presenting with an atypical fracture should also be assessed for symptoms and signs of fracture in the contralateral limb. Interruption of bisphosphonate therapy should be considered, pending a risk/benefit assessment, on an individual basis.

5.6 Renal Impairment

FOSAMAX PLUS D is not recommended for patients with renal impairment (creatinine clearance less than 35 mL/min).

6 ADVERSE REACTIONS

6.1 Clinical Trials Experience

Because clinical trials are conducted under widely varying conditions, adverse reaction rates observed in the clinical trials of a drug cannot be directly compared to rates in the clinical trials of another drug and may not reflect the rates observed in clinical practice.

FOSAMAX

FOSAMAX has been evaluated for safety in approximately 8000 postmenopausal women in clinical studies.

Postmenopausal Women

FOSAMAX daily

In two identically designed, three-year, placebo-controlled, double-blind, multicenter studies (United States and Multinational; n=994), discontinuation of therapy due to any clinical adverse experience occurred in 4.1% of 196 patients treated with FOSAMAX 10 mg/day and 6.0% of 397 patients treated with placebo. In the Fracture Intervention Trial (n=6459), discontinuation of therapy due to any clinical adverse experience occurred in 9.1% of 3236 patients treated with FOSAMAX 5 mg/day for 2 years and 10 mg/day for either one or two additional years and 10.1% of 3223 patients treated with placebo. Discontinuations due to upper gastrointestinal adverse experiences were: FOSAMAX, 3.2%; placebo, 2.7%. In these study populations, 49-54% had a history of gastrointestinal disorders at baseline and 54-89% used nonsteroidal anti-inflammatory drugs or aspirin at some time during the studies. Adverse experiences from these studies considered by the investigators as possibly, probably, or definitely drug related in greater than or equal to 1% of patients treated with either FOSAMAX or placebo are presented in Table 1.

[See table 1 above]

Rash and erythema have occurred.

The adverse experience profile was similar for the 401 patients treated with either 5- or 20-mg doses of FOSAMAX in the United States and Multinational studies. The adverse experience profile for the 296 patients who received continued treatment with either 5- or 10-mg doses of FOSAMAX in the two-year extension of these studies (treatment years 4 and 5) was similar to that observed during the three-year placebo-controlled period. During the extension period, of the 151 patients treated with FOSAMAX 10 mg/day, the proportion of patients who discontinued therapy due to any clinical adverse experience was similar to that during the first three years of the study.

FOSAMAX Once-Weekly

In a one-year, double-blind, multicenter study, the overall safety and tolerability profiles of once weekly FOSAMAX 70 mg and FOSAMAX 10 mg daily were similar. The adverse experiences considered by the investigators as possibly, probably, or definitely drug related in greater than or equal to 1% of patients in either treatment group are presented in Table 2.

Table 2: Osteoporosis Treatment Studies in Postmenopausal Women: Adverse Experiences Considered Possibly, Probably, or Definitely Drug Related by the Investigators and Reported in Greater Than or Equal to 1% of Patients

	Once Weekly FOSAMAX 70 mg % (n=519)	FOSAMAX 10 mg/day % (n=370)
Gastrointestinal		
abdominal pain	3.7	3.0
dyspepsia	2.7	2.2
acid regurgitation	1.9	2.4
nausea	1.9	2.4
abdominal distention	1.0	1.4
constipation	0.8	1.6
flatulence	0.4	1.6
gastritis	0.2	1.1
gastric ulcer	0.0	1.1
Musculoskeletal		
musculoskeletal (bone, muscle, joint) pain	2.9	3.2
muscle cramp	0.2	1.1

Concomitant Use With Estrogen or Estrogen/Progestin Products

In two studies (of one and two years' duration) of postmenopausal osteoporotic women (total: n=853), the safety and tolerability profile of combined treatment with FOSAMAX 10 mg once daily and estrogen ± progestin (n=354) was consistent with those of the individual treatments.

Men

In two placebo-controlled, double-blind, multicenter studies in men (a two-year study of FOSAMAX 10 mg/day and a one-year study of once weekly FOSAMAX 70 mg) the rates of discontinuation of therapy due to any clinical adverse experience were 2.7% for FOSAMAX 10 mg/day vs. 10.5% for placebo, and 6.4% for once weekly FOSAMAX 70 mg vs. 8.6% for placebo. The adverse experiences considered by the investigators as possibly, probably, or definitely drug related in greater than or equal to 2% of patients treated with either FOSAMAX or placebo are presented in Table 3.

[See table 3 above]

Laboratory Test Findings

In double-blind, multicenter, controlled studies, asymptomatic, mild, and transient decreases in serum calcium and phosphate were observed in approximately 18% and 10%, respectively, of patients taking FOSAMAX versus approximately 12% and 3% of those taking placebo. However, the incidences of decreases in serum calcium to less than 8.0 mg/dL (2.0 mM) and serum phosphate to less than or equal to 2.0 mg/dL (0.65 mM) were similar in both treatment groups.

FOSAMAX PLUS D

In a fifteen-week double-blind, multinational study in osteoporotic postmenopausal women (n=682) and men (n=35), the safety profile of FOSAMAX PLUS D (70 mg/2800 international units) was similar to that of FOSAMAX once weekly 70 mg. In the 24-week double-blind extension study in women (n=619) and men (n=33), the safety profile of FOSAMAX PLUS D (70 mg/2800 international units) administered with an additional 2800 international units vitamin D_3 was similar to that of FOSAMAX PLUS D (70 mg/2800 international units).

6.2 Post-Marketing Experience

The following adverse reactions have been identified during post-approval use of FOSAMAX and FOSAMAX PLUS D. Because these reactions are reported voluntarily from a population of uncertain size, it is not always possible to reliably estimate their frequency or establish a causal relationship to drug exposure.

Body as a Whole: hypersensitivity reactions including urticaria and angioedema. Transient symptoms of myalgia, malaise, asthenia and rarely, fever have been reported with alendronate, typically in association with initiation of treatment. Symptomatic hypocalcemia has occurred, generally in association with predisposing conditions. Peripheral edema.

Gastrointestinal: esophagitis, esophageal erosions, esophageal ulcers, esophageal stricture or perforation, and oropharyngeal ulceration. Gastric or duodenal ulcers, some severe and with complications have also been reported *[see Dosage and Administration (2.3); Warnings and Precautions (5.1); Medication Guide]*.

Localized osteonecrosis of the jaw, generally associated with tooth extraction and/or local infection with delayed healing, has been reported *[see Warnings and Precautions (5.4)]*.

Musculoskeletal: bone, joint, and/or muscle pain, occasionally severe, and incapacitating *[see Warnings and Precautions (5.3)]*; joint swelling; low-energy femoral shaft and subtrochanteric fractures *[see Warnings and Precautions (5.5)]*.

Nervous System: dizziness and vertigo.
Pulmonary: acute asthma exacerbations.
Skin: rash (occasionally with photosensitivity), pruritus, alopecia, severe skin reactions, including Stevens-Johnson syndrome and toxic epidermal necrolysis.
Special Senses: uveitis, scleritis or episcleritis.

7 DRUG INTERACTIONS

7.1 Calcium Supplements/Antacids

It is likely that calcium supplements, antacids, and some oral medications will interfere with absorption of alendronate. Therefore, instruct patients to wait at least one-half hour after taking FOSAMAX PLUS D before taking any other oral medications.

7.2 Aspirin

In clinical studies, the incidence of upper gastrointestinal adverse events was increased in patients receiving concomitant therapy with daily doses of FOSAMAX greater than 10 mg and aspirin-containing products.

7.3 Nonsteroidal Anti-Inflammatory Drugs (NSAIDs)

FOSAMAX PLUS D may be administered to patients taking NSAIDs. In a 3-year, controlled, clinical study (n=2027) during which a majority of patients received concomitant NSAIDs, the incidence of upper gastrointestinal adverse events was similar in patients taking FOSAMAX 5 or 10 mg/day compared to those taking placebo. However, since NSAID use is associated with gastrointestinal irritation, caution should be used during concomitant use with FOSAMAX PLUS D.

7.4 Drugs that May Impair the Absorption of Cholecalciferol

Olestra, mineral oils, orlistat, and bile acid sequestrants (e.g., cholestyramine, colestipol) may impair the absorption of vitamin D. Additional vitamin D supplementation should be considered *[see Clinical Pharmacology (12.3)]*.

7.5 Drugs that May Increase the Catabolism of Cholecalciferol

Anticonvulsants, cimetidine, and thiazides may increase the catabolism of vitamin D. Additional vitamin D supplementation should be considered *[see Clinical Pharmacology (12.3)]*.

8 USE IN SPECIFIC POPULATIONS

8.1 Pregnancy

Pregnancy Category C:
Alendronate Sodium

Reproduction studies in rats showed decreased postimplantation survival at 2 mg/kg/day and decreased body weight gain in normal pups at 1 mg/kg/day. Sites of incomplete fetal ossification were statistically significantly increased in rats beginning at 10 mg/kg/day in vertebral (cervical, thoracic, and lumbar), skull, and sternebral bones. The above doses ranged from one time (1 mg/kg) to 10 times (10 mg/kg) a maximum recommended daily dose of 10 mg/day based on surface area, mg/m^2. No similar fetal effects were seen when pregnant rabbits were treated at doses up to 35 mg/kg/day (40 times a 10 mg human daily dose based on surface area, mg/m^2).

Both total and ionized calcium decreased in pregnant rats at 15 mg/kg/day (13 times a 10-mg human daily dose based on surface area, mg/m^2) resulting in delays and failures of delivery. Protracted parturition due to maternal hypocalcemia occurred in rats at doses as low as 0.5 mg/kg/day (0.5 times a 10 mg human daily dose based on surface area, mg/m^2) when rats were treated from before mating through gestation. Maternotoxicity (late pregnancy deaths) occurred in the female rats treated with 15 mg/kg/day for varying periods of time ranging from treatment only during pre-mating to treatment only during early, middle, or late gestation; these deaths were lessened but not eliminated by cessation of treatment. Calcium supplementation either in the drinking water or by minipump could not ameliorate the hypocalcemia or prevent maternal and neonatal deaths due to delays in delivery; intravenous calcium supplementation prevented maternal, but not fetal deaths.

Bisphosphonates are incorporated into the bone matrix, from which they are gradually released over a period of years. The amount of bisphosphonate incorporated into adult bone, and hence, the amount available for release back into the systemic circulation, is directly related to the dose and duration of bisphosphonate use. There are no data on fetal risk in humans. However, there is a theoretical risk of fetal harm, predominantly skeletal, if a woman becomes pregnant after completing a course of bisphosphonate therapy. The impact of variables such as time between cessation of bisphosphonate therapy to conception, the particular bisphosphonate used, and the route of administration (intravenous versus oral) on the risk has not been studied.

Cholecalciferol

No data are available for cholecalciferol (vitamin D_3). Administration of high doses (greater than or equal to 10,000 international units/every other day) of ergocalciferol (vitamin D_2) to pregnant rabbits resulted in abortions and an increased incidence of fetal aortic stenosis. Administration of vitamin D_2 (40,000 international units/day) to pregnant rats resulted in neonatal death, decreased fetal weight, and impaired osteogenesis of long bones postnatally.

There are no studies in pregnant women. FOSAMAX PLUS D should be used during pregnancy only if the potential benefit justifies the potential risk to the mother and fetus.

8.3 Nursing Mothers

Cholecalciferol and some of its active metabolites pass into breast milk. It is not known whether alendronate is excreted in human milk. Because many drugs are excreted in human milk, caution should be exercised when FOSAMAX PLUS D is administered to nursing women.

8.4 Pediatric Use

FOSAMAX PLUS D is not indicated for use in children.

The efficacy and safety of alendronate were examined in a randomized, double-blind, placebo-controlled two-year study of 139 pediatric patients, aged 4-18 years, with severe osteogenesis imperfecta. One-hundred-and-nine patients were randomized to 5 mg alendronate daily (weight less than 40 kg) or 10 mg alendronate daily (weight greater than or equal to 40 kg) and 30 patients to placebo. The mean baseline lumbar spine BMD Z-score of the patients was -4.5. The mean change in lumbar spine BMD Z-score from baseline to Month 24 was 1.3 in the alendronate-treated patients and 0.1 in the placebo-treated patients. Treatment with alendronate did not reduce the risk of fracture. Sixteen percent of the alendronate patients who sustained a radiologically-confirmed fracture by Month 12 of the study had delayed fracture healing (callus remodeling) or fracture non-union when assessed radiographically at Month 24 compared with 9% of the placebo-treated patients. In alendronate-treated patients, bone histomorphometry data obtained at Month 24 demonstrated decreased bone turnover and delayed mineralization time; however, there were no mineralization defects. There were no statistically significant differences between the alendronate and placebo groups in reduction of bone pain.

8.5 Geriatric Use

Of the patients receiving FOSAMAX in the Fracture Intervention Trial (FIT), 71% (n=2302) were greater than or equal to 65 years of age and 17% (n=550) were greater than or equal to 75 years of age. Of the patients receiving FOSAMAX in the United States and Multinational osteoporosis treatment studies in women, and osteoporosis studies in men *[see Clinical Studies (14.1, 14.2)]*, 45% and 54%, respectively, were 65 years of age or over. No overall differences in efficacy or safety were observed between these patients and younger patients, but greater sensitivity of some older individuals cannot be ruled out. Dietary requirements of vitamin D_3 are increased in the elderly.

10 OVERDOSAGE

Alendronate Sodium

Significant lethality after single oral doses with alendronate was seen in female rats and mice at 552 mg/kg (3256 mg/m^2) and 966 mg/kg (2898 mg/m^2), respectively. In males, these values were slightly higher, 626 and 1280 mg/kg, respectively. There was no lethality in dogs at oral doses up to 200 mg/kg (4000 mg/m^2).

No specific information is available on the treatment of overdosage with alendronate. Hypocalcemia, hypophosphatemia, and upper gastrointestinal adverse events, such as upset stomach, heartburn, esophagitis, gastritis, or ulcer, may result from oral overdosage. Milk or antacids should be given to bind alendronate. Due to the risk of esophageal irritation, vomiting should not be induced and the patient should remain fully upright.

Dialysis would not be beneficial.

Cholecalciferol

Significant lethality occurred in mice treated with a single high oral dose of calcitriol (4 mg/kg), the hormonal metabolite of cholecalciferol.

There is limited information regarding doses of cholecalciferol associated with acute toxicity, although intermittent (yearly or twice yearly) single doses of ergocalciferol (vitamin D_2) as high as 600,000 international units have been given without reports of toxicity. Signs and symptoms of vitamin D toxicity include hypercalcemia, hypercalciuria, anorexia, nausea, vomiting, polyuria, polydipsia, weakness, and lethargy. Serum and urine calcium levels should be monitored in patients with suspected vitamin D toxicity. Standard therapy includes restriction of dietary calcium, hydration, and systemic glucocorticoids in patients with severe hypercalcemia.

Dialysis to remove vitamin D would not be beneficial.

11 DESCRIPTION

FOSAMAX PLUS D contains alendronate sodium, a bisphosphonate, and cholecalciferol (vitamin D_3).

Alendronate sodium is a bisphosphonate that acts as a specific inhibitor of osteoclast-mediated bone resorption. Bisphosphonates are synthetic analogs of pyrophosphate that bind to the hydroxyapatite found in bone.

Alendronate sodium is chemically described as (4-amino-1-hydroxybutylidene) bisphosphonic acid monosodium salt trihydrate.

The empirical formula of alendronate sodium is $C_4H_{12}NNaO_7P_2 \bullet 3H_2O$ and its formula weight is 325.12. The structural formula is:

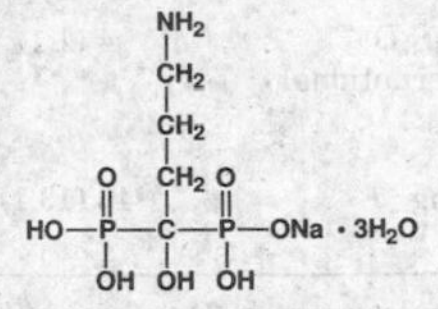

Alendronate sodium is a white, crystalline, nonhygroscopic powder. It is soluble in water, very slightly soluble in alcohol, and practically insoluble in chloroform.

Cholecalciferol (vitamin D_3) is a secosterol that is the natural precursor of the calcium-regulating hormone calcitriol (1,25 dihydroxyvitamin D_3).

The chemical name of cholecalciferol is (3β,5*Z*,7*E*)-9,10-secocholesta-5,7,10(19)-trien-3-ol. The empirical formula of cholecalciferol is $C_{27}H_{44}O$ and its molecular weight is 384.6. The structural formula is:

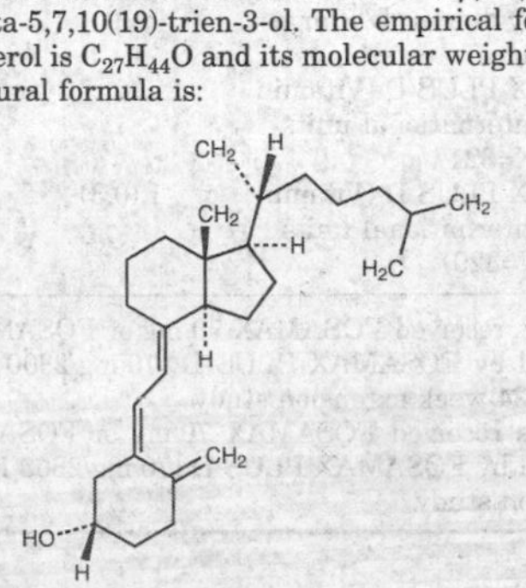

Cholecalciferol is a white, crystalline, odorless powder. Cholecalciferol is practically insoluble in water, freely soluble in usual organic solvents, and slightly soluble in vegetable oils.

FOSAMAX PLUS D for oral administration contains 91.37 mg of alendronate monosodium salt trihydrate, the molar equivalent of 70 mg of free acid, and 70 or 140 mcg of cholecalciferol, equivalent to 2800 or 5600 international units vitamin D, respectively. Each tablet contains the following inactive ingredients: microcrystalline cellulose, lactose anhydrous, medium chain triglycerides, gelatin, croscarmellose sodium, sucrose, colloidal silicon dioxide, magnesium stearate, butylated hydroxytoluene, modified food starch, and sodium aluminum silicate.

12 CLINICAL PHARMACOLOGY

12.1 Mechanism of Action

Alendronate Sodium

Animal studies have indicated the following mode of action. At the cellular level, alendronate shows preferential localization to sites of bone resorption, specifically under osteoclasts. The osteoclasts adhere normally to the bone surface but lack the ruffled border that is indicative of active resorption. Alendronate does not interfere with osteoclast recruitment or attachment, but it does inhibit osteoclast activity. Studies in mice on the localization of radioactive [^{3}H]alendronate in bone showed about 10-fold higher uptake on osteoclast surfaces than on osteoblast surfaces. Bones examined 6 and 49 days after [^{3}H]alendronate administration in rats and mice, respectively, showed that normal bone was formed on top of the alendronate, which was incorporated inside the matrix. While incorporated in bone matrix, alendronate is not pharmacologically active. Thus, alendronate must be continuously administered to suppress osteoclasts on newly formed resorption surfaces. Histomorphometry in baboons and rats showed that alendronate treatment reduces bone turnover (i.e., the number of sites at which bone is remodeled). In addition, bone formation exceeds bone resorption at these remodeling sites, leading to progressive gains in bone mass.

Cholecalciferol

Vitamin D_3 is produced in the skin by photochemical conversion of 7-dehydrocholesterol to previtamin D_3 by ultraviolet light. This is followed by non-enzymatic isomerization to vitamin D_3. In the absence of adequate sunlight exposure, vitamin D_3 is an essential dietary nutrient. Vitamin D_3 in skin and dietary vitamin D_3 (absorbed into chylomicrons) is converted to 25-hydroxyvitamin D_3 in the liver. Conversion to the active calcium-mobilizing hormone 1,25-dihydroxyvitamin D_3 (calcitriol) in the kidney is stimulated by both parathyroid hormone and hypophosphatemia. The principal action of 1,25-dihydroxyvitamin D_3 is to increase intestinal absorption of both calcium and phosphate as well as regulate serum calcium, renal calcium and phosphate excretion, bone formation and bone resorption.

Table 4: 25-hydroxyvitamin D Levels after Treatment with FOSAMAX PLUS D (70 mg/2800 international units) or FOSAMAX 70 mg at Week 15*

	Number (%) of Patients					
25-hydroxyvitamin D Ranges (ng/mL)	**<9**	**9-14**	**15-19**	**20-24**	**25-29**	**30-62**
FOSAMAX PLUS D (70 mg/2800 international units) (N=357)	4 (1.1)	37 (10.4)	87 (24.4)	84 (23.5)	82 (23.0)	63 (17.7)
FOSAMAX 70 mg (N=351)	46 (13.1)	66 (18.8)	108 (30.8)	58 (16.5)	37 (10.5)	36 (10.3)

* Patients who were vitamin D deficient (25-hydroxyvitamin D <9 ng/mL) at baseline were excluded.

Table 5: 25-hydroxyvitamin D Levels after Treatment with FOSAMAX PLUS D at Week 39

	Number (%) of Patients					
25-hydroxyvitamin D Ranges (ng/mL)	**<9**	**9-14**	**15-19**	**20-24**	**25-29**	**30-59**
FOSAMAX PLUS D (Vitamin D_3 5600 international units group)* (N=321)	0	10 (3.1)	29 (9.0)	79 (24.6)	87 (27.1)	116 (36.1)
FOSAMAX PLUS D (Vitamin D_3 2800 international units group)† (N=320)	1 (0.3)	17 (5.3)	56 (17.5)	80 (25.0)	74 (23.1)	92 (28.8)

* Patients received FOSAMAX 70 mg or FOSAMAX PLUS D (70 mg/2800 international units) for the 15-week base study followed by FOSAMAX PLUS D (70 mg/2800 international units) and 2800 international units additional vitamin D_3 for the 24-week extension study.

† Patients received FOSAMAX 70 mg or FOSAMAX PLUS D (70 mg/2800 international units) for 15-week base study followed by FOSAMAX PLUS D (70 mg/2800 international units) and placebo for the additional vitamin D_3 for 24-week extension study.

Vitamin D is required for normal bone formation. Vitamin D insufficiency develops when both sunlight exposure and dietary intake are inadequate. Insufficiency is associated with negative calcium balance, increased parathyroid hormone levels, bone loss, and increased risk of skeletal fracture. In severe cases, deficiency results in more severe hyperparathyroidism, hypophosphatemia, proximal muscle weakness, bone pain and osteomalacia.

12.2 Pharmacodynamics

Alendronate Sodium

Alendronate is a bisphosphonate that binds to bone hydroxyapatite and specifically inhibits the activity of osteoclasts, the bone-resorbing cells. Alendronate reduces bone resorption with no direct effect on bone formation, although the latter process is ultimately reduced because bone resorption and formation are coupled during bone turnover.

Daily oral doses of alendronate (5, 20, and 40 mg for six weeks) in postmenopausal women produced biochemical changes indicative of dose-dependent inhibition of bone resorption, including decreases in urinary calcium and urinary markers of bone collagen degradation (such as deoxypyridinoline and cross-linked N-telopeptides of type I collagen). These biochemical changes tended to return toward baseline values as early as 3 weeks following the discontinuation of therapy with alendronate and did not differ from placebo after 7 months.

Long-term treatment of osteoporosis with FOSAMAX 10 mg/day (for up to five years) reduced urinary excretion of markers of bone resorption, deoxypyridinoline and cross-linked N-telopeptides of type l collagen, by approximately 50% and 70%, respectively, to reach levels similar to those seen in healthy premenopausal women. The decrease in the rate of bone resorption indicated by these markers was evident as early as one month and at three to six months reached a plateau that was maintained for the entire duration of treatment with FOSAMAX. In osteoporosis treatment studies FOSAMAX 10 mg/day decreased the markers of bone formation, osteocalcin and bone specific alkaline phosphatase by approximately 50%, and total serum alkaline phosphatase by approximately 25 to 30% to reach a plateau after 6 to 12 months. Similar reductions in the rate of bone turnover were observed in postmenopausal women during one-year studies with once weekly FOSAMAX 70 mg for the treatment of osteoporosis. These data indicate that the rate of bone turnover reached a new steady-state, despite the progressive increase in the total amount of alendronate deposited within bone.

As a result of inhibition of bone resorption, asymptomatic reductions in serum calcium and phosphate concentrations were also observed following treatment with FOSAMAX. In the long-term studies, reductions from baseline in serum calcium (approximately 2%) and phosphate (approximately 4 to 6%) were evident the first month after the initiation of FOSAMAX 10 mg. No further decreases in serum calcium were observed for the five-year duration of treatment; however, serum phosphate returned toward prestudy levels during years three through five. In one-year studies with once weekly FOSAMAX 70 mg, similar reductions were observed at 6 and 12 months. The reduction in serum phosphate may reflect not only the positive bone mineral balance due to FOSAMAX but also a decrease in renal phosphate reabsorption.

Osteoporosis in Men

Treatment of men with osteoporosis with FOSAMAX 10 mg/day for two years reduced urinary excretion of cross-linked N-telopeptides of type I collagen by approximately 60% and bone-specific alkaline phosphatase by approximately 40%. Similar reductions were observed in a one-year study in men with osteoporosis receiving once weekly FOSAMAX 70 mg.

Cholecalciferol

Vitamin D is required for normal bone formation. Vitamin D insufficiency is associated with negative calcium balance, leading to increased parathyroid hormone levels and worsening of bone loss associated with osteoporosis. When taken without vitamin D, alendronate is also associated with a reduction in serum calcium concentrations and increased parathyroid hormone levels. In a 15-week trial, 717 postmenopausal women and men, mean age 67 years, with osteoporosis (lumbar spine bone mineral density [BMD] of at least 2.5 standard deviations below the premenopausal mean) were randomized to receive either weekly FOSAMAX PLUS D 70 mg/2800 international units vitamin D or weekly FOSAMAX 70 mg alone with no vitamin D supplementation. Patients who were vitamin D deficient (25-hydroxyvitamin D less than 9 ng/mL) at baseline were excluded. Treatment with FOSAMAX PLUS D 70 mg/2800 international units resulted in a smaller reduction in serum calcium levels (-0.9%) when compared to FOSAMAX 70 mg alone (-1.4%). As well, treatment with FOSAMAX PLUS D 70 mg/2800 international units resulted in a significantly smaller increase in parathyroid hormone levels when compared to FOSAMAX 70 mg alone (14% and 24%, respectively).

The sufficiency of patients' vitamin D status is best assessed by measuring 25-hydroxyvitamin D levels. In the 15-week trial mentioned above, baseline 25-hydroxyvitamin D levels were 22.2 ng/mL in the FOSAMAX PLUS D group and 22.1 ng/mL in the FOSAMAX only group. After 15 weeks of treatment, the mean levels were 23.1 ng/mL and 18.4 ng/mL in the FOSAMAX PLUS D and FOSAMAX only groups, respectively. The final levels of 25-hydroxyvitamin D at Week 15 are summarized in Table 4.

[See table 4 above]

Patients (n=652) who completed the above 15-week trial continued in a 24-week extension in which all received FOSAMAX PLUS D (70 mg/2800 international units) and were randomly assigned to receive either additional once weekly vitamin D_3 2800 international units (Vitamin D_3 5600 international units group) or matching placebo (Vitamin D_3 2800 international units group). After 24 weeks of extended treatment (Week 39 from original baseline), the mean levels of 25-hydroxyvitamin D were 27.9 ng/mL and 25.6 ng/mL in the vitamin D_3 5600 international units group and vitamin D_3 2800 international units group, respectively. The percentage of patients with hypercalciuria at Week 39 was not statistically different between treatment groups.

The distribution of the final levels of 25-hydroxyvitamin D at Week 39 is summarized in Table 5.

[See table 5 below]

12.3 Pharmacokinetics

Absorption

Alendronate Sodium

Relative to an intravenous reference dose, the mean oral bioavailability of alendronate in women was 0.64% for doses ranging from 5 to 70 mg when administered after an overnight fast and two hours before a standardized breakfast. Oral bioavailability of the 10-mg tablet in men (0.59%) was similar to that in women when administered after an overnight fast and 2 hours before breakfast.

In a study, the alendronate in the FOSAMAX PLUS D (70 mg/2800 international units) tablet and the FOSAMAX (alendronate sodium) 70-mg tablet were found to be equally bioavailable. In a separate study, the alendronate in the FOSAMAX PLUS D (70 mg/5600 international units) tablet was found to be equally bioavailable to the alendronate in the FOSAMAX (alendronate sodium) 70-mg tablet.

A study examining the effect of timing of a meal on the bioavailability of alendronate was performed in 49 postmenopausal women. Bioavailability was decreased (by approximately 40%) when 10 mg alendronate was administered either 0.5 or 1 hour before a standardized breakfast, when compared to dosing 2 hours before eating. In studies of treatment and prevention of osteoporosis, alendronate was effective when administered at least 30 minutes before breakfast.

Bioavailability was negligible whether alendronate was administered with or up to two hours after a standardized breakfast. Concomitant administration of alendronate with coffee or orange juice reduced bioavailability by approximately 60%.

Cholecalciferol

Following administration of FOSAMAX PLUS D (70 mg/2800 international units) after an overnight fast and two hours before a standard meal, the baseline adjusted mean area under the serum-concentration-time curve ($AUC_{0\text{-}120\ hrs}$) for vitamin D_3 was 120.7 ng-hr/mL. The baseline adjusted mean maximal serum concentration (C_{max}) of vitamin D_3 was 4.0 ng/mL, and the baseline adjusted mean time to maximal serum concentration (T_{max}) was 10.6 hrs. The bioavailability of the 2800 international units vitamin D_3 in FOSAMAX PLUS D is similar to 2800 international units vitamin D_3 administered alone.

In a separate study, the baseline adjusted mean $AUC_{0\text{-}80\ hrs}$ and baseline adjusted mean C_{max} for vitamin D_3 were 355.6 ng-hr/mL and 10.8 ng/mL, respectively. The baseline adjusted mean T_{max} was 9.2 hrs. The bioavailability of the 5600 international units vitamin D_3 in the FOSAMAX PLUS D is similar to 5600 international units vitamin D_3 administered as two 2800 international units vitamin D_3 tablets.

Distribution

Alendronate Sodium

Preclinical studies (in male rats) show that alendronate transiently distributes to soft tissues following 1 mg/kg intravenous administration but is then rapidly redistributed to bone or excreted in the urine. The mean steady-state volume of distribution, exclusive of bone, is at least 28 L in humans. Concentrations of drug in plasma following therapeutic oral doses are too low (less than 5 ng/mL) for analytical detection. Protein binding in human plasma is approximately 78%.

Cholecalciferol

Following absorption, vitamin D_3 enters the blood as part of chylomicrons. Vitamin D_3 is rapidly distributed mostly to the liver where it undergoes metabolism to 25-hydroxyvitamin D_3, the major storage form. Lesser amounts are distributed to adipose tissue and stored as vitamin D_3 at these sites for later release into the circulation. Circulating vitamin D_3 is bound to vitamin D-binding protein.

Metabolism

Alendronate Sodium

There is no evidence that alendronate is metabolized in animals or humans.

Cholecalciferol

Vitamin D_3 is rapidly metabolized by hydroxylation in the liver to 25-hydroxyvitamin D_3, and subsequently metabolized in the kidney to 1,25-dihydroxyvitamin D_3, which represents the biologically active form. Further hydroxylation occurs prior to elimination. A small percentage of vitamin D_3 undergoes glucuronidation prior to elimination.

Excretion
Alendronate Sodium
Following a single intravenous dose of [^{14}C]alendronate, approximately 50% of the radioactivity was excreted in the urine within 72 hours and little or no radioactivity was recovered in the feces. Following a single 10-mg intravenous dose, the renal clearance of alendronate was 71 mL/min (64, 78; 90% confidence interval [CI]), and systemic clearance did not exceed 200 mL/min. Plasma concentrations fell by more than 95% within 6 hours following intravenous administration. The terminal half-life in humans is estimated to exceed 10 years, probably reflecting release of alendronate from the skeleton. Based on the above, it is estimated that after 10 years of oral treatment with FOSAMAX (10 mg daily) the amount of alendronate released daily from the skeleton is approximately 25% of that absorbed from the gastrointestinal tract.
Cholecalciferol
When radioactive vitamin D_3 was intravenously administered to healthy subjects, the mean urinary excretion of radioactivity after 48 hours was 2.4% of the administered dose, and the mean fecal excretion of radioactivity after 48 hours was 4.9% of the administered dose. In both cases, the excreted radioactivity was almost exclusively as metabolites of the parent. The mean half-life of baseline adjusted vitamin D_3 in the serum following an oral dose of FOSAMAX PLUS D is approximately 14 hours.
Special Populations
Pediatric: The oral bioavailability of alendronate in children was similar to that observed in adults; however, FOSAMAX PLUS D is not indicated for use in children *[see Use in Specific Populations (8.4)]*.
Gender: Bioavailability and the fraction of an intravenous dose of alendronate excreted in urine were similar in men and women.
Geriatric:
Alendronate Sodium
Bioavailability and disposition of alendronate (urinary excretion) were similar in elderly and younger patients. No dosage adjustment of alendronate is necessary.
Cholecalciferol
Dietary requirements of vitamin D_3 are increased in the elderly.
Race: Pharmacokinetic differences due to race have not been studied.
Renal Impairment:
Alendronate Sodium
Preclinical studies show that, in rats with kidney failure, increasing amounts of drug are present in plasma, kidney, spleen, and tibia. In healthy controls, drug that is not deposited in bone is rapidly excreted in the urine. No evidence of saturation of bone uptake was found after 3 weeks dosing with cumulative intravenous doses of 35 mg/kg in young male rats. Although no clinical information is available, it is likely that, as in animals, elimination of alendronate via the kidney will be reduced in patients with impaired renal function. Therefore, somewhat greater accumulation of alendronate in bone might be expected in patients with impaired renal function.
No dosage adjustment is necessary for patients with mild-to-moderate renal insufficiency (creatinine clearance 35 to 60 mL/min). FOSAMAX PLUS D is not recommended for patients with more severe renal insufficiency (creatinine clearance less than 35 mL/min) due to lack of experience with alendronate in renal failure.
Cholecalciferol
Patients with renal insufficiency will have decreased ability to form the active 1,25-dihydroxyvitamin D_3 metabolite.
Hepatic Impairment:
Alendronate Sodium
As there is evidence that alendronate is not metabolized or excreted in the bile, no studies were conducted in patients with hepatic insufficiency. No dosage adjustment is necessary.
Cholecalciferol
Vitamin D_3 may not be adequately absorbed in patients who have malabsorption due to inadequate bile production.
Drug Interactions
Alendronate Sodium
Intravenous ranitidine was shown to double the bioavailability of oral alendronate. The clinical significance of this increased bioavailability and whether similar increases will occur in patients given oral H_2-antagonists is unknown.
In healthy subjects, oral prednisone (20 mg three times daily for five days) did not produce a clinically meaningful change in the oral bioavailability of alendronate (a mean increase ranging from 20 to 44%).
Products containing calcium and other multivalent cations are likely to interfere with absorption of alendronate.
Cholecalciferol
Olestra, mineral oils, orlistat, and bile acid sequestrants (e.g., cholestyramine, colestipol) may impair the absorption of vitamin D. Anticonvulsants, cimetidine, and thiazides may increase the catabolism of vitamin D.

Table 6: Effect of FOSAMAX on Fracture Incidence in the Three-Year Study of FIT (patients with vertebral fracture at baseline)

	Percent of Patients			
	FOSAMAX (n=1022)	Placebo (n=1005)	Absolute Reduction in Fracture Incidence	Relative Reduction in Fracture Risk %
Patients with:				
Vertebral fractures (diagnosed by X-ray)*				
≥1 new vertebral fracture	7.9	15.0	7.1	47†
≥2 new vertebral fractures	0.5	4.9	4.4	90†
Clinical (symptomatic) fractures				
Any clinical (symptomatic) fracture	13.8	18.1	4.3	26‡
≥1 clinical (symptomatic) vertebral fracture	2.3	5.0	2.7	54§
Hip fracture	1.1	2.2	1.1	51¶
Wrist (forearm) fracture	2.2	4.1	1.9	48¶

* Number evaluable for vertebral fractures: FOSAMAX, n=984; placebo, n=966
† $p<0.001$
‡ $p=0.007$
§ $p<0.01$
¶ $p<0.05$

13 NONCLINICAL TOXICOLOGY

13.1 Carcinogenesis, Mutagenesis, Impairment of Fertility

The following data are based on findings for the individual components of FOSAMAX PLUS D.
Alendronate Sodium
Harderian gland (a retro-orbital gland not present in humans) adenomas were increased in high-dose female mice (p=0.003) in a 92-week oral carcinogenicity study at doses of alendronate of 1, 3, and 10 mg/kg/day (males) or 1, 2, and 5 mg/kg/day (females). These doses are equivalent to 0.5 to 4 times a maximum recommended daily dose of 10 mg based on surface area, mg/m^2. The relevance of this finding to humans is unknown.
Parafollicular cell (thyroid) adenomas were increased in high-dose male rats (p=0.003) in a 2-year oral carcinogenicity study at doses of 1 and 3.75 mg/kg body weight. These doses are equivalent to 1 and 4 times a 10-mg human daily dose based on surface area, mg/m^2. The relevance of this finding to humans is unknown.
Alendronate was not genotoxic in the *in vitro* microbial mutagenesis assay with and without metabolic activation, in an *in vitro* mammalian cell mutagenesis assay, in an *in vitro* alkaline elution assay in rat hepatocytes, and in an *in vivo* chromosomal aberration assay in mice. In an *in vitro* chromosomal aberration assay in Chinese hamster ovary cells, however, alendronate gave equivocal results.
Alendronate had no effect on fertility (male or female) in rats at oral doses up to 5 mg/kg/day (4 times a 10-mg human daily dose based on surface area, mg/m^2).
Cholecalciferol
The carcinogenic potential of cholecalciferol (vitamin D_3) has not been studied in rodents. Calcitriol, the hormonal metabolite of cholecalciferol, was not genotoxic in the Ames microbial mutagenesis assay with or without metabolic activation, and in an *in vivo* micronucleus assay in mice.
Ergocalciferol (vitamin D_2) at high doses (150,000 to 200,000 international units/kg/day) administered prior to mating resulted in altered estrous cycle and inhibition of pregnancy in rats. The potential effect of cholecalciferol on male fertility is unknown in rats.

13.2 Animal Toxicology and/or Pharmacology

The relative inhibitory activities on bone resorption and mineralization of alendronate and etidronate were compared in the Schenk assay, which is based on histological examination of the epiphyses of growing rats. In this assay, the lowest dose of alendronate that interfered with bone mineralization (leading to osteomalacia) was 6000-fold the antiresorptive dose. The corresponding ratio for etidronate was one to one. These data suggest that alendronate administered in therapeutic doses is highly unlikely to induce osteomalacia.

14 CLINICAL STUDIES

14.1 Treatment of Postmenopausal Osteoporosis

Effect on Fracture Incidence
Data on the effects of FOSAMAX on fracture incidence are derived from three clinical studies of postmenopausal women, 44 to 84 years of age, with osteoporosis: 1) U.S. and Multinational combined: a study of patients with a lumbar spine BMD T-score at or below minus 2.5 with or without a prior vertebral fracture, 2) Three-Year Study of the Fracture Intervention Trial (FIT): a study of patients with at least one baseline vertebral fracture, and 3) Four-Year Study of FIT: a study of patients with low bone mass but without a baseline vertebral fracture.
To assess the effects of FOSAMAX on the incidence of vertebral fractures (detected by digitized radiography; approximately one third of these were clinically symptomatic), the U.S. (478 patients) and Multinational (516 patients in 15 countries) studies (of virtually identical design) were combined in an analysis that compared placebo to the pooled dosage groups of FOSAMAX (5 or 10 mg for three years or 20 mg for two years followed by 5 mg for one year). There was a statistically significant reduction in the proportion of patients treated with FOSAMAX experiencing one or more new vertebral fractures relative to those treated with placebo (3.2% vs. 6.2%; a 48% relative risk reduction). A reduction in the total number of new vertebral fractures (4.2 vs. 11.3 per 100 patients) was also observed. In the pooled analysis, patients who received FOSAMAX had a loss in stature that was statistically significantly less than was observed in those who received placebo (-3.0 mm vs. -4.6 mm).
The Fracture Intervention Trial (FIT) consisted of two studies in postmenopausal women: the Three-Year Study of patients who had at least one baseline radiographic vertebral fracture and the Four-Year Study of patients with low bone mass but without a baseline vertebral fracture. In both studies of FIT, 96% of randomized patients completed the studies (i.e., had a closeout visit at the scheduled end of the study); approximately 80% of patients were still taking study medication upon completion.
Fracture Intervention Trial: Three-Year Study (patients with at least one baseline radiographic vertebral fracture)
This randomized, double-blind, placebo-controlled, 2027-patient study (FOSAMAX, n=1022; placebo, n=1005) demonstrated that treatment with FOSAMAX resulted in statistically significant reductions in fracture incidence at three years as shown in Table 6.
[See table 6 above]
Furthermore, in this population of patients with baseline vertebral fracture, treatment with FOSAMAX significantly reduced the incidence of hospitalizations (25.0% vs. 30.7%).
In the Three-Year Study of FIT, fractures of the hip occurred in 22 (2.2%) of 1005 patients on placebo and 11 (1.1%) of 1022 patients on FOSAMAX, p=0.047. Figure 1 displays the cumulative incidence of hip fractures in this study.

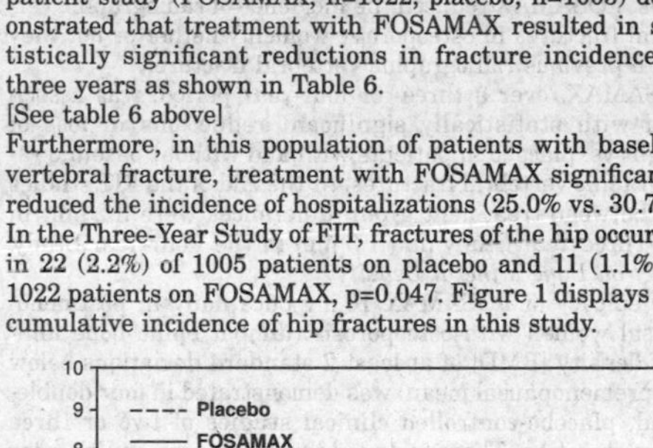

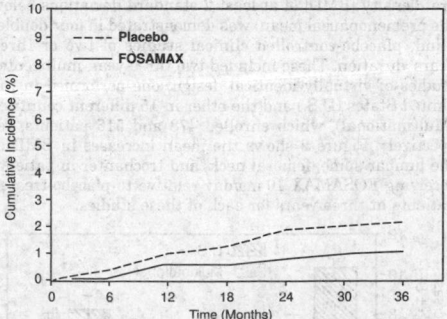

Figure 1: Cumulative Incidence of Hip Fractures in the Three-Year Study of FIT (patients with radiographic vertebral fracture at baseline)

Fracture Intervention Trial: Four-Year Study (patients with low bone mass but without a baseline radiographic vertebral fracture)
This randomized, double-blind, placebo-controlled, 4432-patient study (FOSAMAX, n=2214; placebo, n=2218) further investigated the reduction in fracture incidence due to FOSAMAX. The intent of the study was to recruit women with osteoporosis, defined as a baseline femoral neck BMD at least two standard deviations below the mean for young

Table 7: Effect of FOSAMAX on Fracture Incidence in Osteoporotic* Patients in the Four-Year Study of FIT (patients without vertebral fracture at baseline)

	Percent of Patients			
	FOSAMAX (n=1545)	Placebo (n=1521)	Absolute Reduction in Fracture Incidence	Relative Reduction in Fracture Risk (%)
Patients with:				
Vertebral fractures (diagnosed by X-ray)†				
≥1 new vertebral fracture	2.5	4.8	2.3	48‡
≥2 new vertebral fractures	0.1	0.6	0.5	78§
Clinical (symptomatic) fractures				
Any clinical (symptomatic) fracture	12.9	16.2	3.3	22¶
≥1 clinical (symptomatic) vertebral fracture	1.0	1.6	0.6	41 (NS)#
Hip fracture	1.0	1.4	0.4	29 (NS)#
Wrist (forearm) fracture	3.9	3.8	-0.1	NS#

* Baseline femoral neck BMD at least 2 SD below the mean for young adult women
† Number evaluable for vertebral fractures: FOSAMAX, n=1426; placebo, n=1428
‡ p<0.001
§ p=0.035
¶ p=0.01
# Not significant. This study was not powered to detect differences at these sites.

adult women. However, due to subsequent revisions to the normative values for femoral neck BMD, 31% of patients were found not to meet this entry criterion and thus this study included both osteoporotic and non-osteoporotic women. The results are shown in Table 7 below for the patients with osteoporosis.

[See table 7 above]

Fracture Results Across Studies

In the Three-Year Study of FIT, FOSAMAX reduced the percentage of women experiencing at least one new radiographic vertebral fracture from 15.0% to 7.9% (47% relative risk reduction, p<0.001); in the Four-Year Study of FIT, the percentage was reduced from 3.8% to 2.1% (44% relative risk reduction, p=0.001); and in the combined U.S./Multinational studies, from 6.2% to 3.2% (48% relative risk reduction, p=0.034).

FOSAMAX reduced the percentage of women experiencing multiple (two or more) new vertebral fractures from 4.2% to 0.6% (87% relative risk reduction, p<0.001) in the combined U.S./Multinational studies and from 4.9% to 0.5% (90% relative risk reduction, p<0.001) in the Three-Year Study of FIT. In the Four-Year Study of FIT, FOSAMAX reduced the percentage of osteoporotic women experiencing multiple vertebral fractures from 0.6% to 0.1% (78% relative risk reduction, p=0.035).

Thus, FOSAMAX reduced the incidence of radiographic vertebral fractures in osteoporotic women whether or not they had a previous radiographic vertebral fracture.

FOSAMAX, over a three- or four-year period, was associated with statistically significant reductions in loss of height vs. placebo in patients with and without baseline radiographic vertebral fractures. At the end of the FIT studies the between-treatment group differences were 3.2 mm in the Three-Year Study and 1.3 mm in the Four-Year Study.

Effect on Bone Mineral Density

The efficacy of FOSAMAX 10 mg once daily in postmenopausal women with osteoporosis (lumbar spine bone mineral density [BMD] of at least 2 standard deviations below the premenopausal mean) was demonstrated in four double-blind, placebo-controlled clinical studies of two or three years' duration. These included two three-year, multicenter studies of virtually identical design, one performed in the United States (U.S.) and the other in 15 different countries (Multinational), which enrolled 478 and 516 patients, respectively. Figure 2 shows the mean increases in BMD of the lumbar spine, femoral neck, and trochanter in patients receiving FOSAMAX 10 mg/day relative to placebo-treated patients at three years for each of these studies.

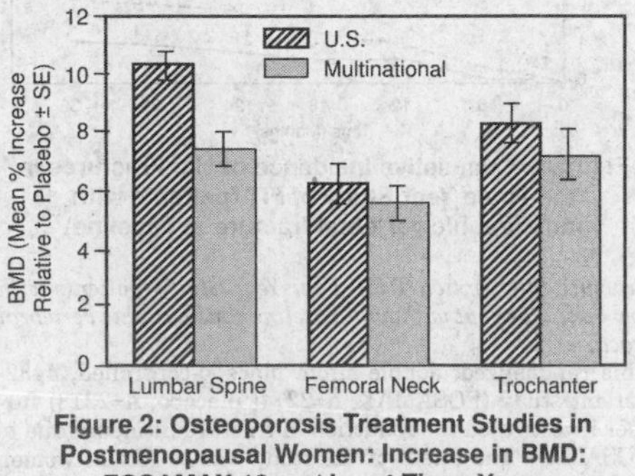

Figure 2: Osteoporosis Treatment Studies in Postmenopausal Women: Increase in BMD: FOSAMAX 10 mg/day at Three Years

At three years significant increases in BMD, relative both to baseline and placebo, were seen at each measurement site in each study in patients who received FOSAMAX 10 mg/day. Total body BMD also increased significantly in each study, suggesting that the increases in bone mass of the spine and hip did not occur at the expense of other skeletal sites. Increases in BMD were evident as early as three months and continued throughout the three years of treatment. (See figure 3 for lumbar spine results.) In the two-year extension of these studies, treatment of 147 patients with FOSAMAX 10 mg/day resulted in continued increases in BMD at the lumbar spine and trochanter (absolute additional increases between years 3 and 5: lumbar spine, 0.94%; trochanter, 0.88%). BMD at the femoral neck, forearm and total body were maintained. FOSAMAX was similarly effective regardless of age, race, baseline rate of bone turnover, and baseline BMD in the range studied (at least 2 standard deviations below the premenopausal mean).

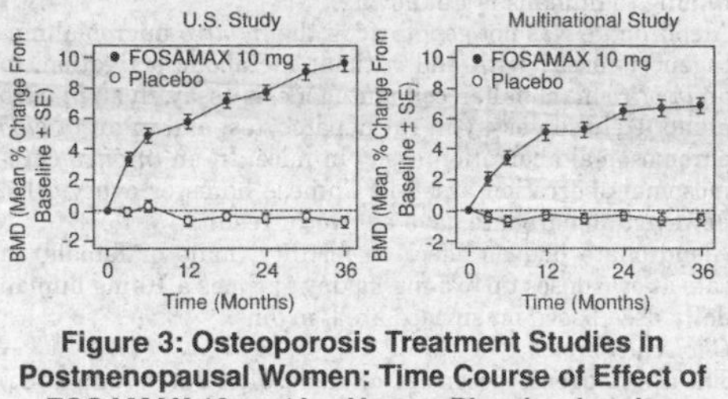

Figure 3: Osteoporosis Treatment Studies in Postmenopausal Women: Time Course of Effect of FOSAMAX 10 mg/day Versus Placebo: Lumbar Spine BMD Percent Change From Baseline

In patients with postmenopausal osteoporosis treated with FOSAMAX 10 mg/day for one or two years, the effects of treatment withdrawal were assessed. Following discontinuation, there were no further increases in bone mass and the rates of bone loss were similar to those of the placebo groups.

The therapeutic equivalence of once weekly FOSAMAX 70 mg (n=519) and FOSAMAX 10 mg daily (n=370) was demonstrated in a one-year, double-blind, multicenter study of postmenopausal women with osteoporosis. In the primary analysis of completers, the mean increases from baseline in lumbar spine BMD at one year were 5.1% (4.8, 5.4%; 95% CI) in the 70-mg once-weekly group (n=440) and 5.4% (5.0, 5.8%; 95% CI) in the 10-mg daily group (n=330). The two treatment groups were also similar with regard to BMD increases at other skeletal sites. The results of the intention-to-treat analysis were consistent with the primary analysis of completers.

Bone Histology

Bone histology in 270 postmenopausal patients with osteoporosis treated with FOSAMAX at doses ranging from 1 to 20 mg/day for one, two, or three years revealed normal mineralization and structure, as well as the expected decrease in bone turnover relative to placebo. These data, together with the normal bone histology and increased bone strength observed in rats and baboons exposed to long-term alendronate treatment, support the conclusion that bone formed during therapy with FOSAMAX is of normal quality.

Concomitant Use with Estrogen Hormone Replacement Therapy

The effects on BMD of treatment with FOSAMAX 10 mg once daily and conjugated estrogen (0.625 mg/day) either alone or in combination were assessed in a two-year, double-blind, placebo-controlled study of hysterectomized postmenopausal osteoporotic women (n=425). At two years, the increases in lumbar spine BMD from baseline were significantly greater with the combination (8.3%) than with either estrogen or FOSAMAX alone (both 6.0%).

The effects on BMD when FOSAMAX was added to stable doses (for at least one year) of HRT (estrogen ± progestin) were assessed in a one-year, double-blind, placebo-controlled study in postmenopausal osteoporotic women (n=428). The addition of FOSAMAX 10 mg once daily to HRT produced, at one year, significantly greater increases in lumbar spine BMD (3.7%) vs. HRT alone (1.1%).

In these studies, significant increases or favorable trends in BMD for combined therapy compared with HRT alone were seen at the total hip, femoral neck, and trochanter. No significant effect was seen for total body BMD.

Histomorphometric studies of transiliac biopsies in 92 subjects showed normal bone architecture. Compared to placebo there was a 98% suppression of bone turnover (as assessed by mineralizing surface) after 18 months of combined treatment with FOSAMAX and HRT, 94% on FOSAMAX alone, and 78% on HRT alone. The long-term effects of combined FOSAMAX and HRT on fracture occurrence and fracture healing have not been studied.

14.2 Treatment to Increase Bone Mass in Men with Osteoporosis

The efficacy of FOSAMAX in men with hypogonadal or idiopathic osteoporosis was demonstrated in two clinical studies.

A two-year, double-blind, placebo-controlled, multicenter study of FOSAMAX 10 mg once daily enrolled a total of 241 men between the ages of 31 and 87 (mean, 63). All patients in the trial had either: 1) a BMD T-score less than or equal to -2 at the femoral neck and less than or equal to -1 at the lumbar spine, or 2) a baseline osteoporotic fracture and a BMD T-score less than or equal to -1 at the femoral neck. At two years, the mean increases relative to placebo in BMD in men receiving FOSAMAX 10 mg/day were significant at the following sites: lumbar spine, 5.3%; femoral neck, 2.6%; trochanter, 3.1%; and total body, 1.6%. Treatment with FOSAMAX also reduced height loss (FOSAMAX, -0.6 mm vs. placebo, -2.4 mm).

A one-year, double-blind, placebo-controlled, multicenter study of once weekly FOSAMAX 70 mg enrolled a total of 167 men between the ages of 38 and 91 (mean, 66). Patients in the study had either: 1) a BMD T-score less than or equal to -2 at the femoral neck and less than or equal to -1 at the lumbar spine, 2) a BMD T-score less than or equal to -2 at the lumbar spine and less than or equal to -1 at the femoral neck, or 3) a baseline osteoporotic fracture and a BMD T-score less than or equal to -1 at the femoral neck. At one year, the mean increases relative to placebo in BMD in men receiving FOSAMAX 70 mg once weekly were significant at the following sites: lumbar spine, 2.8%; femoral neck, 1.9%; trochanter, 2.0%; and total body, 1.2%. These increases in BMD were similar to those seen at one year in the 10 mg once-daily study.

In both studies, BMD responses were similar regardless of age (greater than or equal to 65 years vs. less than 65 years), gonadal function (baseline testosterone less than 9 ng/dL vs. greater than or equal to 9 ng/dL), or baseline BMD (femoral neck and lumbar spine T-score less than or equal to -2.5 vs. greater than -2.5).

16 HOW SUPPLIED/STORAGE AND HANDLING

No. 3870 — Tablets FOSAMAX PLUS D 70 mg/2800 international units are white to off-white, modified capsule-shaped tablets with code 710 on one side and an outline of a bone image on the other. They are supplied as follows:

NDC 0006-0710-44 unit of use blister packages of 4.

No. 6746 — Tablets FOSAMAX PLUS D 70 mg/5600 international units are white to off-white, modified rectangle-shaped tablets with code 270 on one side and an outline of a bone image on the other. They are supplied as follows:

NDC 0006-0270-44 unit of use blister packages of 4

NDC 0006-0270-21 unit dose packages of 20.

Storage

Store at 20-25°C (68-77°F), excursions between 15-30°C (59-86°F) are allowed. [See USP Controlled Room Temperature.] Protect from moisture and light. Store tablets in the original blister package until use.

17 PATIENT COUNSELING INFORMATION

See FDA-Approved Medication Guide.

Instruct patients to read the Medication Guide before starting therapy with FOSAMAX PLUS D and to reread it each time the prescription is renewed.

17.1 Osteoporosis Recommendations, Including Calcium and Vitamin D Supplementation

Instruct patients to take supplemental calcium if intake is inadequate. Patients at increased risk for vitamin D insufficiency (e.g., over the age of 70 years, nursing home bound, or chronically ill) should take additional vitamin D if needed *[see Dosage and Administration (2.4)]*. Patients with gastrointestinal malabsorption syndromes may require additional vitamin D supplementation. Weight-bearing exercise should be considered along with the modification of certain behavioral factors, such as cigarette smoking and/or excessive alcohol consumption, if these factors exist.

17.2 Dosing Instructions

Instruct patients that the expected benefits of FOSAMAX PLUS D may only be obtained when it is taken with plain water the first thing upon arising for the day at least 30 minutes before the first food, beverage, or medication of the day. Even dosing with orange juice or coffee has been shown to markedly reduce the absorption of alendronate *[see Clinical Pharmacology (12.3)]*.

Instruct patients to swallow each tablet of FOSAMAX PLUS D with a full glass of water (6-8 ounces) and not to lie down for at least 30 minutes and until after their first food of the day to facilitate delivery to the stomach and thus reduce the potential for esophageal irritation.

Instruct patients not to chew or suck on the tablet because of a potential for oropharyngeal ulceration.

Instruct patients not to take FOSAMAX PLUS D at bedtime or before arising for the day. Patients should be informed that failure to follow these instructions may increase their risk of esophageal problems.

Instruct patients that if they develop symptoms of esophageal disease (such as difficulty or pain upon swallowing, retrosternal pain or new or worsening heartburn) they should stop taking FOSAMAX PLUS D and consult their physician.

If patients miss a dose of FOSAMAX PLUS D, instruct patients to take one tablet on the morning after they remember. They should not take two tablets on the same day but should return to taking one tablet once a week, as originally scheduled on their chosen day.

Manuf. for: Merck Sharp & Dohme Corp., a subsidiary of **MERCK & CO., INC.**, Whitehouse Station, NJ 08889, USA
By:
FROSST IBERICA, S.A.
28805 Alcalá de Henares
Madrid, Spain

Revised: 04/2013
uspi-0217a1304r014

MEDICATION GUIDE

FOSAMAX® PLUS D (FOSS-ah-max PLUS D)
(alendronate sodium/cholecalciferol)
Tablets

Read the Medication Guide that comes with FOSAMAX® PLUS D before you start taking it and each time you get a refill. There may be new information. This Medication Guide does not take the place of talking with your doctor about your medical condition or your treatment. Talk to your doctor if you have any questions about FOSAMAX PLUS D.

What is the most important information I should know about FOSAMAX PLUS D?

FOSAMAX PLUS D can cause serious side effects including:

1. Esophagus problems
2. Low calcium levels in your blood (hypocalcemia)
3. Bone, joint, or muscle pain
4. Severe jaw bone problems (osteonecrosis)
5. Unusual thigh bone fractures

1. **Esophagus problems.**
   Some people who take FOSAMAX PLUS D may develop problems in the esophagus (the tube that connects the mouth and the stomach). These problems include irritation, inflammation, or ulcers of the esophagus which may sometimes bleed.
   - **It is important that you take FOSAMAX PLUS D exactly as prescribed to help lower your chance of getting esophagus problems. (See the section "How should I take FOSAMAX PLUS D?")**
   - **Stop taking FOSAMAX PLUS D and call your doctor right away if you get chest pain, new or worsening heartburn, or have trouble or pain when you swallow.**
2. **Low calcium levels in your blood (hypocalcemia).**
   FOSAMAX PLUS D may lower the calcium levels in your blood. If you have low blood calcium before you start taking FOSAMAX PLUS D, it may get worse during treatment. Your low blood calcium must be treated before you take FOSAMAX PLUS D. Most people with low blood calcium levels do not have symptoms, but some people may have symptoms. Call your doctor right away if you have symptoms of low blood calcium such as:
   - Spasms, twitches, or cramps in your muscles
   - Numbness or tingling in your fingers, toes, or around your mouth

   Your doctor may prescribe calcium and vitamin D to help prevent low calcium levels in your blood, while you take FOSAMAX PLUS D. Take calcium and vitamin D as your doctor tells you to.
3. **Bone, joint, or muscle pain.**
   Some people who take FOSAMAX PLUS D develop severe bone, joint, or muscle pain.
4. **Severe jaw bone problems (osteonecrosis).**
   Severe jaw bone problems may happen when you take FOSAMAX PLUS D. Your doctor should examine your mouth before you start FOSAMAX PLUS D. Your doctor may tell you to see your dentist before you start FOSAMAX PLUS D. It is important for you to practice good mouth care during treatment with FOSAMAX PLUS D.
5. **Unusual thigh bone fractures.**
   Some people have developed unusual fractures in their thigh bone. Symptoms of a fracture may include new or unusual pain in your hip, groin, or thigh.

Call your doctor right away if you have any of these side effects.

What is FOSAMAX PLUS D?

FOSAMAX PLUS D is a prescription medicine used to:
- Treat osteoporosis in women after menopause. FOSAMAX PLUS D helps increase bone mass and reduces the chance of having a hip or spinal fracture (break).
- Increase bone mass in men with osteoporosis.

FOSAMAX PLUS D should not be used to treat vitamin D deficiency.

It is not known how long FOSAMAX PLUS D works for the treatment and prevention of osteoporosis. You should see your doctor regularly to determine if FOSAMAX PLUS D is still right for you.

FOSAMAX PLUS D is not for use in children.

Who should not take FOSAMAX PLUS D?

Do not take FOSAMAX PLUS D if you:
- Have certain problems with your esophagus, the tube that connects your mouth with your stomach
- Cannot stand or sit upright for at least 30 minutes
- Have low levels of calcium in your blood
- Are allergic to FOSAMAX PLUS D or any of its ingredients. A list of ingredients is at the end of this leaflet.

What should I tell my doctor before taking FOSAMAX PLUS D?

Before you start FOSAMAX PLUS D, be sure to talk to your doctor if you:
- Have problems with swallowing
- Have stomach or digestive problems
- Have low blood calcium
- Plan to have dental surgery or teeth removed
- Have kidney problems
- Have sarcoidosis, leukemia, lymphoma. These conditions may cause changes in vitamin D.
- Have been told you have trouble absorbing minerals in your stomach or intestines (malabsorption syndrome)
- Are pregnant or plan to become pregnant. It is not known if FOSAMAX PLUS D can harm your unborn baby.
- Are breast-feeding or plan to breast-feed. It is not known if FOSAMAX PLUS D passes into your milk and may harm your baby.

Especially tell your doctor if you take:
- antacids
- aspirin
- Nonsteroidal Anti-Inflammatory (NSAID) medicines

Tell your doctor about all the medicines you take, including prescription and non-prescription medicines, vitamins, and herbal supplements. Certain medicines may affect how FOSAMAX PLUS D works.

Know the medicines you take. Keep a list of them and show it to your doctor and pharmacist each time you get a new medicine.

How should I take FOSAMAX PLUS D tablet?
- Take FOSAMAX PLUS D exactly as your doctor tells you.
- **FOSAMAX PLUS D works only if taken on an empty stomach.**
- Take 1 dose of FOSAMAX PLUS D 1 time a week, **after** you get up for the day and **before** taking your first food, drink, or other medicine.
- Take FOSAMAX PLUS D while you are sitting or standing.
- Take your FOSAMAX PLUS D tablet with a full glass (6-8 oz) of plain water.
- **Do not chew or suck on a tablet of FOSAMAX PLUS D.**
- **Do not** take FOSAMAX PLUS D with mineral water, coffee, tea, soda, or juice.
- Do not take FOSAMAX PLUS D at bedtime.

After swallowing FOSAMAX PLUS D, wait at least 30 minutes:
- Before you lie down. You may sit, stand or walk, and do normal activities like reading.
- Before you take your first food or drink except for plain water.
- Before you take other medicines, including antacids, calcium, and other supplements and vitamins.

Do not lie down for at least 30 minutes after you take FOSAMAX PLUS D and after you eat your first food of the day.

If you miss a dose of FOSAMAX PLUS D, do not take it later in the day. Take your missed dose on the next morning after you remember and then return to your normal schedule. Do not take 2 doses on the same day.

If you take too much FOSAMAX PLUS D, call your doctor. Do not try to vomit. Do not lie down.

What are the possible side effects of FOSAMAX PLUS D?

FOSAMAX PLUS D may cause serious side effects.
- See **"What is the most important information I should know about FOSAMAX PLUS D?"**

The most common side effects of FOSAMAX PLUS D are:
- Stomach area (abdominal) pain
- Heartburn
- Constipation
- Diarrhea
- Upset stomach
- Pain in your bones, joints, or muscles
- Nausea

You may get allergic reactions, such as hives or swelling of your face, lips, tongue, or throat.

Worsening of asthma has been reported.

Tell your doctor if you have any side effect that bothers you or that does not go away.

These are not all the possible side effects of FOSAMAX PLUS D. For more information, ask your doctor or pharmacist.

Call your doctor for medical advice about side effects. You may report side effects to FDA at 1-800-FDA-1088.

How do I store FOSAMAX PLUS D?
- Store FOSAMAX PLUS D at room temperature, 68°F to 77°F (20°C to 25°C).
- Keep FOSAMAX PLUS D away from light.
- Keep FOSAMAX PLUS D package and tablets dry.
- Store FOSAMAX PLUS D in the original package.

Keep FOSAMAX PLUS D and all medicines out of the reach of children.

General information about the safe and effective use of FOSAMAX PLUS D.

Medicines are sometimes prescribed for purposes other than those listed in a Medication Guide. Do not use FOSAMAX PLUS D for a condition for which it was not prescribed. Do not give FOSAMAX PLUS D to other people, even if they have the same symptoms you have. It may harm them.

This Medication Guide summarizes the most important information about FOSAMAX PLUS D. If you would like more information, talk with your doctor. You can ask your doctor or pharmacist for information about FOSAMAX PLUS D that is written for health professionals. For more information, go to: www.fosamaxplusd.com or call 1-800-622-4477 (toll-free).

What are the ingredients in FOSAMAX PLUS D?

Active ingredients: alendronate sodium and cholecalciferol (vitamin D_3).

Inactive ingredients: cellulose, lactose, medium chain triglycerides, gelatin, croscarmellose sodium, sucrose, colloidal silicon dioxide, magnesium stearate, butylated hydroxytoluene, modified food starch, and sodium aluminum silicate.

Manuf. for: Merck Sharp & Dohme Corp., a subsidiary of **MERCK & CO., INC.**, Whitehouse Station, NJ 08889, USA
By:
FROSST IBERICA, S.A.
28805 Alcalá de Henares
Madrid, Spain

Revised: 04/2013
usmg-0217a1304r014

This Medication Guide has been approved by the U.S. Food and Drug Administration.

Shown in Product Identification Guide, page 308

GANIRELIX ACETATE INJECTION ℞

FOR SUBCUTANEOUS USE ONLY

DESCRIPTION

Ganirelix Acetate Injection is a synthetic decapeptide with high antagonistic activity against naturally occurring gonadotropin-releasing hormone (GnRH). Ganirelix Acetate is derived from native GnRH with substitutions of amino acids at positions 1, 2, 3, 6, 8, and 10 to form the following molecular formula of the peptide: N-acetyl-3-(2-naphthyl)-D-alanyl-4-chloro-D-phenylalanyl-3-(3-pyridyl)-D-alanyl-L-seryl-L-tyrosyl-N^9,N^{10}-diethyl-D-homoarginyl-L-leucyl-N^9,N^{10}-diethyl-L-homoarginyl-L-prolyl-D-alanylamide acetate. The molecular weight for Ganirelix Acetate is 1570.4 as an anhydrous free base. The structural formula is as follows:

Ganirelix Acetate

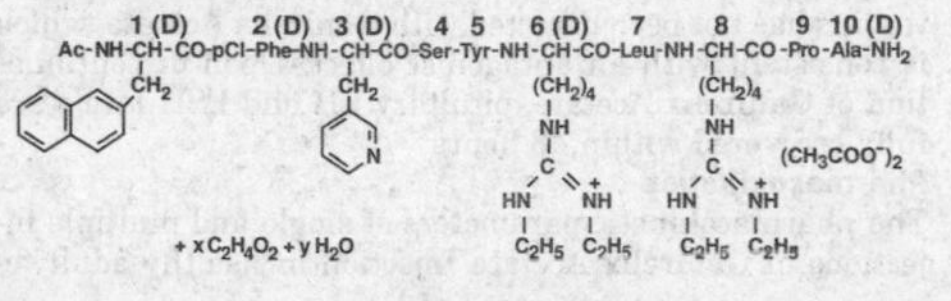

TABLE I: Mean (SD) pharmacokinetic parameters of 250 mcg of Ganirelix Acetate following a single subcutaneous (SC) injection (n=15) and daily SC injections (n=15) for seven days.

	t_{max} h	$t_{1/2}$ h	C_{max} ng/mL	AUC ng•h/mL	CL/F L/h	V_d/F L
Ganirelix Acetate single dose	1.1 (0.3)	12.8 (4.3)	14.8 (3.2)	96 (12)	2.4 (0.2)*	43.7 (11.4)*
Ganirelix Acetate multiple dose	1.1 (0.2)	16.2 (1.6)	11.2 (2.4)	77.1 (9.8)	3.3 (0.4)	76.5 (10.3)

t_{max} Time to maximum concentration
$t_{1/2}$ Elimination half-life
C_{max} Maximum serum concentration
AUC Area under the curve; Single dose: $AUC_{0-\infty}$; multiple dose: AUC_{0-24}
V_d Volume of distribution
CL Clearance = Dose/$AUC_{0-\infty}$
F Absolute bioavailability
* Based on intravenous administration

TABLE II: Results from the multicenter, double-blind, randomized, dose-finding study to assess the efficacy of Ganirelix Acetate Injection to prevent premature LH surges in women undergoing COH with recombinant FSH.

	Daily dose (mcg) of Ganirelix Acetate Injection					
	62.5 mcg	125 mcg	250 mcg	500 mcg	1000 mcg	2000 mcg
No. subjects receiving Ganirelix Acetate	31	66	70	69	66	30
No. subjects with ET*	27	61	62	54	61	27
No. of subjects with LH rise ≥ 10 mIU/mL†	4	6	1	0	0	0
Serum LH (mIU/mL) on day of hCG‡	3.6	2.5	1.7	1.0	0.6	0.3
5th–95th percentiles	0.6–19.9	0.6–11.4	< 0.25–6.4	0.4–4.7	< 0.25–2.2	< 0.25–0.8
Serum E_2 (pg/mL) on day of hCG‡	1475	1110	1160	823	703	441
5th–95th percentiles	645–3720	424–3780	384–3910	279–2720	284–2360	166–1940
Vital pregnancy rate§						
per attempt, n (%)	7 (22.6)	17 (25.8)	25 (35.7)	8 (11.6)	9 (13.6)	2 (6.7)
per transfer, n (%)	7 (25.9)	17 (27.9)	25 (40.3)	8 (14.8)	9 (14.8)	2 (7.4)
Implantation rate (%)¶	14.2 (26.8)	16.3 (30.5)	21.9 (30.6)	9.0 (23.7)	8.5 (21.7)	4.9 (20.1)

(Protocol 38602)
* ET: Embryo Transfer
† Following initiation of Ganirelix Acetate therapy. Includes subjects who have complied with daily injections
‡ Median values
§ As evidenced by ultrasound at 5–6 weeks following ET
¶ Mean (standard deviation)

Ganirelix Acetate Injection is supplied as a colorless, sterile, ready-to-use, aqueous solution intended for SUBCUTANEOUS administration only. Each sterile, prefilled syringe contains 250 mcg/0.5 mL of Ganirelix Acetate, 0.1 mg glacial acetic acid, 23.5 mg mannitol, and water for injection adjusted to pH 5.0 with acetic acid, NF and/or sodium hydroxide, NF.

CLINICAL PHARMACOLOGY

The pulsatile release of GnRH stimulates the synthesis and secretion of luteinizing hormone (LH) and follicle-stimulating hormone (FSH). The frequency of LH pulses in the mid and late follicular phase is approximately 1 pulse per hour. These pulses can be detected as transient rises in serum LH. At midcycle, a large increase in GnRH release results in an LH surge. The midcycle LH surge initiates several physiologic actions including: ovulation, resumption of meiosis in the oocyte, and luteinization. Luteinization results in a rise in serum progesterone with an accompanying decrease in estradiol levels.

Ganirelix Acetate acts by competitively blocking the GnRH receptors on the pituitary gonadotroph and subsequent transduction pathway. It induces a rapid, reversible suppression of gonadotropin secretion. The suppression of pituitary LH secretion by Ganirelix Acetate is more pronounced than that of FSH. An initial release of endogenous gonadotropins has not been detected with Ganirelix Acetate, which is consistent with an antagonist effect. Upon discontinuation of Ganirelix Acetate, pituitary LH and FSH levels are fully recovered within 48 hours.

Pharmacokinetics

The pharmacokinetic parameters of single and multiple injections of Ganirelix Acetate Injection in healthy adult females are summarized in Table I. Steady-state serum concentrations are reached after 3 days of treatment. The pharmacokinetics of Ganirelix Acetate are dose-proportional in the dose range of 125 to 500 mcg.

[See table I above]

Absorption

Ganirelix Acetate is rapidly absorbed following subcutaneous injection with maximum serum concentrations reached approximately one hour after dosing. The mean absolute bioavailability of Ganirelix Acetate following a single 250 mcg subcutaneous injection to healthy female volunteers is 91.1%.

Distribution

The mean (SD) volume of distribution of Ganirelix Acetate in healthy females following intravenous administration of a single 250-mcg dose is 43.7 (11.4) liters (L). *In vitro* protein binding to human plasma is 81.9%.

Metabolism

Following single-dose intravenous administration of radiolabeled Ganirelix Acetate to healthy female volunteers, Ganirelix Acetate is the major compound present in the plasma (50–70% of total radioactivity in the plasma) up to 4 hours and urine (17.1–18.4% of administered dose) up to 24 hours. Ganirelix Acetate is not found in the feces. The 1–4 peptide and 1–6 peptide of Ganirelix Acetate are the primary metabolites observed in the feces.

Excretion

On average, 97.2% of the total radiolabeled Ganirelix Acetate dose is recovered in the feces and urine (75.1% and 22.1%, respectively) over 288 h following intravenous single dose administration of 1 mg [^{14}C]-Ganirelix Acetate. Urinary excretion is virtually complete in 24 h, whereas fecal excretion starts to plateau 192 h after dosing.

Special Populations

The pharmacokinetics of Ganirelix Acetate Injection have not been determined in special populations such as geriatric, pediatric, renally impaired and hepatically impaired patients (see PRECAUTIONS).

Drug-Drug Interactions

Formal *in vivo* or *in vitro* drug-drug interaction studies have not been conducted (see PRECAUTIONS). Since Ganirelix Acetate can suppress the secretion of pituitary gonadotropins, dose adjustments of exogenous gonadotropins may be necessary when used during controlled ovarian hyperstimulation (COH).

Clinical Studies

The efficacy of Ganirelix Acetate Injection was established in two adequate and well-controlled clinical studies which included women with normal endocrine and pelvic ultrasound parameters. The studies intended to exclude subjects with polycystic ovary syndrome (PCOS) and subjects with low or no ovarian reserve. One cycle of study medication was administered to each randomized subject. For both studies, the administration of exogenous recombinant FSH [Follistim® (follitropin beta for injection)] 150 IU daily was initiated on the morning of Day 2 or 3 of a natural menstrual cycle. Ganirelix Acetate Injection was administered on the morning of Day 7 or 8 (Day 6 of recombinant FSH administration). The dose of recombinant FSH administered was adjusted according to individual responses starting on the day of initiation of Ganirelix Acetate. Both recombinant FSH and Ganirelix Acetate were continued daily until at least three follicles were 17 mm or greater in diameter at which time hCG [Pregnyl® (chorionic gonadotropin for injection, USP)] was administered. Following hCG administration, Ganirelix Acetate and recombinant FSH administration were discontinued. Oocyte retrieval, followed by *in vitro* fertilization (IVF) or intracytoplasmic sperm injection (ICSI), was subsequently performed.

In a multicenter, double-blind, randomized, dose-finding study, the safety and efficacy of Ganirelix Acetate Injection were evaluated for the prevention of LH surges in women undergoing COH with recombinant FSH. Ganirelix Acetate Injection doses ranging from 62.5 mcg to 2000 mcg and recombinant FSH were administered to 332 patients undergoing COH for IVF (see TABLE II). Median serum LH on the day of hCG administration decreased with increasing doses of Ganirelix Acetate. Median serum E_2 (17β-estradiol) on the day of hCG administration was 1475, 1110, and 1160 pg/mL for the 62.5-, 125-, and 250-mcg doses, respectively. Lower peak serum E_2 levels of 823, 703, and 441 pg/mL were seen at higher doses of Ganirelix Acetate 500, 1000, and 2000 mcg, respectively. The highest pregnancy and implantation rates were achieved with the 250-mcg dose of Ganirelix Acetate Injection as summarized in Table II.

[See table II above]

Transient LH rises alone were not deleterious to achieving pregnancy with Ganirelix Acetate at doses of 125 mcg (3/6 subjects) and 250 mcg (1/1 subjects). In addition, none of the subjects with LH rises ≥ 10 mIU/mL had premature luteinization indicated by a serum progesterone above 2 ng/mL.

A multicenter, open-label, randomized study was conducted to assess the efficacy and safety of Ganirelix Acetate Injection in women undergoing COH. Follicular phase treatment with Ganirelix Acetate 250 mcg was studied using a luteal phase GnRH agonist as a reference treatment. A total of 463 subjects were treated with Ganirelix Acetate by subcutaneous injection once daily starting on Day 6 of recombinant FSH treatment. Recombinant FSH was maintained at 150 IU for the first 5 days of ovarian stimulation and was then adjusted by the investigator on the sixth day of gonadotropin use according to individual responses. The results for the Ganirelix Acetate arm are summarized in Table III.

TABLE III: Results from the multicenter, open-label, randomized study to assess the efficacy and safety of Ganirelix Acetate Injection in women undergoing COH.

	Ganirelix Acetate 250 mcg
No. subjects treated	463
Duration of GnRH analog (days)*†	5.4 (2.0)
Duration of recombinant FSH (days)*†	9.6 (2.0)
Serum E_2 (pg/mL) on day of hCG‡ 5th–95th percentiles	1190 373–3105
Serum LH (mIU/mL) on day of hCG‡ 5th–95th percentiles	1.6 0.6–6.9
No. of subjects with LH rise ≥ 10 mIU/mL§	13

No. of follicles > 11 mm*†	10.7 (5.3)
No. of subjects with oocyte retrieval	440
No. of oocytes†	8.7 (5.6)
Fertilization rate	62.1%
No. subjects with ET¶	399
No. of embryos transferred†	2.2 (0.6)
No. of embryos†	6.0 (4.5)
Ongoing pregnancy rate#*	
per attempt, n (%)Þ	94 (20.3)
per transfer, n (%)	93 (23.3)
Implantation rate (%)†	15.7 (29)

(Protocol 38607)
Some centers were limited to the transfer of ≤ 2 embryos based on local practice standards
* Restricted to subjects with hCG injection
† Mean (standard deviation)
‡ Median values
§ Following initiation of Ganirelix Acetate therapy
¶ ET: Embryo Transfer
\# As evidenced by ultrasound at 12–16 weeks following ET
Þ Includes one patient who achieved pregnancy with intrauterine induction

The mean number of days of Ganirelix Acetate treatment was 5.4 (2–14).

LH Surges

The midcycle LH surge initiates several physiologic actions including: ovulation, resumption of meiosis in the oocyte, and luteinization. In 463 subjects administered Ganirelix Acetate Injection 250 mcg, a premature LH surge prior to hCG administration, (LH rise ≥ 10 mIU/mL with a significant rise in serum progesterone > 2 ng/mL, or a significant decline in serum estradiol) occurred in less than 1% of subjects.

INDICATIONS AND USAGE

Ganirelix Acetate Injection is indicated for the inhibition of premature LH surges in women undergoing controlled ovarian hyperstimulation.

CONTRAINDICATIONS

Ganirelix Acetate Injection is contraindicated under the following conditions:

- Known hypersensitivity to Ganirelix Acetate or to any of its components.
- Known hypersensitivity to GnRH or any other GnRH analog.
- Known or suspected pregnancy (see PRECAUTIONS).

WARNINGS

Ganirelix Acetate Injection should be prescribed by physicians who are experienced in infertility treatment. Before starting treatment with Ganirelix Acetate, pregnancy must be excluded. Safe use of Ganirelix Acetate during pregnancy has not been established (see CONTRAINDICATIONS and PRECAUTIONS).

PRECAUTIONS

General

Special care should be taken in women with signs and symptoms of active allergic conditions. Cases of hypersensitivity reactions, including anaphylactoid reactions, have been reported, as early as with the first dose, during post-marketing surveillance (see ADVERSE REACTIONS). In the absence of clinical experience, Ganirelix Acetate treatment is not advised in women with severe allergic conditions.

The packaging of this product contains natural rubber latex which may cause allergic reactions (see HOW SUPPLIED).

Information for Patients

Prior to therapy with Ganirelix Acetate Injection, patients should be informed of the duration of treatment and monitoring procedures that will be required. The risk of possible adverse reactions should be discussed (see ADVERSE REACTIONS).

Ganirelix Acetate should not be prescribed if the patient is pregnant.

Laboratory Tests

A neutrophil count ≥ 8.3 ($\times 10^9$/L) was noted in 11.9% (up to 16.8 $\times 10^9$/L) of all subjects treated within the adequate and well-controlled clinical trials. In addition, downward shifts within the Ganirelix Acetate Injection group were observed for hematocrit and total bilirubin. The clinical significance of these findings was not determined.

Drug Interactions

No formal drug-drug interaction studies have been performed.

Carcinogenesis and Mutagenesis, Impairment of Fertility

Long-term toxicity studies in animals have not been performed with Ganirelix Acetate Injection to evaluate the carcinogenic potential of the drug. Ganirelix Acetate did not induce a mutagenic response in the Ames test *(S. typhimurium* and *E. coli)* or produce chromosomal aberrations in *in vitro* assay using Chinese Hamster Ovary cells.

Pregnancy

Pregnancy Category X

Ganirelix Acetate Injection is contraindicated in pregnant women. When administered from Day 7 to near term to pregnant rats and rabbits at doses up to 10 and 30 mcg/day (approximately 0.4 to 3.2 times the human dose based on body surface area), Ganirelix Acetate increased the incidence of litter resorption. There was no increase in fetal abnormalities. No treatment-related changes in fertility, physical, or behavioral characteristics were observed in the offspring of female rats treated with Ganirelix Acetate during pregnancy and lactation.

The effects on fetal resorption are logical consequences of the alteration in hormonal levels brought about by the antigonadotropic properties of this drug and could result in fetal loss in humans. Therefore, this drug should not be used in pregnant women (see CONTRAINDICATIONS).

Nursing Mothers

Ganirelix Acetate Injection should not be used by lactating women. It is not known whether this drug is excreted in human milk.

Geriatric Use

Clinical studies with Ganirelix Acetate Injection did not include a sufficient number of subjects aged 65 and over.

ADVERSE REACTIONS

The safety of Ganirelix Acetate Injection was evaluated in two randomized, parallel-group, multicenter controlled clinical studies. Treatment duration for Ganirelix Acetate ranged from 1 to 14 days. Table IV represents adverse events (AEs) from first day of Ganirelix Acetate administration until confirmation of pregnancy by ultrasound at an incidence of ≥ 1% in Ganirelix Acetate-treated subjects without regard to causality.

TABLE IV: Incidence of common adverse events (Incidence ≥ 1% in Ganirelix Acetate-treated subjects). Completed controlled clinical studies (All-subjects-treated group).

Adverse Events Occurring in ≥ 1%	Ganirelix Acetate N=794 % (n)
Abdominal Pain (gynecological)	4.8 (38)
Death Fetal	3.7 (29)
Headache	3.0 (24)
Ovarian Hyperstimulation Syndrome	2.4 (19)
Vaginal Bleeding	1.8 (14)
Injection Site Reaction	1.1 (9)
Nausea	1.1 (9)
Abdominal Pain (gastrointestinal)	1.0 (8)

During post-marketing surveillance, rare cases of hypersensitivity reactions, including anaphylactoid reactions, have been reported, as early as with the first dose (see PRECAUTIONS).

Congenital Anomalies

Ongoing clinical follow-up studies of 283 newborns of women administered Ganirelix Acetate Injection were reviewed. There were three neonates with major congenital anomalies and 18 neonates with minor congenital anomalies. The major congenital anomalies were: hydrocephalus/meningocele, omphalocele, and Beckwith-Wiedemann Syndrome. The minor congenital anomalies were: nevus, skin tags, sacral sinus, hemangioma, torticollis/asymmetric skull, talipes, supernumerary digit finger, hip subluxation, torticollis/high palate, occiput/abnormal hand crease, hernia umbilicalis, hernia inguinalis, hydrocele, undescended testis, and hydronephrosis. The causal relationship between these congenital anomalies and Ganirelix Acetate is unknown. Multiple factors, genetic and others (including, but not limited to ICSI, IVF, gonadotropins, progesterone) may confound ART (Assisted Reproductive Technology) procedures.

OVERDOSAGE

There have been no reports of overdosage with Ganirelix Acetate Injection in humans.

DOSAGE AND ADMINISTRATION

After initiating FSH therapy on Day 2 or 3 of the cycle, Ganirelix Acetate Injection 250 mcg may be administered subcutaneously once daily during the mid to late portion of the follicular phase. By taking advantage of endogenous pituitary FSH secretion, the requirement for exogenously administered FSH may be reduced. Treatment with Ganirelix Acetate should be continued daily until the day of hCG administration. When a sufficient number of follicles of adequate size are present, as assessed by ultrasound, final maturation of follicles is induced by administering hCG. The administration of hCG should be withheld in cases where the ovaries are abnormally enlarged on the last day of FSH therapy to reduce the chance of developing OHSS (Ovarian Hyperstimulation Syndrome).

Directions for Using Ganirelix Acetate Injection

1. Ganirelix Acetate Injection is supplied in a sterile, prefilled syringe and is intended for SUBCUTANEOUS administration only.
2. Wash hands thoroughly with soap and water.
3. The most convenient sites for SUBCUTANEOUS injection are in the abdomen around the navel or upper thigh.
4. The injection site should be swabbed with a disinfectant to remove any surface bacteria. Clean about two inches around the point where the needle will be inserted and let the disinfectant dry for at least one minute before proceeding.
5. With syringe held upward, remove needle cover.
6. Pinch up a large area of skin between the finger and thumb. Vary the injection site a little with each injection.
7. The needle should be inserted at the base of the pinched-up skin at an angle of 45–90° to the skin surface.
8. When the needle is correctly positioned, it will be difficult to draw back on the plunger. If any blood is drawn into the syringe, the needle tip has penetrated a vein or artery. If this happens, withdraw the needle slightly and reposition the needle without removing it from the skin. Alternatively, remove the needle and use a new, sterile, prefilled syringe. Cover the injection site with a swab containing disinfectant and apply pressure; the site should stop bleeding within one or two minutes.
9. Once the needle is correctly placed, depress the plunger slowly and steadily, so the solution is correctly injected and the skin is not damaged.
10. Pull the syringe out quickly and apply pressure to the site with a swab containing disinfectant.
11. Use the sterile, prefilled syringe only once and dispose of it properly.

HOW SUPPLIED

Ganirelix Acetate Injection is supplied in:

Disposable, sterile, ready for use, prefilled 1 mL glass syringes containing 250 mcg/0.5 mL aqueous solution of Ganirelix Acetate closed with a rubber piston that does not contain latex. Each Ganirelix Acetate sterile, prefilled syringe is affixed with a 27 gauge × ½-inch needle **closed by a needle shield of natural rubber latex** and is blister-packed. (See PRECAUTIONS, General.)

Single syringe NDC 0052-0301-51

Storage

Store at 25°C (77°F); excursions permitted to 15–30°C (59–86°F) [see USP Controlled Room Temperature]. Protect from light.

Rx only

Manufactured for: Merck Sharp & Dohme Corp., a subsidiary of
MERCK & CO., INC., Whitehouse Station, NJ 08889, USA
Manufactured by: Vetter Pharma-Fertigung GmbH & Co. KG, Ravensburg, Germany
US Patent No. 5,767,082.

Revised: 05/2012
900761-GNR-SOi-USPI.2

GARDASIL ℞

[GARD-ah-sill]

[Human Papillomavirus Quadrivalent (Types 6, 11, 16, and 18) Vaccine, Recombinant]
Suspension for Intramuscular Injection

HIGHLIGHTS OF PRESCRIBING INFORMATION
These highlights do not include all the information needed to use GARDASIL safely and effectively. See full prescribing information for GARDASIL.

GARDASIL
[Human Papillomavirus Quadrivalent (Types 6, 11, 16, and 18) Vaccine, Recombinant]
Suspension for intramuscular injection
Initial U.S. Approval: 2006

INDICATIONS AND USAGE

GARDASIL is a vaccine indicated in girls and women 9 through 26 years of age for the prevention of the following diseases caused by Human Papillomavirus (HPV) types included in the vaccine:

- Cervical, vulvar, vaginal, and anal cancer caused by HPV types 16 and 18
- Genital warts (condyloma acuminata) caused by HPV types 6 and 11

And the following precancerous or dysplastic lesions caused by HPV types 6, 11, 16, and 18:

- Cervical intraepithelial neoplasia (CIN) grade 2/3 and Cervical adenocarcinoma *in situ* (AIS)
- Cervical intraepithelial neoplasia (CIN) grade 1
- Vulvar intraepithelial neoplasia (VIN) grade 2 and grade 3
- Vaginal intraepithelial neoplasia (VaIN) grade 2 and grade 3
- Anal intraepithelial neoplasia (AIN) grades 1, 2, and 3

GARDASIL is indicated in boys and men 9 through 26 years of age for the prevention of the following diseases caused by HPV types included in the vaccine:

- Anal cancer caused by HPV types 16 and 18
- Genital warts (condyloma acuminata) caused by HPV types 6 and 11

And the following precancerous or dysplastic lesions caused by HPV types 6, 11, 16, and 18:

- Anal intraepithelial neoplasia (AIN) grades 1, 2, and 3. (1)

Limitations of GARDASIL Use and Effectiveness:

- GARDASIL does not eliminate the necessity for women to continue to undergo recommended cervical cancer screening. (1.3) (17)
- Recipients of GARDASIL should not discontinue anal cancer screening if it has been recommended by a health care provider. (1.3) (17)
- GARDASIL has not been demonstrated to provide protection against disease from vaccine and non-vaccine HPV types to which a person has previously been exposed through sexual activity. (1.3) (14.4) (14.5)
- GARDASIL is not intended to be used for treatment of active external genital lesions; cervical, vulvar, vaginal, and anal cancers; CIN; VIN; VaIN, or AIN. (1.3)
- GARDASIL has not been demonstrated to protect against diseases due to HPV types not contained in the vaccine. (1.3) (14.4) (14.5)
- Not all vulvar, vaginal, and anal cancers are caused by HPV, and GARDASIL protects only against those vulvar, vaginal, and anal cancers caused by HPV 16 and 18. (1.3)
- GARDASIL does not protect against genital diseases not caused by HPV. (1.3)
- Vaccination with GARDASIL may not result in protection in all vaccine recipients. (1.3)
- GARDASIL has not been demonstrated to prevent HPV-related CIN 2/3 or worse in women older than 26 years of age. (14.7)

DOSAGE AND ADMINISTRATION

0.5-mL suspension for intramuscular injection at the following schedule: 0, 2 months, 6 months. (2.1)

DOSAGE FORMS AND STRENGTHS

- 0.5-mL suspension for injection as a single-dose vial and prefilled syringe. (3) (11)

CONTRAINDICATIONS

- Hypersensitivity, including severe allergic reactions to yeast (a vaccine component), or after a previous dose of GARDASIL. (4) (11)

WARNINGS AND PRECAUTIONS

- Because vaccinees may develop syncope, sometimes resulting in falling with injury, observation for 15 minutes after administration is recommended. Syncope, sometimes associated with tonic-clonic movements and other seizure-like activity, has been reported following vaccination with GARDASIL. When syncope is associated with tonic-clonic movements, the activity is usually transient and typically responds to restoring cerebral perfusion by maintaining a supine or Trendelenburg position. (5.1)

ADVERSE REACTIONS

The most common adverse reaction was headache. Common adverse reactions (frequency of at least 1.0% and greater than AAHS control or saline placebo) are fever, nausea, dizziness; and injection-site pain, swelling, erythema, pruritus, and bruising. (6.1)

To report SUSPECTED ADVERSE REACTIONS, contact Merck Sharp & Dohme Corp., a subsidiary of Merck & Co., Inc., at 1-877-888-4231 or VAERS at 1-800-822-7967 or www.vaers.hhs.gov.

DRUG INTERACTIONS

GARDASIL may be administered concomitantly with RECOMBIVAX HB (7.1) or with Menactra and Adacel. (7.2)

USE IN SPECIFIC POPULATIONS

Safety and effectiveness of GARDASIL have not been established in the following populations:

- Pregnant women. Physicians are encouraged to register pregnant women exposed to GARDASIL by calling 1-800-986-8999 so that Merck Sharp & Dohme Corp., a subsidiary of Merck & Co., Inc., can monitor maternal and fetal outcomes. (8.1)
- Children below the age of 9 years. (8.4)
- Immunocompromised individuals. Response to GARDASIL may be diminished. (8.6)

See 17 for PATIENT COUNSELING INFORMATION and FDA-approved patient labeling

Revised: 06/2013

FULL PRESCRIBING INFORMATION: CONTENTS*

*** Sections or subsections omitted from the full prescribing information are not listed**

FULL PRESCRIBING INFORMATION

1 INDICATIONS AND USAGE

1.1 Girls and Women

GARDASIL®[1] is a vaccine indicated in girls and women 9 through 26 years of age for the prevention of the following diseases caused by Human Papillomavirus (HPV) types included in the vaccine:

- Cervical, vulvar, vaginal, and anal cancer caused by HPV types 16 and 18
- Genital warts (condyloma acuminata) caused by HPV types 6 and 11

And the following precancerous or dysplastic lesions caused by HPV types 6, 11, 16, and 18:

- Cervical intraepithelial neoplasia (CIN) grade 2/3 and Cervical adenocarcinoma *in situ* (AIS)
- Cervical intraepithelial neoplasia (CIN) grade 1
- Vulvar intraepithelial neoplasia (VIN) grade 2 and grade 3
- Vaginal intraepithelial neoplasia (VaIN) grade 2 and grade 3
- Anal intraepithelial neoplasia (AIN) grades 1, 2, and 3

1.2 Boys and Men

GARDASIL is indicated in boys and men 9 through 26 years of age for the prevention of the following diseases caused by HPV types included in the vaccine:

- Anal cancer caused by HPV types 16 and 18
- Genital warts (condyloma acuminata) caused by HPV types 6 and 11

And the following precancerous or dysplastic lesions caused by HPV types 6, 11, 16, and 18:

- Anal intraepithelial neoplasia (AIN) grades 1, 2, and 3

1.3 Limitations of GARDASIL Use and Effectiveness

The health care provider should inform the patient, parent, or guardian that vaccination does not eliminate the necessity for women to continue to undergo recommended cervical cancer screening. Women who receive GARDASIL should continue to undergo cervical cancer screening per standard of care. *[See Patient Counseling Information (17).]*

Recipients of GARDASIL should not discontinue anal cancer screening if it has been recommended by a health care provider. *[See Patient Counseling Information (17).]*

GARDASIL has not been demonstrated to provide protection against disease from vaccine and non-vaccine HPV types to which a person has previously been exposed through sexual activity. *[See Clinical Studies (14.4, 14.5).]*

GARDASIL is not intended to be used for treatment of active external genital lesions; cervical, vulvar, vaginal, and anal cancers; CIN; VIN; VaIN; or AIN.

GARDASIL has not been demonstrated to protect against diseases due to HPV types not contained in the vaccine. *[See Clinical Studies (14.4, 14.5).]*

Not all vulvar, vaginal, and anal cancers are caused by HPV, and GARDASIL protects only against those vulvar, vaginal, and anal cancers caused by HPV 16 and 18.

GARDASIL does not protect against genital diseases not caused by HPV.

Vaccination with GARDASIL may not result in protection in all vaccine recipients.

GARDASIL has not been demonstrated to prevent HPV-related CIN 2/3 or worse in women older than 26 years of age. *[See Clinical Studies (14.7).]*

2 DOSAGE AND ADMINISTRATION

2.1 Dosage

GARDASIL should be administered intramuscularly as a 0.5-mL dose at the following schedule: 0, 2 months, 6 months. *[See Clinical Studies (14.8).]*

2.2 Method of Administration

For intramuscular use only.

Shake well before use. Thorough agitation immediately before administration is necessary to maintain suspension of the vaccine. GARDASIL should not be diluted or mixed with other vaccines. After thorough agitation, GARDASIL is a white, cloudy liquid. Parenteral drug products should be inspected visually for particulate matter and discoloration prior to administration. Do not use the product if particulates are present or if it appears discolored.

GARDASIL should be administered intramuscularly in the deltoid region of the upper arm or in the higher anterolateral area of the thigh.

Syncope has been reported following vaccination with GARDASIL and may result in falling with injury; observation for 15 minutes after administration is recommended. *[See Warnings and Precautions (5.1).]*

Single-Dose Vial Use

Withdraw the 0.5-mL dose of vaccine from the single-dose vial using a sterile needle and syringe and use promptly.

Prefilled Syringe Use

This package does not contain a needle. Shake well before use. Attach the needle by twisting in a clockwise direction until the needle fits securely on the syringe. Administer the entire dose as per standard protocol.

3 DOSAGE FORMS AND STRENGTHS

GARDASIL is a suspension for intramuscular administration available in 0.5-mL single dose vials and prefilled syringes. See *Description (11)* for the complete listing of ingredients.

4 CONTRAINDICATIONS

Hypersensitivity, including severe allergic reactions to yeast (a vaccine component), or after a previous dose of GARDASIL. *[See Description (11).]*

5 WARNINGS AND PRECAUTIONS

5.1 Syncope

Because vaccinees may develop syncope, sometimes resulting in falling with injury, observation for 15 minutes after administration is recommended. Syncope, sometimes associated with tonic-clonic movements and other seizure-like activity, has been reported following vaccination with

GARDASIL. When syncope is associated with tonic-clonic movements, the activity is usually transient and typically responds to restoring cerebral perfusion by maintaining a supine or Trendelenburg position.

5.2 Managing Allergic Reactions

Appropriate medical treatment and supervision must be readily available in case of anaphylactic reactions following the administration of GARDASIL.

6 ADVERSE REACTIONS

Overall Summary of Adverse Reactions

Headache, fever, nausea, and dizziness; and local injection site reactions (pain, swelling, erythema, pruritus, and bruising) occurred after administration with GARDASIL.

Syncope, sometimes associated with tonic-clonic movements and other seizure-like activity, has been reported following vaccination with GARDASIL and may result in falling with injury; observation for 15 minutes after administration is recommended. *[See Warnings and Precautions (5.1).]*

Anaphylaxis has been reported following vaccination with GARDASIL.

6.1 Clinical Trials Experience

Because clinical trials are conducted under widely varying conditions, adverse reaction rates observed in the clinical trials of a vaccine cannot be directly compared to rates in the clinical trials of another vaccine and may not reflect the rates observed in practice.

Studies in Girls and Women (9 Through 45 Years of Age) and Boys and Men (9 Through 26 Years of Age)

In 7 clinical trials (5 Amorphous Aluminum Hydroxyphosphate Sulfate [AAHS]-controlled, 1 saline placebo-controlled, and 1 uncontrolled), 18,083 individuals were administered GARDASIL or AAHS control or saline placebo on the day of enrollment, and approximately 2 and 6 months thereafter, and safety was evaluated using vaccination report cards (VRC)-aided surveillance for 14 days after each injection of GARDASIL or AAHS control or saline placebo in these individuals. The individuals who were monitored using VRC-aided surveillance included 10,088 individuals 9 through 45 years of age at enrollment who received GARDASIL and 7,995 individuals who received AAHS control or saline placebo. Few individuals (0.2%) discontinued due to adverse reactions. The race distribution of the 9- through 26-year-old girls and women in the safety population was as follows: 62.3% White; 17.6% Hispanic (Black and White); 6.8% Asian; 6.7% Other; 6.4% Black; and 0.3% American Indian. The race distribution of the 24- through 45-year-old women in the safety population of Study 6 was as follows: 20.6% White; 43.2% Hispanic (Black and White); 0.2% Other; 4.8% Black; 31.2% Asian; and 0.1% American Indian. The race distribution of the 9- through 26-year-old boys and men in the safety population was as follows: 42.0% White; 19.7% Hispanic (Black and White); 11.0% Asian; 11.2% Other; 15.9% Black; and 0.1% American Indian.

Common Injection-Site Adverse Reactions in Girls and Women 9 Through 26 Years of Age

The injection site adverse reactions that were observed among recipients of GARDASIL at a frequency of at least 1.0% and also at a greater frequency than that observed among AAHS control or saline placebo recipients are shown in Table 1.

Table 1
Injection-Site Adverse Reactions in Girls and Women 9 Through 26 Years of Age*

Adverse Reaction (1 to 5 Days Postvaccination)	GARDASIL (N = 5088) %	AAHS Control† (N = 3470) %	Saline Placebo (N = 320) %
Injection Site			
Pain	83.9	75.4	48.6
Swelling	25.4	15.8	7.3
Erythema	24.7	18.4	12.1
Pruritus	3.2	2.8	0.6
Bruising	2.8	3.2	1.6

* The injection-site adverse reactions that were observed among recipients of GARDASIL were at a frequency of at least 1.0% and also at a greater frequency than that observed among AAHS control or saline placebo recipients.
† AAHS Control = Amorphous Aluminum Hydroxyphosphate Sulfate

Common Injection-Site Adverse Reactions in Boys and Men 9 Through 26 Years of Age

The injection site adverse reactions that were observed among recipients of GARDASIL at a frequency of at least 1.0% and also at a greater frequency than that observed among AAHS control or saline placebo recipients are shown in Table 2.

Table 3
Postdose Evaluation of Injection-Site Adverse Reactions in Girls and Women 9 Through 26 Years of Age (1 to 5 Days Postvaccination)

Adverse Reaction	GARDASIL (% occurrence)			AAHS Control* (% occurrence)			Saline Placebo (% occurrence)		
	Post-dose 1 N† = 5011	Post-dose 2 N = 4924	Post-dose 3 N = 4818	Post-dose 1 N = 3410	Post-dose 2 N = 3351	Post-dose 3 N = 3295	Post-dose 1 N = 315	Post-dose 2 N = 301	Post-dose 3 N = 300
Pain	63.4	60.7	62.7	57.0	47.8	49.6	33.7	20.3	27.3
Mild/Moderate	62.5	59.7	61.2	56.6	47.3	48.9	33.3	20.3	27.0
Severe	0.9	1.0	1.5	0.4	0.5	0.6	0.3	0.0	0.3
Swelling‡	10.2	12.8	15.1	8.2	7.5	7.6	4.4	3.0	3.3
Mild/Moderate	9.6	11.9	14.2	8.1	7.2	7.3	4.4	3.0	3.3
Severe	0.6	0.8	0.9	0.2	0.2	0.2	0.0	0.0	0.0
Erythema‡	9.2	12.1	14.7	9.8	8.4	8.9	7.3	5.3	5.7
Mild/Moderate	9.0	11.7	14.3	9.5	8.4	8.8	7.3	5.3	5.7
Severe	0.2	0.3	0.4	0.3	0.1	0.1	0.0	0.0	0.0

* AAHS Control = Amorphous Aluminum Hydroxyphosphate Sulfate
† N = Number of individuals with follow-up
‡ Intensity of swelling and erythema was measured by size (inches): Mild = 0 to ≤1; Moderate = >1 to ≤2; Severe = >2.

Table 4
Postdose Evaluation of Injection-Site Adverse Reactions in Boys and Men 9 Through 26 Years of Age (1 to 5 Days Postvaccination)

Adverse Reaction	GARDASIL (% occurrence)			AAHS Control* (% occurrence)			Saline Placebo (% occurrence)		
	Post-dose 1 N† = 3003	Post-dose 2 N = 2898	Post-dose 3 N = 2826	Post-dose 1 N = 1950	Post-dose 2 N = 1854	Post-dose 3 N = 1799	Post-dose 1 N = 269	Post-dose 2 N = 263	Post-dose 3 N = 259
Pain	44.7	36.9	34.4	38.4	28.2	25.8	27.5	20.5	16.2
Mild/Moderate	44.5	36.4	34.1	37.9	28.2	25.5	27.5	20.2	16.2
Severe	0.2	0.5	0.3	0.4	0.1	0.3	0.0	0.4	0.0
Swelling‡	5.6	6.6	7.7	5.6	4.5	4.1	4.8	1.5	3.5
Mild/Moderate	5.3	6.2	7.1	5.4	4.5	4.0	4.8	1.5	3.1
Severe	0.2	0.3	0.5	0.2	0.0	0.1	0.0	0.0	0.4
Erythema‡	7.2	8.0	8.7	8.3	6.3	5.7	7.1	5.7	5.0
Mild/Moderate	6.8	7.7	8.3	8.0	6.2	5.6	7.1	5.7	5.0
Severe	0.3	0.2	0.3	0.2	0.1	0.1	0.0	0.0	0.0

* AAHS Control = Amorphous Aluminum Hydroxyphosphate Sulfate
† N = Number of individuals with follow-up
‡ Intensity of swelling and erythema was measured by size (inches): Mild = 0 to ≤1; Moderate = >1 to ≤2; Severe = >2.

Table 2
Injection-Site Adverse Reactions in Boys and Men 9 Through 26 Years of Age*

Adverse Reaction (1 to 5 Days Postvaccination)	GARDASIL (N = 3093) %	AAHS Control† (N = 2029) %	Saline Placebo (N = 274) %
Injection Site			
Pain	61.4	50.8	41.6
Erythema	16.7	14.1	14.5
Swelling	13.9	9.6	8.2
Hematoma	1.0	0.3	3.3

* The injection-site adverse reactions that were observed among recipients of GARDASIL were at a frequency of at least 1.0% and also at a greater frequency than that observed among AAHS control or saline placebo recipients.
† AAHS Control = Amorphous Aluminum Hydroxyphosphate Sulfate

Evaluation of Injection-Site Adverse Reactions by Dose in Girls and Women 9 Through 26 Years of Age

An analysis of injection-site adverse reactions in girls and women by dose is shown in Table 3. Of those girls and women who reported an injection-site reaction, 94.3% judged their injection-site adverse reaction to be mild or moderate in intensity.

[See table 3 above]

Evaluation of Injection-Site Adverse Reactions by Dose in Boys and Men 9 Through 26 Years of Age

An analysis of injection-site adverse reactions in boys and men by dose is shown in Table 4. Of those boys and men who reported an injection-site reaction, 96.4% judged their injection-site adverse reaction to be mild or moderate in intensity.

[See table 4 above]

Common Systemic Adverse Reactions in Girls and Women 9 Through 26 Years of Age

Headache was the most commonly reported systemic adverse reaction in both treatment groups (GARDASIL = 28.2% and AAHS control or saline placebo = 28.4%). Fever was the next most commonly reported systemic adverse reaction in both treatment groups (GARDASIL = 13.0% and AAHS control or saline placebo = 11.2%).

Adverse reactions that were observed among recipients of GARDASIL, at a frequency of greater than or equal to 1.0% where the incidence in the GARDASIL group was greater than or equal to the incidence in the AAHS control or saline placebo group, are shown in Table 5.

Table 5
Common Systemic Adverse Reactions in Girls and Women 9 Through 26 Years of Age (GARDASIL ≥Control)*

Adverse Reactions (1 to 15 Days Postvaccination)	GARDASIL (N = 5088) %	AAHS Control† or Saline Placebo (N = 3790) %
Pyrexia	13.0	11.2
Nausea	6.7	6.5
Dizziness	4.0	3.7
Diarrhea	3.6	3.5
Vomiting	2.4	1.9
Cough	2.0	1.5
Toothache	1.5	1.4

Upper respiratory tract infection	1.5	1.5
Malaise	1.4	1.2
Arthralgia	1.2	0.9
Insomnia	1.2	0.9
Nasal congestion	1.1	0.9

* The adverse reactions in this table are those that were observed among recipients of GARDASIL at a frequency of at least 1.0% and greater than or equal to those observed among AAHS control or saline placebo recipients.
† AAHS Control = Amorphous Aluminum Hydroxyphosphate Sulfate

Common Systemic Adverse Reactions in Boys and Men 9 Through 26 Years of Age
Headache was the most commonly reported systemic adverse reaction in both treatment groups (GARDASIL = 12.3% and AAHS control or saline placebo = 11.2%). Fever was the next most commonly reported systemic adverse reaction in both treatment groups (GARDASIL = 8.3% and AAHS control or saline placebo = 6.5%).
Adverse reactions that were observed among recipients of GARDASIL, at a frequency of greater than or equal to 1.0% where the incidence in the group that received GARDASIL was greater than or equal to the incidence in the AAHS control or saline placebo group, are shown in Table 6.

Table 6
Common Systemic Adverse Reactions in Boys and Men 9 Through 26 Years of Age (GARDASIL ≥Control)*

Adverse Reactions (1 to 15 Days Postvaccination)	**GARDASIL** (N = 3093) %	**AAHS Control† or Saline Placebo** (N = 2303) %
Headache	12.3	11.2
Pyrexia	8.3	6.5
Oropharyngeal pain	2.8	2.1
Diarrhea	2.7	2.2
Nasopharyngitis	2.6	2.6
Nausea	2.0	1.0
Upper respiratory tract infection	1.5	1.0
Abdominal pain upper	1.4	1.4
Myalgia	1.3	0.7
Dizziness	1.2	0.9
Vomiting	1.0	0.8

* The adverse reactions in this table are those that were observed among recipients of GARDASIL at a frequency of at least 1.0% and greater than or equal to those observed among AAHS control or saline placebo recipients.
† AAHS Control = Amorphous Aluminum Hydroxyphosphate Sulfate

Evaluation of Fever by Dose in Girls and Women 9 Through 26 Years of Age
An analysis of fever in girls and women by dose is shown in Table 7.
[See table 7 above]
Evaluation of Fever by Dose in Boys and Men 9 Through 26 Years of Age
An analysis of fever in boys and men by dose is shown in Table 8.
[See table 8 above]
Serious Adverse Reactions in the Entire Study Population
Across the clinical studies, 258 individuals (GARDASIL N = 128 or 0.8%; placebo N = 130 or 1.0%) out of 29,323 (GARDASIL N = 15,706; AAHS control N = 13,023; or saline placebo N = 594) individuals (9- through 45-year-old girls and women; and 9- through 26-year-old boys and men) reported a serious systemic adverse reaction.
Of the entire study population (29,323 individuals), 0.04% of the reported serious systemic adverse reactions were judged to be vaccine related by the study investigator. The most frequently (frequency of 4 cases or greater with either GARDASIL, AAHS control, saline placebo, or the total of all three) reported serious systemic adverse reactions, regardless of causality, were:
Headache [0.02% GARDASIL (3 cases) vs. 0.02% AAHS control (2 cases)],
Gastroenteritis [0.02% GARDASIL (3 cases) vs. 0.02% AAHS control (2 cases)],
Appendicitis [0.03% GARDASIL (5 cases) vs. 0.01% AAHS control (1 case)],
Pelvic inflammatory disease [0.02% GARDASIL (3 cases) vs. 0.03% AAHS control (4 cases)],
Urinary tract infection [0.01% GARDASIL (2 cases) vs. 0.02% AAHS control (2 cases)],
Pneumonia [0.01% GARDASIL (2 cases) vs. 0.02% AAHS control (2 cases)],
Pyelonephritis [0.01% GARDASIL (2 cases) vs. 0.02% AAHS control (3 cases)],
Pulmonary embolism [0.01% GARDASIL (2 cases) vs. 0.02% AAHS control (2 cases)].
One case (0.006% GARDASIL; 0.0% AAHS control or saline placebo) of bronchospasm; and 2 cases (0.01% GARDASIL;

Table 7
Postdose Evaluation of Fever in Girls and Women 9 Through 26 Years of Age (1 to 5 Days Postvaccination)

	GARDASIL (% occurrence)			**AAHS Control* or Saline Placebo** (% occurrence)		
Temperature (°F)	Postdose 1 N† = 4945	Postdose 2 N = 4804	Postdose 3 N = 4671	Postdose 1 N = 3681	Postdose 2 N = 3564	Postdose 3 N = 3467
≥100 to <102	3.7	4.1	4.4	3.1	3.8	3.6
≥102	0.3	0.5	0.5	0.2	0.4	0.5

* AAHS Control = Amorphous Aluminum Hydroxyphosphate Sulfate
† N = Number of subjects with follow-up

Table 8
Postdose Evaluation of Fever in Boys and Men 9 Through 26 Years of Age (1 to 5 Days Postvaccination)

	GARDASIL (% occurrence)			**AAHS Control* or Saline Placebo** (% occurrence)		
Temperature (°F)	Postdose 1 N† = 2972	Postdose 2 N = 2849	Postdose 3 N = 2792	Postdose 1 N = 2194	Postdose 2 N = 2079	Postdose 3 N = 2046
≥100 to <102	2.4	2.5	2.3	2.1	2.2	1.6
≥102	0.6	0.5	0.5	0.5	0.3	0.3

* AAHS Control = Amorphous Aluminum Hydroxyphosphate Sulfate
† N = Number of individuals with follow-up

Table 9
Summary of Girls and Women 9 Through 26 Years of Age Who Reported an Incident Condition Potentially Indicative of a Systemic Autoimmune Disorder After Enrollment in Clinical Trials of GARDASIL, Regardless of Causality

Conditions	**GARDASIL** (N = 10,706) **n (%)**	**AAHS Control* or Saline Placebo** (N = 9412) **n (%)**
Arthralgia/Arthritis/Arthropathy†	120 (1.1)	98 (1.0)
Autoimmune Thyroiditis	4 (0.0)	1 (0.0)
Celiac Disease	10 (0.1)	6 (0.1)
Diabetes Mellitus Insulin-dependent	2 (0.0)	2 (0.0)
Erythema Nodosum	2 (0.0)	4 (0.0)
Hyperthyroidism‡	27 (0.3)	21 (0.2)
Hypothyroidism§	35 (0.3)	38 (0.4)
Inflammatory Bowel Disease¶	7 (0.1)	10 (0.1)
Multiple Sclerosis	2 (0.0)	4 (0.0)
Nephritis#	2 (0.0)	5 (0.1)
Optic Neuritis	2 (0.0)	0 (0.0)
Pigmentation DisorderÞ	4 (0.0)	3 (0.0)
Psoriasisß	13 (0.1)	15 (0.2)
Raynaud's Phenomenon	3 (0.0)	4 (0.0)
Rheumatoid Arthritisà	6 (0.1)	2 (0.0)
Scleroderma/Morphea	2 (0.0)	1 (0.0)
Stevens-Johnson Syndrome	1 (0.0)	0 (0.0)
Systemic Lupus Erythematosus	1 (0.0)	3 (0.0)
Uveitis	3 (0.0)	1 (0.0)
All Conditions	245 (2.3)	218 (2.3)

N = Number of individuals enrolled
n = Number of individuals with specific new Medical Conditions
NOTE: Although an individual may have had two or more new Medical Conditions, the individual is counted only once within a category. The same individual may appear in different categories.
* AAHS Control = Amorphous Aluminum Hydroxyphosphate Sulfate
† Arthralgia/Arthritis/Arthropathy includes the following terms: Arthralgia, Arthritis, Arthritis reactive, and Arthropathy
‡ Hyperthyroidism includes the following terms: Basedow's disease, Goiter, Toxic nodular goiter, and Hyperthyroidism
§ Hypothyroidism includes the following terms: Hypothyroidism and thyroiditis
¶ Inflammatory bowel disease includes the following terms: Colitis ulcerative, Crohn's disease, and Inflammatory bowel disease
\# Nephritis includes the following terms: Nephritis, Glomerulonephritis minimal lesion, Glomerulonephritis proliferative
Þ Pigmentation disorder includes the following terms: Pigmentation disorder, Skin depigmentation, and Vitiligo
ß Psoriasis includes the following terms: Psoriasis, Pustular psoriasis, and Psoriatic arthropathy
à Rheumatoid arthritis includes juvenile rheumatoid arthritis. One woman counted in the rheumatoid arthritis group reported rheumatoid arthritis as an adverse experience at Day 130.

0.0% AAHS control or saline placebo) of asthma were reported as serious systemic adverse reactions that occurred following any vaccination visit.

In addition, there was 1 individual in the clinical trials, in the group that received GARDASIL, who reported two injection-site serious adverse reactions (injection-site pain and injection-site joint movement impairment).

Deaths in the Entire Study Population

Across the clinical studies, 40 deaths (GARDASIL N = 21 or 0.1%; placebo N = 19 or 0.1%) were reported in 29,323 (GARDASIL N = 15,706; AAHS control N = 13,023, saline placebo N = 594) individuals (9- through 45-year-old girls and women; and 9- through 26-year-old boys and men). The events reported were consistent with events expected in healthy adolescent and adult populations. The most common cause of death was motor vehicle accident (5 individuals who received GARDASIL and 4 individuals who received AAHS control), followed by drug overdose/suicide (2 individuals who received GARDASIL and 6 individuals who received AAHS control), gun shot wound (1 individual who received GARDASIL and 3 individuals who received AAHS control), and pulmonary embolus/deep vein thrombosis (1 individual who received GARDASIL and 1 individual who received AAHS control). In addition, there were 2 cases of sepsis, 1 case of pancreatic cancer, 1 case of arrhythmia, 1 case of pulmonary tuberculosis, 1 case of hyperthyroidism, 1 case of post-operative pulmonary embolism and acute renal failure, 1 case of traumatic brain injury/cardiac arrest, 1 case of systemic lupus erythematosus, 1 case of cerebrovascular accident, 1 case of breast cancer, and 1 case of nasopharyngeal cancer in the group that received GARDASIL; 1 case of asphyxia, 1 case of acute lymphocytic leukemia, 1 case of chemical poisoning, and 1 case of myocardial ischemia in the AAHS control group; and 1 case of medulloblastoma in the saline placebo group.

Systemic Autoimmune Disorders in Girls and Women 9 Through 26 Years of Age

In the clinical studies, 9- through 26-year-old girls and women were evaluated for new medical conditions that occurred over the course of follow-up. New medical conditions potentially indicative of a systemic autoimmune disorder seen in the group that received GARDASIL or AAHS control or saline placebo are shown in Table 9. This population includes all girls and women who received at least one dose of GARDASIL or AAHS control or saline placebo, and had safety data available.

[See table 9 at top of previous page]

Systemic Autoimmune Disorders in Boys and Men 9 Through 26 Years of Age

In the clinical studies, 9- through 26-year-old boys and men were evaluated for new medical conditions that occurred over the course of follow-up. New medical conditions potentially indicative of a systemic autoimmune disorder seen in the group that received GARDASIL or AAHS control or saline placebo are shown in Table 10. This population includes all boys and men who received at least one dose of GARDASIL or AAHS control or saline placebo, and had safety data available.

[See table 10 above]

Safety in Concomitant Use with RECOMBIVAX HB [hepatitis B vaccine (recombinant)] in Girls and Women 16 Through 23 Years of Age

The safety of GARDASIL when administered concomitantly with RECOMBIVAX HB®[1] [hepatitis B vaccine (recombinant)] was evaluated in an AAHS-controlled study of 1871 girls and women with a mean age of 20.4 years *[see Clinical Studies (14.9)]*. The race distribution of the study individuals was as follows: 61.6% White; 23.8% Other; 11.9% Black; 1.6% Hispanic (Black and White); 0.8% Asian; and 0.3% American Indian. The rates of systemic and injection-site adverse reactions were similar among girls and women who received concomitant vaccination as compared with those who received GARDASIL or RECOMBIVAX HB [hepatitis B vaccine (recombinant)].

Safety in Concomitant Use with Menactra [Meningococcal (Groups A, C, Y and W-135) Polysaccharide Diphtheria Toxoid Conjugate Vaccine] and Adacel [Tetanus Toxoid, Reduced Diphtheria Toxoid and Acellular Pertussis Vaccine Adsorbed (Tdap)]

The safety of GARDASIL when administered concomitantly with Menactra [Meningococcal (Groups A, C, Y and W-135) Polysaccharide Diphtheria Toxoid Conjugate Vaccine] and Adacel [Tetanus Toxoid, Reduced Diphtheria Toxoid and Acellular Pertussis Vaccine Adsorbed (Tdap)] was evaluated in a randomized study of 1040 boys and girls with a mean age of 12.6 years *[see Clinical Studies (14.10)]*. The race distribution of the study subjects was as follows: 77.7% White; 1.4% Multi-racial; 12.3% Black; 6.8% Hispanic (Black and White); 1.2% Asian; 0.4% American Indian, and 0.2% Indian.

There was an increase in injection-site swelling reported at the injection site for GARDASIL (concomitant = 10.9%, non-concomitant = 6.9%) when GARDASIL was administered concomitantly with Menactra and Adacel as compared to non-concomitant (separated by 1 month) vaccination. The majority of injection-site swelling adverse experiences were reported as being mild to moderate in intensity.

Safety in Women 27 Through 45 Years of Age

The adverse reaction profile in women 27 through 45 years of age was comparable to the profile seen in girls and women 9 through 26 years of age.

Table 10
Summary of Boys and Men 9 Through 26 Years of Age Who Reported an Incident Condition Potentially Indicative of a Systemic Autoimmune Disorder After Enrollment in Clinical Trials of GARDASIL, Regardless of Causality

Conditions	GARDASIL (N = 3093) n (%)	AAHS Control* or Saline Placebo (N = 2303) n (%)
Alopecia Areata	2 (0.1)	0 (0.0)
Ankylosing Spondylitis	1 (0.0)	2 (0.1)
Arthralgia/Arthritis/Reactive Arthritis	30 (1.0)	17 (0.7)
Autoimmune Thrombocytopenia	1 (0.0)	0 (0.0)
Diabetes Mellitus Type 1	3 (0.1)	2 (0.1)
Hyperthyroidism	0 (0.0)	1 (0.0)
Hypothyroidism†	3 (0.1)	0 (0.0)
Inflammatory Bowel Disease‡	1 (0.0)	2 (0.1)
Myocarditis	1 (0.0)	1 (0.0)
Proteinuria	1 (0.0)	0 (0.0)
Psoriasis	0 (0.0)	4 (0.2)
Skin Depigmentation	1 (0.0)	0 (0.0)
Vitiligo	2 (0.1)	5 (0.2)
All Conditions	46 (1.5)	34 (1.5)

N = Number of individuals who received at least one dose of either vaccine or placebo
n = Number of individuals with specific new Medical Conditions
NOTE: Although an individual may have had two or more new Medical Conditions, the individual is counted only once within a category. The same individual may appear in different categories.
* AAHS Control = Amorphous Aluminum Hydroxyphosphate Sulfate
† Hypothyroidism includes the following terms: Hypothyroidism and Autoimmune thyroiditis
‡ Inflammatory bowel disease includes the following terms: Colitis ulcerative and Crohn's disease

Table 11
Analysis of Efficacy of GARDASIL in the PPE* Population† of 16- Through 26-Year-Old Girls and Women for Vaccine HPV Types

Population	GARDASIL N	GARDASIL Number of cases	AAHS Control N	AAHS Control Number of cases	% Efficacy (95% CI)
HPV 16- or 18-related CIN 2/3 or AIS					
Study 1‡	755	0	750	12	100.0 (65.1, 100.0)
Study 2	231	0	230	1	100.0 (-3744.9, 100.0)
Study 3	2201	0	2222	36	100.0 (89.2, 100.0)
Study 4	5306	2	5262	63	96.9 (88.2, 99.6)
Combined Protocols§	8493	2	8464	112	98.2 (93.5, 99.8)
HPV 16-related CIN 2/3 or AIS					
Combined Protocols§	7402	2	7205	93	97.9 (92.3, 99.8)
HPV 18-related CIN 2/3 or AIS					
Combined Protocols§	7382	0	7316	29	100.0 (86.6, 100.0)
HPV 16- or 18-related VIN 2/3					
Study 2	231	0	230	0	Not calculated
Study 3	2219	0	2239	6	100.0 (14.4, 100.0)
Study 4	5322	0	5275	4	100.0 (-50.3, 100.0)
Combined Protocols§	7772	0	7744	10	100.0 (55.5, 100.0)
HPV 16- or 18-related VaIN 2/3					
Study 2	231	0	230	0	Not calculated
Study 3	2219	0	2239	5	100.0 (-10.1, 100.0)
Study 4	5322	0	5275	4	100.0 (-50.3, 100.0)
Combined Protocols§	7772	0	7744	9	100.0 (49.5, 100.0)

(Table continued on next page)

6.2 Postmarketing Experience

The following adverse events have been spontaneously reported during post-approval use of GARDASIL. Because these events were reported voluntarily from a population of uncertain size, it is not possible to reliably estimate their frequency or to establish a causal relationship to vaccine exposure.

Table 11 *(cont.)*
Analysis of Efficacy of GARDASIL in the PPE* Population† of 16- Through 26-Year-Old Girls and Women for Vaccine HPV Types

Population	GARDASIL		AAHS Control		% Efficacy (95% CI)
	N	Number of cases	N	Number of cases	
HPV 6-, 11-, 16-, or 18-related CIN (CIN 1, CIN 2/3) or AIS					
Study 2	235	0	233	3	100.0 (-138.4, 100.0)
Study 3	2241	0	2258	77	100.0 (95.1, 100.0)
Study 4	5388	9	5374	145	93.8 (88.0, 97.2)
Combined Protocols§	7864	9	7865	225	96.0 (92.3, 98.2)
HPV 6-, 11-, 16-, or 18-related Genital Warts					
Study 2	235	0	233	3	100.0 (-139.5, 100.0)
Study 3	2261	0	2279	58	100.0 (93.5, 100.0)
Study 4	5404	2	5390	132	98.5 (94.5, 99.8)
Combined Protocols§	7900	2	7902	193	99.0 (96.2, 99.9)
HPV 6- and 11-related Genital Warts					
Combined Protocols§	6932	2	6856	189	99.0 (96.2, 99.9)

N = Number of individuals with at least 1 follow-up visit after Month 7
CI = Confidence Interval
Note 1: Point estimates and confidence intervals are adjusted for person-time of follow-up.
Note 2: The first analysis in the table (i.e., HPV 16- or 18-related CIN 2/3, AIS or worse) was the primary endpoint of the vaccine development plan.
Note 3: Table 11 does not include cases due to non-vaccine HPV types.
AAHS Control = Amorphous Aluminum Hydroxyphosphate Sulfate
* The PPE population consisted of individuals who received all 3 vaccinations within 1 year of enrollment, did not have major deviations from the study protocol, and were naïve (PCR negative and seronegative) to the relevant HPV type(s) (Types 6, 11, 16, and 18) prior to dose 1 and through 1 month postdose 3 (Month 7).
† See Table 14 for analysis of vaccine impact in the general population.
‡ Evaluated only the HPV 16 L1 VLP vaccine component of GARDASIL
§ Analyses of the combined trials were prospectively planned and included the use of similar study entry criteria.

Table 12
Analysis of Efficacy of GARDASIL in the PPE* Population of 16- Through 26-Year-Old Boys and Men for Vaccine HPV Types

Endpoint	GARDASIL		AAHS Control		% Efficacy (95% CI)
	N†	Number of cases	N	Number of cases	
External Genital Lesions HPV 6-, 11-, 16-, or 18- related					
External Genital Lesions	1394	3	1404	32	90.6 (70.1, 98.2)
Condyloma	1394	3	1404	28	89.3 (65.3, 97.9)
PIN 1/2/3	1394	0	1404	4	100.0 (-52.1, 100.0)

CI = Confidence Interval
AAHS Control = Amorphous Aluminum Hydroxyphosphate Sulfate
* The PPE population consisted of individuals who received all 3 vaccinations within 1 year of enrollment, did not have major deviations from the study protocol, and were naïve (PCR negative and seronegative) to the relevant HPV type(s) (Types 6, 11, 16, and 18) prior to dose 1 and through 1 month postdose 3 (Month 7).
† N = Number of individuals with at least 1 follow-up visit after Month 7

Table 13
Analysis of Efficacy of GARDASIL for Anal Disease in the PPE* Population of 16- Through 26-Year-Old Boys and Men in the MSM Sub-study for Vaccine HPV Types

HPV 6-, 11-, 16-, or 18-related Endpoint	GARDASIL		AAHS Control		% Efficacy (95% CI)
	N†	Number of cases	N	Number of cases	
AIN 1/2/3	194	5	208	24	77.5 (39.6, 93.3)
AIN 2/3	194	3	208	13	74.9 (8.8, 95.4)
AIN 1	194	4	208	16	73.0 (16.3, 93.4)
Condyloma Acuminatum	194	0	208	6	100.0 (8.2, 100.0)
Non-acuminate	194	4	208	11	60.4 (-33.5, 90.8)

CI = Confidence Interval
AAHS Control = Amorphous Aluminum Hydroxyphosphate Sulfate
* The PPE population consisted of individuals who received all 3 vaccinations within 1 year of enrollment, did not have major deviations from the study protocol, and were naïve (PCR negative and seronegative) to the relevant HPV type(s) (Types 6, 11, 16, and 18) prior to dose 1 and through 1 month postdose 3 (month 7).
† N = Number of individuals with at least 1 follow-up visit after Month 7

Blood and lymphatic system disorders: Autoimmune hemolytic anemia, idiopathic thrombocytopenic purpura, lymphadenopathy.
Respiratory, thoracic and mediastinal disorders: Pulmonary embolus.
Gastrointestinal disorders: Nausea, pancreatitis, vomiting.
General disorders and administration site conditions: Asthenia, chills, death, fatigue, malaise.
Immune system disorders: Autoimmune diseases, hypersensitivity reactions including anaphylactic/anaphylactoid reactions, bronchospasm, and urticaria.
Musculoskeletal and connective tissue disorders: Arthralgia, myalgia.
Nervous system disorders: Acute disseminated encephalomyelitis, dizziness, Guillain-Barré syndrome, headache, motor neuron disease, paralysis, seizures, syncope (including syncope associated with tonic-clonic movements and other seizure-like activity) sometimes resulting in falling with injury, transverse myelitis.
Infections and infestations: cellulitis.
Vascular disorders: Deep venous thrombosis.

7 DRUG INTERACTIONS

7.1 Use with RECOMBIVAX HB

Results from clinical studies indicate that GARDASIL may be administered concomitantly (at a separate injection site) with RECOMBIVAX HB [hepatitis B vaccine (recombinant)] *[see Clinical Studies (14.9)]*.

7.2 Use with Menactra and Adacel

Results from clinical studies indicate that GARDASIL may be administered concomitantly (at a separate injection site) with Menactra [Meningococcal (Groups A, C, Y and W-135) Polysaccharide Diphtheria Toxoid Conjugate Vaccine] and Adacel [Tetanus Toxoid, Reduced Diphtheria Toxoid and Acellular Pertussis Vaccine Adsorbed (Tdap)] *[see Clinical Studies (14.10)]*.

7.3 Use with Hormonal Contraceptives

In clinical studies of 16- through 26-year-old women, 13,912 (GARDASIL N = 6952; AAHS control or saline placebo N = 6960) who had post-Month 7 follow-up used hormonal contraceptives for a total of 33,859 person-years (65.8% of the total follow-up time in the studies).
In one clinical study of 24- through 45-year-old women, 1357 (GARDASIL N = 690; AAHS control N = 667) who had post-Month 7 follow-up used hormonal contraceptives for a total of 3400 person-years (31.5% of the total follow-up time in the study). Use of hormonal contraceptives or lack of use of hormonal contraceptives among study participants did not impair the immune response in the per protocol immunogenicity (PPI) population.

7.4 Use with Systemic Immunosuppressive Medications

Immunosuppressive therapies, including irradiation, antimetabolites, alkylating agents, cytotoxic drugs, and corticosteroids (used in greater than physiologic doses), may reduce the immune responses to vaccines *[see Use in Specific Populations (8.6)]*.

8 USE IN SPECIFIC POPULATIONS

8.1 Pregnancy

Pregnancy Category B:
Reproduction studies have been performed in female rats at doses equivalent to the recommended human dose and have revealed no evidence of impaired female fertility or harm to the fetus due to GARDASIL. There are, however, no adequate and well-controlled studies in pregnant women. Because animal reproduction studies are not always predictive of human responses, GARDASIL should be used during pregnancy only if clearly needed.
An evaluation of the effect of GARDASIL on embryo-fetal, pre- and postweaning development was conducted using rats. One group of rats was administered GARDASIL twice prior to gestation, during the period of organogenesis (gestation Day 6) and on lactation Day 7. A second group of pregnant rats was administered GARDASIL during the period of organogenesis (gestation Day 6) and on lactation Day 7 only. GARDASIL was administered at 0.5 mL/rat/occasion (120 mcg total protein which is equivalent to the recommended human dose) by intramuscular injection. No adverse effects on mating, fertility, pregnancy, parturition, lactation, embryo-fetal or pre- and postweaning development were observed. There were no vaccine-related fetal malformations or other evidence of teratogenesis noted in this study. In addition, there were no treatment-related effects on developmental signs, behavior, reproductive performance, or fertility of the offspring.
Clinical Studies in Humans
In clinical studies, women underwent urine pregnancy testing prior to administration of each dose of GARDASIL. Women who were found to be pregnant before completion of a 3-dose regimen of GARDASIL were instructed to defer completion of their vaccination regimen until resolution of the pregnancy.

GARDASIL is not indicated for women 27 years of age or older. However, safety data in women 16 through 45 years of age was collected, and 3819 women (GARDASIL N = 1894 vs. AAHS control or saline placebo N = 1925) reported at least 1 pregnancy each.

The overall proportions of pregnancies that resulted in an adverse outcome, defined as the combined numbers of spontaneous abortion, late fetal death, and congenital anomaly cases out of the total number of pregnancy outcomes for which an outcome was known (and excluding elective terminations), were 22.6% (446/1973) in women who received GARDASIL and 23.1% (460/1994) in women who received AAHS control or saline placebo.

Overall, 55 and 65 women in the group that received GARDASIL or AAHS control or saline placebo, respectively (2.9% and 3.4% of all women who reported a pregnancy in the respective vaccination groups), experienced a serious adverse reaction during pregnancy. The most common events reported were conditions that can result in Caesarean section (e.g., failure of labor, malpresentation, cephalopelvic disproportion), premature onset of labor (e.g., threatened abortions, premature rupture of membranes), and pregnancy-related medical problems (e.g., pre-eclampsia, hyperemesis). The proportions of pregnant women who experienced such events were comparable between the groups receiving GARDASIL and AAHS control or saline placebo.

There were 45 cases of congenital anomaly in pregnancies that occurred in women who received GARDASIL and 34 cases of congenital anomaly in pregnancies that occurred in women who received AAHS control or saline placebo.

Further sub-analyses were conducted to evaluate pregnancies with estimated onset within 30 days or more than 30 days from administration of a dose of GARDASIL or AAHS control or saline placebo. For pregnancies with estimated onset within 30 days of vaccination, 5 cases of congenital anomaly were observed in the group that received GARDASIL compared to 1 case of congenital anomaly in the group that received AAHS control or saline placebo. The congenital anomalies seen in pregnancies with estimated onset within 30 days of vaccination included pyloric stenosis, congenital megacolon, congenital hydronephrosis, hip dysplasia, and club foot. Conversely, in pregnancies with onset more than 30 days following vaccination, 40 cases of congenital anomaly were observed in the group that received GARDASIL compared with 33 cases of congenital anomaly in the group that received AAHS control or saline placebo.

Pregnancy Registry for GARDASIL

Merck Sharp & Dohme Corp., a subsidiary of Merck & Co., Inc., maintains a Pregnancy Registry to monitor fetal outcomes of pregnant women exposed to GARDASIL. Patients and health care providers are encouraged to report any exposure to GARDASIL during pregnancy by calling (800) 986-8999.

8.3 Nursing Mothers

Women 16 Through 45 Years of Age

It is not known whether GARDASIL is excreted in human milk. Because many drugs are excreted in human milk, caution should be exercised when GARDASIL is administered to a nursing woman.

GARDASIL or AAHS control were given to a total of 1133 women (vaccine N = 582, AAHS control N = 551) during the relevant Phase III clinical studies.

Overall, 27 and 13 infants of women who received GARDASIL or AAHS control, respectively (representing 4.6% and 2.4% of the total number of women who were breast-feeding during the period in which they received GARDASIL or AAHS control, respectively), experienced a serious adverse reaction.

In a post-hoc analysis of clinical studies, a higher number of breast-feeding infants (n = 7) whose mothers received GARDASIL had acute respiratory illnesses within 30 days post vaccination of the mother as compared to infants (n = 2) whose mothers received AAHS control.

8.4 Pediatric Use

Safety and effectiveness have not been established in pediatric patients below 9 years of age.

8.5 Geriatric Use

The safety and effectiveness of GARDASIL have not been evaluated in a geriatric population, defined as individuals aged 65 years and over.

8.6 Immunocompromised Individuals

The immunologic response to GARDASIL may be diminished in immunocompromised individuals *[see Drug Interactions (7.4)]*.

10 OVERDOSAGE

There have been reports of administration of higher than recommended doses of GARDASIL.

In general, the adverse event profile reported with overdose was comparable to recommended single doses of GARDASIL.

11 DESCRIPTION

GARDASIL, Human Papillomavirus Quadrivalent (Types 6, 11, 16, and 18) Vaccine, Recombinant, is a non-infectious recombinant quadrivalent vaccine prepared from the purified virus-like particles (VLPs) of the major capsid (L1) protein of HPV Types 6, 11, 16, and 18. The L1 proteins are produced by separate fermentations in recombinant *Saccharomyces cerevisiae* and self-assembled into VLPs. The fermentation process involves growth of *S. cerevisiae* on chemically-defined fermentation media which include vitamins, amino acids, mineral salts, and carbohydrates. The VLPs are released from the yeast cells by cell disruption and purified by a series of chemical and physical methods. The purified VLPs are adsorbed on preformed aluminum-containing adjuvant (Amorphous Aluminum Hydroxyphosphate Sulfate). The quadrivalent HPV VLP vaccine is a sterile liquid suspension that is prepared by combining the adsorbed VLPs of each HPV type and additional amounts of the aluminum-containing adjuvant and the final purification buffer.

GARDASIL is a sterile suspension for intramuscular administration. Each 0.5-mL dose contains approximately 20 mcg of HPV 6 L1 protein, 40 mcg of HPV 11 L1 protein, 40 mcg of HPV 16 L1 protein, and 20 mcg of HPV 18 L1 protein.

Each 0.5-mL dose of the vaccine contains approximately 225 mcg of aluminum (as Amorphous Aluminum Hydroxyphosphate Sulfate adjuvant), 9.56 mg of sodium chloride, 0.78 mg of L-histidine, 50 mcg of polysorbate 80, 35 mcg of sodium borate, <7 mcg yeast protein/dose, and water for injection. The product does not contain a preservative or antibiotics.

After thorough agitation, GARDASIL is a white, cloudy liquid.

12 CLINICAL PHARMACOLOGY

12.1 Mechanism of Action

HPV only infects human beings. Animal studies with analogous animal papillomaviruses suggest that the efficacy of L1 VLP vaccines may involve the development of humoral

Table 14

Effectiveness of GARDASIL in Prevention of HPV 6, 11, 16, or 18-Related Genital Disease in Girls and Women 16 Through 26 Years of Age, Regardless of Current or Prior Exposure to Vaccine HPV Types

Endpoint	Analysis	GARDASIL or HPV 16 L1 VLP Vaccine		AAHS Control		% Reduction (95% CI)
		N	Cases	N	Cases	
HPV 16- or 18-related CIN 2/3 or AIS	Prophylactic Efficacy*	9346	4	9407	155	97.4 (93.3, 99.3)
	HPV 16 and/or HPV 18 Positive at Day 1[†]	2870	142	2898	148[‡]	--[§]
	Girls and Women Regardless of Current or Prior Exposure to HPV 16 or 18[¶]	9836	146	9904	303	51.8 (41.1, 60.7)
HPV 16- or 18-related VIN 2/3 or VaIN 2/3	Prophylactic Efficacy*	8642	1	8673	34	97.0 (82.4, 99.9)
	HPV 16 and/or HPV 18 Positive at Day 1[†]	1880	8	1876	4	--[§]
	Girls and Women Regardless of Current or Prior Exposure to HPV 16 or 18[¶]	8955	9	8968	38	76.3 (50.0, 89.9)
HPV 6-, 11-, 16-, 18-related CIN (CIN 1, CIN 2/3) or AIS	Prophylactic Efficacy*	8630	16	8680	309	94.8 (91.5, 97.1)
	HPV 6, HPV 11, HPV 16, and/or HPV 18 Positive at Day 1[†]	2466	186[#]	2437	213[#]	--[§]
	Girls and Women Regardless of Current or Prior Exposure to Vaccine HPV Types[¶]	8819	202	8854	522	61.5 (54.6, 67.4)
HPV 6-, 11-, 16-, or 18-related Genital Warts	Prophylactic Efficacy*	8761	10	8792	252	96.0 (92.6, 98.1)
	HPV 6, HPV 11, HPV 16, and/or HPV 18 Positive at Day 1[†]	2501	51[Þ]	2475	55[Þ]	--[§]
	Girls and Women Regardless of Current or Prior Exposure to Vaccine HPV Types[¶]	8955	61	8968	307	80.3 (73.9, 85.3)
HPV 6- or 11-related Genital Warts	Prophylactic Efficacy*	7769	9	7792	246	96.4 (93.0, 98.4)
	HPV 6 and/or HPV 11 Positive at Day 1[†]	1186	51	1176	54	--[§]
	Girls and Women Regardless of Current or Prior Exposure to Vaccine HPV Types[¶]	8955	60	8968	300	80.1 (73.7, 85.2)

CI = Confidence Interval

N = Number of individuals who have at least one follow-up visit after Day 1

Note 1: The 16- and 18-related CIN 2/3 or AIS composite endpoint included data from studies 1, 2, 3, and 4. All other endpoints only included data from studies 2, 3, and 4.

Note 2: Positive status at Day 1 denotes PCR positive and/or seropositive for the respective type at Day 1.

Note 3: Table 14 does not include disease due to non-vaccine HPV types.

AAHS Control = Amorphous Aluminum Hydroxyphosphate Sulfate

* Includes all individuals who received at least 1 vaccination and who were HPV-naïve (i.e., seronegative and PCR negative) at Day 1 to the vaccine HPV type being analyzed. Case counting started at 1 month postdose 1.

† Includes all individuals who received at least 1 vaccination and who were HPV positive or had unknown HPV status at Day 1, to at least one vaccine HPV type. Case counting started at Day 1.

‡ Out of the 148 AAHS control cases of 16/18 CIN 2/3, 2 women were missing serology or PCR results for Day 1.

§ There is no expected efficacy since GARDASIL has not been demonstrated to provide protection against disease from vaccine HPV types to which a person has previously been exposed through sexual activity.

¶ Includes all individuals who received at least 1 vaccination (regardless of baseline HPV status at Day 1). Case counting started at 1 month postdose 1.

\# Includes 2 AAHS control women with missing serology/PCR data at Day 1.

Þ Includes 1 woman with missing serology/PCR data at Day 1.

Table 15
Effectiveness of GARDASIL in Prevention of Any HPV Type Related Genital Disease in Girls and Women 16 Through 26 Years of Age, Regardless of Current or Prior Infection with Vaccine or Non-Vaccine HPV Types

Endpoints Caused by Vaccine or Non-vaccine HPV Types	Analysis	GARDASIL		AAHS Control		% Reduction (95% CI)
		N	Cases	N	Cases	
CIN 2/3 or AIS	Prophylactic Efficacy*	4616	77	4680	136	42.7 (23.7, 57.3)
	Girls and Women Regardless of Current or Prior Exposure to Vaccine or Non-Vaccine HPV Types†	8559	421	8592	516	18.4 (7.0, 28.4)
VIN 2/3 and VaIN 2/3	Prophylactic Efficacy*	4688	7	4735	31	77.1 (47.1, 91.5)
	Girls and Women Regardless of Current or Prior Exposure to Vaccine or Non-Vaccine HPV Types†	8688	30	8701	61	50.7 (22.5, 69.3)
CIN (Any Grade) or AIS	Prophylactic Efficacy*	4616	272	4680	390	29.7 (17.7, 40.0)
	Girls and Women Regardless of Current or Prior Exposure to Vaccine or Non-Vaccine HPV Types†	8559	967	8592	1189	19.1 (11.9, 25.8)
Genital Warts	Prophylactic Efficacy*	4688	29	4735	169	82.8 (74.3, 88.8)
	Girls and Women Regardless of Current or Prior Exposure to Vaccine or Non-Vaccine HPV Types†	8688	132	8701	350	62.5 (54.0, 69.5)

CI = Confidence Interval
AAHS Control = Amorphous Aluminum Hydroxyphosphate Sulfate
* Includes all individuals who received at least 1 vaccination and who had a Pap test that was negative for SIL [Squamous Intraepithelial Lesion] at Day 1 and were naïve to 14 common HPV types at Day 1. Case counting started at 1 month postdose 1.
† Includes all individuals who received at least 1 vaccination (regardless of baseline HPV status or Pap test result at Day 1). Case counting started at 1 month postdose 1.

Table 16
Effectiveness of GARDASIL in Prevention of HPV Types 6-, 11-, 16-, or 18-Related Anogenital Disease in Boys and Men 16 Through 26 Years of Age, Regardless of Current or Prior Exposure to Vaccine HPV Types

Endpoint	Analysis	GARDASIL		AAHS Control		% Reduction (95% CI)
		N	Cases	N	Cases	
External Genital Lesions	Prophylactic Efficacy*	1775	13	1770	54	76.3 (56.0, 88.1)
	HPV 6, HPV 11, HPV 16, and/or HPV 18 Positive at Day 1†	460	14	453	26	--‡
	Boys and Men Regardless of Current or Prior Exposure to Vaccine or Non-Vaccine HPV Types§	1943	27	1937	80	66.7 (48.0, 79.3)
Condyloma	Prophylactic Efficacy*	1775	10	1770	49	80.0 (59.9, 90.9)
	HPV 6, HPV 11, HPV 16, and/or HPV 18 Positive at Day 1†	460	14	453	25	--‡
	Boys and Men Regardless of Current or Prior Exposure to Vaccine or Non-Vaccine HPV Types§	1943	24	1937	74	68.1 (48.8, 80.7)

(Table continued on next page)

immune responses. Human beings develop a humoral immune response to the vaccine, although the exact mechanism of protection is unknown.

13 NONCLINICAL TOXICOLOGY

13.1 Carcinogenesis, Mutagenesis, Impairment of Fertility

GARDASIL has not been evaluated for the potential to cause carcinogenicity or genotoxicity.
GARDASIL administered to female rats at a dose of 120 mcg total protein, which is equivalent to the recommended human dose, had no effects on mating performance, fertility, or embryonic/fetal survival.
The effect of GARDASIL on male fertility has been studied in male rats at an intramuscular dose of 0.5 mL/rat/occasion (120 mcg total protein which is equivalent to the recommended human dose). One group of male rats was administered GARDASIL once, 3 days prior to cohabitation, and a second group of male rats was administered GARDASIL three times, at 6 weeks, 3 weeks, and 3 days prior to cohabitation. There were no treatment-related effects on reproductive performance including fertility, sperm count, and sperm motility. There were no treatment-related gross or histomorphologic and weight changes on the testes.

14 CLINICAL STUDIES

CIN 2/3 and AIS are the immediate and necessary precursors of squamous cell carcinoma and adenocarcinoma of the cervix, respectively. Their detection and removal has been shown to prevent cancer; thus, they serve as surrogate markers for prevention of cervical cancer. In the clinical studies in girls and women aged 16 through 26 years, cases of CIN 2/3 and AIS were the efficacy endpoints to assess prevention of cervical cancer. In addition, cases of VIN 2/3 and VaIN 2/3 were the efficacy endpoints to assess prevention of HPV-related vulvar and vaginal cancers, and observations of external genital lesions were the efficacy endpoints for the prevention of genital warts.

In clinical studies in boys and men aged 16 through 26 years, efficacy was evaluated using the following endpoints: external genital warts and penile/perineal/perianal intraepithelial neoplasia (PIN) grades 1/2/3 or penile/perineal/perianal cancer. In addition, cases of AIN grades 1/2/3 and anal cancer made up the composite efficacy endpoint used to assess prevention of HPV-related anal cancer.
Anal HPV infection, AIN, and anal cancer were not endpoints in the studies conducted in women. The similarity of HPV-related anal disease in men and women supports bridging the indication of prevention of AIN and anal cancer to women.
Efficacy was assessed in 6 AAHS-controlled, double-blind, randomized Phase II and III clinical studies. The first Phase II study evaluated the HPV 16 component of GARDASIL (Study 1, N = 2391 16- through 26-year-old girls and women) and the second evaluated all components of GARDASIL (Study 2, N = 551 16- through 26-year-old girls and women). Two Phase III studies evaluated GARDASIL in 5442 (Study 3) and 12,157 (Study 4) 16- through 26-year-old girls and women. A third Phase III study, Study 5, evaluated GARDASIL in 4055 16- through 26-year-old boys and men, including a subset of 598 (GARDASIL = 299; placebo = 299) men who self-identified as having sex with men (MSM population). A fourth Phase III study, Study 6, evaluated GARDASIL in 3817 24- through 45-year-old women. Together, these six studies evaluated 28,413 individuals (20,541 girls and women 16 through 26 years of age at enrollment with a mean age of 20.0 years, 4055 boys and men 16 through 26 years of age at enrollment with a mean age of 20.5 years, and 3817 women 24 through 45 years of age at enrollment with a mean age of 34.3 years). The race distribution of the 16- through 26-year-old girls and women in the clinical trials was as follows: 70.4% White; 12.2% Hispanic (Black and White); 8.8% Other; 4.6% Black; 3.8% Asian; and 0.2% American Indian. The race distribution of the 16- through 26-year-old boys and men in the clinical trials was as follows: 35.2% White; 20.5% Hispanic (Black and White); 14.4% Other; 19.8% Black; 10.0% Asian; and 0.1% American Indian. The race distribution of the 24- through 45-year-old women in the clinical trials was as follows: 20.6% White; 43.2% Hispanic (Black and White); 0.2% Other; 4.8% Black; 31.2% Asian; and 0.1% American Indian.
The median duration of follow-up was 4.0, 3.0, 3.0, 3.0, 2.3, and 4.0 years for Study 1, Study 2, Study 3, Study 4, Study 5, and Study 6, respectively. Individuals received vaccine or AAHS control on the day of enrollment and 2 and 6 months thereafter. Efficacy was analyzed for each study individually and for all studies in girls and women combined according to a prospective clinical plan.
Overall, 73% of 16- through 26-year-old girls and women, 67% of 24- through 45-year-old women, and 83% of 16- through 26-year-old boys and men were naïve (i.e., PCR [Polymerase Chain Reaction] negative and seronegative for all 4 vaccine HPV types) to all 4 vaccine HPV types at enrollment.
A total of 27% of 16- through 26-year-old girls and women, 33% of 24- through 45-year-old women, and 17% of 16- through 26-year-old boys and men had evidence of prior exposure to or ongoing infection with at least 1 of the 4 vaccine HPV types. Among these individuals, 74% of 16- through 26-year-old girls and women, 71% of 24- through 45-year-old women, and 78% of 16- through 26-year-old boys and men had evidence of prior exposure to or ongoing infection with only 1 of the 4 vaccine HPV types and were naïve (PCR negative and seronegative) to the remaining 3 types.
In 24- through 45-year-old individuals, 0.4% had been exposed to all 4 vaccine HPV types.
In individuals who were naïve (PCR negative and seronegative) to all 4 vaccine HPV types, CIN, genital warts, VIN, VaIN, PIN, and persistent infection caused by any of the 4 vaccine HPV types were counted as endpoints.
Among individuals who were positive (PCR positive and/or seropositive) for a vaccine HPV type at Day 1, endpoints related to that type were not included in the analyses of prophylactic efficacy. Endpoints related to the remaining types for which the individual was naïve (PCR negative and seronegative) were counted.
For example, in individuals who were HPV 18 positive (PCR positive and/or seropositive) at Day 1, lesions caused by HPV 18 were not counted in the prophylactic efficacy evaluations. Lesions caused by HPV 6, 11, and 16 were included in the prophylactic efficacy evaluations. The same approach was used for the other types.

14.1 Prophylactic Efficacy – HPV Types 6, 11, 16, and 18 in Girls and Women 16 Through 26 Years of Age

GARDASIL was administered without prescreening for presence of HPV infection and the efficacy trials allowed enrollment of girls and women regardless of baseline HPV status (i.e., PCR status or serostatus). Girls and women with current or prior HPV infection with an HPV type contained in the vaccine were not eligible for prophylactic efficacy evaluations for that type.

The primary analyses of efficacy with respect to HPV types 6, 11, 16, and 18 were conducted in the per-protocol efficacy (PPE) population, consisting of girls and women who received all 3 vaccinations within 1 year of enrollment, did not have major deviations from the study protocol, and were naïve (PCR negative in cervicovaginal specimens and seronegative) to the relevant HPV type(s) (Types 6, 11, 16, and 18) prior to dose 1 and through 1 month Postdose 3 (Month 7). Efficacy was measured starting after the Month 7 visit.

GARDASIL was efficacious in reducing the incidence of CIN (any grade including CIN 2/3); AIS; genital warts; VIN (any grade); and VaIN (any grade) related to vaccine HPV types 6, 11, 16, or 18 in those who were PCR negative and seronegative at baseline (Table 11).

In addition, girls and women who were already infected with 1 or more vaccine-related HPV types prior to vaccination were protected from precancerous cervical lesions and external genital lesions caused by the other vaccine HPV types.

[See table 11 on pages 1523 and 1524]

Prophylactic efficacy against overall cervical and genital disease related to HPV 6, 11, 16, and 18 in an extension phase of Study 2, that included data through Month 60, was noted to be 100% (95% CI: 12.3%, 100.0%) among girls and women in the per protocol population naïve to the relevant HPV types.

GARDASIL was efficacious against HPV disease caused by HPV types 6, 11, 16, and 18 in girls and women who were naïve for those specific HPV types at baseline.

14.2 Prophylactic Efficacy – HPV Types 6, 11, 16, and 18 in Boys and Men 16 Through 26 Years of Age

The primary analyses of efficacy were conducted in the per-protocol efficacy (PPE) population. This population consisted of boys and men who received all 3 vaccinations within 1 year of enrollment, did not have major deviations from the study protocol, and were naïve (PCR negative and seronegative) to the relevant HPV type(s) (Types 6, 11, 16, and 18) prior to dose 1 and through 1 month postdose 3 (Month 7). Efficacy was measured starting after the Month 7 visit.

GARDASIL was efficacious in reducing the incidence of genital warts related to vaccine HPV types 6 and 11 in those boys and men who were PCR negative and seronegative at baseline (Table 12). Efficacy against penile/perineal/perianal intraepithelial neoplasia (PIN) grades 1/2/3 or penile/perineal/perianal cancer was not demonstrated as the number of cases was too limited to reach statistical significance.

[See table 12 at top of page 1524]

14.3 Prophylactic Efficacy – Anal Disease Caused by HPV Types 6, 11, 16, and 18 in Boys and Men 16 Through 26 Years of Age in the MSM Sub-study

A sub-study of Study 5 evaluated the efficacy of GARDASIL against anal disease (anal intraepithelial neoplasia and anal cancer) in a population of 598 MSM. The primary analyses of efficacy were conducted in the per-protocol efficacy (PPE) population of Study 5.

GARDASIL was efficacious in reducing the incidence of anal intraepithelial neoplasia (AIN) grades 1 (both condyloma and non-acuminate), 2, and 3 related to vaccine HPV types 6, 11, 16, and 18 in those boys and men who were PCR negative and seronegative at baseline (Table 13).

[See table 13 at top of page 1524]

14.4 Population Impact in Girls and Women 16 Through 26 Years of Age

Effectiveness of GARDASIL in Prevention of HPV Types 6-, 11-, 16-, or 18-Related Genital Disease in Girls and Women 16 Through 26 Years of Age, Regardless of Current or Prior Exposure to Vaccine HPV Types

The clinical trials included girls and women regardless of current or prior exposure to vaccine HPV types, and additional analyses were conducted to evaluate the impact of GARDASIL with respect to HPV 6-, 11-, 16-, and 18-related cervical and genital disease in these girls and women. Here, analyses included events arising among girls and women regardless of baseline PCR status and serostatus, including HPV infections that were present at the start of vaccination as well as events that arose from infections that were acquired after the start of vaccination.

The impact of GARDASIL in girls and women regardless of current or prior exposure to a vaccine HPV type is shown in Table 14. Impact was measured starting 1 month Postdose 1. Prophylactic efficacy denotes the vaccine's efficacy in girls and women who are naïve (PCR negative and seronegative) to the relevant HPV types at Day 1. Vaccine impact in girls and women who were positive for vaccine HPV infection, as well as vaccine impact among girls and women regardless of baseline vaccine HPV PCR status and serostatus are also presented. The majority of CIN and genital warts, VIN, and VaIN related to a vaccine HPV type detected in the group that received GARDASIL occurred as a consequence of HPV infection with the relevant HPV type that was already present at Day 1.

Table 16 *(cont.)*
Effectiveness of GARDASIL in Prevention of HPV Types 6-, 11-, 16-, or 18-Related Anogenital Disease in Boys and Men 16 Through 26 Years of Age, Regardless of Current or Prior Exposure to Vaccine HPV Types

Endpoint	Analysis	GARDASIL		AAHS Control		% Reduction (95% CI)
		N	Cases	N	Cases	
PIN 1/2/3	Prophylactic Efficacy*	1775	4	1770	5	20.7 (-268.4, 84.3)
	HPV 6, HPV 11, HPV 16, and/or HPV 18 Positive at Day 1†	460	2	453	1	--‡
	Boys and Men Regardless of Current or Prior Exposure to Vaccine or Non-Vaccine HPV Types§	1943	6	1937	6	0.3 (-272.8, 73.4)
AIN 1/2/3	Prophylactic Efficacy*	259	9	261	39	76.9 (51.4, 90.1)
	HPV 6, HPV 11, HPV 16, and/or HPV 18 Positive at Day 1†	103	29	116	38	--‡
	Boys and Men Regardless of Current or Prior Exposure to Vaccine or Non-Vaccine HPV Types§	275	38	276	77	50.3 (25.7, 67.2)
AIN 2/3	Prophylactic Efficacy*	259	7	261	19	62.5 (6.9, 86.7)
	HPV 6, HPV 11, HPV 16, and/or HPV 18 Positive at Day 1†	103	11	116	20	--‡
	Boys and Men Regardless of Current or Prior Exposure to Vaccine or Non-Vaccine HPV Types§	275	18	276	39	54.2 (18.0, 75.3)

CI = Confidence Interval
AAHS Control = Amorphous Aluminum Hydroxyphosphate Sulfate
* Includes all individuals who received at least 1 vaccination and who were HPV-naïve (i.e., seronegative and PCR negative) at Day 1 to the vaccine HPV type being analyzed. Case counting started at Day 1.
† Includes all individuals who received at least 1 vaccination and who were HPV positive or had unknown HPV status at Day 1, to at least one vaccine HPV type. Case counting started at Day 1.
‡ There is no expected efficacy since GARDASIL has not been demonstrated to provide protection against disease from vaccine HPV types to which a person has previously been exposed through sexual activity.
§ Includes all individuals who received at least 1 vaccination. Case counting started at Day 1.

Table 17
Effectiveness of GARDASIL in Prevention of Any HPV Type Related Anogenital Disease in Boys and Men 16 Through 26 Years of Age, Regardless of Current or Prior Infection with Vaccine or Non-Vaccine HPV Types

Endpoint	Analysis	GARDASIL		AAHS Control		% Reduction (95% CI)
		N	Cases	N	Cases	
External Genital Lesions	Prophylactic Efficacy*	1275	7	1270	37	81.5 (58.0, 93.0)
	Boys and Men Regardless of Current or Prior Exposure to Vaccine or Non-Vaccine HPV Types†	1943	38	1937	92	59.3 (40.0, 72.9)
Condyloma	Prophylactic Efficacy*	1275	5	1270	33	85.2 (61.8, 95.5)
	Boys and Men Regardless of Current or Prior Exposure to Vaccine or Non-Vaccine HPV Types†	1943	33	1937	85	61.8 (42.3, 75.3)
PIN 1/2/3	Prophylactic Efficacy*	1275	2	1270	4	50.7 (-244.3, 95.5)
	Boys and Men Regardless of Current or Prior Exposure to Vaccine or Non-Vaccine HPV Types†	1943	8	1937	7	-13.9 (-269.0, 63.9)
AIN 1/2/3	Prophylactic Efficacy*	129	12	126	28	54.9 (8.4, 79.1)
	Boys and Men Regardless of Current or Prior Exposure to Vaccine or Non-Vaccine HPV Types†	275	74	276	103	25.7 (-1.1, 45.6)
AIN 2/3	Prophylactic Efficacy*	129	8	126	18	52.5 (-14.8, 82.1)
	Boys and Men Regardless of Current or Prior Exposure to Vaccine or Non-Vaccine HPV Types†	275	44	276	59	24.3 (-13.8, 50.0)

CI = Confidence Interval
AAHS Control = Amorphous Aluminum Hydroxyphosphate Sulfate
* Includes all individuals who received at least 1 vaccination and who were seronegative and PCR negative at enrollment to HPV 6, 11, 16 and 18, and PCR negative at enrollment to HPV 31, 33, 35, 39, 45, 51, 52, 56, 58 and 59. Case counting started at Day 1.
† Includes all individuals who received at least 1 vaccination. Case counting started at Day 1.

Table 18
Summary of Month 7 Anti-HPV cLIA Geometric Mean Titers in the PPI* Population of Girls and Women

Population	N†	n‡	% Seropositive (95% CI)	GMT (95% CI) mMU§/mL
Anti-HPV 6				
9- through 15-year-old girls	1122	917	99.9 (99.4, 100.0)	929.2 (874.6, 987.3)
16- through 26-year-old girls and women	9859	3329	99.8 (99.6, 99.9)	545.0 (530.1, 560.4)
27- through 34-year-old women	667	439	98.4 (96.7, 99.4)	435.6 (393.4, 482.4)
35- through 45-year-old women	957	644	98.1 (96.8, 99.0)	397.3 (365.2, 432.2)
Anti-HPV 11				
9- through 15-year-old girls	1122	917	99.9 (99.4, 100.0)	1304.6 (1224.7, 1389.7)
16- through 26-year-old girls and women	9859	3353	99.8 (99.5, 99.9)	748.9 (726.0, 772.6)
27- through 34-year-old women	667	439	98.2 (96.4, 99.2)	577.9 (523.8, 637.5)
35- through 45-year-old women	957	644	97.7 (96.2, 98.7)	512.8 (472.9, 556.1)
Anti-HPV 16				
9- through 15-year-old girls	1122	915	99.9 (99.4, 100.0)	4918.5 (4556.6, 5309.1)
16- through 26-year-old girls and women	9859	3249	99.8 (99.6, 100.0)	2409.2 (2309.0, 2513.8)
27- through 34-year-old women	667	435	99.3 (98.0, 99.9)	2342.5 (2119.1, 2589.6)
35- through 45-year-old women	957	657	98.2 (96.8, 99.1)	2129.5 (1962.7, 2310.5)
Anti-HPV 18				
9- through 15-year-old girls	1122	922	99.8 (99.2, 100.0)	1042.6 (967.6, 1123.3)
16- through 26-year-old girls and women	9859	3566	99.4 (99.1, 99.7)	475.2 (458.8, 492.1)
27- through 34-year-old women	667	501	98.0 (96.4, 99.0)	385.8 (347.6, 428.1)
35- through 45-year-old women	957	722	96.4 (94.8, 97.6)	324.6 (297.6, 354.0)

cLIA = Competitive Luminex Immunoassay
CI = Confidence Interval
GMT = Geometric Mean Titers
* The PPI population consisted of individuals who received all 3 vaccinations within pre-defined day ranges, did not have major deviations from the study protocol, met predefined criteria for the interval between the Month 6 and Month 7 visit, and were naïve (PCR negative and seronegative) to the relevant HPV type(s) (types 6, 11, 16, and 18) prior to dose 1 and through 1 month Postdose 3 (Month 7).
† Number of individuals randomized to the respective vaccination group who received at least 1 injection.
‡ Number of individuals contributing to the analysis.
§ mMU = milli-Merck Units

There was no clear evidence of protection from disease caused by HPV types for which girls and women were PCR positive regardless of serostatus at baseline.

[See table 14 at top of page 1525]

Effectiveness of GARDASIL in Prevention of Any HPV Type Related Genital Disease in Girls and Women 16 Through 26 Years of Age, Regardless of Current or Prior Infection with Vaccine or Non-Vaccine HPV Types

The impact of GARDASIL against the overall burden of dysplastic or papillomatous cervical, vulvar, and vaginal disease regardless of HPV detection, results from a combination of prophylactic efficacy against vaccine HPV types, disease contribution from vaccine HPV types present at time of vaccination, the disease contribution from HPV types not contained in the vaccine, and disease in which HPV was not detected.

Additional efficacy analyses were conducted in 2 populations: (1) a generally HPV-naïve population (negative to 14 common HPV types and had a Pap test that was negative for SIL [Squamous Intraepithelial Lesion] at Day 1), approximating a population of sexually-naïve girls and women and (2) the general study population of girls and women regardless of baseline HPV status, some of whom had HPV-related disease at Day 1.

Among generally HPV-naïve girls and women and among all girls and women in the study population (including girls and women with HPV infection at Day 1), GARDASIL reduced the overall incidence of CIN 2/3 or AIS; of VIN 2/3 or VaIN 2/3; of CIN (any grade) or AIS; and of Genital Warts (Table 15). These reductions were primarily due to reductions in lesions caused by HPV types 6, 11, 16, and 18 in girls and women naïve (seronegative and PCR negative) for the specific relevant vaccine HPV type. Infected girls and women may already have CIN 2/3 or AIS at Day 1 and some will develop CIN 2/3 or AIS during follow-up, either related to a vaccine or non-vaccine HPV type present at the time of vaccination or related to a non-vaccine HPV type not present at the time of vaccination.

[See table 15 at top of page 1526]

14.5 Population Impact in Boys and Men 16 Through 26 Years of Age

Effectiveness of GARDASIL in Prevention of HPV Types 6-, 11-, 16-, or 18-Related Anogenital Disease in Boys and Men 16 Through 26 Years of Age, Regardless of Current or Prior Exposure to Vaccine HPV Types

Study 5 included boys and men regardless of current or prior exposure to vaccine HPV types, and additional analyses were conducted to evaluate the impact of GARDASIL with respect to HPV 6-, 11-, 16-, and 18-related anogenital disease in these boys and men. Here, analyses included events arising among boys and men regardless of baseline PCR status and serostatus, including HPV infections that were present at the start of vaccination as well as events that arose from infections that were acquired after the start of vaccination.

The impact of GARDASIL in boys and men regardless of current or prior exposure to a vaccine HPV type is shown in Table 16. Impact was measured starting at Day 1. Prophylactic efficacy denotes the vaccine's efficacy in boys and men who are naïve (PCR negative and seronegative) to the relevant HPV types at Day 1. Vaccine impact in boys and men who were positive for vaccine HPV infection, as well as vaccine impact among boys and men regardless of baseline vaccine HPV PCR status and serostatus are also presented. The majority of anogenital disease related to a vaccine HPV type detected in the group that received GARDASIL occurred as a consequence of HPV infection with the relevant HPV type that was already present at Day 1.

There was no clear evidence of protection from disease caused by HPV types for which boys and men were PCR positive regardless of serostatus at baseline.

[See table 16 on pages 1526 and 1527]

Effectiveness of GARDASIL in Prevention of Any HPV Type Related Anogenital Disease in Boys and Men 16 Through 26 Years of Age, Regardless of Current or Prior Infection with Vaccine or Non-Vaccine HPV Types

The impact of GARDASIL against the overall burden of dysplastic or papillomatous anogenital disease regardless of HPV detection, results from a combination of prophylactic efficacy against vaccine HPV types, disease contribution from vaccine HPV types present at time of vaccination, the disease contribution from HPV types not contained in the vaccine, and disease in which HPV was not detected.

Additional efficacy analyses from Study 5 were conducted in 2 populations: (1) a generally HPV-naïve population that consisted of boys and men who are seronegative and PCR negative to HPV 6, 11, 16, and 18 and PCR negative to HPV 31, 33, 35, 39, 45, 51, 52, 56, 58 and 59 at Day 1, approximating a population of sexually-naïve boys and men and (2) the general study population of boys and men regardless of baseline HPV status, some of whom had HPV-related disease at Day 1.

Among generally HPV-naïve boys and men and among all boys and men in Study 5 (including boys and men with HPV infection at Day 1), GARDASIL reduced the overall incidence of anogenital disease (Table 17). These reductions were primarily due to reductions in lesions caused by HPV types 6, 11, 16, and 18 in boys and men naïve (seronegative and PCR negative) for the specific relevant vaccine HPV type. Infected boys and men may already have anogenital disease at Day 1 and some will develop anogenital disease during follow-up, either related to a vaccine or non-vaccine HPV type present at the time of vaccination or related to a non-vaccine HPV type not present at the time of vaccination.

[See table 17 at top of previous page]

14.6 Overall Population Impact

The subject characteristics (e.g. lifetime sex partners, geographic distribution of the subjects) influence the HPV prevalence of the population and therefore the population benefit can vary widely.

The overall efficacy of GARDASIL will vary with the baseline prevalence of HPV infection and disease, the incidence of infections against which GARDASIL has shown protection, and those infections against which GARDASIL has not been shown to protect.

The efficacy of GARDASIL for HPV types not included in the vaccine (i.e., cross-protective efficacy) is a component of the overall impact of the vaccine on rates of disease caused by HPV. Cross-protective efficacy was not demonstrated against disease caused by non-vaccine HPV types in the combined database of the Study 3 and Study 4 trials.

GARDASIL does not protect against genital disease not related to HPV. One woman who received GARDASIL in Study 3 developed an external genital well-differentiated squamous cell carcinoma at Month 24. No HPV DNA was detected in the lesion or in any other samples taken throughout the study.

In 18,150 girls and women enrolled in Study 2, Study 3, and Study 4, GARDASIL reduced definitive cervical therapy procedures by 23.9% (95% CI: 15.2%, 31.7%).

14.7 Studies in Women 27 Through 45 Years of Age

Study 6 evaluated efficacy in 3253 women 27 through 45 years of age based on a combined endpoint of HPV 6-, 11-, 16- or 18-related persistent infection, genital warts, vulvar and vaginal dysplastic lesions of any grade, CIN of any grade, AIS, and cervical cancer. These women were randomized 1:1 to receive either GARDASIL or AAHS control. The efficacy for the combined endpoint was driven primarily by prevention of persistent infection. There was no statistically significant efficacy demonstrated for CIN 2/3, AIS, or cervical cancer. In post hoc analyses conducted to assess the impact of GARDASIL on the individual components of the combined endpoint, the results in the population of women naïve to the relevant HPV type at baseline were as follows: prevention of HPV 6-, 11-, 16- or 18-related persistent infection (80.5% [95% CI: 68.3, 88.6]), prevention of HPV 6-, 11-, 16- or 18-related CIN (any grade) (85.8% [95% CI: 52.4, 97.3]), and prevention of HPV 6-, 11-, 16- or 18-related genital warts (87.6% [95% CI: 7.3, 99.7]).

Efficacy for disease endpoints was diminished in a population impact assessment of women who were vaccinated regardless of baseline HPV status (full analysis set). In the full analysis set (FAS), efficacy was not demonstrated for the following endpoints: prevention of HPV 16- and 18-related CIN 2/3, AIS, or cervical cancer and prevention of HPV 6- and 11-related condyloma. No efficacy was demonstrated against CIN 2/3, AIS, or cervical cancer in the general population irrespective of HPV type (FAS any type analysis).

14.8 Immunogenicity

Assays to Measure Immune Response

The minimum anti-HPV titer that confers protective efficacy has not been determined.

Because there were few disease cases in individuals naïve (PCR negative and seronegative) to vaccine HPV types at baseline in the group that received GARDASIL, it has not been possible to establish minimum anti-HPV 6, anti-HPV 11, anti-HPV 16, and anti-HPV 18 antibody levels that protect against clinical disease caused by HPV 6, 11, 16, and/or 18.

The immunogenicity of GARDASIL was assessed in 23,951 9- through 45-year-old girls and women (GARDASIL N = 12,634; AAHS control or saline placebo N = 11,317) and 5417 9- through 26-year-old boys and men (GARDASIL N = 3109; AAHS control or saline placebo N = 2308).

Type-specific immunoassays with type-specific standards were used to assess immunogenicity to each vaccine HPV type. These assays measured antibodies against neutralizing epitopes for each HPV type. The scales for these assays are unique to each HPV type; thus, comparisons across types and to other assays are not appropriate.

Immune Response to GARDASIL

The primary immunogenicity analyses were conducted in a per-protocol immunogenicity (PPI) population. This population consisted of individuals who were seronegative and PCR negative to the relevant HPV type(s) at enrollment, remained HPV PCR negative to the relevant HPV type(s) through 1 month postdose 3 (Month 7), received all 3 vaccinations, and did not deviate from the study protocol in ways that could interfere with the effects of the vaccine.

Immunogenicity was measured by (1) the percentage of individuals who were seropositive for antibodies against the relevant vaccine HPV type, and (2) the Geometric Mean Titer (GMT).

In clinical studies in 16- through 26-year-old girls and women, 99.8%, 99.8%, 99.8%, and 99.4% who received GARDASIL became anti-HPV 6, anti-HPV 11, anti-HPV 16, and anti-HPV 18 seropositive, respectively, by 1 month postdose 3 across all age groups tested.

In clinical studies in 27- through 45-year-old women, 98.2%, 97.9%, 98.6%, and 97.1% who received GARDASIL became anti-HPV 6, anti-HPV 11, anti-HPV 16, and anti-HPV 18 seropositive, respectively, by 1 month postdose 3 across all age groups tested.

In clinical studies in 16- through 26-year-old boys and men, 98.9%, 99.2%, 98.8%, and 97.4% who received GARDASIL became anti-HPV 6, anti-HPV 11, anti-HPV 16, and anti-HPV 18 seropositive, respectively, by 1 month postdose 3 across all age groups tested.

Across all populations, anti HPV 6, anti-HPV 11, anti-HPV 16, and anti-HPV 18 GMTs peaked at Month 7 (Table 18 and Table 19). GMTs declined through Month 24 and then stabilized through Month 36 at levels above baseline. Tables 20 and 21 display the persistence of anti-HPV cLIA geometric mean titers by gender and age group. The duration of immunity following a complete schedule of immunization with GARDASIL has not been established.

[See table 18 at top of previous page]
[See table 19 above]
[See table 20 at top of next page]
[See table 21 at top of page 1531]

Tables 18 and 19 display the Month 7 immunogenicity data for girls and women and boys and men. Anti-HPV responses 1 month postdose 3 among 9- through 15-year-old adolescent girls were non-inferior to anti-HPV responses in 16- through 26-year-old girls and women in the combined database of immunogenicity studies for GARDASIL. Anti-HPV responses 1 month postdose 3 among 9- through 15-year-old adolescent boys were non-inferior to anti-HPV responses in 16- through 26-year-old boys and men in Study 5.

On the basis of this immunogenicity bridging, the efficacy of GARDASIL in 9- through 15-year-old adolescent girls and boys is inferred.

GMT Response to Variation in Dosing Regimen in 18- Through 26-Year-Old Women

Girls and women evaluated in the PPE population of clinical studies received all 3 vaccinations within 1 year of enrollment. An analysis of immune response data suggests that flexibility of ±1 month for Dose 2 (i.e., Month 1 to Month 3 in the vaccination regimen) and flexibility of ±2 months for Dose 3 (i.e., Month 4 to Month 8 in the vaccination regimen) do not impact the immune responses to GARDASIL.

Duration of the Immune Response to GARDASIL

The duration of immunity following a complete schedule of immunization with GARDASIL has not been established. The peak anti-HPV GMTs for HPV types 6, 11, 16, and 18 occurred at Month 7. Anti-HPV GMTs for HPV types 6, 11, 16, and 18 were similar between measurements at Month 24 and Month 60 in Study 2.

14.9 Studies with RECOMBIVAX HB [hepatitis B vaccine (recombinant)]

The safety and immunogenicity of co-administration of GARDASIL with RECOMBIVAX HB [hepatitis B vaccine (recombinant)] (same visit, injections at separate sites) were evaluated in a randomized, double-blind, study of 1871 women aged 16 through 24 years at enrollment. The race distribution of the girls and women in the clinical trial was as follows: 61.6% White; 1.6% Hispanic (Black and White); 23.8% Other; 11.9% Black; 0.8% Asian; and 0.3% American Indian.

Table 19
Summary of Month 7 Anti-HPV cLIA Geometric Mean Titers in the PPI* Population of Boys and Men

Population	N†	n‡	% Seropositive (95% CI)	GMT (95% CI) mMU§/mL
Anti-HPV 6				
9- through 15-year-old boys	1072	884	99.9 (99.4, 100.0)	1037.5 (963.5, 1117.3)
16- through 26-year-old boys and men	2026	1093	98.9 (98.1, 99.4)	447.8 (418.9, 478.6)
Anti-HPV 11				
9- through 15-year-old boys	1072	885	99.9 (99.4, 100.0)	1386.8 (1298.5, 1481.0)
16- through 26-year-old boys and men	2026	1093	99.2 (98.4, 99.6)	624.3 (588.4, 662.3)
Anti-HPV 16				
9- through 15-year-old boys	1072	882	99.8 (99.2, 100.0)	6056.5 (5601.3, 6548.7)
16- through 26-year-old boys and men	2026	1136	98.8 (97.9, 99.3)	2403.3 (2243.4, 2574.6)
Anti-HPV 18				
9- through 15-year-old boys	1072	887	99.8 (99.2, 100)	1357.4 (1249.4, 1474.7)
16- through 26-year-old boys and men	2026	1175	97.4 (96.3, 98.2)	402.6 (374.6, 432.7)

cLIA = Competitive Luminex Immunoassay
CI = Confidence Interval
GMT = Geometric Mean Titers
* The PPI population consisted of individuals who received all 3 vaccinations within pre-defined day ranges, did not have major deviations from the study protocol, met predefined criteria for the interval between the Month 6 and Month 7 visit, and were naïve (PCR negative and seronegative) to the relevant HPV type(s) (types 6, 11, 16, and 18) prior to dose 1 and through 1 month Postdose 3 (Month 7).
† Number of individuals randomized to the respective vaccination group who received at least 1 injection.
‡ Number of individuals contributing to the analysis.
§ mMU = milli-Merck Units

Subjects either received GARDASIL and RECOMBIVAX HB (n = 466), GARDASIL and RECOMBIVAX HB-matched placebo (n = 468), RECOMBIVAX HB and GARDASIL-matched placebo (n = 467) or RECOMBIVAX-matched placebo and GARDASIL-matched placebo (n = 470) at Day 1, Month 2 and Month 6. Immunogenicity was assessed for all vaccines 1 month post completion of the vaccination series.

Concomitant administration of GARDASIL with RECOMBIVAX HB [hepatitis B vaccine (recombinant)] did not interfere with the antibody response to any of the vaccine antigens when GARDASIL was given concomitantly with RECOMBIVAX HB or separately.

14.10 Studies with Menactra [Meningococcal (Groups A, C, Y and W-135) Polysaccharide Diphtheria Toxoid Conjugate Vaccine] and Adacel [Tetanus Toxoid, Reduced Diphtheria Toxoid and Acellular Pertussis Vaccine Adsorbed (Tdap)]

The safety and immunogenicity of co-administration of GARDASIL with Menactra [Meningococcal (Groups A, C, Y and W-135) Polysaccharide Diphtheria Toxoid Conjugate Vaccine] and Adacel [Tetanus Toxoid, Reduced Diphtheria Toxoid and Acellular Pertussis Vaccine Adsorbed (Tdap)] (same visit, injections at separate sites) were evaluated in an open-labeled, randomized, controlled study of 1040 boys and girls 11 through 17 years of age at enrollment. The race distribution of the subjects in the clinical trial was as follows: 77.7% White; 6.8% Hispanic (Black and White); 1.4% Multi-racial; 12.3% Black; 1.2% Asian; 0.2% Indian; and 0.4% American Indian.

One group received GARDASIL in one limb and both Menactra and Adacel, as separate injections, in the opposite limb concomitantly on Day 1 (n = 517). The second group received the first dose of GARDASIL on Day 1 in one limb then Menactra and Adacel, as separate injections, at Month 1 in the opposite limb (n = 523). Subjects in both vaccination groups received the second dose of GARDASIL at Month 2 and the third dose at Month 6. Immunogenicity was assessed for all vaccines 1 month post completion of the vaccination series (1 dose for Menactra and Adacel and 3 doses for GARDASIL).

Concomitant administration of GARDASIL with Menactra [Meningococcal (Groups A, C, Y and W-135) Polysaccharide Diphtheria Toxoid Conjugate Vaccine] and Adacel [Tetanus Toxoid, Reduced Diphtheria Toxoid and Acellular Pertussis Vaccine Adsorbed (Tdap)] did not interfere with the antibody response to any of the vaccine antigens when GARDASIL was given concomitantly with Menactra and Adacel or separately.

16 HOW SUPPLIED/STORAGE AND HANDLING

All presentations for GARDASIL contain a suspension of 120 mcg L1 protein from HPV types 6, 11, 16, and 18 in a 0.5-mL dose. GARDASIL is supplied in vials and syringes.

Carton of one 0.5-mL single-dose vial. **NDC** 0006-4045-00.

Carton of ten 0.5-mL single-dose vials. **NDC** 0006-4045-41.

Carton of six 0.5-mL single-dose prefilled Luer Lock syringes with tip caps. **NDC** 0006-4109-09.

Store refrigerated at 2 to 8°C (36 to 46°F). Do not freeze. Protect from light.

GARDASIL should be administered as soon as possible after being removed from refrigeration.

GARDASIL can be out of refrigeration (at temperatures at or below 25°C/77°F), for a total time of not more than 72 hours.

17 PATIENT COUNSELING INFORMATION

[See FDA-Approved Patient Labeling.]

Inform the patient, parent, or guardian:

- Vaccination does not eliminate the necessity for women to continue to undergo recommended cervical cancer screening. Women who receive GARDASIL should continue to undergo cervical cancer screening per standard of care.
- Recipients of GARDASIL should not discontinue anal cancer screening if it has been recommended by a health care provider.
- GARDASIL has not been demonstrated to provide protection against disease from vaccine and non-vaccine HPV types to which a person has previously been exposed through sexual activity.
- Since syncope has been reported following vaccination sometimes resulting in falling with injury, observation for 15 minutes after administration is recommended.
- Vaccine information is required to be given with each vaccination to the patient, parent, or guardian.
- Information regarding benefits and risks associated with vaccination.
- GARDASIL is not recommended for use in pregnant women.
- Importance of completing the immunization series unless contraindicated.
- Report any adverse reactions to their health care provider.

Manuf. and Dist. by: Merck Sharp & Dohme Corp., a subsidiary of
MERCK & CO., INC., Whitehouse Station, NJ 08889, USA
Printed in USA

Table 20
Persistence of Anti-HPV cLIA Geometric Mean Titers in 9- Through 45-Year-Old Girls and Women

Assay (cLIA)/ Time Point	9- to 15-Year-Old Girls (N* = 1122)		16- to 26-Year-Old Girls and Women (N * = 9859)		27- to 34-Year-Old Women (N* = 667)		35- to 45-Year-Old Women (N* = 957)	
	n†	GMT (95% CI) mMU‡/mL	n†	GMT (95% CI) mMU‡/mL	n†	GMT (95% CI) mMU‡/mL	n†	GMT (95% CI) mMU‡/mL
Anti-HPV 6								
Month 07	917	929.2 (874.6, 987.3)	3329	545.0 (530.1, 560.4)	439	435.6 (393.4, 482.4)	644	397.3 (365.2, 432.2)
Month 24	214	156.1 (135.6, 179.6)	2788	109.1 (105.2, 113.1)	421	70.7 (63.8, 78.5)	628	69.3 (63.7, 75.4)
Month 36§	356	129.4 (115.6, 144.8)	-	-	399	79.5 (72.0, 87.7)	618	81.1 (75.0, 87.8)
Month 48¶	-	-	2514	73.8 (70.9, 76.8)	391	58.8 (52.9, 65.3)	616	62.0 (57.0, 67.5)
Anti-HPV 11								
Month 07	917	1304.6 (1224.7, 1389.7)	3353	748.9 (726.0, 772.6)	439	577.9 (523.8, 637.5)	644	512.8 (472.9, 556.1)
Month 24	214	218.0 (188.3, 252.4)	2817	137.1 (132.1, 142.3)	421	79.3 (71.5, 87.8)	628	73.4 (67.4, 79.8)
Month 36§	356	148.0 (131.1, 167.1)	-	-	399	81.8 (74.3, 90.1)	618	77.4 (71.6, 83.6)
Month 48¶	-	-	2538	89.4 (85.9, 93.1)	391	67.4 (60.9, 74.7)	616	62.7 (57.8, 68.0)
Anti-HPV 16								
Month 07	915	4918.5 (4556.6, 5309.1)	3249	2409.2 (2309.0, 2513.8)	435	2342.5 (2119.1, 2589.6)	657	2129.5 (1962.7, 2310.5)
Month 24	211	944.2 (804.4, 1108.3)	2721	442.6 (425.0, 460.9)	416	285.9 (254.4, 321.2)	642	271.4 (247.1, 298.1)
Month 36§	353	642.2 (562.8, 732.8)	-	-	399	291.5 (262.5, 323.8)	631	276.7 (254.5, 300.8)
Month 48¶	-	-	2474	326.2 (311.8, 341.3)	394	211.8 (189.5, 236.8)	628	192.8 (176.5, 210.6)
Anti-HPV 18								
Month 07	922	1042.6 (967.6, 1123.3)	3566	475.2 (458.8, 492.1)	501	385.8 (347.6, 428.1)	722	324.6 (297.6, 354.0)
Month 24	214	137.7 (114.8, 165.1)	3002	50.8 (48.2, 53.5)	478	31.8 (28.1, 36.0)	705	26.0 (23.5, 28.8)
Month 36§	357	87.0 (74.8, 101.2)	-	-	453	32.1 (28.5, 36.3)	689	27.0 (24.5, 29.8)
Month 48¶	-	-	2710	33.2 (31.5, 35.0)	444	25.2 (22.3, 28.5)	688	21.2 (19.2, 23.4)

cLIA = Competitive Luminex Immunoassay
CI = Confidence Interval
GMT = Geometric Mean Titers
* N = Number of individuals randomized in the respective group who received at least 1 injection.
† n = Number of individuals in the indicated immunogenicity population.
‡ mMU = milli-Merck Units
§ Month 37 for 9- to 15-year-old girls. No serology samples were collected at this time point for 16- to 26-year-old girls and women.
¶ Month 48/End-of-study visits for 16- to 26-year-old girls and women were generally scheduled earlier than Month 48. Mean visit timing was Month 44. The studies in 9- to 15-year-old girls were planned to end prior to 48 months and therefore no serology samples were collected.

USPI-I-V5011303R017
[1]Registered trademark of Merck Sharp & Dohme Corp., a subsidiary of **Merck & Co., Inc.**

USPPI
Patient Information about
GARDASIL® (pronounced "gard-Ah-sill")
Generic name: [Human Papillomavirus Quadrivalent (Types 6, 11, 16, and 18) Vaccine, Recombinant]

Read this information with care before getting GARDASIL[2]. You (the person getting GARDASIL) will need 3 doses of the vaccine. It is important to read this leaflet when you get each dose. This leaflet does not take the place of talking with your health care provider about GARDASIL.

What is GARDASIL?

GARDASIL is a vaccine (injection/shot) that is used for girls and women 9 through 26 years of age to help protect against the following diseases caused by Human Papillomavirus (HPV):
- Cervical cancer
- Vulvar and vaginal cancers
- Anal cancer
- Genital warts
- Precancerous cervical, vaginal, vulvar, and anal lesions

GARDASIL is used for boys and men 9 through 26 years of age to help protect against the following diseases caused by HPV:
- Anal cancer
- Genital warts
- Precancerous anal lesions
  - The diseases listed above have many causes, and GARDASIL only protects against diseases caused by certain kinds of HPV (called Type 6, Type 11, Type 16, and Type 18). Most of the time, these 4 types of HPV are responsible for the diseases listed above.
  - GARDASIL cannot protect you from a disease that is caused by other types of HPV, other viruses, or bacteria.
  - GARDASIL does not treat HPV infection.
  - You cannot get HPV or any of the above diseases from GARDASIL.

What important information about GARDASIL should I know?
- You should continue to get routine cervical cancer screening.
- GARDASIL may not fully protect everyone who gets the vaccine.
- GARDASIL will not protect against HPV types that you already have.

Who should not get GARDASIL?

You should not get GARDASIL if you have, or have had:
- an allergic reaction after getting a dose of GARDASIL.
- a severe allergic reaction to yeast, amorphous aluminum hydroxyphosphate sulfate, polysorbate 80.

What should I tell my health care provider before getting GARDASIL?

Tell your health care provider if you:
- are pregnant or planning to get pregnant. GARDASIL is not recommended for use in pregnant women.
- have immune problems, like HIV infection, cancer, or you take medicines that affect your immune system.
- have a fever over 100°F (37.8°C).
- had an allergic reaction to another dose of GARDASIL.
- take any medicines, even those you can buy over the counter.

Your health care provider will help decide if you should get the vaccine.

How is GARDASIL given?

GARDASIL is a shot that is usually given in the arm muscle. You will need 3 shots given on the following schedule:
- Dose 1: at a date you and your health care provider choose.
- Dose 2: 2 months after Dose 1.
- Dose 3: 6 months after Dose 1.

Fainting can happen after getting GARDASIL. Sometimes people who faint can fall and hurt themselves. For this reason, your health care provider may ask you to sit or lie down for 15 minutes after you get GARDASIL. Some people who faint might shake or become stiff. This may require evaluation or treatment by your health care provider.

Make sure that you get all 3 doses on time so that you get the best protection. If you miss a dose, talk to your health care provider.

Can other vaccines and medications be given at the same time as GARDASIL?

GARDASIL can be given at the same time as RECOMBIVAX HB®[1] [hepatitis B vaccine (recombinant)] or Menactra [Meningococcal (Groups A, C, Y and W-135) Polysaccharide Diphtheria Toxoid Conjugate Vaccine] and Adacel [Tetanus Toxoid, Reduced Diphtheria Toxoid and Acellular Pertussis Vaccine Adsorbed (Tdap)].

What are the possible side effects of GARDASIL?

The most common side effects with GARDASIL are:
- pain, swelling, itching, bruising, and redness at the injection site
- headache
- fever
- nausea
- dizziness
- vomiting
- fainting

There was no increase in side effects when GARDASIL was given at the same time as RECOMBIVAX HB [hepatitis B vaccine (recombinant)].

There was more injection-site swelling at the injection site for GARDASIL when GARDASIL was given at the same time as Menactra [Meningococcal (Groups A, C, Y and W-135) Polysaccharide Diphtheria Toxoid Conjugate Vaccine] and Adacel [Tetanus Toxoid, Reduced Diphtheria Toxoid and Acellular Pertussis Vaccine Adsorbed (Tdap)].

Tell your health care provider if you have any of the following problems because these may be signs of an allergic reaction:
- difficulty breathing
- wheezing (bronchospasm)
- hives
- rash

Tell your health care provider if you have:
- swollen glands (neck, armpit, or groin)
- joint pain

Table 21
Persistence of Anti-HPV cLIA Geometric Mean Titers in 9- Through 26-Year-Old Boys and Men

Assay (cLIA)/ Time Point	9- to 15-Year-Old Boys (N* = 1072)		16- to 26-Year-Old Boys and Men (N* = 2026)	
	n†	GMT (95% CI) mMU‡/mL	n†	GMT (95% CI) mMU‡/mL
Anti-HPV 6				
Month 07	884	1037.5 (963.5, 1117.3)	1094	447.2 (418.4, 477.9)
Month 24	323	134.1 (119.5, 150.5)	907	80.3 (74.9, 86.0)
Month 36§	342	126.6 (111.9, 143.2)	654	72.4 (68.0, 77.2)
Month 48¶	-	-	-	-
Anti-HPV 11				
Month 07	885	1386.8 (1298.5, 1481.0)	1094	624.5 (588.6, 662.5)
Month 24	324	188.5 (168.4, 211.1)	907	94.6 (88.4, 101.2)
Month 36§	342	148.8 (131.1, 169.0)	654	80.3 (75.7, 85.2)
Month 48¶	-	-	-	-
Anti-HPV 16				
Month 07	882	6056.5 (5601.4, 6548.6)	1137	2401.5 (2241.8, 2572.6)
Month 24	322	938.2 (825.0, 1067.0)	938	347.7 (322.5, 374.9)
Month 36§	341	708.8 (613.9, 818.3)	672	306.7 (287.5, 327.1)
Month 48¶	-	-	-	-
Anti-HPV 18				
Month 07	887	1357.4 (1249.4, 1474.7)	1176	402.6 (374.6, 432.6)
Month 24	324	131.9 (112.1, 155.3)	967	38.7 (35.2, 42.5)
Month 36§	343	113.0 (94.7, 135.0)	690	33.4 (30.9, 36.1)
Month 48¶	-	-	-	-

cLIA = Competitive Luminex Immunoassay
CI = Confidence Interval
GMT = Geometric Mean Titers

* N = Number of individuals randomized in the respective group who received at least 1 injection.
† n = Number of individuals in the indicated immunogenicity population.
‡ mMU = milli-Merck Units
§ Month 36 time point for 16- to 26-year-old boys and men; Month 37 for 9- to 15-year-old boys.
¶ The studies in 9- to 15-year-old boys and girls and 16- to 26-year-old boys and men were planned to end prior to 48 months and therefore no serology samples were collected.

- unusual tiredness, weakness, or confusion
- chills
- generally feeling unwell
- leg pain
- shortness of breath
- chest pain
- aching muscles
- muscle weakness
- seizure
- bad stomach ache
- bleeding or bruising more easily than normal
- skin infection

Contact your health care provider right away if you get any symptoms that concern you, even several months after getting the vaccine.

For a more complete list of side effects, ask your health care provider.

What are the ingredients in GARDASIL?

The ingredients are proteins of HPV Types 6, 11, 16, and 18, amorphous aluminum hydroxyphosphate sulfate, yeast protein, sodium chloride, L-histidine, polysorbate 80, sodium borate, and water for injection.

This leaflet is a summary of information about GARDASIL. If you would like more information, please talk to your health care provider or visit www.gardasil.com.

Manufactured and Distributed by: Merck Sharp & Dohme Corp., a subsidiary of Merck & Co., Inc.
Whitehouse Station, NJ 08889, USA
Issued April 2011
9883616

[2]Registered trademark of Merck Sharp & Dohme Corp., a subsidiary of **Merck & Co., Inc.**

IMPLANON® ℞
(etonogestrel implant)
for subdermal use

HIGHLIGHTS OF PRESCRIBING INFORMATION

These highlights do not include all the information needed to use IMPLANON safely and effectively. See full prescribing information for IMPLANON.

IMPLANON® (etonogestrel implant), for subdermal use
Initial U.S. Approval: 2001

INDICATIONS AND USAGE

IMPLANON is a progestin indicated for use by women to prevent pregnancy. (1)

DOSAGE AND ADMINISTRATION

Insert one IMPLANON subdermally just under the skin at the inner side of the non-dominant upper arm. IMPLANON must be removed no later than by the end of the third year. (2)

DOSAGE FORMS AND STRENGTHS

IMPLANON consists of a single, rod-shaped implant, containing 68 mg etonogestrel, pre-loaded in the needle of a disposable applicator. (3)

CONTRAINDICATIONS

- Known or suspected pregnancy (4)
- Current or past history of thrombosis or thromboembolic disorders (4, 5.4)
- Liver tumors, benign or malignant, or active liver disease (4, 5.7)
- Undiagnosed abnormal genital bleeding (4, 5.2)
- Known or suspected breast cancer, personal history of breast cancer, or other progestin-sensitive cancer, now or in the past (4, 5.6)
- Allergic reaction to any of the components of IMPLANON (4, 6)

WARNINGS AND PRECAUTIONS

- Insertion and removal complications: Pain, paresthesias, bleeding, hematoma, scarring or infection may occur. (5.1)
- Menstrual bleeding pattern: Counsel women regarding changes in bleeding frequency, intensity, or duration. (5.2)
- Ectopic pregnancies: Be alert to the possibility of an ectopic pregnancy in women using IMPLANON who become pregnant or complain of lower abdominal pain. (5.3)
- Thrombotic and other vascular events: The IMPLANON implant should be removed in the event of a thrombosis. (5.4)
- Liver disease: Remove the IMPLANON implant if jaundice occurs. (5.7)
- Elevated blood pressure: The IMPLANON implant should be removed if blood pressure rises significantly and becomes uncontrolled. (5.9)
- Carbohydrate and lipid metabolic effects: Monitor prediabetic and diabetic women using IMPLANON. (5.11)

ADVERSE REACTIONS

Most common (≥10%) adverse reactions reported in clinical trials were change in menstrual bleeding pattern, headache, vaginitis, weight increase, acne, breast pain, abdominal pain, and pharyngitis. (6.1)

To report SUSPECTED ADVERSE REACTIONS, contact Schering Corporation, a subsidiary of Merck & Co., Inc., at 1-800-526-4099 or FDA at 1-800-FDA-1088 or *www.fda.gov/medwatch.*

DRUG INTERACTIONS

Drugs or herbal products that induce certain enzymes, such as CYP3A4, may decrease the effectiveness of progestin hormonal contraceptives or increase breakthrough bleeding. (7.1)

USE IN SPECIFIC POPULATIONS

- Pregnant women: IMPLANON should be removed if maintaining a pregnancy. (8.1)
- Overweight women: IMPLANON may become less effective in overweight women over time, especially in the presence of other factors that decrease etonogestrel concentrations, such as concomitant use of hepatic enzyme inducers. (8.8)

See 17 for PATIENT COUNSELING INFORMATION and FDA-approved patient labeling

Revised: 03/2012

FULL PRESCRIBING INFORMATION: CONTENTS*

*** Sections or subsections omitted from the full prescribing information are not listed**

FULL PRESCRIBING INFORMATION

1 INDICATIONS AND USAGE

IMPLANON® is indicated for use by women to prevent pregnancy.

2 DOSAGE AND ADMINISTRATION

The efficacy of IMPLANON does not depend on daily, weekly or monthly administration.

All healthcare providers should receive instruction and training prior to performing insertion and/or removal of IMPLANON.

A single IMPLANON implant is inserted subdermally in the upper arm. To reduce the risk of neural or vascular injury, the implant should be inserted at the inner side of the non-dominant upper arm about 8-10 cm (3-4 inches) above the medial epicondyle of the humerus. The implant should be inserted subdermally just under the skin to avoid the large blood vessels and nerves that lie deeper in the subcutaneous tissues in the sulcus between the triceps and biceps muscles. IMPLANON must be inserted by the expiration date stated on the packaging. IMPLANON is a long-acting (up to 3 years), reversible, hormonal contraceptive method. The implant must be removed by the end of the third year and may be replaced by a new implant at the time of removal, if continued contraceptive protection is desired.

2.1 Initiating Contraception with IMPLANON

IMPORTANT: Rule out pregnancy before inserting the implant.

Timing of insertion depends on the woman's recent contraceptive history, as follows:

- No preceding hormonal contraceptive use in the past month
  IMPLANON should be inserted between Day 1 (first day of menstrual bleeding) and Day 5 of the menstrual cycle, even if the woman is still bleeding.
  If inserted as recommended, back-up contraception is not necessary. If deviating from the recommended timing of insertion, the woman should be advised to use a barrier method until 7 days after insertion. If intercourse has already occurred, pregnancy should be excluded.
- Switching contraceptive method to IMPLANON
  Combination hormonal contraceptives:
  IMPLANON should preferably be inserted on the day after the last active tablet of the previous combined oral contraceptive or on the day of the removal of the vaginal ring or transdermal patch. At the latest, IMPLANON should be inserted on the day following the usual tablet-free, ring-free, patch-free or placebo tablet interval of the previous combined hormonal contraceptive.
  If inserted as recommended, back-up contraception is not necessary. If deviating from the recommended timing of insertion, the woman should be advised to use a barrier method until 7 days after insertion. If intercourse has already occurred, pregnancy should be excluded.
  Progestin-only contraceptives:
  There are several types of progestin-only methods. IMPLANON should be inserted as follows:
  - Injectable Contraceptives: Insert IMPLANON on the day the next injection is due.
  - Minipill: A woman may switch to IMPLANON on any day of the month. IMPLANON should be inserted within 24 hours after taking the last tablet.
  - Contraceptive implant or intrauterine system (IUS): Insert IMPLANON on the same day as the previous contraceptive implant or IUS is removed.

  If inserted as recommended, back-up contraception is not necessary. If deviating from the recommended timing of insertion, the woman should be advised to use a barrier method until 7 days after insertion. If intercourse has already occurred, pregnancy should be excluded.
- Following abortion or miscarriage
  - First Trimester: IMPLANON should be inserted within 5 days following a first trimester abortion or miscarriage.
  - Second Trimester: Insert IMPLANON between 21 to 28 days following second trimester abortion or miscarriage.

  If inserted as recommended, back-up contraception is not necessary. If deviating from the recommended timing of insertion, the woman should be advised to use a barrier method until 7 days after insertion. If intercourse has already occurred, pregnancy should be excluded.
- Postpartum
  - Not Breastfeeding: IMPLANON should be inserted between 21 to 28 days postpartum. If inserted as recommended, back-up contraception is not necessary. If deviating from the recommended timing of insertion, the woman should be advised to use a barrier method until 7 days after insertion. If intercourse has already occurred, pregnancy should be excluded.
  - Breastfeeding: IMPLANON should be inserted after the fourth postpartum week *[see Use in Specific Populations (8.3)]*. The woman should be advised to use a barrier method until 7 days after insertion. If intercourse has already occurred, pregnancy should be excluded.

2.2 Insertion of IMPLANON

The basis for successful use and subsequent removal of IMPLANON is a correct and carefully performed subdermal insertion of the single, rod-shaped implant in accordance with the instructions. Both the healthcare provider and the woman should be able to feel the implant under the skin after placement.

All healthcare providers performing insertions and/or removals of IMPLANON should receive instructions and training prior to inserting or removing the implant. Information concerning the insertion and removal of IMPLANON will be sent upon request free of charge [1-877-IMPLANON (1-877-467-5266)].

Preparation

Prior to inserting IMPLANON carefully read the instructions for insertion as well as the full prescribing information.

Before insertion of IMPLANON, the healthcare provider should confirm that:

- The woman is not pregnant nor has any other contraindication for the use of IMPLANON *[see Contraindications (4)]*.
- The woman has had a medical history and physical examination, including a gynecologic examination, performed.
- The woman understands the benefits and risks of IMPLANON.
- The woman has received a copy of the Patient Labeling included in packaging.
- The woman has reviewed and completed a consent form to be maintained with the woman's chart.
- The woman does not have allergies to the antiseptic and anesthetic to be used during insertion.

Insert IMPLANON under aseptic conditions.

The following equipment is needed for the implant insertion:

- An examination table for the woman to lie on
- Sterile surgical drapes, sterile gloves, antiseptic solution, sterile marker (optional)
- Local anesthetic, needles, and syringe
- Sterile gauze, adhesive bandage, pressure bandage

An applicator and its parts are shown below (Figures 1a and 1b).

Figure 1a (Not to scale)

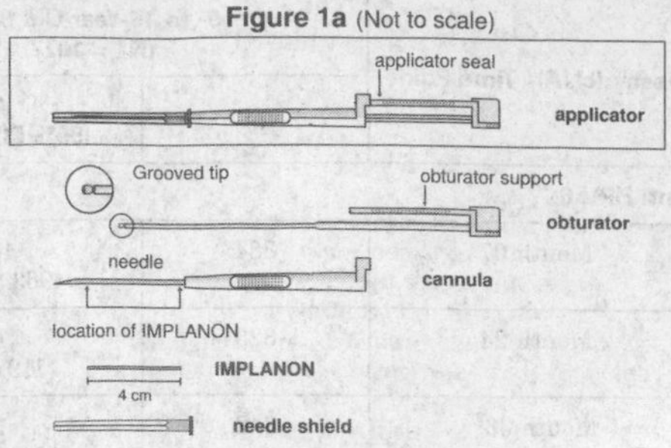

Figure 1b

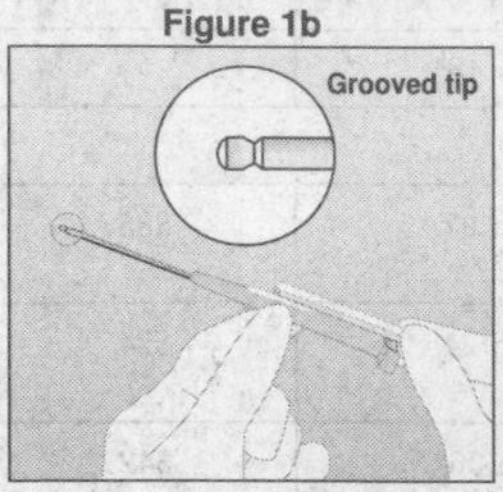

Grooved tip of obturator (enlarged)

The procedure used for IMPLANON insertion is opposite from that of an injection. The obturator keeps IMPLANON in place while the cannula is retracted. The obturator must remain fixed in place while the cannula with needle is retracted from the arm. Do not push the obturator.

Insertion Procedure

Step 1. Have the woman lie on her back on the examination table with her non-dominant arm flexed at the elbow and externally rotated so that her wrist is parallel to her ear or her hand is positioned next to her head (Figure 2).

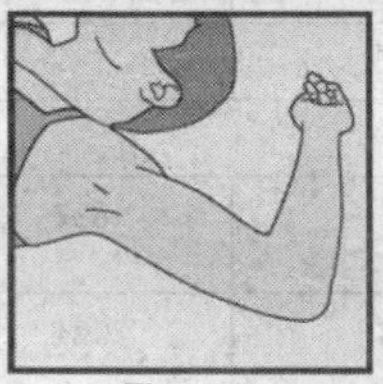

Figure 2

Step 2. Identify the insertion site, which is at the inner side of the non-dominant upper arm about 8-10 cm (3-4 inches) above the medial epicondyle of the humerus (Figure 3). **The implant should be inserted subdermally just under the skin to avoid the large blood vessels and nerves that lie deeper in the subcutaneous tissue in the sulcus between the triceps and biceps muscles** *[see Warnings and Precautions (5.1)]*.

Step 3. Make two marks with a sterile marker: first, mark the spot where the etonogestrel implant will be inserted, and second, mark a spot a few centimeters proximal to the first mark (Figure 3). This second mark will later serve as a direction guide during insertion.

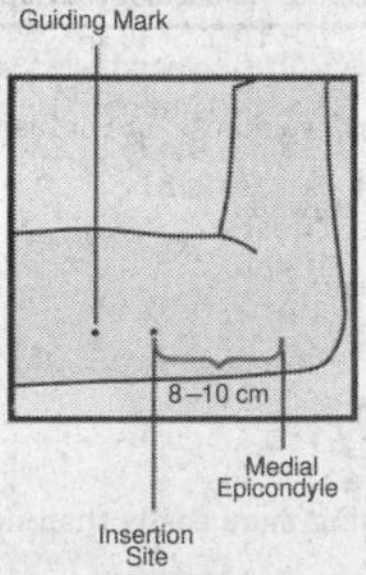

Figure 3

Step 4. Clean the insertion site with an antiseptic solution.

Step 5. Anesthetize the insertion area (for example, with anesthetic spray or by injecting 2 mL of 1% lidocaine just under the skin along the planned insertion tunnel).

Step 6. Remove the sterile pre-loaded disposable IMPLANON applicator carrying the implant from its blister. Keep the IMPLANON needle and rod sterile. The applicator should not be used if sterility is in question. If contamination occurs, use a new package of IMPLANON with a new sterile applicator.

Step 7. Keep the shield on the needle and look for the IMPLANON rod, seen as a white cylinder inside the needle tip.

Step 8. If you don't see the IMPLANON rod, tap the top of the needle shield against a firm surface to bring the implant into the needle tip.

Step 9. Following visual confirmation, lower the IMPLANON rod back into the needle by tapping it back into the needle tip. Then remove the needle shield, while holding the applicator upright.

Step 10. **Note that IMPLANON can fall out of the needle.** Therefore, after you remove the needle shield, keep the applicator in the upright position until the moment of insertion

Step 11. With your free hand, stretch the skin around the insertion site with thumb and index finger (Figure 4).

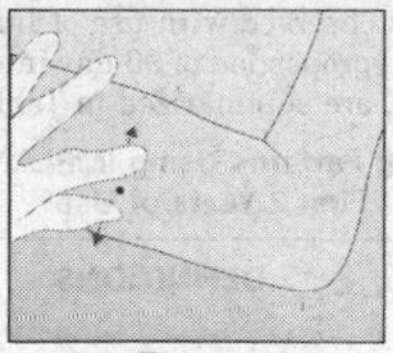

Figure 4

Step 12. At a slight angle (not greater than 20°), insert **only** the tip of the needle with the beveled side up into the insertion site (Figure 5).

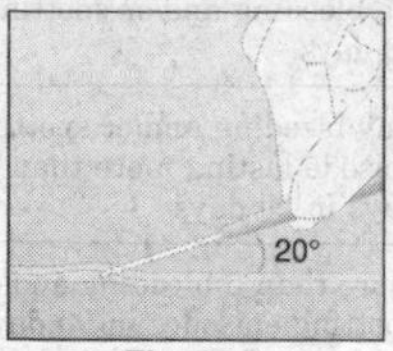

Figure 5

Step 13. Lower the applicator to a horizontal position. Lift the skin up with the tip of the needle, but **keep the needle in the subdermal connective tissue** (Figure 6).

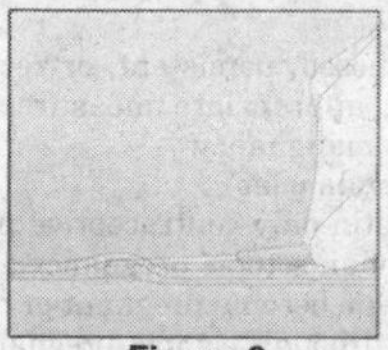

Figure 6

Step 14. While "tenting" (lifting) the skin, gently insert the needle to its full length. Keep the needle parallel to the surface of the skin during insertion (Figure 7).

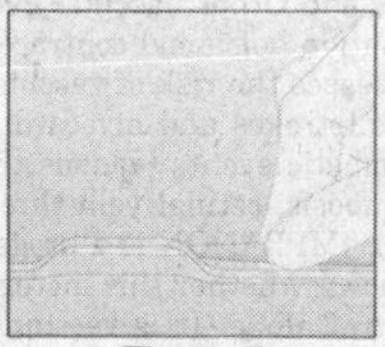

Figure 7

Step 15. **If IMPLANON is placed too deeply, the removal process can be difficult or impossible. If the needle is not inserted to its full length, the implant may protrude from the insertion site and fall out.**

Step 16. Break the seal of the applicator by pressing the obturator support (Figure 8).

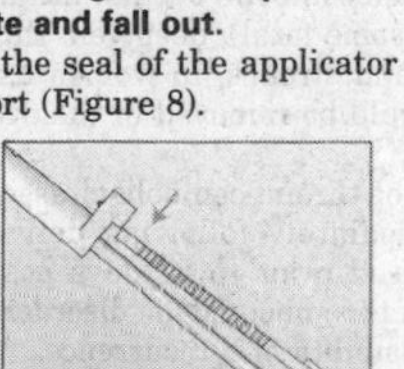

Figure 8

Step 17. Turn the obturator 90° in either direction with respect to the needle (Figure 9).

[See figure 9 at top of next column]

Step 18. While holding the obturator fixed in place on the arm, fully retract the cannula (Figure 10). **Note: This procedure is opposite from an injection. Do not push the obturator. By holding the obturator fixed in place on the**

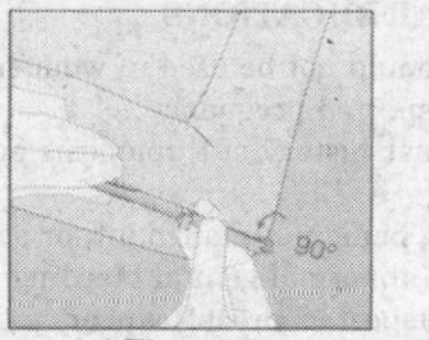

Figure 9

arm and fully retracting the cannula, the implant will be left in its correct subdermal position. Do not simultaneously retract the obturator and cannula from the patient's arm.

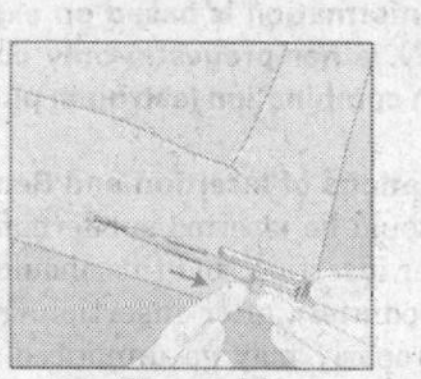

Figure 10

In this figure, the right hand is holding the obturator in place while the left hand is retracting the cannula.

Step 19. Confirm that the implant has been inserted by checking the tip of the needle for the absence of the implant. After insertion of the implant, the grooved tip of the obturator will be visible inside the needle (Figure 11).

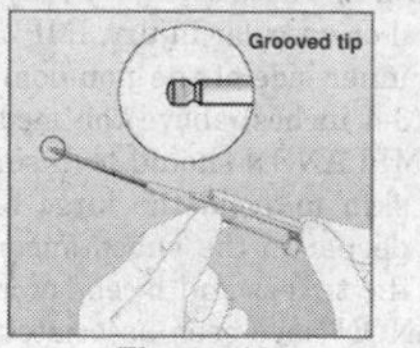

Figure 11

Step 20. **Always verify the presence of the implant in the woman's arm immediately after insertion by palpation.** By palpating both ends of the implant, you should be able to confirm the presence of the 4-cm rod (Figure 12).

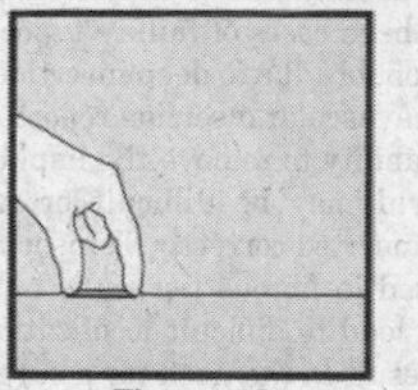

Figure 12

If you cannot feel the implant or are in doubt of its presence,

- Check the tip of the needle for the absence of the implant. After insertion of the implant, the grooved tip of the obturator will be visible inside the needle.
- Use other methods to confirm the presence of the implant. Suitable methods to locate are: ultrasound (US) with a high-frequency linear array transducer (10 MHz or greater) or magnetic resonance imaging (MRI). Please note that the IMPLANON rod is not radiopaque and cannot be seen by X-ray or CT scan. If ultrasound and MRI fail, call 1-877-IMPLANON (1-877-467-5266) for information on the procedure for measuring etonogestrel blood levels.

Until the presence of the implant has been verified, the woman should be advised to use a non-hormonal contraceptive method, such as condoms.

Step 21. Place a small adhesive bandage over the insertion site. Request that the woman palpate the implant.

Step 22. Apply a pressure bandage with sterile gauze to minimize bruising. The woman may remove the pressure bandage in 24 hours and the small bandage over the insertion site in 3 to 5 days.

Step 23. Complete the USER CARD and give it to the woman to keep. Also, complete the PATIENT CHART LABEL and affix it to the woman's medical record.

Step 24. The applicator is for single use only and should be disposed in accordance with the Center for Disease Control and Prevention guidelines for handling of hazardous waste.

2.3 Removal of IMPLANON

Preparation

Before initiating the removal procedure, the healthcare provider should carefully read the instructions for removal and consult the USER CARD and/or the PATIENT CHART LABEL for the location of the implant. The exact location of the implant in the arm should be verified by palpation. If the implant is not palpable, ultrasound with a high-frequency linear array transducer (10 MHz or greater) or magnetic resonance imaging can be performed to verify its presence. A non-palpable implant should always be first located prior to removal. Suitable methods for localization include ultrasound with a high-frequency linear array transducer (10 MHz or greater) or magnetic resonance imaging. If these imaging methods fail to locate the implant, etonogestrel blood level determination can be used for verification of the presence of the implant. For details on etonogestrel blood level determination, call 1-877-IMPLANON (1-877-467-5266) for further instructions.

After localization of a non-palpable implant, consider conducting removal with ultrasound guidance.

There have been occasional reports of migration of the implant; usually this involves minor movement relative to the original position. This may complicate localization of the implant by palpation, ultrasound or magnetic resonance imaging, and removal may require a larger incision and more time.

Exploratory surgery without knowledge of the exact location of the implant is strongly discouraged. Removal of deeply inserted implants should be conducted with caution in order to prevent injury to deeper neural or vascular structures in the arm and be performed by healthcare providers familiar with the anatomy of the arm.

Before removal of the implant, the healthcare provider should confirm that:

- The woman does not have allergies to the antiseptic or anesthetic to be used.

Remove the implant under aseptic conditions.

The following equipment is needed for removal of the implant:

- An examination table for the woman to lie on
- Sterile surgical drapes, sterile gloves, antiseptic solution, sterile marker (optional)
- Local anesthetic, needles, and syringe
- Sterile scalpel, forceps (straight and curved mosquito)
- Skin closure, sterile gauze, adhesive bandage and pressure bandages

Removal Procedure

Step 1. Clean the site where the incision will be made and apply an antiseptic. Locate the implant by palpation and mark the distal end (end closest to the elbow), for example, with a sterile marker (Figure 13).

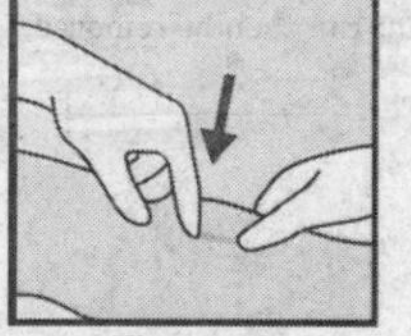

Figure 13

Step 2. Anesthetize the arm, for example, with 0.5 to 1 mL 1% lidocaine at the marked site where the incision will be made (Figure 14). Be sure to inject the local anesthetic **under** the implant to keep it close to the skin surface.

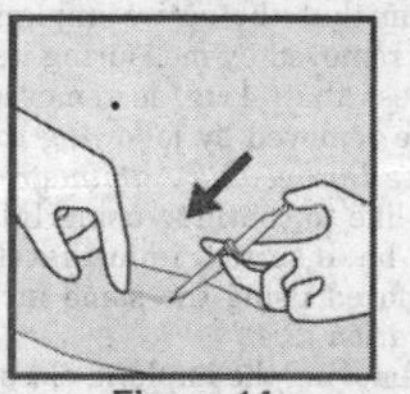

Figure 14

Step 3. Push down the proximal end of the implant (Figure 15) to stabilize it; a bulge may appear indicating the distal end of the implant. Starting at the distal tip of the implant, make a longitudinal incision of 2 mm towards the elbow.

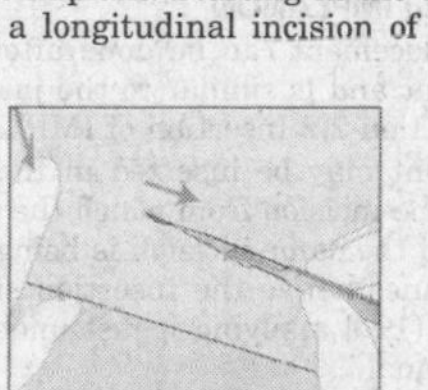

Figure 15

Step 4. Gently push the implant towards the incision until the tip is visible. Grasp the implant with forceps (preferably curved mosquito forceps) and gently remove the implant (Figure 16).

Figure 16

Step 5. If the implant is encapsulated, make an incision into the tissue sheath and then remove the implant with the forceps (Figures 17 and 18).

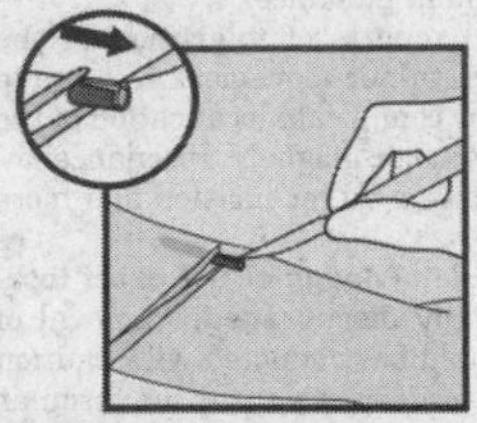

Figure 17

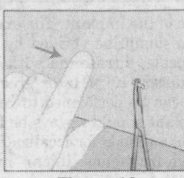

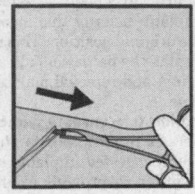

Figure 18

Step 6. If the tip of the implant does not become visible in the incision, gently insert a forceps into the incision (Figure 19). Flip the forceps over into your other hand (Figure 20).

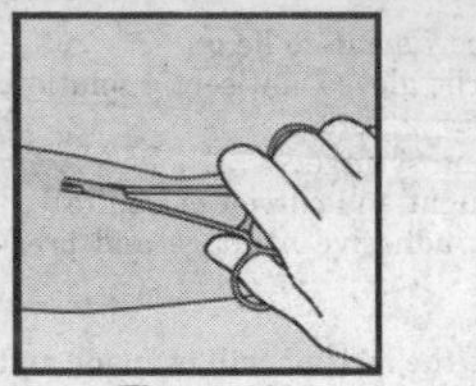

Figure 19

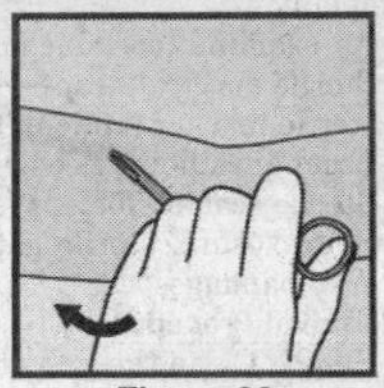

Figure 20

Step 7. With a second pair of forceps carefully dissect the tissue around the implant and grasp the implant (Figure 21). The implant can then be removed.

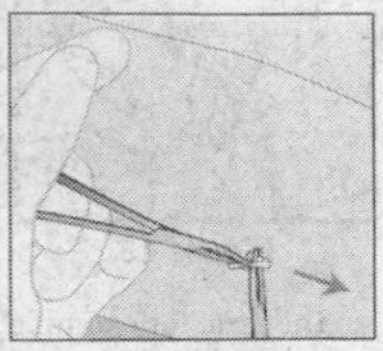

Figure 21

Step 8. Confirm that the entire implant, which is 4 cm long, has been removed by measuring its length. If a partial implant (less than 4 cm) is removed, the remaining piece should be removed by following the instructions in section 2.3. *[See Dosage and Administration (2.3).]* If the woman would like to continue using IMPLANON, a new implant may be inserted immediately after the old implant is removed using the same incision *[see Dosage and Administration (2.4)]*.

Step 9. After removing the implant, close the incision with a steri-strip and apply an adhesive bandage.

Step 10. Apply a pressure bandage with sterile gauze to minimize bruising. The woman may remove the pressure bandage in 24 hours and the small bandage in 3 to 5 days.

2.4 Replacing IMPLANON

Immediate replacement can be done after removal of the previous implant and is similar to the insertion procedure described in section 2.2 Insertion of IMPLANON.

The new implant may be inserted in the same arm, and through the same incision from which the previous implant was removed. If the same incision is being used to insert a new implant, anesthetize the insertion site [for example, 2 mL lidocaine (1%)] applying it just under the skin along the 'insertion canal.'

Follow the subsequent steps in the insertion instructions *[see Dosage and Administration (2.2)]*.

3 DOSAGE FORMS AND STRENGTHS

Single, off-white, soft, flexible, ethylene vinylacetate (EVA) implant, 4 cm in length and 2 mm in diameter containing 68 mg etonogestrel.

4 CONTRAINDICATIONS

IMPLANON should not be used in women who have

- Known or suspected pregnancy
- Current or past history of thrombosis or thromboembolic disorders
- Liver tumors, benign or malignant, or active liver disease
- Undiagnosed abnormal genital bleeding
- Known or suspected breast cancer, personal history of breast cancer, or other progestin-sensitive cancer, now or in the past
- Allergic reaction to any of the components of IMPLANON *[see Adverse Reactions (6)]*

5 WARNINGS AND PRECAUTIONS

The following information is based on experience with either IMPLANON, other progestin-only contraceptives, or experience with combination (estrogen plus progestin) oral contraceptives.

5.1 Complications of Insertion and Removal

IMPLANON should be inserted subdermally so that it will be palpable after insertion, and this should be confirmed by palpation immediately after insertion. Failure to insert IMPLANON properly may go unnoticed unless it is palpated immediately after insertion. Undetected failure to insert the implant may lead to an unintended pregnancy. Complications related to insertion and removal procedures, such as pain, paresthesias, bleeding, hematoma, scarring or infection, may occur. Occasionally in post-marketing use, implant insertions have failed because the implant fell out of the needle or remained in the needle during insertion.

If IMPLANON is inserted too deeply (intramuscular or in the fascia), neural or vascular injury may occur. To reduce the risk of neural or vascular injury, IMPLANON should be inserted at the inner side of the non-dominant upper arm about 8-10 cm (3-4 inches) above the medial epicondyle of the humerus. IMPLANON should be inserted subdermally just under the skin to avoid the large blood vessels and nerves that lie deeper in the subcutaneous tissues in the sulcus between the triceps and biceps muscles. Deep insertions of IMPLANON have been associated with paraesthesia (due to neural injury) and migration of the implant (due to intramuscular or fascial insertion), and in a very few cases with intravascular insertion. If infection develops at the insertion site, start suitable treatment. If the infection persists, the implant should be removed. Incomplete insertions or infections may lead to expulsion. In postmarketing use there have been cases of failure to localize and remove the implant, probably due to deep insertion. There has been 1 case of an intravascular insertion reported post-marketing which led to inability to remove the implant.

Implant removal may be difficult or impossible if the implant is not inserted correctly, is inserted too deeply, not palpable, encased in fibrous tissue, or has migrated. Deep insertions may lead to difficult localization of the implant and may also result in the need for a surgical procedure in an operating room in order to remove the implant. Exploratory surgery without knowledge of the exact location of the implant is strongly discouraged. Removal of deeply inserted implants should be conducted with caution in order to prevent injury to deeper neural or vascular structures in the arm and be performed by healthcare providers familiar with the anatomy of the arm. Failure to remove the implant may result in continued effects of etonogestrel, such as compromised fertility, ectopic pregnancy, or persistence or occurrence of a drug-related adverse event.

5.2 Changes in Menstrual Bleeding Patterns

After starting IMPLANON, women are likely to have a change from their normal menstrual bleeding pattern. These may include changes in bleeding frequency (absent, less, more frequent or continuous), intensity (reduced or increased) or duration. In clinical trials, bleeding patterns ranged from amenorrhea (1 in 5 women) to frequent and/or prolonged bleeding (1 in 5 women). The bleeding pattern experienced during the first three months of IMPLANON use is broadly predictive of the future bleeding pattern for many women. Women should be counseled regarding the bleeding pattern changes they may experience so that they know what to expect. Abnormal bleeding should be evaluated as needed to exclude pathologic conditions or pregnancy.

In clinical studies of IMPLANON, reports of changes in bleeding pattern were the most common reason for stopping treatment (11.1%). Irregular bleeding (10.8%) was the single most common reason women stopped treatment, while amenorrhea (0.3%) was cited less frequently. In these studies, women had an average of 17.7 days of bleeding or spotting every 90 days (based on 3,315 intervals of 90 days recorded by 780 patients). The percentages of patients having 0, 1-7, 8-21, or >21 days of spotting or bleeding over a 90-day interval while using the IMPLANON implant are shown in Table 1.

Table 1: Percentages of Patients with 0, 1 - 7, 8 - 21, or >21 Days of Spotting or Bleeding Over a 90-Day Interval While Using IMPLANON

Total Days of Spotting or Bleeding	Percentage of Patients		
	Treatment Days 91-180 (N = 745)	Treatment Days 271-360 (N = 657)	Treatment Days 631-720 (N = 547)
0 Days	19%	24%	17%
1-7 Days	15%	13%	12%
8-21 Days	30%	30%	37%
>21 Days	35%	33%	35%

Bleeding patterns observed with use of IMPLANON for up to 2 years, and the proportion of 90-day intervals with these bleeding patterns, are summarized in Table 2.

Table 2: Bleeding Patterns Using IMPLANON during the First 2 Years of Use*

BLEEDING PATTERNS	DEFINITIONS	%†
Infrequent	Less than three bleeding and/or spotting episodes in 90 days (excluding amenorrhea)	33.6
Amenorrhea	No bleeding and/or spotting in 90 days	22.2
Prolonged	Any bleeding and/or spotting episode lasting more than 14 days in 90 days	17.7
Frequent	More than 5 bleeding and/or spotting episodes in 90 days	6.7

* Based on 3,315 recording periods of 90 day's duration in 780 women, excluding the first 90 days after implant insertion

† % = Percentage of 90-day intervals with this pattern

In case of undiagnosed, persistent, or recurrent abnormal vaginal bleeding, appropriate measures should be conducted to rule out malignancy.

5.3 Ectopic Pregnancies

As with all progestin-only contraceptive products, be alert to the possibility of an ectopic pregnancy among women using IMPLANON who become pregnant or complain of lower abdominal pain. Although ectopic pregnancies are uncommon among women using IMPLANON, a pregnancy that occurs in a woman using IMPLANON may be more likely to be ectopic than a pregnancy occurring in a woman using no contraception.

5.4 Thrombotic and Other Vascular Events

The use of combination hormonal contraceptives (progestin plus estrogen) increases the risk of vascular events, including arterial events (strokes and myocardial infarctions) or deep venous thrombotic events (venous thromboembolism, deep venous thrombosis, retinal vein thrombosis, and pulmonary embolism). IMPLANON is a progestin-only contraceptive. It is unknown whether this increased risk is applicable to etonogestrel alone. It is recommended, however, that women with risk factors known to increase the risk of venous and arterial thromboembolism be carefully assessed.

There have been postmarketing reports of serious arterial and venous thromboembolic events, including cases of pulmonary emboli (some fatal), deep vein thrombosis, myocardial infarction, and strokes, in women using IMPLANON. IMPLANON should be removed in the event of a thrombosis.

Due to the risk of thromboembolism associated with pregnancy and immediately following delivery, IMPLANON should not be used prior to 21 days postpartum. Women with a history of thromboembolic disorders should be made aware of the possibility of a recurrence.

Evaluate for retinal vein thrombosis immediately if there is unexplained loss of vision, proptosis, diplopia, papilledema, or retinal vascular lesions.

Consider removal of the IMPLANON implant in case of long-term immobilization due to surgery or illness.

5.5 Ovarian Cysts

If follicular development occurs, atresia of the follicle is sometimes delayed, and the follicle may continue to grow beyond the size it would attain in a normal cycle. Generally, these enlarged follicles disappear spontaneously. On rare occasion, surgery may be required.

5.6 Carcinoma of the Breast and Reproductive Organs

Women who currently have or have had breast cancer should not use hormonal contraception because breast cancer may be hormonally sensitive *[see Contraindications (4)]*.

Some studies suggest that the use of combination hormonal contraceptives might increase the incidence of breast cancer; however, other studies have not confirmed such findings.

Some studies suggest that the use of combination hormonal contraceptives is associated with an increase in the risk of cervical cancer or intraepithelial neoplasia. However, there is controversy about the extent to which such findings are due to differences in sexual behavior and other factors.

Women with a family history of breast cancer or who develop breast nodules should be carefully monitored.

5.7 Liver Disease

Disturbances of liver function may necessitate the discontinuation of hormonal contraceptive use until markers of liver function return to normal. Remove IMPLANON if jaundice develops.

Hepatic adenomas are associated with combination hormonal contraceptives use. An estimate of the attributable risk is 3.3 cases per 100,000 for combination hormonal contraceptives users. It is not known whether a similar risk exists with progestin-only methods like IMPLANON.

The progestin in IMPLANON may be poorly metabolized in women with liver impairment. Use of IMPLANON in women with active liver disease or liver cancer is contraindicated *[see Contraindications (4)]*.

5.8 Weight Gain

In clinical studies, mean weight gain in US IMPLANON users was 2.8 pounds after 1 year and 3.7 pounds after 2 years. How much of the weight gain was related to the implant is unknown. In studies, 2.3% of the users reported weight gain as the reason for having the implant removed.

5.9 Elevated Blood Pressure

Women with a history of hypertension-related diseases or renal disease should be discouraged from using hormonal contraception. For women with well-controlled hypertension, use of IMPLANON can be considered. Women with hypertension using IMPLANON should be closely monitored. If sustained hypertension develops during the use of IMPLANON, or if a significant increase in blood pressure does not respond adequately to antihypertensive therapy, IMPLANON should be removed.

5.10 Gallbladder Disease

Studies suggest a small increased relative risk of developing gallbladder disease among combination hormonal contraceptive users. It is not known whether a similar risk exists with progestin-only methods like IMPLANON.

5.11 Carbohydrate and Lipid Metabolic Effects

Use of IMPLANON may induce mild insulin resistance and small changes in glucose concentrations of unknown clinical significance. Carefully monitor prediabetic and diabetic women using IMPLANON.

Women who are being treated for hyperlipidemia should be followed closely if they elect to use IMPLANON. Some progestins may elevate LDL levels and may render the control of hyperlipidemia more difficult.

5.12 Depressed Mood

Women with a history of depressed mood should be carefully observed. Consideration should be given to removing IMPLANON in patients who become significantly depressed.

5.13 Return to Ovulation

In clinical trials with IMPLANON, the etonogestrel levels in blood decreased below sensitivity of the assay by one week after removal of the implant. In addition, pregnancies were observed to occur as early as 7 to 14 days after removal. Therefore, a woman should re-start contraception immediately after removal of the implant if continued contraceptive protection is desired.

5.14 Fluid Retention

Hormonal contraceptives may cause some degree of fluid retention. They should be prescribed with caution, and only with careful monitoring, in patients with conditions which might be aggravated by fluid retention. It is unknown if IMPLANON causes fluid retention.

5.15 Contact Lenses

Contact lens wearers who develop visual changes or changes in lens tolerance should be assessed by an ophthalmologist.

5.16 Monitoring

A woman who is using IMPLANON should have a yearly visit with her healthcare provider for a blood pressure check and for other indicated health care.

5.17 Drug-Laboratory Test Interactions

Sex hormone-binding globulin concentrations may be decreased for the first 6 months after IMPLANON insertion followed by a gradual recovery. Thyroxine concentrations may initially be slightly decreased followed by gradual recovery to baseline.

6 ADVERSE REACTIONS

The following adverse reactions reported with the use of hormonal contraception are discussed elsewhere in the labeling:

- Changes in Menstrual Bleeding Patterns *[see Warnings and Precautions (5.2)]*
- Ectopic Pregnancies *[see Warnings and Precautions (5.3)]*
- Thrombotic and Other Vascular Events *[see Warnings and Precautions (5.4)]*
- Liver Disease *[see Warnings and Precautions (5.7)]*

6.1 Clinical Trials Experience

Because clinical trials are conducted under widely varying conditions, adverse reaction rates observed in the clinical trials of a drug cannot be directly compared to rates in the clinical trials of another drug and may not reflect the rates observed in practice.

In clinical trials including 942 women who were evaluated for safety, change in menstrual bleeding patterns (irregular menses) was the most common adverse reaction causing discontinuation of use of IMPLANON (11.1% of women).

Adverse reactions that resulted in a rate of discontinuation of ≥1% are shown in Table 3.

Table 3: Adverse Reactions Leading to Discontinuation of Treatment in 1% or More of Subjects in Clinical Trials of IMPLANON

Adverse Reactions	All Studies N = 942
Bleeding Irregularities*	11.1%
Emotional Lability†	2.3%
Weight Increase	2.3%
Headache	1.6%
Acne	1.3%
Depression‡	1.0%

* Includes "frequent", "heavy", "prolonged", "spotting", and other patterns of bleeding irregularity.
† Among US subjects (N=330), 6.1% experienced emotional lability that led to discontinuation.
‡ Among US subjects (N=330), 2.4% experienced depression that led to discontinuation.

Other adverse reactions that were reported by at least 5% of subjects in clinical trials of IMPLANON are listed in Table 4.

Table 4: Common Adverse Reactions Reported by ≥5% of Subjects in Clinical Trials with IMPLANON

Adverse Reaction	All Studies N=942
Headache	24.9%
Vaginitis	14.5%
Weight increase	13.7%
Acne	13.5%
Breast pain	12.8%
Abdominal pain	10.9%
Pharyngitis	10.5%
Leukorrhea	9.6%
Influenza-like symptoms	7.6%
Dizziness	7.2%
Dysmenorrhea	7.2%
Back pain	6.8%
Emotional lability	6.5%
Nausea	6.4%
Pain	5.6%
Nervousness	5.6%
Depression	5.5%
Hypersensitivity	5.4%
Insertion site pain	5.2%

Implant site complications were reported by 3.6% of subjects during any of the assessments in clinical trials. Pain was the most frequent implant site complication, reported during and/or after insertion, occurring in 2.9% of subjects. Additionally, hematoma, redness, and swelling were reported by 0.1%, 0.3%, and 0.3% of patients, respectively *[see Warnings and Precautions (5.1)]*.

6.2 Postmarketing Experience

The following additional adverse reactions have been identified during post-approval use of IMPLANON. Because these reactions are reported voluntarily from a population of uncertain size, it is not possible to reliably estimate their frequency or establish a causal relationship to drug exposure.

Gastrointestinal disorders: constipation, diarrhea, flatulence, vomiting.

General disorders and administration site conditions: edema, fatigue, implant site reaction, pyrexia.

Immune system disorders: anaphylactic reactions

Infections and infestations: rhinitis, urinary tract infection.

Investigations: clinically relevant rise in blood pressure, weight decreased.

Metabolism and nutrition disorders: increased appetite.

Musculoskeletal and connective tissue disorders: arthralgia, musculoskeletal pain, myalgia.

Nervous system disorders: convulsions, migraine, somnolence.

Pregnancy, puerperium and perinatal conditions: ectopic pregnancy.

Psychiatric disorders: anxiety, insomnia, libido decreased.

Renal and urinary disorders: dysuria.

Reproductive system and breast disorders: breast discharge, breast enlargement, ovarian cyst, pruritus genital, vulvovaginal discomfort.

Skin and subcutaneous tissue disorders: angioedema, aggravation of angioedema and/or aggravation of hereditary angioedema, alopecia, chloasma, hypertrichosis, pruritus, rash, seborrhea, urticaria.

Vascular disorders: hot flush.

Complications related to insertion or removal of the implant reported include: bruising, slight local irritation, pain or itching, fibrosis at the implant site, paresthesia or paresthesia-like events, scarring and abscess.

7 DRUG INTERACTIONS

7.1 Changes in Contraceptive Effectiveness Associated with Coadministration of Other Products

Drugs or herbal products that induce enzymes, including CYP3A4, that metabolize progestins may decrease the plasma concentrations of progestins, and may decrease the effectiveness of IMPLANON. In women on long-term treatment with hepatic enzyme inducing drugs, it is recommended to remove the implant and to advise a contraceptive method that is unaffected by the interacting drug.

Some of these drugs or herbal products that induce enzymes, including CYP3A4, include:

- barbiturates
- bosentan
- carbamazepine
- felbamate
- griseofulvin
- oxcarbazepine
- phenytoin
- rifampin
- St. John's wort
- Topiramate

HIV Antiretrovirals

Significant changes (increase or decrease) in the plasma levels of progestin have been noted in some cases of coadministration with HIV protease inhibitors or with nonnucleoside reverse transcriptase inhibitors. Consult the labeling of all concurrently-used drugs to obtain further information about interactions with hormonal contraceptives or the potential for enzyme alterations.

7.2 Increase in Plasma Concentrations of Etonogestrel Associated with Coadministered Drugs

CYP3A4 inhibitors such as itraconazole or ketoconazole may increase plasma concentrations of etonogestrel.

7.3 Changes in Plasma Concentrations of Coadministered Drugs

Hormonal contraceptives may affect the metabolism of other drugs. Consequently, plasma concentrations may either increase (for example, cyclosporin) or decrease (for example, lamotrigine). Consult the labeling of all concurrently-used drugs to obtain further information about interactions with hormonal contraceptives or the potential for enzyme alterations.

8 USE IN SPECIFIC POPULATIONS

8.1 Pregnancy

IMPLANON is not indicated for use during pregnancy *[see Contraindications (4)]*.

Teratology studies have been performed in rats and rabbits using oral administration up to 390 and 790 times the human IMPLANON dose (based upon body surface) and revealed no evidence of fetal harm due to etonogestrel exposure.

Studies have revealed no increased risk of birth defects in women who have used combination oral contraceptives before pregnancy or during early pregnancy. There is no evidence that the risk associated with IMPLANON is different from that of combination oral contraceptives.

IMPLANON should be removed if maintaining a pregnancy.

8.3 Nursing Mothers

Based on limited clinical data, IMPLANON may be used during breastfeeding after the fourth postpartum week. Use of IMPLANON before the fourth postpartum week has not been studied. Small amounts of etonogestrel are excreted in breast milk. During the first months after insertion of IMPLANON, when maternal blood levels of etonogestrel are highest, about 100 ng of etonogestrel may be ingested by the child per day based on an average daily milk ingestion of 658 mL. Based on daily milk ingestion of 150 mL/kg, the mean daily infant etonogestrel dose one month after insertion of IMPLANON is about 2.2% of the weight-adjusted maternal daily dose, or about 0.2% of the estimated absolute maternal daily dose. The health of breast-fed infants whose mothers began using IMPLANON during the fourth to eighth week postpartum (n=38) was evaluated in a comparative study with infants of mothers using a non-hormonal IUD (n=33). They were breast-fed for a mean duration of 14 months and followed up to 36 months of age. No significant effects and no differences between the groups were observed on the physical and psychomotor development of these infants. No differences between groups in the production or quality of breast milk were detected.

Healthcare providers should discuss both hormonal and non-hormonal contraceptive options, as steroids may not be the initial choice for these patients.

8.4 Pediatric Use

Safety and efficacy of IMPLANON have been established in women of reproductive age. Safety and efficacy of IMPLANON are expected to be the same for postpubertal adolescents. However, no clinical studies have been conducted in women less than 18 years of age. Use of this product before menarche is not indicated.

8.5 Geriatric Use

This product has not been studied in women over 65 years of age and is not indicated in this population.

8.6 Hepatic Impairment

No studies were conducted to evaluate the effect of hepatic disease on the disposition of IMPLANON. The use of IMPLANON in women with active liver disease is contraindicated *[see Contraindications (4)]*.

8.7 Renal Impairment

No studies were conducted to evaluate the effect of renal disease on the disposition of IMPLANON.

8.8 Overweight Women

The effectiveness of IMPLANON in women who weighed more than 130% of their ideal body weight has not been defined because such women were not studied in clinical trials. Serum concentrations of etonogestrel are inversely related to body weight and decrease with time after implant insertion. It is therefore possible that IMPLANON may be less effective in overweight women, especially in the presence of other factors that decrease serum etonogestrel concentrations such as concomitant use of hepatic enzyme inducers.

10 OVERDOSAGE

Overdosage may result if more than 1 implant is inserted. In case of suspected overdose, the implant should be removed.

11 DESCRIPTION

IMPLANON (etonogestrel implant) is a progestin-only, soft, flexible implant preloaded in a sterile, disposable applicator for subdermal use. The implant is off-white, non-biodegradable and 4 cm in length with a diameter of 2 mm (see Figure 22). Each implant consists of an ethylene vinylacetate (EVA) copolymer core, containing 68 mg of the synthetic progestin etonogestrel, surrounded by an EVA copolymer skin. Once inserted subdermally, the release rate is 60 to 70 mcg/day in Week 5 to 6 and decreases to approximately 35 to 45 mcg/day at the end of the first year, to approximately 30 to 40 mcg/day at the end of the second year, and then to approximately 25 to 30 mcg/day at the end of the third year. IMPLANON is a progestin-only contraceptive and does not contain estrogen. IMPLANON does not contain latex and is not radio-opaque.

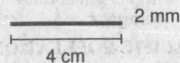

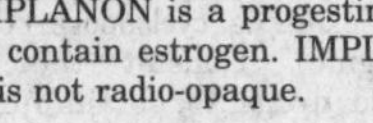

Figure 22 (Not to scale)

Etonogestrel [13-Ethyl-17-hydroxy-11-methylene-18,19-dinor-17α-pregn-4-en-20-yn-3-one], structurally derived from 19-nortestosterone, is the synthetic biologically active metabolite of the synthetic progestin desogestrel. It has a molecular weight of 324.46 and the following structural formula (Figure 23).

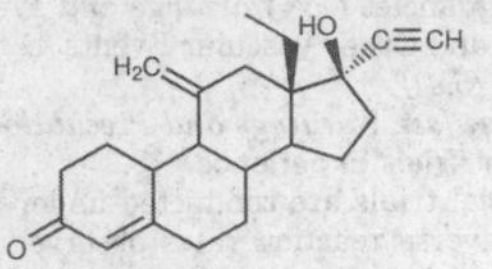

$C_{22}H_{28}O_2$

Figure 23

12 CLINICAL PHARMACOLOGY

12.1 Mechanism of Action

The contraceptive effect of IMPLANON is achieved by suppression of ovulation, increased viscosity of the cervical mucus, and alterations in the endometrium.

12.2 Pharmacodynamics

Exposure-response relationships of IMPLANON are unknown.

12.3 Pharmacokinetics

Absorption

After subdermal insertion of the etonogestrel implant, etonogestrel is released into the circulation and is approximately 100% bioavailable.

The mean peak serum concentrations in 3 pharmacokinetic studies ranged between 781 and 894 pg/mL and were reached within the first few weeks after insertion. The mean serum etonogestrel concentration decreases gradually over time declining to 192 to 261 pg/mL at 12 months (n=41), 154 to 194 pg/mL at 24 months (n=35), and 156 to 177 pg/mL at 36 months (n=17).

The pharmacokinetic profile of IMPLANON from 1 of 3 pharmacokinetic studies is shown in Figure 24.

Figure 24 Mean Serum Concentration-time Profile of Etonogestrel During 2 Years of IMPLANON Use and After Removal in 20 Healthy Women

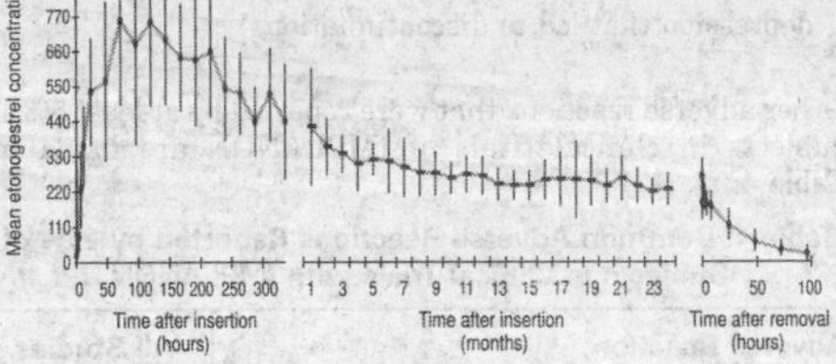

Figure 24

Distribution

The apparent volume of distribution averages about 201 L. Etonogestrel is approximately 32% bound to sex hormone binding globulin (SHBG) and 66% bound to albumin in blood.

Metabolism

In vitro data shows that etonogestrel is metabolized in liver microsomes by the cytochrome P450 3A4 isoenzyme. The biological activity of etonogestrel metabolites is unknown.

Excretion

The elimination half-life of etonogestrel is approximately 25 hours. Excretion of etonogestrel and its metabolites, either as free steroid or as conjugates, is mainly in urine and to a lesser extent in feces. After removal of the implant, etonogestrel concentrations decreased below sensitivity of the assay by 1 week.

13 NONCLINICAL TOXICOLOGY

13.1 Carcinogenesis, Mutagenesis, Impairment of Fertility

In a 24-month carcinogenicity study in rats with subdermal implants releasing 10 and 20 mcg etonogestrel per day (equal to approximately 1.8-3.6 times the systemic steady state exposure in women using IMPLANON), no drug-related carcinogenic potential was observed. Etonogestrel was not genotoxic in the *in vitro* Ames/Salmonella reverse mutation assay, the chromosomal aberration assay in Chinese hamster ovary cells or in the *in vivo* mouse micronucleus test. Fertility returned after withdrawal from treatment.

14 CLINICAL STUDIES

14.1 Pregnancy

In clinical trials of up to 3 years duration that involved 923 subjects, 18 - 40 years of age at entry, and 1,756 women-years of IMPLANON use, the total exposures expressed as 28-day cycle equivalents by study year were:

Year 1: 10,866 cycles
Year 2: 8,581 cycles
Year 3: 3,442 cycles

The clinical trials excluded women who:

- Weighed more than 130% of their ideal body weight
- Were chronically taking medications that induce liver enzymes

In the subgroup of women 18 to 35 years of age at entry, 6 pregnancies during 20,648 cycles of use were reported. Two pregnancies occurred in each of Years 1, 2 and 3. Each conception was likely to have occurred shortly before or within 2 weeks after IMPLANON removal. With these 6 pregnancies, the cumulative Pearl Index was 0.38 pregnancies per 100 women-years of use.

14.2 Return to Ovulation

In clinical trials with IMPLANON, the etonogestrel levels in blood decreased below sensitivity of the assay by one week after removal of the implant. In addition, pregnancies were observed to occur as early as 7 to 14 days after removal. Therefore, a woman should re-start contraception immediately after removal of the implant if continued contraceptive protection is desired.

16 HOW SUPPLIED/STORAGE AND HANDLING

16.1 How Supplied

One IMPLANON package consists of a single implant containing 68 mg etonogestrel that is 4 cm in length and 2 mm in diameter, which is pre-loaded in the needle of a disposable applicator. The sterile applicator containing the implant is packed in a blister pack.

NDC 0052-0272-01

16.2 Storage and Handling

Store IMPLANON (etonogestrel implant) at 25°C (77°F); excursions permitted to 15°-30°C (59°-86°F) [see USP Controlled Room Temperature]. Protect from light. Avoid storing IMPLANON in direct sunlight or at temperatures above 30°C (86°F).

17 PATIENT COUNSELING INFORMATION

"See FDA-Approved Patient Labeling (Patient Information)"

- Counsel women about the insertion and removal procedure of the IMPLANON implant. Provide the woman with a copy of the Patient Labeling and ensure that she understands the information in the Patient Labeling before insertion and removal. A USER CARD and consent form are included in the packaging. Have the woman complete a consent form and retain it in your records. The USER CARD should be filled out and given to the patient after insertion of the IMPLANON implant so that she will have a record of the location of the implant in the upper arm and when it should be removed.
- Counsel women that IMPLANON does not protect against HIV infection (AIDS) or other sexually transmitted diseases.
- Counsel women that the use of IMPLANON may be associated with changes in their normal menstrual bleeding patterns so that they know what to expect.

FDA-Approved Patient Labeling

See the full patient product information for IMPLANON.

Manufactured by: N.V. Organon, Oss,
The Netherlands, a subsidiary of
MERCK & CO., INC., Whitehouse Station, NJ 08889, USA
Distributed by: Schering Corporation, a subsidiary of
MERCK & CO., INC., Whitehouse Station, NJ 08889, USA

Revised: 03/2012
900415-IMP-IPT-USPI.6

FDA-Approved Patient Labeling

IMPLANON® (etonogestrel implant)

Subdermal Use

IMPLANON® does not protect against HIV infection (the virus that causes AIDS) or other sexually transmitted diseases. Read this Patient Information leaflet carefully before you decide if IMPLANON is right for you. This information does not take the place of talking with your healthcare provider. If you have any questions about IMPLANON, ask your healthcare provider.

What is IMPLANON?

IMPLANON is a hormone-releasing birth control implant for use by women to prevent pregnancy for up to 3 years. The implant is a flexible plastic rod about the size of a matchstick that contains a progestin hormone called etonogestrel. Your healthcare provider will insert the implant just under the skin of the inner side of your upper arm. You can use a single IMPLANON implant for up to 3 years. IMPLANON does not contain estrogen.

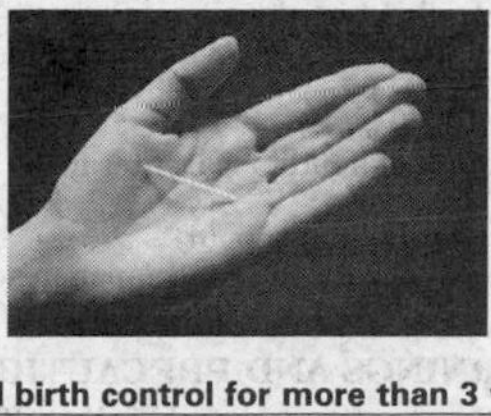

What if I need birth control for more than 3 years?

The IMPLANON implant must be removed after 3 years. Your healthcare provider can insert a new implant under your skin after taking out the old one if you choose to continue using IMPLANON for birth control.

What if I change my mind about birth control and want to stop using IMPLANON before 3 years?

Your healthcare provider can remove the implant at any time. You may become pregnant as early as the first week after removal of the implant. If you do not want to get pregnant after your healthcare provider removes the IMPLANON implant, you should start another birth control method right away.

How does IMPLANON work?

IMPLANON prevents pregnancy in several ways. The most important way is by stopping the release of an egg from your ovary. IMPLANON also thickens the mucus in your cervix and this change may keep sperm from reaching the egg. IMPLANON also changes the lining of your uterus.

How well does IMPLANON work?

When the IMPLANON implant is placed correctly, your chance of getting pregnant is very low (less than 1 pregnancy per 100 women who use IMPLANON for 1 year). It is not known if IMPLANON is as effective in very overweight women because studies did not include many overweight women.

The following chart shows the chance of getting pregnant for women who use different methods of birth control. Each box on the chart contains a list of birth control methods that are similar in effectiveness. The most effective methods are at the top of the chart. The box on the bottom of the chart shows the chance of getting pregnant for women who do not use birth control and are trying to get pregnant.

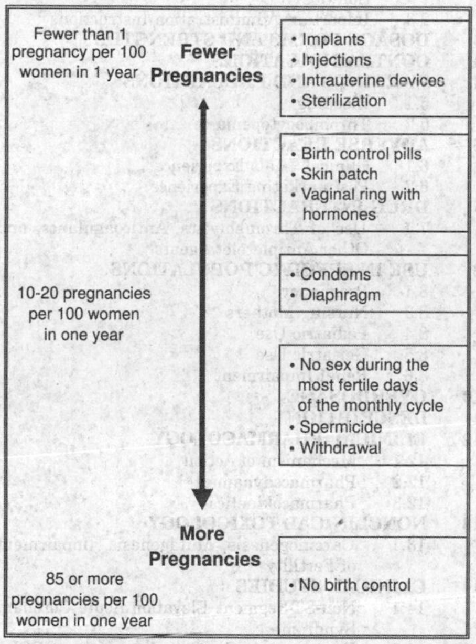

Who should not use IMPLANON?

Do not use IMPLANON if you

- Are pregnant or think you may be pregnant
- Have, or have had serious blood clots, such as blood clots in your legs (deep vein thrombosis), lungs (pulmonary embolism), eyes (total or partial blindness), heart (heart attack), or brain (stroke)
- Have liver disease or a liver tumor
- Have unexplained vaginal bleeding
- Have breast cancer or any other cancer that is sensitive to progestin (a female hormone), now or in the past
- Are allergic to anything in IMPLANON

Tell your healthcare provider if you have or have had any of the conditions listed above. Your healthcare provider can suggest a different method of birth control.

In addition, talk to your healthcare provider about using IMPLANON if you:

- Have diabetes
- Have high cholesterol or triglycerides
- Have headaches
- Have gallbladder or kidney problems
- Have a history of depressed mood
- Have high blood pressure
- Have an allergy to numbing medicines (anesthetics) or medicines used to clean your skin (antiseptics). These medicines will be used when the implant is placed into or removed from your arm.

Interaction with Other Medicines

Tell your healthcare provider about all the medicines you take, including prescription and non-prescription medicines, vitamins and herbal supplements. Certain medicines may make IMPLANON less effective, including:

- barbiturates
- bosentan
- carbamazepine
- felbamate
- griseofulvin
- oxcarbazepine
- phenytoin
- rifampin
- St. John's wort
- topiramate
- HIV medicines

Ask your healthcare provider if you are not sure if your medicine is one listed above.

If there are medicines that you have been taking for a long time, that make IMPLANON less effective, tell your healthcare provider. Your healthcare provider may remove the IMPLANON implant and recommend a birth control method that can be used effectively with these medicines.

When you are using IMPLANON, tell all of your healthcare providers that you have IMPLANON in place in your arm.

How is the IMPLANON implant placed and removed?

Your healthcare provider will place and remove the IMPLANON implant in a minor surgical procedure in his or her office. The implant is placed just under the skin on the inner side of your upper arm.

The timing of insertion is important. Your healthcare provider may:

- Perform a pregnancy test before inserting IMPLANON
- Schedule the insertion at a specific time of your menstrual cycle (for example, within the first days of your regular menstrual bleeding)

Immediately after the IMPLANON implant has been placed, you and your healthcare provider should check that the implant is in your arm by feeling for it.

If you and your healthcare provider cannot feel the IMPLANON implant, use a non-hormonal birth control method (such as condoms) until your healthcare provider confirms that the implant is in place. You may need special tests to check that the implant is in place or to help find the implant when it is time to take it out.

Your healthcare provider will cover the site where IMPLANON was placed with 2 bandages. Leave the top bandage on for 24 hours. Keep the smaller bandage clean, dry, and in place for 3 to 5 days.

You will be asked to review and sign a consent form prior to inserting the IMPLANON implant. You will also get a USER CARD to keep at home with your health records. Your healthcare provider will fill out the USER CARD with the date the implant was inserted and the date the implant is to be removed. Keep track of the date the implant is to be removed. Schedule an appointment with your healthcare provider to remove the implant on or before the removal date.

Be sure to have checkups as advised by your healthcare provider.

What are the most common side effects I can expect while using IMPLANON?

- **Changes in Menstrual Bleeding Patterns (menstrual periods)**

  The most common side effect of IMPLANON is a change in your normal menstrual bleeding pattern. In studies, about one out of ten women stopped using the implant because of an unfavorable change in their bleeding pattern. You may experience longer or shorter bleeding during your periods or have no bleeding at all. The time between periods may vary, and in between periods you may also have spotting.

Talk with your healthcare provider right away if:

- You think you may be pregnant
- Your menstrual bleeding is heavy and prolonged

Besides changes in menstrual bleeding patterns, other frequent side effects that caused women to stop using the implant include:

- Mood swings
- Weight gain
- Headache
- Acne
- Depressed mood

Other common side effects include:

- Headache
- Vaginitis (inflammation of the vagina)
- Weight gain
- Acne
- Breast pain
- Viral infections such as sore throats or flu-like symptoms
- Stomach pain
- Painful periods
- Mood swings, nervousness, or depressed mood
- Back pain
- Nausea
- Dizziness
- Pain
- Pain at the site of insertion

This is not a complete list of possible side effects. For more information, ask your healthcare provider for advice about any side effects that concern you. You may report side effects to the FDA at 1-800-FDA-1088.

What are the possible risks of using IMPLANON?

- **Problems with Insertion and Removal**

  The implant may not be placed in your arm at all due to a failed insertion or if the implant has fallen out of the needle. If this happens, you may become pregnant. Immediately after insertion, and with help from your healthcare provider, you should be able to feel the implant under your skin. If you can't feel the implant, tell your healthcare provider.

  Removal of the implant may be very difficult or impossible because the implant is not where it should be. Special procedures, including surgery in the hospital, may be needed to remove the implant. If the implant is not removed, then the effects of IMPLANON will continue for a longer period of time.

  Other problems related to insertion and removal are:

  - Pain, irritation, swelling, or bruising at the insertion site
  - Scarring, including a thick scar called a keloid around the insertion site
  - Infection
  - Scar tissue may form around the implant making it difficult to remove
  - The implant may come out by itself. You may become pregnant if the implant comes out by itself. Use a back up birth control method and call your healthcare provider right away if the implant comes out.
  - The need for surgery in the hospital to remove the implant
  - Injury to nerves or blood vessels in your arm
  - The implant breaks making removal difficult

- **Ectopic Pregnancy**

  If you become pregnant while using IMPLANON, you have a slightly higher chance that the pregnancy will be ectopic (occurring outside the womb) than do women who do not use birth control. Unusual vaginal bleeding or lower stomach (abdominal) pain may be a sign of ectopic pregnancy. Ectopic pregnancy is a medical emergency that often requires surgery. Ectopic pregnancies can cause serious internal bleeding, infertility, and even death. Call your healthcare provider right away if you think you are pregnant or have unexplained lower stomach (abdominal) pain.

- **Ovarian Cysts**

  Cysts may develop on the ovaries and usually go away without treatment but sometimes surgery is needed to remove them.

- **Breast Cancer**

  It is not known whether IMPLANON use changes a woman's risk for breast cancer. If you have breast cancer now, or have had it in the past, do not use IMPLANON because some breast cancers are sensitive to hormones.

- **Serious Blood Clots**

  IMPLANON may increase your chance of serious blood clots, especially if you have other risk factors such as smoking. It is possible to die from a problem caused by a blood clot, such as a heart attack or a stroke.

  Some examples of serious blood clots are blood clots in the:

  - Legs (deep vein thrombosis)
  - Lung (pulmonary embolism)
  - Brain (stroke)
  - Heart (heart attack)
  - Eyes (total or partial blindness)

  The risk of serious blood clots is increased in women who smoke. If you smoke and want to use IMPLANON, you should quit. Your healthcare provider may be able to help. Tell your healthcare provider at least 4 weeks before if you are going to have surgery or will need to be on bed rest. You have an increased chance of getting blood clots during surgery or bed rest.

- **Other Risks**

  A few women who use birth control that contains hormones may get:

  - High blood pressure
  - Gallbladder problems
  - Rare cancerous or noncancerous liver tumors

When should I call my healthcare provider?

Call your healthcare provider right away if you have:

- Pain in your lower leg that does not go away
- Severe chest pain or heaviness in the chest
- Sudden shortness of breath, sharp chest pain, or coughing blood

- Symptoms of a severe allergic reaction, such as swollen face, tongue or pharynx; trouble swallowing; or hives and trouble breathing
- Sudden severe headache unlike your usual headaches
- Weakness or numbness in your arm, leg, or trouble speaking
- Sudden partial or complete blindness
- Yellowing of your skin or whites of your eyes, especially with fever, tiredness, loss of appetite, dark colored urine, or light colored bowel movements
- Severe pain, swelling, or tenderness in the lower stomach (abdomen)
- Lump in your breast
- Problems sleeping, lack of energy, tiredness, or you feel very sad
- Heavy menstrual bleeding

What if I become pregnant while using IMPLANON?

You should see your healthcare provider right away if you think that you may be pregnant. It is important to remove the implant and make sure that the pregnancy is not ectopic (occurring outside the womb). Based on experience with other hormonal contraceptives, IMPLANON is not likely to cause birth defects.

Can I use IMPLANON when I am breastfeeding?

If you are breastfeeding your child, you may use IMPLANON if 4 weeks have passed since you had your baby. A small amount of the hormone contained in IMPLANON passes into your breast milk. The health of breast-fed children whose mothers were using the implant has been studied up to 3 years of age in a small number of children. No effects on the growth and development of the children were seen. If you are breastfeeding and want to use IMPLANON, talk with your healthcare provider for more information.

Additional Information

This Patient Information leaflet contains important information about IMPLANON. If you would like more information, talk with your healthcare provider. You can ask your healthcare provider for information about IMPLANON that is written for healthcare professionals. You may also call 1-877-IMPLANON (1-877-467-5266) or visit www.IMPLANON-USA.com

Manufactured by: N.V. Organon, Oss, The Netherlands, a subsidiary of **MERCK & CO., INC.**, Whitehouse Station, NJ 08889, USA

Distributed by: Schering Corporation, a subsidiary of **MERCK & CO., INC.**, Whitehouse Station, NJ 08889, USA

Revised: 03/2012
900415-IMP-IPT-PPI.6

IMPLANON®
(etonogestrel implant)
68 mg For Subdermal Use Only
PATIENT CONSENT FORM

I understand the Patient Labeling for IMPLANON®. I have discussed IMPLANON with my healthcare provider who answered all my questions. I understand that there are benefits as well as risks from using IMPLANON. I understand that there are other birth control methods and that each has its own benefits and risks.

I also understand that this Patient Consent Form is important. I understand that I need to sign this form to show that I am making an informed and careful decision to use IMPLANON, and that I have read and understand the following points.

- IMPLANON helps to keep me from getting pregnant.
- No contraceptive method is 100% effective, including IMPLANON.
- IMPLANON is made of a hormone mixed in a plastic rod.
- It is important to have IMPLANON inserted at the right time of my menstrual cycle.
- **After IMPLANON is inserted, I should check that it is in place by gently pressing my fingertips over the skin in my arm where IMPLANON was inserted. I should be able to feel the small rod.**
- IMPLANON must be removed at the end of 3 years. IMPLANON can be removed sooner if I want.
- If I have trouble finding a healthcare provider to remove IMPLANON, I can call (877) 467-5266 for help.
- IMPLANON is placed under the skin of my arm during a procedure done in my healthcare provider's office. There is a slight risk of getting a scar or an infection from this procedure.
- Removal is usually a small office procedure. However, removal may be difficult. Rarely, IMPLANON cannot be found when it is time to remove it. Special procedures, including surgery in the hospital, may be needed. Difficult removals may cause pain and scarring and may result in damage to nerves and blood vessels. If IMPLANON cannot be found, its effects may continue.
- **Most women have changes in their menstrual bleeding while using IMPLANON. I also will likely have changes in my menstrual bleeding while using IMPLANON. My bleeding may be irregular, lighter or heavier, or my bleeding may completely stop. If I think I am pregnant, I should see my healthcare provider as soon as possible.**
- I understand the warning signs for problems with IMPLANON. I should seek medical attention if any warning signs appear.
- I should tell all my healthcare providers that I am using IMPLANON.
- I need to have a medical checkup regularly and at any time I am having problems.
- IMPLANON does not protect me from HIV infection (AIDS) or any other sexually transmitted disease.

After learning about IMPLANON, I choose to use IMPLANON.

____
(Name of Healthcare Provider)

______________________ ____________
(Patient Signature) (Date)

WITNESSED BY:
The patient above has signed this consent in my presence after I counseled her and answered her questions.

______________________ ____________
(Healthcare Provider Signature) (Date)

I have provided an accurate translation of this information to the patient whose signature appears above. She has stated that she understands the information and has had an opportunity to have her questions answered.

______________________ ____________
(Signature of Translator) (Date)

Manufactured by: N.V. Organon, Oss, The Netherlands, a subsidiary of
MERCK & CO., INC.
Whitehouse Station, NJ 08889, USA
Distributed by: Schering Corporation, a subsidiary of
MERCK & CO., INC.
Whitehouse Station, NJ 08889, USA

Revised: March 2012
900415-IMP-IPT-PCF.2

Shown in Product Identification Guide, page 308

INTEGRILIN® ℞

[*ĭn-tĕg-rĭl-in*]
(eptifibatide)
injection, for intravenous use

HIGHLIGHTS OF PRESCRIBING INFORMATION
These highlights do not include all the information needed to use INTEGRILIN safely and effectively. See full prescribing information for INTEGRILIN.
INTEGRILIN® (eptifibatide) injection, for intravenous use
Initial U.S. Approval: 1998

INDICATIONS AND USAGE

INTEGRILIN is a platelet aggregation inhibitor indicated for:

- Treatment of acute coronary syndrome (ACS) managed medically or with percutaneous coronary intervention (PCI) (1.1)
- Treatment of patients undergoing PCI (including intracoronary stenting) (1.2)

DOSAGE AND ADMINISTRATION

ACS or PCI: 180 mcg/kg IV bolus as soon as possible after diagnosis followed by infusion at 2 mcg/kg/min. (2.1, 2.2)
PCI: Add a second 180 mcg/kg bolus at 10 minutes. (2.2)
In patients with creatinine clearance <50 mL/min, reduce the infusion to 1 mcg/kg/min. (2.1, 2.2, 2.3)

DOSAGE FORMS AND STRENGTHS

- 20 mg/10 mL (2 mg/mL) in a single-use vial for bolus injection (3)
- 75 mg/100 mL (0.75 mg/mL) in a single-use vial for infusion (3)
- 200 mg/100 mL (2 mg/mL) in a single-use vial for infusion (3)

CONTRAINDICATIONS

- Bleeding diathesis or bleeding within the previous 30 days (4)
- Severe uncontrolled hypertension (4)
- Major surgery within the preceding 6 weeks (4)
- Stroke within 30 days or any history of hemorrhagic stroke (4)
- Coadministration of another parenteral GP IIb/IIIa inhibitor (4)
- Dependency on renal dialysis (4)
- Known hypersensitivity to any component of the product (4)

WARNINGS AND PRECAUTIONS

- INTEGRILIN can cause serious bleeding. If bleeding cannot be controlled, discontinue INTEGRILIN immediately. Minimize vascular and other traumas. If heparin is given concomitantly, monitor aPTT or ACT. (5.1)
- Thrombocytopenia: Discontinue INTEGRILIN and heparin. Monitor and treat condition appropriately. (5.2)

ADVERSE REACTIONS

Bleeding and hypotension are the most commonly reported adverse reactions. (6.1)
To report SUSPECTED ADVERSE REACTIONS, contact Merck Sharp & Dohme Corp., a subsidiary of Merck & Co., Inc., at 1-877-888-4231 or FDA at 1-800-FDA-1088 or www.fda.gov/medwatch.

DRUG INTERACTIONS

- Coadministration of antiplatelet agents, thrombolytics, heparin, aspirin, and chronic NSAID use increases the risk of bleeding. Avoid concomitant use with other glycoprotein (GP) IIb/IIIa inhibitors. (7.1)

USE IN SPECIFIC POPULATIONS

- *Geriatric Use:* Risk of bleeding increases with age. (8.5)

See 17 for PATIENT COUNSELING INFORMATION
Revised: 08/2013

FULL PRESCRIBING INFORMATION: CONTENTS*

*** Sections or subsections omitted from the full prescribing information are not listed**

FULL PRESCRIBING INFORMATION

1 INDICATIONS AND USAGE

1.1 Acute Coronary Syndrome (ACS)

INTEGRILIN is indicated to decrease the rate of a combined endpoint of death or new myocardial infarction (MI) in patients with ACS (unstable angina [UA]/non-ST-elevation myocardial infarction [NSTEMI]), including patients who are to be managed medically and those undergoing percutaneous coronary intervention (PCI).

1.2 Percutaneous Coronary Intervention (PCI)

INTEGRILIN is indicated to decrease the rate of a combined endpoint of death, new MI, or need for urgent intervention in patients undergoing PCI, including those undergoing intracoronary stenting *[see Clinical Studies (14.1, 14.2)]*.

2 DOSAGE AND ADMINISTRATION

Before infusion of INTEGRILIN, the following laboratory tests should be performed to identify pre-existing hemostatic abnormalities: hematocrit or hemoglobin, platelet count, serum creatinine, and PT/aPTT. In patients undergoing PCI, the activated clotting time (ACT) should also be measured.

The activated partial thromboplastin time (aPTT) should be maintained between 50 and 70 seconds unless PCI is to be performed. In patients treated with heparin, bleeding can be minimized by close monitoring of the aPTT and ACT.

2.1 Dosage in Acute Coronary Syndrome (ACS)

Indication	Normal Renal Function	Creatinine Clearance <50 mL/min
Patients with ACS	180 mcg/kg intravenous (IV) bolus as soon as possible after diagnosis, followed by continuous infusion of 2 mcg/kg/min	180 mcg/kg IV bolus as soon as possible after diagnosis, followed by continuous infusion of 1 mcg/kg/min
	• Infusion should continue until hospital discharge or initiation of coronary artery bypass graft surgery (CABG), up to 72 hours • If a patient is to undergo PCI, the infusion should be continued until hospital discharge or for up to 18 to 24 hours after the procedure, whichever comes first, allowing for up to 96 hours of therapy • Aspirin, 160 to 325 mg, should be given daily	

INTEGRILIN should be given concomitantly with heparin dosed to achieve the following parameters:

<u>During Medical Management</u>: Target aPTT 50 to 70 seconds

- If weight greater than or equal to 70 kg, 5000-unit bolus followed by infusion of 1000 units/h.
- If weight less than 70 kg, 60-units/kg bolus followed by infusion of 12 units/kg/h.

<u>During PCI</u>: Target ACT 200 to 300 seconds

- If heparin is initiated prior to PCI, additional boluses during PCI to maintain an ACT target of 200 to 300 seconds.
- Heparin infusion after the PCI is discouraged.

2.2 Dosage in Percutaneous Coronary Intervention (PCI)

Indication	Normal Renal Function	Creatinine Clearance <50 mL/min
Patients with PCI	180 mcg/kg IV bolus immediately before PCI followed by continuous infusion of 2 mcg/kg/min and a second bolus of 180 mcg/kg (given 10 minutes after the first bolus)	180 mcg/kg IV bolus immediately before PCI followed by continuous infusion of 1 mcg/kg/min and a second bolus of 180 mcg/kg (given 10 minutes after the first bolus)
	• Infusion should be continued until hospital discharge, or for up to 18 to 24 hours, whichever comes first. A minimum of 12 hours of infusion is recommended. • In patients who undergo CABG surgery, INTEGRILIN infusion should be discontinued prior to surgery. • Aspirin, 160 to 325 mg, should be given 1 to 24 hours prior to PCI and daily thereafter	

- INTEGRILIN should be given concomitantly with heparin to achieve a target ACT of 200 to 300 seconds. Administer 60-units/kg bolus initially in patients not treated with heparin within 6 hours prior to PCI.
- Additional boluses during PCI to maintain ACT within target.
- Heparin infusion after the PCI is strongly discouraged.

Patients requiring thrombolytic therapy should discontinue INTEGRILIN.

2.3 Important Administration Instructions

1. Inspect INTEGRILIN for particulate matter and discoloration prior to administration, whenever solution and container permit.
2. May administer INTEGRILIN in the same intravenous line as alteplase, atropine, dobutamine, heparin, lidocaine, meperidine, metoprolol, midazolam, morphine, nitroglycerin, or verapamil. Do not administer INTEGRILIN through the same intravenous line as furosemide.
3. May administer INTEGRILIN in the same IV line with 0.9% NaCl or 0.9% NaCl/5% dextrose. With either vehicle, the infusion may also contain up to 60 mEq/L of potassium chloride.
4. Withdraw the bolus dose(s) of INTEGRILIN from the 10-mL vial into a syringe. Administer the bolus dose(s) by IV push.
5. Immediately following the bolus dose administration, initiate a continuous infusion of INTEGRILIN. When using an intravenous infusion pump, administer INTEGRILIN undiluted directly from the 100-mL vial. Spike the 100-mL vial with a vented infusion set. Center the spike within the circle on the stopper top.
6. Discard any unused portion left in the vial.

Administer INTEGRILIN by volume according to patient weight (see Table 1).

[See table 1 above]

Table 1: INTEGRILIN Dosing Charts by Weight

Patient Weight		180-mcg/kg Bolus Volume	2-mcg/kg/min Infusion Volume (CrCl ≥50 mL/min)		1-mcg/kg/min Infusion Volume (CrCl <50 mL/min)	
(kg)	(lb)	(from 2-mg/mL vial)	(from 2-mg/mL 100-mL vial)	(from 0.75-mg/mL 100-mL vial)	(from 2-mg/mL 100-mL vial)	(from 0.75-mg/mL 100-mL vial)
37-41	81-91	3.4 mL	2 mL/h	6 mL/h	1 mL/h	3 mL/h
42-46	92-102	4 mL	2.5 mL/h	7 mL/h	1.3 mL/h	3.5 mL/h
47-53	103-117	4.5 mL	3 mL/h	8 mL/h	1.5 mL/h	4 mL/h
54-59	118-130	5 mL	3.5 mL/h	9 mL/h	1.8 mL/h	4.5 mL/h
60-65	131-143	5.6 mL	3.8 mL/h	10 mL/h	1.9 mL/h	5 mL/h
66-71	144-157	6.2 mL	4 mL/h	11 mL/h	2 mL/h	5.5 mL/h
72-78	158-172	6.8 mL	4.5 mL/h	12 mL/h	2.3 mL/h	6 mL/h
79-84	173-185	7.3 mL	5 mL/h	13 mL/h	2.5 mL/h	6.5 mL/h
85-90	186-198	7.9 mL	5.3 mL/h	14 mL/h	2.7 mL/h	7 mL/h
91-96	199-212	8.5 mL	5.6 mL/h	15 mL/h	2.8 mL/h	7.5 mL/h
97-103	213-227	9 mL	6 mL/h	16 mL/h	3.0 mL/h	8 mL/h
104-109	228-240	9.5 mL	6.4 mL/h	17 mL/h	3.2 mL/h	8.5 mL/h
110-115	241-253	10.2 mL	6.8 mL/h	18 mL/h	3.4 mL/h	9 mL/h
116-121	254-267	10.7 mL	7 mL/h	19 mL/h	3.5 mL/h	9.5 mL/h
>121	>267	11.3 mL	7.5 mL/h	20 mL/h	3.7 mL/h	10 mL/h

3 DOSAGE FORMS AND STRENGTHS

- Injection: 20 mg of INTEGRILIN in 10 mL (2 mg/mL), for intravenous bolus
- Injection: 75 mg of INTEGRILIN in 100 mL (0.75 mg/mL), for intravenous infusion.
- Injection: 200 mg of INTEGRILIN in 100 mL (2 mg/mL), for intravenous infusion.

4 CONTRAINDICATIONS

Treatment with INTEGRILIN is contraindicated in patients with:

- A history of bleeding diathesis, or evidence of active abnormal bleeding within the previous 30 days
- Severe hypertension (systolic blood pressure >200 mm Hg or diastolic blood pressure >110 mm Hg) not adequately controlled on antihypertensive therapy
- Major surgery within the preceding 6 weeks
- History of stroke within 30 days or any history of hemorrhagic stroke
- Current or planned administration of another parenteral GP IIb/IIIa inhibitor
- Dependency on renal dialysis
- Hypersensitivity to INTEGRILIN or any component of the product (hypersensitivity reactions that occurred included anaphylaxis and urticaria).

5 WARNINGS AND PRECAUTIONS

5.1 Bleeding

Bleeding is the most common complication encountered during INTEGRILIN therapy. Administration of INTEGRILIN is associated with an increase in major and minor bleeding, as classified by the criteria of the Thrombolysis in Myocardial Infarction Study group (TIMI) *[see Adverse Reactions (6.1)]*. Most major bleeding associated with INTEGRILIN has been at the arterial access site for cardiac catheterization or from the gastrointestinal or genitourinary tract. Minimize the use of arterial and venous punctures, intramuscular injections, and the use of urinary catheters, nasotracheal intubation, and nasogastric tubes. When obtaining intravenous access, avoid non-compressible sites (e.g., subclavian or jugular veins).

<u>Use of Thrombolytics, Anticoagulants, and Other Antiplatelet Agents</u>

Risk factors for bleeding include older age, a history of bleeding disorders, and concomitant use of drugs that increase the risk of bleeding (thrombolytics, oral anticoagulants, nonsteroidal anti-inflammatory drugs, and $P2Y_{12}$ inhibitors). Concomitant treatment with other inhibitors of platelet receptor glycoprotein (GP) IIb/IIIa should be avoided. In patients treated with heparin, bleeding can be minimized by close monitoring of the aPTT and ACT *[see Dosage and Administration (2)]*.

<u>Care of the Femoral Artery Access Site in Patients Undergoing Percutaneous Coronary Intervention (PCI)</u>

In patients undergoing PCI, treatment with INTEGRILIN is associated with an increase in major and minor bleeding at the site of arterial sheath placement. After PCI, INTEGRILIN infusion should be continued until hospital discharge or up to 18 to 24 hours, whichever comes first. Heparin use is discouraged after the PCI procedure. Early sheath removal is encouraged while INTEGRILIN is being infused. Prior to removing the sheath, it is recommended that heparin be discontinued for 3 to 4 hours and an aPTT of <45 seconds or ACT <150 seconds be achieved. In any case, both heparin and INTEGRILIN should be discontinued and sheath hemostasis should be achieved at least 2 to 4 hours before hospital discharge. If bleeding at access site cannot be controlled with pressure, infusion of INTEGRILIN and heparin should be discontinued immediately.

5.2 Thrombocytopenia

There have been reports of acute, profound thrombocytopenia (immune-mediated and non-immune mediated) with INTEGRILIN. In the event of acute profound thrombocytopenia or a confirmed platelet decrease to <100,000/mm^3, discontinue INTEGRILIN and heparin (unfractionated or low-molecular weight). Monitor serial platelet counts, assess the presence of drug-dependent antibodies, and treat as appropriate *[see Adverse Reactions (6.1)]*.

There has been no clinical experience with INTEGRILIN initiated in patients with a baseline platelet count <100,000/mm^3. If a patient with low platelet counts is receiving INTEGRILIN, their platelet count should be monitored closely.

6 ADVERSE REACTIONS

The following serious adverse reaction is also discussed elsewhere in the labeling:

- Bleeding *[see Contraindications (4) and Warnings and Precautions (5.1)]*

6.1 Clinical Trials Experience

Because clinical studies are conducted under widely varying conditions, adverse reaction rates observed in the clinical studies of a drug cannot be directly compared to rates in the clinical trials of another drug and may not reflect the rates observed in clinical practice.

A total of 16,782 patients were treated in the Phase III clinical trials (PURSUIT, ESPRIT, and IMPACT II) *[see Clinical Trials (14)]*. These 16,782 patients had a mean age of 62 years (range: 20-94 years). Eighty-nine percent of the patients were Caucasian, with the remainder being predominantly Black (5%) and Hispanic (5%). Sixty-eight percent were men. Because of the different regimens used in PURSUIT, IMPACT II, and ESPRIT, data from the 3 studies were not pooled.

Bleeding and hypotension were the most commonly reported adverse reactions (incidence ≥5% and greater than placebo) in the INTEGRILIN controlled clinical trial database.

<u>Bleeding</u>

The incidence of bleeding and transfusions in the PURSUIT and ESPRIT studies are shown in Table 2. Bleeding was classified as major or minor by the criteria of the TIMI study group. Major bleeding consisted of intracranial hemorrhage and other bleeding that led to decreases in hemoglobin greater than 5 g/dL. Minor bleeding included spontaneous gross hematuria, spontaneous hematemesis, other observed blood loss with a hemoglobin decrease of more than 3 g/dL, and other hemoglobin decreases that were greater than 4 g/dL but less than 5 g/dL. In patients who received transfusions, the corresponding loss in hemoglobin was estimated through an adaptation of the method of Landefeld et al.

Table 2: Bleeding and Transfusions in the PURSUIT and ESPRIT Studies

PURSUIT (ACS)	Placebo n (%)	INTEGRILIN 180/2 n (%)
Patients	4696	4679
Major bleeding*	425 (9.3%)	498 (10.8%)
Minor bleeding*	347 (7.6%)	604 (13.1%)
Requiring transfusions†	490 (10.4%)	601 (12.8%)
ESPRIT (PCI)	**Placebo n (%)**	**INTEGRILIN 180/2/180 n (%)**
Patients	1024	1040
Major bleeding*	4 (0.4%)	13 (1.3%)
Minor bleeding*	18 (2%)	29 (3%)
Requiring transfusions†	11 (1.1%)	16 (1.5%)

Note: Denominator is based on patients for whom data are available.
* For major and minor bleeding, patients are counted only once according to the most severe classification.
† Includes transfusions of whole blood, packed red blood cells, fresh frozen plasma, cryoprecipitate, platelets, and autotransfusion during the initial hospitalization.

The majority of major bleeding reactions in the ESPRIT study occurred at the vascular access site (1 and 8 patients, or 0.1% and 0.8% in the placebo and INTEGRILIN groups, respectively). Bleeding at "other" locations occurred in 0.2% and 0.4% of patients, respectively.

In the PURSUIT study, the greatest increase in major bleeding in INTEGRILIN-treated patients compared to placebo-treated patients was also associated with bleeding at the femoral artery access site (2.8% versus 1.3%). Oropharyngeal (primarily gingival), genitourinary, gastrointestinal, and retroperitoneal bleeding were also seen more commonly in INTEGRILIN-treated patients compared to placebo-treated patients.

Among patients experiencing a major bleed in the IMPACT II study, an increase in bleeding on INTEGRILIN versus placebo was observed only for the femoral artery access site (3.2% versus 2.8%).

Table 3 displays the incidence of TIMI major bleeding according to the cardiac procedures carried out in the PURSUIT study. The most common bleeding complications were related to cardiac revascularization (CABG-related or femoral artery access site bleeding). A corresponding table for ESPRIT is not presented, as every patient underwent PCI in the ESPRIT study and only 11 patients underwent CABG.

Table 3: Major Bleeding by Procedures in the PURSUIT Study

	Placebo n (%)	INTEGRILIN 180/2 n (%)
Patients	4577	4604
Overall incidence of major bleeding	425 (9.3%)	498 (10.8%)
Breakdown by procedure:		
CABG	375 (8.2%)	377 (8.2%)
Angioplasty without CABG	27 (0.6%)	64 (1.4%)
Angiography without angioplasty or CABG	11 (0.2%)	29 (0.6%)
Medical therapy only	12 (0.3%)	28 (0.6%)

Note: Denominators are based on the total number of patients whose TIMI classification was resolved.

In the PURSUIT and ESPRIT studies, the risk of major bleeding with INTEGRILIN increased as patient weight decreased. This relationship was most apparent for patients weighing less than 70 kg.

Bleeding resulting in discontinuation of the study drug was more frequent among patients receiving INTEGRILIN than placebo (4.6% versus 0.9% in ESPRIT, 8% versus 1% in PURSUIT, 3.5% versus 1.9% in IMPACT II).

Intracranial Hemorrhage and Stroke

Intracranial hemorrhage was rare in the PURSUIT, IMPACT II, and ESPRIT clinical studies. In the PURSUIT study, 3 patients in the placebo group, 1 patient in the group treated with INTEGRILIN 180/1.3, and 5 patients in the group treated with INTEGRILIN 180/2 experienced a hemorrhagic stroke. The overall incidence of stroke was 0.5% in patients receiving INTEGRILIN 180/1.3, 0.7% in patients receiving INTEGRILIN 180/2, and 0.8% in placebo patients.

In the IMPACT II study, intracranial hemorrhage was experienced by 1 patient treated with INTEGRILIN 135/0.5, 2 patients treated with INTEGRILIN 135/0.75, and 2 patients in the placebo group. The overall incidence of stroke was 0.5% in patients receiving 135/0.5 INTEGRILIN, 0.7% in patients receiving INTEGRILIN 135/0.75, and 0.7% in the placebo group.

In the ESPRIT study, there were 3 hemorrhagic strokes, 1 in the placebo group and 2 in the INTEGRILIN group. In addition there was 1 case of cerebral infarction in the INTEGRILIN group.

Immunogenicity / Thrombocytopenia

The potential for development of antibodies to eptifibatide has been studied in 433 subjects. INTEGRILIN was nonantigenic in 412 patients receiving a single administration of INTEGRILIN (135-mcg/kg bolus followed by a continuous infusion of either 0.5 mcg/kg/min or 0.75 mcg/kg/min), and in 21 subjects to whom INTEGRILIN (135-mcg/kg bolus followed by a continuous infusion of 0.75 mcg/kg/min) was administered twice, 28 days apart. In both cases, plasma for antibody detection was collected approximately 30 days after each dose. The development of antibodies to eptifibatide at higher doses has not been evaluated.

In patients with suspected INTEGRILIN-related immune-mediated thrombocytopenia, IgG antibodies that react with the GP IIb/IIIa complex were identified in the presence of eptifibatide and in INTEGRILIN-naïve patients. These findings suggest acute thrombocytopenia after the administration of INTEGRILIN can develop as a result of naturally occurring drug-dependent antibodies or those induced by prior exposure to INTEGRILIN. Similar antibodies were identified with other GP IIb/IIIa ligand-mimetic agents. Immune-mediated thrombocytopenia with INTEGRILIN may be associated with hypotension and/or other signs of hypersensitivity.

In the PURSUIT and IMPACT II studies, the incidence of thrombocytopenia (<100,000/mm^3 or ≥50% reduction from baseline) and the incidence of platelet transfusions were similar between patients treated with INTEGRILIN and placebo. In the ESPRIT study, the incidence was 0.6% in the placebo group and 1.2% in the INTEGRILIN group.

Other Adverse Reactions

In the PURSUIT and ESPRIT studies, the incidence of serious nonbleeding adverse reactions was similar in patients receiving placebo or INTEGRILIN (19% and 19%, respectively, in PURSUIT; 6% and 7%, respectively, in ESPRIT). In PURSUIT, the only serious nonbleeding adverse reaction that occurred at a rate of at least 1% and was more common with INTEGRILIN than placebo (7% versus 6%) was hypotension. Most of the serious nonbleeding adverse reactions consisted of cardiovascular reactions typical of a UA population. In the IMPACT II study, serious nonbleeding adverse reactions that occurred in greater than 1% of patients were uncommon and similar in incidence between placebo- and INTEGRILIN-treated patients.

Discontinuation of study drug due to adverse reactions other than bleeding was uncommon in the PURSUIT, IMPACT II, and ESPRIT studies, with no single reaction occurring in >0.5% of the study population (except for "other" in the ESPRIT study).

6.2 Postmarketing Experience

Because the reactions below are reported voluntarily from a population of uncertain size, it is generally not possible to reliably estimate their frequency or establish a causal relationship to drug exposure.

The following adverse reactions have been reported in postmarketing experience, primarily with INTEGRILIN in combination with heparin and aspirin: cerebral, GI, and pulmonary hemorrhage. Fatal bleeding reactions have been reported. Acute profound thrombocytopenia, as well as immune-mediated thrombocytopenia, has been reported *[see Adverse Reactions (6.1)]*.

7 DRUG INTERACTIONS

7.1 Use of Thrombolytics, Anticoagulants, and Other Antiplatelet Agents

Coadministration of antiplatelet agents, thrombolytics, heparin, aspirin, and chronic NSAID use increases the risk of bleeding. Concomitant treatment with other inhibitors of platelet receptor GP IIb/IIIa should be avoided.

8 USE IN SPECIFIC POPULATIONS

8.1 Pregnancy

Pregnancy Category B

Teratology studies have been performed by continuous intravenous infusion of eptifibatide in pregnant rats at total daily doses of up to 72 mg/kg/day (about 4 times the recommended maximum daily human dose on a body surface area basis) and in pregnant rabbits at total daily doses of up to 36 mg/kg/day (also about 4 times the recommended maximum daily human dose on a body surface area basis). These studies revealed no evidence of harm to the fetus due to eptifibatide. There are, however, no adequate and well-controlled studies in pregnant women with INTEGRILIN. Because animal reproduction studies are not always predictive of human response, INTEGRILIN should be used during pregnancy only if clearly needed.

8.3 Nursing Mothers

It is not known whether eptifibatide is excreted in human milk. Because many drugs are excreted in human milk, caution should be exercised when INTEGRILIN is administered to a nursing mother.

8.4 Pediatric Use

Safety and effectiveness of INTEGRILIN in pediatric patients have not been studied.

8.5 Geriatric Use

The PURSUIT and IMPACT II clinical studies enrolled patients up to the age of 94 years (45% were age 65 and over; 12% were age 75 and older). There was no apparent difference in efficacy between older and younger patients treated with INTEGRILIN. The incidence of bleeding complications was higher in the elderly in both placebo and INTEGRILIN groups, and the incremental risk of INTEGRILIN-associated bleeding was greater in the older patients. No dose adjustment was made for elderly patients, but patients over 75 years of age had to weigh at least 50 kg to be enrolled in the PURSUIT study; no such limitation was stipulated in the ESPRIT study *[see Adverse Reactions (6.1)]*.

8.6 Renal Impairment

Approximately 50% of eptifibatide is cleared by the kidney in patients with normal renal function. Total drug clearance is decreased by approximately 50% and steady-state plasma INTEGRILIN concentrations are doubled in patients with an estimated CrCl <50 mL/min (using the Cockcroft-Gault equation). Therefore, the infusion dose should be reduced to 1 mcg/kg/min in such patients *[see Dosage and Administration (2)]*. The safety and efficacy of INTEGRILIN in patients dependent on dialysis has not been established.

10 OVERDOSAGE

There has been only limited experience with overdosage of INTEGRILIN. There were 8 patients in the IMPACT II study, 9 patients in the PURSUIT study, and no patients in the ESPRIT study who received bolus doses and/or infusion doses more than double those called for in the protocols. None of these patients experienced an intracranial bleed or other major bleeding.

Eptifibatide was not lethal to rats, rabbits, or monkeys when administered by continuous intravenous infusion for 90 minutes at a total dose of 45 mg/kg (about 2 to 5 times the recommended maximum daily human dose on a body surface area basis). Symptoms of acute toxicity were loss of righting reflex, dyspnea, ptosis, and decreased muscle tone in rabbits and petechial hemorrhages in the femoral and abdominal areas of monkeys.

From *in vitro* studies, eptifibatide is not extensively bound to plasma proteins and thus may be cleared from plasma by dialysis.

11 DESCRIPTION

Eptifibatide is a cyclic heptapeptide containing 6 amino acids and 1 mercaptopropionyl (des-amino cysteinyl) residue. An interchain disulfide bridge is formed between the cysteine amide and the mercaptopropionyl moieties. Chemically it is N^6-(aminoiminomethyl)-N^2-(3-mercapto-1-oxopropyl)-L-lysylglycyl-L-α-aspartyl-L-tryptophyl-L-prolyl-L-cysteinamide, cyclic (1→6)-disulfide. Eptifibatide binds to the platelet receptor glycoprotein (GP) IIb/IIIa of human platelets and inhibits platelet aggregation.

The eptifibatide peptide is produced by solution-phase peptide synthesis, and is purified by preparative reverse-phase liquid chromatography and lyophilized. The structural formula is:

[See chemical structure at top of next column]

INTEGRILIN Injection is a clear, colorless, sterile, nonpyrogenic solution for intravenous (IV) use with an empirical formula of $C_{35}H_{49}N_{11}O_9S_2$ and a molecular weight of 831.96. Each 10-mL vial contains 2 mg/mL of INTEGRILIN and each 100-mL vial contains either 0.75 mg/mL of INTEGRILIN or 2 mg/mL of INTEGRILIN. Each vial of either size also contains 5.25 mg/mL citric acid and sodium hydroxide to adjust the pH to 5.35.

12 CLINICAL PHARMACOLOGY

12.1 Mechanism of Action

Eptifibatide reversibly inhibits platelet aggregation by preventing the binding of fibrinogen, von Willebrand factor, and other adhesive ligands to GP IIb/IIIa. When administered intravenously, eptifibatide inhibits *ex vivo* platelet aggregation in a dose- and concentration-dependent manner.

Table 5: Clinical Events in the PURSUIT Study

Death or MI	Placebo (n=4739) n (%)	INTEGRILIN (180 mcg/kg bolus then 2 mcg/kg/min infusion) (n=4722) n (%)	p-value
3 days	359 (7.6%)	279 (5.9%)	0.001
7 days	552 (11.6%)	477 (10.1%)	0.016
30 days			
Death or MI (primary endpoint)	745 (15.7%)	672 (14.2%)	0.042
Death	177 (3.7%)	165 (3.5%)	
Nonfatal MI	568 (12%)	507 (10.7%)	

Table 6: Clinical Events (Death or MI) in the PURSUIT Study Within 72 Hours of Randomization

	Placebo	INTEGRILIN (180 mcg/kg bolus then 2 mcg/kg/min infusion)
Overall patient population	n=4739	n=4722
– At 72 hours	7.6%	5.9%
Patients undergoing early PCI	n=631	n=619
– Pre-procedure (nonfatal MI only)	5.5%	1.8%
– At 72 hours	14.4%	9%
Patients not undergoing early PCI	n=4108	n=4103
– At 72 hours	6.5%	5.4%

Table 7: Clinical Events in the IMPACT II Study

	Placebo n (%)	INTEGRILIN (135 mcg/kg bolus then 0.5 mcg/kg/min infusion) n (%)	INTEGRILIN (135 mcg/kg bolus then 0.75 mcg/kg/min infusion) n (%)
Patients	1285	1300	1286
Abrupt Closure	65 (5.1%)	36 (2.8%)	43 (3.3%)
p-value versus placebo		0.003	0.03
Death, MI, or Urgent Intervention			
24 hours	123 (9.6%)	86 (6.6%)	89 (6.9%)
p-value versus placebo		0.006	0.014
48 hours	131 (10.2%)	99 (7.6%)	102 (7.9%)
p-value versus placebo		0.021	0.045
30 days (primary endpoint)	149 (11.6%)	118 (9.1%)	128 (10%)
p-value versus placebo		0.035	0.179
Death or MI			
30 days	110 (8.6%)	89 (6.8%)	95 (7.4%)
p-value versus placebo		0.102	0.272
6 months	151 (11.9%)*	136 (10.6%)*	130 (10.3%)*
p-value versus placebo		0.297	0.182

* Kaplan-Meier estimate of event rate.

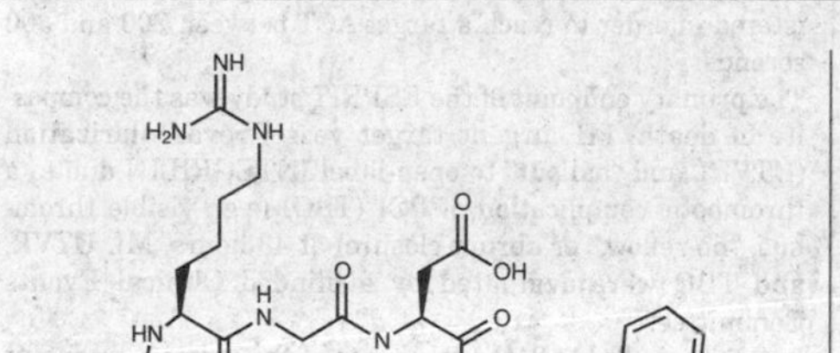

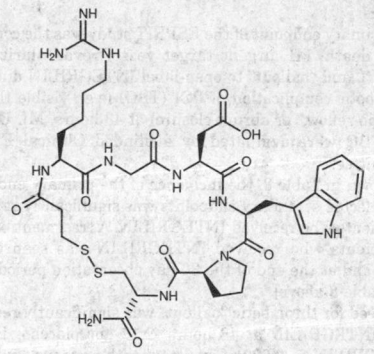

Platelet aggregation inhibition is reversible following cessation of the eptifibatide infusion; this is thought to result from dissociation of eptifibatide from the platelet.

12.2 Pharmacodynamics

Infusion of eptifibatide into baboons caused a dose-dependent inhibition of *ex vivo* platelet aggregation, with complete inhibition of aggregation achieved at infusion rates greater than 5 mcg/kg/min. In a baboon model that is refractory to aspirin and heparin, doses of eptifibatide that inhibit aggregation prevented acute thrombosis with only a modest prolongation (2- to 3-fold) of the bleeding time. Platelet aggregation in dogs was also inhibited by infusions of eptifibatide, with complete inhibition at 2 mcg/kg/min. This infusion dose completely inhibited canine coronary thrombosis induced by coronary artery injury (Folts model). Human pharmacodynamic data were obtained in healthy subjects and in patients presenting with UA or NSTEMI and/or undergoing percutaneous coronary intervention. Studies in healthy subjects enrolled only males; patient studies enrolled approximately one-third women. In these studies, INTEGRILIN inhibited *ex vivo* platelet aggregation induced by adenosine diphosphate (ADP) and other agonists in a dose- and concentration-dependent manner. The effect of INTEGRILIN was observed immediately after administration of a 180-mcg/kg intravenous bolus. Table 4 shows the effects of dosing regimens of INTEGRILIN used in the IMPACT II and PURSUIT studies on *ex vivo* platelet aggregation induced by 20 μM ADP in PPACK-anticoagulated platelet-rich plasma and on bleeding time. The effects of the dosing regimen used in ESPRIT on platelet aggregation have not been studied.

Table 4: Platelet Inhibition and Bleeding Time

	PURSUIT 180/2*
Inhibition of platelet aggregation 15 min after bolus	84%
Inhibition of platelet aggregation at steady state	>90%
Bleeding-time prolongation at steady state	<5×
Inhibition of platelet aggregation 4h after infusion discontinuation	<50%
Bleeding-time prolongation 6h after infusion discontinuation	1.4×

* 180-mcg/kg bolus followed by a continuous infusion of 2 mcg/kg/min.

The INTEGRILIN dosing regimen used in the ESPRIT study included two 180-mcg/kg bolus doses given 10 minutes apart combined with a continuous 2-mcg/kg/min infusion.

When administered alone, INTEGRILIN has no measurable effect on PT or aPTT.

There were no important differences between men and women or between age groups in the pharmacodynamic properties of eptifibatide. Differences among ethnic groups have not been assessed.

12.3 Pharmacokinetics

The pharmacokinetics of eptifibatide are linear and dose-proportional for bolus doses ranging from 90 to 250 mcg/kg and infusion rates from 0.5 to 3 mcg/kg/min. Plasma elimination half-life is approximately 2.5 hours. Administration of a single 180-mcg/kg bolus combined with an infusion produces an early peak level, followed by a small decline prior to attaining steady state (within 4-6 hours). This decline can be prevented by administering a second 180-mcg/kg bolus 10 minutes after the first. The extent of eptifibatide binding to human plasma protein is about 25%. Clearance in patients with coronary artery disease is about 55 mL/kg/h. In healthy subjects, renal clearance accounts for approximately 50% of total body clearance, with the majority of the drug excreted in the urine as eptifibatide, deaminated eptifibatide, and other, more polar metabolites. No major metabolites have been detected in human plasma.

Special Populations

Geriatric

Patients in clinical studies were older (range: 20-94 years) than those in the clinical pharmacology studies. Elderly patients with coronary artery disease demonstrated higher plasma levels and lower total body clearance of eptifibatide when given the same dose as younger patients. Limited data are available on lighter weight (<50 kg) patients over 75 years of age.

Renal Impairment

In patients with moderate to severe renal insufficiency (CrCl <50 mL/min using the Cockcroft-Gault equation), the clearance of eptifibatide is reduced by approximately 50% and steady-state plasma levels approximately doubled *[see Use in Specific Populations (8.6) and Dosage and Administration (2)]*.

Hepatic Impairment

No studies have been conducted in patients with hepatic impairment.

Gender

Males and females have not demonstrated any clinically significant differences in the pharmacokinetics of eptifibatide.

13 NONCLINICAL TOXICOLOGY

13.1 Carcinogenesis, Mutagenesis, Impairment of Fertility

No long-term studies in animals have been performed to evaluate the carcinogenic potential of eptifibatide. Eptifibatide was not genotoxic in the Ames test, the mouse lymphoma cell (L 5178Y, TK+/-) forward mutation test, the human lymphocyte chromosome aberration test, or the mouse micronucleus test. Administered by continuous intravenous infusion at total daily doses up to 72 mg/kg/day (about 4 times the recommended maximum daily human dose on a body surface area basis), eptifibatide had no effect on fertility and reproductive performance of male and female rats.

14 CLINICAL STUDIES

INTEGRILIN was studied in 3 placebo-controlled, randomized studies. PURSUIT evaluated patients with acute coronary syndromes: UA or NSTEMI. Two other studies, ESPRIT and IMPACT II, evaluated patients about to undergo a PCI. Patients underwent primarily balloon angioplasty in IMPACT II and intracoronary stent placement, with or without angioplasty, in ESPRIT.

14.1 Non-ST-Segment Elevation Acute Coronary Syndrome

Non-ST-segment elevation acute coronary syndrome is defined as prolonged (≥10 minutes) symptoms of cardiac ischemia within the previous 24 hours associated with either ST-segment changes (elevations between 0.6 mm and 1 mm or depression >0.5 mm), T-wave inversion (>1 mm), or positive CK-MB. This definition includes "unstable angina" and "NSTEMI" but excludes MI that is associated with Q waves or greater degrees of ST-segment elevation.

PURSUIT (Platelet Glycoprotein IIb/IIIa in Unstable Angina: Receptor Suppression Using INTEGRILIN Therapy)

PURSUIT was a 726-center, 27-country, double-blind, randomized, placebo-controlled study in 10,948 patients presenting with UA or NSTEMI. Patients could be enrolled only if they had experienced cardiac ischemia at rest (≥10 minutes) within the previous 24 hours and had either ST-segment changes (elevations between 0.6 mm and 1 mm or depression >0.5 mm), T-wave inversion (>1 mm), or increased CK-MB. Important exclusion criteria included a history of bleeding diathesis, evidence of abnormal bleeding within the previous 30 days, uncontrolled hypertension, major surgery within the previous 6 weeks, stroke within the previous 30 days, any history of hemorrhagic stroke, serum creatinine >2 mg/dL, dependency on renal dialysis, or platelet count <100,000/mm^3.

Patients were randomized to placebo, to INTEGRILIN 180-mcg/kg bolus followed by a 2-mcg/kg/min infusion (180/2), or to INTEGRILIN 180-mcg/kg bolus followed by a

Table 8: Clinical Events in the ESPRIT Study

	Placebo (n=1024)	INTEGRILIN* (n=1040)	Relative Risk (95% CI)	p-value
Death, MI, UTVR, or Thrombotic "Bailout"				
48 hours (primary endpoint)	108 (10.5%)	69 (6.6%)	0.629 (0.471, 0.84)	0.0015
30 days	120 (11.7%)	78 (7.5%)	0.64 (0.488, 0.84)	0.0011
Death, MI, or UTVR				
48 hours	95 (9.3%)	62 (6%)	0.643 (0.472, 0.875)	0.0045
30 days (key secondary endpoint)	107 (10.4%)	71 (6.8%)	0.653 (0.49, 0.871)	0.0034
Death or MI				
48 hours	94 (9.2%)	57 (5.5%)	0.597 (0.435, 0.82)	0.0013
30 days	104 (10.2%)	66 (6.3%)	0.625 (0.465, 0.84)	0.0016

* INTEGRILIN was administered as 180 mcg/kg boluses at times 0 and 10 minutes and an infusion at 2 mcg/kg/min.

Table 9: Clinical Events at 6 Months and 1 Year in the ESPRIT Study

	Placebo (n=1024)	INTEGRILIN (n=1040)	Hazard Ratio (95% CI)
Death, MI, or Target Vessel Revascularization			
6 months	187 (18.5%)	146 (14.3%)	0.744 (0.599, 0.924)
1 year	222 (22.1%)	178 (17.5%)	0.762 (0.626, 0.929)
Death, MI			
6 months	117 (11.5%)	77 (7.4%)	0.631 (0.473, 0.841)
1 year	126 (12.4%)	83 (8%)	0.63 (0.478, 0.832)

Percentages are Kaplan-Meier event rates.

1.3-mcg/kg/min infusion (180/1.3). The infusion was continued for 72 hours, until hospital discharge, or until the time of CABG, whichever occurred first, except that if PCI was performed, the INTEGRILIN infusion was continued for 24 hours after the procedure, allowing for a duration of infusion up to 96 hours.

The lower-infusion-rate arm was stopped after the first interim analysis when the 2 active-treatment arms appeared to have the same incidence of bleeding.

Patient age ranged from 20 to 94 (mean 63) years, and 65% were male. The patients were 89% Caucasian, 6% Hispanic, and 5% Black, recruited in the United States and Canada (40%), Western Europe (39%), Eastern Europe (16%), and Latin America (5%).

This was a "real world" study; each patient was managed according to the usual standards of the investigational site; frequencies of angiography, PCI, and CABG therefore differed widely from site to site and from country to country. Of the patients in PURSUIT, 13% were managed with PCI during drug infusion, of whom 50% received intracoronary stents; 87% were managed medically (without PCI during drug infusion).

The majority of patients received aspirin (75-325 mg once daily). Heparin was administered intravenously or subcutaneously, at the physician's discretion, most commonly as an intravenous bolus of 5000 units followed by a continuous infusion of 1000 units/h. For patients weighing less than 70 kg, the recommended heparin bolus dose was 60 units/kg followed by a continuous infusion of 12 units/kg/h. A target aPTT of 50 to 70 seconds was recommended. A total of 1250 patients underwent PCI within 72 hours after randomization, in which case they received intravenous heparin to maintain an ACT of 300 to 350 seconds.

The primary endpoint of the study was the occurrence of death from any cause or new MI (evaluated by a blinded Clinical Endpoints Committee) within 30 days of randomization.

Compared to placebo, INTEGRILIN administered as a 180-mcg/kg bolus followed by a 2-mcg/kg/min infusion significantly (p=0.042) reduced the incidence of endpoint events (see Table 6). The reduction in the incidence of endpoint events in patients receiving INTEGRILIN was evident early during treatment, and this reduction was maintained through at least 30 days (see Figure 1). Table 5 also shows the incidence of the components of the primary endpoint, death (whether or not preceded by an MI) and new MI in surviving patients at 30 days.

[See table 5 at top of previous page]

[See figure 1 at top of next column]

Treatment with INTEGRILIN prior to determination of patient management strategy reduced clinical events regardless of whether patients ultimately underwent diagnostic catheterization, revascularization (i.e., PCI or CABG surgery) or continued to receive medical management alone. Table 6 shows the incidence of death or MI within 72 hours.

[See table 6 at top of previous page]

All of the effect of INTEGRILIN was established within 72 hours (during the period of drug infusion), regardless of

Figure 1: Kaplan-Meier Plot of Time to Death or Myocardial Infarction Within 30 Days of Randomization in the PURSUIT Study

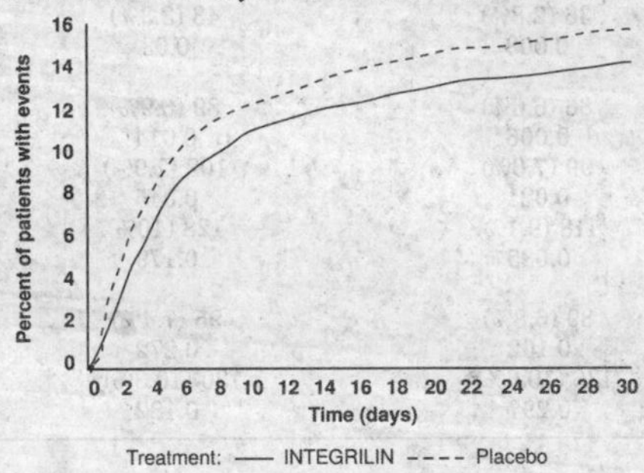

management strategy. Moreover, for patients undergoing early PCI, a reduction in events was evident prior to the procedure.

An analysis of the results by sex suggests that women who would not routinely be expected to undergo PCI receive less benefit from INTEGRILIN (95% confidence limits for relative risk of 0.94 - 1.28) than do men (0.72 - 0.9). This difference may be a true treatment difference, the effect of other differences in these subgroups, or a statistical anomaly. No differential outcomes were seen between male and female patients undergoing PCI (*see results for ESPRIT*).

Follow-up data were available through 165 days for 10,611 patients enrolled in the PURSUIT trial (96.9% of the initial enrollment). This follow-up included 4566 patients who received INTEGRILIN at the 180/2 dose. As reported by the investigators, the occurrence of death from any cause or new MI for patients followed for at least 165 days was reduced from 13.6% with placebo to 12.1% with INTEGRILIN 180/2.

14.2 Percutaneous Coronary Intervention (PCI)

IMPACT II (INTEGRILIN to Minimize Platelet Aggregation and Prevent Coronary Thrombosis II)

IMPACT II was a multicenter, double-blind, randomized, placebo-controlled study conducted in the United States in 4010 patients undergoing PCI. Major exclusion criteria included a history of bleeding diathesis, major surgery within 6 weeks of treatment, gastrointestinal bleeding within 30 days, any stroke or structural CNS abnormality, uncontrolled hypertension, PT >1.2 times control, hematocrit <30%, platelet count <100,000/mm^3, and pregnancy.

Patient age ranged from 24 to 89 (mean 60) years, and 75% were male. The patients were 92% Caucasian, 5% Black, and 3% Hispanic. Forty-one percent of the patients underwent PCI for ongoing ACS. Patients were randomly assigned to 1 of 3 treatment regimens, each incorporating a bolus dose initiated immediately prior to PCI followed by a continuous infusion lasting 20 to 24 hours:

1) 135-mcg/kg bolus followed by a continuous infusion of 0.5 mcg/kg/min of INTEGRILIN (135/0.5);
2) 135-mcg/kg bolus followed by a continuous infusion of 0.75 mcg/kg/min of INTEGRILIN (135/0.75); or
3) a matching placebo bolus followed by a matching placebo continuous infusion.

Each patient received aspirin and an intravenous heparin bolus of 100 units/kg, with additional bolus infusions of up to 2000 additional units of heparin every 15 minutes to maintain an ACT of 300 to 350 seconds.

The primary endpoint was the composite of death, MI, or urgent revascularization, analyzed at 30 days after randomization in all patients who received at least 1 dose of study drug.

As shown in Table 7, each INTEGRILIN regimen reduced the rate of death, MI, or urgent intervention, although at 30 days, this finding was statistically significant only in the lower-dose INTEGRILIN group. As in the PURSUIT study, the effects of INTEGRILIN were seen early and persisted throughout the 30-day period.

[See table 7 at top of previous page]

ESPRIT (Enhanced Suppression of the Platelet IIb/IIIa Receptor with INTEGRILIN Therapy)

The ESPRIT study was a multicenter, double-blind, randomized, placebo-controlled study conducted in the United States and Canada that enrolled 2064 patients undergoing elective or urgent PCI with intended intracoronary stent placement. Exclusion criteria included MI within the previous 24 hours, ongoing chest pain, administration of any oral antiplatelet or oral anticoagulant other than aspirin within 30 days of PCI (although loading doses of thienopyridine on the day of PCI were encouraged), planned PCI of a saphenous vein graft or subsequent "staged" PCI, prior stent placement in the target lesion, PCI within the previous 90 days, a history of bleeding diathesis, major surgery within 6 weeks of treatment, gastrointestinal bleeding within 30 days, any stroke or structural CNS abnormality, uncontrolled hypertension, PT >1.2 times control, hematocrit <30%, platelet count <100,000/mm^3, and pregnancy.

Patient age ranged from 24 to 93 (mean 62) years, and 73% of patients were male. The study enrolled 90% Caucasian, 5% African American, 2% Hispanic, and 1% Asian patients. Patients received a wide variety of stents. Patients were randomized either to placebo or INTEGRILIN administered as an intravenous bolus of 180 mcg/kg followed immediately by a continuous infusion of 2 mcg/kg/min, and a second bolus of 180 mcg/kg administered 10 minutes later (180/2/180). INTEGRILIN infusion was continued for 18 to 24 hours after PCI or until hospital discharge, whichever came first. Each patient received at least 1 dose of aspirin (162-325 mg) and 60 units/kg of heparin as a bolus (not to exceed 6000 units) if not already receiving a heparin infusion. Additional boluses of heparin (10-40 units/kg) could be administered in order to reach a target ACT between 200 and 300 seconds.

The primary endpoint of the ESPRIT study was the composite of death, MI, urgent target vessel revascularization (UTVR), and "bailout" to open-label INTEGRILIN due to a thrombotic complication of PCI (TBO) (e.g., visible thrombus, "no reflow," or abrupt closure) at 48 hours. MI, UTVR, and TBO were evaluated by a blinded Clinical Events Committee.

As shown in Table 8, the incidence of the primary endpoint and selected secondary endpoints was significantly reduced in patients who received INTEGRILIN. A treatment benefit in patients who received INTEGRILIN was seen by 48 hours and at the end of the 30-day observation period.

[See table 8 above]

The need for thrombotic "bailout" was significantly reduced with INTEGRILIN at 48 hours (2.1% for placebo, 1% for INTEGRILIN; p=0.029). Consistent with previous studies of GP IIb/IIIa inhibitors, most of the benefit achieved acutely with INTEGRILIN was in the reduction of MI. INTEGRILIN reduced the occurrence of MI at 48 hours from 9% for placebo to 5.4% (p=0.0015) and maintained that effect with significance at 30 days.

There was no treatment difference with respect to sex in ESPRIT. INTEGRILIN reduced the incidence of the primary endpoint in both men (95% confidence limits for relative risk: 0.54, 1.07) and women (0.24, 0.72) at 48 hours.

Follow-up (12-month) mortality data were available for 2024 patients (1017 on INTEGRILIN) enrolled in the ESPRIT trial (98.1% of the initial enrollment). Twelve-month clinical event data were available for 1964 patients (988 on INTEGRILIN), representing 95.2% of the initial enrollment. As shown in Table 9, the treatment effect of INTEGRILIN seen at 48 hours and 30 days appeared preserved at 6 months and 1 year. Most of the benefit was in reduction of MI.

[See table 9 above]

16 HOW SUPPLIED/STORAGE AND HANDLING

16.1 How Supplied

INTEGRILIN (eptifibatide) injection is supplied as a sterile solution in 10-mL vials containing 20 mg of INTEGRILIN (NDC 0085-1177-01) and 100-mL vials containing either 75 mg of INTEGRILIN (NDC 0085-1136-01) or 200 mg of INTEGRILIN (NDC 0085-1177-02).

16.2 Storage

Vials should be stored refrigerated at 2-8°C (36-46°F). Vials may be transferred to room temperature storage[1] for a period not to exceed 2 months. Upon transfer, vial cartons must be marked by the dispensing pharmacist with a "DISCARD BY" date (2 months from the transfer date or the labeled expiration date, whichever comes first).

Protect from light until administration.

[1] Store at 25°C (77°F); excursions permitted to 15-30°C (59-86°F) [see USP Controlled Room Temperature].

17 PATIENT COUNSELING INFORMATION

Instruct patients to inform the doctor or healthcare provider about any medical conditions, medications, and allergies.

Manufactured for: Merck Sharp & Dohme Corp., a subsidiary of

MERCK & CO., INC., Whitehouse Station, NJ 08889, USA

Manufactured by:

Patheon Italia S.p.A, Ferentino, 03013, Italy

U.S. Patent Nos. 5,686,570; 5,747,447; and 5,756,451.

INTEGRILIN is a registered trademark of Millennium Pharmaceuticals, Inc.

USPI-I-69361303R011

Shown in Product Identification Guide, page 308

INTRON® A ℞

[in' trŏn]

Interferon alfa-2b, recombinant

For Injection

WARNING

Alpha interferons, including INTRON® A, cause or aggravate fatal or life-threatening neuropsychiatric, autoimmune, ischemic, and infectious disorders. Patients should be monitored closely with periodic clinical and laboratory evaluations. Patients with persistently severe or worsening signs or symptoms of these conditions should be withdrawn from therapy. In many but not all cases these disorders resolve after stopping INTRON A therapy. See **WARNINGS** and **ADVERSE REACTIONS.**

Powder for Injection

Vial Strength Million IU	mL Diluent	Final Concentration after Reconstitution million IU/mL*	mg INTRON A† per vial	Route of Administration
10	1	10	0.038	IM, SC, IV, IL
18	1	18	0.069	IM, SC, IV
50	1	50	0.192	IM, SC, IV

* Each mL also contains 20 mg glycine, 2.3 mg sodium phosphate dibasic, 0.55 mg sodium phosphate monobasic, and 1.0 mg human albumin.

† Based on the specific activity of approximately 2.6×10^8 IU/mg protein, as measured by HPLC assay.

Solution Vials for Injection

Vial Strength	Concentration*	mg INTRON A† per vial	Route of Administration
18‡ MIU multidose	3 million IU/0.5 mL	0.088	IM, SC
25§ MIU multidose	5 million IU/0.5 mL	0.123	IM, SC, IL

* Each mL contains 7.5 mg sodium chloride, 1.8 mg sodium phosphate dibasic, 1.3 mg sodium phosphate monobasic, 0.1 mg edetate disodium, 0.1 mg polysorbate 80, and 1.5 mg m-cresol as a preservative.

† Based on the specific activity of approximately 2.6×10^8 IU/mg protein as measured by HPLC assay.

‡ This is a multidose vial which contains a total of 22.8 million IU of interferon alfa-2b, recombinant per 3.8 mL in order to provide the delivery of six 0.5-mL doses, each containing 3 million IU of INTRON A (for a label strength of 18 million IU).

§ This is a multidose vial which contains a total of 32.0 million IU of interferon alfa-2b, recombinant per 3.2 mL in order to provide the delivery of five 0.5-mL doses, each containing 5 million IU of INTRON A (for a label strength of 25 million IU).

Solution in Multidose Pens for Injection

Pen Strength	Concentration*million IU/1.5mL	INTRON A Dose Delivered (6 doses, 0.2 mL each)	mg INTRON A†per 1.5 mL	Route of Administration
3 MIU	22.5	3 MIU/0.2 mL	0.087	SC
5 MIU	37.5	5 MIU/0.2 mL	0.144	SC
10 MIU	75	10 MIU/0.2 mL	0.288	SC

* Each mL also contains 7.5 mg sodium chloride, 1.8 mg sodium phosphate dibasic, 1.3 mg sodium phosphate monobasic, 0.1 mg edetate disodium, 0.1 mg polysorbate 80, and 1.5 mg m-cresol as a preservative.

† Based on the specific activity of approximately 2.6×10^8 IU/mg protein as measured by HPLC assay.

DESCRIPTION

INTRON® A (Interferon alfa-2b) for intramuscular, subcutaneous, intralesional, or intravenous Injection is a purified sterile recombinant interferon product.

INTRON A recombinant for Injection has been classified as an alpha interferon and is a water-soluble protein with a molecular weight of 19,271 daltons produced by recombinant DNA techniques. It is obtained from the bacterial fermentation of a strain of *Escherichia coli* bearing a genetically engineered plasmid containing an interferon alfa-2b gene from human leukocytes. The fermentation is carried out in a defined nutrient medium containing the antibiotic tetracycline hydrochloride at a concentration of 5 to 10 mg/L; the presence of this antibiotic is not detectable in the final product. The specific activity of interferon alfa-2b, recombinant is approximately 2.6×10^8 IU/mg protein as measured by the HPLC assay.

[See first table above]

Prior to administration, the INTRON A Powder for Injection is to be reconstituted with the provided Diluent for INTRON A (Sterile Water for Injection USP) (see **DOSAGE AND ADMINISTRATION**). INTRON A Powder for Injection is a white to cream-colored powder.

[See second table above]
[See third table above]

These packages do not require reconstitution prior to administration (see **DOSAGE AND ADMINISTRATION**). INTRON A Solution for Injection is a clear, colorless solution.

CLINICAL PHARMACOLOGY

General

The interferons are a family of naturally occurring small proteins and glycoproteins with molecular weights of approximately 15,000 to 27,600 daltons produced and secreted by cells in response to viral infections and to synthetic or biological inducers.

Preclinical Pharmacology

Interferons exert their cellular activities by binding to specific membrane receptors on the cell surface. Once bound to the cell membrane, interferons initiate a complex sequence of intracellular events. *In vitro* studies demonstrated that these include the induction of certain enzymes, suppression of cell proliferation, immunomodulating activities such as enhancement of the phagocytic activity of macrophages and augmentation of the specific cytotoxicity of lymphocytes for target cells, and inhibition of virus replication in virus-infected cells.

In a study using human hepatoblastoma cell line HB 611, the *in vitro* antiviral activity of alpha interferon was demonstrated by its inhibition of hepatitis B virus (HBV) replication.

The correlation between these *in vitro* data and the clinical results is unknown. Any of these activities might contribute to interferon's therapeutic effects.

Pharmacokinetics

The pharmacokinetics of INTRON® A were studied in 12 healthy male volunteers following single doses of 5 million IU/m^2 administered intramuscularly, subcutaneously, and as a 30-minute intravenous infusion in a cross-over design.

The mean serum INTRON A concentrations following intramuscular and subcutaneous injections were comparable. The maximum serum concentrations obtained via these routes were approximately 18 to 116 IU/mL and occurred 3 to 12 hours after administration. The elimination half-life of INTRON A following both intramuscular and subcutaneous injections was approximately 2 to 3 hours. Serum concentrations were undetectable by 16 hours after the injections.

After intravenous administration, serum INTRON A concentrations peaked (135–273 IU/mL) by the end of the 30-minute infusion, then declined at a slightly more rapid rate than after intramuscular or subcutaneous drug administration, becoming undetectable 4 hours after the infusion. The elimination half-life was approximately 2 hours.

Urine INTRON A concentrations following a single dose (5 million IU/m^2) were not detectable after any of the parenteral routes of administration. This result was expected since preliminary studies with isolated and perfused rabbit kidneys have shown that the kidney may be the main site of interferon catabolism.

There are no pharmacokinetic data available for the intralesional route of administration.

Serum Neutralizing Antibodies

In INTRON A-treated patients tested for antibody activity in clinical trials, serum anti-interferon neutralizing antibodies were detected in 0% (0/90) of patients with hairy cell leukemia, 0.8% (2/260) of patients treated intralesionally for condylomata acuminata, and 4% (1/24) of patients with AIDS-Related Kaposi's Sarcoma. Serum neutralizing antibodies have been detected in less than 3% of patients treated with higher INTRON A doses in malignancies other than hairy cell leukemia or AIDS-Related Kaposi's Sarcoma. The clinical significance of the appearance of serum anti-interferon neutralizing activity in these indications is not known.

Serum anti-interferon neutralizing antibodies were detected in 7% (12/168) of patients either during treatment or after completing 12 to 48 weeks of treatment with 3 million IU TIW of INTRON A therapy for chronic hepatitis C and in 13% (6/48) of patients who received INTRON A therapy for chronic hepatitis B at 5 million IU QD for 4 months, and in 3% (1/33) of patients treated at 10 million IU TIW. Serum anti-interferon neutralizing antibodies were detected in 9% (5/53) of pediatric patients who received INTRON A therapy for chronic hepatitis B at 6 million IU/m^2 TIW. Among all chronic hepatitis B or C patients, pediatrics and adults with detectable serum neutralizing antibodies, the titers detected were low (22/24 with titers less than or equal to 1:40 and 2/24 with titers less than or equal to 1:160). The appearance of serum anti-interferon neutralizing activity did not appear to affect safety or efficacy.

Hairy Cell Leukemia

In clinical trials in patients with hairy cell leukemia, there was depression of hematopoiesis during the first 1 to 2 months of INTRON A treatment, resulting in reduced numbers of circulating red and white blood cells, and platelets. Subsequently, both splenectomized and nonsplenectomized patients achieved substantial and sustained improvements in granulocytes, platelets, and hemoglobin levels in 75% of treated patients and at least some improvement (minor responses) occurred in 90%. INTRON A treatment resulted in a decrease in bone marrow hypercellularity and hairy cell infiltrates. The hairy cell index (HCI), which represents the percent of bone marrow cellularity times the percent of hairy cell infiltrate, was greater than or equal to 50% at the beginning of the study in 87% of patients. The percentage of patients with such an HCI decreased to 25% after 6 months and to 14% after 1 year. These results indicate that even though hematologic improvement had occurred earlier, prolonged INTRON A treatment may be required to obtain maximal reduction in tumor cell infiltrates in the bone marrow.

The percentage of patients with hairy cell leukemia who required red blood cell or platelet transfusions decreased significantly during treatment and the percentage of patients with confirmed and serious infections declined as granulocyte counts improved. Reversal of splenomegaly and of clinically significant hypersplenism was demonstrated in some patients.

A study was conducted to assess the effects of extended INTRON A treatment on duration of response for patients who responded to initial therapy. In this study, 126 responding patients were randomized to receive additional INTRON A treatment for 6 months or observation for a comparable period, after 12 months of initial INTRON A therapy. During this 6-month period, 3% (2/66) of INTRON A-treated patients relapsed compared with 18% (11/60) who were not treated. This represents a significant difference in time to relapse in favor of continued INTRON A treatment (P=0.006/0.01, Log Rank/Wilcoxon). Since a small proportion of the total population had relapsed, median time to relapse could not be estimated in either group. A similar pattern in relapses was seen when all randomized treatment, including that beyond 6 months, and available follow-up data were assessed. The 15% (10/66) relapses among INTRON A patients occurred over a significantly longer period of time than the 40% (24/60) with observation (P=0.0002/0.0001, Log Rank/Wilcoxon). Median time to relapse was estimated, using the Kaplan-Meier method, to be 6.8 months in the observation group but could not be estimated in the INTRON A group.

Subsequent follow-up with a median time of approximately 40 months demonstrated an overall survival of 87.8%. In a comparable historical control group followed for 24 months, overall median survival was approximately 40%.

Malignant Melanoma

The safety and efficacy of INTRON A was evaluated as adjuvant to surgical treatment in patients with melanoma who were free of disease (post surgery) but at high risk for systemic recurrence. These included patients with lesions of Breslow thickness greater than 4 mm, or patients with lesions of any Breslow thickness with primary or recurrent nodal involvement. In a randomized, controlled trial in 280 patients, 143 patients received INTRON A therapy at 20 million IU/m^2 intravenously five times per week for 4 weeks (induction phase) followed by 10 million IU/m^2 subcutaneously three times per week for 48 weeks (maintenance phase). In the clinical trial, the median daily INTRON A dose administered to patients was 19.1 million IU/m^2 during the induction phase and 9.1 million IU/m^2 during the maintenance phase. INTRON A therapy was begun less than or equal to 56 days after surgical resection. The remaining 137 patients were observed.

INTRON A therapy produced a significant increase in relapse-free and overall survival. Median time to relapse for the INTRON A-treated patients vs observation patients was 1.72 years vs 0.98 years (P<0.01, stratified Log Rank). The estimated 5-year relapse-free survival rate, using the Kaplan-Meier method, was 37% for INTRON A-treated patients vs 26% for observation patients. Median overall survival time for INTRON A-treated patients vs observation patients was 3.82 years vs 2.78 years (P=0.047, stratified Log Rank). The estimated 5-year overall survival rate, using the Kaplan-Meier method, was 46% for INTRON A-treated patients vs 37% for observation patients.

In a second study of 642 resected high-risk melanoma patients, subjects were randomized equally to one of three groups: high-dose INTRON A therapy for 1 year (same schedule as above), low-dose INTRON A therapy for 2 years (3 MU/d TIW SC), and observation. Consistent with the earlier trial, high-dose INTRON A therapy demonstrated an improvement in relapse-free survival (3-year estimated RFS 48% vs 41%; median RFS 2.4 vs 1.6 years, P=not significant). Relapse-free survival in the low-dose INTRON A arm was similar to that seen in the observation arm. Neither high-dose nor low-dose INTRON A therapy showed a benefit in overall survival as compared to observation in this study.

Follicular Lymphoma

The safety and efficacy of INTRON A in conjunction with CHVP, a combination chemotherapy regimen, was evaluated as initial treatment in patients with clinically aggressive, large tumor burden, Stage III/IV follicular Non-Hodgkin's Lymphoma. Large tumor burden was defined by the presence of any one of the following: a nodal or extranodal tumor mass with a diameter of greater than 7 cm; involvement of at least three nodal sites (each with a diameter of greater than 3 cm); systemic symptoms; splenomegaly; serous effusion, orbital or epidural involvement; ureteral compression; or leukemia.

In a randomized, controlled trial, 130 patients received CHVP therapy and 135 patients received CHVP therapy plus INTRON A therapy at 5 million IU subcutaneously three times weekly for the duration of 18 months. CHVP chemotherapy consisted of cyclophosphamide 600 mg/m^2, doxorubicin 25 mg/m^2, and teniposide (VM-26) 60 mg/m^2, administered intravenously on Day 1 and prednisone at a daily dose of 40 mg/m^2 given orally on Days 1 to 5. Treatment consisted of six CHVP cycles administered monthly, followed by an additional six cycles administered every 2 months for 1 year. Patients in both treatment groups received a total of 12 CHVP cycles over 18 months.

The group receiving the combination of INTRON A therapy plus CHVP had a significantly longer progression-free survival (2.9 years vs 1.5 years, P=0.0001, Log Rank test). After a median follow-up of 6.1 years, the median survival for patients treated with CHVP alone was 5.5 years while median survival for patients treated with CHVP plus INTRON A therapy had not been reached (P=0.004, Log Rank test). In three additional published, randomized, controlled studies of the addition of interferon alpha to anthracycline-containing combination chemotherapy regimens,[1–3] the addition of interferon alpha was associated with significantly prolonged progression-free survival. Differences in overall survival were not consistently observed.

Condylomata Acuminata

Condylomata acuminata (venereal or genital warts) are associated with infections of the human papilloma virus (HPV). The safety and efficacy of INTRON A in the treatment of condylomata acuminata were evaluated in three controlled double-blind clinical trials. In these studies, INTRON A doses of 1 million IU per lesion were administered intralesionally three times a week (TIW), in less than or equal to 5 lesions per patient for 3 weeks. The patients were observed for up to 16 weeks after completion of the full treatment course.

INTRON A treatment of condylomata was significantly more effective than placebo, as measured by disappearance of lesions, decreases in lesion size, and by an overall change in disease status. Of 192 INTRON A-treated patients and 206 placebo-treated patients who were evaluable for efficacy at the time of best response during the course of the study, 42% of INTRON A patients vs 17% of placebo patients experienced clearing of all treated lesions. Likewise, 24% of INTRON A patients vs 8% of placebo patients experienced marked (75% to less than 100%) reduction in lesion size, 18% vs 9% experienced moderate (50% to 75%) reduction in lesion size, 10% vs 42% had a slight (less than 50%) reduction in lesion size, 5% vs 24% had no change in lesion size, and 0% vs 1% experienced exacerbation (P<0.001).

In one of these studies, 43% (54/125) of patients in whom multiple (less than or equal to 3) lesions were treated experienced complete clearing of all treated lesions during the course of the study. Of these patients, 81% remained cleared 16 weeks after treatment was initiated.

Patients who did not achieve total clearing of all their treated lesions had these same lesions treated with a second course of therapy. During this second course of treatment, 38% to 67% of patients had clearing of all treated lesions. The overall percentage of patients who had cleared all their treated lesions after two courses of treatment ranged from 57% to 85%.

INTRON A-treated lesions showed improvement within 2 to 4 weeks after the start of treatment in the above study; maximal response to INTRON A therapy was noted 4 to 8 weeks after initiation of treatment.

The response to INTRON A therapy was better in patients who had condylomata for shorter durations than in patients with lesions for a longer duration.

Another study involved 97 patients in whom three lesions were treated with either an intralesional injection of 1.5 million IU of INTRON A per lesion followed by a topical application of 25% podophyllin, or a topical application of 25% podophyllin alone. Treatment was given once a week for 3 weeks. The combined treatment of INTRON A and podophyllin was shown to be significantly more effective than podophyllin alone, as determined by the number of patients whose lesions cleared. This significant difference in response was evident after the second treatment (Week 3) and continued through 8 weeks posttreatment. At the time of the patient's best response, 67% (33/49) of the INTRON A- and podophyllin-treated patients had all three treated lesions clear while 42% (20/48) of the podophyllin-treated patients had all three clear (P=0.003).

AIDS-Related Kaposi's Sarcoma

The safety and efficacy of INTRON A in the treatment of Kaposi's Sarcoma (KS), a common manifestation of the Acquired Immune Deficiency Syndrome (AIDS), were evaluated in clinical trials in 144 patients.

In one study, INTRON A doses of 30 million IU/m^2 were administered subcutaneously three times per week (TIW) to patients with AIDS-Related KS. Doses were adjusted for patient tolerance. The average weekly dose delivered in the first 4 weeks was 150 million IU; at the end of 12 weeks this averaged 110 million IU/week; and by 24 weeks averaged 75 million IU/week.

Forty-four percent of asymptomatic patients responded vs 7% of symptomatic patients. The median time to response was approximately 2 months and 1 month, respectively, for asymptomatic and symptomatic patients. The median duration of response was approximately 3 months and 1 month, respectively, for the asymptomatic and symptomatic patients. Baseline T4/T8 ratios were 0.46 for responders vs 0.33 for nonresponders.

In another study, INTRON A doses of 35 million IU were administered subcutaneously, daily (QD), for 12 weeks. Maintenance treatment, with every other day dosing (QOD), was continued for up to 1 year in patients achieving antitumor and antiviral responses. The median time to response was 2 months and the median duration of response was 5 months in the asymptomatic patients.

In all studies, the likelihood of response was greatest in patients with relatively intact immune systems as assessed by baseline CD4 counts (interchangeable with T4 counts). Results at doses of 30 million IU/m^2 TIW and 35 million IU/QD were subcutaneously similar and are provided together in TABLE 1. This table demonstrates the relationship of response to baseline CD4 count in both asymptomatic and symptomatic patients in the 30 million IU/m^2 TIW and the 35 million IU/QD treatment groups.

In the 30 million IU study group, 7% (5/72) of patients were complete responders and 22% (16/72) of the patients were partial responders. The 35 million IU study had 13% (3/23 patients) complete responders and 17% (4/23) partial responders.

For patients who received 30 million IU TIW, the median survival time was longer in patients with CD4 greater than 200 (30.7 months) than in patients with CD4 less than or equal to 200 (8.9 months). Among responders, the median survival time was 22.6 months vs 9.7 months in nonresponders.

Chronic Hepatitis C

The safety and efficacy of INTRON A in the treatment of chronic hepatitis C was evaluated in 5 randomized clinical studies in which an INTRON A dose of 3 million IU three times a week (TIW) was assessed. The initial three studies were placebo-controlled trials that evaluated a 6-month (24-week) course of therapy. In each of the three studies, INTRON A therapy resulted in a reduction in serum alanine aminotransferase (ALT) in a greater proportion of patients vs control patients at the end of 6 months of dosing. During the 6 months of follow-up, approximately 50% of the patients who responded maintained their ALT response. A combined analysis comparing pretreatment and posttreatment liver biopsies revealed histological improvement in a statistically significantly greater proportion of INTRON A-treated patients compared to controls.

Two additional studies have investigated longer treatment durations (up to 24 months).[5,6] Patients in the two studies to evaluate longer duration of treatment had hepatitis with or without cirrhosis in the absence of decompensated liver disease. Complete response to treatment was defined as normalization of the final two serum ALT levels during the treatment period. A sustained response was defined as a complete response at the end of the treatment period, with sustained normal ALT values lasting at least 6 months following discontinuation of therapy.

In Study 1, all patients were initially treated with INTRON A 3 million IU TIW subcutaneously for 24 weeks (run-in-period). Patients who completed the initial 24-week treatment period were then randomly assigned to receive no further treatment, or to receive 3 million IU TIW for an additional 48 weeks. In Study 2, patients who met the entry criteria were randomly assigned to receive INTRON A 3 million IU TIW subcutaneously for 24 weeks or to receive INTRON A 3 million IU TIW subcutaneously for 96 weeks. In both studies, patient follow-up was variable and some data collection was retrospective.

Results show that longer durations of INTRON A therapy improved the sustained response rate (see TABLE 2). In patients with complete responses (CR) to INTRON A therapy after 6 months of treatment (149/352 [42%]), responses were less often sustained if drug was discontinued (21/70 [30%]) than if it was continued for 18 to 24 months (44/79 [56%]). Of all patients randomized, the sustained response rate in the patients receiving 18 or 24 months of therapy was 22% and 26%, respectively, in the two trials. In patients who did not have a CR by 6 months, additional therapy did not result in significantly more responses, since almost all patients who responded to therapy did so within the first 16 weeks of treatment.

A subset (less than 50%) of patients from the combined extended dosing studies had liver biopsies performed both before and after INTRON A treatment. Improvement in necroinflammatory activity as assessed retrospectively by the Knodell (Study 1) and Scheuer (Study 2) Histology Activity Indices was observed in both studies. A higher number of patients (58%, 45/78) improved with extended therapy than with shorter (6 months) therapy (38%, 34/89) in this subset.

Combination treatment with INTRON A and REBETOL® (ribavirin USP) provided a significant reduction in virologic load and improved histologic response in adult patients with compensated liver disease who were treatment-naïve or had relapsed following therapy with alpha interferon alone; pediatric patients previously untreated with alpha interferon experienced a sustained virologic response. See REBETOL package insert for additional information.

Chronic Hepatitis B

Adults

The safety and efficacy of INTRON A in the treatment of chronic hepatitis B were evaluated in three clinical trials in which INTRON A doses of 30 to 35 million IU per week were administered subcutaneously (SC), as either 5 million IU daily (QD), or 10 million IU three times a week (TIW) for 16 weeks vs no treatment. All patients were 18 years of age or older with compensated liver disease, and had chronic hepatitis B virus (HBV) infection (serum HBsAg positive for at least 6 months) and HBV replication (serum HBeAg positive). Patients were also serum HBV-DNA positive, an additional indicator of HBV replication, as measured by a research assay.[7,8] All patients had elevated serum alanine aminotransferase (ALT) and liver biopsy findings compatible with the diagnosis of chronic hepatitis. Patients with the presence of antibody to human immunodeficiency virus (anti-HIV) or antibody to hepatitis delta virus (anti-HDV) in the serum were excluded from the studies.

Virologic response to treatment was defined in these studies as a loss of serum markers of HBV replication (HBeAg and HBV DNA). Secondary parameters of response included loss of serum HBsAg, decreases in serum ALT, and improvement in liver histology.

In each of two randomized controlled studies, a significantly greater proportion of INTRON A-treated patients exhibited a virologic response compared with untreated control patients (see TABLE 3). In a third study without a concurrent control group, a similar response rate to INTRON A therapy was observed. Pretreatment with prednisone, evaluated in two of the studies, did not improve the response rate and provided no additional benefit.

The response to INTRON A therapy was durable. No patient responding to INTRON A therapy at a dose of 5 million IU QD or 10 million IU TIW relapsed during the follow-up period, which ranged from 2 to 6 months after treatment ended. The loss of serum HBeAg and HBV DNA was maintained in 100% of 19 responding patients followed for 3.5 to 36 months after the end of therapy.

In a proportion of responding patients, loss of HBeAg was followed by the loss of HBsAg. HBsAg was lost in 27% (4/15) of patients who responded to INTRON A therapy at a dose of 5 million IU QD, and 35% (8/23) of patients who responded to 10 million IU TIW. No untreated control patient lost HBsAg in these studies.

In an ongoing study to assess the long-term durability of virologic response, 64 patients responding to INTRON A therapy have been followed for 1.1 to 6.6 years after treatment; 95% (61/64) remain serum HBeAg negative, and 49% (30/61) lost serum HBsAg.

INTRON A therapy resulted in normalization of serum ALT in a significantly greater proportion of treated patients compared to untreated patients in each of two controlled studies (see TABLE 4). In a third study without a concurrent control group, normalization of serum ALT was observed in 50% (12/24) of patients receiving INTRON A therapy.

Virologic response was associated with a reduction in serum ALT to normal or near normal (less than or equal to 1.5 × the upper limit of normal) in 87% (13/15) of patients responding to INTRON A therapy at 5 million IU QD, and 100% (23/23) of patients responding to 10 million IU TIW.

Improvement in liver histology was evaluated in Studies 1 and 3 by comparison of pretreatment and 6-month posttreatment liver biopsies using the semiquantitative Knodell Histology Activity Index.[9] No statistically significant difference in liver histology was observed in treated patients compared to control patients in Study 1. Although statistically significant histological improvement from baseline was observed in treated patients in Study 3 ($P \leq 0.01$), there was no control group for comparison. Of those patients exhibiting a virologic response following treatment with 5 million IU QD or 10 million IU TIW, histological improvement was observed in 85% (17/20) compared to 36% (9/25) of patients who were not virologic responders. The histological improvement was due primarily to decreases in severity of necrosis, degeneration, and inflammation in the periportal, lobular, and portal regions of the liver (Knodell Categories I + II + III). Continued histological improvement was observed in four responding patients who lost serum HBsAg and were followed 2 to 4 years after the end of INTRON A therapy.[10]

Pediatrics

The safety and efficacy of INTRON A in the treatment of chronic hepatitis B was evaluated in one randomized controlled trial of 149 patients ranging from 1 year to 17 years of age. Seventy-two patients were treated with 3 million IU/m² of INTRON A therapy administered subcutaneously three times a week (TIW) for 1 week; the dose was then escalated to 6 million IU/m² TIW for a minimum of 16 weeks

TABLE 1 RESPONSE BY BASELINE CD4 COUNT* IN AIDS-RELATED KS PATIENTS

	30 million IU/m² TIW, SC and 35 million IU QD, SC				
	Asymptomatic			Symptomatic	
CD4<200	4/14	(29%)		0/19	(0%)
200≤CD4≤400	6/12	(50%)	} 58%	0/5	(0%)
CD4>400	5/7	(71%)		0/0	(0%)

* Data for CD4, and asymptomatic and symptomatic classification were not available for all patients.

TABLE 2 SUSTAINED ALT RESPONSE RATE VS DURATION OF THERAPY IN CHRONIC HEPATITIS C PATIENTS INTRON A 3 Million IU TIW

	Treatment Group*- Number of Patients (%)		
Study Number	INTRON A 3 million IU 24 weeks of treatment	INTRON A 3 million IU 72 or 96 weeks of treatment†	Difference (Extended - 24 weeks) (95% CI)‡
	ALT response at the end of follow-up		
1	12/101 (12%)	23/104 (22%)	10% (-3, 24)
2	9/67 (13%)	21/80 (26%)	13% (-4, 30)
Combined Studies	**21/168 (12.5%)**	**44/184 (24%)**	**11.4% (2, 21)**
	ALT response at the end of treatment		
1	40/101 (40%)	51/104 (49%)	--
2	32/67(48%)	35/80 (44%)	--

* Intent-to-treat groups.
† Study 1: 72 weeks of treatment; Study 2: 96 weeks of treatment.
‡ Confidence intervals adjusted for multiple comparisons due to 3 treatment arms in the study.

TABLE 3 VIROLOGIC RESPONSE* IN CHRONIC HEPATITIS B PATIENTS

	Treatment Group† - Number of Patients (%)						
Study Number	INTRON A 5 million IU QD		INTRON A 10 million IU TIW		Untreated Controls		P‡ Value
1[7]	15/38	(39%)	--	--	3/42	(7%)	0.0009
2	--	--	10/24	(42%)	1/22	(5%)	0.005
3[8]	--	--	13/24§	(54%)	2/27	(7%)§	NA§
All Studies	**15/38**	**(39%)**	**23/48**	**(48%)**	**6/91**	**(7%)**	**--**

* Loss of HBeAg and HBV DNA by 6 months posttherapy.
† Patients pretreated with prednisone not shown.
‡ INTRON A treatment group vs untreated control.
§ Untreated control patients evaluated after 24-week observation period. A subgroup subsequently received INTRON A therapy. A direct comparison is not applicable (NA).

up to 24 weeks. The maximum weekly dosage was 10 million IU TIW. Seventy-seven patients were untreated controls. Study entry and response criteria were identical to those described in the adult patient population.

Patients treated with INTRON A therapy had a better response (loss of HBV DNA and HBeAg at 24 weeks of follow-up) compared to the untreated controls (24% [17/72] vs 10% [8/77] $P=0.05$). Sixteen of the 17 responders treated with INTRON A therapy remained HBV DNA and HBeAg negative and had a normal serum ALT 12 to 24 months after completion of treatment. Serum HBsAg became negative in 7 out of 17 patients who responded to INTRON A therapy. None of the control patients who had an HBV DNA and HBeAg response became HBsAg negative. At 24 weeks of follow-up, normalization of serum ALT was similar in patients treated with INTRON A therapy (17%, 12/72) and in untreated control patients (16%, 12/77). Patients with a baseline HBV DNA less than 100 pg/mL were more likely to respond to INTRON A therapy than were patients with a baseline HBV DNA greater than 100 pg/mL (35% vs 9%, respectively). Patients who contracted hepatitis B through maternal vertical transmission had lower response rates than those who contracted the disease by other means (5% vs 31%, respectively). There was no evidence that the effects on HBV DNA and HBeAg were limited to specific subpopulations based on age, gender, or race.

[See table 1 above]
[See table 2 above]
[See table 3 above]
[See table 4 at top of next page]

INDICATIONS AND USAGE

Hairy Cell Leukemia

INTRON® A is indicated for the treatment of patients 18 years of age or older with hairy cell leukemia.

Malignant Melanoma

INTRON A is indicated as adjuvant to surgical treatment in patients 18 years of age or older with malignant melanoma who are free of disease but at high risk for systemic recurrence, within 56 days of surgery.

Follicular Lymphoma

INTRON A is indicated for the initial treatment of clinically aggressive (see **Clinical Pharmacology**) follicular Non-Hodgkin's Lymphoma in conjunction with anthracycline-containing combination chemotherapy in patients 18 years of age or older. Efficacy of INTRON A therapy in patients with low-grade, low-tumor burden follicular Non-Hodgkin's Lymphoma has not been demonstrated.

Condylomata Acuminata

INTRON A is indicated for intralesional treatment of selected patients 18 years of age or older with condylomata acuminata involving external surfaces of the genital and perianal areas (see **DOSAGE AND ADMINISTRATION**). The use of this product in adolescents has not been studied.

AIDS-Related Kaposi's Sarcoma

INTRON A is indicated for the treatment of selected patients 18 years of age or older with AIDS-Related Kaposi's Sarcoma. The likelihood of response to INTRON A therapy is greater in patients who are without systemic symptoms, who have limited lymphadenopathy and who have a relatively intact immune system as indicated by total CD4 count.

Chronic Hepatitis C

INTRON A is indicated for the treatment of chronic hepatitis C in patients 18 years of age or older with compensated liver disease who have a history of blood or blood-product exposure and/or are HCV antibody positive. Studies in these patients demonstrated that INTRON A therapy can produce clinically meaningful effects on this disease, manifested by normalization of serum alanine aminotransferase (ALT) and reduction in liver necrosis and degeneration.

TABLE 4 ALT RESPONSES* IN CHRONIC HEPATITIS B PATIENTS

Study Number	Treatment Group - Number of Patients (%)						P† Value
	INTRON A 5 million IU QD		INTRON A 10 million IU TIW		Untreated Controls		
1	16/38	(42%)	--	--	8/42	(19%)	0.03
2	--	--	10/24	(42%)	1/22	(5%)	0.0034
3	--	--	12/24‡	(50%)	2/27	(7%)‡	NA‡
All Studies	**16/38**	**(42%)**	**22/48**	**(46%)**	**11/91**	**(12%)**	**--**

* Reduction in serum ALT to normal by 6 months posttherapy.
† INTRON A treatment group vs untreated control.
‡ Untreated control patients evaluated after 24-week observation period. A subgroup subsequently received INTRON A therapy. A direct comparison is not applicable (NA).

A liver biopsy should be performed to establish the diagnosis of chronic hepatitis. Patients should be tested for the presence of antibody to HCV. Patients with other causes of chronic hepatitis, including autoimmune hepatitis, should be excluded. Prior to initiation of INTRON A therapy, the physician should establish that the patient has compensated liver disease. The following patient entrance criteria for compensated liver disease were used in the clinical studies and should be considered before INTRON A treatment of patients with chronic hepatitis C:

- No history of hepatic encephalopathy, variceal bleeding, ascites, or other clinical signs of decompensation
- Bilirubin — Less than or equal to 2 mg/dL
- Albumin — Stable and within normal limits
- Prothrombin Time — Less than 3 seconds prolonged
- WBC — Greater than or equal to 3000/mm^3
- Platelets — Greater than or equal to 70,000/mm^3

Serum creatinine should be normal or near normal.
Prior to initiation of INTRON A therapy, CBC and platelet counts should be evaluated in order to establish baselines for monitoring potential toxicity. These tests should be repeated at Weeks 1 and 2 following initiation of INTRON A therapy, and monthly thereafter. Serum ALT should be evaluated at approximately 3-month intervals to assess response to treatment (see **DOSAGE AND ADMINISTRATION**).
Patients with preexisting thyroid abnormalities may be treated if thyroid-stimulating hormone (TSH) levels can be maintained in the normal range by medication. TSH levels must be within normal limits upon initiation of INTRON A treatment and TSH testing should be repeated at 3 and 6 months (see **PRECAUTIONS, Laboratory Tests**).
INTRON A in combination with REBETOL® is indicated for the treatment of chronic hepatitis C in patients 3 years of age and older with compensated liver disease previously untreated with alpha interferon therapy and in patients 18 years of age and older who have relapsed following alpha interferon therapy. See REBETOL package insert for additional information.

Chronic Hepatitis B

INTRON A is indicated for the treatment of chronic hepatitis B in patients 1 year of age or older with compensated liver disease. Patients who have been serum HBsAg positive for at least 6 months and have evidence of HBV replication (serum HBeAg positive) with elevated serum ALT are candidates for treatment. Studies in these patients demonstrated that INTRON A therapy can produce virologic remission of this disease (loss of serum HBeAg) and normalization of serum aminotransferases. INTRON A therapy resulted in the loss of serum HBsAg in some responding patients.
Prior to initiation of INTRON A therapy, it is recommended that a liver biopsy be performed to establish the presence of chronic hepatitis and the extent of liver damage. The physician should establish that the patient has compensated liver disease. The following patient entrance criteria for compensated liver disease were used in the clinical studies and should be considered before INTRON A treatment of patients with chronic hepatitis B:

- No history of hepatic encephalopathy, variceal bleeding, ascites, or other signs of clinical decompensation
- Bilirubin — Normal
- Albumin — Stable and within normal limits
- Prothrombin Time — *Adults* less than 3 seconds prolonged; *Pediatrics* less than or equal to 2 seconds prolonged
- WBC — Greater than or equal to 4000/mm^3
- Platelets — *Adults* greater than or equal to 100,000/mm^3; *Pediatrics* greater than or equal to 150,000/mm^3

Patients with causes of chronic hepatitis other than chronic hepatitis B or chronic hepatitis C should not be treated with INTRON A. CBC and platelet counts should be evaluated prior to initiation of INTRON A therapy in order to establish baselines for monitoring potential toxicity. These tests should be repeated at treatment Weeks 1, 2, 4, 8, 12, and 16. Liver function tests, including serum ALT, albumin, and bilirubin, should be evaluated at treatment Weeks 1, 2, 4, 8, 12, and 16. HBeAg, HBsAg, and ALT should be evaluated at the end of therapy, as well as 3- and 6-months posttherapy, since patients may become virologic responders during the 6-month period following the end of treatment. In clinical studies in adults, 39% (15/38) of responding patients lost HBeAg 1 to 6 months following the end of INTRON A therapy. Of responding patients who lost HBsAg, 58% (7/12) did so 1 to 6 months posttreatment.
A transient increase in ALT greater than or equal to 2 times baseline value (flare) can occur during INTRON A therapy for chronic hepatitis B. In clinical trials in adults and pediatrics, this flare generally occurred 8 to 12 weeks after initiation of therapy and was more frequent in responders (*adults* 63%, 24/38; *pediatrics* 59%, 10/17) than in nonresponders (*adults* 27%, 13/48; *pediatrics* 35%, 19/55). However, in adults and pediatrics, elevations in bilirubin greater than or equal to 3 mg/dL (greater than or equal to 2 times ULN) occurred infrequently (*adults* 2%, 2/86; *pediatrics* 3%, 2/72) during therapy. When ALT flare occurs, in general, INTRON A therapy should be continued unless signs and symptoms of liver failure are observed. During ALT flare, clinical symptomatology and liver function tests including ALT, prothrombin time, alkaline phosphatase, albumin, and bilirubin, should be monitored at approximately 2-week intervals (see **WARNINGS**).

CONTRAINDICATIONS

INTRON® A is contraindicated in patients with:
- Hypersensitivity to interferon alpha or any component of the product
- Autoimmune hepatitis
- Decompensated liver disease

INTRON A and REBETOL® combination therapy is additionally contraindicated in:
- Patients with hypersensitivity to ribavirin or any other component of the product
- Women who are pregnant
- Men whose female partners are pregnant
- Patients with hemoglobinopathies (e.g., thalassemia major, sickle cell anemia)
- Patients with creatinine clearance less than 50 mL/min.

See REBETOL package insert for additional information.

WARNINGS

General

Moderate to severe adverse experiences may require modification of the patient's dosage regimen, or in some cases termination of INTRON® A therapy. Because of the fever and other "flu-like" symptoms associated with INTRON A administration, it should be used cautiously in patients with debilitating medical conditions, such as those with a history of pulmonary disease (e.g., chronic obstructive pulmonary disease) or diabetes mellitus prone to ketoacidosis. Caution should also be observed in patients with coagulation disorders (e.g., thrombophlebitis, pulmonary embolism) or severe myelosuppression.

Cardiovascular Disorders

INTRON A therapy should be used cautiously in patients with a history of cardiovascular disease. Those patients with a history of myocardial infarction and/or previous or current arrhythmic disorder who require INTRON A therapy should be closely monitored (see **PRECAUTIONS, Laboratory Tests**). Cardiovascular adverse experiences, which include hypotension, arrhythmia, or tachycardia of 150 beats per minute or greater, and rarely, cardiomyopathy and myocardial infarction have been observed in some INTRON A-treated patients. Some patients with these adverse events had no history of cardiovascular disease. Transient cardiomyopathy was reported in approximately 2% of the AIDS-Related Kaposi's Sarcoma patients treated with INTRON A. Hypotension may occur during INTRON A administration, or up to 2 days posttherapy, and may require supportive therapy including fluid replacement to maintain intravascular volume.
Supraventricular arrhythmias occurred rarely and appeared to be correlated with preexisting conditions and prior therapy with cardiotoxic agents. These adverse experiences were controlled by modifying the dose or discontinuing treatment, but may require specific additional therapy.

Cerebrovascular Disorders

Ischemic and hemorrhagic cerebrovascular events have been observed in patients treated with interferon alpha-based therapies, including INTRON A. Events occurred in patients with few or no reported risk factors for stroke, including patients less than 45 years of age. Because these are spontaneous reports, estimates of frequency cannot be made and a causal relationship between interferon alpha-based therapies and these events is difficult to establish.

Neuropsychiatric Disorders

DEPRESSION AND SUICIDAL BEHAVIOR INCLUDING SUICIDAL IDEATION, SUICIDAL ATTEMPTS, AND COMPLETED SUICIDES, HOMICIDAL IDEATION, AND AGGRESSIVE BEHAVIOR SOMETIMES DIRECTED TOWARDS OTHERS, HAVE BEEN REPORTED IN ASSOCIATION WITH TREATMENT WITH ALPHA INTERFERONS, INCLUDING INTRON A THERAPY. If patients develop psychiatric problems, including clinical depression, it is recommended that the patients be carefully monitored during treatment and in the 6-month follow-up period.
INTRON A should be used with caution in patients with a history of psychiatric disorders. INTRON A therapy should be discontinued for any patient developing severe psychiatric disorder during treatment. Obtundation and coma have also been observed in some patients, usually elderly, treated at higher doses. While these effects are usually rapidly reversible upon discontinuation of therapy, full resolution of symptoms has taken up to 3 weeks in a few severe episodes. If psychiatric symptoms persist or worsen, or suicidal ideation or aggressive behavior towards others is identified, it is recommended that treatment with INTRON A be discontinued and the patient followed, with psychiatric intervention as appropriate. Narcotics, hypnotics, or sedatives may be used concurrently with caution and patients should be closely monitored until the adverse effects have resolved. Suicidal ideation or attempts occurred more frequently among pediatric patients, primarily adolescents, compared to adult patients (2.4% vs 1%) during treatment and off-therapy follow-up. Cases of encephalopathy have also been observed in some patients, usually elderly, treated with higher doses of INTRON A.
Treatment with interferons may be associated with exacerbated symptoms of psychiatric disorders in patients with co-occurring psychiatric and substance use disorders. If treatment with interferons is initiated in patients with prior history or existence of psychiatric condition or with a history of substance use disorders, treatment considerations should include the need for drug screening and periodic health evaluation, including psychiatric symptom monitoring. Early intervention for re-emergence or development of neuropsychiatric symptoms and substance use is recommended.

Bone Marrow Toxicity

INTRON A therapy suppresses bone marrow function and may result in severe cytopenias including aplastic anemia. It is advised that complete blood counts (CBC) be obtained pretreatment and monitored routinely during therapy (see **PRECAUTIONS, Laboratory Tests**). INTRON A therapy should be discontinued in patients who develop severe decreases in neutrophil (less than 0.5×10^9/L) or platelet counts (less than 25×10^9/L) (see **DOSAGE AND ADMINISTRATION, Guidelines for Dose Modification**).

Ophthalmologic Disorders

Decrease or loss of vision, retinopathy including macular edema, retinal artery or vein thrombosis, retinal hemorrhages and cotton wool spots; optic neuritis, papilledema, and serous retinal detachment may be induced or aggravated by treatment with interferon alfa-2b or other alpha interferons. All patients should receive an eye examination at baseline. Patients with preexisting ophthalmologic disorders (e.g., diabetic or hypertensive retinopathy) should receive periodic ophthalmologic exams during interferon alpha treatment. Any patient who develops ocular symptoms should receive a prompt and complete eye examination. Interferon alfa-2b treatment should be discontinued in patients who develop new or worsening ophthalmologic disorders.

Endocrine Disorders

Infrequently, patients receiving INTRON A therapy developed thyroid abnormalities, either hypothyroid or hyperthyroid. The mechanism by which INTRON A may alter thyroid status is unknown. Patients with preexisting thyroid abnormalities whose thyroid function cannot be maintained in the normal range by medication should not be treated with INTRON A. Prior to initiation of INTRON A therapy, serum TSH should be evaluated. Patients developing symptoms consistent with possible thyroid dysfunction during the course of INTRON A therapy should have their thyroid function evaluated and appropriate treatment instituted. Therapy should be discontinued for patients developing thyroid abnormalities during treatment whose thyroid function cannot be normalized by medication. Discontinuation of INTRON A therapy has not always reversed thyroid dysfunction occurring during treatment. Diabetes mellitus has been observed in patients treated with alpha interferons. Patients with these conditions who cannot be effectively treated by medication should not begin INTRON A therapy. Patients who develop these conditions during treatment and cannot be controlled with medication should not continue INTRON A therapy.

Gastrointestinal Disorders

Hepatotoxicity, including fatality, has been observed in interferon alpha-treated patients, including those treated with INTRON A. Any patient developing liver function abnormalities during treatment should be monitored closely and if appropriate, treatment should be discontinued.

Pulmonary Disorders

Dyspnea, pulmonary infiltrates, pneumonia, bronchiolitis obliterans, interstitial pneumonitis, pulmonary hypertension, and sarcoidosis, some resulting in respiratory failure and/or patient deaths, may be induced or aggravated by INTRON A or other alpha interferons. Recurrence of respiratory failure has been observed with interferon rechallenge. The etiologic explanation for these pulmonary findings has yet to be established. Any patient developing fever, cough, dyspnea, or other respiratory symptoms should have a chest X-ray taken. If the chest X-ray shows pulmonary infiltrates or there is evidence of pulmonary function impairment, the patient should be closely monitored, and, if appropriate, interferon alpha treatment should be discontinued. While this has been reported more often in patients with chronic hepatitis C treated with interferon alpha, it has also been reported in patients with oncologic diseases treated with interferon alpha.

Autoimmune Disorders

Rare cases of autoimmune diseases including thrombocytopenia, vasculitis, Raynaud's phenomenon, rheumatoid arthritis, lupus erythematosus, and rhabdomyolysis have been observed in patients treated with alpha interferons, including patients treated with INTRON A. In very rare cases the event resulted in fatality. The mechanism by which these events developed and their relationship to interferon alpha therapy is not clear. Any patient developing an autoimmune disorder during treatment should be closely monitored and, if appropriate, treatment should be discontinued.

Human Albumin

The powder formulations of this product contain albumin, a derivative of human blood. Based on effective donor screening and product manufacturing processes, it carries an extremely remote risk for transmission of viral diseases. A theoretical risk for transmission of Creutzfeldt-Jakob disease (CJD) also is considered extremely remote. No cases of transmission of viral diseases or CJD have ever been identified for albumin.

AIDS-Related Kaposi's Sarcoma

INTRON A therapy should not be used for patients with rapidly progressive visceral disease (see **CLINICAL PHARMACOLOGY**). Also of note, there may be synergistic adverse effects between INTRON A and zidovudine. Patients receiving concomitant zidovudine have had a higher incidence of neutropenia than that expected with zidovudine alone. Careful monitoring of the WBC count is indicated in all patients who are myelosuppressed and in all patients receiving other myelosuppressive medications. The effects of INTRON A when combined with other drugs used in the treatment of AIDS-related disease are unknown.

Chronic Hepatitis C and Chronic Hepatitis B

Patients with decompensated liver disease, autoimmune hepatitis or a history of autoimmune disease, and patients who are immunosuppressed transplant recipients should not be treated with INTRON A. There are reports of worsening liver disease, including jaundice, hepatic encephalopathy, hepatic failure, and death following INTRON A therapy in such patients. Therapy should be discontinued for any patient developing signs and symptoms of liver failure. Chronic hepatitis B patients with evidence of decreasing hepatic synthetic functions, such as decreasing albumin levels or prolongation of prothrombin time, who nevertheless meet the entry criteria to start therapy, may be at increased risk of clinical decompensation if a flare of aminotransferases occurs during INTRON A treatment. In such patients, if increases in ALT occur during INTRON A therapy for chronic hepatitis B, they should be followed carefully, including close monitoring of clinical symptomatology and liver function tests including ALT, prothrombin time, alkaline phosphatase, albumin, and bilirubin. In considering these patients for INTRON A therapy, the potential risks must be evaluated against the potential benefits of treatment.

Peripheral Neuropathy

Peripheral neuropathy has been reported when alpha interferons were given in combination with telbivudine. In one clinical trial, an increased risk and severity of peripheral neuropathy was observed with the combination use of telbivudine and pegylated interferon alfa-2a as compared to telbivudine alone. The safety and efficacy of telbivudine in combination with interferons for the treatment of chronic hepatitis B has not been demonstrated.

Use with Ribavirin

(See also REBETOL® package insert) REBETOL may cause birth defects and/or death of the unborn child. REBETOL therapy should not be started until a report of a negative pregnancy test has been obtained immediately prior to planned initiation of therapy. Patients should use at least two forms of contraception and have monthly pregnancy tests (see **CONTRAINDICATIONS** and **PRECAUTIONS, Information for Patients**).

Combination treatment with INTRON A and REBETOL was associated with hemolytic anemia. Hemoglobin less than 10 g/dL was observed in approximately 10% of adult and pediatric patients in clinical trials. Anemia occurred within 1 to 2 weeks of initiation of ribavirin therapy. Combination treatment with INTRON A and REBETOL should **not** be used in patients with creatinine clearance less than 50 mL/min. See REBETOL package insert for additional information.

PRECAUTIONS

General

Acute serious hypersensitivity reactions (e.g., urticaria, angioedema, bronchoconstriction, anaphylaxis) have been observed rarely in INTRON® A-treated patients; if such an acute reaction develops, the drug should be discontinued immediately and appropriate medical therapy instituted. Transient rashes have occurred in some patients following injection, but have not necessitated treatment interruption. While fever may be related to the flu-like syndrome reported commonly in patients treated with interferon, other causes of persistent fever should be ruled out.

There have been reports of interferon, including INTRON A, exacerbating preexisting psoriasis and sarcoidosis as well as development of new sarcoidosis. Therefore, INTRON A therapy should be used in these patients only if the potential benefit justifies the potential risk.

Variations in dosage, routes of administration, and adverse reactions exist among different brands of interferon. Therefore, do not use different brands of interferon in any single treatment regimen.

Triglycerides

Elevated triglyceride levels have been observed in patients treated with interferons, including INTRON A therapy. Elevated triglyceride levels should be managed as clinically appropriate. Hypertriglyceridemia may result in pancreatitis. Discontinuation of INTRON A therapy should be considered for patients with persistently elevated triglycerides (e.g., triglycerides greater than 1000 mg/dL) associated with symptoms of potential pancreatitis, such as abdominal pain, nausea, or vomiting.

Drug Interactions

Interactions between INTRON A and other drugs have not been fully evaluated. Caution should be exercised when administering INTRON A therapy in combination with other potentially myelosuppressive agents such as zidovudine. Concomitant use of alpha interferon and theophylline decreases theophylline clearance, resulting in a 100% increase in serum theophylline levels.

Information for Patients

Patients receiving INTRON A alone or in combination with REBETOL® should be informed of the risks and benefits associated with treatment and should be instructed on proper use of the product. To supplement your discussion with a patient, you may wish to provide patients with a copy of the **MEDICATION GUIDE**.

Patients should be informed of, and advised to seek medical attention for, symptoms indicative of serious adverse reactions associated with this product. Such adverse reactions may include depression (suicidal ideation), cardiovascular (chest pain), ophthalmologic toxicity (decrease in/or loss of vision), pancreatitis or colitis (severe abdominal pain), and cytopenias (high persistent fevers, bruising, dyspnea). Patients should be advised that some side effects such as fatigue and decreased concentration might interfere with the ability to perform certain tasks. Patients who are taking INTRON A in combination with REBETOL must be thoroughly informed of the risks to a fetus. Female patients and female partners of male patients must be told to use two forms of birth control during treatment and for six months after therapy is discontinued (see **MEDICATION GUIDE**). Patients should be advised to remain well hydrated during the initial stages of treatment and that use of an antipyretic may ameliorate some of the flu-like symptoms.

If a decision is made to allow a patient to self-administer INTRON A, they should be instructed, based on their treatment, if they should inject a dose of INTRON® A subcutaneously or intramuscularly. If it is too difficult for them to inject themselves, they should be instructed to ask someone who has been trained to give the injection to them. Patients should be instructed on the importance of site selection for self-administering the injection, as well as the importance on rotating the injection sites. A puncture resistant container for the disposal of needles and syringes should be supplied. Patients self-administering INTRON A should be instructed on the proper disposal of needles and syringes and cautioned against reuse.

Dental and Periodontal Disorders

Dental and periodontal disorders have been reported in patients receiving ribavirin and interferon combination therapy. In addition, dry mouth could have a damaging effect on teeth and mucous membranes of the mouth during long-term treatment with the combination of REBETOL and interferon alfa-2b. Patients should brush their teeth thoroughly twice daily and have regular dental examinations. In addition, some patients may experience vomiting. If this reaction occurs, they should be advised to rinse out their mouth thoroughly afterwards.

Laboratory Tests

In addition to those tests normally required for monitoring patients, the following laboratory tests are recommended for all patients on INTRON A therapy, prior to beginning treatment and then periodically thereafter.

- Standard hematologic tests - including hemoglobin, complete and differential white blood cell counts, and platelet count.
- Blood chemistries - electrolytes, liver function tests, and TSH.

Those patients who have preexisting cardiac abnormalities and/or are in advanced stages of cancer should have electrocardiograms taken prior to and during the course of treatment.

Mild-to-moderate leukopenia and elevated serum liver enzyme (SGOT) levels have been reported with intralesional administration of INTRON A (see **ADVERSE REACTIONS**); therefore, the monitoring of these laboratory parameters should be considered.

Baseline chest X-rays are suggested and should be repeated if clinically indicated.

For malignant melanoma patients, differential WBC count and liver function tests should be monitored weekly during the induction phase of therapy and monthly during the maintenance phase of therapy.

For specific recommendations in chronic hepatitis C and chronic hepatitis B, see **INDICATIONS AND USAGE**.

Carcinogenesis, Mutagenesis, Impairment of Fertility

Studies with INTRON A have not been performed to determine carcinogenicity.

Interferon may impair fertility. In studies of interferon administration in nonhuman primates, menstrual cycle abnormalities have been observed. Decreases in serum estradiol and progesterone concentrations have been reported in women treated with human leukocyte interferon.[12] Therefore, fertile women should not receive INTRON A therapy unless they are using effective contraception during the therapy period. INTRON A therapy should be used with caution in fertile men.

Mutagenicity studies have demonstrated that INTRON A is not mutagenic.

Studies in mice (0.1, 1.0 million IU/day), rats (4, 20, 100 million IU/kg/day), and cynomolgus monkeys (1.1 million IU/kg/day; 0.25, 0.75, 2.5 million IU/kg/day) injected with INTRON A for up to 9 days, 3 months, and 1 month, respectively, have revealed no evidence of toxicity. However, in cynomolgus monkeys (4, 20, 100 million IU/kg/day) injected daily for 3 months with INTRON A, toxicity was observed at the mid and high doses and mortality was observed at the high dose.

However, due to the known species-specificity of interferon, the effects in animals are unlikely to be predictive of those in man.

INTRON A in combination with REBETOL should be used with caution in fertile men. See the REBETOL package insert for additional information.

Pregnancy Category C

INTRON A has been shown to have abortifacient effects in *Macaca mulatta* (rhesus monkeys) at 15 and 30 million IU/kg (estimated human equivalent of 5 and 10 million IU/kg, based on body surface area adjustment for a 60-kg adult). There are no adequate and well-controlled studies in pregnant women. INTRON A therapy should be used during pregnancy only if the potential benefit justifies the potential risk to the fetus.

Pregnancy Category X applies to combination treatment with INTRON A and REBETOL (see **CONTRAINDICATIONS**). See REBETOL package insert for additional information. Significant teratogenic and/or embryocidal effects have been demonstrated in all animal species exposed to ri-

TREATMENT-RELATED ADVERSE EXPERIENCES BY INDICATION

Dosing Regimens
Percentage (%) of Patients*

	MALIGNANT MELANOMA	FOLLICULAR LYMPHOMA	HAIRY CELL LEUKEMIA	CONDYLOMATA ACUMINATA	AIDS-RELATED KAPOSI'S SARCOMA		CHRONIC HEPATITIS C†	CHRONIC HEPATITIS B		
								Adults		Pediatrics
	20 MIU/m² Induction (IV) 10 MIU/m² Maintenance (SC)	5 MIU TIW/SC	2 MIU/m² TIW/SC	1 MIU/lesion	30 MIU/m² TIW/SC	35 MIU QD/SC	3 MIU TIW	5 MIU QD	10 MIU TIW	6 MIU/m²TIW
ADVERSE EXPERIENCE	N=143	N=135	N=145	N=352	N=74	N=29	N=183	N=101	N=78	N=116
Application-Site Disorders			20							
injection site inflammation	--	1	--	--	--	--	5	3	--	--
other (≤5%)	burning, injection site bleeding, injection site pain, injection site reaction (5% in chronic hepatitis B pediatrics), itching									
Blood Disorders (<5%)	anemia, anemia hypochromic, granulocytopenia, hemolytic anemia, leukopenia, lymphocytosis, neutropenia (9% in chronic hepatitis C, 14% in chronic hepatitis B pediatrics), thrombocytopenia (10% in chronic hepatitis C) (bleeding 8% in malignant melanoma), thrombocytopenia purpura									
Body as a Whole										
facial edema	--	1	--	<1	--	10	<1	3	1	<1
weight decrease	3	13	<1	<1	5	3	10	2	5	3
other (≤5%)	allergic reaction, cachexia, dehydration, earache, hernia, edema, hypercalcemia, hyperglycemia, hypothermia, inflammation nonspecific, lymphadenitis, lymphadenopathy, mastitis, periorbital edema, poor peripheral circulation, peripheral edema (6% in follicular lymphoma), phlebitis superficial, scrotal/penile edema, thirst, weakness, weight increase									
Cardiovascular System Disorders (<5%)	angina, arrhythmia, atrial fibrillation, bradycardia, cardiac failure, cardiomegaly, cardiomyopathy, coronary artery disorder, extrasystoles, heart valve disorder, hematoma, hypertension (9% in chronic hepatitis C), hypotension, palpitations, phlebitis, postural hypotension, pulmonary embolism, Raynaud's disease, tachycardia, thrombosis, varicose vein									
Endocrine System Disorders (<5%)	aggravation of diabetes mellitus, goiter, gynecomastia, hyperglycemia, hyperthyroidism, hypertriglyceridemia, hypothyroidism, virilism									
Flu-like Symptoms										
fever	81	56	68	56	47	55	34	66	86	94
headache	62	21	39	47	36	21	43	61	44	57
chills	54	--	46	45	--	--	--	--	--	--
myalgia	75	16	39	44	34	28	43	59	40	27
fatigue	96	8	61	18	84	48	23	75	69	71
increased sweating	6	13	8	2	4	21	4	1	1	3
asthenia	--	63	7	--	11	--	40	5	15	5
rigors	2	7	--	--	30	14	16	38	42	30
arthralgia	6	8	8	9	--	3	16	19	8	15
dizziness	23	--	12	9	7	24	9	13	10	8
influenza-like symptoms	10	18	37	--	45	79	26	5	--	<1
back pain	--	15	19	6	1	3	--	--	--	--
dry mouth	1	2	19	--	22	28	5	6	5	--
chest pain	2	8	<1	<1	1	28	4	4	--	--
malaise	6	--	--	14	5	--	13	9	6	3
pain (unspecified)	15	9	18	3	3	3	--	--	--	--
other (<5%)	chest pain substernal, hyperthermia, rhinitis, rhinorrhea									
Gastrointestinal System Disorders										
diarrhea	35	19	18	2	18	45	13	19	8	12
anorexia	69	21	19	1	38	41	14	43	53	43
nausea	66	24	21	17	28	21	19	50	33	18
taste alteration	24	2	13	<1	5	7	2	10	--	--
abdominal pain	2	20	<5	1	5	21	16	5	4	23
loose stools	--	1	--	<1	--	10	2	2	--	2
vomiting	‡	32	6	2	11	14	8	7	10	27
constipation	1	14	<1	--	1	10	4	5	--	2
gingivitis	2§	7§	--	--	--	14	--	1	--	--
dyspepsia	--	2	--	2	4	--	7	3	8	3
other (<5%)	abdominal ascites, abdominal distension, colitis, dysphagia, eructation, esophagitis, flatulence, gallstones, gastric ulcer, gastritis, gastroenteritis, gastrointestinal disorder (7% in follicular lymphoma), gastrointestinal hemorrhage, gastrointestinal mucosal discoloration, gingival bleeding, gum hyperplasia, halitosis, hemorrhoids, increased appetite, increased saliva, intestinal disorder, melena, mouth ulceration, mucositis, oral hemorrhage, oral leukoplakia, rectal bleeding after stool, rectal hemorrhage, stomatitis, stomatitis ulcerative, taste loss, tongue disorder, tooth disorder									
Liver and Biliary System Disorders (<5%)	abnormal hepatic function tests, biliary pain, bilirubinemia, hepatitis, increased lactate dehydrogenase, increased transaminases (SGOT/SGPT) (elevated SGOT 63% in malignant melanoma and 24% in follicular lymphoma), jaundice, right upper quadrant pain (15% in chronic hepatitis C), and very rarely, hepatic encephalopathy, hepatic failure, and death									
Musculoskeletal System Disorders										
musculoskeletal pain	--	18	--	--	--	--	21	9	1	10
other (<5%)	arteritis, arthritis, arthritis aggravated, arthrosis, bone disorder, bone pain, carpal tunnel syndrome, hyporeflexia, leg cramps, muscle atrophy, muscle weakness, polyarteritis nodosa, tendinitis, rheumatoid arthritis, spondylitis									

(Table continued on next page)

bavirin. REBETOL therapy is contraindicated in women who are pregnant and in the male partners of women who are pregnant. See CONTRAINDICATIONS and the REBETOL package insert.

Ribavirin Pregnancy Registry: A Ribavirin Pregnancy Registry has been established to monitor maternal-fetal outcomes of pregnancies in female patients and female partners of male patients exposed to ribavirin during treatment and for 6 months following cessation of treatment. Physicians and patients are encouraged to report such cases by calling 1-800-593-2214.

Nursing Mothers

It is not known whether this drug is excreted in human milk. However, studies in mice have shown that mouse interferons are excreted into the milk. Because of the potential for serious adverse reactions from the drug in nursing infants, a decision should be made whether to discontinue nursing or to discontinue INTRON A therapy, taking into account the importance of the drug to the mother.

Pediatric Use

General

Safety and effectiveness in pediatric patients have not been established for indications other than chronic hepatitis B and chronic hepatitis C.

TREATMENT-RELATED ADVERSE EXPERIENCES BY INDICATION (cont.)

	Dosing Regimens Percentage (%) of Patients*									
	MALIGNANT MELANOMA	FOLLICULAR LYMPHOMA	HAIRY CELL LEUKEMIA	CONDYLOMATA ACUMINATA	AIDS-RELATED KAPOSI'S SARCOMA		CHRONIC HEPATITIS C†	CHRONIC HEPATITIS B		
								Adults		Pediatrics
	20 MIU/m² Induction (IV) 10 MIU/m² Maintenance (SC)	5 MIU TIW/SC	2 MIU/m² TIW/SC	1 MIU/lesion	30 MIU/m² TIW/SC	35 MIU QD/SC	3 MIU TIW	5 MIU QD	10 MIU TIW	6 MIU/m²TIW
ADVERSE EXPERIENCE	N=143	N=135	N=145	N=352	N=74	N=29	N=183	N=101	N=78	N=116
Nervous System and Psychiatric Disorders										
depression	40	9	6	3	9	28	19	17	6	4
paresthesia	13	13	6	1	3	21	5	6	3	<1
impaired concentration	--	1	--	<1	3	14	3	8	5	3
amnesia	¶	1	<5	--	--	14	--	--	--	--
confusion	8	2	<5	4	12	10	1	--	--	2
hypoesthesia	--	1	<5	1	--	10	--	--	--	--
irritability	1	1	--	--	--	--	13	16	12	22
somnolence	1	2	<5	3	3	--	33#	14	9	5
anxiety	1	9	5	<1	1	3	5	2	--	3
insomnia	5	4	--	<1	3	3	12	11	6	8
nervousness	1	1	--	1	--	3	2	3	--	3
decreased libido	1	1	<5	--	--	--	1	5	1	--
other (<5%)	abnormal coordination, abnormal dreaming, abnormal gait, abnormal thinking, aggravated depression, aggressive reaction, agitation (7% in chronic hepatitis B pediatrics), alcohol intolerance, apathy, aphasia, ataxia, Bell's palsy, CNS dysfunction, coma, convulsions, delirium, dysphonia, emotional lability, extrapyramidal disorder, feeling of ebriety, flushing, hearing disorder, hearing impairment, hot flashes, hyperesthesia, hyperkinesia, hypertonia, hypokinesia, impaired consciousness, labyrinthine disorder, loss of consciousness, manic depression, manic reaction, migraine, neuralgia, neuritis, neuropathy, neurosis, paresis, paroniria, parosmia, personality disorder, polyneuropathy, psychosis, speech disorder, stroke, suicidal ideation, suicide attempt, syncope, tinnitus, tremor, twitching, vertigo (8% in follicular lymphoma)									
Reproduction System Disorders (<5%)	amenorrhea (12% in follicular lymphoma), dysmenorrhea, impotence, leukorrhea, menorrhagia, menstrual irregularity, pelvic pain, penis disorder, sexual dysfunction, uterine bleeding, vaginal dryness									
Resistance Mechanism Disorders										
moniliasis	--	1	--	<1	--	17	--	--	--	--
herpes simplex	1	2	--	1	--	3	1	5	--	--
other (<5%)	abscess, conjunctivitis, fungal infection, hemophilus, herpes zoster, infection, infection bacterial, infection nonspecific (7% in follicular lymphoma), infection parasitic, otitis media, sepsis, stye, trichomonas, upper respiratory tract infection, viral infection (7% in chronic hepatitis C)									
Respiratory System Disorders										
dyspnea	15	14	<1	--	1	34	3	5	--	--
coughing	6	13	<1	--	--	31	1	4	--	5
pharyngitis	2	8	<5	1	1	31	3	7	1	7
sinusitis	1	4	--	--	--	21	2	--	--	--
nonproductive coughing	2	7	--	--	--	14	0	1	--	--
nasal congestion	1	7	--	1	--	10	<1	4	--	--
other (≤5%)	asthma, bronchitis (10% in follicular lymphoma), bronchospasm, cyanosis, epistaxis (7% in chronic hepatitis B pediatrics), hemoptysis, hypoventilation, laryngitis, lung fibrosis, pleural effusion, orthopnea, pleural pain, pneumonia, pneumonitis, pneumothorax, rales, respiratory disorder, respiratory insufficiency, sneezing, tonsillitis, tracheitis, wheezing									
Skin and Appendages Disorders										
dermatitis	1	--	8	--	--	--	2	1	--	--
alopecia	29	23	8	--	12	31	28	26	38	17
pruritus	--	10	11	1	7	--	9	6	4	3
rash	19	13	25	--	9	10	5	8	1	5
dry skin	1	3	9	--	9	10	4	3	--	<1
other (<5%)	abnormal hair texture, acne, cellulitis, cyanosis of the hand, cold and clammy skin, dermatitis lichenoides, eczema, epidermal necrolysis, erythema, erythema nodosum, folliculitis, furunculosis, increased hair growth, lacrimal gland disorder, lacrimation, lipoma, maculopapular rash, melanosis, nail disorders, nonherpetic cold sores, pallor, peripheral ischemia, photosensitivity, pruritus genital, psoriasis, psoriasis aggravated, purpura (5% in chronic hepatitis C), rash erythematous, sebaceous cyst, skin depigmentation, skin discoloration, skin nodule, urticaria, vitiligo									
Urinary System Disorders (<5%)	albumin/protein in urine, cystitis, dysuria, hematuria, incontinence, increased BUN, micturition disorder, micturition frequency, nocturia, polyuria (10% in follicular lymphoma), renal insufficiency, urinary tract infection (5% in chronic hepatitis C)									
Vision Disorders (<5%)	abnormal vision, blurred vision, diplopia, dry eyes, eye pain, nystagmus, photophobia									

* Dash (--) indicates not reported
† Percentages based upon a summary of all adverse events during 18 to 24 months of treatment
‡ Vomiting was reported with nausea as a single term
§ Includes stomatitis/mucositis
¶ Amnesia was reported with confusion as a single term
\# Predominantly lethargy

Chronic Hepatitis B
Safety and effectiveness in pediatric patients ranging in age from 1 to 17 years have been established based upon one controlled clinical trial (see **CLINICAL PHARMACOLOGY, INDICATIONS AND USAGE,** and **DOSAGE AND ADMINISTRATION, Chronic Hepatitis B Pediatrics**).
Chronic Hepatitis C
Safety and effectiveness in pediatric patients ranging in age from 3 to 16 years have been established based upon clinical studies in 118 patients. See REBETOL package insert for additional information. Suicidal ideation or attempts occurred more frequently among pediatric patients compared to adult patients (2.4% vs 1%) during treatment and off-therapy follow-up (see **WARNINGS, Neuropsychiatric Disorders**). During a 48-week course of therapy there was a decrease in the rate of linear growth (mean percentile assignment decrease of 7%) and a decrease in the rate of weight gain (mean percentile assignment decrease of 9%). A general reversal of these trends was noted during the 24-week posttreatment period.

Geriatric Use
In all clinical studies of INTRON A, including studies as monotherapy and in combination with REBETOL (ribavirin USP) Capsules, only a small percentage of the subjects were aged 65 and over. These numbers were too few to determine if they respond differently from younger subjects except for the clinical trials of INTRON A in combination with REBETOL, where elderly subjects had a higher frequency of anemia (67%) than did younger patients (28%).

In a database consisting of clinical study and postmarketing reports for various indications, cardiovascular adverse events and confusion were reported more frequently in elderly patients receiving INTRON A therapy compared to younger patients.

In general, INTRON A therapy should be administered to elderly patients cautiously, reflecting the greater frequency of decreased hepatic, renal, bone marrow, and/or cardiac function and concomitant disease or other drug therapy. INTRON A is known to be substantially excreted by the kidney, and the risk of adverse reactions to INTRON A may be greater in patients with impaired renal function. Because elderly patients often have decreased renal function, patients should be carefully monitored during treatment, and dose adjustments made based on symptoms and/or laboratory abnormalities (see **CLINICAL PHARMACOLOGY** and **DOSAGE AND ADMINISTRATION**).

ADVERSE REACTIONS

General

The adverse experiences listed below were reported to be possibly or probably related to INTRON® A therapy during clinical trials. Most of these adverse reactions were mild to moderate in severity and were manageable. Some were transient and most diminished with continued therapy.

The most frequently reported adverse reactions were "flu-like" symptoms, particularly fever, headache, chills, myalgia, and fatigue. More severe toxicities are observed generally at higher doses and may be difficult for patients to tolerate.

[See table on pages 1548 and 1549]

Hairy Cell Leukemia

The adverse reactions most frequently reported during clinical trials in 145 patients with hairy cell leukemia were the "flu-like" symptoms of fever (68%), fatigue (61%), and chills (46%).

Malignant Melanoma

The INTRON A dose was modified because of adverse events in 65% (n=93) of the patients. INTRON A therapy was discontinued because of adverse events in 8% of the patients during induction and 18% of the patients during maintenance. The most frequently reported adverse reaction was fatigue, which was observed in 96% of patients. Other adverse reactions that were recorded in greater than 20% of INTRON A-treated patients included neutropenia (92%), fever (81%), myalgia (75%), anorexia (69%), vomiting/nausea (66%), increased SGOT (63%), headache (62%), chills (54%), depression (40%), diarrhea (35%), alopecia (29%), altered taste sensation (24%), dizziness/vertigo (23%), and anemia (22%).

Adverse reactions classified as severe or life threatening (ECOG Toxicity Criteria grade 3 or 4) were recorded in 66% and 14% of INTRON A-treated patients, respectively. Severe adverse reactions recorded in greater than 10% of INTRON A-treated patients included neutropenia/leukopenia (26%), fatigue (23%), fever (18%), myalgia (17%), headache (17%), chills (16%), and increased SGOT (14%). Grade 4 fatigue was recorded in 4% and grade 4 depression was recorded in 2% of INTRON A-treated patients. No other grade 4 AE was reported in more than 2 INTRON A-treated patients. Lethal hepatotoxicity occurred in 2 INTRON A-treated patients early in the clinical trial. No subsequent lethal hepatotoxicities were observed with adequate monitoring of liver function tests (see **PRECAUTIONS, Laboratory Tests**).

Follicular Lymphoma

Ninety-six percent of patients treated with CHVP plus INTRON A therapy and 91% of patients treated with CHVP alone reported an adverse event of any severity. Asthenia, fever, neutropenia, increased hepatic enzymes, alopecia, headache, anorexia, "flu-like" symptoms, myalgia, dyspnea, thrombocytopenia, paresthesia, and polyuria occurred more frequently in the CHVP plus INTRON A-treated patients than in patients treated with CHVP alone. Adverse reactions classified as severe or life threatening (World Health Organization grade 3 or 4) recorded in greater than 5% of CHVP plus INTRON A-treated patients included neutropenia (34%), asthenia (10%), and vomiting (10%). The incidence of neutropenic infection was 6% in CHVP plus INTRON A vs 2% in CHVP alone. One patient in each treatment group required hospitalization.

Twenty-eight percent of CHVP plus INTRON A-treated patients had a temporary modification/interruption of their INTRON A therapy, but only 13 patients (10%) permanently stopped INTRON A therapy because of toxicity. There were four deaths on study; two patients committed suicide in the CHVP plus INTRON A arm and two patients in the CHVP arm had unwitnessed sudden death. Three patients with hepatitis B (one of whom also had alcoholic cirrhosis) developed hepatotoxicity leading to discontinuation of INTRON A. Other reasons for discontinuation included intolerable asthenia (5/135), severe flu symptoms (2/135), and one patient each with exacerbation of ankylosing spondylitis, psychosis, and decreased ejection fraction.

Condylomata Acuminata

Eighty-eight percent (311/352) of patients treated with INTRON A for condylomata acuminata who were evaluable for safety reported an adverse reaction during treatment. The incidence of the adverse reactions reported increased when the number of treated lesions increased from one to five. All 40 patients who had five warts treated reported some type of adverse reaction during treatment.

Adverse reactions and abnormal laboratory test values reported by patients who were re-treated were qualitatively and quantitatively similar to those reported during the initial INTRON A treatment period.

AIDS-Related Kaposi's Sarcoma

In patients with AIDS-Related Kaposi's Sarcoma, some type of adverse reaction occurred in 100% of the 74 patients treated with 30 million IU/m^2 three times a week and in 97% of the 29 patients treated with 35 million IU per day. Of these adverse reactions, those classified as severe (World Health Organization grade 3 or 4) were reported in 27% to 55% of patients. Severe adverse reactions in the 30 million IU/m^2 TIW study included: fatigue (20%), influenza-like symptoms (15%), anorexia (12%), dry mouth (4%), headache (4%), confusion (3%), fever (3%), myalgia (3%), and nausea and vomiting (1% each). Severe adverse reactions for patients who received the 35 million IU QD included: fever (24%), fatigue (17%), influenza-like symptoms (14%), dyspnea (14%), headache (10%), pharyngitis (7%), and ataxia, confusion, dysphagia, GI hemorrhage, abnormal hepatic function, increased SGOT, myalgia, cardiomyopathy, face edema, depression, emotional lability, suicide attempt, chest pain, and coughing (1 patient each). Overall, the incidence of severe toxicity was higher among patients who received the 35 million IU per day dose.

Chronic Hepatitis C

Two studies of extended treatment (18–24 months) with INTRON A show that approximately 95% of all patients treated experience some type of adverse event and that patients treated for extended duration continue to experience adverse events throughout treatment. Most adverse events reported are mild to moderate in severity. However, 29/152 (19%) of patients treated for 18 to 24 months experienced a serious adverse event compared to 11/163 (7%) of those treated for 6 months. Adverse events which occur or persist during extended treatment are similar in type and severity to those occurring during short-course therapy.

Of the patients achieving a complete response after 6 months of therapy, 12/79 (15%) subsequently discontinued INTRON A treatment during extended therapy because of adverse events, and 23/79 (29%) experienced severe adverse events (WHO grade 3 or 4) during extended therapy.

In patients using combination treatment with INTRON A and REBETOL, the primary toxicity observed was hemolytic anemia. Reductions in hemoglobin levels occurred within the first 1 to 2 weeks of therapy. Cardiac and pulmonary events associated with anemia occurred in approximately 10% of patients treated with INTRON A/REBETOL therapy. See REBETOL package insert for additional information.

Chronic Hepatitis B

Adults

In patients with chronic hepatitis B, some type of adverse reaction occurred in 98% of the 101 patients treated at 5 million IU QD and 90% of the 78 patients treated at 10 million IU TIW. Most of these adverse reactions were mild to moderate in severity, were manageable, and were reversible following the end of therapy.

Adverse reactions classified as severe (causing a significant interference with normal daily activities or clinical state) were reported in 21% to 44% of patients. The severe adverse reactions reported most frequently were the "flu-like" symptoms of fever (28%), fatigue (15%), headache (5%), myalgia (4%), rigors (4%), and other severe "flu-like" symptoms, which occurred in 1% to 3% of patients. Other severe adverse reactions occurring in more than one patient were alopecia (8%), anorexia (6%), depression (3%), nausea (3%), and vomiting (2%).

To manage side effects, the dose was reduced, or INTRON A therapy was interrupted in 25% to 38% of patients. Five percent of patients discontinued treatment due to adverse experiences.

Pediatrics

In pediatric patients, the most frequently reported adverse events were those commonly associated with interferon treatment: flu-like symptoms (100%), gastrointestinal system disorders (46%), and nausea and vomiting (40%). Neutropenia (13%) and thrombocytopenia (3%) were also reported. None of the adverse events were life threatening. The majority were moderate to severe and resolved upon dose reduction or drug discontinuation.

[See table at top of next page]

Postmarketing Experience

The following adverse reactions have been identified during postapproval use of INTRON A alone or in combination with REBETOL. Because these reactions are reported voluntarily from a population of uncertain size, it is not always possible to reliably estimate their frequency or establish a causal relationship to drug exposure.

Blood and Lymphatic System Disorders

pancytopenia (concurrent anemia, leukopenia, thrombocytopenia), aplastic anemia, pure red cell aplasia, thrombotic thrombocytopenic purpura, idiopathic thrombocytopenic purpura

Ear and Labyrinth Disorders

hearing loss

Endocrine Disorders

hypopituitarism

Eye Disorders

Vogt-Koyanagi-Harada syndrome, serous retinal detachment

Gastrointestinal Disorders

pancreatitis

General Disorders and Administration Site Conditions

asthenic conditions (including asthenia, malaise, fatigue)

Immune System Disorders

cases of acute hypersensitivity reactions, including anaphylaxis and angioedema, systemic lupus erythematosus, sarcoidosis or exacerbation of sarcoidosis

Musculoskeletal and Connective Tissue Disorders

myositis

Nervous System Disorders

peripheral neuropathy

Psychiatric Disorders

homicidal ideation, psychosis including hallucinations

Renal and Urinary Disorders

renal failure, renal insufficiency, nephrotic syndrome

Respiratory, Thoracic and Mediastinal Disorders

pulmonary hypertension

Skin and Subcutaneous Tissue Disorders

injection site necrosis, Stevens-Johnson syndrome, toxic epidermal necrolysis, erythema multiforme, urticaria

OVERDOSAGE

There is limited experience with overdosage. Postmarketing surveillance includes reports of patients receiving a single dose as great as 10 times the recommended dose. In general, the primary effects of an overdose are consistent with the effects seen with therapeutic doses of interferon alfa-2b. Hepatic enzyme abnormalities, renal failure, hemorrhage, and myocardial infarction have been reported with single administration overdoses and/or with longer durations of treatment than prescribed (see **ADVERSE REACTIONS**).

Toxic effects after ingestion of interferon alfa-2b are not expected because interferons are poorly absorbed orally. Consultation with a poison center is recommended.

Treatment

There is no specific antidote for interferon alfa-2b. Hemodialysis and peritoneal dialysis are not considered effective for treatment of overdose.

DOSAGE AND ADMINISTRATION

General

IMPORTANT: INTRON® A is supplied as 1) Powder for Injection/Reconstitution; 2) Solution for Injection in Vials; 3) Solution for Injection in Multidose Pens. **Not all dosage forms and strengths are appropriate for some indications.** It is important that you carefully read the instructions below for the indication you are treating to ensure you are using an appropriate dosage form and strength.

To enhance the tolerability of INTRON A, injections should be administered in the evening when possible.

To reduce the incidence of certain adverse reactions, acetaminophen may be administered at the time of injection.

The solution should be allowed to come to room temperature before using.

Hairy Cell Leukemia

(see DOSAGE AND ADMINISTRATION, General)

Dose

The recommended dose for the treatment of hairy cell leukemia is 2 million IU/m^2 administered intramuscularly or subcutaneously 3 times a week for up to 6 months. Patients with platelet counts of less than 50,000/mm^3 should not be administered INTRON A intramuscularly, but instead by subcutaneous administration. Patients who are responding to therapy may benefit from continued treatment.

[see first table at top of page 1552]

NOTE: INTRON A Powder for Injection does not contain a preservative. The vial must be discarded after reconstitution and withdrawal of a single dose.

Dose Adjustment

- If severe adverse reactions develop, the dosage should be modified (50% reduction) or therapy should be temporarily withheld until the adverse reactions abate and then resume at 50% (1 MIU/m^2 TIW).
- If severe adverse reactions persist or recur following dosage adjustment, INTRON A should be permanently discontinued.
- INTRON A should be discontinued for progressive disease or failure to respond after six months of treatment.

ABNORMAL LABORATORY TEST VALUES BY INDICATION

Dosing Regimens
Percentage (%) of Patients

	MALIGNANT MELANOMA	FOLLICULAR LYMPHOMA	HAIRY CELL LEUKEMIA	CONDYLOMATA ACUMINATA	AIDS-RELATED KAPOSI'S SARCOMA		CHRONIC HEPATITIS C	CHRONIC HEPATITIS B		
								Adults		Pediatrics
	20 MIU/m² Induction (IV) 10 MIU/m² Maintenance (SC)	5 MIU TIW/SC	2 MIU/m² TIW/SC	1 MIU/lesion	30 MIU/m² TIW/SC	35 MIU QD/SC	3 MIU TIW	5 MIU QD	10 MIU TIW	6 MIU/m²TIW
Laboratory Tests	N=143	N=135	N=145	N=352	N=69–73	N=26–28	N=140–171	N=96–101	N=75–103	N=113–115
Hemoglobin	22	8	NA	--	1	15	26*	32†	23†	17‡
White Blood Cell Count	§	--	NA	17	10	22	26¶	68¶	34¶	9¶
Platelet Count	15	13	NA	--	0	8	15#	12#	5#	1#
Serum Creatinine	3	2	0	--	--	--	6	3	0	3
Alkaline Phosphatase	13	--	4	--	--	--	--	8	4	0
Lactate Dehydrogenase	1	--	0	--	--	--	--	--	--	--
Serum Urea Nitrogen	12	4	0	--	--	--	--	--	--	--
SGOT	63	24	4	12	11	41	--	2	0	2
SGPT	2	--	13	--	10	15	--	--	--	--
Granulocyte Count										
• Total	92	36	NA	--	31	39	45Þ	75Þ	61Þ	70Þ
• 1000–<1500/mm³	66	--	--	--	--	--	32	30	32	43
• 750–<1000/mm³	--	21	--	--	--	--	10	24	18	18
• 500–<750/mm³	25	--	--	--	--	--	1	17	9	7
• <500/mm³	1	13	--	--	--	--	2	4	2	2

NA - Not Applicable- Patients' initial hematologic laboratory test values were abnormal due to their condition.
* Decrease of ≥2 g/dL; 20% 2–<3 g/dL; 6% ≥3 g/dL
† Decrease of ≥2 g/dL
‡ Decrease of ≥2 g/dL; 14% 2–<3 g/dL; 3% ≥3 g/dL
§ White Blood Cell Count was reported as neutropenia
¶ Decrease to <3000/mm³
\# Decrease to <70,000/mm³
Þ Neutrophils plus bands

Malignant Melanoma
(see DOSAGE AND ADMINISTRATION, General)
INTRON A adjuvant treatment of malignant melanoma is given in two phases, induction and maintenance.
Induction Recommended Dose
The recommended daily dose of INTRON A in induction is 20 million IU/m² as an intravenous infusion, over 20 minutes, 5 consecutive days per week, for 4 weeks (see Dose Adjustment below).

Dosage Forms for This Indication

Dosage Form	Concentration	Route
Powder 10 MIU	10 MIU/mL	IV
Powder 18 MIU	18 MIU/mL	IV
Powder 50 MIU	50 MIU/mL	IV

NOTE: INTRON A Solution for Injection in vials or Multidose Pens is NOT recommended for intravenous administration and should not be used for the induction phase of malignant melanoma.
NOTE: INTRON A Powder for Injection does not contain a preservative. The vial must be discarded after reconstitution and withdrawal of a single dose.
Dose Adjustment
NOTE: Regular laboratory testing should be performed to monitor laboratory abnormalities for the purpose of dose modifications (see **PRECAUTIONS, Laboratory Tests**).
- INTRON A should be withheld for severe adverse reactions, including granulocyte counts greater than 250/mm³ but less than 500/mm³ or SGPT/SGOT greater than 5–10× upper limit of normal, until adverse reactions abate. INTRON A treatment should be restarted at 50% of the previous dose.
- INTRON A should be permanently discontinued for:
  - ◦ Toxicity that does not abate after withholding INTRON A
  - ◦ Severe adverse reactions which recur in patients receiving reduced doses of INTRON A
  - ◦ Granulocyte count less than 250/mm³ or SGPT/SGOT of greater than 10× upper limit of normal

Maintenance Recommended Dose
The recommended dose of INTRON A for maintenance is 10 million IU/m² as a subcutaneous injection three times per week for 48 weeks (see Dose Adjustment below).
[See second table at top of next page]
NOTE: INTRON A Powder for Injection does not contain a preservative. The vial must be discarded after reconstitution and withdrawal of a single dose.

Dose Adjustment
NOTE: Regular laboratory testing should be performed to monitor laboratory abnormalities for the purpose of dose modifications (see **PRECAUTIONS, Laboratory Tests** section).
- INTRON A should be withheld for severe adverse reactions, including granulocyte counts greater than 250/mm³ but less than 500/mm³ or SGPT/SGOT greater than 5–10× upper limit of normal, until adverse reactions abate. INTRON A treatment should be restarted at 50% of the previous dose.
- INTRON A should be permanently discontinued for:
  - ◦ Toxicity that does not abate after withholding INTRON A
  - ◦ Severe adverse reactions which recur in patients receiving reduced doses of INTRON A
  - ◦ Granulocyte count less than 250/mm³ or SGPT/SGOT of greater than 10× upper limit of normal

Follicular Lymphoma
(see DOSAGE and ADMINISTRATION, General)
Dose
The recommended dose of INTRON A for the treatment of follicular lymphoma is 5 million IU subcutaneously three times per week for up to 18 months in conjunction with anthracycline-containing chemotherapy regimen and following completion of the chemotherapy regimen.

Dosage Forms for This Indication

Dosage Form	Concentration	Route	Fixed Doses
Powder 10 MIU (single dose)	10 MIU/mL	SC	N/A
Solution 18 MIU multidose	6 MIU/mL	SC	N/A
Solution 25 MIU multidose	10 MIU/mL	SC	N/A
Pen 5 MIU/dose multidose	25 MIU/mL	SC	2.5, 5.0
Pen 10 MIU/dose multidose	50 MIU/mL	SC	5.0

NOTE: INTRON A Powder for Injection does not contain a preservative. The vial must be discarded after reconstitution and withdrawal of a single dose.
Dose Adjustment
- Doses of myelosuppressive drugs were reduced by 25% from a full-dose CHOP regimen, and cycle length increased by 33% (e.g., from 21 to 28 days) when alpha interferon was added to the regimen.
- Delay chemotherapy cycle if neutrophil count was less than 1500/mm³ or platelet count was less than 75,000/mm³.
- INTRON A should be permanently discontinued if SGOT exceeds greater than 5× the upper limit of normal or serum creatinine greater than 2.0 mg/dL (see **WARNINGS**).
- Administration of INTRON A therapy should be withheld for a neutrophil count less than 1000/mm³, or a platelet count less than 50,000/mm³.
- INTRON A dose should be reduced by 50% (2.5 MIU TIW) for a neutrophil count greater than 1000/mm³, but less than 1500/mm³. The INTRON A dose may be re-escalated to the starting dose (5 million IU TIW) after resolution of hematologic toxicity (ANC greater than 1500/mm³).

Condylomata Acuminata
(see DOSAGE and ADMINISTRATION, General)
Dose
The recommended dose is 1.0 million IU per lesion in a maximum of 5 lesions in a single course. The lesions should be injected three times weekly on alternate days for 3 weeks. An additional course may be administered at 12 to 16 weeks.

Dosage Forms for This Indication

Dosage Form	Concentration	Route
Powder 10 MIU (single dose)	10 MIU/mL	IL
Solution 25 MIU multidose	10 MIU/mL	IL

NOTE: INTRON A Powder for Injection does not contain a preservative. The vial must be discarded after reconstitution and withdrawal of a single dose.
NOTE: Do not use the following formulations for this Indication:
- **the 18 million or 50 million IU Powder for Injection**
- **the 18 million IU multidose INTRON A Solution for Injection**
- **the Multidose Pens**

Dose Adjustment
None
Technique for Injection
The injection should be administered intralesionally using a Tuberculin or similar syringe and a 25-to 30-gauge needle. The needle should be directed at the center of the base of the wart and at an angle almost parallel to the plane of the skin (approximately that in the commonly used PPD test). This will deliver the interferon to the dermal core of the lesion, infiltrating the lesion and causing a small wheal. Care

Dosage Forms for This Indication

Dosage Form	Concentration	Route	Fixed Doses
Powder 10 MIU (single dose)	10 MIU/mL	IM, SC	N/A
Solution 18 MIU multidose	6 MIU/mL	IM, SC	N/A
Solution 25 MIU multidose	10 MIU/mL	IM, SC	N/A
Pen 3 MIU/dose multidose	15 MIU/mL	SC	1.5, 3.0, 4.5
Pen 5 MIU/dose multidose	25 MIU/mL	SC	2.5, 5.0

Dosage Forms for This Indication

Dosage Form	Concentration	Route	Fixed Doses
Powder 10 MIU (single dose)*	10 MIU/mL	SC	N/A
Powder 18 MIU (single dose)†	18 MIU/mL	SC	N/A
Solution 18 MIU multidose	6 MIU/mL	SC	N/A
Solution 25 MIU multidose	10 MIU/mL	SC	N/A
Pen 3 MIU/dose multidose*	15 MIU/mL	SC	1.5, 3.0, 4.5, 6.0
Pen 5 MIU/dose multidose	25 MIU/mL	SC	7.5, 10.0
Pen 10 MIU/dose multidose	50 MIU/mL	SC	10.0, 15.0, 20.0

* Patients receiving 50% dose reduction only
† Patients receiving full dose only

INTRON A Dose	White Blood Cell Count	Granulocyte Count	Platelet Count
Reduce 50%	$<1.5 \times 10^9$ /L	$<0.75 \times 10^9$ /L	$<50 \times 10^9$ /L
Permanently Discontinue	$<1.0 \times 10^9$ /L	$<0.5 \times 10^9$ /L	$<25 \times 10^9$ /L

should be taken not to go beneath the lesion too deeply; subcutaneous injection should be avoided, since this area is below the base of the lesion. Do not inject too superficially since this will result in possible leakage, infiltrating only the keratinized layer and not the dermal core.

AIDS-Related Kaposi's Sarcoma
(see DOSAGE and ADMINISTRATION, General)

Dose

The recommended dose of INTRON A for Kaposi's Sarcoma is 30 million IU/m²/dose administered subcutaneously or intramuscularly three times a week until disease progression or maximal response has been achieved after 16 weeks of treatment. Dose reduction is frequently required (see **Dose Adjustment** below).

Dosage Forms for This Indication

Dosage Form	Concentration	Route
Powder 50 MIU	50 MIU/mL	IM, SC

NOTE: INTRON A Solution for Injection either in vials or in Multidose Pens should NOT be used for AIDS-Related Kaposi's Sarcoma.

NOTE: INTRON A Powder for Injection does not contain a preservative. The vial must be discarded after reconstitution and withdrawal of a single dose.

Dose Adjustment

- INTRON A dose should be reduced by 50% or withheld for severe adverse reactions.
- INTRON A may be resumed at a reduced dose if severe adverse reactions abate with interruption of dosing.
- INTRON A should be permanently discontinued if severe adverse reactions persist or if they recur in patients receiving a reduced dose.

Chronic Hepatitis C
(see DOSAGE and ADMINISTRATION, General)

Dose

The recommended dose of INTRON A for the treatment of chronic hepatitis C is 3 million IU three times a week (TIW) administered subcutaneously or intramuscularly. In patients tolerating therapy with normalization of ALT at 16 weeks of treatment, INTRON A therapy should be extended to 18 to 24 months (72 to 96 weeks) at 3 million IU TIW to improve the sustained response rate (see **CLINICAL PHARMACOLOGY, Chronic Hepatitis C** section). Patients who do not normalize their ALTs or have persistently high levels of HCV RNA after 16 weeks of therapy rarely achieve a sustained response with extension of treatment. Consideration should be given to discontinuing these patients from therapy.

When INTRON A is administered in combination with REBETOL®, patients with impaired renal function and/or those over the age of 50 should be carefully monitored with respect to the development of anemia. See REBETOL package insert for dosing when used in combination with REBETOL for adults and pediatric patients.

Dosage Forms for This Indication

Dosage Form	Concentration	Route	Fixed Doses
Solution 18 MIU multidose	6 MIU/mL	IM, SC	N/A
Pen 3 MIU/dose multidose	15 MIU/mL	SC	1.5, 3.0

Dose Adjustment

If severe adverse reactions develop during INTRON A treatment, the dose should be modified (50% reduction) or therapy should be temporarily discontinued until the adverse reactions abate. If intolerance persists after dose adjustment, INTRON A therapy should be discontinued.

Chronic Hepatitis B Adults
(see **DOSAGE and ADMINISTRATION, General**)

Dose

The recommended dose of INTRON A for the treatment of chronic hepatitis B is 30 to 35 million IU per week, administered subcutaneously or intramuscularly, either as 5 million IU daily (QD) or as 10 million IU three times a week (TIW) for 16 weeks.

Dosage Forms for This Indication

Dosage Form	Concentration	Route	Fixed Doses
Powder 10 MIU (single dose)	10 MIU/mL	IM, SC	N/A
Solution 25 MIU multidose	10 MIU/mL	IM, SC	N/A
Pen 5 MIU/dose multidose	25 MIU/mL	SC	2.5, 5.0, 10.0
Pen 10 MIU/dose multidose	50 MIU/mL	SC	5.0, 10.0

NOTE: INTRON A Powder for Injection does not contain a preservative. The vial must be discarded after reconstitution and withdrawal of a single dose.

Chronic Hepatitis B Pediatrics
(see **DOSAGE and ADMINISTRATION, General**)

Dose

The recommended dose of INTRON A for the treatment of chronic hepatitis B is 3 million IU/m² three times a week (TIW) for the first week of therapy followed by dose escalation to 6 million IU/m² TIW (maximum of 10 million IU TIW) administered subcutaneously for a total duration of 16 to 24 weeks.

Dosage Forms for This Indication

Dosage Form	Concentration	Route	Fixed Doses
Powder 10 MIU (single dose)	10 MIU/mL	SC	N/A
Solution 25 MIU multidose	10 MIU/mL	SC	N/A
Pen 3 MIU/dose multidose	15 MIU/mL	SC	1.5, 3.0, 4.5, 6.0
Pen 5 MIU/dose multidose	25 MIU/mL	SC	2.5, 5.0, 7.5, 10.0
Pen 10 MIU/dose multidose	50 MIU/mL	SC	5.0, 10.0, 15.0, 20.0

NOTE: INTRON A Powder for Injection does not contain a preservative. The vial must be discarded after reconstitution and withdrawal of a single-dose.

Dose Adjustment

If severe adverse reactions or laboratory abnormalities develop during INTRON A therapy, the dose should be modified (50% reduction) or discontinued if appropriate, until the adverse reactions abate. If intolerance persists after dose adjustment, INTRON A therapy should be discontinued.

For patients with decreases in white blood cell, granulocyte or platelet counts, the following guidelines for dose modification should be followed:

[See third table above]

INTRON A therapy was resumed at up to 100% of the initial dose when white blood cell, granulocyte, and/or platelet counts returned to normal or baseline values.

PREPARATION AND ADMINISTRATION

Reconstitution of INTRON® A Powder for Injection

The reconstituted solution is clear and colorless to light yellow. The INTRON A powder reconstituted with Sterile Water for Injection USP is a single-use vial and does not contain a preservative. **DO NOT RE-ENTER VIAL AFTER WITHDRAWING THE DOSE. DISCARD UNUSED PORTION** (see **DOSAGE and ADMINISTRATION**). Once the dose from the single-dose vial has been withdrawn, the sterility of any remaining product can no longer be guaranteed. Pooling of unused portions of some medications has been linked to bacterial contamination and morbidity.

- **Intramuscular, Subcutaneous, or Intralesional Administration**

Inject 1 mL Diluent (Sterile Water for Injection USP) for INTRON A into the INTRON A vial. Swirl gently to hasten complete dissolution of the powder. The appropriate INTRON A dose should then be withdrawn and injected intramuscularly, subcutaneously, or intralesionally (see **MEDICATION GUIDE** for detailed instructions).

Please refer to the **MEDICATION GUIDE** for detailed, step-by-step instructions on how to inject the INTRON A dose. After preparation and administration of the INTRON A injection, it is essential to follow the procedure for proper disposal of syringes and needles (see **MEDICATION GUIDE** for detailed instructions).

Parenteral drug products should be inspected visually for particulate matter and discoloration prior to administration.

- **Intravenous Infusion**

The infusion solution should be prepared immediately prior to use. Based on the desired dose, the appropriate vial strength(s) of INTRON A should be reconstituted with the diluent provided. Inject 1 mL Diluent (Sterile Water for Injection USP) for INTRON A into the INTRON A vial. Swirl gently to hasten complete dissolution of the powder. The appropriate INTRON A dose should then be withdrawn and injected into a 100-mL bag of 0.9% Sodium Chloride Injection USP. The final concentration of INTRON A should not be less than 10 million IU/100 mL.

Please refer to the **MEDICATION GUIDE** for detailed, step-by-step instructions on how to inject the INTRON A dose. After preparation and administration of INTRON A, it is essential to follow the procedure for proper disposal of syringes and needles.

INTRON A Solution for Injection in Vials

INTRON A Solution for Injection is supplied in two multidose vials. The solutions for injection do not require reconstitution prior to administration; the solution is clear and colorless.

The appropriate dose should be withdrawn from the vial and injected intramuscularly, subcutaneously, or intralesionally.

INTRON A Solution for Injection is not recommended for intravenous administration.

Solution for Injection in Multidose Pens

The INTRON A Solution for Injection Multidose Pens are designed to deliver 3 to 12 doses, depending on the individual dose, using a simple dial mechanism, and are for subcutaneous injections only. Only the needles provided in the packaging should be used for the INTRON A Solution for Injection Multidose Pen. A new needle is to be used each time a dose is delivered using the pen. To avoid the possible transmission of disease, each INTRON A Solution for Injection Multidose Pen is for single patient use only.

Please refer to the **MEDICATION GUIDE** for detailed, step-by-step instructions on how to inject the INTRON A dose. After preparation and administration of INTRON A, it is essential to follow the procedure for proper disposal of syringes and needles.

HOW SUPPLIED

INTRON® A Powder for Injection

INTRON A Powder for Injection, 10 million IU per vial and Diluent for INTRON A (Sterile Water for Injection USP) 1.25 mL per vial; boxes containing 1 INTRON A vial and 1 vial of INTRON A Diluent (NDC 0085-0571-02).

INTRON A Powder for Injection, 18 million IU per vial and Diluent for INTRON A (Sterile Water for Injection USP) 1.25 mL per vial; boxes containing 1 vial of INTRON A and 1 vial of INTRON A Diluent (NDC 0085-1110-01).

INTRON A Powder for Injection, 50 million IU per vial and Diluent for INTRON A (Sterile Water for Injection USP) 1.25 mL per vial; boxes containing 1 INTRON A vial and 1 vial of INTRON A Diluent (NDC 0085-0539-01).

INTRON A Solution for Injection in Multidose Pens

INTRON A Solution for Injection, 6 doses of 3 million IU (18 million IU) Multidose Pen (22.5 million IU per 1.5 mL per pen); boxes containing 1 INTRON A Multidose Pen, six disposable needles and alcohol swabs (NDC 0085-1242-01).

INTRON A Solution for Injection, 6 doses of 5 million IU (30 million IU) Multidose Pen (37.5 million IU per 1.5 mL per pen); boxes containing 1 INTRON A Multidose Pen, six disposable needles and alcohol swabs (NDC 0085-1235-01).

INTRON A Solution for Injection, 6 doses of 10 million IU (60 million IU) Multidose Pen (75 million IU per 1.5 mL per pen); boxes containing 1 INTRON A Multidose Pen, six disposable needles and alcohol swabs (NDC 0085-1254-01).

INTRON A Solution for Injection in Vials

INTRON A Solution for Injection, 18 million IU multidose vial (22.8 million IU per 3.8 mL per vial); boxes containing 1 vial of INTRON A Solution for Injection (NDC 0085-1168-01).

INTRON A Solution for Injection, 25 million IU multidose vial (32 million IU per 3.2 mL per vial); boxes containing 1 vial of INTRON A Solution for Injection (NDC 0085-1133-01).

Storage

- **INTRON A Powder for Injection/Reconstitution**
  INTRON A Powder for Injection should be stored in the refrigerator at 2° to 8°C (36°– 46°F). After reconstitution, the solution should be used immediately, but may be stored up to 24 hours at 2° to 8°C (36°– 46°F). Throw away any medicine left in the vial after you withdraw 1 dose.
- **INTRON A Solution for Injection in Vials**
  INTRON A Solution for Injection in vials should be stored in the refrigerator at 2° to 8°C (36°– 46°F).
- **INTRON A Solution for Injection in Multidose Pens**
  INTRON A Solution for Injection in Multidose Pens should be stored in the refrigerator at 2° to 8°C (36°– 46°F).
- **INTRON A Solution for Injection and INTRON A Solution for Injection in the Multidose Pens**
  INTRON A Solution for Injection and INTRON A Solution for Injection in the Multidose Pens should not be frozen and should be kept away from heat. Throw away any unused INTRON A Multidose Pen remaining after 4 weeks. Throw away any unused INTRON A Solution for Injection remaining in the vial after one month.

References

1. Smalley R, et al. *N Engl J Med.* 1992;327:1336–1341.
2. Aviles A, et al. *Leukemia and Lymphoma.* 1996;20:495–499.
3. Unterhalt M, et al. *Blood.* 1996;88(10 Suppl 1):1744A.
4. Schiller J, et al. *J Biol Response Mod.* 1989;8:252–261.
5. Poynard T, et al. *N Engl J Med.* 1995;332(22)1457–1462.
6. Lin R, et al. *J Hepatol.* 1995;23:487–496.
7. Perrillo R, et al. *N Engl J Med.* 1990;323:295–301.
8. Perez V, et al. *J Hepatol.* 1990;11:S113–S117.
9. Knodell R, et al. *Hepatology.* 1981;1:431–435.
10. Perrillo R, et al. *Ann Intern Med.* 1991;115:113–115.
11. Kauppila A, et al. *Int J Cancer.* 1982;29:291–294.

Manufactured by: Schering Corporation, a subsidiary of **MERCK & CO., INC.**
Whitehouse Station, NJ 08889, USA

U.S. Patent Nos. 5,935,566 and 6,610,830.
Rev. 08/12
LRN#030500-INT-MTL-USPI-22

MEDICATION GUIDE

INTRON® A (In-tron-aye)
(Interferon alfa-2b)

Read this Medication Guide before you start taking INTRON A, and each time you get a refill. There may be new information. This information does not take the place of talking with your healthcare provider about your medical condition or your treatment.

If you are taking INTRON A with REBETOL, also read the Medication Guide for REBETOL® (ribavirin) Capsules and Oral Solution.

INTRON A alone is a treatment for certain types of cancers and hepatitis B virus. INTRON A by itself or with REBETOL is a treatment for some people infected with hepatitis C virus.

What is the most important information I should know about INTRON A?

INTRON A can cause serious side effects that:

- **may cause death, or**
- **may worsen certain serious diseases that you may already have.**

Tell your healthcare provider right away if you have any of the symptoms listed below while taking INTRON A. If symptoms get worse, or become severe and continue, your healthcare provider may tell you to stop taking INTRON A permanently. In many, but not all people, these symptoms go away after they stop taking INTRON A.

1. **Heart problems**. Some people who take INTRON A may develop heart problems, including:
   - low blood pressure
   - fast heart rate or abnormal heart beats
   - trouble breathing or chest pain
   - heart attacks or heart muscle problems (cardiomyopathy)
2. **Stroke or symptoms of a stroke. Symptoms may include weakness, loss of coordination, and numbness.** Stroke or symptoms of a stroke may happen in people who have some risk factors **or** no known risk factors for a stroke.
3. **Mental health problems and suicide.** INTRON A may cause you to develop mood or behavior problems that may get worse during treatment with INTRON A or after your last dose, including:
   - irritability (getting upset easily)
   - depression (feeling low, feeling bad about yourself, or feeling hopeless)
   - aggressive behavior
   - thoughts of hurting yourself or others, or suicide
   - former drug addicts may fall back into drug addiction or overdose

   If you have these symptoms, your healthcare provider should carefully monitor you during treatment with INTRON A and for 6 months after your last dose.
4. **New or worsening autoimmune disease**. Some people taking INTRON A develop autoimmune diseases (a condition where the body's immune cells attack other cells or organs in the body), including rheumatoid arthritis, systemic lupus erythematosus, sarcoidosis, and psoriasis. In some people who already have an autoimmune disease, the disease may get worse while on INTRON A.
5. **Infections.** Some people who take INTRON A may get an infection. Symptoms may include:
   - fever
   - chills
   - bloody diarrhea
   - burning or pain with urination
   - urinating often
   - coughing up mucus (phlegm) that is discolored (for example yellow or pink)

While taking INTRON A, you should see a healthcare provider regularly for check-ups and blood tests to make sure that your treatment is working and to check for side effects.

What is INTRON A?

INTRON A is a prescription medicine that is used:

- to treat adults with a blood cancer called hairy cell leukemia
- to treat certain adults with a type of skin cancer called malignant melanoma
- to treat adults with some types of Follicular Non-Hodgkin's Lymphoma along with certain chemotherapy medicines
- to treat certain adults with genital warts (condylomata acuminate), by injecting the medicine directly into the warts
- to treat certain adults with a type of cancer caused by AIDS, called AIDS-related Kaposi's Sarcoma
- alone to treat adults with chronic (lasting a long time) hepatitis C infection with stable liver problems
- with REBETOL to treat chronic (lasting a long time) hepatitis C infection in people 3 years and older with stable liver problems
- to treat chronic (lasting a long time) hepatitis B infection in people 1 year and older with stable liver problems

Who should not take INTRON A?

Do not take INTRON A if you:

- had a serious allergic reaction to another alpha interferon product or are allergic to any of the ingredients in INTRON A. See the end of this Medication Guide for a complete list of ingredients. Ask your healthcare provider if you are not sure.
- have certain types of hepatitis (autoimmune hepatitis)
- have certain other liver problems

Talk to your healthcare provider before taking INTRON A if you have any of these conditions.

What should I tell my healthcare provider before taking INTRON A?

Before you take INTRON A, tell your healthcare provider if you:

- **See "What is the most important information I should know about INTRON A?"**
- have or ever had any problems with your heart, including heart attack or have high blood pressure
- have or ever had bleeding problems or blood clots
- are being treated for a mental illness or had treatment in the past for any mental illness, including depression and suicidal behavior
- have any kind of autoimmune disease (where the body's immune system attacks the body's own cells), such as psoriasis, systemic lupus erythematosus, rheumatoid arthritis
- have or ever had low blood cell counts
- have ever been addicted to drugs or alcohol
- have liver problems (other than hepatitis B or C)
- have or had lung problems, such as chronic obstructive pulmonary disease (COPD)
- have diabetes
- have colitis (inflammation of your intestine)
- have a condition that suppresses your immune system, such as cancer
- have hepatitis B or C infection
- have HIV infection (the virus that causes AIDS)
- have kidney problems
- have high blood triglyceride levels (fat in your blood)
- have an organ transplant and are taking medicine that keeps your body from rejecting your transplant (suppresses your immune system)
- have any other medical conditions
- are pregnant or plan to become pregnant. It is not known if INTRON A will harm your unborn baby. You should use effective birth control during treatment with INTRON A. Talk to your healthcare provider about birth control choices for you during treatment with INTRON A. Tell your healthcare provider if you become pregnant during treatment with INTRON A.
- are breast-feeding or plan to breast-feed. It is not known if INTRON A passes into your breast milk. You and your healthcare provider should decide if you will use INTRON A or breast-feed. You should not do both.

Tell your healthcare provider about all the medicines you take, including prescription and non-prescription medicines, vitamins, and herbal supplements. INTRON A and certain other medicines may affect each other and cause side effects.

Especially tell your healthcare provider if you take:

- the anti-hepatitis B medicine telbivudine (Tyzeka)
- the anti-HIV medicine zidovudine (Retrovir)
- theophylline (Theo-24, Elixophyllin, Uniphyl, Theolair).

Your healthcare provider may need to monitor the amount of theophylline in your body and make changes to your theophylline dose.

Know the medicines you take. Keep a list of them and show it to your healthcare provider and pharmacist when you get a new medicine.

How should I take INTRON A?

- INTRON A is given as an injection under the skin (subcutaneous) or into a muscle (intramuscular), into genital lesions, or as an injection into a vein (intravenous), depending on the condition that is being treated.
- Your healthcare provider will decide your dose of INTRON A and how often you will take it.
- If your healthcare provider decides that you can inject INTRON A for your condition, inject it exactly as prescribed, under your skin (subcutaneous injection) or into your muscle (intramuscular injection). Do not change your dose or how you inject INTRON A unless your healthcare provider tells you to.
- Do not take more than your prescribed dose.
- Your healthcare provider should show you how to prepare and measure your dose of INTRON A and how to inject yourself before you use INTRON A for the first time.
- You should not inject INTRON A until your healthcare provider has shown you how to use INTRON A the right way.
- INTRON A comes as:
  - a powder for injection in a vial that is used only 1 time (single-use vial). The powder must be mixed with water for injection (a diluent) before you inject it.

- a solution for injection in a multi-dose vial
- a solution for injection in a pen that is used more than 1 time (multidose pen)

- See the attached Instructions for Use for detailed instructions for preparing and injecting a dose of INTRON A.
- If you miss a dose of INTRON A, take the missed dose as soon as possible during the same day or the next day, then continue on your regular dosing schedule. If several days go by after you miss a dose, check with your healthcare provider to see what to do.
- Do not inject more than 1 dose or take more than your prescribed dose without talking to your healthcare provider.
- If you take too much INTRON A, call your healthcare provider right away. Your healthcare provider may examine you more closely, and do blood tests.
- Your healthcare provider should do regular blood tests before you start INTRON A, and during your treatment to see how well the treatment is working and to check for side effects.

What are the possible side effects of INTRON A?

INTRON A may cause serious side effects including:

- **See "What is the most important information I should know about INTRON A?"**
- **Blood problems.** INTRON A can affect your bone marrow and cause low white blood cell and platelet counts. In some people, these blood counts may fall to dangerously low levels. If your blood cell counts become very low, you can get infections or have bleeding problems.
- **Serious eye problems.** INTRON A may cause eye problems that may lead to vision loss or blindness. You should have an eye exam before you start taking INTRON A. If you have eye problems or have had them in the past, you may need eye exams while taking INTRON A. Tell your healthcare provider or eye doctor right away if you have any vision changes while taking INTRON A.
- **Thyroid problems.** Some people develop changes in the function of their thyroid. Symptoms of thyroid problems include:
  - problems concentrating
  - feeling cold or hot all the time
  - changes in your weight
  - skin changes
- **Blood sugar problems.** Some people may develop high blood sugar or diabetes. If you have high blood sugar or diabetes before starting INTRON A, talk to your healthcare provider before you take INTRON A. If you develop high blood sugar or diabetes while taking INTRON A, your healthcare provider may tell you to stop INTRON A and prescribe a different medicine for you. Symptoms of high blood sugar or diabetes may include:
  - increased thirst
  - tiredness
  - urinating more often than normal
  - increased appetite
  - weight loss
  - your breath smells like fruit
- **Lung problems including:**
  - trouble breathing
  - pneumonia
  - inflammation of lung tissue
  - new or worse high blood pressure of the lungs (pulmonary hypertension). This can be severe and may lead to death.

  You may need to have a chest X-ray or other tests if you develop fever, cough, shortness of breath, or other symptoms of a lung problem during treatment with INTRON A.
- **Severe liver problems, or worsening of liver problems including liver failure and death.** Symptoms may include:
  - nausea
  - loss of appetite
  - tiredness
  - diarrhea
  - yellowing of your skin or the white part of your eyes
  - bleeding more easily than normal
  - swelling of your stomach area (abdomen)
  - confusion
  - sleepiness
  - you cannot be awakened (coma)
- **Serious allergic reactions and skin reactions. Symptoms may include:**

◦ itching	◦ chest pain
◦ swelling of your face, eyes, lips, tongue, or throat	◦ feeling faint
◦ trouble breathing	◦ skin rash, hives, sores in your mouth, or your skin blisters and peels
◦ anxiousness	

- **Swelling of your pancreas (pancreatitis) and intestines (colitis).** Symptoms may include:
  - severe stomach area (abdomen) pain
  - severe back pain
  - nausea
  - vomiting
  - fever
- **New or worsening autoimmune disease.** Some patients taking INTRON A develop autoimmune diseases (a condition where the body's immune cells attack other cells or organs in the body), including rheumatoid arthritis, systemic lupus erythematosus, sarcoidosis, and psoriasis. In some patients who already have an autoimmune disease, the disease may worsen while on INTRON A.
- **Nerve problems.** People who take INTRON A or other alpha interferon products with telbivudine (Tyzeka) can develop nerve problems such as continuing numbness, tingling, or burning sensation in the arms or legs (peripheral neuropathy). Call your healthcare provider if you have any of these symptoms.
- **Growth problems in children. Weight loss and slowed growth are common in children during treatment with INTRON A.**
- **Dental and gum problems.**

Tell your healthcare provider right away if you have any of the symptoms listed above.

The most common side effects of INTRON A include:

- **Flu-like symptoms.** Symptoms may include: headache, muscle aches, tiredness, and fever. Some of these symptoms may be decreased by injecting your INTRON A dose in the evening. Talk to your healthcare provider about which over-the-counter medicines you can take to help prevent or decrease some of the symptoms.
- **Tiredness.** Many people become very tired during treatment with INTRON A.
- **Appetite problems.** Nausea, loss of appetite, and weight loss can happen with INTRON A.
- **Skin reactions.** Redness, swelling, and itching are common at the injection site.
- **Hair thinning.**

Tell your healthcare provider if you have any side effect that bothers you or that does not go away.

These are not all the side effects of INTRON A. For more information, ask your healthcare provider or pharmacist.

Call your doctor for medical advice about side effects. You may report side effects to the FDA at 1-800-FDA-1088.

How should I store INTRON A?

INTRON A Solution for Injection and INTRON A Solution for Injection in the Multidose Pens:

- Store in the refrigerator between 36°F to 46°F (2°C to 8°C).
- INTRON A Solution for Injection in Multidose vials for injection and INTRON A Solution for Injection in the Multidose Pens may be used to give more than 1 injection of medicine.
- Do not freeze.
- Throw away any unused INTRON A Multidose Pen remaining after 4 weeks.
- Throw away any unused INTRON A Solution for Injection remaining in the vial after one month.

INTRON A Powder for Injection:

Before mixing, store in the refrigerator between 36°F to 46°F (2°C to 8°C).

- After mixing the INTRON A Powder for Injection, use the solution right away or store the solution in the refrigerator for up to 24 hours between 36°F to 46°F (2°C to 8°C).
- Throw away any medicine left in the vial after you withdraw 1 dose.
- Do not freeze.

Keep INTRON A and all medicines out of the reach of children.

General Information about INTRON A

Medicines are sometimes prescribed for purposes other than those listed in a Medication Guide. Do not use INTRON A for a condition for which it was not prescribed. Do not give INTRON A to other people, even if they have the same symptoms that you have. It may harm them.

This Medication Guide summarizes the most important information about INTRON A. If you would like more information, ask your healthcare provider. You can ask your healthcare provider or pharmacist for information about INTRON A that was written for health care professionals.

- For more information, go to www.IntronA.com or call 1-800-622-4477.

What are the ingredients in INTRON A?

Active ingredient: interferon alfa-2b

Inactive ingredients:

- **Powder for injection contains:** glycine, sodium phosphate dibasic, sodium phosphate monobasic, human albumin. Sterile water for injection is provided as a diluent.
- **Solution Multidose vials for injection contain:** sodium chloride, sodium phosphate dibasic, sodium phosphate monobasic, edetate disodium, polysorbate 80, and m-cresol as a preservative.
- **Solution in Multidose Pens for injection contain:** sodium chloride, sodium phosphate dibasic, sodium phosphate monobasic, edetate disodium, polysorbate 80, and m-cresol as a preservative.

The Medication Guide has been approved by the U.S. Food and Drug Administration.

Manufactured by: Schering Corporation, a subsidiary of **Merck & Co., Inc.**, Whitehouse Station, NJ 08889 USA

Revised: 06/2012

LRN#030500-INT-MTL-MG-8

Instructions for Use

INTRON® A (In-tron-aye)

(Interferon alfa-2b, recombinant)

Solution for Injection

Be sure that you read, understand and follow these instructions before injecting INTRON A. Your healthcare provider should show you how to prepare, measure and inject INTRON A properly before you use it for the first time. Ask your healthcare provider if you have any questions.

Before starting, collect all of the supplies that you will need to use for preparing and injecting INTRON A. You will need the following supplies:

- 1 vial of INTRON A solution
- 1 single-use disposable syringe and needle
- 1 cotton ball or gauze
- 2 alcohol swabs

You will also need a puncture-proof disposable container to throw away used syringes, needles and vials.

Important:

- **Never re-use disposable syringes and needles.**
- Make sure you have the right syringe and needle to use with INTRON A. Your healthcare provider should tell you what syringes and needles to use to inject INTRON A.

How should I prepare a dose of INTRON® A?

1 Find a well lit, clean, flat working surface.
2. Before removing INTRON A from the carton, look at the expiration date printed on the carton. Make sure that the expiration date has not passed. Do not use if the expiration date has passed.
3. Wash your hands well with soap and warm water (See Figure 1). Keep your work area, your hands and injection site clean to decrease the risk of infection.

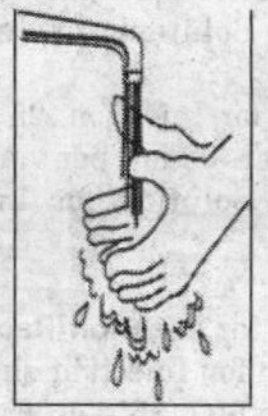

Figure 1

4. Remove 1 vial of INTRON A solution from the carton (See Figure 2).

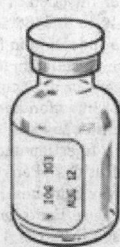

Figure 2

5. Look at the vial of INTRON A. The solution should be clear and colorless, without particles. Do not use the vial of INTRON A if the medicine is cloudy, has particles or is not clear and colorless.
6. Remove the protective plastic cap from the top of the INTRON A vial. Clean the rubber stopper on the top of the INTRON A vial with an alcohol swab (See Figure 3).

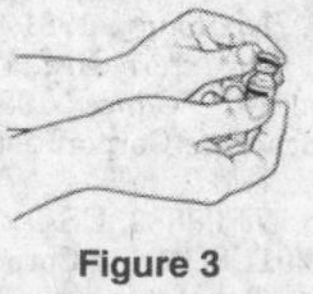

Figure 3

7. Gently warm the INTRON A solution by slowly rolling the vial in the palms of your hands for about one minute (See Figure 4). Do not shake the vial.

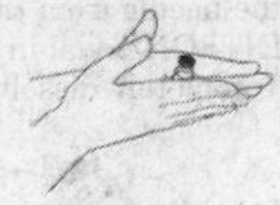

Figure 4

8. Open the package of the syringe you are using (See Figure 5) and if it does not have a needle attached, then attach a new needle to the syringe.

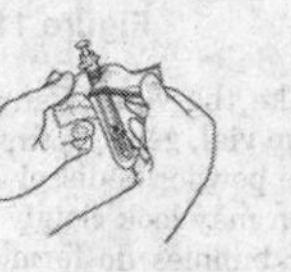

Figure 5

9. Remove the protective cap from the needle of the syringe. Fill the syringe with air by pulling back on the plunger to the mark on the syringe that matches the dose prescribed by your healthcare provider (See Figure 6).

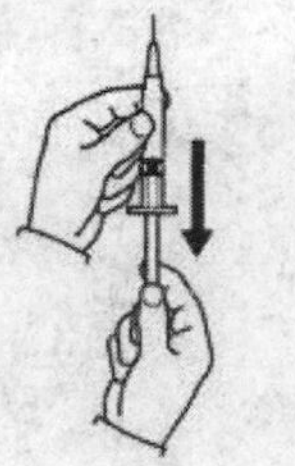

Figure 6

10. Hold the vial of INTRON A Solution for Injection on your flat working surface (See Figure 7). Do not touch the cleaned rubber stopper.

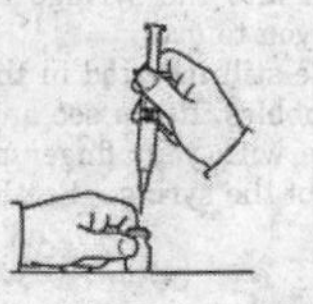

Figure 7

11. Push the needle straight down through the middle of the rubber stopper of the vial containing the INTRON A solution (See Figure 8). Slowly inject all the air from the syringe into the air space above the solution.

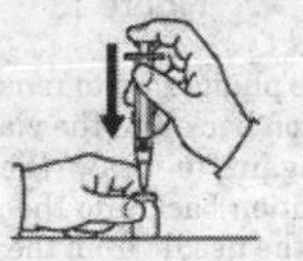

Figure 8

12. Keep the needle in the vial. Turn the vial upside down (See Figure 9).
   - ◦ Make sure the tip of the needle is in the INTRON A solution.
   - ◦ Slowly pull the plunger back to fill the syringe with INTRON A solution to the dose (mL or cc) prescribed by your healthcare provider.

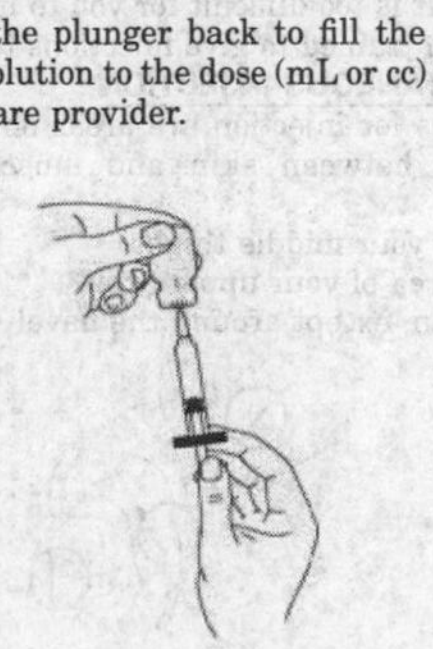

Figure 9

13. With the needle still in the vial, check the syringe for air bubbles (See Figure 10).
   - ◦ If there are any air bubbles, gently tap the syringe with your finger until the air bubbles rise to the top of the syringe.
   - ◦ Slowly push the plunger up to remove the air bubbles.
   - ◦ If you push solution back into the vial, slowly pull back on the plunger to draw the dose prescribed by your healthcare provider.

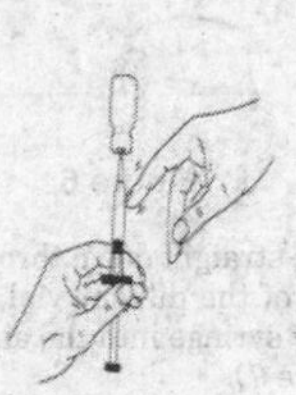

Figure 10

14. Do not remove the needle from the vial. Lay the vial and syringe on its side on your flat work surface until you are ready to inject the INTRON A solution.

How should I choose a site for injection?

Based on your treatment, your healthcare provider will tell you if you should inject a dose of INTRON® A under the skin (subcutaneous injection) or into the muscle (intramuscular injection). If it is too difficult for you to inject, ask someone who has been trained to give injections to help you.

FOR SUBCUTANEOUS INJECTION

The best sites for injection are areas on your body with a layer of fat between skin and muscle such as (See Figure 11):

- the front of your middle thighs
- the outer area of your upper arms
- the abdomen, except around the navel

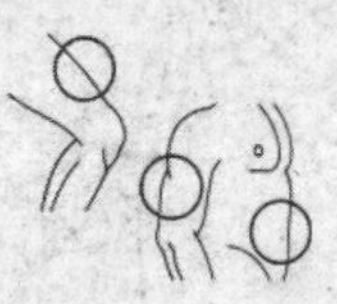

Figure 11

FOR INTRAMUSCULAR INJECTION

The best sites for injection into your muscle are (See Figure 12):

- the front of the middle thighs
- the upper arms
- the upper outer areas of the buttocks

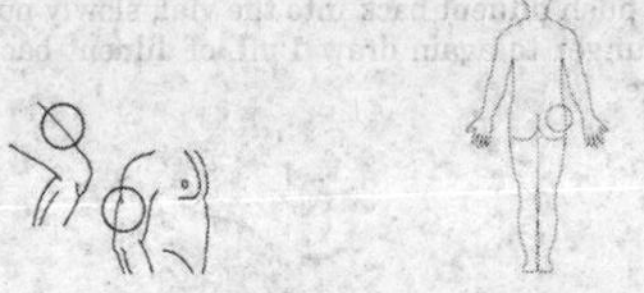

Figure 12

You should use a different site each time you inject INTRON® A to avoid soreness at any one site. Do not inject INTRON A into an area where the skin is irritated, red, bruised, infected or has scars, stretch marks or lumps.

How should I inject a dose of INTRON® A?

15. Clean the injection site with a new alcohol swab. Wait for the area to dry.
16. Pick up the vial and syringe from your flat work surface. Remove the syringe and needle from the vial.
   - ◦ Hold the syringe in the hand that you will use to inject INTRON A.
   - ◦ Do not touch the needle or allow it to touch the work surface.
17. With your other hand, pinch a fold of the skin at the cleaned injection site.

For subcutaneous injection (under the skin):

- ◦ Hold the syringe (like a pencil) at a **45-degree angle** to the skin. With a quick "dart-like" motion, push the needle into the skin (See Figure 13).

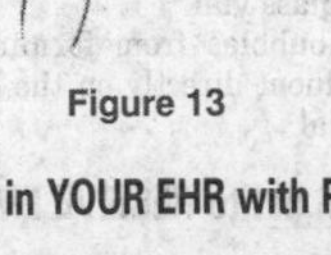

Figure 13

For intramuscular injection (into the muscle):

- ◦ Hold the syringe (like a pencil) at a **90-degree angle** to the skin. With a quick "dart-like" motion, push the needle into the muscle (See Figure 14).

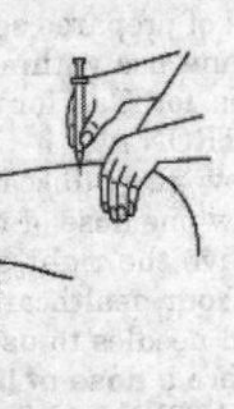

Figure 14

18. After the needle is inserted, remove the hand used to pinch the skin. Use it to hold the syringe barrel.
   - ◦ Pull the plunger back slightly.
   - ◦ **If no blood is present in the syringe,** inject the medicine by gently pressing the plunger all the way down the syringe barrel, until the syringe is empty.
   - ◦ **If blood comes into the syringe,** the needle has entered a blood vessel. Do not inject INTRON® A.
     - ◦ Withdraw the needle and throw away the syringe and needle in the puncture-proof container. See "How should I dispose of used syringes, needles and vials?"
     - ◦ Then, repeat steps 1 through 18 with a new dose of INTRON A and inject the medicine at a new injection site.
19. When the syringe is empty, pull the needle out of the skin.
   - ◦ Place a cotton ball or gauze over the injection site and press for several seconds. Do not massage the injection site.
   - ◦ If there is bleeding, cover the injection site with a bandage.
20. Throw away the used syringe, needle and vial. See "How should I dispose of used syringes, needles and vials?"

How should I dispose of used syringes, needles and vials?

Throw away used syringes, needles and vials in a puncture-proof container, sharps container or a hard container, like a metal can with a lid. Always place needles facing down. Do not use glass or clear plastic containers for disposal of needles and syringes. **Always keep the puncture-proof container out of the reach of children.**

- Check with your healthcare provider for instructions about the right way to throw away used needles and syringes. There may be local or state laws about how to throw away used needles and syringes. Always follow the instructions of your healthcare provider.

Do not throw away used needles, syringes or the puncture-proof container in household trash and do not recycle them.

How should I store INTRON® A?

INTRON A Solution for Injection:

- Store in the refrigerator at 36°F to 46°F (2°C to 8°C).
- Do not freeze Intron A.
- Allow the INTRON A Solution for Injection to come to room temperature before using. INTRON A Solution in Multidose vials for Injection may be used to give more than 1 injection of medicine.
- Throw away any unused INTRON A Solution for Injection remaining in the vial after 1 month
- Keep away from heat.
- **Keep INTRON A and all medicines out of the reach of children.**

Schering Corporation, a subsidiary of **Merck & Co., Inc.**, Whitehouse Station, NJ 08889 USA

U.S. Patent No. 5,935,566 and 6,610,830.
Rev. 02/2011
B-350339708T

Instructions for Use

INTRON® A (In-tron-aye)
(Interferon alfa-2b, recombinant)
Powder for Solution

Be sure that you read, understand, and follow these instructions before injecting INTRON A. Your healthcare provider should show you how to prepare, measure, and inject INTRON A properly before you use it for the first time. Ask your healthcare provider if you have any questions.

Before starting, collect all of the supplies that you will need to use for preparing and injecting INTRON A. For each injection you will need the following supplies:

- ◦ 1 vial of INTRON A powder for solution
- ◦ 1 vial of sterile water for injection (diluent)
- ◦ 1 single-use disposable syringe and needle
- ◦ 1 cotton ball or gauze
- ◦ 2 alcohol swabs

You will also need a puncture-proof disposable container to throw away used syringes, needles and vials.

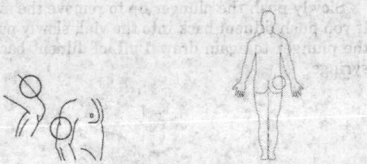

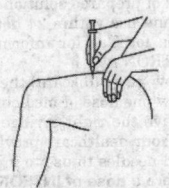

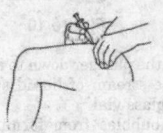

Important:

◦ **Never re-use disposable syringes and needles.**

◦ The vial of mixed INTRON A should be used right away. Do not mix more than 1 vial of INTRON A at a time. If you do not use the vial of prepared solution right away, store it in a refrigerator and use within 24 hours. See the end of these Instructions for Use for information about "How should I store INTRON A?"

◦ After mixing, throw away (discard) the vial of INTRON A after you withdraw one dose of medicine.

◦ Make sure you have the right syringe and needle to use with INTRON A. Your healthcare provider should tell you what syringes and needles to use to inject INTRON A.

How should I prepare a dose of INTRON A?

Before you inject INTRON A, the powder must be mixed with 1 mL (cc) of the sterile water for injection (diluent) from the INTRON A vial package.

1. Find a clean, well-lit, flat work surface.
2. Get one of your INTRON A vial packages. Check the date printed on the carton. Make sure that the expiration date has not passed.
3. Wash your hands well with soap and water. Keep your work area, your hands, and injection site clean to decrease the risk of infection (See Figure 1).

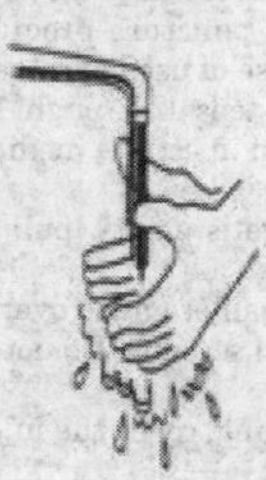

Figure 1

4. Gently warm the vial of diluent by slowly rolling the vial in the palms of your hands for one minute (See Figure 2).

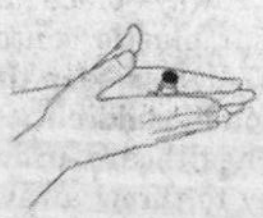

Figure 2

5. Remove the protective plastic cap from the tops of both vials (INTRON A powder and the diluent). Clean the rubber stopper on the top of both vials with an alcohol swab (See Figure 3).

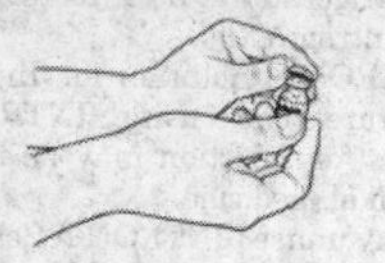

Figure 3

6. Open the package for the syringe (See Figure 4) you are using and if it does not have a needle attached, then attach a new needle to the syringe.

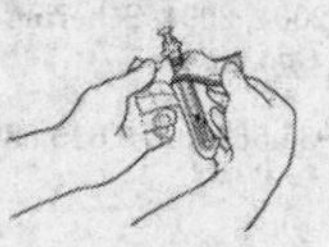

Figure 4

7. Remove the needle cover from the syringe. Fill the syringe with air by pulling the plunger back to 1 mL (See Figure 5).

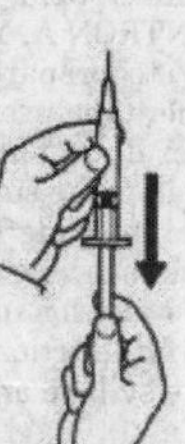

Figure 5

8. Hold the diluent vial on your flat work surface. Do not touch the cleaned rubber stopper (See Figure 6).

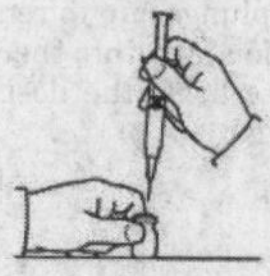

Figure 6

9. Push the needle straight down through the middle of the rubber stopper of the diluent vial and slowly inject all the air from the syringe into the air space above the diluent (See Figure 7).

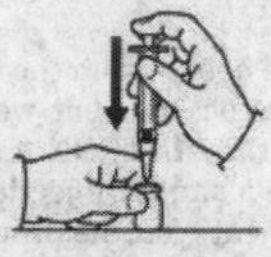

Figure 7

10. Keep the needle in the vial. Turn the vial upside down and make sure the tip of the needle is in the diluent.
    ◦ Slowly pull the plunger back to fill the syringe with diluent to the 1 mL mark on the side of the syringe (See Figure 8).

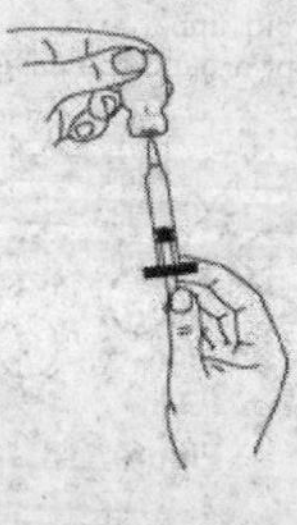

Figure 8

11. With the needle still inserted in the vial, check the syringe for air bubbles (See Figure 9).
    ◦ If there are any air bubbles, gently tap the syringe with your finger until the air bubbles rise to the top of the syringe.
    ◦ Slowly push the plunger up to remove the air bubbles.

If you push diluent back into the vial, slowly pull back on the plunger to again draw 1 mL of diluent back into the syringe.

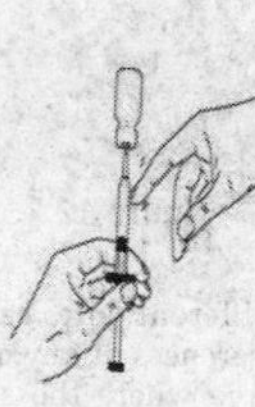

Figure 9

12. Remove the needle from the vial. Do not let the syringe touch anything.
13. Insert the needle through the center of the rubber stopper of the INTRON A powder vial. Do not touch the cleaned rubber stopper.
    ◦ Place the needle tip, at an angle, against the side of the INTRON A powder vial (See Figure 10).

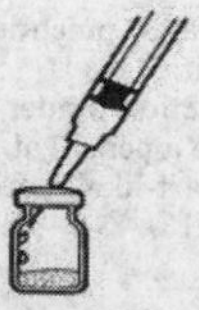

Figure 10

◦ Slowly push the plunger down to inject the diluent into the vial. The stream of liquid should run down the sides of the glass vial.

◦ To prevent bubbles from forming, do not aim the stream of diluent directly on the medicine in the bottom of the vial.

◦ Do not remove the needle from the vial.

14. Gently swirl the INTRON A vial in a circular motion until the powder is completely dissolved (See Figure 11).

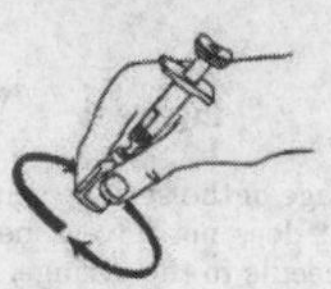

Figure 11

◦ Do not shake the vial. If any powder remains undissolved in the vial, gently turn the vial upside down until all of the powder is dissolved.

◦ The solution may look cloudy or bubbly for a few minutes. If air bubbles do form, wait until the solution settles and all bubbles rise to the top. Then withdraw your dose from the vial.

15. After the INTRON A completely dissolves, the solution should be clear and colorless to light yellow, without particles. Do not use the mixed solution if you see particles in it, or it is not clear and colorless to light yellow.
16. With the needle in the vial, turn the vial upside down (See Figure 12).

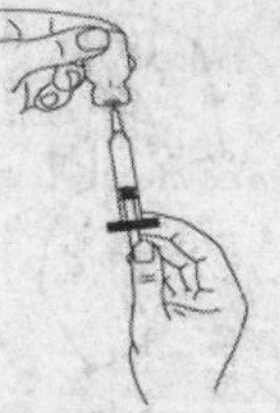

Figure 12

◦ Hold the vial with one hand. Be sure the tip of the needle is in the INTRON A solution. Slowly pull the plunger back to fill the syringe with the exact amount of INTRON A into the syringe that your healthcare provider told you to use.

17. With the needle still inserted in the vial, check the syringe for air bubbles. If you see any air bubbles, gently tap the syringe with your finger until the air bubbles rise to the top of the syringe (See Figure 13).

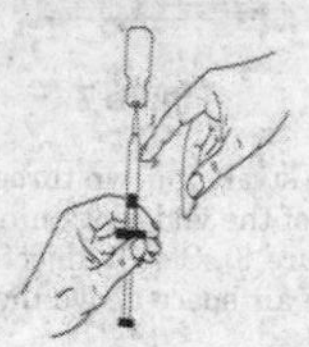

Figure 13

18. Slowly push the plunger up to remove the air bubbles. If you push solution back into the vial, slowly pull back on the plunger again to draw the correct amount of INTRON A solution back into the syringe.
19. Do not remove the needle from the vial. Lay the vial and syringe on its side on your flat work surface until you are ready to inject the INTRON A solution.

How should I choose a site for injection?

Based on your treatment, your healthcare provider will tell you if you should inject a dose of INTRON® A under the skin (subcutaneous injection) or into the muscle (intramuscular injection). If it is too difficult for you to inject, ask someone who has been trained to give injections to help you.

FOR SUBCUTANEOUS INJECTION

The best sites for injection are areas on your body with a layer of fat between skin and muscle, such as (See Figure 14):

- the front of your middle thighs
- the outer area of your upper arms
- the abdomen, except around the navel

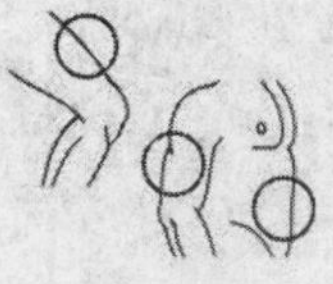

Figure 14

FOR INTRAMUSCULAR INJECTION

The best sites for injection into your muscle are (See Figure 15):

- the front of the middle thighs
- the upper arms
- the upper outer areas of the buttocks

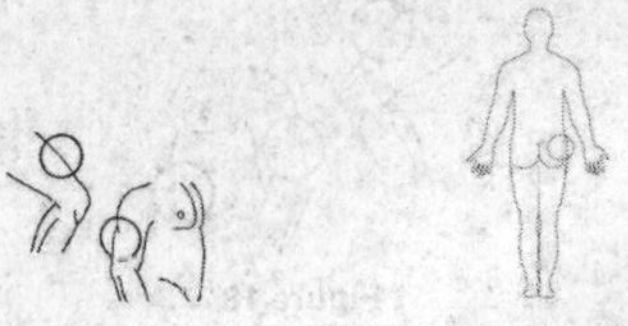

Figure 15

You should use a different site each time you inject INTRON® A to avoid soreness at any one site. Do not inject INTRON A into an area where the skin is irritated, red, bruised, infected or has scars, stretch marks, or lumps.

How should I inject a dose of INTRON® A?

20. Clean the injection site with a new alcohol swab. Wait for the skin to dry.
21. Pick up the vial and syringe from your flat work surface. Remove the syringe and needle from the vial.
    - Hold the syringe in the hand that you will use to inject INTRON A.
    - Do not touch the needle or allow it to touch the work surface.
22. With one hand, pinch a fold of the skin at the cleaned injection site.
23. **For subcutaneous injection (under the skin):**
    - With the other hand, hold the syringe (like a pencil) at a **45-degree angle** to the skin. With a quick "dart-like" motion, push the needle into the skin (See Figure 16).

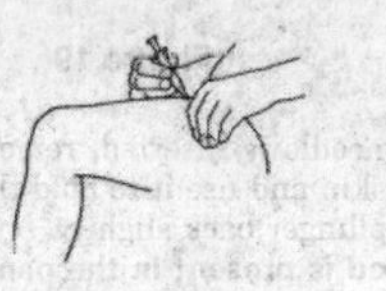

Figure 16

24. **For intramuscular injection (into the muscle):**
    - Hold the syringe (like a pencil) at a **90-degree angle** to the skin.
    - With a quick "dart-like" motion, push the needle into the muscle (See Figure 17).

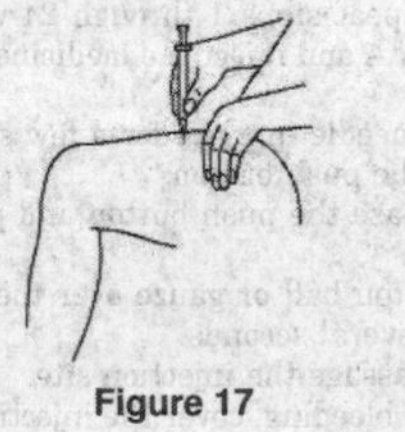

Figure 17

25. After the needle is inserted, remove the hand used to pinch the skin and use it to hold the syringe barrel.
    - Pull the plunger back slightly.
    - **If no blood is present in the syringe**, inject the medicine by gently pushing the plunger all the way down the syringe barrel, until the syringe is empty.
    - **If blood comes into the syringe**, the needle has entered a blood vessel. Do not inject INTRON® A.
      - Withdraw the needle and throw away the syringe and needle in the puncture-proof container. See "How should I dispose of used syringes, needles and vials?".
      - Then, repeat steps 1 through 25 with a new dose of INTRON A and inject the medicine at a new injection site.
26. When the syringe is empty, pull the needle out of the skin.
    - Place a cotton ball or gauze over the injection site and press for several seconds. Do not massage the injection site.
    - If there is bleeding, cover the injection site with a bandage.
27. Throw away the used syringe, needle, and vial. See "How should I dispose of used syringes, needles and vials?".

How should I dispose of used syringes, needles, and vials?

- Throw away used syringes, needles, and vials in a puncture-proof container, such as sharps container, or a hard container like a metal can with a lid. Always place needles facing down. Do not use glass or clear plastic containers for disposal of needles and syringes. **Always keep the puncture-proof container out of the reach of children.**
- Do not throw away used needles, syringes, or the puncture-proof container in household trash and do not recycle them.
- Check with your healthcare provider for instructions about the right way to throw away used needles and syringes. There may be special state and local laws for disposal of used needles and syringes. Always follow the instructions of your healthcare provider.

How should I store INTRON® A?

INTRON A Powder for Injection:

- Before mixing, store in the refrigerator between 36°F to 46°F (2°C to 8°C).
- After mixing the INTRON A Powder for Injection, use the solution right away or store the solution in the refrigerator for up to 24 hours between 36°F to 46°F (2°C to 8°C). Allow the solution to come to room temperature before using.
- Do not freeze Intron A.
- Keep away from heat.
- Throw away any medicine left in the vial after you withdraw 1 dose.

Keep INTRON A and all medicines out of the reach of children.

Schering Corporation, a subsidiary of **Merck & Co., Inc.**, Whitehouse Station, NJ 08889 USA

Rev. 02/2011
U.S. Patent Nos. 5,935,566 and 6,610,830.
35038302T

Instructions for Use

INTRON® A (In-tron-aye)

(Interferon alfa-2b, recombinant)

Solution for Injection Multidose Pen

Be sure that you read, understand, and follow these instructions about the right way to use your Multidose Pen before injecting INTRON A. Your healthcare provider should show you how to prepare, measure, and inject your INTRON A from the Multidose Pen properly before you use it for the first time. Ask your healthcare provider if you have any questions.

Before starting, collect all of the supplies that you will need to use for preparing and injecting INTRON A from your Multidose Pen. Make sure you have the right strength of INTRON A Multidose Pen that your healthcare provider prescribed for you. You will need the following supplies:

- the INTRON A Multidose Pen
- 1 Novofine® needle
- 2 alcohol swabs
- 1 cotton ball or gauze

You will also need a puncture-proof disposable container to throw away your used INTRON A Multidose Pen and the Novofine needle.

Important:

- **Never re-use needles.**
- Make sure that you have the correct INTRON A Multidose Pen prescribed by your healthcare provider. The INTRON A Multidose Pen should only be used with **Novofine** needles. These are the needles that come packaged with the pen. If you use other needles, the pen may not work the right way. You could get the wrong dose of INTRON A.
- INTRON A Multidose Pen may be used to give more than 1 injection of medicine.

To prevent spread of infection, do not allow anyone else to use your multidose pen and needles. Figures 1 and 2 below show the different parts of the INTRON A Multidose Pen and the Novofine needle. The parts of the pen you need to know are:

INTRON A Pen

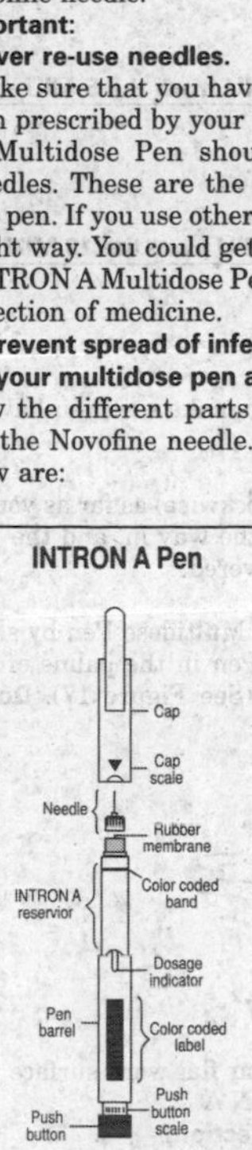

Figure 1

Novofine Needle Assembly

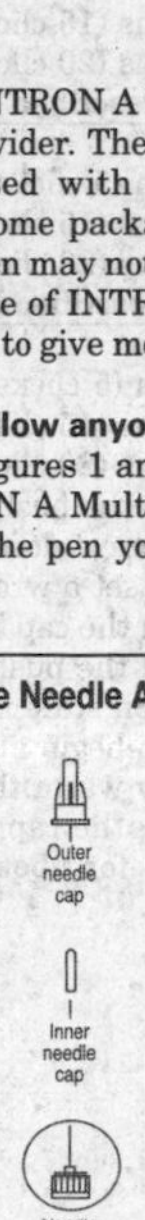

Figure 2

- The **color-coded push button** and **push button scale**. These are located at the bottom of the pen when it is held with the cap side up. This tells you the dose that has been set.
- The **color-coding** band. This is located on the INTRON A reservoir. The band lets you know the dose that you are using.
  - **The 3 MIU INTRON A Multidose Pen**: has a brown push button, a brown color-coding band, and color-coded label.
  - **The 5 MIU INTRON A Multidose Pen**: has a light blue push button, a light blue color-coding band, and color-coded label.
  - **The 10 MIU INTRON A Multidose Pen**: has a pink push button, a pink color-coding band, and color-coded label.
- The **cap**. The cap is used for setting the dose and storing the pen. You will not be able to set the dose or completely close the pen unless you line up the **triangle** on the **cap scale** with the **dosage indicator** on the barrel.

How should I prepare a dose of INTRON® A using a Multidose Pen?

1. Find a clean, well-lit, flat work surface.
2. Get one of your INTRON A Multidose Pen packages. Look at the date printed on the carton to make sure that the expiration date has not passed. Do not use if the expiration date has passed.
3. Wash your hands well with soap and warm water (See Figure 3). It is important to keep your work area, your hands, and injection site clean to decrease the risk of infection.

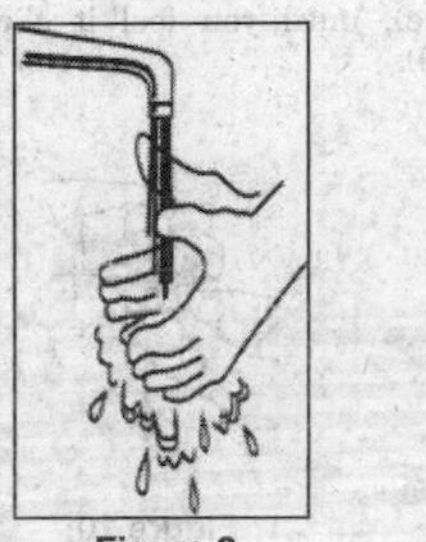

Figure 3

4. Remove the INTRON A Multidose Pen from the carton. Pull the cap off the pen and put the cap on the clean, flat work surface so that the inside of the cap remains clean (you will need to use this cap to recap the INTRON A Multidose pen in step 32 below). Wipe the rubber membrane with one alcohol swab (See Figure 4).

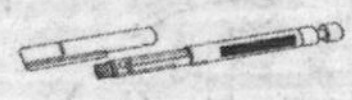

Figure 4

5. Look at the solution inside the pen. The solution should be clear and colorless, without particles. Do not use the INTRON A if the medicine is cloudy, has particles, or is not clear and colorless.
6. Remove the paper backing from the Novofine® needle by pulling the paper tab (See Figure 5). You will see the back of the needle once the paper tab is removed.

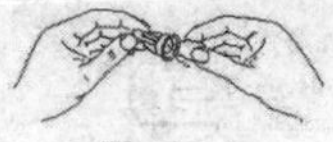

Figure 5

7. Keep the needle in its outer, clear needle cap. Gently push the Novofine needle straight into the pen's rubber membrane that you just cleaned. Screw the needle onto the INTRON A Multidose Pen by turning it in the direction of the arrow in the figure below (clockwise) (See Figure 6).

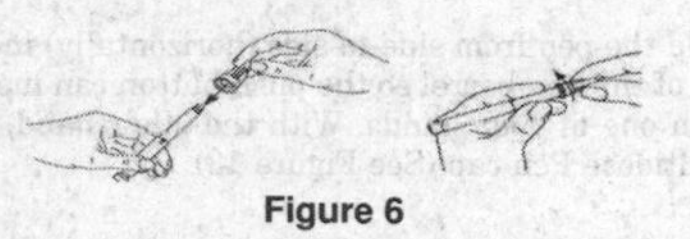

Figure 6

8. With the needle facing up, pull off the outer, clear needle cap (See Figure 7). Set the outer needle cap down on your clean flat work surface for later use and make sure that the inside of the cap remains clean. Next, carefully pull off the white inner needle cap (See Figure 8). The needle can be seen now.

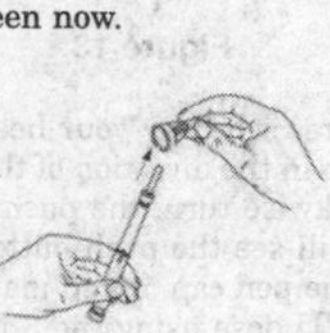

Figure 7

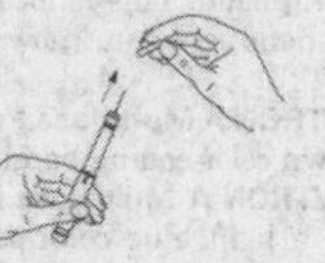

Figure 8

9. Keep the needle facing up and remove any air bubbles that may be in the reservoir by tapping the reservoir with your finger (See Figure 9). If you have any air bubbles, they will rise to the top of the reservoir.

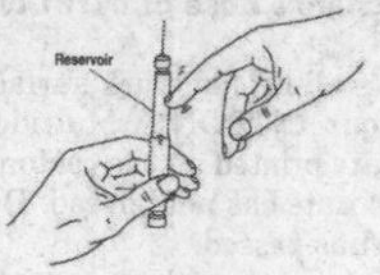

Figure 9

10. Hold the pen by the barrel. Turn the INTRON A reservoir in the direction of the arrow in the figure below (clockwise), until you feel it click into place (See Figure 10).

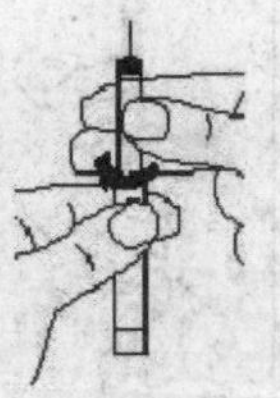

Figure 10

11. Keep the needle facing up and press the push button all the way up. A drop of INTRON A solution should come out of the tip of the needle (See Figure 11).

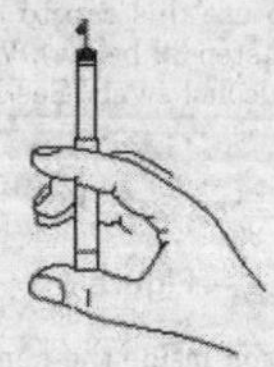

Figure 11

12. Put the outer cap you removed in Step 8 above back on the INTRON A Multidose Pen. Make sure you line up the black triangle on the pen cap with the dosage indicator on the pen barrel (See Figure 12). The pen is now ready to set the dose.

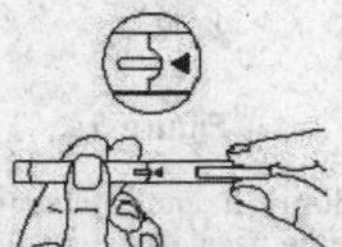

Figure 12

How should I set the dose prescribed by my healthcare provider?

13. Hold the pen from side-to-side (horizontally) in the middle of the pen barrel so the push button can move freely with one of your hands. With the other hand, hold the Multidose Pen cap (See Figure 13).

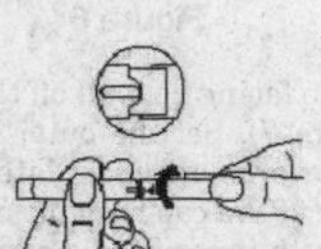

Figure 13

14. Set the dose prescribed by your healthcare provider by turning the cap in the direction of the arrow (clockwise). With each clockwise turn, the push button will start to rise and you will see the push button scale. Do not use force to turn the pen cap or you may damage the pen.
    - To set a 3 MIU dose using the 3 MIU Multidose Pen, turn the cap 2 full turns (10 clicks) = 3 MIU (See Figure 14).

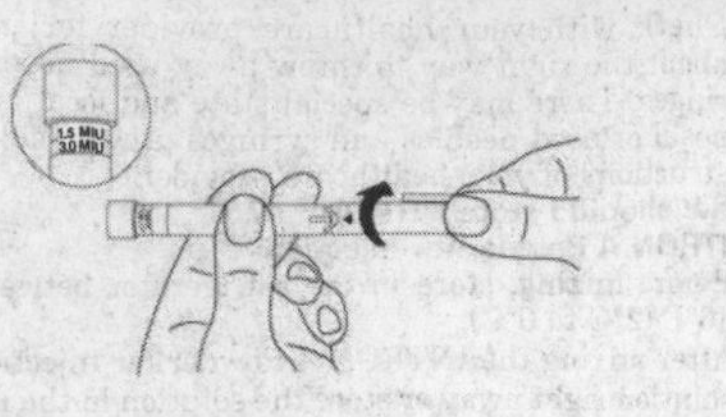

Figure 14

- To set a 5 MIU dose using the 5 MIU Multidose Pen, turn the cap 2 full turns (10 clicks) = 5 MIU (See Figure 15).

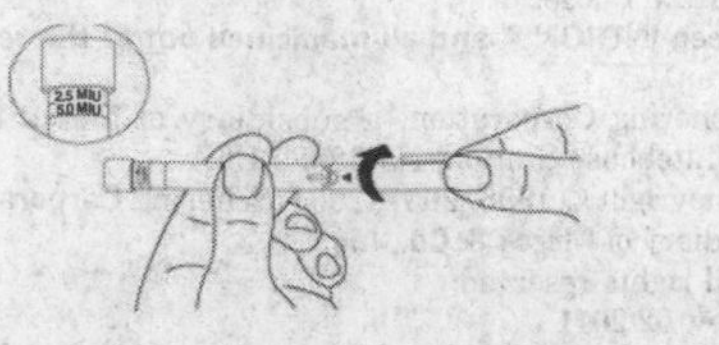

Figure 15

- To set a 10 MIU dose using the 10 MIU Multidose Pen, turn the cap 2 full turns (10 clicks) = 10 MIU (See Figure 16).

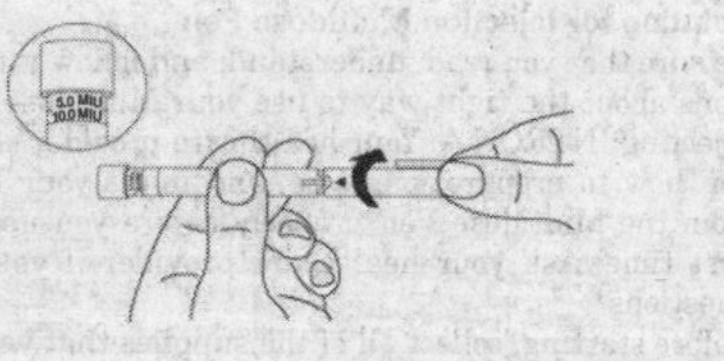

Figure 16

15. After each complete turn, make sure the triangle on the cap is lined up with the dosage indicator on the pen barrel.

If your healthcare provider has prescribed a dose other than 3.0, 5.0, or 10.0 MIU, the dose can be set by turning the cap as many times as shown below:

A dose prescribed other than 3 MIU from the 3 MIU multidose pen

1 full turn (5 clicks) = 1.5 MIU
3 full turns (15 clicks) = 4.5 MIU
4 full turns (20 clicks) = 6 MIU

A dose prescribed other than 5 MIU from the 5 MIU multidose pen

1 full turn (5 clicks) = 2.5 MIU
3 full turns (15 clicks) = 7.5 MIU
4 full turns (20 clicks) = 10 MIU

A dose prescribed other than 10 MIU from the 10 MIU multidose pen

1 full turn (5 clicks) = 5 MIU
3 full turns (15 clicks) = 15 MIU
4 full turns (20 clicks) = 20 MIU

16. Check the push button scale to make sure you have set the correct dose.
17. If you set a wrong dose:
    - Turn the cap back (counterclockwise) as far as you can until the push button is all the way in, and the push button scale is completely covered.
    - Then begin at step 13 again.
18. Gently warm the INTRON® A Multidose Pen by slowly rolling the capped Multidose Pen in the palms of your hands for about one minute (See Figure 17). **Do not shake.**

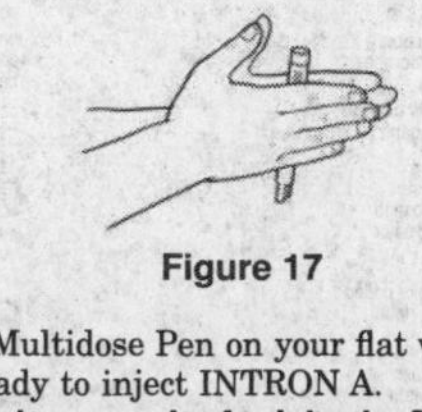

Figure 17

19. Place the Multidose Pen on your flat work surface until you are ready to inject INTRON A.

How should I choose a site for injection?

INTRON® A is given from the Multidose Pen as an injection under the skin (subcutaneous injection). If it is too difficult for you to inject, ask someone who has been trained to give injections to help you.

The best sites for injection are areas on your body with a layer of fat between skin and muscle (See Figure 18), such as:

- the front of the middle thighs
- the outer area of the upper arms
- the abdomen, except around the navel

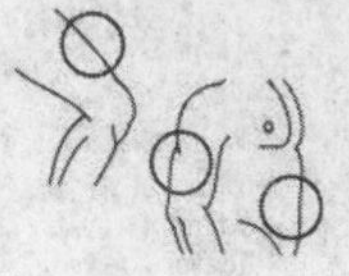

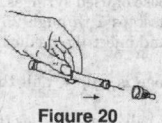

Figure 18

You should use a different site each time you inject INTRON A to avoid soreness at any one site. Do not inject INTRON A into an area where the skin is irritated, red, bruised, infected or has scars, stretch marks, or lumps.

How should I inject a dose of INTRON® A?

20. Clean the injection site with a new alcohol swab.
21. Pick up the Multidose Pen from your flat work surface and remove the cap from the needle.
22. With one hand, pinch a fold of the skin at the cleaned injection site.
23. Hold the Multidose Pen (like a pencil) at a **45-degree angle** to the skin. With a quick "dart-like" motion, push the needle into the skin (See Figure 19).

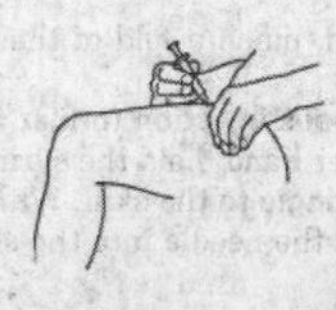

Figure 19

24. After the needle is inserted, remove the hand used to pinch the skin and use it to hold the pen barrel.
    - Pull the plunger back slightly.
    - **If no blood is present in the pen reservoir,** inject the medicine by gently pressing the push button all the way down.
    - **If blood comes into the pen reservoir**, the needle has entered a blood vessel. Do not inject INTRON A.
    - Withdraw the needle and throw away the used INTRON A Multidose Pen and needle in the puncture-proof container. See "How should I dispose of the used INTRON A Multidose Pens and needles?".
    - Then, repeat steps 1 through 24 with a new dose of INTRON A and inject the medicine at a new injection site.
25. Leave the needle in place for a few seconds while holding down the push button.
26. Slowly release the push button and pull the needle out of the skin.
27. Place a cotton ball or gauze over the injection site and press for several seconds.
    - Do not massage the injection site.
    - If there is bleeding, cover the injection site with a bandage.
28. If there is enough solution left in the INTRON A Multidose Pen for another dose of INTRON A, refrigerate the INTRON A Multidose Pen after use.

How should I remove the needle from the Multidose Pen?

29. To remove the needle, you have to recap the needle. Do not hold the cap in your hand, you may hurt yourself. Instead, using a scooping motion, carefully replace the outer, clear needle cap (like capping a pen) (See Figure 20).

Figure 20

30. After you recap the needle, remove the needle by holding the clear outer needle cap with one hand and holding the pen barrel with the other hand. Turn in the direction of the arrow (counterclockwise), as in Figure 21 below.

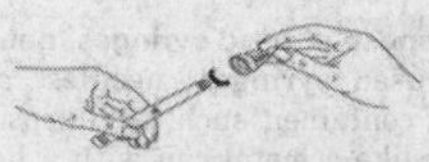

Figure 21

31. Carefully lift the needle off the pen and throw away the capped needle (See Figure 22). See "How should I dispose of the used INTRON A Multidose Pens and needles?"

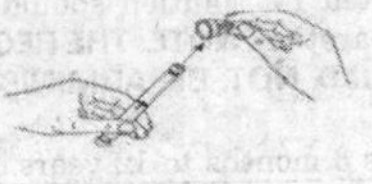

Figure 22

32. Replace the pen cap you removed in Step 4 above over the pen reservoir so that the black triangle is lined up with the dosage indicator (See Figure 23).

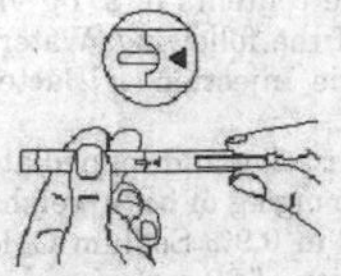

Figure 23

How should I dispose of the used INTRON A Multidose Pens and needles?

- Throw away all used needles and Multidose Pens in a puncture-proof container, sharps container, or a hard container like a metal can with a lid. Always place needles facing down. Do not use glass or clear plastic containers for disposal of needles and syringes. **Always keep the puncture-proof container out of the reach of children.**
- Check with your healthcare provider for instructions about the right way to throw away used needles and used Multidose Pens. There may be local or state laws about how to throw away used needles and Multidose Pens. Always follow the instructions of your healthcare provider.
- Do not throw away used needles and Multidose Pens in household trash and do not recycle them.

How should I store the INTRON® A Multidose Pen?

INTRON A in Multidose Pens:

Store in the refrigerator at 36°F to 46°F (2°C to 8°C).

◦ INTRON A Solution for Injection in the Multidose Pens may be used to give more than 1 injection of medicine.

Do not throw away used needles, syringes or the puncture-proof container in household trash and do not recycle them.

Keep INTRON A and all medicines out of the reach of children.

Schering Corporation, a subsidiary of **Merck & Co., Inc.**, Whitehouse Station, NJ 08889, USA

U.S. Patent Nos. 5,935,566 and 6,610,830

Novofine® is a registered trademark of Novo Nordisk A/S.

B-35038400T

Rev. 02/2011

Shown in Product Identification Guide, page 308

INVANZ® ℞

(ertapenem for injection)
for intravenous (IV) or intramuscular (IM) use

HIGHLIGHTS OF PRESCRIBING INFORMATION

These highlights do not include all the information needed to use INVANZ safely and effectively. See full prescribing information for INVANZ.

INVANZ® (ertapenem for injection) for intravenous (IV) or intramuscular (IM) use

Initial U.S. Approval: 2001

To reduce the development of drug-resistant bacteria and maintain the effectiveness of INVANZ and other antibacterial drugs, INVANZ should be used only to treat or prevent infections that are proven or strongly suspected to be caused by susceptible bacteria. (1)

INDICATIONS AND USAGE

INVANZ is a penem antibacterial indicated in adult patients and pediatric patients (3 months of age and older) for the treatment of the following moderate to severe infections caused by susceptible bacteria:

- Complicated intra-abdominal infections. (1.1)
- Complicated skin and skin structure infections, including diabetic foot infections without osteomyelitis. (1.2)
- Community-acquired pneumonia. (1.3)
- Complicated urinary tract infections including pyelonephritis. (1.4)
- Acute pelvic infections including postpartum endomyometritis, septic abortion and post surgical gynecologic infections. (1.5)

INVANZ is indicated in adults for the prophylaxis of surgical site infection following elective colorectal surgery. (1.6)

DOSAGE AND ADMINISTRATION

Do not mix or co-infuse INVANZ with other medications. Do not use diluents containing dextrose (α–D–glucose). (2.1)

INVANZ should be infused over 30 minutes in both the Treatment and Prophylactic regimens. (2.1)

Dosing considerations should be made in adults with advanced or end-stage renal impairment and those on hemodialysis. (2.4, 2.5)

Treatment regimen:

- Adults and pediatric patients 13 years of age and older. The dosage should be 1 gram once a day intravenously or intramuscularly. (2.2)
- Patients 3 months to 12 years of age should be administered 15 mg/kg twice daily (not to exceed 1 g/day intravenously or intramuscularly.) (2.2)
- Intravenous infusion may be administered in adults and pediatrics for up to 14 days or intramuscular injection for up to 7 days. (2.1)

Prophylaxis regimen for adults:

- 1 gram single dose given 1 hour prior to elective colorectal surgery. (2.3)

DOSAGE FORMS AND STRENGTHS

- Vial 1 gram. (3)
- ADD-Vantage® vial: 1 gram. (3)

CONTRAINDICATIONS

- Known hypersensitivity to product components or anaphylactic reactions to β-lactams. (4)
- Due to the use of lidocaine HCl as a diluent, INVANZ administered intramuscularly is contraindicated in patients with a known hypersensitivity to local anesthetics of the amide type. (4)

WARNINGS AND PRECAUTIONS

- Serious hypersensitivity (anaphylactic) reactions have been reported in patients receiving β-lactams. (5.1)
- Seizures and other central nervous system adverse experiences have been reported during treatment. (5.2)
- Co-administration of INVANZ with valproic acid or divalproex sodium reduces the serum concentration of valproic acid potentially increasing the risk of breakthrough seizures. (5.3)
- *Clostridium difficile*-associated diarrhea (ranging from mild diarrhea to fatal colitis): Evaluate if diarrhea occurs. (5.4)
- Caution should be taken when administering INVANZ intramuscularly to avoid inadvertent injection into a blood vessel. (5.5)

ADVERSE REACTIONS

Adults:

The most common adverse reactions (≥5%) in patients treated with INVANZ, including those who were switched to therapy with an oral antimicrobial, were diarrhea, nausea, headache and infused vein complication. (6.1)

In the prophylaxis indication the overall adverse experience profile was generally comparable to that observed for ertapenem in other clinical trials. (6.1)

Pediatrics:

Adverse reactions in this population were comparable to adults. The most common adverse reactions (≥5%) in pediatric patients treated with INVANZ, including those who were switched to therapy with an oral antimicrobial, were diarrhea, vomiting and infusion site pain. (6.1)

To report SUSPECTED ADVERSE REACTIONS, contact Merck Sharp & Dohme Corp., a subsidiary of Merck & Co., Inc., at 1-877-888-4231 or FDA at 1-800-FDA-1088 or www.fda.gov/medwatch.

DRUG INTERACTIONS

- Co-administration with probenecid inhibits the renal excretion of ertapenem and is therefore not recommended. (7.1)
- The concomitant use of ertapenem and valproic acid/divalproex sodium is generally not recommended. Antibacterials other than carbapenems should be considered to treat infections in patients whose seizures are well controlled on valproic acid or divalproex sodium. (5.2, 7.2)

USE IN SPECIFIC POPULATIONS

- Renal Impairment: Dose adjustment is necessary, if creatinine clearance is ≤30 mL/min/1.73 m². (2.4, 8.6, 12.3)

See 17 for PATIENT COUNSELING INFORMATION

Revised: 06/2013

FULL PRESCRIBING INFORMATION: CONTENTS*

*** Sections or subsections omitted from the full prescribing information are not listed**

FULL PRESCRIBING INFORMATION

1 INDICATIONS AND USAGE

To reduce the development of drug-resistant bacteria and maintain the effectiveness of INVANZ® and other antibacterial drugs, INVANZ should be used only to treat or prevent infections that are proven or strongly suspected to be caused by susceptible bacteria. When culture and susceptibility information are available, they should be considered in selecting or modifying antibacterial therapy. In the absence of such data, local epidemiology and susceptibility patterns may contribute to the empiric selection of therapy.

Treatment

INVANZ is indicated for the treatment of adult patients and pediatric patients (3 months of age and older) with the following moderate to severe infections caused by susceptible isolates of the designated microorganisms *[see Dosage and Administration (2)]*.

1.1 Complicated Intra-Abdominal Infections

INVANZ is indicated for the treatment of complicated intra-abdominal infections due to *Escherichia coli*, *Clostridium clostridioforme*, *Eubacterium lentum*, *Peptostreptococcus* species, *Bacteroides fragilis*, *Bacteroides distasonis*, *Bacteroides ovatus*, *Bacteroides thetaiotaomicron*, or *Bacteroides uniformis*.

1.2 Complicated Skin and Skin Structure Infections, Including Diabetic Foot Infections without Osteomyelitis

INVANZ is indicated for the treatment of complicated skin and skin structure infections, including diabetic foot infections without osteomyelitis due to *Staphylococcus aureus* (methicillin susceptible isolates only), *Streptococcus agalactiae*, *Streptococcus pyogenes*, *Escherichia coli*, *Klebsiella pneumoniae*, *Proteus mirabilis*, *Bacteroides fragilis*, *Peptostreptococcus* species, *Porphyromonas asaccharolytica*, or *Prevotella bivia*. INVANZ has not been studied in diabetic foot infections with concomitant osteomyelitis *[see Clinical Studies (14)]*.

1.3 Community Acquired Pneumonia

INVANZ is indicated for the treatment of community acquired pneumonia due to *Streptococcus pneumoniae* (peni-

Table 1: Treatment Guidelines for Adults and Pediatric Patients With Normal Renal Function* and Body Weight

Infection†	Daily Dose (IV or IM) Adults and Pediatric Patients 13 years of age and older	Daily Dose (IV or IM) Pediatric Patients 3 months to 12 years of age	Recommended Duration of Total Antimicrobial Treatment
Complicated intra-abdominal infections	1 g	15 mg/kg twice daily‡	5 to 14 days
Complicated skin and skin structure infections, including diabetic foot infections§	1 g	15 mg/kg twice daily‡	7 to 14 days¶
Community acquired pneumonia	1 g	15 mg/kg twice daily‡	10 to 14 days#
Complicated urinary tract infections, including pyelonephritis	1 g	15 mg/kg twice daily‡	10 to 14 days#
Acute pelvic infections including postpartum endomyometritis, septic abortion and post surgical gynecologic infections	1 g	15 mg/kg twice daily‡	3 to 10 days

* defined as creatinine clearance >90 mL/min/1.73 m^2
† due to the designated pathogens *[see Indications and Usage (1)]*
‡ not to exceed 1 g/day
§ INVANZ has not been studied in diabetic foot infections with concomitant osteomyelitis *[see Clinical Studies (14.1)]*.
¶ adult patients with diabetic foot infections received up to 28 days of treatment (parenteral or parenteral plus oral switch therapy)
# duration includes a possible switch to an appropriate oral therapy, after at least 3 days of parenteral therapy, once clinical improvement has been demonstrated.

cillin susceptible isolates only) including cases with concurrent bacteremia, *Haemophilus influenzae* (beta-lactamase negative isolates only), or *Moraxella catarrhalis*.

1.4 Complicated Urinary Tract Infections Including Pyelonephritis

INVANZ is indicated for the treatment of complicated urinary tract infections including pyelonephritis due to *Escherichia coli*, including cases with concurrent bacteremia, or *Klebsiella pneumoniae*.

1.5 Acute Pelvic Infections Including Postpartum Endomyometritis, Septic Abortion and Post Surgical Gynecologic Infections

INVANZ is indicated for the treatment of acute pelvic infections including postpartum endomyometritis, septic abortion and post surgical gynecological infections due to *Streptococcus agalactiae, Escherichia coli, Bacteroides fragilis, Porphyromonas asaccharolytica, Peptostreptococcus* species, or *Prevotella bivia*.

Prevention

INVANZ is indicated in adults for:

1.6 Prophylaxis of Surgical Site Infection Following Elective Colorectal Surgery

INVANZ is indicated for the prevention of surgical site infection following elective colorectal surgery.

2 DOSAGE AND ADMINISTRATION

2.1 Instructions for Use in All Patients

For Intravenous or Intramuscular Use

DO NOT MIX OR CO-INFUSE INVANZ WITH OTHER MEDICATIONS. DO NOT USE DILUENTS CONTAINING DEXTROSE (α-D-GLUCOSE).

INVANZ may be administered by intravenous infusion for up to 14 days or intramuscular injection for up to 7 days. When administered intravenously, INVANZ should be infused over a period of 30 minutes. Intramuscular administration of INVANZ may be used as an alternative to intravenous administration in the treatment of those infections for which intramuscular therapy is appropriate.

2.2 Treatment Regimen

13 years of age and older

The dose of INVANZ in patients 13 years of age and older is 1 gram (g) given once a day *[see Clinical Pharmacology (12.3)]*.

3 months to 12 years of age

The dose of INVANZ in patients 3 months to 12 years of age is 15 mg/kg twice daily (not to exceed 1 g/day).

Table 1 presents treatment guidelines for INVANZ.

[See table 1 above]

2.3 Prophylactic Regimen in Adults

Table 2 presents prophylaxis guidelines for INVANZ.

Table 2: Prophylaxis Guidelines for Adults

Indication	Daily Dose (IV) Adults	Recommended Duration of Total Antimicrobial Treatment
Prophylaxis of surgical site infection following elective colorectal surgery	1 g	Single intravenous dose given 1 hour prior to surgical incision

2.4 Patients with Renal Impairment

INVANZ may be used for the treatment of infections in adult patients with renal impairment. In patients whose creatinine clearance is >30 mL/min/1.73 m^2, no dosage adjustment is necessary. Adult patients with severe renal impairment (creatinine clearance ≤30 mL/min/1.73 m^2) and end-stage renal disease (creatinine clearance ≤10 mL/min/1.73 m^2) should receive 500 mg daily. A supplementary dose of 150 mg is recommended if ertapenem is administered within 6 hours prior to hemodialysis. There are no data in pediatric patients with renal impairment.

2.5 Patients on Hemodialysis

When adult patients on hemodialysis are given the recommended daily dose of 500 mg of INVANZ within 6 hours prior to hemodialysis, a supplementary dose of 150 mg is recommended following the hemodialysis session. If INVANZ is given at least 6 hours prior to hemodialysis, no supplementary dose is needed. There are no data in patients undergoing peritoneal dialysis or hemofiltration. There are no data in pediatric patients on hemodialysis.

When only the serum creatinine is available, the following formula[1] may be used to estimate creatinine clearance. The serum creatinine should represent a steady state of renal function.

Males: $\dfrac{(\text{weight in kg}) \times (140\text{-age in years})}{(72) \times \text{serum creatinine (mg/100 mL)}}$

Females: (0.85) × (value calculated for males)

[1]Cockcroft and Gault equation: Cockcroft DW, Gault MH. Prediction of creatinine clearance from serum creatinine. Nephron. 1976

2.6 Patients with Hepatic Impairment

No dose adjustment recommendations can be made in patients with hepatic impairment *[see Use in Specific Populations (8.7) and Clinical Pharmacology (12.3)]*.

2.7 Preparation and Reconstitution for Administration Vials

Adults and pediatric patients 13 years of age and older

Preparation for intravenous administration:

DO NOT MIX OR CO-INFUSE INVANZ WITH OTHER MEDICATIONS. DO NOT USE DILUENTS CONTAINING DEXTROSE (α-D-GLUCOSE).

INVANZ MUST BE RECONSTITUTED AND THEN DILUTED PRIOR TO ADMINISTRATION.

1. Reconstitute the contents of a 1 g vial of INVANZ with 10 mL of one of the following: Water for Injection, 0.9% Sodium Chloride Injection or Bacteriostatic Water for Injection.
2. Shake well to dissolve and immediately transfer contents of the reconstituted vial to 50 mL of 0.9% Sodium Chloride Injection.
3. Complete the infusion within 6 hours of reconstitution.

Preparation for intramuscular administration:

INVANZ MUST BE RECONSTITUTED PRIOR TO ADMINISTRATION.

1. Reconstitute the contents of a 1 g vial of INVANZ with 3.2 mL of 1.0% lidocaine HCl injection[2] (**without epinephrine**). Shake vial thoroughly to form solution.
2. Immediately withdraw the contents of the vial and administer by deep intramuscular injection into a large muscle mass (such as the gluteal muscles or lateral part of the thigh).
3. The reconstituted IM solution should be used within 1 hour after preparation. **NOTE: THE RECONSTITUTED SOLUTION SHOULD NOT BE ADMINISTERED INTRAVENOUSLY.**

Pediatric patients 3 months to 12 years of age

Preparation for intravenous administration:

DO NOT MIX OR CO-INFUSE INVANZ WITH OTHER MEDICATIONS. DO NOT USE DILUENTS CONTAINING DEXTROSE (α-D-GLUCOSE).

INVANZ MUST BE RECONSTITUTED AND THEN DILUTED PRIOR TO ADMINISTRATION.

1. Reconstitute the contents of a 1 g vial of INVANZ with 10 mL of one of the following: Water for Injection, 0.9% Sodium Chloride Injection or Bacteriostatic Water for Injection.
2. Shake well to dissolve and immediately withdraw a volume equal to 15 mg/kg of body weight (not to exceed 1 g/day) and dilute in 0.9% Sodium Chloride Injection to a final concentration of 20 mg/mL or less.
3. Complete the infusion within 6 hours of reconstitution.

Preparation for intramuscular administration:

INVANZ MUST BE RECONSTITUTED PRIOR TO ADMINISTRATION.

1. Reconstitute the contents of a 1 g vial of INVANZ with 3.2 mL of 1.0% lidocaine HCl injection[2] (**without epinephrine**). Shake vial thoroughly to form solution.
2. Immediately withdraw a volume equal to 15 mg/kg of body weight (not to exceed 1 g/day) and administer by deep intramuscular injection into a large muscle mass (such as the gluteal muscles or lateral part of the thigh).
3. The reconstituted IM solution should be used within 1 hour after preparation. **NOTE: THE RECONSTITUTED SOLUTION SHOULD NOT BE ADMINISTERED INTRAVENOUSLY.**

ADD-Vantage®[3] Vials

INVANZ in ADD-Vantage® vials should be reconstituted with ADD-Vantage® diluent containers containing 50 mL or 100 mL of 0.9% Sodium Chloride Injection.

[2]Refer to the prescribing information for lidocaine HCl.
[3]Registered trademark of Hospira Laboratories, Inc.

INSTRUCTIONS FOR USE OF
INVANZ®
(Ertapenem for Injection)
IN ADD-Vantage VIALS
For I.V. Use Only.

To Open Diluent Container:

Peel overwrap from the corner and remove container. Some opacity of the plastic due to moisture absorption during the sterilization process may be observed. This is normal and does not affect the solution quality or safety. The opacity will diminish gradually.

To Assemble Vial and Flexible Diluent Container:

(Use Aseptic Technique)

Remove the protective covers from the top of the vial and the vial port on the diluent container as follows:

To remove the breakaway vial cap, swing the pull ring over the top of the vial and pull down far enough to start the opening. (SEE FIGURE 1.) Pull the ring approximately half way around the cap and then pull straight up to remove the cap. (SEE FIGURE 2.) NOTE: DO NOT ACCESS VIAL WITH SYRINGE.

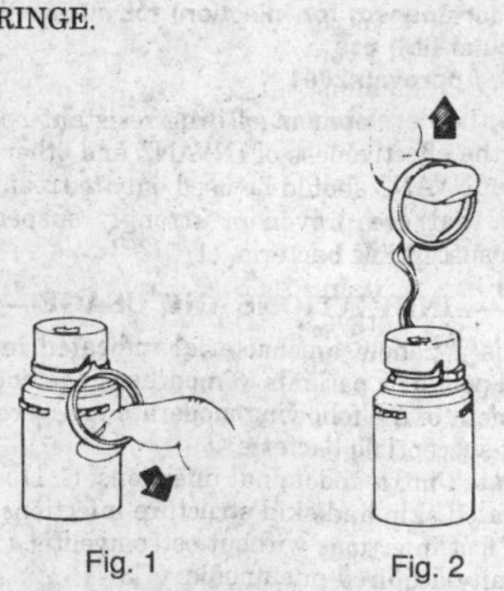

Fig. 1 Fig. 2

To remove the vial port cover, grasp the tab on the pull ring, pull up to break the three tie strings, then pull back to remove the cover. (SEE FIGURE 3.)

Screw the vial into the vial port until it will go no further. THE VIAL MUST BE SCREWED IN TIGHTLY TO ASSURE A SEAL. This occurs approximately ½ turn (180°) after the first audible click. (SEE FIGURE 4.) The clicking sound does not assure a seal; the vial must be turned as far as it will go. NOTE: Once vial is seated, do not attempt to remove. (SEE FIGURE 4.)

Recheck the vial to assure that it is tight by trying to turn it further in the direction of assembly.

Label appropriately.

Fig. 3

Fig. 4

To Prepare Admixture:
Squeeze the bottom of the diluent container gently to inflate the portion of the container surrounding the end of the drug vial.
With the other hand, push the drug vial down into the container telescoping the walls of the container. Grasp the inner cap of the vial through the walls of the container. (SEE FIGURE 5.)
Pull the inner cap from the drug vial. (SEE FIGURE 6.) Verify that the rubber stopper has been pulled out, allowing the drug and diluent to mix.
Mix container contents thoroughly and use within the specified time.

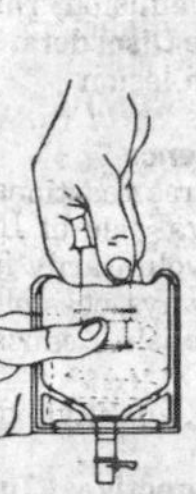

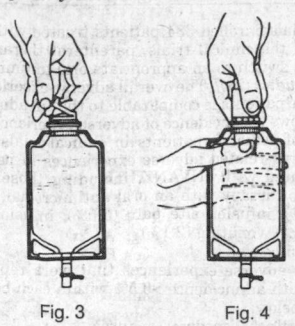
Fig. 5

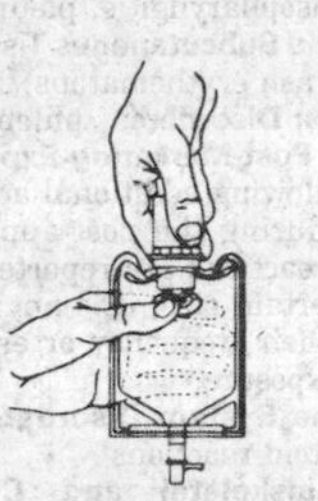
Fig. 6

Preparation for Administration:
(Use Aseptic Technique)
Confirm the activation and admixture of vial contents.
Check for leaks by squeezing container firmly. If leaks are found, discard unit as sterility may be impaired.
Close flow control clamp of administration set.
Remove cover from outlet port at bottom of container.
Insert piercing pin of administration set into port with a twisting motion until the pin is firmly seated. NOTE: See full directions on administration set carton.
Lift the free end of the hanger loop on the bottom of the vial, breaking the two tie strings. Bend the loop outward to lock it in the upright position, then suspend container from hanger.
Squeeze and release drip chamber to establish proper fluid level in chamber.
Open flow control clamp and clear air from set. Close clamp.
Attach set to venipuncture device. If device is not indwelling, prime and make venipuncture.
Regulate rate of administration with flow control clamp.
WARNING: Do not use flexible container in series connections.
Storage
INVANZ (Ertapenem for Injection) 1 g single dose ADD-Vantage® vials should be prepared with ADD-Vantage® diluent containers containing 50 mL or 100 mL of 0.9% Sodium Chloride Injection. When prepared with this diluent, INVANZ (Ertapenem for Injection) maintains satisfactory potency **for 6 hours at room temperature (25°C) or for 24 hours under refrigeration (5°C) and used within 4 hours after removal from refrigeration. Solutions of INVANZ should not be frozen.**
Before administering, see accompanying package circular for INVANZ (Ertapenem for Injection).
Parenteral drug products should be inspected visually for particulate matter and discoloration prior to use, whenever solution and container permit. Solutions of INVANZ range from colorless to pale yellow. Variations of color within this range do not affect the potency of the product.

3 DOSAGE FORMS AND STRENGTHS

Vials
INVANZ is a sterile lyophilized powder in a vial containing 1.046 g ertapenem sodium equivalent to 1 g ertapenem for intravenous infusion or for intramuscular injection.
ADD-Vantage® Vials
INVANZ is a lyophilized powder in an ADD-Vantage® vial containing 1.046 g ertapenem sodium equivalent to 1 g ertapenem for intravenous infusion.

4 CONTRAINDICATIONS

- INVANZ is contraindicated in patients with known hypersensitivity to any component of this product or to other drugs in the same class or in patients who have demonstrated anaphylactic reactions to beta-lactams.
- Due to the use of lidocaine HCl as a diluent, INVANZ administered intramuscularly is contraindicated in patients with a known hypersensitivity to local anesthetics of the amide type.

5 WARNINGS AND PRECAUTIONS

5.1 Hypersensitivity Reactions

Serious and occasionally fatal hypersensitivity (anaphylactic) reactions have been reported in patients receiving therapy with beta-lactams. These reactions are more likely to occur in individuals with a history of sensitivity to multiple allergens. There have been reports of individuals with a history of penicillin hypersensitivity who have experienced severe hypersensitivity reactions when treated with another beta-lactam. Before initiating therapy with INVANZ, careful inquiry should be made concerning previous hypersensitivity reactions to penicillins, cephalosporins, other beta-lactams and other allergens. If an allergic reaction to INVANZ occurs, discontinue the drug immediately. Serious anaphylactic reactions require immediate emergency treatment as clinically indicated.

5.2 Seizure Potential

Seizures and other central nervous system (CNS) adverse experiences have been reported during treatment with INVANZ *[see Adverse Reactions (6.1)]*. During clinical investigations in adult patients treated with INVANZ (1 g once a day), seizures, irrespective of drug relationship, occurred in 0.5% of patients during study therapy plus 14-day follow-up period *[see Adverse Reactions (6.1)]*. These experiences have occurred most commonly in patients with CNS disorders (e.g., brain lesions or history of seizures) and/or compromised renal function. Close adherence to the recommended dosage regimen is urged, especially in patients with known factors that predispose to convulsive activity. Anticonvulsant therapy should be continued in patients with known seizure disorders. If focal tremors, myoclonus, or seizures occur, patients should be evaluated neurologically, placed on anticonvulsant therapy if not already instituted, and the dosage of INVANZ re-examined to determine whether it should be decreased or discontinued.

5.3 Interaction with Valproic Acid

Case reports in the literature have shown that co-administration of carbapenems, including ertapenem, to patients receiving valproic acid or divalproex sodium results in a reduction in valproic acid concentrations. The valproic acid concentrations may drop below the therapeutic range as a result of this interaction, therefore increasing the risk of breakthrough seizures. Increasing the dose of valproic acid or divalproex sodium may not be sufficient to overcome this interaction. The concomitant use of ertapenem and valproic acid/divalproex sodium is generally not recommended. Anti-bacterials other than carbapenems should be considered to treat infections in patients whose seizures are well controlled on valproic acid or divalproex sodium. If administration of INVANZ is necessary, supplemental anticonvulsant therapy should be considered *[see Drug Interactions (7.2)]*.

5.4 *Clostridium difficile*-Associated Diarrhea (CDAD)

CDAD has been reported with use of nearly all antibacterial agents, including ertapenem, and may range in severity from mild diarrhea to fatal colitis. Treatment with antibacterial agents alters the normal flora of the colon leading to overgrowth of *Clostridium difficile*.
Clostridium difficile produces toxins A and B which contribute to the development of CDAD. Hypertoxin producing strains of *Clostridium difficile* cause increased morbidity and mortality, as these infections can be refractory to antimicrobial therapy and may require colectomy. CDAD must be considered in all patients who present with diarrhea following antibiotic use. Careful medical history is necessary since CDAD has been reported to occur over two months after the administration of antibacterial agents.
If CDAD is suspected or confirmed, ongoing antibiotic use not directed against *Clostridium difficile* may need to be discontinued. Appropriate fluid and electrolyte management, protein supplementation, antibiotic treatment of *Clostridium difficile*, and surgical evaluation should be instituted as clinically indicated.

5.5 Caution with Intramuscular Administration

Caution should be taken when administering INVANZ intramuscularly to avoid inadvertent injection into a blood vessel *[see Dosage and Administration (2.7)]*.

5.6 Development of Drug-Resistant Bacteria

As with other antibiotics, prolonged use of INVANZ may result in overgrowth of non-susceptible organisms. Repeated evaluation of the patient's condition is essential. If superinfection occurs during therapy, appropriate measures should be taken.
Prescribing INVANZ in the absence of a proven or strongly suspected bacterial infection or a prophylactic indication is unlikely to provide benefit to the patient and increases the risk of the development of drug-resistant bacteria.

5.7 Laboratory Tests

While INVANZ possesses toxicity similar to the beta-lactam group of antibiotics, periodic assessment of organ system function, including renal, hepatic, and hematopoietic, is advisable during prolonged therapy.

6 ADVERSE REACTIONS

The following are described in greater detail in the Warnings and Precautions section.
- Hypersensitivity Reactions *[see Warnings and Precautions (5.1)]*
- Seizure Potential *[see Warnings and Precautions (5.2)]*
- Interaction with Valproic Acid *[see Warnings and Precautions (5.3)]*
- *Clostridium difficile*-Associated Diarrhea (CDAD) *[see Warnings and Precautions (5.4)]*
- Caution with Intramuscular Administration *[see Warnings and Precautions (5.5)]*
- Development of Drug-Resistant Bacteria *[see Warnings and Precautions (5.6)]*
- Laboratory Tests *[see Warnings and Precautions (5.7)]*

6.1 Clinical Trials Experience

Because clinical trials are conducted under widely varying conditions, adverse reaction rates observed in the clinical trials of a drug cannot be directly compared to rates in the clinical trials of another drug and may not reflect the rates observed in practice.
Adults Receiving INVANZ as a Treatment Regimen
Clinical trials enrolled 1954 patients treated with INVANZ; in some of the clinical trials, parenteral therapy was followed by a switch to an appropriate oral antimicrobial *[see Clinical Studies (14)]*. Most adverse experiences reported in these clinical trials were described as mild to moderate in severity. INVANZ was discontinued due to adverse experiences in 4.7% of patients. Table 3 shows the incidence of adverse experiences reported in ≥2.0% of patients in these trials. The most common drug-related adverse experiences in patients treated with INVANZ, including those who were switched to therapy with an oral antimicrobial, were diarrhea (5.5%), infused vein complication (3.7%), nausea (3.1%), headache (2.2%), and vaginitis in females (2.1%).
[See table 3 at top of next page]
In patients treated for complicated intra-abdominal infections, death occurred in 4.7% (15/316) of patients receiving INVANZ and 2.6% (8/307) of patients receiving comparator drug. These deaths occurred in patients with significant co-morbidity and/or severe baseline infections. Deaths were considered unrelated to study drugs by investigators.
In clinical trials, seizure was reported during study therapy plus 14-day follow-up period in 0.5% of patients treated with INVANZ, 0.3% of patients treated with piperacillin/tazobactam and 0% of patients treated with ceftriaxone *[see Warnings and Precautions (5.2)]*.
Additional adverse experiences that were reported with INVANZ with an incidence >0.1% within each body system are listed below
Body as a Whole: abdominal distention, pain, chills, septicemia, septic shock, dehydration, gout, malaise, asthenia/fatigue, necrosis, candidiasis, weight loss, facial edema, injection site induration, injection site pain, extravasation, phlebitis/thrombophlebitis, flank pain, syncope
Cardiovascular System: heart failure, hematoma, chest pain, hypertension, tachycardia, cardiac arrest, bradycardia, arrhythmia, atrial fibrillation, heart murmur, ventricular tachycardia, asystole, subdural hemorrhage
Digestive System: acid regurgitation, oral candidiasis, dyspepsia, gastrointestinal hemorrhage, anorexia, flatulence, *C. difficile*-associated diarrhea, stomatitis, dysphagia, hemorrhoids, ileus, cholelithiasis, duodenitis, esophagitis, gastritis, jaundice, mouth ulcer, pancreatitis, pyloric stenosis
Musculoskeletal System: leg pain
Nervous System & Psychiatric: anxiety, nervousness, seizure *[see Warnings and Precautions (5.2)]*, tremor, depression, hypesthesia, spasm, paresthesia, aggressive behavior, vertigo
Respiratory System: cough, pharyngitis, rales/rhonchi, respiratory distress, pleural effusion, hypoxemia, bronchoconstriction, pharyngeal discomfort, epistaxis, pleuritic pain, asthma, hemoptysis, hiccups, voice disturbance
Skin & Skin Appendage: erythema, sweating, dermatitis, desquamation, flushing, urticaria
Special Senses: taste perversion
Urogenital System: renal impairment, oliguria/anuria, vaginal pruritus, hematuria, urinary retention, bladder dysfunction, vaginal candidiasis, vulvovaginitis.
In a clinical trial for the treatment of diabetic foot infections in which 289 adult diabetic patients were treated with INVANZ, the adverse experience profile was generally similar to that seen in previous clinical trials.
Prophylaxis of Surgical Site Infection following Elective Colorectal Surgery
In a clinical trial in adults for the prophylaxis of surgical site infection following elective colorectal surgery in which

Table 3: Incidence (%) of Adverse Experiences Reported During Study Therapy Plus 14-Day Follow-Up in ≥2.0% of Adult Patients Treated With INVANZ in Clinical Trials

Adverse Events	INVANZ* 1 g daily (N=802)	Piperacillin/ Tazobactam* 3.375 g q6h (N=774)	INVANZ† 1 g daily (N=1152)	Ceftriaxone† 1 or 2 g daily (N=942)
Local:				
Infused vein complication	7.1	7.9	5.4	6.7
Systemic:				
Death	2.5	1.6	1.3	1.6
Edema/swelling	3.4	2.5	2.9	3.3
Fever	5.0	6.6	2.3	3.4
Abdominal pain	3.6	4.8	4.3	3.9
Hypotension	2.0	1.4	1.0	1.2
Constipation	4.0	5.4	3.3	3.1
Diarrhea	10.3	12.1	9.2	9.8
Nausea	8.5	8.7	6.4	7.4
Vomiting	3.7	5.3	4.0	4.0
Altered mental status‡	5.1	3.4	3.3	2.5
Dizziness	2.1	3.0	1.5	2.1
Headache	5.6	5.4	6.8	6.9
Insomnia	3.2	5.2	3.0	4.1
Dyspnea	2.6	1.8	1.0	2.4
Pruritus	2.0	2.6	1.0	1.9
Rash	2.5	3.1	2.3	1.5
Vaginitis	1.4	1.0	3.3	3.7

* Includes Phase IIb/III Complicated intra-abdominal infections, Complicated skin and skin structure infections and Acute pelvic infections trials
† Includes Phase IIb/III Community acquired pneumonia and Complicated urinary tract infections, and Phase IIa trials
‡ Includes agitation, confusion, disorientation, decreased mental acuity, changed mental status, somnolence, stupor

Table 5: Incidence (%) of Adverse Experiences Reported During Study Therapy Plus 14-Day Follow-Up in ≥2.0% of Pediatric Patients Treated With INVANZ in Clinical Trials

Adverse Events	INVANZ*,† (N=384)	Ceftriaxone* (N=100)	Ticarcillin/Clavulanate† (N=24)
Local:			
Infusion Site Erythema	3.9	3.0	8.3
Infusion Site Pain	7.0	4.0	20.8
Systemic:			
Abdominal Pain	4.7	3.0	4.2
Constipation	2.3	0.0	0.0
Diarrhea	11.7	17.0	4.2
Loose Stools	2.1	0.0	0.0
Vomiting	10.2	11.0	8.3
Pyrexia	4.9	6.0	8.3
Upper Respiratory Tract Infection	2.3	3.0	0.0
Headache	4.4	4.0	0.0
Cough	4.4	3.0	0.0
Diaper Dermatitis	4.7	4.0	0.0
Rash	2.9	2.0	8.3

* Includes Phase IIb Complicated skin and skin structure infections, Community acquired pneumonia and Complicated urinary tract infections trials in which patients 3 months to 12 years of age received INVANZ 15 mg/kg IV twice daily up to a maximum of 1 g or ceftriaxone 50 mg/kg/day IV in two divided doses up to a maximum of 2 g, and patients 13 to 17 years of age received INVANZ 1 g IV daily or ceftriaxone 50 mg/kg/day IV in a single daily dose.
† Includes Phase IIb Acute pelvic infections and Complicated intra-abdominal infections trials in which patients 3 months to 12 years of age received INVANZ 15 mg/kg IV twice daily up to a maximum of 1 g and patients 13 to 17 years of age received INVANZ 1 g IV daily or ticarcillin/clavulanate 50 mg/kg for patients <60 kg or ticarcillin/clavulanate 3.0 g for patients >60 kg, 4 or 6 times a day.

476 patients received a 1 g dose of INVANZ 1 hour prior to surgery and were then followed for safety 14 days post surgery, the overall adverse experience profile was generally comparable to that observed for INVANZ in previous clinical trials. Table 4 shows the incidence of adverse experiences other than those previously described above for INVANZ that were reported regardless of causality in ≥2.0% of patients in this trial.

Table 4: Incidence (%) of Adverse Experiences Reported During Study Therapy Plus 14-Day Follow-Up in ≥2.0% of Adult Patients Treated With INVANZ for Prophylaxis of Surgical Site Infections Following Elective Colorectal Surgery

Adverse Events	INVANZ 1 g (N = 476)	Cefotetan 2 g (N = 476)
Anemia	5.7	6.9
Small intestinal obstruction	2.1	1.9
Pneumonia	2.1	4.0
Postoperative infection	2.3	4.0
Urinary tract infection	3.8	5.5
Wound infection	6.5	12.4
Wound complication	2.9	2.3
Atelectasis	3.4	1.9

Additional adverse experiences that were reported in this prophylaxis trial with INVANZ, regardless of causality, with an incidence >0.5% within each body system are listed below:
Gastrointestinal Disorders: *C. difficile* infection or colitis, dry mouth, hematochezia
General Disorders and Administration Site Condition: crepitations
Infections and Infestations: cellulitis, abdominal abscess, fungal rash, pelvic abscess
Injury, Poisoning and Procedural Complications: incision site complication, incision site hemorrhage, intestinal stoma complication, anastomotic leak, seroma, wound dehiscence, wound secretion
Musculoskeletal and Connective Tissue Disorders: muscle spasms
Nervous System Disorders: cerebrovascular accident
Renal and Urinary Disorders: dysuria, pollakiuria
Respiratory, Thoracic and Mediastinal Disorders: crackles lung, lung infiltration, pulmonary congestion, pulmonary embolism, wheezing.

Pediatric Patients Receiving INVANZ as a Treatment Regimen

Clinical trials enrolled 384 patients treated with INVANZ; in some of the clinical trials, parenteral therapy was followed by a switch to an appropriate oral antimicrobial *[see Clinical Studies (14)]*. The overall adverse experience profile in pediatric patients is comparable to that in adult patients. Table 5 shows the incidence of adverse experiences reported in ≥2.0% of pediatric patients in clinical trials. The most common drug-related adverse experiences in pediatric patients treated with INVANZ, including those who were switched to therapy with an oral antimicrobial, were diarrhea (6.5%), infusion site pain (5.5%), infusion site erythema (2.6%), vomiting (2.1%).

[See table 5 below]

Additional adverse experiences that were reported with INVANZ with an incidence >0.5% within each body system are listed below:
Gastrointestinal Disorders: nausea
General Disorders and Administration Site Condition: hypothermia, chest pain, upper abdominal pain; infusion site pruritus, induration, phlebitis, swelling, and warmth
Infections and Infestations: candidiasis, oral candidiasis, viral pharyngitis, herpes simplex, ear infection, abdominal abscess
Metabolism and Nutrition Disorders: decreased appetite
Musculoskeletal and Connective Tissue Disorders: arthralgia
Nervous System Disorders: dizziness, somnolence
Psychiatric Disorders: insomnia
Reproductive System and Breast Disorders: genital rash
Respiratory, Thoracic and Mediastinal Disorders: wheezing, nasopharyngitis, pleural effusion, rhinitis, rhinorrhea
Skin and Subcutaneous Tissue Disorders: dermatitis, pruritus, rash erythematous, skin lesion
Vascular Disorders: phlebitis.

6.2 Post-Marketing Experience

The following additional adverse reactions have been identified during the post-approval use of INVANZ. Because these reactions are reported voluntarily from a population of uncertain size, it is not always possible to reliably estimate their frequency or establish a causal relationship to drug exposure.
Immune System Disorders: anaphylaxis including anaphylactoid reactions
Musculoskeletal and Connective Tissue Disorders: muscular weakness
Nervous System Disorders: coordination abnormal, depressed level of consciousness, dyskinesia, gait disturbance, myoclonus, tremor
Psychiatric Disorders: altered mental status (including aggression, delirium), hallucinations
Skin and Subcutaneous Tissue Disorders: Drug Rash with Eosinophilia and Systemic Symptoms (DRESS syndrome)

6.3 Adverse Laboratory Changes in Clinical Trials

Adults Receiving INVANZ as Treatment Regimen

Laboratory adverse experiences that were reported during therapy in ≥2.0% of adult patients treated with INVANZ in clinical trials are presented in Table 6. Drug-related laboratory adverse experiences that were reported during therapy in ≥2.0% of adult patients treated with INVANZ, including those who were switched to therapy with an oral antimicrobial, in clinical trials were ALT increased (6.0%), AST increased (5.2%), serum alkaline phosphatase increased (3.4%), and platelet count increased (2.8%). INVANZ was discontinued due to laboratory adverse experiences in 0.3% of patients.

[See table 6 at top of next page]

Additional laboratory adverse experiences that were reported during therapy in >0.1% of patients treated with INVANZ in clinical trials include: increases in serum creatinine, serum glucose, BUN, total, direct and indirect serum bilirubin, serum sodium and potassium, PT and PTT; decreases in serum potassium, serum albumin, WBC, platelet count, and segmented neutrophils.

In a clinical trial for the treatment of diabetic foot infections in which 289 adult diabetic patients were treated with INVANZ, the laboratory adverse experience profile was generally similar to that seen in previous clinical trials.

Prophylaxis of Surgical Site Infection following Elective Colorectal Surgery

In a clinical trial in adults for the prophylaxis of surgical site infection following elective colorectal surgery in which 476 patients received a 1 g dose of INVANZ 1 hour prior to surgery and were then followed for safety 14 days post surgery, the overall laboratory adverse experience profile was generally comparable to that observed for INVANZ in previous clinical trials.

Pediatric Patients Receiving INVANZ as a Treatment Regimen

Laboratory adverse experiences that were reported during therapy in ≥2.0% of pediatric patients treated with INVANZ in clinical trials are presented in Table 7. Drug-related laboratory adverse experiences that were reported during therapy in ≥2.0% of pediatric patients treated with INVANZ, including those who were switched to therapy with an oral antimicrobial, in clinical trials were neutrophil count decreased (3.0%), ALT increased (2.2%), and AST increased (2.1%).

Table 7: Incidence* (%) of Specific Laboratory Adverse Experiences Reported During Study Therapy Plus 14-Day Follow-Up in ≥2.0% of Pediatric Patients Treated With INVANZ in Clinical Trials

Adverse laboratory experiences	INVANZ (n†=379)	Ceftriaxone (n†=97)	Ticarcillin/ Clavulanate (n†=24)
ALT Increased	3.8	1.1	4.3
AST Increased	3.8	1.1	4.3
Neutrophil Count Decreased	5.8	3.1	0.0

* Number of patients with laboratory adverse experiences/Number of patients with the laboratory test; where at least 300 patients had the test
† Number of patients with one or more laboratory tests

Additional laboratory adverse experiences that were reported during therapy in >0.5% of patients treated with INVANZ in clinical trials include: alkaline phosphatase increased, eosinophil count increased, platelet count increased, white blood cell count decreased and urine protein present.

7 DRUG INTERACTIONS

7.1 Probenecid

Probenecid interferes with the active tubular secretion of ertapenem, resulting in increased plasma concentrations of ertapenem *[see Clinical Pharmacology (12.3)]*. Co-administration of probenecid with ertapenem is not recommended.

7.2 Valproic Acid

Case reports in the literature have shown that co-administration of carbapenems, including ertapenem, to patients receiving valproic acid or divalproex sodium results in a reduction of valproic acid concentrations. The valproic acid concentrations may drop below the therapeutic range as a result of this interaction, therefore increasing the risk of breakthrough seizures. Although the mechanism of this interaction is unknown, data from *in vitro* and animal studies suggest that carbapenems may inhibit the hydrolysis of valproic acid's glucuronide metabolite (VPA-g) back to valproic acid, thus decreasing the serum concentrations of valproic acid *[see Warnings and Precautions (5.3)]*.

8 USE IN SPECIFIC POPULATIONS

8.1 Pregnancy

Pregnancy Category B

In mice and rats given intravenous doses of up to 700 mg/kg/day (for mice, approximately 3 times the recommended human dose of 1 g based on body surface area and for rats, approximately 1.2 times the human exposure at the recommended dose of 1 g based on plasma AUCs), there was no evidence of developmental toxicity as assessed by external, visceral, and skeletal examination of the fetuses. However, in mice given 700 mg/kg/day, slight decreases in average fetal weights and an associated decrease in the average number of ossified sacrocaudal vertebrae were observed. Ertapenem crosses the placental barrier in rats.

There are, however, no adequate and well-controlled trials in pregnant women. Because animal reproduction studies are not always predictive of human response, this drug should be used during pregnancy only if clearly needed.

8.2 Labor and Delivery

INVANZ has not been studied for use during labor and delivery.

8.3 Nursing Mothers

Ertapenem is excreted in human breast milk *[see Clinical Pharmacology (12.3)]*. Caution should be exercised when INVANZ is administered to a nursing woman. INVANZ should be administered to nursing mothers only when the expected benefit outweighs the risk.

8.4 Pediatric Use

Safety and effectiveness of INVANZ in pediatric patients 3 months to 17 years of age are supported by evidence from adequate and well-controlled trials in adults, pharmacokinetic data in pediatric patients, and additional data from comparator-controlled trials in pediatric patients 3 months to 17 years of age *[see Indications and Usage (1.1), (1.2), (1.3), (1.4) and (1.5) and Clinical Studies (14.2)]*.

INVANZ is not recommended in infants under 3 months of age as no data are available.

INVANZ is not recommended in the treatment of meningitis in the pediatric population due to lack of sufficient CSF penetration.

8.5 Geriatric Use

Of the 1,835 patients in Phase 2b/3 trials treated with INVANZ, approximately 26 percent were 65 and over, while approximately 12 percent were 75 and over. No overall differences in safety or effectiveness were observed between these patients and younger patients. Other reported clinical experience has not identified differences in responses between the elderly and younger patients, but greater sensitivity of some older individuals cannot be ruled out.

This drug is known to be substantially excreted by the kidney, and the risk of toxic reactions to this drug may be greater in patients with impaired renal function. Because elderly patients are more likely to have decreased renal function, care should be taken in dose selection, and it may be useful to monitor renal function *[see Dosage and Administration (2.2)]*.

Table 6: Incidence* (%) of Laboratory Adverse Experiences Reported During Study Therapy Plus 14-Day Follow-Up in ≥2.0% of Adult Patients Treated With INVANZ in Clinical Trials

Adverse laboratory experiences	INVANZ† 1 g daily (n§=766)	Piperacillin/ Tazobactam† 3.375 g q6h (n§=755)	INVANZ‡ 1 g daily (n§=1122)	Ceftriaxone‡ 1 or 2 g daily (n§=920)
ALT increased	8.8	7.3	8.3	6.9
AST increased	8.4	8.3	7.1	6.5
Serum alkaline phosphatase increased	6.6	7.2	4.3	2.8
Eosinophils increased	1.1	1.1	2.1	1.8
Hematocrit decreased	3.0	2.9	3.4	2.4
Hemoglobin decreased	4.9	4.7	4.5	3.5
Platelet count increased	6.5	6.3	4.3	3.5
Urine RBCs increased	2.5	2.9	1.1	1.0
Urine WBCs increased	2.5	3.2	1.6	1.1

* Number of patients with laboratory adverse experiences/Number of patients with the laboratory test
† Includes Phase IIb/III Complicated intra-abdominal infections, Complicated skin and skin structure infections and Acute pelvic infections trials
‡ Includes Phase IIb/III Community acquired pneumonia and Complicated urinary tract infections, and Phase IIa trials
§ Number of patients with one or more laboratory tests

Table 8: Plasma Concentrations of Ertapenem in Adults After Single Dose Administration

Dose/Route	Average Plasma Concentrations (mcg/mL) 0.5 hr	1 hr	2 hr	4 hr	6 hr	8 hr	12 hr	18 hr	24 hr
1 g IV*	155	115	83	48	31	20	9	3	1
1 g IM	33	53	67	57	40	27	13	4	2

* Infused at a constant rate over 30 minutes

8.6 Patients with Renal Impairment

Dosage adjustment is necessary in patients with creatinine clearance 30 mL/min or less *[see Dosage and Administration (2.4) and Clinical Pharmacology (12.3)]*.

8.7 Patients with Hepatic Impairment

The pharmacokinetics of ertapenem in patients with hepatic impairment have not been established. Of the total number of patients in clinical trials, 37 patients receiving ertapenem 1 g daily and 36 patients receiving comparator drugs were considered to have Child-Pugh Class A, B, or C liver impairment. The incidence of adverse experiences in patients with hepatic impairment was similar between the ertapenem group and the comparator groups.

10 OVERDOSAGE

No specific information is available on the treatment of overdosage with INVANZ. Intentional overdosing of INVANZ is unlikely. Intravenous administration of INVANZ at a dose of 2 g over 30 min or 3 g over 1-2h in healthy adult volunteers resulted in an increased incidence of nausea. In clinical trials in adults, inadvertent administration of three 1 g doses of INVANZ in a 24 hour period resulted in diarrhea and transient dizziness in one patient. In pediatric clinical trials, a single intravenous dose of 40 mg/kg up to a maximum of 2 g did not result in toxicity.

In the event of an overdose, INVANZ should be discontinued and general supportive treatment given until renal elimination takes place.

INVANZ can be removed by hemodialysis; the plasma clearance of the total fraction of ertapenem was increased 30% in subjects with end-stage renal disease when hemodialysis (4 hour session) was performed immediately following administration. However, no information is available on the use of hemodialysis to treat overdosage.

11 DESCRIPTION

INVANZ (Ertapenem for Injection) is a sterile, synthetic, parenteral, 1-β methyl-carbapenem that is structurally related to beta-lactam antibiotics.

Chemically, INVANZ is described as [4*R*-[3(3*S**,5*S**),4α,5β,6β(*R**)]]-3-[[5-[[(3-carboxyphenyl)amino]carbonyl]-3-pyrrolidinyl]thio]-6-(1-hydroxyethyl)-4-methyl-7-oxo-1-azabicyclo[3.2.0]hept-2-ene-2-carboxylic acid monosodium salt. Its molecular weight is 497.50. The empirical formula is $C_{22}H_{24}N_3O_7SNa$, and its structural formula is:

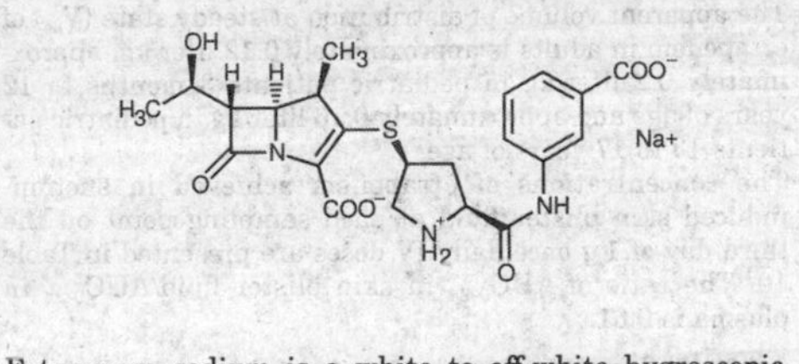

Ertapenem sodium is a white to off-white hygroscopic, weakly crystalline powder. It is soluble in water and 0.9% sodium chloride solution, practically insoluble in ethanol, and insoluble in isopropyl acetate and tetrahydrofuran.

INVANZ is supplied as sterile lyophilized powder for intravenous infusion after reconstitution with appropriate diluent *[see Dosage and Administration (2.7)]* and transfer to 50 mL 0.9% Sodium Chloride Injection or for intramuscular injection following reconstitution with 1% lidocaine hydrochloride. Each vial contains 1.046 grams ertapenem sodium, equivalent to 1 gram ertapenem. The sodium content is approximately 137 mg (approximately 6.0 mEq).

Each vial of INVANZ contains the following inactive ingredients: 175 mg sodium bicarbonate and sodium hydroxide to adjust pH to 7.5.

12 CLINICAL PHARMACOLOGY

12.1 Mechanism of Action

Ertapenem sodium is a carbapenem antibiotic *[see Clinical Pharmacology (12.4)]*.

12.3 Pharmacokinetics

Average plasma concentrations (mcg/mL) of ertapenem following a single 30-minute infusion of a 1 g intravenous (IV) dose and administration of a single 1 g intramuscular (IM) dose in healthy young adults are presented in Table 8.

[See table 8 above]

The area under the plasma concentration-time curve (AUC) of ertapenem in adults increased less-than dose-proportional based on total ertapenem concentrations over the 0.5 to 2 g dose range, whereas the AUC increased greater-than dose-proportional based on unbound ertapenem concentrations. Ertapenem exhibits non-linear pharmacokinetics due to concentration-dependent plasma protein binding at the proposed therapeutic dose *[see Clinical Pharmacology (12.3)]*. There is no accumulation of ertapenem following multiple IV or IM 1 g daily doses in healthy adults.

Average plasma concentrations (mcg/mL) of ertapenem in pediatric patients are presented in Table 9.

[See table 9 at top of next page]

Absorption

Ertapenem, reconstituted with 1% lidocaine HCl injection, USP (in saline without epinephrine), is almost completely absorbed following intramuscular (IM) administration at the recommended dose of 1 g. The mean bioavailability is approximately 90%. Following 1 g daily IM administration, mean peak plasma concentrations (C_{max}) are achieved in approximately 2.3 hours (T_{max}).

Table 9: Plasma Concentrations of Ertapenem in Pediatric Patients After Single IV* Dose Administration

Age Group	Dose	Average Plasma Concentrations (mcg/mL)							
		0.5 hr	1 hr	2 hr	4 hr	6 hr	8 hr	12 hr	24 hr
3 to 23 months									
	15 mg/kg†	103.8	57.3	43.6	23.7	13.5	8.2	2.5	-
	20 mg/kg†	126.8	87.6	58.7	28.4	-	12.0	3.4	0.4
	40 mg/kg‡	199.1	144.1	95.7	58.0	-	20.2	7.7	0.6
2 to 12 years									
	15 mg/kg†	113.2	63.9	42.1	21.9	12.8	7.6	3.0	-
	20 mg/kg†	147.6	97.6	63.2	34.5	-	12.3	4.9	0.5
	40 mg/kg‡	241.7	152.7	96.3	55.6	-	18.8	7.2	0.6
13 to 17 years									
	20 mg/kg†	170.4	98.3	67.8	40.4	-	16.0	7.0	1.1
	1 g§	155.9	110.9	74.8	-	24.0	-	6.2	-
	40 mg/kg‡	255.0	188.7	127.9	76.2	-	31.0	15.3	2.1

* Infused at a constant rate over 30 minutes
† up to a maximum dose of 1 g/day
‡ up to a maximum dose of 2 g/day
§ Based on three patients receiving 1 g ertapenem who volunteered for pharmacokinetic assessment in one of the two safety and efficacy trials

Distribution

Ertapenem is highly bound to human plasma proteins, primarily albumin. In healthy young adults, the protein binding of ertapenem decreases as plasma concentrations increase, from approximately 95% bound at an approximate plasma concentration of <100 micrograms (mcg)/mL to approximately 85% bound at an approximate plasma concentration of 300 mcg/mL.

The apparent volume of distribution at steady state (V_{ss}) of ertapenem in adults is approximately 0.12 liter/kg, approximately 0.2 liter/kg in pediatric patients 3 months to 12 years of age and approximately 0.16 liter/kg in pediatric patients 13 to 17 years of age.

The concentrations of ertapenem achieved in suction-induced skin blister fluid at each sampling point on the third day of 1 g once daily IV doses are presented in Table 10. The ratio of $AUC_{0\text{-}24}$ in skin blister fluid/$AUC_{0\text{-}24}$ in plasma is 0.61.

Table 10: Concentrations (mcg/mL) of Ertapenem in Adult Skin Blister Fluid at each Sampling Point on the Third Day of 1-g Once Daily IV Doses

0.5 hr	1 hr	2 hr	4 hr	8 hr	12 hr	24 hr
7	12	17	24	24	21	8

The concentration of ertapenem in breast milk from 5 lactating women with pelvic infections (5 to 14 days postpartum) was measured at random time points daily for 5 consecutive days following the last 1 g dose of intravenous therapy (3-10 days of therapy). The concentration of ertapenem in breast milk within 24 hours of the last dose of therapy in all 5 women ranged from <0.13 (lower limit of quantitation) to 0.38 mcg/mL; peak concentrations were not assessed. By day 5 after discontinuation of therapy, the level of ertapenem was undetectable in the breast milk of 4 women and below the lower limit of quantitation (<0.13 mcg/mL) in 1 woman.

Metabolism

In healthy young adults, after infusion of 1 g IV radiolabeled ertapenem, the plasma radioactivity consists predominantly (94%) of ertapenem. The major metabolite of ertapenem is the inactive ring-opened derivative formed by hydrolysis of the beta-lactam ring.

Elimination

Ertapenem is eliminated primarily by the kidneys. The mean plasma half-life in healthy young adults is approximately 4 hours and the plasma clearance is approximately 1.8 L/hour. The mean plasma half-life in pediatric patients 13 to 17 years of age is approximately 4 hours and approximately 2.5 hours in pediatric patients 3 months to 12 years of age.

Following the administration of 1 g IV radiolabeled ertapenem to healthy young adults, approximately 80% is recovered in urine and 10% in feces. Of the 80% recovered in urine, approximately 38% is excreted as unchanged drug and approximately 37% as the ring-opened metabolite.

In healthy young adults given a 1 g IV dose, the mean percentage of the administered dose excreted in urine was 17.4% during 0-2 hours postdose, 5.4% during 4-6 hours postdose, and 2.4% during 12-24 hours postdose.

Special Populations

Renal Impairment

Total and unbound fractions of ertapenem pharmacokinetics were investigated in 26 adult subjects (31 to 80 years of age) with varying degrees of renal impairment. Following a single 1 g IV dose of ertapenem, the unbound AUC increased 1.5-fold and 2.3-fold in subjects with mild renal impairment (CL_{CR} 60-90 mL/min/1.73 m^2) and moderate renal impairment (CL_{CR} 31-59 mL/min/1.73 m^2), respectively, compared with healthy young subjects (25 to 45 years of age). No dosage adjustment is necessary in patients with CL_{CR} ≥31 mL/min/1.73 m^2. The unbound AUC increased 4.4-fold and 7.6-fold in subjects with advanced renal impairment (CL_{CR} 5-30 mL/min/1.73 m^2) and end-stage renal disease (CL_{CR} <10 mL/min/1.73 m^2), respectively, compared with healthy young subjects. The effects of renal impairment on AUC of total drug were of smaller magnitude. The recommended dose of ertapenem in adult patients with CL_{CR} ≤30 mL/min/1.73 m^2 is 0.5 grams every 24 hours. Following a single 1 g IV dose given immediately prior to a 4 hour hemodialysis session in 5 adult patients with end-stage renal disease, approximately 30% of the dose was recovered in the dialysate. Dose adjustments are recommended for patients with severe renal impairment and end-stage renal disease *[see Dosage and Administration (2.4)]*. There are no data in pediatric patients with renal impairment.

Hepatic Impairment

The pharmacokinetics of ertapenem in patients with hepatic impairment have not been established. However, ertapenem does not appear to undergo hepatic metabolism based on *in vitro* studies and approximately 10% of an administered dose is recovered in the feces *[see Clinical Pharmacology (12.3)* and *Dosage and Administration (2.6)]*.

Gender

The effect of gender on the pharmacokinetics of ertapenem was evaluated in healthy male (n=8) and healthy female (n=8) subjects. The differences observed could be attributed to body size when body weight was taken into consideration. No dose adjustment is recommended based on gender.

Geriatric Patients

The impact of age on the pharmacokinetics of ertapenem was evaluated in healthy male (n=7) and healthy female (n=7) subjects ≥65 years of age. The total and unbound AUC increased 37% and 67%, respectively, in elderly adults relative to young adults. These changes were attributed to age-related changes in creatinine clearance. No dosage adjustment is necessary for elderly patients with normal (for their age) renal function.

Pediatric Patients

Plasma concentrations of ertapenem are comparable in pediatric patients 13 to 17 years of age and adults following a 1 g once daily IV dose.

Following the 20 mg/kg dose (up to a maximum dose of 1 g), the pharmacokinetic parameter values in patients 13 to 17 years of age (N=6) were generally comparable to those in healthy young adults.

Plasma concentrations at the midpoint of the dosing interval following a single 15 mg/kg IV dose of ertapenem in patients 3 months to 12 years of age are comparable to plasma concentrations at the midpoint of the dosing interval following a 1 g once daily IV dose in adults *[see Clinical Pharmacology (12.3)]*. The plasma clearance (mL/min/kg) of ertapenem in patients 3 months to 12 years of age is approximately 2-fold higher as compared to that in adults. At the 15 mg/kg dose, the AUC value (doubled to model a twice daily dosing regimen, i.e., 30 mg/kg/day exposure) in patients 3 months to 12 years of age was comparable to the AUC value in young healthy adults receiving a 1 g IV dose of ertapenem.

Drug Interactions

When ertapenem is co-administered with probenecid (500 mg p.o. every 6 hours), probenecid competes for active tubular secretion and reduces the renal clearance of ertapenem. Based on total ertapenem concentrations, probenecid increased the AUC of ertapenem by 25%, and reduced the plasma and renal clearance of ertapenem by 20% and 35%, respectively. The half-life of ertapenem was increased from 4.0 to 4.8 hours.

In vitro studies in human liver microsomes indicate that ertapenem does not inhibit metabolism mediated by any of the following cytochrome p450 (CYP) isoforms: 1A2, 2C9, 2C19, 2D6, 2E1 and 3A4.

In vitro studies indicate that ertapenem does not inhibit P-glycoprotein-mediated transport of digoxin or vinblastine and that ertapenem is not a substrate for P-glycoprotein-mediated transport.

12.4 Microbiology

Mechanism of Action

Ertapenem has *in vitro* activity against Gram-positive and Gram-negative aerobic and anaerobic bacteria. The bactericidal activity of ertapenem results from the inhibition of cell wall synthesis and is mediated through ertapenem binding to penicillin binding proteins (PBPs). In *Escherichia coli*, it has strong affinity toward PBPs 1a, 1b, 2, 3, 4 and 5 with preference for PBPs 2 and 3.

Mechanism of Resistance

Ertapenem is stable against hydrolysis by a variety of beta-lactamases, including penicillinases, and cephalosporinases and extended spectrum beta-lactamases. Ertapenem is hydrolyzed by metallo-beta-lactamases.

Ertapenem has been shown to be active against most isolates of the following microorganisms both *in vitro* and in clinical infections as described in the INDICATIONS AND USAGE section:

Gram-positive bacteria:

Staphylococcus aureus (methicillin susceptible isolates only)
Streptococcus agalactiae
Streptococcus pneumoniae (penicillin susceptible isolates only)
Streptococcus pyogenes

Gram-negative bacteria:

Escherichia coli
Haemophilus influenzae (beta-lactamase negative isolates only)
Klebsiella pneumoniae
Moraxella catarrhalis
Proteus mirabilis

Anaerobic bacteria:

Bacteroides fragilis
Bacteroides distasonis
Bacteroides ovatus
Bacteroides thetaiotaomicron
Bacteroides uniformis
Clostridium clostridioforme
Eubacterium lentum
Peptostreptococcus species
Porphyromonas asaccharolytica
Prevotella bivia

The following *in vitro* data are available, **but their clinical significance is unknown**. At least 90% of the following bacteria exhibit an *in vitro* minimum inhibitory concentration (MIC) less than or equal to the susceptible breakpoint for ertapenem. However, the efficacy of ertapenem in treating clinical infections due to these bacteria **has not been** established in adequate and well-controlled clinical trials:

Gram-positive bacteria:

Staphylococcus epidermidis (methicillin susceptible isolates only)
Streptococcus pneumoniae (penicillin-intermediate isolates)

Gram-negative bacteria:

Citrobacter freundii
Citrobacter koseri
Enterobacter aerogenes
Enterobacter cloacae
Haemophilus influenzae (beta-lactamase positive isolates only)
Haemophilus parainfluenzae
Klebsiella oxytoca (excluding ESBL producing isolates)
Morganella morganii
Proteus vulgaris
Providencia rettgeri
Providencia stuartii
Serratia marcescens

Anaerobic bacteria:

Bacteroides vulgatus
Clostridium perfringens
Fusobacterium spp.

Susceptibility Test Methods:

When available, the clinical microbiology laboratory should provide the results of *in vitro* susceptibility tests for antimicrobial drug products used in resident hospitals to the physician as periodic reports which describe the susceptibility profile of nosocomial and community-acquired pathogens. These reports should aid the physician in selecting the most effective antimicrobial.

Dilution Techniques:

Quantitative methods are used to determine antimicrobial minimum inhibitory concentrations (MICs). These MICs provide estimates of the susceptibility of bacteria to antimicrobial compounds. The MICs should be determined using a standardized procedure. Standardized procedures are based on a broth dilution method {1} or equivalent with standardized inoculum concentrations and standardized concentrations of ertapenem powder. The MIC values should be interpreted according to criteria provided in Table 11 and {4}.

Diffusion Techniques:

Quantitative methods that require measurement of zone diameters also provide reproducible estimates of the susceptibility of bacteria to antimicrobial compounds. One such standardized procedure {2} requires the use of standardized inoculum concentrations. This procedure uses paper disks impregnated with 10-μg ertapenem to test the susceptibility of microorganisms to ertapenem. The disk diffusion interpretive criteria should be interpreted according to criteria provided in Table 11 and {4}.

Anaerobic Techniques:

For anaerobic bacteria, the susceptibility to ertapenem as MICs can be determined by standardized test methods {3}. The MIC values obtained should be interpreted according to criteria provided in Table 11 and {4}.

[See table 11 above]

A report of "Susceptible" indicates that the pathogen is likely to be inhibited if the antimicrobial compound at the infection site reaches the concentrations usually achievable. A report of "Intermediate" indicates that the result should be considered equivocal, and, if the microorganism is not fully susceptible to alternative, clinically feasible drugs, the test should be repeated. This category implies possible clinical applicability in body sites where the drug is physiologically concentrated or in situations where high dosage of drug can be used. This category also provides a buffer zone which prevents small uncontrolled technical factors from causing major discrepancies in interpretation. A report of "Resistant" indicates that the pathogen is not likely to be inhibited if the antimicrobial compound at the infection site reaches the concentrations usually achievable; other therapy should be selected.

Quality Control

Standardized susceptibility test procedures require the use of laboratory control microorganisms to ensure the accuracy and precision of supplies and reagents used in the assay, and the techniques of the individuals performing the test. Quality control microorganisms are specific strains of organisms with intrinsic biological properties. QC strains are very stable strains which will give a standard and repeatable susceptibility pattern. The specific strains used for microbiological quality control are not clinically significant. Standard ertapenem powder should provide the following range of values noted in Table 12 and {4,5}.

Table 12: Acceptable Quality Control Ranges for Ertapenem

Microorganism	Minimum Inhibitory Concentrations MIC Range (μg/mL)	Disk Diffusion Zone Diameter (mm)
Escherichia coli ATCC 25922	0.004-0.016	29-36
Haemophilus influenzae ATCC 49766	0.015-0.06	27-33
Staphylococcus aureus ATCC 29213	0.06-0.25	-
Staphylococcus aureus ATCC 25923	-	24-31
Streptococcus pneumoniae ATCC 49619	0.03-0.25	28-35
Bacteroides fragilis ATCC 25285	0.06-0.5 * 0.06-0.25†	-
Bacteroides thetaiotaomicron ATCC 29741	0.5-2.0 * 0.25-1.0 †	-
Eubacterium lentum ATCC 43055	0.5-4.0 * 0.5-2.0 †	-

* Quality control ranges for broth microdilution testing
† Quality control ranges for agar dilution testing

Table 11: Susceptibility Interpretive Criteria for Ertapenem

Pathogen	Minimum Inhibitory Concentrations* MIC (μg/mL)			Disk Diffusion Zone Diameter (mm)		
	S	I	R	S	I	R
Enterobacteriaceae	≤0.5	1	≥2	≥22	19-21	≤18
Staphylococcus aureus†	≤2.0	4.0	≥8.0	≥19	16-18	≤15
Haemophilus spp.*	≤0.5	-	-	≥19	-	-
Streptococcus pneumoniae‡	≤1.0	2	≥4	-	-	-
Streptococcus spp. Beta Hemolytic Group*,‡,§	≤1.0	-	-	-	-	-
Streptococcus spp. Viridans Group*	≤1.0	-	-	-	-	-
Anaerobes	≤4.0	8.0	≥16.0	-	-	-

* For some organism/antimicrobial combinations, the absence or rare occurrence of resistant strains precludes defining any results categories other than "susceptible". For strains yielding results suggestive of a "non-susceptible" category, organism identification and antimicrobial susceptibility test results should be confirmed.

† For oxacillin-susceptible *S. aureus* results for carbapenems, including ertapenem, if tested, should be reported according to the results generated using routine interpretive criteria. For oxacillin-resistant *S. aureus* and coagulase negative staphylococci, other beta lactam agents, including carbapenems, may appear active *in vitro* but are not effective clinically. Results for beta lactam agents other than cephalosporins with anti-MRSA activity should be reported as resistant or should not be reported.

‡ *S. pneumoniae* penicillin MICs ≤2 mcg/mL indicate susceptibility to ertapenem.

§ A beta hemolytic *Streptococcus* spp. (Groups A, B, C, G) isolate susceptible to penicillin (MIC ≤0.12 μg/mL) can be considered susceptible to ertapenem and need not be tested against ertapenem.

13 NONCLINICAL TOXICOLOGY

13.1 Carcinogenesis, Mutagenesis, Impairment of Fertility

No long-term studies in animals have been performed to evaluate the carcinogenic potential of ertapenem.

Ertapenem was neither mutagenic nor genotoxic in the following *in vitro* assays: alkaline elution/rat hepatocyte assay, chromosomal aberration assay in Chinese hamster ovary cells, and TK6 human lymphoblastoid cell mutagenesis assay; and in the *in vivo* mouse micronucleus assay.

In mice and rats, IV doses of up to 700 mg/kg/day (for mice, approximately 3 times the recommended human dose of 1 g based on body surface area and for rats, approximately 1.2 times the human exposure at the recommended dose of 1 g based on plasma AUCs) resulted in no effects on mating performance, fecundity, fertility, or embryonic survival.

13.2 Animal Toxicology and/or Pharmacology

In repeat-dose studies in rats, treatment-related neutropenia occurred at every dose-level tested, including the lowest dose of 2 mg/kg (approximately 2% of the human dose on a body surface area basis).

Studies in rabbits and Rhesus monkeys were inconclusive with regard to the effect on neutrophil counts.

14 CLINICAL STUDIES

14.1 Adults

Complicated Intra-Abdominal Infections

Ertapenem was evaluated in adults for the treatment of complicated intra-abdominal infections in a randomized, double-blind, non-inferiority clinical trial. This trial compared ertapenem (1 g intravenously once a day) with piperacillin/tazobactam (3.375 g intravenously every 6 hours) for 5 to 14 days and enrolled 665 patients with localized complicated appendicitis, and any other complicated intra-abdominal infection including colonic, small intestinal, and biliary infections and generalized peritonitis. The combined clinical and microbiologic success rates in the microbiologically evaluable population at 4 to 6 weeks posttherapy (test-of-cure) were 83.6% (163/195) for ertapenem and 80.4% (152/189) for piperacillin/tazobactam.

Complicated Skin and Skin Structure Infections

Ertapenem was evaluated in adults for the treatment of complicated skin and skin structure infections in a randomized, double-blind, non-inferiority clinical trial. This trial compared ertapenem (1 g intravenously once a day) with piperacillin/tazobactam (3.375 g intravenously every 6 hours) for 7 to 14 days and enrolled 540 patients including patients with deep soft tissue abscess, posttraumatic wound infection and cellulitis with purulent drainage. The clinical success rates at 10 to 21 days posttherapy (test-of-cure) were 83.9% (141/168) for ertapenem and 85.3% (145/170) for piperacillin/tazobactam.

Diabetic Foot Infections

Ertapenem was evaluated in adults for the treatment of diabetic foot infections without concomitant osteomyelitis in a multicenter, randomized, double-blind, non-inferiority clinical trial. This trial compared ertapenem (1 g intravenously once a day) with piperacillin/tazobactam (3.375 g intravenously every 6 hours). Test-of-cure was defined as clinical response between treatment groups in the clinically evaluable population at the 10-day posttherapy follow-up visit. The trial included 295 patients randomized to ertapenem and 291 patients to piperacillin/tazobactam. Both regimens allowed the option to switch to oral amoxicillin/clavulanate for a total of 5 to 28 days of treatment (parenteral and oral). All patients were eligible to receive appropriate adjunctive treatment methods, such as debridement, as is typically required in the treatment of diabetic foot infections, and most patients received these treatments. Patients with suspected osteomyelitis could be enrolled if all the infected bone was removed within 2 days of initiation of study therapy, and preferably within the prestudy period. Investigators had the option to add open-label vancomycin if enterococci or methicillin-resistant *Staphylococcus aureus* (MRSA) were among the pathogens isolated or if patients had a history of MRSA infection and additional therapy was indicated in the opinion of the investigator. Two hundred and four (204) patients randomized to ertapenem and 202 patients randomized to piperacillin/tazobactam were clinically evaluable. The clinical success rates at 10 days posttherapy were 75.0% (153/204) for ertapenem and 70.8% (143/202) for piperacillin/tazobactam.

Community Acquired Pneumonia

Ertapenem was evaluated in adults for the treatment of community acquired pneumonia in two randomized, double-blind, non-inferiority clinical trials. Both trials compared ertapenem (1 g parenterally once a day) with ceftriaxone (1 g parenterally once a day) and enrolled a total of 866 patients. Both regimens allowed the option to switch to oral amoxicillin/clavulanate for a total of 10 to 14 days of treatment (parenteral and oral). In the first trial the primary efficacy parameter was the clinical success rate in the clinically evaluable population and success rates were 92.3% (168/182) for ertapenem and 91.0% (183/201) for ceftriaxone at 7 to 14 days posttherapy (test-of-cure). In the second trial the primary efficacy parameter was the clinical success rate in the microbiologically evaluable population and success rates were 91% (91/100) for ertapenem and 91.8% (45/49) for ceftriaxone at 7 to 14 days posttherapy (test-of-cure).

Complicated Urinary Tract Infections Including Pyelonephritis

Ertapenem was evaluated in adults for the treatment of complicated urinary tract infections including pyelonephritis in two randomized, double-blind, non-inferiority clinical trials. Both trials compared ertapenem (1 g parenterally once a day) with ceftriaxone (1 g parenterally once a day) and enrolled a total of 850 patients. Both regimens allowed the option to switch to oral ciprofloxacin (500 mg twice daily) for a total of 10 to 14 days of treatment (parenteral and oral). The microbiological success rates (combined trials) at 5 to 9 days posttherapy (test-of-cure) were 89.5% (229/256) for ertapenem and 91.1% (204/224) for ceftriaxone.

Acute Pelvic Infections Including Endomyometritis, Septic Abortion and Post-Surgical Gynecological Infections

Ertapenem was evaluated in adults for the treatment of acute pelvic infections in a randomized, double-blind, non-inferiority clinical trial. This trial compared ertapenem (1 g intravenously once a day) with piperacillin/tazobactam (3.375 g intravenously every 6 hours) for 3 to 10 days and enrolled 412 patients including 350 patients with obstetric/

postpartum infections and 45 patients with septic abortion. The clinical success rates in the clinically evaluable population at 2 to 4 weeks posttherapy (test-of-cure) were 93.9% (153/163) for ertapenem and 91.5% (140/153) for piperacillin/tazobactam.

Prophylaxis of Surgical Site Infections Following Elective Colorectal Surgery

Ertapenem was evaluated in adults for prophylaxis of surgical site infection following elective colorectal surgery in a multicenter, randomized, double-blind, non-inferiority clinical trial. This trial compared a single intravenous dose of ertapenem (1 g) versus cefotetan (2 g) administered over 30 minutes, 1 hour before elective colorectal surgery. Test-of-prophylaxis was defined as no evidence of surgical site infection, post-operative anastomotic leak, or unexplained antibiotic use in the clinically evaluable population up to and including at the 4-week posttreatment follow-up visit. The trial included 500 patients randomized to ertapenem and 502 patients randomized to cefotetan. The modified intent-to-treat (MITT) population consisted of 451 ertapenem patients and 450 cefotetan patients and included all patients who were randomized, treated, and underwent elective colorectal surgery with adequate bowel preparation. The clinically evaluable population was a subset of the MITT population and consisted of patients who received a complete dose of study therapy no more than two hours prior to surgical incision and no more than six hours before surgical closure. Clinically evaluable patients had sufficient information to determine outcome at the 4-week follow-up assessment and had no confounding factors that interfered with the assessment of that outcome. Examples of confounding factors included prior or concomitant antibiotic violations, the need for a second surgical procedure during the study period, and identification of a distant site infection with concomitant antibiotic administration and no evidence of subsequent wound infection. Three-hundred forty-six (346) patients randomized to ertapenem and 339 patients randomized to cefotetan were clinically evaluable. The prophylactic success rates at 4 weeks posttreatment in the clinically evaluable population were 70.5% (244/346) for ertapenem and 57.2% (194/339) for cefotetan (difference 13.3%, [95% C.I.: 6.1, 20.4], p<0.001). Prophylaxis failure due to surgical site infections occurred in 18.2% (63/346) ertapenem patients and 31.0% (105/339) cefotetan patients. Post-operative anastomotic leak occurred in 2.9% (10/346) ertapenem patients and 4.1% (14/339) cefotetan patients. Unexplained antibiotic use occurred in 8.4% (29/346) ertapenem patients and 7.7% (26/339) cefotetan patients. Though patient numbers were small in some subgroups, in general, clinical response rates by age, gender, and race were consistent with the results found in the clinically evaluable population. In the MITT analysis, the prophylactic success rates at 4 weeks posttreatment were 58.3% (263/451) for ertapenem and 48.9% (220/450) for cefotetan (difference 9.4%, [95% C.I.: 2.9, 15.9], p=0.002). A statistically significant difference favoring ertapenem over cefotetan with respect to the primary endpoint has been observed at a significance level of 5% in this trial. A second adequate and well-controlled trial to confirm these findings has not been conducted; therefore, the clinical superiority of ertapenem over cefotetan has not been demonstrated.

14.2 Pediatric Patients

Ertapenem was evaluated in pediatric patients 3 months to 17 years of age in two randomized, multicenter clinical trials.

The first trial enrolled 404 patients and compared ertapenem (15 mg/kg intravenous (IV) every 12 hours in patients 3 months to 12 years of age, and 1 g IV once a day in patients 13 to 17 years of age) to ceftriaxone (50 mg/kg/day IV in two divided doses in patients 3 months to 12 years of age and 50 mg/kg/day IV as a single daily dose in patients 13 to 17 years of age) for the treatment of complicated urinary tract infection (UTI), skin and soft tissue infection (SSTI), or community-acquired pneumonia (CAP). Both regimens allowed the option to switch to oral amoxicillin/clavulanate for a total of up to 14 days of treatment (parenteral and oral). The microbiological success rates in the evaluable per protocol (EPP) analysis in patients treated for UTI were 87.0% (40/46) for ertapenem and 90.0% (18/20) for ceftriaxone. The clinical success rates in the EPP analysis in patients treated for SSTI were 95.5% (64/67) for ertapenem and 100% (26/26) for ceftriaxone, and in patients treated for CAP were 96.1% (74/77) for ertapenem and 96.4% (27/28) for ceftriaxone.

The second trial enrolled 112 patients and compared ertapenem (15 mg/kg IV every 12 hours in patients 3 months to 12 years of age, and 1 g IV once a day in patients 13 to 17 years of age) to ticarcillin/clavulanate (50 mg/kg for patients <60 kg or 3.0 g for patients >60 kg, 4 or 6 times a day) up to 14 days for the treatment of complicated intra-abdominal infections (IAI) and acute pelvic infections (API). In patients treated for IAI (primarily patients with perforated or complicated appendicitis), the clinical success rates were 83.7% (36/43) for ertapenem and 63.6% (7/11) for ticarcillin/clavulanate in the EPP analysis. In patients treated for API (post-operative or spontaneous obstetrical endomyometritis, or septic abortion), the clinical success rates were 100% (23/23) for ertapenem and 100% (4/4) for ticarcillin/clavulanate in the EPP analysis.

15 REFERENCES

1. Clinical and Laboratory Standards Institute (CLSI). Methods for Dilution Antimicrobial Susceptibility Tests for Bacteria that Grow Aerobically. 9th Edition; CLSI Document M7-A9. CLSI, Wayne, PA, 2012.
2. Clinical and Laboratory Standards Institute (CLSI). Performance Standards for Antimicrobial Disk Susceptibility Tests. 11th Edition; CLSI Document M2-A11. CLSI, Wayne, PA, 2012.
3. Clinical and Laboratory Standards Institute (CLSI). *Methods for Antimicrobial Susceptibility Testing of Anaerobic Bacteria* – 7th Edition; CLSI Document M11-A7. CLSI, Wayne, PA, 2007.
4. Clinical and Laboratory Standards Institute (CLSI). Performance Standards for Antimicrobial Susceptibility Testing – 22nd Informational Supplement. CLSI Document M100-S22. CLSI, Wayne, PA, 2012.
5. Clinical and Laboratory Standards Institute (CLSI, formerly NCCLS). Performance Standards for Antimicrobial Susceptibility of Anaerobic Bacteria; Informational Supplement. CLSI Document M11-S1. CLSI, Wayne, PA, 2010.

16 HOW SUPPLIED/STORAGE AND HANDLING

16.1 How Supplied

INVANZ is supplied as a sterile lyophilized powder in single dose vials containing ertapenem for intravenous infusion or for intramuscular injection as follows:

No. 3843—1 g ertapenem equivalent

NDC 0006-3843-71 in trays of 10 vials.

INVANZ is supplied as a sterile lyophilized powder in single dose ADD-Vantage® vials containing ertapenem for intravenous infusion as follows:

No. 3845—1 g ertapenem equivalent

NDC 0006-3845-71 in trays of 10 ADD-Vantage® vials.

16.2 Storage and Handling

Before reconstitution

Do not store lyophilized powder above 25°C (77°F).

Reconstituted and infusion solutions

The reconstituted solution, immediately diluted in 0.9% Sodium Chloride Injection *[see Dosage and Administration (2.7)]*, may be stored at room temperature (25°C) and used within 6 hours or stored for 24 hours under refrigeration (5°C) and used within 4 hours after removal from refrigeration. Solutions of INVANZ should not be frozen.

17 PATIENT COUNSELING INFORMATION

17.1 Instructions for Patients

Patients should be advised that allergic reactions, including serious allergic reactions could occur and that serious reactions may require immediate treatment. Advise patients to report any previous hypersensitivity reactions to INVANZ, other beta-lactams or other allergens.

Patients should be counseled to inform their physician if they are taking valproic acid or divalproex sodium. Valproic acid concentrations in the blood may drop below the therapeutic range upon co-administration with INVANZ. If treatment with INVANZ is necessary and continued, alternative or supplemental anti-convulsant medication to prevent and/or treat seizures may be needed.

Patients should be counseled that antibacterial drugs including INVANZ should only be used to treat bacterial infections. They do not treat viral infections (e.g., the common cold). When INVANZ is prescribed to treat a bacterial infection, patients should be told that although it is common to feel better early in the course of therapy, the medication should be taken exactly as directed. Skipping doses or not completing the full course of therapy may (1) decrease the effectiveness of the immediate treatment and (2) increase the likelihood that bacteria will develop resistance and will not be treatable by INVANZ or other antibacterial drugs in the future.

Diarrhea is a common problem caused by antibiotics which usually ends when the antibiotic is discontinued. Sometimes after starting treatment with antibiotics, patients can develop watery and bloody stools (with or without stomach cramps and fever) even as late as two or more months after having taken the last dose of the antibiotic. If this occurs, patients should contact their physician as soon as possible.

Manuf. for: Merck Sharp & Dohme Corp., a subsidiary of **MERCK & CO., INC.**, Whitehouse Station, NJ 08889, USA

By: Laboratoires Merck Sharp & Dohme-Chibret
Clermont Ferrand Cedex 9, 63963, France

US Patent Nos.: 5,478,820; 5,952,323; 5,652,233
Revised 06/2013
uspi-mk0826-i-1306r018

ISENTRESS® ℞
(raltegravir)
Film-Coated Tablets, for oral use

ISENTRESS®
(raltegravir)
Chewable Tablets, for oral use

HIGHLIGHTS OF PRESCRIBING INFORMATION
These highlights do not include all the information needed to use ISENTRESS safely and effectively. See full prescribing information for ISENTRESS.
ISENTRESS® (raltegravir) Film-Coated Tablets, for oral use
ISENTRESS® (raltegravir) Chewable Tablets, for oral use
Initial U.S. Approval: 2007

RECENT MAJOR CHANGES

Indications and Usage (1) 06/2013

INDICATIONS AND USAGE

ISENTRESS is a human immunodeficiency virus integrase strand transfer inhibitor (HIV-1 INSTI) indicated:
- In combination with other antiretroviral agents for the treatment of HIV-1 infection (1).

The safety and efficacy of ISENTRESS have not been established in children less than 2 years of age (1.2).

DOSAGE AND ADMINISTRATION

ISENTRESS can be administered with or without food (2.1).

ISENTRESS 400 mg film-coated tablets cannot be substituted with ISENTRESS 25 mg and 100 mg chewable tablets (2.1).

Adults
- 400 mg film-coated tablet orally, twice daily (2.2).
- During coadministration with rifampin in adults, 800 mg twice daily (2.1).

Children and Adolescents
- 12 years of age and older: One 400 mg film-coated tablet orally, twice daily (2.3).
- 6 to less than 12 years of age:
  - If at least 25 kg in weight:
    One 400 mg film-coated tablet orally, twice daily **OR**
    Chewable tablets: weight based to maximum dose 300 mg twice daily (2.3).
  - If less than 25 kg in weight:
    Chewable tablets: weight based to maximum dose 300 mg twice daily (2.3).
- 2 to less than 6 years of age:
  - If at least 10 kg in weight:
    Chewable tablets: weight based to maximum dose 300 mg twice daily (2.3).

DOSAGE FORMS AND STRENGTHS

- Film-Coated Tablets: 400 mg (3).
- Chewable Tablets: 100 mg scored and 25 mg (3).

CONTRAINDICATIONS

None (4).

WARNINGS AND PRECAUTIONS

- Severe, potentially life-threatening and fatal skin reactions have been reported. This includes cases of Stevens-Johnson syndrome, hypersensitivity reaction and toxic epidermal necrolysis. Immediately discontinue treatment with ISENTRESS and other suspect agents if severe hypersensitivity, severe rash, or rash with systemic symptoms or liver aminotransferase elevations develops and monitor clinical status, including liver aminotransferases closely (5.1).
- Monitor for Immune Reconstitution Syndrome (5.2).
- Inform patients with phenylketonuria that the 100 mg and 25 mg chewable tablets contain phenylalanine (5.3).

ADVERSE REACTIONS

- The most common adverse reactions of moderate to severe intensity (≥2%) are insomnia, headache, dizziness, nausea and fatigue (6.1 and 6.2).
- Creatine kinase elevations were observed in subjects who received ISENTRESS. Myopathy and rhabdomyolysis have been reported. Use with caution in patients at increased risk of myopathy or rhabdomyolysis, such as patients receiving concomitant medications known to cause these conditions and patients with a history of rhabdomyolysis, myopathy or increased serum creatine kinase (6.3).

To report SUSPECTED ADVERSE REACTIONS, contact Merck Sharp & Dohme Corp., a subsidiary of Merck & Co., Inc., at 1-877-888-4231 or FDA at 1-800-FDA-1088 or www.fda.gov/medwatch.

DRUG INTERACTIONS

- Coadministration of ISENTRESS with drugs that are strong inducers of UGT1A1 may result in reduced plasma concentrations of raltegravir (7.2).

USE IN SPECIFIC POPULATIONS

Pregnancy:
- ISENTRESS should be used during pregnancy only if the potential benefit justifies the potential risk to the fetus (8.1).

Nursing Mothers:
- Breastfeeding is not recommended while taking ISENTRESS (8.3).

See 17 for PATIENT COUNSELING INFORMATION and FDA-approved patient labeling

Revised: 08/2013

FULL PRESCRIBING INFORMATION: CONTENTS*

*** Sections or subsections omitted from the full prescribing information are not listed**

FULL PRESCRIBING INFORMATION

1 INDICATIONS AND USAGE

1.1 Adults

ISENTRESS® is indicated in combination with other antiretroviral agents for the treatment of human immunodeficiency virus (HIV-1) infection.

This indication is based on analyses of plasma HIV-1 RNA levels in three double-blind controlled studies of ISENTRESS. Two of these studies were conducted in clinically advanced, 3-class antiretroviral (NNRTI, NRTI, PI) treatment-experienced adults through 96 weeks and one was conducted in treatment-naïve adults through 240 weeks.

The use of other active agents with ISENTRESS is associated with a greater likelihood of treatment response *[see Clinical Studies (14)]*.

1.2 Pediatrics

ISENTRESS is indicated in combination with other antiretroviral agents for the treatment of HIV-1 infection in children and adolescents 2 years of age and older and weighing at least 10 kg *[see Use in Specific Populations (8.4)]*.

This indication is based on the evaluation of safety, tolerability, pharmacokinetic parameters and efficacy of ISENTRESS through at least 24-weeks in a multi-center, open-label, noncomparative study in HIV-1 infected children and adolescents 2 to 18 years of age *[see Clinical Studies (14.3)]*.

The safety and efficacy of ISENTRESS have not been established in children less than 2 years of age.

2 DOSAGE AND ADMINISTRATION

2.1 General Dosing Recommendations

- ISENTRESS Film-Coated Tablets and Chewable Tablets can be administered with or without food *[see Clinical Pharmacology (12.3)]*.
- Maximum dose of chewable tablets is 300 mg twice daily.
- ISENTRESS Chewable Tablets may be chewed or swallowed whole.
- ISENTRESS Film-Coated Tablets must be swallowed whole.
- Because the formulations are not bioequivalent, do not substitute chewable tablets for the 400 mg film-coated tablet.
- During coadministration of ISENTRESS 400 mg film-coated tablets with rifampin, the recommended dosage of ISENTRESS is 800 mg twice daily in adults. There are no data to guide co-administration of ISENTRESS with rifampin in patients below 18 years of age *[see Drug Interactions (7)]*.

2.2 Adults

For the treatment of adult patients with HIV-1 infection, the dosage of ISENTRESS is one 400 mg film-coated tablet administered orally, twice daily.

2.3 Pediatrics

For the treatment of children and adolescents with HIV-1 infection, the dosage of ISENTRESS is as follows:

- **12 years of age and older:** One 400 mg film-coated tablet orally, twice daily
- **6 to less than 12 years of age:**
  If at least 25 kg in weight:
  - One 400 mg film-coated tablet orally, twice daily **OR**
  - Chewable tablets: weight based to maximum dose 300 mg, twice daily as specified in Table 1

  If less than 25 kg in weight:
  - Chewable tablets: weight based to maximum dose 300 mg, twice daily as specified in Table 1
- **2 to less than 6 years of age:**
  If at least 10 kg in weight:
  - Chewable tablets: weight based to maximum dose 300 mg, twice daily as specified in Table 1

Table 1: Recommended Dose* for ISENTRESS Chewable Tablets in Pediatric Patients 2 to Less Than 12 Years of Age

Body Weight (kg)	Dose	Number of Chewable Tablets
10 to less than 14	75 mg twice daily	3 × 25 mg twice daily
14 to less than 20	100 mg twice daily	1 × 100 mg twice daily
20 to less than 28	150 mg twice daily	1.5 × 100 mg† twice daily
28 to less than 40	200 mg twice daily	2 × 100 mg twice daily
at least 40	300 mg twice daily	3 × 100 mg twice daily

* The weight-based dosing recommendation for the chewable tablet is based on approximately 6 mg/kg/dose twice daily.

† The 100 mg chewable tablet can be divided into equal halves.

3 DOSAGE FORMS AND STRENGTHS

- Film-coated Tablets
  400 mg pink, oval-shaped, film-coated tablets with "227" on one side.
- Chewable Tablets
  100 mg pale orange, oval-shaped, orange-banana flavored, chewable tablets scored on both sides and imprinted on one face with the Merck logo and "477" on opposite sides of the score.
  25 mg pale yellow, round, orange-banana flavored, chewable tablets with the Merck logo on one side and "473" on the other side.

4 CONTRAINDICATIONS

None

5 WARNINGS AND PRECAUTIONS

5.1 Severe Skin and Hypersensitivity Reactions

Severe, potentially life-threatening, and fatal skin reactions have been reported. These include cases of Stevens-Johnson syndrome and toxic epidermal necrolysis. Hypersensitivity reactions have also been reported and were characterized by rash, constitutional findings, and sometimes, organ dysfunction, including hepatic failure. Discontinue ISENTRESS and other suspect agents immediately if signs or symptoms of severe skin reactions or hypersensitivity reactions develop (including, but not limited to, severe rash or rash accompanied by fever, general malaise, fatigue, muscle or joint aches, blisters, oral lesions, conjunctivitis, facial edema, hepatitis, eosinophilia, angioedema). Clinical status including liver aminotransferases should be monitored and appropriate therapy initiated. Delay in stopping ISENTRESS treatment or other suspect agents after the onset of severe rash may result in a life-threatening reaction.

5.2 Immune Reconstitution Syndrome

Immune reconstitution syndrome has been reported in patients treated with combination antiretroviral therapy, including ISENTRESS. During the initial phase of combination antiretroviral treatment, patients whose immune systems respond may develop an inflammatory response to indolent or residual opportunistic infections (such as *Mycobacterium avium* infection, cytomegalovirus, *Pneumocystis jiroveci* pneumonia, tuberculosis), which may necessitate further evaluation and treatment.

Autoimmune disorders (such as Graves' disease, polymyositis, and Guillain-Barré syndrome) have also been reported to occur in the setting of immune reconstitution; however, the time to onset is more variable, and can occur many months after initiation of treatment.

5.3 Phenylketonurics

ISENTRESS Chewable Tablets contain phenylalanine, a component of aspartame. Each 25 mg ISENTRESS Chewable Tablet contains approximately 0.05 mg phenylalanine. Each 100 mg ISENTRESS Chewable Tablet contains approximately 0.10 mg phenylalanine. Phenylalanine can be harmful to patients with phenylketonuria.

6 ADVERSE REACTIONS

Because clinical trials are conducted under widely varying conditions, adverse reaction rates observed in the clinical trials of a drug cannot be directly compared to rates in the clinical trials of another drug and may not reflect the rates observed in practice.

6.1 Clinical Trials Experience: Treatment-Naïve Adults

The following safety assessment of ISENTRESS in treatment-naïve subjects is based on the randomized double-blind active controlled study of treatment-naïve subjects, STARTMRK (Protocol 021) with ISENTRESS 400 mg twice daily in combination with a fixed dose of emtricitabine 200 mg (+) tenofovir 300 mg, (N=281) versus efavirenz (EFV) 600 mg at bedtime in combination with emtricitabine (+) tenofovir, (N=282). During double-blind treatment, the total follow-up for subjects receiving ISENTRESS 400 mg twice daily + emtricitabine (+) tenofovir was 1104 patient-years and 1036 patient-years for subjects receiving efavirenz 600 mg at bedtime + emtricitabine (+) tenofovir.

In Protocol 021, the rate of discontinuation of therapy due to adverse events was 5% in subjects receiving ISENTRESS + emtricitabine (+) tenofovir and 10% in subjects receiving efavirenz + emtricitabine (+) tenofovir.

The clinical adverse drug reactions (ADRs) listed below were considered by investigators to be causally related to ISENTRESS + emtricitabine (+) tenofovir or efavirenz + emtricitabine (+) tenofovir. Clinical ADRs of moderate to severe intensity occurring in ≥2% of treatment-naïve subjects treated with ISENTRESS are presented in Table 2.

Table 2: Adverse Drug Reactions* of Moderate to Severe Intensity† Occurring in ≥2% of Treatment-Naïve Adult Subjects Receiving ISENTRESS (240 Week Analysis)

System Organ Class, Preferred Term	Randomized Study Protocol 021	
	ISENTRESS 400 mg Twice Daily + Emtricitabine (+) Tenofovir (n = 281)	Efavirenz 600 mg At Bedtime + Emtricitabine (+) Tenofovir (n = 282)
Gastrointestinal Disorders		
Nausea	3%	4%
General Disorders and Administration		
Fatigue	2%	3%
Nervous System Disorders		
Headache	4%	5%
Dizziness	2%	6%

Psychiatric Disorders

Insomnia	4%	4%

n = total number of subjects per treatment group
* Includes adverse experiences considered by investigators to be at least possibly, probably, or definitely related to the drug.
† Intensities are defined as follows: Moderate (discomfort enough to cause interference with usual activity); Severe (incapacitating with inability to work or do usual activity).

Laboratory Abnormalities

The percentages of adult subjects treated with ISENTRESS 400 mg twice daily or efavirenz in Protocol 021 with selected Grades 2 to 4 laboratory abnormalities that represent a worsening Grade from baseline are presented in Table 3.
[See table 3 above]

Lipids, Change from Baseline

Changes from baseline in fasting lipids are shown in Table 4.
[See table 4 below]

6.2 Clinical Trials Experience: Treatment-Experienced Adults

The safety assessment of ISENTRESS in treatment-experienced subjects is based on the pooled safety data from the randomized, double-blind, placebo-controlled trials, BENCHMRK 1 and BENCHMRK 2 (Protocols 018 and 019) in antiretroviral treatment-experienced HIV-1 infected adult subjects. A total of 462 subjects received the recommended dose of ISENTRESS 400 mg twice daily in combination with optimized background therapy (OBT) compared to 237 subjects taking placebo in combination with OBT. The median duration of therapy in these trials was 96 weeks for subjects receiving ISENTRESS and 38 weeks for subjects receiving placebo. The total exposure to ISENTRESS was 708 patient-years versus 244 patient-years on placebo. The rates of discontinuation due to adverse events were 4% in subjects receiving ISENTRESS and 5% in subjects receiving placebo.

Clinical ADRs were considered by investigators to be causally related to ISENTRESS + OBT or placebo + OBT. Clinical ADRs of moderate to severe intensity occurring in ≥2% of subjects treated with ISENTRESS and occurring at a higher rate compared to placebo are presented in Table 5.

Table 5: Adverse Drug Reactions* of Moderate to Severe Intensity† Occurring in ≥2% of Treatment-Experienced Adult Subjects Receiving ISENTRESS and at a Higher Rate Compared to Placebo (96 Week Analysis)

System Organ Class, Adverse Reactions	Randomized Studies Protocol 018 and 019	
	ISENTRESS 400 mg Twice Daily + OBT (n = 462)	Placebo + OBT (n = 237)
Nervous System Disorders		
Headache	2%	<1%

n=total number of subjects per treatment group.
* Includes adverse reactions at least possibly, probably, or definitely related to the drug.
† Intensities are defined as follows: Moderate (discomfort enough to cause interference with usual activity); Severe (incapacitating with inability to work or do usual activity).

Laboratory Abnormalities

The percentages of adult subjects treated with ISENTRESS 400 mg twice daily or placebo in Protocols 018 and 019 with selected Grade 2 to 4 laboratory abnormalities representing a worsening Grade from baseline are presented in Table 6.
[See table 6 at top of next page]

Less Common Adverse Reactions Observed in Treatment-Naïve and Treatment-Experienced Studies

The following ADRs occurred in <2% of treatment-naïve or treatment-experienced subjects receiving ISENTRESS in a combination regimen. These events have been included because of their seriousness, increased frequency on ISENTRESS compared with efavirenz or placebo, or investigator's assessment of potential causal relationship.

Gastrointestinal Disorders: abdominal pain, gastritis, dyspepsia, vomiting

General Disorders and Administration Site Conditions: asthenia

Hepatobiliary Disorders: hepatitis

Immune System Disorders: hypersensitivity

Infections and Infestations: genital herpes, herpes zoster

Table 3: Selected Grade 2 to 4 Laboratory Abnormalities Reported in Treatment-Naïve Subjects (240 Week Analysis)

Laboratory Parameter Preferred Term (Unit)	Limit	Randomized Study Protocol 021: ISENTRESS 400 mg Twice Daily + Emtricitabine (+) Tenofovir (N = 281)	Efavirenz 600 mg At Bedtime + Emtricitabine (+) Tenofovir (N = 282)
Hematology			
Absolute neutrophil count ($10^3/\mu L$)			
Grade 2	0.75 - 0.999	3%	5%
Grade 3	0.50 - 0.749	3%	1%
Grade 4	<0.50	1%	1%
Hemoglobin (gm/dL)			
Grade 2	7.5 - 8.4	1%	1%
Grade 3	6.5 - 7.4	1%	1%
Grade 4	<6.5	<1%	0%
Platelet count ($10^3/\mu L$)			
Grade 2	50 - 99.999	1%	0%
Grade 3	25 - 49.999	<1%	<1%
Grade 4	<25	0%	0%
Blood chemistry			
Fasting (non-random) serum glucose test (mg/dL)			
Grade 2	126 - 250	7%	6%
Grade 3	251 - 500	2%	1%
Grade 4	>500	0%	0%
Total serum bilirubin			
Grade 2	1.6 - 2.5 × ULN	5%	0%
Grade 3	2.6 - 5.0 × ULN	1%	<1%
Grade 4	>5.0 × ULN	<1%	0%
Serum aspartate aminotransferase			
Grade 2	2.6 - 5.0 × ULN	8%	10%
Grade 3	5.1 - 10.0 × ULN	5%	3%
Grade 4	>10.0 × ULN	1%	<1%
Serum alanine aminotransferase			
Grade 2	2.6 - 5.0 × ULN	11%	12%
Grade 3	5.1 - 10.0 × ULN	2%	2%
Grade 4	>10.0 × ULN	2%	1%
Serum alkaline phosphatase			
Grade 2	2.6 - 5.0 × ULN	1%	3%
Grade 3	5.1 - 10.0 × ULN	0%	1%
Grade 4	>10.0 × ULN	<1%	<1%

ULN = Upper limit of normal range

Table 4: Lipid Values, Mean Change from Baseline, Protocol 021

Laboratory Parameter Preferred Term	ISENTRESS 400 mg Twice Daily + Emtricitabine (+) Tenofovir N = 207		Change from Baseline at Week 240	Efavirenz 600 mg At Bedtime + Emtricitabine (+) Tenofovir N = 187		Change from Baseline at Week 240
	Baseline Mean (mg/dL)	Week 240 Mean (mg/dL)	Mean Change (mg/dL)	Baseline Mean (mg/dL)	Week 240 Mean (mg/dL)	Mean Change (mg/dL)
LDL-Cholesterol*	96	106	10	93	118	25
HDL-Cholesterol*	38	44	6	38	51	13
Total Cholesterol*	159	175	16	157	201	44
Triglyceride*	128	130	2	141	178	37

Notes:
N = total number of subjects per treatment group with at least one lipid test result available. The analysis is based on all available data.
If subjects initiated or increased serum lipid-reducing agents, the last available lipid values prior to the change in therapy were used in the analysis. If the missing data was due to other reasons, subjects were censored thereafter for the analysis. At baseline, serum lipid-reducing agents were used in 5% of subjects in the group receiving ISENTRESS and 3% in the efavirenz group. Through Week 240, serum lipid-reducing agents were used in 9% of subjects in the group receiving ISENTRESS and 15% in the efavirenz group.
* Fasting (non-random) laboratory tests at Week 240.

Psychiatric Disorders: depression (particularly in subjects with a pre-existing history of psychiatric illness), including suicidal ideation and behaviors

Renal and Urinary Disorders: nephrolithiasis, renal failure

6.3 Selected Adverse Events

Cancers were reported in treatment-experienced subjects who initiated ISENTRESS or placebo, both with OBT, and in treatment-naïve subjects who initiated ISENTRESS or efavirenz, both with emtricitabine (+) tenofovir; several were recurrent. The types and rates of specific cancers were those expected in a highly immunodeficient population (many had CD4+ counts below 50 cells/mm^3 and most had prior AIDS diagnoses). The risk of developing cancer in these studies was similar in the group receiving ISENTRESS and the group receiving the comparator.

Grade 2-4 creatine kinase laboratory abnormalities were observed in subjects treated with ISENTRESS (see Table 6). Myopathy and rhabdomyolysis have been reported. Use with caution in patients at increased risk of myopathy or rhabdomyolysis, such as patients receiving concomitant medications known to cause these conditions and patients with a history of rhabdomyolysis, myopathy or increased serum creatine kinase.

Rash occurred more commonly in treatment-experienced subjects receiving regimens containing ISENTRESS + darunavir/ritonavir compared to subjects receiving ISENTRESS without darunavir/ritonavir or darunavir/ritonavir without ISENTRESS. However, rash that was considered drug related occurred at similar rates for all three groups. These rashes were mild to moderate in severity and did not limit therapy; there were no discontinuations due to rash.

6.4 Patients with Co-existing Conditions

Patients Co-infected with Hepatitis B and/or Hepatitis C Virus

In the randomized, double-blind, placebo-controlled trials, treatment-experienced subjects (N = 114/699 or 16%) and treatment-naïve subjects (N = 34/563 or 6%) with chronic (but not acute) active hepatitis B and/or hepatitis C virus co-infection were permitted to enroll provided that baseline liver function tests did not exceed 5 times the upper limit of normal (ULN). In general the safety profile of ISENTRESS in subjects with hepatitis B and/or hepatitis C virus co-infection was similar to that in subjects without hepatitis B and/or hepatitis C virus co-infection, although the rates of AST and ALT abnormalities were higher in the subgroup with hepatitis B and/or hepatitis C virus co-infection for all treatment groups. At 96 weeks, in treatment-experienced subjects, Grade 2 or higher laboratory abnormalities that represent a worsening Grade from baseline of AST, ALT or total bilirubin occurred in 29%, 34% and 13%, respectively, of co-infected subjects treated with ISENTRESS as compared to 11%, 10% and 9% of all other subjects treated with ISENTRESS. At 240 weeks, in treatment-naïve subjects, Grade 2 or higher laboratory abnormalities that represent a worsening Grade from baseline of AST, ALT or total bilirubin occurred in 22%, 44% and 17%, respectively, of co-infected subjects treated with ISENTRESS as compared to 13%, 13% and 5% of all other subjects treated with ISENTRESS.

6.5 Clinical Trials Experience: Pediatrics

ISENTRESS has been studied in 126 antiretroviral treatment-experienced HIV-1 infected children and adolescents 2 through 18 years of age, in combination with other antiretroviral agents in IMPAACT P1066 *[see Use in Specific Populations (8.4) and Clinical Studies (14.3)]*. Of the 126 patients, 96 received the recommended dose of ISENTRESS.

In these 96 children and adolescents, frequency, type and severity of drug related adverse reactions through Week 24 were comparable to those observed in adults.

One patient experienced drug related clinical adverse reactions of Grade 3 psychomotor hyperactivity, abnormal behavior and insomnia; one patient experienced a Grade 2 serious drug related allergic rash.

One patient experienced drug related laboratory abnormalities, Grade 4 AST and Grade 3 ALT, which were considered serious.

6.6 Postmarketing Experience

The following adverse reactions have been identified during postapproval use of ISENTRESS. Because these reactions are reported voluntarily from a population of uncertain size, it is not always possible to reliably estimate their frequency or establish a causal relationship to drug exposure.

Blood and Lymphatic System Disorders: thrombocytopenia

Gastrointestinal Disorders: diarrhea

Hepatobiliary Disorders: hepatic failure (with and without associated hypersensitivity) in patients with underlying liver disease and/or concomitant medications

Musculoskeletal and Connective Tissue Disorders: rhabdomyolysis

Nervous System Disorders: cerebellar ataxia

Psychiatric Disorders: anxiety, paranoia

7 DRUG INTERACTIONS

7.1 Effect of Raltegravir on the Pharmacokinetics of Other Agents

Raltegravir does not inhibit (IC_{50}>100 µM) CYP1A2, CYP2B6, CYP2C8, CYP2C9, CYP2C19, CYP2D6 or CYP3A *in vitro*. Moreover, *in vitro*, raltegravir did not induce CYP1A2, CYP2B6 or CYP3A4. A midazolam drug interaction study confirmed the low propensity of raltegravir to alter the pharmacokinetics of agents metabolized by CYP3A4 *in vivo* by demonstrating a lack of effect of raltegravir on the pharmacokinetics of midazolam, a sensitive CYP3A4 substrate. Similarly, raltegravir is not an inhibitor (IC_{50}>50 µM) of the UDP-glucuronosyltransferases (UGT) tested (UGT1A1, UGT2B7), and raltegravir does not inhibit P-glycoprotein-mediated transport. Based on these data, ISENTRESS is not expected to affect the pharmacokinetics of drugs that are substrates of these enzymes or P-glycoprotein (e.g., protease inhibitors, NNRTIs, opioid analgesics, statins, azole antifungals, proton pump inhibitors and anti-erectile dysfunction agents).

In drug interaction studies, raltegravir did not have a clinically meaningful effect on the pharmacokinetics of the following: hormonal contraceptives, methadone, lamivudine, tenofovir, etravirine, darunavir/ritonavir.

7.2 Effect of Other Agents on the Pharmacokinetics of Raltegravir

Raltegravir is not a substrate of cytochrome P450 (CYP) enzymes. Based on *in vivo* and *in vitro* studies, raltegravir is eliminated mainly by metabolism via a UGT1A1-mediated glucuronidation pathway.

Rifampin, a strong inducer of UGT1A1, reduces plasma concentrations of ISENTRESS. Therefore, in adults the dose of ISENTRESS should be increased during coadministration with rifampin. There are no data to guide co-administration of ISENTRESS with rifampin in patients below 18 years of age *[see Dosage and Administration (2)]*. The impact of other inducers of drug metabolizing enzymes, such as phenytoin and phenobarbital, on UGT1A1 is unknown.

Coadministration of ISENTRESS with drugs that inhibit UGT1A1 may increase plasma levels of raltegravir.

All interaction studies were performed in adults.

Selected drug interactions are presented in Table 7 *[see Clinical Pharmacology (12.3)]*.

[See table 7 at top of next page]

8 USE IN SPECIFIC POPULATIONS

8.1 Pregnancy

Pregnancy Category C

ISENTRESS should be used during pregnancy only if the potential benefit justifies the potential risk to the fetus. There are no adequate and well-controlled studies in pregnant women. In addition, there have been no pharmacokinetic studies conducted in pregnant patients.

Developmental toxicity studies were performed in rabbits (at oral doses up to 1000 mg/kg/day) and rats (at oral doses up to 600 mg/kg/day). The reproductive toxicity study in rats was performed with pre-, peri-, and postnatal evaluation. The highest doses in these studies produced systemic exposures in these species approximately 3- to 4-fold the exposure at the recommended human dose. In both rabbits and rats, no treatment-related effects on embryonic/fetal survival or fetal weights were observed. In addition, no treatment-related external, visceral, or skeletal changes were observed in rabbits. However, treatment-related in-

Table 6: Selected Grade 2 to 4 Laboratory Abnormalities Reported in Treatment-Experienced Subjects (96 Week Analysis)

Laboratory Parameter Preferred Term (Unit)	Limit	Randomized Studies Protocol 018 and 019: ISENTRESS 400 mg Twice Daily + OBT (N = 462)	Placebo + OBT (N = 237)
Hematology			
Absolute neutrophil count (10^3/µL)			
Grade 2	0.75 - 0.999	4%	5%
Grade 3	0.50 - 0.749	3%	3%
Grade 4	<0.50	1%	<1%
Hemoglobin (gm/dL)			
Grade 2	7.5 - 8.4	1%	3%
Grade 3	6.5 - 7.4	1%	1%
Grade 4	<6.5	<1%	0%
Platelet count (10^3/µL)			
Grade 2	50 - 99.999	3%	5%
Grade 3	25 - 49.999	1%	<1%
Grade 4	<25	1%	<1%
Blood chemistry			
Fasting (non-random) serum glucose test (mg/dL)			
Grade 2	126 - 250	10%	7%
Grade 3	251 - 500	3%	1%
Grade 4	>500	0%	0%
Total serum bilirubin			
Grade 2	1.6 - 2.5 × ULN	6%	3%
Grade 3	2.6 - 5.0 × ULN	3%	3%
Grade 4	>5.0 × ULN	1%	0%
Serum aspartate aminotransferase			
Grade 2	2.6 - 5.0 × ULN	9%	7%
Grade 3	5.1 - 10.0 × ULN	4%	3%
Grade 4	>10.0 × ULN	1%	1%
Serum alanine aminotransferase			
Grade 2	2.6 - 5.0 × ULN	9%	9%
Grade 3	5.1 - 10.0 × ULN	4%	2%
Grade 4	>10.0 × ULN	1%	2%
Serum alkaline phosphatase			
Grade 2	2.6 - 5.0 × ULN	2%	<1%
Grade 3	5.1 - 10.0 × ULN	<1%	1%
Grade 4	>10.0 × ULN	1%	<1%
Serum pancreatic amylase test			
Grade 2	1.6 - 2.0 × ULN	2%	1%
Grade 3	2.1 - 5.0 × ULN	4%	3%
Grade 4	>5.0 × ULN	<1%	<1%
Serum lipase test			
Grade 2	1.6 - 3.0 × ULN	5%	4%
Grade 3	3.1 - 5.0 × ULN	2%	1%
Grade 4	>5.0 × ULN	0%	0%
Serum creatine kinase			
Grade 2	6.0 - 9.9 × ULN	2%	2%
Grade 3	10.0 - 19.9 × ULN	4%	3%
Grade 4	≥20.0 × ULN	3%	1%

ULN = Upper limit of normal range

Table 7: Selected Drug Interactions in Adults

Concomitant Drug Class: Drug Name	Effect on Concentration of Raltegravir	Clinical Comment
HIV-1-Antiviral Agents		
atazanavir	↑	Atazanavir, a strong inhibitor of UGT1A1, increases plasma concentrations of raltegravir. However, since concomitant use of ISENTRESS with atazanavir/ritonavir did not result in a unique safety signal in Phase 3 studies, no dose adjustment is recommended.
atazanavir/ritonavir	↑	Atazanavir/ritonavir increases plasma concentrations of raltegravir. However, since concomitant use of ISENTRESS with atazanavir/ritonavir did not result in a unique safety signal in Phase 3 studies, no dose adjustment is recommended.
efavirenz	↓	Efavirenz reduces plasma concentrations of raltegravir. The clinical significance of this interaction has not been directly assessed.
etravirine	↓	Etravirine reduces plasma concentrations of raltegravir. The clinical significance of this interaction has not been directly assessed.
tipranavir/ritonavir	↓	Tipranavir/ritonavir reduces plasma concentrations of raltegravir. However, since comparable efficacy was observed for this combination relative to other ISENTRESS-containing regimens in Phase 3 studies 018 and 019, no dose adjustment is recommended.
Other Agents		
boceprevir	↔	No dose adjustment required for ISENTRESS or boceprevir.
omeprazole	↑	Coadministration of medicinal products that increase gastric pH (e.g., omeprazole) may increase raltegravir levels based on increased raltegravir solubility at higher pH. However, since concomitant use of ISENTRESS with proton pump inhibitors and H2 blockers did not result in a unique safety signal in Phase 3 studies, no dose adjustment is recommended.
rifampin	↓	Rifampin, a strong inducer of UGT1A1, reduces plasma concentrations of raltegravir. The recommended dosage of ISENTRESS is 800 mg twice daily during coadministration with rifampin.

creases over controls in the incidence of supernumerary ribs were seen in rats at 600 mg/kg/day (exposures 3-fold the exposure at the recommended human dose).

Placenta transfer of drug was demonstrated in both rats and rabbits. At a maternal dose of 600 mg/kg/day in rats, mean drug concentrations in fetal plasma were approximately 1.5- to 2.5-fold greater than in maternal plasma at 1 hour and 24 hours postdose, respectively. Mean drug concentrations in fetal plasma were approximately 2% of the mean maternal concentration at both 1 and 24 hours postdose at a maternal dose of 1000 mg/kg/day in rabbits.

Antiretroviral Pregnancy Registry

To monitor maternal-fetal outcomes of pregnant patients exposed to ISENTRESS, an Antiretroviral Pregnancy Registry has been established. Physicians are encouraged to register patients by calling 1-800-258-4263.

8.3 Nursing Mothers

Breastfeeding is not recommended while taking ISENTRESS. In addition, it is recommended that HIV-1-infected mothers not breastfeed their infants to avoid risking postnatal transmission of HIV-1.

It is not known whether raltegravir is secreted in human milk. However, raltegravir is secreted in the milk of lactating rats. Mean drug concentrations in milk were approximately 3-fold greater than those in maternal plasma at a maternal dose of 600 mg/kg/day in rats. There were no effects in rat offspring attributable to exposure of ISENTRESS through the milk.

8.4 Pediatric Use

The safety, tolerability, pharmacokinetic profile, and efficacy of ISENTRESS were evaluated in HIV-1 infected children and adolescents 2 to 18 years of age in an open-label, multicenter clinical trial, IMPAACT P1066 *[see Clinical Pharmacology (12.3)* and *Clinical Studies (14.3)]*. The safety profile was comparable to that observed in adults *[see Adverse Reactions (6.5)]*. See Dosage and Administration (2.3) for dosing recommendations for children 2 years of age and older. Safety and effectiveness of ISENTRESS in children under 2 years of age have not been established.

8.5 Geriatric Use

Clinical studies of ISENTRESS did not include sufficient numbers of subjects aged 65 and over to determine whether they respond differently from younger subjects. Other reported clinical experience has not identified differences in responses between the elderly and younger subjects. In general, dose selection for an elderly patient should be cautious, reflecting the greater frequency of decreased hepatic, renal, or cardiac function, and of concomitant disease or other drug therapy.

8.6 Use in Patients with Hepatic Impairment

No clinically important pharmacokinetic differences between subjects with moderate hepatic impairment and healthy subjects were observed. No dosage adjustment is necessary for patients with mild to moderate hepatic impairment. The effect of severe hepatic impairment on the pharmacokinetics of raltegravir has not been studied *[see Clinical Pharmacology (12.3)]*.

8.7 Use in Patients with Renal Impairment

No clinically important pharmacokinetic differences between subjects with severe renal impairment and healthy subjects were observed. No dosage adjustment is necessary *[see Clinical Pharmacology (12.3)]*.

10 OVERDOSAGE

No specific information is available on the treatment of overdosage with ISENTRESS. Doses as high as 1600-mg single dose and 800-mg twice-daily multiple doses were studied in healthy volunteers without evidence of toxicity. Occasional doses of up to 1800 mg per day were taken in the clinical studies of HIV-1 infected subjects without evidence of toxicity.

In the event of an overdose, it is reasonable to employ the standard supportive measures, e.g., remove unabsorbed material from the gastrointestinal tract, employ clinical monitoring (including obtaining an electrocardiogram), and institute supportive therapy if required. The extent to which ISENTRESS may be dialyzable is unknown.

11 DESCRIPTION

ISENTRESS contains raltegravir potassium, a human immunodeficiency virus integrase strand transfer inhibitor. The chemical name for raltegravir potassium is *N*-[(4-Fluorophenyl)methyl]-1,6-dihydro-5-hydroxy-1-methyl-2-[1-methyl-1-[[(5-methyl-1,3,4-oxadiazol-2-yl)carbonyl]amino]ethyl]-6-oxo-4-pyrimidinecarboxamide monopotassium salt.

The empirical formula is $C_{20}H_{20}FKN_6O_5$ and the molecular weight is 482.51. The structural formula is:

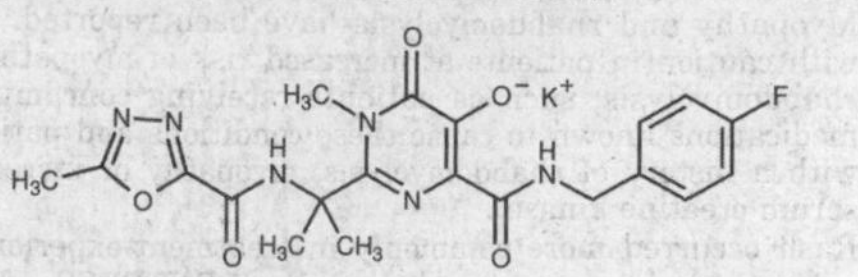

Raltegravir potassium is a white to off-white powder. It is soluble in water, slightly soluble in methanol, very slightly soluble in ethanol and acetonitrile and insoluble in isopropanol.

Each 400 mg film-coated tablet of ISENTRESS for oral administration contains 434.4 mg of raltegravir (as potassium salt), equivalent to 400 mg of raltegravir free phenol and the following inactive ingredients: microcrystalline cellulose, lactose monohydrate, calcium phosphate dibasic anhydrous, hypromellose 2208, poloxamer 407 (contains 0.01% butylated hydroxytoluene as antioxidant), sodium stearyl fumarate, magnesium stearate. In addition, the film coating contains the following inactive ingredients: polyvinyl alcohol, titanium dioxide, polyethylene glycol 3350, talc, red iron oxide and black iron oxide.

Each 100 mg chewable tablet of ISENTRESS for oral administration contains 108.6 mg of raltegravir (as potassium salt), equivalent to 100 mg of raltegravir free phenol and the following inactive ingredients: hydroxypropyl cellulose, sucralose, saccharin sodium, sodium citrate dihydrate, mannitol, red iron oxide, yellow iron oxide, monoammonium glycyrrhizinate, sorbitol, fructose, natural and artificial flavors (orange, banana, and masking that contains aspartame), crospovidone, magnesium stearate, sodium stearyl fumarate, ethylcellulose 20 cP, ammonium hydroxide, medium chain triglycerides, oleic acid, hypromellose 2910/6cP, PEG 400.

Each 25 mg chewable tablet of ISENTRESS for oral administration contains 27.16 mg of raltegravir (as potassium salt), equivalent to 25 mg of raltegravir free phenol and the following inactive ingredients: hydroxypropyl cellulose, sucralose, saccharin sodium, sodium citrate dihydrate, mannitol, yellow iron oxide, monoammonium glycyrrhizinate, sorbitol, fructose, natural and artificial flavors (orange, banana, and masking that contains aspartame), crospovidone, magnesium stearate, sodium stearyl fumarate, ethylcellulose 20 cP, ammonium hydroxide, medium chain triglycerides, oleic acid, hypromellose 2910/6cP, PEG 400.

12 CLINICAL PHARMACOLOGY

12.1 Mechanism of Action

Raltegravir is an HIV-1 antiviral drug *[see Microbiology (12.4)]*.

12.2 Pharmacodynamics

In a monotherapy study raltegravir (400 mg twice daily) demonstrated rapid antiviral activity with mean viral load reduction of 1.66 $\log_{10}$ copies/mL by Day 10.

In the randomized, double-blind, placebo-controlled, dose-ranging trial, Protocol 005, and Protocols 018 and 019, antiviral responses were similar among subjects regardless of dose.

<u>Effects on Electrocardiogram</u>

In a randomized, placebo-controlled, crossover study, 31 healthy subjects were administered a single oral supratherapeutic dose of raltegravir 1600 mg and placebo. Peak raltegravir plasma concentrations were approximately 4-fold higher than the peak concentrations following a 400 mg dose. ISENTRESS did not appear to prolong the QTc interval for 12 hours postdose. After baseline and placebo adjustment, the maximum mean QTc change was -0.4 msec (1-sided 95% upper Cl: 3.1 msec).

12.3 Pharmacokinetics

<u>Adults</u>

<u>Absorption</u>

Raltegravir (film-coated tablet) is absorbed with a T_{max} of approximately 3 hours postdose in the fasted state. Raltegravir AUC and C_{max} increase dose proportionally over the dose range 100 mg to 1600 mg. Raltegravir C_{12hr} increases dose proportionally over the dose range of 100 to 800 mg and increases slightly less than dose proportionally over the dose range 100 mg to 1600 mg. With twice-daily dosing, pharmacokinetic steady state is achieved within approximately the first 2 days of dosing. There is little to no accumulation in AUC and C_{max}. The average accumulation ratio for C_{12hr} ranged from approximately 1.2 to 1.6.

The absolute bioavailability of raltegravir has not been established. Based on a formulation comparison study in healthy adult volunteers, the chewable tablet has higher oral bioavailability compared to the 400 mg film-coated tablet.

In subjects who received 400 mg twice daily alone, raltegravir drug exposures were characterized by a geometric mean $AUC_{0\text{-}12hr}$ of 14.3 μM·hr and C_{12hr} of 142 nM.

Considerable variability was observed in the pharmacokinetics of raltegravir. For observed C_{12hr} in Protocols 018 and

019, the coefficient of variation (CV) for inter-subject variability = 212% and the CV for intra-subject variability = 122%.

Effect of Food on Oral Absorption

ISENTRESS may be administered with or without food. Raltegravir was administered without regard to food in the pivotal safety and efficacy studies in HIV-1-infected patients. The effect of consumption of low-, moderate- and high-fat meals on steady-state raltegravir pharmacokinetics was assessed in healthy volunteers administered the 400 mg film-coated tablet. Administration of multiple doses of raltegravir following a moderate-fat meal (600 Kcal, 21 g fat) did not affect raltegravir AUC to a clinically meaningful degree with an increase of 13% relative to fasting. Raltegravir C_{12hr} was 66% higher and C_{max} was 5% higher following a moderate-fat meal compared to fasting. Administration of raltegravir following a high-fat meal (825 Kcal, 52 g fat) increased AUC and C_{max} by approximately 2-fold and increased C_{12hr} by 4.1-fold. Administration of raltegravir following a low-fat meal (300 Kcal, 2.5 g fat) decreased AUC and C_{max} by 46% and 52%, respectively; C_{12hr} was essentially unchanged. Food appears to increase pharmacokinetic variability relative to fasting.

Administration of the chewable tablet with a high fat meal led to an average 6% decrease in AUC, 62% decrease in C_{max}, and 188% increase in C_{12hr} compared to administration in the fasted state. Administration of the chewable tablet with a high fat meal does not affect raltegravir pharmacokinetics to a clinically meaningful degree and the chewable tablet can be administered without regard to food.

Distribution

Raltegravir is approximately 83% bound to human plasma protein over the concentration range of 2 to 10 µM.

In one study of HIV-1 infected subjects who received raltegravir 400 mg twice daily, raltegravir was measured in the cerebrospinal fluid. In the study (n=18), the median cerebrospinal fluid concentration was 5.8% (range 1 to 53.5%) of the corresponding plasma concentration. This median proportion was approximately 3-fold lower than the free fraction of raltegravir in plasma. The clinical relevance of this finding is unknown.

Metabolism and Excretion

The apparent terminal half-life of raltegravir is approximately 9 hours, with a shorter α-phase half-life (~1 hour) accounting for much of the AUC. Following administration of an oral dose of radiolabeled raltegravir, approximately 51 and 32% of the dose was excreted in feces and urine, respectively. In feces, only raltegravir was present, most of which is likely derived from hydrolysis of raltegravir-glucuronide secreted in bile as observed in preclinical species. Two components, namely raltegravir and raltegravir-glucuronide, were detected in urine and accounted for approximately 9 and 23% of the dose, respectively. The major circulating entity was raltegravir and represented approximately 70% of the total radioactivity; the remaining radioactivity in plasma was accounted for by raltegravir-glucuronide. Studies using isoform-selective chemical inhibitors and cDNA-expressed UDP-glucuronosyltransferases (UGT) show that UGT1A1 is the main enzyme responsible for the formation of raltegravir-glucuronide. Thus, the data indicate that the major mechanism of clearance of raltegravir in humans is UGT1A1-mediated glucuronidation.

Special Populations

Pediatric

The doses recommended for HIV-infected children and adolescents 2 to 18 years of age *[see Dosage and Administration (2.3)]* resulted in a pharmacokinetic profile of raltegravir similar to that observed in adults receiving 400 mg twice daily. Table 8 displays steady state pharmacokinetic parameters in the 400 mg film-coated tablet (6 to 18 years of age) and the chewable tablet (2 to less than 12 years of age).

[See table 8 above]

Table 8: Raltegravir Steady State Pharmacokinetic Parameters Following Administration of Recommended Doses

Age	Formulation	Dose	N*	Geometric Mean (%CV) $AUC_{0\text{-}12hr}$ (µM·hr)	Geometric Mean (%CV) C_{12hr} (nM)
12 to 18 years	Film-coated tablet	400 mg twice daily, regardless of weight†	11	15.7 *(98%)*	333 *(78%)*
6 to less than 12 years	Film-coated tablet	400 mg twice daily, for patients ≥25 kg	11	15.8 *(120%)*	246 *(221%)*
6 to less than 12 years	Chewable tablet	Weight based dosing, see Table 1	10	22.6 *(34%)*	130 *(88%)*
2 to less than 6 years	Chewable tablet	Weight based dosing, see Table 1	12	18.0 *(59%)*	71 *(55%)*

* Number of patients with intensive pharmacokinetic (PK) results at the final recommended dose.

† Patients in this age group received approximately 8 mg/kg/dose at time of intensive PK which met PK and safety targets. Based on review of the individual profiles and receipt of a mean dose of 390 mg, 400 mg twice daily was selected as the recommended dose for this age group.

The pharmacokinetics of raltegravir in children under 2 years of age has not been established.

Age

The effect of age (18 years and older) on the pharmacokinetics of raltegravir was evaluated in the composite analysis. No dosage adjustment is necessary.

Race

The effect of race on the pharmacokinetics of raltegravir in adults was evaluated in the composite analysis. No dosage adjustment is necessary.

Gender

A study of the pharmacokinetics of raltegravir was performed in healthy adult males and females. Additionally, the effect of gender was evaluated in a composite analysis of pharmacokinetic data from 103 healthy subjects and 28 HIV-1 infected subjects receiving raltegravir monotherapy with fasted administration. No dosage adjustment is necessary.

Hepatic Impairment

Raltegravir is eliminated primarily by glucuronidation in the liver. A study of the pharmacokinetics of raltegravir was performed in adult subjects with moderate hepatic impairment. Additionally, hepatic impairment was evaluated in the composite pharmacokinetic analysis. There were no clinically important pharmacokinetic differences between subjects with moderate hepatic impairment and healthy subjects. No dosage adjustment is necessary for patients with mild to moderate hepatic impairment. The effect of severe hepatic impairment on the pharmacokinetics of raltegravir has not been studied.

Renal Impairment

Renal clearance of unchanged drug is a minor pathway of elimination. A study of the pharmacokinetics of raltegravir was performed in adult subjects with severe renal impairment. Additionally, renal impairment was evaluated in the composite pharmacokinetic analysis. There were no clinically important pharmacokinetic differences between subjects with severe renal impairment and healthy subjects. No dosage adjustment is necessary. Because the extent to which ISENTRESS may be dialyzable is unknown, dosing before a dialysis session should be avoided.

UGT1A1 Polymorphism

There is no evidence that common UGT1A1 polymorphisms alter raltegravir pharmacokinetics to a clinically meaningful extent. In a comparison of 30 adult subjects with *28/*28 genotype (associated with reduced activity of UGT1A1) to 27 adult subjects with wild-type genotype, the geometric mean ratio (90% CI) of AUC was 1.41 (0.96, 2.09).

Drug Interactions *[see Drug Interactions (7)]*

[See table 9 above]

Table 9: Effect of Other Agents on the Pharmacokinetics of Raltegravir in Adults

Coadministered Drug	Coadministered Drug Dose/Schedule	Raltegravir Dose/Schedule	Ratio (90% Confidence Interval) of Raltegravir Pharmacokinetic Parameters with/without Coadministered Drug; No Effect = 1.00			
			n	C_{max}	AUC	C_{min}
atazanavir	400 mg daily	100 mg single dose	10	1.53 (1.11, 2.12)	1.72 (1.47, 2.02)	1.95 (1.30, 2.92)
atazanavir/ ritonavir	300 mg/100 mg daily	400 mg twice daily	10	1.24 (0.87, 1.77)	1.41 (1.12, 1.78)	1.77 (1.39, 2.25)
boceprevir	800 mg three times daily	400 mg single dose	22	1.11 (0.91-1.36)	1.04 (0.88-1.22)	0.75 (0.45-1.23)
efavirenz	600 mg daily	400 mg single dose	9	0.64 (0.41, 0.98)	0.64 (0.52, 0.80)	0.79 (0.49, 1.28)
etravirine	200 mg twice daily	400 mg twice daily	19	0.89 (0.68, 1.15)	0.90 (0.68, 1.18)	0.66 (0.34, 1.26)
omeprazole	20 mg daily	400 mg single dose	14 (10 for AUC)	4.15 (2.82, 6.10)	3.12 (2.13, 4.56)	1.46 (1.10, 1.93)
rifampin	600 mg daily	400 mg single dose	9	0.62 (0.37, 1.04)	0.60 (0.39, 0.91)	0.39 (0.30, 0.51)
rifampin	600 mg daily	400 mg twice daily when administered alone; 800 mg twice daily when administered with rifampin	14	1.62 (1.12, 2.33)	1.27 (0.94, 1.71)	0.47 (0.36, 0.61)
ritonavir	100 mg twice daily	400 mg single dose	10	0.76 (0.55, 1.04)	0.84 (0.70, 1.01)	0.99 (0.70, 1.40)
tenofovir	300 mg daily	400 mg twice daily	9	1.64 (1.16, 2.32)	1.49 (1.15, 1.94)	1.03 (0.73, 1.45)
tipranavir/ ritonavir	500 mg/200 mg twice daily	400 mg twice daily	15 (14 for C_{min})	0.82 (0.46, 1.46)	0.76 (0.49, 1.19)	0.45 (0.31, 0.66)

12.4 Microbiology

Mechanism of Action

Raltegravir inhibits the catalytic activity of HIV-1 integrase, an HIV-1 encoded enzyme that is required for viral replication. Inhibition of integrase prevents the covalent insertion, or integration, of unintegrated linear HIV-1 DNA into the host cell genome preventing the formation of the HIV-1 provirus. The provirus is required to direct the production of progeny virus, so inhibiting integration prevents propagation of the viral infection. Raltegravir did not significantly inhibit human phosphoryltransferases including DNA polymerases α, β, and γ.

Table 11: Virologic Outcomes of Randomized Treatment of Protocol 021 at 240 Weeks

	ISENTRESS 400 mg Twice Daily (N = 281)	Efavirenz 600 mg At Bedtime (N = 282)	Difference (ISENTRESS – Efavirenz) (CI)
Subjects with HIV-1 RNA less than 50 copies/mL	66%	60%	6.6% (-1.4%, 14.5%)
Virologic Failure*	8%	15%	
No virologic data at Week 240 Window			
Reasons			
Discontinued study due to AE or death†	5%	10%	
Discontinued study for other reasons‡	15%	14%	
Missing data during window but on study	6%	2%	

* Includes subjects who discontinued prior to Week 240 for lack of efficacy or subjects who are ≥50 copies/mL in the 240-week window (+/- 6-weeks).

† Includes subjects who discontinued due to AE or Death at any time point from Day 1 through the Week 240 window if this resulted in no virologic data on treatment during Week 240 visit window.

‡ Other includes: withdrew consent, loss to follow-up, moved etc., if the viral load at the time of discontinuation was <50 copies/mL.

Antiviral Activity in Cell Culture

Raltegravir at concentrations of 31 ± 20 nM resulted in 95% inhibition (EC_{95}) of viral spread (relative to an untreated virus-infected culture) in human T-lymphoid cell cultures infected with the cell-line adapted HIV-1 variant H9IIIB. In addition, 5 clinical isolates of HIV-1 subtype B had EC_{95} values ranging from 9 to 19 nM in cultures of mitogen-activated human peripheral blood mononuclear cells. In a single-cycle infection assay, raltegravir inhibited infection of 23 HIV-1 isolates representing 5 non-B subtypes (A, C, D, F, and G) and 5 circulating recombinant forms (AE, AG, BF, BG, and cpx) with EC_{50} values ranging from 5 to 12 nM. Raltegravir also inhibited replication of an HIV-2 isolate when tested in CEMx174 cells (EC_{95} value = 6 nM). Additive to synergistic antiretroviral activity was observed when human T-lymphoid cells infected with the H9IIIB variant of HIV-1 were incubated with raltegravir in combination with non-nucleoside reverse transcriptase inhibitors (delavirdine, efavirenz, or nevirapine); nucleoside analog reverse transcriptase inhibitors (abacavir, didanosine, lamivudine, stavudine, tenofovir, zalcitabine, or zidovudine); protease inhibitors (amprenavir, atazanavir, indinavir, lopinavir, nelfinavir, ritonavir, or saquinavir); or the entry inhibitor enfuvirtide.

Resistance

The mutations observed in the HIV-1 integrase coding sequence that contributed to raltegravir resistance (evolved either in cell culture or in subjects treated with raltegravir) generally included an amino acid substitution at either Y143 (changed to C, H, or R) or Q148 (changed to H, K, or R) or N155 (changed to H) plus one or more additional substitutions (i.e., L74M, E92Q, Q95K/R, T97A, E138A/K, G140A/S, V151I, G163R, H183P, Y226C/D/F/H, S230R, and D232N). E92Q and F121C are occasionally seen in the absence of substitutions at Y143, Q148, or N155 in raltegravir-treatment failure subjects.

Treatment-Naïve Adult Subjects: By Week 96 in the STARTMRK trial, the primary raltegravir resistance-associated substitutions were observed in 4 (2 with Y143H/R and 2 with Q148H/R) of the 10 virologic failure subjects with evaluable genotypic data from paired baseline and raltegravir treatment-failure isolates.

Treatment-Experienced Adult Subjects: By Week 96 in the BENCHMRK trials, at least one of the primary raltegravir resistance-associated substitutions, Y143C/H/R, Q148H/K/R, and N155H, was observed in 76 of the 112 virologic failure subjects with evaluable genotypic data from paired baseline and raltegravir treatment-failure isolates. The emergence of the primary raltegravir resistance-associated substitutions was observed cumulatively in 70 subjects by Week 48 and 78 subjects by Week 96, 15.2% and 17% of the raltegravir recipients, respectively. Some (n=58) of those HIV-1 isolates harboring one or more of the primary raltegravir resistance-associated substitutions were evaluated for raltegravir susceptibility yielding a median decrease of 26.3-fold (mean 48.9 ± 44.8-fold decrease, ranging from 0.8- to 159-fold) compared to the wild-type reference.

13 NONCLINICAL TOXICOLOGY

13.1 Carcinogenesis, Mutagenesis, Impairment of Fertility

Carcinogenicity studies of raltegravir in mice did not show any carcinogenic potential. At the highest dose levels, 400 mg/kg/day in females and 250 mg/kg/day in males, systemic exposure was 1.8-fold (females) or 1.2-fold (males) greater than the AUC (54 μM·hr) at the 400-mg twice daily human dose. Treatment-related squamous cell carcinoma of nose/nasopharynx was observed in female rats dosed with 600 mg/kg/day raltegravir for 104 weeks. These tumors were possibly the result of local irritation and inflammation due to local deposition and/or aspiration of drug in the mucosa of the nose/nasopharynx during dosing. No tumors of the nose/nasopharynx were observed in rats dosed with 150 mg/kg/day (males) and 50 mg/kg/day (females) and the systemic exposure in rats was 1.7-fold (males) to 1.4-fold (females) greater than the AUC (54 μM·hr) at the 400-mg twice daily human dose.

No evidence of mutagenicity or genotoxicity was observed in *in vitro* microbial mutagenesis (Ames) tests, *in vitro* alkaline elution assays for DNA breakage, and *in vitro* and *in vivo* chromosomal aberration studies.

No effect on fertility was seen in male and female rats at doses up to 600 mg/kg/day which resulted in a 3-fold exposure above the exposure at the recommended human dose.

14 CLINICAL STUDIES

Description of Clinical Studies

The evidence of durable efficacy of ISENTRESS is based on the analyses of 240-week data from a randomized, double-blind, active-control trial, STARTMRK (Protocol 021) in antiretroviral treatment-naïve HIV-1 infected adult subjects and 96-week data from 2 randomized, double-blind, placebo-controlled studies, BENCHMRK 1 and BENCHMRK 2 (Protocols 018 and 019), in antiretroviral treatment-experienced HIV-1 infected adult subjects.

14.1 Treatment-Naïve Adult Subjects

STARTMRK (Protocol 021) is a Phase 3 study to evaluate the safety and antiretroviral activity of ISENTRESS 400 mg twice daily + emtricitabine (+) tenofovir versus efavirenz 600 mg at bedtime plus emtricitabine (+) tenofovir in treatment-naïve HIV-1-infected subjects with HIV-1 RNA >5000 copies/mL. Randomization was stratified by screening HIV-1 RNA level (≤50,000 copies/mL; and >50,000 copies/mL) and by hepatitis status.

Table 10 shows the demographic characteristics of subjects in the group receiving ISENTRESS 400 mg twice daily and subjects in the comparator group.

Table 10: Baseline Characteristics

Randomized Study Protocol 021	ISENTRESS 400 mg Twice Daily (N = 281)	Efavirenz 600 mg At Bedtime (N = 282)
Gender		
Male	81%	82%
Female	19%	18%
Race		
White	41%	44%
Black	12%	8%
Asian	13%	11%
Hispanic	21%	24%
Native American	<1%	<1%
Multiracial	12%	13%
Region		
Latin America	35%	34%
Southeast Asia	12%	10%
North America	29%	32%
EU/Australia	23%	23%
Age (years)		
18-64	99%	99%
≥65	1%	1%
Mean (SD)	38 (9)	37 (10)
Median (min, max)	37 (19 to 67)	36 (19 to 71)
CD4+ Cell Count (cells/microL)		
Mean (SD)	219 (124)	217 (134)
Median (min, max)	212 (1 to 620)	204 (4 to 807)
Plasma HIV-1 RNA (log_{10} copies/mL)		
Mean (SD)	5 (1)	5 (1)
Median (min, max)	5 (3 to 6)	5 (4 to 6)
Plasma HIV-1 RNA (copies/mL)		
Geometric Mean	103205	106215
Median (min, max)	114000 (400 to 750000)	104000 (4410 to 750000)
History of AIDS*		
Yes	19%	21%
Viral Subtype		
Clade B	78%	82%
Non-Clade B†	21%	17%
Baseline Plasma HIV-1 RNA		
≤100,000 copies/mL	45%	49%
>100,000 copies/mL	55%	51%
Baseline CD4+ Cell Counts		
≤50 cells/mm^3	10%	11%
>50 cells/mm^3 and ≤200 cells/mm^3	37%	37%
>200 cells/mm^3	53%	51%
Hepatitis Status		
Hepatitis B or C Positive‡	6%	6%

Notes:

ISENTRESS and Efavirenz were administered with emtricitabine (+) tenofovir

N = Number of subjects in each group.

* Includes additional subjects identified as having a history of AIDS.

† Non-Clade B Subtypes (# of subjects): Clade A (4), A/C (1), A/G (2), A1 (1), AE (29), AG (12), BF (6), C (37), D (2), F (2), F1 (5), G (2), Complex (3).

‡ Evidence of hepatitis B surface antigen or evidence of HCV RNA by polymerase chain reaction (PCR) quantitative test for hepatitis C Virus.

Week 240 outcomes from Protocol 021 are shown in Table 11.

[See table 11 above]

The mean changes in CD4 count from baseline were 295 cells/mm^3 in the group receiving ISENTRESS 400 mg twice daily and 236 cells/mm^3 in the group receiving Efavirenz 600 mg at bedtime.

14.2 Treatment-Experienced Adult Subjects

BENCHMRK 1 and BENCHMRK 2 are Phase 3 studies to evaluate the safety and antiretroviral activity of ISENTRESS 400 mg twice daily in combination with an optimized background therapy (OBT), versus OBT alone, in HIV-1-infected subjects, 16 years or older, with documented resistance to at least 1 drug in each of 3 classes (NNRTIs, NRTIs, PIs) of antiretroviral therapies. Randomization was stratified by degree of resistance to PI (1PI vs. >1PI) and the use of enfuvirtide in the OBT. Prior to randomization, OBT was selected by the investigator based on genotypic/phenotypic resistance testing and prior ART history.

Table 12 shows the demographic characteristics of subjects in the group receiving ISENTRESS 400 mg twice daily and subjects in the placebo group.

Table 15: Virologic Response at 96 Week Window by Baseline Genotypic/Phenotypic Sensitivity Score

	Percent with HIV-1 RNA <50 copies/mL At Week 96			
	n	ISENTRESS 400 mg Twice Daily + OBT (N = 462)	n	Placebo + OBT (N = 237)
Phenotypic Sensitivity Score (PSS)*				
0	67	43	43	5
1	144	58	71	23
2	142	61	66	32
3 or more	85	48	48	42
Genotypic Sensitivity Score (GSS)*				
0	116	39	65	5
1	177	62	95	26
2	111	61	49	53
3 or more	51	49	23	35

* The Phenotypic Sensitivity Score (PSS) and the Genotypic Sensitivity Score (GSS) were defined as the total oral ARTs in OBT to which a subject's viral isolate showed phenotypic sensitivity and genotypic sensitivity, respectively, based upon phenotypic and genotypic resistance tests. Enfuvirtide use in OBT in enfuvirtide-naïve subjects was counted as one active drug in OBT in the GSS and PSS. Similarly, darunavir use in OBT in darunavir-naïve subjects was counted as one active drug in OBT.

Table 12: Baseline Characteristics

Randomized Studies Protocol 018 and 019	ISENTRESS 400 mg Twice Daily + OBT (N = 462)	Placebo + OBT (N = 237)
Gender		
Male	88%	89%
Female	12%	11%
Race		
White	65%	73%
Black	14%	11%
Asian	3%	3%
Hispanic	11%	8%
Others	6%	5%
Age (years)		
Median (min, max)	45 (16 to 74)	45 (17 to 70)
CD4+ Cell Count		
Median (min, max), cells/mm^3	119 (1 to 792)	123 (0 to 759)
≤50 cells/mm^3	32%	33%
>50 and ≤200 cells/mm^3	37%	36%
Plasma HIV-1 RNA		
Median (min, max), $\log_{10}$ copies/mL	4.8 (2 to 6)	4.7 (2 to 6)
>100,000 copies/mL	36%	33%
History of AIDS		
Yes	92%	91%
Prior Use of ART, Median (1st Quartile, 3rd Quartile)		
Years of ART Use	10 (7 to 12)	10 (8 to 12)
Number of ART	12 (9 to 15)	12 (9 to 14)
Hepatitis Co-infection*		
No Hepatitis B or C virus	83%	84%
Hepatitis B virus only	8%	3%
Hepatitis C virus only	8%	12%
Co-infection of Hepatitis B and C virus	1%	1%
Stratum		
Enfuvirtide in OBT	38%	38%
Resistant to ≥2 PI	97%	95%

* Hepatitis B virus surface antigen positive or hepatitis C virus antibody positive.

Table 13 compares the characteristics of optimized background therapy at baseline in the group receiving ISENTRESS 400 mg twice daily and subjects in the control group.

Table 13: Characteristics of Optimized Background Therapy at Baseline

Randomized Studies Protocol 018 and 019	ISENTRESS 400 mg Twice Daily + OBT (N = 462)	Placebo + OBT (N = 237)
Number of ARTs in OBT		
Median (min, max)	4 (1 to 7)	4 (2 to 7)
Number of Active PI in OBT by Phenotypic Resistance Test*		
0	36%	41%
1 or more	60%	58%
Phenotypic Sensitivity Score (PSS)†		
0	15%	18%
1	31%	30%
2	31%	28%
3 or more	18%	20%
Genotypic Sensitivity Score (GSS)†		
0	25%	27%
1	38%	40%
2	24%	21%
3 or more	11%	10%

* Darunavir use in OBT in darunavir-naïve subjects was counted as one active PI.

† The Phenotypic Sensitivity Score (PSS) and the Genotypic Sensitivity Score (GSS) were defined as the total oral ARTs in OBT to which a subject's viral isolate showed phenotypic sensitivity and genotypic sensitivity, respectively, based upon phenotypic and genotypic resistance tests. Enfuvirtide use in OBT in enfuvirtide-naïve subjects was counted as one active drug in OBT in the GSS and PSS. Similarly, darunavir use in OBT in darunavir-naïve subjects was counted as one active drug in OBT.

Week 96 outcomes for the 699 subjects randomized and treated with the recommended dose of ISENTRESS 400 mg twice daily or placebo in the pooled BENCHMRK 1 and 2 studies are shown in Table 14.

Table 14: Virologic Outcomes of Randomized Treatment of Protocols 018 and 019 at 96 Weeks (Pooled Analysis)

	ISENTRESS 400 mg Twice Daily + OBT (N = 462)	Placebo + OBT (N = 237)
Subjects with HIV-1 RNA less than 50 copies/mL	55%	27%
Virologic Failure*	35%	66%
No virologic data at Week 96 Window		
Reasons		
Discontinued study due to AE or death†	3%	3%
Discontinued study for other reasons‡	4%	4%
Missing data during window but on study	4%	<1%

* Includes subjects who switched to open-label raltegravir after Week 16 due to the protocol-defined virologic failure, subjects who discontinued prior to Week 96 for lack of efficacy, subjects changed OBT due to lack of efficacy prior to Week 96, or subjects who were ≥50 copies in the 96 week window.

† Includes subjects who discontinued due to AE or Death at any time point from Day 1 through the Week 96 window if this resulted in no virologic data on treatment during the Week 96 window.

‡ Other includes: withdrew consent, loss to follow-up, moved etc., if the viral load at the time of discontinuation was <50 copies/mL.

The mean changes in CD4 count from baseline were 118 cells/mm^3 in the group receiving ISENTRESS 400 mg twice daily and 47 cells/mm^3 for the control group.
Treatment-emergent CDC Category C events occurred in 4% of the group receiving ISENTRESS 400 mg twice daily and 5% of the control group.
Virologic responses at Week 96 by baseline genotypic and phenotypic sensitivity score are shown in Table 15.
[See table 15 above]

Switch of Suppressed Subjects from Lopinavir (+) Ritonavir to Raltegravir

The SWITCHMRK 1 & 2 Phase 3 studies evaluated HIV-1 infected subjects receiving suppressive therapy (HIV-1 RNA <50 copies/mL on a stable regimen of lopinavir 200 mg (+) ritonavir 50 mg 2 tablets twice daily plus at least 2 nucleoside reverse transcriptase inhibitors for >3 months) and randomized them 1:1 to either continue lopinavir (+) ritonavir (n=174 and n=178, SWITCHMRK 1 & 2, respectively) or replace lopinavir (+) ritonavir with ISENTRESS 400 mg twice daily (n=174 and n=176, respectively). The primary virology endpoint was the proportion of subjects with HIV-1 RNA less than 50 copies/mL at Week 24 with a prespecified non-inferiority margin of -12% for each study; and the frequency of adverse events up to 24 weeks.
Subjects with a prior history of virological failure were not excluded and the number of previous antiretroviral therapies was not limited.
These studies were terminated after the primary efficacy analysis at Week 24 because they each failed to demonstrate non-inferiority of switching to ISENTRESS versus continuing on lopinavir (+) ritonavir. In the combined analysis of these studies at Week 24, suppression of HIV-1 RNA to less than 50 copies/mL was maintained in 82.3% of the ISENTRESS group versus 90.3% of the lopinavir (+) ritonavir group. Clinical and laboratory adverse events occurred at similar frequencies in the treatment groups.

14.3 Pediatric Subjects

IMPAACT P1066 is a Phase I/II open label multicenter trial to evaluate the pharmacokinetic profile, safety, tolerability, and efficacy of raltegravir in HIV infected children. This study enrolled 126 treatment experienced children and adolescents 2 to 18 years of age. Subjects were stratified by age, enrolling adolescents first and then successively younger children. Subjects received either the 400 mg film-coated tablet formulation (6 to 18 years of age) or the chewable tablet formulation (2 to less than 12 years of age). Raltegravir was administered with an optimized background regimen.

The initial dose finding stage included intensive pharmacokinetic evaluation. Dose selection was based upon achieving similar raltegravir plasma exposure and trough concentration as seen in adults, and acceptable short term safety. After dose selection, additional subjects were enrolled for evaluation of long term safety, tolerability and efficacy. Of the 126 subjects, 96 received the recommended dose of ISENTRESS *[see Dosage and Administration (2.3)]*.

These 96 subjects had a median age of 13 (range 2 to 18) years, were 51% Female, 34% Caucasian, and 59% Black. At baseline, mean plasma HIV-1 RNA was 4.3 log_{10} copies/mL, median CD4 cell count was 481 cells/mm^3 (range: 0 – 2361) and median CD4% was 23.3% (range: 0 – 44). Overall, 8% had baseline plasma HIV-1 RNA >100,000 copies/mL and 59% had a CDC HIV clinical classification of category B or C. Most subjects had previously used at least one NNRTI (78%) or one PI (83%).

Ninety-three (97%) subjects 2 to 18 years of age completed 24 weeks of treatment (3 discontinued due to noncompliance). At Week 24, 54% achieved HIV RNA <50 copies/mL; 72% achieved HIV RNA <400 copies/mL or ≥1 log_{10} HIV RNA drop from baseline. The mean CD4 count (percent) increase from baseline to Week 24 was 119 cells/mm^3 (3.8%).

16 HOW SUPPLIED/STORAGE AND HANDLING

ISENTRESS tablets 400 mg are pink, oval-shaped, film-coated tablets with "227" on one side. They are supplied as follows:

NDC 0006-0227-61 unit-of-use bottles of 60.
No. 3894

ISENTRESS tablets 100 mg are pale orange, oval-shaped, orange-banana flavored, chewable tablets scored on both sides and imprinted on one face with the Merck logo and "477" on opposite sides of the score. They are supplied as follows:

NDC 0006-0477-61 unit-of-use bottles of 60.
No. 3972

ISENTRESS tablets 25 mg are pale yellow, round, orange-banana flavored, chewable tablets with the Merck logo on one side and "473" on the other side. They are supplied as follows:

NDC 0006-0473-61 unit-of-use bottles of 60.
No. 3965

Storage and Handling

400 mg Film-coated Tablets and Chewable Tablets

Store at 20-25°C (68-77°F); excursions permitted to 15-30°C (59-86°F). See USP Controlled Room Temperature.

Chewable Tablets

Store in the original package with the bottle tightly closed. Keep the desiccant in the bottle to protect from moisture.

17 PATIENT COUNSELING INFORMATION

See FDA-approved patient labeling (Patient Information)

Patients should be informed that severe and potentially life-threatening rash has been reported. Patients should be advised to immediately contact their healthcare provider if they develop rash. Instruct patients to immediately stop taking ISENTRESS and other suspect agents, and seek medical attention if they develop a rash associated with any of the following symptoms as it may be a sign of a more serious reaction such as Stevens-Johnson syndrome, toxic epidermal necrolysis or severe hypersensitivity: fever, generally ill feeling, extreme tiredness, muscle or joint aches, blisters, oral lesions, eye inflammation, facial swelling, swelling of the eyes, lips, mouth, breathing difficulty, and/or signs and symptoms of liver problems (e.g., yellowing of the skin or whites of the eyes, dark or tea colored urine, pale colored stools/bowel movements, nausea, vomiting, loss of appetite, or pain, aching or sensitivity on the right side below the ribs). Patients should understand that if severe rash occurs, they will be closely monitored, laboratory tests will be ordered and appropriate therapy will be initiated. Patients should also be told that it is very important that they remain under a physician's care during treatment with ISENTRESS.

Before beginning ISENTRESS, patients should be asked by their healthcare provider if they have a history of rhabdomyolysis, myopathy or increased creatine kinase or if they are taking medications known to cause these conditions such as statins, fenofibrate, gemfibrozil or zidovudine.

Patients should be instructed to immediately report to their healthcare provider any unexplained muscle pain, tenderness, or weakness while taking ISENTRESS.

Patients should be informed that ISENTRESS is not a cure for HIV infection or AIDS. Patients should be told that sustained decreases in plasma HIV RNA have been associated with a reduced risk of progression to AIDS and death. Patients should remain on continuous HIV therapy to control HIV infection and decrease HIV-related illnesses. They should also be told that people taking ISENTRESS may still get infections or other conditions common in people with HIV (opportunistic infections). Patients should be advised to continue to practice safer sex and to use latex or polyurethane condoms to lower the chance of sexual contact with any body fluids such as semen, vaginal secretions or blood. Patients should also be advised to never re-use or share needles or other injection equipment, or share personal items that can have blood or body fluids on them, such as toothbrushes and razor blades.

Physicians should instruct their patients that if they miss a dose, they should take it as soon as they remember. If they do not remember until it is time for the next dose, they should be instructed to skip the missed dose and go back to the regular schedule. Patients should not double their next dose or take more than the prescribed dose.

Patients should be informed that the chewable tablet forms can be chewed or swallowed whole, but the film-coated tablets should only be swallowed whole.

Physicians should alert patients with phenylketonuria that ISENTRESS Chewable Tablets contain phenylalanine *[see Warnings and Precautions (5.3)]*.

Physicians should instruct their patients to read the Patient Information before starting ISENTRESS therapy and to reread each time the prescription is renewed. Patients should be instructed to inform their physician or pharmacist if they develop any unusual symptom, or if any known symptom persists or worsens.

Distributed by:
Merck Sharp & Dohme Corp., a subsidiary of **Merck & Co., Inc.**
Whitehouse Station, NJ 08889, USA
uspi-0518-t-1308r024

For patent information: www.merck.com/product/patent/home.html

Patient Information
ISENTRESS® (eye sen tris)
(raltegravir)
Film-Coated Tablets
ISENTRESS® (eye sen tris)
(raltegravir)
Chewable Tablets

Read this Patient Information before you start taking ISENTRESS and each time you get a refill. There may be new information. This information does not take the place of talking with your doctor about your medical condition or your treatment.

What is ISENTRESS?

ISENTRESS is a prescription HIV medicine used with other HIV medicines to treat adults and children 2 years of age and older weighing at least 10 kg with human immunodeficiency virus (HIV-1) infection. HIV is the virus that causes AIDS (Acquired Immune Deficiency Syndrome).

When used with other HIV medicines, ISENTRESS may reduce the amount of HIV in your blood (called "viral load"). ISENTRESS may also help to increase the number of CD4 (T) cells in your blood which help fight off other infections. Reducing the amount of HIV and increasing the CD4 (T) cell count may improve your immune system. This may reduce your risk of death or infections that can happen when your immune system is weak (opportunistic infections).

It is not known if ISENTRESS is safe and effective in children under 2 years of age.

ISENTRESS does not cure HIV infection or AIDS. People taking ISENTRESS may still develop infections or other conditions associated with HIV infection. Some of these conditions are pneumonia, herpes virus infections, and Mycobacterium avium complex (MAC) infections.

Patients must stay on continuous HIV therapy to control infection and decrease HIV-related illnesses.

Avoid doing things that can spread HIV-1 infection to others:

- **Do not share needles or other injection equipment.**
- **Do not share personal items that can have blood or body fluids on them, like toothbrushes and razor blades.**
- **Do not have any kind of sex without protection.** Always practice safe sex by using a latex or polyurethane condom to lower the chance of sexual contact with semen, vaginal secretions, or blood.

Ask your doctor if you have any questions on how to prevent passing HIV to other people.

What should I tell my doctor before taking ISENTRESS?

Before taking ISENTRESS, tell your doctor if you:

- have liver problems.
- have phenylketonuria (PKU). ISENTRESS Chewable Tablets contain phenylalanine as part of the artificial sweetener, aspartame. The artificial sweetener may be harmful to people with PKU.
- have any other medical conditions.
- are pregnant or plan to become pregnant. It is not known if ISENTRESS can harm your unborn baby.
  Pregnancy Registry: You and your doctor will need to decide if taking ISENTRESS is right for you. If you take ISENTRESS while you are pregnant, talk to your doctor about how you can be included in the Antiretroviral Pregnancy Registry. The purpose of the registry is to follow the health of you and your baby.
- are breastfeeding or plan to breastfeed.
  - Do not breastfeed if you are taking ISENTRESS. You should not breastfeed if you have HIV because of the risk of passing HIV to your baby.
  - Talk with your doctor about the best way to feed your baby.

Tell your doctor about all the medicines you take, including: prescription and non-prescription medicines, vitamins, and herbal supplements. Taking ISENTRESS and certain other medicines may affect each other causing serious side effects. ISENTRESS may affect the way other medicines work and other medicines may affect how ISENTRESS works.

Especially tell your doctor if you take:

- rifampin (Rifadin, Rifamate, Rifater, Rimactane), a medicine commonly used to treat tuberculosis.

Ask your doctor or pharmacist if you are not sure whether any of your medicines are included in the list above.

Know the medicines you take. Keep a list of them to show your doctor and pharmacist when you get a new medicine. Do not start any new medicines while you are taking ISENTRESS without first talking with your doctor.

How should I take ISENTRESS?

- **Take ISENTRESS exactly as prescribed by your doctor.**
- You should stay under the care of your doctor while taking ISENTRESS.
- Do not change your dose of ISENTRESS, switch between the film-coated tablet and the chewable tablet or stop your treatment without talking with your doctor first.
- Take ISENTRESS by mouth, with or without food.
- If your child is taking ISENTRESS, your child's doctor will decide the right dose based on your child's age and weight.
- ISENTRESS Chewable Tablets may be chewed or swallowed whole.
- ISENTRESS Film-Coated Tablets must be swallowed whole.
- If you miss a dose, take it as soon as you remember. If you do not remember until it is time for your next dose, skip the missed dose and go back to your regular schedule. Do not double your next dose or take more than your prescribed dose.
- If you take too much ISENTRESS, call your doctor or go to the nearest emergency room right away.
- Do not run out of ISENTRESS. Get your ISENTRESS refilled from your doctor or pharmacy before you run out.

What are the possible side effects of ISENTRESS?

ISENTRESS can cause serious side effects including:

- **Serious skin reactions and allergic reactions.** Severe, potentially life-threatening and fatal skin reactions and allergic reactions have been reported in some patients taking ISENTRESS. If you develop a rash with any of the following symptoms, stop using ISENTRESS and contact your doctor right away:

  - fever
  - generally ill feeling
  - extreme tiredness
  - muscle or joint aches
  - blisters or sores in mouth
  - blisters or peeling of the skin
  - redness or swelling of the eyes
  - swelling of the mouth or face
  - problems breathing

Sometimes allergic reactions can affect body organs, like the liver. Contact your doctor right away if you have any of the following signs or symptoms of liver problems:

- yellowing of the skin or whites of the eyes
- dark or tea colored urine
- pale colored stools/bowel movements
- nausea/vomiting
- loss of appetite
- pain, aching or tenderness on the right side below the ribs

- **Changes in your immune system (Immune Reconstitution Syndrome)** can happen when you start taking HIV medicines. Your immune system may get stronger and begin to fight infections that have been hidden in your body for a long time. Tell your doctor right away if you start having new symptoms after starting your HIV medicine.
- **Phenylketonuria (PKU). ISENTRESS Chewable Tablets** contain phenylalanine as part of the artificial sweetener, aspartame. The artificial sweetener may be harmful to people with PKU.

In clinical trials, the most common (≥2%) side effects of ISENTRESS include:

- dizziness
- headache

- nausea
- tiredness
- trouble sleeping

In clinical trials, less common (<2%) side effects include:

- allergic reaction
- depression
- hepatitis
- genital herpes
- herpes zoster including shingles
- kidney failure
- kidney stones
- stomach pain
- suicidal thoughts and actions
- vomiting
- weakness

Tell your doctor before beginning ISENTRESS if you have a history of muscle disorders (rhabdomyolysis or myopathy) or increased creatine kinase or if you are taking medications known to cause these conditions such as statins, fenofibrate, gemfibrozil or zidovudine.

Tell your doctor right away if you get unexplained muscle pain, tenderness, or weakness while taking ISENTRESS. This may be a sign of a rare but serious muscle problem that can lead to kidney problems.

Rash occurred more often in patients taking ISENTRESS and darunavir/ritonavir together than with either drug separately, but was generally mild.

Tell your doctor if you have any side effect that bothers you or that does not go away.

These are not all the possible side effects of ISENTRESS. For more information, ask your doctor or pharmacist.

Call your doctor for medical advice about side effects. You may report side effects to FDA at 1-800-FDA-1088.

How should I store ISENTRESS?

Film-Coated Tablets:

- Store ISENTRESS Film-Coated Tablets at room temperature between 68°F to 77°F (20°C to 25°C).

Chewable Tablets:

- Store ISENTRESS Chewable Tablets at room temperature between 68°F to 77°F (20°C to 25°C).
- Store ISENTRESS Chewable Tablets in the original package with the bottle tightly closed.
- Keep the drying agent (desiccant) in the bottle to protect from moisture.

Keep ISENTRESS and all medicines out of the reach of children.

General information about ISENTRESS

Medicines are sometimes prescribed for conditions that are not mentioned in Patient Information Leaflets. Do not use ISENTRESS for a condition for which it was not prescribed. Do not give ISENTRESS to other people, even if they have the same symptoms you have. It may harm them.

This leaflet gives you the most important information about ISENTRESS.

If you would like to know more, talk with your doctor. You can ask your doctor or pharmacist for information about ISENTRESS that is written for health professionals.

For more information go to www.ISENTRESS.com or call 1-800-622-4477.

What are the ingredients in ISENTRESS?

ISENTRESS Film-Coated Tablets:

Active ingredient: raltegravir

Inactive ingredients: microcrystalline cellulose, lactose monohydrate, calcium phosphate dibasic anhydrous, hypromellose 2208, poloxamer 407 (contains 0.01% butylated hydroxytoluene as antioxidant), sodium stearyl fumarate, magnesium stearate.

The film coating contains: polyvinyl alcohol, titanium dioxide, polyethylene glycol 3350, talc, red iron oxide and black iron oxide.

ISENTRESS Chewable Tablets:

Active ingredient: raltegravir

Inactive ingredients: hydroxypropyl cellulose, sucralose, saccharin sodium, sodium citrate dihydrate, mannitol, red iron oxide (100 mg tablet only), yellow iron oxide, monoammonium glycyrrhizinate, sorbitol, fructose, natural and artificial flavors (orange, banana, and masking that contains aspartame), crospovidone, magnesium stearate, sodium stearyl fumarate, ethylcellulose 20 cP, ammonium hydroxide, medium chain triglycerides, oleic acid, hypromellose 2910/6cP, PEG 400.

This Patient Information has been approved by the U.S. Food and Drug Administration.

Distributed by:
Merck Sharp & Dohme Corp., a subsidiary of **Merck & Co., Inc.**
Whitehouse Station, NJ 08889, USA

Revised 08/2013

usppi-0518-t-1308r023

For patent information: www.merck.com/product/patent/home.html

Shown in Product Identification Guide, page 308

JANUMET® ℞
[JAN-you-met]
(sitagliptin/metformin HCl)
tablets

HIGHLIGHTS OF PRESCRIBING INFORMATION
These highlights do not include all the information needed to use JANUMET safely and effectively. See full prescribing information for JANUMET.
JANUMET® (sitagliptin/metformin HCl) tablets
Initial U.S. Approval: 2007

WARNING: LACTIC ACIDOSIS
See full prescribing information for complete boxed warning.

- **Lactic acidosis can occur due to metformin accumulation. The risk increases with conditions such as sepsis, dehydration, excess alcohol intake, hepatic insufficiency, renal impairment, and acute congestive heart failure. (5.1)**
- **Symptoms include malaise, myalgias, respiratory distress, increasing somnolence, and nonspecific abdominal distress. Laboratory abnormalities include low pH, increased anion gap and elevated blood lactate. (5.1)**
- **If acidosis is suspected, discontinue JANUMET and hospitalize the patient immediately. (5.1)**

RECENT MAJOR CHANGES

Dosage and Administration
Recommended Dosing (2.1) 02/2013

INDICATIONS AND USAGE

JANUMET is a dipeptidyl peptidase-4 (DPP-4) inhibitor and biguanide combination product indicated as an adjunct to diet and exercise to improve glycemic control in adults with type 2 diabetes mellitus when treatment with both sitagliptin and metformin is appropriate. (1)

Important Limitations of Use:

- JANUMET should not be used in patients with type 1 diabetes or for the treatment of diabetic ketoacidosis. (1)
- JANUMET has not been studied in patients with a history of pancreatitis. (1, 5.2)

DOSAGE AND ADMINISTRATION

- Individualize the starting dose of JANUMET based on the patient's current regimen. (2.1)
- May adjust the dosing based on effectiveness and tolerability while not exceeding the maximum recommended daily dose of 100 mg sitagliptin and 2000 mg metformin. (2.1)
- JANUMET should be given twice daily with meals, with gradual dose escalation, to reduce the gastrointestinal (GI) side effects due to metformin. (2.1)

DOSAGE FORMS AND STRENGTHS

Tablets: 50 mg sitagliptin/500 mg metformin HCl and 50 mg sitagliptin/1000 mg metformin HCl (3)

CONTRAINDICATIONS

- Renal dysfunction, e.g., serum creatinine ≥1.5 mg/dL [males], ≥1.4 mg/dL [females] or abnormal creatinine clearance. (4, 5.1, 5.4)
- Acute or chronic metabolic acidosis, including diabetic ketoacidosis, with or without coma. (4, 5.1)
- History of a serious hypersensitivity reaction to JANUMET or sitagliptin (one of the components of JANUMET), such as anaphylaxis or angioedema. (5.14, 6.2)
- Temporarily discontinue JANUMET in patients undergoing radiologic studies involving intravascular administration of iodinated contrast materials. (4, 5.1, 5.11)

WARNINGS AND PRECAUTIONS

- Do not use JANUMET in patients with hepatic disease. (5.1, 5.3)
- There have been postmarketing reports of acute renal failure, sometimes requiring dialysis. Before initiating JANUMET and at least annually thereafter, assess renal function and verify as normal. (4, 5.1, 5.4, 5.10, 6.2)
- There have been postmarketing reports of acute pancreatitis, including fatal and non-fatal hemorrhagic or necrotizing pancreatitis. If pancreatitis is suspected, promptly discontinue JANUMET. (5.2)
- Measure hematologic parameters annually. (5.5, 6.1)
- Warn patients against excessive alcohol intake. (5.1, 5.6)
- May need to discontinue JANUMET and temporarily use insulin during periods of stress and decreased intake of fluids and food as may occur with fever, trauma, infection or surgery. (5.7, 5.8, 5.12, 5.13)
- Promptly evaluate patients previously controlled on JANUMET who develop laboratory abnormalities or clinical illness for evidence of ketoacidosis or lactic acidosis. (5.1, 5.8, 5.12, 5.13)
- When used with an insulin secretagogue (e.g., sulfonylurea) or with insulin, a lower dose of the insulin secretagogue or insulin may be required to reduce the risk of hypoglycemia. (2.1, 5.9)
- There have been postmarketing reports of serious allergic and hypersensitivity reactions in patients treated with sitagliptin (one of the components of JANUMET), such as anaphylaxis, angioedema, and exfoliative skin conditions including Stevens-Johnson syndrome. In such cases, promptly stop JANUMET, assess for other potential causes, institute appropriate monitoring and treatment, and initiate alternative treatment for diabetes. (5.14, 6.2)
- There have been no clinical studies establishing conclusive evidence of macrovascular risk reduction with JANUMET or any other anti-diabetic drug. (5.15)

ADVERSE REACTIONS

- The most common adverse reactions reported in ≥5% of patients simultaneously started on sitagliptin and metformin and more commonly than in patients treated with placebo were diarrhea, upper respiratory tract infection, and headache. (6.1)
- Adverse reactions reported in ≥5% of patients treated with sitagliptin in combination with sulfonylurea and metformin and more commonly than in patients treated with placebo in combination with sulfonylurea and metformin were hypoglycemia and headache. (6.1)
- Hypoglycemia was the only adverse reaction reported in ≥5% of patients treated with sitagliptin in combination with insulin and metformin and more commonly than in patients treated with placebo in combination with insulin and metformin. (6.1)
- Nasopharyngitis was the only adverse reaction reported in ≥5% of patients treated with sitagliptin monotherapy and more commonly than in patients given placebo. (6.1)
- The most common (>5%) adverse reactions due to initiation of metformin therapy are diarrhea, nausea/vomiting, flatulence, abdominal discomfort, indigestion, asthenia, and headache. (6.1)

To report SUSPECTED ADVERSE REACTIONS, contact Merck Sharp & Dohme Corp., a subsidiary of Merck & Co., Inc., at 1-877-888-4231 or FDA at 1-800-FDA-1088 or www.fda.gov/medwatch.

DRUG INTERACTIONS

- Cationic drugs eliminated by renal tubular secretion: Use with caution. (5.10, 7.1)

USE IN SPECIFIC POPULATIONS

- Safety and effectiveness of JANUMET in children under 18 years have not been established. (8.4)
- There are no adequate and well-controlled studies in pregnant women. To report drug exposure during pregnancy call 1-800-986-8999. (8.1)

See 17 for PATIENT COUNSELING INFORMATION and Medication Guide

Revised: 03/2013

FULL PRESCRIBING INFORMATION: CONTENTS*

*** Sections or subsections omitted from the full prescribing information are not listed**

FULL PRESCRIBING INFORMATION

WARNING: LACTIC ACIDOSIS

Lactic acidosis is a rare, but serious complication that can occur due to metformin accumulation. The risk increases with conditions such as sepsis, dehydration, excess alcohol intake, hepatic insufficiency, renal impairment, and acute congestive heart failure.

The onset is often subtle, accompanied only by nonspecific symptoms such as malaise, myalgias, respiratory distress, increasing somnolence, and nonspecific abdominal distress.

Laboratory abnormalities include low pH, increased anion gap and elevated blood lactate.

If acidosis is suspected, JANUMET should be discontinued and the patient hospitalized immediately. *[See Warnings and Precautions (5.1).]*

1 INDICATIONS AND USAGE

JANUMET is indicated as an adjunct to diet and exercise to improve glycemic control in adults with type 2 diabetes mellitus when treatment with both sitagliptin and metformin is appropriate. *[See Clinical Studies (14).]*

Important Limitations of Use

JANUMET should not be used in patients with type 1 diabetes or for the treatment of diabetic ketoacidosis, as it would not be effective in these settings.

JANUMET has not been studied in patients with a history of pancreatitis. It is unknown whether patients with a history of pancreatitis are at increased risk for the development of pancreatitis while using JANUMET. *[See Warnings and Precautions (5.2).]*

2 DOSAGE AND ADMINISTRATION

2.1 Recommended Dosing

The dosage of JANUMET should be individualized on the basis of the patient's current regimen, effectiveness, and tolerability while not exceeding the maximum recommended daily dose of 100 mg sitagliptin and 2000 mg metformin. Initial combination therapy or maintenance of combination therapy should be individualized and left to the discretion of the health care provider.

JANUMET should generally be given twice daily with meals, with gradual dose escalation, to reduce the gastrointestinal (GI) side effects due to metformin. JANUMET must not be split or divided before swallowing.

The starting dose of JANUMET should be based on the patient's current regimen. JANUMET should be given twice daily with meals. The following doses are available:

50 mg sitagliptin/500 mg metformin hydrochloride

50 mg sitagliptin/1000 mg metformin hydrochloride.

The recommended starting dose in patients not currently treated with metformin is 50 mg sitagliptin/500 mg metformin hydrochloride twice daily, with gradual dose escalation recommended to reduce gastrointestinal side effects associated with metformin.

The starting dose in patients already treated with metformin should provide sitagliptin dosed as 50 mg twice daily (100 mg total daily dose) and the dose of metformin already being taken. For patients taking metformin 850 mg twice daily, the recommended starting dose of JANUMET is 50 mg sitagliptin/1000 mg metformin hydrochloride twice daily.

Patients treated with an insulin secretagogue or insulin

Co-administration of JANUMET with an insulin secretagogue (e.g., sulfonylurea) or insulin may require lower doses of the insulin secretagogue or insulin to reduce the risk of hypoglycemia *[see Warnings and Precautions (5.9)]*.

No studies have been performed specifically examining the safety and efficacy of JANUMET in patients previously treated with other oral antihyperglycemic agents and switched to JANUMET. Any change in therapy of type 2 diabetes should be undertaken with care and appropriate monitoring as changes in glycemic control can occur.

3 DOSAGE FORMS AND STRENGTHS

- 50 mg/500 mg tablets are light pink, capsule-shaped, film-coated tablets with "575" debossed on one side.
- 50 mg/1000 mg tablets are red, capsule-shaped, film-coated tablets with "577" debossed on one side.

4 CONTRAINDICATIONS

JANUMET (sitagliptin/metformin HCl) is contraindicated in patients with:

- Renal disease or renal dysfunction, e.g., as suggested by serum creatinine levels greater than or equal to 1.5 mg/dL [males], greater than or equal to 1.4 mg/dL [females] or abnormal creatinine clearance which may also result from conditions such as cardiovascular collapse (shock), acute myocardial infarction, and septicemia *[see Warnings and Precautions (5.1)]*.
- Acute or chronic metabolic acidosis, including diabetic ketoacidosis, with or without coma.
- History of a serious hypersensitivity reaction to JANUMET or sitagliptin (one of the components of JANUMET), such as anaphylaxis or angioedema. *[See Warnings and Precautions (5.14); Adverse Reactions (6.2).]*

JANUMET should be temporarily discontinued in patients undergoing radiologic studies involving intravascular administration of iodinated contrast materials, because use of such products may result in acute alteration of renal function *[see Warnings and Precautions (5.11)]*.

5 WARNINGS AND PRECAUTIONS

5.1 Lactic Acidosis

Metformin hydrochloride

Lactic acidosis is a rare, but serious, metabolic complication that can occur due to metformin accumulation during treatment with JANUMET; when it occurs, it is fatal in approximately 50% of cases. Lactic acidosis may also occur in association with a number of pathophysiologic conditions, including diabetes mellitus, and whenever there is significant tissue hypoperfusion and hypoxemia. Lactic acidosis is characterized by elevated blood lactate levels (>5 mmol/L), decreased blood pH, electrolyte disturbances with an increased anion gap, and an increased lactate/pyruvate ratio. When metformin is implicated as the cause of lactic acidosis, metformin plasma levels >5 μg/mL are generally found. The reported incidence of lactic acidosis in patients receiving metformin hydrochloride is very low (approximately 0.03 cases/1000 patient-years, with approximately 0.015 fatal cases/1000 patient-years). In more than 20,000 patient-years exposure to metformin in clinical trials, there were no reports of lactic acidosis. Reported cases have occurred primarily in diabetic patients with significant renal insufficiency, including both intrinsic renal disease and renal hypoperfusion, often in the setting of multiple concomitant medical/surgical problems and multiple concomitant medications. Patients with congestive heart failure requiring pharmacologic management, in particular those with unstable or acute congestive heart failure who are at risk of hypoperfusion and hypoxemia, are at increased risk of lactic acidosis. The risk of lactic acidosis increases with the degree of renal dysfunction and the patient's age. The risk of lactic acidosis may, therefore, be significantly decreased by regular monitoring of renal function in patients taking metformin and by use of the minimum effective dose of metformin. In particular, treatment of the elderly should be accompanied by careful monitoring of renal function. Metformin treatment should not be initiated in patients ≥80 years of age unless measurement of creatinine clearance demonstrates that renal function is not reduced, as these patients are more susceptible to developing lactic acidosis. In addition, metformin should be promptly withheld in the presence of any condition associated with hypoxemia, dehydration, or sepsis. Because impaired hepatic function may significantly limit the ability to clear lactate, metformin should generally be avoided in patients with clinical or laboratory evidence of hepatic disease. Patients should be cautioned against excessive alcohol intake, either acute or chronic, when taking metformin, since alcohol potentiates the effects of metformin hydrochloride on lactate metabolism. In addition, metformin should be temporarily discontinued prior to any intravascular radiocontrast study and for any surgical procedure *[see Warnings and Precautions (5.4, 5.6, 5.7, 5.11)]*.

The onset of lactic acidosis often is subtle, and accompanied only by nonspecific symptoms such as malaise, myalgias, respiratory distress, increasing somnolence, and nonspecific abdominal distress. There may be associated hypothermia, hypotension, and resistant bradyarrhythmias with more marked acidosis. The patient and the patient's physician must be aware of the possible importance of such symptoms and the patient should be instructed to notify the physician immediately if they occur *[see Warnings and Precautions (5.12)]*. Metformin should be withdrawn until the situation is clarified. Serum electrolytes, ketones, blood glucose, and if indicated, blood pH, lactate levels, and even blood metformin levels may be useful. Once a patient is stabilized on any dose level of metformin, gastrointestinal symptoms, which are common during initiation of therapy, are unlikely to be drug related. Later occurrence of gastrointestinal symptoms could be due to lactic acidosis or other serious disease.

Levels of fasting venous plasma lactate above the upper limit of normal but less than 5 mmol/L in patients taking metformin do not necessarily indicate impending lactic acidosis and may be explainable by other mechanisms, such as poorly controlled diabetes or obesity, vigorous physical activity, or technical problems in sample handling *[see Warnings and Precautions (5.8, 5.13)]*.

Lactic acidosis should be suspected in any diabetic patient with metabolic acidosis lacking evidence of ketoacidosis (ketonuria and ketonemia).

Lactic acidosis is a medical emergency that must be treated in a hospital setting. In a patient with lactic acidosis who is taking metformin, the drug should be discontinued immediately and general supportive measures promptly instituted. Because metformin hydrochloride is dialyzable (with a clearance of up to 170 mL/min under good hemodynamic conditions), prompt hemodialysis is recommended to correct the acidosis and remove the accumulated metformin. Such management often results in prompt reversal of symptoms and recovery *[see Contraindications (4); Warnings and Precautions (5.6, 5.7, 5.10, 5.11, 5.12)]*.

5.2 Pancreatitis

There have been postmarketing reports of acute pancreatitis, including fatal and non-fatal hemorrhagic or necrotizing pancreatitis, in patients taking JANUMET. After initiation of JANUMET, patients should be observed carefully for signs and symptoms of pancreatitis. If pancreatitis is suspected, JANUMET should promptly be discontinued and appropriate management should be initiated. It is unknown whether patients with a history of pancreatitis are at increased risk for the development of pancreatitis while using JANUMET.

5.3 Impaired Hepatic Function

Since impaired hepatic function has been associated with some cases of lactic acidosis, JANUMET should generally be avoided in patients with clinical or laboratory evidence of hepatic disease.

5.4 Assessment of Renal Function

Metformin and sitagliptin are known to be substantially excreted by the kidney. The risk of metformin accumulation and lactic acidosis increases with the degree of impairment of renal function. Thus, patients with serum creatinine levels above the upper limit of normal for their age should not receive JANUMET. In the elderly, JANUMET should be carefully titrated to establish the minimum dose for adequate glycemic effect, because aging can be associated with reduced renal function. *[See Warnings and Precautions (5.1); Use in Specific Populations (8.5).]*

There have been postmarketing reports of worsening renal function, including acute renal failure, sometimes requiring dialysis. Before initiation of therapy with JANUMET and at least annually thereafter, renal function should be assessed and verified as normal. In patients in whom development of renal dysfunction is anticipated, particularly in elderly patients, renal function should be assessed more frequently and JANUMET discontinued if evidence of renal impairment is present.

5.5 Vitamin B_{12} Levels

In controlled clinical trials of metformin of 29 weeks duration, a decrease to subnormal levels of previously normal serum Vitamin B_{12} levels, without clinical manifestations, was observed in approximately 7% of patients. Such decrease, possibly due to interference with B_{12} absorption from the B_{12}-intrinsic factor complex, is, however, very rarely associated with anemia and appears to be rapidly reversible with discontinuation of metformin or Vitamin B_{12} supplementation. Measurement of hematologic parameters on an annual basis is advised in patients on JANUMET and any apparent abnormalities should be appropriately investigated and managed. *[See Adverse Reactions (6.1).]*

Certain individuals (those with inadequate Vitamin B_{12} or calcium intake or absorption) appear to be predisposed to developing subnormal Vitamin B_{12} levels. In these patients, routine serum Vitamin B_{12} measurements at two- to three-year intervals may be useful.

5.6 Alcohol Intake

Alcohol is known to potentiate the effect of metformin on lactate metabolism. Patients, therefore, should be warned against excessive alcohol intake, acute or chronic, while receiving JANUMET.

5.7 Surgical Procedures
Use of JANUMET should be temporarily suspended for any surgical procedure (except minor procedures not associated with restricted intake of food and fluids) and should not be restarted until the patient's oral intake has resumed and renal function has been evaluated as normal.

5.8 Change in Clinical Status of Patients with Previously Controlled Type 2 Diabetes
A patient with type 2 diabetes previously well controlled on JANUMET who develops laboratory abnormalities or clinical illness (especially vague and poorly defined illness) should be evaluated promptly for evidence of ketoacidosis or lactic acidosis. Evaluation should include serum electrolytes and ketones, blood glucose and, if indicated, blood pH, lactate, pyruvate, and metformin levels. If acidosis of either form occurs, JANUMET must be stopped immediately and other appropriate corrective measures initiated.

5.9 Use with Medications Known to Cause Hypoglycemia
Sitagliptin
When sitagliptin was used in combination with a sulfonylurea or with insulin, medications known to cause hypoglycemia, the incidence of hypoglycemia was increased over that of placebo used in combination with a sulfonylurea or with insulin *[see Adverse Reactions (6)]*. Therefore, patients also receiving an insulin secretagogue (e.g., sulfonylurea) or insulin may require a lower dose of the insulin secretagogue or insulin to reduce the risk of hypoglycemia *[see Dosage and Administration (2.1)]*.
Metformin hydrochloride
Hypoglycemia does not occur in patients receiving metformin alone under usual circumstances of use, but could occur when caloric intake is deficient, when strenuous exercise is not compensated by caloric supplementation, or during concomitant use with other glucose-lowering agents (such as sulfonylureas and insulin) or ethanol. Elderly, debilitated, or malnourished patients, and those with adrenal or pituitary insufficiency or alcohol intoxication are particularly susceptible to hypoglycemic effects. Hypoglycemia may be difficult to recognize in the elderly, and in people who are taking β-adrenergic blocking drugs.

5.10 Concomitant Medications Affecting Renal Function or Metformin Disposition
Concomitant medication(s) that may affect renal function or result in significant hemodynamic change or may interfere with the disposition of metformin, such as cationic drugs that are eliminated by renal tubular secretion *[see Drug Interactions (7.1)]*, should be used with caution.

5.11 Radiologic Studies with Intravascular Iodinated Contrast Materials
Intravascular contrast studies with iodinated materials (for example, intravenous urogram, intravenous cholangiography, angiography, and computed tomography (CT) scans with intravascular contrast materials) can lead to acute alteration of renal function and have been associated with lactic acidosis in patients receiving metformin *[see Contraindications (4)]*. Therefore, in patients in whom any such study is planned, JANUMET should be temporarily discontinued at the time of or prior to the procedure, and withheld for 48 hours subsequent to the procedure and reinstituted only after renal function has been re-evaluated and found to be normal.

5.12 Hypoxic States
Cardiovascular collapse (shock) from whatever cause, acute congestive heart failure, acute myocardial infarction and other conditions characterized by hypoxemia have been associated with lactic acidosis and may also cause prerenal azotemia. When such events occur in patients on JANUMET therapy, the drug should be promptly discontinued.

5.13 Loss of Control of Blood Glucose
When a patient stabilized on any diabetic regimen is exposed to stress such as fever, trauma, infection, or surgery, a temporary loss of glycemic control may occur. At such times, it may be necessary to withhold JANUMET and temporarily administer insulin. JANUMET may be reinstituted after the acute episode is resolved.

5.14 Hypersensitivity Reactions
There have been postmarketing reports of serious hypersensitivity reactions in patients treated with sitagliptin, one of the components of JANUMET. These reactions include anaphylaxis, angioedema, and exfoliative skin conditions including Stevens-Johnson syndrome. Onset of these reactions occurred within the first 3 months after initiation of treatment with sitagliptin, with some reports occurring after the first dose. If a hypersensitivity reaction is suspected, discontinue JANUMET, assess for other potential causes for the event, and institute alternative treatment for diabetes. *[See Adverse Reactions (6.2).]*
Angioedema has also been reported with other dipeptidyl peptidase-4 (DPP-4) inhibitors. Use caution in a patient with a history of angioedema with another DPP-4 inhibitor because it is unknown whether such patients will be predisposed to angioedema with JANUMET.

Table 1: Sitagliptin and Metformin Co-administered to Patients with Type 2 Diabetes Inadequately Controlled on Diet and Exercise: Adverse Reactions Reported (Regardless of Investigator Assessment of Causality) in ≥5% of Patients Receiving Combination Therapy (and Greater than in Patients Receiving Placebo)*

	Number of Patients (%)			
	Placebo	Sitagliptin 100 mg QD	Metformin 500 mg/ Metformin 1000 mg bid†	Sitagliptin 50 mg bid + Metformin 500 mg/ Metformin 1000 mg bid†
	N = 176	N = 179	N = 364†	N = 372†
Diarrhea	7 (4.0)	5 (2.8)	28 (7.7)	28 (7.5)
Upper Respiratory Tract Infection	9 (5.1)	8 (4.5)	19 (5.2)	23 (6.2)
Headache	5 (2.8)	2 (1.1)	14 (3.8)	22 (5.9)

* Intent-to-treat population.
† Data pooled for the patients given the lower and higher doses of metformin.

Table 2: Pre-selected Gastrointestinal Adverse Reactions (Regardless of Investigator Assessment of Causality) Reported in Patients with Type 2 Diabetes Receiving Sitagliptin and Metformin

	Number of Patients (%)					
	Study of Sitagliptin and Metformin in Patients Inadequately Controlled on Diet and Exercise				Study of Sitagliptin Add-on in Patients Inadequately Controlled on Metformin Alone	
	Placebo	Sitagliptin 100 mg QD	Metformin 500 mg/ Metformin 1000 mg bid*	Sitagliptin 50 mg bid + Metformin 500 mg/ Metformin 1000 mg bid*	Placebo and Metformin ≥1500 mg daily	Sitagliptin 100 mg QD and Metformin ≥1500 mg daily
	N = 176	N = 179	N = 364	N = 372	N = 237	N = 464
Diarrhea	7 (4.0)	5 (2.8)	28 (7.7)	28 (7.5)	6 (2.5)	11 (2.4)
Nausea	2 (1.1)	2 (1.1)	20 (5.5)	18 (4.8)	2 (0.8)	6 (1.3)
Vomiting	1 (0.6)	0 (0.0)	2 (0.5)	8 (2.2)	2 (0.8)	5 (1.1)
Abdominal Pain†	4 (2.3)	6 (3.4)	14 (3.8)	11 (3.0)	9 (3.8)	10 (2.2)

* Data pooled for the patients given the lower and higher doses of metformin.
† Abdominal discomfort was included in the analysis of abdominal pain in the study of initial therapy.

5.15 Macrovascular Outcomes
There have been no clinical studies establishing conclusive evidence of macrovascular risk reduction with JANUMET or any other anti-diabetic drug.

6 ADVERSE REACTIONS

6.1 Clinical Trials Experience
Because clinical trials are conducted under widely varying conditions, adverse reaction rates observed in the clinical trials of a drug cannot be directly compared to rates in the clinical trials of another drug and may not reflect the rates observed in practice.
Sitagliptin and Metformin Co-administration in Patients with Type 2 Diabetes Inadequately Controlled on Diet and Exercise
Table 1 summarizes the most common (≥5% of patients) adverse reactions reported (regardless of investigator assessment of causality) in a 24-week placebo-controlled factorial study in which sitagliptin and metformin were co-administered to patients with type 2 diabetes inadequately controlled on diet and exercise.
[See table 1 above]
Sitagliptin Add-on Therapy in Patients with Type 2 Diabetes Inadequately Controlled on Metformin Alone
In a 24-week placebo-controlled trial of sitagliptin 100 mg administered once daily added to a twice daily metformin regimen, there were no adverse reactions reported regardless of investigator assessment of causality in ≥5% of patients and more commonly than in patients given placebo. Discontinuation of therapy due to clinical adverse reactions was similar to the placebo treatment group (sitagliptin and metformin, 1.9%; placebo and metformin, 2.5%).
Gastrointestinal Adverse Reactions
The incidences of pre-selected gastrointestinal adverse experiences in patients treated with sitagliptin and metformin were similar to those reported for patients treated with metformin alone. See Table 2.
[See table 2 above]
Sitagliptin in Combination with Metformin and Glimepiride
In a 24-week placebo-controlled study of sitagliptin 100 mg as add-on therapy in patients with type 2 diabetes inadequately controlled on metformin and glimepiride (sitagliptin, N=116; placebo, N=113), the adverse reactions reported regardless of investigator assessment of causality in ≥5% of patients treated with sitagliptin and more commonly than in patients treated with placebo were: hypoglycemia (Table 3) and headache (6.9%, 2.7%).
Sitagliptin in Combination with Metformin and Rosiglitazone
In a placebo-controlled study of sitagliptin 100 mg as add-on therapy in patients with type 2 diabetes inadequately controlled on metformin and rosiglitazone (sitagliptin, N=181; placebo, N=97), the adverse reactions reported regardless of investigator assessment of causality through Week 18 in ≥5% of patients treated with sitagliptin and more commonly than in patients treated with placebo were: upper respiratory tract infection (sitagliptin, 5.5%; placebo, 5.2%) and nasopharyngitis (6.1%, 4.1%). Through Week 54, the adverse reactions reported regardless of investigator assessment of causality in ≥5% of patients treated with sitagliptin and more commonly than in patients treated with placebo were: upper respiratory tract infection (sitagliptin, 15.5%; placebo, 6.2%), nasopharyngitis (11.0%, 9.3%), peripheral edema (8.3%, 5.2%), and headache (5.5%, 4.1%).
Sitagliptin in Combination with Metformin and Insulin
In a 24-week placebo-controlled study of sitagliptin 100 mg as add-on therapy in patients with type 2 diabetes inadequately controlled on metformin and insulin (sitagliptin, N=229; placebo, N=233), the only adverse reaction reported regardless of investigator assessment of causality in ≥5% of patients treated with sitagliptin and more commonly than in patients treated with placebo was hypoglycemia (Table 3).
Hypoglycemia
In all (N=5) studies, adverse reactions of hypoglycemia were based on all reports of symptomatic hypoglycemia; a concurrent glucose measurement was not required although most (77%) reports of hypoglycemia were accompanied by a blood glucose measurement ≤70 mg/dL. When the combination of sitagliptin and metformin was co-administered with a sulfonylurea or with insulin, the percentage of patients reporting at least one adverse reaction of hypoglycemia was higher than that observed with placebo and metformin co-administered with a sulfonylurea or with insulin (Table 3).
[See table 3 at top of next page]
The overall incidence of reported adverse reactions of hypoglycemia in patients with type 2 diabetes inadequately con-

Table 3: Incidence and Rate of Hypoglycemia* (Regardless of Investigator Assessment of Causality) in Placebo-Controlled Clinical Studies of Sitagliptin in Combination with Metformin Co-administered with Glimepiride or Insulin

Add-On to Glimepiride + Metformin (24 weeks)	**Sitagliptin 100 mg + Metformin + Glimepiride**	**Placebo + Metformin + Glimepiride**
	N = 116	N = 113
Overall (%)	19 (16.4)	1 (0.9)
Rate (episodes/patient-year)†	0.82	0.02
Severe (%)‡	0 (0.0)	0 (0.0)
Add-On to Insulin + Metformin (24 weeks)	**Sitagliptin 100 mg + Metformin + Insulin**	**Placebo + Metformin + Insulin**
	N = 229	N = 233
Overall (%)	35 (15.3)	19 (8.2)
Rate (episodes/patient-year)†	0.98	0.61
Severe (%)‡	1 (0.4)	1 (0.4)

* Adverse reactions of hypoglycemia were based on all reports of symptomatic hypoglycemia; a concurrent glucose measurement was not required: Intent-to-treat population.
† Based on total number of events (i.e., a single patient may have had multiple events).
‡ Severe events of hypoglycemia were defined as those events requiring medical assistance or exhibiting depressed level/loss of consciousness or seizure.

trolled on diet and exercise was 0.6% in patients given placebo, 0.6% in patients given sitagliptin alone, 0.8% in patients given metformin alone, and 1.6% in patients given sitagliptin in combination with metformin. In patients with type 2 diabetes inadequately controlled on metformin alone, the overall incidence of adverse reactions of hypoglycemia was 1.3% in patients given add-on sitagliptin and 2.1% in patients given add-on placebo.

In the study of sitagliptin and add-on combination therapy with metformin and rosiglitazone, the overall incidence of hypoglycemia was 2.2% in patients given add-on sitagliptin and 0.0% in patients given add-on placebo through Week 18. Through Week 54, the overall incidence of hypoglycemia was 3.9% in patients given add-on sitagliptin and 1.0% in patients given add-on placebo.

With the combination of sitagliptin and metformin, no clinically meaningful changes in vital signs or in ECG (including in QTc interval) were observed.

In a pooled analysis of 19 double-blind clinical trials that included data from 10,246 patients randomized to receive sitagliptin 100 mg/day (N=5429) or corresponding (active or placebo) control (N=4817), the incidence of acute pancreatitis was 0.1 per 100 patient-years in each group (4 patients with an event in 4708 patient-years for sitagliptin and 4 patients with an event in 3942 patient-years for control) *[See Warnings and Precautions (5.2).]*

The most common adverse experience in sitagliptin monotherapy reported regardless of investigator assessment of causality in ≥5% of patients and more commonly than in patients given placebo was nasopharyngitis.

The most common (>5%) established adverse reactions due to initiation of metformin therapy are diarrhea, nausea/vomiting, flatulence, abdominal discomfort, indigestion, asthenia, and headache.

Laboratory Tests

Sitagliptin

The incidence of laboratory adverse reactions was similar in patients treated with sitagliptin and metformin (7.6%) compared to patients treated with placebo and metformin (8.7%). In most but not all studies, a small increase in white blood cell count (approximately 200 cells/microL difference in WBC vs placebo; mean baseline WBC approximately 6600 cells/microL) was observed due to a small increase in neutrophils. This change in laboratory parameters is not considered to be clinically relevant.

Metformin hydrochloride

In controlled clinical trials of metformin of 29 weeks duration, a decrease to subnormal levels of previously normal serum Vitamin B_{12} levels, without clinical manifestations, was observed in approximately 7% of patients. Such decrease, possibly due to interference with B_{12} absorption from the B_{12}-intrinsic factor complex, is, however, very rarely associated with anemia and appears to be rapidly reversible with discontinuation of metformin or Vitamin B_{12} supplementation. *[See Warnings and Precautions (5.5).]*

6.2 Postmarketing Experience

Additional adverse reactions have been identified during postapproval use of JANUMET or sitagliptin, one of the components of JANUMET. These reactions have been reported when JANUMET or sitagliptin have been used alone and/or in combination with other antihyperglycemic agents. Because these reactions are reported voluntarily from a population of uncertain size, it is generally not possible to reliably estimate their frequency or establish a causal relationship to drug exposure.

Hypersensitivity reactions including anaphylaxis, angioedema, rash, urticaria, cutaneous vasculitis, and exfoliative skin conditions including Stevens-Johnson syndrome *[see Warnings and Precautions (5.14)]*; upper respiratory tract infection; hepatic enzyme elevations; acute pancreatitis, including fatal and non-fatal hemorrhagic and necrotizing pancreatitis *[see Indications and Usage (1); Warnings and Precautions (5.2)]*; worsening renal function, including acute renal failure (sometimes requiring dialysis) *[see Warnings and Precautions (5.4)]*; constipation; vomiting; headache; arthralgia; myalgia; pain in extremity; back pain.

7 DRUG INTERACTIONS

7.1 Cationic Drugs

Cationic drugs (e.g., amiloride, digoxin, morphine, procainamide, quinidine, quinine, ranitidine, triamterene, trimethoprim, or vancomycin) that are eliminated by renal tubular secretion theoretically have the potential for interaction with metformin by competing for common renal tubular transport systems. Such interaction between metformin and oral cimetidine has been observed in normal healthy volunteers in both single- and multiple-dose metformin-cimetidine drug interaction studies, with a 60% increase in peak metformin plasma and whole blood concentrations and a 40% increase in plasma and whole blood metformin AUC. There was no change in elimination half-life in the single-dose study. Metformin had no effect on cimetidine pharmacokinetics. Although such interactions remain theoretical (except for cimetidine), careful patient monitoring and dose adjustment of JANUMET and/or the interfering drug is recommended in patients who are taking cationic medications that are excreted via the proximal renal tubular secretory system.

7.2 Digoxin

There was a slight increase in the area under the curve (AUC, 11%) and mean peak drug concentration (C_{max}, 18%) of digoxin with the co-administration of 100 mg sitagliptin for 10 days. These increases are not considered likely to be clinically meaningful. Digoxin, as a cationic drug, has the potential to compete with metformin for common renal tubular transport systems, thus affecting the serum concentrations of either digoxin, metformin or both. Patients receiving digoxin should be monitored appropriately. No dosage adjustment of digoxin or JANUMET is recommended.

7.3 Glyburide

In a single-dose interaction study in type 2 diabetes patients, co-administration of metformin and glyburide did not result in any changes in either metformin pharmacokinetics or pharmacodynamics. Decreases in glyburide AUC and C_{max} were observed, but were highly variable. The single-dose nature of this study and the lack of correlation between glyburide blood levels and pharmacodynamic effects make the clinical significance of this interaction uncertain.

7.4 Furosemide

A single-dose, metformin-furosemide drug interaction study in healthy subjects demonstrated that pharmacokinetic parameters of both compounds were affected by co-administration. Furosemide increased the metformin plasma and blood C_{max} by 22% and blood AUC by 15%, without any significant change in metformin renal clearance. When administered with metformin, the C_{max} and AUC of furosemide were 31% and 12% smaller, respectively, than when administered alone, and the terminal half-life was decreased by 32%, without any significant change in furosemide renal clearance. No information is available about the interaction of metformin and furosemide when co-administered chronically.

7.5 Nifedipine

A single-dose, metformin-nifedipine drug interaction study in normal healthy volunteers demonstrated that co-administration of nifedipine increased plasma metformin C_{max} and AUC by 20% and 9%, respectively, and increased the amount excreted in the urine. T_{max} and half-life were unaffected. Nifedipine appears to enhance the absorption of metformin. Metformin had minimal effects on nifedipine.

7.6 The Use of Metformin with Other Drugs

Certain drugs tend to produce hyperglycemia and may lead to loss of glycemic control. These drugs include the thiazides and other diuretics, corticosteroids, phenothiazines, thyroid products, estrogens, oral contraceptives, phenytoin, nicotinic acid, sympathomimetics, calcium channel blocking drugs, and isoniazid. When such drugs are administered to a patient receiving JANUMET the patient should be closely observed to maintain adequate glycemic control.

In healthy volunteers, the pharmacokinetics of metformin and propranolol, and metformin and ibuprofen were not affected when co-administered in single-dose interaction studies.

Metformin is negligibly bound to plasma proteins and is, therefore, less likely to interact with highly protein-bound drugs such as salicylates, sulfonamides, chloramphenicol, and probenecid, as compared to the sulfonylureas, which are extensively bound to serum proteins.

8 USE IN SPECIFIC POPULATIONS

8.1 Pregnancy

Pregnancy Category B:

JANUMET

There are no adequate and well-controlled studies in pregnant women with JANUMET or its individual components; therefore, the safety of JANUMET in pregnant women is not known. JANUMET should be used during pregnancy only if clearly needed.

Merck Sharp & Dohme Corp., a subsidiary of Merck & Co., Inc., maintains a registry to monitor the pregnancy outcomes of women exposed to JANUMET while pregnant. Health care providers are encouraged to report any prenatal exposure to JANUMET by calling the Pregnancy Registry at 1-800-986-8999.

No animal studies have been conducted with the combined products in JANUMET to evaluate effects on reproduction. The following data are based on findings in studies performed with sitagliptin or metformin individually.

Sitagliptin

Reproduction studies have been performed in rats and rabbits. Doses of sitagliptin up to 125 mg/kg (approximately 12 times the human exposure at the maximum recommended human dose) did not impair fertility or harm the fetus. There are, however, no adequate and well-controlled studies with sitagliptin in pregnant women.

Sitagliptin administered to pregnant female rats and rabbits from gestation day 6 to 20 (organogenesis) was not teratogenic at oral doses up to 250 mg/kg (rats) and 125 mg/kg (rabbits), or approximately 30 and 20 times human exposure at the maximum recommended human dose (MRHD) of 100 mg/day based on AUC comparisons. Higher doses increased the incidence of rib malformations in offspring at 1000 mg/kg, or approximately 100 times human exposure at the MRHD.

Sitagliptin administered to female rats from gestation day 6 to lactation day 21 decreased body weight in male and female offspring at 1000 mg/kg. No functional or behavioral toxicity was observed in offspring of rats.

Placental transfer of sitagliptin administered to pregnant rats was approximately 45% at 2 hours and 80% at 24 hours postdose. Placental transfer of sitagliptin administered to pregnant rabbits was approximately 66% at 2 hours and 30% at 24 hours.

Metformin hydrochloride

Metformin was not teratogenic in rats and rabbits at doses up to 600 mg/kg/day. This represents an exposure of about 2 and 6 times the maximum recommended human daily dose of 2,000 mg based on body surface area comparisons for rats and rabbits, respectively. Determination of fetal concentrations demonstrated a partial placental barrier to metformin.

8.3 Nursing Mothers

No studies in lactating animals have been conducted with the combined components of JANUMET. In studies performed with the individual components, both sitagliptin and metformin are secreted in the milk of lactating rats. It is not known whether sitagliptin is excreted in human milk. Because many drugs are excreted in human milk, caution should be exercised when JANUMET is administered to a nursing woman.

8.4 Pediatric Use

Safety and effectiveness of JANUMET in pediatric patients under 18 years have not been established.

8.5 Geriatric Use

JANUMET

Because sitagliptin and metformin are substantially excreted by the kidney, and because aging can be associated with reduced renal function, JANUMET should be used with caution as age increases. Care should be taken in dose selection and should be based on careful and regular monitoring of renal function. *[See Warnings and Precautions (5.1, 5.4); Clinical Pharmacology (12.3).]*

Sitagliptin

Of the total number of subjects (N=3884) in Phase II and III clinical studies of sitagliptin, 725 patients were 65 years and over, while 61 patients were 75 years and over. No overall differences in safety or effectiveness were observed between subjects 65 years and over and younger subjects. While this and other reported clinical experience have not identified differences in responses between the elderly and younger patients, greater sensitivity of some older individuals cannot be ruled out.

Metformin hydrochloride

Controlled clinical studies of metformin did not include sufficient numbers of elderly patients to determine whether they respond differently from younger patients, although other reported clinical experience has not identified differences in responses between the elderly and young patients. Metformin should only be used in patients with normal renal function. The initial and maintenance dosing of metformin should be conservative in patients with advanced age, due to the potential for decreased renal function in this population. Any dose adjustment should be based on a careful assessment of renal function. *[See Contraindications (4); Warnings and Precautions (5.4); Clinical Pharmacology (12.3).]*

10 OVERDOSAGE

Sitagliptin

During controlled clinical trials in healthy subjects, single doses of up to 800 mg sitagliptin were administered. Maximal mean increases in QTc of 8.0 msec were observed in one study at a dose of 800 mg sitagliptin, a mean effect that is not considered clinically important *[see Clinical Pharmacology (12.2)]*. There is no experience with doses above 800 mg in clinical studies. In Phase I multiple-dose studies, there were no dose-related clinical adverse reactions observed with sitagliptin with doses of up to 400 mg per day for periods of up to 28 days.

In the event of an overdose, it is reasonable to employ the usual supportive measures, e.g., remove unabsorbed material from the gastrointestinal tract, employ clinical monitoring (including obtaining an electrocardiogram), and institute supportive therapy as indicated by the patient's clinical status.

Sitagliptin is modestly dialyzable. In clinical studies, approximately 13.5% of the dose was removed over a 3- to 4-hour hemodialysis session. Prolonged hemodialysis may be considered if clinically appropriate. It is not known if sitagliptin is dialyzable by peritoneal dialysis.

Metformin hydrochloride

Overdose of metformin hydrochloride has occurred, including ingestion of amounts greater than 50 grams. Hypoglycemia was reported in approximately 10% of cases, but no causal association with metformin hydrochloride has been established. Lactic acidosis has been reported in approximately 32% of metformin overdose cases *[see Warnings and Precautions (5.1)]*. Metformin is dialyzable with a clearance of up to 170 mL/min under good hemodynamic conditions. Therefore, hemodialysis may be useful for removal of accumulated drug from patients in whom metformin overdosage is suspected.

11 DESCRIPTION

JANUMET (sitagliptin/metformin HCl) tablets contain two oral antihyperglycemic drugs used in the management of type 2 diabetes: sitagliptin and metformin hydrochloride.

Sitagliptin

Sitagliptin is an orally-active inhibitor of the dipeptidyl peptidase-4 (DPP-4) enzyme. Sitagliptin is present in JANUMET tablets in the form of sitagliptin phosphate monohydrate. Sitagliptin phosphate monohydrate is described chemically as 7-[(3*R*)-3-amino-1-oxo-4-(2,4,5-trifluorophenyl)butyl]-5,6,7,8-tetrahydro-3-(trifluoromethyl)-1,2,4-triazolo[4,3-*a*]pyrazine phosphate (1:1) monohydrate with an empirical formula of $C_{16}H_{15}F_6N_5O \bullet H_3PO_4 \bullet H_2O$ and a molecular weight of 523.32. The structural formula is:

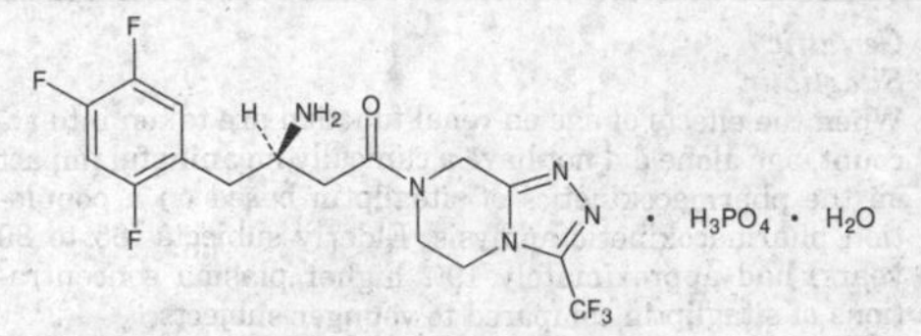

Sitagliptin phosphate monohydrate is a white to off-white, crystalline, non-hygroscopic powder. It is soluble in water and N,N-dimethyl formamide; slightly soluble in methanol; very slightly soluble in ethanol, acetone, and acetonitrile; and insoluble in isopropanol and isopropyl acetate.

Metformin hydrochloride

Metformin hydrochloride (*N,N*-dimethylimidodicarbonimidic diamide hydrochloride) is not chemically or pharmacologically related to any other classes of oral antihyperglycemic agents. Metformin hydrochloride is a white to off-white crystalline compound with a molecular formula of $C_4H_{11}N_5 \bullet HCl$ and a molecular weight of 165.63. Metformin hydrochloride is freely soluble in water and is practically insoluble in acetone, ether, and chloroform. The pK_a of metformin is 12.4. The pH of a 1% aqueous solution of metformin hydrochloride is 6.68. The structural formula is as shown:

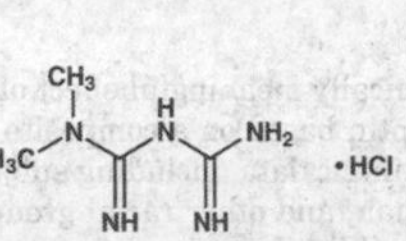

JANUMET

JANUMET is available for oral administration as tablets containing 64.25 mg sitagliptin phosphate monohydrate and metformin hydrochloride equivalent to: 50 mg sitagliptin as free base and 500 mg metformin hydrochloride (JANUMET 50 mg/500 mg) or 1000 mg metformin hydrochloride (JANUMET 50 mg/1000 mg). Each film-coated tablet of JANUMET contains the following inactive ingredients: microcrystalline cellulose, polyvinylpyrrolidone, sodium lauryl sulfate, and sodium stearyl fumarate. In addition, the film coating contains the following inactive ingredients: polyvinyl alcohol, polyethylene glycol, talc, titanium dioxide, red iron oxide, and black iron oxide.

12 CLINICAL PHARMACOLOGY

12.1 Mechanism of Action

JANUMET

JANUMET combines two antihyperglycemic agents with complementary mechanisms of action to improve glycemic control in patients with type 2 diabetes: sitagliptin, a dipeptidyl peptidase-4 (DPP-4) inhibitor, and metformin hydrochloride, a member of the biguanide class.

Sitagliptin

Sitagliptin is a DPP-4 inhibitor, which is believed to exert its actions in patients with type 2 diabetes by slowing the inactivation of incretin hormones. Concentrations of the active intact hormones are increased by sitagliptin, thereby increasing and prolonging the action of these hormones. Incretin hormones, including glucagon-like peptide-1 (GLP-1) and glucose-dependent insulinotropic polypeptide (GIP), are released by the intestine throughout the day, and levels are increased in response to a meal. These hormones are rapidly inactivated by the enzyme DPP-4. The incretins are part of an endogenous system involved in the physiologic regulation of glucose homeostasis. When blood glucose concentrations are normal or elevated, GLP-1 and GIP increase insulin synthesis and release from pancreatic beta cells by intracellular signaling pathways involving cyclic AMP. GLP-1 also lowers glucagon secretion from pancreatic alpha cells, leading to reduced hepatic glucose production. By increasing and prolonging active incretin levels, sitagliptin increases insulin release and decreases glucagon levels in the circulation in a glucose-dependent manner. Sitagliptin demonstrates selectivity for DPP-4 and does not inhibit DPP-8 or DPP-9 activity *in vitro* at concentrations approximating those from therapeutic doses.

Metformin hydrochloride

Metformin is an antihyperglycemic agent which improves glucose tolerance in patients with type 2 diabetes, lowering both basal and postprandial plasma glucose. Its pharmacologic mechanisms of action are different from other classes of oral antihyperglycemic agents. Metformin decreases hepatic glucose production, decreases intestinal absorption of glucose, and improves insulin sensitivity by increasing peripheral glucose uptake and utilization. Unlike sulfonylureas, metformin does not produce hypoglycemia in either patients with type 2 diabetes or normal subjects (except in special circumstances *[see Warnings and Precautions (5.9)]*) and does not cause hyperinsulinemia. With metformin therapy, insulin secretion remains unchanged while fasting insulin levels and day-long plasma insulin response may actually decrease.

12.2 Pharmacodynamics

Sitagliptin

General

In patients with type 2 diabetes, administration of sitagliptin led to inhibition of DPP-4 enzyme activity for a 24-hour period. After an oral glucose load or a meal, this DPP-4 inhibition resulted in a 2- to 3-fold increase in circulating levels of active GLP-1 and GIP, decreased glucagon concentrations, and increased responsiveness of insulin release to glucose, resulting in higher C-peptide and insulin concentrations. The rise in insulin with the decrease in glucagon was associated with lower fasting glucose concentrations and reduced glucose excursion following an oral glucose load or a meal.

Sitagliptin and Metformin hydrochloride Co-administration

In a two-day study in healthy subjects, sitagliptin alone increased active GLP-1 concentrations, whereas metformin alone increased active and total GLP-1 concentrations to similar extents. Co-administration of sitagliptin and metformin had an additive effect on active GLP-1 concentrations. Sitagliptin, but not metformin, increased active GIP concentrations. It is unclear what these findings mean for changes in glycemic control in patients with type 2 diabetes.

In studies with healthy subjects, sitagliptin did not lower blood glucose or cause hypoglycemia.

Cardiac Electrophysiology

In a randomized, placebo-controlled crossover study, 79 healthy subjects were administered a single oral dose of sitagliptin 100 mg, sitagliptin 800 mg (8 times the recommended dose), and placebo. At the recommended dose of 100 mg, there was no effect on the QTc interval obtained at the peak plasma concentration, or at any other time during the study. Following the 800-mg dose, the maximum increase in the placebo-corrected mean change in QTc from baseline at 3 hours postdose was 8.0 msec. This increase is not considered to be clinically significant. At the 800-mg dose, peak sitagliptin plasma concentrations were approximately 11 times higher than the peak concentrations following a 100-mg dose.

In patients with type 2 diabetes administered sitagliptin 100 mg (N=81) or sitagliptin 200 mg (N=63) daily, there were no meaningful changes in QTc interval based on ECG data obtained at the time of expected peak plasma concentration.

12.3 Pharmacokinetics

JANUMET

The results of a bioequivalence study in healthy subjects demonstrated that the JANUMET (sitagliptin/metformin HCl) 50 mg/500 mg and 50 mg/1000 mg combination tablets are bioequivalent to co-administration of corresponding doses of sitagliptin (JANUVIA®) and metformin hydrochloride as individual tablets.

Absorption

Sitagliptin

The absolute bioavailability of sitagliptin is approximately 87%. Co-administration of a high-fat meal with sitagliptin had no effect on the pharmacokinetics of sitagliptin.

Metformin hydrochloride

The absolute bioavailability of a metformin hydrochloride 500-mg tablet given under fasting conditions is approximately 50-60%. Studies using single oral doses of metformin hydrochloride tablets 500 mg to 1500 mg, and 850 mg to 2550 mg, indicate that there is a lack of dose proportionality with increasing doses, which is due to decreased absorption rather than an alteration in elimination. Food decreases the extent of and slightly delays the absorption of metformin, as shown by approximately a 40% lower mean peak plasma concentration (C_{max}), a 25% lower area under the plasma concentration versus time curve (AUC), and a 35-minute prolongation of time to peak plasma concentration (T_{max}) following administration of a single 850-mg tablet of metformin with food, compared to the same tablet strength administered fasting. The clinical relevance of these decreases is unknown.

Distribution

Sitagliptin

The mean volume of distribution at steady state following a single 100-mg intravenous dose of sitagliptin to healthy subjects is approximately 198 liters. The fraction of sitagliptin reversibly bound to plasma proteins is low (38%).

Metformin hydrochloride

The apparent volume of distribution (V/F) of metformin following single oral doses of metformin hydrochloride tablets 850 mg averaged 654 ± 358 L. Metformin is negligibly bound to plasma proteins, in contrast to sulfonylureas, which are more than 90% protein bound. Metformin partitions into erythrocytes, most likely as a function of time. At usual clinical doses and dosing schedules of metformin hydrochloride tablets, steady-state plasma concentrations of metformin are reached within 24-48 hours and are generally <1 mcg/mL. During controlled clinical trials of metformin, maximum metformin plasma levels did not exceed 5 mcg/mL, even at maximum doses.

Metabolism
Sitagliptin
Approximately 79% of sitagliptin is excreted unchanged in the urine with metabolism being a minor pathway of elimination.
Following a [^{14}C]sitagliptin oral dose, approximately 16% of the radioactivity was excreted as metabolites of sitagliptin. Six metabolites were detected at trace levels and are not expected to contribute to the plasma DPP-4 inhibitory activity of sitagliptin. *In vitro* studies indicated that the primary enzyme responsible for the limited metabolism of sitagliptin was CYP3A4, with contribution from CYP2C8.
Metformin hydrochloride
Intravenous single-dose studies in normal subjects demonstrate that metformin is excreted unchanged in the urine and does not undergo hepatic metabolism (no metabolites have been identified in humans) nor biliary excretion.
Excretion
Sitagliptin
Following administration of an oral [^{14}C]sitagliptin dose to healthy subjects, approximately 100% of the administered radioactivity was eliminated in feces (13%) or urine (87%) within one week of dosing. The apparent terminal $t_{1/2}$ following a 100-mg oral dose of sitagliptin was approximately 12.4 hours and renal clearance was approximately 350 mL/min.
Elimination of sitagliptin occurs primarily via renal excretion and involves active tubular secretion. Sitagliptin is a substrate for human organic anion transporter-3 (hOAT-3), which may be involved in the renal elimination of sitagliptin. The clinical relevance of hOAT-3 in sitagliptin transport has not been established. Sitagliptin is also a substrate of p-glycoprotein, which may also be involved in mediating the renal elimination of sitagliptin. However, cyclosporine, a p-glycoprotein inhibitor, did not reduce the renal clearance of sitagliptin.
Metformin hydrochloride
Renal clearance is approximately 3.5 times greater than creatinine clearance, which indicates that tubular secretion is the major route of metformin elimination. Following oral administration, approximately 90% of the absorbed drug is eliminated via the renal route within the first 24 hours, with a plasma elimination half-life of approximately 6.2 hours. In blood, the elimination half-life is approximately 17.6 hours, suggesting that the erythrocyte mass may be a compartment of distribution.
Special Populations
Renal Insufficiency
JANUMET
JANUMET should not be used in patients with renal insufficiency *[see Contraindications (4); Warnings and Precautions (5.4)]*.
Sitagliptin
An approximately 2-fold increase in the plasma AUC of sitagliptin was observed in patients with moderate renal insufficiency, and an approximately 4-fold increase was observed in patients with severe renal insufficiency including patients with ESRD on hemodialysis, as compared to normal healthy control subjects.
Metformin hydrochloride
In patients with decreased renal function (based on measured creatinine clearance), the plasma and blood half-life of metformin is prolonged and the renal clearance is decreased in proportion to the decrease in creatinine clearance.
Hepatic Insufficiency
Sitagliptin
In patients with moderate hepatic insufficiency (Child-Pugh score 7 to 9), mean AUC and C_{max} of sitagliptin increased approximately 21% and 13%, respectively, compared to healthy matched controls following administration of a single 100-mg dose of sitagliptin. These differences are not considered to be clinically meaningful.
There is no clinical experience in patients with severe hepatic insufficiency (Child-Pugh score >9).
Metformin hydrochloride
No pharmacokinetic studies of metformin have been conducted in patients with hepatic insufficiency.
Gender
Sitagliptin
Gender had no clinically meaningful effect on the pharmacokinetics of sitagliptin based on a composite analysis of Phase I pharmacokinetic data and on a population pharmacokinetic analysis of Phase I and Phase II data.
Metformin hydrochloride
Metformin pharmacokinetic parameters did not differ significantly between normal subjects and patients with type 2 diabetes when analyzed according to gender. Similarly, in controlled clinical studies in patients with type 2 diabetes, the antihyperglycemic effect of metformin was comparable in males and females.
Geriatric
Sitagliptin
When the effects of age on renal function are taken into account, age alone did not have a clinically meaningful impact on the pharmacokinetics of sitagliptin based on a population pharmacokinetic analysis. Elderly subjects (65 to 80 years) had approximately 19% higher plasma concentrations of sitagliptin compared to younger subjects.
Metformin hydrochloride
Limited data from controlled pharmacokinetic studies of metformin in healthy elderly subjects suggest that total plasma clearance of metformin is decreased, the half life is prolonged, and C_{max} is increased, compared to healthy young subjects. From these data, it appears that the change in metformin pharmacokinetics with aging is primarily accounted for by a change in renal function (see **GLUCOPHAGE** prescribing information: **CLINICAL PHARMACOLOGY**, Special Populations, Geriatrics).
JANUMET treatment should not be initiated in patients ≥80 years of age unless measurement of creatinine clearance demonstrates that renal function is not reduced *[see Warnings and Precautions (5.1, 5.4)]*.
Pediatric
No studies with JANUMET have been performed in pediatric patients.
Race
Sitagliptin
Race had no clinically meaningful effect on the pharmacokinetics of sitagliptin based on a composite analysis of available pharmacokinetic data, including subjects of white, Hispanic, black, Asian, and other racial groups.
Metformin hydrochloride
No studies of metformin pharmacokinetic parameters according to race have been performed. In controlled clinical studies of metformin in patients with type 2 diabetes, the antihyperglycemic effect was comparable in whites (n=249), blacks (n=51), and Hispanics (n=24).
Body Mass Index (BMI)
Sitagliptin
Body mass index had no clinically meaningful effect on the pharmacokinetics of sitagliptin based on a composite analysis of Phase I pharmacokinetic data and on a population pharmacokinetic analysis of Phase I and Phase II data.
Drug Interactions
Sitagliptin and Metformin hydrochloride
Co-administration of multiple doses of sitagliptin (50 mg) and metformin (1000 mg) given twice daily did not meaningfully alter the pharmacokinetics of either sitagliptin or metformin in patients with type 2 diabetes.
Pharmacokinetic drug interaction studies with JANUMET have not been performed; however, such studies have been conducted with the individual components of JANUMET (sitagliptin and metformin hydrochloride).
Sitagliptin
In Vitro Assessment of Drug Interactions
Sitagliptin is not an inhibitor of CYP isozymes CYP3A4, 2C8, 2C9, 2D6, 1A2, 2C19 or 2B6, and is not an inducer of CYP3A4. Sitagliptin is a p-glycoprotein substrate, but does not inhibit p-glycoprotein mediated transport of digoxin. Based on these results, sitagliptin is considered unlikely to cause interactions with other drugs that utilize these pathways.
Sitagliptin is not extensively bound to plasma proteins. Therefore, the propensity of sitagliptin to be involved in clinically meaningful drug-drug interactions mediated by plasma protein binding displacement is very low.
In Vivo Assessment of Drug Interactions
Effect of Sitagliptin on Other Drugs
In clinical studies, as described below, sitagliptin did not meaningfully alter the pharmacokinetics of metformin, glyburide, simvastatin, rosiglitazone, warfarin, or oral contraceptives, providing *in vivo* evidence of a low propensity for causing drug interactions with substrates of CYP3A4, CYP2C8, CYP2C9, and organic cationic transporter (OCT).
Digoxin: Sitagliptin had a minimal effect on the pharmacokinetics of digoxin. Following administration of 0.25 mg digoxin concomitantly with 100 mg of sitagliptin daily for 10 days, the plasma AUC of digoxin was increased by 11%, and the plasma C_{max} by 18%.
Sulfonylureas: Single-dose pharmacokinetics of glyburide, a CYP2C9 substrate, was not meaningfully altered in subjects receiving multiple doses of sitagliptin. Clinically meaningful interactions would not be expected with other sulfonylureas (e.g., glipizide, tolbutamide, and glimepiride) which, like glyburide, are primarily eliminated by CYP2C9 *[see Warnings and Precautions (5.9)]*.
Simvastatin: Single-dose pharmacokinetics of simvastatin, a CYP3A4 substrate, was not meaningfully altered in subjects receiving multiple daily doses of sitagliptin. Therefore, sitagliptin is not an inhibitor of CYP3A4-mediated metabolism.
Thiazolidinediones: Single-dose pharmacokinetics of rosiglitazone was not meaningfully altered in subjects receiving multiple daily doses of sitagliptin, indicating that sitagliptin is not an inhibitor of CYP2C8-mediated metabolism.
Warfarin: Multiple daily doses of sitagliptin did not meaningfully alter the pharmacokinetics, as assessed by measurement of S(-) or R(+) warfarin enantiomers, or pharmacodynamics (as assessed by measurement of prothrombin INR) of a single dose of warfarin. Because S(-) warfarin is primarily metabolized by CYP2C9, these data also support the conclusion that sitagliptin is not a CYP2C9 inhibitor.
Oral Contraceptives: Co-administration with sitagliptin did not meaningfully alter the steady-state pharmacokinetics of norethindrone or ethinyl estradiol.
Effect of Other Drugs on Sitagliptin
Clinical data described below suggest that sitagliptin is not susceptible to clinically meaningful interactions by co-administered medications.
Cyclosporine: A study was conducted to assess the effect of cyclosporine, a potent inhibitor of p-glycoprotein, on the pharmacokinetics of sitagliptin. Co-administration of a single 100-mg oral dose of sitagliptin and a single 600-mg oral dose of cyclosporine increased the AUC and C_{max} of sitagliptin by approximately 29% and 68%, respectively. These modest changes in sitagliptin pharmacokinetics were not considered to be clinically meaningful. The renal clearance of sitagliptin was also not meaningfully altered. Therefore, meaningful interactions would not be expected with other p-glycoprotein inhibitors.
Metformin hydrochloride
[See Drug Interactions (7.1, 7.3, 7.4, 7.5, 7.6).]

13 NONCLINICAL TOXICOLOGY

13.1 Carcinogenesis, Mutagenesis, Impairment of Fertility

JANUMET
No animal studies have been conducted with the combined products in JANUMET to evaluate carcinogenesis, mutagenesis or impairment of fertility. The following data are based on the findings in studies with sitagliptin and metformin individually.
Sitagliptin
A two-year carcinogenicity study was conducted in male and female rats given oral doses of sitagliptin of 50, 150, and 500 mg/kg/day. There was an increased incidence of combined liver adenoma/carcinoma in males and females and of liver carcinoma in females at 500 mg/kg. This dose results in exposures approximately 60 times the human exposure at the maximum recommended daily adult human dose (MRHD) of 100 mg/day based on AUC comparisons. Liver tumors were not observed at 150 mg/kg, approximately 20 times the human exposure at the MRHD. A two-year carcinogenicity study was conducted in male and female mice given oral doses of sitagliptin of 50, 125, 250, and 500 mg/kg/day. There was no increase in the incidence of tumors in any organ up to 500 mg/kg, approximately 70 times human exposure at the MRHD. Sitagliptin was not mutagenic or clastogenic with or without metabolic activation in the Ames bacterial mutagenicity assay, a Chinese hamster ovary (CHO) chromosome aberration assay, an *in vitro* cytogenetics assay in CHO, an *in vitro* rat hepatocyte DNA alkaline elution assay, and an *in vivo* micronucleus assay.
In rat fertility studies with oral gavage doses of 125, 250, and 1000 mg/kg, males were treated for 4 weeks prior to mating, during mating, up to scheduled termination (approximately 8 weeks total), and females were treated 2 weeks prior to mating through gestation day 7. No adverse effect on fertility was observed at 125 mg/kg (approximately 12 times human exposure at the MRHD of 100 mg/day based on AUC comparisons). At higher doses, nondose-related increased resorptions in females were observed (approximately 25 and 100 times human exposure at the MRHD based on AUC comparison).
Metformin hydrochloride
Long-term carcinogenicity studies have been performed in rats (dosing duration of 104 weeks) and mice (dosing duration of 91 weeks) at doses up to and including 900 mg/kg/day and 1500 mg/kg/day, respectively. These doses are both approximately four times the maximum recommended human daily dose of 2000 mg based on body surface area comparisons. No evidence of carcinogenicity with metformin was found in either male or female mice. Similarly, there was no tumorigenic potential observed with metformin in male rats. There was, however, an increased incidence of benign stromal uterine polyps in female rats treated with 900 mg/kg/day.
There was no evidence of a mutagenic potential of metformin in the following *in vitro* tests: Ames test (*S. typhimurium*), gene mutation test (mouse lymphoma cells), or chromosomal aberrations test (human lymphocytes). Results in the *in vivo* mouse micronucleus test were also negative. Fertility of male or female rats was unaffected by metformin when administered at doses as high as 600 mg/

kg/day, which is approximately three times the maximum recommended human daily dose based on body surface area comparisons.

14 CLINICAL STUDIES

The co-administration of sitagliptin and metformin has been studied in patients with type 2 diabetes inadequately controlled on diet and exercise and in combination with other antihyperglycemic agents.

There have been no clinical efficacy studies conducted with JANUMET; however, bioequivalence of JANUMET with co-administered sitagliptin and metformin hydrochloride tablets was demonstrated.

Sitagliptin and Metformin Co-administration in Patients with Type 2 Diabetes Inadequately Controlled on Diet and Exercise

A total of 1091 patients with type 2 diabetes and inadequate glycemic control on diet and exercise participated in a 24-week, randomized, double-blind, placebo-controlled factorial study designed to assess the efficacy of sitagliptin and metformin co-administration. Patients on an antihyperglycemic agent (N=541) underwent a diet, exercise, and drug washout period of up to 12 weeks duration. After the washout period, patients with inadequate glycemic control (A1C 7.5% to 11%) were randomized after completing a 2-week single-blind placebo run-in period. Patients not on antihyperglycemic agents at study entry (N=550) with inadequate glycemic control (A1C 7.5% to 11%) immediately entered the 2-week single-blind placebo run-in period and then were randomized. Approximately equal numbers of patients were randomized to receive placebo, 100 mg of sitagliptin once daily, 500 mg or 1000 mg of metformin twice daily, or 50 mg of sitagliptin twice daily in combination with 500 mg or 1000 mg of metformin twice daily. Patients who failed to meet specific glycemic goals during the study were treated with glyburide (glibenclamide) rescue.

Sitagliptin and metformin co-administration provided significant improvements in A1C, FPG, and 2-hour PPG compared to placebo, to metformin alone, and to sitagliptin alone (Table 4, Figure 1). Mean reductions from baseline in A1C were generally greater for patients with higher baseline A1C values. For patients not on an antihyperglycemic agent at study entry, mean reductions from baseline in A1C were: sitagliptin 100 mg once daily, -1.1%; metformin 500 mg bid, -1.1%; metformin 1000 mg bid, -1.2%; sitagliptin 50 mg bid with metformin 500 mg bid, -1.6%; sitagliptin 50 mg bid with metformin 1000 mg bid, -1.9%; and for patients receiving placebo, -0.2%. Lipid effects were generally neutral. The decrease in body weight in the groups given sitagliptin in combination with metformin was similar to that in the groups given metformin alone or placebo.

[See table 4 above]

Figure 1: Mean Change from Baseline for A1C (%) over 24 Weeks with Sitagliptin and Metformin, Alone and in Combination in Patients with Type 2 Diabetes Inadequately Controlled with Diet and Exercise*

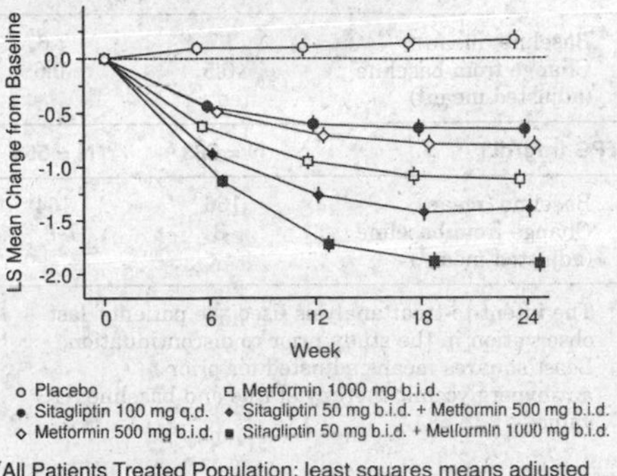

*All Patients Treated Population: least squares means adjusted for prior antihyperglycemic therapy and baseline value.

In addition, this study included patients (N=117) with more severe hyperglycemia (A1C >11% or blood glucose >280 mg/dL) who were treated with twice daily open-label sitagliptin 50 mg and metformin 1000 mg. In this group of patients, the mean baseline A1C value was 11.2%, mean FPG was 314 mg/dL, and mean 2-hour PPG was 441 mg/dL. After 24 weeks, mean decreases from baseline of -2.9% for A1C, -127 mg/dL for FPG, and -208 mg/dL for 2-hour PPG were observed.

Initial combination therapy or maintenance of combination therapy should be individualized and are left to the discretion of the health care provider.

Table 4: Glycemic Parameters at Final Visit (24-Week Study) for Sitagliptin and Metformin, Alone and in Combination in Patients with Type 2 Diabetes Inadequately Controlled on Diet and Exercise*

	Placebo	Sitagliptin 100 mg QD	Metformin 500 mg bid	Metformin 1000 mg bid	Sitagliptin 50 mg bid + Metformin 500 mg bid	Sitagliptin 50 mg bid + Metformin 1000 mg bid
A1C (%)	**N = 165**	**N = 175**	**N = 178**	**N = 177**	**N = 183**	**N = 178**
Baseline (mean)	8.7	8.9	8.9	8.7	8.8	8.8
Change from baseline (adjusted mean†)	0.2	-0.7	-0.8	-1.1	-1.4	-1.9
Difference from placebo (adjusted mean†) (95% CI)		-0.8‡ (-1.1, -0.6)	-1.0‡ (-1.2, -0.8)	-1.3‡ (-1.5, -1.1)	-1.6‡ (-1.8, -1.3)	-2.1‡ (-2.3, -1.8)
Patients (%) achieving A1C <7%	15 (9%)	35 (20%)	41 (23%)	68 (38%)	79 (43%)	118 (66%)
% Patients receiving rescue medication	32	21	17	12	8	2
FPG (mg/dL)	**N = 169**	**N = 178**	**N = 179**	**N = 179**	**N = 183**	**N = 180**
Baseline (mean)	196	201	205	197	204	197
Change from baseline (adjusted mean†)	6	-17	-27	-29	-47	-64
Difference from placebo (adjusted mean†) (95% CI)		-23‡ (-33, -14)	-33‡ (-43, -24)	-35‡ (-45, -26)	-53‡ (-62, -43)	-70‡ (-79, -60)
2-hour PPG (mg/dL)	**N = 129**	**N = 136**	**N = 141**	**N = 138**	**N = 147**	**N = 152**
Baseline (mean)	277	285	293	283	292	287
Change from baseline (adjusted mean†)	0	-52	-53	-78	-93	-117
Difference from placebo (adjusted mean†) (95% CI)		-52‡ (-67, -37)	-54‡ (-69, -39)	-78‡ (-93, -63)	-93‡ (-107, -78)	-117‡ (-131, -102)

* Intent-to-treat population using last observation on study prior to glyburide (glibenclamide) rescue therapy.
† Least squares means adjusted for prior antihyperglycemic therapy status and baseline value.
‡ p<0.001 compared to placebo.

Table 5: Glycemic Parameters at Final Visit (24-Week Study) of Sitagliptin as Add-on Combination Therapy with Metformin*

	Sitagliptin 100 mg QD + Metformin	Placebo + Metformin
A1C (%)	**N = 453**	**N = 224**
Baseline (mean)	8.0	8.0
Change from baseline (adjusted mean†)	-0.7	-0.0
Difference from placebo + metformin (adjusted mean†) (95% CI)	-0.7‡ (-0.8, -0.5)	
Patients (%) achieving A1C <7%	213 (47%)	41 (18%)
FPG (mg/dL)	**N = 454**	**N = 226**
Baseline (mean)	170	174
Change from baseline (adjusted mean†)	-17	9
Difference from placebo + metformin (adjusted mean†) (95% CI)	-25‡ (-31, -20)	
2-hour PPG (mg/dL)	**N = 387**	**N = 182**
Baseline (mean)	275	272
Change from baseline (adjusted mean†)	-62	-11
Difference from placebo + metformin (adjusted mean†) (95% CI)	-51‡ (-61, -41)	

* Intent-to-treat population using last observation on study prior to pioglitazone rescue therapy.
† Least squares means adjusted for prior antihyperglycemic therapy and baseline value.
‡ p<0.001 compared to placebo + metformin.

Sitagliptin Add-on Therapy in Patients with Type 2 Diabetes Inadequately Controlled on Metformin Alone

A total of 701 patients with type 2 diabetes participated in a 24-week, randomized, double-blind, placebo-controlled study designed to assess the efficacy of sitagliptin in combination with metformin. Patients already on metformin (N=431) at a dose of at least 1500 mg per day were randomized after completing a 2-week, single-blind placebo run-in period. Patients on metformin and another antihyperglycemic agent (N=229) and patients not on any antihyperglycemic agents (off therapy for at least 8 weeks, N=41) were randomized after a run-in period of approximately 10 weeks on metformin (at a dose of at least 1500 mg per day) in monotherapy. Patients were randomized to the addition of either 100 mg of sitagliptin or placebo, administered once daily. Patients who failed to meet specific glycemic goals during the studies were treated with pioglitazone rescue.

In combination with metformin, sitagliptin provided significant improvements in A1C, FPG, and 2-hour PPG compared to placebo with metformin (Table 5). Rescue glycemic therapy was used in 5% of patients treated with sitagliptin 100 mg and 14% of patients treated with placebo. A similar decrease in body weight was observed for both treatment groups.

[See table 5 above]

Sitagliptin Add-on Therapy in Patients with Type 2 Diabetes Inadequately Controlled on the Combination of Metformin and Glimepiride

A total of 441 patients with type 2 diabetes participated in a 24-week, randomized, double-blind, placebo-controlled study designed to assess the efficacy of sitagliptin in combination with glimepiride, with or without metformin. Patients entered a run-in treatment period on glimepiride (≥4 mg per day) alone or glimepiride in combination with metformin (≥1500 mg per day). After a dose-titration and dose-stable run-in period of up to 16 weeks and a 2-week placebo run-in period, patients with inadequate glycemic control (A1C 7.5% to 10.5%) were randomized to the addi-

Table 6: Glycemic Parameters at Final Visit (24-Week Study) for Sitagliptin in Combination with Metformin and Glimepiride*

	Sitagliptin 100 mg + Metformin and Glimepiride	Placebo + Metformin and Glimepiride
A1C (%)	**N = 115**	**N = 105**
Baseline (mean)	8.3	8.3
Change from baseline (adjusted mean†)	-0.6	0.3
Difference from placebo (adjusted mean†) (95% CI)	-0.9‡ (-1.1, -0.7)	
Patients (%) achieving A1C <7%	26 (23%)	1 (1%)
FPG (mg/dL)	**N = 115**	**N = 109**
Baseline (mean)	179	179
Change from baseline (adjusted mean†)	-8	13
Difference from placebo (adjusted mean†) (95% CI)	-21‡ (-32, -10)	

* Intent-to-treat population using last observation on study prior to pioglitazone rescue therapy.
† Least squares means adjusted for prior antihyperglycemic therapy status and baseline value.
‡ p<0.001 compared to placebo.

Table 7: Glycemic Parameters at Week 18 for Sitagliptin in Add-on Combination Therapy with Metformin and Rosiglitazone*

	Week 18	
	Sitagliptin 100 mg + Metformin + Rosiglitazone	Placebo + Metformin + Rosiglitazone
A1C (%)	**N =176**	**N = 93**
Baseline (mean)	8.8	8.7
Change from baseline (adjusted mean†)	-1.0	-0.4
Difference from placebo + rosiglitazone + metformin (adjusted mean†) (95% CI)	-0.7‡ (-0.9,-0.4)	
Patients (%) achieving A1C <7%	39 (22%)	9 (10%)
FPG (mg/dL)	**N = 179**	**N =94**
Baseline (mean)	181	182
Change from baseline (adjusted mean†)	-30	-11
Difference from placebo + rosiglitazone + metformin (adjusted mean†) (95% CI)	-18‡ (-26, -10)	
2-hour PPG (mg/dL)	**N = 152**	**N = 80**
Baseline (mean)	256	248
Change from baseline (adjusted mean†)	-59	-21
Difference from placebo + rosiglitazone + metformin (adjusted mean†) (95% CI)	-39‡ (-51, -26)	

* Intent-to-treat population using last observation on study prior to glipizide (or other sulfonylurea) rescue therapy.
† Least squares means adjusted for prior antihyperglycemic therapy status and baseline value.
‡ p<0.001 compared to placebo + metformin + rosiglitazone.

tion of either 100 mg of sitagliptin or placebo, administered once daily. Patients who failed to meet specific glycemic goals during the studies were treated with pioglitazone rescue.

Patients receiving sitagliptin with metformin and glimepiride had significant improvements in A1C and FPG compared to patients receiving placebo with metformin and glimepiride (Table 6), with mean reductions from baseline relative to placebo in A1C of -0.9% and in FPG of -21 mg/dL. Rescue therapy was used in 8% of patients treated with add-on sitagliptin 100 mg and 29% of patients treated with add-on placebo. The patients treated with add-on sitagliptin had a mean increase in body weight of 1.1 kg vs. add-on placebo (+0.4 kg vs. -0.7 kg). In addition, add-on sitagliptin resulted in an increased rate of hypoglycemia compared to add-on placebo. *[See Warnings and Precautions (5.9); Adverse Reactions (6.1).]*

[See table 6 above]

Sitagliptin Add-on Therapy in Patients with Type 2 Diabetes Inadequately Controlled on the Combination of Metformin and Rosiglitazone

A total of 278 patients with type 2 diabetes participated in a 54-week, randomized, double-blind, placebo-controlled study designed to assess the efficacy of sitagliptin in combination with metformin and rosiglitazone. Patients on dual therapy with metformin ≥1500 mg/day and rosiglitazone ≥4 mg/day or with metformin ≥1500 mg/day and pioglitazone ≥30 mg/day (switched to rosiglitazone ≥4 mg/day) entered a dose-stable run-in period of 6 weeks. Patients on other dual therapy were switched to metformin ≥1500 mg/day and rosiglitazone ≥4 mg/day in a dose titration/stabilization run-in period of up to 20 weeks in duration. After the run-in period, patients with inadequate glycemic control (A1C 7.5% to 11%) were randomized 2:1 to the addition of either 100 mg of sitagliptin or placebo, administered once daily. Patients who failed to meet specific glycemic goals during the studies were treated with glipizide (or other sulfonylurea) rescue. The primary time point for evaluation of glycemic parameters was Week 18.

In combination with metformin and rosiglitazone, sitagliptin provided significant improvements in A1C, FPG, and 2-hour PPG compared to placebo with metformin and rosiglitazone (Table 7) at Week 18. At Week 54, mean reduction in A1C was -1.0% for patients treated with sitagliptin and -0.3% for patients treated with placebo in an analysis based on the intent-to-treat population. Rescue therapy was used in 18% of patients treated with sitagliptin 100 mg and 40% of patients treated with placebo. There was no significant difference between sitagliptin and placebo in body weight change.

[See table 7 above]

Sitagliptin Add-on Therapy in Patients with Type 2 Diabetes Inadequately Controlled on the Combination of Metformin and Insulin

A total of 641 patients with type 2 diabetes participated in a 24-week, randomized, double-blind, placebo-controlled study designed to assess the efficacy of sitagliptin as add-on to insulin therapy. Approximately 75% of patients were also taking metformin. Patients entered a 2-week, single-blind run-in treatment period on pre-mixed, long-acting, or intermediate-acting insulin, with or without metformin (≥1500 mg per day). Patients using short-acting insulins were excluded unless the short-acting insulin was administered as part of a pre-mixed insulin. After the run-in period, patients with inadequate glycemic control (A1C 7.5% to 11%) were randomized to the addition of either 100 mg of sitagliptin (N=229) or placebo (N=233), administered once daily. Patients were on a stable dose of insulin prior to enrollment with no changes in insulin dose permitted during the run-in period. Patients who failed to meet specific glycemic goals during the double-blind treatment period were to have uptitration of the background insulin dose as rescue therapy.

Among patients also receiving metformin, the median daily insulin (pre-mixed, intermediate or long acting) dose at baseline was 40 units in the sitagliptin-treated patients and 42 units in the placebo-treated patients. The median change from baseline in daily dose of insulin was zero for both groups at the end of the study. Patients receiving sitagliptin with metformin and insulin had significant improvements in A1C, FPG and 2-hour PPG compared to patients receiving placebo with metformin and insulin (Table 8). The adjusted mean change from baseline in body weight was -0.3 kg in patients receiving sitagliptin with metformin and insulin and -0.2 kg in patients receiving placebo with metformin and insulin. There was an increased rate of hypoglycemia in patients treated with sitagliptin. *[See Warnings and Precautions (5.9); Adverse Reactions (6.1).]*

[See table 8 at top of next page]

Sitagliptin Add-on Therapy vs. Glipizide Add-on Therapy in Patients with Type 2 Diabetes Inadequately Controlled on Metformin

The efficacy of sitagliptin was evaluated in a 52-week, double-blind, glipizide-controlled noninferiority trial in patients with type 2 diabetes. Patients not on treatment or on other antihyperglycemic agents entered a run-in treatment period of up to 12 weeks duration with metformin monotherapy (dose of ≥1500 mg per day) which included washout of medications other than metformin, if applicable. After the run-in period, those with inadequate glycemic control (A1C 6.5% to 10%) were randomized 1:1 to the addition of sitagliptin 100 mg once daily or glipizide for 52 weeks. Patients receiving glipizide were given an initial dosage of 5 mg/day and then electively titrated over the next 18 weeks to a maximum dosage of 20 mg/day as needed to optimize glycemic control. Thereafter, the glipizide dose was to be kept constant, except for down-titration to prevent hypoglycemia. The mean dose of glipizide after the titration period was 10 mg.

After 52 weeks, sitagliptin and glipizide had similar mean reductions from baseline in A1C in the intent-to-treat analysis (Table 9). These results were consistent with the per protocol analysis (Figure 2). A conclusion in favor of the noninferiority of sitagliptin to glipizide may be limited to patients with baseline A1C comparable to those included in the study (over 70% of patients had baseline A1C <8% and over 90% had A1C <9%).

Table 9: Glycemic Parameters in a 52-Week Study Comparing Sitagliptin to Glipizide as Add-On Therapy in Patients Inadequately Controlled on Metformin (Intent-to-Treat Population)*

	Sitagliptin 100 mg + Metformin	Glipizide + Metformin
A1C (%)	**N = 576**	**N = 559**
Baseline (mean)	7.7	7.6
Change from baseline (adjusted mean†)	-0.5	-0.6
FPG (mg/dL)	**N = 583**	**N = 568**
Baseline (mean)	166	164
Change from baseline (adjusted mean†)	-8	-8

* The intent-to-treat analysis used the patients' last observation in the study prior to discontinuation.
† Least squares means adjusted for prior antihyperglycemic therapy status and baseline A1C value.

[See figure 2 at top of next column]

The incidence of hypoglycemia in the sitagliptin group (4.9%) was significantly (p<0.001) lower than that in the glipizide group (32.0%). Patients treated with sitagliptin exhibited a significant mean decrease from baseline in body weight compared to a significant weight gain in patients administered glipizide (-1.5 kg vs. +1.1 kg).

16 HOW SUPPLIED/STORAGE AND HANDLING

No. 6747 — Tablets JANUMET, 50 mg/500 mg, are light pink, capsule-shaped, film-coated tablets with "575" debossed on one side. They are supplied as follows:
NDC 0006-0575-61 unit-of-use bottles of 60
NDC 0006-0575-62 unit-of-use bottles of 180
NDC 0006-0575-52 unit dose blister packages of 50
NDC 0006-0575-82 bulk bottles of 1000.

Table 8: Glycemic Parameters at Final Visit (24-Week Study) for Sitagliptin as Add-on Combination Therapy with Metformin and Insulin*

	Sitagliptin 100 mg + Metformin + Insulin	Placebo + Metformin + Insulin
A1C (%)	**N = 223**	**N = 229**
Baseline (mean)	8.7	8.6
Change from baseline (adjusted mean†,‡)	-0.7	-0.1
Difference from placebo (adjusted mean†) (95% CI)	-0.5§ (-0.7, -0.4)	
Patients (%) achieving A1C (%) <7%	32 (14%)	12 (5%)
FPG (mg/dL)	**N = 225**	**N = 229**
Baseline (mean)	173	176
Change from baseline (adjusted mean†)	-22	-4
Difference from placebo (adjusted mean†) (95% CI)	-18§ (-28, -8.4)	
2-hour PPG (mg/dL)	**N = 182**	**N = 189**
Baseline (mean)	281	281
Change from baseline (adjusted mean†)	-39	1
Difference from placebo (adjusted mean†) (95% CI)	-40§ (-53, -28)	

* Intent-to-treat population using last observation on study prior to rescue therapy.
† Least squares mean adjusted for insulin use at the screening visit, type of insulin used at the screening visit (pre-mixed vs. non pre-mixed [intermediate- or long-acting]), and baseline value.
‡ Treatment by insulin stratum interaction was not significant (p >0.10).
§ p<0.001 compared to placebo.

Figure 2: Mean Change from Baseline for A1C (%) Over 52 Weeks in a Study Comparing Sitagliptin to Glipizide as Add-On Therapy in Patients Inadequately Controlled on Metformin (Per Protocol Population)*

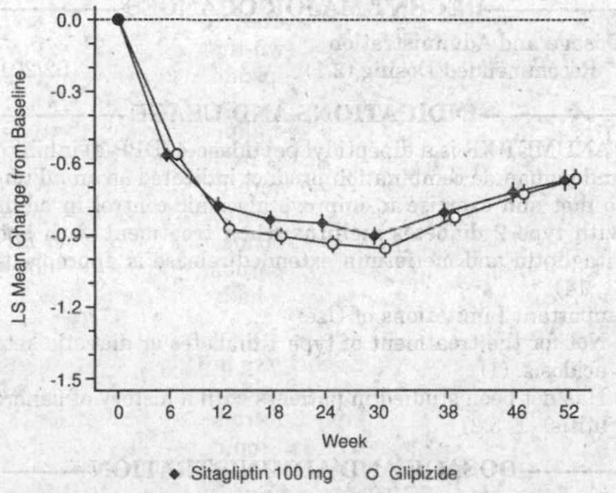

* The per protocol population (mean baseline A1C of 7.5%) included patients without major protocol violations who had observations at baseline and at Week 52.

No. 6749 — Tablets JANUMET, 50 mg/1000 mg, are red, capsule-shaped, film-coated tablets with "577" debossed on one side. They are supplied as follows:
NDC 0006-0577-61 unit-of-use bottles of 60
NDC 0006-0577-62 unit-of-use bottles of 180
NDC 0006-0577-52 unit dose blister packages of 50
NDC 0006-0577-82 bulk bottles of 1000.
Store at 20-25°C (68-77°F), excursions permitted to 15-30°C (59-86°F), [See USP Controlled Room Temperature].

17 PATIENT COUNSELING INFORMATION

See FDA-Approved Patient Labeling (Medication Guide).

17.1 Instructions

Patients should be informed of the potential risks and benefits of JANUMET and of alternative modes of therapy. They should also be informed about the importance of adherence to dietary instructions, regular physical activity, periodic blood glucose monitoring and A1C testing, recognition and management of hypoglycemia and hyperglycemia, and assessment for diabetes complications. During periods of stress such as fever, trauma, infection, or surgery, medication requirements may change and patients should be advised to seek medical advice promptly.

The risks of lactic acidosis due to the metformin component, its symptoms, and conditions that predispose to its development, as noted in Warnings and Precautions (5.1), should be explained to patients. Patients should be advised to discontinue JANUMET immediately and to promptly notify their health practitioner if unexplained hyperventilation, myalgia, malaise, unusual somnolence, dizziness, slow or irregular heart beat, sensation of feeling cold (especially in the extremities) or other nonspecific symptoms occur. Gastrointestinal symptoms are common during initiation of metformin treatment and may occur during initiation of JANUMET therapy; however, patients should consult their physician if they develop unexplained symptoms. Although gastrointestinal symptoms that occur after stabilization are unlikely to be drug related, such an occurrence of symptoms should be evaluated to determine if it may be due to lactic acidosis or other serious disease.

Patients should be counseled against excessive alcohol intake, either acute or chronic, while receiving JANUMET.

Patients should be informed about the importance of regular testing of renal function and hematological parameters when receiving treatment with JANUMET.

Patients should be informed that acute pancreatitis has been reported during postmarketing use of JANUMET. Patients should be informed that persistent severe abdominal pain, sometimes radiating to the back, which may or may not be accompanied by vomiting, is the hallmark symptom of acute pancreatitis. Patients should be instructed to promptly discontinue JANUMET and contact their physician if persistent severe abdominal pain occurs *[see Warnings and Precautions (5.2)]*.

Patients should be informed that the incidence of hypoglycemia is increased when JANUMET is added to an insulin secretagogue (e.g., sulfonylurea) or insulin therapy and that a lower dose of the insulin secretagogue or insulin may be required to reduce the risk of hypoglycemia.

Patients should be informed that allergic reactions have been reported during postmarketing use of sitagliptin, one of the components of JANUMET. If symptoms of allergic reactions (including rash, hives, and swelling of the face, lips, tongue, and throat that may cause difficulty in breathing or swallowing) occur, patients must stop taking JANUMET and seek medical advice promptly.

Patients should be informed that the tablets must never be split or divided before swallowing.

Physicians should instruct their patients to read the Medication Guide before starting JANUMET therapy and to reread each time the prescription is renewed. Patients should be instructed to inform their doctor if they develop any bothersome or unusual symptom, or if any symptom persists or worsens.

17.2 Laboratory Tests

Response to all diabetic therapies should be monitored by periodic measurements of blood glucose and A1C levels, with a goal of decreasing these levels towards the normal range. A1C is especially useful for evaluating long-term glycemic control.

Initial and periodic monitoring of hematologic parameters (e.g., hemoglobin/hematocrit and red blood cell indices) and renal function (serum creatinine) should be performed, at least on an annual basis. While megaloblastic anemia has rarely been seen with metformin therapy, if this is suspected, Vitamin B_{12} deficiency should be excluded.

Dist. by: Merck Sharp & Dohme Corp., a subsidiary of
MERCK & CO., INC., Whitehouse Station, NJ 08889, USA
US Patent Nos.: 6,699,871 and 7,326,708

Revised: 03/2013

USPI-T-0431A1303R007

Medication Guide
JANUMET® (JAN-you-met)
(sitagliptin/metformin hydrochloride)
Tablets

Read this Medication Guide carefully before you start taking JANUMET and each time you get a refill. There may be new information. This information does not take the place of talking with your doctor about your medical condition or your treatment. If you have any questions about JANUMET, ask your doctor or pharmacist.

What is the most important information I should know about JANUMET?

Serious side effects can happen in people taking JANUMET, including:

1. Lactic Acidosis. Metformin, one of the medicines in JANUMET, can cause a rare but serious condition called lactic acidosis (a build-up of lactic acid in the blood) that can cause death. Lactic acidosis is a medical emergency and must be treated in the hospital.

Stop taking JANUMET and call your doctor right away if you get any of the following symptoms, which could be signs of lactic acidosis.

You:
- feel very weak or tired.
- have unusual (not normal) muscle pain.
- have trouble breathing.
- have unusual sleepiness or sleep longer than usual.
- have sudden stomach or intestinal problems with nausea and vomiting or diarrhea.
- feel cold, especially in your arms and legs.
- feel dizzy or lightheaded.
- have a slow or irregular heartbeat.

You have a higher chance of getting lactic acidosis if you:
- have kidney problems. People whose kidneys are not working properly should not take JANUMET.
- have liver problems.
- have congestive heart failure that requires treatment with medicines.
- drink alcohol very often, or drink a lot of alcohol in short-term "binge" drinking.
- get dehydrated (lose a large amount of body fluids). This can happen if you are sick with a fever, vomiting, or diarrhea. Dehydration can also happen when you sweat a lot with activity or exercise and do not drink enough fluids.
- have certain x-ray tests with dyes or contrast agents that are injected into your body.
- have surgery.
- have a heart attack, severe infection, or stroke.
- are 80 years of age or older and have not had your kidneys tested.

2. Pancreatitis (inflammation of the pancreas) which may be severe and lead to death.

Certain medical problems make you more likely to get pancreatitis.

Before you start taking JANUMET:

Tell your doctor if you have ever had
- pancreatitis
- stones in your gallbladder (gallstones)
- a history of alcoholism
- high blood triglyceride levels

Stop taking JANUMET and call your doctor right away if you have pain in your stomach area (abdomen) that is severe and will not go away. The pain may be felt going from your abdomen through to your back. The pain may happen with or without vomiting. These may be symptoms of pancreatitis.

What is JANUMET?
- JANUMET is a prescription medicine that contains two prescription diabetes medicines, sitagliptin (JANUVIA®) and metformin. JANUMET can be used along with diet and exercise to lower blood sugar in adults with type 2 diabetes.
- JANUMET is not for people with type 1 diabetes.
- JANUMET is not for people with diabetic ketoacidosis (increased ketones in your blood or urine).
- If you have had pancreatitis (inflammation of the pancreas) in the past, it is not known if you have a higher chance of getting pancreatitis while you take JANUMET.
- It is not known if JANUMET is safe and effective when used in children under 18 years of age.

Who should not take JANUMET?

Do not take JANUMET if:
- you are allergic to any of the ingredients in JANUMET. See the end of this Medication Guide for a complete list of ingredients in JANUMET.
  Symptoms of a serious allergic reaction to JANUMET may include:
  - rash
  - raised red patches on your skin (hives)
  - swelling of the face, lips, tongue, and throat that may cause difficulty in breathing or swallowing
- you have kidneys which are not working properly.

- you are going to get an injection of dye or contrast agents for an x-ray procedure, JANUMET will need to be stopped for a short time. Talk to your doctor about when you should stop JANUMET and when you should start JANUMET again. See **"What is the most important information I should know about JANUMET?"**.

What should I tell my doctor before taking JANUMET?

Before you take JANUMET, tell your doctor if you:

- have or have had inflammation of your pancreas (pancreatitis).
- have kidney problems.
- have liver problems.
- have heart problems, including congestive heart failure.
- are older than 80 years. If you are over 80 years old you should not take JANUMET unless your kidneys have been checked and they are normal.
- drink alcohol very often, or drink a lot of alcohol in short-term "binge" drinking.
- have any other medical conditions.
- are pregnant or plan to become pregnant. It is not known if JANUMET will harm your unborn baby. If you are pregnant, talk with your doctor about the best way to control your blood sugar while you are pregnant.

  Pregnancy Registry: If you take JANUMET at any time during your pregnancy, talk with your doctor about how you can join the JANUMET pregnancy registry. The purpose of this registry is to collect information about the health of you and your baby. You can enroll in this registry by calling 1-800-986-8999.
- are breast-feeding or plan to breast-feed. It is not known if JANUMET will pass into your breast milk. Talk with your doctor about the best way to feed your baby if you are taking JANUMET.

Tell your doctor about all the medicines you take, including prescription and non-prescription medicines, vitamins, and herbal supplements. JANUMET may affect how well other drugs work and some drugs can affect how well JANUMET works.

Know the medicines you take. Keep a list of your medicines and show it to your doctor and pharmacist when you get a new medicine.

How should I take JANUMET?

- Take JANUMET exactly as your doctor tells you.
- Your doctor may change your dose of JANUMET if needed.
- Your doctor may tell you to take JANUMET along with certain other diabetes medicines. Low blood sugar can happen more often when JANUMET is taken with certain other diabetes medicines. See **"What are the possible side effects of JANUMET?"**.
- Take JANUMET with meals to lower your chance of having an upset stomach.
- Do not break or cut JANUMET tablets before swallowing. If you cannot swallow JANUMET tablets whole, tell your doctor.
- Continue to take JANUMET as long as your doctor tells you.
- If you take too much JANUMET, call your doctor or local Poison Control Center right away.
- If you miss a dose, take it with food as soon as you remember. If you do not remember until it is time for your next dose, skip the missed dose and go back to your regular schedule. Do not take two doses of JANUMET at the same time.
- You may need to stop taking JANUMET for a short time. Call your doctor for instructions if you:
  - are dehydrated (have lost too much body fluid). Dehydration can occur if you are sick with severe vomiting, diarrhea or fever, or if you drink a lot less fluid than normal.
  - plan to have surgery.
  - are going to get an injection of dye or contrast agent for an x-ray procedure. See **"What is the most important information I should know about JANUMET?"** and **"Who should not take JANUMET?"**.
- When your body is under some types of stress, such as fever, trauma (such as a car accident), infection or surgery, the amount of diabetes medicine that you need may change. Tell your doctor right away if you have any of these problems and follow your doctor's instructions.
- Check your blood sugar as your doctor tells you to.
- Stay on your prescribed diet and exercise program while taking JANUMET.
- Talk to your doctor about how to prevent, recognize and manage low blood sugar (hypoglycemia), high blood sugar (hyperglycemia), and problems you have because of your diabetes.
- Your doctor will check your diabetes with regular blood tests, including your blood sugar levels and your hemoglobin A1C.
- Your doctor will do blood tests to check how well your kidneys are working before and during your treatment with JANUMET.

What are the possible side effects of JANUMET?

Serious side effects have happened in people taking JANUMET.

- See **"What is the most important information I should know about JANUMET?"**.
- **Low blood sugar (hypoglycemia).** If you take JANUMET with another medicine that can cause low blood sugar, such as a sulfonylurea or insulin, your risk of getting low blood sugar is higher. The dose of your sulfonylurea medicine or insulin may need to be lowered while you use JANUMET. Signs and symptoms of low blood sugar may include:

• headache	• irritability
• drowsiness	• hunger
• weakness	• fast heart beat
• dizziness	• sweating
• confusion	• feeling jittery

- **Serious allergic reactions.** If you have any symptoms of a serious allergic reaction, stop taking JANUMET and call your doctor right away. See **"Who should not take JANUMET?"**. Your doctor may give you a medicine for your allergic reaction and prescribe a different medicine for your diabetes.
- **Kidney problems**, sometimes requiring dialysis.

The most common side effects of JANUMET include:

- stuffy or runny nose and sore throat
- upper respiratory infection
- diarrhea
- nausea and vomiting
- gas, upset stomach, indigestion
- weakness
- headache

Taking JANUMET with meals can help lessen the common stomach side effects of metformin that usually happen at the beginning of treatment. If you have unusual or sudden stomach problems, talk with your doctor. Stomach problems that start later during treatment may be a sign of something more serious.

JANUMET may have other side effects, including:

- swelling of the hands or legs. Swelling of the hands and legs can happen if you take JANUMET in combination with rosiglitazone (Avandia®). Rosiglitazone is another type of diabetes medicine.

These are not all the possible side effects of JANUMET. For more information, ask your doctor or pharmacist.

Tell your doctor if you have any side effect that bothers you, is unusual, or does not go away.

Call your doctor for medical advice about side effects. You may report side effects to FDA at 1-800-FDA-1088.

How should I store JANUMET?

Store JANUMET at 68°F to 77°F (20°C to 25°C).

Keep JANUMET and all medicines out of the reach of children.

General information about the use of JANUMET

Medicines are sometimes prescribed for purposes other than those listed in Medication Guides. Do not use JANUMET for a condition for which it was not prescribed. Do not give JANUMET to other people, even if they have the same symptoms you have. It may harm them.

This Medication Guide summarizes the most important information about JANUMET. If you would like to know more information, talk with your doctor. You can ask your doctor or pharmacist for additional information about JANUMET that is written for health care professionals. For more information go to www.JANUMET.com or call 1-800-622-4477.

What are the ingredients in JANUMET?

Active ingredients: sitagliptin and metformin hydrochloride

Inactive ingredients: microcrystalline cellulose, polyvinylpyrrolidone, sodium lauryl sulfate, and sodium stearyl fumarate. The tablet film coating contains the following inactive ingredients: polyvinyl alcohol, polyethylene glycol, talc, titanium dioxide, red iron oxide, and black iron oxide.

What is type 2 diabetes?

Type 2 diabetes is a condition in which your body does not make enough insulin, and the insulin that your body produces does not work as well as it should. Your body can also make too much sugar. When this happens, sugar (glucose) builds up in the blood. This can lead to serious medical problems.

High blood sugar can be lowered by diet and exercise, and by certain medicines when necessary.

This Medication Guide has been approved by the U.S. Food and Drug Administration.

Dist. by: Merck Sharp & Dohme Corp., a subsidiary of **MERCK & CO., INC.**, Whitehouse Station, NJ 08889, USA

US Patent Nos.: 6,699,871 and 7,326,708

The trademarks depicted herein are owned by their respective companies.

Revised: 03/2013
USMG-T-0431A1303R007

Shown in Product Identification Guide, page 308

JANUMET® XR ℞

[JAN-you-met]

(sitagliptin and metformin HCl extended-release) tablets

HIGHLIGHTS OF PRESCRIBING INFORMATION

These highlights do not include all the information needed to use JANUMET XR safely and effectively. See full prescribing information for JANUMET XR.

JANUMET® XR (sitagliptin and metformin HCl extended-release) tablets

Initial U.S. Approval: 2012

WARNING: LACTIC ACIDOSIS

See full prescribing information for complete boxed warning.

- **Lactic acidosis can occur due to metformin accumulation. The risk increases with conditions such as sepsis, dehydration, excess alcohol intake, hepatic insufficiency, renal impairment, and acute congestive heart failure. (5.1)**
- **Symptoms include malaise, myalgias, respiratory distress, increasing somnolence, and nonspecific abdominal distress. Laboratory abnormalities include low pH, increased anion gap and elevated blood lactate. (5.1)**
- **If acidosis is suspected, discontinue JANUMET XR and hospitalize the patient immediately. (5.1)**

RECENT MAJOR CHANGES

Dosage and Administration
Recommended Dosing (2.1) 02/2013

INDICATIONS AND USAGE

JANUMET XR is a dipeptidyl peptidase-4 (DPP-4) inhibitor and biguanide combination product indicated as an adjunct to diet and exercise to improve glycemic control in adults with type 2 diabetes mellitus when treatment with both sitagliptin and metformin extended-release is appropriate. (1, 14)

Important Limitations of Use:

- Not for the treatment of type 1 diabetes or diabetic ketoacidosis. (1)
- Has not been studied in patients with a history of pancreatitis. (1, 5.2)

DOSAGE AND ADMINISTRATION

- Individualize the starting dose of JANUMET XR based on the patient's current regimen. (2.1)
- May adjust the dosing based on effectiveness and tolerability while not exceeding the maximum recommended daily dose of 100 mg sitagliptin and 2000 mg metformin extended-release. (2.1)
- Administer once daily with a meal preferably in the evening. Gradually escalate the dose to reduce the gastrointestinal side effects due to metformin. (2.1)
- Maintain the same total daily dose of sitagliptin and metformin when changing between JANUMET and JANUMET XR, without exceeding the maximum recommended daily dose of 2000 mg metformin extended-release. (2.1)

DOSAGE FORMS AND STRENGTHS

JANUMET XR Tablets: 100 mg sitagliptin/1000 mg metformin HCl extended-release, 50 mg sitagliptin/500 mg metformin HCl extended-release, and 50 mg sitagliptin/1000 mg metformin HCl extended-release. (3)

CONTRAINDICATIONS

- Renal dysfunction, e.g., serum creatinine ≥1.5 mg/dL [males], ≥1.4 mg/dL [females] or abnormal creatinine clearance. (4, 5.1, 5.4)
- Metabolic acidosis, including diabetic ketoacidosis. (4, 5.1)
- History of a serious hypersensitivity reaction (e.g., anaphylaxis or angioedema) to JANUMET XR or to one of its components. (5.14, 6.2)

WARNINGS AND PRECAUTIONS

- Lactic acidosis: Warn against excessive alcohol intake. JANUMET XR is not recommended in hepatic impairment and is contraindicated in renal impairment. Ensure normal renal function before initiating and at least annually thereafter.
- Temporarily discontinue JANUMET XR in patients undergoing radiologic studies with intravascular administration

of iodinated contrast materials or any surgical procedures necessitating restricted intake of food or fluids. (5.1, 5.3, 5.4, 5.7)
- There have been postmarketing reports of acute pancreatitis, including fatal and non-fatal hemorrhagic or necrotizing pancreatitis in patients treated with sitagliptin (one of the components of JANUMET XR) with or without metformin. If pancreatitis is suspected, promptly discontinue JANUMET XR. (5.2)
- There have been postmarketing reports of acute renal failure in patients treated with sitagliptin with or without metformin, sometimes requiring dialysis. Before initiating JANUMET XR and at least annually thereafter, assess renal function and verify as normal. (4, 5.1, 5.4, 5.10, 6.2)
- Vitamin B_{12} deficiency: Metformin may lower Vitamin B_{12} levels. Measure hematologic parameters annually. (5.5, 6.1)
- When used with an insulin secretagogue (e.g., sulfonylurea) or with insulin, a lower dose of the insulin secretagogue or insulin may be required to minimize the risk of hypoglycemia. (2.1, 5.9)
- There have been postmarketing reports of serious allergic and hypersensitivity reactions in patients treated with sitagliptin, such as anaphylaxis, angioedema, and exfoliative skin conditions including Stevens-Johnson syndrome. In such cases, promptly stop JANUMET XR, assess for other potential causes, institute appropriate monitoring and treatment, and initiate alternative treatment for diabetes. (5.14, 6.2)
- There have been no clinical studies establishing conclusive evidence of macrovascular risk reduction with JANUMET XR or any other anti-diabetic drug. (5.15)

ADVERSE REACTIONS

- The most common adverse reactions reported in ≥5% of patients simultaneously started on sitagliptin and metformin and more commonly than in patients treated with placebo were diarrhea, upper respiratory tract infection, and headache. (6.1)
- Adverse reactions reported in ≥5% of patients treated with sitagliptin in combination with sulfonylurea and metformin and more commonly than in patients treated with placebo in combination with sulfonylurea and metformin were hypoglycemia and headache. (6.1)
- Hypoglycemia was the only adverse reaction reported in ≥5% of patients treated with sitagliptin in combination with insulin and metformin and more commonly than in patients treated with placebo in combination with insulin and metformin. (6.1)

To report SUSPECTED ADVERSE REACTIONS, contact Merck Sharp & Dohme Corp., a subsidiary of Merck & Co., Inc., at 1-877-888-4231 or FDA at 1-800-FDA-1088 or www.fda.gov/medwatch.

DRUG INTERACTIONS

- Cationic drugs eliminated by renal tubular secretion: Use with caution. (5.10, 7.2)

USE IN SPECIFIC POPULATIONS

- Safety and effectiveness of JANUMET XR in children under 18 years have not been established. (8.4)
- There are no adequate and well-controlled studies in pregnant women. To report drug exposure during pregnancy call 1-800-986-8999. (8.1)

See 17 for PATIENT COUNSELING INFORMATION and Medication Guide

Revised: 07/2013

FULL PRESCRIBING INFORMATION: CONTENTS*

*** Sections or subsections omitted from the full prescribing information are not listed**

FULL PRESCRIBING INFORMATION

WARNING: LACTIC ACIDOSIS

Lactic acidosis is a rare, but serious complication that can occur due to metformin accumulation. The risk increases with conditions such as sepsis, dehydration, excess alcohol intake, hepatic impairment, renal impairment, and acute congestive heart failure.

The onset of lactic acidosis is often subtle, accompanied only by nonspecific symptoms such as malaise, myalgias, respiratory distress, increasing somnolence, and nonspecific abdominal distress.

Laboratory abnormalities include low pH, increased anion gap and elevated blood lactate.

If acidosis is suspected, JANUMET XR (sitagliptin and metformin HCl extended-release) tablets should be discontinued and the patient hospitalized immediately. *[See Warnings and Precautions (5.1).]*

1 INDICATIONS AND USAGE

JANUMET® XR is indicated as an adjunct to diet and exercise to improve glycemic control in adults with type 2 diabetes mellitus when treatment with both sitagliptin and metformin extended-release is appropriate. *[See Clinical Studies (14).]*

Important Limitations of Use

JANUMET XR should not be used in patients with type 1 diabetes mellitus or for the treatment of diabetic ketoacidosis.

JANUMET XR has not been studied in patients with a history of pancreatitis. It is unknown whether patients with a history of pancreatitis are at increased risk for the development of pancreatitis while using JANUMET XR. *[See Warnings and Precautions (5.2).]*

2 DOSAGE AND ADMINISTRATION

2.1 Recommended Dosing

The dose of JANUMET XR should be individualized on the basis of the patient's current regimen, effectiveness, and tolerability while not exceeding the maximum recommended daily dose of 100 mg sitagliptin and 2000 mg metformin. Initial combination therapy or maintenance of combination therapy should be individualized and left to the discretion of the health care provider.

- In patients not currently treated with metformin, the recommended total daily starting dose of JANUMET XR is 100 mg sitagliptin and 1000 mg metformin hydrochloride (HCl) extended-release. Patients with inadequate glycemic control on this dose of metformin can be titrated gradually, to reduce gastrointestinal side effects associated with metformin, up to the maximum recommended daily dose.
- In patients already treated with metformin, the recommended total daily starting dose of JANUMET XR is 100 mg sitagliptin and the previously prescribed dose of metformin.
- For patients taking metformin immediate-release 850 mg twice daily or 1000 mg twice daily, the recommended starting dose of JANUMET XR is two 50 mg sitagliptin/1000 mg metformin hydrochloride extended-release tablets taken together once daily.
- Maintain the same total daily dose of sitagliptin and metformin when changing between JANUMET (sitagliptin and metformin HCl immediate-release) and JANUMET XR. Patients with inadequate glycemic control on this dose of metformin can be titrated gradually, to reduce gastrointestinal side effects associated with metformin, up to the maximum recommended daily dose.

JANUMET XR should be administered with food to reduce the gastrointestinal side effects associated with the metformin component. JANUMET XR should be given once daily with a meal preferably in the evening. JANUMET XR should be swallowed whole. The tablets must not be split, crushed, or chewed before swallowing.

The 100 mg sitagliptin/1000 mg metformin hydrochloride extended-release tablet should be taken as a single tablet once daily. Patients using two JANUMET XR tablets (such as two 50 mg sitagliptin/500 mg metformin hydrochloride extended-release tablets or two 50 mg sitagliptin/1000 mg metformin hydrochloride extended-release tablets) should take the two tablets together once daily.

Patients treated with an insulin secretagogue or insulin

Co-administration of JANUMET XR with an insulin secretagogue (e.g., sulfonylurea) or insulin may require lower doses of the insulin secretagogue or insulin to reduce the risk of hypoglycemia *[see Warnings and Precautions (5.9)]*.

No studies have been performed specifically examining the safety and efficacy of JANUMET XR in patients previously treated with other oral antihyperglycemic agents and switched to JANUMET XR. Any change in therapy of type 2 diabetes should be undertaken with care and appropriate monitoring as changes in glycemic control can occur.

3 DOSAGE FORMS AND STRENGTHS

- 100 mg/1000 mg tablets are blue, bi-convex oval, film-coated tablets with "81" debossed on one side.
- 50 mg/500 mg tablets are light blue, bi-convex oval, film-coated tablets with "78" debossed on one side.
- 50 mg/1000 mg tablets are light green, bi-convex oval, film-coated tablets with "80" debossed on one side.

4 CONTRAINDICATIONS

JANUMET XR is contraindicated in patients with:

- Renal impairment (e.g., serum creatinine levels greater than or equal to 1.5 mg/dL for men, greater than or equal to 1.4 mg/dL for women or abnormal creatinine clearance), which may also result from conditions such as cardiovascular collapse (shock), acute myocardial infarction, and septicemia *[see Warnings and Precautions (5.1)]*.
- Hypersensitivity to metformin hydrochloride.
- Acute or chronic metabolic acidosis, including diabetic ketoacidosis. Diabetic ketoacidosis should be treated with insulin.
- History of a serious hypersensitivity reaction to JANUMET XR or sitagliptin, such as anaphylaxis or angioedema. *[See Warnings and Precautions (5.14); Adverse Reactions (6.2).]*

5 WARNINGS AND PRECAUTIONS

5.1 Lactic Acidosis

Metformin hydrochloride

Lactic acidosis is a serious, metabolic complication that can occur due to metformin accumulation during treatment with JANUMET XR and is fatal in approximately 50% of cases. Lactic acidosis may also occur in association with a number of pathophysiologic conditions, including diabetes mellitus, and whenever there is significant tissue hypoperfusion and hypoxemia. Lactic acidosis is characterized by elevated blood lactate concentrations (>5 mmol/L), decreased blood pH, electrolyte disturbances with an increased anion gap, and an increased lactate/pyruvate ratio. When metformin is implicated as the cause of lactic acidosis, metformin plasma levels >5 μg/mL are generally found. The reported incidence of lactic acidosis in patients receiving metformin hydrochloride is approximately 0.03 cases/1000 patient-years, with approximately 0.015 fatal cases/1000 patient-years. In more than 20,000 patient-years exposure to metformin in clinical trials, there were no reports of lactic acidosis. Reported cases have occurred primarily in diabetic patients with significant renal impairment, including both intrinsic renal disease and renal hypoperfusion, often in the setting of multiple concomitant medical/surgical problems and multiple concomitant medications. Patients with congestive heart failure requiring pharmacologic management, in particular those with unstable or acute congestive heart failure who are at risk of hypoperfusion and hypoxemia, are at increased risk of lactic acidosis. The risk of lactic acidosis increases with the degree of renal dysfunction and the patient's age. The risk of lactic acidosis may, therefore, be significantly decreased by regular monitoring of renal function in patients taking JANUMET XR. In particular, treatment of the elderly should be accompanied by careful monitoring of renal function. JANUMET XR treatment should not be initiated in any patient unless measurement of creatinine clearance demonstrates that renal function is not reduced. In addition, JANUMET XR should be promptly withheld in the presence of any condition associated with hypoxemia, dehydration, or sepsis. Because impaired hepatic function may significantly limit the ability to clear lactate, JANUMET XR should generally be avoided in patients with clinical or laboratory evidence of hepatic impairment. Patients should be cautioned against excessive alcohol intake when taking JANUMET XR, because alcohol potentiates the effects of metformin on lactate metabolism. In addition, JANUMET XR should be temporarily discontinued prior to any intravascular radiocontrast study and for any surgical procedure necessitating restricted intake of food or fluids. Use of topiramate, a carbonic anhydrase inhibitor, in epilepsy and migraine prophylaxis may frequently cause dose-dependent metabolic acidosis (in controlled trials, 32% and 67% for adjunctive treatment in adults and pediatric patients, respectively, and 15 to 25% for monotherapy of epilepsy, with decrease in serum bicarbonate to less than 20 mEq/L; 3% and 11% for adjunctive treatment in adults and pediatric patients, respectively, and 1 to 7% for monotherapy of epilepsy, with decrease in serum bicarbonate to less than 17 mEq/L) and may exacerbate the risk of metformin-induced lactic acidosis. *[See Drug Interactions (7.1); Clinical Pharmacology (12).]* The onset of lactic acidosis often is subtle, and accompanied only by nonspecific symptoms such as malaise, myalgias, respiratory distress, increasing somnolence, and nonspecific abdominal distress. There may be associated hypothermia, hypotension, and resistant bradyarrhythmias with more marked acidosis.

Patients should be educated to promptly report these symptoms to their physician should they occur. If present, JANUMET XR should be withdrawn until lactic acidosis is ruled out. Serum electrolytes, ketones, blood glucose, blood pH, lactate levels, and blood metformin levels may be useful. Once a patient is stabilized on any dose level of JANUMET XR, gastrointestinal symptoms, which are common during initiation of therapy, are unlikely to recur. Later occurrence of gastrointestinal symptoms could be due to lactic acidosis or other serious disease. Levels of fasting venous plasma lactate above the upper limit of normal but less than 5 mmol/L in patients taking JANUMET XR do not necessarily indicate impending lactic acidosis and may be explainable by other mechanisms, such as poorly-controlled diabetes or obesity, vigorous physical activity, or technical problems in sample handling. Lactic acidosis should be suspected in any diabetic patient with metabolic acidosis lacking evidence of ketoacidosis (ketonuria and ketonemia). Lactic acidosis is a medical emergency that must be treated in a hospital setting. In a patient with lactic acidosis who is taking JANUMET XR, the drug should be discontinued immediately and general supportive measures promptly instituted. Because metformin hydrochloride is dialyzable (with a clearance of up to 170 mL/min under good hemodynamic conditions), prompt hemodialysis is recommended to correct the acidosis and remove the accumulated metformin. Such management often results in prompt reversal of symptoms and recovery. *[See Contraindications (4).]*

5.2 Pancreatitis

There have been postmarketing reports of acute pancreatitis, including fatal and non-fatal hemorrhagic or necrotizing pancreatitis, in patients taking sitagliptin with or without metformin. After initiation of JANUMET XR, patients should be observed carefully for signs and symptoms of pancreatitis. If pancreatitis is suspected, JANUMET XR should promptly be discontinued and appropriate management should be initiated. It is unknown whether patients with a history of pancreatitis are at increased risk for the development of pancreatitis while using JANUMET XR.

5.3 Impaired Hepatic Function

Since impaired hepatic function has been associated with some cases of lactic acidosis, JANUMET XR should generally be avoided in patients with clinical or laboratory evidence of hepatic disease.

5.4 Assessment of Renal Function

Metformin and sitagliptin are substantially excreted by the kidney.

Metformin hydrochloride

The risk of metformin accumulation and lactic acidosis increases with the degree of impairment of renal function. Therefore, JANUMET XR is contraindicated in patients with renal impairment.

Before initiation of JANUMET XR and at least annually thereafter, renal function should be assessed and verified as normal. In patients in whom development of renal dysfunction is anticipated (e.g., elderly), renal function should be assessed more frequently and JANUMET XR discontinued if evidence of renal impairment is present.

Sitagliptin

There have been postmarketing reports of worsening renal function in patients taking sitagliptin with or without metformin, including acute renal failure, sometimes requiring dialysis. Before initiation of therapy with JANUMET XR and at least annually thereafter, renal function should be assessed and verified as normal. In patients in whom development of renal dysfunction is anticipated, particularly in elderly patients, renal function should be assessed more frequently and JANUMET XR discontinued if evidence of renal impairment is present.

5.5 Vitamin B_{12} Levels

In controlled clinical trials of metformin of 29 weeks duration, a decrease to subnormal levels of previously normal serum Vitamin B_{12} levels, without clinical manifestations, was observed in approximately 7% of patients. Such decrease, possibly due to interference with B_{12} absorption from the B_{12}-intrinsic factor complex, is, however, very rarely associated with anemia and appears to be rapidly reversible with discontinuation of metformin or Vitamin B_{12} supplementation. Measurement of hematologic parameters on an annual basis is advised in patients on JANUMET XR and any apparent abnormalities should be appropriately investigated and managed. *[See Adverse Reactions (6.1).]*

Certain individuals (those with inadequate Vitamin B_{12} or calcium intake or absorption) appear to be predisposed to developing subnormal Vitamin B_{12} levels. In these patients, routine serum Vitamin B_{12} measurements at two- to three-year intervals may be useful.

5.6 Alcohol Intake

Alcohol potentiates the effect of metformin on lactate metabolism. Patients should be warned against excessive alcohol intake while receiving JANUMET XR.

5.7 Surgical Procedures

Use of JANUMET XR should be temporarily suspended for any surgical procedure (except minor procedures not associated with restricted intake of food and fluids) and should not be restarted until the patient's oral intake has resumed and renal function has been evaluated as normal.

5.8 Change in Clinical Status of Patients with Previously Controlled Type 2 Diabetes

A patient with type 2 diabetes previously well controlled on JANUMET XR who develops laboratory abnormalities or clinical illness (especially vague and poorly defined illness) should be evaluated promptly for evidence of ketoacidosis or lactic acidosis. Evaluation should include serum electrolytes and ketones, blood glucose and, if indicated, blood pH, lactate, pyruvate, and metformin levels. If acidosis of either form occurs, JANUMET XR must be stopped immediately and other appropriate corrective measures initiated.

5.9 Use with Medications Known to Cause Hypoglycemia

Sitagliptin

When sitagliptin was used in combination with a sulfonylurea or with insulin, medications known to cause hypoglycemia, the incidence of hypoglycemia was increased over that of placebo used in combination with a sulfonylurea or with insulin *[see Adverse Reactions (6)]*. Therefore, patients also receiving an insulin secretagogue (e.g., sulfonylurea) or insulin may require a lower dose of the insulin secretagogue or insulin to reduce the risk of hypoglycemia *[see Dosage and Administration (2.1)]*.

Metformin hydrochloride

Hypoglycemia does not occur in patients receiving metformin alone under usual circumstances of use, but could occur when caloric intake is deficient, when strenuous exercise is not compensated by caloric supplementation, or during concomitant use with other glucose-lowering agents (such as sulfonylureas and insulin) or ethanol. Elderly, debilitated, or malnourished patients, and those with adrenal or pituitary insufficiency or alcohol intoxication are particularly susceptible to hypoglycemic effects. Hypoglycemia may be difficult to recognize in the elderly, and in people who are taking β-adrenergic blocking drugs.

5.10 Concomitant Medications Affecting Renal Function or Metformin Disposition

Concomitant medication(s) that may affect renal function or result in significant hemodynamic change or may interfere with the disposition of metformin, such as cationic drugs that are eliminated by renal tubular secretion *[see Drug Interactions (7.2)]*, should be used with caution.

5.11 Radiologic Studies with Intravascular Iodinated Contrast Materials

Intravascular contrast studies with iodinated materials (for example, intravenous urogram, intravenous cholangiography, angiography, and computed tomography (CT) scans with intravascular contrast materials) can lead to acute alteration of renal function and have been associated with lactic acidosis in patients receiving metformin *[see Contraindications (4)]*. Therefore, in patients in whom any such study is planned, JANUMET XR should be temporarily discontinued at the time of or prior to the procedure, and withheld for 48 hours subsequent to the procedure and reinstituted only after renal function has been re-evaluated and found to be normal.

5.12 Hypoxic States

Cardiovascular collapse (shock) from whatever cause, acute congestive heart failure, acute myocardial infarction and other conditions characterized by hypoxemia have been associated with lactic acidosis and may also cause prerenal azotemia. When such events occur in patients on JANUMET XR therapy, the drug should be promptly discontinued.

5.13 Loss of Control of Blood Glucose

When a patient stabilized on any diabetic regimen is exposed to stress such as fever, trauma, infection, or surgery, a temporary loss of glycemic control may occur. At such times, it may be necessary to withhold JANUMET XR and temporarily administer insulin. JANUMET XR may be reinstituted after the acute episode is resolved.

5.14 Hypersensitivity Reactions

There have been postmarketing reports of serious hypersensitivity reactions in patients treated with sitagliptin, one of the components of JANUMET XR. These reactions include anaphylaxis, angioedema, and exfoliative skin conditions including Stevens-Johnson syndrome. Onset of these reactions occurred within the first 3 months after initiation of treatment with sitagliptin, with some reports occurring after the first dose. If a hypersensitivity reaction is suspected, discontinue JANUMET XR, assess for other potential causes for the event, and institute alternative treatment for diabetes. *[See Adverse Reactions (6.2).]*

Use caution in a patient with a history of angioedema to another dipeptidyl peptidase-4 (DPP4) inhibitor because it is unknown whether such patients will be predisposed to angioedema with JANUMET XR.

5.15 Macrovascular Outcomes

There have been no clinical studies establishing conclusive evidence of macrovascular risk reduction with JANUMET XR or any other anti-diabetic drug.

6 ADVERSE REACTIONS

6.1 Clinical Trials Experience

Because clinical trials are conducted under widely varying conditions, adverse reaction rates observed in the clinical trials of a drug cannot be directly compared to rates in the clinical trials of another drug and may not reflect the rates observed in practice.

Sitagliptin and Metformin Immediate-Release Co-administration in Patients with Type 2 Diabetes Inadequately Controlled on Diet and Exercise

Table 1 summarizes the most common (≥5% of patients) adverse reactions reported (regardless of investigator assessment of causality) in a 24-week placebo-controlled factorial study in which sitagliptin and metformin immediate-release were co-administered to patients with type 2 diabetes inadequately controlled on diet and exercise.

[See table 1 below]

Table 1: Sitagliptin and Metformin Immediate-Release Co-administered to Patients with Type 2 Diabetes Inadequately Controlled on Diet and Exercise: Adverse Reactions Reported (Regardless of Investigator Assessment of Causality) in ≥5% of Patients Receiving Combination Therapy (and Greater than in Patients Receiving Placebo) *

	Number of Patients (%)			
	Placebo	Sitagliptin 100 mg once daily	Metformin Immediate-Release 500 mg or 1000 mg twice daily †	Sitagliptin 50 mg twice daily + Metformin Immediate-Release 500 mg or 1000 mg twice daily †
	N = 176	N = 179	N = 364†	N = 372†
Diarrhea	7 (4.0)	5 (2.8)	28 (7.7)	28 (7.5)
Upper Respiratory Tract Infection	9 (5.1)	8 (4.5)	19 (5.2)	23 (6.2)
Headache	5 (2.8)	2 (1.1)	14 (3.8)	22 (5.9)

* Intent-to-treat population.

† Data pooled for the patients given the lower and higher doses of metformin.

Sitagliptin Add-on Therapy in Patients with Type 2 Diabetes Inadequately Controlled on Metformin Immediate-Release Alone

In a 24-week placebo-controlled trial of sitagliptin 100 mg administered once daily added to a twice daily metformin immediate-release regimen, there were no adverse reactions reported regardless of investigator assessment of causality in ≥5% of patients and more commonly than in patients given placebo. Discontinuation of therapy due to clinical adverse reactions was similar to the placebo treatment group (sitagliptin and metformin immediate-release, 1.9%; placebo and metformin immediate-release, 2.5%).

Gastrointestinal Adverse Reactions

The incidences of pre-selected gastrointestinal adverse experiences in patients treated with sitagliptin and metformin immediate-release were similar to those reported for patients treated with metformin immediate-release alone. See Table 2.

[See table 2 above]

Table 2: Pre-selected Gastrointestinal Adverse Reactions (Regardless of Investigator Assessment of Causality) Reported in Patients with Type 2 Diabetes Receiving Sitagliptin and Metformin Immediate-Release

	Number of Patients (%)					
	Study of Sitagliptin and Metformin Immediate-Release in Patients Inadequately Controlled on Diet and Exercise				Study of Sitagliptin Add-on in Patients Inadequately Controlled on Metformin Immediate-Release Alone	
	Placebo	Sitagliptin 100 mg once daily	Metformin Immediate-Release 500 mg or 1000 mg twice daily *	Sitagliptin 50 mg bid + Metformin Immediate-Release 500 mg or 1000 mg twice daily *	Placebo and Metformin Immediate-Release ≥1500 mg daily	Sitagliptin 100 mg once daily and Metformin Immediate-Release ≥1500 mg daily
	N = 176	N = 179	N = 364	N = 372	N = 237	N = 464
Diarrhea	7 (4.0)	5 (2.8)	28 (7.7)	28 (7.5)	6 (2.5)	11 (2.4)
Nausea	2 (1.1)	2 (1.1)	20 (5.5)	18 (4.8)	2 (0.8)	6 (1.3)
Vomiting	1 (0.6)	0 (0.0)	2 (0.5)	8 (2.2)	2 (0.8)	5 (1.1)
Abdominal Pain†	4 (2.3)	6 (3.4)	14 (3.8)	11 (3.0)	9 (3.8)	10 (2.2)

* Data pooled for the patients given the lower and higher doses of metformin.
† Abdominal discomfort was included in the analysis of abdominal pain in the study of initial therapy.

Sitagliptin in Combination with Metformin Immediate-Release and Glimepiride

In a 24-week placebo-controlled study of sitagliptin 100 mg as add-on therapy in patients with type 2 diabetes inadequately controlled on metformin immediate-release and glimepiride (sitagliptin, N=116; placebo, N=113), the adverse reactions reported regardless of investigator assessment of causality in ≥5% of patients treated with sitagliptin and more commonly than in patients treated with placebo were: hypoglycemia (Table 3) and headache (6.9%, 2.7%).

Sitagliptin in Combination with Metformin Immediate-Release and Rosiglitazone

In a placebo-controlled study of sitagliptin 100 mg as add-on therapy in patients with type 2 diabetes inadequately controlled on metformin immediate-release and rosiglitazone (sitagliptin, N=181; placebo, N=97), the adverse reactions reported regardless of investigator assessment of causality through Week 18 in ≥5% of patients treated with sitagliptin and more commonly than in patients treated with placebo were: upper respiratory tract infection (sitagliptin, 5.5%; placebo, 5.2%) and nasopharyngitis (6.1%, 4.1%). Through Week 54, the adverse reactions reported regardless of investigator assessment of causality in ≥5% of patients treated with sitagliptin and more commonly than in patients treated with placebo were: upper respiratory tract infection (sitagliptin, 15.5%; placebo, 6.2%), nasopharyngitis (11.0%, 9.3%), peripheral edema (8.3%, 5.2%), and headache (5.5%, 4.1%).

Sitagliptin in Combination with Metformin Immediate-Release and Insulin

In a 24-week placebo-controlled study of sitagliptin 100 mg as add-on therapy in patients with type 2 diabetes inadequately controlled on metformin immediate-release and insulin (sitagliptin, N=229; placebo, N=233), the only adverse reaction reported regardless of investigator assessment of causality in ≥5% of patients treated with sitagliptin and more commonly than in patients treated with placebo was hypoglycemia (Table 3).

Hypoglycemia

In all (N=5) studies, adverse reactions of hypoglycemia were based on all reports of symptomatic hypoglycemia; a concurrent glucose measurement was not required although most (77%) reports of hypoglycemia were accompanied by a blood glucose measurement ≤70 mg/dL. When the combination of sitagliptin and metformin immediate-release was co-administered with a sulfonylurea or with insulin, the percentage of patients reporting at least one adverse reaction of hypoglycemia was higher than that observed with placebo and metformin immediate-release co-administered with a sulfonylurea or with insulin (Table 3).

[See table 3 above]

Table 3: Incidence and Rate of Hypoglycemia* (Regardless of Investigator Assessment of Causality) in Placebo-Controlled Clinical Studies of Sitagliptin in Combination with Metformin Immediate-Release Co-administered with Glimepiride or Insulin

Add-On to Glimepiride + Metformin Immediate-Release (24 weeks)	Sitagliptin 100 mg + Metformin Immediate-Release + Glimepiride	Placebo + Metformin Immediate-Release + Glimepiride
	N = 116	N = 113
Overall (%)	19 (16.4)	1 (0.9)
Rate (episodes/patient-year) †	0.82	0.02
Severe (%)‡	0 (0.0)	0 (0.0)
Add-On to Insulin + Metformin Immediate-Release (24 weeks)	**Sitagliptin 100 mg + Metformin Immediate-Release + Insulin**	**Placebo + Metformin Immediate-Release + Insulin**
	N = 229	N = 233
Overall (%)	35 (15.3)	19 (8.2)
Rate (episodes/patient-year) †	0.98	0.61
Severe (%)‡	1 (0.4)	1 (0.4)

* Adverse reactions of hypoglycemia were based on all reports of symptomatic hypoglycemia; a concurrent glucose measurement was not required: Intent-to-treat population.
† Based on total number of events (i.e., a single patient may have had multiple events).
‡ Severe events of hypoglycemia were defined as those events requiring medical assistance or exhibiting depressed level/loss of consciousness or seizure.

The overall incidence of reported adverse reactions of hypoglycemia in patients with type 2 diabetes inadequately controlled on diet and exercise was 0.6% in patients given placebo, 0.6% in patients given sitagliptin alone, 0.8% in patients given metformin immediate-release alone, and 1.6% in patients given sitagliptin in combination with metformin immediate-release. In patients with type 2 diabetes inadequately controlled on metformin immediate-release alone, the overall incidence of adverse reactions of hypoglycemia was 1.3% in patients given add-on sitagliptin and 2.1% in patients given add-on placebo.

In the study of sitagliptin and add-on combination therapy with metformin immediate-release and rosiglitazone, the overall incidence of hypoglycemia was 2.2% in patients given add-on sitagliptin and 0.0% in patients given add-on placebo through Week 18. Through Week 54, the overall incidence of hypoglycemia was 3.9% in patients given add-on sitagliptin and 1.0% in patients given add-on placebo.

Vital Signs and Electrocardiograms

With the combination of sitagliptin and metformin immediate-release, no clinically meaningful changes in vital signs or in electrocardiogram parameters (including the QTc interval) were observed.

Pancreatitis

In a pooled analysis of 19 double-blind clinical trials that included data from 10,246 patients randomized to receive sitagliptin 100 mg/day (N=5429) or corresponding (active or placebo) control (N=4817), the incidence of acute pancreatitis was 0.1 per 100 patient-years in each group (4 patients with an event in 4708 patient-years for sitagliptin and 4 patients with an event in 3942 patient-years for control). *[See Warnings and Precautions (5.2).]*

Sitagliptin

The most common adverse experience in sitagliptin monotherapy reported regardless of investigator assessment of causality in ≥5% of patients and more commonly than in patients given placebo was nasopharyngitis.

Metformin Extended-Release

In a 24-week clinical trial in which extended-release metformin or placebo was added to glyburide therapy, the most common (>5% and greater than placebo) adverse reactions in the combined treatment group were hypoglycemia (13.7% vs. 4.9%), diarrhea (12.5% vs. 5.6%), and nausea (6.7% vs. 4.2%).

Laboratory Tests

Sitagliptin

The incidence of laboratory adverse reactions was similar in patients treated with sitagliptin and metformin immediate-release (7.6%) compared to patients treated with placebo and metformin (8.7%). In most but not all studies, a small increase in white blood cell count (approximately 200 cells/microL difference in WBC vs. placebo; mean baseline WBC approximately 6600 cells/microL) was observed due to a small increase in neutrophils. This change in laboratory parameters is not considered to be clinically relevant.

Metformin hydrochloride

In controlled clinical trials of metformin of 29 weeks duration, a decrease to subnormal levels of previously normal serum Vitamin B_{12} levels, without clinical manifestations, was observed in approximately 7% of patients. Such decrease, possibly due to interference with B_{12} absorption from the B_{12}-intrinsic factor complex, is, however, very rarely associated with anemia and appears to be rapidly reversible with discontinuation of metformin or Vitamin B_{12} supplementation. *[See Warnings and Precautions (5.5).]*

6.2 Postmarketing Experience

Additional adverse reactions have been identified during postapproval use of sitagliptin with or without metformin, and/or in combination with other antidiabetic medications. Because these reactions are reported voluntarily from a population of uncertain size, it is generally not possible to reliably estimate their frequency or establish a causal relationship to drug exposure.

Hypersensitivity reactions including anaphylaxis, angioedema, rash, urticaria, cutaneous vasculitis, and exfoliative skin conditions including Stevens-Johnson syndrome *[see Warnings and Precautions (5.14)]*; upper respiratory tract infection; hepatic enzyme elevations; acute pancreatitis, including fatal and non-fatal hemorrhagic and necrotizing pancreatitis *[see Indications and Usage (1); Warnings and Precautions (5.2)]*; worsening renal function, including acute renal failure (sometimes requiring dialysis) *[see Warnings and Precautions (5.4)]*; constipation; vomiting; headache; arthralgia; myalgia; pain in extremity; back pain.

7 DRUG INTERACTIONS

7.1 Carbonic Anhydrase Inhibitors

Topiramate or other carbonic anhydrase inhibitors (e.g., zonisamide, acetazolamide or dichlorphenamide) frequently decrease serum bicarbonate and induce non-anion gap, hyperchloremic metabolic acidosis. Concomitant use of these drugs may induce metabolic acidosis. Use these drugs with caution in patients treated with JANUMET XR, as the risk of lactic acidosis may increase.

7.2 Cationic Drugs

Cationic drugs (e.g., amiloride, digoxin, morphine, procainamide, quinidine, quinine, ranitidine, triamterene, trimethoprim, or vancomycin) that are eliminated by renal tubular secretion theoretically have the potential for interaction with metformin by competing for common renal tubular transport systems. Although such interactions remain theoretical (except for cimetidine), careful patient monitoring and dose adjustment of JANUMET XR and/or the interfering drug is recommended in patients who are taking cationic medications that are excreted via the proximal renal tubular secretory system.

7.3 The Use of Metformin with Other Drugs

Certain drugs tend to produce hyperglycemia and may lead to loss of glycemic control. These drugs include the thiazides and other diuretics, corticosteroids, phenothiazines, thyroid products, estrogens, oral contraceptives, phenytoin, nicotinic acid, sympathomimetics, calcium channel blocking drugs, and isoniazid. When such drugs are administered to a patient receiving JANUMET XR the patient should be closely observed to maintain adequate glycemic control.

8 USE IN SPECIFIC POPULATIONS

8.1 Pregnancy

Pregnancy Category B:

JANUMET XR

There are no adequate and well-controlled studies in pregnant women with JANUMET XR or its individual components; therefore, the safety of JANUMET XR in pregnant women is not known. JANUMET XR should be used during pregnancy only if clearly needed.

Merck Sharp & Dohme Corp., a subsidiary of Merck & Co., Inc., maintains a registry to monitor the pregnancy outcomes of women exposed to JANUMET XR while pregnant. Health care providers are encouraged to report any prenatal exposure to JANUMET XR by calling the Pregnancy Registry at 1-800-986-8999.

No animal studies have been conducted with the combined products in JANUMET XR to evaluate effects on reproduction. The following data are based on findings in studies performed with sitagliptin or metformin individually.

Sitagliptin

Reproduction studies have been performed in rats and rabbits. Doses of sitagliptin up to 125 mg/kg (approximately 12 times the human exposure at the maximum recommended human dose) did not impair fertility or harm the fetus. There are, however, no adequate and well-controlled studies with sitagliptin in pregnant women.

Sitagliptin administered to pregnant female rats and rabbits from gestation day 6 to 20 (organogenesis) was not teratogenic at oral doses up to 250 mg/kg (rats) and 125 mg/kg (rabbits), or approximately 30 and 20 times human exposure at the maximum recommended human dose (MRHD) of 100 mg/day based on AUC comparisons. Higher doses increased the incidence of rib malformations in offspring at 1000 mg/kg, or approximately 100 times human exposure at the MRHD.

Sitagliptin administered to female rats from gestation day 6 to lactation day 21 decreased body weight in male and female offspring at 1000 mg/kg. No functional or behavioral toxicity was observed in offspring of rats.

Placental transfer of sitagliptin administered to pregnant rats was approximately 45% at 2 hours and 80% at 24 hours postdose. Placental transfer of sitagliptin administered to pregnant rabbits was approximately 66% at 2 hours and 30% at 24 hours.

Metformin hydrochloride

Metformin was not teratogenic in rats and rabbits at doses up to 600 mg/kg/day, which represent 3 and 6 times the maximum recommended human daily dose of 2000 mg based on body surface area comparison for rats and rabbits, respectively. However, because animal reproduction studies are not always predictive of human response, metformin hydrochloride should not be used during pregnancy unless clearly needed.

8.3 Nursing Mothers

No studies in lactating animals have been conducted with the combined components of JANUMET XR. In studies performed with the individual components, both sitagliptin and metformin are secreted in the milk of lactating rats. It is not known whether sitagliptin or metformin are excreted in human milk. Because many drugs are excreted in human milk, caution should be exercised when JANUMET XR is administered to a nursing woman.

8.4 Pediatric Use

Safety and effectiveness of JANUMET XR in pediatric patients under 18 years have not been established.

8.5 Geriatric Use

JANUMET XR

Because sitagliptin and metformin are substantially excreted by the kidney, and because aging can be associated with reduced renal function, JANUMET XR should be used with caution as age increases. Care should be taken in dose selection and should be based on careful and regular monitoring of renal function. *[See Warnings and Precautions (5.1, 5.4); Clinical Pharmacology (12.3).]*

Sitagliptin

Of the total number of subjects (N=3884) in premarketing Phase II and III clinical studies of sitagliptin, 725 patients were 65 years and over, while 61 patients were 75 years and over. No overall differences in safety or effectiveness were observed between subjects 65 years and over and younger subjects. While this and other reported clinical experience have not identified differences in responses between the elderly and younger patients, greater sensitivity of some older individuals cannot be ruled out.

Metformin hydrochloride

Controlled clinical studies of metformin did not include sufficient numbers of elderly patients to determine whether they respond differently from younger patients, although other reported clinical experience has not identified differences in responses between the elderly and young patients. Metformin should only be used in patients with normal renal function. The initial and maintenance dosing of metformin should be conservative in patients with advanced age, due to the potential for decreased renal function in this population. Any dose adjustment should be based on a careful assessment of renal function. *[See Contraindications (4); Warnings and Precautions (5.4); Clinical Pharmacology (12.3).]*

10 OVERDOSAGE

Sitagliptin

During controlled clinical trials in healthy subjects, single doses of up to 800 mg sitagliptin were administered. Maximal mean increases in QTc of 8.0 msec were observed in one study at a dose of 800 mg sitagliptin, a mean effect that is not considered clinically important *[see Clinical Pharmacology (12.2)]*. There is no experience with doses above 800 mg in clinical studies. In Phase I multiple-dose studies, there were no dose-related clinical adverse reactions observed with sitagliptin with doses of up to 400 mg per day for periods of up to 28 days.

In the event of an overdose, it is reasonable to employ the usual supportive measures, e.g., remove unabsorbed material from the gastrointestinal tract, employ clinical monitoring (including obtaining an electrocardiogram), and institute supportive therapy as indicated by the patient's clinical status.

Sitagliptin is modestly dialyzable. In clinical studies, approximately 13.5% of the dose was removed over a 3- to 4-hour hemodialysis session. Prolonged hemodialysis may be considered if clinically appropriate. It is not known if sitagliptin is dialyzable by peritoneal dialysis.

Metformin hydrochloride

Overdose of metformin hydrochloride has occurred, including ingestion of amounts greater than 50 grams. Hypoglycemia was reported in approximately 10% of cases, but no causal association with metformin hydrochloride has been established. Lactic acidosis has been reported in approximately 32% of metformin overdose cases *[see Warnings and Precautions (5.1)]*. Metformin is dialyzable with a clearance of up to 170 mL/min under good hemodynamic conditions. Therefore, hemodialysis may be useful for removal of accumulated drug from patients in whom metformin overdosage is suspected.

11 DESCRIPTION

JANUMET XR tablets contain two oral antidiabetic medications used in the management of type 2 diabetes: sitagliptin and metformin hydrochloride extended-release.

Sitagliptin

Sitagliptin is an orally-active inhibitor of the dipeptidyl peptidase-4 (DPP-4) enzyme. Sitagliptin phosphate monohydrate drug substance is used to manufacture JANUMET XR. Sitagliptin phosphate monohydrate is described chemically as 7-[(3R)-3-amino-1-oxo-4-(2,4,5-trifluorophenyl)butyl]-5,6,7,8-tetrahydro-3-(trifluoromethyl)-1,2,4-triazolo[4,3-α]pyrazine phosphate (1:1) monohydrate with an empirical formula of $C_{16}H_{15}F_6N_5O \bullet H_3PO_4 \bullet H_2O$ and a molecular weight of 523.32. The structural formula is:

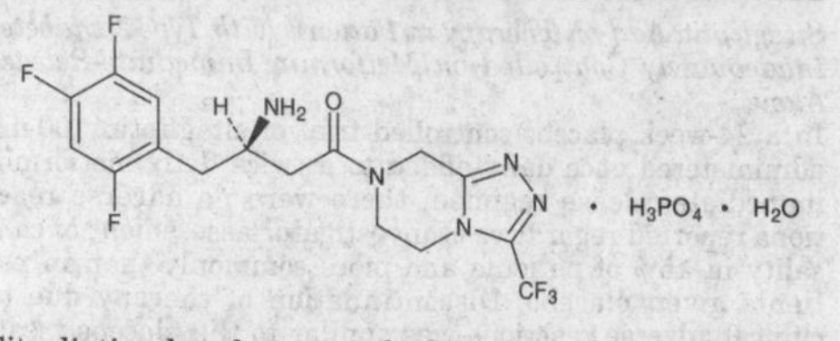

Sitagliptin phosphate monohydrate is a white to off-white, crystalline, non-hygroscopic powder. It is soluble in water and N,N-dimethyl formamide; slightly soluble in methanol; very slightly soluble in ethanol, acetone, and acetonitrile; and insoluble in isopropanol and isopropyl acetate.

Metformin hydrochloride

Metformin hydrochloride (*N,N*-dimethylimidodicarbonimidic diamide hydrochloride) is a white to off-white crystalline compound with a molecular formula of $C_4H_{11}N_5 \bullet HCl$ and a molecular weight of 165.63. Metformin hydrochloride is freely soluble in water and is practically insoluble in acetone, ether, and chloroform. The pK_a of metformin is 12.4. The pH of a 1% aqueous solution of metformin hydrochloride is 6.68. The structural formula is as shown:

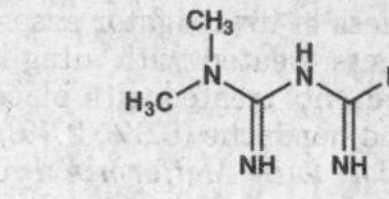

JANUMET XR

JANUMET XR consists of an extended-release metformin core tablet coated with an immediate-release layer of sitagliptin. The sitagliptin layer is coated with a soluble polymeric film. JANUMET XR is available for oral administration as tablets containing 64.25 mg sitagliptin phosphate monohydrate (equivalent to 50 mg sitagliptin as free base) and either 500 mg metformin hydrochloride extended-release (50 mg/500 mg) or 1000 mg metformin hydrochloride extended-release (50 mg/1000 mg). Additionally, JANUMET XR is available for oral administration as tablets containing 128.5 mg sitagliptin phosphate monohydrate (equivalent to 100 mg sitagliptin as free base) and 1000 mg metformin hydrochloride extended-release (100 mg/1000 mg).

All doses of JANUMET XR contain the following inactive ingredients: povidone, hypromellose, colloidal silicon dioxide, sodium stearyl fumarate, propyl gallate, polyethylene glycol, and kaolin. The JANUMET XR 50 mg/500 mg tablet contains the additional inactive ingredient microcrystalline cellulose. In addition, the film coating for all doses contains the following inactive ingredients: hypromellose, hydroxypropyl cellulose, titanium dioxide, FD&C #2/Indigo Carmine Aluminum Lake and carnauba wax. The JANUMET XR 50 mg/1000 mg tablet film coating also contains the inactive ingredient yellow iron oxide.

12 CLINICAL PHARMACOLOGY

12.1 Mechanism of Action

JANUMET XR

JANUMET XR tablets combine two antidiabetic medications with complementary mechanisms of action to improve glycemic control in adults with type 2 diabetes: sitagliptin, a dipeptidyl peptidase-4 (DPP-4) inhibitor, and metformin hydrochloride extended-release, a member of the biguanide class.

Sitagliptin

Sitagliptin is a DPP-4 inhibitor, which exerts its actions in patients with type 2 diabetes by slowing the inactivation of incretin hormones. Concentrations of the active intact hormones are increased by sitagliptin, thereby increasing and prolonging the action of these hormones. Incretin hormones, including glucagon-like peptide-1 (GLP-1) and glucose-dependent insulinotropic polypeptide (GIP), are released by the intestine throughout the day, and levels are increased in response to a meal. These hormones are rapidly inactivated by the enzyme DPP-4. The incretins are part of an endogenous system involved in the physiologic regulation of glucose homeostasis. When blood glucose concentrations are normal or elevated, GLP-1 and GIP increase insulin synthesis and release from pancreatic beta cells by intracellular signaling pathways involving cyclic AMP. GLP-1 also lowers glucagon secretion from pancreatic alpha cells, leading to reduced hepatic glucose production. By increasing and prolonging active incretin levels, sitagliptin increases insulin release and decreases glucagon levels in the circulation in a glucose-dependent manner. Sitagliptin demonstrates selectivity for DPP-4 and does not inhibit DPP-8 or DPP-9 activity *in vitro* at concentrations approximating those from therapeutic doses.

Metformin hydrochloride

Metformin is a biguanide that improves glycemic control in patients with type 2 diabetes, lowering both basal and postprandial plasma glucose. Metformin decreases hepatic glucose production, decreases intestinal absorption of glucose, and improves insulin sensitivity by increasing peripheral glucose uptake and utilization. Metformin does not produce hypoglycemia in either patients with type 2 diabetes or healthy subjects except in certain circumstances *[see Warnings and Precautions (5.9)]* and does not cause hyperinsulinemia. With metformin therapy, insulin secretion remains unchanged while fasting insulin levels and day-long plasma insulin response may actually decrease.

12.2 Pharmacodynamics

Sitagliptin

In patients with type 2 diabetes, administration of sitagliptin led to inhibition of DPP-4 enzyme activity for a 24-hour period. After an oral glucose load or a meal, this DPP-4 inhibition resulted in a 2- to 3-fold increase in circulating levels of active GLP-1 and GIP, decreased glucagon concentrations, and increased responsiveness of insulin release to glucose, resulting in higher C-peptide and insulin concentrations. The rise in insulin with the decrease in glucagon was associated with lower fasting glucose concentrations and reduced glucose excursion following an oral glucose load or a meal.

Sitagliptin and Metformin hydrochloride Co-administration

In a two-day study in healthy subjects, sitagliptin alone increased active GLP-1 concentrations, whereas metformin alone increased active and total GLP-1 concentrations to similar extents. Co-administration of sitagliptin and metformin had an additive effect on active GLP-1 concentrations. Sitagliptin, but not metformin, increased active GIP concentrations. It is unclear what these findings mean for changes in glycemic control in patients with type 2 diabetes.

In studies with healthy subjects, sitagliptin did not lower blood glucose or cause hypoglycemia.

Cardiac Electrophysiology

In a randomized, placebo-controlled crossover study, 79 healthy subjects were administered a single oral dose of sitagliptin 100 mg, sitagliptin 800 mg (8 times the recommended dose), and placebo. At the recommended dose of 100 mg, there was no effect on the QTc interval obtained at the peak plasma concentration, or at any other time during the study. Following the 800-mg dose, the maximum increase in the placebo-corrected mean change in QTc from baseline at 3 hours postdose was 8.0 msec. This increase is not considered to be clinically significant. At the 800-mg dose, peak sitagliptin plasma concentrations were approximately 11 times higher than the peak concentrations following a 100-mg dose.

In patients with type 2 diabetes administered sitagliptin 100 mg (N=81) or sitagliptin 200 mg (N=63) daily, there were no meaningful changes in QTc interval based on ECG data obtained at the time of expected peak plasma concentration.

12.3 Pharmacokinetics

JANUMET XR

The results of a study in healthy subjects demonstrated that the JANUMET XR (sitagliptin and metformin HCl extended-release) 50 mg/500 mg and 100 mg/1000 mg tablets are bioequivalent to co-administration of corresponding doses of sitagliptin and metformin hydrochloride extended-release.

Bioequivalence between two JANUMET XR 50 mg/500 mg tablets and one JANUMET XR 100 mg/1000 mg tablet was also demonstrated.

After administration of two JANUMET XR 50 mg/1000 mg tablets once daily with the evening meal for 7 days in healthy adult subjects, steady-state for sitagliptin and metformin is reached by Day 4 and 5, respectively. The median T_{max} value for sitagliptin and metformin at steady state is approximately 3 and 8 hours postdose, respectively. The median T_{max} value for sitagliptin and metformin after administration of a single tablet of JANUMET is 3 and 3.5 hours postdose, respectively.

Absorption

JANUMET XR

After administration of JANUMET XR tablets with a high-fat breakfast, the AUC for sitagliptin was not altered. The mean C_{max} was decreased by 17%, although the median T_{max} was unchanged relative to the fasted state. After administration of JANUMET XR with a high-fat breakfast, the AUC for metformin increased 62%, the C_{max} for metformin decreased by 9%, and the median T_{max} for metformin occurred 2 hours later relative to the fasted state.

Sitagliptin

The absolute bioavailability of sitagliptin is approximately 87%. Co-administration of a high-fat meal with sitagliptin had no effect on the pharmacokinetics of sitagliptin.

Distribution

Sitagliptin

The mean volume of distribution at steady state following a single 100-mg intravenous dose of sitagliptin to healthy subjects is approximately 198 liters. The fraction of sitagliptin reversibly bound to plasma proteins is low (38%).

Table 4: Effect of Sitagliptin on Systemic Exposure of Coadministered Drugs

Coadministered Drug	Dose of Coadministered Drug*	Dose of Sitagliptin *	Geometric Mean Ratio (ratio with/without sitagliptin) No Effect = 1.00		
				AUC[†]	C_{max}
No dosing adjustments required for the following:					
Digoxin	0.25 mg[‡] once daily for 10 days	100 mg[‡] once daily for 10 days	Digoxin	1.11[§]	1.18
Glyburide	1.25 mg	200 mg[‡] once daily for 6 days	Glyburide	1.09	1.01
Simvastatin	20 mg	200 mg[‡] once daily for 5 days	Simvastatin	0.85[¶]	0.80
			Simvastatin Acid	1.12[¶]	1.06
Rosiglitazone	4 mg	200 mg[‡] once daily for 5 days	Rosiglitazone	0.98	0.99
Warfarin	30 mg single dose on day 5	200 mg[‡] once daily for 11 days	S(-) Warfarin	0.95	0.89
			R(+) Warfarin	0.99	0.89
Ethinyl estradiol and norethindrone	21 days once daily of 35 µg ethinyl estradiol with norethindrone 0.5 mg × 7 days, 0.75 mg × 7 days, 1.0 mg × 7 days	200 mg[‡] once daily for 21 days	Ethinyl estradiol	0.99	0.97
			Norethindrone	1.03	0.98
Metformin	1000 mg[†] twice daily for 14 days	50 mg[‡] twice daily for 7 days	Metformin	1.02[#]	0.97

* All doses administered as single dose unless otherwise specified
† AUC is reported as $AUC_{0-\infty}$ unless otherwise specified
‡ Multiple dose
§ AUC_{0-24hr}
¶ AUC_{0-last}
# AUC_{0-12hr}

Metformin hydrochloride

Distribution studies with extended-release metformin have not been conducted; however, the apparent volume of distribution (V/F) of metformin following single oral doses of immediate-release metformin hydrochloride tablets 850 mg averaged 654 ± 358 L. Metformin is negligibly bound to plasma proteins. Metformin partitions into erythrocytes, most likely as a function of time. At usual clinical doses and dosing schedules of metformin hydrochloride tablets, steady-state plasma concentrations of metformin are reached within 24-48 hours and are generally <1 mcg/mL. During controlled clinical trials of metformin, maximum metformin plasma levels did not exceed 5 mcg/mL, even at maximum doses.

Metabolism

Sitagliptin

Approximately 79% of sitagliptin is excreted unchanged in the urine with metabolism being a minor pathway of elimination.

Following a [^{14}C]sitagliptin oral dose, approximately 16% of the radioactivity was excreted as metabolites of sitagliptin. Six metabolites were detected at trace levels and are not expected to contribute to the plasma DPP-4 inhibitory activity of sitagliptin. *In vitro* studies indicated that the primary enzyme responsible for the limited metabolism of sitagliptin was CYP3A4, with contribution from CYP2C8.

Metformin hydrochloride

Intravenous single-dose studies in normal subjects demonstrate that metformin is excreted unchanged in the urine and does not undergo hepatic metabolism (no metabolites have been identified in humans) or biliary excretion. Metabolism studies with extended-release metformin tablets have not been conducted.

Excretion

Sitagliptin

Following administration of an oral [^{14}C]sitagliptin dose to healthy subjects, approximately 100% of the administered radioactivity was eliminated in feces (13%) or urine (87%) within one week of dosing. The apparent terminal $t_{1/2}$ following a 100-mg oral dose of sitagliptin was approximately 12.4 hours and renal clearance was approximately 350 mL/min.

Elimination of sitagliptin occurs primarily via renal excretion and involves active tubular secretion. Sitagliptin is a substrate for human organic anion transporter-3 (hOAT-3), which may be involved in the renal elimination of sitagliptin. The clinical relevance of hOAT-3 in sitagliptin transport has not been established. Sitagliptin is also a substrate of p-glycoprotein, which may also be involved in mediating the renal elimination of sitagliptin. However, cyclosporine, a p-glycoprotein inhibitor, did not reduce the renal clearance of sitagliptin.

Metformin hydrochloride

Renal clearance is approximately 3.5 times greater than creatinine clearance, which indicates that tubular secretion is the major route of metformin elimination. Following oral administration, approximately 90% of the absorbed drug is eliminated via the renal route within the first 24 hours, with a plasma elimination half-life of approximately 6.2 hours. In blood, the elimination half-life is approximately 17.6 hours, suggesting that the erythrocyte mass may be a compartment of distribution.

Specific Populations

Renal Impairment

JANUMET XR

JANUMET XR should not be used in patients with renal impairment *[see Contraindications (4); Warnings and Precautions (5.4)]*.

Sitagliptin

An approximately 2-fold increase in the plasma AUC of sitagliptin was observed in patients with moderate renal impairment, and an approximately 4-fold increase was observed in patients with severe renal impairment including patients with end-stage renal disease (ESRD) on hemodialysis, as compared to normal healthy control subjects.

Metformin hydrochloride

In patients with decreased renal function (based on measured creatinine clearance), the plasma and blood half-life of metformin is prolonged and the renal clearance is decreased in proportion to the decrease in creatinine clearance.

Hepatic Impairment

Sitagliptin

In patients with moderate hepatic impairment (Child Pugh score 7 to 9), mean AUC and C_{max} of sitagliptin increased approximately 21% and 13%, respectively, compared to healthy matched controls following administration of a single 100-mg dose of sitagliptin. These differences are not considered to be clinically meaningful.

There is no clinical experience in patients with severe hepatic impairment (Child-Pugh score >9).

Metformin hydrochloride

No pharmacokinetic studies of metformin have been conducted in patients with hepatic impairment.

Gender

Sitagliptin

Gender had no clinically meaningful effect on the pharmacokinetics of sitagliptin based on a composite analysis of Phase I pharmacokinetic data and on a population pharmacokinetic analysis of Phase I and Phase II data.

Metformin hydrochloride

Metformin pharmacokinetic parameters did not differ significantly between normal subjects and patients with type 2 diabetes when analyzed according to gender. Similarly, in controlled clinical studies in patients with type 2 diabetes, the antihyperglycemic effect of metformin was comparable in males and females.

Geriatric

Sitagliptin

When the effects of age on renal function are taken into account, age alone did not have a clinically meaningful impact on the pharmacokinetics of sitagliptin based on a population pharmacokinetic analysis. Elderly subjects (65 to 80 years) had approximately 19% higher plasma concentrations of sitagliptin compared to younger subjects.

Metformin hydrochloride

Limited data from controlled pharmacokinetic studies of metformin in healthy elderly subjects suggest that total plasma clearance of metformin is decreased, the half life is prolonged, and C_{max} is increased, compared to healthy young subjects. From these data, it appears that the change in metformin pharmacokinetics with aging is primarily accounted for by a change in renal function.

As is true for all patients, JANUMET XR treatment should not be initiated in geriatric patients unless measurement of creatinine clearance demonstrates that renal function is normal *[see Warnings and Precautions (5.1, 5.4)]*.

Pediatric

No studies with JANUMET XR have been performed in pediatric patients.

Race

Sitagliptin

Race had no clinically meaningful effect on the pharmacokinetics of sitagliptin based on a composite analysis of available pharmacokinetic data, including subjects of white, Hispanic, black, Asian, and other racial groups.

Metformin hydrochloride

No studies of metformin pharmacokinetic parameters according to race have been performed. In controlled clinical studies of metformin in patients with type 2 diabetes, the antihyperglycemic effect was comparable in whites (n=249), blacks (n=51), and Hispanics (n=24).

Body Mass Index (BMI)

Sitagliptin

Body mass index had no clinically meaningful effect on the pharmacokinetics of sitagliptin based on a composite analysis of Phase I pharmacokinetic data and on a population pharmacokinetic analysis of Phase I and Phase II data.

Drug Interactions

Sitagliptin and Metformin hydrochloride

Co-administration of multiple doses of sitagliptin (50 mg) and metformin (1000 mg) given twice daily did not meaningfully alter the pharmacokinetics of either sitagliptin or metformin in patients with type 2 diabetes.

Pharmacokinetic drug interaction studies with JANUMET XR have not been performed; however, such studies have been conducted with the individual components of JANUMET XR (sitagliptin and metformin hydrochloride extended-release).

Sitagliptin

In Vitro Assessment of Drug Interactions

Sitagliptin is not an inhibitor of CYP isozymes CYP3A4, 2C8, 2C9, 2D6, 1A2, 2C19 or 2B6, and is not an inducer of CYP3A4. Sitagliptin is a p-glycoprotein substrate, but does not inhibit p-glycoprotein mediated transport of digoxin. Based on these results, sitagliptin is considered unlikely to cause interactions with other drugs that utilize these pathways.

Sitagliptin is not extensively bound to plasma proteins. Therefore, the propensity of sitagliptin to be involved in clinically meaningful drug-drug interactions mediated by plasma protein binding displacement is very low.

In Vivo Assessment of Drug Interactions

[See table 4 at top of previous page]

[See table 5 above]

[See table 6 above]

[See table 7 above]

Table 5: Effect of Coadministered Drugs on Systemic Exposure of Sitagliptin

Coadministered Drug	Dose of Coadministered Drug*	Dose of Sitagliptin*	Geometric Mean Ratio (ratio with/without coadministered drug) No Effect = 1.00		
				AUC†	C_{max}
No dosing adjustments required for the following:					
Cyclosporine	600 mg once daily	100 mg once daily	Sitagliptin	1.29	1.68
Metformin	1000 mg‡ twice daily for 14 days	50 mg‡ twice daily for 7 days	Sitagliptin	1.02§	1.05

* All doses administered as single dose unless otherwise specified
† AUC is reported as $AUC_{0-\infty}$ unless otherwise specified
‡ Multiple dose
§ AUC_{0-12hr}

Table 6: Effect of Metformin on Systemic Exposure of Coadministered Drugs

Coadministered Drug	Dose of Coadministered Drug*	Dose of Metformin*	Geometric Mean Ratio (ratio with/without metformin) No Effect = 1.00		
				AUC†	C_{max}
No dosing adjustments required for the following:					
Cimetidine	400 mg	850 mg	Cimetidine	0.95‡	1.01
Glyburide	5 mg	500 mg§	Glyburide	0.78¶	0.63¶
Furosemide	40 mg	850 mg	Furosemide	0.87¶	0.69¶
Nifedipine	10 mg	850 mg	Nifedipine	1.10‡	1.08
Propranolol	40 mg	850 mg	Propranolol	1.01‡	0.94
Ibuprofen	400 mg	850 mg	Ibuprofen	0.97#	1.01#

* All doses administered as single dose unless otherwise specified
† AUC is reported as $AUC_{0-\infty}$ unless otherwise specified
‡ AUC_{0-24hr}
§ GLUMETZA (metformin hydrochloride extended-release tablets) 500 mg
¶ Ratio of arithmetic means, p value of difference < 0.05
\# Ratio of arithmetic means

Table 7: Effect of Coadministered Drugs on Systemic Exposure of Metformin

Coadministered Drug	Dose of Coadministered Drug*	Dose of Metformin*	Geometric Mean Ratio (ratio with/without coadministered drug) No Effect = 1.00		
				AUC†	C_{max}
No dosing adjustments required for the following:					
Glyburide	5 mg	500 mg‡	Metformin‡	0.98§	0.99§
Furosemide	40 mg	850 mg	Metformin	1.09§	1.22§
Nifedipine	10 mg	850 mg	Metformin	1.16	1.21
Propranolol	40 mg	850 mg	Metformin	0.90	0.94
Ibuprofen	400 mg	850 mg	Metformin	1.05§	1.07§
Cationic drugs eliminated by renal tubular secretion may reduce metformin elimination: use with caution. *[See Warnings and Precautions (5.10) and Drug Interactions (7.2).]*					
Cimetidine	400 mg	850 mg	Metformin	1.40	1.61
Carbonic anhydrase inhibitors may cause metabolic acidosis: use with caution. *[See Warnings and Precautions (5.1) and Drug Interactions (7.1).]*					
Topiramate	100 mg¶	500 mg¶	Metformin	1.25¶	1.17

* All doses administered as single dose unless otherwise specified
† AUC is reported as $AUC_{0-\infty}$ unless otherwise specified
‡ GLUMETZA (metformin hydrochloride extended-release tablets) 500 mg
§ Ratio of arithmetic means
¶ Steady state 100 mg Topiramate every 12 hr + metformin 500 mg every 12 hr. AUC = AUC_{0-12hr}

13 NONCLINICAL TOXICOLOGY

13.1 Carcinogenesis, Mutagenesis, Impairment of Fertility

JANUMET XR

No animal studies have been conducted with the combined products in JANUMET XR to evaluate carcinogenesis, mutagenesis or impairment of fertility. The following data are based on the findings in studies with sitagliptin and metformin individually.

Sitagliptin

A two-year carcinogenicity study was conducted in male and female rats given oral doses of sitagliptin of 50, 150, and 500 mg/kg/day. There was an increased incidence of combined liver adenoma/carcinoma in males and females and of liver carcinoma in females at 500 mg/kg. This dose results in exposures approximately 60 times the human exposure at the maximum recommended daily adult human dose (MRHD) of 100 mg/day based on AUC comparisons. Liver tumors were not observed at 150 mg/kg, approximately 20 times the human exposure at the MRHD. A two-year carcinogenicity study was conducted in male and female mice given oral doses of sitagliptin of 50, 125, 250, and 500 mg/kg/day. There was no increase in the incidence of tumors in any organ up to 500 mg/kg, approximately 70 times human

exposure at the MRHD. Sitagliptin was not mutagenic or clastogenic with or without metabolic activation in the Ames bacterial mutagenicity assay, a Chinese hamster ovary (CHO) chromosome aberration assay, an *in vitro* cytogenetics assay in CHO, an *in vitro* rat hepatocyte DNA alkaline elution assay, and an *in vivo* micronucleus assay.
In rat fertility studies with oral gavage doses of 125, 250, and 1000 mg/kg, males were treated for 4 weeks prior to mating, during mating, up to scheduled termination (approximately 8 weeks total), and females were treated 2 weeks prior to mating through gestation day 7. No adverse effect on fertility was observed at 125 mg/kg (approximately 12 times human exposure at the MRHD of 100 mg/day based on AUC comparisons). At higher doses, nondose-related increased resorptions in females were observed (approximately 25 and 100 times human exposure at the MRHD based on AUC comparison).
Metformin hydrochloride
Long-term carcinogenicity studies have been performed in Sprague Dawley rats at doses of 150, 300, and 450 mg/kg/day in males and 150, 450, 900, and 1200 mg/kg/day in females. These doses are approximately 2, 4, and 8 times in males, and 3, 7, 12, and 16 times in females of the maximum recommended human daily dose of 2000 mg based on body surface area comparisons. No evidence of carcinogenicity with metformin was found in either male or female rats. A carcinogenicity study was also performed in Tg.AC transgenic mice at doses up to 2000 mg applied dermally. No evidence of carcinogenicity was observed in male or female mice.
Genotoxicity assessments in the Ames test, gene mutation test (mouse lymphoma cells), chromosomal aberrations test (human lymphocytes) and *in vivo* mouse micronucleus tests were negative. Fertility of male or female rats was not affected by metformin when administered at doses up to 600 mg/kg/day, which is approximately 3 times the maximum recommended human daily dose based on body surface area comparisons.

14 CLINICAL STUDIES

The co-administration of sitagliptin and metformin immediate-release has been studied in patients with type 2 diabetes inadequately controlled on diet and exercise and in combination with other antidiabetic medications.
There have been no clinical efficacy or safety studies conducted with JANUMET XR to characterize its effect on hemoglobin A1c (A1C) reduction. Bioequivalence of JANUMET XR tablets with co-administered sitagliptin and extended-release metformin tablets has been demonstrated for all tablet strengths *[see Clinical Pharmacology (12.3)]*.

Metformin Extended-Release Compared to Metformin Immediate-Release in Patients with Type 2 Diabetes

In a multicenter, randomized, double-blind, active-controlled, dose-ranging, parallel group trial extended-release metformin 1500 mg once daily, extended-release metformin 1500 mg per day in divided doses (500 mg in the morning and 1000 mg in the evening), and extended-release metformin 2000 mg once daily were compared to immediate-release metformin 1500 mg per day in divided doses (500 mg in the morning and 1000 mg in the evening). This trial enrolled patients (n = 338) who were newly diagnosed with diabetes, patients treated only with diet and exercise, patients treated with a single antidiabetic medication (sulfonylureas, alpha-glucosidase inhibitors, thiazolidinediones, or meglinitides), and patients (n = 368) receiving metformin up to 1500 mg/day plus a sulfonylurea at a dose equal to or less than one-half the maximum dose. Patients who were enrolled on monotherapy or combination antidiabetic therapy underwent a 6-week washout. Patients randomized to extended-release metformin began titration from 1000 mg/day up to their assigned treatment dose over 3 weeks. Patients randomized to immediate-release metformin initiated 500 mg twice daily for 1 week followed by 500 mg with breakfast and 1000 mg with dinner for the second week. The 3-week treatment period was followed by an additional 21-week period at the randomized dose. For HbA1c and fasting plasma glucose, each of the extended-release metformin regimens was at least as effective as immediate release metformin. Additionally, once daily dosing of extended-release metformin was as effective as twice daily dosing of the immediate-release metformin formulation.

Sitagliptin and Metformin Immediate-Release Co-administration in Patients with Type 2 Diabetes Inadequately Controlled on Diet and Exercise

A total of 1091 patients with type 2 diabetes and inadequate glycemic control on diet and exercise participated in a 24-week, randomized, double-blind, placebo-controlled factorial study designed to assess the efficacy of sitagliptin and metformin immediate-release co-administration. Patients on an antihyperglycemic agent (N=541) underwent a diet, exercise, and drug washout period of up to 12 weeks duration. After the washout period, patients with inadequate glycemic control (A1C 7.5% to 11%) were randomized after completing a 2-week single-blind placebo run-in period. Patients not on antihyperglycemic agents at study entry (N=550) with inadequate glycemic control (A1C 7.5% to 11%) immediately entered the 2-week single-blind placebo run-in period and then were randomized. Approximately equal numbers of patients were randomized to receive placebo, 100 mg of sitagliptin once daily, 500 mg or 1000 mg of metformin immediate-release twice daily, or 50 mg of sitagliptin twice daily in combination with 500 mg or 1000 mg of metformin immediate-release twice daily. Patients who failed to meet specific glycemic goals during the study were treated with glyburide (glibenclamide) rescue.
Sitagliptin and metformin immediate-release co-administration provided significant improvements in A1C, FPG, and 2-hour PPG compared to placebo, to metformin immediate-release alone, and to sitagliptin alone (Table 8, Figure 1). For patients not on an antihyperglycemic agent at study entry, mean reductions from baseline in A1C were: sitagliptin 100 mg once daily, -1.1%; metformin immediate-release 500 mg bid, -1.1%; metformin immediate-release 1000 mg bid, -1.2%; sitagliptin 50 mg bid with metformin immediate-release 500 mg bid, -1.6%; sitagliptin 50 mg bid with metformin immediate-release 1000 mg bid, -1.9%; and for patients receiving placebo, -0.2%. Lipid effects were generally neutral. The decrease in body weight in the groups given sitagliptin in combination with metformin immediate-release was similar to that in the groups given metformin alone or placebo.
[See table 8 above]
[See figure 1 at top of next column]

Table 8: Glycemic Parameters at Final Visit (24-Week Study) for Sitagliptin and Metformin Immediate-Release, Alone and in Combination in Patients with Type 2 Diabetes Inadequately Controlled on Diet and Exercise*

	Placebo	Sitagliptin 100 mg once daily	Metformin Immediate-Release 500 mg twice daily	Metformin Immediate-Release 1000 mg twice daily	Sitagliptin 50 mg bid + Metformin Immediate-Release 500 mg twice daily	Sitagliptin 50 mg bid + Metformin Immediate-Release 1000 mg twice daily
A1C (%)	**N = 165**	**N = 175**	**N = 178**	**N = 177**	**N = 183**	**N = 178**
Baseline (mean)	8.7	8.9	8.9	8.7	8.8	8.8
Change from baseline (adjusted mean†)	0.2	-0.7	-0.8	-1.1	-1.4	-1.9
Difference from placebo (adjusted mean†) (95% CI)		-0.8‡ (-1.1, -0.6)	-1.0‡ (-1.2, -0.8)	-1.3‡ (-1.5, -1.1)	-1.6‡ (-1.8, -1.3)	-2.1‡ (-2.3, -1.8)
Patients (%) achieving A1C <7%	15 (9%)	35 (20%)	41 (23%)	68 (38%)	79 (43%)	118 (66%)
% Patients receiving rescue medication	32	21	17	12	8	2
FPG (mg/dL)	**N = 169**	**N = 178**	**N = 179**	**N = 179**	**N = 183**	**N = 180**
Baseline (mean)	196	201	205	197	204	197
Change from baseline (adjusted mean†)	6	-17	-27	-29	-47	-64
Difference from placebo (adjusted mean†) (95% CI)		-23‡ (-33, -14)	-33‡ (-43, -24)	-35‡ (-45, -26)	-53‡ (-62, -43)	-70‡ (-79, -60)
2-hour PPG (mg/dL)	**N = 129**	**N = 136**	**N = 141**	**N = 138**	**N = 147**	**N = 152**
Baseline (mean)	277	285	293	283	292	287
Change from baseline (adjusted mean†)	0	-52	-53	-78	-93	-117
Difference from placebo (adjusted mean†) (95% CI)		-52‡ (-67, -37)	-54‡ (-69, -39)	-78‡ (-93, -63)	-93‡ (-107, -78)	-117‡ (-131, -102)

* Intent-to-treat population using last observation on study prior to glyburide (glibenclamide) rescue therapy.
† Least squares means adjusted for prior antihyperglycemic therapy status and baseline value.
‡ p<0.001 compared to placebo.

Figure 1: Mean Change from Baseline for A1C (%) over 24 Weeks with Sitagliptin and Metformin Immediate-Release, Alone and in Combination in Patients with Type 2 Diabetes Inadequately Controlled with Diet and Exercise*

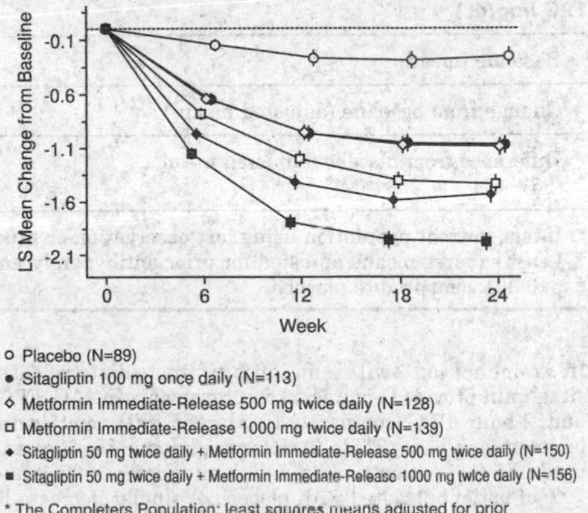

* The Completers Population: least squares means adjusted for prior antihyperglycemic therapy and baseline value.

Initial combination therapy or maintenance of combination therapy should be individualized and are left to the discretion of the health care provider.

Sitagliptin Add-on Therapy in Patients with Type 2 Diabetes Inadequately Controlled on Metformin Immediate-Release Alone

A total of 701 patients with type 2 diabetes participated in a 24-week, randomized, double-blind, placebo-controlled study designed to assess the efficacy of sitagliptin in combination with metformin immediate-release. Patients already on metformin immediate-release (N=431) at a dose of at least 1500 mg per day were randomized after completing a 2-week, single-blind placebo run-in period. Patients on metformin immediate-release and another antihyperglycemic agent (N=229) and patients not on any antihyperglycemic agents (off therapy for at least 8 weeks, N=41) were randomized after a run-in period of approximately 10 weeks on metformin immediate-release (at a dose of at least 1500 mg per day) in monotherapy. Patients were randomized to the addition of either 100 mg of sitagliptin or placebo, administered once daily. Patients who failed to meet specific glycemic goals during the studies were treated with pioglitazone rescue.

Table 9: Glycemic Parameters at Final Visit (24-Week Study) of Sitagliptin as Add-on Combination Therapy with Metformin Immediate-Release*

	Sitagliptin 100 mg once daily + Metformin Immediate-Release	Placebo + Metformin Immediate-Release
A1C (%)	**N = 453**	**N = 224**
Baseline (mean)	8.0	8.0
Change from baseline (adjusted mean†)	-0.7	-0.0
Difference from placebo + metformin immediate-release (adjusted mean†) (95% CI)	-0.7‡ (-0.8, -0.5)	
Patients (%) achieving A1C <7%	213 (47%)	41 (18%)
FPG (mg/dL)	**N = 454**	**N = 226**
Baseline (mean)	170	174
Change from baseline (adjusted mean†)	-17	9
Difference from placebo + metformin immediate-release (adjusted mean†) (95% CI)	-25‡ (-31, -20)	
2-hour PPG (mg/dL)	**N = 387**	**N = 182**
Baseline (mean)	275	272
Change from baseline (adjusted mean†)	-62	-11
Difference from placebo + metformin immediate-release (adjusted mean†) (95% CI)	-51‡ (-61, -41)	

* Intent-to-treat population using last observation on study prior to pioglitazone rescue therapy.
† Least squares means adjusted for prior antihyperglycemic therapy and baseline value.
‡ p<0.001 compared to placebo + metformin.

Table 10: Glycemic Parameters at Final Visit (24-Week Study) for Sitagliptin in Combination with Metformin Immediate-Release and Glimepiride*

	Sitagliptin 100 mg + Metformin Immediate-Release and Glimepiride	Placebo + Metformin Immediate-Release and Glimepiride
A1C (%)	**N = 115**	**N = 105**
Baseline (mean)	8.3	8.3
Change from baseline (adjusted mean†)	-0.6	0.3
Difference from placebo (adjusted mean†) (95% CI)	-0.9‡ (-1.1, -0.7)	
Patients (%) achieving A1C <7%	26 (23%)	1 (1%)
FPG (mg/dL)	**N = 115**	**N = 109**
Baseline (mean)	179	179
Change from baseline (adjusted mean†)	-8	13
Difference from placebo (adjusted mean†) (95% CI)	-21‡ (-32, -10)	

* Intent-to-treat population using last observation on study prior to pioglitazone rescue therapy.
† Least squares means adjusted for prior antihyperglycemic therapy status and baseline value.
‡ p<0.001 compared to placebo.

In combination with metformin immediate-release, sitagliptin provided significant improvements in A1C, FPG, and 2-hour PPG compared to placebo with metformin immediate-release (Table 9). Rescue glycemic therapy was used in 5% of patients treated with sitagliptin 100 mg and 14% of patients treated with placebo. A similar decrease in body weight was observed for both treatment groups.
[See table 9 above]

Sitagliptin Add-on Therapy in Patients with Type 2 Diabetes Inadequately Controlled on the Combination of Metformin Immediate-Release and Glimepiride

A total of 441 patients with type 2 diabetes participated in a 24-week, randomized, double-blind, placebo-controlled study designed to assess the efficacy of sitagliptin in combination with glimepiride, with or without metformin immediate-release. Patients entered a run-in treatment period on glimepiride (≥4 mg per day) alone or glimepiride in combination with metformin immediate-release (≥1500 mg per day). After a dose-titration and dose-stable run-in period of up to 16 weeks and a 2-week placebo run-in period, patients with inadequate glycemic control (A1C 7.5% to 10.5%) were randomized to the addition of either 100 mg of sitagliptin or placebo, administered once daily. Patients who failed to meet specific glycemic goals during the studies were treated with pioglitazone rescue.

Patients receiving sitagliptin with metformin immediate-release and glimepiride had significant improvements in A1C and FPG compared to patients receiving placebo with metformin immediate-release and glimepiride (Table 10), with mean reductions from baseline relative to placebo in A1C of -0.9% and in FPG of -21 mg/dL. Rescue therapy was used in 8% of patients treated with add-on sitagliptin 100 mg and 29% of patients treated with add-on placebo. The patients treated with add-on sitagliptin had a mean increase in body weight of 1.1 kg vs. add-on placebo (+0.4 kg vs. -0.7 kg). In addition, add-on sitagliptin resulted in an increased rate of hypoglycemia compared to add-on placebo. *[See Warnings and Precautions (5.9); Adverse Reactions (6.1).]*
[See table 10 above]

Sitagliptin Add-on Therapy in Patients with Type 2 Diabetes Inadequately Controlled on the Combination of Metformin Immediate-Release and Rosiglitazone

A total of 278 patients with type 2 diabetes participated in a 54-week, randomized, double-blind, placebo-controlled study designed to assess the efficacy of sitagliptin in combination with metformin immediate-release and rosiglitazone. Patients on dual therapy with metformin immediate-release ≥1500 mg/day and rosiglitazone ≥4 mg/day or with metformin immediate-release ≥1500 mg/day and pioglitazone ≥30 mg/day (switched to rosiglitazone ≥4 mg/day) entered a dose-stable run-in period of 6 weeks. Patients on other dual therapy were switched to metformin immediate-release ≥1500 mg/day and rosiglitazone ≥4 mg/day in a dose titration/stabilization run-in period of up to 20 weeks in duration. After the run-in period, patients with inadequate glycemic control (A1C 7.5% to 11%) were randomized 2:1 to the addition of either 100 mg of sitagliptin or placebo, administered once daily. Patients who failed to meet specific glycemic goals during the studies were treated with glipizide (or other sulfonylurea) rescue. The primary time point for evaluation of glycemic parameters was Week 18.

In combination with metformin immediate-release and rosiglitazone, sitagliptin provided significant improvements in A1C, FPG, and 2-hour PPG compared to placebo with metformin immediate-release and rosiglitazone (Table 11) at Week 18. At Week 54, mean reduction in A1C was -1.0% for patients treated with sitagliptin and -0.3% for patients treated with placebo in an analysis based on the intent-to-treat population. Rescue therapy was used in 18% of patients treated with sitagliptin 100 mg and 40% of patients treated with placebo. There was no significant difference between sitagliptin and placebo in body weight change.
[See table 11 at top of next page]

Sitagliptin Add-on Therapy in Patients with Type 2 Diabetes Inadequately Controlled on the Combination of Metformin Immediate-Release and Insulin

A total of 641 patients with type 2 diabetes participated in a 24-week, randomized, double-blind, placebo-controlled study designed to assess the efficacy of sitagliptin as add-on to insulin therapy. Approximately 75% of patients were also taking metformin immediate-release. Patients entered a 2-week, single-blind run-in treatment period on pre-mixed, long-acting, or intermediate-acting insulin, with or without metformin immediate-release (≥1500 mg per day). Patients using short-acting insulins were excluded unless the short-acting insulin was administered as part of a pre-mixed insulin. After the run-in period, patients with inadequate glycemic control (A1C 7.5% to 11%) were randomized to the addition of either 100 mg of sitagliptin (N=229) or placebo (N=233), administered once daily. Patients were on a stable dose of insulin prior to enrollment with no changes in insulin dose permitted during the run-in period. Patients who failed to meet specific glycemic goals during the double-blind treatment period were to have uptitration of the background insulin dose as rescue therapy.

Among patients also receiving metformin immediate-release, the median daily insulin (pre-mixed, intermediate or long acting) dose at baseline was 40 units in the sitagliptin-treated patients and 42 units in the placebo-treated patients. The median change from baseline in daily dose of insulin was zero for both groups at the end of the study. Patients receiving sitagliptin with metformin immediate-release and insulin had significant improvements in A1C, FPG and 2-hour PPG compared to patients receiving placebo with metformin immediate-release and insulin (Table 12). The adjusted mean change from baseline in body weight was -0.3 kg in patients receiving sitagliptin with metformin immediate-release and insulin and -0.2 kg in patients receiving placebo with metformin immediate-release and insulin. There was an increased rate of hypoglycemia in patients treated with sitagliptin. *[See Warnings and Precautions (5.9); Adverse Reactions (6.1).]*
[See table 12 at top of next page]

Sitagliptin Add-on Therapy vs. Glipizide Add-on Therapy in Patients with Type 2 Diabetes Inadequately Controlled on Metformin Immediate-Release

The efficacy of sitagliptin was evaluated in a 52-week, double-blind, glipizide-controlled noninferiority trial in patients with type 2 diabetes. Patients not on treatment or on other antihyperglycemic agents entered a run-in treatment period of up to 12 weeks duration with metformin immediate-release monotherapy (dose of ≥1500 mg per day) which included washout of medications other than metformin immediate-release, if applicable. After the run-in period, those with inadequate glycemic control (A1C 6.5% to 10%) were randomized 1:1 to the addition of sitagliptin 100 mg once daily or glipizide for 52 weeks. Patients receiving glipizide were given an initial dosage of 5 mg/day and then electively titrated over the next 18 weeks to a maximum dosage of 20 mg/day as needed to optimize glycemic control. Thereafter, the glipizide dose was to be kept constant, except for down-titration to prevent hypoglycemia. The mean dose of glipizide after the titration period was 10 mg.

After 52 weeks, sitagliptin and glipizide had similar mean reductions from baseline in A1C in the intent-to-treat analysis (Table 13). These results were consistent with the per protocol analysis (Figure 2). A conclusion in favor of the non-inferiority of sitagliptin to glipizide may be limited to patients with baseline A1C comparable to those included in the study (over 70% of patients had baseline A1C <8% and over 90% had A1C <9%).

[See table 13 at top of next page]

Figure 2: Mean Change from Baseline for A1C (%) Over 52 Weeks in a Study Comparing Sitagliptin to Glipizide as Add-On Therapy in Patients Inadequately Controlled on Metformin Immediate-Release (Per Protocol Population)*

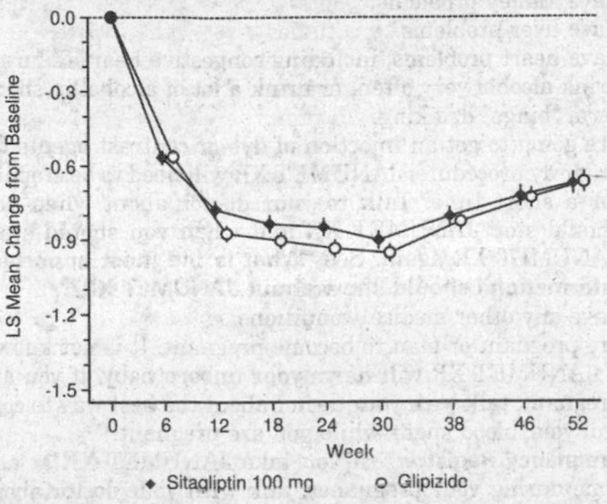

* The per protocol population (mean baseline A1C of 7.5%) included patients without major protocol violations who had observations at baseline and at Week 52.

The incidence of hypoglycemia in the sitagliptin group (4.9%) was significantly (p<0.001) lower than that in the glipizide group (32.0%). Patients treated with sitagliptin exhibited a significant mean decrease from baseline in body weight compared to a significant weight gain in patients administered glipizide (-1.5 kg vs. +1.1 kg).

Table 11: Glycemic Parameters at Week 18 for Sitagliptin in Add-on Combination Therapy with Metformin Immediate-Release and Rosiglitazone*

	Week 18	
	Sitagliptin 100 mg + Metformin Immediate-Release + Rosiglitazone	**Placebo + Metformin Immediate-Release + Rosiglitazone**
A1C (%)	**N = 176**	**N = 93**
Baseline (mean)	8.8	8.7
Change from baseline (adjusted mean†)	-1.0	-0.4
Difference from placebo + rosiglitazone + metformin immediate-release (adjusted mean†) (95% CI)	-0.7‡ (-0.9, -0.4)	
Patients (%) achieving A1C <7%	39 (22%)	9 (10%)
FPG (mg/dL)	**N = 179**	**N = 94**
Baseline (mean)	181	182
Change from baseline (adjusted mean†)	-30	-11
Difference from placebo + rosiglitazone + metformin immediate-release (adjusted mean†) (95% CI)	-18‡ (-26, -10)	
2-hour PPG (mg/dL)	**N = 152**	**N = 80**
Baseline (mean)	256	248
Change from baseline (adjusted mean†)	-59	-21
Difference from placebo + rosiglitazone + metformin immediate-release (adjusted mean†) (95% CI)	-39‡ (-51, -26)	

* Intent-to-treat population using last observation on study prior to glipizide (or other sulfonylurea) rescue therapy.
† Least squares means adjusted for prior antihyperglycemic therapy status and baseline value.
‡ p<0.001 compared to placebo + metformin + rosiglitazone.

Table 12: Glycemic Parameters at Final Visit (24-Week Study) for Sitagliptin as Add-on Combination Therapy with Metformin Immediate-Release and Insulin*

	Sitagliptin 100 mg + Metformin Immediate-Release + Insulin	**Placebo + Metformin Immediate-Release + Insulin**
A1C (%)	**N = 223**	**N = 229**
Baseline (mean)	8.7	8.6
Change from baseline (adjusted mean†, ‡)	-0.7	-0.1
Difference from placebo (adjusted mean†) (95% CI)	-0.5§ (-0.7, -0.4)	
Patients (%) achieving A1C (%) <7%	32 (14%)	12 (5%)
FPG (mg/dL)	**N = 225**	**N = 229**
Baseline (mean)	173	176
Change from baseline (adjusted mean†)	-22	-4
Difference from placebo (adjusted mean†) (95% CI)	-18§ (-28, -8.4)	
2-hour PPG (mg/dL)	**N = 182**	**N = 189**
Baseline (mean)	281	281
Change from baseline (adjusted mean†)	-39	1
Difference from placebo (adjusted mean†) (95% CI)	-40§ (-53, -28)	

* Intent-to-treat population using last observation on study prior to rescue therapy.
† Least squares mean adjusted for insulin use at the screening visit, type of insulin used at the screening visit (pre-mixed vs. non pre-mixed [intermediate- or long-acting]), and baseline value.
‡ Treatment by insulin stratum interaction was not significant (p>0.10).
§ p<0.001 compared to placebo.

16 HOW SUPPLIED/STORAGE AND HANDLING

No. 3961 — Tablets JANUMET XR, 50 mg/500 mg, are light blue, bi-convex oval, film-coated tablets with "78" debossed on one side. They are supplied as follows:
NDC 0006-0078-61 unit-of-use bottles of 60
NDC 0006-0078-62 unit-of-use bottles of 180
NDC 0006-0078-82 bulk bottles of 1000.
No. 3962 — Tablets JANUMET XR, 50 mg/1000 mg, are light green, bi-convex oval, film-coated tablets with "80" debossed on one side. They are supplied as follows:
NDC 0006-0080-61 unit-of-use bottles of 60
NDC 0006-0080-62 unit-of-use bottles of 180
NDC 0006-0080-82 bulk bottles of 1000.
No. 3963 — Tablets JANUMET XR, 100 mg/1000 mg, are blue, bi-convex oval, film-coated tablets with "81" debossed on one side. They are supplied as follows:
NDC 0006-0081-31 unit-of-use bottles of 30
NDC 0006-0081-54 unit-of-use bottles of 90
NDC 0006-0081-82 bulk bottles of 1000.
Store at 20-25°C (68-77°F), excursions permitted to 15-30°C (59-86°F), [See USP Controlled Room Temperature]. Store in a dry place with cap tightly closed. When container is subdivided, dispense into a USP tightly closed, moisture-resistant container.

17 PATIENT COUNSELING INFORMATION

See FDA-approved Medication Guide.

17.1 Instructions

Patients should be informed of the potential risks and benefits of JANUMET XR and of alternative modes of therapy. They should also be informed about the importance of adherence to dietary instructions, regular physical activity, periodic blood glucose monitoring and A1C testing, recognition and management of hypoglycemia and hyperglycemia, and assessment for diabetes complications. During periods of stress such as fever, trauma, infection, or surgery, medication requirements may change and patients should be advised to seek medical advice promptly.

The risks of lactic acidosis due to the metformin component, its symptoms, and conditions that predispose to its development, as noted in *Warnings and Precautions (5.1)*, should be explained to patients. Patients should be advised to discontinue JANUMET XR immediately and to promptly notify their health practitioner if unexplained hyperventilation, myalgia, malaise, unusual somnolence, dizziness, slow or irregular heart beat, sensation of feeling cold (especially in the extremities) or other nonspecific symptoms occur. Gastrointestinal symptoms are common during initiation of metformin treatment and may occur during initiation of JANUMET XR therapy; however, patients should consult their physician if they develop unexplained symptoms. Although gastrointestinal symptoms that occur after stabilization are unlikely to be drug related, such an occurrence of symptoms should be evaluated to determine if it may be due to lactic acidosis or other serious disease.

Patients should be advised to notify their health practitioner or call the Poison Control Center immediately in case of JANUMET XR overdose.

Table 13: Glycemic Parameters in a 52-Week Study Comparing Sitagliptin to Glipizide as Add-On Therapy in Patients Inadequately Controlled on Metformin Immediate-Release (Intent-to-Treat Population) *

	Sitagliptin 100 mg + Metformin Immediate-Release	Glipizide + Metformin Immediate-Release
A1C (%)	**N = 576**	**N = 559**
Baseline (mean)	7.7	7.6
Change from baseline (adjusted mean†)	-0.5	-0.6
FPG (mg/dL)	**N = 583**	**N = 568**
Baseline (mean)	166	164
Change from baseline (adjusted mean†)	-8	-8

* The intent-to-treat analysis used the patients' last observation in the study prior to discontinuation.
† Least squares means adjusted for prior antihyperglycemic therapy status and baseline A1C value.

Patients should be counseled against excessive alcohol intake, either acute or chronic, while receiving JANUMET XR.

Patients should be informed about the importance of regular testing of renal function and hematological parameters when receiving treatment with JANUMET XR.

Patients should be informed that acute pancreatitis has been reported during postmarketing use of JANUMET. Patients should be informed that persistent severe abdominal pain, sometimes radiating to the back, which may or may not be accompanied by vomiting, is the hallmark symptom of acute pancreatitis. Patients should be instructed to promptly discontinue JANUMET XR and contact their physician if persistent severe abdominal pain occurs *[see Warnings and Precautions (5.2)]*.

Patients should be informed that the incidence of hypoglycemia is increased when sitagliptin with or without metformin is added to an insulin secretagogue (e.g., sulfonylurea) or insulin therapy and that a lower dose of the insulin secretagogue or insulin may be required to reduce the risk of hypoglycemia.

Patients should be informed that allergic reactions have been reported during postmarketing use of sitagliptin, one of the components of JANUMET XR. If symptoms of allergic reactions (including rash, hives, and swelling of the face, lips, tongue, and throat that may cause difficulty in breathing or swallowing) occur, patients must stop taking JANUMET XR and seek medical advice promptly.

Patients should be informed that the tablets must be swallowed whole and never split, crushed or chewed.

Physicians should instruct their patients to read the Medication Guide before starting JANUMET XR therapy and to reread each time the prescription is renewed. Patients should be instructed to inform their doctor if they develop any bothersome or unusual symptom, or if any symptom persists or worsens.

17.2 Laboratory Tests

Response to all diabetic therapies should be monitored by periodic measurements of blood glucose and A1C levels, with a goal of decreasing these levels towards the normal range. A1C is especially useful for evaluating long-term glycemic control.

Initial and periodic monitoring of hematologic parameters (e.g., hemoglobin/hematocrit and red blood cell indices) and renal function (serum creatinine) should be performed, at least on an annual basis. While megaloblastic anemia has rarely been seen with metformin therapy, if this is suspected, Vitamin B_{12} deficiency should be excluded.

Manufactured for: Merck Sharp & Dohme Corp., a subsidiary of
MERCK & CO., INC., Whitehouse Station, NJ 08889, USA
Manufactured by:
Merck Sharp & Dohme Corp., a subsidiary of
Merck & Co., Inc., Whitehouse Station, NJ 08889, USA
OR
Patheon Inc., Whitby, Ontario, Canada L1N 5Z5
US Patent Nos.: 6,699,871 and 7,326,708

USPI-XRT-0431A1307R003

Medication Guide
JANUMET® XR (JAN-you-met XR)
(sitagliptin and metformin hydrochloride extended-release) Tablets

Read this Medication Guide carefully before you start taking JANUMET XR and each time you get a refill. There may be new information. This information does not take the place of talking with your doctor about your medical condition or your treatment. If you have any questions about JANUMET XR, ask your doctor or pharmacist.

What is the most important information I should know about JANUMET XR?

Serious side effects can happen in people taking JANUMET XR, including:

1. **Lactic Acidosis.** Metformin, one of the medicines in JANUMET XR, can cause a rare but serious condition called lactic acidosis (a build-up of lactic acid in the blood) that can cause death. Lactic acidosis is a medical emergency and must be treated in the hospital.

   Stop taking JANUMET XR and call your doctor right away if you get any of the following symptoms, which could be signs of lactic acidosis.
   You:
   - feel very weak or tired.
   - have unusual (not normal) muscle pain.
   - have trouble breathing.
   - have unusual sleepiness or sleep longer than usual.
   - have sudden stomach or intestinal problems with nausea and vomiting or diarrhea.
   - feel cold, especially in your arms and legs.
   - feel dizzy or lightheaded.
   - have a slow or irregular heartbeat.

   You have a higher chance of getting lactic acidosis if you:
   - have kidney problems. People whose kidneys are not working properly should not take JANUMET XR.
   - have liver problems.
   - have congestive heart failure that requires treatment with medicines.
   - drink alcohol very often, or drink a lot of alcohol in short-term "binge" drinking.
   - get dehydrated (lose a large amount of body fluids). This can happen if you are sick with a fever, vomiting, or diarrhea. Dehydration can also happen when you sweat a lot with activity or exercise and do not drink enough fluids.
   - have certain x-ray tests with dyes or contrast agents that are injected into your body.
   - have surgery.
   - have a heart attack, severe infection, or stroke.
2. **Pancreatitis** (inflammation of the pancreas) which may be severe and lead to death. Certain medical problems make you more likely to get pancreatitis.

Before you start taking JANUMET XR:
Tell your doctor if you have ever had
- pancreatitis
- stones in your gallbladder (gallstones)
- a history of alcoholism
- high blood triglyceride levels

Stop taking JANUMET XR and call your doctor right away if you have pain in your stomach area (abdomen) that is severe and will not go away. The pain may be felt going from your abdomen through to your back. The pain may happen with or without vomiting. These may be symptoms of pancreatitis.

What is JANUMET XR?
- JANUMET XR is a prescription medicine that contains 2 prescription diabetes medicines, sitagliptin (JANUVIA®) and extended-release metformin hydrochloride. JANUMET XR can be used along with diet and exercise to lower blood sugar in adults with type 2 diabetes.
- JANUMET XR is not for people with type 1 diabetes.
- JANUMET XR is not for people with diabetic ketoacidosis (increased ketones in your blood or urine).
- If you have had pancreatitis (inflammation of the pancreas) in the past, it is not known if you have a higher chance of getting pancreatitis while you take JANUMET XR.
- It is not known if JANUMET XR is safe and effective when used in children under 18 years of age.

Who should not take JANUMET XR?
Do not take JANUMET XR if:
- your kidneys are not working properly.
- you are allergic to any of the ingredients in JANUMET XR. See the end of this Medication Guide for a complete list of ingredients in JANUMET XR.
  Symptoms of a serious allergic reaction to JANUMET XR may include:
  - rash
  - raised red patches on your skin (hives)
  - swelling of the face, lips, tongue, and throat that may cause difficulty in breathing or swallowing
- you have diabetic ketoacidosis. See **"What is JANUMET XR?"**.

What should I tell my doctor before taking JANUMET XR?
Before you take JANUMET XR, tell your doctor if you:
- have or have had inflammation of your pancreas (pancreatitis).
- have kidney problems.
- have liver problems.
- have heart problems, including congestive heart failure.
- drink alcohol very often, or drink a lot of alcohol in short-term "binge" drinking.
- are going to get an injection of dye or contrast agents for an x-ray procedure; JANUMET XR will need to be stopped for a short time. Talk to your doctor about when you should stop JANUMET XR and when you should start JANUMET XR again. See **"What is the most important information I should know about JANUMET XR?"**.
- have any other medical conditions.
- are pregnant or plan to become pregnant. It is not known if JANUMET XR will harm your unborn baby. If you are pregnant, talk with your doctor about the best way to control your blood sugar while you are pregnant.
  Pregnancy Registry: If you take JANUMET XR at any time during your pregnancy, talk with your doctor about how you can join the JANUMET XR pregnancy registry. The purpose of this registry is to collect information about the health of you and your baby. You can enroll in this registry by calling 1-800-986-8999.
- are breast-feeding or plan to breast-feed. It is not known if JANUMET XR will pass into your breast milk. Talk with your doctor about the best way to feed your baby if you are taking JANUMET XR.

Tell your doctor about all the medicines you take, including prescription and non-prescription medicines, vitamins, and herbal supplements. JANUMET XR may affect how well other drugs work and some drugs can affect how well JANUMET XR works.

Know the medicines you take. Keep a list of your medicines and show it to your doctor and pharmacist when you get a new medicine.

How should I take JANUMET XR?
- Take JANUMET XR exactly as your doctor tells you. Your doctor will tell you how many JANUMET XR tablets to take and when you should take them.
- Your doctor may change your dose of JANUMET XR if needed.
- Your doctor may tell you to take JANUMET XR along with certain other diabetes medicines. Low blood sugar (hypoglycemia) can happen more often when JANUMET XR is taken with certain other diabetes medicines. See **"What are the possible side effects of JANUMET XR?"**.
- Take JANUMET XR 1 time each day with a meal to help to lower your chance of having an upset stomach. It is better to take JANUMET XR with your evening meal.
- Take JANUMET XR tablets whole. Do not break, cut, crush, dissolve, or chew JANUMET XR tablets before swallowing. If you cannot swallow JANUMET XR tablets whole, tell your doctor.
- Continue to take JANUMET XR as long as your doctor tells you.
- If you take too much JANUMET XR, call your doctor or local Poison Control Center right away.
- If you miss a dose, take it with food as soon as you remember. If you do not remember until it is time for your next dose, skip the missed dose and go back to your regular schedule. Do not take 2 doses of JANUMET XR at the same time.
- You may need to stop taking JANUMET XR for a short time. Call your doctor for instructions if you:
  - are dehydrated (have lost too much body fluid). Dehydration can occur if you are sick with severe vomiting, diarrhea or fever, or if you drink a lot less fluid than normal.
  - plan to have surgery.
  - are going to get an injection of dye or contrast agent for an x-ray procedure. See **"What is the most important information I should know about JANUMET XR?"** and **"What should I tell my doctor before taking JANUMET XR?"**.
- When your body is under some types of stress, such as fever, trauma (such as a car accident), infection or surgery, the amount of diabetes medicine that you need may change. Tell your doctor right away if you have any of these problems and follow your doctor's instructions.

- Check your blood sugar as your doctor tells you to.
- Stay on your prescribed diet and exercise program while taking JANUMET XR.
- Talk to your doctor about how to prevent, recognize and manage low blood sugar (hypoglycemia), high blood sugar (hyperglycemia), and problems you have because of your diabetes.
- Your doctor will check your diabetes with regular blood tests, including your blood sugar levels and your hemoglobin A1C.
- Your doctor will do blood tests to check how well your kidneys are working before and during your treatment with JANUMET XR.

What are the possible side effects of JANUMET XR?

Serious side effects have happened in people taking JANUMET XR or the individual medicines in JANUMET XR.

- See **"What is the most important information I should know about JANUMET XR?"**.
- **Low blood sugar (hypoglycemia).** If you take JANUMET XR with another medicine that can cause low blood sugar, such as a sulfonylurea or insulin, your risk of getting low blood sugar is higher. The dose of your sulfonylurea medicine or insulin may need to be lowered while you use JANUMET XR. Signs and symptoms of low blood sugar may include:

• headache	• irritability
• drowsiness	• hunger
• weakness	• fast heart beat
• dizziness	• sweating
• confusion	• feeling jittery

- **Serious allergic reactions.** If you have any symptoms of a serious allergic reaction, stop taking JANUMET XR and call your doctor right away. See **"Who should not take JANUMET XR?"**. Your doctor may give you a medicine for your allergic reaction and prescribe a different medicine for your diabetes.
- **Kidney problems,** sometimes requiring dialysis.

The most common side effects of JANUMET XR include:

- stuffy or runny nose and sore throat
- upper respiratory infection
- diarrhea
- nausea and vomiting
- gas, upset stomach, indigestion
- weakness
- headache
- low blood sugar (hypoglycemia) when used in combination with certain medications, such as a sulfonylurea or insulin.

Taking JANUMET XR with meals can help lessen the common stomach side effects of metformin that usually happen at the beginning of treatment. If you have unusual or sudden stomach problems, talk with your doctor. Stomach problems that start later during treatment may be a sign of something more serious.

JANUMET XR may have other side effects, including:

- swelling of the hands or legs. Swelling of the hands and legs can happen if you take JANUMET XR in combination with rosiglitazone (Avandia®). Rosiglitazone is another type of diabetes medicine.

These are not all the possible side effects of JANUMET XR. For more information, ask your doctor or pharmacist.

Tell your doctor if you have any side effect that bothers you, is unusual, or does not go away.

Call your doctor for medical advice about side effects. You may report side effects to FDA at 1-800-FDA-1088.

How should I store JANUMET XR?

Store JANUMET XR at 68°F to 77°F (20°C to 25°C). Store in a dry place and keep cap tightly closed.

Keep JANUMET XR and all medicines out of the reach of children.

General information about the use of JANUMET XR.

Medicines are sometimes prescribed for purposes other than those listed in Medication Guides. Do not use JANUMET XR for a condition for which it was not prescribed. Do not give JANUMET XR to other people, even if they have the same symptoms you have. It may harm them.

This Medication Guide summarizes the most important information about JANUMET XR. If you would like to know more information, talk with your doctor. You can ask your doctor or pharmacist for additional information about JANUMET XR that is written for health care professionals. For more information go to www.janumetxr.com or call 1-800-622-4477.

What are the ingredients in JANUMET XR?

Active ingredients: sitagliptin and metformin hydrochloride extended-release

Inactive ingredients:

- **All doses of JANUMET XR Tablets contain:** povidone, hypromellose, colloidal silicon dioxide, sodium stearyl fumarate, propyl gallate, polyethylene glycol, and kaolin. Film coating contains hypromellose, hydroxypropyl cellulose, titanium dioxide, FD&C #2/Indigo Carmine Aluminum Lake and carnauba wax.
- **In addition the JANUMET XR 50 mg/500 mg Tablets also contain:** microcrystalline cellulose.
- **In addition the JANUMET XR 50 mg/1000 mg Tablets also contain:** yellow iron oxide.

What is type 2 diabetes?

Type 2 diabetes is a condition in which your body does not make enough insulin, and the insulin that your body produces does not work as well as it should. Your body can also make too much sugar. When this happens, sugar (glucose) builds up in the blood. This can lead to serious medical problems.

High blood sugar can be lowered by diet and exercise, and by certain medicines when necessary.

This Medication Guide has been approved by the U.S. Food and Drug Administration.

Manufactured for: Merck Sharp & Dohme Corp., a subsidiary of
MERCK & CO., INC., Whitehouse Station, NJ 08889, USA

Manufactured by:
Merck Sharp & Dohme Corp., a subsidiary of
Merck & Co., Inc., Whitehouse Station, NJ 08889, USA
OR
Patheon Inc., Whitby, Ontario, Canada L1N 5Z5

US Patent Nos.: 6,699,871 and 7,326,708

The trademarks depicted herein are owned by their respective companies.

Revised: 07/2013
USMG-XRT-0431A1307R003

Shown in Product Identification Guide, page 308

JANUVIA® ℞

[ja-new'-vee-a]
(sitagliptin)
Tablets

HIGHLIGHTS OF PRESCRIBING INFORMATION
These highlights do not include all the information needed to use JANUVIA safely and effectively. See full prescribing information for JANUVIA.
JANUVIA® (sitagliptin) Tablets
Initial U.S. Approval: 2006

RECENT MAJOR CHANGES

Dosage and Administration
Recommended Dosing (2.1) 02/2013

INDICATIONS AND USAGE

JANUVIA is a dipeptidyl peptidase-4 (DPP-4) inhibitor indicated as an adjunct to diet and exercise to improve glycemic control in adults with type 2 diabetes mellitus. (1.1)

Important Limitations of Use:

- JANUVIA should not be used in patients with type 1 diabetes or for the treatment of diabetic ketoacidosis. (1.2)
- JANUVIA has not been studied in patients with a history of pancreatitis. (1.2, 5.1)

DOSAGE AND ADMINISTRATION

The recommended dose of JANUVIA is 100 mg once daily. JANUVIA can be taken with or without food. (2.1)

Dosage adjustment is recommended for patients with moderate or severe renal insufficiency or end-stage renal disease. (2.2)

Dosage Adjustment in Patients With Moderate, Severe and End Stage Renal Disease (ESRD) (2.2)

50 mg once daily	25 mg once daily
Moderate CrCl ≥30 to <50 mL/min ~Serum Cr levels [mg/dL] Men: >1.7– ≤3.0; Women: >1.5– ≤2.5	Severe and ESRD CrCl <30 mL/min ~Serum Cr levels [mg/dL] Men: >3.0; Women: >2.5; or on dialysis

DOSAGE FORMS AND STRENGTHS

Tablets: 100 mg, 50 mg, and 25 mg (3)

CONTRAINDICATIONS

History of a serious hypersensitivity reaction to sitagliptin, such as anaphylaxis or angioedema (5.4, 6.2)

WARNINGS AND PRECAUTIONS

- There have been postmarketing reports of acute pancreatitis, including fatal and non-fatal hemorrhagic or necrotizing pancreatitis. If pancreatitis is suspected, promptly discontinue JANUVIA. (5.1)
- There have been postmarketing reports of acute renal failure, sometimes requiring dialysis. Dosage adjustment is recommended in patients with moderate or severe renal insufficiency and in patients with ESRD. Assessment of renal function is recommended prior to initiating JANUVIA and periodically thereafter. (2.2, 5.2, 6.2)
- There is an increased risk of hypoglycemia when JANUVIA is added to an insulin secretagogue (e.g., sulfonylurea) or insulin therapy. Consider lowering the dose of the sulfonylurea or insulin to reduce the risk of hypoglycemia. (2.3, 5.3)
- There have been postmarketing reports of serious allergic and hypersensitivity reactions in patients treated with JANUVIA such as anaphylaxis, angioedema, and exfoliative skin conditions including Stevens-Johnson syndrome. In such cases, promptly stop JANUVIA, assess for other potential causes, institute appropriate monitoring and treatment, and initiate alternative treatment for diabetes. (5.4, 6.2)
- There have been no clinical studies establishing conclusive evidence of macrovascular risk reduction with JANUVIA or any other anti-diabetic drug. (5.5)

ADVERSE REACTIONS

Adverse reactions reported in ≥5% of patients treated with JANUVIA and more commonly than in patients treated with placebo are: upper respiratory tract infection, nasopharyngitis and headache. In the add-on to sulfonylurea and add-on to insulin studies, hypoglycemia was also more commonly reported in patients treated with JANUVIA compared to placebo. (6.1)

To report SUSPECTED ADVERSE REACTIONS, contact Merck Sharp & Dohme Corp., a subsidiary of Merck & Co., Inc., at 1-877-888-4231 or FDA at 1-800-FDA-1088 or www.fda.gov/medwatch.

USE IN SPECIFIC POPULATIONS

- Safety and effectiveness of JANUVIA in children under 18 years have not been established. (8.4)
- There are no adequate and well-controlled studies in pregnant women. To report drug exposure during pregnancy call 1-800-986-8999. (8.1)

See 17 for PATIENT COUNSELING INFORMATION and Medication Guide

Revised: 05/2013

FULL PRESCRIBING INFORMATION: CONTENTS*

*** Sections or subsections omitted from the full prescribing information are not listed**

FULL PRESCRIBING INFORMATION

1 INDICATIONS AND USAGE

1.1 Monotherapy and Combination Therapy

JANUVIA® is indicated as an adjunct to diet and exercise to improve glycemic control in adults with type 2 diabetes mellitus. *[See Clinical Studies (14).]*

1.2 Important Limitations of Use

JANUVIA should not be used in patients with type 1 diabetes or for the treatment of diabetic ketoacidosis, as it would not be effective in these settings.

JANUVIA has not been studied in patients with a history of pancreatitis. It is unknown whether patients with a history of pancreatitis are at increased risk for the development of pancreatitis while using JANUVIA. *[See Warnings and Precautions (5.1).]*

2 DOSAGE AND ADMINISTRATION

2.1 Recommended Dosing

The recommended dose of JANUVIA is 100 mg once daily. JANUVIA can be taken with or without food.

2.2 Patients with Renal Insufficiency

For patients with mild renal insufficiency (creatinine clearance [CrCl] greater than or equal to 50 mL/min, approximately corresponding to serum creatinine levels of less than or equal to 1.7 mg/dL in men and less than or equal to 1.5 mg/dL in women), no dosage adjustment for JANUVIA is required.

For patients with moderate renal insufficiency (CrCl greater than or equal to 30 to less than 50 mL/min, approximately corresponding to serum creatinine levels of greater than 1.7 to less than or equal to 3.0 mg/dL in men and greater than 1.5 to less than or equal to 2.5 mg/dL in women), the dose of JANUVIA is 50 mg once daily.

For patients with severe renal insufficiency (CrCl less than 30 mL/min, approximately corresponding to serum creatinine levels of greater than 3.0 mg/dL in men and greater than 2.5 mg/dL in women) or with end-stage renal disease (ESRD) requiring hemodialysis or peritoneal dialysis, the dose of JANUVIA is 25 mg once daily. JANUVIA may be administered without regard to the timing of dialysis.

Because there is a need for dosage adjustment based upon renal function, assessment of renal function is recommended prior to initiation of JANUVIA and periodically thereafter. Creatinine clearance can be estimated from serum creatinine using the Cockcroft-Gault formula. *[See Clinical Pharmacology (12.3).]* There have been postmarketing reports of worsening renal function in patients with renal insufficiency, some of whom were prescribed inappropriate doses of sitagliptin.

2.3 Concomitant Use with an Insulin Secretagogue (e.g., Sulfonylurea) or with Insulin

When JANUVIA is used in combination with an insulin secretagogue (e.g., sulfonylurea) or with insulin, a lower dose of the insulin secretagogue or insulin may be required to reduce the risk of hypoglycemia. *[See Warnings and Precautions (5.3).]*

3 DOSAGE FORMS AND STRENGTHS

- 100 mg tablets are beige, round, film-coated tablets with "277" on one side.
- 50 mg tablets are light beige, round, film-coated tablets with "112" on one side.
- 25 mg tablets are pink, round, film-coated tablets with "221" on one side.

4 CONTRAINDICATIONS

History of a serious hypersensitivity reaction to sitagliptin, such as anaphylaxis or angioedema. *[See Warnings and Precautions (5.4); Adverse Reactions (6.2).]*

5 WARNINGS AND PRECAUTIONS

5.1 Pancreatitis

There have been postmarketing reports of acute pancreatitis, including fatal and non-fatal hemorrhagic or necrotizing pancreatitis, in patients taking JANUVIA. After initiation of JANUVIA, patients should be observed carefully for signs and symptoms of pancreatitis. If pancreatitis is suspected, JANUVIA should promptly be discontinued and appropriate management should be initiated. It is unknown whether patients with a history of pancreatitis are at increased risk for the development of pancreatitis while using JANUVIA.

5.2 Renal Impairment

Assessment of renal function is recommended prior to initiating JANUVIA and periodically thereafter. A dosage adjustment is recommended in patients with moderate or severe renal insufficiency and in patients with ESRD requiring hemodialysis or peritoneal dialysis. *[See Dosage and Administration (2.2); Clinical Pharmacology (12.3).]* Caution should be used to ensure that the correct dose of JANUVIA is prescribed for patients with moderate (creatinine clearance ≥30 to <50 mL/min) or severe (creatinine clearance <30 mL/min) renal impairment.

There have been postmarketing reports of worsening renal function, including acute renal failure, sometimes requiring dialysis. A subset of these reports involved patients with renal insufficiency, some of whom were prescribed inappropriate doses of sitagliptin. A return to baseline levels of renal insufficiency has been observed with supportive treatment and discontinuation of potentially causative agents. Consideration can be given to cautiously reinitiating JANUVIA if another etiology is deemed likely to have precipitated the acute worsening of renal function.

JANUVIA has not been found to be nephrotoxic in preclinical studies at clinically relevant doses, or in clinical trials.

5.3 Use with Medications Known to Cause Hypoglycemia

When JANUVIA was used in combination with a sulfonylurea or with insulin, medications known to cause hypoglycemia, the incidence of hypoglycemia was increased over that of placebo used in combination with a sulfonylurea or with insulin. *[See Adverse Reactions (6.1).]* Therefore, a lower dose of sulfonylurea or insulin may be required to reduce the risk of hypoglycemia. *[See Dosage and Administration (2.3).]*

5.4 Hypersensitivity Reactions

There have been postmarketing reports of serious hypersensitivity reactions in patients treated with JANUVIA. These reactions include anaphylaxis, angioedema, and exfoliative skin conditions including Stevens-Johnson syndrome. Onset of these reactions occurred within the first 3 months after initiation of treatment with JANUVIA, with some reports occurring after the first dose. If a hypersensitivity reaction is suspected, discontinue JANUVIA, assess for other potential causes for the event, and institute alternative treatment for diabetes. *[See Adverse Reactions (6.2).]*

Angioedema has also been reported with other dipeptidyl peptidase-4 (DPP-4) inhibitors. Use caution in a patient with a history of angioedema with another DPP-4 inhibitor because it is unknown whether such patients will be predisposed to angioedema with JANUVIA.

5.5 Macrovascular Outcomes

There have been no clinical studies establishing conclusive evidence of macrovascular risk reduction with JANUVIA or any other anti-diabetic drug.

6 ADVERSE REACTIONS

6.1 Clinical Trials Experience

Because clinical trials are conducted under widely varying conditions, adverse reaction rates observed in the clinical trials of a drug cannot be directly compared to rates in the clinical trials of another drug and may not reflect the rates observed in practice.

In controlled clinical studies as both monotherapy and combination therapy with metformin, pioglitazone, or rosiglitazone and metformin, the overall incidence of adverse reactions, hypoglycemia, and discontinuation of therapy due to clinical adverse reactions with JANUVIA were similar to placebo. In combination with glimepiride, with or without metformin, the overall incidence of clinical adverse reactions with JANUVIA was higher than with placebo, in part related to a higher incidence of hypoglycemia (see Table 3); the incidence of discontinuation due to clinical adverse reactions was similar to placebo.

Two placebo-controlled monotherapy studies, one of 18- and one of 24-week duration, included patients treated with JANUVIA 100 mg daily, JANUVIA 200 mg daily, and placebo. Five placebo-controlled add-on combination therapy studies were also conducted: one with metformin; one with pioglitazone; one with metformin and rosiglitazone; one with glimepiride (with or without metformin); and one with insulin (with or without metformin). In these trials, patients with inadequate glycemic control on a stable dose of the background therapy were randomized to add-on therapy with JANUVIA 100 mg daily or placebo. The adverse reactions, excluding hypoglycemia, reported regardless of investigator assessment of causality in ≥5% of patients treated with JANUVIA 100 mg daily and more commonly than in patients treated with placebo, are shown in Table 1 for the clinical trials of at least 18 weeks duration. Incidences of hypoglycemia are shown in Table 3.

Table 1: Placebo-Controlled Clinical Studies of JANUVIA Monotherapy or Add-on Combination Therapy with Pioglitazone, Metformin + Rosiglitazone, or Glimepiride +/- Metformin: Adverse Reactions (Excluding Hypoglycemia) Reported in ≥5% of Patients and More Commonly than in Patients Given Placebo, Regardless of Investigator Assessment of Causality*

	Number of Patients (%)	
Monotherapy (18 or 24 weeks)	**JANUVIA 100 mg**	**Placebo**
	N = 443	N = 363
Nasopharyngitis	23 (5.2)	12 (3.3)
Combination with Pioglitazone (24 weeks)	**JANUVIA 100 mg + Pioglitazone**	**Placebo + Pioglitazone**
	N = 175	N = 178
Upper Respiratory Tract Infection	11 (6.3)	6 (3.4)
Headache	9 (5.1)	7 (3.9)
Combination with Metformin + Rosiglitazone (18 weeks)	**JANUVIA 100 mg + Metformin + Rosiglitazone**	**Placebo + Metformin + Rosiglitazone**
	N = 181	N = 97
Upper Respiratory Tract Infection	10 (5.5)	5 (5.2)
Nasopharyngitis	11 (6.1)	4 (4.1)
Combination with Glimepiride (+/- Metformin) (24 weeks)	**JANUVIA 100 mg + Glimepiride (+/- Metformin)**	**Placebo + Glimepiride (+/- Metformin)**
	N = 222	N = 219
Nasopharyngitis	14 (6.3)	10 (4.6)
Headache	13 (5.9)	5 (2.3)

* Intent-to-treat population

In the 24-week study of patients receiving JANUVIA as add-on combination therapy with metformin, there were no adverse reactions reported regardless of investigator assessment of causality in ≥5% of patients and more commonly than in patients given placebo.

In the 24-week study of patients receiving JANUVIA as add-on therapy to insulin (with or without metformin), there were no adverse reactions reported regardless of investigator assessment of causality in ≥5% of patients and more commonly than in patients given placebo, except for hypoglycemia (see Table 3).

In the study of JANUVIA as add-on combination therapy with metformin and rosiglitazone (Table 1), through Week 54 the adverse reactions reported regardless of investigator assessment of causality in ≥5% of patients treated with JANUVIA and more commonly than in patients treated with placebo were: upper respiratory tract infection (JANUVIA, 15.5%; placebo, 6.2%), nasopharyngitis (11.0%, 9.3%), peripheral edema (8.3%, 5.2%), and headache (5.5%, 4.1%).

In a pooled analysis of the two monotherapy studies, the add-on to metformin study, and the add-on to pioglitazone study, the incidence of selected gastrointestinal adverse reactions in patients treated with JANUVIA was as follows: abdominal pain (JANUVIA 100 mg, 2.3%; placebo, 2.1%), nausea (1.4%, 0.6%), and diarrhea (3.0%, 2.3%).

In an additional, 24-week, placebo-controlled factorial study of initial therapy with sitagliptin in combination with metformin, the adverse reactions reported (regardless of investigator assessment of causality) in ≥5% of patients are shown in Table 2.

[See table 2 at left]

In a 24-week study of initial therapy with JANUVIA in combination with pioglitazone, there were no adverse reactions reported (regardless of investigator assessment of causality) in ≥5% of patients and more commonly than in patients given pioglitazone alone.

Table 2: Initial Therapy with Combination of Sitagliptin and Metformin: Adverse Reactions Reported (Regardless of Investigator Assessment of Causality) in ≥5% of Patients Receiving Combination Therapy (and Greater than in Patients Receiving Metformin alone, Sitagliptin alone, and Placebo)*

	Number of Patients (%)			
	Placebo	**Sitagliptin (JANUVIA) 100 mg QD**	**Metformin 500 or 1000 mg bid†**	**Sitagliptin 50 mg bid + Metformin 500 or 1000 mg bid†**
	N = 176	N = 179	N = 364†	N = 372†
Upper Respiratory Infection	9 (5.1)	8 (4.5)	19 (5.2)	23 (6.2)
Headache	5 (2.8)	2 (1.1)	14 (3.8)	22 (5.9)

* Intent-to-treat population.
† Data pooled for the patients given the lower and higher doses of metformin.

No clinically meaningful changes in vital signs or in ECG (including in QTc interval) were observed in patients treated with JANUVIA.

In a pooled analysis of 19 double-blind clinical trials that included data from 10,246 patients randomized to receive sitagliptin 100 mg/day (N=5429) or corresponding (active or placebo) control (N=4817), the incidence of acute pancreatitis was 0.1 per 100 patient-years in each group (4 patients with an event in 4708 patient-years for sitagliptin and 4 patients with an event in 3942 patient-years for control). *[See Warnings and Precautions (5.1).]*

Hypoglycemia

In all (N=9) studies, adverse reactions of hypoglycemia were based on all reports of symptomatic hypoglycemia. A concurrent blood glucose measurement was not required although most (74%) reports of hypoglycemia were accompanied by a blood glucose measurement ≤70 mg/dL. When JANUVIA was co-administered with a sulfonylurea or with insulin, the percentage of patients with at least one adverse reaction of hypoglycemia was higher than in the corresponding placebo group (Table 3).

Table 3: Incidence and Rate of Hypoglycemia* in Placebo-Controlled Clinical Studies when JANUVIA was used as Add-On Therapy to Glimepiride (with or without Metformin) or Insulin (with or without Metformin), Regardless of Investigator Assessment of Causality

Add-On to Glimepiride (+/- Metformin) (24 weeks)	**JANUVIA 100 mg + Glimepiride (+/- Metformin)**	**Placebo + Glimepiride (+/- Metformin)**
	N = 222	N = 219
Overall (%)	27 (12.2)	4 (1.8)
Rate (episodes/patient-year)†	0.59	0.24
Severe (%)‡	0 (0.0)	0 (0.0)
Add-On to Insulin (+/- Metformin) (24 weeks)	**JANUVIA 100 mg + Insulin (+/- Metformin)**	**Placebo + Insulin (+/- Metformin)**
	N = 322	N = 319
Overall (%)	50 (15.5)	25 (7.8)
Rate (episodes/patient-year)†	1.06	0.51
Severe (%)‡	2 (0.6)	1 (0.3)

* Adverse reactions of hypoglycemia were based on all reports of symptomatic hypoglycemia; a concurrent glucose measurement was not required; intent-to-treat population.

† Based on total number of events (i.e., a single patient may have had multiple events).

‡ Severe events of hypoglycemia were defined as those events requiring medical assistance or exhibiting depressed level/loss of consciousness or seizure.

In a pooled analysis of the two monotherapy studies, the add-on to metformin study, and the add-on to pioglitazone study, the overall incidence of adverse reactions of hypoglycemia was 1.2% in patients treated with JANUVIA 100 mg and 0.9% in patients treated with placebo.

In the study of JANUVIA as add-on combination therapy with metformin and rosiglitazone, the overall incidence of hypoglycemia was 2.2% in patients given add-on JANUVIA and 0.0% in patients given add-on placebo through Week 18. Through Week 54, the overall incidence of hypoglycemia was 3.9% in patients given add-on JANUVIA and 1.0% in patients given add-on placebo.

In the 24-week, placebo-controlled factorial study of initial therapy with JANUVIA in combination with metformin, the incidence of hypoglycemia was 0.6% in patients given placebo, 0.6% in patients given JANUVIA alone, 0.8% in patients given metformin alone, and 1.6% in patients given JANUVIA in combination with metformin.

In the study of JANUVIA as initial therapy with pioglitazone, one patient taking JANUVIA experienced a severe episode of hypoglycemia. There were no severe hypoglycemia episodes reported in other studies except in the study involving co-administration with insulin.

Laboratory Tests

Across clinical studies, the incidence of laboratory adverse reactions was similar in patients treated with JANUVIA 100 mg compared to patients treated with placebo. A small increase in white blood cell count (WBC) was observed due to an increase in neutrophils. This increase in WBC (of approximately 200 cells/microL vs placebo, in four pooled placebo-controlled clinical studies, with a mean baseline WBC count of approximately 6600 cells/microL) is not considered to be clinically relevant. In a 12-week study of 91 patients with chronic renal insufficiency, 37 patients with moderate renal insufficiency were randomized to JANUVIA 50 mg daily, while 14 patients with the same magnitude of renal impairment were randomized to placebo. Mean (SE) increases in serum creatinine were observed in patients treated with JANUVIA [0.12 mg/dL (0.04)] and in patients treated with placebo [0.07 mg/dL (0.07)]. The clinical significance of this added increase in serum creatinine relative to placebo is not known.

6.2 Postmarketing Experience

Additional adverse reactions have been identified during postapproval use of JANUVIA as monotherapy and/or in combination with other antihyperglycemic agents. Because these reactions are reported voluntarily from a population of uncertain size, it is generally not possible to reliably estimate their frequency or establish a causal relationship to drug exposure.

Hypersensitivity reactions including anaphylaxis, angioedema, rash, urticaria, cutaneous vasculitis, and exfoliative skin conditions including Stevens-Johnson syndrome *[see Warnings and Precautions (5.4)]*; hepatic enzyme elevations; acute pancreatitis, including fatal and non-fatal hemorrhagic and necrotizing pancreatitis *[see Indications and Usage (1.2); Warnings and Precautions (5.1)]*; worsening renal function, including acute renal failure (sometimes requiring dialysis) *[see Warnings and Precautions (5.2)]*; constipation; vomiting; headache; arthralgia; myalgia; pain in extremity; back pain.

7 DRUG INTERACTIONS

7.1 Digoxin

There was a slight increase in the area under the curve (AUC, 11%) and mean peak drug concentration (C_{max}, 18%) of digoxin with the co-administration of 100 mg sitagliptin for 10 days. Patients receiving digoxin should be monitored appropriately. No dosage adjustment of digoxin or JANUVIA is recommended.

8 USE IN SPECIFIC POPULATIONS

8.1 Pregnancy

Pregnancy Category B:

Reproduction studies have been performed in rats and rabbits. Doses of sitagliptin up to 125 mg/kg (approximately 12 times the human exposure at the maximum recommended human dose) did not impair fertility or harm the fetus. There are, however, no adequate and well-controlled studies in pregnant women. Because animal reproduction studies are not always predictive of human response, this drug should be used during pregnancy only if clearly needed.

Merck Sharp & Dohme Corp., a subsidiary of Merck & Co., Inc., maintains a registry to monitor the pregnancy outcomes of women exposed to JANUVIA while pregnant. Health care providers are encouraged to report any prenatal exposure to JANUVIA by calling the Pregnancy Registry at 1-800-986-8999.

Sitagliptin administered to pregnant female rats and rabbits from gestation day 6 to 20 (organogenesis) was not teratogenic at oral doses up to 250 mg/kg (rats) and 125 mg/kg (rabbits), or approximately 30- and 20-times human exposure at the maximum recommended human dose (MRHD) of 100 mg/day based on AUC comparisons. Higher doses increased the incidence of rib malformations in offspring at 1000 mg/kg, or approximately 100 times human exposure at the MRHD.

Sitagliptin administered to female rats from gestation day 6 to lactation day 21 decreased body weight in male and female offspring at 1000 mg/kg. No functional or behavioral toxicity was observed in offspring of rats.

Placental transfer of sitagliptin administered to pregnant rats was approximately 45% at 2 hours and 80% at 24 hours postdose. Placental transfer of sitagliptin administered to pregnant rabbits was approximately 66% at 2 hours and 30% at 24 hours.

8.3 Nursing Mothers

Sitagliptin is secreted in the milk of lactating rats at a milk to plasma ratio of 4:1. It is not known whether sitagliptin is excreted in human milk. Because many drugs are excreted in human milk, caution should be exercised when JANUVIA is administered to a nursing woman.

8.4 Pediatric Use

Safety and effectiveness of JANUVIA in pediatric patients under 18 years of age have not been established.

8.5 Geriatric Use

Of the total number of subjects (N=3884) in pre-approval clinical safety and efficacy studies of JANUVIA, 725 patients were 65 years and over, while 61 patients were 75 years and over. No overall differences in safety or effectiveness were observed between subjects 65 years and over and younger subjects. While this and other reported clinical experience have not identified differences in responses between the elderly and younger patients, greater sensitivity of some older individuals cannot be ruled out.

This drug is known to be substantially excreted by the kidney. Because elderly patients are more likely to have decreased renal function, care should be taken in dose selection in the elderly, and it may be useful to assess renal function in these patients prior to initiating dosing and periodically thereafter *[see Dosage and Administration (2.2); Clinical Pharmacology (12.3)]*.

10 OVERDOSAGE

During controlled clinical trials in healthy subjects, single doses of up to 800 mg JANUVIA were administered. Maximal mean increases in QTc of 8.0 msec were observed in one study at a dose of 800 mg JANUVIA, a mean effect that is not considered clinically important *[see Clinical Pharmacology (12.2)]*. There is no experience with doses above 800 mg in clinical studies. In Phase I multiple-dose studies, there were no dose-related clinical adverse reactions observed with JANUVIA with doses of up to 600 mg per day for periods of up to 10 days and 400 mg per day for up to 28 days.

In the event of an overdose, it is reasonable to employ the usual supportive measures, e.g., remove unabsorbed material from the gastrointestinal tract, employ clinical monitoring (including obtaining an electrocardiogram), and institute supportive therapy as dictated by the patient's clinical status.

Sitagliptin is modestly dialyzable. In clinical studies, approximately 13.5% of the dose was removed over a 3- to 4-hour hemodialysis session. Prolonged hemodialysis may be considered if clinically appropriate. It is not known if sitagliptin is dialyzable by peritoneal dialysis.

11 DESCRIPTION

JANUVIA Tablets contain sitagliptin phosphate, an orally-active inhibitor of the dipeptidyl peptidase-4 (DPP-4) enzyme.

Sitagliptin phosphate monohydrate is described chemically as 7-[(3*R*)-3-amino-1-oxo-4-(2,4,5-trifluorophenyl)butyl]-5,6,7,8-tetrahydro-3-(trifluoromethyl)-1,2,4-triazolo[4,3-*a*]-pyrazine phosphate (1:1) monohydrate.

The empirical formula is $C_{16}H_{15}F_6N_5O \bullet H_3PO_4 \bullet H_2O$ and the molecular weight is 523.32. The structural formula is:

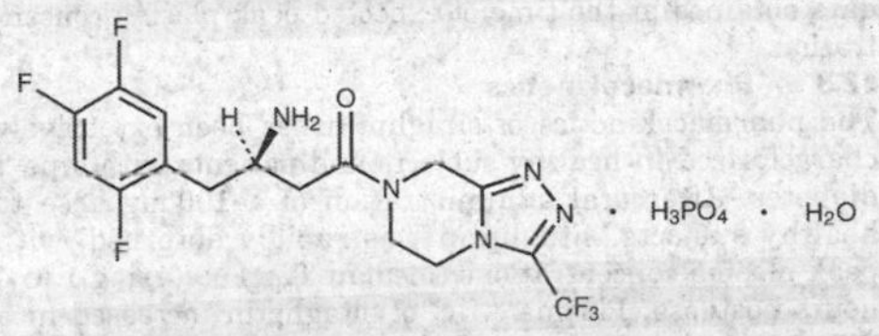

Sitagliptin phosphate monohydrate is a white to off-white, crystalline, non-hygroscopic powder. It is soluble in water and N,N-dimethyl formamide; slightly soluble in methanol; very slightly soluble in ethanol, acetone, and acetonitrile; and insoluble in isopropanol and isopropyl acetate.

Each film-coated tablet of JANUVIA contains 32.13, 64.25, or 128.5 mg of sitagliptin phosphate monohydrate, which is equivalent to 25, 50, or 100 mg, respectively, of free base and the following inactive ingredients: microcrystalline cellulose, anhydrous dibasic calcium phosphate, croscarmellose sodium, magnesium stearate, and sodium stearyl fumarate. In addition, the film coating contains the following inactive ingredients: polyvinyl alcohol, polyethylene glycol, talc, titanium dioxide, red iron oxide, and yellow iron oxide.

12 CLINICAL PHARMACOLOGY

12.1 Mechanism of Action

Sitagliptin is a DPP-4 inhibitor, which is believed to exert its actions in patients with type 2 diabetes by slowing the inactivation of incretin hormones. Concentrations of the active intact hormones are increased by JANUVIA, thereby increasing and prolonging the action of these hormones. Incretin hormones, including glucagon-like peptide-1 (GLP-1) and glucose-dependent insulinotropic polypeptide (GIP), are released by the intestine throughout the day, and levels are increased in response to a meal. These hormones are rapidly inactivated by the enzyme, DPP-4. The incretins are part of an endogenous system involved in the physiologic regulation of glucose homeostasis. When blood glucose concentrations are normal or elevated, GLP-1 and GIP increase insulin synthesis and release from pancreatic beta cells by intracellular signaling pathways involving cyclic AMP. GLP-1 also lowers glucagon secretion from pancreatic alpha cells, leading to reduced hepatic glucose production. By increasing and prolonging active incretin levels, JANUVIA increases insulin release and decreases glucagon levels in the circulation in a glucose-dependent manner. Sitagliptin demonstrates selectivity for DPP-4 and does not inhibit DPP-8 or DPP-9 activity *in vitro* at concentrations approximating those from therapeutic doses.

12.2 Pharmacodynamics

General

In patients with type 2 diabetes, administration of JANUVIA led to inhibition of DPP-4 enzyme activity for a 24-hour period. After an oral glucose load or a meal, this DPP-4 inhibition resulted in a 2- to 3-fold increase in circu-

$$CrCl = \frac{[140 - \text{age (years)}] \times \text{weight (kg)}}{[72 \times \text{serum creatinine (mg/dL)}]} \quad [\times 0.85 \text{ for female patients}]$$

lating levels of active GLP-1 and GIP, decreased glucagon concentrations, and increased responsiveness of insulin release to glucose, resulting in higher C-peptide and insulin concentrations. The rise in insulin with the decrease in glucagon was associated with lower fasting glucose concentrations and reduced glucose excursion following an oral glucose load or a meal.

In a two-day study in healthy subjects, sitagliptin alone increased active GLP-1 concentrations, whereas metformin alone increased active and total GLP-1 concentrations to similar extents. Co-administration of sitagliptin and metformin had an additive effect on active GLP-1 concentrations. Sitagliptin, but not metformin, increased active GIP concentrations. It is unclear how these findings relate to changes in glycemic control in patients with type 2 diabetes.

In studies with healthy subjects, JANUVIA did not lower blood glucose or cause hypoglycemia.

Cardiac Electrophysiology

In a randomized, placebo-controlled crossover study, 79 healthy subjects were administered a single oral dose of JANUVIA 100 mg, JANUVIA 800 mg (8 times the recommended dose), and placebo. At the recommended dose of 100 mg, there was no effect on the QTc interval obtained at the peak plasma concentration, or at any other time during the study. Following the 800 mg dose, the maximum increase in the placebo-corrected mean change in QTc from baseline was observed at 3 hours postdose and was 8.0 msec. This increase is not considered to be clinically significant. At the 800 mg dose, peak sitagliptin plasma concentrations were approximately 11 times higher than the peak concentrations following a 100 mg dose.

In patients with type 2 diabetes administered JANUVIA 100 mg (N=81) or JANUVIA 200 mg (N=63) daily, there were no meaningful changes in QTc interval based on ECG data obtained at the time of expected peak plasma concentration.

12.3 Pharmacokinetics

The pharmacokinetics of sitagliptin has been extensively characterized in healthy subjects and patients with type 2 diabetes. After oral administration of a 100 mg dose to healthy subjects, sitagliptin was rapidly absorbed, with peak plasma concentrations (median T_{max}) occurring 1 to 4 hours postdose. Plasma AUC of sitagliptin increased in a dose-proportional manner. Following a single oral 100 mg dose to healthy volunteers, mean plasma AUC of sitagliptin was 8.52 μM•hr, C_{max} was 950 nM, and apparent terminal half-life ($t_{1/2}$) was 12.4 hours. Plasma AUC of sitagliptin increased approximately 14% following 100 mg doses at steady-state compared to the first dose. The intra-subject and inter-subject coefficients of variation for sitagliptin AUC were small (5.8% and 15.1%). The pharmacokinetics of sitagliptin was generally similar in healthy subjects and in patients with type 2 diabetes.

Absorption

The absolute bioavailability of sitagliptin is approximately 87%. Because coadministration of a high-fat meal with JANUVIA had no effect on the pharmacokinetics, JANUVIA may be administered with or without food.

Distribution

The mean volume of distribution at steady state following a single 100 mg intravenous dose of sitagliptin to healthy subjects is approximately 198 liters. The fraction of sitagliptin reversibly bound to plasma proteins is low (38%).

Metabolism

Approximately 79% of sitagliptin is excreted unchanged in the urine with metabolism being a minor pathway of elimination.

Following a [^{14}C]sitagliptin oral dose, approximately 16% of the radioactivity was excreted as metabolites of sitagliptin. Six metabolites were detected at trace levels and are not expected to contribute to the plasma DPP-4 inhibitory activity of sitagliptin. *In vitro* studies indicated that the primary enzyme responsible for the limited metabolism of sitagliptin was CYP3A4, with contribution from CYP2C8.

Excretion

Following administration of an oral [^{14}C]sitagliptin dose to healthy subjects, approximately 100% of the administered radioactivity was eliminated in feces (13%) or urine (87%) within one week of dosing. The apparent terminal $t_{1/2}$ following a 100 mg oral dose of sitagliptin was approximately 12.4 hours and renal clearance was approximately 350 mL/min.

Elimination of sitagliptin occurs primarily via renal excretion and involves active tubular secretion. Sitagliptin is a substrate for human organic anion transporter-3 (hOAT-3), which may be involved in the renal elimination of sitagliptin. The clinical relevance of hOAT-3 in sitagliptin transport has not been established. Sitagliptin is also a substrate of p-glycoprotein, which may also be involved in mediating the renal elimination of sitagliptin. However, cyclosporine, a p-glycoprotein inhibitor, did not reduce the renal clearance of sitagliptin.

Special Populations

Renal Insufficiency

A single-dose, open-label study was conducted to evaluate the pharmacokinetics of JANUVIA (50 mg dose) in patients with varying degrees of chronic renal insufficiency compared to normal healthy control subjects. The study included patients with renal insufficiency classified on the basis of creatinine clearance as mild (50 to <80 mL/min), moderate (30 to <50 mL/min), and severe (<30 mL/min), as well as patients with ESRD on hemodialysis. In addition, the effects of renal insufficiency on sitagliptin pharmacokinetics in patients with type 2 diabetes and mild or moderate renal insufficiency were assessed using population pharmacokinetic analyses. Creatinine clearance was measured by 24-hour urinary creatinine clearance measurements or estimated from serum creatinine based on the Cockcroft-Gault formula:

[See table above]

Compared to normal healthy control subjects, an approximate 1.1- to 1.6-fold increase in plasma AUC of sitagliptin was observed in patients with mild renal insufficiency. Because increases of this magnitude are not clinically relevant, dosage adjustment in patients with mild renal insufficiency is not necessary. Plasma AUC levels of sitagliptin were increased approximately 2-fold and 4-fold in patients with moderate renal insufficiency and in patients with severe renal insufficiency, including patients with ESRD on hemodialysis, respectively. Sitagliptin was modestly removed by hemodialysis (13.5% over a 3- to 4-hour hemodialysis session starting 4 hours postdose). To achieve plasma concentrations of sitagliptin similar to those in patients with normal renal function, lower dosages are recommended in patients with moderate and severe renal insufficiency, as well as in ESRD patients requiring dialysis. *[See Dosage and Administration (2.2).]*

Hepatic Insufficiency

In patients with moderate hepatic insufficiency (Child-Pugh score 7 to 9), mean AUC and C_{max} of sitagliptin increased approximately 21% and 13%, respectively, compared to healthy matched controls following administration of a single 100 mg dose of JANUVIA. These differences are not considered to be clinically meaningful. No dosage adjustment for JANUVIA is necessary for patients with mild or moderate hepatic insufficiency.

There is no clinical experience in patients with severe hepatic insufficiency (Child-Pugh score >9).

Body Mass Index (BMI)

No dosage adjustment is necessary based on BMI. Body mass index had no clinically meaningful effect on the pharmacokinetics of sitagliptin based on a composite analysis of Phase I pharmacokinetic data and on a population pharmacokinetic analysis of Phase I and Phase II data.

Gender

No dosage adjustment is necessary based on gender. Gender had no clinically meaningful effect on the pharmacokinetics of sitagliptin based on a composite analysis of Phase I pharmacokinetic data and on a population pharmacokinetic analysis of Phase I and Phase II data.

Geriatric

No dosage adjustment is required based solely on age. When the effects of age on renal function are taken into account, age alone did not have a clinically meaningful impact on the pharmacokinetics of sitagliptin based on a population pharmacokinetic analysis. Elderly subjects (65 to 80 years) had approximately 19% higher plasma concentrations of sitagliptin compared to younger subjects.

Pediatric

Studies characterizing the pharmacokinetics of sitagliptin in pediatric patients have not been performed.

Race

No dosage adjustment is necessary based on race. Race had no clinically meaningful effect on the pharmacokinetics of sitagliptin based on a composite analysis of available pharmacokinetic data, including subjects of white, Hispanic, black, Asian, and other racial groups.

Drug Interactions

In Vitro Assessment of Drug Interactions

Sitagliptin is not an inhibitor of CYP isozymes CYP3A4, 2C8, 2C9, 2D6, 1A2, 2C19 or 2B6, and is not an inducer of CYP3A4. Sitagliptin is a p-glycoprotein substrate, but does not inhibit p-glycoprotein mediated transport of digoxin. Based on these results, sitagliptin is considered unlikely to cause interactions with other drugs that utilize these pathways.

Sitagliptin is not extensively bound to plasma proteins. Therefore, the propensity of sitagliptin to be involved in clinically meaningful drug-drug interactions mediated by plasma protein binding displacement is very low.

In Vivo Assessment of Drug Interactions

Effects of Sitagliptin on Other Drugs

In clinical studies, as described below, sitagliptin did not meaningfully alter the pharmacokinetics of metformin, glyburide, simvastatin, rosiglitazone, warfarin, or oral contraceptives, providing *in vivo* evidence of a low propensity for causing drug interactions with substrates of CYP3A4, CYP2C8, CYP2C9, and organic cationic transporter (OCT).

Digoxin: Sitagliptin had a minimal effect on the pharmacokinetics of digoxin. Following administration of 0.25 mg digoxin concomitantly with 100 mg of JANUVIA daily for 10 days, the plasma AUC of digoxin was increased by 11%, and the plasma C_{max} by 18%.

Metformin: Co-administration of multiple twice-daily doses of sitagliptin with metformin, an OCT substrate, did not meaningfully alter the pharmacokinetics of metformin in patients with type 2 diabetes. Therefore, sitagliptin is not an inhibitor of OCT-mediated transport.

Sulfonylureas: Single-dose pharmacokinetics of glyburide, a CYP2C9 substrate, was not meaningfully altered in subjects receiving multiple doses of sitagliptin. Clinically meaningful interactions would not be expected with other sulfonylureas (e.g., glipizide, tolbutamide, and glimepiride) which, like glyburide, are primarily eliminated by CYP2C9.

Simvastatin: Single-dose pharmacokinetics of simvastatin, a CYP3A4 substrate, was not meaningfully altered in subjects receiving multiple daily doses of sitagliptin. Therefore, sitagliptin is not an inhibitor of CYP3A4-mediated metabolism.

Thiazolidinediones: Single-dose pharmacokinetics of rosiglitazone was not meaningfully altered in subjects receiving multiple daily doses of sitagliptin, indicating that JANUVIA is not an inhibitor of CYP2C8-mediated metabolism.

Warfarin: Multiple daily doses of sitagliptin did not meaningfully alter the pharmacokinetics, as assessed by measurement of S(-) or R(+) warfarin enantiomers, or pharmacodynamics (as assessed by measurement of prothrombin INR) of a single dose of warfarin. Because S(-) warfarin is primarily metabolized by CYP2C9, these data also support the conclusion that sitagliptin is not a CYP2C9 inhibitor.

Oral Contraceptives: Co-administration with sitagliptin did not meaningfully alter the steady-state pharmacokinetics of norethindrone or ethinyl estradiol.

Effects of Other Drugs on Sitagliptin

Clinical data described below suggest that sitagliptin is not susceptible to clinically meaningful interactions by co-administered medications.

Metformin: Co-administration of multiple twice-daily doses of metformin with sitagliptin did not meaningfully alter the pharmacokinetics of sitagliptin in patients with type 2 diabetes.

Cyclosporine: A study was conducted to assess the effect of cyclosporine, a potent inhibitor of p-glycoprotein, on the pharmacokinetics of sitagliptin. Co-administration of a single 100 mg oral dose of JANUVIA and a single 600 mg oral dose of cyclosporine increased the AUC and C_{max} of sitagliptin by approximately 29% and 68%, respectively. These modest changes in sitagliptin pharmacokinetics were not considered to be clinically meaningful. The renal clearance of sitagliptin was also not meaningfully altered. Therefore, meaningful interactions would not be expected with other p-glycoprotein inhibitors.

13 NONCLINICAL TOXICOLOGY

13.1 Carcinogenesis, Mutagenesis, Impairment of Fertility

A two-year carcinogenicity study was conducted in male and female rats given oral doses of sitagliptin of 50, 150, and 500 mg/kg/day. There was an increased incidence of combined liver adenoma/carcinoma in males and females and of liver carcinoma in females at 500 mg/kg. This dose results in exposures approximately 60 times the human exposure at the maximum recommended daily adult human dose (MRHD) of 100 mg/day based on AUC comparisons. Liver tumors were not observed at 150 mg/kg, approximately 20 times the human exposure at the MRHD. A two-year carcinogenicity study was conducted in male and female mice given oral doses of sitagliptin of 50, 125, 250, and 500 mg/kg/day. There was no increase in the incidence of tumors in any organ up to 500 mg/kg, approximately 70 times human exposure at the MRHD. Sitagliptin was not mutagenic or clastogenic with or without metabolic activation in the Ames bacterial mutagenicity assay, a Chinese hamster ovary (CHO) chromosome aberration assay, an *in vitro* cytogenetics assay in CHO, an *in vitro* rat hepatocyte DNA alkaline elution assay, and an *in vivo* micronucleus assay.

In rat fertility studies with oral gavage doses of 125, 250, and 1000 mg/kg, males were treated for 4 weeks prior to mating, during mating, up to scheduled termination (approximately 8 weeks total) and females were treated 2 weeks prior to mating through gestation day 7. No adverse effect on fertility was observed at 125 mg/kg (approximately 12 times human exposure at the MRHD of 100 mg/day based on AUC comparisons). At higher doses, nondose-related increased resorptions in females were observed (approximately 25 and 100 times human exposure at the MRHD based on AUC comparison).

14 CLINICAL STUDIES

There were approximately 5200 patients with type 2 diabetes randomized in nine double-blind, placebo-controlled clinical safety and efficacy studies conducted to evaluate the effects of sitagliptin on glycemic control. In a pooled analysis of seven of these studies, the ethnic/racial distribution was approximately 59% white, 20% Hispanic, 10% Asian, 6% black, and 6% other groups. Patients had an overall mean age of approximately 55 years (range 18 to 87 years). In addition, an active (glipizide)-controlled study of 52-weeks duration was conducted in 1172 patients with type 2 diabetes who had inadequate glycemic control on metformin.

In patients with type 2 diabetes, treatment with JANUVIA produced clinically significant improvements in hemoglobin A1C, fasting plasma glucose (FPG) and 2-hour post-prandial glucose (PPG) compared to placebo.

14.1 Monotherapy

A total of 1262 patients with type 2 diabetes participated in two double-blind, placebo-controlled studies, one of 18-week and another of 24-week duration, to evaluate the efficacy and safety of JANUVIA monotherapy. In both monotherapy studies, patients currently on an antihyperglycemic agent discontinued the agent, and underwent a diet, exercise, and drug washout period of about 7 weeks. Patients with inadequate glycemic control (A1C 7% to 10%) after the washout period were randomized after completing a 2-week single-blind placebo run-in period; patients not currently on antihyperglycemic agents (off therapy for at least 8 weeks) with inadequate glycemic control (A1C 7% to 10%) were randomized after completing the 2-week single-blind placebo run-in period. In the 18-week study, 521 patients were randomized to placebo, JANUVIA 100 mg, or JANUVIA 200 mg, and in the 24-week study 741 patients were randomized to placebo, JANUVIA 100 mg, or JANUVIA 200 mg. Patients who failed to meet specific glycemic goals during the studies were treated with metformin rescue, added on to placebo or JANUVIA.

Treatment with JANUVIA at 100 mg daily provided significant improvements in A1C, FPG, and 2-hour PPG compared to placebo (Table 4). In the 18-week study, 9% of patients receiving JANUVIA 100 mg and 17% who received placebo required rescue therapy. In the 24-week study, 9% of patients receiving JANUVIA 100 mg and 21% of patients receiving placebo required rescue therapy. The improvement in A1C compared to placebo was not affected by gender, age, race, prior antihyperglycemic therapy, or baseline BMI. As is typical for trials of agents to treat type 2 diabetes, the mean reduction in A1C with JANUVIA appears to be related to the degree of A1C elevation at baseline. In these 18- and 24-week studies, among patients who were not on an antihyperglycemic agent at study entry, the reductions from baseline in A1C were -0.7% and -0.8%, respectively, for those given JANUVIA, and -0.1% and -0.2%, respectively, for those given placebo. Overall, the 200 mg daily dose did not provide greater glycemic efficacy than the 100 mg daily dose. The effect of JANUVIA on lipid endpoints was similar to placebo. Body weight did not increase from baseline with JANUVIA therapy in either study, compared to a small reduction in patients given placebo.

[See table 4 above]

Table 4: Glycemic Parameters in 18- and 24-Week Placebo-Controlled Studies of JANUVIA in Patients with Type 2 Diabetes*

	18-Week Study		24-Week Study	
	JANUVIA 100 mg	Placebo	JANUVIA 100 mg	Placebo
A1C (%)	N = 193	N = 103	N = 229	N = 244
Baseline (mean)	8.0	8.1	8.0	8.0
Change from baseline (adjusted mean†)	-0.5	0.1	-0.6	0.2
Difference from placebo (adjusted mean†)	-0.6‡		-0.8‡	
(95% CI)	(-0.8, -0.4)		(-1.0, -0.6)	
Patients (%) achieving A1C <7%	69 (36%)	16 (16%)	93 (41%)	41 (17%)
FPG (mg/dL)	N = 201	N = 107	N = 234	N = 247
Baseline (mean)	180	184	170	176
Change from baseline (adjusted mean†)	-13	7	-12	5
Difference from placebo (adjusted mean†)	-20‡		-17‡	
(95% CI)	(-31, -9)		(-24, -10)	
2-hour PPG (mg/dL)	§	§	N = 201	N = 204
Baseline (mean)			257	271
Change from baseline (adjusted mean†)			-49	-2
Difference from placebo (adjusted mean†)			-47‡	
(95% CI)			(-59, -34)	

* Intent-to-treat population using last observation on study prior to metformin rescue therapy.
† Least squares means adjusted for prior antihyperglycemic therapy status and baseline value.
‡ p<0.001 compared to placebo.
§ Data not available.

Additional Monotherapy Study

A multinational, randomized, double-blind, placebo-controlled study was also conducted to assess the safety and tolerability of JANUVIA in 91 patients with type 2 diabetes and chronic renal insufficiency (creatinine clearance <50 mL/min). Patients with moderate renal insufficiency received 50 mg daily of JANUVIA and those with severe renal insufficiency or with ESRD on hemodialysis or peritoneal dialysis received 25 mg daily. In this study, the safety and tolerability of JANUVIA were generally similar to placebo. A small increase in serum creatinine was reported in patients with moderate renal insufficiency treated with JANUVIA relative to those on placebo. In addition, the reductions in A1C and FPG with JANUVIA compared to placebo were generally similar to those observed in other monotherapy studies. *[See Clinical Pharmacology (12.3).]*

14.2 Combination Therapy

Add-on Combination Therapy with Metformin

A total of 701 patients with type 2 diabetes participated in a 24-week, randomized, double-blind, placebo-controlled study designed to assess the efficacy of JANUVIA in combination with metformin. Patients already on metformin (N=431) at a dose of at least 1500 mg per day were randomized after completing a 2-week single-blind placebo run-in period. Patients on metformin and another antihyperglycemic agent (N=229) and patients not on any antihyperglycemic agents (off therapy for at least 8 weeks, N=41) were randomized after a run-in period of approximately 10 weeks on metformin (at a dose of at least 1500 mg per day) in monotherapy. Patients with inadequate glycemic control (A1C 7% to 10%) were randomized to the addition of either 100 mg of JANUVIA or placebo, administered once daily. Patients who failed to meet specific glycemic goals during the studies were treated with pioglitazone rescue.

In combination with metformin, JANUVIA provided significant improvements in A1C, FPG, and 2-hour PPG compared to placebo with metformin (Table 5). Rescue glycemic therapy was used in 5% of patients treated with JANUVIA 100 mg and 14% of patients treated with placebo. A similar decrease in body weight was observed for both treatment groups.

[See table 5 above]

Table 5: Glycemic Parameters at Final Visit (24-Week Study) for JANUVIA in Add-on Combination Therapy with Metformin*

	JANUVIA 100 mg + Metformin	Placebo + Metformin
A1C (%)	N = 453	N = 224
Baseline (mean)	8.0	8.0
Change from baseline (adjusted mean†)	-0.7	-0.0
Difference from placebo + metformin (adjusted mean†)	-0.7‡	
(95% CI)	(-0.8, -0.5)	
Patients (%) achieving A1C <7%	213 (47%)	41 (18%)
FPG (mg/dL)	N = 454	N = 226
Baseline (mean)	170	174
Change from baseline (adjusted mean†)	-17	9
Difference from placebo + metformin (adjusted mean†)	-25‡	
(95% CI)	(-31, -20)	
2-hour PPG (mg/dL)	N = 387	N = 182
Baseline (mean)	275	272
Change from baseline (adjusted mean†)	-62	-11
Difference from placebo + metformin (adjusted mean†)	-51‡	
(95% CI)	(-61, -41)	

* Intent-to-treat population using last observation on study prior to pioglitazone rescue therapy.
† Least squares means adjusted for prior antihyperglycemic therapy and baseline value.
‡ p<0.001 compared to placebo + metformin.

Initial Combination Therapy with Metformin

A total of 1091 patients with type 2 diabetes and inadequate glycemic control on diet and exercise participated in a 24-week, randomized, double-blind, placebo-controlled factorial study designed to assess the efficacy of sitagliptin as initial therapy in combination with metformin. Patients on an antihyperglycemic agent (N=541) discontinued the agent, and underwent a diet, exercise, and drug washout period of up to 12 weeks duration. After the washout period, patients with inadequate glycemic control (A1C 7.5% to 11%) were randomized after completing a 2-week single-blind placebo run-in period. Patients not on antihyperglycemic agents at study entry (N=550) with inadequate glycemic control (A1C 7.5% to 11%) immediately entered the 2-week single-blind placebo run-in period and then were randomized. Approximately equal numbers of patients were randomized to receive initial therapy with placebo, 100 mg of JANUVIA once daily, 500 mg or 1000 mg of metformin twice daily, or 50 mg of sitagliptin twice daily in combination with 500 mg or 1000 mg of metformin twice daily. Patients who failed to meet specific glycemic goals during the study were treated with glyburide (glibenclamide) rescue.

Initial therapy with the combination of JANUVIA and metformin provided significant improvements in A1C, FPG, and 2-hour PPG compared to placebo, to metformin alone, and to JANUVIA alone (Table 6, Figure 1). Mean reductions from baseline in A1C were generally greater for patients with higher baseline A1C values. For patients not on an antihyperglycemic agent at study entry, mean reductions from baseline in A1C were: JANUVIA 100 mg once daily, -1.1%; metformin 500 mg bid, -1.1%; metformin 1000 mg bid, -1.2%; sitagliptin 50 mg bid with metformin 500 mg bid, -1.6%; sitagliptin 50 mg bid with metformin 1000 mg bid, -1.9%; and for patients receiving placebo, -0.2%. Lipid ef-

fects were generally neutral. The decrease in body weight in the groups given sitagliptin in combination with metformin was similar to that in the groups given metformin alone or placebo.
[See table 6 above]

Figure 1: Mean Change from Baseline for A1C (%) over 24 Weeks with Sitagliptin and Metformin, Alone and in Combination as Initial Therapy in Patients with Type 2 Diabetes*

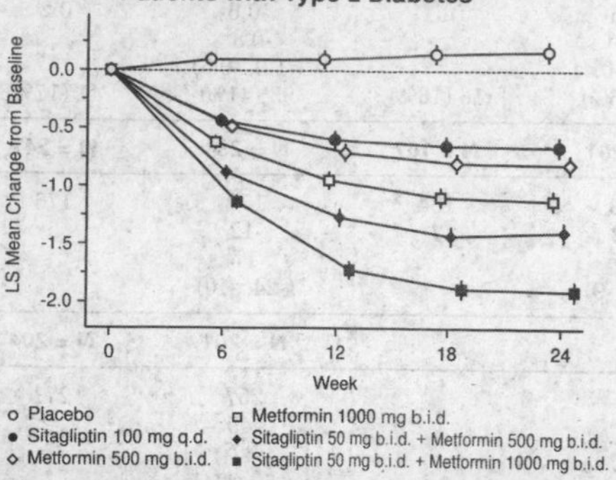

* All Patients Treated Population: least squares means adjusted for prior antihyperglycemic therapy and baseline value.

In addition, this study included patients (N=117) with more severe hyperglycemia (A1C >11% or blood glucose >280 mg/dL) who were treated with twice daily open-label JANUVIA 50 mg and metformin 1000 mg. In this group of patients, the mean baseline A1C value was 11.2%, mean FPG was 314 mg/dL, and mean 2-hour PPG was 441 mg/dL. After 24 weeks, mean decreases from baseline of -2.9% for A1C, -127 mg/dL for FPG, and -208 mg/dL for 2-hour PPG were observed.
Initial combination therapy or maintenance of combination therapy may not be appropriate for all patients. These management options are left to the discretion of the health care provider.

Active-Controlled Study vs Glipizide in Combination with Metformin

The efficacy of JANUVIA was evaluated in a 52-week, double-blind, glipizide-controlled noninferiority trial in patients with type 2 diabetes. Patients not on treatment or on other antihyperglycemic agents entered a run-in treatment period of up to 12 weeks duration with metformin monotherapy (dose of ≥1500 mg per day) which included washout of medications other than metformin, if applicable. After the run-in period, those with inadequate glycemic control (A1C 6.5% to 10%) were randomized 1:1 to the addition of JANUVIA 100 mg once daily or glipizide for 52 weeks. Patients receiving glipizide were given an initial dosage of 5 mg/day and then electively titrated over the next 18 weeks to a maximum dosage of 20 mg/day as needed to optimize glycemic control. Thereafter, the glipizide dose was to be kept constant, except for down-titration to prevent hypoglycemia. The mean dose of glipizide after the titration period was 10 mg.
After 52 weeks, JANUVIA and glipizide had similar mean reductions from baseline in A1C in the intent-to-treat analysis (Table 7). These results were consistent with the per protocol analysis (Figure 2). A conclusion in favor of the noninferiority of JANUVIA to glipizide may be limited to patients with baseline A1C comparable to those included in the study (over 70% of patients had baseline A1C <8% and over 90% had A1C <9%).

Table 7: Glycemic Parameters in a 52-Week Study Comparing JANUVIA to Glipizide as Add-On Therapy in Patients Inadequately Controlled on Metformin (Intent-to-Treat Population)*

	JANUVIA 100 mg	Glipizide
A1C (%)	**N = 576**	**N = 559**
Baseline (mean)	7.7	7.6
Change from baseline (adjusted mean†)	-0.5	-0.6
FPG (mg/dL)	**N = 583**	**N = 568**
Baseline (mean)	166	164
Change from baseline (adjusted mean†)	-8	-8

* The intent-to-treat analysis used the patients' last observation in the study prior to discontinuation.

Table 6: Glycemic Parameters at Final Visit (24-Week Study) for Sitagliptin and Metformin, Alone and in Combination as Initial Therapy*

	Placebo	Sitagliptin (JANUVIA) 100 mg QD	Metformin 500 mg bid	Metformin 1000 mg bid	Sitagliptin 50 mg bid + Metformin 500 mg bid	Sitagliptin 50 mg bid + Metformin 1000 mg bid
A1C (%)	**N = 165**	**N = 175**	**N = 178**	**N = 177**	**N = 183**	**N = 178**
Baseline (mean)	8.7	8.9	8.9	8.7	8.8	8.8
Change from baseline (adjusted mean†)	0.2	-0.7	-0.8	-1.1	-1.4	-1.9
Difference from placebo (adjusted mean†) (95% CI)		-0.8‡ (-1.1, -0.6)	-1.0‡ (-1.2, -0.8)	-1.3‡ (-1.5, -1.1)	-1.6‡ (-1.8, -1.3)	-2.1‡ (-2.3, -1.8)
Patients (%) achieving A1C <7%	15 (9%)	35 (20%)	41 (23%)	68 (38%)	79 (43%)	118 (66%)
% Patients receiving rescue medication	32	21	17	12	8	2
FPG (mg/dL)	**N = 169**	**N = 178**	**N = 179**	**N = 179**	**N = 183**	**N = 180**
Baseline (mean)	196	201	205	197	204	197
Change from baseline (adjusted mean†)	6	-17	-27	-29	-47	-64
Difference from placebo (adjusted mean†) (95% CI)		-23‡ (-33, -14)	-33‡ (-43, -24)	-35‡ (-45, -26)	-53‡ (-62, -43)	-70‡ (-79, -60)
2-hour PPG (mg/dL)	**N = 129**	**N = 136**	**N = 141**	**N = 138**	**N = 147**	**N = 152**
Baseline (mean)	277	285	293	283	292	287
Change from baseline (adjusted mean†)	0	-52	-53	-78	-93	-117
Difference from placebo (adjusted mean†) (95% CI)		-52‡ (-67, -37)	-54‡ (-69, -39)	-78‡ (-93, -63)	-93‡ (-107, -78)	-117‡ (-131, -102)

* Intent-to-treat population using last observation on study prior to glyburide (glibenclamide) rescue therapy.
† Least squares means adjusted for prior antihyperglycemic therapy status and baseline value.
‡ p<0.001 compared to placebo.

† Least squares means adjusted for prior antihyperglycemic therapy status and baseline A1C value.

Figure 2: Mean Change from Baseline for A1C (%) Over 52 Weeks in a Study Comparing JANUVIA to Glipizide as Add-On Therapy in Patients Inadequately Controlled on Metformin (Per Protocol Population)*

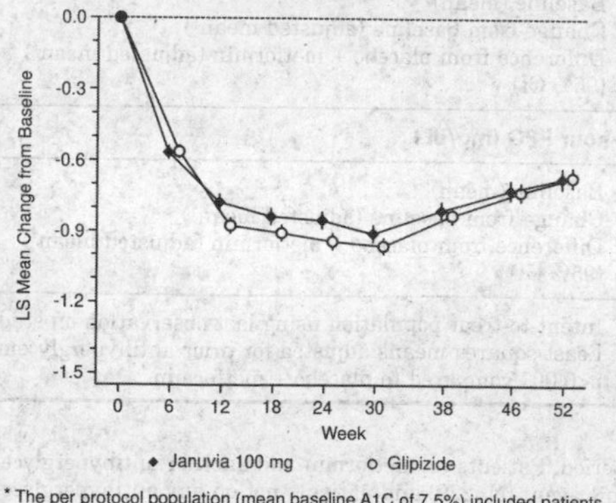

* The per protocol population (mean baseline A1C of 7.5%) included patients without major protocol violations who had observations at baseline and at Week 52.

The incidence of hypoglycemia in the JANUVIA group (4.9%) was significantly (p<0.001) lower than that in the glipizide group (32.0%). Patients treated with JANUVIA exhibited a significant mean decrease from baseline in body weight compared to a significant weight gain in patients administered glipizide (-1.5 kg vs +1.1 kg).

Add-on Combination Therapy with Pioglitazone

A total of 353 patients with type 2 diabetes participated in a 24-week, randomized, double-blind, placebo-controlled study designed to assess the efficacy of JANUVIA in combination with pioglitazone. Patients on any oral antihyperglycemic agent in monotherapy (N=212) or on a PPARγ agent in combination therapy (N=106) or not on an antihyperglycemic agent (off therapy for at least 8 weeks, N=34) were switched to monotherapy with pioglitazone (at a dose of 30-45 mg per day), and completed a run-in period of approximately 12 weeks in duration. After the run-in period on pioglitazone monotherapy, patients with inadequate glycemic control (A1C 7% to 10%) were randomized to the addition of either 100 mg of JANUVIA or placebo, administered once daily. Patients who failed to meet specific glycemic goals during the studies were treated with metformin rescue. Glycemic endpoints measured were A1C and fasting glucose.
In combination with pioglitazone, JANUVIA provided significant improvements in A1C and FPG compared to placebo with pioglitazone (Table 8). Rescue therapy was used in 7% of patients treated with JANUVIA 100 mg and 14% of patients treated with placebo. There was no significant difference between JANUVIA and placebo in body weight change.
[See table 8 at top of next page]

Initial Combination Therapy with Pioglitazone

A total of 520 patients with type 2 diabetes and inadequate glycemic control on diet and exercise participated in a 24-week, randomized, double-blind study designed to assess the efficacy of JANUVIA as initial therapy in combination with pioglitazone. Patients not on antihyperglycemic agents at study entry (<4 weeks cumulative therapy over the past 2 years, and with no treatment over the prior 4 months) with inadequate glycemic control (A1C 8% to 12%) immediately entered the 2-week single-blind placebo run-in period and then were randomized. Approximately equal numbers of patients were randomized to receive initial therapy with 100 mg of JANUVIA in combination with 30 mg of pioglitazone once daily or 30 mg of pioglitazone once daily as monotherapy. There was no glycemic rescue therapy in this study. Initial therapy with the combination of JANUVIA and pioglitazone provided significant improvements in A1C, FPG, and 2-hour PPG compared to pioglitazone monotherapy (Table 9). The improvement in A1C was generally consistent across subgroups defined by gender, age, race, baseline BMI, baseline A1C, or duration of disease. In this study, patients treated with JANUVIA in combination with pioglitazone had a mean increase in body weight of 1.1 kg compared to pioglitazone alone (3.0 kg vs. 1.9 kg). Lipid effects were generally neutral.
[See table 9 at top of next page]

Add-on Combination Therapy with Metformin and Rosiglitazone

A total of 278 patients with type 2 diabetes participated in a 54-week, randomized, double-blind, placebo-controlled study designed to assess the efficacy of JANUVIA in combination with metformin and rosiglitazone. Patients on dual therapy with metformin ≥1500 mg/day and rosiglitazone ≥4 mg/day or with metformin ≥1500 mg/day and pioglitazone ≥30 mg/day (switched to rosiglitazone ≥4 mg/day) entered a dose-stable run-in period of 6 weeks. Patients on other dual therapy were switched to metformin ≥1500 mg/day and rosiglitazone ≥4 mg/day in a dose titration/stabilization run-in period of up to 20 weeks in duration. After the run-in period, patients with inadequate glycemic control (A1C 7.5% to 11%) were randomized 2:1 to the addition of either 100 mg of JANUVIA or placebo, administered once daily. Patients who failed to meet specific glycemic goals during the study were treated with glipizide (or other sulfonylurea) rescue. The primary time point for evaluation of glycemic parameters was Week 18.
In combination with metformin and rosiglitazone, JANUVIA provided significant improvements in A1C, FPG,

and 2-hour PPG compared to placebo with metformin and rosiglitazone (Table 10) at Week 18. At Week 54, mean reduction in A1C was -1.0% for patients treated with JANUVIA and -0.3% for patients treated with placebo in an analysis based on the intent-to-treat population. Rescue therapy was used in 18% of patients treated with JANUVIA 100 mg and 40% of patients treated with placebo. There was no significant difference between JANUVIA and placebo in body weight change.

[See table 10 below]

Add-on Combination Therapy with Glimepiride, with or without Metformin

A total of 441 patients with type 2 diabetes participated in a 24-week, randomized, double-blind, placebo-controlled study designed to assess the efficacy of JANUVIA in combination with glimepiride, with or without metformin. Patients entered a run-in treatment period on glimepiride (≥4 mg per day) alone or glimepiride in combination with metformin (≥1500 mg per day). After a dose-titration and dose-stable run-in period of up to 16 weeks and a 2-week placebo run-in period, patients with inadequate glycemic control (A1C 7.5% to 10.5%) were randomized to the addition of either 100 mg of JANUVIA or placebo, administered once daily. Patients who failed to meet specific glycemic goals during the studies were treated with pioglitazone rescue.

In combination with glimepiride, with or without metformin, JANUVIA provided significant improvements in A1C and FPG compared to placebo (Table 11). In the entire study population (patients on JANUVIA in combination with glimepiride and patients on JANUVIA in combination with glimepiride and metformin), a mean reduction from baseline relative to placebo in A1C of -0.7% and in FPG of -20 mg/dL was seen. Rescue therapy was used in 12% of patients treated with JANUVIA 100 mg and 27% of patients treated with placebo. In this study, patients treated with JANUVIA had a mean increase in body weight of 1.1 kg vs. placebo (+0.8 kg vs. -0.4 kg). In addition, there was an increased rate of hypoglycemia. *[See Warnings and Precautions (5.3); Adverse Reactions (6.1).]*

[See table 11 at top of next page]

Add-on Combination Therapy with Insulin (with or without Metformin)

A total of 641 patients with type 2 diabetes participated in a 24-week, randomized, double-blind, placebo controlled study designed to assess the efficacy of JANUVIA as add-on to insulin therapy (with or without metformin). The racial distribution in this study was approximately 70% white, 18% Asian, 7% black, and 5% other groups. Approximately 14% of the patients in this study were Hispanic. Patients entered a 2-week, single-blind run-in treatment period on pre-mixed, long-acting, or intermediate-acting insulin, with or without metformin (≥1500 mg per day). Patients using short-acting insulins were excluded unless the short-acting insulin was administered as part of a pre-mixed insulin. After the run-in period, patients with inadequate glycemic control (A1C 7.5% to 11%) were randomized to the addition of either 100 mg of JANUVIA or placebo, administered once daily. Patients were on a stable dose of insulin prior to enrollment with no changes in insulin dose permitted during the run-in period. Patients who failed to meet specific glycemic goals during the double-blind treatment period were to have uptitration of the background insulin dose as rescue therapy.

The median daily insulin dose at baseline was 42 units in the patients treated with JANUVIA and 45 units in the placebo-treated patients. The median change from baseline in daily dose of insulin was zero for both groups at the end of the study. In combination with insulin (with or without metformin), JANUVIA provided significant improvements in A1C, FPG, and 2-hour PPG compared to placebo (Table 12). Both treatment groups had an adjusted mean increase in body weight of 0.1 kg from baseline to Week 24. There was an increased rate of hypoglycemia in patients treated with JANUVIA. *[See Warnings and Precautions (5.3); Adverse Reactions (6.1).]*

[See table 12 at top of next page]

Table 8: Glycemic Parameters at Final Visit (24-Week Study) for JANUVIA in Add-on Combination Therapy with Pioglitazone*

	JANUVIA 100 mg + Pioglitazone	Placebo + Pioglitazone
A1C (%)	**N = 163**	**N = 174**
Baseline (mean)	8.1	8.0
Change from baseline (adjusted mean†)	-0.9	-0.2
Difference from placebo + pioglitazone (adjusted mean†) (95% CI)	-0.7‡ (-0.9, -0.5)	
Patients (%) achieving A1C <7%	74 (45%)	40 (23%)
FPG (mg/dL)	**N = 163**	**N = 174**
Baseline (mean)	168	166
Change from baseline (adjusted mean†)	-17	1
Difference from placebo + pioglitazone (adjusted mean†) (95% CI)	-18‡ (-24, -11)	

* Intent-to-treat population using last observation on study prior to metformin rescue therapy.
† Least squares means adjusted for prior antihyperglycemic therapy status and baseline value.
‡ p<0.001 compared to placebo + pioglitazone.

Table 9: Glycemic Parameters at Final Visit (24-Week Study) for JANUVIA in Combination with Pioglitazone as Initial Therapy*

	JANUVIA 100 mg + Pioglitazone	Pioglitazone
A1C (%)	**N = 251**	**N = 246**
Baseline (mean)	9.5	9.4
Change from baseline (adjusted mean†)	-2.4	-1.5
Difference from pioglitazone (adjusted mean†) (95% CI)	-0.9‡ (-1.1, -0.7)	
Patients (%) achieving A1C <7%	151 (60%)	68 (28%)
FPG (mg/dL)	**N = 256**	**N = 253**
Baseline (mean)	203	201
Change from baseline (adjusted mean†)	-63	-40
Difference from pioglitazone (adjusted mean†) (95% CI)	-23‡ (-30, -15)	
2-hour PPG (mg/dL)	**N = 216**	**N = 211**
Baseline (mean)	283	284
Change from baseline (adjusted mean†)	-114	-69
Difference from pioglitazone (adjusted mean†) (95% CI)	-45‡ (-57, -32)	

* Intent-to-treat population using last observation on study.
† Least squares means adjusted for baseline value.
‡ p<0.001 compared to placebo + pioglitazone.

Table 10: Glycemic Parameters at Week 18 for JANUVIA in Add-on Combination Therapy with Metformin and Rosiglitazone*

	JANUVIA 100 mg + Metformin + Rosiglitazone	Placebo + Metformin + Rosiglitazone
A1C (%)	**N = 176**	**N = 93**
Baseline (mean)	8.8	8.7
Change from baseline (adjusted mean†)	-1.0	-0.4
Difference from placebo + rosiglitazone + metformin (adjusted mean†) (95% CI)	-0.7‡ (-0.9, -0.4)	
Patients (%) achieving A1C <7%	39 (22%)	9 (10%)
FPG (mg/dL)	**N = 179**	**N = 94**
Baseline (mean)	181	182
Change from baseline (adjusted mean†)	-30	-11
Difference from placebo + rosiglitazone + metformin (adjusted mean†) (95% CI)	-18‡ (-26, -10)	
2-hour PPG (mg/dL)	**N = 152**	**N = 80**
Baseline (mean)	256	248
Change from baseline (adjusted mean†)	-59	-21
Difference from placebo + rosiglitazone + metformin (adjusted mean†) (95% CI)	-39‡ (-51, -26)	

* Intent-to-treat population using last observation on study prior to glipizide (or other sulfonylurea) rescue therapy.
† Least squares means adjusted for prior antihyperglycemic therapy status and baseline value.
‡ p<0.001 compared to placebo + metformin + rosiglitazone.

16 HOW SUPPLIED/STORAGE AND HANDLING

No. 6737 — Tablets JANUVIA, 25 mg, are pink, round, film-coated tablets with "221" on one side. They are supplied as follows:

NDC 0006-0221-31 unit-of-use bottles of 30
NDC 0006-0221-54 unit-of-use bottles of 90
NDC 0006-0221-28 unit dose blister packages of 100.

No. 6738 — Tablets JANUVIA, 50 mg, are light beige, round, film-coated tablets with "112" on one side. They are supplied as follows:

NDC 0006-0112-31 unit-of-use bottles of 30
NDC 0006-0112-54 unit-of-use bottles of 90
NDC 0006-0112-28 unit dose blister packages of 100.

No. 6739 — Tablets JANUVIA, 100 mg, are beige, round, film-coated tablets with "277" on one side. They are supplied as follows:

NDC 0006-0277-31 unit-of-use bottles of 30
NDC 0006-0277-54 unit-of-use bottles of 90
NDC 0006-0277-33 unit-of-use blister calendar package of 30

Table 11: Glycemic Parameters at Final Visit (24-Week Study) for JANUVIA as Add-On Combination Therapy with Glimepiride, with or without Metformin*

	JANUVIA 100 mg + Glimepiride	Placebo + Glimepiride	JANUVIA 100 mg + Glimepiride + Metformin	Placebo + Glimepiride + Metformin
A1C (%)	**N = 102**	**N = 103**	**N = 115**	**N = 105**
Baseline (mean)	8.4	8.5	8.3	8.3
Change from baseline (adjusted mean†)	-0.3	0.3	-0.6	0.3
Difference from placebo (adjusted mean†) (95% CI)	-0.6‡ (-0.8, -0.3)		-0.9‡ (-1.1, -0.7)	
Patients (%) achieving A1C <7%	11 (11%)	9 (9%)	26 (23%)	1 (1%)
FPG (mg/dL)	**N = 104**	**N = 104**	**N = 115**	**N = 109**
Baseline (mean)	183	185	179	179
Change from baseline (adjusted mean†)	-1	18	-8	13
Difference from placebo (adjusted mean†) (95% CI)	-19§ (-32, -7)		-21‡ (-32, -10)	

* Intent-to-treat population using last observation on study prior to pioglitazone rescue therapy.
† Least squares means adjusted for prior antihyperglycemic therapy status and baseline value.
‡ p<0.001 compared to placebo.
§ p<0.01 compared to placebo.

Table 12: Glycemic Parameters at Final Visit (24-Week Study) for JANUVIA as Add-on Combination Therapy with Insulin*

	JANUVIA 100 mg + Insulin (+/- Metformin)	Placebo + Insulin (+/- Metformin)
A1C (%)	**N = 305**	**N = 312**
Baseline (mean)	8.7	8.6
Change from baseline (adjusted mean†)	-0.6	-0.1
Difference from placebo (adjusted mean†,‡) (95% CI)	-0.6§ (-0.7, -0.4)	
Patients (%) achieving A1C <7%	39 (12.8%)	16 (5.1%)
FPG (mg/dL)	**N = 310**	**N = 313**
Baseline (mean)	176	179
Change from baseline (adjusted mean†)	-18	-4
Difference from placebo (adjusted mean†) (95% CI)	-15§ (-23, -7)	
2-hour PPG (mg/dL)	**N = 240**	**N = 257**
Baseline (mean)	291	292
Change from baseline (adjusted mean†)	-31	5
Difference from placebo (adjusted mean†) (95% CI)	-36§ (-47, -25)	

* Intent-to-treat population using last observation on study prior to rescue therapy.
† Least squares means adjusted for metformin use at the screening visit (yes/no), type of insulin used at the screening visit (pre-mixed vs. non-pre-mixed [intermediate- or long-acting]), and baseline value.
‡ Treatment by stratum interaction was not significant (p>0.10) for metformin stratum and for insulin stratum.
§ p<0.001 compared to placebo.

NDC 0006-0277-28 unit dose blister packages of 100
NDC 0006-0277-82 bottles of 1000.

Storage

Store at 20-25°C (68-77°F), excursions permitted to 15-30°C (59-86°F), [see USP Controlled Room Temperature].

17 PATIENT COUNSELING INFORMATION

See FDA-Approved Patient Labeling (Medication Guide).

17.1 Instructions

Patients should be informed of the potential risks and benefits of JANUVIA and of alternative modes of therapy. Patients should also be informed about the importance of adherence to dietary instructions, regular physical activity, periodic blood glucose monitoring and A1C testing, recognition and management of hypoglycemia and hyperglycemia, and assessment for diabetes complications. During periods of stress such as fever, trauma, infection, or surgery, medication requirements may change and patients should be advised to seek medical advice promptly.

Patients should be informed that acute pancreatitis has been reported during postmarketing use of JANUVIA. Patients should be informed that persistent severe abdominal pain, sometimes radiating to the back, which may or may not be accompanied by vomiting, is the hallmark symptom of acute pancreatitis. Patients should be instructed to promptly discontinue JANUVIA and contact their physician if persistent severe abdominal pain occurs *[see Warnings and Precautions (5.1)]*.

Patients should be informed that the incidence of hypoglycemia is increased when JANUVIA is added to a sulfonylurea or insulin and that a lower dose of the sulfonylurea or insulin may be required to reduce the risk of hypoglycemia.

Patients should be informed that allergic reactions have been reported during postmarketing use of JANUVIA. If symptoms of allergic reactions (including rash, hives, and swelling of the face, lips, tongue, and throat that may cause difficulty in breathing or swallowing) occur, patients must stop taking JANUVIA and seek medical advice promptly.

Physicians should instruct their patients to read the Medication Guide before starting JANUVIA therapy and to reread each time the prescription is renewed. Patients should be instructed to inform their doctor or pharmacist if they develop any unusual symptom, or if any known symptom persists or worsens.

17.2 Laboratory Tests

Patients should be informed that response to all diabetic therapies should be monitored by periodic measurements of blood glucose and A1C levels, with a goal of decreasing these levels towards the normal range. A1C is especially useful for evaluating long-term glycemic control. Patients should be informed of the potential need to adjust dose based on changes in renal function tests over time.

Distributed by: Merck Sharp & Dohme Corp., a subsidiary of
MERCK & CO., INC., Whitehouse Station, NJ 08889, USA
US Patent Nos.: 6,699,871 and 7,326,708

Revised: 05/2013
USPI-T-04311305R011

Medication Guide
JANUVIA® (jah-NEW-vee-ah)
(sitagliptin)
Tablets

Read this Medication Guide carefully before you start taking JANUVIA and each time you get a refill. There may be new information. This information does not take the place of talking with your doctor about your medical condition or your treatment. If you have any questions about JANUVIA, ask your doctor or pharmacist.

What is the most important information I should know about JANUVIA?

Serious side effects can happen in people taking JANUVIA, including inflammation of the pancreas (pancreatitis) which may be severe and lead to death.

Certain medical problems make you more likely to get pancreatitis.

Before you start taking JANUVIA:

Tell your doctor if you have ever had

- pancreatitis
- stones in your gallbladder (gallstones)
- a history of alcoholism
- high blood triglyceride levels
- kidney problems

Stop taking JANUVIA and call your doctor right away if you have pain in your stomach area (abdomen) that is severe and will not go away. The pain may be felt going from your abdomen through to your back. The pain may happen with or without vomiting. These may be symptoms of pancreatitis.

What is JANUVIA?

- JANUVIA is a prescription medicine used along with diet and exercise to lower blood sugar in adults with type 2 diabetes.
- JANUVIA is not for people with type 1 diabetes.
- JANUVIA is not for people with diabetic ketoacidosis (increased ketones in your blood or urine).
- If you have had pancreatitis (inflammation of the pancreas) in the past, it is not known if you have a higher chance of getting pancreatitis while you take JANUVIA.
- It is not known if JANUVIA is safe and effective when used in children under 18 years of age.

Who should not take JANUVIA?

Do not take JANUVIA if:

- you are allergic to any of the ingredients in JANUVIA. See the end of this Medication Guide for a complete list of ingredients in JANUVIA.

  Symptoms of a serious allergic reaction to JANUVIA may include:
  - rash
  - raised red patches on your skin (hives)
  - swelling of the face, lips, tongue, and throat that may cause difficulty in breathing or swallowing

What should I tell my doctor before taking JANUVIA?

Before you take JANUVIA, tell your doctor if you:

- have or have had inflammation of your pancreas (pancreatitis).
- have kidney problems.
- have any other medical conditions.
- are pregnant or plan to become pregnant. It is not known if JANUVIA will harm your unborn baby. If you are pregnant, talk with your doctor about the best way to control your blood sugar while you are pregnant.

  Pregnancy Registry: If you take JANUVIA at any time during your pregnancy, talk with your doctor about how you can join the JANUVIA pregnancy registry. The purpose of this registry is to collect information about the health of you and your baby. You can enroll in this registry by calling 1-800-986-8999.
- are breast-feeding or plan to breast-feed. It is not known if JANUVIA will pass into your breast milk. Talk with your doctor about the best way to feed your baby if you are taking JANUVIA.

Tell your doctor about all the medicines you take, including prescription and non-prescription medicines, vitamins, and herbal supplements.

Know the medicines you take. Keep a list of your medicines and show it to your doctor and pharmacist when you get a new medicine.

How should I take JANUVIA?

- Take JANUVIA 1 time each day exactly as your doctor tells you.
- You can take JANUVIA with or without food.
- Your doctor may do blood tests from time to time to see how well your kidneys are working. Your doctor may change your dose of JANUVIA based on the results of your blood tests.

- Your doctor may tell you to take JANUVIA along with other diabetes medicines. Low blood sugar can happen more often when JANUVIA is taken with certain other diabetes medicines. See **"What are the possible side effects of JANUVIA?"**.
- If you miss a dose, take it as soon as you remember. If you do not remember until it is time for your next dose, skip the missed dose and go back to your regular schedule. Do not take two doses of JANUVIA at the same time.
- If you take too much JANUVIA, call your doctor or local Poison Control Center right away.
- When your body is under some types of stress, such as fever, trauma (such as a car accident), infection or surgery, the amount of diabetes medicine that you need may change. Tell your doctor right away if you have any of these conditions and follow your doctor's instructions.
- Check your blood sugar as your doctor tells you to.
- Stay on your prescribed diet and exercise program while taking JANUVIA.
- Talk to your doctor about how to prevent, recognize and manage low blood sugar (hypoglycemia), high blood sugar (hyperglycemia), and problems you have because of your diabetes.
- Your doctor will check your diabetes with regular blood tests, including your blood sugar levels and your hemoglobin A1C.

What are the possible side effects of JANUVIA?

Serious side effects have happened in people taking JANUVIA.

- See **"What is the most important information I should know about JANUVIA?"**.
- **Low blood sugar (hypoglycemia).** If you take JANUVIA with another medicine that can cause low blood sugar, such as a sulfonylurea or insulin, your risk of getting low blood sugar is higher. The dose of your sulfonylurea medicine or insulin may need to be lowered while you use JANUVIA. Signs and symptoms of low blood sugar may include:

- headache
- drowsiness
- weakness
- dizziness
- confusion
- irritability
- hunger
- fast heart beat
- sweating
- feeling jittery

- **Serious allergic reactions.** If you have any symptoms of a serious allergic reaction, stop taking JANUVIA and call your doctor right away. See **"Who should not take JANUVIA?"**. Your doctor may give you a medicine for your allergic reaction and prescribe a different medicine for your diabetes.
- **Kidney problems**, sometimes requiring dialysis

The most common side effects of JANUVIA include:

- upper respiratory infection
- stuffy or runny nose and sore throat
- headache

JANUVIA may have other side effects, including:

- stomach upset and diarrhea
- swelling of the hands or legs, when JANUVIA is used with rosiglitazone (Avandia®). Rosiglitazone is another type of diabetes medicine.

These are not all the possible side effects of JANUVIA. For more information, ask your doctor or pharmacist.

Tell your doctor if you have any side effect that bothers you, is unusual or does not go away.

Call your doctor for medical advice about side effects. You may report side effects to FDA at 1-800-FDA-1088.

How should I store JANUVIA?

Store JANUVIA at 68°F to 77°F (20°C to 25°C).

Keep JANUVIA and all medicines out of the reach of children.

General information about the use of JANUVIA

Medicines are sometimes prescribed for purposes that are not listed in Medication Guides. Do not use JANUVIA for a condition for which it was not prescribed. Do not give JANUVIA to other people, even if they have the same symptoms you have. It may harm them.

This Medication Guide summarizes the most important information about JANUVIA. If you would like to know more information, talk with your doctor. You can ask your doctor or pharmacist for additional information about JANUVIA that is written for health professionals. For more information, go to www.JANUVIA.com or call 1-800-622-4477.

What are the ingredients in JANUVIA?

Active ingredient: sitagliptin

Inactive ingredients: microcrystalline cellulose, anhydrous dibasic calcium phosphate, croscarmellose sodium, magnesium stearate, and sodium stearyl fumarate. The tablet film coating contains the following inactive ingredients: polyvinyl alcohol, polyethylene glycol, talc, titanium dioxide, red iron oxide, and yellow iron oxide.

What is type 2 diabetes?

Type 2 diabetes is a condition in which your body does not make enough insulin, and the insulin that your body produces does not work as well as it should. Your body can also make too much sugar. When this happens, sugar (glucose) builds up in the blood. This can lead to serious medical problems.

High blood sugar can be lowered by diet and exercise, and by certain medicines when necessary.

This Medication Guide has been approved by the U.S. Food and Drug Administration.

Distributed by: Merck Sharp & Dohme Corp., a subsidiary of

MERCK & CO., INC., Whitehouse Station, NJ 08889, USA

US Patent Nos.: 6,699,871 and 7,326,708

Revised: 05/2013

USMG-T-04311305R011

Shown in Product Identification Guide, page 308

JUVISYNC™ ℞

(sitagliptin and simvastatin)
Tablets

HIGHLIGHTS OF PRESCRIBING INFORMATION

These highlights do not include all the information needed to use JUVISYNC safely and effectively. See full prescribing information for JUVISYNC.

JUVISYNC™ (sitagliptin and simvastatin) Tablets
Initial U.S. Approval: 2011

RECENT MAJOR CHANGES

Indications and Usage	
Important Limitations of Use (1.3)	09/2012
Dosage and Administration	
Recommended Dosing (2.1)	02/2013
Patients with Renal Impairment (2.2)	09/2012
Coadministration with Other Drugs (2.4)	10/2012
Patients with Homozygous Familial Hypercholesterolemia (2.5)	09/2012
Chinese Patients Taking Lipid-Modifying Doses (greater than or equal to 1 g/day Niacin) of Niacin-Containing Products (2.6)	09/2012
Contraindications (4)	10/2012
Warnings and Precautions	
Myopathy/Rhabdomyolysis (5.2)	10/2012
Renal Impairment (5.4)	09/2012

INDICATIONS AND USAGE

JUVISYNC (sitagliptin and simvastatin) is indicated in patients for whom treatment with both sitagliptin and simvastatin is appropriate. (1) Sitagliptin is a dipeptidyl peptidase-4 (DPP-4) inhibitor indicated as an adjunct to diet and exercise to improve glycemic control in adults with type 2 diabetes mellitus. (1.1)

Simvastatin is an HMG-CoA reductase inhibitor (statin) indicated as an adjunctive therapy to diet to:

- Reduce the risk of total mortality by reducing CHD deaths and reduce the risk of non-fatal myocardial infarction, stroke, and the need for revascularization procedures in patients at high risk of coronary events. (1.2)
- Reduce elevated total-C, LDL-C, Apo B, TG and increase HDL-C in patients with primary hyperlipidemia (heterozygous familial and nonfamilial) and mixed dyslipidemia. (1.2)
- Reduce elevated TG in patients with hypertriglyceridemia and reduce TG and VLDL-C in patients with primary dysbeta-lipoproteinemia. (1.2)
- Reduce total-C and LDL-C in adult patients with homozygous familial hypercholesterolemia. (1.2)

Important Limitations of Use:

- JUVISYNC should not be used in patients with type 1 diabetes or for the treatment of diabetic ketoacidosis. (1.3)
- JUVISYNC has not been studied in patients with a history of pancreatitis. (1.3, 5.1)
- JUVISYNC has not been studied in Fredrickson types I and V dyslipidemias. (1.3)
- Patients with severe renal impairment who require sitagliptin 25 mg should not use JUVISYNC due to the unavailability of this dosage strength for JUVISYNC. (1.3)

DOSAGE AND ADMINISTRATION

- Doses are 100 mg/10 mg, 100 mg/20 mg, 100 mg/40 mg, 50 mg/10 mg, 50 mg/20 mg, and 50 mg/40 mg per day. (2.1)
- Recommended usual starting dose for patients with normal or mildly impaired renal function is 100 mg/40 mg once a day in the evening. (2.1)
- Adjustment of the starting dose to 50 mg/40 mg once a day is recommended for patients with moderate renal impairment (CrCl greater than or equal to 30 to less than 50 mL/min, equivalent to serum Cr levels greater than 1.7 to less than or equal to 3.0 mg/dL for men and greater than 1.5 to less than or equal to 2.5 mg/dL for women). (2.2)
- Patients already taking simvastatin (10, 20, or 40 mg) can initiate JUVISYNC at a dose of 100 or 50 mg sitagliptin and the dose of simvastatin already being taken. (2.1)

DOSAGE FORMS AND STRENGTHS

Tablets (sitagliptin/simvastatin): 100 mg/10 mg, 100 mg/20 mg, 100 mg/40 mg, 50 mg/10 mg, 50 mg/20 mg, and 50 mg/40 mg (3)

CONTRAINDICATIONS

- History of a serious hypersensitivity reaction, such as anaphylaxis or angioedema, to any component of this medication. (4, 5.6, 6.2)
- Concomitant administration of strong CYP3A4 inhibitors. (4, 5.2)
- Concomitant administration of gemfibrozil, cyclosporine, or danazol. (4, 5.2)
- Active liver disease, which may include unexplained persistent elevations in hepatic transaminase levels. (4, 5.3)
- Women who are pregnant or may become pregnant. (4, 8.1)
- Nursing mothers. (4, 8.3)

WARNINGS AND PRECAUTIONS

- There have been postmarketing reports of acute pancreatitis, including fatal and non-fatal hemorrhagic or necrotizing pancreatitis. If pancreatitis is suspected, promptly discontinue JUVISYNC. (5.1)
- Skeletal muscle effects (e.g., myopathy and rhabdomyolysis): Risks increase with higher doses and concomitant use of certain medicines. Predisposing factors include advanced age (≥65), female gender, uncontrolled hypothyroidism, and renal impairment. (4, 5.2, 8.5)
- Patients should be advised to report promptly any unexplained and/or persistent muscle pain, tenderness, or weakness. JUVISYNC therapy should be discontinued immediately if myopathy is diagnosed or suspected. See Drug Interaction table. (5.2)
- Liver enzyme abnormalities: Persistent elevations in hepatic transaminase can occur. Check liver enzyme tests before initiating therapy and as clinically indicated thereafter. (5.3)
- There have been postmarketing reports of acute renal failure, sometimes requiring dialysis, in patients treated with sitagliptin. Assessment of renal function is recommended prior to initiation of JUVISYNC and periodically thereafter. (5.4, 6.2)
- There is an increased risk of hypoglycemia when JUVISYNC is added to an insulin secretagogue (e.g., sulfonylurea) or insulin therapy. Consider lowering the dose of the sulfonylurea or insulin to reduce the risk of hypoglycemia. (2.3, 5.5)
- There have been postmarketing reports of serious allergic and hypersensitivity reactions in patients treated with sitagliptin such as anaphylaxis, angioedema, and exfoliative skin conditions including Stevens-Johnson syndrome. In such cases, promptly stop JUVISYNC, assess for other potential causes, institute appropriate monitoring and treatment, and initiate alternative treatment. (5.6, 6.2)

ADVERSE REACTIONS

Most common adverse reactions (incidence ≥5%) with simvastatin are: upper respiratory infection, headache, abdominal pain, constipation, and nausea. Adverse reactions reported in ≥5% of patients treated with sitagliptin and more commonly than in patients treated with placebo are: upper respiratory tract infection, nasopharyngitis and headache. In the add-on to sulfonylurea and add-on to insulin studies, hypoglycemia was also more commonly reported in patients treated with sitagliptin compared to placebo. (6.1)

To report SUSPECTED ADVERSE REACTIONS, contact Merck Sharp & Dohme Corp., a subsidiary of Merck & Co., Inc., at 1-877-888-4231 or FDA at 1-800-FDA-1088 or www.fda.gov/medwatch.

DRUG INTERACTIONS

Drug Interactions Associated with Increased Risk of Myopathy/Rhabdomyolysis (2.4, 4, 5.2, 7.1, 7.2, 7.3, 12.3)

Interacting Agents	Prescribing Recommendations
Strong CYP3A4 inhibitors (e.g., itraconazole, ketoconazole, posaconazole, voriconazole, erythromycin, clarithromycin, telithromycin, HIV protease inhibitors, boceprevir, telaprevir, nefazodone), gemfibrozil, cyclosporine, danazol	Contraindicated with JUVISYNC
Verapamil, diltiazem, dronedarone	Do not exceed 10 mg simvastatin (100 mg/10 mg or 50 mg/10 mg JUVISYNC) daily
Amiodarone, amlodipine, ranolazine	Do not exceed 20 mg simvastatin (100 mg/20 mg or 50 mg/20 mg JUVISYNC) daily
Grapefruit juice	Avoid grapefruit juice

- Coumarin anticoagulants: Concomitant use with simvastatin prolongs INR. Achieve stable INR prior to starting JUVISYNC. Monitor INR frequently until stable upon initiation or alteration of JUVISYNC therapy. (7.6)
- Other lipid-lowering medications: Use with other fibrate products or lipid-modifying doses (≥1 g/day) of niacin increases the risk of adverse skeletal muscle effects. Caution should be used when prescribing with JUVISYNC. (5.2, 7.2, 7.4).

USE IN SPECIFIC POPULATIONS

- Safety and effectiveness of JUVISYNC in children under 18 years have not been established. (8.4)
- There are no adequate and well-controlled studies in pregnant women. (8.1)

See 17 for PATIENT COUNSELING INFORMATION and Medication Guide

Revised: 02/2013

FULL PRESCRIBING INFORMATION: CONTENTS*

*** Sections or subsections omitted from the full prescribing information are not listed**

FULL PRESCRIBING INFORMATION

1 INDICATIONS AND USAGE

JUVISYNC™ (sitagliptin and simvastatin) is indicated in patients for whom treatment with both sitagliptin and simvastatin is appropriate.

1.1 Sitagliptin

Sitagliptin is indicated as an adjunct to diet and exercise to improve glycemic control in adults with type 2 diabetes mellitus. *[See Clinical Studies (14.1).]*

1.2 Simvastatin

Therapy with lipid-altering agents should be only one component of multiple risk factor intervention in individuals at significantly increased risk for atherosclerotic vascular disease due to hypercholesterolemia. Drug therapy is indicated as an adjunct to diet when the response to a diet restricted in saturated fat and cholesterol and other nonpharmacologic measures alone has been inadequate. In patients with coronary heart disease (CHD) or at high risk of CHD, simvastatin can be started simultaneously with diet.

Reductions in Risk of CHD Mortality and Cardiovascular Events

In patients at high risk of coronary events because of existing coronary heart disease, diabetes, peripheral vessel disease, history of stroke or other cerebrovascular disease, simvastatin is indicated to:

- Reduce the risk of total mortality by reducing CHD deaths.
- Reduce the risk of non-fatal myocardial infarction and stroke.
- Reduce the need for coronary and non-coronary revascularization procedures.

Hyperlipidemia

Simvastatin is indicated to:

- Reduce elevated total cholesterol (total-C), low-density lipoprotein cholesterol (LDL-C), apolipoprotein B (Apo B), and triglycerides (TG), and to increase high-density lipoprotein cholesterol (HDL-C) in patients with primary hyperlipidemia (Fredrickson type IIa, heterozygous familial and nonfamilial) or mixed dyslipidemia (Fredrickson type IIb).
- Reduce elevated TG in patients with hypertriglyceridemia (Fredrickson type IV hyperlipidemia).
- Reduce elevated TG and VLDL-C in patients with primary dysbetalipoproteinemia (Fredrickson type lll hyperlipidemia).
- Reduce total-C and LDL-C in patients with homozygous familial hypercholesterolemia as an adjunct to other lipid-lowering treatments (e.g., LDL apheresis) or if such treatments are unavailable.

1.3 Important Limitations of Use

JUVISYNC should not be used in patients with type 1 diabetes or for the treatment of diabetic ketoacidosis, as it would not be effective in these settings.

JUVISYNC has not been studied in patients with a history of pancreatitis. It is unknown whether patients with a history of pancreatitis are at increased risk for the development of pancreatitis while using JUVISYNC. *[See Warnings and Precautions (5.1).]*

JUVISYNC has not been studied in conditions where the major abnormality is elevation of chylomicrons (i.e., hyperlipidemia Fredrickson types I and V).

Because doses of JUVISYNC appropriate for patients with severe renal impairment (CrCl <30 mL/min, approximately corresponding to serum creatinine levels of >3.0 mg/dL in men and >2.5 mg/dL in women) or end-stage renal disease (ESRD) are not available in this combination product, JUVISYNC is not recommended in patients with severe renal impairment or ESRD.

2 DOSAGE AND ADMINISTRATION

2.1 Recommended Dosing

The dosages for therapy with JUVISYNC are 100 mg/10 mg, 100 mg/20 mg, 100 mg/40 mg, 50 mg/10 mg, 50 mg/20 mg, and 50 mg/40 mg (sitagliptin/simvastatin) once daily. JUVISYNC should be taken as a single daily dose in the evening. JUVISYNC must not be split or divided before swallowing.

The recommended starting dose is 100 mg/40 mg per day. For patients already taking simvastatin (10, 20, or 40 mg daily) with or without sitagliptin 100 mg daily, JUVISYNC may be initiated at the dose of 100 mg sitagliptin and the dose of simvastatin already being taken.

After initiation or titration of JUVISYNC, lipid levels may be analyzed after 4 or more weeks and dosage adjusted, if needed.

2.2 Patients with Renal Impairment

JUVISYNC is not recommended in patients with severe renal impairment or ESRD. JUVISYNC can be used in patients with normal renal function or mild renal impairment (creatinine clearance [CrCl] greater than or equal to 50 mL/min, approximately corresponding to serum creatinine levels of less than or equal to 1.7 mg/dL in men and less than or equal to 1.5 mg/dL in women), without adjustment of the sitagliptin dose. Because simvastatin does not undergo significant renal excretion, modification of the dose of the simvastatin component should not be necessary in patients with mild renal impairment.

For patients with moderate renal impairment (CrCl greater than or equal to 30 to less than 50 mL/min, approximately corresponding to serum creatinine levels of greater than 1.7 to less than or equal to 3.0 mg/dL in men and greater than 1.5 to less than or equal to 2.5 mg/dL in women), the recommended starting dose of JUVISYNC is 50 mg/40 mg once daily. For patients with moderate renal impairment who are already taking simvastatin (10, 20, or 40 mg daily) with or without sitagliptin 50 mg daily, JUVISYNC may be initiated at the dose of 50 mg sitagliptin and the dose of simvastatin already being taken.

Assessment of renal function is recommended prior to initiation of JUVISYNC and periodically thereafter. Creatinine clearance can be estimated from serum creatinine using the Cockcroft-Gault formula. *[See Warnings and Precautions (5.4); Clinical Pharmacology (12.3).]* There have been postmarketing reports of worsening renal function in patients with renal impairment treated with sitagliptin, some of whom were prescribed inappropriate doses of sitagliptin.

2.3 Concomitant Use with an Insulin Secretagogue (e.g., Sulfonylurea) or with Insulin

When JUVISYNC is used in combination with an insulin secretagogue (e.g., sulfonylurea) or with insulin, a lower dose of the insulin secretagogue or insulin may be required to reduce the risk of hypoglycemia. *[See Warnings and Precautions (5.5).]*

2.4 Coadministration with Other Drugs

Patients taking Verapamil, Diltiazem, or Dronedarone

- The dose of simvastatin should not exceed 10 mg per day (100 mg/10 mg or 50 mg/10 mg per day of JUVISYNC) *[see Warnings and Precautions (5.2); Drug Interactions (7.3); Clinical Pharmacology (12.3)].*

Patients taking Amiodarone, Amlodipine or Ranolazine

- The dose of simvastatin should not exceed 20 mg per day (100 mg/20 mg or 50 mg/20 mg per day of JUVISYNC) *[see Warnings and Precautions (5.2); Drug Interactions (7.3); Clinical Pharmacology (12.3)].*

2.5 Patients with Homozygous Familial Hypercholesterolemia

The recommended dosage is 100 mg/40 mg (for patients with normal or mildly impaired renal function) or 50 mg/40 mg (for patients with moderately impaired renal function) per day in the evening. JUVISYNC should be used as an adjunct to other lipid-lowering treatments (e.g., LDL apheresis) in these patients or if such treatments are unavailable.

2.6 Chinese Patients Taking Lipid-Modifying Doses (greater than or equal to 1 g/day Niacin) of Niacin-Containing Products

Because of an increased risk for myopathy in Chinese patients taking simvastatin 40 mg coadministered with lipid-modifying doses (greater than or equal to 1 g/day niacin) of niacin-containing products, caution should be used when treating Chinese patients with JUVISYNC 100 mg/40 mg or 50 mg/40 mg per day coadministered with lipid-modifying doses of niacin-containing products. The cause of the increased risk of myopathy is not known. It is also unknown if the risk for myopathy with coadministration of JUVISYNC with lipid-modifying doses of niacin-containing products observed in Chinese patients applies to other Asian patients. *[See Warnings and Precautions (5.2).]*

3 DOSAGE FORMS AND STRENGTHS

- JUVISYNC 100 mg/10 mg tablets are pink-beige, biconvex round, film-coated tablets, coded with the Merck logo and "753" on one side and plain on the other.

- JUVISYNC 100 mg/20 mg tablets are pink-beige, biconvex modified capsule-shaped, film-coated tablets, coded with the Merck logo and "757" on one side and plain on the other.
- JUVISYNC 100 mg/40 mg tablets are orange-beige, biconvex modified capsule-shaped, film-coated tablets, coded with the Merck logo and "773" on one side and plain on the other.
- JUVISYNC 50 mg/10 mg tablets are red, bi-convex modified capsule-shaped, film-coated tablets, coded with the Merck logo and "533" on one side and plain on the other.
- JUVISYNC 50 mg/20 mg tablets are orange-beige, biconvex modified capsule-shaped, film-coated tablets, coded with the Merck logo and "535" on one side and plain on the other.
- JUVISYNC 50 mg/40 mg tablets are red, bi-convex modified capsule-shaped, film-coated tablets, coded with the Merck logo and "537" on one side and plain on the other.

4 CONTRAINDICATIONS

JUVISYNC is contraindicated in the following conditions:

- History of a serious hypersensitivity reaction, such as anaphylaxis or angioedema, to any component of this medication. *[See Warnings and Precautions (5.6); Adverse Reactions (6.2).]*
- Concomitant administration of strong CYP3A4 inhibitors (e.g., itraconazole, ketoconazole, posaconazole, voriconazole, HIV protease inhibitors, boceprevir, telaprevir, erythromycin, clarithromycin, telithromycin and nefazodone) *[see Warnings and Precautions (5.2)]*.
- Concomitant administration of gemfibrozil, cyclosporine, or danazol *[see Warnings and Precautions (5.2)]*.
- Active liver disease, which may include unexplained persistent elevations in hepatic transaminase levels *[see Warnings and Precautions (5.3)]*.
- Women who are pregnant or may become pregnant. Serum cholesterol and triglycerides increase during normal pregnancy, and cholesterol or cholesterol derivatives are essential for fetal development. Because HMG-CoA reductase inhibitors (statins) decrease cholesterol synthesis and possibly the synthesis of other biologically active substances derived from cholesterol, simvastatin may cause fetal harm when administered to a pregnant woman. Atherosclerosis is a chronic process and the discontinuation of lipid-lowering drugs during pregnancy should have little impact on the outcome of long-term therapy of primary hypercholesterolemia. There are no adequate and well-controlled studies of use with JUVISYNC during pregnancy; however, in rare reports congenital anomalies were observed following intrauterine exposure to statins. In rat and rabbit animal reproduction studies, simvastatin revealed no evidence of teratogenicity. **JUVISYNC should be administered to women of childbearing age only when such patients are highly unlikely to conceive.** If the patient becomes pregnant while taking this drug, JUVISYNC should be discontinued immediately and the patient should be apprised of the potential hazard to the fetus *[see Use in Specific Populations (8.1)]*.
- Nursing mothers. Because statins have the potential for serious adverse reactions in nursing infants, women who require treatment with JUVISYNC should not breastfeed their infants. A small amount of another drug in the statin class passes into breast milk. It is not known whether simvastatin is excreted into human milk *[see Use in Specific Populations (8.3)]*.

5 WARNINGS AND PRECAUTIONS

5.1 Pancreatitis

There have been postmarketing reports of acute pancreatitis, including fatal and non-fatal hemorrhagic or necrotizing pancreatitis, in patients taking sitagliptin. After initiation of JUVISYNC, patients should be observed carefully for signs and symptoms of pancreatitis. If pancreatitis is suspected, JUVISYNC should promptly be discontinued and appropriate management should be initiated. It is unknown whether patients with a history of pancreatitis are at increased risk for the development of pancreatitis while using JUVISYNC. *[See also Adverse Reactions (6.2).]*

5.2 Myopathy/Rhabdomyolysis

Simvastatin occasionally causes myopathy manifested as muscle pain, tenderness or weakness with creatine kinase (CK) above ten times the upper limit of normal (ULN). Myopathy sometimes takes the form of rhabdomyolysis with or without acute renal failure secondary to myoglobinuria, and rare fatalities have occurred. The risk of myopathy is increased by high levels of statin activity in plasma. Predisposing factors for myopathy include advanced age (≥65 years), female gender, uncontrolled hypothyroidism, and renal impairment.

The risk of myopathy, including rhabdomyolysis, is dose related. In a clinical trial database in which 41,413 patients were treated with simvastatin, 24,747 (approximately 60%) of whom were enrolled in studies with a median follow-up of at least 4 years, the incidence of myopathy was approximately 0.03% and 0.08% at 20 and 40 mg/day, respectively. The incidence of myopathy with 80 mg (0.61%) was disproportionately higher than that observed at the lower doses. In these trials, patients were carefully monitored and some interacting medicinal products were excluded.

In a clinical trial in which 12,064 patients with a history of myocardial infarction were treated with simvastatin (mean follow-up 6.7 years), the incidence of myopathy (defined as unexplained muscle weakness or pain with a serum creatine kinase [CK] >10 times upper limit of normal [ULN]) in patients on 20 mg/day was approximately 0.02%; in patients treated with 80 mg/day, the incidence was 0.9%. The incidence of rhabdomyolysis (defined as myopathy with a CK >40 times ULN) in patients on 20 mg/day was 0%; in patients on 80 mg/day, the incidence was approximately 0.4%. The incidence of myopathy, including rhabdomyolysis, was highest during the first year and then notably decreased during the subsequent years of treatment. In this trial, patients were carefully monitored and some interacting medicinal products were excluded.

There have been rare reports of immune-mediated necrotizing myopathy (IMNM), an autoimmune myopathy, associated with statin use. IMNM is characterized by: proximal muscle weakness and elevated serum creatine kinase, which persist despite discontinuation of statin treatment; muscle biopsy showing necrotizing myopathy without significant inflammation; improvement with immunosuppressive agents.

All patients starting therapy with JUVISYNC, or whose dose of JUVISYNC is being increased, should be advised of the risk of myopathy, including rhabdomyolysis, and told to report promptly any unexplained muscle pain, tenderness or weakness particularly if accompanied by malaise or fever or if muscle signs and symptoms persist after discontinuing JUVISYNC. JUVISYNC therapy should be discontinued immediately if myopathy is diagnosed or suspected. In most cases, muscle symptoms and CK increases resolved when treatment was promptly discontinued. Periodic CK determinations may be considered in patients starting therapy with JUVISYNC or whose dose is being increased, but there is no assurance that such monitoring will prevent myopathy.

Many of the patients who have developed rhabdomyolysis on therapy with simvastatin have had complicated medical histories, including renal impairment usually as a consequence of long-standing diabetes mellitus. Such patients merit closer monitoring. JUVISYNC therapy should be discontinued if markedly elevated CPK levels occur or myopathy is diagnosed or suspected. JUVISYNC therapy should also be temporarily withheld in any patient experiencing an acute or serious condition predisposing to the development of renal failure secondary to rhabdomyolysis, e.g., sepsis; hypotension; major surgery; trauma; severe metabolic, endocrine, or electrolyte disorders; or uncontrolled epilepsy.

Drug Interactions

The risk of myopathy and rhabdomyolysis is increased by high levels of statin activity in plasma. Simvastatin is metabolized by the cytochrome P450 isoform 3A4. Certain drugs which inhibit this metabolic pathway can raise the plasma levels of simvastatin and may increase the risk of myopathy. These include itraconazole, ketoconazole, posaconazole, and voriconazole, the macrolide antibiotics erythromycin and clarithromycin, the ketolide antibiotic telithromycin, HIV protease inhibitors, boceprevir, telaprevir, the antidepressant nefazodone, and grapefruit juice *[see Clinical Pharmacology (12.3)]*. Combination of these drugs with JUVISYNC is contraindicated. If short-term treatment with strong CYP3A4 inhibitors is unavoidable, therapy with JUVISYNC must be suspended during the course of treatment. *[See Contraindications (4); Drug Interactions (7.1).]*

The combined use of JUVISYNC with gemfibrozil, cyclosporine, or danazol is contraindicated *[see Contraindications (4); Drug Interactions (7.1, 7.2)]*.

Caution should be used when prescribing other fibrates with JUVISYNC, as these agents can cause myopathy when given alone and the risk is increased when they are coadministered *[see Drug Interactions (7.2)]*.

Cases of myopathy, including rhabdomyolysis, have been reported with simvastatin coadministered with colchicine, and caution should be exercised when prescribing JUVISYNC with colchicine *[see Drug Interactions (7.7)]*.

The benefits of the combined use of JUVISYNC with the following drugs should be carefully weighed against the potential risks of combinations: amiodarone, dronedarone, verapamil, diltiazem, amlodipine, ranolazine and lipid-lowering drugs other than gemfibrozil (other fibrates or ≥1 g/day of niacin), *[see Drug Interactions (7.2, 7.3, 7.4); Table 6 in Clinical Pharmacology (12.3)]*.

Cases of myopathy, including rhabdomyolysis, have been observed with simvastatin coadministered with lipid-modifying doses (≥1 g/day niacin) of niacin-containing products. In an ongoing, double-blind, randomized cardiovascular outcomes trial, an independent safety monitoring committee identified that the incidence of myopathy is higher in Chinese compared with non-Chinese patients taking simvastatin 40 mg coadministered with lipid-modifying doses of a niacin-containing product. Caution should be used when treating Chinese patients with JUVISYNC 100 mg/40 mg or 50 mg/40 mg per day coadministered with lipid-modifying doses of niacin-containing products. It is unknown if the risk for myopathy with coadministration of JUVISYNC with lipid-modifying doses of niacin-containing products observed in Chinese patients applies to other Asian patients *[see Drug Interactions (7.4)]*.

Prescribing recommendations for interacting agents are summarized in Table 1 *[see also Dosage and Administration (2.4); Drug Interactions (7.1, 7.2, 7.3); Clinical Pharmacology (12.3)]*.

Table 1: Drug Interactions Associated with Increased Risk of Myopathy/Rhabdomyolysis

Interacting Agents	Prescribing Recommendations
Strong CYP3A4 Inhibitors, e.g.: Itraconazole, Ketoconazole, Posaconazole, Voriconazole, Erythromycin, Clarithromycin, Telithromycin, HIV protease inhibitors, Boceprevir, Telaprevir, Nefazodone Gemfibrozil Cyclosporine Danazol	Contraindicated with JUVISYNC
Verapamil Diltiazem Dronedarone	Do not exceed 10 mg simvastatin (100 mg/10 mg or 50 mg/10 mg JUVISYNC) daily
Amiodarone Amlodipine Ranolazine	Do not exceed 20 mg simvastatin (100 mg/20 mg or 50 mg/20 mg JUVISYNC) daily
Grapefruit juice	Avoid grapefruit juice

5.3 Liver Dysfunction

Persistent increases (to more than 3× the ULN) in serum transaminases have occurred in approximately 1% of patients who received simvastatin in clinical studies. When drug treatment was interrupted or discontinued in these patients, the transaminase levels usually fell slowly to pretreatment levels. The increases were not associated with jaundice or other clinical signs or symptoms. There was no evidence of hypersensitivity.

In the Scandinavian Simvastatin Survival Study (4S) *[see Clinical Studies (14.2)]*, the number of patients with more than one transaminase elevation to >3× ULN, over the course of the study, was not significantly different between the simvastatin and placebo groups (14 [0.7%] vs. 12 [0.6%]). Elevated transaminases resulted in the discontinuation of 8 patients from therapy in the simvastatin group (n=2221) and 5 in the placebo group (n=2223). Of the 1986 simvastatin treated patients in 4S with normal liver function tests (LFTs) at baseline, 8 (0.4%) developed consecutive LFT elevations to >3× ULN and/or were discontinued due to transaminase elevations during the 5.4 years (median follow-up) of the study. Among these 8 patients, 5 initially developed these abnormalities within the first year. All of the patients in this study received a starting dose of 20 mg of simvastatin; 37% were titrated to 40 mg.

In 2 controlled clinical studies in 1105 patients, the 12-month incidence of persistent hepatic transaminase elevation without regard to drug relationship was 0.9% and 2.1% at the 40 and 80 mg dose, respectively. No patients developed persistent liver function abnormalities following the initial 6 months of treatment at a given dose.

It is recommended that liver function tests be performed before the initiation of treatment, and thereafter when clinically indicated. There have been rare postmarketing reports of fatal and non-fatal hepatic failure in patients taking statins, including simvastatin. If serious liver injury with clinical symptoms and/or hyperbilirubinemia or jaundice occurs during treatment with JUVISYNC, promptly interrupt therapy. If an alternate etiology is not found do not restart JUVISYNC. Note that ALT may emanate from muscle, therefore ALT rising with CK may indicate myopathy *[see Warnings and Precautions (5.2)]*.

The drug should be used with caution in patients who consume substantial quantities of alcohol and/or have a past history of liver disease. Active liver diseases or unexplained transaminase elevations are contraindications to the use of JUVISYNC.

Table 3: Initial Therapy with Combination of Sitagliptin and Metformin: Adverse Reactions Reported (Regardless of Investigator Assessment of Causality) in ≥5% of Patients Receiving Combination Therapy (and Greater than in Patients Receiving Metformin alone, Sitagliptin alone, and Placebo)*

	Number of Patients (%)			
	Placebo	Sitagliptin 100 mg QD	Metformin 500 or 1000 mg bid†	Sitagliptin 50 mg bid + Metformin 500 or 1000 mg bid†
	N = 176	N = 179	N = 364†	N = 372†
Upper Respiratory Infection	9 (5.1)	8 (4.5)	19 (5.2)	23 (6.2)
Headache	5 (2.8)	2 (1.1)	14 (3.8)	22 (5.9)

* Intent-to-treat population.
† Data pooled for the patients given the lower and higher doses of metformin.

As with other lipid-lowering agents, moderate (less than 3× ULN) elevations of serum transaminases have been reported following therapy with simvastatin. These changes appeared soon after initiation of therapy with simvastatin, were often transient, were not accompanied by any symptoms and did not require interruption of treatment. *[See also Adverse Reactions (6.1).]*

5.4 Renal Impairment

Assessment of renal function is recommended prior to initiating JUVISYNC and periodically thereafter. JUVISYNC is not recommended for use in patients with severe renal impairment or ESRD because doses of JUVISYNC appropriate for patients with severe renal impairment or ESRD are not available in this combination product. *[See Dosage and Administration (2.2); Clinical Pharmacology (12.3).]*

A dosage adjustment is recommended in patients with moderate renal impairment. *[See Dosage and Administration (2.2); Clinical Pharmacology (12.3).]* Caution should be used to ensure that the correct dose of JUVISYNC is prescribed for patients with moderate renal impairment (creatinine clearance ≥30 to <50 mL/min).

There have been postmarketing reports of worsening renal function, including acute renal failure, sometimes requiring dialysis, in patients treated with sitagliptin. A subset of these reports involved patients with renal impairment, some of whom were prescribed inappropriate doses of sitagliptin. A return to baseline levels of renal impairment has been observed with supportive treatment and discontinuation of potentially causative agents.

Sitagliptin has not been found to be nephrotoxic in preclinical studies at clinically relevant doses, or in clinical trials.

5.5 Use with Medications Known to Cause Hypoglycemia

When sitagliptin was used in combination with a sulfonylurea or with insulin, medications known to cause hypoglycemia, the incidence of hypoglycemia was increased over that of placebo used in combination with a sulfonylurea or with insulin. *[See Adverse Reactions (6.1).]* Therefore, a lower dose of sulfonylurea or insulin may be required to reduce the risk of hypoglycemia. *[See Dosage and Administration (2.3).]*

5.6 Hypersensitivity Reactions

[See also Adverse Reactions (6.2).]

There have been postmarketing reports of serious hypersensitivity reactions in patients treated with sitagliptin. These reactions include anaphylaxis, angioedema, and exfoliative skin conditions including Stevens-Johnson syndrome. Onset of these reactions occurred within the first 3 months after initiation of treatment with sitagliptin, with some reports occurring after the first dose.

If a hypersensitivity reaction is suspected, discontinue JUVISYNC, assess for other potential causes for the event, and institute alternative treatment.

Angioedema has also been reported with other dipeptidyl peptidase-4 (DPP-4) inhibitors. Use caution in a patient with a history of angioedema with another DPP-4 inhibitor because it is unknown whether such patients will be predisposed to angioedema with JUVISYNC.

5.7 Endocrine Function

Increases in A1C and fasting serum glucose levels have been reported with HMG-CoA reductase inhibitors, including simvastatin.

6 ADVERSE REACTIONS

6.1 Clinical Trials Experience

JUVISYNC

Because clinical trials are conducted under widely varying conditions, adverse reaction rates observed in the clinical trials of a drug cannot be directly compared to rates in the clinical trials of another drug and may not reflect the rates observed in practice.

In a pooled subgroup analysis of 19 controlled clinical studies of sitagliptin involving 1582 patients whose background therapy included simvastatin, incidences of adverse reactions for patients treated with sitagliptin and simvastatin (n=827) were similar to those for patients treated with control therapy (placebo or active comparator) and simvastatin (n=755). Among these patients, 3.3% of the sitagliptin-treated group and 4.2% of controls discontinued due to adverse reactions.

Sitagliptin

In controlled clinical studies as both monotherapy and combination therapy with metformin, pioglitazone, or rosiglitazone and metformin, the overall incidence of adverse reactions, hypoglycemia, and discontinuation of therapy due to clinical adverse reactions with sitagliptin were similar to placebo. In combination with glimepiride, with or without metformin, the overall incidence of clinical adverse reactions with sitagliptin was higher than with placebo, in part related to a higher incidence of hypoglycemia (see Table 4); the incidence of discontinuation due to clinical adverse reactions was similar to placebo.

Two placebo-controlled monotherapy studies, one of 18- and one of 24-week duration, included patients treated with sitagliptin 100 mg daily, sitagliptin 200 mg daily, and placebo. Five placebo-controlled add-on combination therapy studies were also conducted: one with metformin; one with pioglitazone; one with metformin and rosiglitazone; one with glimepiride (with or without metformin); and one with insulin (with or without metformin). In these trials, patients with inadequate glycemic control on a stable dose of the background therapy were randomized to add-on therapy with sitagliptin 100 mg daily or placebo. The adverse reactions, excluding hypoglycemia, reported regardless of investigator assessment of causality in ≥5% of patients treated with sitagliptin 100 mg daily and more commonly than in patients treated with placebo, are shown in Table 2 for the clinical trials of at least 18 weeks duration. Incidences of hypoglycemia are shown in Table 4.

Table 2: Placebo-Controlled Clinical Studies of Sitagliptin Monotherapy or Add-on Combination Therapy with Pioglitazone, Metformin + Rosiglitazone, or Glimepiride +/- Metformin: Adverse Reactions (Excluding Hypoglycemia) Reported in ≥5% of Patients and More Commonly than in Patients Given Placebo, Regardless of Investigator Assessment of Causality*

	Number of Patients (%)	
Monotherapy (18 or 24 weeks)	**Sitagliptin 100 mg**	**Placebo**
	N = 443	N = 363
Nasopharyngitis	23 (5.2)	12 (3.3)
Combination with Pioglitazone (24 weeks)	**Sitagliptin 100 mg + Pioglitazone**	**Placebo + Pioglitazone**
	N = 175	N = 178
Upper Respiratory Tract Infection	11 (6.3)	6 (3.4)
Headache	9 (5.1)	7 (3.9)
Combination with Metformin + Rosiglitazone (18 weeks)	**Sitagliptin 100 mg + Metformin + Rosiglitazone**	**Placebo + Metformin + Rosiglitazone**
	N = 181	N = 97
Upper Respiratory Tract Infection	10 (5.5)	5 (5.2)
Nasopharyngitis	11 (6.1)	4 (4.1)
Combination with Glimepiride (+/- Metformin) (24 weeks)	**Sitagliptin 100 mg + Glimepiride (+/- Metformin)**	**Placebo + Glimepiride (+/- Metformin)**
	N = 222	N = 219
Nasopharyngitis	14 (6.3)	10 (4.6)
Headache	13 (5.9)	5 (2.3)

* Intent-to-treat population

In the 24-week study of patients receiving sitagliptin as add-on combination therapy with metformin, there were no adverse reactions reported regardless of investigator assessment of causality in ≥5% of patients and more commonly than in patients given placebo.

In the 24-week study of patients receiving sitagliptin as add-on therapy to insulin (with or without metformin), there were no adverse reactions reported regardless of investigator assessment of causality in ≥5% of patients and more commonly than in patients given placebo, except for hypoglycemia (see Table 4).

In the study of sitagliptin as add-on combination therapy with metformin and rosiglitazone (Table 2), through Week 54 the adverse reactions reported regardless of investigator assessment of causality in ≥5% of patients treated with sitagliptin and more commonly than in patients treated with placebo were: upper respiratory tract infection (sitagliptin, 15.5%; placebo, 6.2%), nasopharyngitis (11.0%, 9.3%), peripheral edema (8.3%, 5.2%), and headache (5.5%, 4.1%).

In a pooled analysis of the two monotherapy studies, the add-on to metformin study, and the add-on to pioglitazone study, the incidence of selected gastrointestinal adverse reactions in patients treated with sitagliptin was as follows: abdominal pain (sitagliptin 100 mg, 2.3%; placebo, 2.1%), nausea (1.4%, 0.6%), and diarrhea (3.0%, 2.3%).

In an additional, 24-week, placebo-controlled factorial study of initial therapy with sitagliptin in combination with metformin, the adverse reactions reported (regardless of investigator assessment of causality) in ≥5% of patients are shown in Table 3.

[See table 3 above]

In a 24-week study of initial therapy with sitagliptin in combination with pioglitazone, there were no adverse reactions reported (regardless of investigator assessment of causality) in ≥5% of patients and more commonly than in patients given pioglitazone alone.

No clinically meaningful changes in vital signs or in ECG (including in QTc interval) were observed in patients treated with sitagliptin.

In a pooled analysis of 19 double-blind clinical trials that included data from 10,246 patients randomized to receive sitagliptin 100 mg/day (N=5429) or corresponding (active or placebo) control (N=4817), the incidence of acute pancreatitis was 0.1 per 100 patient-years in each group (4 patients with an event in 4708 patient-years for sitagliptin and 4 patients with an event in 3942 patient-years for control). *[See Warnings and Precautions (5.1).]*

Hypoglycemia

In the sitagliptin clinical trial program, adverse reactions of hypoglycemia were based on all reports of symptomatic hypoglycemia. A concurrent blood glucose measurement was not required although most (74%) reports of hypoglycemia were accompanied by a blood glucose measurement ≤70 mg/dL. When sitagliptin was coadministered with a sulfonylurea or with insulin, the percentage of patients with at least one adverse reaction of hypoglycemia was higher than in the corresponding placebo group (Table 4).

Table 4: Incidence and Rate of Hypoglycemia* in Placebo-Controlled Clinical Studies when Sitagliptin was used as Add-On Therapy to Glimepiride (with or without Metformin) or Insulin (with or without Metformin), Regardless of Investigator Assessment of Causality

Add-On to Glimepiride (+/- Metformin) (24 weeks)	**Sitagliptin 100 mg + Glimepiride (+/- Metformin)**	**Placebo + Glimepiride (+/- Metformin)**
	N = 222	N = 219
Overall (%)	27 (12.2)	4 (1.8)
Rate (episodes/ patient-year)†	0.59	0.24
Severe (%)‡	0 (0.0)	0 (0.0)

Add-On to Insulin (+/- Metformin) (24 weeks)	Sitagliptin 100 mg + Insulin (+/- Metformin)	Placebo + Insulin (+/- Metformin)
	N = 322	N = 319
Overall (%)	50 (15.5)	25 (7.8)
Rate (episodes/ patient-year)†	1.06	0.51
Severe (%)‡	2 (0.6)	1 (0.3)

* Adverse reactions of hypoglycemia were based on all reports of symptomatic hypoglycemia; a concurrent glucose measurement was not required; intent-to-treat population.
† Based on total number of events (i.e., a single patient may have had multiple events).
‡ Severe events of hypoglycemia were defined as those events requiring medical assistance or exhibiting depressed level/loss of consciousness or seizure.

In a pooled analysis of the two monotherapy studies, the add-on to metformin study, and the add-on to pioglitazone study, the overall incidence of adverse reactions of hypoglycemia was 1.2% in patients treated with sitagliptin 100 mg and 0.9% in patients treated with placebo.

In the study of sitagliptin as add-on combination therapy with metformin and rosiglitazone, the overall incidence of hypoglycemia was 2.2% in patients given add-on sitagliptin and 0.0% in patients given add-on placebo through Week 18. Through Week 54, the overall incidence of hypoglycemia was 3.9% in patients given add-on sitagliptin and 1.0% in patients given add-on placebo.

In the 24-week, placebo-controlled factorial study of initial therapy with sitagliptin in combination with metformin, the incidence of hypoglycemia was 0.6% in patients given placebo, 0.6% in patients given sitagliptin alone, 0.8% in patients given metformin alone, and 1.6% in patients given sitagliptin in combination with metformin.

In the study of sitagliptin as initial therapy with pioglitazone, one patient taking sitagliptin experienced a severe episode of hypoglycemia. There were no severe hypoglycemia episodes reported in other studies except in the study involving coadministration with insulin.

Simvastatin

In the pre-marketing controlled clinical studies and their open-label extensions (2423 patients with median duration of follow-up of approximately 18 months), 1.4% of patients were discontinued due to adverse reactions. The most common adverse reactions that led to treatment discontinuation were: gastrointestinal disorders (0.5%), myalgia (0.1%), and arthralgia (0.1%). The most commonly reported adverse reactions (incidence ≥5%) in simvastatin controlled clinical trials were: upper respiratory infections (9.0%), headache (7.4%), abdominal pain (7.3%), constipation (6.6%), and nausea (5.4%).

Scandinavian Simvastatin Survival Study

In 4S involving 4444 patients (age range 35-71 years, 19% women, 100% Caucasians) treated with 20-40 mg/day of simvastatin (n=2221) or placebo (n=2223) over a median of 5.4 years, adverse reactions reported in ≥2% of patients and at a rate greater than placebo are shown in Table 5.

Table 5: Adverse Reactions Reported Regardless of Causality by ≥2% of Patients Treated with Simvastatin and Greater than Placebo in 4S

	Simvastatin (N = 2221) %	Placebo (N = 2223) %
Body as a Whole		
Edema/swelling	2.7	2.3
Abdominal pain	5.9	5.8
Cardiovascular System Disorders		
Atrial fibrillation	5.7	5.1
Digestive System Disorders		
Constipation	2.2	1.6
Gastritis	4.9	3.9
Endocrine Disorders		
Diabetes mellitus	4.2	3.6
Musculoskeletal Disorders		
Myalgia	3.7	3.2
Nervous System / Psychiatric Disorders		
Headache	2.5	2.1
Insomnia	4.0	3.8
Vertigo	4.5	4.2
Respiratory System Disorders		
Bronchitis	6.6	6.3
Sinusitis	2.3	1.8
Skin / Skin Appendage Disorders		
Eczema	4.5	3.0
Urogenital System Disorders		
Infection, urinary tract	3.2	3.1

Heart Protection Study

In the Heart Protection Study (HPS), involving 20,536 patients (age range 40-80 years, 25% women, 97% Caucasians, 3% other races) treated with simvastatin 40 mg/day (n=10,269) or placebo (n=10,267) over a mean of 5 years, only serious adverse reactions and discontinuations due to any adverse reactions were recorded. Discontinuation rates due to adverse reactions were 4.8% in patients treated with simvastatin compared with 5.1% in patients treated with placebo. The incidence of myopathy/rhabdomyolysis was <0.1% in patients treated with simvastatin.

Other Clinical Studies

In a clinical trial in which 12,064 patients with a history of myocardial infarction were treated with simvastatin (mean follow-up 6.7 years), the incidence of myopathy (defined as unexplained muscle weakness or pain with a serum creatine kinase [CK] >10 times upper limit of normal [ULN]) in patients on 20 mg/day was approximately 0.02%; in patients treated with 80 mg/day, the incidence was 0.9%. The incidence of rhabdomyolysis (defined as myopathy with a CK >40 times ULN) in patients on 20 mg/day was 0%; in patients on 80 mg/day, the incidence was approximately 0.4%. The incidence of myopathy, including rhabdomyolysis, was highest during the first year and then notably decreased during the subsequent years of treatment. In this trial, patients were carefully monitored and some interacting medicinal products were excluded.

Other adverse reactions reported in clinical trials were: diarrhea, rash, dyspepsia, flatulence, and asthenia.

Laboratory Tests

Sitagliptin

Across clinical studies, the incidence of laboratory adverse reactions was similar in patients treated with sitagliptin 100 mg compared to patients treated with placebo. A small increase in white blood cell count (WBC) was observed due to an increase in neutrophils. This increase in WBC (of approximately 200 cells/microL vs placebo, in four pooled placebo-controlled clinical studies, with a mean baseline WBC count of approximately 6600 cells/microL) is not considered to be clinically relevant. In a 12-week study of 91 patients with chronic renal impairment, 37 patients with moderate renal impairment were randomized to sitagliptin 50 mg daily, while 14 patients with the same magnitude of renal impairment were randomized to placebo. Mean (SE) increases in serum creatinine were observed in patients treated with sitagliptin [0.12 mg/dL (0.04)] and in patients treated with placebo [0.07 mg/dL (0.07)]. The clinical significance of this added increase in serum creatinine relative to placebo is not known.

Simvastatin

Marked persistent increases of hepatic transaminases have been noted *[see Warnings and Precautions (5.3)]*. Elevated alkaline phosphatase and γ-glutamyl transpeptidase have also been reported. About 5% of patients had elevations of CK levels of 3 or more times the normal value on one or more occasions. This was attributable to the noncardiac fraction of CK. *[See Warnings and Precautions (5.2).]*

6.2 Postmarketing Experience

Additional adverse reactions have been identified during postapproval use of sitagliptin (as monotherapy and/or in combination with other antihyperglycemic agents) or simvastatin. Because these reactions are reported voluntarily from a population of uncertain size, it is generally not possible to reliably estimate their frequency or establish a causal relationship to drug exposure.

Anemia; depression; headache; dizziness; paresthesia; peripheral neuropathy; interstitial lung disease; pancreatitis; acute pancreatitis, including fatal and non-fatal hemorrhagic and necrotizing pancreatitis *[see Indications and Usage (1.3); Warnings and Precautions (5.1)]*; constipation; vomiting; hepatitis/jaundice; fatal and non-fatal hepatic failure; hepatic enzyme elevations; pruritus; alopecia; a variety of skin changes (e.g., nodules, discoloration, dryness of skin/mucous membranes, changes to hair/nails); muscle cramps; myalgia; rhabdomyolysis; arthralgia; pain in extremity; back pain; worsening renal function, including acute renal failure (sometimes requiring dialysis); erectile dysfunction.

There have been rare reports of immune-mediated necrotizing myopathy associated with statin use *[see Warnings and Precautions (5.2)]*.

There have been rare postmarketing reports of cognitive impairment (e.g., memory loss, forgetfulness, amnesia, memory impairment, confusion) associated with statin use. These cognitive issues have been reported for all statins. The reports are generally nonserious, and reversible upon statin discontinuation, with variable times to symptom onset (1 day to years) and symptom resolution (median of 3 weeks).

Hypersensitivity reactions including anaphylaxis, angioedema, rash, urticaria, cutaneous vasculitis, and exfoliative skin conditions including Stevens-Johnson syndrome have been reported with sitagliptin *[see Warnings and Precautions (5.6)]*.

An apparent hypersensitivity syndrome has been reported rarely with simvastatin which has included some of the following features: anaphylaxis, angioedema, lupus erythematous-like syndrome, polymyalgia rheumatica, dermatomyositis, vasculitis, purpura, thrombocytopenia, leukopenia, hemolytic anemia, positive ANA, ESR increase, eosinophilia, arthritis, arthralgia, urticaria, asthenia, photosensitivity, fever, chills, flushing, malaise, dyspnea, toxic epidermal necrolysis, erythema multiforme, including Stevens-Johnson syndrome.

7 DRUG INTERACTIONS

[See Clinical Pharmacology (12.3).]

7.1 Strong CYP3A4 Inhibitors, Cyclosporine, or Danazol

Strong CYP3A4 inhibitors: Simvastatin, like several other inhibitors of HMG-CoA reductase, is a substrate of CYP3A4. Simvastatin is metabolized by CYP3A4 but has no CYP3A4 inhibitory activity; therefore it is not expected to affect the plasma concentrations of other drugs metabolized by CYP3A4.

Elevated plasma levels of HMG-CoA reductase inhibitory activity increase the risk of myopathy and rhabdomyolysis, particularly with higher doses of simvastatin. *[See Warnings and Precautions (5.2); Clinical Pharmacology (12.3).]*

Concomitant use of drugs labeled as having a strong inhibitory effect on CYP3A4 is contraindicated *[see Contraindications (4)]*. If treatment with itraconazole, ketoconazole, posaconazole, voriconazole, erythromycin, clarithromycin or telithromycin is unavoidable, therapy with JUVISYNC must be suspended during the course of treatment. If JUVISYNC is suspended during treatment with any of these agents, consideration should be given to the use of sitagliptin to maintain glycemic control until JUVISYNC can be reinstated.

Cyclosporine or Danazol: The risk of myopathy, including rhabdomyolysis, is increased by concomitant administration of cyclosporine or danazol. Therefore, concomitant use of these drugs is contraindicated *[see Contraindications (4); Warnings and Precautions (5.2); Clinical Pharmacology (12.3)]*.

7.2 Lipid-Lowering Drugs That Can Cause Myopathy When Given Alone

Gemfibrozil: Contraindicated with JUVISYNC *[see Contraindications (4); Warnings and Precautions (5.2)]*.

Other fibrates: Caution should be used when prescribing with JUVISYNC *[see Warnings and Precautions (5.2)]*.

7.3 Amiodarone, Dronedarone, Ranolazine, or Calcium Channel Blockers

The risk of myopathy, including rhabdomyolysis, is increased by concomitant administration of amiodarone, dronedarone, ranolazine, or calcium channel blockers such as verapamil, diltiazem, or amlodipine *[see Dosage and Administration (2.4); Warnings and Precautions (5.2); Table 6 in Clinical Pharmacology (12.3)]*.

7.4 Niacin

Cases of myopathy, including rhabdomyolysis, have been observed with simvastatin coadministered with lipid-modifying doses (≥1 g/day niacin) of niacin-containing products. In particular, caution should be used when treating Chinese patients with JUVISYNC 100 mg/40 mg or 50 mg/40 mg coadministered with lipid-modifying doses of niacin-containing products. *[See Warnings and Precautions (5.2); Clinical Pharmacology (12.3).]*

7.5 Digoxin

No dosage adjustment of digoxin or JUVISYNC is recommended. Patients receiving digoxin should be monitored.

7.6 Coumarin Anticoagulants

In two clinical studies, one in normal volunteers and the other in hypercholesterolemic patients, simvastatin 20-40 mg/day modestly potentiated the effect of coumarin anticoagulants: the prothrombin time, reported as International Normalized Ratio (INR), increased from a baseline of 1.7 to 1.8 and from 2.6 to 3.4 in the volunteer and patient studies, respectively. With other statins, clinically evident bleeding and/or increased prothrombin time has been reported in a few patients taking coumarin anticoagulants concomitantly. In such patients, prothrombin time should be determined before starting JUVISYNC and frequently enough during early therapy to ensure that no significant alteration of prothrombin time occurs. Once a stable prothrombin time has been documented, prothrombin times can be monitored at the intervals usually recommended for patients on coumarin anticoagulants. If the dose of JUVISYNC is changed or JUVISYNC is discontinued, the same procedure should be repeated. Simvastatin therapy has not been associated with bleeding or with changes in prothrombin time in patients not taking anticoagulants.

7.7 Colchicine

Cases of myopathy, including rhabdomyolysis, have been reported with simvastatin coadministered with colchicine, and caution should be exercised when prescribing JUVISYNC with colchicine.

8 USE IN SPECIFIC POPULATIONS

8.1 Pregnancy

Pregnancy Category X [See Contraindications (4).]

JUVISYNC

JUVISYNC is contraindicated in women who are or may become pregnant. Lipid-lowering drugs offer no benefit during pregnancy, because cholesterol and cholesterol derivatives are needed for normal fetal development. Atherosclerosis is a chronic process, and discontinuation of lipid-lowering drugs during pregnancy should have little impact on long-term outcomes of primary hypercholesterolemia therapy. There are no adequate and well-controlled studies of use of JUVISYNC during pregnancy; however, there are rare reports of congenital anomalies in infants exposed to statins *in utero*. Animal reproduction studies of simvastatin in rats and rabbits showed no evidence of teratogenicity. Serum cholesterol and triglycerides increase during normal pregnancy, and cholesterol or cholesterol derivatives are essential for fetal development. Because statins decrease cholesterol synthesis and possibly the synthesis of other biologically active substances derived from cholesterol, JUVISYNC may cause fetal harm when administered to a pregnant woman. If JUVISYNC is used during pregnancy or if the patient becomes pregnant while taking this drug, the patient should be apprised of the potential hazard to the fetus.

Women of childbearing potential, who require treatment with JUVISYNC for a lipid disorder, should be advised to use effective contraception. For women trying to conceive, discontinuation of JUVISYNC should be considered. If pregnancy occurs, JUVISYNC should be immediately discontinued.

Sitagliptin

Reproduction studies have been performed in rats and rabbits. Doses of sitagliptin up to 125 mg/kg (approximately 12 times the human exposure at the maximum recommended human dose) did not impair fertility or harm the fetus. There are, however, no adequate and well-controlled studies in pregnant women.

Sitagliptin administered to pregnant female rats and rabbits from gestation day 6 to 20 (organogenesis) was not teratogenic at oral doses up to 250 mg/kg (rats) and 125 mg/kg (rabbits), or approximately 30- and 20-times human exposure at the maximum recommended human dose (MRHD) of 100 mg/day based on AUC comparisons. Higher doses increased the incidence of rib malformations in offspring at 1000 mg/kg, or approximately 100 times human exposure at the MRHD.

Sitagliptin administered to female rats from gestation day 6 to lactation day 21 decreased body weight in male and female offspring at 1000 mg/kg. No functional or behavioral toxicity was observed in offspring of rats.

Placental transfer of sitagliptin administered to pregnant rats was approximately 45% at 2 hours and 80% at 24 hours postdose. Placental transfer of sitagliptin administered to pregnant rabbits was approximately 66% at 2 hours and 30% at 24 hours.

Simvastatin

Simvastatin was not teratogenic in rats or rabbits at doses (25, 10 mg/kg/day, respectively) that resulted in 6 times the human exposure based on mg/m^2 surface area. However, in studies with another structurally-related statin, skeletal malformations were observed in rats and mice.

There are rare reports of congenital anomalies following intrauterine exposure to statins. In a review of approximately 100 prospectively followed pregnancies in women exposed to simvastatin or another structurally related statin, the incidences of congenital anomalies, spontaneous abortions, and fetal deaths/stillbirths did not exceed those expected in the general population. However, the study was only able to exclude a 3- to 4-fold increased risk of congenital anomalies over the background rate. In 89% of these cases, drug treatment was initiated prior to pregnancy and was discontinued during the first trimester when pregnancy was identified.

8.3 Nursing Mothers

JUVISYNC

It is not known whether simvastatin is excreted in human milk. Because a small amount of another drug in the same class as simvastatin is excreted in human milk and because of the potential for serious adverse reactions in nursing infants, women taking JUVISYNC should not nurse their infants. A decision should be made whether to discontinue nursing or discontinue JUVISYNC, taking into account the importance of the drug to the mother *[see Contraindications (4)]*.

Sitagliptin

Sitagliptin is secreted in the milk of lactating rats at a milk to plasma ratio of 4:1. It is not known whether sitagliptin is excreted in human milk.

8.4 Pediatric Use

Safety and effectiveness of JUVISYNC in pediatric patients under 18 years of age have not been established.

8.5 Geriatric Use

JUVISYNC

Because advanced age (≥65 years) is a predisposing factor for myopathy, including rhabdomyolysis, JUVISYNC should be prescribed with caution in the elderly *[see Clinical Pharmacology (12.3)]*.

Sitagliptin is known to be substantially excreted by the kidney. Because elderly patients are more likely to have decreased renal function, it may be useful to assess renal function in these patients prior to initiating dosing and periodically thereafter *[see Dosage and Administration (2.2); Clinical Pharmacology (12.3)]*.

Sitagliptin

Of the total number of subjects (N=3884) in pre-approval clinical safety and efficacy studies of sitagliptin, 725 patients were 65 years and over, while 61 patients were 75 years and over. No overall differences in safety or effectiveness were observed between subjects 65 years and over and younger subjects. While this and other reported clinical experience have not identified differences in responses between the elderly and younger patients, greater sensitivity of some older individuals cannot be ruled out.

Simvastatin

Of the 2423 patients who received simvastatin in Phase III clinical studies and the 10,269 patients in the Heart Protection Study who received simvastatin, 363 (15%) and 5366 (52%), respectively were ≥65 years old. In HPS, 615 (6%) were ≥75 years old. No overall differences in safety or effectiveness were observed between these subjects and younger subjects.

A pharmacokinetic study with simvastatin showed the mean plasma level of statin activity to be approximately 45% higher in elderly patients between 70-78 years of age compared with patients between 18-30 years of age. In 4S, 1021 (23%) of 4444 patients were 65 or older. Lipid-lowering efficacy was at least as great in elderly patients compared with younger patients, and simvastatin significantly reduced total mortality and CHD mortality in elderly patients with a history of CHD. In HPS, 52% of patients were elderly (4891 patients 65-69 years and 5806 patients 70 years or older). The relative risk reductions of CHD death, non-fatal MI, coronary and non-coronary revascularization procedures, and stroke were similar in older and younger patients *[see Clinical Studies (14.2)]*. In HPS, among 32,145 patients entering the active run-in period, there were 2 cases of myopathy/rhabdomyolysis; these patients were aged 67 and 73. Of the 7 cases of myopathy/rhabdomyolysis among 10,269 patients allocated to simvastatin, 4 were aged 65 or more (at baseline), of whom one was over 75. There were no overall differences in safety between older and younger patients in either 4S or HPS.

Because advanced age (≥65 years) is a predisposing factor for myopathy, including rhabdomyolysis, simvastatin should be prescribed with caution in the elderly. In a clinical trial of patients treated with simvastatin 80 mg/day, patients ≥65 years of age had an increased risk of myopathy, including rhabdomyolysis, compared to patients <65 years of age. *[See Warnings and Precautions (5.2); Clinical Pharmacology (12.3).]*

8.6 Renal Impairment

JUVISYNC is not recommended for use in patients with severe renal impairment or ESRD *[see Dosage and Administration (2.2)]*.

8.7 Hepatic Impairment

JUVISYNC is contraindicated in patients with active liver disease which may include unexplained persistent elevations in hepatic transaminase levels *[see Contraindications (4) and Warnings and Precautions (5.3)]*.

10 OVERDOSAGE

Sitagliptin

During controlled clinical trials in healthy subjects, single doses of up to 800 mg sitagliptin were administered. Maximal mean increases in QTc of 8.0 msec were observed in one study at a dose of 800 mg sitagliptin, a mean effect that is not considered clinically important *[see Clinical Pharmacology (12.2)]*. There is no experience with doses above 800 mg in humans. In Phase I multiple-dose studies, there were no dose-related clinical adverse reactions observed with sitagliptin with doses of up to 600 mg per day for periods of up to 10 days and 400 mg per day for up to 28 days.

In the event of an overdose, it is reasonable to employ the usual supportive measures, e.g., remove unabsorbed material from the gastrointestinal tract, employ clinical monitoring (including obtaining an electrocardiogram), and institute supportive therapy as dictated by the patient's clinical status.

Sitagliptin is modestly dialyzable. In clinical studies, approximately 13.5% of the dose was removed over a 3- to 4-hour hemodialysis session. Prolonged hemodialysis may be considered if clinically appropriate. It is not known if sitagliptin is dialyzable by peritoneal dialysis.

Simvastatin

Significant lethality was observed in mice after a single oral dose of 9 g/m^2. No evidence of lethality was observed in rats or dogs treated with doses of 30 and 100 g/m^2, respectively. No specific diagnostic signs were observed in rodents. At these doses the only signs seen in dogs were emesis and mucoid stools.

A few cases of overdosage with simvastatin have been reported; the maximum dose taken was 3.6 g. All patients recovered without sequelae. Supportive measures should be taken in the event of an overdose. The dialyzability of simvastatin and its metabolites in man is not known at present.

11 DESCRIPTION

JUVISYNC Tablets contain sitagliptin phosphate, an orally-active inhibitor of the dipeptidyl peptidase-4 (DPP-4) enzyme, and simvastatin, a lipid-lowering agent that is derived synthetically from a fermentation product of *Aspergillus terreus*.

Sitagliptin phosphate monohydrate is described chemically as 7-[(3*R*)-3-amino-1-oxo-4-(2,4,5-trifluorophenyl)butyl]-5,6,7,8-tetrahydro-3-(trifluoromethyl)-1,2,4-triazolo[4,3-*a*]pyrazine phosphate (1:1) monohydrate.

The empirical formula is $C_{16}H_{15}F_6N_5O \bullet H_3PO_4 \bullet H_2O$ and the molecular weight is 523.32. The structural formula is:

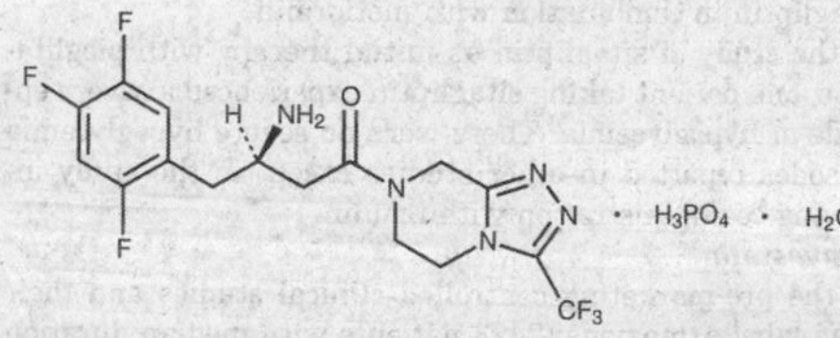

Sitagliptin phosphate monohydrate is a white to off-white, crystalline, non-hygroscopic powder. It is soluble in water and N,N-dimethyl formamide; slightly soluble in methanol; very slightly soluble in ethanol, acetone, and acetonitrile; and insoluble in isopropanol and isopropyl acetate.

After oral ingestion, simvastatin, which is an inactive lactone, is hydrolyzed to the corresponding β-hydroxyacid form. This is an inhibitor of 3-hydroxy-3-methylglutaryl-coenzyme A (HMG-CoA) reductase. This enzyme catalyzes the conversion of HMG-CoA to mevalonate, which is an early and rate-limiting step in the biosynthesis of cholesterol.

Simvastatin is butanoic acid, 2,2-dimethyl-,1,2,3,7,8,8a-hexahydro-3,7-dimethyl-8-[2-(tetrahydro-4-hydroxy-6-oxo-2*H*-pyran-2-yl)-ethyl]-1-naphthalenyl ester, [1*S*-[1α,3α, 7β,8β(2*S**,4*S**),-8aβ]]. The empirical formula of simvastatin is $C_{25}H_{38}O_5$ and its molecular weight is 418.57. Its structural formula is:

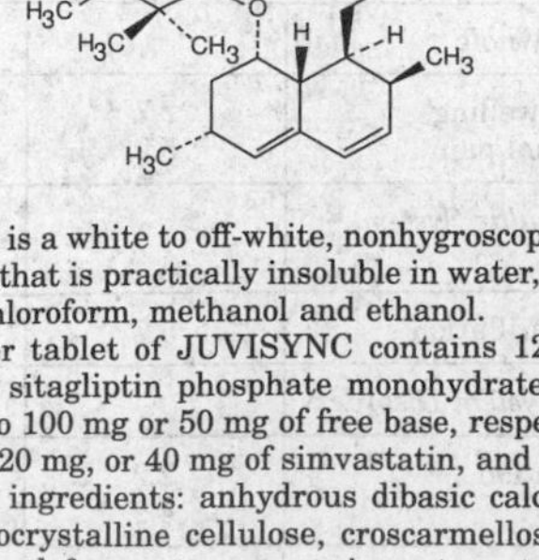

Simvastatin is a white to off-white, nonhygroscopic, crystalline powder that is practically insoluble in water, and freely soluble in chloroform, methanol and ethanol.

Each bilayer tablet of JUVISYNC contains 128.5 mg or 64.25 mg of sitagliptin phosphate monohydrate, which is equivalent to 100 mg or 50 mg of free base, respectively, either 10 mg, 20 mg, or 40 mg of simvastatin, and the following inactive ingredients: anhydrous dibasic calcium phosphate, microcrystalline cellulose, croscarmellose sodium, sodium stearyl fumarate, magnesium stearate, ascorbic acid, citric acid monohydrate, lactose monohydrate, and pre-gelatinized corn starch. In addition, the film coating contains the following inactive ingredients for all tablet strengths: polyvinyl alcohol, polyethylene glycol, talc, titanium dioxide, and red iron oxide. The film coating for the 100 mg/10 mg, 100 mg/20 mg, 100 mg/40 mg, and 50 mg/20 mg tablet strengths also contains yellow iron oxide and black iron oxide. Butylated hydroxyanisole is added as a preservative.

12 CLINICAL PHARMACOLOGY

12.1 Mechanism of Action

Sitagliptin

Sitagliptin is a DPP-4 inhibitor, which is believed to exert its actions in patients with type 2 diabetes by slowing the inactivation of incretin hormones. Concentrations of the active intact hormones are increased by JUVISYNC, thereby increasing and prolonging the action of these hormones. Incretin hormones, including glucagon-like peptide-1 (GLP-1) and glucose-dependent insulinotropic polypeptide (GIP), are released by the intestine throughout the day, and levels are increased in response to a meal. These hormones are rapidly inactivated by the enzyme, DPP-4. The incretins are part of an endogenous system involved in the physiologic regulation of glucose homeostasis. When blood glucose concentrations are normal or elevated, GLP-1 and GIP increase insulin synthesis and release from pancreatic beta cells by intracellular signaling pathways involving cyclic AMP. GLP-1 also lowers glucagon secretion from pancreatic alpha cells, leading to reduced hepatic glucose production. By increasing and prolonging active incretin levels, JUVISYNC increases insulin release and decreases glucagon levels in the circulation in a glucose-dependent manner. Sitagliptin demonstrates selectivity for DPP-4 and does not inhibit DPP-8 or DPP-9 activity *in vitro* at concentrations approximating those from therapeutic doses.

Simvastatin

Simvastatin is a prodrug and is hydrolyzed to its active β-hydroxyacid form, simvastatin acid, after administration. Simvastatin is a specific inhibitor of 3-hydroxy-3-methylglutaryl-coenzyme A (HMG-CoA) reductase, the enzyme that catalyzes the conversion of HMG-CoA to mevalonate, an early and rate limiting step in the biosynthetic pathway for cholesterol. In addition, simvastatin reduces VLDL and TG and increases HDL-C.

12.2 Pharmacodynamics

Sitagliptin

General

In patients with type 2 diabetes, administration of sitagliptin led to inhibition of DPP-4 enzyme activity for a 24-hour period. After an oral glucose load or a meal, this DPP-4 inhibition resulted in a 2- to 3-fold increase in circulating levels of active GLP-1 and GIP, decreased glucagon concentrations, and increased responsiveness of insulin release to glucose, resulting in higher C-peptide and insulin concentrations. The rise in insulin with the decrease in glucagon was associated with lower fasting glucose concentrations and reduced glucose excursion following an oral glucose load or a meal.

In a two-day study in healthy subjects, sitagliptin alone increased active GLP-1 concentrations, whereas metformin alone increased active and total GLP-1 concentrations to similar extents. Coadministration of sitagliptin and metformin had an additive effect on active GLP-1 concentrations. Sitagliptin, but not metformin, increased active GIP concentrations. It is unclear how these findings relate to changes in glycemic control in patients with type 2 diabetes.

In studies with healthy subjects, sitagliptin did not lower blood glucose or cause hypoglycemia.

Cardiac Electrophysiology

In a randomized, placebo-controlled crossover study, 79 healthy subjects were administered a single oral dose of sitagliptin 100 mg, sitagliptin 800 mg (8 times the recommended dose), and placebo. At the recommended dose of 100 mg, there was no effect on the QTc interval obtained at the peak plasma concentration, or at any other time during the study. Following the 800 mg dose, the maximum increase in the placebo-corrected mean change in QTc from baseline was observed at 3 hours postdose and was 8.0 msec. This increase is not considered to be clinically significant. At the 800 mg dose, peak sitagliptin plasma concentrations were approximately 11 times higher than the peak concentrations following a 100 mg dose.

In patients with type 2 diabetes administered sitagliptin 100 mg (N=81) or sitagliptin 200 mg (N=63) daily, there were no meaningful changes in QTc interval based on ECG data obtained at the time of expected peak plasma concentration.

Simvastatin

Epidemiological studies have demonstrated that elevated levels of total-C, LDL-C, as well as decreased levels of HDL-C are associated with the development of atherosclerosis and increased cardiovascular risk. Lowering LDL-C decreases this risk. However, the independent effect of raising HDL-C or lowering TG on the risk of coronary and cardiovascular morbidity and mortality has not been determined.

$$CrCl = \frac{[140 - \text{age (years)}] \times \text{weight (kg)}}{[72 \times \text{serum creatinine (mg/dL)}]} \quad (\times\ 0.85 \text{ for female patients})$$

12.3 Pharmacokinetics

General

JUVISYNC

The results of bioequivalence studies in healthy subjects demonstrated that JUVISYNC (sitagliptin and simvastatin) is bioequivalent to coadministration of sitagliptin and simvastatin as individual tablets.

Sitagliptin and simvastatin do not have a clinically meaningful pharmacokinetic interaction.

Absorption

JUVISYNC

A high-fat breakfast did not affect sitagliptin exposure following administration of JUVISYNC, while simvastatin AUC decreased by 24%, simvastatin C_{max} increased by 20%, and simvastatin acid AUC and C_{max} increased by 37% and 116%, respectively. The clinical significance of the above exposure changes in simvastatin and simvastatin acid is not known. JUVISYNC is recommended to be taken in the evening as indicated in simvastatin labeling.

Sitagliptin

The pharmacokinetics of sitagliptin has been extensively characterized in healthy subjects and patients with type 2 diabetes. After oral administration of a 100 mg dose to healthy subjects, sitagliptin was rapidly absorbed, with peak plasma concentrations (median T_{max}) occurring 1 to 4 hours postdose. Plasma AUC of sitagliptin increased in a dose-proportional manner. Following a single oral 100 mg dose to healthy volunteers, mean plasma AUC of sitagliptin was 8.52 μM·hr, C_{max} was 950 nM, and apparent terminal half-life ($t_{1/2}$) was 12.4 hours. Plasma AUC of sitagliptin increased approximately 14% following 100 mg doses at steady-state compared to the first dose. The intra-subject and inter-subject coefficients of variation for sitagliptin AUC were small (5.8% and 15.1%). The pharmacokinetics of sitagliptin was generally similar in healthy subjects and in patients with type 2 diabetes.

The absolute bioavailability of sitagliptin is approximately 87%.

Simvastatin

Simvastatin is a lactone that is readily hydrolyzed *in vivo* to the corresponding β-hydroxyacid (simvastatin acid), a potent inhibitor of HMG-CoA reductase.

Peak plasma concentrations of simvastatin lactone and simvastatin acid were attained within 1.5 and 4-6 hours postdose, respectively. For simvastatin no substantial deviation from linearity of AUC of inhibitors in the general circulation was observed at doses up to 120 mg.

Distribution

Sitagliptin

The mean volume of distribution at steady state following a single 100 mg intravenous dose of sitagliptin to healthy subjects is approximately 198 liters. The fraction of sitagliptin reversibly bound to plasma proteins is low (38%).

Simvastatin

Both simvastatin and its β-hydroxyacid metabolite are highly bound (approximately 95%) to human plasma proteins. Rat studies indicate that when radiolabeled simvastatin was administered, simvastatin-derived radioactivity crossed the blood-brain barrier.

Metabolism

Sitagliptin

Approximately 79% of sitagliptin is excreted unchanged in the urine with metabolism being a minor pathway of elimination.

Following a [^{14}C]sitagliptin oral dose, approximately 16% of the radioactivity was excreted as metabolites of sitagliptin. Six metabolites were detected at trace levels and are not expected to contribute to the plasma DPP-4 inhibitory activity of sitagliptin. *In vitro* studies indicated that the primary enzyme responsible for the limited metabolism of sitagliptin was CYP3A4, with contribution from CYP2C8.

Simvastatin

The major active metabolites of simvastatin present in human plasma are the β-hydroxyacid of simvastatin and its 6′-hydroxy, 6′-hydroxymethyl, and 6′-exomethylene derivatives. Since simvastatin undergoes extensive first-pass extraction in the liver, the availability of the drug to the general circulation is low (<5%).

Excretion

Sitagliptin

Following administration of an oral [^{14}C]sitagliptin dose to healthy subjects, approximately 100% of the administered radioactivity was eliminated in feces (13%) or urine (87%) within one week of dosing. The apparent terminal $t_{1/2}$ following a 100 mg oral dose of sitagliptin was approximately 12.4 hours and renal clearance was approximately 350 mL/min.

Elimination of sitagliptin occurs primarily via renal excretion and involves active tubular secretion. Sitagliptin is a substrate for human organic anion transporter-3 (hOAT-3), which may be involved in the renal elimination of sitagliptin. The clinical relevance of hOAT-3 in sitagliptin transport has not been established. Sitagliptin is also a substrate of p-glycoprotein, which may also be involved in mediating the renal elimination of sitagliptin. However, cyclosporine, a p-glycoprotein inhibitor, did not reduce the renal clearance of sitagliptin.

Simvastatin

Following an oral dose of ^{14}C-labeled simvastatin in man, 13% of the dose was excreted in urine and 60% in feces. Plasma concentrations of total radioactivity (simvastatin plus ^{14}C-metabolites) peaked at 4 hours and declined rapidly to about 10% of peak by 12 hours postdose.

Special Populations

Renal Impairment

Sitagliptin

A single-dose, open-label study was conducted to evaluate the pharmacokinetics of sitagliptin (50 mg dose) in patients with varying degrees of chronic renal impairment compared to normal healthy control subjects. The study included patients with renal impairment classified on the basis of creatinine clearance as mild (50 to <80 mL/min), moderate (30 to <50 mL/min), and severe (<30 mL/min), as well as patients with ESRD on hemodialysis. In addition, the effects of renal impairment on sitagliptin pharmacokinetics in patients with type 2 diabetes and mild or moderate renal impairment were assessed using population pharmacokinetic analyses. Creatinine clearance was measured by 24-hour urinary creatinine clearance measurements or estimated from serum creatinine based on the Cockcroft-Gault formula:

[See table above]

Compared to normal healthy control subjects, an approximate 1.1- to 1.6-fold increase in plasma AUC of sitagliptin was observed in patients with mild renal impairment. Because increases of this magnitude are not clinically relevant, dosage adjustment in patients with mild renal impairment is not necessary. Plasma AUC levels of sitagliptin were increased approximately 2-fold and 4-fold in patients with moderate renal impairment and in patients with severe renal impairment, including patients with ESRD on hemodialysis, respectively. To achieve plasma concentrations of sitagliptin similar to those in patients with normal renal function, a lower dosage is recommended in patients with moderate renal impairment. JUVISYNC should not be used in patients with severe renal impairment. *[See Dosage and Administration (2.2); Warnings and Precautions (5.4).]*

Hepatic Impairment

Sitagliptin

In patients with moderate hepatic impairment (Child-Pugh score 7 to 9), mean AUC and C_{max} of sitagliptin increased approximately 21% and 13%, respectively, compared to healthy matched controls following administration of a single 100 mg dose of sitagliptin. These differences are not considered to be clinically meaningful.

There is no clinical experience in patients with severe hepatic impairment (Child-Pugh score >9).

Body Mass Index (BMI)

Sitagliptin

Body mass index had no clinically meaningful effect on the pharmacokinetics of sitagliptin based on a composite analysis of Phase I pharmacokinetic data and on a population pharmacokinetic analysis of Phase I and Phase II data.

Gender

Sitagliptin

Gender had no clinically meaningful effect on the pharmacokinetics of sitagliptin based on a composite analysis of Phase I pharmacokinetic data and on a population pharmacokinetic analysis of Phase I and Phase II data.

Geriatric

Sitagliptin

When the effects of age on renal function are taken into account, age alone did not have a clinically meaningful impact on the pharmacokinetics of sitagliptin based on a population pharmacokinetic analysis. Elderly subjects (65 to 80 years) had approximately 19% higher plasma concentrations of sitagliptin compared to younger subjects.

Simvastatin

In a study including 16 elderly patients between 70 and 78 years of age who received simvastatin 40 mg/day, the mean plasma level of HMG-CoA reductase inhibitory activity was increased approximately 45% compared with 18 patients between 18-30 years of age *[see Warnings and Precautions (5.2); Use in Specific Populations (8.5)]*.

Pediatric

Sitagliptin

Studies characterizing the pharmacokinetics of sitagliptin in pediatric patients have not been performed.

Table 6: Effect of Coadministered Drugs or Grapefruit Juice on Simvastatin Systemic Exposure

Coadministered Drug or Grapefruit Juice	Dosing of Coadministered Drug or Grapefruit Juice	Dosing of Simvastatin	Geometric Mean Ratio (Ratio* with / without coadministered drug) No Effect = 1.00		
				AUC	C_{max}
Contraindicated with JUVISYNC *[see Contraindications (4); Warnings and Precautions (5.2)]*					
Telithromycin†	200 mg QD for 4 days	80 mg	simvastatin acid‡ simvastatin	12 8.9	15 5.3
Nelfinavir†	1250 mg BID for 14 days	20 mg QD for 28 days	simvastatin acid‡ simvastatin	6	6.2
Itraconazole†	200 mg QD for 4 days	80 mg	simvastatin acid‡ simvastatin		13.1 13.1
Posaconazole	100 mg (oral suspension) QD for 13 days	40 mg	simvastatin acid simvastatin	7.3 10.3	9.2 9.4
	200 mg (oral suspension) QD for 13 days	40 mg	simvastatin acid simvastatin	8.5 10.6	9.5 11.4
Gemfibrozil	600 mg BID for 3 days	40 mg	simvastatin acid simvastatin	2.85 1.35	2.18 0.91
Avoid grapefruit juice *[see Warnings and Precautions (5.2)]*					
Grapefruit Juice§ (high dose)	200 mL of double-strength TID¶	60 mg single dose	simvastatin acid simvastatin	7 16	
Grapefruit Juice§ (low dose)	8 oz (about 237 mL) of single-strength#	20 mg single dose	simvastatin acid simvastatin	1.3 1.9	
Avoid taking with >10 mg simvastatin (100 mg/10 mg or 50 mg/10 mg JUVISYNC), based on clinical and/or postmarketing experience *[see Warnings and Precautions (5.2)]*					
Verapamil SR	240 mg QD Days 1-7 then 240 mg BID on Days 8-10	80 mg on Day 10	simvastatin acid simvastatin	2.3 2.5	2.4 2.1
Diltiazem	120 mg BID for 10 days	80 mg on Day 10	simvastatin acid simvastatin	2.69 3.10	2.69 2.88
Diltiazem	120 mg BID for 14 days	20 mg on Day 14	simvastatin	4.6	3.6
Dronedarone	400 mg BID for 14 days	40 mg QD for 14 days	simvastatin acid simvastatin	1.96 3.90	2.14 3.75
Avoid taking with >20 mg simvastatin (100 mg/20 mg or 50 mg/20 mg JUVISYNC), based on clinical and/or postmarketing experience *[see Warnings and Precautions (5.2)]*					
Amlodipine	10 mg QD for 10 days	80 mg on Day 10	simvastatin acid simvastatin	1.58 1.77	1.56 1.47
Ranolazine SR	1000 mg BID for 7 days	80 mg on Day 1 and Days 6-9	simvastatin acid simvastatin	2.26 1.86	2.28 1.75
Amiodarone	400 mg QD for 3 days	40 mg on Day 3	simvastatin acid simvastatin	1.75 1.76	1.72 1.79

(Table continued on next page)

Race

Sitagliptin

Race had no clinically meaningful effect on the pharmacokinetics of sitagliptin based on a composite analysis of available pharmacokinetic data, including subjects of white, Hispanic, black, Asian, and other racial groups.

Drug Interactions

Sitagliptin

In Vitro Assessment of Drug Interactions

Sitagliptin is not an inhibitor of CYP isozymes CYP3A4, 2C8, 2C9, 2D6, 1A2, 2C19 or 2B6, and is not an inducer of CYP3A4. Sitagliptin is a p-glycoprotein substrate, but does not inhibit p-glycoprotein mediated transport of digoxin. Based on these results, sitagliptin is considered unlikely to cause interactions with other drugs that utilize these pathways.

Sitagliptin is not extensively bound to plasma proteins. Therefore, the propensity of sitagliptin to be involved in clinically meaningful drug-drug interactions mediated by plasma protein binding displacement is very low.

In Vivo Assessment of Drug Interactions

Effects of Coadministered Sitagliptin and Simvastatin on Other Drugs

Digoxin: There was an increase in the area under the curve (AUC, 26%) and mean peak drug concentration (C_{max}, 41%) of digoxin with the coadministration of 100 mg sitagliptin and 80 mg simvastatin for 5 days. Patients receiving digoxin and JUVISYNC should be monitored.

Effects of Sitagliptin on Other Drugs

In clinical studies, as described below, sitagliptin did not meaningfully alter the pharmacokinetics of metformin, glyburide, simvastatin, rosiglitazone, warfarin, or oral contraceptives, providing *in vivo* evidence of a low propensity for causing drug interactions with substrates of CYP3A4, CYP2C8, CYP2C9, and organic cationic transporter (OCT).

Metformin: Coadministration of multiple twice-daily doses of sitagliptin with metformin, an OCT substrate, did not meaningfully alter the pharmacokinetics of metformin in patients with type 2 diabetes. Therefore, sitagliptin is not an inhibitor of OCT-mediated transport.

Sulfonylureas: Single-dose pharmacokinetics of glyburide, a CYP2C9 substrate, was not meaningfully altered in subjects receiving multiple doses of sitagliptin. Clinically meaningful interactions would not be expected with other sulfonylureas (e.g., glipizide, tolbutamide, and glimepiride) which, like glyburide, are primarily eliminated by CYP2C9.

Thiazolidinediones: Single-dose pharmacokinetics of rosiglitazone was not meaningfully altered in subjects receiving multiple daily doses of sitagliptin, indicating that sitagliptin is not an inhibitor of CYP2C8-mediated metabolism.

Warfarin: Multiple daily doses of sitagliptin did not meaningfully alter the pharmacokinetics, as assessed by measurement of S(-) or R(+) warfarin enantiomers, or pharmacodynamics (as assessed by measurement of prothrombin INR) of a single dose of warfarin. Because S(-) warfarin is primarily metabolized by CYP2C9, these data also support the conclusion that sitagliptin is not a CYP2C9 inhibitor.

Oral Contraceptives: Coadministration with sitagliptin did not meaningfully alter the steady-state pharmacokinetics of norethindrone or ethinyl estradiol.

Effects of Other Drugs on Sitagliptin

Clinical data described below suggest that sitagliptin is not susceptible to clinically meaningful interactions by coadministered medications.

Metformin: Coadministration of multiple twice-daily doses of metformin with sitagliptin did not meaningfully alter the pharmacokinetics of sitagliptin in patients with type 2 diabetes.

Cyclosporine: A study was conducted to assess the effect of cyclosporine, a potent inhibitor of p-glycoprotein, on the pharmacokinetics of sitagliptin. Coadministration of a single 100 mg oral dose of sitagliptin and a single 600 mg oral dose of cyclosporine increased the AUC and C_{max} of sitagliptin by approximately 29% and 68%, respectively. These modest changes in sitagliptin pharmacokinetics were not considered to be clinically meaningful. The renal clearance of sitagliptin was also not meaningfully altered. Therefore, meaningful interactions would not be expected with other p-glycoprotein inhibitors.

Effects of Simvastatin on Other Drugs

CYP3A4 Inhibitors: In a study of 12 healthy volunteers, simvastatin at the 80 mg dose had no effect on the metabolism of the probe cytochrome P450 isoform 3A4 (CYP3A4) substrates midazolam and erythromycin. This indicates that simvastatin is not an inhibitor of CYP3A4, and, therefore, is not expected to affect the plasma levels of other drugs metabolized by CYP3A4.

Effects of Other Drugs on Simvastatin

Cyclosporine: Although the mechanism is not fully understood, cyclosporine has been shown to increase the AUC of statins. The increase in AUC for simvastatin acid is presumably due, in part, to inhibition of CYP3A4.

CYP3A4 Inhibitors: The risk of myopathy is increased by high levels of HMG-CoA reductase inhibitory activity in plasma. Inhibitors of CYP3A4 can raise the plasma levels of HMG-CoA reductase inhibitory activity and increase the risk of myopathy *[see Warnings and Precautions (5.2); Drug Interactions (7.1)]*.

[See table 6 above and on next page]

13 NONCLINICAL TOXICOLOGY

13.1 Carcinogenesis, Mutagenesis, Impairment of Fertility

Sitagliptin

A two-year carcinogenicity study was conducted in male and female rats given oral doses of sitagliptin of 50, 150, and 500 mg/kg/day. There was an increased incidence of combined liver adenoma/carcinoma in males and females and of liver carcinoma in females at 500 mg/kg. This dose results in exposures approximately 60 times the human exposure at the maximum recommended daily adult human dose (MRHD) of 100 mg/day based on AUC comparisons. Liver tumors were not observed at 150 mg/kg, approximately 20 times the human exposure at the MRHD. A two-year carcinogenicity study was conducted in male and female mice given oral doses of sitagliptin of 50, 125, 250, and 500 mg/kg/day. There was no increase in the incidence of tumors in any organ up to 500 mg/kg, approximately 70 times human exposure at the MRHD. Sitagliptin was not mutagenic or clastogenic with or without metabolic activation in the Ames bacterial mutagenicity assay, a Chinese hamster ovary (CHO) chromosome aberration assay, an *in vitro* cytogenetics assay in CHO, an *in vitro* rat hepatocyte DNA alkaline elution assay, and an *in vivo* micronucleus assay.

In rat fertility studies with oral gavage doses of 125, 250, and 1000 mg/kg, males were treated for 4 weeks prior to mating, during mating, up to scheduled termination (approximately 8 weeks total) and females were treated 2 weeks prior to mating through gestation day 7. No adverse effect on fertility was observed at 125 mg/kg (approximately 12 times human exposure at the MRHD of 100 mg/day based on AUC comparisons). At higher doses, nondose-related increased resorptions in females were observed (approximately 25 and 100 times human exposure at the MRHD based on AUC comparison).

Simvastatin

In a 72-week carcinogenicity study, mice were administered daily doses of simvastatin of 25, 100, and 400 mg/kg body weight, which resulted in mean plasma drug levels approximately 2, 8, and 16 times higher than the mean human plasma drug level, respectively (as total inhibitory activity based on AUC) after a 40 mg oral dose. Liver carcinomas were significantly increased in high-dose females and mid- and high-dose males with a maximum incidence of 90% in males. The incidence of adenomas of the liver was significantly increased in mid- and high-dose females. Drug treatment also significantly increased the incidence of lung adenomas in mid- and high-dose males and females. Adenomas of the Harderian gland (a gland of the eye of rodents) were significantly higher in high-dose mice than in controls. No evidence of a tumorigenic effect was observed at 25 mg/kg/day.

In a separate 92-week carcinogenicity study in mice at doses up to 25 mg/kg/day, no evidence of a tumorigenic effect was observed (mean plasma drug levels were approximately 2 times higher than humans given 40 mg simvastatin as measured by AUC).

In a two-year study in rats at 25 mg/kg/day, there was a statistically significant increase in the incidence of thyroid follicular adenomas in female rats exposed to approximately 22 times higher levels of simvastatin than in humans given 40 mg simvastatin (as measured by AUC).

A second two-year rat carcinogenicity study with doses of 50 and 100 mg/kg/day produced hepatocellular adenomas and carcinomas (in female rats at both doses and in males at 100 mg/kg/day). Thyroid follicular cell adenomas were increased in males and females at both doses; thyroid follicular cell carcinomas were increased in females at 100 mg/kg/day. The increased incidence of thyroid neoplasms appears to be consistent with findings from other statins. These treatment levels represented plasma drug levels (AUC) of approximately 14 and 30 times (males) and 44 and 50 times (females) the mean human plasma drug exposure after a 40 milligram daily dose.

No evidence of mutagenicity was observed in a microbial mutagenicity (Ames) test with or without rat or mouse liver metabolic activation. In addition, no evidence of damage to genetic material was noted in an *in vitro* alkaline elution assay using rat hepatocytes, a V-79 mammalian cell forward mutation study, an *in vitro* chromosome aberration study in CHO cells, or an *in vivo* chromosomal aberration assay in mouse bone marrow.

There was decreased fertility in male rats treated with simvastatin for 34 weeks at 25 mg/kg body weight (8 times the maximum human exposure level, based on AUC, in patients receiving 40 mg/day); however, this effect was not observed during a subsequent fertility study in which simvastatin was administered at this same dose level to male rats for 11 weeks (the entire cycle of spermatogenesis including epididymal maturation). No microscopic changes were observed in the testes of rats from either study. At 180 mg/kg/day, (which produces exposure levels 44 times higher than those in humans taking 40 mg/day based on surface area, mg/m^2), seminiferous tubule degeneration (necrosis and loss of spermatogenic epithelium) was observed. In dogs, there was drug-related testicular atrophy, decreased spermatogenesis, spermatocytic degeneration and giant cell formation at 10 mg/kg/day, (approximately 4 times the human exposure, based on AUC, at 40 mg/day). The clinical significance of these findings is unclear.

13.2 Animal Toxicology and/or Pharmacology

Simvastatin

Optic nerve degeneration was seen in clinically normal dogs treated with simvastatin for 14 weeks at 180 mg/kg/day, a dose that produced mean plasma drug levels about 24 times higher than the mean plasma drug level in humans taking 40 mg/day.

A chemically similar drug in this class also produced optic nerve degeneration (Wallerian degeneration of retinogeniculate fibers) in clinically normal dogs in a dose-dependent fashion starting at 60 mg/kg/day, a dose that produced mean plasma drug levels about 30 times higher than the mean plasma drug level in humans taking the highest recommended dose (as measured by total enzyme inhibitory activity). This same drug also produced vestibulocochlear Wallerian-like degeneration and retinal ganglion cell chromatolysis in dogs treated for 14 weeks at 180 mg/kg/day, a dose that resulted in a mean plasma drug level similar to that seen with the 60 mg/kg/day dose.

CNS vascular lesions, characterized by perivascular hemorrhage and edema, mononuclear cell infiltration of perivascular spaces, perivascular fibrin deposits and necrosis of small vessels were seen in dogs treated with simvastatin at a dose of 360 mg/kg/day, a dose that produced mean plasma drug levels that were about 28 times higher than the mean plasma drug levels in humans taking 40 mg/day. Similar CNS vascular lesions have been observed with several other drugs of this class.

There were cataracts in female rats after two years of treatment with 50 and 100 mg/kg/day (44 and 50 times the human AUC at 40 mg/day, respectively) and in dogs after three months at 90 mg/kg/day (38 times) and at two years at 50 mg/kg/day (10 times).

14 CLINICAL STUDIES

14.1 Sitagliptin Clinical Studies

There were approximately 5200 patients with type 2 diabetes randomized in nine double-blind, placebo-controlled clinical safety and efficacy studies conducted to evaluate the effects of sitagliptin on glycemic control. In a pooled analysis of seven of these studies, the ethnic/racial distribution was approximately 59% white, 20% Hispanic, 10% Asian, 6% black, and 6% other groups. Patients had an overall mean age of approximately 55 years (range 18 to 87 years). In addition, an active (glipizide)-controlled study of 52 weeks duration was conducted in 1172 patients with type 2 diabetes who had inadequate glycemic control on metformin.

Table 6 *(cont.)*: Effect of Coadministered Drugs or Grapefruit Juice on Simvastatin Systemic Exposure

Coadministered Drug or Grapefruit Juice	Dosing of Coadministered Drug or Grapefruit Juice	Dosing of Simvastatin	Geometric Mean Ratio (Ratio* with / without coadministered drug) No Effect = 1.00		
				AUC	C_{max}
No dosing adjustments required for the following:					
Fenofibrate	160 mg QD for 14 days	80 mg QD on Days 8-14	simvastatin acid simvastatin	0.64 0.89	0.89 0.83
Niacin extended-release Þ	2 g single dose	20 mg single dose	simvastatin acid simvastatin	1.6 1.4	1.84 1.08
Propranolol	80 mg single dose	80 mg single dose	total inhibitor	0.79	↓ from 33.6 to 21.1 ng·eq/mL
			active inhibitor	0.79	↓ from 7.0 to 4.7 ng·eq/mL

* Results based on a chemical assay except results with propranolol as indicated.
† Results could be representative of the following CYP3A4 inhibitors: ketoconazole, erythromycin, clarithromycin, HIV protease inhibitors, and nefazodone.
‡ Simvastatin acid refers to the β-hydroxyacid of simvastatin.
§ The effect of amounts of grapefruit juice between those used in these two studies on simvastatin pharmacokinetics has not been studied.
¶ Double-strength: one can of frozen concentrate diluted with one can of water. Grapefruit juice was administered TID for 2 days, and 200 mL together with single dose simvastatin and 30 and 90 minutes following single dose simvastatin on Day 3.
# Single-strength: one can of frozen concentrate diluted with 3 cans of water. Grapefruit juice was administered with breakfast for 3 days, and simvastatin was administered in the evening on Day 3.
Þ Chinese patients have an increased risk for myopathy with simvastatin coadministered with lipid-modifying doses (≥ 1 gram/day niacin) of niacin-containing products, and the risk is dose-related *[see Warnings and Precautions (5.2); Drug Interactions (7.4)]*.

In patients with type 2 diabetes, treatment with sitagliptin produced clinically significant improvements in hemoglobin A1C, fasting plasma glucose (FPG) and 2-hour postprandial glucose (PPG) compared to placebo.

Monotherapy

A total of 1262 patients with type 2 diabetes participated in two double-blind, placebo-controlled studies, one of 18-week and another of 24-week duration, to evaluate the efficacy and safety of sitagliptin monotherapy. In both monotherapy studies, patients currently on an antihyperglycemic agent discontinued the agent, and underwent a diet, exercise, and drug washout period of about 7 weeks. Patients with inadequate glycemic control (A1C 7% to 10%) after the washout period were randomized after completing a 2-week single-blind placebo run-in period; patients not currently on antihyperglycemic agents (off therapy for at least 8 weeks) with inadequate glycemic control (A1C 7% to 10%) were randomized after completing the 2-week single-blind placebo run-in period. In the 18-week study, 521 patients were randomized to placebo, sitagliptin 100 mg, or sitagliptin 200 mg, and in the 24-week study 741 patients were randomized to placebo, sitagliptin 100 mg, or sitagliptin 200 mg. Patients who failed to meet specific glycemic goals during the studies were treated with metformin rescue, added on to placebo or sitagliptin.

Treatment with sitagliptin at 100 mg daily provided significant improvements in A1C, FPG, and 2-hour PPG compared to placebo (Table 7). In the 18-week study, 9% of patients receiving sitagliptin 100 mg and 17% who received placebo required rescue therapy. In the 24-week study, 9% of patients receiving sitagliptin 100 mg and 21% of patients receiving placebo required rescue therapy. The improvement in A1C compared to placebo was not affected by gender, age, race, prior antihyperglycemic therapy, or baseline BMI. As is typical for trials of agents to treat type 2 diabetes, the mean reduction in A1C with sitagliptin appears to be related to the degree of A1C elevation at baseline. In these 18- and 24-week studies, among patients who were not on an antihyperglycemic agent at study entry, the reductions from baseline in A1C were -0.7% and -0.8%, respectively, for those given sitagliptin, and -0.1% and -0.2%, respectively, for those given placebo. Overall, the 200 mg daily dose did not provide greater glycemic efficacy than the 100 mg daily dose. Body weight did not increase from baseline with sitagliptin therapy in either study, compared to a small reduction in patients given placebo.

[See table 7 at top of next page]

Add-on Combination Therapy with Metformin

A total of 701 patients with type 2 diabetes participated in a 24-week, randomized, double-blind, placebo-controlled study designed to assess the efficacy of sitagliptin in combination with metformin. Patients already on metformin (N=431) at a dose of at least 1500 mg per day were randomized after completing a 2-week single-blind placebo run-in period. Patients on metformin and another antihyperglycemic agent (N=229) and patients not on any antihyperglycemic agents (off therapy for at least 8 weeks, N=41) were randomized after a run-in period of approximately 10 weeks on metformin (at a dose of at least 1500 mg per day) in monotherapy. Patients with inadequate glycemic control (A1C 7% to 10%) were randomized to the addition of either 100 mg of sitagliptin or placebo, administered once daily. Patients who failed to meet specific glycemic goals during the studies were treated with pioglitazone rescue.

In combination with metformin, sitagliptin provided significant improvements in A1C, FPG, and 2-hour PPG compared to placebo with metformin (Table 8). Rescue glycemic therapy was used in 5% of patients treated with sitagliptin 100 mg and 14% of patients treated with placebo. A similar decrease in body weight was observed for both treatment groups.

[See table 8 at top of next page]

Initial Combination Therapy with Metformin

A total of 1091 patients with type 2 diabetes and inadequate glycemic control on diet and exercise participated in a 24-week, randomized, double-blind, placebo-controlled factorial study designed to assess the efficacy of sitagliptin as initial therapy in combination with metformin. Patients on an antihyperglycemic agent (N=541) discontinued the agent, and underwent a diet, exercise, and drug washout period of up to 12 weeks duration. After the washout period, patients with inadequate glycemic control (A1C 7.5% to 11%) were randomized after completing a 2-week single-blind placebo run-in period. Patients not on antihyperglycemic agents at study entry (N=550) with inadequate glycemic control (A1C 7.5% to 11%) immediately entered the 2-week single-blind placebo run-in period and then were randomized. Approximately equal numbers of patients were randomized to receive initial therapy with placebo, 100 mg of sitagliptin once daily, 500 mg or 1000 mg of metformin twice daily, or 50 mg of sitagliptin twice daily in combination with 500 mg or 1000 mg of metformin twice daily. Patients who failed to meet specific glycemic goals during the study were treated with glyburide (glibenclamide) rescue.

Initial therapy with the combination of sitagliptin and metformin provided significant improvements in A1C, FPG, and 2-hour PPG compared to placebo, to metformin alone, and to

Table 7: Glycemic Parameters in 18- and 24-Week Placebo-Controlled Studies of Sitagliptin in Patients with Type 2 Diabetes*

	18-Week Study		24-Week Study	
	Sitagliptin 100 mg	**Placebo**	**Sitagliptin 100 mg**	**Placebo**
A1C (%)	**N = 193**	**N = 103**	**N = 229**	**N = 244**
Baseline (mean)	8.0	8.1	8.0	8.0
Change from baseline (adjusted mean†)	-0.5	0.1	-0.6	0.2
Difference from placebo (adjusted mean†) (95% CI)	-0.6‡ (-0.8, -0.4)		-0.8‡ (-1.0, -0.6)	
Patients (%) achieving A1C <7%	69 (36%)	16 (16%)	93 (41%)	41 (17%)
FPG (mg/dL)	**N = 201**	**N = 107**	**N = 234**	**N = 247**
Baseline (mean)	180	184	170	176
Change from baseline (adjusted mean†)	-13	7	-12	5
Difference from placebo (adjusted mean†) (95% CI)	-20‡ (-31, -9)		-17‡ (-24, -10)	
2-hour PPG (mg/dL)	§	§	**N = 201**	**N = 204**
Baseline (mean)			257	271
Change from baseline (adjusted mean†)			-49	-2
Difference from placebo (adjusted mean†) (95% CI)			-47‡ (-59, -34)	

* Intent-to-treat population using last observation on study prior to metformin rescue therapy.
† Least squares means adjusted for prior antihyperglycemic therapy status and baseline value.
‡ p<0.001 compared to placebo.
§ Data not available.

Table 8: Glycemic Parameters at Final Visit (24-Week Study) for Sitagliptin in Add-on Combination Therapy with Metformin*

	Sitagliptin 100 mg + Metformin	**Placebo + Metformin**
A1C (%)	**N = 453**	**N = 224**
Baseline (mean)	8.0	8.0
Change from baseline (adjusted mean†)	-0.7	-0.0
Difference from placebo + metformin (adjusted mean†) (95% CI)	-0.7‡ (-0.8, -0.5)	
Patients (%) achieving A1C <7%	213 (47%)	41 (18%)
FPG (mg/dL)	**N = 454**	**N = 226**
Baseline (mean)	170	174
Change from baseline (adjusted mean†)	-17	9
Difference from placebo + metformin (adjusted mean†) (95% CI)	-25‡ (-31, -20)	
2-hour PPG (mg/dL)	**N = 387**	**N = 182**
Baseline (mean)	275	272
Change from baseline (adjusted mean†)	-62	-11
Difference from placebo + metformin (adjusted mean†) (95% CI)	-51‡ (-61, -41)	

* Intent-to-treat population using last observation on study prior to pioglitazone rescue therapy.
† Least squares means adjusted for prior antihyperglycemic therapy and baseline value.
‡ p<0.001 compared to placebo + metformin.

sitagliptin alone (Table 9, Figure 1). Mean reductions from baseline in A1C were generally greater for patients with higher baseline A1C values. For patients not on an antihyperglycemic agent at study entry, mean reductions from baseline in A1C were: sitagliptin 100 mg once daily, -1.1%; metformin 500 mg bid, -1.1%; metformin 1000 mg bid, -1.2%; sitagliptin 50 mg bid with metformin 500 mg bid, -1.6%; sitagliptin 50 mg bid with metformin 1000 mg bid, -1.9%; and for patients receiving placebo, -0.2%. The decrease in body weight in the groups given sitagliptin in combination with metformin was similar to that in the groups given metformin alone or placebo.

[See table 9 at top of next page]

[See figure 1 at top of next column]

In addition, this study included patients (N=117) with more severe hyperglycemia (A1C >11% or blood glucose >280 mg/dL) who were treated with twice daily open-label sitagliptin 50 mg and metformin 1000 mg. In this group of patients, the mean baseline A1C value was 11.2%, mean FPG was 314 mg/dL, and mean 2-hour PPG was 441 mg/dL. After 24 weeks, mean decreases from baseline of -2.9% for A1C, -127 mg/dL for FPG, and -208 mg/dL for 2-hour PPG were observed.

Figure 1: Mean Change from Baseline for A1C (%) over 24 Weeks with Sitagliptin and Metformin, Alone and in Combination as Initial Therapy in Patients with Type 2 Diabetes*

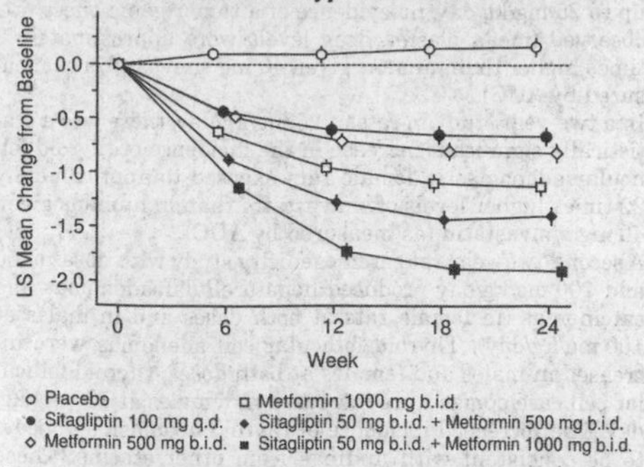

* All Patients Treated Population; least squares means adjusted for prior antihyperglycemic therapy and baseline value.

Initial combination therapy or maintenance of combination therapy may not be appropriate for all patients. These management options are left to the discretion of the health care provider.

Active-Controlled Study vs Glipizide in Combination with Metformin

The efficacy of sitagliptin was evaluated in a 52-week, double-blind, glipizide-controlled noninferiority trial in patients with type 2 diabetes. Patients not on treatment or on other antihyperglycemic agents entered a run-in treatment period of up to 12 weeks duration with metformin monotherapy (dose of ≥1500 mg per day) which included washout of medications other than metformin, if applicable. After the run-in period, those with inadequate glycemic control (A1C 6.5% to 10%) were randomized 1:1 to the addition of sitagliptin 100 mg once daily or glipizide for 52 weeks. Patients receiving glipizide were given an initial dosage of 5 mg/day and then electively titrated over the next 18 weeks to a maximum dosage of 20 mg/day as needed to optimize glycemic control. Thereafter, the glipizide dose was to be kept constant, except for down-titration to prevent hypoglycemia. The mean dose of glipizide after the titration period was 10 mg.

After 52 weeks, sitagliptin and glipizide had similar mean reductions from baseline in A1C in the intent-to-treat analysis (Table 10). These results were consistent with the per protocol analysis (Figure 2). A conclusion in favor of the non-inferiority of sitagliptin to glipizide may be limited to patients with baseline A1C comparable to those included in the study (over 70% of patients had baseline A1C <8% and over 90% had A1C <9%).

Table 10: Glycemic Parameters in a 52-Week Study Comparing Sitagliptin to Glipizide as Add-On Therapy in Patients Inadequately Controlled on Metformin (Intent-to-Treat Population)*

	Sitagliptin 100 mg	**Glipizide**
A1C (%)	**N = 576**	**N = 559**
Baseline (mean)	7.7	7.6
Change from baseline (adjusted mean†)	-0.5	-0.6
FPG (mg/dL)	**N = 583**	**N = 568**
Baseline (mean)	166	164
Change from baseline (adjusted mean†)	-8	-8

* The intent-to-treat analysis used the patients' last observation in the study prior to discontinuation.
† Least squares means adjusted for prior antihyperglycemic therapy status and baseline A1C value.

[See figure 2 at top of next column]

The incidence of hypoglycemia in the sitagliptin group (4.9%) was significantly (p<0.001) lower than that in the glipizide group (32.0%). Patients treated with sitagliptin exhibited a significant mean decrease from baseline in body weight compared to a significant weight gain in patients administered glipizide (-1.5 kg vs +1.1 kg).

Add-on Combination Therapy with Pioglitazone

A total of 353 patients with type 2 diabetes participated in a 24-week, randomized, double-blind, placebo-controlled study designed to assess the efficacy of sitagliptin in combi-

Table 9: Glycemic Parameters at Final Visit (24-Week Study) for Sitagliptin and Metformin, Alone and in Combination as Initial Therapy*

	Placebo	Sitagliptin 100 mg QD	Metformin 500 mg bid	Metformin 1000 mg bid	Sitagliptin 50 mg bid + Metformin 500 mg bid	Sitagliptin 50 mg bid + Metformin 1000 mg bid
A1C (%)	**N = 165**	**N = 175**	**N = 178**	**N = 177**	**N = 183**	**N = 178**
Baseline (mean)	8.7	8.9	8.9	8.7	8.8	8.8
Change from baseline (adjusted mean†)	0.2	-0.7	-0.8	-1.1	-1.4	-1.9
Difference from placebo (adjusted mean†) (95% CI)		-0.8‡ (-1.1, -0.6)	-1.0‡ (-1.2, -0.8)	-1.3‡ (-1.5, -1.1)	-1.6‡ (-1.8, -1.3)	-2.1‡ (-2.3, -1.8)
Patients (%) achieving A1C <7%	15 (9%)	35 (20%)	41 (23%)	68 (38%)	79 (43%)	118 (66%)
% Patients receiving rescue medication	32	21	17	12	8	2
FPG (mg/dL)	**N = 169**	**N = 178**	**N = 179**	**N = 179**	**N = 183**	**N = 180**
Baseline (mean)	196	201	205	197	204	197
Change from baseline (adjusted mean†)	6	-17	-27	-29	-47	-64
Difference from placebo (adjusted mean†) (95% CI)		-23‡ (-33, -14)	-33‡ (-43, -24)	-35‡ (-45, -26)	-53‡ (-62, -43)	-70‡ (-79, -60)
2-hour PPG (mg/dL)	**N = 129**	**N = 136**	**N = 141**	**N = 138**	**N = 147**	**N = 152**
Baseline (mean)	277	285	293	283	292	287
Change from baseline (adjusted mean†)	0	-52	-53	-78	-93	-117
Difference from placebo (adjusted mean†) (95% CI)		-52‡ (-67, -37)	-54‡ (-69, -39)	-78‡ (-93, -63)	-93‡ (-107, -78)	-117‡ (-131, -102)

* Intent-to-treat population using last observation on study prior to glyburide (glibenclamide) rescue therapy.
† Least squares means adjusted for prior antihyperglycemic therapy status and baseline value.
‡ p<0.001 compared to placebo.

Figure 2: Mean Change from Baseline for A1C (%) Over 52 Weeks in a Study Comparing Sitagliptin to Glipizide as Add-On Therapy in Patients Inadequately Controlled on Metformin (Per Protocol Population)*

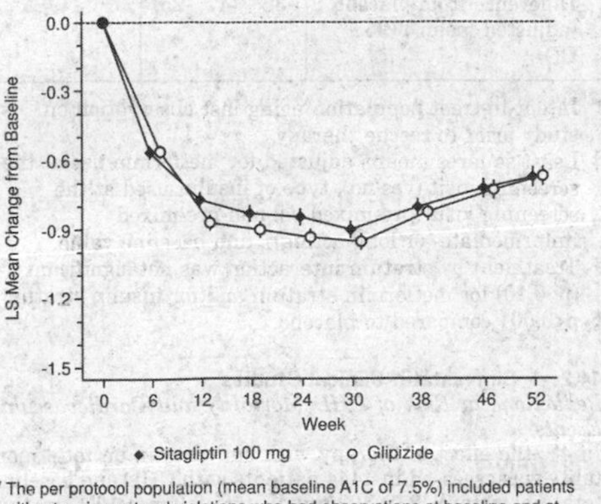

* The per protocol population (mean baseline A1C of 7.5%) included patients without major protocol violations who had observations at baseline and at Week 52.

nation with pioglitazone. Patients on any oral antihyperglycemic agent in monotherapy (N=212) or on a PPARγ agent in combination therapy (N=106) or not on an antihyperglycemic agent (off therapy for at least 8 weeks, N=34) were switched to monotherapy with pioglitazone (at a dose of 30-45 mg per day), and completed a run-in period of approximately 12 weeks in duration. After the run-in period on pioglitazone monotherapy, patients with inadequate glycemic control (A1C 7% to 10%) were randomized to the addition of either 100 mg of sitagliptin or placebo, administered once daily. Patients who failed to meet specific glycemic goals during the studies were treated with metformin rescue. Glycemic endpoints measured were A1C and fasting glucose. In combination with pioglitazone, sitagliptin provided significant improvements in A1C and FPG compared to placebo with pioglitazone (Table 11). Rescue therapy was used in 7% of patients treated with sitagliptin 100 mg and 14% of patients treated with placebo. There was no significant difference between sitagliptin and placebo in body weight change.

Table 11: Glycemic Parameters at Final Visit (24-Week Study) for Sitagliptin in Add-on Combination Therapy with Pioglitazone*

	Sitagliptin 100 mg + Pioglitazone	Placebo + Pioglitazone
A1C (%)	**N = 163**	**N = 174**
Baseline (mean)	8.1	8.0
Change from baseline (adjusted mean†)	-0.9	-0.2
Difference from placebo + pioglitazone (adjusted mean†) (95% CI)	-0.7‡ (-0.9, -0.5)	
Patients (%) achieving A1C <7%	74 (45%)	40 (23%)
FPG (mg/dL)	**N = 163**	**N = 174**
Baseline (mean)	168	166
Change from baseline (adjusted mean†)	-17	1
Difference from placebo + pioglitazone (adjusted mean†) (95% CI)	-18‡ (-24, -11)	

* Intent-to-treat population using last observation on study prior to metformin rescue therapy.

† Least squares means adjusted for prior antihyperglycemic therapy status and baseline value.

‡ p<0.001 compared to placebo + pioglitazone.

Initial Combination Therapy with Pioglitazone

A total of 520 patients with type 2 diabetes and inadequate glycemic control on diet and exercise participated in a 24-week, randomized, double-blind study designed to assess the efficacy of sitagliptin as initial therapy in combination with pioglitazone. Patients not on antihyperglycemic agents at study entry (<4 weeks cumulative therapy over the past 2 years, and with no treatment over the prior 4 months) with inadequate glycemic control (A1C 8% to 12%) immediately entered the 2-week single-blind placebo run-in period and then were randomized. Approximately equal numbers of patients were randomized to receive initial therapy with 100 mg of sitagliptin in combination with 30 mg of pioglitazone once daily or 30 mg of pioglitazone once daily as monotherapy. There was no glycemic rescue therapy in this study. Initial therapy with the combination of sitagliptin and pioglitazone provided significant improvements in A1C, FPG, and 2-hour PPG compared to pioglitazone monotherapy (Table 12). The improvement in A1C was generally consistent across subgroups defined by gender, age, race, baseline BMI, baseline A1C, or duration of disease. In this study, patients treated with sitagliptin in combination with pioglitazone had a mean increase in body weight of 1.1 kg compared to pioglitazone alone (3.0 kg vs. 1.9 kg).

Table 12: Glycemic Parameters at Final Visit (24-Week Study) for Sitagliptin in Combination with Pioglitazone as Initial Therapy*

	Sitagliptin 100 mg + Pioglitazone	Pioglitazone
A1C (%)	**N = 251**	**N = 246**
Baseline (mean)	9.5	9.4
Change from baseline (adjusted mean†)	-2.4	-1.5
Difference from pioglitazone (adjusted mean†) (95% CI)	-0.9‡ (-1.1, -0.7)	
Patients (%) achieving A1C <7%	151 (60%)	68 (28%)
FPG (mg/dL)	**N = 256**	**N = 253**
Baseline (mean)	203	201
Change from baseline (adjusted mean†)	-63	-40
Difference from pioglitazone (adjusted mean†) (95% CI)	-23‡ (-30, -15)	
2-hour PPG (mg/dL)	**N = 216**	**N = 211**
Baseline (mean)	283	284
Change from baseline (adjusted mean†)	-114	-69
Difference from pioglitazone (adjusted mean†) (95% CI)	-45‡ (-57, -32)	

* Intent-to-treat population using last observation on study.
† Least squares means adjusted for baseline value.
‡ p<0.001 compared to placebo + pioglitazone.

Add-on Combination Therapy with Metformin and Rosiglitazone

A total of 278 patients with type 2 diabetes participated in a 54-week, randomized, double-blind, placebo-controlled study designed to assess the efficacy of sitagliptin in combination with metformin and rosiglitazone. Patients on dual therapy with metformin ≥1500 mg/day and rosiglitazone ≥4 mg/day or with metformin ≥1500 mg/day and pioglitazone ≥30 mg/day (switched to rosiglitazone ≥4 mg/day) entered a dose-stable run-in period of 6 weeks. Patients on other dual therapy were switched to metformin ≥1500 mg/day and rosiglitazone ≥4 mg/day in a dose titration/stabilization run-in period of up to 20 weeks in duration. After the run-in period, patients with inadequate glycemic control (A1C 7.5% to 11%) were randomized 2:1 to the addition of either 100 mg of sitagliptin or placebo, administered once daily. Patients who failed to meet specific glycemic goals during the study were treated with glipizide (or other sulfonylurea) rescue. The primary time point for evaluation of glycemic parameters was Week 18.

In combination with metformin and rosiglitazone, sitagliptin provided significant improvements in A1C, FPG, and 2-hour PPG compared to placebo with metformin and rosiglitazone (Table 13) at Week 18. At Week 54, mean reduction in A1C was -1.0% for patients treated with sitagliptin and -0.3% for patients treated with placebo in an analysis based on the intent-to-treat population. Rescue therapy was used in 18% of patients treated with sitagliptin 100 mg and 40% of patients treated with placebo. There was no significant difference between sitagliptin and placebo in body weight change.

Table 13: Glycemic Parameters at Week 18 for Sitagliptin in Add-on Combination Therapy with Metformin and Rosiglitazone*

	Sitagliptin 100 mg + Metformin + Rosiglitazone	Placebo + Metformin + Rosiglitazone
A1C (%)	**N = 176**	**N = 93**
Baseline (mean)	8.8	8.7
Change from baseline (adjusted mean†)	-1.0	-0.4
Difference from placebo + rosiglitazone + metformin (adjusted mean†) (95% CI)	-0.7‡ (-0.9, -0.4)	
Patients (%) achieving A1C <7%	39 (22%)	9 (10%)
FPG (mg/dL)	**N = 179**	**N = 94**
Baseline (mean)	181	182
Change from baseline (adjusted mean†)	-30	-11
Difference from placebo + rosiglitazone + metformin (adjusted mean†) (95% CI)	-18‡ (-26, -10)	
2-hour PPG (mg/dL)	**N = 152**	**N = 80**
Baseline (mean)	256	248
Change from baseline (adjusted mean†)	-59	-21
Difference from placebo + rosiglitazone + metformin (adjusted mean†) (95% CI)	-39‡ (-51, -26)	

* Intent-to-treat population using last observation on study prior to glipizide (or other sulfonylurea) rescue therapy.
† Least squares means adjusted for prior antihyperglycemic therapy status and baseline value.
‡ p<0.001 compared to placebo + metformin + rosiglitazone.

Add-on Combination Therapy with Glimepiride, with or without Metformin

A total of 441 patients with type 2 diabetes participated in a 24-week, randomized, double-blind, placebo-controlled study designed to assess the efficacy of sitagliptin in combination with glimepiride, with or without metformin. Patients entered a run-in treatment period on glimepiride (≥4 mg per day) alone or glimepiride in combination with metformin (≥1500 mg per day). After a dose-titration and dose-stable run-in period of up to 16 weeks and a 2-week placebo run-in period, patients with inadequate glycemic control (A1C 7.5% to 10.5%) were randomized to the addition of either 100 mg of sitagliptin or placebo, administered once daily. Patients who failed to meet specific glycemic goals during the studies were treated with pioglitazone rescue.

In combination with glimepiride, with or without metformin, sitagliptin provided significant improvements in A1C and FPG compared to placebo (Table 14). In the entire study population (patients on sitagliptin in combination with glimepiride and patients on sitagliptin in combination with glimepiride and metformin), a mean reduction from baseline relative to placebo in A1C of -0.7% and in FPG of -20 mg/dL was seen. Rescue therapy was used in 12% of patients treated with sitagliptin 100 mg and 27% of patients treated with placebo. In this study, patients treated with sitagliptin had a mean increase in body weight of 1.1 kg vs. placebo (+0.8 kg vs. -0.4 kg). In addition, there was an increased rate of hypoglycemia. *[See Warnings and Precautions (5.5); Adverse Reactions (6.1).]*

[See table 14 above]

Table 14: Glycemic Parameters at Final Visit (24-Week Study) for Sitagliptin as Add-On Combination Therapy with Glimepiride, with or without Metformin*

	Sitagliptin 100 mg + Glimepiride	Placebo + Glimepiride	Sitagliptin 100 mg + Glimepiride + Metformin	Placebo + Glimepiride + Metformin
A1C (%)	**N = 102**	**N = 103**	**N = 115**	**N = 105**
Baseline (mean)	8.4	8.5	8.3	8.3
Change from baseline (adjusted mean†)	-0.3	0.3	-0.6	0.3
Difference from placebo (adjusted mean†) (95% CI)	-0.6‡ (-0.8, -0.3)		-0.9‡ (-1.1, -0.7)	
Patients (%) achieving A1C <7%	11 (11%)	9 (9%)	26 (23%)	1 (1%)
FPG (mg/dL)	**N = 104**	**N = 104**	**N = 115**	**N = 109**
Baseline (mean)	183	185	179	179
Change from baseline (adjusted mean†)	-1	18	-8	13
Difference from placebo (adjusted mean†) (95% CI)	-19§ (-32, -7)		-21‡ (-32, -10)	

* Intent-to-treat population using last observation on study prior to pioglitazone rescue therapy.
† Least squares means adjusted for prior antihyperglycemic therapy status and baseline value.
‡ p<0.001 compared to placebo.
§ p<0.01 compared to placebo.

Add-on Combination Therapy with Insulin (with or without Metformin)

A total of 641 patients with type 2 diabetes participated in a 24-week, randomized, double-blind, placebo-controlled study designed to assess the efficacy of sitagliptin as add-on to insulin therapy (with or without metformin). The racial distribution in this study was approximately 70% white, 18% Asian, 7% black, and 5% other groups. Approximately 14% of the patients in this study were Hispanic. Patients entered a 2-week, single-blind run-in treatment period on pre-mixed, long-acting, or intermediate-acting insulin, with or without metformin (≥1500 mg per day). Patients using short-acting insulins were excluded unless the short-acting insulin was administered as part of a pre-mixed insulin. After the run-in period, patients with inadequate glycemic control (A1C 7.5% to 11%) were randomized to the addition of either 100 mg of sitagliptin or placebo, administered once daily. Patients were on a stable dose of insulin prior to enrollment with no changes in insulin dose permitted during the run-in period. Patients who failed to meet specific glycemic goals during the double-blind treatment period were to have uptitration of the background insulin dose as rescue therapy.

The median daily insulin dose at baseline was 42 units in the patients treated with sitagliptin and 45 units in the placebo-treated patients. The median change from baseline in daily dose of insulin was zero for both groups at the end of the study. In combination with insulin (with or without metformin), sitagliptin provided significant improvements in A1C, FPG, and 2-hour PPG compared to placebo (Table 15). Both treatment groups had an adjusted mean increase in body weight of 0.1 kg from baseline to Week 24. There was an increased rate of hypoglycemia in patients treated with sitagliptin. *[See Warnings and Precautions (5.5); Adverse Reactions (6.1).]*

Table 15: Glycemic Parameters at Final Visit (24-Week Study) for Sitagliptin as Add-on Combination Therapy with Insulin*

	Sitagliptin 100 mg + Insulin (+/- Metformin)	Placebo + Insulin (+/- Metformin)
A1C (%)	**N = 305**	**N = 312**
Baseline (mean)	8.7	8.6
Change from baseline (adjusted mean†)	-0.6	-0.1
Difference from placebo (adjusted mean†,‡) (95% CI)	-0.6§ (-0.7, -0.4)	
Patients (%) achieving A1C <7%	39 (12.8%)	16 (5.1%)
FPG (mg/dL)	**N = 310**	**N = 313**
Baseline (mean)	176	179
Change from baseline (adjusted mean†)	-18	-4
Difference from placebo (adjusted mean†) (95% CI)	-15§ (-23, -7)	
2-hour PPG (mg/dL)	**N = 240**	**N = 257**
Baseline (mean)	291	292
Change from baseline (adjusted mean†)	-31	5
Difference from placebo (adjusted mean†) (95% CI)	-36§ (-47, -25)	

* Intent-to-treat population using last observation on study prior to rescue therapy.
† Least squares means adjusted for metformin use at the screening visit (yes/no), type of insulin used at the screening visit (pre-mixed vs. non-pre-mixed [intermediate- or long-acting]), and baseline value.
‡ Treatment by stratum interaction was not significant (p>0.10) for metformin stratum and for insulin stratum.
§ p<0.001 compared to placebo.

14.2 Simvastatin Clinical Studies

Reductions in Risk of CHD Mortality and Cardiovascular Events

In 4S, the effect of therapy with simvastatin on total mortality was assessed in 4444 patients with CHD and baseline total cholesterol 212-309 mg/dL (5.5-8.0 mmol/L). In this multicenter, randomized, double-blind, placebo-controlled study, patients were treated with standard care, including diet, and either simvastatin 20-40 mg/day (n=2221) or placebo (n=2223) for a median duration of 5.4 years. Over the course of the study, treatment with simvastatin led to mean reductions in total-C, LDL-C and TG of 25%, 35%, and 10%, respectively, and a mean increase in HDL-C of 8%. Simvastatin significantly reduced the risk of mortality by 30% (p=0.0003, 182 deaths in the simvastatin group vs 256 deaths in the placebo group). The risk of CHD mortality was significantly reduced by 42% (p=0.00001, 111 vs 189 deaths). There was no statistically significant difference between groups in non-cardiovascular mortality. Simvastatin significantly decreased the risk of having major coronary events (CHD mortality plus hospital-verified and silent nonfatal myocardial infarction [MI]) by 34% (p<0.00001, 431 vs 622 patients with one or more events). The risk of having a hospital-verified non-fatal MI was reduced by 37%. Simvastatin significantly reduced the risk for undergoing myocardial revascularization procedures (coronary artery bypass grafting or percutaneous transluminal coronary angioplasty) by 37% (p<0.00001, 252 vs 383 patients).

Simvastatin significantly reduced the risk of fatal plus non-fatal cerebrovascular events (combined stroke and transient ischemic attacks) by 28% (p=0.033, 75 vs 102 patients). Simvastatin reduced the risk of major coronary events to a similar extent across the range of baseline total and LDL cholesterol levels. Because there were only 53 female deaths, the effect of simvastatin on mortality in women could not be adequately assessed. However, simvastatin significantly lessened the risk of having major coronary events by 34% (60 vs 91 women with one or more event). The randomization was stratified by angina alone (21% of each treatment group) or a previous MI. Because there were only 57 deaths among the patients with angina alone at baseline, the effect of simvastatin on mortality in this subgroup could not be adequately assessed. However, trends in reduced coronary mortality, major coronary events and revascularization procedures were consistent between this group and the total study cohort. Additionally, simvastatin resulted in similar decreases in relative risk for total mortality, CHD mortality, and major coronary events in elderly patients (≥65 years), compared with younger patients.

The Heart Protection Study (HPS) was a large, multi-center, placebo-controlled, double-blind study with a mean duration of 5 years conducted in 20,536 patients (10,269 on simvastatin 40 mg and 10,267 on placebo), including 5963 patients with diabetes mellitus (2978 on simvastatin and 2985 on placebo). Patients were allocated to treatment using a covariate adaptive method which took into account the distribution of 10 important baseline characteristics of patients already enrolled and minimized the imbalance of those characteristics across the groups. Patients had a mean age of 64 years (range 40-80 years), were 97% Caucasian and were at high risk of developing a major coronary event because of existing CHD (65%), diabetes (Type 2, 26%; Type 1, 3%), history of stroke or other cerebrovascular disease (16%), peripheral vessel disease (33%), or hypertension in males ≥65 years (6%). At baseline, 3421 patients (17%) had LDL-C levels below 100 mg/dL, of whom 953 (5%) had LDL-C levels below 80 mg/dL; 7068 patients (34%) had levels between 100 and 130 mg/dL; and 10,047 patients (49%) had levels greater than 130 mg/dL.

The HPS results showed that simvastatin 40 mg/day significantly reduced: total and CHD mortality; non-fatal MI, stroke, and revascularization procedures (coronary and non-coronary) (see Table 16).

[See table 16 above]

Two composite endpoints were defined in order to have sufficient events to assess relative risk reductions across a range of baseline characteristics (see Figure 3). A composite of major coronary events (MCE) was comprised of CHD mortality and non-fatal MI (analyzed by time-to-first event; 898 patients treated with simvastatin had events and 1212 patients on placebo had events). A composite of major vascular events (MVE) was comprised of MCE, stroke and revascularization procedures including coronary, peripheral and other non-coronary procedures (analyzed by time-to-first event; 2033 patients treated with simvastatin had events and 2585 patients on placebo had events). Significant relative risk reductions were observed for both composite endpoints (27% for MCE and 24% for MVE, p<0.0001). Treatment with simvastatin produced significant relative risk reductions for all components of the composite endpoints. The risk reductions produced by simvastatin in both MCE and MVE were evident and consistent regardless of cardiovascular disease related medical history at study entry (i.e., CHD alone; or peripheral vascular disease, cerebrovascular disease, diabetes or treated hypertension, with or without CHD), gender, age, creatinine levels up to the entry limit of 2.3 mg/dL, baseline levels of LDL-C, HDL-C, apolipoprotein B and A-1, baseline concomitant cardiovascular medications (i.e., aspirin, beta blockers, or calcium channel blockers), smoking status, alcohol intake, or obesity. Diabetic patients showed risk reductions for MCE and MVE (27% and 22%, respectively; p<0.0001) due to simvastatin treatment regardless of baseline A1C levels or obesity with the greatest effects seen for diabetic patients without CHD.

[See figure 3 above]

Modifications of Lipid Profiles

Primary Hyperlipidemia (Fredrickson type lla and llb)

Simvastatin has been shown to be effective in reducing total-C and LDL-C in heterozygous familial and non-familial forms of hyperlipidemia and in mixed hyperlipidemia. Maximal to near maximal response is generally achieved within 4-6 weeks and maintained during chronic therapy. Simvastatin consistently and significantly decreased total-C, LDL-C, total-C/HDL-C ratio, and LDL-C/HDL-C ratio; simvastatin also decreased TG and increased HDL-C (see Table 17).

[See table 17 at top of next page]

Hypertriglyceridemia (Fredrickson type lV)

The results of a subgroup analysis in 74 patients with type IV hyperlipidemia from a 130-patient, double-blind, placebo-controlled, 3-period crossover study are presented in Table 18.

Table 16: Summary of Heart Protection Study Results

Endpoint	Simvastatin (N=10,269) n (%)*	Placebo (N=10,267) n (%)*	Risk Reduction (%) (95% CI)	p-Value
Primary				
Mortality	1328 (12.9)	1507 (14.7)	13 (6-19)	p=0.0003
CHD mortality	587 (5.7)	707 (6.9)	18 (8-26)	p=0.0005
Secondary				
Non-fatal MI	357 (3.5)	574 (5.6)	38 (30-46)	p<0.0001
Stroke	444 (4.3)	585 (5.7)	25 (15-34)	p<0.0001
Tertiary				
Coronary revascularization	513 (5)	725 (7.1)	30 (22-38)	p<0.0001
Peripheral and other non-coronary revascularization	450 (4.4)	532 (5.2)	16 (5-26)	p=0.006

* n = number of patients with indicated event

Figure 3: The Effects of Treatment with Simvastatin on Major Vascular Events and Major Coronary Events in HPS

Baseline Characteristics	N	Major Vascular Events Incidence (%) Simvastatin	Major Vascular Events Incidence (%) Placebo	Major Coronary Events Incidence (%) Simvastatin	Major Coronary Events Incidence (%) Placebo
All patients	20,536	19.8	25.2	8.7	11.8
Without CHD	7,150	16.1	20.8	5.1	8.0
With CHD	13,386	21.8	27.5	10.7	13.9
Diabetes mellitus	5,963	20.2	25.1	9.4	12.6
Without CHD	3,982	13.8	18.6	5.5	8.4
With CHD	1,981	33.4	37.8	17.4	21.0
Without diabetes mellitus	14,573	19.6	25.2	8.5	11.5
Peripheral vascular disease	6,748	26.4	32.7	10.9	13.8
Without CHD	2,701	24.7	30.5	7.0	10.1
With CHD	4,047	27.6	34.3	13.4	16.4
Cerebrovascular disease	3,280	24.7	29.8	10.4	13.3
Without CHD	1,820	18.7	23.6	5.9	8.7
With CHD	1,460	32.4	37.4	16.2	19.0
Gender					
Female	5,082	14.4	17.7	5.2	7.8
Male	15,454	21.6	27.6	9.9	13.1
Age (years)					
≥ 40 to < 65	9,839	16.9	22.1	6.2	9.2
≥ 65 to < 70	4,891	20.9	27.2	9.5	13.1
≥ 70	5,806	23.6	28.7	12.4	15.2
LDL-cholesterol (mg/dL)					
< 100	3,421	16.4	21.0	7.5	9.8
≥ 100 to < 130	7,068	18.9	24.7	7.9	11.9
≥ 130	10,047	21.6	26.9	9.7	12.4
HDL-cholesterol (mg/dL)					
< 35	7,176	22.6	29.9	10.2	14.4
≥ 35 to < 43	5,666	20.0	25.1	8.9	11.7
≥ 43	7,694	17.0	20.9	7.3	9.4

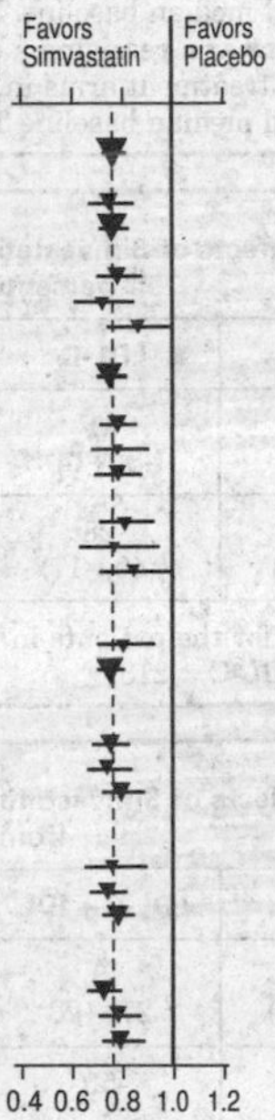

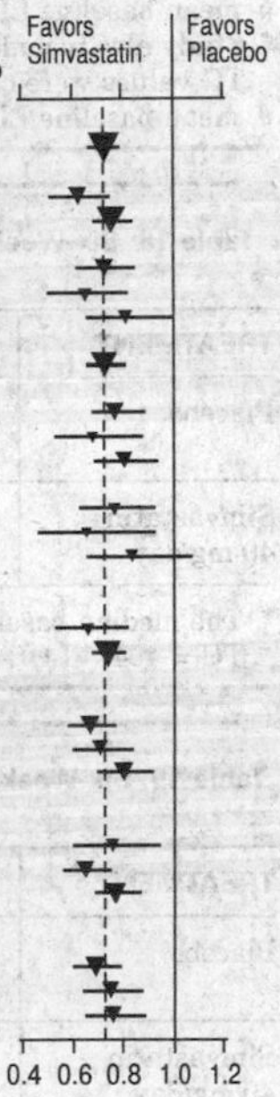

N = number of patients in each subgroup. The inverted triangles are point estimates of the relative risk, with their 95% confidence intervals represented as a line. The area of a triangle is proportional to the number of patients with MVE or MCE in the subgroup relative to the number with MVE or MCE, respectively, in the entire study population. The vertical solid line represents a relative risk of one. The vertical dashed line represents the point estimate of relative risk in the entire study population.

[See table 18 at top of next page]

Dysbetalipoproteinemia (Fredrickson type lll)

The results of a subgroup analysis in 7 patients with type lll hyperlipidemia (dysbetalipoproteinemia) (apo E2/2) (VLDL-C/TG>0.25) from a 130-patient, double-blind, placebo-controlled, 3-period crossover study are presented in Table 19.

[See table 19 at top of next page]

Homozygous Familial Hypercholesterolemia

In a controlled clinical study, 4 patients, 19-27 years of age, with homozygous familial hypercholesterolemia received simvastatin 40 mg/day in a single dose or in 3 divided doses. Reductions in LDL-C were observed for all patients. The mean LDL-C reduction for the 40 mg dose was 14% (range 8% to 23%, median 12%).

Endocrine Function

In clinical studies, simvastatin did not impair adrenal reserve or significantly reduce basal plasma cortisol concentration. Small reductions from baseline in basal plasma testosterone in men were observed in clinical studies with simvastatin, an effect also observed with other statins and the bile acid sequestrant cholestyramine. There was no effect on plasma gonadotropin levels. In a placebo-controlled, 12-week study there was no significant effect of simvastatin 80 mg on the plasma testosterone response to human chorionic gonadotropin. In another 24-week study, simvastatin 20-40 mg had no detectable effect on spermatogenesis. In 4S, in which 4444 patients were randomized to simvastatin 20-40 mg/day or placebo for a median duration of 5.4 years, the incidence of male sexual adverse events in the two treatment groups was not significantly different. Because of these factors, the small changes in plasma testosterone are unlikely to be clinically significant. The effects, if any, on the pituitary-gonadal axis in pre-menopausal women are unknown.

16 HOW SUPPLIED/STORAGE AND HANDLING

JUVISYNC 100 mg/10 mg tablets are pink-beige, bi-convex round, film-coated tablets, coded with the Merck logo and "753" on one side and plain on the other. They are supplied as follows:

NDC 0006-0753-31 unit of use bottles of 30
NDC 0006-0753-54 unit of use bottles of 90
NDC 0006-0753-82 bottles of 1000.

JUVISYNC 100 mg/20 mg tablets are pink-beige, bi-convex modified capsule-shaped, film-coated tablets, coded with the Merck logo and "757" on one side and plain on the other. They are supplied as follows:

NDC 0006-0757-31 unit of use bottles of 30
NDC 0006-0757-54 unit of use bottles of 90
NDC 0006-0757-82 bottles of 1000.

JUVISYNC 100 mg/40 mg tablets are orange-beige, bi-convex modified capsule-shaped, film-coated tablets, coded with the Merck logo and "773" on one side and plain on the other. They are supplied as follows:

NDC 0006-0773-31 unit of use bottles of 30
NDC 0006-0773-54 unit of use bottles of 90
NDC 0006-0773-82 bottles of 1000.

Table 17: Mean Response in Patients with Primary Hyperlipidemia and Combined (mixed) Hyperlipidemia (Mean Percent Change from Baseline After 6 to 24 Weeks)

TREATMENT	N	TOTAL-C	LDL-C	HDL-C	TG*
Lower Dose Comparative Study† (Mean % Change at Week 6)					
Simvastatin 5 mg q.p.m.	109	-19	-26	10	-12
Simvastatin 10 mg q.p.m.	110	-23	-30	12	-15
Scandinavian Simvastatin Survival Study‡ (Mean % Change at Week 6)					
Placebo	2223	-1	-1	0	-2
Simvastatin 20 mg q.p.m.	2221	-28	-38	8	-19
Upper Dose Comparative Study§, ¶ (Mean % Change Averaged at Weeks 18 and 24)					
Simvastatin 40 mg q.p.m.	433	-31	-41	9	-18
Multi-Center Combined Hyperlipidemia Study# (Mean % Change at Week 6)					
Placebo	125	1	2	3	-4
Simvastatin 40 mg q.p.m.	123	-25	-29	13	-28

* median percent change
† mean baseline LDL-C 244 mg/dL and median baseline TG 168 mg/dL
‡ mean baseline LDL-C 188 mg/dL and median baseline TG 128 mg/dL
§ mean baseline LDL-C 226 mg/dL and median baseline TG 156 mg/dL
¶ Study also included another treatment arm receiving a different dose of simvastatin; baseline mean LDL-C and median TG values were calculated across all treatment arms in study
\# mean baseline LDL-C 156 mg/dL and median baseline TG 391 mg/dL.

Table 18: Six-Week, Lipid-Lowering Effects of Simvastatin in Type IV Hyperlipidemia Median Percent Change (25th and 75th percentile) from Baseline*

TREATMENT	N	Total-C	LDL-C	HDL-C	TG	VLDL-C	Non-HDL-C
Placebo	74	+2 (-7, +7)	+1 (-8, +14)	+3 (-3, +10)	-9 (-25, +13)	-7 (-25, +11)	+1 (-9, +8)
Simvastatin 40 mg/day	74	-25 (-34, -19)	-28 (-40, -17)	+11 (+5, +23)	-29 (-43, -16)	-37 (-54, -23)	-32 (-42, -23)

* The median baseline values (mg/dL) for the patients in this study were: total-C = 254, LDL-C = 135, HDL-C = 36, TG = 404, VLDL-C = 83, and non-HDL-C = 215.

Table 19: Six-Week, Lipid-Lowering Effects of Simvastatin in Type III Hyperlipidemia Median Percent Change (min, max) from Baseline*

TREATMENT	N	Total-C	LDL-C + IDL	HDL-C	TG	VLDL-C + IDL	Non-HDL-C
Placebo	7	-8 (-24, +34)	-8 (-27, +23)	-2 (-21, +16)	+4 (-22, +90)	-4 (-28, +78)	-8 (-26, -39)
Simvastatin 40 mg/day	7	-50 (-66, -39)	-50 (-60, -31)	+7 (-8, +23)	-41 (-74, -16)	-58 (-90, -37)	-57 (-72, -44)

* The median baseline values (mg/dL) were: total-C = 324, LDL-C = 121, HDL-C = 31, TG = 411, VLDL-C = 170, and non-HDL-C = 291.

JUVISYNC 50 mg/10 mg tablets are red, bi-convex modified capsule-shaped, film-coated tablets, coded with the Merck logo and "533" on one side and plain on the other. They are supplied as follows:
NDC 0006-0533-31 unit of use bottles of 30
NDC 0006-0533-54 unit of use bottles of 90
JUVISYNC 50 mg/20 mg tablets are orange-beige, bi-convex modified capsule-shaped, film-coated tablets, coded with the Merck logo and "535" on one side and plain on the other. They are supplied as follows:
NDC 0006-0535-31 unit of use bottles of 30
NDC 0006-0535-54 unit of use bottles of 90
JUVISYNC 50 mg/40 mg tablets are red, bi-convex modified capsule-shaped, film-coated tablets, coded with the Merck logo and "537" on one side and plain on the other. They are supplied as follows:
NDC 0006-0537-31 unit of use bottles of 30
NDC 0006-0537-54 unit of use bottles of 90

Storage
Store at 20-25°C (68-77°F), excursions permitted to 15-30°C (59-86°F). [See USP Controlled Room Temperature.] Store in a dry place with cap tightly closed.

Storage of 1000 count bottles
Dispense into a USP tightly closed, moisture-resistant container.

17 PATIENT COUNSELING INFORMATION

See FDA-Approved Patient Labeling (Medication Guide).

17.1 Instructions

Patients should be informed of the potential risks and benefits of JUVISYNC and of alternative modes of therapy. Patients should also be informed about the importance of adherence to dietary instructions, regular physical activity, periodic blood glucose monitoring and A1C testing, recognition and management of hypoglycemia and hyperglycemia, and assessment for diabetes complications. During periods of stress such as fever, trauma, infection, or surgery, medication requirements may change and patients should be advised to seek medical advice promptly.

Patients should be informed that acute pancreatitis has been reported during postmarketing use of sitagliptin. Patients should be informed that persistent severe abdominal pain, sometimes radiating to the back, which may or may not be accompanied by vomiting, is the hallmark symptom of acute pancreatitis. Patients should be instructed to promptly discontinue JUVISYNC and contact their physician if persistent severe abdominal pain occurs *[see Warnings and Precautions (5.1)]*.

Patients should be informed that the incidence of hypoglycemia is increased when sitagliptin is added to a sulfonylurea or insulin and that a lower dose of the sulfonylurea or insulin may be required to reduce the risk of hypoglycemia.

Patients should be informed that allergic reactions have been reported during postmarketing use of sitagliptin. If symptoms of allergic reactions (including rash, hives, and swelling of the face, lips, tongue, and throat that may cause difficulty in breathing or swallowing) occur, patients must stop taking JUVISYNC and seek medical advice promptly.

Patients should be informed that the tablets must never be split or divided before swallowing.

Physicians should instruct their patients to read the Medication Guide before starting JUVISYNC therapy and to reread each time the prescription is renewed. Patients should be instructed to inform their doctor or pharmacist if they develop any unusual symptom, or if any known symptom persists or worsens.

Patients should be advised to adhere to their National Cholesterol Education Program (NCEP)-recommended diet, a regular exercise program, and periodic testing of a fasting lipid panel.

Patients should be advised about substances they should not take concomitantly with JUVISYNC *[see Contraindications (4); Warnings and Precautions (5.2)]*. Patients should also be advised to inform other healthcare professionals prescribing a new medication or increasing the dose of an existing medication that they are taking JUVISYNC.

17.2 Laboratory Tests

Patients should be informed that response to JUVISYNC should be monitored by periodic measurements of blood glucose, A1C, and cholesterol levels, with a goal of decreasing these levels towards the normal range. A1C is especially useful for evaluating long-term glycemic control. Patients should be informed of the potential need to adjust the dose or discontinue JUVISYNC based on changes in renal function test results over time.

It is recommended that liver function tests be performed before the initiation of JUVISYNC, and thereafter when clinically indicated. All patients treated with JUVISYNC should be advised to report promptly any symptoms that may indicate liver injury, including fatigue, anorexia, right upper abdominal discomfort, dark urine or jaundice.

17.3 Muscle Pain

All patients starting therapy with JUVISYNC should be advised of the risk of myopathy, including rhabdomyolysis, and told to report promptly any unexplained muscle pain, tenderness or weakness particularly if accompanied by malaise or fever or if these muscle signs or symptoms persist after discontinuing JUVISYNC. The risk of myopathy, including rhabdomyolysis, occurring with use of JUVISYNC is increased when taking certain types of medication or consuming grapefruit juice. Patients should discuss all medication, both prescription and over the counter, with their healthcare professional.

17.4 Pregnancy

Women of childbearing age should be advised to use an effective method of birth control to prevent pregnancy while using JUVISYNC. Discuss future pregnancy plans with your patients, and discuss when to stop taking JUVISYNC if they are trying to conceive. Patients should be advised that if they become pregnant they should stop taking JUVISYNC and call their healthcare professional.

17.5 Breastfeeding

Women who are breastfeeding should not use JUVISYNC. Patients who have a lipid disorder and are breastfeeding should be advised to discuss the options with their healthcare professional.

Manufactured for:
Merck Sharp & Dohme Corp., a subsidiary of
MERCK & CO., INC., Whitehouse Station, NJ 08889, USA
Manufactured by:
MSD International GmbH
Clonmel, Co. Tipperary,
Ireland
US Patent Nos.: 6,699,871 and 7,326,708

Revised: 02/2013
USPI-T-0431D1302R005

Medication Guide
JUVISYNC™ (JU-vih-sink)
(sitagliptin and simvastatin)
Tablets

Read this Medication Guide carefully before you start taking JUVISYNC and each time you get a refill. There may be new information. This information does not take the place of talking with your doctor about your medical condition or your treatment. If you have any questions about JUVISYNC, ask your doctor or pharmacist.

What is the most important information I should know about JUVISYNC?

Serious side effects can happen in people taking JUVISYNC, including inflammation of the pancreas (pancreatitis) which may be severe and lead to death. Certain medical problems make you more likely to get pancreatitis.

Before you start taking JUVISYNC:
Tell your doctor if you have ever had
- pancreatitis
- stones in your gallbladder (gallstones)
- a history of alcoholism
- high blood triglyceride levels
- kidney problems

Stop taking JUVISYNC and call your doctor right away if you have pain in your stomach area (abdomen) that is severe and will not go away. The pain may be felt going from your abdomen through to your back. The pain may happen with or without vomiting. These may be symptoms of pancreatitis.

What is JUVISYNC?

- JUVISYNC is a prescription medicine that contains two medicines, sitagliptin and simvastatin, in one pill. JUVISYNC can be used in adults who need both sitagliptin and simvastatin.
- Sitagliptin can be used along with diet and exercise to lower blood sugar in adults with type 2 diabetes.
- Simvastatin can be used with diet and exercise in adults at high risk for heart attack or stroke to lower your chance of:
  - death from heart problems
  - having a heart attack or stroke
  - needing certain blood vessel procedures
- Simvastatin can be used in adults with certain cholesterol problems to lower levels of total cholesterol, LDL (bad) cholesterol, and fatty substances called triglycerides in the blood. In addition, simvastatin raises levels of HDL (good) cholesterol. Simvastatin is for people who cannot control their cholesterol levels by diet and exercise alone. You should stay on a cholesterol-lowering diet while taking this medicine.
- Sitagliptin is not for people with type 1 diabetes.
- Sitagliptin is not for people with diabetic ketoacidosis (increased ketones in your blood or urine).
- If you have had inflammation of your pancreas (pancreatitis) in the past, it is not known if you have a higher chance of getting pancreatitis while you take sitagliptin.
- JUVISYNC has not been studied in people who have an increase of chylomicrons (Fredrickson types I and V).
- JUVISYNC is not for people with certain kidney problems.
- It is not known if JUVISYNC is safe and effective when used in children under 18 years of age.

For more information, see the sections called **"What is type 2 diabetes?"** and **"What should I know about high cholesterol?"**.

Who should not take JUVISYNC?

Do not take JUVISYNC if you:

- are allergic to any of the ingredients in JUVISYNC. See the end of this Medication Guide for a complete list of ingredients in JUVISYNC.
  Symptoms of a serious allergic reaction to JUVISYNC may include:
  - rash
  - raised red patches on your skin (hives)
  - swelling of the face, lips, tongue, and throat that may cause difficulty in breathing or swallowing
- take certain medicines such as:
  - anti-fungal medicines including:
    - itraconazole
    - ketoconazole
    - posaconazole
    - voriconazole
  - HIV protease inhibitors, including:
    - indinavir
    - nelfinavir
    - ritonavir
    - saquinavir
    - tipranavir
    - atazanavir
  - certain hepatitis C virus protease inhibitors, including:
    - boceprevir
    - telaprevir
  - certain antibiotics, including:
    - erythromycin
    - clarithromycin
    - telithromycin
  - nefazodone
  - a fibrate medicine for lowering cholesterol called gemfibrozil
  - cyclosporine
  - danazol

  Ask your doctor if you are not sure whether your medicine is listed above.
- have active liver disease or repeated blood tests indicating possible liver problems.
- are pregnant or think you may be pregnant, or you are planning to become pregnant.
- are a woman of childbearing age, you should use an effective method of birth control to prevent pregnancy while using JUVISYNC.
- are breastfeeding or plan to breastfeed.

What should I tell my doctor before taking JUVISYNC?

Before you take JUVISYNC, tell your doctor if you:

- have or have had inflammation of your pancreas (pancreatitis).
- have kidney problems.
- drink substantial quantities of alcohol or ever had liver problems.
- have any other medical conditions.
- are taking drugs that prevent blood clots, such as warfarin.

Taking JUVISYNC with certain substances can increase the risk of muscle problems. It is especially important to tell your doctor if you take:

- fibric acid derivatives (such as fenofibrate)
- amiodarone or dronedarone (drugs used to treat an irregular heartbeat)
- the following medicines used to treat high blood pressure, chest pain with heart disease, or other heart problems:
  - verapamil
  - diltiazem
  - amlodipine
  - ranolazine
- grapefruit juice (which should be avoided while taking JUVISYNC)
- colchicine (a medicine used to treat gout)
- large doses of niacin or nicotinic acid

Tell your doctor if you are taking niacin or a niacin-containing product, as this may increase your risk of muscle problems, especially if you are Chinese.

Tell all of your doctors about all the medicines you take, including prescription and non-prescription medicines, vitamins, and herbal supplements.

Know the medicines you take. Keep a list of your medicines and show it to your doctor and pharmacist when you get a new medicine.

How should I take JUVISYNC?

- Take one JUVISYNC tablet each day, in the evening, exactly as your doctor tells you.
- Do not break or cut JUVISYNC tablets before swallowing. If you cannot swallow JUVISYNC tablets whole, tell your doctor.
- Your doctor may tell you to take JUVISYNC along with other diabetes medicines. Low blood sugar can happen more often when JUVISYNC is taken with certain other diabetes medicines. See **"What are the possible side effects of JUVISYNC?"**.
- If you take too much JUVISYNC, call your doctor or go to the nearest hospital emergency room right away.
- When your body is under some types of stress, such as fever, trauma (such as a car accident), infection or surgery, the amount of diabetes medicine that you need may change. Tell your doctor right away if you have any of these conditions and follow your doctor's instructions.
- Check your blood sugar as your doctor tells you to.
- Stay on your prescribed diet and exercise program while taking JUVISYNC.
- Talk to your doctor about how to prevent, recognize and manage low blood sugar (hypoglycemia), high blood sugar (hyperglycemia), and problems you have because of your diabetes.
- Your doctor will monitor your condition with regular blood tests, including your blood sugar levels, hemoglobin A1C, and cholesterol levels, and to check for side effects.
- Your doctor will do blood tests to check how well your kidneys are working before and during your treatment with JUVISYNC. Your doctor may change your dose or discontinue JUVISYNC based on the results of your blood tests.

What are the possible side effects of JUVISYNC?

Serious side effects have happened in people taking JUVISYNC.

- See **"What is the most important information I should know about JUVISYNC?"**.
- **myopathy (muscle weakness) and rhabdomyolysis (muscle breakdown).** Tell your doctor right away if you have unexplained muscle pain, tenderness, or weakness especially with fever while you take JUVISYNC.
  - Muscle problems, including muscle breakdown, can be serious in some people and on rare occasions may cause kidney damage that can lead to death.
  - The risk of muscle breakdown is greater at higher doses of JUVISYNC.
  - The risk of muscle breakdown is greater in people 65 years of age and older, females, and people with kidney or thyroid problems.

  If you have muscle problems that do not go away even after your doctor has advised you to stop taking JUVISYNC, notify your doctor. Your doctor may do further tests to diagnose the cause of your muscle problems.
- **liver problems.** Your doctor should do blood tests to check your liver before you start taking JUVISYNC and if you have any symptoms of liver problems while you take JUVISYNC. Call your doctor right away if you have the following symptoms of liver problems:
  - feel tired or weak
  - loss of appetite
  - upper belly pain
  - dark urine
  - yellowing of your skin or the whites of your eyes
- **kidney problems,** sometimes requiring dialysis
- **low blood sugar (hypoglycemia).** If you take JUVISYNC with another medicine that can cause low blood sugar, such as a sulfonylurea or insulin, your risk of getting low blood sugar is higher. The dose of your sulfonylurea medicine or insulin may need to be lowered while you use JUVISYNC. Signs and symptoms of low blood sugar may include:
  - headache
  - drowsiness
  - weakness
  - dizziness
  - confusion
  - irritability
  - hunger
  - fast heart beat
  - sweating
  - feeling jittery
- **Serious allergic reactions.** If you have any symptoms of a serious allergic reaction, stop taking JUVISYNC and call your doctor right away. See **"Who should not take JUVISYNC?"**. Your doctor may give you a medicine for your allergic reaction and prescribe a different medicine for your diabetes.

The most common side effects of JUVISYNC include:

- upper respiratory infection
- stuffy or runny nose and sore throat
- headache
- stomach pain
- constipation
- nausea

JUVISYNC may have other side effects, including:

- swelling of the hands or legs. Swelling of the hands or legs can happen if you take JUVISYNC in combination with rosiglitazone (Avandia®). Rosiglitazone is another type of diabetes medicine.
- joint pain
- muscle pain
- alterations in some laboratory blood tests
- liver problems (sometimes serious)
- nausea
- dizziness
- tingling sensation
- depression
- trouble sleeping
- poor memory
- erectile dysfunction
- breathing problems including persistent cough and/or shortness of breath or fever.

These are not all the possible side effects of JUVISYNC. For more information, ask your doctor or pharmacist.

Tell your doctor if you have any side effect that bothers you, is unusual or does not go away.

Call your doctor for medical advice about side effects. You may report side effects to FDA at 1-800-FDA-1088.

How should I store JUVISYNC?

Store JUVISYNC at 68°F to 77°F (20°C to 25°C). Store in a dry place with cap tightly closed.

Keep JUVISYNC and all medicines out of the reach of children.

General information about the use of JUVISYNC

Medicines are sometimes prescribed for purposes that are not listed in Medication Guides. Do not use JUVISYNC for a condition for which it was not prescribed. Do not give JUVISYNC to other people, even if they have the same symptoms you have. It may harm them.

This Medication Guide summarizes the most important information about JUVISYNC. If you would like to know more information, talk with your doctor. You can ask your doctor or pharmacist for additional information about JUVISYNC that is written for health professionals. For more information, go to www.JUVISYNC.com or call 1-800-622-4477.

What are the ingredients in JUVISYNC?

Active ingredients: sitagliptin and simvastatin

Inactive ingredients: anhydrous dibasic calcium phosphate, microcrystalline cellulose, croscarmellose sodium, sodium stearyl fumarate, magnesium stearate, ascorbic acid, citric acid monohydrate, lactose monohydrate, pregelatinized corn starch, butylated hydroxyanisole. The tablet film coating contains the following inactive ingredients: polyvinyl alcohol, polyethylene glycol, talc, titanium dioxide, and red iron oxide. The film coating for certain tablet strengths also contains yellow iron oxide and black iron oxide.

What is type 2 diabetes?

Type 2 diabetes is a condition in which your body does not make enough insulin, and the insulin that your body produces does not work as well as it should. Your body can also make too much sugar. When this happens, sugar (glucose) builds up in the blood. This can lead to serious medical problems.

High blood sugar can be lowered by diet and exercise, and by certain medicines when necessary.

What should I know about high cholesterol?

Cholesterol is a type of fat found in your blood. Cholesterol comes from two sources. It is produced by your body and it comes from the food you eat. Your total cholesterol is made up of both LDL and HDL cholesterol.

LDL cholesterol is called "bad" cholesterol because it can build up in the wall of your arteries and form plaque, which can slow or block blood flow to your heart, brain, and other organs.

HDL cholesterol is called "good" cholesterol because it keeps the bad cholesterol from building up in the arteries.
Triglycerides also are fats found in your body.
Manufactured for: Merck Sharp & Dohme Corp., a subsidiary of
MERCK & CO., INC., Whitehouse Station, NJ 08889, USA
Manufactured by:
MSD International GmbH
Clonmel, Co. Tipperary,
Ireland
US Patent Nos.: 6,699,871 and 7,326,708
The trademarks depicted herein are owned by their respective companies.

Revised: 02/2013
USMG-T-0431D1302R005
This Medication Guide has been approved by the U.S. Food and Drug Administration.
Shown in Product Identification Guide, page 308

LIPTRUZET™ ℞

[LIP-true-zett]
(ezetimibe and atorvastatin)
tablets for oral use

HIGHLIGHTS OF PRESCRIBING INFORMATION
These highlights do not include all the information needed to use LIPTRUZET safely and effectively. See full prescribing information for LIPTRUZET.
LIPTRUZET™ (ezetimibe and atorvastatin) tablets for oral use
Initial U.S. Approval: 2013

INDICATIONS AND USAGE

LIPTRUZET, which contains a cholesterol absorption inhibitor and an HMG-CoA reductase inhibitor (statin), is indicated as adjunctive therapy to diet to:
- reduce elevated total-C, LDL-C, Apo B, TG, and non-HDL-C, and to increase HDL-C in patients with primary (heterozygous familial and non-familial) hyperlipidemia or mixed hyperlipidemia. (1.1)
- reduce elevated total-C and LDL-C in patients with homozygous familial hypercholesterolemia (HoFH), as an adjunct to other lipid-lowering treatments. (1.2)

Limitations of Use
- No incremental benefit of LIPTRUZET on cardiovascular morbidity and mortality over and above that demonstrated for atorvastatin has been established. LIPTRUZET has not been studied in Fredrickson Type I, III, IV, and V dyslipidemias. (1.3)

DOSAGE AND ADMINISTRATION

- Dosage range is 10/10 mg/day through 10/80 mg/day. (2.1)
- Recommended starting dose is 10/10 mg/day or 10/20 mg/day. (2.1)
- Recommended starting dose is 10/40 mg/day for patients requiring a >55% reduction in LDL-C. (2.1)
- Dosing of LIPTRUZET should occur either ≥2 hours before or ≥4 hours after administration of a bile acid sequestrant. (2.3, 7.11)

DOSAGE FORMS AND STRENGTHS

- Tablets (ezetimibe mg/atorvastatin mg): 10/10, 10/20, 10/40, 10/80. (3)

CONTRAINDICATIONS

- Active liver disease or unexplained persistent elevations of hepatic transaminase levels. (4, 5.2)
- Hypersensitivity to any component of LIPTRUZET. (4, 6.2)
- Women who are pregnant or may become pregnant. (4, 8.1)
- Nursing mothers. (4, 8.3)

WARNINGS AND PRECAUTIONS

- Patients should be advised to report promptly any unexplained and/or persistent muscle pain, tenderness, or weakness. LIPTRUZET should be discontinued immediately if myopathy is diagnosed or suspected. (5.1)
- Skeletal muscle effects (e.g., myopathy and rhabdomyolysis): Risks increase with higher doses and concomitant use of certain CYP3A4 inhibitors, fibric acid derivatives, and cyclosporine. Predisposing factors include advanced age (>65), uncontrolled hypothyroidism, and renal impairment. Rare cases of rhabdomyolysis with acute renal failure secondary to myoglobinuria have been reported. (5.1, 8.5)
- Liver enzyme abnormalities: Persistent elevations in hepatic transaminase can occur. Check liver enzyme tests before initiating therapy and as clinically indicated thereafter. (5.2)

ADVERSE REACTIONS

- Common adverse reactions (incidence ≥2% and greater than placebo) are: increased ALT, increased AST, and musculoskeletal pain. (6.1)

To report SUSPECTED ADVERSE REACTIONS, contact Merck Sharp & Dohme Corp., a subsidiary of Merck & Co., Inc., at 1-877-888-4231 or FDA at 1-800-FDA-1088 or www.fda.gov/medwatch.

DRUG INTERACTIONS

Drug Interactions Associated with Increased Risk of Myopathy/Rhabdomyolysis with Atorvastatin (2.3, 5.1, 7, 12.3)

Interacting Agents	Prescribing Recommendations for LIPTRUZET
Cyclosporine, HIV protease inhibitors (tipranavir plus ritonavir), hepatitis C protease inhibitor (telaprevir), gemfibrozil	Avoid LIPTRUZET
HIV protease inhibitor (lopinavir plus ritonavir)	Use with caution and lowest dose necessary.
Clarithromycin, itraconazole, HIV protease inhibitors (saquinavir plus ritonavir, darunavir plus ritonavir, fosamprenavir, fosamprenavir plus ritonavir)	Do not exceed 10/20 mg LIPTRUZET daily.
HIV protease inhibitor (nelfinavir), hepatitis C protease inhibitor (boceprevir)	Do not exceed 10/40 mg LIPTRUZET daily.

- Other lipid-lowering medications: Use with fenofibrates or lipid-modifying doses (≥1 g/day) of niacin increases the risk of adverse skeletal muscle effects. Caution should be used when prescribing with LIPTRUZET. (7)
- Fenofibrates: Combination increases exposure of ezetimibe. If cholelithiasis is suspected in a patient receiving ezetimibe and a fenofibrate, gallbladder studies are indicated and alternative lipid-lowering therapy should be considered. (7.5, 12.3)
- Cholestyramine: Combination decreases exposure of ezetimibe. (2.3, 12.3)
- Digoxin: Patients should be monitored appropriately. (7.7)
- Oral contraceptives: Values for norethindrone and ethinyl estradiol may be increased. (7.8)
- Rifampin should be simultaneously coadministered with LIPTRUZET. (7.9)

USE IN SPECIFIC POPULATIONS

- Hepatic impairment: Plasma concentrations of atorvastatin are markedly increased in patients with chronic alcoholic liver disease. (8.6, 12.3)

See 17 for PATIENT COUNSELING INFORMATION and FDA-approved patient labeling

Revised: 05/2013

FULL PRESCRIBING INFORMATION: CONTENTS*

*** Sections or subsections omitted from the full prescribing information are not listed**

FULL PRESCRIBING INFORMATION

1 INDICATIONS AND USAGE

Therapy with lipid-altering agents should be only one component of multiple risk factor intervention in individuals at significantly increased risk for atherosclerotic vascular disease due to hypercholesterolemia. Drug therapy is indicated as an adjunct to diet when the response to a diet restricted in saturated fat and cholesterol and other nonpharmacologic measures alone has been inadequate.

1.1 Primary Hyperlipidemia

LIPTRUZET™ is indicated for the reduction of elevated total cholesterol (total-C), low-density lipoprotein cholesterol (LDL-C), apolipoprotein B (Apo B), triglycerides (TG), and non-high-density lipoprotein cholesterol (non-HDL-C), and to increase high-density lipoprotein cholesterol (HDL-C) in patients with primary (heterozygous familial and non-familial) hyperlipidemia or mixed hyperlipidemia.

1.2 Homozygous Familial Hypercholesterolemia (HoFH)

LIPTRUZET is indicated for the reduction of elevated total-C and LDL-C in patients with homozygous familial hypercholesterolemia, as an adjunct to other lipid-lowering treatments (e.g., LDL apheresis) or if such treatments are unavailable.

1.3 Limitations of Use

No incremental benefit of LIPTRUZET on cardiovascular morbidity and mortality over and above that demonstrated for atorvastatin has been established. LIPTRUZET has not been studied in Fredrickson type I, III, IV, and V dyslipidemias.

2 DOSAGE AND ADMINISTRATION

2.1 Recommended Dosing

The dosage range of LIPTRUZET is 10/10 mg/day to 10/80 mg/day. The recommended starting dose of LIPTRUZET is 10/10 mg/day or 10/20 mg/day. LIPTRUZET can be administered as a single dose at any time of the day, with or without food. The recommended starting dose for patients who require a larger reduction in LDL-C (greater than 55%) is 10/40 mg/day. After initiation and/or upon titration of LIPTRUZET, lipid levels should be analyzed within 2 or more weeks and dosage adjusted accordingly.
Patients should swallow LIPTRUZET tablets whole. Tablets should not be crushed, dissolved, or chewed.

2.2 Patients with Homozygous Familial Hypercholesterolemia

The dosage of LIPTRUZET in patients with homozygous familial hypercholesterolemia is 10/40 mg/day or 10/80 mg/day. LIPTRUZET should be used as an adjunct to other lipid-lowering treatments (e.g., LDL apheresis) in these patients or if such treatments are unavailable.

2.3 Coadministration with Other Drugs

Bile Acid Sequestrants

Dosing of LIPTRUZET should occur either ≥2 hours before or ≥4 hours after administration of a bile acid sequestrant *[see Drug Interactions (7.11)]*.

Cyclosporine, Clarithromycin, Itraconazole, or Certain Protease Inhibitors

In patients taking cyclosporine or the HIV protease inhibitors (tipranavir plus ritonavir) or the hepatitis C protease inhibitor (telaprevir), therapy with LIPTRUZET should be avoided. In patients with HIV taking lopinavir plus ritonavir, caution should be used when prescribing LIPTRUZET and the lowest dose necessary employed. In patients taking clarithromycin, itraconazole, or in patients with HIV taking a combination of saquinavir plus ritonavir, darunavir plus ritonavir, fosamprenavir, or fosamprenavir plus ritonavir, therapy with LIPTRUZET should be limited to 10/20 mg, and appropriate clinical assessment is recommended to ensure that the lowest dose necessary of LIPTRUZET is employed. In patients taking the HIV protease inhibitor nelfinavir or the hepatitis C protease inhibitor boceprevir, therapy with LIPTRUZET should be limited to 10/40 mg, and appropriate clinical assessment is recommended to ensure that the lowest dose necessary of LIPTRUZET is employed. *[See Warnings and Precautions (5.1) and Drug Interactions (7).]*

Other Concomitant Lipid-Lowering Therapy

The combination of LIPTRUZET and gemfibrozil is not recommended *[see Warnings and Precautions (5.1) and Drug Interactions (7.4)]*.

3 DOSAGE FORMS AND STRENGTHS

- LIPTRUZET™ 10 mg/10 mg (ezetimibe 10 mg/ atorvastatin 10 mg) tablets are white to off-white capsule-shaped, biconvex film-coated tablets with code "320" on one side.
- LIPTRUZET™ 10 mg/20 mg (ezetimibe 10 mg/ atorvastatin 20 mg) tablets are white to off-white round, biconvex film-coated tablets with code "321" on one side.
- LIPTRUZET™ 10 mg/40 mg (ezetimibe 10 mg/ atorvastatin 40 mg) tablets are white to off-white oval, biconvex film-coated tablets with code "322" on one side.
- LIPTRUZET™ 10 mg/80 mg (ezetimibe 10 mg/ atorvastatin 80 mg) tablets are white to off-white capsule-shaped, biconvex film-coated tablets with code "323" on one side.

4 CONTRAINDICATIONS

Active liver disease or unexplained persistent elevations of hepatic transaminase levels.

Hypersensitivity to any component of LIPTRUZET *[see Adverse Reactions (6.2)]*.

Women who are pregnant or may become pregnant. LIPTRUZET may cause fetal harm when administered to a pregnant woman. Serum cholesterol and triglycerides increase during normal pregnancy, and cholesterol or cholesterol derivatives are essential for fetal development. Atherosclerosis is a chronic process and discontinuation of lipid-lowering drugs during pregnancy should have little impact on the outcome of long-term therapy of primary hypercholesterolemia. There are no adequate and well-controlled studies of LIPTRUZET use during pregnancy; however in rare reports, congenital anomalies were observed following intrauterine exposure to statins. In rat and rabbit animal reproduction studies, atorvastatin revealed no evidence of teratogenicity. LIPTRUZET should be administered to women of childbearing age only when such patients are highly unlikely to conceive and have been informed of the potential hazards. If the patient becomes pregnant while taking this drug, LIPTRUZET should be discontinued immediately, and the patient should be apprised of the potential hazard to the fetus *[see Use in Specific Populations (8.1)]*.

Nursing mothers. It is not known whether atorvastatin is excreted into human milk; however, a small amount of another drug in this class does pass into breast milk. Because statins have the potential for serious adverse reactions in nursing infants, women who require LIPTRUZET treatment should not breast-feed their infants *[see Use in Specific Populations (8.3)]*.

5 WARNINGS AND PRECAUTIONS

5.1 Myopathy/Rhabdomyolysis

Atorvastatin

Rare cases of rhabdomyolysis with acute renal failure secondary to myoglobinuria have been reported with atorvastatin and with other drugs in this class. A history of renal impairment may be a risk factor for the development of rhabdomyolysis. Such patients merit closer monitoring for skeletal muscle effects.

Atorvastatin, like other statins, occasionally causes myopathy, defined as muscle aches or muscle weakness in conjunction with increases in creatine phosphokinase (CPK) values >10 times upper limit of normal (ULN). The concomitant use of higher doses of atorvastatin with certain drugs such as cyclosporine and strong CYP3A4 inhibitors (e.g., clarithromycin, itraconazole, and HIV protease inhibitors) increases the risk of myopathy/rhabdomyolysis.

There have been rare reports of immune-mediated necrotizing myopathy (IMNM), an autoimmune myopathy, associated with statin use. IMNM is characterized by: proximal muscle weakness and elevated serum creatinine kinase, which persist despite discontinuation of statin treatment; muscle biopsy showing necrotizing myopathy without significant inflammation; improvement with immunosuppressive agents.

Myopathy should be considered in any patient with diffuse myalgias, muscle tenderness or weakness, and/or marked elevation of CPK. Patients should be advised to report promptly unexplained muscle pain, tenderness or weakness, particularly if accompanied by malaise or fever or if muscle signs and symptoms persist after discontinuing LIPTRUZET. LIPTRUZET therapy should be discontinued if markedly elevated CPK levels occur or myopathy is diagnosed or suspected.

The risk of myopathy during treatment with statins is increased with concurrent administration of cyclosporine, fibric acid derivatives, erythromycin, clarithromycin, the hepatitis C protease inhibitor telaprevir, combinations of HIV protease inhibitors, including saquinavir plus ritonavir, lopinavir plus ritonavir, tipranavir plus ritonavir, darunavir plus ritonavir, fosamprenavir, and fosamprenavir plus ritonavir, niacin, or azole antifungals. Physicians considering combined therapy with LIPTRUZET and fibric acid derivatives, erythromycin, clarithromycin, a combination of saquinavir plus ritonavir, lopinavir plus ritonavir, darunavir plus ritonavir, fosamprenavir, or fosamprenavir plus ritonavir, azole antifungals, or lipid-modifying doses of niacin should carefully weigh the potential benefits and risks and should carefully monitor patients for any signs or symptoms of muscle pain, tenderness, or weakness, particularly during the initial months of therapy and during any periods of upward dosage titration of either drug. Lower starting and maintenance doses of LIPTRUZET should be considered when taken concomitantly with the aforementioned drugs. *[See Drug Interactions (7).]* Periodic CPK determinations may be considered in such situations, but there is no assurance that such monitoring will prevent the occurrence of severe myopathy.

Prescribing recommendations for interacting agents are summarized in Table 1 *[see also Dosage and Administration (2.3), Drug Interactions (7), Clinical Pharmacology (12.3)]*.

Table 1: Drug Interactions Associated with Increased Risk of Myopathy/Rhabdomyolysis with Atorvastatin

Interacting Agents	Prescribing Recommendations for LIPTRUZET
Cyclosporine, HIV protease inhibitors (tipranavir plus ritonavir), hepatitis C protease inhibitor (telaprevir), gemfibrozil	Avoid LIPTRUZET.
HIV protease inhibitor (lopinavir plus ritonavir)	Use with caution and lowest dose necessary.
Clarithromycin, itraconazole, HIV protease inhibitors (saquinavir plus ritonavir*, darunavir plus ritonavir, fosamprenavir, fosamprenavir plus ritonavir)	Do not exceed 10/20 mg LIPTRUZET daily.
HIV protease inhibitor (nelfinavir), hepatitis C protease inhibitor (boceprevir)	Do not exceed 10/40 mg LIPTRUZET daily.

* Use with caution and with the lowest dose necessary *[see Clinical Pharmacology (12.3)]*

Cases of myopathy, including rhabdomyolysis, have been reported with atorvastatin coadministered with colchicine, and caution should be exercised when prescribing LIPTRUZET with colchicine *[see Drug Interactions (7.10)]*.

LIPTRUZET therapy should be temporarily withheld or discontinued in any patient with an acute, serious condition suggestive of a myopathy or having a risk factor predisposing to the development of renal failure secondary to rhabdomyolysis (e.g., severe acute infection, hypotension, major surgery, trauma, severe metabolic, endocrine and electrolyte disorders, and uncontrolled seizures).

Ezetimibe

In clinical trials, there was no excess of myopathy or rhabdomyolysis associated with ezetimibe compared with the relevant control arm (placebo or statin alone). However, myopathy and rhabdomyolysis are known adverse reactions to statins and other lipid-lowering drugs. In clinical trials, the incidence of creatine phosphokinase (CPK) >10 times ULN was 0.2% for ezetimibe vs. 0.1% for placebo, and 0.1% for ezetimibe coadministered with a statin vs. 0.4% for statins alone. Risk for skeletal muscle toxicity increases with higher doses of statin, advanced age (>65), hypothyroidism, renal impairment, and depending on the statin used, concomitant use of other drugs.

In post-marketing experience with ezetimibe, cases of myopathy and rhabdomyolysis have been reported. Most patients who developed rhabdomyolysis were taking a statin prior to initiating ezetimibe. However, rhabdomyolysis has been reported with ezetimibe monotherapy and with the addition of ezetimibe to agents known to be associated with increased risk of rhabdomyolysis, such as fibric acid derivatives. LIPTRUZET and a fenofibrate, if taking concomitantly, should both be immediately discontinued if myopathy is diagnosed or suspected. The presence of muscle symptoms and a CPK level >10 times the ULN indicates myopathy.

5.2 Liver Enzymes

Atorvastatin

Statins, like some other lipid-lowering therapies, have been associated with biochemical abnormalities of liver function. Persistent elevations (>3 times ULN occurring on 2 or more occasions) in serum transaminases occurred in 0.7% of patients who received atorvastatin in clinical trials. The incidence of these abnormalities was 0.2%, 0.2%, 0.6%, and 2.3% for 10, 20, 40, and 80 mg atorvastatin, respectively.

One patient in clinical trials of atorvastatin developed jaundice. Increases in liver function tests (LFT) in other patients were not associated with jaundice or other clinical signs or symptoms. Upon dose reduction, drug interruption, or discontinuation, transaminase levels returned to or near pretreatment levels without sequelae. Eighteen of 30 patients with persistent LFT elevations continued treatment with a reduced dose of atorvastatin.

Ezetimibe

In controlled clinical studies, the incidence of consecutive elevations (≥3 times ULN) in hepatic transaminase levels was similar between ezetimibe (0.5%) and placebo (0.3%).

In controlled clinical combination studies of ezetimibe coadministered with atorvastatin, the incidence of consecutive elevations (≥3 times ULN) in hepatic transaminase levels was 0.6% for patients treated with ezetimibe administered with atorvastatin. These elevations in transaminases were generally asymptomatic, not associated with cholestasis, and returned to baseline after discontinuation of therapy or with continued treatment.

LIPTRUZET

It is recommended that liver enzyme tests be obtained prior to initiating therapy with LIPTRUZET and repeated as clinically indicated. There have been rare postmarketing reports of fatal and non-fatal hepatic failure in patients taking statins, including atorvastatin. If serious liver injury with clinical symptoms and/or hyperbilirubinemia or jaundice occurs during treatment with LIPTRUZET, promptly interrupt therapy. If an alternate etiology is not found, do not restart LIPTRUZET.

LIPTRUZET should be used with caution in patients who consume substantial quantities of alcohol and/or have a history of liver disease. Active liver disease or unexplained persistent transaminase elevations are contraindications to the use of LIPTRUZET *[see Contraindications (4)]*.

5.3 Endocrine Function

Increases in HbA1c and fasting serum glucose levels have been reported with HMG-CoA reductase inhibitors, including atorvastatin.

Statins interfere with cholesterol synthesis and theoretically might blunt adrenal and/or gonadal steroid production. Clinical studies have shown that atorvastatin does not reduce basal plasma cortisol concentration or impair adrenal reserve and that ezetimibe did not impair adrenocortical steroid hormone production. The effects of statins on male fertility have not been studied in adequate numbers of patients. The effects, if any, on the pituitary-gonadal axis in premenopausal women are unknown. Caution should be exercised if LIPTRUZET is administered concomitantly with drugs that may decrease the levels or activity of endogenous steroid hormones, such as ketoconazole, spironolactone, and cimetidine.

5.4 Use in Patients with Recent Stroke or TIA

In a post-hoc analysis of the Stroke Prevention by Aggressive Reduction in Cholesterol Levels (SPARCL) study where atorvastatin 80 mg vs. placebo was administered in 4,731 subjects without CHD who had a stroke or TIA within the preceding 6 months, a higher incidence of hemorrhagic stroke was seen in the atorvastatin 80 mg group compared to placebo (55, 2.3% atorvastatin vs. 33, 1.4% placebo; HR: 1.68, 95% CI: 1.09, 2.59; p=0.0168). The incidence of fatal hemorrhagic stroke was similar across treatment groups (17 vs. 18 for the atorvastatin and placebo groups, respectively). The incidence of nonfatal hemorrhagic stroke was significantly higher in the atorvastatin (38, 1.6%) group as compared to the placebo group (16, 0.7%). Some baseline

Table 2*: Clinical and Selected Laboratory Adverse Reactions Occurring in ≥2% of Patients Treated with LIPTRUZET and at an Incidence Greater than Placebo, Regardless of Causality

Body System/Organ Class Adverse Reaction	Placebo (%) n=60	Ezetimibe 10 mg (%) n=65	Atorvastatin† (%) n=248	LIPTRUZET† (%) n=255
Nervous system disorders				
Dizziness	0	6	<1	2
Respiratory, thoracic, and mediastinal disorders				
Coughing	0	3	<1	2
Gastrointestinal disorders				
Abdominal pain	2	2	4	3
Nausea	0	2	5	3
Musculoskeletal and connective tissue disorders				
Arthralgia	0	5	6	3
Muscle weakness	0	2	0	2
Musculoskeletal pain	3	8	5	4
Metabolism and nutrition disorders				
Hyperkalemia	0	0	<1	2
Infections and infestations				
Bronchitis	0	2	2	2
Sinusitis	0	3	2	2
Vascular disorders				
Hot flushes	0	0	<1	2
Investigations				
ALT increased	0	0	2	5
AST increased	0	0	<1	4

* Placebo-controlled combination study in which the active ingredients equivalent to LIPTRUZET were coadministered.
† All doses.

Table 4: Clinical Adverse Reactions Occurring in > 2% in Patents Treated with any dose of Atorvastatin and at an Incidence Greater than Placebo Regardless of Causality (% of patients).

Adverse Reaction*	Any dose n=8755	Atorvastatin 10 mg n=3908	Atorvastatin 20 mg n=188	Atorvastatin 40 mg n=604	Atorvastatin 80 mg n=4055	Placebo n=7311
Nasopharyngitis	8.3	12.9	5.3	7.0	4.2	8.2
Arthralgia	6.9	8.9	11.7	10.6	4.3	6.5
Diarrhea	6.8	7.3	6.4	14.1	5.2	6.3
Pain in extremity	6.0	8.5	3.7	9.3	3.1	5.9
Urinary tract infection	5.7	6.9	6.4	8.0	4.1	5.6
Dyspepsia	4.7	5.9	3.2	6.0	3.3	4.3
Nausea	4.0	3.7	3.7	7.1	3.8	3.5
Musculoskeletal pain	3.8	5.2	3.2	5.1	2.3	3.6
Muscle spasms	3.6	4.6	4.8	5.1	2.4	3.0
Myalgia	3.5	3.6	5.9	8.4	2.7	3.1
Insomnia	3.0	2.8	1.1	5.3	2.8	2.9
Pharyngolaryngeal pain	2.3	3.9	1.6	2.8	0.7	2.1

* Adverse Reaction >2% in any dose greater than placebo

characteristics, including hemorrhagic and lacunar stroke on study entry, were associated with a higher incidence of hemorrhagic stroke in the atorvastatin group.

5.5 CNS Toxicity

Atorvastatin

Brain hemorrhage was seen in a female dog treated for 3 months at 120 mg/kg/day. Brain hemorrhage and optic nerve vacuolation were seen in another female dog that was sacrificed in moribund condition after 11 weeks of escalating doses up to 280 mg/kg/day. The 120 mg/kg dose resulted in a systemic exposure approximately 16 times the human plasma area-under-the-curve (AUC, 0-24 hours) based on the maximum human dose of 80 mg/day. A single tonic convulsion was seen in each of 2 male dogs (one treated at 10 mg/kg/day and one at 120 mg/kg/day) in a 2-year study. No CNS lesions have been observed in mice after chronic treatment for up to 2 years at doses up to 400 mg/kg/day or in rats at doses up to 100 mg/kg/day. These doses were 6 to 11 times (mouse) and 8 to 16 times (rat) the human $AUC_{(0-24)}$ based on the maximum recommended human dose of 80 mg/day.

CNS vascular lesions, characterized by perivascular hemorrhages, edema, and mononuclear cell infiltration of perivascular spaces, have been observed in dogs treated with other members of this class. A chemically similar drug in this class produced optic nerve degeneration (Wallerian degeneration of retinogeniculate fibers) in clinically normal dogs in a dose-dependent fashion at a dose that produced plasma drug levels about 30 times higher than the mean drug level in humans taking the highest recommended dose.

6 ADVERSE REACTIONS

The following serious adverse reactions are discussed in greater detail in other sections of the label:

- Rhabdomyolysis and myopathy *[see Warnings and Precautions (5.1)]*
- Liver enzyme abnormalities *[see Warnings and Precautions (5.2)]*

6.1 Clinical Trials Experience

LIPTRUZET

Because clinical studies are conducted under widely varying conditions, adverse reaction rates observed in the clinical studies of a drug cannot be directly compared to rates in the clinical studies of another drug and may not reflect the rates observed in clinical practice.

In a LIPTRUZET (ezetimibe and atorvastatin) placebo-controlled clinical trial, 628 patients (age range 18-86 years, 59% women, 85% Caucasians, 6% Blacks, 5% Hispanics, 3% Asians) with a median treatment duration of 12 weeks, 6% of patients on LIPTRUZET and 5% of patients on placebo discontinued due to adverse reactions.

The most common adverse reactions in the group treated with LIPTRUZET that led to treatment discontinuation and occurred at a rate greater than placebo were:

- Myalgia (0.8%)
- Abdominal pain (0.8%)
- Increased hepatic enzymes (0.8%)

The most commonly reported adverse reactions (incidence ≥2% and greater than placebo) in this trial were: increased ALT (5%), increased AST (4%), and musculoskeletal pain (4%).

LIPTRUZET has been evaluated for safety in 2403 patients in 7 clinical trials (one placebo-controlled trial and six active-controlled trials).

Table 2 summarizes the frequency of clinical adverse reactions reported in ≥2% of patients treated with LIPTRUZET (n=255) and at an incidence greater than placebo, regardless of causality assessment, from the placebo-controlled trial.

[See table 2 at left]

After completing the 12-week study, eligible patients were assigned to coadministered ezetimibe and atorvastatin equivalent to LIPTRUZET (10/10-10/80) or atorvastatin (10-80 mg/day) for an additional 48 weeks. The long-term coadministration of ezetimibe plus atorvastatin had an overall safety profile similar to that of atorvastatin alone.

Ezetimibe

In 10 double-blind, placebo-controlled clinical trials, 2396 patients with primary hyperlipidemia (age range 9-86 years, 50% women, 90% Caucasians, 5% Blacks, 3% Hispanics, 2% Asians) and elevated LDL-C were treated with ezetimibe 10 mg/day for a median treatment duration of 12 weeks (range 0 to 39 weeks).

Adverse reactions reported in ≥2% of patients treated with ezetimibe and at an incidence greater than placebo regardless of causality assessment are shown in Table 3.

Table 3: Clinical Adverse Reactions Occurring in ≥2% of Patients Treated with Ezetimibe and at an Incidence Greater than Placebo, Regardless of Causality

Body System/ Organ Class Adverse Reaction	Ezetimibe 10 mg (%) n=2396	Placebo (%) n=1159
Gastrointestinal disorders		
Diarrhea	4.1	3.7
General disorders and administration site conditions		
Fatigue	2.4	1.5
Infections and infestations		
Influenza	2.0	1.5
Sinusitis	2.8	2.2
Upper respiratory tract infection	4.3	2.5
Musculoskeletal and connective tissue disorders		
Arthralgia	3.0	2.2
Pain in extremity	2.7	2.5

Atorvastatin

In an atorvastatin placebo-controlled clinical trial database of 16,066 patients (8755 atorvastatin vs. 7311 placebo; age range 10–93 years, 39% women, 91% Caucasians, 3% Blacks, 2% Asians, 4% other) with a median treatment duration of 53 weeks, 9.7% of patients on atorvastatin and 9.5% of the patients on placebo discontinued due to adverse reactions regardless of causality.

The most commonly reported adverse reactions (incidence ≥2% and greater than placebo) regardless of causality, in patients treated with atorvastatin in placebo controlled trials (n=8755) were: nasopharyngitis (8.3%), arthralgia (6.9%), diarrhea (6.8%), pain in extremity (6.0%), and urinary tract infection (5.7%).

Table 4 summarizes the frequency of clinical adverse reactions, regardless of causality, reported in ≥2% and at a rate greater than placebo in patients treated with atorvastatin (n=8755), from seventeen placebo-controlled trials.

[See table 4 above]

6.2 Postmarketing Experience

Because the reactions below are reported voluntarily from a population of uncertain size, it is generally not possible to reliably estimate their frequency or establish a causal relationship to drug exposure.

The additional events described below have been identified during post-approval use of ezetimibe and/or atorvastatin.

Blood and lymphatic system disorders: thrombocytopenia

Nervous system disorders: headache; paresthesia; peripheral neuropathy

There have been rare postmarketing reports of cognitive impairment (e.g., memory loss, forgetfulness, amnesia, memory impairment, confusion) associated with statin use. These cognitive issues have been reported for all statins. The reports are generally nonserious, and reversible upon statin discontinuation, with variable times to symptom onset (1 day to years) and symptom resolution (median of 3 weeks).

Gastrointestinal disorders: pancreatitis

Skin and subcutaneous tissue disorders: angioedema; bullous rashes (including erythema multiforme, Stevens-Johnson syndrome, and toxic epidermal necrolysis); rash; urticaria

Musculoskeletal and connective tissue disorders: myopathy/rhabdomyolysis *[see Warnings and Precautions (5.1)]*

There have been rare reports of immune-mediated necrotizing myopathy associated with statin use *[see Warnings and Precautions (5.1)]*.

Injury, poisoning and procedural complications: tendon rupture

Immune system disorders: anaphylaxis; hypersensitivity reactions
Hepatobiliary disorders: hepatitis; cholelithiasis; cholecystitis; fatal and nonfatal hepatic failure
Psychiatric disorders: depression
Laboratory abnormalities: elevated creatine phosphokinase

7 DRUG INTERACTIONS

[See Clinical Pharmacology (12.3).]
LIPTRUZET
The risk of myopathy during treatment with statins is increased with concurrent administration of fibric acid derivatives, lipid-modifying doses of niacin, cyclosporine, or strong CYP3A4 inhibitors (e.g., clarithromycin, HIV protease inhibitors, and itraconazole) *[see Warnings and Precautions (5.1)* and *Clinical Pharmacology (12.3)]*.

7.1 Strong Inhibitors of Cytochrome P450 3A4

Atorvastatin is metabolized by cytochrome P450 3A4. Concomitant administration of atorvastatin with strong inhibitors of CYP3A4 can lead to increases in plasma concentrations of atorvastatin. The extent of interaction and potentiation of effects depend on the variability of effect on CYP3A4. Because LIPTRUZET contains atorvastatin, the risk of myopathy during treatment with LIPTRUZET is increased with concurrent administration of:
Clarithromycin: Atorvastatin AUC was significantly increased with concomitant administration of 80 mg atorvastatin with clarithromycin (500 mg twice daily) compared to that of atorvastatin alone *[see Clinical Pharmacology (12.3)]*. Therefore, in patients taking clarithromycin, caution should be used when the LIPTRUZET dose exceeds 10/20 mg *[see Warnings and Precautions (5.1) and Dosage and Administration (2.3)]*.
Combination of Protease Inhibitors: Atorvastatin AUC was significantly increased with concomitant administration of atorvastatin with several combinations of HIV protease inhibitors, as well as with the hepatitis C protease inhibitor telaprevir, compared to that of atorvastatin alone *[see Clinical Pharmacology (12.3)]*. Therefore, in patients taking the HIV protease inhibitor tipranavir plus ritonavir, or the hepatitis C protease inhibitor telaprevir, concomitant use of LIPTRUZET should be avoided. In patients taking the HIV protease inhibitor lopinavir plus ritonavir, caution should be used when prescribing LIPTRUZET and the lowest dose necessary should be used. In patients taking the HIV protease inhibitors saquinavir plus ritonavir, darunavir plus ritonavir, fosamprenavir, or fosamprenavir plus ritonavir, the dose of LIPTRUZET should not exceed 10/20 mg and should be used with caution *[see Warnings and Precautions (5.1)* and *Dosage and Administration (2.3)]*. In patients taking the HIV protease inhibitor nelfinavir or the hepatitis C protease inhibitor boceprevir, the dose of LIPTRUZET should not exceed 10/40 mg daily and close clinical monitoring is recommended.
Itraconazole: Atorvastatin AUC was significantly increased with concomitant administration of atorvastatin 40 mg and itraconazole 200 mg *[see Clinical Pharmacology (12.3)]*. Therefore, in patients taking itraconazole, do not use a LIPTRUZET dose that exceeds 10/20 mg *[see Warnings and Precautions (5.1)* and *Dosage and Administration (2.3)]*.

7.2 Cyclosporine

Atorvastatin and atorvastatin-metabolites are substrates of the OATP1B1 transporter. Inhibitors of the OATP1B1 (e.g., cyclosporine) can increase the bioavailability of atorvastatin. Atorvastatin AUC was significantly increased with concomitant administration of atorvastatin 10 mg and cyclosporine 5.2 mg/kg/day compared to that of atorvastatin alone *[see Clinical Pharmacology (12.3)]*.
In addition, ezetimibe and cyclosporine used concomitantly can increase exposure to both ezetimibe and cyclosporine. The degree of increase in ezetimibe exposure may be greater in patients with severe renal impairment.
The coadministration of LIPTRUZET with cyclosporine should be avoided *[see Warnings and Precautions (5.1)]*.

7.3 Grapefruit Juice

Grapefruit juice contains one or more components that inhibit CYP3A4 and can increase plasma concentrations of atorvastatin, especially with excessive grapefruit juice consumption (>1.2 liters per day).

7.4 Gemfibrozil

Due to an increased risk of myopathy/rhabdomyolysis when HMG-CoA reductase inhibitors are coadministered with gemfibrozil, concomitant administration of LIPTRUZET with gemfibrozil should be avoided *[see Warnings and Precautions (5.1)]*.

7.5 Fenofibrates (e.g., fenofibrate and fenofibric acid)

Because it is known that the risk of myopathy during treatment with HMG-CoA reductase inhibitors is increased with concurrent administration of fenofibrates, LIPTRUZET should be administered with caution when used concomitantly with a fenofibrate *[see Warnings and Precautions (5.1)]*.
Fenofibrates may increase cholesterol excretion into the bile, leading to cholelithiasis. If cholelithiasis is suspected in a patient receiving LIPTRUZET and a fenofibrate, gallbladder studies are indicated and alternative lipid-lowering therapy should be considered *[see the product labeling for fenofibrate and fenofibric acid]*.

7.6 Niacin

The risk of skeletal muscle effects may be enhanced when LIPTRUZET is used in combination with niacin; a reduction in LIPTRUZET dosage should be considered in this setting *[see Warnings and Precautions (5.1)]*.

7.7 Digoxin

When multiple doses of atorvastatin and digoxin were coadministered, steady state plasma digoxin concentrations increased by approximately 20%. Patients taking digoxin should be monitored appropriately.

7.8 Oral Contraceptives

Coadministration of atorvastatin and an oral contraceptive increased AUC values for norethindrone and ethinyl estradiol *[see Clinical Pharmacology (12.3)]*. These increases should be considered when selecting an oral contraceptive for a woman taking LIPTRUZET.

7.9 Rifampin or Other Inducers of Cytochrome P450 3A4

Concomitant administration of atorvastatin with inducers of cytochrome P450 3A4 (e.g., efavirenz, rifampin) can lead to variable reductions in plasma concentrations of atorvastatin. Due to the dual interaction mechanism of rifampin, simultaneous coadministration of LIPTRUZET with rifampin is recommended, as delayed administration of atorvastatin after administration of rifampin has been associated with a significant reduction in atorvastatin plasma concentrations.

7.10 Colchicine

Cases of myopathy, including rhabdomyolysis, have been reported with atorvastatin coadministered with colchicine, and caution should be exercised when prescribing LIPTRUZET with colchicine.

7.11 Cholestyramine

Concomitant cholestyramine administration decreased the mean area under the curve (AUC) of total ezetimibe approximately 55%. The incremental LDL-C reduction due to adding ezetimibe to cholestyramine may be reduced by this interaction.

7.12 Coumarin Anticoagulants

If LIPTRUZET is added to warfarin, a coumarin anticoagulant, the International Normalized Ratio (INR) should be appropriately monitored.

8 USE IN SPECIFIC POPULATIONS

8.1 Pregnancy

Pregnancy Category X.
[See Contraindications (4).]
LIPTRUZET
LIPTRUZET is contraindicated in women who are or may become pregnant. Serum cholesterol and triglycerides increase during normal pregnancy. Lipid-lowering drugs offer no benefit during pregnancy, because cholesterol and cholesterol derivatives are needed for normal fetal development. Atherosclerosis is a chronic process, and discontinuation of lipid-lowering drugs during pregnancy should have little impact on long-term outcomes of primary hypercholesterolemia therapy.
There are no adequate and well-controlled studies of LIPTRUZET use during pregnancy. There have been rare reports of congenital anomalies following intrauterine exposure to statins. In a review of about 100 prospectively followed pregnancies in women exposed to other statins, the incidences of congenital anomalies, spontaneous abortions, and fetal deaths/stillbirths did not exceed the rate expected in the general population. However, this study was only able to exclude a three-to-four-fold increased risk of congenital anomalies over background incidence. In 89% of these cases, drug treatment started before pregnancy and stopped during the first trimester when pregnancy was identified.
Statins may cause fetal harm when administered to a pregnant woman. Because LIPTRUZET contains atorvastatin, LIPTRUZET should be administered to women of childbearing potential only when such patients are highly unlikely to conceive and have been informed of the potential hazards. If the woman becomes pregnant while taking LIPTRUZET, it should be discontinued immediately and the patient advised again as to the potential hazards to the fetus and the lack of known clinical benefit with continued use during pregnancy.
Ezetimibe
In oral (gavage) embryo-fetal development studies of ezetimibe conducted in rats and rabbits during organogenesis, there was no evidence of embryolethal effects at the doses tested (250, 500, 1000 mg/kg/day). In rats, increased incidences of common fetal skeletal findings (extra pair of thoracic ribs, unossified cervical vertebral centra, shortened ribs) were observed at 1000 mg/kg/day (~10 times the human exposure at 10 mg daily based on $AUC_{0\text{-}24hr}$ for total ezetimibe). In rabbits treated with ezetimibe, an increased incidence of extra thoracic ribs was observed at 1000 mg/kg/day (150 times the human exposure at 10 mg daily based on $AUC_{0\text{-}24hr}$ for total ezetimibe). Ezetimibe crossed the placenta when pregnant rats and rabbits were given multiple oral doses.
Multiple-dose studies of ezetimibe given in combination with statins in rats and rabbits during organogenesis result in higher ezetimibe and statin exposures. Reproductive findings occur at lower doses in combination therapy compared to monotherapy.
Atorvastatin
Atorvastatin crosses the rat placenta and reaches a level in fetal liver equivalent to that of maternal plasma. Atorvastatin was not teratogenic in rats at doses up to 300 mg/kg/day or in rabbits at doses up to 100 mg/kg/day. These doses resulted in multiples of about 30 times (rat) or 20 times (rabbit) the human exposure based on surface area (mg/m^2).
In a study in rats given 20, 100, or 225 mg/kg/day, from gestation Day 7 through to lactation Day 21 (weaning), there was decreased pup survival at birth, neonate, weaning, and maturity in pups of mothers dosed with 225 mg/kg/day. Body weight was decreased on Days 4 and 21 in pups of mothers dosed at 100 mg/kg/day; pup body weight was decreased at birth and at Days 4, 21, and 91 at 225 mg/kg/day. Pup development was delayed (rotorod performance at 100 mg/kg/day and acoustic startle at 225 mg/kg/day; pinnae detachment and eye opening at 225 mg/kg/day). These doses correspond to 6 times (100 mg/kg) and 22 times (225 mg/kg) the human AUC at 80 mg/day. Rare reports of congenital anomalies have been received following intrauterine exposure to statin reductase inhibitors.

8.3 Nursing Mothers

In rat studies, exposure to total ezetimibe in nursing pups was up to half of that observed in maternal plasma. It is not known whether ezetimibe is excreted into human breast milk.
It is not known whether atorvastatin is excreted in human milk, but a small amount of another drug in this class does pass into breast milk. Nursing rat pups had plasma and liver atorvastatin levels of 50% and 40%, respectively, of that in their mother's milk. Because of the potential for adverse reactions in nursing infants, women taking LIPTRUZET should not breast-feed *[see Contraindications (4)]*.

8.4 Pediatric Use

LIPTRUZET
Safety and effectiveness have not been established in pediatric patients.
Ezetimibe
Based on total ezetimibe (ezetimibe + ezetimibe-glucuronide) there are no pharmacokinetic differences between adolescents and adults. Pharmacokinetic data in the pediatric population <10 years of age are not available.
Atorvastatin
Pharmacokinetic data in the pediatric population are not available.

8.5 Geriatric Use

Of the patients who received ezetimibe coadministered with atorvastatin in clinical studies, 1166 were 65 and older (this included 291 who were 75 and older). The effectiveness and safety of LIPTRUZET were similar between these patients and younger subjects. Greater sensitivity of some older individuals cannot be ruled out. Since advanced age (≥65 years) is a predisposing factor for myopathy, LIPTRUZET should be prescribed with caution in the elderly. *[See Clinical Pharmacology (12.3).]*
In geriatric patients, no dosage adjustment of LIPTRUZET is necessary.

8.6 Hepatic Impairment

LIPTRUZET is contraindicated in patients with active liver disease or unexplained persistent elevations in hepatic transaminase levels *[see Contraindications (4), Warnings and Precautions (5.2), and Clinical Pharmacology (12.3)]*.

8.7 Renal Impairment

A history of renal impairment may be a risk factor for statin-associated myopathy. These patients merit closer monitoring for skeletal muscle effects *[see Warnings and Precautions (5.1)]*.
In patients with renal impairment, no dosage adjustment of LIPTRUZET is necessary.

10 OVERDOSAGE

LIPTRUZET
No specific treatment of overdosage with LIPTRUZET can be recommended. In the event of an overdose, the patient should be treated symptomatically, and supportive measures instituted as required.
Ezetimibe
In clinical studies, administration of ezetimibe, 50 mg/day to 15 healthy subjects for up to 14 days, 40 mg/day to 18 patients with primary hyperlipidemia for up to 56 days, and 40 mg/day to 27 patients with homozygous sitosterolemia for 26 weeks, was generally well tolerated. One female pa-

tient with homozygous sitosterolemia took an accidental overdose of ezetimibe 120 mg/day for 28 days with no reported clinical or laboratory adverse events.

Atorvastatin

Due to extensive drug binding to plasma proteins, hemodialysis is not expected to significantly enhance atorvastatin clearance.

11 DESCRIPTION

LIPTRUZET contains ezetimibe, a selective inhibitor of intestinal cholesterol and related phytosterol absorption, and atorvastatin, a 3-hydroxy-3-methylglutaryl-coenzyme A (HMG-CoA) reductase inhibitor.

The chemical name of ezetimibe is 1-(4-fluorophenyl)-3(R)-[3-(4-fluorophenyl)-3(S)-hydroxypropyl]-4(S)-(4-hydroxyphenyl)-2-azetidinone. The empirical formula is $C_{24}H_{21}F_2NO_3$. Its molecular weight is 409.4.

Ezetimibe is a white, crystalline powder that is freely to very soluble in ethanol, methanol, and acetone and practically insoluble in water. Its structural formula is:

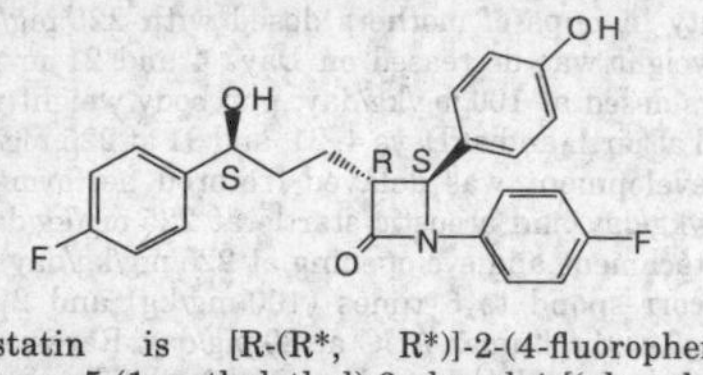

Atorvastatin is [R-(R*, R*)]-2-(4-fluorophenyl)-ß, δ-dihydroxy-5-(1-methylethyl)-3-phenyl-4-[(phenylamino) carbonyl]-1H-pyrrole-1-heptanoic acid, calcium salt (2:1).

Atorvastatin calcium is a white to off-white amorphous powder that is very slightly soluble in water, insoluble in acetonitrile, and soluble in methanol. The empirical formula of atorvastatin calcium is $(C_{33}H_{34}FN_2O_5)_2Ca$. The molecular weight of atorvastatin calcium is 1155.37. Its structural formula is:

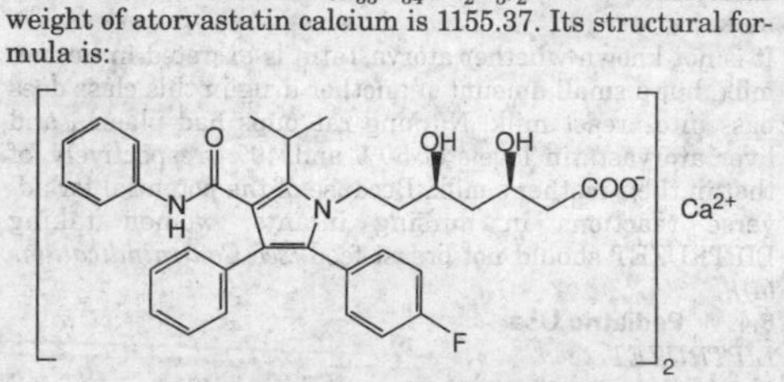

LIPTRUZET is available for oral use as tablets containing 10 mg of ezetimibe and: 10.34 mg of atorvastatin calcium, equivalent to 10 mg of atorvastatin (LIPTRUZET 10 mg/10 mg); 20.68 mg of atorvastatin calcium, equivalent to 20 mg of atorvastatin (LIPTRUZET 10 mg/20 mg); 41.37 mg of atorvastatin calcium, equivalent to 40 mg of atorvastatin (LIPTRUZET 10 mg/40 mg); or 82.73 mg of atorvastatin calcium, equivalent to 80 mg of atorvastatin (LIPTRUZET 10 mg/80 mg). Each film-coated tablet of LIPTRUZET contains the following inactive ingredients: lactose monohydrate, microcrystalline cellulose, croscarmellose sodium, povidone, sodium lauryl sulfate, magnesium stearate, lactose anhydrous, hydroxypropyl cellulose, and sodium bicarbonate. In addition, the film coating contains the following inactive ingredients: hydroxypropyl cellulose, hypromellose, titanium dioxide, and carnauba wax.

12 CLINICAL PHARMACOLOGY

12.1 Mechanism of Action

LIPTRUZET

Plasma cholesterol is derived from intestinal absorption and endogenous synthesis. LIPTRUZET contains ezetimibe and atorvastatin, two lipid-lowering compounds with complementary mechanisms of action.

Ezetimibe

Ezetimibe reduces blood cholesterol by inhibiting the absorption of cholesterol by the small intestine. The molecular target of ezetimibe has been shown to be the sterol transporter, Niemann-Pick C1-Like 1 (NPC1L1), which is involved in the intestinal uptake of cholesterol and phytosterols. In a 2-week clinical study in 18 hypercholesterolemic patients, ezetimibe inhibited intestinal cholesterol absorption by 54%, compared with placebo. Ezetimibe had no clinically meaningful effect on the plasma concentrations of the fat-soluble vitamins A, D, and E and did not impair adrenocortical steroid hormone production.

Ezetimibe does not inhibit cholesterol synthesis in the liver or increase bile acid excretion. Ezetimibe localizes at the brush border of the small intestine and inhibits the absorption of cholesterol, leading to a decrease in the delivery of intestinal cholesterol to the liver. This causes a reduction of hepatic cholesterol stores and an increase in clearance of cholesterol from the blood; this distinct mechanism is complementary to that of statins *[see Clinical Studies (14)]*.

Atorvastatin

In animal models, atorvastatin lowers plasma cholesterol and lipoprotein levels by inhibiting HMG-CoA reductase and cholesterol synthesis in the liver and by increasing the number of hepatic LDL receptors on the cell-surface to enhance uptake and catabolism of LDL; atorvastatin also reduces LDL production and the number of LDL particles.

12.2 Pharmacodynamics

Clinical studies have demonstrated that elevated levels of total-C, LDL-C and Apo B, the major protein constituent of LDL, promote human atherosclerosis. In addition, decreased levels of HDL-C are associated with the development of atherosclerosis. Epidemiologic studies have established that cardiovascular morbidity and mortality vary directly with the level of total-C and LDL-C and inversely with the level of HDL-C. Like LDL, cholesterol-enriched triglyceride-rich lipoproteins, including very-low-density lipoproteins (VLDL), intermediate-density lipoproteins (IDL), and remnants, can also promote atherosclerosis. The independent effect of raising HDL-C or lowering TG on the risk of coronary and cardiovascular morbidity and mortality has not been determined.

Atorvastatin as well as some of its metabolites are pharmacologically active in humans. The liver is the primary site of action and the principal site of cholesterol synthesis and LDL clearance. Drug dosage, rather than systemic drug concentration, correlates better with LDL-C reduction. Individualization of drug dosage should be based on therapeutic response *[see Dosage and Administration (2)]*.

12.3 Pharmacokinetics

LIPTRUZET

LIPTRUZET 10/10 and 10/80 tablets have been shown to be bioequivalent to coadministration of corresponding doses of ezetimibe and atorvastatin tablets. LIPTRUZET 10/20 and 10/40 tablets have been shown to be clinically equivalent in LDL-C response to the corresponding coadministered doses of ezetimibe and atorvastatin tablets. *[See Clinical Studies (14.1).]*

Absorption

Ezetimibe

After oral administration, ezetimibe is absorbed and extensively conjugated to a pharmacologically active phenolic glucuronide (ezetimibe-glucuronide).

Atorvastatin

Maximum plasma atorvastatin concentrations after oral administration occur within 1 to 2 hours. Extent of absorption increases in proportion to atorvastatin dose. The absolute bioavailability of atorvastatin (parent drug) is approximately 14% and the systemic availability of HMG-CoA reductase inhibitory activity is approximately 30%. The low systemic availability is attributed to presystemic clearance in gastrointestinal mucosa and/or hepatic first-pass metabolism. Plasma atorvastatin concentrations are lower (approximately 30% for C_{max} and AUC) following evening drug administration compared with morning. However, LDL-C reduction is the same regardless of the time of day of drug administration.

Effect of Food on Oral Absorption

LIPTRUZET

A high-fat meal decreased atorvastatin AUC and C_{max} 11% and 35%, respectively, of the LIPTRUZET 10/80 tablet. A high-fat meal decreased unconjugated ezetimibe AUC 2% and increased unconjugated ezetimibe C_{max} 10% of the LIPTRUZET 10/80 tablet.

LIPTRUZET can be taken with or without food *[see Dosage and Administration (2.1)]*.

Distribution

Ezetimibe

Ezetimibe and ezetimibe-glucuronide are highly bound (>90%) to human plasma proteins.

Atorvastatin

Mean volume of distribution of atorvastatin is approximately 381 liters. Atorvastatin is ≥98% bound to plasma proteins. A blood/plasma ratio of approximately 0.25 indicates poor drug penetration into red blood cells. Based on observations in rats, atorvastatin is likely to be secreted in human milk *[see Contraindications (4); Use in Specific Populations (8.3)]*.

Metabolism and Excretion

Ezetimibe

Ezetimibe is primarily metabolized in the small intestine and liver via glucuronide conjugation with subsequent biliary and renal excretion. Minimal oxidative metabolism has been observed in all species evaluated.

In humans, ezetimibe is rapidly metabolized to ezetimibe-glucuronide. Ezetimibe and ezetimibe-glucuronide are the major drug-derived compounds detected in plasma, constituting approximately 10 to 20% and 80 to 90% of the total drug in plasma, respectively. Both ezetimibe and ezetimibe-glucuronide are eliminated from plasma with a half-life of approximately 22 hours for both ezetimibe and ezetimibe-glucuronide. Plasma concentration-time profiles exhibit multiple peaks, suggesting enterohepatic recycling.

Following oral administration of ^{14}C-ezetimibe (20 mg) to human subjects, total ezetimibe (ezetimibe + ezetimibe-glucuronide) accounted for approximately 93% of the total radioactivity in plasma. After 48 hours, there were no detectable levels of radioactivity in the plasma.

Approximately 78% and 11% of the administered radioactivity were recovered in the feces and urine, respectively, over a 10-day collection period. Ezetimibe was the major component in feces and accounted for 69% of the administered dose, while ezetimibe-glucuronide was the major component in urine and accounted for 9% of the administered dose.

Atorvastatin

Atorvastatin is extensively metabolized to ortho- and parahydroxylated derivatives and various beta-oxidation products. *In vitro* inhibition of HMG-CoA reductase by ortho- and parahydroxylated metabolites is equivalent to that of atorvastatin. Approximately 70% of circulating inhibitory activity for HMG-CoA reductase is attributed to active metabolites. *In vitro* studies suggest the importance of atorvastatin metabolism by cytochrome P450 3A4, consistent with increased plasma concentrations of atorvastatin in humans following coadministration with erythromycin, a known inhibitor of this isozyme *[see Drug Interactions (7.1)]*. In animals, the ortho-hydroxy metabolite undergoes further glucuronidation.

Atorvastatin and its metabolites are eliminated primarily in bile following hepatic and/or extra-hepatic metabolism; however, the drug does not appear to undergo enterohepatic recirculation. Mean plasma elimination half-life of atorvastatin in humans is approximately 14 hours, but the half-life of inhibitory activity for HMG-CoA reductase is 20 to 30 hours due to the contribution of active metabolites. Less than 2% of a dose of atorvastatin is recovered in urine following oral administration.

Specific Populations

Geriatric Patients

Ezetimibe

In a multiple-dose study with ezetimibe given 10 mg once daily for 10 days, plasma concentrations for total ezetimibe were about 2-fold higher in older (≥65 years) healthy subjects compared to younger subjects.

Atorvastatin

Plasma concentrations of atorvastatin are higher (approximately 40% for C_{max} and 30% for AUC) in healthy elderly subjects (age ≥65 years) than in young adults. Clinical data suggest a greater degree of LDL-lowering at any dose of drug in the elderly patient population compared to younger adults.

Pediatric Patients: *[See Use in Specific Populations (8.4).]*

Gender

Ezetimibe

In a multiple-dose study with ezetimibe given 10 mg once daily for 10 days, plasma concentrations for total ezetimibe were slightly higher (<20%) in women than in men.

Atorvastatin

Plasma concentrations of atorvastatin in women differ from those in men (approximately 20% higher for C_{max} and 10% lower for AUC); however, there is no clinically significant difference in LDL-C reduction with atorvastatin between men and women.

Race

Ezetimibe

Based on a meta-analysis of multiple-dose pharmacokinetic studies, there were no pharmacokinetic differences between Black and Caucasian subjects. Studies in Asian subjects indicated that the pharmacokinetics of ezetimibe were similar to those seen in Caucasian subjects.

Hepatic Impairment

Ezetimibe

After a single 10-mg dose of ezetimibe, the mean AUC for total ezetimibe was increased approximately 1.7-fold in patients with mild hepatic impairment (Child-Pugh score 5 to 6), compared to healthy subjects. The mean AUC values for total ezetimibe and ezetimibe increased approximately 3- to 4-fold and 5- to 6-fold, respectively, in patients with moderate (Child-Pugh score 7 to 9) or severe hepatic impairment (Child-Pugh score 10 to 15). In a 14-day, multiple-dose study (10 mg daily) in patients with moderate hepatic impairment, the mean AUC for total ezetimibe and ezetimibe increased approximately 4-fold on both Day 1 and Day 14 when compared to healthy subjects.

Atorvastatin

In patients with chronic alcoholic liver disease, plasma concentrations of atorvastatin are markedly increased. C_{max} and AUC are each 4-fold greater in patients with Child-Pugh A disease. C_{max} and AUC are approximately 16-fold and 11-fold increased, respectively, in patients with Child-Pugh B disease *[see Contraindications (4)]*.

Renal Impairment

[See Warnings and Precautions (5.1), Use in Specific Populations (8.7)]

Ezetimibe

After a single 10-mg dose of ezetimibe in patients with severe renal disease (n=8; mean CrCl ≤30 mL/min/1.73 m^2), the mean AUC values for total ezetimibe, ezetimibe-glucuronide, and ezetimibe were increased approximately 1.5-fold, compared to healthy subjects (n=9).

Atorvastatin

Renal disease has no influence on the plasma concentrations or LDL-C reduction of atorvastatin.

Hemodialysis

Atorvastatin

While studies have not been conducted in patients with end-stage renal disease, hemodialysis is not expected to significantly enhance clearance of atorvastatin since the drug is extensively bound to plasma proteins.

Drug Interactions [See also Drug Interactions (7).]

No clinically significant pharmacokinetic interaction was seen when ezetimibe was coadministered with atorvastatin. Specific pharmacokinetic drug interaction studies with LIPTRUZET have not been performed.

Cytochrome P450: Ezetimibe had no significant effect on a series of probe drugs (caffeine, dextromethorphan, tolbutamide, and IV midazolam) known to be metabolized by cytochrome P450 (1A2, 2D6, 2C8/9 and 3A4) in a "cocktail" study of twelve healthy adult males. This indicates that ezetimibe is neither an inhibitor nor an inducer of these cytochrome P450 isozymes, and it is unlikely that ezetimibe will affect the metabolism of drugs that are metabolized by these enzymes.

Atorvastatin is metabolized by cytochrome P450 3A4. Concomitant administration of LIPTRUZET with inhibitors of cytochrome P450 3A4 can lead to increases in plasma concentrations of the atorvastatin component of LIPTRUZET. The extent of interaction and potentiation of effects depends on the variability of effect on cytochrome P450 3A4.

Ezetimibe

Table 5: Effect of Coadministered Drugs on Total Ezetimibe

Coadministered Drug and Dosing Regimen	Total Ezetimibe*	
	Change in AUC	Change in C_{max}
Cyclosporine-stable dose required (75-150 mg BID)†,‡	↑240%	↑290%
Fenofibrate, 200 mg QD, 14 days‡	↑48%	↑64%
Gemfibrozil, 600 mg BID, 7 days‡	↑64%	↑91%
Cholestyramine, 4 g BID, 14 days‡	↓55%	↓4%
Aluminum & magnesium hydroxide combination antacid, single dose§	↓4%	↓30%
Cimetidine, 400 mg BID, 7 days	↑6%	↑22%
Glipizide, 10 mg, single dose	↑4%	↓8%
Statins		
Lovastatin 20 mg QD, 7 days	↑9%	↑3%
Pravastatin 20 mg QD, 14 days	↑7%	↑23%
Atorvastatin 10 mg QD, 14 days	↓2%	↑12%
Rosuvastatin 10 mg QD, 14 days	↑13%	↑18%
Fluvastatin 20 mg QD, 14 days	↓19%	↑7%

* Based on 10-mg dose of ezetimibe

† Post-renal transplant patients with mild impaired or normal renal function. In a different study, a renal transplant patient with severe renal impairment (creatinine clearance of 13.2 mL/min/1.73 m^2) who was receiving multiple medications, including cyclosporine, demonstrated a 12-fold greater exposure to total ezetimibe compared to healthy subjects.

‡ *See Drug Interactions (7)*

§ Supralox®, 20 mL

[See table 6 above]

Atorvastatin

[See table 7 at top of next page]

[See table 8 at top of page 1625]

Table 6: Effect of Ezetimibe Coadministration on Systemic Exposure to Other Drugs

Coadministered Drug and its Dosage Regimen	Ezetimibe Dosage Regimen	Change in AUC of Coadministered Drug	Change in C_{max} of Coadministered Drug
Warfarin, 25 mg single dose on Day 7	10 mg QD, 11 days	↓2% (R-warfarin) ↓4% (S-warfarin)	↑3% (R-warfarin) ↑1% (S-warfarin)
Digoxin, 0.5 mg single dose	10 mg QD, 8 days	↑2%	↓7%
Gemfibrozil, 600 mg BID, 7 days*	10 mg QD, 7 days	↓1%	↓11%
Ethinyl estradiol & Levonorgestrel, QD, 21 days	10 mg QD, Days 8-14 of 21 d oral contraceptive cycle	Ethinyl estradiol 0% Levonorgestrel 0%	Ethinyl estradiol ↓9% Levonorgestrel ↓5%
Glipizide, 10 mg on Days 1 and 9	10 mg QD, Days 2-9	↓3%	↓5%
Fenofibrate, 200 mg QD, 14 days*	10 mg QD, 14 days	↑11%	↑7%
Cyclosporine, 100 mg single dose Day 7*	20 mg QD, 8 days	↑15%	↑10%
Statins			
Lovastatin 20 mg QD, 7 days	10 mg QD, 7 days	↑19%	↑3%
Pravastatin 20 mg QD, 14 days	10 mg QD, 14 days	↓20%	↓24%
Atorvastatin 10 mg QD, 14 days	10 mg QD, 14 days	↓4%	↑7%
Rosuvastatin 10 mg QD, 14 days	10 mg QD, 14 days	↑19%	↑17%
Fluvastatin 20 mg QD, 14 days	10 mg QD, 14 days	↓39%	↓27%

* *See Drug Interactions (7)*

13 NONCLINICAL TOXICOLOGY

13.1 Carcinogenesis, Mutagenesis, Impairment of Fertility

No animal carcinogenicity or fertility studies have been conducted with the combination of ezetimibe and atorvastatin. The combination of ezetimibe with atorvastatin did not show evidence of mutagenicity *in vitro* in a microbial mutagenicity (Ames) test with *Salmonella typhimurium* and *Escherichia coli* with or without metabolic activation. No evidence of clastogenicity was observed *in vitro* in a chromosomal aberration assay in human peripheral blood lymphocytes with ezetimibe and atorvastatin with or without metabolic activation. There was no evidence of genotoxicity at doses up to 250 mg/kg with the combination of ezetimibe and atorvastatin (1:1) in the *in vivo* mouse micronucleus test.

Ezetimibe

A 104-week dietary carcinogenicity study with ezetimibe was conducted in rats at doses up to 1500 mg/kg/day (males) and 500 mg/kg/day (females) (~20 times the human exposure at 10 mg daily based on $AUC_{0\text{-}24hr}$ for total ezetimibe). A 104-week dietary carcinogenicity study with ezetimibe was also conducted in mice at doses up to 500 mg/kg/day (>150 times the human exposure at 10 mg daily based on $AUC_{0\text{-}24hr}$ for total ezetimibe). There were no statistically significant increases in tumor incidences in drug-treated rats or mice.

No evidence of mutagenicity was observed *in vitro* in a microbial mutagenicity (Ames) test with *Salmonella typhimurium* and *Escherichia coli* with or without metabolic activation. No evidence of clastogenicity was observed *in vitro* in a chromosomal aberration assay in human peripheral blood lymphocytes with or without metabolic activation. In addition, there was no evidence of genotoxicity in the *in vivo* mouse micronucleus test.

In oral (gavage) fertility studies of ezetimibe conducted in rats, there was no evidence of reproductive toxicity at doses up to 1000 mg/kg/day in male or female rats (~7 times the human exposure at 10 mg daily based on $AUC_{0\text{-}24hr}$ for total ezetimibe).

Atorvastatin

In a 2-year carcinogenicity study in rats at dose levels of 10, 30, and 100 mg/kg/day, 2 rare tumors were found in muscle in high-dose females: in one, there was a rhabdomyosarcoma and, in another, there was a fibrosarcoma. This dose represents a plasma $AUC_{0\text{-}24hr}$ value of approximately 16 times the mean human plasma drug exposure after an 80-mg oral dose.

A 2-year carcinogenicity study in mice given 100, 200, or 400 mg/kg/day resulted in a significant increase in liver adenomas in high-dose males and liver carcinomas in high-dose females. These findings occurred at plasma $AUC_{0\text{-}24hr}$ values of approximately 6 times the mean human plasma drug exposure after an 80-mg oral dose.

In vitro, atorvastatin was not mutagenic or clastogenic in the following tests with and without metabolic activation: the Ames test with *Salmonella typhimurium* and *Escherichia coli*, the HGPRT forward mutation assay in Chinese hamster lung cells, and the chromosomal aberration assay in Chinese hamster lung cells. Atorvastatin was negative in the *in vivo* mouse micronucleus test.

Studies in rats performed at doses up to 175 mg/kg (15 times the human exposure) produced no changes in fertility. There was aplasia and aspermia in the epididymis of 2 of 10 rats treated with 100 mg/kg/day of atorvastatin for 3 months (16 times the human AUC at the 80-mg dose); testis weights were significantly lower at 30 and 100 mg/kg and epididymal weight was lower at 100 mg/kg. Male rats given 100 mg/kg/day for 11 weeks prior to mating had decreased sperm motility, spermatid head concentration, and increased abnormal sperm. Atorvastatin caused no adverse effects on semen parameters, or reproductive organ histopathology in dogs given doses of 10, 40, or 120 mg/kg for two years.

13.2 Animal Toxicology and/or Pharmacology

Ezetimibe

In a rat model, where the glucuronide metabolite of ezetimibe (ezetimibe-glucuronide) was administered intraduodenally, the metabolite was as potent as ezetimibe in inhibiting the absorption of cholesterol, suggesting that the glucuronide metabolite had activity similar to the parent drug.

In 1-month studies in dogs given ezetimibe (0.03 to 300 mg/kg/day), the concentration of cholesterol in gallbladder bile increased ~2- to 4-fold. However, a dose of 300 mg/kg/day administered to dogs for one year did not result in gallstone formation or any other adverse hepatobiliary effects. In a 14-day study in mice given ezetimibe (0.3 to 5 mg/kg/day) and fed a low-fat or cholesterol-rich diet, the concentration of cholesterol in gallbladder bile was either unaffected or reduced to normal levels, respectively.

A series of acute preclinical studies was performed to determine the selectivity of ezetimibe for inhibiting cholesterol absorption. Ezetimibe inhibited the absorption of ^{14}C-cholesterol with no effect on the absorption of triglycerides, fatty acids, bile acids, progesterone, ethinyl estradiol, or the fat-soluble vitamins A and D.

Table 7: Effect of Coadministered Drugs on the Pharmacokinetics of Atorvastatin

Coadministered Drug and Dosing Regimen	Atorvastatin		
	Dose (mg)	Change in AUC*	Change in C_{max}*
Cyclosporine 5.2 mg/kg/day, stable dose†	10 mg QD for 28 days	↑8.7 fold	↑10.7 fold
Tipranavir 500 mg BID/ ritonavir 200 mg BID, 7 days†	10 mg, SD	↑9.4 fold	↑8.6 fold
Telaprevir 750 mg q8h, 10 days†	20 mg, SD	↑7.88 fold	↑10.6 fold
Saquinavir 400 mg BID/ ritonavir 400 mg BID, 15 days†,‡	40 mg QD for 4 days	↑3.9 fold	↑4.3 fold
Clarithromycin 500 mg BID, 9 days†	80 mg QD for 8 days	↑4.4 fold	↑5.4 fold
Darunavir 300 mg BID/ ritonavir 100 mg BID, 9 days†	10 mg QD for 4 days	↑3.4 fold	↑2.25 fold
Itraconazole 200 mg QD, 4 days†	40 mg, SD	↑3.3 fold	↑20%
Fosamprenavir 700 mg BID/ritonavir 100 mg BID, 14 days†	10 mg QD for 4 days	↑2.53 fold	↑2.84 fold
Fosamprenavir 1400 mg BID, 14 days†	10 mg QD for 4 days	↑2.3 fold	↑4.04 fold
Nelfinavir 1250 mg BID, 14 days†	10 mg QD for 28 days	↑74%	↑2.2 fold
Grapefruit Juice, 240 mL QD†,§	40 mg, SD	↑37%	↑16%
Diltiazem 240 mg QD, 28 days	40 mg, SD	↑51%	No change
Erythromycin 500 mg QID, 7 days	10 mg, SD	↑33%	↑38%
Amlodipine 10 mg, single dose	80 mg, SD	↑15%	↓12%
Cimetidine 300 mg QD, 4 weeks	10 mg QD for 2 weeks	↓Less than 1%	↓11%
Colestipol 10 mg BID, 28 weeks	40 mg QD for 28 weeks	Not determined	↓26%¶
Maalox TC® 30 mL QD, 17 days	10 mg QD for 15 days	↓33%	↓34%
Efavirenz 600 mg QD, 14 days	10 mg for 3 days	↓41%	↓1%
Rifampin 600 mg QD, 7 days (coadministered) †,#	40 mg, SD	↑30%	↑2.7 fold
Rifampin 600 mg QD, 5 days (doses separated) †,#	40 mg, SD	↓80%	↓40%
Gemfibrozil 600 mg BID, 7 days†	40 mg, SD	↑35%	↓Less than 1%
Fenofibrate 160 mg QD, 7 days†	40 mg, SD	↑3%	↑2%
Boceprevir 800 mg TID, 7 days	40 mg, SD	↑2.30 fold	↑2.66 fold

* Data given as x-fold change represent a simple ratio between coadministration and atorvastatin alone (i.e., 1-fold = no change). Data given as % change represent % difference relative to atorvastatin alone (i.e., 0% = no change).
† *See Warnings and Precautions (5.1)* and *Drug Interactions (7)* for clinical significance.
‡ The dose of saquinavir plus ritonavir in this study is not the clinically used dose. The increase in atorvastatin exposure when used clinically is likely to be higher than what was observed in this study. Therefore, caution should be applied and the lowest dose necessary should be used.
§ Greater increases in AUC (up to 2.5 fold) and/or C_{max} (up to 71%) have been reported with excessive grapefruit consumption (≥ 750 mL - 1.2 liters per day).
¶ Single sample taken 8-16 h post-dose.
\# Due to the dual interaction mechanism of rifampin, simultaneous coadministration of atorvastatin with rifampin is recommended, as delayed administration of atorvastatin after administration of rifampin has been associated with a significant reduction in atorvastatin plasma concentrations.

In 4- to 12-week toxicity studies in mice, ezetimibe did not induce cytochrome P450 drug metabolizing enzymes. In toxicity studies, a pharmacokinetic interaction of ezetimibe with statins (parents or their active hydroxy acid metabolites) was seen in rats, dogs, and rabbits.

14 CLINICAL STUDIES

14.1 Primary Hyperlipidemia

LIPTRUZET – Lipid Efficacy

LIPTRUZET reduces total-C, LDL-C, Apo B, TG, and non-HDL-C, and increases HDL-C in patients with hypercholesterolemia.

LIPTRUZET is effective in men and women with hyperlipidemia. Experience in non-Caucasians is limited and does not permit a precise estimate of the magnitude of the effects of LIPTRUZET.

In a multicenter, double-blind, placebo-controlled, clinical study in patients with hyperlipidemia, 628 patients were treated for up to 12 weeks and 246 for up to an additional 48 weeks. Patients were randomized to receive placebo, ezetimibe (10 mg), atorvastatin (10 mg, 20 mg, 40 mg, or 80 mg), or coadministered ezetimibe and atorvastatin equivalent to LIPTRUZET (10/10, 10/20, 10/40, and 10/80) in the 12-week study. After completing the 12-week study, patients who agreed to participate in the study extension were assigned to coadministered ezetimibe and atorvastatin equivalent to LIPTRUZET (10/10-10/80) or atorvastatin (10-80 mg/day) for an additional 48 weeks.

The patient population was: 59% female; 85% Caucasian, 6% Black, 3% Asian, 5% Hispanic, 1% American Indian, <1% other; 18 to 86 years of age (mean age 57 years).

Patients receiving all doses of LIPTRUZET were compared to those receiving all doses of atorvastatin. LIPTRUZET lowered total-C, LDL-C, Apo B, TG, and non-HDL-C, and increased HDL-C significantly more than atorvastatin alone. (See Table 9.)

[See table 9 at top of next page]

The changes in lipid endpoints after an additional 48 weeks of treatment with LIPTRUZET (all doses) or with atorvastatin (all doses) were generally consistent with the 12-week data displayed above in the 245 subjects (out of the 576 who completed the 12-week study) who agreed to participate in the study extension.

A multicenter, double-blind, controlled, 14-week study was conducted in 621 patients with heterozygous familial hypercholesterolemia (HeFH), coronary heart disease (CHD), or multiple cardiovascular risk factors (≥2), adhering to an NCEP Step I or stricter diet. All patients received atorvastatin 10 mg for a minimum of 4 weeks prior to randomization. Patients were then randomized to receive either coadministered ezetimibe and atorvastatin (equivalent to LIPTRUZET 10/10) or atorvastatin 20 mg/day monotherapy. Patients who did not achieve their LDL-C target goal after 4 and/or 9 weeks of randomized treatment were titrated to double the atorvastatin dose.

The patient population was: 47% female; 91% Caucasian, 2% Black, 2% Asian, 5% Hispanic, <1% other; 18 to 82 years of age (mean age 61 years).

LIPTRUZET 10/10 was significantly more effective than doubling the dose of atorvastatin to 20 mg in further reducing total-C, LDL-C, TG, and non-HDL-C. Results for HDL-C between the two treatment groups were not significantly different. (See Table 10.) In addition, at Week 4 significantly more patients receiving LIPTRUZET 10/10 attained LDL-C <100 mg/dL (<2.6 mmol/L) compared to those receiving atorvastatin 20 mg, 12% vs. 2%. The baseline mean LDL-C levels for patients receiving LIPTRUZET 10/10 and atorvastatin 20 mg were 186 mg/dL and 187 mg/dL, respectively.

[See table 10 at top of next page]

The Titration of Atorvastatin Versus Ezetimibe Add-On to Atorvastatin in Patients with Hypercholesterolemia (TEMPO) study, a multicenter, double-blind, controlled, 6-week study, included 184 patients with an LDL-C level ≥100 mg/dL and ≤160 mg/dL (≥2.6 mmol/L and ≤4.1 mmol/L) and at moderate high risk for coronary heart disease (CHD). All patients received atorvastatin 20 mg for a minimum of 4 weeks prior to randomization. Patients not at the optional NCEP ATP III LDL-C level (<100 mg/dL [<2.6 mmol/L]) were randomized to receive either coadministered ezetimibe and atorvastatin (equivalent to LIPTRUZET 10/20) or atorvastatin 40 mg for 6 weeks.

The patient population was: 45% female; 60% Caucasian, 26% Multi-racial, 6% Black, 8% Asian, <1% American Indian or Alaska native; 24 to 78 years of age (mean age 58 years).

LIPTRUZET 10/20 was significantly more effective than doubling the dose of atorvastatin to 40 mg in further reducing total-C, LDL-C, Apo B and non-HDL-C. Results for HDL-C and TG between the two treatment groups were not significantly different. (See Table 11.) In addition, significantly more patients receiving LIPTRUZET 10/20 attained LDL-C <100 mg/dL (<2.6 mmol/L) compared to those receiving atorvastatin 40 mg, 84% vs. 49%.

[See table 11 at top of next page]

The Ezetimibe Plus Atorvastatin Versus Atorvastatin Titration in Achieving Lower LDL-C Targets in Hypercholesterolemic Patients (EZ-PATH) study, a multicenter, double-blind, controlled, 6-week study, included 556 patients with an LDL-C level ≥70 mg/dL and ≤160 mg/dL (≥1.8 mmol/L and ≤4.1 mmol/L) and at high risk for coronary heart disease (CHD). All patients received atorvastatin 40 mg for a minimum of 4 weeks prior to randomization. Patients not at the optional NCEP ATP III LDL-C level <70 mg/dL (<1.8 mmol/L) were randomized to receive either coadministered ezetimibe and atorvastatin (equivalent to LIPTRUZET 10/40) or atorvastatin 80 mg for 6 weeks.

The patient population was: 39% female; 81% Caucasian, 11% Black, 6% Multi-racial, 2% Asian; 31 to 80 years of age (mean age 52 years).

LIPTRUZET 10/40 was significantly more effective than doubling the dose of atorvastatin to 80 mg in further reducing total-C, LDL-C, Apo B, TG, and non-HDL-C. Results for HDL-C between the two treatment groups were not significantly different. (See Table 12.) In addition, significantly more patients receiving LIPTRUZET 10/40 attained LDL-C <70 mg/dL (<1.8 mmol/L) compared to those receiving atorvastatin 80 mg, 74% vs. 32%.

[See table 12 at top of next page]

LIPTRUZET 10/20 and 10/40 - Clinical Equivalence to Coadministered Components

LIPTRUZET has been shown to be bioequivalent to coadministration of corresponding doses of its ezetimibe and atorvastatin components with the exception of slightly lower atorvastatin C_{max} for the 10/20 and 10/40 mg doses *[see Clinical Pharmacology (12.3)]*, which, in two separate studies, have been shown to be clinically equivalent in LDL-C response after six weeks of treatment to their corresponding coadministered components.

In these two multicenter, double-blind, controlled, crossover studies, patients with primary hypercholesterolemia and low, moderate, or moderately high cardiovascular risk received LIPTRUZET 10/20-mg (Study 1) or 10/40-mg (Study 2) tablets or the corresponding coadministered components once daily for 6 weeks. They then crossed over, after a 6-week washout, to the coadministered components or LIPTRUZET at corresponding doses for an additional 6 weeks. From untreated baseline, mean changes in LDL-C for LIPTRUZET vs. the coadministered components, respectively, were -54.0% vs. -53.8% for 10/20-mg (Study 1), and -58.9% vs. -58.7% for 10/40-mg (Study 2). Mean changes for total-C, Apo B, TG, non-HDL-C, and HDL C were also similar between the two treatment groups and supported the conclusion of clinical equivalence.

14.2 Homozygous Familial Hypercholesterolemia (HoFH)

A double-blind, randomized, 12-week study was performed in patients with a clinical and/or genotypic diagnosis of HoFH. Data were analyzed from a subgroup of patients (n=36) receiving atorvastatin 40 mg at baseline. Increasing the dose of atorvastatin from 40 to 80 mg (n=12) produced a reduction of LDL-C of 2% from baseline on atorvastatin 40 mg. Coadministered ezetimibe and atorvastatin equivalent to LIPTRUZET (10/40 and 10/80 pooled, n=24), produced a reduction of LDL-C of 19% from baseline on atorvastatin 40 mg. In those patients coadministered ezetimibe and atorvastatin equivalent to LIPTRUZET (10/80, n=12), a reduction of LDL-C of 25% from baseline on atorvastatin 40 mg was produced.

After completing the 12-week study, eligible patients (n=35), who were receiving atorvastatin 40 mg at baseline, were assigned to coadministered ezetimibe and atorvastatin equivalent to LIPTRUZET 10/40 for up to an additional 24 months. Following at least 4 weeks of treatment, the atorvastatin dose could be doubled to a maximum dose of 80 mg.

At the end of the 24 months, LIPTRUZET (10/40 and 10/80 pooled) produced a reduction of LDL-C that was consistent with that seen in the 12-week study.

Table 8: Effect of Atorvastatin on the Pharmacokinetics of Coadministered Drugs

Atorvastatin	Coadministered Drug and Dosing Regimen		
	Drug/Dose (mg)	Change in AUC	Change in C_{max}
80 mg QD for 15 days	Antipyrine, 600 mg SD	↑3%	↓11%
80 mg QD for 14 days	Digoxin 0.25 mg QD, 20 days*	↑15%	↑20%
40 mg QD for 22 days	Oral contraceptive QD, 2 months - norethindrone 1 mg - ethinyl estradiol 35 µg	↑28% ↑19%	↑23% ↑30%
10 mg, SD	Tipranavir 500 mg BID/ ritonavir 200 mg BID, 7 days	No change	No change
10 mg QD for 4 days	Fosamprenavir 1400 mg BID, 14 days	↓27%	↓18%
10 mg QD for 4 days	Fosamprenavir 700 mg BID/ritonavir 100 mg BID, 14 days	No change	No change

* *See Drug Interactions (7)* for clinical significance.

Table 9: Response to LIPTRUZET in Patients with Primary Hyperlipidemia (Mean* % Change from Untreated Baseline† at 12 weeks)

Treatment (Daily Dose)	N	Total-C [Baseline‡]	LDL-C [Baseline‡]	Apo B [Baseline‡]	TG* [Baseline‡]	HDL-C [Baseline‡]	Non-HDL-C [Baseline‡]
Pooled data (All LIPTRUZET doses)§	255	-41% [267]	-56% [182]	-45% [170]	-33% [165]	+7% [50.8]	-52% [217]
Pooled data (All atorvastatin doses)§	248	-32% [269]	-44% [181]	-36% [168]	-24% [155]	+4% [53.7]	-41% [215]
Ezetimibe 10 mg	65	-14% [259]	-20% [177]	-15% [167]	-5% [145]	+4% [50.6]	-18% [209]
Placebo	60	+4% [262]	+4% [180]	+3% [168]	-6% [143]	+4% [50.4]	+4% [212]
LIPTRUZET by dose							
10/10	65	-38% [262]	-53% [177]	-43% [165]	-31% [158]	+9% [51.9]	-49% [211]
10/20	62	-39% [269]	-54% [184]	-44% [174]	-30% [165]	+9% [49.3]	-50% [220]
10/40	65	-42% [271]	-56% [184]	-45% [173]	-34% [180]	+5% [51.1]	-52% [220]
10/80	63	-46% [267]	-61% [183]	-50% [169]	-40% [146]	+7% [50.9]	-58% [216]
Atorvastatin by dose							
10 mg	60	-26% [271]	-37% [185]	-28% [168]	-21% [153]	+6% [53.7]	-34% [217]
20 mg	60	-30% [267]	-42% [177]	-34% [164]	-23% [147]	+4% [55.5]	-39% [211]
40 mg	66	-32% [266]	-45% [180]	-37% [167]	-24% [159]	+4% [53.0]	-41% [213]
80 mg	62	-40% [270]	-54% [184]	-46% [171]	-31% [163]	+3% [52.7]	-51% [218]

* For triglycerides, median % change from baseline
† Baseline - on no lipid-lowering drug
‡ Baseline units: mg/dL; medians for TG, means for all other values
§ LIPTRUZET pooled (10/10-10/80) significantly reduced total-C, LDL-C, Apo B, TG, non-HDL-C, and significantly increased HDL-C compared to all doses of atorvastatin pooled (10-80 mg).

16 HOW SUPPLIED/STORAGE AND HANDLING

Tablets LIPTRUZET 10 mg/10 mg are white to off-white capsule-shaped, biconvex film-coated tablets with code "320" on one side.

They are supplied as follows:

NDC 66582-320-30 unit of use packages of 30 (three foil pouches each containing one 10-count blister card)

NDC 66582-320-54 unit of use packages of 90 (nine foil pouches each containing one 10-count blister card)

Tablets LIPTRUZET 10 mg/20 mg are white to off-white round, biconvex film-coated tablets with code "321" on one side.

They are supplied as follows:

NDC 66582-321-30 unit of use packages of 30 (three foil pouches each containing one 10-count blister card)

NDC 66582-321-54 unit of use packages of 90 (nine foil pouches each containing one 10-count blister card)

Tablets LIPTRUZET 10 mg/40 mg are white to off-white oval, biconvex film-coated tablets with code "322" on one side.

They are supplied as follows:

NDC 66582-322-30 unit of use packages of 30 (three foil pouches each containing one 10-count blister card)

NDC 66582-322-54 unit of use packages of 90 (nine foil pouches each containing one 10-count blister card)

Tablets LIPTRUZET 10 mg/80 mg are white to off-white capsule-shaped, biconvex film-coated tablets with code "323" on one side.

They are supplied as follows:

NDC 66582-323-30 unit of use packages of 30 (three foil pouches each containing one 10-count blister card)

NDC 66582-323-54 unit of use packages of 90 (nine foil pouches each containing one 10-count blister card)

Storage of Unit of Use Packages of 30 and 90

Store LIPTRUZET at 20-25°C (68-77°F), excursions permitted to 15-30°C (59-86°F) [see USP Controlled Room Temper-

Table 10: Response to LIPTRUZET after 4 Weeks in Patients with CHD or Multiple Cardiovascular Risk Factors and an LDL-C ≥130 mg/dL (Mean* % Change from Baseline†)

Treatment (Daily Dose)	N	Total-C [Baseline‡]	LDL-C [Baseline‡]	HDL-C [Baseline‡]	TG* [Baseline‡]	Non-HDL-C [Baseline‡]
LIPTRUZET 10/10	305	-17%§ [262]	-24%§ [186]	+2% [50.0]	-9%§ [117]	-22%§ [212]
Atorvastatin 20 mg	316	-6% [264]	-9% [187]	+1% [49.9]	-4% [119]	-8% [214]

* For triglycerides, median % change from baseline
† Patients on atorvastatin 10 mg, then switched to LIPTRUZET 10/10 or titrated to atorvastatin 20 mg
‡ Baseline units: mg/dL; medians for TG, means for all other values
§ $p<0.05$ for difference with atorvastatin

Table 11: Response to LIPTRUZET in Patients with Primary Hypercholesterolemia (Mean* % Change from Baseline†)

Treatment (Daily Dose)	N	Total-C [Baseline‡]	LDL-C [Baseline‡]	Apo B [Baseline‡]	HDL-C [Baseline‡]	TG* [Baseline‡]	Non-HDL-C [Baseline‡]
LIPTRUZET 10/20	92	-20%§ [203]	-31%§ [120]	-21%§ [123]	+3% [50.9]	-18% [155]	-27%§ [152]
Atorvastatin 40 mg	92	-7% [201]	-11% [118]	-8% [120]	+1% [52.1]	-6% [148]	-10% [149]

* For triglycerides, median % change from baseline
† Patients on atorvastatin 20 mg, then switched to LIPTRUZET 10/20 or titrated to atorvastatin 40 mg
‡ Baseline units: mg/dL; medians for TG, means for all other values
§ $p<0.05$ for difference with atorvastatin

Table 12: Response to LIPTRUZET in Patients with Primary Hypercholesterolemia (Mean* % Change from Baseline†)

Treatment (Daily Dose)	N	Total-C [Baseline‡]	LDL-C [Baseline‡]	Apo B [Baseline‡]	HDL-C [Baseline‡]	TG* [Baseline‡]	Non-HDL-C [Baseline‡]
LIPTRUZET 10/40	277	-17%§ [165]	-27%§ [89]	-18%§ [101]	0% [47.7]	-12%§ [131]	-23%§ [117]
Atorvastatin 80 mg	279	-7% [165]	-11% [90]	-8% [102]	-1% [46.9]	-6% [136]	-9% [118]

* For triglycerides, median % change from baseline
† Patients on atorvastatin 20 mg, then switched to LIPTRUZET 10/40 or titrated to atorvastatin 80 mg
‡ Baseline units: mg/dL; medians for TG, means for all other values
§ $p<0.05$ for difference with atorvastatin

ature]. Store in the foil pouch until use. After the foil pouch is opened, protect LIPTRUZET from moisture and light. Once a tablet is removed, slide blister card back into case. Store the case in a dry place, and discard any unused tablets 30 days after the pouch is opened.

17 PATIENT COUNSELING INFORMATION

See FDA-Approved Patient Labeling (Patient Information). Patients should be advised to adhere to their National Cholesterol Education Program (NCEP)-recommended diet, a regular exercise program, and periodic testing of a fasting lipid panel.

17.1 Muscle Pain

All patients starting therapy with LIPTRUZET should be advised of the risk of myopathy and told to report promptly any unexplained muscle pain, tenderness or weakness particularly if accompanied by malaise or fever or if these muscle signs or symptoms persist after discontinuing LIPTRUZET. The risk of this occurring is increased when taking certain types of medication or consuming larger quantities (>1 liter) of grapefruit juice. Patients should discuss all medication, both prescription and over-the-counter, with their physician.

17.2 Liver Enzymes

It is recommended that liver enzyme tests be performed before the initiation of LIPTRUZET and if signs or symptoms of liver injury occur. All patients treated with LIPTRUZET should be advised to report promptly any symptoms that may indicate liver injury, including fatigue, anorexia, right upper abdominal discomfort, dark urine, or jaundice.

17.3 Pregnancy

Women of childbearing age should be advised to use an effective method of birth control to prevent pregnancy while using LIPTRUZET. Discuss future pregnancy plans with your patients, and discuss when to stop taking LIPTRUZET if they are trying to conceive. Patients should be advised that if they become pregnant they should stop taking LIPTRUZET and call their healthcare professional.

17.4 Breast-Feeding

Women who are breast-feeding should be advised to not use LIPTRUZET. Patients who have a lipid disorder and are breast-feeding should be advised to discuss the options with their healthcare professionals.

17.5 Important Storage and Administration Instructions

Patients should be advised to store LIPTRUZET at room temperature, 20-25°C (68-77°F). They should also be advised:

- not to open a pouch until they are ready to use LIPTRUZET
- that after the foil pouch is opened, LIPTRUZET should be protected from moisture and light, and stored in a dry place
- that for packages containing a plastic case (unit of use packages of 30 and 90), once they remove a tablet from the blister card, they should slide the blister card back into the plastic case
- to discard any unused tablets 30 days after the pouch is opened

Tablets should be swallowed whole. Do not crush, dissolve, or chew tablets.

If a dose is missed, the patient should not take an extra dose. Just resume the usual schedule.

Manufactured by:
Merck Sharp & Dohme Corp., a subsidiary of
MERCK & CO., INC., Whitehouse Station, NJ 08889, USA
U.S. Patent Nos. 5,846,966 and RE37,721.
USPI-T-0653C1305R000

Patient Information
LIPTRUZET™ (LIP-true-zett)
(ezetimibe and atorvastatin)
Tablets

Generic name: ezetimibe and atorvastatin tablets

Read this information carefully before you start taking LIPTRUZET™ and each time you get more LIPTRUZET. There may be new information. This information does not take the place of talking with your doctor about your medical condition or your treatment. If you have any questions about LIPTRUZET, ask your doctor. Only your doctor can determine if LIPTRUZET is right for you.

What is LIPTRUZET?

LIPTRUZET contains 2 cholesterol-lowering medications, ezetimibe and atorvastatin.

LIPTRUZET is a prescription medicine used to lower levels of total cholesterol, LDL (bad) cholesterol and fatty substances called triglycerides in the blood. In addition, LIPTRUZET raises levels of HDL (good) cholesterol. LIPTRUZET is for patients who cannot control their cholesterol levels by diet and exercise alone. You should stay on a cholesterol-lowering diet while taking this medicine.

LIPTRUZET has not been shown to reduce heart attacks or strokes more than atorvastatin alone.

It is not known if LIPTRUZET is safe and effective in children.

Who should not take LIPTRUZET?

Do not take LIPTRUZET if you:

- have active liver problems or repeated blood tests showing possible liver problems.
- are allergic to ezetimibe or atorvastatin or any of the ingredients in LIPTRUZET. See the end of this leaflet for a complete list of ingredients in LIPTRUZET.
- are pregnant or plan to become pregnant. LIPTRUZET may harm your unborn baby. If you are a woman of childbearing age, you should use an effective method of birth control while taking LIPTRUZET. Stop taking LIPTRUZET and call your doctor right away if you get pregnant while taking LIPTRUZET.
- are breastfeeding or plan to breastfeed. LIPTRUZET can pass into your breast milk and may harm your baby. Talk to your doctor about the best way to feed your baby if you take LIPTRUZET. Do not breastfeed while taking LIPTRUZET.

What should I tell my doctor before taking LIPTRUZET?

Before you take LIPTRUZET, tell your doctor if you:

- have a thyroid problem
- have kidney problems
- have diabetes
- have unexplained muscle aches or weakness
- drink more than 2 glasses of alcohol daily or have or have had liver problems
- have any other medical conditions

Tell your doctor about all the medicines you take, including prescription and non-prescription medicines, vitamins, and herbal supplements.

Taking LIPTRUZET with certain other medicines or substances can increase the risk of muscle problems or other side effects.

Especially tell your doctor if you take medicines for:

- your immune system
- cholesterol
- infections
- birth control
- heart failure
- HIV or AIDS
- hepatitis C
- gout

Also tell your doctor if you drink large amounts of grapefruit juice.

How should I take LIPTRUZET?

- Take LIPTRUZET exactly as your doctor tells you to take it.
- Your doctor will tell you how much LIPTRUZET to take and when to take it.
- Your doctor may change your dose if needed.
- Do not open your LIPTRUZET pouch until you are ready to take LIPTRUZET.
- Take LIPTRUZET 1 time each day, with or without food. It may be easier to remember to take your dose if you do it at the same time every day, such as with breakfast, dinner, or at bedtime.
- Tablets should be swallowed whole. Do not crush, dissolve, or chew tablets.
- Keep taking LIPTRUZET unless your doctor tells you to stop. If you stop taking LIPTRUZET, your cholesterol may rise again.
- If you miss a dose, do not take an extra dose. Just resume your usual schedule.
- If you take too much LIPTRUZET, call your doctor or Poison Control Center at 1-800-222-1222 or go to the nearest hospital emergency room right away.
- See your doctor regularly to check your cholesterol level and to check for side effects. Your doctor may do blood tests to check your liver before you start taking LIPTRUZET and during treatment.

What should I avoid while taking LIPTRUZET?

- Do not start any new medicines before talking to your doctor. This includes prescription and non-prescription medicines, vitamins, and herbal supplements. LIPTRUZET and certain other medicines can interact causing serious side effects.
- Do not drink more than 2 glasses of alcohol daily.
- Do not get pregnant. If you get pregnant, stop taking LIPTRUZET right away and call your doctor.

What are the possible side effects of LIPTRUZET?

LIPTRUZET may cause serious side effects, including:

- **muscle problems.** LIPTRUZET can cause serious muscle problems that can lead to kidney problems, including kidney failure. You have a higher chance for muscle problems if you are taking certain other medicines with LIPTRUZET.

Tell your doctor right away if:

- **you have unexplained muscle pain, tenderness, or weakness, especially if you have a fever or feel more tired than usual, while you take LIPTRUZET.**
- you have muscle problems that do not go away even after your doctor has advised you to stop taking LIPTRUZET. Your doctor may do further tests to diagnose the cause of your muscle problems.

- **liver problems.** Your doctor should do blood tests to check your liver before you start taking LIPTRUZET and if you have symptoms of liver problems while you take LIPTRUZET. Call your doctor right away if you have the following symptoms of liver problems:
  - feel tired or weak
  - loss of appetite
  - upper belly pain
  - dark urine
  - yellowing of your skin or the whites of your eyes

Also call your doctor right away if you have:

- allergic reactions including swelling of the face, lips, tongue, and/or throat that may cause difficulty in breathing or swallowing which may require treatment right away
- nausea and vomiting
- passing brown or dark-colored urine
- you feel more tired than usual
- stomach pain
- allergic skin reactions

The most common side effects of LIPTRUZET include:

- muscle and body pain
- changes in your liver function tests

Additional side effects that have been reported in people taking LIPTRUZET, ezetimibe or atorvastatin in clinical studies or general use include: joint pain; diarrhea; tendon problems; memory loss; confusion; depression.

Tell your doctor if you have any side effect that bothers you or that does not go away.

These are not all the possible side effects of LIPTRUZET. For more information, ask your doctor or pharmacist.

Call your doctor for medical advice about side effects. You may report side effects to FDA at 1-800-FDA-1088.

How should I store LIPTRUZET?

- Store LIPTRUZET at room temperature between 68°F to 77°F (20°C to 25°C).
- Keep LIPTRUZET in the foil pouch until you are ready to take it.
- After you remove a LIPTRUZET tablet from the blister card, slide the blister card back into the case (where a case is provided) and store in a dry place.
- Write down the date the foil pouch was opened in the space provided.
- Keep LIPTRUZET tablets dry and out of the light.
- Safely throw away unused LIPTRUZET tablets **30 days** after the foil pouch is opened.

Keep LIPTRUZET and all medicines out of the reach of children.

General information about the safe and effective use of LIPTRUZET.

LIPTRUZET may help to reduce your cholesterol in 2 ways. It reduces the cholesterol absorbed in your digestive tract, as well as the cholesterol your body makes by itself. LIPTRUZET does not help you lose weight.

Medicines are sometimes prescribed for purposes other than those listed in the Patient Information leaflet. Do not use LIPTRUZET for a condition for which it was not prescribed. Do not give LIPTRUZET to other people, even if they have the same problem that you have. It may harm them.

This Patient Information leaflet summarizes the most important information about LIPTRUZET. If you would like more information, talk with your doctor. You can ask your pharmacist or doctor for information about LIPTRUZET that is written for health professionals.

For more information, go to www.LIPTRUZET.com or call 1-800-672-6372.

What are the ingredients in LIPTRUZET?

Active ingredients: ezetimibe and atorvastatin

Inactive ingredients: lactose monohydrate, microcrystalline cellulose, croscarmellose sodium, povidone, sodium lauryl sulfate, magnesium stearate, lactose anhydrous, hydroxypropyl cellulose, sodium bicarbonate. The tablet film coating contains the following inactive ingredients: hydroxypropyl cellulose, hypromellose, titanium dioxide, and carnauba wax

This Patient Information has been approved by the U.S. Food and Drug Administration

Manufactured by:
Merck Sharp & Dohme Corp., a subsidiary of
MERCK & CO., INC., Whitehouse Station, NJ 08889, USA
U.S. Patent Nos. 5,846,966 and RE37,721.
Issued: 05/2013
USPPI-T-0653C1305R000

Shown in Product Identification Guide, page 308

LOTRISONE® CREAM ℞
(clotrimazole and betamethasone dipropionate)

FOR TOPICAL USE ONLY. NOT FOR OPHTHALMIC, ORAL, OR INTRAVAGINAL USE. NOT RECOMMENDED FOR PATIENTS UNDER THE AGE OF 17 YEARS AND NOT RECOMMENDED FOR DIAPER DERMATITIS.

DESCRIPTION

LOTRISONE® Cream contains combinations of clotrimazole, a synthetic antifungal agent, and betamethasone dipropionate, a synthetic corticosteroid, for dermatologic use.

Chemically, clotrimazole is 1-(*o*-chloro-α,α-diphenylbenzyl) imidazole, with the empirical formula $C_{22}H_{17}ClN_2$, a molecular weight of 344.84, and the following structural formula:

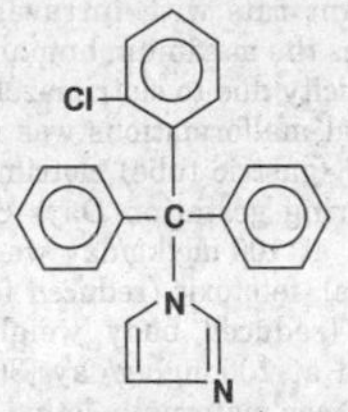

Clotrimazole is an odorless, white crystalline powder, insoluble in water and soluble in ethanol.

Betamethasone dipropionate has the chemical name 9-fluoro-11β,17,21-trihydroxy-16β-methylpregna-1,4-diene-3,20-dione 17,21-dipropionate, with the empirical formula $C_{28}H_{37}FO_7$, a molecular weight of 504.59, and the following structural formula:

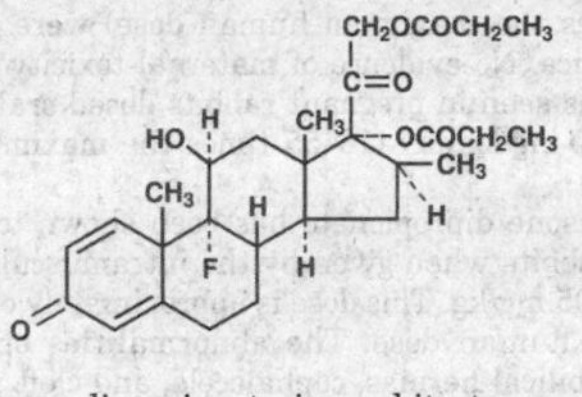

Betamethasone dipropionate is a white to creamy white, odorless crystalline powder, insoluble in water.

Each gram of **LOTRISONE Cream** contains 10 mg clotrimazole and 0.643 mg betamethasone dipropionate (equivalent to 0.5 mg betamethasone), in a hydrophilic cream consisting of purified water, mineral oil, white petrolatum, cetyl alcohol plus stearyl alcohol, ceteareth-30, propylene glycol, sodium phosphate monobasic monohydrate, and phosphoric acid; benzyl alcohol as a preservative.

LOTRISONE Cream may contain sodium hydroxide. LOTRISONE Cream is smooth, uniform, and white to off-white in color.

CLINICAL PHARMACOLOGY

Clotrimazole and Betamethasone Dipropionate

LOTRISONE® Cream has been shown to be at least as effective as clotrimazole alone in a different cream vehicle. Use of corticosteroids in the treatment of a fungal infection may lead to suppression of host inflammation leading to worsening or decreased cure rate.

Clotrimazole

Skin penetration and systemic absorption of clotrimazole following topical application of LOTRISONE Cream has not been studied. The following information was obtained using 1% clotrimazole cream and solution formulations. Six hours after the application of radioactive clotrimazole 1% cream and 1% solution onto intact and acutely inflamed skin, the concentration of clotrimazole varied from 100 mcg/cm³ in the stratum corneum, to 0.5 to 1 mcg/cm³ in the reticular dermis, and 0.1 mcg/cm³ in the subcutis. No measurable amount of radioactivity (<0.001 mcg/mL) was found in the serum within 48 hours after application under occlusive dressing of 0.5 mL of the solution or 0.8 g of the cream. Only 0.5% or less of the applied radioactivity was excreted in the urine.

Microbiology

Mechanism of Action: Clotrimazole is an imidazole antifungal agent. Imidazoles inhibit 14-α-demethylation of lanosterol in fungi by binding to one of the cytochrome P-450 enzymes. This leads to the accumulation of 14-α-methylsterols and reduced concentrations of ergosterol, a sterol essential for a normal fungal cytoplasmic membrane. The methylsterols may affect the electron transport system, thereby inhibiting growth of fungi.

Activity *In Vivo*: Clotrimazole has been shown to be active against most strains of the following dermatophytes, both *in vitro* and in clinical infections as described in the **INDICATIONS AND USAGE** section: *Epidermophyton floccosum, Trichophyton mentagrophytes,* and *Trichophyton rubrum.*

Activity *In Vitro*: *In vitro*, clotrimazole has been shown to have activity against many dermatophytes, **but the clinical significance of this information is unknown.**

Drug Resistance: Strains of dermatophytes having a natural resistance to clotrimazole have not been reported. Resistance to azoles including clotrimazole has been reported in some *Candida* species.

No single-step or multiple-step resistance to clotrimazole has developed during successive passages of *Trichophyton mentagrophytes*.

Betamethasone Dipropionate

Betamethasone dipropionate, a corticosteroid, has been shown to have topical (dermatologic) and systemic pharmacologic and metabolic effects characteristic of this class of drugs.

Pharmacokinetics

The extent of percutaneous absorption of topical corticosteroids is determined by many factors, including the vehicle, the integrity of the epidermal barrier, and the use of occlusive dressings (see **DOSAGE AND ADMINISTRATION**). Topical corticosteroids can be absorbed from normal intact skin. Inflammation and/or other disease processes in the skin may increase percutaneous absorption of topical corticosteroids. Occlusive dressings substantially increase the percutaneous absorption of topical corticosteroids (see **DOSAGE AND ADMINISTRATION**).

Once absorbed through the skin, the pharmacokinetics of topical corticosteroids are similar to systemically administered corticosteroids. Corticosteroids are bound to plasma proteins in varying degrees. Corticosteroids are metabolized primarily in the liver and are then excreted by the kidneys. Some of the topical corticosteroids and their metabolites are also excreted into the bile.

Studies performed with LOTRISONE Cream indicate that these topical combination antifungal/corticosteroids may have vasoconstrictor potencies in a range that is comparable to high-potency topical corticosteroids. Therefore, use is not recommended in patients less than 17 years of age, in diaper dermatitis, and under occlusion.

CLINICAL STUDIES (LOTRISONE® CREAM)

In clinical studies of tinea corporis, tinea cruris, and tinea pedis, patients treated with LOTRISONE Cream showed a better clinical response at the first return visit than patients treated with clotrimazole cream. In tinea corporis and tinea cruris, the patient returned 3 to 5 days after starting treatment, and in tinea pedis, after 1 week. Mycological cure rates observed in patients treated with LOTRISONE Cream were as good as or better than in those patients treated with clotrimazole cream. In these same clinical studies, patients treated with LOTRISONE Cream showed better clinical responses and mycological cure rates when compared with patients treated with betamethasone dipropionate cream.

INDICATIONS AND USAGE

LOTRISONE® Cream is indicated in patients 17 years and older for the topical treatment of symptomatic inflammatory tinea pedis, tinea cruris, and tinea corporis due to *Epidermophyton floccosum, Trichophyton mentagrophytes,* and *Trichophyton rubrum.* Effective treatment without the risks associated with topical corticosteroid use may be obtained using a topical antifungal agent that does not contain a corticosteroid, especially for noninflammatory tinea infections. The efficacy of LOTRISONE Cream for the treatment of infections caused by zoophilic dermatophytes (e.g., *Microsporum canis*) has not been established. Several cases of treatment failure of LOTRISONE Cream in the treatment of infections caused by *Microsporum canis* have been reported.

CONTRAINDICATIONS

LOTRISONE® Cream is contraindicated in patients who are sensitive to clotrimazole, betamethasone dipropionate, other corticosteroids or imidazoles, or to any ingredient in these preparations.

PRECAUTIONS

General

Systemic absorption of topical corticosteroids can produce reversible hypothalamic-pituitary-adrenal (HPA) axis suppression with the potential for glucocorticosteroid insufficiency after withdrawal of treatment. Manifestations of Cushing's syndrome, hyperglycemia, and glucosuria can also be produced in some patients by systemic absorption of topical corticosteroids while on treatment.

Conditions which augment systemic absorption include use over large surface areas, prolonged use, and use under occlusive dressings. Use of more than one corticosteroid-containing product at the same time may increase total systemic glucocorticoid exposure. Patients applying LOTRISONE® Cream to a large surface area or to areas under occlusion should be evaluated periodically for evidence of HPA axis suppression. This may be done by using the ACTH stimulation, morning plasma cortisol, and urinary-free cortisol tests.

If HPA axis suppression is noted, an attempt should be made to withdraw the drug, to reduce the frequency of application, or to substitute a less potent corticosteroid. Recovery of HPA axis function is generally prompt upon discontinuation of topical corticosteroids. Infrequently, signs and symptoms of glucocorticosteroid insufficiency may occur, requiring supplemental systemic corticosteroids.

In a small study, LOTRISONE Cream was applied using large dosages, 7 g daily for 14 days (BID) to the crural area of normal adult subjects. Three of the 8 normal subjects on whom LOTRISONE Cream was applied exhibited low morning plasma cortisol levels during treatment. One of these subjects had an abnormal Cortrosyn test. The effect on morning plasma cortisol was transient and subjects recovered 1 week after discontinuing dosing. In addition, 2 separate studies in pediatric patients demonstrated adrenal suppression as determined by cosyntropin testing (see **PRECAUTIONS, Pediatric Use** section).

Pediatric patients may be more susceptible to systemic toxicity from equivalent doses due to their larger skin surface to body mass ratios (see **PRECAUTIONS, Pediatric Use** section).

If irritation develops, LOTRISONE Cream should be discontinued and appropriate therapy instituted.

THE SAFETY OF LOTRISONE CREAM HAS NOT BEEN DEMONSTRATED IN THE TREATMENT OF DIAPER DERMATITIS. ADVERSE EVENTS CONSISTENT WITH CORTICOSTEROID USE HAVE BEEN OBSERVED IN PATIENTS TREATED WITH LOTRISONE CREAM FOR DIAPER DERMATITIS. THE USE OF LOTRISONE CREAM IN THE TREATMENT OF DIAPER DERMATITIS IS NOT RECOMMENDED.

Information for Patients

Patients using LOTRISONE Cream should receive the following information and instructions:

1. The medication is to be used as directed by the physician and is not recommended for use longer than the prescribed time period. It is for external use only. Avoid contact with the eyes, the mouth, or intravaginally.
2. This medication is to be used for the full prescribed treatment time, even though the symptoms may have improved. Notify the physician if there is no improvement after 1 week of treatment for tinea cruris or tinea corporis, or after 2 weeks for tinea pedis.
3. This medication should only be used for the disorder for which it was prescribed.
4. Other corticosteroid-containing products should not be used with LOTRISONE without first talking with your physician.
5. The treated skin area should not be bandaged, covered, or wrapped so as to be occluded (see **DOSAGE AND ADMINISTRATION**).
6. Any signs of local adverse reactions should be reported to your physician.
7. Patients should avoid sources of infection or reinfection.
8. When using LOTRISONE Cream in the groin area, patients should use the medication for 2 weeks only, and apply the cream sparingly. Patients should wear loose-fitting clothing. Notify the physician if the condition persists after 2 weeks.
9. The safety of LOTRISONE Cream has not been demonstrated in the treatment of diaper dermatitis. Adverse events consistent with corticosteroid use have been observed in patients treated with LOTRISONE Cream for diaper dermatitis. The use of LOTRISONE Cream in the treatment of diaper dermatitis is not recommended.

Laboratory Tests

If there is a lack of response to LOTRISONE Cream, appropriate confirmation of the diagnosis, including possible mycological studies, is indicated before instituting another course of therapy.

The following tests may be helpful in evaluating HPA axis suppression due to the corticosteroid components:

Urinary-free cortisol test
Morning plasma cortisol test
ACTH (cosyntropin) stimulation test

Carcinogenesis, Mutagenesis, Impairment of Fertility

There are no adequate laboratory animal studies with either the combination of clotrimazole and betamethasone dipropionate or with either component individually to evaluate carcinogenesis.

Betamethasone was negative in the bacterial mutagenicity assay (*Salmonella typhimurium* and *Escherichia coli*) and in the mammalian cell mutagenicity assay (CHO/HGPRT). It was positive in the *in vitro* human lymphocyte chromosome aberration assay, and equivocal in the *in vivo* mouse bone marrow micronucleus assay. This pattern of response is similar to that of dexamethasone and hydrocortisone.

Reproductive studies with betamethasone dipropionate carried out in rabbits at doses of 1.0 mg/kg by the intramuscular route and in mice up to 33 mg/kg by the intramuscular route indicated no impairment of fertility except for dose-related increases in fetal resorption rates in both species. These doses are approximately 5- and 38-fold the maximum human dose based on body surface areas, respectively.

In a combined study of the effects of clotrimazole on fertility, teratogenicity, and postnatal development, male and female rats were dosed orally (diet admixture) with levels of 5, 10, 25, or 50 mg/kg/day (approximately 1–8 times the maximum dose in a 60-kg adult based on body surface area) from 10 weeks prior to mating until 4 weeks postpartum. No adverse effects on the duration of estrous cycle, fertility, or duration of pregnancy were noted.

Pregnancy

Teratogenic Effects: Pregnancy Category C

There have been no teratogenic studies performed in animals or humans with the combination of clotrimazole and betamethasone dipropionate. Corticosteroids are generally teratogenic in laboratory animals when administered at relatively low dosage levels.

Studies in pregnant rats with intravaginal doses up to 100 mg/kg (15 times the maximum human dose) revealed no evidence of fetotoxicity due to clotrimazole exposure.

No increase in fetal malformations was noted in pregnant rats receiving oral (gastric tube) clotrimazole doses up to 100 mg/kg/day during gestation Days 6 to 15. However, clotrimazole dosed at 100 mg/kg/day was embryotoxic (increased resorptions), fetotoxic (reduced fetal weights), and maternally toxic (reduced body weight gain) to rats. Clotrimazole dosed at 200 mg/kg/day (30 times the maximum human dose) was maternally lethal, and therefore, fetuses were not evaluated in this group. Also in this study, doses up to 50 mg/kg/day (8 times the maximum human dose) had no adverse effects on dams or fetuses. However, in the combined fertility, teratogenicity, and postnatal development study described above, 50 mg/kg clotrimazole was associated with reduced maternal weight gain and reduced numbers of offspring reared to 4 weeks.

Oral clotrimazole doses of 25, 50, 100, and 200 mg/kg/day (2–15 times the maximum human dose) were not teratogenic in mice. No evidence of maternal toxicity or embryotoxicity was seen in pregnant rabbits dosed orally with 60, 120, or 180 mg/kg/day (18–55 times the maximum human dose).

Betamethasone dipropionate has been shown to be teratogenic in rabbits when given by the intramuscular route at doses of 0.05 mg/kg. This dose is approximately one-fifth the maximum human dose. The abnormalities observed included umbilical hernias, cephalocele, and cleft palates.

Betamethasone dipropionate has not been tested for teratogenic potential by the dermal route of administration. Some corticosteroids have been shown to be teratogenic after dermal application to laboratory animals.

There are no adequate and well-controlled studies in pregnant women of the teratogenic effects of topically applied corticosteroids. Therefore, LOTRISONE Cream should be used during pregnancy only if the potential benefit justifies the potential risk to the fetus.

Nursing Mothers

Systemically administered corticosteroids appear in human milk and could suppress growth, interfere with endogenous corticosteroid production, or cause other untoward effects. It is not known whether topical administration of corticosteroids could result in sufficient systemic absorption to produce detectable quantities in human milk. Because many drugs are excreted in human milk, caution should be exercised when LOTRISONE Cream is administered to a nursing woman.

Pediatric Use

Adverse events consistent with corticosteroid use have been observed in patients under 12 years of age treated with LOTRISONE Cream. In open-label studies, 17 of 43 (39.5%) evaluable pediatric patients (aged 12-16 years old) using LOTRISONE Cream for treatment of tinea pedis demonstrated adrenal suppression as determined by cosyntropin testing. In another open-label study, 8 of 17 (47.1%) evaluable pediatric patients (aged 12-16 years old) using LOTRISONE Cream for treatment of tinea cruris demonstrated adrenal suppression as determined by cosyntropin testing. **THE USE OF LOTRISONE CREAM IN THE TREATMENT OF PATIENTS UNDER 17 YEARS OF AGE OR PATIENTS WITH DIAPER DERMATITIS IS NOT RECOMMENDED.**

Because of a higher ratio of skin surface area to body mass, pediatric patients under the age of 12 years are at a higher risk with LOTRISONE Cream. The studies described above suggest that pediatric patients under the age of 17 years may also have this risk. They are at increased risk of developing Cushing's syndrome while on treatment and adrenal insufficiency after withdrawal of treatment. Adverse effects, including striae and growth retardation, have been reported with inappropriate use of LOTRISONE Cream in infants and children (see **PRECAUTIONS** and **ADVERSE REACTIONS**).

Hypothalamic-pituitary-adrenal (HPA) axis suppression, Cushing's syndrome, linear growth retardation, delayed weight gain, and intracranial hypertension have been reported in children receiving topical corticosteroids. Manifestations of adrenal suppression in children include low plasma cortisol levels and absence of response to ACTH stimulation. Manifestations of intracranial hypertension include bulging fontanelles, headaches, and bilateral papilledema.

Geriatric Use

Clinical studies of LOTRISONE Cream did not include sufficient numbers of subjects aged 65 and over to determine whether they respond differently from younger subjects. Postmarket adverse event reporting for LOTRISONE Cream in patients aged 65 and above includes reports of skin atrophy and rare reports of skin ulceration. Caution should be exercised with the use of these corticosteroid-containing topical products on thinning skin. **THE USE OF LOTRISONE CREAM UNDER OCCLUSION, SUCH AS IN DIAPER DERMATITIS, IS NOT RECOMMENDED.**

ADVERSE REACTIONS

Adverse reactions reported for LOTRISONE® Cream in clinical trials were paresthesia in 1.9% of patients, and rash, edema, and secondary infection, each in less than 1% of patients.

The following local adverse reactions have been reported with topical corticosteroids and may occur more frequently with the use of occlusive dressings. These reactions are listed in an approximate decreasing order of occurrence: itching, irritation, dryness, folliculitis, hypertrichosis, acneiform eruptions, hypopigmentation, perioral dermatitis, allergic contact dermatitis, maceration of the skin, secondary infection, skin atrophy, striae, miliaria, capillary fragility (ecchymoses), telangiectasia, and sensitization (local reactions upon repeated application of product). In the pediatric population, reported adverse events for LOTRISONE Cream include growth retardation, benign intracranial hypertension, Cushing's syndrome (HPA axis suppression), and local cutaneous reactions, including skin atrophy.

Systemic absorption of topical corticosteroids has produced reversible hypothalamic-pituitary-adrenal (HPA) axis suppression, manifestations of Cushing's syndrome, hyperglycemia, and glucosuria in some patients.

Adverse reactions reported with the use of clotrimazole are as follows: erythema, stinging, blistering, peeling, edema, pruritus, urticaria, and general irritation of the skin.

OVERDOSAGE

Amounts greater than 45 g/week of LOTRISONE® Cream should not be used. Acute overdosage with topical application of LOTRISONE Cream is unlikely and would not be expected to lead to a life-threatening situation. LOTRISONE Cream should not be used for longer than the prescribed time period.

Topically applied corticosteroids, such as the one contained in LOTRISONE Cream can be absorbed in sufficient amounts to produce systemic effects (see **PRECAUTIONS**).

DOSAGE AND ADMINISTRATION

Gently massage sufficient LOTRISONE® Cream into the affected skin areas twice a day, in the morning and evening. **LOTRISONE Cream should not be used longer than 2 weeks in the treatment of tinea corporis or tinea cruris, and amounts greater than 45 g per week of LOTRISONE Cream should not be used.** If a patient with tinea corporis or tinea cruris shows no clinical improvement after 1 week of treatment with LOTRISONE Cream, the diagnosis should be reviewed.

LOTRISONE Cream should not be used longer than 4 weeks in the treatment of tinea pedis and amounts greater than 45 g per week of LOTRISONE Cream should not be used. If a patient with tinea pedis shows no clinical improvement after 2 weeks of treatment with LOTRISONE Cream, the diagnosis should be reviewed.

LOTRISONE Cream should not be used with occlusive dressings.

HOW SUPPLIED

LOTRISONE® Cream is supplied in 15-g (NDC 0085-0924-01) and 45-g tubes (NDC 0085-0924-02), boxes of one. **Store at 25°C (77°F); excursions permitted to 15–30°C (59–86°F) [see USP Controlled Room Temperature].**

Rx only

Manufactured for:
Merck Sharp & Dohme Corp., a subsidiary of
MERCK & CO., INC., Whitehouse Station, NJ 08889, USA
Manufactured by:
Schering Plough Canada Inc., Pointe Claire, Quebec H9R 1B4, Canada

Revised: 01/2013
LRN# 000370-LOS-CR-USPI.3

LOTRISONE® Cream
(clotrimazole and betamethasone dipropionate)
Patient's Instructions for Use
Patient Information Leaflet

What is LOTRISONE® Cream?

LOTRISONE Cream is a medication used on the skin to treat fungal infections of the feet, groin, and body, as diagnosed by your doctor. LOTRISONE Cream should be used for fungal infections that are inflamed and have symptoms of redness and/or itching. Talk to your doctor if your fungal infection does not have these symptoms. LOTRISONE Cream contains a corticosteroid. Notify your doctor if you notice side effects with the use of LOTRISONE Cream (see **"What are the possible side effects of LOTRISONE Cream?"** below). LOTRISONE Cream is not to be used in the eyes, in the mouth, or in the vagina.

How does LOTRISONE® Cream work?

LOTRISONE Cream is a combination of an antifungal agent (clotrimazole) and a corticosteroid (betamethasone dipropionate). Clotrimazole works against fungus. Betamethasone dipropionate, a corticosteroid, is used to help relieve redness, swelling, itching, and other discomforts of fungal infections.

Who should NOT use LOTRISONE® Cream?

LOTRISONE Cream is not recommended for use in patients under the age of 17 years. LOTRISONE Cream is not recommended for use in diaper rash.

Patients who are sensitive to clotrimazole and betamethasone dipropionate, other imidazoles or corticosteroids, or any ingredients in the preparation should not use LOTRISONE Cream.

How should I use LOTRISONE® Cream?

Gently massage sufficient LOTRISONE Cream into the affected and surrounding skin areas twice a day, in the morning and evening. Treatment for 2 weeks on the groin or on the body, and for 4 weeks on the feet is recommended. The use of LOTRISONE Cream for longer than 4 weeks is not recommended for any condition. Prolonged use of LOTRISONE Cream may lead to unwanted side effects.

What other important information should I know about LOTRISONE® Cream?

1. This medication is to be used for the full prescribed treatment time, even though the symptoms may have improved. Notify your doctor if there is no improvement after 1 week of treatment on the groin or body or after 2 weeks on the feet.
2. This medication should only be used for the disorder for which it was prescribed.
3. The treated skin area should not be bandaged or otherwise covered or wrapped.
4. Other corticosteroid-containing products should not be used with LOTRISONE without first talking with your physician.
5. Any signs of side effects where LOTRISONE Cream is applied should be reported to your doctor.
6. When using LOTRISONE Cream in the groin area, it is especially important to use the medication for 2 weeks only, and to apply the cream sparingly. You should tell your doctor if your problem persists after 2 weeks. You should also wear loose-fitting clothing so as to avoid tightly covering the area where LOTRISONE Cream is applied.
7. This medication is not recommended for use in diaper rash.

What are the possible side effects of LOTRISONE® Cream?

The following side effects have been reported with topical corticosteroid medications: itching, irritation, dryness, infection of the hair follicles, increased hair, acne, fragile blood vessels, spider veins, sensitization (local reactions upon repeated application of product), change in skin color, allergic skin reaction, skin thinning, and stretch marks. In children, reported adverse events for LOTRISONE Cream include slower growth, Cushing's syndrome (a type of hormone imbalance that can be very serious), and local skin reactions, including thinning skin and stretch marks. Hormone imbalance (adrenal suppression) was demonstrated in clinical studies in children.

Can LOTRISONE® Cream be used if I am pregnant or plan to become pregnant or if I am nursing?

Before using LOTRISONE Cream, tell your doctor if you are pregnant or plan to become pregnant. Also, tell your doctor if you are nursing.

How should LOTRISONE® Cream be stored?

LOTRISONE Cream should be stored at 25°C (77°F); excursions permitted to 15–30°C (59–86°F) [see USP Controlled Room Temperature].

General advice about prescription medicines

This medicine was prescribed for your particular condition. Only use LOTRISONE® Cream to treat the condition for which your doctor has prescribed. Do not give LOTRISONE Cream to other people. It may harm them.

This leaflet summarizes the most important information about LOTRISONE Cream. If you would like more information, talk with your doctor. You can ask your pharmacist or doctor for information about LOTRISONE Cream that is written for health professionals.

Rx only

Manufactured for:
Merck Sharp & Dohme Corp., a subsidiary of
MERCK & CO., INC., Whitehouse Station, NJ 08889, USA
Manufactured by:
Schering Plough Canada Inc., Pointe Claire, Quebec H9R 1B4, Canada

Revised: 08/2012
LRN# 000370-LOS-CR-PPI.2.

M-M-R® II ℞

[em em ar too]

(MEASLES, MUMPS, and RUBELLA VIRUS VACCINE LIVE)

DESCRIPTION

M-M-R[1] II (Measles, Mumps, and Rubella Virus Vaccine Live) is a live virus vaccine for vaccination against measles (rubeola), mumps, and rubella (German measles).

M-M-R II is a sterile lyophilized preparation of (1) ATTENUVAX[1] (Measles Virus Vaccine Live), a more attenuated line of measles virus, derived from Enders' attenuated Edmonston strain and propagated in chick embryo cell culture; (2) MUMPSVAX[1] (Mumps Virus Vaccine Live), the Jeryl Lynn[2] (B level) strain of mumps virus propagated in chick embryo cell culture; and (3) MERUVAX[1] II (Rubella Virus Vaccine Live), the Wistar RA 27/3 strain of live attenuated rubella virus propagated in WI-38 human diploid lung fibroblasts.{1,2}

The growth medium for measles and mumps is Medium 199 (a buffered salt solution containing vitamins and amino acids and supplemented with fetal bovine serum) containing SPGA (sucrose, phosphate, glutamate, and recombinant human albumin) as stabilizer and neomycin.

The growth medium for rubella is Minimum Essential Medium (MEM) [a buffered salt solution containing vitamins and amino acids and supplemented with fetal bovine serum] containing recombinant human albumin and neomycin. Sorbitol and hydrolyzed gelatin stabilizer are added to the individual virus harvests.

The cells, virus pools, and fetal bovine serum are all screened for the absence of adventitious agents.

The reconstituted vaccine is for subcutaneous administration. Each 0.5 mL dose contains not less than 1,000 $TCID_{50}$ (tissue culture infectious doses) of measles virus; 12,500 $TCID_{50}$ of mumps virus; and 1,000 $TCID_{50}$ of rubella virus. Each dose of the vaccine is calculated to contain sorbitol (14.5 mg), sodium phosphate, sucrose (1.9 mg), sodium chloride, hydrolyzed gelatin (14.5 mg), recombinant human albumin (≤0.3 mg), fetal bovine serum (<1 ppm), other buffer and media ingredients and approximately 25 mcg of neomycin. The product contains no preservative.

Before reconstitution, the lyophilized vaccine is a light yellow compact crystalline plug. M-M-R II, when reconstituted as directed, is clear yellow.

[1]Registered trademark of Merck Sharp & Dohme Corp., a subsidiary of **Merck & Co., Inc.**

[2]Trademark of Merck Sharp & Dohme Corp., a subsidiary of **Merck & Co., Inc.**

CLINICAL PHARMACOLOGY

Measles, mumps, and rubella are three common childhood diseases, caused by measles virus, mumps virus (paramyxoviruses), and rubella virus (togavirus), respectively, that may be associated with serious complications and/or death. For example, pneumonia and encephalitis are caused by measles. Mumps is associated with aseptic meningitis, deafness and orchitis; and rubella during pregnancy may cause congenital rubella syndrome in the infants of infected mothers.

The impact of measles, mumps, and rubella vaccination on the natural history of each disease in the United States can be quantified by comparing the maximum number of measles, mumps, and rubella cases reported in a given year prior to vaccine use to the number of cases of each disease reported in 1995. For measles, 894,134 cases reported in 1941 compared to 288 cases reported in 1995 resulted in a 99.97% decrease in reported cases; for mumps, 152,209 cases reported in 1968 compared to 840 cases reported in 1995 resulted in a 99.45% decrease in reported cases; and for rubella, 57,686 cases reported in 1969 compared to 200 cases reported in 1995 resulted in a 99.65% decrease.{3}

Clinical studies of 284 triple seronegative children, 11 months to 7 years of age, demonstrated that M-M-R II is highly immunogenic and generally well tolerated. In these studies, a single injection of the vaccine induced measles hemagglutination-inhibition (HI) antibodies in 95%, mumps neutralizing antibodies in 96%, and rubella HI antibodies in 99% of susceptible persons. However, a small percentage (1-5%) of vaccinees may fail to seroconvert after the primary dose (see also INDICATIONS AND USAGE, Recommended Vaccination Schedule).

A study{4} of 6-month-old and 15-month-old infants born to vaccine-immunized mothers demonstrated that, following vaccination with ATTENUVAX, 74% of the 6-month-old infants developed detectable neutralizing antibody (NT) titers while 100% of the 15-month-old infants developed NT. This rate of seroconversion is higher than that previously reported for 6-month-old infants born to naturally immune mothers tested by HI assay. When the 6-month-old infants of immunized mothers were revaccinated at 15 months, they developed antibody titers equivalent to the 15-month-old vaccinees. The lower seroconversion rate in 6-month-olds has two possible explanations: 1) Due to the limit of the detection level of the assays (NT and enzyme immunoassay [EIA]), the presence of trace amounts of undetectable maternal antibody might interfere with the seroconversion of infants; or 2) The immune system of 6-month-olds is not always capable of mounting a response to measles vaccine as measured by the two antibody assays.

There is some evidence to suggest that infants who are born to mothers who had wild-type measles and who are vaccinated at less than one year of age may not develop sustained antibody levels when later revaccinated. The advantage of early protection must be weighed against the chance for failure to respond adequately on reimmunization.{5,6}

Efficacy of measles, mumps, and rubella vaccines was established in a series of double-blind controlled field trials which demonstrated a high degree of protective efficacy afforded by the individual vaccine components.{7-12} These studies also established that seroconversion in response to vaccination against measles, mumps, and rubella paralleled protection from these diseases.{13-15}

Following vaccination, antibodies associated with protection can be measured by neutralization assays, HI, or ELISA (enzyme linked immunosorbent assay) tests. Neutralizing and ELISA antibodies to measles, mumps, and rubella viruses are still detectable in most individuals 11 to 13 years after primary vaccination.{16-18} See INDICATIONS AND USAGE, Non-Pregnant Adolescent and Adult Females, for Rubella Susceptibility Testing.

The RA 27/3 rubella strain in M-M-R II elicits higher immediate post-vaccination HI, complement-fixing and neutralizing antibody levels than other strains of rubella vaccine{19-25} and has been shown to induce a broader profile of circulating antibodies including anti-theta and anti-iota precipitating antibodies.{26,27} The RA 27/3 rubella strain immunologically simulates natural infection more closely than other rubella vaccine viruses.{27-29} The increased levels and broader profile of antibodies produced by RA 27/3 strain rubella virus vaccine appear to correlate with greater resistance to subclinical reinfection with the wild virus,{27,29-31} and provide greater confidence for lasting immunity.

INDICATIONS AND USAGE

Recommended Vaccination Schedule

M-M-R II is indicated for simultaneous vaccination against measles, mumps, and rubella in individuals 12 months of age or older.

Individuals first vaccinated at 12 months of age or older should be revaccinated prior to elementary school entry. Revaccination is intended to seroconvert those who do not respond to the first dose. The Advisory Committee on Immunization Practices (ACIP) recommends administration of the first dose of M-M-R II at 12 to 15 months of age and administration of the second dose of M-M-R II at 4 to 6 years of age.{59} In addition, some public health jurisdictions mandate the age for revaccination. Consult the complete text of applicable guidelines regarding routine revaccination including that of high-risk adult populations.

Measles Outbreak Schedule

Infants Between 6 to 12 Months of Age

Local health authorities may recommend measles vaccination of infants between 6 to 12 months of age in outbreak situations. This population may fail to respond to the components of the vaccine. Safety and effectiveness of mumps and rubella vaccine in infants less than 12 months of age have not been established. The younger the infant, the lower the likelihood of seroconversion (see CLINICAL PHARMACOLOGY). Such infants should receive a second dose of M-M-R II between 12 to 15 months of age followed by revaccination at elementary school entry.{59}

Unnecessary doses of a vaccine are best avoided by ensuring that written documentation of vaccination is preserved and a copy given to each vaccinee's parent or guardian.

Other Vaccination Considerations

Non-Pregnant Adolescent and Adult Females

Immunization of susceptible non-pregnant adolescent and adult females of childbearing age with live attenuated rubella virus vaccine is indicated if certain precautions are observed (see below and PRECAUTIONS). Vaccinating susceptible postpubertal females confers individual protection against subsequently acquiring rubella infection during pregnancy, which in turn prevents infection of the fetus and consequent congenital rubella injury.(33)

Women of childbearing age should be advised not to become pregnant for 3 months after vaccination and should be informed of the reasons for this precaution.

The ACIP has stated "If it is practical and if reliable laboratory services are available, women of childbearing age who are potential candidates for vaccination can have serologic tests to determine susceptibility to rubella. However, with the exception of premarital and prenatal screening, routinely performing serologic tests for all women of childbearing age to determine susceptibility (so that vaccine is given only to proven susceptible women) can be effective but is expensive. Also, 2 visits to the health-care provider would be necessary — one for screening and one for vaccination. Accordingly, rubella vaccination of a woman who is not known to be pregnant and has no history of vaccination is justifiable without serologic testing — and may be preferable, particularly when costs of serology are high and follow-up of identified susceptible women for vaccination is not assured."(33)

Postpubertal females should be informed of the frequent occurrence of generally self-limited arthralgia and/or arthritis beginning 2 to 4 weeks after vaccination (see ADVERSE REACTIONS).

Postpartum Women

It has been found convenient in many instances to vaccinate rubella-susceptible women in the immediate postpartum period (see PRECAUTIONS, Nursing Mothers).

Other Populations

Previously unvaccinated children older than 12 months who are in contact with susceptible pregnant women should receive live attenuated rubella vaccine (such as that contained in monovalent rubella vaccine or in M-M-R II) to reduce the risk of exposure of the pregnant woman.

Individuals planning travel outside the United States, if not immune, can acquire measles, mumps, or rubella and import these diseases into the United States. Therefore, prior to international travel, individuals known to be susceptible to one or more of these diseases can either receive the indicated monovalent vaccine (measles, mumps, or rubella), or a combination vaccine as appropriate. However, M-M-R II is preferred for persons likely to be susceptible to mumps and rubella; and if monovalent measles vaccine is not readily available, travelers should receive M-M-R II regardless of their immune status to mumps or rubella.(34-36)

Vaccination is recommended for susceptible individuals in high-risk groups such as college students, health-care workers, and military personnel.(33,34,37)

According to ACIP recommendations, most persons born in 1956 or earlier are likely to have been infected with measles naturally and generally need not be considered susceptible. All children, adolescents, and adults born after 1956 are considered susceptible and should be vaccinated, if there are no contraindications. This includes persons who may be immune to measles but who lack adequate documentation of immunity such as: (1) physician-diagnosed measles, (2) laboratory evidence of measles immunity, or (3) adequate immunization with live measles vaccine on or after the first birthday.(34)

The ACIP recommends that "Persons vaccinated with inactivated vaccine followed within 3 months by live vaccine should be revaccinated with two doses of live vaccine. Revaccination is particularly important when the risk of exposure to wild-type measles virus is increased, as may occur during international travel."(34)

Post-Exposure Vaccination

Vaccination of individuals exposed to wild-type measles may provide some protection if the vaccine can be administered within 72 hours of exposure. If, however, vaccine is given a few days before exposure, substantial protection may be afforded.(34,38,39) There is no conclusive evidence that vaccination of individuals recently exposed to wild-type mumps or wild-type rubella will provide protection.(33,37)

Use With Other Vaccines

See DOSAGE AND ADMINISTRATION, Use With Other Vaccines.

CONTRAINDICATIONS

Hypersensitivity to any component of the vaccine, including gelatin.(40)

Do not give M-M-R II to pregnant females; the possible effects of the vaccine on fetal development are unknown at this time. If vaccination of postpubertal females is undertaken, pregnancy should be avoided for three months following vaccination (see INDICATIONS AND USAGE, Non-Pregnant Adolescent and Adult Females and PRECAUTIONS, Pregnancy).

Anaphylactic or anaphylactoid reactions to neomycin (each dose of reconstituted vaccine contains approximately 25 mcg of neomycin).

Febrile respiratory illness or other active febrile infection. However, the ACIP has recommended that all vaccines can be administered to persons with minor illnesses such as diarrhea, mild upper respiratory infection with or without low-grade fever, or other low-grade febrile illness.(41)

Patients receiving immunosuppressive therapy. This contraindication does not apply to patients who are receiving corticosteroids as replacement therapy, e.g., for Addison's disease.

Individuals with blood dyscrasias, leukemia, lymphomas of any type, or other malignant neoplasms affecting the bone marrow or lymphatic systems.

Primary and acquired immunodeficiency states, including patients who are immunosuppressed in association with AIDS or other clinical manifestations of infection with human immunodeficiency viruses;(41-43) cellular immune deficiencies; and hypogammaglobulinemic and dysgammaglobulinemic states. Measles inclusion body encephalitis(60) (MIBE), pneumonitis(61) and death as a direct consequence of disseminated measles vaccine virus infection have been reported in immunocompromised individuals inadvertently vaccinated with measles-containing vaccine.

Individuals with a family history of congenital or hereditary immunodeficiency, until the immune competence of the potential vaccine recipient is demonstrated.

WARNINGS

Due caution should be employed in administration of M-M-R II to persons with a history of cerebral injury, individual or family histories of convulsions, or any other condition in which stress due to fever should be avoided. The physician should be alert to the temperature elevation which may occur following vaccination (see ADVERSE REACTIONS).

Hypersensitivity to Eggs

Live measles vaccine and live mumps vaccine are produced in chick embryo cell culture. Persons with a history of anaphylactic, anaphylactoid, or other immediate reactions (e.g., hives, swelling of the mouth and throat, difficulty breathing, hypotension, or shock) subsequent to egg ingestion may be at an enhanced risk of immediate-type hypersensitivity reactions after receiving vaccines containing traces of chick embryo antigen. The potential risk to benefit ratio should be carefully evaluated before considering vaccination in such cases. Such individuals may be vaccinated with extreme caution, having adequate treatment on hand should a reaction occur (see PRECAUTIONS).(45)

However, the AAP has stated, "Most children with a history of anaphylactic reactions to eggs have no untoward reactions to measles or MMR vaccine. Persons are not at increased risk if they have egg allergies that are not anaphylactic, and they should be vaccinated in the usual manner. In addition, skin testing of egg-allergic children with vaccine has not been predictive of which children will have an immediate hypersensitivity reaction...Persons with allergies to chickens or chicken feathers are not at increased risk of reaction to the vaccine."(44)

Hypersensitivity to Neomycin

The AAP states, "Persons who have experienced anaphylactic reactions to topically or systemically administered neomycin should not receive measles vaccine. Most often, however, neomycin allergy manifests as a contact dermatitis, which is a delayed-type (cell-mediated) immune response rather than anaphylaxis. In such persons, an adverse reaction to neomycin in the vaccine would be an erythematous, pruritic nodule or papule, 48 to 96 hours after vaccination. A history of contact dermatitis to neomycin is not a contraindication to receiving measles vaccine."(44)

Thrombocytopenia

Individuals with current thrombocytopenia may develop more severe thrombocytopenia following vaccination. In addition, individuals who experienced thrombocytopenia with the first dose of M-M-R II (or its component vaccines) may develop thrombocytopenia with repeat doses. Serologic status may be evaluated to determine whether or not additional doses of vaccine are needed. The potential risk to benefit ratio should be carefully evaluated before considering vaccination in such cases (see ADVERSE REACTIONS).

PRECAUTIONS

General

Adequate treatment provisions including epinephrine injection (1:1000), should be available for immediate use should an anaphylactic or anaphylactoid reaction occur.

Special care should be taken to ensure that the injection does not enter a blood vessel.

Children and young adults who are known to be infected with human immunodeficiency viruses and are not immunosuppressed may be vaccinated. However, vaccinees who are infected with HIV should be monitored closely for vaccine-preventable diseases because immunization may be less effective than for uninfected persons (see CONTRAINDICATIONS).(42,43)

Vaccination should be deferred for 3 months or longer following blood or plasma transfusions, or administration of immune globulin (human).(44)

Excretion of small amounts of the live attenuated rubella virus from the nose or throat has occurred in the majority of susceptible individuals 7 to 28 days after vaccination. There is no confirmed evidence to indicate that such virus is transmitted to susceptible persons who are in contact with the vaccinated individuals. Consequently, transmission through close personal contact, while accepted as a theoretical possibility, is not regarded as a significant risk.(33) However, transmission of the rubella vaccine virus to infants via breast milk has been documented (see Nursing Mothers).

There are no reports of transmission of live attenuated measles or mumps viruses from vaccinees to susceptible contacts.

It has been reported that live attenuated measles, mumps and rubella virus vaccines given individually may result in a temporary depression of tuberculin skin sensitivity. Therefore, if a tuberculin test is to be done, it should be administered either before or simultaneously with M-M-R II.

Children under treatment for tuberculosis have not experienced exacerbation of the disease when immunized with live measles virus vaccine;(46) no studies have been reported to date of the effect of measles virus vaccines on untreated tuberculous children. However, individuals with active untreated tuberculosis should not be vaccinated.

As for any vaccine, vaccination with M-M-R II may not result in protection in 100% of vaccinees.

The health-care provider should determine the current health status and previous vaccination history of the vaccinee.

The health-care provider should question the patient, parent, or guardian about reactions to a previous dose of M-M-R II or other measles-, mumps-, or rubella-containing vaccines.

Information for Patients

The health-care provider should provide the vaccine information required to be given with each vaccination to the patient, parent, or guardian.

The health-care provider should inform the patient, parent, or guardian of the benefits and risks associated with vaccination. For risks associated with vaccination see WARNINGS, PRECAUTIONS, and ADVERSE REACTIONS.

Patients, parents, or guardians should be instructed to report any serious adverse reactions to their health-care provider who in turn should report such events to the U.S. Department of Health and Human Services through the Vaccine Adverse Event Reporting System (VAERS), 1-800-822-7967.(47)

Pregnancy should be avoided for 3 months following vaccination, and patients should be informed of the reasons for this precaution (see INDICATIONS AND USAGE, Non-Pregnant Adolescent and Adult Females, CONTRAINDICATIONS, and PRECAUTIONS, Pregnancy).

Laboratory Tests

See INDICATIONS AND USAGE, Non-Pregnant Adolescent and Adult Females, for Rubella Susceptibility Testing, and CLINICAL PHARMACOLOGY.

Drug Interactions

See DOSAGE AND ADMINISTRATION, Use With Other Vaccines.

Immunosuppressive Therapy

The immune status of patients about to undergo immunosuppressive therapy should be evaluated so that the physician can consider whether vaccination prior to the initiation of treatment is indicated (see CONTRAINDICATIONS and PRECAUTIONS).

The ACIP has stated that "patients with leukemia in remission who have not received chemotherapy for at least 3 months may receive live virus vaccines. Short-term (<2 weeks), low- to moderate-dose systemic corticosteroid therapy, topical steroid therapy (e.g. nasal, skin), long-term alternate-day treatment with low to moderate doses of short-acting systemic steroid, and intra-articular, bursal, or tendon injection of corticosteroids are not immunosuppressive in their usual doses and do not contraindicate the administration of [measles, mumps, or rubella vaccine]."(33,34,37)

Immune Globulin

Administration of immune globulins concurrently with M-M-R II may interfere with the expected immune response.(33,34,44)

See also PRECAUTIONS, General.

Carcinogenesis, Mutagenesis, Impairment of Fertility

M-M-R II has not been evaluated for carcinogenic or mutagenic potential, or potential to impair fertility.

Pregnancy

Pregnancy Category C

Animal reproduction studies have not been conducted with M-M-R II. It is also not known whether M-M-R II can cause fetal harm when administered to a pregnant woman or can affect reproduction capacity. Therefore, the vaccine should not be administered to pregnant females; furthermore, pregnancy should be avoided for 3 months following vaccination (see INDICATIONS AND USAGE, Non-Pregnant Adolescent and Adult Females and CONTRAINDICATIONS).

In counseling women who are inadvertently vaccinated when pregnant or who become pregnant within 3 months of vaccination, the physician should be aware of the following: (1) In a 10-year survey involving over 700 pregnant women who received rubella vaccine within 3 months before or after conception (of whom 189 received the Wistar RA 27/3 strain), none of the newborns had abnormalities compatible with congenital rubella syndrome;{48} (2) Mumps infection during the first trimester of pregnancy may increase the rate of spontaneous abortion. Although mumps vaccine virus has been shown to infect the placenta and fetus, there is no evidence that it causes congenital malformations in humans;{37} and (3) Reports have indicated that contracting wild-type measles during pregnancy enhances fetal risk. Increased rates of spontaneous abortion, stillbirth, congenital defects and prematurity have been observed subsequent to infection with wild-type measles during pregnancy.{57,58} There are no adequate studies of the attenuated (vaccine) strain of measles virus in pregnancy. However, it would be prudent to assume that the vaccine strain of virus is also capable of inducing adverse fetal effects.

Nursing Mothers

It is not known whether measles or mumps vaccine virus is secreted in human milk. Recent studies have shown that lactating postpartum women immunized with live attenuated rubella vaccine may secrete the virus in breast milk and transmit it to breast-fed infants.{49} In the infants with serological evidence of rubella infection, none exhibited severe disease; however, one exhibited mild clinical illness typical of acquired rubella.{50,51} Caution should be exercised when M-M-R II is administered to a nursing woman.

Pediatric Use

Safety and effectiveness of measles vaccine in infants below the age of 6 months have not been established (see also CLINICAL PHARMACOLOGY). Safety and effectiveness of mumps and rubella vaccine in infants less than 12 months of age have not been established.

Geriatric Use

Clinical studies of M-M-R II did not include sufficient numbers of seronegative subjects aged 65 and over to determine whether they respond differently from younger subjects. Other reported clinical experience has not identified differences in responses between the elderly and younger subjects.

ADVERSE REACTIONS

The following adverse reactions are listed in decreasing order of severity, without regard to causality, within each body system category and have been reported during clinical trials, with use of the marketed vaccine, or with use of monovalent or bivalent vaccine containing measles, mumps, or rubella:

Body as a Whole

Panniculitis; atypical measles; fever; syncope; headache; dizziness; malaise; irritability.

Cardiovascular System

Vasculitis.

Digestive System

Pancreatitis; diarrhea; vomiting; parotitis; nausea.

Endocrine System

Diabetes mellitus.

Hemic and Lymphatic System

Thrombocytopenia (see WARNINGS, Thrombocytopenia); purpura; regional lymphadenopathy; leukocytosis.

Immune System

Anaphylaxis and anaphylactoid reactions have been reported as well as related phenomena such as angioneurotic edema (including peripheral or facial edema) and bronchial spasm in individuals with or without an allergic history.

Musculoskeletal System

Arthritis; arthralgia; myalgia.

Arthralgia and/or arthritis (usually transient and rarely chronic), and polyneuritis are features of infection with wild-type rubella and vary in frequency and severity with age and sex, being greatest in adult females and least in prepubertal children. This type of involvement as well as myalgia and paresthesia, have also been reported following administration of MERUVAX II.

Chronic arthritis has been associated with wild-type rubella infection and has been related to persistent virus and/or viral antigen isolated from body tissues. Only rarely have vaccine recipients developed chronic joint symptoms.

Following vaccination in children, reactions in joints are uncommon and generally of brief duration. In women, incidence rates for arthritis and arthralgia are generally higher than those seen in children (children: 0-3%; women: 12-26%),{17,52,53} and the reactions tend to be more marked and of longer duration. Symptoms may persist for a matter of months or on rare occasions for years. In adolescent girls, the reactions appear to be intermediate in incidence between those seen in children and in adult women. Even in women older than 35 years, these reactions are generally well tolerated and rarely interfere with normal activities.

Nervous System

Encephalitis; encephalopathy; measles inclusion body encephalitis (MIBE) (see CONTRAINDICATIONS); subacute sclerosing panencephalitis (SSPE); Guillain-Barré Syndrome (GBS); febrile convulsions; afebrile convulsions or seizures; ataxia; polyneuritis; polyneuropathy; ocular palsies; paresthesia.

Experience from more than 80 million doses of all live measles vaccines given in the U.S. through 1975 indicates that significant central nervous system reactions such as encephalitis and encephalopathy, occurring within 30 days after vaccination, have been temporally associated with measles vaccine very rarely.{54} In no case has it been shown that reactions were actually caused by vaccine. The Centers for Disease Control and Prevention has pointed out that "a certain number of cases of encephalitis may be expected to occur in a large childhood population in a defined period of time even when no vaccines are administered". However, the data suggest the possibility that some of these cases may have been caused by measles vaccines. The risk of such serious neurological disorders following live measles virus vaccine administration remains far less than that for encephalitis and encephalopathy with wild-type measles (one per two thousand reported cases).

Post-marketing surveillance of the more than 200 million doses of M-M-R and M-M-R II that have been distributed worldwide over 25 years (1971 to 1996) indicates that serious adverse events such as encephalitis and encephalopathy continue to be rarely reported.{17}

There have been reports of subacute sclerosing panencephalitis (SSPE) in children who did not have a history of infection with wild-type measles but did receive measles vaccine. Some of these cases may have resulted from unrecognized measles in the first year of life or possibly from the measles vaccination. Based on estimated nationwide measles vaccine distribution, the association of SSPE cases to measles vaccination is about one case per million vaccine doses distributed. This is far less than the association with infection with wild-type measles, 6-22 cases of SSPE per million cases of measles. The results of a retrospective case-controlled study conducted by the Centers for Disease Control and Prevention suggest that the overall effect of measles vaccine has been to protect against SSPE by preventing measles with its inherent higher risk of SSPE.{55}

Cases of aseptic meningitis have been reported to VAERS following measles, mumps, and rubella vaccination. Although a causal relationship between the Urabe strain of mumps vaccine and aseptic meningitis has been shown, there is no evidence to link Jeryl Lynn™ mumps vaccine to aseptic meningitis.

Respiratory System

Pneumonia; pneumonitis (see CONTRAINDICATIONS); sore throat; cough; rhinitis.

Skin

Stevens-Johnson syndrome; erythema multiforme; urticaria; rash; measles-like rash; pruritis.

Local reactions including burning/stinging at injection site; wheal and flare; redness (erythema); swelling; induration; tenderness; vesiculation at injection site.

Special Senses — Ear

Nerve deafness; otitis media.

Special Senses — Eye

Retinitis; optic neuritis; papillitis; retrobulbar neuritis; conjunctivitis.

Urogenital System

Epididymitis; orchitis.

Other

Death from various, and in some cases unknown, causes has been reported rarely following vaccination with measles, mumps, and rubella vaccines; however, a causal relationship has not been established in healthy individuals (see CONTRAINDICATIONS). No deaths or permanent sequelae were reported in a published post-marketing surveillance study in Finland involving 1.5 million children and adults who were vaccinated with M-M-R II during 1982 to 1993.{56}

Under the National Childhood Vaccine Injury Act of 1986, health-care providers and manufacturers are required to record and report certain suspected adverse events occurring within specific time periods after vaccination. However, the U.S. Department of Health and Human Services (DHHS) has established a Vaccine Adverse Event Reporting System (VAERS) which will accept all reports of suspected events.{47} A VAERS report form as well as information regarding reporting requirements can be obtained by calling VAERS 1-800-822-7967.

DOSAGE AND ADMINISTRATION

FOR SUBCUTANEOUS ADMINISTRATION

Do not inject intravascularly.

The dose for any age is 0.5 mL administered subcutaneously, preferably into the outer aspect of the upper arm.

The recommended age for primary vaccination is 12 to 15 months.

Revaccination with M-M-R II is recommended prior to elementary school entry. See also INDICATIONS AND USAGE, Recommended Vaccination Schedule.

Children first vaccinated when younger than 12 months of age should receive another dose between 12 to 15 months of age followed by revaccination prior to elementary school entry.{59} See also INDICATIONS AND USAGE, Measles Outbreak Schedule.

Immune Globulin (IG) is not to be given concurrently with M-M-R II (see PRECAUTIONS, General and PRECAUTIONS, Drug Interactions).

CAUTION: A sterile syringe free of preservatives, antiseptics, and detergents should be used for each injection and/or reconstitution of the vaccine because these substances may inactivate the live virus vaccine. A 25 gauge, 5/8″ needle is recommended.

To reconstitute, use only the diluent supplied, since it is free of preservatives or other antiviral substances which might inactivate the vaccine.

Single Dose Vial — First withdraw the entire volume of diluent into the syringe to be used for reconstitution. Inject all the diluent in the syringe into the vial of lyophilized vaccine, and agitate to mix thoroughly. If the lyophilized vaccine cannot be dissolved, discard. Withdraw the entire contents into a syringe and inject the total volume of restored vaccine subcutaneously.

It is important to use a separate sterile syringe and needle for each individual patient to prevent transmission of hepatitis B and other infectious agents from one person to another.

Parenteral drug products should be inspected visually for particulate matter and discoloration prior to administration whenever solution and container permit. M-M-R II, when reconstituted, is clear yellow.

Use With Other Vaccines

M-M-R II should be given one month before or after administration of other live viral vaccines.

M-M-R II has been administered concurrently with VARIVAX[1] [Varicella Virus Vaccine Live (Oka/Merck)], and PedvaxHIB[1] [*Haemophilus b* Conjugate Vaccine (Meningococcal Protein Conjugate)] using separate injection sites and syringes. No impairment of immune response to individually tested vaccine antigens was demonstrated. The type, frequency, and severity of adverse experiences observed with M-M-R II were similar to those seen when each vaccine was given alone.

Routine administration of DTP (diphtheria, tetanus, pertussis) and/or OPV (oral poliovirus vaccine) concurrently with measles, mumps and rubella vaccines is not recommended because there are limited data relating to the simultaneous administration of these antigens.

However, other schedules have been used. The ACIP has stated "Although data are limited concerning the simultaneous administration of the entire recommended vaccine series (i.e., DTaP [or DTwP], IPV [or OPV], Hib with or without Hepatitis B vaccine, and varicella vaccine), data from numerous studies have indicated no interference between routinely recommended childhood vaccines (either live, attenuated, or killed). These findings support the simultaneous use of all vaccines as recommended."{32}

HOW SUPPLIED

No. 4681 — M-M-R II is supplied as follows: (1) a box of 10 single-dose vials of lyophilized vaccine (package A), **NDC** 0006-4681-00; and (2) a box of 10 vials of diluent (package B). To conserve refrigerator space, the diluent may be stored separately at room temperature.

Storage

To maintain potency, M-M-R II must be stored between -58°F and +46°F (-50°C to +8°C). Use of dry ice may subject M-M-R II to temperatures colder than -58°F (-50°C).

Protect the vaccine from light at all times, since such exposure may inactivate the viruses.

Before reconstitution, store the lyophilized vaccine at 36°F to 46°F (2°C to 8°C). The diluent may be stored in the refrigerator with the lyophilized vaccine or separately at room temperature. **Do not freeze the diluent.**

It is recommended that the vaccine be used as soon as possible after reconstitution. Store reconstituted vaccine in the vaccine vial in a dark place at 36°F to 46°F (2°C to 8°C) and discard if not used within 8 hours.

For information regarding stability under conditions other than those recommended, call 1-800-MERCK-90.

REFERENCES

1. Plotkin, S.A.; Cornfeld, D.; Ingalls, T.H.: Studies of immunization with living rubella virus: Trials in children with a strain cultured from an aborted fetus, Am. J. Dis. Child. *110:* 381-389, 1965.
2. Plotkin, S.A.; Farquhar, J.; Katz, M.; Ingalls, T.H.: A new attenuated rubella virus grown in human fibroblasts: Evidence for reduced nasopharyngeal excretion, Am. J. Epidemiol. *86:* 468-477, 1967.
3. Monthly Immunization Table, MMWR *45*(1): 24-25, January 12, 1996.
4. Johnson, C.E.; et al: Measles Vaccine Immunogenicity in 6- Versus 15-Month-Old Infants Born to Mothers in the Measles Vaccine Era, Pediatrics, *93*(6): 939-943, 1994.
5. Linneman, C.C.; et al: Measles Immunity After Vaccination: Results in Children Vaccinated Before 10 Months of Age, Pediatrics, *69*(3): 332-335, March 1982.
6. Stetler, H.C.; et al: Impact of Revaccinating Children Who Initially Received Measles Vaccine Before 10 Months of Age, Pediatrics *77*(4): 471-476, April 1986.
7. Hilleman, M.R.; Buynak, E.B.; Weibel, R.E.; et al: Development and Evaluation of the Moraten Measles Virus Vaccine, JAMA *206*(3): 587-590, 1968.
8. Weibel, R.E.; Stokes, J.; Buynak, E.B.; et al: Live, Attenuated Mumps Virus Vaccine 3. Clinical and Serologic Aspects in a Field Evaluation, N. Engl. J. Med. *276:* 245-251, 1967.
9. Hilleman, M.R.; Weibel, R.E.; Buynak, E.B.; et al: Live, Attenuated Mumps Virus Vaccine 4. Protective Efficacy as Measured in a Field Evaluation, N. Engl. J. Med. *276:* 252-258, 1967.
10. Cutts, F.T.; Henderson, R.H.; Clements, C.J.; et al: Principles of measles control, Bull WHO *69*(1): 1-7, 1991.
11. Weibel, R.E.; Buynak, E.B.; Stokes, J.; et al: Evaluation Of Live Attenuated Mumps Virus Vaccine, Strain Jeryl Lynn, First International Conference on Vaccines Against Viral and Rickettsial Diseases of Man, World Health Organization, No. 147, May 1967.
12. Leibhaber, H.; Ingalls, T.H.; LeBouvier, G.L.; et al: Vaccination With RA 27/3 Rubella Vaccine, Am. J. Dis. Child. *123:* 133-136, February 1972.
13. Rosen, L.: Hemagglutination and Hemagglutination-Inhibition with Measles Virus, Virology *13:* 139-141, January 1961.
14. Brown, G.C.; et al: Fluorescent-Antibody Marker for Vaccine-Induced Rubella Antibodies, Infection and Immunity *2*(4): 360-363, 1970.
15. Buynak, E.B.; et al: Live Attenuated Mumps Virus Vaccine 1. Vaccine Development, Proceedings of the Society for Experimental Biology and Medicine, *123:* 768-775, 1966.
16. Weibel, R.E.; Carlson, A.J.; Villarejos, V.M.; Buynak, E.B.; McLean, A.A.; Hilleman, M.R.: Clinical and Laboratory Studies of Combined Live Measles, Mumps, and Rubella Vaccines Using the RA 27/3 Rubella Virus, Proc. Soc. Exp. Biol. Med. *165:* 323-326, 1980.
17. Unpublished data from the files of Merck Research Laboratories.
18. Watson, J.C.; Pearson, J.S.; Erdman, D.D.; et al: An Evaluation of Measles Revaccination Among School-Entry Age Children, 31st Interscience Conference on Antimicrobial Agents and Chemotherapy, Abstract #268, 143, 1991.
19. Fogel, A.; Moshkowitz, A.; Rannon, L.; Gerichter, Ch.B.: Comparative trials of RA 27/3 and Cendehill rubella vaccines in adult and adolescent females, Am. J. Epidemiol. *93:* 392-393, 1971.
20. Andzhaparidze, O.G.; Desyatskova, R.G.; Chervonski, G.I.; Pryanichnikova, L.V.: Immunogenicity and reactogenicity of live attenuated rubella virus vaccines, Am. J. Epidemiol. *91:* 527-530, 1970.
21. Freestone, D.S.; Reynolds, G.M.; McKinnon, J.A.; Prydie, J.: Vaccination of schoolgirls against rubella. Assessment of serological status and a comparative trial of Wistar RA 27/3 and Cendehill strain live attenuated rubella vaccines in 13-year-old schoolgirls in Dudley, Br. J. Prev. Soc. Med. *29:* 258-261, 1975.
22. Grillner, L.; Hedstrom, C.E.; Bergstrom, H.; Forssman, L.; Rigner, A.; Lycke, E.: Vaccination against rubella of newly delivered women, Scand. J. Infect. Dis. *5:* 237-241, 1973.
23. Grillner, L.: Neutralizing antibodies after rubella vaccination of newly delivered women: a comparison between three vaccines, Scand. J. Infect. Dis. *7:* 169-172, 1975.
24. Wallace, R.B.; Isacson, P.: Comparative trial of HPV-77, DE-5 and RA 27/3 live-attenuated rubella vaccines, Am. J. Dis. Child. *124:* 536-538, 1972.
25. Lalla, M.; Vesikari, T.; Virolainen, M.: Lymphoblast proliferation and humoral antibody response after rubella vaccination, Clin. Exp. Immunol. *15:* 193-202, 1973.
26. LeBouvier, G.L.; Plotkin, S.A.: Precipitin responses to rubella vaccine RA 27/3, J. Infect. Dis. *123:* 220-223, 1971.
27. Horstmann, D.M.: Rubella: The challenge of its control, J. Infect. Dis. *123:* 640-654, 1971.
28. Ogra, P.L.; Kerr-Grant, D.; Umana, G.; Dzierba, J.; Weintraub, D.: Antibody response in serum and nasopharynx after naturally acquired and vaccine-induced infection with rubella virus, N. Engl. J. Med. *285:* 1333-1339, 1971.
29. Plotkin, S.A.; Farquhar, J.D.; Ogra, P.L.: Immunologic properties of RA 27/3 rubella virus vaccine, J. Am. Med. Assoc. *225:* 585-590, 1973.
30. Liebhaber, H.; Ingalls, T.H.; LeBouvier, G.L.; Horstmann, D.M.: Vaccination with RA 27/3 rubella vaccine. Persistence of immunity and resistance to challenge after two years, Am. J. Dis. Child. *123:* 133-136, 1972.
31. Farquhar, J.D.: Follow-up on rubella vaccinations and experience with subclinical reinfection, J. Pediatr. *81:* 460-465, 1972.
32. Centers for Disease Control and Prevention. Recommended childhood immunization schedule — United States, January-June 1996, MMWR *44*(51 & 52): 940-943, January 5, 1996.
33. Rubella Prevention: Recommendation of the Immunization Practices Advisory Committee (ACIP), MMWR *39*(RR-15): 1-18, November 23, 1990.
34. Measles Prevention: Recommendations of the Immunization Practices Advisory Committee (ACIP), MMWR *38*(S-9): 5-22, December 29, 1989.
35. Jong, E.C., The Travel and Tropical Medicine Manual, W.B. Saunders Company, p. 12-16, 1987.
36. Committee on Immunization Council of Medical Societies, American College of Physicians, Phila., PA, Guide for Adult Immunization, First Edition, 1985.
37. Recommendations of the Immunization Practices Advisory Committee (ACIP), Mumps Prevention, MMWR *38*(22): 388-400, June 9, 1989.
38. King, G.E.; Markowitz, L.E.; Patriarca, P.A.; et al: Clinical Efficacy of Measles Vaccine During the 1990 Measles Epidemic, Pediatr. Infect. Dis. J. *10*(12): 883-888, December 1991.
39. Krasinski, K.; Borkowsky, W.: Measles and Measles Immunity in Children Infected With Human Immunodeficiency Virus, JAMA *261*(17): 2512-2516, 1989.
40. Kelso, J.M.; Jones, R.T.; Yunginger, J.W.: Anaphylaxis to measles, mumps, and rubella vaccine mediated by IgE to gelatin, J. Allergy Clin. Immunol. *91:* 867-872, 1993.
41. General Recommendations on Immunization, Recommendations of the Advisory Committee on Immunization Practices, MMWR *43*(RR-1): 1-38, January 28, 1994.
42. Center for Disease Control: Immunization of Children Infected with Human T-Lymphotropic Virus Type III/Lymphadenopathy-Associated Virus, Annals of Internal Medicine, *106:* 75-78, 1987.
43. Krasinski, K.; Borkowsky, W.; Krugman, S.: Antibody following measles immunization in children infected with human T-cell lymphotropic virus-type III/lymphadenopathy associated virus (HTLV-III/LAV) [Abstract]. In: Program and abstracts of the International Conference on Acquired Immunodeficiency Syndrome, Paris, France, June 23-25, 1986.
44. Peter, G.; et al (eds): Report of the Committee on Infectious Diseases, Twenty-fourth Edition, American Academy of Pediatrics, 344-357, 1997.
45. Isaacs, D.; Menser, M.: Modern Vaccines, Measles, Mumps, Rubella, and Varicella, Lancet *335:* 1384-1387, June 9, 1990.
46. Starr, S.; Berkovich, S.: The effect of measles, gamma globulin modified measles, and attenuated measles vaccine on the course of treated tuberculosis in children, Pediatrics *35:* 97-102, January 1965.
47. Vaccine Adverse Event Reporting System — United States, MMWR *39*(41): 730-733, October 19, 1990.
48. Rubella vaccination during pregnancy — United States, 1971-1981. MMWR *31*(35): 477-481, September 10, 1982.
49. Losonsky, G.A.; Fishaut, J.M.; Strussenber, J.; Ogra, P.L.: Effect of immunization against rubella on lactation products. II. Maternal-neonatal interactions, J. Infect. Dis. *145:* 661-666, 1982.
50. Landes, R.D.; Bass, J.W.; Millunchick, E.W.; Oetgen, W.J.: Neonatal rubella following postpartum maternal immunization, J. Pediatr. *97:* 465-467, 1980.
51. Lerman, S.J.: Neonatal rubella following postpartum maternal immunization, J. Pediatr. *98:* 668, 1981. (Letter)
52. Gershon, A.; et al: Live attenuated rubella virus vaccine: comparison of responses to HPV-77-DE5 and RA 27/3 strains, Am. J. Med. Sci. *279*(2): 95-97, 1980.
53. Weibel, R.E.; et al: Clinical and laboratory studies of live attenuated RA 27/3 and HPV-77-DE rubella virus vaccines, Proc. Soc. Exp. Biol. Med. *165:* 44-49, 1980.
54. CDC. Important Information about Measles, Mumps, and Rubella, and Measles, Mumps, and Rubella Vaccines. 1980. 1983.
55. CDC, Measles Surveillance, Report No. 11, p. 14, September 1982.
56. Peltola, H.; et al: The elimination of indigenous measles, mumps, and rubella from Finland by a 12-year, two dose vaccination program. N. Engl. J. Med. *331:* 1397-1402, 1994.
57. Eberhart-Phillips, J.E.; et al: Measles in pregnancy: a descriptive study of 58 cases. Obstetrics and Gynecology, *82*(5): 797-801, November 1993.
58. Jespersen, C.S.; et al: Measles as a cause of fetal defects: A retrospective study of ten measles epidemics in Greenland. Acta Paediatr Scand. *66:* 367-372, May 1977.
59. Measles, Mumps, and Rubella — Vaccine Use and Strategies for Elimination of Measles, Rubella, and Congenital Rubella Syndrome and Control of Mumps: Recommendations of the Advisory Committee on Immunization Practices (ACIP), MMWR *47*(RR-8): May 22, 1998.
60. Bitnum, A.; et al: Measles Inclusion Body Encephalitis Caused by the Vaccine Strain of Measles Virus. Clin. Infect. Dis. *29:* 855-861, 1999.
61. Angel, J.B.; et al: Vaccine Associated Measles Pneumonitis in an Adult with AIDS. Annals of Internal Medicine, *129:* 104-106, 1998.

Dist. by: Merck Sharp & Dohme Corp., a subsidiary of **MERCK & CO., INC.**, Whitehouse Station, NJ 08889, USA
Issued December 2010
Printed in USA
9912202

PATIENT PACKAGE INSERT

Patient Information about
M-M-R® II (pronounced "em em ar too")
Generic name: Measles, Mumps, and Rubella Virus Vaccine Live

This is a summary of information about M-M-R II[1]. You should read it before you or your child receives the vaccine. If you have any questions about the vaccine after reading this leaflet, you should ask your health care provider. This is a summary only. It does not take the place of talking about M-M-R II with your doctor, nurse, or other health care provider. Only your health care provider can decide if M-M-R II is right for you or your child.

What is M-M-R II and how does it work?

M-M-R II is also known as Measles, Mumps, and Rubella Virus Vaccine Live. It is a live virus vaccine that is given as a shot. This vaccine is usually given to people one year old or older. It is meant to help prevent measles (rubeola), mumps, and rubella (German measles).

M-M-R II contains weakened forms of measles virus, mumps virus, and rubella virus.

M-M-R II works by helping the immune system protect you or your child from getting measles, mumps, or rubella.

M-M-R II may not protect everyone who gets the vaccine.

M-M-R II does not treat measles, mumps, or rubella once you or your child has them.

What do I need to know about measles, mumps, and rubella?

Measles is also known as rubeola. It is a serious illness. Measles virus can be passed to others if you have it. Measles can give you a high fever, cough, and a rash. The illness can last for 1 to 2 weeks. In rare cases, it can also cause an infection of the brain. This could lead to seizures, hearing loss, mental retardation, and even death.

Mumps can also be passed to others. This virus can cause fever and headache. It also makes the glands under your jaw swell and be painful. The illness often lasts for several days. Sometimes, mumps can make the testicles swell and be painful. In some cases, it can cause meningitis, which is a mild swelling of the coverings of the brain and spinal cord.

Rubella is also known as German measles. It is often a mild illness. Rubella virus can cause a mild fever, swollen glands in the neck, pain and swelling in the joints, and a rash that lasts for a short time. It can be very dangerous if a pregnant woman catches it. Women who catch German measles when they are pregnant can have babies who are stillborn. Also, the babies may be blind or deaf, or have heart disease or mental retardation.

Who should not get M-M-R II?

Do not get M-M-R II if you or your child:

- are allergic to any of its ingredients (This includes gelatin or neomycin. See the ingredient list at the end of this leaflet.);
- have a weakened immune system, such as an immune deficiency, an inherited immune disorder, leukemia, lymphoma, or HIV/AIDS;
- take high doses of steroids by mouth or in a shot;
- have a fever higher than 101.3°F (38.5°C);
- are pregnant or plan to get pregnant within the next three months.

How is M-M-R II given?

M-M-R II is given as a shot to people one year old or older. The dose of the vaccine is the same for everyone. If your child gets the shot when he or she is one year old or older, a second dose is recommended. Often, the second dose is given right before the child goes to elementary school (4 to 6 years of age). If your child is less than one year old when he or she first gets the shot, a second dose should be given when they are 12 to 15 months old. Then, a third shot should be given between 4 and 6 years of age. Your doctor will decide the best time and number of shots by using official recommendations.

If a dose is missed, your health care provider will let you know when you should have it.

Non-pregnant adolescent and adult females of childbearing age who are susceptible to rubella can be vaccinated with M-M-R II (or live attenuated rubella virus vaccine) if certain precautions are taken. In many cases, it is convenient to give the vaccine to women at risk for rubella right after they give birth.

What are the possible side effects of M-M-R II?

The most common side effect of vaccination with M-M-R II is burning and/or stinging at the site of the shot for a short time.

Other side effects may include:
- Fever
- Rash

Less common side effects may also include:
- Swelling of the testicles
- Joint pain and/or swelling

Some side effects are rare but may be serious. You should call your health care provider if you notice any of the following problems:
- Difficulty breathing, wheezing, hives, or a skin rash may be signs of an allergic reaction.
- Bleeding or bruising under the skin.
- Seizures, a severe headache, or a change in behavior or consciousness.

Other side effects may also occur. Your doctor has a more complete list of side effects for M-M-R II.

Contact your doctor or health care provider if you or your child have any new or unusual symptoms after receiving M-M-R II.

You may also report any adverse reactions to your doctor or your child's health care provider or submit a report directly to the Vaccine Adverse Event Reporting System (VAERS). The VAERS toll-free number is 1-800-822-7967 or you may report online to www.vaers.hhs.gov.

What are the ingredients of M-M-R II?

Active Ingredients: weakened forms of the measles, mumps, and rubella viruses.

Inactive Ingredients: sorbitol, sodium phosphate, potassium phosphate, sucrose, sodium chloride, hydrolyzed gelatin, recombinant human albumin, fetal bovine serum, other buffer and media ingredients, neomycin.

What else should I know about M-M-R II?

If you get M-M-R II while you are pregnant, please call 1-800-986-8999. Or, you can have your health care provider call.

This leaflet summarizes important information about M-M-R II.

If you would like more information, talk to your health care provider or call 1-800-622-4477.

Rx Only

Issued December 2010

9912202

Dist. by: Merck Sharp & Dohme Corp., a subsidiary of **MERCK & CO., INC.**,Whitehouse Station, NJ 08889, USA

MAXALT ℞

[max-awlt]

(rizatriptan benzoate)

tablets, for oral use

MAXALT-MLT

(rizatriptan benzoate)

orally disintegrating tablets

HIGHLIGHTS OF PRESCRIBING INFORMATION

These highlights do not include all the information needed to use MAXALT and MAXALT-MLT safely and effectively. See full prescribing information for MAXALT and MAXALT-MLT.

MAXALT (rizatriptan benzoate) tablets, for oral use

MAXALT-MLT (rizatriptan benzoate) orally disintegrating tablets

Initial U.S. Approval: 1998

INDICATIONS AND USAGE

MAXALT is a serotonin (5-HT) 1B/1D receptor agonist (triptan) indicated for the acute treatment of migraine with or without aura in adults and in pediatric patients 6 to 17 years of age (1)

Limitations of Use:
- Use only after clear diagnosis of migraine has been established (1)
- Not indicated for the prophylactic therapy of migraine (1)
- Not indicated for the treatment of cluster headache (1)

DOSAGE AND ADMINISTRATION

- Adults: 5 or 10 mg single dose; separate repeat doses by at least two hours; maximum dose in a 24-hour period: 30 mg (2.1)
- Pediatric patients 6 to 17 years: 5 mg single dose in patients less than 40 kg (88 lb); 10 mg single dose in patients 40 kg (88 lb) or more (2.2)
- Adjust dose if co-administered with propranolol (2.4)

DOSAGE FORMS AND STRENGTHS

- MAXALT Tablets: 5 and 10 mg (3)
- MAXALT-MLT Orally Disintegrating Tablets: 5 and 10 mg (3)

CONTRAINDICATIONS

- History of ischemic heart disease or coronary artery vasospasm (4)
- History of stroke or transient ischemic attack (4)
- Peripheral vascular disease (4)
- Ischemic bowel disease (4)
- Uncontrolled hypertension (4)
- Recent (within 24 hours) use of another 5-HT_1 agonist (e.g., another triptan), or of an ergotamine-containing medication (4)
- Hemiplegic or basilar migraine (4)
- MAO-A inhibitor used in the past 2 weeks (4)
- Hypersensitivity to MAXALT or MAXALT-MLT (4)

WARNINGS AND PRECAUTIONS

- Myocardial ischemia, myocardial infarction, and Prinzmetal's angina: Perform cardiac evaluation in patients with multiple cardiovascular risk factors (5.1)
- Arrhythmias: Discontinue dosing if occurs (5.2)
- Chest/throat/neck/jaw pain, tightness, pressure, or heaviness; Generally not associated with myocardial ischemia; Evaluate patients at high risk (5.3)
- Cerebral hemorrhage, subarachnoid hemorrhage, and stroke: Discontinue dosing if occurs (5.4)
- Gastrointestinal ischemic events, peripheral vasospastic reactions: Discontinue dosing if occurs (5.5)
- Medication overuse headache: Detoxification may be necessary (5.6)
- Serotonin syndrome: Discontinue dosing if occurs (5.7)

ADVERSE REACTIONS

The most common adverse reactions in adults were (incidence ≥5% and greater than placebo): asthenia/fatigue, somnolence, pain/pressure sensation and dizziness (6.1)

To report SUSPECTED ADVERSE REACTIONS, contact Merck Sharp & Dohme Corp., a subsidiary of Merck & Co., Inc., at 1-877-888-4231 or FDA at 1-800-FDA-1088 or www.fda.gov/medwatch.

USE IN SPECIFIC POPULATIONS

- Pregnancy: Based on animal data, may cause fetal harm (8.1)
- Phenylketonurics: MAXALT-MLT contains phenylalanine (8.6)

See 17 for PATIENT COUNSELING INFORMATION and FDA-approved patient labeling

Revised: 01/2013

FULL PRESCRIBING INFORMATION: CONTENTS*

*** Sections or subsections omitted from the full prescribing information are not listed**

FULL PRESCRIBING INFORMATION

1 INDICATIONS AND USAGE

MAXALT® and MAXALT-MLT® are indicated for the acute treatment of migraine with or without aura in adults and in pediatric patients 6 to 17 years old.

Limitations of Use
- MAXALT should only be used where a clear diagnosis of migraine has been established. If a patient has no response for the first migraine attack treated with MAXALT, the diagnosis of migraine should be reconsidered before MAXALT is administered to treat any subsequent attacks.
- MAXALT is not indicated for use in the management of hemiplegic or basilar migraine *[see Contraindications (4)]*.
- MAXALT is not indicated for the prevention of migraine attacks.
- Safety and effectiveness of MAXALT have not been established for cluster headache.

2 DOSAGE AND ADMINISTRATION

2.1 Dosing Information in Adults

The recommended starting dose of MAXALT is either 5 mg or 10 mg for the acute treatment of migraines in adults. The 10-mg dose may provide a greater effect than the 5-mg dose, but may have a greater risk of adverse reactions *[see Clinical Studies (14.1)]*.

Redosing in Adults

Although the effectiveness of a second dose or subsequent doses has not been established in placebo-controlled trials, if the migraine headache returns, a second dose may be administered 2 hours after the first dose. The maximum daily dose should not exceed 30 mg in any 24-hour period. The safety of treating, on average, more than four headaches in a 30-day period has not been established.

2.2 Dosing Information in Pediatric Patients (Age 6 to 17 Years)

Dosing in pediatric patients is based on the patient's body weight. The recommended dose of MAXALT is 5 mg in patients weighing less than 40 kg (88 lb), and 10 mg in patients weighing 40 kg (88 lb) or more.

The efficacy and safety of treatment with more than one dose of MAXALT within 24 hours in pediatric patients 6 to 17 years of age have not been established.

2.3 Administration of MAXALT-MLT Orally Disintegrating Tablets

For MAXALT-MLT Orally Disintegrating Tablets, administration with liquid is not necessary. Orally disintegrating tablets are packaged in a blister within an outer aluminum pouch and patients should not remove the blister from the outer pouch until just prior to dosing. The blister pack should then be peeled open with dry hands and the orally disintegrating tablet placed on the tongue, where it will dissolve and be swallowed with the saliva.

2.4 Dosage Adjustment for Patients on Propranolol

Adult Patients

In adult patients taking propranolol, only the 5-mg dose of MAXALT is recommended, up to a maximum of 3 doses in any 24-hour period (15 mg) *[see Drug Interactions (7.1) and Clinical Pharmacology (12.3)]*.

Pediatric Patients

For pediatric patients weighing 40 kg (88 lb) or more, taking propranolol, only a single 5-mg dose of MAXALT is recommended (maximum dose of 5 mg in a 24-hour period). MAXALT should not be prescribed to propranolol-treated pediatric patients who weigh less than 40 kg (88 lb) *[see Drug Interactions (7.1) and Clinical Pharmacology (12.3)]*.

3 DOSAGE FORMS AND STRENGTHS

MAXALT Tablets
- 5 mg tablets are pale pink, capsule-shaped, compressed tablets coded MRK on one side and 266 on the other.
- 10 mg tablets are pale pink, capsule-shaped, compressed tablets coded MAXALT on one side and MRK 267 on the other.

MAXALT-MLT Orally Disintegrating Tablets

- 5 mg orally disintegrating tablets are white to off-white, round lyophilized tablets debossed with a modified triangle on one side.
- 10 mg orally disintegrating tablets are white to off-white, round lyophilized tablets debossed with a modified square on one side.

4 CONTRAINDICATIONS

MAXALT is contraindicated in patients with:

- Ischemic coronary artery disease (angina pectoris, history of myocardial infarction, or documented silent ischemia), or other significant underlying cardiovascular disease *[see Warnings and Precautions (5.1)]*.
- Coronary artery vasospasm including Prinzmetal's angina *[see Warnings and Precautions (5.1)]*.
- History of stroke or transient ischemic attack (TIA) *[see Warnings and Precautions (5.4)]*.
- Peripheral vascular disease (PVD) *[see Warnings and Precautions (5.5)]*.
- Ischemic bowel disease *[see Warnings and Precautions (5.5)]*.
- Uncontrolled hypertension *[see Warnings and Precautions (5.8)]*.
- Recent use (i.e., within 24 hours) of another 5-HT_1 agonist, ergotamine-containing medication, or ergot-type medication (such as dihydroergotamine or methysergide) *[see Drug Interactions (7.2 and 7.3)]*.
- Hemiplegic or basilar migraine *[see Indications and Usage (1)]*.
- Concurrent administration or recent discontinuation (i.e., within 2 weeks) of a MAO-A inhibitor *[see Drug Interactions (7.5) and Clinical Pharmacology (12.3)]*.
- Hypersensitivity to MAXALT or MAXALT-MLT (angioedema and anaphylaxis seen) *[see Adverse Reactions (6.2)]*.

5 WARNINGS AND PRECAUTIONS

5.1 Myocardial Ischemia, Myocardial Infarction, and Prinzmetal's Angina

MAXALT should not be given to patients with ischemic or vasospastic coronary artery disease. There have been rare reports of serious cardiac adverse reactions, including acute myocardial infarction, occurring within a few hours following administration of MAXALT. Some of these reactions occurred in patients without known coronary artery disease (CAD). 5-HT_1 agonists, including MAXALT may cause coronary artery vasospasm (Prinzmetal's Angina), even in patients without a history of CAD.

Triptan-naïve patients who have multiple cardiovascular risk factors (e.g., increased age, diabetes, hypertension, smoking, obesity, strong family history of CAD) should have a cardiovascular evaluation prior to receiving MAXALT. If there is evidence of CAD or coronary artery vasospasm, MAXALT should not be administered *[see Contraindications (4)]*. For patients who have a negative cardiovascular evaluation, consideration should be given to administration of the first MAXALT dose in a medically-supervised setting and performing an electrocardiogram (ECG) immediately following MAXALT administration. Periodic cardiovascular evaluation should be considered in intermittent long-term users of MAXALT who have cardiovascular risk factors.

5.2 Arrhythmias

Life-threatening disturbances of cardiac rhythm, including ventricular tachycardia and ventricular fibrillation leading to death, have been reported within a few hours following the administration of 5-HT_1 agonists. Discontinue MAXALT if these disturbances occur.

5.3 Chest, Throat, Neck and/or Jaw Pain/Tightness/Pressure

As with other 5-HT_1 agonists, sensations of tightness, pain, pressure, and heaviness in the precordium, throat, neck and jaw commonly occur after treatment with MAXALT and are usually non-cardiac in origin. However, if a cardiac origin is suspected, patients should be evaluated. Patients shown to have CAD and those with Prinzmetal's variant angina should not receive 5-HT_1 agonists.

5.4 Cerebrovascular Events

Cerebral hemorrhage, subarachnoid hemorrhage, and stroke have occurred in patients treated with 5-HT_1 agonists, and some have resulted in fatalities. In a number of cases, it appears possible that the cerebrovascular events were primary, the 5-HT_1 agonist having been administered in the incorrect belief that the symptoms experienced were a consequence of migraine, when they were not. Also, patients with migraine may be at increased risk of certain cerebrovascular events (e.g., stroke, hemorrhage, transient ischemic attack). Discontinue MAXALT if a cerebrovascular event occurs.

As with other acute migraine therapies, before treating headaches in patients not previously diagnosed as migraineurs, and in migraineurs who present with atypical symptoms, care should be taken to exclude other potentially serious neurological conditions. MAXALT should not be administered to patients with a history of stroke or transient ischemic attack *[see Contraindications (4)]*.

5.5 Other Vasospasm Reactions

5-HT_1 agonists, including MAXALT, may cause non-coronary vasospastic reactions, such as peripheral vascular ischemia, gastrointestinal vascular ischemia and infarction (presenting with abdominal pain and bloody diarrhea), splenic infarction, and Raynaud's syndrome. In patients who experience symptoms or signs suggestive of non-coronary vasospasm reaction following the use of any 5-HT_1 agonist, the suspected vasospasm reaction should be ruled out before receiving additional MAXALT doses.

Reports of transient and permanent blindness and significant partial vision loss have been reported with the use of 5-HT_1 agonists. Since visual disorders may be part of a migraine attack, a causal relationship between these events and the use of 5-HT_1 agonists have not been clearly established.

5.6 Medication Overuse Headache

Overuse of acute migraine drugs (e.g., ergotamine, triptans, opioids, or a combination of drugs for 10 or more days per month) may lead to exacerbation of headache (medication overuse headache). Medication overuse headache may present as migraine-like daily headaches, or as a marked increase in frequency of migraine attacks. Detoxification of patients, including withdrawal of the overused drugs, and treatment of withdrawal symptoms (which often includes a transient worsening of headache) may be necessary.

5.7 Serotonin Syndrome

Serotonin syndrome may occur with triptans, including MAXALT particularly during co-administration with selective serotonin reuptake inhibitors (SSRIs), serotonin norepinephrine reuptake inhibitors (SNRIs), tricyclic antidepressants (TCAs), and MAO inhibitors *[see Drug Interactions (7.5)]*. Serotonin syndrome symptoms may include mental status changes (e.g., agitation, hallucinations, coma), autonomic instability (e.g., tachycardia, labile blood pressure, hyperthermia), neuromuscular aberrations (e.g., hyperreflexia, incoordination) and/or gastrointestinal symptoms (e.g., nausea, vomiting, diarrhea). The onset of symptoms can occur within minutes to hours of receiving a new or a greater dose of a serotonergic medication. MAXALT treatment should be discontinued if serotonin syndrome is suspected *[see Drug Interactions (7.4) and Patient Counseling Information (17)]*.

5.8 Increase in Blood Pressure

Significant elevation in blood pressure, including hypertensive crisis with acute impairment of organ systems, has been reported on rare occasions in patients with and without a history of hypertension receiving 5-HT_1 agonists, including MAXALT. In healthy young adult male and female patients who received maximal doses of MAXALT (10 mg every 2 hours for 3 doses), slight increases in blood pressure (approximately 2-3 mmHg) were observed. MAXALT is contraindicated in patients with uncontrolled hypertension *[see Contraindications (4)]*.

6 ADVERSE REACTIONS

The following adverse reactions are discussed in more detail in other sections of the labeling:

- Myocardial Ischemia, Myocardial Infarction, and Prinzmetal's Angina *[see Warnings and Precautions (5.1)]*.
- Arrhythmias *[see Warnings and Precautions (5.2)]*.
- Chest, Throat, Neck and/or Jaw Pain/Tightness/Pressure *[see Warnings and Precautions (5.3)]*.
- Cerebrovascular Events *[see Warnings and Precautions (5.4)]*.
- Other Vasospasm Reactions *[see Warnings and Precautions (5.5)]*.
- Medication Overuse Headache *[see Warnings and Precautions (5.6)]*.
- Serotonin Syndrome *[see Warnings and Precautions (5.7)]*.
- Increase in Blood Pressure *[see Warnings and Precautions (5.8)]*.

6.1 Clinical Trials Experience

Because clinical studies are conducted under widely varying conditions, adverse reaction rates observed in the clinical studies of a drug cannot be directly compared to rates in the clinical studies of another drug and may not reflect the rates observed in practice.

Adults

Incidence in Controlled Clinical Trials

Adverse reactions to MAXALT were assessed in controlled clinical trials that included over 3700 adult patients who received single or multiple doses of MAXALT Tablets. The most common adverse reactions during treatment with MAXALT (≥5% in either treatment group and greater than placebo) were asthenia/fatigue, somnolence, pain/pressure sensation and dizziness. These adverse reactions appeared to be dose related.

Table 1 lists the adverse reactions (incidence ≥2% and greater than placebo) after a single dose of MAXALT in adults.

Table 1: Incidence (≥2% and Greater than Placebo) of Adverse Reactions After a Single Dose of MAXALT Tablets or Placebo in Adults

Adverse Reactions	% of Patients MAXALT 5 mg (N=977)	MAXALT 10 mg (N=1167)	Placebo (N=627)
Atypical Sensations	4	5	4
Paresthesia	3	4	<2
Pain and other Pressure Sensations	6	9	3
Chest Pain: tightness/pressure and/or heaviness	<2	3	1
Neck/throat/jaw: pain/tightness/ pressure	<2	2	1
Regional Pain: tightness/pressure and/or heaviness	<1	2	0
Pain, location unspecified	3	3	<2
Digestive	9	13	8
Dry Mouth	3	3	1
Nausea	4	6	4
Neurological	14	20	11
Dizziness	4	9	5
Headache	<2	2	<1
Somnolence	4	8	4
Other			
Asthenia/fatigue	4	7	2

The frequencies of adverse reactions in clinical trials did not increase when up to three doses were taken within 24 hours. Adverse reaction frequencies were also unchanged by concomitant use of drugs commonly taken for migraine prophylaxis (including propranolol), oral contraceptives, or analgesics. The incidences of adverse reactions were not affected by age or gender. There were insufficient data to assess the impact of race on the incidence of adverse reactions.

Other Events Observed in Association with the Administration of MAXALT in Adults

In the following section, the frequencies of less commonly reported adverse events are presented that were not reported in other sections of the labeling. Because the reports include events observed in open studies, the role of MAXALT in their causation cannot be reliably determined. Furthermore, variability associated with adverse event reporting, the terminology used to describe adverse events, limit the value of the quantitative frequency estimates provided. Event frequencies are calculated as the number of patients who used MAXALT and reported an event divided by the total number of patients exposed to MAXALT (N=3716). All reported events occurred at an incidence ≥1%, or are believed to be reasonably associated with the use of the drug. Events are further classified within body system categories and enumerated in order of decreasing frequency using the following definitions: frequent adverse events are those defined as those occurring in at least (>)1/100 patients; infrequent adverse experiences are those occurring in 1/100 to 1/1000 patients; and rare adverse experiences are those occurring in fewer than 1/1000 patients.

General: Infrequent was facial edema. Rare were syncope and edema/swelling.

Atypical Sensations: Frequent were warm sensations.

Cardiovascular: Frequent was palpitation. Infrequent were tachycardia, cold extremities, and bradycardia.

Digestive: Frequent were diarrhea and vomiting. Infrequent were dyspepsia, tongue edema and abdominal distention.

Musculoskeletal: Infrequent were muscle weakness, stiffness, myalgia and muscle cramp/spasm.

Neurological/Psychiatric: Frequent were hypoesthesia, euphoria and tremor. Infrequent were vertigo, insomnia, confusion/disorientation, gait abnormality, memory impairment, and agitation.

Respiratory: Frequent was dyspnea. Infrequent was pharyngeal edema.

Special Senses: Infrequent were blurred vision and tinnitus. Rare was eye swelling.

Skin and Skin Appendage: Frequent was flushing. Infrequent were sweating, pruritus, rash, and urticaria. Rare was erythema, hot flashes.

The adverse reaction profile seen with MAXALT-MLT Orally Disintegrating Tablets was similar to that seen with MAXALT Tablets.

Pediatric Patients 6 to 17 Years of Age

Incidence in Controlled Clinical Trials in Pediatric Patients

Adverse reactions to MAXALT-MLT were assessed in a controlled clinical trial in the acute treatment of migraines (Study 7) that included a total of 1382 pediatric patients 6-17 years of age, of which 977 (72%) administered at least one dose of study treatment (MAXALT-MLT and/or placebo) *[see Clinical Studies (14.2)]*. The incidence of adverse reactions reported for pediatric patients in the acute clinical trial was similar in patients who received MAXALT to those who received placebo. The adverse reaction pattern in pediatric patients is expected to be similar to that in adults.

Other Events Observed in Association with the Administration of MAXALT-MLT in Pediatric Patients

In the following section, the frequencies of less commonly reported adverse events are presented. Because the reports include events observed in open studies, the role of MAXALT-MLT in their causation cannot be reliably determined. Furthermore, variability associated with adverse event reporting, the terminology used to describe adverse events, limit the value of the quantitative frequency estimates provided.

Event frequencies are calculated as the number of pediatric patients 6 to 17 years of age who used MAXALT-MLT and reported an event divided by the total number of patients exposed to MAXALT-MLT (N=1068). All reported events occurred at an incidence ≥1%, or are believed to be reasonably associated with the use of the drug. Events are further classified within system organ class and enumerated in order of decreasing frequency using the following definitions: frequent adverse events are those occurring in (>)1/100 pediatric patients; infrequent adverse experiences are those occurring in 1/100 to 1/1000 pediatric patients; and rare adverse experiences are those occurring in fewer than 1/1000 patients.

General: Frequent was fatigue.

Ear and labyrinth disorders: Infrequent was hypoacusis.

Gastrointestinal disorders: Frequent was abdominal discomfort.

Nervous system disorders: Infrequent were coordination abnormal, disturbance in attention, and presyncope.

Psychiatric disorders: Infrequent was hallucination.

6.2 Postmarketing Experience

The following section enumerates potentially important adverse events that have occurred in clinical practice and which have been reported spontaneously to various surveillance systems. The events enumerated include all except those already listed in other sections of the labeling or those too general to be informative. Because the reports cite events reported spontaneously from worldwide postmarketing experience, frequency of events and the role of MAXALT in their causation cannot be reliably determined.

Neurological/Psychiatric: Seizure.

General: Allergic conditions including anaphylaxis/anaphylactoid reaction, angioedema, wheezing, and toxic epidermal necrolysis *[see Contraindications (4)].*

Special Senses: Dysgeusia.

7 DRUG INTERACTIONS

7.1 Propranolol

The dose of MAXALT should be adjusted in propranolol-treated patients, as propranolol has been shown to increase the plasma AUC of rizatriptan by 70% *[see Dosage and Administration (2.4) and Clinical Pharmacology (12.3)].*

7.2 Ergot-Containing Drugs

Ergot-containing drugs have been reported to cause prolonged vasospastic reactions. Because these effects may be additive, use of ergotamine-containing or ergot-type medications (like dihydroergotamine or methysergide) and MAXALT within 24 hours is contraindicated *[see Contraindications (4)].*

7.3 Other 5-HT$_1$ Agonists

Because their vasospastic effects may be additive, coadministration of MAXALT and other 5-HT$_1$ agonists within 24 hours of each other is contraindicated *[see Contraindications (4)].*

7.4 SSRIs/SNRIs and Serotonin Syndrome

Cases of serotonin syndrome have been reported during coadministration of triptans and selective serotonin reuptake inhibitors (SSRIs) or serotonin norepinephrine reuptake inhibitors (SNRIs) *[see Warnings and Precautions (5.7)].*

7.5 Monoamine Oxidase Inhibitors

MAXALT is contraindicated in patients taking MAO-A inhibitors and non-selective MAO inhibitors. A specific MAO-A inhibitor increased the systemic exposure of rizatriptan and its metabolite *[see Contraindications (4) and Clinical Pharmacology (12.3)].*

8 USE IN SPECIFIC POPULATIONS

8.1 Pregnancy

Pregnancy Category C

There are no adequate and well-controlled studies in pregnant women. MAXALT should be used during pregnancy only if the potential benefit justifies the potential risk to the fetus.

In a general reproductive study in rats, birth weights and pre- and post-weaning weight gain were reduced in the offspring of females treated prior to and during mating and throughout gestation and lactation with doses of 10 and 100 mg/kg/day. In a pre- and post-natal developmental toxicity study in rats, an increase in mortality of the offspring at birth and for the first three days after birth, a decrease in pre- and post-weaning weight gain, and decreased performance in a passive avoidance test (which indicates a decrease in learning capacity of the offspring) were observed at doses of 100 and 250 mg/kg/day. The no-effect dose for all of these effects was 5 mg/kg/day, associated with a maternal plasma exposure (AUC) approximately 7.5 times that in humans receiving the MRDD. With doses of 100 and 250 mg/kg/day, the decreases in average weight of both the male and female offspring persisted into adulthood. All effects on the offspring in both studies occurred in the absence of any apparent maternal toxicity.

In embryofetal development studies, no teratogenic effects were observed when pregnant rats and rabbits were administered doses of 100 and 50 mg/kg/day, respectively, during organogenesis. Fetal weights were decreased in conjunction with decreased maternal weight gain at the highest doses tested. The developmental no-effect dose in these studies was 10 mg/kg/day in both rats and rabbits (maternal exposures approximately 15 times human exposure at the MRDD). Toxicokinetic studies demonstrated placental transfer of drug in both species.

Merck Sharp & Dohme Corp., a subsidiary of Merck & Co., Inc., maintains a registry to monitor the pregnancy outcomes of women exposed to MAXALT while pregnant. Healthcare providers are encouraged to report any prenatal exposure to MAXALT by calling the Pregnancy Registry at 1-800-986-8999.

8.3 Nursing Mothers

It is not known whether this drug is excreted in human milk. Because many drugs are excreted in human milk, caution should be exercised when MAXALT is administered to a nursing woman. Rizatriptan is extensively excreted in rat milk, with levels in milk at least 5-fold higher than levels in maternal plasma.

8.4 Pediatric Use

Safety and effectiveness in pediatric patients under 6 years of age have not been established.

The efficacy and safety of MAXALT in the acute treatment of migraine in patients aged 6 to 17 years was established in an adequate and well-controlled study *[see Clinical Studies (14.2)].*

The incidence of adverse reactions reported for pediatric patients in the acute clinical trial was similar in patients who received MAXALT to those who received placebo. The adverse reaction pattern in pediatric patients is expected to be similar to that in adults.

8.5 Geriatric Use

Clinical studies of MAXALT did not include sufficient numbers of subjects aged 65 and over to determine whether they respond differently from younger subjects. Other reported clinical experience has not identified differences in responses between the elderly and younger patients.

Although the pharmacokinetics of rizatriptan were similar in elderly (aged ≥65 years) and in younger adults (n=17), in general, dose selection for an elderly patient should be cautious, starting at the low end of the dosing range. This reflects the greater frequency of decreased hepatic, renal, or cardiac function, and of concomitant disease or other drug therapy.

Geriatric patients who have other cardiovascular risk factors (e.g., diabetes, hypertension, smoking, obesity, strong family history of coronary artery disease) should have a cardiovascular evaluation prior to receiving MAXALT *[see Warnings and Precautions (5.1)].*

8.6 Patients with Phenylketonuria

Orally Disintegrating Tablets contain phenylalanine (a component of aspartame). The 5- and 10-mg orally disintegrating tablets contain 1.1 and 2.1 mg phenylalanine, respectively.

10 OVERDOSAGE

No overdoses of MAXALT were reported during clinical trials in adults.

Some adult patients who received 40 mg of MAXALT either a single dose or as two doses with a 2-hour interdose interval had dizziness and somnolence.

In a clinical pharmacology study in which 12 adult subjects received MAXALT, at total cumulative doses of 80 mg (given within four hours), two of the subjects experienced syncope, dizziness, bradycardia including third degree AV block, vomiting, and/or incontinence.

In the long-term, open label study, involving 606 treated pediatric migraineurs 12 to 17 years of age (of which 432 were treated for at least 12 months), 151 patients (25%) took two 10-mg doses of MAXALT-MLT within a 24 hour period. Adverse reactions for 3 of these patients included abdominal discomfort, fatigue, and dyspnea.

In addition, based on the pharmacology of MAXALT, hypertension or myocardial ischemia could occur after overdosage. Gastrointestinal decontamination, (i.e., gastric lavage followed by activated charcoal) should be considered in patients suspected of an overdose with MAXALT. Clinical and electrocardiographic monitoring should be continued for at least 12 hours, even if clinical symptoms are not observed.

The effects of hemo- or peritoneal dialysis on serum concentrations of rizatriptan are unknown.

11 DESCRIPTION

MAXALT contains rizatriptan benzoate, a selective 5-hydroxytryptamine$_{1B/1D}$ (5-HT$_{1B/1D}$) receptor agonist. Rizatriptan benzoate is described chemically as: *N,N*-dimethyl-5-(1*H*-1,2,4-triazol-1-ylmethyl)-1*H*-indole-3-ethanamine monobenzoate and its structural formula is:

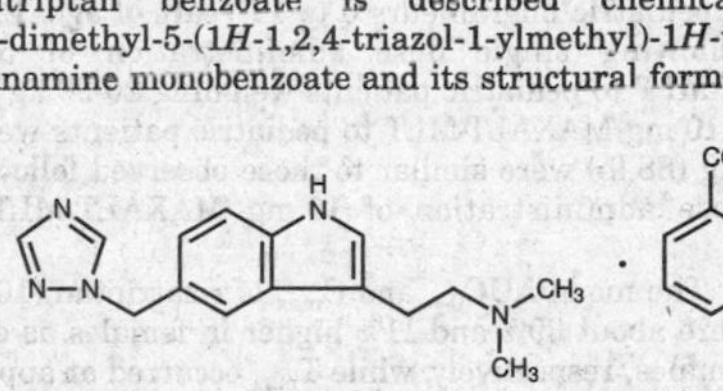

Its empirical formula is $C_{15}H_{19}N_5 \bullet C_7H_6O_2$, representing a molecular weight of the free base of 269.4. Rizatriptan benzoate is a white to off-white, crystalline solid that is soluble in water at about 42 mg per mL (expressed as free base) at 25°C.

MAXALT Tablets and MAXALT-MLT Orally Disintegrating Tablets are available for oral administration in strengths of 5 and 10 mg (corresponding to 7.265 mg or 14.53 mg of the benzoate salt, respectively). Each compressed tablet contains the following inactive ingredients: lactose monohydrate, microcrystalline cellulose, pregelatinized starch, ferric oxide (red), and magnesium stearate.

Each lyophilized orally disintegrating tablet contains the following inactive ingredients: gelatin, mannitol, glycine, aspartame, and peppermint flavor.

12 CLINICAL PHARMACOLOGY

12.1 Mechanism of Action

Rizatriptan binds with high affinity to human cloned 5-HT$_{1B/1D}$ receptors. MAXALT presumably exerts its therapeutic effects in the treatment of migraine headache by binding to 5-HT$_{1B/1D}$ receptors located on intracranial blood vessels and sensory nerves of the trigeminal system.

12.3 Pharmacokinetics

Absorption

Rizatriptan is completely absorbed following oral administration. The mean oral absolute bioavailability of the MAXALT Tablet is about 45%, and mean peak plasma concentrations (C_{max}) are reached in approximately 1-1.5 hours (T_{max}). The presence of a migraine headache did not appear to affect the absorption or pharmacokinetics of rizatriptan. Food has no significant effect on the bioavailability of rizatriptan but delays the time to reach peak concentration by an hour. In clinical trials, MAXALT was administered without regard to food.

The bioavailability and C_{max} of rizatriptan were similar following administration of MAXALT Tablets and MAXALT-MLT Orally Disintegrating Tablets, but the rate of absorption is somewhat slower with MAXALT-MLT, with T_{max} delayed by up to 0.7 hour. AUC of rizatriptan is approximately 30% higher in females than in males. No accumulation occurred on multiple dosing.

Distribution

The mean volume of distribution is approximately 140 liters in male subjects and 110 liters in female subjects. Rizatriptan is minimally bound (14%) to plasma proteins.

Metabolism

The primary route of rizatriptan metabolism is via oxidative deamination by monoamine oxidase-A (MAO-A) to the indole acetic acid metabolite, which is not active at the 5-HT$_{1B/1D}$ receptor. N-monodesmethyl-rizatriptan, a metabolite with activity similar to that of parent compound at the 5-HT$_{1B/1D}$ receptor, is formed to a minor degree. Plasma concentrations of N-monodesmethyl-rizatriptan are approximately 14% of those of parent compound, and it is eliminated at a similar rate. Other minor metabolites, the N-oxide, the 6-hydroxy compound, and the sulfate conjugate of the 6-hydroxy metabolite are not active at the 5-HT$_{1B/1D}$ receptor.

Elimination

The total radioactivity of the administered dose recovered over 120 hours in urine and feces was 82% and 12%, respectively, following a single 10-mg oral administration of ^{14}C-rizatriptan. Following oral administration of ^{14}C-rizatriptan, rizatriptan accounted for about 17% of circulating plasma radioactivity. Approximately 14% of an oral dose is excreted in urine as unchanged rizatriptan while 51% is excreted as indole acetic acid metabolite, indicating substantial first pass metabolism.

The plasma half-life of rizatriptan in males and females averages 2-3 hours.

Cytochrome P450 Isoforms

Rizatriptan is not an inhibitor of the activities of human liver cytochrome P450 isoforms 3A4/5, 1A2, 2C9, 2C19, or 2E1; rizatriptan is a competitive inhibitor (K_i=1400 nM) of cytochrome P450 2D6, but only at high, clinically irrelevant concentrations.

Special Populations

Geriatric: Rizatriptan pharmacokinetics in healthy elderly non-migraineur volunteers (age 65-77 years) were similar to those in younger non-migraineur volunteers (age 18-45 years).

Pediatric: The pharmacokinetics of rizatriptan was determined in pediatric migraineurs 6 to 17 years of age. Exposures following single dose administration of 5 mg MAXALT-MLT to pediatric patients weighing 20-39 kg (44-87 lb) or 10 mg MAXALT-MLT to pediatric patients weighing ≥40 kg (88 lb) were similar to those observed following single dose administration of 10 mg MAXALT-MLT to adults.

Gender: The mean $AUC_{0-\infty}$ and C_{max} of rizatriptan (10 mg orally) were about 30% and 11% higher in females as compared to males, respectively, while T_{max} occurred at approximately the same time.

Hepatic impairment: Following oral administration in patients with hepatic impairment caused by mild to moderate alcoholic cirrhosis of the liver, plasma concentrations of rizatriptan were similar in patients with mild hepatic insufficiency compared to a control group of subjects with normal hepatic function; plasma concentrations of rizatriptan were approximately 30% greater in patients with moderate hepatic insufficiency.

Renal impairment: In patients with renal impairment (creatinine clearance 10-60 mL/min/1.73 m^2), the $AUC_{0-\infty}$ of rizatriptan was not significantly different from that in subjects with normal renal function. In hemodialysis patients, (creatinine clearance <2 mL/min/1.73 m^2), however, the AUC for rizatriptan was approximately 44% greater than that in patients with normal renal function.

Race: Pharmacokinetic data revealed no significant differences between African American and Caucasian subjects.

Drug Interactions

[See also Drug Interactions (7).]

Monoamine oxidase inhibitors: Rizatriptan is principally metabolized via monoamine oxidase, 'A' subtype (MAO-A). Plasma concentrations of rizatriptan may be increased by drugs that are selective MAO-A inhibitors (e.g., moclobemide) or nonselective MAO inhibitors [type A and B] (e.g., isocarboxazid, phenelzine, tranylcypromine, and pargyline). In a drug interaction study, when MAXALT 10 mg was administered to subjects (n=12) receiving concomitant therapy with the selective, reversible MAO-A inhibitor, moclobemide 150 mg t.i.d., there were mean increases in rizatriptan AUC and C_{max} of 119% and 41% respectively; and the AUC of the active N-monodesmethyl metabolite of rizatriptan was increased more than 400%. The interaction would be expected to be greater with irreversible MAO inhibitors. No pharmacokinetic interaction is anticipated in patients receiving selective MAO-B inhibitors *[see Contraindications (4) and Drug Interactions (7.5)]*.

Propranolol: In a study of concurrent administration of propranolol 240 mg/day and a single dose of rizatriptan 10 mg in healthy adult subjects (n=11), mean plasma AUC for rizatriptan was increased by 70% during propranolol administration, and a four-fold increase was observed in one subject. The AUC of the active N-monodesmethyl metabolite of rizatriptan was not affected by propranolol *[see Dosage and Administration (2.4) and Drug Interactions (7.1)]*.

Nadolol/Metoprolol: In a drug interactions study, effects of multiple doses of nadolol 80 mg or metoprolol 100 mg every 12 hours on the pharmacokinetics of a single dose of 10 mg rizatriptan were evaluated in healthy subjects (n=12). No pharmacokinetic interactions were observed.

Paroxetine: In a study of the interaction between the selective serotonin reuptake inhibitor (SSRI) paroxetine 20 mg/day for two weeks and a single dose of MAXALT 10 mg in healthy subjects (n=12), neither the plasma concentrations of rizatriptan nor its safety profile were affected by paroxetine *[see Warnings and Precautions (5.7), Drug Interactions (7.4), and Patient Counseling Information (17)]*.

Oral contraceptives: In a study of concurrent administration of an oral contraceptive during 6 days of administration of MAXALT (10-30 mg/day) in healthy female volunteers (n=18), rizatriptan did not affect plasma concentrations of ethinyl estradiol or norethindrone.

13 NONCLINICAL TOXICOLOGY

13.1 Carcinogenesis, Mutagenesis, Impairment of Fertility

Carcinogenesis: Oral carcinogenicity studies were conducted in mice (100 weeks) and rats (106 weeks) at doses of up to 125 mg/kg/day. Plasma exposures (AUC) at the highest dose tested were approximately 150 (mice) and 240 times (rats) that in humans at the maximum recommended daily dose (MRDD) of 30 mg/day. There was no evidence of an increase in tumor incidence related to rizatriptan in either species.

Mutagenesis: Rizatriptan was neither mutagenic nor clastogenic in a battery of *in vitro* and *in vivo* genetic toxicity studies, including: the microbial mutagenesis (Ames) assay, *in vitro* mammalian cell mutagenesis and chromosomal aberration assays, and the *in vivo* chromosomal aberration assay in mouse.

Impairment of Fertility: In a fertility study in rats, altered estrus cyclicity and delays in time to mating were observed in females treated orally with 100 mg/kg/day rizatriptan. The no-effect dose was 10 mg/kg/day (approximately 15 times the human exposure at the MRDD). There were no other fertility-related effects in the female rats. There was no impairment of fertility or reproductive performance in male rats treated with up to 250 mg/kg/day (approximately 550 times the human exposure at the MRDD).

14 CLINICAL STUDIES

14.1 Adults

The efficacy of MAXALT Tablets was established in four multicenter, randomized, placebo-controlled trials. Patients enrolled in these studies were primarily female (84%) and Caucasian (88%), with a mean age of 40 years (range of 18 to 71). Patients were instructed to treat a moderate to severe headache. Headache response, defined as a reduction of moderate or severe headache pain to no or mild headache pain, was assessed for up to 2 hours (Study 1) or up to 4 hours after dosing (Studies 2, 3 and 4). Associated symptoms of nausea, photophobia, and phonophobia and maintenance of response up to 24 hours post-dose were evaluated. A second dose of MAXALT Tablets was allowed 2 to 24 hours after dosing for treatment of recurrent headache in Studies 1 and 2. Additional analgesics and/or antiemetics were allowed 2 hours after initial treatment for rescue in all four studies.

In all studies, the percentage of patients achieving headache response 2 hours after treatment was significantly greater in patients who received either MAXALT 5 or 10 mg compared to those who received placebo. In a separate study, doses of 2.5 mg were not different from placebo. Doses greater than 10 mg were associated with an increased incidence of adverse effects. The results from the four controlled studies are summarized in Table 2.

Table 2: Response Rates 2 Hours Following Treatment of Initial Headache in Studies 1, 2, 3, and 4

Study	Placebo	MAXALT Tablets 5 mg	MAXALT Tablets 10 mg
1	35% (n=304)	62%* (n=458)	71%*,† (n=456)
2‡	37% (n=82)	—	77%* (n=320)
3	23% (n=80)	63%* (n=352)	—
4	40% (n=159)	60%* (n=164)	67%* (n=385)

* p-value <0.05 in comparison with placebo.
† p-value <0.05 in comparison with 5 mg.
‡ Results for initial headache only.

Comparisons of drug performance based upon results obtained in different clinical trials may not be reliable. Because studies are conducted at different times, with different samples of patients, by different investigators, employing different criteria and/or different interpretations of the same criteria, under different conditions (dose, dosing regimen, etc.), quantitative estimates of treatment response and the timing of response may be expected to vary considerably from study to study.

The estimated probability of achieving an initial headache response within 2 hours following treatment in pooled Studies 1, 2, 3, and 4 is depicted in Figure 1.

Figure 1: Estimated Probability of Achieving an Initial Headache Response by 2 Hours in Pooled Studies 1, 2, 3, and 4*

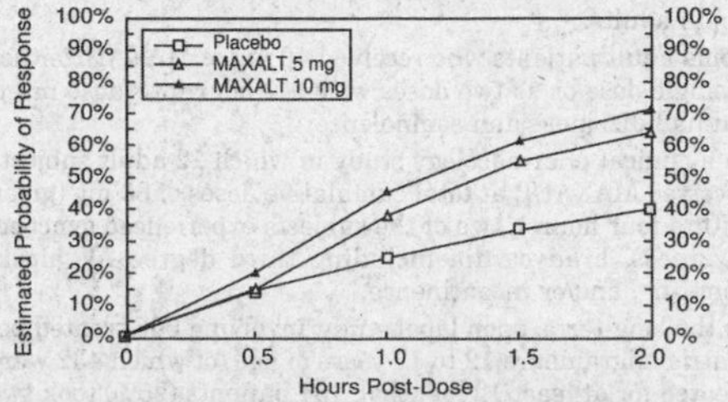

* Figure 1 shows the Kaplan-Meier plot of the probability over time of obtaining headache response (no or mild pain) following treatment with MAXALT or placebo. The averages displayed are based on pooled data from 4 placebo-controlled, outpatient trials providing evidence of efficacy (Studies 1, 2, 3, and 4). Patients taking additional treatment or not achieving headache response prior to 2 hours were censored at 2 hours.

For patients with migraine-associated photophobia, phonophobia, and nausea at baseline, there was a decreased incidence of these symptoms following administration of MAXALT compared to placebo.

Two to 24 hours following the initial dose of study treatment, patients were allowed to use additional treatment for pain response in the form of a second dose of study treatment or other medication. The estimated probability of patients taking a second dose or other medication for migraine over the 24 hours following the initial dose of study treatment is summarized in Figure 2.

Figure 2: Estimated Probability of Patients Taking a Second Dose of MAXALT Tablets or Other Medication for Migraines Over the 24 Hours Following the Initial Dose of Study Treatment in Pooled Studies 1, 2, 3, and 4*

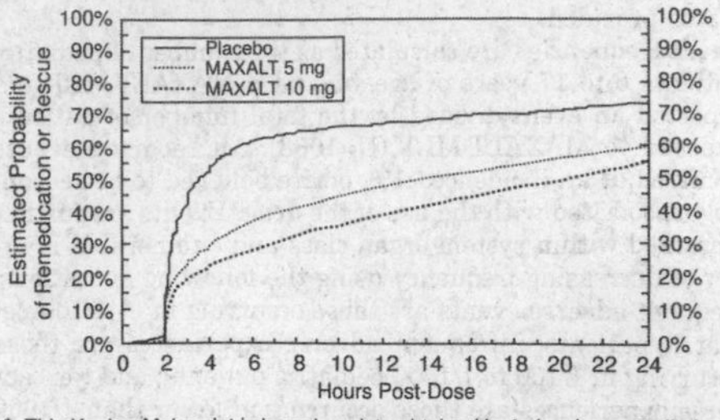

* This Kaplan-Meier plot is based on data obtained in 4 placebo-controlled outpatient clinical trials (Studies 1, 2, 3, and 4). Patients not using additional treatments were censored at 24 hours. The plot includes both patients who had headache response at 2 hours and those who had no response to the initial dose. Remedication was not allowed within 2 hours post-dose.

Efficacy was unaffected by the presence of aura; by the gender, or age of the patient; or by concomitant use of common migraine prophylactic drugs (e.g., beta-blockers, calcium channel blockers, tricyclic antidepressants) or oral contraceptives. In two additional similar studies, efficacy was unaffected by relationship to menses. There were insufficient data to assess the impact of race on efficacy.

MAXALT-MLT Orally Disintegrating Tablets

The efficacy of MAXALT-MLT was established in two multicenter, randomized, placebo-controlled trials that were similar in design to the trials of MAXALT Tablets (Studies 5 and 6). Patients were instructed to treat a moderate to severe headache. Patients treated in these studies were primarily female (88%) and Caucasian (95%), with a mean age of 42 years (range 18-72).

In both studies, the percentage of patients achieving headache response 2 hours after treatment was significantly greater in patients who received either MAXALT-MLT 5 or 10 mg compared to those who received placebo. The results from Studies 5 and 6 are summarized in Table 3.

Table 3: Response Rates 2 Hours Following Treatment of Initial Headache in Studies 5 and 6

Study	Placebo	MAXALT-MLT 5 mg	MAXALT-MLT 10 mg
5	47% (n=98)	66%* (n=100)	66%* (n=113)
6	28% (n=180)	59%* (n=181)	74%*,† (n=186)

* p-value <0.01 in comparison with placebo.
† p-value <0.01 in comparison with 5 mg.

The estimated probability of achieving an initial headache response by 2 hours following treatment with MAXALT-MLT in pooled Studies 5 and 6 is depicted in Figure 3.

Figure 3: Estimated Probability of Achieving an Initial Headache Response with MAXALT-MLT by 2 Hours in Pooled Studies 5 and 6*

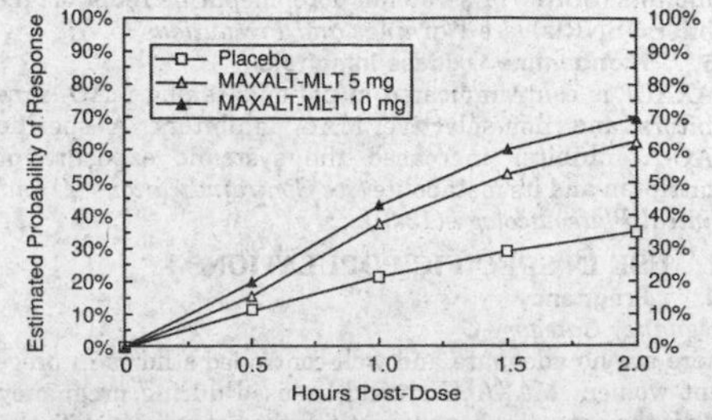

* Figure 3 shows the Kaplan-Meier plot of the probability over time of obtaining headache response (no or mild pain) following treatment with MAXALT-MLT or placebo. The averages displayed are based on pooled data from 2 placebo-controlled, outpatient trials providing evidence of efficacy (Studies 5 and 6). Patients taking additional treatment or not achieving headache response prior to 2 hours were censored at 2 hours.

For patients with migraine-associated photophobia and phonophobia at baseline, there was a decreased incidence of these symptoms following administration of MAXALT-MLT as compared to placebo.

Two to 24 hours following the initial dose of study treatment, patients were allowed to use additional treatment for pain response in the form of a second dose of study treatment or other medication. The estimated probability of patients taking a second dose or other medication for migraine over the 24 hours following the initial dose of study treatment is summarized in Figure 4.

Figure 4: Estimated Probability of Patients Taking a Second Dose of MAXALT-MLT or Other Medication for Migraines Over the 24 Hours Following the Initial Dose of Study Treatment in Pooled Studies 5 and 6*

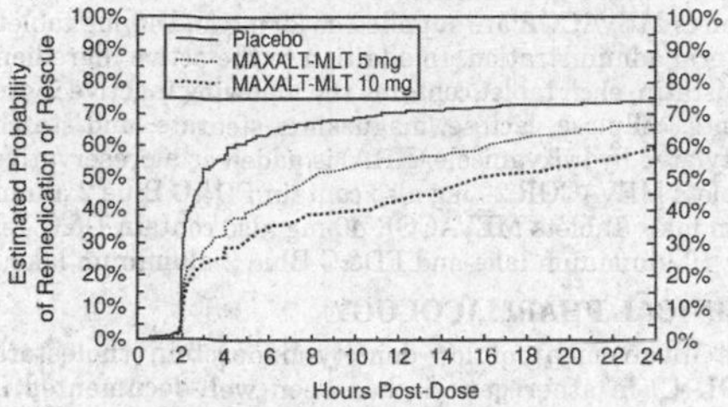

* This Kaplan-Meier plot is based on data obtained in 2 placebo-controlled outpatient clinical trials (Studies 5 and 6). Patients not using additional treatments were censored at 24 hours. The plot includes both patients who had headache response at 2 hours and those who had no response to the initial dose. Remedication was not allowed within 2 hours post-dose.

14.2 Pediatric Patients 6 to 17 Years of Age

The efficacy of MAXALT-MLT in pediatric patients 6 to 17 years was evaluated in a multicenter, randomized, double-blind, placebo-controlled, parallel group clinical trial (Study 7). Patients had to have at least a 6-month history of migraine attacks (with or without aura) usually lasting 3 hours or more (when untreated). The patient population was historically non-responsive to NSAIDs and acetaminophen therapy.

Patients were instructed to treat a single migraine attack with headache pain of moderate to severe intensity. The treatment phase of the study had two stages. Stage 1 was used to identify placebo non-responders, who then entered into Stage 2, in which patients were randomized to MAXALT-MLT or placebo. Using a weight-based dosing strategy, patients 20 kg to <40 kg (44 lb to <88 lb) received MAXALT-MLT 5 mg or placebo, and patients ≥40 kg (88 lb) received MAXALT-MLT 10 mg or placebo.

The mean age for the studied patient population was 13 years. Sixty-one percent of the patients were Caucasian, and fifty-six percent of the patients were female. The percentage of patients achieving the primary efficacy endpoint of no headache pain at 2 hours after treatment was significantly greater in patients who received MAXALT-MLT, compared with those who received placebo (33% vs. 24%). Study 7 results are summarized in Table 4.

Table 4: Response Rates 2 Hours Following Treatment of Initial Headache in Pediatric Patients 6 to 17 Years of Age in Study 7

Endpoint	Placebo	MAXALT-MLT	p-Value
No headache pain at 2 hours post-dose	24% (n/m=94/388)	33% (n/m=126/382)	0.01

n = Number of evaluable patients with no headache pain at 2 hours post-dose.
m = Number of evaluable patients in population.

The observed percentage of pediatric patients achieving no headache pain within 2 hours following initial treatment with MAXALT-MLT is shown in Figure 5.

[See figure 5 at top of next column]

The prevalence of the exploratory endpoints of absence of migraine-associated symptoms (nausea, photophobia, and phonophobia) at 2 hours after taking the dose was not statistically significantly different between patients who received MAXALT-MLT and those who received placebo.

Figure 5: Observed Percentage of Patients Reporting No Headache Pain by 2 Hours Post-Dose in Study 7

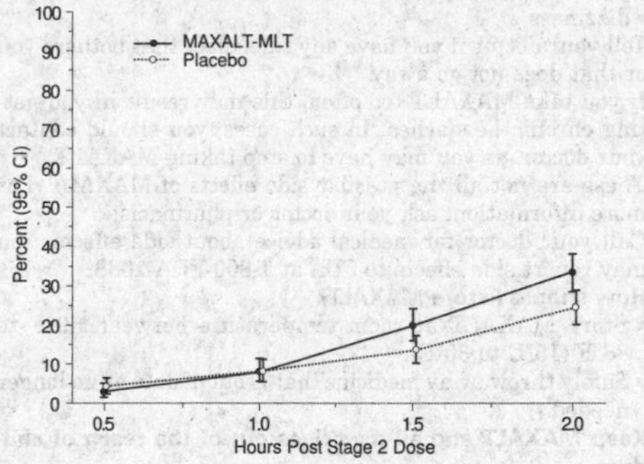

16 HOW SUPPLIED/STORAGE AND HANDLING

No. 3732 — MAXALT Tablets, 5 mg, are pale pink, capsule-shaped, compressed tablets coded MRK on one side and 266 on the other:

NDC 0006-0266-18, carton of 18 tablets.

No. 3733 — MAXALT Tablets, 10 mg, are pale pink, capsule-shaped, compressed tablets coded MAXALT on one side and MRK 267 on the other:

NDC 0006-0267-18, carton of 18 tablets.

No. 3800 — MAXALT-MLT Orally Disintegrating Tablets, 5 mg, are white to off-white, round lyophilized orally disintegrating tablets debossed with a modified triangle on one side, and measuring 10.0-11.5 mm (side-to-side) with a peppermint flavor. Each orally disintegrating tablet is individually packaged in a blister inside an aluminum pouch (sachet). They are supplied as follows:

NDC 0006-3800-18, 6 × unit of use carrying case of 3 orally disintegrating tablets (18 tablets total).

No. 3801 — MAXALT-MLT Orally Disintegrating Tablets, 10 mg, are white to off-white, round lyophilized orally disintegrating tablets debossed with a modified square on one side, and measuring 12.0-13.8 mm (side-to-side) with a peppermint flavor. Each orally disintegrating tablet is individually packaged in a blister inside an aluminum pouch (sachet). They are supplied as follows:

NDC 0006-3801-18, 6 × unit of use carrying case of 3 orally disintegrating tablets (18 tablets total).

Storage

Store MAXALT Tablets at room temperature, 59-86°F (15-30°C).

Store MAXALT-MLT Orally Disintegrating Tablets at room temperature, 59-86°F (15-30°C).

17 PATIENT COUNSELING INFORMATION

See FDA-Approved Patient Labeling (Patient Information).

Risk of Myocardial Ischemia and/or Infarction, Prinzmetal's Angina, Other Vasospasm-Related Events, and Cerebrovascular Events

Inform patients that MAXALT may cause serious cardiovascular side effects such as myocardial infarction or stroke. Although serious cardiovascular events can occur without warning symptoms, patients should be alert for the signs and symptoms of chest pain, shortness of breath, weakness, slurring of speech, and should ask for medical advice when observing any indicative sign or symptoms. Patients should be apprised of the importance of this follow-up *[see Warnings and Precautions (5.1, 5.2, 5.4, 5.5)]*.

Serotonin Syndrome

Patients should be cautioned about the risk of serotonin syndrome with the use of MAXALT or other triptans, particularly during combined use with selective serotonin reuptake inhibitors (SSRIs) or serotonin norepinephrine reuptake inhibitors (SNRIs) *[see Warnings and Precautions (5.7), Drug Interactions (7.4), and Clinical Pharmacology (12.3)]*.

Pregnancy

Inform patients that MAXALT should not be used during pregnancy unless the potential benefit justifies the potential risk to the fetus *[see Use in Specific Populations (8.1)]*.

Nursing Mothers

Advise patients to notify their healthcare provider if they are breastfeeding or plan to breastfeed *[see Use in Specific Populations (8.3)]*.

Ability to Perform Complex Tasks

Since migraines or treatment with MAXALT may cause somnolence and dizziness, instruct patients to evaluate their ability to perform complex tasks during migraine attacks and after administration of MAXALT.

Medication Overuse Headache

Inform patients that use of acute migraine drugs for 10 or more days per month may lead to an exacerbation of headache, and encourage patients to record headache frequency and drug use (e.g., by keeping a headache diary) *[see Warnings and Precautions (5.6)]*.

Handling of Orally Disintegrating Tablets Packages

Instruct patients not to remove the blister from the outer aluminum pouch until ready to use the orally disintegrating tablet inside *[see Dosage and Administration (2.3)]*.

Patients with Phenylketonuria

Inform phenylketonuric patients that MAXALT-MLT Orally Disintegrating Tablets contain phenylalanine (a component of aspartame). Each 5-mg orally disintegrating tablet contains 1.1 mg phenylalanine, and each 10-mg orally disintegrating tablet contains 2.1 mg phenylalanine *[see Use in Specific Populations (8.6)]*.

MAXALT Tablets and MAXALT-MLT Orally Disintegrating Tablets are manufactured for:
Merck Sharp & Dohme Corp., a subsidiary of
MERCK & CO., INC., Whitehouse Station, NJ 08889, USA
MAXALT Tablets are manufactured by:
Merck Sharp & Dohme Ltd.
Cramlington, Northumberland NE23 3JU, United Kingdom
MAXALT-MLT Orally Disintegrating Tablets are manufactured by:
Catalent UK Swindon, Zydis Ltd.
Swindon, Wiltshire, SN5 8RU, United Kingdom

Revised: 01/2013
USPI-T-MLT-04621301R011

Patient Information
MAXALT® (max-awlt) and MAXALT-MLT®
rizatriptan benzoate
Tablets and Orally Disintegrating Tablets

Read this Patient Information before you start taking MAXALT® and each time you get a refill. There may be new information. This information does not take the place of talking to your doctor about your medical condition or your treatment.

Unless otherwise stated, the information in this Patient Information leaflet applies to both MAXALT Tablets and to MAXALT-MLT® Orally Disintegrating Tablets.

What is MAXALT?

MAXALT is a prescription medicine that belongs to a class of medicines called Triptans. MAXALT is available as a traditional tablet (MAXALT) and as an orally disintegrating tablet (MAXALT-MLT).

MAXALT and MAXALT-MLT are used to treat migraine attacks with or without aura in adults and in children 6 to 17 years of age.

MAXALT is not to be used to prevent migraine attacks.

MAXALT is not for the treatment of hemiplegic or basilar migraines.

It is not known if MAXALT is safe and effective for the treatment of cluster headaches.

It is not known if taking more than 1 dose of MAXALT in 24 hours is safe and effective in children 6 to 17 years of age.

It is not known if MAXALT is safe and effective in children under 6 years of age.

Who should not take MAXALT?

Do not take MAXALT if you:

- have or have had heart problems
- have or have had a stroke or a transient ischemic attack (TIA)
- have or have had blood vessel problems including ischemic bowel disease
- have uncontrolled high blood pressure
- have taken other Triptan medicines in the last 24 hours
- have taken ergot-containing medicines in the last 24 hours
- have hemiplegic or basilar migraines
- take monoamine oxidase (MAO) inhibitor or have taken a MAO inhibitor within the last 2 weeks
- are allergic to rizatriptan benzoate or any of the ingredients in MAXALT. See the end of this leaflet for a complete list of ingredients in MAXALT.

Talk to your doctor before taking this medicine if you have any of the conditions listed above or if you are not sure if you take any of these medicines.

What should I tell my doctor before taking MAXALT?

Before you take MAXALT, tell your doctor if you:

- have or have had heart problems, high blood pressure, chest pain, or shortness of breath
- have any risk factors for heart problems or blood vessel problems such as:
  - high blood pressure
  - high cholesterol
  - smoking
  - obesity
  - diabetes
  - family history of heart problems
  - you are post menopausal
  - you are a male over 40
- have phenylketonuria (PKU). MAXALT-MLT orally disintegrating tablets contain phenylalanine.
- have kidney or liver problems
- have any other medical condition
- are pregnant or plan to become pregnant. It is not known if MAXALT will harm your unborn baby. If you become pregnant while taking MAXALT, talk to your healthcare provider about registering with the pregnancy registry at the Merck National Service Center. You can enroll in this registry by calling 1-800-986-8999. The purpose of this registry is to collect information about the safety of MAXALT in pregnancy.
- are breastfeeding or plan to breastfeed. It is not known if MAXALT passes into your breast milk. Talk to your doctor about the best way to feed your baby if you take MAXALT.

Tell your doctor about all the medicines you take, including prescription and nonprescription medicines, vitamins, and herbal supplements.
MAXALT and other medicines may affect each other causing side effects. MAXALT may affect the way other medicines work, and other medicines may affect how MAXALT works.
Especially tell your doctor if you take:
- propranolol containing medicines such as Inderal®, Inderal® LA, or Innopran® XL
- medicines used to treat mood disorders, including selective serotonin reuptake inhibitors (SSRIs) or serotonin norepinephrine reuptake inhibitors (SNRIs).

Ask your doctor or pharmacist for a list of these medicines, if you are not sure.
Know the medicines you take. Keep a list of them to show your doctor and pharmacist when you get a new medicine.
How should I take MAXALT?
- Take MAXALT exactly as your doctor tells you to take it.
- Your doctor will tell you how much MAXALT to take and when to take it.
- **To take MAXALT-MLT:**
  - Leave MAXALT-MLT orally disintegrating tablets in the package it comes in until you are ready to take it. When you are ready to take it:
    - Remove the blister from the foil pouch. Do not push the MAXALT-MLT orally disintegrating tablet through the blister.
    - Peel open the blister pack with dry hands and place the MAXALT-MLT orally disintegrating tablet on your tongue. The tablet will dissolve and be swallowed with your saliva. No liquid is needed to take the orally disintegrating tablet.
- If your headache comes back after your first MAXALT dose:
  - For adults: a second dose may be taken 2 hours after the first dose. Do not take more than 30 mg of MAXALT in a 24-hour period (for example, do not take more than 3 10-mg tablets in a 24-hour period).
  - For children 6 to 17 years of age: It is not known if taking more than 1 dose of MAXALT in 24 hours is safe and effective. Talk to your doctor about what to do if your headache does not go away or comes back.
- If you take too much MAXALT, call your doctor or go to the nearest hospital emergency room right away.

What should I avoid while taking MAXALT?
MAXALT may cause dizziness, weakness, or fainting. If you have these symptoms, do not drive a car, use machinery, or do anything that needs you to be alert.
What are the possible side effects of MAXALT?
MAXALT may cause serious side effects. Call your doctor or go to the nearest hospital emergency room right away if you think you are having any of the serious side effects of MAXALT including:
- **heart attack.** Symptoms of a heart attack may include:
  - chest discomfort in the center of your chest that lasts for more than a few minutes or that goes away and comes back
  - chest discomfort that feels like uncomfortable pressure, squeezing, fullness or pain
  - pain or discomfort in your arms, back, neck, jaw or stomach
  - shortness of breath with or without chest discomfort
  - breaking out in a cold sweat
  - nausea or vomiting
  - feeling lightheaded
- **stroke.** Symptoms of a stroke may include the following sudden symptoms:
  - numbness or weakness in your face, arm or leg, especially on one side of your body
  - confusion, problems speaking or understanding
  - problems seeing in 1 or both of your eyes
  - problems walking, dizziness, loss of balance or coordination
  - severe headache with no known cause
- **blood vessel problems.** Symptoms of blood vessel problems may include:
  - stomach pain
  - bloody diarrhea
  - vision problems
  - coldness and numbness of hands and feet
- **serotonin syndrome.** A condition called serotonin syndrome can happen when Triptan medicines such as MAXALT are taken with certain other medicines. Symptoms of serotonin syndrome may include:
  - agitation
  - hallucinations
  - coma
  - fast heartbeat
  - fast changes in your blood pressure
  - increased body temperature
  - muscle spasm
  - loss of coordination
  - nausea, vomiting or diarrhea
- **increased blood pressure.**

The most common side effects of MAXALT in adults include:
- feeling sleepy or tired
- pain or pressure in your chest or throat
- dizziness

Tell your doctor if you have any side effect that bothers you or that does not go away.
If you take MAXALT too often, this may result in you getting chronic headaches. In such cases, you should contact your doctor, as you may have to stop taking MAXALT.
These are not all the possible side effects of MAXALT. For more information, ask your doctor or pharmacist.
Call your doctor for medical advice about side effects. You may report side effects to FDA at 1-800-FDA-1088.
How should I store MAXALT?
- Store MAXALT at room temperature between 59°F to 86°F (15°C to 30°C).
- Safely throw away medicine that is out of date or no longer needed.

Keep MAXALT and all medicines out of the reach of children.
General Information about the safe and effective use of MAXALT.
Medicines are sometimes prescribed for purposes other than those listed in a Patient Information leaflet. Do not use MAXALT for a condition for which it was not prescribed. Do not give MAXALT to other people, even if they have the same symptoms that you have. It may harm them.
This Patient Information leaflet summarizes the most important information about MAXALT. If you would like more information, talk to your doctor. You can ask your pharmacist or doctor for information about MAXALT that is written for health professionals.
For more information, go to www.maxalt.com or call 1-800-986-8999.
What are the ingredients in MAXALT?
Active ingredient in MAXALT and MAXALT-MLT orally disintegrating tablets:
rizatriptan benzoate.
Inactive ingredients in MAXALT: lactose monohydrate, microcrystalline cellulose, pregelatinized starch, ferric oxide (red), and magnesium stearate.
Inactive ingredients in MAXALT-MLT orally disintegrating tablets: gelatin, mannitol, glycine, aspartame, and peppermint flavor.
MAXALT-MLT orally disintegrating tablets contain aspartame, a source of phenylalanine.
Phenylketonurics:
MAXALT-MLT orally disintegrating tablets 5-mg contain 1.1 mg of phenylalanine. MAXALT-MLT orally disintegrating tablets 10-mg contain 2.1 mg of phenylalanine.
This Patient Information has been approved by the U.S. Food and Drug Administration.
MAXALT Tablets and MAXALT-MLT Orally Disintegrating Tablets are manufactured for:
Merck Sharp & Dohme Corp., a subsidiary of
MERCK & CO., INC., Whitehouse Station, NJ 08889, USA
MAXALT Tablets are manufactured by:
Merck Sharp & Dohme Ltd.
Cramlington, Northumberland NE23 3JU, United Kingdom
MAXALT-MLT Orally Disintegrating Tablets are manufactured by:
Catalent UK Swindon, Zydis Ltd.
Swindon, Wiltshire, SN5 8RU, United Kingdom
The brands listed are the trademarks of their respective owners.

Revised: 01/2013
USPPI-T-MLT-04621301R011
Shown in Product Identification Guide, page 308

MEVACOR® (LOVASTATIN) TABLETS

℞

DESCRIPTION

MEVACOR® (Lovastatin) is a cholesterol lowering agent isolated from a strain of *Aspergillus terreus*. After oral ingestion, lovastatin, which is an inactive lactone, is hydrolyzed to the corresponding β–hydroxyacid form. This is a principal metabolite and an inhibitor of 3–hydroxy-3–methylglutaryl-coenzyme A (HMG–CoA) reductase. This enzyme catalyzes the conversion of HMG–CoA to mevalonate, which is an early and rate limiting step in the biosynthesis of cholesterol.
Lovastatin is [1*S*-[1α(*R**),3α,7β,8β(2*S**,4*S**), 8aβ]]-1,2,3,7,8,8a–hexahydro-3,7–dimethyl-8-[2–(tetrahydro-4-hydroxy-6-oxo-2*H*-pyran-2–yl)ethyl]-1-naphthalenyl 2-methylbutanoate. The empirical formula of lovastatin is $C_{24}H_{36}O_5$ and its molecular weight is 404.55. Its structural formula is:

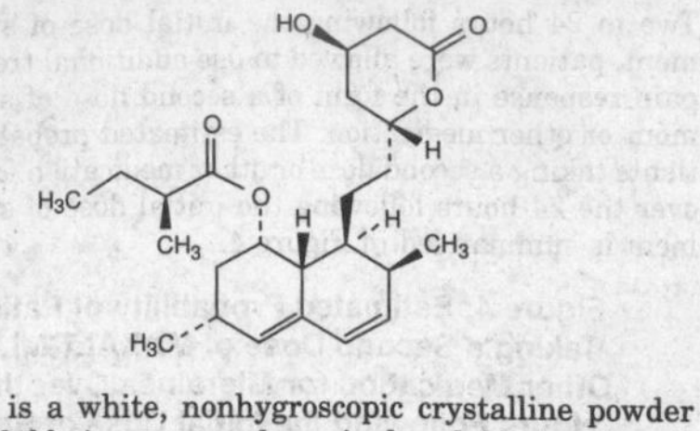

Lovastatin is a white, nonhygroscopic crystalline powder that is insoluble in water and sparingly soluble in ethanol, methanol, and acetonitrile.
Tablets MEVACOR are supplied as 20 mg and 40 mg tablets for oral administration. In addition to the active ingredient lovastatin, each tablet contains the following inactive ingredients: cellulose, lactose, magnesium stearate, and starch. Butylated hydroxyanisole (BHA) is added as a preservative. Tablets MEVACOR 20 mg also contain FD&C Blue 2 aluminum lake. Tablets MEVACOR 40 mg also contain D&C Yellow 10 aluminum lake and FD&C Blue 2 aluminum lake.

CLINICAL PHARMACOLOGY

The involvement of low-density lipoprotein cholesterol (LDL–C) in atherogenesis has been well-documented in clinical and pathological studies, as well as in many animal experiments. Epidemiological and clinical studies have established that high LDL–C and low high-density lipoprotein cholesterol (HDL–C) are both associated with coronary heart disease. However, the risk of developing coronary heart disease is continuous and graded over the range of cholesterol levels and many coronary events do occur in patients with total cholesterol (total–C) and LDL–C in the lower end of this range.
MEVACOR has been shown to reduce both normal and elevated LDL–C concentrations. LDL is formed from very low-density lipoprotein (VLDL) and is catabolized predominantly by the high affinity LDL receptor. The mechanism of the LDL-lowering effect of MEVACOR may involve both reduction of VLDL–C concentration, and induction of the LDL receptor, leading to reduced production and/or increased catabolism of LDL–C. Apolipoprotein B also falls substantially during treatment with MEVACOR. Since each LDL particle contains one molecule of apolipoprotein B, and since little apolipoprotein B is found in other lipoproteins, this strongly suggests that MEVACOR does not merely cause cholesterol to be lost from LDL, but also reduces the concentration of circulating LDL particles. In addition, MEVACOR can produce increases of variable magnitude in HDL–C, and modestly reduces VLDL–C and plasma triglycerides (TG) (see Tables II-IV under Clinical Studies). The effects of MEVACOR on Lp(a), fibrinogen, and certain other independent biochemical risk markers for coronary heart disease are unknown.
MEVACOR is a specific inhibitor of HMG–CoA reductase, the enzyme which catalyzes the conversion of HMG–CoA to mevalonate. The conversion of HMG–CoA to mevalonate is an early step in the biosynthetic pathway for cholesterol.
Pharmacokinetics
Lovastatin is a lactone which is readily hydrolyzed *in vivo* to the corresponding β–hydroxyacid, a strong inhibitor of HMG–CoA reductase. Inhibition of HMG–CoA reductase is the basis for an assay in pharmacokinetic studies of the β–hydroxyacid metabolites (active inhibitors) and, following base hydrolysis, active plus latent inhibitors (total inhibitors) in plasma following administration of lovastatin.
Following an oral dose of ^{14}C–labeled lovastatin in man, 10% of the dose was excreted in urine and 83% in feces. The latter represents absorbed drug equivalents excreted in bile, as well as any unabsorbed drug. Plasma concentrations of total radioactivity (lovastatin plus ^{14}C–metabolites) peaked at 2 hours and declined rapidly to about 10% of peak by 24 hours postdose. Absorption of lovastatin, estimated relative to an intravenous reference dose, in each of four animal species tested, averaged about 30% of an oral dose. In animal studies, after oral dosing, lovastatin had high selectivity for the liver, where it achieved substantially higher concentrations than in non-target tissues. Lovastatin undergoes extensive first-pass extraction in the liver, its primary site of action, with subsequent excretion of drug equivalents in the bile. As a consequence of extensive hepatic extraction of lovastatin, the availability of drug to the general circulation is low and variable. In a single dose study in four hypercholesterolemic patients, it was estimated that less than 5% of an oral dose of lovastatin reaches the general circulation as active inhibitors. Following administration of lovastatin tablets the coefficient of variation, based on between-subject variability, was approximately 40% for the area under the curve (AUC) of total inhibitory activity in the general circulation.
Both lovastatin and its β–hydroxyacid metabolite are highly bound (>95%) to human plasma proteins. Animal studies demonstrated that lovastatin crosses the blood-brain and placental barriers.

The major active metabolites present in human plasma are the β–hydroxyacid of lovastatin, its 6′–hydroxy derivative, and two additional metabolites. Peak plasma concentrations of both active and total inhibitors were attained within 2 to 4 hours of dose administration. While the recommended therapeutic dose range is 10 to 80 mg/day, linearity of inhibitory activity in the general circulation was established by a single dose study employing lovastatin tablet dosages from 60 to as high as 120 mg. With a once-a-day dosing regimen, plasma concentrations of total inhibitors over a dosing interval achieved a steady state between the second and third days of therapy and were about 1.5 times those following a single dose. When lovastatin was given under fasting conditions, plasma concentrations of total inhibitors were on average about two-thirds those found when lovastatin was administered immediately after a standard test meal.

In a study of patients with severe renal insufficiency (creatinine clearance 10–30 mL/min), the plasma concentrations of total inhibitors after a single dose of lovastatin were approximately two-fold higher than those in healthy volunteers.

In a study including 16 elderly patients between 70–78 years of age who received MEVACOR 80 mg/day, the mean plasma level of HMG–CoA reductase inhibitory activity was increased approximately 45% compared with 18 patients between 18–30 years of age (see PRECAUTIONS, Geriatric Use).

Although the mechanism is not fully understood, cyclosporine has been shown to increase the AUC of HMG-CoA reductase inhibitors. The increase in AUC for lovastatin and lovastatin acid is presumably due, in part, to inhibition of CYP3A4.

The risk of myopathy is increased by high levels of HMG–CoA reductase inhibitory activity in plasma. Strong inhibitors of CYP3A4 can raise the plasma levels of HMG–CoA reductase inhibitory activity and increase the risk of myopathy (see WARNINGS, Myopathy/Rhabdomyolysis and PRECAUTIONS, Drug Interactions).

Lovastatin is a substrate for cytochrome P450 isoform 3A4 (CYP3A4) (see PRECAUTIONS, Drug Interactions). Grapefruit juice contains one or more components that inhibit CYP3A4 and can increase the plasma concentrations of drugs metabolized by CYP3A4. In one study[1], 10 subjects consumed 200 mL of double-strength grapefruit juice (one can of frozen concentrate diluted with one rather than 3 cans of water) three times daily for 2 days and an additional 200 mL double-strength grapefruit juice together with and 30 and 90 minutes following a single dose of 80 mg lovastatin on the third day. This regimen of grapefruit juice resulted in a mean increase in the serum concentration of lovastatin and its β–hydroxyacid metabolite (as measured by the area under the concentration-time curve) of 15–fold and 5–fold, respectively [as measured using a chemical assay — high performance liquid chromatography]. In a second study, 15 subjects consumed one 8 oz glass of single-strength grapefruit juice (one can of frozen concentrate diluted with 3 cans of water) with breakfast for 3 consecutive days and a single dose of 40 mg lovastatin in the evening of the third day. This regimen of grapefruit juice resulted in a mean increase in the plasma concentration (as measured by the area under the concentration-time curve) of active and total HMG–CoA reductase inhibitory activity [using an enzyme inhibition assay both before (for active inhibitors) and after (for total inhibitors) base hydrolysis] of 1.34–fold and 1.36–fold, respectively, and of lovastatin and its β–hydroxyacid metabolite [measured using a chemical assay — liquid chromatography/tandem mass spectrometry — different from that used in the first[1] study] of 1.94–fold and 1.57–fold, respectively. The effect of amounts of grapefruit juice between those used in these two studies on lovastatin pharmacokinetics has not been studied.

[See table I above]

[1]Kantola, T, et al., Clin Pharmacol Ther 1998; 63(4):397–402.

TABLE I: The Effect of Other Drugs on Lovastatin Exposure When Both Were Co-administered

	Number of Subjects	Dosing of Coadministered Drug or Grapefruit Juice	Dosing of Lovastatin	AUC Ratio* (with / without coadministered drug) No Effect = 1.00	
				Lovastatin	Lovastatin acid†
Gemfibrozil	11	600 mg BID for 3 days	40 mg	0.96	2.80
Itraconazole‡	12	200 mg QD for 4 days	40 mg on Day 4	> 36§	22
	10	100 mg QD for 4 days	40 mg on Day 4	> 14.8§	15.4
Grapefruit Juice¶ (high dose)	10	200 mL of double-strength TID#	80 mg single dose	15.3	5.0
Grapefruit Juice¶ (low dose)	16	8 oz (about 250 mL) of single-strengthÞ for 4 days	40 mg single dose	1.94	1.57
Cyclosporine	16	Not describedß	10 mg QD for 10 days	5- to 8-fold	NDà
	Number of Subjects	Dosing of Coadministered Drug or Grapefruit Juice	Dosing of Lovastatin	AUC Ratio* (with / without coadministered drug) No Effect = 1.00	
				Total Lovastatin acidè	
Diltiazem	10	120 mg BID for 14 days	20 mg	3.57è	

* Results based on a chemical assay.
† Lovastatin acid refers to the β-hydroxyacid of lovastatin.
‡ The mean total AUC of lovastatin without itraconazole phase could not be determined accurately. Results could be representative of strong CYP3A4 inhibitors such as ketoconazole, posaconazole, clarithromycin, telithromycin, HIV protease inhibitors, and nefazodone.
§ Estimated minimum change.
¶ The effect of amounts of grapefruit juice between those used in these two studies on lovastatin pharmacokinetics has not been studied.
# Double-strength: one can of frozen concentrate diluted with one can of water. Grapefruit juice was administered TID for 2 days, and 200 mL together with single dose lovastatin and 30 and 90 minutes following single dose lovastatin on Day 3.
Þ Single-strength: one can of frozen concentrate diluted with 3 cans of water. Grapefruit juice was administered with breakfast for 3 days, and lovastatin was administered in the evening on Day 3.
ß Cyclosporine-treated patients with psoriasis or post kidney or heart transplant patients with stable graft function, transplanted at least 9 months prior to study.
à ND = Analyte not determined.
è Lactone converted to acid by hydrolysis prior to analysis. Figure represents total unmetabolized acid and lactone.

Clinical Studies in Adults

MEVACOR has been shown to be highly effective in reducing total–C and LDL–C in heterozygous familial and non-familial forms of primary hypercholesterolemia and in mixed hyperlipidemia. A marked response was seen within 2 weeks, and the maximum therapeutic response occurred within 4–6 weeks. The response was maintained during continuation of therapy. Single daily doses given in the evening were more effective than the same dose given in the morning, perhaps because cholesterol is synthesized mainly at night.

In multicenter, double-blind studies in patients with familial or non-familial hypercholesterolemia, MEVACOR, administered in doses ranging from 10 mg q.p.m. to 40 mg b.i.d., was compared to placebo. MEVACOR consistently and significantly decreased plasma total–C, LDL–C, total–C/HDL–C ratio and LDL–C/HDL–C ratio. In addition, MEVACOR produced increases of variable magnitude in HDL–C, and modestly decreased VLDL–C and plasma TG (see Tables II through IV for dose response results).

The results of a study in patients with primary hypercholesterolemia are presented in Table II.

[See table II at top of next page]

MEVACOR was compared to cholestyramine in a randomized open parallel study. The study was performed with patients with hypercholesterolemia who were at high risk of myocardial infarction. Summary results are presented in Table III.

[See table III at top of next page]

MEVACOR was studied in controlled trials in hypercholesterolemic patients with well-controlled non-insulin dependent diabetes mellitus with normal renal function. The effect of MEVACOR on lipids and lipoproteins and the safety profile of MEVACOR were similar to that demonstrated in studies in nondiabetics. MEVACOR had no clinically important effect on glycemic control or on the dose requirement of oral hypoglycemic agents.

Expanded Clinical Evaluation of Lovastatin (EXCEL) Study

MEVACOR was compared to placebo in 8,245 patients with hypercholesterolemia (total-C 240-300 mg/dL [6.2 mmol/L - 7.6 mmol/L], LDL–C >160 mg/dL [4.1 mmol/L]) in the randomized, double-blind, parallel, 48–week EXCEL study. All changes in the lipid measurements (Table IV) in MEVACOR treated patients were dose-related and significantly different from placebo (p≤0.001). These results were sustained throughout the study.

[See table IV at top of next page]

Air Force/Texas Coronary Atherosclerosis Prevention Study (AFCAPS/TexCAPS)

The Air Force/Texas Coronary Atherosclerosis Prevention Study (AFCAPS/TexCAPS), a double blind, randomized, placebo-controlled, primary prevention study, demonstrated that treatment with MEVACOR decreased the rate of acute major coronary events (composite endpoint of myocardial infarction, unstable angina, and sudden cardiac death) compared with placebo during a median of 5.1 years of follow-up. Participants were middle-aged and elderly men (ages 45-73) and women (ages 55-73) without symptomatic cardiovascular disease with average to moderately elevated total–C and LDL–C, below average HDL–C, and who were at high risk based on elevated total–C/HDL–C. In addition to age, 63% of the participants had at least one other risk factor (baseline HDL–C <35 mg/dL, hypertension, family history, smoking and diabetes).

AFCAPS/TexCAPS enrolled 6,605 participants (5,608 men, 997 women) based on the following lipid entry criteria: total–C range of 180-264 mg/dL, LDL–C range of 130-190 mg/dL, HDL–C of ≤45 mg/dL for men and ≤47 mg/dL for women, and TG of ≤400 mg/dL. Participants were treated with standard care, including diet, and either MEVACOR 20-40 mg daily (n=3,304) or placebo (n=3,301). Approximately 50% of the participants treated with MEVACOR were titrated to 40 mg daily when their LDL–C remained >110 mg/dL at the 20–mg starting dose.

MEVACOR reduced the risk of a first acute major coronary event, the primary efficacy endpoint, by 37% (MEVACOR 3.5%, placebo 5.5%; p<0.001; Figure 1). A first acute major coronary event was defined as myocardial infarction (54 participants on MEVACOR, 94 on placebo) or unstable angina (54 vs. 80) or sudden cardiac death (8 vs. 9). Furthermore, among the secondary endpoints, MEVACOR reduced the risk of unstable angina by 32% (1.8 vs. 2.6%; p=0.023), of myocardial infarction by 40% (1.7 vs. 2.9%; p=0.002), and of undergoing coronary revascularization procedures (e.g., coronary artery bypass grafting or percutaneous transluminal coronary angioplasty) by 33% (3.2 vs. 4.8%; p=0.001). Trends in risk reduction associated with treatment with MEVACOR were consistent across men and women, smokers and non-smokers, hypertensives and non-hypertensives, and older and younger participants. Participants with ≥2 risk factors had risk reductions (RR) in both acute major coronary events (RR 43%) and coronary revascularization procedures (RR 37%). Because there were too few events among those participants with age as their only risk factor in this study, the effect of MEVACOR on outcomes could not be adequately assessed in this subgroup.

TABLE II: MEVACOR vs. Placebo (Mean Percent Change from Baseline After 6 Weeks)

DOSAGE	N	TOTAL-C	LDL-C	HDL-C	LDL-C/ HDL-C	TOTAL-C/ HDL-C	TG.
Placebo	33	−2	−1	−1	0	+1	+9
MEVACOR							
10 mg q.p.m.	33	−16	−21	+5	−24	−19	−10
20 mg q.p.m.	33	−19	−27	+6	−30	−23	+9
10 mg b.i.d.	32	−19	−28	+8	−33	−25	−7
40 mg q.p.m.	33	−22	−31	+5	−33	−25	−8
20 mg b.i.d.	36	−24	−32	+2	−32	−24	−6

TABLE III: MEVACOR vs. Cholestyramine (Percent Change from Baseline After 12 Weeks)

TREATMENT	N	TOTAL-C (mean)	LDL-C (mean)	HDL-C (mean)	LDL-C/ HDL-C (mean)	TOTAL-C/ HDL-C (mean)	VLDL-C (median)	TG. (mean)
MEVACOR								
20 mg b.i.d.	85	−27	−32	+9	−36	−31	−34	−21
40 mg b.i.d.	88	−34	−42	+8	−44	−37	−31	−27
Cholestyramine								
12 g b.i.d.	88	−17	−23	+8	−27	−21	+2	+11

TABLE IV: MEVACOR vs. Placebo (Percent Change from Baseline — Average Values Between Weeks 12 and 48)

DOSAGE	N*	TOTAL-C (mean)	LDL-C (mean)	HDL-C (mean)	LDL-C/ HDL-C (mean)	TOTAL-C/ HDL-C (mean)	TG. (median)
Placebo	1663	+0.7	+0.4	+2.0	+0.2	+0.6	+4
MEVACOR							
20 mg q.p.m.	1642	−17	−24	+6.6	−27	−21	−10
40 mg q.p.m.	1645	−22	−30	+7.2	−34	−26	−14
20 mg b.i.d.	1646	−24	−34	+8.6	−38	−29	−16
40 mg b.i.d.	1649	−29	−40	+9.5	−44	−34	−19

* Patients enrolled

TABLE V: Lipid-lowering Effects of Lovastatin in Adolescent Boys with Heterozygous Familial Hypercholesterolemia (Mean Percent Change from Baseline at Week 48 in Intention-to-Treat Population)

DOSAGE	N	TOTAL-C	LDL-C	HDL-C	TG.*	Apolipoprotein B
Placebo	61	−1.1	−1.4	−2.2	−1.4	−4.4
MEVACOR	64	−19.3	−24.2	+1.1	−1.9	−21

* data presented as median percent changes

TABLE VI: Lipid-lowering Effects of Lovastatin in Post-Menarchal Girls with Heterozygous Familial Hypercholesterolemia (Mean Percent Change from Baseline at Week 24 in Intention-to-Treat Population)

DOSAGE	N	TOTAL-C	LDL-C	HDL-C	TG.*	Apolipoprotein B
Placebo	18	+3.6	+2.5	+4.8	−3.0	+6.4
MEVACOR	35	−22.4	−29.2	+2.4	−22.7	−24.4

* data presented as median percent changes

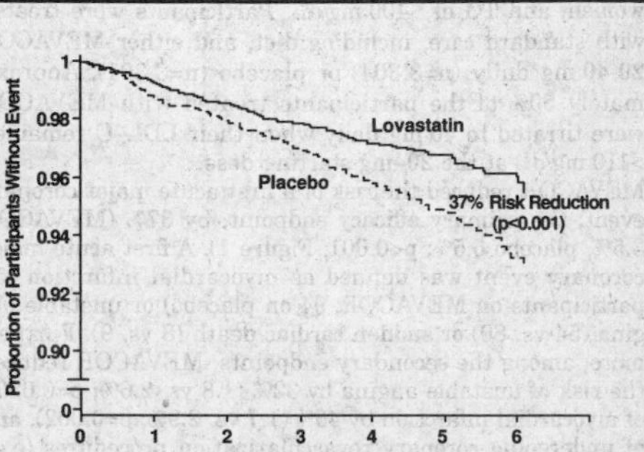

Figure 1: Acute Major Coronary Events (Primary Endpoint)

Atherosclerosis

In the Canadian Coronary Atherosclerosis Intervention Trial (CCAIT), the effect of therapy with lovastatin on coronary atherosclerosis was assessed by coronary angiography in hyperlipidemic patients. In the randomized, double-blind, controlled clinical trial, patients were treated with conventional measures (usually diet and 325 mg of aspirin every other day) and either lovastatin 20-80 mg daily or placebo. Angiograms were evaluated at baseline and at two years by computerized quantitative coronary angiography (QCA). Lovastatin significantly slowed the progression of lesions as measured by the mean change per-patient in minimum lumen diameter (the primary endpoint) and percent diameter stenosis, and decreased the proportions of patients categorized with disease progression (33% vs. 50%) and with new lesions (16% vs. 32%).

In a similarly designed trial, the Monitored Atherosclerosis Regression Study (MARS), patients were treated with diet and either lovastatin 80 mg daily or placebo. No statistically significant difference between lovastatin and placebo was seen for the primary endpoint (mean change per patient in percent diameter stenosis of all lesions), or for most secondary QCA endpoints. Visual assessment by angiographers who formed a consensus opinion of overall angiographic change (Global Change Score) was also a secondary endpoint. By this endpoint, significant slowing of disease was seen, with regression in 23% of patients treated with lovastatin compared to 11% of placebo patients.

In the Familial Atherosclerosis Treatment Study (FATS), either lovastatin or niacin in combination with a bile acid sequestrant for 2.5 years in hyperlipidemic subjects significantly reduced the frequency of progression and increased the frequency of regression of coronary atherosclerotic lesions by QCA compared to diet and, in some cases, low-dose resin.

The effect of lovastatin on the progression of atherosclerosis in the coronary arteries has been corroborated by similar findings in another vasculature. In the Asymptomatic Carotid Artery Progression Study (ACAPS), the effect of therapy with lovastatin on carotid atherosclerosis was assessed by B–mode ultrasonography in hyperlipidemic patients with early carotid lesions and without known coronary heart disease at baseline. In this double-blind, controlled clinical trial, 919 patients were randomized in a 2 × 2 factorial design to placebo, lovastatin 10-40 mg daily and/or warfarin. Ultrasonograms of the carotid walls were used to determine the change per patient from baseline to three years in mean maximum intimal-medial thickness (IMT) of 12 measured segments. There was a significant regression of carotid lesions in patients receiving lovastatin alone compared to those receiving placebo alone (p=0.001). The predictive value of changes in IMT for stroke has not yet been established. In the lovastatin group there was a significant reduction in the number of patients with major cardiovascular events relative to the placebo group (5 vs. 14) and a significant reduction in all-cause mortality (1 vs. 8).

Eye

There was a high prevalence of baseline lenticular opacities in the patient population included in the early clinical trials with lovastatin. During these trials the appearance of new opacities was noted in both the lovastatin and placebo groups. There was no clinically significant change in visual acuity in the patients who had new opacities reported nor was any patient, including those with opacities noted at baseline, discontinued from therapy because of a decrease in visual acuity.

A three–year, double-blind, placebo-controlled study in hypercholesterolemic patients to assess the effect of lovastatin on the human lens demonstrated that there were no clinically or statistically significant differences between the lovastatin and placebo groups in the incidence, type or progression of lenticular opacities. There are no controlled clinical data assessing the lens available for treatment beyond three years.

Clinical Studies in Adolescent Patients

Efficacy of Lovastatin in Adolescent Boys with Heterozygous Familial Hypercholesterolemia

In a double-blind, placebo-controlled study, 132 boys 10-17 years of age (mean age 12.7 yrs) with heterozygous familial hypercholesterolemia (heFH) were randomized to lovastatin (n=67) or placebo (n=65) for 48 weeks. Inclusion in the study required a baseline LDL–C level between 189 and 500 mg/dL and at least one parent with an LDL–C level >189 mg/dL. The mean baseline LDL–C value was 253.1 mg/dL (range: 171-379 mg/dL) in the MEVACOR group compared to 248.2 mg/dL (range: 158.5-413.5 mg/dL) in the placebo group. The dosage of lovastatin (once daily in the evening) was 10 mg for the first 8 weeks, 20 mg for the second 8 weeks, and 40 mg thereafter.

MEVACOR significantly decreased plasma levels of total–C, LDL–C and apolipoprotein B (see Table V).

[See table V above]

The mean achieved LDL–C value was 190.9 mg/dL (range: 108-336 mg/dL) in the MEVACOR group compared to 244.8 mg/dL (range: 135-404 mg/dL) in the placebo group.

Efficacy of Lovastatin in Post-Menarchal Girls with Heterozygous Familial Hypercholesterolemia

In a double-blind, placebo-controlled study, 54 girls 10-17 years of age who were at least 1 year post-menarche with heFH were randomized to lovastatin (n=35) or placebo (n=19) for 24 weeks. Inclusion in the study required a baseline LDL–C level of 160-400 mg/dL and a parental history of familial hypercholesterolemia. The mean baseline LDL–C value was 218.3 mg/dL (range: 136.3-363.7 mg/dL) in the MEVACOR group compared to 198.8 mg/dL (range: 151.1-283.1 mg/dL) in the placebo group. The dosage of lovastatin (once daily in the evening) was 20 mg for the first 4 weeks, and 40 mg thereafter.

MEVACOR significantly decreased plasma levels of total–C, LDL–C, and apolipoprotein B (see Table VI).

[See table VI above]

The mean achieved LDL–C value was 154.5 mg/dL (range: 82-286 mg/dL) in the MEVACOR group compared to 203.5 mg/dL (range: 135-304 mg/dL) in the placebo group.

The safety and efficacy of doses above 40 mg daily have not been studied in children. The long-term efficacy of lovastatin therapy in childhood to reduce morbidity and mortality in adulthood has not been established.

INDICATIONS AND USAGE

Therapy with MEVACOR should be a component of multiple risk factor intervention in those individuals with dyslipidemia at risk for atherosclerotic vascular disease. MEVACOR should be used in addition to a diet restricted in saturated fat and cholesterol as part of a treatment strategy to lower total–C and LDL–C to target levels when the response to diet and other nonpharmacological measures alone has been inadequate to reduce risk.

Primary Prevention of Coronary Heart Disease

In individuals without symptomatic cardiovascular disease, average to moderately elevated total–C and LDL–C, and below average HDL–C, MEVACOR is indicated to reduce the risk of:
- Myocardial infarction
- Unstable angina
- Coronary revascularization procedures

(See CLINICAL PHARMACOLOGY, Clinical Studies.)

Coronary Heart Disease

MEVACOR is indicated to slow the progression of coronary atherosclerosis in patients with coronary heart disease as part of a treatment strategy to lower total–C and LDL–C to target levels.

Hypercholesterolemia

Therapy with lipid-altering agents should be a component of multiple risk factor intervention in those individuals at significantly increased risk for atherosclerotic vascular disease due to hypercholesterolemia. MEVACOR is indicated as an adjunct to diet for the reduction of elevated total–C and LDL–C levels in patients with primary hypercholesterolemia (Types IIa and IIb[2]), when the response to diet restricted in saturated fat and cholesterol and to other nonpharmacological measures alone has been inadequate.

[2]Classification of Hyperlipoproteinemias

Type	Lipoproteins elevated	Lipid Elevations major	minor
I	chylomicrons	TG	↑→C
IIa	LDL	C	—
IIb	LDL, VLDL	C	TG
III (rare)	IDL	C/TG	—
IV	VLDL	TG	↑→C
V (rare)	chylomicrons, VLDL	TG	↑→C

IDL = intermediate-density lipoprotein.

Adolescent Patients with Heterozygous Familial Hypercholesterolemia

MEVACOR is indicated as an adjunct to diet to reduce total–C, LDL–C and apolipoprotein B levels in adolescent boys and girls who are at least one year post-menarche, 10-17 years of age, with heFH if after an adequate trial of diet therapy the following findings are present:

1. LDL-C remains >189 mg/dL or
2. LDL-C remains >160 mg/dL and:
   - there is a positive family history of premature cardiovascular disease or
   - two or more other CVD risk factors are present in the adolescent patient

General Recommendations

Prior to initiating therapy with lovastatin, secondary causes for hypercholesterolemia (e.g., poorly controlled diabetes mellitus, hypothyroidism, nephrotic syndrome, dysproteinemias, obstructive liver disease, other drug therapy, alcoholism) should be excluded, and a lipid profile performed to measure total–C, HDL–C, and TG. For patients with TG less than 400 mg/dL (<4.5 mmol/L), LDL–C can be estimated using the following equation:

LDL-C = total-C – [0.2 × (TG) + HDL-C]

For TG levels >400 mg/dL (>4.5 mmol/L), this equation is less accurate and LDL–C concentrations should be determined by ultracentrifugation. In hypertriglyceridemic patients, LDL–C may be low or normal despite elevated total–C. In such cases, MEVACOR is not indicated.

The National Cholesterol Education Program (NCEP) Treatment Guidelines are summarized below:

[See table above]

NCEP Treatment Guidelines: LDL–C Goals and Cutpoints for Therapeutic Lifestyle Changes and Drug Therapy in Different Risk Categories

Risk Category	LDL Goal (mg/dL)	LDL Level at Which to Initiate Therapeutic Lifestyle Changes (mg/dL)	LDL Level at Which to Consider Drug Therapy (mg/dL)
CHD* or CHD risk equivalents (10-year risk >20%)	<100	≥100	≥130 (100–129: drug optional)†
2+ Risk factors (10 year risk ≤20%)	<130	≥130	10-year risk 10–20%: ≥130 10-year risk <10%: ≥ 160
0–1 Risk factor‡	<160	≥160	≥190 (160–189: LDL-lowering drug optional)

* CHD, coronary heart disease

† Some authorities recommend use of LDL-lowering drugs in this category if an LDL–C level of <100 mg/dL cannot be achieved by therapeutic lifestyle changes. Others prefer use of drugs that primarily modify triglycerides and HDL–C, e.g., nicotinic acid or fibrate. Clinical judgment also may call for deferring drug therapy in this subcategory.

‡ Almost all people with 0–1 risk factor have a 10-year risk<10%; thus, 10-year risk assessment in people with 0–1 risk factor is not necessary.

After the LDL–C goal has been achieved, if the TG is still ≥200 mg/dL, non-HDL–C (total–C minus HDL–C) becomes a secondary target of therapy. Non-HDL–C goals are set 30 mg/dL higher than LDL–C goals for each risk category.

At the time of hospitalization for an acute coronary event, consideration can be given to initiating drug therapy at discharge if the LDL–C is ≥130 mg/dL (see NCEP Guidelines above).

Since the goal of treatment is to lower LDL–C, the NCEP recommends that LDL–C levels be used to initiate and assess treatment response. Only if LDL–C levels are not available, should the total–C be used to monitor therapy.

Although MEVACOR may be useful to reduce elevated LDL–C levels in patients with combined hypercholesterolemia and hypertriglyceridemia where hypercholesterolemia is the major abnormality (Type IIb hyperlipoproteinemia), it has not been studied in conditions where the major abnormality is elevation of chylomicrons, VLDL or IDL (i.e., hyperlipoproteinemia types I, III, IV, or V).[2]

The NCEP classification of cholesterol levels in pediatric patients with a familial history of hypercholesterolemia or premature cardiovascular disease is summarized below:

Category	Total-C (mg/dL)	LDL-C (mg/dL)
Acceptable	<170	<110
Borderline	170–199	110–129
High	≥200	≥130

Children treated with lovastatin in adolescence should be re-evaluated in adulthood and appropriate changes made to their cholesterol-lowering regimen to achieve adult goals for LDL–C.

CONTRAINDICATIONS

Hypersensitivity to any component of this medication.

Active liver disease or unexplained persistent elevations of serum transaminases (see WARNINGS).

Concomitant administration with strong CYP3A4 inhibitors (e.g., itraconazole, ketoconazole, posaconazole, voriconazole, HIV protease inhibitors, boceprevir, telaprevir, erythromycin, clarithromycin, telithromycin and nefazodone) (see WARNINGS, Myopathy/Rhabdomyolysis).

Pregnancy and lactation (see PRECAUTIONS, Pregnancy and Nursing Mothers). Atherosclerosis is a chronic process and the discontinuation of lipid-lowering drugs during pregnancy should have little impact on the outcome of long-term therapy of primary hypercholesterolemia. Moreover, cholesterol and other products of the cholesterol biosynthesis pathway are essential components for fetal development, including synthesis of steroids and cell membranes. Because of the ability of inhibitors of HMG–CoA reductase such as MEVACOR to decrease the synthesis of cholesterol and possibly other products of the cholesterol biosynthesis pathway, MEVACOR is contraindicated during pregnancy and in nursing mothers. **MEVACOR should be administered to women of childbearing age only when such patients are highly unlikely to conceive.** If the patient becomes pregnant while taking this drug, MEVACOR should be discontinued immediately and the patient should be apprised of the potential hazard to the fetus (see PRECAUTIONS, Pregnancy).

WARNINGS

Myopathy/Rhabdomyolysis

Lovastatin, like other inhibitors of HMG–CoA reductase, occasionally causes myopathy manifested as muscle pain, tenderness or weakness with creatine kinase (CK) above ten times the upper limit of normal (ULN). Myopathy sometimes takes the form of rhabdomyolysis with or without acute renal failure secondary to myoglobinuria, and rare fatalities have occurred. The risk of myopathy is increased by high levels of HMG–CoA reductase inhibitory activity in plasma.

As with other HMG-CoA reductase inhibitors, the risk of myopathy/rhabdomyolysis is dose related. In a clinical study (EXCEL) in which patients were carefully monitored and some interacting drugs were excluded, there was one case of myopathy among 4933 patients randomized to lovastatin 20-40 mg daily for 48 weeks, and 4 among 1649 patients randomized to 80 mg daily.

There have been rare reports of immune-mediated necrotizing myopathy (IMNM), an autoimmune myopathy, associated with statin use. IMNM is characterized by: proximal muscle weakness and elevated serum creatine kinase, which persist despite discontinuation of statin treatment; muscle biopsy showing necrotizing myopathy without significant inflammation; improvement with immunosuppressive agents.

All patients starting therapy with MEVACOR, or whose dose of MEVACOR is being increased, should be advised of the risk of myopathy and told to report promptly any unexplained muscle pain, tenderness or weakness particularly if accompanied by malaise or fever or if muscle signs and symptoms persist after discontinuing MEVACOR. MEVACOR therapy should be discontinued immediately if myopathy is diagnosed or suspected. In most cases, muscle symptoms and CK increases resolved when treatment was promptly discontinued. Periodic CK determinations may be considered in patients starting therapy with MEVACOR or whose dose is being increased, but there is no assurance that such monitoring will prevent myopathy.

Many of the patients who have developed rhabdomyolysis on therapy with lovastatin have had complicated medical histories, including renal insufficiency usually as a consequence of long-standing diabetes mellitus. Such patients merit closer monitoring. MEVACOR therapy should be discontinued if markedly elevated CPK levels occur or myopathy is diagnosed or suspected. MEVACOR therapy should also be temporarily withheld in any patient experiencing an acute or serious condition predisposing to the development of renal failure secondary to rhabdomyolysis, e.g., sepsis; hypotension; major surgery; trauma; severe metabolic, endocrine, or electrolyte disorders; or uncontrolled epilepsy.

The risk of myopathy/rhabdomyolysis is increased by concomitant use of lovastatin with the following:

Strong inhibitors of CYP3A4: Lovastatin, like several other inhibitors of HMG-CoA reductase, is a substrate of cytochrome P450 3A4 (CYP3A4). Certain drugs which inhibit this metabolic pathway can raise the plasma levels of lovastatin and may increase the risk of myopathy. These include itraconazole, ketoconazole, posaconazole, voriconazole, the macrolide antibiotics erythromycin and clarithromycin, the ketolide antibiotic telithromycin, HIV protease inhibitors, boceprevir, telaprevir, or the antidepressant nefazodone. Combination of these drugs with lovastatin is contraindicated. If short-term treatment with strong CYP3A4 inhibitors is unavoidable, therapy with lovastatin should be suspended during the course of treatment (see CONTRAINDICATIONS; PRECAUTIONS, Drug Interactions).

Gemfibrozil: The combined use of lovastatin with gemfibrozil should be avoided.

Other lipid-lowering drugs (other fibrates or ≥1 g/day of niacin): Caution should be used when prescribing other fibrates or lipid-lowering doses (≥1 g/day) of niacin with lovastatin, as these agents can cause myopathy when given alone. **The benefit of further alterations in lipid levels by the combined use of lovastatin with other fibrates or niacin should be carefully weighed against the potential risks of these combinations.**

Cyclosporine: The use of lovastatin with cyclosporine should be avoided.

Danazol, diltiazem, dronedarone or verapamil with higher doses of lovastatin: The dose of lovastatin should not exceed 20 mg daily in patients receiving concomitant medication with danazol, diltiazem, dronedarone, or verapamil. The benefits of the use of lovastatin in patients receiving danazol, diltiazem, dronedarone, or verapamil should be carefully weighed against the risks of these combinations.

Amiodarone: The dose of lovastatin should not exceed 40 mg daily in patients receiving concomitant medication with amiodarone. The combined use of lovastatin at doses higher than 40 mg daily with amiodarone should be avoided unless the clinical benefit is likely to outweigh the increased risk of myopathy. The risk of myopathy/rhabdomyolysis is increased when amiodarone is used concomitantly with higher doses of a closely related member of the HMG-CoA reductase inhibitor class.

Colchicine: Cases of myopathy, including rhabdomyolysis, have been reported with lovastatin coadministered with colchicine, and caution should be exercised when prescribing lovastatin with colchicine (see PRECAUTIONS, Drug Interactions).

Ranolazine: The risk of myopathy, including rhabdomyolysis, may be increased by concomitant administration of ranolazine. Dose adjustment of lovastatin may be considered during co-administration with ranolazine.
Prescribing recommendations for interacting agents are summarized in Table VII (see also CLINICAL PHARMACOLOGY, Pharmacokinetics; PRECAUTIONS, Drug Interactions; DOSAGE AND ADMINISTRATION).

Table VII: Drug Interactions Associated with Increased Risk of Myopathy/Rhabdomyolysis

Interacting Agents	Prescribing Recommendations
Strong CYP3A4 inhibitors, e.g.: Ketoconazole Itraconazole Posaconazole Voriconazole Erythromycin Clarithromycin Telithromycin HIV protease inhibitors Boceprevir Telaprevir Nefazodone	Contraindicated with lovastatin
Gemfibrozil Cyclosporine	Avoid with lovastatin
Danazol Diltiazem Dronedarone Verapamil	Do not exceed 20 mg lovastatin daily
Amiodarone	Do not exceed 40 mg lovastatin daily
Grapefruit juice	Avoid grapefruit juice

Liver Dysfunction

Persistent increases (to more than 3 times the upper limit of normal) in serum transaminases occurred in 1.9% of adult patients who received lovastatin for at least one year in early clinical trials (see ADVERSE REACTIONS). When the drug was interrupted or discontinued in these patients, the transaminase levels usually fell slowly to pretreatment levels. The increases usually appeared 3 to 12 months after the start of therapy with lovastatin, and were not associated with jaundice or other clinical signs or symptoms. There was no evidence of hypersensitivity. In the EXCEL study (see CLINICAL PHARMACOLOGY, Clinical Studies), the incidence of persistent increases in serum transaminases over 48 weeks was 0.1% for placebo, 0.1% at 20 mg/day, 0.9% at 40 mg/day, and 1.5% at 80 mg/day in patients on lovastatin. However, in post-marketing experience with MEVACOR, symptomatic liver disease has been reported rarely at all dosages (see ADVERSE REACTIONS).
In AFCAPS/TexCAPS, the number of participants with consecutive elevations of either alanine aminotransferase (ALT) or aspartate aminotransferase (AST) (> 3 times the upper limit of normal), over a median of 5.1 years of follow-up, was not significantly different between the MEVACOR and placebo groups (18 [0.6%] vs. 11 [0.3%]). The starting dose of MEVACOR was 20 mg/day; 50% of the MEVACOR treated participants were titrated to 40 mg/day at Week 18. Of the 18 participants on MEVACOR with consecutive elevations of either ALT or AST, 11 (0.7%) elevations occurred in participants taking 20 mg/day, while 7 (0.4%) elevations occurred in participants titrated to 40 mg/day. Elevated transaminases resulted in discontinuation of 6 (0.2%) participants from therapy in the MEVACOR group (n=3,304) and 4 (0.1%) in the placebo group (n=3,301).
It is recommended that liver enzyme tests be obtained prior to initiating therapy with MEVACOR and repeated as clinically indicated.
There have been rare postmarketing reports of fatal and non-fatal hepatic failure in patients taking statins, including lovastatin. If serious liver injury with clinical symptoms and/or hyperbilirubinemia or jaundice occurs during treatment with MEVACOR, promptly interrupt therapy. If an alternate etiology is not found do not restart MEVACOR.
The drug should be used with caution in patients who consume substantial quantities of alcohol and/or have a past history of liver disease. Active liver disease or unexplained transaminase elevations are contraindications to the use of lovastatin.
As with other lipid-lowering agents, moderate (less than three times the upper limit of normal) elevations of serum transaminases have been reported following therapy with MEVACOR (see ADVERSE REACTIONS). These changes appeared soon after initiation of therapy with MEVACOR, were often transient, were not accompanied by any symptoms and interruption of treatment was not required.

PRECAUTIONS

General

Lovastatin may elevate creatine phosphokinase and transaminase levels (see WARNINGS and ADVERSE REACTIONS). This should be considered in the differential diagnosis of chest pain in a patient on therapy with lovastatin.

Homozygous Familial Hypercholesterolemia

MEVACOR is less effective in patients with the rare homozygous familial hypercholesterolemia, possibly because these patients have no functional LDL receptors. MEVACOR appears to be more likely to raise serum transaminases (see ADVERSE REACTIONS) in these homozygous patients.

Information for Patients

Patients should be advised about substances they should not take concomitantly with MEVACOR and be advised to report promptly unexplained muscle pain, tenderness, or weakness particularly if accompanied by malaise or fever or if muscle signs and symptoms persist after discontinuing MEVACOR (see list below and WARNINGS, Myopathy/Rhabdomyolysis). Patients should also be advised to inform other physicians prescribing a new medication that they are taking MEVACOR.
It is recommended that liver enzymes be checked before starting therapy, and if signs or symptoms of liver injury occur. All patients treated with MEVACOR should be advised to report promptly any symptoms that may indicate liver injury, including fatigue, anorexia, right upper abdominal discomfort, dark urine or jaundice.

Drug Interactions

CYP3A4 Interactions
Lovastatin is metabolized by CYP3A4 but has no CYP3A4 inhibitory activity; therefore it is not expected to affect the plasma concentrations of other drugs metabolized by CYP3A4. Strong inhibitors of CYP3A4 (e.g., itraconazole, ketoconazole, posaconazole, voriconazole, clarithromycin, telithromycin, HIV protease inhibitors, boceprevir, telaprevir, nefazodone, and erythromycin), and grapefruit juice increase the risk of myopathy by reducing the elimination of lovastatin. **(See CONTRAINDICATIONS, WARNINGS, Myopathy/Rhabdomyolysis, and CLINICAL PHARMACOLOGY, Pharmacokinetics.)**
Interactions With Lipid-Lowering Drugs That Can Cause Myopathy When Given Alone
The risk of myopathy is also increased by the following lipid-lowering drugs that are not strong CYP3A4 inhibitors, but which can cause myopathy when given alone.
See WARNINGS, Myopathy/Rhabdomyolysis.
Gemfibrozil
Other fibrates
Niacin (nicotinic acid) (≥1 g/day)
Other Drug Interactions
Cyclosporine: The risk of myopathy/rhabdomyolysis is increased by concomitant administration of cyclosporine (see WARNINGS, Myopathy/Rhabdomyolysis).
Danazol, Diltiazem, Dronedarone or Verapamil: The risk of myopathy/rhabdomyolysis is increased by concomitant administration of danazol, diltiazem, dronedarone or verapamil particularly with higher doses of lovastatin (see WARNINGS, Myopathy/Rhabdomyolysis; CLINICAL PHARMACOLOGY, Pharmacokinetics).
Amiodarone: The risk of myopathy/rhabdomyolysis is increased when amiodarone is used concomitantly with a closely related member of the HMG–CoA reductase inhibitor class (see WARNINGS, Myopathy/Rhabdomyolysis).
Coumarin Anticoagulants: In a small clinical trial in which lovastatin was administered to warfarin treated patients, no effect on prothrombin time was detected. However, another HMG–CoA reductase inhibitor has been found to produce a less than two-second increase in prothrombin time in healthy volunteers receiving low doses of warfarin. Also, bleeding and/or increased prothrombin time have been reported in a few patients taking coumarin anticoagulants concomitantly with lovastatin. It is recommended that in patients taking anticoagulants, prothrombin time be determined before starting lovastatin and frequently enough during early therapy to insure that no significant alteration of prothrombin time occurs. Once a stable prothrombin time has been documented, prothrombin times can be monitored at the intervals usually recommended for patients on coumarin anticoagulants. If the dose of lovastatin is changed, the same procedure should be repeated. Lovastatin therapy has not been associated with bleeding or with changes in prothrombin time in patients not taking anticoagulants.
Colchicine: Cases of myopathy, including rhabdomyolysis, have been reported with lovastatin coadministered with colchicine. See WARNINGS, Myopathy/Rhabdomyolysis.
Ranolazine: The risk of myopathy, including rhabdomyolysis, may be increased by concomitant administration of ranolazine. See WARNINGS, Myopathy/Rhabdomyolysis.
Propranolol: In normal volunteers, there was no clinically significant pharmacokinetic or pharmacodynamic interaction with concomitant administration of single doses of lovastatin and propranolol.
Digoxin: In patients with hypercholesterolemia, concomitant administration of lovastatin and digoxin resulted in no effect on digoxin plasma concentrations.
Oral Hypoglycemic Agents: In pharmacokinetic studies of MEVACOR in hypercholesterolemic non-insulin dependent diabetic patients, there was no drug interaction with glipizide or with chlorpropamide (see CLINICAL PHARMACOLOGY, Clinical Studies).

Endocrine Function

Increases in HbA1c and fasting serum glucose levels have been reported with HMG-CoA reductase inhibitors, including MEVACOR.
HMG–CoA reductase inhibitors interfere with cholesterol synthesis and as such might theoretically blunt adrenal and/or gonadal steroid production. Results of clinical trials with drugs in this class have been inconsistent with regard to drug effects on basal and reserve steroid levels. However, clinical studies have shown that lovastatin does not reduce basal plasma cortisol concentration or impair adrenal reserve, and does not reduce basal plasma testosterone concentration. Another HMG–CoA reductase inhibitor has been shown to reduce the plasma testosterone response to HCG. In the same study, the mean testosterone response to HCG was slightly but not significantly reduced after treatment with lovastatin 40 mg daily for 16 weeks in 21 men. The effects of HMG-CoA reductase inhibitors on male fertility have not been studied in adequate numbers of male patients. The effects, if any, on the pituitary-gonadal axis in pre-menopausal women are unknown. Patients treated with lovastatin who develop clinical evidence of endocrine dysfunction should be evaluated appropriately. Caution should also be exercised if an HMG–CoA reductase inhibitor or other agent used to lower cholesterol levels is administered to patients also receiving other drugs (e.g., spironolactone, cimetidine) that may decrease the levels or activity of endogenous steroid hormones.

CNS Toxicity

Lovastatin produced optic nerve degeneration (Wallerian degeneration of retinogeniculate fibers) in clinically normal dogs in a dose-dependent fashion starting at 60 mg/kg/day, a dose that produced mean plasma drug levels about 30 times higher than the mean drug level in humans taking the highest recommended dose (as measured by total enzyme inhibitory activity). Vestibulocochlear Wallerian-like degeneration and retinal ganglion cell chromatolysis were also seen in dogs treated for 14 weeks at 180 mg/kg/day, a dose which resulted in a mean plasma drug level (C_{max}) similar to that seen with the 60 mg/kg/day dose.
CNS vascular lesions, characterized by perivascular hemorrhage and edema, mononuclear cell infiltration of perivascular spaces, perivascular fibrin deposits and necrosis of small vessels, were seen in dogs treated with lovastatin at a dose of 180 mg/kg/day, a dose which produced plasma drug levels (C_{max}) which were about 30 times higher than the mean values in humans taking 80 mg/day.
Similar optic nerve and CNS vascular lesions have been observed with other drugs of this class.
Cataracts were seen in dogs treated for 11 and 28 weeks at 180 mg/kg/day and 1 year at 60 mg/kg/day.

Carcinogenesis, Mutagenesis, Impairment of Fertility

In a 21-month carcinogenic study in mice, there was a statistically significant increase in the incidence of hepatocellular carcinomas and adenomas in both males and females at 500 mg/kg/day. This dose produced a total plasma drug exposure 3 to 4 times that of humans given the highest recommended dose of lovastatin (drug exposure was measured as total HMG–CoA reductase inhibitory activity in extracted plasma). Tumor increases were not seen at 20 and 100 mg/kg/day, doses that produced drug exposures of 0.3 to 2 times that of humans at the 80 mg/day dose. A statistically significant increase in pulmonary adenomas was seen in female mice at approximately 4 times the human drug exposure. (Although mice were given 300 times the human dose [HD] on a mg/kg body weight basis, plasma levels of total inhibitory activity were only 4 times higher in mice than in humans given 80 mg of MEVACOR.)
There was an increase in incidence of papilloma in the non-glandular mucosa of the stomach of mice beginning at exposures of 1 to 2 times that of humans. The glandular mucosa was not affected. The human stomach contains only glandular mucosa.
In a 24-month carcinogenicity study in rats, there was a positive dose response relationship for hepatocellular carcinogenicity in males at drug exposures between 2-7 times that of human exposure at 80 mg/day (doses in rats were 5, 30 and 180 mg/kg/day).
An increased incidence of thyroid neoplasms in rats appears to be a response that has been seen with other HMG–CoA reductase inhibitors.
A chemically similar drug in this class was administered to mice for 72 weeks at 25, 100, and 400 mg/kg body weight, which resulted in mean serum drug levels approximately 3, 15, and 33 times higher than the mean human serum drug concentration (as total inhibitory activity) after a 40 mg oral

dose. Liver carcinomas were significantly increased in high dose females and mid- and high dose males, with a maximum incidence of 90 percent in males. The incidence of adenomas of the liver was significantly increased in mid- and high dose females. Drug treatment also significantly increased the incidence of lung adenomas in mid- and high dose males and females. Adenomas of the Harderian gland (a gland of the eye of rodents) were significantly higher in high dose mice than in controls.

No evidence of mutagenicity was observed in a microbial mutagen test using mutant strains of *Salmonella typhimurium* with or without rat or mouse liver metabolic activation. In addition, no evidence of damage to genetic material was noted in an *in vitro* alkaline elution assay using rat or mouse hepatocytes, a V–79 mammalian cell forward mutation study, an *in vitro* chromosome aberration study in CHO cells, or an *in vivo* chromosomal aberration assay in mouse bone marrow.

Drug-related testicular atrophy, decreased spermatogenesis, spermatocytic degeneration and giant cell formation were seen in dogs starting at 20 mg/kg/day. Similar findings were seen with another drug in this class. No drug-related effects on fertility were found in studies with lovastatin in rats. However, in studies with a similar drug in this class, there was decreased fertility in male rats treated for 34 weeks at 25 mg/kg body weight, although this effect was not observed in a subsequent fertility study when this same dose was administered for 11 weeks (the entire cycle of spermatogenesis, including epididymal maturation). In rats treated with this same reductase inhibitor at 180 mg/kg/day, seminiferous tubule degeneration (necrosis and loss of spermatogenic epithelium) was observed. No microscopic changes were observed in the testes from rats of either study. The clinical significance of these findings is unclear.

Pregnancy

Pregnancy Category X

See CONTRAINDICATIONS.

Safety in pregnant women has not been established.

Lovastatin has been shown to produce skeletal malformations in offspring of pregnant mice and rats dosed during gestation at 80 mg/kg/day (affected mouse fetuses/total: 8/307 compared to 4/289 in the control group; affected rat fetuses/total: 6/324 compared to 2/308 in the control group). Female rats dosed before mating through gestation at 80 mg/kg/day also had fetuses with skeletal malformations (affected fetuses/total: 1/152 compared to 0/171 in the control group). The 80 mg/kg/day dose in mice is 7 times the human dose based on body surface area and in rats results in 5 times the human exposure based on AUC. In pregnant rats given doses of 2, 20, or 200 mg/kg/day and treated through lactation, the following effects were observed: neonatal mortality (4.1%, 3.5%, and 46%, respectively, compared to 0.6% in the control group), decreased pup body weights throughout lactation (up to 5%, 8%, and 38%, respectively, below control), supernumerary ribs in dead pups (affected fetuses/total: 0/7, 1/17, and 11/79, respectively, compared to 0/5 in the control group), delays in ossification in dead pups (affected fetuses/total: 0/7, 0/17, and 1/79, respectively, compared to 0/5 in the control group) and delays in pup development (delays in the appearance of an auditory startle response at 200 mg/kg/day and free-fall righting reflexes at 20 and 200 mg/kg/day).

Direct dosing of neonatal rats by subcutaneous injection with 10 mg/kg/day of the open hydroxyacid form of lovastatin resulted in delayed passive avoidance learning in female rats (mean of 8.3 trials to criterion, compared to 7.3 and 6.4 in untreated and vehicle-treated controls; no effects on retention 1 week later) at exposures 4 times the human systemic exposure at 80 mg/day based on AUC. No effect was seen in male rats. No evidence of malformations was observed when pregnant rabbits were given 5 mg/kg/day (doses equivalent to a human dose of 80 mg/day based on body surface area) or a maternally toxic dose of 15 mg/kg/day (3 times the human dose of 80 mg/day based on body surface area).

Rare clinical reports of congenital anomalies following intrauterine exposure to HMG-CoA reductase inhibitors have been received. However, in an analysis[3] of greater than 200 prospectively followed pregnancies exposed during the first trimester to MEVACOR or another closely related HMG-CoA reductase inhibitor, the incidence of congenital anomalies was comparable to that seen in the general population. This number of pregnancies was sufficient to exclude a 3-fold or greater increase in congenital anomalies over the background incidence.

Maternal treatment with MEVACOR may reduce the fetal levels of mevalonate, which is a precursor of cholesterol biosynthesis. Atherosclerosis is a chronic process, and ordinarily discontinuation of lipid-lowering drugs during pregnancy should have little impact on the long-term risk associated with primary hypercholesterolemia. For these reasons, MEVACOR should not be used in women who are pregnant, or can become pregnant (see CONTRAINDICATIONS). MEVACOR should be administered to women of child-bearing potential only when such patients are highly unlikely to conceive and have been informed of the potential hazards. Treatment should be immediately discontinued as soon as pregnancy is recognized.

	Placebo (N = 1663) %	MEVACOR 20 mg q.p.m. (N = 1642) %	MEVACOR 40 mg q.p.m. (N = 1645) %	MEVACOR 20 mg b.i.d. (N = 1646) %	MEVACOR 40 mg b.i.d. (N = 1649) %
Body As a Whole					
Asthenia	1.4	1.7	1.4	1.5	1.2
Gastrointestinal					
Abdominal pain	1.6	2.0	2.0	2.2	2.5
Constipation	1.9	2.0	3.2	3.2	3.5
Diarrhea	2.3	2.6	2.4	2.2	2.6
Dyspepsia	1.9	1.3	1.3	1.0	1.6
Flatulence	4.2	3.7	4.3	3.9	4.5
Nausea	2.5	1.9	2.5	2.2	2.2
Musculoskeletal					
Muscle cramps	0.5	0.6	0.8	1.1	1.0
Myalgia	1.7	2.6	1.8	2.2	3.0
Nervous System / Psychiatric					
Dizziness	0.7	0.7	1.2	0.5	0.5
Headache	2.7	2.6	2.8	2.1	3.2
Skin					
Rash	0.7	0.8	1.0	1.2	1.3
Special Senses					
Blurred vision	0.8	1.1	0.9	0.9	1.2

[3]Manson, J.M., Freyssinges, C., Ducrocq, M.B., Stephenson, W.P., Postmarketing Surveillance of Lovastatin and Simvastatin Exposure During Pregnancy. *Reproductive Toxicology*. 10(6):439-446. 1996.

Nursing Mothers

It is not known whether lovastatin is excreted in human milk. Because a small amount of another drug in this class is excreted in human breast milk and because of the potential for serious adverse reactions in nursing infants, women taking MEVACOR should not nurse their infants (see CONTRAINDICATIONS).

Pediatric Use

Safety and effectiveness in patients 10-17 years of age with heFH have been evaluated in controlled clinical trials of 48 weeks duration in adolescent boys and controlled clinical trials of 24 weeks duration in girls who were at least 1 year post-menarche. Patients treated with lovastatin had an adverse experience profile generally similar to that of patients treated with placebo. **Doses greater than 40 mg have not been studied in this population.** In these limited controlled studies, there was no detectable effect on growth or sexual maturation in the adolescent boys or on menstrual cycle length in girls. See CLINICAL PHARMACOLOGY, Clinical Studies in Adolescent Patients; ADVERSE REACTIONS, Adolescent Patients; and DOSAGE AND ADMINISTRATION, Adolescent Patients (10-17 years of age) with Heterozygous Familial Hypercholesterolemia. Adolescent females should be counseled on appropriate contraceptive methods while on lovastatin therapy (see CONTRAINDICATIONS and PRECAUTIONS, Pregnancy). **Lovastatin has not been studied in pre-pubertal patients or patients younger than 10 years of age.**

Geriatric Use

A pharmacokinetic study with lovastatin showed the mean plasma level of HMG–CoA reductase inhibitory activity to be approximately 45% higher in elderly patients between 70-78 years of age compared with patients between 18-30 years of age; however, clinical study experience in the elderly indicates that dosage adjustment based on this age-related pharmacokinetic difference is not needed. In the two large clinical studies conducted with lovastatin (EXCEL and AFCAPS/TexCAPS), 21% (3094/14850) of patients were ≥65 years of age. Lipid-lowering efficacy with lovastatin was at least as great in elderly patients compared with younger patients, and there were no overall differences in safety over the 20 to 80 mg/day dosage range (see CLINICAL PHARMACOLOGY).

ADVERSE REACTIONS

MEVACOR is generally well tolerated; adverse reactions usually have been mild and transient.

Phase III Clinical Studies

In Phase III controlled clinical studies involving 613 patients treated with MEVACOR, the adverse experience profile was similar to that shown below for the 8,245–patient EXCEL study (see Expanded Clinical Evaluation of Lovastatin (EXCEL) Study).

Persistent increases of serum transaminases have been noted (see WARNINGS, Liver Dysfunction). About 11% of patients had elevations of CK levels of at least twice the normal value on one or more occasions. The corresponding values for the control agent cholestyramine was 9 percent. This was attributable to the noncardiac fraction of CK. Large increases in CK have sometimes been reported (see WARNINGS, Myopathy/Rhabdomyolysis).

Expanded Clinical Evaluation of Lovastatin (EXCEL) Study

MEVACOR was compared to placebo in 8,245 patients with hypercholesterolemia (total-C 240-300 mg/dL [6.2-7.8 mmol/L]) in the randomized, double-blind, parallel, 48-week EXCEL study. Clinical adverse experiences reported as possibly, probably or definitely drug-related in ≥1% in any treatment group are shown in the table below. For no event was the incidence on drug and placebo statistically different.

[See table above]

Other clinical adverse experiences reported as possibly, probably or definitely drug-related in 0.5 to 1.0 percent of patients in any drug treated group are listed below. In all these cases the incidence on drug and placebo was not statistically different. *Body as a Whole*: chest pain; *Gastrointestinal:* acid regurgitation, dry mouth, vomiting; *Musculoskeletal:* leg pain, shoulder pain, arthralgia; *Nervous System / Psychiatric*: insomnia, paresthesia; *Skin*: alopecia, pruritus; *Special Senses*: eye irritation.

In the EXCEL study (see CLINICAL PHARMACOLOGY, Clinical Studies), 4.6% of the patients treated up to 48 weeks were discontinued due to clinical or laboratory adverse experiences which were rated by the investigator as possibly, probably or definitely related to therapy with MEVACOR. The value for the placebo group was 2.5%.

Air Force/Texas Coronary Atherosclerosis Prevention Study (AFCAPS/TexCAPS)

In AFCAPS/TexCAPS (see CLINICAL PHARMACOLOGY, Clinical Studies) involving 6,605 participants treated with 20-40 mg/day of MEVACOR (n=3,304) or placebo (n=3,301), the safety and tolerability profile of the group treated with MEVACOR was comparable to that of the group treated with placebo during a median of 5.1 years of follow-up. The adverse experiences reported in AFCAPS/TexCAPS were similar to those reported in EXCEL (see ADVERSE REACTIONS, Expanded Clinical Evaluation of Lovastatin (EXCEL) Study).

Concomitant Therapy

In controlled clinical studies in which lovastatin was administered concomitantly with cholestyramine, no adverse reactions peculiar to this concomitant treatment were observed. The adverse reactions that occurred were limited to those reported previously with lovastatin or cholestyramine. Other lipid-lowering agents were not administered concomitantly with lovastatin during controlled clinical studies. Preliminary data suggests that the addition of gemfibrozil to therapy with lovastatin is not associated with greater reduction in LDL–C than that achieved with lovastatin alone. In uncontrolled clinical studies, most of the patients who have developed myopathy were receiving concomitant therapy with cyclosporine, gemfibrozil or niacin (nicotinic acid). The combined use of lovastatin with cyclosporine or gemfibrozil should be avoided. Caution should be used when prescribing other fibrates or lipid-lowering doses (≥1 g/day) of niacin with lovastatin (see WARNINGS, Myopathy/Rhabdomyolysis).

The following effects have been reported with drugs in this class. Not all the effects listed below have necessarily been associated with lovastatin therapy.

Skeletal: muscle cramps, myalgia, myopathy, rhabdomyolysis, arthralgias.

There have been rare reports of immune-mediated necrotizing myopathy associated with statin use (see WARNINGS, Myopathy/Rhabdomyolysis).

Neurological: dysfunction of certain cranial nerves (including alteration of taste, impairment of extra-ocular movement, facial paresis), tremor, dizziness, vertigo, paresthesia, peripheral neuropathy, peripheral nerve palsy, psychic disturbances, anxiety, insomnia, depression.

There have been rare postmarketing reports of cognitive impairment (e.g., memory loss, forgetfulness, amnesia, memory impairment, confusion) associated with statin use. These cognitive issues have been reported for all statins. The reports are generally nonserious, and reversible upon statin discontinuation, with variable times to symptom onset (1 day to years) and symptom resolution (median of 3 weeks).

Hypersensitivity Reactions: An apparent hypersensitivity syndrome has been reported rarely which has included one or more of the following features: anaphylaxis, angioedema, lupus erythematous-like syndrome, polymyalgia rheumatica, dermatomyositis, vasculitis, purpura, thrombocytopenia, leukopenia, hemolytic anemia, positive ANA, ESR increase, eosinophilia, arthritis, arthralgia, urticaria, asthenia, photosensitivity, fever, chills, flushing, malaise, dyspnea, toxic epidermal necrolysis, erythema multiforme, including Stevens-Johnson syndrome.

Gastrointestinal: pancreatitis, hepatitis, including chronic active hepatitis, cholestatic jaundice, fatty change in liver; and rarely, cirrhosis, fulminant hepatic necrosis, and hepatoma; anorexia, vomiting, fatal and non-fatal hepatic failure.

Skin: alopecia, pruritus. A variety of skin changes (e.g., nodules, discoloration, dryness of skin/mucous membranes, changes to hair/nails) have been reported.

Reproductive: gynecomastia, loss of libido, erectile dysfunction.

Eye: progression of cataracts (lens opacities), ophthalmoplegia.

Laboratory Abnormalities: elevated transaminases, alkaline phosphatase, γ-glutamyl transpeptidase, and bilirubin; thyroid function abnormalities.

Adolescent Patients (ages 10–17 years)

In a 48–week controlled study in adolescent boys with heFH (n=132) and a 24–week controlled study in girls who were at least 1 year post-menarche with heFH (n=54), the safety and tolerability profile of the groups treated with MEVACOR (10 to 40 mg daily) was generally similar to that of the groups treated with placebo (see CLINICAL PHARMACOLOGY, Clinical Studies in Adolescent Patients and PRECAUTIONS, Pediatric Use).

OVERDOSAGE

After oral administration of MEVACOR to mice, the median lethal dose observed was >15 g/m².

Five healthy human volunteers have received up to 200 mg of lovastatin as a single dose without clinically significant adverse experiences. A few cases of accidental overdosage have been reported; no patients had any specific symptoms, and all patients recovered without sequelae. The maximum dose taken was 5-6 g.

Until further experience is obtained, no specific treatment of overdosage with MEVACOR can be recommended.

The dialyzability of lovastatin and its metabolites in man is not known at present.

DOSAGE AND ADMINISTRATION

The patient should be placed on a standard cholesterol-lowering diet before receiving MEVACOR and should continue on this diet during treatment with MEVACOR (see NCEP Treatment Guidelines for details on dietary therapy). MEVACOR should be given with meals.

Adult Patients

The usual recommended starting dose is 20 mg once a day given with the evening meal. The recommended dosing range of lovastatin is 10-80 mg/day in single or two divided doses; the maximum recommended dose is 80 mg/day. Doses should be individualized according to the recommended goal of therapy (see NCEP Guidelines and CLINICAL PHARMACOLOGY). Patients requiring reductions in LDL–C of 20% or more to achieve their goal (see INDICATIONS AND USAGE) should be started on 20 mg/day of MEVACOR. A starting dose of 10 mg of lovastatin may be considered for patients requiring smaller reductions. Adjustments should be made at intervals of 4 weeks or more. The 10 mg dosage is provided for information purposes only. Although lovastatin tablets 10 mg are available in the marketplace, MEVACOR is no longer marketed in the 10 mg strength.

Cholesterol levels should be monitored periodically and consideration should be given to reducing the dosage of MEVACOR if cholesterol levels fall significantly below the targeted range.

Dosage in Patients taking Danazol, Diltiazem, Dronedarone or Verapamil

In patients taking danazol, diltiazem, dronedarone or verapamil concomitantly with lovastatin, therapy should begin with 10 mg of lovastatin and should not exceed 20 mg/day (see CLINICAL PHARMACOLOGY, Pharmacokinetics, WARNINGS, Myopathy/Rhabdomyolysis, PRECAUTIONS, Drug Interactions, Other Drug Interactions).

Dosage in Patients taking Amiodarone

In patients taking amiodarone concomitantly with MEVACOR, the dose should not exceed 40 mg/day (see WARNINGS, Myopathy/Rhabdomyolysis and PRECAUTIONS, Drug Interactions, Other Drug Interactions).

Adolescent Patients (10-17 years of age) with Heterozygous Familial Hypercholesterolemia

The recommended dosing range of lovastatin is 10-40 mg/day; the maximum recommended dose is 40 mg/day. Doses should be individualized according to the recommended goal of therapy (see NCEP Pediatric Panel Guidelines[4], CLINICAL PHARMACOLOGY, and INDICATIONS AND USAGE). Patients requiring reductions in LDL–C of 20% or more to achieve their goal should be started on 20 mg/day of MEVACOR. A starting dose of 10 mg of lovastatin may be considered for patients requiring smaller reductions. Adjustments should be made at intervals of 4 weeks or more.

[4]National Cholesterol Education Program (NCEP): Highlights of the Report of the Expert Panel on Blood Cholesterol Levels in Children and Adolescents. *Pediatrics.* 89(3):495-501. 1992.

Concomitant Lipid-Lowering Therapy

MEVACOR is effective alone or when used concomitantly with bile-acid sequestrants (see WARNINGS, Myopathy/Rhabdomyolysis and PRECAUTIONS, Drug Interactions).

Dosage in Patients with Renal Insufficiency

In patients with severe renal insufficiency (creatinine clearance <30 mL/min), dosage increases above 20 mg/day should be carefully considered and, if deemed necessary, implemented cautiously (see CLINICAL PHARMACOLOGY and WARNINGS, Myopathy/Rhabdomyolysis).

HOW SUPPLIED

No. 8123 — Tablets MEVACOR 20 mg are blue, octagonal tablets, coded MSD 731 on one side and plain on the other. They are supplied as follows:

NDC 0006-0731-61 unit of use bottles of 60.

No. 8124 — Tablets MEVACOR 40 mg are green, octagonal tablets, coded MSD 732 on one side and plain on the other. They are supplied as follows:

NDC 0006-0732-61 unit of use bottles of 60.

Storage

Store at 20-25°C (68-77°F). [See USP Controlled Room Temperature.] Tablets MEVACOR must be protected from light and stored in a well-closed, light-resistant container.

Manuf. for: Merck Sharp & Dohme Corp., a subsidiary of **MERCK & CO., INC.**, Whitehouse Station, NJ 08889, USA
By:
Mylan Pharmaceuticals Inc.
Morgantown, WV 26505, USA
OR
Mylan Pharmaceuticals ULC
Etobicoke, Ontario, Canada M8Z 2S6

Revised: 10/2012
USPI-T-08031210R063

Shown in Product Identification Guide, page 308

NASONEX® ℞

[*nā-sō-nĕks*]
(mometasone furoate monohydrate)
Nasal Spray, 50 mcg†

HIGHLIGHTS OF PRESCRIBING INFORMATION
These highlights do not include all the information needed to use NASONEX safely and effectively. See full prescribing information for NASONEX.
NASONEX® (mometasone furoate monohydrate) Nasal Spray, 50 mcg†
†calculated on the anhydrous basis
Initial U.S. Approval: 1997

INDICATIONS AND USAGE

NASONEX is a corticosteroid indicated for:

1. Treatment of Nasal Symptoms of Allergic Rhinitis in patients ≥2 years of age (1.1)
2. Treatment of Nasal Congestion Associated with Seasonal Allergic Rhinitis in patients ≥2 years of age (1.2)
3. Prophylaxis of Seasonal Allergic Rhinitis in patients ≥12 years of age (1.3)
4. Treatment of Nasal Polyps in patients ≥18 years of age (1.4)

DOSAGE AND ADMINISTRATION

For Intranasal Use Only

- Treatment of Nasal Symptoms of Allergic Rhinitis (2.1)
  Adults & Adolescents (12 yrs. and older): 2 sprays in each nostril once daily
  Children (2-11 yrs.): 1 spray in each nostril once daily
- Treatment of Nasal Congestion Associated with Seasonal Allergic Rhinitis (2.2)
  Adults & Adolescents (12 yrs. and older): 2 sprays in each nostril once daily
  Children (2-11 yrs.): 1 spray in each nostril once daily
- Prophylaxis of Seasonal Allergic Rhinitis (2.3)
  Adults & Adolescents (12 yrs. and older): 2 sprays in each nostril once daily
- Treatment of Nasal Polyps (2.4)

Adults (18 yrs. and older): 2 sprays in each nostril twice daily. 2 sprays in each nostril once daily may also be effective in some patients.

DOSAGE FORMS AND STRENGTHS

Nasal Spray: 50 mcg of mometasone furoate in each 100-microliter spray (3)

CONTRAINDICATIONS

Patients with known hypersensitivity to mometasone furoate or any of the ingredients of NASONEX. (4)

WARNINGS AND PRECAUTIONS

- Epistaxis, nasal ulceration, *Candida albicans* infection, nasal septal perforation, impaired wound healing. Monitor patients periodically for signs of adverse effects on the nasal mucosa. Avoid use in patients with recent nasal ulcers, nasal surgery, or nasal trauma. (5.1)
- Development of glaucoma or cataracts. Monitor patients closely with a change in vision or with a history of increased intraocular pressure, glaucoma, and/or cataracts. (5.2)
- Potential worsening of existing tuberculosis; fungal, bacterial, viral, or parasitic infections; or ocular herpes simplex. More serious or even fatal course of chickenpox or measles in susceptible patients. Use caution in patients with the above because of the potential for worsening of these infections. (5.4)
- Hypercorticism and adrenal suppression with higher than recommended dosages or at the regular dosage in susceptible individuals. If such changes occur, discontinue NASONEX Nasal Spray slowly. (5.5)
- Potential reduction in growth velocity in children. Monitor growth routinely in pediatric patients receiving NASONEX Nasal Spray. (5.6, 8.4)

ADVERSE REACTIONS

The most common adverse reactions (≥5%) included headache, viral infection, pharyngitis, epistaxis and cough. (6)

To report SUSPECTED ADVERSE REACTIONS, contact Merck Sharp & Dohme Corp., a subsidiary of Merck & Co., Inc., at 1-877-888-4231 or FDA at 1-800-FDA-1088 or www.fda.gov/medwatch.

See 17 for PATIENT COUNSELING INFORMATION and FDA-approved patient labeling

Revised: 03/2013

FULL PRESCRIBING INFORMATION: CONTENTS*

*** Sections or subsections omitted from the full prescribing information are not listed**

FULL PRESCRIBING INFORMATION

1 INDICATIONS AND USAGE

1.1 Treatment of Allergic Rhinitis

NASONEX® Nasal Spray 50 mcg is indicated for the treatment of the nasal symptoms of seasonal allergic and perennial allergic rhinitis, in adults and pediatric patients 2 years of age and older.

1.2 Treatment of Nasal Congestion Associated with Seasonal Allergic Rhinitis

NASONEX Nasal Spray 50 mcg is indicated for the relief of nasal congestion associated with seasonal allergic rhinitis, in adults and pediatric patients 2 years of age and older.

1.3 Prophylaxis of Seasonal Allergic Rhinitis

NASONEX Nasal Spray 50 mcg is indicated for the prophylaxis of the nasal symptoms of seasonal allergic rhinitis in adult and adolescent patients 12 years and older.

1.4 Treatment of Nasal Polyps

NASONEX Nasal Spray 50 mcg is indicated for the treatment of nasal polyps in patients 18 years of age and older.

2 DOSAGE AND ADMINISTRATION

Administer NASONEX Nasal Spray 50 mcg by the intranasal route only. Prior to initial use of NASONEX Nasal Spray, 50 mcg, the pump must be primed by actuating ten times or until a fine spray appears. The pump may be stored unused for up to 1 week without repriming. If unused for more than 1 week, reprime by actuating two times, or until a fine spray appears.

2.1 Treatment of Allergic Rhinitis

Adults and Adolescents 12 Years of Age and Older:
The recommended dose for treatment of the nasal symptoms of seasonal allergic and perennial allergic rhinitis is 2 sprays (50 mcg of mometasone furoate in each spray) in each nostril once daily (total daily dose of 200 mcg).

Children 2 to 11 Years of Age:
The recommended dose for treatment of the nasal symptoms of seasonal allergic and perennial allergic rhinitis is 1 spray (50 mcg of mometasone furoate in each spray) in each nostril once daily (total daily dose of 100 mcg).

2.2 Treatment of Nasal Congestion Associated with Seasonal Allergic Rhinitis

Adults and Adolescents 12 Years of Age and Older:
The recommended dose for treatment of nasal congestion associated with seasonal allergic rhinitis is two sprays (50 mcg of mometasone furoate in each spray) in each nostril once daily (total daily dose of 200 mcg).

Children 2 to 11 Years of Age:
The recommended dose for treatment of nasal congestion associated with seasonal allergic rhinitis is one spray (50 mcg of mometasone furoate in each spray) in each nostril once daily (total daily dose of 100 mcg).

2.3 Prophylaxis of Seasonal Allergic Rhinitis

Adults and Adolescents 12 Years of Age and Older:
The recommended dose for prophylaxis treatment of nasal symptoms of seasonal allergic rhinitis is 2 sprays (50 mcg of mometasone furoate in each spray) in each nostril once daily (total daily dose of 200 mcg).

In patients with a known seasonal allergen that precipitates nasal symptoms of seasonal allergic rhinitis, prophylaxis with NASONEX Nasal Spray 50 mcg (200 mcg/day) is recommended 2 to 4 weeks prior to the anticipated start of the pollen season.

2.4 Treatment of Nasal Polyps

Adults 18 Years of Age and Older:
The recommended dose for the treatment of nasal polyps is 2 sprays (50 mcg of mometasone furoate in each spray) in each nostril twice daily (total daily dose of 400 mcg). A dose of 2 sprays (50 mcg of mometasone furoate in each spray) in each nostril once daily (total daily dose of 200 mcg) is also effective in some patients.

3 DOSAGE FORMS AND STRENGTHS

NASONEX Nasal Spray 50 mcg is a metered-dose, manual pump spray unit containing an aqueous suspension of mometasone furoate monohydrate equivalent to 0.05% w/w mometasone furoate calculated on the anhydrous basis.

After initial priming (10 actuations), each actuation of the pump delivers a metered spray containing 100 mg or 100 microliter of suspension containing mometasone furoate monohydrate equivalent to 50 mcg of mometasone furoate calculated on the anhydrous basis. Each bottle of NASONEX Nasal Spray 50 mcg provides 120 sprays.

4 CONTRAINDICATIONS

NASONEX Nasal Spray is contraindicated in patients with known hypersensitivity to mometasone furoate or any of its ingredients.

5 WARNINGS AND PRECAUTIONS

5.1 Local Nasal Effects

Epistaxis

In clinical studies, epistaxis was observed more frequently in patients with allergic rhinitis with NASONEX Nasal Spray than those who received placebo *[see Adverse Reactions (6)]*.

Candida Infection

In clinical studies with NASONEX Nasal Spray 50 mcg, the development of localized infections of the nose and pharynx with *Candida albicans* has occurred. When such an infection develops, use of NASONEX Nasal Spray 50 mcg should be discontinued and appropriate local or systemic therapy instituted, if needed.

Nasal Septum Perforation

Instances of nasal septum perforation have been reported following the intranasal application of corticosteroids. As with any long-term topical treatment of the nasal cavity, patients using NASONEX Nasal Spray 50 mcg over several months or longer should be examined periodically for possible changes in the nasal mucosa.

Impaired Wound Healing

Because of the inhibitory effect of corticosteroids on wound healing, patients who have experienced recent nasal septum ulcers, nasal surgery, or nasal trauma should not use a nasal corticosteroid until healing has occurred.

5.2 Glaucoma and Cataracts

Nasal and inhaled corticosteroids may result in the development of glaucoma and/or cataracts. Therefore, close monitoring is warranted in patients with a change in vision or with a history of increased intraocular pressure, glaucoma, and/or cataracts.

Glaucoma and cataract formation was evaluated in one controlled study of 12 weeks' duration and one uncontrolled study of 12 months' duration in patients treated with NASONEX Nasal Spray, 50 mcg at 200 mcg/day, using intraocular pressure measurements and slit lamp examination. No significant change from baseline was noted in the mean intraocular pressure measurements for the 141 NASONEX-treated patients in the 12-week study, as compared with 141 placebo-treated patients. No individual NASONEX-treated patient was noted to have developed a significant elevation in intraocular pressure or cataracts in this 12-week study. Likewise, no significant change from baseline was noted in the mean intraocular pressure measurements for the 139 NASONEX-treated patients in the 12-month study and again, no cataracts were detected in these patients. Nonetheless, nasal and inhaled corticosteroids have been associated with the development of glaucoma and/or cataracts.

5.3 Hypersensitivity Reactions

Hypersensitivity reactions including instances of wheezing may occur after the intranasal administration of mometasone furoate monohydrate. Discontinue NASONEX Nasal Spray if such reactions occur *[see Contraindications (4)]*.

5.4 Immunosuppression

Persons who are on drugs which suppress the immune system are more susceptible to infections than healthy individuals. Chickenpox and measles, for example, can have a more serious or even fatal course in nonimmune children or adults on corticosteroids. In such children or adults who have not had these diseases, particular care should be taken to avoid exposure. How the dose, route, and duration of corticosteroid administration affect the risk of developing a disseminated infection is not known. The contribution of the underlying disease and/or prior corticosteroid treatment to the risk is also not known. If exposed to chickenpox, prophylaxis with varicella zoster immune globin (VZIG) may be indicated. If exposed to measles, prophylaxis with pooled intramuscular immunoglobulin (IG) may be indicated. (See the respective package inserts for complete VZIG and IG prescribing information.) If chickenpox develops, treatment with antiviral agents may be considered.

Corticosteroids should be used with caution, if at all, in patients with active or quiescent tuberculous infection of the respiratory tract, or in untreated fungal, bacterial, systemic viral infections, or ocular herpes simplex because of the potential for worsening of these infections.

5.5 Hypothalamic-Pituitary-Adrenal Axis Effect

Hypercorticism and Adrenal Suppression

When intranasal steroids are used at higher than recommended dosages or in susceptible individuals at recommended dosages, systemic corticosteroid effects such as hypercorticism and adrenal suppression may appear. If such changes occur, the dosage of NASONEX Nasal Spray should be discontinued slowly, consistent with accepted procedures for discontinuing oral corticosteroid therapy.

5.6 Effect on Growth

Corticosteroids may cause a reduction in growth velocity when administered to pediatric patients. Monitor the growth routinely of pediatric patients receiving NASONEX Nasal Spray. To minimize the systemic effects of intranasal corticosteroids, including NASONEX Nasal Spray, titrate each patient's dose to the lowest dosage that effectively controls his/her symptoms *[see Use in Specific Populations (8.4)]*.

6 ADVERSE REACTIONS

Systemic and local corticosteroid use may result in the following:

- Epistaxis, ulcerations, *Candida albicans* infection, impaired wound healing *[see Warnings and Precautions (5.1)]*
- Cataracts and glaucoma *[see Warnings and Precautions (5.2)]*
- Immunosuppression *[see Warnings and Precautions (5.4)]*
- Hypothalamic-pituitary-adrenal (HPA) axis effects, including growth reduction *[see Warnings and Precautions (5.5, 5.6), Use in Specific Populations (8.4)]*

6.1 Clinical Trials Experience

Because clinical trials are conducted under widely varying conditions, adverse reaction rates observed in the clinical trials of a drug cannot be directly compared to rates in the clinical trials of another drug and may not reflect the rates observed in practice.

Allergic Rhinitis

Adults and adolescents 12 years of age and older

In controlled US and international clinical studies, a total of 3210 adult and adolescent patients 12 years and older with allergic rhinitis received treatment with NASONEX Nasal Spray 50 mcg at doses of 50 to 800 mcg/day. The majority of patients (n=2103) were treated with 200 mcg/day. A total of 350 adult and adolescent patients have been treated for one year or longer. Adverse events did not differ significantly based on age, sex, or race. Four percent or less of patients in clinical trials discontinued treatment because of adverse events and the discontinuation rate was similar for the vehicle and active comparators.

All adverse events (regardless of relationship to treatment) reported by 5% or more of adult and adolescent patients ages 12 years and older who received NASONEX Nasal Spray 50 mcg, 200 mcg/day vs. placebo and that were more common with NASONEX Nasal Spray 50 mcg than placebo, are displayed in TABLE 1 below.

TABLE 1: ADULT AND ADOLESCENT PATIENTS 12 YEARS AND OLDER – ADVERSE EVENTS FROM CONTROLLED CLINICAL TRIALS IN SEASONAL ALLERGIC AND PERENNIAL ALLERGIC RHINITIS (PERCENT OF PATIENTS REPORTING)

	NASONEX 200 mcg (n=2103)	VEHICLE PLACEBO (n=1671)
Headache	26	22
Viral Infection	14	11
Pharyngitis	12	10
Epistaxis/Blood-Tinged Mucus	11	6
Coughing	7	6
Upper Respiratory Tract Infection	6	2
Dysmenorrhea	5	3
Musculoskeletal Pain	5	3
Sinusitis	5	3

Other adverse events which occurred in less than 5% but greater than or equal to 2% of adult and adolescent patients (ages 12 years and older) treated with NASONEX Nasal Spray 50 mcg, 200-mcg/day (regardless of relationship to treatment), and more frequently than in the placebo group included: arthralgia, asthma, bronchitis, chest pain, conjunctivitis, diarrhea, dyspepsia, earache, flu-like symptoms, myalgia, nausea, and rhinitis.

Pediatric patients <12 years of age

In controlled US and international studies, a total of 990 pediatric patients (ages 3 to 11 years) with allergic rhinitis received treatment with NASONEX Nasal Spray 50 mcg, at doses of 25 to 200 mcg/day. The majority of pediatric patients (n=720) were treated with 100 mcg/day. A total of 163 pediatric patients have been treated for one year or longer. Two percent or less of patients in clinical trials who received NASONEX Nasal Spray 50 mcg discontinued treatment because of adverse events and the discontinuation rate was similar for the placebo and active comparators.

Adverse events which occurred in ≥5% of pediatric patients (ages 3 to 11 years) treated with NASONEX Nasal Spray 50 mcg, 100 mcg/day vs. placebo (regardless of relationship to treatment) and more frequently than in the placebo group included upper respiratory tract infection (5% in NASONEX Nasal Spray 50 mcg group vs. 4% in placebo) and vomiting (5% in NASONEX Nasal Spray 50 mcg group vs. 4% in placebo).

Other adverse events which occurred in less than 5% but greater than or equal to 2% of pediatric patients (ages 3 to 11 years) treated with NASONEX Nasal Spray 50 mcg, 100 mcg/day vs. placebo (regardless of relationship to treatment) and more frequently than in the placebo group included: diarrhea, nasal irritation, otitis media, and wheezing.

The adverse event (regardless of relationship to treatment) reported by 5% of pediatric patients ages 2 to 5 years who received NASONEX Nasal Spray, 50 mcg, 100 mcg/day in a clinical trial vs. placebo including 56 subjects (28 each NASONEX Nasal Spray, 50 mcg and placebo) and that was more common with NASONEX Nasal Spray, 50 mcg than placebo, included: upper respiratory tract infection (7% vs. 0%, respectively). The other adverse event which occurred in less than 5% but greater than or equal to 2% of mometasone furoate pediatric patients ages 2 to 5 years treated with 100 mcg doses vs. placebo (regardless of relationship to treatment) and more frequently than in the placebo group included: skin trauma.

Nasal Polyps

Adults 18 years of age and older

In controlled clinical studies, the types of adverse events observed in patients with nasal polyps were similar to those observed for patients with allergic rhinitis. A total of 594 adult patients (ages 18 to 86 years) received NASONEX Nasal Spray 50 mcg at doses of 200 mcg once or twice daily for up to 4 months for treatment of nasal polyps. The overall incidence of adverse events for patients treated with NASONEX Nasal Spray 50 mcg was comparable to patients with the placebo except for epistaxis, which was 9% for 200 mcg once daily, 13% for 200 mcg twice daily, and 5% for the placebo.

Nasal ulcers and nasal and oral candidiasis were also reported in patients treated with NASONEX Nasal Spray 50 mcg primarily in patients treated for longer than 4 weeks.

Nasal Congestion Associated with Seasonal Allergic Rhinitis

A total of 1008 patients aged 12 years and older received NASONEX Nasal Spray 50 mcg 200 mcg/day (n=506) or placebo (n=502) for 15 days. Adverse events that occurred more frequently in patients treated with NASONEX Nasal Spray 50 mcg than in patients with the placebo included sinus headache (1.2% in NASONEX Nasal Spray 50 mcg group vs. 0.2% in placebo) and epistaxis (1% in NASONEX Nasal Spray 50 mcg group vs. 0.2% in placebo) and the overall adverse event profile was similar to that observed in the other allergic rhinitis trials.

6.2 Post-Marketing Experience

The following adverse reactions have been identified during the post-marketing period for NASONEX Nasal Spray 50 mcg: nasal burning and irritation, anaphylaxis and angioedema, disturbances in taste and smell and nasal septal perforation. Because these reactions are reported voluntarily from a population of uncertain size, it is not always possible to reliably estimate their frequency or establish a causal relationship to drug exposure.

7 DRUG INTERACTIONS

No formal drug-drug interaction studies have been conducted with NASONEX Nasal Spray 50 mcg.

Inhibitors of Cytochrome P450 3A4: Studies have shown that mometasone furoate is primarily and extensively metabolized in the liver of all species investigated and undergoes extensive metabolism to multiple metabolites. *In vitro* studies have confirmed the primary role of cytochrome CYP 3A4 in the metabolism of this compound. Coadministration with ketoconazole, a potent CYP 3A4 inhibitor, may increase the plasma concentrations of mometasone furoate *[see Clinical Pharmacology (12.3)]*.

8 USE IN SPECIFIC POPULATIONS

8.1 Pregnancy

Teratogenic Effects: Pregnancy Category C: There are no adequate and well-controlled studies in pregnant women. NASONEX Nasal Spray 50 mcg, like other corticosteroids, should be used during pregnancy only if the potential benefits justify the potential risk to the fetus. Experience with oral corticosteroids since their introduction in pharmacologic, as opposed to physiologic, doses suggests that rodents are more prone to teratogenic effects from corticosteroids than humans. In addition, because there is a natural increase in corticosteroid production during pregnancy, most women will require a lower exogenous corticosteroid dose and many will not need corticosteroid treatment during pregnancy.

In mice, mometasone furoate caused cleft palate at subcutaneous doses (less than the MRDID in adults on a mcg/m^2 basis). Fetal survival was reduced at approximately 2 times the MRDID in adults on a mcg/m^2 basis. No toxicity was observed at less than the MRDID in adults on a mcg/m^2 basis.

In rats, mometasone furoate produced umbilical hernia at topical dermal doses approximately 10 times the MRDID in adults on a mcg/m^2 basis. A topical dermal dose approximately 6 times the MRDID in adults on a mcg/m^2 basis produced delays in ossification, but no malformations.

In rabbits, mometasone furoate caused multiple malformations (e.g., flexed front paws, gallbladder agenesis, umbilical hernia, and hydrocephaly) at topical dermal doses approximately 6 times the MRDID in adults on a mcg/m^2 basis. In an oral study, mometasone furoate increased resorptions and caused cleft palate and/or head malformations (hydrocephaly or domed head) at approximately 30 times the MRDID in adults on a mcg/m^2 basis. At approximately 110 times the MRDID in adults on a mcg/m^2 basis, most litters were aborted or resorbed. No toxicity was observed at approximately 6 times the MRDID in adults on a mcg/m^2 basis.

When rats received subcutaneous doses of mometasone furoate throughout pregnancy or during the later stages of pregnancy, a dose less than the MRDID in adults on a mcg/m^2 basis caused prolonged and difficult labor and reduced the number of live births, birth weight, and early pup survival.

Nonteratogenic Effects: Hypoadrenalism may occur in infants born to women receiving corticosteroids during pregnancy. Such infants should be carefully monitored.

8.3 Nursing Mothers

It is not known if mometasone furoate is excreted in human milk. Because other corticosteroids are excreted in human milk, caution should be used when NASONEX Nasal Spray, 50 mcg is administered to nursing women.

8.4 Pediatric Use

The safety and effectiveness of NASONEX Nasal Spray 50 mcg for allergic rhinitis in children 12 years of age and older have been established *[see Adverse Reactions (6.1) and Clinical Studies (14.1)]*. Use of NASONEX Nasal Spray 50 mcg for allergic rhinitis in pediatric patients 2 to 11 years of age is supported by safety and efficacy data from clinical studies. Seven hundred and twenty (720) patients 3 to 11 years of age with allergic rhinitis were treated with mometasone furoate nasal spray 50 mcg (100 mcg total daily dose) in controlled clinical trials *[see Adverse Reactions (6.1) and Clinical Studies (14.2)]*. Twenty-eight (28) patients 2 to 5 years of age with allergic rhinitis were treated with mometasone furoate nasal spray 50 mcg (100 mcg total daily dose) in a controlled trial to evaluate safety *[see Adverse Reactions (6.1)]*. Safety and effectiveness of NASONEX Nasal Spray 50 mcg for allergic rhinitis in children less than 2 years of age have not been established.

The safety and effectiveness of NASONEX Nasal Spray for the treatment of nasal polyps in children less than 18 years of age have not been established. One 4-month trial was conducted to evaluate the safety and efficacy of NASONEX in the treatment of nasal polyps in pediatric patients 6 to 17 years of age. The primary objective of the study was to evaluate safety; efficacy parameters were collected as secondary endpoints. A total of 127 patients with nasal polyps were randomized to placebo or NASONEX Nasal Spray 100 mcg once or twice daily (patients 6 to 11 years of age) or 200 mcg once or twice daily (patients 12 to 17 years of age). The results of this trial did not support the efficacy of NASONEX Nasal Spray in the treatment of nasal polyps in pediatric patients. The adverse events reported in this trial were similar to the adverse events reported in patients 18 years of age and older with nasal polyps.

Controlled clinical studies have shown intranasal corticosteroids may cause a reduction in growth velocity in pediatric patients. This effect has been observed in the absence of laboratory evidence of hypothalamic-pituitary-adrenal (HPA) axis suppression, suggesting that growth velocity is a more sensitive indicator of systemic corticosteroid exposure in pediatric patients than some commonly used tests of HPA axis function. The long-term effects of this reduction in growth velocity associated with intranasal corticosteroids, including the impact on final adult height, are unknown. The potential for "catch up" growth following discontinuation of treatment with intranasal corticosteroids has not been adequately studied. The growth of pediatric patients receiving intranasal corticosteroids, including NASONEX Nasal Spray, 50 mcg, should be monitored routinely (e.g., via stadiometry). The potential growth effects of prolonged treatment should be weighed against clinical benefits obtained and the availability of safe and effective noncorticosteroid treatment alternatives. To minimize the systemic effects of intranasal corticosteroids, including NASONEX Nasal Spray, 50 mcg, each patient should be titrated to his/her lowest effective dose.

A clinical study to assess the effect of NASONEX Nasal Spray 50 mcg (100 mcg total daily dose) on growth velocity has been conducted in pediatric patients 3 to 9 years of age with allergic rhinitis. No statistically significant effect on growth velocity was observed for NASONEX Nasal Spray 50 mcg compared to placebo following one year of treatment. No evidence of clinically relevant HPA axis suppression was observed following a 30-minute cosyntropin infusion.

The potential of NASONEX Nasal Spray 50 mcg to cause growth suppression in susceptible patients or when given at higher doses cannot be ruled out.

8.5 Geriatric Use

A total of 280 patients above 64 years of age with allergic rhinitis or nasal polyps (age range 64 to 86 years) have been treated with NASONEX Nasal Spray 50 mcg for up to 3 or 4 months, respectively. The adverse reactions reported in this population were similar in type and incidence to those reported by younger patients.

8.6 Hepatic Impairment

Concentrations of mometasone furoate appear to increase with severity of hepatic impairment *[see Clinical Pharmacology (12.3)]*.

10 OVERDOSAGE

There are no data available on the effects of acute or chronic overdosage with NASONEX Nasal Spray 50 mcg. Because of low systemic bioavailability, and an absence of acute drug-related systemic findings in clinical studies, overdose is unlikely to require any therapy other than observation. Intranasal administration of 1600 mcg (4 times the recommended dose of NASONEX Nasal Spray 50 mcg for the treatment of nasal polyps in patients 18 years of age and older) daily for 29 days, to healthy human volunteers, showed no increased incidence of adverse events. Single intranasal doses up to 4000 mcg and oral inhalation doses up to 8000 mcg have been studied in human volunteers with no adverse effects reported. Chronic over dosage with any corticosteroid may result in signs or symptoms of hypercorticism *[see Warnings and Precautions (5.4)]*. Acute overdosage with this dosage form is unlikely since one bottle of NASONEX Nasal Spray 50 mcg contains approximately 8500 mcg of mometasone furoate.

11 DESCRIPTION

Mometasone furoate monohydrate, the active component of NASONEX Nasal Spray, 50 mcg, is an anti-inflammatory corticosteroid having the chemical name, 9,21-Dichloro-11ß,17-dihydroxy-16α-methylpregna-1,4-diene-3,20-dione 17-(2 furoate) monohydrate, and the following chemical structure:

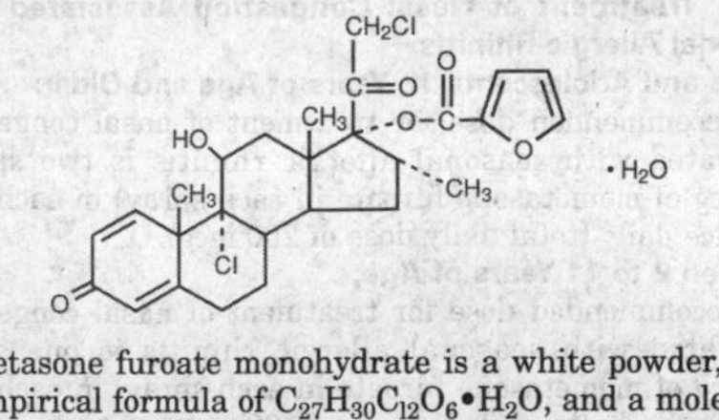

Mometasone furoate monohydrate is a white powder, with an empirical formula of $C_{27}H_{30}C_{12}O_6 \cdot H_2O$, and a molecular weight of 539.45. It is practically insoluble in water; slightly soluble in methanol, ethanol, and isopropanol; soluble in acetone and chloroform; and freely soluble in tetrahydrofuran. Its partition coefficient between octanol and water is greater than 5000.

NASONEX Nasal Spray 50 mcg is a metered-dose, manual pump spray unit containing an aqueous suspension of mometasone furoate monohydrate equivalent to 0.05% w/w mometasone furoate calculated on the anhydrous basis; in an aqueous medium containing glycerin, microcrystalline cellulose and carboxymethylcellulose sodium, sodium citrate, citric acid, benzalkonium chloride, and polysorbate 80. The pH is between 4.3 and 4.9.

12 CLINICAL PHARMACOLOGY

12.1 Mechanism of Action

NASONEX Nasal Spray 50 mcg is a corticosteroid demonstrating potent anti-inflammatory properties. The precise mechanism of corticosteroid action on allergic rhinitis is not known. Corticosteroids have been shown to have a wide range of effects on multiple cell types (e.g., mast cells, eosinophils, neutrophils, macrophages, and lymphocytes) and mediators (e.g., histamine, eicosanoids, leukotrienes, and cytokines) involved in inflammation.

In two clinical studies utilizing nasal antigen challenge, NASONEX Nasal Spray, 50 mcg decreased some markers of the early- and late-phase allergic response. These observations included decreases (vs. placebo) in histamine and eosinophil cationic protein levels, and reductions (vs. baseline) in eosinophils, neutrophils, and epithelial cell adhesion proteins. The clinical significance of these findings is not known.

The effect of NASONEX Nasal Spray, 50 mcg on nasal mucosa following 12 months of treatment was examined in 46 patients with allergic rhinitis. There was no evidence of atrophy and there was a marked reduction in intraepithelial eosinophilia and inflammatory cell infiltration (e.g., eosinophils, lymphocytes, monocytes, neutrophils, and plasma cells).

12.2 Pharmacodynamics

Adrenal Function in Adults: Four clinical pharmacology studies have been conducted in humans to assess the effect of NASONEX Nasal Spray, 50 mcg at various doses on adrenal function. In one study, daily doses of 200 and 400 mcg of NASONEX Nasal Spray, 50 mcg and 10 mg of prednisone were compared to placebo in 64 patients (22 to 44 years of age) with allergic rhinitis. Adrenal function before and after 36 consecutive days of treatment was assessed by measuring plasma cortisol levels following a 6-hour Cortrosyn (ACTH) infusion and by measuring 24-hour urinary free cortisol levels. NASONEX Nasal Spray, 50 mcg, at both the 200- and 400-mcg dose, was not associated with a statistically significant decrease in mean plasma cortisol levels post-Cortrosyn infusion or a statistically significant decrease in the 24-hour urinary free cortisol levels compared to placebo. A statistically significant decrease in the mean plasma cortisol levels post-Cortrosyn infusion and 24-hour urinary free cortisol levels was detected in the prednisone treatment group compared to placebo.

A second study assessed adrenal response to NASONEX Nasal Spray, 50 mcg (400 and 1600 mcg/day), prednisone (10 mg/day), and placebo, administered for 29 days in 48 male volunteers (21 to 40 years of age). The 24-hour plasma cortisol area under the curve (AUC_{0-24}), during and after an 8-hour Cortrosyn infusion and 24-hour urinary free cortisol levels were determined at baseline and after 29 days of treatment. No statistically significant differences in adrenal function were observed with NASONEX Nasal Spray, 50 mcg compared to placebo.

A third study evaluated single, rising doses of NASONEX Nasal Spray, 50 mcg (1000, 2000, and 4000 mcg/day), orally administered mometasone furoate (2000, 4000, and 8000 mcg/day), orally administered dexamethasone (200, 400, and 800 mcg/day), and placebo (administered at the end of each series of doses) in 24 male volunteers (22 to 39 years of age). Dose administrations were separated by at least 72 hours. Determination of serial plasma cortisol levels at 8 AM and for the 24-hour period following each treatment were used to calculate the plasma cortisol area under the curve (AUC_{0-24}). In addition, 24-hour urinary free cortisol levels were collected prior to initial treatment administration and during the period immediately following each dose. No statistically significant decreases in the plasma cortisol AUC, 8 AM cortisol levels, or 24-hour urinary free cortisol levels were observed in volunteers treated with either NASONEX Nasal Spray, 50 mcg or oral mometasone, as compared with placebo treatment. Conversely, nearly all volunteers treated with the three doses of dexamethasone demonstrated abnormal 8 AM cortisol levels (defined as a cortisol level <10 mcg/dL), reduced 24-hour plasma AUC values, and decreased 24-hour urinary free cortisol levels, as compared to placebo treatment.

In a fourth study, adrenal function was assessed in 213 patients (18 to 81 years of age) with nasal polyps before and after 4 months of treatment with either NASONEX Nasal Spray, 50 mcg, (200 mcg once or twice daily) or placebo by measuring 24-hour urinary free cortisol levels. NASONEX Nasal Spray, 50 mcg, at both doses (200 and 400 mcg/day), was not associated with statistically significant decreases in the 24-hour urinary free cortisol levels compared to placebo.

Three clinical pharmacology studies have been conducted in pediatric patients to assess the effect of mometasone furoate nasal spray on the adrenal function at daily doses of 50, 100, and 200 mcg vs. placebo. In one study, adrenal function before and after 7 consecutive days of treatment was assessed in 48 pediatric patients with allergic rhinitis (ages 6 to 11 years) by measuring morning plasma cortisol and 24-hour urinary free cortisol levels. Mometasone furoate nasal spray, at all three doses, was not associated with a statistically significant decrease in mean plasma cortisol levels or a statistically significant decrease in the 24-hour urinary free cortisol levels compared to placebo. In the second study, adrenal function before and after 14 consecutive days of treatment was assessed in 48 pediatric patients (ages 3 to 5 years) with allergic rhinitis by measuring plasma cortisol levels following a 30-minute Cortrosyn infusion. Mometasone furoate nasal spray, 50 mcg, at all three doses (50, 100, and 200 mcg/day), was not associated with a statistically significant decrease in mean plasma cortisol levels post-Cortrosyn infusion compared to placebo. All patients had a normal response to Cortrosyn. In the third study, adrenal function before and after up to 42 consecutive days of once-daily treatment was assessed in 52 patients with allergic rhinitis (ages 2 to 5 years), 28 of whom received mometasone furoate nasal spray, 50 mcg per nostril (total daily dose 100 mcg), by measuring morning plasma cortisol and 24-hour urinary free cortisol levels. Mometasone furoate nasal spray was not associated with a statistically significant decrease in mean plasma cortisol levels or a statistically significant decrease in the 24-hour urinary free cortisol levels compared to placebo.

12.3 Pharmacokinetics

Absorption:

Mometasone furoate monohydrate administered as a nasal spray suspension has very low bioavailability (<1%) in plasma using a sensitive assay with a lower quantitation limit (LOQ) of 0.25 pcg/mL.

Distribution:

The *in vitro* protein binding for mometasone furoate was reported to be 98% to 99% in concentration range of 5 to 500 ng/mL.

Metabolism:

Studies have shown that any portion of a mometasone furoate dose which is swallowed and absorbed undergoes extensive metabolism to multiple metabolites. There are no major metabolites detectable in plasma. Upon *in vitro* incubation, one of the minor metabolites formed is 6ß-hydroxy-mometasone furoate. In human liver microsomes, the formation of the metabolite is regulated by cytochrome P-450 3A4 (CYP3A4).

Elimination:

Following intravenous administration, the effective plasma elimination half-life of mometasone furoate is 5.8 hours. Any absorbed drug is excreted as metabolites mostly via the bile, and to a limited extent, into the urine.

Specific Populations:

Hepatic Impairment: Administration of a single inhaled dose of 400 mcg mometasone furoate to subjects with mild (n=4), moderate (n=4), and severe (n=4) hepatic impairment resulted in only 1 or 2 subjects in each group having detectable peak plasma concentrations of mometasone furoate (ranging from 50 to 105 pcg/mL). The observed peak plasma concentrations appear to increase with severity of hepatic impairment, however, the numbers of detectable levels were few.

Renal Impairment: The effects of renal impairment on mometasone furoate pharmacokinetics have not been adequately investigated.

Pediatric: Mometasone furoate pharmacokinetics have not been investigated in the pediatric population *[see Use in Specific Populations (8.4)]*.

Gender: The effects of gender on mometasone furoate pharmacokinetics have not been adequately investigated.

Race: The effects of race on mometasone furoate pharmacokinetics have not been adequately investigated.

Drug-Drug Interactions:

Inhibitors of Cytochrome P450 3A4: In a drug interaction study, an inhaled dose of mometasone furoate 400 mcg was given to 24 healthy subjects twice daily for 9 days and ketoconazole 200 mg (as well as placebo) were given twice daily concomitantly on Days 4 to 9. Mometasone furoate plasma concentrations were <150 pcg/mL on Day 3 prior to coadministration of ketoconazole or placebo. Following concomitant administration of ketoconazole, 4 out of 12 subjects in the ketoconazole treatment group (n=12) had peak plasma concentrations of mometasone furoate >200 pcg/mL on Day 9 (211-324 pcg/mL).

13 NONCLINICAL TOXICOLOGY

13.1 Carcinogenesis, Mutagenesis, Impairment of Fertility

In a 2-year carcinogenicity study in Sprague Dawley rats, mometasone furoate demonstrated no statistically significant increase in the incidence of tumors at inhalation doses up to 67 mcg/kg (approximately 1 and 2 times the maximum recommended daily intranasal dose [MRDID] in adults [400 mcg] and children [100 mcg], respectively, on a mcg/m^2 basis). In a 19-month carcinogenicity study in Swiss CD-1 mice, mometasone furoate demonstrated no statistically significant increase in the incidence of tumors at inhalation doses up to 160 mcg/kg (approximately 2 times the MRDID in adults and children, respectively, on a mcg/m^2 basis).

Mometasone furoate increased chromosomal aberrations in an *in vitro* Chinese hamster ovary-cell assay, but did not increase chromosomal aberrations in an *in vitro* Chinese hamster lung cell assay. Mometasone furoate was not mutagenic in the Ames test or mouse-lymphoma assay, and was not clastogenic in an *in vivo* mouse micronucleus assay and a rat bone marrow chromosomal aberration assay or a mouse male germ-cell chromosomal aberration assay. Mometasone furoate also did not induce unscheduled DNA synthesis *in vivo* in rat hepatocytes.

In reproductive studies in rats, impairment of fertility was not produced by subcutaneous doses up to 15 mcg/kg (less than the MRDID in adults on a mcg/m^2 basis).

13.2 Animal Toxicology and/or Pharmacology
Reproduction Toxicology Studies

In mice, mometasone furoate caused cleft palate at subcutaneous doses of 60 mcg/kg and above (less than the MRDID in adults on a mcg/m^2 basis). Fetal survival was reduced at 180 mcg/kg (approximately 2 times the MRDID in adults on a mcg/m^2 basis). No toxicity was observed at 20 mcg/kg (less than the MRDID in adults on a mcg/m^2 basis).

In rats, mometasone furoate produced umbilical hernia at topical dermal doses of 600 mcg/kg and above (approximately 10 times the MRDID in adults on a mcg/m^2 basis). A dose of 300 mcg/kg (approximately 6 times the MRDID in adults on a mcg/m^2 basis) produced delays in ossification, but no malformations. In rabbits, mometasone furoate caused multiple malformations (e.g., flexed front paws, gallbladder agenesis, umbilical hernia, hydrocephaly) at topical dermal doses of 150 mcg/kg and above (approximately 6 times the MRDID in adults on a mcg/m^2 basis). In an oral study, mometasone furoate increased resorptions and caused cleft palate and/or head malformations (hydrocephaly or domed head) at 700 mcg/kg (approximately 30 times the MRDID in adults on a mcg/m^2 basis). At 2800 mcg/kg (approximately 110 times the MRDID in adults on a mcg/m^2 basis), most litters were aborted or resorbed. No toxicity was observed at 140 mcg/kg (approximately 6 times the MRDID in adults on a mcg/m^2 basis).

When rats received subcutaneous doses of mometasone furoate throughout pregnancy or during the later stages of pregnancy, 15 mcg/kg (less than the MRDID in adults on a mcg/m^2 basis) caused prolonged and difficult labor and reduced the number of live births, birth weight, and early pup survival. Similar effects were not observed at 7.5 mcg/kg (less than the MRDID in adults on a mcg/m^2 basis).

14 CLINICAL STUDIES

14.1 Allergic Rhinitis in Adults and Adolescents

The efficacy and safety of NASONEX Nasal Spray, 50 mcg in the prophylaxis and treatment of seasonal allergic rhinitis and the treatment of perennial allergic rhinitis have been evaluated in 18 controlled trials, and one uncontrolled clinical trial, in approximately 3000 adults (ages 17 to 85 years) and adolescents (ages 12 to 16 years). Of the total number of patients, there were 1757 males and 1453 females, including a total of 283 adolescents (182 boys and 101 girls) with seasonal allergic or perennial allergic rhinitis. Patients were treated with NASONEX Nasal Spray 50 mcg at doses ranging from 50 to 800 mcg/day. The majority of patients were treated with 200 mcg/day. The allergic rhinitis trials evaluated the total nasal symptom scores that included stuffiness, rhinorrhea, itching, and sneezing. Patients treated with NASONEX Nasal Spray 50 mcg, 200 mcg/day had a statistically significant decrease in total nasal symptom scores compared to placebo-treated patients. No additional benefit was observed for mometasone furoate doses greater than 200 mcg/day. A total of 350 patients have been treated with NASONEX Nasal Spray 50 mcg for 1 year or longer.

In patients with seasonal allergic rhinitis, NASONEX Nasal Spray 50 mcg, demonstrated improvement in nasal symptoms (vs. placebo) within 11 hours after the first dose based on one single-dose, parallel-group study of patients in an outdoor "park" setting (park study) and one environmental exposure unit (EEU) study, and within 2 days in two randomized, double-blind, placebo-controlled, parallel-group seasonal allergic rhinitis studies. Maximum benefit is usually achieved within 1 to 2 weeks after initiation of dosing.

Prophylaxis of seasonal allergic rhinitis for patients 12 years of age and older with NASONEX Nasal Spray 50 mcg, given at a dose of 200 mcg/day, was evaluated in two clinical studies in 284 patients. These studies were designed such that patients received 4 weeks of prophylaxis with NASONEX Nasal Spray 50 mcg prior to the anticipated onset of the pollen season; however, some patients received only 2 to 3 weeks of prophylaxis. Patients receiving 2 to 4 weeks of prophylaxis with NASONEX Nasal Spray 50 mcg demonstrated a statistically significantly smaller mean increase in total nasal symptom scores with onset of the pollen season as compared to placebo patients.

14.2 Allergic Rhinitis in Pediatrics

The efficacy and safety of NASONEX Nasal Spray 50 mcg in the treatment of seasonal allergic and perennial allergic rhinitis in pediatric patients (ages 3 to 11 years) have been evaluated in four controlled trials. This included approximately 990 pediatric patients ages 3 to 11 years (606 males and 384 females) with seasonal allergic or perennial allergic rhinitis treated with mometasone furoate nasal spray at doses ranging from 25 to 200 mcg/day. Pediatric patients treated with NASONEX Nasal Spray 50 mcg (100 mcg total daily dose, 374 patients) had a significant decrease in total nasal symptom (nasal congestion, rhinorrhea, itching, and sneezing) scores, compared to placebo-treated patients. No additional benefit was observed for the 200-mcg mometasone furoate total daily dose in pediatric patients (ages 3 to 11 years). A total of 163 pediatric patients have been treated for 1 year.

TABLE 2: EFFECT OF NASONEX NASAL SPRAY IN TWO RANDOMIZED, PLACEBO-CONTROLLED TRIALS IN PATIENTS WITH NASAL POLYPS

	NASONEX 200 mcg qd	NASONEX 200 mcg bid	Placebo	*P*-value for NASONEX 200 mcg qd vs. placebo	*P*-value for NASONEX 200 mcg bid vs. placebo
Study 1	N=115	N=122	N=117		
Baseline bilateral polyp grade*	4.21	4.27	4.25		
Mean change from baseline in bilateral polyps grade	-1.15	-0.96	-0.50	<0.001	0.01
Baseline nasal congestion†	2.29	2.35	2.28		
Mean change from baseline in nasal congestion	-0.47	-0.61	-0.24	0.001	<0.001
Study 2	N=102	N=102	N=106		
Baseline bilateral polyp grade*	4.00	4.10	4.17		
Mean change from baseline in bilateral polyps grade	-0.78	-0.96	-0.62	0.33	0.04
Baseline nasal congestion†	2.23	2.20	2.18		
Mean change from baseline in nasal congestion	-0.42	-0.66	-0.23	0.01	<0.001

* polyps in each nasal fossa were graded by the investigator based on endoscopic visualization, using a scale of 0-3 where 0=no polyps; 1=polyps in the middle meatus, not reaching below the inferior border of the middle turbinate; 2=polyps reaching below the inferior border of the middle turbinate but not the inferior border of the inferior turbinate; 3=polyps reaching to or below the border of the inferior turbinate, or polyps medial to the middle turbinate (score reflects sum of left and right nasal fossa grades).

† nasal congestion/obstruction was scored daily by the patient using a 0-3 categorical scale where 0=no symptoms, 1=mild symptoms, 2=moderate symptoms and 3=severe symptoms.

TABLE 3: EFFECT OF NASONEX NASAL SPRAY IN TWO RANDOMIZED, PLACEBO-CONTROLLED TRIALS ON NASAL CONGESTION IN PATIENTS WITH SEASONAL ALLERGIC RHINITIS

Treatment (Patient Number)	Baseline * LS Mean †	Change from Baseline LS Mean †	Difference from Placebo LS Mean †	*P*-value for NASONEX 200 mcg qd vs. placebo
Study 1				
NASONEX 200 mcg qd (N=176)	2.63	-0.64	-0.15	0.006
Placebo (N=175)	2.62	-0.49		
Study 2				
NASONEX 200 mcg qd (N=168)	2.62	-0.71	-0.31	<0.001
Placebo (N=164)	2.60	-0.40		

* nasal congestion/obstruction was scored daily by the patient using a 0-3 categorical scale where 0=no symptoms, 1=mild symptoms, 2=moderate symptoms and 3=severe symptoms.

† LS Mean and p-value was from an ANCOVA model with treatment, baseline value, and center effects.

TABLE 4: EFFECT OF NASONEX NASAL SPRAY ON TNSS IN TWO RANDOMIZED, PLACEBO-CONTROLLED TRIALS IN PATIENTS WITH SEASONAL ALLERGIC RHINITIS

Treatment (Patient Number)	Baseline * LS Mean †	Change from Baseline LS Mean †	Difference from Placebo LS Mean †	*P*-value for NASONEX 200 mcg qd vs. placebo
Study 1				
NASONEX 200 mcg qd (N=176)	9.60	-2.68	-0.83	<0.001
Placebo (N=175)	9.66	-1.85		
Study 2				
NASONEX 200 mcg qd (N=168)	9.39	-3.00	-1.27	<0.001
Placebo (N=164)	9.50	-1.73		

* TNSS was the sum of four individual symptom scores: rhinorrhea, nasal congestion/stuffiness, nasal itching and sneezing. Each symptom was to be rated on a scale of 0=none, 1=mild, 2=moderate, 3=severe.

† LS Mean and p-value was from an ANCOVA model with treatment, baseline value, and center effects.

14.3 Nasal Polyps in Adults 18 Years of Age and Older

Two studies were performed to evaluate the efficacy and safety of NASONEX Nasal Spray in the treatment of nasal polyps. These studies involved 664 patients with nasal polyps, 441 of whom received NASONEX Nasal Spray. These studies were randomized, double-blind, placebo-controlled, parallel-group, multicenter studies in patients 18 to 86 years of age with bilateral nasal polyps. Patients were randomized to receive NASONEX Nasal Spray 200 mcg once daily, 200 mcg twice daily or placebo for a period of 4 months. The co-primary efficacy endpoints were 1) change from baseline in nasal congestion/obstruction averaged over the first month of treatment; and 2) change from baseline to last assessment in bilateral polyp grade during the entire 4 months of treatment as assessed by endoscopy. Efficacy was demonstrated in both studies at a dose of 200 mcg twice daily and in one study at a dose of 200 mcg once a day (see TABLE 2 below).

[See table 2 at left]

There were no clinically relevant differences in the effectiveness of NASONEX Nasal Spray, 50 mcg, in the studies evaluating treatment of nasal polyps across subgroups of patients defined by gender, age, or race.

14.4 Nasal Congestion Associated with Seasonal Allergic Rhinitis

The efficacy and safety of NASONEX Nasal Spray 50 mcg for nasal congestion associated with seasonal allergic rhinitis were evaluated in three randomized, placebo-controlled, double blind clinical trials of 15 days duration. The three trials included a total of 1008 patients 12 years of age and older with nasal congestion associated with seasonal allergic rhinitis, of whom 506 received NASONEX Nasal Spray 200 mcg daily and 502 received placebo. Of the 1008 patients, the majority 784 (78 %) were Caucasians. The majority of the patients were between 18 to < 65 years of age with a mean age of 38.8 years and were predominantly women (66%). The primary efficacy endpoint was the change from baseline in average morning and evening reflective nasal congestion score over treatment day 1 to day 15. The key secondary efficacy endpoint was the change from baseline in average morning and evening reflective total nasal symptom score (TNSS=rhinorrhea [nasal discharge/runny nose or postnasal drip], nasal congestion/stuffiness, nasal itching, sneezing) averaged over treatment day 1 to 15. Two out of three studies demonstrated that treatment with NASONEX Nasal Spray significantly reduced the nasal congestion symptom score and the TNSS compared to placebo in patients 12 years of age and older with seasonal allergic rhinitis (see TABLE 3 and 4 below).

[See table 3 below]

[See table 4 below]

Based on results in other studies with NASONEX Nasal Spray in pediatric patients, effects on nasal congestion associated with seasonal allergic rhinitis in patients below 12 years of age is similar to those seen in adults and adolescents *[see Clinical Studies (14.2)]*.

16 HOW SUPPLIED/STORAGE AND HANDLING

NASONEX (mometasone furoate monohydrate) Nasal Spray, 50 mcg is supplied in a white, high-density, polyethylene bottle fitted with a white metered-dose, manual spray pump, and blue cap. It contains 17 g of product formulation, 120 sprays, each delivering 50 mcg of mometasone furoate per actuation.

(NDC 0085-1288-01).

Store at 25°C (77°F); excursions permitted to 15-30°C (59-86°F) [see USP Controlled Room Temperature]. Protect from light.

When NASONEX Nasal Spray, 50 mcg is removed from its cardboard container, prolonged exposure of the product to direct light should be avoided. Brief exposure to light, as with normal use, is acceptable.

SHAKE WELL BEFORE EACH USE.

Keep out of reach of children.

17 PATIENT COUNSELING INFORMATION

See FDA-approved labeling

17.1 Local Nasal Effect

Patients should be informed that treatment with NASONEX Nasal Spray 50 mcg may be associated with adverse reactions which include epistaxis (nose bleed) and nasal septum perforation. *Candida* infection may also occur. Because of the inhibitory effect of corticosteroids on wound healing, patients who have experienced recent nasal septum ulcers, nasal surgery, or nasal trauma should not use a nasal corticosteroid until healing has occurred *[see Warnings and Precautions (5.1)]*. Patients should be cautioned not to spray NASONEX Nasal Spray 50 mcg directly onto the nasal septum.

17.2 Glaucoma and Cataracts

Patients should be informed that nasal and inhaled corticosteroids may result in the development of glaucoma and/or cataracts. Therefore, close monitoring is warranted in patients with a change in vision or with a history of increased intraocular pressure, glaucoma, and/or cataracts. Patients should be cautioned not to spray NASONEX Nasal Spray 50 mcg into the eyes *[see Warnings and Precautions (5.2)]*.

17.3 Immunosuppression

Persons who are on immunosuppressant doses of corticosteroids should be warned to avoid exposure to chickenpox or measles, and patients should also be advised that if they are exposed, medical advice should be sought without delay *[see Warnings and Precautions (5.4)]*.

17.4 Use Regularly for Best Effect

Patients should use NASONEX Nasal Spray 50 mcg on a regular basis for optimal effect. Improvement in nasal symptoms of allergic rhinitis has been shown to occur within 1 to 2 days after initiation of dosing. Maximum benefit is usually achieved within 1 to 2 weeks after initiation of dosing. Patients should not increase the prescribed dosage but should contact their physician if symptoms do not improve, or if the condition worsens. Administration to young children should be aided by an adult.

If a patient missed a dose, the patient should be advised to take the dose as soon as they remember. The patient should not take more than the recommended dose for the day.

Manufactured for: Merck Sharp & Dohme Corp., a subsidiary of
MERCK & CO., INC., Whitehouse Station, NJ 08889, USA
Manufactured by:
MSD International GmbH (Singapore Branch),
Singapore 638414, Singapore
U.S. Patent No. 6,127,353.

Revised: 03/2013
032088-NSX-NS-USPI.13

Patient Information

NASONEX® **[nā-zə-neks]** (mometasone furoate monohydrate) **Nasal Spray, 50 mcg**

FOR INTRANASAL USE ONLY

Read the Patient Information that comes with NASONEX before you start using it and each time you get a refill. There may be new information. This Patient Information does not take the place of talking to your healthcare provider about your medical condition or treatment. If you have any questions about NASONEX, ask your healthcare provider.

What is NASONEX?

NASONEX Nasal Spray is a man-made (synthetic) corticosteroid medicine that is used to:

- treat the nasal symptoms of seasonal and year-round allergic rhinitis (inflammation of the lining of the nose) in adults and children 2 years of age and older.
- treat nasal congestion that happens with seasonal allergic rhinitis in adults and children 2 years of age and older.
- prevent nasal symptoms of seasonal allergic rhinitis in people 12 years of age and older.
- treat nasal polyps in people 18 years and older.

The safety and effectiveness of NASONEX has not been shown:

- in children under 2 years of age to treat allergic rhinitis.
- in children under 18 years of age to treat nasal polyps.

Who should not use NASONEX?

Do not use NASONEX if you are allergic to any of the ingredients in NASONEX. See the end of this leaflet for a complete list of ingredients in NASONEX.

What should I tell my healthcare provider before using NASONEX?

Before you take NASONEX, tell your healthcare provider if you:

- have had recent nasal sores, nasal surgery, or nasal injury.
- have eye or vision problems, such as cataracts or glaucoma (increased pressure in your eye).
- have tuberculosis or any untreated fungal, bacterial, viral infections, or eye infections caused by herpes.
- have been near someone who has chickenpox or measles.
- are not feeling well or have any other symptoms that you do not understand.
- have any other medical conditions.
- **are pregnant or planning to become pregnant.** It is not known if NASONEX will harm your unborn baby. Talk to your doctor if you are pregnant or plan to become pregnant.
- **are breastfeeding or planning to breastfeed.** It is not known whether NASONEX passes into your breast milk.

Tell your healthcare provider about all the medicines you take including prescription and non-prescription medicines, vitamins, and herbal supplements.

NASONEX and other medicines may affect each other and cause side effects. NASONEX may affect the way other medicines work, and other medicines may affect how NASONEX works.

Know the list of medicine you take. Keep a list of your medications with you to show your healthcare provider and pharmacist when a new medication is prescribed.

How should I use NASONEX?

- Use NASONEX exactly as prescribed by your healthcare provider.
- This medicine is for use in the nose only. Do not spray it into your mouth or eyes.
- An adult should help a young child use this medicine.
- For best results, you should keep using NASONEX regularly each day without missing a dose. If you do miss a dose of NASONEX, take it as soon as you remember. However, do not take more than the daily dose prescribed by your doctor.
- Do not use NASONEX more often than prescribed. Ask your healthcare provider if you have any questions.
- For detailed instructions on how to use NASONEX Nasal Spray, see the **"Patient Instructions for Use"** at the end of this leaflet.

See your healthcare provider regularly to assess your symptoms while taking NASONEX and to check for side effects.

What should I avoid while taking NASONEX?

If you are taking other corticosteroid medicines for allergy, either by mouth or injection, your healthcare provider may advise you to stop taking them once you begin using NASONEX.

What are the possible side effects of NASONEX?

NASONEX may cause serious side effects, including:

- **Thrush *(candida)*, a fungal infection in your nose and throat.** Tell your doctor if you have any redness or white colored patches in your nose or throat.
- **Slow wound healing. Do not** use NASONEX until your nose has healed if you have a sore in your nose, if you have surgery on your nose, or if your nose has been injured.
- **Some people may have eye problems, including glaucoma and cataracts.** You should have regular eye exams.
- **Immune system problems that may increase your risk of infections.** You are more likely to get infections if you take medicines that weaken your immune system. Avoid contact with people who have contagious diseases such as chicken pox or measles while using NASONEX. Symptoms of infection may include: fever, pain, aches, chills, feeling tired, nausea and vomiting. Tell your doctor about any signs of infection while you are using NASONEX.
- **Adrenal insufficiency.** Adrenal insufficiency is a condition in which the adrenal glands do not make enough steroid hormones. Symptoms of adrenal insufficiency can include: tiredness, weakness, nausea and vomiting and low blood pressure.

The most common side effects of NASONEX include:

- headache
- viral infection
- sore throat
- nosebleeds
- cough

Tell your healthcare provider if you have any side effect that bothers you or that does not go away.

These are not all the possible side effects of NASONEX. For more information ask your healthcare provider or pharmacist.

Call your doctor for medical advice about side effects. You may report side effects to FDA at 1-800-FDA-1088.

How should I store NASONEX?

- Store NASONEX at room temperature between 59°F to 86°F (15°C to 30°C).
- Avoid prolonged exposure of NASONEX container to bright light.
- Shake well before each use.

Keep NASONEX and all medicines out of the reach of children.

General information about NASONEX

Medicines are sometimes prescribed for conditions that are not listed in a Patient Information leaflet. Do not use NASONEX for a condition for which it was not prescribed. Do not give NASONEX to other people even if they have the same symptoms you have. It may harm them.

This Patient Information leaflet provides a summary of the most important information about NASONEX. If you would like more information, talk with your healthcare provider. You can ask your healthcare provider or pharmacist for information about NASONEX that is written for health professionals.

For more information, go to www.NASONEX.com or call 1-800-622-4477.

What are the ingredients in NASONEX?

Active Ingredients: mometasone furoate monohydrate

Inactive Ingredients: glycerin, microcrystalline cellulose and carboxymethylcellulose sodium, sodium citrate, citric acid, benzalkonium chloride, and polysorbate 80.

Patient Instructions for Use

For use in your nose only.

Read the Patient Instructions for Use carefully before you start to use your NASONEX Nasal Spray. If you have any questions, ask your healthcare provider.

Shake the bottle well before each use.

1. Remove the plastic cap (**See** Figure 1).

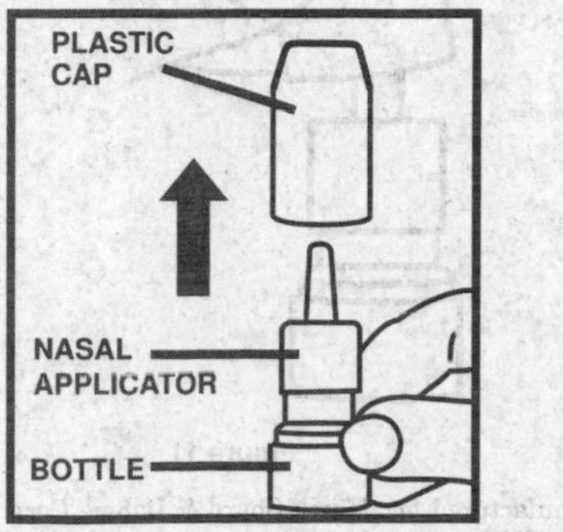

Figure 1

2. Before you use NASONEX for the first time, prime the pump by pressing downward on the shoulders of the white nasal applicator using your index finger and middle finger while holding the base of the bottle with your thumb (**See** Figure 2). **Do Not** pierce the nasal applicator. Press down and release the pump 10 times or until a fine spray appears. **Do Not** spray into eyes. The pump is now ready to use. The pump may be stored unused for up to 1 week without repriming. If unused for more than 1 week, reprime by spraying 2 times or until a fine spray appears.

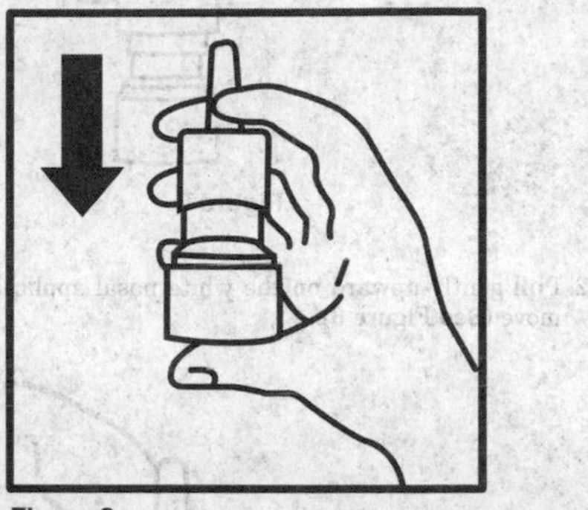

Figure 2

3. Gently blow your nose to clear the nostrils. Close 1 nostril. Tilt your head forward slightly, keep the bottle upright, carefully insert the nasal applicator into the other nostril (**See** Figure 3). **Do Not** spray directly onto the nasal septum (the wall between the two nostrils).

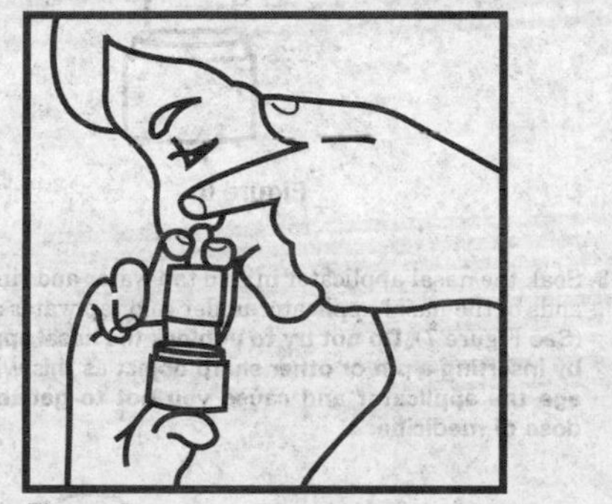

Figure 3

4. For each spray, hold the spray bottle upright and press firmly downward 1 time on the shoulders of the white nasal applicator using your index and middle fingers while supporting the base of the bottle with your thumb. Breathe gently inward through the nostril (**See** Figure 4).

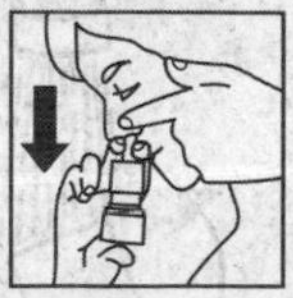

Figure 4

Note: It is important to keep the NASONEX unit in an upright orientation (as seen in Figure 4). Failure to do so may result in an incomplete or non-existent spray.

5. Then breathe out through the mouth.
6. Repeat in the other nostril.
7. Wipe the nasal applicator with a clean tissue and replace the plastic cap.

Each bottle of NASONEX Nasal Spray contains enough medicine for you to spray medicine from the bottle 120 times. Do not use the bottle of NASONEX Nasal Spray after 120 sprays. Additional sprays after the 120 sprays may not contain the right amount of medicine, **you should keep track of the number of sprays used from each bottle of NASONEX Nasal Spray,** and throw away the bottle even if it has medicine still left in. **Do not count any sprays used for priming the device.** Talk with your healthcare provider before your supply runs out to see if you should get a refill of your medicine.

Pediatric Use: Administration to young children should be done by an adult. Steps 1 through 7 from the **Patient Instructions for Use,** should be followed.

Cleaning: Do not try to unblock the nasal applicator with a sharp object. Please see **Patient Instructions for Cleaning Applicator.**

Patient Instructions for Cleaning Applicator

1. To clean the nasal applicator, remove the plastic cap (**See** Figure 5).

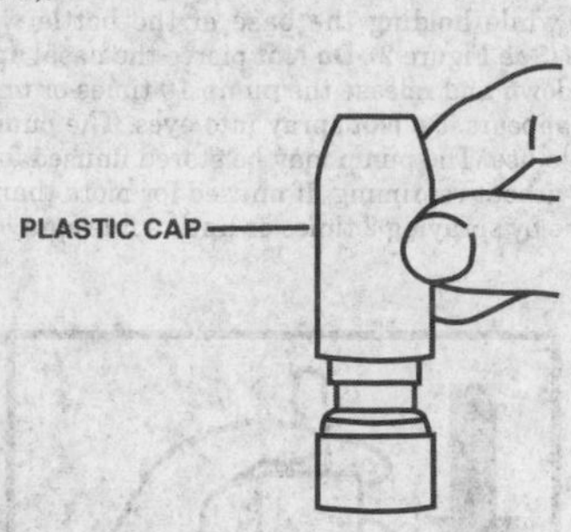

Figure 5

2. Pull gently upward on the white nasal applicator to remove (**See** Figure 6).

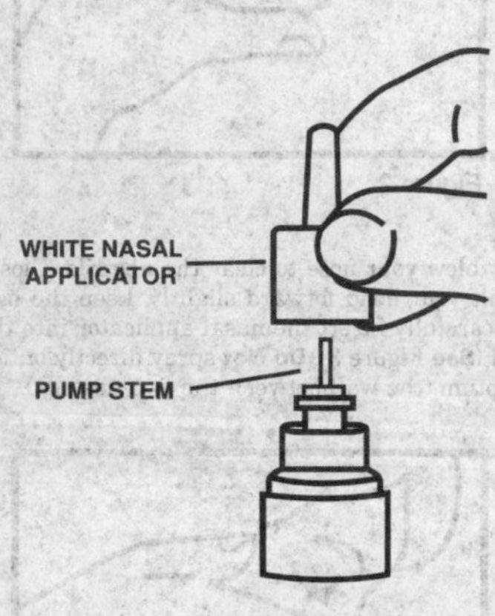

Figure 6

3. Soak the nasal applicator in cold tap water and rinse both ends of the nasal applicator under cold tap water and dry (**See** Figure 7). **Do not try to unblock the nasal applicator by inserting a pin or other sharp object as this will damage the applicator and cause you not to get the right dose of medicine.**

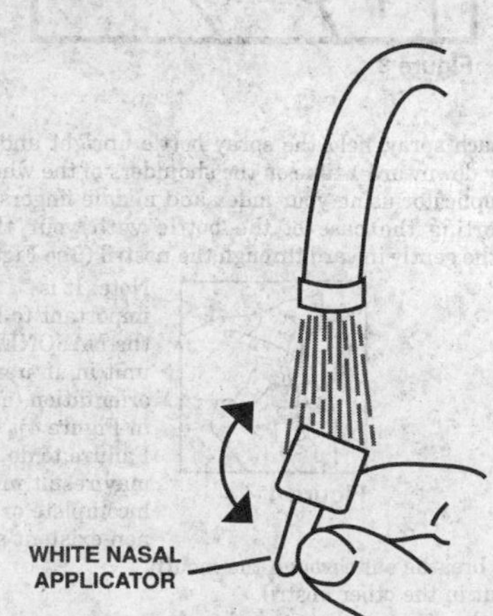

Figure 7

4. Rinse the plastic cap under cold water and dry (**See** Figure 8).

[See figure 8 at top of next column]

5. Put the nasal applicator back together making sure the pump stem is reinserted into the applicator's center hole (**See** Figure 9).

[See figure 9 at top of next column]

6. Reprime the pump by pressing downward on the shoulders of the white nasal applicator using your index and middle fingers while holding the base of the bottle with your thumb. Press down and release the pump 2 times or until a fine spray appears. **Do Not** spray into eyes. The pump is now ready to use. The pump may be stored unused for up to 1 week without repriming. If unused for

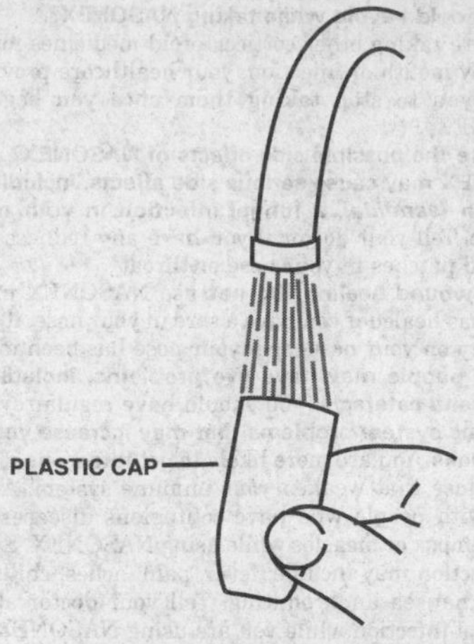

Figure 8

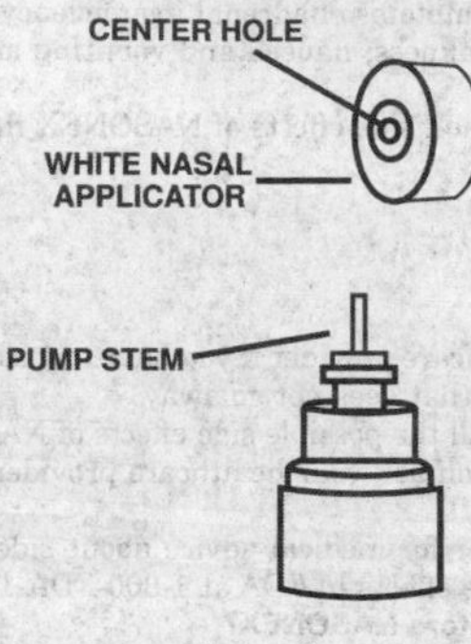

Figure 9

more than 1 week, reprime by spraying 2 times or until a fine spray appears (**See** Figure 10).

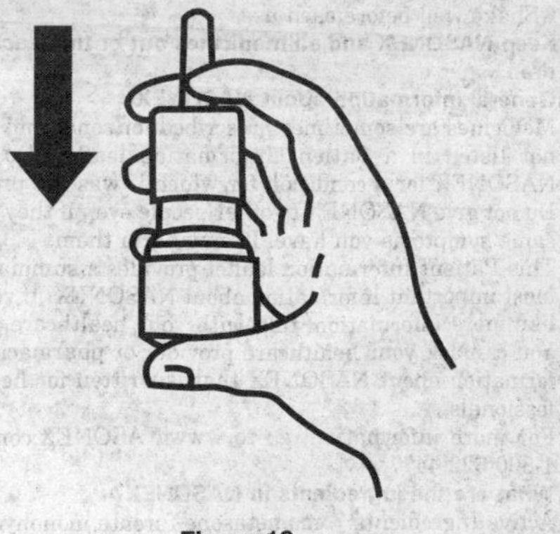

Figure 10

7. Replace the plastic cap (**See** Figure 11).

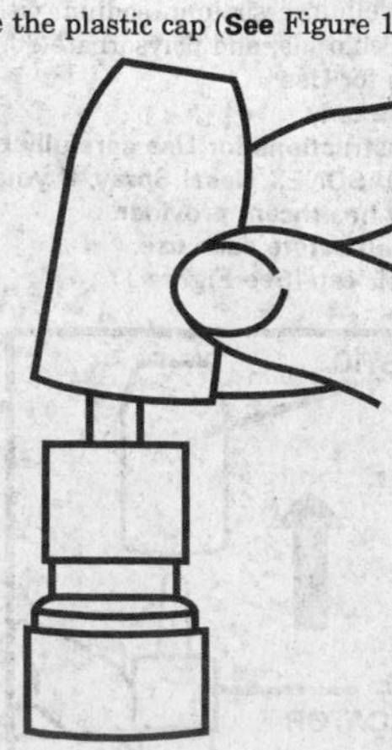

Figure 11

Manufactured for: Merck Sharp & Dohme Corp., a subsidiary of
MERCK & CO., INC., Whitehouse Station, NJ 08889, USA

Manufactured by:
MSD International GmbH (Singapore Branch),
Singapore 638414, Singapore
U.S. Patent No. 6,127,353.

Revised: 03/2013
032088-NSX-NS-PPI.8

Shown in Product Identification Guide, page 308

NEXPLANON® ℞

(etonogestrel implant)
Radiopaque
Subdermal Use Only

HIGHLIGHTS OF PRESCRIBING INFORMATION
These highlights do not include all the information needed to use NEXPLANON safely and effectively. See full prescribing information for NEXPLANON.
NEXPLANON® (etonogestrel implant)
Radiopaque
Subdermal Use Only
Initial U.S. Approval: 2001

INDICATIONS AND USAGE

NEXPLANON is a progestin indicated for use by women to prevent pregnancy. (1)

DOSAGE AND ADMINISTRATION

Insert one NEXPLANON subdermally just under the skin at the inner side of the non-dominant upper arm. NEXPLANON must be removed no later than by the end of the third year. (2)

DOSAGE FORMS AND STRENGTHS

NEXPLANON consists of a single, radiopaque, rod-shaped implant, containing 68 mg etonogestrel, pre-loaded in the needle of a disposable applicator. (3)

CONTRAINDICATIONS

- Known or suspected pregnancy. (4)
- Current or past history of thrombosis or thromboembolic disorders. (4, 5.4)
- Liver tumors, benign or malignant, or active liver disease. (4, 5.7)
- Undiagnosed abnormal genital bleeding. (4, 5.2)
- Known or suspected breast cancer, personal history of breast cancer, or other progestin-sensitive cancer, now or in the past. (4, 5.6)
- Allergic reaction to any of the components of NEXPLANON. (4, 6)

WARNINGS AND PRECAUTIONS

- Insertion and removal complications: Pain, paresthesias, bleeding, hematoma, scarring or infection may occur. (5.1)
- Menstrual bleeding pattern: Counsel women regarding changes in bleeding frequency, intensity, or duration. (5.2)
- Ectopic pregnancies: Be alert to the possibility of an ectopic pregnancy in women using NEXPLANON who become pregnant or complain of lower abdominal pain. (5.3)
- Thrombotic and other vascular events: The NEXPLANON implant should be removed in the event of a thrombosis. (5.4)
- Liver disease: Remove the NEXPLANON implant if jaundice occurs. (5.7)
- Elevated blood pressure: The NEXPLANON implant should be removed if blood pressure rises significantly and becomes uncontrolled. (5.9)
- Carbohydrate and lipid metabolic effects: Monitor prediabetic and diabetic women using NEXPLANON. (5.11)

ADVERSE REACTIONS

Most common (≥10%) adverse reactions reported in clinical trials were change in menstrual bleeding pattern, headache, vaginitis, weight increase, acne, breast pain, abdominal pain, and pharyngitis. (6.1)

To report SUSPECTED ADVERSE REACTIONS, contact Merck Sharp & Dohme Corp., a subsidiary of Merck & Co., Inc., at 1-877-888-4231 or FDA at 1-800-FDA-1088 or *www.fda.gov/medwatch.*

DRUG INTERACTIONS

Drugs or herbal products that induce certain enzymes, such as CYP3A4, may decrease the effectiveness of progestin hormonal contraceptives or increase breakthrough bleeding. (7.1)

USE IN SPECIFIC POPULATIONS

- Pregnant women: NEXPLANON should be removed if maintaining a pregnancy. (8.1)
- Overweight women: NEXPLANON may become less effective in overweight women over time, especially in the presence of other factors that decrease etonogestrel concentrations, such as concomitant use of hepatic enzyme inducers. (8.8)

See 17 for PATIENT COUNSELING INFORMATION and FDA-approved patient labeling

Revised: 05/2012

FULL PRESCRIBING INFORMATION: CONTENTS*

*** Sections or subsections omitted from the full prescribing information are not listed**

FULL PRESCRIBING INFORMATION

1 INDICATIONS AND USAGE

NEXPLANON® is indicated for use by women to prevent pregnancy.

2 DOSAGE AND ADMINISTRATION

The efficacy of NEXPLANON does not depend on daily, weekly or monthly administration.

All healthcare providers should receive instruction and training prior to performing insertion and/or removal of NEXPLANON.

A single NEXPLANON implant is inserted subdermally in the upper arm. To reduce the risk of neural or vascular injury, the implant should be inserted at the inner side of the non-dominant upper arm about 8-10 cm (3-4 inches) above the medial epicondyle of the humerus. The implant should be inserted subdermally just under the skin to avoid the large blood vessels and nerves that lie deeper in the subcutaneous tissues in the sulcus between the triceps and biceps muscles. NEXPLANON must be inserted by the expiration date stated on the packaging. NEXPLANON is a long-acting (up to 3 years), reversible, hormonal contraceptive method. The implant must be removed by the end of the third year and may be replaced by a new implant at the time of removal, if continued contraceptive protection is desired.

2.1 Initiating Contraception With NEXPLANON

IMPORTANT: Rule out pregnancy before inserting the implant.

Timing of insertion depends on the woman's recent contraceptive history, as follows:

- <u>No preceding hormonal contraceptive use in the past month</u>

NEXPLANON should be inserted between Day 1 (first day of menstrual bleeding) and Day 5 of the menstrual cycle, even if the woman is still bleeding.

If inserted as recommended, back-up contraception is not necessary. If deviating from the recommended timing of insertion, the woman should be advised to use a barrier method until 7 days after insertion. If intercourse has already occurred, pregnancy should be excluded.

- <u>Switching contraceptive method to NEXPLANON</u>

<u>Combination hormonal contraceptives:</u>

NEXPLANON should preferably be inserted on the day after the last active tablet of the previous combined oral contraceptive or on the day of removal of the vaginal ring or transdermal patch. At the latest, NEXPLANON should be inserted on the day following the usual tablet-free, ring-free, patch-free or placebo tablet interval of the previous combined hormonal contraceptive.

If inserted as recommended, back-up contraception is not necessary. If deviating from the recommended timing of insertion, the woman should be advised to use a barrier method until 7 days after insertion. If intercourse has already occurred, pregnancy should be excluded.

<u>Progestin-only contraceptives:</u>

There are several types of progestin-only methods. NEXPLANON should be inserted as follows:

- Injectable Contraceptives: Insert NEXPLANON on the day the next injection is due.
- Minipill: A woman may switch to NEXPLANON on any day of the month. NEXPLANON should be inserted within 24 hours after taking the last tablet.
- Contraceptive implant or intrauterine system (IUS): Insert NEXPLANON on the same day the previous contraceptive implant or IUS is removed.

If inserted as recommended, back-up contraception is not necessary. If deviating from the recommended timing of insertion, the woman should be advised to use a barrier method until 7 days after insertion. If intercourse has already occurred, pregnancy should be excluded.

- <u>Following abortion or miscarriage</u>
- First Trimester: NEXPLANON should be inserted within 5 days following a first trimester abortion or miscarriage.
- Second Trimester: Insert NEXPLANON between 21 to 28 days following second trimester abortion or miscarriage.

If inserted as recommended, back-up contraception is not necessary. If deviating from the recommended timing of insertion, the woman should be advised to use a barrier method until 7 days after insertion. If intercourse has already occurred, pregnancy should be excluded.

- <u>Postpartum</u>
- Not Breastfeeding: NEXPLANON should be inserted between 21 to 28 days postpartum. If inserted as recommended, back-up contraception is not necessary. If deviating from the recommended timing of insertion, the woman should be advised to use a barrier method until 7 days after insertion. If intercourse has already occurred, pregnancy should be excluded.
- Breastfeeding: NEXPLANON should be inserted after the fourth postpartum week *[see Use in Specific Populations (8.3)]*. The woman should be advised to use a barrier method until 7 days after insertion. If intercourse has already occurred, pregnancy should be excluded.

2.2 Insertion of NEXPLANON

The basis for successful use and subsequent removal of NEXPLANON is a correct and carefully performed subdermal insertion of the single, rod-shaped implant in accordance with the instructions. Both the healthcare provider and the woman should be able to feel the implant under the skin after placement.

All healthcare providers performing insertions and/or removals of NEXPLANON should receive instructions and training prior to inserting or removing the implant. Information concerning the insertion and removal of NEXPLANON will be sent upon request free of charge [1-877-467-5266].

<u>Preparation</u>

Prior to inserting NEXPLANON carefully read the instructions for insertion as well as the full prescribing information.

Before insertion of NEXPLANON, the healthcare provider should confirm that:

- The woman is not pregnant nor has any other contraindication for the use of NEXPLANON *[see Contraindications (4)]*.
- The woman has had a medical history and physical examination, including a gynecologic examination, performed.
- The woman understands the benefits and risks of NEXPLANON.
- The woman has received a copy of the Patient Labeling included in packaging.
- The woman has reviewed and completed a consent form to be maintained with the woman's chart.
- The woman does not have allergies to the antiseptic and anesthetic to be used during insertion.

Insert NEXPLANON under aseptic conditions.

The following equipment is needed for the implant insertion:

- An examination table for the woman to lie on
- Sterile surgical drapes, sterile gloves, antiseptic solution, sterile marker (optional)
- Local anesthetic, needles, and syringe
- Sterile gauze, adhesive bandage, pressure bandage

Insertion Procedure

Step 1. Have the woman lie on her back on the examination table with her non-dominant arm flexed at the elbow and externally rotated so that her wrist is parallel to her ear or her hand is positioned next to her head (Figure 1).

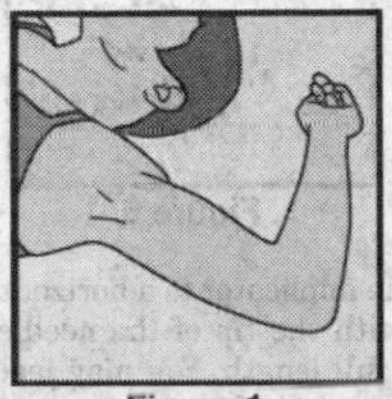

Figure 1

Step 2. Identify the insertion site, which is at the inner side of the non-dominant upper arm about 8-10 cm (3-4 inches) above the medial epicondyle of the humerus (Figure 2). **The implant should be inserted subdermally just under the skin to avoid the large blood vessels and nerves that lie deeper in the subcutaneous tissue in the sulcus between the triceps and biceps muscles** *[see Warnings and Precautions (5.1)]*.

Step 3. Make two marks with a sterile marker: first, mark the spot where the etonogestrel implant will be inserted, and second, mark a spot a few centimeters proximal to the first mark (Figure 2). This second mark will later serve as a direction guide during insertion.

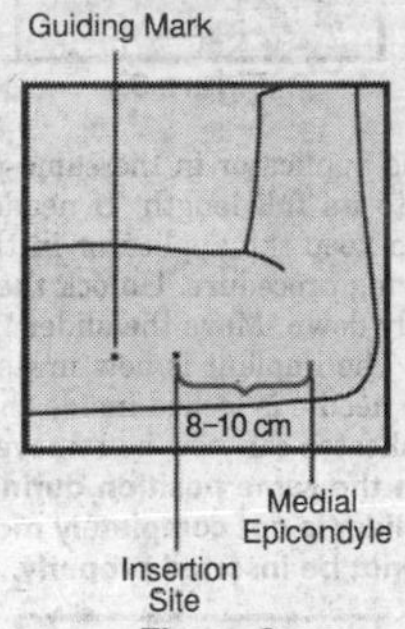

Figure 2

Step 4. Clean the insertion site with an antiseptic solution.

Step 5. Anesthetize the insertion area (for example, with anesthetic spray or by injecting 2 mL of 1% lidocaine just under the skin along the planned insertion tunnel).

Step 6. Remove the sterile preloaded disposable NEXPLANON applicator carrying the implant from its blister. The applicator should not be used if sterility is in question.

Step 7. Hold the applicator just above the needle at the textured surface area. Remove the transparent protection cap by sliding it horizontally in the direction of the arrow away from the needle (Figure 3). If the cap does not come off easily, the applicator should not be used. You can see the white colored implant by looking into the tip of the needle. **Do not touch the purple slider until you have fully inserted the needle subdermally, as it will retract the needle and prematurely release the implant from the applicator.**

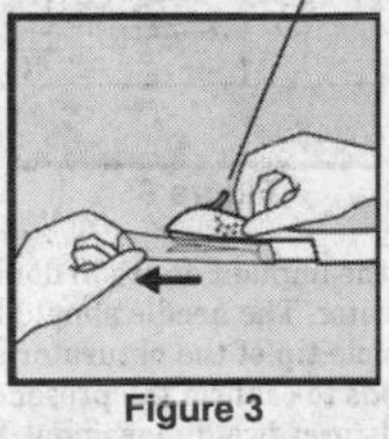

Figure 3

Step 8. With your free hand, stretch the skin around the insertion site with thumb and index finger (Figure 4).

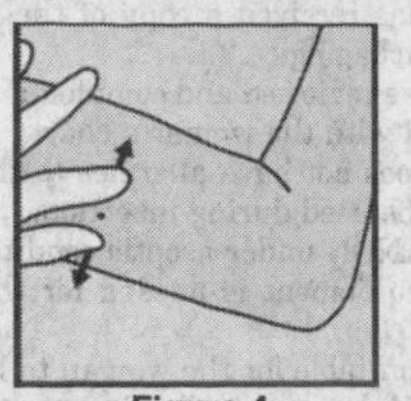

Figure 4

Step 9. Puncture the skin with the tip of the needle angled about 30° (Figure 5).

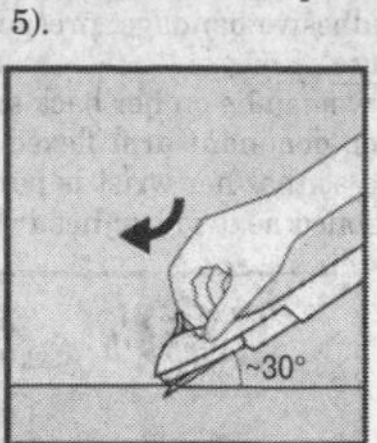

Figure 5

Step 10. Lower the applicator to a horizontal position. While lifting the skin with the tip of the needle (Figure 6), slide the needle to its full length. You may feel slight resistance but do not exert excessive force. **If the needle is not inserted to its full length, the implant will not be inserted properly. You can best see movement of the needle if you are seated and are looking at the applicator from the side and NOT from above. In this position, you can clearly see the insertion site and the movement of the needle just under the skin.**

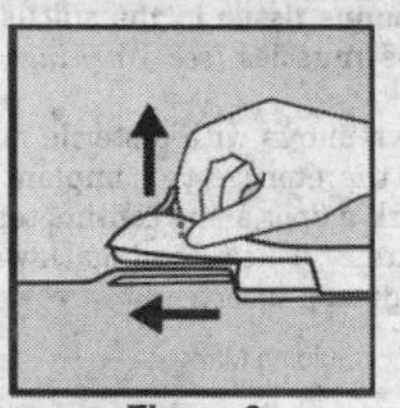

Figure 6

Step 11. Keep the applicator in the same position with the needle inserted to its full length. If needed, you may use your free hand to keep the applicator in the same position during the following procedure. Unlock the purple slider by pushing it slightly down. Move the slider fully back until it stops (Figure 7). The implant is now in its final subdermal position, and the needle is locked inside the body of the applicator. The applicator can now be removed. **If the applicator is not kept in the same position during this procedure or if the purple slider is not completely moved to the back, the implant will not be inserted properly.**

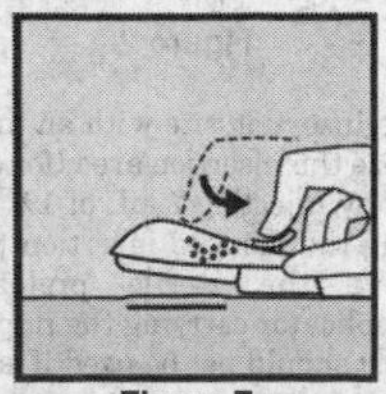

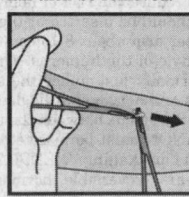

Figure 7

Step 12. **Always verify the presence of the implant in the woman's arm immediately after insertion by palpation.** By palpating both ends of the implant, you should be able to confirm the presence of the 4 cm rod (Figure 8).

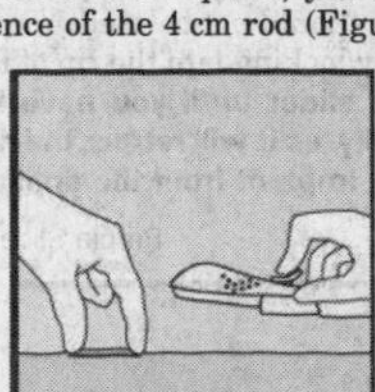

Figure 8

If you cannot feel the implant or are in doubt of its presence,

- Check the applicator. The needle should be fully retracted and only the purple tip of the obturator should be visible.
- Use other methods to confirm the presence of the implant. Suitable methods are: two-dimensional X-ray, X-ray computerized tomography (CT scan), ultrasound scanning (USS) with a high-frequency linear array transducer (10 MHz or greater) or magnetic resonance imaging (MRI).

  If these methods fail, call 1-877-467-5266 for information on the procedure for measuring etonogestrel blood levels.

Until the presence of the implant has been verified, the woman should be advised to use a non-hormonal contraceptive method, such as condoms.

Step 13. Place a small adhesive bandage over the insertion site. Request that the woman palpate the implant.

Step 14. Apply a pressure bandage with sterile gauze to minimize bruising. The woman may remove the pressure bandage in 24 hours and the small bandage over the insertion site after 3 to 5 days.

Step 15. Complete the USER CARD and give it to the woman to keep. Also, complete the PATIENT CHART LABEL and affix it to the woman's medical record.

Step 16. The applicator is for single use only and should be disposed in accordance with the Center for Disease Control and Prevention guidelines for handling of hazardous waste.

2.3 Removal of NEXPLANON

Preparation

Before initiating the removal procedure, the healthcare provider should carefully read the instructions for removal and consult the USER CARD and/or the PATIENT CHART LABEL for the location of the implant. The exact location of the implant in the arm should be verified by palpation. If the implant is not palpable, two-dimensional X-ray can be performed to verify its presence.

A non-palpable implant should always be first located prior to removal. Suitable methods for localization include: two-dimensional X-ray, X-ray computer tomography (CT), ultrasound scanning (USS) with a high-frequency linear array transducer (10 MHz or greater) or magnetic resonance imaging (MRI). If these imaging methods fail to locate the implant, etonogestrel blood level determination can be used for verification of the presence of the implant. For details on etonogestrel blood level determination, call 1-877-467-5266 for further instructions.

After localization of a non-palpable implant, consider conducting removal with ultrasound guidance.

There have been occasional reports of migration of the implant; usually this involves minor movement relative to the original position. This may complicate localization of the implant by palpation, CT, USS and/or MRI, and removal may require a larger incision and more time.

Exploratory surgery without knowledge of the exact location of the implant is strongly discouraged. Removal of deeply inserted implants should be conducted with caution in order to prevent injury to deeper neural or vascular structures in the arm and be performed by healthcare providers familiar with the anatomy of the arm.

Before removal of the implant, the healthcare provider should confirm that:

- The woman does not have allergies to the antiseptic or anesthetic to be used.

Remove the implant under aseptic conditions.

The following equipment is needed for removal of the implant:

- An examination table for the woman to lie on
- Sterile surgical drapes, sterile gloves, antiseptic solution, sterile marker (optional)
- Local anesthetic, needles, and syringe
- Sterile scalpel, forceps (straight and curved mosquito)
- Skin closure, sterile gauze, adhesive bandage and pressure bandages

Removal Procedure

Step 1. Clean the site where the incision will be made and apply an antiseptic. Locate the implant by palpation and mark the distal end (end closest to the elbow), for example, with a sterile marker (Figure 9).

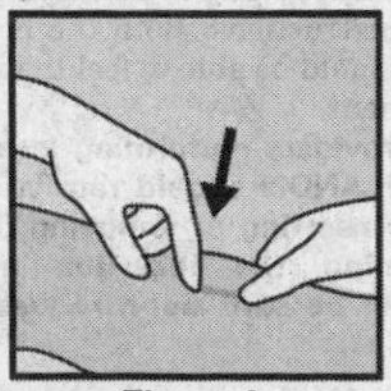

Figure 9

Step 2. Anesthetize the arm, for example, with 0.5 to 1 mL 1% lidocaine at the marked site where the incision will be made (Figure 10). Be sure to inject the local anesthetic under the implant to keep it close to the skin surface.

[See figure 10 at top of next column]

Step 3. Push down the proximal end of the implant (Figure 11) to stabilize it; a bulge may appear indicating the distal

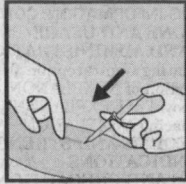

Figure 10

end of the implant. Starting at the distal tip of the implant, make a longitudinal incision of 2 mm towards the elbow.

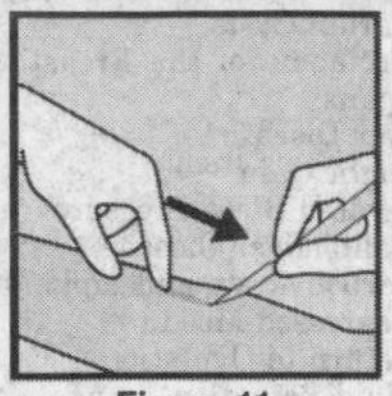

Figure 11

Step 4. Gently push the implant towards the incision until the tip is visible. Grasp the implant with forceps (preferably curved mosquito forceps) and gently remove the implant (Figure 12).

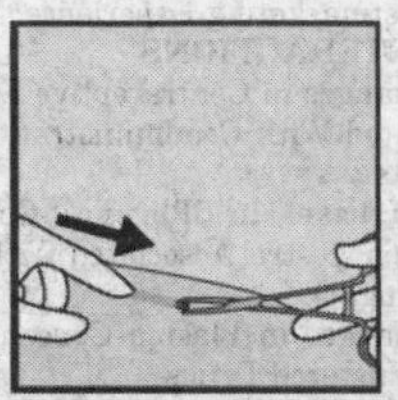

Figure 12

Step 5. If the implant is encapsulated, make an incision into the tissue sheath and then remove the implant with the forceps (Figures 13 and 14).

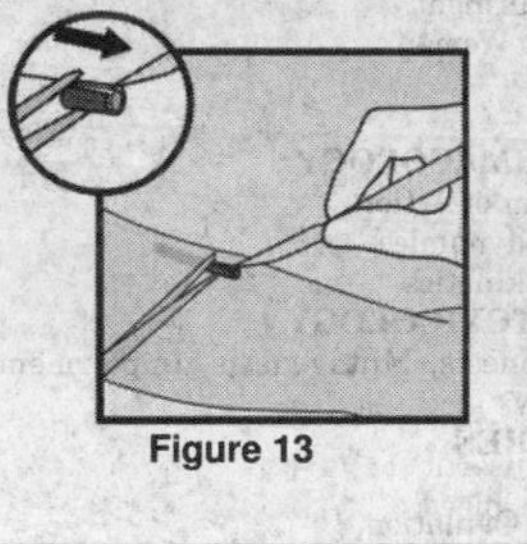

Figure 13

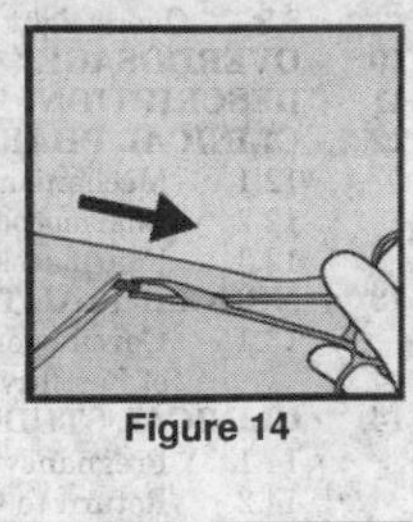

Figure 14

Step 6. If the tip of the implant does not become visible in the incision, gently insert a forceps into the incision (Figure 15). Flip the forceps over into your other hand (Figure 16).

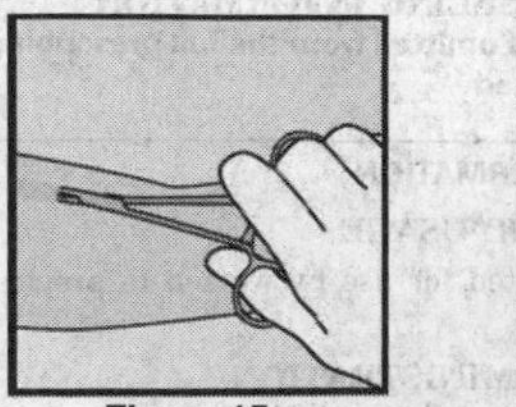

Figure 15

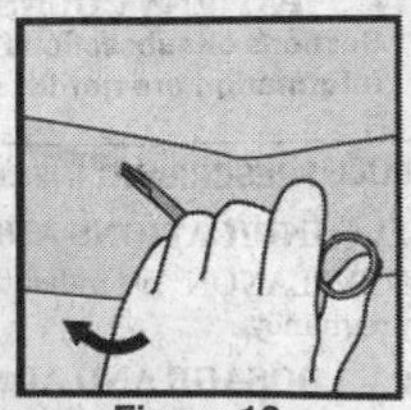

Figure 16

Step 7. With a second pair of forceps carefully dissect the tissue around the implant and grasp the implant (Figure 17). The implant can then be removed.

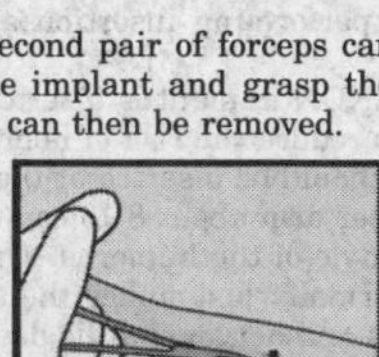

Figure 17

Step 8. Confirm that the entire implant, which is 4 cm long, has been removed by measuring its length. If a partial implant (less than 4 cm) is removed, the remaining piece should be removed by following the instructions in section 2.3. *[See Dosage and Administration (2.3).]* If the woman would like to continue using NEXPLANON, a new implant may be inserted immediately after the old implant is removed using the same incision *[see Dosage and Administration (2.4)]*.

Step 9. After removing the implant, close the incision with a steri-strip and apply an adhesive bandage.

Step 10. Apply a pressure bandage with sterile gauze to minimize bruising. The woman may remove the pressure bandage in 24 hours and the small bandage in 3 to 5 days.

2.4 Replacing NEXPLANON

Immediate replacement can be done after removal of the previous implant and is similar to the insertion procedure described in section 2.2 Insertion of NEXPLANON.

The new implant may be inserted in the same arm, and through the same incision from which the previous implant was removed. If the same incision is being used to insert a new implant, anesthetize the insertion site [for example, 2 mL lidocaine (1%)] applying it just under the skin along the 'insertion canal.'

Follow the subsequent steps in the insertion instructions *[see Dosage and Administration (2.2)]*.

3 DOSAGE FORMS AND STRENGTHS

Single, white/off-white, soft, radiopaque, flexible, ethylene vinylacetate (EVA) implant, 4 cm in length and 2 mm in diameter containing 68 mg etonogestrel and 15 mg of barium sulfate.

4 CONTRAINDICATIONS

NEXPLANON should not be used in women who have

- Known or suspected pregnancy
- Current or past history of thrombosis or thromboembolic disorders
- Liver tumors, benign or malignant, or active liver disease
- Undiagnosed abnormal genital bleeding
- Known or suspected breast cancer, personal history of breast cancer, or other progestin-sensitive cancer, now or in the past
- Allergic reaction to any of the components of NEXPLANON *[see Adverse Reactions (6)]*

5 WARNINGS AND PRECAUTIONS

The following information is based on experience with either the non-radiopaque etonogestrel implant (IMPLANON), other progestin-only contraceptives, or experience with combination (estrogen plus progestin) oral contraceptives.

5.1 Complications of Insertion and Removal

NEXPLANON should be inserted subdermally so that it will be palpable after insertion, and this should be confirmed by palpation immediately after insertion. Failure to insert NEXPLANON properly may go unnoticed unless it is palpated immediately after insertion. Undetected failure to insert the implant may lead to an unintended pregnancy. Complications related to insertion and removal procedures, such as pain, paresthesias, bleeding, hematoma, scarring or infection, may occur.

If NEXPLANON is inserted too deeply (intramuscular or in the fascia), neural or vascular injury may occur. To reduce the risk of neural or vascular injury, NEXPLANON should be inserted at the inner side of the non-dominant upper arm about 8-10 cm (3-4 inches) above the medial epicondyle of the humerus. NEXPLANON should be inserted subdermally just under the skin to avoid the large blood vessels and nerves that lie deeper in the subcutaneous tissues in the sulcus between the triceps and biceps muscles. Deep insertions of the non-radiopaque etonogestrel implant (IMPLANON) have been associated with paraesthesia (due to neural injury) and migration of the implant (due to intramuscular or fascial insertion), and in a very few cases with intravascular insertion. If infection develops at the insertion site, start suitable treatment. If the infection persists, the implant should be removed. Incomplete insertions or infections may lead to expulsion.

Implant removal may be difficult or impossible if the implant is not inserted correctly, is inserted too deeply, not palpable, encased in fibrous tissue, or has migrated. Deep insertions may lead to difficult localization of the implant and may also result in the need for a surgical procedure in an operating room in order to remove the implant. Exploratory surgery without knowledge of the exact location of the implant is strongly discouraged. Removal of deeply inserted implants should be conducted with caution in order to prevent injury to deeper neural or vascular structures in the arm and be performed by healthcare providers familiar with the anatomy of the arm. Failure to remove the implant may result in continued effects of etonogestrel, such as compromised fertility, ectopic pregnancy, or persistence or occurrence of a drug-related adverse event.

5.2 Changes in Menstrual Bleeding Patterns

After starting NEXPLANON, women are likely to have a change from their normal menstrual bleeding pattern. These may include changes in bleeding frequency (absent, less, more frequent or continuous), intensity (reduced or increased) or duration. In clinical trials of the non-radiopaque etonogestrel implant (IMPLANON), bleeding patterns ranged from amenorrhea (1 in 5 women) to frequent and/or prolonged bleeding (1 in 5 women). The bleeding pattern experienced during the first three months of NEXPLANON use is broadly predictive of the future bleeding pattern for many women. Women should be counseled regarding the bleeding pattern changes they may experience so that they know what to expect. Abnormal bleeding should be evaluated as needed to exclude pathologic conditions or pregnancy.

In clinical studies of the non-radiopaque etonogestrel implant, reports of changes in bleeding pattern were the most common reason for stopping treatment (11.1%). Irregular bleeding (10.8%) was the single most common reason women stopped treatment, while amenorrhea (0.3%) was cited less frequently. In these studies, women had an average of 17.7 days of bleeding or spotting every 90 days (based on 3,315 intervals of 90 days recorded by 780 patients). The percentages of patients having 0, 1-7, 8-21, or >21 days of spotting or bleeding over a 90-day interval while using the non-radiopaque etonogestrel implant are shown in Table 1.

Table 1: Percentages of Patients With 0, 1-7, 8-21, or >21 Days of Spotting or Bleeding Over a 90-Day Interval While Using the Non-Radiopaque Etonogestrel Implant (IMPLANON)

Total Days of Spotting or Bleeding	Percentage of Patients		
	Treatment Days 91-180 (N = 745)	Treatment Days 271-360 (N = 657)	Treatment Days 631-720 (N = 547)
0 Days	19%	24%	17%
1-7 Days	15%	13%	12%
8-21 Days	30%	30%	37%
>21 Days	35%	33%	35%

Bleeding patterns observed with use of the non-radiopaque etonogestrel implant for up to 2 years, and the proportion of 90-day intervals with these bleeding patterns, are summarized in Table 2.

Table 2: Bleeding Patterns Using the Non-Radiopaque Etonogestrel Implant (IMPLANON) During the First 2 Years of Use*

BLEEDING PATTERNS	DEFINITIONS	%†
Infrequent	Less than three bleeding and/or spotting episodes in 90 days (excluding amenorrhea)	33.6
Amenorrhea	No bleeding and/or spotting in 90 days	22.2
Prolonged	Any bleeding and/or spotting episode lasting more than 14 days in 90 days	17.7
Frequent	More than 5 bleeding and/or spotting episodes in 90 days	6.7

* Based on 3315 recording periods of 90 days duration in 780 women, excluding the first 90 days after implant insertion

† % = Percentage of 90-day intervals with this pattern

In case of undiagnosed, persistent, or recurrent abnormal vaginal bleeding, appropriate measures should be conducted to rule out malignancy.

5.3 Ectopic Pregnancies

As with all progestin-only contraceptive products, be alert to the possibility of an ectopic pregnancy among women using NEXPLANON who become pregnant or complain of lower abdominal pain. Although ectopic pregnancies are uncommon among women using NEXPLANON, a pregnancy that occurs in a woman using NEXPLANON may be more likely to be ectopic than a pregnancy occurring in a woman using no contraception.

5.4 Thrombotic and Other Vascular Events

The use of combination hormonal contraceptives (progestin plus estrogen) increases the risk of vascular events, including arterial events (strokes and myocardial infarctions) or deep venous thrombotic events (venous thromboembolism, deep venous thrombosis, retinal vein thrombosis, and pulmonary embolism). NEXPLANON is a progestin-only contraceptive. It is unknown whether this increased risk is applicable to etonogestrel alone. It is recommended, however, that women with risk factors known to increase the risk of venous and arterial thromboembolism be carefully assessed.

There have been postmarketing reports of serious arterial and venous thromboembolic events, including cases of pulmonary emboli (some fatal), deep vein thrombosis, myocardial infarction, and strokes, in women using the non-radiopaque etonogestrel implant. NEXPLANON should be removed in the event of a thrombosis.

Due to the risk of thromboembolism associated with pregnancy and immediately following delivery, NEXPLANON should not be used prior to 21 days postpartum. Women with a history of thromboembolic disorders should be made aware of the possibility of a recurrence.

Evaluate for retinal vein thrombosis immediately if there is unexplained loss of vision, proptosis, diplopia, papilledema, or retinal vascular lesions.

Consider removal of the NEXPLANON implant in case of long-term immobilization due to surgery or illness.

5.5 Ovarian Cysts

If follicular development occurs, atresia of the follicle is sometimes delayed, and the follicle may continue to grow beyond the size it would attain in a normal cycle. Generally, these enlarged follicles disappear spontaneously. On rare occasion, surgery may be required.

5.6 Carcinoma of the Breast and Reproductive Organs

Women who currently have or have had breast cancer should not use hormonal contraception because breast cancer may be hormonally sensitive *[see Contraindications (4)]*. Some studies suggest that the use of combination hormonal contraceptives might increase the incidence of breast cancer; however, other studies have not confirmed such findings.

Some studies suggest that the use of combination hormonal contraceptives is associated with an increase in the risk of cervical cancer or intraepithelial neoplasia. However, there is controversy about the extent to which these findings are due to differences in sexual behavior and other factors.

Women with a family history of breast cancer or who develop breast nodules should be carefully monitored.

5.7 Liver Disease

Disturbances of liver function may necessitate the discontinuation of hormonal contraceptive use until markers of liver function return to normal. Remove NEXPLANON if jaundice develops.

Hepatic adenomas are associated with combination hormonal contraceptives use. An estimate of the attributable risk is 3.3 cases per 100,000 for combination hormonal contraceptives users. It is not known whether a similar risk exists with progestin-only methods like NEXPLANON.

The progestin in NEXPLANON may be poorly metabolized in women with liver impairment. Use of NEXPLANON in women with active liver disease or liver cancer is contraindicated *[see Contraindications (4)]*.

5.8 Weight Gain

In clinical studies, mean weight gain in U.S. non-radiopaque etonogestrel implant (IMPLANON) users was 2.8 pounds after one year and 3.7 pounds after two years. How much of the weight gain was related to the non-radiopaque etonogestrel implant is unknown. In studies, 2.3% of the users reported weight gain as the reason for having the non-radiopaque etonogestrel implant removed.

5.9 Elevated Blood Pressure

Women with a history of hypertension-related diseases or renal disease should be discouraged from using hormonal contraception. For women with well-controlled hypertension, use of NEXPLANON can be considered. Women with hypertension using NEXPLANON should be closely monitored. If sustained hypertension develops during the use of NEXPLANON, or if a significant increase in blood pressure does not respond adequately to antihypertensive therapy, NEXPLANON should be removed.

5.10 Gallbladder Disease

Studies suggest a small increased relative risk of developing gallbladder disease among combination hormonal contraceptive users. It is not known whether a similar risk exists with progestin-only methods like NEXPLANON.

5.11 Carbohydrate and Lipid Metabolic Effects

Use of NEXPLANON may induce mild insulin resistance and small changes in glucose concentrations of unknown clinical significance. Carefully monitor prediabetic and diabetic women using NEXPLANON.

Women who are being treated for hyperlipidemia should be followed closely if they elect to use NEXPLANON. Some progestins may elevate LDL levels and may render the control of hyperlipidemia more difficult.

5.12 Depressed Mood

Women with a history of depressed mood should be carefully observed. Consideration should be given to removing NEXPLANON in patients who become significantly depressed.

5.13 Return to Ovulation

In clinical trials with the non-radiopaque etonogestrel implant (IMPLANON), the etonogestrel levels in blood decreased below sensitivity of the assay by one week after removal of the implant. In addition, pregnancies were observed to occur as early as 7 to 14 days after removal. Therefore, a woman should re-start contraception immediately after removal of the implant if continued contraceptive protection is desired.

5.14 Fluid Retention

Hormonal contraceptives may cause some degree of fluid retention. They should be prescribed with caution, and only with careful monitoring, in patients with conditions which might be aggravated by fluid retention. It is unknown if NEXPLANON causes fluid retention.

5.15 Contact Lenses

Contact lens wearers who develop visual changes or changes in lens tolerance should be assessed by an ophthalmologist.

5.16 Monitoring

A woman who is using NEXPLANON should have a yearly visit with her healthcare provider for a blood pressure check and for other indicated health care.

5.17 Drug-Laboratory Test Interactions

Sex hormone-binding globulin concentrations may be decreased for the first six months after NEXPLANON insertion followed by gradual recovery. Thyroxine concentrations may initially be slightly decreased followed by gradual recovery to baseline.

6 ADVERSE REACTIONS

The following adverse reactions reported with the use of hormonal contraception are discussed elsewhere in the labeling:

- Changes in Menstrual Bleeding Patterns *[see Warnings and Precautions (5.2)]*
- Ectopic Pregnancies *[see Warnings and Precautions (5.3)]*
- Thrombotic and Other Vascular Events *[see Warnings and Precautions (5.4)]*
- Liver Disease *[see Warnings and Precautions (5.7)]*

6.1 Clinical Trials Experience

Because clinical trials are conducted under widely varying conditions, adverse reaction rates observed in the clinical trials of a drug cannot be directly compared to rates in the clinical trials of another drug and may not reflect the rates observed in practice.

In clinical trials involving 942 women who were evaluated for safety, change in menstrual bleeding patterns (irregular menses) was the most common adverse reaction causing discontinuation of use of the non-radiopaque etonogestrel implant (IMPLANON) (11.1% of women).

Adverse reactions that resulted in a rate of discontinuation of ≥1% are shown in Table 3.

Table 3: Adverse Reactions Leading to Discontinuation of Treatment in 1% or More of Subjects in Clinical Trials of the Non-Radiopaque Etonogestrel Implant (IMPLANON)

Adverse Reactions	All Studies N = 942
Bleeding Irregularities*	11.1%
Emotional Lability†	2.3%
Weight Increase	2.3%
Headache	1.6%
Acne	1.3%
Depression‡	1.0%

* Includes "frequent", "heavy", "prolonged", "spotting", and other patterns of bleeding irregularity.
† Among US subjects (N=330), 6.1% experienced emotional lability that led to discontinuation.
‡ Among US subjects (N=330), 2.4% experienced depression that led to discontinuation.

Other adverse reactions that were reported by at least 5% of subjects in the non-radiopaque etonogestrel implant clinical trials are listed in Table 4.

Table 4: Common Adverse Reactions Reported by ≥5% of Subjects in Clinical Trials With the Non-Radiopaque Etonogestrel Implant (IMPLANON)

Adverse Reactions	All Studies N = 942
Headache	24.9%
Vaginitis	14.5%
Weight increase	13.7%
Acne	13.5%
Breast pain	12.8%
Abdominal pain	10.9%
Pharyngitis	10.5%
Leukorrhea	9.6%
Influenza-like symptoms	7.6%
Dizziness	7.2%
Dysmenorrhea	7.2%
Back pain	6.8%
Emotional lability	6.5%
Nausea	6.4%
Pain	5.6%
Nervousness	5.6%
Depression	5.5%
Hypersensitivity	5.4%
Insertion site pain	5.2%

In a clinical trial of NEXPLANON, in which investigators were asked to examine the implant site after insertion, implant site reactions were reported in 8.6% of women. Erythema was the most frequent implant site complication, reported during and/or shortly after insertion, occurring in 3.3% of subjects. Additionally, hematoma (3.0%), bruising (2.0%), pain (1.0%), and swelling (0.7%) were reported.

6.2 Postmarketing Experience

The following additional adverse reactions have been identified during post-approval use of the non-radiopaque etonogestrel implant (IMPLANON). Because these reactions are reported voluntarily from a population of uncertain size, it is not possible to reliably estimate their frequency or establish a causal relationship to drug exposure.

Gastrointestinal disorders: constipation, diarrhea, flatulence, vomiting.
General disorders and administration site conditions: edema, fatigue, implant site reaction, pyrexia.
Immune system disorders: anaphylactic reactions.
Infections and infestations: rhinitis, urinary tract infection.
Investigations: clinically relevant rise in blood pressure, weight decreased.
Metabolism and nutrition disorders: increased appetite.
Musculoskeletal and connective tissue disorders: arthralgia, musculoskeletal pain, myalgia.
Nervous system disorders: convulsions, migraine, somnolence.
Pregnancy, puerperium and perinatal conditions: ectopic pregnancy.
Psychiatric disorders: anxiety, insomnia, libido decreased.
Renal and urinary disorders: dysuria.
Reproductive system and breast disorders: breast discharge, breast enlargement, ovarian cyst, pruritus genital, vulvovaginal discomfort.
Skin and subcutaneous tissue disorders: angioedema, aggravation of angioedema and/or aggravation of hereditary angioedema, alopecia, chloasma, hypertrichosis, pruritus, rash, seborrhea, urticaria.
Vascular disorders: hot flush.

Complications related to insertion or removal of the non-radiopaque etonogestrel implant reported include: bruising, slight local irritation, pain or itching, fibrosis at the implant site, paresthesia or paresthesia-like events, scarring and abscess.

7 DRUG INTERACTIONS

7.1 Changes in Contraceptive Effectiveness Associated With Coadministration of Other Products

Drugs or herbal products that induce enzymes, including CYP3A4, that metabolize progestins may decrease the plasma concentrations of progestins, and may decrease the effectiveness of NEXPLANON. In women on long-term treatment with hepatic enzyme inducing drugs, it is recommended to remove the implant and to advise a contraceptive method that is unaffected by the interacting drug.

Some of these drugs or herbal products that induce enzymes, including CYP3A4, include:

- barbiturates
- bosentan
- carbamazepine
- felbamate
- griseofulvin
- oxcarbazepine
- phenytoin
- rifampin
- St. John's wort
- topiramate

HIV Antiretrovirals

Significant changes (increase or decrease) in the plasma levels of progestin have been noted in some cases of coadministration with HIV protease inhibitors or with non-nucleoside reverse transcriptase inhibitors. Consult the labeling of all concurrently-used drugs to obtain further information about interactions with hormonal contraceptives or the potential for enzyme alterations.

7.2 Increase in Plasma Concentrations of Etonogestrel Associated With Coadministered Drugs

CYP3A4 inhibitors such as itraconazole or ketoconazole may increase plasma concentrations of etonogestrel.

7.3 Changes in Plasma Concentrations of Coadministered Drugs

Hormonal contraceptives may affect the metabolism of other drugs. Consequently, plasma concentrations may either increase (for example, cyclosporin) or decrease (for example, lamotrigine). Consult the labeling of all concurrently-used drugs to obtain further information about interactions with hormonal contraceptives or the potential for enzyme alterations.

8 USE IN SPECIFIC POPULATIONS

8.1 Pregnancy

NEXPLANON is not indicated for use during pregnancy *[see Contraindications (4)]*.

Teratology studies have been performed in rats and rabbits using oral administration up to 390 and 790 times the human etonogestrel dose (based upon body surface), respectively, and revealed no evidence of fetal harm due to etonogestrel exposure.

Studies have revealed no increased risk of birth defects in women who have used combination oral contraceptives before pregnancy or during early pregnancy. There is no evidence that the risk associated with etonogestrel is different from that of combination oral contraceptives.

NEXPLANON should be removed if maintaining a pregnancy.

8.3 Nursing Mothers

Based on limited clinical data, NEXPLANON may be used during breastfeeding after the fourth postpartum week. Use of NEXPLANON before the fourth postpartum week has not been studied. Small amounts of etonogestrel are excreted in breast milk. During the first months after insertion of NEXPLANON, when maternal blood levels of etonogestrel are highest, about 100 ng of etonogestrel may be ingested by the child per day based on an average daily milk ingestion of 658 mL. Based on daily milk ingestion of 150 mL/kg, the mean daily infant etonogestrel dose one month after insertion of the non-radiopaque etonogestrel implant (IMPLANON) is about 2.2% of the weight-adjusted maternal daily dose, or about 0.2% of the estimated absolute maternal daily dose. The health of breastfed infants whose mothers began using the non-radiopaque etonogestrel implant during the fourth to eighth week postpartum (n=38) was evaluated in a comparative study with infants of mothers using a non-hormonal IUD (n=33). They were breastfed for a mean duration of 14 months and followed up to 36 months of age. No significant effects and no differences between the groups were observed on the physical and psychomotor development of these infants. No differences between groups in the production or quality of breast milk were detected.

Healthcare providers should discuss both hormonal and non-hormonal contraceptive options, as steroids may not be the initial choice for these patients.

8.4 Pediatric Use

Safety and efficacy of NEXPLANON have been established in women of reproductive age. Safety and efficacy of NEXPLANON are expected to be the same for postpubertal adolescents. However, no clinical studies have been conducted in women less than 18 years of age. Use of this product before menarche is not indicated.

8.5 Geriatric Use

This product has not been studied in women over 65 years of age and is not indicated in this population.

8.6 Hepatic Impairment

No studies were conducted to evaluate the effect of hepatic disease on the disposition of NEXPLANON. The use of NEXPLANON in women with active liver disease is contraindicated *[see Contraindications (4)]*.

8.7 Renal Impairment

No studies were conducted to evaluate the effect of renal disease on the disposition of NEXPLANON.

8.8 Overweight Women

The effectiveness of the etonogestrel implant in women who weighed more than 130% of their ideal body weight has not been defined because such women were not studied in clinical trials. Serum concentrations of etonogestrel are inversely related to body weight and decrease with time after implant insertion. It is therefore possible that NEXPLANON may be less effective in overweight women, especially in the presence of other factors that decrease serum etonogestrel concentrations such as concomitant use of hepatic enzyme inducers.

10 OVERDOSAGE

Overdosage may result if more than one implant is inserted. In case of suspected overdose, the implant should be removed.

11 DESCRIPTION

NEXPLANON is a radiopaque, progestin-only, soft, flexible implant preloaded in a sterile, disposable applicator for subdermal use. The implant is white/off-white, non-biodegradable and 4 cm in length with a diameter of 2 mm (see Figure 18). Each implant consists of an ethylene vinylacetate (EVA) copolymer core, containing 68 mg of the synthetic progestin etonogestrel and barium sulfate (radiopaque ingredient), surrounded by an EVA copolymer skin. Once inserted subdermally, the release rate is 60-70 mcg/day in week 5-6 and decreases to approximately 35-45 mcg/day at the end of the first year, to approximately 30-40 mcg/day at the end of the second year, and then to approximately 25-30 mcg/day at the end of the third year. NEXPLANON is a progestin-only contraceptive and does not contain estrogen. NEXPLANON does not contain latex.

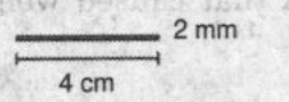

Figure 18 (Not to scale)

Etonogestrel [13-Ethyl-17-hydroxy-11-methylene-18,19-dinor-17α-pregn-4-en-20-yn-3-one], structurally derived from 19-nortestosterone, is the synthetic biologically active metabolite of the synthetic progestin desogestrel. It has a molecular weight of 324.46 and the following structural formula (Figure 19).

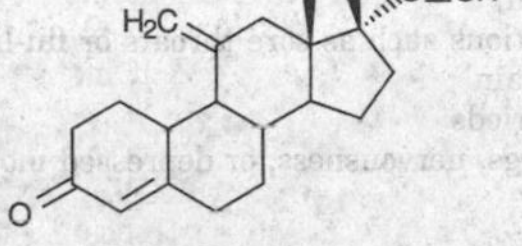

$C_{22}H_{28}O_2$

Figure 19

12 CLINICAL PHARMACOLOGY

12.1 Mechanism of Action

The contraceptive effect of NEXPLANON is achieved by suppression of ovulation, increased viscosity of the cervical mucus, and alterations in the endometrium.

12.2 Pharmacodynamics

Exposure-response relationships of NEXPLANON are unknown.

12.3 Pharmacokinetics

Absorption

After subdermal insertion of the etonogestrel implant, etonogestrel is released into the circulation and is approximately 100% bioavailable.

In a three year clinical trial, NEXPLANON and the non-radiopaque etonogestrel implant (IMPLANON) yielded comparable systemic exposure to etonogestrel. For NEXPLANON, the mean (± SD) maximum serum etonogestrel concentrations were 1200 (± 604) pg/mL and were reached within the first two weeks after insertion (n=50). The mean (± SD) serum etonogestrel concentration decreased gradually over time, declining to 202 (± 55) pg/mL at 12 months (n=41), 164 (± 58) pg/mL at 24 months (n=37), and 138 (± 43) pg/mL at 36 months (n=32). For the non-radiopaque etonogestrel implant (IMPLANON), the mean (± SD) maximum serum etonogestrel concentrations were 1145 (± 577) pg/mL and were reached within the first two weeks after insertion (n=53). The mean (± SD) serum etonogestrel concentration decreased gradually over time, declining to 223 (± 73) pg/mL at 12 months (n=40), 172 (± 77) pg/mL at 24 months (n=32), and 153 (± 52) pg/mL at 36 months (n=30).

The pharmacokinetic profile of NEXPLANON is shown in Figure 20.

[See figure 20 above]

Distribution

The apparent volume of distribution averages about 201 L. Etonogestrel is approximately 32% bound to sex hormone binding globulin (SHBG) and 66% bound to albumin in blood.

Metabolism

In vitro data shows that etonogestrel is metabolized in liver microsomes by the cytochrome P450 3A4 isoenzyme. The biological activity of etonogestrel metabolites is unknown.

Figure 20: Mean (± SD) Serum Concentration-Time Profile of Etonogestrel After Insertion of NEXPLANON During 3 Years of Use

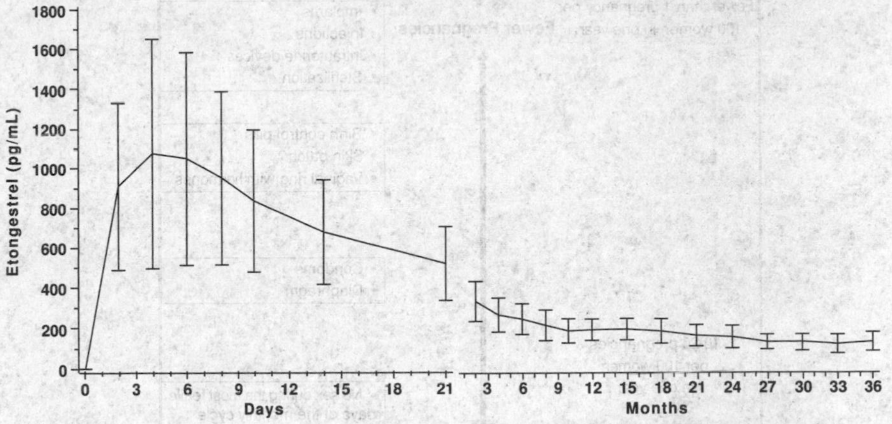

Excretion

The elimination half-life of etonogestrel is approximately 25 hours. Excretion of etonogestrel and its metabolites, either as free steroid or as conjugates, is mainly in urine and to a lesser extent in feces. After removal of the implant, etonogestrel concentrations decreased below sensitivity of the assay by one week.

13 NONCLINICAL TOXICOLOGY

13.1 Carcinogenesis, Mutagenesis, Impairment of Fertility

In a 24-month carcinogenicity study in rats with subdermal implants releasing 10 and 20 mcg etonogestrel per day (equal to approximately 1.8-3.6 times the systemic steady state exposure in women using NEXPLANON), no drug-related carcinogenic potential was observed. Etonogestrel was not genotoxic in the *in vitro* Ames/Salmonella reverse mutation assay, the chromosomal aberration assay in Chinese hamster ovary cells or in the *in vivo* mouse micronucleus test. Fertility returned after withdrawal from treatment.

14 CLINICAL STUDIES

14.1 Pregnancy

In clinical trials of up to 3 years duration that involved 923 subjects, 18-40 years of age at entry, and 1756 women-years of use with the non-radiopaque etonogestrel implant (IMPLANON), the total exposures expressed as 28-day cycle equivalents by study year were:

Year 1: 10,866 cycles
Year 2: 8581 cycles
Year 3: 3442 cycles

The clinical trials excluded women who:

- Weighed more than 130% of their ideal body weight
- Were chronically taking medications that induce liver enzymes

In the subgroup of women, 18-35 years of age at entry, 6 pregnancies during 20,648 cycles of use were reported. Two pregnancies occurred in each of Years 1, 2, and 3. Each conception was likely to have occurred shortly before or within 2 weeks after removal of the non-radiopaque etonogestrel implant. With these 6 pregnancies, the cumulative Pearl Index was 0.38 pregnancies per 100 women-years of use.

14.2 Return to Ovulation

In clinical trials with the non-radiopaque etonogestrel implant (IMPLANON), the etonogestrel levels in blood decreased below sensitivity of the assay by one week after removal of the implant. In addition, pregnancies were observed to occur as early as 7 to 14 days after removal. Therefore, a woman should re-start contraception immediately after removal of the implant if continued contraceptive protection is desired.

14.3 Implant Insertion and Removal Characteristics

Out of 301 insertions of the NEXPLANON implant in a clinical trial, the mean insertion time (from the removal of the protection cap of the applicator until retraction of the needle from the arm) was 27.9 ± 29.3 seconds. After insertion, 300 out of 301 (99.7%) NEXPLANON implants were palpable. The single, non-palpable implant was not inserted according to the instructions.

For 112 out of 114 (98.2%) subjects in 2 clinical trials for whom insertion and removal data were available, NEXPLANON implants were clearly visible with use of two-dimensional x-ray after insertion. The two implants that were not clearly visible after insertion were clearly visible with two-dimensional x-ray before removal.

16 HOW SUPPLIED/STORAGE AND HANDLING

16.1 How Supplied

One NEXPLANON package consists of a single implant containing 68 mg etonogestrel that is 4 cm in length and 2 mm in diameter, which is pre-loaded in the needle of a disposable applicator. The sterile applicator containing the implant is packed in a blister pack.

NDC 0052-0274-01

16.2 Storage and Handling

Store NEXPLANON (etonogestrel implant) Radiopaque at 25°C (77°F); excursions permitted to 15-30°C (59-86°F) [see USP Controlled Room Temperature]. Avoid storing NEXPLANON at temperatures above 30°C (86°F).

17 PATIENT COUNSELING INFORMATION

See FDA-Approved Patient Labeling.

Information for Patients

- Counsel women about the insertion and removal procedure of the NEXPLANON implant. Provide the woman with a copy of the Patient Labeling and ensure that she understands the information in the Patient Labeling before insertion and removal. A USER CARD and consent form are included in the packaging. Have the woman complete a consent form and retain it in your records. The USER CARD should be filled out and given to the woman after insertion of the NEXPLANON implant so that she will have a record of the location of the implant in the upper arm and when it should be removed.
- Counsel women that NEXPLANON does not protect against HIV infection (AIDS) or other sexually transmitted diseases.
- Counsel women that the use of NEXPLANON may be associated with changes in their normal menstrual bleeding patterns so that they know what to expect.

FDA-Approved Patient Labeling

See the full patient product information for NEXPLANON.

Manufactured for: Merck Sharp & Dohme Corp., a subsidiary of

MERCK & CO., INC., Whitehouse Station, NJ 08889, USA

Manufactured by: N.V. Organon, Oss, The Netherlands, a subsidiary of **Merck & Co., Inc.**, Whitehouse Station, NJ 08889, USA

Revised: 05/2012
900415-IMPx-IPT-USPI.11

FDA-Approved Patient Labeling

NEXPLANON® (etonogestrel implant)

Radiopaque

Subdermal Use Only

NEXPLANON® does not protect against HIV infection (the virus that causes AIDS) or other sexually transmitted diseases. Read this Patient Information leaflet carefully before you decide if NEXPLANON is right for you. This information does not take the place of talking with your healthcare provider. If you have any questions about NEXPLANON, ask your healthcare provider.

What is NEXPLANON?

NEXPLANON is a hormone-releasing birth control implant for use by women to prevent pregnancy for up to 3 years. The implant is a flexible plastic rod about the size of a matchstick that contains a progestin hormone called etonogestrel. It also contains a small amount of barium sulfate so that the implant can be seen by X-ray. Your healthcare provider will insert the implant just under the

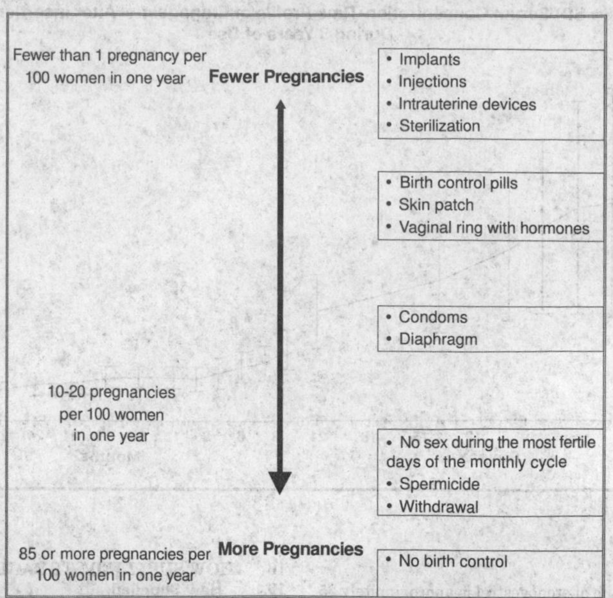

skin of the inner side of your upper arm. You can use a single NEXPLANON implant for up to 3 years. NEXPLANON does not contain estrogen.

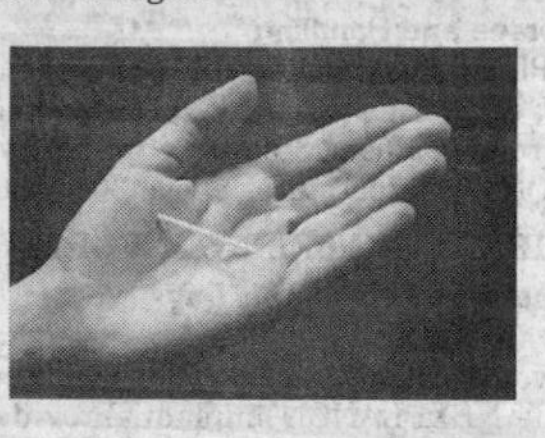

What if I need birth control for more than 3 years?

The NEXPLANON implant must be removed after 3 years. Your healthcare provider can insert a new implant under your skin after taking out the old one if you choose to continue using NEXPLANON for birth control.

What if I change my mind about birth control and want to stop using NEXPLANON before 3 years?

Your healthcare provider can remove the implant at any time. You may become pregnant as early as the first week after removal of the implant. If you do not want to get pregnant after your healthcare provider removes the NEXPLANON implant, you should start another birth control method right away.

How does NEXPLANON work?

NEXPLANON prevents pregnancy in several ways. The most important way is by stopping the release of an egg from your ovary. NEXPLANON also thickens the mucus in your cervix and this change may keep sperm from reaching the egg. NEXPLANON also changes the lining of your uterus.

How well does NEXPLANON work?

When the NEXPLANON implant is placed correctly, your chance of getting pregnant is very low (less than 1 pregnancy per 100 women who use NEXPLANON for 1 year). It is not known if NEXPLANON is as effective in very overweight women because studies did not include many overweight women.

The following chart shows the chance of getting pregnant for women who use different methods of birth control. Each box on the chart contains a list of birth control methods that are similar in effectiveness. The most effective methods are at the top of the chart. The box on the bottom of the chart shows the chance of getting pregnant for women who do not use birth control and are trying to get pregnant.

[See figure above]

Who should not use NEXPLANON?

Do not use NEXPLANON if you:
- Are pregnant or think you may be pregnant
- Have, or have had blood clots, such as blood clots in your legs (deep venous thrombosis), lungs (pulmonary embolism), eyes (total or partial blindness), heart (heart attack), or brain (stroke)
- Have liver disease or a liver tumor
- Have unexplained vaginal bleeding
- Have breast cancer or any other cancer that is sensitive to progestin (a female hormone), now or in the past
- Are allergic to anything in NEXPLANON

Tell your healthcare provider if you have or have had any of the conditions listed above. Your healthcare provider can suggest a different method of birth control.

In addition, talk to your healthcare provider about using NEXPLANON if you:
- Have diabetes
- Have high cholesterol or triglycerides
- Have headaches
- Have gallbladder or kidney problems
- Have a history of depressed mood
- Have high blood pressure
- Have an allergy to numbing medicines (anesthetics) or medicines used to clean your skin (antiseptics). These medicines will be used when the implant is placed into or removed from your arm.

Interaction with Other Medicines

Tell your healthcare provider about all the medicines you take, including prescription and non-prescription medicines, vitamins and herbal supplements. Certain medicines may make NEXPLANON less effective, including:
- barbiturates
- bosentan
- carbamazepine
- felbamate
- griseofulvin
- oxcarbazepine
- phenytoin
- rifampin
- St. John's wort
- topiramate
- HIV medicines

Ask your healthcare provider if you are not sure if your medicine is one listed above.

If there are medicines that you have been taking for a long time, that make NEXPLANON less effective, tell your healthcare provider. Your healthcare provider may remove the NEXPLANON implant and recommend a birth control method that can be used effectively with these medicines.

When you are using NEXPLANON, tell all of your healthcare providers that you have NEXPLANON in place in your arm.

How is the NEXPLANON implant placed and removed?

Your healthcare provider will place and remove the NEXPLANON implant in a minor surgical procedure in his or her office. The implant is placed just under the skin on the inner side of your upper arm.

The timing of insertion is important. Your healthcare provider may:
- Perform a pregnancy test before inserting NEXPLANON
- Schedule the insertion at a specific time of your menstrual cycle (for example, within the first days of your regular menstrual bleeding)

Immediately after the NEXPLANON implant has been placed, you and your healthcare provider should check that the implant is in your arm by feeling for it.

If you and your healthcare provider cannot feel the NEXPLANON implant, use a non-hormonal birth control method (such as condoms) until your healthcare provider confirms that the implant is in place. You may need special tests to check that the implant is in place or to help find the implant when it is time to take it out.

Your healthcare provider will cover the site where NEXPLANON was placed with 2 bandages. Leave the top bandage on for 24 hours. Keep the smaller bandage clean, dry, and in place for 3 to 5 days.

You will be asked to review and sign a consent form prior to inserting the NEXPLANON implant. You will also get a USER CARD to keep at home with your health records. Your healthcare provider will fill out the USER CARD with the date the implant was inserted and the date the implant is to be removed. Keep track of the date the implant is to be removed. Schedule an appointment with your healthcare provider to remove the implant on or before the removal date.

Be sure to have checkups as advised by your healthcare provider.

What are the most common side effects I can expect while using NEXPLANON?

• Changes in Menstrual Bleeding Patterns (menstrual periods)

The most common side effect of NEXPLANON is a change in your normal menstrual bleeding pattern. In studies, one out of ten women stopped using the implant because of an unfavorable change in their bleeding pattern. You may experience longer or shorter bleeding during your periods or have no bleeding at all. The time between periods may vary, and in between periods you may also have spotting.

Tell your healthcare provider right away if:
- You think you may be pregnant
- Your menstrual bleeding is heavy and prolonged

Besides changes in menstrual bleeding patterns, other frequent side effects that caused women to stop using the implant include:
- Mood swings
- Weight gain
- Headache
- Acne
- Depressed mood

Other common side effects include:
- Headache
- Vaginitis (inflammation of the vagina)
- Weight gain
- Acne
- Breast pain
- Viral infections such as sore throats or flu-like symptoms
- Stomach pain
- Painful periods
- Mood swings, nervousness, or depressed mood
- Back pain
- Nausea
- Dizziness
- Pain
- Pain at the site of insertion

This is not a complete list of possible side effects. For more information, ask your healthcare provider for advice about any side effects that concern you. You may report side effects to the FDA at 1-800-FDA-1088.

What are the possible risks of using NEXPLANON?

• Problems with Insertion and Removal

The implant may not be placed in your arm at all due to a failed insertion. If this happens, you may become pregnant. Immediately after insertion, and with help from your healthcare provider, you should be able to feel the implant under your skin. If you can't feel the implant, tell your healthcare provider.

Removal of the implant may be very difficult or impossible because the implant is not where it should be. Special procedures, including surgery in the hospital, may be needed to remove the implant. If the implant is not removed, then the effects of NEXPLANON will continue for a longer period of time.

Other problems related to insertion and removal are:
- Pain, irritation, swelling, or bruising at the insertion site
- Scarring, including a thick scar called a keloid around the insertion site
- Infection
- Scar tissue may form around the implant making it difficult to remove
- The implant may come out by itself. You may become pregnant if the implant comes out by itself. Use a back up birth control method and call your healthcare provider right away if the implant comes out.
- The need for surgery in the hospital to remove the implant
- Injury to nerves or blood vessels in your arm
- The implant breaks making removal difficult

• Ectopic Pregnancy

If you become pregnant while using NEXPLANON, you have a slightly higher chance that the pregnancy will be ectopic (occurring outside the womb) than do women who do not use birth control. Unusual vaginal bleeding or lower stomach (abdominal) pain may be a sign of ectopic pregnancy. Ectopic pregnancy is a medical emergency that often requires surgery. Ectopic pregnancies can cause serious internal bleeding, infertility, and even death. Call your healthcare provider right away if you think you are pregnant or have unexplained lower stomach (abdominal) pain.

- **Ovarian Cysts**

Cysts may develop on the ovaries and usually go away without treatment but sometimes surgery is needed to remove them.

- **Breast Cancer**

It is not known whether NEXPLANON use changes a woman's risk for breast cancer. If you have breast cancer now, or have had it in the past, do not use NEXPLANON because some breast cancers are sensitive to hormones.

- **Serious Blood Clots**

NEXPLANON may increase your chance of serious blood clots, especially if you have other risk factors such as smoking. It is possible to die from a problem caused by a blood clot, such as a heart attack or a stroke.

Some examples of serious blood clots are blood clots in the:
- Legs (deep vein thrombosis)
- Lungs (pulmonary embolism)
- Brain (stroke)
- Heart (heart attack)
- Eyes (total or partial blindness)

The risk of serious blood clots is increased in women who smoke. If you smoke and want to use NEXPLANON, you should quit. Your healthcare provider may be able to help. Tell your healthcare provider at least 4 weeks before if you are going to have surgery or will need to be on bed rest. You have an increased chance of getting blood clots during surgery or bed rest.

- **Other Risks**

A few women who use birth control that contains hormones may get:
- High blood pressure
- Gallbladder problems
- Rare cancerous or noncancerous liver tumors

When should I call my healthcare provider?

Call your healthcare provider right away if you have:
- Pain in your lower leg that does not go away
- Severe chest pain or heaviness in the chest
- Sudden shortness of breath, sharp chest pain, or coughing blood
- Symptoms of a severe allergic reaction, such as swollen face, tongue or pharynx; trouble swallowing; or hives and trouble breathing
- Sudden severe headache unlike your usual headaches
- Weakness or numbness in your arm, leg, or trouble speaking
- Sudden partial or complete blindness
- Yellowing of your skin or whites of your eyes, especially with fever, tiredness, loss of appetite, dark colored urine, or light colored bowel movements
- Severe pain, swelling, or tenderness in the lower stomach (abdomen)
- Lump in your breast
- Problems sleeping, lack of energy, tiredness, or you feel very sad
- Heavy menstrual bleeding

What if I become pregnant while using NEXPLANON?

You should see your healthcare provider right away if you think that you may be pregnant. It is important to remove the implant and make sure that the pregnancy is not ectopic (occurring outside the womb). Based on experience with other hormonal contraceptives, NEXPLANON is not likely to cause birth defects.

Can I use NEXPLANON when I am breastfeeding?

If you are breastfeeding your child, you may use NEXPLANON if 4 weeks have passed since you had your baby. A small amount of the hormone contained in NEXPLANON passes into your breast milk. The health of breast-fed children whose mothers were using the implant has been studied up to 3 years of age in a small number of children. No effects on the growth and development of the children were seen. If you are breastfeeding and want to use NEXPLANON, talk with your healthcare provider for more information.

Additional Information

This Patient Information leaflet contains important information about NEXPLANON. If you would like more information, talk with your healthcare provider. You can ask your healthcare provider for information about NEXPLANON that is written for healthcare professionals. You may also call 1-877-467-5266 or visit www.NEXPLANON-USA.com.

Manufactured for: Merck Sharp & Dohme Corp., a subsidiary of

MERCK & CO., INC., Whitehouse Station, NJ 08889, USA

Manufactured by: N.V. Organon, Oss, The Netherlands, a subsidiary of **Merck & Co., Inc.**, Whitehouse Station, NJ 08889, USA

Revised: 05/2012

900415-IMPx-IPT-PPI.10

NEXPLANON® (etonogestrel implant)

Radiopaque

Subdermal Use Only

PATIENT CONSENT FORM

I understand the Patient Labeling for NEXPLANON®. I have discussed NEXPLANON with my healthcare provider who answered all my questions. I understand that there are benefits as well as risks with using NEXPLANON. I understand that there are other birth control methods and that each has its own benefits and risks.

I also understand that this Patient Consent Form is important. I understand that I need to sign this form to show that I am making an informed and careful decision to use NEXPLANON, and that I have read and understand the following points.

- NEXPLANON helps to keep me from getting pregnant.
- No contraceptive method is 100% effective, including NEXPLANON.
- NEXPLANON has an implant that contains a hormone.
- It is important to have the NEXPLANON implant **placed in my arm** at the right time of my menstrual cycle.
- **After the implant is placed in my arm, I should check that it is in place by gently pressing my fingertips over the skin where the implant was placed. I should be able to feel the implant.**
- The implant must be removed at the end of three years. The implant can be removed sooner if I want.
- If I have trouble finding a healthcare provider to remove the implant, I can call 1-877-467-5266 for help.
- The implant is placed under the skin of my arm during a procedure done in my healthcare provider's office. There is a slight risk of getting a scar or an infection from this procedure.
- Removal is usually a minor procedure. Sometimes, removal may be more difficult. Special procedures, including surgery in the hospital, may be needed. Difficult removals may cause pain and scarring and may result in injury to nerves and blood vessels. If the implant is not removed, its effects may continue.
- **Most women have changes in their menstrual bleeding patterns while using NEXPLANON. I also will likely have changes in my menstrual bleeding pattern while using NEXPLANON. My bleeding may be irregular, lighter or heavier, or my bleeding may completely stop. If I think I am pregnant, I should contact my healthcare provider as soon as possible.**
- I understand the warning signs for problems with NEXPLANON. I should seek medical attention if any warning signs appear.
- I should tell all my healthcare providers that I am using NEXPLANON.
- I need to have a medical checkup regularly and at any time I am having problems.
- NEXPLANON does not protect me from HIV infection (AIDS) or any other sexually transmitted diseases.

After learning about NEXPLANON, I choose to use NEXPLANON.

____

(Name of Healthcare Provider)

____

(Patient Signature) (Date)

WITNESSED BY:

The patient above has signed this consent in my presence after I counseled her and answered her questions.

____

(Healthcare Provider Signature) (Date)

I have provided an accurate translation of this information to the patient whose signature appears above. She has stated that she understands the information and has had an opportunity to have her questions answered.

____

(Signature of Translator) (Date)

Manufactured for: Merck Sharp & Dohme Corp., a subsidiary of

MERCK & CO., INC., Whitehouse Station, NJ 08889, USA

Manufactured by: N.V. Organon, Oss, The Netherlands, a subsidiary of **Merck & Co., Inc.**, Whitehouse Station, NJ 08889, USA

Revised: 05/2012

900415-IMPx-IPT-PCF.2

NITRO-DUR® ℞

[*nī-trō-dŭr*]

(nitroglycerin)

Transdermal Infusion System

DESCRIPTION

Nitroglycerin is 1,2,3-propanetriol trinitrate, an organic nitrate whose structural formula is:

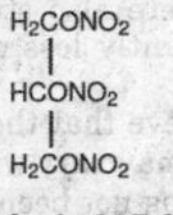

and whose molecular weight is 227.09. The organic nitrates are vasodilators, active on both arteries and veins.

The NITRO-DUR® (nitroglycerin) Transdermal Infusion System is a flat unit designed to provide continuous controlled release of nitroglycerin through intact skin. The rate of release of nitroglycerin is linearly dependent upon the area of the applied system; each cm^2 of applied system delivers approximately 0.02 mg of nitroglycerin per hour. Thus, the 5-, 10-, 15-, 20-, 30-, and 40-cm^2 systems deliver approximately 0.1, 0.2, 0.3, 0.4, 0.6, and 0.8 mg of nitroglycerin per hour, respectively.

The remainder of the nitroglycerin in each system serves as a reservoir and is not delivered in normal use. After 12 hours, for example, each system has delivered approximately 6% of its original content of nitroglycerin.

The NITRO-DUR transdermal system contains nitroglycerin in acrylic-based polymer adhesives with a resinous cross-linking agent to provide a continuous source of active ingredient. Each unit is sealed in a paper polyethylene-foil pouch.

Cross section of the system.

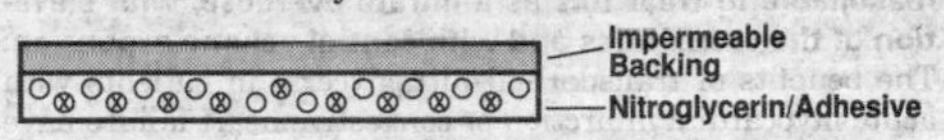

CLINICAL PHARMACOLOGY

The principal pharmacological action of nitroglycerin is relaxation of vascular smooth muscle and consequent dilatation of peripheral arteries and veins, especially the latter. Dilatation of the veins promotes peripheral pooling of blood and decreases venous return to the heart, thereby reducing left ventricular end-diastolic pressure and pulmonary capillary wedge pressure (preload). Arteriolar relaxation reduces systemic vascular resistance, systolic arterial pressure, and mean arterial pressure (afterload). Dilatation of the coronary arteries also occurs. The relative importance of preload reduction, afterload reduction, and coronary dilatation remains undefined.

Dosing regimens for most chronically used drugs are designed to provide plasma concentrations that are continuously greater than a minimally effective concentration. This strategy is inappropriate for organic nitrates. Several well-controlled clinical trials have used exercise testing to assess the antianginal efficacy of continuously delivered nitrates. In the large majority of these trials, active agents were indistinguishable from placebo after 24 hours (or less) of continuous therapy. Attempts to overcome nitrate tolerance by dose escalation, even to doses far in excess of those used acutely, have consistently failed. Only after nitrates have been absent from the body for several hours has their antianginal efficacy been restored.

Pharmacokinetics

The volume of distribution of nitroglycerin is about 3 L/kg, and nitroglycerin is cleared from this volume at extremely rapid rates, with a resulting serum half-life of about 3 minutes. The observed clearance rates (close to 1 L/kg/min) greatly exceed hepatic blood flow; known sites of extrahepatic metabolism include red blood cells and vascular walls. The first products in the metabolism of nitroglycerin are inorganic nitrate and the 1,2- and 1,3-dinitroglycerols. The dinitrates are less effective vasodilators than nitroglycerin, but they are longer-lived in the serum, and their net contribution to the overall effect of chronic nitroglycerin regimens is not known. The dinitrates are further metabolized to (nonvasoactive) mononitrates and, ultimately, to glycerol and carbon dioxide.

To avoid development of tolerance to nitroglycerin, drug-free intervals of 10 to 12 hours are known to be sufficient; shorter intervals have not been well studied. In one well-controlled clinical trial, subjects receiving nitroglycerin appeared to exhibit a rebound or withdrawal effect, so that their exercise tolerance at the end of the daily drug-free interval was less than that exhibited by the parallel group receiving placebo.

In healthy volunteers, steady-state plasma concentrations of nitroglycerin are reached by about 2 hours after application of a patch and are maintained for the duration of wearing the system (observations have been limited to 24 hours). Upon removal of the patch, the plasma concentration declines with a half-life of about an hour.

Clinical Trials

Regimens in which nitroglycerin patches were worn for 12 hours daily have been studied in well-controlled trials up to 4 weeks in duration. Starting about 2 hours after application and continuing until 10 to 12 hours after application, patches that deliver at least 0.4 mg of nitroglycerin per hour have consistently demonstrated greater antianginal activity than placebo. Lower-dose patches have not been as well studied, but in one large, well-controlled trial in which higher-dose patches were also studied, patches delivering 0.2 mg/hr had significantly less antianginal activity than placebo.

It is reasonable to believe that the rate of nitroglycerin absorption from patches may vary with the site of application, but this relationship has not been adequately studied.

INDICATIONS AND USAGE

Transdermal nitroglycerin is indicated for the prevention of angina pectoris due to coronary artery disease. The onset of action of transdermal nitroglycerin is not sufficiently rapid for this product to be useful in aborting an acute attack.

CONTRAINDICATIONS

Allergic reactions to organic nitrates are extremely rare, but they do occur. Nitroglycerin is contraindicated in patients who are allergic to it. Allergy to the adhesives used in nitroglycerin patches has also been reported, and it similarly constitutes a contraindication to the use of this product.

WARNINGS

Amplification of the vasodilatory effects of the NITRO-DUR patch by phosphodiesterase inhibitors, eg, sildenafil can result in severe hypotension. The time course and dose dependence of this interaction have not been studied. Appropriate supportive care has not been studied, but it seems reasonable to treat this as a nitrate overdose, with elevation of the extremities and with central volume expansion.

The benefits of transdermal nitroglycerin in patients with acute myocardial infarction or congestive heart failure have not been established. If one elects to use nitroglycerin in these conditions, careful clinical or hemodynamic monitoring must be used to avoid the hazards of hypotension and tachycardia.

A cardioverter/defibrillator should not be discharged through a paddle electrode that overlies a NITRO-DUR patch. The arcing that may be seen in this situation is harmless in itself, but it may be associated with local current concentration that can cause damage to the paddles and burns to the patient.

PRECAUTIONS

General

Severe hypotension, particularly with upright posture, may occur with even small doses of nitroglycerin, particularly in the elderly. The NITRO-DUR Transdermal Infusion System should therefore be used with caution in elderly patients who may be volume-depleted, are on multiple medications, or who, for whatever reason, are already hypotensive. Hypotension induced by nitroglycerin may be accompanied by paradoxical bradycardia and increased angina pectoris.

Elderly patients may be more susceptible to hypotension and may be at greater risk of falling at the therapeutic doses of nitroglycerin.

Nitrate therapy may aggravate the angina caused by hypertrophic cardiomyopathy, particularly in the elderly.

In industrial workers who have had long-term exposure to unknown (presumably high) doses of organic nitrates, tolerance clearly occurs. Chest pain, acute myocardial infarction, and even sudden death have occurred during temporary withdrawal of nitrates from these workers, demonstrating the existence of true physical dependence.

Several clinical trials in patients with angina pectoris have evaluated nitroglycerin regimens which incorporated a 10- to 12-hour, nitrate-free interval. In some of these trials, an increase in the frequency of anginal attacks during the nitrate-free interval was observed in a small number of patients. In one trial, patients had decreased exercise tolerance at the end of the nitrate-free interval. Hemodynamic rebound has been observed only rarely; on the other hand, few studies were so designed that rebound, if it had occurred, would have been detected. The importance of these observations to the routine, clinical use of transdermal nitroglycerin is unknown.

Information for Patients

Daily headaches sometimes accompany treatment with nitroglycerin. In patients who get these headaches, the headaches may be a marker of the activity of the drug. Patients should resist the temptation to avoid headaches by altering the schedule of their treatment with nitroglycerin, since loss of headache may be associated with simultaneous loss of antianginal efficacy.

Treatment with nitroglycerin may be associated with lightheadedness on standing, especially just after rising from a recumbent or seated position. This effect may be more frequent in patients who have also consumed alcohol.

After normal use, there is enough residual nitroglycerin in discarded patches that they are a potential hazard to children and pets.

A patient leaflet is supplied with the systems.

Drug Interactions

The vasodilating effects of nitroglycerin may be additive with those of other vasodilators. Alcohol, in particular, has been found to exhibit additive effects of this variety.

Carcinogenesis, Mutagenesis, Impairment of Fertility

Animal carcinogenesis studies with topically applied nitroglycerin have not been performed.

Rats receiving up to 434 mg/kg/day of dietary nitroglycerin for 2 years developed dose-related fibrotic and neoplastic changes in liver, including carcinomas, and interstitial cell tumors in testes. At high dose, the incidences of hepatocellular carcinomas in both sexes were 52% vs 0% in controls, and incidences of testicular tumors were 52% vs 8% in controls. Lifetime dietary administration of up to 1058 mg/kg/day of nitroglycerin was not tumorigenic in mice.

Nitroglycerin was weakly mutagenic in Ames tests performed in two different laboratories. Nevertheless, there was no evidence of mutagenicity in an *in vivo* dominant lethal assay with male rats treated with doses up to about 363 mg/kg/day, po, or in *in vitro* cytogenetic tests in rat and dog tissues.

In a three-generation reproduction study, rats received dietary nitroglycerin at doses up to about 434 mg/kg/day for 6 months prior to mating of the F_0 generation with treatment continuing through successive F_1 and F_2 generations. The high dose was associated with decreased feed intake and body weight gain in both sexes at all matings. No specific effect on the fertility of the F_0 generation was seen. Infertility noted in subsequent generations, however, was attributed to increased interstitial cell tissue and aspermatogenesis in the high-dose males. In this three-generation study there was no clear evidence of teratogenicity.

Pregnancy

Pregnancy Category C

Animal teratology studies have not been conducted with nitroglycerin transdermal systems. Teratology studies in rats and rabbits, however, were conducted with topically applied nitroglycerin ointment at doses up to 80 mg/kg/day and 240 mg/kg/day, respectively. No toxic effects on dams or fetuses were seen at any dose tested. There are no adequate and well-controlled studies in pregnant women. Nitroglycerin should be given to a pregnant woman only if clearly needed.

Nursing Mothers

It is not known whether nitroglycerin is excreted in human milk. Because many drugs are excreted in human milk, caution should be exercised when nitroglycerin is administered to a nursing woman.

Pediatric Use

Safety and effectiveness in pediatric patients have not been established.

Geriatric Use

Clinical studies of NITRO-DUR Transdermal Infusion System did not include sufficient information to determine whether subjects 65 years and older respond differently from younger subjects. Additional clinical data from the published literature indicate that the elderly demonstrate increased sensitivity to nitrates, which may result in hypotension and increased risk of falling. In general, dose selection for an elderly patient should be cautious, usually starting at the low end of the dosing range, reflecting the greater frequency of the decreased hepatic, renal, or cardiac function, and of concomitant disease or other drug therapy.

ADVERSE REACTIONS

Adverse reactions to nitroglycerin are generally dose related, and almost all of these reactions are the result of nitroglycerin's activity as a vasodilator. Headache, which may be severe, is the most commonly reported side effect. Headache may be recurrent with each daily dose, especially at higher doses. Transient episodes of lightheadedness, occasionally related to blood pressure changes, may also occur. Hypotension occurs infrequently, but in some patients it may be severe enough to warrant discontinuation of therapy. Syncope, crescendo angina, and rebound hypertension have been reported but are uncommon.

Allergic reactions to nitroglycerin are also uncommon, and the great majority of those reported have been cases of contact dermatitis or fixed drug eruptions in patients receiving nitroglycerin in ointments or patches. There have been a few reports of genuine anaphylactoid reactions, and these reactions can probably occur in patients receiving nitroglycerin by any route.

Extremely rarely, ordinary doses of organic nitrates have caused methemoglobinemia in normal-seeming patients. Methemoglobinemia is so infrequent at these doses that further discussion of its diagnosis and treatment is deferred (see **OVERDOSAGE**).

Application-site irritation may occur but is rarely severe.

In two placebo-controlled trials of intermittent therapy with nitroglycerin patches at 0.2 to 0.8 mg/hr, the most frequent adverse reactions among 307 subjects were as follows:

	Placebo	Patch
Headache	18%	63%
Lightheadedness	4%	6%
Hypotension, and/or Syncope	0%	4%
Increased Angina	2%	2%

OVERDOSAGE

Hemodynamic Effects

Nitroglycerin toxicity is generally mild. The estimated adult oral lethal dose of nitroglycerin is 200 mg to 1,200 mg. Infants may be more susceptible to toxicity from nitroglycerin. Consultation with a poison center should be considered.

Laboratory determinations of serum levels of nitroglycerin and its metabolites are not widely available, and such determinations have, in any event, no established role in the management of nitroglycerin overdose.

No data are available to suggest physiological maneuvers (eg, maneuvers to change the pH of the urine) that might accelerate elimination of nitroglycerin and its active metabolites. Similarly, it is not known which – if any – of these substances can usefully be removed from the body by hemodialysis.

No specific antagonist to the vasodilator effects of nitroglycerin is known, and no intervention has been subject to controlled study as a therapy of nitroglycerin overdose. Because the hypotension associated with nitroglycerin overdose is the result of venodilatation and arterial hypovolemia, prudent therapy in this situation should be directed toward increase in central fluid volume. Passive elevation of the patient's legs may be sufficient, but intravenous infusion of normal saline or similar fluid may also be necessary. The use of epinephrine or other arterial vasoconstrictors in this setting is likely to do more harm than good.

In patients with renal disease or congestive heart failure, therapy resulting in central volume expansion is not without hazard. Treatment of nitroglycerin overdose in these patients may be subtle and difficult, and invasive monitoring may be required.

Methemoglobinemia

Nitrate ions liberated during metabolism of nitroglycerin can oxidize hemoglobin into methemoglobin. Even in patients totally without cytochrome b5 reductase activity, however, and even assuming that the nitrate moieties of nitroglycerin are quantitatively applied to oxidation of hemoglobin, about 1 mg/kg of nitroglycerin should be required before any of these patients manifests clinically significant (^{3}10%) methemoglobinemia. In patients with normal reductase function, significant production of methemoglobin should require even larger doses of nitroglycerin. In one study in which 36 patients received 2 to 4 weeks of continuous nitroglycerin therapy at 3.1 to 4.4 mg/hr, the average methemoglobin level measured was 0.2%; this was comparable to that observed in parallel patients who received placebo.

Notwithstanding these observations, there are case reports of significant methemoglobinemia in association with moderate overdoses of organic nitrates. None of the affected patients had been thought to be unusually susceptible.

Methemoglobin levels are available from most clinical laboratories. The diagnosis should be suspected in patients who exhibit signs of impaired oxygen delivery despite adequate cardiac output and adequate arterial PO_2. Classically, methemoglobinemic blood is described as chocolate brown, without color change on exposure to air.

Methemoglobinemia should be treated with methylene blue if the patient develops cardiac or CNS effects of hypoxia. The initial dose is 1 to 2 mg/kg infused intravenously over 5 minutes. Repeat methemoglobin levels should be obtained 30 minutes later and a repeat dose of 0.5 to 1.0 mg/kg may be used if the level remains elevated and the patient is still symptomatic. Relative contraindications for methylene blue include known NADH methemoglobin reductase deficiency or G-6-PD deficiency. Infants under the age of 4 months may not respond to methylene blue due to immature NADH methemoglobin reductase. Exchange transfusion has been used successfully in critically ill patients when methemoglobinemia is refractory to treatment.

DOSAGE AND ADMINISTRATION

The suggested starting dose is between 0.2 mg/hr[1] and 0.4 mg/hr[1]. Doses between 0.4 mg/hr[1] and 0.8 mg/hr[1] have shown continued effectiveness for 10 to 12 hours daily for at least 1 month (the longest period studied) of intermittent administration. Although the minimum nitrate-free interval has not been defined, data show that a nitrate-free interval of 10 to 12 hours is sufficient (see **CLINICAL PHARMACOLOGY**). Thus, an appropriate dosing schedule for nitroglycerin patches would include a daily patch-on period of 12 to 14 hours and a daily patch-off period of 10 to 12 hours.

Although some well-controlled clinical trials using exercise tolerance testing have shown maintenance of effectiveness when patches are worn continuously, the large majority of such controlled trials have shown the development of tolerance (ie, complete loss of effect) within the first 24 hours after therapy was initiated. Dose adjustment, even to levels much higher than generally used, did not restore efficacy.

[1]Release rates were formerly described in terms of drug delivered per 24 hours. In these terms, the supplied NITRO-DUR systems would be rated at 2.5 mg/24 hours (0.1 mg/hour), 5 mg/24 hours (0.2 mg/hour), 7.5 mg/24 hours (0.3 mg/hour), 10 mg/24 hours (0.4 mg/hour), and 15 mg/24 hours (0.6 mg/hour).

HOW SUPPLIED

NITRO-DUR System Rated Release *In Vivo**	Total Nitroglycerin Content	System Size	Package Size
0.1 mg/hr	20 mg	5 cm^2	Unit Dose 30 (NDC 0085-3305-30) Institutional Package 30 (NDC 0085-3305-35)
0.2 mg/hr	40 mg	10 cm^2	Unit Dose 30 (NDC 0085-3310-30) Institutional Package 30 (NDC 0085-3310-35)
0.3 mg/hr	60 mg	15 cm^2	Unit Dose 30 (NDC 0085-3315-30) Institutional Package 30 (NDC 0085-3315-35)
0.4 mg/hr	80 mg	20 cm^2	Unit Dose 30 (NDC 0085-3320-30) Institutional Package 30 (NDC 0085-3320-35)
0.6 mg/hr	120 mg	30 cm^2	Unit Dose 30 (NDC 0085-3330-30) Institutional Package 30 (NDC 0085-3330-35)
0.8 mg/hr	160 mg	40 cm^2	Unit Dose 30 (NDC 0085-0819-30) Institutional Package 30 (NDC 0085-0819-35)

* Release rates were formerly described in terms of drug delivered per 24 hours. In these terms, the supplied NITRO-DUR systems would be rated at 2.5 mg/24 hours (0.1 mg/hour), 5 mg/24 hours (0.2 mg/hour), 7.5 mg/24 hours (0.3 mg/hour), 10 mg/24 hours (0.4 mg/hour), and 15 mg/24 hours (0.6 mg/hour).

Store at 25°C (77°F); excursions permitted to 15-30°C (59-86°F) [see USP Controlled Room Temperature]. Do not refrigerate.

Rx only

Merck Sharp & Dohme Corp., a subsidiary of
MERCK & CO.,INC., Whitehouse Station, NJ 08889, USA

Revised: 05/2012
35208003T

Please read this instruction sheet carefully before using NITRO-DUR

Information for the Patient About—
Nitro-Dur®
(nitroglycerin)
Transdermal Infusion System

Summary

NITRO-DUR® is a unique method of administering nitroglycerin to the bloodstream. NITRO-DUR eliminates the swallowing of pills or the application of a messy ointment. Nitroglycerin is a medication your doctor has prescribed for you to help reduce the frequency and severity of angina attacks (chest pain).

How your NITRO-DUR Transdermal Infusion System works

Nitroglycerin causes the veins (vessels that return blood to the heart) to relax so that the work load of the heart is reduced. This lowers the heart's oxygen needs.

As a result, the heart muscle is well nourished and the frequency of angina attacks is reduced. NITRO-DUR is applied directly to the skin. The nitroglycerin passes from the adhesive surface through the skin—allowing medication to be absorbed directly into the bloodstream. This manner of delivering medicine to your bloodstream provides you with nitroglycerin with one daily application of a NITRO-DUR unit.

Instructions for use

Placement area

Select a reasonably hair-free application site. Avoid extremities below the knee or elbow, skin folds, scar tissue, burned or irritated areas.

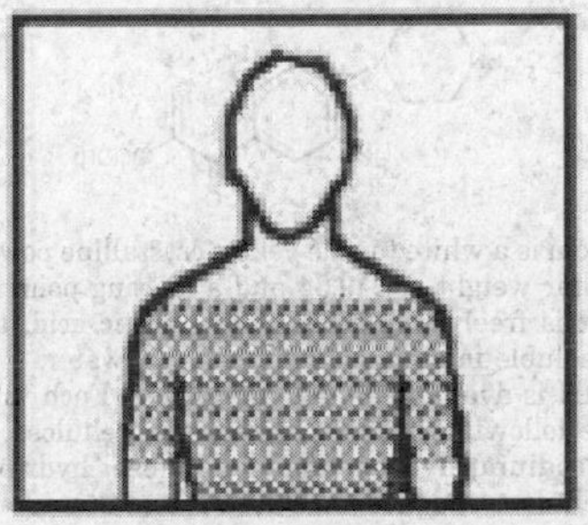

Application

Wash hands before applying.

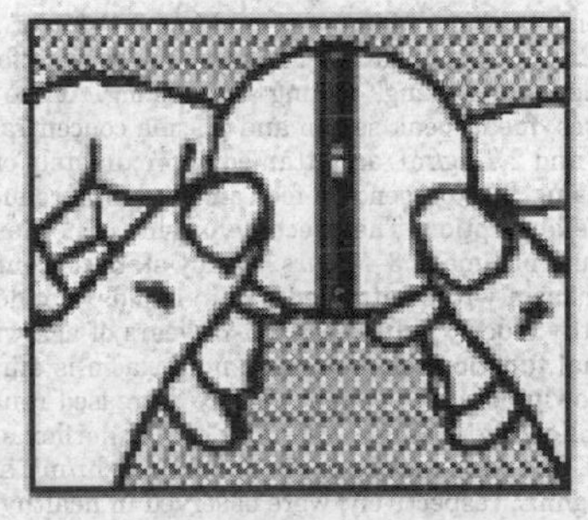

Hold the unit with brown lines facing you, in an up and down position.

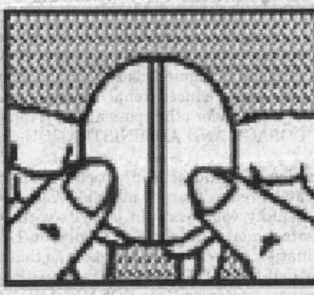

Bend the sides of unit away from you, then toward you until you hear the "SNAP".

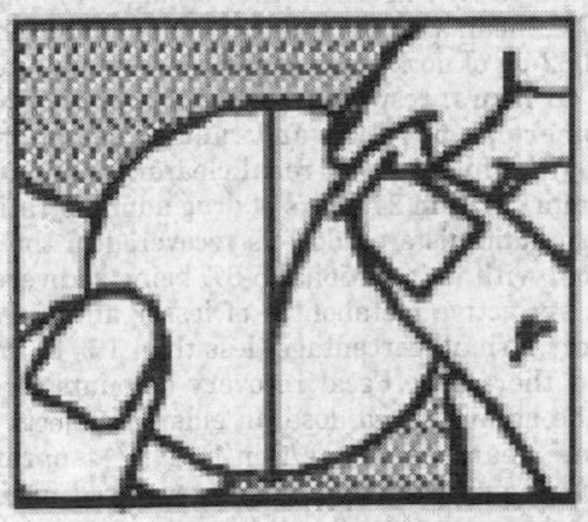

Peel off one side of the plastic backing.

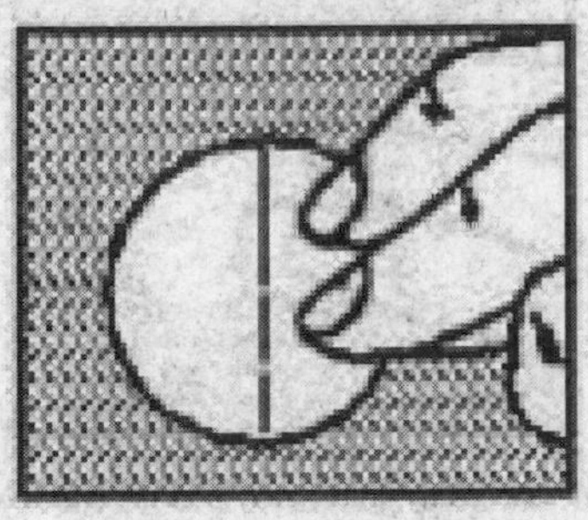

Using the other half of the backing as a handle, apply the sticky side of the patch to the skin.

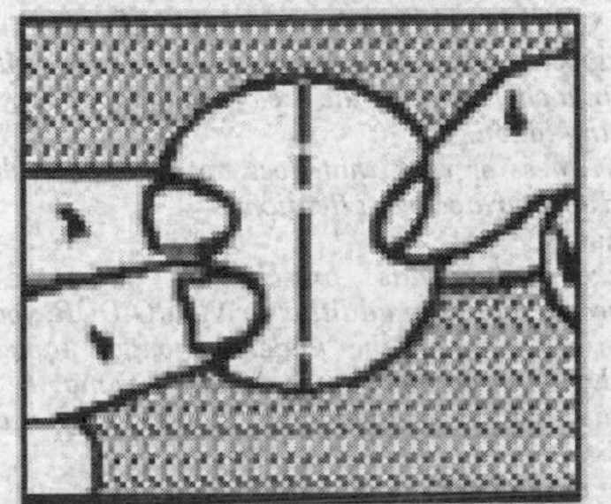

Press the sticky side on the skin, and smooth down.

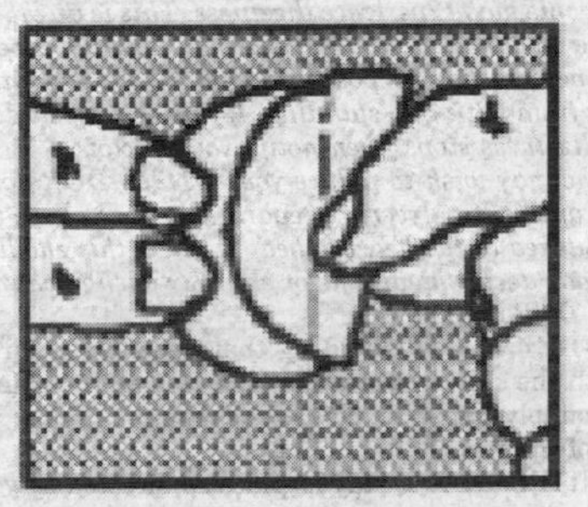

Fold back the remaining side of the patch. Grasp the edge of the plastic applicator by the stripe, and pull it across the skin.

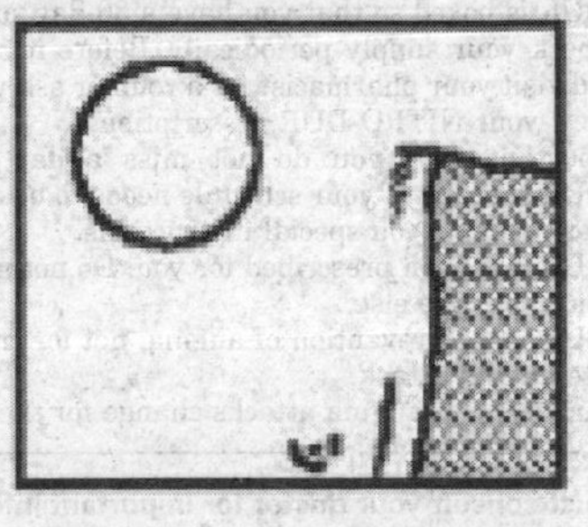

Wash hands to remove any drug.

Removal

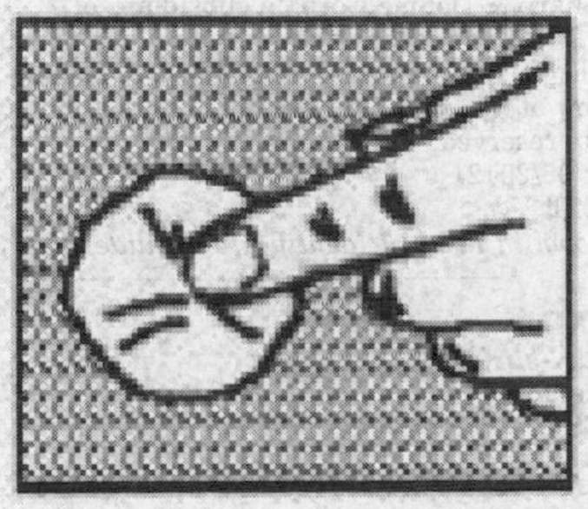

Press down on the center of the system to raise its outer edge away from the skin.

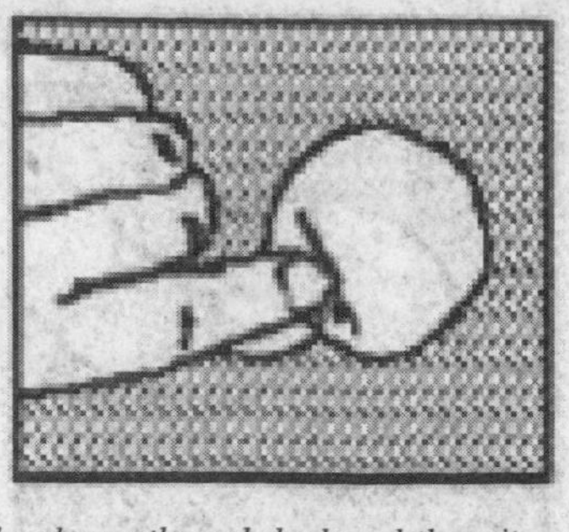

Grasp the edge gently, and slowly peel the unit away from skin.

Wash skin area with soap and water. Towel dry. Wash hands. You may use a different application site every day.

Skin care

1. *After you remove NITRO-DUR, your skin may feel warm and appear red. This is normal. The redness will disappear in a short time. If the area feels dry, you may apply a soothing lotion.*
2. *Any redness or rash that does not disappear should be called to your doctor's attention.*

Cautions

If your doctor has prescribed "under-the-tongue" nitroglycerin tablets in addition to NITRO-DUR, you should sit down before taking the "under-the-tongue" tablet. If dizziness should occur, notify your doctor. This may be an indication that the "under-the-tongue" tablet dosage needs to be reduced.

Possible side effects

The most common side effect experienced by people taking nitroglycerin is headache. Your doctor may tell you to take a mild analgesic to relieve the headache.

Some people may experience dizziness. This is due to a slight decrease in blood pressure, which is usually experienced when a person changes position, from lying flat to sitting upright or from sitting to standing. If this occurs, sit down until the dizziness stops, then notify your doctor.

He or she may wish to reduce your NITRO-DUR dosage. In some people, nitroglycerin preparations may cause the skin to feel flushed or the heart to beat faster. If this should occur, notify your doctor; again, he or she may wish to change your NITRO-DUR dosage.

NITRO-DUR is a unique drug that depends on direct contact with the skin to work. For this reason, the skin should be reasonably hair-free, clean, and dry.

Other information

Allow NITRO-DUR to stay in place as directed by your doctor.

Showering is permitted with NITRO-DUR in place.

NITRO-DUR should be kept out of reach of children and pets.

Store at room temperature 77°F (25°C).

NITRO-DUR is boxed so that you have a 30-day supply. Be sure to check your supply periodically. Before it runs low, you should visit your pharmacist for a refill or ask your doctor to renew your NITRO-DUR prescription.

It is important that you do not miss a day of your NITRO-DUR therapy. If your schedule needs to be changed, your doctor will give you special instructions.

NITRO-DUR has been prescribed for you. Do not give your medication to anyone else.

NITRO-DUR is for prevention of angina; not for treatment of an acute angina attack.

Notify your doctor if angina attacks change for the worse.

You must consult your doctor for important information before using this drug.

Merck Sharp & Dohme Corp., a subsidiary of
MERCK & CO.,INC., Whitehouse Station, NJ 08889, USA

Revised: 05/2012
35207902T

Shown in Product Identification Guide, page 308

NOROXIN® ℞

[nor-AHK-sin]
(norfloxacin)
TABLETS

WARNING:
Fluoroquinolones, including NOROXIN, are associated with an increased risk of tendinitis and tendon rupture in all ages. This risk is further increased in older patients usually over 60 years of age, in patients taking corticosteroid drugs, and in patients with kidney, heart or lung transplants (see WARNINGS). Fluoroquinolones, including NOROXIN, may exacerbate muscle weakness in persons with myasthenia gravis. Avoid NOROXIN in patients with known history of myasthenia gravis (see WARNINGS).

To reduce the development of drug-resistant bacteria and maintain the effectiveness of NOROXIN® and other antibacterial drugs, NOROXIN should be used only to treat or prevent infections that are proven or strongly suspected to be caused by bacteria.

DESCRIPTION

NOROXIN (Norfloxacin) is a synthetic, broad-spectrum antibacterial agent for oral administration. Norfloxacin, a fluoroquinolone, is 1-ethyl-6-fluoro-1,4-dihydro-4-oxo-7-(1-piperazinyl)-3-quinolinecarboxylic acid. Its empirical formula is $C_{16}H_{18}FN_3O_3$ and the structural formula is:

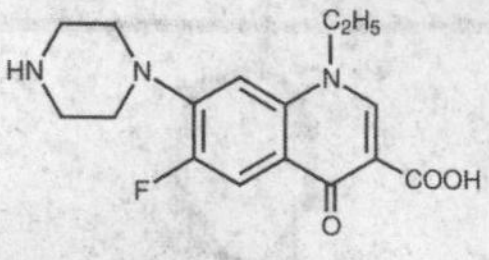

Norfloxacin is a white to pale yellow crystalline powder with a molecular weight of 319.34 and a melting point of about 221°C. It is freely soluble in glacial acetic acid, and very slightly soluble in ethanol, methanol and water.

NOROXIN is available in 400-mg tablets. Each tablet contains the following inactive ingredients: cellulose, croscarmellose sodium, hydroxypropyl cellulose, hydroxypropyl methylcellulose, magnesium stearate, and titanium dioxide. Norfloxacin, a fluoroquinolone, differs from non-fluorinated quinolones by having a fluorine atom at the 6 position and a piperazine moiety at the 7 position.

CLINICAL PHARMACOLOGY

In fasting healthy volunteers, at least 30-40% of an oral dose of NOROXIN is absorbed. Absorption is rapid following single doses of 200 mg, 400 mg and 800 mg. At the respective doses, mean peak serum and plasma concentrations of 0.8, 1.5 and 2.4 μg/mL are attained approximately one hour after dosing. The presence of food and/or dairy products may decrease absorption. The effective half-life of norfloxacin in serum and plasma is 3-4 hours. Steady-state concentrations of norfloxacin will be attained within two days of dosing.

In healthy elderly volunteers (65-75 years of age with normal renal function for their age), norfloxacin is eliminated more slowly because of their slightly decreased renal function. Following a single 400-mg dose of norfloxacin, the mean (± SD) AUC and C_{max} of 9.8 (2.83) μg•hr/mL and 2.02 (0.77) μg/mL, respectively, were observed in healthy elderly volunteers. The extent of systemic exposure was slightly higher than that seen in younger adults (AUC 6.4 μg•hr/mL and C_{max} 1.5 μg/mL). Drug absorption appears unaffected. However, the effective half-life of norfloxacin in these elderly subjects is 4 hours.

There is no information on accumulation of norfloxacin with repeated administration in elderly patients. However, no dosage adjustment is required based on age alone. In elderly patients with reduced renal function, the dosage should be adjusted as for other patients with renal impairment (see DOSAGE AND ADMINISTRATION, Renal Impairment).

The disposition of norfloxacin in patients with creatinine clearance rates greater than 30 mL/min/1.73 m^2 is similar to that in healthy volunteers. In patients with creatinine clearance rates equal to or less than 30 mL/min/1.73 m^2, the renal elimination of norfloxacin decreases so that the effective serum half-life is 6.5 hours. In these patients, alteration of dosage is necessary (see DOSAGE AND ADMINISTRATION). Drug absorption appears unaffected by decreasing renal function.

Norfloxacin is eliminated through metabolism, biliary excretion, and renal excretion. After a single 400-mg dose of NOROXIN, mean antimicrobial activities equivalent to 278, 773, and 82 μg of norfloxacin/g of feces were obtained at 12, 24, and 48 hours, respectively. Renal excretion occurs by both glomerular filtration and tubular secretion as evidenced by the high rate of renal clearance (approximately 275 mL/min). Within 24 hours of drug administration, 26 to 32% of the administered dose is recovered in the urine as norfloxacin with an additional 5-8% being recovered in the urine as six active metabolites of lesser antimicrobial potency. Only a small percentage (less than 1%) of the dose is recovered thereafter. Fecal recovery accounts for another 30% of the administered dose. In elderly subjects (average creatinine clearance 91 mL/min/1.73 m^2) approximately 22% of the administered dose was recovered in urine and renal clearance averaged 154 mL/min.

Two to three hours after a single 400-mg dose, urinary concentrations of 200 μg/mL or more are attained in the urine. In healthy volunteers, mean urinary concentrations of norfloxacin remain above 30 μg/mL for at least 12 hours following a 400-mg dose. The urinary pH may affect the solubility of norfloxacin. Norfloxacin is least soluble at urinary pH of 7.5 with greater solubility occurring at pHs above and below this value. The serum protein binding of norfloxacin is between 10 and 15%.

The following are mean concentrations of norfloxacin in various fluids and tissues measured 1 to 4 hours post-dose after two 400-mg doses, unless otherwise indicated:

Renal Parenchyma	7.3 μg/g
Prostate	2.5 μg/g
Seminal Fluid	2.7 μg/mL
Testicle	1.6 μg/g
Uterus/Cervix	3.0 μg/g
Vagina	4.3 μg/g
Fallopian Tube	1.9 μg/g
Bile	6.9 μg/mL (after two 200-mg doses)

Microbiology

Mechanism of Action

Norfloxacin inhibits bacterial deoxyribonucleic acid synthesis and is bactericidal. At the molecular level, three specific events are attributed to norfloxacin in *E. coli* cells:

1. inhibition of the ATP-dependent DNA supercoiling reaction catalyzed by DNA gyrase,
2. inhibition of the relaxation of supercoiled DNA,
3. promotion of double-stranded DNA breakage.

The fluorine atom at the 6 position provides increased potency against gram-negative organisms, and the piperazine moiety at the 7 position is responsible for antipseudomonal activity.

Drug Resistance

Resistance to norfloxacin due to spontaneous mutation *in vitro* is a rare occurrence (range: 10^{-9} to 10^{-12} cells). Resistant organisms have emerged during therapy with norfloxacin in less than 1% of patients treated. Organisms in which development of resistance is greatest are the following:

Pseudomonas aeruginosa
Klebsiella pneumoniae
Acinetobacter spp.
Enterococcus spp.

For this reason, when there is a lack of satisfactory clinical response, repeat culture and susceptibility testing should be done. Nalidixic acid-resistant organisms are generally susceptible to norfloxacin *in vitro*; however, these organisms may have higher minimum inhibitory concentrations (MICs) to norfloxacin than nalidixic acid-susceptible strains. There is generally no cross-resistance between norfloxacin and other classes of antibacterial agents. Therefore, norfloxacin may demonstrate activity against indicated organisms resistant to some other antimicrobial agents including the aminoglycosides, penicillins, cephalosporins, tetracyclines, macrolides, and sulfonamides, including combinations of sulfamethoxazole and trimethoprim. Antagonism has been demonstrated *in vitro* between norfloxacin and nitrofurantoin.

Activity *in vitro* and *in vivo*

Norfloxacin has *in vitro* activity against a broad range of gram-positive and gram-negative aerobic bacteria.

Norfloxacin has been shown to be active against most strains of the following microorganisms both *in vitro* and in clinical infections as described in the **INDICATIONS AND USAGE** section.

Gram-positive aerobes:
Enterococcus faecalis
Staphylococcus aureus
Staphylococcus epidermidis
Staphylococcus saprophyticus
Streptococcus agalactiae

Gram-negative aerobes:
Citrobacter freundii
Enterobacter aerogenes
Enterobacter cloacae
Escherichia coli
Klebsiella pneumoniae
Neisseria gonorrhoeae
Proteus mirabilis
Proteus vulgaris
Pseudomonas aeruginosa
Serratia marcescens

The following *in vitro* data are available, **but their clinical significance is unknown.**

Norfloxacin exhibits *in vitro* MICs of ≤4 μg/mL against most (≥90%) strains of the following microorganisms; however, the safety and effectiveness of norfloxacin in treating clinical infections due to these microorganisms have not been established in adequate and well-controlled clinical trials.

Gram-negative aerobes:

Citrobacter diversus
Edwardsiella tarda
Enterobacter agglomerans
Haemophilus ducreyi
Klebsiella oxytoca
Morganella morganii
Providencia alcalifaciens
Providencia rettgeri
Providencia stuartii
Pseudomonas fluorescens
Pseudomonas stutzeri

Other:

Ureaplasma urealyticum

NOROXIN is not generally active against obligate anaerobes.

Norfloxacin has not been shown to be active against *Treponema pallidum* (see WARNINGS).

Susceptibility Tests

Dilution Techniques

Quantitative methods are used to determine antimicrobial MICs. These MICs provide estimates of the susceptibility of bacteria to antimicrobial compounds. The MICs should be determined using a standardized procedure. Standardized procedures are based on a dilution method{1} (broth, agar, or microdilution) or equivalent with standardized inoculum concentrations and standardized concentrations of norfloxacin powder. The MIC values should be interpreted according to the criteria outlined in Table 1.

Diffusion Techniques

Quantitative methods that require measurement of zone diameters also provide reproducible estimates of the susceptibility of bacteria to antimicrobial compounds. One such standardized procedure{2} requires the use of standardized inoculum concentrations. This procedure uses paper disks impregnated with 10-μg norfloxacin to test the susceptibility of microorganisms to norfloxacin. Reports from the laboratory providing results of the standard single-disk susceptibility test with a 10-μg norfloxacin disk should be interpreted according to the criteria outlined in Table 1. Interpretation involves correlation of the diameter obtained in the disk test with the MIC for norfloxacin.

Table 1: Susceptibility Interpretive Criteria for Norfloxacin

MIC (μg/mL)			Zone Diameter (mm)		
S	I	R	S	I	R
≤4	8	≥16	≥17	13-16	≤12

These interpretative criteria apply only to isolates from urinary tract infections. There are no established norfloxacin interpretive criteria for *Neisseria gonorrhoeae* or organisms isolated from other infection sites.
S=Susceptible, I=Intermediate, and R=Resistant

A report of "Susceptible" indicates that the pathogen is likely to be inhibited if the antimicrobial compound in the blood reaches the concentrations usually achievable. A report of "Intermediate" indicates that the result should be considered equivocal, and, if the microorganism is not fully susceptible to alternative, clinically feasible drugs, the test should be repeated. This category implies possible clinical applicability in body sites where the drug is physiologically concentrated or in situations where high dosage of drug can be used. This category also provides a buffer zone which prevents small uncontrolled technical factors from causing major discrepancies in interpretation. A report of "Resistant" indicates that the pathogen is not likely to be inhibited if the antimicrobial compound in the blood reaches the concentrations usually achievable; other therapy should be selected.

Quality Control

Standardized susceptibility test procedures require the use of laboratory control microorganisms to control the technical aspects of the laboratory procedures. Standard norfloxacin powder should provide the MIC values outlined in Table 2. For the diffusion techniques, the 10-μg norfloxacin disk should provide the zone diameters outlined in Table 2.

Table 2: Quality Control for Susceptibility Testing

Strains	MIC Range (μg/mL)	Zone Diameter (mm)
Enterococcus faecalis (ATCC 29212)	2 – 8	Not applicable
Escherichia coli (ATCC 25922)	0.03 – 0.12	28 – 35
P. aeruginosa (ATCC 27853)	1 – 4	22 – 29
Staphylococcus aureus (ATCC 29213)	0.5 – 2	Not applicable
Staphylococcus aureus (ATCC 25923)	Not applicable	17 – 28

INDICATIONS AND USAGE

NOROXIN is indicated for the treatment of adults with the following infections caused by susceptible strains of the designated microorganisms:

Urinary tract infections

Uncomplicated urinary tract infections (including cystitis) due to *Enterococcus faecalis, Escherichia coli, Klebsiella pneumoniae, Proteus mirabilis, Pseudomonas aeruginosa, Staphylococcus epidermidis, Staphylococcus saprophyticus, Citrobacter freundii*[1], *Enterobacter aerogenes*[1], *Enterobacter cloacae*[1], *Proteus vulgaris*[1], *Staphylococcus aureus*[1], or *Streptococcus agalactiae*[1].

Complicated urinary tract infections due to *Enterococcus faecalis, Escherichia coli, Klebsiella pneumoniae, Proteus mirabilis, Pseudomonas aeruginosa*, or *Serratia marcescens*[1].

[1]Efficacy for this organism in this organ system was studied in fewer than 10 infections.

Sexually transmitted diseases

(see WARNINGS)

Uncomplicated urethral and cervical gonorrhea due to *Neisseria gonorrhoeae.*

Prostatitis

Prostatitis due to *Escherichia coli.*

(See DOSAGE AND ADMINISTRATION for appropriate dosing instructions.)

Penicillinase production should have no effect on norfloxacin activity.

Appropriate culture and susceptibility tests should be performed before treatment in order to isolate and identify organisms causing the infection and to determine their susceptibility to norfloxacin. Therapy with norfloxacin may be initiated before results of these tests are known; once results become available, appropriate therapy should be given. Repeat culture and susceptibility testing performed periodically during therapy will provide information not only on the therapeutic effect of the antimicrobial agents but also on the possible emergence of bacterial resistance.

To reduce the development of drug-resistant bacteria and maintain the effectiveness of NOROXIN and other antibacterial drugs, NOROXIN should be used only to treat or prevent infections that are proven or strongly suspected to be caused by susceptible bacteria. When culture and susceptibility information are available, they should be considered in selecting or modifying antibacterial therapy. In the absence of such data, local epidemiology and susceptibility patterns may contribute to the empiric selection of therapy.

CONTRAINDICATIONS

NOROXIN (norfloxacin) is contraindicated in persons with a history of hypersensitivity, tendinitis, or tendon rupture associated with the use of norfloxacin or any member of the quinolone group of antimicrobial agents.

WARNINGS

Tendinopathy and Tendon Rupture: Fluoroquinolones, including NOROXIN, are associated with an increased risk of tendinitis and tendon rupture in all ages. This adverse reaction most frequently involves the Achilles tendon, and rupture of the Achilles tendon may require surgical repair. Tendinitis and tendon rupture in the rotator cuff (the shoulder), the hand, the biceps, the thumb, and other tendon sites have also been reported. The risk of developing fluoroquinolone-associated tendinitis and tendon rupture is further increased in older patients usually over 60 years of age, in patients taking corticosteroid drugs, and in patients with kidney, heart or lung transplants. Factors, in addition to age and corticosteroid use, that may independently increase the risk of tendon rupture include strenuous physical activity, renal failure, and previous tendon disorders such as rheumatoid arthritis. Tendinitis and tendon rupture have also occurred in patients taking fluoroquinolones who do not have the above risk factors. Tendon rupture can occur during or after completion of therapy; cases occurring up to several months after completion of therapy have been reported. NOROXIN should be discontinued if the patient experiences pain, swelling, inflammation or rupture of a tendon. Patients should be advised to rest at the first sign of tendinitis or tendon rupture, and to contact their healthcare provider regarding changing to a non-quinolone antimicrobial drug.

Exacerbation of Myasthenia Gravis: Fluoroquinolones, including NOROXIN, have neuromuscular blocking activity and may exacerbate muscle weakness in persons with myasthenia gravis. Post-marketing serious adverse events, including deaths and requirement for ventilatory support, have been associated with fluoroquinolone use in persons with myasthenia gravis. Avoid NOROXIN in patients with known history of myasthenia gravis. (See PRECAUTIONS, Information for Patients and ADVERSE REACTIONS, Post-Marketing, Musculoskeletal.)

Safety in Children, Adolescents, Nursing mothers, and during Pregnancy: THE SAFETY AND EFFICACY OF ORAL NORFLOXACIN IN PEDIATRIC PATIENTS, ADOLESCENTS (UNDER THE AGE OF 18), PREGNANT WOMEN, AND NURSING MOTHERS HAVE NOT BEEN ESTABLISHED. (See PRECAUTIONS, Pediatric Use, Pregnancy, and Nursing Mothers subsections.) The oral administration of single doses of norfloxacin, 6 times[2] the recommended human clinical dose (on a mg/kg basis), caused lameness in immature dogs. Histologic examination of the weight-bearing joints of these dogs revealed permanent lesions of the cartilage. Other quinolones also produced erosions of the cartilage in weight-bearing joints and other signs of arthropathy in immature animals of various species (see ANIMAL PHARMACOLOGY).

Central Nervous System Effects/Disorders: Convulsions have been reported in patients receiving norfloxacin. Convulsions, increased intracranial pressure (including pseudotumor cerebri), and toxic psychoses have been reported in patients receiving drugs in this class. Quinolones may also cause central nervous system (CNS) stimulation which may lead to tremors, restlessness, lightheadedness, confusion, and hallucinations. If these reactions occur in patients receiving norfloxacin, the drug should be discontinued and appropriate measures instituted.

The effects of norfloxacin on brain function or on the electrical activity of the brain have not been tested. Therefore, until more information becomes available, norfloxacin, like all other quinolones, should be used with caution in patients with known or suspected CNS disorders, such as severe cerebral arteriosclerosis, epilepsy, and other factors which predispose to seizures (see ADVERSE REACTIONS).

Hypersensitivity Reactions: Serious and occasionally fatal hypersensitivity (anaphylactic) reactions, some following the first dose, have been reported in patients receiving quinolone therapy, including NOROXIN. Some reactions were accompanied by cardiovascular collapse, loss of consciousness, tingling, pharyngeal or facial edema, dyspnea, urticaria and itching. Only a few patients had a history of hypersensitivity reactions. If an allergic reaction to norfloxacin occurs, discontinue the drug. Serious acute hypersensitivity reactions require immediate emergency treatment with epinephrine. Oxygen, intravenous fluids, antihistamines, corticosteroids, pressor amines, and airway management, including intubation, should be administered as indicated.

Other serious and sometimes fatal events, some due to hypersensitivity, and some due to uncertain etiology, have been reported rarely in patients receiving therapy with quinolones, including NOROXIN. These events may be severe and generally occur following the administration of multiple doses. Clinical manifestations may include one or more of the following:

- fever, rash or severe dermatologic reactions (e.g., toxic epidermal necrolysis, Stevens-Johnson syndrome);
- vasculitis; arthralgia; myalgia; serum sickness;
- allergic pneumonitis;
- interstitial nephritis; acute renal insufficiency or failure;
- hepatitis; jaundice; acute hepatic necrosis or failure;
- anemia, including hemolytic and aplastic; thrombocytopenia, including thrombotic thrombocytopenic purpura; leukopenia; agranulocytosis; pancytopenia; and/or other hematologic abnormalities.

The drug should be discontinued immediately at the first appearance of a skin rash, jaundice, or any other sign of hypersensitivity, and supportive measures should be instituted (see PRECAUTIONS, Information for Patients and ADVERSE REACTIONS).

Clostridium Difficile Associated Diarrhea: Clostridium difficile associated diarrhea (CDAD) has been reported with use of nearly all antibacterial agents, including NOROXIN and may range in severity from mild diarrhea to fatal colitis. Treatment with antibacterial agents alters the normal flora of the colon leading to overgrowth of *C. difficile*.

C. difficile produces toxins A and B which contribute to the development of CDAD.

Hypertoxin producing strains of *C. difficile* cause increased morbidity and mortality, as these infections can be refractory to antimicrobial therapy and may require colectomy. CDAD must be considered in all patients who present with diarrhea following antibiotic use. Careful medical history is necessary since CDAD has been reported to occur over two months after the administration of antibacterial agents.

If CDAD is suspected or confirmed, ongoing antibiotic use not directed against *C. difficile* may need to be discontinued. Appropriate fluid and electrolyte management, protein supplementation, antibiotic treatment of *C. difficile,* and surgical evaluation should be instituted as clinically indicated.

Peripheral Neuropathy: Rare cases of sensory or sensorimotor axonal polyneuropathy affecting small and/or large axons resulting in paresthesias, hypoesthesias, dysesthesias and weakness have been reported in patients receiving quinolones, including norfloxacin. Norfloxacin should be discontinued if the patient experiences symptoms of neuropathy including pain, burning, tingling, numbness, and/or weakness, or is found to have deficits in light touch, pain, temperature, position sense, vibratory sensation, and/or motor strength in order to prevent the development of an irreversible condition.

*Syphilis Treatment: Norfloxacin has **not** been shown to be effective in the treatment of syphilis.* Antimicrobial agents used in high doses for short periods of time to treat gonorrhea may mask or delay the symptoms of incubating syphilis. All patients with gonorrhea should have a serologic test for syphilis at the time of diagnosis. Patients treated with norfloxacin should have a follow-up serologic test for syphilis after three months.

[2]Based on a patient weight of 50 kg.

PRECAUTIONS

General

Needle-shaped crystals were found in the urine of some volunteers who received either placebo, 800 mg norfloxacin, or 1600 mg norfloxacin (at or twice the recommended daily dose, respectively) while participating in a double-blind, crossover study comparing single doses of norfloxacin with placebo. While crystalluria is not expected to occur under usual conditions with a dosage regimen of 400 mg b.i.d., as a precaution, the daily recommended dosage should not be exceeded and the patient should drink sufficient fluids to ensure a proper state of hydration and adequate urinary output.

Alteration in dosage regimen is necessary for patients with impaired renal function (see DOSAGE AND ADMINISTRATION).

Moderate to severe photosensitivity/phototoxicity reactions, the latter of which may manifest as exaggerated sunburn reactions (e.g., burning, erythema, exudation, vesicles, blistering, edema) involving areas exposed to light (typically the face, "V" area of the neck, extensor surfaces of the forearms, dorsa of the hands), can be associated with the use of quinolone antibiotics after sun or UV light exposure. Therefore, excessive exposure to these sources of light should be avoided. Drug therapy should be discontinued if phototoxicity occurs (see ADVERSE REACTIONS, Post-Marketing).

Rarely, hemolytic reactions have been reported in patients with latent or actual defects in glucose-6-phosphate dehydrogenase activity who take quinolone antibacterial agents, including norfloxacin (see ADVERSE REACTIONS).

Prescribing NOROXIN in the absence of a proven or strongly suspected bacterial infection or a prophylactic indication is unlikely to provide benefit to the patient and increases the risk of the development of drug-resistant bacteria.

Information for Patients

Patients should be advised:

— to contact their healthcare provider if they experience pain, swelling, or inflammation of a tendon, or weakness or inability to use one of their joints; rest and refrain from exercise; and discontinue NOROXIN treatment. The risk of severe tendon disorders with fluoroquinolones is higher in older patients usually over 60 years of age, in patients taking corticosteroid drugs, and in patients with kidney, heart or lung transplants.

— that fluoroquinolones like NOROXIN may cause worsening of myasthenia gravis symptoms, including muscle weakness and breathing problems. Patients should call their healthcare provider right away if they have any worsening muscle weakness or breathing problems.

— that norfloxacin may cause changes in the electrocardiogram (QTc interval prolongation).

— that norfloxacin should be avoided in patients receiving class IA (e.g., quinidine, procainamide) or class III (e.g., amiodarone, sotalol) antiarrhythmic agents.

— that norfloxacin should be used with caution in subjects receiving drugs that affect the QTc interval such as cisapride, erythromycin, antipsychotics, and tricyclic antidepressants.

— to inform their physicians of any personal or family history of QTc prolongation or proarrhythmic conditions such as hypokalemia, bradycardia or recent myocardial ischemia.

— that peripheral neuropathies have been associated with norfloxacin use. If symptoms of peripheral neuropathy including pain, burning, tingling, numbness, and/or weakness develop, they should discontinue treatment and contact their physicians.

— to drink fluids liberally.

— that norfloxacin should be taken at least one hour before or at least two hours after a meal or ingestion of milk and/or other dairy products.

— that multivitamins or other products containing iron or zinc, antacids or Videx®[3] (Didanosine), chewable/buffered tablets or the pediatric powder for oral solution, should not be taken within the two-hour period before or within the two-hour period after taking norfloxacin (see PRECAUTIONS, Drug Interactions).

— that norfloxacin can cause dizziness and lightheadedness and, therefore, patients should know how they react to norfloxacin before they operate an automobile or machinery or engage in activities requiring mental alertness and coordination.

— that norfloxacin may be associated with hypersensitivity reactions, even following the first dose, and to discontinue the drug at the first sign of a skin rash or other allergic reaction.

— that photosensitivity/phototoxicity has been reported in patients receiving quinolones. Patients should minimize or avoid exposure to natural or artificial sunlight (tanning beds or UVA/B treatment) while taking quinolones. If patients need to be outdoors while using quinolones, they should wear loose-fitting clothes that protect skin from sun exposure and discuss other sun protection measures with their physician. If a sunburn-like reaction or skin eruption occurs, patients should contact their physician.

— that some quinolones may increase the effects of theophylline and/or caffeine (see PRECAUTIONS, Drug Interactions).

— that convulsions have been reported in patients taking quinolones, including norfloxacin, and to notify their physician before taking this drug if there is a history of this condition.

— that diarrhea is a common problem caused by antibiotics, which usually ends when the antibiotic is discontinued. Sometimes after starting the treatment with antibiotics, patients can develop watery and bloody stools (with or without stomach cramps and fever) even as late as two or more months after having taken the last dose of the antibiotic. If this occurs, patients should contact their physician as soon as possible.

Patients should be counseled that antibacterial drugs including NOROXIN should only be used to treat bacterial infections. They do not treat viral infections (e.g., the common cold). When NOROXIN is prescribed to treat a bacterial infection, patients should be told that although it is common to feel better early in the course of therapy, the medication should be taken exactly as directed. Skipping doses or not completing the full course of therapy may (1) decrease the effectiveness of the immediate treatment and (2) increase the likelihood that bacteria will develop resistance and will not be treatable by NOROXIN or other antibacterial drugs in the future.

[3]Registered trademark of Bristol-Myers Squibb Company

Laboratory Tests

As with any potent antibacterial agent, periodic assessment of organ system functions, including renal, hepatic, and hematopoietic, is advisable during prolonged therapy.

Drug Interactions

Quinolones, including norfloxacin, have been shown *in vitro* to inhibit CYP1A2. Concomitant use with drugs metabolized by CYP1A2 (e.g., caffeine, clozapine, ropinirole, tacrine, theophylline, tizanidine) may result in increased substrate drug concentrations when given in usual doses. Patients taking any of these drugs concomitantly with norfloxacin should be carefully monitored.

Elevated plasma levels of theophylline have been reported with concomitant quinolone use. There have been reports of theophylline-related side effects in patients on concomitant therapy with norfloxacin and theophylline. Therefore, monitoring of theophylline plasma levels should be considered and dosage of theophylline adjusted as required.

Elevated serum levels of cyclosporine have been reported with concomitant use of cyclosporine with norfloxacin. Therefore, cyclosporine serum levels should be monitored and appropriate cyclosporine dosage adjustments made when these drugs are used concomitantly.

Quinolones, including norfloxacin, may enhance the effects of oral anticoagulants, including warfarin or its derivatives or similar agents. When these products are administered concomitantly, prothrombin time or other suitable coagulation tests should be closely monitored.

The concomitant administration of quinolones including norfloxacin with glyburide (a sulfonylurea agent) has, on rare occasions, resulted in severe hypoglycemia. Therefore, monitoring of blood glucose is recommended when these agents are co-administered.

Diminished urinary excretion of norfloxacin has been reported during the concomitant administration of probenecid and norfloxacin.

The concomitant use of nitrofurantoin is not recommended since nitrofurantoin may antagonize the antibacterial effect of NOROXIN in the urinary tract.

Multivitamins, or other products containing iron or zinc, antacids or sucralfate, should not be administered concomitantly with, or within 2 hours of, the administration of norfloxacin, because they may interfere with absorption resulting in lower serum and urine levels of norfloxacin.

Videx® (Didanosine) chewable/buffered tablets or the pediatric powder for oral solution should not be administered concomitantly with, or within 2 hours of, the administration of norfloxacin, because these products may interfere with absorption resulting in lower serum and urine levels of norfloxacin.

Some quinolones have also been shown to interfere with the metabolism of caffeine. This may lead to reduced clearance of caffeine and a prolongation of the plasma half-life that may lead to accumulation of caffeine in plasma when products containing caffeine are consumed while taking norfloxacin.

The concomitant administration of a non-steroidal anti-inflammatory drug (NSAID) with a quinolone, including norfloxacin, may increase the risk of CNS stimulation and convulsive seizures. Therefore, NOROXIN should be used with caution in individuals receiving NSAIDS concomitantly.

Carcinogenesis, Mutagenesis, Impairment of Fertility

No increase in neoplastic changes was observed with norfloxacin as compared to controls in a study in rats, lasting up to 96 weeks at doses 8-9 times[2] the usual human dose (on a mg/kg basis).

Norfloxacin was tested for mutagenic activity in a number of *in vivo* and *in vitro* tests. Norfloxacin had no mutagenic effect in the dominant lethal test in mice and did not cause chromosomal aberrations in hamsters or rats at doses 30-60 times[2] the usual human dose (on a mg/kg basis). Norfloxacin had no mutagenic activity *in vitro* in the Ames microbial mutagen test, Chinese hamster fibroblasts and V-79 mammalian cell assay. Although norfloxacin was weakly positive in the Rec-assay for DNA repair, all other mutagenic assays were negative including a more sensitive test (V-79).

Norfloxacin did not adversely affect the fertility of male and female mice at oral doses up to 30 times[2] the usual human dose (on a mg/kg basis).

Pregnancy

Teratogenic Effects

Pregnancy Category C

Norfloxacin has been shown to produce embryonic loss in monkeys when given in doses 10 times[2] the maximum daily total human dose (on a mg/kg basis). At this dose, peak plasma levels obtained in monkeys were approximately 2 times those obtained in humans. There has been no evidence of a teratogenic effect in any of the animal species tested (rat, rabbit, mouse, monkey) at 6-50 times[2] the maximum daily human dose (on a mg/kg basis). There are, however, no adequate and well-controlled studies in pregnant women. Norfloxacin should be used during pregnancy only if the potential benefit justifies the potential risk to the fetus.

Nursing Mothers

It is not known whether norfloxacin is excreted in human milk.

When a 200-mg dose of NOROXIN was administered to nursing mothers, norfloxacin was not detected in human milk. However, because the dose studied was low, because other drugs in this class are secreted in human milk, and because of the potential for serious adverse reactions from norfloxacin in nursing infants, a decision should be made to discontinue nursing or to discontinue the drug, taking into account the importance of the drug to the mother.

Pediatric Use

The safety and effectiveness of oral norfloxacin in pediatric patients and adolescents below the age of 18 years have not been established. Norfloxacin causes arthropathy in juvenile animals of several animal species. (See WARNINGS and ANIMAL PHARMACOLOGY.)

Geriatric Use

Geriatric patients are at increased risk for developing severe tendon disorders including tendon rupture when being treated with a fluoroquinolone such as NOROXIN. This risk is further increased in patients receiving concomitant corticosteroid therapy. Tendinitis or tendon rupture can involve the Achilles, hand, shoulder, or other tendon sites and can occur during or after completion of therapy; cases occurring up to several months after fluoroquinolone treatment have been reported. Caution should be used when prescribing NOROXIN to elderly patients, especially those on corticosteroids. Patients should be informed of this potential side effect and advised to discontinue NOROXIN and contact their healthcare provider if any symptoms of tendinitis or tendon rupture occur (see Boxed Warning; WARNINGS; and ADVERSE REACTIONS, Post-Marketing).

Of the 340 subjects in one large clinical study of NOROXIN for treatment of urinary tract infections, 103 patients were 65 and older, 77 of whom were 70 and older; no overall differences in safety and effectiveness were evident between these subjects and younger subjects. In clinical practice, no difference in the type of reported adverse experiences have been observed between the elderly and younger patients except for a possible increased risk of tendon rupture in elderly patients receiving concomitant corticosteroids (see WARNINGS). In addition, increased risk for other adverse experiences in some older individuals cannot be ruled out (see ADVERSE REACTIONS).

This drug is known to be substantially excreted by the kidney, and the risk of toxic reactions to this drug may be greater in patients with impaired renal function. Because elderly patients are more likely to have decreased renal function, care should be taken in dose selection, and it may be useful to monitor renal function (see DOSAGE AND ADMINISTRATION).

A pharmacokinetic study of NOROXIN in elderly volunteers (65 to 75 years of age with normal renal function for their age) was carried out (see CLINICAL PHARMACOLOGY).

In general, elderly patients may be more susceptible to drug-associated effects of the QTc interval. Therefore, precaution should be taken when using NOROXIN concomitantly with drugs that can result in prolongation of the QTc interval (e.g., class IA or class III antiarrhythmics) or in patients with risk factors for torsades de pointes (e.g., known QTc prolongation, uncorrected hypokalemia).

ADVERSE REACTIONS

Single-Dose Studies

In clinical trials involving 82 healthy subjects and 228 patients with gonorrhea, treated with a single dose of norfloxacin, 6.5% reported drug-related adverse experiences. However, the following incidence figures were calculated without reference to drug relationship.

The most common adverse experiences (>1.0%) were: dizziness (2.6%), nausea (2.6%), headache (2.0%), and abdominal cramping (1.6%).

Additional reactions (0.3%-1.0%) were: anorexia, diarrhea, hyperhidrosis, asthenia, anal/rectal pain, constipation, dyspepsia, flatulence, tingling of the fingers, and vomiting.

Laboratory adverse changes considered drug-related were reported in 4.5% of patients/subjects. These laboratory changes were: increased AST (SGOT) (1.6%), decreased WBC (1.3%), decreased platelet count (1.0%), increased urine protein (1.0%), decreased hematocrit and hemoglobin (0.6%), and increased eosinophils (0.6%).

Multiple-Dose Studies

In clinical trials involving 52 healthy subjects and 1980 patients with urinary tract infections or prostatitis treated with multiple doses of norfloxacin, 3.6% reported drug-related adverse experiences. However, the incidence figures below were calculated without reference to drug relationship.

The most common adverse experiences (>1.0%) were: nausea (4.2%), headache (2.8%), dizziness (1.7%), and asthenia (1.3%).

Additional reactions (0.3%-1.0%) were: abdominal pain, back pain, constipation, diarrhea, dry mouth, dyspepsia/heartburn, fever, flatulence, hyperhidrosis, loose stools, pruritus, rash, somnolence, and vomiting.

Less frequent reactions (0.1%-0.2%) included: abdominal swelling, allergies, anorexia, anxiety, bitter taste, blurred vision, bursitis, chest pain, chills, depression, dysmenorrhea, edema, erythema, foot or hand swelling, insomnia, mouth ulcer, myocardial infarction, palpitation, pruritus ani, renal colic, sleep disturbances, and urticaria.

Abnormal laboratory values observed in these patients/subjects were: eosinophilia (1.5%), elevation of ALT (SGPT) (1.4%), decreased WBC and/or neutrophil count (1.4%), elevation of AST (SGOT) (1.4%), and increased alkaline phosphatase (1.1%). Those occurring less frequently included increased BUN, increased LDH, increased serum creatinine, decreased hematocrit, and glycosuria.

Post-Marketing

The most frequently reported adverse reaction in post-marketing experience is rash.

CNS effects characterized as generalized seizures, myoclonus and tremors have been reported with NOROXIN (see WARNINGS). Visual disturbances have been reported with drugs in this class.

The following additional adverse reactions have been reported since the drug was marketed:

Hypersensitivity Reactions

Hypersensitivity reactions have been reported including anaphylactoid reactions, angioedema, dyspnea, vasculitis, urticaria, arthritis, arthralgia and myalgia (see WARNINGS).

Skin

Toxic epidermal necrolysis, Stevens-Johnson syndrome and erythema multiforme, exfoliative dermatitis, photosensitivity/phototoxicity reactions (see PRECAUTIONS), leukocytoclastic vasculitis, drug rash with eosinophilia and systemic symptoms (DRESS syndrome).

Gastrointestinal

Pseudomembranous colitis, hepatitis, jaundice including cholestatic jaundice and elevated liver function tests, pancreatitis (rare), stomatitis. The onset of pseudomembranous colitis symptoms may occur during or after antibacterial treatment (see WARNINGS).

Hepatic

Hepatic failure, including fatal cases.

Cardiovascular

On rare occasions, prolonged QTc interval and ventricular arrhythmia including torsades de pointes.

Renal

Interstitial nephritis, renal failure.

Nervous System/Psychiatric

Peripheral neuropathy, Guillain-Barré syndrome, ataxia, paresthesia, hypoesthesia, psychic disturbances including psychotic reactions and confusion.

Musculoskeletal

Tendinitis, tendon rupture; exacerbation of myasthenia gravis (see WARNINGS, Exacerbation of myasthenia gravis); elevated creatine kinase (CK), muscle spasms.

Hematologic

Neutropenia; leukopenia; agranulocytosis; hemolytic anemia, sometimes associated with glucose-6-phosphate dehydrogenase deficiency; thrombocytopenia.

Special Senses

Hearing loss, tinnitus, diplopia, dysgeusia.

Other adverse events reported with quinolones include: agranulocytosis, albuminuria, candiduria, crystalluria, cylindruria, dysphagia, elevation of blood glucose, elevation of serum cholesterol, elevation of serum potassium, elevation of serum triglycerides, hematuria, hepatic necrosis, symptomatic hypoglycemia, nystagmus, postural hypotension, prolongation of prothrombin time, and vaginal candidiasis.

OVERDOSAGE

No significant lethality was observed in male and female mice and rats at single oral doses up to 4 g/kg.

In the event of acute overdosage, the stomach should be emptied by inducing vomiting or by gastric lavage, and the patient carefully observed and given symptomatic and supportive treatment. Adequate hydration must be maintained.

DOSAGE AND ADMINISTRATION

Tablets NOROXIN should be taken at least one hour before or at least two hours after a meal or ingestion of milk and/or other dairy products. Multivitamins, other products containing iron or zinc, antacids containing magnesium and aluminum, sucralfate, or Videx® (Didanosine), chewable/buffered tablets or the pediatric powder for oral solution, should not be taken within 2 hours of administration of norfloxacin. Tablets NOROXIN should be taken with a glass of water. Patients receiving NOROXIN should be well hydrated (see PRECAUTIONS).

Normal Renal Function

The recommended daily dose of NOROXIN is as described in the following chart:

[See table above]

Infection	Description	Unit Dose	Frequency	Duration	Daily Dose
Urinary Tract	Uncomplicated UTI's (cystitis) due to *E. coli*, *K. pneumoniae*, or *P. mirabilis*	400 mg	q12h	3 days	800 mg
	Uncomplicated UTI's due to other indicated organisms	400 mg	q12h	7-10 days	800 mg
	Complicated UTI's	400 mg	q12h	10-21 days	800 mg
Sexually Transmitted Diseases	Uncomplicated Gonorrhea	800 mg	single dose	1 day	800 mg
Prostatitis	Acute or Chronic	400 mg	q12h	28 days	800 mg

Renal Impairment

NOROXIN may be used for the treatment of urinary tract infections in patients with renal insufficiency. In patients with a creatinine clearance rate of 30 mL/min/1.73 m^2 or less, the recommended dosage is one 400-mg tablet once daily for the duration given above. At this dosage, the urinary concentration exceeds the MICs for most urinary pathogens susceptible to norfloxacin, even when the creatinine clearance is less than 10 mL/min/1.73 m^2.

When only the serum creatinine level is available, the following formula (based on sex, weight, and age of the patient) may be used to convert this value into creatinine clearance. The serum creatinine should represent a steady state of renal function.

$$\text{Males: } \frac{(\text{weight in kg}) \times (140 - \text{age})}{(72) \times \text{serum creatinine (mg/100 mL)}}$$

Females: (0.85) × (above value)

Elderly

Elderly patients being treated for urinary tract infections who have a creatinine clearance of greater than 30 mL/min/1.73 m^2 should receive the dosages recommended under *Normal Renal Function*.

Elderly patients being treated for urinary tract infections who have a creatinine clearance of 30 mL/min/1.73 m^2 or less should receive 400 mg once daily as recommended under *Renal Impairment*.

HOW SUPPLIED

No. 8338 — Tablets NOROXIN 400 mg are white to off-white, oval shaped, film-coated tablets, coded 705 on one side and plain on the other. They are supplied as follows:

NDC 0006-0705-20 unit of use bottles of 20.

Storage

Store at 25°C (77°F); excursions permitted to 15-30°C (59-86°F) [see USP Controlled Room Temperature]. Keep container tightly closed.

ANIMAL PHARMACOLOGY

Norfloxacin and related drugs have been shown to cause arthropathy in immature animals of most species tested (see WARNINGS).

Crystalluria has occurred in laboratory animals tested with norfloxacin. In dogs, needle-shaped drug crystals were seen in the urine at doses of 50 mg/kg/day. In rats, crystals were reported following doses of 200 mg/kg/day.

Embryo lethality and slight maternotoxicity (vomiting and anorexia) were observed in cynomolgus monkeys at doses of 150 mg/kg/day or higher.

Ocular toxicity, seen with some related drugs, was not observed in any norfloxacin-treated animals.

REFERENCES

1. Clinical and Laboratory Standards Institute, Methods for dilution antimicrobial susceptibility tests for bacteria that grow aerobically - Eighth edition, Approved Standard CLSI Document M7-A8, Vol. 29, No. 2, CLSI, Wayne, PA, 2009.
2. Clinical and Laboratory Standards Institute, Performance standards for antimicrobial disk susceptibility tests - Tenth edition, Approved Standard CLSI Document M2-A10, Vol. 29, No. 1, CLSI, Wayne, PA, 2009.

Manufactured for: Merck Sharp & Dohme Corp., a subsidiary of
MERCK & CO., INC., Whitehouse Station, NJ 08889, USA
Manufactured by: Merck Sharp & Dohme (Italia) S.p.A.
Via Emilia, 21
27100 Pavia, Italy

Revised: 12/2012
USPI-T-03661212R010

MEDICATION GUIDE

NOROXIN® [nor-AHK-sin]
(norfloxacin)
Tablets

Read the Medication Guide that comes with NOROXIN® before you start taking it and each time you get a refill. There may be new information. This Medication Guide does not take the place of talking to your healthcare provider about your medical condition or your treatment.

What is the most important information I should know about NOROXIN?

NOROXIN belongs to a class of antibiotics called fluoroquinolones. NOROXIN can cause side effects that may be serious or even cause death. If you develop any of the following serious side effects, get medical help right away. Talk with your healthcare provider about whether you should continue to take NOROXIN.

1. **Tendon rupture or swelling of the tendon (tendinitis)**
   - **Tendon problems can happen in people of all ages who take NOROXIN.** Tendons are tough cords of tissue that connect muscle to bones. Symptoms of tendon problems may include:
     - Pain, swelling, tears and inflammation of tendons including the back of the ankle (Achilles), shoulder, hand, or other tendon sites.

- **The risk of getting tendon problems while you take NOROXIN is higher if you:**
  - are over 60 years of age
  - are taking steroids (corticosteroids)
  - have had a kidney, heart or lung transplant
- **Tendon problems can happen in people who do not have the above risk factors when they take NOROXIN. Other reasons that can increase your risk of tendon problems can include:**
  - physical activity or exercise
  - kidney failure
  - tendon problems in the past, such as in people with rheumatoid arthritis (RA)
- **Call your healthcare provider right away at the first sign of tendon pain, swelling or inflammation.** Stop taking NOROXIN until tendinitis or tendon rupture has been ruled out by your healthcare provider. Avoid exercise and using the affected area. The most common area of pain and swelling is the Achilles tendon at the back of your ankle. This can also happen with other tendons.
- **Talk to your healthcare provider about the risk of tendon rupture with continued use of NOROXIN.** You may need a different antibiotic that is not a fluoroquinolone to treat your infection.
- **Tendon rupture can happen while you are taking or after you have finished taking NOROXIN.** Tendon ruptures have happened up to several months after patients have finished taking their fluoroquinolone.
- **Get medical help right away if you get any of the following signs or symptoms of a tendon rupture:**
  - hear or feel a snap or pop in a tendon area
  - bruising right after an incident in a tendon area
  - unable to move the affected area or bear weight

2. **Worsening of myasthenia gravis (a disease which causes muscle weakness)**
   Fluoroquinolones like NOROXIN may cause worsening of myasthenia gravis symptoms, including muscle weakness and breathing problems. Call your healthcare provider right away if you have any worsening muscle weakness or breathing problems.

See the section "What are the possible side effects of NOROXIN?" for more information about side effects.

What is NOROXIN?

NOROXIN is a fluoroquinolone antibiotic medicine used in adults to treat certain infections caused by certain germs called bacteria. It is not known if NOROXIN is safe and works in children under 18 years of age. Children have a higher chance of getting bone and joint (musculoskeletal) problems while taking NOROXIN.

Sometimes infections are caused by viruses rather than by bacteria. Examples include viral infections in the sinuses and lungs, such as the common cold or flu. Antibiotics including NOROXIN do not kill viruses.

Call your healthcare provider if you think your condition is not getting better while you are taking NOROXIN.

Who should not take NOROXIN?

Do not take NOROXIN if you:

- have ever had a severe allergic reaction to an antibiotic known as a fluoroquinolone, or are allergic to any of the ingredients in NOROXIN. Ask your healthcare provider if you are not sure. See the list of ingredients in NOROXIN at the end of this Medication Guide.
- have had tendinitis or tendon rupture with the use of NOROXIN or another fluoroquinolone antibiotic.

What should I tell my healthcare provider before taking NOROXIN?

See **"What is the most important information I should know about NOROXIN?"**

Tell your healthcare provider about all your medical conditions, including if you:

- have tendon problems
- have a disease that causes muscle weakness (myasthenia gravis)
- have central nervous system problems (such as epilepsy)
- have nerve problems
- have or anyone in your family has an irregular heartbeat, especially a condition called "QTc prolongation"
- have low potassium (hypokalemia)
- have a slow heartbeat called bradycardia
- have a history of seizures
- have kidney problems. You may need a lower dose of NOROXIN if your kidneys do not work well.
- have rheumatoid arthritis (RA) or other history of joint problems
- are pregnant or planning to become pregnant. It is not known if NOROXIN will harm your unborn child.
- are breast-feeding or planning to breast-feed. It is not known if NOROXIN passes into breast milk. You and your healthcare provider should decide whether you will take NOROXIN or breast-feed.

Tell your healthcare provider about all the medicines you take, including prescription and nonprescription medicines, vitamins, and herbal and dietary supplements. NOROXIN and other medicines[4] can affect each other causing side effects. Especially tell your healthcare provider if you take:

- an NSAID (Non-Steroidal Anti-Inflammatory Drug). Many common medicines for pain relief are NSAIDs. Taking an NSAID while you take NOROXIN or other fluoroquinolones may increase your risk of central nervous system effects and seizures. See **"What are the possible side effects of NOROXIN?"**
- glyburide (Micronase, Glynase, Diabeta, Glucovance). See **"What are the possible side effects of NOROXIN?"**
- a blood thinner (warfarin, Coumadin, Jantoven)
- a medicine to control your heart rate or rhythm (antiarrhythmics). See **"What are the possible side effects of NOROXIN?"**
- an anti-psychotic medicine
- a tricyclic antidepressant
- erythromycin
- a water pill (diuretic)
- a steroid medicine. Corticosteroids taken by mouth or by injection may increase the chance of tendon injury.
- probenecid (Probalan, Col-probenecid)
- cyclosporine (Gengraf, Sandimmune, Neoral)
- products that contain caffeine
- clozapine (Fazaclo ODT, Clozaril)
- ropinirole (Requip, Requip XL)
- tacrine (Cognex)
- tizanidine (Zanaflex)
- theophylline (Theo-24, Elixophyllin, Theochron, Uniphyl, Theolair)
- cisapride (Propulsid)
- certain medicines may keep NOROXIN from working correctly. Take NOROXIN either 2 hours before or 2 hours after taking these products:
  - an antacid, multivitamin or other product that has iron or zinc
  - sucralfate (Carafate)
  - didanosine (Videx, Videx EC)
- You should not take the medicine nitrofurantoin (Furadantin, Macrodantin, Macrobid) while taking NOROXIN.

Ask your healthcare provider if you are not sure if your medicine is listed above.

Know the medicines you take. Keep a list of your medicines and show it to your healthcare provider and pharmacist when you get a new medicine.

How should I take NOROXIN?

- Take NOROXIN exactly as prescribed by your healthcare provider.
- NOROXIN is usually taken every 12 hours for patients with normal kidney function.
- Take NOROXIN with a glass of water.
- Drink plenty of fluids while taking NOROXIN.
- Take NOROXIN at least one hour before or 2 hours after a meal or having milk or other dairy products.
- Do not skip any doses, or stop taking NOROXIN even if you begin to feel better, until you finish your prescribed treatment, unless:
  - you have tendon effects (see **"What is the most important information I should know about NOROXIN?"**),
  - you have a serious allergic reaction (see **"What are the possible side effects of NOROXIN?"**), or
  - your healthcare provider tells you to stop. This will help make sure that all of the bacteria are killed and lower the chance that the bacteria will become resistant to NOROXIN. If this happens, NOROXIN and other antibiotic medicines may not work in the future.
- If you miss a dose of NOROXIN, take it as soon as you remember. Do not take two doses of NOROXIN at the same time. Do not take more than 2 doses of NOROXIN in one day.
- If you take too much, call your healthcare provider or get medical help immediately.

What should I avoid while taking NOROXIN?

- NOROXIN can make you feel dizzy and lightheaded. Do not drive, operate machinery, or do other activities that require mental alertness or coordination until you know how NOROXIN affects you.
- Avoid sunlamps and tanning beds, and try to limit your time in the sun. NOROXIN can make your skin sensitive to the sun (photosensitivity) and the light from sunlamps and tanning beds. You could get severe sunburn, blisters or swelling of your skin. If you get any of these symptoms while taking NOROXIN, call your healthcare provider right away. You should use sunscreen and wear a hat and clothes that cover your skin if you have to be in sunlight.

What are the possible side effects of NOROXIN?

NOROXIN can cause side effects that may be serious or even cause death. See **"What is the most important information I should know about NOROXIN?"**

Other serious side effects of NOROXIN include:

- **Central Nervous System Effects.** Seizures have been reported in people who take fluoroquinolone antibiotics including NOROXIN. Tell your healthcare provider if you have a history of seizures. Ask your healthcare provider whether taking NOROXIN will change your risk of having a seizure.
  Central Nervous System (CNS) side effects may happen as soon as after taking the first dose of NOROXIN. Talk to your healthcare provider right away if you get any of these side effects, or other changes in mood or behavior:
  - feel lightheaded
  - seizures
  - hear voices, see things, or sense things that are not there (hallucinations)
  - feel restless
  - tremors
  - feel anxious or nervous
  - confusion
  - feel more suspicious (paranoia)
- **Serious allergic reactions.** Allergic reactions can happen in people who take fluoroquinolones, including NOROXIN, even after only one dose. Stop taking NOROXIN and get emergency medical help right away if you get any of the following symptoms of a severe allergic reaction:
  - hives
  - trouble breathing or swallowing
  - swelling of the lips, tongue, face
  - throat tightness, hoarseness
  - rapid heartbeat
  - faint
  - skin rash accompanied by fever and feeling unwell
  - yellowing of the skin or eyes. Stop taking NOROXIN and tell your healthcare provider right away if you get yellowing of your skin or white part of your eyes, or if you have dark urine. These can be signs of a serious reaction to NOROXIN (a liver problem).
- **Skin rash.** Skin rash may happen in people taking NOROXIN, even after only one dose. Stop taking NOROXIN at the first sign of a skin rash and call your healthcare provider. Skin rash may be sign of a more serious reaction to NOROXIN.
- **Serious heart rhythm changes (QTc prolongation and torsade de pointes).** Tell your healthcare provider right away if you have a change in your heart beat (a fast or irregular heartbeat), or if you faint. NOROXIN may cause a rare heart problem known as prolongation of the QTc interval. This condition can cause an abnormal heartbeat and can be very dangerous. The chances of this happening are higher in people:
  - who are elderly
  - with a family history of prolonged QTc interval
  - with low blood potassium (hypokalemia)
  - who take certain medicines to control heart rhythm (antiarrhythmics)
- **Intestine infection (Pseudomembranous colitis).** Pseudomembranous colitis can happen with most antibiotics, including NOROXIN. Call your healthcare provider right away if you get watery diarrhea, diarrhea that does not go away, or bloody stools. You may have stomach cramps and a fever. Pseudomembranous colitis can happen 2 or more months after you have finished your antibiotic.
- **Changes in sensation and possible nerve damage (Peripheral Neuropathy).** Damage to the nerves in arms, hands, legs, or feet can happen in people taking fluoroquinolones, including NOROXIN. Talk with your healthcare provider right away if you get any of the following symptoms of peripheral neuropathy in your arms, hands, legs, or feet:
  - pain
  - burning
  - tingling
  - numbness
  - weakness

  NOROXIN may need to be stopped to prevent permanent nerve damage.
- **Low blood sugar (hypoglycemia).** People taking NOROXIN and other fluoroquinolone medicines with the oral anti-diabetes medicine glyburide (Micronase, Glynase, Diabeta, Glucovance) can get low blood sugar (hypoglycemia) which can sometimes be severe. Tell your healthcare provider if you get low blood sugar while taking NOROXIN. Your antibiotic medicine may need to be changed.
- **Sensitivity to sunlight (photosensitivity).** See **"What should I avoid while taking NOROXIN?"**

The most common side effects of NOROXIN include:

- dizziness
- nausea
- diarrhea
- heartburn
- headache
- stomach (abdominal) cramping
- weakness
- changes in certain liver function tests

These are not all the possible side effects of NOROXIN. Tell your healthcare provider about any side effect that bothers you or that does not go away.

Call your healthcare provider for medical advice about side effects. You may report side effects to FDA at 1-800-FDA-1088.

How should I store NOROXIN?

Store between 59-86°F (15-30°C).

Keep container closed tightly.

Keep NOROXIN and all medicines out of the reach of children.

General Information about NOROXIN

Medicines are sometimes prescribed for purposes other than those listed in a Medication Guide. Do not use NOROXIN for a condition for which it is not prescribed. Do not give NOROXIN to other people, even if they have the same symptoms that you have. It may harm them.

This Medication Guide summarizes the most important information about NOROXIN. If you would like more information about NOROXIN, talk with your healthcare provider. You can ask your healthcare provider or pharmacist for information about NOROXIN that is written for healthcare professionals. For more information call 1-800-622-4477.

What are the ingredients in NOROXIN?

Active ingredient: norfloxacin

Inactive ingredients: cellulose, croscarmellose sodium, hydroxypropyl cellulose, hydroxypropyl methylcellulose, magnesium stearate and titanium dioxide

This Medication Guide has been approved by the U.S. Food and Drug Administration.

[4]Other brands listed are the trademarks of their respective owners and are not trademarks of Merck Sharp & Dohme Corp.

Manufactured for: Merck Sharp & Dohme Corp., a subsidiary of

MERCK & CO., INC., Whitehouse Station, NJ 08889, USA

Manufactured by:

Merck Sharp & Dohme (Italia) S.p.A.

Via Emilia, 21

27100 Pavia, Italy

Revised: 06/2012

USMG-T-03661206R009

Shown in Product Identification Guide, page 308

NOXAFIL® ℞

(Posaconazole)

ORAL SUSPENSION 40 mg/mL

HIGHLIGHTS OF PRESCRIBING INFORMATION

These highlights do not include all the information needed to use NOXAFIL ORAL SUSPENSION safely and effectively. See full prescribing information for NOXAFIL ORAL SUSPENSION.

NOXAFIL® (Posaconazole) ORAL SUSPENSION 40 mg/mL

Initial U.S. Approval: 2006

RECENT MAJOR CHANGES

Contraindications, HMG-CoA Reductase Inhibitors Primarily Metabolized Through CYP3A4 (4.4) 06/2012

INDICATIONS AND USAGE

NOXAFIL is a triazole antifungal agent indicated for:

- prophylaxis of invasive *Aspergillus* and *Candida* infections in patients, 13 years of age and older, who are at high risk of developing these infections due to being severely immunocompromised, such as HSCT recipients with GVHD or those with hematologic malignancies with prolonged neutropenia from chemotherapy. (1.1)
- the treatment of oropharyngeal candidiasis (OPC), including OPC refractory (rOPC) to itraconazole and/or fluconazole. (1.2)

DOSAGE AND ADMINISTRATION

Indication	Dose and Duration of Therapy
Prophylaxis of Invasive Fungal Infections	200 mg (5 mL) three times a day. Duration of therapy is based on recovery from neutropenia or immunosuppression. (2.1)
Oropharyngeal Candidiasis (OPC)	Loading dose of 100 mg (2.5 mL) twice a day on the first day, then 100 mg (2.5 mL) once a day for 13 days. (2.1)
OPC Refractory (rOPC) to Itraconazole and/or Fluconazole	400 mg (10 mL) twice a day. Duration of therapy should be based on the severity of the patient's underlying disease and clinical response. (2.1)

DOSAGE FORMS AND STRENGTHS

NOXAFIL Oral Suspension 40 mg per mL (3)

CONTRAINDICATIONS

- Do not administer to persons with known hypersensitivity to posaconazole, any component of NOXAFIL, or other azole antifungal agents. (4.1)
- Do not coadminister NOXAFIL with the following drugs; NOXAFIL increases concentrations of:
  - Sirolimus: can result in sirolimus toxicity (4.2, 7.1)
  - CYP3A4 substrates (pimozide, quinidine): can result in QTc interval prolongation and rare occurrences of TdP (4.3, 7.2)
  - HMG-CoA Reductase Inhibitors Primarily Metabolized Through CYP3A4: can lead to rhabdomyolysis (4.4, 7.3)
  - Ergot alkaloids: can result in ergotism (4.5, 7.4)

WARNINGS AND PRECAUTIONS

- Calcineurin Inhibitor Toxicity: NOXAFIL increases concentrations of cyclosporine or tacrolimus; reduce dose of cyclosporine and tacrolimus and monitor concentrations frequently. (5.1)
- Arrhythmias and QTc Prolongation: NOXAFIL has been shown to prolong the QTc interval and cause rare occurrences of TdP. Administer with caution to patients with potentially proarrhythmic conditions. Do not administer with drugs known to prolong QTc interval and metabolized through CYP3A4. Correct K^+, Mg^{++}, and Ca^{++} before starting NOXAFIL. (5.2)
- Hepatic Toxicity: elevations in LFTs (generally reversible on discontinuation) may occur. Discontinuation should be considered in patients who develop abnormal LFTs or monitor LFTs during treatment. (5.3)
- Midazolam: NOXAFIL can prolong hypnotic/sedative effects. Monitor patients and benzodiazepine receptor antagonists should be available. (5.4, 7.5)

ADVERSE REACTIONS

- Common treatment-emergent adverse reactions (>30%) in prophylaxis studies are fever, diarrhea and nausea. (6.2)
- Common treatment-emergent adverse reactions (>5%) in controlled OPC pool are diarrhea, nausea, headache, vomiting, and fever. Common adverse reactions (>20%) in the refractory OPC pool are fever, diarrhea, nausea, vomiting, and coughing. (6.2)

To report SUSPECTED ADVERSE REACTIONS, contact Merck Sharp & Dohme Corp., a subsidiary of Merck & Co., Inc., at 1-877-888-4231 or FDA at 1-800-FDA-1088 or *www.fda.gov/medwatch.*

DRUG INTERACTIONS

Interaction Drug	Interaction
Rifabutin, phenytoin, efavirenz, cimetidine, esomeprazole	Avoid coadministration unless the benefit outweighs the risks (7.6, 7.7, 7.8, 7.9)
Other drugs metabolized by CYP3A4 (tacrolimus, cyclosporine, vinca alkaloids, calcium channel blockers)	Consider dosage adjustment and monitor for adverse effects and toxicity (7.1, 7.10, 7.11)
Digoxin	Monitor digoxin plasma concentrations (7.12)
Fosamprenavir, metoclopramide	Monitor for breakthrough fungal infections (7.6, 7.13)

USE IN SPECIFIC POPULATIONS

- Pregnancy: Based on animal data, may cause fetal harm. (8.1)
- Nursing Mothers: Discontinue drug or nursing, taking in to consideration the importance of drug to the mother. (8.3)
- Severe renal impairment: Monitor closely for breakthrough fungal infections. (8.6)

See 17 for PATIENT COUNSELING INFORMATION

Revised: 12/2012

FULL PRESCRIBING INFORMATION: CONTENTS*

*** Sections or subsections omitted from the full prescribing information are not listed**

FULL PRESCRIBING INFORMATION

1. INDICATIONS AND USAGE

1.1 Prophylaxis of Invasive *Aspergillus* and *Candida* Infections

NOXAFIL® Oral Suspension is indicated for prophylaxis of invasive *Aspergillus* and *Candida* infections in patients, 13 years of age and older, who are at high risk of developing these infections due to being severely immunocompromised, such as hematopoietic stem cell transplant (HSCT) recipients with graft-versus-host disease (GVHD) or those with hematologic malignancies with prolonged neutropenia from chemotherapy.

1.2 Treatment of Oropharyngeal Candidiasis Including Oropharyngeal Candidiasis Refractory to Itraconazole and/or Fluconazole

NOXAFIL is indicated for the treatment of oropharyngeal candidiasis, including oropharyngeal candidiasis refractory to itraconazole and/or fluconazole.

2. DOSAGE AND ADMINISTRATION

2.1 Dosage

Table 1

Indication	Dose and Duration of Therapy
Prophylaxis of Invasive Fungal Infections	200 mg (5 mL) three times a day. The duration of therapy is based on recovery from neutropenia or immunosuppression.
Oropharyngeal Candidiasis	Loading dose of 100 mg (2.5 mL) twice a day on the first day, then 100 mg (2.5 mL) once a day for 13 days.
Oropharyngeal Candidiasis Refractory to itraconazole and/or fluconazole	400 mg (10 mL) twice a day. Duration of therapy should be based on the severity of the patient's underlying disease and clinical response.

2.2 Administration Instructions

Shake NOXAFIL Oral Suspension well before use.

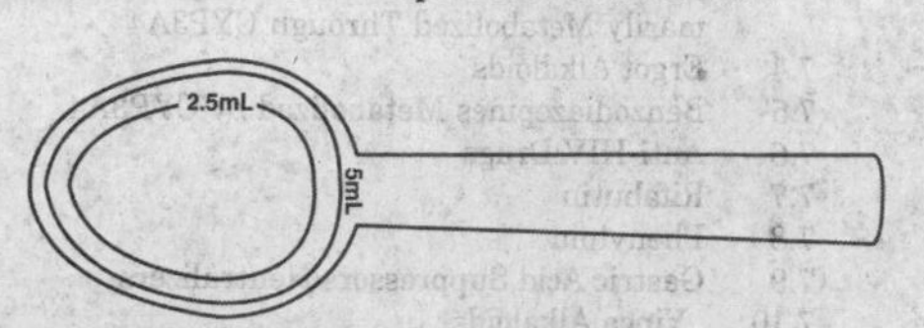

Figure 1: A measured dosing spoon is provided, marked for doses of 2.5 mL and 5 mL.

It is recommended that the spoon is rinsed with water after each administration and before storage.

Each dose of NOXAFIL should be administered with a full meal or with a liquid nutritional supplement or an acidic carbonated beverage (e.g., ginger ale) in patients who cannot eat a full meal.

To enhance the oral absorption of posaconazole and optimize plasma concentrations:

- Each dose of NOXAFIL should be administered during or immediately (i.e., within 20 minutes) following a full meal. In patients who cannot eat a full meal, each dose of NOXAFIL should be administered with a liquid nutritional supplement or an acidic carbonated beverage. For patients who cannot eat a full meal or tolerate an oral nutritional supplement or an acidic carbonated beverage, alternative antifungal therapy should be considered or patients should be monitored closely for breakthrough fungal infections.
- Patients who have severe diarrhea or vomiting should be monitored closely for breakthrough fungal infections.
- Coadministration of drugs that can decrease the plasma concentrations of posaconazole should generally be avoided unless the benefit outweighs the risk. If such drugs are necessary, patients should be monitored closely for breakthrough fungal infections *[see Drug Interactions (7.6, 7.7, 7.8, 7.9, 7.13)]*.

3. DOSAGE FORMS AND STRENGTHS

NOXAFIL Oral Suspension is available in 4-ounce (123 mL) amber glass bottles with child-resistant closures (NDC 0085-1328-01) containing 105 mL of suspension (40 mg of posaconazole per mL).

4. CONTRAINDICATIONS

4.1 Hypersensitivity

NOXAFIL is contraindicated in persons with known hypersensitivity to posaconazole, any component of NOXAFIL, or other azole antifungal agents.

4.2 Use with Sirolimus

NOXAFIL is contraindicated with sirolimus. Concomitant administration of NOXAFIL with sirolimus increases the sirolimus blood concentrations by approximately 9 fold and can result in sirolimus toxicity *[see Drug Interactions (7.1) and Clinical Pharmacology (12.3)]*.

4.3 QT Prolongation with Concomitant Use with CYP3A4 Substrates

NOXAFIL is contraindicated with CYP3A4 substrates that prolong the QT interval. Concomitant administration of NOXAFIL with the CYP3A4 substrates, pimozide and quinidine may result in increased plasma concentrations of these drugs, leading to QTc prolongation and rare occurrences of torsades de pointes *[see Warnings and Precautions (5.2) and Drug Interactions (7.2)]*.

4.4 HMG-CoA Reductase Inhibitors Primarily Metabolized Through CYP3A4

Coadministration with the HMG-CoA reductase inhibitors that are primarily metabolized through CYP3A4 (e.g., atorvastatin, lovastatin, and simvastatin) is contraindicated since increased plasma concentration of these drugs can lead to rhabdomyolysis *[see Drug Interactions (7.3) and Clinical Pharmacology (12.3)]*.

Table 2: Study 1 and Study 2. Number (%) of Randomized Subjects Reporting Treatment-Emergent Adverse Reactions: Frequency of at Least 10% in the Posaconazole or Fluconazole Treatment Groups (Pooled Prophylaxis Safety Analysis)

Body System Preferred Term	Posaconazole (n=605)		Fluconazole (n=539)		Itraconazole (n=58)	
Subjects Reporting any Adverse Reaction	**595**	**(98)**	**531**	**(99)**	**58**	**(100)**
Body as a Whole - General Disorders						
Fever	274	(45)	254	(47)	32	(55)
Headache	171	(28)	141	(26)	23	(40)
Rigors	122	(20)	87	(16)	17	(29)
Fatigue	101	(17)	98	(18)	5	(9)
Edema Legs	93	(15)	67	(12)	11	(19)
Anorexia	92	(15)	94	(17)	16	(28)
Dizziness	64	(11)	56	(10)	5	(9)
Edema	54	(9)	68	(13)	8	(14)
Weakness	51	(8)	52	(10)	2	(3)
Cardiovascular Disorders, General						
Hypertension	106	(18)	88	(16)	3	(5)
Hypotension	83	(14)	79	(15)	10	(17)
Disorders of Blood and Lymphatic System						
Anemia	149	(25)	124	(23)	16	(28)
Neutropenia	141	(23)	122	(23)	23	(40)
Febrile Neutropenia	118	(20)	85	(16)	23	(40)
Disorders of the Reproductive System and Breast						
Vaginal Hemorrhage*	24	(10)	20	(9)	3	(12)
Gastrointestinal System Disorders						
Diarrhea	256	(42)	212	(39)	35	(60)
Nausea	232	(38)	198	(37)	30	(52)
Vomiting	174	(29)	173	(32)	24	(41)
Abdominal Pain	161	(27)	147	(27)	21	(36)
Constipation	126	(21)	94	(17)	10	(17)
Mucositis NOS	105	(17)	68	(13)	15	(26)
Dyspepsia	61	(10)	50	(9)	6	(10)
Heart Rate and Rhythm Disorders						
Tachycardia	72	(12)	75	(14)	3	(5)
Infection and Infestations						
Bacteremia	107	(18)	98	(18)	16	(28)
Herpes Simplex	88	(15)	61	(11)	10	(17)
Cytomegalovirus Infection	82	(14)	69	(13)	0	
Pharyngitis	71	(12)	60	(11)	12	(21)
Upper Respiratory Tract Infection	44	(7)	54	(10)	5	(9)
Liver and Biliary System Disorders						
Bilirubinemia	59	(10)	51	(9)	11	(19)

(Table continued on next page)

4.5 Use with Ergot Alkaloids

Posaconazole may increase the plasma concentrations of ergot alkaloids (ergotamine and dihydroergotamine) which may lead to ergotism *[see Drug Interactions (7.4)]*.

5. WARNINGS AND PRECAUTIONS

5.1 Calcineurin-Inhibitor Drug Interactions

Concomitant administration of NOXAFIL with cyclosporine or tacrolimus increases the whole blood trough concentrations of these calcineurin-inhibitors *[see Drug Interactions (7.1) and Clinical Pharmacology (12.3)]*. Nephrotoxicity and leukoencephalopathy (including isolated deaths) have been reported in clinical efficacy studies in patients with elevated cyclosporine concentrations. Frequent monitoring of tacrolimus or cyclosporine whole blood trough concentrations should be performed during and at discontinuation of posaconazole treatment and the tacrolimus or cyclosporine dose adjusted accordingly.

5.2 Arrhythmias and QT Prolongation

Some azoles, including posaconazole, have been associated with prolongation of the QT interval on the electrocardiogram. In addition, rare cases of torsades de pointes have been reported in patients taking posaconazole.

Results from a multiple time-matched ECG analysis in healthy volunteers did not show any increase in the mean of the QTc interval. Multiple, time-matched ECGs collected over a 12-hour period were recorded at baseline and steady-state from 173 healthy male and female volunteers (18–85 years of age) administered posaconazole 400 mg BID with a high-fat meal. In this pooled analysis, the mean QTc (Fridericia) interval change from baseline was –5 msec following administration of the recommended clinical dose. A decrease in the QTc(F) interval (–3 msec) was also observed in a small number of subjects (n=16) administered placebo. The placebo-adjusted mean maximum QTc(F) interval change from baseline was <0 msec (–8 msec). No healthy subject administered posaconazole had a QTc(F) interval ≥500 msec or an increase ≥60 msec in their QTc(F) interval from baseline.

Posaconazole should be administered with caution to patients with potentially proarrhythmic conditions. Do not administer with drugs that are known to prolong the QTc interval and are metabolized through CYP3A4 *[see Contraindications (4.3) and Drug Interactions (7.2)]*. Rigorous attempts to correct potassium, magnesium, and calcium should be made before starting posaconazole.

5.3 Hepatic Toxicity

Hepatic reactions (e.g., mild to moderate elevations in alanine aminotransferase (ALT), aspartate aminotransferase (AST), alkaline phosphatase, total bilirubin, and/or clinical hepatitis) have been reported in clinical trials. The elevations in liver function tests were generally reversible on discontinuation of therapy, and in some instances these tests normalized without drug interruption and rarely required drug discontinuation. Isolated cases of more severe hepatic reactions including cholestasis or hepatic failure including deaths have been reported in patients with serious underlying medical conditions (e.g., hematologic malignancy) during treatment with posaconazole. These severe hepatic reactions were seen primarily in subjects receiving the 800 mg daily (400 mg BID or 200 mg QID) in clinical trials. Liver function tests should be evaluated at the start of and during the course of posaconazole therapy. Patients who develop abnormal liver function tests during posaconazole therapy should be monitored for the development of more severe hepatic injury. Patient management should include laboratory evaluation of hepatic function (particularly liver function tests and bilirubin). Discontinuation of posaconazole must be considered if clinical signs and symptoms consistent with liver disease develop that may be attributable to posaconazole.

5.4 Use with Midazolam

Concomitant administration of NOXAFIL with midazolam increases the midazolam plasma concentrations by approximately 5 fold. Increased plasma midazolam concentrations could potentiate and prolong hypnotic and sedative effects. Patients must be monitored closely for adverse effects associated with high plasma concentrations of midazolam and benzodiazepine receptor antagonists must be available to reverse these effects *[see Drug Interactions (7.5) and Clinical Pharmacology (12.3)]*.

6. ADVERSE REACTIONS

6.1 Serious and Otherwise Important Adverse Reactions

The following serious and otherwise important adverse reactions are discussed in detail in another section of the labeling:

- Hypersensitivity *[see Contraindications (4.1)]*
- Arrhythmias and QT Prolongation *[see Warnings and Precautions (5.2)]*
- Hepatic Toxicity *[see Warnings and Precautions (5.3)]*

6.2 Clinical Trials Experience

Because clinical trials are conducted under widely varying conditions, adverse reaction rates observed in clinical trials of NOXAFIL cannot be directly compared to rates in the clinical trials of another drug and may not reflect the rates observed in practice.

The safety of posaconazole therapy has been assessed in 1844 patients in clinical trials. This includes 605 patients in the active-controlled prophylaxis studies, 557 patients in the active-controlled OPC studies, 239 patients in refractory OPC studies, and 443 patients from other indications. This represents a heterogeneous population, including immunocompromised patients, e.g., patients with hematological malignancy, neutropenia post-chemotherapy, graft vs. host disease post hematopoietic stem cell transplant, and HIV infection, as well as non-neutropenic patients. This patient population was 71% male, had a mean age of 42 years (range 8–84 years, 6% of patients were ≥65 years of age and 1% was <18 years of age), and were 64% white, 16% Hispanic, and 36% non-white (including 14% black). Posaconazole therapy was given to 171 patients for ≥6 months, with 58 patients receiving posaconazole therapy for ≥12 months. **Table 2** presents treatment-emergent adverse reactions observed at an incidence of >10% in posaconazole prophylaxis studies. **Table 3** presents treatment-emergent adverse reactions observed at an incidence of at least 10% in the OPC/rOPC studies.

Table 2 *(cont.)*: Study 1 and Study 2. Number (%) of Randomized Subjects Reporting Treatment-Emergent Adverse Reactions: Frequency of at Least 10% in the Posaconazole or Fluconazole Treatment Groups (Pooled Prophylaxis Safety Analysis)

Body System Preferred Term	Posaconazole (n=605)		Fluconazole (n=539)		Itraconazole (n=58)	
Subjects Reporting any Adverse Reaction	595	(98)	531	(99)	58	(100)
Metabolic and Nutritional Disorders						
Hypokalemia	181	(30)	142	(26)	30	(52)
Hypomagnesemia	110	(18)	84	(16)	11	(19)
Hyperglycemia	68	(11)	76	(14)	2	(3)
Hypocalcemia	56	(9)	55	(10)	5	(9)
Musculoskeletal System Disorders						
Musculoskeletal Pain	95	(16)	82	(15)	9	(16)
Arthralgia	69	(11)	67	(12)	5	(9)
Back Pain	63	(10)	66	(12)	4	(7)
Platelet, Bleeding and Clotting Disorders						
Thrombocytopenia	175	(29)	146	(27)	20	(34)
Petechiae	64	(11)	54	(10)	9	(16)
Psychiatric Disorders						
Insomnia	103	(17)	92	(17)	11	(19)
Anxiety	52	(9)	61	(11)	9	(16)
Respiratory System Disorders						
Coughing	146	(24)	130	(24)	14	(24)
Dyspnea	121	(20)	116	(22)	15	(26)
Epistaxis	82	(14)	73	(14)	12	(21)
Skin and Subcutaneous Tissue Disorders						
Rash	113	(19)	96	(18)	25	(43)
Pruritus	69	(11)	62	(12)	11	(19)

NOS = not otherwise specified.

* Percentages of sex-specific adverse reactions are based on the number of males/females.

Prophylaxis of Aspergillus and Candida: In the 2 randomized, comparative prophylaxis studies, the safety of posaconazole 200 mg three times a day was compared to fluconazole 400 mg once daily or itraconazole 200 mg twice a day in severely immunocompromised patients.

The most frequently reported adverse reactions (>30%) in the prophylaxis clinical trials were fever, diarrhea and nausea.

The most common adverse reactions leading to discontinuation of posaconazole in the prophylaxis studies were associated with GI disorders, specifically, nausea (2%), vomiting (2%), and hepatic enzymes increased (2%).

[See table 2 on previous page and above]

HIV Infected Subjects with OPC: In 2 randomized comparative studies in OPC, the safety of posaconazole at a dose of less than or equal to 400 mg QD in 557 HIV-infected patients was compared to the safety of fluconazole in 262 HIV-infected patients at a dose of 100 mg QD.

An additional 239 HIV-infected patients with refractory OPC received posaconazole in 2 non-comparative trials for refractory OPC (rOPC).

Of these subjects, 149 received the 800-mg/day dose and the remainder received the less than or equal to 400-mg QD dose.

In the OPC/rOPC studies, the most common adverse reactions were fever, diarrhea, nausea, headache, and vomiting.

The most common adverse reactions that led to treatment discontinuation of posaconazole in the Controlled OPC Pool included respiratory insufficiency (1%) and pneumonia (1%).

In the refractory OPC pool, the most common adverse reactions that led to treatment discontinuation of posaconazole were AIDS (7%) and respiratory insufficiency (3%).

[See table 3 at top of next page]

Adverse reactions were reported more frequently in the pool of patients with refractory OPC. Among these highly immunocompromised patients with advanced HIV disease, serious adverse reactions (SARs) were reported in 55% (132/239). The most commonly reported SARs were fever (13%) and neutropenia (10%).

Less Common Adverse Reactions: Clinically significant adverse reactions reported during clinical trials in prophylaxis, OPC/rOPC or other trials with posaconazole which occurred in less than 5% of patients are listed below:

- **Blood and lymphatic system disorders:** hemolytic uremic syndrome, thrombotic thrombocytopenic purpura, neutropenia aggravated
- **Endocrine disorders:** adrenal insufficiency
- **Nervous system disorders:** paresthesia
- **Immune system disorders:** allergic reaction *[see Contraindications (4.1)]*
- **Cardiac disorders:** Torsades de pointes *[see Warnings and Precautions (5.2)]*
- **Vascular disorders:** pulmonary embolism
- **Liver and Biliary System Disorders:** bilirubinemia, hepatic enzymes increased, hepatic function abnormal, hepatitis, hepatomegaly, jaundice, SGOT Increased, SGPT Increased
- **Metabolic and Nutritional Disorders:** hypokalemia
- **Platelet, Bleeding, and Clotting Disorders:** thrombocytopenia
- **Renal & Urinary System Disorders:** renal failure acute

Clinical Laboratory Values: In healthy volunteers and patients, elevation of liver function test values did not appear to be associated with higher plasma concentrations of posaconazole. The majority of abnormal liver function tests were minor, transient, and did not lead to discontinuation of therapy.

For the prophylaxis studies, the number of patients with changes in liver function tests from Common Toxicity Criteria (CTC) Grade 0, 1, or 2 at baseline to Grade 3 or 4 during the study is presented in **Table 4**.

Table 4: Study 1 and Study 2. Changes in Liver Function Test Results from CTC Grade 0, 1, or 2 at Baseline to Grade 3 or 4

Number (%) of Patients With Change*		
Study 1		
Laboratory Parameter	**Posaconazole n=301**	**Fluconazole n=299**
AST	11/266 (4)	13/266 (5)
ALT	47/271 (17)	39/272 (14)
Bilirubin	24/271 (9)	20/275 (7)
Alkaline Phosphatase	9/271 (3)	8/271 (3)
Study 2		
Laboratory Parameter	**Posaconazole (n=304)**	**Fluconazole/ Itraconazole (n=298)**
AST	9/286 (3)	5/280 (2)
ALT	18/289 (6)	13/284 (5)
Bilirubin	20/290 (7)	25/285 (9)
Alkaline Phosphatase	4/281 (1)	1/276 (<1)

CTC = Common Toxicity Criteria; AST= Aspartate Aminotransferase; ALT= Alanine Aminotransferase.

* Change from Grade 0 to 2 at baseline to Grade 3 or 4 during the study. These data are presented in the form X/Y, where X represents the number of patients who met the criterion as indicated, and Y represents the number of patients who had a baseline observation and at least one post-baseline observation.

The number of patients treated for OPC with clinically significant liver function test (LFT) abnormalities at any time during the studies is provided in **Table 5**. (LFT abnormalities were present in some of these patients prior to initiation of the study drug).

[See table 5 at top of next page]

6.3 Postmarketing Experience

No clinically significant postmarketing adverse reactions were identified that have not previously been reported during clinical trials experience.

7. DRUG INTERACTIONS

Posaconazole is primarily metabolized via UDP glucuronidation and is a substrate of p-glycoprotein efflux. Therefore, inhibitors or inducers of these clearance pathways may affect posaconazole plasma concentrations. Posaconazole is also a strong inhibitor of CYP3A4. Therefore, plasma concentrations of drugs predominantly metabolized by CYP3A4 may be increased by posaconazole *[see Clinical Pharmacology (12.3)]*.

7.1 Immunosuppressants Metabolized by CYP3A4

Sirolimus: Concomitant administration of posaconazole with sirolimus increases the sirolimus blood concentrations by approximately 9 fold and can result in sirolimus toxicity. Therefore, posaconazole is contraindicated with sirolimus *[see Contraindications (4.2) and Clinical Pharmacology (12.3)]*.

Tacrolimus: Posaconazole has been shown to significantly increase the C_{max} and AUC of tacrolimus. At initiation of posaconazole treatment, reduce the tacrolimus dose to approximately one-third of the original dose. Frequent monitoring of tacrolimus whole blood trough concentrations should be performed during and at discontinuation of posaconazole treatment and the tacrolimus dose adjusted accordingly *[see Warnings and Precautions (5.1) and Clinical Pharmacology (12.3)]*.

Cyclosporine: Posaconazole has been shown to increase cyclosporine whole blood concentrations in heart transplant patients upon initiation of posaconazole treatment. It is recommended to reduce cyclosporine dose to approximately three-fourths of the original dose upon initiation of posaconazole treatment. Frequent monitoring of cyclosporine whole blood trough concentrations should be performed during and at discontinuation of posaconazole treatment and the cyclosporine dose adjusted accordingly *[see Warnings and Precautions (5.1) and Clinical Pharmacology (12.3)]*.

7.2 CYP3A4 Substrates

Concomitant administration of posaconazole with CYP3A4 substrates such as pimozide and quinidine may result in increased plasma concentrations of these drugs, leading to QTc prolongation and rare occurrences of torsades de pointes. Therefore, posaconazole is contraindicated with these drugs *[see Contraindications (4.3) and Warnings and Precautions (5.2)]*.

Table 3: Treatment-Emergent Adverse Reactions with Frequency of at Least 10% in OPC Studies (Treated Population)

Body System Preferred Term	Number (%) of Subjects: Controlled OPC Pool: Posaconazole n=557	Controlled OPC Pool: Fluconazole n=262	Refractory OPC Pool: Posaconazole n=239
Subjects Reporting any Adverse Reaction*	356 (64)	175 (67)	221 (92)
Body as a Whole – General Disorders			
Fever	34 (6)	22 (8)	82 (34)
Headache	44 (8)	23 (9)	47 (20)
Anorexia	10 (2)	4 (2)	46 (19)
Fatigue	18 (3)	12 (5)	31 (13)
Asthenia	9 (2)	5 (2)	31 (13)
Rigors	2 (<1)	4 (2)	29 (12)
Pain	4 (1)	2 (1)	27 (11)
Disorders of Blood and Lymphatic System			
Neutropenia	21 (4)	8 (3)	39 (16)
Anemia	11 (2)	5 (2)	34 (14)
Gastrointestinal System Disorders			
Diarrhea	58 (10)	34 (13)	70 (29)
Nausea	48 (9)	30 (11)	70 (29)
Vomiting	37 (7)	18 (7)	67 (28)
Abdominal Pain	27 (5)	17 (6)	43 (18)
Infection and Infestations			
Candidiasis, Oral	3 (1)	1 (<1)	28 (12)
Herpes Simplex	16 (3)	8 (3)	26 (11)
Pneumonia	17 (3)	6 (2)	25 (10)
Metabolic and Nutritional Disorders			
Weight Decrease	4 (1)	2 (1)	33 (14)
Dehydration	4 (1)	7 (3)	27 (11)
Psychiatric Disorders			
Insomnia	8 (1)	3 (1)	39 (16)
Respiratory System Disorders			
Coughing	18 (3)	11 (4)	60 (25)
Dyspnea	8 (1)	8 (3)	28 (12)
Skin and Subcutaneous Tissue Disorders			
Rash	15 (3)	10 (4)	36 (15)
Sweating Increased	13 (2)	5 (2)	23 (10)

OPC=oropharyngeal candidiasis; SGOT=serum glutamic oxaloacetic transaminase (same as AST); SGPT=serum glutamic pyruvic transaminase (same as ALT).

* Number of subjects reporting treatment-emergent adverse reactions at least once during the study, without regard to relationship to treatment. Subjects may have reported more than 1 event.

7.3 HMG-CoA Reductase Inhibitors (Statins) Primarily Metabolized Through CYP3A4

Concomitant administration of posaconazole with simvastatin increases the simvastatin plasma concentrations by approximately 10 fold. Therefore, posaconazole is contraindicated with HMG-CoA reductase inhibitors primarily metabolized through CYP3A4 *[see Contraindications (4.4) and Clinical Pharmacology (12.3)]*.

7.4 Ergot Alkaloids

Most of the ergot alkaloids are substrates of CYP3A4. Posaconazole may increase the plasma concentrations of ergot alkaloids (ergotamine and dihydroergotamine) which may lead to ergotism. Therefore, posaconazole is contraindicated with ergot alkaloids *[see Contraindications (4.5)]*.

7.5 Benzodiazepines Metabolized by CYP3A4

Concomitant administration of posaconazole with midazolam increases the midazolam plasma concentrations by approximately 5 fold. Increased plasma midazolam concentrations could potentiate and prolong hypnotic and sedative effects. Concomitant use of posaconazole and other benzodiazepines metabolized by CYP3A4 (e.g., alprazolam, triazolam) could result in increased plasma concentrations of these benzodiazepines. Patients must be monitored closely for adverse effects associated with high plasma concentrations of benzodiazepines metabolized by CYP3A4 and benzodiazepine receptor antagonists must be available to reverse these effects *[see Warnings and Precautions (5.4) and Clinical Pharmacology (12.3)]*.

7.6 Anti-HIV Drugs

Efavirenz: Efavirenz induces UDP-glucuronidase and significantly decreases posaconazole plasma concentrations *[see Clinical Pharmacology (12.3)]*. It is recommended to avoid concomitant use of efavirenz with posaconazole unless the benefit outweighs the risks.

Ritonavir and Atazanavir: Ritonavir and atazanavir are metabolized by CYP3A4 and posaconazole increases plasma concentrations of these drugs *[see Clinical Pharmacology (12.3)]*. Frequent monitoring of adverse effects and toxicity of ritonavir and atazanavir should be performed during coadministration with posaconazole.

Fosamprenavir: Combining fosamprenavir with posaconazole may lead to decreased posaconazole plasma concentrations. If concomitant administration is required, close monitoring for breakthrough fungal infections is recommended *[see Clinical Pharmacology (12.3)]*.

7.7 Rifabutin

Rifabutin induces UDP-glucuronidase and decreases posaconazole plasma concentrations. Rifabutin is also metabolized by CYP3A4. Therefore, coadministration of rifabutin with posaconazole increases rifabutin plasma concentrations *[see Clinical Pharmacology (12.3)]*. Concomitant use of posaconazole and rifabutin should be avoided unless the benefit to the patient outweighs the risk. However, if concomitant administration is required, close monitoring for breakthrough fungal infections as well as frequent monitoring of full blood counts and adverse reactions due to increased rifabutin plasma concentrations (e.g., uveitis, leukopenia) are recommended.

7.8 Phenytoin

Phenytoin induces UDP-glucuronidase and decreases posaconazole plasma concentrations. Phenytoin is also metabolized by CYP3A4. Therefore, coadministration of phenytoin with posaconazole increases phenytoin plasma concentrations *[see Clinical Pharmacology (12.3)]*. Concomitant use of posaconazole and phenytoin should be avoided unless the benefit to the patient outweighs the risk. However, if concomitant administration is required, close monitoring for breakthrough fungal infections is recommended and frequent monitoring of phenytoin concentrations should be performed while coadministered with posaconazole and dose reduction of phenytoin should be considered.

7.9 Gastric Acid Suppressors/Neutralizers

Cimetidine (an H_2-receptor antagonist) and esomeprazole (a proton pump inhibitor) decrease posaconazole plasma concentrations *[see Clinical Pharmacology (12.3)]*. It is recommended to avoid concomitant use of cimetidine and esomeprazole with posaconazole unless the benefit outweighs the risks. However, if concomitant administration is required, close monitoring for breakthrough fungal infections is recommended.

No clinically relevant effects were observed when posaconazole is concomitantly used with antacids and H_2-receptor antagonists other than cimetidine. No dosage adjustment of posaconazole is required when posaconazole is concomitantly used with antacids and H_2-receptor antagonists other than cimetidine.

7.10 Vinca Alkaloids

Most of the vinca alkaloids are substrates of CYP3A4. Posaconazole may increase the plasma concentrations of vinca alkaloids (e.g., vincristine and vinblastine) which may lead to neurotoxicity. Therefore, it is recommended that dose adjustment of the vinca alkaloid be considered.

7.11 Calcium Channel Blockers Metabolized by CYP3A4

Posaconazole may increase the plasma concentrations of calcium channel blockers metabolized by CYP3A4 (e.g., verapamil, diltiazem, nifedipine, nicardipine, felodipine). Frequent monitoring for adverse reactions and toxicity related to calcium channel blockers is recommended during coadministration. Dose reduction of calcium channel blockers may be needed.

7.12 Digoxin

Increased plasma concentrations of digoxin have been reported in patients receiving digoxin and posaconazole. Therefore, monitoring of digoxin plasma concentrations is recommended during coadministration.

7.13 Gastrointestinal Motility Agents

Metoclopramide decreases posaconazole plasma concentrations *[see Clinical Pharmacology (12.3)]*. If metoclopramide is concomitantly administered, it is recommended to closely monitor for breakthrough fungal infections.

Loperamide does not affect posaconazole plasma concentrations *[see Clinical Pharmacology (12.3)]*. No dosage adjustment of posaconazole is required when loperamide and posaconazole are used concomitantly.

7.14 Glipizide

Although no dosage adjustment of glipizide is required, it is recommended to monitor glucose concentrations when posaconazole and glipizide are concomitantly used.

Table 5: Clinically Significant Laboratory Test Abnormalities without Regard to Baseline Value

	Controlled		Refractory
	Posaconazole	Fluconazole	Posaconazole
Laboratory Test	n=557(%)	n=262(%)	n=239(%)
ALT > 3.0 × ULN	16/537 (3)	13/254 (5)	25/226 (11)
AST > 3.0 × ULN	33/537 (6)	26/254 (10)	39/223 (17)
Total Bilirubin > 1.5 × ULN	15/536 (3)	5/254 (2)	9/197 (5)
Alkaline Phosphatase > 3.0 × ULN	17/535 (3)	15/253 (6)	24/190 (13)

ALT= Alanine Aminotransferase; AST= Aspartate Aminotransferase.

Table 6: The Mean (%CV) [min-max] Posaconazole Pharmacokinetic Parameters Following Single-Dose Suspension Administration of 200 mg and 400 mg Under Fed and Fasted Conditions

Dose (mg)	C_{max} (ng/mL)	T_{max}* (hr)	AUC (I) (ng·hr/mL)	CL/F (L/hr)	t½ (hr)
200 mg fasted (n=20)†	132 (50) [45–267]	3.50 [1.5–36‡]	4179 (31) [2705–7269]	51 (25) [28–74]	23.5 (25) [15.3–33.7]
200 mg nonfat (n=20)†	378 (43) [131–834]	4 [3–5]	10,753 (35) [4579–17,092]	21 (39) [12–44]	22.2 (18) [17.4–28.7]
200 mg high fat (54 gm fat) (n=20)†	512 (34) [241–1016]	5 [4–5]	15,059 (26) [10,341–24,476]	14 (24) [8.2–19]	23.0 (19) [17.2–33.4]
400 mg fasted (n=23)§	121 (75) [27–366]	4 [2–12]	5258 (48) [2834–9567]	91 (40) [42–141]	27.3 (26) [16.8–38.9]
400 mg with liquid nutritional supplement (14 gm fat) (n=23)§	355 (43) [145–720]	5 [4–8]	11,295 (40) [3865–20,592]	43 (56) [19–103]	26.0 (19) [18.2–35.0]

* Median [min-max].

† n=15 for AUC (I), CL/F, and t ½

‡ The subject with T_{max} of 36 hrs had relatively constant plasma levels over 36 hrs (1.7 ng/mL difference between 4 hrs and 36 hrs).

§ n=10 for AUC (I), CL/F, and t ½

8. USE IN SPECIFIC POPULATIONS

8.1 Pregnancy

Pregnancy Category C: There are no adequate and well-controlled studies in pregnant women. NOXAFIL should be used in pregnancy only if the potential benefit outweighs the potential risk to the fetus.

Posaconazole has been shown to cause skeletal malformations (cranial malformations and missing ribs) in rats when given in doses ≥27 mg/kg (≥1.4 times the 400-mg BID regimen based on steady-state plasma concentrations of drug in healthy volunteers). The no-effect dose for malformations in rats was 9 mg/kg, which is 0.7 times the exposure achieved with the 400-mg BID regimen. No malformations were seen in rabbits at doses up to 80 mg/kg. In the rabbit, the no-effect dose was 20 mg/kg, while high doses of 40 mg/kg and 80 mg/kg, 2.9 or 5.2 times the exposure achieved with the 400-mg BID regimen, caused an increase in resorptions. In rabbits dosed at 80 mg/kg, a reduction in body weight gain of females and a reduction in litter size were seen.

8.3 Nursing Mothers

Posaconazole is excreted in milk of lactating rats. It is not known whether NOXAFIL is excreted in human milk. Because of the potential for serious adverse reactions from NOXAFIL in nursing infants, a decision should be made whether to discontinue nursing or to discontinue the drug, taking into account the importance of the drug to the mother.

8.4 Pediatric Use

The safety and effectiveness of posaconazole have been established in the age groups 13 to 17 years of age. The safety and effectiveness of posaconazole in pediatric patients below the age of 13 years have not been established. Use of posaconazole in these age groups is supported by evidence from adequate and well-controlled studies of posaconazole in adults with additional data.

A total of 12 patients 13 to 17 years of age received 600 mg/day (200 mg three times a day) for prophylaxis of invasive fungal infections. The safety profile in these patients <18 years of age appears similar to the safety profile observed in adults. Based on pharmacokinetic data in 10 of these pediatric patients, the mean steady-state average posaconazole concentration (Cav) was similar between these patients and adults (≥18 years of age).

A total of 16 patients 8 to 17 years of age were treated with 800 mg/day (400 mg twice a day or 200 mg four times a day) in a study for another indication. Based on pharmacokinetic data in 12 of these pediatric patients, the mean steady-state average posaconazole concentration (Cav) was similar between these patients and adults (≥18 years of age).

In the prophylaxis studies, the mean steady-state posaconazole average concentration (Cav) was similar among ten adolescents (13 to 17 years of age) and adults (≥18 years of age). This is consistent with pharmacokinetic data from another study in which mean steady-state posaconazole Cav from 12 adolescent patients (8–17 years of age) was similar to that in the adults (≥18 years of age).

8.5 Geriatric Use

Of the 605 patients randomized to posaconazole in the prophylaxis clinical trials, 63 (10%) were ≥65 years of age. In addition, 48 patients treated with greater than or equal to 800-mg/day posaconazole in another indication were ≥65 years of age. No overall differences in safety were observed between the geriatric patients and younger patients; therefore, no dosage adjustment is recommended for geriatric patients.

The pharmacokinetics of posaconazole are comparable in young and elderly subjects (≥65 years of age). No adjustment in the dosage of NOXAFIL is necessary in elderly patients (≥65 years of age) based on age.

No overall differences in the pharmacokinetics and safety were observed between elderly and young subjects during clinical trials, but greater sensitivity of some older individuals cannot be ruled out.

8.6 Renal Insufficiency

Following single-dose administration of 400 mg of the oral suspension, there was no significant effect of mild (CLcr: 50–80 mL/min/1.73m^2, n=6) and moderate (CLcr: 20–49 mL/min/1.73m^2, n=6) renal insufficiency on posaconazole pharmacokinetics; therefore, no dose adjustment is required in patients with mild to moderate renal impairment. In subjects with severe renal insufficiency (CLcr: <20 mL/min/1.73m^2), the mean plasma exposure (AUC) was similar to that in patients with normal renal function (CLcr: >80 mL/min/1.73m^2); however, the range of the AUC estimates was highly variable (CV=96%) in these subjects with severe renal insufficiency as compared to that in the other renal impairment groups (CV<40%). Due to the variability in exposure, patients with severe renal impairment should be monitored closely for breakthrough fungal infections *[see Dosage and Administration (2)]*.

Table 7: The Effect of Varying Gastric Administration Conditions on the C_{max} and AUC of Posaconazole in Healthy Volunteers

Study Description	Administration Arms	Change in C_{max} (ratio estimate*; 90% CI of the ratio estimate)	Change in AUC (ratio estimate*; 90% CI of the ratio estimate)
400-mg single dose with a high-fat meal relative to fasted state (n=12)	5 minutes before high-fat meal	↑96% (1.96; 1.48–2.59)	↑111% (2.11; 1.60–2.78)
	During high-fat meal	↑339% (4.39; 3.32–5.80)	↑382% (4.82; 3.66–6.35)
	20 minutes after high-fat meal	↑333% (4.33; 3.28–5.73)	↑387% (4.87; 3.70–6.42)
400 mg BID and 200 mg QID for 7 days in fasted state and with liquid nutritional supplement (BOOST®) (n=12)	400 mg BID with BOOST	↑65% (1.65; 1.29–2.11)	↑66% (1.66; 1.30–2.13)
	200 mg QID with BOOST	No Effect	No Effect
Divided daily dose from 400 mg BID to 200 mg QID for 7 days regardless of fasted conditions or with BOOST (n=12)	Fasted state	↑136% (2.36; 1.84–3.02)	↑161% (2.61; 2.04–3.35)
	With BOOST	↑137% (2.37; 1.86–3.04)	↑157% (2.57; 2.00–3.30)
400-mg single dose with carbonated acidic beverage (ginger ale) and/or proton pump inhibitor (esomeprazole) (n=12)	Ginger ale	↑92% (1.92; 1.51–2.44)	↑70% (1.70; 1.43–2.03)
	Esomeprazole	↓32% (0.68; 0.53–0.86)	↓30% (0.70; 0.59–0.83)
400-mg single dose with a prokinetic agent (metoclopramide 10 mg TID for 2 days) + BOOST or a antikinetic agent (loperamide 4- mg single dose) + BOOST (n=12)	With metoclopramide + BOOST	↓21% (0.79; 0.72–0.87)	↓19% (0.81; 0.72–0.91)
	With loperamide + BOOST	↓3% (0.97; 0.88–1.07)	↑11% (1.11; 0.99–1.25)
400-mg single dose either orally with BOOST or via an NG tube with BOOST (n=16)	Via NG tube†	↓19% (0.81; 0.71–0.91)	↓23% (0.77; 0.69–0.86)

* Ratio Estimate is the ratio of coadministered drug plus posaconazole to coadministered drug alone for C_{max} or AUC.
† In 5 subjects, the C_{max} and AUC decreased substantially (range: -27% to -53% and -33% to -51%, respectively) when NOXAFIL was administered via an NG tube compared to when NOXAFIL was administered orally. It is recommended to closely monitor patients for breakthrough fungal infections when NOXAFIL is administered via an NG tube because a lower plasma exposure may be associated with an increase risk of treatment failure.

Table 8: The Mean (%CV) [min-max] Posaconazole Steady-State Pharmacokinetic Parameters in Patients Following Oral Administration of Posaconazole 200 mg TID and 400 mg BID

Dose*	Cav (ng/mL)	AUC† (ng·hr/mL)	CL/F (L/hr)	V/F (L)	$t_{½}$ (hr)
200 mg TID‡ (n=252)	1103 (67) [21.5–3650]	ND§	ND§	ND§	ND§
200 mg TID¶ (n=215)	583 (65) [89.7–2200]	15,900 (62) [4100–56,100]	51.2 (54) [10.7–146]	2425 (39) [828–5702]	37.2 (39) [19.1–148]
400 mg BID# (n=23)	723 (86) [6.70–2256]	9093 (80) [1564–26,794]	76.1 (78) [14.9–256]	3088 (84) [407–13,140]	31.7 (42) [12.4–67.3]

Note: Cav based on observed data; other pharmacokinetic parameters based on estimates from population pharmacokinetic analyses
* Oral suspension administration
† AUC $_{(0–24\ hr)}$ for 200 mg TID and AUC $_{(0–12\ hr)}$ for 400 mg BID
‡ Allogeneic hematopoietic stem cell transplant (HSCT) recipients with graft-versus-host disease
§ Not done
The variability in average plasma posaconazole concentrations in patients was relatively higher than that in healthy subjects.
¶ Neutropenic patients who were receiving cytotoxic chemotherapy for acute myelogenous leukemia or myelodysplastic syndromes
\# Febrile neutropenic patients or patients with refractory invasive fungal infections, Cav n=24

8.7 Hepatic Insufficiency

After a single oral dose of posaconazole 400 mg, the mean AUC was 43%, 27%, and 21% higher in subjects with mild (Child-Pugh Class A, N=6), moderate (Child-Pugh Class B, N=6), and severe (Child-Pugh Class C, N=6) hepatic insufficiency, respectively, compared to subjects with normal hepatic function (N=18). Compared to subjects with normal hepatic function, the mean C_{max} was 1% higher, 40% higher, and 34% lower in subjects with mild, moderate, and severe hepatic insufficiency, respectively. The mean apparent oral clearance (CL/F) was reduced by 18%, 36%, and 28% in subjects with mild, moderate, and severe hepatic insufficiency, respectively, compared to subjects with normal hepatic function. The elimination half-life ($t_{1/2}$) was 27 hours, 39 hours, 27 hours, and 43 hours in subjects with normal hepatic function and mild, moderate, and severe hepatic insufficiency, respectively.

It is recommended that no dose adjustment of NOXAFIL is needed in patients with mild to severe hepatic insufficiency (Child-Pugh Class A, B, and C) *[see Dosage and Administration (2)* and *Warnings and Precautions (5)]*.

8.8 Gender

The pharmacokinetics of posaconazole are comparable in men and women. No adjustment in the dosage of NOXAFIL is necessary based on gender.

8.9 Race

The pharmacokinetic profile of posaconazole is not significantly affected by race. No adjustment in the dosage of NOXAFIL is necessary based on race.

10. OVERDOSAGE

During the clinical trials, some patients received posaconazole up to 1600 mg/day with no adverse reactions noted that were different from the lower doses. In addition, accidental overdose was noted in one patient who took 1200 mg BID for 3 days. No related adverse reactions were noted by the investigator.

Posaconazole is not removed by hemodialysis.

11. DESCRIPTION

NOXAFIL is a triazole antifungal agent available as a suspension for oral administration.

Posaconazole is designated chemically as 4-[4-[4-[4-[[(3*R*,5*R*)-5-(2,4-difluorophenyl)tetrahydro-5-(1*H*-1,2,4-triazol-1-ylmethyl)-3-furanyl]methoxy]phenyl]-1-piperazinyl]phenyl]-2-[(1*S*,2*S*)-1-ethyl-2-hydroxypropyl]-2,4-dihydro-3*H*-1,2,4-triazol-3-one with an empirical formula of $C_{37}H_{42}F_2N_8O_4$ and a molecular weight of 700.8. The chemical structure is:

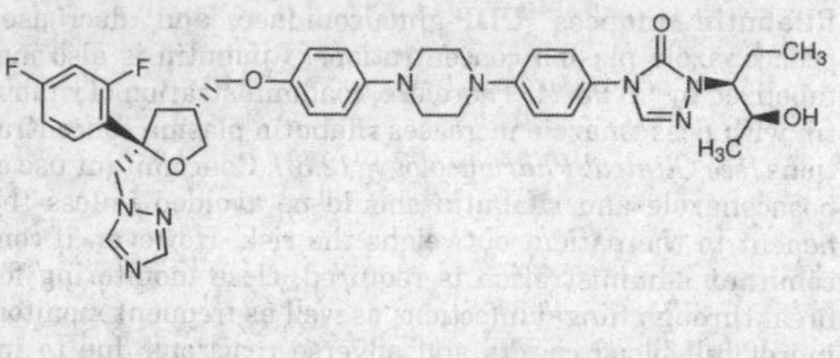

Posaconazole is a white powder and is insoluble in water.

NOXAFIL Oral Suspension is a white, cherry-flavored immediate-release suspension containing 40 mg of posaconazole per mL and the following inactive ingredients: polysorbate 80, simethicone, sodium benzoate, sodium citrate dihydrate, citric acid monohydrate, glycerin, xanthan gum, liquid glucose, titanium dioxide, artificial cherry flavor, and purified water.

12. CLINICAL PHARMACOLOGY

12.1 Mechanism of Action

Posaconazole is a triazole antifungal agent *[see Clinical Pharmacology (12.4)]*.

12.2 Pharmacodynamics

Exposure Response Relationship: In clinical studies of immunocompromised patients, a wide range of plasma exposures to posaconazole was noted. A pharmacokinetic-pharmacodynamic analysis of patient data revealed an apparent association between average posaconazole concentrations (Cav) and prophylactic efficacy. A lower Cav may be associated with an increased risk of treatment failure [defined in the study as treatment discontinuation, use of empiric systemic antifungal therapy (SAF), or invasive fungal infections (IFI)].

To enhance the oral absorption of posaconazole and optimize plasma concentrations:

- Each dose of NOXAFIL should be administered during or immediately (i.e., within 20 minutes) following a full meal. In patients who cannot eat a full meal, each dose of NOXAFIL should be administered with a liquid nutritional supplement or an acidic carbonated beverage. For patients who cannot eat a full meal or tolerate an oral nutritional supplement or an acidic carbonated beverage, alternative antifungal therapy should be considered or patients should be monitored closely for breakthrough fungal infections.
- Patients who have severe diarrhea or vomiting should be monitored closely for breakthrough fungal infections.
- Coadministration of drugs that can decrease the plasma concentrations of posaconazole should generally be avoided unless the benefit outweighs the risk. If such drugs are necessary, patients should be monitored closely for breakthrough fungal infections *[see Drug Interactions (7.2)]*.

12.3 Pharmacokinetics

Absorption: In clinical studies of immunocompromised patients, a wide range of plasma exposures to posaconazole was noted. A pharmacokinetic-pharmacodynamic analysis of patient data revealed an apparent association between average posaconazole concentrations (Cav) and prophylactic efficacy. A lower Cav may be associated with an increased risk of treatment failure [defined in the study as treatment discontinuation, use of empiric systemic antifungal therapy (SAF), or invasive fungal infections (IFI)].

Posaconazole is absorbed with a median T_{max} of ~3 to 5 hours. Dose proportional increases in plasma exposure (AUC) to posaconazole were observed following single oral doses from 50 mg to 800 mg and following multiple-dose administration from 50 mg BID to 400 mg BID. No further increases in exposure were observed when the dose was increased from 400 mg BID to 600 mg BID in febrile neutropenic patients or those with refractory invasive fungal infections. Steady-state plasma concentrations are attained at 7 to 10 days following multiple-dose administration.

Following single-dose administration of 200 mg, the mean AUC and C_{max} of posaconazole are approximately 3 times higher when administered with a nonfat meal and approximately 4 times higher when administered with a high-fat meal (~50 gm fat) relative to the fasted state. Following single-dose administration of 400 mg, the mean AUC and C_{max} of posaconazole are approximately 3 times higher when administered with a liquid nutritional supplement (14 gm fat) relative to the fasted state (see **Table 6**). In order to assure attainment of adequate plasma concentrations, it is recommended to administer posaconazole with food or a nutritional supplement.

[See table 6 at top of page 1669]
[See table 7 at top of previous page]

The mean (%CV) [min-max] posaconazole average steady-state plasma concentrations (Cav) and steady-state pharmacokinetic parameters in patients following administration of 200 mg TID and 400 mg BID of the oral suspension are provided in **Table 8.**

[See table 8 at top of previous page]

Distribution: Posaconazole has an apparent volume of distribution of 1774 L, suggesting extensive extravascular distribution and penetration into the body tissues.

Posaconazole is highly protein bound (>98%), predominantly to albumin.

Metabolism: Posaconazole primarily circulates as the parent compound in plasma. Of the circulating metabolites, the majority are glucuronide conjugates formed via UDP glucuronidation (phase 2 enzymes). Posaconazole does not have any major circulating oxidative (CYP450 mediated) metabolites. The excreted metabolites in urine and feces account for ~17% of the administered radiolabeled dose.

Posaconazole is primarily metabolized via UDP glucuronidation (phase 2 enzymes) and is a substrate for p-glycoprotein (P-gp) efflux. Therefore, inhibitors or inducers of these clearance pathways may affect posaconazole plasma concentrations. A summary of drugs studied clinically, which affect posaconazole concentrations, is provided in **Table 9.**

[See table 9 above]

In vitro studies with human hepatic microsomes and clinical studies indicate that posaconazole is an inhibitor primarily of CYP3A4. A clinical study in healthy volunteers also indicates that posaconazole is a strong CYP3A4 inhibitor as evidenced by a >5-fold increase in midazolam AUC. Therefore, plasma concentrations of drugs predominantly metabolized by CYP3A4 may be increased by posaconazole. A summary of the drugs studied clinically, for which plasma concentrations were affected by posaconazole, is provided in **Table 10** *[see Contraindications (4)* and *Drug Interactions (7.1) including recommendations]*.

[See table 10 above and on next page]

Additional clinical studies demonstrated that no clinically significant effects on zidovudine, lamivudine, indinavir, or caffeine were observed when administered with posaconazole 200 mg QD; therefore, no dose adjustments are required for these coadministered drugs when coadministered with posaconazole 200 mg QD.

Excretion: Posaconazole is eliminated with a mean half-life ($t_{1/2}$) of 35 hours (range: 20–66 hours) and a total body clearance (CL/F) of 32 L/hr. Posaconazole is predominantly eliminated in the feces (71% of the radiolabeled dose up to 120 hours) with the major component eliminated as parent drug (66% of the radiolabeled dose). Renal clearance is a minor elimination pathway, with 13% of the radiolabeled dose excreted in urine up to 120 hours (<0.2% of the radiolabeled dose is parent drug).

12.4 Microbiology

Mechanism of Action:

Posaconazole blocks the synthesis of ergosterol, a key component of the fungal cell membrane, through the inhibition of cytochrome P-450 dependent enzyme lanosterol 14α-demethylase responsible for the conversion of lanosterol to ergosterol in the fungal cell membrane. This results in an accumulation of methylated sterol precursors and a depletion of ergosterol within the cell membrane thus weakening the structure and function of the fungal cell membrane. This may be responsible for the antifungal activity of posaconazole.

Activity in vitro:

Posaconazole has *in vitro* activity against *Aspergillus fumigatus* and *Candida albicans*, including *Candida albicans* isolates from patients refractory to itraconazole or fluconazole or both drugs *[see Clinical Studies (14), Indications and Usage (1) and Dosage and Administration (2)]*.

13. NONCLINICAL TOXICOLOGY

13.1 Carcinogenesis, Mutagenesis, Impairment of Fertility

No drug-related neoplasms were recorded in rats or mice treated with posaconazole for 2 years at doses higher than

Table 9: Summary of the Effect of Coadministered Drugs on Posaconazole in Healthy Volunteers

Coadministered Drug (Postulated Mechanism of Interaction)	Coadministered Drug Dose/Schedule	Posaconazole Dose/ Schedule	Effect on Bioavailability of Posaconazole: Change in Mean C_{max} (ratio estimate*; 90% CI of the ratio estimate)	Effect on Bioavailability of Posaconazole: Change in Mean AUC (ratio estimate*; 90% CI of the ratio estimate)
Efavirenz (UDP-G Induction)	400 mg QD × 10 and 20 days	400 mg (oral suspension) BID × 10 and 20 days	↓45% (0.55; 0.47–0.66)	↓ 50% (0.50; 0.43–0.60)
Fosamprenavir (unknown mechanism)	700 mg BID × 10 days	200 mg QD on the 1st day, 200 mg BID on the 2nd day, then 400 mg BID × 8 Days	↓21% 0.79 (0.71–0.89)	↓23% 0.77 (0.68–0.87)
Rifabutin (UDP-G Induction)	300 mg QD × 17 days	200 mg (tablets) QD × 10 days	↓ 43% (0.57; 0.43–0.75)	↓ 49% (0.51; 0.37–0.71)
Phenytoin (UDP-G Induction)	200 mg QD × 10 days	200 mg (tablets) QD × 10 days	↓ 41% (0.59; 0.44–0.79)	↓ 50% (0.50; 0.36–0.71)
Cimetidine (Alteration of Gastric pH)	400 mg BID × 10 days	200 mg (tablets) QD × 10 days	↓ 39% (0.61; 0.53–0.70)	↓ 39% (0.61; 0.54–0.69)
Esomeprazole (Increase in gastric pH)	40 mg QAM × 3 days	400 mg (oral suspension) single dose	↓ 46% (0.54; 0.43–0.69)	↓ 32% (0.68; 0.57–0.81)
Metoclopramide (Increase in gastric motility)	10 mg TID × 2 days	400 mg (oral suspension) single dose	↓ 21% (0.79; 0.72–0.87)	↓ 19% (0.81; 0.72–0.91)

* Ratio Estimate is the ratio of coadministered drug plus posaconazole to posaconazole alone for C_{max} or AUC.

Table 10: Summary of the Effect of Posaconazole on Coadministered Drugs in Healthy Volunteers and Patients

Coadministered Drug (Postulated Mechanism of Interaction is Inhibition of CYP3A4 by posaconazole)	Coadministered Drug Dose/Schedule	Posaconazole Dose/ Schedule	Effect on Bioavailability of Coadministered Drugs: Change in Mean C_{max} (ratio estimate*; 90% CI of the ratio estimate)	Effect on Bioavailability of Coadministered Drugs: Change in Mean AUC (ratio estimate*; 90% CI of the ratio estimate)
Sirolimus	2-mg single oral dose	400 mg (oral suspension) BID × 16 days	↑ 572% (6.72; 5.62–8.03)	↑ 788% (8.88; 7.26–10.9)
Cyclosporin	Stable maintenance dose in heart transplant recipients	200 mg (tablets) QD × 10 days	↑ cyclosporine whole blood trough concentrations Cyclosporine dose reductions of up to 29% were required	
Tacrolimus	0.05-mg/kg single oral dose	400 mg (oral suspension) BID × 7 days	↑ 121% (2.21; 2.01–2.42)	↑ 358% (4.58; 4.03–5.19)
Simvastatin	40-mg single oral dose	100 mg (oral suspension) QD × 13 days	Simvastatin ↑ 841% (9.41, 7.13–12.44) Simvastatin Acid ↑ 817% (9.17, 7.36–11.43)	Simvastatin ↑ 931% (10.31, 8.40–12.67) Simvastatin Acid ↑634% (7.34, 5.82–9.25)
		200 mg (oral suspension) QD × 13 days	Simvastatin ↑ 1041% (11.41, 7.99–16.29) Simvastatin Acid ↑ 851% (9.51, 8.15–11.10)	Simvastatin ↑ 960% (10.60, 8.63–13.02) Simvastatin Acid ↑748% (8.48, 7.04–10.23)

(Table continued on next page)

the clinical dose. In a 2-year carcinogenicity study, rats were given posaconazole orally at doses up to 20 mg/kg (females), or 30 mg/kg (males). These doses are equivalent to 3.9 or 3.5 times the exposure achieved with a 400-mg BID regimen, respectively, based on steady-state AUC in healthy volunteers administered a high-fat meal (400-mg BID regimen). In the mouse study, mice were treated at oral doses up to 60 mg/kg/day or 4.8 times the exposure achieved with a 400-mg BID regimen.

Posaconazole was not genotoxic or clastogenic when evaluated in bacterial mutagenicity (Ames), a chromosome aberration study in human peripheral blood lymphocytes, a Chinese hamster ovary cell mutagenicity study, and a mouse bone marrow micronucleus study.

Posaconazole had no effect on fertility of male rats at a dose up to 180 mg/kg (1.7 × the 400-mg BID regimen based on steady-state plasma concentrations in healthy volunteers) or female rats at a dose up to 45 mg/kg (2.2 × the 400-mg BID regimen).

14. CLINICAL STUDIES

14.1 Prophylaxis of *Aspergillus* and *Candida* Infections

Two randomized, controlled studies were conducted using posaconazole as prophylaxis for the prevention of invasive fungal infections (IFIs) among patients at high risk due to severely compromised immune systems.

The first study (Study 1) was a randomized, double-blind trial that compared posaconazole oral suspension (200 mg three times a day) with fluconazole capsules (400 mg once daily) as prophylaxis against invasive fungal infections in allogeneic hematopoietic stem cell transplant (HSCT) recipients with Graft versus Host Disease (GVHD). Efficacy of prophylaxis was evaluated using a composite endpoint of

Table 10 *(cont.)*: Summary of the Effect of Posaconazole on Coadministered Drugs in Healthy Volunteers and Patients

Coadministered Drug (Postulated Mechanism of Interaction is Inhibition of CYP3A4 by posaconazole)	Coadministered Drug Dose/Schedule	Posaconazole Dose/Schedule	Effect on Bioavailability of Coadministered Drugs: Change in Mean C_{max} (ratio estimate*; 90% CI of the ratio estimate)	Effect on Bioavailability of Coadministered Drugs: Change in Mean AUC (ratio estimate*; 90% CI of the ratio estimate)
Midazolam	0.4-mg single IV dose†	200 mg (oral suspension) BID × 7 days	↑ 30% (1.3; 1.13–1.48)	↑ 362% (4.62; 4.02–5.3)
	0.4-mg single IV dose†	400 mg (oral suspension) BID × 7 days	↑62% (1.62; 1.41–1.86)	↑524% (6.24; 5.43–7.16)
	2-mg single oral dose†	200 mg (oral suspension) QD × 7 days	↑ 169% (2.69; 2.46–2.93)	↑ 470% (5.70; 4.82–6.74)
	2-mg single oral dose†	400 mg (oral suspension) BID × 7 days	↑ 138% (2.38; 2.13–2.66)	↑ 397% (4.97; 4.46–5.54)
Rifabutin	300 mg QD × 17 days	200 mg (tablets) QD × 10 days	↑ 31% (1.31; 1.10–1.57)	↑ 72% (1.72;1.51–1.95)
Phenytoin	200 mg QD PO × 10 days	200 mg (tablets) QD × 10 days	↑ 16% (1.16; 0.85–1.57)	↑ 16% (1.16; 0.84–1.59)
Ritonavir	100 mg QD × 14 days	400 mg (oral suspension) BID × 7 days	↑ 49% (1.49; 1.04–2.15)	↑ 80% (1.8;1.39–2.31)
Atazanavir	300 mg QD × 14 days	400 mg (oral suspension) BID × 7 days	↑ 155% (2.55; 1.89–3.45)	↑ 268% (3.68; 2.89–4.70)
Atazanavir/ritonavir boosted regimen	300 mg/100 mg QD × 14 days	400 mg (oral suspension) BID × 7 days	↑ 53% (1.53; 1.13–2.07)	↑ 146% (2.46; 1.93–3.13)

* Ratio Estimate is the ratio of coadministered drug plus posaconazole to coadministered drug alone for C_{max} or AUC.
† The mean terminal half-life of midazolam was increased from 3 hours to 7 to 11 hours during coadministration with posaconazole.

proven/probable IFIs, death, or treatment with systemic antifungal therapy (patients may have met more than one of these criteria). Study 1 assessed all patients while on study therapy plus 7 days and at 16 weeks post-randomization. The mean duration of therapy was comparable between the 2 treatment groups (80 days, posaconazole; 77 days, fluconazole). **Table 11** contains the results from Study 1.

Table 11: Results from Blinded Clinical Study 1 in Prophylaxis of IFI in All Randomized Patients with Hematopoietic Stem Cell Transplant (HSCT) and Graft-vs.-Host Disease (GVHD)

	Posaconazole n=301	Fluconazole n=299
On therapy plus 7 days		
Clinical Failure*	50 (17%)	55 (18%)
Failure due to:		
Proven/Probable IFI	7 (2%)	22 (7%)
(*Aspergillus*)	3 (1%)	17 (6%)
(*Candida*)	1 (<1%)	3 (1%)
(Other)	3 (1%)	2 (1%)
All Deaths	22 (7%)	24 (8%)
Proven/probable fungal infection prior to death	2 (<1%)	6 (2%)
SAF†	27 (9%)	25 (8%)
Through 16 weeks		
Clinical Failure*,‡	99 (33%)	110 (37%)
Failure due to:		
Proven/Probable IFI	16 (5%)	27 (9%)
(*Aspergillus*)	7 (2%)	21 (7%)
(*Candida*)	4 (1%)	4 (1%)
(Other)	5 (2%)	2 (1%)
All Deaths	58 (19%)	59 (20%)
Proven/probable fungal infection prior to death	10 (3%)	16 (5%)
SAF†	26 (9%)	30 (10%)
Event free lost to follow-up§	24 (8%)	30 (10%)

* Patients may have met more than one criterion defining failure.
† Use of systemic antifungal therapy (SAF) criterion is based on protocol definitions (empiric/IFI usage >4 consecutive days).
‡ 95% confidence interval (posaconazole-fluconazole) = (-11.5%, +3.7%).
§ Patients who are lost to follow-up (not observed for 112 days), and who did not meet another clinical failure endpoint. These patients were considered failures.

The second study (Study 2) was a randomized, open-label study that compared posaconazole oral suspension (200 mg 3 times a day) with fluconazole suspension (400 mg once daily) or itraconazole oral solution (200 mg twice a day) as prophylaxis against IFIs in neutropenic patients who were receiving cytotoxic chemotherapy for acute myelogenous leukemia or myelodysplastic syndromes. As in Study 1, efficacy of prophylaxis was evaluated using a composite endpoint of proven/probable IFIs, death, or treatment with systemic antifungal therapy (Patients might have met more than one of these criteria). Study 2 assessed patients while on treatment plus 7 days and 100 days postrandomization. The mean duration of therapy was comparable between the 2 treatment groups (29 days, posaconazole; 25 days, fluconazole or itraconazole). **Table 12** contains the results from Study 2.

Table 12: Results from Open-Label Clinical Study 2 in Prophylaxis of IFI in All Randomized Patients with Hematologic Malignancy and Prolonged Neutropenia

	Posaconazole n=304	Fluconazole/ Itraconazole n=298
On therapy plus 7 days		
Clinical Failure*,†	82 (27%)	126 (42%)
Failure due to:		
Proven/Probable IFI	7 (2%)	25 (8%)
(*Aspergillus*)	2 (1%)	20 (7%)
(*Candida*)	3 (1%)	2 (1%)
(Other)	2 (1%)	3 (1%)
All Deaths	17 (6%)	25 (8%)
Proven/probable fungal infection prior to death	1 (<1%)	2 (1%)
SAF‡	67 (22%)	98 (33%)
Through 100 days postrandomization		
Clinical Failure†	158 (52%)	191 (64%)
Failure due to:		
Proven/Probable IFI	14 (5%)	33 (11%)
(*Aspergillus*)	2 (1%)	26 (9%)
(*Candida*)	10 (3%)	4 (1%)
(Other)	2 (1%)	3 (1%)
All Deaths	44 (14%)	64 (21%)
Proven/probable fungal infection prior to death	2 (1%)	16 (5%)
SAF‡	98 (32%)	125 (42%)
Event free lost to follow-up§	34 (11%)	24 (8%)

* 95% confidence interval (posaconazole-fluconazole/itraconazole) = (-22.9%, -7.8%).
† Patients may have met more than one criterion defining failure.
‡ Use of systemic antifungal therapy (SAF) criterion is based on protocol definitions (empiric/IFI usage >3 consecutive days).
§ Patients who are lost to follow-up (not observed for 100 days), and who did not meet another clinical failure endpoint. These patients were considered failures.

In summary, 2 clinical studies of prophylaxis were conducted. As seen in the accompanying tables (Tables 11 and 12), clinical failure represented a composite endpoint of breakthrough IFI, mortality and use of systemic antifungal therapy. In Study 1 (Table 11), the clinical failure rate of posaconazole (33%) was similar to fluconazole (37%), (95% CI for the difference posaconazole–comparator -11.5% to 3.7%) while in Study 2 (Table 12) clinical failure was lower for patients treated with posaconazole (27%) when compared to patients treated with fluconazole or itraconazole (42%), (95% CI for the difference posaconazole–comparator -22.9% to -7.8%).

All-cause mortality was similar at 16 weeks for both treatment arms in Study 1 [POS 58/301 (19%) vs. FLU 59/299 (20%)]; all-cause mortality was lower at 100 days for posaconazole-treated patients in Study 2 [POS 44/304 (14%) vs. FLU/ITZ 64/298 (21%)]. Both studies demonstrated substantially fewer breakthrough infections caused by *Aspergillus* species in patients receiving posaconazole prophylaxis when compared to patients receiving fluconazole or itraconazole.

14.2 Treatment of Oropharyngeal Candidiasis

Study 3 was a randomized, controlled, evaluator-blinded study in HIV-infected patients with oropharyngeal candidiasis. Patients were treated with posaconazole or fluconazole oral suspension (both posaconazole and fluconazole were given as follows: 100 mg twice a day for 1 day followed by 100 mg once a day for 13 days).

Clinical and mycological outcomes were assessed after 14 days of treatment and at 4 weeks after the end of treatment. Patients who received at least 1 dose of study medication and had a positive oral swish culture of *Candida* species at baseline were included in the analyses (see **Table 13**). The majority of the subjects had *C. albicans* as the baseline pathogen.

Clinical success at Day 14 (complete or partial resolution of all ulcers and/or plaques and symptoms) and clinical relapse rates (recurrence of signs or symptoms after initial cure or improvement) 4 weeks after the end of treatment were similar between the treatment arms (see **Table 13**).

Mycologic eradication rates (absence of colony forming units in quantitative culture at the end of therapy, Day 14), as well as mycologic relapse rates (4 weeks after the end of treatment) were also similar between the treatment arms (see **Table 13**).

Table 13: Clinical Success, Mycological Eradication, and Relapse Rates in Oropharyngeal Candidiasis

	Posaconazole	Fluconazole
Clinical Success at End of Therapy (Day 14)	155/169 (91.7%)	148/160 (92.5%)
Clinical Relapse (4 Weeks after End of Therapy)	45/155 (29.0%)	52/148 (35.1%)

Mycological Eradication (absence of CFU) at End of Therapy (Day 14)	88/169 (52.1%)	80/160 (50.0%)
Mycological Relapse (4 Weeks after End of Treatment)	49/88 (55.6%)	51/80 (63.7%)

Mycologic response rates, using a criterion for success as a posttreatment quantitative culture with ≤20 colony forming units (CFU/mL) were also similar between the two groups (posaconazole 68.0%, fluconazole 68.1%). The clinical significance of this finding is unknown.

14.3 Treatment of Oropharyngeal Candidiasis Refractory to Treatment with Fluconazole or Itraconazole

Study 4 was a noncomparative study of posaconazole oral suspension in HIV-infected subjects with OPC that was refractory to treatment with fluconazole or itraconazole. An episode of OPC was considered refractory if there was failure to improve or worsening of OPC after a standard course of therapy with fluconazole greater than or equal to 100 mg/day for at least 10 consecutive days or itraconazole 200 mg/day for at least 10 consecutive days and treatment with either fluconazole or itraconazole had not been discontinued for more than 14 days prior to treatment with posaconazole. Of the 199 subjects enrolled in this study, 89 subjects met these strict criteria for refractory infection.

Forty-five subjects with refractory OPC were treated with posaconazole 400 mg BID for 3 days, followed by 400 mg QD for 25 days with an option for further treatment during a 3-month maintenance period. Following a dosing amendment, a further 44 subjects were treated with posaconazole 400 mg BID for 28 days. The efficacy of posaconazole was assessed by the clinical success (cure or improvement) rate after 4 weeks of treatment. The clinical success rate was 74.2% (66/89). The clinical success rates for both the original and the amended dosing regimens were similar (73.3% and 75.0%, respectively).

15 REFERENCES

1. Clinical and Laboratory Standards Institute (CLSI) Reference Method for Broth Dilution Antifungal Susceptibility Testing of Yeasts; Approved Standard - 3rd edition. CLSI document M 27- A3. CLSI, 940 West Valley Rd. Suite 1400, Wayne, PA 19087-1898, 2008.
2. CLSI. Method for Antifungal Disk Diffusion Susceptibility Testing of Yeasts; Approved Guideline - 2nd edition. M44 - A2, CLSI, Wayne, PA, 2009.
3. CLSI. Reference Method for Broth Dilution Antifungal Susceptibility Testing of M38 - A2, CLSI, Wayne, PA, 2008.
4. CLSI. Method for Antifungal Disc Diffusion Susceptibility Testing of Nondermatophyte Filamentous Fungi; Approved Standard - 2nd edition. M51-A, CLSI, Wayne, PA, 2010.

16. HOW SUPPLIED/STORAGE AND HANDLING

Supplied with each bottle is a plastic dosing spoon calibrated for measuring 2.5-mL and 5-mL doses.

Store at 25°C (77°F); excursions permitted to 15°–30°C (59°–86°F). DO NOT FREEZE.

17. PATIENT COUNSELING INFORMATION

17.1 Administration with Food

Take each dose of NOXAFIL Oral Suspension during or immediately (i.e., within 20 minutes) following a full meal. In patients who cannot eat a full meal each dose of NOXAFIL should be administered with a liquid nutritional supplement or an acidic carbonated beverage (e.g., ginger ale) in order to enhance absorption.

17.2 Drug Interactions

Patients should be advised to inform their physician immediately if they:

- develop severe diarrhea or vomiting.
- are currently taking drugs that are known to prolong the QTc interval and are metabolized through CYP3A4.
- are currently taking a cyclosporine or tacrolimus, or if you notice swelling of 1 leg or shortness of breath.
- are taking other drugs or before they begin taking other drugs as certain drugs can decrease or increase the plasma concentrations of posaconazole.

17.3 Serious and Potentially Serious Adverse Reactions

Patients should be advised to inform their physician immediately if they:

- notice a change in heart rate or heart rhythm, or have a heart condition or circulatory disease. Posaconazole can be administered with caution to patients with potentially proarrhythmic conditions.
- are pregnant, plan to become pregnant, or are nursing.
- have liver disease or you develop itching, your eyes or skin turn yellow, you feel more tired than usual or feel like you have the flu.
- have ever had an allergic reaction to other antifungal medicines such as ketoconazole, fluconazole, itraconazole, or voriconazole.

Manuf. for: Merck Sharp & Dohme Corp., a subsidiary of **MERCK & CO., INC.**, Whitehouse Station, NJ 08889, USA

Manuf. by: Patheon Inc., Whitby, Ontario, Canada L1N 5Z5

U.S. Patent Nos. 5,661,151; 5,703,079; and 6,958,337.

BOOST® is a registered trademark of Société des Produits Nestlé, S.A.

Revised: 11/2012

056592-POS-SUo-USPI-27

PATIENT INFORMATION

NOXAFIL®

(posaconazole) ORAL SUSPENSION

Read the Patient Information that comes with NOXAFIL Oral Suspension before you start taking it and each time you get a refill. There may be new information. This information does not replace talking with your doctor about your condition or treatment. Only your doctor can prescribe NOXAFIL and determine if it is right for you.

What is NOXAFIL?

- NOXAFIL is a prescription medicine that is used to prevent invasive fungal infections (infections that can spread throughout the body) caused by *Aspergillus* or *Candida* in patients with weak immune systems because of medicines or diseases [such as stem cell transplantation with graft-vs.-host disease or chemotherapy for hematologic malignancy (blood cancers)].
- NOXAFIL is also used to treat fungal infections in the mouth or throat area (known as "thrush") caused by fungi called *Candida*. NOXAFIL can be used as initial treatment or as a treatment after itraconazole and/or fluconazole have failed.

NOXAFIL is for adults and children over 13 years of age.

What should I tell my doctor before taking NOXAFIL?

Tell your doctor about all your health conditions, including if you:

- are taking certain drugs that suppress your immune system like **cyclosporine (Neoral®)**, or **tacrolimus (Prograf®)**. Serious and rare fatal toxicity from cyclosporine has occurred when taken in combination with posaconazole, and, therefore, reduction of the dose of drugs like **cyclosporine** or **tacrolimus** and frequent monitoring of drug levels of these medicines is necessary when taking them in combination with NOXAFIL.
- are taking certain drugs for HIV infection, such as **ritonavir, atazanavir, efavirenz,** or **fosamprenavir**. Efavirenz can cause a decrease in NOXAFIL levels in the body, and, therefore, it is recommended that efavirenz should not be administered with NOXAFIL. Similarly to efavirenz, fosamprenavir may also decrease levels of NOXAFIL in the body.
- are taking **midazolam**, a hypnotic and sedative medication. NOXAFIL in combination with midazolam increases the midazolam plasma concentrations, which could increase and prolong sleepiness.
- have ever had an allergic reaction to other antifungal medicines such as ketoconazole, fluconazole, itraconazole, or voriconazole.
- are taking any other medicines, including prescription and nonprescription medicines, vitamins, and herbal supplements.
- have, or have had, liver problems. Your doctor may do blood tests to make sure you should take NOXAFIL.
- have, or have had, an abnormal heart rate or rhythm.
- are, or think you are, pregnant. Do not use NOXAFIL during pregnancy unless specifically advised by your doctor. You should use effective birth control while you are taking NOXAFIL if you are a woman who could become pregnant.

Contact your doctor immediately if you become pregnant while being treated with NOXAFIL.

Do not breastfeed while being treated with NOXAFIL, unless specifically advised by your doctor.

Who should not take NOXAFIL?

- Do NOT take NOXAFIL if you are taking any of the medicines listed below. If any of these medicines are taken together with NOXAFIL, serious or life-threatening side effects from these medicines, or a decrease in the effect of NOXAFIL can occur. Tell your doctor right away if you are taking any of these medicines:
  - sirolimus
  - ergot alkaloids (ergotamine, dihydroergotamine, methylsergide, methylergonovine, ergonovine, or bromocriptine)
  - pimozide
  - quinidine
  - certain statin medicines (medicines that lower cholesterol), (atorvastatin, lovastatin, and simvastatin)
  - rifabutin
  - phenytoin
  - cimetidine
- If you have questions or are uncertain about your medicines, talk with your doctor or pharmacist.
- Do not take NOXAFIL if you are allergic to anything in it. There is a list of what is in NOXAFIL at the end of this leaflet.

Can I take other medicines with NOXAFIL?

NOXAFIL and many medicines can interact with each other, and some must not be taken together (see **"Who should not take NOXAFIL?"**). The dose of other medicines may need to be adjusted when taken with NOXAFIL [for example, **cyclosporine (Neoral®), tacrolimus (Prograf®)**] (see **"What should I tell my doctor before taking NOXAFIL?"**).

Knowing the medicines that you are taking is important. **Tell your doctor** about all the medicines you take including prescription and nonprescription medicines, vitamins, and herbal supplements. Keep a list of them with you to show your doctor or pharmacist. Do not take any new medicine without talking to your doctor.

What are possible side effects of NOXAFIL?

The most commonly reported side effects were fever, nausea, diarrhea, vomiting, and headache.

Rarely, NOXAFIL may cause serious or life-threatening side effects. It may also cause severe drug interactions as discussed above. Call your doctor right away if you have any of the symptoms listed below.

Changes in heart rate or rhythm. People who have certain heart conditions or who take certain other medicines have a higher chance for this problem.

Rarely, very serious liver problems were reported in patients with serious underlying medical conditions. Your doctor may test your liver function while you are taking NOXAFIL. Call your doctor if you have any of these symptoms, as these may be signs of liver problems: you have itching, your eyes or skin turn yellow, you feel more tired than usual or feel like you have the flu, or you have nausea or vomiting.

Rarely, an increase in blood clots may occur in patients with blood cancers or post-stem cell transplantation. These events may or may not be further increased in patients also on posaconazole and primarily occurred in patients also receiving cyclosporine or tacrolimus. If you notice swelling of one leg or shortness of breath, notify your doctor immediately.

These are not all the side effects associated with NOXAFIL. For more information, ask your doctor or pharmacist. If you experience any unusual effects while taking NOXAFIL, contact your doctor immediately.

How do I take NOXAFIL?

- NOXAFIL comes in cherry-flavored liquid form. Shake NOXAFIL Oral Suspension well before use.
- Take NOXAFIL for as long as your doctor tells you. Take each dose of NOXAFIL during or immediately (i.e., within 20 minutes) following a full meal. In patients who cannot eat a full meal, each dose of NOXAFIL should be administered with a liquid nutritional supplement or an acidic carbonated beverage (e.g., ginger ale).
- Follow your doctor's instructions on how much NOXAFIL you should take and when.

If you miss a dose of NOXAFIL, take it as soon as you remember.

- If you take too much NOXAFIL, call your doctor or poison control center immediately.
- Tell your doctor right away if you develop severe diarrhea or vomiting.

A measured dosing spoon is provided, marked for doses of 2.5 mL and 5 mL.

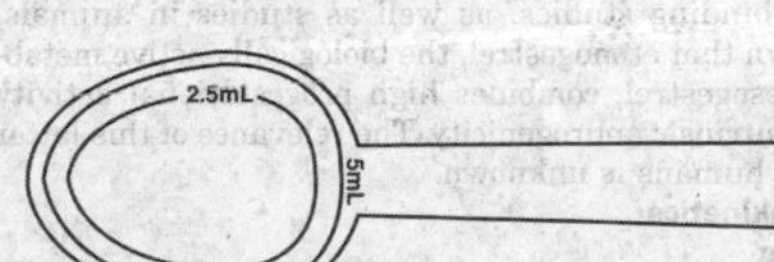

It is recommended that the spoon is rinsed with water after each administration and before storage.

How do I store NOXAFIL?

- **Store at 25°C (77°F); excursions permitted to 15°–30°C (59°–86°F) [see USP Controlled Room Temperature]. DO NOT FREEZE. Keep all containers tightly closed.**
- **Keep NOXAFIL, as well as other medicines, out of the reach of children.**

General information about NOXAFIL

Doctors can prescribe medicines for conditions that are not in this leaflet. Use NOXAFIL only as directed by your doctor. Do not give it to other people, even if they have the same symptoms as you. It may harm them.

This leaflet gives the most important information about NOXAFIL. For more information, talk to your doctor. You can ask your doctor or pharmacist for information about NOXAFIL that is written for health care professionals.

What is in NOXAFIL?
Active ingredient: posaconazole.
Inactive ingredients: polysorbate 80, simethicone, sodium benzoate, sodium citrate dihydrate, citric acid monohydrate, glycerin, xanthan gum, liquid glucose, titanium dioxide, artificial cherry flavor, and purified water.
Manuf. for: Merck Sharp & Dohme Corp., a subsidiary of **MERCK & CO., INC.,** Whitehouse Station, NJ 08889, USA
Manuf. by: Patheon Inc., Whitby, Ontario, Canada L1N 5Z5
U.S. Patent Nos. 5,661,151; 5,703,079; and 6,958,337.

Revised: 12/2012
056592-POS-SUo-PPI-11
Rx only

NUVARING® ℞

(etonogestrel/ethinyl estradiol vaginal ring)

delivers 0.120 mg/0.015 mg per day

Women should be counseled that this product does not protect against HIV infection (AIDS) and other sexually transmitted diseases.

FOR VAGINAL USE ONLY

DESCRIPTION

NuvaRing® (etonogestrel/ethinyl estradiol vaginal ring) is a non-biodegradable, flexible, transparent, colorless to almost colorless, combination contraceptive vaginal ring containing two active components, a progestin, etonogestrel (13-ethyl-17-hydroxy-11-methylene-18,19-dinor-17α-pregn-4-en-20-yn-3-one) and an estrogen, ethinyl estradiol (19-nor-17α-pregna-1,3,5(10)-trien-20-yne-3, 17-diol). When placed in the vagina, each ring releases on average 0.120 mg/day of etonogestrel and 0.015 mg/day of ethinyl estradiol over a three-week period of use. NuvaRing® is made of ethylene vinylacetate copolymers (28% and 9% vinylacetate) and magnesium stearate and contains 11.7 mg etonogestrel and 2.7 mg ethinyl estradiol. NuvaRing® is latex-free. NuvaRing® has an outer diameter of 54 mm and a cross-sectional diameter of 4 mm. The molecular weights for etonogestrel and ethinyl estradiol are 324.46 and 296.40, respectively.

The structural formulas are as follows:

ETONOGESTREL

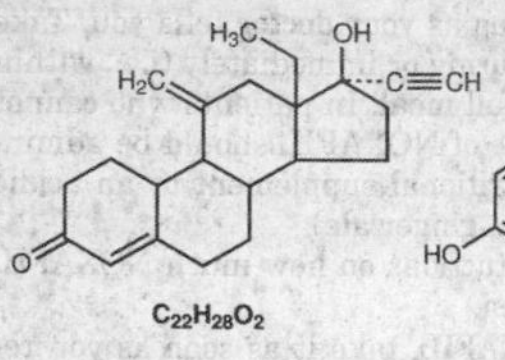

$C_{22}H_{28}O_2$

ETHINYL ESTRADIOL

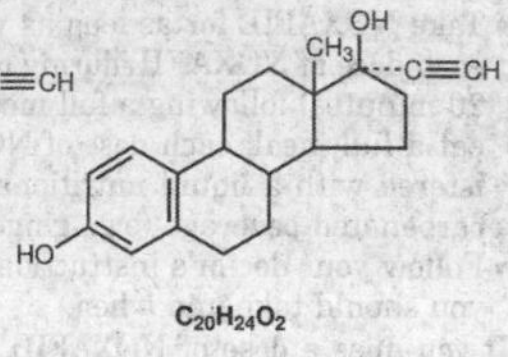

$C_{20}H_{24}O_2$

CLINICAL PHARMACOLOGY

Combination hormonal contraceptives act by suppression of gonadotropins. Although the primary effect of this action is inhibition of ovulation, other alterations include changes in the cervical mucus (which increase the difficulty of sperm entry into the uterus) and the endometrium (which reduce the likelihood of implantation).

Receptor binding studies, as well as studies in animals, have shown that etonogestrel, the biologically active metabolite of desogestrel, combines high progestational activity with low intrinsic androgenicity. The relevance of this latter finding in humans is unknown.

Pharmacokinetics

Absorption

Etonogestrel

Etonogestrel released by NuvaRing® is rapidly absorbed. The bioavailability of etonogestrel after vaginal administration is approximately 100%. The serum etonogestrel and ethinyl estradiol concentrations observed during three weeks of NuvaRing® use are summarized in Table I.

Ethinyl estradiol

Ethinyl estradiol released by NuvaRing® is rapidly absorbed. The bioavailability of ethinyl estradiol after vaginal administration is approximately 56%, which is comparable to that with oral administration of ethinyl estradiol. The serum ethinyl estradiol concentrations observed during three weeks of NuvaRing® use are summarized in Table I.

TABLE I: MEAN (SD) SERUM ETONOGESTREL AND ETHINYL ESTRADIOL CONCENTRATIONS (n=16).

	1 week	2 weeks	3 weeks
etonogestrel (pg/mL)	1578 (408)	1476 (362)	1374 (328)
ethinyl estradiol (pg/mL)	19.1 (4.5)	18.3 (4.3)	17.6 (4.3)

The pharmacokinetic profile of etonogestrel and ethinyl estradiol during use of NuvaRing® is shown in Figure 1.

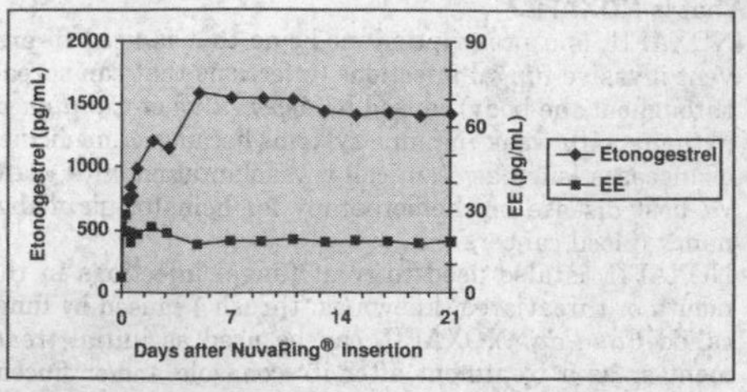

Figure 1. Mean serum concentration-time profile of etonogestrel and ethinyl estradiol during three weeks of NuvaRing® use.

The pharmacokinetic parameters of etonogestrel and ethinyl estradiol were determined during one cycle of NuvaRing® use in 16 healthy female subjects and are summarized in Table II.

[See table II below]

Distribution

Etonogestrel

Etonogestrel is approximately 32% bound to sex hormone-binding globulin (SHBG) and approximately 66% bound to albumin in blood.

Ethinyl estradiol

Ethinyl estradiol is highly but not specifically bound to serum albumin (98.5%) and induces an increase in the serum concentrations of SHBG.

Metabolism

In vitro data shows that both etonogestrel and ethinyl estradiol are metabolized in liver microsomes by the cytochrome P450 3A4 isoenzyme. Ethinyl estradiol is primarily metabolized by aromatic hydroxylation, but a wide variety of hydroxylated and methylated metabolites are formed. These are present as free metabolites and as sulfate and glucuronide conjugates. The hydroxylated ethinyl estradiol metabolites have weak estrogenic activity. The biological activity of etonogestrel metabolites is unknown.

Excretion

Etonogestrel and ethinyl estradiol are primarily eliminated in urine, bile and feces.

Special Populations

Race

No formal studies were conducted to evaluate the effect of race on the pharmacokinetics of NuvaRing®.

Hepatic Insufficiency

No formal studies were conducted to evaluate the effect of hepatic disease on the pharmacokinetics, safety, and efficacy of NuvaRing®. However, steroid hormones may be poorly metabolized in women with impaired liver function (see PRECAUTIONS).

Renal Insufficiency

No formal studies were conducted to evaluate the effect of renal disease on the pharmacokinetics, safety, and efficacy of NuvaRing®.

TABLE II: MEAN (SD) PHARMACOKINETIC PARAMETERS OF NuvaRing® (n=16).

Hormone	C_{max} pg/mL	T_{max} hr	$t_{1/2}$ hr	CL L/hr
etonogestrel	1716 (445)	200.3 (69.6)	29.3 (6.1)	3.4 (0.8)
ethinyl estradiol	34.7 (17.5)	59.3 (67.5)	44.7 (28.8)	34.8 (11.6)

C_{max}- maximum serum drug concentration
T_{max}- time at which maximum serum drug concentration occurs
$t_{1/2}$- elimination half-life, calculated by $0.693/K_{elim}$
CL - apparent clearance

Drug-Drug Interactions

Interactions between contraceptive steroids and other drugs have been reported in the literature (see PRECAUTIONS). The drug interactions of NuvaRing® were evaluated in several studies.

A single-dose vaginal administration of an oil-based 1200 mg miconazole nitrate capsule increased the serum concentrations of etonogestrel and ethinyl estradiol by approximately 17% and 16%, respectively. Following multiple doses of 200 mg miconazole nitrate by vaginal suppository or vaginal cream, the mean serum concentrations of etonogestrel and ethinyl estradiol increased by up to 40%.

A single-dose vaginal administration of 100 mg water-based nonoxynol-9 spermicide gel did not affect the serum concentrations of etonogestrel or ethinyl estradiol.

The serum concentrations of etonogestrel and ethinyl estradiol were not affected by concomitant administration of oral amoxicillin or doxycycline in standard dosages during 10 days of antibiotic treatment.

Tampon Use

The use of tampons had no effect on serum concentrations of etonogestrel and ethinyl estradiol during use of NuvaRing®.

INDICATIONS AND USAGE

NuvaRing® is indicated for the prevention of pregnancy in women who elect to use this product as a method of contraception. Like oral contraceptives, NuvaRing® is highly effective if used as recommended in this label.

In three large clinical trials of 13 cycles of NuvaRing® use, pregnancy rates were between one and two per 100 women-years of use. Table III lists the pregnancy rates for users of various contraceptive methods.

[See table III at top of next page]

CONTRAINDICATIONS

NuvaRing® should not be used in women who currently have the following conditions:

- Thrombophlebitis or thromboembolic disorders
- A past history of deep vein thrombophlebitis or thromboembolic disorders
- Cerebral vascular or coronary artery disease (current or history)
- Valvular heart disease with thrombogenic complications
- Severe hypertension
- Diabetes with vascular involvement
- Headaches with focal neurological symptoms
- Major surgery with prolonged immobilization
- Known or suspected carcinoma of the breast or personal history of breast cancer
- Carcinoma of the endometrium or other known or suspected estrogen-dependent neoplasia
- Undiagnosed abnormal genital bleeding
- Cholestatic jaundice of pregnancy or jaundice with prior hormonal contraceptive use
- Hepatic tumors (benign or malignant) or active liver disease
- Known or suspected pregnancy
- Heavy smoking (≥15 cigarettes per day) and over age 35
- Hypersensitivity to any of the components of NuvaRing®

WARNINGS

Cigarette smoking increases the risk of serious cardiovascular side effects from combination oral contraceptive use. This risk increases with age and with heavy smoking (15 or more cigarettes per day) and is quite marked in women over 35 years of age. Women who use combination hormonal contraceptives, including NuvaRing®, should be strongly advised not to smoke.

NuvaRing® and other contraceptives that contain both an estrogen and a progestin are called combination hormonal contraceptives. There is no epidemiologic data available to determine whether safety and efficacy with the vaginal route of administration of combination hormonal contraceptives would be different than the oral route.

The use of oral contraceptives is associated with increased risks of several serious conditions including venous and arterial thrombotic and thromboembolic events (such as myocardial infarction, thromboembolism, and stroke), hepatic neoplasia, gallbladder disease, and hypertension, although the risk of serious morbidity or mortality is very small in healthy women without underlying risk factors. The risk of morbidity and mortality increases significantly in the presence of other underlying risk factors such as certain inherited thrombophilias, hypertension, hyperlipidemias, obesity, and diabetes.

The information contained in this package insert is principally based on studies carried out in women who used oral contraceptives with formulations of higher doses of estrogens and progestogens than those in common use today. The effect of long-term use of oral contraceptives with lower doses of both estrogens and progestogens remains to be determined.

Throughout this labeling, epidemiologic studies reported are of two types: retrospective or case control studies and prospective or cohort studies. Case control studies provide a measure of the relative risk of a disease, namely, a *ratio* of the incidence of a disease among oral contraceptive users to that among non-users. The relative risk does not provide information on the actual clinical occurrence of a disease. Cohort studies provide a measure of attributable risk, which is the *difference* in the incidence of disease between oral contraceptive users and non-users. The attributable risk does provide information about the actual occurrence of a disease in the population. For further information, the reader is referred to a text on epidemiologic methods.

1. THROMBOEMBOLIC DISORDERS AND OTHER VASCULAR PROBLEMS

a. Thromboembolism

An increased risk of thromboembolic and thrombotic disease associated with the use of oral contraceptives is well established. Case control studies have found the relative risk of users compared to non-users to be three for the first episode of superficial venous thrombosis, four to 11 for deep vein thrombosis or pulmonary embolism, and 1.5 to six for women with predisposing conditions for venous thromboembolic disease. Cohort studies have shown the relative risk to be somewhat lower, about three for new cases and about 4.5 for new cases requiring hospitalization. The risk of thromboembolic disease associated with oral contraceptives is not related to length of use and disappears after pill use is stopped.

Several epidemiology studies indicate that third generation oral contraceptives, including those containing desogestrel (etonogestrel, the progestin in NuvaRing®, is the biologically active metabolite of desogestrel), are associated with a higher risk of venous thromboembolism than certain second generation oral contraceptives. In general, these studies indicate an approximate two-fold increased risk, which corresponds to an additional one to two cases of venous thromboembolism per 10,000 women-years of use. However, data from additional studies have not shown this two-fold increase in risk. It is unknown if NuvaRing® has a different risk of venous thromboembolism than second generation oral contraceptives.

A two- to four-fold increase in relative risk of post-operative thromboembolic complications has been reported with the use of oral contraceptives. The relative risk of venous thrombosis in women who have predisposing conditions is twice that of women without such medical conditions. If feasible, combination hormonal contraceptives, including NuvaRing®, should be discontinued at least four weeks prior to and for two weeks after elective surgery of a type associated with an increase in risk of thromboembolism and during and following prolonged immobilization. Since the immediate postpartum period is also associated with an increased risk of thromboembolism, combination hormonal contraceptives, such as NuvaRing®, should be started no earlier than four to six weeks after delivery in women who elect not to breastfeed.

The clinician should be alert to the earliest manifestations of thrombotic disorders (thrombophlebitis, pulmonary embolism, cerebrovascular disorders, and retinal thrombosis). Should any of these occur or be suspected, NuvaRing® should be discontinued immediately.

b. Myocardial infarction

An increased risk of myocardial infarction has been attributed to oral contraceptive use. This risk is primarily in smokers or women with other underlying risk factors for coronary artery disease such as hypertension, hypercholesterolemia, morbid obesity, and diabetes. The relative risk of heart attack for current combination oral contraceptive users has been estimated to be two to six. The risk is very low in women under the age of 30.

Smoking in combination with oral contraceptive use has been shown to contribute substantially to the incidence of myocardial infarction in women in their mid-thirties or older with smoking accounting for the majority of excess cases. Mortality rates associated with circulatory disease have been shown to increase substantially in smokers, over the age of 35 and non-smokers over the age of 40 among women who use oral contraceptives (see Table IV).

[See table IV above]

Oral contraceptives may compound the effects of well-known risk factors, such as hypertension, diabetes, hyperlipidemias, age, and obesity. In particular, some progestogens are known to decrease HDL cholesterol and cause glucose intolerance, while estrogens may create a state of hyperinsulinism. Oral contraceptives have been shown to increase blood pressure among users (see WARNINGS). Similar effects on risk factors have been associated with an increased risk of heart disease. NuvaRing® must be used with caution in women with cardiovascular disease risk factors.

c. Cerebrovascular diseases

Oral contraceptives have been shown to increase both the relative and attributable risks of cerebrovascular events (thrombotic and hemorrhagic strokes), although, in general, the risk is greatest among older (>35 years), hypertensive women who also smoke. Hypertension was found to be a risk factor for both users and non-users, for both types of strokes, while smoking interacted to increase the risk for hemorrhagic strokes.

In a large study, the relative risk of thrombotic strokes has been shown to range from three for normotensive users to 14 for users with severe hypertension. The relative risk of hemorrhagic stroke is reported to be 1.2 for non-smokers who used oral contraceptives, 2.6 for smokers who did not use oral contraceptives, 7.6 for smokers who used oral contraceptives, 1.8 for normotensive users and 25.7 for users with severe hypertension. The attributable risk is also greater in older women. Oral contraceptives also increase the risk for stroke in women with other underlying risk factors such as certain inherited or acquired thrombophilias, hyperlipidemias, and obesity. Women with migraine (particularly migraine with aura) who take combination oral contraceptives may be at an increased risk of stroke.

TABLE III: PERCENTAGE OF WOMEN EXPERIENCING AN UNINTENDED PREGNANCY DURING THE FIRST YEAR OF TYPICAL USE AND THE FIRST YEAR OF PERFECT USE OF CONTRACEPTION AND THE PERCENTAGE CONTINUING USE AT THE END OF THE FIRST YEAR: UNITED STATES.

	% of Women Experiencing an Unintended Pregnancy within the First Year of Use		% of Women Continuing Use at One Year*
Method (1)	Typical Use† (2)	Perfect Use‡ (3)	(4)
Chance#	85	85	
SpermicidesÞ	26	6	40
Periodic abstinence	25		63
Calendar		9	
Ovulation Method		3	
Sympto-Thermalß		2	
Post-Ovulation		1	
Capà			
Parous Women	40	26	42
Nulliparous Women	20	9	56
Sponge			
Parous Women	40	20	42
Nulliparous Women	20	9	56
Diaphragmà	20	6	56
Withdrawal	19	4	
Condomè			
Female (Reality)	21	5	56
Male	14	3	61
Pill	5		71
Progestin Only		0.5	
Combined		0.1	
IUD			
Progesterone T	2.0	1.5	81
Copper T 380A	0.8	0.6	78
LNg 20	0.1	0.1	81
Depo-Provera	0.3	0.3	70
Norplant and Norplant-2	0.05	0.05	88
Female sterilization	0.5	0.5	100
Male sterilization	0.15	0.10	100

Emergency Contraceptive Pills: Treatment initiated within 72 hours after unprotected intercourse reduces the risk of pregnancy by at least 75%.§

Lactation Amenorrhea Method: LAM is a highly effective, temporary method of contraception.¶

Adapted from Hatcher et al., Contraceptive Technology, 17th Revised Edition. New York, NY: Irvington Publishers, 1998.

* Among couples attempting to avoid pregnancy, the percentage who continue to use a method for one year.

† Among *typical* couples who initiate use of a method (not necessarily for the first time), the percentage who experience an accidental pregnancy during the first year if they do not stop use for any other reason.

‡ Among couples who initiate use of a method (not necessarily for the first time) and who use it *perfectly* (both consistently and correctly), the percentage who experience an accidental pregnancy during the first year if they do not stop use for any other reason.

§ The treatment schedule is one dose within 72 hours after unprotected intercourse, and a second dose 12 hours after the first dose. The FDA has declared the following brands of oral contraceptives to be safe and effective for emergency contraception: Ovral (one dose is two white pills), Alesse (one dose is five pink pills), Nordette or Levlen (one dose is four yellow pills).

¶ However, to maintain effective protection against pregnancy, another method of contraception must be used as soon as menstruation resumes, the frequency or duration of breastfeeds is reduced, bottle feeds are introduced, or the baby reaches six months of age.

The percents becoming pregnant in columns (2) and (3) are based on data from populations where contraception is not used and from women who cease using contraception in order to become pregnant. Among such populations, about 89% become pregnant within one year. This estimate was lowered slightly (to 85%) to represent the percent who would become pregnant within one year among women now relying on reversible methods of contraception if they abandoned contraception altogether.

Þ Foams, creams, gels, vaginal suppositories, and vaginal film.

ß Cervical mucus (ovulation) method supplemented by calendar in the pre-ovulatory and basal body temperature in the post-ovulatory phases.

à With spermicidal cream or jelly.

è Without spermicides.

TABLE IV: CIRCULATORY DISEASE MORTALITY RATES PER 100,000 WOMAN-YEARS BY AGE, SMOKING STATUS, AND COMBINATION ORAL CONTRACEPTIVE USE.

AGE	EVER-USERS NON-SMOKERS	EVER-USERS SMOKERS	CONTROLS NON-SMOKERS	CONTROLS SMOKERS
15–24	0.0	10.5	0.0	0.0
25–34	4.4	14.2	2.7	4.2
35–44	21.5	63.4	6.4	15.2
45+	52.4	206.7	11.4	27.9

(Adapted from P.M. Layde and V. Beral, Lancet, 1981;1:541–546.)

TABLE V: ANNUAL NUMBER OF BIRTH-RELATED OR METHOD-RELATED DEATHS ASSOCIATED WITH CONTROL OF FERTILITY PER 100,000 NON-STERILE WOMEN, BY FERTILITY CONTROL METHOD ACCORDING TO AGE.

Method of control and outcome	15–19	20–24	25–29	30–34	35–39	40–44
No fertility control methods*	7.0	7.4	9.1	14.8	25.7	28.2
Oral contraceptives non-smoker†	0.3	0.5	0.9	1.9	13.8	31.6
Oral contraceptives smoker†	2.2	3.4	6.6	13.5	51.1	117.2
IUD†	0.8	0.8	1.0	1.0	1.4	1.4
Condom*	1.1	1.6	0.7	0.2	0.3	0.4
Diaphragm/spermicide*	1.9	1.2	1.2	1.3	2.2	2.8
Periodic abstinence*	2.5	1.6	1.6	1.7	2.9	3.6

(Adapted from H.W. Ory, Family Planning Perspectives 1983;15:50–56.)
* Deaths are birth related
† Deaths are method related

d. Dose-related risk of vascular disease from oral contraceptives

A positive association has been observed between the amount of estrogen and progestogen in oral contraceptives and the risk of vascular disease. A decline in serum high-density lipoproteins (HDL) has been reported with many progestational agents. A decline in serum high-density lipoproteins has been associated with an increased incidence of ischemic heart disease. Because estrogens increase HDL cholesterol, the net effect of an oral contraceptive depends on a balance achieved between doses of estrogen and progestogen and the nature and absolute amount of progestogens used in the contraceptives. The activity and amount of both hormones should be considered in the choice of a hormonal contraceptive.

Minimizing exposure to estrogen and progestogen is in keeping with good principles of therapeutics. For any particular estrogen/progestogen combination, the dosage regimen prescribed should be one which contains the least amount of estrogen and progestogen that is compatible with a low failure rate and the needs of the individual patient. New acceptors of hormonal contraceptive agents should be started on a product containing the lowest hormone content that provides satisfactory results in the individual.

e. Persistence of risk of vascular disease

There are two studies that have shown persistence of risk of vascular disease for ever-users of oral contraceptives. In a study in the United States, the risk of developing myocardial infarction after discontinuing oral contraceptives persists for at least nine years for women 40–49 years old who had used oral contraceptives for five or more years, but this increased risk was not demonstrated in other age groups. In another study in Great Britain, the risk of developing cerebrovascular disease persisted for at least six years after discontinuation of oral contraceptives, although excess risk was very small. However, both studies were performed with oral contraceptive formulations containing 50 micrograms or more of estrogen.

It is unknown whether NuvaRing® is distinct from combination oral contraceptives with regard to the occurrence of venous or arterial thrombosis.

2. ESTIMATES OF MORTALITY FROM CONTRACEPTIVE USE

One study gathered data from a variety of sources that have estimated the mortality rate associated with different methods of contraception at different ages (Table V). These estimates include the combined risk of death associated with contraceptive methods plus the risk attributable to pregnancy in the event of method failure. Each method of contraception has its specific benefits and risks. The study concluded that with the exception of oral contraceptive users age 35 and older who smoke and age 40 and older who do not smoke, mortality associated with all methods of birth control is low and below that associated with childbirth.

The observation of a possible increase in risk of mortality with age for oral contraceptive users is based on data gathered in the 1970's, but not reported until 1983. However, current clinical practice involves the use of lower estrogen-dose formulations combined with careful restriction of hormonal contraceptive use to women who do not have the various risk factors listed in this labeling.

Because of these changes in practice and, also, because of some limited new data which suggest that the risk of cardiovascular disease with the use of oral contraceptives may now be less than previously observed, the Fertility and Maternal Health Drugs Advisory Committee was asked to review the topic in 1989. The Committee concluded that although cardiovascular disease risks may be increased with oral contraceptive use after age 40 in healthy non-smoking women (even with the newer low-dose formulations), there are also greater potential health risks associated with pregnancy in older women and with the alternative surgical and medical procedures which may be necessary if such women do not have access to effective and acceptable means of contraception. Therefore, the Committee recommended that the benefits of low-dose hormonal oral contraceptive use by healthy non-smoking women over 40 may outweigh the possible risks. Older women, as all women who take hormonal contraceptives, should take the lowest possible dose formulation that is effective and meets the individual patient needs.

[See table V above]

3. CARCINOMA OF THE REPRODUCTIVE ORGANS AND BREASTS

Numerous epidemiologic studies have been performed on the incidence of breast, endometrial, ovarian, and cervical cancer in women using combination oral contraceptives. Although the risk of breast cancer may be slightly increased among current users of oral contraceptives (RR = 1.24), this excess risk decreases over time after oral contraceptive discontinuation and by 10 years after cessation the increased risk disappears. The risk does not increase with duration of use, and no relationships have been found with dose or type of steroid. The patterns of risk are also similar regardless of a woman's reproductive history or her family breast cancer history. The subgroup for whom risk has been found to be significantly elevated is women who first used oral contraceptives before age 20, but because breast cancer is so rare at these young ages, the number of cases attributable to this early oral contraceptive use is extremely small. Breast cancers diagnosed in current or previous oral contraceptive users tend to be less advanced clinically than in never-users. Women who currently have or have had breast cancer should not use hormonal contraceptives because breast cancer is a hormone-sensitive tumor.

Some studies suggest that combination oral contraceptive use has been associated with an increase in the risk of cervical intraepithelial neoplasia in some populations of women. However, there continues to be controversy about the extent to which such findings may be due to differences in sexual behavior and other factors.

In spite of many studies of the relationship between oral contraceptive use and breast and cervical cancers, a cause-and-effect relationship has not been established.

It is unknown whether NuvaRing® is distinct from oral contraceptives with regard to the above statements.

4. HEPATIC NEOPLASIA

Benign hepatic adenomas are associated with oral contraceptive use, although the incidence of benign tumors is rare in the United States. Indirect calculations have estimated the attributable risk to be in the range of 3.3 cases per 100,000 for users, a risk that increases after four or more years of use. Rupture of rare, benign, hepatic adenomas may cause death through intra-abdominal hemorrhage.

Studies from Britain have shown an increased risk of developing hepatocellular carcinoma in long term (>8 years) oral contraceptive users. However, these cancers are extremely rare in the US and the attributable risk (the excess incidence) of liver cancers in oral contraceptive users approaches less than one per million users. It is unknown whether NuvaRing® is distinct from oral contraceptives in this regard.

5. OCULAR LESIONS

There have been clinical case reports of retinal thrombosis associated with the use of oral contraceptives. NuvaRing® should be discontinued if there is unexplained partial or complete loss of vision, onset of proptosis or diplopia, papilledema, or retinal vascular lesions. Appropriate diagnostic and therapeutic measures should be undertaken immediately.

6. HORMONAL CONTRACEPTIVE USE BEFORE OR DURING EARLY PREGNANCY

Hormonal contraceptives should not be used during pregnancy.

Extensive epidemiologic studies have revealed no increased risk of birth defects in women who have used oral contraceptives prior to pregnancy. Studies also do not suggest a teratogenic effect, particularly in so far as cardiac anomalies and limb reduction defects are concerned, when oral contraceptives are taken inadvertently during early pregnancy.

Combination hormonal contraceptives, such as NuvaRing®, should not be used to induce withdrawal bleeding as a test for pregnancy. NuvaRing® should not be used during pregnancy to treat threatened or habitual abortion. It is recommended that for any woman who has not adhered to the prescribed regimen for use of NuvaRing® and has missed a menstrual period or who has missed two consecutive periods, pregnancy should be ruled out.

7. GALLBLADDER DISEASE

Combination hormonal contraceptives, such as NuvaRing®, may worsen existing gallbladder disease and may accelerate the development of this disease in previously asymptomatic women. Women with a history of combination hormonal contraceptive-related cholestasis are more likely to have the condition recur with subsequent combination hormonal contraceptive use.

8. CARBOHYDRATE AND LIPID METABOLIC EFFECTS

Hormonal contraceptives have been shown to cause a decrease in glucose tolerance in some users. However, in the non-diabetic woman, combination hormonal contraceptives appear to have no effect on fasting blood glucose. Prediabetic and diabetic women should be carefully observed while taking combination hormonal contraceptives, such as NuvaRing®. In a clinical study involving 37 NuvaRing®-treated subjects, glucose tolerance tests showed no clinically significant changes in serum glucose levels from baseline to cycle six.

A small proportion of women will have persistent hypertriglyceridemia while using oral contraceptives. Changes in serum triglycerides and lipoprotein levels have been reported in combination hormonal contraceptive users.

9. ELEVATED BLOOD PRESSURE

Women with severe hypertension should not be started on hormonal contraceptives. An increase in blood pressure has been reported in women taking oral contraceptives and this increase is more likely in older oral contraceptive users and with continued use. Data from the Royal College of General Practitioners and subsequent randomized trials have shown that the incidence of hypertension increases with increasing concentrations of progestogens.

Women with a history of hypertension or hypertension-related diseases, or renal disease should be encouraged to use another method of contraception. If these women elect to use NuvaRing®, they should be monitored closely and if significant elevation of blood pressure occurs, NuvaRing® should be discontinued. For most women, elevated blood pressure will return to normal after stopping hormonal contraceptives, and there is no difference in the occurrence of hypertension between former and never-users.

10. HEADACHE

The onset or exacerbation of migraine or development of headache with a new pattern which is recurrent, persistent, or severe requires discontinuation of NuvaRing® and evaluation of the cause.

11. BLEEDING IRREGULARITIES

Bleeding Patterns

Breakthrough bleeding and spotting are sometimes encountered in women using NuvaRing®. If abnormal bleeding while using NuvaRing® persists or is severe, appropriate investigation should be instituted to rule out the possibility of organic pathology or pregnancy, and appropriate treatment should be instituted when necessary. In the event of amenorrhea, pregnancy should be ruled out.

Bleeding patterns were evaluated in three large clinical studies. In the US-Canadian study (n=1177), the percentages of subjects with breakthrough bleeding/spotting ranged from 7.2 to 11.7% during cycles 1–13. In the two non-US studies, the percentages of subjects with breakthrough bleeding/spotting ranged from 2.6 to 6.4% (Study 1, n=1145 European and Israeli subjects) and from 2.0 to 8.7% (Study 2, n=512 European and South American subjects). In these three studies, the percentages of women who did not have withdrawal bleeding in a given cycle ranged from 0.3 to 3.8%.

Some women may encounter amenorrhea or oligomenorrhea after discontinuing use of NuvaRing®, especially when such a condition was pre-existent.

12. ECTOPIC PREGNANCY

Ectopic as well as intrauterine pregnancy may occur in contraceptive failures.

PRECAUTIONS

1. SEXUALLY TRANSMITTED DISEASES

Women should be counseled that this product does not protect against HIV infection (AIDS) and other sexually transmitted diseases.

2. PHYSICAL EXAMINATION AND FOLLOW-UP

It is routine medical practice for women using NuvaRing®, as for all women, to have an annual medical evaluation including physical examination and relevant laboratory tests. The physical examination should include special reference to blood pressure, breasts, abdomen, pelvic organs and vagina (including cervical cytology). In case of undiagnosed, persistent or recurrent abnormal vaginal bleeding, appropriate measures should be conducted to rule out malignancy. Women with a family history of breast cancer or who have breast nodules should be monitored with particular care.

3. LIPID DISORDERS

Women who are being treated for hyperlipidemias should be followed closely if they elect to use NuvaRing®. Some progestogens may elevate LDL levels and may render the control of hyperlipidemias more difficult.

In women with familial defects of lipoprotein metabolism receiving estrogen-containing preparations, there have been case reports of significant elevations of plasma triglycerides leading to pancreatitis.

4. LIVER FUNCTION

If jaundice develops in any woman using NuvaRing®, product use should be discontinued. The hormones in NuvaRing® may be poorly metabolized in women with impaired liver function.

5. FLUID RETENTION

Steroid hormones like those in NuvaRing®, may cause some degree of fluid retention. NuvaRing® should be prescribed with caution, and only with careful monitoring, in women with conditions which might be aggravated by fluid retention.

6. EMOTIONAL DISORDERS

Women becoming significantly depressed while taking hormonal contraceptives should stop the medication and use an alternate method of contraception in an attempt to determine whether the symptom is drug related. Women with a history of depression should be carefully observed and the drug discontinued if depression recurs to a serious degree.

7. TAMPON USE

On rare occasions, NuvaRing® may be expelled while removing a tampon (see EXPULSION). Pharmacokinetic data show that the use of tampons has no effect on the systemic absorption of the hormones released by NuvaRing®.

8. TOXIC SHOCK SYNDROME (TSS)

Cases of toxic shock syndrome have been associated with tampons and certain barrier contraceptives. Very rare cases of TSS have been reported by NuvaRing® users; in some cases the women were also using tampons. No causal relationship between the use of NuvaRing® and TSS has been established. If a patient exhibits signs or symptoms of TSS, the possibility of this diagnosis should not be excluded and appropriate medical evaluation and treatment initiated.

9. CONTACT LENSES

Contact lens wearers who develop visual changes or changes in lens tolerance should be assessed by an ophthalmologist.

10. DRUG INTERACTIONS

Changes in contraceptive effectiveness associated with co-administration of other drugs:

a. Anti-infective agents and anticonvulsants

Contraceptive effectiveness may be reduced when hormonal contraceptives are co-administered with some antifungals, anticonvulsants, and other drugs that increase metabolism of contraceptive steroids. This could result in unintended pregnancy or breakthrough bleeding. Examples include barbiturates, griseofulvin, rifampin, phenylbutazone, phenytoin, carbamazepine, felbamate, oxcarbazepine, topiramate, and modafinil. Women may need to use an additional contraceptive method when taking such medications.

b. Anti-HIV protease inhibitors

Several of the anti-HIV protease inhibitors have been studied with co-administration of oral combination hormonal contraceptives; significant changes (increases and decreases) in the plasma levels of the estrogen and progestin have been noted in some cases. The efficacy and safety of hormonal contraceptive products may be affected with co-administration of anti-HIV protease inhibitors. Healthcare providers should refer to the label of the individual anti-HIV protease inhibitors for further drug-drug interaction information.

c. Herbal products

Herbal products containing St. John's wort (hypericum perforatum) may induce hepatic enzymes (cytochrome P450) and p-glycoprotein transporter and may reduce the effectiveness of contraceptive steroids. This may also result in breakthrough bleeding.

Increase in plasma hormone levels associated with co-administered drugs

Co-administration of atorvastatin and certain oral contraceptives containing ethinyl estradiol increase AUC values for ethinyl estradiol by approximately 20%. Ascorbic acid and acetaminophen may increase plasma ethinyl estradiol levels, possibly by inhibition of conjugation. CYP 3A4 inhibitors such as itraconazole or ketoconazole may increase plasma hormone levels. Co-administration of vaginal miconazole nitrate and NuvaRing® increases the serum concentrations of etonogestrel and ethinyl estradiol by up to 40%.

Changes in plasma levels of co-administered drugs

Combination hormonal contraceptives containing some synthetic estrogens (e.g., ethinyl estradiol) may inhibit the metabolism of other compounds. Increased plasma concentrations of cyclosporine, prednisolone, and theophylline have been reported with concomitant administration of oral contraceptives. In addition, oral contraceptives may induce the conjugation of other compounds. Decreased plasma concentrations of acetaminophen and increased clearance of temazepam, salicylic acid, morphine and clofibric acid have been noted when these drugs were administered with oral contraceptives.

11. INTERACTIONS WITH LABORATORY TESTS

Certain endocrine and liver function tests and blood components may be affected by combined hormonal contraceptives:

a. Increased prothrombin and factors VII, VIII, IX, and X; decreased antithrombin 3, increased norepinephrine-induced platelet aggregability.

b. Increased thyroid-binding globulin (TBG) leading to increased circulating total thyroid hormone, as measured by protein-bound iodine (PBI), T4 by column or by radioimmunoassay. Free T3 resin uptake is decreased, reflecting the elevated TBG; free T4 concentration is unaltered.

c. Other binding proteins may be elevated in serum.

d. Sex hormone-binding globulins are increased and result in elevated levels of total circulating sex steroids; however, free or biologically active levels either decrease or remain unchanged.

e. Triglycerides may be increased and levels of various other lipids and lipoproteins may be affected.

f. Glucose tolerance may be decreased.

g. Serum folate levels may be depressed by oral contraceptive therapy. This may be of clinical significance if a woman becomes pregnant shortly after discontinuing NuvaRing®.

12. CARCINOGENESIS, MUTAGENESIS, IMPAIRMENT OF FERTILITY

In a 24-month carcinogenicity study in rats with subdermal implants releasing 10 and 20 mcg etonogestrel per day, (approximately 0.3 and 0.6 times the systemic steady-state exposure of women using NuvaRing®), no drug-related carcinogenic potential was observed. Etonogestrel was not genotoxic in the *in vitro* Ames/Salmonella reverse mutation assay, the chromosomal aberration assay in Chinese hamster ovary cells or in the *in vivo* mouse micronucleus test. Fertility returned after withdrawal from treatment (see WARNINGS).

13. PREGNANCY

Pregnancy Category X
(see CONTRAINDICATIONS and WARNINGS).

Teratology studies have been performed in rats and rabbits using the oral route of administration at doses up to 130 and 260 times, respectively, the human NuvaRing® dose (based on body surface area) and have revealed no evidence of harm to the fetus due to etonogestrel.

14. NURSING MOTHERS

The effects of NuvaRing® in nursing mothers have not been evaluated and are unknown. Small amounts of contraceptive steroids have been identified in the milk of nursing mothers and a few adverse effects on the child have been reported, including jaundice and breast enlargement. In addition, contraceptive steroids given in the postpartum period may interfere with lactation by decreasing the quantity and quality of breast milk. Long-term follow-up of children whose mothers used combination hormonal contraceptives while breastfeeding has shown no deleterious effects on infants. However, women who are breastfeeding should be advised not to use NuvaRing® but to use other forms of contraception until the child is weaned.

15. PEDIATRIC USE

Safety and efficacy of NuvaRing® have been established in women of reproductive age. Safety and efficacy are expected to be the same for postpubertal adolescents under the age of 16 and for users 16 years and older. Use of this product before menarche is not indicated.

16. GERIATRIC USE

This product has not been studied in women over 65 years of age and is not indicated in this population.

17. VAGINAL USE

NuvaRing® may not be suitable for women with conditions that make the vagina more susceptible to vaginal irritation or ulceration. Vaginal/cervical erosion or ulceration in women using NuvaRing® has been rarely reported. In some cases, the ring adhered to vaginal tissue, necessitating removal by a healthcare provider.

Some women are aware of the ring at random times during the 21 days of use or during intercourse. During intercourse some sexual partners may feel NuvaRing® in the vagina. However, clinical studies revealed that 90% of couples did not find this to be a problem.

NuvaRing® may interfere with the correct placement and position of a diaphragm. A diaphragm is therefore not recommended as a back-up method with NuvaRing® use.

18. URINARY BLADDER INSERTION

There have been rare reports of inadvertent insertions of NuvaRing® into the urinary bladder, which required cystoscopic removal. Healthcare providers should assess for ring insertion into the urinary bladder in NuvaRing® users who present with persistent urinary symptoms and are unable to locate the ring.

19. EXPULSION

NuvaRing® can be accidentally expelled, for example, while removing a tampon, during intercourse, or with straining during a bowel movement. NuvaRing® should be left in the vagina for a continuous period of three weeks. If the ring is accidentally expelled and is left outside of the vagina for **less than three hours** contraceptive efficacy is not reduced. NuvaRing® can be rinsed with cool to lukewarm (not hot) water and reinserted as soon as possible, but at the latest within three hours. If NuvaRing® is lost, a new vaginal ring should be inserted and the regimen should be continued without alteration.

If NuvaRing® is out of the vagina for more than three continuous hours:

During Weeks 1 and 2

If NuvaRing® has been out of the vagina for more than three continuous hours during the 1st or 2nd week of use, contraceptive efficacy may be reduced. The woman should reinsert the ring as soon as she remembers. A barrier method such as condoms or spermicides must be used until the ring has been used continuously for seven days.

During Week 3

If NuvaRing® has been out of the vagina for more than three continuous hours during the 3rd week of the three-week use period, the woman should discard that ring. One of the following two options should be chosen:

1. Insert a new ring immediately. Inserting a new ring will start the next three-week use period. The woman may not experience a withdrawal bleed from her previous cycle. However, breakthrough spotting or bleeding may occur.
2. Have a withdrawal bleeding and insert a new ring no later than seven days (7×24 hours) from the time the previous ring was removed or expelled. This option should only be chosen if the ring was used continuously for the preceding seven days.

A barrier method such as condoms or spermicides must be used until the new ring has been used continuously for seven days.

20. DISCONNECTED RING

There have been reported cases of NuvaRing® disconnecting at the weld joint. This is not expected to affect the contraceptive effectiveness of NuvaRing®. In the event of a disconnected ring, vaginal discomfort or expulsion (slipping out) is more likely to occur (see EXPULSION). If a woman discovers that her NuvaRing® has disconnected, she should discard the ring and replace it with a new ring.

INFORMATION FOR THE PATIENT

The woman should be instructed regarding the proper use of NuvaRing® (see PATIENT INFORMATION printed below).

ADVERSE REACTIONS

The most common adverse events reported by five to 14% of women using NuvaRing® in clinical trials (n=2501) were the following: vaginitis, headache, upper respiratory tract infection, vaginal secretion, sinusitis, weight gain, and nausea. The most frequent system-organ class adverse events leading to discontinuation in one to 2.5% of women using NuvaRing® in the trials included the following: device-related events (foreign body sensation, coital problems, device expulsion), vaginal symptoms (discomfort/vaginitis/vaginal secretion), headache, emotional lability, and weight gain.

Listed below are adverse reactions that have been associated with the use of combination hormonal contraceptives. These are also likely to apply to combination vaginal hormonal contraceptives, such as NuvaRing®.

An increased risk of the following serious adverse reactions has been associated with the use of combination hormonal contraceptives (see CONTRAINDICATIONS and WARNINGS):

• Thrombophlebitis and venous thrombosis with or without embolism	• Cerebral hemorrhage
• Arterial thromboembolism	• Cerebral thrombosis
• Pulmonary embolism	• Hypertension
• Myocardial infarction	• Gallbladder disease
	• Hepatic adenomas or benign liver tumors

There is evidence of an association between the following conditions and the use of combination hormonal contraceptives:

• Mesenteric thrombosis	• Retinal thrombosis

The following additional adverse reactions have been reported in users of combination hormonal contraceptives and are believed to be drug-related:

• Nausea	• Change in weight or appetite (increase or decrease)
• Vomiting	• Change in cervical ectropion and secretion
• Gastrointestinal symptoms (such as abdominal pain, cramps and bloating)	• Possible diminution in lactation when given immediately postpartum
• Breakthrough bleeding	• Cholestatic jaundice
• Spotting	• Migraine headache
• Change in menstrual flow	• Rash (allergic)
• Amenorrhea	• Mood changes, including depression
• Temporary infertility after discontinuation of treatment	• Vaginitis, including candidiasis
• Edema/fluid retention	• Change in corneal curvature (steepening)
• Melasma/chloasma which may persist	• Intolerance to contact lenses
• Breast changes: tenderness, pain, enlargement, and secretion	• Exacerbation of systemic lupus erythematosus
• Decrease in serum folate levels	• Exacerbation of chorea
• Exacerbation of porphyria	• Anaphylactic/anaphylactoid reactions, including urticaria, angioedema, and severe reactions with respiratory and circulatory symptoms
• Aggravation of varicose veins	

The following additional adverse reactions have been reported in users of combination hormonal contraceptives and a causal association has been neither confirmed nor refuted:

• Pre-menstrual syndrome	• Erythema nodosum
• Cataracts	• Hemorrhagic eruption
• Cystitis-like syndrome	• Impaired renal function
• Headache	• Hemolytic uremic syndrome
• Nervousness	• Acne
• Dizziness	• Changes in libido
• Hirsutism	• Colitis
• Loss of scalp hair	• Budd-Chiari Syndrome
• Erythema multiforme	• Optic neuritis, which may lead to partial or complete loss of vision
• Dysmenorrhea	
• Pancreatitis	

OVERDOSAGE

Overdosage of combination hormonal contraceptives may cause nausea, vomiting, vaginal bleeding, or other menstrual irregularities. Given the nature and design of NuvaRing® it is unlikely that overdosage will occur. If NuvaRing® is broken, it does not release a higher dose of hormones. Serious ill effects have not been reported following acute ingestion of large doses of oral contraceptives by young children. There are no antidotes and further treatment should be symptomatic.

DOSAGE AND ADMINISTRATION

To achieve maximum contraceptive effectiveness, NuvaRing® must be used as directed (see When to Start NuvaRing® below). One NuvaRing® is inserted in the vagina. **The ring is to remain in place continuously for three weeks.** It is removed for a one-week break, during which a withdrawal bleed usually occurs. A new ring is inserted one week after the last ring was removed.

The user can choose the insertion position that is most comfortable to her, for example, standing with one leg up, squatting, or lying down. The ring is to be compressed and inserted into the vagina. The exact position of NuvaRing® inside the vagina is not critical for its function. The vaginal ring must be inserted on the appropriate day and left in place for three consecutive weeks. This means that the ring is removed three weeks later on the same day of the week as it was inserted and at about the same time. NuvaRing® can be removed by hooking the index finger under the forward rim or by grasping the rim between the index and middle finger and pulling it out. The used ring should be placed in the sachet (foil pouch) and discarded in a waste receptacle out of the reach of children and pets (do not flush in toilet).

After a one-week break, during which a withdrawal bleed usually occurs, a new ring is inserted on the same day of the week as it was inserted in the previous cycle. The withdrawal bleed usually starts on day 2–3 after removal of the ring and may not have finished before the next ring is inserted. In order to maintain contraceptive effectiveness, the new ring must be inserted one week after the previous one was removed even if menstrual bleeding has not finished.

When to Start NuvaRing®

IMPORTANT: The possibility of ovulation and conception prior to the first use of NuvaRing® should be considered.

No hormonal contraceptive use in the preceding cycle

Insert NuvaRing® on the first day of the woman's natural cycle (i.e., the first day of her menstrual bleeding). NuvaRing® may also be started on days 2–5 of the woman's cycle, but in this case a barrier method, such as male condoms or spermicide, is recommended for the first seven days of NuvaRing® use in the first cycle.

Changing from a combined hormonal contraceptive

The woman may switch from her previous combined hormonal contraceptive on any day, but at the latest on the day following the usual hormone-free interval, if she has been using her hormonal method consistently and correctly, or if it is reasonably certain that she is not pregnant.

Changing from a progestagen-only method (minipill, implant, or injection) or from a progestagen-releasing intrauterine system (IUS)

The woman may switch on any day from the minipill. She should switch from an implant or the IUS on the day of its removal and from an injectable on the day when the next injection would be due. In all of these cases, the woman should use an additional barrier method such as a male condom or spermicide, for the first seven days.

Following complete first trimester abortion

The woman may start using NuvaRing® within the first five days following a complete first trimester abortion and does not need to use an additional method of contraception. If use of NuvaRing® is not started within five days following a first trimester abortion, the woman should follow the instructions for "No hormonal contraceptive use in the preceding cycle." In the meantime she should be advised to use a non-hormonal contraceptive method.

Following delivery or second trimester abortion

The use of NuvaRing® for contraception may be initiated four weeks postpartum in women who elect not to breastfeed. Women who are breastfeeding should be advised not to use NuvaRing® but to use other forms of contraception until the child is weaned. NuvaRing® use may be initiated four weeks after a second trimester abortion. When NuvaRing® is used postpartum or postabortion, the increased risk of thromboembolic disease must be considered. (See CONTRAINDICATIONS and WARNINGS concerning thromboembolic disease. See PRECAUTIONS for "Nursing Mothers".) If a woman begins using NuvaRing® postpartum, she should be instructed to use an additional method of contraception, such as male condoms or spermicide, for the first seven days. If she has not yet had a period, the possibility of ovulation and conception occurring prior to initiation of NuvaRing® should be considered.

Deviations from the Recommended Regimen

To prevent loss of contraceptive efficacy, women should not deviate from the recommended regimen. NuvaRing® should be left in the vagina for a continuous period of three weeks.

Inadvertent removal, expulsion, or prolonged ring-free interval

If the ring is accidentally expelled and is left outside of the vagina for **less than three hours** contraceptive efficacy is not reduced. NuvaRing® can be rinsed with cool to lukewarm (not hot) water and **reinserted as soon as possible**, but at the latest within three hours. If NuvaRing® is lost, a new vaginal ring should be inserted and the regimen should be continued without alteration. If NuvaRing® is out of the vagina for more than three hours, the directions listed under PRECAUTIONS, EXPULSION should be followed.

If the ring-free interval has been extended beyond one week, the possibility of pregnancy should be considered, and an additional method of contraception, such as male condoms or spermicide, **MUST** be used until NuvaRing® has been used **continuously for seven days.**

Prolonged Use of NuvaRing®

If NuvaRing® has been left in place for up to one extra week (i.e., up to four weeks total), the woman will remain protected. NuvaRing® should be removed and the woman should insert a new ring after a one-week ring-free interval. The mean serum etonogestrel concentration during the fourth week of continuous use of NuvaRing® was 1272 ± 311 pg/mL compared to a mean concentration range of 1578 ± 408 to 1374 ± 328 pg/mL during weeks one to three. The mean serum ethinyl estradiol concentration during the fourth week of continuous use of NuvaRing® was 16.8 ± 4.6 pg/mL compared to a mean concentration range of 19.1 ± 4.5 to 17.6 ± 4.3 pg/mL during weeks one to three. If NuvaRing® has been left in place for longer than four weeks, pregnancy should be ruled out, and an additional method of contraception, such as male condoms or spermicide, **MUST** be used until a new NuvaRing® has been used **continuously for seven days.**

In the event of a missed menstrual period

1. If the woman has not adhered to the prescribed regimen (NuvaRing® has been out of the vagina for more than three hours or the preceding ring-free interval was extended beyond one week) the possibility of pregnancy should be considered at the time of the first missed period and NuvaRing® use should be discontinued if pregnancy is confirmed.
2. If the woman has adhered to the prescribed regimen and misses two consecutive periods, pregnancy should be ruled out.
3. If the woman has retained one NuvaRing® for longer than four weeks, pregnancy should be ruled out.

HOW SUPPLIED

Each NuvaRing® (etonogestrel/ethinyl estradiol vaginal ring) is individually packaged in a reclosable aluminum laminate sachet consisting of three layers, from outside to inside: polyester, aluminum foil, and low-density polyethylene. The ring should be replaced in this reclosable sachet after use for convenient disposal.

Box of 3 sachets	NDC 0052-0273-03

Storage

Prior to dispensing to the user, store refrigerated 2–8°C (36–46°F). After dispensing to the user, NuvaRing® can be stored for up to 4 months at 25°C (77°F); excursions permitted to 15–30°C (59–86°F) [see USP Controlled Room Temperature]. Avoid storing NuvaRing® in direct sunlight or at temperatures above 30°C (86°F). For the Dispenser: When NuvaRing® is dispensed to the user, place an expiration date on the label. The date should not exceed either 4 months from the date of dispensing or the expiration date, whichever comes first.

Rx only

REFERENCES FURNISHED UPON REQUEST

Manufactured for: Merck Sharp & Dohme Corp., a subsidiary of

MERCK & CO., INC., Whitehouse Station, NJ 08889, USA

Manufactured by: N.V. Organon, Oss, The Netherlands, a subsidiary of

Merck & Co., Inc., Whitehouse Station, NJ 08889, USA

U.S. Patent No. 5,989,581.

Revised: 05/2012

900702-EE/ENG-RNG-USPI.2

NUVARING®

(etonogestrel/ethinyl estradiol vaginal ring)

delivers 0.120 mg/0.015 mg per day

PATIENT INFORMATION

Rx only

Read this leaflet carefully before you use NuvaRing® so that you understand the benefits and risks of using this form of birth control. The leaflet gives you information about the possible serious side effects of NuvaRing®. This leaflet will also tell you how to use NuvaRing® properly so that it will give you the best possible protection against pregnancy. Read the information you get whenever you get a new prescription or refill, because there may be new information. This information does not take the place of talking with your healthcare provider.

What is NuvaRing®?

NuvaRing® (NEW-vah-ring) is a flexible combined contraceptive vaginal ring. It is used to prevent pregnancy. **It does not protect against HIV infection (AIDS) and other sexually transmitted diseases (STDs) such as chlamydia, genital herpes, genital warts, gonorrhea, hepatitis B, and syphilis.** NuvaRing® contains a combination of a progestin and estrogen, two kinds of female hormones. You insert the ring in your vagina and leave it there for three weeks. After the ring is inserted, it releases a continuous low dose of hormones into your body. You then remove it for a one-week ring-free period.

Contraceptives that contain both an estrogen and a progestin are called combination hormonal contraceptives. Most studies on combination contraceptives have used oral (taken by mouth) contraceptives. NuvaRing® may have the same risks that have been found for combination oral contraceptives. This leaflet will tell you about risks of taking combination oral contraceptives that may also apply to NuvaRing® users. In addition, it will tell you how to use NuvaRing® properly so that it will give you the best possible protection against pregnancy.

Who should not use NuvaRing®?

Cigarette smoking increases the risk of serious cardiovascular side effects when you use combination oral contraceptives. This risk increases even more if you are over age 35 and if you smoke 15 or more cigarettes a day. Women who use combination hormonal contraceptives, including NuvaRing®, are strongly advised not to smoke.

Do not use **NuvaRing®** if you have any of the following conditions:

• a history of heart attack or stroke

- a history of blood clots in your legs (thrombophlebitis), lungs (pulmonary embolism), or eyes
- a history of blood clots in the deep veins of your legs
- chest pain (angina pectoris)
- severe high blood pressure
- diabetes with complications of the kidneys, eyes, nerves, or blood vessels
- headaches with neurological symptoms
- known or suspected breast cancer or cancer of the lining of the uterus, cervix, or vagina (now or in the past)
- unexplained vaginal bleeding (until a diagnosis is reached by your healthcare provider)
- yellowing of the whites of the eyes or of the skin (jaundice) during pregnancy or during previous use of hormonal birth control of any kind (the pill, patch, vaginal ring, injection, or implant)
- liver tumor (benign or cancerous)
- heart valve or heart rhythm disorders that may be associated with formation of blood clots
- need for a long period of bed rest following major surgery
- known or suspected pregnancy
- active liver disease with abnormal liver function tests
- an allergy or hypersensitivity to any of the components of NuvaRing®

Tell your healthcare provider if you have ever had any of the conditions just listed. Your healthcare provider can suggest another method of birth control.

Talk with your healthcare provider about using NuvaRing® if you:

- smoke
- recently had a baby
- recently had a miscarriage or abortion
- are breastfeeding
- are taking other medications

In addition, talk to your healthcare provider about using NuvaRing® if you have any of the following conditions. Women with any of these conditions should be checked often by their doctor or healthcare provider if they choose to use NuvaRing®.

- a family history of breast cancer
- breast nodules, fibrocystic disease, an abnormal breast x-ray, or abnormal mammogram
- diabetes
- elevated cholesterol or triglycerides
- high blood pressure
- migraine or other headaches or epilepsy
- depression
- gallbladder, liver, heart, or kidney disease
- scanty or irregular menstrual periods
- plan to have major surgery (You may need to stop using NuvaRing® for a while to reduce your chance of getting blood clots.)
- any condition that makes the vagina get irritated easily
- prolapsed (dropped) uterus, dropped bladder (cystocele), or rectal prolapse (rectocele)
- severe constipation
- history of toxic shock syndrome

How should I use NuvaRing®?

For the best protection from pregnancy, use NuvaRing® exactly as directed. Insert one NuvaRing® in the vagina and **keep it in place for three weeks in a row.** Remove it for a one-week break and then insert a new ring. During the one-week break, you will usually have your menstrual period. Your healthcare provider should examine you at least once a year to see if there are any signs of side effects of NuvaRing® use.

When should I start NuvaRing®?

Follow the instructions in one of the sections below to find out when to start using NuvaRing®:

If you **did not** use a hormonal contraceptive in the preceding cycle

Insert NuvaRing® on the first day of your cycle, (i.e., the first day of menstrual bleeding). NuvaRing® will work immediately, it is not necessary to use an additional contraceptive method. You may also start on days 2–5 of your cycle, but in this case make sure you also use an extra method of birth control (barrier method), such as male condoms or spermicide for the first seven days of NuvaRing® use in the first cycle.

If you are changing from a combined hormonal contraceptive pill or patch (containing both progestin and estrogen)

Switch from your previous combined hormonal contraceptive on any day, but at the latest on the day following the usual hormone-free interval by inserting NuvaRing®. If you have been using your hormonal contraceptive method consistently and correctly, no extra birth control method should be needed.

If you are changing from a progestagen-only method (minipill, implant or injection) or from a progestagen-releasing intrauterine system (IUS)

You may switch on any day from a minipill. You should switch from an implant or the IUS on the day of its removal and from an injectable on the day when the next injection would be due. In all of these cases, you should use an extra method of birth control, such as a male condom or spermicide, for the first seven days of ring use.

Following first trimester abortion or miscarriage

If you start using NuvaRing® within five days after a complete first trimester abortion or miscarriage, you do not need to use an extra method of contraception.

If NuvaRing® is not started within five days after a first trimester abortion or miscarriage, begin NuvaRing® at the time of your next menstrual period. Counting the first day of your menstrual period as "Day 1", insert NuvaRing® on or before Day 5 of the cycle, even if you have not finished bleeding. During this first cycle, use an extra method of birth control, such as male condoms or spermicide, for the first seven days of ring use.

How do I insert NuvaRing®?

1. Each NuvaRing® comes in a reclosable foil pouch. After washing and drying your hands, remove NuvaRing® from its foil pouch. Keep the foil pouch for proper disposal of the ring after use. Choose the position that is most comfortable for you. For example, lying down, squatting, or standing with one leg up (Figures 1a, 1b, and 1c, respectively).

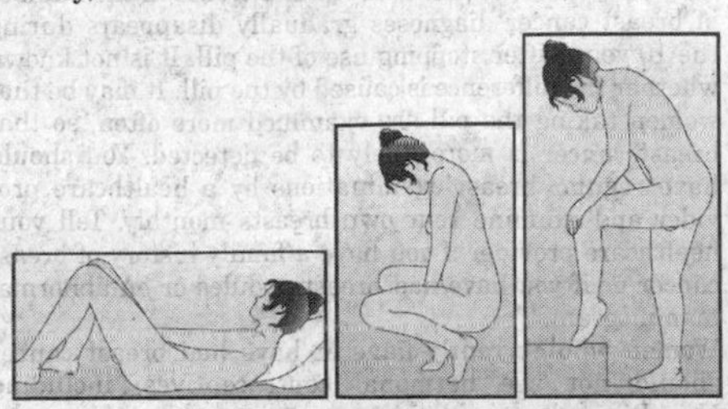

Figures 1a, 1b, and 1c. Positions for NuvaRing® insertion.

2. Hold NuvaRing® between your thumb and index finger (Figure 2a) and press the opposite sides of the ring together (Figure 2b).

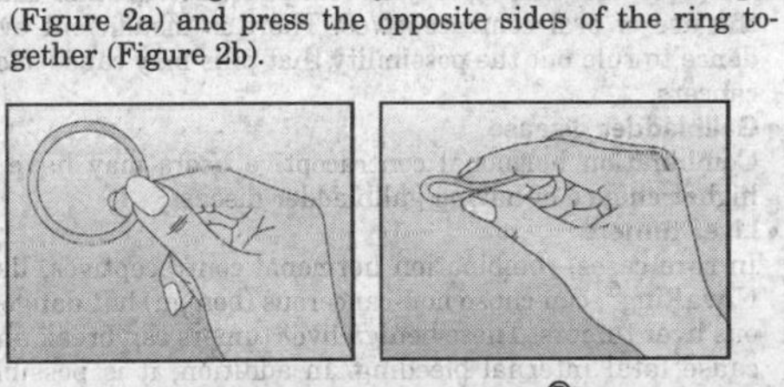

Figures 2a and 2b. Holding NuvaRing® and pressing the sides together.

3. Gently push the folded ring into your vagina (Figures 3a and 3b). The exact position of NuvaRing® in the vagina is not important for it to work (Figures 3c and 3d).

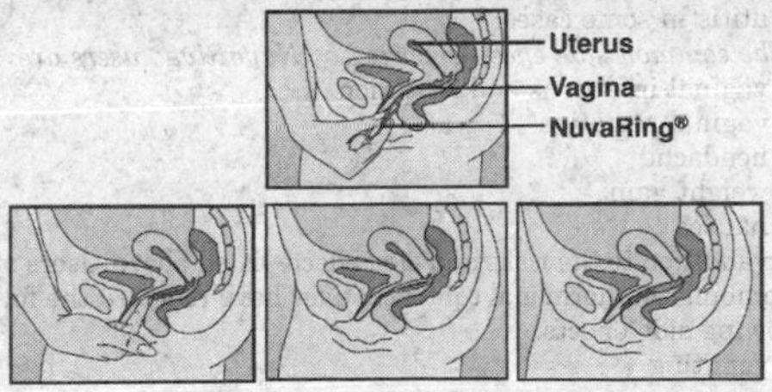

Figures 3a, 3b, 3c, and 3d. Inserting and positioning of NuvaRing®.

Although some women may be aware of NuvaRing® in the vagina, most women do not feel it once it is in place. If you feel discomfort, NuvaRing® is probably not inserted back far enough in the vagina. Use your finger to gently push the NuvaRing® farther into your vagina. **There is no danger of NuvaRing® being pushed too far up in the vagina or getting lost.** NuvaRing® can be inserted only as far as the end of the vagina, where the cervix (the narrow, lower end of the uterus) will block NuvaRing® from going any farther.

4. Once inserted, keep NuvaRing® in place for three weeks in a row.

How do I remove NuvaRing®?

[See figure 4 at top of next column]

1. Remove the ring three weeks after insertion on the same day of the week as it was inserted, at about the same time of day.

   You can remove NuvaRing® by hooking the index finger under the forward rim or by holding the rim between the index and middle finger and pulling it out (Figure 4).
2. Place the used ring in the foil pouch and properly dispose of it in a waste receptacle out of the reach of children and pets. Do not throw it in the toilet.

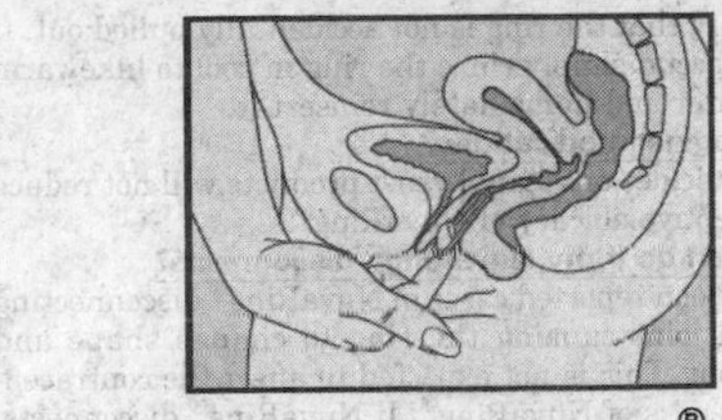

Figure 4. Removing NuvaRing®.

Your menstrual period will usually start two to three days after the ring is removed and may not have finished before the next ring is inserted. **To continue to have pregnancy protection, you must insert the new ring one week after the last one was removed, even if your menstrual period has not stopped.**

If you locate the ring in your vagina, but are unable to remove it, please contact your healthcare provider.

When do I insert a new ring?

After no more than a one-week ring-free break, insert a new ring on the same day of the week as it was removed in the last cycle. If the ring-free interval has been extended beyond one week, the possibility of pregnancy should be considered, and an extra method of birth control, such as male condoms or spermicide, **MUST** be used until NuvaRing® has been used **continuously for seven days.**

If NuvaRing® slips out:

NuvaRing® can accidentally slip out of the vagina while removing a tampon, during intercourse, or straining during a bowel movement. If NuvaRing® slips out of the vagina **and it has been out for less than three hours,** you should still be protected from pregnancy. NuvaRing® can be rinsed with cool to lukewarm (not hot) water and reinserted as soon as possible, and at the latest within three hours of removal or expulsion (slipping out).

If NuvaRing® is out of the vagina for more than three continuous hours:

During Weeks 1 and 2: If the ring **has been out of the vagina for more than three continuous hours** during the 1st or 2nd week of use, contraceptive effectiveness may be reduced. Reinsert ring as soon as you remember and use an extra method of birth control, such as male condoms or spermicide, until the ring has been used continuously for seven days.

During Week 3: If NuvaRing® slips **out of the vagina for more than three continuous hours** during the 3rd week of the three-week use period, throw the ring away and choose one of the following two options.

1. Insert a new ring immediately. Inserting a new ring will start the next three-week use period. You may not experience a period from your previous cycle. However, breakthrough spotting or bleeding may occur.
2. Have your period and insert a new ring no later than seven days (7×24 hours) from the time the previous ring was removed or expelled. This option should only be chosen if the ring was used continuously for the preceding seven days.

In addition, a barrier method such as condoms or spermicides must be used until the ring has been used continuously for seven days.

Women with conditions affecting the vagina, such as a prolapsed (dropped) uterus, may be more likely to have NuvaRing® slip out of the vagina. If NuvaRing® slips out repeatedly, you should consult with your healthcare provider.

If NuvaRing® is in your vagina too long:

If NuvaRing® has been left in your vagina for an extra week or less (four weeks total or less), you will remain protected. Remove NuvaRing® and insert a new ring after a one-week ring-free break.

If NuvaRing® has been left in place for more than four weeks, you may not be adequately protected from pregnancy and you must check to be sure you are not pregnant. You **MUST** use an extra method of birth control, such as male condoms or spermicide, until the new NuvaRing® has been in place for **seven days in a row.**

If you miss a menstrual period:

You must check to be sure that you are not pregnant if:

1. you miss a period and NuvaRing® was out of the vagina for more than three hours during the three weeks of ring use
2. you miss a period and waited longer than one week to insert a new ring
3. you have followed the instructions and you miss two periods in a row
4. you have left NuvaRing® in place for longer than four weeks

Can I use tampons when using NuvaRing®?

Use of tampons will not reduce the contraceptive efficacy of NuvaRing®. Insert NuvaRing® before inserting a tampon. You should pay particular attention when removing a tampon to be sure that the ring is not accidentally pulled out. If this should occur, simply rinse the ring in cool to lukewarm (not hot) water and immediately reinsert it.

Can I use vaginal medications?

Use of spermicides or vaginal yeast products will not reduce the contraceptive efficacy of NuvaRing®.

What should I do if my NuvaRing® disconnects?

There have been reported cases of NuvaRing® disconnecting at the weld joint causing the ring to change shape and straighten out. This is not expected to affect the contraceptive effectiveness of NuvaRing®. If NuvaRing® disconnects, expulsion (slipping out) is more likely to occur (see "If NuvaRing® slips out"). If you discover the ring has disconnected, you should discard the ring and replace it with a new ring.

Overdose

NuvaRing® is unlikely to cause an overdose because the ring holding the medicine releases a steady amount of contraceptive hormones. Do not use more than one ring at a time. Overdose of combination hormonal contraceptives may cause nausea, vomiting, or vaginal bleeding.

What should I avoid while using NuvaRing®?

Cigarette smoking increases the risk of serious cardiovascular side effects when you use combination oral contraceptives, including NuvaRing®. This risk increases even more if you are over age 35 and if you smoke 15 or more cigarettes a day. Women who use combination hormonal contraceptives, like NuvaRing®, are strongly advised not to smoke.

Do not breastfeed while using NuvaRing®. Some of the medicine may pass through the milk to the baby and could cause yellowing of the skin (jaundice) and breast enlargement in your baby. NuvaRing® could also decrease the amount and quality of your breast milk.

The hormones in NuvaRing® can interact with many other medicines and herbal supplements. Tell your healthcare provider about any medicines you are taking, including prescription medicines, over-the-counter medicines, herbal remedies, and vitamins.

The blood levels of the hormones released by NuvaRing® were increased when women used a vaginal medication (miconazole nitrate) for a yeast infection while NuvaRing® was in place. The pregnancy protection of NuvaRing® is not likely to be changed by use of these products. The blood levels of these hormones were not changed when women used vaginal, water-based spermicides (nonoxynol or N-9 products) along with NuvaRing®.

Certain drugs and herbal supplements may interact with combined hormonal contraceptives to make them less effective in preventing pregnancy or cause an increase in breakthrough bleeding. Such drugs include rifampin, drugs used for epilepsy such as barbiturates (for example, phenobarbital), carbamazepine, and phenytoin, primidone, topiramate, phenylbutazone, modafinil, and some drugs used for HIV such as ritonavir. Pregnancies and breakthrough bleeding have been reported by users of combined hormonal contraceptives who also used the herbal supplement St. John's wort. You may need to use a nonhormonal method of contraception during any cycle in which you take drugs that can make oral contraceptives less effective. Be sure to tell your healthcare provider if you are taking or start taking any other medications, including nonprescription products or herbal products while using NuvaRing®.

While using NuvaRing®, you should not rely upon a diaphragm when you need a back-up method of birth control because NuvaRing® may interfere with the correct placement and position of a diaphragm.

If you are scheduled for any laboratory tests, tell your doctor or healthcare provider you are using NuvaRing®. Contraceptive hormones may change certain blood tests results.

What are the possible risks and side effects of NuvaRing®?

- **Blood clots**

  The hormones in NuvaRing® may cause changes in your blood clotting system which may allow your blood to clot more easily. If blood clots form in your legs, they can travel to the lungs and cause a sudden blockage of a vessel carrying blood to the lungs. Rarely, clots occur in the blood vessels of the eye and may cause blindness, double vision, or other vision problems. The risk of getting blood clots may be greater with the type of progestin in NuvaRing® than with some other progestins in certain low-dose birth control pills. It is unknown if the risk of blood clots is different with NuvaRing® use than with the use of certain birth control pills.

  If you take hormonal contraceptives and need elective surgery, need to stay in bed for a prolonged illness or have recently delivered a baby, you may be at risk of developing blood clots. You should consult your doctor or healthcare provider about stopping hormonal contraceptives three to four weeks before surgery and not taking hormonal contraceptives for two weeks after surgery or during bed rest. You should also not take hormonal contraceptives soon after delivery of a baby. It is advisable to wait for at least four weeks after delivery if you are not breastfeeding. If you are breastfeeding, you should wait until you have weaned your child before using the pill (see PRECAUTIONS, NURSING MOTHERS).

- **Strokes and heart attacks**

  Hormonal contraceptives may increase your risk of strokes (blockage of blood flow to the brain) or heart attacks (blockage of blood flow to the heart). Any of these conditions can cause death or serious disability. Smoking greatly increases the risk of having strokes and heart attacks. Furthermore, smoking and the use of combination hormonal contraceptives, like NuvaRing®, greatly increases the chances of developing and dying of heart disease. If you use combination hormonal contraceptives, including NuvaRing®, you should not smoke.

- **High blood pressure and heart disease**

  Combination hormonal contraceptives, including NuvaRing®, can worsen conditions like high blood pressure, diabetes, and problems with cholesterol and triglycerides.

- **Cancer of the reproductive organs and breast**

  Breast cancer has been diagnosed slightly more often in women who use the pill than in women of the same age who do not use the pill. This small increase in the number of breast cancer diagnoses gradually disappears during the 10 years after stopping use of the pill. It is not known whether the difference is caused by the pill. It may be that women taking the pill are examined more often, so that breast cancer is more likely to be detected. You should have regular breast examinations by a healthcare provider and examine your own breasts monthly. Tell your healthcare provider if you have a family history of breast cancer or if you have had breast nodules or an abnormal mammogram.

  Women who currently have or have had breast cancer should not use hormonal contraceptives, including NuvaRing®, because breast cancer is usually a hormone-sensitive tumor.

  Some studies have found an increase in the incidence of cancer of the cervix in women who use oral contraceptives. However, this finding may be related to factors other than the use of oral contraceptives. There is insufficient evidence to rule out the possibility that pills may cause such cancers.

- **Gallbladder disease**

  Combination hormonal contraceptive users may have a higher chance of having gallbladder disease.

- **Liver tumors**

  In rare cases, combination hormonal contraceptives, like NuvaRing®, can cause non-cancerous (benign) but dangerous liver tumors. These benign liver tumors can break and cause fatal internal bleeding. In addition, it is possible that women who use combination hormonal contraceptives, like NuvaRing®, have a higher chance of getting liver cancer. However, liver cancers are extremely rare.

- **Lipid metabolism and inflammation of the pancreas**

  In women with inherited defects of lipid metabolism, there have been reports of significant elevations of plasma triglycerides during estrogen therapy. This has led to pancreatitis in some cases.

The common side effects reported by NuvaRing® users are:

- vaginal infections and irritation
- vaginal secretion
- headache
- weight gain
- nausea

In addition to the risks and side effects listed above, users of combination hormonal contraceptives have reported the following side effects:

- vomiting
- change in appetite
- abdominal cramps and bloating
- breast tenderness or enlargement
- irregular vaginal bleeding or spotting
- changes in menstrual cycle
- temporary infertility after treatment
- fluid retention (edema)
- spotty darkening of the skin, particularly on the face
- rash
- weight changes
- depression
- intolerance to contact lenses
- nervousness
- dizziness
- loss of scalp hair

Call your healthcare provider right away if you get any of the symptoms listed below. They may be signs of a serious problem:

- sharp chest pain, coughing blood, or sudden shortness of breath (possible clot in the lung)
- pain in the calf (back of lower leg; possible clot in the leg)
- crushing chest pain or heaviness in the chest (possible heart attack)
- sudden severe headache or vomiting, dizziness or fainting, problems with vision or speech, weakness, or numbness in an arm or leg (possible stroke)
- sudden partial or complete loss of vision (possible clot in the eye)
- yellowing of the skin or whites of the eyes (jaundice), especially with fever, tiredness, loss of appetite, dark colored urine, or light colored bowel movements (possible liver problems)
- severe pain, swelling, or tenderness in the abdomen (gallbladder or liver problems)
- sudden fever (usually 102°F or more), vomiting, diarrhea, dizziness, fainting, or a sunburn-like rash on the face or body (very rarely, toxic shock syndrome)
- breast lumps (possible breast cancer or benign breast disease)
- irregular vaginal bleeding or spotting that happens in more than one menstrual cycle or lasts for more than a few days
- urgent, frequent, burning and/or painful urination, and cannot locate the ring in the vagina (rarely, accidental placement of NuvaRing® into the urinary bladder)
- swelling (edema) of your fingers or ankles
- difficulty in sleeping, weakness, lack of energy, fatigue, or a change in mood (possible severe depression)

How effective is NuvaRing®?

If NuvaRing® is used according to the directions, your chance of getting pregnant is about 1 to 2% a year. This means that, for every 100 women who use NuvaRing® for a year, one or two will become pregnant. Your chance of getting pregnant increases if NuvaRing® is not used exactly according to the directions.

By comparison, the chances of getting pregnant in the first year of typical use (not always following directions exactly) of other methods of birth control are as follows:

No birth control method:	85%
Spermicides alone:	26%
Periodic abstinence methods (calendar, ovulation, thermometer):	25%
Withdrawal:	19%
Cervical Cap with spermicides:	20 to 40%
Vaginal sponge:	20 to 40%
Diaphragm with spermicides:	20%
Condom alone (male):	14%
Condom alone (female):	21%
Oral contraceptives:	5%
IUD:	less than 1 to 2%
Implants:	less than 1%
Injection:	less than 1%
Sterilization:	less than 1%

Other Information

- **Store NuvaRing® at room temperature, 25°C (77°F). Temperatures can be from 15-30°C (59-86°F). Avoid direct sunlight or storing above 30°C (86°F).**
- Medicines are sometimes prescribed for conditions that are not mentioned in patient information leaflets. Do not use NuvaRing® for a condition for which it was not prescribed. Do not give NuvaRing® to anyone else who may want to use it.
- Place the used ring in the reclosable foil pouch and properly dispose of it in a waste receptacle out of the reach of children and pets.

This leaflet summarizes the most important information about NuvaRing®. If you would like more information, talk with your healthcare provider. You can ask your pharmacist or healthcare provider for information about NuvaRing® that is written for health professionals.

1-877-NUVARING

Manufactured for: Merck Sharp & Dohme Corp., a subsidiary of

MERCK & CO., INC., Whitehouse Station, NJ 08889, USA

Manufactured by: N.V. Organon, Oss, The Netherlands, a subsidiary of

Merck & Co., Inc., Whitehouse Station, NJ 08889, USA

U.S. Patent No. 5,989,581.

Revised: 05/2012

900702-EE/ENG-RNG-PPI.2

Shown in Product Identification Guide, page 308

PEDVAXHIB® LIQUID ℞

[*ped-vax-hib*]

[Haemophilus b Conjugate Vaccine (Meningococcal Protein Conjugate)]

DESCRIPTION

PedvaxHIB® [Haemophilus b Conjugate Vaccine (Meningococcal Protein Conjugate)] is a highly purified capsular polysaccharide (polyribosylribitol phosphate or PRP) of *Haemophilus influenzae* type b (Haemophilus b, Ross strain) that is covalently bound to an outer membrane protein complex

(OMPC) of the B11 strain of *Neisseria meningitidis* serogroup B. The covalent bonding of the PRP to the OMPC which is necessary for enhanced immunogenicity of the PRP is confirmed by quantitative analysis of the conjugate's components following chemical treatment which yields a unique amino acid. The potency of PedvaxHIB is determined by assay of PRP.

Haemophilus influenzae type b and *Neisseria meningitidis* serogroup B are grown in complex fermentation media. The PRP is purified from the culture broth by purification procedures which include ethanol fractionation, enzyme digestion, phenol extraction and diafiltration. The OMPC from *Neisseria meningitidis* is purified by detergent extraction, ultracentrifugation, diafiltration and sterile filtration.

Liquid PedvaxHIB is ready to use and does not require a diluent. Each 0.5 mL dose of Liquid PedvaxHIB is a sterile product formulated to contain: 7.5 mcg of Haemophilus b PRP, 125 mcg of *Neisseria meningitidis* OMPC and 225 mcg of aluminum as amorphous aluminum hydroxyphosphate sulfate (previously referred to as aluminum hydroxide), in 0.9% sodium chloride, but does not contain lactose or thimerosal. Liquid PedvaxHIB is a slightly opaque white suspension.

This vaccine is for intramuscular administration and not for intravenous injection. (See DOSAGE AND ADMINISTRATION.)

CLINICAL PHARMACOLOGY

Prior to the introduction of Haemophilus b Conjugate Vaccines, *Haemophilus influenzae* type b (Hib) was the most frequent cause of bacterial meningitis and a leading cause of serious, systemic bacterial disease in young children worldwide.(1,2,3,4)

Hib disease occurred primarily in children under 5 years of age in the United States prior to the initiation of a vaccine program and was estimated to account for nearly 20,000 cases of invasive infections annually, approximately 12,000 of which were meningitis. The mortality rate from Hib meningitis is about 5%. In addition, up to 35% of survivors develop neurologic sequelae including seizures, deafness, and mental retardation.(5,6) Other invasive diseases caused by this bacterium include cellulitis, epiglottitis, sepsis, pneumonia, septic arthritis, osteomyelitis and pericarditis.

Prior to the introduction of the vaccine, it was estimated that 17% of all cases of Hib disease occurred in infants less than 6 months of age.(7) The peak incidence of Hib meningitis occurs between 6 to 11 months of age. Forty-seven percent of all cases occur by one year of age with the remaining 53% of cases occurring over the next four years.(2,20)

Among children under 5 years of age, the risk of invasive Hib disease is increased in certain populations including the following:

- Daycare attendees(8,9)
- Lower socio-economic groups(10)
- Blacks(11) (especially those who lack the Km(1) immunoglobulin allotype)(12)
- Caucasians who lack the G2m(n or 23) immunoglobulin allotype(13)
- Native Americans(14,15,16)
- Household contacts of cases(17)
- Individuals with asplenia, sickle cell disease, or antibody deficiency syndromes(18,19)

An important virulence factor of the Hib bacterium is its polysaccharide capsule (PRP). Antibody to PRP (anti-PRP) has been shown to correlate with protection against Hib disease.(3,21) While the anti-PRP level associated with protection using conjugated vaccines has not yet been determined, the level of anti-PRP associated with protection in studies using bacterial polysaccharide immune globulin or nonconjugated PRP vaccines ranged from >0.15 to >1.0 mcg/mL.(22-28)

Nonconjugated PRP vaccines are capable of stimulating B-lymphocytes to produce antibody without the help of T-lymphocytes (T-independent). The responses to many other antigens are augmented by helper T-lymphocytes (T-dependent). PedvaxHIB is a PRP-conjugate vaccine in which the PRP is covalently bound to the OMPC carrier(29) producing an antigen which is postulated to convert the T-independent antigen (PRP alone) into a T-dependent antigen resulting in both an enhanced antibody response and immunologic memory.

Clinical Evaluation of PedvaxHIB

PedvaxHIB, in a lyophilized formulation (lyophilized PedvaxHIB), was initially evaluated in 3,486 Native American (Navajo) infants, who completed the primary two-dose regimen in a randomized, double-blind, placebo-controlled study (The Protective Efficacy Study). At the time of the study, this population had a much higher incidence of Hib disease than the United States population as a whole and also had a lower antibody response to Haemophilus b Conjugate Vaccines, including PedvaxHIB.(14,15,16,30,33)

Each infant in this study received two doses of either placebo or lyophilized PedvaxHIB with the first dose administered at a mean of 8 weeks of age and the second administered approximately two months later; DTP and OPV were administered concomitantly. Antibody levels were measured in a subset of each group (TABLE 1).

TABLE 1: Antibody Responses in Navajo Infants

Vaccine	No. of Subjects	Time	% Subjects with >0.15 mcg/mL	% Subjects with >1.0 mcg/mL	Anti-PRP GMT (mcg/mL)
Lyophilized PedvaxHIB*	416†	Pre-Vaccination	44	10	0.16
	416	Post-Dose 1	88	52	0.95
	416	Post-Dose 2	91	60	1.43
Placebo*	461†	Pre-Vaccination	44	9	0.16
	461	Post-Dose 1	21	2	0.09
	461	Post-Dose 2	14	1	0.08
Lyophilized PedvaxHIB	27‡	Prebooster	70	33	0.51
	27	Postbooster§	100	89	8.39

* Post-Vaccination values obtained approximately 1–3 months after each dose.
† The Protective Efficacy Study
‡ Immunogenicity Trial(34)
§ Booster given at 12 months of age; Post-Vaccination values obtained 1 month after administration of booster dose.

TABLE 2: Antibody Responses to Liquid and Lyophilized PedvaxHIB in Infants From the General U.S. Population

Formulation	Age (Months)	Time	No. of Subjects	% Subjects with anti-PRP >0.15 mcg/mL	% Subjects with anti-PRP >1.0 mcg/mL	Anti-PRP GMT (mcg/mL)
Liquid PedvaxHIB (7.5 mcg PRP)	2-3	Pre-Vaccination	487	32	7	0.12
		Post-Dose 1*	480	94	64	1.55
		Post-Dose 2†	393	97	80	3.22
	12-15	Prebooster	284	80	30	0.49
		Postbooster†	284	99	95	10.23
	24‡	Persistence	94	97	55	1.29
Lyophilized PedvaxHIB (15 mcg PRP)	2-3	Pre-Vaccination	171	37	6	0.13
		Post-Dose 1*	169	97	72	1.88
		Post-Dose 2†	133	99	81	2.69
	12-15	Prebooster	87	71	28	0.39
		Postbooster†	87	99	91	7.64
	24‡	Persistence	37	97	54	1.10

* Approximately two months Post-Vaccination
† Approximately one month Post-Vaccination
‡ Approximately

[See table 1 above]

Most subjects were initially followed until 15 to 18 months of age. During this time, 22 cases of invasive Hib disease occurred in the placebo group (8 cases after the first dose and 14 cases after the second dose) and only 1 case in the vaccine group (none after the first dose and 1 after the second dose). Following the primary two-dose regimen, the protective efficacy of lyophilized PedvaxHIB was calculated to be 93% with a 95% confidence interval of 57%-98% (p=0.001, two-tailed). In the two months between the first and second doses, the difference in number of cases of disease between placebo and vaccine recipients (8 vs. 0 cases, respectively) was statistically significant (p=0.008, two-tailed); however, a primary two-dose regimen is required for infants 2-14 months of age.

At termination of the study, placebo recipients were offered vaccine. All original participants were then followed two years and nine months from termination of the study. During this extended follow-up, invasive Hib disease occurred in an additional seven of the original placebo recipients prior to receiving vaccine and in one of the original vaccine recipients (who had received only one dose of vaccine). No cases of invasive Hib disease were observed in placebo recipients after they received at least one dose of vaccine. Efficacy for this follow-up period, estimated from person-days at risk, was 96.6% (95 C.I., 72.2-99.9%) in children under 18 months of age and 100% (95 C.I., 23.5-100%) in children over 18 months of age.(33)

Since protective efficacy with lyophilized PedvaxHIB was demonstrated in such a high risk population, it would be expected to be predictive of efficacy in other populations.

The safety and immunogenicity of lyophilized PedvaxHIB were evaluated in infants and children in other clinical studies that were conducted in various locations throughout the United States. PedvaxHIB was highly immunogenic in all age groups studied.(31,32)

Lyophilized PedvaxHIB induced antibody levels greater than 1.0 mcg/mL in children who were poor responders to nonconjugated PRP vaccines. In a study involving such a subpopulation,(33,34) 34 children ranging in age from 27 to 61 months who developed invasive Hib disease despite previous vaccination with nonconjugated PRP vaccines were randomly assigned to 2 groups. One group (n=14) was vaccinated with lyophilized PedvaxHIB and the other group (n=20) with a nonconjugated PRP vaccine at a mean interval of approximately 12 months after recovery from disease. All 14 children vaccinated with lyophilized PedvaxHIB but only 6 of 20 children re-vaccinated with a nonconjugated PRP vaccine achieved an antibody level of >1.0 mcg/mL. The 14 children who had not responded to revaccination with the nonconjugated PRP vaccine were then vaccinated with a single dose of lyophilized PedvaxHIB; following this vaccination, all achieved antibody levels of >1.0 mcg/mL.

In addition, lyophilized PedvaxHIB has been studied in children at high risk of Hib disease because of genetically-related deficiencies [Blacks who were Km(1) allotype negative and Caucasians who were G2m(23) allotype negative] and are considered hyporesponsive to nonconjugated PRP vaccines on this basis.(35) The hyporesponsive children had anti-PRP responses comparable to those of allotype positive children of similar age range when vaccinated with lyophilized PedvaxHIB. All children achieved anti-PRP levels of >1.0 mcg/mL.

The safety and immunogenicity of Liquid PedvaxHIB were compared with those of lyophilized PedvaxHIB in a randomized clinical study involving 903 infants 2 to 6 months of age from the general U.S. population. DTP and OPV were administered concomitantly to most subjects. The antibody responses induced by each formulation of PedvaxHIB were similar. TABLE 2 shows antibody responses from this clinical study in subjects who received their first dose at 2 to 3 months of age.

[See table 2 above]

A booster dose of PedvaxHIB is required in infants who complete the primary two-dose regimen before 12 months of age. This booster dose will help maintain antibody levels during the first two years of life when children are at highest risk for invasive Hib disease. (See TABLE 2 and DOSAGE AND ADMINISTRATION.)

In four United States studies, antibody responses to lyophilized PedvaxHIB were evaluated in several subpopulations of infants initially vaccinated between 2 to 3 months of age. (See TABLE 3.)

[See table 3 at top of next page]

In two United States studies, antibody responses to Liquid PedvaxHIB were evaluated in several subpopulations of infants initially vaccinated between 2 to 3 months of age. (See TABLE 4.)

[See table 4 at top of next page]

Antibodies to the OMPC of *N. meningitidis* have been demonstrated in vaccinee sera, but the clinical relevance of these antibodies has not been established.(33)

TABLE 3: Antibody Responses* After Two Doses of Lyophilized PedvaxHIB Among Infants Initially Vaccinated at 2–3 Months of Age By Racial/Ethnic Group

Racial/Ethnic Groups	No. of Subjects	LYOPHILIZED % Subjects With Anti-PRP >0.15 mcg/mL	>1.0 mcg/mL	Anti-PRP GMT (mcg/mL)
Native American†	54	96	70	2.47
Caucasian	201	99	82	3.52
Hispanic	76	99	88	3.54
Black	23	100	96	5.40

* One month after the second dose
† Apache and Navajo

TABLE 4: Antibody Responses* After Two Doses of Liquid PedvaxHIB Among Infants Initially Vaccinated at 2–3 Months of Age By Racial/Ethnic Group

Racial/Ethnic Groups	No. of Subjects	LIQUID % Subjects With Anti-PRP >0.15 mcg/mL	>1.0 mcg/mL	Anti-PRP GMT (mcg/mL)
Native American†	90	97	78	2.76
Caucasian	143	94	72	2.16
Hispanic	184	98	85	4.34
Black	18	100	94	7.58

* One month after the second dose
† Apache and Navajo

TABLE 5: Fever or Local Reactions in Subjects First Vaccinated at 2 to 6 Months of Age with Liquid PedvaxHIB*

Reaction	No. of Subjects Evaluated	Post-Dose 1 (hr) 6	24	48	No. of Subjects Evaluated	Post-Dose 2 (hr) 6	24	48
		Percentage				Percentage		
Fever† >38.3°C (≥101°F) Rectal	222	18.1	4.4	0.5	206	14.1	9.4	2.8
Erythema >2.5 cm diameter	674	2.2	1.0	0.5	562	1.6	1.1	0.4
Swelling >2.5 cm diameter	674	2.5	1.9	0.9	562	0.9	0.9	1.3

* DTP and OPV were administered concomitantly to most subjects.
† Fever was also measured by another method or reported as normal for an additional 345 infants after dose 1 and for an additional 249 infants after dose 2; however, these data are not included in this table.

Interchangeability of Licensed Haemophilus b Conjugate Vaccines and PedvaxHIB

Published studies have examined the interchangeability of other licensed Haemophilus b Conjugate Vaccines and PedvaxHIB.(42,43,44,45,52) According to the American Academy of Pediatrics, excellent immune responses have been achieved when different vaccines have been interchanged in the primary series. If PedvaxHIB is given in a series with one of the other products licensed for infants, the recommended number of doses to complete the series is determined by the other product and not by PedvaxHIB. PedvaxHIB may be interchanged with other licensed Haemophilus b Conjugate Vaccines for the booster dose.(52)

Use with Other Vaccines

Results from clinical studies indicate that Liquid PedvaxHIB can be administered concomitantly with DTP, OPV, eIPV (enhanced inactivated poliovirus vaccine), VARIVAX® [Varicella Virus Vaccine Live (Oka/Merck)], M-M-R® II (Measles, Mumps, and Rubella Virus Vaccine Live) or RECOMBIVAX HB® [Hepatitis B Vaccine (Recombinant)].(33) No impairment of immune response to individual tested vaccine antigens was demonstrated.

The type, frequency and severity of adverse experiences observed in these studies with PedvaxHIB were similar to those seen when the other vaccines were given alone.

In addition, a PRP-OMPC-containing product, COMVAX® [Haemophilus b Conjugate (Meningococcal Protein Conjugate) and Hepatitis B (Recombinant) Vaccine], was given concomitantly with a booster dose of DTaP [diphtheria, tetanus, acellular pertussis] at approximately 15 months of age, using separate sites and syringes for injectable vaccines. No impairment of immune response to these individually tested vaccine antigens was demonstrated. COMVAX has also been administered concomitantly with the primary series of DTaP to a limited number of infants. PRP antibody responses are satisfactory for COMVAX, but immune responses are currently unavailable for DTaP (see Manufacturer's Product Circular for COMVAX). No serious vaccine-related adverse events were reported.(33)

INDICATIONS AND USAGE

Liquid PedvaxHIB is indicated for routine vaccination against invasive disease caused by *Haemophilus influenzae* type b in infants and children 2 to 71 months of age.

Liquid PedvaxHIB will not protect against disease caused by *Haemophilus influenzae* other than type b or against other microorganisms that cause invasive disease such as meningitis or sepsis. As with any vaccine, vaccination with Liquid PedvaxHIB may not result in a protective antibody response in all individuals given the vaccine.

BECAUSE OF THE POTENTIAL FOR IMMUNE TOLERANCE, Liquid PedvaxHIB IS NOT RECOMMENDED FOR USE IN INFANTS YOUNGER THAN 6 WEEKS OF AGE. (See PRECAUTIONS.)

Revaccination

Infants completing the primary two-dose regimen before 12 months of age should receive a booster dose (see DOSAGE AND ADMINISTRATION).

CONTRAINDICATIONS

Hypersensitivity to any component of the vaccine or the diluent.

Persons who develop symptoms suggestive of hypersensitivity after an injection should not receive further injections of the vaccine.

PRECAUTIONS

General

As for any vaccine, adequate treatment provisions, including epinephrine, should be available for immediate use should an anaphylactoid reaction occur.

Use caution when vaccinating latex-sensitive individuals since the vial stopper contains dry natural latex rubber that may cause allergic reactions.

Special care should be taken to ensure that the injection does not enter a blood vessel.

It is important to use a separate sterile syringe and needle for each patient to prevent transmission of hepatitis B or other infectious agents from one person to another.

As with other vaccines, Liquid PedvaxHIB may not induce protective antibody levels immediately following vaccination.

As reported with Haemophilus b Polysaccharide Vaccine(36) and another Haemophilus b Conjugate Vaccine(37), cases of Hib disease may occur in the week after vaccination, prior to the onset of the protective effects of the vaccines.

There is insufficient evidence that Liquid PedvaxHIB given immediately after exposure to natural *Haemophilus influenzae* type b will prevent illness.

The decision to administer or delay vaccination because of current or recent febrile illness depends on the severity of symptoms and on the etiology of the disease. The Advisory Committee on Immunization Practices (ACIP) has recommended that vaccination should be delayed during the course of an acute febrile illness. All vaccines can be administered to persons with minor illnesses such as diarrhea, mild upper-respiratory infection with or without low-grade fever, or other low-grade febrile illness. Persons with moderate or severe febrile illness should be vaccinated as soon as they have recovered from the acute phase of the illness.(46)

If PedvaxHIB is used in persons with malignancies or those receiving immunosuppressive therapy or who are otherwise immunocompromised, the expected immune response may not be obtained.

Instructions to Healthcare Provider

The healthcare provider should determine the current health status and previous vaccination history of the vaccinee.

The healthcare provider should question the patient, parent, or guardian about reactions to a previous dose of PedvaxHIB or other Haemophilus b Conjugate Vaccines.

Information for Patients

The healthcare provider should provide the vaccine information required to be given with each vaccination to the patient, parent, or guardian.

The healthcare provider should inform the patient, parent, or guardian of the benefits and risks associated with vaccination. For risks associated with vaccination, see ADVERSE REACTIONS.

Patients, parents, and guardians should be instructed to report any serious adverse reactions to their healthcare provider who in turn should report such events to the U. S. Department of Health and Human Services through the Vaccine Adverse Event Reporting System (VAERS), 1-800-822-7967.(47)

Laboratory Test Interactions

Sensitive tests (e.g., Latex Agglutination Kits) may detect PRP derived from the vaccine in urine of some vaccinees for at least 30 days following vaccination with lyophilized PedvaxHIB;(38) in clinical studies with lyophilized PedvaxHIB, such children demonstrated normal immune response to the vaccine.

Carcinogenesis, Mutagenesis, Impairment of Fertility

Liquid PedvaxHIB has not been evaluated for carcinogenic or mutagenic potential, or potential to impair fertility.

Pregnancy

Pregnancy Category C

Animal reproduction studies have not been conducted with PedvaxHIB. Liquid PedvaxHIB is not recommended for use in individuals 6 years of age and older.

Pediatric Use

Safety and effectiveness in infants below the age of 2 months and in children 6 years of age and older have not been established. In addition, Liquid PedvaxHIB should not be used in infants younger than 6 weeks of age because this will lead to a reduced anti-PRP response and may lead to immune tolerance (impaired ability to respond to subsequent exposure to the PRP antigen).(49-51) Liquid PedvaxHIB is not recommended for use in individuals 6 years of age and older because they are generally not at risk of Hib disease.

Geriatric Use

This vaccine is NOT recommended for use in adult populations.

ADVERSE REACTIONS

Liquid PedvaxHIB

In a multicenter clinical study (n=903) comparing the effects of Liquid PedvaxHIB with those of lyophilized PedvaxHIB, 1,699 doses of Liquid PedvaxHIB were administered to 678 healthy infants 2 to 6 months of age from the general U.S. population. DTP and OPV were administered concomitantly to most subjects. Both formulations of PedvaxHIB were generally well tolerated and no serious vaccine-related adverse reactions were reported.

During a three-day period following primary vaccination with Liquid PedvaxHIB in these infants, the most frequently reported (>1%) adverse reactions, without regard to causality, excluding those shown in TABLE 5, in decreasing order of frequency, were: irritability, sleepiness, injection site pain/soreness, injection site erythema (≤2.5 cm diameter, see also TABLE 5), injection site swelling/induration (≤2.5 cm diameter, see also TABLE 5), unusual high-pitched crying, prolonged crying (>4 hr), diarrhea, vomiting, crying, pain, otitis media, rash, and upper respiratory infection.

Selected objective observations reported by parents over a 48-hour period in these infants following primary vaccination with Liquid PedvaxHIB are summarized in TABLE 5. [See table 5 at top of previous page]

Adverse reactions during a three-day period following administration of the booster dose were generally similar in type and frequency to those seen following primary vaccination.

Lyophilized PedvaxHIB

In The Protective Efficacy Study (see CLINICAL PHARMACOLOGY), 4,459 healthy Navajo infants 6 to 12 weeks of age received lyophilized PedvaxHIB or placebo. Most of these infants received DTP/OPV concomitantly. No differences were seen in the type and frequency of serious health problems expected in this Navajo population or in serious adverse experiences reported among those who received lyophilized PedvaxHIB and those who received placebo, and none was reported to be related to lyophilized PedvaxHIB. Only one serious reaction (tracheitis) was reported as possibly related to lyophilized PedvaxHIB and only one (diarrhea) as possibly related to placebo. Seizures occurred infrequently in both groups (9 occurred in vaccine recipients, 8 of whom also received DTP; 8 occurred in placebo recipients, 7 of whom also received DTP) and were not reported to be related to lyophilized PedvaxHIB.

In early clinical studies involving the administration of 8,086 doses of lyophilized PedvaxHIB alone to 5,027 healthy infants and children 2 months to 71 months of age, lyophilized PedvaxHIB was generally well tolerated. No serious adverse reactions were reported. In a subset of these infants, urticaria was reported in two children, and thrombocytopenia was seen in one child. A cause and effect relationship between these side effects and the vaccination has not been established.

Potential Adverse Reactions

The use of Haemophilus b Polysaccharide Vaccines and another Haemophilus b Conjugate Vaccine has been associated with the following additional adverse effects: early onset Hib disease and Guillain-Barré syndrome. A cause and effect relationship between these side effects and the vaccination was not established.{36,37,39,40,41,49}

Post-Marketing Adverse Reactions

The following additional adverse reactions have been reported with the use of the lyophilized and liquid formulations of PedvaxHIB:

Hemic and Lymphatic System
Lymphadenopathy
Hypersensitivity
Rarely, angioedema
Nervous System
Febrile seizures
Skin
Sterile injection site abscess

DOSAGE AND ADMINISTRATION

Liquid PedvaxHIB

FOR INTRAMUSCULAR ADMINISTRATION
DO NOT INJECT INTRAVENOUSLY

If there is an interruption or delay between doses in the primary series, there is no need to repeat the series, but dosing should be continued at the next clinic visit. (See CONTRAINDICATIONS and PRECAUTIONS.)

2 to 14 Months of Age

Infants 2 to 14 months of age should receive a 0.5 mL dose of vaccine ideally beginning at 2 months of age followed by a 0.5 mL dose 2 months later (or as soon as possible thereafter). When the primary two-dose regimen is completed before 12 months of age, a booster dose is required (see below and TABLE 6). Infants born prematurely, regardless of birth weight, should be vaccinated at the same chronological age and according to the same schedule and precautions as full-term infants and children.{46}

15 Months of Age and Older

Children 15 months of age and older previously unvaccinated against Hib disease should receive a single 0.5 mL dose of vaccine.

Booster Dose

In infants completing the primary two-dose regimen before 12 months of age, a booster dose (0.5 mL) should be administered at 12 to 15 months of age, but not earlier than 2 months after the second dose.

Vaccination regimens for Liquid PedvaxHIB by age group are outlined in TABLE 6.

TABLE 6: Vaccination Regimens for Liquid PedvaxHIB By Age Groups

Age (Months) at First Dose	Primary	Age (Months) at Booster Dose
2–10	2 doses, 2 mo. apart	12–15
11–14	2 doses, 2 mo. apart	—
15–71	1 dose	—

Interchangeability

PedvaxHIB may be interchanged with other licensed Haemophilus b Conjugate Vaccines for the primary and booster doses.{52} (See CLINICAL PHARMACOLOGY.)

Use with Other Vaccines

Results from clinical studies indicate that Liquid PedvaxHIB can be administered concomitantly with DTP, OPV, eIPV (enhanced inactivated poliovirus vaccine), VARIVAX [Varicella Virus Vaccine Live (Oka/Merck)], M-M-R II (Measles, Mumps, and Rubella Virus Vaccine Live) or RECOMBIVAX HB [Hepatitis B Vaccine (Recombinant)]. No impairment of immune response to these individually tested vaccine antigens was demonstrated.

The type, frequency and severity of adverse experiences observed in these studies with PedvaxHIB were similar to those seen with the other vaccines when given alone. (See CLINICAL PHARMACOLOGY.)

In addition, a PRP-OMPC-containing product, COMVAX [Haemophilus b Conjugate (Meningococcal Protein Conjugate) and Hepatitis B (Recombinant) Vaccine], was given concomitantly with a booster dose of DTaP [diphtheria, tetanus, acellular pertussis] at approximately 15 months of age, using separate sites and syringes for injectable vaccines. No impairment of immune response to these individually tested vaccine antigens was demonstrated. COMVAX has also been administered concomitantly with the primary series of DTaP to a limited number of infants. PRP antibody responses are satisfactory for COMVAX, but immune responses are currently unavailable for DTaP (see Manufacturer's Product Circular for COMVAX). No serious vaccine-related adverse events were reported.{33}

Parenteral drug products should be inspected visually for extraneous particulate matter and discoloration prior to administration whenever solution and container permit.

Liquid PedvaxHIB is a slightly opaque white suspension. (See DESCRIPTION.)

The vaccine should be used as supplied; no reconstitution is necessary.

Shake well before withdrawal and use. Thorough agitation is necessary to maintain suspension of the vaccine.

Inject 0.5 mL intramuscularly, preferably into the anterolateral thigh or the outer aspect of the upper arm. The buttocks should not be used for active vaccination of infants and children, because of the potential risk of injury to the sciatic nerve.

HOW SUPPLIED

Liquid PedvaxHIB is supplied as follows:

No. 4897 — A box of 10 single-dose vials of liquid vaccine, **NDC** 0006-4897-00.

Storage

Store vaccine at 2-8°C (36-46°F).
DO NOT FREEZE.

REFERENCES

1. Cochi, S. L., et al: Immunization of U.S. children with *Haemophilus influenzae* type b polysaccharide vaccine: A cost-effectiveness model of strategy assessment. JAMA *253:* 521-529, 1985.
2. Schlech, W. F., III, et al: Bacterial meningitis in the United States, 1978 through 1981. The National Bacterial Meningitis Surveillance Study. JAMA *253:* 1749-1754, 1985.
3. Peltola, H., et al: Prevention of *Haemophilus influenzae* type b bacteremic infections with the capsular polysaccharide vaccine. N Engl J Med *310:* 1561-1566, 1984.
4. Cadoz, M., et al: Etude epidemiologique des cas de meningitis purulentes hospitalises a Dakar pendant la decemie 1970-1979. Bull WHO *59:* 575-584, 1981.
5. Sell, S. H., et al: Long-term Sequelae of *Haemophilus influenzae* meningitis. Pediatr *49:* 206-217, 1972.
6. Taylor, H. G., et al: Intellectual, neuropsychological, and achievement outcomes in children six to eight years after recovery from *Haemophilus influenzae* meningitis. Pediatr *74:* 198-205, 1984.
7. Hay, J. W., et al: Cost-benefit analysis of two strategies for prevention of *Haemophilus influenzae* type b infection. Pediatr *80*(3): 319-329, 1987.
8. Redmond, S. R., et al: *Haemophilus influenzae* type b disease: an epidemiologic study with special reference to daycare centers. JAMA *252:* 2581-2584, 1984.
9. Istre, G. R., et al: Risk factors for primary invasive *Haemophilus influenzae* disease: increased risk from daycare attendance and school age household members. J Pediatr *106:* 190-195, 1985.
10. Fraser, D.W., et al: Risk factors in bacterial meningitis: Charleston County, South Carolina. J Infect Dis *127:* 271-277, 1973.
11. Tarr, P. I., et al: Demographic factors in the epidemiology of *Haemophilus influenzae* meningitis in young children. J Pediatr *92:* 884-888, 1978.
12. Granoff, D. M., et al: Response to immunization with *Haemophilus influenzae* type b polysaccharide-pertussis vaccine and risk of Haemophilus meningitis in children with Km(1) immunoglobulin allotype. J Clin Invest *74:* 1708-1714, 1984.
13. Ambrosino, D. M., et al: Correlation between G2m(n) immunoglobulin allotype and human antibody response and susceptibility to polysaccharide encapsulated bacteria. J Clin Invest *75:* 1935-1942, 1985.
14. Coulehan, J. L., et al: Epidemiology of *Haemophilus influenzae* type b disease among Navajo Indians. Pub Health Rep *99:* 404-409, 1984.
15. Losonsky, G. A., et al: *Haemophilus influenzae* disease in the White Mountain Apaches: molecular epidemiology of a high risk population. Pediatr Infect Dis J *3:* 539-547, 1985.
16. Ward, J. I., et al: *Haemophilus influenzae* disease in Alaskan Eskimos: characteristics of a population with an unusual incidence of disease. Lancet *1:* 1281-1285, 1981.
17. Ward, J. I., et al: *Haemophilus influenzae* meningitis: a national study of secondary spread in household contacts. N Engl J Med *301:* 122-126, 1979.
18. Ward, J., et al: *Haemophilus influenzae* bacteremia in children with sickle cell disease. J Pediatr *88:* 261-263, 1976.
19. Bartlett, A. V., et al: Unusual presentations of *Haemophilus influenzae* infections in immunocompromised patients. J Pediatr *102:* 55-58, 1983.
20. Recommendations of the Immunization Practices Advisory Committee. Polysaccharide vaccine for prevention of *Haemophilus influenzae* type b disease. MMWR *34*(15): 201-205, 1985.
21. Santosham, M., et al: Prevention of *Haemophilus influenzae* type b infections in high-risk infants treated with bacterial polysaccharide immune globulin. N Engl J Med *317:* 923-929, 1987.
22. Siber, G. R., et al: Preparation of human hyperimmune globulin to *Haemophilus influenzae* b, *Streptococcus pneumoniae*, and *Neisseria meningitidis*. Infect Immun *45:* 248-254, 1984.
23. Smith, D. H., et al: Responses of children immunized with the capsular polysaccharide of *Haemophilus influenzae* type b. Pediatr *52:* 637-645, 1973.
24. Robbins, J. B., et al: Quantitative measurement of 'natural' and immunization-induced *Haemophilus influenzae* type b capsular polysaccharide antibodies. Pediatr Res *7:* 103-110, 1973.
25. Kaythy, H., et al: The protective level of serum antibodies to the capsular polysaccharide of *Haemophilus influenzae* type b. J Infect Dis *147:* 1100, 1983.
26. Peltola, H., et al: *Haemophilus influenzae* type b capsular polysaccharide vaccine in children: a double-blind field study of 100,000 vaccinees 3 months to 5 years of age in Finland. Pediatr *60:* 730-737, 1977.
27. Ward, J. I., et al: *Haemophilus influenzae* type b vaccines: Lessons For the Future. Pediatr *81:* 886-893, 1988.
28. Daum, R. S., et al: *Haemophilus influenzae* type b vaccines: Lessons From the Past. Pediatr *81:* 893-897, 1988.
29. Marburg, S., et al: Bimolecular chemistry of macromolecules: Synthesis of bacterial polysaccharide conjugates with *Neisseria meningitidis* membrane protein. J Am Chem Soc *108:* 5282-5287, 1986.
30. Letson, G. W., et al: Comparison of active and combined passive/active immunization of Navajo children against *Haemophilus influenzae* type b. Pediatr Infect Dis J 7(111): 747-752, 1988.
31. Einhorn, M. S., et al: Immunogenicity in infants of *Haemophilus influenzae* type b polysaccharide in a conjugate vaccine with *Neisseria meningitidis* outer-membrane protein. Lancet *2:* 299-302, 1986.
32. Ahonkhai, V.I., et al: *Haemophilus influenzae* type b Conjugate Vaccine (Meningococcal Protein Conjugate) (PedvaxHIB TM): Clinical Evaluation. Pediatr *85*(4): 676-681, 1990.
33. Data on file at Merck Research Laboratories.
34. Granoff, D. M., et al: Immunogenicity of *Haemophilus influenzae* type b polysaccharide—outer membrane protein conjugate vaccine in patients who acquired Haemophilus disease despite previous vaccination with type b polysaccharide vaccine. J. Pediatr. *114*(6): 925-933, June 1989.
35. Lenoir, A. A., et al: Response to *Haemophilus influenzae* type b (*H. influenzae* type b) polysaccharide *N. meningitidis* outer membrane protein (PS-OMP) conjugate vaccine in relation to Km(1) and G2m(23) allotypes. Twenty-sixth Interscience Conference on Antimicrobial Agents and Chemotherapy (Abstract #216) 133, 1986.
36. Mortimer, E. A.: Efficacy of Haemophilus b polysaccharide vaccine: An enigma. JAMA *260:* 1454, 1988.
37. Meekison, W., et al: Post-marketing surveillance of adverse effects following ProHIBiT vaccine. British Columbia Canada Diseases Weekly Report *15-28:* 143-145, 1989.
38. Goepp, J. G., et al: Persistent urinary antigen excretion in infants vaccinated with *Haemophilus influenzae* type

b capsular polysaccharide conjugated with outer membrane protein from *Neisseria meningitidis*. Pediatr Infect Dis J *11*(1): 2-5, 1992.

39. Milstein, J. B., et al: Adverse reactions reported following receipt of *Haemophilus influenzae* type b vaccine: An analysis after one year of marketing. Pediatr *80:* 270, 1987.
40. Black, S., et al: b-CAPSA 1 *Haemophilus influenzae* type b capsular polysaccharide vaccine safety. Pediatr *79:* 321-325, 1987.
41. D'Cruz, O. F., et al: Acute inflammatory demyelinating polyradiculoneuropathy (Guillain-Barré syndrome) after immunization with *Haemophilus influenzae* type b Conjugate Vaccine. J Pediatr *115:* 743-746, 1989.
42. Recommendations of the Immunization Practices Advisory Committee. Recommendations for use of Haemophilus b Conjugate Vaccines and a combined diphtheria, tetanus, pertussis, and Haemophilus b vaccine. MMWR *42*(RR-13): 1-15, 1993.
43. Daum, R. S., et al: Interchangeability of *Haemophilus influenzae* type b vaccines for the primary series (mix and match): a preliminary analysis [Abstract 976]. Pediatr Res *33:* 166A, 1993.
44. Greenberg, D. P., et al: Enhanced antibody responses in infants given different sequences of heterogenous *Haemophilus influenzae* type b Conjugate Vaccines. J Pediatr *126:* 206-211, 1995.
45. Anderson, E. L., et al: Interchangeability of Conjugated *Haemophilus influenzae* type b Vaccines in Infants. JAMA *273:* 849-853, 1995.
46. Recommendations of the Immunization Practices Advisory Committee. General Recommendations on Immunization. MMWR *43*(RR-1), 1994.
47. Vaccine Adverse Event Reporting System - United States. MMWR *39*(41): 730-733, October 19, 1990.
48. Institute of Medicine Adverse Events Associated With Childhood Vaccines Evidence Bearing on Causality. National Academy Press, Washington, D.C., 260-261, 1994.
49. Keyserling, H.L., et al: Program and Abstracts of the 30th ICAAC, (Abstract #63), 1990.
50. Ward, J.I., et al: Program and Abstracts of the 32nd ICAAC, (Abstract #984), 1992.
51. Lieberman, J.M., et al: Infect Dis, (Abstract #1028), 1993.
52. American Academy of Pediatrics. Recommended Childhood Immunization Schedule - United States, January-December 1998. Pediatr *101*(1): 154-157, 1998.

Manuf. and Dist. by: Merck Sharp & Dohme Corp., a subsidiary of **MERCK & CO., INC.**, Whitehouse Station, NJ 08889, USA
Issued December 2010
Printed in USA
9877903

PEGINTRON ℞

[pĕg-ĭn-trŏn]
(Peginterferon alfa-2b)
for Injection, for Subcutaneous Use

HIGHLIGHTS OF PRESCRIBING INFORMATION
These highlights do not include all the information needed to use PegIntron safely and effectively. See full prescribing information for PegIntron.
PegIntron® (Peginterferon alfa-2b) for Injection, for Subcutaneous Use
Initial U.S. Approval: 2001

WARNING: RISK OF SERIOUS DISORDERS AND RIBAVIRIN-ASSOCIATED EFFECTS
See full prescribing information for complete boxed warning.
- **May cause or aggravate fatal or life-threatening neuropsychiatric, autoimmune, ischemic, and infectious disorders. Monitor closely and withdraw therapy with persistently severe or worsening signs or symptoms of the above disorders. (5)**

Use with Ribavirin
- **Ribavirin may cause birth defects and fetal death; avoid pregnancy in female patients and female partners of male patients. (5.1)**

RECENT MAJOR CHANGES

Dosage and Administration,
Dose Reduction (2.3) 05/2013

INDICATIONS AND USAGE

PegIntron is an antiviral indicated for treatment of Chronic Hepatitis C (CHC) in patients with compensated liver disease. (1.1)

	PegIntron Dose (Adults)*	PegIntron Dose (Pediatric Patients)	REBETOL Dose* (Adults)	REBETOL Dose (Pediatric Patients)
PegIntron Combination Therapy (2.1)	1.5 mcg/kg/week	60 mcg/m²/week	800-1400 mg orally daily with food	15 mg/kg/day orally with food in 2 divided doses

* Refer to Tables 1-7 of the full Prescribing Information.

DOSAGE AND ADMINISTRATION

- PegIntron is administered by subcutaneous injection. [See table above]
- Dose reduction is recommended in patients experiencing certain adverse reactions or renal dysfunction. (2.3, 2.5)

DOSAGE FORMS AND STRENGTHS

Single-use vial (with 1.25 mL diluent) and REDIPEN® (3):
- 50 mcg per 0.5 mL, 80 mcg per 0.5 mL, 120 mcg per 0.5 mL, 150 mcg per 0.5 mL.

CONTRAINDICATIONS

- Known hypersensitivity reactions, such as urticaria, angioedema, bronchoconstriction, anaphylaxis, Stevens-Johnson syndrome, and toxic epidermal necrolysis to interferon alpha or any other product component. (4)
- Autoimmune hepatitis. (4)
- Hepatic decompensation (Child-Pugh score greater than 6 [class B and C]) in cirrhotic CHC patients before or during treatment. (4)

Additional contraindications for combination therapy with ribavirin:
- Pregnant women and men whose female partners are pregnant. (4, 8.1)
- Hemoglobinopathies (e.g., thalassemia major, sickle-cell anemia). (4)
- Creatinine clearance less than 50 mL/min. (4)

WARNINGS AND PRECAUTIONS

- Birth defects and fetal death with ribavirin: Patients must have a negative pregnancy test prior to therapy, use at least 2 forms of contraception, and undergo monthly pregnancy tests. (5.1)

Patients exhibiting the following conditions should be closely monitored and may require dose reduction or discontinuation of therapy:
- Hemolytic anemia with ribavirin. (5.1)
- Neuropsychiatric events. (5.2)
- History of significant or unstable cardiac disease. (5.3)
- Hypothyroidism, hyperthyroidism, hyperglycemia, diabetes mellitus that cannot be effectively treated by medication. (5.4)
- New or worsening ophthalmologic disorders. (5.5)
- Ischemic and hemorrhagic cerebrovascular events. (5.6)
- Severe decreases in neutrophil or platelet counts. (5.7)
- History of autoimmune disorders. (5.8)
- Pancreatitis and ulcerative or hemorrhagic/ischemic colitis and pancreatitis. (5.9, 5.10)
- Pulmonary infiltrates or pulmonary function impairment. (5.11)
- Child-Pugh score greater than 6 (class B and C). (4, 5.12)
- Increased creatinine levels in patients with renal insufficiency. (5.13)
- Serious, acute hypersensitivity reactions and cutaneous eruptions. (5.14)
- Dental/periodontal disorders reported with combination therapy. (5.16)
- Hypertriglyceridemia may result in pancreatitis (e.g., triglycerides greater than 1000 mg/dL). (5.17)
- Weight loss and growth inhibition reported with combination therapy in pediatric patients. (5.18)
- Peripheral neuropathy when used in combination with telbivudine. (5.19)

ADVERSE REACTIONS

Most common adverse reactions (greater than 40%) in adult patients receiving either PegIntron or PegIntron/REBETOL are injection site inflammation/reaction, fatigue/asthenia, headache, rigors, fevers, nausea, myalgia and anxiety/emotional lability/irritability (6.1). Most common adverse reactions (greater than 25%) in pediatric patients receiving PegIntron/REBETOL are pyrexia, headache, neutropenia, fatigue, anorexia, injection-site erythema, vomiting (6.1).

To report SUSPECTED ADVERSE REACTIONS, contact Schering Corporation, a subsidiary of Merck & Co., Inc., at 1-800-526-4099 or FDA at 1-800-FDA-1088 or *www.fda.gov/medwatch.*

DRUG INTERACTIONS

- Drug metabolized by CYP450: Caution with drugs metabolized by CYP2C8/9 (e.g., warfarin, phenytoin) or CYP2D6 (e.g., flecainide). (7.1)
- Methadone: Monitor for increased narcotic effect. (7.2)
- Nucleoside analogues: Closely monitor for toxicities. Discontinue nucleoside reverse transcriptase inhibitors or reduce dose or discontinue interferon, ribavirin, or both with worsening toxicities. (7.3)
- Didanosine: Concurrent use with REBETOL is not recommended. (7.3)

USE IN SPECIFIC POPULATIONS

- Ribavirin Pregnancy Registry (8.1)
- Pediatrics: safety and efficacy in pediatrics less than 3 years old have not been established. (8.4)
- Geriatrics: neuropsychiatric, cardiac, pulmonary, GI, and systemic (flu-like) adverse reactions may be more severe. (8.5)
- Organ transplant: safety and efficacy have not been studied. (8.6)
- HIV or HBV co-infection: safety and efficacy have not been established. (8.7)

See 17 for PATIENT COUNSELING INFORMATION and Medication Guide

Revised: 05/2013

FULL PRESCRIBING INFORMATION: CONTENTS*

*** Sections or subsections omitted from the full prescribing information are not listed**

FULL PRESCRIBING INFORMATION

WARNING: RISK OF SERIOUS DISORDERS AND RIBAVIRIN-ASSOCIATED EFFECTS

Alpha interferons, including PegIntron, may cause or aggravate fatal or life-threatening neuropsychiatric, autoimmune, ischemic, and infectious disorders. Patients should be monitored closely with periodic clinical and laboratory evaluations. Patients with persistently severe or worsening signs or symptoms of these conditions should be withdrawn from therapy. In many, but not all cases, these disorders resolve after stopping PegIntron therapy *[see Warnings and Precautions (5) and Adverse Reactions (6.1)]*.

Use with Ribavirin

Ribavirin may cause birth defects and death of the unborn child. Extreme care must be taken to avoid pregnancy in female patients and in female partners of male patients. Ribavirin causes hemolytic anemia. The anemia associated with ribavirin therapy may result in a worsening of cardiac disease. *[See ribavirin labeling.]*

1 INDICATIONS AND USAGE

1.1 Chronic Hepatitis C (CHC)

PegIntron®, as part of a combination regimen, is indicated for the treatment of Chronic Hepatitis C (CHC) in patients with compensated liver disease.

- PegIntron in combination with REBETOL® (ribavirin) and an approved Hepatitis C Virus (HCV) NS3/4A protease inhibitor is indicated in adult patients (18 years of age and older) with HCV genotype 1 infection (see labeling of the specific HCV NS3/4A protease inhibitor for further information).
- PegIntron in combination with REBETOL is indicated in patients with genotypes other than 1, pediatric patients (3-17 years of age), or in patients with genotype 1 infection where use of an HCV NS3/4A protease inhibitor is not warranted based on tolerability, contraindications or other clinical factors.

PegIntron monotherapy should only be used in the treatment of CHC in patients with compensated liver disease if there are contraindications to or significant intolerance of REBETOL and is indicated for use only in previously untreated adult patients. Combination therapy provides substantially better response rates than monotherapy *[see Clinical Studies (14)]*.

2 DOSAGE AND ADMINISTRATION

2.1 PegIntron Combination Therapy

Adults

The recommended dose of PegIntron is 1.5 mcg/kg/week. The volume of PegIntron to be injected depends on the strength of PegIntron and patient's body weight *(see **Table 1**)*.

The recommended dose of REBETOL for use with PegIntron is 800 to 1400 mg orally based on patient body weight. REBETOL should be taken with food. REBETOL should not be used in patients with creatinine clearance less than 50 mL/min.

See labeling of the specific HCV NS3/4A protease inhibitor for information regarding dosing regimen and administration of the protease inhibitor in combination with PegIntron and ribavirin.

Duration of Treatment – Treatment with PegIntron/REBETOL of Interferon Alpha-naïve Patients

The treatment duration for patients with genotype 1 is 48 weeks. Discontinuation of therapy should be considered in patients who do not achieve at least a 2 $\log_{10}$ drop or loss of HCV-RNA at 12 weeks, or if HCV-RNA remains detectable after 24 weeks of therapy. Patients with genotype 2 and 3 should be treated for 24 weeks.

Duration of Treatment – Re-treatment with PegIntron/REBETOL of Prior Treatment Failures

For patients with genotype 1 infection, PegIntron and REBETOL without an HCV NS3/4A protease inhibitor should only be used if there are contraindications, significant intolerance or other clinical factors that would not warrant use of an HCV NS3/4A protease inhibitor. The treatment duration for patients who previously failed therapy is 48 weeks, regardless of HCV genotype. Re-treated patients who fail to achieve undetectable HCV-RNA at Week 12 of therapy, or whose HCV-RNA remains detectable after 24 weeks of therapy, are highly unlikely to achieve SVR and discontinuation of therapy should be considered *[see Clinical Studies (14.1)]*.

[See table 1 above]

Table 1: Recommended PegIntron Combination Therapy Dosing (Adults)

Body Weight kg (lbs)	PegIntron REDIPEN® or Vial Strength to Use	Amount of PegIntron (mcg) to Administer	Volume (mL)* of PegIntron to Administer	REBETOL Daily Dose	REBETOL Number of Capsules
<40 (<88)	50 mcg per 0.5 mL	50	0.5	800 mg/day	2 × 200 mg capsules A.M. 2 × 200 mg capsules P.M.
40-50 (88-111)	80 mcg per 0.5 mL	64	0.4	800 mg/day	2 × 200 mg capsules A.M. 2 × 200 mg capsules P.M.
51-60 (112-133)		80	0.5	800 mg/day	2 × 200 mg capsules A.M. 2 × 200 mg capsules P.M.
61-65 (134-144)	120 mcg per 0.5 mL	96	0.4	800 mg/day	2 × 200 mg capsules A.M. 2 × 200 mg capsules P.M.
66-75 (145-166)		96	0.4	1000 mg/day	2 × 200 mg capsules A.M. 3 × 200 mg capsules P.M.
76-80 (167-177)		120	0.5	1000 mg/day	2 × 200 mg capsules A.M. 3 × 200 mg capsules P.M.
81-85 (178-187)				1200 mg/day	3 × 200 mg capsules A.M. 3 × 200 mg capsules P.M.
86-105 (188-231)	150 mcg per 0.5 mL	150	0.5	1200 mg/day	3 × 200 mg capsules A.M. 3 × 200 mg capsules P.M.
>105 (>231)	†	†	†	1400 mg/day	3 × 200 mg capsules A.M. 4 × 200 mg capsules P.M.

* When reconstituted as directed.

† For patients weighing greater than 105 kg (greater than 231 pounds), the PegIntron dose of 1.5 mcg/kg/week should be calculated based on the individual patient weight. Two vials of PegIntron may be necessary to provide the dose.

Pediatric Patients

Dosing for pediatric patients is determined by body surface area for PegIntron and by body weight for REBETOL. The recommended dose of PegIntron is 60 mcg/m²/week subcutaneously in combination with 15 mg/kg/day of REBETOL orally in 2 divided doses *(see **Table 2**)* for pediatric patients ages 3 to 17 years. Patients who reach their 18th birthday while receiving PegIntron/REBETOL should remain on the pediatric dosing regimen. The treatment duration for patients with genotype 1 is 48 weeks. Patients with genotype 2 and 3 should be treated for 24 weeks.

Table 2: Recommended REBETOL* Dosing in Combination Therapy (Pediatrics)

Body Weight kg (lbs)	REBETOL Daily Dose	REBETOL Number of Capsules
<47 (<103)	15 mg/kg/day	Use REBETOL oral solution†
47-59 (103-131)	800 mg/day	2 × 200 mg capsules A.M. 2 × 200 mg capsules P.M.
60-73 (132-162)	1000 mg/day	2 × 200 mg capsules A.M. 3 × 200 mg capsules P.M.
>73 (>162)	1200 mg/day	3 × 200 mg capsules A.M. 3 × 200 mg capsules P.M.

* REBETOL to be used in combination with PegIntron 60 mcg/m² weekly.

† REBETOL oral solution may be used for any patient regardless of body weight.

2.2 PegIntron Monotherapy

The recommended dose of PegIntron regimen is 1 mcg/kg/week subcutaneously for 1 year administered on the same day of the week. Discontinuation of therapy should be considered in patients who do not achieve at least a 2 $\log_{10}$ drop or loss of HCV-RNA at 12 weeks of therapy, or whose HCV-RNA levels remain detectable after 24 weeks of therapy. The volume of PegIntron to be injected depends on patient weight *(see **Table 3**)*.

Table 3: Recommended PegIntron Monotherapy Dosing

Body Weight kg (lbs)	PegIntron REDIPEN or Vial Strength to Use	Amount of PegIntron (mcg) to Administer	Volume (mL)* of PegIntron to Administer
≤45 (≤100)	50 mcg per 0.5 mL	40	0.4
46-56 (101-124)		50	0.5
57-72 (125-159)	80 mcg per 0.5 mL	64	0.4
73-88 (160-195)		80	0.5
89-106 (196-234)	120 mcg per 0.5 mL	96	0.4
107-136 (235-300)		120	0.5
137-160 (301-353)	150 mcg per 0.5 mL	150	0.5

* When reconstituted as directed.

2.3 Dose Reduction

If a serious adverse reaction develops during the course of treatment *[see Warnings and Precautions (5)]* discontinue or modify the dosage of PegIntron and REBETOL until the adverse event abates or decreases in severity. If persistent or recurrent serious adverse events develop despite adequate dosage adjustment, discontinue treatment. For guidelines for dose modifications and discontinuation based on depression or laboratory parameters see **Tables 4** and **5**. Dose reduction of PegIntron in adult patients on PegIntron/REBETOL combination therapy is accomplished in a two-step process from the original starting dose of 1.5 mcg/kg/week, to 1 mcg/kg/week, then to 0.5 mcg/kg/week, if needed. Dose reduction in patients on PegIntron monotherapy is accomplished by reducing the original starting dose of 1 mcg/kg/week to 0.5 mcg/kg/week. Dose reduction of PegIntron in adults may be accomplished by utilizing a lower dose strength or administering a lesser volume as shown in Table 6 or 7.

In the adult combination therapy Study 2, dose reductions occurred in 42% of subjects receiving PegIntron 1.5 mcg/kg plus REBETOL 800 mg daily, including 57% of those subjects weighing 60 kg or less. In Study 4, 16% of subjects had a dose reduction of PegIntron to 1 mcg/kg in combination with REBETOL, with an additional 4% requiring the second dose reduction of PegIntron to 0.5 mcg/kg due to adverse events *[see Adverse Reactions (6.1)]*.

Dose reduction in pediatric patients is accomplished by modifying the recommended dose in a 2-step process from the original starting dose of 60 mcg/m²/week, to 40 mcg/m²/week, then to 20 mcg/m²/week, if needed *(see **Tables 4** and **5**)*. In the pediatric combination therapy trial, dose reductions occurred in 25% of subjects receiving PegIntron 60 mcg/m² weekly plus REBETOL 15 mg/kg daily.

[See table 4 above]

[See table 5 below]

Table 6: Reduced PegIntron Dose (0.5 mcg/kg) for (1 mcg/kg) Monotherapy in Adults

Body Weight kg (lbs)	PegIntron REDIPEN/Vial Strength to Use	Amount of PegIntron (mcg) to Administer	Volume (mL) * of PegIntron to Administer
≤45 (≤100)	50 mcg per 0.5 mL†	20	0.2
46-56 (101-124)		25	0.25
57-72 (125-159)	50 mcg per 0.5 mL	30	0.3
73-88 (160-195)		40	0.4
89-106 (196-234)	50 mcg per 0.5 mL	50	0.5
107-136 (235-300)	80 mcg per 0.5 mL	64	0.4
≥137 (≥301)		80	0.5

* When reconstituted as directed.

† Must use vial. Minimum delivery for REDIPEN 0.3 mL.

[See table 7 at top of next page]

2.4 Discontinuation of Dosing

Adults

See labeling of the specific HCV NS3/4A protease inhibitor for information regarding discontinuation of dosing based on treatment futility.

In HCV genotype 1, interferon-alfa-naïve patients receiving PegIntron, alone or in combination with REBETOL, discontinuation of therapy is recommended if there is not at least a 2 $\log_{10}$ drop or loss of HCV-RNA at 12 weeks of therapy, or if HCV-RNA levels remain detectable after 24 weeks of therapy. Regardless of genotype, previously treated patients who have detectable HCV-RNA at Week 12 or 24, are highly unlikely to achieve SVR and discontinuation of therapy is recommended.

Pediatrics (3-17 years of age)

It is recommended that patients receiving PegIntron/REBETOL combination (excluding those with HCV genotype 2 and 3) be discontinued from therapy at 12 weeks if their treatment Week 12 HCV-RNA dropped less than 2 $\log_{10}$ compared to pretreatment or at 24 weeks if they have detectable HCV-RNA at treatment Week 24.

2.5 Renal Function

In patients with moderate renal dysfunction (creatinine clearance 30-50 mL/min), the PegIntron dose should be reduced by 25%. Patients with severe renal dysfunction (creatinine clearance 10-29 mL/min), including those on hemodialysis, should have the PegIntron dose reduced by 50%. If renal function decreases during treatment, PegIntron therapy should be discontinued. When PegIntron is administered in combination with REBETOL, subjects with impaired renal function or those over the age of 50 should be more carefully monitored with respect to the development of anemia. PegIntron/REBETOL should not be used in patients with creatinine clearance less than 50 mL/min.

2.6 Preparation and Administration

PegIntron REDIPEN

PegIntron REDIPEN consists of a dual-chamber glass cartridge with sterile, lyophilized peginterferon alfa-2b in the active chamber and Sterile Water for Injection USP in the diluent chamber. The PegIntron in the glass cartridge should appear as a white to off-white tablet-shaped solid that is whole or in pieces, or powder.

To reconstitute the lyophilized peginterferon alfa-2b in the REDIPEN:

- Hold the REDIPEN upright (dose button down) and press the 2 halves of the pen together until there is an audible click.

Table 4: Guidelines for Modification or Discontinuation of PegIntron or PegIntron/REBETOL and for Scheduling Visits for Patients with Depression

Depression Severity*	Initial Management (4-8 weeks)		Depression Status		
	Dose Modification	Visit Schedule	Remains Stable	Improves	Worsens
Mild	No change	Evaluate once weekly by visit or phone	Continue weekly visit schedule	Resume normal visit schedule	See moderate or severe depression
Moderate	Adults: Adjust Dose* Pediatrics: Decrease dose to 40 mcg/m²/week, then to 20 mcg/m²/week, if needed	Evaluate once weekly (office visit at least every other week)	Consider psychiatric consultation. Continue reduced dosing	If symptoms improve and are stable for 4 weeks, may resume normal visit schedule. Continue reduced dosing or return to normal dose	See severe depression
Severe	Discontinue PegIntron/REBETOL permanently	Obtain immediate psychiatric consultation	Psychiatric therapy as necessary		

* See DSM-IV for definitions. For patients on PegIntron/REBETOL combination therapy: 1st dose reduction of PegIntron is to 1 mcg/kg/week, 2nd dose reduction (if needed) of PegIntron is to 0.5 mcg/kg/week. For patients on PegIntron monotherapy: decrease PegIntron dose to 0.5 mcg/kg/week.

Table 5: Guidelines for Dose Modification and Discontinuation of PegIntron or PegIntron/REBETOL Based on Laboratory Parameters in Adults and Pediatrics

Laboratory Parameters	Reduce PegIntron Dose (see note 1) if:	Reduce ribavirin Daily Dose (see note 2) if:	Discontinue Therapy if:
WBC	1.0 to <1.5 × 10^9/L	N/A	<1.0 × 10^9/L
Neutrophils	0.5 to <0.75 × 10^9/L	N/A	<0.5 × 10^9/L
Platelets	25 to <50 × 10^9/L (adults)	N/A	<25 × 10^9/L (adults)
	50 to <70 × 10^9/L (pediatrics)	N/A	<50 × 10^9/L (pediatrics)
Creatinine	N/A	N/A	>2 mg/dL (pediatrics)
Hemoglobin in patients without history of cardiac disease	N/A	8.5 to <10 g/dL	<8.5 g/dL
	Reduce PegIntron Dose by Half and the Ribavirin Dose by 200 mg/day if:		
Hemoglobin in patients with history of cardiac disease*†	≥2 g/dL decrease in hemoglobin during any four week period during treatment		<8.5 g/dL or <12 g/dL after four weeks of dose reduction

Note 1: *Adult patients on combination therapy*: 1st dose reduction of PegIntron is to 1 mcg/kg/week. If needed, 2nd dose reduction of PegIntron is to 0.5 mcg/kg/week.

Adult patients on PegIntron monotherapy: decrease PegIntron dose to 0.5 mcg/kg/week.

Pediatric patients: 1st dose reduction of PegIntron is to 40 mcg/m²/week, 2nd dose reduction of PegIntron is to 20 mcg/m²/week.

Note 2: *Adult patients*: 1st dose reduction of ribavirin is by 200 mg/day (except in patients receiving the 1400 mg, dose reduction should be by 400 mg/day). If needed, 2nd dose reduction of ribavirin is by an additional 200 mg/day. Patients whose dose of ribavirin is reduced to 600 mg daily receive one 200 mg capsule in the morning and two 200 mg capsules in the evening.

Pediatric patients: 1st dose reduction of ribavirin is to 12 mg/kg/day, 2nd dose reduction of ribavirin is to 8 mg/kg/day.

* Pediatric patients who have pre-existing cardiac conditions and experience a hemoglobin decrease greater than or equal to 2 g/dL during any 4-week period during treatment should have weekly evaluations and hematology testing.

† These guidelines are for patients with stable cardiac disease. Patients with a history of significant or unstable cardiac disease should not be treated with PegIntron /REBETOL combination therapy *[see Warnings and Precautions (5.3)]*.

- Gently invert the pen to mix the solution. **DO NOT SHAKE.** The reconstituted solution has a concentration of either 50 mcg per 0.5 mL, 80 mcg per 0.5 mL, 120 mcg per 0.5 mL, or 150 mcg per 0.5 mL for a single subcutaneous injection.
- Visually inspect the solution for particulate matter and discoloration prior to administration. The reconstituted solution should be clear and colorless. Do not use the solution if it is discolored or not clear, or if particulates are present.

Keeping the pen upright, attach the supplied needle and select the appropriate PegIntron dose by pulling back on the dosing button until the dark bands are visible and turning the button until the dark band is aligned with the correct dose. The prepared PegIntron solution is to be injected subcutaneously.

The PegIntron REDIPEN is a single-use pen and does not contain a preservative. The reconstituted solution should be used immediately and cannot be stored for more than 24 hours at 2-8°C *[see How Supplied/Storage and Handling (16)]*. **DO NOT REUSE THE REDIPEN.** The sterility of any remaining product can no longer be guaranteed. **DISCARD THE UNUSED PORTION.** Pooling of unused portions of some medications has been linked to bacterial contamination and morbidity.

PegIntron Vials

Two BD® Safety-Lok® syringes are provided in the package; one syringe is for the reconstitution steps and one for the patient injection. There is a plastic safety sleeve to be pulled over the needle after use. The syringe locks with an audible click when the green stripe on the safety sleeve covers the red stripe on the needle. Instructions for the preparation and administration of PegIntron Powder for Injection are provided below.

- **Reconstitute the PegIntron lyophilized product with only 0.7 mL of the 1.25 mL of supplied diluent (Sterile Water for Injection USP). The diluent vial is for single use only. The remaining diluent should be discarded.** No other medications should be added to solutions containing PegIntron, and PegIntron should not be reconstituted with other diluents.
- Swirl gently to hasten complete dissolution of the powder. The reconstituted solution should be clear and colorless.

- Visually inspect the solution for particulate matter and discoloration prior to administration. The solution should not be used if discolored or cloudy, or if particulates are present.
- The appropriate PegIntron dose should be withdrawn and injected subcutaneously. PegIntron vials are for single use only and do not contain a preservative.

The reconstituted solution should be used immediately and cannot be stored for more than 24 hours at 2-8°C *[see How Supplied/Storage and Handling (16)]*. **DO NOT REUSE THE VIAL.** The sterility of any remaining product can no longer be guaranteed. **DISCARD THE UNUSED PORTION.** Pooling of unused portions of some medications has been linked to bacterial contamination and morbidity.

3 DOSAGE FORMS AND STRENGTHS

- Single-use vial: 1.25 mL diluent vial: 50 mcg per 0.5 mL, 80 mcg per 0.5 mL, 120 mcg per 0.5 mL, 150 mcg per 0.5 mL.
- Single-use REDIPEN: 50 mcg per 0.5 mL, 80 mcg per 0.5 mL, 120 mcg per 0.5 mL, 150 mcg per 0.5 mL.

4 CONTRAINDICATIONS

PegIntron is contraindicated in patients with:

- known hypersensitivity reactions, such as urticaria, angioedema, bronchoconstriction, anaphylaxis, Stevens-Johnson syndrome, and toxic epidermal necrolysis to interferon alpha or any other component of the product
- autoimmune hepatitis
- hepatic decompensation (Child-Pugh score greater than 6 [class B and C]) in cirrhotic CHC patients before or during treatment

PegIntron/ribavirin combination therapy is additionally contraindicated in:

- women who are pregnant. Ribavirin may cause fetal harm when administered to a pregnant woman. Ribavirin is contraindicated in women who are or may become pregnant. If ribavirin is used during pregnancy, or if the patient becomes pregnant while taking ribavirin, the patient should be apprised of the potential hazard to her fetus *[see Use in Specific Populations (8.1)]*.
- men whose female partners are pregnant
- patients with hemoglobinopathies (e.g., thalassemia major, sickle-cell anemia)
- patients with creatinine clearance less than 50 mL/min

5 WARNINGS AND PRECAUTIONS

Patients should be monitored for the following serious conditions, some of which may become life threatening. Patients with persistently severe or worsening signs or symptoms should be withdrawn from therapy.

5.1 Use with Ribavirin

Pregnancy

Ribavirin may cause birth defects and death of the unborn child. Ribavirin therapy should not be started until a report of a negative pregnancy test has been obtained immediately prior to planned initiation of therapy. Patients should use at least 2 forms of contraception and have monthly pregnancy tests during treatment and during the 6-month period after treatment has been stopped *[see BOXED WARNING, Contraindications (4), Patient Counseling Information (17), and ribavirin labeling]*.

Anemia

Ribavirin caused hemolytic anemia in 10% of PegIntron/REBETOL-treated subjects within 1 to 4 weeks of initiation of therapy. Complete blood counts should be obtained pretreatment and at Week 2 and Week 4 of therapy or more frequently if clinically indicated. Anemia associated with ribavirin therapy may result in a worsening of cardiac disease. Decrease in dosage or discontinuation of ribavirin may be necessary *[see Dosage and Administration (2.3)* and *ribavirin labeling]*.

5.2 Neuropsychiatric Events

Life-threatening or fatal neuropsychiatric events, including suicide, suicidal and homicidal ideation, depression, relapse of drug addiction/overdose, and aggressive behavior sometimes directed towards others have occurred in patients with and without a previous psychiatric disorder during PegIntron treatment and follow-up. Psychoses, hallucinations, bipolar disorders, and mania have been observed in patients treated with interferon alpha.

PegIntron should be used with caution in patients with a history of psychiatric disorders. Treatment with interferons may be associated with exacerbated symptoms of psychiatric disorders in patients with co-occurring psychiatric and substance use disorders. If treatment with interferons is initiated in patients with prior history or existence of psychiatric condition or with a history of substance use disorders, treatment considerations should include the need for drug screening and periodic health evaluation, including psychiatric symptom monitoring. Early intervention for re-emergence or development of neuropsychiatric symptoms and substance use is recommended.

Patients should be advised to report immediately any symptoms of depression or suicidal ideation to their prescribing physicians. Physicians should monitor all patients for evidence of depression and other psychiatric symptoms. If patients develop psychiatric problems, including clinical depression, it is recommended that the patients be carefully monitored during treatment and in the 6-month follow-up period. If psychiatric symptoms persist or worsen, or suicidal ideation or aggressive behavior towards others is identified, it is recommended that treatment with PegIntron be discontinued, and the patient followed, with psychiatric intervention as appropriate. In severe cases, PegIntron should be stopped immediately and psychiatric intervention instituted *[see Dosage and Administration (2.3)]*. Cases of encephalopathy have been observed in some patients, usually elderly, treated at higher doses of PegIntron.

Table 7: Two-Step Dose Reduction of PegIntron in Combination Therapy in Adults

First Dose Reduction to PegIntron 1 mcg/kg				Second Dose Reduction to PegIntron 0.5 mcg/kg			
Body weight kg (lbs)	PegIntron REDIPEN/Vial Strength to Use	Amount of PegIntron (mcg) to Administer	Volume (mL) * of PegIntron to Administer	Body weight kg (lbs)	PegIntron REDIPEN/ Vial Strength to Use	Amount of PegIntron (mcg) to Administer	Volume (mL) * of PegIntron to Administer
<40 (<88)	50 mcg per 0.5 mL	35	0.35	<40 (<88)	50 mcg per 0.5 mL†	20	0.2
40-50 (88-111)		45	0.45	40-50 (88-111)		25	0.25
51-60 (112-133)		50	0.5	51-60 (112-133)	50 mcg per 0.5 mL	30	0.3
61-75 (134-166)	80 mcg per 0.5 mL	64	0.4	61-75 (134-166)		35	0.35
76-85 (167-187)		80	0.5	76-85 (167-187)		45	0.45
86-104 (188-230)	120 mcg per 0.5 mL	96	0.4	86-104 (188-230)		50	0.5
105-125 (231-275)		108	0.45	105-125 (231-275)	80 mcg per 0.5 mL	64	0.4
>125 (>275)	150 mcg per 0.5 mL	135	0.45	>125 (>275)		72	0.45

* When reconstituted as directed.
† Must use vial. Minimum delivery for REDIPEN 0.3 mL.

5.3 Cardiovascular Events

Cardiovascular events, which include hypotension, arrhythmia, tachycardia, cardiomyopathy, angina pectoris, and myocardial infarction, have been observed in patients treated with PegIntron. PegIntron should be used cautiously in patients with cardiovascular disease. Patients with a history of myocardial infarction and arrhythmic disorder who require PegIntron therapy should be closely monitored *[see Warnings and Precautions (5.15)]*. Patients with a history of significant or unstable cardiac disease should not be treated with PegIntron/ribavirin combination therapy *[see ribavirin labeling]*.

5.4 Endocrine Disorders

PegIntron causes or aggravates hypothyroidism and hyperthyroidism. Hyperglycemia has been observed in patients treated with PegIntron. Diabetes mellitus, including cases of new onset Type 1 diabetes, has been observed in patients treated with alpha interferons, including PegIntron. Patients with these conditions who cannot be effectively treated by medication should not begin PegIntron therapy. Patients who develop these conditions during treatment and cannot be controlled with medication should not continue PegIntron therapy.

5.5 Ophthalmologic Disorders

Decrease or loss of vision, retinopathy including macular edema, retinal artery or vein thrombosis, retinal hemorrhages and cotton wool spots, optic neuritis, papilledema, and serous retinal detachment may be induced or aggravated by treatment with peginterferon alfa-2b or other alpha interferons. All patients should receive an eye examination at baseline. Patients with preexisting ophthalmologic disorders (e.g., diabetic or hypertensive retinopathy) should receive periodic ophthalmologic exams during interferon alpha treatment. Any patient who develops ocular symptoms should receive a prompt and complete eye examination. Peginterferon alfa 2b treatment should be discontinued in patients who develop new or worsening ophthalmologic disorders.

5.6 Cerebrovascular Disorders

Ischemic and hemorrhagic cerebrovascular events have been observed in patients treated with interferon alfa-based therapies, including PegIntron. Events occurred in patients with few or no reported risk factors for stroke, including patients less than 45 years of age. Because these are spontaneous reports, estimates of frequency cannot be made, and a causal relationship between interferon alfa-based therapies and these events is difficult to establish.

5.7 Bone Marrow Toxicity

PegIntron suppresses bone marrow function, sometimes resulting in severe cytopenias. PegIntron should be discontinued in patients who develop severe decreases in neutrophil or platelet counts *[see Dosage and Administration (2.3)]*. Ribavirin may potentiate the neutropenia induced by interferon alpha. Very rarely alpha interferons may be associated with aplastic anemia.

5.8 Autoimmune Disorders

Development or exacerbation of autoimmune disorders (e.g., thyroiditis, thrombotic thrombocytopenic purpura, idiopathic thrombocytopenic purpura, rheumatoid arthritis, interstitial nephritis, systemic lupus erythematosus, and psoriasis) has been observed in patients receiving PegIntron. PegIntron should be used with caution in patients with autoimmune disorders.

5.9 Pancreatitis

Fatal and nonfatal pancreatitis has been observed in patients treated with alpha interferon. PegIntron therapy should be suspended in patients with signs and symptoms suggestive of pancreatitis and discontinued in patients diagnosed with pancreatitis.

5.10 Colitis

Fatal and nonfatal ulcerative or hemorrhagic/ischemic colitis have been observed within 12 weeks of the start of alpha interferon treatment. Abdominal pain, bloody diarrhea, and fever are the typical manifestations. PegIntron treatment should be discontinued immediately in patients who develop these signs and symptoms. The colitis usually resolves within 1 to 3 weeks of discontinuation of alpha interferons.

5.11 Pulmonary Disorders

Dyspnea, pulmonary infiltrates, pneumonia, bronchiolitis obliterans, interstitial pneumonitis, pulmonary hypertension, and sarcoidosis, some resulting in respiratory failure or patient deaths, may be induced or aggravated by PegIntron or alpha interferon therapy. Recurrence of respiratory failure has been observed with interferon rechallenge. PegIntron combination treatment should be suspended in patients who develop pulmonary infiltrates or pulmonary function impairment. Patients who resume interferon treatment should be closely monitored.

Because of the fever and other "flu-like" symptoms associated with PegIntron administration, it should be used cautiously in patients with debilitating medical conditions, such as those with a history of pulmonary disease (e.g., chronic obstructive pulmonary disease).

5.12 Hepatic Failure

Chronic Hepatitis C (CHC) patients with cirrhosis may be at risk of hepatic decompensation and death when treated

Table 8: Adverse Reactions Occurring in Greater than 5% of Subjects

Adverse Reactions	Percentage of Subjects Reporting Adverse Reactions* Study 1		Study 2	
	PegIntron 1 mcg/kg (N=297)	INTRON A 3 MIU (N=303)	PegIntron 1.5 mcg/kg/ REBETOL (N=511)	INTRON A/ REBETOL (N=505)
Application Site				
Injection Site	47	20	75	49
Inflammation/Reaction				
Autonomic Nervous System				
Dry Mouth	6	7	12	8
Increased Sweating	6	7	11	7
Flushing	6	3	4	3
Body as a Whole				
Fatigue/Asthenia	52	54	66	63
Headache	56	52	62	58
Rigors	23	19	48	41
Fever	22	12	46	33
Weight Loss	11	13	29	20
Right Upper Quadrant Pain	8	8	12	6
Chest Pain	6	4	8	7
Malaise	7	6	4	6
Central/Peripheral Nervous System				
Dizziness	12	10	21	17
Endocrine				
Hypothyroidism	5	3	5	4
Gastrointestinal				
Nausea	26	20	43	33
Anorexia	20	17	32	27
Diarrhea	18	16	22	17
Vomiting	7	6	14	12
Abdominal Pain	15	11	13	13
Dyspepsia	6	7	9	8
Constipation	1	3	5	5
Hematologic Disorders				
Neutropenia	6	2	26	14
Anemia	0	0	12	17
Leukopenia	<1	0	6	5
Thrombocytopenia	7	<1	5	2
Liver and Biliary System				
Hepatomegaly	6	5		4
Musculoskeletal				
Myalgia	54	53	56	50
Arthralgia	23	27	34	28
Musculoskeletal Pain	28	22	21	19

(Table continued on next page)

with alpha interferons, including PegIntron. Cirrhotic CHC patients co-infected with HIV receiving highly active antiretroviral therapy (HAART) and alpha interferons with or without ribavirin appear to be at increased risk for the development of hepatic decompensation compared to patients not receiving HAART. During treatment, patients' clinical status and hepatic function should be closely monitored, and PegIntron treatment should be immediately discontinued if decompensation (Child-Pugh score greater than 6) is observed *[see Contraindications (4)]*.

5.13 Patients with Renal Insufficiency

Increases in serum creatinine levels have been observed in patients with renal insufficiency receiving interferon alpha products, including PegIntron. Patients with impaired renal function should be closely monitored for signs and symptoms of interferon toxicity, including increases in serum creatinine, and PegIntron dosing should be adjusted accordingly or discontinued *[see Clinical Pharmacology (12.3) and Dosage and Administration (2.3)]*. PegIntron monotherapy should be used with caution in patients with creatinine clearance less than 50 mL/min; the potential risks should be weighed against the potential benefits in these patients. Combination therapy with ribavirin must not be used in patients with creatinine clearance less than 50 mL/min *[see ribavirin labeling]*.

5.14 Hypersensitivity

Serious, acute hypersensitivity reactions (e.g., urticaria, angioedema, bronchoconstriction, anaphylaxis) and cutaneous eruptions (Stevens-Johnson syndrome, toxic epidermal necrolysis) have been rarely observed during alpha interferon therapy. If such a reaction develops during treatment with PegIntron, discontinue treatment and institute appropriate medical therapy immediately. Transient rashes do not necessitate interruption of treatment.

5.15 Laboratory Tests

PegIntron alone or in combination with ribavirin may cause severe decreases in neutrophil and platelet counts, and hematologic, endocrine (e.g., TSH), and hepatic abnormalities. Transient elevations in ALT (2- to 5-fold above baseline) were observed in 10% of subjects treated with PegIntron, and were not associated with deterioration of other liver functions. Triglyceride levels are frequently elevated in patients receiving alpha interferon therapy including PegIntron and should be periodically monitored.

Patients on PegIntron or PegIntron/REBETOL combination therapy should have hematology and blood chemistry testing before the start of treatment and then periodically thereafter. In the adult clinical trial, complete blood counts (including hemoglobin, neutrophil, and platelet counts) and chemistries (including AST, ALT, bilirubin, and uric acid) were measured during the treatment period at Weeks 2, 4, 8, and 12, and then at 6-week intervals, or more frequently if abnormalities developed. In pediatric subjects, the same laboratory parameters were evaluated with additional assessment of hemoglobin at treatment Week 6. TSH levels were measured every 12 weeks during the treatment period. HCV-RNA should be measured periodically during treatment *[see Dosage and Administration (2)]*.

Patients who have pre-existing cardiac abnormalities should have electrocardiograms done before treatment with PegIntron/ribavirin.

5.16 Dental and Periodontal Disorders

Dental and periodontal disorders have been reported in patients receiving PegIntron/REBETOL combination therapy. In addition, dry mouth could have a damaging effect on teeth and mucous membranes of the mouth during long-term treatment with the combination of REBETOL and PegIntron. Patients should brush their teeth thoroughly twice daily and have regular dental examinations. If vomiting occurs, patients should be advised to rinse out their mouth thoroughly afterwards.

5.17 Triglycerides

Elevated triglyceride levels have been observed in patients treated with interferon alpha, including PegIntron therapy. Hypertriglyceridemia may result in pancreatitis *[see Warnings and Precautions (5.9)]*. Elevated triglyceride levels should be managed as clinically appropriate. Discontinuation of PegIntron therapy should be considered for patients with symptoms of potential pancreatitis, such as abdominal pain, nausea, or vomiting, and persistently elevated triglycerides (e.g., triglycerides greater than 100 mg/dL).

5.18 Impact on Growth — Pediatric Use

Data on the effects of PegIntron plus REBETOL on growth come from an open-label trial in subjects 3 through 17 years of age, and weight and height changes are compared to US normative population data. In general, the weight and height gain of pediatric subjects treated with PegIntron plus REBETOL lags behind that predicted by normative population data for the entire length of treatment. After about 6 months post-treatment (follow-up Week 24), subjects had weight gain rebounds and regained their weight to 53rd percentile, above the average of the normative population and similar to that predicted by their average baseline weight (57th percentile). After about 6 months post-treatment, height gain stabilized and subjects treated with PegIntron plus REBETOL had an average height percentile of 44th percentile, which was less than the average of the normative population and less than their average baseline height (51st percentile). Severely inhibited growth velocity (less than 3rd percentile) was observed in 70% of the subjects while on treatment. Of the subjects experiencing severely inhibited growth, 20% had continued inhibited growth velocity (less than 3rd percentile) after 6 months of follow-up.

Table 8 *(cont.)*: Adverse Reactions Occurring in Greater than 5% of Subjects

Adverse Reactions	*Percentage of Subjects Reporting Adverse Reactions** Study 1		Study 2	
	PegIntron 1 mcg/kg (N=297)	INTRON A 3 MIU (N=303)	PegIntron 1.5 mcg/kg/ REBETOL (N=511)	INTRON A/ REBETOL (N=505)
Psychiatric				
Insomnia	23	23	40	41
Depression	29	25	31	34
Anxiety/Emotional Lability/Irritability	28	34	47	47
Concentration Impaired	10	8	17	21
Agitation	2	2	8	5
Nervousness	4	3	6	6
Reproductive, Female				
Menstrual Disorder	4	3	7	6
Resistance Mechanism				
Viral Infection	11	10	12	12
Fungal Infection	<1	3	6	1
Respiratory System				
Dyspnea	4	2	26	24
Coughing	8	5	23	16
Pharyngitis	10	7	12	13
Rhinitis	2	2	8	6
Sinusitis	7	7	6	5
Skin and Appendages				
Alopecia	22	22	36	32
Pruritus	12	8	29	28
Rash	6	7	24	23
Skin Dry	11	9	24	23
Special Senses, Other				
Taste Perversion	<1	2	9	4
Vision Disorders				
Vision Blurred	2	3	5	6
Conjunctivitis	4	2	4	5

* Subjects reporting one or more adverse reactions. A subject may have reported more than one adverse reaction within a body system/organ class category.

Among the boys studied, the age groups of 3-11 years old and 12-17 years old had similar height percentile decreases of approximately 5 percentiles after 6 months post-treatment; weight gain continued to be similar to their average baseline percentile. Girls who were 3-11 years old and treated for 48 weeks had the largest average drop in height and weight percentiles (13 percentiles and 7 percentiles, respectively), whereas girls 12-17 years old continued along their average baseline height and weight percentiles after 6 months post-treatment.

5.19 Peripheral Neuropathy

Peripheral neuropathy has been reported when alpha interferons were given in combination with telbivudine. In one clinical trial, an increased risk and severity of peripheral neuropathy was observed with the combination use of telbivudine and pegylated interferon alfa-2a as compared to telbivudine alone. The safety and efficacy of telbivudine in combination with interferons for the treatment of chronic hepatitis B has not been demonstrated.

6 ADVERSE REACTIONS

Clinical trials with PegIntron alone or in combination with REBETOL have been conducted in over 6900 subjects from 3 to 75 years of age.

Serious adverse reactions have occurred in approximately 12% of subjects in clinical trials with PegIntron with or without REBETOL *[see BOXED WARNING, Warnings and Precautions (5)]*. The most common serious events occurring in subjects treated with PegIntron and REBETOL were depression and suicidal ideation *[see Warnings and Precautions (5.2)]*, each occurring at a frequency of less than 1%. The most common fatal events occurring in subjects treated with PegIntron and REBETOL were cardiac arrest, suicidal ideation, and suicide attempt *[see Warnings and Precautions (5.2, 5.3)]*, all occurring in less than 1% of subjects.

Greater than 96% of all subjects in clinical trials experienced one or more adverse events. The most commonly reported adverse reactions in adult subjects receiving either PegIntron or PegIntron/REBETOL were injection-site inflammation/reaction, fatigue/asthenia, headache, rigors, fevers, nausea, myalgia, and emotional lability/irritability. The most common adverse events in pediatric subjects, ages 3 and older, were pyrexia, headache, vomiting, neutropenia, fatigue, anorexia, injection-site erythema, and abdominal pain.

6.1 Clinical Trials Experience

Because clinical trials are conducted under widely varying conditions, adverse reaction rates observed in the clinical trials of a drug cannot be directly compared to rates in the clinical trials of another drug and may not reflect the rates observed in clinical practice.

Adults

Study 1 compared PegIntron monotherapy with INTRON® A monotherapy. Study 2 compared combination therapy of PegIntron/REBETOL with combination therapy with INTRON A/REBETOL. In these clinical trials, nearly all subjects experienced one or more adverse reactions. Study 3 compared a PegIntron/weight-based REBETOL combination to a PegIntron/flat dose REBETOL regimen. Study 4 compared two PegIntron (1.5 mcg/kg/week and 1 mcg/kg/week) doses in combination with REBETOL and a third treatment group receiving Pegasys® (180 mcg/week)/Copegus® (1000-1200 mg/day).

Adverse reactions that occurred in Studies 1 and 2 at greater than 5% incidence are provided in **Table 8** by treatment group. Due to potential differences in ascertainment procedures, adverse reaction rate comparisons across trials should not be made. **Table 9** summarizes the treatment-related adverse reactions in Study 4 that occurred at a greater than or equal to 10% incidence.

[See table 8 on previous page and above]

Table 9: Treatment-Related Adverse Reactions (Greater than or Equal to 10% Incidence) By Descending Frequency

Adverse Reactions	*Percentage of Subjects Reporting Treatment-Related Adverse Reactions* Study 4 PegIntron 1.5 mcg/ kg with REBETOL (N=1019)	PegIntron 1 mcg/kg with REBETOL (N=1016)	Pegasys 180 mcg with Copegus (N=1035)
Fatigue	67	68	64
Headache	50	47	41
Nausea	40	35	34
Chills	39	36	23
Insomnia	38	37	41
Anemia	35	30	34
Pyrexia	35	32	21
Injection Site Reactions	34	35	23
Anorexia	29	25	21
Rash	29	25	34
Myalgia	27	26	22
Neutropenia	26	19	31
Irritability	25	25	25
Depression	25	19	20
Alopecia	23	20	17
Dyspnea	21	20	22
Arthralgia	21	22	22
Pruritus	18	15	19
Influenza-like Illness	16	15	15
Dizziness	16	14	13
Diarrhea	15	16	14
Cough	15	16	17
Weight Decreased	13	10	10
Vomiting	12	10	9
Unspecified Pain	12	13	9
Dry Skin	11	11	12
Anxiety	11	11	10
Abdominal Pain	10	10	10
Leukopenia	9	7	10

The adverse reaction profile in Study 3, which compared PegIntron/weight-based REBETOL combination to a PegIntron/flat-dose REBETOL regimen, revealed an increased rate of anemia with weight-based dosing (29% vs. 19% for weight-based vs. flat-dose regimens, respectively). However, the majority of cases of anemia were mild and responded to dose reductions.

The incidence of serious adverse reactions was comparable in all trials. In the PegIntron monotherapy trial (Study 1) the incidence of serious adverse reactions was similar (about 12%) in all treatment groups. In Study 2, the incidence of serious adverse reactions was 17% in the PegIntron/REBETOL groups compared to 14% in the INTRON A/REBETOL group. In Study 3, there was a similar incidence of serious adverse reactions reported for the weight-based REBETOL group (12%) and for the flat-dose REBETOL regimen.

In many but not all cases, adverse reactions resolved after dose reduction or discontinuation of therapy. Some subjects experienced ongoing or new serious adverse reactions during the 6-month follow-up period.

There have been 31 subject deaths that occurred during treatment or during follow-up in these clinical trials. In Study 1, there was 1 suicide in a subject receiving PegIntron monotherapy and 2 deaths among subjects receiving INTRON A monotherapy (1 murder/suicide and 1 sudden death). In Study 2, there was 1 suicide in a subject receiving PegIntron/REBETOL combination therapy, and 1 subject death in the INTRON A/REBETOL group (motor vehicle accident). In Study 3, there were 14 deaths, 2 of which were probable suicides, and 1 was an unexplained death in a person with a relevant medical history of depression. In Study 4, there were 12 deaths, 6 of which occurred in subjects receiving PegIntron/REBETOL combination therapy; 5 in the PegIntron 1.5 mcg/REBETOL arm (N=1019) and 1 in the PegIntron 1 mcg/REBETOL arm (n=1016); and 6 of which occurred in subjects receiving Pegasys/Copegus (N=1035). There were 3 suicides that occurred during the off-treatment follow-up period in subjects who received PegIntron (1.5 mcg/kg)/REBETOL combination therapy.

In Studies 1 and 2, 10% to 14% of subjects receiving PegIntron, alone or in combination with REBETOL, discontinued therapy compared with 6% treated with INTRON A alone and 13% treated with INTRON A in combination with REBETOL. Similarly in Study 3, 15% of subjects receiving PegIntron in combination with weight-based REBETOL and 14% of subjects receiving PegIntron and flat-dose REBETOL discontinued therapy due to an adverse reaction. The most common reasons for discontinuation of therapy were related to known interferon effects of psychiatric, systemic (e.g., fatigue, headache), or gastrointestinal adverse reactions. In Study 4, 13% of subjects in the PegIntron 1.5 mcg/REBETOL arm, 10% in the PegIntron 1 mcg/REBETOL arm, and 13% in the Pegasys 180 mcg/Copegus arm discontinued therapy due to adverse events.

In Study 2, dose reductions due to adverse reactions occurred in 42% of subjects receiving PegIntron (1.5 mcg/kg)/REBETOL and in 34% of those receiving INTRON A/REBETOL. The majority of subjects (57%) weighing 60 kg or less receiving PegIntron (1.5 mcg/kg)/REBETOL required dose reduction. Reduction of interferon was dose-related (PegIntron 1.5 mcg/kg more than PegIntron 0.5 mcg/kg or INTRON A), 40%, 27%, 28%, respectively. Dose reduction for REBETOL was similar across all three groups, 33% to 35%. The most common reasons for dose modifications were neutropenia (18%) or anemia (9%). Other common reasons included depression, fatigue, nausea, and thrombocytopenia. In Study 3, dose modifications due to adverse reactions occurred more frequently with weight-based dosing (WBD) compared to flat dosing (29% and 23%, respectively). In Study 4, 16% of subjects had a dose reduction of PegIntron to 1 mcg/kg in combination with REBETOL, with an additional 4% requiring the second dose reduction of PegIntron to 0.5 mcg/kg due to adverse events, compared to 15% of subjects in the Pegasys/Copegus arm, who required a dose reduction to 135 mcg/week with Pegasys, with an additional 7% requiring a second dose reduction to 90 mcg/week with Pegasys.

In the PegIntron/REBETOL combination trials the most common adverse reactions were psychiatric, which occurred among 77% of subjects in Study 2 and 68% to 69% of subjects in Study 3. These psychiatric adverse reactions included most commonly depression, irritability, and insomnia, each reported by approximately 30% to 40% of subjects in all treatment groups. Suicidal behavior (ideation, attempts, and suicides) occurred in 2% of all subjects during treatment or during follow-up after treatment cessation *[see Warnings and Precautions (5.2)]*. In Study 4, psychiatric adverse reactions occurred in 58% of subjects in the PegIntron 1.5 mcg/REBETOL arm, 55% of subjects in the PegIntron 1 mcg/REBETOL arm, and 57% of subjects in the Pegasys 180 mcg/Copegus arm.

PegIntron induced fatigue or headache in approximately two-thirds of subjects, with fever or rigors in approximately half of the subjects. The severity of some of these systemic symptoms (e.g., fever and headache) tended to decrease as treatment continued. In Studies 1 and 2, application site inflammation and reaction (e.g., bruise, itchiness, and irritation) occurred at approximately twice the incidence with PegIntron therapies (in up to 75% of subjects) compared with INTRON A. However, injection-site pain was infrequent (2-3%) in all groups. In Study 3, there was a 23% to 24% incidence overall for injection-site reactions or inflammation.

In Study 2, many subjects continued to experience adverse reactions several months after discontinuation of therapy. By the end of the 6-month follow-up period, the incidence of ongoing adverse reactions by body class in the PegIntron 1.5/REBETOL group was 33% (psychiatric), 20% (musculoskeletal), and 10% (for endocrine and for GI). In approximately 10% to 15% of subjects, weight loss, fatigue, and headache had not resolved.

Individual serious adverse reactions in Study 2 occurred at a frequency less than or equal to 1% and included suicide attempt, suicidal ideation, severe depression; psychosis, aggressive reaction, relapse of drug addiction/overdose; nerve palsy (facial, oculomotor); cardiomyopathy, myocardial infarction, angina, pericardial effusion, retinal ischemia, retinal artery or vein thrombosis, blindness, decreased visual acuity, optic neuritis, transient ischemic attack, supraventricular arrhythmias, loss of consciousness; neutropenia, infection (sepsis, pneumonia, abscess, cellulitis); emphysema, bronchiolitis obliterans, pleural effusion, gastroenteritis, pancreatitis, gout, hyperglycemia, hyperthyroidism and hypothyroidism, autoimmune thrombocytopenia with or without purpura, rheumatoid arthritis, interstitial nephritis, lupus-like syndrome, sarcoidosis, aggravated psoriasis; urticaria, injection-site necrosis, vasculitis, and phototoxicity.

Subjects receiving PegIntron/REBETOL as re-treatment after failing a previous interferon combination regimen reported adverse reactions similar to those previously associated with this regimen during clinical trials of treatment-naïve subjects.

Pediatric Subjects

In general, the adverse-reaction profile in the pediatric population was similar to that observed in adults. In the pediatric trial, the most prevalent adverse reactions in all subjects were pyrexia (80%), headache (62%), neutropenia (33%), fatigue (30%), anorexia (29%), injection-site erythema (29%), and vomiting (27%). The majority of adverse reactions reported in the trial were mild or moderate in severity. Severe adverse reactions were reported in 7% (8/107) of all subjects and included injection-site pain (1%), pain in extremity (1%), headache (1%), neutropenia (1%), and pyrexia (4%). Important adverse reactions that occurred in this subject population were nervousness (7%; 7/107), aggression (3%; 3/107), anger (2%; 2/107), and depression (1%; 1/107). Five subjects received levothyroxine treatment; three with clinical hypothyroidism and two with asymptomatic TSH elevations.

Dose modifications were required in 25% of subjects, most commonly for anemia, neutropenia, and weight loss. Two subjects (2%; 2/107) discontinued therapy as the result of an adverse reaction.

Adverse reactions that occurred with a greater than or equal to 10% incidence in the pediatric trial subjects are provided in **Table 10**.

Table 10: Percentage of Pediatric Subjects with Treatment-related Adverse Reactions (in At Least 10% of All Subjects)

System Organ Class Preferred Term	All Subjects N=107
Blood and Lymphatic System Disorders	
Neutropenia	33%
Anemia	11%
Leukopenia	10%
Gastrointestinal Disorders	
Abdominal Pain	21%
Abdominal Pain Upper	12%
Vomiting	27%
Nausea	18%
General Disorders and Administration Site Conditions	
Pyrexia	80%
Fatigue	30%
Injection-site Erythema	29%
Chills	21%
Asthenia	15%
Irritability	14%
Investigations	
Weight Decreased	19%
Metabolism and Nutrition Disorders	
Anorexia	29%
Decreased Appetite	22%
Musculoskeletal and Connective Tissue Disorders	
Arthralgia	17%
Myalgia	17%
Nervous System Disorders	
Headache	62%
Dizziness	14%
Skin and Subcutaneous Tissue Disorders	
Alopecia	17%

Laboratory Values

Adults

Changes in selected laboratory values during treatment with PegIntron alone or in combination with REBETOL treatment are described below. **Decreases in hemoglobin, neutrophils, and platelets may require dose reduction or permanent discontinuation from therapy** *[see Dosage and Administration (2.3) and Warnings and Precautions (5.1, 5.7)]*.

Hemoglobin. Hemoglobin levels decreased to less than 11 g/dL in about 30% of subjects in Study 2. In Study 3, 47% of subjects receiving WBD REBETOL and 33% on flat-dose REBETOL had decreases in hemoglobin levels less than 11 g/dL. Reductions in hemoglobin to less than 9 g/dL occurred more frequently in subjects receiving WBD compared to flat dosing (4% and 2%, respectively). In Study 2, dose modification was required in 9% and 13% of subjects in the PegIntron/REBETOL and INTRON A/REBETOL groups. In Study 4, subjects receiving PegIntron (1.5 mcg/kg)/REBETOL had decreases in hemoglobin levels to between 8.5 to less than 10 g/dL (28%) and to less than 8.5 g/dL (3%), whereas in subjects receiving Pegasys 180 mcg/Copegus these decreases occurred in 26% and 4% of subjects, respectively. Hemoglobin levels became stable by treatment Weeks 4 to 6 on average. The typical pattern observed was a decrease in hemoglobin levels by treatment Week 4 followed by stabilization and a plateau, which was maintained to the end of treatment. In the PegIntron monotherapy trial, hemoglobin decreases were generally mild and dose modifications were rarely necessary *[see Dosage and Administration (2.3)]*.

Neutrophils. Decreases in neutrophil counts were observed in a majority of subjects treated with PegIntron alone (70%) or as combination therapy with REBETOL in Study 2 (85%) and INTRON A/REBETOL (60%). Severe potentially life-threatening neutropenia (less than 0.5×10^9/L) occurred in 1% of subjects treated with PegIntron monotherapy, 2% of subjects treated with INTRON A/REBETOL, and in approximately 4% of subjects treated with PegIntron/REBETOL in Study 2. Two percent of subjects receiving PegIntron monotherapy and 18% of subjects receiving PegIntron/REBETOL in Study 2 required modification of interferon dosage. Few subjects (less than 1%) required permanent discontinuation of treatment. Neutrophil counts generally returned to pretreatment levels 4 weeks after cessation of therapy *[see Dosage and Administration (2.3)]*.

Platelets. Platelet counts decreased to less than 100,000/mm^3 in approximately 20% of subjects treated with PegIntron alone or with REBETOL and in 6% of subjects treated with INTRON A/REBETOL. Severe decreases in platelet counts (less than 50,000/mm^3) occur in less than 4% of subjects. Patients may require discontinuation or dose modification as a result of platelet decreases *[see Dosage and Administration (2.3)]*. In Study 2, 1% or 3% of subjects required dose modification of INTRON A or PegIntron, respectively. Platelet counts generally returned to pretreatment levels 4 weeks after the cessation of therapy.

Triglycerides. Elevated triglyceride levels have been observed in patients treated with interferon alphas, including PegIntron *[see Warnings and Precautions (5.17)]*.

Thyroid Function. Development of TSH abnormalities, with or without clinical manifestations, is associated with interferon therapies. In Study 2, clinically apparent thyroid disorders occurred among subjects treated with either INTRON A or PegIntron (with or without REBETOL) at a similar incidence (5% for hypothyroidism and 3% for hyperthyroidism). Subjects developed new-onset TSH abnormalities while on treatment and during the follow-up period. At the end of the follow-up period, 7% of subjects still had abnormal TSH values *[see Warnings and Precautions (5.4)]*.

Bilirubin and Uric Acid. In Study 2, 10% to 14% of subjects developed hyperbilirubinemia and 33% to 38% developed hyperuricemia in association with hemolysis. Six subjects developed mild to moderate gout.

Pediatric Subjects

Decreases in hemoglobin, white blood cells, platelets, and neutrophils may require dose reduction or permanent discontinuation from therapy *[see Dosage and Administration (2.3)]*. Changes in selected laboratory values during treatment of 107 pediatric subjects with PegIntron/REBETOL combination therapy are described in **Table 11.** Most of the changes in laboratory values in this trial were mild or moderate.

Table 11: Selected Laboratory Abnormalities during Treatment Phase with PegIntron Plus REBETOL in Previously Untreated Pediatric Subjects

Laboratory Parameter*	All Subjects (N=107)
Hemoglobin (g/dL)	
9.5 to <11.0	30%
8.0 to <9.5	2%
WBC ($\times 10^9$/L)	
2.0-2.9	39%
1.5 to <2.0	3%
Platelets ($\times 10^9$/L)	
70-100	1%
50 to <70	—
25 to <50	1%
Neutrophils ($\times 10^9$/L)	
1.0-1.5	35%
0.75 to <1.0	26%
0.5 to <0.75	13%
<0.5	3%
Total Bilirubin	
1.26-2.59 × ULN†	7%
Evidence of Hepatic Failure	—

* The table summarizes the worst category observed within the period per subject per laboratory test. Only subjects with at least one treatment value for a given laboratory test are included.

† ULN=Upper limit of normal.

6.2 Immunogenicity

As with all therapeutic proteins, there is potential for immunogenicity. Approximately 2% of subjects receiving PegIntron (32/1759) or INTRON A (11/728) with or without REBETOL developed low-titer (less than or equal to 160) neutralizing antibodies to PegIntron or INTRON A. The clinical and pathological significance of the appearance of serum-neutralizing antibodies is unknown. The incidence of antibody formation is highly dependent on the sensitivity and specificity of the assay. Additionally, the observed incidence of antibody (including neutralizing antibody) positivity in an assay may be influenced by several factors, including assay methodology, sample handling, timing of sample collection, concomitant medications, and underlying disease. For these reasons, comparison of the incidence of antibodies to PegIntron with the incidence of antibodies to other products may be misleading.

6.3 Postmarketing Experience

The following adverse reactions have been identified during post-approval use of PegIntron therapy. Because these reactions are reported voluntarily from a population of uncertain size, it is not always possible to reliably estimate their frequency or establish a causal relationship to drug exposure.

Blood and Lymphatic System Disorders
Pure red cell aplasia, thrombotic thrombocytopenic purpura

Cardiac Disorders
Palpitations

Ear and Labyrinth Disorders
Hearing loss, vertigo, hearing impairment

Endocrine Disorders
Diabetic ketoacidosis, diabetes

Eye Disorders
Vogt-Koyanagi-Harada syndrome, serous retinal detachment

Gastrointestinal Disorders
Aphthous stomatitis

General Disorders and Administration Site Conditions
Asthenic conditions (including asthenia, malaise, fatigue)

Immune System Disorders
Cases of acute hypersensitivity reactions (including anaphylaxis, angioedema, urticaria); Stevens-Johnson syndrome, toxic epidermal necrolysis, systemic lupus erythematosus, erythema multiforme

Infections and Infestations
Bacterial infection including sepsis

Metabolism and Nutrition Disorders
Dehydration, hypertriglyceridemia

Musculoskeletal and Connective Tissue Disorders
Rhabdomyolysis, myositis

Nervous System Disorders
Seizures, memory loss, peripheral neuropathy, paraesthesia, migraine headache

Psychiatric Disorders
Homicidal ideation

Respiratory, Thoracic, and Mediastinal Disorders
Pulmonary hypertension

Renal and Urinary Disorders
Renal failure, renal insufficiency

Skin and Subcutaneous Tissue Disorders
Psoriasis

Vascular Disorders
Hypertension, hypotension

7 DRUG INTERACTIONS

7.1 Drugs Metabolized by Cytochrome P-450

When administering PegIntron with medications metabolized by CYP2C8/9 (e.g., warfarin and phenytoin) or CYP2D6 (e.g., flecainide), the therapeutic effect of these substrates may be decreased *[see Clinical Pharmacology (12.3)]*.

7.2 Methadone

PegIntron may increase methadone concentrations *[see Clinical Pharmacology (12.3)]*. The clinical significance of this finding is unknown; however, patients should be monitored for signs and symptoms of increased narcotic effect.

7.3 Use with Ribavirin (Nucleoside Analogues)

Hepatic decompensation (some fatal) has occurred in cirrhotic HIV/HCV co-infected patients receiving combination antiretroviral therapy for HIV and interferon alpha and ribavirin. Adding treatment with alpha interferons alone or in combination with ribavirin may increase the risk in this patient subset. Patients receiving interferon with ribavirin and nucleoside reverse transcriptase inhibitors (NRTIs) should be closely monitored for treatment- associated toxicities, especially hepatic decompensation and anemia. Discontinuation of NRTIs should be considered as medically appropriate *[see labeling for individual NRTI product]*. Dose reduction or discontinuation of interferon, ribavirin, or both should also be considered if worsening clinical toxicities are observed, including hepatic decompensation (e.g., Child-Pugh greater than 6).

Stavudine, Lamivudine, and Zidovudine

In vitro studies have shown ribavirin can reduce the phosphorylation of pyrimidine nucleoside analogues such as stavudine, lamivudine, and zidovudine. In a trial with another pegylated interferon alpha, no evidence of a pharmacokinetic or pharmacodynamic (e.g., loss of HIV/HCV virologic suppression) interaction was seen when ribavirin was coadministered with zidovudine, lamivudine, or stavudine in HIV/HCV co-infected subjects *[see Clinical Pharmacology (12.3)]*.

HIV/HCV co-infected subjects who were administered zidovudine in combination with pegylated interferon alpha and ribavirin developed severe neutropenia (ANC less than 500) and severe anemia (hemoglobin less than 8 g/dL) more frequently than similar subjects not receiving zidovudine.

Didanosine

Co-administration of ribavirin and didanosine is not recommended. Reports of fatal hepatic failure, as well as peripheral neuropathy, pancreatitis, and symptomatic hyperlactatemia/lactic acidosis have been reported in clinical trials *[see Clinical Pharmacology (12.3)]*.

8 USE IN SPECIFIC POPULATIONS

8.1 Pregnancy

PegIntron Monotherapy

Pregnancy Category C: Nonpegylated interferon alfa-2b has been shown to have abortifacient effects in *Macaca mulatta* (rhesus monkeys) at 15 and 30 million IU/kg (estimated human equivalent of 5 and 10 million IU/kg, based on body surface area adjustment for a 60-kg adult). PegIntron should be assumed to also have abortifacient potential. There are no adequate and well-controlled trials in pregnant women. PegIntron therapy is to be used during pregnancy only if the potential benefit justifies the potential risk to the fetus. Therefore, PegIntron is recommended for use in fertile women only when they are using effective contraception during the treatment period.

Use with Ribavirin

Pregnancy Category X: Significant teratogenic and/or embryocidal effects have been demonstrated in all animal species exposed to ribavirin. Ribavirin therapy is contraindicated in women who are pregnant and in the male partners of women who are pregnant *[see Contraindications (4) and ribavirin labeling]*.

A Ribavirin Pregnancy Registry has been established to monitor maternal-fetal outcomes of pregnancies in female patients and female partners of male patients exposed to ribavirin during treatment and for 6 months following cessation of treatment. Physicians and patients are encouraged to report such cases by calling 1-800-593-2214.

8.3 Nursing Mothers

It is not known whether the components of PegIntron and/or ribavirin are excreted in human milk. Studies in mice have shown that mouse interferons are excreted in breast milk. Because of the potential for adverse reactions from the drug in nursing infants, a decision must be made whether to discontinue nursing or discontinue the PegIntron and ribavirin treatment, taking into account the importance of the therapy to the mother.

8.4 Pediatric Use

Safety and effectiveness in pediatric patients below the age of 3 years have not been established. Clinical trials in pediatric subjects less than 3 years of age are not considered feasible due to the small proportion of patients in this age group requiring treatment for CHC.

8.5 Geriatric Use

In general, younger patients tend to respond better than older patients to interferon-based therapies. Clinical trials of PegIntron alone or in combination with REBETOL did not include sufficient numbers of subjects aged 65 and over to determine whether they respond differently than younger subjects. Treatment with alpha interferons, including PegIntron, is associated with neuropsychiatric, cardiac, pulmonary, GI, and systemic (flu-like) adverse effects. Because these adverse reactions may be more severe in the elderly, caution should be exercised in the use of PegIntron in this population. This drug is known to be substantially excreted by the kidney. Because elderly patients are more likely to have decreased renal function, the risk of toxic reactions to this drug may be greater in patients with impaired renal function *[see Clinical Pharmacology (12.3)]*. When using PegIntron/ ribavirin therapy, refer also to the ribavirin labeling.

8.6 Organ Transplant Recipients

The safety and efficacy of PegIntron alone or in combination with ribavirin for the treatment of hepatitis C in liver or other organ transplant recipients have not been studied. In a small (n=16) single-center, uncontrolled case experience, renal failure in renal allograft recipients receiving interferon alpha and ribavirin combination therapy was more frequent than expected from the center's previous experience with renal allograft recipients not receiving combination therapy. The relationship of the renal failure to renal allograft rejection is not clear.

8.7 HIV or HBV Co-infection

The safety and efficacy of PegIntron/ ribavirin for the treatment of patients with HCV co-infected with HIV or HBV have not been established.

10 OVERDOSAGE

There is limited experience with overdosage. In the clinical trials, a few subjects accidentally received a dose greater than that prescribed. There were no instances in which a participant in the monotherapy or combination therapy trials received more than 10.5 times the intended dose of PegIntron. The maximum dose received by any subject was 3.45 mcg/kg weekly over a period of approximately 12 weeks. The maximum known overdosage of ribavirin was an intentional ingestion of 10 g (fifty 200 mg capsules). There were no serious reactions attributed to these overdosages. In cases of overdosing, symptomatic treatment and close observation of the patient are recommended.

11 DESCRIPTION

PegIntron, peginterferon alfa-2b, is a covalent conjugate of recombinant alfa-2b interferon with monomethoxy polyethylene glycol (PEG). The average molecular weight of the PEG portion of the molecule is 12,000 daltons. The average molecular weight of the PegIntron molecule is approximately 31,000 daltons. The specific activity of peginterferon alfa-2b is approximately 0.7×10^8 IU/mg protein.

Interferon alfa-2b is a water-soluble protein with a molecular weight of 19,271 daltons produced by recombinant DNA techniques. It is obtained from the bacterial fermentation of a strain of *Escherichia coli* bearing a genetically engineered plasmid containing an interferon gene from human leukocytes.

PegIntron is supplied in both vials and the REDIPEN for subcutaneous use.

Vials

Each vial contains either 74 mcg, 118.4 mcg, 177.6 mcg, or 222 mcg of PegIntron as a white to off-white tablet-like solid that is whole/in pieces or as a loose powder, and 1.11 mg dibasic sodium phosphate anhydrous, 1.11 mg monobasic sodium phosphate dihydrate, 59.2 mg sucrose, and 0.074 mg polysorbate 80. Following reconstitution with 0.7 mL of the supplied Sterile Water for Injection USP, each vial contains PegIntron at strengths of either 50 mcg per 0.5 mL, 80 mcg per 0.5 mL, 120 mcg per 0.5 mL, or 150 mcg per 0.5 mL.

REDIPEN

REDIPEN is a dual-chamber glass cartridge containing lyophilized PegIntron as a white to off-white tablet or powder that is whole or in pieces in the sterile active chamber and a second chamber containing Sterile Water for Injection USP. Each PegIntron REDIPEN contains either 67.5 mcg, 108 mcg, 162 mcg, or 202.5 mcg of PegIntron, and 1.013 mg dibasic sodium phosphate anhydrous, 1.013 mg monobasic sodium phosphate dihydrate, 54 mg sucrose, and 0.0675 mg polysorbate 80. Each cartridge is reconstituted to allow for the administration of up to 0.5 mL of solution. Following reconstitution, each REDIPEN contains PegIntron at strengths of either 50 mcg per 0.5 mL, 80 mcg per 0.5 mL, 120 mcg per 0.5 mL, or 150 mcg per 0.5 mL for a single use. Because a small volume of reconstituted solution is lost during preparation of PegIntron, each REDIPEN contains an excess amount of PegIntron powder and diluent to ensure delivery of the labeled dose.

12 CLINICAL PHARMACOLOGY

12.1 Mechanism of Action

Pegylated recombinant human interferon alfa-2b is an inducer of the innate antiviral immune response *[see Microbiology (12.4)]*.

12.2 Pharmacodynamics

The pharmacodynamic effects of peginterferon alfa-2b include inhibition of viral replication in virus-infected cells, the suppression of cell cycle progression/cell proliferation, induction of apoptosis, anti-angiogenic activities, and numerous immunomodulating activities, such as enhancement of the phagocytic activity of macrophages, activation of NK cells, stimulation of cytotoxic T-lymphocytes, and the upregulation of the Th1 T-helper cell subset.

PegIntron raises concentrations of effector proteins such as serum neopterin and 2′5′ oligoadenylate synthetase, raises body temperature, and causes reversible decreases in leukocyte and platelet counts. The correlation between the *in vitro* and *in vivo* pharmacologic and pharmacodynamic and clinical effects is unknown.

12.3 Pharmacokinetics

Following a single subcutaneous dose of PegIntron, the mean absorption half-life ($t\ ½\ k_a$) was 4.6 hours. Maximal serum concentrations (C_{max}) occur between 15 and 44 hours postdose, and are sustained for up to 48 to 72 hours. The C_{max} and AUC measurements of PegIntron increase in a dose-related manner. After multiple dosing, there is an increase in bioavailability of PegIntron. Week 48 mean trough concentrations (320 pg/mL; range 0, 2960) are approximately 3-fold higher than Week 4 mean trough concentrations (94 pg/mL; range 0, 416). The mean PegIntron elimination half-life is approximately 40 hours (range 22-60 hours) in patients with HCV infection. The apparent clearance of PegIntron is estimated to be approximately 22 mL/hr•kg. Renal elimination accounts for 30% of the clearance.

Pegylation of interferon alfa-2b produces a product (PegIntron) whose clearance is lower than that of nonpegylated interferon alfa-2b. When compared to INTRON A, PegIntron (1 mcg/kg) has approximately a 7-fold lower mean apparent clearance and a 5-fold greater mean half-life, permitting a reduced dosing frequency. At effective therapeutic doses, PegIntron has approximately 10-fold greater C_{max} and 50-fold greater AUC than interferon alfa-2b.

Renal Dysfunction

Following multiple dosing of PegIntron (1 mcg/kg subcutaneously given every week for 4 weeks) the clearance of PegIntron is reduced by a mean of 17% in subjects with moderate renal impairment (creatinine clearance 30-49 mL/min) and by a mean of 44% in subjects with severe renal impairment (creatinine clearance 10-29 mL/min) compared to subjects with normal renal function. Clearance was similar in subjects with severe renal impairment not on dialysis and subjects who are receiving hemodialysis. The dose of PegIntron for monotherapy should be reduced in patients with moderate or severe renal impairment *[see Dosage and Administration (2.3)* and *REBETOL labeling]*. REBETOL should not be used in patients with creatinine clearance less than 50 mL/min *[see REBETOL labeling, WARNINGS]*.

Gender

During the 48-week treatment period with PegIntron, no differences in the pharmacokinetic profiles were observed between male and female subjects with chronic hepatitis C infection.

Geriatric Patients

The pharmacokinetics of geriatric subjects (65 years of age and older) treated with a single subcutaneous dose of 1 mcg/kg of PegIntron were similar in C_{max}, AUC, clearance, or elimination half-life as compared to younger subjects (28-44 years of age).

Pediatric Patients

Population pharmacokinetics for PegIntron and REBETOL (capsules and oral solution) were evaluated in pediatric subjects with chronic hepatitis C between 3 and 17 years of age. In pediatric patients receiving PegIntron 60 mcg/m²/week subcutaneously, exposure may be approximately 50% higher than observed in adults receiving 1.5 mcg/kg/week subcutaneously. The pharmacokinetics of REBETOL (dose-normalized) in this trial were similar to those reported in a prior trial of REBETOL in combination with INTRON A in pediatric subjects and in adults.

Effect of Food on Absorption of Ribavirin

Both AUC_{tf} and C_{max} increased by 70% when REBETOL capsules were administered with a high-fat meal (841 kcal, 53.8 g fat, 31.6 g protein, and 57.4 g carbohydrate) in a single-dose pharmacokinetic trial *[see Dosage and Administration (2.1)]*.

Drug Interactions

Drugs Metabolized by Cytochrome P-450

The pharmacokinetics of representative drugs metabolized by CYP1A2 (caffeine), CYP2C8/9 (tolbutamide), CYP2D6 (dextromethorphan), CYP3A4 (midazolam), and N-acetyltransferase (dapsone) were studied in 22 subjects with chronic hepatitis C who received PegIntron (1.5 mcg/kg) once weekly for 4 weeks. PegIntron treatment resulted in a 28% (mean) increase in a measure of CYP2C8/9 activity. PegIntron treatment also resulted in a 66% (mean) increase in a measure of CYP2D6 activity; however, the effect was variable as 13 subjects had an increase, 5 subjects had a decrease, and 4 subjects had no significant change *[see Drug Interactions (7.1)]*.

No significant effect was observed on the pharmacokinetics of representative drugs metabolized by CYP1A2, CYP3A4, or N-acetyltransferase. The effects of PegIntron on CYP2C19 activity were not assessed.

Methadone

The pharmacokinetics of concomitant administration of methadone and PegIntron were evaluated in 18 PegIntron-naïve chronic hepatitis C subjects receiving 1.5 mcg/kg PegIntron subcutaneously weekly. All subjects were on stable methadone maintenance therapy receiving greater than or equal to 40 mg/day prior to initiating PegIntron. Mean methadone AUC was approximately 16% higher after 4 weeks of PegIntron treatment as compared to baseline. In 2 subjects, methadone AUC was approximately double after 4 weeks of PegIntron treatment as compared to baseline *[see Drug Interactions (7.2)]*.

Use with Ribavirin

Zidovudine, Lamivudine, and Stavudine

Ribavirin has been shown *in vitro* to inhibit phosphorylation of zidovudine, lamivudine, and stavudine. However, in a trial with another pegylated interferon in combination with ribavirin, no pharmacokinetic (e.g., plasma concentrations or intracellular triphosphorylated active metabolite concentrations) or pharmacodynamic (e.g., loss of HIV/HCV virologic suppression) interaction was observed when ribavirin and lamivudine (n=18), stavudine (n=10), or zidovudine (n=6) were co-administered as part of a multi-drug regimen to HIV/HCV co-infected subjects *[see Drug Interactions (7.3)]*.

Didanosine

Exposure to didanosine or its active metabolite (dideoxyadenosine 5′- triphosphate) is increased when didanosine is co-administered with ribavirin, which could cause or worsen clinical toxicities *[see Drug Interactions (7.3)]*.

12.4 Microbiology

Mechanism of Action

The biological activity of PegIntron is derived from its interferon alfa-2b moiety. Peginterferon alfa-2b binds to and activates the human type 1 interferon receptor. Upon binding, the receptor subunits dimerize, and activate multiple intracellular signal transduction pathways. Signal transduction is initially mediated by the JAK/STAT activation, which may occur in a wide variety of cells. Interferon receptor activation also activates NFκB in many cell types. Given the diversity of cell types that respond to interferon alfa-2b, and the multiplicity of potential intracellular responses to interferon receptor activation, peginterferon alfa-2b is expected to have pleiotropic biological effects in the body.

The mechanism by which ribavirin contributes to its antiviral efficacy in the clinic is not fully understood. Ribavirin has direct antiviral activity in tissue culture against many RNA viruses. Ribavirin increases the mutation frequency in the genomes of several viruses and ribavirin triphosphate inhibits HCV polymerase in a biochemical reaction.

Antiviral Activity

The anti-HCV activity of interferon was demonstrated in cell culture using self-replicating HCV-RNA (HCV replicon cells) or HCV infection and resulted in an effective concentration (EC_{50}) value of 1 to 10 IU/mL.

The antiviral activity of ribavirin in the HCV-replicon is not well understood and has not been defined because of the cellular toxicity of ribavirin.

Resistance

HCV genotypes show wide variability in their response to pegylated recombinant human interferon/ribavirin therapy. Genetic changes associated with the variable response have not been identified.

Cross-resistance

There is no reported cross-resistance between pegylated/nonpegylated interferons and ribavirin.

12.5 Pharmacogenomics

A retrospective genome-wide association analysis[1,2] of 1671 subjects (1604 subjects from Study 4 *[see Clinical Studies (14.1)]* and 67 subjects from another clinical trial) was performed to identify human genetic contributions to anti-HCV treatment response in previously untreated HCV genotype 1 subjects. A single nucleotide polymorphism near the gene encoding interferon-lambda-3 (*IL28B rs12979860*) was associated with variable SVR rates. The *rs12979860* genotype was categorized as CC, CT and TT. In the pooled analysis of Caucasian, African-American, and Hispanic subjects from these trials (n=1587), SVR rates by *rs12979860* genotype were as follows: CC 66% vs. CT 30% vs. TT 22%. The genotype frequencies differed depending on racial/ethnic background, but the relationship of SVR to *IL28B* genotype was consistent across various racial/ethnic groups *(see* ***Table 12****)*. Other variants near the *IL28B* gene (e.g., *rs8099917* and *rs8103142*) have been identified; however, they have not been shown to independently influence SVR rates during treatment with pegylated interferon alpha therapies combined with ribavirin.[1]

Table 12: SVR Rates by IL28B Genotype*

Population	CC	CT	TT
Caucasian	69% (301/436)	33% (196/596)	27% (38/139)
African-American	48% (20/42)	15% (22/146)	13% (15/112)
Hispanic	56% (19/34)	38% (21/56)	27% (7/26)

* The SVR rates are the overall rates for subjects treated with PegIntron 1.0 mcg/kg/REBETOL, PegIntron 1.5 mcg/kg/REBETOL and Pegasys 180 mcg/Copegus according to self-reported race/ethnicity.

13 NONCLINICAL TOXICOLOGY

13.1 Carcinogenesis, Mutagenesis, Impairment of Fertility

Carcinogenesis and Mutagenesis

PegIntron has not been tested for its carcinogenic potential. Neither PegIntron nor its components, interferon or methoxypolyethylene glycol, caused damage to DNA when tested in the standard battery of mutagenesis assays, in the presence and absence of metabolic activation.

Use with Ribavirin: See ribavirin labeling for additional warnings relevant to PegIntron therapy in combination with ribavirin.

Impairment of Fertility

PegIntron may impair human fertility. Irregular menstrual cycles were observed in female cynomolgus monkeys given subcutaneous injections of 4239 mcg/m² PegIntron alone every other day for 1 month (approximately 345 times the recommended weekly human dose based upon body surface area). These effects included transiently decreased serum levels of estradiol and progesterone, suggestive of anovulation. Normal menstrual cycles and serum hormone levels resumed in these animals 2 to 3 months following cessation of PegIntron treatment. Every other day dosing with 262 mcg/m² (approximately 21 times the weekly human dose) had no effects on cycle duration or reproductive hormone status. The effects of PegIntron on male fertility have not been studied.

14 CLINICAL STUDIES

14.1 Chronic Hepatitis C in Adults

PegIntron Monotherapy — Study 1

A randomized trial compared treatment with PegIntron (0.5, 1, or 1.5 mcg/kg once weekly subcutaneously) to treatment with INTRON A (3 million units 3 times weekly subcutaneously) in 1219 adults with chronic hepatitis from HCV infection. The subjects were not previously treated with interferon alpha, had compensated liver disease, detectable HCV-RNA, elevated ALT, and liver histopathology consistent with chronic hepatitis. Subjects were treated for 48 weeks and were followed for 24 weeks post-treatment.

Seventy percent of all subjects were infected with HCV genotype 1, and 74 percent of all subjects had high baseline levels of HCV-RNA (more than 2 million copies per mL of serum), two factors known to predict poor response to treatment.

Response to treatment was defined as undetectable HCV-RNA and normalization of ALT at 24 weeks post-treatment. The response rates to the 1 and 1.5 mcg/kg PegIntron doses were similar (approximately 24%) to each other and were both higher than the response rate to INTRON A (12%) *(see **Table 13**)*.

[See table 13 above]

Table 13: Rates of Response to Treatment – Study 1

	A PegIntron 0.5 mcg/kg (N=315)	B PegIntron 1 mcg/kg (N=298)	C INTRON A 3 MIU three times weekly (N=307)	B - C (95% CI) Difference between PegIntron 1 mcg/kg and INTRON A
Treatment Response (Combined Virologic Response and ALT Normalization)	17%	24%	12%	11 (5, 18)
Virologic Response*	18%	25%	12%	12 (6, 19)
ALT Normalization	24%	29%	18%	11 (5, 18)

*Serum HCV is measured by a research-based quantitative polymerase chain reaction assay by a central laboratory.

Subjects with both viral genotype 1 and high serum levels of HCV-RNA at baseline were less likely to respond to treatment with PegIntron. Among subjects with the two unfavorable prognostic variables, 8% (12/157) responded to PegIntron treatment and 2% (4/169) responded to INTRON A. Doses of PegIntron higher than the recommended dose did not result in higher response rates in these subjects.

Subjects receiving PegIntron with viral genotype 1 had a response rate of 14% (28/199) while subjects with other viral genotypes had a 45% (43/96) response rate.

Ninety-six percent of the responders in the PegIntron groups and 100% of responders in the INTRON A group first cleared their viral RNA by Week 24 of treatment *[see Dosage and Administration (2)]*.

The treatment response rates were similar in men and women. Response rates were lower in African-American and Hispanic subjects and higher in Asians compared to Caucasians. Although African Americans had a higher proportion of poor prognostic factors compared to Caucasians, the number of non-Caucasians studied (9% of the total) was insufficient to allow meaningful conclusions about differences in response rates after adjusting for prognostic factors.

Liver biopsies were obtained before and after treatment in 60% of subjects. A modest reduction in inflammation compared to baseline that was similar in all 4 treatment groups was observed.

PegIntron / REBETOL Combination Therapy — Study 2

A randomized trial compared treatment with two PegIntron/REBETOL regimens [PegIntron 1.5 mcg/kg subcutaneously once weekly/REBETOL 800 mg orally daily (in divided doses); PegIntron 1.5 mcg/kg subcutaneously once weekly for 4 weeks then 0.5 mcg/kg subcutaneously once weekly for 44 weeks/REBETOL 1000 or 1200 mg orally daily (in divided doses)] with INTRON A [3 MIU subcutaneously thrice weekly/REBETOL 1000 or 1200 mg orally daily (in divided doses)] in 1530 adults with chronic hepatitis C. Interferon-naïve subjects were treated for 48 weeks and followed for 24 weeks post-treatment. Eligible subjects had compensated liver disease, detectable HCV-RNA, elevated ALT, and liver histopathology consistent with chronic hepatitis.

Response to treatment was defined as undetectable HCV-RNA at 24 weeks post-treatment. The response rate to the PegIntron 1.5 mcg/kg plus REBETOL 800 mg dose was higher than the response rate to INTRON A/REBETOL *(see **Table 14**)*. The response rate to PegIntron 1.5→0.5 mcg/kg/REBETOL was essentially the same as the response to INTRON A/REBETOL (data not shown).

Table 14: Rates of Response to Treatment – Study 2

	PegIntron 1.5 mcg/kg once weekly REBETOL 800 mg daily	INTRON A 3 MIU three times weekly REBETOL 1000/ 1200 mg daily
Overall response * †	52% (264/511)	46% (231/505)
Genotype 1	41% (141/348)	33% (112/343)
Genotype 2-6	75% (123/163)	73% (119/162)

* Serum HCV-RNA is measured with a research-based quantitative polymerase chain reaction assay by a central laboratory.

† Difference in overall treatment response (PegIntron/REBETOL vs. INTRON A/REBETOL) is 6% with 95% confidence interval of (0.18, 11.63) adjusted for viral genotype and presence of cirrhosis at baseline. Response to treatment was defined as undetectable HCV-RNA at 24 weeks post-treatment.

Subjects with viral genotype 1, regardless of viral load, had a lower response rate to PegIntron (1.5 mcg/kg)/REBETOL (800 mg) compared to subjects with other viral genotypes. Subjects with both poor prognostic factors (genotype 1 and high viral load) had a response rate of 30% (78/256) compared to a response rate of 29% (71/247) with INTRON A/REBETOL.

Subjects with lower body weight tended to have higher adverse reaction rates *[see Adverse Reactions (6.1)]* and higher response rates than subjects with higher body weights. Differences in response rates between treatment arms did not substantially vary with body weight.

Treatment response rates with PegIntron/REBETOL were 49% in men and 56% in women. Response rates were lower in African American and Hispanic subjects and higher in Asians compared to Caucasians. Although African Americans had a higher proportion of poor prognostic factors compared to Caucasians, the number of non-Caucasians studied (11% of the total) was insufficient to allow meaningful conclusions about differences in response rates after adjusting for prognostic factors in this trial.

Liver biopsies were obtained before and after treatment in 68% of subjects. Compared to baseline, approximately two-thirds of subjects in all treatment groups were observed to have a modest reduction in inflammation.

PegIntron / REBETOL Combination Therapy — Study 3

In a large United States community-based trial, 4913 subjects with chronic hepatitis C were randomized to receive PegIntron 1.5 mcg/kg subcutaneously once weekly in combination with a REBETOL dose of 800 to 1400 mg (weight-based dosing [WBD]) or 800 mg (flat) orally daily (in divided doses) for 24 or 48 weeks based on genotype. Response to treatment was defined as undetectable HCV-RNA (based on an assay with a lower limit of detection of 125 IU/mL) at 24 weeks post-treatment.

Treatment with PegIntron 1.5 mcg/kg and REBETOL 800 to 1400 mg resulted in a higher sustained virologic response compared to PegIntron in combination with a flat 800 mg daily dose of REBETOL. Subjects weighing greater than 105 kg obtained the greatest benefit with WBD, although a modest benefit was also observed in subjects weighing greater than 85 to 105 kg *(see **Table 15**)*. The benefit of WBD in subjects weighing greater than 85 kg was observed with HCV genotypes 1-3. Insufficient data were available to reach conclusions regarding other genotypes. Use of WBD resulted in an increased incidence of anemia *[see Adverse Reactions (6.1)]*.

[See table 15 above]

Table 15: SVR Rates by Treatment and Baseline Weight – Study 3

Treatment Group	Subject Baseline Weight			
	<65 kg (<143 lb)	65-85 kg (143-188 lb)	>85-105 kg (>188-231 lb)	>105 kg (>231 lb)
WBD*	50% (173/348)	45% (449/994)	42% (351/835)	47% (138/292)
Flat	51% (173/342)	44% (443/1011)	39% (318/819)	33% (91/272)

* *P*=0.01, primary efficacy comparison (based on data from subjects weighing 65 kg or higher at baseline and utilizing a logistic regression analysis that includes treatment [WBD or Flat], genotype and presence/absence of advanced fibrosis, in the model).

A total of 1552 subjects weighing greater than 65 kg in Study 3 had genotype 2 or 3 and were randomized to 24 or 48 weeks of therapy. No additional benefit was observed with the longer treatment duration.

PegIntron / REBETOL Combination Therapy — Study 4

A large randomized trial compared the safety and efficacy of treatment for 48 weeks with two PegIntron/REBETOL regimens [PegIntron 1.5 mcg/kg and 1 mcg/kg subcutaneously once weekly both in combination with REBETOL 800 to 1400 mg PO daily (in two divided doses)] and Pegasys 180 mcg subcutaneously once weekly in combination with Copegus 1000 to 1200 mg PO daily (in two divided doses) in 3070 treatment-naïve adults with chronic hepatitis C genotype 1. In this trial, lack of early virologic response (undetectable HCV-RNA or greater than or equal to 2 $\log_{10}$ reduction from baseline) by treatment Week 12 was the criterion for discontinuation of treatment. SVR was defined as undetectable HCV-RNA (Roche COBAS TaqMan assay, a lower limit of quantitation of 27 IU/mL) at 24 weeks post-treatment *(see **Table 16**)*.

Table 16: SVR Rates by Treatment – Study 4

	PegIntron 1.5 mcg/kg/ REBETOL	PegIntron 1 mcg/kg/ REBETOL	Pegasys 180 mcg/ Copegus
SVR	40% (406/1019)	38% (386/1016)	41% (423/1035)

Overall SVR rates were similar among the three treatment groups. Regardless of treatment group, SVR rates were lower in subjects with poor prognostic factors. Subjects with poor prognostic factors randomized to PegIntron (1.5 mcg/kg)/REBETOL or Pegasys/Copegus, however, achieved higher SVR rates compared to similar subjects randomized to PegIntron 1 mcg/kg/REBETOL. For the PegIntron 1.5 mcg/kg plus REBETOL dose, SVR rates for subjects with and without the following prognostic factors were as follows: cirrhosis (10% vs. 42%), normal ALT levels (32% vs. 42%), baseline viral load greater than 600,000 IU/mL (35% vs. 61%), 40 years of age and older (38% vs. 50%), and African American race (23% vs. 44%). In subjects with undetectable HCV-RNA at Week 12 who received PegIntron (1.5 mcg/kg)/REBETOL, the SVR rate was 81% (328/407).

PegIntron / REBETOL Combination Therapy in Prior Treatment Failures — Study 5

In a noncomparative trial, 2293 subjects with moderate to severe fibrosis who failed previous treatment with combination alpha interferon/ribavirin were re-treated with PegIntron, 1.5 mcg/kg subcutaneously, once weekly, in combination with weight adjusted ribavirin. Eligible subjects included prior nonresponders (subjects who were HCV-RNA positive at the end of a minimum 12 weeks of treatment) and prior relapsers (subjects who were HCV-RNA negative at the end of a minimum 12 weeks of treatment and subsequently relapsed after post-treatment follow-up). Subjects who were negative at Week 12 were treated for 48 weeks and followed for 24 weeks post-treatment. Response to treatment was defined as undetectable HCV-RNA at 24 weeks post-treatment (measured using a research-based test, limit of detection 125 IU/mL). The overall response rate was 22% (497/2293) (99% CI: 19.5, 23.9). Subjects with the following characteristics were less likely to benefit from

Table 17: SVR Rates by Baseline Characteristics of Prior Treatment Failures

HCV Genotype/ Metavir Fibrosis Score	Overall SVR by Previous Response and Treatment			
	Nonresponder		Relapser	
	alfa interferon/ ribavirin % (number of subjects)	peginterferon (2a and 2b combined)/ ribavirin % (number of subjects)	alfa interferon/ ribavirin % (number of subjects)	peginterferon (2a and 2b combined)/ ribavirin % (number of subjects)
Overall	18 (158/903)	6 (30/476)	43 (130/300)	35 (113/344)
HCV 1	13 (98/761)	4 (19/431)	32 (67/208)	23 (56/243)
F2	18 (36/202)	6 (7/117)	42 (33/79)	32 (23/72)
F3	16 (38/233)	4 (4/112)	28 (16/58)	21 (14/67)
F4	7 (24/325)	4 (8/202)	26 (18/70)	18 (19/104)
HCV 2/3	49 (53/109)	36 (10/28)	67 (54/81)	57 (52/92)
F2	68 (23/34)	56 (5/9)	76 (19/25)	61 (11/18)
F3	39 (11/28)	38 (3/8)	67 (18/27)	62 (18/29)
F4	40 (19/47)	18 (2/11)	59 (17/29)	51 (23/45)
HCV 4	17 (5/29)	7 (1/15)	88 (7/8)	50 (4/8)

re-treatment: previous nonresponse, previous pegylated interferon treatment, significant bridging fibrosis or cirrhosis, and genotype 1 infection.

The re-treatment sustained virologic response rates by baseline characteristics are summarized in **Table 17**.

[See table 17 above]

Achievement of an undetectable HCV-RNA at treatment Week 12 was a strong predictor of SVR. In this trial, 1470 (64%) subjects did not achieve an undetectable HCV-RNA at treatment Week 12, and were offered enrollment into long-term treatment trials, due to an inadequate treatment response. Of the 823 (36%) subjects who were HCV-RNA undetectable at treatment Week 12, those infected with genotype 1 had an SVR of 48% (245/507), with a range of responses by fibrosis scores (F4-F2) of 39-55%. Subjects infected with genotype 2/3 who were HCV-RNA undetectable at treatment Week 12 had an overall SVR of 70% (196/281), with a range of responses by fibrosis scores (F4-F2) of 60-83%. For all genotypes, higher fibrosis scores were associated with a decreased likelihood of achieving SVR.

14.2 Chronic Hepatitis C in Pediatrics

PegIntron/REBETOL Combination Therapy — Pediatric Trial

Previously untreated pediatric subjects 3 to 17 years of age with compensated chronic hepatitis C and detectable HCV-RNA were treated with REBETOL 15 mg/kg/day plus PegIntron 60 mcg/m^2 once weekly for 24 or 48 weeks based on HCV genotype and baseline viral load. All subjects were to be followed for 24 weeks post-treatment. A total of 107 subjects received treatment, of which 52% were female, 89% were Caucasian, and 67% were infected with HCV genotype 1. Subjects infected with genotype 1, 4 or genotype 3 with HCV-RNA greater than or equal to 600,000 IU/mL received 48 weeks of therapy while those infected with genotype 2 or genotype 3 with HCV-RNA less than 600,000 IU/mL received 24 weeks of therapy. The trial results are summarized in **Table 18**.

Table 18: SVR Rates by Genotype and Treatment Duration - Pediatric Trial

	All Subjects N=107	
	24 Weeks	48 Weeks
Genotype	Virologic Response N* † (%)	Virologic Response N* † (%)
All	26/27 (96.3)	44/80 (55.0)
1	—	38/72 (52.8)
2	14/15 (93.3)	—
3‡	12/12 (100)	2/3 (66.7)
4	—	4/5 (80.0)

* Response to treatment was defined as undetectable HCV-RNA at 24 weeks post-treatment.
† N = number of responders/number of subjects with given genotype, and assigned treatment duration.
‡ Subjects with genotype 3 low viral load (less than 600,000 IU/mL) were to receive 24 weeks of treatment while those with genotype 3 and high viral load were to receive 48 weeks of treatment.

15 REFERENCES

1. Ge, D., Fellay, J., Thompson, A.J., Simon, J.S., Shianna, K.V., Urban, T.J., Heinzen, E.L., Qiu, P., Bertelsen, A.H., Muir, A.J., Sulkowski, M., McHutchison, J.G., Goldstein, D.B., Genetic variation in IL28B predicts hepatitis C treatment-induced viral clearance, Nature 2009;461(7262):399-401.
2. Thompson, A.J., Muir, A.J., Sulkowski, M.S., Ge, D., Fellay, J., Shianna, K.V., Urban, T., Afdhal, N.H., Jacobson, I.M., Esteban, R., Poordad, F., Lawitz, E.J., McCone, J., Shiffman, M.L., Galler, G.W., Lee, W.M., Reindollar, R., King, J.W., Kwo, P.Y., Ghalib, R.H., Freilich, B., Nyberg, L.M., Zeuzem, S., Poynard, T., Vock, D.M., Pieper, K.S., Patel, K., Tillmann, H.L., Noviello, S., Koury, K., Pedicone, L.D., Brass, C.A., Albrecht, J.K., Goldstein, D.B., McHutchison, J.G., Interlukin-28B polymorphism improves viral kinetics and is the strongest pretreatment predictor of sustained virologic response in genotype 1 hepatitis C virus, Gastroenterology 2010;139:120-129.

16 HOW SUPPLIED/STORAGE AND HANDLING

PegIntron REDIPEN

Each PegIntron REDIPEN Package Contains:	
A box containing one 50 mcg per 0.5 mL PegIntron REDIPEN and 1 BD needle and 2 alcohol swabs.	(NDC 0085-1323-01)
A box containing one 80 mcg per 0.5 mL PegIntron REDIPEN and 1 BD needle and 2 alcohol swabs.	(NDC 0085-1316-01)
A box containing one 120 mcg per 0.5 mL PegIntron REDIPEN and 1 BD needle and 2 alcohol swabs.	(NDC 0085-1297-01)
A box containing one 150 mcg per 0.5 mL PegIntron REDIPEN and 1 BD needle and 2 alcohol swabs.	(NDC 0085-1370-01)

Each PegIntron REDIPEN PAK 4 Contains:	
A box containing four 50 mcg per 0.5 mL PegIntron REDIPEN Units, each containing 1 BD needle and 2 alcohol swabs.	(NDC 0085-1323-02)
A box containing four 80 mcg per 0.5 mL PegIntron REDIPEN Units, each containing 1 BD needle and 2 alcohol swabs.	(NDC 0085-1316-02)
A box containing four 120 mcg per 0.5 mL PegIntron REDIPEN Units, each containing 1 BD needle and 2 alcohol swabs.	(NDC 0085-1297-02)
A box containing four 150 mcg per 0.5 mL PegIntron REDIPEN Units, each containing 1 BD needle and 2 alcohol swabs.	(NDC 0085-1370-02)

PegIntron Vials

Each PegIntron Package Contains:	
A box containing one 50 mcg per 0.5 mL vial of PegIntron Powder for Injection and one 1.25 mL vial of Diluent (Sterile Water for Injection USP), 2 BD Safety Lok syringes with a safety sleeve and 2 alcohol swabs.	(NDC 0085-1368-01)
A box containing one 80 mcg per 0.5 mL vial of PegIntron Powder for Injection and one 1.25 mL vial of Diluent (Sterile Water for Injection USP), 2 BD Safety Lok syringes with a safety sleeve and 2 alcohol swabs.	(NDC 0085-1291-01)
A box containing one 120 mcg per 0.5 mL vial of PegIntron Powder for Injection and one 1.25 mL vial of Diluent (Sterile Water for Injection USP), 2 BD Safety Lok syringes with a safety sleeve and 2 alcohol swabs.	(NDC 0085-1304-01)
A box containing one 150 mcg per 0.5 mL vial of PegIntron Powder for Injection and one 1.25 mL vial of Diluent (Sterile Water for Injection USP), 2 BD Safety Lok syringes with a safety sleeve and 2 alcohol swabs.	(NDC 0085-1279-01)

Storage

PegIntron REDIPEN

PegIntron REDIPEN should be stored at 2-8°C (36-46°F). After reconstitution, the solution should be used immediately, but may be stored up to 24 hours at 2-8°C (36-46°F). The reconstituted solution contains no preservative, and is clear and colorless. **DO NOT FREEZE. Keep away from heat.**

PegIntron Vials

PegIntron should be stored at 25°C (77°F); excursions permitted to 15-30°C (59-86°F) [see USP Controlled Room Temperature]. After reconstitution with supplied diluent, the solution should be used immediately but may be stored up to 24 hours at 2-8°C (36-46°F). The reconstituted solution contains no preservative, and is clear and colorless. **DO NOT FREEZE. Keep away from heat.**

Disposal Instructions

Patients should be thoroughly instructed in the importance of proper disposal. After preparation and administration of PegIntron for Injection, patients should be advised to use a puncture-resistant container for the disposal of used syringes, needles, and the REDIPEN. The full container should be disposed of in accordance with state and local laws. Patients should also be cautioned against reusing or sharing needles, syringes, or the REDIPEN.

17 PATIENT COUNSELING INFORMATION

See FDA-approved patient labeling (Medication Guide and Instructions for Use)

A patient should self-inject PegIntron only if it has been determined that it is appropriate, the patient agrees to medical follow-up as necessary, and training in proper injection technique has been given to him/her.

17.1 Pregnancy

Patients must be informed that REBETOL (ribavirin) may cause birth defects and death of the unborn child. Extreme care must be taken to avoid pregnancy in female patients and in female partners of male patients during treatment with combination PegIntron/ribavirin therapy and for 6 months post-therapy. Combination PegIntron/ribavirin therapy should not be initiated until a report of a negative pregnancy test has been obtained immediately prior to initiation of therapy. It is recommended that patients undergo monthly pregnancy tests during therapy and for 6 months post-therapy *[see Contraindications (4), Use in Specific Populations (8.1),* and *ribavirin labeling].*

17.2 HCV Transmission

Inform patients that there are no data regarding whether PegIntron therapy will prevent transmission of HCV infection to others. Also, it is not known if treatment with PegIntron will cure hepatitis C or prevent cirrhosis, liver failure, or liver cancer that may be the result of infection with the hepatitis C virus.

17.3 Laboratory Evaluations, Hydration, "Flu-like" Symptoms

Patients should be advised that laboratory evaluations are required before starting therapy and periodically thereafter *[see Warnings and Precautions (5.15)].* It is advised that patients be well hydrated, especially during the initial stages of treatment. "Flu-like" symptoms associated with administration of PegIntron may be minimized by bedtime administration of PegIntron or by use of antipyretics.

Patients developing fever, cough, shortness of breath or other symptoms of a lung problem during treatment with PegIntron may need to have a chest X-ray or other tests to adequately treat them.

17.4 Instructions for Use

Patients receiving PegIntron should be directed in its appropriate preparation, handling, measurement, and injection, and referred to the Instructions for Use for PegIntron Powder for Solution and PegIntron REDIPEN.

Patients should be directed to store PegIntron before mixing as follows:

- PegIntron REDIPEN: store in the refrigerator between 36-46°F (2-8°C)
- PegIntron Powder for Solution: store at room temperature between 59-86°F (15-30°C)

Patients should be instructed on the importance of site selection for self-administering the injection, as well as the importance on rotating the injection sites.

Manufactured by: Schering Corporation, a subsidiary of **MERCK & CO., INC.**, Whitehouse Station, NJ 08889, USA

U.S. Patent Nos. 5,951,974; 6,180,096; and 6,610,830.

BD and Safety-Lok are registered trademarks of Becton, Dickinson and Company.

054031-PGI-MTL-USPI.74

MEDICATION GUIDE

PegIntron® (peg-In-tron)

(Peginterferon alfa-2b) for injection, for subcutaneous use

Read this Medication Guide before you start taking PegIntron®, and each time you get a refill. There may be new information. This information does not take the place of talking with your healthcare provider about your medical condition or your treatment.

If you are taking PegIntron with REBETOL (ribavirin) with or without an approved hepatitis C virus (HCV) protease inhibitor, also read the Medication Guides for those medicines.

PegIntron, by itself or in combination with other approved medicines, is a treatment for some people who are infected with hepatitis C virus.

What is the most important information I should know about PegIntron?

PegIntron can cause serious side effects that:

- **may cause death, or**
- **may worsen certain serious diseases that you may already have.**

Tell your healthcare provider right away if you have any of the symptoms listed below while taking PegIntron. If symptoms get worse, or become severe and continue, your healthcare provider may tell you to stop taking PegIntron permanently. In many, but not all, people, these symptoms go away after they stop taking PegIntron.

1. **Mental health problems and suicide.** PegIntron may cause you to develop mood or behavior problems that may get worse during treatment with PegIntron or after your last dose, including:
   - irritability (getting upset easily)
   - depression (feeling low, feeling bad about yourself, or feeling hopeless)
   - aggressive behavior
   - thoughts of hurting yourself or others, or suicide
   - former drug addicts may fall back into drug addiction or overdose

   If you have these symptoms, your healthcare provider should carefully monitor you during treatment with PegIntron and for 6 months after your last dose.
2. **Heart problems.** Some people who take PegIntron may get heart problems, including:
   - low blood pressure
   - fast heart rate or abnormal heart beat
   - trouble breathing or chest pain
   - heart attacks or heart muscle problems (cardiomyopathy)
3. **Stroke or symptoms of a stroke. Symptoms may include weakness, loss of coordination, and numbness.** Stroke or symptoms of a stroke may happen in people who have some risk factors **or** no known risk factors for a stroke.
4. **New or worsening autoimmune problems.** Some people taking PegIntron develop autoimmune problems (a condition where the body's immune cells attack other cells or organs in the body), including rheumatoid arthritis, systemic lupus erythematosus, and psoriasis. In some people who already have an autoimmune problem, it may get worse during your treatment with PegIntron.
5. **Infections.** Some people who take PegIntron may get an infection. Symptoms may include:
   - fever
   - chills
   - bloody diarrhea
   - burning or pain with urination
   - urinating often
   - coughing up mucus (phlegm) that is discolored (for example, yellow or pink)

PegIntron in combination with REBETOL (ribavirin) may cause birth defects or the death of your unborn baby. Do not take PegIntron and ribavirin combination therapy if you or your sexual partner is pregnant or plan to be come pregnant. Do not become pregnant within 6 months after discontinuing PegIntron and ribavirin combination therapy. You must use 2 forms of birth control when you take PegIntron and ribavirin and for the 6 months after treatment.

- Females must have a pregnancy test before starting the PegIntron and ribavirin combination therapy, every month while on the combination therapy, and every month for the 6 months after the last dose of combination therapy.
- If you or your female sexual partner becomes pregnant while taking the PegIntron and ribavirin combination therapy or within 6 months after you stop taking the combination therapy, tell your healthcare provider right away. You or your healthcare provider should contact the Ribavirin pregnancy registry by calling 1-800-593-2214. The Ribavirin pregnancy registry collects information about what happens to mothers and their babies if the mother takes ribavirin while she is pregnant.

While taking PegIntron, you should see a healthcare provider regularly for check-ups and blood tests to make sure that your treatment is working, and to check for side effects.

What is PegIntron?

PegIntron is a prescription medicine that is used:

- with REBETOL (ribavirin) and an approved hepatitis C virus (HCV) protease inhibitor to treat chronic (lasting a long time) hepatitis C infection in adults.
- with REBETOL (ribavirin) to treat chronic (lasting a long time) hepatitis C infection in people 3 years and older with stable liver problems.
- alone, sometimes to treat adults who have chronic (lasting a long time) hepatitis C infection with stable liver problems and who can not take REBETOL (ribavirin).

People with hepatitis C have the virus in their blood and in their liver. PegIntron reduces the amount of virus in the body and helps the body's immune system fight the virus. REBETOL (ribavirin) is a drug that helps to fight the viral infection but does not work when used by itself to treat chronic hepatitis C.

It is not known if PegIntron use for longer than 1 year is safe and will work.

It is not known if PegIntron use in children younger than 3 years old is safe and will work.

Who should not take PegIntron?

Do not take PegIntron:

- if you have had a serious allergic reaction to another alpha interferon or to any of the ingredients in PegIntron. See the end of this Medication Guide for a complete list of ingredients. Ask your healthcare provider if you are not sure.
- if you have certain types of hepatitis (autoimmune hepatitis).
- if you have certain other liver problems.
- with REBETOL (ribavirin) if you are pregnant, planning to get pregnant, or breastfeeding. See "What is the most important information I should know about PegIntron?"

Talk to your healthcare provider before taking PegIntron if you have any of these conditions.

What should I tell my healthcare provider before taking PegIntron?

Before you take PegIntron, see **"What is the most important information I should know about PegIntron?"**, and tell your healthcare provider if you:

- are being treated for a mental illness or had treatment in the past for any mental illness, including depression and suicidal behavior
- have or ever had any problems with your heart, including heart attack or high blood pressure
- have any kind of autoimmune disease (where the body's immune system attacks the body's own cells), such as psoriasis, systemic lupus erythematosus, rheumatoid arthritis
- have or ever had bleeding problems or a blood clot
- have or ever had low blood cell counts
- have ever been addicted to drugs or alcohol
- have liver disease (other than hepatitis C infection)
- have or had lung disease such as chronic obstructive pulmonary disease (COPD)
- have thyroid problems
- have diabetes
- have colitis (inflammation of your intestine)
- have a condition that suppresses your immune system, such as cancer
- have hepatitis B infection
- have HIV infection
- have kidney problems
- have high blood triglyceride levels (fat in your blood)
- have an organ transplant and are taking medicine that keeps your body from rejecting your transplant (suppresses your immune system)
- have any other medical conditions
- are pregnant or plan to become pregnant. PegIntron may harm your unborn baby. You should use effective birth control during treatment with PegIntron. Talk to your healthcare provider about birth control choices for you during treatment with PegIntron. Tell your healthcare provider if you become pregnant during treatment with PegIntron.
- are breastfeeding or plan to breastfeed. It is not known if PegIntron passes into your breast milk. You and your healthcare provider should decide if you will use PegIntron or breastfeed.

Tell your healthcare provider about all the medicines you take, including prescription and non-prescription medicines, vitamins, and herbal supplements. PegIntron and certain other medicines may affect each other and cause side effects.

Especially tell your healthcare provider if you take the anti-hepatitis B medicine telbivudine (Tyzeka).

Know the medicines you take. Keep a list of them and show it to your healthcare provider and pharmacist when you get a new medicine.

How should I take PegIntron?

- Take PegIntron exactly as your healthcare provider tells you to. Your healthcare provider will tell you how much PegIntron to take and when to take it. Do not take more than your prescribed dose.
- Take your prescribed dose of PegIntron every week, on the same day of each week and at the same time.
- PegIntron is given as an injection under your skin (subcutaneous injection). Your healthcare provider should show you how to prepare and measure your dose of PegIntron, and how to inject yourself before you use PegIntron for the first time.
- You should not inject PegIntron until your healthcare provider has shown you how to use PegIntron the right way.
- PegIntron comes as a powder in a single-use vial and as a single-use REDIPEN. Your healthcare provider will prescribe the PegIntron that is right for you. See the Instructions for Use that comes with your PegIntron for detailed instructions for preparing and injecting a dose of PegIntron.
- If you miss a dose of PegIntron, take the missed dose as soon as possible during the same day or the next day, then continue on your regular dosing schedule. If several days go by after you miss a dose, check with your healthcare provider about what to do.
- Do not inject more than 1 dose of PegIntron in one week without talking to your healthcare provider.
- If you take too much PegIntron, call your healthcare provider right away. Your healthcare provider may examine you more closely, and do blood tests.
- Your healthcare provider should do regular blood tests before you start PegIntron, and during treatment to see how well the treatment is working and to check you for side effects.

What are the possible side effects of PegIntron?

PegIntron may cause serious side effects including:

See "What is the most important information I should know about PegIntron?"

- **Serious eye problems.** PegIntron may cause eye problems that may lead to vision loss or blindness. You should have an eye exam before you start taking PegIntron. If you have eye problems or have had them in the past, you may need eye exams while you are taking PegIntron. Tell your healthcare provider or eye doctor right away if you have any vision changes while taking PegIntron.
- **Blood problems.** PegIntron can affect your bone marrow and cause low white blood cell and platelet counts. In some people, these blood counts may fall to dangerously low levels. If your blood counts become very low, you can get infections, and problems with bleeding and bruising.

- **Swelling of your pancreas (pancreatitis) or intestines (colitis).**
  Symptoms may include:
  - severe stomach area (abdomen) pain
  - severe back pain
  - nausea and vomiting
  - bloody diarrhea
  - fever
- **Lung problems including:**
  - trouble breathing
  - pneumonia
  - inflammation of lung tissue
  - new or worse high blood pressure of the lungs (pulmonary hypertension). This can be severe and may lead to death.

  You may need to have a chest X-ray or other tests if you develop fever, cough, shortness of breath or other symptoms of a lung problem during treatment with PegIntron.
- **Severe liver problems, or worsening of liver problems, including liver failure and death.** Symptoms may include:
  - nausea
  - loss of appetite
  - tiredness
  - diarrhea
  - yellowing of your skin or the white part of your eyes
  - bleeding more easily than normal
  - swelling of your stomach area (abdomen)
  - confusion
  - sleepiness
  - you cannot be awakened (coma)
- **Thyroid problems.** Some people develop changes in their thyroid function. Symptoms of thyroid changes include:
  - problems concentrating
  - feeling cold or hot all of the time
  - weight changes
  - skin changes
- **Blood sugar problems.** Some people may develop high blood sugar or diabetes. If you have high blood sugar or diabetes that is not controlled before starting PegIntron, talk to your healthcare provider before you take PegIntron. If you develop high blood sugar or diabetes while taking PegIntron, your healthcare provider may tell you to stop PegIntron and prescribe a different medicine for you. Symptoms of high blood sugar or diabetes may include:
  - increased thirst
  - tiredness
  - urinating more often than normal
  - increased appetite
  - weight loss
  - your breath smells like fruit
- **Serious allergic reactions and skin reactions. Symptoms may include:**
  - itching
  - swelling of the face, eyes, lips, tongue, or throat
  - trouble breathing
  - anxiousness
  - chest pain
  - feeling faint
  - skin rash, hives, sores in your mouth, or your skin blisters and peels
- **Growth problems in children. Weight loss and slowed growth are common in children during treatment with PegIntron.**
- **Nerve problems.** People who take PegIntron or other alpha interferon products with telbivudine (Tyzeka) can develop nerve problems such as continuing numbness, tingling, or burning sensation in the arms or legs (peripheral neuropathy). Call your healthcare provider if you have any of these symptoms.
- **Dental and gum problems.**

Tell your healthcare provider right away if you have any of the symptoms listed above.

The most common side effects of PegIntron include:

- **Flu-like symptoms.** Symptoms may include: headache, muscle aches, tiredness, and fever. Some of these symptoms may be decreased by injecting your PegIntron dose at bedtime. Talk to your healthcare provider about which over-the-counter medicines you can take to help prevent or decrease some of these symptoms.
- **Tiredness.** Many people become very tired during treatment with PegIntron.
- **Appetite problems.** Nausea, loss of appetite, and weight loss can happen with PegIntron.
- **Skin reactions.** Redness, swelling, and itching are common at the site of injection.
- **Hair thinning.**

Tell your healthcare provider if you have any side effect that bothers you or that does not go away.

These are not all of the possible side effects of PegIntron. For more information, ask your healthcare provider or pharmacist.

Call your doctor for medical advice about side effects. You may report side effects to FDA at 1–800–FDA–1088.

How should I store PegIntron?

- Before mixing, store PegIntron REDIPEN in the refrigerator between 36°F to 46°F (2°C to 8°C).
- Before mixing, store PegIntron vials at room temperature between 59°F to 86°F (15°C to 30°C).
- Keep PegIntron away from heat.
- After mixing, use PegIntron right away or store it in the refrigerator for up to 24 hours between 36°F to 46°F (2°C to 8°C).
- Do not freeze PegIntron.
- **Keep PegIntron and all medicines out of the reach of children.**

General Information about PegIntron

Medicines are sometimes prescribed for purposes other than those listed in a Medication Guide. Do not use PegIntron for a condition for which it was not prescribed. Do not give PegIntron to other people, even if they have the same symptoms that you have. It may harm them.

This Medication Guide summarizes the most important information about PegIntron. If you would like more information, ask your healthcare provider. You can ask your healthcare provider or pharmacist for information about PegIntron that was written for healthcare professionals.

For more information, go to www.PegIntron.com or call 1-800-526-4099.

What are the ingredients in PegIntron?

Active ingredients: peginterferon alfa-2b

Inactive ingredients: dibasic sodium phosphate anhydrous, monobasic sodium phosphate dihydrate, sucrose, polysorbate 80. Sterile water for injection is supplied as a diluent.

The Medication Guide has been approved by the U.S. Food and Drug Administration.

Manufactured by: Schering Corporation, a subsidiary of **MERCK & CO., INC.**, Whitehouse Station, NJ 08889, USA.

U.S. Patent Nos. 5,951,974; 6,180,096; and 6,610,830.

Revised: 05/2013

054031-PGI-MTL-MG.15

Instructions for Use

PegIntron ® (peg-In-tron)

(Peginterferon alfa-2b)

Solution for Injection REDIPEN

How to Use the PegIntron® REDIPEN® Single-dose Delivery System.

Be sure that you read, understand, and follow these instructions before injecting PegIntron Solution. Your healthcare provider should show you how to prepare, measure, and inject PegIntron properly before you use it for the first time. Ask your healthcare provider if you have any questions.

Before starting, collect all of the supplies that you will need to use for preparing and injecting PegIntron. For each injection you will need a PegIntron REDIPEN package that contains:

- the PegIntron REDIPEN single-dose delivery system
- 1 disposable needle
- 2 alcohol swabs
- dosing tray (the dosing tray is the bottom half of the REDIPEN package)

- You will need gauze or a cotton ball to press to the injection site after injecting. You will also need a puncture-proof disposable container to throw away your used REDIPEN.

Important:

- **Never re-use needles.**
- Make sure that you have the correct PegIntron REDIPEN prescribed by your healthcare provider. The PegIntron REDIPEN system is for a single use, by one person only, 1 time a week. **The REDIPEN must not be shared.**

  The PegIntron REDIPEN should only be used with the injection needle that is provided in the packaging for the PegIntron REDIPEN system. If you use other needles, the pen may not work the right way.
  - Figures 1 and 2 below show the different parts of the PegIntron REDIPEN Delivery System and the injection needle. Figure 3 below shows the dosing tray with the REDIPEN. The parts of the pen you need to know are:

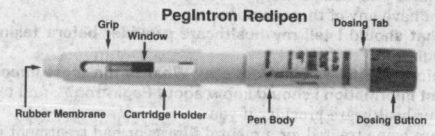

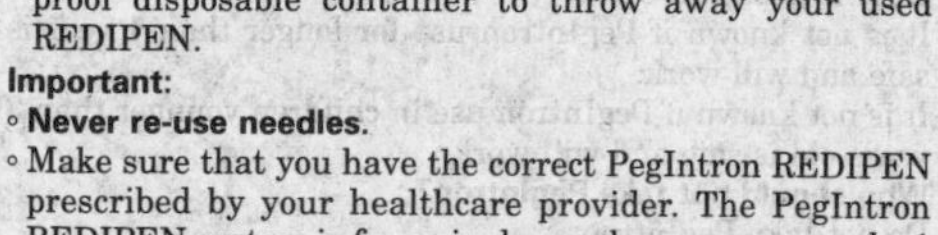

Figure 1

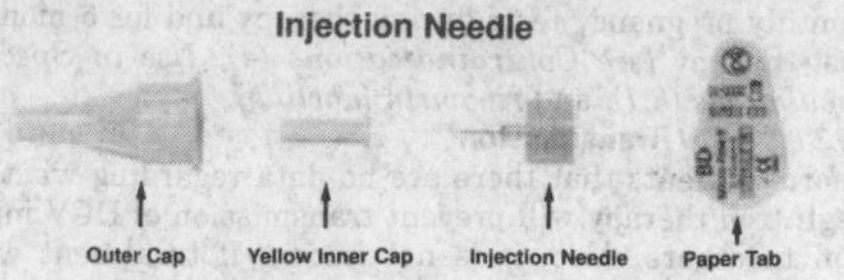

Figure 2

Figure 3

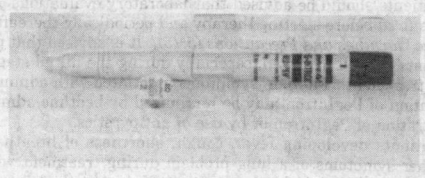

How should I prepare a dose of PegIntron using the REDIPEN?

1. Find a clean, well-lit, flat work surface.
2. Take the PegIntron REDIPEN out of the refrigerator and allow the medicine to come to room temperature. Look at the date printed on the PegIntron REDIPEN carton to make sure that the expiration date has not passed. Do not use if the expiration date has passed.
3. After taking the PegIntron REDIPEN out of the carton, look in the window of the REDIPEN and make sure the PegIntron in the cartridge holder window is a white to off-white tablet that is whole, or in pieces, or powdered.
4. Wash your hands well with soap and water. It is important to keep your work area, your hands, and the injection site clean to decrease the risk of infection (see Figure 4).

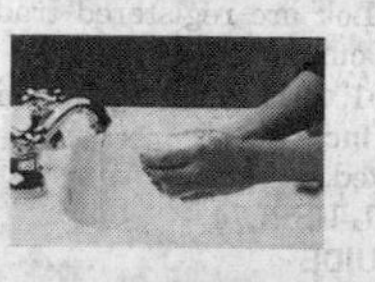

Figure 4

Mix the Drug

5. **Place the PegIntron REDIPEN upright** in the dosing tray on a hard, flat, non-slip surface with the dosing button down (see Figure 5). You may want to hold the REDIPEN using the grip.

Figure 5

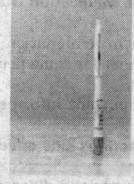

6. To mix the powder and the liquid, keep the REDIPEN upright in the dosing tray and press the top half of the REDIPEN downward toward the hard, flat, non-slip surface **until you hear the "click" sound** (see Figure 6). When you hear the click, you will notice in the window that both dark stoppers are now touching. The dosing button should be flat with the pen body.

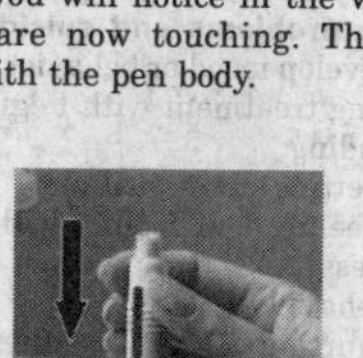

Figure 6

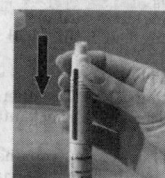

7. Wait several seconds for the powder to completely dissolve. Do not shake. If the solution does not dissolve, gently turn the PegIntron REDIPEN upside down two times (see Figure 7).

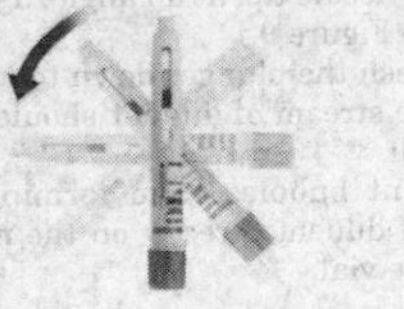

Figure 7

8. Keep the PegIntron REDIPEN **UPRIGHT**, with the dosing button down. Look through the REDIPEN window to see that the mixed PegIntron solution is completely dissolved. The solution should be clear and colorless **before use**. It is normal to see some small bubbles in the REDIPEN window, near the top of the solution. Do not use the PegIntron REDIPEN solution if it is discolored, or not clear, or if it has particles in it.
9. Place the PegIntron REDIPEN back into the dosing tray provided in the packaging (see Figure 8). The dosing button will be on the bottom.

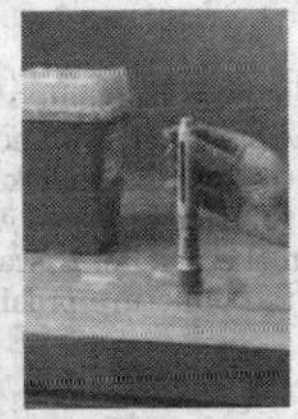

Figure 8

Attach the Needle

10. Before you attach the needle to the PegIntron REDIPEN, wipe the rubber membrane of the PegIntron REDIPEN with an alcohol swab.
11. Remove the protective paper tab from the injection needle, but do not remove either the outer cap or the yellow inner cap from the injection needle.
12. Keep the PegIntron REDIPEN upright in the dosing tray and push the injection needle straight into the REDIPEN rubber membrane. Screw the needle onto the PegIntron REDIPEN by turning it in a clockwise direction (see Figure 9).
    - Remember to leave the needle caps in place when you attach the needle to the REDIPEN. Pushing the needle through the rubber membrane "primes" the needle and allows the extra liquid and air in the pen to be removed.

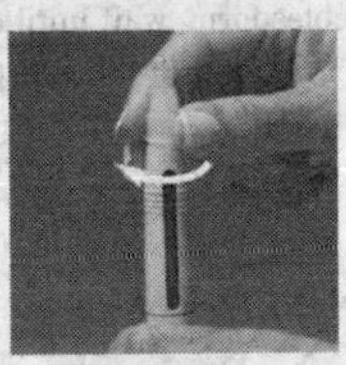

Figure 9

NOTE: Some fluid will trickle out. This is **normal**. The dark stoppers move up and you will no longer see the fluid in the window once the needle is successfully primed.

- Remove the outer clear needle cap on the REDIPEN, but leave the yellow cap on (see Figure 10).

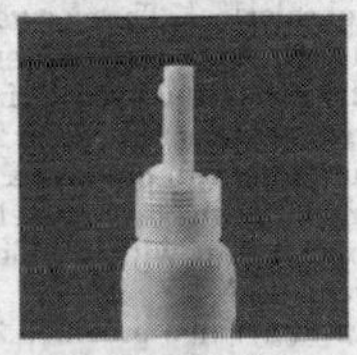

Figure 10

How should I set the dose prescribed by my healthcare provider?

Dial the Dose

13. Holding the PegIntron REDIPEN firmly, pull the dosing button out as far as it will go (see Figure 11). You will see a dark band.
    Do not push the dosing button in until you are ready to self-inject the PegIntron dose.

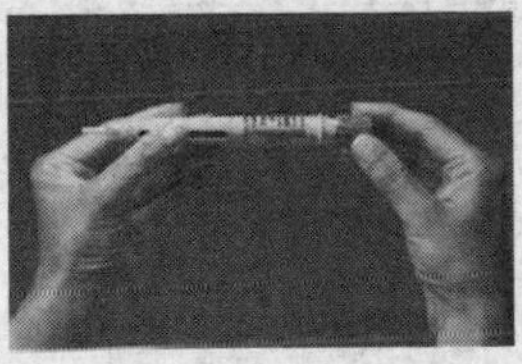

Figure 11

14. Turn the dosing button until your prescribed dose is lined up with the dosing tab (see Figure 12). The dosing button will turn freely. If you have trouble dialing your dose, check to make sure the dosing button has been pulled out **as far** as it will go (see Figure 13).

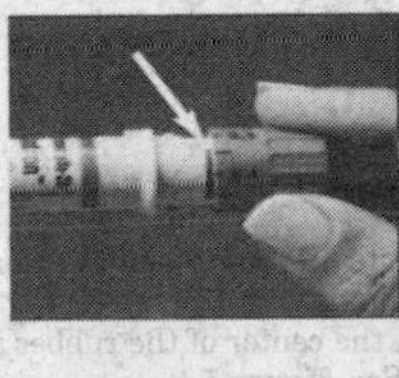

Figure 12

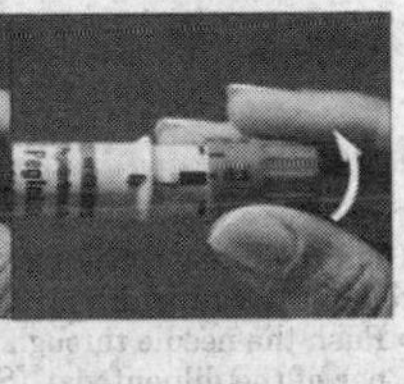

Figure 13

15. Carefully lay the PegIntron REDIPEN down on the dosing tray or on a hard, flat, non-slip surface. Do not remove the yellow needle cap and do not push the dosing button in until you are ready to self-inject the PegIntron dose.

Choosing an Injection Site

The best sites for giving yourself an injection are those areas with a layer of fat between the skin and muscle, like your thigh, the outer surface of your upper arm, and abdomen (see Figure 14). Do not inject yourself in the area near your navel or waistline. If you are very thin, you should only use the thigh or outer surface of the arm for injection.

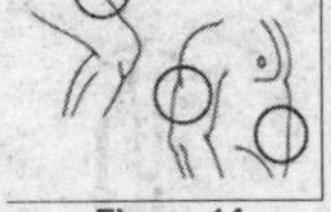

Figure 14

You should use a different site each time you inject PegIntron to avoid soreness at any one site. Do not inject PegIntron into an area where the skin is irritated, red, bruised, infected, or has scars, stretch marks, or lumps.

How should I Inject a dose of PegIntron?

16. Clean the skin where the injection is to be given with the second alcohol swab provided, and wait for the skin to dry.
17. There may be some liquid around the yellow inner needle cap (see Figure 15). This is normal.

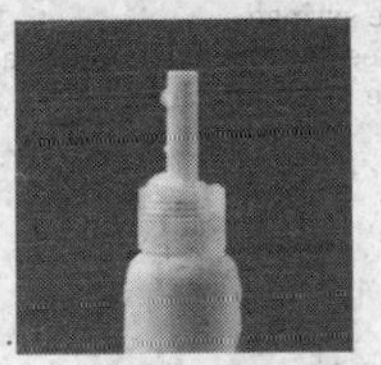

Figure 15

18. Remove the **yellow** inner needle cap when the injection site is dry (see Figure 16). You are now ready to inject.

[See figure 16 at top of next column]

19. Hold the PegIntron REDIPEN with your fingers wrapped around the pen body barrel and your thumb on the dosing button (see Figure 17).

[See figure 17 at top of next column]

20. With your other hand, pinch the skin in the area you have cleaned for injection.

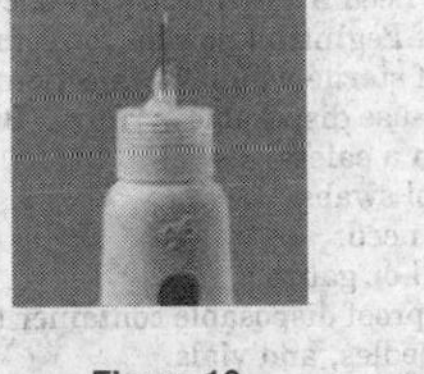

Figure 16

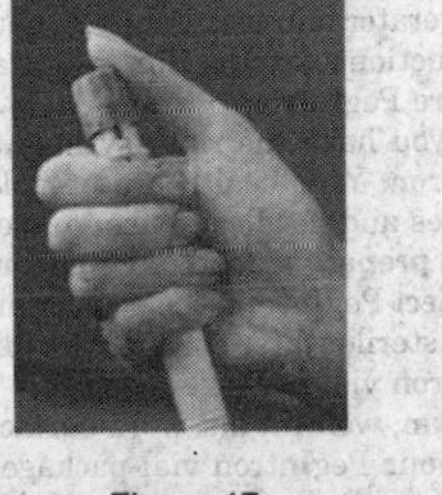

Figure 17

21. Insert the needle into the pinched skin at an angle of 45° to 90° (see Figure 18).

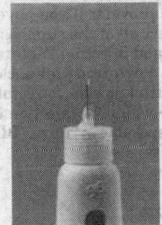

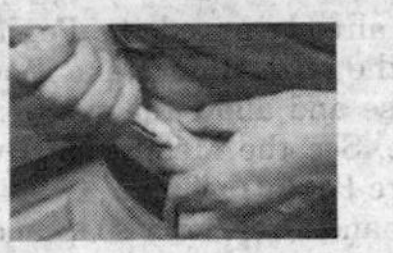

Figure 18

22. Press the dosing button down slowly and firmly until you can not push it any further. Keep your thumb pressed down on the dosing button for an additional 5 seconds to make sure that you get the complete dose.
23. Slowly release the dosing button and remove the needle from your skin.
24. Gently press the injection site with a small bandage or sterile gauze if needed for a few seconds but do not massage the injection site. If there is bleeding, cover with an adhesive bandage. Do not recap the needle and do not reuse the REDIPEN.

How do I dispose of the REDIPEN?

- Throw away the REDIPEN and needle and any solution remaining in the REDIPEN in a puncture-proof container, sharps container, or a hard container like a metal can with a lid. Always place needles facing down. Do not use glass or clear plastic containers. **Always keep the puncture-proof container out of reach of children.**
- Do not throw away used REDIPENS and needles in household trash and do not recycle them.
- Check with your healthcare provider for instructions about the right way to throw away used REDIPENS and needles. There may be local or state laws about how to throw away used REDIPENS and needles. Always follow the instructions of your healthcare provider.

How should I store PegIntron?

- Before mixing, store PegIntron REDIPEN in the refrigerator between 36°F to 46°F (2°C to 8°C).
- After mixing, use PegIntron right away or store it in the refrigerator for up to 24 hours between 36°F to 46°F (2°C to 8°C).
- Do not freeze PegIntron.
- Keep PegIntron away from heat.
- **Keep PegIntron and all medicines out of the reach of children.**

Manufactured by: Schering Corporation, a subsidiary of **Merck & Co., Inc.,** Whitehouse Station, NJ 08889, USA.

Rev February/2011

35038809T

Instructions for Use

PegIntron ® (peg-In-tron)

(Peginterferon alfa-2b)

Powder for Solution

Be sure that you read, understand and follow these instructions before injecting PegIntron Solution. Your healthcare provider should show you how to prepare, measure, and inject PegIntron properly before you use it for the first time. Ask your healthcare provider if you have any questions.

Before starting, collect all of the supplies that you will need to use for preparing and injecting PegIntron. For each injection you will need a PegIntron vial package that contains:

- 1 vial of PegIntron powder for solution
- 1 vial of sterile water for injection (diluent)
- 2 single-use disposable syringes (BD Safety Lok syringes with a safety sleeve)
- 2 alcohol swabs

You will also need:

- 1 cotton ball or gauze
- a puncture-proof disposable container to throw away used syringes, needles, and vials.

Important:

- **Never re-use disposable syringes and needles.**
- The vial of mixed PegIntron should be used right away. Do not mix more than 1 vial of PegIntron at a time. If you do not use the vial of the prepared solution right away, store it in a refrigerator and use within 24 hours. See the end of these Instructions for Use for information about "How should I store PegIntron?"
- Make sure you have the right syringe and needle to use with PegIntron. Your healthcare provider should tell you what syringes and needles to use to inject PegIntron.

How should I prepare a dose of PegIntron?

Before you inject PegIntron, the powder must be mixed with 0.7 mL of the sterile water for injection (diluent) that comes in the PegIntron vial package.

1. Find a clean, well-lit, flat work surface.
2. Get 1 of your PegIntron vial packages. Check the date printed on the PegIntron carton. Make sure that the expiration date has not passed. Do not use your PegIntron vial packages if the expiration date has passed. The medicine in the PegIntron vial should look like a white to off-white tablet that is whole, or in pieces, or powdered.
   If you have already mixed the PegIntron solution and stored it in the refrigerator, take it out of the refrigerator before use and allow the solution to come to room temperature. See the Medication Guide section "How should I store PegIntron?"
3. Wash your hands well with soap and water, rinse and towel dry (see Figure 1). Keep your work area, your hands, and injection site clean to decrease the risk of infection.

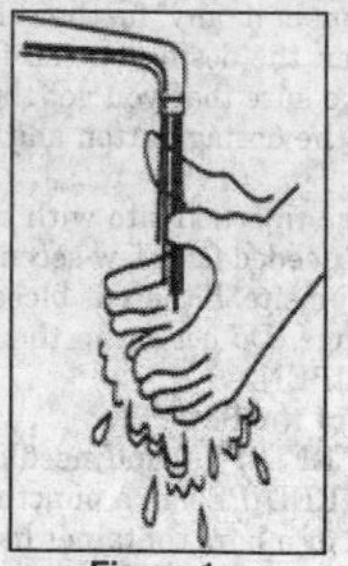

Figure 1

The disposable syringes have needles that are already attached and cannot be removed. Each syringe has a clear plastic safety sleeve that is pulled over the needle for disposal after use. The safety sleeve should remain tight against the flange while using the syringe and moved over the needle only when ready for disposal. (See Figure 2.)

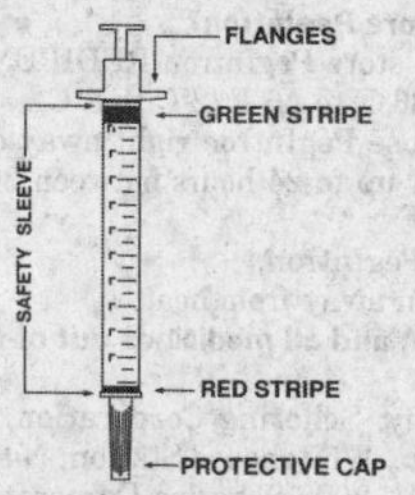

Figure 2

4. Remove the protective wrapper from one of the syringes provided. Use the syringe for steps 4 through 15. Make sure that the syringe safety sleeve is sitting against the flange. (See Figure 2.)
5. Remove the protective plastic cap from the tops of both the sterile water for injection (diluent) and the PegIntron vials (see Figure 3). Clean the rubber stopper on the top of both vials with an alcohol swab.

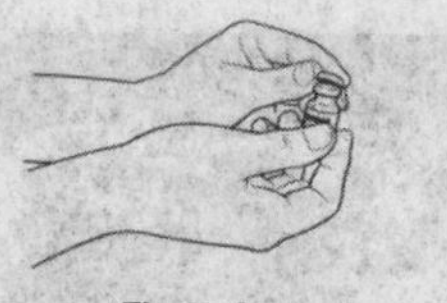

Figure 3

6. Carefully remove the protective cap straight off of the needle to avoid damaging the needle point.
7. Fill the syringe with air by pulling back on the plunger to 0.7 mL. (See Figure 4.)

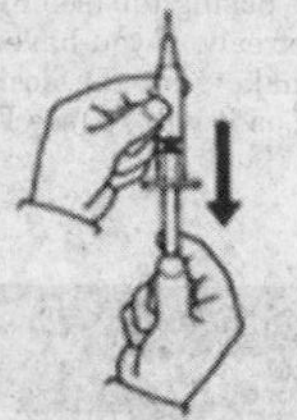

Figure 4

8. Hold the diluent vial upright. Do not touch the cleaned top of the vial with your hands.
   - Push the needle through the center of the rubber stopper of the diluent vial. (See Figure 5.)
   - Slowly inject all the air from the syringe into the air space above the diluent in the vial. (See Figure 6.)

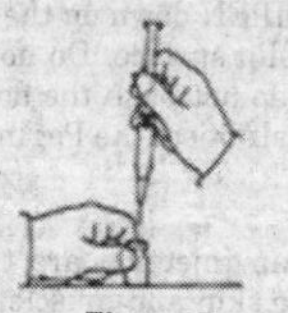

Figure 5

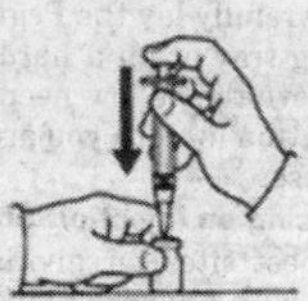

Figure 6

9. Turn the vial upside down and make sure the tip of the needle is in the liquid.
10. Withdraw only 0.7 mL of diluent by pulling the plunger back to the 0.7 mL mark on the side of the syringe. (See Figure 7.)

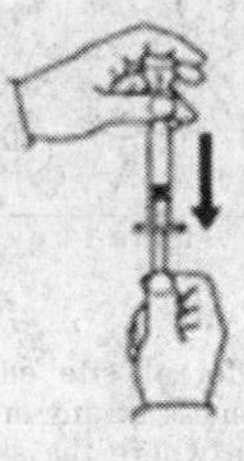

Figure 7

11. With the needle still inserted in the vial, check the syringe for air bubbles.
    - If there are any air bubbles, gently tap the syringe with your finger until the air bubbles rise to the top of the syringe.
    - Slowly push the plunger up to remove the air bubbles.
    - If you push diluent back into the vial, slowly pull back on the plunger to draw the correct amount of diluent back into the syringe.
12. Remove the needle from the vial. (See Figure 8.) Do not let the syringe touch anything.

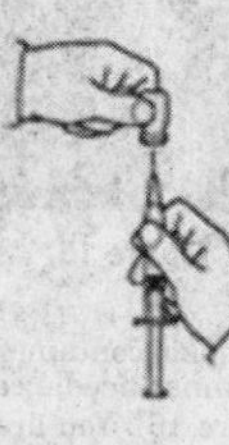

Figure 8

13. Throw away any diluent that is left over in the vial.
14. Insert the needle through the center of the rubber stopper of the PegIntron powder vial. Do not touch the cleaned rubber stopper.
    - Place the needle tip, at an angle, against the side of the vial. (See Figure 9.)
    - Slowly push the plunger down to inject the 0.7 mL diluent. The stream of diluent should run down the side of the vial.
    - To prevent bubbles from forming, do not aim the stream of diluent directly on the medicine in the bottom of the vial.

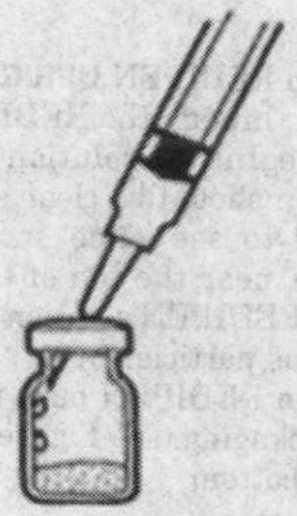

Figure 9

15. Remove the needle from the vial.
    - Firmly grasp the safety sleeve and pull it over the exposed needle until you hear a click (see Figure 10). The green stripe on the safety sleeve will completely cover the red stripe on the needle. Discard the syringe, needle, and vial in the puncture-proof container.

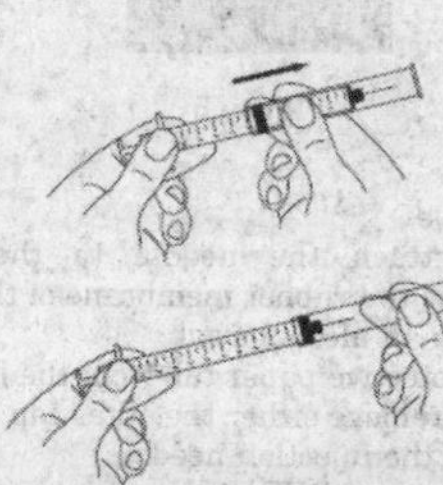

Figure 10

16. Gently swirl the vial in a gentle circular motion, until the PegIntron is completely dissolved (mixed together). (See Figure 11.)
    - Do not shake the vial. If any powder remains undissolved in the vial, gently turn the vial upside down until all of the powder is dissolved.
    - The solution may look cloudy or bubbly for a few minutes. If air bubbles form, wait until the solution settles and all bubbles rise to the top.

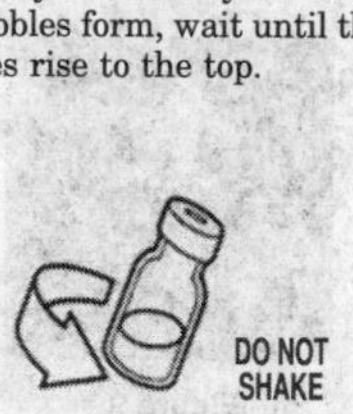

Figure 11

17. After the PegIntron completely dissolves, the solution should be clear, colorless and without particles. It is normal to see a ring of foam or bubbles on the surface.
    Do not use the mixed solution if you see particles in it, or it is not clear and colorless. Throw away the syringe and needle in the puncture-proof container. (See the section "How should I dispose of the used syringes, needles, and vials?".) Then, repeat steps 1 through 23 with a new vial of PegIntron and diluent to prepare a new syringe.
18. After the PegIntron powder completely dissolves, clean the rubber stopper again with an alcohol swab before you withdraw your dose.
19. Unwrap the second syringe provided. You will use it to give yourself the injection.
    - Carefully remove the protective cap from the needle. Fill the syringe with air by pulling the plunger to the number on the side of the syringe (mL) that matches your prescribed dose. (See Figure 12.)

[See figure 12 at top of next column]

- Hold the PegIntron vial upright. Do not touch the cleaned top of the vial with your hands. (See Figure 13.)

[See figure 13 at top of next column]

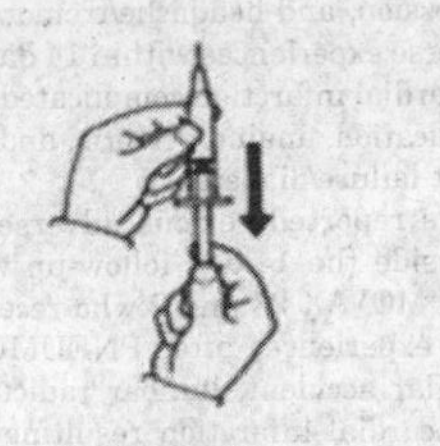

Figure 12

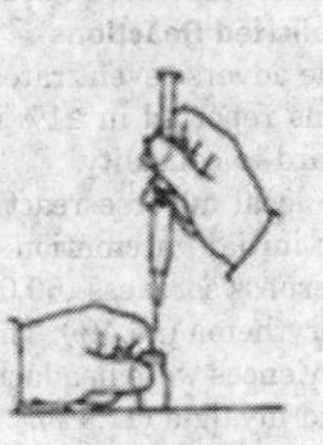

Figure 13

◦ Insert the needle into the vial containing the PegIntron solution. Inject the air into the center of the vial. (See Figure 14.)

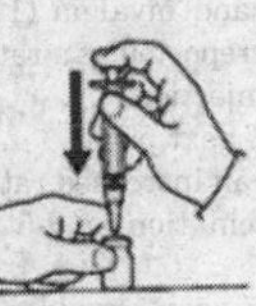

Figure 14

20. Turn the PegIntron vial upside down. Be sure the tip of the needle is in the PegIntron solution.
    ◦ Hold the vial and syringe with one hand. Be sure the tip of the needle is in the PegIntron Solution. With the other hand, slowly pull the plunger back to fill the syringe with the exact amount of PegIntron into the syringe your healthcare provider told you to use. (See Figure 15.)

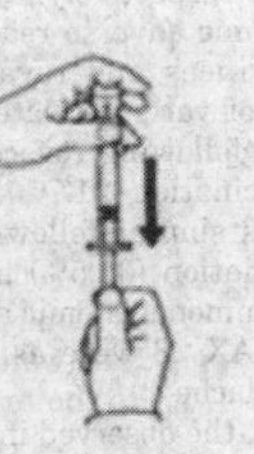

Figure 15

21. Check for air bubbles in the syringe. If you see any air bubbles, hold the syringe with the needle pointing up. Gently tap the syringe until the air bubbles rise. Then, slowly push the plunger up to remove any air bubbles. If you push solution into the vial, slowly pull back on the plunger again to draw the correct amount of PegIntron back into the syringe. When you are ready to inject the medicine, remove the needle from the vial. (See Figure 16.)

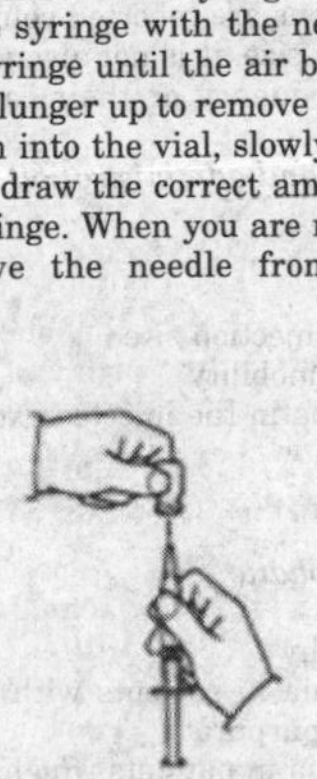

Figure 16

How should I choose a site for injection?

The best sites for giving yourself an injection are those areas with a layer of fat between the skin and muscle, like your thigh, the outer surface of your upper arm, and abdomen (see Figure 17). Do not inject yourself in the area near your navel or waistline. If you are very thin, you should only use the thigh or outer surface of the arm for injection.

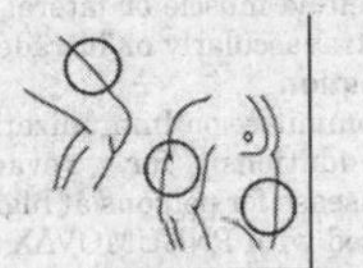

Figure 17

You should use a different site each time you inject PegIntron to avoid soreness at any one site. Do not inject PegIntron solution into an area where the skin is irritated, red, bruised, infected or has scars, stretch marks, or lumps.

How should I inject a dose of PegIntron?

22. Clean the skin where the injection is to be given with an alcohol swab. Wait for the area to dry.
    ◦ Make sure the safety sleeve of the syringe is pushed firmly against the syringe flange so that the needle is fully exposed. (See Figure 2.)
23. With one hand, pinch a fold of skin. With your other hand, pick up the syringe and hold it like a pencil.
    ◦ Insert the needle into the pinched skin at a 45- to 90-degree angle with a quick dart-like motion (see Figure 18).

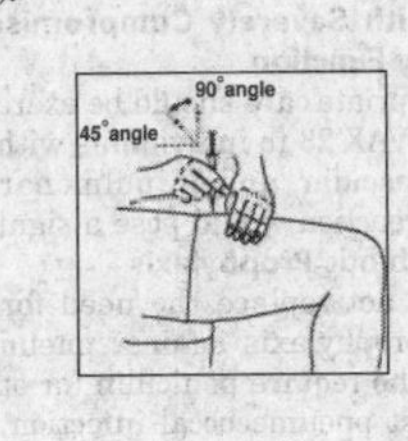

Figure 18

◦ After the needle is inserted, remove the hand that you used to pinch your skin. Use it to hold the syringe barrel.
◦ Pull the plunger of the syringe back very slightly.
◦ **If no blood is present in the syringe**, inject the medicine by gently pressing the plunger all the way down the syringe barrel, until the syringe is empty.
◦ **If blood comes into the syringe**, the needle has entered a blood vessel. Do not inject.
    ◦ Withdraw the needle and throw away the syringe and needle in the puncture-proof container. (See step 24 and the disposal steps below.)
    ◦ Then, repeat steps 1 through 23 with a new vial of PegIntron and diluent to prepare a new syringe, and inject the medicine at a new site.

24. When the syringe is empty, pull the needle out of the skin.
    ◦ Place a cotton ball or gauze over the injection site and press for several seconds. Do not massage the injection site.
    ◦ If there is bleeding, cover it with a bandage.
25. After injecting your dose:
    ◦ Firmly grasp the safety sleeve and pull it over the exposed needle until you hear a click, and the green stripe on the safety sleeve covers the red stripe on the needle (see Figure 19).

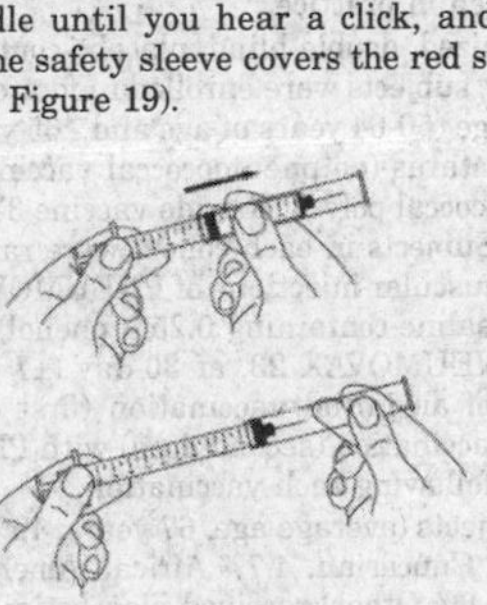

Figure 19

26. Throw away the used syringe, needle, and vials in the puncture-proof disposable container. (See "How should I dispose of the used syringes, needles, and vials?")

How should I dispose of the used syringes, needles, and vials?

- Throw away used syringes, needles, and vials in a puncture-proof container, sharps container, or a hard container like a metal can with a lid. Always place needles facing down. Do not use glass or clear plastic containers. **Always keep the puncture-proof container out of the reach of children.**
- Do not throw away used needles, syringes, or the puncture-proof container in household trash and do not recycle them.
- Check with your healthcare provider for instructions about the right way to throw away used needles and syringes. There may be local or state laws about how to throw away used needles and syringes. Always follow the instructions of your healthcare provider.

How should I store PegIntron?

- Before mixing, store PegIntron vials at room temperature, between 59°F to 86°F (15°C to 30°C).
- After mixing, use PegIntron right away or store it in the refrigerator for up to 24 hours between 36°F to 46°F (2°C to 8°C).
- Do not freeze PegIntron.
- Keep PegIntron away from heat.
- **Keep PegIntron and all medicines out of the reach of children.**

Manufactured by: Schering Corporation, a subsidiary of **Merck & Co., Inc.**, Whitehouse Station, NJ 08889, USA.

Rev February/2011

35038906T

Shown in Product Identification Guide, page 308

PNEUMOVAX® 23 ℞

(pneumococcal vaccine polyvalent)
Sterile, Liquid Vaccine for Intramuscular or Subcutaneous Injection

HIGHLIGHTS OF PRESCRIBING INFORMATION

These highlights do not include all the information needed to use PNEUMOVAX 23 safely and effectively. See full prescribing information for PNEUMOVAX 23.

PNEUMOVAX® 23 (pneumococcal vaccine polyvalent)
Sterile, Liquid Vaccine for Intramuscular or Subcutaneous Injection
Initial U.S. Approval: 1983

INDICATIONS AND USAGE

PNEUMOVAX 23 is a vaccine indicated for active immunization for the prevention of pneumococcal disease caused by the 23 serotypes contained in the vaccine (1, 2, 3, 4, 5, 6B, 7F, 8, 9N, 9V, 10A, 11A, 12F, 14, 15B, 17F, 18C, 19F, 19A, 20, 22F, 23F, and 33F).

PNEUMOVAX 23 is approved for use in persons 50 years of age or older and persons aged ≥2 years who are at increased risk for pneumococcal disease. (1.1, 14.1)

DOSAGE AND ADMINISTRATION

Single 0.5-mL dose of PNEUMOVAX 23 administered intramuscularly or subcutaneously only. (2.2)

DOSAGE FORMS AND STRENGTHS

Clear, sterile solution supplied in a (0.5-mL dose) single-dose vial and a multidose (5-dose) vial. (3)

CONTRAINDICATIONS

Severe allergic reaction (e.g., anaphylaxis) to any component of PNEUMOVAX 23. (4.1)

WARNINGS AND PRECAUTIONS

- Use caution and appropriate care for individuals with severely compromised cardiovascular and/or pulmonary function in whom a systemic reaction would pose a significant risk. (5.2)

ADVERSE REACTIONS

The most common adverse reactions, reported in >10% of subjects vaccinated with PNEUMOVAX 23 in clinical trials, were: injection-site pain/soreness/tenderness (60.0%), injection-site swelling/induration (20.3%), headache (17.6%), injection-site erythema (16.4%), asthenia and fatigue (13.2%), and myalgia (11.9%). (6.1)

To report SUSPECTED ADVERSE REACTIONS, contact Merck Sharp & Dohme Corp., a subsidiary of Merck & Co., Inc., at 1-877-888-4231 or VAERS at 1-800-822-7967 or www.vaers.hhs.gov.

DRUG INTERACTIONS

In a randomized clinical study, a reduced immune response to ZOSTAVAX® as measured by gpELISA was observed in individuals who received concurrent administration of PNEUMOVAX 23 and ZOSTAVAX compared with individuals who received these vaccines 4 weeks apart. Consider administration of the two vaccines separated by at least 4 weeks. (7.1, 14.3)

USE IN SPECIFIC POPULATIONS

Pregnancy: No human or animal data are available. Use only if clearly needed. (8.1)

Pediatrics: PNEUMOVAX 23 is not approved for use in children younger than 2 years of age because children in this age group do not develop an effective immune response to capsular types contained in the polysaccharide vaccine. (8.4)

Geriatrics: For subjects aged 65 years or older in a clinical study systemic adverse reactions, determined by the investigator to be vaccine-related, were higher following revaccination (33.1%) than following initial vaccination (21.7%). Routine revaccination of immunocompetent persons previously vaccinated with a 23-valent vaccine, is not recommended.[1] (8.5)

Immunocompromised Individuals: Response to vaccination may be diminished. (5.4, 8.6)

See 17 for PATIENT COUNSELING INFORMATION and FDA-approved patient labeling

Revised: 04/2013

FULL PRESCRIBING INFORMATION: CONTENTS*

*** Sections or subsections omitted from the full prescribing information are not listed**

FULL PRESCRIBING INFORMATION

1 INDICATIONS AND USAGE

1.1 Indications and Use

PNEUMOVAX® 23 is a vaccine indicated for active immunization for the prevention of pneumococcal disease caused by the 23 serotypes contained in the vaccine (1, 2, 3, 4, 5, 6B, 7F, 8, 9N, 9V, 10A, 11A, 12F, 14, 15B, 17F, 18C, 19F, 19A, 20, 22F, 23F, and 33F). PNEUMOVAX 23 is approved for use in persons 50 years of age or older and persons aged ≥2 years who are at increased risk for pneumococcal disease.

1.2 Limitations of Use

PNEUMOVAX 23 will not prevent disease caused by capsular types of pneumococcus other than those contained in the vaccine.

2 DOSAGE AND ADMINISTRATION

For intramuscular or subcutaneous injection using a sterile needle and syringe.

2.1 Preparation

- Parenteral drug products should be inspected visually for particulate matter and discoloration prior to administration. If either of these two conditions exists, the vaccine should not be administered.
- Use a separate sterile syringe and needle for each individual patient to prevent transmission of infectious agents from one person to another. Withdraw 0.5 mL from the vial using a sterile needle and syringe free of preservatives, antiseptics, and detergents.
- Do not mix PNEUMOVAX 23 with other vaccines in the same syringe or vial.

2.2 Administration

Administer a single 0.5-mL dose of PNEUMOVAX 23 intramuscularly or subcutaneously using a sterile needle and syringe into the deltoid muscle or lateral mid-thigh.

Do not inject intravascularly or intradermally.

2.3 Revaccination

The Advisory Committee on Immunization Practices (ACIP) has recommendations for revaccination against pneumococcal disease for persons at high risk who were previously vaccinated with PNEUMOVAX 23. Routine revaccination of immunocompetent persons previously vaccinated with a 23-valent vaccine, is not recommended.[1,2]

3 DOSAGE FORMS AND STRENGTHS

PNEUMOVAX 23 is a clear, sterile solution supplied in a (0.5-mL dose) single-dose vial and a 5-dose vial. *[See Description (11) and How Supplied/Storage and Handling (16).]*

4 CONTRAINDICATIONS

4.1 Hypersensitivity

Do not administer PNEUMOVAX 23 to individuals with a history of anaphylactic/anaphylactoid or severe allergic reaction to any component of the vaccine *[See Description (11)]*.

5 WARNINGS AND PRECAUTIONS

5.1 Persons with Moderate or Severe Acute Illness

Defer vaccination with PNEUMOVAX 23 in persons with moderate or severe acute illness.

5.2 Persons with Severely Compromised Cardiovascular or Pulmonary Function

Caution and appropriate care should be exercised in administering PNEUMOVAX 23 to individuals with severely compromised cardiovascular and/or pulmonary function in whom a systemic reaction would pose a significant risk.

5.3 Use of Antibiotic Prophylaxis

This vaccine does not replace the need for penicillin (or other antibiotic) prophylaxis against pneumococcal infection. In patients who require penicillin (or other antibiotic) prophylaxis against pneumococcal infection, such prophylaxis should not be discontinued after vaccination with PNEUMOVAX 23.

5.4 Persons with Altered Immunocompetence

Persons who are immunocompromised, including persons receiving immunosuppressive therapy, may have a diminished immune response to PNEUMOVAX 23. *[See Use in Specific Populations (8.6).]*

5.5 Persons with Chronic Cerebrospinal Fluid Leakage

PNEUMOVAX 23 may not be effective in preventing pneumococcal meningitis in patients who have chronic cerebrospinal fluid (CSF) leakage resulting from congenital lesions, skull fractures, or neurosurgical procedures.

6 ADVERSE REACTIONS

The most common adverse reactions, reported in >10% of subjects vaccinated with PNEUMOVAX 23 in clinical trials were: injection-site pain/soreness/tenderness (60.0%), injection-site swelling/induration (20.3%), headache (17.6%), injection-site erythema (16.4%), asthenia/fatigue (13.2%), and myalgia (11.9%). *[See Adverse Reactions (6.1).]*

6.1 Clinical Trials Experience

Because clinical trials are conducted under widely varying conditions, adverse reaction rates observed in the clinical trials of a vaccine cannot be directly compared to rates in the clinical trials of another vaccine and may not reflect the rates observed in practice.

In a randomized, double-blind, placebo-controlled crossover clinical trial, subjects were enrolled in four different cohorts defined by age (50-64 years of age and ≥65 years of age) and vaccination status (no pneumococcal vaccination or receipt of a pneumococcal polysaccharide vaccine 3-5 years prior to the study). Subjects in each cohort were randomized to receive intramuscular injections of PNEUMOVAX 23 followed by placebo (saline containing 0.25% phenol), or placebo followed by PNEUMOVAX 23, at 30-day (±7 days) intervals. The safety of an initial vaccination (first dose) was compared to revaccination (second dose) with PNEUMOVAX 23 for 14 days following each vaccination.

All 1008 subjects (average age, 67 years; 49% male and 51% female; 91% Caucasian, 4.7% African-American, 3.5% Hispanic, and 0.8% Other) received placebo injections.

Initial vaccination was evaluated in a total of 444 subjects (average age 65 years; 32% male and 68% female; 93% Caucasian, 3.2% African-American, 3.4% Hispanic, and 1.1% Other).

Revaccination was evaluated in 564 subjects (average age 69 years; 53% male and 47% female; 90% Caucasian, 3.5% Hispanic, 6.0% African-American, and 0.5% Other).

Serious Adverse Experiences

In this study, 10 subjects had serious adverse experiences within 14 days of vaccination: 6 who received PNEUMOVAX 23 and 4 who received placebo. Serious adverse experiences within 14 days after PNEUMOVAX 23 included angina pectoris, heart failure, chest pain, ulcerative colitis, depression, and headache/tremor/stiffness/sweating. Serious adverse experiences within 14 days after placebo included myocardial infarction complicated with heart failure, alcohol intoxication, angina pectoris, and edema/urinary retention/heart failure/diabetes.

Five subjects reported serious adverse experiences that occurred outside the 14-day follow-up window: 3 who received PNEUMOVAX 23 and 2 who received placebo. Serious adverse experiences after PNEUMOVAX 23 included cerebrovascular accident, lumbar radiculopathy, and pancreatitis/myocardial infarction resulting in death. Serious adverse experiences after placebo included heart failure and motor vehicle accident resulting in death.

Solicited and Unsolicited Reactions

Table 1 presents the adverse event rates for all solicited and unsolicited reactions reported in ≥1% in any group in this study, without regard to causality.

The most common local adverse reactions reported at the injection site after initial vaccination with PNEUMOVAX 23 were pain/tenderness/soreness (60.0%), swelling/induration (20.3%), and erythema (16.4%). The most common systemic adverse experiences were headache (17.6%), asthenia/fatigue (13.2%), and myalgia (11.9%).

The most common local adverse reactions reported at the injection site after revaccination with PNEUMOVAX 23 were pain/soreness/tenderness (77.2%), swelling (39.8%), and erythema (34.5%). The most common systemic adverse reactions with revaccination were headache (18.1%), asthenia/fatigue (17.9%), and myalgia (17.3%). All of these adverse reactions were reported at a rate lower than 10% after receiving a placebo injection.

[See table 1 at top of next page]

In this clinical study an increased rate of local reactions was observed with revaccination at 3-5 years following initial vaccination.

For subjects aged 65 years or older, injection-site adverse reaction rate was higher following revaccination (79.3%) than following initial vaccination (52.9%). The proportion of subjects reporting injection site discomfort that interfered with or prevented usual activity or injection site induration ≥4 inches was higher following revaccination (30.6%) than following initial vaccination (10.4%). Injection site reactions typically resolved by 5 days following vaccination.

For subjects aged 50-64 years, the injection-site adverse reaction rate for revaccinees and initial vaccinees was similar (79.6% and 72.8% respectively).

The rate of systemic adverse reactions was similar among both initial vaccinees and revaccinees within each age group. The rate of vaccine-related systemic adverse reactions was higher following revaccination (33.1%) than following initial vaccination (21.7%) in subjects 65 years of age or older, and was similar following revaccination (37.5%) and initial vaccination (35.5%) in subjects 50-64 years of age. The most common systemic adverse reactions reported after PNEUMOVAX 23 were as follows: asthenia/fatigue, myalgia and headache.

Regardless of age, the observed increase in post vaccination use of analgesics (≤13% in the revaccinees and ≤4% in the initial vaccinees) returned to baseline by day 5.

6.2 Post-Marketing Experience

The following list of adverse reactions includes those identified during post approval use of PNEUMOVAX 23. Because these reactions are reported voluntarily from a population of uncertain size, it is not always possible to reliably estimate their frequency or their causal relationship to product exposure.

General disorders and administration site conditions
- Cellulitis
- Malaise
- Fever (>102°F)
- Warmth at the injection site
- Decreased limb mobility
- Peripheral edema in the injected extremity

Digestive System
- Nausea
- Vomiting

Hematologic/Lymphatic
- Lymphadenitis
- Lymphadenopathy
- Thrombocytopenia in patients with stabilized idiopathic thrombocytopenic purpura[3]
- Hemolytic anemia in patients who have had other hematologic disorders
- Leukocytosis

Hypersensitivity reactions including
- Anaphylactoid reactions
- Serum Sickness
- Angioneurotic edema

Musculoskeletal System
- Arthralgia
- Arthritis

Nervous System
Paresthesia
Radiculoneuropathy
Guillain-Barré syndrome
Febrile convulsion
Skin
Rash
Urticaria
Cellulitis-like reactions
Erythema multiforme
Investigations
Increased serum C-reactive protein

7 DRUG INTERACTIONS

7.1 Concomitant Administration with Other Vaccines

In a randomized clinical study, a reduced immune response to ZOSTAVAX® as measured by gpELISA was observed in individuals who received concurrent administration of PNEUMOVAX 23 and ZOSTAVAX compared with individuals who received these vaccines 4 weeks apart. Consider administration of the two vaccines separated by at least 4 weeks. *[See Clinical Studies (14.3).]*

Limited safety and immunogenicity data from clinical trials are available on the concurrent administration of PNEUMOVAX 23 and vaccines other than ZOSTAVAX.

8 USE IN SPECIFIC POPULATIONS

8.1 Pregnancy

Pregnancy Category C: Animal reproduction studies have not been conducted with PNEUMOVAX 23. It is also not known whether PNEUMOVAX 23 can cause fetal harm when administered to a pregnant woman or can affect reproduction capacity. PNEUMOVAX 23 should be given to a pregnant woman only if clearly needed.

8.3 Nursing Mothers

It is not known whether this drug is excreted in human milk. Because many drugs are excreted in human milk, caution should be exercised when PNEUMOVAX 23 is administered to a nursing woman.

8.4 Pediatric Use

PNEUMOVAX 23 is not approved for use in children less than 2 years of age. Children in this age group do not develop an effective immune response to the capsular types contained in this polysaccharide vaccine.

The ACIP has recommendations for use of PNEUMOVAX 23 in children 2 years of age or older, who have previously received pneumococcal vaccines, and who are at increased risk for pneumococcal disease.[2]

8.5 Geriatric Use

In one clinical trial of PNEUMOVAX 23, conducted post-licensure, a total of 629 subjects who were aged ≥65 years and 201 subjects who were aged ≥75 years were enrolled.

In this trial, the safety of PNEUMOVAX 23 in adults 65 years of age and older (N=629) was compared to the safety of PNEUMOVAX 23 in adults 50 to 64 years of age (N=379). The subjects in this study had underlying chronic illness but were in stable condition; at least 1 medical condition at enrollment was reported by 86.3% of subjects who were 50 to 64 years old, and by 96.7% of subjects who were 65 to 91 years old. The rate of vaccine-related systemic adverse experiences was higher following revaccination (33.1%) than following primary vaccination (21.7%) in subjects ≥65 years of age, and was similar following revaccination (37.5%) and primary vaccination (35.5%) in subjects 50 to 64 years of age.

Since elderly individuals may not tolerate medical interventions as well as younger individuals, a higher frequency and/or a greater severity of reactions in some older individuals cannot be ruled out.

Post-marketing reports have been received in which some elderly individuals had severe adverse experiences and a complicated clinical course following vaccination. Some individuals with underlying medical conditions of varying severity experienced local reactions and fever associated with clinical deterioration requiring hospital care.

8.6 Immunocompromised Individuals

Persons who are immunocompromised, including persons receiving immunosuppressive therapy, may have a diminished immune response to PNEUMOVAX 23.

11 DESCRIPTION

PNEUMOVAX 23 (Pneumococcal Vaccine Polyvalent) is a sterile, liquid vaccine consisting of a mixture of purified capsular polysaccharides from *Streptococcus pneumoniae* types (1, 2, 3, 4, 5, 6B, 7F, 8, 9N, 9V, 10A, 11A, 12F, 14, 15B, 17F, 18C, 19F, 19A, 20, 22F, 23F, and 33F).

PNEUMOVAX 23 is a clear, colorless solution. Each 0.5-mL dose of vaccine contains 25 micrograms of each polysaccharide type in isotonic saline solution containing 0.25% phenol as a preservative. The vaccine is used directly as supplied. No dilution or reconstitution is necessary.

12 CLINICAL PHARMACOLOGY

12.1 Mechanism of Action

PNEUMOVAX 23 induces type-specific antibodies that enhance opsonization, phagocytosis, and killing of pneumococci by leukocytes and other phagocytic cells. The levels of antibodies that correlate with protection against pneumococcal disease have not been clearly defined.

Table 1: Incidence of Injection-Site and Systemic Complaints in Adults ≥50 Years of Age Receiving Their First (Initial) or Second (Revaccination) Dose of PNEUMOVAX 23 (Pneumococcal Polysaccharide Vaccine, 23 Valent) or Placebo Occurring at ≥1% in Any Group

	PNEUMOVAX 23 Initial Vaccination N=444	PNEUMOVAX 23 Revaccination* N=564	Placebo Injection† N=1008
Number Followed for Safety	438	548	984‡
	AE Rate	AE Rate	AE Rate
Injection-Site Complaints			
Solicited Events			
Pain/Soreness/Tenderness	60.0%	77.2%	7.7%
Swelling/Induration	20.3%	39.8%	2.8%
Erythema	16.4%	34.5%	3.3%
Unsolicited Events			
Ecchymosis	0%	1.1%	0.3%
Pruritus	0.2%	1.6%	0.0%
Systemic Complaints			
Solicited Events			
Asthenia/Fatigue	13.2%	17.9%	6.7%
Chills	2.7%	7.8%	1.8%
Myalgia	11.9%	17.3%	3.3%
Headache	17.6%	18.1%	8.9%
Unsolicited Events			
Fever§	1.4%	2.0%	0.7%
Diarrhea	1.1%	0.7%	0.5%
Dyspepsia	1.1%	1.1%	0.9%
Nausea	1.8%	1.8%	0.9%
Back Pain	0.9%	0.9%	1.0%
Neck Pain	0.7%	1.5%	0.2%
Upper Respiratory Infection	1.8%	2.6%	1.8%
Pharyngitis	1.1%	0.4%	1.3%

* Subjects receiving their second dose of pneumococcal polysaccharide vaccine as PNEUMOVAX 23 approximately 3-5 years after their first dose.
† Subjects receiving placebo injection from this study combined over periods.
‡ The number of subjects receiving placebo followed for injection-site complaints. The corresponding number of subjects followed for systemic complaints was 981.
§ Fever events include subjects who felt feverish in addition to subjects with elevated temperature.

14 CLINICAL STUDIES

14.1 Effectiveness

The protective efficacy of pneumococcal vaccines containing six (types 1, 2, 4, 8, 12F, and 25) or twelve (types 1, 2, 3, 4, 6A, 8, 9N, 12F, 25, 7F, 18C, and 46) capsular polysaccharides was investigated in two controlled studies in South Africa in male novice gold miners ranging in age from 16 to 58 years, in whom there was a high attack rate for pneumococcal pneumonia and bacteremia.[4] In both studies, participants in the control groups received either meningococcal polysaccharide serogroup A vaccine or saline placebo. In both studies, attack rates for vaccine type pneumococcal pneumonia were observed for the period from 2 weeks through about 1 year after vaccination. Protective efficacy was 76% and 92%, respectively, for the 6- and 12-valent vaccines, for the capsular types represented.

Three similar studies in South African young adult male novice gold miners were carried out by Dr. R. Austrian and associates[5] using similar pneumococcal vaccines prepared for the National Institute of Allergy and Infectious Diseases, with pneumococcal vaccines containing a 6-valent formulation (types 1, 3, 4, 7, 8, and 12) or a 13-valent formulation (types 1, 2, 3, 4, 6, 7, 8, 9, 12, 14, 18, 19, and 25) capsular polysaccharides. The reduction in pneumococcal pneumonia caused by the capsular types contained in the vaccines was 79%. Reduction in type-specific pneumococcal bacteremia was 82%.

A prospective study in France found a pneumococcal vaccine containing fourteen (types 1, 2, 3, 4, 6A, 7F, 8, 9N, 12F, 14, 18C, 19F, 23F, and 25) capsular polysaccharides to be 77% (95%CI: 51% to 89%) effective in reducing the incidence of pneumonia among male and female nursing home residents with a mean age of 74 (standard deviation of 4 years).[6]

In a study using a pneumococcal vaccine containing eight (types 1, 3, 6, 7, 14, 18, 19, and 23) capsular polysaccharides, vaccinated children and young adults aged 2 to 25 years who had sickle cell disease, congenital asplenia, or undergone a splenectomy experienced significantly less bacteremic pneumococcal disease than patients who were not vaccinated.[7]

In the United States, one post-licensure randomized controlled trial, in the elderly or patients with chronic medical conditions who received a 14-valent pneumococcal polysaccharide vaccine (types 1, 2, 3, 4, 6A, 8, 9N, 12F, 14, 19F, 23F, 25, 7F, and 18C), did not support the efficacy of the vaccine for nonbacteremic pneumonia.[8]

A retrospective cohort analysis study based on the U.S. Centers for Disease Control and Prevention (CDC) pneumococcal surveillance system, showed 57% (95%CI: 45% to 66%) overall protective effectiveness against invasive infections caused by serotypes included in PNEUMOVAX 23 in persons ≥6 years of age, 65 to 84% effectiveness among specific patient groups (e.g., persons with diabetes mellitus, coronary vascular disease, congestive heart failure, chronic pulmonary disease, and anatomic asplenia) and 75% (95%CI: 57% to 85%) effectiveness in immunocompetent persons aged ≥65 years of age. Vaccine effectiveness could not be confirmed for certain groups of immunocompromised patients.[9]

14.2 Immunogenicity

The levels of antibodies that correlate with protection against pneumococcal disease have not been clearly defined. Antibody responses to most pneumococcal capsular types are generally low or inconsistent in children less than 2 years of age.

14.3 Concomitant Administration with Other Vaccines

In a double-blind, controlled clinical trial, 473 adults, 60 years of age or older, were randomized to receive ZOSTAVAX and PNEUMOVAX 23 concomitantly (N=237), or PNEUMOVAX 23 alone followed 4 weeks later by ZOSTAVAX alone (N=236). At four weeks postvaccination, the varicella-zoster virus (VZV) antibody levels following concomitant use were significantly lower than the VZV antibody levels following nonconcomitant administration (GMTs of 338 vs. 484 gp ELISA units/mL, respectively; GMT ratio = 0.70 (95% CI: [0.61, 0.80]).

Limited safety and immunogenicity data from clinical trials are available on the concurrent administration of PNEUMOVAX 23 and vaccines other than ZOSTAVAX.

15 REFERENCES

1. Centers for Disease Control and Prevention. Prevention of Pneumococcal Disease. Recommendations of the Advisory Committee on Immunization Practices (ACIP). MMWR. *46*(No. RR-8): 1-25, 1997. Available from: http://www.cdc.gov/mmwr/PDF/rr/rr4608.pdf
2. Centers for Disease Control and Prevention. Prevention of Pneumococcal Disease Among Infants and Children --- Use of 13-Valent Pneumococcal Conjugate Vaccine and 23-Valent Pneumococcal Polysaccharide Vaccine, MMWR *59*(RR11): 1-18, 2010. http://www.cdc.gov/mmwr/preview/mmwrhtml/rr5911a1.htm?s_cid=rr5911a1_e
3. Kelton, J.G.: Vaccination-associated relapse of immune thrombocytopenia, JAMA. *245*(4): 369-371, 1981.
4. Smit, P.; Oberholzer, D.; Hayden-Smith, S.; Koornhof, H.J.; Hilleman, M.R.: Protective efficacy of pneumococcal polysaccharide vaccines, JAMA. *238:* 2613-2616, 1977.
5. Austrian, R.; Douglas, R.M.; Schiffman, G.; Coetzee, A.M.; Koornhof, H.J.; Hayden-Smith, S.; Reid, R.D.W.: Prevention of pneumococcal pneumonia by vaccination, Trans. Assoc. Am. Physicians. *89:* 184-194, 1976.
6. Gaillat, J.; Zmirou, D.; Mallaret, M.R.: Essai clinique du vaccin antipneumococcique chez des personnes agees vivant en institution, Rev. Epidemiol. Sante Publique. *33:* 437-44, 1985.
7. Ammann, A.J.; Addiego, J.; Wara, D.W.; Lubin, B.; Smith, W.B.; Mentzer, W.C.: Polyvalent pneumococcal-polysaccharide immunization of patients with sickle-cell anemia and patients with splenectomy, N. Engl. J. Med. *297:* 897-900, 1977.
8. Simberkoff, M.S.; Cross, A.P.; Al-Ibrahim, M.: Efficacy of pneumococcal vaccine in high risk patients: results of a Veterans Administration cooperative study, N. Engl. J. Med. *315:* 1318-27, 1986.
9. Butler, J.C.; Breiman, R.F.; Campbell, J.F.; Lipman, H.B.; Broome, C.V.; Facklam, R.R.: Pneumococcal polysaccharide vaccine efficacy. An evaluation of current recommendations, JAMA. *270:* 1826-31, 1993.
10. Vaccine Adverse Event Reporting System - United States, MMWR. *39*(41): 730-33, October 19, 1990.

16 HOW SUPPLIED/STORAGE AND HANDLING

PNEUMOVAX 23 is supplied as follows:

NDC 0006-4739-00 — one 5-dose vial, color coded with a purple cap and stripe on the vial labels and cartons.

NDC 0006-4943-00 — a box of 10 single-dose vials, color coded with a purple cap and stripe on the vial labels and cartons.

16.1 Storage and Handling

- Store unopened and opened vials at 2-8°C (36-46°F).
- All vaccine must be discarded after the expiration date.

17 PATIENT COUNSELING INFORMATION

See FDA-Approved Patient Labeling (Patient Information).

- Inform the patient, parent or guardian of the benefits and risks associated with vaccination.
- Tell the patient, parent or guardian that vaccination with PNEUMOVAX 23 may not offer 100% protection from pneumococcal infection.
- Provide the patient, parent or guardian with the vaccine information statements required by the National Childhood Vaccine Injury Act of 1986, with each immunization.
- Instruct the patient, parent or guardian to report any serious adverse reactions to their health care provider who in turn should report such events to the vaccine manufacturer or the U.S. Department of Health and Human Services through the Vaccine Adverse Event Reporting System (VAERS), 1-800-822-7967, or report online at www.vaers.hhs.gov.[10]

Manuf. and Dist. by: Merck Sharp & Dohme Corp., a subsidiary of

MERCK & CO., INC., Whitehouse Station, NJ 08889, USA

Revised: 03/2013

Printed in USA

USPI-I-V1101303R038

Patient Information about

PNEUMOVAX® 23 (pronounced "noo-mo-vax 23")

Generic Name: pneumococcal vaccine polyvalent

Read this leaflet before you or your child gets the vaccine called PNEUMOVAX 23. If you have any questions about the vaccine after you read this, you should ask your health care provider. This is a summary only. It does not take the place of talking to your doctor, nurse or other health care provider about the vaccine. Only your health care provider can decide if PNEUMOVAX 23 is right for you or your child.

What is PNEUMOVAX 23?

PNEUMOVAX 23 is a vaccine that is given as a shot. It helps protect you from infection by certain germs or bacteria which are called pneumococcus (pronounced "noo-mo-ca-cus"). PNEUMOVAX 23 is for people 50 years of age and older. It is also for people who are 2 years of age and older if they have certain medical conditions that put them at increased risk for infection.

Illnesses or health problems may allow these germs to spread into the blood, lungs, or brain where they can cause serious diseases such as:

- An infection in the blood
- A lung infection (pneumonia) that can also come with an infection in the blood
- An infection of the coverings of the brain and spinal cord (meningitis).

PNEUMOVAX 23 may not protect everyone who gets it. It will not protect against diseases that are caused by bacteria types that are not in the vaccine.

Who should not get PNEUMOVAX 23?

You should not get this vaccine if you (or your child):

- are allergic to any of its ingredients
- had an allergic reaction to PNEUMOVAX 23 in the past
- are less than 2 years old.

What should I tell my health care provider before getting PNEUMOVAX 23?

Tell your health care provider if you (or your child):

- are allergic to PNEUMOVAX 23
- have heart or lung problems
- have a fever
- have immune problems or are receiving radiation treatment for chemotherapy
- are pregnant or breast-feeding

How is PNEUMOVAX 23 given?

Most often, just one shot is given.

If you or your child is in a high-risk group for pneumococcal infection, then your health care provider will decide if it would be helpful to give a second shot of PNEUMOVAX 23 at a later time.

Can PNEUMOVAX 23 be given with other vaccines?

Talk to your health care provider if you plan to get ZOSTAVAX at the same time as PNEUMOVAX 23 because it may be better to get these vaccines at least 4 weeks apart. Talk to your health care provider if you plan to get PNEUMOVAX 23 at the same time as other vaccines.

What are the possible side effects of PNEUMOVAX 23?

The most common side effects are:

- pain, warmth, soreness, redness, swelling, and hardening at the injection site
- headache
- weakness, feeling tired
- muscle pain

Tell your health care provider or get emergency help right away if you get any of the following problems after vaccination because these may be signs of an allergic reaction or other serious conditions:

- difficulty breathing
- wheezing
- rash
- hives

Side effects at the site where you get the shot may be more common and may feel worse after a second shot than after the first shot.

Tell your health care provider if you or your child has a side effect that bothers you or that does not go away.

For a more complete list of side effects, ask your health care provider.

You may also report any side effect to your or your child's health care provider, or directly to the Vaccine Adverse Event Reporting System (VAERS). You may call the VAERS number 1-800-822-7967 at no charge, or report online to www.vaers.hhs.gov.

What are the ingredients of PNEUMOVAX 23?

Active Ingredients:	Bacterial sugars from 23 pneumococcal types: 1, 2, 3, 4, 5, 6B, 7F, 8, 9N, 9V, 10A, 11A, 12F, 14, 15B, 17F, 18C, 19F, 19A, 20, 22F, 23F, and 33F
Inactive Ingredients:	Phenol (a preservative)

What else should I know about PNEUMOVAX 23?

Some adults and children have problems with leakage of spinal fluid after the skull is cracked or injured or after medical operations and this may increase their risk for pneumococcal infection. PNEUMOVAX 23 may not be able to prevent all of these infections.

This leaflet is a summary of information about PNEUMOVAX 23. If you would like more information, talk to your health care provider. You can also call the Merck National Service Center at 1-800-622-4477.

Manuf. and Dist. by: Merck Sharp & Dohme Corp., a subsidiary of

MERCK & CO., INC., Whitehouse Station, NJ 08889, USA

Revised: 03/2013

USPPI-I-V1101303R038

Printed in USA

Rx Only

PREGNYL® ℞

(chorionic gonadotropin for injection, USP)

DESCRIPTION

Human chorionic gonadotropin (HCG), a polypeptide hormone produced by the human placenta, is composed of an alpha and a beta subunit. The alpha sub-unit is essentially identical to the alpha subunits of the human pituitary gonadotropins, luteinizing hormone (LH) and follicle-stimulating hormone (FSH), as well as to the alpha subunit of human thyroid-stimulating hormone (TSH). The beta subunits of these hormones differ in amino acid sequence.

PREGNYL® (chorionic gonadotropin for injection USP) is a highly purified pyrogen-free preparation obtained from the urine of pregnant females. It is standardized by a biological assay procedure. It is available for intramuscular injection in multiple dose vials containing 10,000 USP units of sterile dried powder with 5 mg monobasic sodium phosphate and 4.4 mg dibasic sodium phosphate. If required, pH is adjusted with sodium hydroxide and/or phosphoric acid. Each package also contains a 10-mL vial of solvent containing: water for injection with 0.56% sodium chloride and 0.9% BENZYL ALCOHOL, WHICH IS NOT FOR USE IN NEWBORNS. If required, pH is adjusted with sodium hydroxide and/or hydrochloric acid.

CLINICAL PHARMACOLOGY

The action of HCG is virtually identical to that of pituitary LH, although HCG appears to have a small degree of FSH activity as well. It stimulates production of gonadal steroid hormones by stimulating the interstitial cells (Leydig cells) of the testis to produce androgens and the corpus luteum of the ovary to produce progesterone.

Androgen stimulation in the male leads to the development of secondary sex characteristics and may stimulate testicular descent when no anatomical impediment to descent is present. This descent is usually reversible when HCG is discontinued.

During the normal menstrual cycle, LH participates with FSH in the development and maturation of the normal ovarian follicle, and the mid-cycle LH surge triggers ovulation. HCG can substitute for LH in this function. During a normal pregnancy, HCG secreted by the placenta maintains the corpus luteum after LH secretion decreases, supporting continued secretion of estrogen and progesterone and preventing menstruation. HCG HAS NO KNOWN EFFECT ON FAT MOBILIZATION, APPETITE OR SENSE OF HUNGER, OR BODY FAT DISTRIBUTION.

INDICATIONS AND USAGE

HCG HAS NOT BEEN DEMONSTRATED TO BE EFFECTIVE ADJUNCTIVE THERAPY IN THE TREATMENT OF OBESITY. THERE IS NO SUBSTANTIAL EVIDENCE THAT IT INCREASES WEIGHT LOSS BEYOND THAT RESULTING FROM CALORIC RESTRICTION, THAT IT CAUSES A MORE ATTRACTIVE OR "NORMAL" DISTRIBUTION OF FAT, OR THAT IT DECREASES THE HUNGER AND DISCOMFORT ASSOCIATED WITH CALORIE-RESTRICTED DIETS.

1. Prepubertal cryptorchidism not due to anatomical obstruction. In general, HCG is thought to induce testicular descent in situations when descent would have occurred

at puberty. HCG thus may help predict whether or not orchiopexy will be needed in the future. Although, in some cases, descent following HCG administration is permanent, in most cases, the response is temporary. Therapy is usually instituted in children between the ages of 4 and 9.
2. Selected cases of hypogonadotropic hypogonadism (hypogonadism secondary to a pituitary deficiency) in males.
3. Induction of ovulation and pregnancy in the anovulatory, infertile woman in whom the cause of anovulation is secondary and not due to primary ovarian failure, and who has been appropriately pretreated with human menotropins.

CONTRAINDICATIONS

Precocious puberty, prostatic carcinoma or other androgen-dependent neoplasm, prior allergic reaction to HCG.

WARNINGS

HCG should be used in conjunction with human menopausal gonadotropins only by physicians experienced with infertility problems who are familiar with the criteria for patient selection, contraindications, warnings, precautions, and adverse reactions described in the package insert for menotropins.
Anaphylaxis has been reported with urinary-derived HCG products.
The principal serious adverse reactions during this use are: (1) ovarian hyperstimulation, a syndrome of sudden ovarian enlargement, ascites with or without pain, and/or pleural effusion, (2) rupture of ovarian cysts with resultant hemoperitoneum, (3) multiple births, and (4) arterial thromboembolism.

PRECAUTIONS

General
Since androgens may cause fluid retention, HCG should be used with caution in patients with cardiac or renal disease, epilepsy, migraine, or asthma.
Pediatric Use
Induction of androgen secretion by HCG may induce precocious puberty in pediatric patients treated for cryptorchidism. Therapy should be discontinued if signs of precocious puberty occur.
Geriatric Use
Clinical studies of PREGNYL® (chorionic gonadotropin for injection USP) did not include subjects aged 65 and over.

ADVERSE REACTIONS

Headache, irritability, restlessness, depression, fatigue, edema, precocious puberty, gynecomastia, pain at the site of injection.
Hypersensitivity reactions, both localized and systemic in nature, have been reported.

DOSAGE AND ADMINISTRATION

For intramuscular use only. The dosage regimen employed in any particular case will depend upon the indication for the use, the age and weight of the patient, and the physician's preference. The following regimens have been advocated by various authorities:
Prepubertal cryptorchidism not due to anatomical obstruction. Therapy is usually instituted in children between the ages of 4 and 9.
1. 4000 USP units 3 times weekly for 3 weeks.
2. 5000 USP units every second day for 4 injections.
3. 15 injections for 500 to 1000 USP units over a period of 6 weeks.
4. 500 USP units 3 times weekly for 4 to 6 weeks. If this course of treatment is not successful, another series is begun 1 month later, giving 1000 USP units per injection.

Selected cases of hypogonadotropic hypogonadism in males.
1. 500 to 1000 USP units 3 times a week for 3 weeks, followed by the same dose twice a week for 3 weeks.
2. 4000 USP units 3 times weekly for 6 to 9 months, following which the dosage may be reduced to 2000 USP units 3 times weekly for an additional 3 months.

Induction of ovulation and pregnancy in the anovulatory, infertile woman in whom the cause of anovulation is secondary and not due to primary ovarian failure and who has been appropriately pretreated with human menotropins.
(See prescribing information for menotropins for dosage and administration for that drug product.)
5000 to 10,000 USP units 1 day following the last dose of menotropins. (A dosage of 10,000 USP units is recommended in the labeling for menotropins.)
Directions for Reconstitution
Two-vial package: Withdraw sterile air from lyophilized vial and inject into diluent vial. Remove 1–10 mL from diluent and add to lyophilized vial; agitate gently until powder is completely dissolved in solution.
Parenteral drug products should be inspected visually for particulate matter and discoloration prior to administration, whenever solution and container permit.

IMPORTANT: USE COMPLETELY AFTER RECONSTITUTION. RECONSTITUTED SOLUTION IS STABLE FOR 60 DAYS WHEN REFRIGERATED.

HOW SUPPLIED

Two-vial package containing:
1-10 mL lyophilized multiple dose vial containing: 10,000 USP units chorionic gonadotropin per vial, NDC 0052-0315-10.
1 10 mL vial of solvent containing: water for injection with sodium chloride 0.56% and benzyl alcohol 0.9%, NDC 0052-0325-10.
When reconstituted, each 10 mL vial contains:

Chorionic gonadotropin	10,000 USP Units
Monobasic sodium phosphate	5 mg
Dibasic sodium phosphate	4.4 mg
Sodium chloride	0.56%
Benzyl alcohol	0.9%

If required pH adjusted with sodium hydroxide and/or phosphoric acid.
Storage
Store at controlled room temperature 15–30°C (59–86°F). Reconstituted solution is stable for 60 days when refrigerated.
Rx only
Manufactured for: Merck Sharp & Dohme Corp., a subsidiary of **MERCK & CO., INC.**, Whitehouse Station, NJ 08889, USA
Manufactured by: Baxter Pharmaceutical Solutions LLC, Bloomington, IN 47403, USA

Revised: 08/2012
900829-HCG-PWi-USPI.5

PRIMAXIN® I.V. ℞
(IMIPENEM AND CILASTATIN FOR INJECTION)

To reduce the development of drug-resistant bacteria and maintain the effectiveness of PRIMAXIN® I.V. and other antibacterial drugs, PRIMAXIN I.V. should be used only to treat or prevent infections that are proven or strongly suspected to be caused by bacteria.
For Intravenous Injection Only

DESCRIPTION

PRIMAXIN I.V. (Imipenem and Cilastatin for Injection) is a sterile formulation of imipenem (a thienamycin antibiotic) and cilastatin sodium (the inhibitor of the renal dipeptidase, dehydropeptidase I), with sodium bicarbonate added as a buffer. PRIMAXIN I.V. is a potent broad spectrum antibacterial agent for intravenous administration.
Imipenem (N-formimidoylthienamycin monohydrate) is a crystalline derivative of thienamycin, which is produced by *Streptomyces cattleya*. Its chemical name is (5*R*,6*S*)-3-[[2-(formimidoylamino)ethyl]thio]-6-[(*R*)-1-hydroxyethyl]-7-oxo-1-azabicyclo[3.2.0]hept-2-ene-2-carboxylic acid monohydrate. It is an off-white, nonhygroscopic crystalline compound with a molecular weight of 317.37. It is sparingly soluble in water and slightly soluble in methanol. Its empirical formula is $C_{12}H_{17}N_3O_4S \cdot H_2O$, and its structural formula is:

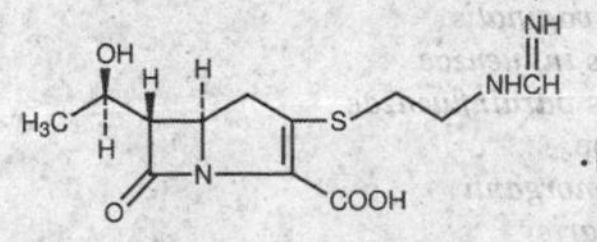

Cilastatin sodium is the sodium salt of a derivatized heptenoic acid. Its chemical name is sodium (*Z*)-7-[[(*R*)-2-amino-2-carboxyethyl]thio]-2-[(*S*)-2,2-dimethylcyclopropanecarboxamido]-2-heptenoate. It is an off-white to yellowish-white, hygroscopic, amorphous compound with a molecular weight of 380.43. It is very soluble in water and in methanol. Its empirical formula is $C_{16}H_{25}N_2O_5SNa$, and its structural formula is:

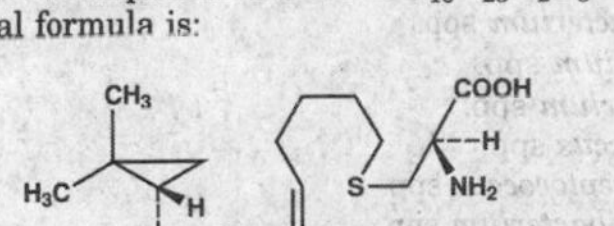

PRIMAXIN I.V. is buffered to provide solutions in the pH range of 6.5 to 8.5. There is no significant change in pH when solutions are prepared and used as directed. (See COMPATIBILITY AND STABILITY.) PRIMAXIN I.V. 250 contains 18.8 mg of sodium (0.8 mEq) and PRIMAXIN I.V. 500 contains 37.5 mg of sodium (1.6 mEq). Solutions of PRIMAXIN I.V. range from colorless to yellow. Variations of color within this range do not affect the potency of the product.

CLINICAL PHARMACOLOGY

Adults
Intravenous Administration
Intravenous infusion of PRIMAXIN I.V. over 20 minutes results in peak plasma levels of imipenem antimicrobial activity that range from 14 to 24 μg/mL for the 250 mg dose, from 21 to 58 μg/mL for the 500 mg dose, and from 41 to 83 μg/mL for the 1000 mg dose. At these doses, plasma levels of imipenem antimicrobial activity decline to below 1 μg/mL or less in 4 to 6 hours. Peak plasma levels of cilastatin following a 20-minute intravenous infusion of PRIMAXIN I.V. range from 15 to 25 μg/mL for the 250 mg dose, from 31 to 49 μg/mL for the 500 mg dose, and from 56 to 88 μg/mL for the 1000 mg dose.
The plasma half-life of each component is approximately 1 hour. The binding of imipenem to human serum proteins is approximately 20% and that of cilastatin is approximately 40%. Approximately 70% of the administered imipenem is recovered in the urine within 10 hours after which no further urinary excretion is detectable. Urine concentrations of imipenem in excess of 10 μg/mL can be maintained for up to 8 hours with PRIMAXIN I.V. at the 500-mg dose. Approximately 70% of the cilastatin sodium dose is recovered in the urine within 10 hours of administration of PRIMAXIN I.V. No accumulation of imipenem/cilastatin in plasma or urine is observed with regimens administered as frequently as every 6 hours in patients with normal renal function.
In healthy elderly volunteers (65 to 75 years of age with normal renal function for their age), the pharmacokinetics of a single dose of imipenem 500 mg and cilastatin 500 mg administered intravenously over 20 minutes are consistent with those expected in subjects with slight renal impairment for which no dosage alteration is considered necessary. The mean plasma half-lives of imipenem and cilastatin are 91 ± 7.0 minutes and 69 ± 15 minutes, respectively. Multiple dosing has no effect on the pharmacokinetics of either imipenem or cilastatin, and no accumulation of imipenem/cilastatin is observed.
Imipenem, when administered alone, is metabolized in the kidneys by dehydropeptidase I resulting in relatively low levels in urine. Cilastatin sodium, an inhibitor of this enzyme, effectively prevents renal metabolism of imipenem so that when imipenem and cilastatin sodium are given concomitantly, fully adequate antibacterial levels of imipenem are achieved in the urine.
After a 1 gram dose of PRIMAXIN I.V., the following average levels of imipenem were measured (usually at 1 hour post dose except where indicated) in the tissues and fluids listed:

Tissue or Fluid	N	Imipenem Level μg/mL or μg/g	Range
Vitreous Humor	3	3.4 (3.5 hours post dose)	2.88–3.6
Aqueous Humor	5	2.99 (2 hours post dose)	2.4–3.9
Lung Tissue	8	5.6 (median)	3.5–15.5
Sputum	1	2.1	—
Pleural	1	22.0	—
Peritoneal	12	23.9 S.D.±5.3 (2 hours post dose)	—
Bile	2	5.3 (2.25 hours post dose)	4.6–6.0
CSF (uninflamed)	5	1.0 (4 hours post dose)	0.26–2.0
CSF (inflamed)	7	2.6 (2 hours post dose)	0.5–5.5
Fallopian Tubes	1	13.6	—
Endometrium	1	11.1	—
Myometrium	1	5.0	—
Bone	10	2.6	0.4–5.4
Interstitial Fluid	12	16.4	10.0–22.6
Skin	12	4.4	NA
Fascia	12	4.4	NA

Imipenem-cilastatin sodium is hemodialyzable. However, usefulness of this procedure in the overdosage setting is questionable. (See OVERDOSAGE.)
Microbiology
The bactericidal activity of imipenem results from the inhibition of cell wall synthesis. Its greatest affinity is for penicillin binding proteins (PBPs) 1A, 1B, 2, 4, 5 and 6 of *Escherichia coli*, and 1A, 1B, 2, 4 and 5 of *Pseudomonas aeruginosa*. The lethal effect is related to binding to PBP 2 and PBP 1B.
Imipenem has a high degree of stability in the presence of beta-lactamases, both penicillinases and cephalosporinases produced by gram-negative and gram-positive bacteria. It is a potent inhibitor of beta-lactamases from certain gram-

Table 1: Susceptibility Interpretive Criteria for Imipenem

Pathogen	Minimum Inhibitory Concentrations MIC (μg/mL)			Disk Diffusion Zone Diameter (mm)		
	S	I	R	S	I	R
Enterobacteriaceae	≤1.0	2.0	≥4.0	≥23	20-22	≤19
Pseudomonas aeruginosa	≤2	4	≥8	≥19	16-18	≤15
Acinetobacter spp.	≤4	8	≥16	≥16	14-15	≤13
Staphylococcus spp.*	≤4	8	≥16	≥16	14-15	≤13
Haemophilus influenzae and *H. parainfluenzae*†	≤4	-	-	≥16	-	-
Streptococcus pneumoniae‡	≤0.12	0.25-0.5	≥1	-	-	-
Anaerobes	≤4.0	8.0	≥16.0	-	-	-

* For oxacillin-susceptible *S. aureus* and coagulase negative staphylococci results for carbapenems, including imipenem, if tested, should be reported according to the results generated using routine interpretive criteria. For oxacillin-resistant *S. aureus* and coagulase negative staphylococci, other beta lactam agents, including carbapenems, may appear active *in vitro* but are not effective clinically. Results for beta lactam agents other than cephalosporins with anti-MRSA activity should be reported as resistant or should not be reported.
† For some organism/antimicrobial combinations, the absence or rare occurrence of resistant strains precludes defining any results categories other than "susceptible". For strains yielding results suggestive of a "non-susceptible" category, organism identification and antimicrobial susceptibility test results should be confirmed.
‡ For non-meningitis *S. pneumoniae* isolates, penicillin MICs ≤0.06 μg/mL (or oxacillin zones ≥20 mm) indicate susceptibility to imipenem.

Table 2: Acceptable Quality Control Ranges for Imipenem

Microorganism	Minimum Inhibitory Concentrations MIC Range (μg/mL)	Disk Diffusion Zone Diameter (mm)
Pseudomonas aeruginosa ATCC 27853	1-4	20-28
Escherichia coli ATCC 25922	0.06-0.25	26-32
Haemophilus influenzae ATCC 49247	-	21-29
Haemophilus influenzae ATCC 49766	0.25-1.0	-
Staphylococcus aureus ATCC 29213	0.015-0.06	-
Enterococcus faecalis ATCC 29212	0.5-2.0	-
Streptococcus pneumoniae ATCC 49619	0.03-0.12	-
Bacteroides fragilis ATCC 25285	0.03-0.25* 0.03-0.125†	-
Bacteroides thetaiotaomicron ATCC 29741	0.25-1.0* 0.125-0.5†	-
Eubacterium lentum ATCC 43055	0.25-2.0* 0.125-0.5†	-

* Quality control ranges for broth microdilution testing
† Quality control ranges for agar dilution testing

negative bacteria which are inherently resistant to most beta-lactam antibiotics, e.g., *Pseudomonas aeruginosa*, *Serratia* spp., and *Enterobacter* spp.

Imipenem has *in vitro* activity against a wide range of gram-positive and gram-negative organisms. Imipenem has been shown to be active against most strains of the following microorganisms, both *in vitro* and in clinical infections treated with the intravenous formulation of imipenem-cilastatin sodium as described in the INDICATIONS AND USAGE section.

Gram-positive aerobes:
Enterococcus faecalis (formerly *S. faecalis*)
(NOTE: Imipenem is inactive *in vitro* against *Enterococcus faecium* [formerly *S. faecium*].)
Staphylococcus aureus including penicillinase-producing strains
Staphylococcus epidermidis including penicillinase-producing strains
(NOTE: Methicillin-resistant staphylococci should be reported as resistant to imipenem.)
Streptococcus agalactiae (Group B streptococci)
Streptococcus pneumoniae
Streptococcus pyogenes
Gram-negative aerobes:
Acinetobacter spp.
Citrobacter spp.
Enterobacter spp.
Escherichia coli
Gardnerella vaginalis
Haemophilus influenzae
Haemophilus parainfluenzae
Klebsiella spp.
Morganella morganii
Proteus vulgaris
Providencia rettgeri
Pseudomonas aeruginosa
(NOTE: Imipenem is inactive *in vitro* against *Stenotrophomonas* [formerly *Xanthomonas*, formerly *Pseudomonas*] *maltophilia* and some strains of *Burkholderia cepacia*.)
Serratia spp., including *S. marcescens*
Gram-positive anaerobes:
Bifidobacterium spp.
Clostridium spp.
Eubacterium spp.
Peptococcus spp.
Peptostreptococcus spp.
Propionibacterium spp.
Gram-negative anaerobes:
Bacteroides spp., including *B. fragilis*
Fusobacterium spp.

The following *in vitro* data are available, **but their clinical significance is unknown**.

Imipenem exhibits *in vitro* minimum inhibitory concentrations (MICs) of 4 μg/mL or less against most (≥90%) strains of the following microorganisms; however, the safety and effectiveness of imipenem in treating clinical infections due to these microorganisms have not been established in adequate and well-controlled clinical trials.

Gram-positive aerobes:
Bacillus spp.
Listeria monocytogenes
Nocardia spp.
Staphylococcus saprophyticus
Group C streptococci
Group G streptococci
Viridans group streptococci
Gram-negative aerobes:
Aeromonas hydrophila
Alcaligenes spp.
Capnocytophaga spp.
Haemophilus ducreyi
Neisseria gonorrhoeae including penicillinase-producing strains
Pasteurella spp.
Providencia stuartii
Gram-negative anaerobes:
Prevotella bivia
Prevotella disiens
Prevotella melaninogenica
Veillonella spp.

In vitro tests show imipenem to act synergistically with aminoglycoside antibiotics against some isolates of *Pseudomonas aeruginosa*.

Susceptibility Test Methods

When available, the clinical microbiology laboratory should provide to the physician the results of *in vitro* susceptibility tests for antimicrobial drug products used in resident hospitals as periodic reports which describe the susceptibility profile of nosocomial and community-acquired pathogens. These reports should aid the physician in selecting the most effective antimicrobial.

Dilution Techniques

Quantitative methods are used to determine antimicrobial minimum inhibitory concentrations (MICs). These MICs provide estimates of the susceptibility of bacteria to antimicrobial compounds. The MICs should be determined using a standardized procedure. Standardized procedures are based on a broth dilution method{1,2} or equivalent with standardized inoculum concentrations and standardized concentrations of imipenem powder. The MIC values should be interpreted according to criteria provided in Table 1.

Diffusion Techniques

Quantitative methods that require measurement of zone diameters also provide reproducible estimates of the susceptibility of bacteria to antimicrobial compounds. One such standardized procedure requires the use of standardized inoculum concentrations {2,3}. This procedure uses paper disks impregnated with 10-μg imipenem to test the susceptibility of microorganisms to imipenem. The disk diffusion interpretive criteria should be interpreted according to criteria provided in Table 1.

Anaerobic Techniques

For anaerobic bacteria, the susceptibility to imipenem as MICs can be determined by standardized test methods.{2,4} The MIC values obtained should be interpreted according to criteria provided in Table 1.

The MIC and disk diffusion values obtained should be interpreted according to the following criteria:
[See table 1 above]

A report of "Susceptible" indicates that the pathogen is likely to be inhibited if the antimicrobial compound at the infection site reaches the concentrations usually achievable. A report of "Intermediate" indicates that the result should be considered equivocal, and, if the microorganism is not fully susceptible to alternative, clinically feasible drugs, the test should be repeated. This category implies possible clinical applicability in body sites where the drug is physiologically concentrated or in situations where high dosage of drug can be used. This category also provides a buffer zone which prevents small uncontrolled technical factors from causing major discrepancies in interpretation. A report of "Resistant" indicates that the pathogen is not likely to be inhibited if the antimicrobial compound at the infection site reaches the concentrations usually achievable, and that other therapy should be selected.

Quality Control

Standardized susceptibility test procedures require the use of laboratory control microorganisms to ensure the accuracy and precision of supplies and reagents used in the assay, and the techniques of the individuals performing the test. Quality control microorganisms are specific strains of organisms with intrinsic biological properties. QC strains are very stable strains which will give a standard and repeatable susceptibility pattern. The specific strains used for microbiological quality control are not clinically significant. Standard imipenem powder should provide the following range of values noted in Table 2.{2}
[See table 2 above]

INDICATIONS AND USAGE

PRIMAXIN I.V. is indicated for the treatment of serious infections caused by susceptible strains of the designated microorganisms in the conditions listed below:

1. **Lower respiratory tract infections.** *Staphylococcus aureus* (penicillinase-producing strains), *Acinetobacter* species, *Enterobacter* species, *Escherichia coli*, *Haemophilus influenzae*, *Haemophilus parainfluenzae*[1], *Klebsiella* species, *Serratia marcescens*
2. **Urinary tract infections** (complicated and uncomplicated). *Enterococcus faecalis*, *Staphylococcus aureus* (penicillinase-producing strains)[1], *Enterobacter* species, *Escherichia coli*, *Klebsiella* species, *Morganella morganii*[1], *Proteus vulgaris*[1], *Providencia rettgeri*[1], *Pseudomonas aeruginosa*
3. **Intra-abdominal infections.** *Enterococcus faecalis*, *Staphylococcus aureus* (penicillinase-producing strains)[1], *Staphylococcus epidermidis*, *Citrobacter* species, *Enterobacter* species, *Escherichia coli*, *Klebsiella* species, *Morganella morganii*[1], *Proteus* species, *Pseudomonas aeruginosa*, *Bifidobacterium* species, *Clostridium* species, *Eubacterium* species, *Peptococcus* species, *Peptostreptococcus* species, *Propionibacterium* species[1], *Bacteroides* species including *B. fragilis*, *Fusobacterium* species
4. **Gynecologic infections.** *Enterococcus faecalis*, *Staphylococcus aureus* (penicillinase-producing strains)[1], *Staphylococcus epidermidis*, *Streptococcus agalactiae* (Group B streptococci), *Enterobacter* species[1], *Escherichia coli*, *Gardnerella vaginalis*, *Klebsiella* species[1], *Proteus* species, *Bifidobacterium* species[1], *Peptococcus* species[1], *Peptostreptococcus* species, *Propionibacterium* species[1], *Bacteroides* species including *B. fragilis*[1]
5. **Bacterial septicemia.** *Enterococcus faecalis*, *Staphylococcus aureus* (penicillinase-producing strains), *Enterobacter* species, *Escherichia coli*, *Klebsiella* species, *Pseudomonas aeruginosa*, *Serratia* species[1], *Bacteroides* species including *B. fragilis*[1]
6. **Bone and joint infections.** *Enterococcus faecalis*, *Staphylococcus aureus* (penicillinase-producing strains), *Staphylococcus epidermidis*, *Enterobacter* species, *Pseudomonas aeruginosa*
7. **Skin and skin structure infections.** *Enterococcus faecalis*, *Staphylococcus aureus* (penicillinase-producing strains), *Staphylococcus epidermidis*, *Acinetobacter* species, *Citrobacter* species, *Enterobacter* species, *Escherichia coli*, *Klebsiella* species, *Morganella morganii*, *Proteus vulgaris*, *Providencia rettgeri*[1], *Pseudomonas aeruginosa*, *Serratia* species, *Peptococcus* species, *Peptostreptococcus* species, *Bacteroides* species including *B. fragilis*, *Fusobacterium* species[1]
8. **Endocarditis.** *Staphylococcus aureus* (penicillinase-producing strains)
9. **Polymicrobic infections.** PRIMAXIN I.V. is indicated for polymicrobic infections including those in which *S. pneumoniae* (pneumonia, septicemia), *S. pyogenes* (skin and skin structure), or nonpenicillinase-producing *S. aureus* is one of the causative organisms. However, monobacterial infections due to these organisms are usually treated with narrower spectrum antibiotics, such as penicillin G.

PRIMAXIN I.V. is not indicated in patients with meningitis because safety and efficacy have not been established.

For Pediatric Use information, see PRECAUTIONS, Pediatric Use, and DOSAGE AND ADMINISTRATION sections.

Because of its broad spectrum of bactericidal activity against gram-positive and gram-negative aerobic and anaerobic bacteria, PRIMAXIN I.V. is useful for the treatment of mixed infections and as presumptive therapy prior to the identification of the causative organisms.

Although clinical improvement has been observed in patients with cystic fibrosis, chronic pulmonary disease, and lower respiratory tract infections caused by *Pseudomonas aeruginosa*, bacterial eradication may not necessarily be achieved.

As with other beta-lactam antibiotics, some strains of *Pseudomonas aeruginosa* may develop resistance fairly rapidly during treatment with PRIMAXIN I.V. During therapy of *Pseudomonas aeruginosa* infections, periodic susceptibility testing should be done when clinically appropriate.

Infections resistant to other antibiotics, for example, cephalosporins, penicillin, and aminoglycosides, have been shown to respond to treatment with PRIMAXIN I.V.

To reduce the development of drug-resistant bacteria and maintain the effectiveness of PRIMAXIN I.V. and other antibacterial drugs, PRIMAXIN I.V. should be used only to treat or prevent infections that are proven or strongly suspected to be caused by susceptible bacteria. When culture and susceptibility information are available, they should be considered in selecting or modifying antibacterial therapy. In the absence of such data, local epidemiology and susceptibility patterns may contribute to the empiric selection of therapy.

[1]Efficacy for this organism in this organ system was studied in fewer than 10 infections.

CONTRAINDICATIONS

PRIMAXIN I.V. is contraindicated in patients who have shown hypersensitivity to any component of this product.

WARNINGS

SERIOUS AND OCCASIONALLY FATAL HYPERSENSITIVITY (ANAPHYLACTIC) REACTIONS HAVE BEEN REPORTED IN PATIENTS RECEIVING THERAPY WITH BETA-LACTAMS. THESE REACTIONS ARE MORE APT TO OCCUR IN PERSONS WITH A HISTORY OF SENSITIVITY TO MULTIPLE ALLERGENS.

THERE HAVE BEEN REPORTS OF PATIENTS WITH A HISTORY OF PENICILLIN HYPERSENSITIVITY WHO HAVE EXPERIENCED SEVERE HYPERSENSITIVITY REACTIONS WHEN TREATED WITH ANOTHER BETA-LACTAM. BEFORE INITIATING THERAPY WITH PRIMAXIN I.V., CAREFUL INQUIRY SHOULD BE MADE CONCERNING PREVIOUS HYPERSENSITIVITY REACTIONS TO PENICILLINS, CEPHALOSPORINS, OTHER BETA-LACTAMS, AND OTHER ALLERGENS. IF AN ALLERGIC REACTION OCCURS, PRIMAXIN SHOULD BE DISCONTINUED.

SERIOUS ANAPHYLACTIC REACTIONS REQUIRE IMMEDIATE EMERGENCY TREATMENT WITH EPINEPHRINE. OXYGEN, INTRAVENOUS STEROIDS, AND AIRWAY MANAGEMENT, INCLUDING INTUBATION, MAY ALSO BE ADMINISTERED AS INDICATED.

Seizure Potential

Seizures and other CNS adverse experiences, such as confusional states and myoclonic activity, have been reported during treatment with PRIMAXIN I.V. (See PRECAUTIONS and ADVERSE REACTIONS.)

Case reports in the literature have shown that co-administration of carbapenems, including imipenem, to patients receiving valproic acid or divalproex sodium results in a reduction in valproic acid concentrations. The valproic acid concentrations may drop below the therapeutic range as a result of this interaction, therefore increasing the risk of breakthrough seizures. Increasing the dose of valproic acid or divalproex sodium may not be sufficient to overcome this interaction. The concomitant use of imipenem and valproic acid/divalproex sodium is generally not recommended. Anti-bacterials other than carbapenems should be considered to treat infections in patients whose seizures are well controlled on valproic acid or divalproex sodium. If administration of PRIMAXIN I.V. is necessary, supplemental anti-convulsant therapy should be considered (see PRECAUTIONS, Drug Interactions).

Clostridium difficile associated diarrhea (CDAD) has been reported with use of nearly all antibacterial agents, including PRIMAXIN I.V., and may range in severity from mild diarrhea to fatal colitis. Treatment with antibacterial agents alters the normal flora of the colon leading to overgrowth of *C. difficile*.

C. difficile produces toxins A and B which contribute to the development of CDAD.

Hypertoxin producing strains of *C. difficile* cause increased morbidity and mortality, as these infections can be refractory to antimicrobial therapy and may require colectomy. CDAD must be considered in all patients who present with diarrhea following antibiotic use. Careful medical history is necessary since CDAD has been reported to occur over two months after the administration of antibacterial agents.

If CDAD is suspected or confirmed, ongoing antibiotic use not directed against *C. difficile* may need to be discontinued. Appropriate fluid and electrolyte management, protein supplementation, antibiotic treatment of *C. difficile*, and surgical evaluation should be instituted as clinically indicated.

PRECAUTIONS

General

CNS adverse experiences such as confusional states, myoclonic activity, and seizures have been reported during treatment with PRIMAXIN I.V., especially when recommended dosages were exceeded. These experiences have occurred most commonly in patients with CNS disorders (e.g., brain lesions or history of seizures) and/or compromised renal function. However, there have been reports of CNS adverse experiences in patients who had no recognized or documented underlying CNS disorder or compromised renal function.

When recommended doses were exceeded, adult patients with creatinine clearances of $\leq$20 mL/min/1.73 m^2, whether or not undergoing hemodialysis, had a higher risk of seizure activity than those without impairment of renal function. Therefore, close adherence to the dosing guidelines for these patients is recommended. (See DOSAGE AND ADMINISTRATION.)

Patients with creatinine clearances of $\leq$5 mL/min/1.73 m^2 should not receive PRIMAXIN I.V. unless hemodialysis is instituted within 48 hours.

For patients on hemodialysis, PRIMAXIN I.V. is recommended only when the benefit outweighs the potential risk of seizures.

Close adherence to the recommended dosage and dosage schedules is urged, especially in patients with known factors that predispose to convulsive activity. Anticonvulsant therapy should be continued in patients with known seizure disorders. If focal tremors, myoclonus, or seizures occur, patients should be evaluated neurologically, placed on anticonvulsant therapy if not already instituted, and the dosage of PRIMAXIN I.V. re-examined to determine whether it should be decreased or the antibiotic discontinued.

As with other antibiotics, prolonged use of PRIMAXIN I.V. may result in overgrowth of nonsusceptible organisms. Repeated evaluation of the patient's condition is essential. If superinfection occurs during therapy, appropriate measures should be taken.

Prescribing PRIMAXIN I.V. in the absence of a proven or strongly suspected bacterial infection or a prophylactic indication is unlikely to provide benefit to the patient and increases the risk of the development of drug-resistant bacteria.

Information for Patients

Patients should be counseled to inform their physician if they are taking valproic acid or divalproex sodium. Valproic acid concentrations in the blood may drop below the therapeutic range upon co-administration with PRIMAXIN I.V. If treatment with PRIMAXIN I.V. is necessary and continued, alternative or supplemental anti-convulsant medication to prevent and/or treat seizures may be needed.

Patients should be counseled that antibacterial drugs including PRIMAXIN I.V. should only be used to treat bacterial infections. They do not treat viral infections (e.g., the common cold). When PRIMAXIN I.V. is prescribed to treat a bacterial infection, patients should be told that although it is common to feel better early in the course of therapy, the medication should be taken exactly as directed. Skipping doses or not completing the full course of therapy may (1) decrease the effectiveness of the immediate treatment and (2) increase the likelihood that bacteria will develop resistance and will not be treatable by PRIMAXIN I.V. or other antibacterial drugs in the future.

Diarrhea is a common problem caused by antibiotics, which usually ends when the antibiotic is discontinued. Sometimes after starting treatment with antibiotics, patients can develop watery and bloody stools (with or without stomach cramps and fever) even as late as two or more months after having taken the last dose of the antibiotic. If this occurs, patients should contact their physician as soon as possible.

Laboratory Tests

While PRIMAXIN I.V. possesses the characteristic low toxicity of the beta-lactam group of antibiotics, periodic assessment of organ system functions, including renal, hepatic, and hematopoietic, is advisable during prolonged therapy.

Drug Interactions

Generalized seizures have been reported in patients who received ganciclovir and PRIMAXIN. These drugs should not be used concomitantly unless the potential benefits outweigh the risks.

Since concomitant administration of PRIMAXIN and probenecid results in only minimal increases in plasma levels of imipenem and plasma half-life, it is not recommended that probenecid be given with PRIMAXIN.

PRIMAXIN should not be mixed with or physically added to other antibiotics. However, PRIMAXIN may be administered concomitantly with other antibiotics, such as aminoglycosides.

Case reports in the literature have shown that co-administration of carbapenems, including imipenem, to patients receiving valproic acid or divalproex sodium results in a reduction in valproic acid concentrations. The valproic acid concentrations may drop below the therapeutic range as a result of this interaction, therefore increasing the risk of breakthrough seizures. Although the mechanism of this interaction is unknown, data from *in vitro* and animal studies suggest that carbapenems may inhibit the hydrolysis of valproic acid's glucuronide metabolite (VPA-g) back to valproic acid, thus decreasing the serum concentrations of valproic acid (see WARNINGS, Seizure Potential).

Carcinogenesis, Mutagenesis, Impairment of Fertility

Long term studies in animals have not been performed to evaluate carcinogenic potential of imipenem-cilastatin. Genetic toxicity studies were performed in a variety of bacterial and mammalian tests *in vivo* and *in vitro*. The tests used were: V79 mammalian cell mutagenesis assay (imipenem-cilastatin sodium alone and imipenem alone), Ames test (cilastatin sodium alone and imipenem alone), unscheduled DNA synthesis assay (imipenem-cilastatin sodium) and *in vivo* mouse cytogenetics test (imipenem-cilastatin sodium). None of these tests showed any evidence of genetic alterations.

Reproductive tests in male and female rats were performed with imipenem-cilastatin sodium at intravenous doses up to 80 mg/kg/day and at a subcutaneous dose of 320 mg/kg/day, approximately equal to the highest recommended human dose of the intravenous formulation (on a mg/m^2 body surface area basis). Slight decreases in live fetal body weight were restricted to the highest dosage level. No other adverse effects were observed on fertility, reproductive performance, fetal viability, growth or postnatal development of pups.

Pregnancy

Teratogenic Effects

Pregnancy Category C:

Teratology studies with cilastatin sodium at doses of 30, 100, and 300 mg/kg/day administered intravenously to rabbits and 40, 200, and 1000 mg/kg/day administered subcutaneously to rats, up to approximately 1.9 and 3.2 times[2] the maximum recommended daily human dose (on a mg/m^2 body surface area basis) of the intravenous formulation of imipenem-cilastatin sodium (50 mg/kg/day) in the two species, respectively, showed no evidence of adverse effect on the fetus. No evidence of teratogenicity was observed in rabbits given imipenem at intravenous doses of 15, 30 or 60 mg/kg/day and rats given imipenem at intravenous doses of 225, 450, or 900 mg/kg/day, up to approximately 0.4 and 2.9 times[2] the maximum recommended daily human dose (on a mg/m^2 body surface area basis) in the two species, respectively.

Teratology studies with imipenem-cilastatin sodium at intravenous doses of 20 and 80, and a subcutaneous dose of 320 mg/kg/day, up to 0.5 times[2] (mice) to approximately equal to (rats) the highest recommended daily intravenous human dose (on a mg/m^2 body surface area basis) in pregnant rodents during the period of major organogenesis, revealed no evidence of teratogenicity.

Imipenem-cilastatin sodium, when administered subcutaneously to pregnant rabbits at dosages equivalent to the usual human dose of the intravenous formulation and higher (1000-4000 mg/day), caused body weight loss, diarrhea, and maternal deaths. When comparable doses of imipenem-cilastatin sodium were given to non-pregnant rabbits, body weight loss, diarrhea, and deaths were also observed. This intolerance is not unlike that seen with other beta-lactam antibiotics in this species and is probably due to alteration of gut flora.

A teratology study in pregnant cynomolgus monkeys given imipenem-cilastatin sodium at doses of 40 mg/kg/day (bolus intravenous injection) or 160 mg/kg/day (subcutaneous injection) resulted in maternal toxicity including emesis, inappetence, body weight loss, diarrhea, abortion, and death in some cases. In contrast, no significant toxicity was observed when non-pregnant cynomolgus monkeys were given doses of imipenem-cilastatin sodium up to 180 mg/kg/day (subcutaneous injection). When doses of imipenem-cilastatin sodium (approximately 100 mg/kg/day or approximately 0.6 times[2] the maximum recommended daily human dose of the intravenous formulation) were administered to pregnant cynomolgus monkeys at an intravenous infusion rate which mimics human clinical use, there was minimal maternal intolerance (occasional emesis), no maternal deaths, no evidence of teratogenicity, but an increase in embryonic loss relative to control groups.

No adverse effects on the fetus or on lactation were observed when imipenem-cilastatin sodium was administered subcutaneously to rats late in gestation at dosages up to 320 mg/kg/day, approximately equal to the highest recommended human dose (on a mg/m^2 body surface area basis).

There are, however, no adequate and well-controlled studies in pregnant women. PRIMAXIN I.V. should be used during pregnancy only if the potential benefit justifies the potential risk to the mother and fetus.

[2]Based on patient body surface area of 1.6 m^2 (weight of 60 kg).

Nursing Mothers

It is not known whether imipenem-cilastatin sodium is excreted in human milk. Because many drugs are excreted in human milk, caution should be exercised when PRIMAXIN I.V. is administered to a nursing woman.

Pediatric Use

Use of PRIMAXIN I.V. in pediatric patients, neonates to 16 years of age, is supported by evidence from adequate and well-controlled studies of PRIMAXIN I.V. in adults and by the following clinical studies and published literature in pediatric patients: Based on published studies of 178[3] pediatric patients ≥3 months of age (with non-CNS infections), the recommended dose of PRIMAXIN I.V. is 15-25 mg/kg/dose administered every six hours. Doses of 25 mg/kg/dose in patients 3 months to <3 years of age, and 15 mg/kg/dose in patients 3-12 years of age were associated with mean trough plasma concentrations of imipenem of 1.1±0.4 µg/mL and 0.6±0.2 µg/mL following multiple 60-minute infusions, respectively; trough urinary concentrations of imipenem were in excess of 10 µg/mL for both doses. These doses have provided adequate plasma and urine concentrations for the treatment of non-CNS infections. Based on studies in adults, the maximum daily dose for treatment of infections with fully susceptible organisms is 2.0 g per day, and of infections with moderately susceptible organisms (primarily some strains of *P. aeruginosa*) is 4.0 g/day. (See DOSAGE AND ADMINISTRATION, Table 3.) Higher doses (up to 90 mg/kg/day in older children) have been used in patients with cystic fibrosis. (See DOSAGE AND ADMINISTRATION.)

Based on studies of 135[4] pediatric patients ≤3 months of age (weighing ≥1,500 g), the following dosage schedule is recommended for non-CNS infections:

<1 wk of age: 25 mg/kg every 12 hrs
1-4 wks of age: 25 mg/kg every 8 hrs
4 wks-3 mos. of age: 25 mg/kg every 6 hrs.

In a published dose-ranging study of smaller premature infants (670-1,890 g) in the first week of life, a dose of 20 mg/kg q12h by 15-30 minutes infusion was associated with mean peak and trough plasma imipenem concentrations of 43 µg/mL and 1.7 µg/mL after multiple doses, respectively. However, moderate accumulation of cilastatin in neonates may occur following multiple doses of PRIMAXIN I.V. The safety of this accumulation is unknown.

PRIMAXIN I.V. is not recommended in pediatric patients with CNS infections because of the risk of seizures.

PRIMAXIN I.V. is not recommended in pediatric patients <30 kg with impaired renal function, as no data are available.

[3]Two patients were less than 3 months of age.
[4]One patient was greater than 3 months of age.

Geriatric Use

Of the approximately 3600 subjects ≥18 years of age in clinical studies of PRIMAXIN I.V., including postmarketing studies, approximately 2800 received PRIMAXIN I.V. Of the subjects who received PRIMAXIN I.V., data are available on approximately 800 subjects who were 65 and over, including approximately 300 subjects who were 75 and over. No overall differences in safety or effectiveness were observed between these subjects and younger subjects. Other reported clinical experience has not identified differences in responses between the elderly and younger patients, but greater sensitivity of some older individuals cannot be ruled out.

This drug is known to be substantially excreted by the kidney, and the risk of toxic reactions to this drug may be greater in patients with impaired renal function. Because elderly patients are more likely to have decreased renal function, care should be taken in dose selection, and it may be useful to monitor renal function.

No dosage adjustment is required based on age (see CLINICAL PHARMACOLOGY, Adults). Dosage adjustment in the case of renal impairment is necessary (see DOSAGE AND ADMINISTRATION, Reduced Intravenous Schedule for Adults with Impaired Renal Function and/or Body Weight <70 kg).

ADVERSE REACTIONS

Adults

PRIMAXIN I.V. is generally well tolerated. Many of the 1,723 patients treated in clinical trials were severely ill and had multiple background diseases and physiological impairments, making it difficult to determine causal relationship of adverse experiences to therapy with PRIMAXIN I.V.

Local Adverse Reactions

Adverse local clinical reactions that were reported as possibly, probably, or definitely related to therapy with PRIMAXIN I.V. were:

Phlebitis/thrombophlebitis — 3.1%
Pain at the injection site — 0.7%
Erythema at the injection site — 0.4%
Vein induration — 0.2%
Infused vein infection — 0.1%

Systemic Adverse Reactions

The most frequently reported systemic adverse clinical reactions that were reported as possibly, probably, or definitely related to PRIMAXIN I.V. were nausea (2.0%), diarrhea (1.8%), vomiting (1.5%), rash (0.9%), fever (0.5%), hypotension (0.4%), seizures (0.4%) (see PRECAUTIONS), dizziness (0.3%), pruritus (0.3%), urticaria (0.2%), somnolence (0.2%).

Additional adverse systemic clinical reactions reported as possibly, probably, or definitely drug related occurring in less than 0.2% of the patients or reported since the drug was marketed are listed within each body system in order of decreasing severity: *Gastrointestinal* — pseudomembranous colitis (the onset of pseudomembranous colitis symptoms may occur during or after antibacterial treatment, see WARNINGS), hemorrhagic colitis, hepatitis (including fulminant hepatitis), hepatic failure, jaundice, gastroenteritis, abdominal pain, glossitis, tongue papillar hypertrophy, staining of the teeth and/or tongue, heartburn, pharyngeal pain, increased salivation; *Hematologic* — pancytopenia, bone marrow depression, thrombocytopenia, neutropenia, leukopenia, hemolytic anemia; *CNS* — encephalopathy, tremor, confusion, myoclonus, paresthesia, vertigo, headache, psychic disturbances including hallucinations; *Special Senses* — hearing loss, tinnitus, taste perversion; *Respiratory* — chest discomfort, dyspnea, hyperventilation, thoracic spine pain; *Cardiovascular* — palpitations, tachycardia; *Skin* — Stevens-Johnson syndrome, toxic epidermal necrolysis, erythema multiforme, angioneurotic edema, flushing, cyanosis, hyperhidrosis, skin texture changes, candidiasis, pruritus vulvae; *Body as a whole* — polyarthralgia, asthenia/weakness, drug fever; *Renal* — acute renal failure, oliguria/anuria, polyuria, urine discoloration. The role of PRIMAXIN I.V. in changes in renal function is difficult to assess, since factors predisposing to pre-renal azotemia or to impaired renal function usually have been present.

Adverse Laboratory Changes

Adverse laboratory changes without regard to drug relationship that were reported during clinical trials or reported since the drug was marketed were:

Hepatic: Increased ALT (SGPT), AST (SGOT), alkaline phosphatase, bilirubin, and LDH

Hemic: Increased eosinophils, positive Coombs test, increased WBC, increased platelets, decreased hemoglobin and hematocrit, agranulocytosis, increased monocytes, abnormal prothrombin time, increased lymphocytes, increased basophils

Electrolytes: Decreased serum sodium, increased potassium, increased chloride

Renal: Increased BUN, creatinine

Urinalysis: Presence of urine protein, urine red blood cells, urine white blood cells, urine casts, urine bilirubin, and urine urobilinogen.

Pediatric Patients

In studies of 178 pediatric patients ≥3 months of age, the following adverse events were noted:

The Most Common Clinical Adverse Experiences Without Regard to Drug Relationship (Patient Incidence >1%)

Adverse Experience	No. of Patients (%)
Digestive System	
Diarrhea	7* (3.9)
Gastroenteritis	2 (1.1)
Vomiting	2* (1.1)
Skin	
Rash	4 (2.2)
Irritation, I.V. site	2 (1.1)
Urogenital System	
Urine discoloration	2 (1.1)
Cardiovascular System	
Phlebitis	4 (2.2)

*One patient had both vomiting and diarrhea and is counted in each category.

In studies of 135 patients (newborn to 3 months of age), the following adverse events were noted:

The Most Common Clinical Adverse Experiences Without Regard to Drug Relationship (Patient Incidence >1%)

Adverse Experience	No. of Patients (%)
Digestive System	
Diarrhea	4 (3.0%)
Oral Candidiasis	2 (1.5%)
Skin	
Rash	2 (1.5%)
Urogenital System	
Oliguria/anuria	3 (2.2%)
Cardiovascular System	
Tachycardia	2 (1.5%)
Nervous System	
Convulsions	8 (5.9%)

[See first table at top of next page]

Patients (<3 Months of Age) With Normal Pretherapy but Abnormal During Therapy Laboratory Values

Laboratory Parameter	No. of Patients With Abnormalities* (%)
Eosinophil Count↑	11 (9.0%)
Hematocrit↓	3 (2.0%)
Hematocrit↑	1 (1.0%)
Platelet Count↑	5 (4.0%)
Platelet Count↓	2 (2.0%)
Serum Creatinine↑	5 (5.0%)
Bilirubin↑	3 (3.0%)
Bilirubin↓	1 (1.0%)
AST (SGOT)↑	5 (6.0%)
ALT (SGPT)↑	3 (3.0%)
Serum Alkaline Phosphate↑	2 (3.0%)

* The denominator used for percentages was the number of patients for whom the test was performed during or post-treatment and, therefore, varies by test.

Examination of published literature and spontaneous adverse event reports suggested a similar spectrum of adverse events in adult and pediatric patients.

OVERDOSAGE

The acute intravenous toxicity of imipenem-cilastatin sodium in a ratio of 1:1 was studied in mice at doses of 751 to 1359 mg/kg. Following drug administration, ataxia was rapidly produced and clonic convulsions were noted in about 45 minutes. Deaths occurred within 4-56 minutes at all doses.

The acute intravenous toxicity of imipenem-cilastatin sodium was produced within 5-10 minutes in rats at doses of 771 to 1583 mg/kg. In all dosage groups, females had decreased activity, bradypnea, and ptosis with clonic convulsions preceding death; in males, ptosis was seen at all dose levels while tremors and clonic convulsions were seen at all but the lowest dose (771 mg/kg). In another rat study, female rats showed ataxia, bradypnea, and decreased activity in all but the lowest dose (550 mg/kg); deaths were preceded by clonic convulsions. Male rats showed tremors at all doses and clonic convulsions and ptosis were seen at the two highest doses (1130 and 1734 mg/kg). Deaths occurred between 6 and 88 minutes with doses of 771 to 1734 mg/kg.

In the case of overdosage, discontinue PRIMAXIN I.V., treat symptomatically, and institute supportive measures as required. Imipenem-cilastatin sodium is hemodialyzable. However, usefulness of this procedure in the overdosage setting is questionable.

DOSAGE AND ADMINISTRATION

Adults

The dosage recommendations for PRIMAXIN I.V. represent the quantity of imipenem to be administered. An equivalent amount of cilastatin is also present in the solution. Each 125 mg, 250 mg, or 500 mg dose should be given by intravenous administration over 20 to 30 minutes. Each 750 mg or 1000 mg dose should be infused over 40 to 60 minutes. In patients who develop nausea during the infusion, the rate of infusion may be slowed.

The total daily dosage for PRIMAXIN I.V. should be based on the type or severity of infection and given in equally divided doses based on consideration of degree of susceptibility of the pathogen(s), renal function, and body weight. Adult patients with impaired renal function, as judged by creatinine clearance ≤70 mL/min/1.73 m^2, require adjustment of dosage as described in the succeeding section of these guidelines.

Intravenous Dosage Schedule for Adults with Normal Renal Function and Body Weight ≥70 kg

Doses cited in Table 3 are based on a patient with normal renal function and a body weight of 70 kg. These doses should be used for a patient with a creatinine clearance of ≥71 mL/min/1.73 m^2 and a body weight of ≥70 kg. A reduction in dose must be made for a patient with a creatinine clearance of ≤70 mL/min/1.73 m^2 and/or a body weight less than 70 kg. (See Tables 4 and 5.)

Dosage regimens in column A of Table 3 are recommended for infections caused by fully susceptible organisms which represent the majority of pathogenic species. Dosage regimens in column B of Table 3 are recommended for infections caused by organisms with moderate susceptibility to imipenem, primarily some strains of *P. aeruginosa*.

TABLE 3: INTRAVENOUS DOSAGE SCHEDULE FOR ADULTS WITH NORMAL RENAL FUNCTION AND BODY WEIGHT ≥70 kg

Type or Severity of Infection	A Fully susceptible organisms including gram-positive and gram-negative aerobes and anaerobes	B Moderately susceptible organisms, primarily some strains of *P. aeruginosa*
Mild	250 mg q6h (TOTAL DAILY DOSE = 1.0g)	500 mg q6h (TOTAL DAILY DOSE = 2.0g)
Moderate	500 mg q8h (TOTAL DAILY DOSE = 1.5g) or 500 mg q6h (TOTAL DAILY DOSE = 2.0g)	500 mg q6h (TOTAL DAILY DOSE = 2.0g) or 1 g q8h (TOTAL DAILY DOSE = 3.0g)
Severe, life threatening only	500 mg q6h (TOTAL DAILY DOSE = 2.0g)	1 g q8h (TOTAL DAILY DOSE = 3.0g) or 1 g q6h (TOTAL DAILY DOSE = 4.0g)
Uncomplicated urinary tract infection	250 mg q6h (TOTAL DAILY DOSE = 1.0g)	250 mg q6h (TOTAL DAILY DOSE = 1.0g)
Complicated urinary tract infection	500 mg q6h (TOTAL DAILY DOSE = 2.0g)	500 mg q6h (TOTAL DAILY DOSE = 2.0g)

Patients (≥3 Months of Age) With Normal Pretherapy but Abnormal During Therapy Laboratory Values

Laboratory Parameter	Abnormality			No. of Patients With Abnormalities/No. of Patients With Lab Done	(%)
Hemoglobin	Age	<5 mos.: 6 mos. – 12 yrs.:	<10 gm % <11.5 gm %	19/129	(14.7)
Hematocrit	Age	<5 mos.: 6 mos. – 12 yrs.:	<30 vol % <34.5 vol %	23/129	(17.8)
Neutrophils		≤1000/mm^3 (absolute)		4/123	(3.3)
Eosinophils		≥7%		15/117	(12.8)
Platelet Count		≥500 ths/mm^3		16/119	(13.4)
Urine Protein		≥1		8/97	(8.2)
Serum Creatinine		>1.2 mg/dL		0/105	(0)
BUN		>22 mg/dL		0/108	(0)
AST (SGOT)		>36 IU/L		14/78	(17.9)
ALT (SGPT)		>30 IU/L		10/93	(10.8)

TABLE 4: REDUCED INTRAVENOUS DOSAGE OF PRIMAXIN I.V. IN ADULT PATIENTS WITH IMPAIRED RENAL FUNCTION AND/OR BODY WEIGHT <70 kg

	If TOTAL DAILY DOSE from TABLE 3 is: 1.0 g/day				1.5 g/day				2.0 g/day			
And Body Weight (kg) is:	and creatinine clearance (mL/min/1.73 m^2) is: ≥71	41-70	21-40	6-20	and creatinine clearance (mL/min/1.73 m^2) is: ≥71	41-70	21-40	6-20	and creatinine clearance (mL/min/1.73 m^2) is: ≥71	41-70	21-40	6-20
	then the reduced dosage regimen (mg) is:				then the reduced dosage regimen (mg) is:				then the reduced dosage regimen (mg) is:			
≥70	250 q6h	250 q8h	250 q12h	250 q12h	500 q8h	250 q6h	250 q8h	250 q12h	500 q6h	500 q8h	250 q6h	250 q12h
60	250 q8h	125 q6h	250 q12h	125 q12h	250 q6h	250 q8h	250 q8h	250 q12h	500 q8h	250 q6h	250 q8h	250 q12h
50	125 q6h	125 q6h	125 q8h	125 q12h	250 q6h	250 q8h	250 q12h	250 q12h	250 q6h	250 q6h	250 q8h	250 q12h
40	125 q6h	125 q8h	125 q12h	125 q12h	250 q8h	125 q6h	125 q8h	125 q12h	250 q6h	250 q8h	250 q12h	250 q12h
30	125 q8h	125 q8h	125 q12h	125 q12h	125 q6h	125 q8h	125 q8h	125 q12h	250 q8h	125 q6h	125 q8h	125 q12h

Due to the high antimicrobial activity of PRIMAXIN I.V., it is recommended that the maximum total daily dosage not exceed 50 mg/kg/day or 4.0 g/day, whichever is lower. There is no evidence that higher doses provide greater efficacy. However, patients over twelve years of age with cystic fibrosis and normal renal function have been treated with PRIMAXIN I.V. at doses up to 90 mg/kg/day in divided doses, not exceeding 4.0 g/day.

Reduced Intravenous Schedule for Adults with Impaired Renal Function and/or Body Weight <70 kg

Patients with creatinine clearance of ≤70 mL/min/1.73 m^2 and/or body weight less than 70 kg require dosage reduction of PRIMAXIN I.V. as indicated in the tables below. Creatinine clearance may be calculated from serum creatinine concentration by the following equation:

$$T_{cc} \text{ (Males)} = \frac{\text{(wt. in kg) (140 - age)}}{\text{(72) (creatinine in mg/dL)}}$$

$$T_{cc} \text{ (Females)} = 0.85 \times \text{(above value)}$$

To determine the dose for adults with impaired renal function and/or reduced body weight:

1. Choose a total daily dose from Table 3 based on infection characteristics.
2. a) If the total daily dose is 1.0 g, 1.5 g, or 2.0 g, use the appropriate subsection of Table 4 and continue with step 3.
   b) If the total daily dose is 3.0 g or 4.0 g, use the appropriate subsection of Table 5 and continue with step 3.
3. From Table 4 or 5:
   a) Select the body weight on the far left which is closest to the patient's body weight (kg).
   b) Select the patient's creatinine clearance category.
   c) Where the row and column intersect is the reduced dosage regimen.

[See table 4 above]
[See table 5 at top of next page]

Patients with creatinine clearances of 6 to 20 mL/min/1.73 m^2 should be treated with PRIMAXIN I.V. 125 mg or 250 mg every 12 hours for most pathogens. There may be an increased risk of seizures when doses of 500 mg every 12 hours are administered to these patients.

Patients with creatinine clearance ≤5 mL/min/1.73 m^2 should not receive PRIMAXIN I.V. unless hemodialysis is instituted within 48 hours. There is inadequate information to recommend usage of PRIMAXIN I.V. for patients undergoing peritoneal dialysis.

Hemodialysis

When treating patients with creatinine clearances of ≤5 mL/min/1.73 m^2 who are undergoing hemodialysis, use the dosage recommendations for patients with creatinine clearances of 6-20 mL/min/1.73 m^2. (See Reduced Intravenous Dosage Schedule for Adults with Impaired Renal Function and/or Body Weight <70 kg.) Both imipenem and cilastatin are cleared from the circulation during hemodialysis. The patient should receive PRIMAXIN I.V. after hemodialysis and at 12 hour intervals timed from the end of that hemodialysis session. Dialysis patients, especially those with background CNS disease, should be carefully monitored; for patients on hemodialysis, PRIMAXIN I.V. is recommended only when the benefit outweighs the potential risk of seizures. (See PRECAUTIONS.)

Pediatric Patients

See PRECAUTIONS, Pediatric Patients.

For pediatric patients ≥3 months of age, the recommended dose for non-CNS infections is 15-25 mg/kg/dose administered every six hours. Based on studies in adults, the maximum daily dose for treatment of infections with fully susceptible organisms is 2.0 g per day, and of infections with moderately susceptible organisms (primarily some strains of *P. aeruginosa*) is 4.0 g/day. Higher doses (up to 90 mg/kg/day in older children) have been used in patients with cystic fibrosis.

For pediatric patients ≤3 months of age (weighing ≥1,500 g), the following dosage schedule is recommended for non-CNS infections:

<1 wk of age: 25 mg/kg every 12 hrs
1-4 wks of age: 25 mg/kg every 8 hrs
4 wks-3 mos. of age: 25 mg/kg every 6 hrs.

Doses less than or equal to 500 mg should be given by intravenous infusion over 15 to 30 minutes. Doses greater than 500 mg should be given by intravenous infusion over 40 to 60 minutes.

PRIMAXIN I.V. is not recommended in pediatric patients with CNS infections because of the risk of seizures.

PRIMAXIN I.V. is not recommended in pediatric patients <30 kg with impaired renal function, as no data are available.

TABLE 5: REDUCED INTRAVENOUS DOSAGE OF PRIMAXIN I.V. IN ADULT PATIENTS WITH IMPAIRED RENAL FUNCTION AND/OR BODY WEIGHT <70 kg

	If TOTAL DAILY DOSE from TABLE 3 is: 3.0 g/day				4.0 g/day			
And Body Weight (kg) is:	and creatinine clearance ($mL/min/1.73\ m^2$) is: ≥71	41-70	21-40	6-20	and creatinine clearance ($mL/min/1.73\ m^2$) is: ≥71	41-70	21-40	6-20
	then the reduced dosage regimen (mg) is:				then the reduced dosage regimen (mg) is:			
≥70	1000 q8h	500 q6h	500 q8h	500 q12h	1000 q6h	750 q8h	500 q6h	500 q12h
60	750 q8h	500 q8h	500 q8h	500 q12h	1000 q8h	750 q8h	500 q8h	500 q12h
50	500 q6h	500 q8h	250 q6h	250 q12h	750 q8h	500 q6h	500 q8h	500 q12h
40	500 q8h	250 q6h	250 q8h	250 q12h	500 q6h	500 q8h	250 q6h	250 q12h
30	250 q6h	250 q8h	250 q8h	250 q12h	500 q8h	250 q6h	250 q8h	250 q12h

PREPARATION OF SOLUTION

Vials

Contents of the vials must be suspended and transferred to 100 mL of an appropriate infusion solution.

A suggested procedure is to add approximately 10 mL from the appropriate infusion solution (see list of diluents under COMPATIBILITY AND STABILITY) to the vial. Shake well and transfer the resulting suspension to the infusion solution container.

Benzyl alcohol as a preservative has been associated with toxicity in neonates. While toxicity has not been demonstrated in pediatric patients greater than three months of age, small pediatric patients in this age range may also be at risk for benzyl alcohol toxicity. Therefore, diluents containing benzyl alcohol should not be used when PRIMAXIN I.V. is constituted for administration to pediatric patients in this age range.

CAUTION: THE SUSPENSION IS NOT FOR DIRECT INFUSION.

Repeat with an additional 10 mL of infusion solution to ensure complete transfer of vial contents to the infusion solution. **The resulting mixture should be agitated until clear.**

ADD-Vantage®[5] Vials

See separate INSTRUCTIONS FOR USE OF 'PRIMAXIN I.V.' IN ADD-Vantage® VIALS. PRIMAXIN I.V. in ADD-Vantage® vials should be reconstituted with ADD-Vantage® diluent containers containing 100 mL of either 0.9% Sodium Chloride Injection or 100 mL 5% Dextrose Injection.

[5]Registered trademark of Abbott Laboratories, Inc.

COMPATIBILITY AND STABILITY

Before Reconstitution:

The dry powder should be stored at a temperature below 25°C (77°F).

Reconstituted Solutions:

Solutions of PRIMAXIN I.V. range from colorless to yellow. Variations of color within this range do not affect the potency of the product.

Vials

PRIMAXIN I.V., as supplied in single use vials and reconstituted with the following diluents (see PREPARATION OF SOLUTION), maintains satisfactory potency for 4 hours at room temperature or for 24 hours under refrigeration (5°C). Solutions of PRIMAXIN I.V. should not be frozen.

0.9% Sodium Chloride Injection
5% or 10% Dextrose Injection
5% Dextrose and 0.9% Sodium Chloride Injection
5% Dextrose Injection with 0.225% or 0.45% saline solution
5% Dextrose Injection with 0.15% potassium chloride solution
Mannitol 5% and 10%

ADD-Vantage® vials

PRIMAXIN I.V., as supplied in single dose ADD-Vantage® vials and reconstituted with the following diluents (see PREPARATION OF SOLUTION), maintains satisfactory potency for 4 hours at room temperature.

0.9% Sodium Chloride Injection
5% Dextrose Injection

PRIMAXIN I.V. should not be mixed with or physically added to other antibiotics. However, PRIMAXIN I.V. may be administered concomitantly with other antibiotics, such as aminoglycosides.

HOW SUPPLIED

PRIMAXIN I.V. is supplied as a sterile powder mixture in single dose containers including vials and ADD-Vantage® vials containing imipenem (anhydrous equivalent) and cilastatin sodium as follows:

No. 3514 — 250 mg imipenem equivalent and 250 mg cilastatin equivalent and 10 mg sodium bicarbonate as a buffer

NDC 0006-3514-58 in trays of 25 vials.

No. 3516 — 500 mg imipenem equivalent and 500 mg cilastatin equivalent and 20 mg sodium bicarbonate as a buffer

NDC 0006-3516-59 in trays of 25 vials.

No. 3551 — 250 mg imipenem equivalent and 250 mg cilastatin equivalent and 10 mg sodium bicarbonate as a buffer

NDC 0006-3551-58 in trays of 25 ADD-Vantage® vials.

No. 3552 — 500 mg imipenem equivalent and 500 mg cilastatin equivalent and 20 mg sodium bicarbonate as a buffer

NDC 0006-3552-59 in trays of 25 ADD-Vantage® vials.

REFERENCES

1. Clinical and Laboratory Standards Institute (CLSI). Methods for Dilution Antimicrobial Susceptibility Tests for Bacteria that Grow Aerobically; Approved Standard - 9th ed. CLSI document M07-A9. CLSI, 950 West Valley Rd., Suite 2500, Wayne, PA 19087, 2012.
2. CLSI. Performance Standards for Antimicrobial Susceptibility Testing; 22nd Informational Supplement. CLSI document M100-S22, 2012.
3. CLSI. Performance Standards for Antimicrobial Disk Susceptibility Tests; Approved Standard – 11th ed. CLSI document M02-A11, 2012.
4. CLSI. Methods for Antimicrobial Susceptibility Testing of Anaerobic Bacteria; Approved Standard – 8th ed. CLSI document M11-A8, 2012.

Merck Sharp & Dohme Corp., a subsidiary of
MERCK & CO., INC., Whitehouse Station, NJ 08889, USA

Revised: April 2012
USPI-IV-0787B1204R037

INSTRUCTIONS FOR USE OF PRIMAXIN® I.V.

(Imipenem and Cilastatin for Injection)
(Formerly called Imipenem-Cilastatin Sodium for Injection)
IN ADD-Vantage®[5] VIALS
For IV Use Only.

INSTRUCTIONS FOR USE

To Open Diluent Container:

Peel overwrap from the corner and remove container. Some opacity of the plastic due to moisture absorption during the sterilization process may be observed. This is normal and does not affect the solution quality or safety. The opacity will diminish gradually.

To Assemble Vial and Flexible Diluent Container:

(Use Aseptic Technique)

1. Remove the protective covers from the top of the vial and the vial port on the diluent container as follows:
   a. To remove the breakaway vial cap, swing the pull ring over the top of the vial and pull down far enough to start the opening. (SEE FIGURE 1.) Pull the ring approximately half way around the cap and then pull straight up to remove the cap. (SEE FIGURE 2.) NOTE: DO NOT ACCESS VIAL WITH SYRINGE.

[See figures 1 and 2 at top of next column]

   b. To remove the vial port cover, grasp the tab on the pull ring, pull up to break the three tie strings, then pull back to remove the cover. (SEE FIGURE 3.)
2. Screw the vial into the vial port until it will go no further. THE VIAL MUST BE SCREWED IN TIGHTLY TO ASSURE A SEAL. This occurs approximately ½ turn (180°) after the first audible click. (SEE FIGURE 4.) The clicking sound does not assure a seal; the vial must be turned as far as it will go. NOTE: Once vial is seated, do not attempt to remove. (SEE FIGURE 4.)

Fig. 1

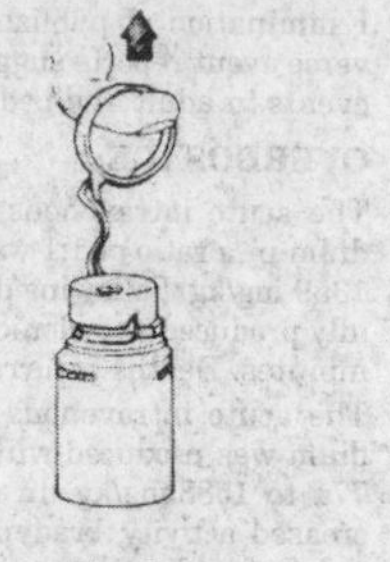

Fig. 2

3. Recheck the vial to assure that it is tight by trying to turn it further in the direction of assembly.
4. Label appropriately.

Fig. 3

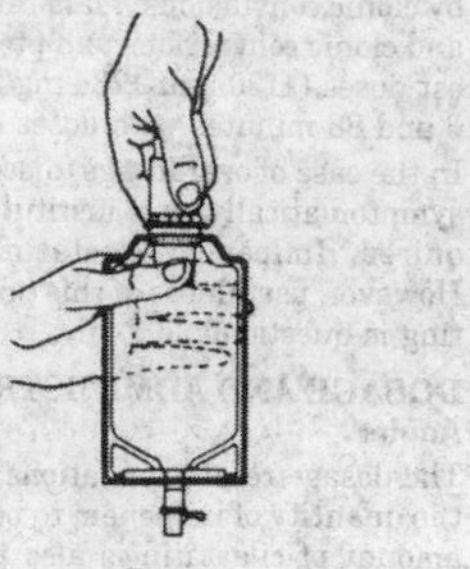

Fig. 4

To Prepare Admixture:

1. Squeeze the bottom of the diluent container gently to inflate the portion of the container surrounding the end of the drug vial.
2. With the other hand, push the drug vial down into the container telescoping the walls of the container. Grasp the inner cap of the vial through the walls of the container. (SEE FIGURE 5.)
3. Pull the inner cap from the drug vial. (SEE FIGURE 6.) Verify that the rubber stopper has been pulled out, allowing the drug and diluent to mix.
4. Mix container contents thoroughly and use within the specified time.

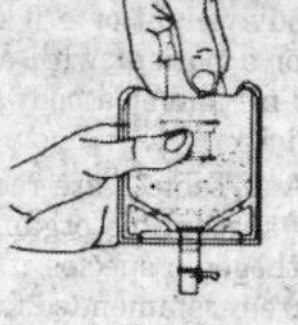

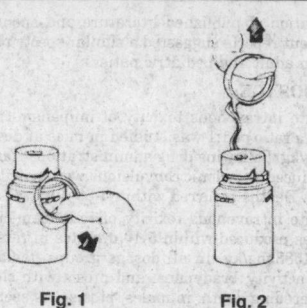

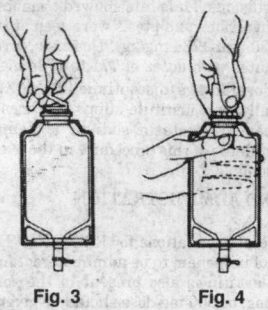

Fig. 5

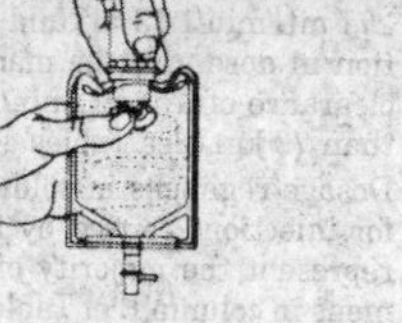

Fig. 6

Preparation for Administration:

(Use Aseptic Technique)

1. Confirm the activation and admixture of vial contents.
2. Check for leaks by squeezing container firmly. If leaks are found, discard unit as sterility may be impaired.
3. Close flow control clamp of administration set.
4. Remove cover from outlet port at bottom of container.
5. Insert piercing pin of administration set into port with a twisting motion until the pin is firmly seated. NOTE: See full directions on administration set carton.
6. Lift the free end of the hanger loop on the bottom of the vial, breaking the two tie strings. Bend the loop outward to lock it in the upright position, then suspend container from hanger.
7. Squeeze and release drip chamber to establish proper fluid level in chamber.
8. Open flow control clamp and clear air from set. Close clamp.
9. Attach set to venipuncture device. If device is not indwelling, prime and make venipuncture.
10. Regulate rate of administration with flow control clamp.

WARNING: Do not use flexible container in series connections.

Stability

PRIMAXIN I.V.[6] (Imipenem and Cilastatin for Injection) 250 or 500 single dose ADD-Vantage® vials should be prepared with ADD-Vantage® diluent containers containing 100 mL of either 0.9 percent Sodium Chloride Injection or 5 percent Dextrose Injection. When prepared with either of these diluents, PRIMAXIN I.V. (Imipenem and Cilastatin for Injection) maintains satisfactory potency for 4 hours at room temperature.

Before administering, see accompanying package circular for PRIMAXIN I.V. (Imipenem and Cilastatin for Injection).
Issued February 2010
Printed In USA
9805601

[6]Registered trademark of Merck Sharp & Dohme Corp., a subsidiary of **Merck & Co., Inc.**

PRINIVIL® TABLETS ℞

[pri-ni-vil]
(LISINOPRIL)

WARNING: FETAL TOXICITY
- **When pregnancy is detected, discontinue PRINIVIL as soon as possible.**
- **Drugs that act directly on the renin-angiotensin system can cause injury and death to the developing fetus. See WARNINGS, Fetal Toxicity**

DESCRIPTION

PRINIVIL® (Lisinopril), a synthetic peptide derivative, is an oral long-acting angiotensin converting enzyme inhibitor. Lisinopril is chemically described as (*S*)-1-[N^2-(1-carboxy-3-phenylpropyl)-L-lysyl]-L-proline dihydrate. Its empirical formula is $C_{21}H_{31}N_3O_5 \bullet 2H_2O$ and its structural formula is:

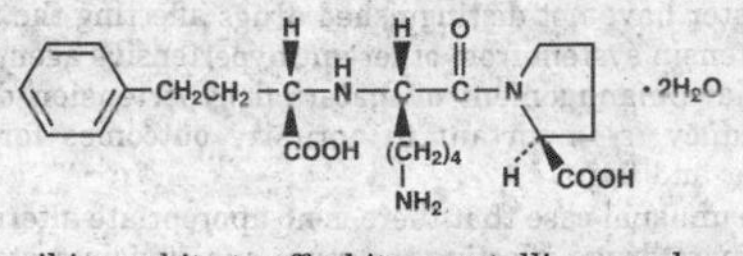

Lisinopril is a white to off-white, crystalline powder, with a molecular weight of 441.52. It is soluble in water and sparingly soluble in methanol and practically insoluble in ethanol.

PRINIVIL is supplied as 5 mg, 10 mg, and 20 mg tablets for oral administration. In addition to the active ingredient lisinopril, each tablet contains the following inactive ingredients: calcium phosphate, mannitol, magnesium stearate, and starch. The 10 mg and 20 mg tablets also contain iron oxide.

CLINICAL PHARMACOLOGY

Mechanism of Action

Lisinopril inhibits angiotensin converting enzyme (ACE) in human subjects and animals. ACE is a peptidyl dipeptidase that catalyzes the conversion of angiotensin I to the vasoconstrictor substance, angiotensin II. Angiotensin II also stimulates aldosterone secretion by the adrenal cortex. The beneficial effects of lisinopril in hypertension and heart failure appear to result primarily from suppression of the renin-angiotensin-aldosterone system. Inhibition of ACE results in decreased plasma angiotensin II which leads to decreased vasopressor activity and to decreased aldosterone secretion. The latter decrease may result in a small increase of serum potassium. In hypertensive patients with normal renal function treated with PRINIVIL alone for up to 24 weeks, the mean increase in serum potassium was approximately 0.1 mEq/L; however, approximately 15 percent of patients had increases greater than 0.5 mEq/L and approximately six percent had a decrease greater than 0.5 mEq/L. In the same study, patients treated with PRINIVIL and hydrochlorothiazide for up to 24 weeks had a mean decrease in serum potassium of 0.1 mEq/L; approximately 4 percent of patients had increases greater than 0.5 mEq/L and approximately 12 percent had a decrease greater than 0.5 mEq/L. (See PRECAUTIONS.) Removal of angiotensin II negative feedback on renin secretion leads to increased plasma renin activity.

ACE is identical to kininase, an enzyme that degrades bradykinin. Whether increased levels of bradykinin, a potent vasodepressor peptide, play a role in the therapeutic effects of PRINIVIL remains to be elucidated.

While the mechanism through which PRINIVIL lowers blood pressure is believed to be primarily suppression of the renin-angiotensin-aldosterone system, PRINIVIL is antihypertensive even in patients with low-renin hypertension. Although PRINIVIL was antihypertensive in all races studied, Black hypertensive patients (usually a low-renin hypertensive population) had a smaller average response to monotherapy than non-Black patients.

Concomitant administration of PRINIVIL and hydrochlorothiazide further reduced blood pressure in Black and non-Black patients and any racial difference in blood pressure response was no longer evident.

Pharmacokinetics and Metabolism

Adult Patients: Following oral administration of PRINIVIL, peak serum concentrations of lisinopril occur within about 7 hours, although there was a trend to a small delay in time taken to reach peak serum concentrations in acute myocardial infarction patients. Declining serum concentrations exhibit a prolonged terminal phase which does not contribute to drug accumulation. This terminal phase probably represents saturable binding to ACE and is not proportional to dose. Lisinopril does not appear to be bound to other serum proteins.

Lisinopril does not undergo metabolism and is excreted unchanged entirely in the urine. Based on urinary recovery, the mean extent of absorption of lisinopril is approximately 25 percent, with large inter-subject variability (6-60 percent) at all doses tested (5-80 mg). Lisinopril absorption is not influenced by the presence of food in the gastrointestinal tract. The absolute bioavailability of lisinopril is reduced to about 16 percent in patients with stable NYHA Class II-IV congestive heart failure, and the volume of distribution appears to be slightly smaller than that in normal subjects. The oral bioavailability of lisinopril in patients with acute myocardial infarction is similar to that in healthy volunteers.

Upon multiple dosing, lisinopril exhibits an effective half-life of accumulation of 12 hours.

Impaired renal function decreases elimination of lisinopril, which is excreted principally through the kidneys, but this decrease becomes clinically important only when the glomerular filtration rate is below 30 mL/min. Above this glomerular filtration rate, the elimination half-life is little changed. With greater impairment, however, peak and trough lisinopril levels increase, time to peak concentration increases and time to attain steady state is prolonged. Older patients, on average, have (approximately doubled) higher blood levels and area under the plasma concentration time curve (AUC) than younger patients. (See DOSAGE AND ADMINISTRATION.) Lisinopril can be removed by hemodialysis.

Studies in rats indicate that lisinopril crosses the blood-brain barrier poorly. Multiple doses of lisinopril in rats do not result in accumulation in any tissues. Milk of lactating rats contains radioactivity following administration of ^{14}C lisinopril. By whole body autoradiography, radioactivity was found in the placenta following administration of labeled drug to pregnant rats, but none was found in the fetuses.

Pediatric Patients: The pharmacokinetics of lisinopril were studied in 29 pediatric hypertensive patients between 6 years and 16 years with glomerular filtration rate >30 mL/min/1.73 m^2. After doses of 0.1 to 0.2 mg/kg, steady state peak plasma concentrations of lisinopril occurred within 6 hours and the extent of absorption based on urinary recovery was about 28%. These values are similar to those obtained previously in adults. The typical value of lisinopril oral clearance (systemic clearance/absolute bioavailability) in a child weighing 30 kg is 10 L/h, which increases in proportion to renal function.

Pharmacodynamics and Clinical Effects

Hypertension:

Adult Patients: Administration of PRINIVIL to patients with hypertension results in a reduction of supine and standing blood pressure to about the same extent with no compensatory tachycardia. Symptomatic postural hypotension is usually not observed although it can occur and should be anticipated in volume and/or salt-depleted patients. (See WARNINGS.) When given together with thiazide-type diuretics, the blood pressure lowering effects of the two drugs are approximately additive.

In most patients studied, onset of antihypertensive activity was seen at one hour after oral administration of an individual dose of PRINIVIL, with peak reduction of blood pressure achieved by six hours. Although an antihypertensive effect was observed 24 hours after dosing with recommended single daily doses, the effect was more consistent and the mean effect was considerably larger in some studies with doses of 20 mg or more than with lower doses. However, at all doses studied, the mean antihypertensive effect was substantially smaller 24 hours after dosing than it was six hours after dosing.

In some patients achievement of optimal blood pressure reduction may require two to four weeks of therapy.

The antihypertensive effects of PRINIVIL are maintained during long-term therapy. Abrupt withdrawal of PRINIVIL has not been associated with a rapid increase in blood pressure or a significant increase in blood pressure compared to pretreatment levels.

Two dose-response studies utilizing a once daily regimen were conducted in 438 mild to moderate hypertensive patients not on a diuretic. Blood pressure was measured 24 hours after dosing. An antihypertensive effect of PRINIVIL was seen with 5 mg in some patients. However, in both studies blood pressure reduction occurred sooner and was greater in patients treated with 10, 20, or 80 mg of PRINIVIL. In controlled clinical studies, PRINIVIL 20-80 mg has been compared in patients with mild to moderate hypertension to hydrochlorothiazide 12.5-50 mg and with atenolol 50-500 mg; and in patients with moderate to severe hypertension to metoprolol 100-200 mg. It was superior to hydrochlorothiazide in effects on systolic and diastolic blood pressure in a population that was ¾ Caucasian. PRINIVIL was approximately equivalent to atenolol and metoprolol in effects on diastolic blood pressure and had somewhat greater effects on systolic blood pressure.

PRINIVIL had similar effectiveness and adverse effects in younger and older (>65 years) patients. It was less effective in Blacks than in Caucasians.

In hemodynamic studies in patients with essential hypertension, blood pressure reduction was accompanied by a reduction in peripheral arterial resistance with little or no change in cardiac output and in heart rate. In a study in nine hypertensive patients, following administration of PRINIVIL, there was an increase in mean renal blood flow that was not significant. Data from several small studies are inconsistent with respect to the effect of PRINIVIL on glomerular filtration rate in hypertensive patients with normal renal function, but suggest that changes, if any, are not large.

In patients with renovascular hypertension PRINIVIL has been shown to be well tolerated and effective in controlling blood pressure (see PRECAUTIONS).

Pediatric Patients: In a clinical study involving 115 hypertensive pediatric patients 6 to 16 years of age, patients who weighed <50 kg received either 0.625, 2.5, or 20 mg of lisinopril daily and patients who weighed ≥50 kg received either 1.25, 5, or 40 mg of lisinopril daily. At the end of 2 weeks, lisinopril administered once daily lowered trough blood pressure in a dose-dependent manner with consistent antihypertensive efficacy demonstrated at doses >1.25 mg (0.02 mg/kg). This effect was confirmed in a withdrawal phase, where the diastolic pressure rose by about 9 mmHg more in patients randomized to placebo than it did in patients who were randomized to remain on the middle and high doses of lisinopril. The dose-dependent antihypertensive effect of lisinopril was consistent across several demographic subgroups: age, Tanner stage, gender, race. In this study, lisinopril was generally well-tolerated.

In the above pediatric studies, lisinopril was given either as tablets or in a suspension for those children and infants who were unable to swallow tablets or who required a lower dose than is available in tablet form (see DOSAGE AND ADMINISTRATION, Preparation of Suspension).

Heart Failure:

During baseline-controlled clinical trials, in patients receiving digitalis and diuretics, single doses of PRINIVIL resulted in decreases in pulmonary capillary wedge pressure, systemic vascular resistance and blood pressure accompanied by an increase in cardiac output and no change in heart rate.

In two placebo-controlled, 12-week clinical studies using doses of PRINIVIL up to 20 mg, PRINIVIL as adjunctive therapy to digitalis and diuretics improved the following signs and symptoms due to congestive heart failure: edema, rales, paroxysmal nocturnal dyspnea and jugular venous distention. In one of the studies beneficial response was also noted for: orthopnea, presence of third heart sound and the number of patients classified as NYHA Class III and IV. Exercise tolerance was also improved in this study. The effect of lisinopril on mortality in patients with heart failure has not been evaluated.

The once daily dosing for the treatment of congestive heart failure was the only dosage regimen used during clinical trial development and was determined by the measurement of hemodynamic responses.

Acute Myocardial Infarction:

The Gruppo Italiano per lo Studio della Sopravvivenza nell'Infarto Miocardico (GISSI - 3) study was a multicenter, controlled, randomized, unblinded clinical trial conducted in 19,394 patients with acute myocardial infarction admitted to a coronary care unit. It was designed to examine the effects of short-term (6 week) treatment with lisinopril, nitrates, their combination, or no therapy on short-term (6 week) mortality and on long-term death and markedly impaired cardiac function. Patients presenting within 24 hours of the onset of symptoms who were hemodynamically stable were randomized, in a 2 × 2 factorial design, to six weeks of either

1. PRINIVIL alone (n=4841),
2. nitrates alone (n=4869),
3. PRINIVIL plus nitrates (n=4841), or
4. open control (n=4843).

All patients received routine therapies, including thrombolytics (72%), aspirin (84%), and a beta-blocker (31%), as appropriate, normally utilized in acute myocardial infarction (MI) patients.

The protocol excluded patients with hypotension (systolic blood pressure ≤100 mmHg), severe heart failure, cardiogenic shock and renal dysfunction (serum creatinine >2 mg/dL and/or proteinuria >500 mg/24 h). Doses of PRINIVIL were adjusted as necessary according to protocol. (See DOSAGE AND ADMINISTRATION.)

Study treatment was withdrawn at six weeks except where clinical conditions indicated continuation of treatment.

The primary outcomes of the trial were the overall mortality at six weeks and a combined endpoint at six months after the myocardial infarction, consisting of the number of patients who died, had late (day 4) clinical congestive heart failure, or had extensive left ventricular damage defined as ejection fraction ≤35%, or an akinetic-dyskinetic [A-D] score ≥45%. Patients receiving PRINIVIL (n=9646) alone or with nitrates, had an 11 percent lower risk of death (2p [two-tailed]=0.04) compared to patients receiving no PRINIVIL (n=9672) (6.4 percent versus 7.2 percent, respectively) at six weeks. Although patients randomized to receive PRINIVIL for up to six weeks also fared numerically better on the combined end-point at 6 months, the open nature of the assessment of heart failure, substantial loss to follow-up echocardiography, and substantial excess use of lisinopril between 6 weeks and 6 months in the group randomized to 6 weeks of lisinopril, preclude any conclusion about this endpoint.

Patients with acute myocardial infarction, treated with PRINIVIL had a higher (9.0 percent versus 3.7 percent, respectively) incidence of persistent hypotension (systolic blood pressure <90 mmHg for more than 1 hour) and renal dysfunction (2.4 percent versus 1.1 percent) in-hospital and at six weeks (increasing creatinine concentration to over 3 mg/dL or a doubling or more of the baseline serum creatinine concentration). (See ADVERSE REACTIONS, ACUTE MYOCARDIAL INFARCTION.)

INDICATIONS AND USAGE

Hypertension

PRINIVIL is indicated for the treatment of hypertension. It may be used alone as initial therapy or concomitantly with other classes of antihypertensive agents.

Heart Failure

PRINIVIL is indicated as adjunctive therapy in the management of heart failure in patients who are not responding adequately to diuretics and digitalis.

Acute Myocardial Infarction

PRINIVIL is indicated for the treatment of hemodynamically stable patients within 24 hours of acute myocardial infarction, to improve survival. Patients should receive, as appropriate, the standard recommended treatments such as thrombolytics, aspirin and beta-blockers.

In using PRINIVIL, consideration should be given to the fact that another angiotensin converting enzyme inhibitor, captopril, has caused agranulocytosis, particularly in patients with renal impairment or collagen vascular disease, and that available data are insufficient to show that PRINIVIL does not have a similar risk. (See WARNINGS.)

In considering use of PRINIVIL, it should be noted that in controlled clinical trials ACE inhibitors have an effect on blood pressure that is less in Black patients than in non-Blacks. In addition, it should be noted that Black patients receiving ACE inhibitors have been reported to have a higher incidence of angioedema compared to non-Blacks (see WARNINGS, Anaphylactoid and Possibly Related Reactions, Head and Neck Angioedema).

CONTRAINDICATIONS

PRINIVIL is contraindicated in patients who are hypersensitive to this product and in patients with a history of angioedema related to previous treatment with an angiotensin converting enzyme inhibitor and in patients with hereditary or idiopathic angioedema.

Do not coadminister aliskiren with PRINIVIL in patients with diabetes.

WARNINGS

Anaphylactoid and Possibly Related Reactions

Presumably because angiotensin converting enzyme inhibitors affect the metabolism of eicosanoids and polypeptides, including endogenous bradykinin, patients receiving ACE inhibitors (including PRINIVIL) may be subject to a variety of adverse reactions, some of them serious.

Head and Neck Angioedema: Angioedema of the face, extremities, lips, tongue, glottis and/or larynx has been reported in patients treated with angiotensin converting enzyme inhibitors, including PRINIVIL. This may occur at any time during treatment. ACE inhibitors have been associated with a higher rate of angioedema in Black than in non-Black patients. In such cases PRINIVIL should be promptly discontinued and appropriate therapy and monitoring should be provided until complete and sustained resolution of signs and symptoms has occurred. Even in those instances where swelling of only the tongue is involved, without respiratory distress, patients may require prolonged observation since treatment with antihistamines and corticosteroids may not be sufficient. Very rarely, fatalities have been reported due to angioedema associated with laryngeal edema or tongue edema. Patients with involvement of the tongue, glottis or larynx are likely to experience airway obstruction, especially those with a history of airway surgery. **Where there is involvement of the tongue, glottis or larynx, likely to cause airway obstruction, appropriate therapy, e.g., subcutaneous epinephrine solution 1:1000 (0.3 mL to 0.5 mL) and/or measures necessary to ensure a patent airway, should be promptly provided.** (See ADVERSE REACTIONS.)

Patients with a history of angioedema unrelated to ACE inhibitor therapy may be at increased risk of angioedema while receiving an ACE inhibitor (see also INDICATIONS AND USAGE and CONTRAINDICATIONS).

Intestinal Angioedema: Intestinal angioedema has been reported in patients treated with ACE inhibitors. These patients presented with abdominal pain (with or without nausea or vomiting); in some cases there was no prior history of facial angioedema and C-1 esterase levels were normal. The angioedema was diagnosed by procedures including abdominal CT scan or ultrasound, or at surgery, and symptoms resolved after stopping the ACE inhibitor. Intestinal angioedema should be included in the differential diagnosis of patients on ACE inhibitors presenting with abdominal pain.

Anaphylactoid reactions during desensitization: Two patients undergoing desensitizing treatment with hymenoptera venom while receiving ACE inhibitors sustained life-threatening anaphylactoid reactions. In the same patients, these reactions were avoided when ACE inhibitors were temporarily withheld, but they reappeared upon inadvertent rechallenge.

Anaphylactoid reactions during membrane exposure: Sudden and potentially life-threatening anaphylactoid reactions have been reported in some patients dialyzed with high-flux membranes (e.g., AN69®) and treated concomitantly with an ACE inhibitor. In such patients, dialysis must be stopped immediately, and aggressive therapy for anaphylactoid reactions be initiated. Symptoms have not been relieved by antihistamines in these situations. In these patients, consideration should be given to using a different type of dialysis membrane or a different class of antihypertensive agent. Anaphylactoid reactions have also been reported in patients undergoing low-density lipoprotein apheresis with dextran sulfate absorption.

Hypotension

Excessive hypotension is rare in patients with uncomplicated hypertension treated with PRINIVIL alone.

Patients with heart failure given PRINIVIL commonly have some reduction in blood pressure with peak blood pressure reduction occurring 6 to 8 hours post dose, but discontinuation of therapy because of continuing symptomatic hypotension usually is not necessary when dosing instructions are followed; caution should be observed when initiating therapy. (See DOSAGE AND ADMINISTRATION.)

Patients at risk of excessive hypotension, sometimes associated with oliguria and/or progressive azotemia, and rarely with acute renal failure and/or death, include those with the following conditions or characteristics: heart failure with systolic blood pressure below 100 mmHg, hyponatremia, high-dose diuretic therapy, recent intensive diuresis or increase in diuretic dose, renal dialysis, or severe volume and/or salt depletion of any etiology. It may be advisable to eliminate the diuretic (except in patients with heart failure), reduce the diuretic dose or increase salt intake cautiously before initiating therapy with PRINIVIL in patients at risk for excessive hypotension who are able to tolerate such adjustments. (See PRECAUTIONS, Drug Interactions, and ADVERSE REACTIONS.)

Patients with acute myocardial infarction in the GISSI - 3 study had a higher (9.0 percent versus 3.7 percent) incidence of persistent hypotension (systolic blood pressure <90 mmHg for more than 1 hour) when treated with PRINIVIL. Treatment with PRINIVIL must not be initiated in acute myocardial infarction patients at risk of further serious hemodynamic deterioration after treatment with a vasodilator (e.g., systolic blood pressure of 100 mmHg or lower) or cardiogenic shock.

In patients at risk of excessive hypotension, therapy should be started under very close medical supervision and such patients should be followed closely for the first two weeks of treatment and whenever the dose of PRINIVIL and/or diuretic is increased. Similar considerations may apply to patients with ischemic heart or cerebrovascular disease, or in patients with acute myocardial infarction, in whom an excessive fall in blood pressure could result in a myocardial infarction or cerebrovascular accident.

If excessive hypotension occurs, the patient should be placed in the supine position and, if necessary, receive an intravenous infusion of normal saline. A transient hypotensive response is not a contraindication to further doses of PRINIVIL which usually can be given without difficulty once the blood pressure has stabilized. If symptomatic hypotension develops, a dose reduction or discontinuation of PRINIVIL or concomitant diuretic may be necessary.

Leukopenia/Neutropenia/Agranulocytosis

Another angiotensin converting enzyme inhibitor, captopril, has been shown to cause agranulocytosis and bone marrow depression, rarely in uncomplicated patients but more frequently in patients with renal impairment especially if they also have a collagen vascular disease. Available data from clinical trials of PRINIVIL are insufficient to show that PRINIVIL does not cause agranulocytosis at similar rates. Marketing experience has revealed rare cases of leukopenia/neutropenia and bone marrow depression in which a causal relationship to lisinopril cannot be excluded. Periodic monitoring of white blood cell counts in patients with collagen vascular disease and renal disease should be considered.

Hepatic Failure

Rarely, ACE inhibitors have been associated with a syndrome that starts with cholestatic jaundice or hepatitis and progresses to fulminant hepatic necrosis, and (sometimes) death. The mechanism of this syndrome is not understood. Patients receiving ACE inhibitors who develop jaundice or marked elevations of hepatic enzymes should discontinue the ACE inhibitor and receive appropriate medical follow-up.

Fetal Toxicity

Pregnancy Category D

Use of drugs that act on the renin-angiotensin system during the second and third trimesters of pregnancy reduces fetal renal function and increases fetal and neonatal morbidity and death. Resulting oligohydramnios can be associated with fetal lung hypoplasia and skeletal deformations. Potential neonatal adverse effects include skull hypoplasia, anuria, hypotension, renal failure, and death. When pregnancy is detected, discontinue PRINIVIL as soon as possible. These adverse outcomes are usually associated with the use of these drugs in the second and third trimester of pregnancy. Most epidemiologic studies examining fetal abnormalities after exposure to antihypertensive use in the first trimester have not distinguished drugs affecting the renin-angiotensin system from other antihypertensive agents. Appropriate management of maternal hypertension during pregnancy is important to optimize outcomes for both mother and fetus.

In the unusual case that there is no appropriate alternative therapy to drugs affecting the renin-angiotensin system for a particular patient, apprise the mother of the potential risk to the fetus. Perform serial ultrasound examinations to assess the intra-amniotic environment. If oligohydramnios is observed, discontinue PRINIVIL, unless it is considered lifesaving for the mother. Fetal testing may be appropriate, based on the week of pregnancy. Patients and physicians should be aware, however, that oligohydramnios may not appear until after the fetus has sustained irreversible injury. Closely observe infants with histories of *in utero* exposure to PRINIVIL for hypotension, oliguria, and hyperkalemia (see Precautions, Pediatric Use).

No teratogenic effects of lisinopril were seen in studies of pregnant mice, rats, and rabbits. On a body surface area basis, the doses used were 55 times, 33 times, and 0.15 times, respectively, the maximum recommended human daily dose (MRHDD).

PRECAUTIONS

General

Aortic Stenosis/Hypertrophic Cardiomyopathy: As with all vasodilators, lisinopril should be given with caution to patients with obstruction in the outflow tract of the left ventricle.

Impaired Renal Function: As a consequence of inhibiting the renin-angiotensin-aldosterone system, changes in renal function may be anticipated in susceptible individuals. In patients with severe congestive heart failure whose renal function may depend on the activity of the renin-angiotensin-aldosterone system, treatment with angiotensin converting enzyme inhibitors, including PRINIVIL, may be associated with oliguria and/or progressive azotemia and rarely with acute renal failure and/or death.

In hypertensive patients with unilateral or bilateral renal artery stenosis, increases in blood urea nitrogen and serum creatinine may occur. Experience with another angiotensin converting enzyme inhibitor suggests that these increases are usually reversible upon discontinuation of PRINIVIL and/or diuretic therapy. In such patients renal function should be monitored during the first few weeks of therapy.

Some patients with hypertension or heart failure with no apparent pre-existing renal vascular disease have developed increases in blood urea nitrogen and serum creatinine, usually minor and transient, especially when PRINIVIL has been given concomitantly with a diuretic. This is more likely to occur in patients with pre-existing renal impairment. Dosage reduction and/or discontinuation of the diuretic and/or PRINIVIL may be required.

Patients with acute myocardial infarction in the GISSI - 3 study, treated with PRINIVIL, had a higher (2.4 percent versus 1.1 percent) incidence of renal dysfunction in-hospital and at six weeks (increasing creatinine concentration to over 3 mg/dL or a doubling or more of the baseline serum creatinine concentration). In acute myocardial infarction, treatment with PRINIVIL should be initiated with caution in patients with evidence of renal dysfunction, defined as serum creatinine concentration exceeding 2 mg/dL. If renal dysfunction develops during treatment with

PRINIVIL (serum creatinine concentration exceeding 3 mg/dL or a doubling from the pre-treatment value) then the physician should consider withdrawal of PRINIVIL.

Evaluation of patients with hypertension, heart failure, or myocardial infarction should always include assessment of renal function. (See DOSAGE AND ADMINISTRATION.)

Hyperkalemia: In clinical trials hyperkalemia (serum potassium greater than 5.7 mEq/L) occurred in approximately 2.2 percent of hypertensive patients and 4.8 percent of patients with heart failure. In most cases these were isolated values which resolved despite continued therapy. Hyperkalemia was a cause of discontinuation of therapy in approximately 0.1 percent of hypertensive patients, 0.6 percent of patients with heart failure and 0.1 percent of patients with myocardial infarction. Risk factors for the development of hyperkalemia include renal insufficiency, diabetes mellitus, and the concomitant use of potassium-sparing diuretics, potassium supplements and/or potassium-containing salt substitutes. Hyperkalemia can cause serious, sometimes fatal, arrhythmias. PRINIVIL should be used cautiously, if at all, with these agents and with frequent monitoring of serum potassium. (See Drug Interactions.)

Cough: Presumably due to the inhibition of the degradation of endogenous bradykinin, persistent nonproductive cough has been reported with all ACE inhibitors, always resolving after discontinuation of therapy. ACE inhibitor-induced cough should be considered in the differential diagnosis of cough.

Surgery/Anesthesia: In patients undergoing major surgery or during anesthesia with agents that produce hypotension, PRINIVIL may block angiotensin II formation secondary to compensatory renin release. If hypotension occurs and is considered to be due to this mechanism, it can be corrected by volume expansion.

Information for Patients

Angioedema: Angioedema, including laryngeal edema, may occur at any time during treatment with angiotensin converting enzyme inhibitors, including lisinopril. Patients should be so advised and told to report immediately any signs or symptoms suggesting angioedema (swelling of face, extremities, eyes, lips, tongue, difficulty in swallowing or breathing) and to take no more drug until they have consulted with the prescribing physician.

Symptomatic Hypotension: Patients should be cautioned to report lightheadedness especially during the first few days of therapy. If actual syncope occurs, the patients should be told to discontinue the drug until they have consulted with the prescribing physician.

All patients should be cautioned that excessive perspiration and dehydration may lead to an excessive fall in blood pressure because of reduction in fluid volume. Other causes of volume depletion such as vomiting or diarrhea may also lead to a fall in blood pressure; patients should be advised to consult with their physician.

Hyperkalemia: Patients should be told not to use salt substitutes containing potassium without consulting their physician.

Hypoglycemia: Diabetic patients treated with oral antidiabetic agents or insulin starting an ACE inhibitor should be told to closely monitor for hypoglycemia, especially during the first month of combined use. (See Drug Interactions.)

Leukopenia/Neutropenia: Patients should be told to report promptly any indication of infection (e.g., sore throat, fever) which may be a sign of leukopenia/neutropenia.

Pregnancy: Female patients of childbearing age should be told about the consequences of exposure to PRINIVIL during pregnancy. Discuss treatment options with women planning to become pregnant. Patients should be asked to report pregnancies to their physicians as soon as possible.

Drug Interactions

Hypotension - Patients on Diuretic Therapy: Patients on diuretics, and especially those in whom diuretic therapy was recently instituted, may occasionally experience an excessive reduction of blood pressure after initiation of therapy with PRINIVIL. The possibility of hypotensive effects with PRINIVIL can be minimized by either discontinuing the diuretic or increasing the salt intake prior to initiation of treatment with PRINIVIL. If it is necessary to continue the diuretic, initiate therapy with PRINIVIL at a dose of 5 mg daily, and provide close medical supervision after the initial dose until blood pressure has stabilized. (See WARNINGS and DOSAGE AND ADMINISTRATION.) When a diuretic is added to the therapy of a patient receiving PRINIVIL, an additional antihypertensive effect is usually observed. Studies with ACE inhibitors in combination with diuretics indicate that the dose of the ACE inhibitor can be reduced when it is given with a diuretic. (See DOSAGE AND ADMINISTRATION.)

Antidiabetics: Epidemiological studies have suggested that concomitant administration of ACE inhibitors and antidiabetic medicines (insulins, oral hypoglycemic agents) may cause an increased blood-glucose-lowering effect with risk of hypoglycemia. This phenomenon appeared to be more likely to occur during the first weeks of combined treatment and in patients with renal impairment. In diabetic patients treated with oral antidiabetic agents or insulin, glycemic control should be closely monitored for hypoglycemia, especially during the first month of treatment with an ACE inhibitor.

Non-steroidal Anti-inflammatory Agents Including Selective Cyclooxygenase-2 (COX-2) Inhibitors: Reports suggest that NSAIDs including selective COX-2 inhibitors may diminish the antihypertensive effect of ACE inhibitors, including lisinopril. This interaction should be given consideration in patients taking NSAIDs or selective COX-2 inhibitors concomitantly with ACE inhibitors.

In a study in 36 patients with mild to moderate hypertension where the antihypertensive effects of PRINIVIL alone were compared to PRINIVIL given concomitantly with indomethacin, the use of indomethacin was associated with a reduced antihypertensive effect, although the difference between the two regimens was not significant.

In some patients with compromised renal function (e.g., elderly patients or patients who are volume-depleted including those on diuretic therapy) who are being treated with non-steroidal anti-inflammatory drugs, including selective COX-2 inhibitors, the co-administration of angiotensin II receptor antagonists or ACE inhibitors may result in a further deterioration of renal function, including possible acute renal failure. These effects are usually reversible.

These interactions should be considered in patients taking NSAIDS including selective COX-2 inhibitors concomitantly with diuretics and angiotensin II antagonists or ACE inhibitors. Therefore, monitor effects on blood pressure and renal function when administering the combination, especially in the elderly.

Dual Blockade of the Renin-angiotensin-aldosterone System: Dual blockade of the renin-angiotensin-aldosterone system (RAAS) with angiotensin receptor blockers, ACE inhibitors, or direct renin inhibitors (such as aliskiren) is associated with increased risks of hypotension, syncope, hyperkalemia, and changes in renal function (including acute renal failure) compared to monotherapy. Closely monitor blood pressure, renal function, and electrolytes in patients on PRINIVIL and other agents that affect the RAAS. Do not coadminister aliskiren with PRINIVIL in patients with diabetes. Avoid use of aliskiren with PRINIVIL in patients with renal impairment (GFR <60ml/min).

Other Agents: PRINIVIL has been used concomitantly with nitrates and/or digoxin without evidence of clinically significant adverse interactions. This included post myocardial infarction patients who were receiving intravenous or transdermal nitroglycerin. No clinically important pharmacokinetic interactions occurred when PRINIVIL was used concomitantly with propranolol or hydrochlorothiazide. The presence of food in the stomach does not alter the bioavailability of PRINIVIL.

Agents Increasing Serum Potassium: PRINIVIL attenuates potassium loss caused by thiazide-type diuretics. Use of PRINIVIL with potassium-sparing diuretics (e.g., spironolactone, eplerenone, triamterene, or amiloride), potassium supplements, or potassium-containing salt substitutes may lead to significant increases in serum potassium. Therefore, if concomitant use of these agents is indicated because of demonstrated hypokalemia, they should be used with caution and with frequent monitoring of serum potassium. Potassium-sparing agents should generally not be used in patients with heart failure who are receiving PRINIVIL.

Lithium: Lithium toxicity has been reported in patients receiving lithium concomitantly with drugs which cause elimination of sodium, including ACE inhibitors. Lithium toxicity was usually reversible upon discontinuation of lithium and the ACE inhibitor. It is recommended that serum lithium levels be monitored frequently if PRINIVIL is administered concomitantly with lithium.

Gold: Nitritoid reactions (symptoms include facial flushing, nausea, vomiting and hypotension) have been reported rarely in patients on therapy with injectable gold (sodium aurothiomalate) and concomitant ACE inhibitor therapy including PRINIVIL.

Carcinogenesis, Mutagenesis, Impairment of Fertility

There was no evidence of a tumorigenic effect when lisinopril was administered orally for 105 weeks to male and female rats at doses up to 90 mg/kg/day or for 92 weeks to male and female mice at doses up to 135 mg/kg/day. These doses are 10 times and 7 times, respectively, the maximum recommended human daily dose (MRHDD) when compared on a body surface area basis.

Lisinopril was not mutagenic in the Ames microbial mutagen test with or without metabolic activation. It was also negative in a forward mutation assay using Chinese hamster lung cells. Lisinopril did not produce single strand DNA breaks in an *in vitro* alkaline elution rat hepatocyte assay. In addition, lisinopril did not produce increases in chromosomal aberrations in an *in vitro* test in Chinese hamster ovary cells or in an *in vivo* study in mouse bone marrow.

There were no adverse effects on reproductive performance in male and female rats treated with up to 300 mg/kg/day of lisinopril (33 times the MRHDD when compared on a body surface area basis).

Nursing Mothers

Milk of lactating rats contains radioactivity following administration of ^{14}C lisinopril. It is not known whether this drug is secreted in human milk. Because many drugs are secreted in human milk, and because of the potential for serious adverse reactions in nursing infants from ACE inhibitors, a decision should be made whether to discontinue nursing or discontinue PRINIVIL, taking into account the importance of the drug to the mother.

Pediatric Use

Neonates with a history of *in utero* exposure to PRINIVIL:

If oliguria or hypotension occurs, direct attention toward support of blood pressure and renal perfusion. Exchange transfusions or dialysis may be required as a means of reversing hypotension and/or substituting for disordered renal function. Lisinopril, which crosses the placenta, has been removed from neonatal circulation by peritoneal dialysis with some clinical benefit, and theoretically may be removed by exchange transfusion, although there is no experience with the latter procedure.

Antihypertensive effects of PRINIVIL have been established in hypertensive pediatric patients aged 6 to 16 years. There are no data on the effect of PRINIVIL on blood pressure in pediatric patients under the age of 6 or in pediatric patients with glomerular filtration rate <30 mL/min/1.73 m^2 (see CLINICAL PHARMACOLOGY, Pharmacokinetics and Metabolism and Pharmacodynamics and Clinical Effects, and DOSAGE AND ADMINISTRATION).

Geriatric Use

Clinical studies of PRINIVIL in patients with hypertension and congestive heart failure did not include sufficient numbers of subjects aged 65 and over to determine whether they respond differently from younger subjects. Other clinical experience in this population has not identified differences in responses between the elderly and younger patients. In general, dose selection for an elderly patient should be cautious, usually starting at the low end of the dosing range, reflecting the greater frequency of decreased hepatic, renal, or cardiac function, and of concomitant disease or other drug therapy.

In a clinical study of PRINIVIL in patients with myocardial infarctions 4413 (47 percent) were 65 and over, while 1656 (18 percent) were 75 and over. No overall differences in safety or efficacy were observed between elderly and younger patients.

Other reported clinical experience has not identified differences in responses between elderly and younger patients, but greater sensitivity of some older individuals cannot be ruled out.

Pharmacokinetic studies indicate that maximum blood levels and area under plasma concentration time curve (AUC) are doubled in elderly patients.

This drug is known to be substantially excreted by the kidney, and the risk of toxic reactions to this drug may be greater in patients with impaired renal function. Because elderly patients are more likely to have decreased renal function, care should be taken in dose selection. Evaluation of patients with hypertension, congestive heart failure, or myocardial infarction should always include assessment of renal function. (See DOSAGE AND ADMINISTRATION.)

ADVERSE REACTIONS

PRINIVIL has been found to be generally well tolerated in controlled clinical trials involving 1969 patients with hypertension or heart failure. For the most part, adverse experiences were mild and transient.

HYPERTENSION

In clinical trials in patients with hypertension treated with PRINIVIL, discontinuation of therapy due to clinical adverse experiences occurred in 5.7 percent of patients. The overall frequency of adverse experiences could not be related to total daily dosage within the recommended therapeutic dosage range.

For adverse experiences occurring in greater than one percent of patients with hypertension treated with PRINIVIL or PRINIVIL plus hydrochlorothiazide in controlled clinical trials and more frequently with PRINIVIL and/or PRINIVIL plus hydrochlorothiazide than placebo, comparative incidence data are listed in table 1 below:

[See table 1 at top of next page]

Chest pain and back pain were also seen but were more common on placebo than PRINIVIL.

HEART FAILURE

In patients with heart failure treated with PRINIVIL for up to four years, discontinuation of therapy due to clinical adverse experiences occurred in 11.0 percent of patients. In controlled studies in patients with heart failure, therapy was discontinued in 8.1 percent of patients treated with PRINIVIL for up to 12 weeks, compared to 7.7 percent of patients treated with placebo for 12 weeks.

The following table lists those adverse experiences which occurred in greater than one percent of patients with heart failure treated with PRINIVIL or placebo for up to 12 weeks in controlled clinical trials and more frequently on PRINIVIL than placebo.

Table 1: Percent of Patients in Controlled Studies

	PRINIVIL (n=1349) Incidence (discontinuation)	PRINIVIL/ Hydrochlorothiazide (n=629) Incidence (discontinuation)	Placebo (n=207) Incidence (discontinuation)
Body As A Whole			
Fatigue	2.5 (0.3)	4.0 (0.5)	1.0 (0.0)
Asthenia	1.3 (0.5)	2.1 (0.2)	1.0 (0.0)
Orthostatic Effects	1.2 (0.0)	3.5 (0.2)	1.0 (0.0)
Cardiovascular			
Hypotension	1.2 (0.5)	1.6 (0.5)	0.5 (0.5)
Digestive			
Diarrhea	2.7 (0.2)	2.7 (0.3)	2.4 (0.0)
Nausea	2.0 (0.4)	2.5 (0.2)	2.4 (0.0)
Vomiting	1.1 (0.2)	1.4 (0.1)	0.5 (0.0)
Dyspepsia	0.9 (0.0)	1.9 (0.0)	0.0 (0.0)
Musculoskeletal			
Muscle Cramps	0.5 (0.0)	2.9 (0.8)	0.5 (0.0)
Nervous/Psychiatric			
Headache	5.7 (0.2)	4.5 (0.5)	1.9 (0.0)
Dizziness	5.4 (0.4)	9.2 (1.0)	1.9 (0.0)
Paresthesia	0.8 (0.1)	2.1 (0.2)	0.0 (0.0)
Decreased Libido	0.4 (0.1)	1.3 (0.1)	0.0 (0.0)
Vertigo	0.2 (0.1)	1.1 (0.2)	0.0 (0.0)
Respiratory			
Cough	3.5 (0.7)	4.6 (0.8)	1.0 (0.0)
Upper Respiratory Infection	2.1 (0.1)	2.7 (0.1)	0.0 (0.0)
Common Cold	1.1 (0.1)	1.3 (0.1)	0.0 (0.0)
Nasal Congestion	0.4 (0.1)	1.3 (0.1)	0.0 (0.0)
Influenza	0.3 (0.1)	1.1 (0.1)	0.0 (0.0)
Skin			
Rash	1.3 (0.4)	1.6 (0.2)	0.5 (0.5)
Urogenital			
Impotence	1.0 (0.4)	1.6 (0.5)	0.0 (0.0)

Table 2: Controlled Trials

	PRINIVIL (n=407) Incidence (discontinuation)	Placebo (n=155) Incidence (discontinuation)
	12 weeks	12 weeks
Body As A Whole		
Chest Pain	3.4 (0.2)	1.3 (0.0)
Abdominal Pain	2.2 (0.7)	1.9 (0.0)
Cardiovascular		
Hypotension	4.4 (1.7)	0.6 (0.6)
Digestive		
Diarrhea	3.7 (0.5)	1.9 (0.0)
Nervous/Psychiatric		
Dizziness	11.8 (1.2)	4.5 (1.3)
Headache	4.4 (0.2)	3.9 (0.0)
Respiratory		
Upper Respiratory Infection	1.5 (0.0)	1.3 (0.0)
Skin		
Rash	1.7 (0.5)	0.6 (0.6)

Also observed at >1% with PRINIVIL but more frequent or as frequent on placebo than PRINIVIL in controlled trials were asthenia, angina pectoris, nausea, dyspnea, cough and pruritus.

Worsening of heart failure, anorexia, increased salivation, muscle cramps, back pain, myalgia, depression, chest sound abnormalities and pulmonary edema were also seen in controlled clinical trials, but were more common on placebo than PRINIVIL.

ACUTE MYOCARDIAL INFARCTION

In the GISSI - 3 trial, in patients treated with PRINIVIL for six weeks following acute myocardial infarction, discontinuation of therapy occurred in 17.6 percent of patients.

Patients treated with PRINIVIL had a significantly higher incidence of hypotension and renal dysfunction compared with patients not taking PRINIVIL.

In the GISSI - 3 trial, hypotension (9.7 percent), renal dysfunction (2.0 percent), cough (0.5 percent), post-infarction angina (0.3 percent), skin rash and generalized edema (0.01 percent), and angioedema (0.01 percent) resulted in withdrawal of treatment. In elderly patients treated with PRINIVIL, discontinuation due to renal dysfunction was 4.2 percent.

Other clinical adverse experiences occurring in 0.3 to 1.0 percent of patients with hypertension or heart failure treated with PRINIVIL in controlled trials and rarer, serious, possibly drug-related events reported in uncontrolled studies or marketing experience are listed below, and within each category, are in order of decreasing severity:

Body as a Whole: Anaphylactoid reactions (see WARNINGS, Anaphylactoid and Possibly Related Reactions), syncope, orthostatic effects, chest discomfort, pain, pelvic pain, flank pain, edema, facial edema, virus infection, fever, chills, malaise.

Cardiovascular: Cardiac arrest; myocardial infarction or cerebrovascular accident, possibly secondary to excessive hypotension in high-risk patients (see WARNINGS, Hypotension); pulmonary embolism and infarction, arrhythmias (including ventricular tachycardia, atrial tachycardia, atrial fibrillation, bradycardia and premature ventricular contractions), palpitations, transient ischemic attacks, paroxysmal nocturnal dyspnea, orthostatic hypotension, decreased blood pressure, peripheral edema, vasculitis.

Digestive: Pancreatitis, hepatitis (hepatocellular or cholestatic jaundice) (see WARNINGS, Hepatic Failure), vomiting, gastritis, dyspepsia, heartburn, gastrointestinal cramps, constipation, flatulence, dry mouth.

Hematologic: Rare cases of bone marrow depression, hemolytic anemia, leukopenia/neutropenia, and thrombocytopenia.

Endocrine: Diabetes mellitus, syndrome of inappropriate antidiuretic hormone secretion (SIADH).

Metabolic: Weight loss, dehydration, fluid overload, gout, weight gain. Cases of hypoglycemia in diabetic patients on oral antidiabetic agents or insulin have been reported (see PRECAUTIONS, Drug Interactions).

Musculoskeletal: Arthritis, arthralgia, neck pain, hip pain, low back pain, joint pain, leg pain, knee pain, shoulder pain, arm pain, lumbago.

Nervous System/Psychiatric: Stroke, ataxia, memory impairment, tremor, peripheral neuropathy (e.g., dysesthesia), spasm, paresthesia, confusion, insomnia, somnolence, hypersomnia, irritability, and nervousness.

Respiratory System: Malignant lung neoplasms, hemoptysis, pulmonary infiltrates, eosinophilic pneumonitis, bronchospasm, asthma, pleural effusion, pneumonia, bronchitis, wheezing, orthopnea, painful respiration, epistaxis, laryngitis, sinusitis, pharyngeal pain, pharyngitis, rhinitis, rhinorrhea.

Skin: Urticaria, alopecia, herpes zoster, photosensitivity, skin lesions, skin infections, pemphigus, erythema, flushing, diaphoresis. Other severe skin reactions (including toxic epidermal necrolysis, Stevens-Johnson syndrome and cutaneous pseudolymphoma) have been reported rarely; causal relationship has not been established.

Special Senses: Visual loss, diplopia, blurred vision, tinnitus, photophobia, taste disturbances.

Urogenital System: Acute renal failure, oliguria, anuria, uremia, progressive azotemia, renal dysfunction (see PRECAUTIONS and DOSAGE AND ADMINISTRATION), pyelonephritis, dysuria, urinary tract infection, breast pain.

Miscellaneous: A symptom complex has been reported which may include a positive ANA, an elevated erythrocyte sedimentation rate, arthralgia/arthritis, myalgia, fever, vasculitis, eosinophilia and leukocytosis. Rash, photosensitivity or other dermatological manifestations may occur alone or in combination with these symptoms.

Angioedema: Angioedema has been reported in patients receiving PRINIVIL (0.1%) with an incidence higher in Black than in non-Black patients. Angioedema associated with laryngeal edema may be fatal. If angioedema of the face, extremities, lips, tongue, glottis and/or larynx occurs, treatment with PRINIVIL should be discontinued and appropriate therapy instituted immediately. In rare cases, intestinal angioedema has been reported with angiotensin converting enzyme inhibitors including lisinopril. (See WARNINGS.)

Hypotension: In hypertensive patients, hypotension occurred in 1.2 percent and syncope occurred in 0.1 percent of patients. Hypotension or syncope was a cause for discontinuation of therapy in 0.5 percent of hypertensive patients. In patients with heart failure, hypotension occurred in 5.3 percent and syncope occurred in 1.8 percent of patients. These adverse experiences were causes for discontinuation of therapy in 1.8 percent of these patients. In patients treated with PRINIVIL for six weeks after acute myocardial infarction, hypotension (systolic blood pressure ≤100 mmHg) resulted in discontinuation of therapy in 9.7 percent of the patients. (See WARNINGS.)

Fetal/Neonatal Morbidity and Mortality: See WARNINGS, Fetal/Neonatal Morbidity and Mortality.

Cough: See PRECAUTIONS, Cough.

Pediatric Patients: No relevant differences between the adverse experience profile for pediatric patients and that previously reported for adult patients were identified.

Clinical Laboratory Test Findings

Serum Electrolytes: Hyperkalemia (see PRECAUTIONS), hyponatremia.

Creatinine, Blood Urea Nitrogen: Minor increases in blood urea nitrogen and serum creatinine, reversible upon discontinuation of therapy, were observed in about 2.0 percent of patients with essential hypertension treated with PRINIVIL alone. Increases were more common in patients receiving concomitant diuretics and in patients with renal artery stenosis. (See PRECAUTIONS.) Reversible minor increases in blood urea nitrogen and serum creatinine were observed in approximately 11.6 percent of patients with heart failure on concomitant diuretic therapy. Frequently, these abnormalities resolved when the dosage of the diuretic was decreased.

Hemoglobin and Hematocrit: Small decreases in hemoglobin and hematocrit (mean decreases of approximately 0.4 g percent and 1.3 vol percent, respectively) occurred frequently in patients treated with PRINIVIL but were rarely of clinical importance in patients without some other cause of anemia. In clinical trials, less than 0.1 percent of patients discontinued therapy due to anemia. Hemolytic anemia has been reported; a causal relationship to lisinopril cannot be excluded.

Liver Function Tests: Rarely, elevations of liver enzymes and/or serum bilirubin have occurred (see WARNINGS, Hepatic Failure).

In hypertensive patients, 2.0 percent discontinued therapy due to laboratory adverse experiences, principally elevations in blood urea nitrogen (0.6 percent), serum creatinine (0.5 percent) and serum potassium (0.4 percent). In the heart failure trials, 3.4 percent of patients discontinued therapy due to laboratory adverse experiences, 1.8 percent due to elevations in blood urea nitrogen and/or creatinine and 0.6 percent due to elevations in serum potassium. In the myocardial infarction trial, 2.0 percent of patients receiving PRINIVIL discontinued therapy due to renal dysfunction (increasing creatinine concentration to over 3 mg/dL or a doubling or more of the baseline serum creatinine concentration); less than 1.0 percent of patients discontinued therapy due to other laboratory adverse experiences: 0.1 percent with hyperkalemia and less than 0.1 percent with hepatic enzyme alterations.

OVERDOSAGE

Following a single oral dose of 20 g/kg, no lethality occurred in rats and death occurred in one of 20 mice receiving the same dose. The most likely manifestation of overdosage would be hypotension, for which the usual treatment would be intravenous infusion of normal saline solution.

Lisinopril can be removed by hemodialysis. (See WARNINGS, Anaphylactoid reactions during membrane exposure.)

DOSAGE AND ADMINISTRATION

Hypertension

Initial Therapy: In patients with uncomplicated essential hypertension not on diuretic therapy, the recommended initial dose is 10 mg once a day. Dosage should be adjusted according to blood pressure response. The usual dosage range is 20 to 40 mg per day administered in a single daily dose. The antihypertensive effect may diminish toward the end of the dosing interval regardless of the administered dose, but most commonly with a dose of 10 mg daily. This can be evaluated by measuring blood pressure just prior to dosing to determine whether satisfactory control is being maintained for 24 hours. If it is not, an increase in dose should be considered. Doses up to 80 mg have been used but do not appear to give a greater effect. If blood pressure is not controlled with PRINIVIL alone, a low dose of a diuretic may be added. Hydrochlorothiazide 12.5 mg has been shown to provide an additive effect. After the addition of a diuretic, it may be possible to reduce the dose of PRINIVIL.

Diuretic Treated Patients: In hypertensive patients who are currently being treated with a diuretic, symptomatic hypotension may occur occasionally following the initial dose of PRINIVIL. The diuretic should be discontinued, if possible, for two to three days before beginning therapy with PRINIVIL to reduce the likelihood of hypotension. (See WARNINGS.) The dosage of PRINIVIL should be adjusted according to blood pressure response. If the patient's blood pressure is not controlled with PRINIVIL alone, diuretic therapy may be resumed as described above.

If the diuretic cannot be discontinued, an initial dose of 5 mg should be used under medical supervision for at least two hours and until blood pressure has stabilized for at least an additional hour. (See WARNINGS and PRECAUTIONS, Drug Interactions.)

Concomitant administration of PRINIVIL with potassium supplements, potassium salt substitutes, or potassium-sparing diuretics may lead to increases of serum potassium (see PRECAUTIONS).

Dosage Adjustment in Renal Impairment: The usual dose of PRINIVIL (10 mg) is recommended for patients with a creatinine clearance greater than 30 mL/min (serum creatinine of up to approximately 3 mg/dL). For patients with creatinine clearance greater than or equal to 10 mL/min and less than or equal to 30 mL/min (serum creatinine greater than or equal to 3 mg/dL), the first dose is 5 mg once daily. For patients with creatinine clearance less than 10 mL/min (usually on hemodialysis) the recommended initial dose is 2.5 mg. The dosage may be titrated upward until blood pressure is controlled or to a maximum of 40 mg daily.

Table 3

Renal Status	Creatinine-Clearance mL/min	Initial Dose mg/day
Normal Renal Function to Mild Impairment	>30 mL/min	10 mg
Moderate to Severe Impairment	≥10 ≤30 mL/min	5 mg
Dialysis Patients*	<10 mL/min	2.5 mg†

* See WARNINGS, Anaphylactoid reactions during membrane exposure.

† *Dosage or dosing interval should be adjusted depending on the blood pressure response.*

Heart Failure

PRINIVIL is indicated as adjunctive therapy with diuretics and (usually) digitalis. The recommended starting dose is 5 mg once a day.

When initiating treatment with lisinopril in patients with heart failure, the initial dose should be administered under medical observation, especially in those patients with low blood pressure (systolic blood pressure below 100 mmHg). The mean peak blood pressure lowering occurs six to eight hours after dosing. Observation should continue until blood pressure is stable. The concomitant diuretic dose should be reduced, if possible, to help minimize hypovolemia which may contribute to hypotension. (See WARNINGS and PRECAUTIONS, Drug Interactions.) The appearance of hypotension after the initial dose of PRINIVIL does not preclude subsequent careful dose titration with the drug, following effective management of the hypotension.

The usual effective dosage range is 5 to 20 mg per day administered as a single daily dose.

Dosage Adjustment in Patients with Heart Failure and Renal Impairment or Hyponatremia: In patients with heart failure who have hyponatremia (serum sodium less than 130 mEq/L) or moderate to severe renal impairment (creatinine clearance less than or equal to 30 mL/min or serum creatinine greater than 3 mg/dL), therapy with PRINIVIL should be initiated at a dose of 2.5 mg once a day under close medical supervision. (See WARNINGS and PRECAUTIONS, Drug Interactions.)

Acute Myocardial Infarction

In hemodynamically stable patients within 24 hours of the onset of symptoms of acute myocardial infarction, the first dose of PRINIVIL is 5 mg given orally, followed by 5 mg after 24 hours, 10 mg after 48 hours and then 10 mg of PRINIVIL once daily. Dosing should continue for six weeks. Patients should receive, as appropriate, the standard recommended treatments such as thrombolytics, aspirin and beta-blockers. Patients with a low systolic blood pressure (less than or equal to 120 mmHg) when treatment is started or during the first 3 days after the infarct should be given a lower 2.5 mg oral dose of PRINIVIL (see WARNINGS). If hypotension occurs (systolic blood pressure less than or equal to 100 mmHg) a daily maintenance dose of 5 mg may be given with temporary reductions to 2.5 mg if needed. If prolonged hypotension occurs (systolic blood pressure less than 90 mmHg for more than 1 hour) PRINIVIL should be withdrawn. For patients who develop symptoms of heart failure, see DOSAGE AND ADMINISTRATION, Heart Failure.

Dosage Adjustment in Patients with Myocardial Infarction with Renal Impairment: In acute myocardial infarction, treatment with PRINIVIL should be initiated with caution in patients with evidence of renal dysfunction, defined as serum creatinine concentration exceeding 2 mg/dL. No evaluation of dosage adjustment in myocardial infarction patients with severe renal impairment has been performed.

Use in Elderly

In general, blood pressure response and adverse experiences were similar in younger and older patients given similar doses of PRINIVIL. Pharmacokinetic studies, however, indicate that maximum blood levels and area under the plasma concentration time curve (AUC) are doubled in older patients, so that dosage adjustments should be made with particular caution.

Pediatric Hypertensive Patients 6 years of age and older

The usual recommended starting dose is 0.07 mg/kg once daily (up to 5 mg total). Dosage should be adjusted according to blood pressure response. Doses above 0.61 mg/kg (or in excess of 40 mg) have not been studied in pediatric patients. (See CLINICAL PHARMACOLOGY, Pharmacokinetics and Metabolism and Pharmacodynamics and Clinical Effects.)

PRINIVIL is not recommended in pediatric patients younger than 6 years or in pediatric patients with glomerular filtration rate less than 30 mL/min/1.73 m^2 (see CLINICAL PHARMACOLOGY, Pharmacokinetics and Metabolism, Pharmacodynamics and Clinical Effects and PRECAUTIONS).

Preparation of Suspension (for 200 mL of a 1.0 mg/mL suspension)

Add 10 mL of Purified Water USP to a polyethylene terephthalate (PET) bottle containing ten 20-mg tablets of PRINIVIL and shake for at least one minute. Add 30 mL of Bicitra® diluent and 160 mL of Ora-Sweet SF™ to the concentrate in the PET bottle and gently shake for several seconds to disperse the ingredients. The suspension should be stored at or below 25°C (77°F) and can be stored for up to four weeks. Shake the suspension before each use.

HOW SUPPLIED

No. 8110 — Tablets PRINIVIL, 5 mg, are white, oval shaped compressed tablets with code MSD 19 on one side and scored on the other side. They are supplied as follows:

NDC 0006-0019-54 unit of use bottles of 90.

No. 8111 — Tablets PRINIVIL, 10 mg, are light yellow, oval shaped compressed tablets with code MSD 106 on one side and scored on the other side. They are supplied as follows:

NDC 0006-0106-54 unit of use bottles of 90.

No. 8112 — Tablets PRINIVIL, 20 mg, are peach, oval shaped compressed tablets with code MSD 207 on one side and scored on the other side. They are supplied as follows:

NDC 0006-0207-54 unit of use bottles of 90.

Storage

Store at controlled room temperature, 15-30°C (59-86°F), and protect from moisture.

Dispense in a tight container, if product package is subdivided.

Manuf. for: Merck Sharp & Dohme Corp., a subsidiary of **MERCK & CO., INC.**, Whitehouse Station, NJ 08889, USA

Manufactured by:

MERCK SHARP & DOHME LTD.

Cramlington, Northumberland, UK NE23 3JU

Revised: 12/2012

USPI-T-05211212R008

Shown in Product Identification Guide, page 308

PROPECIA® ℞

[*Pro-pee-sha*]

(finasteride)

tablets for oral use

HIGHLIGHTS OF PRESCRIBING INFORMATION

These highlights do not include all the information needed to use PROPECIA safely and effectively. See full prescribing information for PROPECIA.

PROPECIA® (finasteride) tablets for oral use

Initial U.S. Approval: 1992

RECENT MAJOR CHANGES

Warnings and Precautions, Increased Risk of High-Grade Prostate Cancer with 5α-Reductase Inhibitors (5.3) 06/2011

INDICATIONS AND USAGE

- PROPECIA is a 5α-reductase inhibitor indicated for the treatment of male pattern hair loss (androgenetic alopecia) in **MEN ONLY** (1).
- PROPECIA is not indicated for use in women (1, 4, 5.1).

DOSAGE AND ADMINISTRATION

- PROPECIA may be administered with or without meals (2).
- One tablet (1 mg) taken once daily (2.1).
- In general, daily use for three months or more is necessary before benefit is observed (2.2).

DOSAGE FORMS AND STRENGTHS

1 mg tablets (3).

CONTRAINDICATIONS

- Pregnancy (4, 5.1, 8.1, 16).
- Hypersensitivity to any components of this product (4).

WARNINGS AND PRECAUTIONS

- PROPECIA is not indicated for use in women or pediatric patients (5.1, 5.4).
- Women should not handle crushed or broken PROPECIA tablets when they are pregnant or may potentially be pregnant due to potential risk to a male fetus (5.1, 8.1, 16).
- PROPECIA causes a decrease in serum PSA levels. Any confirmed increase in PSA while on PROPECIA may signal the presence of prostate cancer and should be evaluated, even if those values are still within the normal range for men not taking a 5α-reductase inhibitor (5.2).
- 5α-reductase inhibitors may increase the risk of high-grade prostate cancer (5.3, 6.1).

ADVERSE REACTIONS

The most common adverse reactions, reported in ≥1% of patients treated with PROPECIA and greater than in patients treated with placebo are: decreased libido, erectile dysfunction and ejaculation disorder (6.1).

To report SUSPECTED ADVERSE REACTIONS, contact Merck Sharp & Dohme Corp., a subsidiary of Merck & Co., Inc., at 1-877-888-4231 or FDA at 1-800-FDA-1088 or www.fda.gov/medwatch.

See 17 for PATIENT COUNSELING INFORMATION and FDA-approved patient labeling

Revised: 04/2012

FULL PRESCRIBING INFORMATION: CONTENTS*

*** Sections or subsections omitted from the full prescribing information are not listed**

FULL PRESCRIBING INFORMATION

1 INDICATIONS AND USAGE

PROPECIA® is indicated for the treatment of male pattern hair loss (androgenetic alopecia) in **MEN ONLY**.
Efficacy in bitemporal recession has not been established.
PROPECIA is not indicated for use in women.

2 DOSAGE AND ADMINISTRATION

PROPECIA may be administered with or without meals.
The recommended dose of PROPECIA is one tablet (1 mg) taken once daily.
In general, daily use for three months or more is necessary before benefit is observed. Continued use is recommended to sustain benefit, which should be re-evaluated periodically. Withdrawal of treatment leads to reversal of effect within 12 months.

3 DOSAGE FORMS AND STRENGTHS

PROPECIA tablets (1 mg) are tan, octagonal, film-coated convex tablets with "stylized P" logo on one side and PROPECIA on the other.

4 CONTRAINDICATIONS

PROPECIA is contraindicated in the following:

- Pregnancy. Finasteride use is contraindicated in women when they are or may potentially be pregnant. Because of the ability of Type II 5α-reductase inhibitors to inhibit the conversion of testosterone to 5α-dihydrotestosterone (DHT), finasteride may cause abnormalities of the external genitalia of a male fetus of a pregnant woman who receives finasteride. If this drug is used during pregnancy, or if pregnancy occurs while taking this drug, the pregnant woman should be apprised of the potential hazard to the male fetus. *[See Warnings and Precautions (5.1), Use in Specific Populations (8.1), How Supplied/Storage and Handling (16) and Patient Counseling Information (17.1).]*
  In female rats, low doses of finasteride administered during pregnancy have produced abnormalities of the external genitalia in male offspring.
- Hypersensitivity to any component of this medication.

5 WARNINGS AND PRECAUTIONS

5.1 Exposure of Women — Risk to Male Fetus

PROPECIA is not indicated for use in women. Women should not handle crushed or broken PROPECIA tablets when they are pregnant or may potentially be pregnant because of the possibility of absorption of finasteride and the subsequent potential risk to a male fetus. PROPECIA tablets are coated and will prevent contact with the active ingredient during normal handling, provided that the tablets have not been broken or crushed. *[See Indications and Usage (1), Contraindications (4), Use in Specific Populations (8.1), How Supplied/Storage and Handling (16) and Patient Counseling Information (17.1).]*

5.2 Effects on Prostate Specific Antigen (PSA)

In clinical studies with PROPECIA (finasteride, 1 mg) in men 18-41 years of age, the mean value of serum prostate specific antigen (PSA) decreased from 0.7 ng/mL at baseline to 0.5 ng/mL at Month 12. Further, in clinical studies with PROSCAR (finasteride, 5 mg) when used in older men who have benign prostatic hyperplasia (BPH), PSA levels are decreased by approximately 50%. Other studies with PROSCAR showed it may also cause decreases in serum PSA in the presence of prostate cancer. These findings should be taken into account for proper interpretation of serum PSA when evaluating men treated with finasteride. Any confirmed increase from the lowest PSA value while on PROPECIA may signal the presence of prostate cancer and should be evaluated, even if PSA levels are still within the normal range for men not taking a 5α-reductase inhibitor. Non-compliance to therapy with PROPECIA may also affect PSA test results.

5.3 Increased Risk of High-Grade Prostate Cancer with 5α-Reductase Inhibitors

Men aged 55 and over with a normal digital rectal examination and PSA ≤3.0 ng/mL at baseline taking finasteride 5 mg/day (5 times the dose of PROPECIA) in the 7-year Prostate Cancer Prevention Trial (PCPT) had an increased risk of Gleason score 8-10 prostate cancer (finasteride 1.8% vs placebo 1.1%). *[See Adverse Reactions (6.1).]* Similar results were observed in a 4-year placebo-controlled clinical trial with another 5α-reductase inhibitor (dutasteride, AVODART) (1% dutasteride vs 0.5% placebo). 5α-reductase inhibitors may increase the risk of development of high-grade prostate cancer. Whether the effect of 5α-reductase inhibitors to reduce prostate volume, or study-related factors, impacted the results of these studies has not been established.

5.4 Pediatric Patients

PROPECIA is not indicated for use in pediatric patients *[see Use in Specific Populations (8.4)]*.

6 ADVERSE REACTIONS

6.1 Clinical Trials Experience

Because clinical trials are conducted under widely varying conditions, adverse reaction rates observed in the clinical trials of a drug cannot be directly compared to rates in the clinical trials of another drug and may not reflect the rates observed in clinical practice.

Clinical Studies for PROPECIA (finasteride 1 mg) in the Treatment of Male Pattern Hair Loss

In three controlled clinical trials for PROPECIA of 12-month duration, 1.4% of patients taking PROPECIA (n=945) were discontinued due to adverse experiences that were considered to be possibly, probably or definitely drug-related (1.6% for placebo; n=934).
Clinical adverse experiences that were reported as possibly, probably or definitely drug-related in ≥1% of patients treated with PROPECIA or placebo are presented in Table 1.

TABLE 1 Drug-Related Adverse Experiences for PROPECIA (finasteride 1 mg) in Year 1 (%) MALE PATTERN HAIR LOSS

	PROPECIA N=945	Placebo N=934
Decreased Libido	1.8	1.3
Erectile Dysfunction	1.3	0.7
Ejaculation Disorder *(Decreased Volume of Ejaculate)*	1.2 *(0.8)*	0.7 *(0.4)*
Discontinuation due to drug-related sexual adverse experiences	1.2	0.9

Integrated analysis of clinical adverse experiences showed that during treatment with PROPECIA, 36 (3.8%) of 945 men had reported one or more of these adverse experiences as compared to 20 (2.1%) of 934 men treated with placebo (p=0.04). Resolution occurred in men who discontinued therapy with PROPECIA due to these side effects and in most of those who continued therapy. The incidence of each of the above adverse experiences decreased to ≤0.3% by the fifth year of treatment with PROPECIA.
In a study of finasteride 1 mg daily in healthy men, a median decrease in ejaculate volume of 0.3 mL (-11%) compared with 0.2 mL (-8%) for placebo was observed after 48 weeks of treatment. Two other studies showed that finasteride at 5 times the dosage of PROPECIA (5 mg daily) produced significant median decreases of approximately 0.5 mL (-25%) compared to placebo in ejaculate volume, but this was reversible after discontinuation of treatment.
In the clinical studies with PROPECIA, the incidences for breast tenderness and enlargement, hypersensitivity reactions, and testicular pain in finasteride-treated patients were not different from those in patients treated with placebo.

Controlled Clinical Trials and Long-Term Open Extension Studies for PROSCAR® (finasteride 5 mg) and AVODART (dutasteride) in the Treatment of Benign Prostatic Hyperplasia

In the PROSCAR Long-Term Efficacy and Safety Study (PLESS), a 4-year controlled clinical study, 3040 patients between the ages of 45 and 78 with symptomatic BPH and an enlarged prostate were evaluated for safety over a period of 4 years (1524 on PROSCAR 5 mg/day and 1516 on placebo). 3.7% (57 patients) treated with PROSCAR 5 mg and 2.1% (32 patients) treated with placebo discontinued therapy as a result of adverse reactions related to sexual function, which are the most frequently reported adverse reactions.
Table 2 presents the only clinical adverse reactions considered possibly, probably or definitely drug related by the investigator, for which the incidence on PROSCAR was ≥1% and greater than placebo over the 4 years of the study. In years 2-4 of the study, there was no significant difference between treatment groups in the incidences of impotence, decreased libido and ejaculation disorder.
[See table 2 above]

TABLE 2 Drug-Related Adverse Experiences for PROSCAR (finasteride 5 mg) BENIGN PROSTATIC HYPERPLASIA

	Year 1 (%)		Years 2, 3 and 4* (%)	
	Finasteride, 5 mg	Placebo	Finasteride, 5 mg	Placebo
Impotence	8.1	3.7	5.1	5.1
Decreased Libido	6.4	3.4	2.6	2.6
Decreased Volume of Ejaculate	3.7	0.8	1.5	0.5
Ejaculation Disorder	0.8	0.1	0.2	0.1
Breast Enlargement	0.5	0.1	1.8	1.1
Breast Tenderness	0.4	0.1	0.7	0.3
Rash	0.5	0.2	0.5	0.1

N = 1524 and 1516, finasteride vs placebo, respectively
* Combined Years 2-4

The adverse experience profiles in the 1-year, placebo-controlled, Phase III BPH studies and the 5-year open extensions with PROSCAR 5 mg and PLESS were similar.
There is no evidence of increased sexual adverse experiences with increased duration of treatment with PROSCAR 5 mg. New reports of drug-related sexual adverse experiences decreased with duration of therapy.
During the 4- to 6-year placebo- and comparator-controlled Medical Therapy of Prostatic Symptoms (MTOPS) study that enrolled 3047 men, there were 4 cases of breast cancer in men treated with PROSCAR but no cases in men not treated with PROSCAR. During the 4-year placebo-controlled PLESS study that enrolled 3040 men, there were 2 cases of breast cancer in placebo-treated men, but no cases were reported in men treated with PROSCAR.
During the 7-year placebo-controlled Prostate Cancer Prevention Trial (PCPT) that enrolled 18,882 men, there was 1 case of breast cancer in men treated with PROSCAR, and 1 case of breast cancer in men treated with placebo. The relationship between long-term use of finasteride and male breast neoplasia is currently unknown.
The PCPT trial was a 7-year randomized, double-blind, placebo-controlled trial that enrolled 18,882 healthy men ≥55 years of age with a normal digital rectal examination and a PSA ≤3.0 ng/mL. Men received either PROSCAR (finasteride 5 mg) or placebo daily. Patients were evaluated annually with PSA and digital rectal exams. Biopsies were performed for elevated PSA, an abnormal digital rectal exam, or the end of study. The incidence of Gleason score 8-10 prostate cancer was higher in men treated with finasteride (1.8%) than in those treated with placebo (1.1%). In a 4-year placebo-controlled clinical trial with another 5α-reductase inhibitor [AVODART (dutasteride)], similar results for Gleason score 8-10 prostate cancer were observed (1% dutasteride vs 0.5% placebo). The clinical significance of these findings with respect to use of PROPECIA by men is unknown.
No clinical benefit has been demonstrated in patients with prostate cancer treated with PROSCAR. PROSCAR is not approved to reduce the risk of developing prostate cancer.

6.2 Postmarketing Experience

The following adverse reactions have been identified during post approval use of PROPECIA. Because these reactions are reported voluntarily from a population of uncertain size, it is not always possible to reliably estimate their frequency or establish a causal relationship to drug exposure:

Hypersensitivity Reaction: hypersensitivity reactions including rash, pruritus, urticaria, and swelling of the lips and face;

Reproductive System: sexual dysfunction that continued after discontinuation of treatment, including erectile dysfunction, libido disorders, ejaculation disorders, and orgasm disorders; male infertility and/or poor seminal quality (normalization or improvement of seminal quality has been reported after discontinuation of finasteride); testicular pain. *[See Adverse Reactions (6.1).]*

Neoplasms: male breast cancer;

Breast disorders: breast tenderness and enlargement;

Nervous System / Psychiatric: depression

7 DRUG INTERACTIONS

7.1 Cytochrome P450-Linked Drug Metabolizing Enzyme System

No drug interactions of clinical importance have been identified. Finasteride does not appear to affect the cytochrome P450-linked drug-metabolizing enzyme system. Compounds that have been tested in man include antipyrine, digoxin, propranolol, theophylline, and warfarin and no clinically meaningful interactions were found.

7.2 Other Concomitant Therapy

Although specific interaction studies were not performed, finasteride doses of 1 mg or more were concomitantly used in clinical studies with acetaminophen, acetylsalicylic acid, α-blockers, analgesics, angiotensin-converting enzyme (ACE) inhibitors, anticonvulsants, benzodiazepines, beta blockers, calcium-channel blockers, cardiac nitrates, diuretics, H_2 antagonists, HMG-CoA reductase inhibitors, prostaglandin synthetase inhibitors (also referred to as NSAIDs), and quinolone anti-infectives without evidence of clinically significant adverse interactions.

8 USE IN SPECIFIC POPULATIONS

8.1 Pregnancy

Pregnancy Category X *[see Contraindications (4)]*. PROPECIA is contraindicated for use in women who are or may become pregnant. PROPECIA is a Type II 5α-reductase inhibitor that prevents conversion of testosterone to 5α-dihydrotestosterone (DHT), a hormone necessary for normal development of male genitalia. In animal studies, finasteride caused abnormal development of external genitalia in male fetuses. If this drug is used during pregnancy, or if the patient becomes pregnant while taking this drug, the patient should be apprised of the potential hazard to the male fetus.

Abnormal male genital development is an expected consequence when conversion of testosterone to 5α-dihydrotestosterone (DHT) is inhibited by 5α-reductase inhibitors. These outcomes are similar to those reported in male infants with genetic 5α-reductase deficiency. Women could be exposed to finasteride through contact with crushed or broken PROPECIA tablets or semen from a male partner taking PROPECIA. With regard to finasteride exposure through the skin, PROPECIA tablets are coated and will prevent skin contact with finasteride during normal handling if the tablets have not been crushed or broken. Women who are pregnant or may become pregnant should not handle crushed or broken PROPECIA tablets because of possible exposure of a male fetus. If a pregnant woman comes in contact with crushed or broken PROPECIA tablets, the contact area should be washed immediately with soap and water. With regard to potential finasteride exposure through semen, a study has been conducted in men receiving PROPECIA 1 mg/day that measured finasteride concentrations in semen *[see Clinical Pharmacology (12.3)]*.

In an embryo-fetal development study, pregnant rats received finasteride during the period of major organogenesis (gestation days 6 to 17). At maternal doses of oral finasteride approximately 1 to 684 times the recommended human dose (RHD) of 1 mg/day (based on AUC at animal doses of 0.1 to 100 mg/kg/day) there was a dose-dependent increase in hypospadias that occurred in 3.6 to 100% of male offspring. Exposure multiples were estimated using data from nonpregnant rats. Days 16 to 17 of gestation is a critical period in male fetal rats for differentiation of the external genitalia. At oral maternal doses approximately 0.2 times the RHD (based on AUC at animal dose of 0.03 mg/kg/day), male offspring had decreased prostatic and seminal vesicular weights, delayed preputial separation and transient nipple development. Decreased anogenital distance occurred in male offspring of pregnant rats that received approximately 0.02 times the RHD (based on AUC at animal dose of 0.003 mg/kg/day). No abnormalities were observed in female offspring exposed to any dose of finasteride *in utero*.

No developmental abnormalities were observed in the offspring of untreated females mated with finasteride-treated male rats that received approximately 488 times the RHD (based on AUC at animal dose of 80 mg/kg/day). Slightly decreased fertility was observed in male offspring after administration of about 20 times the RHD (based on AUC at animal dose of 3 mg/kg/day) to female rats during late gestation and lactation. No effects on fertility were seen in female offspring under these conditions.

No evidence of male external genital malformations or other abnormalities were observed in rabbit fetuses exposed to finasteride during the period of major organogenesis (gestation days 6-18) at maternal doses up to 100 mg/kg/day (finasteride exposure levels were not measured in rabbits). However, this study may not have included the critical period for finasteride effects on development of male external genitalia in the rabbit.

The fetal effects of maternal finasteride exposure during the period of embryonic and fetal development were evaluated in the rhesus monkey (gestation days 20-100), in a species and development period more predictive of specific effects in humans than the studies in rats and rabbits. Intravenous administration of finasteride to pregnant monkeys at doses as high as 800 ng/day (estimated maximal blood concentration of 1.86 ng/mL or about 930 times the highest estimated exposure of pregnant women to finasteride from semen of men taking 1 mg/day) resulted in no abnormalities in male fetuses. In confirmation of the relevance of the rhesus model for human fetal development, oral administration of a dose of finasteride (2 mg/kg/day or approximately 120,000 times the highest estimated blood levels of finasteride from semen of men taking 1 mg/day) to pregnant monkeys resulted in external genital abnormalities in male fetuses. No other abnormalities were observed in male fetuses and no finasteride-related abnormalities were observed in female fetuses at any dose.

8.3 Nursing Mothers

PROPECIA is not indicated for use in women.

It is not known whether finasteride is excreted in human milk.

8.4 Pediatric Use

PROPECIA is not indicated for use in pediatric patients. Safety and effectiveness in pediatric patients have not been established.

8.5 Geriatric Use

Clinical efficacy studies with PROPECIA did not include subjects aged 65 and over. Based on the pharmacokinetics of finasteride 5 mg, no dosage adjustment is necessary in the elderly for PROPECIA *[see Clinical Pharmacology (12.3)]*. However the efficacy of PROPECIA in the elderly has not been established.

8.6 Hepatic Impairment

Caution should be exercised in the administration of PROPECIA in those patients with liver function abnormalities, as finasteride is metabolized extensively in the liver *[see Clinical Pharmacology (12.3)]*.

8.7 Renal Impairment

No dosage adjustment is necessary in patients with renal impairment *[see Clinical Pharmacology (12.3)]*.

10 OVERDOSAGE

In clinical studies, single doses of finasteride up to 400 mg and multiple doses of finasteride up to 80 mg/day for three months did not result in adverse reactions. Until further experience is obtained, no specific treatment for an overdose with finasteride can be recommended.

Significant lethality was observed in male and female mice at single oral doses of 1500 mg/m^2 (500 mg/kg) and in female and male rats at single oral doses of 2360 mg/m^2 (400 mg/kg) and 5900 mg/m^2 (1000 mg/kg), respectively.

11 DESCRIPTION

PROPECIA (finasteride) tablets contain finasteride as the active ingredient. Finasteride, a synthetic 4-azasteroid compound, is a specific inhibitor of steroid Type II 5α-reductase, an intracellular enzyme that converts the androgen testosterone into 5α-dihydrotestosterone (DHT).

The chemical name of finasteride is *N-tert*-Butyl-3-oxo-4-aza-5α-androst-1-ene-17β-carboxamide. The empirical formula of finasteride is $C_{23}H_{36}N_2O_2$ and its molecular weight is 372.55. Its structural formula is:

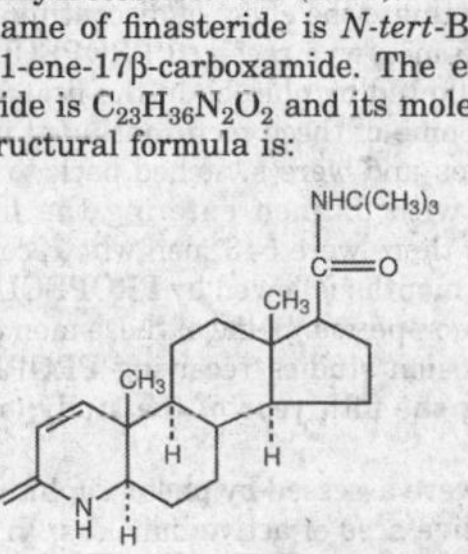

Finasteride is a white crystalline powder with a melting point near 250°C. It is freely soluble in chloroform and in lower alcohol solvents but is practically insoluble in water.

PROPECIA (finasteride) tablets are film-coated tablets for oral administration. Each tablet contains 1 mg of finasteride and the following inactive ingredients: lactose monohydrate, microcrystalline cellulose, pregelatinized starch, sodium starch glycolate, hydroxypropyl methylcellulose, hydroxypropyl cellulose, titanium dioxide, magnesium stearate, talc, docusate sodium, yellow ferric oxide, and red ferric oxide.

12 CLINICAL PHARMACOLOGY

12.1 Mechanism of Action

Finasteride is a competitive and specific inhibitor of Type II 5α-reductase, an intracellular enzyme that converts the androgen testosterone into DHT. Two distinct isozymes are found in mice, rats, monkeys, and humans: Type I and II. Each of these isozymes is differentially expressed in tissues and developmental stages. In humans, Type I 5α-reductase is predominant in the sebaceous glands of most regions of skin, including scalp, and liver. Type I 5α-reductase is responsible for approximately one-third of circulating DHT. The Type II 5α-reductase isozyme is primarily found in prostate, seminal vesicles, epididymides, and hair follicles as well as liver, and is responsible for two-thirds of circulating DHT.

In humans, the mechanism of action of finasteride is based on its preferential inhibition of the Type II isozyme. Using native tissues (scalp and prostate), *in vitro* binding studies examining the potential of finasteride to inhibit either isozyme revealed a 100-fold selectivity for the human Type II 5α-reductase over Type I isozyme (IC_{50}=500 and 4.2 nM for Type I and II, respectively). For both isozymes, the inhibition by finasteride is accompanied by reduction of the inhibitor to dihydrofinasteride and adduct formation with NADP+. The turnover for the enzyme complex is slow ($t_{1/2}$ approximately 30 days for the Type II enzyme complex and 14 days for the Type I complex). Inhibition of Type II 5α-reductase blocks the peripheral conversion of testosterone to DHT, resulting in significant decreases in serum and tissue DHT concentrations.

In men with male pattern hair loss (androgenetic alopecia), the balding scalp contains miniaturized hair follicles and increased amounts of DHT compared with hairy scalp. Administration of finasteride decreases scalp and serum DHT concentrations in these men. The relative contributions of these reductions to the treatment effect of finasteride have not been defined. By this mechanism, finasteride appears to interrupt a key factor in the development of androgenetic alopecia in those patients genetically predisposed.

12.2 Pharmacodynamics

Finasteride produces a rapid reduction in serum DHT concentration, reaching 65% suppression within 24 hours of oral dosing with a 1-mg tablet. Mean circulating levels of testosterone and estradiol were increased by approximately 15% as compared to baseline, but these remained within the physiologic range.

Finasteride has no affinity for the androgen receptor and has no androgenic, antiandrogenic, estrogenic, antiestrogenic, or progestational effects. In studies with finasteride, no clinically meaningful changes in luteinizing hormone (LH), follicle-stimulating hormone (FSH) or prolactin were detected. In healthy volunteers, treatment with finasteride did not alter the response of LH and FSH to gonadotropin-releasing hormone indicating that the hypothalamic-pituitary-testicular axis was not affected. Finasteride had no effect on circulating levels of cortisol, thyroid-stimulating hormone, or thyroxine, nor did it affect the plasma lipid profile (e.g., total cholesterol, low-density lipoproteins, high-density lipoproteins and triglycerides) or bone mineral density.

12.3 Pharmacokinetics

Absorption

In a study in 15 healthy young male subjects, the mean bioavailability of finasteride 1-mg tablets was 65% (range 26-170%), based on the ratio of area under the curve (AUC) relative to an intravenous (IV) reference dose. At steady state following dosing with 1 mg/day (n=12), maximum finasteride plasma concentration averaged 9.2 ng/mL (range, 4.9-13.7 ng/mL) and was reached 1 to 2 hours postdose; $AUC_{(0\text{-}24\ hr)}$ was 53 ng·hr/mL (range, 20-154 ng·hr/mL). Bioavailability of finasteride was not affected by food.

Distribution

Mean steady-state volume of distribution was 76 liters (range, 44-96 liters; n=15). Approximately 90% of circulating finasteride is bound to plasma proteins. There is a slow accumulation phase for finasteride after multiple dosing.

Finasteride has been found to cross the blood-brain barrier. Semen levels have been measured in 35 men taking finasteride 1 mg/day for 6 weeks. In 60% (21 of 35) of the samples, finasteride levels were undetectable (<0.2 ng/mL). The mean finasteride level was 0.26 ng/mL and the highest level measured was 1.52 ng/mL. Using the highest semen level measured and assuming 100% absorption from a 5-mL ejaculate per day, human exposure through vaginal absorption would be up to 7.6 ng per day, which is 650-fold less than the dose of finasteride (5 µg) that had no effect on circulating DHT levels in men. *[See Use in Specific Populations (8.1).]*

Metabolism

Finasteride is extensively metabolized in the liver, primarily via the cytochrome P450 3A4 enzyme subfamily. Two metabolites, the t-butyl side chain monohydroxylated and monocarboxylic acid metabolites, have been identified that possess no more than 20% of the 5α-reductase inhibitory activity of finasteride.

Excretion

Following intravenous infusion in healthy young subjects (n=15), mean plasma clearance of finasteride was 165 mL/min (range, 70-279 mL/min). Mean terminal half-life in plasma was 4.5 hours (range, 3.3-13.4 hours; n=12). Following an oral dose of ^{14}C-finasteride in man (n=6), a mean of 39% (range, 32-46%) of the dose was excreted in the urine in the form of metabolites; 57% (range, 51-64%) was excreted in the feces.

Mean terminal half-life is approximately 5-6 hours in men 18-60 years of age and 8 hours in men more than 70 years of age.

TABLE 3 Mean (SD) Pharmacokinetic Parameters in Healthy Men (ages 18-26)

	Mean (± SD) n=15
Bioavailability	65% (26-170%)*
Clearance (mL/min)	165 (55)
Volume of Distribution (L)	76 (14)

* Range

TABLE 4 Mean (SD) Noncompartmental Pharmacokinetic Parameters After Multiple Doses of 1 mg/day in Healthy Men (ages 19-42)

	Mean (± SD) (n=12)
AUC (ng·hr/mL)	53 (33.8)
Peak Concentration (ng/mL)	9.2 (2.6)
Time to Peak (hours)	1.3 (0.5)
Half-Life (hours)*	4.5 (1.6)

* First-dose values; all other parameters are last-dose values

Renal Impairment

No dosage adjustment is necessary in patients with renal impairment. In patients with chronic renal impairment, with creatinine clearances ranging from 9.0 to 55 mL/min, AUC, maximum plasma concentration, half-life, and protein binding after a single dose of ^{14}C-finasteride were similar to those obtained in healthy volunteers. Urinary excretion of metabolites was decreased in patients with renal impairment. This decrease was associated with an increase in fecal excretion of metabolites. Plasma concentrations of metabolites were significantly higher in patients with renal impairment (based on a 60% increase in total radioactivity AUC). However, finasteride has been tolerated in men with normal renal function receiving up to 80 mg/day for 12 weeks where exposure of these patients to metabolites would presumably be much greater.

Hepatic Impairment

The effect of hepatic impairment on finasteride pharmacokinetics has not been studied. Caution should be used in the administration of PROPECIA in patients with liver function abnormalities, as finasteride is metabolized extensively in the liver.

13   NONCLINICAL TOXICOLOGY

13.1   Carcinogenesis, Mutagenesis, Impairment of Fertility

No evidence of a tumorigenic effect was observed in a 24-month study in Sprague-Dawley rats receiving doses of finasteride up to 160 mg/kg/day in males and 320 mg/kg/day in females. These doses produced respective systemic exposure in rats of 888 and 2192 times those observed in man receiving the recommended human dose of 1 mg/day. All exposure calculations were based on calculated AUC$_{(0-24 hr)}$ for animals and mean AUC$_{(0-24 hr)}$ for man (0.05 µg·hr/mL).

In a 19-month carcinogenicity study in CD-1 mice, a statistically significant (p≤0.05) increase in the incidence of testicular Leydig cell adenomas was observed at 1824 times the human exposure (250 mg/kg/day). In mice at 184 times the human exposure, estimated (25 mg/kg/day) and in rats

at 312 times the human exposure (≥40 mg/kg/day) an increase in the incidence of Leydig cell hyperplasia was observed. A positive correlation between the proliferative changes in the Leydig cells and an increase in serum LH levels (2- to 3-fold above control) has been demonstrated in both rodent species treated with high doses of finasteride. No drug-related Leydig cell changes were seen in either rats or dogs treated with finasteride for 1 year at 240 and 2800 times (20 mg/kg/day and 45 mg/kg/day, respectively), or in mice treated for 19 months at 18.4 times the human exposure, estimated (2.5 mg/kg/day).

No evidence of mutagenicity was observed in an *in vitro* bacterial mutagenesis assay, a mammalian cell mutagenesis assay, or in an *in vitro* alkaline elution assay. In an *in vitro* chromosome aberration assay, using Chinese hamster ovary cells, there was a slight increase in chromosome aberrations. In an *in vivo* chromosome aberration assay in mice, no treatment-related increase in chromosome aberration was observed with finasteride at the maximum tolerated dose of 250 mg/kg/day (1824 times the human exposure) as determined in the carcinogenicity studies.

In sexually mature male rabbits treated with finasteride at 4344 times the human exposure (80 mg/kg/day) for up to 12 weeks, no effect on fertility, sperm count, or ejaculate volume was seen. In sexually mature male rats treated with 488 times the human exposure (80 mg/kg/day), there were no significant effects on fertility after 6 or 12 weeks of treatment; however, when treatment was continued for up to 24 or 30 weeks, there was an apparent decrease in fertility, fecundity, and an associated significant decrease in the weights of the seminal vesicles and prostate. All these effects were reversible within 6 weeks of discontinuation of treatment. No drug-related effect on testes or on mating performance has been seen in rats or rabbits. This decrease in fertility in finasteride-treated rats is secondary to its effect on accessory sex organs (prostate and seminal vesicles) resulting in failure to form a seminal plug. The seminal plug is essential for normal fertility in rats but is not relevant in man.

14   CLINICAL STUDIES

14.1   Studies in Men

The efficacy of PROPECIA was demonstrated in men (88% Caucasian) with mild to moderate androgenetic alopecia (male pattern hair loss) between 18 and 41 years of age. In order to prevent seborrheic dermatitis which might confound the assessment of hair growth in these studies, all men, whether treated with finasteride or placebo, were instructed to use a specified, medicated, tar-based shampoo (Neutrogena T/Gel®[1] Shampoo) during the first 2 years of the studies.

There were three double-blind, randomized, placebo-controlled studies of 12-month duration. The two primary endpoints were hair count and patient self-assessment; the two secondary endpoints were investigator assessment and ratings of photographs. In addition, information was collected regarding sexual function (based on a self-administered questionnaire) and non-scalp body hair growth. The three studies were conducted in 1879 men with mild to moderate, but not complete, hair loss. Two of the studies enrolled men with predominantly mild to moderate vertex hair loss (n=1553). The third enrolled men having mild to moderate hair loss in the anterior mid-scalp area with or without vertex balding (n=326).

[1]Registered trademark of Johnson & Johnson

Studies in Men with Vertex Baldness

Of the men who completed the first 12 months of the two vertex baldness trials, 1215 elected to continue in double-blind, placebo-controlled, 12-month extension studies. There were 547 men receiving PROPECIA for both the initial study and first extension periods (up to 2 years of treatment) and 60 men receiving placebo for the same periods. The extension studies were continued for 3 additional years, with 323 men on PROPECIA and 23 on placebo entering the fifth year of the study.

In order to evaluate the effect of discontinuation of therapy, there were 65 men who received PROPECIA for the initial 12 months followed by placebo in the first 12-month extension period. Some of these men continued in additional extension studies and were switched back to treatment with PROPECIA, with 32 men entering the fifth year of the study. Lastly, there were 543 men who received placebo for the initial 12 months followed by PROPECIA in the first 12-month extension period. Some of these men continued in additional extension studies receiving PROPECIA, with 290 men entering the fifth year of the study (see Figure 1 below).

Hair counts were assessed by photographic enlargements of a representative area of active hair loss. In these two studies in men with vertex baldness, significant increases in hair count were demonstrated at 6 and 12 months in men treated with PROPECIA, while significant hair loss from baseline was demonstrated in those treated with placebo. At

12 months there was a 107-hair difference from placebo (p<0.001, PROPECIA [n=679] vs placebo [n=672]) within a 1-inch diameter circle (5.1 cm²). Hair count was maintained in those men taking PROPECIA for up to 2 years, resulting in a 138-hair difference between treatment groups (p<0.001, PROPECIA [n=433] vs placebo [n=47]) within the same area. In men treated with PROPECIA, the maximum improvement in hair count compared to baseline was achieved during the first 2 years. Although the initial improvement was followed by a slow decline, hair count was maintained above baseline throughout the 5 years of the studies. Furthermore, because the decline in the placebo group was more rapid, the difference between treatment groups also continued to increase throughout the studies, resulting in a 277-hair difference (p<0.001, PROPECIA [n=219] vs placebo [n=15]) at 5 years (see Figure 1 below).

Patients who switched from placebo to PROPECIA (n=425) had a decrease in hair count at the end of the initial 12-month placebo period, followed by an increase in hair count after 1 year of treatment with PROPECIA. This increase in hair count was less (56 hairs above original baseline) than the increase (91 hairs above original baseline) observed after 1 year of treatment in men initially randomized to PROPECIA. Although the increase in hair count, relative to when therapy was initiated, was comparable between these two groups, a higher absolute hair count was achieved in patients who were started on treatment with PROPECIA in the initial study. This advantage was maintained through the remaining 3 years of the studies. A change of treatment from PROPECIA to placebo (n=48) at the end of the initial 12 months resulted in reversal of the increase in hair count 12 months later, at 24 months (see Figure 1 below).

At 12 months, 58% of men in the placebo group had further hair loss (defined as any decrease in hair count from baseline), compared with 14% of men treated with PROPECIA. In men treated for up to 2 years, 72% of men in the placebo group demonstrated hair loss, compared with 17% of men treated with PROPECIA. At 5 years, 100% of men in the placebo group demonstrated hair loss, compared with 35% of men treated with PROPECIA.

Figure 1

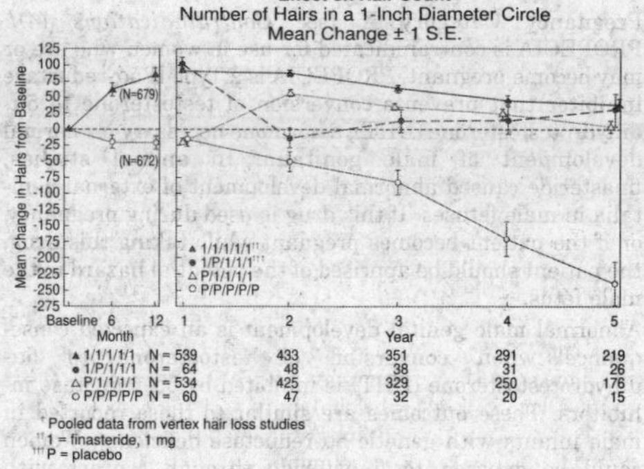

Effect on Hair Count[1]
Number of Hairs in a 1-Inch Diameter Circle
Mean Change ± 1 S.E.

	▲ 1/1/1/1/1 N =	■ 1/P/1/1/1 N =	△ P/1/1/1/1 N =	○ P/P/P/P/P N =
	539	64	534	60
	433	48	425	47
	351	38	329	32
	291	31	250	20
	219	26	176	15

* Pooled data from vertex hair loss studies
1 = finasteride, 1 mg
P = placebo

Patient self-assessment was obtained at each clinic visit from a self-administered questionnaire, which included questions on their perception of hair growth, hair loss, and appearance. This self-assessment demonstrated an increase in amount of hair, a decrease in hair loss, and improvement in appearance in men treated with PROPECIA. Overall improvement compared with placebo was seen as early as 3 months (p<0.05), with improvement maintained over 5 years.

Investigator assessment was based on a 7-point scale evaluating increases or decreases in scalp hair at each patient visit. This assessment showed significantly greater increases in hair growth in men treated with PROPECIA compared with placebo as early as 3 months (p<0.001). At 12 months, the investigators rated 65% of men treated with PROPECIA as having increased hair growth compared with 37% in the placebo group. At 2 years, the investigators rated 80% of men treated with PROPECIA as having increased hair growth compared with 47% of men treated with placebo. At 5 years, the investigators rated 77% of men treated with PROPECIA as having increased hair growth, compared with 15% of men treated with placebo.

An independent panel rated standardized photographs of the head in a blinded fashion based on increases or decreases in scalp hair using the same 7-point scale as the investigator assessment. At 12 months, 48% of men treated with PROPECIA had an increase as compared with 7% of men treated with placebo. At 2 years, an increase in hair growth was demonstrated in 66% of men treated with PROPECIA, compared with 7% of men treated with placebo. At 5 years, 48% of men treated with PROPECIA demonstrated an increase in hair growth, 42% were rated as having no change (no further visible progression of hair loss from baseline) and 10% were rated as having lost hair when compared to baseline. In comparison, 6% of men treated with placebo demonstrated an increase in hair growth, 19% were rated as having no change and 75% were rated as having lost hair when compared to baseline.

A 48-week, placebo-controlled study designed to assess by phototrichogram the effect of PROPECIA on total and actively growing (anagen) scalp hairs in vertex baldness enrolled 212 men with androgenetic alopecia. At baseline and 48 weeks, total and anagen hair counts were obtained in a 1-cm^2 target area of the scalp. Men treated with PROPECIA showed increases from baseline in total and anagen hair counts of 7 hairs and 18 hairs, respectively, whereas men treated with placebo had decreases of 10 hairs and 9 hairs, respectively. These changes in hair counts resulted in a between-group difference of 17 hairs in total hair count (p<0.001) and 27 hairs in anagen hair count (p<0.001), and an improvement in the proportion of anagen hairs from 62% at baseline to 68% for men treated with PROPECIA.

Other Results in Vertex Baldness Studies

A sexual function questionnaire was self-administered by patients participating in the two vertex baldness trials to detect more subtle changes in sexual function. At Month 12, statistically significant differences in favor of placebo were found in 3 of 4 domains (sexual interest, erections, and perception of sexual problems). However, no significant difference was seen in the question on overall satisfaction with sex life.

In one of the two vertex baldness studies, patients were questioned on non-scalp body hair growth. PROPECIA did not appear to affect non-scalp body hair.

Study in Men with Hair Loss in the Anterior Mid-Scalp Area

A study of 12-month duration, designed to assess the efficacy of PROPECIA in men with hair loss in the anterior mid-scalp area, also demonstrated significant increases in hair count compared with placebo. Increases in hair count were accompanied by improvements in patient self-assessment, investigator assessment, and ratings based on standardized photographs. Hair counts were obtained in the anterior mid-scalp area, and did not include the area of bitemporal recession or the anterior hairline.

Summary of Clinical Studies in Men

Clinical studies were conducted in men aged 18 to 41 with mild to moderate degrees of androgenetic alopecia. All men treated with PROPECIA or placebo received a tar-based shampoo (Neutrogena T/Gel® Shampoo) during the first 2 years of the studies. Clinical improvement was seen as early as 3 months in the patients treated with PROPECIA and led to a net increase in scalp hair count and hair regrowth. In clinical studies for up to 5 years, treatment with PROPECIA slowed the further progression of hair loss observed in the placebo group. In general, the difference between treatment groups continued to increase throughout the 5 years of the studies.

Ethnic Analysis of Clinical Data from Men

In a combined analysis of the two studies on vertex baldness, mean hair count changes from baseline were 91 vs -19 hairs (PROPECIA vs placebo) among Caucasians (n=1185), 49 vs -27 hairs among Blacks (n=84), 53 vs -38 hairs among Asians (n=17), 67 vs 5 hairs among Hispanics (n=45) and 67 vs -15 hairs among other ethnic groups (n=20). Patient self-assessment showed improvement across racial groups with PROPECIA treatment, except for satisfaction of the frontal hairline and vertex in Black men, who were satisfied overall.

14.2 Study in Women

In a study involving 137 postmenopausal women with androgenetic alopecia who were treated with PROPECIA (n=67) or placebo (n=70) for 12 months, effectiveness could not be demonstrated. There was no improvement in hair counts, patient self-assessment, investigator assessment, or ratings of standardized photographs in the women treated with PROPECIA when compared with the placebo group *[see Indications and Usage (1.1)]*.

16 HOW SUPPLIED/STORAGE AND HANDLING

No. 6642 — PROPECIA tablets, 1 mg, are tan, octagonal, film-coated convex tablets with "stylized P" logo on one side and PROPECIA on the other. They are supplied as follows:

NDC 0006-0071-31 bottles of 30 (with desiccant)

NDC 0006-0071-54 PROPAK® bottles of 90 (with desiccant).

Storage and Handling

Store at room temperature, 15-30°C (59-86°F). Keep container closed and protect from moisture.

Women should not handle crushed or broken PROPECIA tablets when they are pregnant or may potentially be pregnant because of the possibility of absorption of finasteride and the subsequent potential risk to a male fetus. PROPECIA tablets are coated and will prevent contact with the active ingredient during normal handling, provided that the tablets are not broken or crushed *[see Warnings and Precautions (5.1), Use in Specific Populations (8.1) and Patient Counseling Information (17.1)]*.

17 PATIENT COUNSELING INFORMATION

"See FDA-approved patient labeling (Patient Information)"

17.1 Exposure of Women — Risk to Male Fetus

Physicians should inform patients that women who are pregnant or may potentially be pregnant should not handle crushed or broken PROPECIA tablets because of the possibility of absorption of finasteride and the subsequent potential risk to a male fetus. PROPECIA tablets are coated and will prevent contact with the active ingredient during normal handling, provided that the tablets have not been broken or crushed. If a woman who is pregnant or may potentially be pregnant comes in contact with crushed or broken PROPECIA tablets, the contact area should be washed immediately with soap and water *[see Contraindications (4), Warnings and Precautions (5.1), Use in Specific Populations (8.1) and How Supplied/Storage and Handling (16)]*.

17.2 Increased Risk of High-Grade Prostate Cancer

Patients should be informed that there was an increase in high-grade prostate cancer in men treated with 5α-reductase inhibitors indicated for BPH treatment, compared to those treated with placebo in studies looking at the use of these drugs to prevent prostate cancer *[see Warnings and Precautions (5.3) and Adverse Reactions (6.1)]*.

17.3 Additional Instructions

Physicians should instruct their patients to promptly report any changes in their breasts such as lumps, pain or nipple discharge. Breast changes including breast enlargement, tenderness and neoplasm have been reported *[see Adverse Reactions (6.1)]*.

Physicians should instruct their patients to read the patient package insert before starting therapy with PROPECIA and to read it again each time the prescription is renewed so that they are aware of current information for patients regarding PROPECIA.

Dist. by: Merck Sharp & Dohme Corp., a subsidiary of **MERCK & CO., INC., Whitehouse Station, NJ 08889, USA**

US Patent Nos.: 5,547,957; 5,571,817

Revised: 04/2012
USPI-1T-09061204R010

Patient Information
PROPECIA (Pro-pee-sha)
(finasteride)
Tablets

PROPECIA® is for use by **MEN ONLY** and should **NOT** be used by women or children.

Read this Patient Information before you start taking PROPECIA and each time you get a refill. There may be new information. This information does not take the place of talking with your healthcare provider about your medical condition or treatment.

What is PROPECIA?

PROPECIA is a prescription medicine used for the treatment of male pattern hair loss (androgenetic alopecia).

It is not known if PROPECIA works for a receding hairline on either side of and above your forehead (temporal area).

PROPECIA is not for use by women and children.

Who should not take PROPECIA?

Do not take PROPECIA if you:

- are pregnant or may become pregnant. PROPECIA may harm your unborn baby.
  - PROPECIA tablets are coated and will prevent contact with the medicine during handling, as long as the tablets are not broken or crushed. Females who are pregnant or who may become pregnant should not come in contact with broken or crushed PROPECIA tablets. If a pregnant woman comes in contact with crushed or broken PROPECIA tablets, wash the contact area right away with soap and water. If a woman who is pregnant comes into contact with the active ingredient in PROPECIA, a healthcare provider should be consulted.
  - If a woman who is pregnant with a male baby swallows or comes in contact with the medicine in PROPECIA, the male baby may be born with sex organs that are not normal.
- are allergic to any of the ingredients in PROPECIA. See the end of this leaflet for a complete list of ingredients in PROPECIA.

What should I tell my healthcare provider before taking PROPECIA?

Before taking PROPECIA, tell your healthcare provider if you:

- have any other medical conditions, including problems with your prostate or liver

Tell your healthcare provider about all the medicines you take, including prescription and non-prescription medicines, vitamins, and herbal supplements.

Know the medicines you take. Keep a list of them to show your healthcare provider and pharmacist when you get a new medicine.

How should I take PROPECIA?

- Take PROPECIA exactly as your healthcare provider tells you to take it.
- You may take PROPECIA with or without food.
- If you forget to take PROPECIA, do not take an extra tablet. Just take the next tablet as usual.

PROPECIA will not work faster or better if you take it more than once a day.

What are the possible side effects of PROPECIA?

- **decrease in your blood Prostate Specific Antigen (PSA) levels.** PROPECIA can affect a blood test called PSA (Prostate-Specific Antigen) for the screening of prostate cancer. If you have a PSA test done you should tell your healthcare provider that you are taking PROPECIA because PROPECIA decreases PSA levels. Changes in PSA levels will need to be evaluated by your healthcare provider. Any increase in follow-up PSA levels from their lowest point may signal the presence of prostate cancer and should be evaluated, even if the test results are still within the normal range for men not taking PROPECIA. You should also tell your healthcare provider if you have not been taking PROPECIA as prescribed because this may affect the PSA test results. For more information, talk to your healthcare provider.
- There may be an increased risk of a more serious form of prostate cancer in men taking finasteride at 5 times the dose of PROPECIA.

The most common side effects of PROPECIA include:

- decrease in sex drive
- trouble getting or keeping an erection
- a decrease in the amount of semen

The following have been reported in general use with PROPECIA:

- breast tenderness and enlargement. Tell your healthcare provider about any changes in your breasts such as lumps, pain or nipple discharge.
- depression;
- decrease in sex drive that continued after stopping the medication;
- allergic reactions including rash, itching, hives and swelling of the lips and face;
- problems with ejaculation that continued after stopping medication;
- testicular pain;
- difficulty in achieving an erection that continued after stopping the medication;
- male infertility and/or poor quality of semen.
- in rare cases, male breast cancer.

Tell your healthcare provider if you have any side effect that bothers you or that does not go away.

These are not all the possible side effects of PROPECIA. For more information, ask your healthcare provider or pharmacist.

Call your doctor for medical advice about side effects. You may report side effects to FDA at 1-800-FDA-1088.

How should I store PROPECIA?

- Store PROPECIA at room temperature between 59°F to 86°F (15°C to 30°C).
- Keep PROPECIA in a closed container and keep PROPECIA tablets dry (protect from moisture).

Keep PROPECIA and all medicines out of the reach of children.

General information about the safe and effective use of PROPECIA.

Medicines are sometimes prescribed for purposes other than those listed in this Patient Information leaflet. Do not use PROPECIA for a condition for which it was not prescribed. Do not give PROPECIA to other people, even if they have the same symptoms you have. It may harm them.

This Patient Information leaflet summarizes the most important information about PROPECIA. If you would like more information, talk with your healthcare provider. You can ask your pharmacist or healthcare provider for information about PROPECIA that is written for health professionals. For more information, **call 1-888-637-2522.**

What are the ingredients in PROPECIA?

Active ingredient: finasteride.

Inactive ingredients: lactose monohydrate, microcrystalline cellulose, pregelatinized starch, sodium starch glycolate, hydroxypropyl methylcellulose, hydroxypropyl cellulose, titanium dioxide, magnesium stearate, talc, docusate sodium, yellow ferric oxide, and red ferric oxide.

This Patient Information has been approved by the U.S. Food and Drug Administration.

Dist. by: Merck Sharp & Dohme Corp., a subsidiary of **MERCK & CO., INC., Whitehouse Station, NJ 08889, USA**

US Patent Nos.: 5,547,957; 5,571,817

Revised: 04/2012
USPPI-1T-09061204R010

Shown in Product Identification Guide, page 308

PROQUAD® ℞
[*prō-kwăd*]
Measles, Mumps, Rubella and Varicella Virus Vaccine Live
Lyophilized preparation for subcutaneous injection

HIGHLIGHTS OF PRESCRIBING INFORMATION
These highlights do not include all the information needed to use ProQuad safely and effectively. See full prescribing information for ProQuad.
ProQuad®
Measles, Mumps, Rubella and Varicella Virus Vaccine Live
Lyophilized preparation for subcutaneous injection
Initial U.S. Approval: 2005

INDICATIONS AND USAGE

ProQuad is a vaccine indicated for active immunization for the prevention of measles, mumps, rubella, and varicella in children 12 months through 12 years of age. (1)

DOSAGE AND ADMINISTRATION

A 0.5-mL dose for subcutaneous injection only. (2.1)
- The first dose is usually administered at 12 to 15 months of age. (2.1)
- A second dose, if needed, is usually administered at 4 to 6 years of age. (2.1)

DOSAGE FORMS AND STRENGTHS

Suspension for injection (0.5-mL dose) supplied as a lyophilized vaccine to be reconstituted using only accompanying sterile diluent. (2.2, 3)

CONTRAINDICATIONS

- History of anaphylactic reaction to neomycin or hypersensitivity to gelatin or any other component of the vaccine. (4.1)
- Primary or acquired immunodeficiency states. (4.2)
- Family history of congenital or hereditary immunodeficiency. (4.2)
- Immunosuppressive therapy. (4.2, 7.3)
- Active untreated tuberculosis or febrile illness (>101.3°F or >38.5°C). (4.3)
- Pregnancy. (4.4, 8.1, 17.1)

WARNINGS AND PRECAUTIONS

- Administration of ProQuad (dose 1) to children 12 to 23 months old who have not been previously vaccinated against measles, mumps, rubella, or varicella, nor had a history of the wild-type infections, is associated with higher rates of fever and febrile seizures at 5 to 12 days after vaccination when compared to children vaccinated with M-M-R® II and VARIVAX® administered separately. (5.1, 6.1, 6.3)
- Use caution when administering ProQuad to children with a history of cerebral injury or seizures or any other condition in which stress due to fever should be avoided. (5.2)
- Use caution when administering ProQuad to children with anaphylaxis or immediate hypersensitivity to eggs (5.3) or contact hypersensitivity to neomycin. (5.4)
- Use caution when administering ProQuad to children with thrombocytopenia. (5.5)
- Avoid close contact with high-risk individuals susceptible to varicella since transmission of varicella vaccine virus may occur between vaccinees and susceptible contacts. (5.8)
- Avoid pregnancy for 3 months following vaccination with measles, mumps, rubella, and/or varicella vaccines. (8.1, 17.1)
- Defer vaccination for at least 3 months following blood or plasma transfusions, or administration of immune globulins (IG). (5.9, 7.1)
- Avoid using salicylates for 6 weeks after vaccination with ProQuad. (6.1, 7.2, 17.1)

ADVERSE REACTIONS

- The most frequent vaccine-related adverse events reported in ≥5% of subjects vaccinated with ProQuad were:
  - injection-site reactions (pain/tenderness/soreness, erythema, and swelling)
  - fever
  - irritability. (6.1)
- Systemic vaccine-related adverse events that were reported at a significantly greater rate in recipients of ProQuad than in recipients of the component vaccines administered concomitantly were:
  - fever
  - measles-like rash. (6.1)

To report SUSPECTED ADVERSE REACTIONS, contact Merck Sharp & Dohme Corp., a subsidiary of Merck & Co., Inc., at 1-877-888-4231 or VAERS at 1-800-822-7967 or www.vaers.hhs.gov.

DRUG INTERACTIONS

- Tuberculin testing should be administered anytime before, simultaneously with, or at least 4 to 6 weeks after ProQuad. (7.4)
- ProQuad may be administered concomitantly with *Haemophilus influenzae* type b conjugate vaccine and/or hepatitis B vaccine at separate injection sites. (7.5)
- ProQuad may be administered concomitantly with pneumococcal 7-valent conjugate vaccine and/or hepatitis A vaccine (inactivated) at separate injection sites. (7.5)

USE IN SPECIFIC POPULATIONS

Pregnancy: Do not administer ProQuad to females who are pregnant; the possible effects of the vaccine on fetal development are unknown at this time. (8.1)
To report vaccine exposure during pregnancy call 1-800-986-8999.

See 17 for PATIENT COUNSELING INFORMATION
Revised: 08/2011

FULL PRESCRIBING INFORMATION: CONTENTS*

*** Sections or subsections omitted from the full prescribing information are not listed**

FULL PRESCRIBING INFORMATION

1 INDICATIONS AND USAGE

ProQuad® is a vaccine indicated for active immunization for the prevention of measles, mumps, rubella, and varicella in children 12 months through 12 years of age.

2 DOSAGE AND ADMINISTRATION

2.1 Recommended Dose and Schedule

FOR SUBCUTANEOUS ADMINISTRATION ONLY

Each 0.5-mL dose of ProQuad is administered subcutaneously.
The first dose is usually administered at 12 to 15 months of age but may be given anytime through 12 years of age.
If a second dose of measles, mumps, rubella, and varicella vaccine is needed, ProQuad may be used. This dose is usually administered at 4 to 6 years of age. At least 1 month should elapse between a dose of a measles-containing vaccine such as M-M-R® II (measles, mumps, and rubella virus vaccine live) and a dose of ProQuad. At least 3 months should elapse between a dose of varicella-containing vaccine and ProQuad.

2.2 Preparation for Administration

CAUTION: Preservatives, antiseptics, detergents, and other anti-viral substances may inactivate the vaccine. Use only sterile syringes that are free of preservatives, antiseptics, detergents, and other anti-viral substances for reconstitution and injection of ProQuad.
Withdraw the entire volume of the supplied diluent into a syringe. Use only the diluent supplied with the vaccine since it is free of preservatives or other anti-viral substances.
Inject the entire content of the syringe into the vial containing the powder. Gently agitate to dissolve completely.
Parenteral drug products should be inspected visually for particulate matter and discoloration prior to administration. Visually inspect the vaccine before and after reconstitution prior to administration. Before reconstitution, the lyophilized vaccine is a white to pale yellow compact crystalline plug. ProQuad, when reconstituted, is a clear pale yellow to light pink liquid.
Withdraw the entire amount of the reconstituted vaccine from the vial into the same syringe and inject the entire volume.

TO MINIMIZE LOSS OF POTENCY, THE VACCINE SHOULD BE ADMINISTERED IMMEDIATELY AFTER RECONSTITUTION. IF NOT USED IMMEDIATELY, THE RECONSTITUTED VACCINE MAY BE STORED AT ROOM TEMPERATURE, PROTECTED FROM LIGHT, FOR UP TO 30 MINUTES. DISCARD RECONSTITUTED VACCINE IF IT IS NOT USED WITHIN 30 MINUTES.

2.3 Method of Administration

Inject the vaccine subcutaneously into the outer aspect of the deltoid region of the upper arm or into the higher anterolateral area of the thigh.

Use With Other Vaccines

Use different injection sites to administer each vaccine if other vaccines are administered concomitantly. *[See Drug Interactions (7.5).]*

3 DOSAGE FORMS AND STRENGTHS

ProQuad is a suspension for injection supplied as a 0.5-mL single dose vial of lyophilized vaccine to be reconstituted using the sterile diluent supplied *[see How Supplied/Storage and Handling (16)]*.

4 CONTRAINDICATIONS

4.1 Hypersensitivity

Do not administer ProQuad to individuals with a history of anaphylactic reactions to neomycin. If vaccination with ProQuad is medically necessary for such individuals, they are advised to consult an allergist or immunologist and should receive ProQuad only in settings where anaphylactic reactions can be appropriately managed.
Do not administer ProQuad to individuals with a history of hypersensitivity to gelatin or any other component of the vaccine or following previous vaccination with ProQuad, VARIVAX® (varicella virus vaccine live), or any measles-, mumps-, or rubella-containing vaccine *[see Description (11) and Warnings and Precautions (5) for exceptions]*.

4.2 Immunosuppression

Do not administer ProQuad to individuals with blood dyscrasias, leukemia, lymphomas of any type, or other malignant neoplasms affecting the bone marrow or lymphatic system; or to individuals on immunosuppressive therapy (including high-dose systemic corticosteroids) *[see Drug Interactions (7.3)]*. Vaccination with a live, attenuated vaccine, such as varicella, can result in a more extensive vaccine-associated rash or disseminated disease in individuals on immunosuppressive drugs. ProQuad may be used by individuals who are receiving topical corticosteroids or low-dose corticosteroids, as are commonly used for asthma prophylaxis or in patients who are receiving corticosteroids as replacement therapy, *e.g.*, for Addison's disease.
Do not administer ProQuad to individuals with primary and acquired immunodeficiency states, including AIDS or other clinical manifestations of infection with human immunodeficiency viruses; cellular immune deficiencies; and hypogammaglobulinemic and dysgammaglobulinemic states. Measles inclusion body encephalitis, pneumonitis, and death as a direct consequence of disseminated measles vaccine virus infection have been reported in severely immunocompromised individuals inadvertently vaccinated with measles-containing vaccine. In addition, disseminated varicella vaccine virus infection has been reported in children with underlying immunodeficiency disorders who were inadvertently vaccinated with a varicella-containing vaccine.[1]
Do not administer ProQuad to individuals with a family history of congenital or hereditary immunodeficiency, unless the immune competence of the potential vaccine recipient is demonstrated.

4.3 Concurrent Illness

Do not administer ProQuad to individuals with active untreated tuberculosis or to individuals with an active febrile illness with fever >101.3°F (>38.5°C).

4.4 Pregnancy
Do not administer ProQuad to individuals who are pregnant; the possible effects of the vaccine on fetal development are unknown at this time *[see Use in Specific Populations (8.1)]*.

5 WARNINGS AND PRECAUTIONS

5.1 Fever and Febrile Seizures
Administration of ProQuad (dose 1) to children 12 to 23 months old who have not been previously vaccinated against measles, mumps, rubella, or varicella, nor had a history of the wild-type infections, is associated with higher rates of fever and febrile seizures at 5 to 12 days after vaccination when compared to children vaccinated with dose 1 of both M-M-R II and VARIVAX administered separately *[see Adverse Reactions (6.3)]*.

5.2 History of Cerebral Injury or Seizures
Exercise caution when administering ProQuad to persons with a history of cerebral injury, individual or family history of convulsions, or any other condition in which stress due to fever should be avoided. Healthcare providers should be alert to the temperature elevations that may occur following vaccination.

5.3 Hypersensitivity to Eggs
Live measles vaccine and live mumps vaccine are produced in chick embryo cell culture. Persons with a history of anaphylactic or other immediate hypersensitivity reactions (*e.g.*, hives, swelling of the mouth and throat, difficulty breathing, hypotension, or shock) subsequent to egg ingestion may be at an enhanced risk of immediate-type hypersensitivity reactions after receiving vaccines containing traces of chick embryo antigen. Carefully evaluate the potential risk-to-benefit ratio before considering vaccination in such cases. Such individuals may be vaccinated with extreme caution; adequate treatment should be readily available should a reaction occur *[see Contraindications (4.1)]*.{2}
Children with egg allergy are at low risk for anaphylactic reactions to measles-containing vaccines (including M-M-R II), and skin testing of children allergic to eggs is not predictive of reactions to M-M-R II vaccine. Persons with allergies to chickens or feathers are not at increased risk of reaction to the vaccine.{2}

5.4 Contact Hypersensitivity to Neomycin
Most often, neomycin allergy manifests as a contact dermatitis, which is not a contraindication to receiving measles-, mumps-, rubella-, or varicella-containing vaccine.

5.5 Thrombocytopenia
Carefully evaluate the potential risk-to-benefit ratio before considering vaccination with ProQuad in children with thrombocytopenia or in those who experienced thrombocytopenia after vaccination with a previous dose of measles, mumps, rubella, and/or varicella vaccine. No clinical data are available regarding the development or worsening of thrombocytopenia in individuals vaccinated with ProQuad. Cases of thrombocytopenia have been reported after primary vaccination with measles vaccine, measles, mumps, and rubella vaccine, after varicella vaccination, and following re-vaccination with measles vaccine or M-M-R II *[see Adverse Reactions (6.2)]*.

5.6 Use for Post-Exposure Prophylaxis
The safety and efficacy of ProQuad for use after exposure to measles, mumps, rubella, or varicella have not been established.

5.7 Use in HIV-Infected Children
The safety and efficacy of ProQuad for use in children known to be infected with human immunodeficiency viruses have not been established.

5.8 Risk of Vaccine Virus Transmission
Post-licensing experience with VARIVAX suggests that transmission of varicella vaccine virus may occur between healthy vaccine recipients (who develop or do not develop a varicella-like rash) and contacts susceptible to varicella, as well as high-risk individuals susceptible to varicella.
High-risk individuals susceptible to varicella include:
- Immunocompromised individuals;
- Pregnant women without documented positive history of varicella (chickenpox) or laboratory evidence of prior infection;
- Newborn infants of mothers without documented positive history of varicella or laboratory evidence of prior infection and all newborn infants born at <28 weeks gestation regardless of maternal varicella immunity.

Vaccine recipients should attempt to avoid, to the extent possible, close association with high-risk individuals susceptible to varicella for up to 6 weeks following vaccination. In circumstances where contact with high-risk individuals susceptible to varicella is unavoidable, the potential risk of transmission of the varicella vaccine virus should be weighed against the risk of acquiring and transmitting wild-type varicella virus.
Excretion of small amounts of the live, attenuated rubella virus from the nose or throat has occurred in the majority of susceptible individuals 7 to 28 days after vaccination. There is no confirmed evidence to indicate that such virus is transmitted to susceptible persons who are in contact with the vaccinated individuals. Consequently, transmission through close personal contact, while accepted as a theoretical possibility, is not regarded as a significant risk. However, transmission of the rubella vaccine virus to infants via breast milk has been documented *[see Use in Specific Populations (8.3)]*.
There are no reports of transmission of the more attenuated Enders' Edmonston strain of measles virus or the Jeryl Lynn™ strain of mumps virus from vaccine recipients to susceptible contacts.

5.9 Immune Globulins and Transfusions
Immune globulins (IG) administered concomitantly with ProQuad contain antibodies that may interfere with vaccine virus replication and decrease the expected immune response. Vaccination should be deferred for at least 3 months following blood or plasma transfusions, or administration of IG.
The appropriate suggested interval between transfusion or IG administration and vaccination will vary with the type of transfusion or indication for, and dose of, IG (*e.g.*, 5 months for Varicella Zoster Immune Globulin [VZIG]).{2} Following administration of ProQuad, any IG including VZIG should not be given for 1 month thereafter unless its use outweighs the benefits of vaccination.{2} *[See Drug Interactions (7.1).]*

5.10 Risk of Transmission of Creutzfeldt-Jakob Disease and other Adventitious Agents
This product contains albumin, a derivative of human blood. Based on effective donor screening and product manufacturing processes, it carries an extremely remote risk for transmission of viral diseases. Although there is a theoretical risk for transmission of Creutzfeldt-Jakob disease (CJD), no cases of transmission of CJD or viral disease have ever been identified that were associated with the use of albumin. The cells, virus pools, bovine serum, and human albumin used in manufacturing are all evaluated and tested to provide assurance that the final product is free of potential adventitious agents *[see Description (11)]*.

6 ADVERSE REACTIONS

6.1 Clinical Trials Experience
Because clinical trials are conducted under widely varying conditions, adverse reaction rates observed in the clinical trials of a vaccine cannot be directly compared to rates in the clinical trials of another vaccine and may not reflect the rates observed in clinical practice. Vaccine-related adverse reactions reported during clinical trials were assessed by the study investigators to be possibly, probably, or definitely vaccine-related and are summarized below.

Children 12 Through 23 Months of Age Who Received a Single Dose of ProQuad
ProQuad was administered to 4497 children 12 through 23 months of age involved in 4 randomized clinical trials without concomitant administration with other vaccines. The safety of ProQuad was compared with the safety of M-M-R II and VARIVAX given concomitantly (N=2038) at separate injection sites. The safety profile for ProQuad was similar to the component vaccines. Children in these studies were monitored for up to 42 days postvaccination using vaccination report card-aided surveillance. Safety follow-up was obtained for 98% of children in each group. Few subjects (<0.1%) who received ProQuad discontinued the study due to an adverse reaction. The race distribution of the study subjects across these studies following a first dose of ProQuad was as follows: 65.2% White; 13.1% African-American; 11.1% Hispanic; 5.8% Asian/Pacific; 4.5% other; and 0.2% American Indian. The racial distribution of the control group was similar to that of the group who received ProQuad. The gender distribution across the studies following a first dose of ProQuad was 52.5% male and 47.5% female. The gender distribution of the control group was similar to that of the group who received ProQuad. Vaccine-related injection-site and systemic adverse reactions observed among recipients of ProQuad or M-M-R II and VARIVAX at a rate of at least 1% are shown in Table 1. Systemic vaccine-related adverse reactions that were reported at a significantly greater rate in individuals who received a first dose of ProQuad than in individuals who received first doses of M-M-R II and VARIVAX concomitantly at separate injection sites were fever (≥102°F [≥38.9°C] oral equivalent or abnormal) (21.5% versus 14.9%, respectively, risk difference 6.6%, 95% CI: 4.6, 8.5), and measles-like rash (3.0% versus 2.1%, respectively, risk difference 1.0%, 95% CI: 0.1, 1.8). Both fever and measles-like rash usually occurred within 5 to 12 days following the vaccination, were of short duration, and resolved with no long-term sequelae. Pain/tenderness/soreness at the injection site was reported at a statistically lower rate in individuals who received ProQuad than in individuals who received M-M-R II and VARIVAX concomitantly at separate injection sites (22.0% versus 26.8%, respectively, risk difference -4.8%, 95% CI: -7.1, -2.5). The only vaccine-related injection-site adverse reaction that was more frequent among recipients of ProQuad than recipients of M-M-R II and VARIVAX was rash at the injection site (2.4% versus 1.6%, respectively, risk difference 0.9%, 95% CI: 0.1, 1.5).

Table 1: Vaccine-Related Injection-Site and Systemic Adverse Reactions Reported in ≥1% of Children Who Received ProQuad Dose 1 or M-M-R II and VARIVAX at 12 to 23 Months of Age (0 to 42 Days Postvaccination)

Adverse Reactions	ProQuad (N=4497) (n=4424) %	M-M-R II and VARIVAX (N=2038) (n=1997) %
*Injection Site**		
Pain/tenderness/soreness†	22.0	26.7
Erythema†	14.4	15.8
Swelling†	8.4	9.8
Ecchymosis	1.5	2.3
Rash	2.3	1.5
Systemic		
Fever†,‡	21.5	14.9
Irritability	6.7	6.7
Measles-like rash†	3.0	2.1
Varicella-like rash†	2.1	2.2
Rash (not otherwise specified)	1.6	1.4
Upper respiratory infection	1.3	1.1
Viral exanthema	1.2	1.1
Diarrhea	1.2	1.3

N = number of subjects vaccinated.
n = number of subjects with safety follow-up.
* Injection-site adverse reactions for M-M-R II and VARIVAX are based on occurrence with either of the vaccines administered.
† Designates a solicited adverse reaction. Injection-site adverse reactions were solicited only from Days 0 to 4 postvaccination.
‡ Temperature reported as elevated (≥102°F, oral equivalent) or abnormal.

Rubella-like rashes were observed in <1% of subjects following a first dose of ProQuad.
In these clinical trials, two cases of herpes zoster were reported among 2108 healthy subjects 12 through 23 months of age who were vaccinated with their first dose of ProQuad and followed for 1 year. Both cases were unremarkable and no sequelae were reported.

Children 15 to 31 Months of Age Who Received a Second Dose of ProQuad
In 5 clinical trials, 2780 healthy children were vaccinated with ProQuad (dose 1) at 12 to 23 months of age and then administered a second dose approximately 3 to 9 months later. The race distribution of the study subjects across these studies following a second dose of ProQuad was as follows: 64.4% White; 14.1% African-American; 12.0% Hispanic; 5.9% other; 3.5% Asian/Pacific; and 0.1% American Indian. The gender distribution across the studies following a second dose of ProQuad was 51.5% male and 48.5% female. Children in these open-label studies were monitored for at least 28 days postvaccination using vaccination report card-aided surveillance. Safety follow-up was obtained for approximately 97% of children overall. Vaccine-related injection-site and systemic adverse reactions observed after Dose 1 and 2 of ProQuad at a rate of at least 1% are shown in Table 2. In these trials, the overall rates of systemic adverse reactions after ProQuad (dose 2) were comparable to, or lower than, those seen with the first dose. In the subset of children who received both ProQuad dose 1 and dose 2 in these trials (N=2408) with follow-up for fever, fever ≥102.2°F (≥38.9°C) was observed significantly less frequently days 1 to 28 after the second dose (10.8%) than after the first dose (19.1%) (risk difference 8.3%, 95% CI: 6.4, 10.3). Fevers ≥102.2°F (≥38.9°C) days 5 to 12 after vaccinations were also reported significantly less frequently after dose 2 (3.9%) than after dose 1 (13.6%) (risk difference 9.7%, 95% CI: 8.1, 11.3). In the subset of children who received both doses and for whom injection-site reactions were reported (N=2679), injection-site erythema was noted significantly more frequently after ProQuad (dose 2) as compared to ProQuad (dose 1) (12.6% and 10.8%, respectively, risk difference -1.8, 95% CI: -3.3, -0.3); however, pain and tenderness at the injection site was significantly lower after dose 2 (16.1%) as compared with after dose 1 (21.9%) (risk difference, 5.8%, 95% CI: 4.1, 7.6). Two children had febrile seizures after ProQuad (dose 2); both febrile seizures were

Table 3: Vaccine-Related Injection-Site and Systemic Adverse Reactions Reported in ≥1% of Children Previously Vaccinated with M-M-R II and VARIVAX Who Received ProQuad + Placebo, M-M-R II + Placebo, or M-M-R II + VARIVAX at 4 to 6 Years of Age (1 to 43 Days Postvaccination)

Adverse Reactions	ProQuad + Placebo (N=399) (n=397) %	M-M-R II + Placebo (N=205) (n=205) %	M-M-R II + VARIVAX (N=195) (n=193) %
Systemic			
Fever*,†	2.5	2.0	4.1
Cough	1.3	0.5	0.5
Irritability	1.0	0.5	1.0
Headache	0.8	1.5	1.6
Rhinorrhea	0.5	1.0	0.5
Nasopharyngitis	0.3	1.0	1.0
Vomiting	0.3	1.0	0.5
Upper respiratory infection	0.0	0.0	1.0

	ProQuad %	Placebo %	M-M-R II %	Placebo %	M-M-R II %	VARIVAX %
Injection-Site						
Pain*	41.1	34.5	36.6	34.1	35.2	36.8
Erythema*	24.4	13.4	15.6	14.1	14.5	15.5
Swelling*	15.6	8.1	10.2	8.8	7.8	10.9
Bruising	3.5	3.8	2.4	3.4	1.6	2.1
Rash	1.5	1.3	0.0	0.0	0.5	0.0
Pruritus	1.0	0.3	0.0	0.0	0.0	1.0
Nodule	0.0	0.0	0.0	0.0	0.0	1.0

N = number of subjects vaccinated.
n = number of subjects with safety follow-up.
* Designates a solicited adverse reaction. Injection-site adverse reactions were solicited only from Days 1 to 5 postvaccination.
† Temperature reported as elevated (≥102°F, oral equivalent) or abnormal.

thought to be related to a concurrent viral illness *[see Adverse Reactions (6.3) and Clinical Studies (14)]*. These studies were not designed or statistically powered to detect a difference in rates of febrile seizure between recipients of ProQuad as compared to M-M-R II and VARIVAX. The risk of febrile seizure has not been evaluated in a clinical study comparing the incidence rate after ProQuad (dose 2) with the incidence rate after concomitant M-M-R II (dose 2) and VARIVAX (dose 2). *[See Adverse Reactions (6.1), Children 4 to 6 Years of Age Who Received ProQuad After Primary Vaccination with M-M-R II and VARIVAX.]*

Table 2: Vaccine-Related Injection-Site and Systemic Adverse Reactions Reported in ≥1% of Children Who Received ProQuad Dose 1 at 12 to 23 Months of Age and Dose 2 at 15 to 31 Months of Age (1 to 28 Days Postvaccination)

Adverse Reactions	ProQuad Dose 1 (N=3112) (n=3019) %	ProQuad Dose 2 (N=2780) (n=2695) %
*Injection-Site**		
Pain/tenderness/soreness*	21.4	15.9
Erythema*	10.7	12.4
Swelling*	8.0	8.5
Injection-site bruising	1.1	0.0
Systemic		
Fever*,†	20.4	8.3
Irritability	6.0	2.4
Measles-like/Rubella-like rash	4.3	0.9
Varicella-like/Vesicular rash	1.5	0.1
Diarrhea	1.3	0.6
Upper respiratory infection	1.3	1.4
Rash (not otherwise specified)	1.2	0.6
Rhinorrhea	1.1	1.0

N = number of subjects vaccinated.
n = number of subjects with safety follow-up
* Designates a solicited adverse reaction. Injection-site adverse reactions were solicited only from Days 1 to 5 postvaccination.
† Temperature reported as elevated or abnormal.

Children 4 to 6 Years of Age Who Received ProQuad After Primary Vaccination with M-M-R II and VARIVAX

In a double-blind clinical trial, 799 healthy 4- to 6-year-old children who received M-M-R II and VARIVAX at least 1 month prior to study entry were randomized to receive ProQuad and placebo (N=399), M-M-R II and placebo concomitantly (N=205) at separate injection sites, or M-M-R II and VARIVAX (N=195) concomitantly at separate injection sites *[see Clinical Studies (14)]*. Children in these studies were monitored for up to 42 days postvaccination using vaccination report card-aided surveillance. Safety follow-up was obtained for >98% of children in each group. The race distribution of the study subjects following a dose of ProQuad was as follows: 78.4% White; 12.3% African-American; 3.8% Hispanic; 3.5% other; and 2.0% Asian/Pacific. The gender distribution following a dose of ProQuad was 52.1% male and 47.9% female. Injection-site and systemic adverse reactions observed after Dose 1 and 2 of ProQuad at a rate of at least 1% are shown in Table 3. *[See Clinical Studies (14).]*

[See table 3 above]

Safety in Trials that Evaluated Concomitant Use with Other Vaccines

ProQuad Administered with Diphtheria and Tetanus Toxoids and Acellular Pertussis Vaccine Adsorbed (DTaP) and Haemophilus influenzae type b Conjugate (Meningococcal Protein Conjugate) and Hepatitis B (Recombinant) Vaccine

In an open-label clinical trial, 1434 children were randomized to receive ProQuad given with diphtheria and tetanus toxoids and acellular pertussis vaccine adsorbed (DTaP) and *Haemophilus influenzae* type b conjugate (meningococcal protein conjugate) and hepatitis B (recombinant) vaccine concomitantly (N=949) or non-concomitantly with ProQuad given first and the other vaccines 6 weeks later (N=485). No clinically significant differences in adverse events were reported between treatment groups *[see Clinical Studies (14)]*. The race distribution of the study subjects who received ProQuad was as follows: 70.7% White; 10.9% Asian/Pacific; 10.7% African-American; 4.5% Hispanic; 3.0% other; and 0.2% American Indian. The gender distribution of the study subjects who received ProQuad was 53.6% male and 46.4% female.

ProQuad Administered with Pneumococcal 7-valent Conjugate Vaccine and/or Hepatitis A Vaccine, Inactivated

In an open-label clinical trial, 1027 healthy children 12 to 23 months of age were randomized to receive ProQuad (dose 1) and pneumococcal 7-valent conjugate vaccine (dose 4) concomitantly (N=510) or non-concomitantly at different clinic visits (N=517). The race distribution of the study subjects was as follows: 65.2% White; 15.1% African-American; 10.0% Hispanic; 6.6% other; and 3.0% Asian/Pacific. The gender distribution of the study subjects was 54.5% male and 45.5% female. Injection-site and systemic adverse reactions observed among recipients of ProQuad administered concomitantly or non-concomitantly with pneumococcal 7-valent conjugate vaccine at a rate of at least 1% are shown in Table 4. No clinically significant differences in adverse reactions were reported between the concomitant and non-concomitant treatment groups *[see Clinical Studies (14)]*.

Table 4: Vaccine-Related Injection-Site and Systemic Adverse Reactions Reported in ≥1% of Children Who Received ProQuad (dose 1) Concomitantly or Non-Concomitantly with PCV7* (dose 4) at the First Visit (1 to 28 Days Postvaccination)

Adverse Reactions	ProQuad + PCV7 (N=510) (n=498) %	PCV7 (N=258) (n=250) %	ProQuad (N=259) (n=255) %
Injection-Site - ProQuad			
Pain†	24.9	N/A	24.7
Erythema†	12.4	N/A	11.0
Swelling†	10.8	N/A	7.5
Bruising	2.0	N/A	1.6
Injection-Site - PCV7			
Pain†	30.5	29.6	N/A
Erythema†	21.1	24.4	N/A
Swelling†	17.9	20.0	N/A
Bruising	1.6	1.2	N/A
Systemic			
Fever†,‡	15.5	10.0	15.3
Measles-like rash	4.4	0.8	5.1
Irritability	3.8	3.6	3.5
Upper respiratory infection	1.6	0.8	1.2
Varicella-like/vesicular rash	1.6	0.0	1.2
Diarrhea	0.8	1.2	1.2
Vomiting	0.6	0.8	1.2
Rash	0.4	0.0	1.2
Somnolence	0.0	0.0	1.2

N/A = Not applicable.
N = number of subjects vaccinated.
n = number of subjects with safety follow-up.
* PCV7 = Pneumococcal 7-valent conjugate vaccine, dose 4.
† Designates a solicited adverse reaction. Injection-site adverse reactions were solicited only from Days 1 to 5 postvaccination.
‡ Temperature reported as elevated (≥102°F, oral equivalent) or abnormal.

In an open-label clinical trial, 699 healthy children 12 to 23 months of age were randomized to receive 2 doses of VAQTA® (hepatitis A vaccine, inactivated) (N=352) or 2 doses of VAQTA concomitantly with 2 doses of ProQuad (N=347) at least 6 months apart. An additional 1101 subjects received 2 doses of VAQTA alone at least 6 months apart (non-randomized), resulting in 1453 subjects receiving 2 doses of VAQTA alone (1101 non-randomized and 352 randomized) and 347 subjects receiving 2 doses of VAQTA concomitantly with ProQuad (all randomized). The race distribution of the study subjects following a dose of ProQuad was as follows: 47.3% White; 42.7% Hispanic; 5.5% other; 2.9% African-American; and 1.7% Asian/Pacific. The gender distribution of the study subjects following a dose of ProQuad was 49.3% male and 50.7% female. Vaccine-related injection-site adverse reactions (days 1 to 5 postvaccination) and systemic adverse events (days 1 to 14 post VAQTA and days 1 to 28 post ProQuad vaccination) observed among recipients of VAQTA and ProQuad administered concomitantly with VAQTA at a rate of at least 1% are shown in Tables 5 and 6, respectively. In addition, among the randomized cohort, in the 14 days after each vaccination, the rates of fever (including all vaccine- and non-vaccine-related reports) were significantly higher in subjects who received ProQuad with VAQTA concomitantly after dose 1 (22.0%) as compared to subjects given dose 1 of VAQTA without ProQuad (10.8%). However, rates of fever were not significantly higher in subjects who received ProQuad with VAQTA concomitantly after dose 2 (12.5%) as compared to subjects given dose 2 of VAQTA without ProQuad (9.4%). In post-hoc analyses, these rates were significantly different for dose 1 (RR 2.03 [95% CI: 1.42, 2.94]), but not dose 2 (RR 1.32 [95% CI: 0.82, 2.13]). Rates of injection-site adverse reactions and other systemic adverse events were lower following a second dose than following the first dose of both vaccines given concomitantly.

[See table 5 at top of next page]

[See table 6 at top of next page]

In an open-label clinical trial, 653 children 12 to 23 months of age were randomized to receive a first dose of ProQuad with VAQTA and pneumococcal 7-valent conjugate vaccine concomitantly (N=330) or a first dose of ProQuad and pneumococcal 7-valent conjugate vaccine concomitantly and then vaccinated with VAQTA 6 weeks later (N=323). Approximately 6 months later, subjects received either the second doses of ProQuad and VAQTA concomitantly or the second

Table 5: Vaccine-Related Injection-Site Adverse Reactions Reported in ≥1% of Children Who Received VAQTA or ProQuad Concomitantly with VAQTA 1 to 5 Days After Vaccination with VAQTA or VAQTA and ProQuad

Adverse Reactions	Dose 1		Dose 2	
	VAQTA (N=1453) (n=1412) %	ProQuad + VAQTA (N=347) (n=328) %	VAQTA (N=1301) (n=1254) %	ProQuad + VAQTA (N=292) (n=264) %
Injection-Site VAQTA				
Pain/tenderness*	29.2	27.1	30.1	25.0
Erythema*	13.5	12.5	14.3	11.7
Swelling*	7.1	9.1	9.0	8.0
Injection-site bruising	1.9	2.4	1.0	0.8
Injection-Site ProQuad				
Pain/tenderness*	N/A	30.5	N/A	26.2
Erythema*	N/A	13.4	N/A	12.9
Swelling*	N/A	6.7	N/A	6.5
Injection-site bruising	N/A	1.5	N/A	0.4

N/A = Not applicable.
N = number of subjects vaccinated.
n = number of subjects with safety follow-up.
* Designates a solicited adverse reaction. Injection-site adverse reactions were solicited only from Days 1 to 5 postvaccination.

Table 6: Vaccine-Related Systemic Adverse Reactions Reported in ≥1% of Children Who Received VAQTA* or ProQuad Concomitantly with VAQTA 1 to 14 Days After VAQTA or Vaccination with ProQuad and VAQTA and 1 to 28 Days After Vaccination with ProQuad and VAQTA

Adverse Reactions	Dose 1			Dose 2		
	Days 1 to 14		Days 1 to 28	Days 1 to 14		Days 1 to 28
	VAQTA† (N=1453) (n=1412) %	ProQuad + VAQTA† (N=347) (n=328) %	ProQuad + VAQTA (N=347) (n=328) %	VAQTA (N=1301) (n=1254) %	ProQuad + VAQTA† (N=292) (n=264) %	ProQuad + VAQTA† (N=291) (n=263) %
Fever‡,§	5.7	14.9	15.2	4.1	8.0	8.4
Irritability	5.8	7.0	7.3	3.5	5.3	5.3
Measles-like rash	0.0	3.4	3.4	0.0	1.1	1.1
Rhinorrhea	0.6	2.7	3.0	0.6	1.1	2.7
Diarrhea	1.5	1.8	2.4	1.7	0.4	0.8
Cough	0.6	2.1	2.1	0.2	0.8	1.5
Vomiting	1.1	0.3	0.9	0.6	0.8	1.1

N = number of subjects vaccinated.
n = number of subjects with safety follow-up.
* Systemic adverse events for subjects given VAQTA alone were collected for 14 days postvaccination.
† Safety follow-up for systemic adverse reactions was 14 days for VAQTA and 28 days for ProQuad + VAQTA.
‡ Designates a solicited adverse reaction.
§ Temperature reported as elevated or abnormal.

doses of ProQuad and VAQTA separately. The race distribution of the study subjects was as follows: 60.3% White; 21.6% African-American; 9.5% Hispanic; 7.2% other, 1.1% Asian/Pacific; and 0.3% American Indian. The gender distribution of the study subjects was 50.7% male and 49.3% female. Vaccine-related injection-site and systemic adverse reactions observed among recipients of concomitant ProQuad, VAQTA, and pneumococcal 7-valent conjugate vaccine and ProQuad and pneumococcal 7-valent conjugate vaccine at a rate of at least 1% are shown in Tables 7 and 8. In the 28 days after vaccination with the first dose of ProQuad, the rates of fever (including all vaccine- and non-vaccine-related reports) were comparable in subjects who received the 3 vaccines together (38.6%) as compared with subjects given ProQuad and pneumococcal 7-valent conjugate vaccine (42.7%). The rates of fever in the 28 days following the second dose of ProQuad were also comparable in subjects who received ProQuad and VAQTA together (17.4%) as compared with subjects given ProQuad separately from VAQTA (17.0%). In a post-hoc analysis, these differences were not statistically significant after ProQuad (dose 1) (RR 0.90 [95% CI: 0.75, 1.09]) nor after dose 2 (RR 1.02 [95% CI: 0.70, 1.51]). No clinically significant differences in adverse reactions were reported among treatment groups *[see Clinical Studies (14)]*.

[See table 7 at top of next page]
[See table 8 at top of next page]

Reye's syndrome following wild-type varicella infection has occurred in children and adolescents, the majority of whom had received salicylates. In all clinical studies of ProQuad or VARIVAX, the recommendation was made to avoid the use of salicylates for 6 weeks after vaccination. There were no reports of Reye's syndrome in recipients of ProQuad or VARIVAX during these studies *[see Drug Interactions (7.2) and Patient Counseling Information (17.1)]*.

6.2 Post-Marketing Experience

The following adverse events have been identified during post-approval use of either the components of ProQuad or ProQuad. Because the reactions are in some cases described in the literature or reported voluntarily from a population of uncertain size, it is not always possible to reliably estimate their frequency or establish a causal relationship.

Post-Marketing Reports

Adverse events reported with post-marketing use of ProQuad and/or in clinical studies and/or post-marketing use of M-M-R II, the component vaccines, and VARIVAX without regard to causality or frequency are summarized below.

Infections and infestations

Atypical measles, candidiasis, cellulitis, herpes zoster, infection, influenza, measles, orchitis, parotitis, respiratory infection, skin infection, varicella (vaccine strain).

Blood and the lymphatic system disorders

Aplastic anemia, lymphadenitis, regional lymphadenopathy, thrombocytopenia.

Immune system disorders

Anaphylactoid reaction, anaphylaxis and related phenomena such as angioneurotic edema, facial edema, and peripheral edema, anaphylaxis in individuals with or without an allergic history.

Psychiatric disorders

Agitation, apathy, nervousness.

Nervous system disorders

Afebrile convulsions or seizures, aseptic meningitis (see below), ataxia, Bell's palsy, cerebrovascular accident, convulsion, dizziness, dream abnormality, encephalitis (see below), encephalopathy (see below), febrile seizure, Guillain-Barré syndrome, headache, hypersomnia, measles inclusion body encephalitis *[see Contraindications (4.2)]*, ocular palsies, paraesthesia, polyneuritis, polyneuropathy, subacute sclerosing panencephalitis (see below), syncope, transverse myelitis, tremor.

Eye disorders

Edema of the eyelid, irritation, optic neuritis, retinitis, retrobulbar neuritis.

Ear and labyrinth disorders

Ear pain, nerve deafness.

Vascular disorders

Extravasation.

Respiratory, thoracic and mediastinal disorders

Bronchial spasm, bronchitis, epistaxis, pneumonitis *[see Contraindications (4.3)]*, pneumonia, pulmonary congestion, rhinitis, sinusitis, sneezing, sore throat, wheezing.

Gastrointestinal disorders

Abdominal pain, flatulence, hematochezia, mouth ulcer.

Skin and subcutaneous tissue disorders

Erythema multiforme, Henoch-Schönlein purpura, herpes simplex, impetigo, panniculitis, pruritus, purpura, skin induration, Stevens-Johnson syndrome, sunburn.

Musculoskeletal, connective tissue and bone disorders

Arthritis and/or arthralgia (usually transient and rarely chronic, see below), musculoskeletal pain, myalgia, pain of the hip, leg, or neck, swelling.

Reproductive system and breast disorders

Epididymitis.

General disorders and administration site conditions

Injection-site complaints (burning and/or stinging of short duration, eczema, edema/swelling, hive-like rash, discoloration, hematoma, induration, lump, vesicles, wheal and flare), inflammation, lip abnormality, papillitis, roughness/dryness, stiffness, trauma, varicella-like rash, venipuncture site hemorrhage, warm sensation, warm to touch.

Deaths have been reported following vaccination with measles, mumps, and rubella vaccines; however, a causal relationship has not been established in healthy individuals. Death as a direct consequence of disseminated measles vaccine virus infection has been reported in severely immunocompromised individuals in whom a measles-containing vaccine is contraindicated and who were inadvertently vaccinated. However, there were no deaths or permanent sequelae reported in a published post-marketing surveillance study in Finland involving 1.5 million children and adults who were vaccinated with M-M-R II during 1982 to 1993.{3}

Encephalitis and encephalopathy have been reported approximately once for every 3 million doses of the combination of measles, mumps, and rubella vaccine contained in M-M-R II. In no case has it been shown conclusively that reactions were actually caused by the vaccine; however, the data suggest the possibility that some of these cases may have been caused by measles vaccines. The risk of such serious neurological disorders following live measles virus vaccine administration remains far less than that for encephalitis and encephalopathy with wild-type measles (1 per 2000 reported cases).

Recipients of rubella vaccine may develop chronic joint symptoms. Arthralgia and/or arthritis, and polyneuritis after wild-type rubella virus infection vary in frequency and severity with age and gender, being greatest in adult females and least in pre-pubertal children. Following vaccination in children, reactions in joints are uncommon (0 to 3%) and of brief duration. In women, incidence rates for arthritis and arthralgia are higher than those seen in children (12 to 26%), and the reactions tend to be more marked and of longer duration (*e.g.*, months or years). In adolescent girls, the reactions appear to be intermediate in incidence between those seen in children and adult women.

Chronic arthritis has been associated with wild-type rubella infection and has been related to persistent virus and/or viral antigen isolated from body tissues. Chronic joint symptoms have been reported following administration of rubella-containing vaccine.

There have been reports of subacute sclerosing panencephalitis (SSPE) in children who did not have a history of infection with wild-type measles but did receive measles vaccine. Some of these cases may have resulted from unrecognized measles in the first year of life or possibly from the measles vaccination. Based on estimated measles vaccine distribution in the United States (US), the association of SSPE cases to measles vaccination is about one case per million vaccine doses distributed. The association with wild-type measles virus infection is 6 to 22 cases of SSPE per million cases of measles. The results of a retrospective case-controlled study suggest that the overall effect of measles vaccine has been to protect against SSPE by preventing measles with its inherent higher risk of SSPE.

Cases of aseptic meningitis have been reported to VAERS following measles, mumps, and rubella vaccination. Although a causal relationship between other strains of mumps vaccine and aseptic meningitis has been shown, there is no evidence to link Jeryl Lynn™ mumps vaccine to aseptic meningitis.

Table 7: Vaccine-Related Injection-Site Adverse Reactions Reported in ≥1% of Children Who Received ProQuad + VAQTA + PCV7* Concomitantly or VAQTA Alone Followed by ProQuad + PCV7 Concomitantly (1 to 5 Days After a Dose of ProQuad)

Adverse Reactions	Dose 1		Dose 2	
	VAQTA + ProQuad + PCV7 (N=330) (n=311) %	VAQTA Alone Followed by ProQuad + PCV7 (N=323) (n=302) %	VAQTA + ProQuad (N=273) (n=265) %	VAQTA Alone Followed by ProQuad (N=240) (n=230) %
Injection-Site - ProQuad				
Pain/tenderness†	21.2	24.2	18.1	17.0
Erythema†	13.5	11.9	10.6	13.0
Swelling†	7.4	10.9	8.3	11.7
Bruising	1.9	1.3	0.8	0.4
Injection-Site - VAQTA				
Pain/tenderness†	20.6	15.3	17.5	20.3
Erythema†	9.6	11.7	9.1	12.7
Swelling†	6.8	9.5	6.1	7.6
Bruising	1.3	1.1	1.1	1.6
Rash	1.0	0.0	0.4	0.4
Injection-Site - PCV7				
Pain/tenderness†	25.4	27.6	N/A	N/A
Erythema†	16.4	16.6	N/A	N/A
Swelling†	13.2	14.3	N/A	N/A
Bruising	0.6	1.7	N/A	N/A

N/A = Not applicable.
N = number of subjects vaccinated.
n = number of subjects with safety follow-up.
* PCV7 = Pneumococcal 7-valent conjugate vaccine.
† Designates a solicited adverse reaction. Injection-site adverse reactions were solicited only from Days 1 to 5 postvaccination at each vaccine injection site.

Table 8: Vaccine-Related Systemic Adverse Reactions Reported in ≥1% of Children Who Received ProQuad + VAQTA + PCV7* Concomitantly, or VAQTA Alone Followed By ProQuad + PCV7 Concomitantly (1 to 28 Days After a Dose of ProQuad)

Adverse Reactions	Dose 1		Dose 2	
	VAQTA + ProQuad + PCV7 (N=330) (n=311) %	VAQTA Alone Followed by ProQuad + PCV7 (N=323) (n=302) %	VAQTA + ProQuad (N=273) (n=265) %	VAQTA Alone Followed by ProQuad (N=240) (n=230) %
Fever†,‡	26.4	27.2	9.1	9.6
Irritability	4.8	6.3	1.9	1.3
Measles-like rash†	2.3	4.0	0.0	0.0
Varicella-like rash†	1.0	1.7	0.0	0.0
Rash (not otherwise specified)	1.3	1.3	0.0	0.9
Diarrhea	1.3	1.3	0.4	1.3
Upper respiratory infection	1.0	1.3	1.1	0.9
Viral infection	1.0	0.7	0.0	0.0
Rhinorrhea	0.0	0.7	1.1	0.0

N = number of subjects vaccinated.
n = number of subjects with safety follow-up.
* PCV7 = Pneumococcal 7-valent conjugate vaccine.
† Designates a solicited adverse reaction.
‡ Temperature reported as elevated or abnormal.

Table 9: Confirmed Febrile Seizures Days 5 to 12 and 0 to 30 After Vaccination with ProQuad (dose 1) Compared to Concomitant Vaccination with M-M-R II and VARIVAX (dose 1) in Children 12 to 60 Months of Age

Time Period	ProQuad cohort (N=31,298)		MMR+V cohort (N=31,298)		Relative risk (95% CI)
	n	Incidence per 1,000	n	Incidence per 1,000	
5 to 12 Days	22	0.70	10	0.32	2.20 (1.04, 4.65)
0 to 30 Days	44	1.41	40	1.28	1.10 (0.72, 1.69)

Cases of thrombocytopenia have been reported after use of measles vaccine, measles, mumps, and rubella vaccine, and after varicella vaccination. Post-marketing experience with live measles, mumps, and rubella vaccine indicates that individuals with current thrombocytopenia may develop more severe thrombocytopenia following vaccination. In addition, individuals who experienced thrombocytopenia following the first dose of a live measles, mumps, and rubella vaccine may develop thrombocytopenia with repeat doses. Serologic testing for antibody to measles, mumps, or rubella should be considered in order to determine if additional doses of vaccine are needed *[see Warnings and Precautions (5.5)]*.

The reported rate of zoster in recipients of VARIVAX appears not to exceed that previously determined in a population-based study of healthy children who had experienced wild-type varicella.{4} In clinical trials, 8 cases of herpes zoster were reported in 9454 vaccinated individuals 12 months to 12 years of age during 42,556 person-years of follow-up. This resulted in a calculated incidence of at least 18.8 cases per 100,000 person-years. All 8 cases reported after VARIVAX were mild and no sequelae were reported. The long-term effect of VARIVAX on the incidence of herpes zoster is unknown at present.

6.3 Post-Marketing Observational Safety Surveillance Study

Safety was evaluated in an observational study that included 69,237 children vaccinated with ProQuad 12 months to 12 years old. A historical comparison group included 69,237 age-, gender-, and date-of-vaccination (day and month) matched subjects who were given M-M-R II and VARIVAX concomitantly. The primary objective was to assess the incidence of febrile seizures occurring within various time intervals after vaccination in 12- to 60-month-old children who had neither been vaccinated against measles, mumps, rubella, or varicella, nor had a history of the wild-type infections (N=31,298 vaccinated with ProQuad, including 31,043 who were 12 to 23 months old). The incidence of febrile seizures was also assessed in a historical control group of children who had received their first vaccination with M-M-R II and VARIVAX concomitantly (N=31,298, including 31,019 who were 12 to 23 months old). The secondary objective was to assess the general safety of ProQuad in the 30-day period after vaccination in children 12 months to 12 years old.

In pre-licensure clinical studies, an increase in fever was observed 5 to 12 days after vaccination with ProQuad (dose 1) compared to M-M-R II and VARIVAX (dose 1) given concomitantly. In the post-marketing observational surveillance study, results from the primary safety analysis revealed an approximate two-fold increase in the risk of febrile seizures in the same 5 to 12 day timeframe after vaccination with ProQuad (dose 1). The incidence of febrile seizures 5 to 12 days after ProQuad (dose 1) (0.70 per 1000 children) was higher than that in children receiving M-M-R II and VARIVAX concomitantly (0.32 per 1000 children) [relative risk (RR) 2.20, 95% confidence interval (CI): 1.04, 4.65]. The incidence of febrile seizures 0 to 30 days after ProQuad (dose 1) (1.41 per 1000 children) was similar to that observed in children receiving M-M-R II and VARIVAX concomitantly [RR 1.10 (95% CI: 0.72, 1.69)]. See Table 9. General safety analyses revealed that the risks of fever (RR=1.89; 95% CI: 1.67, 2.15) and skin eruption (RR=1.68; 95% CI: 1.07, 2.64) were significantly higher after ProQuad (dose 1) compared with those who received concomitant first doses of M-M-R II and VARIVAX, respectively. All medical events that resulted in hospitalization or emergency room visits were compared between the group given ProQuad and the historical comparison group, and no other safety concerns were identified in this study.

[See table 9 above]

In this observational post-marketing study, no case of febrile seizure was observed during the 5 to 12 day post-vaccination time period among 26,455 children who received ProQuad as a second dose of M-M-R II and VARIVAX. In addition, detailed general safety data were available from more than 25,000 children who received ProQuad as a second dose of M-M-R II and VARIVAX, most of them (95%) between 4 and 6 years of age, and an analysis of these data by an independent, external safety monitoring committee did not identify any specific safety concern.

7 DRUG INTERACTIONS

7.1 Immune Globulins and Transfusions

Immune globulins (IG) administered concomitantly with ProQuad contain antibodies that may interfere with vaccine virus replication and decrease the expected immune response. Vaccination should be deferred for at least 3 months following blood or plasma transfusions, or administration of IG.

The appropriate suggested interval between transfusion or IG administration and vaccination will vary with the type of transfusion or indication for, and dose of, IG (*e.g.*, 5 months for Varicella Zoster Immune Globulin [VZIG]).{2} Following administration of ProQuad, any IG including VZIG should not be given for 1 month thereafter unless its use outweighs the benefits of vaccination.{2} *[See Warnings and Precautions (5.9).]*

7.2 Salicylates

Reye's syndrome has been reported following the use of salicylates during wild-type varicella infection. Vaccine recipients should avoid use of salicylates for 6 weeks after vaccination with ProQuad. *[See Adverse Reactions (6.1) and Patient Counseling Information (17.1).]*

7.3 Corticosteroids and Immunosuppressive Drugs

ProQuad may be used in individuals who are receiving topical corticosteroids or low-dose corticosteroids for asthma prophylaxis or replacement therapy, *e.g.*, for Addison's disease. ProQuad should not be given to individuals receiving immunosuppressive doses of corticosteroids or other immunosuppressive drugs. Vaccination with a live, attenuated vaccine, such as varicella or measles, can result in a more extensive vaccine-associated rash or disseminated disease in individuals on immunosuppressive drugs *[see Contraindications (4.2)]*.

7.4 Drug/Laboratory Test Interactions

Live, attenuated measles, mumps, and rubella virus vaccines given individually may result in a temporary depression of tuberculin skin sensitivity. Therefore, if a tuberculin test is to be done, it should be administered either any time before, simultaneously with, or at least 4 to 6 weeks after ProQuad.

7.5 Use With Other Vaccines

At least 1 month should elapse between a dose of a measles-containing vaccine such as M-M-R II and a dose of ProQuad, and at least 3 months should elapse between administration of 2 doses of ProQuad or varicella-containing vaccines.

ProQuad may be administered concomitantly with *Haemophilus influenzae* type b conjugate (meningococcal protein conjugate) and hepatitis B (recombinant). Additionally, ProQuad may be administered concomitantly with pneumococcal 7-valent conjugate vaccine, and/or hepatitis A (inactivated) vaccines. *[See Clinical Studies (14).]*

There are no data regarding the administration of ProQuad with inactivated poliovirus vaccine or with other live virus vaccines.

There are insufficient data to support concomitant vaccination with diphtheria and tetanus toxoids and acellular pertussis vaccine adsorbed. *[See Clinical Studies (14).]*

Children under treatment for tuberculosis have not experienced exacerbation of the disease when vaccinated with live measles virus vaccine; no studies have been reported to date of the effect of measles virus vaccines on children with untreated tuberculosis.

8 USE IN SPECIFIC POPULATIONS

8.1 Pregnancy

Pregnancy Category C: Animal reproduction studies have not been conducted with ProQuad.

Do not administer ProQuad to pregnant females. It is also not known whether ProQuad can cause fetal harm when administered to a pregnant woman or can affect reproduction capacity. If vaccination of post-pubertal females is undertaken, pregnancy should be avoided for 3 months following vaccination. *[See Contraindications (4.4).]*

In counseling women who are inadvertently vaccinated when pregnant or who become pregnant within 3 months of vaccination, the healthcare provider should be aware of the following: (1) Reports have indicated that contracting wild-type measles during pregnancy enhances fetal risk. Increased rates of spontaneous abortion, stillbirth, congenital defects, and prematurity have been observed subsequent to wild-type measles during pregnancy. There are no adequate studies of the attenuated (vaccine) strain of measles virus in pregnancy. However, it would be prudent to assume that the vaccine strain of virus is also capable of inducing adverse fetal effects; (2) Mumps infection during the first trimester of pregnancy may increase the rate of spontaneous abortion. Although mumps vaccine virus has been shown to infect the placenta and fetus, there is no evidence that it causes congenital malformations in humans;{5} (3) In a 10-year survey involving over 700 pregnant women who received rubella vaccine within 3 months before or after conception (of whom 189 received the Wistar RA 27/3 strain), none of the newborns had abnormalities compatible with congenital rubella syndrome;{6} and (4) Wild-type varicella can sometimes cause congenital varicella infection.

Merck Sharp & Dohme Corp., a subsidiary of Merck & Co., Inc., maintains a Pregnancy Registry to monitor fetal outcomes of pregnant women exposed to varicella-containing vaccine (Oka/Merck). In the first 9 years of the Pregnancy Registry for varicella vaccine (Oka/Merck), of 129 seronegative women and 423 women of unknown serostatus who received varicella vaccine during pregnancy or within 3 months before pregnancy, none had newborns with abnormalities compatible with congenital varicella syndrome.

Patients and health care providers are encouraged to report any exposure to varicella-containing vaccine (Oka/Merck) during pregnancy by calling 1-800-986-8999.

8.3 Nursing Mothers

Do not administer ProQuad to nursing women. It is not known whether ProQuad is excreted in human milk. Because many drugs are excreted in human milk, caution should be exercised when ProQuad is administered to a nursing woman. The secretion of measles and mumps viruses in human milk has not been studied; however, studies have shown that lactating postpartum women vaccinated with live rubella vaccine may secrete the virus in breast milk and transmit it to breast fed infants. Limited evidence in the literature suggests that virus, viral DNA, or viral antigen could not be detected in the breast milk of women who were vaccinated postpartum with the vaccine strain of varicella virus.{7,8} *[See Warnings and Precautions (5.8).]*

8.4 Pediatric Use

Do not administer ProQuad to infants younger than 12 months of age or to children 13 years and older. Safety and effectiveness of ProQuad in infants younger than 12 months of age and in children 13 years and older have not been studied. ProQuad is not approved for use in persons in these age groups. *[See Adverse Reactions (6) and Clinical Studies (14).]*

Table 10: Summary of Combined Immunogenicity Results 6 Weeks Following the Administration of a Single Dose of ProQuad (Varicella Virus Potency ≥3.97 $\log_{10}$ PFU) or M-M-R II and VARIVAX (Per-Protocol Population)

Group	Antigen	n	Observed Response Rate (95% CI)	Observed GMT (95% CI)
ProQuad (N=5446*)	Varicella	4381	91.2% (90.3%, 92.0%)	15.5 (15.0, 15.9)
	Measles	4733	97.4% (96.9%, 97.9%)	3124.9 (3038.9, 3213.3)
	Mumps (OD cutoff)†	973	98.8% (97.9%, 99.4%)	105.3 (98.0, 113.1)
	Mumps (wild-type ELISA)†	3735	95.8% (95.1%, 96.4%)	93.1 (90.2, 96.0)
	Rubella	4773	98.5% (98.1%, 98.8%)	91.8 (89.6, 94.1)
M-M-R II + VARIVAX (N=2038*)	Varicella	1417	94.1% (92.8%, 95.3%)	16.6 (15.9, 17.4)
	Measles	1516	98.2% (97.4%, 98.8%)	2239.6 (2138.3, 2345.6)
	Mumps (OD cutoff)†	501	99.4% (98.3%, 99.9%)	87.5 (79.7, 96.0)
	Mumps (wild-type ELISA)†	1017	98.0% (97.0%, 98.8%)	90.8 (86.2, 95.7)
	Rubella	1528	98.5% (97.7%, 99.0%)	102.2 (97.8, 106.7)

n = Number of per-protocol subjects with evaluable serology.
CI = Confidence interval.
GMT = Geometric mean titer.
ELISA = Enzyme-linked immunosorbent assay.
PFU = Plaque-forming units.
OD = Optical density.
* Includes ProQuad + Placebo followed by ProQuad (Visit 1) (Protocol 009), ProQuad Middle and High Doses (Visit 1) (Protocol 011), ProQuad (Lot 1, Lot 2, Lot 3) (Protocol 012), both the Concomitant and Non-concomitant groups (Protocol 013).
† The mumps antibody response was assessed by a vaccine-strain ELISA in Protocols 009 and 011 and by a wild-type ELISA in Protocols 012 and 013. In the former assay, the serostatus was based on the OD cutoff of the assay. In the latter assay, 10 mumps ELISA units was used as the serostatus cutoff.

Table 11: Summary of Immune Response to a First and Second Dose of ProQuad in Subjects < 3 Years of Age Who Received ProQuad with a Varicella Virus Dose ≥3.97 Log_{10} PFU*

		Dose 1 N=1097			Dose 2 N=1097		
Antigen	Serostatus Cutoff/ Response Criteria	n	Observed Response Rate (95% CI)	Observed GMT (95% CI)	n	Observed Response Rate (95% CI)	Observed GMT (95% CI)
Measles	≥120 mIU/mL†	915	98.1% (97.0%, 98.9%)	2956.8 (2786.3, 3137.7)	915	99.5% (98.7%, 99.8%)	5958.0 (5518.9, 6432.1)
	≥255 mIU/mL	943	97.8% (96.6%, 98.6%)	2966.0 (2793.4, 3149.2)	943	99.4% (98.6%, 99.8%)	5919.3 (5486.2, 6386.6)
Mumps	≥OD Cutoff (ELISA antibody units)	920	98.7% (97.7%, 99.3%)	106.7 (99.1, 114.8)	920	99.9% (99.4%, 100%)	253.1 (237.9, 269.2)
Rubella	≥10 IU/mL	937	97.7% (96.5%, 98.5%)	91.1 (85.9, 96.6)	937	98.3% (97.2%, 99.0%)	158.8 (149.1, 169.2)

(Table continued on next page)

8.5 Geriatric Use

ProQuad is not indicated for use in the geriatric population (≥age 65).

11 DESCRIPTION

ProQuad (Measles, Mumps, Rubella and Varicella Virus Vaccine Live) is a combined, attenuated, live virus vaccine containing measles, mumps, rubella, and varicella viruses. ProQuad is a sterile lyophilized preparation of (1) the components of M-M-R II (Measles, Mumps, and Rubella Virus Vaccine Live): Measles Virus Vaccine Live, a more attenuated line of measles virus, derived from Enders' attenuated Edmonston strain and propagated in chick embryo cell culture; Mumps Virus Vaccine Live, the Jeryl Lynn™ (B level) strain of mumps virus propagated in chick embryo cell culture; Rubella Virus Vaccine Live, the Wistar RA 27/3 strain of live attenuated rubella virus propagated in WI-38 human diploid lung fibroblasts; and (2) Varicella Virus Vaccine Live (Oka/Merck), the Oka/Merck strain of varicella-zoster virus propagated in MRC-5 cells. The cells, virus pools, bovine serum, and human albumin used in manufacturing are all tested to provide assurance that the final product is free of potential adventitious agents.

ProQuad, when reconstituted as directed, is a sterile suspension for subcutaneous administration. Each 0.5-mL dose contains not less than 3.00 $\log_{10}$ TCID_{50} of measles virus; 4.30 $\log_{10}$ TCID_{50} of mumps virus; 3.00 $\log_{10}$ TCID_{50} of rubella virus; and a minimum of 3.99 $\log_{10}$ PFU of Oka/Merck varicella virus.

Each 0.5-mL dose of the vaccine contains no more than 21 mg of sucrose, 11 mg of hydrolyzed gelatin, 2.4 mg of sodium chloride, 1.8 mg of sorbitol, 0.40 mg of monosodium L-glutamate, 0.34 mg of sodium phosphate dibasic, 0.31 mg of human albumin, 0.17 mg of sodium bicarbonate, 72 mcg of potassium phosphate monobasic, 60 mcg of potassium chloride; 36 mcg of potassium phosphate dibasic; residual components of MRC-5 cells including DNA and protein; <16 mcg of neomycin, bovine calf serum (0.5 mcg), and other buffer and media ingredients. The product contains no preservative.

12 CLINICAL PHARMACOLOGY

12.1 Mechanism of Action

ProQuad has been shown to induce measles-, mumps-, rubella-, and varicella-specific immunity, which is thought to be the mechanism by which it protects against these four childhood diseases.

The efficacy of ProQuad was established through the use of immunological correlates for protection against measles, mumps, rubella, and varicella. Results from efficacy studies or field effectiveness studies that were previously conducted for the component vaccines were used to define levels of serum antibodies that correlated with protection against measles, mumps, and rubella. Also, in previous studies with varicella vaccine, antibody responses against varicella virus ≥5 gpELISA units/mL in a glycoprotein enzyme-linked immunosorbent assay (gpELISA) (not commercially available) similarly correlated with long-term protection. In these efficacy studies, the clinical endpoint for measles and mumps was a clinical diagnosis of either disease confirmed by a 4-fold or greater rise in serum antibody titers between either postvaccination or acute and convalescent titers; for rubella, a 4-fold or greater rise in antibody titers with or without clinical symptoms of rubella; and for varicella, varicella-like rash that occurred >42 days postvaccination and for which varicella was not excluded by either viral cultures of the lesion or serological tests. Specific laboratory evidence of varicella either by serology or culture was not required to confirm the diagnosis of varicella. Clinical studies with a single dose of ProQuad have shown that vaccination elicited rates of antibody responses against measles, mumps, and rubella that were similar to those observed after vaccination with a single dose of M-M-R II *[see Clinical Studies (14)]* and seroresponse rates for varicella virus were similar to those observed after vaccination with a single dose of VARIVAX *[see Clinical Studies (14)]*. The duration of protection from measles, mumps, rubella, and varicella infections after vaccination with ProQuad is unknown.

12.4 Persistence of Antibody Responses After Vaccination

The persistence of antibody at 1 year after vaccination was evaluated in a subset of 2107 children enrolled in the clinical trials. Antibody was detected in 98.9% (1722/1741) for measles, 96.7% (1676/1733) for mumps, 99.6% (1796/1804) for rubella, and 97.5% (1512/1550) for varicella (≥5 gpELISA units/mL) of vaccinees following a single dose of ProQuad.

Experience with M-M-R II demonstrates that antibodies to measles, mumps, and rubella viruses are still detectable in most individuals 11 to 13 years after primary vaccination.{9} Varicella antibodies were present for up to ten years postvaccination in most of the individuals tested who received 1 dose of VARIVAX.

13 NONCLINICAL TOXICOLOGY

13.1 Carcinogenesis, Mutagenesis, Impairment of Fertility

ProQuad has not been evaluated for its carcinogenic, mutagenic, or teratogenic potential, or its potential to impair fertility.

14 CLINICAL STUDIES

Formal studies to evaluate the clinical efficacy of ProQuad have not been performed.

Efficacy of the measles, mumps, rubella, and varicella components of ProQuad was previously established in a series of clinical studies with the monovalent vaccines. A high degree of protection from infection was demonstrated in these studies.{10-17}

Immunogenicity in Children 12 Months to 6 Years of Age

Prior to licensure, immunogenicity was studied in 5845 healthy children 12 months to 6 years of age with a negative clinical history of measles, mumps, rubella, and varicella who participated in 5 randomized clinical trials. The immunogenicity of ProQuad was similar to that of its individual component vaccines (M-M-R II and VARIVAX), which are currently used in routine vaccination.

The presence of detectable antibody was assessed by an appropriately sensitive enzyme-linked immunosorbent assay (ELISA) for measles, mumps (wild-type and vaccine-type strains), and rubella, and by gpELISA for varicella. For evaluation of vaccine response rates, a positive result in the measles ELISA corresponded to measles antibody concentrations of ≥255 mIU/mL when compared to the WHO II (66/202) Reference Immunoglobulin for Measles.

Children were positive for mumps antibody if the antibody level was ≥10 ELISA units/mL. A positive result in the rubella ELISA corresponded to concentrations of ≥10 IU rubella antibody/mL when compared to the WHO International Reference Serum for Rubella; children with varicella antibody levels ≥5 gpELISA units/mL were considered to be seropositive since a response rate based on ≥5 gpELISA units/mL has been shown to be highly correlated with long-term protection.

Table 11 *(cont.)*: Summary of Immune Response to a First and Second Dose of ProQuad in Subjects < 3 Years of Age Who Received ProQuad with a Varicella Virus Dose ≥3.97 Log_{10} PFU*

		Dose 1 N=1097			Dose 2 N=1097		
Antigen	Serostatus Cutoff/ Response Criteria	n	Observed Response Rate (95% CI)	Observed GMT (95% CI)	n	Observed Response Rate (95% CI)	Observed GMT (95% CI)
Varicella	<1.25 to ≥5 gpELISA units	864	86.6% (84.1%, 88.8%)	11.6 (10.9, 12.3)	864	99.4% (98.7%, 99.8%)	477.5 (437.8, 520.7)
	≥OD Cutoff (gpELISA units)	695	87.2% (84.5%, 89.6%)	11.6 (10.9, 12.4)	695	99.4% (98.5%, 99.8%)	478.7 (434.8, 527.1)

ProQuad (Middle Dose) = ProQuad containing a varicella virus dose of 3.97 log_{10} PFU.
ProQuad (High Dose) = ProQuad containing a varicella virus dose of 4.25 log_{10} PFU.
ELISA = Enzyme-linked immunosorbent assay.
gpELISA = Glycoprotein enzyme-linked immunosorbent assay.
N = Number vaccinated at baseline.
n = Number of subjects who were per-protocol Postdose 1 and Postdose 2 and satisfied the given prevaccination serostatus cutoff.
CI = Confidence interval.
GMT = Geometric mean titer.
PFU = Plaque-forming units.

* Includes the following treatment groups: ProQuad + Placebo followed by ProQuad (Visit 1) (Protocol 009) and ProQuad (Middle and High Dose) (Protocol 011).

† Samples from Protocols 009 and 011 were assayed in the legacy format Measles ELISA, which reported antibody titers in Measles ELISA units. To convert titers from ELISA units to mIU/mL, titers for these 2 protocols were divided by 0.1025. The lowest measurable titer postvaccination is 207.5 mIU/mL. The response rate for measles in the legacy format is the percent of subjects with a negative baseline measles antibody titer, as defined by the optical density (OD) cutoff, with a postvaccination measles antibody titer ≥207.5 mIU/mL. Samples from Protocols 009 and 011 were assayed in the legacy format Rubella ELISA, which reported antibody titers in Rubella ELISA units. To convert titers from ELISA units to IU/mL, titers for these 2 protocols were divided by 1.28.

Table 12: Summary of Antibody Responses to Measles, Mumps, Rubella, and Varicella at 6 Weeks Postvaccination in Subjects 4 to 6 Years of Age Who Had Previously Received M-M-R II and VARIVAX (Per-Protocol Population)

Group Number (Description)	n	GMT (95% CI)	Seropositivity Rate (95% CI)	% ≥4-Fold Rise in Titer (95% CI)	Geometric Mean Fold Rise (95% CI)
			Measles*		
Group 1 (N=399) (ProQuad + placebo)	367	1985.9 (1817.6, 2169.9)	100% (99.0%, 100%)	4.9% (2.9%, 7.6%)	1.21 (1.13, 1.30)
Group 2 (N=205) (M-M-R II + placebo)	185	2046.9 (1815.2, 2308.2)	100% (98.0%, 100%)	4.3% (1.9%, 8.3%)	1.28 (1.17, 1.40)
Group 3 (N=195) (M-M-R II + VARIVAX)	171	2084.3 (1852.3, 2345.5)	99.4% (96.8%, 100%)	4.7% (2.0%, 9.0%)	1.31 (1.17, 1.46)
			Mumps†		
Group 1 (N=399) (ProQuad + placebo)	367	206.0 (188.2, 225.4)	99.5% (98.0%, 99.9%)	27.2% (22.8%, 32.1%)	2.43 (2.19, 2.69)
Group 2 (N=205) (M-M-R II + placebo)	185	308.5 (269.6, 352.9)	100% (98.0%, 100%)	41.1% (33.9%, 48.5%)	3.69 (3.14, 4.32)
Group 3 (N=195) (M-M-R II + VARIVAX)	171	295.9 (262.5, 333.5)	100% (97.9%, 100%)	41.5% (34.0%, 49.3%)	3.36 (2.84, 3.97)
			Rubella‡		
Group 1 (N=399) (ProQuad + placebo)	367	217.3 (200.1, 236.0)	100% (99.0%, 100%)	32.7% (27.9%, 37.8%)	3.00 (2.72, 3.31)
Group 2 (N=205) (M-M-R II + placebo)	185	174.0 (157.3, 192.6)	100% (98.0%, 100%)	31.9% (25.2%, 39.1%)	2.81 (2.41, 3.27)
Group 3 (N=195) (M-M-R II + VARIVAX)	171	154.1 (138.9, 170.9)	99.4% (96.8%, 100%)	26.9% (20.4%, 34.2%)	2.47 (2.17, 2.81)
			Varicella§		
Group 1 (N=399) (ProQuad + placebo)	367	322.2 (278.9, 372.2)	98.9% (97.2%, 99.7%)	80.7 (76.2%, 84.6%)	12.43 (10.63, 14.53)
Group 2 (N=205) (M-M-R II + placebo)	185	N/A	N/A	N/A	N/A
Group 3 (N=195) (M-M-R II + VARIVAX)	171	209.3 (171.2, 255.9)	99.4% (96.8%, 100%)	71.9% (64.6%, 78.5%)	8.50 (6.69, 10.81)

gpELISA = Glycoprotein enzyme-linked immunosorbent assay; ELISA = Enzyme-linked immunosorbent assay; CI = Confidence interval; GMT = Geometric mean titer; N/A = Not applicable; N = Number of subjects vaccinated; n = number of subjects in the per-protocol analysis.

* Measles GMTs are reported in mIU/mL; seropositivity corresponds to ≥120 mIU/mL.

† Mumps GMTs are reported in mumps Ab units/mL; seropositivity corresponds to ≥10 Ab units/mL.

‡ Rubella titers obtained by the legacy format were converted to their corresponding titers in the modified format. Rubella serostatus was determined after the conversion to IU/mL: seropositivity corresponds to ≥10 IU/mL.

§ Varicella GMTs are reported in gpELISA units/mL; seropositivity rate is reported by % of subjects with postvaccination antibody titers ≥5 gpELISA units/mL. Percentages are calculated as the number of subjects who met the criterion divided by the number of subjects contributing to the per-protocol analysis.

Immunogenicity in Children 12 to 23 Months of Age After a Single Dose

In 4 randomized clinical trials, 5446 healthy children 12 to 23 months of age were administered ProQuad, and 2038 children were vaccinated with M-M-R II and VARIVAX given concomitantly at separate injection sites. Subjects enrolled in each of these trials had a negative clinical history, no known recent exposure, and no vaccination history for varicella, measles, mumps, and rubella. Children were excluded from study participation if they had an immune impairment or had a history of allergy to components of the vaccine(s). Except for in 1 trial *[see ProQuad Administered with Diphtheria and Tetanus Toxoids and Acellular Pertussis Vaccine Adsorbed (DTaP) and Haemophilus influenzae type b Conjugate (Meningococcal Protein Conjugate) and Hepatitis B (Recombinant) Vaccine below]*, no concomitant vaccines were permitted during study participation. The race distribution of the study subjects across these studies following a first dose of ProQuad was as follows: 66.3% White; 12.7% African-American; 9.9% Hispanic; 6.7% Asian/Pacific; 4.2% other; and 0.2% American Indian. The gender distribution of the study subjects across these studies following a first dose of ProQuad was 52.6% male and 47.4% female. A summary of combined immunogenicity results 6 weeks following administration of a single dose of ProQuad or M-M-R II and VARIVAX is shown in Table 10. These results were similar to the immune response rates induced by concomitant administration of single doses of M-M-R II and VARIVAX at separate injection sites (lower bound of the 95% CI for the risk difference in measles, mumps, and rubella seroconversion rates were >-5.0 percentage points and the lower bound of the 95% CI for the risk difference in varicella seroprotection rates was either >-15 percentage points [one study] or >-10.0 percentage points [three studies]).

[See table 10 at top of page 1723]

Immunogenicity in Children 15 to 31 Months of Age After a Second Dose of ProQuad

In 2 of the 4 randomized clinical trials described above, a subgroup (N=1035) of the 5446 children administered a single dose of ProQuad were administered a second dose of ProQuad approximately 3 to 9 months after the first dose. Children were excluded from receiving a second dose of ProQuad if they were recently exposed to or developed varicella, measles, mumps, and/or rubella prior to receipt of the second dose. No concomitant vaccines were administered to these children. The race distribution across these studies following a second dose of ProQuad was as follows: 67.3% White; 14.3% African-American; 8.3% Hispanic; 5.4% Asian/Pacific; 4.4% other; 0.2% American Indian; and 0.10% mixed. The gender distribution of the study subjects across these studies following a second dose of ProQuad was 50.4% male and 49.6% female. A summary of immune responses following a second dose of ProQuad is presented in Table 11. Results from this study showed that 2 doses of ProQuad administered at least 3 months apart elicited a positive antibody response to all four antigens in greater than 98% of subjects. The geometric mean titers (GMTs) following the second dose of ProQuad increased approximately 2-fold each for measles, mumps, and rubella, and approximately 41-fold for varicella.

[See table 11 at top of pages 1723 and 1724]

Immunogenicity in Children 4 to 6 Years of Age Who Received a First Dose of ProQuad After Primary Vaccination With M-M-R II and VARIVAX

In a clinical trial, 799 healthy 4- to 6-year-old children who had received M-M-R II and VARIVAX at least 1 month prior to study entry were randomized to receive ProQuad and placebo (N=399), M-M-R II and placebo concomitantly at separate injection sites (N=205), or M-M-R II and VARIVAX concomitantly at separate injection sites (N=195). Children were eligible if they were previously administered primary doses of M-M-R II and VARIVAX, either concomitantly or non-concomitantly, at 12 months of age or older. Children were excluded if they were recently exposed to measles, mumps, rubella, and/or varicella, had an immune impairment, or had a history of allergy to components of the vaccine(s). No concomitant vaccines were permitted during study participation. *[See Adverse Reactions (6.1) for ethnicity and gender information.]*

A summary of antibody responses to measles, mumps, rubella, and varicella at 6 weeks postvaccination in subjects who had previously received M-M-R II and VARIVAX is shown in Table 12. Results from this study showed that a first dose of ProQuad after primary vaccination with M-M-R II and VARIVAX elicited a positive antibody response to all four antigens in greater than 98% of subjects. Postvaccination GMTs for recipients of ProQuad were similar to those following a second dose of M-M-R II and VARIVAX administered concomitantly at separate injection sites (the lower bound of the 95% CI around the fold difference in measles, mumps, rubella, and varicella GMTs excluded 0.5). Additionally, GMTs for measles, mumps, and rubella were similar to those following a second dose of M-M-R II given concomitantly with placebo (the lower bound of the 95% CI around the fold difference for the comparison of measles, mumps, and rubella GMTs excluded 0.5).

[See table 12 at top of previous page]

Immunogenicity Following Concomitant Use with Other Vaccines

ProQuad with Pneumococcal 7-valent Conjugate Vaccine and/or VAQTA

In a clinical trial, 1027 healthy children 12 to 15 months of age were randomized to receive ProQuad and pneumococcal 7-valent conjugate vaccine concomitantly (N=510) at separate injection sites or ProQuad and pneumococcal 7-valent conjugate vaccine non-concomitantly (N=517) at separate clinic visits. *[See Adverse Reactions (6.1) for ethnicity and gender information.]* The statistical analysis of non-inferiority in antibody response rates to measles, mumps, rubella, and varicella at 6 weeks postvaccination for subjects are shown in Table 13. In the per-protocol population, seroconversion rates were not inferior in children given ProQuad and pneumococcal 7-valent conjugate vaccine concomitantly when compared to seroconversion rates seen in children given these vaccines non-concomitantly for measles, mumps, and rubella. In children with baseline varicella antibody titers <1.25 gpELISA units/mL, the varicella seroprotection rates were not inferior when rates after concomitant and non-concomitant vaccination were compared 6 weeks postvaccination. Statistical analysis of non-inferiority in GMTs to *S. pneumoniae* serotypes at 6 weeks postvaccination are shown in Table 14. Geometric mean antibody titers (GMTs) for *S. pneumoniae* types 4, 6B, 9V, 14, 18C, 19F, and 23F were not inferior when antibody titers in the concomitant and non-concomitant groups were compared 6 weeks postvaccination.

[See table 13 above]

Table 13: Statistical Analysis of Non-Inferiority in Antibody Response Rates to Measles, Mumps, Rubella, and Varicella at 6 Weeks Postvaccination for Subjects Initially Seronegative to Measles, Mumps, or Rubella, or With Varicella Antibody Titer <1.25 gpELISA units at Baseline in the ProQuad + PCV7* Treatment Group and the ProQuad followed by PCV7 Control Group (Per-Protocol Analysis)

Assay Parameter	ProQuad + PCV7 (N=510) n	ProQuad + PCV7 (N=510) Estimated Response†	ProQuad followed by PCV7 (N=259) n	ProQuad followed by PCV7 (N=259) Estimated Response†	Difference (percentage points)†, ‡ (95% CI)
Measles % ≥255 mIU/mL	406	97.3%	204	99.5%	-2.2 (-4.6, 0.2)
Mumps % ≥10 Ab units/mL	403	96.6%	208	98.6%	-1.9 (-4.5, 1.0)
Rubella % ≥10 IU/mL	377	98.7%	195	97.9%	0.9 (-1.3, 4.1)
Varicella % ≥5 gpELISA units/mL	379	92.5%	192	87.9%	4.5 (-0.4, 10.4)

Seronegative defined as baseline measles antibody titer <255 mIU/mL for measles, baseline mumps antibody titer <10 ELISA Ab units/mL for mumps, and baseline rubella antibody titer <10 IU/mL for rubella.
The conclusion of non-inferiority is based on the lower bound of the 2-sided 95% CI on the risk difference being greater than -10 percentage points (*i.e.*excluding a decrease equal to or more than the prespecified criterion of 10.0 percentage points). This indicates that the difference is statistically significantly less than the prespecified clinically relevant decrease of 10.0 percentage points at the 1-sided alpha = 0.025 level.
N = Number of subjects vaccinated in each treatment group.
n = Number of subjects with measles antibody titer <255 mIU/mL, mumps antibody titer <10 ELISA Ab units/mL, rubella antibody titer <10 IU/mL, or varicella antibody titer <1.25 gpELISA units/mL at baseline and with postvaccination serology contributing to the per-protocol analysis.
Ab = antibody; ELISA = Enzyme-linked immunosorbent assay; gpELISA = Glycoprotein enzyme-linked immunosorbent assay; CI = Confidence interval.

* PCV7 = Pneumococcal 7-valent conjugate vaccine.
† Estimated responses and their differences were based on statistical analysis models adjusting for study center.
‡ ProQuad + PCV7 - ProQuad followed by PCV7.

Table 14: Statistical Analysis of Non-Inferiority in GMTs to S. pneumoniae Serotypes at 6 Weeks Postvaccination in the ProQuad + PCV7* Treatment Group and the PCV7 Followed by ProQuad Control Group (Per-Protocol Analysis)

Serotype	Parameter	Group 1 ProQuad + PCV7 (N=510) n	Group 1 Estimated Response‡	Group 2 PCV7 followed by ProQuad (N=258) n	Group 2 Estimated Response‡	Fold-Difference†* (95% CI)
4	GMT	410	1.5	193	1.3	1.2 (1.0, 1.4)
6B	GMT	410	8.9	192	8.4	1.1 (0.9, 1.2)
9V	GMT	409	2.9	193	2.5	1.2 (1.0, 1.3)
14	GMT	408	6.5	193	5.7	1.1 (1.0, 1.3)
18C	GMT	408	2.3	193	2.0	1.2 (1.0, 1.3)
19F	GMT	408	3.5	192	3.1	1.1 (1.0, 1.3)
23F	GMT	413	4.1	197	3.7	1.1 (1.0, 1.3)

The conclusion of non-inferiority is based on the lower bound of the 2-sided 95% CI on the fold-difference being greater than 0.5, (*i.e.* excluding a decrease of 2-fold or more). This indicates that the fold-difference is statistically significantly less than the pre-specified clinically relevant 2-fold difference at the 1-sided alpha = 0.025 level.
N = Number of subjects vaccinated in each treatment group; n = Number of subjects contributing to the per-protocol analysis for the given serotype; GMT = geometric mean titer; CI = Confidence interval.

* PCV7 = Pneumococcal 7-valent conjugate vaccine.
† ProQuad + PCV7 / PCV7 followed by ProQuad.
‡ Estimated responses and their fold-difference were based on statistical analysis models adjusting for study center and prevaccination titer.

Table 15: Statistical Analysis of Non-Inferiority of the Response Rate for Varicella Antibody at 6 Weeks Postvaccination Among Subjects Who Received VAQTA Concomitantly or Non-Concomitantly With ProQuad and PCV7* (Per-Protocol Analysis Set)

Parameter	Group 1: Concomitant VAQTA with ProQuad + PCV7 (N=330)		Group 2: Non-concomitant VAQTA separate from ProQuad + PCV7 (N=323)		Difference† (percentage points): Group 1 – Group 2 (95% CI)
	n	Estimated Response†	n	Estimated Response†	
% ≥5 gpELISA units/mL‡	225§	93.2%	232§	98.3%	-5.1 (-9.3, -1.4)

N = Number of subjects enrolled/randomized; n = Number of subjects contributing to the per protocol analysis for varicella; CI = Confidence interval.
The conclusion of similarity (non-inferiority) was based on the lower bound of the 2-sided 95% CI on the risk difference excluding a decrease of 10 percentage points or more (lower bound >-10.0). This indicated that the risk difference was statistically significantly greater than the pre-specified clinically relevant difference of -10 percentage points at the 1-sided alpha = 0.025 level.

* PCV7 = Pneumococcal 7-valent conjugate vaccine
† Estimated responses and their differences were based on a statistical analysis model adjusting for combined study center.
‡ 6 weeks following Dose 1.
§ Initial Serostatus <1.25 gpELISA units/ mL.

Table 16: Statistical Analysis of Non-Inferiority of the Seropositivity Rate (SPR) for Hepatitis A Antibody at 4 Weeks Postdose 2 of VAQTA Among Subjects Who Received VAQTA Concomitantly or Non-Concomitantly With ProQuad and PCV7* (Per-Protocol Analysis Set)

Parameter	Group 1: Concomitant VAQTA with ProQuad + PCV7 (N=330)		Group 2: Non-concomitant VAQTA separate from ProQuad + PCV7 (N=323)		Difference† (percentage points): Group 1 - Group 2 (95% CI)
	n	Estimated Response†	n	Estimated Response†	
% ≥10 mIU/mL‡	182§	100.0%	159§	99.3%	0.7 (-1.4, 3.8)

CI = Confidence interval; N = Number of subjects enrolled/randomized; n = Number of subjects contributing to the per-protocol analysis for hepatitis A.
The conclusion of non-inferiority was based on the lower bound of the 2-sided 95% CI on the risk difference being greater than -10 percentage points (*i.e.* excluding a decrease of 10 percentage points or more) (lower bound >-10.0). This indicated that the risk difference was statistically significantly greater than the pre-specified clinically relevant difference of -10 percentage points at the 1-sided alpha = 0.025 level.

* PCV7 = Pneumococcal 7-valent conjugate vaccine.
† Estimated responses and their differences were based on a statistical analysis model adjusting for combined study center.
‡ 4 weeks following receipt of 2 doses of VAQTA.
§ Regardless of initial serostatus.

Table 17: Statistical Analysis of Non-Inferiority in Geometric Mean Titers (GMT) to S. pneumoniae Serotypes at 6 Weeks Postvaccination Among Subjects Who Received VAQTA Concomitantly or Non-Concomitantly With ProQuad and PCV7* (Per-Protocol Analysis Set)

Serotype	Group 1: Concomitant VAQTA with ProQuad + PCV7 (N=330)		Group 2: Non-concomitant VAQTA separate from ProQuad + PCV7 (N=323)		Fold-Difference† (95% CI)
	n	Estimated Response†	n	Estimated Response†	
4	246	1.9	247	1.7	1.1 (0.9, 1.3)
6B	246	9.9	246	9.9	1.0 (0.8, 1.2)
9V	247	3.7	247	4.2	0.9 (0.8, 1.0)
14	248	7.8	247	7.6	1.0 (0.9, 1.2)
18C	247	2.9	247	2.7	1.1 (0.9, 1.3)
19F	248	4.0	248	3.8	1.1 (0.9, 1.2)
23F	247	5.1	247	4.4	1.1 (1.0, 1.3)

CI = Confidence interval; GMT = Geometric mean titer; N = Number of subjects enrolled/randomized; n = Number of subjects contributing to the per-protocol analysis for *S. pneumoniae* serotypes.
The conclusion of non-inferiority was based on the lower bound of the 2-sided 95% CI on the fold-difference being greater than 0.5 (*i.e.* excluding a decrease of 2-fold or more). This indicates that the fold-difference was statistically significantly less than the prespecified clinically relevant 2-fold difference at the 1-sided alpha = 0.025 level.

* PCV7 = Pneumococcal 7-valent conjugate vaccine.
† Estimated responses and their fold-difference were based on statistical analysis models adjusting for combined study center and prevaccination titer.

[See table 14 at top of previous page]
In a clinical trial, 653 healthy children 12 to 15 months of age were randomized to receive VAQTA, ProQuad, and pneumococcal 7-valent conjugate vaccine concomitantly (N=330) or ProQuad and pneumococcal 7-valent conjugate vaccine concomitantly followed by VAQTA 6 weeks later (N=323). *[See Adverse Reactions (6.1) for ethnicity and gender information.]* Statistical analysis of non-inferiority of the response rate for varicella antibody at 6 weeks postvaccination among subjects who received VAQTA concomitantly or non-concomitantly with ProQuad and pneumococcal 7-valent conjugate vaccine is shown in Table 15. For the varicella component of ProQuad, in subjects with baseline antibody titers <1.25 gpELISA units/mL, the proportion with a titer ≥5 gpELISA units/mL 6 weeks after their first dose of ProQuad was non-inferior when ProQuad was administered with VAQTA and pneumococcal 7-valent conjugate vaccine as compared to the proportion with a titer ≥5 gpELISA units/mL when ProQuad was administered with pneumococcal 7-valent conjugate vaccine alone. Statistical analysis of non-inferiority of the seropositivity rate for hepatitis A antibody at 4 weeks postdose 2 of VAQTA among subjects who received VAQTA concomitantly or non-concomitantly with ProQuad and pneumococcal 7-valent conjugate vaccine is shown in Table 16. The seropositivity rate to hepatitis A 4 weeks after a second dose of VAQTA given concomitantly with ProQuad and pneumococcal 7-valent conjugate vaccine (defined as the percent of subjects with a titer ≥10 mIU/mL) was non-inferior to the seropositivity rate observed when VAQTA was administered separately from ProQuad and pneumococcal 7-valent conjugate vaccine. Statistical analysis of non-inferiority in GMT to *S. pneumoniae* serotypes at 6 weeks postvaccination among subjects who received VAQTA concomitantly or non-concomitantly with ProQuad and pneumococcal 7-valent conjugate vaccine is shown in Table 17. Additionally, the GMTs for *S. pneumoniae* types 4, 6B, 9V, 14, 18C, 19F, and 23F 6 weeks after vaccination with pneumococcal 7-valent conjugate vaccine administered concomitantly with ProQuad and VAQTA were non-inferior as compared to GMTs observed in the group given pneumococcal 7-valent conjugate vaccine with ProQuad alone. An earlier clinical study involving 617 healthy children provided data that indicated that the seroresponse rates 6 weeks post vaccination for measles, mumps, and rubella in those given M-M-R II and VAQTA concomitantly (N=309) were non-inferior as compared to historical controls.
[See table 15 above]
[See table 16 above]
[See table 17 below]

ProQuad Administered with Diphtheria and Tetanus Toxoids and Acellular Pertussis Vaccine Adsorbed (DTaP) and Haemophilus influenzae type b Conjugate (Meningococcal Protein Conjugate) and Hepatitis B (Recombinant) Vaccine
In a clinical trial, 1913 healthy children 12 to 15 months of age were randomized to receive ProQuad plus diphtheria and tetanus toxoids and acellular pertussis vaccine adsorbed (DTaP) and *Haemophilus influenzae* type b conjugate (meningococcal protein conjugate) and hepatitis B (recombinant) vaccine concomitantly at separate injection sites (N=949), ProQuad at the initial visit followed by DTaP and *Haemophilus* b conjugate and hepatitis B (recombinant) vaccine given concomitantly 6 weeks later (N=485), or M-M-R II and VARIVAX given concomitantly at separate injection sites (N=479) at the first visit. *[See Adverse Reactions (6.1) for ethnicity and gender information.]* Seroconversion rates and antibody titers for measles, mumps, rubella, varicella, anti-PRP, and hepatitis B were comparable between the 2 groups given ProQuad at approximately 6 weeks postvaccination indicating that ProQuad and *Haemophilus* b conjugate (meningococcal protein conjugate) and hepatitis B (recombinant) vaccine may be administered concomitantly at separate injection sites (see Table 18 below). Response rates for measles, mumps, rubella, varicella, *Haemophilus influenzae* type b, and hepatitis B were not inferior in children given ProQuad plus *Haemophilus influenzae* type b conjugate (meningococcal protein conjugate) and hepatitis B (recombinant) vaccines concomitantly when compared to ProQuad at the initial visit and *Haemophilus influenzae* type b conjugate (meningococcal protein conjugate) and hepatitis B (recombinant) vaccines given concomitantly 6 weeks later. There are insufficient data to support concomitant vaccination with diphtheria and tetanus toxoids and acellular pertussis vaccine adsorbed (data not shown).
[See table 18 at top of next page]

15 REFERENCES

1. Levy O, et al. Disseminated varicella infection due to the vaccine strain of varicella-zoster virus, in a patient with a novel deficiency in natural killer T cells. *J Infect Dis.* 188(7):948-53, 2003.
2. Committee on Infectious Diseases, American Academy of Pediatrics. In: Pickering LK, Baker CJ, Overturf GD, et al., eds. Red Book: 2003 Report of the Committee on Infectious Diseases. 26th ed. Elk Grove Village, IL: American Academy of Pediatrics. 419-29, 2003.
3. Peltola H, et al. The elimination of indigenous measles, mumps, and rubella from Finland by a 12-year, two-dose vaccination program. *N Engl J Med.* 331(21):1397-1402, 1994.
4. Guess HA, et al. Population-based studies of varicella complications. *Pediatrics.* 78(4 Pt 2):723-727, 1986.

Table 18: Summary of the Comparison of the Immunogenicity Endpoints for Measles, Mumps, Rubella, Varicella, Haemophilus influenzae type b, and Hepatitis B Responses Following Vaccination with ProQuad, Haemophilus influenzae type b Conjugate (Meningococcal Protein Conjugate), and Hepatitis B (Recombinant) Vaccine and DTaP Administered Concomitantly Versus Non-Concomitant Vaccination with ProQuad Followed by These Vaccines

		Concomitant Group	Non-Concomitant Group		
		N=949	N=485		
Vaccine Antigen	Parameter	Response	Response	Risk Difference (95% CI)	Criterion for Non-inferiority
Measles	% ≥120 mIU/mL	97.8%	98.7%	-0.9 (-2.3, 0.6)	LB >-5.0
Mumps	% ≥10 ELISA Ab units/mL	95.4%	95.1%	0.3 (-1.7, 2.6)	LB >-5.0
Rubella	% ≥10 IU/mL	98.6%	99.3%	-0.7 (-1.8, 0.5)	LB >-5.0
Varicella	% ≥5 gpELISA units/mL	89.6%	90.8%	-1.2 (-4.1, 2.0)	LB >-10.0
HiB-PRP	% ≥1.0 mcg/mL	94.6%	96.5%	-1.9 (-4.1, 0.8)	LB >-10 0
HepB	% ≥10 mIU/mL	95.9%	98.8%	-2.8 (-4.8, -0.8)	LB >10.0

HiB-PRP = *Haemophilus influenzae* type b, polyribosyl phosphate; HepB = hepatitis B; LB = lower bound, limit for non-inferiority comparison.

5. Recommendations of the Immunization Practices Advisory Committee (ACIP), Mumps Prevention. *MMWR*. 38(22):388-392, 397-400, 1989.
6. Rubella vaccination during pregnancy--United States, 1971-1986. *MMWR Morb Mortal Wkly Rep*. 36(28):457-61, 1987.
7. Bohlke K, Galil K, Jackson LA, et al. Postpartum varicella vaccination: Is the vaccine virus excreted in breast milk? *Obstetrics and Gynecology*. 102(5):970-977, 2003.
8. Dolbear GL, Moffat J, Falkner C and Wojtowycz M. A Pilot Study: Is attenuated varicella virus present in breast milk after postpartum immunization? *Obstetrics and Gynecology*. 101(4 Suppl.):47S-47S, 2003.
9. Weibel RE, et al. Clinical and laboratory studies of combined live measles, mumps, and rubella vaccines using the RA 27/3 rubella virus. *Proc Soc Exp Biol Med*. 165(2):323-326, 1980.
10. Hilleman MR, Stokes J, Jr., Buynak EB, Weibel R, Halenda R, Goldner H. Studies of live attenuated measles virus vaccine in man: II. appraisal of efficacy. *Am J Public Health*. 52(2):44-56, 1962.
11. Krugman S, Giles JP, Jacobs AM. Studies on an attenuated measles-virus vaccine: VI. clinical, antigenic and prophylactic effects of vaccine in institutionalized children. *N Engl J Med*. 263(4):174-7, 1960.
12. Hilleman MR, Weibel RE, Buynak EB, Stokes J, Jr., Whitman JE, Jr. Live, attenuated mumps-virus vaccine. 4. Protective efficacy as measured in a field evaluation. *N Engl J Med*. 276(5):252-8, 1967.
13. Sugg WC, Finger JA, Levine RH, Pagano JS. Field evaluation of live virus mumps vaccine. *J Pediatr*. 72(4):461-6, 1968.
14. The Benevento and Compobasso Pediatricians Network for the Control of Vaccine-Preventable Diseases, D'Argenio P, Citarella A, Selvaggi MTM. Field evaluation of the clinical effectiveness of vaccines against pertussis, measles, rubella and mumps. *Vaccine*. 16(8):818-22, 1998.
15. Furukawa T, Miyata T, Kondo K, Kuno K, Isomura S, Takekoshi T. Rubella vaccination during an epidemic. *JAMA*. 213(6):987-90, 1970.
16. Vazquez M, et al. The effectiveness of the varicella vaccine in clinical practice. *N Engl J Med*. 344(13):955-960, 2001.
17. Kuter B, et al. Ten year follow up of healthy children who received one or two injections of varicella vaccine. *Pediatr Infect Dis J*. 23(2):132-137, 2004.

16 HOW SUPPLIED/STORAGE AND HANDLING

No. 4999 — ProQuad is supplied as follows:
(1) a package of 10 single-dose vials of lyophilized vaccine, NDC 0006-4999-00 (package A)
(2) a separate package of 10 vials of sterile water diluent (package B).

Storage

To maintain potency, ProQuad must be stored frozen between -58°F and +5°F (-50°C to -15°C). Use of dry ice may subject ProQuad to temperatures colder than -58°F (-50°C).

Before reconstitution, store the lyophilized vaccine continuously in a reliably maintained freezer (*e.g.,* chest, frost-free) for up to 18 months.

ProQuad may be stored at refrigerator temperature (36° to 46°F, 2° to 8°C) for up to 72 hours prior to reconstitution. Discard any ProQuad vaccine stored at 36° to 46°F which is not used within 72 hours of removal from 5°F (-15°C) storage.

Protect the vaccine from light at all times since such exposure may inactivate the vaccine viruses.

IF NOT USED IMMEDIATELY, THE RECONSTITUTED VACCINE MAY BE STORED AT ROOM TEMPERATURE, PROTECTED FROM LIGHT, FOR UP TO 30 MINUTES.

DISCARD RECONSTITUTED VACCINE IF IT IS NOT USED WITHIN 30 MINUTES.

DO NOT FREEZE RECONSTITUTED VACCINE.

Diluent should be stored separately at room temperature (68° to 77°F, 20° to 25°C), or in a refrigerator (36° to 46°F, 2° to 8°C).

For information regarding stability under conditions other than those recommended, call 1-800-MERCK-90.

17 PATIENT COUNSELING INFORMATION

17.1 Instructions

Provide the required vaccine information to the patient, parent, or guardian.

Inform the patient, parent, or guardian of the benefits and risks associated with vaccination.

Inform the patient, parent, or guardian that the vaccine recipient should avoid use of salicylates for 6 weeks after vaccination with ProQuad *[see Adverse Reactions (6.1) and Drug Interactions (7.2)]*.

Instruct post-pubertal females to avoid pregnancy for 3 months following vaccination *[see Indications and Usage (1) and Use In Specific Populations (8.1)]*.

Inform patients, parents, or guardians that vaccination with ProQuad may not offer 100% protection from measles, mumps, rubella, and varicella infection.

Instruct patients, parents, or guardians to report any adverse reactions to their health care provider. The U.S. Department of Health and Human Services has established a Vaccine Adverse Event Reporting System (VAERS) to accept all reports of suspected adverse events after the administration of any vaccine, including but not limited to the reporting of events required by the National Childhood Vaccine Injury Act of 1986. For information or a copy of the vaccine reporting form, call the VAERS toll free number at 1-800-822-7967, or report online at http://www.vaers.hhs.gov.

Dist. by: Merck Sharp & Dohme Corp., a subsidiary of **MERCK & CO., INC.**, Whitehouse Station, NJ 08889, USA
Issued August 2011
Printed in USA
9950905

PROSCAR®

(finasteride)
Tablets

℞

HIGHLIGHTS OF PRESCRIBING INFORMATION

These highlights do not include all the information needed to use PROSCAR safely and effectively. See full prescribing information for PROSCAR.

PROSCAR® (finasteride) Tablets
Initial U.S. Approval: 1992

RECENT MAJOR CHANGES

Indications and Usage, Limitations of Use (1.3) 06/2011
Warnings and Precautions
Increased Risk of High-Grade Prostate Cancer (5.2) 06/2011

INDICATIONS AND USAGE

PROSCAR, is a 5α-reductase inhibitor, indicated for the treatment of symptomatic benign prostatic hyperplasia (BPH) in men with an enlarged prostate to (1.1):

- Improve symptoms
- Reduce the risk of acute urinary retention
- Reduce the risk of the need for surgery including transurethral resection of the prostate (TURP) and prostatectomy.

PROSCAR administered in combination with the alpha-blocker doxazosin is indicated to reduce the risk of symptomatic progression of BPH (a confirmed ≥4 point increase in American Urological Association (AUA) symptom score) (1.2).

Limitations of Use: PROSCAR is not approved for the prevention of prostate cancer (1.3).

DOSAGE AND ADMINISTRATION

PROSCAR may be administered with or without meals (2).
Monotherapy: One tablet (5 mg) taken once a day (2.1).
Combination with Doxazosin: One tablet (5 mg) taken once a day in combination with the alpha-blocker doxazosin (2.2).

DOSAGE FORMS AND STRENGTHS

5-mg film-coated tablets (3).

CONTRAINDICATIONS

Hypersensitivity to any components of this product (4).
Women who are or may potentially be pregnant (4, 5.4, 8.1, 16).

WARNINGS AND PRECAUTIONS

- PROSCAR reduces serum prostate specific antigen (PSA) levels by approximately 50%. However, any confirmed increase in PSA while on PROSCAR may signal the presence of prostate cancer and should be evaluated, even if those values are still within the normal range for men not taking a 5α-reductase inhibitor (5.1).
- PROSCAR may increase the risk of high-grade prostate cancer (5.2, 6.1).
- Women should not handle crushed or broken PROSCAR tablets when they are pregnant or may potentially be pregnant due to potential risk to a male fetus (5.3, 8.1, 16).
- PROSCAR is not indicated for use in pediatric patients or women (5.4, 8.1, 8.3, 8.4, 12.3).
- Prior to initiating treatment with PROSCAR for BPH, consideration should be given to other urological conditions that may cause similar symptoms (5.6).

ADVERSE REACTIONS

The drug-related adverse reactions, reported in ≥1% in patients treated with PROSCAR and greater than in patients treated with placebo over a 4-year study are: impotence, decreased libido, decreased volume of ejaculate, breast enlargement, breast tenderness and rash (6.1).

To report SUSPECTED ADVERSE REACTIONS, contact Merck Sharp & Dohme Corp., a subsidiary of Merck & Co., Inc., at 1-877-888-4231 or FDA at 1-800-FDA-1088 or www.fda.gov/medwatch.

See 17 for PATIENT COUNSELING INFORMATION and FDA-approved patient labeling

Revised: 01/2013

FULL PRESCRIBING INFORMATION: CONTENTS*

*** Sections or subsections omitted from the full prescribing information are not listed**

FULL PRESCRIBING INFORMATION

1 INDICATIONS AND USAGE

1.1 Monotherapy

PROSCAR® is indicated for the treatment of symptomatic benign prostatic hyperplasia (BPH) in men with an enlarged prostate to:

- Improve symptoms
- Reduce the risk of acute urinary retention
- Reduce the risk of the need for surgery including transurethral resection of the prostate (TURP) and prostatectomy.

1.2 Combination with Alpha-Blocker

PROSCAR administered in combination with the alpha-blocker doxazosin is indicated to reduce the risk of symptomatic progression of BPH (a confirmed ≥4 point increase in American Urological Association (AUA) symptom score).

1.3 Limitations of Use

PROSCAR is not approved for the prevention of prostate cancer.

2 DOSAGE AND ADMINISTRATION

PROSCAR may be administered with or without meals.

2.1 Monotherapy

The recommended dose of PROSCAR is one tablet (5 mg) taken once a day *[see Clinical Studies (14.1)]*.

2.2 Combination with Alpha-Blocker

The recommended dose of PROSCAR is one tablet (5 mg) taken once a day in combination with the alpha-blocker doxazosin *[see Clinical Studies (14.2)]*.

3 DOSAGE FORMS AND STRENGTHS

5-mg blue, modified apple-shaped, film-coated tablets, with the code MSD 72 on one side and PROSCAR on the other.

4 CONTRAINDICATIONS

PROSCAR is contraindicated in the following:

- Hypersensitivity to any component of this medication.
- Pregnancy. Finasteride use is contraindicated in women when they are or may potentially be pregnant. Because of the ability of Type II 5α-reductase inhibitors to inhibit the conversion of testosterone to 5α-dihydrotestosterone (DHT), finasteride may cause abnormalities of the external genitalia of a male fetus of a pregnant woman who receives finasteride. If this drug is used during pregnancy, or if pregnancy occurs while taking this drug, the pregnant woman should be apprised of the potential hazard to the male fetus. *[See also Warnings and Precautions (5.3), Use in Specific Populations (8.1), How Supplied/Storage and Handling (16) and Patient Counseling Information (17.2).]*
  In female rats, low doses of finasteride administered during pregnancy have produced abnormalities of the external genitalia in male offspring.

5 WARNINGS AND PRECAUTIONS

5.1 Effects on Prostate Specific Antigen (PSA) and the Use of PSA in Prostate Cancer Detection

In clinical studies, PROSCAR reduced serum PSA concentration by approximately 50% within six months of treatment. This decrease is predictable over the entire range of PSA values in patients with symptomatic BPH, although it may vary in individuals.

For interpretation of serial PSAs in men taking PROSCAR, a new PSA baseline should be established at least six months after starting treatment and PSA monitored periodically thereafter. Any confirmed increase from the lowest PSA value while on PROSCAR may signal the presence of prostate cancer and should be evaluated, even if PSA levels are still within the normal range for men not taking a 5α-reductase inhibitor. Non-compliance with PROSCAR therapy may also affect PSA test results. To interpret an isolated PSA value in patients treated with PROSCAR for six months or more, PSA values should be doubled for comparison with normal ranges in untreated men. These adjustments preserve the utility of PSA to detect prostate cancer in men treated with PROSCAR.

PROSCAR may also cause decreases in serum PSA in the presence of prostate cancer.

The ratio of free to total PSA (percent free PSA) remains constant even under the influence of PROSCAR. If clinicians elect to use percent free PSA as an aid in the detection of prostate cancer in men undergoing finasteride therapy, no adjustment to its value appears necessary.

5.2 Increased Risk of High-Grade Prostate Cancer

Men aged 55 and over with a normal digital rectal examination and PSA ≤3.0 ng/mL at baseline taking finasteride 5 mg/day in the 7-year Prostate Cancer Prevention Trial (PCPT) had an increased risk of Gleason score 8-10 prostate cancer (finasteride 1.8% vs placebo 1.1%). *[See Indications and Usage (1.3) and Adverse Reactions (6.1).]* Similar results were observed in a 4-year placebo-controlled clinical trial with another 5α-reductase inhibitor (dutasteride, AVODART) (1% dutasteride vs 0.5% placebo). 5α-reductase inhibitors may increase the risk of development of high-grade prostate cancer. Whether the effect of 5α-reductase inhibitors to reduce prostate volume, or study-related factors, impacted the results of these studies has not been established.

5.3 Exposure of Women — Risk to Male Fetus

Women should not handle crushed or broken PROSCAR tablets when they are pregnant or may potentially be pregnant because of the possibility of absorption of finasteride and the subsequent potential risk to a male fetus. PROSCAR tablets are coated and will prevent contact with the active ingredient during normal handling, provided that the tablets have not been broken or crushed. *[See Contraindications (4), Use in Specific Populations (8.1), Clinical Pharmacology (12.3), How Supplied/Storage and Handling (16) and Patient Counseling Information (17.2).]*

5.4 Pediatric Patients and Women

PROSCAR is not indicated for use in pediatric patients *[see Use in Specific Populations (8.4) and Clinical Pharmacology (12.3)]* or women *[see also Warnings and Precautions (5.3), Use in Specific Populations (8.1), Clinical Pharmacology (12.3), How Supplied/Storage and Handling (16) and Patient Counseling Information (17.2)]*.

5.5 Effect on Semen Characteristics

Treatment with PROSCAR for 24 weeks to evaluate semen parameters in healthy male volunteers revealed no clinically meaningful effects on sperm concentration, mobility, morphology, or pH. A 0.6 mL (22.1%) median decrease in ejaculate volume with a concomitant reduction in total sperm per ejaculate was observed. These parameters remained within the normal range and were reversible upon discontinuation of therapy with an average time to return to baseline of 84 weeks.

5.6 Consideration of Other Urological Conditions

Prior to initiating treatment with PROSCAR, consideration should be given to other urological conditions that may cause similar symptoms. In addition, prostate cancer and BPH may coexist.

Patients with large residual urinary volume and/or severely diminished urinary flow should be carefully monitored for obstructive uropathy. These patients may not be candidates for finasteride therapy.

6 ADVERSE REACTIONS

6.1 Clinical Trials Experience

PROSCAR is generally well tolerated; adverse reactions usually have been mild and transient.

4-Year Placebo-Controlled Study (PLESS)

In PLESS, 1524 patients treated with PROSCAR and 1516 patients treated with placebo were evaluated for safety over a period of 4 years. The most frequently reported adverse reactions were related to sexual function. 3.7% (57 patients) treated with PROSCAR and 2.1% (32 patients) treated with placebo discontinued therapy as a result of adverse reactions related to sexual function, which are the most frequently reported adverse reactions.

Table 1 presents the only clinical adverse reactions considered possibly, probably or definitely drug related by the investigator, for which the incidence on PROSCAR was ≥1% and greater than placebo over the 4 years of the study. In years 2-4 of the study, there was no significant difference between treatment groups in the incidences of impotence, decreased libido and ejaculation disorder.

[See table 1 below]

Phase III Studies and 5-Year Open Extensions

The adverse experience profile in the 1-year, placebo-controlled, Phase III studies, the 5-year open extensions, and PLESS were similar.

Medical Therapy of Prostatic Symptoms (MTOPS) Study

In the MTOPS study, 3047 men with symptomatic BPH were randomized to receive PROSCAR 5 mg/day (n=768), doxazosin 4 or 8 mg/day (n=756), the combination of PROSCAR 5 mg/day and doxazosin 4 or 8 mg/day (n=786), or placebo (n=737) for 4 to 6 years. *[See Clinical Studies (14.2).]*

The incidence rates of drug-related adverse experiences reported by ≥2% of patients in any treatment group in the MTOPS Study are listed in Table 2.

The individual adverse effects which occurred more frequently in the combination group compared to either drug alone were: asthenia, postural hypotension, peripheral edema, dizziness, decreased libido, rhinitis, abnormal ejaculation, impotence and abnormal sexual function (see Table 2). Of these, the incidence of abnormal ejaculation in patients receiving combination therapy was comparable to the sum of the incidences of this adverse experience reported for the two monotherapies.

Combination therapy with finasteride and doxazosin was associated with no new clinical adverse experience.

Four patients in MTOPS reported the adverse experience breast cancer. Three of these patients were on finasteride only and one was on combination therapy. *[See Long Term Data.]*

The MTOPS Study was not specifically designed to make statistical comparisons between groups for reported adverse experiences. In addition, direct comparisons of safety data

Table 1: Drug-Related Adverse Experiences

	Year 1 (%)		Years 2, 3 and 4* (%)	
	Finasteride	Placebo	Finasteride	Placebo
Impotence	8.1	3.7	5.1	5.1
Decreased Libido	6.4	3.4	2.6	2.6
Decreased Volume of Ejaculate	3.7	0.8	1.5	0.5
Ejaculation Disorder	0.8	0.1	0.2	0.1
Breast Enlargement	0.5	0.1	1.8	1.1
Breast Tenderness	0.4	0.1	0.7	0.3
Rash	0.5	0.2	0.5	0.1

N = 1524 and 1516, finasteride vs placebo, respectively
* Combined Years 2-4

between the MTOPS study and previous studies of the single agents may not be appropriate based upon differences in patient population, dosage or dose regimen, and other procedural and study design elements.
[See table 2 above]

Long-Term Data

High-Grade Prostate Cancer

The PCPT trial was a 7-year randomized, double-blind, placebo-controlled trial that enrolled 18,882 men ≥55 years of age with a normal digital rectal examination and a PSA ≤3.0 ng/mL. Men received either PROSCAR (finasteride 5 mg) or placebo daily. Patients were evaluated annually with PSA and digital rectal exams. Biopsies were performed for elevated PSA, an abnormal digital rectal exam, or the end of study. The incidence of Gleason score 8-10 prostate cancer was higher in men treated with finasteride (1.8%) than in those treated with placebo (1.1%) *[see Indications and Usage (1.3) and Warnings and Precautions (5.2)]*. In a 4-year placebo-controlled clinical trial with another 5α-reductase inhibitor (dutasteride, AVODART), similar results for Gleason score 8-10 prostate cancer were observed (1% dutasteride vs 0.5% placebo).
No clinical benefit has been demonstrated in patients with prostate cancer treated with PROSCAR.

Breast Cancer

During the 4- to 6-year placebo- and comparator-controlled MTOPS study that enrolled 3047 men, there were 4 cases of breast cancer in men treated with finasteride but no cases in men not treated with finasteride. During the 4-year, placebo-controlled PLESS study that enrolled 3040 men, there were 2 cases of breast cancer in placebo-treated men but no cases in men treated with finasteride. During the 7-year placebo-controlled Prostate Cancer Prevention Trial (PCPT) that enrolled 18,882 men, there was 1 case of breast cancer in men treated with finasteride, and 1 case of breast cancer in men treated with placebo. The relationship between long-term use of finasteride and male breast neoplasia is currently unknown.

Sexual Function

There is no evidence of increased sexual adverse experiences with increased duration of treatment with PROSCAR. New reports of drug-related sexual adverse experiences decreased with duration of therapy.

6.2 Postmarketing Experience

The following additional adverse events have been reported in postmarketing experience with PROSCAR. Because these events are reported voluntarily from a population of uncertain size, it is not always possible to reliably estimate their frequency or establish a causal relationship to drug exposure:
- hypersensitivity reactions, including pruritus, urticaria, and swelling of the lips and face
- testicular pain
- sexual dysfunction that continued after discontinuation of treatment, including erectile dysfunction, decreased libido and ejaculation disorders (e.g. reduced ejaculate volume). These events were reported rarely in men taking PROSCAR for the treatment of BPH. Most men were older and were taking concomitant medications and/or had comorbid conditions. The independent role of PROSCAR in these events is unknown.
- male infertility and/or poor seminal quality were reported rarely in men taking PROSCAR for the treatment of BPH. Normalization or improvement of poor seminal quality has been reported after discontinuation of finasteride. The independent role of PROSCAR in these events is unknown.
- depression
- male breast cancer.

The following additional adverse event related to sexual dysfunction that continued after discontinuation of treatment has been reported in postmarketing experience with finasteride at lower doses used to treat male pattern baldness. Because the event is reported voluntarily from a population of uncertain size, it is not always possible to reliably estimate its frequency or establish a causal relationship to drug exposure:
- orgasm disorders

7 DRUG INTERACTIONS

7.1 Cytochrome P450-Linked Drug Metabolizing Enzyme System

No drug interactions of clinical importance have been identified. Finasteride does not appear to affect the cytochrome P450-linked drug metabolizing enzyme system. Compounds that have been tested in man have included antipyrine, digoxin, propranolol, theophylline, and warfarin and no clinically meaningful interactions were found.

7.2 Other Concomitant Therapy

Although specific interaction studies were not performed, PROSCAR was concomitantly used in clinical studies with acetaminophen, acetylsalicylic acid, α-blockers, angiotensin-converting enzyme (ACE) inhibitors, analgesics, anti-convulsants, beta-adrenergic blocking agents, diuretics, calcium channel blockers, cardiac nitrates, HMG-CoA reductase inhibitors, nonsteroidal anti-inflammatory drugs (NSAIDs), benzodiazepines, H_2 antagonists and quinolone anti-infectives without evidence of clinically significant adverse interactions.

Table 2: Incidence ≥2% in One or More Treatment Groups: Drug-Related Clinical Adverse Experiences in MTOPS

Adverse Experience	Placebo (N=737) (%)	Doxazosin 4 mg or 8 mg* (N=756) (%)	Finasteride (N=768) (%)	Combination (N=786) (%)
Body as a whole				
Asthenia	7.1	15.7	5.3	16.8
Headache	2.3	4.1	2.0	2.3
Cardiovascular				
Hypotension	0.7	3.4	1.2	1.5
Postural Hypotension	8.0	16.7	9.1	17.8
Metabolic and Nutritional				
Peripheral Edema	0.9	2.6	1.3	3.3
Nervous				
Dizziness	8.1	17.7	7.4	23.2
Libido Decreased	5.7	7.0	10.0	11.6
Somnolence	1.5	3.7	1.7	3.1
Respiratory				
Dyspnea	0.7	2.1	0.7	1.9
Rhinitis	0.5	1.3	1.0	2.4
Urogenital				
Abnormal Ejaculation	2.3	4.5	7.2	14.1
Gynecomastia	0.7	1.1	2.2	1.5
Impotence	12.2	14.4	18.5	22.6
Sexual Function Abnormal	0.9	2.0	2.5	3.1

* Doxazosin dose was achieved by weekly titration (1 to 2 to 4 to 8 mg). The final tolerated dose (4 mg or 8 mg) was administered at end-Week 4. Only those patients tolerating at least 4 mg were kept on doxazosin. The majority of patients received the 8-mg dose over the duration of the study.

8 USE IN SPECIFIC POPULATIONS

8.1 Pregnancy

Pregnancy Category X. *[See Contraindications (4).]*
PROSCAR is contraindicated for use in women who are or may become pregnant. PROSCAR is a Type II 5α-reductase inhibitor that prevents conversion of testosterone to 5α-dihydrotestosterone (DHT), a hormone necessary for normal development of male genitalia. In animal studies, finasteride caused abnormal development of external genitalia in male fetuses. If this drug is used during pregnancy, or if the patient becomes pregnant while taking this drug, the patient should be apprised of the potential hazard to the male fetus.
Abnormal male genital development is an expected consequence when conversion of testosterone to 5α-dihydrotestosterone (DHT) is inhibited by 5α-reductase inhibitors. These outcomes are similar to those reported in male infants with genetic 5α-reductase deficiency. Women could be exposed to finasteride through contact with crushed or broken PROSCAR tablets or semen from a male partner taking PROSCAR. With regard to finasteride exposure through the skin, PROSCAR tablets are coated and will prevent skin contact with finasteride during normal handling if the tablets have not been crushed or broken. Women who are pregnant or may become pregnant should not handle crushed or broken PROSCAR tablets because of possible exposure of a male fetus. If a pregnant woman comes in contact with crushed or broken PROSCAR tablets, the contact area should be washed immediately with soap and water. With regard to potential finasteride exposure through semen, two studies have been conducted in men receiving PROSCAR 5 mg/day that measured finasteride concentrations in semen *[see Clinical Pharmacology (12.3)]*.
In an embryo-fetal development study, pregnant rats received finasteride during the period of major organogenesis (gestation days 6 to 17). At maternal doses of oral finasteride approximately 0.1 to 86 times the maximum recommended human dose (MRHD) of 5 mg/day (based on AUC at animal doses of 0.1 to 100 mg/kg/day) there was a dose-dependent increase in hypospadias that occurred in 3.6 to 100% of male offspring. Exposure multiples were estimated using data from nonpregnant rats. Days 16 to 17 days of gestation is a critical period in male fetal rats for differentiation of the external genitalia. At oral maternal doses approximately 0.03 times the MRHD (based on AUC at animal dose of 0.03 mg/kg/day), male offspring had decreased prostatic and seminal vesicular weights, delayed preputial separation and transient nipple development. Decreased anogenital distance occurred in male offspring of pregnant rats that received approximately 0.003 times the MRHD (based on AUC at animal dose of 0.003 mg/kg/day). No abnormalities were observed in female offspring at any maternal dose of finasteride.
No developmental abnormalities were observed in the offspring of untreated females mated with finasteride treated male rats that received approximately 61 times the MRHD (based on AUC at animal dose of 80 mg/kg/day). Slightly decreased fertility was observed in male offspring after administration of about 3 times the MRHD (based on AUC at animal dose of 3 mg/kg/day) to female rats during late gestation and lactation. No effects on fertility were seen in female offspring under these conditions.
No evidence of male external genital malformations or other abnormalities were observed in rabbit fetuses exposed to finasteride during the period of major organogenesis (gestation days 6-18) at maternal oral doses up to 100 mg/kg /day, (finasteride exposure levels were not measured in rabbits). However, this study may not have included the critical period for finasteride effects on development of male external genitalia in the rabbit.
The fetal effects of maternal finasteride exposure during the period of embryonic and fetal development were evaluated in the rhesus monkey (gestation days 20-100), in a species and development period more predictive of specific effects in humans than the studies in rats and rabbits. Intravenous administration of finasteride to pregnant monkeys at doses as high as 800 ng/day (estimated maximal blood concentration of 1.86 ng/mL or about 143 times the highest estimated exposure of pregnant women to finasteride from semen of men taking 5 mg/day) resulted in no abnormalities in male fetuses. In confirmation of the relevance of the rhesus model for human fetal development, oral administration of a dose of finasteride (2 mg/kg/day or approximately 18,000 times the highest estimated blood levels of finasteride from semen of men taking 5 mg/day) to pregnant monkeys resulted in external genital abnormalities in male fetuses. No other abnormalities were observed in male fetuses and no finasteride-related abnormalities were observed in female fetuses at any dose.

8.3 Nursing Mothers

PROSCAR is not indicated for use in women.
It is not known whether finasteride is excreted in human milk.

8.4 Pediatric Use

PROSCAR is not indicated for use in pediatric patients.
Safety and effectiveness in pediatric patients have not been established.

8.5 Geriatric Use

Of the total number of subjects included in PLESS, 1480 and 105 subjects were 65 and over and 75 and over, respectively. No overall differences in safety or effectiveness were observed between these subjects and younger subjects, and other reported clinical experience has not identified differences in responses between the elderly and younger patients. No dosage adjustment is necessary in the elderly *[see Clinical Pharmacology (12.3) and Clinical Studies (14)]*.

8.6 Hepatic Impairment

Caution should be exercised in the administration of PROSCAR in those patients with liver function abnormalities, as finasteride is metabolized extensively in the liver *[see Clinical Pharmacology (12.3)]*.

8.7 Renal Impairment

No dosage adjustment is necessary in patients with renal impairment *[see Clinical Pharmacology (12.3)]*.

10 OVERDOSAGE

Patients have received single doses of PROSCAR up to 400 mg and multiple doses of PROSCAR up to 80 mg/day for three months without adverse effects. Until further experience is obtained, no specific treatment for an overdose with PROSCAR can be recommended.

Significant lethality was observed in male and female mice at single oral doses of 1500 mg/m^2 (500 mg/kg) and in female and male rats at single oral doses of 2360 mg/m^2 (400 mg/kg) and 5900 mg/m^2 (1000 mg/kg), respectively.

11 DESCRIPTION

PROSCAR (finasteride), a synthetic 4-azasteroid compound, is a specific inhibitor of steroid Type II 5α-reductase, an intracellular enzyme that converts the androgen testosterone into 5α-dihydrotestosterone (DHT).

Finasteride is 4-azaandrost-1-ene-17-carboxamide, N-(1,1-dimethylethyl)-3-oxo-,(5α,17ß)-. The empirical formula of finasteride is $C_{23}H_{36}N_2O_2$ and its molecular weight is 372.55. Its structural formula is:

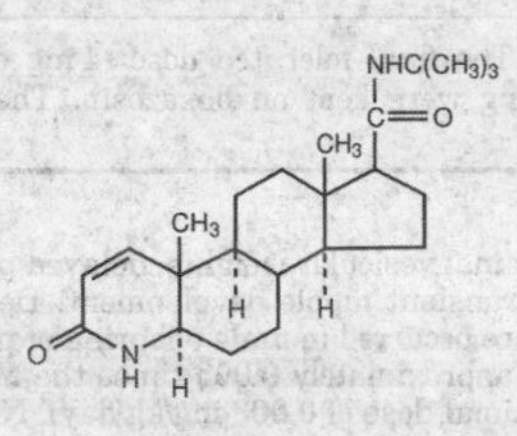

Finasteride is a white crystalline powder with a melting point near 250°C. It is freely soluble in chloroform and in lower alcohol solvents, but is practically insoluble in water. PROSCAR (finasteride) tablets for oral administration are film-coated tablets that contain 5 mg of finasteride and the following inactive ingredients: hydrous lactose, microcrystalline cellulose, pregelatinized starch, sodium starch glycolate, hydroxypropyl cellulose LF, hydroxypropyl methylcellulose, titanium dioxide, magnesium stearate, talc, docusate sodium, FD&C Blue 2 aluminum lake and yellow iron oxide.

12 CLINICAL PHARMACOLOGY

12.1 Mechanism of Action

The development and enlargement of the prostate gland is dependent on the potent androgen, 5α-dihydrotestosterone (DHT). Type II 5α-reductase metabolizes testosterone to DHT in the prostate gland, liver and skin. DHT induces androgenic effects by binding to androgen receptors in the cell nuclei of these organs.

Finasteride is a competitive and specific inhibitor of Type II 5α-reductase with which it slowly forms a stable enzyme complex. Turnover from this complex is extremely slow ($t_{1/2}$ ~ 30 days). This has been demonstrated both *in vivo* and *in vitro*. Finasteride has no affinity for the androgen receptor. In man, the 5α-reduced steroid metabolites in blood and urine are decreased after administration of finasteride.

12.2 Pharmacodynamics

In man, a single 5-mg oral dose of PROSCAR produces a rapid reduction in serum DHT concentration, with the maximum effect observed 8 hours after the first dose. The suppression of DHT is maintained throughout the 24-hour dosing interval and with continued treatment. Daily dosing of PROSCAR at 5 mg/day for up to 4 years has been shown to reduce the serum DHT concentration by approximately 70%. The median circulating level of testosterone increased by approximately 10-20% but remained within the physiologic range. In a separate study in healthy men treated with finasteride 1 mg per day (n=82) or placebo (n=69), mean circulating levels of testosterone and estradiol were increased by approximately 15% as compared to baseline, but these remained within the physiologic range.

In patients receiving PROSCAR 5 mg/day, increases of about 10% were observed in luteinizing hormone (LH) and follicle-stimulating hormone (FSH), but levels remained within the normal range. In healthy volunteers, treatment with PROSCAR did not alter the response of LH and FSH to gonadotropin-releasing hormone indicating that the hypothalamic-pituitary-testicular axis was not affected.

In patients with BPH, PROSCAR has no effect on circulating levels of cortisol, prolactin, thyroid-stimulating hormone, or thyroxine. No clinically meaningful effect was observed on the plasma lipid profile (i.e., total cholesterol, low density lipoproteins, high density lipoproteins and triglycerides) or bone mineral density.

Adult males with genetically inherited Type II 5α-reductase deficiency also have decreased levels of DHT. Except for the associated urogenital defects present at birth, no other clinical abnormalities related to Type II 5α-reductase deficiency have been observed in these individuals. These individuals have a small prostate gland throughout life and do not develop BPH.

In patients with BPH treated with finasteride (1-100 mg/day) for 7-10 days prior to prostatectomy, an approximate 80% lower DHT content was measured in prostatic tissue removed at surgery, compared to placebo; testosterone tissue concentration was increased up to 10 times over pretreatment levels, relative to placebo. Intraprostatic content of PSA was also decreased.

In healthy male volunteers treated with PROSCAR for 14 days, discontinuation of therapy resulted in a return of DHT levels to pretreatment levels in approximately 2 weeks. In patients treated for three months, prostate volume, which declined by approximately 20%, returned to close to baseline value after approximately three months of discontinuation of therapy.

12.3 Pharmacokinetics

Absorption

In a study of 15 healthy young subjects, the mean bioavailability of finasteride 5-mg tablets was 63% (range 34-108%), based on the ratio of area under the curve (AUC) relative to an intravenous (IV) reference dose. Maximum finasteride plasma concentration averaged 37 ng/mL (range, 27-49 ng/mL) and was reached 1-2 hours postdose. Bioavailability of finasteride was not affected by food.

Distribution

Mean steady-state volume of distribution was 76 liters (range, 44-96 liters). Approximately 90% of circulating finasteride is bound to plasma proteins. There is a slow accumulation phase for finasteride after multiple dosing. After dosing with 5 mg/day of finasteride for 17 days, plasma concentrations of finasteride were 47 and 54% higher than after the first dose in men 45-60 years old (n=12) and ≥70 years old (n=12), respectively. Mean trough concentrations after 17 days of dosing were 6.2 ng/mL (range, 2.4-9.8 ng/mL) and 8.1 ng/mL (range, 1.8-19.7 ng/mL), respectively, in the two age groups. Although steady state was not reached in this study, mean trough plasma concentration in another study in patients with BPH (mean age, 65 years) receiving 5 mg/day was 9.4 ng/mL (range, 7.1-13.3 ng/mL; n=22) after over a year of dosing.

Finasteride has been shown to cross the blood brain barrier but does not appear to distribute preferentially to the CSF.

In 2 studies of healthy subjects (n=69) receiving PROSCAR 5 mg/day for 6-24 weeks, finasteride concentrations in semen ranged from undetectable (<0.1 ng/mL) to 10.54 ng/mL. In an earlier study using a less sensitive assay, finasteride concentrations in the semen of 16 subjects receiving PROSCAR 5 mg/day ranged from undetectable (<1.0 ng/mL) to 21 ng/mL. Thus, based on a 5-mL ejaculate volume, the amount of finasteride in semen was estimated to be 50- to 100-fold less than the dose of finasteride (5 μg) that had no effect on circulating DHT levels in men *[see also Use in Specific Populations (8.1)]*.

Metabolism

Finasteride is extensively metabolized in the liver, primarily via the cytochrome P450 3A4 enzyme subfamily. Two metabolites, the t-butyl side chain monohydroxylated and monocarboxylic acid metabolites, have been identified that possess no more than 20% of the 5α-reductase inhibitory activity of finasteride.

Excretion

In healthy young subjects (n=15), mean plasma clearance of finasteride was 165 mL/min (range, 70-279 mL/min) and mean elimination half-life in plasma was 6 hours (range, 3-16 hours). Following an oral dose of ^{14}C-finasteride in man (n=6), a mean of 39% (range, 32-46%) of the dose was excreted in the urine in the form of metabolites; 57% (range, 51-64%) was excreted in the feces.

The mean terminal half-life of finasteride in subjects ≥70 years of age was approximately 8 hours (range, 6-15 hours; n=12), compared with 6 hours (range, 4-12 hours; n=12) in subjects 45-60 years of age. As a result, mean $AUC_{(0-24\ hr)}$ after 17 days of dosing was 15% higher in subjects ≥70 years of age than in subjects 45-60 years of age (p=0.02).

Table 3: Mean (SD) Pharmacokinetic Parameters in Healthy Young Subjects (n=15)

	Mean (±SD)
Bioavailability	63% (34-108%)*
Clearance (mL/min)	165 (55)
Volume of Distribution (L)	76 (14)
Half-Life (hours)	6.2 (2.1)

* Range

Pediatric

Finasteride pharmacokinetics have not been investigated in patients <18 years of age.

Finasteride is not indicated for use in pediatric patients *[see Warnings and Precautions (5.4), Use in Specific Populations (8.4)]*.

Gender

Finasteride is not indicated for use in women *[see Contraindications (4), Warnings and Precautions (5.3 and 5.4), Use in Specific Populations (8.1), How Supplied/Storage and Handling (16) and Patient Counseling Information (17.2)]*.

Geriatric

No dosage adjustment is necessary in the elderly. Although the elimination rate of finasteride is decreased in the elderly, these findings are of no clinical significance. *[See Clinical Pharmacology (12.3) and Use in Specific Populations (8.5).]*

Table 4: Mean (SD) Noncompartmental Pharmacokinetic Parameters After Multiple Doses of 5 mg/day in Older Men

	Mean (± SD) 45-60 years old (n=12)	≥70 years old (n=12)
AUC (ng•hr/mL)	389 (98)	463 (186)
Peak Concentration (ng/mL)	46.2 (8.7)	48.4 (14.7)
Time to Peak (hours)	1.8 (0.7)	1.8 (0.6)
Half-Life (hours)*	6.0 (1.5)	8.2 (2.5)

* First-dose values; all other parameters are last-dose values

Race

The effect of race on finasteride pharmacokinetics has not been studied.

Hepatic Impairment

The effect of hepatic impairment on finasteride pharmacokinetics has not been studied. Caution should be exercised in the administration of PROSCAR in those patients with liver function abnormalities, as finasteride is metabolized extensively in the liver.

Renal Impairment

No dosage adjustment is necessary in patients with renal impairment. In patients with chronic renal impairment, with creatinine clearances ranging from 9.0 to 55 mL/min, AUC, maximum plasma concentration, half-life, and protein binding after a single dose of ^{14}C-finasteride were similar to values obtained in healthy volunteers. Urinary excretion of metabolites was decreased in patients with renal impairment. This decrease was associated with an increase in fecal excretion of metabolites. Plasma concentrations of metabolites were significantly higher in patients with renal impairment (based on a 60% increase in total radioactivity AUC). However, finasteride has been well tolerated in BPH patients with normal renal function receiving up to 80 mg/day for 12 weeks, where exposure of these patients to metabolites would presumably be much greater.

13 NONCLINICAL TOXICOLOGY

13.1 Carcinogenesis, Mutagenesis, Impairment of Fertility

No evidence of a tumorigenic effect was observed in a 24-month study in Sprague-Dawley rats receiving doses of finasteride up to 160 mg/kg/day in males and 320 mg/kg/day in females. These doses produced respective systemic exposure in rats of 111 and 274 times those observed in man receiving the recommended human dose of 5 mg/day. All exposure calculations were based on calculated $AUC_{(0-24\ hr)}$ for animals and mean $AUC_{(0-24\ hr)}$ for man (0.4 μg•hr/mL).

In a 19-month carcinogenicity study in CD-1 mice, a statistically significant (p≤0.05) increase in the incidence of testicular Leydig cell adenomas was observed at 228 times the human exposure (250 mg/kg/day). In mice at 23 times the human exposure, estimated (25 mg/kg/day) and in rats at 39 times the human exposure (40 mg/kg/day) an increase in the incidence of Leydig cell hyperplasia was observed. A positive correlation between the proliferative changes in the Leydig cells and an increase in serum LH levels (2- to 3-fold above control) has been demonstrated in both rodent species treated with high doses of finasteride. No drug-related Leydig cell changes were seen in either rats or dogs treated with finasteride for 1 year at 30 and 350 times (20 mg/kg/

day and 45 mg/kg/day, respectively) or in mice treated for 19 months at 2.3 times the human exposure, estimated (2.5 mg/kg/day).

No evidence of mutagenicity was observed in an *in vitro* bacterial mutagenesis assay, a mammalian cell mutagenesis assay, or in an *in vitro* alkaline elution assay. In an *in vitro* chromosome aberration assay, using Chinese hamster ovary cells, there was a slight increase in chromosome aberrations. These concentrations correspond to 4000-5000 times the peak plasma levels in man given a total dose of 5 mg. In an *in vivo* chromosome aberration assay in mice, no treatment-related increase in chromosome aberration was observed with finasteride at the maximum tolerated dose of 250 mg/kg/day (228 times the human exposure) as determined in the carcinogenicity studies.

In sexually mature male rabbits treated with finasteride at 543 times the human exposure (80 mg/kg/day) for up to 12 weeks, no effect on fertility, sperm count, or ejaculate volume was seen. In sexually mature male rats treated with 61 times the human exposure (80 mg/kg/day), there were no significant effects on fertility after 6 or 12 weeks of treatment; however, when treatment was continued for up to 24 or 30 weeks, there was an apparent decrease in fertility, fecundity and an associated significant decrease in the weights of the seminal vesicles and prostate. All these effects were reversible within 6 weeks of discontinuation of treatment. No drug-related effect on testes or on mating performance has been seen in rats or rabbits. This decrease in fertility in finasteride-treated rats is secondary to its effect on accessory sex organs (prostate and seminal vesicles) resulting in failure to form a seminal plug. The seminal plug is essential for normal fertility in rats and is not relevant in man.

14 CLINICAL STUDIES

14.1 Monotherapy

PROSCAR 5 mg/day was initially evaluated in patients with symptoms of BPH and enlarged prostates by digital rectal examination in two 1-year, placebo-controlled, randomized, double-blind studies and their 5-year open extension studies.

PROSCAR was further evaluated in the PROSCAR Long-Term Efficacy and Safety Study (PLESS), a double-blind, randomized, placebo-controlled, 4-year, multicenter study. 3040 patients between the ages of 45 and 78, with moderate to severe symptoms of BPH and an enlarged prostate upon digital rectal examination, were randomized into the study (1524 to finasteride, 1516 to placebo) and 3016 patients were evaluable for efficacy. 1883 patients completed the 4-year study (1000 in the finasteride group, 883 in the placebo group).

Effect on Symptom Score

Symptoms were quantified using a score similar to the American Urological Association Symptom Score, which evaluated both obstructive symptoms (impairment of size and force of stream, sensation of incomplete bladder emptying, delayed or interrupted urination) and irritative symptoms (nocturia, daytime frequency, need to strain or push the flow of urine) by rating on a 0 to 5 scale for six symptoms and a 0 to 4 scale for one symptom, for a total possible score of 34.

Patients in PLESS had moderate to severe symptoms at baseline (mean of approximately 15 points on a 0-34 point scale). Patients randomized to PROSCAR who remained on therapy for 4 years had a mean (± 1 SD) decrease in symptom score of 3.3 (± 5.8) points compared with 1.3 (± 5.6) points in the placebo group. (See Figure 1.) A statistically significant improvement in symptom score was evident at 1 year in patients treated with PROSCAR vs placebo (–2.3 vs –1.6), and this improvement continued through Year 4.

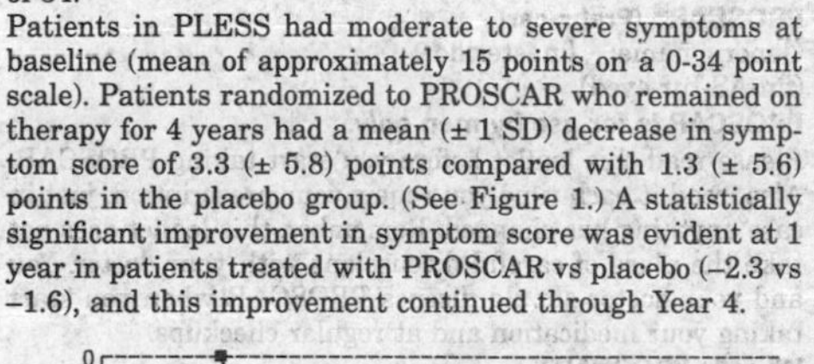

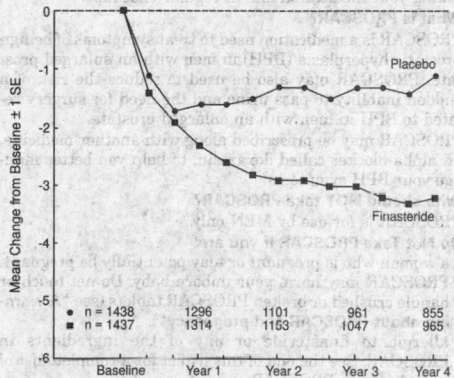

Figure 1: Symptom Score in PLESS

Results seen in earlier studies were comparable to those seen in PLESS. Although an early improvement in urinary symptoms was seen in some patients, a therapeutic trial of at least 6 months was generally necessary to assess whether a beneficial response in symptom relief had been achieved. The improvement in BPH symptoms was seen during the first year and maintained throughout an additional 5 years of open extension studies.

Effect on Acute Urinary Retention and the Need for Surgery

In PLESS, efficacy was also assessed by evaluating treatment failures. Treatment failure was prospectively defined as BPH-related urological events or clinical deterioration, lack of improvement and/or the need for alternative therapy. BPH-related urological events were defined as urological surgical intervention and acute urinary retention requiring catheterization. Complete event information was available for 92% of the patients. The following table (Table 5) summarizes the results.

Table 5: All Treatment Failures in PLESS

Event	Patients (%)* Placebo N=1503	Finasteride N=1513	Relative Risk†	95% CI	P Value†
All Treatment Failures	37.1	26.2	0.68	(0.57 to 0.79)	<0.001
Surgical Interventions for BPH	10.1	4.6	0.45	(0.32 to 0.63)	<0.001
Acute Urinary Retention Requiring Catheterization	6.6	2.8	0.43	(0.28 to 0.66)	<0.001
Two consecutive symptom scores ≥20	9.2	6.7			
Bladder Stone	0.4	0.5			
Incontinence	2.1	1.7			
Renal Failure	0.5	0.6			
UTI	5.7	4.9			
Discontinuation due to worsening of BPH, lack of improvement, or to receive other medical treatment	21.8	13.3			

* patients with multiple events may be counted more than once for each type of event
† Hazard ratio based on log rank test

[See table 5 above]

Compared with placebo, PROSCAR was associated with a significantly lower risk for acute urinary retention or the need for BPH-related surgery [13.2% for placebo vs 6.6% for PROSCAR; 51% reduction in risk, 95% CI: (34 to 63%)]. Compared with placebo, PROSCAR was associated with a significantly lower risk for surgery [10.1% for placebo vs 4.6% for PROSCAR; 55% reduction in risk, 95% CI: (37 to 68%)] and with a significantly lower risk of acute urinary retention [6.6% for placebo vs 2.8% for PROSCAR; 57% reduction in risk, 95% CI: (34 to 72%)]; see Figures 2 and 3.

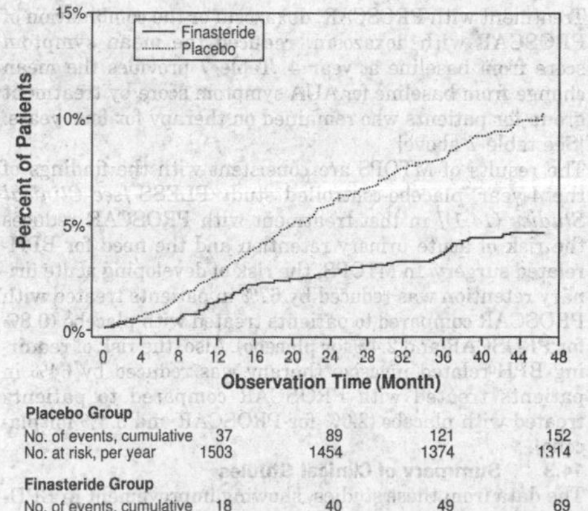

Figure 2: Percent of Patients Having Surgery for BPH, Including TURP

[See figure 3 at top of next column]

Effect on Maximum Urinary Flow Rate

In the patients in PLESS who remained on therapy for the duration of the study and had evaluable urinary flow data, PROSCAR increased maximum urinary flow rate by 1.9 mL/sec compared with 0.2 mL/sec in the placebo group. There was a clear difference between treatment groups in maximum urinary flow rate in favor of PROSCAR by month

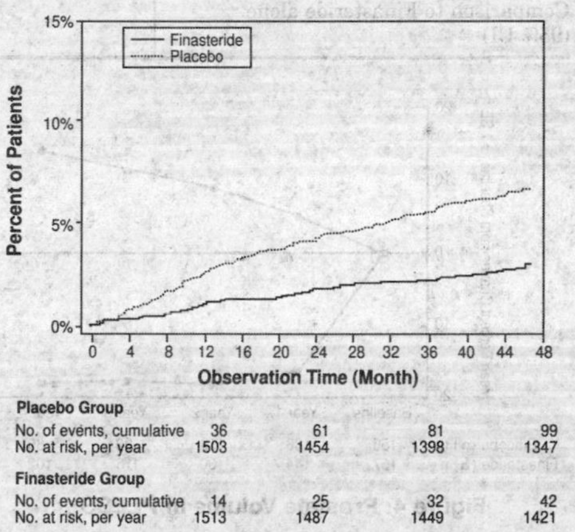

Figure 3: Percent of Patients Developing Acute Urinary Retention (Spontaneous and Precipitated)

4 (1.0 vs 0.3 mL/sec) which was maintained throughout the study. In the earlier 1-year studies, increase in maximum urinary flow rate was comparable to PLESS and was maintained through the first year and throughout an additional 5 years of open extension studies.

Effect on Prostate Volume

In PLESS, prostate volume was assessed yearly by magnetic resonance imaging (MRI) in a subset of patients. In patients treated with PROSCAR who remained on therapy, prostate volume was reduced compared with both baseline and placebo throughout the 4-year study. PROSCAR decreased prostate volume by 17.9% (from 55.9 cc at baseline to 45.8 cc at 4 years) compared with an increase of 14.1% (from 51.3 cc to 58.5 cc) in the placebo group (p<0.001). (See Figure 4.)

Results seen in earlier studies were comparable to those seen in PLESS. Mean prostate volume at baseline ranged between 40-50 cc. The reduction in prostate volume was seen during the first year and maintained throughout an additional five years of open extension studies.

[See figure 4 at top of next column]

Prostate Volume as a Predictor of Therapeutic Response

A meta-analysis combining 1-year data from seven double-blind, placebo-controlled studies of similar design, including 4491 patients with symptomatic BPH, demonstrated that, in patients treated with PROSCAR, the magnitude of symptom response and degree of improvement in maximum urinary flow rate were greater in patients with an enlarged prostate at baseline.

14.2 Combination with Alpha-Blocker Therapy

The Medical Therapy of Prostatic Symptoms (MTOPS) Trial was a double-blind, randomized, placebo-controlled, multicenter, 4- to 6-year study (average 5 years) in 3047 men with symptomatic BPH, who were randomized to receive PROSCAR 5 mg/day (n=768), doxazosin 4 or 8 mg/day (n=756), the combination of PROSCAR 5 mg/day and doxa-

Table 6: Count and Percent Incidence of Primary Outcome Events by Treatment Group in MTOPS

	Treatment Group				
Event	Placebo N=737 N (%)	Doxazosin N=756 N (%)	Finasteride N=768 N (%)	Combination N=786 N (%)	Total N=3047 N (%)
AUA 4-point rise	100 (13.6)	59 (7.8)	74 (9.6)	41 (5.2)	274 (9.0)
Acute urinary retention	18 (2.4)	13 (1.7)	6 (0.8)	4 (0.5)	41 (1.3)
Incontinence	8 (1.1)	11 (1.5)	9 (1.2)	3 (0.4)	31 (1.0)
Recurrent UTI/urosepsis	2 (0.3)	2 (0.3)	0 (0.0)	1 (0.1)	5 (0.2)
Creatinine rise	0 (0.0)	0 (0.0)	0 (0.0)	0 (0.0)	0 (0.0)
Total Events	128 (17.4)	85 (11.2)	89 (11.6)	49 (6.2)	351 (11.5)

Table 7: Change From Baseline in AUA Symptom Score by Treatment Group at Year 4 in MTOPS

	Placebo N=534	Doxazosin N=582	Finasteride N=565	Combination N=598
Baseline Mean (SD)	16.8 (6.0)	17.0 (5.9)	17.1 (6.0)	16.8 (5.8)
Mean Change AUA Symptom Score (SD)	-4.9 (5.8)	-6.6 (6.1)	-5.6 (5.9)	-7.4 (6.3)
Comparison to Placebo (95% CI)		-1.8 (-2.5, -1.1)	-0.7 (-1.4, 0.0)	-2.5 (-3.2, -1.8)
Comparison to Doxazosin alone (95% CI)				-0.7 (-1.4, 0.0)
Comparison to Finasteride alone (95% CI)				-1.8 (-2.5, -1.1)

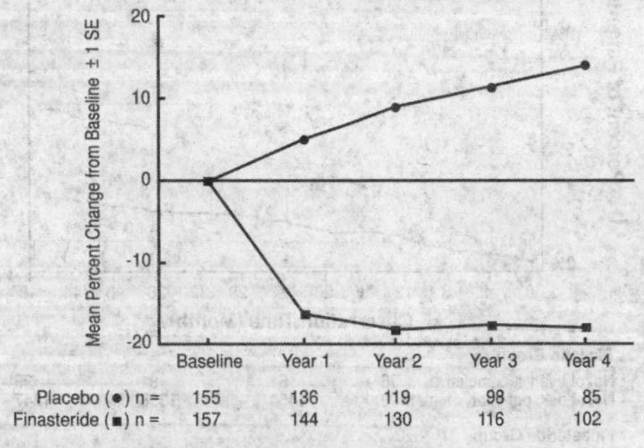

Figure 4: Prostate Volume in PLESS

zosin 4 or 8 mg/day (n=786), or placebo (n=737). All participants underwent weekly titration of doxazosin (or its placebo) from 1 to 2 to 4 to 8 mg/day. Only those who tolerated the 4 or 8 mg dose level were kept on doxazosin (or its placebo) in the study. The participant's final tolerated dose (either 4 mg or 8 mg) was administered beginning at end-Week 4. The final doxazosin dose was administered once per day, at bedtime.

The mean patient age at randomization was 62.6 years (±7.3 years). Patients were Caucasian (82%), African American (9%), Hispanic (7%), Asian (1%) or Native American (<1%). The mean duration of BPH symptoms was 4.7 years (±4.6 years). Patients had moderate to severe BPH symptoms at baseline with a mean AUA symptom score of approximately 17 out of 35 points. Mean maximum urinary flow rate was 10.5 mL/sec (±2.6 mL/sec). The mean prostate volume as measured by transrectal ultrasound was 36.3 mL (±20.1 mL). Prostate volume was ≤20 mL in 16% of patients, ≥50 mL in 18% of patients and between 21 and 49 mL in 66% of patients.

The primary endpoint was a composite measure of the first occurrence of any of the following five outcomes: a ≥4 point confirmed increase from baseline in symptom score, acute urinary retention, BPH-related renal insufficiency (creatinine rise), recurrent urinary tract infections or urosepsis, or incontinence. Compared to placebo, treatment with PROSCAR, doxazosin, or combination therapy resulted in a reduction in the risk of experiencing one of these five outcome events by 34% (p=0.002), 39% (p<0.001), and 67% (p<0.001), respectively. Combination therapy resulted in a significant reduction in the risk of the primary endpoint compared to treatment with PROSCAR alone (49%; p≤0.001) or doxazosin alone (46%; p≤0.001). (See Table 6.)

[See table 6 above]

The majority of the events (274 out of 351; 78%) was a confirmed ≥4 point increase in symptom score, referred to as symptom score progression. The risk of symptom score progression was reduced by 30% (p=0.016), 46% (p<0.001), and 64% (p<0.001) in patients treated with PROSCAR, doxazosin, or the combination, respectively, compared to patients treated with placebo (see Figure 5). Combination therapy significantly reduced the risk of symptom score progression compared to the effect of PROSCAR alone (p<0.001) and compared to doxazosin alone (p=0.037).

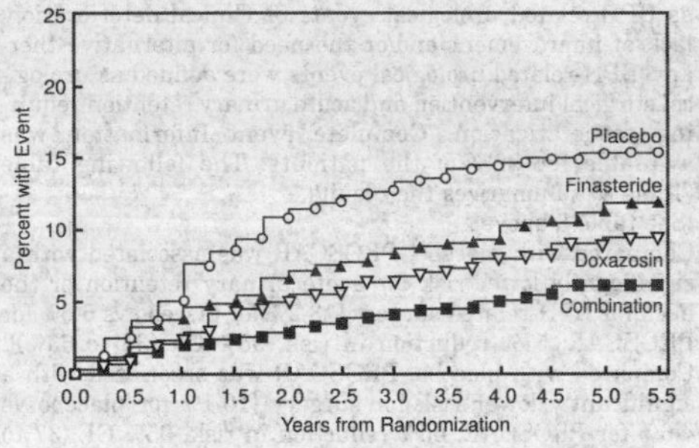

Figure 5: Cumulative Incidence of a 4-Point Rise in AUA Symptom Score by Treatment Group

Treatment with PROSCAR, doxazosin or the combination of PROSCAR with doxazosin, reduced the mean symptom score from baseline at year 4. Table 7 provides the mean change from baseline for AUA symptom score by treatment group for patients who remained on therapy for four years.

[See table 7 above]

The results of MTOPS are consistent with the findings of the 4-year, placebo-controlled study PLESS *[see Clinical Studies (14.1)]* in that treatment with PROSCAR reduces the risk of acute urinary retention and the need for BPH-related surgery. In MTOPS, the risk of developing acute urinary retention was reduced by 67% in patients treated with PROSCAR compared to patients treated with placebo (0.8% for PROSCAR and 2.4% for placebo). Also, the risk of requiring BPH-related invasive therapy was reduced by 64% in patients treated with PROSCAR compared to patients treated with placebo (2.0% for PROSCAR and 5.4% for placebo).

14.3 Summary of Clinical Studies

The data from these studies, showing improvement in BPH-related symptoms, reduction in treatment failure (BPH-related urological events), increased maximum urinary flow rates, and decreasing prostate volume, suggest that PROSCAR arrests the disease process of BPH in men with an enlarged prostate.

16 HOW SUPPLIED/STORAGE AND HANDLING

No. 3094 — PROSCAR tablets 5 mg are blue, modified apple-shaped, film-coated tablets, with the code MSD 72 on one side and PROSCAR on the other. They are supplied as follows:

NDC 0006-0072-31 unit of use bottles of 30
NDC 0006-0072-58 unit of use bottles of 100.

Storage and Handling

Store at room temperatures below 30°C (86°F). Protect from light and keep container tightly closed.

Women should not handle crushed or broken PROSCAR tablets when they are pregnant or may potentially be pregnant because of the possibility of absorption of finasteride and the subsequent potential risk to a male fetus *[see Warnings and Precautions (5.3), Use in Specific Populations (8.1) and Patient Counseling Information (17.2)].*

17 PATIENT COUNSELING INFORMATION

See FDA-Approved Patient Labeling (Patient Information).

17.1 Increased Risk of High-Grade Prostate Cancer

Patients should be informed that there was an increase in high-grade prostate cancer in men treated with 5α-reductase inhibitors indicated for BPH treatment, including PROSCAR, compared to those treated with placebo in studies looking at the use of these drugs to prevent prostate cancer *[see Indications and Usage (1.3), Warnings and Precautions (5.2), and Adverse Reactions (6.1)].*

17.2 Exposure of Women – Risk to Male Fetus

Physicians should inform patients that women who are pregnant or may potentially be pregnant should not handle crushed or broken PROSCAR tablets because of the possibility of absorption of finasteride and the subsequent potential risk to the male fetus. PROSCAR tablets are coated and will prevent contact with the active ingredient during normal handling, provided that the tablets have not been broken or crushed. If a woman who is pregnant or may potentially be pregnant comes in contact with crushed or broken PROSCAR tablets, the contact area should be washed immediately with soap and water *[see Contraindications (4), Warnings and Precautions (5.3), Use in Specific Populations (8.1) and How Supplied/Storage and Handling (16)].*

17.3 Additional Instructions

Physicians should inform patients that the volume of ejaculate may be decreased in some patients during treatment with PROSCAR. This decrease does not appear to interfere with normal sexual function. However, impotence and decreased libido may occur in patients treated with PROSCAR *[see Adverse Reactions (6.1)].*

Physicians should instruct their patients to promptly report any changes in their breasts such as lumps, pain or nipple discharge. Breast changes including breast enlargement, tenderness and neoplasm have been reported *[see Adverse Reactions (6.1)].*

Physicians should instruct their patients to read the patient package insert before starting therapy with PROSCAR and to reread it each time the prescription is renewed so that they are aware of current information for patients regarding PROSCAR.

Dist. by: Merck Sharp & Dohme Corp., a subsidiary of **MERCK & CO., INC.**, Whitehouse Station, NJ 08889, USA

Revised: 01/2013
USPI-5T-09061301R010

PROSCAR® (finasteride) Tablets
Patient Information about
PROSCAR® (Prahs-car)

Generic name: finasteride
(fin-AS-tur-eyed)

PROSCAR is for use by men only.

Please read this leaflet before you start taking PROSCAR. Also, read it each time you renew your prescription, just in case anything has changed. Remember, this leaflet does not take the place of careful discussions with your doctor. You and your doctor should discuss PROSCAR when you start taking your medication and at regular checkups.

What is PROSCAR?

PROSCAR is a medication used to treat symptoms of benign prostatic hyperplasia (BPH) in men with an enlarged prostate. PROSCAR may also be used to reduce the risk of a sudden inability to pass urine and the need for surgery related to BPH in men with an enlarged prostate.

PROSCAR may be prescribed along with another medicine, an alpha-blocker called doxazosin, to help you better manage your BPH symptoms.

Who should NOT take PROSCAR?

PROSCAR is for use by MEN only.

Do Not Take PROSCAR if you are:

- a woman who is pregnant or may potentially be pregnant. PROSCAR may harm your unborn baby. Do not touch or handle crushed or broken PROSCAR tablets (see **"A warning about PROSCAR and pregnancy"**).
- allergic to finasteride or any of the ingredients in PROSCAR. See the end of this leaflet for a complete list of ingredients in PROSCAR.

A warning about PROSCAR and pregnancy:

Women who are or may potentially be pregnant must not use PROSCAR. They should also not handle crushed or broken tablets of PROSCAR. PROSCAR tablets are coated and will prevent contact with the active ingredient during normal handling, provided that the tablets are not broken or crushed.

If a woman who is pregnant with a male baby absorbs the active ingredient in PROSCAR after oral use or through the skin, it may cause the male baby to be born with abnormalities of the sex organs. If a woman who is pregnant comes into contact with the active ingredient in PROSCAR, a doctor should be consulted.

How should I take PROSCAR?

Follow your doctor's instruction.

- Take one tablet by mouth each day. To avoid forgetting to take PROSCAR, you can take it at the same time every day.
- If you forget to take PROSCAR, do not take an extra tablet. Just take the next tablet as usual.
- You may take PROSCAR with or without food.
- Do not share PROSCAR with anyone else; it was prescribed only for you.

What are the possible side effects of PROSCAR?

PROSCAR may increase the chance of a more serious form of prostate cancer.

The most common side effects of PROSCAR include:

- trouble getting or keeping an erection (impotence)
- decrease in sex drive
- decreased volume of ejaculate
- ejaculation disorders
- enlarged or painful breast. You should promptly report to your doctor any changes in your breasts such as lumps, pain or nipple discharge.

The following have been reported in general use with PROSCAR and/or finasteride at lower doses:

- allergic reactions, including rash, itching, hives, and swelling of the lips and face
- rarely, some men may have testicular pain
- trouble getting or keeping an erection that continued after stopping the medication
- problems with ejaculation that continued after stopping the medication
- male infertility and/or poor quality of semen. Improvement in the quality of semen has been reported after stopping the medication.
- depression
- decrease in sex drive that continued after stopping the medication
- in rare cases, male breast cancer has been reported.

You should discuss side effects with your doctor before taking PROSCAR and anytime you think you are having a side effect. These are not all the possible side effects with PROSCAR. For more information, ask your doctor or pharmacist.

Call your doctor for medical advice about side effects. You may report side effects to FDA at: 1-800-FDA-1088.

What you need to know while taking PROSCAR:

- **You should see your doctor regularly while taking PROSCAR.** Follow your doctor's advice about when to have these checkups.
- **Checking for prostate cancer.** Your doctor has prescribed PROSCAR for BPH and not for treatment of prostate cancer — but a man can have BPH and prostate cancer at the same time. Your doctor may continue checking for prostate cancer while you take PROSCAR.
- **About Prostate-Specific Antigen (PSA).** Your doctor may have done a blood test called PSA for the screening of prostate cancer. Because PROSCAR decreases PSA levels, you should tell your doctor(s) that you are taking PROSCAR. Changes in PSA levels will need to be evaluated by your doctor(s). Any increase in follow-up PSA levels from their lowest point may signal the presence of prostate cancer and should be evaluated, even if the test results are still within the normal range. You should also tell your doctor if you have not been taking PROSCAR as prescribed because this may affect the PSA test results. For more information, talk to your doctor.

How should I store PROSCAR?

- Store PROSCAR tablets in a dry place at room temperature.
- Keep PROSCAR in the original container and keep the container closed.

PROSCAR tablets are coated and will prevent contact with the active ingredient during normal handling, provided that the tablets are not broken or crushed.

Keep PROSCAR and all medications out of the reach of children.

Do not give your PROSCAR tablets to anyone else. It has been prescribed only for you.

For more information call 1-800-622-4477.

What are the ingredients in PROSCAR?

Active ingredients: finasteride

Inactive ingredients: hydrous lactose, microcrystalline cellulose, pregelatinized starch, sodium starch glycolate, hydroxypropyl cellulose LF, hydroxypropyl methylcellulose, titanium dioxide, magnesium stearate, talc, docusate sodium, FD&C Blue 2 aluminum lake and yellow iron oxide.

What is BPH?

BPH is an enlargement of the prostate gland. The prostate is located below the bladder. As the prostate enlarges, it may slowly restrict the flow of urine. This can lead to symptoms such as:

- a weak or interrupted urinary stream
- a feeling that you cannot empty your bladder completely
- a feeling of delay or hesitation when you start to urinate
- a need to urinate often, especially at night
- a feeling that you must urinate right away.

In some men, BPH can lead to serious problems, including urinary tract infections, a sudden inability to pass urine (acute urinary retention), as well as the need for surgery.

What PROSCAR does:

PROSCAR lowers levels of a hormone called DHT (dihydrotestosterone), which is a cause of prostate growth. Lowering DHT leads to shrinkage of the enlarged prostate gland in most men. This can lead to gradual improvement in urine flow and symptoms over the next several months. PROSCAR will help reduce the risk of developing a sudden inability to pass urine and the need for surgery related to an enlarged prostate. However, since each case of BPH is different, you should know that:

- Even though the prostate shrinks, you may NOT notice an improvement in urine flow or symptoms.
- You may need to take PROSCAR for six (6) months or more to see whether it improves your symptoms.
- Therapy with PROSCAR may reduce your risk for a sudden inability to pass urine and the need for surgery for an enlarged prostate.

Dist. by: Merck Sharp & Dohme Corp., a subsidiary of **MERCK & CO., INC.**, Whitehouse Station, NJ 08889, USA

Revised: 01/2013
USPPI-5T-09061301R010

Shown in Product Identification Guide, page 308

PROVENTIL® HFA ℞

[prō-vĕn-tĕl H-F-A]
(albuterol sulfate)
Inhalation Aerosol

FOR ORAL INHALATION ONLY
Prescribing Information

DESCRIPTION

The active component of PROVENTIL® HFA (albuterol sulfate) Inhalation Aerosol is albuterol sulfate, USP racemic α^1 [(*tert*-Butylamino)methyl]-4-hydroxy-*m*-xylene-α,α'-diol sulfate (2:1)(salt), a relatively selective beta$_2$-adrenergic bronchodilator having the following chemical structure:

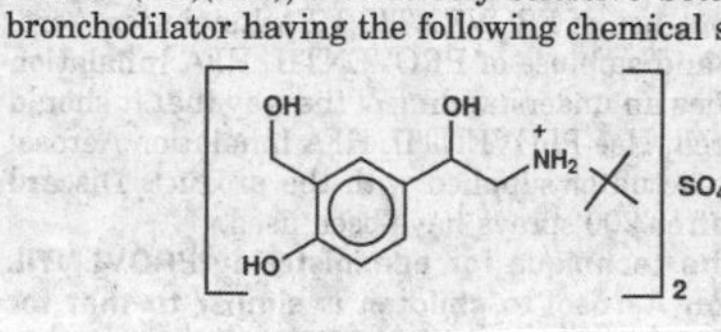

Albuterol sulfate is the official generic name in the United States. The World Health Organization recommended name for the drug is salbutamol sulfate. The molecular weight of albuterol sulfate is 576.7, and the empirical formula is (C13H21 NO3)2•H2SO4. Albuterol sulfate is a white to off-white crystalline solid. It is soluble in water and slightly soluble in ethanol. PROVENTIL HFA Inhalation Aerosol is a pressurized metered-dose aerosol unit for oral inhalation. It contains a microcrystalline suspension of albuterol sulfate in propellant HFA-134a (1,1,1,2-tetrafluoroethane), ethanol, and oleic acid.

Each actuation delivers 120 mcg albuterol sulfate, USP from the valve and 108 mcg albuterol sulfate, USP from the mouthpiece (equivalent to 90 mcg of albuterol base from the mouthpiece). Each canister provides 200 inhalations. It is recommended to prime the inhaler before using for the first time and in cases where the inhaler has not been used for more than 2 weeks by releasing four "test sprays" into the air, away from the face.

This product does not contain chlorofluorocarbons (CFCs) as the propellant.

CLINICAL PHARMACOLOGY

Mechanism of Action *In vitro* studies and *in vivo* pharmacologic studies have demonstrated that albuterol has a preferential effect on beta$_2$-adrenergic receptors compared with isoproterenol. While it is recognized that beta$_2$-adrenergic receptors are the predominant receptors on bronchial smooth muscle, data indicate that there is a population of beta$_2$-receptors in the human heart existing in a concentration between 10% and 50% of cardiac beta-adrenergic receptors. The precise function of these receptors has not been established. (See **WARNINGS, Cardiovascular Effects** section.)

Activation of beta$_2$-adrenergic receptors on airway smooth muscle leads to the activation of adenylcyclase and to an increase in the intracellular concentration of cyclic-3′,5′-adenosine monophosphate (cyclic AMP). This increase of cyclic AMP leads to the activation of protein kinase A, which inhibits the phosphorylation of myosin and lowers intracellular ionic calcium concentrations, resulting in relaxation. Albuterol relaxes the smooth muscles of all airways, from the trachea to the terminal bronchioles. Albuterol acts as a functional antagonist to relax the airway irrespective of the spasmogen involved, thus protecting against all bronchoconstrictor challenges. Increased cyclic AMP concentrations are also associated with the inhibition of release of mediators from mast cells in the airway.

Albuterol has been shown in most clinical trials to have more effect on the respiratory tract, in the form of bronchial smooth muscle relaxation, than isoproterenol at comparable doses while producing fewer cardiovascular effects. Controlled clinical studies and other clinical experience have shown that inhaled albuterol, like other beta-adrenergic agonist drugs, can produce a significant cardiovascular effect in some patients, as measured by pulse rate, blood pressure, symptoms, and/or electrocardiographic changes.

Preclinical Intravenous studies in rats with albuterol sulfate have demonstrated that albuterol crosses the blood-brain barrier and reaches brain concentrations amounting to approximately 5% of the plasma concentrations. In structures outside the blood-brain barrier (pineal and pituitary glands), albuterol concentrations were found to be 100 times those in the whole brain.

Studies in laboratory animals (minipigs, rodents, and dogs) have demonstrated the occurrence of cardiac arrhythmias and sudden death (with histologic evidence of myocardial necrosis) when beta$_2$-agonist and methylxanthines were administered concurrently. The clinical significance of these findings is unknown.

Propellant HFA-134a is devoid of pharmacological activity except at very high doses in animals (380-1300 times the maximum human exposure based on comparisons of AUC values), primarily producing ataxia, tremors, dyspnea, or salivation. These are similar to effects produced by the structurally related chlorofluorocarbons (CFCs), which have been used extensively in metered dose inhalers.

In animals and humans, propellant HFA-134a was found to be rapidly absorbed and rapidly eliminated, with an elimination half-life of 3 to 27 minutes in animals and 5 to 7 minutes in humans. Time to maximum plasma concentration (Tmax) and mean residence time are both extremely short, leading to a transient appearance of HFA-134a in the blood with no evidence of accumulation.

Pharmacokinetics In a single-dose bioavailability study which enrolled six healthy, male volunteers, transient low albuterol levels (close to the lower limit of quantitation) were observed after administration of two puffs from both PROVENTIL® HFA Inhalation Aerosol and a CFC 11/12 propelled albuterol inhaler. No formal pharmacokinetic analyses were possible for either treatment, but systemic albuterol levels appeared similar.

Clinical Trials In a 12-week, randomized, double-blind, double-dummy, active- and placebo-controlled trial, 565 patients with asthma were evaluated for the bronchodilator efficacy of PROVENTIL HFA Inhalation Aerosol (193 patients) in comparison to a CFC 11/12 propelled albuterol inhaler (186 patients) and an HFA-134a placebo inhaler (186 patients).

Serial FEV1 measurements (shown below as percent change from test-day baseline) demonstrated that two inhalations of PROVENTIL HFA Inhalation Aerosol produced significantly greater improvement in pulmonary function than placebo and produced outcomes which were clinically comparable to a CFC 11/12 propelled albuterol inhaler.

The mean time to onset of a 15% increase in FEV1 was 6 minutes and the mean time to peak effect was 50 to 55 minutes. The mean duration of effect as measured by a 15% increase in FEV1 was 3 hours. In some patients, duration of effect was as long as 6 hours.

In another clinical study in adults, two inhalations of PROVENTIL HFA Inhalation Aerosol taken 30 minutes before exercise prevented exercise-induced bronchospasm as demonstrated by the maintenance of FEV1 within 80% of baseline values in the majority of patients.

In a 4-week, randomized, open-label trial, 63 children, 4 to 11 years of age, with asthma were evaluated for the bronchodilator efficacy of PROVENTIL HFA Inhalation Aerosol (33 pediatric patients) in comparison to a CFC 11/12 propelled albuterol inhaler (30 pediatric patients).

[See figure at top of next column]

Serial FEV1 measurements as percent change from test-day baseline demonstrated that two inhalations of PROVENTIL HFA Inhalation Aerosol produced outcomes which were clinically comparable to a CFC 11/12 propelled albuterol inhaler.

The mean time to onset of a 12% increase in FEV1 for PROVENTIL HFA Inhalation Aerosol was 7 minutes and the mean time to peak effect was approximately 50 minutes.

FEV_1 as Percent Change from Predose in a Large 12-Week Clinical Trial

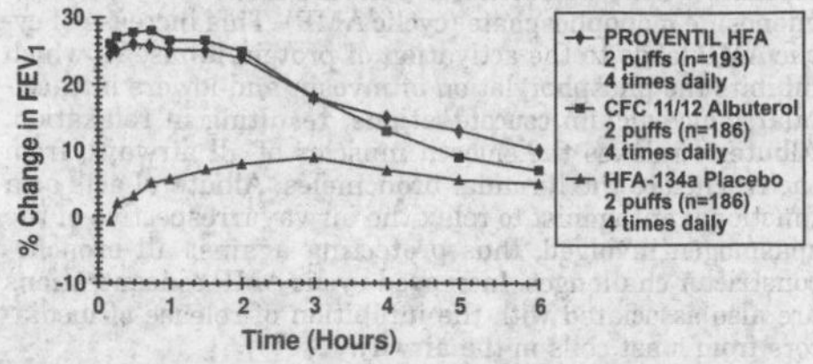

The mean duration of effect as measured by a 12% increase in FEV1 was 2.3 hours. In some pediatric patients, duration of effect was as long as 6 hours.

In another clinical study in pediatric patients, two inhalations of PROVENTIL HFA Inhalation Aerosol taken 30 minutes before exercise provided comparable protection against exercise-induced bronchospasm as a CFC 11/12 propelled albuterol inhaler.

INDICATIONS AND USAGE

PROVENTIL® HFA Inhalation Aerosol is indicated in adults and children 4 years of age and older for the treatment or prevention of bronchospasm with reversible obstructive airway disease and for the prevention of exercise-induced bronchospasm.

CONTRAINDICATIONS

PROVENTIL® HFA Inhalation Aerosol is contraindicated in patients with a history of hypersensitivity to albuterol or any other PROVENTIL HFA components.

WARNINGS

1. **Paradoxical Bronchospasm:** Inhaled albuterol sulfate can produce paradoxical bronchospasm that may be life threatening. If paradoxical bronchospasm occurs, PROVENTIL® HFA Inhalation Aerosol should be discontinued immediately and alternative therapy instituted. It should be recognized that paradoxical bronchospasm, when associated with inhaled formulations, frequently occurs with the first use of a new canister.
2. **Deterioration of Asthma:** Asthma may deteriorate acutely over a period of hours or chronically over several days or longer. If the patient needs more doses of PROVENTIL HFA Inhalation Aerosol than usual, this may be a marker of destabilization of asthma and requires re-evaluation of the patient and treatment regimen, giving special consideration to the possible need for anti-inflammatory treatment, e.g., corticosteroids.
3. **Use of Anti-inflammatory Agents:** The use of beta-adrenergic-agonist bronchodilators alone may not be adequate to control asthma in many patients. Early consideration should be given to adding anti-inflammatory agents, e.g., corticosteroids, to the therapeutic regimen.
4. **Cardiovascular Effects:** PROVENTIL HFA Inhalation Aerosol, like other beta-adrenergic agonists, can produce clinically significant cardiovascular effects in some patients as measured by pulse rate, blood pressure, and/or symptoms. Although such effects are uncommon after administration of PROVENTIL HFA Inhalation Aerosol at recommended doses, if they occur, the drug may need to be discontinued. In addition, beta-agonists have been reported to produce ECG changes, such as flattening of the T wave, prolongation of the QTc interval, and ST segment depression. The clinical significance of these findings is unknown. Therefore, PROVENTIL HFA Inhalation Aerosol, like all sympathomimetic amines, should be used with caution in patients with cardiovascular disorders, especially coronary insufficiency, cardiac arrhythmias, and hypertension.
5. **Do Not Exceed Recommended Dose:** Fatalities have been reported in association with excessive use of inhaled sympathomimetic drugs in patients with asthma. The exact cause of death is unknown, but cardiac arrest following an unexpected development of a severe acute asthmatic crisis and subsequent hypoxia is suspected.
6. **Immediate Hypersensitivity Reactions:** Immediate hypersensitivity reactions may occur after administration of albuterol sulfate, as demonstrated by rare cases of urticaria, angioedema, rash, bronchospasm, anaphylaxis, and oropharyngeal edema.

PRECAUTIONS

General Albuterol sulfate, as with all sympathomimetic amines, should be used with caution in patients with cardiovascular disorders, especially coronary insufficiency, cardiac arrhythmias, and hypertension; in patients with convulsive disorders, hyperthyroidism, or diabetes mellitus; and in patients who are unusually responsive to sympathomimetic amines. Clinically significant changes in systolic and diastolic blood pressure have been seen in individual patients and could be expected to occur in some patients after use of any beta-adrenergic bronchodilator.

Large doses of intravenous albuterol have been reported to aggravate preexisting diabetes mellitus and ketoacidosis. As with other beta-agonists, albuterol may produce significant hypokalemia in some patients, possibly through intracellular shunting, which has the potential to produce adverse cardiovascular effects. The decrease is usually transient, not requiring supplementation.

Information for Patients See illustrated Patient's Instructions for Use. SHAKE WELL BEFORE USING. Patients should be given the following information:

It is recommended to prime the inhaler before using for the first time and in cases where the inhaler has not been used for more than 2 weeks by releasing four "test sprays" into the air, away from the face.

KEEPING THE PLASTIC MOUTHPIECE CLEAN IS VERY IMPORTANT TO PREVENT MEDICATION BUILDUP AND BLOCKAGE. THE MOUTHPIECE SHOULD BE WASHED, SHAKEN TO REMOVE EXCESS WATER, AND AIR DRIED THOROUGHLY AT LEAST ONCE A WEEK. INHALER MAY CEASE TO DELIVER MEDICATION IF NOT PROPERLY CLEANED.

The mouthpiece should be cleaned (with the canister removed) by running warm water through the top and bottom for 30 seconds at least once a week. The mouthpiece must be shaken to remove excess water, then air dried thoroughly (such as overnight). Blockage from medication buildup or improper medication delivery may result from failure to thoroughly air dry the mouthpiece.

If the mouthpiece should become blocked (little or no medication coming out of the mouthpiece), the blockage may be removed by washing as described above.

If it is necessary to use the inhaler before it is completely dry, shake off excess water, replace canister, test spray twice away from face, and take the prescribed dose. After such use, the mouthpiece should be rewashed and allowed to air dry thoroughly.

The action of PROVENTIL® HFA Inhalation Aerosol should last up to 4 to 6 hours. PROVENTIL HFA Inhalation Aerosol should not be used more frequently than recommended. Do not increase the dose or frequency of doses of PROVENTIL HFA Inhalation Aerosol without consulting your physician. If you find that treatment with PROVENTIL HFA Inhalation Aerosol becomes less effective for symptomatic relief, your symptoms become worse, and/or you need to use the product more frequently than usual, medical attention should be sought immediately. While you are taking PROVENTIL HFA Inhalation Aerosol, other inhaled drugs and asthma medications should be taken only as directed by your physician.

Common adverse effects of treatment with inhaled albuterol include palpitations, chest pain, rapid heart rate, tremor, or nervousness. If you are pregnant or nursing, contact your physician about use of PROVENTIL HFA Inhalation Aerosol. Effective and safe use of PROVENTIL HFA Inhalation Aerosol includes an understanding of the way that it should be administered. Use PROVENTIL HFA Inhalation Aerosol only with the actuator supplied with the product. Discard the canister after 200 sprays have been used.

In general, the technique for administering PROVENTIL HFA Inhalation Aerosol to children is similar to that for adults. Children should use PROVENTIL HFA Inhalation Aerosol under adult supervision, as instructed by the patient's physician. (See **Patient's Instructions for Use.**)

Drug Interactions

1. **Beta-Blockers:** Beta-adrenergic-receptor blocking agents not only block the pulmonary effect of beta-agonists, such as PROVENTIL HFA Inhalation Aerosol, but may produce severe bronchospasm in asthmatic patients. Therefore, patients with asthma should not normally be treated with beta-blockers. However, under certain circumstances, e.g., as prophylaxis after myocardial infarction, there may be no acceptable alternatives to the use of beta-adrenergic blocking agents in patients with asthma. In this setting, cardioselective beta-blockers should be considered, although they should be administered with caution.
2. **Diuretics:** The ECG changes and/or hypokalemia which may result from the administration of nonpotassium-sparing diuretics (such as loop or thiazide diuretics) can be acutely worsened by beta-agonists, especially when the recommended dose of the beta-agonist is exceeded. Although the clinical significance of these effects is not known, caution is advised in the coadministration of beta-agonists with nonpotassium-sparing diuretics.
3. **Albuterol-Digoxin:** Mean decreases of 16% and 22% in serum digoxin levels were demonstrated after single-dose intravenous and oral administration of albuterol, respectively, to normal volunteers who had received digoxin for 10 days. The clinical significance of these findings for patients with obstructive airway disease who are receiving albuterol and digoxin on a chronic basis is unclear; nevertheless, it would be prudent to carefully evaluate the serum digoxin levels in patients who are currently receiving digoxin and albuterol.
4. **Monoamine Oxidase Inhibitors or Tricyclic Antidepressants:** PROVENTIL HFA Inhalation Aerosol should be administered with extreme caution to patients being treated with monoamine oxidase inhibitors or tricyclic antidepressants, or within 2 weeks of discontinuation of such agents, because the action of albuterol on the cardiovascular system may be potentiated.

Carcinogenesis, Mutagenesis, and Impairment of Fertility

In a 2-year study in SPRAGUE-DAWLEY® rats, albuterol sulfate caused a dose-related increase in the incidence of benign leiomyomas of the mesovarium at the above dietary doses of 2 mg/kg (approximately 15 times the maximum recommended daily inhalation dose for adults on a mg/m^2 basis and approximately 6 times the maximum recommended daily inhalation dose for children on a mg/m^2 basis). In another study this effect was blocked by the coadministration of propranolol, a nonselective beta-adrenergic antagonist. In an 18-month study in CD-1 mice, albuterol sulfate showed no evidence of tumorigenicity at dietary doses of up to 500 mg/kg (approximately 1700 times the maximum recommended daily inhalation dose for adults on a mg/m^2 basis and approximately 800 times the maximum recommended daily inhalation dose for children on a mg/m^2 basis). In a 22-month study in Golden Hamsters, albuterol sulfate showed no evidence of tumorigenicity at dietary doses of up to 50 mg/kg (approximately 225 times the maximum recommended daily inhalation dose for adults on a mg/m^2 basis and approximately 110 times the maximum recommended daily inhalation dose for children on a mg/m^2 basis).

Albuterol sulfate was not mutagenic in the Ames test or a mutation test in yeast. Albuterol sulfate was not clastogenic in a human peripheral lymphocyte assay or in an AH1 strain mouse micronucleus assay.

Reproduction studies in rats demonstrated no evidence of impaired fertility at oral doses up to 50 mg/kg (approximately 340 times the maximum recommended daily inhalation dose for adults on a mg/m^2 basis).

Pregnancy *Teratogenic Effects* Pregnancy Category C

Albuterol sulfate has been shown to be teratogenic in mice. A study in CD-1 mice given albuterol sulfate subcutaneously showed cleft palate formation in 5 of 111 (4.5%) fetuses at 0.25 mg/kg (less than the maximum recommended daily inhalation dose for adults on a mg/m^2 basis) and in 10 of 108 (9.3%) fetuses at 2.5 mg/kg (approximately 8 times the maximum recommended daily inhalation dose for adults on a mg/m^2 basis). The drug did not induce cleft palate formation at a dose of 0.025 mg/kg (less than the maximum recommended daily inhalation dose for adults on a mg/m^2 basis). Cleft palate also occurred in 22 of 72 (30.5%) fetuses from females treated subcutaneously with 2.5 mg/kg of isoproterenol (positive control).

A reproduction study in Stride Dutch rabbits revealed cranioschisis in 7 of 19 (37%) fetuses when albuterol sulfate was administered orally at 50 mg/kg dose (approximately 680 times the maximum recommended daily inhalation dose for adults on a mg/m^2 basis).

In an inhalation reproduction study in SPRAGUE-DAWLEY rats, the albuterol sulfate/HFA-134a formulation did not exhibit any teratogenic effects at 10.5 mg/kg (approximately 70 times the maximum recommended daily inhalation dose for adults on a mg/m^2 basis).

A study in which pregnant rats were dosed with radiolabeled albuterol sulfate demonstrated that drug-related material is transferred from the maternal circulation to the fetus.

There are no adequate and well-controlled studies of PROVENTIL HFA Inhalation Aerosol or albuterol sulfate in pregnant women. PROVENTIL HFA Inhalation Aerosol should be used during pregnancy only if the potential benefit justifies the potential risk to the fetus.

During worldwide marketing experience, various congenital anomalies, including cleft palate and limb defects, have been reported in the offspring of patients being treated with albuterol. Some of the mothers were taking multiple medications during their pregnancies. Because no consistent pattern of defects can be discerned, a relationship between albuterol use and congenital anomalies has not been established.

Use in Labor and Delivery

Because of the potential for beta-agonist interference with uterine contractility, use of PROVENTIL HFA Inhalation Aerosol for relief of bronchospasm during labor should be restricted to those patients in whom the benefits clearly outweigh the risk.

Tocolysis: Albuterol has not been approved for the management of preterm labor. The benefit:risk ratio when albuterol is administered for tocolysis has not been established. Serious adverse reactions, including pulmonary edema, have been reported during or following treatment of premature labor with $beta_2$-agonists, including albuterol.

Nursing Mothers

Plasma levels of albuterol sulfate and HFA-134a after inhaled therapeutic doses are very low in humans, but it is not known whether the components of PROVENTIL HFA Inhalation Aerosol are excreted in human milk.

Because of the potential for tumorigenicity shown for albuterol in animal studies and lack of experience with the use of PROVENTIL HFA Inhalation Aerosol by nursing mothers, a decision should be made whether to discontinue nursing or to discontinue the drug, taking into account the importance of the drug to the mother. Caution should be exercised when albuterol sulfate is administered to a nursing woman.

Pediatrics

The safety and effectiveness of PROVENTIL HFA Inhalation Aerosol in pediatric patients below the age of 4 years have not been established.

Geriatrics

PROVENTIL HFA Inhalation Aerosol has not been studied in a geriatric population. As with other $beta_2$-agonists, special caution should be observed when using PROVENTIL HFA Inhalation Aerosol in elderly patients who have concomitant cardiovascular disease that could be adversely affected by this class of drug.

ADVERSE REACTIONS

Adverse reaction information concerning PROVENTIL® HFA Inhalation Aerosol is derived from a 12-week, double-blind, double-dummy study which compared PROVENTIL HFA Inhalation Aerosol, a CFC 11/12 propelled albuterol inhaler, and an HFA-134a placebo inhaler in 565 asthmatic patients. The following table lists the incidence of all adverse events (whether considered by the investigator drug related or unrelated to drug) from this study which occurred at a rate of 3% or greater in the PROVENTIL HFA Inhalation Aerosol treatment group and more frequently in the PROVENTIL HFA Inhalation Aerosol treatment group than in the placebo group. Overall, the incidence and nature of the adverse reactions reported for PROVENTIL HFA Inhalation Aerosol and a CFC 11/12 propelled albuterol inhaler were comparable.

[See table above]

Adverse Experience Incidences (% of patients) in a Large 12-week Clinical Trial*

Body System/ Adverse Event (Preferred Term)		PROVENTIL® HFA Inhalation Aerosol (N=193)	CFC 11/12 Propelled Albuterol Inhaler (N=186)	HFA-134a Placebo Inhaler (N=186)
Application Site Disorders	Inhalation Site Sensation	6	9	2
	Inhalation Taste Sensation	4	3	3
Body as a Whole	Allergic Reaction/Symptoms	6	4	<1
	Back Pain	4	2	3
	Fever	6	2	5
Central and Peripheral Nervous System	Tremor	7	8	2
Gastrointestinal System	Nausea	10	9	5
	Vomiting	7	2	3
Heart Rate and Rhythm Disorder	Tachycardia	7	2	<1
Psychiatric Disorders	Nervousness	7	9	3
Respiratory System Disorders	Respiratory Disorder (unspecified)	6	4	5
	Rhinitis	16	22	14
	Upper Resp Tract Infection	21	20	18
Urinary System Disorder	Urinary Tract Infection	3	4	2

*This table includes all adverse events (whether considered by the investigator drug related or unrelated to drug) which occurred at an incidence rate of at least 3.0% in the PROVENTIL HFA Inhalation Aerosol group and more frequently in the PROVENTIL HFA Inhalation Aerosol group than in the HFA-134a placebo inhaler group.

Adverse events reported by less than 3% of the patients receiving PROVENTIL HFA Inhalation Aerosol, and by a greater proportion of PROVENTIL HFA Inhalation Aerosol patients than placebo patients, which have the potential to be related to PROVENTIL HFA Inhalation Aerosol include: dysphonia, increased sweating, dry mouth, chest pain, edema, rigors, ataxia, leg cramps, hyperkinesia, eructation, flatulence, tinnitus, diabetes mellitus, anxiety, depression, somnolence, rash. Palpitation and dizziness have also been observed with PROVENTIL HFA Inhalation Aerosol.

Adverse events reported in a 4-week pediatric clinical trial comparing PROVENTIL HFA Inhalation Aerosol and a CFC 11/12 propelled albuterol inhaler occurred at a low incidence rate and were similar to those seen in the adult trials.

In small, cumulative dose studies, tremor, nervousness, and headache appeared to be dose related.

Rare cases of urticaria, angioedema, rash, bronchospasm, and oropharyngeal edema have been reported after the use of inhaled albuterol. In addition, albuterol, like other sympathomimetic agents, can cause adverse reactions such as hypertension, angina, vertigo, central nervous system stimulation, insomnia, headache, metabolic acidosis, and drying or irritation of the oropharynx.

OVERDOSAGE

The expected symptoms with overdosage are those of excessive beta-adrenergic stimulation and/or occurrence or exaggeration of any of the symptoms listed under **ADVERSE REACTIONS**, e.g., seizures, angina, hypertension or hypotension, tachycardia with rates up to 200 beats per minute, arrhythmias, nervousness, headache, tremor, dry mouth, palpitation, nausea, dizziness, fatigue, malaise, and insomnia.

Hypokalemia may also occur. As with all sympathomimetic medications, cardiac arrest and even death may be associated with abuse of PROVENTIL® HFA Inhalation Aerosol. Treatment consists of discontinuation of PROVENTIL HFA Inhalation Aerosol together with appropriate symptomatic therapy. The judicious use of a cardioselective beta-receptor blocker may be considered, bearing in mind that such medication can produce bronchospasm. There is insufficient evidence to determine if dialysis is beneficial for overdosage of PROVENTIL HFA Inhalation Aerosol.

The oral median lethal dose of albuterol sulfate in mice is greater than 2000 mg/kg (approximately 6800 times the maximum recommended daily inhalation dose for adults on a mg/m^2 basis and approximately 3200 times the maximum recommended daily inhalation dose for children on a mg/m^2 basis). In mature rats, the subcutaneous median lethal dose of albuterol sulfate is approximately 450 mg/kg (approximately 3000 times the maximum recommended daily inhalation dose for adults on a mg/m^2 basis and approximately 1400 times the maximum recommended daily inhalation dose for children on a mg/m^2 basis). In young rats, the subcutaneous median lethal dose is approximately 2000 mg/kg (approximately 14,000 times the maximum recommended daily inhalation dose for adults on a mg/m^2 basis and approximately 6400 times the maximum recommended daily inhalation dose for children on a mg/m^2 basis). The inhalation median lethal dose has not been determined in animals.

DOSAGE AND ADMINISTRATION

For treatment of acute episodes of bronchospasm or prevention of asthmatic symptoms, the usual dosage for adults and children 4 years of age and older is two inhalations repeated every 4 to 6 hours. More frequent administration or a larger number of inhalations is not recommended. In some patients, one inhalation every 4 hours may be sufficient. Each actuation of PROVENTIL® HFA Inhalation Aerosol delivers 108 mcg of albuterol sulfate (equivalent to 90 mcg of albuterol base) from the mouthpiece. It is recommended to prime the inhaler before using for the first time and in cases where the inhaler has not been used for more than 2 weeks by releasing four "test sprays" into the air, away from the face.

Exercise Induced Bronchospasm Prevention: The usual dosage for adults and children 4 years of age and older is two inhalations 15 to 30 minutes before exercise.

To maintain proper use of this product, it is important that the mouthpiece be washed and dried thoroughly at least once a week. The inhaler may cease to deliver medication if not properly cleaned and dried thoroughly (see **PRECAUTIONS, Information for Patients** section). Keeping the plastic mouthpiece clean is very important to prevent medication buildup and blockage. The inhaler may cease to deliver medication if not properly cleaned and air dried thoroughly. If the mouthpiece becomes blocked, washing the mouthpiece will remove the blockage.

If a previously effective dose regimen fails to provide the usual response, this may be a marker of destabilization of asthma and requires reevaluation of the patient and the treatment regimen, giving special consideration to the possible need for anti-inflammatory treatment, e.g., corticosteroids.

HOW SUPPLIED

PROVENTIL® HFA (albuterol sulfate) Inhalation Aerosol is supplied as a pressurized aluminum canister with a yellow plastic actuator and orange dust cap each in boxes of one. Each actuation delivers 120 mcg of albuterol sulfate from the valve and 108 mcg of albuterol sulfate from the mouthpiece (equivalent to 90 mcg of albuterol base). Canisters with a labeled net weight of 6.7 g contain 200 inhalations (NDC 0085-1132-01).

Rx only. Store between 15°-25°C (59°-77°F). For best results, canister should be at room temperature before use. SHAKE WELL BEFORE USING.

The yellow actuator supplied with PROVENTIL HFA Inhalation Aerosol should not be used with any other product canisters, and actuator from other products should not be used with a PROVENTIL HFA Inhalation Aerosol canister. The correct amount of medication in each canister cannot be assured after 200 actuations, even though the canister is not completely empty. The canister should be discarded when the labeled number of actuations have been used.

WARNING: Avoid spraying in eyes. Contents under pressure. Do not puncture or incinerate. Exposure to temperatures above 120°F may cause bursting. Keep out of reach of children.

PROVENTIL® HFA Inhalation Aerosol does not contain chlorofluorocarbons (CFCs) as the propellant.

Developed and Manufactured by:
3M Health Care Limited
Loughborough UK
or
3M Drug Delivery Systems
Northridge, CA 91324, USA
Distributed by:
Schering Corporation, a subsidiary of
MERCK & CO., INC.
Whitehouse Station, NJ 08889, USA

658000
Rev. 06/12

Attention Health Care Professional:
Detach Patient's Instructions for Use from package insert and dispense with the product.

PROVENTIL® HFA
(albuterol sulfate)
Inhalation Aerosol
FOR ORAL INHALATION ONLY
Patient's Instructions for Use

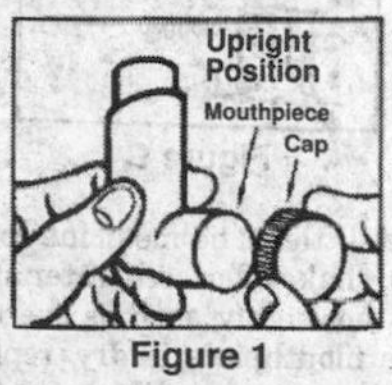

Figure 1

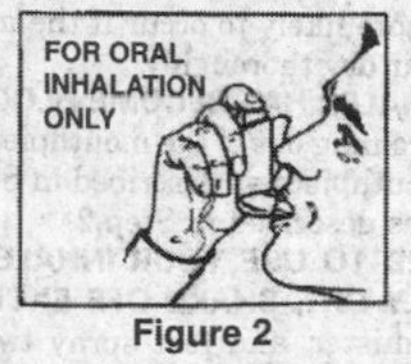

Figure 2

Before using your PROVENTIL® HFA (albuterol sulfate) Inhalation Aerosol, read complete instructions carefully. Children should use PROVENTIL HFA Inhalation Aerosol under adult supervision, as instructed by the patient's doctor

Please note that (CFC) indicates that this inhalation aerosol does not contain chlorofluorocarbons (CFCs) as the propellant.

1. SHAKE THE INHALER WELL immediately before each use. **Then remove the cap from the mouthpiece** (see Figure 1). **Check mouthpiece for foreign objects prior to use.** Make sure the canister is fully inserted into the actuator.
2. As with all aerosol medications, it is recommended to prime the inhaler before using for the first time and in cases where the inhaler has not been used for more than 2 weeks. Prime by releasing four "test sprays" into the air, away from your face.
3. BREATHE OUT FULLY THROUGH THE MOUTH, expelling as much air from your lungs as possible. Place the mouthpiece fully into the mouth, holding the inhaler in its upright position (see Figure 2) and closing the lips around it.
4. WHILE BREATHING IN DEEPLY AND SLOWLY THROUGH THE MOUTH, FULLY DEPRESS THE TOP OF THE METAL CANISTER with your index finger (see Figure 2).
5. HOLD YOUR BREATH AS LONG AS POSSIBLE, up to 10 seconds. Before breathing out, remove the inhaler from your mouth and release your finger from the canister.
6. If your physician has prescribed additional puffs, wait 1 minute, shake the inhaler again, and repeat steps 3 through 5. Replace the cap after use.
7. KEEPING THE PLASTIC MOUTHPIECE CLEAN IS EXTREMELY IMPORTANT TO PREVENT MEDICATION BUILDUP AND BLOCKAGE. THE MOUTHPIECE SHOULD BE WASHED, SHAKEN TO REMOVE EXCESS WATER, AND AIR DRIED THOROUGHLY AT LEAST ONCE A WEEK. INHALER MAY STOP SPRAYING IF NOT PROPERLY CLEANED.

Routine cleaning instructions:

Step 1. To clean, remove the canister and mouthpiece cap. Wash the mouthpiece through the top and bottom with warm running water for 30 seconds at least once a week (see Figure A). **Never immerse the metal canister in water.**

Figure A

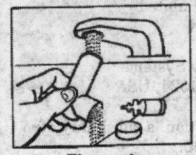

Wash mouthpiece under warm running water.

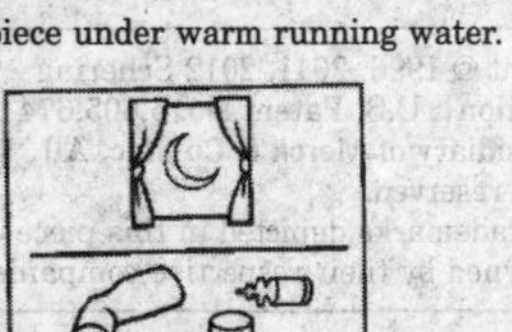

Figure B

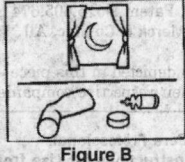

Allow mouthpiece to air dry, such as overnight.

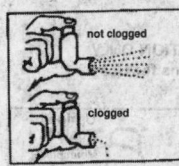

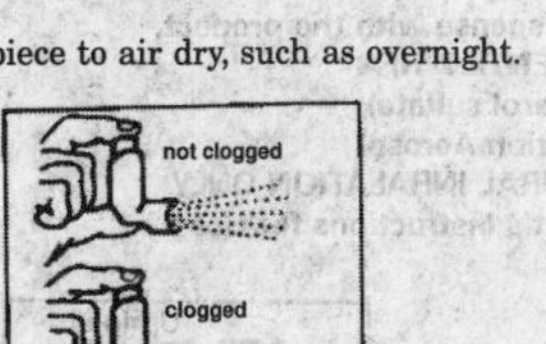

Figure C

When blocked, little or no medicine comes out.

Step 2. To dry, shake off excess water and let the mouthpiece air dry thoroughly, such as overnight (see Figure B). When the mouthpiece is dry, replace the canister and the mouthpiece cap. Blockage from medication buildup is more likely to occur if the mouthpiece is not allowed to air dry thoroughly.

IF YOUR INHALER HAS BECOME BLOCKED (little or no medication coming out of the mouthpiece, see Figure C), wash the mouthpiece as described in Step 1 and air dry thoroughly as described in Step 2.

IF YOU NEED TO USE YOUR INHALER BEFORE IT IS COMPLETELY DRY, SHAKE OFF EXCESS WATER, replace the canister, and test spray twice into the air, away from your face, to remove most of the water remaining in the mouthpiece. Then take your dose as prescribed. **After such use, rewash and air dry thoroughly as described in Steps 1 and 2.**

8. The correct amount of medication in each inhalation cannot be assured after 200 actuations, even though the canister is not completely empty. The canister should be discarded when the labeled number of actuations have been used. Before you reach the specific number of actuations, you should consult your physician to determine whether a refill is needed. Just as you should not take extra doses without consulting your physician, you also should not stop using PROVENTIL HFA Inhalation Aerosol without consulting your physician.

You may notice a slightly different taste or spray force than you are used to with PROVENTIL HFA Inhalation Aerosol, compared to other albuterol inhalation aerosol products.

DOSAGE:

Use only as directed by your physician.

WARNINGS:

The action of PROVENTIL® HFA Inhalation Aerosol should last up to 4 to 6 hours. PROVENTIL HFA Inhalation Aerosol should not be used more frequently than recommended. Do not increase the number of puffs or frequency of doses of PROVENTIL HFA Inhalation Aerosol without consulting your physician. If you find that treatment with PROVENTIL HFA Inhalation Aerosol becomes less effective for symptomatic relief, your symptoms become worse, and/or you need to use the product more frequently than usual, medical attention should be sought immediately. While you are taking PROVENTIL HFA Inhalation Aerosol, other inhaled drugs should be taken only as directed by your physician. If you are pregnant or nursing, contact your physician about the use of PROVENTIL HFA Inhalation Aerosol.

Common adverse effects of treatment with PROVENTIL HFA Inhalation Aerosol include palpitations, chest pain, rapid heart rate, tremor, or nervousness. Effective and safe use of PROVENTIL HFA Inhalation Aerosol includes an understanding of the way that it should be administered. Use PROVENTIL HFA Inhalation Aerosol only with the yellow actuator supplied with the product. The PROVENTIL HFA Inhalation Aerosol actuator should not be used with other aerosol medications.

For best results, use at room temperature. Avoid exposing product to extreme heat and cold.

Shake well before use.

Contents Under Pressure.

Do not puncture. Do not store near heat or open flame. Exposure to temperatures above 120°F may cause bursting. Never throw container into fire or incinerator. Store between 15° - 25°C (59° - 77°F). Avoid spraying in eyes. Keep out of reach of children.

Further Information: Your PROVENTIL® HFA (albuterol sulfate) Inhalation Aerosol does not contain chlorofluorocarbons (CFCs) as the propellant. Instead, the inhaler contains a hydrofluoroalkane (HFA-134a) as the propellant.

Developed and Manufactured by:
3M Health Care Limited
Loughborough UK
or
3M Drug Delivery Systems
Northridge, CA 91324, USA
Distributed by:
Schering Corporation, a subsidiary of
MERCK & CO., INC.
Whitehouse Station, NJ 08889, USA

Rev. 06/12 658000

U.S. Patent No. 5,605,674.

REBETOL® ℞

[rē' bə-tōl]
(ribavirin, USP)
Capsules, Oral Solution

HIGHLIGHTS OF PRESCRIBING INFORMATION

These highlights do not include all the information needed to use REBETOL safely and effectively. See full prescribing information for REBETOL.

REBETOL® (ribavirin USP) Capsules, Oral Solution
Initial U.S. Approval: 1998

WARNING: RISK OF SERIOUS DISORDERS AND RIBAVIRIN-ASSOCIATED EFFECTS

See full prescribing information for complete boxed warning.

- **REBETOL monotherapy is not effective for the treatment of chronic hepatitis C (5.10).**
- **The hemolytic anemia associated with REBETOL therapy may result in worsening of cardiac disease that has led to fatal and nonfatal myocardial infarctions. Patients with a history of significant or unstable cardiac disease should not be treated with REBETOL (2.4, 5.2, 6.1).**
- **Significant teratogenic and embryocidal effects have been demonstrated in all animal species exposed to ribavirin. Therefore, REBETOL therapy is contraindicated in women who are pregnant and in the male partners of women who are pregnant. Extreme care must be taken to avoid pregnancy during therapy and for 6 months after completion of treatment in both female patients and in female partners of male patients who are taking REBETOL therapy (4, 5.1, 8.1, 13.1, 17.2).**

RECENT MAJOR CHANGES

Dosage and Administration
REBETOL/PegIntron Combination Therapy (2.1) 05/2013
Dose Modifications (2.4) 05/2013

INDICATIONS AND USAGE

REBETOL is a nucleoside analogue indicated in combination with interferon alfa-2b (pegylated and nonpegylated) for the treatment of Chronic Hepatitis C (CHC) in patients 3 years of age or older with compensated liver disease. (1.1)

Patients with the following characteristics are less likely to benefit from re-treatment after failing a course of therapy: previous nonresponse, previous pegylated interferon treatment, significant bridging fibrosis or cirrhosis, and genotype 1 infection.

DOSAGE AND ADMINISTRATION

REBETOL is administered according to body weight. (2.1, 2.2)

Dose reduction or discontinuation is recommended in patients experiencing certain adverse reactions or renal dysfunction. (2.4, 2.5, 12.3)

DOSAGE FORMS AND STRENGTHS

REBETOL Capsules 200 mg (3)
REBETOL Oral Solution 40 mg per mL (3)

CONTRAINDICATIONS

- Pregnant women and men whose female partners are pregnant (4, 8.1)
- Known hypersensitivity reactions such as Stevens-Johnson syndrome, toxic, epidermal necrolysis, and erythema multiforme to ribavirin or any component of the product (4)
- Autoimmune hepatitis (4)
- Hemoglobinopathies (4)
- Creatinine clearance less than 50 mL/min (4)
- Coadministration with didanosine (4, 7.1)

WARNINGS AND PRECAUTIONS

- *Pregnancy Category X* (5.1, 8.1, 8.3)
  - Birth defects and fetal death with ribavirin: Patients must have a negative pregnancy test prior to therapy; use at least 2 forms of contraception and undergo monthly pregnancy tests.

Patients exhibiting the following conditions should be closely monitored and may require dose reduction or discontinuation of therapy:

- Monotherapy with ribavirin is not permitted. (5.10)
- Hemolytic anemia may occur with a significant initial drop in hemoglobin. (5.2)
- Pancreatitis. (5.3)
- Pulmonary infiltrates or pulmonary function impairment. (5.4)
- New or worsening ophthalmologic disorders. (5.5)
- Severe decreases in neutrophil and platelet counts, and hematologic, endocrine (e.g., TSH), and hepatic abnormalities. (5.6)
- Dental/periodontal disorders reported with combination therapy. (5.7)
- Concomitant administration of azathioprine. (5.8)
- Weight loss and growth inhibition reported with combination therapy in pediatric patients. (5.9)

ADVERSE REACTIONS

Hemolytic anemia. (6.1)

Most common adverse reactions (approximately 40%) in adult patients receiving REBETOL/PegIntron or INTRON A combination therapy are injection site reaction, fatigue/asthenia, headache, rigors, fevers, nausea, myalgia and anxiety/emotional lability/irritability. (6.1, 6.2) Most common adverse reactions (greater than 25%) in pediatric patients receiving REBETOL/PegIntron therapy are: pyrexia, headache, neutropenia, fatigue, anorexia, injection site erythema, and vomiting. (6.1)

To report SUSPECTED ADVERSE REACTIONS, contact Merck Sharp & Dohme Corp., a subsidiary of Merck & Co. Inc. at 1-877-888-4231 or FDA at 1-800-FDA-1088 or *www.fda.gov/medwatch*.

DRUG INTERACTIONS

Nucleoside analogues: Closely monitor for toxicities. Discontinue nucleoside reverse transcriptase inhibitors or reduce dose or discontinue interferon, ribavirin or both with worsening toxicities. (7.2)

USE IN SPECIFIC POPULATIONS

- Nursing mothers: Potential adverse reactions from the drug in nursing infants. (8.1, 8.3)
- Pediatrics: Safety and efficacy in patients less than 3 years old have not been established. (8.4)
- Organ transplant recipients: Safety and efficacy not studied. (8.6)
- Co-infected Patients: Safety and efficacy with HIV or HBV co-infection have not been established. (8.7)

See 17 for PATIENT COUNSELING INFORMATION and Medication Guide

Revised: 05/2013

FULL PRESCRIBING INFORMATION: CONTENTS*

*** Sections or subsections omitted from the full prescribing information are not listed**

FULL PRESCRIBING INFORMATION

WARNING: RISK OF SERIOUS DISORDERS AND RIBAVIRIN-ASSOCIATED EFFECTS

- **REBETOL monotherapy is not effective for the treatment of chronic hepatitis C virus infection and should not be used alone for this indication *[see Warnings and Precautions (5.10)]*.**
- **The primary toxicity of ribavirin is hemolytic anemia. The anemia associated with REBETOL therapy may result in worsening of cardiac disease that has led to fatal and nonfatal myocardial infarctions. Patients with a history of significant or unstable cardiac disease should not be treated with REBETOL *[see Dosage and Administration (2.4), Warnings and Precautions (5.2), and Adverse Reactions (6.1)]*.**
- **Significant teratogenic and embryocidal effects have been demonstrated in all animal species exposed to ribavirin. In addition, ribavirin has a multiple-dose half-life of 12 days, and so it may persist in nonplasma compartments for as long as 6 months. Therefore, REBETOL therapy is contraindicated in women who are pregnant and in the male partners of women who are pregnant. Extreme care must be taken to avoid pregnancy during therapy and for 6 months after completion of treatment in both female patients and in female partners of male patients who are taking REBETOL therapy. At least two reliable forms of effective contraception must be utilized during treatment and during the 6-month post-treatment follow-up period *[see Contraindications (4), Warnings and Precautions (5.1), Use in Specific Populations (8.1), Nonclinical Toxicology (13.1), and Patient Counseling Information (17.2)]*.**

1 INDICATIONS AND USAGE

1.1 Chronic Hepatitis C (CHC)

REBOTOL® (ribavirin) in combination with interferon alfa-2b (pegylated and nonpegylated) is indicated for the treatment of Chronic Hepatitis C (CHC) in patients 3 years of age and older with compensated liver disease *[see Warnings and Precautions (5.9, 5.10), and Use in Specific Populations (8.4)]*.

The following points should be considered when initiating REBETOL combination therapy with PegIntron® or INTRON A®:

- These indications are based on achieving undetectable HCV-RNA after treatment for 24 or 48 weeks and maintaining a Sustained Virologic Response (SVR) 24 weeks after the last dose.
- Combination therapy with REBETOL/PegIntron is preferred over REBETOL/INTRON A as this combination provides substantially better response rates *[see Clinical Studies (14)]*.
- Patients with the following characteristics are less likely to benefit from re-treatment after failing a course of therapy: previous nonresponse, previous pegylated interferon treatment, significant bridging fibrosis or cirrhosis, and genotype 1 infection *[see Clinical Studies (14)]*.
- No safety and efficacy data are available for treatment of longer than one year.

2 DOSAGE AND ADMINISTRATION

Under no circumstances should REBETOL capsules be opened, crushed, or broken. REBETOL should be taken with food *[see Clinical Pharmacology (12.3)]*. REBETOL should not be used in patients with creatinine clearance less than 50 mL/min.

2.1 REBETOL/PegIntron Combination Therapy

Adult Patients

The recommended dose of PegIntron is 1.5 mcg/kg/week subcutaneously in combination with 800 to 1400 mg REBETOL capsules orally based on patient body weight (see **Table 1**). The volume of PegIntron to be injected depends on the strength of PegIntron and patient's body weight, refer to labeling for PegIntron for additional dosing information.

Duration of Treatment – Interferon Alpha-naïve Patients

The treatment duration for patients with genotype 1 is 48 weeks. Discontinuation of therapy should be considered in patients who do not achieve at least a 2 $\log_{10}$ drop or loss of HCV-RNA at 12 weeks, or if HCV-RNA remains detectable after 24 weeks of therapy. Patients with genotype 2 and 3 should be treated for 24 weeks.

Duration of Treatment – Re-treatment with PegIntron/REBETOL of Prior Treatment Failures

The treatment duration for patients who previously failed therapy is 48 weeks, regardless of HCV genotype. Re-treated patients who fail to achieve undetectable HCV-RNA at Week 12 of therapy, or whose HCV-RNA remains detectable after 24 weeks of therapy, are highly unlikely to achieve SVR and discontinuation of therapy should be considered *[see Clinical Studies (14.1)]*.

Table 1: Recommended Dosing for REBETOL in Combination Therapy with PegIntron (Adults)

Body Weight kg (lbs)	REBETOL Daily Dose	REBETOL Number of Capsules
<66 (<144)	800 mg/day	2 × 200-mg capsules A.M. 2 × 200-mg capsules P.M.
66-80 (145-177)	1000 mg/day	2 × 200-mg capsules A.M. 3 × 200-mg capsules P.M.
81-105 (178-231)	1200 mg/day	3 × 200-mg capsules A.M. 3 × 200-mg capsules P.M.
>105 (231)	1400 mg/day	3 × 200-mg capsules A.M. 4 × 200-mg capsules P.M.

Pediatric Patients

Dosing for pediatric patients is determined by body surface area for PegIntron and by body weight for REBETOL. The recommended dose of PegIntron is 60 mcg/m^2/week subcutaneously in combination with 15 mg/kg/day of REBETOL orally in two divided doses (see **Table 2**) for pediatric patients ages 3-17 years. Patients who reach their 18th birthday while receiving PegIntron/REBETOL should remain on the pediatric dosing regimen. The treatment duration for patients with genotype 1 is 48 weeks. Patients with genotype 2 and 3 should be treated for 24 weeks.

Table 2: Recommended REBETOL* Dosing in Combination Therapy (Pediatrics)

Body Weight kg (lbs)	REBETOL Daily Dose	REBETOL Number of Capsules
<47 (<103)	15 mg/kg/day	Use REBETOL Oral Solution†
47-59 (103-131)	800 mg/day	2 × 200-mg capsules A.M. 2 × 200-mg capsules P.M.
60-73 (132-162)	1000 mg/day	2 × 200-mg capsules A.M. 3 × 200-mg capsules P.M.
>73 (>162)	1200 mg/day	3 × 200-mg capsules A.M. 3 × 200-mg capsules P.M.

* REBETOL to be used in combination with PegIntron 60 mcg/m^2 weekly.

† REBETOL Oral Solution may be used for any patient regardless of body weight.

2.2 REBETOL/INTRON A Combination Therapy

Adults

Duration of Treatment – Interferon Alpha-naïve Patients

The recommended dose of INTRON A is 3 million IU three times weekly subcutaneously. The recommended dose of REBETOL capsules depends on the patient's body weight (refer to **Table 3**). The recommended duration of treatment for patients previously untreated with interferon is 24 to 48 weeks. The duration of treatment should be individualized to the patient depending on baseline disease characteristics, response to therapy, and tolerability of the regimen *[see Indications and Usage (1.1), Adverse Reactions (6.1), and Clinical Studies (14)]*. After 24 weeks of treatment, virologic response should be assessed. Treatment discontinuation should be considered in any patient who has not achieved an HCV-RNA below the limit of detection of the assay by 24 weeks. There are no safety and efficacy data on treatment for longer than 48 weeks in the previously untreated patient population.

Duration of Treatment – Re-treatment with INTRON A/REBETOL in Relapse Patients

In patients who relapse following nonpegylated interferon monotherapy, the recommended duration of treatment is 24 weeks.

Table 3: Recommended Dosing

Body Weight	REBETOL Capsules
≤75 kg	2 × 200-mg capsules AM 3 × 200-mg capsules PM daily orally
>75 kg	3 × 200-mg capsules AM 3 × 200-mg capsules PM daily orally

Pediatrics

The recommended dose of REBETOL is 15 mg/kg per day orally (divided dose AM and PM). Refer to **Table 2** for Pediatric Dosing of REBETOL in combination with INTRON A. INTRON A for Injection by body weight of 25 kg to 61 kg is 3 million IU/m^2 three times weekly subcutaneously. Refer to adult dosing table for greater than 61 kg body weight.

The recommended duration of treatment is 48 weeks for pediatric patients with genotype 1. After 24 weeks of treatment, virologic response should be assessed. Treatment discontinuation should be considered in any patient who has not achieved an HCV-RNA below the limit of detection of the assay by this time. The recommended duration of treatment for pediatric patients with genotype 2/3 is 24 weeks.

2.3 Laboratory Tests

The following laboratory tests are recommended for all patients treated with REBETOL, prior to beginning treatment and then periodically thereafter.

- Standard hematologic tests - including hemoglobin (pretreatment, Week 2 and Week 4 of therapy, and as clinically appropriate *[see Warnings and Precautions (5.2, 5.7)]*, complete and differential white blood cell counts, and platelet count.
- Blood chemistries - liver function tests and TSH.
- Pregnancy - including monthly monitoring for women of childbearing potential.
- ECG *[see Warnings and Precautions (5.2)]*.

2.4 Dose Modifications

If severe adverse reactions or laboratory abnormalities develop during combination REBETOL/INTRON A therapy or REBETOL/PegIntron therapy, modify, or discontinue the dose until the adverse reaction abates or decreases in severity *[see Warnings and Precautions (5)]*. If intolerance persists after dose adjustment, combination therapy should be discontinued. Dose reduction of PegIntron in adult patients on REBETOL/PegIntron combination therapy is accomplished in a two-step process from the original starting dose of 1.5 mcg/kg/week, to 1 mcg/kg/week, then to 0.5 mcg/kg/week, if needed. Refer to labeling for PegIntron for additional information regarding dose reduction of PegIntron.

In the adult combination therapy Study 2, dose reductions occurred in 42% of subjects receiving PegIntron 1.5 mcg/kg and REBETOL 800 mg daily, including 57% of those subjects weighing 60 kg or less. In Study 4, 16% of subjects had a dose reduction of PegIntron to 1 mcg/kg in combination with REBETOL, with an additional 4% requiring the second dose reduction of PegIntron to 0.5 mcg/kg due to adverse events *[see Adverse Reactions (6.1)]*.

Dose reduction in pediatric patients is accomplished by modifying the recommended PegIntron dose in a two-step process from the original starting dose of 60 mcg/m^2/week, to 40 mcg/m^2/week, then to 20 mcg/m^2/week, if needed (see **Table 4**). In the pediatric combination therapy trial, dose reductions occurred in 25% of subjects receiving PegIntron 60 mcg/m^2 weekly and REBETOL 15 mg/kg daily. Dose reduction in pediatric patients is accomplished by modifying the recommended REBETOL dose from the original starting dose of 15 mg/kg daily in a two-step process to 12 mg/kg/day, then to 8 mg/kg/day, if needed (see **Table 4**).

REBETOL should not be used in patients with creatinine clearance less than 50 mL/min. Patients with impaired renal function and those over the age of 50 should be carefully monitored with respect to development of anemia *[see Warnings and Precautions (5.2), Use in Specific Populations (8.5), and Clinical Pharmacology (12.3)]*.

REBETOL should be administered with caution to patients with pre-existing cardiac disease. Patients should be assessed before commencement of therapy and should be appropriately monitored during therapy. If there is any deterioration of cardiovascular status, therapy should be stopped *[see Warnings and Precautions (5.2)]*.

For patients with a history of stable cardiovascular disease, a permanent dose reduction is required if the hemoglobin decreases by greater than or equal to 2 g/dL during any 4-week period. In addition, for these cardiac history patients, if the hemoglobin remains less than 12 g/dL after 4 weeks on a reduced dose, the patient should discontinue combination therapy.

It is recommended that a patient whose hemoglobin level falls below 10 g/dL have his/her REBETOL dose modified or discontinued per **Table 4** *[see Warnings and Precautions (5.2)]*.

[See table 4 below]

Refer to labeling for INTRON A or PegIntron for additional information about how to reduce an INTRON A or PegIntron dose.

Table 4: Guidelines for Dose Modification and Discontinuation of REBETOL in combination with PegIntron or INTRON A Based on Laboratory Parameters in Adults and Pediatrics

Laboratory Parameters	Reduce REBETOL Daily Dose (see note 1) if:	Reduce PegIntron or INTRON A Dose (see note 2) if:	Discontinue Therapy if:
WBC	N/A	1.0 to <1.5 × 10^9/L	<1.0 × 10^9/L
Neutrophils	N/A	0.5 to <0.75 × 10^9/L	<0.5 × 10^9/L
Platelets	N/A	25 to < 50 × 10^9/L (adults)	<25 × 10^9/L (adults)
	N/A	50 to <70 × 10^9/L (pediatrics)	<50 × 10^9/L (pediatrics)
Creatinine	N/A	N/A	>2 mg/dL (pediatrics)
Hemoglobin in patients without history of cardiac disease	8.5 to <10 g/dL	N/A	<8.5 g/dL
	Reduce REBETOL Dose by 200 mg/day and PegIntron or INTRON A Dose by Half if:		
Hemoglobin in patients with history of stable cardiac disease*†	≥2 g/dL decrease in hemoglobin during any four week period during treatment		<8.5 g/dL or <12 g/dL after four weeks of dose reduction

Note 1: *Adult patients: 1st dose reduction of ribavirin is by 200 mg/day (except in patients receiving the 1,400 mg, dose reduction should be by 400 mg/day). If needed, 2nd dose reduction of ribavirin is by an additional 200 mg/day. Patients whose dose of ribavirin is reduced to 600 mg daily receive one 200 mg capsule in the morning and two 200 mg capsules in the evening.*

Pediatric patients: 1st dose reduction of ribavirin is to 12 mg/kg/day, 2nd dose reduction of ribavirin is to 8 mg/kg/day.

Note 2: *Adult patients treated with REBETOL and PegIntron: 1st dose reduction of PegIntron is to 1 mcg/kg/week. If needed, 2nd dose reduction of PegIntron is to 0.5 mcg/kg/week.*

Pediatric patients treated with REBETOL and PegIntron: 1st dose reduction of PegIntron is to 40 mcg/m^2/week, 2nd dose reduction of PegIntron is to 20 mcg/m^2/week.

For patients on REBETOL/INTRON A combination therapy: reduce INTRON A dose by 50%.

* Pediatric patients who have pre-existing cardiac conditions and experience a hemoglobin decrease greater than or equal to 2 g/dL during any 4-week period during treatment should have weekly evaluations and hematology testing.

† These guidelines are for patients with stable cardiac disease. Patients with a history of significant or unstable cardiac disease should not be treated with PegIntron /REBETOL combination therapy *[see Warnings and Precautions (5.2)]*.

2.5 Discontinuation of Dosing

Adults In HCV genotype 1, interferon-alfa-naïve patients receiving PegIntron in combination with ribavirin, discontinuation of therapy is recommended if there is not at least a 2 log$_{10}$ drop or loss of HCV-RNA at 12 weeks of therapy, or if HCV-RNA levels remain detectable after 24 weeks of therapy. Regardless of genotype, previously treated patients who have detectable HCV-RNA at Week 12 or 24 are highly unlikely to achieve SVR and discontinuation of therapy should be considered.

Pediatrics (3-17 years of age) It is recommended that patients receiving PegIntron/REBETOL combination (excluding HCV Genotype 2 and 3) be discontinued from therapy at 12 weeks if their treatment Week 12 HCV-RNA dropped less than 2 log$_{10}$ compared to a pretreatment or at 24 weeks if they have detectable HCV-RNA at treatment Week 24.

3 DOSAGE FORMS AND STRENGTHS

REBETOL Capsules 200 mg

REBETOL Oral Solution 40 mg per mL

4 CONTRAINDICATIONS

REBETOL combination therapy is contraindicated in:

- women who are pregnant. REBETOL may cause fetal harm when administered to a pregnant woman. REBETOL is contraindicated in women who are or may become pregnant. If REBETOL is used during pregnancy, or if the patient becomes pregnant while taking REBETOL, the patient should be apprised of the potential hazard to her fetus *[see Warnings and Precautions (5.1), Use in Specific Populations (8.1), and Patient Counseling Information (17.2)]*
- men whose female partners are pregnant
- patients with known hypersensitivity reactions such as Stevens-Johnson syndrome, toxic, epidermal necrolysis, and erythema multiforme to ribavirin or any component of the product
- patients with autoimmune hepatitis
- patients with hemoglobinopathies (e.g., thalassemia major, sickle-cell anemia)
- patients with creatinine clearance less than 50 mL/min. *[see Use in Specific Populations (8.5) and Clinical Pharmacology (12.3)]*
- Coadministration of REBETOL and didanosine is contraindicated because exposure to the active metabolite of didanosine (dideoxyadenosine 5'-triphosphate) is increased. Fatal hepatic failure, as well as peripheral neuropathy, pancreatitis, and symptomatic hyperlactatemia/lactic acidosis have been reported in patients receiving didanosine in combination with ribavirin *[see Drug Interactions (7.1)]*.

5 WARNINGS AND PRECAUTIONS

5.1 Pregnancy

REBETOL capsules and oral solution may cause birth defects and death of the unborn child. REBETOL therapy should not be started until a report of a negative pregnancy test has been obtained immediately prior to planned initiation of therapy. Patients should use at least two forms of contraception and have monthly pregnancy tests during treatment and during the 6-month period after treatment has been stopped. Extreme care must be taken to avoid pregnancy in female patients and in female partners of male patients. REBETOL has demonstrated significant teratogenic and embryocidal effects in all animal species in which adequate studies have been conducted. These effects occurred at doses as low as one twentieth of the recommended human dose of ribavirin. REBETOL therapy should not be started until a report of a negative pregnancy test has been obtained immediately prior to planned initiation of therapy *[see Boxed Warning, Contraindications (4), Use in Specific Populations (8.1), and Patient Counseling Information (17.2)]*.

5.2 Anemia

The primary toxicity of ribavirin is hemolytic anemia, which was observed in approximately 10% of REBETOL/INTRON A-treated subjects in clinical trials. The anemia associated with REBETOL capsules occurs within 1 to 2 weeks of initiation of therapy. Because the initial drop in hemoglobin may be significant, it is advised that hemoglobin or hematocrit be obtained before the start of treatment and at Week 2 and Week 4 of therapy, or more frequently if clinically indicated. Patients should then be followed as clinically appropriate *[see Dosage and Administration (2.4, 2.5)]*.

Fatal and nonfatal myocardial infarctions have been reported in patients with anemia caused by REBETOL. Patients should be assessed for underlying cardiac disease before initiation of ribavirin therapy. Patients with preexisting cardiac disease should have electrocardiograms administered before treatment, and should be appropriately monitored during therapy. If there is any deterioration of cardiovascular status, therapy should be suspended or discontinued *[see Dosage and Administration (2.4, 2.5)]*. Because cardiac disease may be worsened by drug-induced anemia, patients with a history of significant or unstable cardiac disease should not use REBETOL.

5.3 Pancreatitis
REBETOL and INTRON A or PegIntron therapy should be suspended in patients with signs and symptoms of pancreatitis and discontinued in patients with confirmed pancreatitis.

5.4 Pulmonary Disorders
Pulmonary symptoms, including dyspnea, pulmonary infiltrates, pneumonitis, pulmonary hypertension, and pneumonia, have been reported during therapy with REBETOL with alpha interferon combination therapy; occasional cases of fatal pneumonia have occurred. In addition, sarcoidosis or the exacerbation of sarcoidosis has been reported. If there is evidence of pulmonary infiltrates or pulmonary function impairment, the patient should be closely monitored, and if appropriate, combination therapy should be discontinued.

5.5 Ophthalmologic Disorders
Ribavirin is used in combination therapy with alpha interferons. Decrease or loss of vision, retinopathy including macular edema, retinal artery or vein, thrombosis, retinal hemorrhages and cotton wool spots, optic neuritis, papilledema, and serous retinal detachment are induced or aggravated by treatment with alpha interferons. All patients should receive an eye examination at baseline. Patients with pre-existing ophthalmologic disorders (e.g., diabetic or hypertensive retinopathy) should receive periodic ophthalmologic exams during combination therapy with alpha interferon treatment. Any patient who develops ocular symptoms should receive a prompt and complete eye examination. Combination therapy with alpha interferons should be discontinued in patients who develop new or worsening ophthalmologic disorders.

5.6 Laboratory Tests
PegIntron in combination with ribavirin may cause severe decreases in neutrophil and platelet counts, and hematologic, endocrine (e.g., TSH), and hepatic abnormalities.
Patients on PegIntron/REBETOL combination therapy should have hematology and blood chemistry testing before the start of treatment and then periodically thereafter. In the adult clinical trial, complete blood counts (including hemoglobin, neutrophil, and platelet counts) and chemistries (including AST, ALT, bilirubin, and uric acid) were measured during the treatment period at Weeks 2, 4, 8, 12, and then at 6-week intervals, or more frequently if abnormalities developed. In pediatric subjects, the same laboratory parameters were evaluated with additional assessment of hemoglobin at treatment Week 6. TSH levels were measured every 12 weeks during the treatment period. HCV-RNA should be measured periodically during treatment *[see Dosage and Administration (2)]*.

5.7 Dental and Periodontal Disorders
Dental and periodontal disorders have been reported in patients receiving ribavirin and interferon or peginterferon combination therapy. In addition, dry mouth could have a damaging effect on teeth and mucous membranes of the mouth during long-term treatment with the combination of REBETOL and pegylated or nonpegylated interferon alfa-2b. Patients should brush their teeth thoroughly twice daily and have regular dental examinations. If vomiting occurs, they should be advised to rinse out their mouth thoroughly afterwards.

5.8 Concomitant Administration of Azathioprine
Pancytopenia (marked decreases in red blood cells, neutrophils, and platelets) and bone marrow suppression have been reported in the literature to occur within 3 to 7 weeks after the concomitant administration of pegylated interferon/ribavirin and azathioprine. In this limited number of patients (n=8), myelotoxicity was reversible within 4 to 6 weeks upon withdrawal of both HCV antiviral therapy and concomitant azathioprine and did not recur upon reintroduction of either treatment alone. PegIntron, REBETOL, and azathioprine should be discontinued for pancytopenia, and pegylated interferon/ribavirin should not be reintroduced with concomitant azathioprine *[see Drug Interactions (7.4)]*.

5.9 Impact on Growth - Pediatric Use
Data on the effects of PegIntron and REBETOL on growth come from an open-label study in subjects 3 through 17 years of age, and weight and height changes are compared to US normative population data. In general, the weight and height gain of pediatric subjects treated with PegIntron and REBETOL lags behind that predicted by normative population data for the entire length of treatment. After about 6 months post-treatment (follow-up Week 24), subjects had weight gain rebounds and regained their weight to 53rd percentile, above the average of the normative population and similar to that predicted by their average baseline weight (57th percentile). After about 6 months post-treatment, height gain stabilized and subjects treated with PegIntron and REBETOL had an average height percentile of 44th percentile, which was less than the average of the normative population and less than their average baseline height (51st percentile). Severely inhibited growth velocity (less than 3rd percentile) was observed in 70% of the subjects while on treatment. Of the subjects experiencing severely inhibited growth, 20% had continued inhibited growth velocity (less than 3rd percentile) after 6 months of follow-up.

Table 5: Adverse Reactions Occurring in Greater Than 5% of Adult Subjects

Adverse Reactions	Percentage of Subjects Reporting Adverse Reactions*: PegIntron 1.5 mcg/kg/ REBETOL (N=511)	INTRON A/ REBETOL (N=505)
Application Site		
Injection Site Inflammation	25	18
Injection Site Reaction	58	36
Autonomic Nervous System		
Dry Mouth	12	8
Increased Sweating	11	7
Flushing	4	3
Body as a Whole		
Fatigue/Asthenia	66	63
Headache	62	58
Rigors	48	41
Fever	46	33
Weight Loss	29	20
Right Upper Quadrant Pain	12	6
Chest Pain	8	7
Malaise	4	6
Central/Peripheral Nervous System		
Dizziness	21	17
Endocrine		
Hypothyroidism	5	4
Gastrointestinal		
Nausea	43	33
Anorexia	32	27
Diarrhea	22	17
Vomiting	14	12
Abdominal Pain	13	13
Dyspepsia	9	8
Constipation	5	5
Hematologic Disorders		
Neutropenia	26	14
Anemia	12	17
Leukopenia	6	5
Thrombocytopenia	5	2
Liver and Biliary System		
Hepatomegaly	4	4
Musculoskeletal		
Myalgia	56	50
Arthralgia	34	28
Musculoskeletal Pain	21	19
Psychiatric		
Insomnia	40	41
Depression	31	34
Anxiety/Emotional Lability/Irritability	47	47
Concentration Impaired	17	21
Agitation	8	5
Nervousness	6	6
Reproductive, Female		
Menstrual Disorder	7	6
Resistance Mechanism		
Viral Infection	12	12
Fungal Infection	6	1
Respiratory System		
Dyspnea	26	24
Coughing	23	16
Pharyngitis	12	13
Rhinitis	8	6
Sinusitis	6	5
Skin and Appendages		
Alopecia	36	32
Pruritus	29	28
Rash	24	23
Skin Dry	24	23
Special Senses, Other		
Taste Perversion	9	4
Vision Disorders		
Vision Blurred	5	6
Conjunctivitis	4	5

* A subject may have reported more than one adverse reaction within a body system/organ class category.

Among the boys studied, the age groups of 3-11 years old and 12-17 years old had similar height percentile decreases of approximately 5 percentiles after 6 months post-treatment; weight gain continued to be similar to their average baseline percentile. Girls who were 3-11 years old and treated for 48 weeks had the largest average drop in height and weight percentiles (13 percentiles and 7 percentiles, respectively), whereas girls 12-17 years old continued along their average baseline height and weight percentiles after 6 months post-treatment.

Table 6: Treatment-Related Adverse Reactions (Greater Than or Equal to 10% Incidence) By Descending Frequency

Adverse Reactions	Study 4 *Percentage of Subjects Reporting Treatment-Related Adverse Reactions* PegIntron 1.5 mcg/kg with REBETOL (N=1019)	PegIntron 1 mcg/kg with REBETOL (N=1016)	Pegasys 180 mcg with Copegus (N=1035)
Fatigue	67	68	64
Headache	50	47	41
Nausea	40	35	34
Chills	39	36	23
Insomnia	38	37	41
Anemia	35	30	34
Pyrexia	35	32	21
Injection Site Reactions	34	35	23
Anorexia	29	25	21
Rash	29	25	34
Myalgia	27	26	22
Neutropenia	26	19	31
Irritability	25	25	25
Depression	25	19	20
Alopecia	23	20	17
Dyspnea	21	20	22
Arthralgia	21	22	22
Pruritus	18	15	19
Influenza-like Illness	16	15	15
Dizziness	16	14	13
Diarrhea	15	16	14
Cough	15	16	17
Weight Decreased	13	10	10
Vomiting	12	10	9
Unspecified Pain	12	13	9
Dry Skin	11	11	12
Anxiety	11	11	10
Abdominal Pain	10	10	10
Leukopenia	9	7	10

5.10 Usage Safeguards

Based on results of clinical trials, ribavirin monotherapy is not effective for the treatment of chronic hepatitis C virus infection; therefore, REBETOL capsules or oral solution must not be used alone. The safety and efficacy of REBETOL capsules and oral solution have only been established when used together with INTRON A or PegIntron (not other interferons) as combination therapy.

The safety and efficacy of REBETOL/INTRON A and PegIntron therapy for the treatment of HIV infection, adenovirus, RSV, parainfluenza, or influenza infections have not been established. REBETOL capsules should not be used for these indications. Ribavirin for inhalation has separate labeling, which should be consulted if ribavirin inhalation therapy is being considered.

There are significant adverse reactions caused by REBETOL/INTRON A or PegIntron therapy, including severe depression and suicidal ideation, hemolytic anemia, suppression of bone marrow function, autoimmune and infectious disorders, pulmonary dysfunction, pancreatitis, and diabetes. Suicidal ideation or attempts occurred more frequently among pediatric patients, primarily adolescents, compared to adult patients (2.4% versus 1%) during treatment and off-therapy follow-up. Labeling for INTRON A and PegIntron should be reviewed in their entirety for additional safety information prior to initiation of combination treatment.

6 ADVERSE REACTIONS

Clinical trials with REBETOL in combination with PegIntron or INTRON A have been conducted in over 7800 subjects from 3 to 76 years of age.

The primary toxicity of ribavirin is hemolytic anemia. Reductions in hemoglobin levels occurred within the first 1 to 2 weeks of oral therapy. Cardiac and pulmonary reactions associated with anemia occurred in approximately 10% of patients *[see Warnings and Precautions (5.2)]*.

Greater than 96% of all subjects in clinical trials experienced one or more adverse reactions. The most commonly reported adverse reactions in adult subjects receiving PegIntron or INTRON A in combination with REBETOL were injection site inflammation/reaction, fatigue/asthenia, headache, rigors, fevers, nausea, myalgia and anxiety/emotional lability/irritability. The most common adverse reactions in pediatric subjects, ages 3 and older, receiving REBETOL in combination with PegIntron or INTRON A were pyrexia, headache, neutropenia, fatigue, anorexia, injection site erythema, and vomiting.

The Adverse Reactions section references the following clinical trials:

- REBETOL/PegIntron Combination therapy trials:
  - Clinical Study 1 – evaluated PegIntron monotherapy (not further described in this label; see labeling for PegIntron for information about this trial).
  - Study 2 – evaluated REBETOL 800 mg/day flat dose in combination with 1.5 mcg/kg/week PegIntron or with INTRON A.
  - Study 3 – evaluated PegIntron/weight-based REBETOL in combination with PegIntron/flat dose REBETOL regimen.
  - Study 4 – compared two PegIntron (1.5 mcg/kg/week and 1 mcg/kg/week) doses in combination with REBETOL and a third treatment group receiving Pegasys® (180 mcg/week)/Copegus® (1000-1200 mg/day).
  - Study 5 – evaluated PegIntron (1.5 mcg/kg/week) in combination with weight-based REBETOL in prior treatment failure subjects.
- PegIntron/REBETOL Combination Therapy in Pediatric Patients
- REBETOL/INTRON A Combination Therapy trials for adults and pediatrics

Serious adverse reactions have occurred in approximately 12% of subjects in clinical trials with PegIntron with or without REBETOL *[see BOXED WARNING, Warnings and Precautions (5)]*. The most common serious events occurring in subjects treated with PegIntron and REBETOL were depression and suicidal ideation *[see Warnings and Precautions (5.2)]*, each occurring at a frequency of less than 1%. Suicidal ideation or attempts occurred more frequently among pediatric patients, primarily adolescents, compared to adult patients (2.4% versus 1%) during treatment and off-therapy follow-up *[see Warnings and Precautions (5.10)]*. The most common fatal reaction occurring in subjects treated with PegIntron and REBETOL was cardiac arrest, suicide ideation, and suicide attempt *[see Warnings and Precautions (5.10)]*, all occurring in less than 1% of subjects.

Because clinical trials are conducted under widely varying conditions, adverse reactions rates observed in the clinical trials of a drug cannot be directly compared to rates in the clinical trials of another drug and may not reflect the rates observed in clinical practice.

6.1 Clinical Trials Experience – REBETOL/PegIntron Combination Therapy

Adult Subjects

Adverse reactions that occurred in the clinical trial at greater than 5% incidence are provided by treatment group from the REBETOL/PegIntron Combination Therapy (Study 2) in **Table 5**.

[See table 5 at top of previous page]

Table 6 summarizes the treatment-related adverse reactions in Study 4 that occurred at a greater than or equal to 10% incidence.

[See table 6 above]

The incidence of serious adverse reactions was comparable in all trials. In Study 3, there was a similar incidence of serious adverse reactions reported for the weight-based REBETOL group (12%) and for the flat-dose REBETOL regimen. In Study 2, the incidence of serious adverse reactions was 17% in the PegIntron/REBETOL groups compared to 14% in the INTRON A/REBETOL group.

In many but not all cases, adverse reactions resolved after dose reduction or discontinuation of therapy. Some subjects experienced ongoing or new serious adverse reactions during the 6-month follow-up period. In Study 2, many subjects continued to experience adverse reactions several months after discontinuation of therapy. By the end of the 6-month follow-up period, the incidence of ongoing adverse reactions by body class in the PegIntron 1.5/REBETOL group was 33% (psychiatric), 20% (musculoskeletal), and 10% (for endocrine and for GI). In approximately 10 to 15% of subjects, weight loss, fatigue, and headache had not resolved.

There have been 31 subject deaths that occurred during treatment or during follow-up in these clinical trials. In Study 1, there was 1 suicide in a subject receiving PegIntron monotherapy and 2 deaths among subjects receiving INTRON A monotherapy (1 murder/suicide and 1 sudden death). In Study 2, there was 1 suicide in a subject receiving PegIntron/REBETOL combination therapy; and 1 subject death in the INTRON A/REBETOL group (motor vehicle accident). In Study 3, there were 14 deaths, 2 of which were probable suicides and 1 was an unexplained death in a person with a relevant medical history of depression. In Study 4, there were 12 deaths, 6 of which occurred in subjects who received PegIntron/REBETOL combination therapy, 5 in the PegIntron 1.5 mcg/REBETOL arm (N=1019) and 1 in the PegIntron 1 mcg/REBETOL arm (N=1016), and 6 of which occurred in subjects receiving Pegasys/Copegus (N=1035); there were 3 suicides that occurred during the off treatment follow-up period in subjects who received PegIntron (1.5 mcg/kg)/REBETOL combination therapy.

In Studies 1 and 2, 10 to 14% of subjects receiving PegIntron, alone or in combination with REBETOL, discontinued therapy compared with 6% treated with INTRON A alone and 13% treated with INTRON A in combination with REBETOL. Similarly in Study 3, 15% of subjects receiving

PegIntron in combination with weight-based REBETOL and 14% of subjects receiving PegIntron and flat dose REBETOL discontinued therapy due to an adverse reaction. The most common reasons for discontinuation of therapy were related to known interferon effects of psychiatric, systemic (e.g., fatigue, headache), or gastrointestinal adverse reactions. In Study 4, 13% of subjects in the PegIntron 1.5 mcg/REBETOL arm, 10% in the PegIntron 1 mcg/REBETOL arm and 13% in the Pegasys 180 mcg/Copegus arm discontinued due to adverse events.

In Study 2, dose reductions due to adverse reactions occurred in 42% of subjects receiving PegIntron (1.5 mcg/kg)/REBETOL and in 34% of those receiving INTRON A/REBETOL. The majority of subjects (57%) weighing 60 kg or less receiving PegIntron (1.5 mcg/kg)/REBETOL required dose reduction. Reduction of interferon was dose-related (PegIntron 1.5 mcg/kg greater than PegIntron 0.5 mcg/kg or INTRON A), 40%, 27%, 28%, respectively. Dose reduction for REBETOL was similar across all three groups, 33 to 35%. The most common reasons for dose modifications were neutropenia (18%), or anemia (9%) *(see **Laboratory Values**)*. Other common reasons included depression, fatigue, nausea, and thrombocytopenia. In Study 3, dose modifications due to adverse reactions occurred more frequently with weight-based dosing (WBD) compared to flat dosing (29% and 23%, respectively). In Study 4, 16% of subjects had a dose reduction of PegIntron to 1 mcg/kg in combination with REBETOL, with an additional 4% requiring the second dose reduction of PegIntron to 0.5 mcg/kg due to adverse events compared to 15% of subjects in the Pegasys/Copegus arm, who required a dose reduction to 135 mcg/week with Pegasys, with an additional 7% in the Pegasys/Copegus arm requiring second dose reduction to 90 mcg/week with Pegasys.

In the PegIntron/REBETOL combination trials the most common adverse reactions were psychiatric, which occurred among 77% of subjects in Study 2 and 68% to 69% of subjects in Study 3. These psychiatric adverse reactions included most commonly depression, irritability, and insomnia, each reported by approximately 30% to 40% of subjects in all treatment groups. Suicidal behavior (ideation, attempts, and suicides) occurred in 2% of all subjects during treatment or during follow-up after treatment cessation *[see Warnings and Precautions (5)]*. In Study 4, psychiatric adverse reactions occurred in 58% of subjects in the PegIntron 1.5 mcg/REBETOL arm, 55% of subjects in the PegIntron 1 mcg/REBETOL arm, and 57% of subjects in the Pegasys 180 mcg/Copegus arm.

PegIntron induced fatigue or headache in approximately two-thirds of subjects, with fever or rigors in approximately half of the subjects. The severity of some of these systemic symptoms (e.g., fever and headache) tended to decrease as treatment continued. In Studies 1 and 2, application site inflammation and reaction (e.g., bruise, itchiness, and irritation) occurred at approximately twice the incidence with PegIntron therapies (in up to 75% of subjects) compared with INTRON A. However, injection site pain was infrequent (2 to 3%) in all groups. In Study 3, there was a 23% to 24% incidence overall for injection site reactions or inflammation.

Subjects receiving REBETOL/PegIntron as re-treatment after failing a previous interferon combination regimen reported adverse reactions similar to those previously associated with this regimen during clinical trials of treatment-naïve subjects.

Pediatric Subjects

In general, the adverse-reaction profile in the pediatric population was similar to that observed in adults. In the pediatric trial, the most prevalent adverse reactions in all subjects were pyrexia (80%), headache (62%), neutropenia (33%), fatigue (30%), anorexia (29%), injection-site erythema (29%) and vomiting (27%). The majority of adverse reactions reported in the trial were mild or moderate in severity. Severe adverse reactions were reported in 7% (8/107) of all subjects and included injection site pain (1%), pain in extremity (1%), headache (1%), neutropenia (1%), and pyrexia (4%). Important adverse reactions that occurred in this subject population were nervousness (7%; 7/107), aggression (3%; 3/107), anger (2%; 2/107), and depression (1%; 1/107). Five subjects received levothyroxine treatment, three with clinical hypothyroidism and two with asymptomatic TSH elevations.

Dose modifications of PegIntron and/or ribavirin were required in 25% of subjects due to treatment-related adverse reactions, most commonly for anemia, neutropenia and weight loss. Two subjects (2%; 2/107) discontinued therapy as the result of an adverse reaction.

Adverse reactions that occurred with a greater than or equal to 10% incidence in the pediatric trial subjects are provided in **Table 7**.

Table 7: Percentage of Pediatric Subjects with Treatment-Related Adverse Reactions (in At Least 10% of All Subjects)

System Organ Class Preferred Term	All Subjects (N=107)
Blood and Lymphatic System Disorders	
Neutropenia	33%
Anemia	11%
Leukopenia	10%
Gastrointestinal Disorders	
Abdominal Pain	21%
Abdominal Pain Upper	12%
Vomiting	27%
Nausea	18%
General Disorders and Administration Site Conditions	
Pyrexia	80%
Fatigue	30%
Injection-site Erythema	29%
Chills	21%
Asthenia	15%
Irritability	14%
Investigations	
Weight Loss	19%
Metabolism and Nutrition Disorders	
Anorexia	29%
Decreased Appetite	22%
Musculoskeletal and Connective Tissue Disorders	
Arthralgia	17%
Myalgia	17%
Nervous System Disorders	
Headache	62%
Dizziness	14%
Skin and Subcutaneous Tissue Disorders	
Alopecia	17%

Laboratory Values

Adult and Pediatric Subjects

The adverse reaction profile in Study 3, which compared PegIntron/weight-based REBETOL combination to a PegIntron/flat dose REBETOL regimen, revealed an increased rate of anemia with weight-based dosing (29% vs. 19% for weight-based vs. flat dose regimens, respectively). However, the majority of cases of anemia were mild and responded to dose reductions.

Changes in selected laboratory values during treatment in combination with REBETOL treatment are described below. **Decreases in hemoglobin, leukocytes, neutrophils, and platelets may require dose reduction or permanent discontinuation from therapy** *[see Dosage and Administration (2.4)]*. Changes in selected laboratory values during therapy are described in **Table 8**. Most of the changes in laboratory values in the PegIntron/REBETOL trial with pediatrics were mild or moderate.

[See table 8 at top of next page]

Hemoglobin. Hemoglobin levels decreased to less than 11 g/dL in about 30% of subjects in Study 2. In Study 3, 47% of subjects receiving WBD REBETOL and 33% on flat-dose REBETOL had decreases in hemoglobin levels less than 11 g/dl. Reductions in hemoglobin to less than 9 g/dL occurred more frequently in subjects receiving WBD compared to flat dosing (4% and 2%, respectively). In Study 2, dose modification was required in 9% and 13% of subjects in the PegIntron/REBETOL and INTRON A/REBETOL groups. In Study 4, subjects receiving PegIntron (1.5 mcg/kg)/REBETOL had decreases in hemoglobin levels to between 8.5 to less than 10 g/dL (28%) and to less than 8.5 g/dL (3%), whereas in patients receiving Pegasys 180 mcg/Copegus these decreases occurred in 26% and 4% of subjects respectively. Hemoglobin levels became stable by treatment Weeks 4-6 on average. The typical pattern observed was a decrease in hemoglobin levels by treatment Week 4 followed by stabilization and a plateau, which was maintained to the end of treatment. In the PegIntron monotherapy trial, hemoglobin decreases were generally mild and dose modifications were rarely necessary *[see Dosage and Administration (2.4)]*.

Neutrophils. Decreases in neutrophil counts were observed in a majority of adult subjects treated with combination therapy with REBETOL in Study 2 (85%) and INTRON A/REBETOL (60%). Severe potentially life-threatening neutropenia (less than 0.5×10^9/L) occurred in 2% of subjects treated with INTRON A/REBETOL and in approximately 4% of subjects treated with PegIntron/REBETOL in Study 2. Eighteen percent of subjects receiving PegIntron/REBETOL in Study 2 required modification of interferon dosage. Few subjects (less than 1%) required permanent discontinuation of treatment. Neutrophil counts generally returned to pre-treatment levels 4 weeks after cessation of therapy *[see Dosage and Administration (2.4)]*.

Platelets. Platelet counts decreased to less than 100,000/mm^3 in approximately 20% of subjects treated with PegIntron alone or with REBETOL and in 6% of adult subjects treated with INTRON A/REBETOL. Severe decreases in platelet counts (less than 50,000/mm^3) occur in less than 4% of adult subjects. Patients may require discontinuation or dose modification as a result of platelet decreases *[see Dosage and Administration (2.4)]*. In Study 2, 1% or 3% of subjects required dose modification of INTRON A or PegIntron, respectively. Platelet counts generally returned to pretreatment levels 4 weeks after the cessation of therapy.

Thyroid Function. Development of TSH abnormalities, with or without clinical manifestations, is associated with interferon therapies. In Study 2, clinically apparent thyroid disorders occurred among subjects treated with either INTRON A or PegIntron (with or without REBETOL) at a similar incidence (5% for hypothyroidism and 3% for hyperthyroidism). Subjects developed new onset TSH abnormalities while on treatment and during the follow-up period. At the end of the follow-up period 7% of subjects still had abnormal TSH values.

Bilirubin and uric acid. In Study 2, 10 to 14% of subjects developed hyperbilirubinemia and 33 to 38% developed hyperuricemia in association with hemolysis. Six subjects developed mild to moderate gout.

6.2 Clinical Trials Experience – REBETOL/INTRON A Combination Therapy

Adult Subjects

In clinical trials, 19% and 6% of previously untreated and relapse subjects, respectively, discontinued therapy due to adverse reactions in the combination arms compared to 13% and 3% in the interferon arms. Selected treatment-related adverse reactions that occurred in the US trials with greater than or equal to 5% incidence are provided by treatment group (see **Table 9**). In general, the selected treatment-related adverse reactions were reported with lower incidence in the international trials as compared to the US trials, with the exception of asthenia, influenza-like symptoms, nervousness, and pruritus.

Pediatric Subjects

In clinical trials of 118 pediatric subjects 3 to 16 years of age, 6% discontinued therapy due to adverse reactions. Dose modifications were required in 30% of subjects, most commonly for anemia and neutropenia. In general, the adverse-reaction profile in the pediatric population was similar to that observed in adults. Injection site disorders, fever, anorexia, vomiting, and emotional lability occurred more frequently in pediatric subjects compared to adult subjects. Conversely, pediatric subjects experienced less fatigue, dyspepsia, arthralgia, insomnia, irritability, impaired concentration, dyspnea, and pruritus compared to adult subjects. Selected treatment-related adverse reactions that occurred with greater than or equal to 5% incidence among all pediatric subjects who received the recommended dose of REBETOL/INTRON A combination therapy are provided in **Table 9**.

[See table 9 on pages 1743 and 1744]

Laboratory Values

Changes in selected hematologic values (hemoglobin, white blood cells, neutrophils, and platelets) during therapy are described below (see **Table 10**).

Hemoglobin. Hemoglobin decreases among subjects receiving REBETOL therapy began at Week 1, with stabilization by Week 4. In previously untreated subjects treated for 48 weeks, the mean maximum decrease from baseline was 3.1 g/dL in the US trial and 2.9 g/dL in the international trial. In relapse subjects, the mean maximum decrease from baseline was 2.8 g/dL in the US trial and 2.6 g/dL in the international trial. Hemoglobin values returned to pretreatment levels within 4 to 8 weeks of cessation of therapy in most subjects.

Table 8: Selected Laboratory Abnormalities During Treatment with REBETOL and PegIntron or REBETOL and INTRON A in Previously Untreated Subjects

Laboratory Parameters*	Percentage of Subjects		
	Adults (Study 2)		Pediatrics
	PegIntron/ REBETOL (N=511)	INTRON A/ REBETOL (N=505)	PegIntron/ REBETOL (N=107)*
Hemoglobin (g/dL)			
9.5 to <11.0	26	27	30
8.0 to <9.5	3	3	2
6.5-7.9	0.2	0.2	-
Leukocytes (× 10⁹/L)			
2.0-2.9	46	41	39
1.5 to <2.0	24	8	3
1.0-1.4	5	1	-
Neutrophils (× 10⁹/L)			
1.0-1.5	33	37	35
0.75 to <1.0	25	13	26
0.5 to <0.75	18	7	13
<0.5	4	2	3
Platelets (× 10⁹/L)			
70-100	15	5	1
50 to <70	3	0.8	-
30-49	0.2	0.2	-
25 to <50	-	-	1
Total Bilirubin	(mg/dL)		(μmole/L)
1.5-3.0	10	13	-
1.26-2.59 × ULN†	-	-	7
3.1-6.0	0.6	0.2	-
2.6-5 × ULN†	-	-	-
6.1-12.0	0	0.2	-
ALT (U/L)			
2 × Baseline	0.6	0.2	1
2.1-5 × Baseline	3	1	5
5.1-10 × Baseline	0	0	3

* The table summarizes the worst category observed within the period per subject per laboratory test. Only subjects with at least one treatment value for a given laboratory test are included.
† ULN=Upper limit of normal.

Bilirubin and Uric Acid. Increases in both bilirubin and uric acid, associated with hemolysis, were noted in clinical trials. Most were moderate biochemical changes and were reversed within 4 weeks after treatment discontinuation. This observation occurred most frequently in subjects with a previous diagnosis of Gilbert's syndrome. This has not been associated with hepatic dysfunction or clinical morbidity.

[See table 10 at top of page 1744]

6.3 Postmarketing Experiences

The following adverse reactions have been identified and reported during post approval use of REBETOL in combination with INTRON A or PegIntron. Because these reactions are reported voluntarily from a population of uncertain size, it is not always possible to reliably estimate their frequency or establish a causal relationship to drug exposure.

Blood and Lymphatic System disorders
Pure red cell aplasia, aplastic anemia
Ear and Labyrinth disorders
Hearing disorder, vertigo
Respiratory, Thoracic and Mediastinal disorders
Pulmonary hypertension
Eye disorders
Serous retinal detachment
Endocrine disorders
Diabetes

7 DRUG INTERACTIONS

7.1 Didanosine

Exposure to didanosine or its active metabolite (dideoxyadenosine 5′-triphosphate) is increased when didanosine is coadministered with ribavirin, which could cause or worsen clinical toxicities; therefore, coadministration of REBETOL capsules or oral solution and didanosine is contraindicated. Reports of fatal hepatic failure, as well as peripheral neuropathy, pancreatitis, and symptomatic hyperlactatemia/lactic acidosis have been reported in clinical trials.

7.2 Nucleoside Analogues

Hepatic decompensation (some fatal) has occurred in cirrhotic HIV/HCV co-infected patients receiving combination antiretroviral therapy for HIV and interferon alpha and ribavirin. Adding treatment with alpha interferons alone or in combination with ribavirin may increase the risk in this patient population. Patients receiving interferon with ribavirin and nucleoside reverse transcriptase inhibitors (NRTIs) should be closely monitored for treatment-associated toxicities, especially hepatic decompensation and anemia. Discontinuation of NRTIs should be considered as medically appropriate *(see labeling for individual NRTI product)*. Dose reduction or discontinuation of interferon, ribavirin, or both should also be considered if worsening clinical toxicities are observed, including hepatic decompensation (e.g., Child-Pugh greater than 6).

Ribavirin may antagonize the cell culture antiviral activity of stavudine and zidovudine against HIV. Ribavirin has been shown in cell culture to inhibit phosphorylation of lamivudine, stavudine, and zidovudine, which could lead to decreased antiretroviral activity. However, in a study with another pegylated interferon in combination with ribavirin, no pharmacokinetic (e.g., plasma concentrations or intracellular triphosphorylated active metabolite concentrations) or pharmacodynamic (e.g., loss of HIV/HCV virologic suppress) interaction was observed when ribavirin and lamivudine (n=18), stavudine (n=10), or zidovudine (n=6) were coadministered as part of a multidrug regimen in HIV/HCV co-infected subjects. Therefore, concomitant use of ribavirin with either of these drugs should be used with caution.

7.3 Drugs Metabolized by Cytochrome P-450

Results of *in vitro* studies using both human and rat liver microsome preparations indicated little or no cytochrome P-450 enzyme-mediated metabolism of ribavirin, with minimal potential for P-450 enzyme-based drug interactions.

No pharmacokinetic interactions were noted between INTRON A and REBETOL capsules in a multiple-dose pharmacokinetic study.

7.4 Azathioprine

The use of ribavirin for the treatment of chronic hepatitis C in patients receiving azathioprine has been reported to induce severe pancytopenia and may increase the risk of azathioprine-related myelotoxicity. Inosine monophosphate dehydrogenase (IMDH) is required for one of the metabolic pathways of azathioprine. Ribavirin is known to inhibit IMDH, thereby leading to accumulation of an azathioprine metabolite, 6-methylthioinosine monophosphate (6-MTITP), which is associated with myelotoxicity (neutropenia, thrombocytopenia, and anemia). Patients receiving azathioprine with ribavirin should have complete blood counts, including platelet counts, monitored weekly for the first month, twice monthly for the second and third months of treatment, then monthly or more frequently if dosage or other therapy changes are necessary *[see Warnings and Precautions (5.8)]*.

8 USE IN SPECIFIC POPULATIONS

8.1 Pregnancy

Pregnancy Category X

[See Contraindications (4), Warnings and Precautions (5.1), and Nonclinical Toxicology (13.1)].

Treatment and Post-treatment:

Potential Risk to the Fetus:

Ribavirin is known to accumulate in intracellular components from where it is cleared very slowly. It is not known whether ribavirin contained in sperm will exert a potential teratogenic effect upon fertilization of the ova. In a study in rats, it was concluded that dominant lethality was not induced by ribavirin at doses up to 200 mg/kg for 5 days (estimated human equivalent doses of 7.14 to 28.6 mg/kg, based on body surface area adjustment for a 60 kg adult; up to 1.7 times the maximum recommended human dose of ribavirin). However, because of the potential human teratogenic effects of ribavirin, male patients should be advised to take every precaution to avoid risk of pregnancy for their female partners.

Women of childbearing potential should not receive REBETOL unless they are using effective contraception (two reliable forms) during the therapy period. In addition, effective contraception should be utilized for 6 months post-therapy based on a multiple-dose half-life ($t_{1/2}$) of ribavirin of 12 days.

Male patients and their female partners must practice effective contraception (two reliable forms) during treatment with REBETOL and for the 6-month post-therapy period (e.g., 15 half-lives for ribavirin clearance from the body).

A Ribavirin Pregnancy Registry has been established to monitor maternal-fetal outcomes of pregnancies in female patients and female partners of male patients exposed to ribavirin during treatment and for 6 months following cessation of treatment. Physicians and patients are encouraged to report such cases by calling 1-800-593-2214.

8.3 Nursing Mothers

It is not known whether the REBETOL product is excreted in human milk. Because of the potential for serious adverse reactions from the drug in nursing infants, a decision should be made whether to discontinue nursing or to delay or discontinue REBETOL.

8.4 Pediatric Use

Safety and effectiveness of REBETOL in combination with PegIntron has not been established in pediatric patients below the age of 3 years. For treatment with REBETOL/ INTRON A, evidence of disease progression, such as hepatic inflammation and fibrosis, as well as prognostic factors for response, HCV genotype and viral load should be considered when deciding to treat a pediatric patient. The benefits of treatment should be weighed against the safety findings observed.

Table 9: Selected Treatment-Related Adverse Reactions: Previously Untreated and Relapse Adult Subjects and Previously Untreated Pediatric Subjects

	Percentage of Subjects						
	US Previously Untreated Study				US Relapse Study		Pediatric Subjects
	24 weeks of treatment		48 weeks of treatment		24 weeks of treatment		48 weeks of treatment
Subjects Reporting Adverse Reactions*	INTRON A/ REBETOL (N=228)	INTRON A/ Placebo (N=231)	INTRON A/ REBETOL (N=228)	INTRON A/ Placebo (N=225)	INTRON A/ REBETOL (N=77)	INTRON A/ Placebo (N=76)	INTRON A/ REBETOL (N=118)
Application Site Disorders							
Injection Site Inflammation	13	10	12	14	6	8	14
Injection Site Reaction	7	9	8	9	5	3	19
Body as a Whole - General Disorders							
Headache	63	63	66	67	66	68	69
Fatigue	68	62	70	72	60	53	58
Rigors	40	32	42	39	43	37	25
Fever	37	35	41	40	32	36	61
Influenza-like Symptoms	14	18	18	20	13	13	31
Asthenia	9	4	9	9	10	4	5
Chest Pain	5	4	9	8	6	7	5
Central & Peripheral Nervous System Disorders							
Dizziness	17	15	23	19	26	21	20
Gastrointestinal System Disorders							
Nausea	38	35	46	33	47	33	33
Anorexia	27	16	25	19	21	14	51
Dyspepsia	14	6	16	9	16	9	<1
Vomiting	11	10	9	13	12	8	42
Musculoskeletal System Disorders							
Myalgia	61	57	64	63	61	58	32
Arthralgia	30	27	33	36	29	29	15
Musculoskeletal Pain	20	26	28	32	22	28	21
Psychiatric Disorders							
Insomnia	39	27	39	30	26	25	14
Irritability	23	19	32	27	25	20	10
Depression	32	25	36	37	23	14	13
Emotional Lability	7	6	11	8	12	8	16
Concentration Impaired	11	14	14	14	10	12	5
Nervousness	4	2	4	4	5	4	3
Respiratory System Disorders							
Dyspnea	19	9	18	10	17	12	5
Sinusitis	9	7	10	14	12	7	<1
Skin and Appendages Disorders							
Alopecia	28	27	32	28	27	26	23

(Table continued on next page)

Suicidal ideation or attempts occurred more frequently among pediatric patients, primarily adolescents, compared to adult patients (2.4% vs. 1%) during treatment and off-therapy follow-up *[see Warnings and Precautions (5.10)]*. As in adult patients, pediatric patients experienced other psychiatric adverse reactions (e.g., depression, emotional lability, somnolence), anemia, and neutropenia *[see Warnings and Precautions (5.2)]*.

8.5 Geriatric Use

Clinical trials of REBETOL/INTRON A or PegIntron therapy did not include sufficient numbers of subjects aged 65 and over to determine if they respond differently from younger subjects.

REBETOL is known to be substantially excreted by the kidney, and the risk of toxic reactions to this drug may be greater in patients with impaired renal function. Because elderly patients often have decreased renal function, care should be taken in dose selection. Renal function should be monitored and dosage adjustments should be made accordingly. REBETOL should not be used in patients with creatinine clearance less than 50 mL/min *[see Contraindications (4)]*.

In general, REBETOL capsules should be administered to elderly patients cautiously, starting at the lower end of the dosing range, reflecting the greater frequency of decreased hepatic and cardiac function, and of concomitant disease or other drug therapy. In clinical trials, elderly subjects had a higher frequency of anemia (67%) than younger patients (28%) *[see Warnings and Precautions (5.2)]*.

8.6 Organ Transplant Recipients

The safety and efficacy of INTRON A and PegIntron alone or in combination with REBETOL for the treatment of hepatitis C in liver or other organ transplant recipients have not been established. In a small (n=16) single-center, uncontrolled case experience, renal failure in renal allograft recipients receiving interferon alpha and ribavirin combination therapy was more frequent than expected from the center's previous experience with renal allograft recipients not receiving combination therapy. The relationship of the renal failure to renal allograft rejection is not clear.

8.7 HIV or HBV Co-infection

The safety and efficacy of PegIntron/REBETOL and INTRON A/REBETOL for the treatment of patients with HCV co-infected with HIV or HBV have not been established.

10 OVERDOSAGE

There is limited experience with overdosage. Acute ingestion of up to 20 g of REBETOL capsules, INTRON A ingestion of up to 120 million units, and subcutaneous doses of INTRON A up to 10 times the recommended doses have been reported. Primary effects that have been observed are increased incidence and severity of the adverse reactions related to the therapeutic use of INTRON A and REBETOL. However, hepatic enzyme abnormalities, renal failure, hemorrhage, and myocardial infarction have been reported with administration of single subcutaneous doses of INTRON A that exceed dosing recommendations.

There is no specific antidote for INTRON A or REBETOL overdose, and hemodialysis and peritoneal dialysis are not effective for treatment of overdose of these agents.

11 DESCRIPTION

REBETOL (ribavirin), is a synthetic nucleoside analogue (purine analogue). The chemical name of ribavirin is 1-β-D-ribofuranosyl-1H-1,2,4-triazole-3-carboxamide and has the following structural formula (see **Figure 1**).

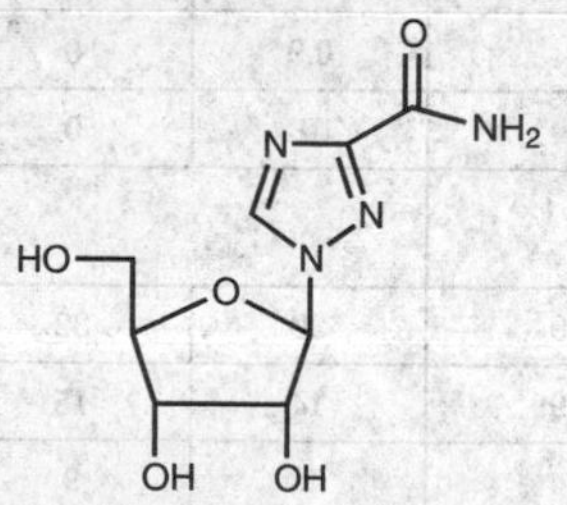

Figure 1: Structural Formula

Ribavirin is a white, crystalline powder. It is freely soluble in water and slightly soluble in anhydrous alcohol. The empirical formula is $C_8H_{12}N_4O_5$ and the molecular weight is 244.21.

REBETOL capsules consist of a white powder in a white, opaque, gelatin capsule. Each capsule contains 200 mg ribavirin and the inactive ingredients microcrystalline cellulose, lactose monohydrate, croscarmellose sodium, and magnesium stearate. The capsule shell consists of gelatin, sodium lauryl sulfate, silicon dioxide, and titanium dioxide. The capsule is printed with edible blue pharmaceutical ink which is made of shellac, anhydrous ethyl alcohol, isopropyl alcohol, n-butyl alcohol, propylene glycol, ammonium hydroxide, and FD&C Blue #2 aluminum lake.

REBETOL oral solution is a clear, colorless to pale or light yellow bubble gum-flavored liquid. Each milliliter of the solution contains 40 mg of ribavirin and the inactive ingredients sucrose, glycerin, sorbitol, propylene glycol, sodium citrate, citric acid, sodium benzoate, natural and artificial flavor for bubble gum #15864, and water.

Table 9: Selected Treatment-Related Adverse Reactions: Previously Untreated and Relapse Adult Subjects and Previously Untreated Pediatric Subjects

Subjects Reporting Adverse Reactions*	Percentage of Subjects						
	US Previously Untreated Study				US Relapse Study		Pediatric Subjects
	24 weeks of treatment		48 weeks of treatment		24 weeks of treatment		48 weeks of treatment
	INTRON A/ REBETOL (N=228)	INTRON A/ Placebo (N=231)	INTRON A/ REBETOL (N=228)	INTRON A/ Placebo (N=225)	INTRON A/ REBETOL (N=77)	INTRON A/ Placebo (N=76)	INTRON A/ REBETOL (N=118)
Rash	20	9	28	8	21	5	17
Pruritus	21	9	19	8	13	4	12
Special Senses, Other Disorders							
Taste Perversion	7	4	8	4	6	5	<1

* Subjects reporting one or more adverse reactions. A subject may have reported more than one adverse reaction within a body system/organ class category.

Table 10: Selected Laboratory Abnormalities During Treatment With REBETOL and INTRON A: Previously Untreated and Relapse Adult Subjects and Previously Untreated Pediatric Subjects

	Percentage of Subjects						
	US Previously Untreated Study				US Relapse Study		Pediatric Subjects
	24 weeks of treatment		48 weeks of treatment		24 weeks of treatment		48 weeks of treatment
	INTRON A/ REBETOL (N=228)	INTRON A/ Placebo (N=231)	INTRON A/ REBETOL (N=228)	INTRON A/ Placebo (N=225)	INTRON A/ REBETOL (N=77)	INTRON A/ Placebo (N=76)	INTRON A/ REBETOL (N=118)
Hemoglobin (g/dL)							
9.5 to 10.9	24	1	32	1	21	3	24
8.0 to 9.4	5	0	4	0	4	0	3
6.5 to 7.9	0	0	0	0.4	0	0	0
<6.5	0	0	0	0	0	0	0
Leukocytes (× 10^9/L)							
2.0 to 2.9	40	20	38	23	45	26	35
1.5 to 1.9	4	1	9	2	5	3	8
1.0 to 1.4	0.9	0	2	0	0	0	0
<1.0	0	0	0	0	0	0	0
Neutrophils (× 10^9/L)							
1.0 to 1.49	30	32	31	44	42	34	37
0.75 to 0.99	14	15	14	11	16	18	15
0.5 to 0.74	9	9	14	7	8	4	16
<0.5	11	8	11	5	5	8	3
Platelets (× 10^9/L)							
70 to 99	9	11	11	14	6	12	0.8
50 to 69	2	3	2	3	0	5	2
30 to 49	0	0.4	0	0.4	0	0	0
<30	0.9	0	1	0.9	0	0	0
Total Bilirubin (mg/dL)							
1.5 to 3.0	27	13	32	13	21	7	2
3.1 to 6.0	0.9	0.4	2	0	3	0	0
6.1 to 12.0	0	0	0.4	0	0	0	0
>12.0	0	0	0	0	0	0	0

12 CLINICAL PHARMACOLOGY

12.1 Mechanism of Action

Ribavirin is an antiviral agent *[see Clinical Pharmacology (12.4)]*.

12.3 Pharmacokinetics

Single- and multiple-dose pharmacokinetic properties in adults are summarized in **Table 11**. Ribavirin was rapidly and extensively absorbed following oral administration. However, due to first-pass metabolism, the absolute bioavailability averaged 64% (44%). There was a linear relationship between dose and AUC_{tf} (AUC from time zero to last measurable concentration) following single doses of 200 to 1200 mg ribavirin. The relationship between dose and C_{max} was curvilinear, tending to asymptote above single doses of 400 to 600 mg.

Upon multiple oral dosing, based on AUC_{12hr}, a 6-fold accumulation of ribavirin was observed in plasma. Following oral dosing with 600 mg twice daily, steady-state was reached by approximately 4 weeks, with mean steady-state plasma concentrations of 2200 ng/mL (37%). Upon discontinuation of dosing, the mean half-life was 298 (30%) hours, which probably reflects slow elimination from nonplasma compartments.

Effect of Antacid on Absorption of Ribavirin:

Coadministration of REBETOL capsules with an antacid containing magnesium, aluminum, and simethicone resulted in a 14% decrease in mean ribavirin AUC_{tf}. The clinical relevance of results from this single-dose study is unknown.

[See table 11 at top of next page]

Tissue Distribution:

Ribavirin transport into nonplasma compartments has been most extensively studied in red blood cells, and has been identified to be primarily via an e_s-type equilibrative nucleoside transporter. This type of transporter is present on virtually all cell types and may account for the extensive volume of distribution. Ribavirin does not bind to plasma proteins.

Metabolism and Excretion:

Ribavirin has two pathways of metabolism: (i) a reversible phosphorylation pathway in nucleated cells; and (ii) a degradative pathway involving deribosylation and amide hydrolysis to yield a triazole carboxylic acid metabolite. Ribavirin and its triazole carboxamide and triazole carboxylic acid metabolites are excreted renally. After oral administration of 600 mg of ^{14}C-ribavirin, approximately 61% and 12% of the radioactivity was eliminated in the urine and feces, respectively, in 336 hours. Unchanged ribavirin accounted for 17% of the administered dose.

Special Populations:

<u>Renal Dysfunction</u>

The pharmacokinetics of ribavirin were assessed after administration of a single oral dose (400 mg) of ribavirin to non HCV-infected subjects with varying degrees of renal dysfunction. The mean AUC_{tf} value was threefold greater in subjects with creatinine clearance values between 10 to 30 mL/min when compared to control subjects (creatinine clearance greater than 90 mL/min). In subjects with creatinine clearance values between 30 to 60 mL/min, AUC_{tf} was twofold greater when compared to control subjects. The increased AUC_{tf} appears to be due to reduction of renal and nonrenal clearance in these subjects. Phase 3 efficacy trials included subjects with creatinine clearance values greater than 50 mL/min. The multiple-dose pharmacokinetics of ribavirin cannot be accurately predicted in patients with renal dysfunction. Ribavirin is not effectively removed by hemodialysis. Patients with creatinine clearance less than 50 mL/min should not be treated with REBETOL *[see Contraindications (4)]*.

<u>Hepatic Dysfunction</u>

The effect of hepatic dysfunction was assessed after a single oral dose of ribavirin (600 mg). The mean AUC_{tf} values were not significantly different in subjects with mild, moderate, or severe hepatic dysfunction (Child-Pugh Classification A, B, or C) when compared to control subjects. However, the mean C_{max} values increased with severity of hepatic dysfunction and was twofold greater in subjects with severe hepatic dysfunction when compared to control subjects.

<u>Elderly Patients</u>

Pharmacokinetic evaluations in elderly subjects have not been performed.

<u>Gender</u>

There were no clinically significant pharmacokinetic differences noted in a single-dose trial of 18 male and 18 female subjects.

<u>Pediatric Patients</u>

Multiple-dose pharmacokinetic properties for REBETOL capsules and INTRON A in pediatric subjects with chronic hepatitis C between 5 and 16 years of age are summarized in **Table 12**. The pharmacokinetics of REBETOL and INTRON A (dose-normalized) are similar in adults and pediatric subjects.

Complete pharmacokinetic characteristics of REBETOL oral solution have not been determined in pediatric sub-

Table 11: Mean (% CV) Pharmacokinetic Parameters for REBETOL When Administered Individually to Adults

Parameter	REBETOL		
	Single-Dose 600 mg Oral Solution (N=14)	Single-Dose 600 mg Capsules (N=12)	Multiple-Dose 600 mg Capsules twice daily (N=12)
T_{max} (hr)	1.00 (34)	1.7 (46)*	3 (60)
C_{max} (ng/mL)	872 (42)	782 (37)	3680 (85)
AUC_{tf} (ng·hr/mL)	14,098 (38)	13,400 (48)	228,000 (25)
$T_{1/2}$ (hr)		43.6 (47)	298 (30)
Apparent Volume of Distribution (L)		2825 (9)†	
Apparent Clearance (L/hr)		38.2 (40)	
Absolute Bioavailability		64% (44)‡	

* N=11.
† Data obtained from a single-dose pharmacokinetic study using ^{14}C labeled ribavirin; N=5.
‡ N=6.

jects. Ribavirin C_{min} values were similar following administration of REBETOL oral solution or REBETOL capsules during 48 weeks of therapy in pediatric subjects (3 to 16 years of age).

Table 12: Mean (% CV) Multiple-dose Pharmacokinetic Parameters for INTRON A and REBETOL Capsules When Administered to Pediatric Subjects with Chronic Hepatitis C

Parameter	REBETOL 15 mg/kg/day as 2 divided doses (N=17)	INTRON A 3 MIU/m² three times weekly (N=54)
T_{max} (hr)	1.9 (83)	5.9 (36)
C_{max} (ng/mL)	3275 (25)	51 (48)
AUC*	29,774 (26)	622 (48)
Apparent Clearance L/hr/kg	0.27 (27)	ND†

Note: numbers in parenthesis indicate % coefficient of variation.
* AUC_{12} (ng·hr/mL) for REBETOL; AUC_{0-24} (IU·hr/mL) for INTRON A.
† ND=not done.

A clinical trial in pediatric subjects with chronic hepatitis C between 3 and 17 years of age was conducted in which pharmacokinetics for PegIntron and REBETOL (capsules and oral solution) were evaluated. In pediatric subjects receiving body surface area-adjusted dosing of PegIntron at 60 mcg/m²/week, the log transformed ratio estimate of exposure during the dosing interval was predicted to be 58% [90% CI: 141%, 177%] higher than observed in adults receiving 1.5 mcg/kg/week. The pharmacokinetics of REBETOL (dose-normalized) in this trial were similar to those reported in a prior study of REBETOL in combination with INTRON A in pediatric subjects and in adults.

Effect of Food on Absorption of Ribavirin

Both AUC_{tf} and C_{max} increased by 70% when REBETOL capsules were administered with a high-fat meal (841 kcal, 53.8 g fat, 31.6 g protein, and 57.4 g carbohydrate) in a single-dose pharmacokinetic study *[see Dosage and Administration (2)]*.

12.4 Microbiology

Mechanism of Action

The mechanism by which ribavirin contributes to its antiviral efficacy in the clinic is not fully understood. Ribavirin has direct antiviral activity in tissue culture against many RNA viruses. Ribavirin increases the mutation frequency in the genomes of several viruses and ribavirin triphosphate inhibits HCV polymerase in a biochemical reaction.

Antiviral Activity in Cell Culture

The antiviral activity of ribavirin in the HCV-replicon is not well understood and has not been defined because of the cellular toxicity of ribavirin. Direct antiviral activity has been observed in tissue culture of other RNA viruses. The anti-HCV activity of interferon was demonstrated in cell containing self-replicating HCV-RNS (HCV replicon cells) or HCV infection.

Resistance

HCV genotypes show wide variability in their response to pegylated recombinant human interferon/ribavirin therapy. Genetic changes associated with the variable response have not been identified.

Cross-resistance

There is no reported cross-resistance between pegylated/non-pegylated interferons and ribavirin.

13 NONCLINICAL TOXICOLOGY

13.1 Carcinogenesis, Mutagenesis, Impairment of Fertility

Carcinogenesis

Ribavirin did not cause an increase in any tumor type when administered for 6 months in the transgenic p53 deficient mouse model at doses up to 300 mg/kg (estimated human equivalent of 25 mg/kg based on body surface area adjustment for a 60 kg adult; approximately 1.9 times the maximum recommended human daily dose). Ribavirin was non-carcinogenic when administered for 2 years to rats at doses up to 40 mg/kg (estimated human equivalent of 5.71 mg/kg based on body surface area adjustment for a 60 kg adult).

Mutagenesis

Ribavirin demonstrated increased incidences of mutation and cell transformation in multiple genotoxicity assays. Ribavirin was active in the Balb/3T3 *In Vitro* Cell Transformation Assay. Mutagenic activity was observed in the mouse lymphoma assay, and at doses of 20 to 200 mg/kg (estimated human equivalent of 1.67 to 16.7 mg/kg, based on body surface area adjustment for a 60 kg adult; 0.1 to 1 times the maximum recommended human 24-hour dose of ribavirin) in a mouse micronucleus assay. A dominant lethal assay in rats was negative, indicating that if mutations occurred in rats they were not transmitted through male gametes.

Impairment of Fertility

Ribavirin demonstrated significant embryocidal and teratogenic effects at doses well below the recommended human dose in all animal species in which adequate studies have been conducted. Malformations of the skull, palate, eye, jaw, limbs, skeleton, and gastrointestinal tract were noted. The incidence and severity of teratogenic effects increased with escalation of the drug dose. Survival of fetuses and offspring was reduced. In conventional embryotoxicity/teratogenicity studies in rats and rabbits, observed no-effect dose levels were well below those for proposed clinical use (0.3 mg/kg/day for both the rat and rabbit; approximately 0.06 times the recommended human 24-hour dose of ribavirin). No maternal toxicity or effects on offspring were observed in a peri/postnatal toxicity study in rats dosed orally at up to 1 mg/kg/day (estimated human equivalent dose of 0.17 mg/kg based on body surface area adjustment for a 60 kg adult; approximately 0.01 times the maximum recommended human 24-hour dose of ribavirin) *[see Contraindications (4), and Warnings and Precautions (5.1)]*.

Fertile women and partners of fertile women should not receive REBETOL unless the patient and his/her partner are using effective contraception (two reliable forms). Based on a multiple-dose half-life ($t_{1/2}$) of ribavirin of 12 days, effective contraception must be utilized for 6 months post-therapy (e.g., 15 half-lives of clearance for ribavirin).

REBETOL should be used with caution in fertile men. In studies in mice to evaluate the time course and reversibility of ribavirin-induced testicular degeneration at doses of 15 to 150 mg/kg/day (estimated human equivalent of 1.25 to 12.5 mg/kg/day, based on body surface area adjustment for a 60-kg adult; 0.1-0.8 times the maximum human 24-hour dose of ribavirin) administered for 3 or 6 months, abnormalities in sperm occurred. Upon cessation of treatment, essentially total recovery from ribavirin-induced testicular toxicity was apparent within 1 or 2 spermatogenesis cycles.

13.2 Animal Toxicology and Pharmacology

Long-term studies in the mouse and rat [18 to 24 months; doses of 20 to 75 and 10 to 40 mg/kg/day, respectively (estimated human equivalent doses of 1.67 to 6.25 and 1.43 to 5.71 mg/kg/day, respectively, based on body surface area adjustment for a 60 kg adult; approximately 0.1 to 0.4 times the maximum human 24-hour dose of ribavirin)] have demonstrated a relationship between chronic ribavirin exposure and increased incidences of vascular lesions (microscopic hemorrhages) in mice. In rats, retinal degeneration occurred in controls, but the incidence was increased in ribavirin-treated rats.

In a study in which rat pups were dosed postnatally with ribavirin at doses of 10, 25, and 50 mg/kg/day, drug-related deaths occurred at 50 mg/kg (at rat pup plasma concentrations below human plasma concentrations at the human therapeutic dose) between study Days 13 and 48. Rat pups dosed from postnatal Days 7 through 63 demonstrated a minor, dose-related decrease in overall growth at all doses, which was subsequently manifested as slight decreases in body weight, crown-rump length, and bone length. These effects showed evidence of reversibility, and no histopathological effects on bone were observed. No ribavirin effects were observed regarding neurobehavioral or reproductive development.

14 CLINICAL STUDIES

Clinical Study 1 evaluated PegIntron monotherapy. See PegIntron labeling for information about this trial.

14.1 REBETOL/PegIntron Combination Therapy

Adult Subjects

Study 2

A randomized trial compared treatment with two PegIntron/REBETOL regimens [PegIntron 1.5 mcg/kg subcutaneously once weekly/REBETOL 800 mg orally daily (in divided doses); PegIntron 1.5 mcg/kg subcutaneously once weekly for 4 weeks then 0.5 mcg/kg subcutaneously once weekly for 44 weeks/REBETOL 1000 or 1200 mg orally daily (in divided doses)] with INTRON A [3 MIU subcutaneously three times weekly/REBETOL 1000 or 1200 mg orally daily (in divided doses)] in 1530 adults with chronic hepatitis C. Interferon-naïve subjects were treated for 48 weeks and followed for 24 weeks post-treatment. Eligible subjects had compensated liver disease, detectable HCV-RNA, elevated ALT, and liver histopathology consistent with chronic hepatitis.

Response to treatment was defined as undetectable HCV-RNA at 24 weeks post-treatment (see **Table 13**). The response rate to the PegIntron 1.5 mcg/kg and ribavirin 800 mg dose was higher than the response rate to INTRON A/REBETOL (see **Table 13**).The response rate to PegIntron 1.5→0.5 mcg/kg/REBETOL was essentially the same as the response to INTRON A/REBETOL (data not shown).

Table 13: Rates of Response to Combination Treatment – Study 2

	PegIntron 1.5 mcg/kg once weekly REBETOL 800 mg once daily	INTRON A 3 MIU three times weekly REBETOL 1000/1200 mg once daily
Overall response*,†	52% (264/511)	46% (231/505)
Genotype 1	41% (141/348)	33% (112/343)
Genotype 2-6	75% (123/163)	73% (119/162)

* Serum HCV-RNA was measured with a research-based quantitative polymerase chain reaction assay by a central laboratory.
† Difference in overall treatment response (PegIntron/REBETOL vs. INTRON A/REBETOL) is 6% with 95% confidence interval of (0.18, 11.63) adjusted for viral genotype and presence of cirrhosis at baseline. Response to treatment was defined as undetectable HCV-RNA at 24 weeks post-treatment.

Subjects with viral genotype 1, regardless of viral load, had a lower response rate to PegIntron (1.5 mcg/kg)/REBETOL (800 mg) compared to subjects with other viral genotypes. Subjects with both poor prognostic factors (genotype 1 and high viral load) had a response rate of 30% (78/256) compared to a response rate of 29% (71/247) with INTRON A/REBETOL combination therapy.

Subjects with lower body weight tended to have higher adverse-reaction rates *[see Adverse Reactions (6.1)]* and

Table 14: SVR Rate by Treatment and Baseline Weight - Study 3

Treatment Group	Subject Baseline Weight			
	<65 kg (<143 lb)	65-85 kg (143-188 lb)	>85-105 kg (>188-231 lb)	>105 kg (>231 lb)
WBD*	50% (173/348)	45% (449/994)	42% (351/835)	47% (138/292)
Flat	51% (173/342)	44% (443/1011)	39% (318/819)	33% (91/272)

* *P*=0.01, primary efficacy comparison (based on data from subjects weighing 65 kg or higher at baseline and utilizing a logistic regression analysis that includes treatment [WBD or Flat], genotype and presence/absence of advanced fibrosis, in the model).

Table 16: SVR Rates by Baseline Characteristics of Prior Treatment Failures - Study 5

HCV Genotype / Metavir Fibrosis Score	Overall SVR by Previous Response and Treatment: Nonresponder — interferon alfa/ribavirin % (number of subjects)	Nonresponder — peginterferon (2a and 2b combined)/ribavirin % (number of subjects)	Relapser — interferon alfa/ribavirin % (number of subjects)	Relapser — peginterferon (2a and 2b combined)/ribavirin % (number of subjects)
Overall	18 (158/903)	6 (30/476)	43 (130/300)	35 (113/344)
HCV 1	13 (98/761)	4 (19/431)	32 (67/208)	23 (56/243)
F2	18 (36/202)	6 (7/117)	42 (33/79)	32 (23/72)
F3	16 (38/233)	4 (4/112)	28 (16/58)	21 (14/67)
F4	7 (24/325)	4 (8/202)	26 (18/70)	18 (19/104)
HCV 2/3	49 (53/109)	36 (10/28)	67 (54/81)	57 (52/92)
F2	68 (23/34)	56 (5/9)	76 (19/25)	61 (11/18)
F3	39 (11/28)	38 (3/8)	67 (18/27)	62 (18/29)
F4	40 (19/47)	18 (2/11)	59 (17/29)	51 (23/45)
HCV 4	17 (5/29)	7 (1/15)	88 (7/8)	50 (4/8)

higher response rates than subjects with higher body weights. Differences in response rates between treatment arms did not substantially vary with body weight.

Treatment response rates with PegIntron/REBETOL combination therapy were 49% in men and 56% in women. Response rates were lower in African American and Hispanic subjects and higher in Asians compared to Caucasians. Although African Americans had a higher proportion of poor prognostic factors compared to Caucasians, the number of non-Caucasians studied (11% of the total) was insufficient to allow meaningful conclusions about differences in response rates after adjusting for prognostic factors in this trial.

Liver biopsies were obtained before and after treatment in 68% of subjects. Compared to baseline, approximately two-thirds of subjects in all treatment groups were observed to have a modest reduction in inflammation.

Study 3

In a large United States community-based trial, 4913 subjects with chronic hepatitis C were randomized to receive PegIntron 1.5 mcg/kg subcutaneously once weekly in combination with a REBETOL dose of 800 to 1400 mg (weight-based dosing [WBD]) or 800 mg (flat) orally daily (in divided doses) for 24 or 48 weeks based on genotype. Response to treatment was defined as undetectable HCV-RNA (based on an assay with a lower limit of detection of 125 IU/mL) at 24 weeks post-treatment.

Treatment with PegIntron 1.5 mcg/kg and REBETOL 800 to 1400 mg resulted in a higher sustained virologic response compared to PegIntron in combination with a flat 800 mg daily dose of REBETOL. Subjects weighing greater than 105 kg obtained the greatest benefit with WBD, although a modest benefit was also observed in subjects weighing greater than 85 to 105 kg (see **Table 14**). The benefit of WBD in subjects weighing greater than 85 kg was observed with HCV genotypes 1-3. Insufficient data were available to reach conclusions regarding other genotypes. Use of WBD resulted in an increased incidence of anemia *[see Adverse Reactions (6.1)]*.

[See table 14 above]

A total of 1552 subjects weighing greater than 65 kg in Study 3 had genotype 2 or 3 and were randomized to 24 or 48 weeks of therapy. No additional benefit was observed with the longer treatment duration.

Study 4

A large randomized trial compared the safety and efficacy of treatment for 48 weeks with two PegIntron/REBETOL regimens [PegIntron 1.5 mcg/kg and 1 mcg/kg subcutaneously once weekly both in combination with REBETOL 800 to 1400 mg PO daily (in two divided doses)] and Pegasys 180 mcg subcutaneously once weekly in combination with Copegus 1000 to 1200 mg PO daily (in two divided doses) in 3070 treatment-naïve adults with chronic hepatitis C genotype 1. In this trial, lack of early virologic response (undetectable HCV-RNA or greater than or equal to 2 $\log_{10}$ reduction from baseline) by treatment Week 12 was the criterion for discontinuation of treatment. SVR was defined as undetectable HCV-RNA (Roche COBAS TaqMan assay, a lower limit of quantitation of 27 IU/mL) at 24 weeks post-treatment (see **Table 15**).

Table 15: Response Rate by Treatment – Study 4

% (number) of Subjects		
PegIntron 1.5 mcg/kg/ REBETOL	PegIntron 1 mcg/kg/ REBETOL	Pegasys 180 mcg/ Copegus
40 (406/ 1019)	38 (386/ 1016)	41 (423/ 1035)

Overall SVR rates were similar among the three treatment groups. Regardless of treatment group, SVR rates were lower in subjects with poor prognostic factors. Subjects with poor prognostic factors randomized to PegIntron (1.5 mcg/kg)/REBETOL or Pegasys/Copegus, however, achieved higher SVR rates compared to similar subjects randomized to PegIntron 1 mcg/kg/REBETOL. For the PegIntron 1.5 mcg/kg and REBETOL dose, SVR rates for subjects with and without the following prognostic factors were as follows: cirrhosis (10% vs. 42%), normal ALT levels (32% vs. 42%), baseline viral load greater than 600,000 IU/mL (35% vs. 61%), 40 years of age and older (38% vs. 50%), and African American race (23% vs. 44%). In subjects with undetectable HCV-RNA at treatment Week 12 who received PegIntron (1.5 mcg/kg)/REBETOL, the SVR rate was 81% (328/407).

Study 5 - REBETOL/PegIntron Combination Therapy in Prior Treatment Failures

In a noncomparative trial, 2293 subjects with moderate to severe fibrosis who failed previous treatment with combination alpha interferon/ribavirin were re-treated with PegIntron, 1.5 mcg/kg subcutaneously, once weekly, in combination with weight adjusted ribavirin. Eligible subjects included prior nonresponders (subjects who were HCV-RNA positive at the end of a minimum 12 weeks of treatment) and prior relapsers (subjects who were HCV-RNA negative at the end of a minimum 12 weeks of treatment and subsequently relapsed after post-treatment follow-up). Subjects who were negative at Week 12 were treated for 48 weeks and followed for 24 weeks post-treatment. Response to treatment was defined as undetectable HCV-RNA at 24 weeks post-treatment (measured using a research-based test, limit of detection 125 IU/mL). The overall response rate was 22% (497/2293) (99% CI: 19.5, 23.9). Subjects with the following characteristics were less likely to benefit from re-treatment: previous nonresponse, previous pegylated interferon treatment, significant bridging fibrosis or cirrhosis, and genotype 1 infection.

The re-treatment sustained virologic response rates by baseline characteristics are summarized in **Table 16**.

[See table 16 above]

Achievement of an undetectable HCV-RNA at treatment Week 12 was a strong predictor of SVR. In this trial, 1470 (64%) subjects did not achieve an undetectable HCV-RNA at treatment Week 12, and were offered enrollment into long-term treatment trials, due to an inadequate treatment response. Of the 823 (36%) subjects who were HCV-RNA undetectable at treatment Week 12, those infected with genotype 1 had an SVR of 48% (245/507), with a range of responses by fibrosis scores (F4-F2) of 39-55%. Subjects infected with genotype 2/3 who were HCV-RNA undetectable at treatment Week 12 had an overall SVR of 70% (196/281), with a range of responses by fibrosis scores (F4-F2) of 60-83%. For all genotypes, higher fibrosis scores were associated with a decreased likelihood of achieving SVR.

Pediatric Subjects

Previously untreated pediatric subjects 3 to 17 years of age with compensated chronic hepatitis C and detectable HCV-RNA were treated with REBETOL 15 mg/kg per day and PegIntron 60 mcg/m^2 once weekly for 24 or 48 weeks based on HCV genotype and baseline viral load. All subjects were to be followed for 24 weeks post-treatment. A total of 107 subjects received treatment, of which 52% were female, 89% were Caucasian, and 67% were infected with HCV Genotype 1. Subjects infected with Genotypes 1, 4 or Genotype 3 with HCV-RNA greater than or equal to 600,000 IU/mL received 48 weeks of therapy while those infected with Genotype 2 or Genotype 3 with HCV-RNA less than 600,000 IU/mL received 24 weeks of therapy. The trial results are summarized in **Table 17**.

Table 17: Sustained Virologic Response Rates by Genotype and Assigned Treatment Duration – Pediatric Trial

Genotype	All Subjects N=107: 24 Weeks — Virologic Response N*,† (%)	48 Weeks — Virologic Response N*,† (%)
All	26/27 (96.3)	44/80 (55.0)
1	-	38/72 (52.8)
2	14/15 (93.3)	-
3‡	12/12 (100)	2/3 (66.7)
4	-	4/5 (80.0)

* Response to treatment was defined as undetectable HCV-RNA at 24 weeks post-treatment.

† N=number of responders/number of subjects with given genotype, and assigned treatment duration.

‡ Subjects with genotype 3 low viral load (less than 600,000 IU/mL) were to receive 24 weeks of treatment while those with genotype 3 and high viral load were to receive 48 weeks of treatment.

14.2 REBETOL/INTRON A Combination Therapy

Adult Subjects

Previously Untreated Subjects

Adults with compensated chronic hepatitis C and detectable HCV-RNA (assessed by a central laboratory using a research-based RT-PCR assay) who were previously untreated with alpha interferon therapy were enrolled into two multicenter, double-blind trials (US and international) and randomized to receive REBETOL capsules 1200 mg/day (1000 mg/day for subjects weighing less than or equal to 75 kg) and INTRON A 3 MIU three times weekly or INTRON A and placebo for 24 or 48 weeks followed by 24

weeks of off-therapy follow-up. The international trial did not contain a 24-week INTRON A and placebo treatment arm. The US trial enrolled 912 subjects who, at baseline, were 67% male, 89% Caucasian with a mean Knodell HAI score (I+II+III) of 7.5, and 72% genotype 1. The international trial, conducted in Europe, Israel, Canada, and Australia, enrolled 799 subjects (65% male, 95% Caucasian, mean Knodell score 6.8, and 58% genotype 1).
Trial results are summarized in **Table 18.**
[See table 18 above]
Of subjects who had not achieved HCV-RNA below the limit of detection of the research-based assay by Week 24 of REBETOL/INTRON A treatment, less than 5% responded to an additional 24 weeks of combination treatment.
Among subjects with HCV Genotype 1 treated with REBETOL/INTRON A therapy who achieved HCV-RNA below the detection limit of the research-based assay by 24 weeks, those randomized to 48 weeks of treatment had higher virologic responses compared to those in the 24-week treatment group. There was no observed increase in response rates for subjects with HCV non-genotype 1 randomized to REBETOL/INTRON A therapy for 48 weeks compared to 24 weeks.

Relapse Subjects

Subjects with compensated chronic hepatitis C and detectable HCV-RNA (assessed by a central laboratory using a research-based RT-PCR assay) who had relapsed following one or two courses of interferon therapy (defined as abnormal serum ALT levels) were enrolled into two multicenter, double-blind trials (US and international) and randomized to receive REBETOL 1200 mg/day (1000 mg/day for subjects weighing ≤75 kg) and INTRON A 3 MIU three times weekly or INTRON A and placebo for 24 weeks followed by 24 weeks of off-therapy follow-up. The US trial enrolled 153 subjects who, at baseline, were 67% male, 92% Caucasian with a mean Knodell HAI score (I+II+III) of 6.8, and 58% genotype 1. The international trial, conducted in Europe, Israel, Canada, and Australia, enrolled 192 subjects (64% male, 95% Caucasian, mean Knodell score 6.6, and 56% genotype 1). Trial results are summarized in **Table 19.**
[See table 19 at right]
Virologic and histologic responses were similar among male and female subjects in both the previously untreated and relapse trials.

Pediatric Subjects

Pediatric subjects 3 to 16 years of age with compensated chronic hepatitis C and detectable HCV-RNA (assessed by a central laboratory using a research-based RT-PCR assay) were treated with REBETOL 15 mg/kg per day and INTRON A 3 MIU/m^2 three times weekly for 48 weeks followed by 24 weeks of off-therapy follow-up. A total of 118 subjects received treatment, of which 57% were male, 80% Caucasian, and 78% genotype 1. Subjects less than 5 years of age received REBETOL oral solution and those 5 years of age or older received either REBETOL oral solution or capsules.
Trial results are summarized in **Table 20.**

Table 20: Virologic Response: Previously Untreated Pediatric Subjects*

	INTRON A 3 MIU/m^2 three times weekly/ REBETOL 15 mg/kg/day
Overall Response† (N=118)	54 (46)
Genotype 1 (N=92)	33 (36)
Genotype non-1 (N=26)	21 (81)

* Number (%) of subjects.
† Defined as HCV-RNA below limit of detection using a research-based RT-PCR assay at end of treatment and during follow-up period.

Subjects with viral genotype 1, regardless of viral load, had a lower response rate to INTRON A/REBETOL combination therapy compared to subjects with genotype non-1, 36% vs. 81%. Subjects with both poor prognostic factors (genotype 1 and high viral load) had a response rate of 26% (13/50).

16 HOW SUPPLIED/STORAGE AND HANDLING

REBETOL 200 mg Capsules are white, opaque capsules with REBETOL, 200 mg, and the Schering Corporation logo imprinted on the capsule shell; the capsules are packaged in a bottle containing 56 capsules (NDC 0085-1351-05), 70 capsules (NDC 0085-1385-07), and 84 capsules (NDC 0085-1194-03).
REBETOL Oral Solution 40 mg per mL is a clear, colorless to pale or light yellow bubble gum-flavored liquid and it is packaged in 4-oz amber glass bottles (100 mL/bottle) with child-resistant closures (NDC 0085-1318-01).

Table 18: Virologic and Histologic Responses: Previously Untreated Subjects*

	US Trial				International Trial		
	24 weeks of treatment		48 weeks of treatment		24 weeks of treatment	48 weeks of treatment	
	INTRON A/ REBETOL (N=228)	INTRON A/ Placebo (N=231)	INTRON A/ REBETOL (N=228)	INTRON A/ Placebo (N=225)	INTRON A/ REBETOL (N=265)	INTRON A/ REBETOL (N=268)	INTRON A/ Placebo (N=266)
Virologic Response							
Responder†	65 (29)	13 (6)	85 (37)	27 (12)	86 (32)	113 (42)	46 (17)
Nonresponder	147 (64)	194 (84)	110 (48)	168 (75)	158 (60)	120 (45)	196 (74)
Missing Data	16 (7)	24 (10)	33 (14)	30 (13)	21 (8)	35 (13)	24 (9)
Histologic Response							
Improvement‡	102 (45)	77 (33)	96 (42)	65 (29)	103 (39)	102 (38)	69 (26)
No improvement	77 (34)	99 (43)	61 (27)	93 (41)	85 (32)	58 (22)	111 (41)
Missing Data	49 (21)	55 (24)	71 (31)	67 (30)	77 (29)	108 (40)	86 (32)

* Number (%) of subjects.
† Defined as HCV-RNA below limit of detection using a research-based RT-PCR assay at end of treatment and during follow-up period.
‡ Defined as post-treatment (end of follow-up) minus pretreatment liver biopsy Knodell HAI score (I+II+III) improvement of greater than or equal to 2 points.

Table 19: Virologic and Histologic Responses: Relapse Subjects*

	US Trial		International Trial	
	INTRON A/ REBETOL (N=77)	INTRON A/ Placebo (N=76)	INTRON A/ REBETOL (N=96)	INTRON A/ Placebo (N=96)
Virologic Response				
Responder†	33 (43)	3 (4)	46 (48)	5 (5)
Nonresponder	36 (47)	66 (87)	45 (47)	91 (95)
Missing Data	8 (10)	7 (9)	5 (5)	0 (0)
Histologic Response				
Improvement‡	38 (49)	27 (36)	49 (51)	30 (31)
No improvement	23 (30)	37 (49)	29 (30)	44 (46)
Missing Data	16 (21)	12 (16)	18 (19)	22 (23)

* Number (%) of subjects.
† Defined as HCV-RNA below limit of detection using a research-based RT-PCR assay at end of treatment and during follow-up period.
‡ Defined as post-treatment (end of follow-up) minus pretreatment liver biopsy Knodell HAI score (I+II+III) improvement of greater than or equal to 2 points.

The bottle of REBETOL Capsules should be stored at 25°C (77°F); excursions permitted to 15-30°C (59-86°F) [see USP Controlled Room Temperature].
REBETOL Oral Solution should be stored between 2-8°C (36-46°F) or at 25°C (77°F); excursions permitted to 15-30°C (59-86°F) [see USP Controlled Room Temperature].

17 PATIENT COUNSELING INFORMATION

See FDA-Approved Patient Labeling (Medication Guide).

17.1 Anemia

The most common adverse experience occurring with REBETOL capsules is anemia, which may be severe *[see Warnings and Precautions (5.2) and Adverse Reactions (6)]*. Patients should be advised that laboratory evaluations are required prior to starting therapy and periodically thereafter *[see Dosage and Administration (2.3)]*. It is advised that patients be well hydrated, especially during the initial stages of treatment.

17.2 Pregnancy

Patients must be informed that REBETOL capsules and oral solution may cause birth defects and death of the unborn child. REBETOL must not be used by women who are pregnant or by men whose female partners are pregnant. Extreme care must be taken to avoid pregnancy in female patients and in female partners of male patients taking REBETOL. REBETOL should not be initiated until a report of a negative pregnancy test has been obtained immediately prior to initiation of therapy. Patients must perform a pregnancy test monthly during therapy and for 6 months post therapy. Women of childbearing potential must be counseled about use of effective contraception (two reliable forms) prior to initiating therapy. Patients (male and female) must be advised of the teratogenic/embryocidal risks and must be instructed to practice effective contraception during REBETOL and for 6 months post therapy. Patients (male and female) should be advised to notify the physician immediately in the event of a pregnancy *[see Contraindications (4), Warnings and Precautions (5.1), and Use in Specific Populations (8.1)]*.
If pregnancy does occur during treatment or during 6 months post therapy, the patient must be advised of the teratogenic risk of REBETOL therapy to the fetus. Patients, or partners of patients, should immediately report any pregnancy that occurs during treatment or within 6 months after treatment cessation to their physician. Prescribers should report such cases by calling 1-800-593-2214.

17.3 Risks versus Benefits

Patients receiving REBETOL capsules should be informed of the benefits and risks associated with treatment, directed in its appropriate use, and referred to the patient **MEDICATION GUIDE**. Patients should be informed that the effect of treatment of hepatitis C infection on transmission is not known, and that appropriate precautions to prevent transmission of the hepatitis C virus should be taken.
Patients should be informed about what to do in the event they miss a dose of REBETOL; the missed dose should be taken as soon as possible during the same day. Patients should not double the next dose. Patients should be advised to contact their healthcare provider if they have questions.

REBETOL Oral Solution manufactured for:
Merck Sharp & Dohme Corp., a subsidiary of
MERCK & CO., INC.
Whitehouse Station, NJ 08889, USA
Manufactured by:
Schering-Plough Canada, Inc.
Pointe Claire, Quebec, Canada
REBETOL Capsules manufactured by:
Merck Sharp & Dohme Corp., a subsidiary of
MERCK & CO., INC.
Whitehouse Station, NJ 08889, USA
U.S. Patent No. 6,790,837.

USPI-MTL-89081305R026

MEDICATION GUIDE
REBETOL® (REB-eh-tol)
(ribavirin)
Capsules and Oral Solution

Read this Medication Guide before you start taking REBETOL, and each time you get a refill. There may be new information. This information does not take the place of talking to your health care provider about your medical condition or your treatment.

What is the most important information I should know about REBETOL®?

1. **Do Not take REBETOL alone to treat chronic hepatitis C infection.** REBETOL should be used in combination with **either interferon alfa-2b (Intron® A) or peginterferon alfa-2b (PegIntron®)** to treat chronic hepatitis C infection.
2. **REBETOL may cause a significant drop in your red blood cell count and cause anemia in some cases. Anemia has been associated with worsening of Heart Problems, and in rare cases can cause a Heart Attack and Death.** Tell your health care provider if you have ever had any heart problems. REBETOL may not be right for you. **Seek medical attention right away if you experience chest pain.**
3. **REBETOL may cause Birth Defects or the Death of your unborn baby. Do Not Take REBETOL if you or your sexual partner is pregnant or plan to become pregnant. Do Not become Pregnant within 6 months after discontinuing REBETOL therapy.** You must use 2 forms of birth control when you take REBETOL and for the 6 months after treatment.
   - Females must have a pregnancy test before starting REBETOL, every month while taking REBETOL, and every month for the 6 months after the last dose of REBETOL.
   - **If you or your female sexual partner becomes pregnant while taking REBETOL or within 6 months after you stop taking REBETOL, tell your health care provider right away. You or your health care provider should contact the REBETOL pregnancy registry by calling 1-800-593-2214. The REBETOL pregnancy registry collects information about what happens to mothers and their babies if the mother takes REBETOL while she is pregnant.**

What is REBETOL®?

REBETOL is a medicine used with either interferon alfa-2b (Intron A) or peginterferon alfa-2b (PegIntron) to treat chronic (lasting a long time) hepatitis C infection in people 3 years and older with liver disease.

It is not known if REBETOL use for longer than 1 year is safe and will work.

It is not known if REBETOL use in children younger than 3 years old is safe and will work.

Who should not take REBETOL®?

See "What is the most important information I should know about REBETOL?"

Do not take REBETOL if you have:
- or ever had serious allergic reactions to the ingredients in REBETOL. See the end of this Medication Guide for a complete list of ingredients.
- certain types of hepatitis (autoimmune hepatitis).
- certain blood disorders (hemoglobinopathies).
- severe kidney disease.
- taken or currently take didanosine (VIDEX®).

Talk to your health care provider before taking REBETOL if you have any of these conditions.

What should I tell my health care provider before taking REBETOL®?

Before you take REBETOL, tell your health care provider if you have or ever had:
- treatment for hepatitis C that did not work for you.
- breathing problems. REBETOL may cause or worsen breathing problems you already have.
- vision problems. REBETOL may cause eye problems or worsen eye problems you already have. You should have an eye exam before you start treatment with REBETOL.
- certain blood disorders such as anemia (low red blood cell count).
- high blood pressure, heart problems, or have had a heart attack. Your health care provider should check your blood and heart before you start treatment with REBETOL.
- thyroid problems.
- liver problems other than hepatitis C infection.
- human immunodeficiency virus (HIV) or any immunity problems.
- mental health problems, including depression or thoughts of suicide.
- kidney problems.
- an organ transplant.
- diabetes. REBETOL may make your diabetes worse or harder to treat.
- any other medical condition.
- are breastfeeding. It is not known if REBETOL passes into your breast milk. You and your health care provider should decide if you will take REBETOL or breastfeed.

Tell your health care provider about all the medicines you take, including prescription medicines, vitamins, and herbal supplements. REBETOL may affect the way other medicines work.

Especially tell your health care provider if you take didanosine (VIDEX®) or azathioprine (Imuran and Azasan).

Know the medicines you take. Keep a list of them to show your health care provider or pharmacist when you get a new medicine.

How should I take REBETOL®?
- Take REBETOL exactly as your health care provider tells you. Your health care provider will tell you how much REBETOL to take and when to take it.
- Take REBETOL with food.
- Take **REBETOL Capsules** whole. Do not open, break, or crush **REBETOL Capsules** before swallowing. If you cannot swallow **REBETOL Capsules** whole, tell your health care provider.
- If you miss a dose of REBETOL, take the missed dose as soon as possible during the same day. Do not double the next dose. If you have questions about what to do, call your health care provider.
- If you take too much REBETOL, call your health care provider or Poison Control Center at 1-800-222-1222, or go to the nearest hospital emergency room right away.

What are the possible side effects of REBETOL®?

REBETOL may cause serious side effects, including:

See "What is the most important information I should know about REBETOL?"
- **Swelling and irritation of your pancreas (pancreatitis).** You may have stomach pain, nausea, vomiting, or diarrhea.
- **Serious breathing problems.** Difficulty breathing may be a sign of a serious lung infection (pneumonia) that can lead to death.
- **Serious eye problems** that may lead to vision loss or blindness.
- **Dental problems.** Your mouth may be very dry, which can lead to problems with your teeth and gums.
- **Severe depression.**
- **Suicidal thoughts and attempts.** Adults and children who take REBETOL, especially teenagers, are more likely to have suicidal thoughts or attempt to hurt themselves while taking REBETOL. Call your health care provider right away or go to the nearest hospital emergency room if you have new or worse depression or thoughts about suicide or dying.
- **Severe blood disorders.** An increased risk when used in combination with pegylated alpha interferons and azathioprine.
- **Weight loss and slowed growth in children.**

Tell your health care provider right away if you have any side effect that bothers you or that does not go away.

The most common side effects of REBETOL include:
- flu-like symptoms - feeling tired, headache, shaking along with high temperature (fever), nausea, and muscle aches.
- mood changes, feeling irritable.

The most common side effects of REBETOL in children include:
- a decrease in the blood cells that fight infection (neutropenia).
- a decrease in appetite.
- stomach pain and vomiting.

Tell your health care provider if you have any side effect that bothers you or that does not go away.

These are not all the possible side effects of REBETOL. For more information ask your health care provider or pharmacist.

Call your doctor for medical advice about side effects. You may report side effects to FDA at 1-800-FDA-1088.

How should I store REBETOL®?
- Store **REBETOL Capsules** between 59-86°F (15-30°C).
- Store **REBETOL Oral Solution** between 59-86°F (15-30°C) or in the refrigerator between 36-46°F (2-8°C).

Keep REBETOL and all medicines out of the reach of children.

GENERAL INFORMATION ABOUT THE SAFE AND EFFECTIVE USE OF REBETOL®.

It is not known if treatment with REBETOL will cure hepatitis C virus infections or prevent cirrhosis, liver failure, or liver cancer that can be caused by hepatitis C virus infections. It is not known if taking REBETOL will prevent you from infecting another person with the hepatitis C virus.

Medicines are sometimes prescribed for purposes other than those listed in a Medication Guide. Do not use REBETOL for a condition for which it was not prescribed. Do not give REBETOL to other people, even if they have the same symptoms that you have. It may harm them.

This Medication Guide summarizes the most important information about REBETOL. If you would like more information, talk with your health care provider. You can ask your pharmacist or health care provider for information about REBETOL that is written for health professionals.

What are the ingredients in REBETOL®?

Active ingredients: ribavirin

REBETOL Capsules

Inactive ingredients: microcrystalline cellulose, lactose monohydrate, croscarmellose sodium, and magnesium stearate. The capsule shell consists of gelatin, sodium lauryl sulfate, silicon dioxide, and titanium dioxide. The capsule is printed with edible blue pharmaceutical ink which is made of shellac, anhydrous ethyl alcohol, isopropyl alcohol, n-butyl alcohol, propylene glycol, ammonium hydroxide, and FD&C Blue #2 aluminum lake.

REBETOL Oral Solution

Inactive ingredients: sucrose, glycerin, sorbitol, propylene glycol, sodium citrate, citric acid, sodium benzoate, natural and artificial flavor for bubble gum # 15864, and water.

This Medication Guide has been approved by the U.S. Food and Drug Administration.

REBETOL Oral Solution manufactured for:
Merck Sharp & Dohme Corp., a subsidiary of
MERCK & CO., INC.
Whitehouse Station, NJ 08889, USA
Manufactured by: Schering-Plough Canada, Inc., Pointe Claire, Quebec, Canada
REBETOL Capsules manufactured by:
Merck Sharp & Dohme Corp., a subsidiary of
MERCK & CO., INC.
Whitehouse Station, NJ 08889, USA
VIDEX® is a registered trademark of Bristol-Myers Squibb Company.

Revised: 05/2013
MG-MTL-89081305R016

Shown in Product Identification Guide, page 308

RECOMBIVAX HB® ℞
[re-com-biv-ax]
HEPATITIS B VACCINE (RECOMBINANT)

DESCRIPTION

RECOMBIVAX HB® Hepatitis B Vaccine (Recombinant) is a non-infectious subunit viral vaccine derived from hepatitis B surface antigen (HBsAg) produced in yeast cells. A portion of the hepatitis B virus gene, coding for HBsAg, is cloned into yeast, and the vaccine for hepatitis B is produced from cultures of this recombinant yeast strain according to methods developed in the Merck Research Laboratories.

The antigen is harvested and purified from fermentation cultures of a recombinant strain of the yeast *Saccharomyces cerevisiae* containing the gene for the *adw* subtype of HBsAg. The fermentation process involves growth of *Saccharomyces cerevisiae* on a complex fermentation medium which consists of an extract of yeast, soy peptone, dextrose, amino acids and mineral salts. The HBsAg protein is released from the yeast cells by cell disruption and purified by a series of physical and chemical methods. The purified protein is treated in phosphate buffer with formaldehyde and then coprecipitated with alum (potassium aluminum sulfate) to form bulk vaccine adjuvanted with amorphous aluminum hydroxyphosphate sulfate. Each dose contains less than 1% yeast protein. The vaccine produced by the Merck method has been shown to be comparable to the plasma-derived vaccine in terms of animal potency (mouse, monkey, and chimpanzee) and protective efficacy (chimpanzee and human).

The vaccine against hepatitis B, prepared from recombinant yeast cultures, is free of association with human blood or blood products.

Each lot of hepatitis B vaccine is tested for sterility.

RECOMBIVAX HB is a sterile suspension for intramuscular injection. However, for persons at risk of hemorrhage following intramuscular injection, the vaccine may be administered subcutaneously. (See DOSAGE AND ADMINISTRATION).

RECOMBIVAX HB Hepatitis B Vaccine (Recombinant) is supplied in three formulations. (See HOW SUPPLIED.)

Pediatric/Adolescent Formulation (Without Preservative), 10 mcg/mL: each 0.5 mL dose contains 5 mcg of hepatitis B surface antigen.

Adult Formulation (Without Preservative), 10 mcg/mL: each 1 mL dose contains 10 mcg of hepatitis B surface antigen.

Dialysis Formulation (Without Preservative), 40 mcg/mL: each 1 mL dose contains 40 mcg of hepatitis B surface antigen.

All formulations contain approximately 0.5 mg of aluminum (provided as amorphous aluminum hydroxyphosphate sulfate, previously referred to as aluminum hydroxide) per mL of vaccine. In each formulation, hepatitis B surface antigen is adsorbed onto approximately 0.5 mg of aluminum (provided as amorphous aluminum hydroxyphosphate sulfate) per mL of vaccine. The vaccine contains <15 mcg/mL residual formaldehyde. The vaccine is of the *adw* subtype. RECOMBIVAX HB is indicated for vaccination of persons at risk of infection from hepatitis B virus including all known subtypes. RECOMBIVAX HB Dialysis Formulation is indicated for vaccination of adult predialysis and dialysis patients against infection caused by all known subtypes of hepatitis B virus.

CLINICAL PHARMACOLOGY

Hepatitis B virus is one of several hepatitis viruses that cause a systemic infection, with a major pathology in the liver. These include hepatitis A virus, hepatitis D virus, and hepatitis C and E viruses, previously referred to as non-A, non-B hepatitis viruses.

Hepatitis B virus is an important cause of viral hepatitis. There is no specific treatment for this disease. The incubation period for hepatitis B is relatively long; six weeks to six months may elapse between exposure and the onset of clinical symptoms. The prognosis following infection with hepatitis B virus is variable and dependent on at least three factors: (1) Age — Infants and younger children usually experience milder initial disease than older persons;{1} (2) Dose of virus — The higher the dose, the more likely acute icteric hepatitis B will result;{1} and, (3) Severity of associated underlying disease — Underlying malignancy or preexisting hepatic disease predisposes to increased morbidity and mortality.{1}

Persistence of viral infection (the chronic hepatitis B virus carrier state) occurs in 5-10% of persons following acute hepatitis B, and occurs more frequently after initial anicteric hepatitis B than after initial icteric disease. Consequently, carriers of hepatitis B surface antigen (HBsAg) frequently give no history of having had recognized acute hepatitis. The Centers for Disease Control and Prevention (CDC) estimates that there are more than 300 million chronic carriers worldwide and 1.25 million chronic carriers of hepatitis B virus in the USA.{29,30} Chronic carriers represent the largest human reservoir of hepatitis B virus.

Serious complications and sequelae of hepatitis B virus infection include massive hepatic necrosis, cirrhosis of the liver and chronic active hepatitis. More than one million people worldwide die each year of hepatitis B-associated acute and chronic liver disease.{33} In the United States, hepatitis B-virus-related acute and chronic liver disease causes approximately 4-5000 deaths annually.{29,30}

Reduced Risk of Hepatocellular Carcinoma

Hepatocellular carcinoma is another serious complication of hepatitis B virus infection. Studies have demonstrated the link between chronic hepatitis B infection and hepatocellular carcinoma; 80% of primary liver cancers are caused by hepatitis B virus infection. The CDC has recognized hepatitis B vaccine as the first anti-cancer vaccine because it can prevent primary liver cancer.{34}

There is also evidence that several diseases other than hepatitis have been associated with hepatitis B virus infection through an immunologic mechanism involving antigen-antibody complexes. Such diseases include a syndrome with rash, urticaria, and arthralgia resembling serum sickness; periarteritis nodosa; membranous glomerulonephritis; and infantile papular acrodermatitis.{3,4}

Although the vehicles for transmission of the virus are often blood and blood products, viral antigen has also been found in tears, saliva, breast milk, urine, semen and vaginal secretions. Hepatitis B virus is capable of surviving at least a month{29} on environmental surfaces exposed to body fluids containing hepatitis B virus. Infection may occur when hepatitis B virus, transmitted by infected body fluids, is implanted via mucous surfaces or percutaneously introduced through accidental or deliberate breaks in the skin.

Transmission of hepatitis B virus infection is often associated with close interpersonal contact with an infected individual and with crowded living conditions. In such circumstances, transmission by inoculation via routes other than overt percutaneous ones may be quite common.{1} Perinatal transmission of hepatitis B infection from infected mother to child, at or shortly after birth, can occur if the mother is a hepatitis B surface antigen (HBsAg) carrier or if the mother has an acute hepatitis B infection in the third trimester. Infection in infancy by the hepatitis B virus usually leads to the chronic carrier state. Without prophylaxis, infants born to women whose sera are positive for both the hepatitis B surface antigen and the e antigen have an 85-90% likelihood of being infected and becoming a chronic carrier.{5,6} Well-controlled studies have shown that administration of three 0.5 mL doses of Hepatitis B Immune Globulin (Human) - HBIG starting at birth is 75% effective in preventing establishment of the chronic carrier state in these infants during the first year of life.{6} However, the protective effect of HBIG is transient.

Hepatitis B is endemic throughout the world and is a serious medical problem in population groups at increased risk. Because vaccination limited to high-risk individuals has failed to substantially lower the overall incidence of hepatitis B infection, both the Advisory Committee on Immunization Practices (ACIP) and the Committee on Infectious Diseases of the American Academy of Pediatrics (AAP) have also endorsed universal infant immunization as part of a comprehensive strategy for the control of hepatitis B infection.{7,8} In addition, the ACIP also recommends hepatitis B vaccination for all infants and children born after November 21, 1991 and catch-up vaccination of children at high risk of infection (children <11 years of age in households of Pacific Islander ethnicity or of first generation immigrants/refugees from countries with an intermediate or high endemicity of infection).{30} These advisory groups further recommend broad-based vaccination of adolescents. The ACIP recommends that all individuals not previously vaccinated with hepatitis B vaccine be vaccinated at 11-12 years of age with the age-appropriate dose of vaccine and that the vaccination schedule take into account the feasibility of delivering three doses of vaccine to this age group. In addition, older unvaccinated adolescents with identified risk factors for hepatitis B virus infection should also be vaccinated.{30} Similarly, the AAP recommends that universal immunization of all adolescents should be implemented when resources permit with emphasis on those individuals in high-risk settings.{8} A National Institutes of Health Consensus Development Conference Panel on the management of hepatitis C recommends the immunization of all hepatitis C virus (HCV) positive individuals with hepatitis B vaccine.{35} (Refer to INDICATIONS AND USAGE.)

Numerous epidemiological studies have shown that persons who develop anti-HBs following active infection with the hepatitis B virus are protected against the disease on reexposure to the virus.{9}

Clinical studies have shown that RECOMBIVAX HB when injected into the deltoid muscle induced protective levels of antibody in 96% of 1213 healthy adults who received the recommended 3-dose regimen. Antibody responses varied with age; a protective level of antibody was induced in 98% of 787 young adults 20-29 years of age, 94% of 249 adults 30-39 years of age and in 89% of 177 adults ≥40 years of age.{10} Studies with hepatitis B vaccine derived from plasma have shown that a lower response rate (81%) to vaccine may be obtained if the vaccine is administered as a buttock injection.{11} Seroconversion rates and geometric mean antibody titers were measured 1 to 2 months after the third dose. Multiple clinical studies have defined a protective antibody (anti-HBs) level as 1) 10 or more sample ratio units (SRU) as determined by radioimmunoassay or 2) a positive result as determined by enzyme immunoassay.{2} Note: 10 SRU is comparable to 10 mIU/mL of antibody.{12,13,14,15}

RECOMBIVAX HB was shown to be highly immunogenic in clinical studies involving infants, children, and adolescents. Three 5 mcg doses of vaccine induced a protective level of antibody in 100% of 92 infants, 99% of 129 children, and in 99% of 112 adolescents{10} (see DOSAGE AND ADMINISTRATION).

The protective efficacy of three 5 mcg doses of RECOMBIVAX HB has been demonstrated in neonates born of mothers positive for both HBsAg and HBeAg (a core-associated antigenic complex which correlates with high infectivity). In a clinical study of infants who received one dose of HBIG at birth followed by the recommended three-dose regimen of RECOMBIVAX HB, chronic infection had not occurred in 96% of 130 infants after nine months of follow-up.{16} The estimated efficacy in prevention of chronic hepatitis B infection was 95% as compared to the infection rate in untreated historical controls.{17} Significantly fewer neonates became chronically infected when given one dose of HBIG at birth followed by the recommended three-dose regimen of RECOMBIVAX HB when compared to historical controls who received only a single dose of HBIG.{6} Testing for HBsAg and anti-HBs is recommended at 12-15 months of age. If HBsAg is not detectable, and anti-HBs is present, the child has been protected.

As demonstrated in the above study, HBIG, when administered simultaneously with RECOMBIVAX HB at separate body sites, did not interfere with the induction of protective antibodies against hepatitis B virus elicited by the vaccine.

For adolescents (11 through 15 years of age), the immunogenicity of a two-dose regimen (10 mcg at 0 and 4-6 months) was compared with that of the standard three-dose regimen (5 mcg at 0, 1, and 6 months) in an open, randomized, multicenter study. The proportion of adolescents receiving the two-dose regimen who developed a protective level of antibody one month after the last dose (99% of 255 subjects) appears similar to that among adolescents who received the three-dose regimen (98% of 121 subjects). After adolescents (11 through 15 years of age) received the first 10-mcg dose of the two-dose regimen, the proportion who developed a protective level of antibody was approximately 72%.{10}

In one published study, the seroprotection rates in individuals with chronic HCV infection given the standard regimen of RECOMBIVAX HB was approximately 70%.{36} In a second published study of intravenous drug users given an accelerated schedule of RECOMBIVAX HB, infection with HCV did not affect the response to RECOMBIVAX HB.{37}

As with other hepatitis B vaccines, the duration of the protective effect of RECOMBIVAX HB in healthy vaccinees is unknown at present, and the need for booster doses is not yet defined. However, long-term follow-up (5 to 9 years) of approximately 3000 high-risk vaccinees (infants of carrier mothers, male homosexuals, Alaskan Natives) who developed an anti-HBs titer of ≥10 mIU/mL when given a similar plasma-derived vaccine at intervals of 0, 1, and 6 months showed that no subjects developed clinically apparent hepatitis B infection and that 5 subjects developed antigenemia, even though up to half of the subjects failed to maintain a titer at this level.{18-21} Persistence of vaccine-induced immunologic memory among healthy vaccinees who responded to a primary course of plasma-derived or recombinant hepatitis B vaccine has been demonstrated by an anamnestic antibody response to a booster dose of RECOMBIVAX HB given 5-12 years later.{22}

Predialysis and Dialysis Patients

Predialysis and dialysis adult patients respond less well to hepatitis B vaccines than do healthy individuals; however, vaccination of adult patients early in the course of their renal disease produces higher seroconversion rates than vaccination after dialysis has been initiated.{30} In addition, the responses to these vaccines may be lower if the vaccine is administered as a buttock injection. When 40 mcg of Hepatitis B Vaccine (Recombinant), was administered in the deltoid muscle, 89% of 28 participants developed anti-HBs with 86% achieving levels ≥10 mIU/mL. However, when the same dosage of this vaccine was administered inappropriately either in the buttock or a combination of buttock and deltoid, 62% of 47 participants developed anti-HBs with 55% achieving levels of ≥10 mIU/mL.{10}

A booster dose or revaccination with RECOMBIVAX HB Dialysis Formulation may be considered in predialysis/dialysis patients if the anti-HBs level is less than 10 mIU/mL.{23}

Reports in the literature describe a more virulent form of hepatitis B associated with superinfections or coinfections by delta virus, an incomplete RNA virus. Delta virus can only infect and cause illness in persons infected with hepatitis B virus since the delta agent requires a coat of HBsAg in order to become infectious. Therefore, persons immune to hepatitis B virus infection should also be immune to delta virus infection.{2}

Interchangeability of Plasma-Derived and Recombinant Hepatitis B Vaccines

Although there have been no clinical studies in which a three-dose vaccine series was initiated with HEPTAVAX-B® (Hepatitis B Vaccine) and completed with RECOMBIVAX HB, or vice versa, extensive *in vitro* and *in vivo* studies have demonstrated that these two vaccines are immunologically comparable.{22,24-28}

INDICATIONS AND USAGE

RECOMBIVAX HB is indicated for vaccination against infection caused by all known subtypes of hepatitis B virus.

RECOMBIVAX HB Dialysis Formulation is indicated for vaccination of adult predialysis and dialysis patients against infection caused by all known subtypes of hepatitis B virus.

Vaccination with RECOMBIVAX HB is recommended for:

1. Infants including those born to HBsAg positive mothers (high-risk infants).
2. Children born after November 21, 1991.{30}
3. Adolescents (see CLINICAL PHARMACOLOGY).
4. Other persons of all ages in areas of high prevalence or those who are or may be at increased risk of infection with hepatitis B virus, such as:{30}

• *Health Care Personnel*

Dentists and oral surgeons.
Physicians and surgeons.
Nurses.
Paramedical personnel and custodial staff who may be exposed to the virus via blood or other patient specimens.
Dental hygienists and dental nurses.
Laboratory personnel handling blood, blood products, and other patient specimens.
Dental, medical and nursing students.

- *Selected Patients and Patient Contacts*
  Staff in hemodialysis units and hematology/oncology units.
  Hemodialysis patients and patients with early renal failure before they require hemodialysis.
  Patients requiring frequent and/or large volume blood transfusions or clotting factor concentrates (e.g., persons with hemophilia, thalassemia).
  Individuals with hepatitis C virus infection.{35}
  Clients (residents) and staff of institutions for the mentally handicapped.
  Classroom contacts of deinstitutionalized mentally handicapped persons who have persistent hepatitis B surface antigenemia and who show aggressive behavior.
  Household and other intimate contacts of persons with persistent hepatitis B surface antigenemia.
- *Sub-populations with a known high incidence of the disease, such as:*
  Alaskan Natives.
  Pacific Islanders.
  Refugees from areas where hepatitis B virus infection is endemic.
  Adoptees from countries where hepatitis B virus infection is endemic.
- *International Travelers*
- *Military Personnel identified as being at increased risk*
- *Morticians and Embalmers*
- *Blood bank and plasma fractionation workers*
- *Persons at Increased Risk of the Disease Due to Their Sexual Practices, such as:*
  Persons who have heterosexual activity with multiple partners.
  Persons who repeatedly contract sexually transmitted diseases.
  Homosexual and bisexual adolescent and adult men.
  Female prostitutes.
- *Prisoners*
- *Injection drug users*

Neither dosage strength will prevent hepatitis caused by other agents, such as hepatitis A virus, hepatitis C virus, hepatitis E virus or other viruses known to infect the liver.

Revaccination

See CLINICAL PHARMACOLOGY.

Use with Other Vaccines

Results from clinical studies indicate that RECOMBIVAX HB can be administered concomitantly with DTP (Diphtheria, Tetanus and whole cell Pertussis), OPV (oral Poliomyelitis vaccine), M-M-R® II (Measles, Mumps, and Rubella Virus Vaccine Live), Liquid PedvaxHIB® [Haemophilus b Conjugate Vaccine (Meningococcal Protein Conjugate)] or a booster dose of DTaP [Diphtheria, Tetanus, acellular Pertussis], using separate sites and syringes for injectable vaccines. No impairment of immune response to individually tested vaccine antigens was demonstrated.

The type, frequency and severity of adverse experiences observed in these studies with RECOMBIVAX HB were similar to those seen when the other vaccines were given alone.

In addition, an HBsAg-containing product, COMVAX® [Haemophilus b Conjugate (Meningococcal Protein Conjugate) and Hepatitis B (Recombinant) Vaccine], was given concomitantly with eIPV (enhanced inactivated Poliovirus vaccine) or VARIVAX® [Varicella Virus Vaccine Live (Oka/Merck)], using separate sites and syringes for injectable vaccines. No impairment of immune response to these individually tested vaccine antigens was demonstrated. No serious vaccine-related adverse events were reported.

COMVAX has also been administered concomitantly with the primary series of DTaP to a limited number of infants. No serious vaccine-related adverse events were reported.{10}

Separate sites and syringes should be used for simultaneous administration of injectable vaccines.

CONTRAINDICATIONS

Hypersensitivity to yeast or any component of the vaccine.

WARNINGS

Patients who develop symptoms suggestive of hypersensitivity after an injection should not receive further injections of the vaccine (see CONTRAINDICATIONS).

Because of the long incubation period for hepatitis B, it is possible for unrecognized infection to be present at the time the vaccine is given. The vaccine may not prevent hepatitis B in such patients.

PRECAUTIONS

General

As with any percutaneous vaccine, epinephrine (1:1000) should be available for immediate use should an anaphylactoid reaction occur.

Use caution when vaccinating latex-sensitive individuals since the vial stopper and the syringe plunger stopper and tip cap contain dry natural latex rubber that may cause allergic reactions.

Any serious active infection including febrile illness is reason for delaying use of the vaccine except when in the opinion of the physician, withholding the vaccine entails a greater risk.

Caution and appropriate care should be exercised in administering the vaccine to individuals with severely compromised cardiopulmonary status or to others in whom a febrile or systemic reaction could pose a significant risk.

Instructions to Healthcare Provider

The healthcare provider should determine the current health status and previous vaccination history of the vaccinee.

The healthcare provider should question the patient, parent or guardian about reactions to a previous dose of RECOMBIVAX HB or other hepatitis B vaccines.

The healthcare provider must record in the patient's permanent record: the manufacturer, lot number, date of administration, and the name and address of the person administering the vaccine.

Injection of a blood vessel should be avoided.

Information for Vaccine Recipients and Parents/Guardians

The healthcare provider should provide the vaccine information required to be given with each vaccination to the patient, parent or guardian.

The healthcare provider should inform the patient, parent or guardian of the benefits and risks associated with vaccination, as well as the importance of completing the immunization series. For risks associated with vaccination, see WARNINGS, PRECAUTIONS, and ADVERSE REACTIONS.

Patients, parents and guardians should be instructed to report any serious adverse reactions to their healthcare provider, who in turn should report such events to the U.S. Department of Health and Human Services through the Vaccine Adverse Event Reporting System (VAERS), 1-800-822-7967.{31} The healthcare provider should inform the parent or guardian of the National Vaccine Injury Compensation Program (NVICP), 1-800-338-2382.

Drug Interactions

There are no known drug interactions. (See INDICATIONS AND USAGE, Use with Other Vaccines.)

Carcinogenesis, Mutagenesis, Impairment of Fertility

RECOMBIVAX HB has not been evaluated for its carcinogenic or mutagenic potential, or its potential to impair fertility.

Pregnancy

Pregnancy Category C: Animal reproduction studies have not been conducted with the vaccine. It is also not known whether the vaccine can cause fetal harm when administered to a pregnant woman or can affect reproduction capacity. The vaccine should be given to a pregnant woman only if clearly needed.

Nursing Mothers

It is not known whether the vaccine is excreted in human milk. Because many drugs are excreted in human milk, caution should be exercised when the vaccine is administered to a nursing woman.

Pediatric Use

RECOMBIVAX HB has been shown to be usually well-tolerated and highly immunogenic in infants and children of all ages. Newborns also respond well; maternally transferred antibodies do not interfere with the active immune response to the vaccine. See DOSAGE AND ADMINISTRATION for recommended pediatric dosage and for recommended dosage for infants born to HBsAg positive mothers.

The safety and effectiveness of RECOMBIVAX HB Dialysis Formulation in children have not been established.

Geriatric Use

Clinical studies of RECOMBIVAX HB used for licensure did not include sufficient numbers of subjects 65 years of age and older to determine whether they respond differently from younger subjects. However, in later studies it has been shown that a diminished antibody response and seroprotective levels can be expected in persons older than 60 years of age.{38}

ADVERSE REACTIONS

RECOMBIVAX HB and RECOMBIVAX HB Dialysis Formulation are generally well-tolerated. No adverse experiences were reported during clinical trials which could be related to changes in the titers of antibodies to yeast. As with any vaccine, there is the possibility that broad use of the vaccine could reveal adverse reactions not observed in clinical trials.

In three clinical studies, 434 doses of RECOMBIVAX HB, 5 mcg, were administered to 147 healthy infants and children (up to 10 years of age) who were monitored for 5 days after each dose. Injection site reactions and systemic complaints were reported following 0.2% and 10.4% of the injections, respectively. The most frequently reported systemic adverse reactions (>1% injections), in decreasing order of frequency, were irritability, fever (≥101°F oral equivalent), diarrhea, fatigue/weakness, diminished appetite, and rhinitis.{10}

In a study that compared the three-dose regimen (5 mcg) with the two-dose regimen (10 mcg) of RECOMBIVAX HB in adolescents, the overall frequency of adverse reactions was generally similar.

In a group of studies, 3258 doses of RECOMBIVAX HB, 10 mcg, were administered to 1252 healthy adults who were monitored for 5 days after each dose. Injection site reactions and systemic complaints were reported following 17% and 15% of the injections, respectively. The following adverse reactions were reported:

Incidence Equal To or Greater Than 1% of Injections

LOCAL REACTION (INJECTION SITE)

Injection site reactions consisting principally of soreness, and including pain, tenderness, pruritus, erythema, ecchymosis, swelling, warmth, and nodule formation.

BODY AS A WHOLE

The most frequent systemic complaints include fatigue/weakness; headache; fever (≥100°F); and malaise.

DIGESTIVE SYSTEM

Nausea; and diarrhea

RESPIRATORY SYSTEM

Pharyngitis; and upper respiratory infection

Incidence Less Than 1% of Injections

BODY AS A WHOLE

Sweating; achiness; sensation of warmth; lightheadedness; chills; and flushing

DIGESTIVE SYSTEM

Vomiting; abdominal pains/cramps; dyspepsia; and diminished appetite

RESPIRATORY SYSTEM

Rhinitis; influenza; and cough

NERVOUS SYSTEM

Vertigo/dizziness; and paresthesia

INTEGUMENTARY SYSTEM

Pruritus; rash (non-specified); angioedema; and urticaria

MUSCULOSKELETAL SYSTEM

Arthralgia including monoarticular; myalgia; back pain; neck pain; shoulder pain; and neck stiffness

HEMIC/LYMPHATIC SYSTEM

Lymphadenopathy

PSYCHIATRIC/BEHAVIORAL

Insomnia/disturbed sleep

SPECIAL SENSES

Earache

UROGENITAL SYSTEM

Dysuria

CARDIOVASCULAR SYSTEM

Hypotension

Marketed Experience

The following additional adverse reactions have been reported with use of the marketed vaccine. In many instances, the relationship to the vaccine was unclear.

Hypersensitivity

Anaphylaxis and symptoms of immediate hypersensitivity reactions including rash, pruritus, urticaria, edema, angioedema, dyspnea, chest discomfort, bronchial spasm, palpitation, or symptoms consistent with a hypotensive episode have been reported within the first few hours after vaccination. An apparent hypersensitivity syndrome (serum-sickness-like) of delayed onset has been reported days to weeks after vaccination, including: arthralgia/arthritis (usually transient), fever, and dermatologic reactions such as urticaria, erythema multiforme, ecchymoses and erythema nodosum (see WARNINGS and PRECAUTIONS).

Digestive System

Elevation of liver enzymes; constipation

Nervous System

Guillain-Barré Syndrome; multiple sclerosis; exacerbation of multiple sclerosis; myelitis including transverse myelitis; seizure; febrile seizure; peripheral neuropathy including Bell's Palsy; radiculopathy; herpes zoster; migraine; muscle weakness; hypesthesia; encephalitis

Integumentary System

Stevens-Johnson Syndrome; alopecia; petechiae; eczema

Musculoskeletal System

Arthritis

Pain in extremity

Hematologic

Increased erythrocyte sedimentation rate; thrombocytopenia

Immune System

Systemic lupus erythematosus (SLE); lupus-like syndrome; vasculitis; polyarteritis nodosa

Psychiatric/Behavioral

Irritability; agitation; somnolence

Special Senses

Optic neuritis; tinnitus; conjunctivitis; visual disturbances; uveitis

Cardiovascular System

Syncope; tachycardia.

The following adverse reaction has been reported with another Hepatitis B Vaccine (Recombinant) but not with RECOMBIVAX HB: keratitis.

Patients, parents and guardians should be instructed to report any serious adverse reactions to their healthcare provider, who in turn should report such events to the U.S. Department of Health and Human Services through the Vaccine Adverse Event Reporting System (VAERS), 1-800-822-7967.{31}

DOSAGE AND ADMINISTRATION

Do not inject intravenously or intradermally.

RECOMBIVAX HB Hepatitis B Vaccine (Recombinant) DIALYSIS FORMULATION [(40 mcg/mL) (WITHOUT PRESERVATIVE)] IS INTENDED ONLY FOR ADULT PREDIALYSIS/DIALYSIS PATIENTS.

RECOMBIVAX HB Hepatitis B Vaccine (Recombinant) PEDIATRIC/ADOLESCENT (WITHOUT PRESERVATIVE) and ADULT FORMULATIONS (WITHOUT PRESERVATIVE) ARE NOT INTENDED FOR USE IN PREDIALYSIS/DIALYSIS PATIENTS.

Three-Dose Regimen

The vaccination regimen for each population consists of 3 doses of vaccine given according to the following schedule:

First dose: at elected date
Second dose: 1 month later
Third dose: 6 months after the first dose

For infants born of mothers who are HBsAg positive or mothers of unknown HBsAg status, treatment recommendations are described in the subsection titled: Guidelines for Treatment of Infants Born of HBsAg Positive Mothers or Mothers of Unknown HBsAg Status.

Two-Dose Regimen – Adolescents (11 through 15 years of age)

An alternate two-dose regimen is available for routine vaccination of adolescents (11 through 15 years of age). The regimen consists of two doses of vaccine (10 mcg) given according to the following schedule:

First injection: at elected date
Second injection: 4-6 months later

Table 1 summarizes the dose and formulation of RECOMBIVAX HB for specific populations, regardless of the risk of infection with hepatitis B virus.

[See table 1 above]

Table 1

Group	Dose/Regimen	Formulation	Color Code
Infants, Children and Adolescents 0-19 years of age	5 mcg (0.5 mL) 3×5 mcg	Pediatric/Adolescent	Yellow
Adolescents* 11 through 15 years of age	10 mcg† (1.0 mL) 2×10 mcg	Adult	Green
Adults ≥20 years of age	10 mcg† (1.0 mL) 3×10 mcg	Adult	Green
Predialysis and Dialysis Patients‡	40 mcg (1.0 mL) 3×40 mcg	Dialysis	Blue

* Adolescents (11 through 15 years of age) may receive either regimen: the 3×5 mcg (Pediatric/Adolescent Formulation) or the 2×10 mcg (Adult Formulation).

† If the suggested formulation is not available, the appropriate dosage can be achieved from another formulation provided that the total volume of vaccine administered does not exceed 1 mL. However, the Dialysis Formulation may be used only for adult predialysis/dialysis patients.

‡ See also recommendations for revaccination of predialysis and dialysis patients in DOSAGE AND ADMINISTRATION, Revaccination.

RECOMBIVAX HB is for intramuscular injection. The *deltoid muscle* is the preferred site for intramuscular injection in adults. Data suggest that injections given in the buttocks frequently are given into fatty tissue instead of into muscle. Such injections have resulted in a lower seroconversion rate than was expected. The *anterolateral thigh* is the recommended site for intramuscular injection in infants and young children.

For persons at risk of hemorrhage following intramuscular injection, RECOMBIVAX HB may be administered subcutaneously. However, when other aluminum-adsorbed vaccines have been administered subcutaneously, an increased incidence of local reactions including subcutaneous nodules has been observed. Therefore, subcutaneous administration should be used only in persons (e.g., hemophiliacs) who are at risk of hemorrhage following intramuscular injections.

The vaccine should be used as supplied; no dilution or reconstitution is necessary. The full recommended dose of the vaccine should be used.

For All Formulations: Since none of the formulations contain a preservative, once the single-dose vial has been penetrated, the withdrawn vaccine should be used promptly, and the vial must be discarded.

Shake well before use. Thorough agitation at the time of administration is necessary to maintain suspension of the vaccine.

Parenteral drug products should be inspected visually for particulate matter and discoloration prior to administration. After thorough agitation, the vaccine is a slightly opaque, white suspension.

Withdraw the recommended dose from the vial using a sterile needle and syringe free of preservatives, antiseptics, and detergents.

It is important to use a separate sterile syringe and needle for each individual patient to prevent transmission of hepatitis and other infectious agents from one person to another. Needles should be disposed of properly and should not be recapped.

Injection must be accomplished with a needle long enough to ensure intramuscular deposition of the vaccine.

Guidelines for Treatment of Infants Born of HBsAg Positive Mothers or Mothers of Unknown HBsAg Status

Each infant should receive three 5 mcg doses of RECOMBIVAX HB irrespective of the mother's HBsAg status (see Table 1). The ACIP recommends that if the mother is determined to be HBsAg positive within 7 days of delivery, the infant also should be given a dose of HBIG (0.5 mL) immediately. The first dose of RECOMBIVAX HB may be given at the same time as HBIG, but it should be administered in the opposite anterolateral thigh.{7}

Revaccination

The duration of the protective effect of RECOMBIVAX HB in healthy vaccinees is unknown at present and the need for booster doses is not yet defined (see CLINICAL PHARMACOLOGY).

A booster dose or revaccination with RECOMBIVAX HB Dialysis Formulation (blue color code) may be considered in predialysis/dialysis patients if the anti-HBs level is less than 10 mIU/mL 1 to 2 months after the third dose.{23} The ACIP recommends that the need for booster doses of vaccine should be assessed by annual antibody testing and a booster dose given when antibody levels decline to <10 mIU/mL.{30}

Known or Presumed Exposure to HBsAg

There are no prospective studies directly testing the efficacy of a combination of HBIG and RECOMBIVAX HB in preventing clinical hepatitis B following percutaneous, ocular or mucous membrane exposure to hepatitis B virus. However, since most persons with such exposures (e.g., healthcare workers) are candidates for RECOMBIVAX HB and since combined HBIG plus vaccine is more efficacious than HBIG alone in perinatal exposures, the following guidelines are recommended for persons who have been exposed to hepatitis B virus such as through (1) percutaneous (needlestick), ocular, mucous membrane exposure to blood known or presumed to contain HBsAg, (2) human bites by known or presumed HBsAg carriers, that penetrate the skin, or (3) following intimate sexual contact with known or presumed HBsAg carriers.

HBIG (0.06 mL/kg) should be given intramuscularly as soon as possible after exposure and within 24 hours if possible. RECOMBIVAX HB (see dosage recommendation) should be given intramuscularly at a separate site within 7 days of exposure and second and third doses given one and six months, respectively, after the first dose.

Prefilled Syringe

Shake well before use. Attach the needle by twisting in a clockwise direction until the needle fits securely on the syringe. Administer the entire dose as per standard protocol.

HOW SUPPLIED

PEDIATRIC/ADOLESCENT FORMULATION (PRESERVATIVE FREE)

Vials

No. 4980 — RECOMBIVAX HB for use in infants, children, and adolescents is supplied as 5 mcg/0.5 mL of HBsAg in a 0.5 mL single-dose vial, color coded with a yellow cap and stripe on the vial labels and cartons and an orange banner on the vial labels and cartons stating "Preservative Free", **NDC** 0006-4980-00.

No. 4981 — RECOMBIVAX HB for use in infants, children, and adolescents is supplied as 5 mcg/0.5 mL of HBsAg in a 0.5 mL single-dose vial, in a box of 10 single-dose vials, color coded with a yellow cap and stripe on the vial labels and cartons and an orange banner on the vial labels and cartons stating "Preservative Free", **NDC** 0006-4981-00.

Syringes

No. 4093 — RECOMBIVAX HB for use in infants, children and adolescents is supplied as 5 mcg/0.5 mL of HBsAg in a carton of 6 prefilled single-dose Luer Lock syringes with tip caps, color coded with a yellow plunger rod and stripe on the peel-off syringe labels and cartons and an orange banner on the cartons stating "Preservative Free", **NDC** 0006-4093-09.

ADULT FORMULATION (PRESERVATIVE FREE)

Vials

No. 4995 — RECOMBIVAX HB for use in adults and adolescents (11 through 15 years of age) is supplied as 10 mcg/mL of HBsAg in a 1 mL single-dose vial, color coded with a green cap and stripe on the vial labels and cartons and an orange banner on the vial labels and cartons stating "Preservative Free", **NDC** 0006-4995-00.

No. 4995 — RECOMBIVAX HB for use in adults and adolescents (11 through 15 years of age) is supplied as 10 mcg/mL of HBsAg in a 1 mL single-dose vial, in a box of 10 single-dose vials, color coded with a green cap and stripe on the vial labels and cartons and an orange banner on the vial labels and cartons stating "Preservative Free", **NDC** 0006-4995-41.

Syringes

No. 4094 — RECOMBIVAX HB for use in adults and adolescents (11 through 15 years of age) is supplied as 10 mcg/1.0 mL HBsAg in a carton of 6 single-dose prefilled Luer Lock syringes with tip caps, color coded with a green plunger rod and stripe on the peel-off syringe labels and cartons and an orange banner on the carton stating "Preservative Free", **NDC** 0006-4094-09.

DIALYSIS FORMULATION (PRESERVATIVE FREE)

Vials

No. 4992 — RECOMBIVAX HB Dialysis Formulation is supplied as 40 mcg/mL of HBsAg in a 1 mL single-dose vial, color coded with a blue cap and stripe on the vial labels and cartons and an orange banner on the vial labels and cartons stating "Preservative Free", **NDC** 0006-4992-00.

Storage

Store vials and syringes at 2-8°C (36-46°F). Storage above or below the recommended temperature may reduce potency.

Do not freeze since freezing destroys potency.

REFERENCES

1. Robinson, W.S.: Hepatitis B Virus and the Delta Virus, in "Principles and Practice of Infectious Diseases," G.L. Mandell; R.G. Douglas; J.E. Bennett (eds), vol. 2, New York, John Wiley & Sons, 1002-1029, 1985.
2. Recommendation of the Immunization Practices Advisory Committee (ACIP): Protection Against Viral Hepatitis, MMWR *39*(RR-2): 5-22, Feb. 9, 1990.
3. Balistreri, W.F.: Viral Hepatitis, Unique Aspects of Infection During Childhood, Consultant *24*(4): 131-153 passim, April 1984.
4. Robinson, W.S.: Hepatitis B Virus and Hepatitis Delta Virus, in "Principles and Practice of Infectious Diseases," G.L. Mandell, R.G. Douglas, and J.E. Bennett (eds), Churchill Livingstone, 1204-1231, 1990.
5. Stevens, C.E.; Toy, P.T.; Tong, M.J.; Taylor, P.E.; Vyas, G.N.; Nair, P.V.; Gudavalli, M.; Krugman, S.: Perinatal Hepatitis B Virus Transmission in the United States, JAMA *253*(12): 1740-1745, 1985.
6. Beasley, R.P.; Hwang, L.; Stevens, C.E.; Lin, C.; Hsieh, F.; Wang, K.; Sun, T.; Szmuness, W.: Efficacy of Hepatitis B Immune Globulin for Prevention of Perinatal Transmission of the Hepatitis B Virus Carrier State: Final Report of a Randomized Double-Blind, Placebo-Controlled Trial, Hepatology *3:* 135-141, 1983.
7. Recommendations of the Immunization Practices Advisory Committee (ACIP): Hepatitis B Virus: A Comprehensive Strategy for Eliminating Transmission in the United States Through Universal Childhood Vaccination, MMWR *40*(RR-13): 1-25, November 22, 1991.
8. Universal Hepatitis B Immunization, Committee on Infectious Diseases, Pediatrics *89*(4): 795-800, 1992.
9. Melnick, J.L.: Historical Aspects of Hepatitis B Vaccine, in "Hepatitis B Vaccine INSERM Symposium No. 18," P. Maupas and P. Guesry (eds), Elsevier/North-Holland Biomedical Press, 23-31, 1981.
10. Data on file at Merck Research Laboratories.
11. Centers for Disease Control: Suboptimal Response to Hepatitis B Vaccine Given by Injection into the Buttock. MMWR *34*(8): 105-113, March 1, 1985.
12. Hadler, S.C., et al.: Long-term Immunogenicity and Efficacy of Hepatitis B Vaccine in Homosexual Men, NEJM *315:* 209-214, 1986.
13. Szmuness, W.; Stevens, C.E.; Horley, H.J., et al.: Hepatitis B Vaccine. Demonstration of Efficacy in a Controlled Clinical Trial in a High-risk Population in the United States. NEJM *303:* 833-841, 1980.

14. Francis, D.P.; Hadler, S.C.; Thompson, S.E., et al.: The Prevention of Hepatitis B with Vaccine. Report of the Centers for Disease Control Multi-center Efficacy Trial among Homosexual Men. Ann. Int. Med. *97:* 362-366, 1982.
15. Szmuness, W.; Stevens, C.E.; Horley, H.J., et al.: Hepatitis B Vaccine in Medical Staff of Hemodialysis Units. Efficacy and Subtype Cross-protection, NEJM *307:* 1481-1486, 1982.
16. Stevens, C.E.; Taylor, P.E.; Tong, M.J., et al.: Prevention of Perinatal Hepatitis B Virus Infection with Hepatitis B Immune Globulin and Hepatitis B Vaccine, in Zuckerman, A.J. (ed.), "Viral Hepatitis and Liver Diseases", Alan R. Liss, 982-983, 1988.
17. Stevens, C.E.; Taylor, P.E.; Tong, M.J., et al.: Yeast-Recombinant Hepatitis B Vaccine, Efficacy with Hepatitis B Immune Globulin in Prevention of Perinatal Hepatitis B Virus Transmission, JAMA *257*(19): 2612-2616, 1987.
18. Wainwright, R.B.; McMahon, B.J.; Bulkow, L.R., et al.: Duration of Immunogenicity and Efficacy of Hepatitis B Vaccine in a Yupik Eskimo Population, Preliminary Results of an 8-Year Study, in "Viral Hepatitis and Liver Disease," F.B. Hollinger, S.M. Lemon, and H. Margolis (eds), Williams & Wilkins, 762-766, 1990.
19. Hadler, S.C.; Coleman, P.J.; O'Malley, P., et al.: Evaluation of Long-Term Protection by Hepatitis B Vaccine for Seven to Nine Years in Homosexual Men, in "Viral Hepatitis and Liver Disease," F.B. Hollinger, S.M. Lemon, and H. Margolis (eds), Williams & Wilkins, 766-768, 1990.
20. Tong, M.J.; Stevens, C.E.; Taylor, P.E., et al.: Prevention of Hepatitis B Infection in Infants Born to HBeAg Positive HBsAg Carrier Mothers in the United States, in "An Update, 1989, Progress in Hepatitis B Immunization," P. Coursaget and M.J. Tong (eds), Colloque INSERM/John Libbey Eurotext Ltd., Vol. 194, 339-345, 1990.
21. Hwang, L-Y.; Lee, C-Y.; and Beasley, R.P.: Five-Year Follow-up of HBV Vaccination with Plasma-derived Vaccine in Neonates: Evaluation of Immunogenicity and Efficacy Against Perinatal Transmission, in "Viral Hepatitis and Liver Disease," F.B. Hollinger, S.M. Lemon, and H. Margolis (eds), Williams & Wilkins, 759-761, 1990.
22. West, D.J.; Calandra, G.B.: Vaccine Induced Immunologic Memory for Hepatitis B Surface Antigen; Implications for Policy on Booster Vaccination, Vaccine, *14*(11): 1019-1027, 1996.
23. Recommendations of the Immunization Practices Advisory Committee (ACIP); Update on Hepatitis B Prevention, MMWR *36*(23): 353-366, June 19, 1987.
24. Emini, E.A.; Ellis, R.W.; Miller, W.J.; McAleer, W.J.; Scolnick, E.M. and Gerety, R.J.: Production and Immunological Analysis of Recombinant Hepatitis B Vaccine, J. Infection, *13*(Sup. A): 3-9, 1986.
25. Brown, S.E.; Stanley, C.; Howard, C.R.; Zuckerman, A.J.; Steward, M.W.: Antibody Responses to Recombinant and Plasma- derived Hepatitis B Vaccines, Brit. Med. J., *292:* 159-161, 1986.
26. Yamamoto, S.; Kuroki, T.; Kurai, K.; Iino, S.: Comparison of Results for Phase I Studies with Recombinant and Plasma-derived Hepatitis B Vaccines, and Controlled Study Comparing Intramuscular and Subcutaneous Injections of Recombinant Hepatitis B Vaccine, J. Infection, *13*(Sup. A): 53-60, 1986.
27. Jilg, W.; Schmidt, M.; Zoulek, G.; Lorbeer, B.; Wilske, B.; Deinhardt, F.: Clinical Evaluation of a Recombinant Hepatitis B Vaccine, Lancet, 1174-1175, Nov. 24, 1984.
28. Schalm, S.W.; Heytink, R.A.; Kruining, H.; Bakker-Bendik, M.: Immunogenicity of Recombinant Yeast Hepatitis-B Vaccine, Neth. J. Med. *29:* 28, 1986.
29. Centers for Disease Control: Epidemiology and Prevention of Vaccine-preventative Diseases, W. Atkinson, L. Furphy, J. Gantt, M. Mayfield, G. Phyne (eds), chapter 9.
30. Recommendations of the Advisory Committee on Immunization Practices (ACIP): Hepatitis B Virus Infection: A Comprehensive Strategy to Eliminate Transmission in the United States, 1996 update, MMWR (draft January 13, 1996).
31. Vaccine Adverse Event Reporting System - United States. MMWR *39*(41): 730-733, October 19, 1990.
32. Zajac, B.A.; West, D.J.; McAleer, W.J.; Scolnick, E.M.: Overview of Clinical Studies with Hepatitis B Vaccine Made by Recombinant DNA, J. Infection, *13*(Sup. A): 39-45, July 1986.
33. WHO Bulletin, Expanded Programme on Immunization, Hepatitis B Vaccine – Making Global Progress. October, 1996.
34. Centers for Disease Control and Prevention, Federal Register, February 23, 1999, *64*(35): 9044-9045.
35. National Institutes of Health, National Institutes of Health Consensus Development Conference Panel Statement: Management of Hepatitis C, Hepatology, *26*(Suppl. 1): 2S-10S, 1997.
36. Wiedmann, M.; Liebert, U.G.; Oesen, U.; Porst, H.; Wiese, M.; Schroeder, S.; Halm, U.; Mossner, J.; Berr, F.: Decreased Immunogenicity of Recombinant Hepatitis B Vaccine in Chronic Hepatitis C, Hepatology, *31:* 230-234, 2000.
37. Minniti, F.; Baldo, V.; Trivello, R.; Bricolo, R.; Di Furia, L.; Renzulli, G.; Chiaramonte, M.: Response to HBV vaccine in Relation to anti-HCV and anti-HBc Positivity: a Study in Intravenous Drug Addicts, Vaccine, *17:* 3083-3085, 1999.
38. Centers for Disease Control and Prevention. A Comprehensive Immunization Strategy to Eliminate Transmission of Hepatitis B Virus Infection in the United States. Recommendations of the Advisory Committee on Immunization Practices (ACIP). Part 2: Immunization of Adults, MMWR 2006;*55*(RR-16);1-25.

Manuf. and Dist. by: Merck Sharp & Dohme Corp., a subsidiary of
MERCK & CO., INC., Whitehouse Station, NJ 08889, USA
Issued July 2011
Printed in USA
9987435

REMERON® ℞

[rem-er-on]
(mirtazapine)
Tablets

> **Suicidality and Antidepressant Drugs**
> **Antidepressants increased the risk compared to placebo of suicidal thinking and behavior (suicidality) in children, adolescents, and young adults in short-term studies of major depressive disorder (MDD) and other psychiatric disorders. Anyone considering the use of REMERON® (mirtazapine) Tablets or any other antidepressant in a child, adolescent, or young adult must balance this risk with the clinical need. Short-term studies did not show an increase in the risk of suicidality with antidepressants compared to placebo in adults beyond age 24; there was a reduction in risk with antidepressants compared to placebo in adults aged 65 and older. Depression and certain other psychiatric disorders are themselves associated with increases in the risk of suicide. Patients of all ages who are started on antidepressant therapy should be monitored appropriately and observed closely for clinical worsening, suicidality, or unusual changes in behavior. Families and caregivers should be advised of the need for close observation and communication with the prescriber. REMERON is not approved for use in pediatric patients. (See WARNINGS: Clinical Worsening and Suicide Risk, PRECAUTIONS: Information for Patients, and PRECAUTIONS: Pediatric Use)**

DESCRIPTION

REMERON® (mirtazapine) Tablets are an orally administered drug. Mirtazapine has a tetracyclic chemical structure and belongs to the piperazino-azepine group of compounds. It is designated 1,2,3,4,10,14b-hexahydro-2-methylpyrazino [2,1-a] pyrido [2,3-c] benzazepine and has the empirical formula of $C_{17}H_{19}N_3$. Its molecular weight is 265.36. The structural formula is the following and it is the racemic mixture:

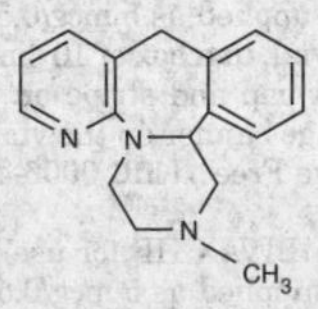

Mirtazapine is a white to creamy white crystalline powder which is slightly soluble in water.
REMERON is supplied for oral administration as scored film-coated tablets containing 15 or 30 mg of mirtazapine, and unscored film-coated tablets containing 45 mg of mirtazapine. Each tablet also contains corn starch, hydroxypropyl cellulose, magnesium stearate, colloidal silicon dioxide, lactose, and other inactive ingredients.

CLINICAL PHARMACOLOGY

Pharmacodynamics

The mechanism of action of REMERON (mirtazapine) Tablets, as with other drugs effective in the treatment of major depressive disorder, is unknown.
Evidence gathered in preclinical studies suggests that mirtazapine enhances central noradrenergic and serotonergic activity. These studies have shown that mirtazapine acts as an antagonist at central presynaptic α_2–adrenergic inhibitory autoreceptors and heteroreceptors, an action that is postulated to result in an increase in central noradrenergic and serotonergic activity.
Mirtazapine is a potent antagonist of $5\text{-}HT_2$ and $5\text{-}HT_3$ receptors. Mirtazapine has no significant affinity for the $5\text{-}HT_{1A}$ and $5\text{-}HT_{1B}$ receptors.
Mirtazapine is a potent antagonist of histamine (H_1) receptors, a property that may explain its prominent sedative effects.
Mirtazapine is a moderate peripheral α_1–adrenergic antagonist, a property that may explain the occasional orthostatic hypotension reported in association with its use.
Mirtazapine is a moderate antagonist at muscarinic receptors, a property that may explain the relatively low incidence of anticholinergic side effects associated with its use.

Pharmacokinetics

REMERON (mirtazapine) Tablets are rapidly and completely absorbed following oral administration and have a half-life of about 20 to 40 hours. Peak plasma concentrations are reached within about 2 hours following an oral dose. The presence of food in the stomach has a minimal effect on both the rate and extent of absorption and does not require a dosage adjustment.
Mirtazapine is extensively metabolized after oral administration. Major pathways of biotransformation are demethylation and hydroxylation followed by glucuronide conjugation. *In vitro* data from human liver microsomes indicate that cytochrome 2D6 and 1A2 are involved in the formation of the 8-hydroxy metabolite of mirtazapine, whereas cytochrome 3A is considered to be responsible for the formation of the N-desmethyl and N-oxide metabolite. Mirtazapine has an absolute bioavailability of about 50%. It is eliminated predominantly via urine (75%) with 15% in feces. Several unconjugated metabolites possess pharmacological activity but are present in the plasma at very low levels. The (–) enantiomer has an elimination half-life that is approximately twice as long as the (+) enantiomer and therefore achieves plasma levels that are about 3 times as high as that of the (+) enantiomer.
Plasma levels are linearly related to dose over a dose range of 15 to 80 mg. The mean elimination half-life of mirtazapine after oral administration ranges from approximately 20 to 40 hours across age and gender subgroups, with females of all ages exhibiting significantly longer elimination half-lives than males (mean half-life of 37 hours for females vs. 26 hours for males). Steady state plasma levels of mirtazapine are attained within 5 days, with about 50% accumulation (accumulation ratio = 1.5).
Mirtazapine is approximately 85% bound to plasma proteins over a concentration range of 0.01 to 10 mcg/mL.

Special Populations

Geriatric
Following oral administration of REMERON (mirtazapine) Tablets 20 mg/day for 7 days to subjects of varying ages (range, 25–74), oral clearance of mirtazapine was reduced in the elderly compared to the younger subjects. The differences were most striking in males, with a 40% lower clearance in elderly males compared to younger males, while the clearance in elderly females was only 10% lower compared to younger females. Caution is indicated in administering REMERON to elderly patients (see PRECAUTIONS and DOSAGE AND ADMINISTRATION).
Pediatrics
Safety and effectiveness of mirtazapine in the pediatric population have not been established (see PRECAUTIONS).
Gender
The mean elimination half-life of mirtazapine after oral administration ranges from approximately 20 to 40 hours across age and gender subgroups, with females of all ages exhibiting significantly longer elimination half-lives than males (mean half-life of 37 hours for females vs. 26 hours for males) (see Pharmacokinetics).
Race
There have been no clinical studies to evaluate the effect of race on the pharmacokinetics of REMERON.
Renal Insufficiency
The disposition of mirtazapine was studied in patients with varying degrees of renal function. Elimination of mirtazapine is correlated with creatinine clearance. Total body clearance of mirtazapine was reduced approximately 30% in patients with moderate (Clcr=11–39 mL/min/1.73 m^2) and approximately 50% in patients with severe (Clcr=<10 mL/min/1.73 m^2) renal impairment when compared to normal subjects. Caution is indicated in administering REMERON to patients with compromised renal function (see PRECAUTIONS and DOSAGE AND ADMINISTRATION).
Hepatic Insufficiency
Following a single 15-mg oral dose of REMERON, the oral clearance of mirtazapine was decreased by approximately 30% in hepatically impaired patients compared to subjects with normal hepatic function. Caution is indicated in ad-

ministering REMERON to patients with compromised hepatic function (see PRECAUTIONS and DOSAGE AND ADMINISTRATION).

Clinical Trials Showing Effectiveness

The efficacy of REMERON (mirtazapine) Tablets as a treatment for major depressive disorder was established in 4 placebo-controlled, 6-week trials in adult outpatients meeting DSM-III criteria for major depressive disorder. Patients were titrated with mirtazapine from a dose range of 5 mg up to 35 mg/day. Overall, these studies demonstrated mirtazapine to be superior to placebo on at least 3 of the following 4 measures: 21-Item Hamilton Depression Rating Scale (HDRS) total score; HDRS Depressed Mood Item; CGI Severity score; and Montgomery and Asberg Depression Rating Scale (MADRS). Superiority of mirtazapine over placebo was also found for certain factors of the HDRS, including anxiety/somatization factor and sleep disturbance factor. The mean mirtazapine dose for patients who completed these 4 studies ranged from 21 to 32 mg/day. A fifth study of similar design utilized a higher dose (up to 50 mg) per day and also showed effectiveness.

Examination of age and gender subsets of the population did not reveal any differential responsiveness on the basis of these subgroupings.

In a longer-term study, patients meeting (DSM-IV) criteria for major depressive disorder who had responded during an initial 8 to 12 weeks of acute treatment on REMERON were randomized to continuation of REMERON or placebo for up to 40 weeks of observation for relapse. Response during the open phase was defined as having achieved a HAM-D 17 total score of ≤8 and a CGI-Improvement score of 1 or 2 at 2 consecutive visits beginning with week 6 of the 8 to 12 weeks in the open-label phase of the study. Relapse during the double-blind phase was determined by the individual investigators. Patients receiving continued REMERON treatment experienced significantly lower relapse rates over the subsequent 40 weeks compared to those receiving placebo. This pattern was demonstrated in both male and female patients.

INDICATIONS AND USAGE

REMERON (mirtazapine) Tablets are indicated for the treatment of major depressive disorder.

The efficacy of REMERON in the treatment of major depressive disorder was established in 6-week controlled trials of outpatients whose diagnoses corresponded most closely to the Diagnostic and Statistical Manual of Mental Disorders – 3rd edition (DSM-III) category of major depressive disorder (see CLINICAL PHARMACOLOGY).

A major depressive episode (DSM-IV) implies a prominent and relatively persistent (nearly every day for at least 2 weeks) depressed or dysphoric mood that usually interferes with daily functioning, and includes at least 5 of the following 9 symptoms: depressed mood, loss of interest in usual activities, significant change in weight and/or appetite, insomnia or hypersomnia, psychomotor agitation or retardation, increased fatigue, feelings of guilt or worthlessness, slowed thinking or impaired concentration, a suicide attempt, or suicidal ideation.

The effectiveness of REMERON in hospitalized depressed patients has not been adequately studied.

The efficacy of REMERON in maintaining a response in patients with major depressive disorder for up to 40 weeks following 8 to 12 weeks of initial open-label treatment was demonstrated in a placebo-controlled trial. Nevertheless, the physician who elects to use REMERON for extended periods should periodically re-evaluate the long-term usefulness of the drug for the individual patient (see CLINICAL PHARMACOLOGY).

CONTRAINDICATIONS

Hypersensitivity

REMERON (mirtazapine) Tablets are contraindicated in patients with a known hypersensitivity to mirtazapine or to any of the excipients.

Monoamine Oxidase Inhibitors

The use of monoamine oxidase inhibitors (MAOIs) intended to treat psychiatric disorders with REMERON Tablets or within 14 days of stopping treatment with REMERON is contraindicated because of an increased risk of serotonin syndrome. The use of REMERON within 14 days of stopping an MAOI intended to treat psychiatric disorders is also contraindicated (see WARNINGS and DOSAGE AND ADMINISTRATION).

Starting REMERON in a patient who is being treated with MAOIs such as linezolid or intravenous methylene blue is also contraindicated because of an increased risk of serotonin syndrome (see WARNINGS and DOSAGE AND ADMINISTRATION).

WARNINGS

Clinical Worsening and Suicide Risk

Patients with major depressive disorder (MDD), both adult and pediatric, may experience worsening of their depression and/or the emergence of suicidal ideation and behavior (suicidality) or unusual changes in behavior, whether or not they are taking antidepressant medications, and this risk may persist until significant remission occurs. Suicide is a known risk of depression and certain other psychiatric disorders, and these disorders themselves are the strongest predictors of suicide. There has been a long-standing concern, however, that antidepressants may have a role in inducing worsening of depression and the emergence of suicidality in certain patients during the early phases of treatment. Pooled analyses of short-term placebo-controlled trials of antidepressant drugs (SSRIs and others) showed that these drugs increase the risk of suicidal thinking and behavior (suicidality) in children, adolescents, and young adults (ages 18–24) with major depressive disorder (MDD) and other psychiatric disorders. Short-term studies did not show an increase in the risk of suicidality with antidepressants compared to placebo in adults beyond age 24; there was a reduction in risk with antidepressants compared to placebo in adults aged 65 and older.

The pooled analyses of placebo-controlled trials in children and adolescents with MDD, obsessive compulsive disorder (OCD), or other psychiatric disorders included a total of 24 short-term trials of 9 antidepressant drugs in over 4400 patients. The pooled analyses of placebo-controlled trials in adults with MDD or other psychiatric disorders included a total of 295 short-term trials (median duration of 2 months) of 11 antidepressant drugs in over 77,000 patients. There was considerable variation in risk of suicidality among drugs, but a tendency toward an increase in the younger patients for almost all drugs studied. There were differences in absolute risk of suicidality across different indications, with the highest incidence in MDD. The risk differences (drug vs. placebo), however, were relatively stable within age strata and across indications. These risk differences (drug-placebo difference in the number of cases of suicidality per 1000 patients treated) are provided in Table 1.

Table 1

Age Range	Drug-Placebo Difference in Number of Cases of Suicidality per 1000 Patients Treated
Increases Compared to Placebo	
<18	14 additional cases
18–24	5 additional cases
Decreases Compared to Placebo	
25–64	1 fewer case
≥65	6 fewer cases

No suicides occurred in any of the pediatric trials. There were suicides in the adult trials, but the number was not sufficient to reach any conclusion about drug effect on suicide.

It is unknown whether the suicidality risk extends to longer-term use, i.e., beyond several months. However, there is substantial evidence from placebo-controlled maintenance trials in adults with depression that the use of antidepressants can delay the recurrence of depression.

All patients being treated with antidepressants for any indication should be monitored appropriately and observed closely for clinical worsening, suicidality, and unusual changes in behavior, especially during the initial few months of a course of drug therapy, or at times of dose changes, either increases or decreases.

The following symptoms, anxiety, agitation, panic attacks, insomnia, irritability, hostility, aggressiveness, impulsivity, akathisia (psychomotor restlessness), hypomania, and mania, have been reported in adult and pediatric patients being treated with antidepressants for major depressive disorder as well as for other indications, both psychiatric and nonpsychiatric. Although a causal link between the emergence of such symptoms and either the worsening of depression and/or the emergence of suicidal impulses has not been established, there is concern that such symptoms may represent precursors to emerging suicidality.

Consideration should be given to changing the therapeutic regimen, including possibly discontinuing the medication, in patients whose depression is persistently worse, or who are experiencing emergent suicidality or symptoms that might be precursors to worsening depression or suicidality, especially if these symptoms are severe, abrupt in onset, or were not part of the patient's presenting symptoms.

Families and caregivers of patients being treated with antidepressants for major depressive disorder or other indications, both psychiatric and nonpsychiatric, should be alerted about the need to monitor patients for the emergence of agitation, irritability, unusual changes in behavior, and the other symptoms described above, as well as the emergence of suicidality, and to report such symptoms immediately to health care providers. Such monitoring should include daily observation by families and caregivers. Prescriptions for REMERON (mirtazapine) Tablets should be written for the smallest quantity of tablets consistent with good patient management, in order to reduce the risk of overdose.

Screening Patients for Bipolar Disorder

A major depressive episode may be the initial presentation of bipolar disorder. It is generally believed (though not established in controlled trials) that treating such an episode with an antidepressant alone may increase the likelihood of precipitation of a mixed/manic episode in patients at risk for bipolar disorder. Whether any of the symptoms described above represent such a conversion is unknown. However, prior to initiating treatment with an antidepressant, patients with depressive symptoms should be adequately screened to determine if they are at risk for bipolar disorder; such screening should include a detailed psychiatric history, including a family history of suicide, bipolar disorder, and depression. It should be noted that REMERON (mirtazapine) Tablets are not approved for use in treating bipolar depression.

Agranulocytosis

In premarketing clinical trials, 2 (1 with Sjögren's Syndrome) out of 2796 patients treated with REMERON (mirtazapine) Tablets developed agranulocytosis [absolute neutrophil count (ANC) <500/mm^3 with associated signs and symptoms, e.g., fever, infection, etc.] and a third patient developed severe neutropenia (ANC <500/mm^3 without any associated symptoms). For these 3 patients, onset of severe neutropenia was detected on days 61, 9, and 14 of treatment, respectively. All 3 patients recovered after REMERON was stopped. These 3 cases yield a crude incidence of severe neutropenia (with or without associated infection) of approximately 1.1 per thousand patients exposed, with a very wide 95% confidence interval, i.e., 2.2 cases per 10,000 to 3.1 cases per 1000. If a patient develops a sore throat, fever, stomatitis, or other signs of infection, along with a low WBC count, treatment with REMERON should be discontinued and the patient should be closely monitored.

Serotonin Syndrome

The development of a potentially life-threatening serotonin syndrome has been reported with SNRIs and SSRIs, including REMERON, alone but particularly with concomitant use of other serotonergic drugs (including triptans, tricyclic antidepressants, fentanyl, lithium, tramadol, tryptophan, buspirone, and St. John's wort), and with drugs that impair metabolism of serotonin (in particular, MAOIs, both those intended to treat psychiatric disorders and also others, such as linezolid and intravenous methylene blue).

Serotonin syndrome symptoms may include mental status changes (e.g., agitation, hallucinations, delirium, and coma), autonomic instability (e.g., tachycardia, labile blood pressure, dizziness, diaphoresis, flushing, hyperthermia), neuromuscular symptoms (e.g., tremor, rigidity, myoclonus, hyperreflexia, incoordination), seizures, and/or gastrointestinal symptoms (e.g., nausea, vomiting, diarrhea). Patients should be monitored for the emergence of serotonin syndrome.

The concomitant use of REMERON with MAOIs intended to treat psychiatric disorders is contraindicated. REMERON should also not be started in a patient who is being treated with MAOIs such as linezolid or intravenous methylene blue. All reports with methylene blue that provided information on the route of administration involved intravenous administration in the dose range of 1 mg/kg to 8 mg/kg. No reports involved the administration of methylene blue by other routes (such as oral tablets or local tissue injection) or at lower doses. There may be circumstances when it is necessary to initiate treatment with an MAOI such as linezolid or intravenous methylene blue in a patient taking REMERON. REMERON should be discontinued before initiating treatment with the MAOI (see CONTRAINDICATIONS and DOSAGE AND ADMINISTRATION).

If concomitant use of REMERON with other serotonergic drugs, including triptans, tricyclic antidepressants, fentanyl, lithium, tramadol, buspirone, tryptophan, and St. John's wort, is clinically warranted, be aware of a potential increased risk for serotonin syndrome, particularly during treatment initiation and dose increases.

Treatment with REMERON and any concomitant serotonergic agents should be discontinued immediately if the above events occur and supportive symptomatic treatment should be initiated.

PRECAUTIONS

General

Discontinuation Symptoms

There have been reports of adverse reactions upon the discontinuation of REMERON (mirtazapine) Tablets (particularly when abrupt), including but not limited to the following: dizziness, abnormal dreams, sensory disturbances (including paresthesia and electric shock sensations), agitation, anxiety, fatigue, confusion, headache, tremor, nausea, vomiting, and sweating, or other symptoms which may be of clinical significance. The majority of the reported cases are mild and self-limiting. Even though these have been reported as adverse reactions, it should be realized that these symptoms may be related to underlying disease.

Patients currently taking REMERON should NOT discontinue treatment abruptly, due to risk of discontinuation symptoms. At the time that a medical decision is made to discontinue treatment with REMERON, a gradual reduction in the dose, rather than an abrupt cessation, is recommended.

Akathisia/Psychomotor Restlessness

The use of antidepressants has been associated with the development of akathisia, characterized by a subjectively unpleasant or distressing restlessness and need to move, often accompanied by an inability to sit or stand still. This is most likely to occur within the first few weeks of treatment. In patients who develop these symptoms, increasing the dose may be detrimental.

Hyponatremia

Hyponatremia has been reported very rarely with the use of mirtazapine. Caution should be exercised in patients at risk, such as elderly patients or patients concomitantly treated with medications known to cause hyponatremia.

Somnolence

In US controlled studies, somnolence was reported in 54% of patients treated with REMERON (mirtazapine) Tablets, compared to 18% for placebo and 60% for amitriptyline. In these studies, somnolence resulted in discontinuation for 10.4% of REMERON-treated patients, compared to 2.2% for placebo. It is unclear whether or not tolerance develops to the somnolent effects of REMERON. Because of the potentially significant effects of REMERON on impairment of performance, patients should be cautioned about engaging in activities requiring alertness until they have been able to assess the drug's effect on their own psychomotor performance (see PRECAUTIONS: Information for Patients).

Dizziness

In US controlled studies, dizziness was reported in 7% of patients treated with REMERON, compared to 3% for placebo and 14% for amitriptyline. It is unclear whether or not tolerance develops to the dizziness observed in association with the use of REMERON.

Increased Appetite/Weight Gain

In US controlled studies, appetite increase was reported in 17% of patients treated with REMERON, compared to 2% for placebo and 6% for amitriptyline. In these same trials, weight gain of ≥7% of body weight was reported in 7.5% of patients treated with mirtazapine, compared to 0% for placebo and 5.9% for amitriptyline. In a pool of premarketing US studies, including many patients for long-term, open-label treatment, 8% of patients receiving REMERON discontinued for weight gain. In an 8-week-long pediatric clinical trial of doses between 15 to 45 mg/day, 49% of REMERON-treated patients had a weight gain of at least 7%, compared to 5.7% of placebo-treated patients (see PRECAUTIONS: Pediatric Use).

Cholesterol/Triglycerides

In US controlled studies, nonfasting cholesterol increases to ≥20% above the upper limits of normal were observed in 15% of patients treated with REMERON, compared to 7% for placebo and 8% for amitriptyline. In these same studies, nonfasting triglyceride increases to ≥500 mg/dL were observed in 6% of patients treated with mirtazapine, compared to 3% for placebo and 3% for amitriptyline.

Transaminase Elevations

Clinically significant ALT (SGPT) elevations (≥3 times the upper limit of the normal range) were observed in 2.0% (8/424) of patients exposed to REMERON in a pool of short-term US controlled trials, compared to 0.3% (1/328) of placebo patients and 2.0% (3/181) of amitriptyline patients. Most of these patients with ALT increases did not develop signs or symptoms associated with compromised liver function. While some patients were discontinued for the ALT increases, in other cases, the enzyme levels returned to normal despite continued REMERON treatment. REMERON should be used with caution in patients with impaired hepatic function (see CLINICAL PHARMACOLOGY and DOSAGE AND ADMINISTRATION).

Activation of Mania/Hypomania

Mania/hypomania occurred in approximately 0.2% (3/1299 patients) of REMERON-treated patients in US studies. Although the incidence of mania/hypomania was very low during treatment with mirtazapine, it should be used carefully in patients with a history of mania/hypomania.

Seizure

In premarketing clinical trials, only 1 seizure was reported among the 2796 US and non-US patients treated with REMERON. However, no controlled studies have been carried out in patients with a history of seizures. Therefore, care should be exercised when mirtazapine is used in these patients.

Use in Patients with Concomitant Illness

Clinical experience with REMERON in patients with concomitant systemic illness is limited. Accordingly, care is advisable in prescribing mirtazapine for patients with diseases or conditions that affect metabolism or hemodynamic responses.

REMERON has not been systematically evaluated or used to any appreciable extent in patients with a recent history of myocardial infarction or other significant heart disease. REMERON was associated with significant orthostatic hypotension in early clinical pharmacology trials with normal volunteers. Orthostatic hypotension was infrequently observed in clinical trials with depressed patients. REMERON should be used with caution in patients with known cardiovascular or cerebrovascular disease that could be exacerbated by hypotension (history of myocardial infarction, angina, or ischemic stroke) and conditions that would predispose patients to hypotension (dehydration, hypovolemia, and treatment with antihypertensive medication).

Mirtazapine clearance is decreased in patients with moderate [glomerular filtration rate (GFR)=11–39 mL/min/1.73 m^2] and severe [GFR <10 mL/min/1.73 m^2] renal impairment, and also in patients with hepatic impairment. Caution is indicated in administering REMERON to such patients (see CLINICAL PHARMACOLOGY and DOSAGE AND ADMINISTRATION).

Information for Patients

Prescribers or other health professionals should inform patients, their families, and their caregivers about the benefits and risks associated with treatment with REMERON (mirtazapine) Tablets and should counsel them in its appropriate use. A patient Medication Guide about "Antidepressant Medicines, Depression and other Serious Mental Illnesses, and Suicidal Thoughts or Actions" is available for REMERON. The prescriber or health professional should instruct patients, their families, and their caregivers to read the Medication Guide and should assist them in understanding its contents. Patients should be given the opportunity to discuss the contents of the Medication Guide and to obtain answers to any questions they may have. The complete text of the Medication Guide is reprinted at the end of this document.

Patients should be advised of the following issues and asked to alert their prescriber if these occur while taking REMERON.

Clinical Worsening and Suicide Risk

Patients, their families, and their caregivers should be encouraged to be alert to the emergence of anxiety, agitation, panic attacks, insomnia, irritability, hostility, aggressiveness, impulsivity, akathisia (psychomotor restlessness), hypomania, mania, other unusual changes in behavior, worsening of depression, and suicidal ideation, especially early during antidepressant treatment and when the dose is adjusted up or down. Families and caregivers of patients should be advised to look for the emergence of such symptoms on a day-to-day basis, since changes may be abrupt. Such symptoms should be reported to the patient's prescriber or health professional, especially if they are severe, abrupt in onset, or were not part of the patient's presenting symptoms. Symptoms such as these may be associated with an increased risk for suicidal thinking and behavior and indicate a need for very close monitoring and possibly changes in the medication.

Agranulocytosis

Patients who are to receive REMERON should be warned about the risk of developing agranulocytosis. Patients should be advised to contact their physician if they experience any indication of infection such as fever, chills, sore throat, mucous membrane ulceration, or other possible signs of infection. Particular attention should be paid to any flu-like complaints or other symptoms that might suggest infection.

Interference with Cognitive and Motor Performance

REMERON may impair judgment, thinking, and particularly, motor skills, because of its prominent sedative effect. The drowsiness associated with mirtazapine use may impair a patient's ability to drive, use machines, or perform tasks that require alertness. Thus, patients should be cautioned about engaging in hazardous activities until they are reasonably certain that REMERON therapy does not adversely affect their ability to engage in such activities.

Completing Course of Therapy

While patients may notice improvement with REMERON therapy in 1 to 4 weeks, they should be advised to continue therapy as directed.

Concomitant Medication

Patients should be advised to inform their physician if they are taking, or intend to take, any prescription or over-the-counter drugs, since there is a potential for REMERON to interact with other drugs.

Patients should be made aware of a potential increased risk for serotonin syndrome if concomitant use of REMERON with other serotonergic drugs, including triptans, tricyclic antidepressants, fentanyl, lithium, tramadol, buspirone, tryptophan, and St. John's wort, is clinically warranted, particularly during treatment initiation and dose increases.

Alcohol

The impairment of cognitive and motor skills produced by REMERON has been shown to be additive with those produced by alcohol. Accordingly, patients should be advised to avoid alcohol while taking mirtazapine.

Pregnancy

Patients should be advised to notify their physician if they become pregnant or intend to become pregnant during REMERON therapy.

Nursing

Patients should be advised to notify their physician if they are breastfeeding an infant.

Laboratory Tests

There are no routine laboratory tests recommended.

Drug Interactions

As with other drugs, the potential for interaction by a variety of mechanisms (e.g., pharmacodynamic, pharmacokinetic inhibition or enhancement, etc.) is a possibility (see CLINICAL PHARMACOLOGY).

Monoamine Oxidase Inhibitors

(See CONTRAINDICATIONS, WARNINGS, and DOSAGE AND ADMINISTRATION.)

Serotonergic Drugs

(See CONTRAINDICATIONS and WARNINGS.)

Drugs Affecting Hepatic Metabolism

The metabolism and pharmacokinetics of REMERON (mirtazapine) Tablets may be affected by the induction or inhibition of drug-metabolizing enzymes.

Drugs that are Metabolized by and/or Inhibit Cytochrome P450 Enzymes

CYP Enzyme Inducers

(these studies used both drugs at steady state)

Phenytoin

In healthy male patients (n=18), phenytoin (200 mg daily) increased mirtazapine (30 mg daily) clearance about 2-fold, resulting in a decrease in average plasma mirtazapine concentrations of 45%. Mirtazapine did not significantly affect the pharmacokinetics of phenytoin.

Carbamazepine

In healthy male patients (n=24), carbamazepine (400 mg b.i.d.) increased mirtazapine (15 mg b.i.d.) clearance about 2-fold, resulting in a decrease in average plasma mirtazapine concentrations of 60%.

When phenytoin, carbamazepine, or another inducer of hepatic metabolism (such as rifampicin) is added to mirtazapine therapy, the mirtazapine dose may have to be increased. If treatment with such a medicinal product is discontinued, it may be necessary to reduce the mirtazapine dose.

CYP Enzyme Inhibitors

Cimetidine

In healthy male patients (n=12), when cimetidine, a weak inhibitor of CYP1A2, CYP2D6, and CYP3A4, given at 800 mg b.i.d. at steady state was coadministered with mirtazapine (30 mg daily) at steady state, the Area Under the Curve (AUC) of mirtazapine increased more than 50%. Mirtazapine did not cause relevant changes in the pharmacokinetics of cimetidine. The mirtazapine dose may have to be decreased when concomitant treatment with cimetidine is started, or increased when cimetidine treatment is discontinued.

Ketoconazole

In healthy, male, Caucasian patients (n=24), coadministration of the potent CYP3A4 inhibitor ketoconazole (200 mg b.i.d. for 6.5 days) increased the peak plasma levels and the AUC of a single 30-mg dose of mirtazapine by approximately 40% and 50%, respectively.

Caution should be exercised when coadministering mirtazapine with potent CYP3A4 inhibitors, HIV protease inhibitors, azole antifungals, erythromycin, or nefazodone.

Paroxetine

In an *in vivo* interaction study in healthy, CYP2D6 extensive metabolizer patients (n=24), mirtazapine (30 mg/day), at steady state, did not cause relevant changes in the pharmacokinetics of steady state paroxetine (40 mg/day), a CYP2D6 inhibitor.

Other Drug-Drug Interactions

Amitriptyline

In healthy, CYP2D6 extensive metabolizer patients (n=32), amitriptyline (75 mg daily), at steady state, did not cause relevant changes in the pharmacokinetics of steady state mirtazapine (30 mg daily); mirtazapine also did not cause relevant changes to the pharmacokinetics of amitriptyline.

Warfarin

In healthy male subjects (n=16), mirtazapine (30 mg daily), at steady state, caused a small (0.2) but statistically significant increase in the International Normalized Ratio (INR) in subjects treated with warfarin. As at a higher dose of mirtazapine, a more pronounced effect can not be excluded, it is advisable to monitor the INR in case of concomitant treatment of warfarin with mirtazapine.

Lithium
No relevant clinical effects or significant changes in pharmacokinetics have been observed in healthy male subjects on concurrent treatment with subtherapeutic levels of lithium (600 mg/day for 10 days) at steady state and a single 30-mg dose of mirtazapine. The effects of higher doses of lithium on the pharmacokinetics of mirtazapine are unknown.

Risperidone
In an *in vivo*, nonrandomized, interaction study, subjects (n=6) in need of treatment with an antipsychotic and antidepressant drug, showed that mirtazapine (30 mg daily) at steady state did not influence the pharmacokinetics of risperidone (up to 3 mg b.i.d.).

Alcohol
Concomitant administration of alcohol (equivalent to 60 g) had a minimal effect on plasma levels of mirtazapine (15 mg) in 6 healthy male subjects. However, the impairment of cognitive and motor skills produced by REMERON were shown to be additive with those produced by alcohol. Accordingly, patients should be advised to avoid alcohol while taking REMERON.

Diazepam
Concomitant administration of diazepam (15 mg) had a minimal effect on plasma levels of mirtazapine (15 mg) in 12 healthy subjects. However, the impairment of motor skills produced by REMERON has been shown to be additive with those caused by diazepam. Accordingly, patients should be advised to avoid diazepam and other similar drugs while taking REMERON.

Carcinogenesis, Mutagenesis, Impairment of Fertility

Carcinogenesis
Carcinogenicity studies were conducted with mirtazapine given in the diet at doses of 2, 20, and 200 mg/kg/day to mice and 2, 20, and 60 mg/kg/day to rats. The highest doses used are approximately 20 and 12 times the maximum recommended human dose (MRHD) of 45 mg/day on an mg/m^2 basis in mice and rats, respectively. There was an increased incidence of hepatocellular adenoma and carcinoma in male mice at the high dose. In rats, there was an increase in hepatocellular adenoma in females at the mid and high doses and in hepatocellular tumors and thyroid follicular adenoma/cystadenoma and carcinoma in males at the high dose. The data suggest that the above effects could possibly be mediated by non-genotoxic mechanisms, the relevance of which to humans is not known.
The doses used in the mouse study may not have been high enough to fully characterize the carcinogenic potential of REMERON (mirtazapine) Tablets.

Mutagenesis
Mirtazapine was not mutagenic or clastogenic and did not induce general DNA damage as determined in several genotoxicity tests: Ames test, *in vitro* gene mutation assay in Chinese hamster V 79 cells, *in vitro* sister chromatid exchange assay in cultured rabbit lymphocytes, *in vivo* bone marrow micronucleus test in rats, and unscheduled DNA synthesis assay in HeLa cells.

Impairment of Fertility
In a fertility study in rats, mirtazapine was given at doses up to 100 mg/kg [20 times the maximum recommended human dose (MRHD) on an mg/m^2 basis]. Mating and conception were not affected by the drug, but estrous cycling was disrupted at doses that were 3 or more times the MRHD, and pre-implantation losses occurred at 20 times the MRHD.

Pregnancy
Teratogenic Effects
Pregnancy Category C
Reproduction studies in pregnant rats and rabbits at doses up to 100 mg/kg and 40 mg/kg, respectively [20 and 17 times the maximum recommended human dose (MRHD) on an mg/m^2 basis, respectively], have revealed no evidence of teratogenic effects. However, in rats, there was an increase in postimplantation losses in dams treated with mirtazapine. There was an increase in pup deaths during the first 3 days of lactation and a decrease in pup birth weights. The cause of these deaths is not known. The effects occurred at doses that were 20 times the MRHD, but not at 3 times the MRHD, on an mg/m^2 basis. There are no adequate and well-controlled studies in pregnant women. Because animal reproduction studies are not always predictive of human response, this drug should be used during pregnancy only if clearly needed.

Nursing Mothers
Because some REMERON may be excreted into breast milk, caution should be exercised when REMERON (mirtazapine) Tablets are administered to nursing women.

Pediatric Use
Safety and effectiveness in the pediatric population have not been established (see BOXED WARNING and WARNINGS: Clinical Worsening and Suicide Risk). Two placebo-controlled trials in 258 pediatric patients with MDD have been conducted with REMERON (mirtazapine) Tablets, and the data were not sufficient to support a claim for use in pediatric patients. Anyone considering the use of REMERON in a child or adolescent must balance the potential risks with the clinical need.
In an 8-week-long pediatric clinical trial of doses between 15 to 45 mg/day, 49% of REMERON-treated patients had a weight gain of at least 7%, compared to 5.7% of placebo-treated patients. The mean increase in weight was 4 kg (2 kg SD) for REMERON-treated patients versus 1 kg (2 kg SD) for placebo-treated patients (see PRECAUTIONS: Increased Appetite/Weight Gain).

Geriatric Use
Approximately 190 elderly individuals (≥65 years of age) participated in clinical studies with REMERON (mirtazapine) Tablets. This drug is known to be substantially excreted by the kidney (75%), and the risk of decreased clearance of this drug is greater in patients with impaired renal function. Because elderly patients are more likely to have decreased renal function, care should be taken in dose selection. Sedating drugs may cause confusion and over-sedation in the elderly. No unusual adverse age-related phenomena were identified in this group. Pharmacokinetic studies revealed a decreased clearance in the elderly. Caution is indicated in administering REMERON to elderly patients (see CLINICAL PHARMACOLOGY and DOSAGE AND ADMINISTRATION).

ADVERSE REACTIONS

Associated with Discontinuation of Treatment
Approximately 16% of the 453 patients who received REMERON (mirtazapine) Tablets in US 6-week controlled clinical trials discontinued treatment due to an adverse experience, compared to 7% of the 361 placebo-treated patients in those studies. The most common events (≥1%) associated with discontinuation and considered to be drug related (i.e., those events associated with dropout at a rate at least twice that of placebo) are included in Table 2.

Table 2: Common Adverse Events Associated With Discontinuation of Treatment in 6-Week US REMERON Trials

Adverse Event	Percentage of Patients Discontinuing With Adverse Event	
	REMERON (n=453)	Placebo (n=361)
Somnolence	10.4%	2.2%
Nausea	1.5%	0%

Commonly Observed Adverse Events in US Controlled Clinical Trials
The most commonly observed adverse events associated with the use of REMERON (mirtazapine) Tablets (incidence of 5% or greater) and not observed at an equivalent incidence among placebo-treated patients (REMERON incidence at least twice that for placebo) are listed in Table 3.

Table 3: Common Treatment-Emergent Adverse Events Associated With the Use of REMERON in 6-Week US Trials

Adverse Event	Percentage of Patients Reporting Adverse Event	
	REMERON (n=453)	Placebo (n=361)
Somnolence	54%	18%
Increased Appetite	17%	2%
Weight Gain	12%	2%
Dizziness	7%	3%

Adverse Events Occurring at an Incidence of 1% or More Among REMERON-Treated Patients
Table 4 enumerates adverse events that occurred at an incidence of 1% or more, and were more frequent than in the placebo group, among REMERON (mirtazapine) Tablets-treated patients who participated in short-term US placebo-controlled trials in which patients were dosed in a range of 5 to 60 mg/day. This table shows the percentage of patients in each group who had at least 1 episode of an event at some time during their treatment. Reported adverse events were classified using a standard COSTART-based dictionary terminology.
The prescriber should be aware that these figures cannot be used to predict the incidence of side effects in the course of usual medical practice where patient characteristics and other factors differ from those which prevailed in the clinical trials. Similarly, the cited frequencies cannot be compared with figures obtained from other investigations involving different treatments, uses, and investigators. The cited figures, however, do provide the prescribing physician with some basis for estimating the relative contribution of drug and nondrug factors to the side-effect incidence rate in the population studied.

Table 4: Incidence of Adverse Clinical Experiences* (≥1%) in Short-Term US Controlled Studies

Body System / Adverse Clinical Experience	REMERON (n=453)	Placebo (n=361)
Body as a Whole		
Asthenia	8%	5%
Flu Syndrome	5%	3%
Back Pain	2%	1%
Digestive System		
Dry Mouth	25%	15%
Increased Appetite	17%	2%
Constipation	13%	7%
Metabolic and Nutritional Disorders		
Weight Gain	12%	2%
Peripheral Edema	2%	1%
Edema	1%	0%
Musculoskeletal System		
Myalgia	2%	1%
Nervous System		
Somnolence	54%	18%
Dizziness	7%	3%
Abnormal Dreams	4%	1%
Thinking Abnormal	3%	1%
Tremor	2%	1%
Confusion	2%	0%
Respiratory System		
Dyspnea	1%	0%
Urogenital System		
Urinary Frequency	2%	1%

* Events reported by at least 1% of patients treated with REMERON are included, except the following events, which had an incidence on placebo greater than or equal to REMERON: headache, infection, pain, chest pain, palpitation, tachycardia, postural hypotension, nausea, dyspepsia, diarrhea, flatulence, insomnia, nervousness, libido decreased, hypertonia, pharyngitis, rhinitis, sweating, amblyopia, tinnitus, taste perversion.

ECG Changes
The electrocardiograms for 338 patients who received REMERON (mirtazapine) Tablets and 261 patients who received placebo in 6-week, placebo-controlled trials were analyzed. Prolongation in QTc ≥500 msec was not observed among mirtazapine-treated patients; mean change in QTc was +1.6 msec for mirtazapine and –3.1 msec for placebo. Mirtazapine was associated with a mean increase in heart rate of 3.4 bpm, compared to 0.8 bpm for placebo. The clinical significance of these changes is unknown.

Other Adverse Events Observed During the Premarketing Evaluation of REMERON
During its premarketing assessment, multiple doses of REMERON (mirtazapine) Tablets were administered to 2796 patients in clinical studies. The conditions and duration of exposure to mirtazapine varied greatly, and included (in overlapping categories) open and double-blind studies, uncontrolled and controlled studies, inpatient and outpatient studies, fixed-dose and titration studies. Untoward events associated with this exposure were recorded by clinical investigators using terminology of their own choosing. Consequently, it is not possible to provide a meaningful estimate of the proportion of individuals experiencing adverse events without first grouping similar types of untoward events into a smaller number of standardized event categories.

In the tabulations that follow, reported adverse events were classified using a standard COSTART-based dictionary terminology. The frequencies presented, therefore, represent the proportion of the 2796 patients exposed to multiple doses of REMERON who experienced an event of the type cited on at least 1 occasion while receiving REMERON. All reported events are included except those already listed in Table 4, those adverse experiences subsumed under COSTART terms that are either overly general or excessively specific so as to be uninformative, and those events for which a drug cause was very remote.

It is important to emphasize that, although the events reported occurred during treatment with REMERON, they were not necessarily caused by it.

Events are further categorized by body system and listed in order of decreasing frequency according to the following definitions: frequent adverse events are those occurring on 1 or more occasions in at least 1/100 patients; infrequent adverse events are those occurring in 1/100 to 1/1000 patients; rare events are those occurring in fewer than 1/1000 patients. Only those events not already listed in Table 4 appear in this listing. Events of major clinical importance are also described in the WARNINGS and PRECAUTIONS sections.

Body as a Whole: *frequent:* malaise, abdominal pain, abdominal syndrome acute; *infrequent:* chills, fever, face edema, ulcer, photosensitivity reaction, neck rigidity, neck pain, abdomen enlarged; *rare:* cellulitis, chest pain substernal.

Cardiovascular System: *frequent:* hypertension, vasodilatation; *infrequent:* angina pectoris, myocardial infarction, bradycardia, ventricular extrasystoles, syncope, migraine, hypotension; *rare:* atrial arrhythmia, bigeminy, vascular headache, pulmonary embolus, cerebral ischemia, cardiomegaly, phlebitis, left heart failure.

Digestive System: *frequent:* vomiting, anorexia; *infrequent:* eructation, glossitis, cholecystitis, nausea and vomiting, gum hemorrhage, stomatitis, colitis, liver function tests abnormal; *rare:* tongue discoloration, ulcerative stomatitis, salivary gland enlargement, increased salivation, intestinal obstruction, pancreatitis, aphthous stomatitis, cirrhosis of liver, gastritis, gastroenteritis, oral moniliasis, tongue edema.

Endocrine System: *rare:* goiter, hypothyroidism.

Hemic and Lymphatic System: *rare:* lymphadenopathy, leukopenia, petechia, anemia, thrombocytopenia, lymphocytosis, pancytopenia.

Metabolic and Nutritional Disorders: *frequent:* thirst; *infrequent:* dehydration, weight loss; *rare:* gout, SGOT increased, healing abnormal, acid phosphatase increased, SGPT increased, diabetes mellitus, hyponatremia.

Musculoskeletal System: *frequent:* myasthenia, arthralgia; *infrequent:* arthritis, tenosynovitis; *rare:* pathologic fracture, osteoporosis fracture, bone pain, myositis, tendon rupture, arthrosis, bursitis.

Nervous System: *frequent:* hypesthesia, apathy, depression, hypokinesia, vertigo, twitching, agitation, anxiety, amnesia, hyperkinesia, paresthesia; *infrequent:* ataxia, delirium, delusions, depersonalization, dyskinesia, extrapyramidal syndrome, libido increased, coordination abnormal, dysarthria, hallucinations, manic reaction, neurosis, dystonia, hostility, reflexes increased, emotional lability, euphoria, paranoid reaction; *rare:* aphasia, nystagmus, akathisia (psychomotor restlessness), stupor, dementia, diplopia, drug dependence, paralysis, grand mal convulsion, hypotonia, myoclonus, psychotic depression, withdrawal syndrome, serotonin syndrome.

Respiratory System: *frequent:* cough increased, sinusitis; *infrequent:* epistaxis, bronchitis, asthma, pneumonia; *rare:* asphyxia, laryngitis, pneumothorax, hiccup.

Skin and Appendages: *frequent:* pruritus, rash; *infrequent:* acne, exfoliative dermatitis, dry skin, herpes simplex, alopecia; *rare:* urticaria, herpes zoster, skin hypertrophy, seborrhea, skin ulcer.

Special Senses: *infrequent:* eye pain, abnormality of accommodation, conjunctivitis, deafness, keratoconjunctivitis, lacrimation disorder, glaucoma, hyperacusis, ear pain; *rare:* blepharitis, partial transitory deafness, otitis media, taste loss, parosmia.

Urogenital System: *frequent:* urinary tract infection; *infrequent:* kidney calculus, cystitis, dysuria, urinary incontinence, urinary retention, vaginitis, hematuria, breast pain, amenorrhea, dysmenorrhea, leukorrhea, impotence; *rare:* polyuria, urethritis, metrorrhagia, menorrhagia, abnormal ejaculation, breast engorgement, breast enlargement, urinary urgency.

Other Adverse Events Observed During Postmarketing Evaluation of REMERON

Adverse events reported since market introduction, which were temporally (but not necessarily causally) related to mirtazapine therapy, include 4 cases of the ventricular arrhythmia torsades de pointes. In 3 of the 4 cases, however, concomitant drugs were implicated. All patients recovered. Cases of severe skin reactions, including Stevens-Johnson syndrome, bullous dermatitis, erythema multiforme and toxic epidermal necrolysis have also been reported.

DRUG ABUSE AND DEPENDENCE

Controlled Substance Class

REMERON (mirtazapine) Tablets are not a controlled substance.

Physical and Psychologic Dependence

REMERON (mirtazapine) Tablets have not been systematically studied in animals or humans for its potential for abuse, tolerance, or physical dependence. While the clinical trials did not reveal any tendency for any drug-seeking behavior, these observations were not systematic and it is not possible to predict on the basis of this limited experience the extent to which a CNS-active drug will be misused, diverted and/or abused once marketed. Consequently, patients should be evaluated carefully for history of drug abuse, and such patients should be observed closely for signs of REMERON misuse or abuse (e.g., development of tolerance, incrementations of dose, drug-seeking behavior).

OVERDOSAGE

Human Experience

There is very limited experience with REMERON (mirtazapine) Tablets overdose. In premarketing clinical studies, there were 8 reports of REMERON overdose alone or in combination with other pharmacological agents. The only drug overdose death reported while taking REMERON was in combination with amitriptyline and chlorprothixene in a non-US clinical study. Based on plasma levels, the REMERON dose taken was 30 to 45 mg, while plasma levels of amitriptyline and chlorprothixene were found to be at toxic levels. All other premarketing overdose cases resulted in full recovery. Signs and symptoms reported in association with overdose included disorientation, drowsiness, impaired memory, and tachycardia. There were no reports of ECG abnormalities, coma, or convulsions following overdose with REMERON alone.

Overdose Management

Treatment should consist of those general measures employed in the management of overdose with any drug effective in the treatment of major depressive disorder. Ensure an adequate airway, oxygenation, and ventilation. Monitor cardiac rhythm and vital signs. General supportive and symptomatic measures are also recommended. Induction of emesis is not recommended. Gastric lavage with a large-bore orogastric tube with appropriate airway protection, if needed, may be indicated if performed soon after ingestion, or in symptomatic patients. Activated charcoal should be administered. There is no experience with the use of forced diuresis, dialysis, hemoperfusion, or exchange transfusion in the treatment of mirtazapine overdosage. No specific antidotes for mirtazapine are known.

In managing overdosage, consider the possibility of multiple-drug involvement. The physician should consider contacting a poison control center for additional information on the treatment of any overdose. Telephone numbers for certified poison control centers are listed in the *Physicians' Desk Reference* (PDR).

DOSAGE AND ADMINISTRATION

Initial Treatment

The recommended starting dose for REMERON (mirtazapine) Tablets is 15 mg/day, administered in a single dose, preferably in the evening prior to sleep. In the controlled clinical trials establishing the efficacy of REMERON in the treatment of major depressive disorder, the effective dose range was generally 15 to 45 mg/day. While the relationship between dose and satisfactory response in the treatment of major depressive disorder for REMERON has not been adequately explored, patients not responding to the initial 15-mg dose may benefit from dose increases up to a maximum of 45 mg/day. REMERON has an elimination half-life of approximately 20 to 40 hours; therefore, dose changes should not be made at intervals of less than 1 to 2 weeks in order to allow sufficient time for evaluation of the therapeutic response to a given dose.

Elderly and Patients with Renal or Hepatic Impairment

The clearance of mirtazapine is reduced in elderly patients and in patients with moderate to severe renal or hepatic impairment. Consequently, the prescriber should be aware that plasma mirtazapine levels may be increased in these patient groups, compared to levels observed in younger adults without renal or hepatic impairment (see PRECAUTIONS and CLINICAL PHARMACOLOGY).

Maintenance/Extended Treatment

It is generally agreed that acute episodes of depression require several months or longer of sustained pharmacological therapy beyond response to the acute episode. Systematic evaluation of REMERON (mirtazapine) Tablets has demonstrated that its efficacy in major depressive disorder is maintained for periods of up to 40 weeks following 8 to 12 weeks of initial treatment at a dose of 15 to 45 mg/day (see CLINICAL PHARMACOLOGY). Based on these limited data, it is unknown whether or not the dose of REMERON needed for maintenance treatment is identical to the dose needed to achieve an initial response. Patients should be periodically reassessed to determine the need for maintenance treatment and the appropriate dose for such treatment.

Switching a Patient To or From a Monoamine Oxidase Inhibitor (MAOI) Intended to Treat Psychiatric Disorders

At least 14 days should elapse between discontinuation of an MAOI intended to treat psychiatric disorders and initiation of therapy with REMERON (mirtazapine) Tablets. Conversely, at least 14 days should be allowed after stopping REMERON before starting an MAOI intended to treat psychiatric disorders (see CONTRAINDICATIONS).

Use of REMERON With Other MAOIs, Such as Linezolid or Methylene Blue

Do not start REMERON in a patient who is being treated with linezolid or intravenous methylene blue because there is an increased risk of serotonin syndrome. In a patient who requires more urgent treatment of a psychiatric condition, other interventions, including hospitalization, should be considered (see CONTRAINDICATIONS).

In some cases, a patient already receiving therapy with REMERON may require urgent treatment with linezolid or intravenous methylene blue. If acceptable alternatives to linezolid or intravenous methylene blue treatment are not available and the potential benefits of linezolid or intravenous methylene blue treatment are judged to outweigh the risks of serotonin syndrome in a particular patient, REMERON should be stopped promptly, and linezolid or intravenous methylene blue can be administered. The patient should be monitored for symptoms of serotonin syndrome for 2 weeks or until 24 hours after the last dose of linezolid or intravenous methylene blue, whichever comes first. Therapy with REMERON may be resumed 24 hours after the last dose of linezolid or intravenous methylene blue (see WARNINGS).

The risk of administering methylene blue by non-intravenous routes (such as oral tablets or by local injection) or in intravenous doses much lower than 1 mg/kg with REMERON is unclear. The clinician should, nevertheless, be aware of the possibility of emergent symptoms of serotonin syndrome with such use (see WARNINGS).

Discontinuation of Remeron Treatment

Symptoms associated with the discontinuation or dose reduction of REMERON Tablets have been reported. Patients should be monitored for these and other symptoms when discontinuing treatment or during dosage reduction. A gradual reduction in the dose over several weeks, rather than abrupt cessation, is recommended whenever possible. If intolerable symptoms occur following a decrease in the dose or upon discontinuation of treatment, dose titration should be managed on the basis of the patient's clinical response (see PRECAUTIONS and ADVERSE REACTIONS).

HOW SUPPLIED

REMERON (mirtazapine) Tablets are supplied as:

15 mg Tablets — oval, scored, yellow, coated, with "Organon" debossed on 1 side and "$^{T}{}_{3}{}^{Z}$" on the other side.

Bottles of 30 NDC 0052-0105-30

30 mg Tablets — oval, scored, red-brown, coated, with "Organon" debossed on 1 side and "$^{T}{}_{5}{}^{Z}$" on the other side.

Bottles of 30 NDC 0052-0107-30

45 mg Tablets — oval, white, coated, with "Organon" debossed on 1 side and "$^{T}{}_{7}{}^{Z}$" on the other side.

Bottles of 30 NDC 0052-0109-30

Storage

Store at 25°C (77°F); excursions permitted to 15-30°C (59-86°F) [see USP Controlled Room Temperature]. Protect from light and moisture.

Rx only

Manufactured for: Merck Sharp & Dohme Corp., a subsidiary of

MERCK & CO., INC., Whitehouse Station, NJ 08889, USA

Manufactured by: N.V. Organon, Oss, The Netherlands, a subsidiary of

Merck & Co., Inc., Whitehouse Station, NJ 08889, USA

Revised: 11/2012

900246-REM-TB-USPI.5

Medication Guide

REMERON® (rĕm' - ĕ – rŏn)

(mirtazapine)

Tablets

Read the Medication Guide that comes with REMERON before you start taking it and each time you get a refill. There may be new information. This Medication Guide does not take the place of talking to your healthcare provider about your medical condition or treatment. If you have any questions about REMERON, talk to your healthcare provider.

What is the most important information I should know about REMERON®?
REMERON and other antidepressant medicines may cause serious side effects, including:
1. **Suicidal thoughts or actions:**
   - **REMERON and other antidepressant medicines may increase suicidal thoughts or actions in some children, teenagers, or young adults within the first few months of treatment or when the dose is changed.**
   - Depression or other serious mental illnesses are the most important causes of suicidal thoughts or actions.
   - Watch for these changes and call your healthcare provider right away if you notice:
     - New or sudden changes in mood, behavior, actions, thoughts, or feelings, especially if severe.
     - Pay particular attention to such changes when REMERON is started or when the dose is changed.

Keep all follow-up visits with your healthcare provider and call between visits if you are worried about symptoms.

Call your healthcare provider right away if you have any of the following symptoms, or call 911 if an emergency, especially if they are new, worse, or worry you:
- attempts to commit suicide
- acting on dangerous impulses
- acting aggressive or violent
- thoughts about suicide or dying
- new or worse depression
- new or worse anxiety or panic attacks
- feeling agitated, restless, angry or irritable
- trouble sleeping
- an increase in activity or talking more than what is normal for you
- other unusual changes in behavior or mood

Call your healthcare provider right away if you have any of the following symptoms, or call 911 if an emergency. REMERON may be associated with these serious side effects:

2. **Manic episodes:**
   - greatly increased energy
   - severe trouble sleeping
   - racing thoughts
   - reckless behavior
   - unusually grand ideas
   - excessive happiness or irritability
   - talking more or faster than usual
3. **Decreased White Blood Cells** called neutrophils, which are needed to fight infections. Tell your doctor if you have any indication of infection such as fever, chills, sore throat, or mouth or nose sores, especially symptoms which are flu-like.
4. **Serotonin Syndrome. This condition can be life-threatening and may include:**
   - agitation, hallucinations, coma or other changes in mental status
   - coordination problems or muscle twitching (overactive reflexes)
   - racing heartbeat, high or low blood pressure
   - sweating or fever
   - nausea, vomiting, or diarrhea
   - muscle rigidity
5. **Seizures**
6. **Low salt (sodium) levels in the blood.** Elderly people may be at greater risk for this. Symptoms may include:
   - headache
   - weakness or feeling unsteady
   - confusion, problems concentrating or thinking or memory problems
7. **Sleepiness.** It is best to take **REMERON** close to bedtime.
8. **Severe skin reactions:** Call your doctor right away if you have any or all of the following symptoms:
   - severe rash with skin swelling (including on the palms of the hands and soles of the feet)
   - painful reddening of the skin and/or blisters/ulcers on the body or in the mouth
9. **Severe allergic reactions: trouble breathing, swelling of the face, tongue, eyes or mouth**
   - rash, itchy welts (hives) or blisters, alone or with fever or joint pain
10. **Increases in appetite or weight.** Children and adolescents should have height and weight monitored during treatment.
11. **Increased cholesterol and triglyceride levels in your blood**

Do not stop REMERON without first talking to your healthcare provider. Stopping REMERON too quickly may cause potentially serious symptoms including:
- dizziness
- abnormal dreams
- agitation
- anxiety
- fatigue
- confusion
- headache
- shaking
- tingling sensation
- nausea, vomiting
- sweating

What is REMERON?
REMERON is a prescription medicine used to treat depression. It is important to talk with your healthcare provider about the risks of treating depression and also the risks of not treating it. You should discuss all treatment choices with your healthcare provider.
Talk to your healthcare provider if you do not think that your condition is getting better with REMERON treatment.

Who should not take REMERON?
Do not take REMERON:
- if you are allergic to mirtazapine or any of the ingredients in REMERON. See the end of this Medication Guide for a complete list of ingredients in REMERON.
- If you take a monoamine oxidase inhibitor (MAOI). Ask your healthcare provider or pharmacist if you are not sure if you take an MAOI, including the antibiotic linezolid.
- Do not take an MAOI within 2 weeks of stopping REMERON unless directed to do so by your physician.
- Do not start REMERON if you stopped taking an MAOI in the last 2 weeks unless directed to do so by your physician.

People who take REMERON close in time to an MAOI may have serious or even life-threatening side effects. Get medical help right away if you have any of these symptoms:
- high fever
- uncontrolled muscle spasms
- stiff muscles
- rapid changes in heart rate or blood pressure
- confusion
- loss of consciousness (pass out)

What should I tell my healthcare provider before taking REMERON?
Ask if you are not sure.
Before starting REMERON, tell your healthcare provider if you:
- Are taking certain drugs such as:
  - Triptans used to treat migraine headache
  - Medicines used to treat mood, anxiety, psychotic or thought disorders, including tricyclics, lithium, SSRIs, SNRIs, or antipsychotics
  - Tramadol used to treat pain
  - Over-the-counter supplements such as tryptophan or St. John's wort
  - Phenytoin, carbamazepine, or rifampicin (these drugs can decrease your blood level of REMERON)
  - Cimetidine or ketoconazole (these drugs can increase your blood level of REMERON)
- Have or had:
  - liver problems
  - kidney problems
  - heart problems
  - seizures or convulsions
  - bipolar disorder or mania
  - a tendency to get dizzy or faint
- are pregnant or plan to become pregnant. It is not known if REMERON will harm your unborn baby. Talk to your healthcare provider about the benefits and risks of treating depression during pregnancy
- are breastfeeding or plan to breastfeed. Some REMERON may pass into your breast milk. Talk to your healthcare provider about the best way to feed your baby while taking REMERON

Tell your healthcare provider about all the medicines that you take, including prescription and non-prescription medicines, vitamins, and herbal supplements. REMERON and some medicines may interact with each other, may not work as well, or may cause serious side effects.
Your healthcare provider or pharmacist can tell you if it is safe to take REMERON with your other medicines. Do not start or stop any medicine while taking REMERON without talking to your healthcare provider first.

> If you take REMERON, you should not take any other medicines that contain mirtazapine including REMERONSolTab®.

How should I take REMERON?
- Take REMERON exactly as prescribed. Your healthcare provider may need to change the dose of REMERON until it is the right dose for you.
- Take REMERON at the same time each day, preferably in the evening at bedtime.
- Swallow REMERON as directed.
- It is common for antidepressant medicines such as REMERON to take up to a few weeks before you start to feel better. Do not stop taking REMERON if you do not feel results right away.
- Do not stop taking or change the dose of REMERON without first talking to your doctor, even if you feel better.
- REMERON may be taken with or without food.
- If you miss a dose of REMERON, take the missed dose as soon as you remember. If it is almost time for the next dose, skip the missed dose and take your next dose at the regular time. Do not take two doses of REMERON at the same time.
- If you take too much REMERON, call your healthcare provider or poison control center right away, or get emergency treatment.

What should I avoid while taking REMERON?
- REMERON can cause sleepiness or may affect your ability to make decisions, think clearly, or react quickly. You should not drive, operate heavy machinery, or do other dangerous activities until you know how REMERON affects you.
- Avoid drinking alcohol or taking diazepam (a medicine used for anxiety, insomnia and seizures, for example) or similar medicines while taking REMERON. If you are uncertain about whether certain medication can be taken with REMERON, please discuss with your doctor.

What are the possible side effects of REMERON?
REMERON may cause serious side effects, including all of those described in the section entitled "What is the most important information I should know about REMERON?"
Common possible side effects in people who take REMERON include:
- sleepiness
- increased appetite, weight gain
- dry mouth
- constipation
- dizziness
- abnormal dreams

Tell your healthcare provider if you have any side effect that bothers you or that does not go away. These are not all the possible side effects of REMERON. For more information, ask your healthcare provider or pharmacist.

CALL YOUR DOCTOR FOR MEDICAL ADVICE ABOUT SIDE EFFECTS. YOU MAY REPORT SIDE EFFECTS TO THE FDA AT 1-800-FDA-1088.

How should I store REMERON?
- Store REMERON at room temperature 25°C (77°F). Storage at 15°C-30°C (59°F-86°F) is permitted occasionally.
- Keep REMERON away from light.
- Keep REMERON bottle closed tightly.

Keep REMERON and all medicines out of the reach of children.

General information about REMERON
Medicines are sometimes prescribed for purposes other than those listed in a Medication Guide. Do not use REMERON for a condition for which it was not prescribed. Do not give REMERON to other people, even if they have the same condition. It may harm them.
This Medication Guide summarizes the most important information about REMERON. If you would like more information, talk with your healthcare provider. You may ask your healthcare provider or pharmacist for information about REMERON that is written for healthcare professionals.
For more information about REMERON call 1-800-526-4099 or go to www.REMERON.com.

What are the ingredients in REMERON?
Active ingredient: mirtazapine
Inactive ingredients:
- **15 mg tablets:** Starch (corn), hydroxypropyl cellulose, magnesium stearate, colloidal silicon dioxide, lactose, hypromellose, polyethylene glycol 8000, titanium dioxide, ferric oxide (yellow).
- **30 mg tablets:** Starch (corn), hydroxypropyl cellulose, magnesium stearate, colloidal silicon dioxide, lactose, hypromellose, polyethylene glycol 8000, titanium dioxide, ferric oxide (yellow), ferric oxide (red).
- **45 mg tablets:** Starch (corn), hydroxypropyl cellulose, magnesium stearate, colloidal silicon dioxide, lactose, hypromellose, polyethylene glycol 8000, titanium dioxide.

This Medication Guide has been approved by the U.S. Food and Drug Administration.
Manufactured for: Merck Sharp & Dohme Corp., a subsidiary of
MERCK & CO., INC., Whitehouse Station, NJ 08889, USA
Manufactured by: N.V. Organon, Oss, The Netherlands, a subsidiary of **Merck & Co., Inc.**, Whitehouse Station, NJ 08889, USA

Revised: 11/2012
900246-REM-TB-MG.5
Shown in Product Identification Guide, page 309

REMERONSolTab® ℞
[rem-er-on]
(mirtazapine)
Orally Disintegrating Tablets
ONCE-A-DAY

Suicidality and Antidepressant Drugs
Antidepressants increased the risk compared to placebo of suicidal thinking and behavior (suicidality) in children, adolescents, and young adults in short-term studies of major depressive disorder (MDD) and other psychiatric disorders. Anyone considering the use of REMERONSolTab® (mirtazapine) Orally Disintegrating Tablets or any other antidepressant in a child, adolescent, or young adult must balance this risk with the clinical need. Short-term studies did not show an increase in the risk of suicidality with antidepressants compared to placebo in adults beyond age 24; there was a reduction in risk with antidepressants compared to placebo in adults aged 65 and older. Depression and certain other psychiatric disorders are themselves associated with increases in the risk of suicide. Patients of all ages who are started on antidepressant therapy should be monitored appropriately and observed closely for clinical worsening, suicidality, or unusual changes in behavior. Families and caregivers should be advised of the need for close observation and communication with the prescriber. REMERONSolTab is not approved for use in pediatric patients. (See WARNINGS: Clinical Worsening and Suicide Risk, PRECAUTIONS: Information for Patients, and PRECAUTIONS: Pediatric Use.)

DESCRIPTION

REMERONSolTab® (mirtazapine) Orally Disintegrating Tablets are an orally administered drug. Mirtazapine has a tetracyclic chemical structure and belongs to the piperazino-azepine group of compounds. It is designated 1,2,3,4,10,14b-hexahydro-2-methylpyrazino [2,1-a] pyrido [2,3-c] benzazepine and has the empirical formula of $C_{17}H_{19}N_3$. Its molecular weight is 265.36. The structural formula is the following and it is the racemic mixture:

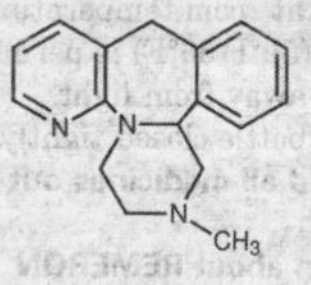

Mirtazapine is a white to creamy white crystalline powder which is slightly soluble in water. REMERONSolTab is available for oral administration as an orally disintegrating tablet containing 15, 30, or 45 mg of mirtazapine. It disintegrates in the mouth within seconds after placement on the tongue, allowing its contents to be subsequently swallowed with or without water. REMERONSolTab also contains the following inactive ingredients: aspartame, citric acid, crospovidone, hypromellose, magnesium stearate, mannitol, microcrystalline cellulose, natural and artificial orange flavor, polymethacrylate, povidone, sodium bicarbonate, starch, and sucrose.

CLINICAL PHARMACOLOGY

Pharmacodynamics

The mechanism of action of REMERONSolTab (mirtazapine) Orally Disintegrating Tablets, as with other drugs effective in the treatment of major depressive disorder, is unknown.

Evidence gathered in preclinical studies suggests that mirtazapine enhances central noradrenergic and serotonergic activity. These studies have shown that mirtazapine acts as an antagonist at central presynaptic α_2-adrenergic inhibitory autoreceptors and heteroreceptors, an action that is postulated to result in an increase in central noradrenergic and serotonergic activity.

Mirtazapine is a potent antagonist of 5-HT_2 and 5-HT_3 receptors. Mirtazapine has no significant affinity for the 5-HT_{1A} and 5-HT_{1B} receptors.

Mirtazapine is a potent antagonist of histamine (H_1) receptors, a property that may explain its prominent sedative effects.

Mirtazapine is a moderate peripheral α_1-adrenergic antagonist, a property that may explain the occasional orthostatic hypotension reported in association with its use.

Mirtazapine is a moderate antagonist at muscarinic receptors, a property that may explain the relatively low incidence of anticholinergic side effects associated with its use.

Pharmacokinetics

REMERONSolTab (mirtazapine) Orally Disintegrating Tablets are rapidly and completely absorbed following oral administration and have a half-life of about 20 to 40 hours. Peak plasma concentrations are reached within about 2 hours following an oral dose. The presence of food in the stomach has a minimal effect on both the rate and extent of absorption and does not require a dosage adjustment. REMERONSolTab Orally Disintegrating Tablets are bioequivalent to REMERON® (mirtazapine) Tablets.

Mirtazapine is extensively metabolized after oral administration. Major pathways of bio-transformation are demethylation and hydroxylation followed by glucuronide conjugation. *In vitro* data from human liver microsomes indicate that cytochrome 2D6 and 1A2 are involved in the formation of the 8-hydroxy metabolite of mirtazapine, whereas cytochrome 3A is considered to be responsible for the formation of the N-desmethyl and N-oxide metabolite. Mirtazapine has an absolute bioavailability of about 50%. It is eliminated predominantly via urine (75%) with 15% in feces. Several unconjugated metabolites possess pharmacological activity but are present in the plasma at very low levels. The (−) enantiomer has an elimination half-life that is approximately twice as long as the (+) enantiomer and therefore achieves plasma levels that are about 3 times as high as that of the (+) enantiomer.

Plasma levels are linearly related to dose over a dose range of 15 to 80 mg. The mean elimination half-life of mirtazapine after oral administration ranges from approximately 20 to 40 hours across age and gender subgroups, with females of all ages exhibiting significantly longer elimination half-lives than males (mean half-life of 37 hours for females vs. 26 hours for males). Steady state plasma levels of mirtazapine are attained within 5 days, with about 50% accumulation (accumulation ratio=1.5).

Mirtazapine is approximately 85% bound to plasma proteins over a concentration range of 0.01 to 10 mcg/mL.

Special Populations

Geriatric

Following oral administration of REMERON (mirtazapine) Tablets 20 mg/day for 7 days to subjects of varying ages (range, 25–74), oral clearance of mirtazapine was reduced in the elderly compared to the younger subjects. The differences were most striking in males, with a 40% lower clearance in elderly males compared to younger males, while the clearance in elderly females was only 10% lower compared to younger females. Caution is indicated in administering REMERONSolTab (mirtazapine) Orally Disintegrating Tablets to elderly patients (see PRECAUTIONS and DOSAGE AND ADMINISTRATION).

Pediatrics

Safety and effectiveness of mirtazapine in the pediatric population have not been established (see PRECAUTIONS).

Gender

The mean elimination half-life of mirtazapine after oral administration ranges from approximately 20 to 40 hours across age and gender subgroups, with females of all ages exhibiting significantly longer elimination half-lives than males (mean half-life of 37 hours for females vs. 26 hours for males) (see Pharmacokinetics).

Race

There have been no clinical studies to evaluate the effect of race on the pharmacokinetics of REMERONSolTab.

Renal Insufficiency

The disposition of mirtazapine was studied in patients with varying degrees of renal function. Elimination of mirtazapine is correlated with creatinine clearance. Total body clearance of mirtazapine was reduced approximately 30% in patients with moderate (Clcr=11–39 mL/min/1.73 m^2) and approximately 50% in patients with severe (Clcr=<10 mL/min/1.73 m^2) renal impairment when compared to normal subjects. Caution is indicated in administering REMERONSolTab to patients with compromised renal function (see PRECAUTIONS and DOSAGE AND ADMINISTRATION).

Hepatic Insufficiency

Following a single 15-mg oral dose of REMERON, the oral clearance of mirtazapine was decreased by approximately 30% in hepatically impaired patients compared to subjects with normal hepatic function. Caution is indicated in administering REMERONSolTab to patients with compromised hepatic function (see PRECAUTIONS and DOSAGE AND ADMINISTRATION).

Clinical Trials Showing Effectiveness

The efficacy of REMERON (mirtazapine) Tablets as a treatment for major depressive disorder was established in 4 placebo-controlled, 6-week trials in adult outpatients meeting DSM-III criteria for major depressive disorder. Patients were titrated with mirtazapine from a dose range of 5 mg up to 35 mg/day. Overall, these studies demonstrated mirtazapine to be superior to placebo on at least 3 of the following 4 measures: 21-Item Hamilton Depression Rating Scale (HDRS) total score; HDRS Depressed Mood Item; CGI Severity score; and Montgomery and Asberg Depression Rating Scale (MADRS). Superiority of mirtazapine over placebo was also found for certain factors of the HDRS, including anxiety/somatization factor and sleep disturbance factor. The mean mirtazapine dose for patients who completed these 4 studies ranged from 21 to 32 mg/day. A fifth study of similar design utilized a higher dose (up to 50 mg) per day and also showed effectiveness.

Examination of age and gender subsets of the population did not reveal any differential responsiveness on the basis of these subgroupings.

In a longer-term study, patients meeting (DSM-IV) criteria for major depressive disorder who had responded during an initial 8 to 12 weeks of acute treatment on REMERON were randomized to continuation of REMERON or placebo for up to 40 weeks of observation for relapse. Response during the open phase was defined as having achieved a HAM-D 17 total score of ≤8 and a CGI-Improvement score of 1 or 2 at 2 consecutive visits beginning with week 6 of the 8 to 12 weeks in the open-label phase of the study. Relapse during the double-blind phase was determined by the individual investigators. Patients receiving continued REMERON treatment experienced significantly lower relapse rates over the subsequent 40 weeks compared to those receiving placebo. This pattern was demonstrated in both male and female patients.

INDICATIONS AND USAGE

REMERONSolTab (mirtazapine) Orally Disintegrating Tablets are indicated for the treatment of major depressive disorder.

The efficacy of REMERON (mirtazapine) Tablets in the treatment of major depressive disorder was established in 6-week controlled trials of outpatients whose diagnoses corresponded most closely to the Diagnostic and Statistical Manual of Mental Disorders – 3rd edition (DSM-III) category of major depressive disorder (see CLINICAL PHARMACOLOGY).

A major depressive episode (DSM-IV) implies a prominent and relatively persistent (nearly every day for at least 2 weeks) depressed or dysphoric mood that usually interferes with daily functioning, and includes at least 5 of the following 9 symptoms: depressed mood, loss of interest in usual activities, significant change in weight and/or appetite, insomnia or hypersomnia, psychomotor agitation or retardation, increased fatigue, feelings of guilt or worthlessness, slowed thinking or impaired concentration, a suicide attempt, or suicidal ideation.

The effectiveness of REMERONSolTab in hospitalized depressed patients has not been adequately studied.

The efficacy of REMERON in maintaining a response in patients with major depressive disorder for up to 40 weeks following 8 to 12 weeks of initial open-label treatment was demonstrated in a placebo-controlled trial. Nevertheless, the physician who elects to use REMERON for extended periods should periodically re-evaluate the long-term usefulness of the drug for the individual patient (see CLINICAL PHARMACOLOGY).

CONTRAINDICATIONS

Hypersensitivity

REMERONSolTab (mirtazapine) Orally Disintegrating Tablets are contraindicated in patients with a known hypersensitivity to mirtazapine or to any of the excipients.

Monoamine Oxidase Inhibitors

The use of monoamine oxidase inhibitors (MAOIs) intended to treat psychiatric disorders with REMERONSolTab Orally Disintegrating Tablets or within 14 days of stopping treatment with REMERONSolTab is contraindicated because of an increased risk of serotonin syndrome. The use of REMERONSolTab within 14 days of stopping an MAOI intended to treat psychiatric disorders is also contraindicated (see WARNINGS and DOSAGE AND ADMINISTRATION).

Starting REMERONSolTab in a patient who is being treated with MAOIs such as linezolid or intravenous methylene blue is also contraindicated because of an increased risk of serotonin syndrome (see WARNINGS and DOSAGE AND ADMINISTRATION).

WARNINGS

Clinical Worsening and Suicide Risk

Patients with major depressive disorder (MDD), both adult and pediatric, may experience worsening of their depression and/or the emergence of suicidal ideation and behavior (suicidality) or unusual changes in behavior, whether or not they are taking antidepressant medications, and this risk may persist until significant remission occurs. Suicide is a known risk of depression and certain other psychiatric disorders, and these disorders themselves are the strongest predictors of suicide. There has been a long-standing concern, however, that antidepressants may have a role in inducing worsening of depression and the emergence of suicidality in certain patients during the early phases of treatment. Pooled analyses of short-term placebo-controlled trials of antidepressant drugs (SSRIs and others) showed that these drugs increase the risk of suicidal thinking and behavior (suicidality) in children, adolescents, and young adults (ages 18–24) with major depressive disorder (MDD) and other psychiatric disorders. Short-term studies did not show an increase in the risk of suicidality with antidepressants compared to placebo in adults beyond age 24; there was a reduction in risk with antidepressants compared to placebo in adults aged 65 and older.

The pooled analyses of placebo-controlled trials in children and adolescents with MDD, obsessive compulsive disorder (OCD), or other psychiatric disorders included a total of 24 short-term trials of 9 antidepressant drugs in over 4400 patients. The pooled analyses of placebo-controlled trials in adults with MDD or other psychiatric disorders included a total of 295 short-term trials (median duration of 2 months) of 11 antidepressant drugs in over 77,000 patients. There was considerable variation in risk of suicidality among drugs, but a tendency toward an increase in the younger patients for almost all drugs studied. There were differences in absolute risk of suicidality across different indications, with the highest incidence in MDD. The risk differences (drug vs. placebo), however, were relatively stable within age strata and across indications. These risk differences (drug-placebo difference in the number of cases of suicidality per 1000 patients treated) are provided in Table 1.

Table 1

Age Range	Drug-Placebo Difference in Number of Cases of Suicidality per 1000 Patients Treated
	Increases Compared to Placebo
<18	14 additional cases
18–24	5 additional cases
	Decreases Compared to Placebo
25–64	1 fewer case
≥65	6 fewer cases

No suicides occurred in any of the pediatric trials. There were suicides in the adult trials, but the number was not sufficient to reach any conclusion about drug effect on suicide.

It is unknown whether the suicidality risk extends to longer-term use, i.e., beyond several months. However, there is substantial evidence from placebo-controlled maintenance trials in adults with depression that the use of antidepressants can delay the recurrence of depression.

All patients being treated with antidepressants for any indication should be monitored appropriately and observed closely for clinical worsening, suicidality, and unusual changes in behavior, especially during the initial few months of a course of drug therapy, or at times of dose changes, either increases or decreases.

The following symptoms, anxiety, agitation, panic attacks, insomnia, irritability, hostility, aggressiveness, impulsivity, akathisia (psychomotor restlessness), hypomania, and mania, have been reported in adult and pediatric patients being treated with antidepressants for major depressive disorder as well as for other indications, both psychiatric and nonpsychiatric. Although a causal link between the emergence of such symptoms and either the worsening of depression and/or the emergence of suicidal impulses has not been established, there is concern that such symptoms may represent precursors to emerging suicidality.

Consideration should be given to changing the therapeutic regimen, including possibly discontinuing the medication, in patients whose depression is persistently worse, or who are experiencing emergent suicidality or symptoms that might be precursors to worsening depression or suicidality, especially if these symptoms are severe, abrupt in onset, or were not part of the patient's presenting symptoms.

Families and caregivers of patients being treated with antidepressants for major depressive disorder or other indications, both psychiatric and nonpsychiatric, should be alerted about the need to monitor patients for the emergence of agitation, irritability, unusual changes in behavior, and the other symptoms described above, as well as the emergence of suicidality, and to report such symptoms immediately to health care providers. Such monitoring should include daily observation by families and caregivers. Prescriptions for REMERONSolTab (mirtazapine) Orally Disintegrating Tablets should be written for the smallest quantity of tablets consistent with good patient management, in order to reduce the risk of overdose.

Screening Patients for Bipolar Disorder

A major depressive episode may be the initial presentation of bipolar disorder. It is generally believed (though not established in controlled trials) that treating such an episode with an antidepressant alone may increase the likelihood of precipitation of a mixed/manic episode in patients at risk for bipolar disorder. Whether any of the symptoms described above represent such a conversion is unknown. However, prior to initiating treatment with an antidepressant, patients with depressive symptoms should be adequately screened to determine if they are at risk for bipolar disorder; such screening should include a detailed psychiatric history, including a family history of suicide, bipolar disorder, and depression. It should be noted that REMERONSolTab (mirtazapine) Orally Disintegrating Tablets are not approved for use in treating bipolar depression.

Agranulocytosis

In premarketing clinical trials, 2 (1 with Sjögren's Syndrome) out of 2796 patients treated with REMERON (mirtazapine) Tablets developed agranulocytosis [absolute neutrophil count (ANC) <500/mm^3 with associated signs and symptoms, e.g., fever, infection, etc.] and a third patient developed severe neutropenia (ANC <500/mm^3 without any associated symptoms). For these 3 patients, onset of severe neutropenia was detected on days 61, 9, and 14 of treatment, respectively. All 3 patients recovered after REMERON was stopped. These 3 cases yield a crude incidence of severe neutropenia (with or without associated infection) of approximately 1.1 per thousand patients exposed, with a very wide 95% confidence interval, i.e., 2.2 cases per 10,000 to 3.1 cases per 1000. If a patient develops a sore throat, fever, stomatitis, or other signs of infection, along with a low WBC count, treatment with REMERONSolTab (mirtazapine) Orally Disintegrating Tablets should be discontinued and the patient should be closely monitored.

Serotonin Syndrome

The development of a potentially life-threatening serotonin syndrome has been reported with SNRIs and SSRIs, including REMERONSolTab, alone but particularly with concomitant use of other serotonergic drugs (including triptans, tricyclic antidepressants, fentanyl, lithium, tramadol, tryptophan, buspirone, and St. John's wort) and with drugs that impair metabolism of serotonin (in particular, MAOIs, both those intended to treat psychiatric disorders and also others, such as linezolid and intravenous methylene blue).

Serotonin syndrome symptoms may include mental status changes (e.g., agitation, hallucinations, delirium, and coma), autonomic instability (e.g., tachycardia, labile blood pressure, dizziness, diaphoresis, flushing, hyperthermia), neuromuscular symptoms (e.g., tremor, rigidity, myoclonus, hyperreflexia, incoordination), seizures, and/or gastrointestinal symptoms (e.g., nausea, vomiting, diarrhea). Patients should be monitored for the emergence of serotonin syndrome.

The concomitant use of REMERONSolTab with MAOIs intended to treat psychiatric disorders is contraindicated. REMERONSolTab should also not be started in a patient who is being treated with MAOIs such as linezolid or intravenous methylene blue. All reports with methylene blue that provided information on the route of administration involved intravenous administration in the dose range of 1 mg/kg to 8 mg/kg. No reports involved the administration of methylene blue by other routes (such as oral tablets or local tissue injection) or at lower doses. There may be circumstances when it is necessary to initiate treatment with an MAOI such as linezolid or intravenous methylene blue in a patient taking REMERONSolTab. REMERONSolTab should be discontinued before initiating treatment with the MAOI (see CONTRAINDICATIONS and DOSAGE AND ADMINISTRATION).

If concomitant use of REMERONSolTab with other serotonergic drugs, including triptans, tricyclic antidepressants, fentanyl, lithium, tramadol, buspirone, tryptophan, and St. John's wort, is clinically warranted, be aware of a potential increased risk for serotonin syndrome, particularly during treatment initiation and dose increases.

Treatment with REMERONSolTab and any concomitant serotonergic agents should be discontinued immediately if the above events occur and supportive symptomatic treatment should be initiated.

PRECAUTIONS

General

Discontinuation Symptoms

There have been reports of adverse reactions upon the discontinuation of REMERON/ REMERONSolTab (mirtazapine) Orally Disintegrating Tablets (particularly when abrupt), including but not limited to the following: dizziness, abnormal dreams, sensory disturbances (including paresthesia and electric shock sensations), agitation, anxiety, fatigue, confusion, headache, tremor, nausea, vomiting, and sweating, or other symptoms which may be of clinical significance. The majority of the reported cases are mild and self-limiting. Even though these have been reported as adverse reactions, it should be realized that these symptoms may be related to underlying disease.

Patients currently taking REMERONSolTab should NOT discontinue treatment abruptly, due to risk of discontinuation symptoms. At the time that a medical decision is made to discontinue treatment with REMERON, a gradual reduction in the dose, rather than an abrupt cessation, is recommended.

Akathisia/Psychomotor Restlessness

The use of antidepressants has been associated with the development of akathisia, characterized by a subjectively unpleasant or distressing restlessness and need to move, often accompanied by an inability to sit or stand still. This is most likely to occur within the first few weeks of treatment. In patients who develop these symptoms, increasing the dose may be detrimental.

Hyponatremia

Hyponatremia has been reported very rarely with the use of mirtazapine. Caution should be exercised in patients at risk, such as elderly patients or patients concomitantly treated with medications known to cause hyponatremia.

Somnolence

In US controlled studies, somnolence was reported in 54% of patients treated with REMERON (mirtazapine) Tablets, compared to 18% for placebo and 60% for amitriptyline. In these studies, somnolence resulted in discontinuation for 10.4% of REMERON-treated patients, compared to 2.2% for placebo. It is unclear whether or not tolerance develops to the somnolent effects of REMERON. Because of the potentially significant effects of REMERON on impairment of performance, patients should be cautioned about engaging in activities requiring alertness until they have been able to assess the drug's effect on their own psychomotor performance (see PRECAUTIONS: Information for Patients).

Dizziness

In US controlled studies, dizziness was reported in 7% of patients treated with REMERON, compared to 3% for placebo and 14% for amitriptyline. It is unclear whether or not tolerance develops to the dizziness observed in association with the use of REMERON.

Increased Appetite/Weight Gain

In US controlled studies, appetite increase was reported in 17% of patients treated with REMERON, compared to 2% for placebo and 6% for amitriptyline. In these same trials, weight gain of ≥7% of body weight was reported in 7.5% of patients treated with mirtazapine, compared to 0% for placebo and 5.9% for amitriptyline. In a pool of premarketing US studies, including many patients for long-term, open-label treatment, 8% of patients receiving REMERON discontinued for weight gain. In an 8-week-long pediatric clinical trial of doses between 15 to 45 mg/day, 49% of REMERON-treated patients had a weight gain of at least 7%, compared to 5.7% of placebo-treated patients (see PRECAUTIONS: Pediatric Use).

Cholesterol/Triglycerides

In US controlled studies, nonfasting cholesterol increases to ≥20% above the upper limits of normal were observed in 15% of patients treated with REMERON, compared to 7% for placebo and 8% for amitriptyline. In these same studies, nonfasting triglyceride increases to ≥500 mg/dL were observed in 6% of patients treated with mirtazapine, compared to 3% for placebo and 3% for amitriptyline.

Transaminase Elevations

Clinically significant ALT (SGPT) elevations (≥3 times the upper limit of the normal range) were observed in 2.0% (8/424) of patients exposed to REMERON in a pool of short-term US controlled trials, compared to 0.3% (1/328) of placebo patients and 2.0% (3/181) of amitriptyline patients. Most of these patients with ALT increases did not develop signs or symptoms associated with compromised liver function. While some patients were discontinued for the ALT increases, in other cases, the enzyme levels returned to normal despite continued REMERON treatment. REMERONSolTab (mirtazapine) Orally Disintegrating Tablets should be used with caution in patients with impaired hepatic function (see CLINICAL PHARMACOLOGY and DOSAGE AND ADMINISTRATION).

Activation of Mania/Hypomania

Mania/hypomania occurred in approximately 0.2% (3/1299 patients) of REMERON-treated patients in US studies. Although the incidence of mania/hypomania was very low during treatment with mirtazapine, it should be used carefully in patients with a history of mania/hypomania.

Seizure

In premarketing clinical trials, only 1 seizure was reported among the 2796 US and non-US patients treated with REMERON. However, no controlled studies have been carried out in patients with a history of seizures. Therefore, care should be exercised when mirtazapine is used in these patients.

Use in Patients with Concomitant Illness

Clinical experience with REMERONSolTab in patients with concomitant systemic illness is limited. Accordingly, care is advisable in prescribing mirtazapine for patients with diseases or conditions that affect metabolism or hemodynamic responses.

REMERONSolTab has not been systematically evaluated or used to any appreciable extent in patients with a recent history of myocardial infarction or other significant heart disease. REMERON was associated with significant orthostatic hypotension in early clinical pharmacology trials with normal volunteers. Orthostatic hypotension was infrequently observed in clinical trials with depressed patients. REMERONSolTab should be used with caution in patients with known cardiovascular or cerebrovascular disease that could be exacerbated by hypotension (history of myocardial infarction, angina, or ischemic stroke) and conditions that would predispose patients to hypotension (dehydration, hypovolemia, and treatment with antihypertensive medication).

Mirtazapine clearance is decreased in patients with moderate [glomerular filtration rate (GFR)=11–39 mL/min/1.73 m^2] and severe [GFR <10 mL/min/1.73 m^2] renal impairment, and also in patients with hepatic impairment. Caution is indicated in administering REMERONSolTab to such patients (see CLINICAL PHARMACOLOGY and DOSAGE AND ADMINISTRATION).

Information for Patients

Prescribers or other health professionals should inform patients, their families, and their caregivers about the benefits and risks associated with treatment with REMERONSolTab (mirtazapine) Orally Disintegrating Tablets and should counsel them in its appropriate use. A patient Medication Guide about "Antidepressant Medicines, Depression and other Serious Mental Illnesses, and Suicidal Thoughts or Actions" is available for REMERONSolTab. The prescriber or health professional should instruct patients, their families, and their caregivers to read the Medication Guide and should assist them in understanding its contents. Patients should be given the opportunity to discuss the contents of the Medication Guide and to obtain answers to any questions they may have. The complete text of the Medication Guide is reprinted at the end of this document.

Patients should be advised of the following issues and asked to alert their prescriber if these occur while taking REMERONSolTab.

Clinical Worsening and Suicide Risk

Patients, their families, and their caregivers should be encouraged to be alert to the emergence of anxiety, agitation, panic attacks, insomnia, irritability, hostility, aggressiveness, impulsivity, akathisia (psychomotor restlessness), hypomania, mania, other unusual changes in behavior, worsening of depression, and suicidal ideation, especially early during antidepressant treatment and when the dose is adjusted up or down. Families and caregivers of patients should be advised to look for the emergence of such symptoms on a day-to-day basis, since changes may be abrupt. Such symptoms should be reported to the patient's prescriber or health professional, especially if they are severe, abrupt in onset, or were not part of the patient's presenting symptoms. Symptoms such as these may be associated with an increased risk for suicidal thinking and behavior and indicate a need for very close monitoring and possibly changes in the medication.

Agranulocytosis

Patients who are to receive REMERONSolTab should be warned about the risk of developing agranulocytosis. Patients should be advised to contact their physician if they experience any indication of infection such as fever, chills, sore throat, mucous membrane ulceration, or other possible signs of infection. Particular attention should be paid to any flu-like complaints or other symptoms that might suggest infection.

Interference with Cognitive and Motor Performance

REMERONSolTab may impair judgment, thinking, and particularly, motor skills, because of its prominent sedative effect. The drowsiness associated with mirtazapine use may impair a patient's ability to drive, use machines, or perform tasks that require alertness. Thus, patients should be cautioned about engaging in hazardous activities until they are reasonably certain that REMERONSolTab therapy does not adversely affect their ability to engage in such activities.

Completing Course of Therapy

While patients may notice improvement with REMERONSolTab therapy in 1 to 4 weeks, they should be advised to continue therapy as directed.

Concomitant Medication

Patients should be advised to inform their physician if they are taking, or intend to take, any prescription or over-the-counter drugs, since there is a potential for REMERONSolTab to interact with other drugs.

Patients should be made aware of a potential increased risk for serotonin syndrome if concomitant use of REMERONSolTab with other serotonergic drugs, including triptans, tricyclic antidepressants, fentanyl, lithium, tramadol, buspirone, tryptophan, and St. John's wort, is clinically warranted, particularly during treatment initiation and dose increases.

Alcohol

The impairment of cognitive and motor skills produced by REMERON has been shown to be additive with those produced by alcohol. Accordingly, patients should be advised to avoid alcohol while taking any dosage form of mirtazapine.

Phenylalanine

Phenylketonuric patients should be informed that REMERONSolTab contains phenylalanine 2.6 mg per 15-mg tablet, 5.2 mg per 30-mg tablet, and 7.8 mg per 45-mg tablet.

Pregnancy

Patients should be advised to notify their physician if they become pregnant or intend to become pregnant during REMERONSolTab therapy.

Nursing

Patients should be advised to notify their physician if they are breastfeeding an infant.

Laboratory Tests

There are no routine laboratory tests recommended.

Drug Interactions

As with other drugs, the potential for interaction by a variety of mechanisms (e.g., pharmacodynamic, pharmacokinetic inhibition or enhancement, etc.) is a possibility (see CLINICAL PHARMACOLOGY).

Monoamine Oxidase Inhibitors

(See CONTRAINDICATIONS, WARNINGS, and DOSAGE AND ADMINISTRATION.)

Serotonergic Drugs

(See CONTRAINDICATIONS and WARNINGS.)

Drugs Affecting Hepatic Metabolism

The metabolism and pharmacokinetics of REMERONSolTab (mirtazapine) Orally Disintegrating Tablets may be affected by the induction or inhibition of drug-metabolizing enzymes.

Drugs that are Metabolized by and/or Inhibit Cytochrome P450 Enzymes

CYP Enzyme Inducers (these studies used both drugs at steady state)

Phenytoin

In healthy male patients (n=18), phenytoin (200 mg daily) increased mirtazapine (30 mg daily) clearance about 2-fold, resulting in a decrease in average plasma mirtazapine concentrations of 45%. Mirtazapine did not significantly affect the pharmacokinetics of phenytoin.

Carbamazepine

In healthy male patients (n=24), carbamazepine (400 mg b.i.d.) increased mirtazapine (15 mg b.i.d.) clearance about 2-fold, resulting in a decrease in average plasma mirtazapine concentrations of 60%.

When phenytoin, carbamazepine, or another inducer of hepatic metabolism (such as rifampicin) is added to mirtazapine therapy, the mirtazapine dose may have to be increased. If treatment with such a medicinal product is discontinued, it may be necessary to reduce the mirtazapine dose.

CYP Enzyme Inhibitors

Cimetidine

In healthy male patients (n=12), when cimetidine, a weak inhibitor of CYP1A2, CYP2D6, and CYP3A4, given at 800 mg b.i.d. at steady state was coadministered with mirtazapine (30 mg daily) at steady state, the Area Under the Curve (AUC) of mirtazapine increased more than 50%. Mirtazapine did not cause relevant changes in the pharmacokinetics of cimetidine. The mirtazapine dose may have to be decreased when concomitant treatment with cimetidine is started, or increased when cimetidine treatment is discontinued.

Ketoconazole

In healthy, male, Caucasian patients (n=24), coadministration of the potent CYP3A4 inhibitor ketoconazole (200 mg b.i.d. for 6.5 days) increased the peak plasma levels and the AUC of a single 30-mg dose of mirtazapine by approximately 40% and 50%, respectively.

Caution should be exercised when coadministering mirtazapine with potent CYP3A4 inhibitors, HIV protease inhibitors, azole antifungals, erythromycin, or nefazodone.

Paroxetine

In an *in vivo* interaction study in healthy, CYP2D6 extensive metabolizer patients (n=24), mirtazapine (30 mg/day), at steady state, did not cause relevant changes in the pharmacokinetics of steady state paroxetine (40 mg/day), a CYP2D6 inhibitor.

Other Drug-Drug Interactions

Amitriptyline

In healthy, CYP2D6 extensive metabolizer patients (n=32), amitriptyline (75 mg daily), at steady state, did not cause relevant changes to the pharmacokinetics of steady state mirtazapine (30 mg daily); mirtazapine also did not cause relevant changes to the pharmacokinetics of amitriptyline.

Warfarin

In healthy male subjects (n=16), mirtazapine (30 mg daily), at steady state, caused a small (0.2) but statistically significant increase in the International Normalized Ratio (INR) in subjects treated with warfarin. As at a higher dose of mirtazapine, a more pronounced effect can not be excluded, it is advisable to monitor the INR in case of concomitant treatment of warfarin with mirtazapine.

Lithium

No relevant clinical effects or significant changes in pharmacokinetics have been observed in healthy male subjects on concurrent treatment with subtherapeutic levels of lithium (600 mg/day for 10 days) at steady state and a single 30 mg dose of mirtazapine. The effects of higher doses of lithium on the pharmacokinetics of mirtazapine are unknown.

Risperidone

In an *in vivo*, nonrandomized, interaction study, subjects (n=6) in need of treatment with an antipsychotic and antidepressant drug, showed that mirtazapine (30 mg daily) at steady state did not influence the pharmacokinetics of risperidone (up to 3 mg b.i.d.).

Alcohol

Concomitant administration of alcohol (equivalent to 60 g) had a minimal effect on plasma levels of mirtazapine (15 mg) in 6 healthy male subjects. However, the impairment of cognitive and motor skills produced by REMERON were shown to be additive with those produced by alcohol. Accordingly, patients should be advised to avoid alcohol while taking REMERONSolTab.

Diazepam

Concomitant administration of diazepam (15 mg) had a minimal effect on plasma levels of mirtazapine (15 mg) in 12 healthy subjects. However, the impairment of motor skills produced by REMERON has been shown to be additive with those caused by diazepam. Accordingly, patients should be advised to avoid diazepam and other similar drugs while taking REMERONSolTab.

Carcinogenesis, Mutagenesis, Impairment of Fertility

Carcinogenesis

Carcinogenicity studies were conducted with mirtazapine given in the diet at doses of 2, 20, and 200 mg/kg/day to mice and 2, 20, and 60 mg/kg/day to rats. The highest doses used are approximately 20 and 12 times the maximum recommended human dose (MRHD) of 45 mg/day on an mg/m^2 basis in mice and rats, respectively. There was an increased incidence of hepatocellular adenoma and carcinoma in male mice at the high dose. In rats, there was an increase in hepatocellular adenoma in females at the mid and high doses and in hepatocellular tumors and thyroid follicular adenoma/cystadenoma and carcinoma in males at the high dose. The data suggest that the above effects could possibly be mediated by non-genotoxic mechanisms, the relevance of which to humans is not known.

The doses used in the mouse study may not have been high enough to fully characterize the carcinogenic potential of REMERON (mirtazapine) Tablets.

Mutagenesis

Mirtazapine was not mutagenic or clastogenic and did not induce general DNA damage as determined in several genotoxicity tests: Ames test, *in vitro* gene mutation assay in Chinese hamster V 79 cells, *in vitro* sister chromatid exchange assay in cultured rabbit lymphocytes, *in vivo* bone marrow micronucleus test in rats, and unscheduled DNA synthesis assay in HeLa cells.

Impairment of Fertility

In a fertility study in rats, mirtazapine was given at doses up to 100 mg/kg [20 times the maximum recommended human dose (MRHD) on an mg/m^2 basis]. Mating and conception were not affected by the drug, but estrous cycling was disrupted at doses that were 3 or more times the MRHD, and pre-implantation losses occurred at 20 times the MRHD.

Pregnancy

Teratogenic Effects

Pregnancy Category C

Reproduction studies in pregnant rats and rabbits at doses up to 100 mg/kg and 40 mg/kg, respectively [20 and 17 times the maximum recommended human dose (MRHD) on an mg/m^2 basis, respectively], have revealed no evidence of teratogenic effects. However, in rats, there was an increase in postimplantation losses in dams treated with mirtazapine. There was an increase in pup deaths during the first 3 days of lactation and a decrease in pup birth weights. The cause of these deaths is not known. The effects occurred at doses that were 20 times the MRHD, but not at 3 times the MRHD, on an mg/m^2 basis. There are no adequate and well-controlled studies in pregnant women. Because animal reproduction studies are not always predictive of human response, this drug should be used during pregnancy only if clearly needed.

Nursing Mothers

Because some REMERONSolTab may be excreted in breast milk, caution should be exercised when REMERONSolTab (mirtazapine) Orally Disintegrating Tablets are administered to nursing women.

Pediatric Use

Safety and effectiveness in the pediatric population have not been established (see BOXED WARNING and WARNINGS: Clinical Worsening and Suicide Risk). Two placebo-controlled trials in 258 pediatric patients with MDD have been conducted with REMERON (mirtazapine) Tablets, and the data were not sufficient to support a claim for use in pediatric patients. Anyone considering the use of REMERONSolTab (mirtazapine) Orally Disintegrating Tablets in a child or adolescent must balance the potential risks with the clinical need.

In an 8-week-long pediatric clinical trial of doses between 15 to 45 mg/day, 49% of REMERON-treated patients had a weight gain of at least 7%, compared to 5.7% of placebo-treated patients. The mean increase in weight was 4 kg (2 kg SD) for REMERON-treated patients versus 1 kg (2 kg SD) for placebo-treated patients (see PRECAUTIONS: Increased Appetite/Weight Gain).

Geriatric Use

Approximately 190 elderly individuals (≥65 years of age) participated in clinical studies with REMERON (mirtazapine) Tablets. This drug is known to be substantially excreted by the kidney (75%), and the risk of decreased clearance of this drug is greater in patients with impaired renal function. Because elderly patients are more likely to have decreased renal function, care should be taken in dose selection. Sedating drugs may cause confusion and over-sedation in the elderly. No unusual adverse age-related phenomena were identified in this group. Pharmacokinetic studies revealed a decreased clearance in the elderly. Caution is indicated in administering REMERONSolTab (mirtazapine) Orally Disintegrating Tablets to elderly patients (see CLINICAL PHARMACOLOGY and DOSAGE AND ADMINISTRATION).

ADVERSE REACTIONS

Associated with Discontinuation of Treatment

Approximately 16% of the 453 patients who received REMERON (mirtazapine) Tablets in US 6-week controlled clinical trials discontinued treatment due to an adverse experience, compared to 7% of the 361 placebo-treated patients in those studies. The most common events (≥1%) associated with discontinuation and considered to be drug related (i.e., those events associated with dropout at a rate at least twice that of placebo) are included in Table 2.

Table 2: Common Adverse Events Associated With Discontinuation of Treatment in 6-Week US REMERON Trials

Adverse Event	Percentage of Patients Discontinuing with Adverse Event	
	REMERON (n=453)	Placebo (n=361)
Somnolence	10.4%	2.2%
Nausea	1.5%	0%

Commonly Observed Adverse Events in US Controlled Clinical Trials

The most commonly observed adverse events associated with the use of REMERON (mirtazapine) Tablets (incidence of 5% or greater) and not observed at an equivalent incidence among placebo-treated patients (REMERON incidence at least twice that for placebo) are listed in Table 3.

Table 3: Common Treatment-Emergent Adverse Events Associated With the Use of REMERON in 6-Week US Trials

Adverse Event	Percentage of Patients Reporting Adverse Event	
	REMERON (n=453)	Placebo (n=361)
Somnolence	54%	18%
Increased Appetite	17%	2%
Weight Gain	12%	2%
Dizziness	7%	3%

Adverse Events Occurring at an Incidence of 1% or More Among REMERON-Treated Patients

Table 4 enumerates adverse events that occurred at an incidence of 1% or more, and were more frequent than in the placebo group, among REMERON (mirtazapine) Tablets-treated patients who participated in short-term US placebo-controlled trials in which patients were dosed in a range of 5 to 60 mg/day. This table shows the percentage of patients in each group who had at least 1 episode of an event at some time during their treatment. Reported adverse events were classified using a standard COSTART-based dictionary terminology.

The prescriber should be aware that these figures cannot be used to predict the incidence of side effects in the course of usual medical practice where patient characteristics and other factors differ from those which prevailed in the clinical trials. Similarly, the cited frequencies cannot be compared with figures obtained from other investigations involving different treatments, uses, and investigators. The cited figures, however, do provide the prescribing physician with some basis for estimating the relative contribution of drug and nondrug factors to the side-effect incidence rate in the population studied.

Table 4: Incidence of Adverse Clinical Experiences* (≥1%) in Short-Term US Controlled Studies

Body System Adverse Clinical Experience	REMERON (n=453)	Placebo (n=361)
Body as a Whole		
Asthenia	8%	5%
Flu Syndrome	5%	3%
Back Pain	2%	1%
Digestive System		
Dry Mouth	25%	15%
Increased Appetite	17%	2%
Constipation	13%	7%
Metabolic and Nutritional Disorders		
Weight Gain	12%	2%
Peripheral Edema	2%	1%
Edema	1%	0%
Musculoskeletal System		
Myalgia	2%	1%
Nervous System		
Somnolence	54%	18%
Dizziness	7%	3%
Abnormal Dreams	4%	1%
Thinking Abnormal	3%	1%
Tremor	2%	1%
Confusion	2%	0%
Respiratory System		
Dyspnea	1%	0%
Urogenital System		
Urinary Frequency	2%	1%

* Events reported by at least 1% of patients treated with REMERON are included, except the following events, which had an incidence on placebo greater than or equal to REMERON: headache, infection, pain, chest pain, palpitation, tachycardia, postural hypotension, nausea, dyspepsia, diarrhea, flatulence, insomnia, nervousness, libido decreased, hypertonia, pharyngitis, rhinitis, sweating, amblyopia, tinnitus, taste perversion.

ECG Changes

The electrocardiograms for 338 patients who received REMERON (mirtazapine) Tablets and 261 patients who received placebo in 6-week, placebo-controlled trials were analyzed. Prolongation in QTc ≥500 msec was not observed among mirtazapine-treated patients; mean change in QTc was +1.6 msec for mirtazapine and −3.1 msec for placebo. Mirtazapine was associated with a mean increase in heart rate of 3.4 bpm, compared to 0.8 bpm for placebo. The clinical significance of these changes is unknown.

Other Adverse Events Observed During the Premarketing Evaluation of REMERON

During its premarketing assessment, multiple doses of REMERON (mirtazapine) Tablets were administered to 2796 patients in clinical studies. The conditions and duration of exposure to mirtazapine varied greatly, and included (in overlapping categories) open and double-blind studies, uncontrolled and controlled studies, inpatient and outpatient studies, fixed-dose and titration studies. Untoward events associated with this exposure were recorded by clinical investigators using terminology of their own choosing. Consequently, it is not possible to provide a meaningful estimate of the proportion of individuals experiencing adverse events without first grouping similar types of untoward events into a smaller number of standardized event categories.

In the tabulations that follow, reported adverse events were classified using a standard COSTART-based dictionary terminology. The frequencies presented, therefore, represent the proportion of the 2796 patients exposed to multiple doses of REMERON who experienced an event of the type cited on at least 1 occasion while receiving REMERON. All reported events are included except those already listed in Table 4, those adverse experiences subsumed under COSTART terms that are either overly general or excessively specific so as to be uninformative, and those events for which a drug cause was very remote. It is important to emphasize that, although the events reported occurred during treatment with REMERON, they were not necessarily caused by it.

Events are further categorized by body system and listed in order of decreasing frequency according to the following definitions: frequent adverse events are those occurring on 1 or more occasions in at least 1/100 patients; infrequent adverse events are those occurring in 1/100 to 1/1000 patients; rare events are those occurring in fewer than 1/1000 patients. Only those events not already listed in Table 4 appear in this listing. Events of major clinical importance are also described in the WARNINGS and PRECAUTIONS sections.

Body as a Whole: *frequent:* malaise, abdominal pain, abdominal syndrome acute; *infrequent:* chills, fever, face edema, ulcer, photosensitivity reaction, neck rigidity, neck pain, abdomen enlarged; *rare:* cellulitis, chest pain substernal.

Cardiovascular System: *frequent:* hypertension, vasodilatation; *infrequent:* angina pectoris, myocardial infarction, bradycardia, ventricular extrasystoles, syncope, migraine, hypotension; *rare:* atrial arrhythmia, bigeminy, vascular headache, pulmonary embolus, cerebral ischemia, cardiomegaly, phlebitis, left heart failure.

Digestive System: *frequent:* vomiting, anorexia; *infrequent:* eructation, glossitis, cholecystitis, nausea and vomiting, gum hemorrhage, stomatitis, colitis, liver function tests abnormal; *rare:* tongue discoloration, ulcerative stomatitis, salivary gland enlargement, increased salivation, intestinal obstruction, pancreatitis, aphthous stomatitis, cirrhosis of liver, gastritis, gastroenteritis, oral moniliasis, tongue edema.

Endocrine System: *rare:* goiter, hypothyroidism.

Hemic and Lymphatic System: *rare:* lymphadenopathy, leukopenia, petechia, anemia, thrombocytopenia, lymphocytosis, pancytopenia.

Metabolic and Nutritional Disorders: *frequent:* thirst; *infrequent:* dehydration, weight loss; *rare:* gout, SGOT increased, healing abnormal, acid phosphatase increased, SGPT increased, diabetes mellitus, hyponatremia.

Musculoskeletal System: *frequent:* myasthenia, arthralgia; *infrequent:* arthritis, tenosynovitis; *rare:* pathologic fracture, osteoporosis fracture, bone pain, myositis, tendon rupture, arthrosis, bursitis.

Nervous System: *frequent:* hypesthesia, apathy, depression, hypokinesia, vertigo, twitching, agitation, anxiety, amnesia, hyperkinesia, paresthesia; *infrequent:* ataxia, delirium, delusions, depersonalization, dyskinesia, extrapyramidal syndrome, libido increased, coordination abnormal, dysarthria, hallucinations, manic reaction, neurosis, dystonia, hostility, reflexes increased, emotional lability, euphoria, paranoid reaction; *rare:* aphasia, nystagmus, akathisia (psychomotor restlessness), stupor, dementia, diplopia, drug dependence, paralysis, grand mal convulsion, hypotonia, myoclonus, psychotic depression, withdrawal syndrome, serotonin syndrome.

Respiratory System: *frequent:* cough increased, sinusitis; *infrequent:* epistaxis, bronchitis, asthma, pneumonia; *rare:* asphyxia, laryngitis, pneumothorax, hiccup.

Skin and Appendages: *frequent:* pruritus, rash; *infrequent:* acne, exfoliative dermatitis, dry skin, herpes simplex, alopecia; *rare:* urticaria, herpes zoster, skin hypertrophy, seborrhea, skin ulcer.

Special Senses: *infrequent:* eye pain, abnormality of accommodation, conjunctivitis, deafness, keratoconjunctivitis, lacrimation disorder, glaucoma, hyperacusis, ear pain; *rare:* blepharitis, partial transitory deafness, otitis media, taste loss, parosmia.

Urogenital System: *frequent:* urinary tract infection; *infrequent:* kidney calculus, cystitis, dysuria, urinary incontinence, urinary retention, vaginitis, hematuria, breast pain, amenorrhea, dysmenorrhea, leukorrhea, impotence; *rare:* polyuria, urethritis, metrorrhagia, menorrhagia, abnormal ejaculation, breast engorgement, breast enlargement, urinary urgency.

Other Adverse Events Observed During Postmarketing Evaluation of REMERON

Adverse events reported since market introduction, which were temporally (but not necessarily causally) related to mirtazapine therapy, include 4 cases of the ventricular arrhythmia torsades de pointes. In 3 of the 4 cases, however, concomitant drugs were implicated. All patients recovered. Cases of severe skin reactions, including Stevens-Johnson syndrome, bullous dermatitis, erythema multiforme and toxic epidermal necrolysis have also been reported.

DRUG ABUSE AND DEPENDENCE

Controlled Substance Class

REMERONSolTab (mirtazapine) Orally Disintegrating Tablets are not a controlled substance.

Physical and Psychologic Dependence

REMERONSolTab (mirtazapine) Orally Disintegrating Tablets have not been systematically studied in animals or humans for its potential for abuse, tolerance, or physical dependence. While the clinical trials did not reveal any tendency for any drug-seeking behavior, these observations were not systematic and it is not possible to predict on the basis of this limited experience the extent to which a CNS-active drug will be misused, diverted and/or abused once marketed. Consequently, patients should be evaluated carefully for history of drug abuse, and such patients should be observed closely for signs of REMERONSolTab misuse or abuse (e.g., development of tolerance, incrementations of dose, drug-seeking behavior).

OVERDOSAGE

Human Experience

There is very limited experience with REMERONSolTab (mirtazapine) Orally Disintegrating Tablets overdose. In premarketing clinical studies, there were 8 reports of REMERON overdose alone or in combination with other pharmacological agents. The only drug overdose death reported while taking REMERON was in combination with amitriptyline and chlorprothixene in a non-US clinical study. Based on plasma levels, the REMERON dose taken was 30 to 45 mg, while plasma levels of amitriptyline and chlorprothixene were found to be at toxic levels. All other premarketing overdose cases resulted in full recovery. Signs and symptoms reported in association with overdose included disorientation, drowsiness, impaired memory, and tachycardia. There were no reports of ECG abnormalities, coma, or convulsions following overdose with REMERON alone.

Overdose Management

Treatment should consist of those general measures employed in the management of overdose with any drug effective in the treatment of major depressive disorder. Ensure an adequate airway, oxygenation, and ventilation. Monitor cardiac rhythm and vital signs. General supportive and symptomatic measures are also recommended. Induction of emesis is not recommended. Gastric lavage with a large-bore orogastric tube with appropriate airway protection, if needed, may be indicated if performed soon after ingestion, or in symptomatic patients. Because of the rapid disintegration of REMERONSolTab (mirtazapine) Orally Disintegrating Tablets, pill fragments may not appear in gastric contents obtained with lavage. Activated charcoal should be administered. There is no experience with the use of forced diuresis, dialysis, hemoperfusion, or exchange transfusion in the treatment of mirtazapine overdosage. No specific antidotes for mirtazapine are known.

In managing overdosage, consider the possibility of multiple-drug involvement. The physician should consider contacting a poison control center for additional information on the treatment of any overdose. Telephone numbers for certified poison control centers are listed in the *Physicians' Desk Reference* (PDR).

DOSAGE AND ADMINISTRATION

Initial Treatment

The recommended starting dose for REMERONSolTab (mirtazapine) Orally Disintegrating Tablets is 15 mg/day, administered in a single dose, preferably in the evening prior to sleep. In the controlled clinical trials establishing the efficacy of REMERON in the treatment of major depressive disorder, the effective dose range was generally 15 to 45 mg/day. While the relationship between dose and satisfactory response in the treatment of major depressive disorder for REMERON has not been adequately explored, patients not responding to the initial 15-mg dose may benefit from dose increases up to a maximum of 45 mg/day. REMERON has an elimination half-life of approximately 20 to 40 hours; therefore, dose changes should not be made at intervals of less than 1 to 2 weeks in order to allow sufficient time for evaluation of the therapeutic response to a given dose.

Administration of REMERONSolTab (mirtazapine) Orally Disintegrating Tablets

Patients should be instructed to open tablet blister pack with dry hands and place the tablet on the tongue. The tablet should be used immediately after removal from its blister; once removed, it cannot be stored. REMERONSolTab (mirtazapine) Orally Disintegrating Tablets will disintegrate rapidly on the tongue and can be swallowed with saliva. No water is needed for taking the tablet. Patients should not attempt to split the tablet.

Elderly and Patients with Renal or Hepatic Impairment

The clearance of mirtazapine is reduced in elderly patients and in patients with moderate to severe renal or hepatic impairment. Consequently, the prescriber should be aware that plasma mirtazapine levels may be increased in these patient groups, compared to levels observed in younger adults without renal or hepatic impairment (see PRECAUTIONS and CLINICAL PHARMACOLOGY).

Maintenance/Extended Treatment

It is generally agreed that acute episodes of depression require several months or longer of sustained pharmacological therapy beyond response to the acute episode. Systematic evaluation of REMERON (mirtazapine) Tablets has demonstrated that its efficacy in major depressive disorder is maintained for periods of up to 40 weeks following 8 to 12 weeks of initial treatment at a dose of 15 to 45 mg/day (see CLINICAL PHARMACOLOGY). Based on these limited data, it is unknown whether or not the dose of REMERON needed for maintenance treatment is identical to the dose needed to achieve an initial response. Patients should be periodically reassessed to determine the need for maintenance treatment and the appropriate dose for such treatment.

Switching a Patient To or From a Monoamine Oxidase Inhibitor (MAOI) Intended to Treat Psychiatric Disorders

At least 14 days should elapse between discontinuation of an MAOI intended to treat psychiatric disorders and initiation of therapy with REMERONSolTab Orally Disintegrating Tablets. Conversely, at least 14 days should be allowed after stopping REMERONSolTab before starting an MAOI intended to treat psychiatric disorders (see CONTRAINDICATIONS).

Use of REMERONSolTab With Other MAOIs, Such as Linezolid or Methylene Blue

Do not start REMERONSolTab in a patient who is being treated with linezolid or intravenous methylene blue because there is an increased risk of serotonin syndrome. In a patient who requires more urgent treatment of a psychiatric condition, other interventions, including hospitalization, should be considered (see CONTRAINDICATIONS).

In some cases, a patient already receiving therapy with REMERONSolTab may require urgent treatment with linezolid or intravenous methylene blue. If acceptable alternatives to linezolid or intravenous methylene blue treatment are not available and the potential benefits of linezolid or intravenous methylene blue treatment are judged to outweigh the risks of serotonin syndrome in a particular patient, REMERONSolTab should be stopped promptly, and linezolid or intravenous methylene blue can be administered. The patient should be monitored for symptoms of serotonin syndrome for 2 weeks or until 24 hours after the last dose of linezolid or intravenous methylene blue, whichever comes first. Therapy with REMERONSolTab may be resumed 24 hours after the last dose of linezolid or intravenous methylene blue (see WARNINGS).

The risk of administering methylene blue by non-intravenous routes (such as oral tablets or by local injection) or in intravenous doses much lower than 1 mg/kg with REMERONSolTab is unclear. The clinician should, nevertheless, be aware of the possibility of emergent symptoms of serotonin syndrome with such use (see WARNINGS).

Discontinuation of Remeron Treatment

Symptoms associated with the discontinuation or dose reduction of REMERONSolTab Orally Disintegrating Tablets have been reported. Patients should be monitored for these and other symptoms when discontinuing treatment or during dosage reduction. A gradual reduction in the dose over several weeks, rather than abrupt cessation, is recommended whenever possible. If intolerable symptoms occur following a decrease in the dose or upon discontinuation of treatment, dose titration should be managed on the basis of the patient's clinical response (see PRECAUTIONS and ADVERSE REACTIONS).

HOW SUPPLIED

REMERONSolTab (mirtazapine) Orally Disintegrating Tablets are supplied as:

15 mg Tablets — round, white, with "T_1^Z" debossed on 1 side.

Box of 30 5 × 6 Unit Dose Blisters NDC 0052-0106-30

30 mg Tablets — round, white, with "T_2^Z" debossed on 1 side.

Box of 30 5 × 6 Unit Dose Blisters NDC 0052-0108-30

45 mg Tablets — round, white, with "T_4^Z" debossed on 1 side.

Box of 30 5 × 6 Unit Dose Blisters NDC 0052-0110-30

Storage

Store at 25°C (77°F); excursions permitted to 15-30°C (59-86°F) [see USP Controlled Room Temperature]. Protect from light and moisture. Use immediately upon opening individual tablet blister.

Rx only

Manufactured for: Merck Sharp & Dohme Corp., a subsidiary of

MERCK & CO., INC., Whitehouse Station, NJ 08889, USA

Manufactured by:

Cephalon, Inc.

Salt Lake City, UT 84116, USA

Revised: 11/2012

900246-REMST-TBfd-USPI.5

Medication Guide

REMERONSolTab® (rĕm′ - ĕ - rŏn - sōl′ – tăb)

(mirtazapine)

Orally Disintegrating Tablets

Read the Medication Guide that comes with REMERONSolTab before you start taking it and each time you get a refill. There may be new information. This Medication Guide does not take the place of talking to your healthcare provider about your medical condition or treatment. If you have any questions about REMERONSolTab, talk to your healthcare provider.

What is the most important information I should know about REMERONSolTab®?

REMERONSolTab and other antidepressant medicines may cause serious side effects, including:

1. Suicidal thoughts or actions:
- **REMERONSolTab and other antidepressant medicines may increase suicidal thoughts or actions in some children, teenagers, or young adults within the first few months of treatment or when the dose is changed.**
- Depression or other serious mental illnesses are the most important causes of suicidal thoughts or actions.
- Watch for these changes and call your healthcare provider right away if you notice:
  - New or sudden changes in mood, behavior, actions, thoughts, or feelings, especially if severe.
  - Pay particular attention to such changes when REMERONSolTab is started or when the dose is changed.

Keep all follow-up visits with your healthcare provider and call between visits if you are worried about symptoms.

Call your healthcare provider right away if you have any of the following symptoms, or call 911 if an emergency, especially if they are new, worse, or worry you:
- attempts to commit suicide
- acting on dangerous impulses
- acting aggressive or violent
- thoughts about suicide or dying
- new or worse depression
- new or worse anxiety or panic attacks
- feeling agitated, restless, angry or irritable
- trouble sleeping
- an increase in activity or talking more than what is normal for you
- other unusual changes in behavior or mood

Call your healthcare provider right away if you have any of the following symptoms, or call 911 if an emergency. REMERONSolTab may be associated with these serious side effects:

2. Manic episodes:
- greatly increased energy
- severe trouble sleeping
- racing thoughts
- reckless behavior
- unusually grand ideas
- excessive happiness or irritability
- talking more or faster than usual

3. Decreased White Blood Cells called neutrophils, which are needed to fight infections. Tell your doctor if you have any indication of infection such as fever, chills, sore throat, or mouth or nose sores, especially symptoms which are flu-like.

4. Serotonin Syndrome. This condition can be life-threatening and may include:
- agitation, hallucinations, coma or other changes in mental status
- coordination problems or muscle twitching (overactive reflexes)
- racing heartbeat, high or low blood pressure
- sweating or fever
- nausea, vomiting, or diarrhea
- muscle rigidity

5. Seizures

6. Low salt (sodium) levels in the blood. Elderly people may be at greater risk for this. Symptoms may include:
- headache
- weakness or feeling unsteady
- confusion, problems concentrating or thinking or memory problems

7. Sleepiness. It is best to take **REMERONSolTab** close to bedtime.

8. Severe skin reactions: Call your doctor right away if you have any or all of the following symptoms:
- severe rash with skin swelling (including on the palms of the hands and soles of the feet)
- painful reddening of the skin and/or blisters/ulcers on the body or in the mouth

9. Severe allergic reactions: trouble breathing, swelling of the face, tongue, eyes or mouth
- rash, itchy welts (hives) or blisters, alone or with fever or joint pain

10. Increases in appetite or weight. Children and adolescents should have height and weight monitored during treatment.

11. Increased cholesterol and triglyceride levels in your blood

Do not stop REMERONSolTab without first talking to your healthcare provider. Stopping REMERONSolTab too quickly may cause potentially serious symptoms including:
- dizziness
- abnormal dreams
- agitation
- anxiety
- fatigue
- confusion
- headache
- shaking
- tingling sensation
- nausea, vomiting
- sweating

What is REMERONSolTab?

REMERONSolTab is a prescription medicine used to treat depression. It is important to talk with your healthcare provider about the risks of treating depression and also the risks of not treating it. You should discuss all treatment choices with your healthcare provider.

Talk to your healthcare provider if you do not think that your condition is getting better with REMERONSolTab treatment.

Who should not take REMERONSolTab?

Do not take REMERONSolTab:
- if you are allergic to mirtazapine or any of the ingredients in REMERONSolTab. See the end of this Medication Guide for a complete list of ingredients in REMERONSolTab.
- if you take a monoamine oxidase inhibitor (MAOI). Ask your healthcare provider or pharmacist if you are not sure if you take an MAOI, including the antibiotic linezolid.
- Do not take an MAOI within 2 weeks of stopping REMERONSolTab unless directed to do so by your physician.
- Do not start REMERONSolTab if you stopped taking an MAOI in the last 2 weeks unless directed to do so by your physician.

People who take REMERONSolTab close in time to an MAOI may have serious or even life-threatening side effects. Get medical help right away if you have any of these symptoms:
- high fever
- uncontrolled muscle spasms
- stiff muscles
- rapid changes in heart rate or blood pressure
- confusion
- loss of consciousness (pass out)

What should I tell my healthcare provider before taking REMERONSolTab?

Ask if you are not sure.

Before starting REMERONSolTab, tell your healthcare provider if you:
- are taking certain drugs such as:
  - Triptans used to treat migraine headache
  - Medicines used to treat mood, anxiety, psychotic or thought disorders, including tricyclics, lithium, SSRIs, SNRIs, or antipsychotics
  - Tramadol used to treat pain
  - Over-the-counter supplements such as tryptophan or St. John's wort
  - Phenytoin, carbamazepine, or rifampicin (these drugs can decrease your blood level of REMERONSolTab)
  - Cimetidine or ketoconazole (these drugs can increase your blood level of REMERONSolTab)
- Have or had:
  - liver problems
  - kidney problems
  - heart problems
  - seizures or convulsions
  - bipolar disorder or mania
  - a tendency to get dizzy or faint
- are pregnant or plan to become pregnant. It is not known if REMERONSolTab will harm your unborn baby. Talk to your healthcare provider about the benefits and risks of treating depression during pregnancy
- are breastfeeding or plan to breastfeed. Some REMERONSolTab may pass into your breast milk. Talk to your healthcare provider about the best way to feed your baby while taking REMERONSolTab

Tell your healthcare provider about all the medicines that you take, including prescription and non-prescription medicines, vitamins, and herbal supplements. REMERONSolTab and some medicines may interact with each other, may not work as well, or may cause serious side effects.

Your healthcare provider or pharmacist can tell you if it is safe to take REMERONSolTab with your other medicines. Do not start or stop any medicine while taking REMERONSolTab without talking to your healthcare provider first.

> If you take REMERONSolTab, you should not take any other medicines that contain mirtazapine including REMERON® Tablets.

How should I take REMERONSolTab?
- Take REMERONSolTab exactly as prescribed. Your healthcare provider may need to change the dose of REMERONSolTab until it is the right dose for you.
- Take REMERONSolTab at the same time each day, preferably in the evening at bedtime.
- Open the tablet blister pack with dry hands and place the tablet whole on the tongue, immediately after removal from the blister pack.
- REMERONSolTab will disintegrate rapidly on the tongue and can be swallowed with saliva. No water is needed for taking it.
- Do not attempt to split the REMERONSolTab.
- It is common for antidepressant medicines such as REMERONSolTab to take up to a few weeks before you start to feel better. Do not stop taking REMERONSolTab if you do not feel results right away.
- Do not stop taking or change the dose of REMERONSolTab without first talking to your doctor, even if you feel better.
- REMERONSolTab may be taken with or without food.
- If you miss a dose of REMERONSolTab, take the missed dose as soon as you remember. If it is almost time for the next dose, skip the missed dose and take your next dose at the regular time. Do not take two doses of REMERONSolTab at the same time.
- If you take too much REMERONSolTab, call your healthcare provider or poison control center right away, or get emergency treatment.

What should I avoid while taking REMERONSolTab?
- REMERONSolTab can cause sleepiness or may affect your ability to make decisions, think clearly, or react quickly. You should not drive, operate heavy machinery, or do other dangerous activities until you know how REMERONSolTab affects you.
- Avoid drinking alcohol or taking diazepam (a medicine used for anxiety, insomnia and seizures, for example) or similar medicines while taking REMERONSolTab. If you are uncertain about whether certain medication can be taken with REMERONSolTab, please discuss with your doctor.

What are the possible side effects of REMERONSolTab?

REMERONSolTab may cause serious side effects, including all of those described in the section entitled "What is the most important information I should know about REMERONSolTab?"

Common possible side effects in people who take REMERONSolTab include:
- sleepiness
- increased appetite, weight gain
- dry mouth
- constipation
- dizziness
- abnormal dreams

Tell your healthcare provider if you have any side effect that bothers you or that does not go away. These are not all the possible side effects of REMERONSolTab. For more information, ask your healthcare provider or pharmacist.

CALL YOUR DOCTOR FOR MEDICAL ADVICE ABOUT SIDE EFFECTS. YOU MAY REPORT SIDE EFFECTS TO THE FDA AT 1-800-FDA-1088.

How should I store REMERONSolTab?
- Store REMERONSolTab at room temperature 25°C (77°F). Storage at 15°C-30°C (59°F-86°F) is permitted occasionally.
- Keep REMERONSolTab away from light and moisture.
- Use immediately upon opening individual tablet blister.

Keep REMERONSolTab and all medicines out of the reach of children.

General information about REMERONSolTab

Medicines are sometimes prescribed for purposes other than those listed in a Medication Guide. Do not use REMERONSolTab for a condition for which it was not prescribed. Do not give REMERONSolTab to other people, even if they have the same condition. It may harm them.

This Medication Guide summarizes the most important information about REMERONSolTab. If you would like more information, talk with your healthcare provider. You may ask your healthcare provider or pharmacist for information about REMERONSolTab that is written for healthcare professionals.

For more information about REMERONSolTab call 1-800-526-4099 or go to www.REMERONSolTab.com.

What are the ingredients in REMERONSolTab?

Active ingredient: mirtazapine

Inactive ingredients 15mg, 30mg and 45mg tablets: Aspartame, citric acid anhydrous, crospovidone, magnesium stearate, mannitol, microcrystalline cellulose, natural and artificial orange flavor, sodium bicarbonate, hypromellose, povidone, sugar spheres, Eudragit E100.

This Medication Guide has been approved by the U.S. Food and Drug Administration.

Manufactured for: Merck Sharp & Dohme Corp., a subsidiary of

MERCK & Co., INC., Whitehouse Station, NJ 08889, USA

Manufactured by:

Cephalon, Inc.

Salt Lake City, UT 84116, USA

Revised: 11/2012

900246-REMST-TBfd-MG.5

Shown in Product Identification Guide, page 309

ROTATEQ ℞

[Row-ta-tech]

(Rotavirus Vaccine, Live, Oral, Pentavalent)

Oral Solution

HIGHLIGHTS OF PRESCRIBING INFORMATION

These highlights do not include all the information needed to use RotaTeq safely and effectively. See full prescribing information for RotaTeq.

RotaTeq (Rotavirus Vaccine, Live, Oral, Pentavalent) Oral Solution

Initial U.S. Approval: 2006

RECENT MAJOR CHANGES

Warnings and Precautions

Managing Allergic Reactions (5.1)	12/2012
Intussusception (5.3)	06/2013

INDICATIONS AND USAGE

RotaTeq® is indicated for the prevention of rotavirus gastroenteritis caused by the G1, G2, G3 and G4 serotypes contained in the vaccine. (1)

RotaTeq is approved for use in infants 6 weeks to 32 weeks of age.

DOSAGE AND ADMINISTRATION

- FOR ORAL USE ONLY. NOT FOR INJECTION. (2)
- The vaccination series consists of three ready-to-use liquid doses of RotaTeq administered orally starting at 6 to 12 weeks of age, with the subsequent doses administered at 4- to 10-week intervals. The third dose should not be given after 32 weeks of age. (2)

DOSAGE FORMS AND STRENGTHS

2 mL solution for oral administration of 5 live human-bovine reassortant rotaviruses which contains a minimum of $2.0 - 2.8 \times 10^6$ infectious units (IU) per reassortant dose, depending on the serotype, and not greater than 116×10^6 IU per aggregate dose. (3)

CONTRAINDICATIONS

- A demonstrated history of hypersensitivity to the vaccine or any component of the vaccine. (4.1)
- History of Severe Combined Immunodeficiency Disease (SCID). (4.2) (6.2)
- History of intussusception. (4.3)

WARNINGS AND PRECAUTIONS

- No safety or efficacy data are available from clinical trials regarding the administration of RotaTeq to infants who are potentially immunocompromised (e.g., HIV/AIDS). (5.2)
- In a post-marketing study, cases of intussusception were observed in temporal association within 21 days following the first dose of RotaTeq, with a clustering of cases in the first 7 days. (5.3, 6.2)
- No safety or efficacy data are available for the administration of RotaTeq to infants with a history of gastrointestinal disorders (e.g., active acute gastrointestinal illness, chronic diarrhea, failure to thrive, history of congenital abdominal disorders, and abdominal surgery). (5.4)
- Vaccine virus transmission from vaccine recipient to non-vaccinated contacts has been reported. Caution is advised when considering whether to administer RotaTeq to individuals with immunodeficient contacts. (5.5)

ADVERSE REACTIONS

Most common adverse events included diarrhea, vomiting, irritability, otitis media, nasopharyngitis, and bronchospasm. (6.1)

To report SUSPECTED ADVERSE REACTIONS, contact Merck Sharp & Dohme Corp., a subsidiary of Merck & Co., Inc., at 1-877-888-4231 or VAERS at 1-800-822-7967 or www.vaers.hhs.gov(4).

USE IN SPECIFIC POPULATIONS

Pediatric Use: Safety and efficacy have not been established in infants less than 6 weeks of age or greater than 32 weeks of age. Data are available from clinical studies to support the use of RotaTeq in:

- Pre-term infants according to their age in weeks since birth
- Infants with controlled gastroesophageal reflux disease. (8.4)

See 17 for PATIENT COUNSELING INFORMATION and FDA-approved patient labeling

Revised: 06/2013

FULL PRESCRIBING INFORMATION: CONTENTS*

*** Sections or subsections omitted from the full prescribing information are not listed**

FULL PRESCRIBING INFORMATION

1 INDICATIONS AND USAGE

RotaTeq® is indicated for the prevention of rotavirus gastroenteritis in infants and children caused by the serotypes G1, G2, G3, and G4 when administered as a 3-dose series to infants between the ages of 6 to 32 weeks. The first dose of RotaTeq should be administered between 6 and 12 weeks of age *[see Dosage and Administration (2)]*.

2 DOSAGE AND ADMINISTRATION

FOR ORAL USE ONLY. NOT FOR INJECTION.

The vaccination series consists of three ready-to-use liquid doses of RotaTeq administered orally starting at 6 to 12 weeks of age, with the subsequent doses administered at 4- to 10-week intervals. The third dose should not be given after 32 weeks of age *[see Clinical Studies (14)]*.

There are no restrictions on the infant's consumption of food or liquid, including breast milk, either before or after vaccination with RotaTeq.

Do not mix the RotaTeq vaccine with any other vaccines or solutions. Do not reconstitute or dilute *[see Dosage and Administration (2.2)]*.

For storage instructions *[see How Supplied/Storage and Handling (16.1)]*.

Each dose is supplied in a container consisting of a squeezable plastic dosing tube with a twist-off cap, allowing for direct oral administration. The dosing tube is contained in a pouch *[see Dosage and Administration (2.2)]*.

2.1 Use with Other Vaccines

In clinical trials, RotaTeq was administered concomitantly with other licensed pediatric vaccines *[see Adverse Reactions (6.1), Drug Interactions (7.1), and Clinical Studies (14)]*.

2.2 Instructions for Use

To administer the vaccine:

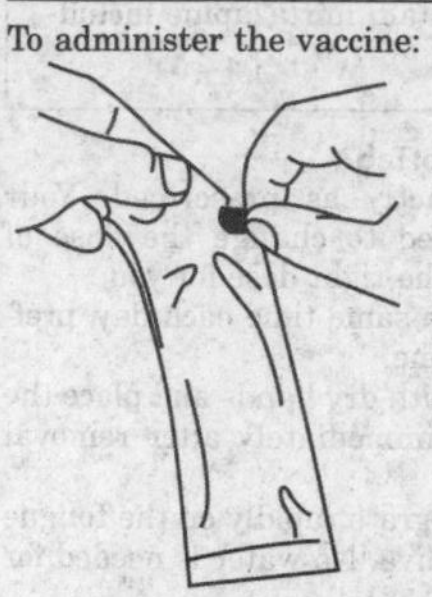

Tear open the pouch and remove the dosing tube.

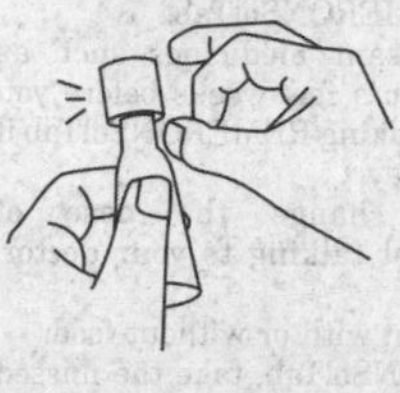

Clear the fluid from the dispensing tip by holding tube vertically and tapping cap.

Open the dosing tube in 2 easy motions:

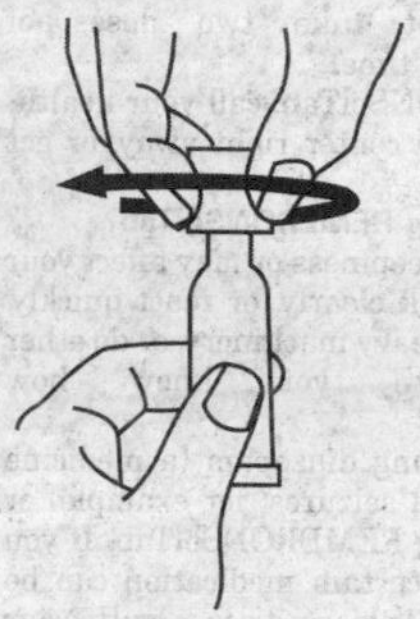

1. Puncture the dispensing tip by screwing cap ***clockwise*** until it becomes tight.

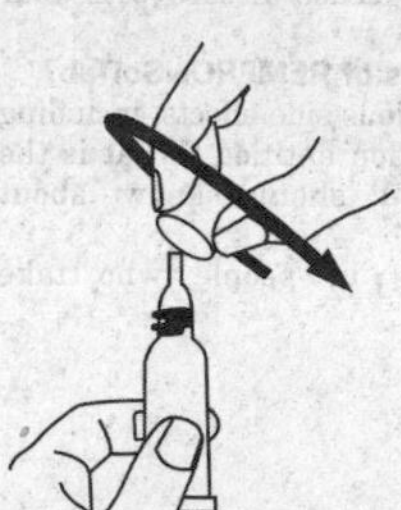

2. Remove cap by turning it ***counterclockwise***.

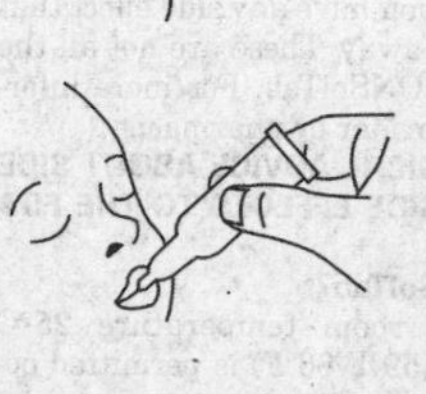

Administer dose by gently squeezing liquid into infant's mouth toward the inner cheek until dosing tube is empty. (A residual drop may remain in the tip of the tube.)

If for any reason an incomplete dose is administered (e.g., infant spits or regurgitates the vaccine), a replacement dose is not recommended, since such dosing was not studied in the clinical trials. The infant should continue to receive any remaining doses in the recommended series.

Discard the empty tube and cap in approved biological waste containers according to local regulations.

3 DOSAGE FORMS AND STRENGTHS

RotaTeq, 2 mL for oral use, is a ready-to-use solution of live reassortant rotaviruses, containing G1, G2, G3, G4 and P1A[8] which contains a minimum of $2.0 - 2.8 \times 10^6$ infectious units (IU) per individual reassortant dose, depending on the serotype, and not greater than 116×10^6 IU per aggregate dose.

Each dose is supplied in a container consisting of a squeezable plastic dosing tube with a twist-off cap, allowing for direct oral administration. The dosing tube is contained in a pouch.

4 CONTRAINDICATIONS

4.1 Hypersensitivity

A demonstrated history of hypersensitivity to any component of the vaccine.

Infants who develop symptoms suggestive of hypersensitivity after receiving a dose of RotaTeq should not receive further doses of RotaTeq.

4.2 Severe Combined Immunodeficiency Disease

Infants with Severe Combined Immunodeficiency Disease (SCID) should not receive RotaTeq. Post-marketing reports of gastroenteritis, including severe diarrhea and prolonged shedding of vaccine virus, have been reported in infants who were administered RotaTeq and later identified as having SCID *[see Adverse Reactions (6.2)]*.

4.3 History of Intussusception

Infants with a history of intussusception should not receive RotaTeq.

5 WARNINGS AND PRECAUTIONS

5.1 Managing Allergic Reactions

Appropriate medical treatment and supervision must be available to manage possible anaphylactic reactions following administration of the vaccine.

5.2 Immunocompromised Populations

No safety or efficacy data are available from clinical trials regarding the administration of RotaTeq to infants who are potentially immunocompromised including:

- Infants with blood dyscrasias, leukemia, lymphomas of any type, or other malignant neoplasms affecting the bone marrow or lymphatic system.
- Infants on immunosuppressive therapy (including high-dose systemic corticosteroids). RotaTeq may be administered to infants who are being treated with topical corticosteroids or inhaled steroids.
- Infants with primary and acquired immunodeficiency states, including HIV/AIDS or other clinical manifestations of infection with human immunodeficiency viruses; cellular immune deficiencies; and hypogammaglobulinemic and dysgammaglobulinemic states. There are insufficient data from the clinical trials to support administration of RotaTeq to infants with indeterminate HIV status who are born to mothers with HIV/AIDS.
- Infants who have received a blood transfusion or blood products, including immunoglobulins within 42 days.

Vaccine virus transmission from vaccine recipient to non-vaccinated contacts has been reported *[see Warnings and Precautions (5.5)]*.

5.3 Intussusception

Following administration of a previously licensed live rhesus rotavirus reassortant vaccine, an increased risk of intussusception was observed.(1)

In a post-marketing observational study in the US cases of intussusception were observed in temporal association within 21 days following the first dose of RotaTeq, with a clustering of cases in the first 7 days. *[See Adverse Reactions (6.2)]*

In worldwide passive post-marketing surveillance, cases of intussusception have been reported in temporal association with RotaTeq. *[See Adverse Reactions (6.2)]*

5.4 Gastrointestinal Illness

No safety or efficacy data are available for administration of RotaTeq to infants with a history of gastrointestinal disorders including infants with active acute gastrointestinal illness, infants with chronic diarrhea and failure to thrive, and infants with a history of congenital abdominal disorders, and abdominal surgery. Caution is advised when considering administration of RotaTeq to these infants.

5.5 Shedding and Transmission

Shedding of vaccine virus was evaluated among a subset of subjects in the Rotavirus Efficacy and Safety Trial (REST) 4 to 6 days after each dose and among all subjects who submitted a stool antigen rotavirus positive sample at any time. RotaTeq was shed in the stools of 32 of 360 [8.9%, 95% CI (6.2%, 12.3%)] vaccine recipients tested after dose 1; 0 of 249 [0.0%, 95% CI (0.0%, 1.5%)] vaccine recipients tested after dose 2; and in 1 of 385 [0.3%, 95% CI (<0.1%, 1.4%)] vaccine recipients after dose 3. In phase 3 studies, shedding was observed as early as 1 day and as late as 15 days after a dose. Transmission of vaccine virus was not evaluated in phase 3 studies.

Transmission of vaccine virus strains from vaccinees to non-vaccinated contacts has been observed post-marketing.

The potential risk of transmission of vaccine virus should be weighed against the risk of acquiring and transmitting natural rotavirus.

Caution is advised when considering whether to administer RotaTeq to individuals with immunodeficient close contacts such as:

- Individuals with malignancies or who are otherwise immunocompromised;
- Individuals with primary immunodeficiency; or
- Individuals receiving immunosuppressive therapy.

5.6 Febrile Illness

Febrile illness may be reason for delaying use of RotaTeq except when, in the opinion of the physician, withholding the vaccine entails a greater risk. Low-grade fever (<100.5°F [38.1°C]) itself and mild upper respiratory infection do not preclude vaccination with RotaTeq.

5.7 Incomplete Regimen

The clinical studies were not designed to assess the level of protection provided by only one or two doses of RotaTeq.

5.8 Limitations of Vaccine Effectiveness

RotaTeq may not protect all vaccine recipients against rotavirus.

5.9 Post-Exposure Prophylaxis

No clinical data are available for RotaTeq when administered after exposure to rotavirus.

6 ADVERSE REACTIONS

6.1 Clinical Studies Experience

71,725 infants were evaluated in 3 placebo-controlled clinical trials including 36,165 infants in the group that received RotaTeq and 35,560 infants in the group that received placebo. Parents/guardians were contacted on days 7, 14, and 42 after each dose regarding intussusception and any other serious adverse events. The racial distribution was as follows: White (69% in both groups); Hispanic-American (14% in both groups); Black (8% in both groups); Multiracial (5% in both groups); Asian (2% in both groups); Native American (RotaTeq 2%, placebo 1%); and Other (<1% in both groups). The gender distribution was 51% male and 49% female in both vaccination groups.

Because clinical trials are conducted under conditions that may not be typical of those observed in clinical practice, the adverse reaction rates presented below may not be reflective of those observed in clinical practice.

Serious Adverse Events

Serious adverse events occurred in 2.4% of recipients of RotaTeq when compared to 2.6% of placebo recipients within the 42-day period of a dose in the phase 3 clinical studies of RotaTeq. The most frequently reported serious adverse events for RotaTeq compared to placebo were:

bronchiolitis	(0.6% RotaTeq vs. 0.7% Placebo),
gastroenteritis	(0.2% RotaTeq vs. 0.3% Placebo),
pneumonia	(0.2% RotaTeq vs. 0.2% Placebo),
fever	(0.1% RotaTeq vs. 0.1% Placebo), and
urinary tract infection	(0.1% RotaTeq vs. 0.1% Placebo).

Deaths

Across the clinical studies, 52 deaths were reported. There were 25 deaths in the RotaTeq recipients compared to 27 deaths in the placebo recipients. The most commonly reported cause of death was sudden infant death syndrome, which was observed in 8 recipients of RotaTeq and 9 placebo recipients.

Intussusception

In REST, 34,837 vaccine recipients and 34,788 placebo recipients were monitored by active surveillance to identify potential cases of intussusception at 7, 14, and 42 days after each dose, and every 6 weeks thereafter for 1 year after the first dose.

For the primary safety outcome, cases of intussusception occurring within 42 days of any dose, there were 6 cases among RotaTeq recipients and 5 cases among placebo recipients (see Table 1). The data did not suggest an increased risk of intussusception relative to placebo.

Table 1: Confirmed cases of intussusception in recipients of RotaTeq as compared with placebo recipients during REST

	RotaTeq (n=34,837)	Placebo (n=34,788)
Confirmed intussusception cases within 42 days of any dose	6	5
Relative risk (95% CI) *	1.6 (0.4, 6.4)	
Confirmed intussusception cases within 365 days of dose 1	13	15
Relative risk (95% CI)	0.9 (0.4, 1.9)	

* Relative risk and 95% confidence interval based upon group sequential design stopping criteria employed in REST.

Among vaccine recipients, there were no confirmed cases of intussusception within the 42-day period after the first dose, which was the period of highest risk for the rhesus rotavirus-based product (see Table 2).

Table 2: Intussusception cases by day range in relation to dose in REST

	Dose 1		Dose 2		Dose 3		Any Dose	
Day Range	RotaTeq	Placebo	RotaTeq	Placebo	RotaTeq	Placebo	RotaTeq	Placebo
1-7	0	0	1	0	0	0	1	0
1-14	0	0	1	0	0	1	1	1
1-21	0	0	3	0	0	1	3	1
1-42	0	1	4	1	2	3	6	5

Table 4: Solicited adverse experiences within the first week after doses 1, 2, and 3 (Detailed Safety Cohort)

Adverse experience	Dose 1 RotaTeq	Dose 1 Placebo	Dose 2 RotaTeq	Dose 2 Placebo	Dose 3 RotaTeq	Dose 3 Placebo
	n=5,616	n=5,077	n=5,215	n=4,725	n=4,865	n=4,382
Elevated temperature*	17.1%	16.2%	20.0%	19.4%	18.2%	17.6%
	n=6,130	n=5,560	n=5,703	n=5,173	n=5,496	n=4,989
Vomiting	6.7%	5.4%	5.0%	4.4%	3.6%	3.2%
Diarrhea	10.4%	9.1%	8.6%	6.4%	6.1%	5.4%
Irritability	7.1%	7.1%	6.0%	6.5%	4.3%	4.5%

* Temperature ≥100.5°F [38.1°C] rectal equivalent obtained by adding 1 degree F to otic and oral temperatures and 2 degrees F to axillary temperatures

Table 6: Solicited adverse experiences within the first week of doses 1, 2, and 3 among pre-term infants

Adverse event	Dose 1 RotaTeq	Dose 1 Placebo	Dose 2 RotaTeq	Dose 2 Placebo	Dose 3 RotaTeq	Dose 3 Placebo
	N=127	N=133	N=124	N=121	N=115	N=108
Elevated temperature*	18.1%	17.3%	25.0%	28.1%	14.8%	20.4%
	N=154	N=154	N=137	N=137	N=135	N=129
Vomiting	5.8%	7.8%	2.9%	2.2%	4.4%	4.7%
Diarrhea	6.5%	5.8%	7.3%	7.3%	3.7%	3.9%
Irritability	3.9%	5.2%	2.9%	4.4%	8.1%	5.4%

* Temperature ≥100.5°F [38.1°C] rectal equivalent obtained by adding 1 degree F to otic and oral temperatures and 2 degrees F to axillary temperatures

[See table 2 above]

All of the children who developed intussusception recovered without sequelae with the exception of a 9-month-old male who developed intussusception 98 days after dose 3 and died of post-operative sepsis. There was a single case of intussusception among 2,470 recipients of RotaTeq in a 7-month-old male in the phase 1 and 2 studies (716 placebo recipients).

Hematochezia

Hematochezia reported as an adverse experience occurred in 0.6% (39/6,130) of vaccine and 0.6% (34/5,560) of placebo recipients within 42 days of any dose. Hematochezia reported as a serious adverse experience occurred in <0.1% (4/36,150) of vaccine and <0.1% (7/35,536) of placebo recipients within 42 days of any dose.

Seizures

All seizures reported in the phase 3 trials of RotaTeq (by vaccination group and interval after dose) are shown in Table 3.

Table 3: Seizures reported by day range in relation to any dose in the phase 3 trials of RotaTeq

Day range	1-7	1-14	1-42
RotaTeq	10	15	33
Placebo	5	8	24

Seizures reported as serious adverse experiences occurred in <0.1% (27/36,150) of vaccine and <0.1% (18/35,536) of placebo recipients (not significant). Ten febrile seizures were reported as serious adverse experiences, 5 were observed in vaccine recipients and 5 in placebo recipients.

Kawasaki Disease

In the phase 3 clinical trials, infants were followed for up to 42 days of vaccine dose. Kawasaki disease was reported in 5 of 36,150 vaccine recipients and in 1 of 35,536 placebo recipients with unadjusted relative risk 4.9 (95% CI 0.6, 239.1).

Most Common Adverse Events

Solicited Adverse Events

Detailed safety information was collected from 11,711 infants (6,138 recipients of RotaTeq) which included a subset of subjects in REST and all subjects from Studies 007 and 009 (Detailed Safety Cohort). A Vaccination Report Card was used by parents/guardians to record the child's temperature and any episodes of diarrhea and vomiting on a daily basis during the first week following each vaccination. Table 4 summarizes the frequencies of these adverse events and irritability.

[See table 4 above]

Other Adverse Events

Parents/guardians of the 11,711 infants were also asked to report the presence of other events on the Vaccination Report Card for 42 days after each dose.

Fever was observed at similar rates in vaccine (N=6,138) and placebo (N=5,573) recipients (42.6% vs. 42.8%). Adverse events that occurred at a statistically higher incidence (i.e., 2-sided p-value <0.05) within the 42 days of any dose among recipients of RotaTeq as compared with placebo recipients are shown in Table 5.

Table 5: Adverse events that occurred at a statistically higher incidence within 42 days of any dose among recipients of RotaTeq as compared with placebo recipients

Adverse event	RotaTeq N=6,138	Placebo N=5,573
	n (%)	n (%)
Diarrhea	1,479 (24.1%)	1,186 (21.3%)
Vomiting	929 (15.2%)	758 (13.6%)
Otitis media	887 (14.5%)	724 (13.0%)
Nasopharyngitis	422 (6.9%)	325 (5.8%)
Bronchospasm	66 (1.1%)	40 (0.7%)

Safety in Pre-Term Infants

RotaTeq or placebo was administered to 2,070 pre-term infants (25 to 36 weeks gestational age, median 34 weeks) according to their age in weeks since birth in REST. All pre-term infants were followed for serious adverse experiences; a subset of 308 infants was monitored for all adverse experiences. There were 4 deaths throughout the study, 2 among vaccine recipients (1 SIDS and 1 motor vehicle accident) and 2 among placebo recipients (1 SIDS and 1 unknown cause). No cases of intussusception were reported. Serious adverse experiences occurred in 5.5% of vaccine and 5.8% of

Table 7

Name of Reassortant	Human Rotavirus Parent Strains and Outer Surface Protein Compositions	Bovine Rotavirus Parent Strain and Outer Surface Protein Composition	Reassortant Outer Surface Protein Composition (Human Rotavirus Component in Bold)	Minimum Dose Levels (10^6 infectious units)
G1	WI79 – G1P1A[8]	WC3 - G6, P7[5]	**G1**P7[5]	2.2
G2	SC2 – G2P2[6]		**G2**P7[5]	2.8
G3	WI78 – G3P1A[8]		**G3**P7[5]	2.2
G4	BrB – G4P2[6]		**G4**P7[5]	2.0
P1A[8]	WI79 – G1P1A[8]		G6**P1A[8]**	2.3

Table 8: Efficacy of RotaTeq against any grade of severity of and severe* G1-4 rotavirus gastroenteritis through the first rotavirus season postvaccination in REST

	Per Protocol		Intent-to-Treat†	
	RotaTeq	Placebo	RotaTeq	Placebo
Subjects vaccinated	2,834	2,839	2,834	2,839
	Gastroenteritis cases			
Any grade of severity	82	315	150	371
Severe*	1	51	2	55
	Efficacy estimate % and (95% confidence interval)			
Any grade of severity	74.0 (66.8, 79.9)		60.0 (51.5, 67.1)	
Severe*	98.0 (88.3, 100.0)		96.4 (86.2, 99.6)	

* Severe gastroenteritis defined by a clinical scoring system based on the intensity and duration of symptoms of fever, vomiting, diarrhea, and behavioral changes

† ITT analysis includes all subjects in the efficacy cohort who received at least one dose of vaccine.

placebo recipients. The most common serious adverse experience was bronchiolitis, which occurred in 1.4% of vaccine and 2.0% of placebo recipients. Parents/guardians were asked to record the child's temperature and any episodes of vomiting and diarrhea daily for the first week following vaccination. The frequencies of these adverse experiences and irritability within the week after dose 1 are summarized in Table 6.

[See table 6 at top of previous page]

6.2 Post-Marketing Experience

The following adverse events have been identified during post-approval use of RotaTeq from reports to the Vaccine Adverse Event Reporting System (VAERS).

Reporting of adverse events following immunization to VAERS is voluntary, and the number of doses of vaccine administered is not known; therefore, it is not always possible to reliably estimate the adverse event frequency or establish a causal relationship to vaccine exposure using VAERS data.

In post-marketing experience, the following adverse events have been reported following the use of RotaTeq:

Immune system disorders:
- Anaphylactic reaction

Gastrointestinal disorders:
- Intussusception (including death)
- Hematochezia
- Gastroenteritis with vaccine viral shedding in infants with Severe Combined Immunodeficiency Disease (SCID)

Skin and subcutaneous tissue disorders:
- Urticaria
- Angioedema

Infections and infestations:
- Kawasaki disease
- Transmission of vaccine virus strains from vaccine recipient to non-vaccinated contacts.

Post-Marketing Observational Safety Surveillance Studies

The temporal association between vaccination with RotaTeq and intussusception was evaluated in the Post-licensure Rapid Immunization Safety Monitoring (PRISM) program {2}, an electronic active surveillance program comprised of 3 US health insurance plans.

More than 1.2 million RotaTeq vaccinations (507,000 of which were first doses) administered to infants 5 through 36 weeks of age were evaluated. From 2004 through 2011, potential cases of intussusception in either the inpatient or emergency department setting and vaccine exposures were identified through electronic procedure and diagnosis codes. Medical records were reviewed to confirm intussusception and rotavirus vaccination status.

The risk of intussusception was assessed using self-controlled risk interval and cohort designs, with adjustment for age. Risk windows of 1-7 and 1-21 days were evaluated. Cases of intussusception were observed in temporal association within 21 days following the first dose of RotaTeq, with a clustering of cases in the first 7 days. Based on the results, approximately 1 to 1.5 excess cases of intussusception occur per 100,000 vaccinated US infants within 21 days following the first dose of RotaTeq. In the first year of life, the background rate of intussusception hospitalizations in the US has been estimated to be approximately 34 per 100,000 infants.{3}

In an earlier prospective post-marketing observational cohort study conducted using a large US medical claims database, the risks of intussusception or Kawasaki disease resulting in emergency department visits or hospitalizations during the 30 days following any dose of vaccine were analyzed among 85,150 infants receiving one or more doses of RotaTeq from February 2006 through March 2009. Medical charts were reviewed to confirm these diagnoses. Evaluation included concurrent (n = 62,617) and historical (n=100,000 from 2001-2005) control groups of infants who received diphtheria, tetanus and acellular pertussis vaccine (DTaP) but not RotaTeq.

Confirmed intussusception cases in the RotaTeq group were compared with those in the concurrent DTaP control group and in the historical control group. The data were analyzed post-dose 1 and post any dose, in both 7 day and 30 day risk windows. A statistically significant increased risk of intussusception after RotaTeq vaccination was not observed.

One confirmed case of Kawasaki disease (23 days post-dose 3) was identified among infants vaccinated with RotaTeq and one confirmed case of Kawasaki disease (22 days post-dose 2) was identified among concurrent DTaP controls (relative risk = 0.7; 95% CI: 0.01-55.56).

In addition, general safety was monitored by electronic search of the automated records database for all emergency department visits and hospitalizations in the 30-day period after each dose of RotaTeq compared with: 1) days 31-60 after each dose of RotaTeq (self-matched controls) and 2) the 30-day period after each dose of DTaP vaccine (historical control subset from 2004-2005, n=40,000). In safety analyses which evaluated multiple follow-up windows after vaccination (days: 0-7, 1-7, 8-14 and 0-30), no safety concerns were identified for infants vaccinated with RotaTeq when compared with self-matched controls and the historical control subset.

Reporting Adverse Events

Parents or guardians should be instructed to report any adverse reactions to their health care provider.

Health care providers should report all adverse events to the U.S. Department of Health and Human Services' Vaccine Adverse Events Reporting System (VAERS). VAERS accepts all reports of suspected adverse events after the administration of any vaccine, including but not limited to the reporting of events required by the National Childhood Vaccine Injury Act of 1986. For information or a copy of the vaccine reporting form, call the VAERS toll-free number at 1-800-822-7967 or report on line to www.vaers.hhs.gov.{4}

7 DRUG INTERACTIONS

Immunosuppressive therapies including irradiation, antimetabolites, alkylating agents, cytotoxic drugs and corticosteroids (used in greater than physiologic doses), may reduce the immune response to vaccines.

7.1 Concomitant Vaccine Administration

In clinical trials, RotaTeq was administered concomitantly with diphtheria and tetanus toxoids and acellular pertussis (DTaP), inactivated poliovirus vaccine (IPV), H. influenzae type b conjugate (Hib), hepatitis B vaccine, and pneumococcal conjugate vaccine *[see Clinical Studies (14)]*. The safety data available are in the ADVERSE REACTIONS section *[see Adverse Reactions (6.1)]*. There was no evidence for reduced antibody responses to the vaccines that were concomitantly administered with RotaTeq.

8 USE IN SPECIFIC POPULATIONS

8.1 Pregnancy

Pregnancy Category C: Animal reproduction studies have not been conducted with RotaTeq. It is also not known whether RotaTeq can cause fetal harm when administered to a pregnant woman or can affect reproduction capacity. RotaTeq is not indicated in women of child-bearing age and should not be administered to pregnant females.

8.4 Pediatric Use

Safety and efficacy have not been established in infants less than 6 weeks of age or greater than 32 weeks of age.

Data are available from clinical studies to support the use of RotaTeq in pre-term infants according to their age in weeks since birth *[see Adverse Reactions (6.1)]*.

Data are available from clinical studies to support the use of RotaTeq in infants with controlled gastroesophageal reflux disease.

10 OVERDOSAGE

There have been post-marketing reports of infants who received more than one dose or a replacement dose of RotaTeq after regurgitation *[see Dosage and Administration (2.2)]*. In limited post-marketing experience of reported overdosage, the adverse events reported after incorrect administration of higher than recommended doses of RotaTeq were similar to adverse events observed with the approved dosage and schedule.

11 DESCRIPTION

RotaTeq is a live, oral pentavalent vaccine that contains 5 live reassortant rotaviruses. The rotavirus parent strains of the reassortants were isolated from human and bovine hosts. Four reassortant rotaviruses express one of the outer capsid proteins (G1, G2, G3, or G4) from the human rotavirus parent strain and the attachment protein (serotype P7) from the bovine rotavirus parent strain. The fifth reassortant virus expresses the attachment protein, P1A (genotype P[8]), herein referred to as serotype P1A[8], from the human rotavirus parent strain and the outer capsid protein of serotype G6 from the bovine rotavirus parent strain (see Table 7).

[See table 7 above]

The reassortants are propagated in Vero cells using standard cell culture techniques in the absence of antifungal agents.

The reassortants are suspended in a buffered stabilizer solution. Each vaccine dose contains sucrose, sodium citrate, sodium phosphate monobasic monohydrate, sodium hydroxide, polysorbate 80, cell culture media, and trace amounts of fetal bovine serum. RotaTeq contains no preservatives.

In the manufacturing process for RotaTeq, a porcine-derived material is used. DNA from porcine circoviruses (PCV) 1 and 2 has been detected in RotaTeq. PCV-1 and PCV-2 are not known to cause disease in humans.

RotaTeq is a pale yellow clear liquid that may have a pink tint.

The plastic dosing tube and cap do not contain latex.

12 CLINICAL PHARMACOLOGY

Rotavirus is a leading cause of severe acute gastroenteritis in infants and young children, with over 95% of these children infected by the time they are 5 years old.{5} The most severe cases occur among infants and young children between 6 months and 24 months of age.{6}

12.1 Mechanism of Action

The exact immunologic mechanism by which RotaTeq protects against rotavirus gastroenteritis is unknown *[see Clinical Studies (14.6)]*. RotaTeq is a live viral vaccine that replicates in the small intestine and induces immunity.

13 NONCLINICAL TOXICOLOGY

13.1 Carcinogenesis, Mutagenesis, Impairment of Fertility

RotaTeq has not been evaluated for its carcinogenic or mutagenic potential or its potential to impair fertility.

14 CLINICAL STUDIES

Overall, 72,324 infants were randomized in 3 placebo-controlled, phase 3 studies conducted in 11 countries on 3 continents. The data demonstrating the efficacy of RotaTeq in preventing rotavirus gastroenteritis come from 6,983 of these infants from the US (including Navajo and White Mountain Apache Nations) and Finland who were enrolled in 2 of these studies: REST and Study 007. The third trial, Study 009, provided clinical evidence supporting the consistency of manufacture and contributed data to the overall safety evaluation.

The racial distribution of the efficacy subset was as follows: White (RotaTeq 68%, placebo 69%); Hispanic-American (RotaTeq 10%, placebo 9%); Black (2% in both groups); Multiracial (RotaTeq 4%, placebo 5%); Asian (<1% in both groups); Native American (RotaTeq 15%, placebo 14%); and Other (<1% in both groups). The gender distribution was 52% male and 48% female in both vaccination groups.

The efficacy evaluations in these studies included: 1) Prevention of any grade of severity of rotavirus gastroenteritis; 2) Prevention of severe rotavirus gastroenteritis, as defined by a clinical scoring system; and 3) Reduction in hospitalizations due to rotavirus gastroenteritis.

The vaccine was given as a three-dose series to healthy infants with the first dose administered between 6 and 12 weeks of age and followed by two additional doses administered at 4- to 10-week intervals. The age of infants receiving the third dose was 32 weeks of age or less. Oral polio vaccine administration was not permitted; however, other childhood vaccines could be concomitantly administered. Breast-feeding was permitted in all studies.

The case definition for rotavirus gastroenteritis used to determine vaccine efficacy required that a subject meet both of the following clinical and laboratory criteria: (1) greater than or equal to 3 watery or looser-than-normal stools within a 24-hour period and/or forceful vomiting; and (2) rotavirus antigen detection by enzyme immunoassay (EIA) in a stool specimen taken within 14 days of onset of symptoms. The severity of rotavirus acute gastroenteritis was determined by a clinical scoring system that took into account the intensity and duration of symptoms of fever, vomiting, diarrhea, and behavioral changes.

The primary efficacy analyses included cases of rotavirus gastroenteritis caused by serotypes G1, G2, G3, and G4 that occurred at least 14 days after the third dose through the first rotavirus season post vaccination.

Analyses were also done to evaluate the efficacy of RotaTeq against rotavirus gastroenteritis caused by serotypes G1, G2, G3, and G4 at any time following the first dose through the first rotavirus season postvaccination among infants who received at least one vaccination (Intent-to-treat, ITT).

14.1 Rotavirus Efficacy and Safety Trial

Primary efficacy against any grade of severity of rotavirus gastroenteritis caused by naturally occurring serotypes G1, G2, G3, or G4 through the first rotavirus season after vaccination was 74.0% (95% CI: 66.8, 79.9) and the ITT efficacy was 60.0% (95% CI: 51.5, 67.1). Primary efficacy against severe rotavirus gastroenteritis caused by naturally occurring serotypes G1, G2, G3, or G4 through the first rotavirus season after vaccination was 98.0% (95% CI: 88.3, 100.0), and ITT efficacy was 96.4% (95% CI: 86.2, 99.6). See Table 8.

[See table 8 at top of previous page]

The efficacy of RotaTeq against severe disease was also demonstrated by a reduction in hospitalizations for rotavirus gastroenteritis among all subjects enrolled in REST. RotaTeq reduced hospitalizations for rotavirus gastroenteritis caused by serotypes G1, G2, G3, and G4 through the first two years after the third dose by 95.8% (95% CI: 90.5, 98.2). The ITT efficacy in reducing hospitalizations was 94.7% (95% CI: 89.3, 97.3) as shown in Table 9.

[See table 9 above]

Table 9: Efficacy of RotaTeq in reducing G1-4 rotavirus-related hospitalizations in REST

	Per Protocol		Intent-to-Treat*	
	RotaTeq	Placebo	RotaTeq	Placebo
Subjects vaccinated	34,035	34,003	34,035	34,003
Number of hospitalizations	6	144	10	187
Efficacy estimate % and (95% confidence interval)	95.8 (90.5, 98.2)		94.7 (89.3, 97.3)	

* ITT analysis includes all subjects who received at least one dose of vaccine.

14.2 Study 007

Primary efficacy against any grade of severity of rotavirus gastroenteritis caused by naturally occurring serotypes G1, G2, G3, or G4 through the first rotavirus season after vaccination was 72.5% (95% CI: 50.6, 85.6) and the ITT efficacy was 58.4% (95% CI: 33.8, 74.5). Primary efficacy against severe rotavirus gastroenteritis caused by naturally occurring serotypes G1, G2, G3, or G4 through the first rotavirus season after vaccination was 100% (95% CI: 13.0, 100.0) and ITT efficacy against severe rotavirus disease was 100% (95% CI: 30.2, 100.0) as shown in Table 10.

[See table 10 above]

Table 10: Efficacy of RotaTeq against any grade of severity of and severe* G1-4 rotavirus gastroenteritis through the first rotavirus season postvaccination in Study 007

	Per Protocol		Intent-to-Treat†	
	RotaTeq	Placebo	RotaTeq	Placebo
Subjects vaccinated	650	660	650	660
Gastroenteritis cases				
Any grade of severity	15	54	27	64
Severe*	0	6	0	7
Efficacy estimate % and (95% confidence interval)				
Any grade of severity	72.5 (50.6, 85.6)		58.4 (33.8, 74.5)	
Severe*	100.0 (13.0, 100.0)		100.0 (30.2, 100.0)	

* Severe gastroenteritis defined by a clinical scoring system based on the intensity and duration of symptoms of fever, vomiting, diarrhea, and behavioral change

† ITT analysis includes all subjects in the efficacy cohort who received at least one dose of vaccine.

14.3 Multiple Rotavirus Seasons

The efficacy of RotaTeq through a second rotavirus season was evaluated in a single study (REST). Efficacy against any grade of severity of rotavirus gastroenteritis caused by rotavirus serotypes G1, G2, G3, and G4 through the two rotavirus seasons after vaccination was 71.3% (95% CI: 64.7, 76.9). The efficacy of RotaTeq in preventing cases occurring only during the second rotavirus season postvaccination was 62.6% (95% CI: 44.3, 75.4). The efficacy of RotaTeq beyond the second season postvaccination was not evaluated.

14.4 Rotavirus Gastroenteritis Regardless of Serotype

The rotavirus serotypes identified in the efficacy subset of REST and Study 007 were G1P1A[8]; G2P1[4]; G3P1A[8]; G4P1A[8]; and G9P1A[8].

In REST, the efficacy of RotaTeq against any grade of severity of naturally occurring rotavirus gastroenteritis regardless of serotype was 71.8% (95% CI: 64.5, 77.8) and efficacy against severe rotavirus disease was 98.0% (95% CI: 88.3, 99.9). The ITT efficacy starting at dose 1 was 50.9% (95% CI: 41.6, 58.9) for any grade of severity of rotavirus disease and was 96.4% (95% CI: 86.3, 99.6) for severe rotavirus disease.

In Study 007, the primary efficacy of RotaTeq against any grade of severity of rotavirus gastroenteritis regardless of serotype was 72.7% (95% CI: 51.9, 85.4) and efficacy against severe rotavirus disease was 100% (95% CI: 12.7, 100). The ITT efficacy starting at dose 1 was 48.0% (95% CI: 21.6, 66.1) for any grade of severity of rotavirus disease and was 100% (95% CI: 30.4, 100.0) for severe rotavirus disease.

14.5 Rotavirus Gastroenteritis by Serotype

The efficacy against any grade of severity of rotavirus gastroenteritis by serotype in the REST efficacy cohort is shown in Table 11.

[See table 11 above]

Table 11: Serotype-specific efficacy of RotaTeq against any grade of severity of rotavirus gastroenteritis among infants in the REST efficacy cohort through the first rotavirus season postvaccination (Per Protocol)

	Number of cases		
Serotype identified by PCR	RotaTeq (N=2,834)	Placebo (N=2,839)	% Efficacy (95% Confidence Interval)
Serotypes present in RotaTeq			
G1P1A[8]	72	286	74.9 (67.3, 80.9)
G2P1[4]	6	17	63.4 (2.6, 88.2)
G3P1A[8]	1	6	NS
G4P1A[8]	3	6	NS
Serotypes not present in RotaTeq			
G9P1A[8]	1	3	NS
Unidentified*	11	15	NS

N=number vaccinated
NS=not significant

* Includes rotavirus antigen-positive samples in which the specific serotype could not be identified by PCR

In a separate post hoc analysis of health care utilization data from 68,038 infants (RotaTeq 34,035 and placebo 34,003) in REST, using a case definition that included culture confirmation, hospitalization and emergency departments visits due to G9P1A[8] rotavirus gastroenteritis were reduced (RotaTeq 0 cases: placebo 14 cases) by 100% (95% CI: 69.6%, 100.0%).

14.6 Immunogenicity

A relationship between antibody responses to RotaTeq and protection against rotavirus gastroenteritis has not been established. In phase 3 studies, 92.9% to 100% of 439 recipients of RotaTeq achieved a 3-fold or more rise in serum anti-rotavirus IgA after a three-dose regimen when compared to 12.3%-20.0% of 397 placebo recipients.

15 REFERENCES

1. Murphy TV, Gargiullo PM, Massoudi MS et al. Intussusception among infants given an oral rotavirus vaccine. N Engl J Med 2001;344:564-572.
2. Yih WK, Lieu TA, Kulldorff M, et al. Intussusception risk after rotavirus vaccination in US infants. Mini-Sentinel. www.mini-sentinel.org.

3. Tate JE, Simonsen L, Viboud C, et al. Trends in intussusception hospitalizations among US infants, 1993-2004: implications for monitoring the safety of the new rotavirus vaccination program. Pediatrics 2008;121(5):e1125-e1132.
4. Centers for Disease Control and Prevention. General recommendations on immunization: recommendations of the Advisory Committee on Immunization Practices (ACIP) and the American Academy of Family Physicians (AAFP). MMWR 2002;51(RR-2):1-35.
5. Parashar UD et al. Global illness and deaths caused by rotavirus disease in children. Emerg Infect Dis 2003;9(5):565-572.
6. Parashar UD, Holman RC, Clarke MJ, Bresee JS, Glass RI. Hospitalizations associated with rotavirus diarrhea in the United States, 1993 through 1995: surveillance based on the new ICD-9-CM rotavirus-specific diagnostic code. J Infect Dis 1998;177:13-7.

16 HOW SUPPLIED/STORAGE AND HANDLING

RotaTeq, 2 mL, a solution for oral use, is a pale yellow clear liquid that may have a pink tint. It is supplied as follows:
NDC 0006-4047-41 package of 10 individually pouched single-dose tubes.
NDC 0006-4047-20 package of 25 individually pouched single-dose tubes.
The plastic dosing tube and cap do not contain latex.

16.1 Storage and Handling

Store and transport refrigerated at 2-8°C (36-46°F). RotaTeq should be administered as soon as possible after being removed from refrigeration. For information regarding stability under conditions other than those recommended, call 1-800-MERCK-90.
Protect from light.
RotaTeq should be discarded in approved biological waste containers according to local regulations.
The product must be used before the expiration date.

17 PATIENT COUNSELING INFORMATION

See FDA-Approved Patient Labeling (Patient Information).
Parents or guardians should be given a copy of the required vaccine information and be given the "Patient Information" appended to this insert. Parents and/or guardians should be encouraged to read the patient information that describes the benefits and risks associated with the vaccine and ask any questions they may have during the visit *[see Warnings and Precautions (5) and Patient Information]*.
Manuf. and Dist. by: Merck Sharp & Dohme Corp., a subsidiary of
MERCK & CO., INC., Whitehouse Station, NJ 08889, USA

Revised: 06/2013
Printed in USA
USPI-OS-V2601306R020

Patient Information
RotaTeq®(pronounced "RŌ-tuh-tek")
rotavirus vaccine, live, oral, pentavalent

Read this information carefully before your child receives each dose of RotaTeq® in case any information about the vaccine changes. Your child will need 3 doses of the vaccine over the course of a few months. This leaflet is a summary of certain information about RotaTeq and does not take the place of talking with your child's doctor, who can give you more complete information written for health care professionals.

What is RotaTeq?
RotaTeq is an oral vaccine used to help prevent rotavirus infection in children. Rotavirus infection can cause fever, vomiting, and diarrhea that can be severe and can lead to loss of body fluids (dehydration), hospitalization and even death in some children. RotaTeq may not fully protect all children that get the vaccine, and if your child already has the virus it will not help them.

Who should not receive RotaTeq?
Your child should not get RotaTeq if:
- He or she had an allergic reaction after getting a dose of this vaccine.
- He or she is allergic to any of the ingredients of the vaccine. A list of ingredients can be found at the end of this leaflet.
- He or she has Severe Combined Immunodeficiency Disease (SCID).
- He or she has ever had intussusception, a form of blockage of the intestines.

What should I tell the doctor before my child gets RotaTeq?
Tell your doctor if your child:
- Has illness with fever. A mild fever or cold by itself is not reason to delay taking the vaccine.
- Has diarrhea or has been vomiting.
- Has not been gaining weight or is not growing as expected.
- Has a blood disorder.
- Has any type of cancer.
- Has a weak immune system because of a disease (this includes HIV/AIDS).
- Gets treatment or takes medicines that may weaken the immune system (such as high doses of steroids) or has received a blood transfusion or blood products within the past 42 days.
- Was born with gastrointestinal problems, or has had a blockage or abdominal surgery.
- Has regular close contact with a member of family or household who has a weak immune system such as someone with cancer or someone taking medicines that weaken their immune system.

What are the possible side effects of RotaTeq?
The most common side effects reported after taking RotaTeq were diarrhea, vomiting, fever, runny nose and sore throat, wheezing or coughing, and ear infection.
Call your child's doctor or go to the emergency department right away if your child has any of the following problems after getting RotaTeq, even if it has been several weeks since the last dose because these may be signs of a serious problem called intussusception:
- bad vomiting
- bad diarrhea
- severe stomach pain
- blood in the stool.

Intussusception happens when a part of the intestine gets blocked or twisted.
Since FDA approval, reports of infants with intussusception following RotaTeq have been received by the Vaccine Adverse Event Reporting System (VAERS). Intussusception occurred days and sometimes weeks after vaccination. Some infants needed hospitalization, surgery on their intestines, or a special enema to treat this problem. Death due to intussusception has occurred.
A study conducted after approval of RotaTeq showed an increased risk of intussusception in the 21 days after the first dose of RotaTeq, but especially in the first 7 days.
Other reported side effects include:
- allergic reactions, which may be severe and may include face and mouth swelling, difficulty breathing, wheezing, hives, and/or skin rash; and
- Kawasaki disease (a serious condition that can affect the heart; symptoms may include fever, rash, red eyes, red mouth, swollen glands, swollen hands and feet and, if not treated, death can occur).

Call your doctor right away if your child has any side effects that concern you or seem to get worse.
These are NOT all the possible side effects of RotaTeq. You can ask your doctor for a more complete list.
You, as a parent or guardian, may also report any adverse reactions to your child's doctor or directly to VAERS. The VAERS toll-free number is 1-800-822-7967 or report online to www.vaers.hhs.gov.
Events that have been identified or reported as side effects following RotaTeq can happen when no vaccine has been given.

What other important information should I know?
Since FDA approval, the spread of vaccine virus to non-vaccinated contacts has been reported. Tell your doctor if you have someone in your household who has a weak immune system, cancer or is taking medications that can weaken the immune system so that your doctor can provide further advice. Hand washing is recommended after diaper changes to help prevent the spread of vaccine virus.

Can RotaTeq be given with other vaccines?
Your child may get RotaTeq at the same time as other childhood vaccines.

How is RotaTeq given?
The vaccine is given by mouth. Your child will receive 3 doses of the vaccine. The first dose is given when your child is 6 to 12 weeks of age, the second dose is given 4 to 10 weeks later and the third dose is given 4 to 10 weeks after the second dose. The last (third) dose should be given to your child by 32 weeks of age.
Your doctor will gently squeeze the vaccine into your child's mouth (see Figure 1). Your infant may spit out some or all of it. If this happens, the dose does not need to be given again during that visit.

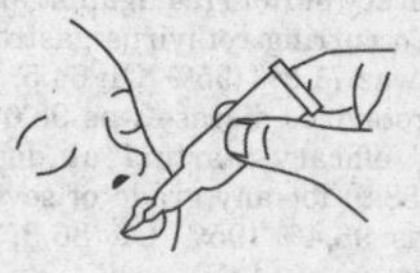

Figure 1

What do I do if my child misses a dose of RotaTeq?
All 3 doses of the vaccine should be given to your child by 32 weeks of age. Your doctor will tell you when your child should come for the follow-up doses. It is important to keep those appointments. If you forget or are not able to go back at the planned time, ask your doctor for advice.

What else should I know about RotaTeq?
This leaflet gives a summary of certain information about the vaccine. If you have any questions or concerns about RotaTeq, talk to your doctor.

What are the ingredients in RotaTeq?
5 live rotavirus strains (G1, G2, G3, G4, and P1).
Sucrose, sodium citrate, sodium phosphate monobasic monohydrate, sodium hydroxide, polysorbate 80 and also fetal bovine serum.
Parts of porcine circovirus (a virus that infects pigs) types 1 and 2 have been found in RotaTeq. Porcine circovirus type 1 (PCV-1) and porcine circovirus type 2 (PCV-2) are not known to cause disease in humans.

Rx only
Manuf. and Dist. by: Merck Sharp & Dohme Corp., a subsidiary of
MERCK & CO., INC., Whitehouse Station, NJ 08889, USA

Revised: 06/2013
USPPI-OS-V2601306R019

SAPHRIS® ℞

[sa-ph-ris]
(asenapine)
sublingual tablets

HIGHLIGHTS OF PRESCRIBING INFORMATION
These highlights do not include all the information needed to use SAPHRIS (asenapine) safely and effectively. See full prescribing information for SAPHRIS.
SAPHRIS® (asenapine) sublingual tablets
Initial U.S. Approval: 2009

> **WARNING: INCREASED MORTALITY IN ELDERLY PATIENTS WITH DEMENTIA-RELATED PSYCHOSIS**
> ***See full prescribing information for complete boxed warning.***
> **Elderly patients with dementia-related psychosis treated with antipsychotic drugs are at an increased risk of death. SAPHRIS is not approved for the treatment of patients with dementia-related psychosis. (5.1)**

INDICATIONS AND USAGE

SAPHRIS is an atypical antipsychotic indicated for:
- Treatment of schizophrenia. (1.1)
  Efficacy was established in two 6-week clinical trials and one maintenance trial in patients with schizophrenia in adults. (14.1)
- Acute treatment, as monotherapy or adjunctive therapy, of manic or mixed episodes associated with bipolar I disorder. (1.2)
  Efficacy was established in two 3-week monotherapy trials and in one 3-week adjunctive trial in patients with manic or mixed episodes associated with bipolar I disorder in adults. (14.2)

DOSAGE AND ADMINISTRATION

[See table at top of next page]
Administration: Do not swallow tablet. SAPHRIS sublingual tablets should be placed under the tongue and left to dissolve completely. The tablet will dissolve in saliva within seconds. Eating and drinking should be avoided for 10 minutes after administration. (2.1, 17.1)

DOSAGE FORMS AND STRENGTHS

Sublingual tablets: 5 mg and 10 mg (3)
Sublingual tablets, black cherry flavor: 5 mg and 10 mg (3)

CONTRAINDICATIONS

Known hypersensitivity to SAPHRIS (asenapine), or to any components in the formulation. (4, 5.7, 17.3)

WARNINGS AND PRECAUTIONS

- *Cerebrovascular Adverse Events:* An increased incidence of cerebrovascular adverse events (e.g., stroke, transient ischemic attack) has been seen in elderly patients with dementia-related psychoses treated with atypical antipsychotic drugs. (5.2)
- *Neuroleptic Malignant Syndrome:* Manage with immediate discontinuation and close monitoring. (5.3)
- *Tardive Dyskinesia:* Discontinue if clinically appropriate. (5.4)
- *Hyperglycemia and Diabetes Mellitus:* Monitor patients for symptoms of hyperglycemia including polydipsia, polyuria, polyphagia, and weakness. Monitor glucose regularly in patients with, and at risk for, diabetes. (5.5)
- *Weight Gain:* Patients should receive regular monitoring of weight. (5.6)

	Starting Dose	Recommended Dose	Maximum Dose
Schizophrenia – acute treatment in adults (2.2)	5 mg sublingually twice daily	5 mg sublingually twice daily	10 mg sublingually twice daily
Schizophrenia – maintenance treatment in adults (2.2)	5 mg sublingually twice daily for one week	10 mg sublingually twice daily	10 mg sublingually twice daily
Bipolar mania – adults: monotherapy (2.3)	10 mg sublingually twice daily	5–10 mg sublingually twice daily	10 mg sublingually twice daily
Bipolar mania – adults: as an adjunct to lithium or valproate (2.3)	5 mg sublingually twice daily	5–10 mg sublingually twice daily	10 mg sublingually twice daily

- *Hypersensitivity Reactions:* Hypersensitivity reactions, including anaphylaxis and angioedema, have been observed. (5.7)
- *Orthostatic Hypotension and Syncope:* Dizziness, tachycardia or bradycardia, and syncope may occur, especially early in treatment. Use with caution in patients with known cardiovascular or cerebrovascular disease, and in antipsychotic-naïve patients. (5.8)
- *Leukopenia, Neutropenia, and Agranulocytosis* have been reported with antipsychotics. Patients with a pre-existing low white blood cell count (WBC) or a history of leukopenia/neutropenia should have their complete blood count (CBC) monitored frequently during the first few months of therapy and SAPHRIS should be discontinued at the first sign of a decline in WBC in the absence of other causative factors. (5.9)
- *QT Prolongation:* Increases in QT interval; avoid use with drugs that also increase the QT interval and in patients with risk factors for prolonged QT interval. (5.10)
- *Seizures:* Use cautiously in patients with a history of seizures or with conditions that lower the seizure threshold. (5.12)
- *Potential for Cognitive and Motor Impairment:* Use caution when operating machinery. (5.13)
- *Suicide:* The possibility of a suicide attempt is inherent in schizophrenia and bipolar disorder. Closely supervise high-risk patients. (5.15)

ADVERSE REACTIONS

Commonly observed adverse reactions (incidence ≥5% and at least twice that for placebo) were (6.1):

- Schizophrenia: akathisia, oral hypoesthesia, and somnolence.
- Bipolar Disorder (Monotherapy): somnolence, dizziness, extrapyramidal symptoms other than akathisia, and weight increased.
- Bipolar Disorder (Adjunctive): somnolence and oral hypoesthesia.

To report SUSPECTED ADVERSE REACTIONS, contact Merck Sharp & Dohme Corp., a subsidiary of Merck & Co., Inc., at 1-877-888-4231 or FDA at 1-800-FDA-1088 or www.fda.gov/medwatch.

DRUG INTERACTIONS

- *Fluvoxamine (strong CYP1A2 inhibitor) and Paroxetine (CYP2D6 substrate and inhibitor):* cautiously approach coadministration with SAPHRIS. (7.1, 7.2)

USE IN SPECIFIC POPULATIONS

- *Pregnancy:* Use SAPHRIS during pregnancy only if the potential benefit justifies the potential risk. (8.1)
- *Nursing Mothers:* Breast feeding is not recommended. (8.3)
- *Pediatric Use:* Safety and effectiveness have not been established. (8.4)
- *Renal Impairment:* No dose adjustment needed. (8.6)
- *Hepatic Impairment:* SAPHRIS is not recommended in patients with severe hepatic impairment (Child-Pugh C). (2.4, 8.7, 12.3)

See 17 for PATIENT COUNSELING INFORMATION

Revised: 03/2013

FULL PRESCRIBING INFORMATION: CONTENTS*

*** Sections or subsections omitted from the full prescribing information are not listed**

FULL PRESCRIBING INFORMATION

WARNING: INCREASED MORTALITY IN ELDERLY PATIENTS WITH DEMENTIA-RELATED PSYCHOSIS

Elderly patients with dementia-related psychosis treated with antipsychotic drugs are at an increased risk of death. Analyses of 17 placebo-controlled trials (modal duration of 10 weeks), largely in patients taking atypical antipsychotic drugs, revealed a risk of death in the drug-treated patients of between 1.6 to 1.7 times that seen in placebo-treated patients. Over the course of a typical 10-week controlled trial, the rate of death in drug-treated patients was about 4.5%, compared to a rate of about 2.6% in the placebo group. Although the causes of death were varied, most of the deaths appeared to be either cardiovascular (e.g., heart failure, sudden death) or infectious (e.g., pneumonia) in nature. Observational studies suggest that, similar to atypical antipsychotic drugs, treatment with conventional antipsychotic drugs may increase mortality. The extent to which the findings of increased mortality in observational studies may be attributed to the antipsychotic drug as opposed to some characteristic(s) of the patients is not clear. SAPHRIS® (asenapine) is not approved for the treatment of patients with dementia-related psychosis *[see Warnings and Precautions (5.1)]*.

1 INDICATIONS AND USAGE

1.1 Schizophrenia

SAPHRIS is indicated for the treatment of schizophrenia. The efficacy of SAPHRIS was established in two 6-week trials and one maintenance trial in adults *[see Clinical Studies (14.1)]*.

1.2 Bipolar Disorder

Monotherapy: SAPHRIS is indicated for the acute treatment of manic or mixed episodes associated with bipolar I disorder. Efficacy was established in two 3-week monotherapy trials in adults *[see Clinical Studies (14.2)]*.

Adjunctive Therapy: SAPHRIS is indicated as adjunctive therapy with either lithium or valproate for the acute treatment of manic or mixed episodes associated with bipolar I disorder. Efficacy was established in one 3-week adjunctive trial in adults *[see Clinical Studies (14.2)]*.

2 DOSAGE AND ADMINISTRATION

2.1 Administration Instructions

SAPHRIS is a sublingual tablet. To ensure optimal absorption, patients should be instructed to place the tablet under the tongue and allow it to dissolve completely. The tablet will dissolve in saliva within seconds. SAPHRIS sublingual tablets should not be crushed, chewed, or swallowed *[see Clinical Pharmacology (12.3)]*. Patients should be instructed to not eat or drink for 10 minutes after administration *[see Clinical Pharmacology (12.3) and Patient Counseling Information (17.1)]*.

2.2 Schizophrenia

Usual Dose for Acute Treatment in Adults: The recommended starting and target dose of SAPHRIS is 5 mg given twice daily. In short term controlled trials, there was no suggestion of added benefit with a 10 mg twice daily dose, but there was a clear increase in certain adverse reactions. The safety of doses above 10 mg twice daily has not been evaluated in clinical studies.

Maintenance Treatment: Efficacy was demonstrated with SAPHRIS in a maintenance trial in patients with schizophrenia. The starting dose in this study was 5 mg twice daily with an increase up to 10 mg twice daily after 1 week based on tolerability *[see Clinical Studies (14.1)]*. While there is no body of evidence available to answer the question of how long the schizophrenic patient should remain on SAPHRIS, patients should be periodically reassessed to determine the need for maintenance treatment.

2.3 Bipolar Disorder

Usual Dose for Acute Treatment of Manic or Mixed Episodes Associated with Bipolar I Disorder in Adults:

Monotherapy: The recommended starting dose of SAPHRIS, and the dose maintained by 90% of the patients studied, is 10 mg twice daily. The dose can be decreased to 5 mg twice daily if warranted by adverse effects or based on individual tolerability.

In controlled monotherapy trials, the starting dose for SAPHRIS was 10 mg twice daily. On the second and subsequent days of the trials, the dose could be lowered to 5 mg twice daily, based on tolerability, but less than 10% of patients had their dose reduced. The safety of doses above 10 mg twice daily has not been evaluated in clinical trials.

Adjunctive Therapy: The recommended starting dose of SAPHRIS is 5 mg twice daily when administered as adjunctive therapy with either lithium or valproate. Depending on the clinical response and tolerability in the individual patient, the dose can be increased to 10 mg twice daily. The safety of doses above 10 mg twice daily as adjunctive therapy with lithium or valproate has not been evaluated in clinical trials.

Maintenance Treatment: While there is no body of evidence available to answer the question of how long the bipolar patient should remain on SAPHRIS, whether used as monotherapy or as adjunctive therapy with lithium or valproate, it is generally recommended that responding patients be continued beyond the acute response. If SAPHRIS is used for extended periods in bipolar disorder, the physician should periodically re-evaluate the long-term risks and benefits of the drug for the individual patient.

2.4 Dosage in Special Populations

In a study of subjects with hepatic impairment who were treated with a single dose of SAPHRIS 5 mg, there were increases in asenapine exposures (compared to subjects with normal hepatic function), that correlated with the degree of hepatic impairment. While the results indicated that no dosage adjustments are required in patients with mild (Child-Pugh A) or moderate (Child-Pugh B) hepatic impairment, there was a 7-fold increase (on average) in asenapine concentrations in subjects with severe hepatic impairment (Child-Pugh C) compared to the concentrations of those in subjects with normal hepatic function. Therefore, SAPHRIS is not recommended in patients with severe hepatic impairment *[see Use in Special Populations (8.7)]*. Dosage adjustments are not routinely required on the basis of age, gender, race, or renal impairment status *[see Use in Specific Populations (8.4, 8.5, 8.6) and Clinical Pharmacology (12.3)]*.

2.5 Switching from Other Antipsychotics

There are no systematically collected data to specifically address switching patients with schizophrenia or bipolar mania from other antipsychotics to SAPHRIS or concerning concomitant administration with other antipsychotics. While immediate discontinuation of the previous antipsychotic treatment may be acceptable for some patients with schizophrenia, more gradual discontinuation may be most appropriate for others. In all cases, the period of overlapping antipsychotic administration should be minimized.

3 DOSAGE FORMS AND STRENGTHS

- SAPHRIS 5-mg tablets are round, white to off-white sublingual tablets, with "5" on one side.
- SAPHRIS 10-mg tablets are round, white to off-white sublingual tablets, with "10" on one side.
- SAPHRIS 5-mg tablets, black cherry flavor, are round, white to off-white sublingual tablets, with "5" on one side within a circle.
- SAPHRIS 10-mg tablets, black cherry flavor, are round, white to off-white sublingual tablets, with "10" on one side within a circle.

4 CONTRAINDICATIONS

Hypersensitivity reactions, including anaphylaxis and angioedema, have been observed in patients treated with asenapine. Therefore, SAPHRIS is contraindicated in patients with a known hypersensitivity to the product *[see Warnings and Precautions (5.7), Adverse Reactions (6) and Patient Counseling Information (17.3)]*.

5 WARNINGS AND PRECAUTIONS

5.1 Increased Mortality in Elderly Patients with Dementia-Related Psychosis

Elderly patients with dementia-related psychosis treated with antipsychotic drugs are at an increased risk of death. SAPHRIS is not approved for the treatment of patients with dementia-related psychosis *[see Boxed Warning]*.

5.2 Cerebrovascular Adverse Events, Including Stroke, In Elderly Patients with Dementia-Related Psychosis

In placebo-controlled trials with risperidone, aripiprazole, and olanzapine in elderly subjects with dementia, there was a higher incidence of cerebrovascular adverse reactions (cerebrovascular accidents and transient ischemic attacks) including fatalities compared to placebo-treated subjects. SAPHRIS is not approved for the treatment of patients with dementia-related psychosis *[see also Boxed Warning and Warnings and Precautions (5.1)]*.

5.3 Neuroleptic Malignant Syndrome

A potentially fatal symptom complex sometimes referred to as Neuroleptic Malignant Syndrome (NMS) has been reported in association with administration of antipsychotic drugs, including SAPHRIS. Clinical manifestations of NMS are hyperpyrexia, muscle rigidity, altered mental status, and evidence of autonomic instability (irregular pulse or blood pressure, tachycardia, diaphoresis, and cardiac dysrhythmia). Additional signs may include elevated creatine phosphokinase, myoglobinuria (rhabdomyolysis), and acute renal failure.

The diagnostic evaluation of patients with this syndrome is complicated. It is important to exclude cases where the clinical presentation includes both serious medical illness (e.g. pneumonia, systemic infection) and untreated or inadequately treated extrapyramidal signs and symptoms (EPS). Other important considerations in the differential diagnosis include central anticholinergic toxicity, heat stroke, drug fever, and primary central nervous system pathology.

The management of NMS should include: 1) immediate discontinuation of antipsychotic drugs and other drugs not essential to concurrent therapy; 2) intensive symptomatic treatment and medical monitoring; and 3) treatment of any concomitant serious medical problems for which specific treatments are available. There is no general agreement about specific pharmacological treatment regimens for NMS.

If a patient requires antipsychotic drug treatment after recovery from NMS, the potential reintroduction of drug therapy should be carefully considered. The patient should be carefully monitored, since recurrences of NMS have been reported.

5.4 Tardive Dyskinesia

A syndrome of potentially irreversible, involuntary, dyskinetic movements can develop in patients treated with antipsychotic drugs. Although the prevalence of the syndrome appears to be highest among the elderly, especially elderly women, it is impossible to rely upon prevalence estimates to predict, at the inception of antipsychotic treatment, which patients are likely to develop the syndrome. Whether antipsychotic drug products differ in their potential to cause Tardive Dyskinesia (TD) is unknown.

The risk of developing TD and the likelihood that it will become irreversible are believed to increase as the duration of treatment and the total cumulative dose of antipsychotic drugs administered to the patient increase. However, the syndrome can develop, although much less commonly, after relatively brief treatment periods at low doses.

There is no known treatment for established cases of TD, although the syndrome may remit, partially or completely, if antipsychotic treatment is withdrawn. Antipsychotic treatment, itself, however, may suppress (or partially suppress) the signs and symptoms of the syndrome and thereby may possibly mask the underlying process. The effect that symptomatic suppression has upon the long-term course of the syndrome is unknown.

Given these considerations, SAPHRIS should be prescribed in a manner that is most likely to minimize the occurrence of TD. Chronic antipsychotic treatment should generally be reserved for patients who suffer from a chronic illness that (1) is known to respond to antipsychotic drugs, and (2) for whom alternative, equally effective, but potentially less harmful treatments are not available or appropriate. In patients who do require chronic treatment, the smallest dose and the shortest duration of treatment producing a satisfactory clinical response should be sought. The need for continued treatment should be reassessed periodically.

If signs and symptoms of TD appear in a patient on SAPHRIS, drug discontinuation should be considered. However, some patients may require treatment with SAPHRIS despite the presence of the syndrome.

5.5 Hyperglycemia and Diabetes Mellitus

Hyperglycemia, in some cases extreme and associated with ketoacidosis or hyperosmolar coma or death, has been reported in patients treated with atypical antipsychotics. Assessment of the relationship between atypical antipsychotic use and glucose abnormalities is complicated by the possibility of an increased background risk of diabetes mellitus in patients with schizophrenia and the increasing incidence of diabetes mellitus in the general population. Given these confounders, the relationship between atypical antipsychotic use and hyperglycemia-related adverse reactions is not completely understood. However, epidemiological studies suggest an increased risk of treatment-emergent hyperglycemia-related adverse events in patients treated with the atypical antipsychotics included in these studies. Because SAPHRIS was not marketed at the time these studies were performed, it is not known if SAPHRIS is associated with this increased risk. Precise risk estimates for hyperglycemia-related adverse events in patients treated with atypical antipsychotics are not available.

Patients with an established diagnosis of diabetes mellitus who are started on atypical antipsychotics should be monitored regularly for worsening of glucose control. Patients with risk factors for diabetes mellitus (e.g., obesity, family history of diabetes) who are starting treatment with atypical antipsychotics should undergo fasting blood glucose testing at the beginning of treatment and periodically during treatment. Any patient treated with atypical antipsychotics should be monitored for symptoms of hyperglycemia including polydipsia, polyuria, polyphagia, and weakness. Patients who develop symptoms of hyperglycemia during treatment with atypical antipsychotics should undergo fasting blood glucose testing. In some cases, hyperglycemia has resolved when the atypical antipsychotic was discontinued; however, some patients required continuation of antidiabetic treatment despite discontinuation of the antipsychotic drug.

5.6 Weight Gain

Increases in weight have been observed in pre-marketing clinical trials with SAPHRIS. Patients receiving SAPHRIS should receive regular monitoring of weight *[see Patient Counseling Information (17.7)]*.

In short-term schizophrenia and bipolar mania trials, there were differences in mean weight gain between SAPHRIS-treated and placebo-treated patients. In short-term, placebo-controlled schizophrenia trials, the mean weight gain was 1.1 kg for SAPHRIS-treated patients compared to 0.1 kg for placebo-treated patients. The proportion of patients with a ≥7% increase in body weight (at Endpoint) was 4.9% for SAPHRIS-treated patients versus 2% for placebo-treated patients. In short-term, placebo-controlled bipolar mania trials, the mean weight gain for SAPHRIS-treated patients was 1.3 kg compared to 0.2 kg for placebo-treated patients. The proportion of patients with a ≥7% increase in body weight (at Endpoint) was 5.8% for SAPHRIS-treated patients versus 0.5% for placebo-treated patients.

In a 52-week, double-blind, comparator-controlled trial of patients with schizophrenia or schizoaffective disorder, the mean weight gain from baseline was 0.9 kg. The proportion of patients with a ≥7% increase in body weight (at Endpoint) was 14.7%. **Table 1** provides the mean weight change from baseline and the proportion of patients with a weight gain of ≥7% categorized by Body Mass Index (BMI) at baseline:

Table 1: Weight Change Results Categorized by BMI at Baseline: Comparator-Controlled 52-Week Study in Schizophrenia

	BMI <23 SAPHRIS N=295	BMI 23 - ≤27 SAPHRIS N=290	BMI >27 SAPHRIS N=302
Mean change from Baseline (kg)	1.7	1	0
% with ≥7% increase in body weight	22%	13%	9%

5.7 Hypersensitivity Reactions

Hypersensitivity reactions, including anaphylaxis and angioedema, have been observed in patients treated with asenapine. In several cases, these reactions occurred after the first dose. These hypersensitivity reactions included: anaphylaxis, angioedema, hypotension, tachycardia, swollen tongue, dyspnea, wheezing and rash.

5.8 Orthostatic Hypotension, Syncope, and Other Hemodynamic Effects

SAPHRIS may induce orthostatic hypotension and syncope in some patients, especially early in treatment, because of its α_1-adrenergic antagonist activity. In short-term schizophrenia trials, syncope was reported in 0.2% (1/572) of patients treated with therapeutic doses (5 mg or 10 mg twice daily) of SAPHRIS, compared to 0.3% (1/378) of patients treated with placebo. In short-term bipolar mania trials, syncope was reported in 0.3% (1/379) of patients treated with therapeutic doses (5 mg or 10 mg twice daily) of SAPHRIS, compared to 0% (0/203) of patients treated with placebo. During pre-marketing clinical trials with SAPHRIS, including long-term trials without comparison to placebo, syncope was reported in 0.6% (11/1953) of patients treated with SAPHRIS.

Four normal volunteers in clinical pharmacology studies treated with either intravenous, oral, or sublingual SAPHRIS experienced hypotension, bradycardia, and sinus pauses. These spontaneously resolved in 3 cases, but the fourth subject received external cardiac massage. The risk of this sequence of hypotension, bradycardia, and sinus pause might be greater in nonpsychiatric patients compared to psychiatric patients who are possibly more adapted to certain effects of psychotropic drugs.

Patients should be instructed about nonpharmacologic interventions that help to reduce the occurrence of orthostatic hypotension (e.g., sitting on the edge of the bed for several minutes before attempting to stand in the morning and slowly rising from a seated position). SAPHRIS should be used with caution in (1) patients with known cardiovascular disease (history of myocardial infarction or ischemic heart disease, heart failure or conduction abnormalities), cerebrovascular disease, or conditions which would predispose patients to hypotension (dehydration, hypovolemia, and treatment with antihypertensive medications); and (2) in the elderly. SAPHRIS should be used cautiously when treating patients who receive treatment with other drugs that can induce hypotension, bradycardia, respiratory or central nervous system depression *[see Drug Interactions (7)]*. Monitoring of orthostatic vital signs should be considered in all such patients, and a dose reduction should be considered if hypotension occurs.

5.9 Leukopenia, Neutropenia, and Agranulocytosis

In clinical trial and postmarketing experience, events of leukopenia/neutropenia have been reported temporally related to antipsychotic agents, including SAPHRIS. Agranulocytosis (including fatal cases) has been reported with other agents in the class.

Possible risk factors for leukopenia/neutropenia include pre-existing low white blood cell count (WBC) and history of drug induced leukopenia/neutropenia. Patients with a pre-existing low WBC or a history of drug induced leukopenia/neutropenia should have their complete blood count (CBC) monitored frequently during the first few months of therapy and SAPHRIS should be discontinued at the first sign of decline in WBC in the absence of other causative factors.

Patients with neutropenia should be carefully monitored for fever or other symptoms or signs of infection and treated promptly if such symptoms or signs occur. Patients with severe neutropenia (absolute neutrophil count <1000/mm^3) should discontinue SAPHRIS and have their WBC followed until recovery.

5.10 QT Prolongation

The effects of SAPHRIS on the QT/QTc interval were evaluated in a dedicated QT study. This trial involved SAPHRIS doses of 5 mg, 10 mg, 15 mg, and 20 mg twice daily, and placebo, and was conducted in 151 clinically stable patients with schizophrenia, with electrocardiographic assessments throughout the dosing interval at baseline and steady state. At these doses, SAPHRIS was associated with increases in QTc interval ranging from 2 to 5 msec compared to placebo. No patients treated with SAPHRIS experienced QTc increases ≥60 msec from baseline measurements, nor did any patient experience a QTc of ≥500 msec.

Electrocardiogram (ECG) measurements were taken at various time points during the SAPHRIS clinical trial program (5-mg or 10-mg twice daily doses). Post-baseline QT prolongations exceeding 500 msec were reported at comparable rates for SAPHRIS and placebo in these short-term trials. There were no reports of Torsade de Pointes or any other adverse reactions associated with delayed ventricular repolarization.

The use of SAPHRIS should be avoided in combination with other drugs known to prolong QTc including Class 1A antiarrhythmics (e.g., quinidine, procainamide) or Class 3 antiarrhythmics (e.g., amiodarone, sotalol), antipsychotic medications (e.g., ziprasidone, chlorpromazine, thioridazine), and antibiotics (e.g., gatifloxacin, moxifloxacin). SAPHRIS should also be avoided in patients with a history of cardiac arrhythmias and in other circumstances that may increase the risk of the occurrence of torsade de pointes and/or sudden death in association with the use of drugs that prolong the QTc interval, including bradycardia; hypokalemia or hypomagnesemia; and presence of congenital prolongation of the QT interval.

5.11 Hyperprolactinemia

Like other drugs that antagonize dopamine D_2 receptors, SAPHRIS can elevate prolactin levels, and the elevation can persist during chronic administration. Hyperprolactinemia may suppress hypothalamic GnRH, resulting in reduced pituitary gonadotropin secretion. This, in turn, may inhibit reproductive function by impairing gonadal steroidogenesis in both female and male patients. Galactorrhea, amenorrhea, gynecomastia, and impotence have been reported in patients receiving prolactin-elevating compounds. Long-standing hyperprolactinemia when associated with hypogonadism may lead to decreased bone density in both female and male subjects. In SAPHRIS clinical trials, the incidences of adverse events related to abnormal prolactin levels were 0.4% versus 0% for placebo *[see Adverse Reactions (6.1)]*.

Tissue culture experiments indicate that approximately one-third of human breast cancers are prolactin-dependent *in vitro*, a factor of potential importance if the prescription of these drugs is considered in a patient with previously-detected breast cancer. Neither clinical studies nor epidemiologic studies conducted to date have shown an association between chronic administration of this class of drugs and tumorigenesis in humans, but the available evidence is too limited to be conclusive.

5.12 Seizures

Seizures were reported in 0% and 0.3% (0/572, 1/379) of patients treated with doses of 5 mg and 10 mg twice daily of SAPHRIS, respectively, compared to 0% (0/503, 0/203) of patients treated with placebo in short-term schizophrenia and bipolar mania trials, respectively. During pre-marketing clinical trials with SAPHRIS, including long-term trials without comparison to placebo, seizures were reported in 0.3% (5/1953) of patients treated with SAPHRIS. As with other antipsychotic drugs, SAPHRIS should be used with caution in patients with a history of seizures or with conditions that potentially lower the seizure threshold, e.g., Alzheimer's dementia. Conditions that lower the seizure threshold may be more prevalent in patients 65 years or older.

5.13 Potential for Cognitive and Motor Impairment

Somnolence was reported in patients treated with SAPHRIS. It was usually transient with the highest incidence reported during the first week of treatment. In short-term, fixed-dose, placebo-controlled schizophrenia trials, somnolence was reported in 15% (41/274) of patients on SAPHRIS 5 mg twice daily and in 13% (26/208) of patients on SAPHRIS 10 mg twice daily compared to 7% (26/378) of placebo patients. In short-term, placebo-controlled bipolar mania trials of therapeutic doses (5-10 mg twice daily), somnolence was reported in 24% (90/379) of patients on SAPHRIS compared to 6% (13/203) of placebo patients. During pre-marketing clinical trials with SAPHRIS, including long-term trials without comparison to placebo, somnolence was reported in 18% (358/1953) of patients treated with SAPHRIS. Somnolence (including sedation) led to discontinuation in 0.6% (12/1953) of patients in short-term, placebo-controlled trials.

Patients should be cautioned about performing activities requiring mental alertness, such as operating hazardous machinery or operating a motor vehicle, until they are reasonably certain that SAPHRIS therapy does not affect them adversely.

5.14 Body Temperature Regulation

Disruption of the body's ability to reduce core body temperature has been attributed to antipsychotic agents. In the short-term placebo-controlled trials for both schizophrenia and acute bipolar disorder, the incidence of adverse reactions suggestive of body temperature increases was low (≤1%) and comparable to placebo. During pre-marketing clinical trials with SAPHRIS, including long-term trials without comparison to placebo, the incidence of adverse reactions suggestive of body temperature increases (pyrexia and feeling hot) was ≤1%. Appropriate care is advised when prescribing SAPHRIS for patients who will be experiencing conditions that may contribute to an elevation in core body temperature, e.g., exercising strenuously, exposure to extreme heat, receiving concomitant medication with anticholinergic activity, or being subject to dehydration.

5.15 Suicide

The possibility of a suicide attempt is inherent in psychotic illnesses and bipolar disorder, and close supervision of high-risk patients should accompany drug therapy. Prescriptions for SAPHRIS should be written for the smallest quantity of tablets consistent with good patient management in order to reduce the risk of overdose.

5.16 Dysphagia

Esophageal dysmotility and aspiration have been associated with antipsychotic drug use. Dysphagia was reported in 0.2% and 0% (1/572, 0/379) of patients treated with therapeutic doses (5-10 mg twice daily) of SAPHRIS as compared to 0% (0/378, 0/203) of patients treated with placebo in short-term schizophrenia and bipolar mania trials, respectively. During pre-marketing clinical trials with SAPHRIS, including long-term trials without comparison to placebo, dysphagia was reported in 0.1% (2/1953) of patients treated with SAPHRIS.

Aspiration pneumonia is a common cause of morbidity and mortality in elderly patients, in particular those with advanced Alzheimer's dementia. SAPHRIS is not indicated for the treatment of dementia-related psychosis, and should not be used in patients at risk for aspiration pneumonia *[see also Warnings and Precautions (5.1)]*.

5.17 Use in Patients with Concomitant Illness

Clinical experience with SAPHRIS in patients with certain concomitant systemic illnesses is limited *[see Clinical Pharmacology (12.3)]*.

SAPHRIS has not been evaluated in patients with a recent history of myocardial infarction or unstable heart disease. Patients with these diagnoses were excluded from pre-marketing clinical trials. Because of the risk of orthostatic hypotension with SAPHRIS, caution should be observed in cardiac patients *[see Warnings and Precautions (5.6)]*.

6 ADVERSE REACTIONS

The following adverse reactions are discussed in more detail in other sections of the labeling:

- Use in Elderly Patients with Dementia-Related Psychosis *[see Boxed Warning and Warnings and Precautions (5.1 and 5.2)]*
- Neuroleptic Malignant Syndrome *[see Warnings and Precautions (5.3)]*
- Tardive Dyskinesia *[see Warnings and Precautions (5.4)]*
- Hyperglycemia and Diabetes Mellitus *[see Warnings and Precautions (5.5)]*
- Weight Gain *[see Warnings and Precautions (5.6)]*
- Hypersensitivity Reactions *[see Warnings and Precautions (5.7) and Patient Counseling Information (17.3)]*
- Application site reactions including oral ulcers, blisters, peeling/sloughing and inflammation *[see Adverse Reactions (6.2)]*
- Orthostatic Hypotension, Syncope, and other Hemodynamic Effects *[see Warnings and Precautions (5.8)]*
- Leukopenia, Neutropenia, and Agranulocytosis *[see Warnings and Precautions (5.9)]*
- QT Interval Prolongation *[see Warnings and Precautions (5.10)]*
- Hyperprolactinemia *[see Warnings and Precautions (5.11)]*
- Seizures *[see Warnings and Precautions (5.12)]*
- Potential for Cognitive and Motor Impairment *[see Warnings and Precautions (5.13)]*
- Body Temperature Regulation *[see Warnings and Precautions (5.14)]*
- Suicide *[see Warnings and Precautions (5.15)]*
- Dysphagia *[see Warnings and Precautions (5.16)]*
- Use in Patients with Concomitant Illness *[see Warnings and Precautions (5.17)]*

The most common adverse reactions (≥5% and at least twice the rate of placebo) reported with acute treatment in schizophrenia were akathisia, oral hypoesthesia, and somnolence. The safety profile of SAPHRIS in the maintenance treatment of schizophrenia was similar to that seen with acute treatment.

The most common adverse reactions (≥5% and at least twice the rate of placebo) reported with acute monotherapy treatment of manic or mixed episodes associated with bipolar I disorder were somnolence, dizziness, extrapyramidal symptoms other than akathisia, and weight increased and during the adjunctive therapy trial in bipolar disorder were somnolence and oral hypoesthesia.

The information below is derived from a clinical trial database for SAPHRIS consisting of over 4565 patients and/or normal subjects exposed to one or more sublingual doses of SAPHRIS. A total of 1314 SAPHRIS-treated patients were treated for at least 24 weeks and 785 SAPHRIS-treated patients had at least 52 weeks of exposure at therapeutic doses.

The stated frequencies of adverse reactions represent the proportion of individuals who experienced a treatment-emergent adverse event of the type listed. A reaction was considered treatment emergent if it occurred for the first time or worsened while receiving therapy following baseline evaluation.

The figures in the tables and tabulations cannot be used to predict the incidence of side effects in the course of usual medical practice where patient characteristics and other factors differ from those that prevailed in the clinical trials. Similarly, the cited frequencies cannot be compared with figures obtained from other clinical investigations involving different treatment, uses, and investigators. The cited figures, however, do provide the prescriber with some basis for estimating the relative contribution of drug and nondrug factors to the adverse reaction incidence in the population studied.

6.1 Clinical Studies Experience

Adult Patients with Schizophrenia: The following findings are based on the short-term placebo-controlled premarketing trials for schizophrenia (a pool of three 6-week fixed-dose trials and one 6-week flexible-dose trial) in which sublingual SAPHRIS was administered in doses ranging from 5 to 10 mg twice daily.

Adverse Reactions Associated with Discontinuation of Treatment: A total of 9% of SAPHRIS-treated subjects and 10% of placebo subjects discontinued due to adverse reactions. There were no drug-related adverse reactions associated with discontinuation in subjects treated with SAPHRIS at the rate of at least 1% and at least twice the placebo rate.

Adverse Reactions Occurring at an Incidence of 2% or More in SAPHRIS-Treated Schizophrenic Patients: Adverse reactions associated with the use of SAPHRIS (incidence of 2% or greater, rounded to the nearest percent, and SAPHRIS incidence greater than placebo) that occurred during acute therapy (up to 6-weeks in patients with schizophrenia) are shown in **Table 2**.

[See table 2 at top of next page]

Dose-Related Adverse Reactions: Of all the adverse reactions listed in **Table 2**, the only apparent dose-related adverse reaction was akathisia.

Monotherapy in Adult Patients with Bipolar Mania: The following findings are based on the short-term placebo-controlled trials for bipolar mania (a pool of two 3-week flexible-dose trials) in which sublingual SAPHRIS was administered in doses of 5 mg or 10 mg twice daily.

Adverse Reactions Associated with Discontinuation of Treatment: Approximately 10% (38/379) of SAPHRIS-treated patients in short-term, placebo-controlled trials discontinued treatment due to an adverse reaction, compared with about 6% (12/203) on placebo. The most common adverse reactions associated with discontinuation in subjects treated with SAPHRIS (rates at least 1% and at least twice the placebo rate) were anxiety (1.1%) and oral hypoesthesia (1.1%) compared to placebo (0%).

Adverse Reactions Occurring at an Incidence of 2% or More Among SAPHRIS-Treated (Monotherapy) Bipolar Patients: Adverse reactions associated with the use of SAPHRIS (incidence of 2% or greater, rounded to the nearest percent, and SAPHRIS incidence greater than placebo) that occurred during acute monotherapy (up to 3-weeks in patients with bipolar mania) are shown in **Table 3**.

Table 3: Adverse Reactions Reported in 2% or More of Subjects in One of the SAPHRIS Dose Groups and Which Occurred at Greater Incidence Than in the Placebo Group in 3-Week Bipolar Mania Trials

System Organ Class/ Preferred Term	Placebo N=203	SAPHRIS 5 mg or 10 mg twice daily* N=379
Gastrointestinal disorders		
Dry mouth	1%	3%
Dyspepsia	2%	4%
Oral hypoesthesia	<1%	4%
Toothache	2%	3%
General disorders		
Fatigue	2%	4%
Investigations		
Weight increased	<1%	5%
Metabolism disorders		
Increased appetite	1%	4%
Musculoskeletal and connective tissue disorders		
Arthralgia	1%	3%
Pain in extremity	<1%	2%
Nervous system disorders		
Akathisia	2%	4%
Dizziness	3%	11%
Dysgeusia	<1%	3%
Headache	11%	12%
Other extrapyramidal symptoms (excluding akathisia)†	2%	7%
Somnolence‡	6%	24%
Psychiatric disorders		
Anxiety	2%	4%
Depression	1%	2%
Insomnia	5%	6%

* SAPHRIS 5 mg to 10 mg twice daily with flexible dosing.

† Extrapyramidal symptoms included: dystonia, blepharospasm, torticollis, dyskinesia, tardive dyskinesia, muscle rigidity, parkinsonism, gait disturbance, masked facies, and tremor (excluding akathisia).

‡ Somnolence includes the following events: somnolence, sedation, and hypersomnia.

Adjunctive Therapy in Adult Patients with Bipolar Mania: The following findings are based on a 12 week placebo-controlled trial (with a 3 week efficacy endpoint) in adult patients with bipolar mania in which sublingual SAPHRIS was administered in doses of 5 mg or 10 mg twice daily as adjunctive therapy with lithium or valproate.

Adverse Reactions Associated with Discontinuation of Treatment: Approximately 16% (25/158) of SAPHRIS-treated patients discontinued treatment due to an adverse reaction, compared with about 11% (18/166) on placebo. The most common adverse reactions associated with discontinuation in subjects treated with SAPHRIS (rates at least 1% and at least twice the placebo rate) were depression (2.5%), suicidal ideation (2.5%), bipolar 1 disorder (1.9%), insomnia (1.9%) and depressive symptoms (1.3%).

Adverse Reactions Occurring at an Incidence of 2% or More Among SAPHRIS-Treated (Adjunctive) Bipolar Patients: Adverse reactions associated with the use of SAPHRIS (incidence of 2% or greater, rounded to the nearest percent, and SAPHRIS incidence greater than placebo) that occurred during acute adjunctive therapy at 3 weeks, a time when most of the patients were still participating in the trial, are shown in **Table 4**.

Table 4: Adverse Reactions Reported in 2% or More Among SAPHRIS-Treated (Adjunctive) Bipolar Mania Patients and Which Occurred at Greater Incidence Than in the Placebo Group at 3 Weeks

System Organ Class/ Preferred Term	Placebo N=166	SAPHRIS 5 mg or 10 mg twice daily* N=158
Gastrointestinal disorders		
Dyspepsia	2%	3%
Oral hypoesthesia	0%	5%
General disorders		
Fatigue	2%	4%
Edema peripheral	<1%	3%
Investigations		
Weight increased	0%	3%
Nervous system disorders		
Dizziness	2%	4%
Other extrapyramidal symptoms (excluding akathisia)†	5%	6%
Somnolence‡	10%	22%
Psychiatric disorders		
Insomnia	8%	10%
Vascular disorders		
Hypertension	<1%	3%

* SAPHRIS 5 mg to 10 mg twice daily with flexible dosing.

† Extrapyramidal symptoms included: dystonia, parkinsonism, oculogyration, and tremor (excluding akathisia).

‡ Somnolence includes the following events: somnolence and sedation.

Table 2: Adverse Reactions Reported in 2% or More of Subjects in One of the SAPHRIS Dose Groups and Which Occurred at Greater Incidence Than in the Placebo Group in 6-Week Schizophrenia Trials

System Organ Class/ Preferred Term	Placebo N=378	SAPHRIS 5 mg twice daily N=274	SAPHRIS 10 mg twice daily N=208	All SAPHRIS* 5 mg or 10 mg twice daily N=572
Gastrointestinal disorders				
Constipation	6%	7%	4%	5%
Dry mouth	1%	3%	1%	2%
Oral hypoesthesia	1%	6%	7%	5%
Salivary hypersecretion	0%	<1%	4%	2%
Stomach discomfort	1%	<1%	3%	2%
Vomiting	5%	4%	7%	5%
General disorders				
Fatigue	3%	4%	3%	3%
Irritability	<1%	2%	1%	2%
Investigations				
Weight increased	<1%	2%	2%	3%
Metabolism disorders				
Increased appetite	<1%	3%	0%	2%
Nervous system disorders				
Akathisia†	3%	4%	11%	6%
Dizziness	4%	7%	3%	5%
Extrapyramidal symptoms (excluding akathisia)‡	7%	9%	12%	10%
Somnolence§	7%	15%	13%	13%
Psychiatric disorders				
Insomnia	13%	16%	15%	15%
Vascular disorders				
Hypertension	2%	2%	3%	2%

* Also includes the Flexible-dose trial (N=90).

† Akathisia includes: akathisia and hyperkinesia.

‡ Extrapyramidal symptoms included dystonia, oculogyration, dyskinesia, tardive dyskinesia, muscle rigidity, parkinsonism, tremor, and extrapyramidal disorder (excluding akathisia).

§ Somnolence includes the following events: somnolence, sedation, and hypersomnia.

Dystonia: *Antipsychotic Class Effect:* Symptoms of dystonia, prolonged abnormal contractions of muscle groups, may occur in susceptible individuals during the first few days of treatment. Dystonic symptoms include: spasm of the neck muscles, sometimes progressing to tightness of the throat, swallowing difficulty, difficulty breathing, and/or protrusion of the tongue. While these symptoms can occur at low doses, they occur more frequently and with greater severity with high potency and at higher doses of first generation antipsychotic drugs. An elevated risk of acute dystonia is observed in males and younger age groups.

Extrapyramidal Symptoms: In the short-term, placebo-controlled schizophrenia and bipolar mania trials, data was objectively collected on the Simpson Angus Rating Scale for extrapyramidal symptoms (EPS), the Barnes Akathisia Scale (for akathisia) and the Assessments of Involuntary Movement Scales (for dyskinesias). The mean change from baseline for the all-SAPHRIS 5 mg or 10 mg twice daily treated group was comparable to placebo in each of the rating scale scores.

In the short-term, placebo-controlled schizophrenia trials, the incidence of reported EPS-related events, excluding events related to akathisia, for SAPHRIS-treated patients was 10% versus 7% for placebo; and the incidence of akathisia-related events for SAPHRIS-treated patients was 6% versus 3% for placebo. In short-term placebo-controlled bipolar mania trials, the incidence of EPS-related events, excluding events related to akathisia, for SAPHRIS-treated patients was 7% versus 2% for placebo; and the incidence of akathisia-related events for SAPHRIS-treated patients was 4% versus 2% for placebo.

Other Findings: Oral hypoesthesia and/or oral paraesthesia may occur directly after administration of asenapine and usually resolves within 1 hour.

Laboratory Test Abnormalities:

Glucose: The effects on fasting serum glucose levels in the short-term schizophrenia and bipolar mania trials revealed no clinically relevant mean changes *[see also Warnings and Precautions (5.5)]*. In the short-term placebo-controlled schizophrenia trials, the mean increase in fasting glucose levels for SAPHRIS-treated patients was 3.2 mg/dL compared to a decrease of 1.6 mg/dL for placebo-treated patients. The proportion of patients with fasting glucose elevations ≥126 mg/dL (at Endpoint), was 7.4% for SAPHRIS-treated patients versus 6% for placebo-treated patients. In the short-term, placebo-controlled bipolar mania trials, the mean decreases in fasting glucose levels for both SAPHRIS-treated and placebo-treated patients were 0.6 mg/dL. The proportion of patients with fasting glucose elevations ≥126 mg/dL (at Endpoint), was 4.9% for SAPHRIS-treated patients versus 2.2% for placebo-treated patients.

In a 52-week, double-blind, comparator-controlled trial of patients with schizophrenia and schizoaffective disorder, the mean increase from baseline of fasting glucose was 2.4 mg/dL.

Lipids: The effects on total cholesterol and fasting triglycerides in the short-term schizophrenia and bipolar mania trials revealed no clinically relevant mean changes. In short-term, placebo-controlled schizophrenia trials, the mean increase in total cholesterol levels for SAPHRIS-treated patients was 0.4 mg/dL compared to a decrease of 3.6 mg/dL for placebo-treated patients. The proportion of patients with total cholesterol elevations ≥240 mg/dL (at Endpoint) was 8.3% for SAPHRIS-treated patients versus 7% for placebo-treated patients. In short-term, placebo-controlled bipolar mania trials, the mean increase in total cholesterol levels for SAPHRIS-treated patients was 1.1 mg/dL compared to a decrease of 1.5 mg/dL in placebo-treated patients. The proportion of patients with total cholesterol elevations ≥240 mg/dL (at Endpoint) was 8.7% for SAPHRIS-treated patients versus 8.6% for placebo-treated patients. In short-term, placebo-controlled schizophrenia trials, the mean increase in triglyceride levels for SAPHRIS-treated patients was 3.8 mg/dL compared to a decrease of 13.5 mg/dL for placebo-treated patients. The proportion of patients with elevations in triglycerides ≥200 mg/dL (at Endpoint) was 13.2% for SAPHRIS-treated patients versus 10.5% for placebo-treated patients. In short-term, placebo-controlled bipolar mania trials, the mean decrease in triglyceride levels for SAPHRIS-treated patients was 3.5 mg/dL versus 17.9 mg/dL for placebo-treated subjects. The proportion of patients with elevations in triglycerides ≥200 mg/dL (at Endpoint) was 15.2% for SAPHRIS-treated patients versus 11.4% for placebo-treated patients.

In a 52-week, double-blind, comparator-controlled trial of patients with schizophrenia and schizoaffective disorder, the mean decrease from baseline of total cholesterol was 6 mg/dL and the mean decrease from baseline of fasting triglycerides was 9.8 mg/dL.

Transaminases: Transient elevations in serum transaminases (primarily ALT) in the short-term schizophrenia and bipolar mania trials were more common in treated patients but mean changes were not clinically relevant. In short-term, placebo-controlled schizophrenia trials, the mean increase in transaminase levels for SAPHRIS-treated patients was 1.6 units/L compared to a decrease of 0.4 units/L for placebo-treated patients. The proportion of patients with transaminase elevations ≥3 times ULN (at Endpoint) was 0.9% for SAPHRIS-treated patients versus 1.3% for placebo-treated patients. In short-term, placebo-controlled bipolar mania trials, the mean increase in transaminase levels for SAPHRIS-treated patients was 8.9 units/L compared to a decrease of 4.9 units/L in placebo-treated patients. The proportion of patients with transaminase elevations >3 times upper limit of normal (ULN) (at Endpoint) was 2.5% for SAPHRIS-treated patients versus 0.6% for placebo-treated patients. No cases of more severe liver injury were seen.

In a 52-week, double-blind, comparator-controlled trial of patients with schizophrenia and schizoaffective disorder, the mean increase from baseline of ALT was 1.7 units/L.

Prolactin: The effects on prolactin levels in the short-term schizophrenia and bipolar mania trials revealed no clinically relevant mean changes in baseline. In short-term, placebo-controlled schizophrenia trials, the mean decreases in prolactin levels were 6.5 ng/mL for SAPHRIS-treated patients compared to 10.7 ng/mL for placebo-treated patients. The proportion of patients with prolactin elevations ≥4 times ULN (at Endpoint) were 2.6% for SAPHRIS-treated patients versus 0.6% for placebo-treated patients. In short-term, placebo-controlled bipolar mania trials, the mean increase in prolactin levels was 4.9 ng/mL for SAPHRIS-treated patients compared to a decrease of 0.2 ng/mL for placebo-treated patients. The proportion of patients with prolactin elevations ≥4 times ULN (at Endpoint) were 2.3% for SAPHRIS-treated patients versus 0.7% for placebo-treated patients.

In a long-term (52-week), double-blind, comparator-controlled trial of patients with schizophrenia and schizoaffective disorder, the mean decrease in prolactin from baseline for SAPHRIS-treated patients was 26.9 ng/mL.

Creatine Kinase (CK): The proportion of patients with CK elevations >3 times ULN at any time were 6.4% and 11.1% for patients treated with SAPHRIS 5 mg bid and 10 mg bid, respectively, as compared to 6.7% for placebo-treated patients in short-term, fixed-dose trials in schizophrenia and bipolar mania. The clinical relevance of this finding is unknown.

Other Adverse Reactions Observed During the Premarketing Evaluation of SAPHRIS: Following is a list of MedDRA terms that reflect adverse reactions reported by patients treated with sublingual SAPHRIS at multiple doses of ≥5 mg twice daily during any phase of a trial within the database of adult patients. The reactions listed are those that could be of clinical importance, as well as reactions that are plausibly drug-related on pharmacologic or other grounds. Reactions already listed in other parts of *Adverse Reactions (6)*, or those considered in *Warnings and Precautions (5)* or *Overdosage (10)* are not included. Although the reactions reported occurred during treatment with SAPHRIS, they were not necessarily caused by it. Reactions are further categorized by MedDRA system organ class and listed in order of decreasing frequency according to the following definitions: those occurring in at least 1/100 patients (only those not already listed in the tabulated results from placebo-controlled trials appear in this listing); those occurring in 1/100 to 1/1000 patients; and those occurring in fewer than 1/1000 patients.

Blood and lymphatic disorders: *≥1/1000 patients:* thrombocytopenia; *≥1/1000 patients and <1/100 patients:* anemia

Cardiac disorders: *≥1/1000 patients and <1/100 patients:* tachycardia, temporary bundle branch block

Eye disorders: *≥1/1000 patients and <1/100 patients:* accommodation disorder

Gastrointestinal disorders: *≥1/1000 patients and <1/100 patients:* oral paraesthesia, glossodynia, swollen tongue

General disorders: *<1/1000 patients:* idiosyncratic drug reaction

Investigations: *≥1/1000 patients and <1/100 patients:* hyponatremia

Nervous system disorders: *≥1/1000 patients and <1/100 patients:* dysarthria

6.2 Postmarketing Experience

The following adverse reactions have been identified during post-approval use of SAPHRIS. Application site reactions, primarily in the sublingual area, have been reported. These application site reactions included oral ulcers, blisters, peeling/sloughing, and inflammation. In many cases, the occurrence of these application site reactions led to discontinuation of therapy.

7 DRUG INTERACTIONS

The risks of using SAPHRIS in combination with other drugs have not been extensively evaluated. Given the primary CNS effects of SAPHRIS, caution should be used when it is taken in combination with other centrally acting drugs or alcohol.

Because of its α_1-adrenergic antagonism with potential for inducing hypotension, SAPHRIS may enhance the effects of certain antihypertensive agents.

7.1 Potential for Other Drugs to Affect SAPHRIS

Asenapine is cleared primarily through direct glucuronidation by UGT1A4 and oxidative metabolism by cytochrome P450 isoenzymes (predominantly CYP1A2). The potential effects of inhibitors of several of these enzyme pathways on asenapine clearance were studied.

[See table 5 above]

Table 5: Summary of Effect of Coadministered Drugs on Exposure to Asenapine in Healthy Volunteers

Coadministered drug (Postulated effect on CYP450/UGT)	Dose schedules		Effect on asenapine pharmacokinetics		Recommendation
	Coadministered drug	Asenapine	C_{max}	$AUC_{0-\infty}$	
Fluvoxamine (CYP1A2 inhibitor)	25 mg twice daily for 8 days	5-mg Single Dose	+13%	+29%	Coadminister with caution*
Paroxetine (CYP2D6 inhibitor)	20 mg once daily for 9 days	5-mg Single Dose	–13%	–9%	No SAPHRIS dose adjustment required *[see Drug Interactions (7.2)]*
Imipramine (CYP1A2/2C19/3A4 inhibitor)	75-mg Single Dose	5-mg Single Dose	+17%	+10%	No SAPHRIS dose adjustment required
Cimetidine (CYP3A4/2D6/1A2 inhibitor)	800 mg twice daily for 8 days	5-mg Single Dose	–13%	+1%	No SAPHRIS dose adjustment required
Carbamazepine (CYP3A4 inducer)	400 mg twice daily for 15 days	5-mg Single Dose	–16%	–16%	No SAPHRIS dose adjustment required
Valproate (UGT1A4 inhibitor)	500 mg twice daily for 9 days	5-mg Single Dose	2%	–1%	No SAPHRIS dose adjustment required

* The full therapeutic dose of fluvoxamine would be expected to cause a greater increase in asenapine plasma concentrations. AUC: Area under the curve.

A population pharmacokinetic analysis indicated that the concomitant administration of lithium had no effect on the pharmacokinetics of asenapine.

7.2 Potential for SAPHRIS to Affect Other Drugs

Coadministration with CYP2D6 Substrates: *In vitro* studies indicate that asenapine weakly inhibits CYP2D6. Following coadministration of dextromethorphan and SAPHRIS in healthy subjects, the ratio of dextrorphan/dextromethorphan (DX/DM) as a marker of CYP2D6 activity was measured. Indicative of CYP2D6 inhibition, treatment with SAPHRIS 5 mg twice daily decreased the DX/DM ratio to 0.43. In the same study, treatment with paroxetine 20 mg daily decreased the DX/DM ratio to 0.032. In a separate study, coadministration of a single 75-mg dose of imipramine with a single 5-mg dose of SAPHRIS did not affect the plasma concentrations of the metabolite desipramine (a CYP2D6 substrate). Thus, *in vivo*, SAPHRIS appears to be at most a weak inhibitor of CYP2D6. Coadministration of a

single 20-mg dose of paroxetine (a CYP2D6 substrate and inhibitor) during treatment with 5 mg SAPHRIS twice daily in 15 healthy male subjects resulted in an almost 2-fold increase in paroxetine exposure. Asenapine may enhance the inhibitory effects of paroxetine on its own metabolism. SAPHRIS should be coadministered cautiously with drugs that are both substrates and inhibitors for CYP2D6.
Valproic acid and lithium pre-dose serum concentrations collected from an adjunctive therapy study were comparable between asenapine treated patients and placebo treated patients indicating a lack of effect of asenapine on valproic and lithium plasma levels.

8 USE IN SPECIFIC POPULATIONS

8.1 Pregnancy

Pregnancy Category C: There are no adequate and well-controlled studies of SAPHRIS in pregnant women.
In animal studies, asenapine increased post-implantation loss and decreased pup weight and survival at doses similar to or less than recommended clinical doses. In these studies there was no increase in the incidence of structural abnormalities caused by asenapine.
Asenapine was not teratogenic in reproduction studies in rats and rabbits at intravenous doses up to 1.5 mg/kg in rats and 0.44 mg/kg in rabbits. These doses are 0.7 and 0.4 times, respectively, the maximum recommended human dose (MRHD) of 10 mg twice daily given sublingually on a mg/m^2 basis. Plasma levels of asenapine were measured in the rabbit study, and the area under the curve (AUC) at the highest dose tested was 2 times that in humans receiving the MRHD.
In a study in which rats were treated from day 6 of gestation through day 21 postpartum with intravenous doses of asenapine of 0.3, 0.9, and 1.5 mg/kg/day (0.15, 0.4, and 0.7 times the MRHD of 10 mg twice daily given sublingually on a mg/m^2 basis), increases in post-implantation loss and early pup deaths were seen at all doses, and decreases in subsequent pup survival and weight gain were seen at the two higher doses. A cross-fostering study indicated that the decreases in pup survival were largely due to prenatal drug effects. Increases in post-implantation loss and decreases in pup weight and survival were also seen when pregnant rats were dosed orally with asenapine.

Non-teratogenic Effects

Neonates exposed to antipsychotic drugs during the third trimester of pregnancy are at risk for extrapyramidal and/or withdrawal symptoms following delivery. There have been reports of agitation, hypertonia, hypotonia, tremor, somnolence, respiratory distress and feeding disorder in these neonates. These complications have varied in severity; while in some cases symptoms have been self-limited, in other cases neonates have required intensive care unit support and prolonged hospitalization. SAPHRIS (asenapine) should be used during pregnancy only if the potential benefit justifies the potential risk to the fetus.

8.2 Labor and Delivery

The effect of SAPHRIS on labor and delivery in humans is unknown.

8.3 Nursing Mothers

Asenapine is excreted in milk of rats during lactation. It is not known whether asenapine or its metabolites are excreted in human milk. Because many drugs are excreted in human milk, caution should be exercised when SAPHRIS is administered to a nursing woman. It is recommended that women receiving SAPHRIS should not breast feed.

8.4 Pediatric Use

Safety and effectiveness in pediatric patients have not been established.

8.5 Geriatric Use

Clinical studies of SAPHRIS in the treatment of schizophrenia and bipolar mania did not include sufficient numbers of patients aged 65 and over to determine whether or not they respond differently than younger patients. Of the approximately 2250 patients in pre-marketing clinical studies of SAPHRIS, 1.1% (25) were 65 years of age or over. Multiple factors that might increase the pharmacodynamic response to SAPHRIS, causing poorer tolerance or orthostasis, could be present in elderly patients, and these patients should be monitored carefully.
In elderly patients with psychosis, asenapine exposure (AUC) was on average 40% higher compared to younger adult patients *[see Clinical Pharmacology (12.3)]*.
Elderly patients with dementia-related psychosis treated with SAPHRIS are at an increased risk of death compared to placebo. SAPHRIS is not approved for the treatment of patients with dementia-related psychosis *[see Boxed Warning]*.

8.6 Renal Impairment

The exposure of asenapine following a single dose of 5 mg was similar among subjects with varying degrees of renal impairment and subjects with normal renal function *[see Clinical Pharmacology (12.3)]*.

8.7 Hepatic Impairment

In subjects with severe hepatic impairment who were treated with a single dose of SAPHRIS 5 mg, asenapine exposures (on average), were 7-fold higher than the exposures observed in subjects with normal hepatic function. Thus, SAPHRIS is not recommended in patients with severe hepatic impairment (Child-Pugh C) *[see Dosage and Administration (2.4) and Clinical Pharmacology (12.3)]*.

9 DRUG ABUSE AND DEPENDENCE

9.1 Controlled Substance

SAPHRIS is not a controlled substance.

9.2 Abuse

SAPHRIS has not been systematically studied in animals or humans for its abuse potential or its ability to induce tolerance or physical dependence. Thus, it is not possible to predict the extent to which a CNS-active drug will be misused, diverted and/or abused once it is marketed. Patients should be evaluated carefully for a history of drug abuse, and such patients should be observed carefully for signs that they are misusing or abusing SAPHRIS (e.g., drug-seeking behavior, increases in dose).

10 OVERDOSAGE

Human Experience: In pre-marketing clinical studies involving more than 3350 patients and/or healthy subjects, accidental or intentional acute overdosage of SAPHRIS was identified in 3 patients. Among these few reported cases of overdose, the highest estimated ingestion of SAPHRIS was 400 mg. Reported adverse reactions at the highest dosage included agitation and confusion.
Management of Overdosage: There is no specific antidote to SAPHRIS. The possibility of multiple drug involvement should be considered. An electrocardiogram should be obtained and management of overdose should concentrate on supportive therapy, maintaining an adequate airway, oxygenation and ventilation, and management of symptoms.
Hypotension and circulatory collapse should be treated with appropriate measures, such as intravenous fluids and/or sympathomimetic agents (epinephrine and dopamine should not be used, since beta stimulation may worsen hypotension in the setting of SAPHRIS-induced alpha blockade). In case of severe extrapyramidal symptoms, anticholinergic medication should be administered. Close medical supervision and monitoring should continue until the patient recovers.

11 DESCRIPTION

SAPHRIS is a psychotropic agent that is available for sublingual administration. Asenapine belongs to the class dibenzo-oxepino pyrroles. The chemical designation is (3a*RS*,12b*RS*)-5-Chloro-2-methyl-2,3,3a,12b-tetrahydro-1*H*dibenzo[2,3:6,7]oxepino[4,5-*c*]pyrrole (2*Z*)-2-butenedioate (1:1). Its molecular formula is $C_{17}H_{16}ClNO \bullet C_4H_4O_4$ and its molecular weight is 401.84 (free base: 285.8). The chemical structure is:

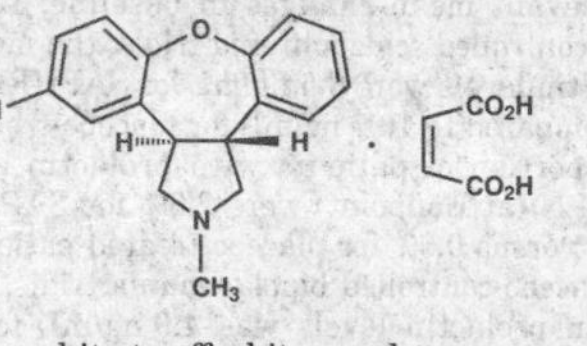

Asenapine is a white to off-white powder.
SAPHRIS is supplied for sublingual administration in tablets containing 5-mg or 10-mg asenapine; inactive ingredients include gelatin and mannitol.
SAPHRIS, black cherry flavor, is supplied for sublingual administration in tablets containing 5-mg or 10-mg asenapine; inactive ingredients include gelatin, mannitol, sucralose, and black cherry flavor.

12 CLINICAL PHARMACOLOGY

12.1 Mechanism of Action

The mechanism of action of asenapine, as with other drugs having efficacy in schizophrenia and bipolar disorder, is unknown. It has been suggested that the efficacy of asenapine in schizophrenia is mediated through a combination of antagonist activity at D_2 and $5\text{-}HT_{2A}$ receptors.

12.2 Pharmacodynamics

Asenapine exhibits high affinity for serotonin $5\text{-}HT_{1A}$, $5\text{-}HT_{1B}$, $5\text{-}HT_{2A}$, $5\text{-}HT_{2B}$, $5\text{-}HT_{2C}$, $5\text{-}HT_5$, $5\text{-}HT_6$, and $5\text{-}HT_7$ receptors (Ki values of 2.5, 4.0, 0.06, 0.16, 0.03, 1.6, 0.25, and 0.13 nM), dopamine D_2, D_3, D_4, and D_1 receptors (Ki values of 1.3, 0.42, 1.1, and 1.4 nM), α_1 and α_2-adrenergic receptors (Ki values of 1.2 and 1.2 nM), and histamine H_1 receptors (Ki value 1.0 nM), and moderate affinity for H_2 receptors (Ki value of 6.2 nM). In *in vitro* assays asenapine acts as an antagonist at these receptors. Asenapine has no appreciable affinity for muscarinic cholinergic receptors (e.g., Ki value of 8128 nM for M_1).

12.3 Pharmacokinetics

Following a single 5-mg dose of SAPHRIS, the mean C_{max} was approximately 4 ng/mL and was observed at a mean t_{max} of 1 hour. Elimination of asenapine is primarily through direct glucuronidation by UGT1A4 and oxidative metabolism by cytochrome P450 isoenzymes (predominantly CYP1A2). Following an initial more rapid distribution phase, the mean terminal half-life is approximately 24 hrs. With multiple-dose twice-daily dosing, steady-state is attained within 3 days. Overall, steady-state asenapine pharmacokinetics are similar to single-dose pharmacokinetics.
Absorption: Following sublingual administration, asenapine is rapidly absorbed with peak plasma concentrations occurring within 0.5 to 1.5 hours. The absolute bioavailability of sublingual asenapine at 5 mg is 35%. Increasing the dose from 5 mg to 10 mg twice daily (a two-fold increase) results in less than linear (1.7 times) increases in both the extent of exposure and maximum concentration. The absolute bioavailability of asenapine when swallowed is low (<2% with an oral tablet formulation).
The intake of water several (2 or 5) minutes after asenapine administration resulted in decreased asenapine exposure. Therefore, eating and drinking should be avoided for 10 minutes after administration *[see Dosage and Administration (2.1)]*.
Distribution: Asenapine is rapidly distributed and has a large volume of distribution (approximately 20 - 25 L/kg), indicating extensive extravascular distribution. Asenapine is highly bound (95%) to plasma proteins, including albumin and α_1-acid glycoprotein.
Metabolism and Elimination: Direct glucuronidation by UGT1A4 and oxidative metabolism by cytochrome P450 isoenzymes (predominantly CYP1A2) are the primary metabolic pathways for asenapine.
Asenapine is a high clearance drug with a clearance after intravenous administration of 52 L/h. In this circumstance, hepatic clearance is influenced primarily by changes in liver blood flow rather than by changes in the intrinsic clearance, i.e., the metabolizing enzymatic activity. Following an initial more rapid distribution phase, the terminal half life of asenapine is approximately 24 hours. Steady-state concentrations of asenapine are reached within 3 days of twice daily dosing.
After administration of a single dose of [^{14}C]-labeled asenapine, about 90% of the dose was recovered; approximately 50% was recovered in urine, and 40% recovered in feces. About 50% of the circulating species in plasma have been identified. The predominant species was asenapine N^+-glucuronide; others included N-desmethylasenapine, N-desmethylasenapine N-carbamoyl glucuronide, and unchanged asenapine in smaller amounts. SAPHRIS activity is primarily due to the parent drug.
In vitro studies indicate that asenapine is a substrate for UGT1A4, CYP1A2 and to a lesser extent CYP3A4 and CYP2D6. Asenapine is a weak inhibitor of CYP2D6. Asenapine does not cause induction of CYP1A2 or CYP3A4 activities in cultured human hepatocytes. Coadministration of asenapine with known inhibitors, inducers or substrates of these metabolic pathways has been studied in a number of drug-drug interaction studies *[see Drug Interactions (7)]*.
Smoking: A population pharmacokinetic analysis indicated that smoking, which induces CYP1A2, had no effect on the clearance of asenapine in smokers. In a crossover study in which 24 healthy male subjects (who were smokers) were administered a single 5-mg sublingual dose, concomitant smoking had no effect on the pharmacokinetics of asenapine.
Food: A crossover study in 26 healthy male subjects was performed to evaluate the effect of food on the pharmacokinetics of a single 5-mg dose of asenapine. Consumption of food immediately prior to sublingual administration decreased asenapine exposure by 20%; consumption of food 4 hours after sublingual administration decreased asenapine exposure by about 10%. These effects are probably due to increased hepatic blood flow.
In clinical trials establishing the efficacy and safety of SAPHRIS, patients were instructed to avoid eating for 10 minutes following sublingual dosing. There were no other restrictions with regard to the timing of meals in these trials *[see Dosage and Administration (2.1) and Patient Counseling Information (17.1)]*.
Water: In clinical trials establishing the efficacy and safety of SAPHRIS, patients were instructed to avoid drinking for 10 minutes following sublingual dosing. The effect of water administration following 10-mg sublingual SAPHRIS dosing was studied at different time points of 2, 5, 10, and 30 minutes in 15 healthy male subjects. The exposure of asenapine following administration of water 10 minutes after sublingual dosing was equivalent to that when water was administered 30 minutes after dosing. Reduced exposure to asenapine was observed following water administration at 2 minutes (19% decrease) and 5 minutes (10% decrease) *[see Dosage and Administration (2.1) and Patient Counseling Information (17.1)]*.
Special Populations:
<u>Hepatic Impairment:</u> The effect of decreased hepatic function on the pharmacokinetics of asenapine, administered as a single 5-mg sublingual dose, was studied in 30 subjects (8 each in those with normal hepatic function and Child-Pugh

A and B groups, and 6 in the Child-Pugh C group). In subjects with mild or moderate hepatic impairment (Child-Pugh A or B), asenapine exposure was 12% higher than that in subjects with normal hepatic function, indicating that dosage adjustment is not required for these subjects. In subjects with severe hepatic impairment, asenapine exposures were on average 7 times higher than the exposures of those in subjects with normal hepatic function. Thus, SAPHRIS is not recommended in patients with severe hepatic impairment (Child-Pugh C) *[see Dosage in Specific Populations (2.4) and Use in Specific Populations (8.7) and Warnings and Precautions (5.14)].*

Renal Impairment: The effect of decreased renal function on the pharmacokinetics of asenapine was studied in subjects with mildly (creatinine clearance (CrCl) 51 to 80 mL/min; N=8), moderately (CrCl 30 to 50 mL/min; N=8), and severely (CrCl less than 30 mL/min but not on dialysis; N=8) impaired renal function and compared to normal subjects (CrCl greater than 80 mL/min; N=8). The exposure of asenapine following a single dose of 5 mg was similar among subjects with varying degrees of renal impairment and subjects with normal renal function. Dosage adjustment based upon degree of renal impairment is not required. The effect of renal function on the excretion of other metabolites and the effect of dialysis on the pharmacokinetics of asenapine has not been studied *[see Use in Specific Populations (8.6)].*

Geriatric Patients: In elderly patients (N=96) with psychosis (65-85 years of age), asenapine exposure (AUC) was on average 40% higher compared to younger adult patients. No dosage adjustment is necessary. In a population pharmacokinetic analysis, a decrease in clearance with increasing age was observed, implying a 30% higher exposure in elderly as compared to adult patients *[see Use in Specific Populations (8.5)].*

Gender: The potential difference in asenapine pharmacokinetics between males and females was not studied in a dedicated trial. In a population pharmacokinetic analysis, no significant differences between genders were observed.

Race: In a population pharmacokinetic analysis, no effect of race on asenapine concentrations was observed. In a dedicated study, the pharmacokinetics of SAPHRIS were similar in Caucasian and Japanese subjects.

13 NONCLINICAL TOXICOLOGY

13.1 Carcinogenesis, Mutagenesis, Impairment of Fertility

Carcinogenesis: In a lifetime carcinogenicity study in CD-1 mice asenapine was administered subcutaneously at doses up to those resulting in plasma levels (AUC) estimated to be 5 times those in humans receiving the MRHD of 10 mg twice daily. The incidence of malignant lymphomas was increased in female mice, with a no-effect dose resulting in plasma levels estimated to be 1.5 times those in humans receiving the MRHD. The mouse strain used has a high and variable incidence of malignant lymphomas, and the significance of these results to humans is unknown. There were no increases in other tumor types in female mice. In male mice, there were no increases in any tumor type.

In a lifetime carcinogenicity study in Sprague-Dawley rats, asenapine did not cause any increases in tumors when administered subcutaneously at doses up to those resulting in plasma levels (AUC) estimated to be 5 times those in humans receiving the MRHD.

Mutagenesis: No evidence for genotoxic potential of asenapine was found in the *in vitro* bacterial reverse mutation assay, the *in vitro* forward gene mutation assay in mouse lymphoma cells, the *in vitro* chromosomal aberration assays in human lymphocytes, the *in vitro* sister chromatid exchange assay in rabbit lymphocytes, or the *in vivo* micronucleus assay in rats.

Impairment of Fertility: Asenapine did not impair fertility in rats when tested at doses up to 11 mg/kg twice daily given orally. This dose is 10 times the maximum recommended human dose of 10 mg twice daily given sublingually on a mg/m² basis.

14 CLINICAL STUDIES

14.1 Schizophrenia

The efficacy of SAPHRIS in the treatment of schizophrenia in adults was evaluated in three fixed-dose, short-term (6 week), randomized, double-blind, placebo-controlled, and active-controlled (haloperidol, risperidone, and olanzapine) trials of adult patients who met DSM-IV criteria for schizophrenia and were having an acute exacerbation of their schizophrenic illness. In two of the three trials SAPHRIS demonstrated superior efficacy to placebo. In a third trial, SAPHRIS could not be distinguished from placebo; however, an active control in that trial was superior to placebo.

In the two positive trials for SAPHRIS, the primary efficacy rating scale was the Positive and Negative Syndrome Scale (PANSS), which assesses the symptoms of schizophrenia. The primary endpoint was change from baseline to endpoint on the PANSS total score. The results of the SAPHRIS trials in schizophrenia follow:

In trial 1, a 6-week trial (n=174), comparing SAPHRIS (5 mg twice daily) to placebo, SAPHRIS 5 mg twice daily was statistically superior to placebo on the PANSS total score.

In trial 2, a 6-week trial (n=448), comparing two fixed doses of SAPHRIS (5 mg and 10 mg twice daily) to placebo, SAPHRIS 5 mg twice daily was statistically superior to placebo on the PANSS total score. SAPHRIS 10 mg twice daily showed no added benefit compared to 5 mg twice daily and was not significantly different from placebo.

An examination of population subgroups did not reveal any clear evidence of differential responsiveness on the basis of age, gender or race.

Maintenance of efficacy has been demonstrated in a placebo-controlled, double-blind, multicenter, flexible dose (5 mg or 10 mg twice daily based on tolerability) clinical trial with a randomized withdrawal design. A total of 700 patients entered open-label treatment with SAPHRIS for a period of 26 weeks. Of these, a total of 386 patients who met pre-specified criteria for continued stability (mean length of stabilization was 22 weeks) were randomized to a double-blind, placebo-controlled, randomized withdrawal phase. SAPHRIS was statistically superior to placebo in time to relapse or impending relapse defined as increase in PANSS ≥20% from baseline and a Clinical Global Impression–Severity of Illness (CGI-S) score ≥4 (at least 2 days within 1 week) or PANSS score ≥5 on "hostility" or "uncooperativeness" items and CGI-S score ≥4 (≥2 days within a week), or PANSS score ≥5 on any two of the following items: "unusual thought content," "conceptual disorganization," or "hallucinatory behavior" items, and CGI-S score ≥4 (≥2 days within 1 week) or investigator judgment of worsening symptoms or increased risk of violence to self (including suicide) or other persons. The Kaplan-Meier curves of the time to relapse or impending relapse during the double-blind, placebo-controlled, randomized withdrawal phase of this trial for SAPHRIS and placebo are shown in Figure 1.

Figure 1: Kaplan-Meier Estimation of Percent Relapse/Impending Relapse for SAPHRIS and placebo

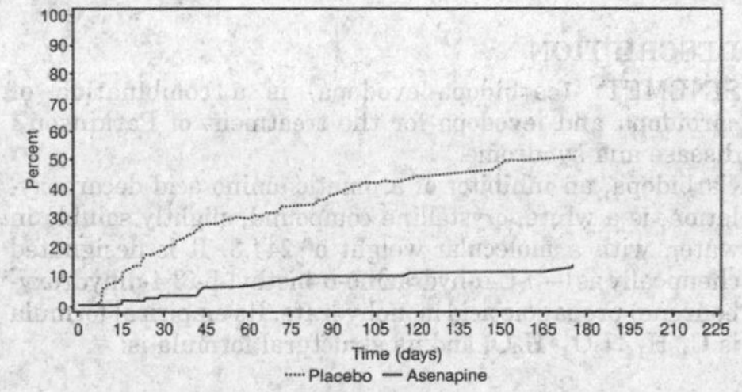

Time(days) represents the number of days from randomization to the first date of achieving relapse/impending relapse status.
The product limit estimators are based on the Kaplan-Meier distribution with censoring at last double-blind dose date.

14.2 Bipolar Disorder

Monotherapy: The efficacy of SAPHRIS in the treatment of acute mania was established in two similarly designed 3-week, randomized, double-blind, placebo-controlled, and active-controlled (olanzapine) trials of adult patients who met DSM-IV criteria for Bipolar I Disorder with an acute manic or mixed episode with or without psychotic features. The primary rating instrument used for assessing manic symptoms in these trials was the Young Mania Rating Scale (YMRS). Patients were also assessed on the Clinical Global Impression – Bipolar (CGI-BP) scale. In both trials, all patients randomized to SAPHRIS were initially administered 10 mg twice daily, and the dose could be adjusted within the dose range of 5 to 10 mg twice daily from Day 2 onward based on efficacy and tolerability. Ninety percent of patients remained on the 10-mg twice daily dose. SAPHRIS was statistically superior to placebo on the YMRS total score and the CGI-BP Severity of Illness score (mania) in both studies. An examination of subgroups did not reveal any clear evidence of differential responsiveness on the basis of age, gender or race.

Adjunctive Therapy: The efficacy of SAPHRIS as an adjunctive therapy in acute mania was established in a 12-week, placebo-controlled trial with a 3-week primary efficacy endpoint involving 326 patients with a manic or mixed episode of Bipolar I Disorder, with or without psychotic features, who were partially responsive to lithium or valproate monotherapy after at least 2 weeks of treatment. SAPHRIS was statistically superior to placebo in the reduction of manic symptoms (measured by the YMRS total score) as an adjunctive therapy to lithium or valproate monotherapy at week 3.

16 HOW SUPPLIED/STORAGE AND HANDLING

SAPHRIS (asenapine) sublingual tablets are supplied as:

5-mg Tablets
Round, white to off-white sublingual tablets, with "5" on one side.
Child-resistant packaging

Box of 60	6 blisters with 10 tablets	NDC 0052-0118-06

Hospital Unit Dose

Box of 100	10 blisters with 10 tablets	NDC 0052-0118-90

10-mg Tablets
Round, white to off-white sublingual tablets, with "10" on one side.
Child-resistant packaging

Box of 60	6 blisters with 10 tablets	NDC 0052-0119-06

Hospital Unit Dose

Box of 100	10 blisters with 10 tablets	NDC 0052-0119-90

5-mg Tablets, black cherry flavor
Round, white to off-white sublingual tablets, with "5" on one side within a circle.
Child-resistant packaging

Box of 60	6 blisters with 10 tablets	NDC 0052-2139-03

Hospital Unit Dose

Box of 100	10 blisters with 10 tablets	NDC 0052-2139-04

10-mg Tablets, black cherry flavor
Round, white to off-white sublingual tablets, with "10" on one side within a circle.
Child-resistant packaging

Box of 60	6 blisters with 10 tablets	NDC 0052-2142-03

Hospital Unit Dose

Box of 100	10 blisters with 10 tablets	NDC 0052-2142-04

Storage
Store at 15°-30°C (59°-86°F) [see USP Controlled Room Temperature].

17 PATIENT COUNSELING INFORMATION

17.1 Tablet Administration

IMPORTANT:
- **Do not remove tablet until ready to administer.**
- **Use dry hands when handling tablet.**

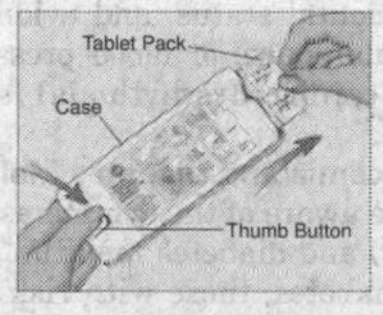

Step 1. Firmly press and hold thumb button, then pull out tablet pack.
Do not push tablet through tablet pack.
Do not cut or tear tablet pack.

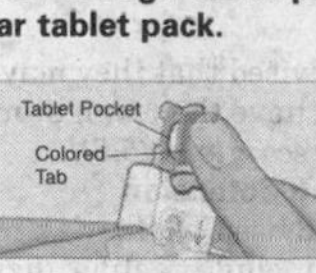

Step 2. Peel back colored tab.

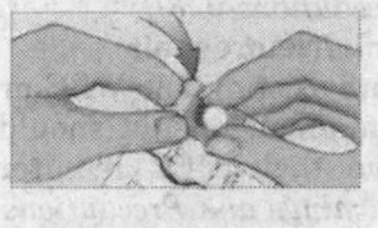

Step 3. Gently remove tablet.
Do not crush tablet.

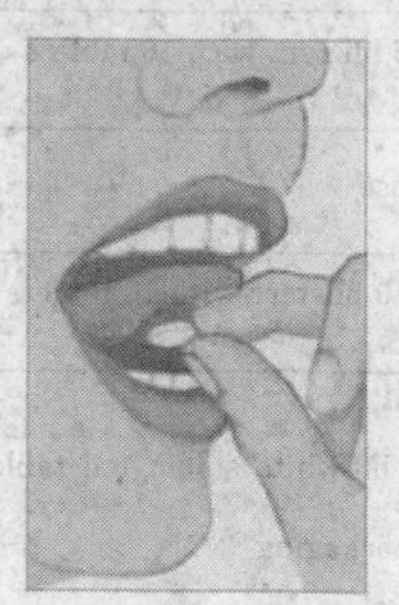

Step 4. Place tablet **under** tongue and allow it to dissolve completely.

Do not chew or swallow tablet.
Do not eat or drink for 10 minutes.

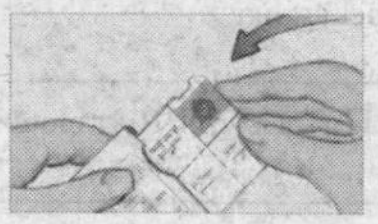

Step 5. Slide tablet pack into case until it clicks.
[see Drug Interactions (7) and Clinical Pharmacology (12.3)].

17.2 Increased Mortality in Elderly Patients with Dementia-Related Psychosis
Patients and caregivers should be advised that elderly patients with dementia-related psychoses treated with atypical antipsychotic drugs are at increased risk of death compared with placebo. SAPHRIS is not approved for elderly patients with dementia-related psychosis *[see Warnings and Precautions (5.1)]*.

17.3 Hypersensitivity Reactions
Patients should be informed of the signs and symptoms of a serious allergic reaction (e.g., difficulty breathing, itching, swelling of the face, tongue or throat, feeling lightheaded etc.). Patients should be instructed to seek immediate emergency assistance if they develop any of these signs and symptoms *[see Warnings and Precautions (5.7) and Adverse Reactions (6)]*.

17.4 Application Site Reactions
Inform patients that application site reactions including oral ulcers, blisters, peeling/sloughing and inflammation have been reported. Instruct patients to monitor for these reactions *[see Adverse Reactions (6.2)]*.

17.5 Neuroleptic Malignant Syndrome
Patients and caregivers should be counseled that a potentially fatal symptom complex sometimes referred to as Neuroleptic Malignant Syndrome (NMS) has been reported in association with administration of antipsychotic drugs. Signs and symptoms of NMS include hyperpyrexia, muscle rigidity, altered mental status, and evidence of autonomic instability (irregular pulse or blood pressure, tachycardia, diaphoresis, and cardiac dysrhythmia) *[see Warnings and Precautions (5.3)]*.

17.6 Hyperglycemia and Diabetes Mellitus
Patients should be aware of the symptoms of hyperglycemia (high blood sugar) and diabetes mellitus. Patients who are diagnosed with diabetes, those with risk factors for diabetes, or those that develop these symptoms during treatment should have their blood glucose monitored at the beginning of and periodically during treatment *[see Warnings and Precautions (5.5)]*.

17.7 Weight Gain
Patients should be advised that they may experience weight gain. Patients should have their weight monitored regularly *[see Warnings and Precautions (5.6)]*.

17.8 Orthostatic Hypotension
Patients should be advised of the risk of orthostatic hypotension (symptoms include feeling dizzy or lightheaded upon standing) especially early in treatment, and also at times of re-initiating treatment or increases in dose *[see Warnings and Precautions (5.8)]*.

17.9 Leukopenia/Neutropenia
Patients with a pre-existing low WBC or a history of drug induced leukopenia/neutropenia should be advised that they should have their CBC monitored while taking SAPHRIS *[see Warnings and Precautions (5.9)]*.

17.10 Interference with Cognitive and Motor Performance
Patients should be cautioned about performing activities requiring mental alertness, such as operating hazardous machinery or operating a motor vehicle, until they are reasonably certain that SAPHRIS therapy does not affect them adversely *[see Warnings and Precautions (5.13)]*.

17.11 Heat Exposure and Dehydration
Patients should be advised regarding appropriate care in avoiding overheating and dehydration *[see Warnings and Precautions (5.14)]*.

17.12 Concomitant Medication and Alcohol
Patients should be advised to inform their physicians if they are taking, or plan to take, any prescription or over-the-counter medications since there is a potential for interactions. Patients should be advised to avoid alcohol while taking SAPHRIS *[see Drug Interactions (7)]*.

17.13 Pregnancy and Nursing
Patients should be advised to notify their physician if they become pregnant or intend to become pregnant during therapy with SAPHRIS. Patients should be advised not to breast feed if they are taking SAPHRIS *[see Use in Special Populations (8.1, 8.3)]*.

Manufactured for: Merck Sharp & Dohme Corp., a subsidiary of
MERCK & CO., INC., Whitehouse Station, NJ 08889, USA
Manufactured by: Catalent UK Swindon Zydis Ltd., Blagrove, Swindon, Wiltshire, SN5 8RU, UK
U.S. Patent Nos. 5,763,476 and 7,741,358.

Revised: 03/2013
900274-ASP-TB-USPI.25
Shown in Product Identification Guide, page 309

SINEMET®
(carbidopa-levodopa)
Tablets ℞

DESCRIPTION
SINEMET® (carbidopa-levodopa) is a combination of carbidopa and levodopa for the treatment of Parkinson's disease and syndrome.
Carbidopa, an inhibitor of aromatic amino acid decarboxylation, is a white, crystalline compound, slightly soluble in water, with a molecular weight of 244.3. It is designated chemically as (—)-L-α-hydrazino-α-methyl-β-(3,4-dihydroxybenzene) propanoic acid monohydrate. Its empirical formula is $C_{10}H_{14}N_2O_4 \bullet H_2O$, and its structural formula is:

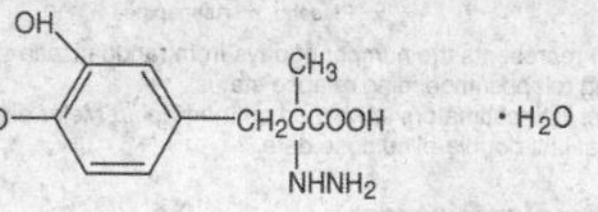

Tablet content is expressed in terms of anhydrous carbidopa which has a molecular weight of 226.3.
Levodopa, an aromatic amino acid, is a white, crystalline compound, slightly soluble in water, with a molecular weight of 197.2. It is designated chemically as (—)-L-α-amino-β-(3,4-dihydroxybenzene) propanoic acid. Its empirical formula is $C_9H_{11}NO_4$, and its structural formula is:

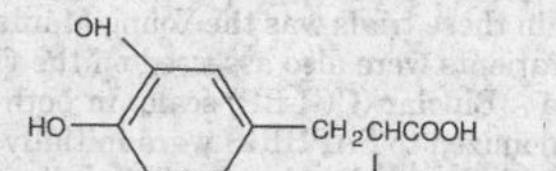

SINEMET is supplied as tablets in three strengths:
SINEMET 25-100, containing 25 mg of carbidopa and 100 mg of levodopa.
SINEMET 10-100, containing 10 mg of carbidopa and 100 mg of levodopa.
SINEMET 25-250, containing 25 mg of carbidopa and 250 mg of levodopa.
Inactive ingredients are hydroxypropyl cellulose, pregelatinized starch, crospovidone, microcrystalline cellulose, and magnesium stearate. SINEMET 10-100 and 25-250 Tablets also contain FD&C Blue #2/Indigo Carmine AL. SINEMET 25-100 Tablets also contain D&C Yellow #10 Lake.

CLINICAL PHARMACOLOGY
Mechanism of Action
Parkinson's disease is a progressive, neurodegenerative disorder of the extrapyramidal nervous system affecting the mobility and control of the skeletal muscular system. Its characteristic features include resting tremor, rigidity, and bradykinetic movements. Symptomatic treatments, such as levodopa therapies, may permit the patient better mobility. Current evidence indicates that symptoms of Parkinson's disease are related to depletion of dopamine in the corpus striatum. Administration of dopamine is ineffective in the treatment of Parkinson's disease apparently because it does not cross the blood-brain barrier. However, levodopa, the metabolic precursor of dopamine, does cross the blood-brain barrier, and presumably is converted to dopamine in the brain. This is thought to be the mechanism whereby levodopa relieves symptoms of Parkinson's disease.

Pharmacodynamics
When levodopa is administered orally, it is rapidly decarboxylated to dopamine in extracerebral tissues so that only a small portion of a given dose is transported unchanged to the central nervous system. For this reason, large doses of levodopa are required for adequate therapeutic effect, and these may often be accompanied by nausea and other adverse reactions, some of which are attributable to dopamine formed in extracerebral tissues.
Since levodopa competes with certain amino acids for transport across the gut wall, the absorption of levodopa may be impaired in some patients on a high protein diet.
Carbidopa inhibits decarboxylation of peripheral levodopa. It does not cross the blood-brain barrier and does not affect the metabolism of levodopa within the central nervous system.
The incidence of levodopa-induced nausea and vomiting is less with SINEMET than with levodopa. In many patients, this reduction in nausea and vomiting will permit more rapid dosage titration.
Since its decarboxylase inhibiting activity is limited to extracerebral tissues, administration of carbidopa with levodopa makes more levodopa available for transport to the brain.

Pharmacokinetics
Carbidopa reduces the amount of levodopa required to produce a given response by about 75% and, when administered with levodopa, increases both plasma levels and the plasma half-life of levodopa, and decreases plasma and urinary dopamine and homovanillic acid.
The plasma half-life of levodopa is about 50 minutes, without carbidopa. When carbidopa and levodopa are administered together, the half-life of levodopa is increased to about 1.5 hours. At steady state, the bioavailability of carbidopa from SINEMET tablets is approximately 99% relative to the concomitant administration of carbidopa and levodopa.
In clinical pharmacologic studies, simultaneous administration of carbidopa and levodopa produced greater urinary excretion of levodopa in proportion to the excretion of dopamine than administration of the two drugs at separate times.
Pyridoxine hydrochloride (vitamin B_6), in oral doses of 10 mg to 25 mg, may reverse the effects of levodopa by increasing the rate of aromatic amino acid decarboxylation. Carbidopa inhibits this action of pyridoxine; therefore, SINEMET can be given to patients receiving supplemental pyridoxine (vitamin B_6).

INDICATIONS AND USAGE
SINEMET is indicated in the treatment of the symptoms of idiopathic Parkinson's disease (paralysis agitans), postencephalitic parkinsonism, and symptomatic parkinsonism which may follow injury to the nervous system by carbon monoxide intoxication and/or manganese intoxication. SINEMET is indicated in these conditions to permit the administration of lower doses of levodopa with reduced nausea and vomiting, with more rapid dosage titration, with a somewhat smoother response, and with supplemental pyridoxine (vitamin B_6).
In some patients a somewhat smoother antiparkinsonian effect results from therapy with SINEMET than with levodopa. However, patients with markedly irregular ("on-off") responses to levodopa have not been shown to benefit from SINEMET.
Although the administration of carbidopa permits control of parkinsonism and Parkinson's disease with much lower doses of levodopa, there is no conclusive evidence at present that this is beneficial other than in reducing nausea and vomiting, permitting more rapid titration, and providing a somewhat smoother response to levodopa.
Certain patients who responded poorly to levodopa have improved when SINEMET was substituted. This is most likely due to decreased peripheral decarboxylation of levodopa which results from administration of carbidopa rather than to a primary effect of carbidopa on the nervous system. Carbidopa has not been shown to enhance the intrinsic efficacy of levodopa in parkinsonian syndromes.
In considering whether to give SINEMET to patients already on levodopa who have nausea and/or vomiting, the practitioner should be aware that, while many patients may be expected to improve, some do not. Since one cannot predict which patients are likely to improve, this can only be determined by a trial of therapy. It should be further noted that in controlled trials comparing SINEMET with levodopa, about half of the patients with nausea and/or vomiting on levodopa improved spontaneously despite being retained on the same dose of levodopa during the controlled portion of the trial.

CONTRAINDICATIONS

Nonselective monoamine oxidase (MAO) inhibitors are contraindicated for use with SINEMET. These inhibitors must be discontinued at least two weeks prior to initiating therapy with SINEMET. SINEMET may be administered concomitantly with the manufacturer's recommended dose of an MAO inhibitor with selectivity for MAO type B (e.g., selegiline HCl) (see PRECAUTIONS, Drug Interactions).

SINEMET is contraindicated in patients with known hypersensitivity to any component of this drug, and in patients with narrow-angle glaucoma.

Because levodopa may activate a malignant melanoma, SINEMET should not be used in patients with suspicious, undiagnosed skin lesions or a history of melanoma.

WARNINGS

When SINEMET is to be given to patients who are being treated with levodopa, levodopa must be discontinued at least twelve hours before therapy with SINEMET is started. In order to reduce adverse reactions, it is necessary to individualize therapy. See DOSAGE AND ADMINISTRATION section before initiating therapy.

The addition of carbidopa with levodopa in the form of SINEMET reduces the peripheral effects (nausea, vomiting) due to decarboxylation of levodopa; however, carbidopa does not decrease the adverse reactions due to the central effects of levodopa. Because carbidopa permits more levodopa to reach the brain and more dopamine to be formed, certain adverse CNS effects, e.g., dyskinesias (involuntary movements), may occur at lower dosages and sooner with SINEMET than with levodopa alone.

Levodopa alone, as well as SINEMET, is associated with dyskinesias. The occurrence of dyskinesias may require dosage reduction.

As with levodopa, SINEMET may cause mental disturbances. These reactions are thought to be due to increased brain dopamine following administration of levodopa. All patients should be observed carefully for the development of depression with concomitant suicidal tendencies. Patients with past or current psychoses should be treated with caution.

SINEMET should be administered cautiously to patients with severe cardiovascular or pulmonary disease, bronchial asthma, renal, hepatic or endocrine disease.

As with levodopa, care should be exercised in administering SINEMET to patients with a history of myocardial infarction who have residual atrial, nodal, or ventricular arrhythmias. In such patients, cardiac function should be monitored with particular care during the period of initial dosage adjustment, in a facility with provisions for intensive cardiac care.

As with levodopa, treatment with SINEMET may increase the possibility of upper gastrointestinal hemorrhage in patients with a history of peptic ulcer.

Neuroleptic Malignant Syndrome (NMS)

Sporadic cases of a symptom complex resembling NMS have been reported in association with dose reductions or withdrawal of therapy with SINEMET. Therefore, patients should be observed carefully when the dosage of SINEMET is reduced abruptly or discontinued, especially if the patient is receiving neuroleptics.

NMS is an uncommon but life-threatening syndrome characterized by fever or hyperthermia. Neurological findings, including muscle rigidity, involuntary movements, altered consciousness, mental status changes; other disturbances, such as autonomic dysfunction, tachycardia, tachypnea, sweating, hyper- or hypotension; laboratory findings, such as creatine phosphokinase elevation, leukocytosis, myoglobinuria, and increased serum myoglobin have been reported.

The early diagnosis of this condition is important for the appropriate management of these patients. Considering NMS as a possible diagnosis and ruling out other acute illnesses (e.g., pneumonia, systemic infection, etc.) is essential. This may be especially complex if the clinical presentation includes both serious medical illness and untreated or inadequately treated extrapyramidal signs and symptoms (EPS). Other important considerations in the differential diagnosis include central anticholinergic toxicity, heat stroke, drug fever, and primary central nervous system (CNS) pathology.

The management of NMS should include: 1) intensive symptomatic treatment and medical monitoring and 2) treatment of any concomitant serious medical problems for which specific treatments are available. Dopamine agonists, such as bromocriptine, and muscle relaxants, such as dantrolene, are often used in the treatment of NMS, however, their effectiveness has not been demonstrated in controlled studies.

PRECAUTIONS

General

As with levodopa, periodic evaluations of hepatic, hematopoietic, cardiovascular, and renal function are recommended during extended therapy.

Patients with chronic wide-angle glaucoma may be treated cautiously with SINEMET provided the intraocular pressure is well-controlled and the patient is monitored carefully for changes in intraocular pressure during therapy.

Dopaminergic agents, including levodopa, may be associated with somnolence and very rarely episodes of sudden onset of sleep. In some cases, these episodes may occur without awareness or warning during daily activities. Patients must be informed of this and advised to exercise caution while driving or operating machines while being treated with dopaminergic agents, including levodopa. Patients who have experienced somnolence and/or an episode of sudden sleep onset must refrain from driving or operating machines (see Information for Patients).

Melanoma

Epidemiological studies have shown that patients with Parkinson's disease have a higher risk (2- to approximately 6-fold higher) of developing melanoma than the general population. Whether the increased risk observed was due to Parkinson's disease or other factors, such as drugs used to treat Parkinson's disease, is unclear.

For the reasons stated above, patients and providers are advised to monitor for melanomas frequently and on a regular basis when using SINEMET for any indication. Ideally, periodic skin examinations should be performed by appropriately qualified individuals (e.g., dermatologists).

Information for Patients

The patient should be informed that SINEMET is an immediate-release formulation of carbidopa-levodopa that is designed to begin release of ingredients within 30 minutes. It is important that SINEMET be taken at regular intervals according to the schedule outlined by the physician. The patient should be cautioned not to change the prescribed dosage regimen and not to add any additional antiparkinson medications, including other carbidopa-levodopa preparations, without first consulting the physician.

Patients should be advised that sometimes a 'wearing-off' effect may occur at the end of the dosing interval. The physician should be notified if such response poses a problem to lifestyle.

Patients should be advised that occasionally, dark color (red, brown, or black) may appear in saliva, urine, or sweat after ingestion of SINEMET. Although the color appears to be clinically insignificant, garments may become discolored.

The patient should be advised that a change in dict to foods that are high in protein may delay the absorption of levodopa and may reduce the amount taken up in the circulation. Excessive acidity also delays stomach emptying, thus delaying the absorption of levodopa. Iron salts (such as in multivitamin tablets) may also reduce the amount of levodopa available to the body. The above factors may reduce the clinical effectiveness of the levodopa or carbidopa-levodopa therapy.

Patients should be alerted to the possibility of sudden onset of sleep during daily activities, in some cases without awareness or warning signs, when they are taking dopaminergic agents, including levodopa. Patients should be advised to exercise caution while driving or operating machinery and that if they have experienced somnolence and/or sudden sleep onset, they must refrain from these activities. (See PRECAUTIONS, General.)

There have been reports of patients experiencing intense urges to gamble, increased sexual urges, and other intense urges, and the inability to control these urges while taking one or more of the medications that increase central dopaminergic tone and that are generally used for the treatment of Parkinson's disease, including SINEMET. Although it is not proven that the medications caused these events, these urges were reported to have stopped in some cases when the dose was reduced or the medication was stopped. Prescribers should ask patients about the development of new or increased gambling urges, sexual urges or other urges while being treated with SINEMET. Patients should inform their physician if they experience new or increased gambling urges, increased sexual urges, or other intense urges while taking SINEMET. Physicians should consider dose reduction or stopping the medication if a patient develops such urges while taking SINEMET.

NOTE: The suggested advice to patients being treated with SINEMET is intended to aid in the safe and effective use of this medication. It is not a disclosure of all possible adverse or intended effects.

Laboratory Tests

Abnormalities in laboratory tests may include elevations of liver function tests such as alkaline phosphatase, SGOT (AST), SGPT (ALT), lactic dehydrogenase, and bilirubin. Abnormalities in blood urea nitrogen and positive Coombs test have also been reported. Commonly, levels of blood urea nitrogen, creatinine, and uric acid are lower during administration of SINEMET than with levodopa.

SINEMET may cause a false-positive reaction for urinary ketone bodies when a test tape is used for determination of ketonuria. This reaction will not be altered by boiling the urine specimen. False-negative tests may result with the use of glucose-oxidase methods of testing for glucosuria.

Cases of falsely diagnosed pheochromocytoma in patients on carbidopa-levodopa therapy have been reported very rarely. Caution should be exercised when interpreting the plasma and urine levels of catecholamines and their metabolites in patients on levodopa or carbidopa-levodopa therapy.

Drug Interactions

Caution should be exercised when the following drugs are administered concomitantly with SINEMET.

Symptomatic postural hypotension occurred when SINEMET was added to the treatment of a patient receiving antihypertensive drugs. Therefore, when therapy with SINEMET is started, dosage adjustment of the antihypertensive drug may be required.

For patients receiving MAO inhibitors (Type A or B), see CONTRAINDICATIONS. Concomitant therapy with selegiline and carbidopa-levodopa may be associated with severe orthostatic hypotension not attributable to carbidopa-levodopa alone (see CONTRAINDICATIONS).

There have been rare reports of adverse reactions, including hypertension and dyskinesia, resulting from the concomitant use of tricyclic antidepressants and SINEMET.

Dopamine D_2 receptor antagonists (e.g., phenothiazines, butyrophenones, risperidone) and isoniazid may reduce the therapeutic effects of levodopa. In addition, the beneficial effects of levodopa in Parkinson's disease have been reported to be reversed by phenytoin and papaverine. Patients taking these drugs with SINEMET should be carefully observed for loss of therapeutic response.

Iron salts may reduce the bioavailability of levodopa and carbidopa. The clinical relevance is unclear.

Although metoclopramide may increase the bioavailability of levodopa by increasing gastric emptying, metoclopramide may also adversely affect disease control by its dopamine receptor antagonistic properties.

Carcinogenesis, Mutagenesis, Impairment of Fertility

In a two-year bioassay of SINEMET, no evidence of carcinogenicity was found in rats receiving doses of approximately two times the maximum daily human dose of carbidopa and four times the maximum daily human dose of levodopa.

In reproduction studies with SINEMET, no effects on fertility were found in rats receiving doses of approximately two times the maximum daily human dose of carbidopa and four times the maximum daily human dose of levodopa.

Pregnancy

Pregnancy Category C. No teratogenic effects were observed in a study in mice receiving up to 20 times the maximum recommended human dose of SINEMET. There was a decrease in the number of live pups delivered by rats receiving approximately two times the maximum recommended human dose of carbidopa and approximately five times the maximum recommended human dose of levodopa during organogenesis. SINEMET caused both visceral and skeletal malformations in rabbits at all doses and ratios of carbidopa/levodopa tested, which ranged from 10 times/5 times the maximum recommended human dose of carbidopa/levodopa to 20 times/10 times the maximum recommended human dose of carbidopa/levodopa.

There are no adequate or well-controlled studies in pregnant women. It has been reported from individual cases that levodopa crosses the human placental barrier, enters the fetus, and is metabolized. Carbidopa concentrations in fetal tissue appeared to be minimal. Use of SINEMET in women of childbearing potential requires that the anticipated benefits of the drug be weighed against possible hazards to mother and child.

Nursing Mothers

In a study of one nursing mother with Parkinson's disease, excretion of levodopa in human breast milk was reported. Therefore, caution should be exercised when SINEMET is administered to a nursing woman.

Pediatric Use

Safety and effectiveness in pediatric patients have not been established. Use of the drug in patients below the age of 18 is not recommended.

ADVERSE REACTIONS

The most common adverse reactions reported with SINEMET have included dyskinesias, such as choreiform, dystonic, and other involuntary movements, and nausea.

The following other adverse reactions have been reported with SINEMET:

Body as a Whole

Chest pain, asthenia.

Cardiovascular

Cardiac irregularities, hypotension, orthostatic effects including orthostatic hypotension, hypertension, syncope, phlebitis, palpitation.

Gastrointestinal

Dark saliva, gastrointestinal bleeding, development of duodenal ulcer, anorexia, vomiting, diarrhea, constipation, dyspepsia, dry mouth, taste alterations.

Hematologic

Agranulocytosis, hemolytic and non-hemolytic anemia, thrombocytopenia, leukopenia.

Hypersensitivity
Angioedema, urticaria, pruritus, Henoch-Schonlein purpura, bullous lesions (including pemphigus-like reactions).
Musculoskeletal
Back pain, shoulder pain, muscle cramps.
Nervous System/Psychiatric
Psychotic episodes including delusions, hallucinations, and paranoid ideation, neuroleptic malignant syndrome (NMS, see WARNINGS), bradykinetic episodes ("on-off" phenomenon), confusion, agitation, dizziness, somnolence, dream abnormalities including nightmares, insomnia, paresthesia, headache, depression with or without development of suicidal tendencies, dementia, pathological gambling, increased libido including hypersexuality, impulse control symptoms. Convulsions also have occurred; however, a causal relationship with SINEMET has not been established.
Respiratory
Dyspnea, upper respiratory infection.
Skin
Rash, increased sweating, alopecia, dark sweat.
Urogenital
Urinary tract infection, urinary frequency, dark urine.
Laboratory Tests
Decreased hemoglobin and hematocrit; abnormalities in alkaline phosphatase, SGOT (AST), SGPT (ALT), lactic dehydrogenase, bilirubin, blood urea nitrogen (BUN), Coombs test; elevated serum glucose; white blood cells, bacteria, and blood in the urine.
Other adverse reactions that have been reported with levodopa alone and with various carbidopa-levodopa formulations, and may occur with SINEMET are:
Body as a Whole
Abdominal pain and distress, fatigue.
Cardiovascular
Myocardial infarction.
Gastrointestinal
Gastrointestinal pain, dysphagia, sialorrhea, flatulence, bruxism, burning sensation of the tongue, heartburn, hiccups.
Metabolic
Edema, weight gain, weight loss.
Musculoskeletal
Leg pain.
Nervous System/Psychiatric
Ataxia, extrapyramidal disorder, falling, anxiety, gait abnormalities, nervousness, decreased mental acuity, memory impairment, disorientation, euphoria, blepharospasm (which may be taken as an early sign of excess dosage; consideration of dosage reduction may be made at this time), trismus, increased tremor, numbness, muscle twitching, activation of latent Horner's syndrome, peripheral neuropathy.
Respiratory
Pharyngeal pain, cough.
Skin
Malignant melanoma (see also CONTRAINDICATIONS), flushing.
Special Senses
Oculogyric crises, diplopia, blurred vision, dilated pupils.
Urogenital
Urinary retention, urinary incontinence, priapism.
Miscellaneous
Bizarre breathing patterns, faintness, hoarseness, malaise, hot flashes, sense of stimulation.
Laboratory Tests
Decreased white blood cell count and serum potassium; increased serum creatinine and uric acid; protein and glucose in urine.

OVERDOSAGE

Management of acute overdosage with SINEMET is the same as management of acute overdosage with levodopa. Pyridoxine is not effective in reversing the actions of SINEMET.
General supportive measures should be employed, along with immediate gastric lavage. Intravenous fluids should be administered judiciously and an adequate airway maintained. Electrocardiographic monitoring should be instituted and the patient carefully observed for the development of arrhythmias; if required, appropriate antiarrhythmic therapy should be given. The possibility that the patient may have taken other drugs as well as SINEMET should be taken into consideration. To date, no experience has been reported with dialysis; hence, its value in overdosage is not known.
Based on studies in which high doses of levodopa and/or carbidopa were administered, a significant proportion of rats and mice given single oral doses of levodopa of approximately 1500-2000 mg/kg are expected to die. A significant proportion of infant rats of both sexes are expected to die at a dose of 800 mg/kg. A significant proportion of rats are expected to die after treatment with similar doses of carbidopa. The addition of carbidopa in a 1:10 ratio with levodopa increases the dose at which a significant proportion of mice are expected to die to 3360 mg/kg.

DOSAGE AND ADMINISTRATION

The optimum daily dosage of SINEMET must be determined by careful titration in each patient. SINEMET tablets are available in a 1:4 ratio of carbidopa to levodopa (SINEMET 25-100) as well as 1:10 ratio (SINEMET 25-250 and SINEMET 10-100). Tablets of the two ratios may be given separately or combined as needed to provide the optimum dosage.
Studies show that peripheral dopa decarboxylase is saturated by carbidopa at approximately 70 to 100 mg a day. Patients receiving less than this amount of carbidopa are more likely to experience nausea and vomiting.

Usual Initial Dosage

Dosage is best initiated with one tablet of SINEMET 25-100 three times a day. This dosage schedule provides 75 mg of carbidopa per day. Dosage may be increased by one tablet every day or every other day, as necessary, until a dosage of eight tablets of SINEMET 25-100 a day is reached.
If SINEMET 10-100 is used, dosage may be initiated with one tablet three or four times a day. However, this will not provide an adequate amount of carbidopa for many patients. Dosage may be increased by one tablet every day or every other day until a total of eight tablets (2 tablets q.i.d.) is reached.

How to Transfer Patients from Levodopa

Levodopa must be discontinued at least twelve hours before starting SINEMET. A daily dosage of SINEMET should be chosen that will provide approximately 25% of the previous levodopa dosage. Patients who are taking less than 1500 mg of levodopa a day should be started on one tablet of SINEMET 25-100 three or four times a day. The suggested starting dosage for most patients taking more than 1500 mg of levodopa is one tablet of SINEMET 25-250 three or four times a day.

Maintenance

Therapy should be individualized and adjusted according to the desired therapeutic response. At least 70 to 100 mg of carbidopa per day should be provided. When a greater proportion of carbidopa is required, one tablet of SINEMET 25-100 may be substituted for each tablet of SINEMET 10-100. When more levodopa is required, SINEMET 25-250 should be substituted for SINEMET 25-100 or SINEMET 10-100. If necessary, the dosage of carbidopa/levodopa 25-250 may be increased by one-half or one tablet every day or every other day to a maximum of eight tablets a day. Experience with total daily dosages of carbidopa greater than 200 mg is limited.
Because both therapeutic and adverse responses occur more rapidly with SINEMET than with levodopa alone, patients should be monitored closely during the dose adjustment period. Specifically, involuntary movements will occur more rapidly with SINEMET than with levodopa. The occurrence of involuntary movements may require dosage reduction. Blepharospasm may be a useful early sign of excess dosage in some patients.

Addition of Other Antiparkinsonian Medications

Standard drugs for Parkinson's disease, other than levodopa without a decarboxylase inhibitor, may be used concomitantly while SINEMET is being administered, although dosage adjustments may be required.

Interruption of Therapy

Sporadic cases of a symptom complex resembling Neuroleptic Malignant Syndrome (NMS) have been associated with dose reductions and withdrawal of SINEMET. Patients should be observed carefully if abrupt reduction or discontinuation of SINEMET is required, especially if the patient is receiving neuroleptics. (See WARNINGS.)
If general anesthesia is required, SINEMET may be continued as long as the patient is permitted to take fluids and medication by mouth. If therapy is interrupted temporarily, the patient should be observed for symptoms resembling NMS, and the usual daily dosage may be administered as soon as the patient is able to take oral medication.

HOW SUPPLIED

No. 3916A — SINEMET 25-100 Tablets are yellow, round, uncoated tablets that are coded "650" on one side and plain on the other. They are supplied as follows:
NDC 0006-3916-68 bottles of 100.
No. 3915 — SINEMET 10-100 Tablets are light dapple-blue, round, uncoated tablets that are coded "647" on one side and plain on the other. They are supplied as follows:
NDC 0006-3915-68 bottles of 100.
No. 3917 — SINEMET 25-250 Tablets are light dapple-blue, round, uncoated tablets that are coded "654" on one side and plain on the other. They are supplied as follows:
NDC 0006-3917-68 bottles of 100.

Storage and Handling

Store at 25°C (77°F), excursions permitted to 15-30°C (59-86°F) [see USP Controlled Room Temperature]. Store in a tightly closed container, protected from light and moisture. Dispense in a tightly closed, light-resistant container.
Rx Only
Manufactured for:
Merck Sharp & Dohme Corp., a subsidiary of **MERCK & CO., INC.**, Whitehouse Station, NJ 08889, USA
By:
Mylan Pharmaceuticals, Inc.
Morgantown, WV 26505, USA
Issued February 2011
9998301

SINEMET® CR SUSTAINED-RELEASE TABLETS ℞

(carbidopa-levodopa)

DESCRIPTION

SINEMET® CR (carbidopa-levodopa) is a sustained-release combination of carbidopa and levodopa for the treatment of Parkinson's disease and syndrome.
Carbidopa, an inhibitor of aromatic amino acid decarboxylation, is a white, crystalline compound, slightly soluble in water, with a molecular weight of 244.3. It is designated chemically as (—)-L-α-hydrazino-α-methyl-β-(3,4-dihydroxybenzene) propanoic acid monohydrate. Its empirical formula is $C_{10}H_{14}N_2O_4 \bullet H_2O$, and its structural formula is:

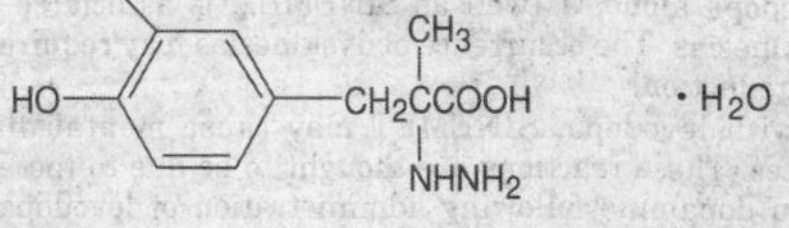

Tablet content is expressed in terms of anhydrous carbidopa, which has a molecular weight of 226.3.
Levodopa, an aromatic amino acid, is a white, crystalline compound, slightly soluble in water, with a molecular weight of 197.2. It is designated chemically as (—)-L-α-amino-β-(3,4-dihydroxybenzene) propanoic acid. Its empirical formula is $C_9H_{11}NO_4$, and its structural formula is:

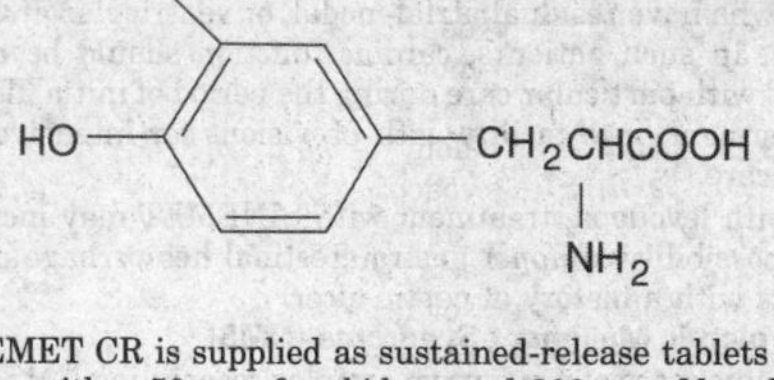

SINEMET CR is supplied as sustained-release tablets containing either 50 mg of carbidopa and 200 mg of levodopa, or 25 mg of carbidopa and 100 mg of levodopa. Inactive ingredients are hydroxypropyl cellulose, magnesium stearate, and hypromellose. SINEMET CR 25-100 and SINEMET CR 50-200 also contain FD&C Blue #2/Indigo Carmine AL and FD&C Red #40/Allura Red AC AL.
The 50-200 tablet is supplied as an oval, compressed tablet that is dappled-purple in color and is coded "521" on one side and plain on the other. The 25-100 tablet is supplied as an oval, compressed tablet that is dappled-purple in color and is coded "601" on one side and plain on the other. The SINEMET CR tablet is a polymeric-based drug delivery system that controls the release of carbidopa and levodopa as it slowly erodes. SINEMET CR 25-100 is available to facilitate titration when 100 mg steps are required.

CLINICAL PHARMACOLOGY

Mechanism of Action

Parkinson's disease is a progressive, neurodegenerative disorder of the extrapyramidal nervous system affecting the mobility and control of the skeletal muscular system. Its characteristic features include resting tremor, rigidity, and bradykinetic movements. Symptomatic treatments, such as levodopa therapies, may permit the patient better mobility. Current evidence indicates that symptoms of Parkinson's disease are related to depletion of dopamine in the corpus striatum. Administration of dopamine is ineffective in the treatment of Parkinson's disease apparently because it does not cross the blood-brain barrier. However, levodopa, the metabolic precursor of dopamine, does cross the blood-brain barrier, and presumably is converted to dopamine in the brain. This is thought to be the mechanism whereby levodopa relieves symptoms of Parkinson's disease.

Pharmacodynamics

When levodopa is administered orally, it is rapidly decarboxylated to dopamine in extracerebral tissues so that only a small portion of a given dose is transported unchanged to the central nervous system. For this reason, large doses of levodopa are required for adequate therapeutic effect, and these may often be accompanied by nausea and other adverse reactions, some of which are attributable to dopamine formed in extracerebral tissues.

Since levodopa competes with certain amino acids for transport across the gut wall, the absorption of levodopa may be impaired in some patients on a high protein diet.

Carbidopa inhibits decarboxylation of peripheral levodopa. It does not cross the blood-brain barrier and does not affect the metabolism of levodopa within the central nervous system.

Since its decarboxylase inhibiting activity is limited to extracerebral tissues, administration of carbidopa with levodopa makes more levodopa available for transport to the brain.

Patients treated with levodopa therapy for Parkinson's disease may develop motor fluctuations characterized by end-of-dose failure, peak dose dyskinesia, and akinesia. The advanced form of motor fluctuations ('on-off' phenomenon) is characterized by unpredictable swings from mobility to immobility. Although the causes of the motor fluctuations are not completely understood, in some patients they may be attenuated by treatment regimens that produce steady plasma levels of levodopa.

SINEMET CR contains either 50 mg of carbidopa and 200 mg of levodopa, or 25 mg of carbidopa and 100 mg of levodopa in a sustained-release dosage form designed to release these ingredients over a 4- to 6-hour period. With SINEMET CR there is less variation in plasma levodopa levels than with SINEMET® (carbidopa-levodopa) immediate release tablets, the conventional formulation. *However, SINEMET CR is less systemically bioavailable than SINEMET and may require increased daily doses to achieve the same level of symptomatic relief as provided by SINEMET.*

In clinical trials, patients with moderate to severe motor fluctuations who received SINEMET CR *did not experience quantitatively significant reductions* in 'off' time when compared to SINEMET. However, global ratings of improvement as assessed by both patient and physician were better during therapy with SINEMET CR than with SINEMET. In patients without motor fluctuations, SINEMET CR, under controlled conditions, provided the same therapeutic benefit with less frequent dosing when compared to SINEMET.

Pharmacokinetics

Carbidopa reduces the amount of levodopa required to produce a given response by about 75% and, when administered with levodopa, increases both plasma levels and the plasma half-life of levodopa, and decreases plasma and urinary dopamine and homovanillic acid.

Elimination half-life of levodopa in the presence of carbidopa is about 1.5 hours. Following SINEMET CR, the apparent half-life of levodopa may be prolonged because of continuous absorption.

In healthy elderly subjects (56-67 years old) the mean time-to-peak concentration of levodopa after a single dose of SINEMET CR 50-200 was about 2 hours as compared to 0.5 hours after standard SINEMET. The maximum concentration of levodopa after a single dose of SINEMET CR was about 35% of the standard SINEMET (1151 vs. 3256 ng/mL). The extent of availability of levodopa from SINEMET CR was about 70-75% relative to intravenous levodopa or standard SINEMET in the elderly. The absolute bioavailability of levodopa from SINEMET CR (relative to I.V.) in young subjects was shown to be only about 44%. The extent of availability and the peak concentrations of levodopa were comparable in the elderly after a single dose and at steady state after t.i.d. administration of SINEMET CR 50-200. In elderly subjects, the average trough levels of levodopa at steady state after the CR tablet were about 2-fold higher than after the standard SINEMET (163 vs. 74 ng/mL).

In these studies, using similar total daily doses of levodopa, plasma levodopa concentrations with SINEMET CR fluctuated in a narrower range than with SINEMET. Because the bioavailability of levodopa from SINEMET CR relative to SINEMET is approximately 70-75%, the daily dosage of levodopa necessary to produce a given clinical response with the sustained-release formulation will usually be higher.

The extent of availability and peak concentrations of levodopa after a single dose of SINEMET CR 50-200 increased by about 50% and 25%, respectively, when administered with food.

At steady state, the bioavailability of carbidopa from SINEMET Tablets is approximately 99% relative to the concomitant administration of carbidopa and levodopa. At steady state, carbidopa bioavailability from SINEMET CR 50-200 is approximately 58% relative to that from SINEMET.

Pyridoxine hydrochloride (vitamin B_6), in oral doses of 10 mg to 25 mg, may reverse the effects of levodopa by increasing the rate of aromatic amino acid decarboxylation. Carbidopa inhibits this action of pyridoxine.

INDICATIONS AND USAGE

SINEMET CR is indicated in the treatment of the symptoms of idiopathic Parkinson's disease (paralysis agitans), post-encephalitic parkinsonism, and symptomatic parkinsonism which may follow injury to the nervous system by carbon monoxide intoxication and/or manganese intoxication.

CONTRAINDICATIONS

Nonselective MAO inhibitors are contraindicated for use with SINEMET CR. These inhibitors must be discontinued at least two weeks prior to initiating therapy with SINEMET CR. SINEMET CR may be administered concomitantly with the manufacturer's recommended dose of an MAO inhibitor with selectivity for MAO type B (e.g., selegiline HCl) (see PRECAUTIONS, Drug Interactions).

SINEMET CR is contraindicated in patients with known hypersensitivity to any component of this drug, and in patients with narrow-angle glaucoma.

Because levodopa may activate a malignant melanoma, SINEMET CR should not be used in patients with suspicious, undiagnosed skin lesions or a history of melanoma.

WARNINGS

When patients are receiving levodopa without a decarboxylase inhibitor, levodopa must be discontinued at least twelve hours before SINEMET CR is started. In order to reduce adverse reactions, it is necessary to individualize therapy. SINEMET CR should be substituted at a dosage that will provide approximately 25% of the previous levodopa dosage (see DOSAGE AND ADMINISTRATION).

Carbidopa does not decrease adverse reactions due to central effects of levodopa. By permitting more levodopa to reach the brain, particularly when nausea and vomiting is not a dose-limiting factor, certain adverse CNS effects, e.g., dyskinesias, will occur at lower dosages and sooner during therapy with SINEMET CR than with levodopa alone.

Patients receiving SINEMET CR may develop increased dyskinesias compared to SINEMET. Dyskinesias are a common side effect of carbidopa-levodopa treatment. The occurrence of dyskinesias may require dosage reduction.

As with levodopa, SINEMET CR may cause mental disturbances. These reactions are thought to be due to increased brain dopamine following administration of levodopa. All patients should be observed carefully for the development of depression with concomitant suicidal tendencies. Patients with past or current psychoses should be treated with caution.

SINEMET CR should be administered cautiously to patients with severe cardiovascular or pulmonary disease, bronchial asthma, renal, hepatic or endocrine disease.

As with levodopa, care should be exercised in administering SINEMET CR to patients with a history of myocardial infarction who have residual atrial, nodal, or ventricular arrhythmias. In such patients, cardiac function should be monitored with particular care during the period of initial dosage adjustment, in a facility with provisions for intensive cardiac care.

As with levodopa, treatment with SINEMET CR may increase the possibility of upper gastrointestinal hemorrhage in patients with a history of peptic ulcer.

Neuroleptic Malignant Syndrome (NMS)

Sporadic cases of a symptom complex resembling NMS have been reported in association with dose reductions or withdrawal of SINEMET and SINEMET CR.

Therefore, patients should be observed carefully when the dosage of SINEMET CR is reduced abruptly or discontinued, especially if the patient is receiving neuroleptics.

NMS is an uncommon but life-threatening syndrome characterized by fever or hyperthermia. Neurological findings, including muscle rigidity, involuntary movements, altered consciousness, mental status changes; other disturbances, such as autonomic dysfunction, tachycardia, tachypnea, sweating, hyper- or hypotension; laboratory findings, such as creatine phosphokinase elevation, leukocytosis, myoglobinuria, and increased serum myoglobin have been reported.

The early diagnosis of this condition is important for the appropriate management of these patients. Considering NMS as a possible diagnosis and ruling out other acute illnesses (e.g., pneumonia, systemic infection, etc.) is essential. This may be especially complex if the clinical presentation includes both serious medical illness and untreated or inadequately treated extrapyramidal signs and symptoms (EPS). Other important considerations in the differential diagnosis include central anticholinergic toxicity, heat stroke, drug fever, and primary central nervous system (CNS) pathology.

The management of NMS should include: 1) intensive symptomatic treatment and medical monitoring and 2) treatment of any concomitant serious medical problems for which specific treatments are available. Dopamine agonists, such as bromocriptine, and muscle relaxants, such as dantrolene, are often used in the treatment of NMS; however, their effectiveness has not been demonstrated in controlled studies.

PRECAUTIONS

General

As with levodopa, periodic evaluations of hepatic, hematopoietic, cardiovascular, and renal function are recommended during extended therapy.

Patients with chronic wide-angle glaucoma may be treated cautiously with SINEMET CR provided the intraocular pressure is well-controlled and the patient is monitored carefully for changes in intraocular pressure during therapy.

Dopaminergic agents, including levodopa, may be associated with somnolence and very rarely episodes of sudden onset of sleep. In some cases, these episodes may occur without awareness or warning during daily activities. Patients must be informed of this and advised to exercise caution while driving or operating machines while being treated with dopaminergic agents, including levodopa. Patients who have experienced somnolence and/or an episode of sudden sleep onset must refrain from driving or operating machines (see Information for Patients).

Melanoma

Epidemiological studies have shown that patients with Parkinson's disease have a higher risk (2- to approximately 6-fold higher) of developing melanoma than the general population. Whether the increased risk observed was due to Parkinson's disease or other factors, such as drugs used to treat Parkinson's disease, is unclear.

For the reasons stated above, patients and providers are advised to monitor for melanomas frequently and on a regular basis when using SINEMET CR for any indication. Ideally, periodic skin examinations should be performed by appropriately qualified individuals (e.g., dermatologists).

Information for Patients

The patient should be informed that SINEMET CR is a sustained-release formulation of carbidopa-levodopa which releases these ingredients over a 4- to 6-hour period. It is important that SINEMET CR be taken at regular intervals according to the schedule outlined by the physician. The patient should be cautioned not to change the prescribed dosage regimen and not to add any additional antiparkinson medications, including other carbidopa-levodopa preparations, without first consulting the physician.

If abnormal involuntary movements appear or get worse during treatment with SINEMET CR, the physician should be notified, as dosage adjustment may be necessary.

Patients should be advised that sometimes the onset of effect of the first morning dose of SINEMET CR may be delayed for up to 1 hour compared with the response usually obtained from the first morning dose of SINEMET. The physician should be notified if such delayed responses pose a problem in treatment.

Patients should be advised that, occasionally, dark color (red, brown, or black) may appear in saliva, urine, or sweat after ingestion of SINEMET CR. Although the color appears to be clinically insignificant, garments may become discolored.

The patient should be informed that a change in diet to foods that are high in protein may delay the absorption of levodopa and may reduce the amount taken up in the circulation. Excessive acidity also delays stomach emptying, thus delaying the absorption of levodopa. Iron salts (such as in multivitamin tablets) may also reduce the amount of levodopa available to the body. The above factors may reduce the clinical effectiveness of the levodopa or carbidopa-levodopa therapy.

Patients must be advised that the whole or half tablet should be swallowed without chewing or crushing.

Patients should be alerted to the possibility of sudden onset of sleep during daily activities, in some cases without awareness or warning signs, when they are taking dopaminergic agents, including levodopa. Patients should be advised to exercise caution while driving or operating machinery and that if they have experienced somnolence and/or sudden sleep onset, they must refrain from these activities. (See PRECAUTIONS, General.)

There have been reports of patients experiencing intense urges to gamble, increased sexual urges, and other intense urges, and the inability to control these urges while taking one or more of the medications that increase central dopaminergic tone and that are generally used for the treatment of Parkinson's disease, including SINEMET CR. Although it is not proven that the medications caused these events, these urges were reported to have stopped in some cases when the dose was reduced or the medication was stopped. Prescribers should ask patients about the development of new or increased gambling urges, sexual urges or other urges while being treated with SINEMET CR. Patients should inform their physician if they experience new or increased gambling urges, increased sexual urges, or other intense urges while taking SINEMET CR. Physicians should consider dose reduction or stopping the medication if a patient develops such urges while taking SINEMET CR.

NOTE: The suggested advice to patients being treated with SINEMET CR is intended to aid in the safe and effective use of this medication. It is not a disclosure of all possible adverse or intended effects.

Laboratory Tests

Abnormalities in laboratory tests may include elevations of liver function tests such as alkaline phosphatase, SGOT

(AST), SGPT (ALT), lactic dehydrogenase, and bilirubin. Abnormalities in blood urea nitrogen and positive Coombs test have also been reported. Commonly, levels of blood urea nitrogen, creatinine, and uric acid are lower during administration of carbidopa-levodopa preparations than with levodopa.
Carbidopa-levodopa preparations, such as SINEMET and SINEMET CR, may cause a false-positive reaction for urinary ketone bodies when a test tape is used for determination of ketonuria. This reaction will not be altered by boiling the urine specimen. False-negative tests may result with the use of glucose-oxidase methods of testing for glucosuria.
Cases of falsely diagnosed pheochromocytoma in patients on carbidopa-levodopa therapy have been reported very rarely. Caution should be exercised when interpreting the plasma and urine levels of catecholamines and their metabolites in patients on levodopa or carbidopa-levodopa therapy.

Drug Interactions

Caution should be exercised when the following drugs are administered concomitantly with SINEMET CR.
Symptomatic postural hypotension has occurred when carbidopa-levodopa preparations were added to the treatment of patients receiving some antihypertensive drugs. Therefore, when therapy with SINEMET CR is started, dosage adjustment of the antihypertensive drug may be required.
For patients receiving monoamine oxidase (MAO) inhibitors (Type A or B), see CONTRAINDICATIONS. Concomitant therapy with selegiline and carbidopa-levodopa may be associated with severe orthostatic hypotension not attributable to carbidopa-levodopa alone (see CONTRAINDICATIONS).
There have been rare reports of adverse reactions, including hypertension and dyskinesia, resulting from the concomitant use of tricyclic antidepressants and carbidopa-levodopa preparations.
Dopamine D_2 receptor antagonists (e.g., phenothiazines, butyrophenones, risperidone) and isoniazid may reduce the therapeutic effects of levodopa. In addition, the beneficial effects of levodopa in Parkinson's disease have been reported to be reversed by phenytoin and papaverine. Patients taking these drugs with SINEMET CR should be carefully observed for loss of therapeutic response.
Iron salts may reduce the bioavailability of levodopa and carbidopa. The clinical relevance is unclear.
Although metoclopramide may increase the bioavailability of levodopa by increasing gastric emptying, metoclopramide may also adversely affect disease control by its dopamine receptor antagonistic properties.

Carcinogenesis, Mutagenesis, Impairment of Fertility

In a two-year bioassay of SINEMET, no evidence of carcinogenicity was found in rats receiving doses of approximately two times the maximum daily human dose of carbidopa and four times the maximum daily human dose of levodopa (equivalent to 8 SINEMET CR tablets).
In reproduction studies with SINEMET, no effects on fertility were found in rats receiving doses of approximately two times the maximum daily human dose of carbidopa and four times the maximum daily human dose of levodopa (equivalent to 8 SINEMET CR tablets).

Pregnancy

Pregnancy Category C. No teratogenic effects were observed in a study in mice receiving up to 20 times the maximum recommended human dose of SINEMET. There was a decrease in the number of live pups delivered by rats receiving approximately two times the maximum recommended human dose of carbidopa and approximately five times the maximum recommended human dose of levodopa during organogenesis. SINEMET caused both visceral and skeletal malformations in rabbits at all doses and ratios of carbidopa/levodopa tested, which ranged from 10 times/5 times the maximum recommended human dose of carbidopa/levodopa to 20 times/10 times the maximum recommended human dose of carbidopa/levodopa.
There are no adequate or well-controlled studies in pregnant women. It has been reported from individual cases that levodopa crosses the human placental barrier, enters the fetus, and is metabolized. Carbidopa concentrations in fetal tissue appeared to be minimal. Use of SINEMET CR in women of childbearing potential requires that the anticipated benefits of the drug be weighed against possible hazards to mother and child.

Nursing Mothers

In a study of one nursing mother with Parkinson's disease, excretion of levodopa in human breast milk was reported. Therefore, caution should be exercised when SINEMET CR is administered to a nursing woman.

Pediatric Use

Safety and effectiveness in pediatric patients have not been established. Use of the drug in patients below the age of 18 is not recommended.

ADVERSE REACTIONS

In controlled clinical trials, patients predominantly with moderate to severe motor fluctuations while on SINEMET were randomized to therapy with either SINEMET or SINEMET CR. The adverse experience frequency profile of SINEMET CR did not differ substantially from that of SINEMET, as shown in Table 1.

Table 1: Clinical Adverse Experiences Occurring in 1% or Greater of Patients

Adverse Experience	SINEMET CR n = 491 %	SINEMET n = 524 %
Dyskinesia	16.5	12.2
Nausea	5.5	5.7
Hallucinations	3.9	3.2
Confusion	3.7	2.3
Dizziness	2.9	2.3
Depression	2.2	1.3
Urinary tract infection	2.2	2.3
Headache	2.0	1.9
Dream abnormalities	1.8	0.8
Dystonia	1.8	0.8
Vomiting	1.8	1.9
Upper respiratory infection	1.8	1.0
Dyspnea	1.6	0.4
'On-Off' phenomena	1.6	1.1
Back pain	1.6	0.6
Dry mouth	1.4	1.1
Anorexia	1.2	1.1
Diarrhea	1.2	0.6
Insomnia	1.2	1.0
Orthostatic hypotension	1.0	1.1
Shoulder pain	1.0	0.6
Chest pain	1.0	0.8
Muscle cramps	0.8	1.0
Paresthesia	0.8	1.1
Urinary frequency	0.8	1.1
Dyspepsia	0.6	1.1
Constipation	0.2	1.5

Abnormal laboratory findings occurring at a frequency of 1% or greater in approximately 443 patients who received SINEMET CR and 475 who received SINEMET during controlled clinical trials included: decreased hemoglobin and hematocrit; elevated serum glucose; white blood cells, bacteria and blood in the urine.
The adverse experiences observed in patients in uncontrolled studies were similar to those seen in controlled clinical studies.
Other adverse experiences reported overall in clinical trials in 748 patients treated with SINEMET CR, listed by body system in order of decreasing frequency, include:
Body as a Whole
Asthenia, fatigue, abdominal pain, orthostatic effects.
Cardiovascular
Palpitation, hypertension, hypotension, myocardial infarction.
Gastrointestinal
Gastrointestinal pain, dysphagia, heartburn.
Metabolic
Weight loss.
Musculoskeletal
Leg pain.
Nervous System / Psychiatric
Chorea, somnolence, falling, anxiety, disorientation, decreased mental acuity, gait abnormalities, extrapyramidal disorder, agitation, nervousness, sleep disorders, memory impairment.
Respiratory
Cough, pharyngeal pain, common cold.
Skin
Rash.
Special Senses
Blurred vision.
Urogenital
Urinary incontinence.
Laboratory Tests
Decreased white blood cell count and serum potassium; increased BUN, serum creatinine and serum LDH; protein and glucose in the urine.
The following adverse experiences have been reported in post-marketing experience with SINEMET CR:
Cardiovascular
Cardiac irregularities, syncope.
Gastrointestinal
Taste alterations, dark saliva.
Hypersensitivity
Angioedema, urticaria, pruritus, bullous lesions (including pemphigus-like reactions).
Nervous System / Psychiatric
Neuroleptic malignant syndrome (NMS, see WARNINGS), increased tremor, peripheral neuropathy, psychotic episodes including delusions and paranoid ideation, pathological gambling, increased libido including hypersexuality, impulse control symptoms.
Skin
Alopecia, flushing, dark sweat.
Urogenital
Dark urine.
Other adverse reactions that have been reported with levodopa alone and with various carbidopa-levodopa formulations and may occur with SINEMET CR are:
Cardiovascular
Phlebitis.
Gastrointestinal
Gastrointestinal bleeding, development of duodenal ulcer, sialorrhea, bruxism, hiccups, flatulence, burning sensation of tongue.
Hematologic
Hemolytic and non-hemolytic anemia, thrombocytopenia, leukopenia, agranulocytosis.
Hypersensitivity
Henoch-Schonlein purpura.
Metabolic
Weight gain, edema.
Nervous System / Psychiatric
Ataxia, depression with suicidal tendencies, dementia, euphoria, convulsions (however, a causal relationship has not been established); bradykinetic episodes, numbness, muscle twitching, blepharospasm (which may be taken as an early sign of excess dosage; consideration of dosage reduction may be made at this time), trismus, activation of latent Horner's syndrome, nightmares.
Skin
Malignant melanoma (see also CONTRAINDICATIONS), increased sweating.
Special Senses
Oculogyric crises, mydriasis, diplopia.
Urogenital
Urinary retention, priapism.
Miscellaneous
Faintness, hoarseness, malaise, hot flashes, sense of stimulation, bizarre breathing patterns.
Laboratory Tests
Abnormalities in alkaline phosphatase, SGOT (AST), SGPT (ALT), bilirubin, Coombs test, uric acid.

OVERDOSAGE

Management of acute overdosage with SINEMET CR is the same as with levodopa. Pyridoxine is not effective in reversing the actions of SINEMET CR.
General supportive measures should be employed, along with immediate gastric lavage. Intravenous fluids should be administered judiciously and an adequate airway maintained. Electrocardiographic monitoring should be instituted and the patient carefully observed for the development of arrhythmias; if required, appropriate antiarrhythmic therapy should be given. The possibility that the patient may have taken other drugs as well as SINEMET CR should be taken into consideration. To date, no experience has been reported with dialysis; hence, its value in overdosage is not known.
Based on studies in which high doses of levodopa and/or carbidopa were administered, a significant proportion of rats and mice given single oral doses of levodopa of approximately 1500-2000 mg/kg are expected to die. A significant proportion of infant rats of both sexes are expected to die at a dose of 800 mg/kg. A significant proportion of rats are expected to die after treatment with similar doses of carbidopa. The addition of carbidopa in a 1:10 ratio with levodopa increases the dose at which a significant proportion of mice are expected to die to 3360 mg/kg.

DOSAGE AND ADMINISTRATION

SINEMET CR contains carbidopa and levodopa in a 1:4 ratio as either the 50-200 tablet or the 25-100 tablet. The daily dosage of SINEMET CR must be determined by careful titration. Patients should be monitored closely during the dose adjustment period, particularly with regard to appearance or worsening of involuntary movements, dyskinesias or nausea. SINEMET CR should not be chewed or crushed.
Standard drugs for Parkinson's disease, other than levodopa without a decarboxylase inhibitor, may be used concomitantly while SINEMET CR is being administered, although their dosage may have to be adjusted.
Since carbidopa prevents the reversal of levodopa effects caused by pyridoxine, SINEMET CR can be given to patients receiving supplemental pyridoxine (vitamin B_6).

Initial Dosage

Patients currently treated with conventional carbidopa-levodopa preparations: Studies show that peripheral dopa-decarboxylase is saturated by the bioavailable carbidopa at doses of 70 mg a day and greater. Because the bioavailabilities of carbidopa and levodopa in SINEMET and SINEMET CR are different, appropriate adjustments should be made, as shown in Table 2.

Table 2: Approximate Bioavailabilities at Steady State*

Tablet	Amount of Levodopa (mg) in Each Tablet	Approximate Bioavailability	Approximate Amount of Bioavailable Levodopa (mg) in Each Tablet
SINEMET CR 50-200	200	0.70-0.75†	140-150
SINEMET 25-100	100	0.99‡	99

* This table is only a guide to bioavailabilities since other factors such as food, drugs, and inter-patient variabilities may affect the bioavailability of carbidopa and levodopa.
† The extent of availability of levodopa from SINEMET CR was about 70-75% relative to intravenous levodopa or standard SINEMET in the elderly.
‡ The extent of availability of levodopa from SINEMET was 99% relative to intravenous levodopa in the healthy elderly.

[See table 2 above]
Dosage with SINEMET CR should be substituted at an amount that provides approximately 10% more levodopa per day, although this may need to be increased to a dosage that provides up to 30% more levodopa per day depending on clinical response (see DOSAGE AND ADMINISTRATION, Titration with SINEMET CR). The interval between doses of SINEMET CR should be 4-8 hours during the waking day. (See CLINICAL PHARMACOLOGY, Pharmacodynamics.)
A guideline for initiation of SINEMET CR is shown in Table 3.

Table 3: Guidelines for Initial Conversion from SINEMET to SINEMET CR

SINEMET Total Daily Dose* Levodopa (mg)	SINEMET CR Suggested Dosage Regimen
300-400	200 mg b.i.d.
500-600	300 mg b.i.d. or 200 mg t.i.d.
700-800	A total of 800 mg in 3 or more divided doses (e.g., 300 mg a.m., 300 mg early p.m., and 200 mg later p.m.)
900-1000	A total of 1000 mg in 3 or more divided doses (e.g., 400 mg a.m., 400 mg early p.m., and 200 mg later p.m.)

* For dosing ranges not shown in the table see DOSAGE AND ADMINISTRATION, Initial Dosage — *Patients currently treated with conventional carbidopa-levodopa preparations.*

Patients currently treated with levodopa without a decarboxylase inhibitor: Levodopa must be discontinued at least twelve hours before therapy with SINEMET CR is started. SINEMET CR should be substituted at a dosage that will provide approximately 25% of the previous levodopa dosage. In patients with mild to moderate disease, the initial dose is usually 1 tablet of SINEMET CR 50-200 b.i.d.
Patients not receiving levodopa: In patients with mild to moderate disease, the initial recommended dose is 1 tablet of SINEMET CR 50-200 b.i.d. Initial dosage should not be given at intervals of less than 6 hours.

Titration with SINEMET CR
Following initiation of therapy, doses and dosing intervals may be increased or decreased depending upon therapeutic response. Most patients have been adequately treated with doses of SINEMET CR that provide 400 to 1600 mg of levodopa per day, administered as divided doses at intervals ranging from 4 to 8 hours during the waking day. Higher doses of SINEMET CR (2400 mg or more of levodopa per day) and shorter intervals (less than 4 hours) have been used, but are not usually recommended.
When doses of SINEMET CR are given at intervals of less than 4 hours, and/or if the divided doses are not equal, it is recommended that the smaller doses be given at the end of the day.
An interval of at least 3 days between dosage adjustments is recommended.

Maintenance
Because Parkinson's disease is progressive, periodic clinical evaluations are recommended; adjustment of the dosage regimen of SINEMET CR may be required.

Addition of Other Antiparkinson Medications
Anticholinergic agents, dopamine agonists, and amantadine can be given with SINEMET CR. Dosage adjustment of SINEMET CR may be necessary when these agents are added.
A dose of carbidopa-levodopa immediate release 25-100 or 10-100 (one half or a whole tablet) can be added to the dosage regimen of SINEMET CR in selected patients with advanced disease who need additional immediate-release levodopa for a brief time during daytime hours.

Interruption of Therapy
Sporadic cases of a symptom complex resembling Neuroleptic Malignant Syndrome (NMS) have been associated with dose reductions and withdrawal of SINEMET or SINEMET CR.
Patients should be observed carefully if abrupt reduction or discontinuation of SINEMET CR is required, especially if the patient is receiving neuroleptics. (See WARNINGS.)
If general anesthesia is required, SINEMET CR may be continued as long as the patient is permitted to take oral medication. If therapy is interrupted temporarily, the patient should be observed for symptoms resembling NMS, and the usual dosage should be administered as soon as the patient is able to take oral medication.

HOW SUPPLIED
No. 3919 — SINEMET CR 50-200 (carbidopa-levodopa) Sustained-Release Tablets containing 50 mg of carbidopa and 200 mg of levodopa are dappled-purple in color, oval, compressed tablets that are coded "521" on one side and plain on the other. They are supplied as follows:
NDC 0006-3919-68 bottles of 100.
No. 3918 — SINEMET CR 25-100 (carbidopa-levodopa) Sustained-Release Tablets containing 25 mg of carbidopa and 100 mg of levodopa are dappled-purple in color, oval, compressed tablets that are coded "601" on one side and plain on the other. They are supplied as follows:
NDC 0006-3918-68 bottles of 100.

Storage and Handling
Store at 25°C (77°F), excursions permitted to 15-30°C (59-86°F) [see USP Controlled Room Temperature]. Store in a tightly closed container, protected from light and moisture. Dispense in a tightly closed, light-resistant container.

Rx Only
Manufactured for:
Merck Sharp & Dohme Corp., a subsidiary of
MERCK & CO., INC., Whitehouse Station, NJ 08889, USA
By:
Mylan Pharmaceuticals, Inc.
Morgantown, WV 26505, USA
Issued February 2011
9998401

SINGULAIR® ℞
[sing-u-lair]
(montelukast sodium)
Tablets, Chewable Tablets, and Oral Granules

HIGHLIGHTS OF PRESCRIBING INFORMATION
These highlights do not include all the information needed to use SINGULAIR safely and effectively. See full prescribing information for SINGULAIR.
SINGULAIR® (montelukast sodium) Tablets, Chewable Tablets, and Oral Granules
Initial U.S. Approval: 1998

RECENT MAJOR CHANGES

Warnings and Precautions

Neuropsychiatric Events (5.4)	03/2013
Eosinophilic Conditions (5.5)	06/2013

INDICATIONS AND USAGE
SINGULAIR is a leukotriene receptor antagonist indicated for:
- Prophylaxis and chronic treatment of asthma in patients 12 months of age and older (1.1).
- Acute prevention of exercise-induced bronchoconstriction (EIB) in patients 6 years of age and older (1.2).
- Relief of symptoms of allergic rhinitis (AR): seasonal allergic rhinitis (SAR) in patients 2 years of age and older, and perennial allergic rhinitis (PAR) in patients 6 months of age and older (1.3).

DOSAGE AND ADMINISTRATION
Administration (by indications):
- Asthma (2.1): Once daily in the evening for patients 12 months and older.
- Acute prevention of EIB (2.2): One tablet at least 2 hours before exercise for patients 6 years of age and older.
- Seasonal allergic rhinitis (2.3): Once daily for patients 2 years and older.
- Perennial allergic rhinitis (2.3): Once daily for patients 6 months and older.

Dosage (by age) (2):
- 15 years and older: one 10-mg tablet.
- 6 to 14 years: one 5-mg chewable tablet.
- 2 to 5 years: one 4-mg chewable tablet or one packet of 4-mg oral granules.
- 6 to 23 months: one packet of 4-mg oral granules.

Patients with both asthma and allergic rhinitis should take only one dose daily in the evening (2.4). For oral granules: Must administer within 15 minutes after opening the packet (with or without mixing with food) (2.5).

DOSAGE FORMS AND STRENGTHS
- SINGULAIR 10-mg Film-Coated Tablets
- SINGULAIR 5-mg and 4-mg Chewable Tablets
- SINGULAIR 4-mg Oral Granules (3)

CONTRAINDICATIONS
- Hypersensitivity to any component of this product (4).

WARNINGS AND PRECAUTIONS
- Do not prescribe SINGULAIR to treat an acute asthma attack (5.1).
- Advise patients to have appropriate rescue medication available (5.1).
- Inhaled corticosteroid may be reduced gradually. Do not abruptly substitute SINGULAIR for inhaled or oral corticosteroids (5.2).
- Patients with known aspirin sensitivity should continue to avoid aspirin or non-steroidal anti-inflammatory agents while taking SINGULAIR (5.3).
- Neuropsychiatric events have been reported with SINGULAIR. Instruct patients to be alert for neuropsychiatric events. Evaluate the risks and benefits of continuing treatment with SINGULAIR if such events occur (5.4 and 6.2).
- Systemic eosinophilia, sometimes presenting with clinical features of vasculitis consistent with Churg-Strauss syndrome, has been reported. These events have been sometimes associated with the reduction of oral corticosteroid therapy (5.5 and 6.2).
- Inform patients with phenylketonuria that the 4-mg and 5-mg chewable tablets contain phenylalanine (5.6).

ADVERSE REACTIONS
Most common adverse reactions (incidence ≥5% and greater than placebo listed in descending order of frequency): upper respiratory infection, fever, headache, pharyngitis, cough, abdominal pain, diarrhea, otitis media, influenza, rhinorrhea, sinusitis, otitis (6.1).
To report SUSPECTED ADVERSE REACTIONS, contact Merck Sharp & Dohme Corp., a subsidiary of Merck & Co., Inc., at 1-877-888-4231 or FDA at 1-800-FDA-1088 or www.fda.gov/medwatch.
See 17 for PATIENT COUNSELING INFORMATION and FDA-approved patient labeling
Revised: 06/2013

FULL PRESCRIBING INFORMATION: CONTENTS*

*** Sections or subsections omitted from the full prescribing information are not listed**

FULL PRESCRIBING INFORMATION

1 INDICATIONS AND USAGE

1.1 Asthma

SINGULAIR® is indicated for the prophylaxis and chronic treatment of asthma in adults and pediatric patients 12 months of age and older.

1.2 Exercise-Induced Bronchoconstriction (EIB)

SINGULAIR is indicated for prevention of exercise-induced bronchoconstriction (EIB) in patients 6 years of age and older.

1.3 Allergic Rhinitis

SINGULAIR is indicated for the relief of symptoms of seasonal allergic rhinitis in patients 2 years of age and older and perennial allergic rhinitis in patients 6 months of age and older.

2 DOSAGE AND ADMINISTRATION

2.1 Asthma

SINGULAIR should be taken once daily in the evening. The following doses are recommended:

For adults and adolescents 15 years of age and older: one 10-mg tablet.

For pediatric patients 6 to 14 years of age: one 5-mg chewable tablet.

For pediatric patients 2 to 5 years of age: one 4-mg chewable tablet or one packet of 4-mg oral granules.

For pediatric patients 12 to 23 months of age: one packet of 4-mg oral granules.

Safety and effectiveness in pediatric patients less than 12 months of age with asthma have not been established.

There have been no clinical trials in patients with asthma to evaluate the relative efficacy of morning versus evening dosing. The pharmacokinetics of montelukast are similar whether dosed in the morning or evening. Efficacy has been demonstrated for asthma when montelukast was administered in the evening without regard to time of food ingestion.

2.2 Exercise-Induced Bronchoconstriction (EIB)

For prevention of EIB, a single dose of SINGULAIR should be taken at least 2 hours before exercise. The following doses are recommended:

For adults and adolescents 15 years of age and older: one 10-mg tablet.

For pediatric patients 6 to 14 years of age: one 5-mg chewable tablet.

An additional dose of SINGULAIR should not be taken within 24 hours of a previous dose. Patients already taking SINGULAIR daily for another indication (including chronic asthma) should not take an additional dose to prevent EIB. All patients should have available for rescue a short-acting β-agonist. Safety and efficacy in patients younger than 6 years of age have not been established. Daily administration of SINGULAIR for the chronic treatment of asthma has not been established to prevent acute episodes of EIB.

2.3 Allergic Rhinitis

For allergic rhinitis, SINGULAIR should be taken once daily. Efficacy was demonstrated for seasonal allergic rhinitis when montelukast was administered in the morning or the evening without regard to time of food ingestion. The time of administration may be individualized to suit patient needs.

The following doses for the treatment of symptoms of seasonal allergic rhinitis are recommended:

For adults and adolescents 15 years of age and older: one 10-mg tablet.

For pediatric patients 6 to 14 years of age: one 5-mg chewable tablet.

For pediatric patients 2 to 5 years of age: one 4-mg chewable tablet or one packet of 4-mg oral granules.

Safety and effectiveness in pediatric patients younger than 2 years of age with seasonal allergic rhinitis have not been established.

The following doses for the treatment of symptoms of perennial allergic rhinitis are recommended:

For adults and adolescents 15 years of age and older: one 10-mg tablet.

For pediatric patients 6 to 14 years of age: one 5-mg chewable tablet.

For pediatric patients 2 to 5 years of age: one 4-mg chewable tablet or one packet of 4-mg oral granules.

For pediatric patients 6 to 23 months of age: one packet of 4-mg oral granules.

Safety and effectiveness in pediatric patients younger than 6 months of age with perennial allergic rhinitis have not been established.

2.4 Asthma and Allergic Rhinitis

Patients with both asthma and allergic rhinitis should take only one SINGULAIR dose daily in the evening.

2.5 Instructions for Administration of Oral Granules

SINGULAIR 4-mg oral granules can be administered either directly in the mouth, dissolved in 1 teaspoonful (5 mL) of cold or room temperature baby formula or breast milk, or mixed with a spoonful of cold or room temperature soft foods; based on stability studies, only applesauce, carrots, rice, or ice cream should be used. The packet should not be opened until ready to use. After opening the packet, the full dose (with or without mixing with baby formula, breast milk, or food) must be administered within 15 minutes. If mixed with baby formula, breast milk, or food, SINGULAIR oral granules must not be stored for future use. Discard any unused portion. SINGULAIR oral granules are not intended to be dissolved in any liquid other than baby formula or breast milk for administration. However, liquids may be taken subsequent to administration. SINGULAIR oral granules can be administered without regard to the time of meals.

3 DOSAGE FORMS AND STRENGTHS

- SINGULAIR 10-mg Film-Coated Tablets are beige, rounded square-shaped tablets, with code MRK 117 or MSD 117 on one side and SINGULAIR on the other.
- SINGULAIR 5-mg Chewable Tablets are pink, round, biconvex-shaped tablets, with code MRK 275 or MSD 275 on one side and SINGULAIR on the other.
- SINGULAIR 4-mg Chewable Tablets are pink, oval, biconvex-shaped tablets, with code MRK 711 or MSD 711 on one side and SINGULAIR on the other.
- SINGULAIR 4-mg Oral Granules are white granules with 500 mg net weight, packed in a child-resistant foil packet.

4 CONTRAINDICATIONS

- Hypersensitivity to any component of this product.

5 WARNINGS AND PRECAUTIONS

5.1 Acute Asthma

SINGULAIR is not indicated for use in the reversal of bronchospasm in acute asthma attacks, including status asthmaticus. Patients should be advised to have appropriate rescue medication available. Therapy with SINGULAIR can be continued during acute exacerbations of asthma. Patients who have exacerbations of asthma after exercise should have available for rescue a short-acting inhaled β-agonist.

5.2 Concomitant Corticosteroid Use

While the dose of inhaled corticosteroid may be reduced gradually under medical supervision, SINGULAIR should not be abruptly substituted for inhaled or oral corticosteroids.

5.3 Aspirin Sensitivity

Patients with known aspirin sensitivity should continue avoidance of aspirin or non-steroidal anti-inflammatory agents while taking SINGULAIR. Although SINGULAIR is effective in improving airway function in asthmatics with documented aspirin sensitivity, it has not been shown to truncate bronchoconstrictor response to aspirin and other non-steroidal anti-inflammatory drugs in aspirin-sensitive asthmatic patients *[see Clinical Studies (14.1)]*.

5.4 Neuropsychiatric Events

Neuropsychiatric events have been reported in adult, adolescent, and pediatric patients taking SINGULAIR. Post-marketing reports with SINGULAIR use include agitation, aggressive behavior or hostility, anxiousness, depression, disorientation, disturbance in attention, dream abnormalities, hallucinations, insomnia, irritability, memory impairment, restlessness, somnambulism, suicidal thinking and behavior (including suicide), and tremor. The clinical details of some post-marketing reports involving SINGULAIR appear consistent with a drug-induced effect.

Patients and prescribers should be alert for neuropsychiatric events. Patients should be instructed to notify their prescriber if these changes occur. Prescribers should carefully evaluate the risks and benefits of continuing treatment with SINGULAIR if such events occur *[see Adverse Reactions (6.2)]*.

5.5 Eosinophilic Conditions

Patients with asthma on therapy with SINGULAIR may present with systemic eosinophilia, sometimes presenting with clinical features of vasculitis consistent with Churg-Strauss syndrome, a condition which is often treated with systemic corticosteroid therapy. These events have been sometimes associated with the reduction of oral corticosteroid therapy. Physicians should be alert to eosinophilia, vasculitic rash, worsening pulmonary symptoms, cardiac complications, and/or neuropathy presenting in their patients. A causal association between SINGULAIR and these underlying conditions has not been established *[see Adverse Reactions (6.2)]*.

5.6 Phenylketonuria

Phenylketonuric patients should be informed that the 4-mg and 5-mg chewable tablets contain phenylalanine (a component of aspartame), 0.674 and 0.842 mg per 4-mg and 5-mg chewable tablet, respectively.

6 ADVERSE REACTIONS

6.1 Clinical Trials Experience

Because clinical trials are conducted under widely varying conditions, adverse reaction rates observed in the clinical trials of a drug cannot be directly compared to rates in the clinical trials of another drug and may not reflect the rates observed in clinical practice. In the following description of clinical trials experience, adverse reactions are listed regardless of causality assessment.

The most common adverse reactions (incidence ≥5% and greater than placebo; listed in descending order of frequency) in controlled clinical trials were: upper respiratory infection, fever, headache, pharyngitis, cough, abdominal pain, diarrhea, otitis media, influenza, rhinorrhea, sinusitis, otitis.

Adults and Adolescents 15 Years of Age and Older with Asthma

SINGULAIR has been evaluated for safety in approximately 2950 adult and adolescent patients 15 years of age and older in clinical trials. In placebo-controlled clinical trials, the following adverse experiences reported with SINGULAIR occurred in greater than or equal to 1% of patients and at an incidence greater than that in patients treated with placebo:

Table 1: Adverse Experiences Occurring in ≥1% of Patients with an Incidence Greater than that in Patients Treated with Placebo

	SINGULAIR 10 mg/day (%) (n=1955)	Placebo (%) (n=1180)
Body As A Whole		
Pain, abdominal	2.9	2.5
Asthenia/fatigue	1.8	1.2
Fever	1.5	0.9
Trauma	1.0	0.8
Digestive System Disorders		
Dyspepsia	2.1	1.1
Pain, dental	1.7	1.0
Gastroenteritis, infectious	1.5	0.5
Nervous System/Psychiatric		
Headache	18.4	18.1
Dizziness	1.9	1.4
Respiratory System Disorders		
Influenza	4.2	3.9
Cough	2.7	2.4
Congestion, nasal	1.6	1.3
Skin/Skin Appendages Disorder		
Rash	1.6	1.2
*Laboratory Adverse Experiences**		
ALT increased	2.1	2.0
AST increased	1.6	1.2
Pyuria	1.0	0.9

* Number of patients tested (SINGULAIR and placebo, respectively): ALT and AST, 1935, 1170; pyuria, 1924, 1159.

The frequency of less common adverse events was comparable between SINGULAIR and placebo.

The safety profile of SINGULAIR, when administered as a single dose for prevention of EIB in adult and adolescent patients 15 years of age and older, was consistent with the safety profile previously described for SINGULAIR.

Cumulatively, 569 patients were treated with SINGULAIR for at least 6 months, 480 for one year, and 49 for two years in clinical trials. With prolonged treatment, the adverse experience profile did not significantly change.

Pediatric Patients 6 to 14 Years of Age with Asthma

SINGULAIR has been evaluated for safety in 476 pediatric patients 6 to 14 years of age. Cumulatively, 289 pediatric patients were treated with SINGULAIR for at least 6 months, and 241 for one year or longer in clinical trials. The safety profile of SINGULAIR in the 8-week, double-blind, pediatric efficacy trial was generally similar to the adult safety profile. In pediatric patients 6 to 14 years of age receiving SINGULAIR, the following events occurred with a frequency ≥2% and more frequently than in pediatric patients who received placebo: pharyngitis, influenza, fever, sinusitis, nausea, diarrhea, dyspepsia, otitis, viral infection, and laryngitis. The frequency of less common adverse events was comparable between SINGULAIR and placebo. With prolonged treatment, the adverse experience profile did not significantly change.

The safety profile of SINGULAIR, when administered as a single dose for prevention of EIB in pediatric patients 6 years of age and older, was consistent with the safety profile previously described for SINGULAIR.

In studies evaluating growth rate, the safety profile in these pediatric patients was consistent with the safety profile previously described for SINGULAIR. In a 56-week, double-blind study evaluating growth rate in pediatric patients 6 to 8 years of age receiving SINGULAIR, the following events not previously observed with the use of SINGULAIR in this age group occurred with a frequency ≥2% and more frequently than in pediatric patients who received placebo: headache, rhinitis (infective), varicella, gastroenteritis, atopic dermatitis, acute bronchitis, tooth infection, skin infection, and myopia.

Pediatric Patients 2 to 5 Years of Age with Asthma

SINGULAIR has been evaluated for safety in 573 pediatric patients 2 to 5 years of age in single- and multiple-dose studies. Cumulatively, 426 pediatric patients 2 to 5 years of age were treated with SINGULAIR for at least 3 months, 230 for 6 months or longer, and 63 patients for one year or longer in clinical trials. In pediatric patients 2 to 5 years of age receiving SINGULAIR, the following events occurred with a frequency ≥2% and more frequently than in pediatric patients who received placebo: fever, cough, abdominal pain, diarrhea, headache, rhinorrhea, sinusitis, otitis, influenza, rash, ear pain, gastroenteritis, eczema, urticaria, varicella, pneumonia, dermatitis, and conjunctivitis.

Pediatric Patients 6 to 23 Months of Age with Asthma

Safety and effectiveness in pediatric patients younger than 12 months of age with asthma have not been established.

SINGULAIR has been evaluated for safety in 175 pediatric patients 6 to 23 months of age. The safety profile of SINGULAIR in a 6-week, double-blind, placebo-controlled clinical study was generally similar to the safety profile in adults and pediatric patients 2 to 14 years of age. In pediatric patients 6 to 23 months of age receiving SINGULAIR, the following events occurred with a frequency ≥2% and more frequently than in pediatric patients who received placebo: upper respiratory infection, wheezing; otitis media; pharyngitis, tonsillitis, cough; and rhinitis. The frequency of less common adverse events was comparable between SINGULAIR and placebo.

Adults and Adolescents 15 Years of Age and Older with Seasonal Allergic Rhinitis

SINGULAIR has been evaluated for safety in 2199 adult and adolescent patients 15 years of age and older in clinical trials. SINGULAIR administered once daily in the morning or in the evening had a safety profile similar to that of placebo. In placebo-controlled clinical trials, the following event was reported with SINGULAIR with a frequency ≥1% and at an incidence greater than placebo: upper respiratory infection, 1.9% of patients receiving SINGULAIR vs. 1.5% of patients receiving placebo. In a 4-week, placebo-controlled clinical study, the safety profile was consistent with that observed in 2-week studies. The incidence of somnolence was similar to that of placebo in all studies.

Pediatric Patients 2 to 14 Years of Age with Seasonal Allergic Rhinitis

SINGULAIR has been evaluated in 280 pediatric patients 2 to 14 years of age in a 2-week, multicenter, double-blind, placebo-controlled, parallel-group safety study. SINGULAIR administered once daily in the evening had a safety profile similar to that of placebo. In this study, the following events occurred with a frequency ≥2% and at an incidence greater than placebo: headache, otitis media, pharyngitis, and upper respiratory infection.

Adults and Adolescents 15 Years of Age and Older with Perennial Allergic Rhinitis

SINGULAIR has been evaluated for safety in 3357 adult and adolescent patients 15 years of age and older with perennial allergic rhinitis of whom 1632 received SINGULAIR in two, 6-week, clinical studies. SINGULAIR administered once daily had a safety profile consistent with that observed in patients with seasonal allergic rhinitis and similar to that of placebo. In these two studies, the following events were reported with SINGULAIR with a frequency ≥1% and at an incidence greater than placebo: sinusitis, upper respiratory infection, sinus headache, cough, epistaxis, and increased ALT. The incidence of somnolence was similar to that of placebo.

Pediatric Patients 6 Months to 14 Years of Age with Perennial Allergic Rhinitis

The safety in patients 2 to 14 years of age with perennial allergic rhinitis is supported by the safety in patients 2 to 14 years of age with seasonal allergic rhinitis. The safety in patients 6 to 23 months of age is supported by data from pharmacokinetic and safety and efficacy studies in asthma in this pediatric population and from adult pharmacokinetic studies.

6.2 Post-Marketing Experience

The following adverse reactions have been identified during post-approval use of SINGULAIR. Because these reactions are reported voluntarily from a population of uncertain size, it is not always possible to reliably estimate their frequency or establish a causal relationship to drug exposure.

Blood and lymphatic system disorders: increased bleeding tendency, thrombocytopenia.

Immune system disorders: hypersensitivity reactions including anaphylaxis, hepatic eosinophilic infiltration.

Psychiatric disorders: agitation including aggressive behavior or hostility, anxiousness, depression, disorientation, disturbance in attention, dream abnormalities, hallucinations, insomnia, irritability, memory impairment, restlessness, somnambulism, suicidal thinking and behavior (including suicide), and tremor *[see Warnings and Precautions (5.4)]*.

Nervous system disorders: drowsiness, paraesthesia/hypoesthesia, seizures.

Cardiac disorders: palpitations.

Respiratory, thoracic and mediastinal disorders: epistaxis, pulmonary eosinophilia.

Gastrointestinal disorders: diarrhea, dyspepsia, nausea, pancreatitis, vomiting.

Hepatobiliary disorders: Cases of cholestatic hepatitis, hepatocellular liver-injury, and mixed-pattern liver injury have been reported in patients treated with SINGULAIR. Most of these occurred in combination with other confounding factors, such as use of other medications, or when SINGULAIR was administered to patients who had underlying potential for liver disease such as alcohol use or other forms of hepatitis.

Skin and subcutaneous tissue disorders: angioedema, bruising, erythema multiforme, erythema nodosum, pruritus, Stevens-Johnson syndrome/toxic epidermal necrolysis, urticaria.

Musculoskeletal and connective tissue disorders: arthralgia, myalgia including muscle cramps.

General disorders and administration site conditions: edema.

Patients with asthma on therapy with SINGULAIR may present with systemic eosinophilia, sometimes presenting with clinical features of vasculitis consistent with Churg-Strauss syndrome, a condition which is often treated with systemic corticosteroid therapy. These events have been sometimes associated with the reduction of oral corticosteroid therapy. Physicians should be alert to eosinophilia, vasculitic rash, worsening pulmonary symptoms, cardiac complications, and/or neuropathy presenting in their patients *[see Warnings and Precautions (5.5)]*.

7 DRUG INTERACTIONS

No dose adjustment is needed when SINGULAIR is coadministered with theophylline, prednisone, prednisolone, oral contraceptives, terfenadine, digoxin, warfarin, gemfibrozil, itraconazole, thyroid hormones, sedative hypnotics, non-steroidal anti-inflammatory agents, benzodiazepines, decongestants, and Cytochrome P450 (CYP) enzyme inducers *[see Clinical Pharmacology (12.3)]*.

8 USE IN SPECIFIC POPULATIONS

8.1 Pregnancy

Pregnancy Category B: There are no adequate and well-controlled studies in pregnant women. Because animal reproduction studies are not always predictive of human response, SINGULAIR should be used during pregnancy only if clearly needed.

Teratogenic Effect: No teratogenicity was observed in rats and rabbits at doses approximately 100 and 110 times, respectively, the maximum recommended daily oral dose in adults based on AUCs *[see Nonclinical Toxicology (13.2)]*.

During worldwide marketing experience, congenital limb defects have been rarely reported in the offspring of women being treated with SINGULAIR during pregnancy. Most of these women were also taking other asthma medications during their pregnancy. A causal relationship between these events and SINGULAIR has not been established.

8.3 Nursing Mothers

Studies in rats have shown that montelukast is excreted in milk. It is not known if montelukast is excreted in human milk. Because many drugs are excreted in human milk, caution should be exercised when SINGULAIR is given to a nursing mother.

8.4 Pediatric Use

Safety and efficacy of SINGULAIR have been established in adequate and well-controlled studies in pediatric patients with asthma 6 to 14 years of age. Safety and efficacy profiles in this age group are similar to those seen in adults *[see Adverse Reactions (6.1), Clinical Pharmacology, Special Populations (12.3), and Clinical Studies (14.1, 14.2)]*.

The efficacy of SINGULAIR for the treatment of seasonal allergic rhinitis in pediatric patients 2 to 14 years of age and for the treatment of perennial allergic rhinitis in pediatric patients 6 months to 14 years of age is supported by extrapolation from the demonstrated efficacy in patients 15 years of age and older with allergic rhinitis as well as the assumption that the disease course, pathophysiology and the drug's effect are substantially similar among these populations.

The safety of SINGULAIR 4-mg chewable tablets in pediatric patients 2 to 5 years of age with asthma has been demonstrated by adequate and well-controlled data *[see Adverse Reactions (6.1)]*. Efficacy of SINGULAIR in this age group is extrapolated from the demonstrated efficacy in patients 6 years of age and older with asthma and is based on similar pharmacokinetic data, as well as the assumption that the disease course, pathophysiology and the drug's effect are substantially similar among these populations. Efficacy in this age group is supported by exploratory efficacy assessments from a large, well-controlled safety study conducted in patients 2 to 5 years of age.

The safety of SINGULAIR 4-mg oral granules in pediatric patients 12 to 23 months of age with asthma has been demonstrated in an analysis of 172 pediatric patients, 124 of whom were treated with SINGULAIR, in a 6-week, double-blind, placebo-controlled study *[see Adverse Reactions (6.1)]*. Efficacy of SINGULAIR in this age group is extrapolated from the demonstrated efficacy in patients 6 years of age and older with asthma based on similar mean systemic exposure (AUC), and that the disease course, pathophysiology and the drug's effect are substantially similar among these populations, supported by efficacy data from a safety trial in which efficacy was an exploratory assessment.

The safety of SINGULAIR 4-mg and 5-mg chewable tablets in pediatric patients aged 2 to 14 years with allergic rhinitis is supported by data from studies conducted in pediatric patients aged 2 to 14 years with asthma. A safety study in pediatric patients 2 to 14 years of age with seasonal allergic rhinitis demonstrated a similar safety profile *[see Adverse Reactions (6.1)]*. The safety of SINGULAIR 4-mg oral granules in pediatric patients as young as 6 months of age with perennial allergic rhinitis is supported by extrapolation from safety data obtained from studies conducted in pediatric patients 6 months to 23 months of age with asthma and from pharmacokinetic data comparing systemic exposures in patients 6 months to 23 months of age to systemic exposures in adults.

The safety and effectiveness in pediatric patients below the age of 12 months with asthma, 6 months with perennial allergic rhinitis, and 6 years with exercise-induced bronchoconstriction have not been established.

Growth Rate in Pediatric Patients

A 56-week, multi-center, double-blind, randomized, active- and placebo-controlled parallel group study was conducted to assess the effect of SINGULAIR on growth rate in 360 patients with mild asthma, aged 6 to 8 years. Treatment groups included SINGULAIR 5 mg once daily, placebo, and beclomethasone dipropionate administered as 168 mcg twice daily with a spacer device. For each subject, a growth rate was defined as the slope of a linear regression line fit to the height measurements over 56 weeks. The primary comparison was the difference in growth rates between SINGULAIR and placebo groups. Growth rates, expressed as least-squares (LS) mean (95% CI) in cm/year, for the SINGULAIR, placebo, and beclomethasone treatment groups were 5.67 (5.46, 5.88), 5.64 (5.42, 5.86), and 4.86 (4.64, 5.08), respectively. The differences in growth rates, expressed as least-squares (LS) mean (95% CI) in cm/year, for SINGULAIR minus placebo, beclomethasone minus placebo, and SINGULAIR minus beclomethasone treatment groups were 0.03 (-0.26, 0.31), -0.78 (-1.06, -0.49); and 0.81 (0.53, 1.09), respectively. Growth rate (expressed as mean change in height over time) for each treatment group is shown in FIGURE 1.

[See figure 1 at top of next column]

8.5 Geriatric Use

Of the total number of subjects in clinical studies of montelukast, 3.5% were 65 years of age and over, and 0.4% were 75 years of age and over. No overall differences in safety or effectiveness were observed between these subjects and younger subjects, and other reported clinical experience has not identified differences in responses between the elderly and younger patients, but greater sensitivity of some

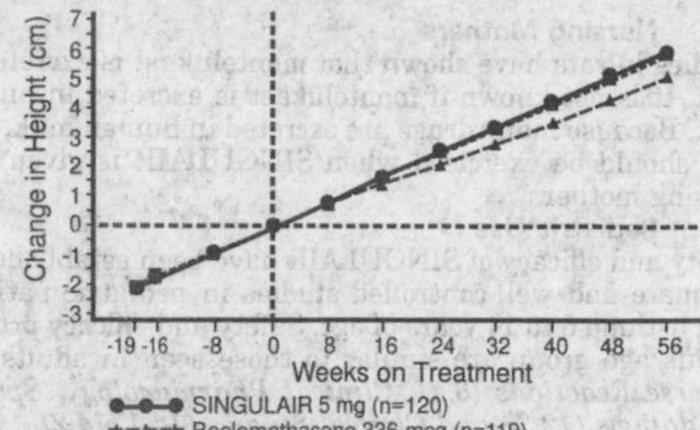

*The standard errors of the treatment group means in change in height are too small to be visible on the plot

Figure 1: Change in Height (cm) from Randomization Visit by Scheduled Week (Treatment Group Mean ± Standard Error* of the Mean)

older individuals cannot be ruled out. The pharmacokinetic profile and the oral bioavailability of a single 10-mg oral dose of montelukast are similar in elderly and younger adults. The plasma half-life of montelukast is slightly longer in the elderly. No dosage adjustment in the elderly is required.

8.6 Hepatic Insufficiency

No dosage adjustment is required in patients with mild-to-moderate hepatic insufficiency *[see Clinical Pharmacology (12.3)]*.

8.7 Renal Insufficiency

No dosage adjustment is recommended in patients with renal insufficiency *[see Clinical Pharmacology (12.3)]*.

10 OVERDOSAGE

No specific information is available on the treatment of overdosage with SINGULAIR. In chronic asthma studies, montelukast has been administered at doses up to 200 mg/day to adult patients for 22 weeks and, in short-term studies, up to 900 mg/day to patients for approximately a week without clinically important adverse experiences. In the event of overdose, it is reasonable to employ the usual supportive measures; e.g., remove unabsorbed material from the gastrointestinal tract, employ clinical monitoring, and institute supportive therapy, if required.

There have been reports of acute overdosage in post-marketing experience and clinical studies with SINGULAIR. These include reports in adults and children with a dose as high as 1000 mg. The clinical and laboratory findings observed were consistent with the safety profile in adults and pediatric patients. There were no adverse experiences in the majority of overdosage reports. The most frequently occurring adverse experiences were consistent with the safety profile of SINGULAIR and included abdominal pain, somnolence, thirst, headache, vomiting and psychomotor hyperactivity.

It is not known whether montelukast is removed by peritoneal dialysis or hemodialysis.

11 DESCRIPTION

Montelukast sodium, the active ingredient in SINGULAIR, is a selective and orally active leukotriene receptor antagonist that inhibits the cysteinyl leukotriene $CysLT_1$ receptor.

Montelukast sodium is described chemically as [*R*-(*E*)]-1-[[[1-[3-[2-(7-chloro-2-quinolinyl)ethenyl]phenyl]-3-[2-(1-hydroxy-1-methylethyl)phenyl]propyl]thio]methyl]cyclopropaneacetic acid, monosodium salt.

The empirical formula is $C_{35}H_{35}ClNNaO_3S$, and its molecular weight is 608.18. The structural formula is:

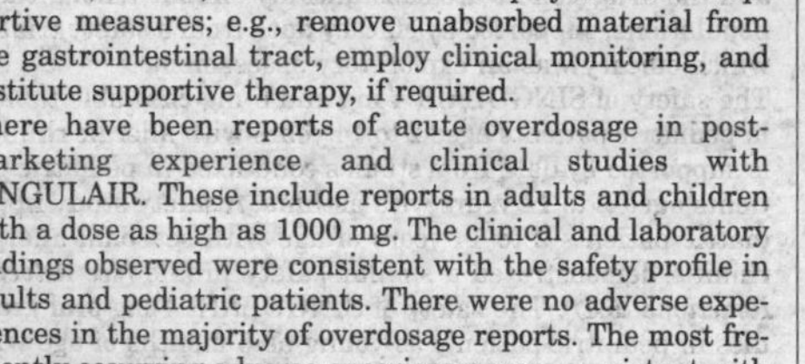

Montelukast sodium is a hygroscopic, optically active, white to off-white powder. Montelukast sodium is freely soluble in ethanol, methanol, and water and practically insoluble in acetonitrile.

Each 10-mg film-coated SINGULAIR tablet contains 10.4 mg montelukast sodium, which is equivalent to 10 mg of montelukast, and the following inactive ingredients: microcrystalline cellulose, lactose monohydrate, croscarmellose sodium, hydroxypropyl cellulose, and magnesium stearate. The film coating consists of: hydroxypropyl methylcellulose, hydroxypropyl cellulose, titanium dioxide, red ferric oxide, yellow ferric oxide, and carnauba wax.

Each 4-mg and 5-mg chewable SINGULAIR tablet contains 4.2 and 5.2 mg montelukast sodium, respectively, which are equivalent to 4 and 5 mg of montelukast, respectively. Both chewable tablets contain the following inactive ingredients: mannitol, microcrystalline cellulose, hydroxypropyl cellulose, red ferric oxide, croscarmellose sodium, cherry flavor, aspartame, and magnesium stearate.

Each packet of SINGULAIR 4-mg oral granules contains 4.2 mg montelukast sodium, which is equivalent to 4 mg of montelukast. The oral granule formulation contains the following inactive ingredients: mannitol, hydroxypropyl cellulose, and magnesium stearate.

12 CLINICAL PHARMACOLOGY

12.1 Mechanism of Action

The cysteinyl leukotrienes (LTC_4, LTD_4, LTE_4) are products of arachidonic acid metabolism and are released from various cells, including mast cells and eosinophils. These eicosanoids bind to cysteinyl leukotriene (CysLT) receptors. The CysLT type-1 ($CysLT_1$) receptor is found in the human airway (including airway smooth muscle cells and airway macrophages) and on other pro-inflammatory cells (including eosinophils and certain myeloid stem cells). CysLTs have been correlated with the pathophysiology of asthma and allergic rhinitis. In asthma, leukotriene-mediated effects include airway edema, smooth muscle contraction, and altered cellular activity associated with the inflammatory process. In allergic rhinitis, CysLTs are released from the nasal mucosa after allergen exposure during both early- and late-phase reactions and are associated with symptoms of allergic rhinitis.

Montelukast is an orally active compound that binds with high affinity and selectivity to the $CysLT_1$ receptor (in preference to other pharmacologically important airway receptors, such as the prostanoid, cholinergic, or β-adrenergic receptor). Montelukast inhibits physiologic actions of LTD_4 at the $CysLT_1$ receptor without any agonist activity.

12.2 Pharmacodynamics

Montelukast causes inhibition of airway cysteinyl leukotriene receptors as demonstrated by the ability to inhibit bronchoconstriction due to inhaled LTD_4 in asthmatics. Doses as low as 5 mg cause substantial blockage of LTD_4-induced bronchoconstriction. In a placebo-controlled, crossover study (n=12), SINGULAIR inhibited early- and late-phase bronchoconstriction due to antigen challenge by 75% and 57%, respectively.

The effect of SINGULAIR on eosinophils in the peripheral blood was examined in clinical trials. In patients with asthma aged 2 years and older who received SINGULAIR, a decrease in mean peripheral blood eosinophil counts ranging from 9% to 15% was noted, compared with placebo, over the double-blind treatment periods. In patients with seasonal allergic rhinitis aged 15 years and older who received SINGULAIR, a mean increase of 0.2% in peripheral blood eosinophil counts was noted, compared with a mean increase of 12.5% in placebo-treated patients, over the double-blind treatment periods; this reflects a mean difference of 12.3% in favor of SINGULAIR. The relationship between these observations and the clinical benefits of montelukast noted in the clinical trials is not known *[see Clinical Studies (14)]*.

12.3 Pharmacokinetics

Absorption

Montelukast is rapidly absorbed following oral administration. After administration of the 10-mg film-coated tablet to fasted adults, the mean peak montelukast plasma concentration (C_{max}) is achieved in 3 to 4 hours (T_{max}). The mean oral bioavailability is 64%. The oral bioavailability and C_{max} are not influenced by a standard meal in the morning.

For the 5-mg chewable tablet, the mean C_{max} is achieved in 2 to 2.5 hours after administration to adults in the fasted state. The mean oral bioavailability is 73% in the fasted state versus 63% when administered with a standard meal in the morning.

For the 4-mg chewable tablet, the mean C_{max} is achieved 2 hours after administration in pediatric patients 2 to 5 years of age in the fasted state.

The 4-mg oral granule formulation is bioequivalent to the 4-mg chewable tablet when administered to adults in the fasted state. The co-administration of the oral granule formulation with applesauce did not have a clinically significant effect on the pharmacokinetics of montelukast. A high fat meal in the morning did not affect the AUC of montelukast oral granules; however, the meal decreased C_{max} by 35% and prolonged T_{max} from 2.3 ± 1.0 hours to 6.4 ± 2.9 hours.

The safety and efficacy of SINGULAIR in patients with asthma were demonstrated in clinical trials in which the 10-mg film-coated tablet and 5-mg chewable tablet formulations were administered in the evening without regard to the time of food ingestion. The safety of SINGULAIR in patients with asthma was also demonstrated in clinical trials in which the 4-mg chewable tablet and 4-mg oral granule formulations were administered in the evening without regard to the time of food ingestion. The safety and efficacy of SINGULAIR in patients with seasonal allergic rhinitis were demonstrated in clinical trials in which the 10-mg film-coated tablet was administered in the morning or evening without regard to the time of food ingestion.

The comparative pharmacokinetics of montelukast when administered as two 5-mg chewable tablets versus one 10-mg film-coated tablet have not been evaluated.

Distribution

Montelukast is more than 99% bound to plasma proteins. The steady state volume of distribution of montelukast averages 8 to 11 liters. Studies in rats with radiolabeled montelukast indicate minimal distribution across the blood-brain barrier. In addition, concentrations of radiolabeled material at 24 hours postdose were minimal in all other tissues.

Metabolism

Montelukast is extensively metabolized. In studies with therapeutic doses, plasma concentrations of metabolites of montelukast are undetectable at steady state in adults and pediatric patients.

In vitro studies using human liver microsomes indicate that CYP3A4, 2C8, and 2C9 are involved in the metabolism of montelukast. At clinically relevant concentrations, 2C8 appears to play a major role in the metabolism of montelukast.

Elimination

The plasma clearance of montelukast averages 45 mL/min in healthy adults. Following an oral dose of radiolabeled montelukast, 86% of the radioactivity was recovered in 5-day fecal collections and <0.2% was recovered in urine. Coupled with estimates of montelukast oral bioavailability, this indicates that montelukast and its metabolites are excreted almost exclusively via the bile.

In several studies, the mean plasma half-life of montelukast ranged from 2.7 to 5.5 hours in healthy young adults. The pharmacokinetics of montelukast are nearly linear for oral doses up to 50 mg. During once-daily dosing with 10-mg montelukast, there is little accumulation of the parent drug in plasma (14%).

Special Populations

Hepatic Insufficiency: Patients with mild-to-moderate hepatic insufficiency and clinical evidence of cirrhosis had evidence of decreased metabolism of montelukast resulting in 41% (90% CI=7%, 85%) higher mean montelukast AUC following a single 10-mg dose. The elimination of montelukast was slightly prolonged compared with that in healthy subjects (mean half-life, 7.4 hours). No dosage adjustment is required in patients with mild-to-moderate hepatic insufficiency. The pharmacokinetics of SINGULAIR in patients with more severe hepatic impairment or with hepatitis have not been evaluated.

Renal Insufficiency: Since montelukast and its metabolites are not excreted in the urine, the pharmacokinetics of montelukast were not evaluated in patients with renal insufficiency. No dosage adjustment is recommended in these patients.

Gender: The pharmacokinetics of montelukast are similar in males and females.

Race: Pharmacokinetic differences due to race have not been studied.

Adolescents and Pediatric Patients: Pharmacokinetic studies evaluated the systemic exposure of the 4-mg oral granule formulation in pediatric patients 6 to 23 months of age, the 4-mg chewable tablets in pediatric patients 2 to 5 years of age, the 5-mg chewable tablets in pediatric patients 6 to 14 years of age, and the 10-mg film-coated tablets in young adults and adolescents ≥15 years of age.

The plasma concentration profile of montelukast following administration of the 10-mg film-coated tablet is similar in adolescents ≥15 years of age and young adults. The 10-mg film-coated tablet is recommended for use in patients ≥15 years of age.

The mean systemic exposure of the 4-mg chewable tablet in pediatric patients 2 to 5 years of age and the 5-mg chewable tablets in pediatric patients 6 to 14 years of age is similar to the mean systemic exposure of the 10-mg film-coated tablet in adults. The 5-mg chewable tablet should be used in pediatric patients 6 to 14 years of age and the 4-mg chewable tablet should be used in pediatric patients 2 to 5 years of age.

In children 6 to 11 months of age, the systemic exposure to montelukast and the variability of plasma montelukast concentrations were higher than those observed in adults. Based on population analyses, the mean AUC (4296 ng•hr/mL [range 1200 to 7153]) was 60% higher and the mean C_{max} (667 ng/mL [range 201 to 1058]) was 89% higher than those observed in adults (mean AUC 2689 ng•hr/mL [range 1521 to 4595]) and mean C_{max} (353 ng/mL [range 180 to 548]). The systemic exposure in children 12 to 23 months of age was less variable, but was still higher than that observed in adults. The mean AUC (3574 ng•hr/mL [range 2229 to 5408]) was 33% higher and the mean C_{max} (562 ng/mL [range 296 to 814]) was 60% higher than those observed in adults. Safety and tolerability of montelukast in a single-dose pharmacokinetic study in 26 children 6 to 23 months of age were similar to that of patients two years and above *[see Adverse Reactions (6.1)]*. The 4-mg oral granule formulation should be used for pediatric patients 12 to 23 months of age for the treatment of asthma, or for pediatric patients 6 to 23 months of age for the treatment of perennial allergic rhinitis. Since the 4-mg oral granule formulation is bioequivalent to the 4-mg chewable tablet, it can also be used as an alternative formulation to the 4-mg chewable tablet in pediatric patients 2 to 5 years of age.

Drug-Drug Interactions

Theophylline, Prednisone, and Prednisolone: SINGULAIR has been administered with other therapies routinely used in the prophylaxis and chronic treatment of asthma with no apparent increase in adverse reactions. In drug-interaction studies, the recommended clinical dose of montelukast did not have clinically important effects on the pharmacokinetics of the following drugs: theophylline, prednisone, and prednisolone.

Montelukast at a dose of 10 mg once daily dosed to pharmacokinetic steady state, did not cause clinically significant changes in the kinetics of a single intravenous dose of theophylline [predominantly a cytochrome P450 (CYP) 1A2 substrate]. Montelukast at doses of ≥100 mg daily dosed to pharmacokinetic steady state, did not cause any clinically significant change in plasma profiles of prednisone or prednisolone following administration of either oral prednisone or intravenous prednisolone.

Oral Contraceptives, Terfenadine, Digoxin, and Warfarin: In drug interaction studies, the recommended clinical dose of montelukast did not have clinically important effects on the pharmacokinetics of the following drugs: oral contraceptives (norethindrone 1 mg/ethinyl estradiol 35 mcg), terfenadine, digoxin, and warfarin. Montelukast at doses of ≥100 mg daily dosed to pharmacokinetic steady state did not significantly alter the plasma concentrations of either component of an oral contraceptive containing norethindrone 1 mg/ethinyl estradiol 35 mcg. Montelukast at a dose of 10 mg once daily dosed to pharmacokinetic steady state did not change the plasma concentration profile of terfenadine (a substrate of CYP3A4) or fexofenadine, the carboxylated metabolite, and did not prolong the QTc interval following co-administration with terfenadine 60 mg twice daily; did not change the pharmacokinetic profile or urinary excretion of immunoreactive digoxin; did not change the pharmacokinetic profile of warfarin (primarily a substrate of CYP2C9, 3A4 and 1A2) or influence the effect of a single 30-mg oral dose of warfarin on prothrombin time or the International Normalized Ratio (INR).

Thyroid Hormones, Sedative Hypnotics, Non-Steroidal Anti-Inflammatory Agents, Benzodiazepines, and Decongestants: Although additional specific interaction studies were not performed, SINGULAIR was used concomitantly with a wide range of commonly prescribed drugs in clinical studies without evidence of clinical adverse interactions. These medications included thyroid hormones, sedative hypnotics, non-steroidal anti-inflammatory agents, benzodiazepines, and decongestants.

Cytochrome P450 (CYP) Enzyme Inducers: Phenobarbital, which induces hepatic metabolism, decreased the area under the plasma concentration curve (AUC) of montelukast approximately 40% following a single 10-mg dose of montelukast. No dosage adjustment for SINGULAIR is recommended. It is reasonable to employ appropriate clinical monitoring when potent CYP enzyme inducers, such as phenobarbital or rifampin, are co-administered with SINGULAIR.

Effect of Montelukast on Cytochrome P450 (CYP) Enzymes: Montelukast is a potent inhibitor of CYP2C8 *in vitro.* However, data from a clinical drug-drug interaction study involving montelukast and rosiglitazone (a probe substrate representative of drugs primarily metabolized by CYP2C8) in 12 healthy individuals demonstrated that the pharmacokinetics of rosiglitazone are not altered when the drugs are coadministered, indicating that montelukast does not inhibit CYP2C8 *in vivo*. Therefore, montelukast is not anticipated to alter the metabolism of drugs metabolized by this enzyme (e.g., paclitaxel, rosiglitazone, and repaglinide). Based on further *in vitro* results in human liver microsomes, therapeutic plasma concentrations of montelukast do not inhibit CYP 3A4, 2C9, 1A2, 2A6, 2C19, or 2D6.

Cytochrome P450 (CYP) Enzyme Inhibitors: In vitro studies have shown that montelukast is a substrate of CYP 2C8, 2C9, and 3A4. Co-administration of montelukast with itraconazole, a strong CYP 3A4 inhibitor, resulted in no significant increase in the systemic exposure of montelukast. Data from a clinical drug-drug interaction study involving montelukast and gemfibrozil (an inhibitor of both CYP 2C8 and 2C9) demonstrated that gemfibrozil, at a therapeutic dose, increased the systemic exposure of montelukast by 4.4-fold. Co-administration of itraconazole, gemfibrozil, and montelukast did not further increase the systemic exposure of montelukast. Based on available clinical experience, no dosage adjustment of montelukast is required upon co-administration with gemfibrozil *[see Overdosage (10)]*.

13 NONCLINICAL TOXICOLOGY

13.1 Carcinogenesis, Mutagenesis, Impairment of Fertility

No evidence of tumorigenicity was seen in carcinogenicity studies of either 2 years in Sprague-Dawley rats or 92 weeks in mice at oral gavage doses up to 200 mg/kg/day or 100 mg/kg/day, respectively. The estimated exposure in rats was approximately 120 and 75 times the AUC for adults and children, respectively, at the maximum recommended daily oral dose. The estimated exposure in mice was approximately 45 and 25 times the AUC for adults and children, respectively, at the maximum recommended daily oral dose.

Montelukast demonstrated no evidence of mutagenic or clastogenic activity in the following assays: the microbial mutagenesis assay, the V-79 mammalian cell mutagenesis assay, the alkaline elution assay in rat hepatocytes, the chromosomal aberration assay in Chinese hamster ovary cells, and in the *in vivo* mouse bone marrow chromosomal aberration assay.

In fertility studies in female rats, montelukast produced reductions in fertility and fecundity indices at an oral dose of 200 mg/kg (estimated exposure was approximately 70 times the AUC for adults at the maximum recommended daily oral dose). No effects on female fertility or fecundity were observed at an oral dose of 100 mg/kg (estimated exposure was approximately 20 times the AUC for adults at the maximum recommended daily oral dose). Montelukast had no effects on fertility in male rats at oral doses up to 800 mg/kg (estimated exposure was approximately 160 times the AUC for adults at the maximum recommended daily oral dose).

13.2 Animal Toxicology and/or Pharmacology

Reproductive Toxicology Studies

No teratogenicity was observed at oral doses up to 400 mg/kg/day and 300 mg/kg/day in rats and rabbits, respectively. These doses were approximately 100 and 110 times the maximum recommended daily oral dose in adults, respectively, based on AUCs. Montelukast crosses the placenta following oral dosing in rats and rabbits *[see Pregnancy (8.1)]*.

14 CLINICAL STUDIES

14.1 Asthma

Adults and Adolescents 15 Years of Age and Older with Asthma

Clinical trials in adults and adolescents 15 years of age and older demonstrated there is no additional clinical benefit to montelukast doses above 10 mg once daily.

The efficacy of SINGULAIR for the chronic treatment of asthma in adults and adolescents 15 years of age and older was demonstrated in two (U.S. and Multinational) similarly designed, randomized, 12-week, double-blind, placebo-controlled trials in 1576 patients (795 treated with SINGULAIR, 530 treated with placebo, and 251 treated with active control). The median age was 33 years (range 15 to 85); 56.8% were females and 43.2% were males. The ethnic/racial distribution in these studies was 71.6% Caucasian, 17.7% Hispanic, 7.2% other origins and 3.5% Black. Patients had mild or moderate asthma and were non-smokers who required approximately 5 puffs of inhaled β-agonist per day on an "as-needed" basis. The patients had a mean baseline percent of predicted forced expiratory volume in 1 second (FEV_1) of 66% (approximate range, 40 to 90%). The co-primary endpoints in these trials were FEV_1 and daytime asthma symptoms. In both studies after 12 weeks, a random subset of patients receiving SINGULAIR was switched to placebo for an additional 3 weeks of double-blind treatment to evaluate for possible rebound effects.

The results of the U.S. trial on the primary endpoint, morning FEV_1, expressed as mean percent change from baseline averaged over the 12-week treatment period, are shown in FIGURE 2. Compared with placebo, treatment with one SINGULAIR 10-mg tablet daily in the evening resulted in a statistically significant increase in FEV_1 percent change from baseline (13.0%-change in the group treated with SINGULAIR vs. 4.2%-change in the placebo group, p<0.001); the change from baseline in FEV_1 for SINGULAIR was 0.32 liters compared with 0.10 liters for placebo, corresponding to a between-group difference of 0.22 liters (p<0.001, 95% CI 0.17 liters, 0.27 liters). The results of the Multinational trial on FEV_1 were similar.

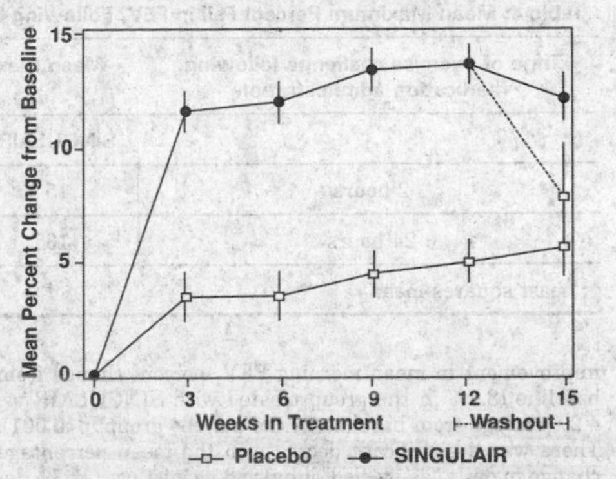

Figure 2: FEV_1 Mean Percent Change from Baseline (U.S. Trial: SINGULAIR N=406; Placebo N=270) (ANOVA Model)

The effect of SINGULAIR on other primary and secondary endpoints, represented by the Multinational study is shown in TABLE 2. Results on these endpoints were similar in the US study.

[See table 2 above]

Table 2: Effect of SINGULAIR on Primary and Secondary Endpoints in a Multinational Placebo-controlled Trial (ANOVA Model)

	SINGULAIR			Placebo		
Endpoint	N	Baseline	Mean Change from Baseline	N	Baseline	Mean Change from Baseline
Daytime Asthma Symptoms (0 to 6 scale)	372	2.35	-0.49*	245	2.40	-0.26
β-agonist (puffs per day)	371	5.35	-1.65*	241	5.78	-0.42
AM PEFR (L/min)	372	339.57	25.03*	244	335.24	1.83
PM PEFR (L/min)	372	355.23	20.13*	244	354.02	-0.49
Nocturnal Awakenings (#/week)	285	5.46	-2.03*	195	5.57	-0.78

* p<0.001, compared with placebo

Both studies evaluated the effect of SINGULAIR on secondary outcomes, including asthma attack (utilization of health-care resources such as an unscheduled visit to a doctor's office, emergency room, or hospital; or treatment with oral, intravenous, or intramuscular corticosteroid), and use of oral corticosteroids for asthma rescue. In the Multinational study, significantly fewer patients (15.6% of patients) on SINGULAIR experienced asthma attacks compared with patients on placebo (27.3%, p<0.001). In the US study, 7.8% of patients on SINGULAIR and 10.3% of patients on placebo experienced asthma attacks, but the difference between the two treatment groups was not significant (p=0.334). In the Multinational study, significantly fewer patients (14.8% of patients) on SINGULAIR were prescribed oral corticosteroids for asthma rescue compared with patients on placebo (25.7%, p<0.001). In the US study, 6.9% of patients on SINGULAIR and 9.9% of patients on placebo were prescribed oral corticosteroids for asthma rescue, but the difference between the two treatment groups was not significant (p=0.196).

Onset of Action and Maintenance of Effects

In each placebo-controlled trial in adults, the treatment effect of SINGULAIR, measured by daily diary card parameters, including symptom scores, "as-needed" β-agonist use, and PEFR measurements, was achieved after the first dose and was maintained throughout the dosing interval (24 hours). No significant change in treatment effect was observed during continuous once-daily evening administration in non-placebo-controlled extension trials for up to one year. Withdrawal of SINGULAIR in asthmatic patients after 12 weeks of continuous use did not cause rebound worsening of asthma.

Pediatric Patients 6 to 14 Years of Age with Asthma

The efficacy of SINGULAIR in pediatric patients 6 to 14 years of age was demonstrated in one 8-week, double-blind, placebo-controlled trial in 336 patients (201 treated with SINGULAIR and 135 treated with placebo) using an inhaled β-agonist on an "as-needed" basis. The patients had a mean baseline percent predicted FEV_1 of 72% (approximate range, 45 to 90%) and a mean daily inhaled β-agonist requirement of 3.4 puffs of albuterol. Approximately 36% of the patients were on inhaled corticosteroids. The median age was 11 years (range 6 to 15); 35.4% were females and 64.6% were males. The ethnic/racial distribution in this study was 80.1% Caucasian, 12.8% Black, 4.5% Hispanic, and 2.7% other origins.

Compared with placebo, treatment with one 5-mg SINGULAIR chewable tablet daily resulted in a significant

Table 3: Mean Maximum Percent Fall in FEV_1 Following Exercise Challenge in Study A (N=47) ANOVA Model

Time of exercise challenge following medication administration	Mean Maximum percent fall in FEV_1*		Treatment difference % for SINGULAIR versus Placebo (95% CI)*
	SINGULAIR	Placebo	
2 hours	13	22	-9 (-12, -5)
8.5 hours	12	17	-5 (-9, -2)
24 hours	10	14	-4 (-7, -1)

* Least squares-mean

Table 4: Mean Maximum Percent Fall in FEV_1 Following Exercise Challenge in Pediatric Patients (N=64) ANOVA Model

Time of exercise challenge following medication administration	Mean Maximum percent fall in FEV_1*		Treatment difference % for SINGULAIR versus Placebo (95% CI)*
	SINGULAIR	Placebo	
2 hours	15	20	-5 (-9, -1)
24 hours	13	17	-4 (-7, -1)

* Least squares-mean

improvement in mean morning FEV_1 percent change from baseline (8.7% in the group treated with SINGULAIR vs. 4.2% change from baseline in the placebo group, p<0.001). There was a significant decrease in the mean percentage change in daily "as-needed" inhaled β-agonist use (11.7% decrease from baseline in the group treated with SINGULAIR vs. 8.2% increase from baseline in the placebo group, p<0.05). This effect represents a mean decrease from baseline of 0.56 and 0.23 puffs per day for the montelukast and placebo groups, respectively. Subgroup analyses indicated that younger pediatric patients aged 6 to 11 had efficacy results comparable to those of the older pediatric patients aged 12 to 14.

Similar to the adult studies, no significant change in the treatment effect was observed during continuous once-daily administration in one open-label extension trial without a concurrent placebo group for up to 6 months.

Pediatric Patients 2 to 5 Years of Age with Asthma

The efficacy of SINGULAIR for the chronic treatment of asthma in pediatric patients 2 to 5 years of age was explored in a 12-week, placebo-controlled safety and tolerability study in 689 patients, 461 of whom were treated with SINGULAIR. The median age was 4 years (range 2 to 6); 41.5% were females and 58.5% were males. The ethnic/racial distribution in this study was 56.5% Caucasian, 20.9% Hispanic, 14.4% other origins, and 8.3% Black.

While the primary objective was to determine the safety and tolerability of SINGULAIR in this age group, the study included exploratory efficacy evaluations, including daytime and overnight asthma symptom scores, β-agonist use, oral corticosteroid rescue, and the physician's global evaluation. The findings of these exploratory efficacy evaluations, along with pharmacokinetics and extrapolation of efficacy data from older patients, support the overall conclusion that SINGULAIR is efficacious in the maintenance treatment of asthma in patients 2 to 5 years of age.

Effects in Patients on Concomitant Inhaled Corticosteroids

Separate trials in adults evaluated the ability of SINGULAIR to add to the clinical effect of inhaled corticosteroids and to allow inhaled corticosteroid tapering when used concomitantly.

One randomized, placebo-controlled, parallel-group trial (n=226) enrolled adults with stable asthma with a mean FEV_1 of approximately 84% of predicted who were previously maintained on various inhaled corticosteroids (delivered by metered-dose aerosol or dry powder inhalers). The median age was 41.5 years (range 16 to 70); 52.2% were females and 47.8% were males. The ethnic/racial distribution in this study was 92.0% Caucasian, 3.5% Black, 2.2% Hispanic, and 2.2% Asian. The types of inhaled corticosteroids and their mean baseline requirements included beclomethasone dipropionate (mean dose, 1203 mcg/day), triamcinolone acetonide (mean dose, 2004 mcg/day), flunisolide (mean dose, 1971 mcg/day), fluticasone propionate (mean dose, 1083 mcg/day), or budesonide (mean dose, 1192 mcg/day). Some of these inhaled corticosteroids were non-U.S.-approved formulations, and doses expressed may not be ex-actuator. The pre-study inhaled corticosteroid requirements were reduced by approximately 37% during a 5- to 7-week placebo run-in period designed to titrate patients toward their lowest effective inhaled corticosteroid dose. Treatment with SINGULAIR resulted in a further 47% reduction in mean inhaled corticosteroid dose compared with a mean reduction of 30% in the placebo group over the 12-week active treatment period (p≤0.05). It is not known whether the results of this study can be generalized to patients with asthma who require higher doses of inhaled corticosteroids or systemic corticosteroids.

In another randomized, placebo-controlled, parallel-group trial (n=642) in a similar population of adult patients previously maintained, but not adequately controlled, on inhaled corticosteroids (beclomethasone 336 mcg/day), the addition of SINGULAIR to beclomethasone resulted in statistically significant improvements in FEV_1 compared with those patients who were continued on beclomethasone alone or those patients who were withdrawn from beclomethasone and treated with montelukast or placebo alone over the last 10 weeks of the 16-week, blinded treatment period. Patients who were randomized to treatment arms containing beclomethasone had statistically significantly better asthma control than those patients randomized to SINGULAIR alone or placebo alone as indicated by FEV_1, daytime asthma symptoms, PEFR, nocturnal awakenings due to asthma, and "as-needed" β-agonist requirements.

In adult patients with asthma with documented aspirin sensitivity, nearly all of whom were receiving concomitant inhaled and/or oral corticosteroids, a 4-week, randomized, parallel-group trial (n=80) demonstrated that SINGULAIR, compared with placebo, resulted in significant improvement in parameters of asthma control. The magnitude of effect of SINGULAIR in aspirin-sensitive patients was similar to the effect observed in the general population of asthma patients studied. The effect of SINGULAIR on the bronchoconstrictor response to aspirin or other non-steroidal anti-inflammatory drugs in aspirin-sensitive asthmatic patients has not been evaluated *[see Warnings and Precautions (5.3)]*.

14.2 Exercise-Induced Bronchoconstriction (EIB)

Exercise-Induced Bronchoconstriction (Adults, Adolescents, and Pediatric Patients 6 years of age and older)

The efficacy of SINGULAIR, 10 mg, when given as a single dose 2 hours before exercise for the prevention of EIB was investigated in three (U.S. and Multinational), randomized, double-blind, placebo-controlled crossover studies that included a total of 160 adult and adolescent patients 15 years of age and older with EIB. Exercise challenge testing was conducted at 2 hours, 8.5 or 12 hours, and 24 hours following administration of a single dose of study drug (SINGULAIR 10 mg or placebo). The primary endpoint was the mean maximum percent fall in FEV_1 following the 2 hours post-dose exercise challenge in all three studies (Study A, Study B, and Study C). In Study A, a single dose of SINGULAIR 10 mg demonstrated a statistically significant protective benefit against EIB when taken 2 hours prior to exercise. Some patients were protected from EIB at 8.5 and 24 hours after administration; however, some patients were not. The results for the mean maximum percent fall at each timepoint in Study A are shown in TABLE 3 and are representative of the results from the other two studies.

[See table 3 above]

The efficacy of SINGULAIR 5-mg chewable tablets, when given as a single dose 2 hours before exercise for the prevention of EIB, was investigated in one multinational, randomized, double-blind, placebo-controlled crossover study that included a total of 64 pediatric patients 6 to 14 years of age with EIB. Exercise challenge testing was conducted at 2 hours and 24 hours following administration of a single dose of study drug (SINGULAIR 5 mg or placebo). The primary endpoint was the mean maximum percent fall in FEV_1 following the 2 hours post-dose exercise challenge. A single dose of SINGULAIR 5 mg demonstrated a statistically significant protective benefit against EIB when taken 2 hours prior to exercise (TABLE 4). Similar results were shown at 24 hours post-dose (a secondary endpoint). Some patients were protected from EIB at 24 hours after administration; however, some patients were not. No timepoints were assessed between 2 and 24 hours post-dose.

[See table 4 above]

The efficacy of SINGULAIR for prevention of EIB in patients below 6 years of age has not been established.

Daily administration of SINGULAIR for the chronic treatment of asthma has not been established to prevent acute episodes of EIB.

In a 12-week, randomized, double-blind, parallel group study of 110 adult and adolescent asthmatics 15 years of age and older, with a mean baseline FEV_1 percent of predicted of 83% and with documented exercise-induced exacerbation of asthma, treatment with SINGULAIR, 10 mg, once daily in the evening, resulted in a statistically significant reduction in mean maximal percent fall in FEV_1 and mean time to recovery to within 5% of the pre-exercise FEV_1. Exercise challenge was conducted at the end of the dosing interval (i.e., 20 to 24 hours after the preceding dose). This effect was maintained throughout the 12-week treatment period indicating that tolerance did not occur. SINGULAIR did not, however, prevent clinically significant deterioration in maximal percent fall in FEV_1 after exercise (i.e., ≥20% decrease from pre-exercise baseline) in 52% of patients studied. In a separate crossover study in adults, a similar effect was observed after two once-daily 10-mg doses of SINGULAIR.

In pediatric patients 6 to 14 years of age, using the 5-mg chewable tablet, a 2-day crossover study demonstrated effects similar to those observed in adults when exercise challenge was conducted at the end of the dosing interval (i.e., 20 to 24 hours after the preceding dose).

14.3 Allergic Rhinitis (Seasonal and Perennial)

Seasonal Allergic Rhinitis

The efficacy of SINGULAIR tablets for the treatment of seasonal allergic rhinitis was investigated in 5 similarly designed, randomized, double-blind, parallel-group, placebo- and active-controlled (loratadine) trials conducted in North America. The 5 trials enrolled a total of 5029 patients, of whom 1799 were treated with SINGULAIR tablets. Patients were 15 to 82 years of age with a history of seasonal allergic rhinitis, a positive skin test to at least one relevant seasonal allergen, and active symptoms of seasonal allergic rhinitis at study entry.

The period of randomized treatment was 2 weeks in 4 trials and 4 weeks in one trial. The primary outcome variable was mean change from baseline in daytime nasal symptoms score (the average of individual scores of nasal congestion, rhinorrhea, nasal itching, sneezing) as assessed by patients on a 0-3 categorical scale.

Four of the five trials showed a significant reduction in daytime nasal symptoms scores with SINGULAIR 10-mg tablets compared with placebo. The results of one trial are shown below. The median age in this trial was 35.0 years (range 15 to 81); 65.4% were females and 34.6% were males. The ethnic/racial distribution in this study was 83.1% Caucasian, 6.4% other origins, 5.8% Black, and 4.8% Hispanic. The mean changes from baseline in daytime nasal symptoms score in the treatment groups that received SINGULAIR tablets, loratadine, and placebo are shown in TABLE 5. The remaining three trials that demonstrated efficacy showed similar results.

[See table 5 at top of next page]

Perennial Allergic Rhinitis

The efficacy of SINGULAIR tablets for the treatment of perennial allergic rhinitis was investigated in 2 randomized, double-blind, placebo-controlled studies conducted in North America and Europe. The two studies enrolled a total of 3357 patients, of whom 1632 received SINGULAIR 10-mg tablets. Patients 15 to 82 years of age with perennial allergic rhinitis as confirmed by history and a positive skin test to at least one relevant perennial allergen (dust mites, animal dander, and/or mold spores), who had active symptoms at the time of study entry, were enrolled.

In the study in which efficacy was demonstrated, the median age was 35 years (range 15 to 81); 64.1% were females and 35.9% were males. The ethnic/racial distribution in this study was 83.2% Caucasian, 8.1% Black, 5.4% Hispanic, 2.3% Asian, and 1.0% other origins. SINGULAIR 10-mg tablets once daily was shown to significantly reduce symptoms of perennial allergic rhinitis over a 6-week treatment period (TABLE 6); in this study the primary outcome variable was mean change from baseline in daytime nasal symptoms score (the average of individual scores of nasal congestion, rhinorrhea, and sneezing).

[See table 6 at top of next page]

The other 6-week study evaluated SINGULAIR 10 mg (n=626), placebo (n=609), and an active-control (cetirizine 10 mg; n=120). The primary analysis compared the mean change from baseline in daytime nasal symptoms score for SINGULAIR vs. placebo over the first 4 weeks of treatment; the study was not designed for statistical comparison between SINGULAIR and the active-control. The primary outcome variable included nasal itching in addition to nasal congestion, rhinorrhea, and sneezing. The estimated difference between SINGULAIR and placebo was -0.04 with a 95% CI of (-0.09, 0.01). The estimated difference between the active-control and placebo was -0.10 with a 95% CI of (-0.19, -0.01).

Table 5: Effects of SINGULAIR on Daytime Nasal Symptoms Score* in a Placebo- and Active-controlled Trial in Patients with Seasonal Allergic Rhinitis (ANCOVA Model)

Treatment Group (N)	Baseline Mean Score	Mean Change from Baseline	Difference Between Treatment and Placebo (95% CI) Least-Squares Mean
SINGULAIR 10 mg (344)	2.09	-0.39	-0.13† (-0.21, -0.06)
Placebo (351)	2.10	-0.26	N.A.
Active Control‡ (Loratadine 10 mg) (599)	2.06	-0.46	-0.24† (-0.31, -0.17)

* Average of individual scores of nasal congestion, rhinorrhea, nasal itching, sneezing as assessed by patients on a 0-3 categorical scale.
† Statistically different from placebo (p≤0.001).
‡ The study was not designed for statistical comparison between SINGULAIR and the active control (loratadine).

Table 6: Effects of SINGULAIR on Daytime Nasal Symptoms Score* in a Placebo-controlled Trial in Patients with Perennial Allergic Rhinitis (ANCOVA Model)

Treatment Group (N)	Baseline Mean Score	Mean Change from Baseline	Difference Between Treatment and Placebo (95% CI) Least-Squares Mean
SINGULAIR 10 mg (1000)	2.09	-0.42	-0.08† (-0.12, -0.04)
Placebo (980)	2.10	-0.35	N.A.

* Average of individual scores of nasal congestion, rhinorrhea, sneezing as assessed by patients on a 0-3 categorical scale.
† Statistically different from placebo (p≤0.001).

16 HOW SUPPLIED/STORAGE AND HANDLING

No. 3841 — SINGULAIR Oral Granules, 4 mg, are white granules with 500 mg net weight, packed in a child-resistant foil packet. They are supplied as follows:
NDC 0006-3841-30 unit of use carton with 30 packets.
SINGULAIR Tablets, 4 mg, are pink, oval, bi-convex-shaped chewable tablets. They are supplied as either No. 3796 or No. 6628:
No. 3796 — with code MRK 711 on one side and SINGULAIR on the other:
NDC 0006-0711-31 unit of use high-density polyethylene (HDPE) bottles of 30 with a polypropylene child-resistant cap, an aluminum foil induction seal, and silica gel desiccant
NDC 0006-0711-54 unit of use high-density polyethylene (HDPE) bottles of 90 with a polypropylene child-resistant cap, an aluminum foil induction seal, and silica gel desiccant
NDC 0006-0711-28 unit dose paper and aluminum foil-backed aluminum foil peelable blister packs of 100.
No. 6628 — with code MSD 711 on one side and SINGULAIR on the other:
NDC 0006-1711-31 unit of use high-density polyethylene (HDPE) bottles of 30 with a polypropylene child-resistant cap, an aluminum foil induction seal, and silica gel desiccant
NDC 0006-1711-54 unit of use high-density polyethylene (HDPE) bottles of 90 with a polypropylene child-resistant cap, an aluminum foil induction seal, and silica gel desiccant.
SINGULAIR Tablets, 5 mg, are pink, round, bi-convex-shaped chewable tablets. They are supplied as either No. 3760 or No. 6543:
No. 3760 — with code MRK 275 on one side and SINGULAIR on the other:
NDC 0006-0275-31 unit of use high-density polyethylene (HDPE) bottles of 30 with a polypropylene child-resistant cap, an aluminum foil induction seal, and silica gel desiccant
NDC 0006-0275-54 unit of use high-density polyethylene (HDPE) bottles of 90 with a polypropylene child-resistant cap, an aluminum foil induction seal, and silica gel desiccant
NDC 0006-0275-28 unit dose paper and aluminum foil-backed aluminum foil peelable blister packs of 100
NDC 0006-0275-82 bulk packaging high-density polyethylene (HDPE) bottles of 1000 with a non-child-resistant white plastic closure with a wax paper/pulp liner, an aluminum foil induction seal, and silica gel desiccant.
No. 6543 — with code MSD 275 on one side and SINGULAIR on the other:
NDC 0006-9275-31 unit of use high-density polyethylene (HDPE) bottles of 30 with a polypropylene child-resistant cap, an aluminum foil induction seal, and silica gel desiccant
NDC 0006-9275-54 unit of use high-density polyethylene (HDPE) bottles of 90 with a polypropylene child-resistant cap, an aluminum foil induction seal, and silica gel desiccant
NDC 0006-9275-82 bulk packaging high-density polyethylene (HDPE) bottles of 1000 with a non-child-resistant white plastic closure with a wax paper/pulp liner, an aluminum foil induction seal, and silica gel desiccant.
SINGULAIR Tablets, 10 mg, are beige, rounded square-shaped, film-coated tablets. They are supplied as either No. 3761 or No. 6558:
No. 3761 — with code MRK 117 on one side and SINGULAIR on the other:
NDC 0006-0117-31 unit of use high-density polyethylene (HDPE) bottles of 30 with a polypropylene child-resistant cap, an aluminum foil induction seal, and silica gel desiccant
NDC 0006-0117-54 unit of use high-density polyethylene (HDPE) bottles of 90 with a polypropylene child-resistant cap, an aluminum foil induction seal, and silica gel desiccant
NDC 0006-0117-28 unit dose paper and aluminum foil-backed aluminum foil peelable blister pack of 100
NDC 0006-0117-80 bulk packaging high-density polyethylene (HDPE) bottles of 8000 with a non-child-resistant white plastic closure with a wax paper/pulp liner, an aluminum foil induction seal, and silica gel desiccant.
No. 6558 — with code MSD 117 on one side and SINGULAIR on the other:
NDC 0006-9117-31 unit of use high-density polyethylene (HDPE) bottles of 30 with a polypropylene child-resistant cap, an aluminum foil induction seal, and silica gel desiccant
NDC 0006-9117-54 unit of use high-density polyethylene (HDPE) bottles of 90 with a polypropylene child-resistant cap, an aluminum foil induction seal, and silica gel desiccant
NDC 0006-9117-80 bulk packaging high-density polyethylene (HDPE) bottles of 8000 with a non-child-resistant white plastic closure with a wax paper/pulp liner, an aluminum foil induction seal, and silica gel desiccant.

Storage
Store SINGULAIR 4-mg oral granules, 4-mg chewable tablets, 5-mg chewable tablets and 10-mg film-coated tablets at 25°C (77°F), excursions permitted to 15-30°C (59-86°F) [see USP Controlled Room Temperature]. Protect from moisture and light. Store in original package.

Storage for Bulk Bottles
Store bottles of 1000 SINGULAIR 5-mg chewable tablets and 8000 SINGULAIR 10-mg film-coated tablets at 25°C (77°F), excursions permitted to 15-30°C (59-86°F) [see USP Controlled Room Temperature]. Protect from moisture and light. Store in original container. When product container is subdivided, repackage into a well-closed, light-resistant container.

17 PATIENT COUNSELING INFORMATION

See FDA-approved patient labeling (Patient Information).

Information for Patients

- Patients should be advised to take SINGULAIR daily as prescribed, even when they are asymptomatic, as well as during periods of worsening asthma, and to contact their physicians if their asthma is not well controlled.
- Patients should be advised that oral SINGULAIR is not for the treatment of acute asthma attacks. They should have appropriate short-acting inhaled β-agonist medication available to treat asthma exacerbations. Patients who have exacerbations of asthma after exercise should be instructed to have available for rescue a short-acting inhaled β-agonist. Daily administration of SINGULAIR for the chronic treatment of asthma has not been established to prevent acute episodes of EIB.
- Patients should be advised that, while using SINGULAIR, medical attention should be sought if short-acting inhaled bronchodilators are needed more often than usual, or if more than the maximum number of inhalations of short-acting bronchodilator treatment prescribed for a 24-hour period are needed.
- Patients receiving SINGULAIR should be instructed not to decrease the dose or stop taking any other anti-asthma medications unless instructed by a physician.
- Patients should be instructed to notify their physician if neuropsychiatric events occur while using SINGULAIR.
- Patients with known aspirin sensitivity should be advised to continue avoidance of aspirin or non-steroidal anti-inflammatory agents while taking SINGULAIR.
- Phenylketonuric patients should be informed that the 4-mg and 5-mg chewable tablets contain phenylalanine (a component of aspartame).

Dist. by: Merck Sharp & Dohme Corp., a subsidiary of **MERCK & CO., INC.**, Whitehouse Station, NJ 08889, USA

uspi-0476-mf-1306r029

Patient Information
SINGULAIR® (SING-u-lair)
(montelukast sodium)
Tablets
SINGULAIR®
(montelukast sodium)
Chewable Tablets
SINGULAIR®
(montelukast sodium)
Oral Granules

Read the Patient Information Leaflet that comes with SINGULAIR® before you start taking it and each time you get a refill. There may be new information. This leaflet does not take the place of talking with your healthcare provider about your medical condition or your treatment.

What is SINGULAIR?

- SINGULAIR is a prescription medicine that blocks substances in the body called leukotrienes. This may help to improve symptoms of asthma and allergic rhinitis. SINGULAIR does not contain a steroid.

SINGULAIR is used to:

1. Prevent asthma attacks and for the long-term treatment of asthma in adults and children ages 12 months and older.
   Do not take SINGULAIR if you need relief right away for a sudden asthma attack. If you get an asthma attack, you should follow the instructions your healthcare provider gave you for treating asthma attacks.
2. Prevent exercise-induced asthma in people 6 years of age and older.
3. Help control the symptoms of allergic rhinitis (sneezing, stuffy nose, runny nose, itching of the nose). SINGULAIR is used to treat:
   - outdoor allergies that happen part of the year (seasonal allergic rhinitis) in adults and children ages 2 years and older, **and**
   - indoor allergies that happen all year (perennial allergic rhinitis) in adults and children ages 6 months and older.

Who should not take SINGULAIR?

Do not take SINGULAIR if you are allergic to any of its ingredients.
See the end of this leaflet for a complete list of the ingredients in SINGULAIR.

What should I tell my healthcare provider before taking SINGULAIR?

Before taking SINGULAIR, tell your healthcare provider if you:

- are allergic to aspirin
- have phenylketonuria. SINGULAIR chewable tablets contain aspartame, a source of phenylalanine

- have any other medical conditions
- are pregnant or plan to become pregnant. Talk to your doctor if you are pregnant or plan to become pregnant, as SINGULAIR may not be right for you.
- are breast-feeding or plan to breast-feed. It is not known if SINGULAIR passes into your breast milk. Talk to your healthcare provider about the best way to feed your baby while taking SINGULAIR.

Tell your healthcare provider about all the medicines you take, including prescription and non-prescription medicines, vitamins, and herbal supplements. Some medicines may affect how SINGULAIR works, or SINGULAIR may affect how your other medicines work.

How should I take SINGULAIR?

For anyone who takes SINGULAIR:

- Take SINGULAIR exactly as prescribed by your healthcare provider. Your healthcare provider will tell you how much SINGULAIR to take, and **when to take it.**
- Do not stop taking SINGULAIR or change when you take it without talking with your healthcare provider.
- You can take SINGULAIR with food or without food. See the information below in the section "How should I give SINGULAIR oral granules to my child?" for information about what foods and liquids can be taken with SINGULAIR oral granules.
- **If you or your child misses a dose of SINGULAIR, just take the next dose at your regular time.** Do not take 2 doses at the same time.
- If you take too much SINGULAIR, call your healthcare provider or a Poison Control Center right away.

For adults and children 12 months of age and older with asthma:

- Take SINGULAIR 1 time each day, in the evening. Continue to take SINGULAIR every day for as long as your healthcare provider prescribes it, even if you have no asthma symptoms.
- Tell your healthcare provider right away if your asthma symptoms get worse, or if you need to use your rescue inhaler medicine more often for asthma attacks.
- **Do not take SINGULAIR if you need relief right away from a sudden asthma attack.** If you get an asthma attack, you should follow the instructions your healthcare provider gave you for treating asthma attacks.
- Always have your rescue inhaler medicine with you for asthma attacks.
- Do not stop taking or lower the dose of your other asthma medicines unless your healthcare provider tells you to.

For patients 6 years of age and older for the prevention of exercise-induced asthma:

- Take SINGULAIR at least 2 hours before exercise.
- Always have your rescue inhaler medicine with you for asthma attacks.
- If you take SINGULAIR every day for chronic asthma or allergic rhinitis, **do not** take another dose to prevent exercise-induced asthma. Talk to your healthcare provider about your treatment for exercise-induced asthma.
- **Do not take 2 doses of SINGULAIR within 24 hours (1 day).**

For adults and children 2 years of age and older with seasonal allergic rhinitis, or for adults and children 6 months of age and older with perennial allergic rhinitis:

- Take SINGULAIR 1 time each day, at about the same time each day.

How should I give SINGULAIR oral granules to my child?

Give SINGULAIR oral granules to your child exactly as instructed by your healthcare provider.

Do not open the packet until ready to use.

SINGULAIR 4-mg oral granules can be given:

- right in the mouth; or
- dissolved in 1 teaspoonful (5 mL) of cold or room temperature baby formula or breast milk; or
- mixed with 1 spoonful of one of the following soft foods at cold or room temperature: applesauce, mashed carrots, rice, or ice cream.

Give the child all of the mixture right away, within 15 minutes.

Do not store any leftover SINGULAIR mixture (oral granules mixed with food, baby formula, or breast milk) for use at a later time. Throw away any unused portion.

Do not mix SINGULAIR oral granules with any liquid drink other than baby formula or breast milk. Your child may drink other liquids after swallowing the mixture.

What is the dose of SINGULAIR?

The dose of SINGULAIR prescribed for your or your child's condition is based on age:

- 6 to 23 months: one packet of 4-mg oral granules.
- 2 to 5 years: one 4-mg chewable tablet or one packet of 4-mg oral granules.
- 6 to 14 years: one 5-mg chewable tablet.
- 15 years and older: one 10-mg tablet.

What should I avoid while taking SINGULAIR?

If you have asthma and aspirin makes your asthma symptoms worse, continue to avoid taking aspirin or other medicines called non-steroidal anti-inflammatory drugs (NSAIDs) while taking SINGULAIR.

What are the possible side effects of SINGULAIR?

SINGULAIR may cause serious side effects.

- **Behavior and mood-related changes.** Tell your healthcare provider right away if you or your child have any of these symptoms while taking SINGULAIR:
  - agitation including aggressive behavior or hostility
  - attention problems
  - bad or vivid dreams
  - depression
  - disorientation (confusion)
  - feeling anxious
  - hallucinations (seeing or hearing things that are not really there)
  - irritability
  - memory problems
  - restlessness
  - sleep walking
  - suicidal thoughts and actions (including suicide)
  - tremor
  - trouble sleeping
- **Increase in certain white blood cells (eosinophils) and possible inflamed blood vessels throughout the body (systemic vasculitis).** Rarely, this can happen in people with asthma who take SINGULAIR. This sometimes happens in people who also take a steroid medicine by mouth that is being stopped or the dose is being lowered.
  Tell your healthcare provider right away if you get one or more of these symptoms:
  - a feeling of pins and needles or numbness of arms or legs
  - a flu-like illness
  - rash
  - severe inflammation (pain and swelling) of the sinuses (sinusitis)

The most common side effects with SINGULAIR include:

- upper respiratory infection
- fever
- headache
- sore throat
- cough
- stomach pain
- diarrhea
- earache or ear infection
- flu
- runny nose
- sinus infection

Other side effects with SINGULAIR include:

- increased bleeding tendency, low blood platelet count
- allergic reactions [including swelling of the face, lips, tongue, and/or throat (which may cause trouble breathing or swallowing), hives and itching]
- dizziness, drowsiness, pins and needles/numbness, seizures (convulsions or fits)
- palpitations
- nose bleed, stuffy nose, swelling (inflammation) of the lungs
- heartburn, indigestion, inflammation of the pancreas, nausea, stomach or intestinal upset, vomiting
- hepatitis
- bruising, rash, severe skin reactions (erythema multiforme, Stevens-Johnson syndrome/toxic epidermal necrolysis) that may occur without warning
- joint pain, muscle aches and muscle cramps
- tiredness, swelling

Tell your healthcare provider if you have any side effect that bothers you or that does not go away.

These are not all the possible side effects of SINGULAIR. For more information ask your healthcare provider or pharmacist.

Call your healthcare provider for medical advice about side effects. You may report side effects to FDA at 1-800-FDA-1088.

How should I store SINGULAIR?

- Store SINGULAIR at 59°F to 86°F (15°C to 30°C).
- Keep SINGULAIR in the container it comes in.
- Keep SINGULAIR in a dry place and away from light.

General Information about the safe and effective use of SINGULAIR

Medicines are sometimes prescribed for purposes other than those mentioned in Patient Information Leaflets. Do not use SINGULAIR for a condition for which it was not prescribed. Do not give SINGULAIR to other people even if they have the same symptoms you have. It may harm them. **Keep SINGULAIR and all medicines out of the reach of children.**

This leaflet summarizes information about SINGULAIR. If you would like more information, talk to your healthcare provider. You can ask your pharmacist or healthcare provider for information about SINGULAIR that is written for health professionals. For more information, call the Merck National Service Center at 1-800-NSC-Merck (1-800-672-6372).

What are the ingredients in SINGULAIR?

Active ingredient: montelukast sodium

Inactive ingredients:

- 4-mg oral granules: mannitol, hydroxypropyl cellulose, and magnesium stearate.
- 4-mg and 5-mg chewable tablets: mannitol, microcrystalline cellulose, hydroxypropyl cellulose, red ferric oxide, croscarmellose sodium, cherry flavor, aspartame, and magnesium stearate.
  People with Phenylketonuria: SINGULAIR 4-mg chewable tablets contain 0.674 mg of phenylalanine, and SINGULAIR 5-mg chewable tablets contain 0.842 mg of phenylalanine.
- 10-mg tablet: microcrystalline cellulose, lactose monohydrate, croscarmellose sodium, hydroxypropyl cellulose, and magnesium stearate. The film coating contains: hydroxypropyl methylcellulose, hydroxypropyl cellulose, titanium dioxide, red ferric oxide, yellow ferric oxide, and carnauba wax.

Dist. by: Merck Sharp & Dohme Corp., a subsidiary of **MERCK & CO., INC.**, Whitehouse Station, NJ 08889, USA

Revised: 06/2013
usppi-0476-mf-1306r029

Shown in Product Identification Guide, page 309

STROMECTOL® ℞

[stro-mec-tol]
(ivermectin)
Tablets

DESCRIPTION

STROMECTOL[1] (Ivermectin) is a semisynthetic, anthelmintic agent for oral administration. Ivermectin is derived from the avermectins, a class of highly active broad-spectrum, anti-parasitic agents isolated from the fermentation products of *Streptomyces avermitilis.* Ivermectin is a mixture containing at least 90% 5-*O*-demethyl-22,23-dihydroavermectin A_{1a} and less than 10% 5-*O*-demethyl-25-de(1-methylpropyl)-22,23-dihydro-25-(1-methylethyl)avermectin A_{1a}, generally referred to as 22,23-dihydroavermectin B_{1a} and B_{1b}, or H_2B_{1a} and H_2B_{1b}, respectively. The respective empirical formulas are $C_{48}H_{74}O_{14}$ and $C_{47}H_{72}O_{14}$, with molecular weights of 875.10 and 861.07, respectively. The structural formulas are:

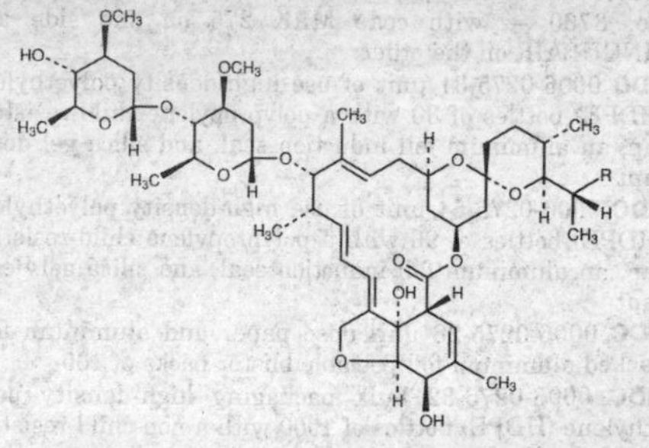

Component B_{1a}, R = C_2H_5 Component B_{1b}, R = CH_3

Ivermectin is a white to yellowish-white, nonhygroscopic, crystalline powder with a melting point of about 155°C. It is insoluble in water but is freely soluble in methanol and soluble in 95% ethanol.

STROMECTOL is available in 3-mg tablets containing the following inactive ingredients: microcrystalline cellulose, pregelatinized starch, magnesium stearate, butylated hydroxyanisole, and citric acid powder (anhydrous).

[1]Registered trademark of Merck Sharp & Dohme Corp., a subsidiary of **Merck & Co., Inc.**

CLINICAL PHARMACOLOGY

Pharmacokinetics

Following oral administration of ivermectin, plasma concentrations are approximately proportional to the dose. In two studies, after single 12-mg doses of STROMECTOL in fasting healthy volunteers (representing a mean dose of 165 mcg/kg), the mean peak plasma concentrations of the major component (H_2B_{1a}) were 46.6 (±21.9) (range: 16.4-101.1) and 30.6 (±15.6) (range: 13.9-68.4) ng/mL, respectively, at approximately 4 hours after dosing. Ivermectin is metabolized in the liver, and ivermectin and/or its metabolites are excreted almost exclusively in the feces over an estimated 12 days, with less than 1% of the administered dose excreted in the urine. The plasma half-life of ivermectin in man is approximately 18 hours following oral administration.

The safety and pharmacokinetic properties of ivermectin were further assessed in a multiple-dose clinical pharmacokinetic study involving healthy volunteers. Subjects received oral doses of 30 to 120 mg (333 to 2000 mcg/kg) ivermectin in a fasted state or 30 mg (333 to 600 mcg/kg) ivermectin following a standard high-fat (48.6 g of fat) meal. Administration of 30 mg ivermectin following a high-fat meal resulted in an approximate 2.5 fold increase in bioavailability relative to administration of 30 mg ivermectin in the fasted state.

In vitro studies using human liver microsomes and recombinant CYP450 enzymes have shown that ivermectin is primarily metabolized by CYP3A4. Depending on the *in vitro* method used, CYP2D6 and CYP2E1 were also shown to be involved in the metabolism of ivermectin but to a significantly lower extent compared to CYP3A4. The findings of *in vitro* studies using human liver microsomes suggest that clinically relevant concentrations of ivermectin do not significantly inhibit the metabolizing activities of CYP3A4, CYP2D6, CYP2C9, CYP1A2, and CYP2E1.

Microbiology

Ivermectin is a member of the avermectin class of broad-spectrum antiparasitic agents which have a unique mode of action. Compounds of the class bind selectively and with high affinity to glutamate-gated chloride ion channels which occur in invertebrate nerve and muscle cells. This leads to an increase in the permeability of the cell membrane to chloride ions with hyperpolarization of the nerve or muscle cell, resulting in paralysis and death of the parasite. Compounds of this class may also interact with other ligand-gated chloride channels, such as those gated by the neurotransmitter gamma-aminobutyric acid (GABA).

The selective activity of compounds of this class is attributable to the facts that some mammals do not have glutamate-gated chloride channels and that the avermectins have a low affinity for mammalian ligand-gated chloride channels. In addition, ivermectin does not readily cross the blood-brain barrier in humans.

Ivermectin is active against various life-cycle stages of many but not all nematodes. It is active against the tissue microfilariae of *Onchocerca volvulus* but not against the adult form. Its activity against *Strongyloides stercoralis* is limited to the intestinal stages.

Clinical Studies

Strongyloidiasis

Two controlled clinical studies using albendazole as the comparative agent were carried out in international sites where albendazole is approved for the treatment of strongyloidiasis of the gastrointestinal tract, and three controlled studies were carried out in the U.S. and internationally using thiabendazole as the comparative agent. Efficacy, as measured by cure rate, was defined as the absence of larvae in at least two follow-up stool examinations 3 to 4 weeks post-therapy. Based on this criterion, efficacy was significantly greater for STROMECTOL (a single dose of 170 to 200 mcg/kg) than for albendazole (200 mg b.i.d. for 3 days). STROMECTOL administered as a single dose of 200 mcg/kg for 1 day was as efficacious as thiabendazole administered at 25 mg/kg b.i.d. for 3 days.

Summary of Cure Rates for Ivermectin Versus Comparative Agents in the Treatment of Strongyloidiasis

	Cure Rate* (%)	
	Ivermectin†	Comparative Agent
Albendazole‡ Comparative		
International Study	24/26 (92)	12/22 (55)
WHO Study	126/152 (83)	67/149 (45)
Thiabendazole§ Comparative		
International Study	9/14 (64)	13/15 (87)
US Studies	14/14 (100)	16/17 (94)

* Number and % of evaluable patients
† 170-200 mcg/kg
‡ 200 mg b.i.d. for 3 days
§ 25 mg/kg b.i.d. for 3 days

In one study conducted in France, a non-endemic area where there was no possibility of reinfection, several patients were observed to have recrudescence of *Strongyloides* larvae in their stool as long as 106 days following ivermectin therapy. Therefore, at least three stool examinations should be conducted over the three months following treatment to ensure eradication. If recrudescence of larvae is observed, retreatment with ivermectin is indicated. Concentration techniques (such as using a Baermann apparatus) should be employed when performing these stool examinations, as the number of *Strongyloides* larvae per gram of feces may be very low.

Onchocerciasis

The evaluation of STROMECTOL in the treatment of onchocerciasis is based on the results of clinical studies involving 1278 patients. In a double-blind, placebo-controlled study involving adult patients with moderate to severe onchocercal infection, patients who received a single dose of 150 mcg/kg STROMECTOL experienced an 83.2% and 99.5% decrease in skin microfilariae count (geometric mean) 3 days and 3 months after the dose, respectively. A marked reduction of >90% was maintained for up to 12 months after the single dose. As with other microfilaricidal drugs, there was an increase in the microfilariae count in the anterior chamber of the eye at day 3 after treatment in some patients. However, at 3 and 6 months after the dose, a significantly greater percentage of patients treated with STROMECTOL had decreases in microfilariae count in the anterior chamber than patients treated with placebo.

In a separate open study involving pediatric patients ages 6 to 13 (n=103; weight range: 17-41 kg), similar decreases in skin microfilariae counts were observed for up to 12 months after dosing.

INDICATIONS AND USAGE

STROMECTOL is indicated for the treatment of the following infections:

Strongyloidiasis of the intestinal tract. STROMECTOL is indicated for the treatment of intestinal (i.e., nondisseminated) strongyloidiasis due to the nematode parasite *Strongyloides stercoralis*.

This indication is based on clinical studies of both comparative and open-label designs, in which 64-100% of infected patients were cured following a single 200-mcg/kg dose of ivermectin. (See CLINICAL PHARMACOLOGY, Clinical Studies.)

Onchocerciasis. STROMECTOL is indicated for the treatment of onchocerciasis due to the nematode parasite *Onchocerca volvulus*.

This indication is based on randomized, double-blind, placebo-controlled and comparative studies conducted in 1427 patients in onchocerciasis-endemic areas of West Africa. The comparative studies used diethylcarbamazine citrate (DEC-C).

NOTE: STROMECTOL has no activity against adult *Onchocerca volvulus* parasites. The adult parasites reside in subcutaneous nodules which are infrequently palpable. Surgical excision of these nodules (nodulectomy) may be considered in the management of patients with onchocerciasis, since this procedure will eliminate the microfilariae-producing adult parasites.

CONTRAINDICATIONS

STROMECTOL is contraindicated in patients who are hypersensitive to any component of this product.

WARNINGS

Historical data have shown that microfilaricidal drugs, such as diethylcarbamazine citrate (DEC-C), might cause cutaneous and/or systemic reactions of varying severity (the Mazzotti reaction) and ophthalmological reactions in patients with onchocerciasis. These reactions are probably due to allergic and inflammatory responses to the death of microfilariae. Patients treated with STROMECTOL for onchocerciasis may experience these reactions in addition to clinical adverse reactions possibly, probably, or definitely related to the drug itself. (See ADVERSE REACTIONS, Onchocerciasis.)

The treatment of severe Mazzotti reactions has not been subjected to controlled clinical trials. Oral hydration, recumbency, intravenous normal saline, and/or parenteral corticosteroids have been used to treat postural hypotension. Antihistamines and/or aspirin have been used for most mild to moderate cases.

PRECAUTIONS

General

After treatment with microfilaricidal drugs, patients with hyperreactive onchodermatitis (sowda) may be more likely than others to experience severe adverse reactions, especially edema and aggravation of onchodermatitis.

Rarely, patients with onchocerciasis who are also heavily infected with *Loa loa* may develop a serious or even fatal encephalopathy either spontaneously or following treatment with an effective microfilaricide. In these patients, the following adverse experiences have also been reported: pain (including neck and back pain), red eye, conjunctival hemorrhage, dyspnea, urinary and/or fecal incontinence, difficulty in standing/walking, mental status changes, confusion, lethargy, stupor, seizures, or coma. This syndrome has been seen very rarely following the use of ivermectin. In individuals who warrant treatment with ivermectin for any reason and have had significant exposure to *Loa loa*-endemic areas of West or Central Africa, pretreatment assessment for loiasis and careful post-treatment follow-up should be implemented.

Information for Patients

STROMECTOL should be taken on an empty stomach with water. (See CLINICAL PHARMACOLOGY, Pharmacokinetics.)

Strongyloidiasis: The patient should be reminded of the need for repeated stool examinations to document clearance of infection with *Strongyloides stercoralis*.

Onchocerciasis: The patient should be reminded that treatment with STROMECTOL does not kill the adult *Onchocerca* parasites, and therefore repeated follow-up and retreatment is usually required.

Drug Interactions

Post-marketing reports of increased INR (International Normalized Ratio) have been rarely reported when ivermectin was co-administered with warfarin.

Carcinogenesis, Mutagenesis, Impairment of Fertility

Long-term studies in animals have not been performed to evaluate the carcinogenic potential of ivermectin.

Ivermectin was not genotoxic *in vitro* in the Ames microbial mutagenicity assay of *Salmonella typhimurium* strains TA1535, TA1537, TA98, and TA100 with and without rat liver enzyme activation, the Mouse Lymphoma Cell Line L5178Y (cytotoxicity and mutagenicity) assays, or the unscheduled DNA synthesis assay in human fibroblasts.

Ivermectin had no adverse effects on the fertility in rats in studies at repeated doses of up to 3 times the maximum recommended human dose of 200 mcg/kg (on a mg/m²/day basis).

Pregnancy

Teratogenic Effects

Pregnancy Category C

Ivermectin has been shown to be teratogenic in mice, rats, and rabbits when given in repeated doses of 0.2, 8.1, and 4.5 times the maximum recommended human dose, respectively (on a mg/m²/day basis). Teratogenicity was characterized in the three species tested by cleft palate; clubbed forepaws were additionally observed in rabbits. These developmental effects were found only at or near doses that were maternotoxic to the pregnant female. Therefore, ivermectin does not appear to be selectively fetotoxic to the developing fetus. There are, however, no adequate and well-controlled studies in pregnant women. Ivermectin should not be used during pregnancy since safety in pregnancy has not been established.

Nursing Mothers

STROMECTOL is excreted in human milk in low concentrations. Treatment of mothers who intend to breast-feed should only be undertaken when the risk of delayed treatment to the mother outweighs the possible risk to the newborn.

Pediatric Use

Safety and effectiveness in pediatric patients weighing less than 15 kg have not been established.

Geriatric Use

Clinical studies of STROMECTOL did not include sufficient numbers of subjects aged 65 and over to determine whether they respond differently from younger subjects. Other reported clinical experience has not identified differences in responses between the elderly and younger patients. In general, treatment of an elderly patient should be cautious, reflecting the greater frequency of decreased hepatic, renal, or cardiac function, and of concomitant disease or other drug therapy.

Strongyloidiasis in Immunocompromised Hosts

In immunocompromised (including HIV-infected) patients being treated for intestinal strongyloidiasis, repeated courses of therapy may be required. Adequate and well-controlled clinical studies have not been conducted in such patients to determine the optimal dosing regimen. Several treatments, i.e., at 2-week intervals, may be required, and cure may not be achievable. Control of extra-intestinal strongyloidiasis in these patients is difficult, and suppressive therapy, i.e., once per month, may be helpful.

ADVERSE REACTIONS

Strongyloidiasis

In four clinical studies involving a total of 109 patients given either one or two doses of 170 to 200 mcg/kg of STROMECTOL, the following adverse reactions were reported as possibly, probably, or definitely related to STROMECTOL:

Body as a Whole: asthenia/fatigue (0.9%), abdominal pain (0.9%)

Gastrointestinal: anorexia (0.9%), constipation (0.9%), diarrhea (1.8%), nausea (1.8%), vomiting (0.9%)

Nervous System/Psychiatric: dizziness (2.8%), somnolence (0.9%), vertigo (0.9%), tremor (0.9%)

Skin: pruritus (2.8%), rash (0.9%), and urticaria (0.9%).

In comparative trials, patients treated with STROMECTOL experienced more abdominal distention and chest discomfort than patients treated with albendazole. However, STROMECTOL was better tolerated than thiabendazole in comparative studies involving 37 patients treated with thiabendazole.

The Mazzotti-type and ophthalmologic reactions associated with the treatment of onchocerciasis or the disease itself would not be expected to occur in strongyloidiasis patients treated with STROMECTOL. (See ADVERSE REACTIONS, Onchocerciasis.)

Laboratory Test Findings

In clinical trials involving 109 patients given either one or two doses of 170 to 200 mcg/kg STROMECTOL, the following laboratory abnormalities were seen regardless of drug relationship: elevation in ALT and/or AST (2%), decrease in leukocyte count (3%). Leukopenia and anemia were seen in one patient.

Onchocerciasis

In clinical trials involving 963 adult patients treated with 100 to 200 mcg/kg STROMECTOL, worsening of the following Mazzotti reactions during the first 4 days post-treatment were reported: arthralgia/synovitis (9.3%), axillary lymph node enlargement and tenderness (11.0% and 4.4%, respectively), cervical lymph node enlargement and tenderness (5.3% and 1.2%, respectively), inguinal lymph node enlargement and tenderness (12.6% and 13.9%, respectively), other lymph node enlargement and tenderness (3.0% and 1.9%, respectively), pruritus (27.5%), skin involvement including edema, papular and pustular or frank urticarial rash (22.7%), and fever (22.6%). (See WARNINGS.)

In clinical trials, ophthalmological conditions were examined in 963 adult patients before treatment, at day 3, and months 3 and 6 after treatment with 100 to 200 mcg/kg STROMECTOL. Changes observed were primarily deterioration from baseline 3 days post-treatment. Most changes either returned to baseline condition or improved over baseline severity at the month 3 and 6 visits. The percentages of patients with worsening of the following conditions at day 3, month 3 and 6, respectively, were: limbitis: 5.5%, 4.8%, and 3.5% and punctate opacity: 1.8%, 1.8%, and 1.4%. The corresponding percentages for patients treated with placebo were: limbitis: 6.2%, 9.9%, and 9.4% and punctate opacity: 2.0%, 6.4%, and 7.2%. (See WARNINGS.)

In clinical trials involving 963 adult patients who received 100 to 200 mcg/kg STROMECTOL, the following clinical adverse reactions were reported as possibly, probably, or definitely related to the drug in ≥1% of the patients: facial edema (1.2%), peripheral edema (3.2%), orthostatic hypotension (1.1%), and tachycardia (3.5%). Drug-related headache and myalgia occurred in <1% of patients (0.2% and 0.4%, respectively). However, these were the most common adverse experiences reported overall during these trials regardless of causality (22.3% and 19.7%, respectively).

A similar safety profile was observed in an open study in pediatric patients ages 6 to 13.

The following ophthalmological side effects do occur due to the disease itself but have also been reported after treatment with STROMECTOL: abnormal sensation in the eyes, eyelid edema, anterior uveitis, conjunctivitis, limbitis, keratitis, and chorioretinitis or choroiditis. These have rarely been severe or associated with loss of vision and have generally resolved without corticosteroid treatment.

Laboratory Test Findings

In controlled clinical trials, the following laboratory adverse experiences were reported as possibly, probably, or definitely related to the drug in ≥1% of the patients: eosinophil-ia (3%) and hemoglobin increase (1%).

Post-Marketing Experience

The following adverse reactions have been reported since the drug was registered overseas:

Onchocerciasis

Conjunctival hemorrhage

All Indications

Hypotension (mainly orthostatic hypotension), worsening of bronchial asthma, toxic epidermal necrolysis, Stevens-Johnson syndrome, seizures, hepatitis, elevation of liver enzymes, and elevation of bilirubin.

OVERDOSAGE

Significant lethality was observed in mice and rats after single oral doses of 25 to 50 mg/kg and 40 to 50 mg/kg, respectively. No significant lethality was observed in dogs after single oral doses of up to 10 mg/kg. At these doses, the treatment-related signs that were observed in these animals include ataxia, bradypnea, tremors, ptosis, decreased activity, emesis, and mydriasis.

In accidental intoxication with, or significant exposure to, unknown quantities of veterinary formulations of ivermectin in humans, either by ingestion, inhalation, injection, or exposure to body surfaces, the following adverse effects have been reported most frequently: rash, edema, headache, dizziness, asthenia, nausea, vomiting, and diarrhea. Other adverse effects that have been reported include: seizure, ataxia, dyspnea, abdominal pain, paresthesia, urticaria, and contact dermatitis.

In case of accidental poisoning, supportive therapy, if indicated, should include parenteral fluids and electrolytes, respiratory support (oxygen and mechanical ventilation if necessary) and pressor agents if clinically significant hypotension is present. Induction of emesis and/or gastric lavage as soon as possible, followed by purgatives and other routine anti-poison measures, may be indicated if needed to prevent absorption of ingested material.

DOSAGE AND ADMINISTRATION

Strongyloidiasis

The recommended dosage of STROMECTOL for the treatment of strongyloidiasis is a single oral dose designed to provide approximately 200 mcg of ivermectin per kg of body weight. See Table 1 for dosage guidelines. Patients should take tablets on an empty stomach with water. (See CLINICAL PHARMACOLOGY, Pharmacokinetics.) In general, additional doses are not necessary. However, follow-up stool examinations should be performed to verify eradication of infection. (See CLINICAL PHARMACOLOGY, Clinical Studies.)

Table 1: Dosage Guidelines for STROMECTOL for Strongyloidiasis

Body Weight (kg)	Single Oral Dose Number of 3-mg Tablets
15-24	1 tablet
25-35	2 tablets
36-50	3 tablets
51-65	4 tablets
66-79	5 tablets
≥80	200 mcg/kg

Onchocerciasis

The recommended dosage of STROMECTOL for the treatment of onchocerciasis is a single oral dose designed to provide approximately 150 mcg of ivermectin per kg of body weight. See Table 2 for dosage guidelines. Patients should take tablets on an empty stomach with water. (See CLINICAL PHARMACOLOGY, Pharmacokinetics.) In mass distribution campaigns in international treatment programs, the most commonly used dose interval is 12 months. For the treatment of individual patients, retreatment may be considered at intervals as short as 3 months.

Table 2: Dosage Guidelines for STROMECTOL for Onchocerciasis

Body Weight (kg)	Single Oral Dose Number of 3-mg Tablets
15-25	1 tablet
26-44	2 tablets
45-64	3 tablets
65-84	4 tablets
≥85	150 mcg/kg

HOW SUPPLIED

No. 8495 — Tablets STROMECTOL 3 mg are white, round, flat, bevel-edged tablets coded MSD on one side and 32 on the other side. They are supplied as follows:

NDC 0006-0032-20 unit dose packages of 20.

Storage

Store at temperatures below 30°C (86°F).

Dist. by: Merck Sharp & Dohme Corp., a subsidiary of **MERCK & CO., INC.**, Whitehouse Station, NJ 08889, USA

Manufactured by:
Merck Sharp & Dohme BV
Waarderweg 39
2031 BN Haarlem
Netherlands
Issued May 2010
Printed in the Netherlands
9032319
87447/080610
8495

SYLATRON™ ℞

(peginterferon alfa-2b)
for injection, for subcutaneous use

HIGHLIGHTS OF PRESCRIBING INFORMATION

These highlights do not include all the information needed to use SYLATRON safely and effectively. See full prescribing information for SYLATRON.

SYLATRON™ (peginterferon alfa-2b)
for injection, for subcutaneous use
Initial U.S. Approval: 2011

WARNING: DEPRESSION AND OTHER NEUROPSYCHIATRIC DISORDERS

See full prescribing information for complete boxed warning.

The risk of serious depression, with suicidal ideation and completed suicides, and other serious neuropsychiatric disorders are increased with alpha interferons, including SYLATRON. Permanently discontinue SYLATRON in patients with persistently severe or worsening signs or symptoms of depression, psychosis, or encephalopathy. These disorders may not resolve after stopping SYLATRON *[see Warnings and Precautions (5.1) and Adverse Reactions (6.1)]*.

INDICATIONS AND USAGE

SYLATRON is an alpha interferon indicated for the adjuvant treatment of melanoma with microscopic or gross nodal involvement within 84 days of definitive surgical resection including complete lymphadenectomy. (1)

DOSAGE AND ADMINISTRATION

- 6 mcg/kg/week subcutaneously for 8 doses followed by;
- 3 mcg/kg/week subcutaneously for up to 5 years. (2.1)

DOSAGE FORMS AND STRENGTHS

- 296 mcg lyophilized powder per single-use vial
- 444 mcg lyophilized powder per single-use vial
- 888 mcg lyophilized powder per single-use vial

CONTRAINDICATIONS

- Known serious hypersensitivity reactions to peginterferon alfa-2b or interferon alfa-2b. (4)
- Autoimmune hepatitis. (4)
- Hepatic decompensation (Child-Pugh score >6 [class B and C]). (4)

WARNINGS AND PRECAUTIONS

- Depression and other serious neuropsychiatric adverse reactions. (5.1)
- History of significant or unstable cardiac disease. (5.2)
- Retinal disorders. (5.3)
- Child-Pugh score >6 (class B and C). (4, 5.4)
- Hypothyroidism, hyperthyroidism, hyperglycemia, diabetes mellitus that cannot be effectively treated by medication. (4, 5.5)

ADVERSE REACTIONS

Most common adverse reactions (>60%) are: fatigue, increased ALT, increased AST, pyrexia, headache, anorexia, myalgia, nausea, chills, and injection site reaction. (6.1)

To report SUSPECTED ADVERSE REACTIONS, contact Schering Corporation at 1-800-526-4099 or FDA at 1-800-FDA-1088 or www.fda.gov/medwatch.

DRUG INTERACTIONS

- Drug metabolized by cytochrome P-450 (CYP) enzymes: Monitor closely when used in combination with drugs metabolized by CYP2C9 or CYP2D6. (7)

USE IN SPECIFIC POPULATIONS

- Pregnancy: Based on animal data, may cause fetal harm. (8.1)
- Pediatrics: Safety and efficacy in patients <18 years old have not been established. (8.4)
- Renal Impairment: Increase frequency of monitoring for SYLATRON toxicity in patients with moderate and severe renal impairment. (8.7)

See 17 for PATIENT COUNSELING INFORMATION and the FDA-approved Medication Guide

Revised: 12/2012

FULL PRESCRIBING INFORMATION: CONTENTS*

16 HOW SUPPLIED/STORAGE AND HANDLING
17 PATIENT COUNSELING INFORMATION
* Sections or subsections omitted from the full prescribing information are not listed

FULL PRESCRIBING INFORMATION

WARNING: DEPRESSION AND OTHER NEUROPSYCHIATRIC DISORDERS

The risk of serious depression, with suicidal ideation and completed suicides, and other serious neuropsychiatric disorders are increased with alpha interferons, including SYLATRON. Permanently discontinue SYLATRON in patients with persistently severe or worsening signs or symptoms of depression, psychosis, or encephalopathy. These disorders may not resolve after stopping SYLATRON *[see Warnings and Precautions (5.1) and Adverse Reactions (6.1)]*.

1 INDICATIONS AND USAGE

SYLATRON™ is an alpha interferon indicated for the adjuvant treatment of melanoma with microscopic or gross nodal involvement within 84 days of definitive surgical resection including complete lymphadenectomy.

2 DOSAGE AND ADMINISTRATION

2.1 Recommended Dose

- 6 mcg/kg/week subcutaneously for 8 doses, followed by 3 mcg/kg/week subcutaneously for up to 5 years.
- Premedicate with acetaminophen 500 to 1000 mg orally 30 minutes prior to the first dose of SYLATRON and as needed for subsequent doses.

2.2 Dose Modification

Guidelines for Dose Modification provided below are based on the National Cancer Institute Common Terminology Criteria for Adverse Events (NCI-CTCAE Version 2.0).

- Permanently discontinue SYLATRON for:
  - Persistent or worsening severe neuropsychiatric disorders
  - Grade 4 non-hematologic toxicity
  - Inability to tolerate a dose of 1 mcg/kg/wk
  - New or worsening retinopathy
- Withhold SYLATRON dose for any of the following:
  - Absolute Neutrophil Count (ANC) <0.5×10^9/L
  - Platelet Count (PLT) <50×10^9/L
  - ECOG PS ≥2
  - Non-hematologic toxicity ≥ Grade 3
- Resume dosing at a reduced dose (see Table 1) when all of the following are present:
  - Absolute Neutrophil Count (ANC) ≥0.5×10^9/L
  - Platelet Count (PLT) ≥50×10^9/L
  - ECOG PS 0–1
  - Non-hematologic toxicity has completely resolved or improved to Grade 1

TABLE 1: SYLATRON Dose Modifications

Starting Dose	Dose Modifications for Doses 1 to 8
6 mcg/kg/week	First Dose Modification: 3 mcg/kg/week
	Second Dose Modification: 2 mcg/kg/week
	Third Dose Modification: 1 mcg/kg/week
	Permanently discontinue if unable to tolerate 1 mcg/kg/week
Starting Dose	**Dose Modifications for Doses 9 to 260**
3 mcg/kg/week	First Dose Modification: 2 mcg/kg/week
	Second Dose Modification: 1 mcg/kg/week
	Permanently discontinue if unable to tolerate 1 mcg/kg/week

2.3 Preparation and Administration

Reconstitute SYLATRON with 0.7 mL of Sterile Water for Injection USP.

Upon reconstitution, the final concentration of SYLATRON will be

- 40 mcg per each 0.1 mL for vials containing 296 mcg of SYLATRON
- 60 mcg per each 0.1 mL for vials containing 444 mcg of SYLATRON
- 120 mcg per each 0.1 mL for vials containing 888 mcg of SYLATRON

- Swirl gently to dissolve the lyophilized powder. **DO NOT SHAKE.**
- Visually inspect the solution for particulate matter and discoloration prior to administration. Discard if solution is discolored, cloudy, or if particulates are present.
- Do not withdraw more than 0.5 mL of reconstituted solution from each vial.
- Administer SYLATRON subcutaneously. Rotate injection sites.
- If reconstituted solution is not used immediately, store at 2°–8°C (36°–46°F) for no more than 24 hours. Discard reconstituted solution after 24 hours. **DO NOT FREEZE.**
- For single-use only. **DISCARD ANY UNUSED PORTION.**

3 DOSAGE FORMS AND STRENGTHS

- 296 mcg lyophilized powder per single-use vial
- 444 mcg lyophilized powder per single-use vial
- 888 mcg lyophilized powder per single-use vial

4 CONTRAINDICATIONS

SYLATRON is contraindicated in patients with:

- A history of anaphylaxis to peginterferon alfa-2b or interferon alfa-2b
- autoimmune hepatitis
- hepatic decompensation (Child-Pugh score >6 [class B and C])

5 WARNINGS AND PRECAUTIONS

5.1 Depression and Other Serious Neuropsychiatric Adverse Reactions

Peginterferon alfa-2b can cause life-threatening or fatal neuropsychiatric reactions. These include suicide, suicidal and homicidal ideation, depression, and an increased risk of relapse of recovering drug addicts. In the clinical trial, depression occurred in 59% of SYLATRON-treated patients and 24% of patients in the observation group. Depression was severe or life threatening in 7% of SYLATRON-treated patients compared with <1% of patients in the observation arm.

In post-marketing experience, neuropsychiatric adverse reactions have been reported up to 6 months after discontinuation of peginterferon alfa-2b. Based on post-marketing experience with peginterferon alfa-2b and interferon alfa-2b, treatment may also result in aggressive behavior, psychoses, hallucinations, bipolar disorders, mania, and encephalopathy.

Advise patients and their caregivers to immediately report any symptoms of depression or suicidal ideation to their healthcare provider. Monitor and evaluate patients for signs and symptoms of depression and other psychiatric symptoms every 3 weeks during the first 8 weeks of treatment and every 6 months thereafter. Monitor patients during treatment and for at least 6 months after the last dose of SYLATRON. Permanently discontinue SYLATRON for persistent severe or worsening psychiatric symptoms or behaviors and refer for psychiatric evaluation.

5.2 Cardiovascular Adverse Reactions

In the clinical trial, cardiac adverse reactions, including myocardial infarction, bundle-branch block, ventricular tachycardia, and supraventricular arrhythmia occurred in 4% of SYLATRON-treated patients compared with 2% of patients in the observation group. In post-marketing experience, hypotension, cardiomyopathy, and angina pectoris have occurred in patients treated with peginterferon alfa-2b. Permanently discontinue SYLATRON for new onset of ventricular arrhythmia or cardiovascular decompensation.

5.3 Retinopathy and Other Serious Ocular Adverse Reactions

Peginterferon alfa-2b can cause decrease in visual acuity or blindness due to retinopathy. Retinal and ocular changes include macular edema, retinal artery or vein thrombosis, retinal hemorrhages and cotton wool spots, optic neuritis, papilledema, and serous retinal detachment may be induced or aggravated by treatment with peginterferon alfa-2b or other alpha interferons. In the clinical study, two SYLATRON-treated patients developed partial loss of vision due to retinal thrombosis (n=1) or retinopathy (n=1). The overall incidence of serious retinal disorders, visual disturbances, blurred vision, and reduction in visual acuity was <1% in both SYLATRON-treated patients and the observation group.

Perform an eye examination that includes assessment of visual acuity and indirect ophthalmoscopy or fundus photography at baseline in patients with preexisting retinopathy and at any time during SYLATRON treatment in patients who experience changes in vision. Permanently discontinue SYLATRON in patients who develop new or worsening retinopathy.

5.4 Hepatic Failure

Peginterferon alfa-2b, increases the risk of hepatic decompensation and death in patients with cirrhosis. Monitor hepatic function with serum bilirubin, ALT, AST, alkaline phosphatase, and LDH at 2 and 8 weeks, and 2 and 3 months following initiation of SYLATRON, then every 6 months while receiving SYLATRON. Permanently discontinue SYLATRON for evidence of severe (Grade 3) hepatic injury or hepatic decompensation (Child-Pugh score >6 [class B and C]) *[see Contraindications (4)]*.

5.5 Endocrinopathies

Peginterferon alfa-2b can cause new onset or worsening of hypothyroidism, hyperthyroidism, and diabetes mellitus. In the clinical study, 1% of patients developed hypothyroidism; the overall incidence of endocrine disorders was 2% in SYLATRON-treated patients compared to <1% for patients in the observation group.

Obtain TSH levels within 4 weeks prior to initiation of SYLATRON, at 3 and 6 months following initiation, then every 6 months thereafter while receiving SYLATRON. Permanently discontinue SYLATRON in patients who develop hypothyroidism, hyperthyroidism or diabetes mellitus that cannot be effectively managed.

6 ADVERSE REACTIONS

The following serious adverse reactions are discussed in greater detail in other sections of the labeling:

- Depression and Other Neuropsychiatric Adverse Reactions *[see Warnings and Precautions (5.1)]*
- Cardiovascular Adverse Reactions *[see Warnings and Precautions (5.2)]*
- Retinopathy and Other Serious Ocular Adverse Reactions *[see Warnings and Precautions (5.3)]*
- Hepatic Failure *[see Warnings and Precautions (5.4)]*
- Endocrinopathies *[see Warnings and Precautions (5.5)]*

6.1 Clinical Trials Experience

The data described below reflect exposure to SYLATRON in 608 patients with surgically resected, AJCC Stage III melanoma. SYLATRON was studied in an open label, multicenter, randomized, observation controlled trial. The median age of the population was 50 years with 10% of patients 65 years or older, and 42% were female. Fourteen percent of patients completed the 5 year treatment schedule.

Patients randomized to SYLATRON were to receive total doses of 48 mcg/kg (6 mcg/kg subcutaneous once weekly for 8 doses), and 780 mcg/kg (3 mcg/kg subcutaneous once weekly until disease recurrence or for up to 5 years), as tolerated. The median total dose received was 42 mcg/kg (range: 6 to 78 mcg/kg) for the first 8 doses, and 136 mcg/kg (range: 1 to 774 mcg/kg) for doses 9 to 260.

Because clinical trials are conducted under widely varying conditions, adverse reaction rates observed in the clinical trials of a drug cannot be directly compared to rates in the clinical trials of another drug and may not reflect the rates observed in clinical practice.

Serious adverse events were reported in 199 (33%) patients who received SYLATRON and 94 (15%) patients in the observation group.

The most common adverse reactions experienced by SYLATRON-treated patients were fatigue (94%), increased ALT (77%), increased AST (77%), pyrexia (75%), headache (70%), anorexia (69%), myalgia (68%), nausea (64%), chills (63%), and injection site reaction (62%). The most common serious adverse reactions were fatigue (7%), increased ALT (3%), increased AST (3%), and pyrexia (3%) in the SYLATRON-treated group vs. <1% in the observation group for these reactions.

Thirty three percent of patients receiving SYLATRON discontinued treatment due to adverse reactions. The most common adverse reactions present at the time of treatment discontinuation were fatigue (27%), depression (17%), anorexia (15%), increased ALT (14%), increased AST (14%), myalgia (13%), nausea (13%), headache (13%), and pyrexia (11%). Adverse events that occurred in the clinical study at ≥ 5% incidence in the SYLATRON-treated group and with a greater incidence in patients receiving SYLATRON as compared to the observation group are presented in **Table 2**.

[See table 2 at top of next page]

6.2 Immunogenicity

As with all therapeutic proteins, there is potential for immunogenicity. In a clinical study conducted in patients with melanoma, the incidence of binding antibodies to peginterferon alfa-2b was approximately 35% (50/144 patients). Among the patients who tested positive for binding antibodies, one patient developed neutralizing antibodies. The impact of antibody formation on pharmacokinetics, safety and efficacy of peg-interferon alfa-2b could not be assessed based on limited available data.

The incidence of antibody formation is highly dependent on the sensitivity and specificity of the assay. Additionally, the observed incidence of antibody (including neutralizing antibody) positivity in an assay may be influenced by several factors, including assay methodology, sample handling, timing of sample collection, concomitant medications, and underlying disease. For these reasons, comparison of the incidence of antibodies to SYLATRON with the incidence of antibodies to other products may be misleading.

6.3 Postmarketing Experience

The following adverse reactions have been identified during post-approval use of peginterferon alfa-2b as monotherapy and in combination with ribavirin in chronic hepatitis C (CHC) patients. Because these reactions are reported voluntarily from a population of uncertain size, it is not always possible to reliably estimate their frequency or establish a causal relationship to drug exposure.

TABLE 2: Incidence of Adverse Reactions[*] Occurring in ≥5% of Melanoma Patients Treated with SYLATRON and with a Greater Incidence as Compared to Observation

Adverse Reaction	SYLATRON N=608		Observation N=628	
	All Grades (%)	Grade 3 and 4 (%)	All Grades (%)	Grade 3 and 4 (%)
Any Adverse Reaction	100	51	82	18
General Disorders and Administrative Site Conditions				
Fatigue	94	16	41	1
Pyrexia	75	4	9	0
Chills	63	1	6	0
Injection Site Reaction	62	1.8	0	0
Metabolic/Laboratory				
ALT or AST Increased	77	11	26	1
Blood Alkaline Phosphatase Increased	23	0	11	<1
Weight Decreased	11	<1	1	<1
GGT Increased	8	4	1	<1
Proteinuria	7	0	3	0
Anemia	6	<1	2	<1
Nervous System Disorders				
Headache	70	4	19	1
Dysgeusia	38	0	1	0
Dizziness	35	2	11	<1
Olfactory Nerve Disorder	23	0	1	0
Paraesthesia	21	<1	14	<1
Metabolism and Nutrition Disorders				
Anorexia	69	3	13	0
Musculoskeletal and Connective Tissue Disorders				
Myalgia	68	4	23	<1
Arthralgia	51	3	22	1
Gastrointestinal Disorders				
Nausea	64	3	11	<1
Diarrhea	37	1	8	<1
Vomiting	26	1	4	0
Psychiatric Disorders				
Depression	59	7	24	<1
Skin and Subcutaneous Tissue Disorders				
Exfoliative Rash	36	1	4	0
Alopecia	34	0	1	0
Respiratory, Thoracic and Mediastinal Disorders				
Dyspnea	6	1	2	1
Cough	5	<1	2	0

* **Adverse reactions were graded using NCI CTCAE, V.2.0.**

Blood and Lymphatic System Disorders
pure red cell aplasia, thrombotic thrombocytopenic purpura

Ear and Labyrinth Disorders
hearing loss, vertigo, hearing impairment

Endocrine Disorders
diabetic ketoacidosis

Eye Disorders
Vogt-Koyanagi-Harada syndrome

Gastrointestinal Disorders
aphthous stomatitis, pancreatitis, colitis

Infusion reactions
angioedema, urticaria, bronchoconstriction

Immune System Disorders
systemic lupus erythematosus, erythema multiforme, thyroiditis, thrombotic thrombocytopenic purpura, idiopathic thrombocytopenic purpura, rheumatoid arthritis, interstitial nephritis, and systemic lupus erythematosus

Infections
sepsis

Metabolism and Nutrition Disorders
hypertriglyceridemia

Musculoskeletal and Connective Tissue Disorders
rhabdomyolysis, myositis

Nervous System Disorders
seizures, memory loss, peripheral neuropathy, paraesthesia, migraine headache

Respiratory, Thoracic and Mediastinal Disorders
dyspnea, pulmonary infiltrates, pneumonia, bronchiolitis obliterans, interstitial pneumonitis, sarcoidosis and pulmonary hypertension

Skin and Subcutaneous Tissue Disorders
Stevens-Johnson syndrome, toxic epidermal necrolysis, psoriasis

Vascular Disorders
hypertension, hypotension, stroke

7 DRUG INTERACTIONS

In healthy subjects who were administered peginterferon alfa-2b subcutaneously at 1 mcg/kg once weekly for four weeks with probe drugs of metabolic enzymes administered before the first dose and after the fourth dose, a measure of CYP2C9 activity increased to 125% of baseline, whereas a measure of CYP2D6 activity decreased to 51% of baseline *[see Clinical Pharmacology (12.3)]*.

When administering SYLATRON with medications metabolized by CYP2C9 or CYP2D6, the therapeutic effect of these drugs may be altered.

The effects of pegylated interferon alfa-2b on the pharmacokinetics of drugs metabolized by cytochrome P-450 enzymes have not been studied at the higher clinical doses for patients with melanoma (3 mcg/kg/week and 6 mcg/kg/week).

8 USE IN SPECIFIC POPULATIONS

8.1 Pregnancy

Pregnancy Category C:

There are no adequate and well-controlled studies of SYLATRON in pregnant women. Nonpegylated interferon alfa-2b was an abortifacient in *Macaca mulatta* (rhesus monkeys) at 15 and 30 million international units (IU)/kg (estimated human equivalent of 5 and 10 million IU/kg, based on body surface area adjustment for a 60-kg adult). The estimated Intron A human equivalent dose of 5 to 10 million IU/kg daily is approximately equal to a human equivalent dose of 79 to 158 mcg/kg/week of SYLATRON. Use SYLATRON during pregnancy only if the potential benefit justifies the potential risk to the fetus.

8.3 Nursing Mothers

It is not known whether the components of SYLATRON are excreted in human milk. Studies in mice have shown that mouse interferons are excreted in breast milk. Because of the potential for adverse reactions from the drug in nursing infants, a decision must be made whether to discontinue nursing or discontinue the SYLATRON treatment, taking into account the importance of the therapy to the mother.

8.4 Pediatric Use

Safety and effectiveness in patients below the age of 18 years have not been established.

8.5 Geriatric Use

Clinical studies of SYLATRON did not include sufficient numbers of subjects aged 65 and over to determine whether they respond differently from younger subjects.

8.6 Hepatic Impairment

SYLATRON has not been studied in patients with melanoma who have hepatic impairment. In patients treated for viral hepatitis, peginterferon alfa-2b treatment is contraindicated in those with moderate or severe hepatic impairment (Child-Pugh scores >6). Discontinue SYLATRON if hepatic decompensation (Child-Pugh scores >6) occurs during treatment. *[See Contraindications (4) and Warnings and Precautions (5.4).]*

8.7 Renal Impairment

The mean area under the concentration-time curve (AUC_{last}) following a single dose of peginterferon alfa-2b at 1 mcg/kg increased by 1.3-, 1.7- and 1.9-fold in subjects with mild (creatinine clearance 50–79 mL/min), moderate (creatinine clearance 30–50 mL/min) and severe (creatinine clearance 10–29 mL/min) renal impairment, respectively. After multiple doses, the mean AUC_{tau} increased by 1.3-fold in moderate and 2.1-fold in severe renal impairment. No clinical meaningful amounts of peginterferon alfa-2b were removed during hemodialysis. Dose reductions of 25% and 50% are recommended in patients with moderate and severe renal impairment, respectively, receiving alpha interferons for chronic hepatitis C.

The effect of varying degrees of renal impairment on the pharmacokinetics of peginterferon alfa-2b at the recommended doses of 3 mcg/kg or 6 mcg/kg for patients with melanoma has not been studied.

10 OVERDOSAGE

The experience with overdose of SYLATRON is limited. Patients who were over dosed experienced the following adverse reactions: severe fatigue, headache, myalgia, neutropenia, and thrombocytopenia. The highest single dose administered was 14 mcg/kg.

11 DESCRIPTION

SYLATRON, peginterferon alfa-2b, is a covalent conjugate of recombinant alfa-2b interferon with monomethoxy polyethylene glycol (PEG). The average molecular weight of the PEG portion of the molecule is 12,000 daltons. The average molecular weight of the SYLATRON molecule is approximately 31,000 daltons. The specific activity of pegylated interferon alfa-2b is approximately 0.7×10^8 international units/mg protein.

Interferon alfa-2b is a protein with a molecular weight of 19,271 daltons produced by recombinant DNA techniques. It is obtained from the bacterial fermentation of a strain of *Escherichia coli* bearing a genetically engineered plasmid containing an interferon gene from human leukocytes.

Each vial contains either 296 mcg, 444 mcg or 888 mcg of peginterferon alfa-2b as a sterile, white to off-white lyophilized powder, and dibasic sodium phosphate anhydrous (1.11 mg), monobasic sodium phosphate dihydrate (1.11 mg), polysorbate 80 (0.074 mg), and sucrose (59.2 mg). Following reconstitution with 0.7 mL of Sterile Water for Injection USP, each vial contains SYLATRON at 40 mcg per 0.1 mL, 60 mcg per 0.1 mL, or 120 mcg per 0.1 mL.

12 CLINICAL PHARMACOLOGY

12.1 Mechanism of Action

Peginterferon alfa-2b is a pleiotropic cytokine; the mechanism by which it exerts its effects in patients with melanoma is unknown.

12.3 Pharmacokinetics

The pharmacokinetics were studied in 32 patients receiving adjuvant therapy for melanoma with SYLATRON according to the recommended dose and schedule (6 mcg/kg/week for 8 doses, followed by 3 mcg/kg/week thereafter). At a dose of 6 mcg/kg/week once weekly, the geometric mean C_{max} was 4.4 ng/mL (CV 51%) and the geometric mean $AUC_{(tau)}$ was 430 ng•hr/mL (CV 35%) at week 8. The mean terminal half-life was approximately 51 hours (CV 18%). The mean accumulation from week 1 to week 8 was 1.7. After administration of 3 mcg/kg/week once weekly, the mean geometric C_{max} was 2.5 ng/mL (CV 33%) and the geometric mean $AUC_{(tau)}$ was 228 ng•hr/mL (CV 24%) at week 4. The mean terminal half-life was approximately 43 hours (CV 19%).

Renal Dysfunction:

The disposition of peginterferon alfa-2b was studied in 26 subjects with varying degrees of renal function after administration of a single subcutaneous dose of peginterferon alfa-2b at 1 mcg/kg. Renal clearance accounts for approximately 30% of total peginterferon alfa-2b clearance. The AUC_{last} increased by 1.3-, 1.7- and 1.9-fold in mild, moderate and severe renal impairment, respectively. The mean elimination half-life and maximal plasma concentration (C_{max}) increased in subjects with renal impairment. The mean AUC_{last} was similar in subjects with severe renal impairment on and not on hemodialysis, suggesting that no clinical meaningful amounts of peginterferon alfa-2b were removed during hemodialysis.

After subcutaneous administration of 1 mcg/kg of peginterferon alfa-2b once weekly for four weeks in 21 subjects with varying degrees of renal function, AUC_{tau} at week 4 increased 1.3-fold in moderate and 2.1-fold in severe renal impairment. The C_{max} at week 4 increased 1.8-fold in severe renal impairment, but no difference was observed in moderate renal impairment *[see Use in Specific Populations (8.7)]*.

The effect of varying degrees of renal impairment on pharmacokinetics of peginterferon alfa-2b at 3 mcg/kg and 6 mcg/kg recommended for patients with melanoma has not been studied.

Drug Interactions:

In a two-way crossover trial, 12 healthy subjects were administered probe drugs of metabolic enzymes: caffeine (CYP1A2), tolbutamide (CYP2C9), dextromethorphan (CYP2D6), midazolam (CYP3A4), and dapsone (N-acetyltransferase, NAT), with or without a single subcutaneous (SC) dose of peginterferon alfa-2b at 1 mcg/kg. The results suggest that single doses of peginterferon alfa-2b do not affect activities of CYP1A2, CYP2C9, CYP2D6, CYP3A4 and NAT enzymes.

In 24 healthy subjects, the effect of subcutaneous doses of peginterferon alfa-2b at 1 mcg/kg/week for 4 weeks on the pharmacokinetics of caffeine, tolbutamide, dextromethorphan and midazolam were studied. A measure of CYP2C9 activity increased to 125% (90% CI: 116% to 135%) of baseline, whereas a measure of CYP2D6 activity decreased to 51% (90% CI: 38% to 67%) of baseline when coadministered with peginterferon alfa-2b at week 4, indicating that peginterferon alfa-2b may affect the metabolism of CYP2C9 and CYP2D6 drugs. A measure of CYP1A2 and CYP3A4 activity did not show clinically meaningful changes.

When patients are administered SYLATRON with medications metabolized by CYP2C9 or CYP2D6, the therapeutic effect of these drugs may be altered.

The effects of peginterferon alfa-2b at the clinical doses for melanoma (3 mcg/kg/week and 6 mcg/kg/week) on the systemic exposure of drugs metabolized by cytochrome P-450 enzymes have not been studied *[see Drug Interactions (7)]*.

13 NONCLINICAL TOXICOLOGY

13.1 Carcinogenesis, Mutagenesis, Impairment of Fertility

Carcinogenesis and Mutagenesis:

SYLATRON has not been tested for its carcinogenic potential. Neither peginterferon alfa-2b nor its components, interferon or methoxypolyethylene glycol, caused damage to DNA when tested in the standard battery of mutagenesis assays, in the presence and absence of metabolic activation.

Impairment of Fertility:

SYLATRON may impair human fertility. Irregular menstrual cycles were observed in female cynomolgus monkeys given subcutaneous injections of 4239 mcg/m^2 peginterferon alfa-2b alone every other day for 1 month (approximately 72 to 144 times the recommended weekly human dose based upon body surface area). These effects included transiently decreased serum levels of estradiol and progesterone, suggestive of anovulation. Normal menstrual cycles and serum hormone levels resumed in these animals 2 to 3 months following cessation of peginterferon alfa-2b treatment. Every other day dosing with 262 mcg/m^2 (approximately 3.5 to 7 times the recommended weekly human dose) had no effects on cycle duration or reproductive hormone status. The effects of SYLATRON on male fertility have not been studied.

14 CLINICAL STUDIES

The safety and effectiveness of SYLATRON were evaluated in an open-label, multicenter, randomized (1:1) study conducted in 1256 patients with surgically resected, AJCC Stage III melanoma within 84 days of regional lymph node dissection. Patients were randomized to observation (no therapy) (n=629) or to SYLATRON (n=627) at a dose of 6 mcg/kg by subcutaneous injection once weekly for 8 doses followed by a 3 mcg/kg subcutaneous injection once weekly for a period of up to 5 years total treatment. The dose of SYLATRON was adjusted to maintain an ECOG Performance Status of 0 to 1.

The median age of the population was 50 years with 11% of patients 65 years or older, and 42% were female. Forty percent of the study population had microscopic, nonpalpable nodal involvement and 59% had clinically palpable nodes prior to lymphadenectomy. A total of 54% of subjects had one pathologically positive lymph node, 34% had 2 to 4 positive nodes, and 12% had 5 or more. Most subjects had no second primary lesion (98%). Ulceration of the primary lesion was present in 30% of subjects (52% had no ulceration of the primary lesion, and the status was missing/unknown for 18% of subjects). The most common sites were the trunk (43%) or the leg (32%). Eighty-four percent had an International Prognostic Index (IPI) score of 0 and 16% had an IPI score of 1. The main outcome measure was relapse-free survival (RFS), defined as the time from randomization to the earliest date of any relapse (local, regional, in-transit, or distant), or death from any cause. Secondary outcome measures included overall survival.

Patients in the SYLATRON arm received 6 mcg/kg/week for a median of 8.0 weeks. Less than 1% of patients took longer than 9 weeks to complete the 6 mcg/kg/week dosing regimen. Approximately one-third (36%) of patients required dose reductions and 29% of patients required a dose delay, with an average delay of 1.2 weeks, during the initial 8 weeks of SYLATRON. Ninety-four patients (16%) did not continue on to the 3 mcg/kg/week dosing regimen.

Patients who continued on SYLATRON after the initial 8 doses, received 3 mcg/kg/week for a median duration of treatment of 14.3 months. Approximately half (52%) of the patients underwent dose reductions and 70% required dose delays (average delay 2.2 weeks).

Based on 696 RFS events, determined by the Independent Review Committee, median RFS was 34.8 months (95% CI: 26.1, 47.4) and 25.5 months (95% CI: 19.6, 30.8) in the SYLATRON and observation arms, respectively. The estimated hazard ratio for RFS was 0.82 (95% CI: 0.71, 0.96; unstratified log-rank p =0.011) in favor of SYLATRON. Figure 1 shows the Kaplan-Meier curves of RFS.

[See figure 1 at top of next column]

There was no statistically significant difference in survival between the SYLATRON and the observation arms. Based on 525 deaths, the estimated hazard ratio of SYLATRON versus observation was 0.98 (95% CI: 0.82, 1.16).

FIGURE 1: Kaplan-Meier Curves for Relapse-Free Survival

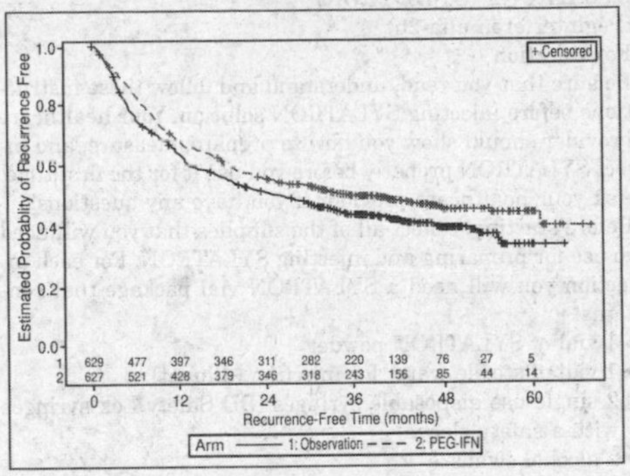

16 HOW SUPPLIED/STORAGE AND HANDLING

Each SYLATRON Package Contains:

A box containing one 296 mcg vial of SYLATRON powder and one 1.25 mL vial of Sterile Water for Injection, USP, 2 B-D Safety Lok syringes with a safety sleeve and 2 alcohol swabs.	(NDC 0085-1388-01)
A box containing one 444 mcg vial of SYLATRON powder and one 1.25 mL vial of Sterile Water for Injection, USP, 2 B-D Safety Lok syringes with a safety sleeve and 2 alcohol swabs.	(NDC 0085-1287-02)
A box containing one 888 mcg vial of SYLATRON powder and one 1.25 mL vial of Sterile Water for Injection, USP, 2 B-D Safety Lok syringes with a safety sleeve and 2 alcohol swabs.	(NDC 0085-1312-01)

Each SYLATRON PACK 4 Contains:

A box containing four 296 mcg vials of SYLATRON powder and four 1.25 mL vials of Sterile Water for Injection, USP, 8 B-D Safety Lok syringes with a safety sleeve and 8 alcohol swabs.	(NDC 0085-1388-02)
A box containing four 444 mcg vials of SYLATRON powder and four 1.25 mL vials of Sterile Water for Injection, USP, 8 B-D Safety Lok syringes with a safety sleeve and 8 alcohol swabs.	(NDC 0085-1287-03)
A box containing four 888 mcg vials of SYLATRON powder and four 1.25 mL vials of Sterile Water for Injection, USP, 8 B-D Safety Lok syringes with a safety sleeve and 8 alcohol swabs.	(NDC 0085-1312-02)

Storage:

SYLATRON should be stored at 25°C (77°F); excursions permitted to 15°–30°C (59–86°F) [see USP Controlled Room Temperature]. **DO NOT FREEZE.**

17 PATIENT COUNSELING INFORMATION

See FDA-approved patient labeling (Instructions for Use and Medication Guide).

- Advise patients that SYLATRON may be administered with antipyretics at bedtime to minimize common "flu-like" symptoms (including chills, fever, muscle aches, joint pain, headaches, tiredness).
- Advise patients to maintain hydration if experiencing "flu-like" symptoms.
- Advise patients and their caregivers to immediately report any symptoms of depression or suicidal ideation to their healthcare provider during treatment and up to 6 months after the last dose.
- Use SYLATRON during pregnancy only if the potential benefit justifies the potential risk to the fetus *[see Use in Specific Populations (8.1)]*.
- Instruct patients to not re-use or share syringes and needles.
- Instruct patients on proper disposal of vials, syringes and needles.

Manufactured by: Schering Corporation, a subsidiary of **MERCK & CO., INC.**, Whitehouse Station, NJ 08889, USA
U.S. Patent Nos. 5,951,974; 6,180,096; and 6,610,830.

Revised: 12/2012
LRN#054031-SYL-PWi-USPI.20

SYLATRON IFU Powder for Injection
Instructions for Use
SYLATRON™ (SY-LA-TRON)
(Peginterferon alfa-2b)
For Injection

Be sure that you read, understand and follow these instructions before injecting SYLATRON solution. Your healthcare provider should show you how to prepare, measure, and inject SYLATRON properly before you use it for the first time. Ask your healthcare provider if you have any questions.

Before starting, collect all of the supplies that you will need to use for preparing and injecting SYLATRON. For each injection you will need a SYLATRON vial package that contains:

- 1 vial of SYLATRON powder
- 1 vial of sterile water for injection (diluent)
- 2 single-use disposable syringes (BD Safety Lok syringes with a safety sleeve)
- 2 alcohol swabs

You will also need:

- 1 cotton ball or gauze
- a puncture-proof disposable container to throw away used syringes, needles, and vials.

Important:

- **Do not re-use or share syringes and needles.**
- The vial of mixed SYLATRON should be used right away. Do not mix more than 1 vial of SYLATRON at a time. If you do not use the vial of the prepared solution right away, store it in a refrigerator and use within 24 hours. See the end of these Instructions for Use for information about "How should I store SYLATRON?"
- Make sure you have the right syringe and needle to use with SYLATRON. Your healthcare provider should tell you what syringes and needles to use to inject SYLATRON.

How should I prepare a dose of SYLATRON?

Before you inject SYLATRON, the powder must be mixed with 0.7 mL of the sterile water for injection (diluent) that comes in the SYLATRON vial package.

1. Find a clean, well-lit, flat work surface.
2. Get 1 of your SYLATRON vial packages. Check the date printed on the SYLATRON carton. Make sure that the expiration date has not passed. Do not use your SYLATRON vial packages if the expiration date has passed. The medicine in the SYLATRON vial should look like a white to off-white tablet that is whole, or in pieces, or powdered.
   If you have already mixed the SYLATRON solution and stored it in the refrigerator, take it out of the refrigerator before use and allow the solution to come to room temperature.
3. Wash your hands well with soap and water, rinse and towel dry (see Figure 1). Keep your work area, your hands, and injection site clean to decrease the risk of infection.

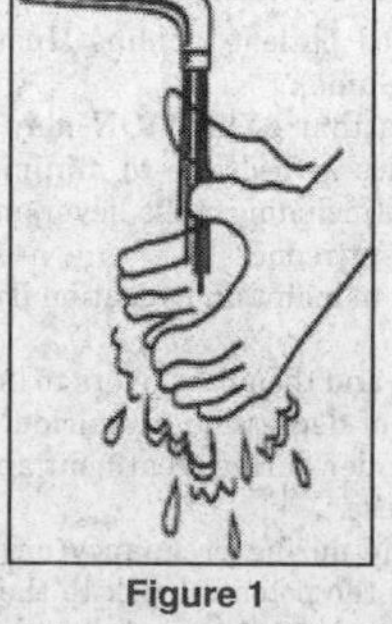

Figure 1

The disposable syringes have needles that are already attached and cannot be removed. Each syringe has a clear plastic safety sleeve that is pulled over the needle for disposal after use. The safety sleeve should remain tight against the flange while using the syringe and moved over the needle only when ready for disposal. (See Figure 2.)

[See figure 2 at top of next column]

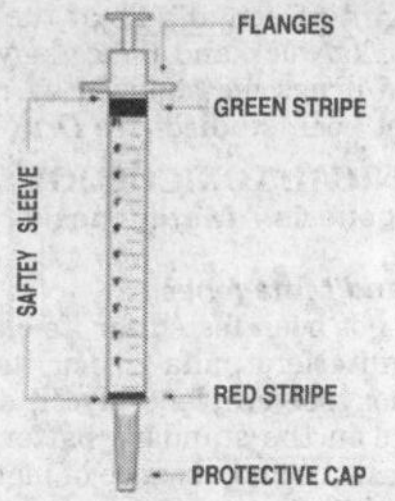

Figure 2

4. Remove the protective wrapper from one of the syringes provided. Use the syringe for steps 4 through 15. Make sure that the syringe safety sleeve is sitting against the flange. (See Figure 2.)
5. Remove the protective plastic cap from the tops of both the sterile water for injection (diluent) and the SYLATRON vials (see Figure 3). Clean the rubber stopper on the top of both vials with an alcohol swab.

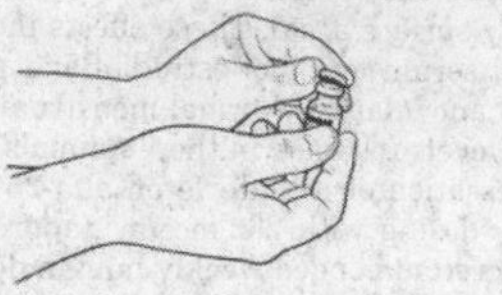

Figure 3

6. Carefully remove the protective cap straight off of the needle to avoid damaging the needle point.
7. Fill the syringe with air by pulling back on the plunger to 0.7 mL. (See Figure 4.)

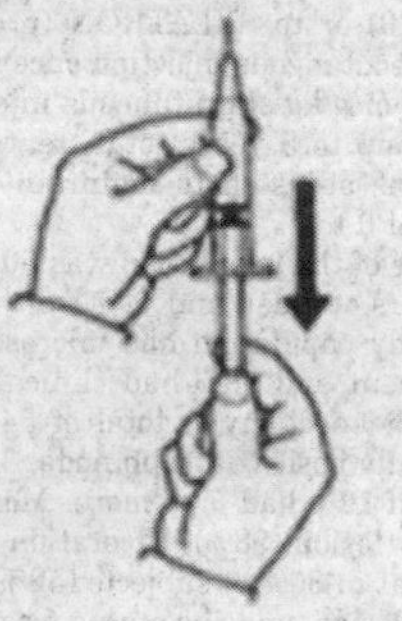

Figure 4

8. Hold the diluent vial upright. Do not touch the cleaned top of the vial with your hands.
   - Push the needle through the center of the rubber stopper of the diluent vial. (See Figure 5.)
   - Slowly inject all the air from the syringe into the air space above the diluent in the vial. (See Figure 6.)

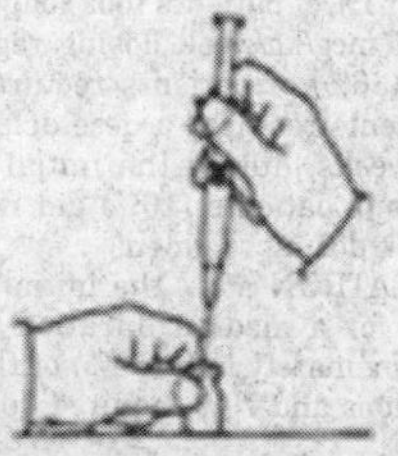

Figure 5

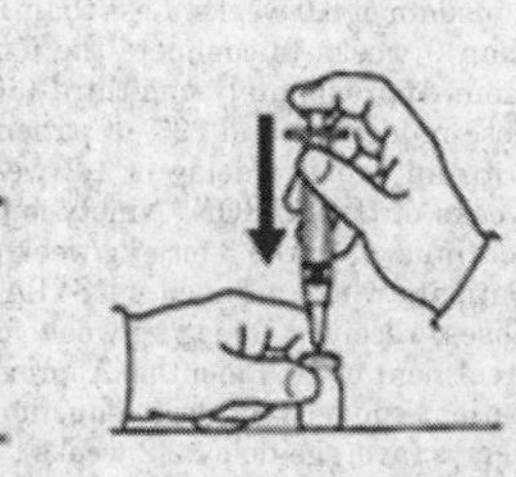

Figure 6

9. Turn the vial upside down and make sure the tip of the needle is in the liquid.
10. Withdraw only 0.7 mL of diluent by pulling the plunger back to the 0.7 mL mark on the side of the syringe. (See Figure 7.)

[See figure 7 at top of next column]

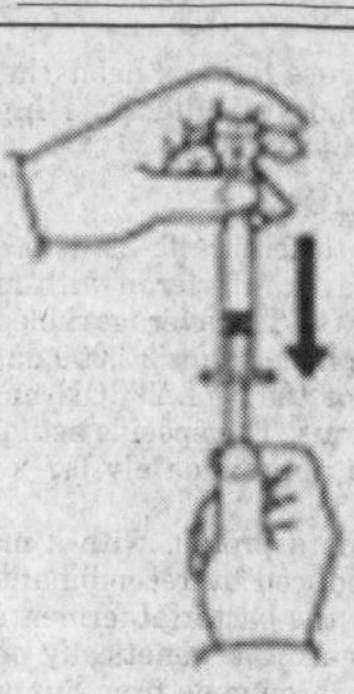

Figure 7

11. With the needle still inserted in the vial, check the syringe for air bubbles.
    - If there are any air bubbles, gently tap the syringe with your finger until the air bubbles rise to the top of the syringe.
    - Slowly push the plunger up to remove the air bubbles.
    - If you push diluent back into the vial, slowly pull back on the plunger to draw the correct amount of diluent back into the syringe.
12. Remove the needle from the vial. (See Figure 8.) Do not let the syringe touch anything.

[See figure 8 at top of next column]

Figure 8

13. Throw away the diluent vial.
14. Insert the needle through the center of the rubber stopper of the SYLATRON powder vial. Do not touch the cleaned rubber stopper.
    - Place the needle tip, at an angle, against the side of the vial. (See Figure 9.)
    - Slowly push the plunger down to inject the 0.7 mL diluent. The stream of diluent should run down the side of the vial.
    - To prevent bubbles from forming, do not aim the stream of diluent directly on the medicine in the bottom of the vial.

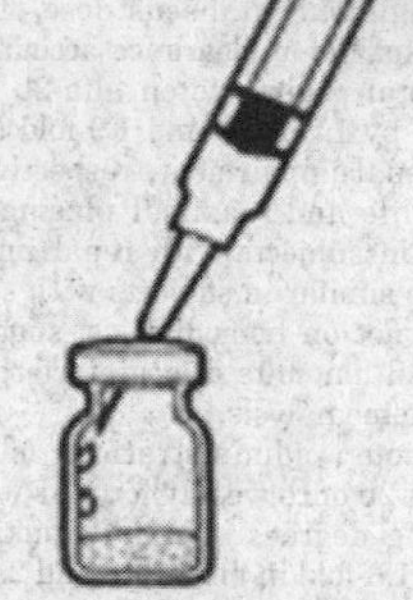

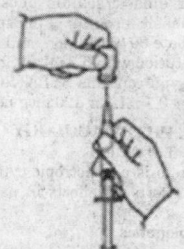

Figure 9

15. Remove the needle from the vial.
    - Firmly grasp the safety sleeve and pull it over the exposed needle until you hear a click (see Figure 10). The green stripe on the safety sleeve will completely cover the red stripe on the needle. Discard the syringe, needle, and vial in the puncture-proof container.

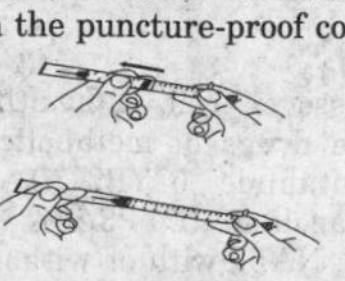

Figure 10

16. Gently swirl the vial in a gentle circular motion, until the SYLATRON is completely dissolved (mixed together). (See Figure 11.)
    - Do not shake the vial. If any powder remains undissolved in the vial, gently turn the vial upside down until all of the powder is dissolved.
    - The solution may look cloudy or bubbly for a few minutes. If air bubbles form, wait until the solution settles and all bubbles rise to the top.

[See figure 11 at top of next column]

17. After the SYLATRON completely dissolves, the solution should be clear, colorless and without particles. It is normal to see a ring of foam or bubbles on the surface.
    - Do not use the mixed solution if you see particles in it, or it is not clear and colorless. Throw away the syringe and needle in the puncture-proof container. (See the

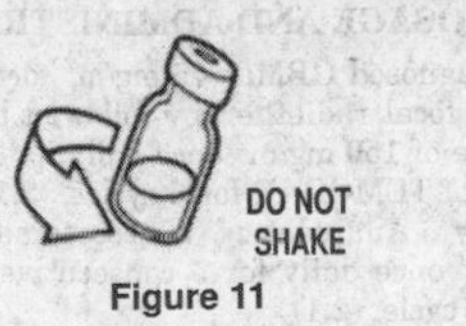

Figure 11

section "How should I dispose of the used syringes, needles, and vials?".) Then, repeat steps 1 through 17 with a new vial of SYLATRON and diluent to prepare a new syringe.

18. After the SYLATRON powder completely dissolves, clean the rubber stopper again with an alcohol swab before you withdraw your dose.
19. Unwrap the second syringe provided. You will use it to give yourself the injection.
    - Carefully remove the protective cap from the needle. Fill the syringe with air by pulling the plunger to the number on the side of the syringe (mL) that matches your prescribed dose. (See Figure 12.)

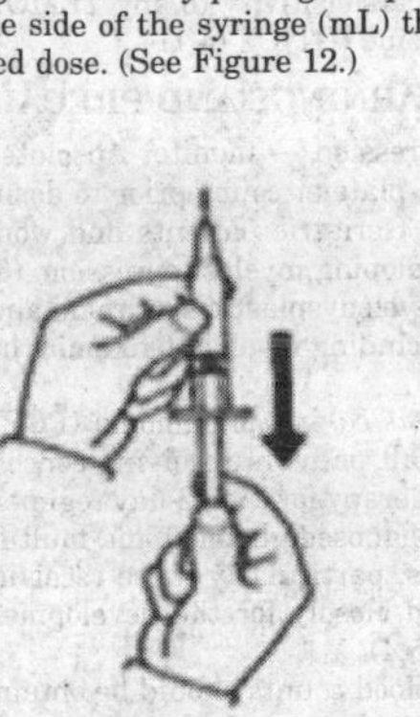
Figure 12

    - Hold the SYLATRON vial upright. Do not touch the cleaned top of the vial with your hands. (See Figure 13.)

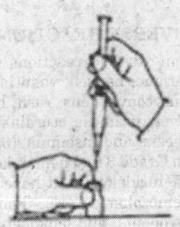

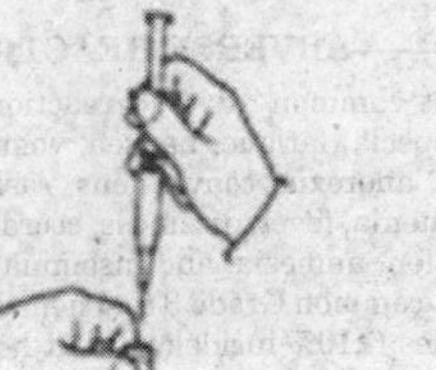
Figure 13

    - Insert the needle into the vial containing the SYLATRON solution. Inject the air into the center of the vial. (See Figure 14.)

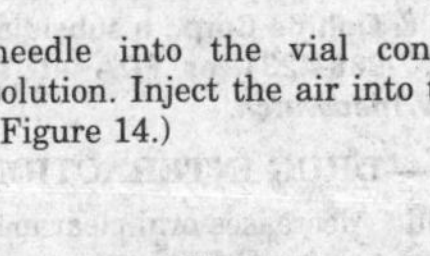
Figure 14

20. Turn the SYLATRON vial upside down. Be sure the tip of the needle is in the SYLATRON solution.
    - Hold the vial and syringe with one hand. Be sure the tip of the needle is in the SYLATRON solution. With the other hand, slowly pull the plunger back to fill the syringe with the exact amount of SYLATRON into the syringe your healthcare provider told you to use. (See Figure 15.)

[See figure 15 at top of next column]

21. Check for air bubbles in the syringe. If you see any air bubbles, hold the syringe with the needle pointing up. Gently tap the syringe until the air bubbles rise. Then, slowly push the plunger up to remove any air bubbles. If you push solution into the vial, slowly pull back on the plunger again to draw the correct amount of SYLATRON back into the syringe. When you are ready

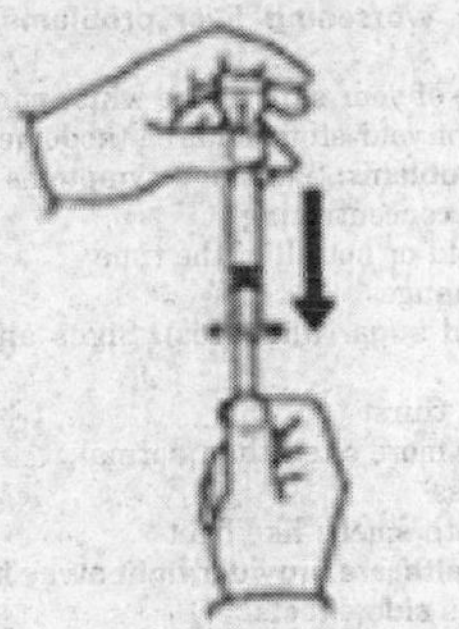
Figure 15

to inject the medicine, remove the needle from the vial. (See Figure 16.)

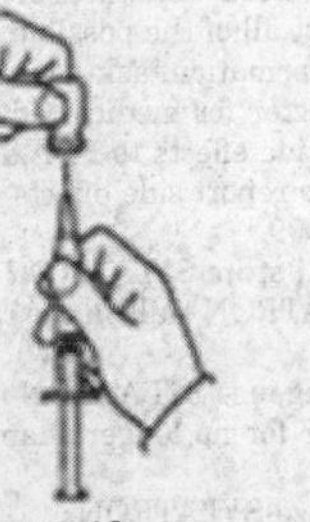
Figure 16

How should I choose a site for injection?

The best sites for giving yourself an injection are those areas with a layer of fat between the skin and muscle, like your thigh, the outer surface of your upper arm, and abdomen (see Figure 17). Do not inject yourself in the area near your navel or waistline. If you are very thin, you should only use the thigh or outer surface of the arm for injection.

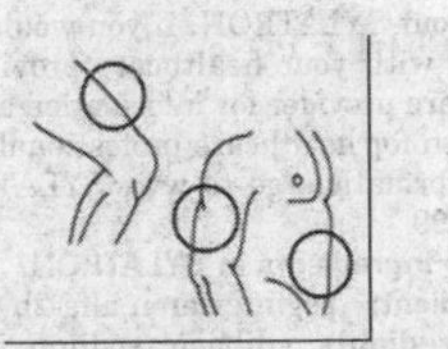
Figure 17

You should use a different site each time you inject SYLATRON to help avoid soreness at any one site. Do not inject SYLATRON solution into an area where the skin is irritated, red, bruised, infected or has scars, stretch marks, or lumps.

How should I inject a dose of SYLATRON?

22. Clean the skin where the injection is to be given with an alcohol swab. Wait for the area to dry.
    - Make sure the safety sleeve of the syringe is pushed firmly against the syringe flange so that the needle is fully exposed. (See Figure 2.)
23. With one hand, pinch a fold of skin. With your other hand, pick up the syringe and hold it like a pencil.
    - Insert the needle into the pinched skin at a 45- to 90-degree angle with a quick dart-like motion (see Figure 18).

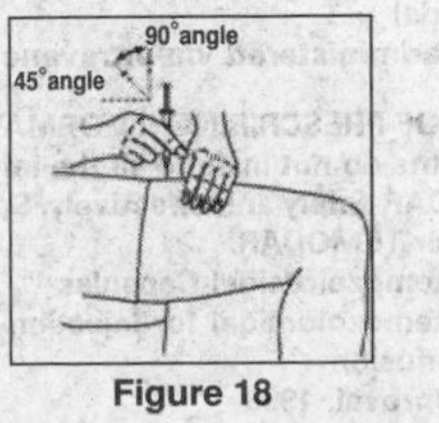

Figure 18

    - After the needle is inserted, remove the hand that you used to pinch your skin. Use it to hold the syringe barrel.
    - Pull the plunger of the syringe back very slightly.
    - **If no blood is present in the syringe**, inject the medicine by gently pressing the plunger all the way down the syringe barrel, until the syringe is empty.
    - **If blood comes into the syringe**, the needle has entered a blood vessel. Do not inject.
        - Withdraw the needle and throw away the syringe and needle in the puncture-proof container. (See step 24 and the disposal steps below.)
        - Then, repeat steps 1 through 23 with a new vial of SYLATRON and diluent to prepare a new syringe, and inject the medicine at a new site.
24. When the syringe is empty, pull the needle out of the skin.
    - Place a cotton ball or gauze over the injection site and press for several seconds. Do not massage the injection site.
    - If there is bleeding, cover it with a bandage.
25. After injecting your dose:
    - Firmly grasp the safety sleeve and pull it over the exposed needle until you hear a click, and the green stripe on the safety sleeve covers the red stripe on the needle (see Figure 19).

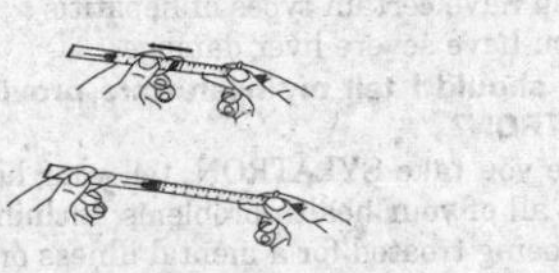
Figure 19

26. Throw away the used syringe, needle, and SYLATRON vial(s) in the puncture-proof disposable container. (See "How should I dispose of the used syringes, needles, and vials?".)

How should I dispose of the used syringes, needles, and vials?

- Throw away used syringes, needles, and vials in a puncture-proof container, sharps container, or a hard container like a metal can with a lid. Always place needles facing down. Do not use glass or clear plastic containers. **Always keep the puncture-proof container out of the reach of children.**
- Do not throw away used needles, syringes, or the puncture-proof container in household trash and do not recycle them.
- Check with your healthcare provider for instructions about the right way to throw away used needles and syringes. There may be local or state laws about how to throw away used needles and syringes. Always follow the instructions of your healthcare provider.

How should I store SYLATRON?

- Before mixing, store SYLATRON vials at 59°F to 86°F (15°C to 30°C).
- After mixing, use SYLATRON right away or store it in the refrigerator for up to 24 hours between 36°F to 46°F (2°C to 8°C). Throw away any mixed SYLATRON that is not used within 24 hours.
- Do not freeze SYLATRON.
- Keep SYLATRON away from heat.
- **Keep SYLATRON and all medicines out of the reach of children.**

These Instructions for Use have been approved by the U.S. Food and Drug Administration.

Manufactured by: Schering Corporation, a subsidiary of **MERCK & CO., INC.**, Whitehouse Station, NJ 08889, USA

U.S. Patent Nos. 5,951,974; 6,180,096; and 6,610,830.

Revised: 07/2012

LRN# 054031-SYL-PWi-IFU.8

MEDICATION GUIDE

SYLATRON™ (SY-LA-TRON)

(Peginterferon alfa-2b)

Read this Medication Guide before you start taking SYLATRON, and each time you get a refill. There may be new information. This Medication Guide does not take the place of talking with your healthcare provider about your medical condition or your treatment.

What is the most important information I should know about SYLATRON?

SYLATRON can cause serious mental health problems which can lead to suicide.

SYLATRON may cause you to develop mood or behavior problems that may get worse during treatment with SYLATRON or after your last dose. Call your healthcare provider right away if you, your family, or caregiver notice any of the following:

- irritability (getting upset easily)
- depression (feeling low, feeling bad about yourself, or feeling hopeless)
- aggressive behavior
- thoughts of hurting yourself or others, or thoughts of suicide

Former drug addicts may fall back into drug addiction or overdose.

If you have these symptoms, your healthcare provider should carefully monitor you during treatment with SYLATRON and for 6 months after your last dose.

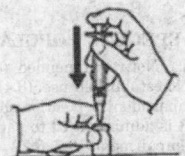

If symptoms get worse or become severe and continue, your healthcare provider may tell you to stop taking SYLATRON permanently. These signs or symptoms may not go away after you stop taking SYLATRON.
See **"What are the possible side effects of SYLATRON?"** for more information about side effects.

What is SYLATRON?

SYLATRON is a prescription medicine that is used to prevent malignant melanoma (a kind of skin cancer) from coming back after it has been removed by surgery. SYLATRON should be started within 84 days of surgery to remove lymph nodes containing cancer.
It is not known if SYLATRON is safe and effective in children less than 18 years of age.

Who should not take SYLATRON?

Do not take SYLATRON:
- if you have had a serious allergic reaction to peginterferon alfa-2b or to interferon alfa-2b
- if you have certain types of hepatitis
- if you have severe liver damage

What should I tell my healthcare provider before taking SYLATRON?

Before you take SYLATRON, tell your healthcare provider about all of your health problems, including if you:
- are being treated for a mental illness or had treatment in the past for mental illness, including depression or thoughts of suicide or suicide attempts. See **"What is the most important information I should know about SYLATRON?"**
- have liver damage from drugs or disease
- have ever been addicted to drugs or alcohol
- have or had an overactive or underactive thyroid gland
- have diabetes
- have any other medical problem(s)
- are pregnant or plan to become pregnant. It is not known if SYLATRON will harm your unborn baby.
- are breastfeeding or plan to breastfeed. You and your healthcare provider should decide if you should use SYLATRON or breastfeed. You should not do both.

Tell your healthcare provider about all the medicines you take, including prescription and non-prescription medicines, vitamins, and herbal supplements.
SYLATRON and certain other medicines may affect each other and cause side effects.
Know the medicines you take. Keep a list of them to show your healthcare providers and pharmacists each time you get a new medicine.
You should not start a new medicine before your talk with the healthcare provider who prescribes you SYLATRON.

How should I take SYLATRON?

- Take SYLATRON exactly as your healthcare provider tells you to. Your healthcare provider will tell you how much SYLATRON to take and when to take it.
- Do not take more than your prescribed dose. Call your healthcare provider right away if you take too much SYLATRON.
- Inject SYLATRON one time each week unless instructed differently by your healthcare provider. Call your healthcare provider for instructions if you miss a dose.
- SYLATRON is given as an injection under your skin (subcutaneous injection). Your healthcare provider should show you how to prepare and measure your dose of SYLATRON, and how to inject yourself before you use SYLATRON for the first time.
- Expect to get "flu-like" symptoms when taking SYLATRON. To help reduce flu-like symptoms:
  - You should take 500 mg to 1,000 mg of acetaminophen 30 minutes before your first dose of SYLATRON.
  - Follow your healthcare provider's instructions about taking acetaminophen before future doses of SYLATRON.
  - Inject SYLATRON at bedtime to help reduce flu-like symptoms.
  - Drink plenty of fluids.

Your healthcare provider should do blood tests before starting and during treatment with SYLATRON.
Your healthcare provider will monitor you while taking SYLATRON. Based on this monitoring, your healthcare provider may:
- Keep your prescribed dose the same;
- Reduce your prescribed dose;
- Tell you to skip a dose or doses; or
- Tell you to stop taking SYLATRON permanently.

What are the possible side effects of SYLATRON?

SYLATRON can cause serious side effects or worsen existing problems, including:
See **"What is the most important information I should know about SYLATRON?"**.
- **Heart problems.** Signs and symptoms can include:
  - fast heart rate or abnormal heart beat
  - trouble breathing or chest pain
- **Serious eye problems.** Symptoms can include:
  - decrease in vision
  - blurred vision
- **Severe or worsening liver problems.** Symptoms can include:
  - yellowing of your skin or the white part of your eyes
  - swelling of your stomach area (abdomen)
- **Thyroid problems.** Signs and symptoms can include:
  - problems concentrating
  - feeling cold or hot all of the time
  - weight changes
- **High blood sugar (diabetes).** Signs and symptoms can include:
  - increased thirst
  - urinating more often than normal
  - weight loss
  - your breath smells like fruit

Call your healthcare provider right away if you have any of these serious side effects.

The most common side effects of SYLATRON include:
- flu-like symptoms, which may include fever, headache, tiredness, muscle or joint aches, chills, nausea, or loss of appetite
- feeling sad or depressed
- redness, swelling, or itching around the injection site
- changes in blood tests measuring how your liver works

These are not all of the possible side effects of SYLATRON. For more information, ask your healthcare provider.
Call your doctor for medical advice about side effects. You may report side effects to FDA at 1–800–FDA–1088.
You may also report side effects to Schering Corporation at 1-800-526-4099.

How should I store SYLATRON?

- Store SYLATRON vials in the carton at 59°F to 86°F (15°C to 30°C).
- After mixing, use SYLATRON right away or store it in the refrigerator for no longer than 24 hours at 36°F to 46°F (2°C to 8°C).
- Do not freeze SYLATRON.

Keep SYLATRON and all medicines out of the reach of children.

General information about the safe and effective use of SYLATRON

Medicines are sometimes prescribed for purposes other than those listed in a Medication Guide. Do not use SYLATRON for a condition for which it was not prescribed. Do not give to other people; it may harm them.
This Medication Guide summarizes the most important information about SYLATRON. If you would like more information, talk with your healthcare provider. You can ask your healthcare provider for information about SYLATRON that is written for healthcare professionals.
For more information, go to www.SYLATRON.com or call 1-800-526-4099.

What are the ingredients in SYLATRON?

Active ingredient: peginterferon alfa-2b
Inactive ingredients: dibasic sodium phosphate anhydrous, monobasic sodium phosphate dihydrate, polysorbate 80, sucrose, sterile water for injection is supplied as a diluent.
The Medication Guide has been approved by the U.S. Food and Drug Administration.
Manufactured by: Schering Corporation, a subsidiary of **MERCK & CO., INC.**, Whitehouse Station, NJ 08889, USA
U.S. Patent Nos. 5,951,974; 6,180,096; and 6,610,830.
Revised: 07/2012
LRN#054031-SYL-PWi-MG.9

TEMODAR® ℞
[*tĕm-ō-dăr*]
(temozolomide)
Capsules

TEMODAR®
(temozolomide)
for Injection administered via intravenous infusion

HIGHLIGHTS OF PRESCRIBING INFORMATION
These highlights do not include all the information needed to use TEMODAR safely and effectively. See full prescribing information for TEMODAR.
TEMODAR® (temozolomide) Capsules
TEMODAR® (temozolomide) for Injection administered via intravenous infusion
Initial U.S. Approval: 1999

INDICATIONS AND USAGE

TEMODAR is an alkylating drug indicated for the treatment of adult patients with:
- Newly diagnosed glioblastoma multiforme (GBM) concomitantly with radiotherapy and then as maintenance treatment. (1.1)
- Refractory anaplastic astrocytoma patients who have experienced disease progression on a drug regimen containing nitrosourea and procarbazine. (1.2)

DOSAGE AND ADMINISTRATION

- Newly Diagnosed GBM: 75 mg/m^2 for 42 days concomitant with focal radiotherapy followed by initial maintenance dose of 150 mg/m^2 once daily for Days 1–5 of a 28-day cycle of TEMODAR for 6 cycles. (2.1)
- Refractory Anaplastic Astrocytoma: Initial dose 150 mg/m^2 once daily for 5 consecutive days per 28-day treatment cycle. (2.1)
- The recommended dose for TEMODAR as an intravenous infusion over 90 minutes is the same as the dose for the oral capsule formulation. Bioequivalence has been established only when TEMODAR for Injection was given over 90 minutes. (2.1, 12.3)

DOSAGE FORMS AND STRENGTHS

- 5-mg, 20-mg, 100-mg, 140-mg, 180-mg, and 250-mg capsules. (3)
- 100-mg powder for injection. (3)

CONTRAINDICATIONS

- Known hypersensitivity to any TEMODAR component or to dacarbazine (DTIC). (4.1)

WARNINGS AND PRECAUTIONS

- Myelosuppression — monitor Absolute Neutrophil Count (ANC) and platelet count prior to dosing and throughout treatment. Geriatric patients and women have a higher risk of developing myelosuppression. (5.1)
- Cases of myelodysplastic syndrome and secondary malignancies, including myeloid leukemia, have been observed. (5.2)
- *Pneumocystis carinii* pneumonia (PCP) – prophylaxis required for all patients receiving concomitant TEMODAR and radiotherapy for the 42-day regimen for the treatment of newly diagnosed glioblastoma multiforme. (5.3)
- All patients, particularly those receiving steroids, should be observed closely for the development of lymphopenia and PCP. (5.4)
- Complete blood counts should be obtained throughout the treatment course as specified. (5.4)
- Fetal harm can occur when administered to a pregnant woman. Women should be advised to avoid becoming pregnant when receiving TEMODAR. (5.5)
- As bioequivalence has been established only when given over 90 minutes, infusion over a shorter or longer period of time may result in suboptimal dosing; the possibility of an increase in infusion-related adverse reactions cannot be ruled out. (5.6)

ADVERSE REACTIONS

- The most common adverse reactions (≥10% incidence) are: alopecia, fatigue, nausea, vomiting, headache, constipation, anorexia, convulsions, rash, hemiparesis, diarrhea, asthenia, fever, dizziness, coordination abnormal, viral infection, amnesia, and insomnia. (6.1)
- The most common Grade 3 to 4 hematologic laboratory abnormalities (≥10% incidence) that have developed during treatment with temozolomide are: lymphopenia, thrombocytopenia, neutropenia, and leukopenia. (6.1)
- Allergic reactions have also been reported. (6)

To report SUSPECTED ADVERSE REACTIONS, contact Merck Sharp & Dohme Corp., a subsidiary of Merck & Co., Inc., at 1-877-888-4231 or FDA at 1-800-FDA-1088 or *www.fda.gov/medwatch*.

DRUG INTERACTIONS

- Valproic acid: decreases oral clearance of temozolomide. (7.1)

USE IN SPECIFIC POPULATIONS

- Nursing mothers: Not recommended. (8.3)
- Pediatric use: No established use. (8.4)
- Hepatic/Renal Impairment: Caution should be exercised when TEMODAR is administered to patients with severe renal or hepatic impairment. (8.6, 8.7)

See 17 for PATIENT COUNSELING INFORMATION and FDA-approved patient labeling

Revised: 06/2013

FULL PRESCRIBING INFORMATION: CONTENTS*

*** Sections or subsections omitted from the full prescribing information are not listed**

FULL PRESCRIBING INFORMATION

1 INDICATIONS AND USAGE

1.1 Newly Diagnosed Glioblastoma Multiforme

TEMODAR® (temozolomide) is indicated for the treatment of adult patients with newly diagnosed glioblastoma multiforme concomitantly with radiotherapy and then as maintenance treatment.

1.2 Refractory Anaplastic Astrocytoma

TEMODAR is indicated for the treatment of adult patients with refractory anaplastic astrocytoma, i.e., patients who have experienced disease progression on a drug regimen containing nitrosourea and procarbazine.

2 DOSAGE AND ADMINISTRATION

2.1 Recommended Dosing and Dose Modification Guidelines

The recommended dose for TEMODAR as an intravenous infusion over 90 minutes is the same as the dose for the oral capsule formulation. Bioequivalence has been established only when TEMODAR for Injection was given over 90 minutes *[see Clinical Pharmacology (12.3)]*. Dosage of TEMODAR must be adjusted according to nadir neutrophil and platelet counts in the previous cycle and the neutrophil and platelet counts at the time of initiating the next cycle. For TEMODAR dosage calculations based on body surface area (BSA) see **Table 5**. For suggested capsule combinations on a daily dose see **Table 6**.

Patients with Newly Diagnosed High Grade Glioma:

Concomitant Phase:

TEMODAR is administered at 75 mg/m^2 daily for 42 days concomitant with focal radiotherapy (60 Gy administered in 30 fractions) followed by maintenance TEMODAR for 6 cycles. Focal RT includes the tumor bed or resection site with a 2- to 3-cm margin. No dose reductions are recommended during the concomitant phase; however, dose interruptions or discontinuation may occur based on toxicity. The TEMODAR dose should be continued throughout the 42-day concomitant period up to 49 days if all of the following conditions are met: absolute neutrophil count greater than or equal to 1.5 × 10^9/L, platelet count greater than or equal to 100 × 10^9/L, common toxicity criteria (CTC) nonhematological toxicity less than or equal to Grade 1 (except for alopecia, nausea, and vomiting). During treatment a complete blood count should be obtained weekly. Temozolomide dosing should be interrupted or discontinued during concomitant phase according to the hematological and nonhematological toxicity criteria as noted in **Table 1**. *Pneumocystis carinii* pneumonia (PCP) prophylaxis is required during the concomitant administration of TEMODAR and radiotherapy, and should be continued in patients who develop lymphocytopenia until recovery from lymphocytopenia (CTC Grade less than or equal to 1).

TABLE 1: Temozolomide Dosing Interruption or Discontinuation During Concomitant Radiotherapy and Temozolomide

Toxicity	TMZ Interruption*	TMZ Discontinuation
Absolute Neutrophil Count	greater than or equal to 0.5 and less than 1.5 × 10^9/L	less than 0.5 × 10^9/L
Platelet Count	greater than or equal to 10 and less than 100 × 10^9/L	less than 10 × 10^9/L
CTC Nonhematological Toxicity (except for alopecia, nausea, vomiting)	CTC Grade 2	CTC Grade 3 or 4

TMZ=temozolomide; CTC=Common Toxicity Criteria.

* Treatment with concomitant TMZ could be continued when all of the following conditions were met: absolute neutrophil count greater than or equal to 1.5 × 10^9/L; platelet count greater than or equal to 100 × 10^9/L; CTC nonhematological toxicity less than or equal to Grade 1 (except for alopecia, nausea, vomiting).

Maintenance Phase:

Cycle 1:

Four weeks after completing the TEMODAR+RT phase, TEMODAR is administered for an additional 6 cycles of maintenance treatment. Dosage in Cycle 1 (maintenance) is 150 mg/m^2 once daily for 5 days followed by 23 days without treatment.

Cycles 2–6:

At the start of Cycle 2, the dose can be escalated to 200 mg/m^2, if the CTC nonhematologic toxicity for Cycle 1 is Grade less than or equal to 2 (except for alopecia, nausea, and vomiting), absolute neutrophil count (ANC) is greater than or equal to 1.5 × 10^9/L, and the platelet count is greater than or equal to 100 × 10^9/L. The dose remains at 200 mg/m^2 per day for the first 5 days of each subsequent cycle except if toxicity occurs. If the dose was not escalated at Cycle 2, escalation should not be done in subsequent cycles.

Dose Reduction or Discontinuation During Maintenance:

Dose reductions during the maintenance phase should be applied according to **Tables 2** and **3**.

During treatment, a complete blood count should be obtained on Day 22 (21 days after the first dose of TEMODAR) or within 48 hours of that day, and weekly until the ANC is above 1.5 × 10^9/L (1500/μL) and the platelet count exceeds 100 × 10^9/L (100,000/μL). The next cycle of TEMODAR should not be started until the ANC and platelet count exceed these levels. Dose reductions during the next cycle should be based on the lowest blood counts and worst nonhematologic toxicity during the previous cycle. Dose reductions or discontinuations during the maintenance phase should be applied according to **Tables 2** and **3**.

TABLE 2: Temozolomide Dose Levels for Maintenance Treatment

Dose Level	Dose (mg/m^2/day)	Remarks
−1	100	Reduction for prior toxicity
0	150	Dose during Cycle 1
1	200	Dose during Cycles 2–6 in absence of toxicity

TABLE 3: Temozolomide Dose Reduction or Discontinuation During Maintenance Treatment

Toxicity	Reduce TMZ by 1 Dose Level*	Discontinue TMZ
Absolute Neutrophil Count	less than 1.0 × 10^9/L	See footnote†
Platelet Count	less than 50 × 10^9/L	See footnote†
CTC Nonhematological Toxicity (except for alopecia, nausea, vomiting)	CTC Grade 3	CTC Grade 4†

TMZ=temozolomide; CTC=Common Toxicity Criteria.

* TMZ dose levels are listed in **Table 2**.

† TMZ is to be discontinued if dose reduction to less than 100 mg/m^2 is required or if the same Grade 3 nonhematological toxicity (except for alopecia, nausea, vomiting) recurs after dose reduction.

Patients with Refractory Anaplastic Astrocytoma:

For adults the initial dose is 150 mg/m^2 once daily for 5 consecutive days per 28-day treatment cycle. For adult patients, if both the nadir and day of dosing (Day 29, Day 1 of next cycle) ANC are greater than or equal to 1.5 × 10^9/L (1500/μL) and both the nadir and Day 29, Day 1 of next cycle platelet counts are greater than or equal to 100 × 10^9/L (100,000/μL), the TEMODAR dose may be increased to 200 mg/m^2/day for 5 consecutive days per 28-day treatment cycle. During treatment, a complete blood count should be obtained on Day 22 (21 days after the first dose) or within 48 hours of that day, and weekly until the ANC is above 1.5 × 10^9/L (1500/μL) and the platelet count exceeds 100 × 10^9/L (100,000/μL). The next cycle of TEMODAR should not be started until the ANC and platelet count exceed these levels. If the ANC falls to less than 1.0 × 10^9/L (1000/μL) or the platelet count is less than 50 × 10^9/L (50,000/μL) during any cycle, the next cycle should be reduced by 50 mg/m^2, but not below 100 mg/m^2, the lowest recommended dose (see **Table 4**). TEMODAR therapy can be continued until disease progression. In the clinical trial, treatment could be continued for a maximum of 2 years, but the optimum duration of therapy is not known.

TABLE 4: Dosing Modification Table

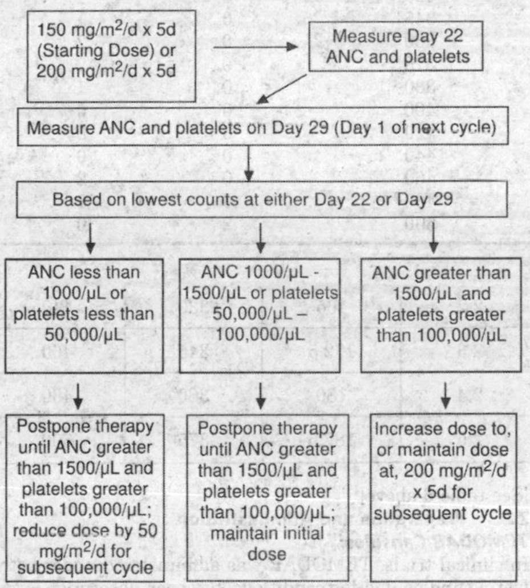

TABLE 5: Daily Dose Calculations by Body Surface Area (BSA)

Total BSA (m^2)	75 mg/m^2 (mg daily)	150 mg/m^2 (mg daily)	200 mg/m^2 (mg daily)
1.0	75	150	200
1.1	82.5	165	220
1.2	90	180	240
1.3	97.5	195	260
1.4	105	210	280
1.5	112.5	225	300
1.6	120	240	320
1.7	127.5	255	340
1.8	135	270	360
1.9	142.5	285	380
2.0	150	300	400
2.1	157.5	315	420

TABLE 6: Suggested Capsule Combinations Based on Daily Dose in Adults

	Number of Daily Capsules by Strength (mg)					
Total Daily Dose (mg)	**250 mg**	**180 mg**	**140 mg**	**100 mg**	**20 mg**	**5 mg**
75	0	0	0	0	3	3
82.5	0	0	0	0	4	0
90	0	0	0	0	4	2
97.5	0	0	0	1	0	0
105	0	0	0	1	0	1
112.5	0	0	0	1	0	2
120	0	0	0	1	1	0
127.5	0	0	0	1	1	1
135	0	0	0	1	1	3
142.5	0	0	1	0	0	0
150	0	0	1	0	0	2
157.5	0	0	1	0	1	0
165	0	0	1	0	1	1
172.5	0	0	1	0	1	2
180	0	1	0	0	0	0
187.5	0	1	0	0	0	1
195	0	1	0	0	0	3
200	0	1	0	0	1	0
210	0	0	0	2	0	2
220	0	0	0	2	1	0
225	0	0	0	2	1	1
240	0	0	1	1	0	0
255	1	0	0	0	0	1
260	1	0	0	0	0	2
270	1	0	0	0	1	0
280	0	0	2	0	0	0
285	0	0	2	0	0	1
300	0	0	0	3	0	0
315	0	0	0	3	0	3
320	0	1	1	0	0	0
330	0	1	1	0	0	2
340	0	1	1	0	1	0
345	0	1	1	0	1	1
360	0	2	0	0	0	0
375	0	2	0	0	0	3
380	0	1	0	2	0	0
400	0	0	0	4	0	0
420	0	0	3	0	0	0
440	0	0	3	0	1	0
460	0	2	0	1	0	0
480	0	1	0	3	0	0
500	2	0	0	0	0	0

2.2	165	330	440
2.3	172.5	345	460
2.4	180	360	480
2.5	187.5	375	500

[See table 6 above]

2.2 Preparation and Administration

TEMODAR Capsules:

In clinical trials, TEMODAR was administered under both fasting and nonfasting conditions; however, absorption is affected by food *[see Clinical Pharmacology (12.3)]*, and consistency of administration with respect to food is recommended. There are no dietary restrictions with TEMODAR. To reduce nausea and vomiting, TEMODAR should be taken on an empty stomach. Bedtime administration may be advised. Antiemetic therapy may be administered prior to and/or following administration of TEMODAR.

TEMODAR (temozolomide) Capsules should not be opened or chewed. They should be swallowed whole with a glass of water.

If capsules are accidentally opened or damaged, precautions should be taken to avoid inhalation or contact with the skin or mucous membranes *[see How Supplied/Storage and Handling (16.1)]*.

TEMODAR for Injection:

Each vial of TEMODAR for Injection contains sterile and pyrogen-free temozolomide lyophilized powder. When reconstituted with 41 mL Sterile Water for Injection, the resulting solution will contain 2.5 mg/mL temozolomide. Bring the vial to room temperature prior to reconstitution with Sterile Water for Injection. The vials should be gently swirled and not shaken. Vials should be inspected, and any vial containing visible particulate matter should not be used. Do not further dilute the reconstituted solution. After reconstitution, store at room temperature (25°C [77°F]). Reconstituted product must be used within 14 hours, including infusion time.

Using aseptic technique, withdraw up to 40 mL from each vial to make up the total dose based on **Table 5** above and transfer into an empty 250 mL infusion bag {2}. TEMODAR for Injection should be infused intravenously using a pump over a period of 90 minutes. TEMODAR for Injection should be administered only by intravenous infusion. Flush the lines before and after each TEMODAR infusion.

TEMODAR for Injection may be administered in the same intravenous line with 0.9% Sodium Chloride injection only. Because no data are available on the compatibility of TEMODAR for Injection with other intravenous substances or additives, other medications should not be infused simultaneously through the same intravenous line.

3 DOSAGE FORMS AND STRENGTHS

- TEMODAR (temozolomide) Capsules for oral administration
  - 5-mg capsules have opaque white bodies with green caps. The capsule body is imprinted with two stripes, the dosage strength, and the Schering-Plough logo. The cap is imprinted with "TEMODAR."
  - 20-mg capsules have opaque white bodies with yellow caps. The capsule body is imprinted with two stripes, the dosage strength, and the Schering-Plough logo. The cap is imprinted with "TEMODAR."
  - 100-mg capsules have opaque white bodies with pink caps. The capsule body is imprinted with two stripes, the dosage strength, and the Schering-Plough logo. The cap is imprinted with "TEMODAR."
  - 140-mg capsules have opaque white bodies with blue caps. The capsule body is imprinted with two stripes, the dosage strength, and the Schering-Plough logo. The cap is imprinted with "TEMODAR."
  - 180-mg capsules have opaque white bodies with orange caps. The capsule body is imprinted with two stripes, the dosage strength, and the Schering-Plough logo. The cap is imprinted with "TEMODAR."
  - 250-mg capsules have opaque white bodies with white caps. The capsule body is imprinted with two stripes, the dosage strength, and the Schering-Plough logo. The cap is imprinted with "TEMODAR."
- TEMODAR (temozolomide) is available as 100-mg/vial powder for injection. The lyophilized powder is white to light tan/light pink.

4 CONTRAINDICATIONS

4.1 Hypersensitivity

TEMODAR (temozolomide) is contraindicated in patients who have a history of hypersensitivity reaction (such as urticaria, allergic reaction including anaphylaxis, toxic epidermal necrolysis, and Stevens-Johnson syndrome) to any of its components. TEMODAR is also contraindicated in patients who have a history of hypersensitivity to dacarbazine (DTIC), since both drugs are metabolized to 5-(3-methyltriazen-1-yl)-imidazole-4-carboxamide (MTIC).

5 WARNINGS AND PRECAUTIONS

5.1 Myelosuppression

Patients treated with TEMODAR may experience myelosuppression, including prolonged pancytopenia, which may result in aplastic anemia, which in some cases has resulted in a fatal outcome. In some cases, exposure to concomitant medications associated with aplastic anemia, including carbamazepine, phenytoin, and sulfamethoxazole/trimethoprim, complicates assessment. Prior to dosing, patients must have an absolute neutrophil count (ANC) greater than or equal to 1.5×10^9/L and a platelet count greater than or equal to 100×10^9/L. A complete blood count should be obtained on Day 22 (21 days after the first dose) or within 48 hours of that day, and weekly until the ANC is above 1.5×10^9/L and platelet count exceeds 100×10^9/L. Geriatric patients and women have been shown in clinical trials to have a higher risk of developing myelosuppression.

5.2 Myelodysplastic Syndrome

Cases of myelodysplastic syndrome and secondary malignancies, including myeloid leukemia, have been observed.

5.3 *Pneumocystis carinii* Pneumonia

For treatment of newly diagnosed glioblastoma multiforme: Prophylaxis against *Pneumocystis carinii* pneumonia (PCP) is required for all patients receiving concomitant TEMODAR and radiotherapy for the 42-day regimen.

There may be a higher occurrence of PCP when temozolomide is administered during a longer dosing regimen. However, all patients receiving temozolomide, particularly patients receiving steroids, should be observed closely for the development of PCP regardless of the regimen.

5.4 Laboratory Tests

For the concomitant treatment phase with RT, a complete blood count should be obtained prior to initiation of treatment and weekly during treatment.

For the 28-day treatment cycles, a complete blood count should be obtained prior to treatment on Day 1 and on Day 22 (21 days after the first dose) of each cycle. Blood counts should be performed weekly until recovery if the ANC falls below 1.5×10^9/L and the platelet count falls below 100×10^9/L *[see Recommended Dosing and Dose Modification Guidelines (2.1)]*.

5.5 Use in Pregnancy

TEMODAR can cause fetal harm when administered to a pregnant woman. Administration of TEMODAR to rats and rabbits during organogenesis at 0.38 and 0.75 times the maximum recommended human dose (75 and 150 mg/m^2), respectively, caused numerous fetal malformations of the external organs, soft tissues, and skeleton in both species *[see Use in Specific Populations (8.1)]*.

5.6 Infusion Time

As bioequivalence has been established only when TEMODAR for Injection was given over 90 minutes, infusion over a shorter or longer period of time may result in suboptimal dosing. Additionally, the possibility of an increase in infusion-related adverse reactions cannot be ruled out.

6 ADVERSE REACTIONS

6.1 Clinical Trials Experience

Because clinical trials are conducted under widely varying conditions, adverse reaction rates observed in the clinical trials of a drug cannot be directly compared to rates in the clinical trials of another drug and may not reflect the rates observed in practice.

Newly Diagnosed Glioblastoma Multiforme:

During the concomitant phase (TEMODAR+radiotherapy), adverse reactions including thrombocytopenia, nausea, vomiting, anorexia, and constipation were more frequent in the TEMODAR+RT arm. The incidence of other adverse reactions was comparable in the two arms. The most common adverse reactions across the cumulative TEMODAR experience were alopecia, nausea, vomiting, anorexia, headache, and constipation (see **Table 7**). Forty-nine percent (49%) of patients treated with TEMODAR reported one or more severe or life-threatening reactions, most commonly fatigue (13%), convulsions (6%), headache (5%), and thrombocytopenia (5%). Overall, the pattern of reactions during the maintenance phase was consistent with the known safety profile of TEMODAR.

[See table 7 at top of next page]

Myelosuppression (neutropenia and thrombocytopenia), which is a known dose-limiting toxicity for most cytotoxic agents, including TEMODAR, was observed. When laboratory abnormalities and adverse reactions were combined, Grade 3 or Grade 4 neutrophil abnormalities including neutropenic reactions were observed in 8% of the patients, and

Grade 3 or Grade 4 platelet abnormalities, including thrombocytopenic reactions, were observed in 14% of the patients treated with TEMODAR.

Refractory Anaplastic Astrocytoma:

Tables 8 and 9 show the incidence of adverse reactions in the 158 patients in the anaplastic astrocytoma study for whom data are available. In the absence of a control group, it is not clear in many cases whether these reactions should be attributed to temozolomide or the patients' underlying conditions, but nausea, vomiting, fatigue, and hematologic effects appear to be clearly drug-related. The most frequently occurring adverse reactions were nausea, vomiting, headache, and fatigue. The adverse reactions were usually NCI Common Toxicity Criteria (CTC) Grade 1 or 2 (mild to moderate in severity) and were self-limiting, with nausea and vomiting readily controlled with antiemetics. The incidence of severe nausea and vomiting (CTC Grade 3 or 4) was 10% and 6%, respectively. Myelosuppression (thrombocytopenia and neutropenia) was the dose-limiting adverse reaction. It usually occurred within the first few cycles of therapy and was not cumulative.

Myelosuppression occurred late in the treatment cycle and returned to normal, on average, within 14 days of nadir counts. The median nadirs occurred at 26 days for platelets (range: 21–40 days) and 28 days for neutrophils (range: 1–44 days). Only 14% (22/158) of patients had a neutrophil nadir and 20% (32/158) of patients had a platelet nadir, which may have delayed the start of the next cycle. Less than 10% of patients required hospitalization, blood transfusion, or discontinuation of therapy due to myelosuppression.

In clinical trial experience with 110 to 111 women and 169 to 174 men (depending on measurements), there were higher rates of Grade 4 neutropenia (ANC less than 500 cells/μL) and thrombocytopenia (less than 20,000 cells/μL) in women than men in the first cycle of therapy (12% vs. 5% and 9% vs. 3%, respectively).

In the entire safety database for which hematologic data exist (N=932), 7% (4/61) and 9.5% (6/63) of patients over age 70 experienced Grade 4 neutropenia or thrombocytopenia in the first cycle, respectively. For patients less than or equal to age 70, 7% (62/871) and 5.5% (48/879) experienced Grade 4 neutropenia or thrombocytopenia in the first cycle, respectively. Pancytopenia, leukopenia, and anemia have also been reported.

TABLE 7: Number (%) of Patients with Adverse Reactions: All and Severe/Life Threatening (Incidence of 5% or Greater)

	Concomitant Phase RT Alone (n=285)		Concomitant Phase RT+TMZ (n=288)*		Maintenance Phase TMZ (n=224)	
	All	Grade ≥3	All	Grade ≥3	All	Grade ≥3
Subjects Reporting any Adverse Reaction	**258 (91)**	**74 (26)**	**266 (92)**	**80 (28)**	**206 (92)**	**82 (37)**
Body as a Whole — General Disorders						
Anorexia	25 (9)	1 (<1)	56 (19)	2 (1)	61 (27)	3 (1)
Dizziness	10 (4)	0	12 (4)	2 (1)	12 (5)	0
Fatigue	139 (49)	15 (5)	156 (54)	19 (7)	137 (61)	20 (9)
Headache	49 (17)	11 (4)	56 (19)	5 (2)	51 (23)	9 (4)
Weakness	9 (3)	3 (1)	10 (3)	5 (2)	16 (7)	4 (2)
Central and Peripheral Nervous System Disorders						
Confusion	12 (4)	6 (2)	11 (4)	4 (1)	12 (5)	4 (2)
Convulsions	20 (7)	9 (3)	17 (6)	10 (3)	25 (11)	7 (3)
Memory Impairment	12 (4)	1 (<1)	8 (3)	1 (<1)	16 (7)	2 (1)
Disorders of the Eye						
Vision Blurred	25 (9)	4 (1)	26 (9)	2 (1)	17 (8)	0
Disorders of the Immune System						
Allergic Reaction	7 (2)	1 (<1)	13 (5)	0	6 (3)	0
Gastrointestinal System Disorders						
Abdominal Pain	2 (1)	0	7 (2)	1 (<1)	11 (5)	1 (<1)
Constipation	18 (6)	0	53 (18)	3 (1)	49 (22)	0
Diarrhea	9 (3)	0	18 (6)	0	23 (10)	2 (1)
Nausea	45 (16)	1 (<1)	105 (36)	2 (1)	110 (49)	3 (1)
Stomatitis	14 (5)	1 (<1)	19 (7)	0	20 (9)	3 (1)
Vomiting	16 (6)	1 (<1)	57 (20)	1 (<1)	66 (29)	4 (2)
Injury and Poisoning						
Radiation Injury NOS	11 (4)	1 (<1)	20 (7)	0	5 (2)	0
Musculoskeletal System Disorders						
Arthralgia	2 (1)	0	7 (2)	1 (<1)	14 (6)	0
Platelet, Bleeding and Clotting Disorders						
Thrombocytopenia	3 (1)	0	11 (4)	8 (3)	19 (8)	8 (4)
Psychiatric Disorders						
Insomnia	9 (3)	1 (<1)	14 (5)	0	9 (4)	0
Respiratory System Disorders						
Coughing	3 (1)	0	15 (5)	2 (1)	19 (8)	1 (<1)
Dyspnea	9 (3)	4 (1)	11 (4)	5 (2)	12 (5)	1 (<1)
Skin and Subcutaneous Tissue Disorders						
Alopecia	179 (63)	0	199 (69)	0	124 (55)	0
Dry Skin	6 (2)	0	7 (2)	0	11 (5)	1 (<1)
Erythema	15 (5)	0	14 (5)	0	2 (1)	0
Pruritus	4 (1)	0	11 (4)	0	11 (5)	0
Rash	42 (15)	0	56 (19)	3 (1)	29 (13)	3 (1)
Special Senses Other, Disorders						
Taste Perversion	6 (2)	0	18 (6)	0	11 (5)	0

RT+TMZ=radiotherapy plus temozolomide; NOS=not otherwise specified.
Note: Grade 5 (fatal) adverse reactions are included in the Grade ≥3 column.
* One patient who was randomized to RT only arm received RT+temozolomide.

TABLE 8: Adverse Reactions in the Anaplastic Astrocytoma Trial in Adults (≥5%)

	No. (%) of TEMODAR Patients (N=158)	
	All Reactions	Grade 3/4
Any Adverse Reaction	**153 (97)**	**79 (50)**
Body as a Whole		
Headache	65 (41)	10 (6)
Fatigue	54 (34)	7 (4)
Asthenia	20 (13)	9 (6)
Fever	21 (13)	3 (2)
Back pain	12 (8)	4 (3)
Cardiovascular		
Edema peripheral	17 (11)	1 (1)
Central and Peripheral Nervous System		
Convulsions	36 (23)	8 (5)
Hemiparesis	29 (18)	10 (6)
Dizziness	19 (12)	1 (1)
Coordination abnormal	17 (11)	2 (1)
Amnesia	16 (10)	6 (4)
Insomnia	16 (10)	0
Paresthesia	15 (9)	1 (1)
Somnolence	15 (9)	5 (3)
Paresis	13 (8)	4 (3)
Urinary incontinence	13 (8)	3 (2)
Ataxia	12 (8)	3 (2)
Dysphasia	11 (7)	1 (1)
Convulsions local	9 (6)	0
Gait abnormal	9 (6)	1 (1)
Confusion	8 (5)	0
Endocrine		
Adrenal hypercorticism	13 (8)	0
Gastrointestinal System		
Nausea	84 (53)	16 (10)
Vomiting	66 (42)	10 (6)
Constipation	52 (33)	1 (1)
Diarrhea	25 (16)	3 (2)
Abdominal pain	14 (9)	2 (1)
Anorexia	14 (9)	1 (1)
Metabolic		
Weight increase	8 (5)	0
Musculoskeletal System		
Myalgia	8 (5)	
Psychiatric Disorders		
Anxiety	11 (7)	1 (1)
Depression	10 (6)	0
Reproductive Disorders		
Breast pain, female	4 (6)	
Resistance Mechanism Disorders		
Infection viral	17 (11)	0
Respiratory System		
Upper respiratory tract infection	13 (8)	0
Pharyngitis	12 (8)	0
Sinusitis	10 (6)	0
Coughing	8 (5)	0
Skin and Appendages		
Rash	13 (8)	0
Pruritus	12 (8)	2 (1)
Urinary System		
Urinary tract infection	12 (8)	0
Micturition increased frequency	9 (6)	0
Vision		
Diplopia	8 (5)	0
Vision abnormal*	8 (5)	

* Blurred vision; visual deficit; vision changes; vision troubles

TABLE 9: Adverse Hematologic Effects (Grade 3 to 4) in the Anaplastic Astrocytoma Trial in Adults

	TEMODAR*
Hemoglobin	7/158 (4%)
Lymphopenia	83/152 (55%)
Neutrophils	20/142 (14%)
Platelets	29/156 (19%)
WBC	18/158 (11%)

* Change from Grade 0 to 2 at baseline to Grade 3 or 4 during treatment.

TEMODAR for injection delivers equivalent temozolomide dose and exposure to both temozolomide and 5-(3-methyltriazen-1-yl)-imidazole-4-carboxamide (MTIC) as the corresponding TEMODAR capsules. Adverse reactions probably related to treatment that were reported from the 2 studies with the intravenous formulation (n=35) that were not reported in studies using the TEMODAR capsules were:

pain, irritation, pruritus, warmth, swelling, and erythema at infusion site as well as the following adverse reactions: petechiae and hematoma.

6.2 Postmarketing Experience

The following adverse reactions have been identified during postapproval use of TEMODAR. Because these reactions are reported voluntarily from a population of uncertain size, it is not always possible to reliably estimate their frequency or establish a causal relationship to the drug exposure.

TEMODAR Capsules: allergic reactions, including anaphylaxis, have been reported. Erythema multiforme has been reported, which resolved after discontinuation of TEMODAR and, in some cases, recurred upon rechallenge. Cases of toxic epidermal necrolysis and Stevens-Johnson syndrome have been reported.

There have been reported cases of hepatotoxicity, including elevations of liver enzymes, hyperbilirubinemia, cholestasis, and hepatitis.

Opportunistic infections including *Pneumocystis carinii* pneumonia (PCP) have also been reported. Cases of interstitial pneumonitis/pneumonitis, alveolitis, and pulmonary fibrosis have been reported. Prolonged pancytopenia, which may result in aplastic anemia, has been reported, and in some cases has resulted in a fatal outcome.

7 DRUG INTERACTIONS

7.1 Valproic Acid

Administration of valproic acid decreases oral clearance of temozolomide by about 5%. The clinical implication of this effect is not known *[see Clinical Pharmacology (12.3)].*

8 USE IN SPECIFIC POPULATIONS

8.1 Pregnancy

Pregnancy Category D. See Warnings and Precautions section.

TEMODAR can cause fetal harm when administered to a pregnant woman. Five consecutive days of oral temozolomide administration of 0.38 and 0.75 times the highest recommended human dose (75 and 150 mg/m^2) in rats and rabbits, respectively, during the period of organogenesis caused numerous malformations of the external and internal soft tissues and skeleton in both species. Doses equivalent to 0.75 times the highest recommended human dose (150 mg/m^2) caused embryolethality in rats and rabbits as indicated by increased resorptions. There are no adequate and well-controlled studies in pregnant women. If this drug is used during pregnancy, or if the patient becomes pregnant while taking this drug, the patient should be apprised of the potential hazard to a fetus. Women of childbearing potential should be advised to avoid becoming pregnant during therapy with TEMODAR.

8.3 Nursing Mothers

It is not known whether this drug is excreted in human milk. Because many drugs are excreted in human milk and because of the potential for serious adverse reactions in nursing infants and tumorigenicity shown for temozolomide in animal studies, a decision should be made whether to discontinue nursing or to discontinue the drug, taking into account the importance of TEMODAR to the mother.

8.4 Pediatric Use

Safety and effectiveness in pediatric patients have not been established. TEMODAR Capsules have been studied in 2 open-label studies in pediatric patients (aged 3–18 years) at a dose of 160 to 200 mg/m^2 daily for 5 days every 28 days. In one trial, 29 patients with recurrent brain stem glioma and 34 patients with recurrent high grade astrocytoma were enrolled. All patients had recurrence following surgery and radiation therapy, while 31% also had disease progression following chemotherapy. In a second study conducted by the Children's Oncology Group (COG), 122 patients were enrolled, including patients with medulloblastoma/PNET (29), high grade astrocytoma (23), low grade astrocytoma (22), brain stem glioma (16), ependymoma (14), other CNS tumors (9), and non-CNS tumors (9). The TEMODAR toxicity profile in pediatric patients is similar to adults. **Table 10** shows the adverse reactions in 122 children in the COG study.

TABLE 10: Adverse Reactions Reported in the Pediatric Cooperative Group Trial (≥10%)

	No. (%) of TEMODAR Patients (N=122)*	
Body System/Organ Class Adverse Reaction	**All Reactions**	**Grade 3/4**
Subjects Reporting an AE	**107 (88)**	**69 (57)**
Body as a Whole		
Central and Peripheral Nervous System		
Central cerebral CNS cortex	22 (18)	13 (11)
Gastrointestinal System		
Nausea	56 (46)	5 (4)
Vomiting	62 (51)	4 (3)
Platelet, Bleeding and Clotting		
Thrombocytopenia	71 (58)	31 (25)
Red Blood Cell Disorders		
Decreased Hemoglobin	62 (51)	7 (6)
White Cell and RES Disorders		
Decreased WBC	71 (58)	21 (17)
Lymphopenia	73 (60)	48 (39)
Neutropenia	62 (51)	24 (20)

* These various tumors included the following: PNET-medulloblastoma, glioblastoma, low grade astrocytoma, brain stem tumor, ependymoma, mixed glioma, oligodendroglioma, neuroblastoma, Ewing's sarcoma, pineoblastoma, alveolar soft part sarcoma, neurofibrosarcoma, optic glioma, and osteosarcoma.

8.5 Geriatric Use

Clinical studies of temozolomide did not include sufficient numbers of subjects aged 65 and over to determine whether they responded differently from younger subjects. Other reported clinical experience has not identified differences in responses between the elderly and younger patients. In general, dose selection for an elderly patient should be cautious, reflecting the greater frequency of decreased hepatic, renal, or cardiac function, and of concomitant disease or other drug therapy.

In the anaplastic astrocytoma study population, patients 70 years of age or older had a higher incidence of Grade 4 neutropenia and Grade 4 thrombocytopenia (2/8; 25%, P=0.31 and 2/10; 20%, P=0.09, respectively) in the first cycle of therapy than patients under 70 years of age *[see Warnings and Precautions (5.1) and Adverse Reactions (6.1)].*

In newly diagnosed patients with glioblastoma multiforme, the adverse reaction profile was similar in younger patients (<65 years) vs. older (≥65 years).

8.6 Renal Impairment

Caution should be exercised when TEMODAR is administered to patients with severe renal impairment *[see Clinical Pharmacology (12.3)].*

8.7 Hepatic Impairment

Caution should be exercised when TEMODAR is administered to patients with severe hepatic impairment *[see Clinical Pharmacology (12.3)].*

10 OVERDOSAGE

Doses of 500, 750, 1000, and 1250 mg/m^2 (total dose per cycle over 5 days) have been evaluated clinically in patients. Dose-limiting toxicity was hematologic and was reported with any dose but is expected to be more severe at higher doses. An overdose of 2000 mg per day for 5 days was taken by one patient and the adverse reactions reported were pancytopenia, pyrexia, multi-organ failure, and death. There are reports of patients who have taken more than 5 days of treatment (up to 64 days), with adverse reactions reported including bone marrow suppression, which in some cases was severe and prolonged, and infections and resulted in death. In the event of an overdose, hematologic evaluation is needed. Supportive measures should be provided as necessary.

11 DESCRIPTION

TEMODAR contains temozolomide, an imidazotetrazine derivative. The chemical name of temozolomide is 3,4-dihydro-3-methyl-4-oxoimidazo[5,1-d]-*as*-tetrazine-8-carboxamide. The structural formula is:

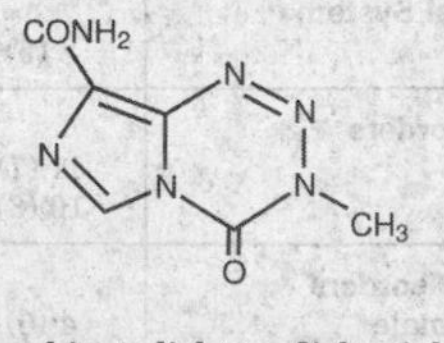

The material is a white to light tan/light pink powder with a molecular formula of $C_6H_6N_6O_2$ and a molecular weight of 194.15. The molecule is stable at acidic pH (<5) and labile at pH >7; hence TEMODAR can be administered orally and intravenously. The prodrug, temozolomide, is rapidly hydrolyzed to the active 5-(3-methyltriazen-1-yl) imidazole-4-carboxamide (MTIC) at neutral and alkaline pH values, with hydrolysis taking place even faster at alkaline pH.

TEMODAR Capsules:

Each capsule for oral use contains either 5 mg, 20 mg, 100 mg, 140 mg, 180 mg, or 250 mg of temozolomide.

The inactive ingredients for TEMODAR Capsules are as follows:

TEMODAR 5 mg: lactose anhydrous (132.8 mg), colloidal silicon dioxide (0.2 mg), sodium starch glycolate (7.5 mg), tartaric acid (1.5 mg), and stearic acid (3 mg).

TEMODAR 20 mg: lactose anhydrous (182.2 mg), colloidal silicon dioxide (0.2 mg), sodium starch glycolate (11 mg), tartaric acid (2.2 mg), and stearic acid (4.4 mg).

TEMODAR 100 mg: lactose anhydrous (175.7 mg), colloidal silicon dioxide (0.3 mg), sodium starch glycolate (15 mg), tartaric acid (3 mg), and stearic acid (6 mg).

TEMODAR 140 mg: lactose anhydrous (246 mg), colloidal silicon dioxide (0.4 mg), sodium starch glycolate (21 mg), tartaric acid (4.2 mg), and stearic acid (8.4 mg).

TEMODAR 180 mg: lactose anhydrous (316.3 mg), colloidal silicon dioxide (0.5 mg), sodium starch glycolate (27 mg), tartaric acid (5.4 mg), and stearic acid (10.8 mg).

TEMODAR 250 mg: lactose anhydrous (154.3 mg), colloidal silicon dioxide (0.7 mg), sodium starch glycolate (22.5 mg), tartaric acid (9 mg), and stearic acid (13.5 mg).

The body of the capsules is made of gelatin, and is opaque white. The cap is also made of gelatin, and the colors vary based on the dosage strength. The capsule body and cap are imprinted with pharmaceutical branding ink, which contains shellac, dehydrated alcohol, isopropyl alcohol, butyl alcohol, propylene glycol, purified water, strong ammonia solution, potassium hydroxide, and ferric oxide.

TEMODAR 5 mg: The green cap contains gelatin, titanium dioxide, iron oxide yellow, sodium lauryl sulfate, and FD&C Blue #2.

TEMODAR 20 mg: The yellow cap contains gelatin, sodium lauryl sulfate, and iron oxide yellow.

TEMODAR 100 mg: The pink cap contains gelatin, titanium dioxide, sodium lauryl sulfate, and iron oxide red.

TEMODAR 140 mg: The blue cap contains gelatin, sodium lauryl sulfate, and FD&C Blue #2.

TEMODAR 180 mg: The orange cap contains gelatin, iron oxide red, iron oxide yellow, titanium dioxide, and sodium lauryl sulfate.

TEMODAR 250 mg: The white cap contains gelatin, titanium dioxide, and sodium lauryl sulfate.

TEMODAR for Injection:

Each vial contains 100 mg of sterile and pyrogen-free temozolomide lyophilized powder for intravenous injection. The inactive ingredients are: mannitol (600 mg), L-threonine (160 mg), polysorbate 80 (120 mg), sodium citrate dihydrate (235 mg), and hydrochloric acid (160 mg).

12 CLINICAL PHARMACOLOGY

12.1 Mechanism of Action

Temozolomide is not directly active but undergoes rapid nonenzymatic conversion at physiologic pH to the reactive compound 5-(3-methyltriazen-1-yl)-imidazole-4-carboxamide (MTIC). The cytotoxicity of MTIC is thought to be primarily due to alkylation of DNA. Alkylation (methylation) occurs mainly at the O^6 and N^7 positions of guanine.

12.3 Pharmacokinetics

Absorption:

Temozolomide is rapidly and completely absorbed after oral administration with a peak plasma concentration (C_{max}) achieved in a median T_{max} of 1 hour. Food reduces the rate and extent of temozolomide absorption. Mean peak plasma concentration and AUC decreased by 32% and 9%, respectively, and median T_{max} increased by 2-fold (from 1–2.25 hours) when temozolomide was administered after a modified high-fat breakfast.

A pharmacokinetic study comparing oral and intravenous temozolomide in 19 patients with primary CNS malignancies showed that 150 mg/m^2 TEMODAR for injection administered over 90 minutes is bioequivalent to 150 mg/m^2 TEMODAR oral capsules with respect to both C_{max} and AUC of temozolomide and MTIC. Following a single 90-minute intravenous infusion of 150 mg/m^2, the geometric mean C_{max} values for temozolomide and MTIC were 7.3 mcg/mL and 276 ng/mL, respectively. Following a single oral dose of 150 mg/m^2, the geometric mean C_{max} values for temozolomide and MTIC were 7.5 mcg/mL and 282 ng/mL, respectively. Following a single 90-minute intravenous infusion of 150 mg/m^2, the geometric mean AUC values for temozolomide and MTIC were 24.6 mcg·hr/mL and 891 ng·hr/mL, respectively. Following a single oral dose of 150 mg/m^2, the geometric mean AUC values for temozolomide and MTIC were 23.4 mcg·hr/mL and 864 ng·hr/mL, respectively.

Distribution:

Temozolomide has a mean apparent volume of distribution of 0.4 L/kg (%CV=13%). It is weakly bound to human plasma proteins; the mean percent bound of drug-related total radioactivity is 15%.

Metabolism and Elimination:

Temozolomide is spontaneously hydrolyzed at physiologic pH to the active species, MTIC and to temozolomide acid metabolite. MTIC is further hydrolyzed to 5-amino-imidazole-4-carboxamide (AIC), which is known to be an intermediate in purine and nucleic acid biosynthesis, and to methylhydrazine, which is believed to be the active alkylating species. Cytochrome P450 enzymes play only a minor role in the metabolism of temozolomide and MTIC. Relative to the AUC of temozolomide, the exposure to MTIC and AIC is 2.4% and 23%, respectively.

Excretion:
About 38% of the administered temozolomide total radioactive dose is recovered over 7 days: 37.7% in urine and 0.8% in feces. The majority of the recovery of radioactivity in urine is unchanged temozolomide (5.6%), AIC (12%), temozolomide acid metabolite (2.3%), and unidentified polar metabolite(s) (17%). Overall clearance of temozolomide is about 5.5 L/hr/m^2. Temozolomide is rapidly eliminated, with a mean elimination half-life of 1.8 hours, and exhibits linear kinetics over the therapeutic dosing range of 75 to 250 mg/m^2/day.

Effect of Age:
A population pharmacokinetic analysis indicated that age (range: 19–78 years) has no influence on the pharmacokinetics of temozolomide.

Effect of Gender:
A population pharmacokinetic analysis indicated that women have an approximately 5% lower clearance (adjusted for body surface area) for temozolomide than men.

Effect of Race:
The effect of race on the pharmacokinetics of temozolomide has not been studied.

Tobacco Use:
A population pharmacokinetic analysis indicated that the oral clearance of temozolomide is similar in smokers and nonsmokers.

Effect of Renal Impairment:
A population pharmacokinetic analysis indicated that creatinine clearance over the range of 36 to 130 mL/min/m^2 has no effect on the clearance of temozolomide after oral administration. The pharmacokinetics of temozolomide have not been studied in patients with severely impaired renal function (CLcr <36 mL/min/m^2). Caution should be exercised when TEMODAR is administered to patients with severe renal impairment *[see Use in Special Populations (8.6)]*. TEMODAR has not been studied in patients on dialysis.

Effect of Hepatic Impairment:
A study showed that the pharmacokinetics of temozolomide in patients with mild-to-moderate hepatic impairment (Child-Pugh Class I – II) were similar to those observed in patients with normal hepatic function. Caution should be exercised when temozolomide is administered to patients with severe hepatic impairment *[see Use in Specific Populations (8.7)]*.

Effect of Other Drugs on Temozolomide Pharmacokinetics:
In a multiple-dose study, administration of TEMODAR Capsules with ranitidine did not change the C_{max} or AUC values for temozolomide or MTIC.

A population analysis indicated that administration of valproic acid decreases the clearance of temozolomide by about 5% *[see Drug Interactions (7.1)]*.

A population analysis did not demonstrate any influence of coadministered dexamethasone, prochlorperazine, phenytoin, carbamazepine, ondansetron, H_2-receptor antagonists, or phenobarbital on the clearance of orally administered temozolomide.

13 NONCLINICAL TOXICOLOGY

13.1 Carcinogenesis, Mutagenesis, Impairment of Fertility

Temozolomide is carcinogenic in rats at doses less than the maximum recommended human dose. Temozolomide induced mammary carcinomas in both males and females at doses 0.13 to 0.63 times the maximum human dose (25–125 mg/m^2) when administered orally on 5 consecutive days every 28 days for 6 cycles. Temozolomide also induced fibrosarcomas of the heart, eye, seminal vesicles, salivary glands, abdominal cavity, uterus, and prostate, carcinomas of the seminal vesicles, schwannomas of the heart, optic nerve, and harderian gland, and adenomas of the skin, lung, pituitary, and thyroid at doses 0.5 times the maximum daily dose. Mammary tumors were also induced following 3 cycles of temozolomide at the maximum recommended daily dose.

Temozolomide is a mutagen and a clastogen. In a reverse bacterial mutagenesis assay (Ames assay), temozolomide increased revertant frequency in the absence and presence of metabolic activation. Temozolomide was clastogenic in human lymphocytes in the presence and absence of metabolic activation.

Temozolomide impairs male fertility. Temozolomide caused syncytial cells/immature sperm formation at 0.25 and 0.63 times the maximum recommended human dose (50 and 125 mg/m^2) in rats and dogs, respectively, and testicular atrophy in dogs at 0.63 times the maximum recommended human dose (125 mg/m^2).

13.2 Animal Toxicology and/or Pharmacology

Toxicology studies in rats and dogs identified a low incidence of hemorrhage, degeneration, and necrosis of the retina at temozolomide doses equal to or greater than 0.63 times the maximum recommended human dose (125 mg/m^2). These changes were most commonly seen at doses where mortality was observed.

14 CLINICAL STUDIES

14.1 Newly Diagnosed Glioblastoma Multiforme

Five hundred and seventy-three patients were randomized to receive either TEMODAR (TMZ)+Radiotherapy (RT) (n=287) or RT alone (n=286). Patients in the TEMODAR+RT arm received concomitant TEMODAR (75 mg/m^2) once daily, starting the first day of RT until the last day of RT, for 42 days (with a maximum of 49 days). This was followed by 6 cycles of TEMODAR alone (150 or 200 mg/m^2) on Days 1 to 5 of every 28-day cycle, starting 4 weeks after the end of RT. Patients in the control arm received RT only. In both arms, focal radiation therapy was delivered as 60 Gy/30 fractions. Focal RT includes the tumor bed or resection site with a 2- to 3-cm margin. *Pneumocystis carinii* pneumonia (PCP) prophylaxis was required during the TMZ+RT, regardless of lymphocyte count, and was to continue until recovery of lymphocyte count to less than or equal to Grade 1.

At the time of disease progression, TEMODAR was administered as salvage therapy in 161 patients of the 282 (57%) in the RT alone arm, and 62 patients of the 277 (22%) in the TEMODAR+RT arm.

The addition of concomitant and maintenance TEMODAR to radiotherapy in the treatment of patients with newly diagnosed GBM showed a statistically significant improvement in overall survival compared to radiotherapy alone (**Figure 1**). The hazard ratio (HR) for overall survival was 0.63 (95% CI for HR=0.52-0.75) with a log-rank P<0.0001 in favor of the TEMODAR arm. The median survival was increased by 2.5 months in the TEMODAR arm.

FIGURE 1: Kaplan-Meier Curves for Overall Survival (ITT Population)

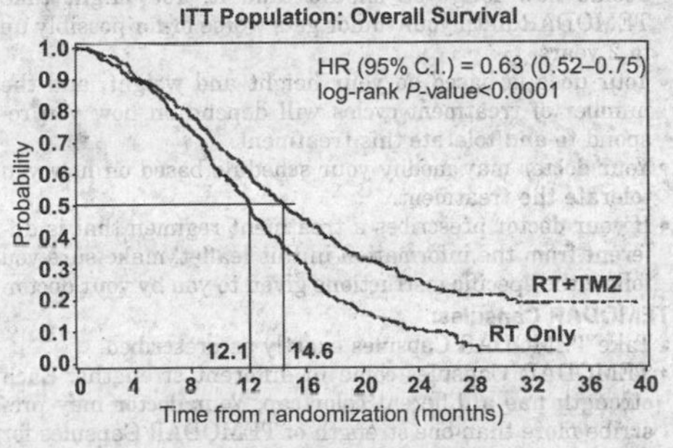

14.2 Refractory Anaplastic Astrocytoma

A single-arm, multicenter study was conducted in 162 patients who had anaplastic astrocytoma at first relapse and who had a baseline Karnofsky performance status of 70 or greater. Patients had previously received radiation therapy and may also have previously received a nitrosourea with or without other chemotherapy. Fifty-four patients had disease progression on prior therapy with both a nitrosourea and procarbazine, and their malignancy was considered refractory to chemotherapy (refractory anaplastic astrocytoma population). Median age of this subgroup of 54 patients was 42 years (19–76). Sixty-five percent were male. Seventy-two percent of patients had a KPS of >80. Sixty-three percent of patients had surgery other than a biopsy at the time of initial diagnosis. Of those patients undergoing resection, 73% underwent a subtotal resection and 27% underwent a gross total resection. Eighteen percent of patients had surgery at the time of first relapse. The median time from initial diagnosis to first relapse was 13.8 months (4.2–75.4).

TEMODAR Capsules were given for the first 5 consecutive days of a 28-day cycle at a starting dose of 150 mg/m^2/day. If the nadir and day of dosing (Day 29, Day 1 of next cycle) absolute neutrophil count was greater than or equal to 1.5 × 10^9/L (1500/μL) and the nadir and Day 29, Day 1 of next cycle platelet count was greater than or equal to 100 × 10^9/L (100,000/μL), the TEMODAR dose was increased to 200 mg/m^2/day for the first 5 consecutive days of a 28-day cycle.

In the refractory anaplastic astrocytoma population, the overall tumor response rate (CR+PR) was 22% (12/54 patients) and the complete response rate was 9% (5/54 patients). The median duration of all responses was 50 weeks (range: 16–114 weeks) and the median duration of complete responses was 64 weeks (range: 52–114 weeks). In this population, progression-free survival at 6 months was 45% (95% CI: 31%–58%) and progression-free survival at 12 months was 29% (95% CI: 16%–42%). Median progression-free survival was 4.4 months. Overall survival at 6 months was 74% (95% CI: 62%–86%) and 12-month overall survival was 65% (95% CI: 52%–78%). Median overall survival was 15.9 months.

15 REFERENCES

1. OSHA Technical Manual, TED 1-0.15A, Section VI: Chapter 2. Controlling Occupational Exposure to Hazardous Drugs. OSHA, 1999.
2. American Society of Health-System Pharmacists. ASHP guidelines on handling hazardous drugs. *Am J Health-Syst Pharm.* 2006; 63:1172–1193.
3. NIOSH Alert: Preventing occupational exposures to antineoplastic and other hazardous drugs in healthcare settings. 2004. U.S. Department of Health and Human Services, Public Health Service, Centers for Disease Control and Prevention, National Institute for Occupational Safety and Health, DHHS (NIOSH) Publication No. 2004-165.[3]
4. Polovich, M., White, J. M., & Kelleher, L.O. (eds.) 2005. Chemotherapy and biotherapy guidelines and recommendations for practice (2nd. ed.) Pittsburgh, PA: Oncology.

16 HOW SUPPLIED/STORAGE AND HANDLING

16.1 Safe Handling and Disposal

Care should be exercised in the handling and preparation of TEMODAR. Vials and capsules should not be opened. If vials or capsules are accidentally opened or damaged, rigorous precautions should be taken with the contents to avoid inhalation or contact with the skin or mucous membranes. The use of gloves and safety glasses is recommended to avoid exposure in case of breakage of the vial or capsules. Procedures for proper handling and disposal of anticancer drugs should be considered [1–4]. Several guidelines on this subject have been published.

16.2 How Supplied

TEMODAR Capsules:
TEMODAR (temozolomide) Capsules are supplied in amber glass bottles with child-resistant polypropylene caps or child-resistant sachets containing the following capsule strengths:

TEMODAR Capsules 5 mg: have opaque white bodies with green caps. The capsule body is imprinted with two stripes, the dosage strength, and the Schering-Plough logo. The cap is imprinted with "TEMODAR".
They are supplied as follows:
Bottles:
5-count – NDC 0085-3004-02
14-count – NDC 0085-3004-01
Sachets:
5-count – NDC 0085-3004-03
14-count – NDC 0085-3004-04

TEMODAR Capsules 20 mg: have opaque white bodies with yellow caps. The capsule body is imprinted with two stripes, the dosage strength, and the Schering-Plough logo. The cap is imprinted with "TEMODAR".
They are supplied as follows:
Bottles:
5-count – NDC 0085-1519-02
14-count – NDC 0085-1519-01
Sachets:
5-count – NDC 0085-1519-03
14-count – NDC 0085-1519-04

TEMODAR Capsules 100 mg: have opaque white bodies with pink caps. The capsule body is imprinted with two stripes, the dosage strength, and the Schering-Plough logo. The cap is imprinted with "TEMODAR".
They are supplied as follows:
Bottles:
5-count – NDC 0085-1366-02
14-count – NDC 0085-1366-01
Sachets:
5-count – NDC 0085-1366-03
14-count – NDC 0085-1366-04

TEMODAR Capsules 140 mg: have opaque white bodies with blue caps. The capsule body is imprinted with two stripes, the dosage strength, and the Schering-Plough logo. The cap is imprinted with "TEMODAR".
They are supplied as follows:
Bottles:
5-count – NDC 0085-1425-01
14-count – NDC 0085-1425-02
Sachets:
5-count – NDC 0085-1425-03
14-count – NDC 0085-1425-04

TEMODAR Capsules 180 mg: have opaque white bodies with orange caps. The capsule body is imprinted with two stripes, the dosage strength, and the Schering-Plough logo. The cap is imprinted with "TEMODAR".
They are supplied as follows:
Bottles:
5-count – NDC 0085-1430-01
14-count – NDC 0085-1430-02
Sachets:
5-count – NDC 0085-1430-03
14-count – NDC 0085-1430-04

TEMODAR Capsules 250 mg: have opaque white bodies with white caps. The capsule body is imprinted with two stripes, the dosage strength, and the Schering-Plough logo. The cap is imprinted with "TEMODAR".
They are supplied as follows:
Bottles:
5-count – NDC 0085-1417-01

Sachets:
5-count – NDC 0085-1417-02

TEMODAR for Injection:

TEMODAR (temozolomide) for Injection is supplied in single-use glass vials containing 100 mg temozolomide. The lyophilized powder is white to light tan/light pink.

TEMODAR for Injection 100 mg:
NDC 0085-1381-01

16.3 Storage

Store TEMODAR Capsules at 25°C (77°F); excursions permitted to 15–30°C (59–86°F) [see USP Controlled Room Temperature].

Store TEMODAR for Injection refrigerated at 2–8°C (36–46°F). After reconstitution, store reconstituted product at room temperature (25°C [77°F]). Reconstituted product must be used within 14 hours, including infusion time.

17 PATIENT COUNSELING INFORMATION

See FDA-Approved Patient Labeling (Patient Information).

17.1 Information for the Patient

Physicians should discuss the following with their patients:

- Nausea and vomiting are the most frequently occurring adverse reactions. Nausea and vomiting are usually either self-limiting or readily controlled with standard antiemetic therapy.
- Capsules should not be opened. If capsules are accidentally opened or damaged, rigorous precautions should be taken with the capsule contents to avoid inhalation or contact with the skin or mucous membranes.
- The medication should be kept away from children and pets.

TEMODAR Capsules

Manufactured by: Merck Sharp & Dohme Corp., a subsidiary of

MERCK & CO., INC., Whitehouse Station, NJ 08889, USA

TEMODAR for Injection

Manufactured by: Merck Sharp & Dohme Corp., a subsidiary of

MERCK & CO., INC., Whitehouse Station, NJ 08889, USA

Manufactured by:
Baxter Oncology GmbH, Halle 33790, Germany

For patent information: www.merck.com/product/patent/home.html

Revised: 06/2013
uspi-mk7365-mtl-1306r015

Patient Information
TEMODAR® (tĕm-ō-dăr)
(temozolomide)
Capsules
TEMODAR® (tĕm-ō-dăr)
(temozolomide)
for Injection

What is the most important information I should know about TEMODAR?

- **TEMODAR may cause birth defects.** Male and female patients who take TEMODAR should use effective birth control. Female patients and female partners of male patients should avoid becoming pregnant while taking TEMODAR.

See the section "What are the possible side effects of TEMODAR?" for more information about side effects.

What is TEMODAR?

TEMODAR (temozolomide) is a prescription medicine used to treat adults with certain brain cancer tumors. TEMODAR blocks cell growth, especially cells that grow fast, such as cancer cells. TEMODAR may decrease the size of certain brain tumors in some patients.

It is not known if TEMODAR is safe and effective in children.

Who should not take TEMODAR?

Do not take TEMODAR if you:

- have had an allergic reaction to dacarbazine (DTIC), another cancer medicine.
- have had a red itchy rash, or a severe allergic reaction, such as trouble breathing, swelling of the face, throat, or tongue, or severe skin reaction to TEMODAR or any of the ingredients in TEMODAR. If you are not sure, ask your doctor. See the end of the leaflet for a list of ingredients in TEMODAR.

What should I tell my doctor before taking TEMODAR?

Tell your doctor about all your medical conditions, including if you:

- are allergic to dacarbazine (DTIC) or have had a severe allergic reaction to TEMODAR. See "Who should not take TEMODAR?"
- have kidney problems
- have liver problems
- are pregnant. See "What is the most important information I should know about TEMODAR?"
- are breast-feeding. It is not known whether TEMODAR passes into breast milk. You and your doctor should decide if you will breast-feed or take TEMODAR. You should not do both without talking with your doctor.

Tell your doctor about all the medicines you take, including prescription and non-prescription medicines, vitamins, and herbal supplements. Especially tell your doctor if you take a medicine that contains valproic acid (Stavzor®, Depakene®).

Know the medicines you take. Keep a list of them and show it to your doctor and pharmacist when you get a new medicine.

How should I take TEMODAR?

TEMODAR may be taken by mouth as a capsule at home, or you may receive TEMODAR by injection into a vein (intravenous). Your doctor will decide the best way for you to take TEMODAR.

There are two common dosing schedules for taking TEMODAR.

- Some people take TEMODAR for 42 days in a row (possibly 49 days depending on side effects) with radiation treatment. This is one cycle of treatment. After this, you may have "maintenance" treatment. Your doctor may prescribe 6 more cycles of TEMODAR. For each of these cycles, you take TEMODAR one time each day for 5 days in a row and then you stop taking it for the next 23 days. This is a 28-day maintenance treatment cycle.
- Another way to take TEMODAR is to take it one time each day for 5 days in a row only, and then you stop taking it for the next 23 days. This is one cycle of treatment (28 days). Your doctor will watch your progress on TEMODAR and decide how long you should take it. You might take TEMODAR until your tumor gets worse or for possibly up to 2 years.
- Your dose is based on your height and weight, and the number of treatment cycles will depend on how you respond to and tolerate this treatment.
- Your doctor may modify your schedule based on how you tolerate the treatment.
- If your doctor prescribes a treatment regimen that is different from the information in this leaflet, make sure you follow the specific instructions given to you by your doctor.

TEMODAR Capsules:

- Take TEMODAR Capsules exactly as prescribed.
- TEMODAR Capsules come in different strengths. Each strength has a different color cap. Your doctor may prescribe more than one strength of TEMODAR Capsules for you, so it is important that you understand how to take your medicine the right way. Be sure that you understand exactly how many capsules you need to take on each day of your treatment, and what strengths to take. This may be different whenever you start a new cycle.
- Talk to your doctor before you take your dose if you are not sure how much to take. This will help to prevent taking too much TEMODAR and decrease your chances of getting serious side effects.
- Take each day's dose of TEMODAR Capsules at one time, with a full glass of water.
- **Swallow TEMODAR Capsules whole. Do not chew, open, or split the capsules.**
- If TEMODAR Capsules are accidentally opened or damaged, be careful not to breathe in (inhale) the powder from the capsules or get the powder on your skin or mucous membranes (for example, in your nose or mouth). If contact with any of these areas happens, flush the area with water.
- If you vomit TEMODAR Capsules, do not take any more capsules. Wait and take your next planned dose.
- The medicine is used best by your body if you take it at the same time every day in relation to a meal.
- To lessen nausea, try to take TEMODAR on an empty stomach or at bedtime. Your doctor may prescribe medicine to prevent or treat nausea, or other medicines to lessen side effects with TEMODAR.
- See your doctor regularly to check your progress. Your doctor will check you for side effects that you might not notice.
- If you miss a dose of TEMODAR, talk with your doctor for instructions about when to take your next dose of TEMODAR.
- Call your doctor right away if you take more than the prescribed amount of TEMODAR. It is important that you do not take more than the amount of TEMODAR prescribed for you.

TEMODAR for Injection:

- You will receive TEMODAR as an infusion directly into your vein. Your treatment will take about 90 minutes.
- Your doctor may prescribe medicine to prevent or treat nausea, or other medicines to relieve side effects with TEMODAR.

What should I avoid while taking TEMODAR?

- Female patients and female partners of male patients should avoid becoming pregnant while taking TEMODAR. See "What is the most important information I should know about TEMODAR?"

What are the possible side effects of TEMODAR?

TEMODAR can cause serious side effects.

- See "What is the most important information I should know about TEMODAR?"
- **Decreased blood cells.** TEMODAR affects cells that grow rapidly, including bone marrow cells. This can cause you to have a decrease in blood cells. Your doctor can monitor your blood for these effects.
  - White blood cells are needed to fight infections. Neutrophils are a type of white blood cell that help prevent bacterial infections. Decreased neutrophils can lead to serious infections that can lead to death. Other white blood cells called lymphocytes may also be decreased.
  - Platelets are blood cells needed for normal blood clotting. Low platelet counts can lead to bleeding. Tell your doctor about any unusual bruising or bleeding.

Your doctor will check your blood regularly while you are taking TEMODAR to see if these side effects are happening. Your doctor may need to change the dose of TEMODAR or when you get it depending on your blood cell counts. People who are age 70 or older and women may be more likely to have their blood cells affected.

- ***Pneumocystis carinii* Pneumonia (PCP).** PCP is an infection that people can get when their immune system is weak. TEMODAR decreases white blood cells, which makes your immune system weaker and can increase your risk of getting PCP. **All patients** taking TEMODAR will be watched carefully by their doctor for this infection, especially patients who take steroids. Tell your doctor if you have any of the following signs and symptoms of PCP infection: shortness of breath and/or fever, chills, dry cough.
- **Secondary cancers.** Blood problems such as myelodysplastic syndrome and secondary cancers, such as a certain kind of leukemia, can happen in people who take TEMODAR. Your doctor will watch you for this.
- **Convulsions.** Convulsions may be severe or life-threatening in people who take TEMODAR.

Common side effects with TEMODAR include:

- nausea and vomiting. Your doctor can prescribe medicines that may help reduce these symptoms.
- headache
- feeling tired
- loss of appetite
- hair loss
- constipation
- bruising
- rash
- paralysis on one side of the body
- diarrhea
- weakness
- fever
- dizziness
- coordination problems
- viral infection
- sleep problems
- memory loss
- pain, irritation, itching, warmth, swelling or redness at the site of infusion
- bruising or small red or purple spots under the skin

Tell your doctor about any side effect that bothers you or that does not go away.

These are not all the possible side effects with TEMODAR. For more information, ask your doctor or pharmacist.

Call your doctor for medical advice about side effects. You may report side effects to FDA at 1-800-FDA-1088.

How should I store TEMODAR Capsules?

- Store TEMODAR Capsules at 77°F (controlled room temperature). Storage at 59°F to 86°F (15°C to 30°C) is permitted occasionally.
- **Keep TEMODAR Capsules out of the reach of children and pets.**

General information about TEMODAR.

Medicines are sometimes prescribed for purposes other than those listed in the Patient Information leaflet. Do not use TEMODAR for a condition for which it was not prescribed. Do not give TEMODAR to other people, even if they have the same symptoms that you have. It may harm them.

This leaflet summarizes the most important information about TEMODAR. If you would like more information, talk with your doctor. You can ask your pharmacist or doctor for information about TEMODAR that is written for health professionals.

For more information, go to www.TEMODAR.com or call 1-877-888-4231.

How are TEMODAR Capsules supplied?

TEMODAR Capsules contain a white capsule body with a color cap and the colors vary based on the dosage strength. The capsules are available in six different strengths.

TEMODAR Capsule Strength	Color
5 mg	Green Cap
20 mg	Yellow Cap
100 mg	Pink Cap
140 mg	Blue Cap
180 mg	Orange Cap
250 mg	White Cap

What are the ingredients in TEMODAR?

TEMODAR Capsules:

Active ingredient: temozolomide.

Inactive ingredients: lactose anhydrous, colloidal silicon dioxide, sodium starch glycolate, tartaric acid, stearic acid. The body of the capsules is made of gelatin and is opaque white. The cap is also made of gelatin, and the colors vary based on the dosage strength. The capsule body and cap are imprinted with pharmaceutical branding ink, which contains shellac, dehydrated alcohol, isopropyl alcohol, butyl alcohol, propylene glycol, purified water, strong ammonia, potassium hydroxide, and ferric oxide.

TEMODAR 5 mg: The green cap contains gelatin, titanium dioxide, iron oxide yellow, sodium lauryl sulfate, and FD&C Blue #2.

TEMODAR 20 mg: The yellow cap contains gelatin, sodium lauryl sulfate, and iron oxide yellow.

TEMODAR 100 mg: The pink cap contains gelatin, titanium dioxide, sodium lauryl sulfate, and iron oxide red.

TEMODAR 140 mg: The blue cap contains gelatin, sodium lauryl sulfate, and FD&C Blue #2.

TEMODAR 180 mg: The orange cap contains gelatin, iron oxide red, iron oxide yellow, titanium dioxide, and sodium lauryl sulfate.

TEMODAR 250 mg: The white cap contains gelatin, titanium dioxide, and sodium lauryl sulfate.

TEMODAR for Injection:

Active ingredient: temozolomide.

Inactive ingredients: mannitol, L-threonine, polysorbate 80, sodium citrate dihydrate, and hydrochloric acid.

TEMODAR Capsules

Manufactured by: Merck Sharp & Dohme Corp., a subsidiary of

MERCK & CO., INC., Whitehouse Station, NJ 08889, USA

TEMODAR for Injection

Manufactured by: Merck Sharp & Dohme Corp., a subsidiary of

MERCK & CO., INC., Whitehouse Station, NJ 08889, USA

Manufactured by:

Baxter Oncology GmbH, Halle 33790, Germany

For patent information: www.merck.com/product/patent/home.html

Revised: 06/2013

ppi-mk7365-mtl-1306r007

TEMODAR® (temozolomide) for Injection

PHARMACIST:

Dispense enclosed Patient Package Insert to each patient.

PHARMACIST INFORMATION SHEET

What is TEMODAR? *[See Full Prescribing Information, Indications and Usage (1)].*

TEMODAR® (temozolomide) is an alkylating drug for the treatment of adult patients with newly diagnosed glioblastoma multiforme and refractory anaplastic astrocytoma.

How is TEMODAR dosed? *[See Full Prescribing Information, Recommended Dosing and Dose Modification Guidelines (2.1)].*

The daily dose of TEMODAR for a given patient is calculated by the physician, based on the patient's body surface area (BSA) *[see* ***Table 5*** *in the Full Prescribing Information, Recommended Dosing and Dose Modification Guidelines (2.1)].* The recommended dose for TEMODAR as an intravenous infusion over 90 minutes is the same as the dose for the oral capsule formulation. Bioequivalence has been established only when TEMODAR for Injection was given over 90 minutes. The dose for subsequent cycles may be adjusted according to nadir neutrophil and platelet counts in the previous cycle and at the time of initiating the next cycle.

Dosing for Patients with Refractory Anaplastic Astrocytoma *[See Full Prescribing Information, Recommended Dosing and Dose Modification Guidelines, Patients with Refractory Anaplastic Astrocytoma (2.1)].*

Dosage of TEMODAR must be adjusted according to nadir neutrophil and platelet counts in the previous cycle and neutrophil and platelet counts at the time of initiating the next cycle. The initial dose is 150 mg/m^2 orally once daily for 5 consecutive days per 28-day treatment cycle. If both the nadir and day of dosing (Day 29, Day 1 of next cycle) absolute neutrophil counts (ANC) are greater than or equal to 1.5×10^9/L (1500/μL) and both the nadir and Day 29, Day 1 of next cycle platelet counts are greater than or equal to 100 $\times 10^9$/L (100,000/μL), the TEMODAR dose may be increased to 200 mg/m^2/day for 5 consecutive days per 28-day treatment cycle. During treatment, a complete blood count should be obtained on Day 22 (21 days after the first dose) or within 48 hours of that day, and weekly until the ANC is above 1.5×10^9/L (1500/μL) and the platelet count exceeds 100×10^9/L (100,000/μL). The next cycle of TEMODAR should not be started until the ANC and platelet count exceed these levels. If the ANC falls to less than 1.0×10^9/L (1000/μL) or the platelet count is less than 50×10^9/L (50,000/μL) during any cycle, the next cycle should be reduced by 50 mg/m^2, but not below 100 mg/m^2, the lowest recommended dose *[see* ***Table 4*** *in the Full Prescribing Information, Recommended Dosing and Dose Modification Guidelines (2.1)].*

Patients should continue to receive TEMODAR until their physician determines that their disease has progressed, or until unacceptable side effects or toxicities occur. Physicians may alter the treatment regimen for a given patient.

Dosing for Patients with Newly Diagnosed Glioblastoma Multiforme *[See Full Prescribing Information, Recommended Dosing and Dose Modification Guidelines, Patients with Newly Diagnosed High Grade Glioma (2.1)].*

Concomitant Phase Treatment Schedule

TEMODAR is administered at 75 mg/m^2 daily for 42 days concomitant with focal radiotherapy (60 Gy administered in 30 fractions), followed by maintenance TEMODAR for 6 cycles. No dose reductions are recommended; however, dose interruptions may occur based on patient tolerance. The TEMODAR dose can be continued throughout the 42-day concomitant period up to 49 days if all of the following conditions are met: absolute neutrophil count greater than or equal to 1.5×10^9/L, platelet count greater than or equal to 100×10^9/L, common toxicity criteria (CTC) non-hematological toxicity less than or equal to Grade 1 (except for alopecia, nausea, and vomiting). During treatment a complete blood count should be obtained weekly. Temozolomide dosing should be interrupted or discontinued during concomitant phase according to the hematological and non-hematological toxicity criteria as noted in **Table 1** of the Full Prescribing Information under 2.1 Recommended Dosing and Dose Modification Guidelines. *Pneumocystis carinii* pneumonia (PCP) prophylaxis is required during the concomitant administration of TEMODAR and radiotherapy, and should be continued in patients who develop lymphocytopenia until recovery from lymphocytopenia (CTC Grade less than or equal to 1).

Maintenance Phase Treatment Schedule

Four weeks after completing the TEMODAR + RT phase, TEMODAR is administered for an additional 6 cycles of maintenance treatment. Dosage in Cycle 1 (maintenance) is 150 mg/m^2 once daily for 5 days followed by 23 days without treatment. At the start of Cycle 2, the dose can be escalated to 200 mg/m^2, if the CTC non-hematologic toxicity for Cycle 1 is Grade less than or equal to 2 (except for alopecia, nausea, and vomiting), absolute neutrophil count (ANC) is greater than or equal to 1.5×10^9/L, and the platelet count is greater than or equal to 100×10^9/L. If the dose was not escalated at Cycle 2, escalation should not be done in subsequent cycles. The dose remains at 200 mg/m^2 per day for the first 5 days of each subsequent cycle except if toxicity occurs.

During treatment a complete blood count should be obtained on Day 22 (21 days after the first dose) or within 48 hours of that day, and weekly until the ANC is above 1.5×10^9/L (1500/μL) and the platelet count exceeds 100×10^9/L (100,000/μL). The next cycle of TEMODAR should not be started until the ANC and platelet count exceed these levels. Dose reductions during the next cycle should be based on the lowest blood counts and worst nonhematologic toxicity during the previous cycle. Dose reductions or discontinuations during the maintenance phase should be applied according to **Tables 2** and **3** in the Full Prescribing Information under 2.1 Recommended Dosing and Dose Modification Guidelines.

How is TEMODAR for Injection prepared? *[See Full Prescribing Information, Preparation and Administration, TEMODAR for Injection (2.2)].*

Care should be exercised in the handling and preparation of TEMODAR. Vials should not be opened. If vials are accidentally opened or damaged, rigorous precautions should be taken with the contents to avoid inhalation or contact with the skin or mucous membranes. The use of gloves and safety glasses is recommended to avoid exposure in case of breakage of the vial. Procedures for proper handling and disposal of anticancer drugs should be considered {1-4}. Several guidelines on this subject have been published.

1. TEMODAR for Injection vials should be stored refrigerated at 2°–8°C (36°–46°F).
2. Bring the vial to room temperature prior to reconstitution with Sterile Water for Injection.
3. Using aseptic technique, reconstitute each vial with 41 mL Sterile Water for Injection. The resulting solution will contain 2.5 mg/mL temozolomide.
4. Vial should be gently swirled and not shaken. Inspect vials, and any vial containing visible particulate matter should not be used. Do not further dilute the reconstituted solution. Upon reconstitution, store at room temperature for up to 14 hours, including infusion time.
5. Using aseptic technique, withdraw up to 40 mL from each vial to make up the total dose and transfer into an empty 250 mL infusion bag.
6. Attach the pump tubing to the bag, purge the tubing and then cap.

How is TEMODAR for Injection administered? *[See Full Prescribing Information, Preparation and Administration, TEMODAR for Injection (2.2)].*

TEMODAR for Injection is administered as an intravenous infusion over 90 minutes. Bioequivalence has been established only when TEMODAR for Injection was given over 90 minutes. TEMODAR for Injection should be administered only by intravenous infusion. Flush the lines before and after each TEMODAR infusion.

TEMODAR for Injection may be administered in the same intravenous line with 0.9% Sodium Chloride injection only. Because no data are available on the compatibility of TEMODAR for Injection with other intravenous substances or additives, other medications should not be infused simultaneously through the same intravenous line.

What should the patient avoid during treatment with TEMODAR? *[See Full Prescribing Information, Use in Specific Populations, Pregnancy (8.1) and Nursing Mothers (8.3)].*

There are no dietary restrictions for patients taking TEMODAR. TEMODAR may affect testicular function, so male patients should exercise adequate birth control measures. TEMODAR may cause birth defects. Female patients should avoid becoming pregnant while receiving this drug. It is not known whether TEMODAR is excreted into breast milk. Because many drugs are excreted in human milk, and because of the potential for serious adverse reactions in nursing infants and tumorigenicity shown for temozolomide in animal studies, a decision should be made whether to discontinue nursing or to discontinue the drug, taking into account the importance of TEMODAR to the mother.

What are the side effects of TEMODAR? *[See Full Prescribing Information, Adverse Reactions (6)].*

Nausea and vomiting are the most common side effects associated with TEMODAR. Noncumulative myelosuppression is the dose-limiting toxicity. Patients should be evaluated periodically by their physician to monitor blood counts.

Other commonly reported side effects reported by patients taking TEMODAR are fatigue, constipation, alopecia, anorexia, headache, and bruising, as well as pain, irritation, itching, warmth, swelling, and redness at the site of infusion.

How is TEMODAR supplied? *[See Full Prescribing Information, How Supplied / Storage and Handling (16)].*

TEMODAR for Injection is supplied in single-use glass vials containing 100 mg temozolomide. TEMODAR is also available as capsules in 5-mg, 20-mg, 100-mg, 140-mg, 180-mg, and 250-mg strengths.

1. OSHA Technical Manual, TED 1-0.15A, Section VI: Chapter 2. Controlling Occupational Exposure to Hazardous Drugs. OSHA, 1999.
2. American Society of Health-System Pharmacists. ASHP guidelines on handling hazardous drugs. *Am J Health-Syst Pharm.* 2006; 63:1172–1193.
3. NIOSH Alert: Preventing occupational exposures to antineoplastic and other hazardous drugs in health care settings. 2004. U.S. Department of Health and Human Services, Public Health Service, Centers for Disease Control and Prevention, National Institute for Occupational Safety and Health, DHHS (NIOSH) Publication No. 2004-165.[3]
4. Polovich, M., White, J. M., & Kelleher, L.O. (eds.) 2005. Chemotherapy and biotherapy guidelines and recommendations for practice (2nd. ed.) Pittsburgh, PA: Oncology.

TEMODAR for Injection

Manufactured for: Merck Sharp & Dohme Corp., a subsidiary of

MERCK & CO., INC., Whitehouse Station, NJ 08889, USA

Manufactured by:

Baxter Oncology GmbH, Halle 33790, Germany

For patent information: www.merck.com/product/patent/home.html

Revised: 06/2013

phi-mk7365-pwi-1306r013

TEMODAR® (temozolomide) Capsules
PHARMACIST:
Dispense enclosed Patient Package Insert to each patient.
PHARMACIST INFORMATION SHEET

IMPORTANT DISPENSING INFORMATION
For every patient, TEMODAR must be dispensed in a separate vial or in its original package making sure each container lists the strength per capsule and that patients take the appropriate number of capsules from each package or vial.
Please see the dispensing instructions below for more information.

What is TEMODAR?
TEMODAR® (temozolomide) is an oral alkylating agent for the treatment of newly diagnosed glioblastoma multiforme and refractory anaplastic astrocytoma.
How is TEMODAR dosed?
The daily dose of TEMODAR Capsules for a given patient is calculated by the physician, based on the patient's body surface area (BSA). The resulting dose is then rounded off to the nearest 5 mg. An example of the dosing may be as follows: the initial daily dose of TEMODAR in milligrams is the BSA multiplied by mg/m^2/day, (a patient with a BSA of 1.84 is 1.84×75 mg = 138, or 140 mg/day). The dose for subsequent cycles may be adjusted according to nadir neutrophil and platelet counts in the previous cycle and at the time of initiating the next cycle.
How might the dose of TEMODAR be modified for Refractory Anaplastic Astrocytoma?
Dosage of TEMODAR must be adjusted according to nadir neutrophil and platelet counts in the previous cycle and neutrophil and platelet counts at the time of initiating the next cycle. The initial dose is 150 mg/m^2 orally once daily for 5 consecutive days per 28-day treatment cycle. If both the nadir and day of dosing (Day 29, Day 1 of next cycle) absolute neutrophil counts (ANC) are greater than or equal to 1.5×10^9/L (1500/µL) and both the nadir and Day 29, Day 1 of next cycle platelet counts are greater than or equal to 100 $\times 10^9$/L (100,000/µL), the TEMODAR dose may be increased to 200 mg/m^2/day for 5 consecutive days per 28-day treatment cycle. During treatment, a complete blood count should be obtained on Day 22 (21 days after the first dose) or within 48 hours of that day, and weekly until the ANC is above 1.5×10^9/L (1500/µL) and the platelet count exceeds 100×10^9/L (100,000/µL). The next cycle of TEMODAR should not be started until the ANC and platelet count exceed these levels. If the ANC falls to less than 1.0×10^9/L (1000/µL) or the platelet count is less than 50×10^9/L (50,000/µL) during any cycle, the next cycle should be reduced by 50 mg/m^2, but not below 100 mg/m^2, the lowest recommended dose (see **Table 1** below).

TABLE 1: Dosing Modification Table for Refractory Anaplastic Astrocytoma

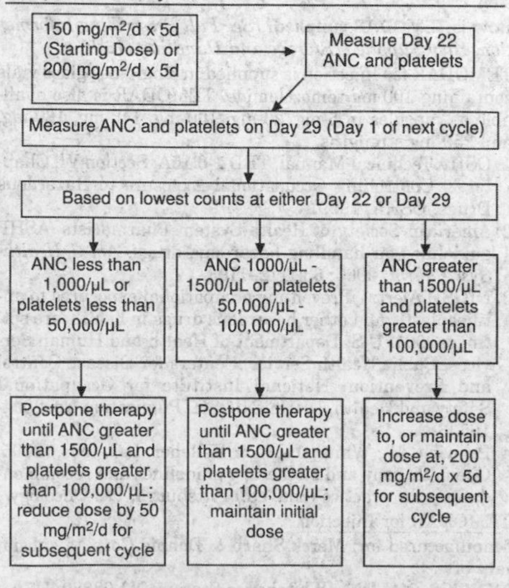

What is the TEMODAR Capsules treatment regimen?
TEMODAR is given for 5 consecutive days on a 28-day cycle. Patients should continue taking TEMODAR until their physician determines that their disease has progressed, up to 2 years, or until unacceptable side effects or toxicities occur. Physicians may alter the treatment regimen for a given patient.
Newly Diagnosed Concomitant Phase Treatment Schedule
TEMODAR is administered orally at 75 mg/m^2 daily for 42 days concomitant with focal radiotherapy (60 Gy administered in 30 fractions), followed by maintenance TEMODAR for 6 cycles. No dose reductions are recommended; however, dose interruptions may occur based on patient tolerance. The TEMODAR dose can be continued throughout the 42-day concomitant period up to 49 days if all of the following conditions are met: absolute neutrophil count greater than or equal to 1.5×10^9/L, platelet count greater than or equal to 100 $\times 10^9$/L, common toxicity criteria (CTC) nonhematological toxicity less than or equal to Grade 1 (except for alopecia, nausea and vomiting). During treatment a complete blood count should be obtained weekly. Temozolomide dosing should be interrupted or discontinued during concomitant phase according to the hematological and nonhematological toxicity criteria as noted in **Table 2**. *Pneumocystis carinii* pneumonia (PCP) prophylaxis is required during the concomitant administration of TEMODAR and radiotherapy, and should be continued in patients who develop lymphocytopenia until recovery from lymphocytopenia (CTC grade less than or equal to 1).

TABLE 2: Temozolomide Dosing Interruption or Discontinuation During Concomitant Radiotherapy and Temozolomide

Toxicity	TMZ Interruption*	TMZ Discontinuation
Absolute Neutrophil Count	greater than or equal to 0.5 and less than 1.5×10^9/L	less than 0.5×10^9/L
Platelet Count	greater than or equal to 10 and less than 100×10^9/L	less than 10×10^9/L
CTC Nonhematological Toxicity (except for alopecia, nausea, vomiting)	CTC Grade 2	CTC Grade 3 or 4

TMZ = temozolomide; CTC = Common Toxicity Criteria.

* Treatment with concomitant TMZ could be continued when all of the following conditions were met: absolute neutrophil count greater than or equal to 1.5×10^9/L; platelet count greater than or equal to 100×10^9/L; CTC nonhematological toxicity less than or equal to Grade 1 (except for alopecia, nausea, vomiting).

Maintenance Phase Treatment Schedule
Four weeks after completing the TEMODAR + RT phase, TEMODAR is administered for an additional 6 cycles of maintenance treatment. Dosage in Cycle 1 (maintenance) is 150 mg/m^2 once daily for 5 days followed by 23 days without treatment. At the start of Cycle 2, the dose is escalated to 200 mg/m^2, if the CTC nonhematologic toxicity for Cycle 1 is Grade less than or equal to 2 (except for alopecia, nausea and vomiting), absolute neutrophil count (ANC) is greater than or equal to 1.5×10^9/L, and the platelet count is greater than or equal to 100×10^9/L. If the dose was not escalated at Cycle 2, escalation should not be done in subsequent cycles. The dose remains at 200 mg/m^2 per day for the first 5 days of each subsequent cycle except if toxicity occurs.
During treatment a complete blood count should be obtained on Day 22 (21 days after the first dose) or within 48 hours of that day, and weekly until the ANC is above 1.5×10^9/L (1500/µL) and the platelet count exceeds 100×10^9/L (100,000/µL). The next cycle of TEMODAR should not be started until the ANC and platelet count exceed these levels. Dose reductions during the next cycle should be based on the lowest blood counts and worst nonhematologic toxicity during the previous cycle. Dose reductions or discontinuations during the maintenance phase should be applied according to **Tables 3** and **4**.

TABLE 3: Temozolomide Dose Levels for Maintenance Treatment

Dose Level	Dose (mg/m^2/day)	Remarks
–1	100	Reduction for prior toxicity
0	150	Dose during Cycle 1
1	200	Dose during Cycles 2–6 in absence of toxicity

TABLE 4: Temozolomide Dose Reduction or Discontinuation During Maintenance Treatment

Toxicity	Reduce TMZ by 1 Dose Level*	Discontinue TMZ
Absolute Neutrophil Count	less than 1.0×10^9/L	See footnote†
Platelet Count	less than 50×10^9/L	See footnote†
CTC Nonhematological Toxicity (except for alopecia, nausea, vomiting)	CTC Grade 3	CTC Grade 4†

TMZ = temozolomide; CTC = Common Toxicity Criteria.
* TMZ dose levels are listed in **Table 3**.
† TMZ is to be discontinued if dose reduction to less than 100 mg/m^2 is required or if the same Grade 3 nonhematological toxicity (except for alopecia, nausea, vomiting) recurs after dose reduction.

How is TEMODAR taken?
Patients should take each day's dose with a full glass of water at the same time each day. Taking the medication on an empty stomach or at bedtime may help ease nausea. If patients are also taking antinausea or other medications to relieve the side effects associated with TEMODAR, they should be advised to take these medications 30 minutes before they take TEMODAR. Temozolomide causes the rapid appearance of malignant tumors in rats. Patients **SHOULD NOT** open or split the capsules. If capsules are accidentally opened or damaged, rigorous precautions should be taken with the capsule contents to avoid inhalation or contact with the skin or mucous membranes. The medication should be kept away from children and pets. The TEMODAR capsules should be swallowed whole and **NEVER CHEWED**.
What should the patient avoid during treatment with TEMODAR?
There are no dietary restrictions for patients taking TEMODAR. TEMODAR may affect testicular function, so male patients should exercise adequate birth control measures. TEMODAR may cause birth defects. Female patients should avoid becoming pregnant while receiving this drug. Women who are nursing prior to receiving TEMODAR should discontinue nursing. It is not known whether TEMODAR is excreted into breast milk.
Because many drugs are excreted in human milk, and because of the potential for serious adverse reactions in nursing infants and tumorigenicity shown for temozolomide in animal studies, a decision should be made whether to discontinue nursing or to discontinue the drug, taking into account the importance of TEMODAR to the mother.
What are the side effects of TEMODAR?
Nausea and vomiting are the most common side effects associated with TEMODAR. Noncumulative myelosuppression is the dose-limiting toxicity. Patients should be evaluated periodically by their physician to monitor blood counts.
Other commonly reported side effects reported by patients taking TEMODAR are fatigue, constipation, alopecia, anorexia, and headache.
How is TEMODAR supplied?
TEMODAR Capsules are available in 5-mg, 20-mg, 100-mg, 140-mg, 180-mg, and 250-mg strengths. The capsules contain a white capsule body with a color cap, and the colors vary based on the dosage strength.

TEMODAR Capsule Strength	Color
5 mg	Green Cap
20 mg	Yellow Cap
100 mg	Pink Cap
140 mg	Blue Cap
180 mg	Orange Cap
250 mg	White Cap

The 5-mg, 20-mg, 100-mg, 140-mg, and 180-mg capsule strengths are available in 5-count and 14-count packages. The 250-mg capsule strength is available in a 5-count package.
How is TEMODAR dispensed?
Each strength of TEMODAR must be dispensed in a separate vial or in its original package (one strength per one container). Follow the instructions below:
Based on the dose prescribed, determine the number of each strength of TEMODAR capsules needed for the full 42- or 5-day cycle as prescribed by the physician. For example, in a 5-day cycle, 275 mg/day would be dispensed as five 250-mg capsules, five 20-mg capsules and five 5-mg capsules. Label

each container with the appropriate number of capsules to be taken each day. Dispense to the patient, making sure each container lists the strength (mg) per capsule and that he or she understands to take the appropriate number of capsules of TEMODAR from each package or vial to equal the total daily dose prescribed by the physician.

How can TEMODAR be ordered?

TEMODAR can be ordered from your wholesaler. It is important to understand if TEMODAR is being used as part of a 42-day regimen or as part of a 5-day course. Remember to order enough TEMODAR for the appropriate cycle.

For example:

- a 5-day course of 360 mg/day would require the following to be ordered: two 5-count packages of 180-mg capsules.
- a 42-day course of 140 mg/day would require the following to be ordered: three 14-count packages of 140-mg capsules.

For examples of other dosing regimens, please refer to the full **Prescribing Information (Table 6)**.

TEMODAR Product	NDC Number
Bottles:	
5-mg capsules (5 count)	0085-3004-02
5-mg capsules (14 count)	0085-3004-01
20-mg capsules (5 count)	0085-1519-02
20-mg capsules (14 count)	0085-1519-01
100-mg capsules (5 count)	0085-1366-02
100-mg capsules (14 count)	0085-1366-01
140-mg capsules (5 count)	0085-1425-01
140-mg capsules (14 count)	0085-1425-02
180-mg capsules (5 count)	0085-1430-01
180-mg capsules (14 count)	0085-1430-02
250-mg capsules (5 count)	0085-1417-01
Sachets:	
5-mg capsules (5 count)	0085-3004-03
5-mg capsules (14 count)	0085-3004-04
20-mg capsules (5 count)	0085-1519-03
20-mg capsules (14 count)	0085-1519-04
100-mg capsules (5 count)	0085-1366-03
100-mg capsules (14 count)	0085-1366-04
140 mg capsules (5 count)	0085-1425-03
140-mg capsules (14 count)	0085-1425-04
180-mg capsules (5 count)	0085-1430-03
180-mg capsules (14 count)	0085-1430-04
250-mg capsules (5 count)	0085-1417-02

TEMODAR Capsules
Manufactured by: Merck Sharp & Dohme Corp., a subsidiary of
MERCK & CO., INC., Whitehouse Station, NJ 08889, USA
For patent information: www.merck.com/product/patent/home.html

Revised: 06/2013
phi-mk7365-cp-1306r009
Shown in Product Identification Guide, page 309

TICE® BCG ℞

[tīss BCG]

BCG LIVE

(FOR INTRAVESICAL USE)

> **WARNING**
>
> **TICE® BCG contains live, attenuated mycobacteria. Because of the potential risk for transmission, it should be prepared, handled, and disposed of as a biohazard material (see PRECAUTIONS and DOSAGE AND ADMINISTRATION sections).**
>
> **BCG infections have been reported in health care workers, primarily from exposures resulting from accidental needle sticks or skin lacerations during the preparation of BCG for administration. Nosocomial infections have been reported in patients receiving parenteral drugs that were prepared in areas in which BCG was reconstituted. BCG is capable of dissemination when administered by the intravesical route, and serious infections, including fatal infections, have been reported in patients receiving intravesical BCG (see WARNINGS, PRECAUTIONS, and ADVERSE REACTIONS sections).**

DESCRIPTION

TICE® BCG for intravesical use, is an attenuated, live culture preparation of the Bacillus of Calmette and Guerin (BCG) strain of *Mycobacterium bovis.*[1] The TICE strain was developed at the University of Illinois from a strain originated at the Pasteur Institute.

The medium in which the BCG organism is grown for preparation of the freeze-dried cake is composed of the following ingredients: glycerin, asparagine, citric acid, potassium phosphate, magnesium sulfate, and iron ammonium citrate. The final preparation prior to freeze drying also contains lactose. The freeze-dried BCG preparation is delivered in glass vials, each containing 1 to 8×10^8 colony forming units (CFU) of TICE BCG which is equivalent to approximately 50 mg wet weight. Determination of *in vitro* potency is achieved through colony counts derived from a serial dilution assay. A single dose consists of 1 reconstituted vial (see **DOSAGE AND ADMINISTRATION**).

For intravesical use the entire vial is reconstituted with sterile saline. TICE BCG is viable upon reconstitution. No preservatives have been added.

CLINICAL PHARMACOLOGY

TICE® BCG induces a granulomatous reaction at the local site of administration. Intravesical TICE BCG has been used as a therapy for, and prophylaxis against, recurrent tumors in patients with carcinoma *in situ* (CIS) of the urinary bladder, and to prevent recurrence of Stage TaT1 papillary tumors of the bladder at high risk of recurrence. The precise mechanism of action is unknown.

CLINICAL STUDIES

To evaluate the efficacy of intravesical administration of TICE® BCG in the treatment of carcinoma *in situ*, patients were identified who had been treated with TICE BCG under 6 different Investigational New Drug (IND) applications in which the most important shared aspect was the use of an induction plus maintenance schedule. Patients received TICE BCG (50 mg; 1 to 8×10^8 CFU) intravesically, once weekly for at least 6 weeks and once monthly thereafter for up to 12 months. A longer maintenance was given in some cases. The study population consisted of 153 patients, 132 males, 19 females, and 2 unidentified as to gender. Thirty patients lacking baseline documentation of CIS and 4 patients lost to follow-up were not evaluable for treatment response. Therefore, 119 patients were available for efficacy evaluation. The mean age was 69 years (range: 38-97 years). There were 2 categories of clinical response: (1) Complete Histological Response (CR), defined as complete resolution of carcinoma *in situ* documented by cystoscopy and cytology, with or without biopsy; and (2) Complete Clinical Response Without Cytology (CRNC), defined as an apparent complete disappearance of tumor upon cystoscopy. The results of a 1987 analysis of the evaluable patients are shown in **Table 1**.

[See table 1 above]

Table 1: The Response of Patients With CIS Bladder Cancer in 6 IND Studies

	Entered	Evaluable	CR	CRNC	Overall response
No. (%) of patients	153	119 (78%)	54 (46%)	36 (30%)	90 (76%)

A 1989 update of these data is presented in **Table 2**. The median duration of follow-up was 47 months.

[See table 2 above]

Table 2: Follow-up Response of Patients With CIS Bladder Cancer in 6 IND Studies

	1989 Status of 90 Responders (CR or CRNC)			
Response	**1987/CR n=54**	**1987/CRNC n=36**	**1987 Response n=90**	**Percent**
CR	30	15	45	50
CRNC	0	0	0	0
Unrelated deaths	6	6	12	13
Failure	18	15	33	37

There was no significant difference in response rates between patients with or without prior intravesical chemotherapy. The median duration of response, calculated from the Kaplan-Meier curve as median time to recurrence, is estimated at 4 years or greater. The incidence of cystectomy for 90 patients who achieved a complete response (CR or CRNC) was 11%. The median time to cystectomy in patients who achieved a complete response (CR or CRNC) exceeded 74 months.

The efficacy of intravesical TICE BCG in preventing the recurrence of a TaT1 bladder cancer after complete transurethral resection of all papillary tumors was evaluated in 2 open-label, randomized phase III clinical trials. Initial diagnosis of patients included in the studies was determined by cystoscopic biopsies. One was conducted by the Southwestern Oncology Group (SWOG) in patients at high risk of recurrence. High risk was defined as 2 occurrences of tumor within 56 weeks, any stage T1 tumor, or 3 or more tumors presenting simultaneously. The second study was conducted at the Nijmegen University Hospital; Nijmegen, The Netherlands. In this study patients were not selected for high risk of recurrence. In both studies treatment was initiated between 1 and 2 weeks after transurethral resection (TUR).

In the SWOG trial (study 8795) patients were randomized to TICE BCG or mitomycin C (MMC). Both drugs were given intravesically weekly for 6 weeks, at 8 and 12 weeks, and then monthly for a total treatment duration of 1 year. Cystoscopy and urinary cytology were performed every 3 months for 2 years. Patients with progressive disease or residual or recurrent disease at or after the 6 month follow-up were removed from the study and were classified as treatment failures.

A total of 469 patients was entered into the study: 237 to the TICE BCG arm and 232 to the MMC arm. Twenty-two patients were subsequently found to be ineligible, and 66 patients had concurrent CIS, and were analyzed separately. Four patients were lost to follow-up, leaving 191 evaluable patients in the TICE BCG arm and 186 in the MMC arm. Of the patients, 84% were male and 16% were female. The average age of these patients was 65 years old.

The Kaplan-Meier estimates of 2-year disease-free survival are shown in **Table 3**. The difference in disease-free survival time between the 2 groups was statistically significant by the log rank test (P=0.03). The 95% confidence interval of the difference in 2-year disease-free survival was 12% ± 10%. No statistically significant differences between the groups were noted in time to tumor progression, tumor invasion, or overall survival.

Table 3: Results of SWOG Study 8795

	TICE BCG Arm N=191	MMC Arm N=186
Estimated disease-free survival at 2 years	57%	45%
95% Confidence Interval (CI)	(50%, 65%)	(38%, 53%)

In the Nijmegen study, the efficacy of 3 treatments was compared: TICE substrain BCG, *Rijksinstituut voor Volksgezondheid en Milieuhygiene* substrain BCG (BCG-RIVM), and MMC.

TICE BCG and BCG-RIVM were given intravesically weekly for 6 weeks. In contrast to the SWOG study, maintenance BCG was not given. Mitomycin C was given intravesically weekly for 4 weeks and then monthly for a total duration of treatment of 6 months. Cystoscopy and urinary cytology were performed every 3 months until recurrence.

A total of 469 patients was enrolled and randomized. Thirty-two patients were not evaluable, 17 were ineligible, 15 were withdrawn before treatment, and 50 had concurrent CIS and were analyzed separately, leaving 387 evaluable patients: 117 in the TICE BCG arm, 134 in the BCG-RIVM arm, and 136 in the MMC arm. Twenty-eight patients (24%) in the TICE BCG arm, 32 patients (24%) in the BCG-RIVM arm, and 24 patients (18%) in the MMC arm had TaG1 tumors. The median duration of follow-up was 22 months (range: 3-54 months).

The Kaplan-Meier estimates of 2-year disease-free survival are shown in **Table 4**. The differences in disease-free survival among the 3 arms were not statistically significant by the log-rank test (P=0.08).

[See table 4 at top of next page]

In both the SWOG 8795 study and the Nijmegen study, acute toxicity was more common, and usually more severe, with TICE BCG than with MMC (see **ADVERSE REACTIONS**).

INDICATIONS AND USAGE

TICE® BCG is indicated for the treatment and prophylaxis of carcinoma *in situ* (CIS) of the urinary bladder, and for the prophylaxis of primary or recurrent stage Ta and/or T1 papillary tumors following transurethral resection (TUR). TICE BCG is not recommended for stage TaG1 papillary tumors, unless they are judged to be at high risk of tumor recurrence.

Table 4: Results of Nijmegen Study

	TICE BCG Arm N=117	BCG-RIVM Arm N=134	MMC Arm N=136
Estimated disease-free survival at 2 years	53%	62%	64%
95% Confidence Interval (CI)	(44%, 64%)	(53%, 72%)	(55%, 74%)

Table 5: Summary of Adverse Effects Seen in 674 Patients With Superficial Bladder Cancer, Including 153 With Carcinoma *in Situ*

Adverse event	Percent of patients N	Overall (Grade ≥3)	Adverse event	Percent of patients N	Overall (Grade ≥3)
Dysuria	401	60% (11%)	Arthritis/myalgia	18	3% (<1%)
Urinary frequency	272	40% (7%)	Headache/dizziness	16	2% (0)
Flu-like syndrome	224	33% (9%)	Urinary incontinence	16	2% (0)
Hematuria	175	26% (7%)	Anorexia/weight loss	15	2% (<1%)
Fever	134	20% (8%)	Urinary debris	15	2% (<1%)
Malaise/fatigue	50	7% (0)	Allergy	14	2% (<1%)
Cystitis	40	6% (2%)	Cardiac (unclassified)	13	2% (1%)
Urgency	39	6% (1%)	Genital inflammation/ abscess	12	2% (<1%)
Nocturia	30	5% (1%)	Respiratory (unclassified)	11	2% (<1%)
Cramps/pain	27	4% (1%)	Urinary tract infection	10	2% (1%)
Rigors	22	3% (1%)	Abdominal pain	10	2% (1%)
Nausea/vomiting	20	3% (<1%)			

TICE BCG is not indicated for papillary tumors of stages higher than T1.

CONTRAINDICATIONS

TICE® BCG should not be used in immunosuppressed patients or persons with congenital or acquired immune deficiencies, whether due to concurrent disease (e.g., AIDS, leukemia, lymphoma) cancer therapy (e.g., cytotoxic drugs, radiation), or immunosuppressive therapy (e.g., corticosteroids).

Treatment should be postponed until resolution of a concurrent febrile illness, urinary tract infection, or gross hematuria. Seven to 14 days should elapse before BCG is administered following biopsy, TUR, or traumatic catheterization.

TICE BCG should not be administered to persons with active tuberculosis. Active tuberculosis should be ruled out in individuals who are PPD positive before starting treatment with TICE BCG.

WARNINGS

BCG LIVE (TICE® BCG) is not a vaccine for the prevention of cancer. BCG Vaccine USP, not BCG LIVE (TICE BCG), should be used for the prevention of tuberculosis. For vaccination use, refer to BCG Vaccine USP prescribing information.

TICE BCG is an infectious agent. Physicians using this product should be familiar with the literature on the prevention and treatment of BCG-related complications, and should be prepared in such emergencies to contact an infectious disease specialist with experience in treating the infectious complications of intravesical BCG. The treatment of the infectious complications of BCG requires long-term, multiple-drug antibiotic therapy. Special culture media are required for mycobacteria, and physicians administering intravesical BCG or those caring for these patients should have these media readily available.

Instillation of TICE BCG with an actively bleeding mucosa may promote systemic BCG infection. Treatment should be postponed for at least 1 week following transurethral resection, biopsy, traumatic catheterization, or gross hematuria. Deaths have been reported as a result of systemic BCG infection and sepsis.[2,3] Patients should be monitored for the presence of symptoms and signs of toxicity after each intravesical treatment. Febrile episodes with flu-like symptoms lasting more than 72 hours, fever ≥103°F, systemic manifestations increasing in intensity with repeated instillations, or persistent abnormalities of liver function tests suggest systemic BCG infection and may require antituberculous therapy. Local symptoms (prostatitis, epididymitis, orchitis) lasting more than 2 to 3 days may also suggest active infection (see **WARNINGS, *Management of Serious BCG Complications*** section).

The use of TICE BCG may cause tuberculin sensitivity. Since this is a valuable aid in the diagnosis of tuberculosis, it is advisable to determine the tuberculin reactivity by PPD skin testing before treatment.

Intravesical instillations of BCG should be postponed during treatment with antibiotics, since antimicrobial therapy may interfere with the effectiveness of TICE BCG (see **PRECAUTIONS**). TICE BCG should not be used in individuals with concurrent infections.

Small bladder capacity has been associated with increased risk of severe local reactions and should be considered in deciding to use TICE BCG therapy.

Management of Serious BCG Complications.

Acute, localized irritative toxicities of TICE BCG may be accompanied by systemic manifestations, consistent with a "flu-like" syndrome. Systemic adverse effects of 1 to 2 days' duration such as malaise, fever, and chills often reflect hypersensitivity reactions. However, **symptoms such as fever of ≥38.5°C (101.3°F), or acute localized inflammation such as epididymitis, prostatitis, or orchitis persisting longer than 2 to 3 days suggest active infection, and evaluation for serious infectious complication should be considered.** In patients who develop persistent fever or experience an acute febrile illness consistent with BCG infection, 2 or more antimycobacterial agents should be administered while diagnostic evaluation, including cultures, is conducted. **BCG treatment should be discontinued.** Negative cultures do not necessarily rule out infection. Physicians using this product should be familiar with the literature on prevention, diagnosis, and treatment of BCG-related complications and, when appropriate, should consult an infectious disease specialist or other physician with experience in the diagnosis and treatment of mycobacterial infections. TICE BCG is sensitive to the most commonly used antituberculous agents (isoniazid, rifampin, and ethambutol). **TICE BCG is not sensitive to pyrazinamide.**

PRECAUTIONS

General

TICE® BCG contains live mycobacteria and should be prepared and handled using aseptic technique (see **DOSAGE AND ADMINISTRATION, Preparation of Agent** section). BCG infections have been reported in health care workers preparing BCG for administration. Needle stick injuries should be avoided during the handling and mixing of TICE BCG. Nosocomial infections have been reported in patients receiving parenteral drugs which were prepared in areas in which BCG was prepared.[4]

BCG is capable of dissemination when administered by intravesical route, and serious reactions, including fatal infections, have been reported in patients receiving intravesical BCG.[3] Care should be taken not to traumatize the urinary tract or to introduce contaminants into the urinary system. Seven to 14 days should elapse before TICE BCG is administered following TUR, biopsy, or traumatic catheterization. TICE BCG should be administered with caution to persons in groups at high risk for HIV infection.

Laboratory Tests

The use of TICE BCG may cause tuberculin sensitivity. It is advisable to determine the tuberculin reactivity of patients receiving TICE BCG by PPD skin testing before treatment is initiated.

Information for Patients

TICE BCG is retained in the bladder for 2 hours and then voided. Patients should void while seated in order to avoid splashing of urine. For the 6 hours after treatment, urine voided should be disinfected for 15 minutes with an equal volume of household bleach before flushing. Patients should be instructed to increase fluid intake in order to "flush" the bladder in the hours following BCG treatment. Patients may experience burning with the first void after treatment. Patients should be attentive to side effects, such as fever, chills, malaise, flu-like symptoms, or increased fatigue. If the patient experiences severe urinary side effects, such as burning or pain on urination, urgency, frequency of urination, blood in urine, or other symptoms such as joint pain, cough, or skin rash, the physician should be notified.

Drug Interaction

Drug combinations containing immunosuppressants and/or bone marrow depressants and/or radiation interfere with the development of the immune response and should not be used in combination with TICE BCG. Antimicrobial therapy for other infections may interfere with the effectiveness of TICE BCG. There are no data to suggest that the acute, local urinary tract toxicity common with BCG is due to mycobacterial infection, and **antituberculosis drugs (e.g., isoniazid) should not be used to prevent or treat the local, irritative toxicities of TICE BCG.**

Carcinogenesis, Mutagenesis, Impairment of Fertility

TICE BCG has not been evaluated for its carcinogenic, mutagenic potentials, or impairment of fertility.

Pregnancy

Teratogenic Effects – Pregnancy Category C

Animal reproduction studies have not been conducted with TICE BCG. It is also not known whether TICE BCG can cause fetal harm when administered to a pregnant woman or can affect reproductive capacity. TICE BCG should not be given to a pregnant woman except when clearly needed. Women should be advised not to become pregnant while on therapy.

Nursing Mothers

It is not known whether TICE BCG is excreted in human milk. Because many drugs are excreted in human milk and because of the potential for serious adverse reactions from TICE BCG in nursing infants, it is advisable to discontinue nursing or to discontinue the drug, taking into account the importance of the drug to the mother.

Pediatric Use

Safety and effectiveness of TICE BCG for the treatment of superficial bladder cancer in pediatric patients have not been established.

Geriatric Use

Of the total number of subjects in clinical studies of TICE BCG, the average age was 66 years old. No overall difference in safety or effectiveness was observed between older and younger subjects. Other reported clinical experience has not identified differences in response between elderly and younger patients, but greater sensitivity of some older individuals to BCG cannot be ruled out.

ADVERSE REACTIONS

Symptoms of bladder irritability, related to the inflammatory response induced, are reported in approximately 60% of patients receiving TICE® BCG. The symptoms typically begin 4 to 6 hours after instillation and last 24 to 72 hours. The irritative side effects are usually seen following the third instillation, and tend to increase in severity after each administration.

The irritative bladder adverse effects can usually be managed symptomatically with products such as pyridium, propantheline bromide, oxybutynin chloride, and acetaminophen. The mechanism of action of the irritative side effects has not been firmly established, but is most consistent with an immunological mechanism.[3] There is no evidence that dose reduction or antituberculous drug therapy can prevent or lessen the irritative toxicity of TICE BCG.

"Flu-like" symptoms (malaise, fever, and chills) which may accompany the localized, irritative toxicities often reflect hypersensitivity reactions which can be treated symptomatically. Antihistamines have also been used.[5]

Adverse reactions to TICE BCG tend to be progressive in frequency and severity with subsequent instillation. Delay or postponement of subsequent treatment may or may not reduce the severity of a reaction during subsequent instillation.

Although uncommon, serious infectious complications of intravesical BCG have been reported.[2,3,6] The most serious infectious complication of BCG is disseminated sepsis with associated mortality. In addition, *M. bovis* infections have been reported in lung, liver, bone, bone marrow, kidney, regional lymph nodes, and prostate in patients who have received intravesical BCG. Some male genitourinary tract infections (orchitis/epididymitis) have been resistant to multiple-drug antituberculous therapy and required orchiectomy.

If a patient develops persistent fever or experiences an acute febrile illness consistent with BCG infection, BCG treatment should be discontinued and the patient immediately evaluated and treated for systemic infection (see WARNINGS).

The local and systemic adverse reactions reported in a review of 674 patients with superficial bladder cancer, including 153 patients with carcinoma *in situ*, are summarized in **Table 5**.

[See table 5 above]

The following adverse events were reported in ≤1% of patients: anemia, BCG sepsis, coagulopathy, contracted bladder, diarrhea, epididymitis/prostatitis, hepatic granuloma, hepatitis, leukopenia, neurologic (unclassified), orchitis, pneumonitis, pyuria, rash, thrombocytopenia, urethritis, and urinary obstruction.

In SWOG study 8795, toxicity evaluations were available on a total of 222 TICE BCG-treated patients and 220 MMC-treated patients. Direct bladder toxicity (cramps, dysuria, frequency, urgency, hematuria, hemorrhagic cystitis, or incontinence) was seen more often with TICE BCG with 356 events, compared to 234 events for MMC. Grade ≤2 toxicity was seen significantly more frequently following TICE BCG treatment (P=0.003). No life-threatening toxicity was seen in either arm. Systemic toxicity with TICE BCG was markedly increased compared to that of MMC, with 181 events for TICE BCG compared to 80 for MMC. The frequency of toxicity was increased in all grades, particularly for grades 2 and 3. The most common complaints were malaise, fatigue and lethargy, fever, and abdominal pain. Thirty-two TICE BCG patients were reported to have been treated with isoniazid. Five TICE BCG patients had liver enzyme elevation, including 2 with grade 3 elevations. Eighteen of the 222 (8.1%) TICE BCG patients failed to complete the prescribed protocol compared to 6.2% in the MMC group. **Table 6** summarizes the most common adverse reactions reported in this trial.[7]

[See table 6 above]

Table 6: Most Common Adverse Reactions in SWOG Study 8795*

	Study arm			
	TICE BCG (N=222)		MMC (N=220)	
Adverse event	**All Grades**	**Grade ≥3**	**All Grades**	**Grade ≥3**
Dysuria	115 (52%)	6 (3%)	77 (35%)	5 (2%)
Urgency/frequency	112 (50%)	5 (2%)	63 (29%)	7 (3%)
Hematuria	85 (38%)	6 (3%)	56 (25%)	5 (2%)
Flu-like symptoms	54 (24%)	1 (<1%)	29 (13%)	0
Fever	37 (17%)	1 (<1%)	7 (3%)	0
Pain (not specified)	37 (17%)	4 (2%)	22 (10%)	1 (<1%)
Hemorrhagic cystitis	19 (9%)	3 (1%)	10 (5%)	0
Chills	19 (9%)	0	2 (1%)	0
Bladder cramps	18 (8%)	0	9 (4%)	0
Nausea	16 (7%)	0	12 (5%)	0
Incontinence	8 (4%)	0	3 (1%)	0
Myalgia/arthralgia	7 (3%)	0	0	0
Diaphoresis	7 (3%)	0	1 (<1%)	0
Rash	6 (3%)	1 (<1%)	16 (7%)	2 (1%)

* The adverse reaction profile of TICE BCG was similar in the Nijmegen study.[8]

OVERDOSAGE

Overdosage occurs if more than 1 vial of TICE® BCG is administered per instillation. If overdosage occurs, the patient should be closely monitored for signs of active local or systemic BCG infection. For acute local or systemic reactions suggesting active infection, an infectious disease specialist experienced in BCG complications should be consulted.

DOSAGE AND ADMINISTRATION

The dose for the intravesical treatment of carcinoma *in situ* and for the prophylaxis of recurrent papillary tumors consists of 1 vial of TICE® BCG suspended in 50 mL preservative-free saline.

Do not inject subcutaneously or intravenously.

Preparation of Agent

The preparation of the TICE BCG suspension should be done using aseptic technique. To avoid cross-contamination, parenteral drugs should not be prepared in areas where BCG has been prepared. A separate area for the preparation of the TICE BCG suspension is recommended. All equipment, supplies, and receptacles in contact with TICE BCG should be handled and disposed of as biohazardous. The pharmacist or individual responsible for mixing the agent should wear gloves and take precautions to avoid contact of BCG with broken skin. If preparation cannot be performed in a biocontainment hood, then a mask and gown should be worn to avoid inhalation of BCG organisms and inadvertent exposure to broken skin.

Option 1 (Using Syringe Method)

Draw 1 mL of sterile, preservative-free saline (0.9% Sodium Chloride Injection USP) at 4-25°C into a small syringe (e.g., 3 mL) and add to 1 vial of TICE BCG to resuspend. Gently swirl the vial until a homogenous suspension is obtained. Avoid forceful agitation which may cause clumping of the mycobacteria. Dispense the cloudy TICE BCG suspension into the top end of a catheter-tip syringe which contains 49 mL of saline diluent, bringing the total volume to 50 mL. To mix, gently rotate the syringe.

Option 2 (Using Reconstitution Accessories)

Reconstitution Accessories may be provided with each TICE BCG product order. Please refer to the Reconstitution Accessories Instructions provided with the accessories for a full description of the product reconstitution procedures using these accessories.

The reconstituted TICE BCG should be kept refrigerated (2-8°C), protected from exposure to direct sunlight, and used within 2 hours. Unused solution should be discarded after 2 hours.

Note: DO NOT filter the contents of the TICE BCG vial. Precautions should be taken to avoid exposing the TICE BCG to direct sunlight. Bacteriostatic solutions must be avoided. In addition, use only sterile, preservative-free saline, 0.9% Sodium Chloride Injection USP as diluent.

Treatment and Schedule

Allow 7 to 14 days to elapse after bladder biopsy before TICE BCG is administered. Patients should not drink fluids for 4 hours before treatment and should empty their bladder prior to TICE BCG administration. The reconstituted TICE BCG is instilled into the bladder by gravity flow via the catheter. **DO NOT** depress plunger and force the flow of the TICE BCG. The TICE BCG is retained in the bladder 2 hours and then voided. Patients unable to retain the suspension for 2 hours should be allowed to void sooner, if necessary.

While the BCG is retained in the bladder, the patient ideally should be repositioned from left side to right side and also should lie upon the back and the abdomen, changing these positions every 15 minutes to maximize bladder surface exposure to the agent.

A standard treatment schedule consists of 1 intravesical instillation per week for 6 weeks. This schedule may be repeated once if tumor remission has not been achieved and if the clinical circumstances warrant. Thereafter, intravesical TICE BCG administration should continue at approximately monthly intervals for at least 6 to 12 months. There are no data to support the interchangeability of BCG LIVE products.

HOW SUPPLIED

TICE® BCG is supplied in a box of 1 vial of TICE BCG. Each vial contains 1 to 8 × 10^8 CFU, which is equivalent to approximately 50 mg (wet weight), as lyophilized (freeze-dried) powder, NDC 0052-0602-02.

STORAGE

The intact vials of TICE® BCG should be stored refrigerated, at 2-8°C (36-46°F).

This agent contains live bacteria and should be protected from **direct** sunlight. The product should not be used after the expiration date printed on the label.

Rx only

REFERENCES

1. DeJager R, Guinan P, Lamm D, Khanna O, Brosman S, DeKernion J, et al. Long-Term Complete Remission in Bladder Carcinoma in Situ with Intravesical TICE Bacillus Calmette Guerin. *Urology* 1991;38:507-513.
2. Rawls WH, Lamm DL, Lowe BA, Crawford ED, Sarosdy MF, Montie JE, Grossman HB, Scardino PT. Fatal Sepsis Following Intravesical Bacillus Calmette-Guerin Administration For Bladder Cancer. *J Urol* 1990;144:1328-1330.
3. Lamm DL, van der Meijden APM, Morales A, Brosman SA, Catalona WJ, Herr HW, et al. Incidence and Treatment of Complications of Bacillus Calmette-Guerin Intravesical Therapy in Superficial Bladder Cancer. *J. Urol* 1992;147:596-600.
4. Stone MM, Vannier AM, Storch SK, Nitta AT, Zhang Y. Brief Report: Meningitis Due to Iatrogenic BCG Infection in Two Immunocompromised Children. *NEJM* 1995:333:561-563.
5. Steg A, Leleu C, Debre B, Gibod-Boccon L, Sicard D. Systemic Bacillus Calmette-Guerin Infection in Patients Treated by Intravesical BCG Therapy for Superficial Bladder Cancer. *EORTC Genitourinary Group Monograph 6: BCG in Superficial Bladder Cancer.* Edited by F.M. J. Debruyne, L. Denis and A.P.M. van der Meijden. New York: Alan R. Liss Inc., pp. 325-334.
6. van der Meijden, APM. Practical Approaches to the Prevention and Treatment of Adverse Reactions to BCG. *Eur Urol* 1995;27(suppl 1):23-28.
7. Lamm DL, Blumenstein BA, Crawford ED, Crissman JD, Lowe BA, Smith JA, Sarosdy MF, Schellhammer PF, Sagalowsky AI, Messing EM, et al. Randomized Intergroup Comparison of Bacillus Calmette-Guerin Immunotherapy and Mitomycin C Chemotherapy Prophylaxis in Superficial Transitional Cell Carcinoma of the Bladder. *Urol Oncol* 1995;1:119-126.
8. Witjes JA, van der Meijden APM, Witjes WPJ, et al. A Randomized Prospective Study Comparing Intravesical Instillations of Mitomycin-C, BCG-Tice, and BCG-RIVM in pTa-pT1 Tumours and Primary Carcinoma *In Situ* of the Urinary Bladder. *Eur J Cancer* 1993;29A(12):1672-1676.

Manufactured for: Merck Sharp & Dohme Corp., a subsidiary of

MERCK & CO., INC.,Whitehouse Station, NJ 08889, USA

Manufactured by: Organon Teknika Corporation LLC, Durham, NC 27712, USA, a subsidiary of **Merck & Co., Inc.**, Whitehouse Station, NJ 08889, USA

U.S. License No. 1747

TICE is a registered trademark of The Board of Trustees of the University of Illinois, used under the license of Organon Teknika Corporation.

Rev. 10/2012

RM129.9

Shown in Product Identification Guide, page 309

TRUSOPT® ℞

(dorzolamide hydrochloride ophthalmic solution)

Sterile Ophthalmic Solution 2%

DESCRIPTION

TRUSOPT® (dorzolamide hydrochloride ophthalmic solution) is a carbonic anhydrase inhibitor formulated for topical ophthalmic use.

Dorzolamide hydrochloride is described chemically as: (4*S*-*trans*)-4-(ethylamino)-5,6-dihydro-6-methyl-4*H*-thieno[2,3-*b*]thiopyran-2-sulfonamide 7,7-dioxide monohydrochloride. Dorzolamide hydrochloride is optically active. The specific rotation is

$$\alpha^{25°}_{405} \text{ (C=1, water) = ~-17°.}$$

Its empirical formula is $C_{10}H_{16}N_2O_4S_3$•HCl and its structural formula is:

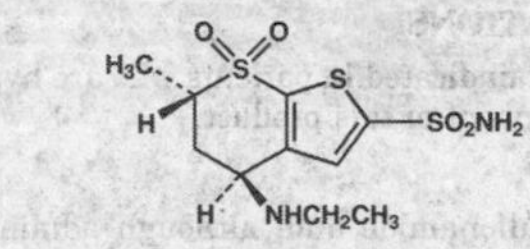

Dorzolamide hydrochloride has a molecular weight of 360.9 and a melting point of about 264°C. It is a white to off-white, crystalline powder, which is soluble in water and slightly soluble in methanol and ethanol.

TRUSOPT Sterile Ophthalmic Solution is supplied as a sterile, isotonic, buffered, slightly viscous, aqueous solution of dorzolamide hydrochloride. The pH of the solution is approximately 5.6, and the osmolarity is 260-330 mOsM. Each mL of TRUSOPT 2% contains 20 mg dorzolamide (22.3 mg of dorzolamide hydrochloride). Inactive ingredients are hydroxyethyl cellulose, mannitol, sodium citrate dihydrate, sodium hydroxide (to adjust pH) and water for injection. Benzalkonium chloride 0.0075% is added as a preservative.

CLINICAL PHARMACOLOGY

Mechanism of Action

Carbonic anhydrase (CA) is an enzyme found in many tissues of the body including the eye. It catalyzes the reversible reaction involving the hydration of carbon dioxide and the dehydration of carbonic acid. In humans, carbonic anhydrase exists as a number of isoenzymes, the most active being carbonic anhydrase II (CA-II), found primarily in red blood cells (RBCs), but also in other tissues. Inhibition of carbonic anhydrase in the ciliary processes of the eye decreases aqueous humor secretion, presumably by slowing the formation of bicarbonate ions with subsequent reduction in sodium and fluid transport. The result is a reduction in intraocular pressure (IOP).

TRUSOPT Ophthalmic Solution contains dorzolamide hydrochloride, an inhibitor of human carbonic anhydrase II. Following topical ocular administration, TRUSOPT reduces elevated intraocular pressure. Elevated intraocular pressure is a major risk factor in the pathogenesis of optic nerve damage and glaucomatous visual field loss.

Pharmacokinetics/Pharmacodynamics

When topically applied, dorzolamide reaches the systemic circulation. To assess the potential for systemic carbonic anhydrase inhibition following topical administration, drug and metabolite concentrations in RBCs and plasma and carbonic anhydrase inhibition in RBCs were measured. Dorzolamide accumulates in RBCs during chronic dosing as a result of binding to CA-II. The parent drug forms a single N-desethyl metabolite, which inhibits CA-II less potently than the parent drug but also inhibits CA-I. The metabolite also accumulates in RBCs where it binds primarily to CA-I. Plasma concentrations of dorzolamide and metabolite are generally below the assay limit of quantitation (15nM). Dorzolamide binds moderately to plasma proteins (approximately 33%). Dorzolamide is primarily excreted unchanged in the urine; the metabolite also is excreted in urine. After dosing is stopped, dorzolamide washes out of RBCs nonlinearly, resulting in a rapid decline of drug concentration initially, followed by a slower elimination phase with a half-life of about four months.

To simulate the systemic exposure after long-term topical ocular administration, dorzolamide was given orally to eight healthy subjects for up to 20 weeks. The oral dose of 2 mg b.i.d. closely approximates the amount of drug delivered by topical ocular administration of TRUSOPT 2% t.i.d. Steady state was reached within 8 weeks. The inhibition of CA-II and total carbonic anhydrase activities was below the degree of inhibition anticipated to be necessary for a pharmacological effect on renal function and respiration in healthy individuals.

Clinical Studies

The efficacy of TRUSOPT was demonstrated in clinical studies in the treatment of elevated intraocular pressure in patients with glaucoma or ocular hypertension (baseline IOP ≥ 23 mmHg). The IOP-lowering effect of TRUSOPT was approximately 3 to 5 mmHg throughout the day and this was consistent in clinical studies of up to one year duration. The efficacy of TRUSOPT when dosed less frequently than three times a day (alone or in combination with other products) has not been established.

In a one year clinical study, the effect of TRUSOPT 2% t.i.d. on the corneal endothelium was compared to that of betaxolol ophthalmic solution b.i.d. and timolol maleate ophthalmic solution 0.5% b.i.d. There were no statistically significant differences between groups in corneal endothelial cell counts or in corneal thickness measurements. There was a mean loss of approximately 4% in the endothelial cell counts for each group over the one year period.

INDICATIONS AND USAGE

TRUSOPT Ophthalmic Solution is indicated in the treatment of elevated intraocular pressure in patients with ocular hypertension or open-angle glaucoma.

CONTRAINDICATIONS

TRUSOPT is contraindicated in patients who are hypersensitive to any component of this product.

WARNINGS

TRUSOPT is a sulfonamide and, although administered topically, is absorbed systemically. Therefore, the same types of adverse reactions that are attributable to sulfonamides may occur with topical administration with TRUSOPT. Fatalities have occurred, although rarely, due to severe reactions to sulfonamides including Stevens-Johnson syndrome, toxic epidermal necrolysis, fulminant hepatic necrosis, agranulocytosis, aplastic anemia, and other blood dyscrasias. Sensitization may recur when a sulfonamide is readministered irrespective of the route of administration. If signs of serious reactions or hypersensitivity occur, discontinue the use of this preparation.

PRECAUTIONS

General

The management of patients with acute angle-closure glaucoma requires therapeutic interventions in addition to ocular hypotensive agents. TRUSOPT has not been studied in patients with acute angle-closure glaucoma.

TRUSOPT has not been studied in patients with severe renal impairment (CrCl < 30 mL/min). Because TRUSOPT and its metabolite are excreted predominantly by the kidney, TRUSOPT is not recommended in such patients.

TRUSOPT has not been studied in patients with hepatic impairment and should therefore be used with caution in such patients.

In clinical studies, local ocular adverse effects, primarily conjunctivitis and lid reactions, were reported with chronic administration of TRUSOPT. Many of these reactions had the clinical appearance and course of an allergic-type reaction that resolved upon discontinuation of drug therapy. If such reactions are observed, TRUSOPT should be discontinued and the patient evaluated before considering restarting the drug. (See ADVERSE REACTIONS.)

There is a potential for an additive effect on the known systemic effects of carbonic anhydrase inhibition in patients receiving an oral carbonic anhydrase inhibitor and TRUSOPT. The concomitant administration of TRUSOPT and oral carbonic anhydrase inhibitors is not recommended.

There have been reports of bacterial keratitis associated with the use of multiple-dose containers of topical ophthalmic products. These containers had been inadvertently contaminated by patients who, in most cases, had a concurrent corneal disease or a disruption of the ocular epithelial surface.

Choroidal detachment has been reported with administration of aqueous suppressant therapy (e.g., dorzolamide) after filtration procedures.

There is an increased potential for developing corneal edema in patients with low endothelial cell counts. Precautions should be used when prescribing TRUSOPT to this group of patients.

Information for Patients

TRUSOPT is a sulfonamide and although administered topically is absorbed systemically. Therefore the same types of adverse reactions that are attributable to sulfonamides may occur with topical administration. Patients should be advised that if serious or unusual reactions including severe skin reactions or signs of hypersensitivity occur, they should discontinue the use of the product (see WARNINGS).

Patients should be advised that if they develop any ocular reactions, particularly conjunctivitis and lid reactions, they should discontinue use and seek their physician's advice.

Patients should be instructed to avoid allowing the tip of the dispensing container to contact the eye or surrounding structures.

Patients should also be instructed that ocular solutions, if handled improperly or if the tip of the dispensing container contacts the eye or surrounding structures, can become contaminated by common bacteria known to cause ocular infections. Serious damage to the eye and subsequent loss of vision may result from using contaminated solutions.

Patients also should be advised that if they have ocular surgery or develop an intercurrent ocular condition (e.g., trauma or infection), they should immediately seek their physician's advice concerning the continued use of the present multidose container.

If more than one topical ophthalmic drug is being used, the drugs should be administered at least ten minutes apart.

Patients should be advised that TRUSOPT contains benzalkonium chloride which may be absorbed by soft contact lenses. Contact lenses should be removed prior to administration of the solution. Lenses may be reinserted 15 minutes following TRUSOPT administration.

Drug Interactions

Although acid-base and electrolyte disturbances were not reported in the clinical trials with TRUSOPT, these disturbances have been reported with oral carbonic anhydrase inhibitors and have, in some instances, resulted in drug interactions (e.g., toxicity associated with high-dose salicylate therapy). Therefore, the potential for such drug interactions should be considered in patients receiving TRUSOPT.

Carcinogenesis, Mutagenesis, Impairment of Fertility

In a two-year study of dorzolamide hydrochloride administered orally to male and female Sprague-Dawley rats, urinary bladder papillomas were seen in male rats in the highest dosage group of 20 mg/kg/day (250 times the recommended human ophthalmic dose). Papillomas were not seen in rats given oral doses equivalent to approximately 12 times the recommended human ophthalmic dose. No treatment-related tumors were seen in a 21-month study in female and male mice given oral doses up to 75 mg/kg/day (~900 times the recommended human ophthalmic dose).

The increased incidence of urinary bladder papillomas seen in the high-dose male rats is a class-effect of carbonic anhydrase inhibitors in rats. Rats are particularly prone to developing papillomas in response to foreign bodies, compounds causing crystalluria, and diverse sodium salts.

No changes in bladder urothelium were seen in dogs given oral dorzolamide hydrochloride for one year at 2 mg/kg/day (25 times the recommended human ophthalmic dose) or monkeys dosed topically to the eye at 0.4 mg/kg/day (~5 times the recommended human ophthalmic dose) for one year.

The following tests for mutagenic potential were negative: (1) *in vivo* (mouse) cytogenetic assay; (2) *in vitro* chromosomal aberration assay; (3) alkaline elution assay; (4) V-79 assay; and (5) Ames test.

In reproduction studies of dorzolamide hydrochloride in rats, there were no adverse effects on the reproductive capacity of males or females at doses up to 188 or 94 times, respectively, the recommended human ophthalmic dose.

Pregnancy

Teratogenic Effects

Pregnancy Category C

Developmental toxicity studies with dorzolamide hydrochloride in rabbits at oral doses of ≥ 2.5 mg/kg/day (31 times the recommended human ophthalmic dose) revealed malformations of the vertebral bodies. These malformations occurred at doses that caused metabolic acidosis with decreased body weight gain in dams and decreased fetal weights. No treatment-related malformations were seen at 1.0 mg/kg/day (13 times the recommended human ophthalmic dose). There are no adequate and well-controlled studies in pregnant women. TRUSOPT should be used during pregnancy only if the potential benefit justifies the potential risk to the fetus.

Nursing Mothers

In a study of dorzolamide hydrochloride in lactating rats, decreases in body weight gain of 5 to 7% in offspring at an oral dose of 7.5 mg/kg/day (94 times the recommended human ophthalmic dose) were seen during lactation. A slight delay in postnatal development (incisor eruption, vaginal canalization and eye openings), secondary to lower fetal body weight, was noted.

It is not known whether this drug is excreted in human milk. Because many drugs are excreted in human milk and because of the potential for serious adverse reactions in nursing infants from TRUSOPT, a decision should be made whether to discontinue nursing or to discontinue the drug, taking into account the importance of the drug to the mother.

Pediatric Use

Safety and IOP-lowering effects of TRUSOPT have been demonstrated in pediatric patients in a 3-month, multicenter, double-masked, active-treatment-controlled trial.

Geriatric Use

No overall differences in safety or effectiveness have been observed between elderly and younger patients.

ADVERSE REACTIONS

Controlled clinical trials

The most frequent adverse events associated with TRUSOPT were ocular burning, stinging, or discomfort immediately following ocular administration (approximately one-third of patients). Approximately one-quarter of patients noted a bitter taste following administration. Superficial punctate keratitis occurred in 10-15% of patients and signs and symptoms of ocular allergic reaction in approximately 10%. Events occurring in approximately 1-5% of patients were conjunctivitis and lid reactions (see PRECAUTIONS, General), blurred vision, eye redness, tearing, dryness, and photophobia. Other ocular events and systemic events were reported infrequently, including headache, nausea, asthenia/fatigue; and, rarely, skin rashes, urolithiasis, and iridocyclitis.

In a 3-month, double-masked, active-treatment-controlled, multicenter study in pediatric patients, the adverse experience profile of TRUSOPT was comparable to that seen in adult patients.

Clinical practice

The following adverse events have occurred either at low incidence (<1%) during clinical trials or have been reported during the use of TRUSOPT in clinical practice where these events were reported voluntarily from a population of unknown size and frequency of occurrence cannot be determined precisely. They have been chosen for inclusion based on factors such as seriousness, frequency of reporting, possible causal connection to TRUSOPT, or a combination of these factors: signs and symptoms of systemic allergic reactions including angioedema, bronchospasm, pruritus, and urticaria; Stevens-Johnson syndrome and toxic epidermal necrolysis; dizziness, paresthesia; ocular pain, transient myopia, choroidal detachment following filtration surgery, eyelid crusting; dyspnea; contact dermatitis, epistaxis, dry mouth and throat irritation.

OVERDOSAGE

Electrolyte imbalance, development of an acidotic state, and possible central nervous system effects may occur. Serum electrolyte levels (particularly potassium) and blood pH levels should be monitored.

DOSAGE AND ADMINISTRATION

The dose is one drop of TRUSOPT Ophthalmic Solution in the affected eye(s) three times daily.

TRUSOPT may be used concomitantly with other topical ophthalmic drug products to lower intraocular pressure. If more than one topical ophthalmic drug is being used, the drugs should be administered at least ten minutes apart.

HOW SUPPLIED

TRUSOPT Ophthalmic Solution is a slightly opalescent, nearly colorless, slightly viscous solution.

No. 3519 — TRUSOPT Ophthalmic Solution 2% is supplied in an OCUMETER® PLUS container, a white, translucent, HDPE plastic ophthalmic dispenser with a controlled drop tip and a white polystyrene cap with orange label as follows:

NDC 0006-3519-36, 10 mL, in an 18 mL capacity bottle.

Storage

Store TRUSOPT Ophthalmic Solution at 15-30°C (59-86°F). Protect from light.

Rx only

Manuf. for: Merck Sharp & Dohme Corp., a subsidiary of **MERCK & CO., INC.**, Whitehouse Station, NJ 08889, USA

By: Laboratoires Merck Sharp & Dohme-Chibret

Clermont Ferrand Cedex 9, 63963, France

Issued August 2011
516358Z/220711-1/3519

9368212

INSTRUCTIONS FOR USE

TRUSOPT®
(dorzolamide hydrochloride ophthalmic solution)
Sterile Ophthalmic Solution 2%

Please follow these instructions carefully when using TRUSOPT®. Use TRUSOPT as prescribed by your doctor.

1. If you use other topically applied ophthalmic medications, they should be administered at least 10 minutes before or after TRUSOPT.
2. Wash hands before each use.
3. Before using the medication for the first time, be sure the Safety Strip on the front of the bottle is unbroken. A gap between the bottle and the cap is normal for an unopened bottle.

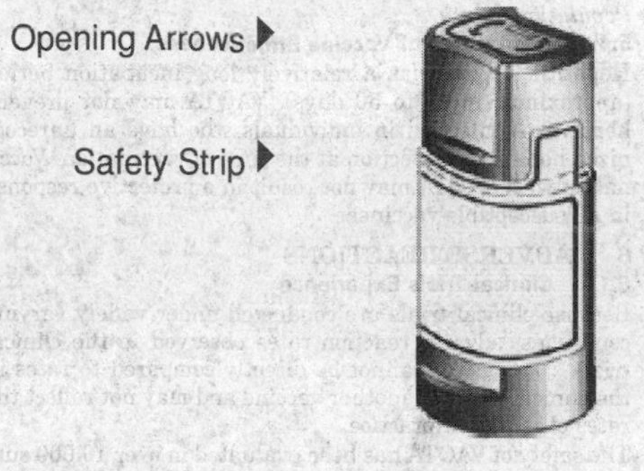

4. Tear off the Safety Strip to break the seal.

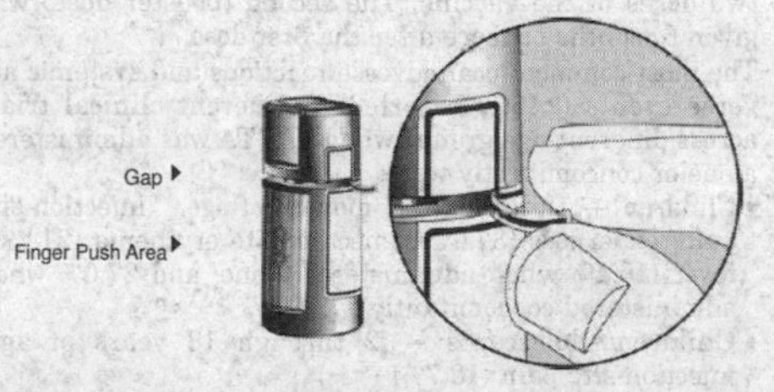

5. To open the bottle, unscrew the cap by turning as indicated by the arrows on the top of the cap. Do not pull the cap directly up and away from the bottle. Pulling the cap directly up will prevent your dispenser from operating properly.

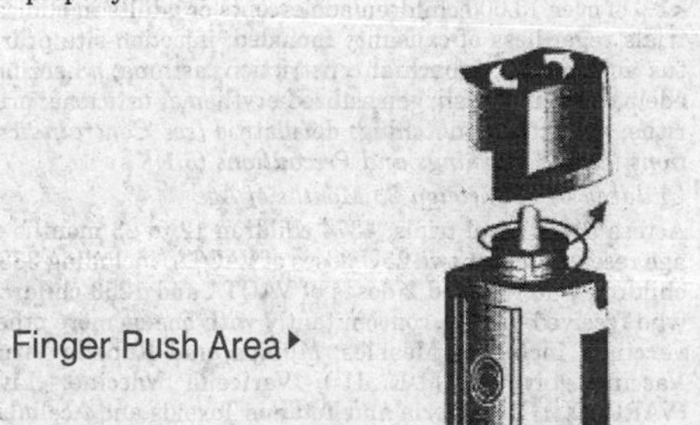

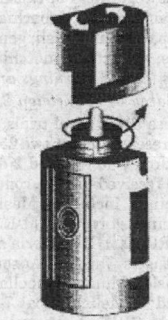

6. Tilt your head back and pull your lower eyelid down slightly to form a pocket between your eyelid and your eye.

[See first figure at top of next column]

7. Invert the bottle, and press lightly with the thumb or index finger over the "Finger Push Area" (as shown) until a single drop is dispensed into the eye as directed by your doctor.

[See second figure at top of next column]

DO NOT TOUCH YOUR EYE OR EYELID WITH THE DROPPER TIP.

OPHTHALMIC MEDICATIONS, IF HANDLED IMPROPERLY, CAN BECOME CONTAMINATED BY COMMON BACTERIA KNOWN TO CAUSE EYE INFECTIONS. SERIOUS DAMAGE TO THE EYE AND SUBSEQUENT LOSS OF VISION MAY RESULT FROM USING CONTAMINATED OPHTHALMIC MEDICATIONS. IF YOU THINK YOUR MEDICATION MAY BE CONTAMINATED, OR IF

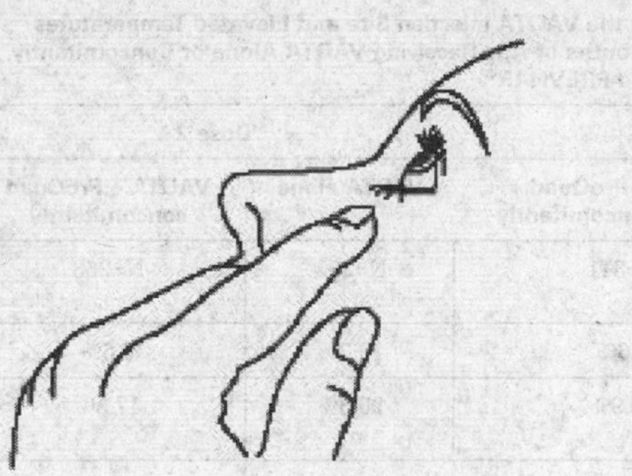

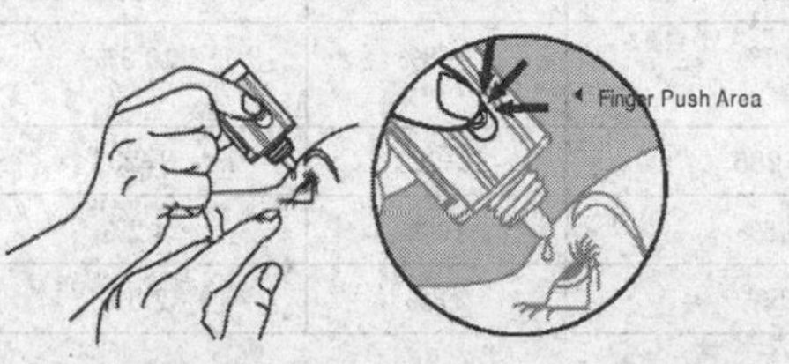

YOU DEVELOP AN EYE INFECTION, CONTACT YOUR DOCTOR IMMEDIATELY CONCERNING CONTINUED USE OF THIS BOTTLE.

8. If drop dispensing is difficult after opening for the first time, replace the cap on the bottle and tighten (DO NOT OVERTIGHTEN) and then remove by turning the cap in the opposite direction as indicated by the arrows on the top of the cap.
9. Repeat steps 6 & 7 with the other eye if instructed to do so by your doctor.
10. Replace the cap by turning until it is firmly touching the bottle. The arrow on the left side of the cap must be aligned with the arrow on the left side of the bottle label for proper closure. Do not overtighten or you may damage the bottle and cap.
11. The dispenser tip is designed to provide a single drop; therefore, do NOT enlarge the hole of the dispenser tip.
12. After you have used all doses, there will be some TRUSOPT left in the bottle. You should not be concerned since an extra amount of TRUSOPT has been added and you will get the full amount of TRUSOPT that your doctor prescribed. Do not attempt to remove excess medicine from the bottle.

WARNING: Keep out of reach of children.

If you have any questions about the use of TRUSOPT, please consult your doctor.

Issued August 2011
Manuf. for: Merck Sharp & Dohme Corp., a subsidiary of **MERCK & CO., Inc.**, Whitehouse Station, NJ 08889, USA
By: Laboratoires Merck Sharp & Dohme-Chibret
Clermont Ferrand Cedex 9, 63963, France

9368212

VAQTA® ℞

[va-q-ta]
(Hepatitis A Vaccine, Inactivated)
Suspension for Intramuscular Injection

HIGHLIGHTS OF PRESCRIBING INFORMATION
These highlights do not include all the information needed to use VAQTA safely and effectively. See full prescribing information for VAQTA.
VAQTA® (Hepatitis A Vaccine, Inactivated)
Suspension for Intramuscular Injection
Initial U.S. Approval: 1996

INDICATIONS AND USAGE

VAQTA is a vaccine indicated for the prevention of disease caused by hepatitis A virus (HAV) in persons 12 months of age and older. The primary dose should be given at least 2 weeks prior to expected exposure to HAV. (1.1)

DOSAGE AND ADMINISTRATION

- For intramuscular administration only. (2)
- Children/Adolescents: vaccination consists of a 0.5-mL primary dose administered intramuscularly, and a 0.5-mL booster dose administered intramuscularly 6 to 18 months later. (2.1)
- Adults: vaccination consists of a 1-mL primary dose administered intramuscularly, and a 1-mL booster dose administered intramuscularly 6 to 18 months later. (2.1)

DOSAGE FORMS AND STRENGTHS

Suspension supplied in four presentations:
- 0.5-mL pediatric dose in single-dose vials and prefilled syringes. (3, 11, 16)
- 1-mL adult dose in single-dose vials and prefilled syringes. (3, 11, 16)

CONTRAINDICATIONS

Do not administer VAQTA to individuals with a history of immediate and/or severe allergic or hypersensitivity reactions (*e.g.*, anaphylaxis) after a previous dose of any hepatitis A vaccine or with an anaphylactic reaction to neomycin. (4, 11)

WARNINGS AND PRECAUTIONS

- Appropriate medical treatment and supervision must be available to manage possible anaphylactic reactions following administration of the vaccine. (5.1)
- The vial stopper and the syringe plunger stopper and tip cap contain dry natural latex rubber that may cause allergic reactions in latex-sensitive individuals. (5.2)

ADVERSE REACTIONS

The most common local adverse reactions and systemic adverse events (≥15%) reported in different clinical trials across different age groups when VAQTA was administered alone or concomitantly were:
- Children — 12 through 23 months of age: injection-site pain/tenderness (37.0%), injection-site erythema (21.2%), fever (16.4% when administered alone, and 27.0% when administered concomitantly)(6.1)
- Children/Adolescents — 2 through 18 years of age: injection-site pain (18.7%) (6.1)
- Adults — 19 years of age and older: injection-site pain, tenderness, or soreness (67.0%), injection-site warmth (18.2%) and headache (16.1%) (6.1)

To report SUSPECTED ADVERSE REACTIONS, contact Merck Sharp & Dohme Corp., a subsidiary of Merck & Co., Inc., at 1-877-888-4231 or VAERS at 1-800-822-7967 or www.vaers.hhs.gov.

DRUG INTERACTIONS

- Do not mix VAQTA with any other vaccine in the same syringe or vial. (7.1)

USE IN SPECIFIC POPULATIONS

- Safety and effectiveness of VAQTA have not been established in children less than 12 months of age. (8.4)
- Pregnancy: No human or animal studies have been conducted. Use only if clearly indicated. (8.1)

See 17 for PATIENT COUNSELING INFORMATION
Revised: 11/2012

FULL PRESCRIBING INFORMATION: CONTENTS*

Table 1 Incidences of Solicited Local Adverse Reactions at the VAQTA Injection Site and Elevated Temperatures Following Each Dose of VAQTA in Healthy Children 12-23 Months of Age Receiving VAQTA Alone or Concomitantly With ProQuad and PREVNAR*

	Dose 1		Dose 2	
Adverse reaction: Days 1-5 unless noted	**VAQTA alone**	**VAQTA + ProQuad + Prevnar concomitantly**	**VAQTA alone**	**VAQTA + ProQuad concomitantly**
Injection site adverse reactions	N=274	N=311	N=251	N=263
Injection site erythema	11.7%	9.6%	12.7%	9.5%
Injection site pain/ tenderness	15.3%	20.9%	20.3%	17.5%
Injection site swelling	9.5%	6.8%	7.6%	6.1%
Temperature > 98.6°F or feverish (Days 1-14)	12.4%	35.7%	10.8%	10.3%
	N=243	N=285	N=221	N=237
Temperature ≥ 100.4°F	10.3%	16.8%	10%	4.2%
Temperature ≥ 102.2 °F	2.1%	3.5%	2.3%	2.5%

N=number of subjects for whom data are available.
* Pneumococcal 7-valent Conjugate Vaccine

Table 2 Incidences of Unsolicited Systemic Adverse Events ≥5% in Any Group Following Each Dose of VAQTA in Healthy Children 12-23 Months of Age Receiving VAQTA Alone or Concomitantly With ProQuad and PREVNAR*

	Dose 1		Dose 2	
Adverse Event: Days 1-14	**VAQTA alone**	**VAQTA + ProQuad + PREVNAR concomitantly**	**VAQTA alone**	**VAQTA + ProQuad concomitantly**
	N=274	N=311	N=251	N=263
General Disorders and Administration Site Conditions				
Irritability	3.6%	6.1%	2.8%	2.7%
Infections and Infestations				
Upper respiratory tract infection	3.3%	6.1%	4.8%	5.7%
Skin and Subcutaneous Tissue Disorders				
Dermatitis diaper	1.1%	6.1%	2.4%	3.4%

* Pneumococcal 7-valent Conjugate Vaccine

*** Sections or subsections omitted from the full prescribing information are not listed**

FULL PRESCRIBING INFORMATION

1 INDICATIONS AND USAGE

1.1 Indications and Use

VAQTA®[1] [Hepatitis A Vaccine, Inactivated] is indicated for the prevention of disease caused by hepatitis A virus (HAV) in persons 12 months of age and older. The primary dose should be given at least 2 weeks prior to expected exposure to HAV.

[1] Registered trademark of Merck Sharp & Dohme Corp., a subsidiary of **Merck & Co., Inc.**

2 DOSAGE AND ADMINISTRATION

FOR INTRAMUSCULAR ADMINISTRATION ONLY.

2.1 Dosage and Schedule

Children/Adolescents (12 months through 18 years of age): The vaccination schedule consists of a primary 0.5-mL dose administered intramuscularly, and a 0.5-mL booster dose administered intramuscularly 6 to 18 months later.

Adults (≥19 *years of age*): The vaccination schedule consists of a primary 1-mL dose administered intramuscularly, and a 1-mL booster dose administered intramuscularly 6 to 18 months later.

Booster Immunization Following Another Manufacturer's Hepatitis A Vaccine: A booster dose of VAQTA may be given at 6 to 12 months following a primary dose of HAVRIX[2] *[see Clinical Studies (14.6)].*

[2] Hepatitis A Vaccine: HAVRIX is a registered trademark of GlaxoSmithKline

2.2 Preparation and Administration

Shake the single-dose vial or single-dose prefilled syringe well to obtain a slightly opaque, white suspension before withdrawal and use. Parenteral drug products should be inspected visually for particulate matter and discoloration prior to administration, whenever solution and container permit. Discard if the suspension does not appear homogeneous or if extraneous particulate matter remains or discoloration is observed.

For single-dose vials, withdraw and administer entire dose of VAQTA intramuscularly using a sterile needle and syringe.

For single-dose prefilled syringes, securely attach a needle by twisting in a clockwise direction and administer dose of VAQTA intramuscularly.

For adults, adolescents, and children older than 2 years of age, the deltoid muscle is the preferred site for intramuscular injection. For children 12 through 23 months of age, the anterolateral area of the thigh is the preferred site for intramuscular injection.

3 DOSAGE FORMS AND STRENGTHS

Suspension for injection available in four presentations:
- 0.5-mL pediatric dose in single-dose vials and prefilled syringes
- 1-mL adult dose in single-dose vials and prefilled syringes

[See Description (11) for listing of vaccine components and How Supplied/Storage and Handling (16).]

4 CONTRAINDICATIONS

Do not administer VAQTA to individuals with a history of immediate and/or severe allergic or hypersensitivity reactions (*e.g.*, anaphylaxis) after a previous dose of any hepatitis A vaccine, or to individuals who have had an anaphylactic reaction to any component of VAQTA, including neomycin *[see Description (11)].*

5 WARNINGS AND PRECAUTIONS

5.1 Prevention and Management of Allergic Vaccine Reactions

Appropriate medical treatment and supervision must be available to manage possible anaphylactic reactions following administration of the vaccine *[see Contraindications (4)].*

5.2 Hypersensitivity to Latex

The vial stopper and the syringe plunger stopper and tip cap contain dry natural latex rubber that may cause allergic reactions in latex-sensitive individuals *[see How Supplied/ Storage and Handling (16)].*

5.3 Altered Immunocompetence

Immunocompromised persons, including individuals receiving immunosuppressive therapy, may have a diminished immune response to VAQTA and may not be protected against HAV infection after vaccination *[see Use in Specific Populations (8.6)].*

5.4 Limitations of Vaccine Effectiveness

Hepatitis A virus has a relatively long incubation period (approximately 20 to 50 days). VAQTA may not prevent hepatitis A infection in individuals who have an unrecognized hepatitis A infection at the time of vaccination. Vaccination with VAQTA may not result in a protective response in all susceptible vaccinees.

6 ADVERSE REACTIONS

6.1 Clinical Trials Experience

Because clinical trials are conducted under widely varying conditions, adverse reaction rates observed in the clinical trials of a vaccine cannot be directly compared to rates in the clinical trials of another vaccine and may not reflect the rates observed in practice.

The safety of VAQTA has been evaluated in over 10,000 subjects 1 year to 85 years of age. Subjects were given one or two doses of the vaccine. The second (booster dose) was given 6 months or more after the first dose.

The most common local adverse reactions and systemic adverse events (≥15%) reported in different clinical trials across different age groups when VAQTA was administered alone or concomitantly were:
- Children — 12 through 23 months of age: injection-site pain/tenderness (37.0%), injection-site erythema (21.2%), fever (16.4% when administered alone, and 27.0% when administered concomitantly).
- Children/Adolescents — 2 through 18 years of age: injection-site pain (18.7%)
- Adults — 19 years of age and older: injection-site pain, tenderness, or soreness (67.0%), injection-site warmth (18.2%) and headache (16.1%)

Allergic Reactions

Local and/or systemic allergic reactions that occurred in <1% of over 10,000 children/adolescents or adults in clinical trials regardless of causality included: injection-site pruritus and/or rash; bronchial constriction; asthma; wheezing; edema/swelling; rash; generalized erythema; urticaria; pruritus; eye irritation/itching; dermatitis *[see Contraindications (4) and Warnings and Precautions (5.1)].*

Children — 12 through 23 Months of Age

Across five clinical trials, 4374 children 12 to 23 months of age received one or two 25U doses of VAQTA, including 3885 children who received 2 doses of VAQTA and 1250 children who received VAQTA concomitantly with one or more other vaccines, including Measles, Mumps, and Rubella Virus Vaccine, Live (M-M-R II[1]), Varicella Vaccine, Live (VARIVAX[1]), Diphtheria and Tetanus Toxoids and Acellular Pertussis Vaccine, Adsorbed (Tripedia[3] or INFANRIX[4]), Measles, Mumps, Rubella, and Varicella Vaccine, Live (ProQuad[1]), Pneumococcal 7-valent Conjugate Vaccine (Diphtheria CRM_{197}, Prevnar[5]), or Haemophilus B Conjugate Vaccine (Meningococcal Protein Conjugate, PedvaxHIB[1]). Overall, the race distribution of study subjects was as follows: 64.7% Caucasian; 15.7% Hispanic-American; 12.3% Black; 4.8% other; 1.4% Asian; and 1.1% Native American. The distribution of subjects by gender was 51.8% male and 48.2% female.

In an open-label clinical trial, 653 children 12 to 23 months of age were randomized to receive a first dose of VAQTA with ProQuad and Prevnar concomitantly (N=330) or a first dose of ProQuad and pneumococcal 7-valent conjugate vaccine concomitantly, followed by a first dose of VAQTA 6 weeks later (N=323). Approximately 6 months later, subjects received either the second doses of ProQuad and VAQTA concomitantly or the second doses of ProQuad and VAQTA separately. The race distribution of the study subjects was as follows: 60.3% Caucasian; 21.6% African-American; 9.5% Hispanic-American; 7.2% other; 1.1% Asian; and 0.3% Native American. The distribution of subjects by gender was 50.7% male and 49.3% female.

Table 3 Incidences of Solicited Local Adverse Reactions at the VAQTA Injection Site and Elevated Temperatures Following Each Dose of VAQTA in Healthy Children 12-23 Months of Age Receiving VAQTA Alone or Concomitantly with PedvaxHIB With or Without INFANRIX (Stage I) and those Receiving VAQTA Alone at Both Doses (Stage II)

	Stage I			Stage II	
	Dose 1		Dose 2	Dose 1	Dose 2
Adverse Reaction: Days 1-5 unless noted	VAQTA alone	VAQTA + PedvaxHIB and Infanrix or VAQTA + PedvaxHIB concomitantly	VAQTA alone	VAQTA alone	VAQTA alone
Injection site adverse reactions	N=256	N=302	N=503	N=647	N=599
Injection site erythema	18.0%	19.9%	21.5%	11.7%	16.2%
Injection site pain/ tenderness	21.9%	36.4%	27.4%	20.1%	22.9%
Injection site swelling	10.2%	14.2%	10.1%	7.1%	7.0%
Temperature > 98.6°F or feverish (Days 1-14)	10.2%	17.2%	10.7%	10.0%	8.2%
	N=234	N=290	N=473	N=631	N=591
Temperature ≥ 100.4°F	9.0%	16.9%	9.1%	9.4%	8.6%
Temperature ≥ 102.2 °F	3.8%	3.1%	3.2%	2.9%	2.4%

N= number of subjects for whom data is available

Table 4 Incidences of Unsolicited Systemic Adverse Events ≥5% in Any Group Following Each Dose of VAQTA in Healthy Children 12-23 Months of Age Receiving VAQTA Alone or Concomitantly with PedvaxHIB With or Without INFANRIX (Stage I) and those Receiving VAQTA Alone at Both Doses (Stage II)

	Stage I			Stage II	
	Dose 1		Dose 2	Dose 1	Dose 2
Adverse Event: Days 1-14	VAQTA alone	VAQTA + PedvaxHIB and Infanrix or VAQTA + PedvaxHIB concomitantly	VAQTA alone	VAQTA alone	VAQTA alone
	N=256	N=302	N=503	N=647	N=599
Gastrointestinal Disorders					
Diarrhea	3.9%	8.3%	3.8%	4.6%	3.8%
Teething	3.1%	2.3%	1.4%	5.7%	4.3%
General Disorders and Administration Site Conditions					
Irritability	6.3%	9.6%	4.0%	8.8%	6.5%
Infections and Infestations					
Upper respiratory tract infection	2.3%	3.3%	3.0%	4.9%	5.2%
Respiratory, Thoracic and Mediastinal Disorders					
Rhinorrhea	2.0%	4.0%	3.8%	6.2%	3.8%

Table 1 presents rates of solicited local reactions at the VAQTA injection site and rates of elevated temperatures (≥100.4°F and ≥102.2°F) that occurred within 5 days following each dose of VAQTA and elevated temperatures >98.6°F for a total of 14 days after vaccination; occurrences of these events were recorded daily on diary cards. Table 2 presents rates of unsolicited systemic adverse events that occurred within 14 days at ≥5% in any group following each dose of VAQTA.

[See table 1 at top of previous page]
[See table 2 at top of previous page]

In Stage I of an open, multicenter, randomized study, children 15 months of age were randomized to receive the first dose of VAQTA alone (N=151) or concomitantly with PedvaxHIB and INFANRIX (N=155); another group of children 15 months of age were randomized to receive the first dose of VAQTA alone (N=152) or concomitantly with PedvaxHIB (N=159). All groups received the second dose of VAQTA alone at least 6 months following the first dose. The race distribution of Stage I study subjects was: 63.9% Caucasian; 17.5% Hispanic-American; 14.7% Black; 2.6% other; and 1.3% Asian. The distribution of subjects by gender was 54.0% male and 46.0% female. In Stage II of this study, an additional 654 children 12-17 months of age received the first dose of VAQTA alone followed by the second dose of VAQTA 6 months later. The race distribution of Stage II of the study subjects was: 66.1% Caucasian; 10.6% Hispanic-American; 16.8% Black; 4.7% other; and 1.5% Asian. The distribution of subjects by gender was 51.2% male and 48.8% female.

Table 3 presents rates of solicited local reactions at the VAQTA injection-site and rates of elevated temperatures (≥100.4°F and ≥102.2°F) that occurred within 5 days following each dose of VAQTA and elevated temperatures >98.6°F for a total of 14 days following each dose of VAQTA. Occurrences of these events were recorded daily on diary cards. Table 4 presents rates of unsolicited systemic adverse events that occurred within 14 days at ≥5% following each dose of VAQTA.

[See table 3 above]
[See table 4 above]

Data presented in Tables 1 through 4 on solicited local reactions, and solicited and unsolicited systemic adverse events with incidence ≥5% following each dose of VAQTA are representative of other clinical trials of VAQTA in children 12 through 23 months of age. Across the five studies conducted in children 12-23 months of age, ≥39.9% of subjects experienced local adverse reactions and ≥55.7% of subjects experienced systemic adverse events. The majority of local and systemic adverse events were mild to moderate in intensity.

The following additional unsolicited local adverse reactions and systemic adverse events were observed at a common frequency of ≥1% to <10% in any individual clinical study. This listing includes only the adverse reactions not reported elsewhere in the label. These local adverse reactions and systemic adverse events occurred among recipients of VAQTA alone or VAQTA given concomitantly within 14 days following any dose of VAQTA across four clinical studies.

Eye disorders: Conjunctivitis

Gastrointestinal disorders: Constipation; vomiting

General disorders and administration site conditions: Injection-site bruising; injection-site ecchymosis

Infections and infestations: Otitis media; nasopharyngitis; rhinitis; viral infection; croup; pharyngitis streptococcal; laryngotracheobronchitis; viral exanthema; gastroenteritis viral; roseola

Metabolism and nutrition disorders: Anorexia

Psychiatric disorders: Insomnia; crying

Respiratory, thoracic and mediastinal disorders: Cough; nasal congestion; respiratory congestion

Skin and subcutaneous tissue disorders: Rash vesicular; measles-like/rubella-like rash; varicella-like rash; rash morbilliform

[3] Registered trademark of Sanofi Pasteur, Inc.
[4] Registered trademark of GlaxoSmithKline
[5] Registered trademark of Wyeth Pharmaceuticals, Inc.

Serious Adverse Events (Children 12 through 23 Months of Age): Across the five studies conducted in subjects 12-23 months of age, 0.7% (32/4374) of subjects reported a serious adverse event following any dose of VAQTA, and 0.1% (5/4374) of subjects reported a serious adverse event judged to be vaccine related by the study investigator. The serious adverse events were collected over the period defined in each protocol (14, 28, or 42 days). Vaccine-related serious adverse events which occurred following any dose of VAQTA with or without concomitant vaccines included febrile seizure (0.05%), dehydration (0.02%), gastroenteritis (0.02%), and cellulitis (0.02%).

Children / Adolescents — 2 Years through 18 Years of Age

In 11 clinical trials, 2615 healthy children 2 years through 18 years of age received at least one dose of VAQTA. These studies included administration of VAQTA in varying doses and regimens (1377 children received one or more 25U doses). The race distribution of the study subjects who received at least one dose of VAQTA in these studies was as follows: 84.7% Caucasian; 10.6% American Indian; 2.3% African-American; 1.5% Hispanic-American; 0.6% other; 0.2% Oriental. The distribution of subjects by gender was 51.2% male and 48.8% female.

In a double-blind, placebo-controlled efficacy trial (i.e. The Monroe Efficacy Study), 1037 healthy children and adolescents 2 through 16 years of age were randomized to receive a primary dose of 25U of VAQTA and a booster dose of VAQTA 6, 12, or 18 months later, or placebo (alum diluent). All study subjects were Caucasian: 51.5% were male and 48.5% were female. Subjects were followed days 1 to 5 post-vaccination for fever and local adverse reactions and days 1 to 14 for systemic adverse events. The most common adverse events/reactions were injection-site reactions, reported by 6.4% of subjects. Table 5 summarizes local adverse reactions and systemic adverse events reported in ≥1% of subjects. There were no significant differences in the rates of any adverse events or adverse reactions between vaccine and placebo recipients after Dose 1.

Table 5 Local Adverse Reactions and Systemic Adverse Events (≥1%) in Healthy Children and Adolescents from the Monroe Efficacy Study

Adverse Event	VAQTA (N=519)		Placebo (Alum Diluent)*,†,‡ (N=518)
	Dose 1* Rate (Percent)	Booster Rate (Percent)	Rate (Percent)
Injection Site§	n=515	n=475	n=510
Pain	6.4%	3.4%	6.3%
Tenderness	4.9%	1.7%	6.1%
Erythema	1.9%	0.8%	1.8%

Swelling	1.7%	1.5%	1.6%
Warmth	1.7%	0.6%	1.6%
Systemic¶	n=519	n=475	n=518
Abdominal pain	1.2%	1.1%	1.0%
Pharyngitis	1.2%	0%	0.8%
Headache	0.4%	0.8%	1.0%

N=Number of subjects enrolled/randomized.

Percent=percentage of subjects for whom data are available with adverse event

n=number of subjects for whom adverse events available

* No statistically significant differences between the two groups.

† Second injection of placebo not administered because code for the trial was broken.

‡ Placebo (Alum diluent) = amorphous aluminum hydroxyphosphate sulfate.

§ Adverse Reactions at the injection site (VAQTA) Days 1-5 after vaccination with VAQTA

¶ Systemic adverse events reported Days 1-15 after vaccination, regardless of causality.

Adults — 19 Years of Age and Older

In an open-label clinical trial, 240 healthy adults 18 to 54 years of age were randomized to receive either VAQTA (50U/1-mL) with Typhim Vi[3] (Typhoid Vi polysaccharide vaccine) and YF-Vax[3] (yellow fever vaccine) concomitantly (N=80), typhoid Vi polysaccharide and yellow fever vaccines concomitantly (N=80), or VAQTA alone (N=80). Approximately 6 months later, subjects who received VAQTA were administered a second dose of VAQTA. The race distribution of the study subjects who received VAQTA with or without typhoid Vi polysaccharide and yellow fever vaccine was as follows: 78.3% Caucasian; 14.2% Oriental; 3.3% other; 2.1% African-American; 1.7% Indian; 0.4% Hispanic-American. The distribution of subjects by gender was 40.8% male and 59.2% female. Subjects were monitored for local adverse reactions and fever for 5 days and systemic adverse events for 14 days after each vaccination. In the 14 days after the first dose of VAQTA, the proportion of subjects with adverse events was similar between recipients of VAQTA given concomitantly with typhoid Vi polysaccharide and yellow fever vaccines compared to recipients of typhoid Vi polysaccharide and yellow fever vaccines without VAQTA. Table 6 summarizes solicited local adverse reactions and Table 7 summarizes unsolicited systemic adverse events reported in ≥5% in adults who received one or two doses of VAQTA alone and for subjects who received VAQTA concomitantly with typhoid Vi polysaccharide and yellow fever vaccines. There were no solicited systemic complaints reported at a rate ≥5%. Fever ≥101°F occurred in 1.3% of subjects in each group.

Table 6 Incidences of Solicited Local Adverse Reactions in Healthy Adults ≥19 Years of Age Occurring at ≥5% After Any Dose

Adverse Event	VAQTA administered alone (N=80)	VAQTA + ViCPS* and Yellow Fever vaccines administered concomitantly† (N=80)
	Rate (Percent)	
Injection-site‡		
Pain/tenderness/ soreness	78.8%	70.3%
Warmth	23.7%	23.7%
Swelling	16.2%	8.8%
Erythema	17.5%	6.3%

N=Number of subjects enrolled/randomized.

Percent=percentage of subjects with adverse event.

* ViCPS=Typhoid Vi polysaccharide vaccine.

† VAQTA administered concomitantly with typhoid Vi polysaccharide (ViCPS) and yellow fever vaccines.

‡ Adverse Reactions at the injection site (VAQTA) Days 1-5 after vaccination

Table 7 Incidences of Unsolicited Systemic Adverse Events in Adults ≥19 Years of Age Occurring at ≥5% After Any Dose

Body System / Adverse Event	VAQTA administered alone (N=80)	VAQTA + ViCPS* and Yellow Fever vaccines administered concomitantly† (N=80)
	Rate (Percent)	
General disorders and administration site reactions‡		
Asthenia/fatigue	7.5%	11.3%
Chills	1.3%	7.5%
Gastrointestinal disorders‡		
Nausea	7.5%	12.5%
Musculoskeletal and connective tissue disorders‡		
Myalgia	5.0%	10.0%
Arm pain	0.0%	6.3%
Nervous system disorders‡		
Headache	23.8%	26.3%
Infections and infestations‡		
Upper respiratory infection	7.5%	3.8%
Pharyngitis	2.5%	6.3%

N=Number of subjects enrolled/randomized with data available.

Percent=percentage of subjects with adverse event for whom data are available.

* ViCPS=Typhoid Vi polysaccharide vaccine.

† VAQTA administered concomitantly with typhoid Vi polysaccharide (ViCPS) and yellow fever vaccines.

‡ Systemic Adverse Events reported Days 1-15 after vaccination, regardless of causality.

In four clinical trials involving 1645 healthy adults 19 years of age and older who received one or more 50U doses of hepatitis A vaccine, subjects were followed for fever and local adverse reactions 1 to 5 days postvaccination and for systemic adverse events 1 to 14 days postvaccination. One single-blind study evaluated doses of VAQTA with varying amounts of viral antigen and/or alum content in healthy adults ≥170 pounds and ≥30 years of age (N=210 adults administered 50U/1-mL dose). One open-label study evaluated VAQTA given with immune globulin or alone (N=164 adults who received VAQTA alone). A third study was single-blind and evaluated 3 different lots of VAQTA (N=1112). The fourth study that was also single-blind evaluated doses of VAQTA with varying amounts of viral antigen in healthy adults ≥170 pounds and ≥30 years of age (N=159 adults administered the 50U/1-mL dose). Overall, the race distribution of the study subjects who received at least one dose of VAQTA was as follows: 94.2% Caucasian; 2.2% Black; 1.5% Hispanic; 1.5% Oriental; 0.4% other; 0.2% American Indian. 47.6% of subjects were male and 52.4% were female. The most common adverse event/reaction was injection-site pain/soreness/tenderness reported by 67.0% of subjects. Of all reported injection-site reactions 99.8% were mild (*i.e.,* easily tolerated with no medical intervention) or moderate (*i.e.,* minimally interfered with usual activity possibly requiring little medical intervention). Listed below in Table 8 are the local adverse reactions and systemic adverse events reported by ≥5% of subjects, in decreasing order of frequency within each body system.

Table 8 Incidences of Local Adverse Reactions and Systemic Adverse Events ≥5% in Adults 19 Years of Age and Older

Body System / Adverse Events	VAQTA (Any Dose) (N=1645) Rate (n/total n)
Nervous system disorders*	n=1641
Headache	16.1%
General disorders and administration site reactions†	n=1640
Injection-site pain/tenderness/ soreness	67.0%
Injection-site warmth	18.2%
Injection-site swelling	14.7%
Injection-site erythema	13.7%

N=Number of subjects enrolled/randomized.

n=Number of subjects in each category with data available.

Percent=percentage of subjects for whom data are available with adverse event.

* Systemic Adverse Events reported Days 1 to 14 after vaccination, regardless of causality.

† Adverse Reactions at the injection site (VAQTA) and measured fever Days 1 to 5 after vaccination.

The following additional unsolicited systemic adverse events were observed among recipients of VAQTA that occurred within 14 days at a common frequency of ≥1% to <10% following any dose not reported elsewhere in the label. These adverse reactions have been reported across 4 clinical studies.

Musculoskeletal and connective tissue disorders: Back pain; stiffness

Reproductive system and breast disorders: Menstruation disorders

6.2 Post-Marketing Experience

The following additional adverse events have been reported with use of the marketed vaccine. Because these reactions are reported voluntarily from a population of uncertain size, it is not possible to reliably estimate their frequency or establish a causal relationship to a vaccine exposure.

Blood and lymphatic disorders: Thrombocytopenia.

Nervous system disorders: Guillain-Barré syndrome; cerebellar ataxia; encephalitis.

Post-Marketing Observational Safety Study

In a post-marketing, 60-day safety surveillance study, conducted at a large health maintenance organization in the United States, a total of 42,110 individuals ≥2 years of age received 1 or 2 doses of VAQTA (13,735 children/adolescents and 28,375 adult subjects). Safety was passively monitored by electronic search of the automated medical records database for emergency room and outpatient visits, hospitalizations, and deaths. Medical charts were reviewed when an event was considered to be possibly vaccine-related by the investigator. None of the serious adverse events identified were assessed as being related to vaccine by the investigator. Diarrhea/gastroenteritis, resulting in outpatient visits, was determined by the investigator to be the only vaccine-related nonserious adverse reaction in the study. There was no vaccine-related adverse reaction identified that had not been reported in earlier clinical trials with VAQTA.

7 DRUG INTERACTIONS

7.1 Use with Other Vaccines

Do not mix VAQTA with any other vaccine in the same syringe or vial. Use separate injection sites and syringes for each vaccine. Please refer to package inserts of coadministered vaccines.

In clinical trials in children, VAQTA was concomitantly administered with one or more of the following US licensed vaccines: Measles, Mumps, and Rubella Virus Vaccine, Live; Varicella Vaccine, Live; Diphtheria and Tetanus Toxoids and Acellular Pertussis Vaccine, Adsorbed; Measles, Mumps, Rubella, and Varicella Vaccine, Live; Pneumococcal 7-valent Conjugate Vaccine (Diphtheria CRM_{197}); and Haemophilus B Conjugate Vaccine (Meningococcal Protein Conjugate). Safety and immunogenicity were similar for concomitantly administered vaccines compared to separately administered vaccines.

In clinical trials in adults, VAQTA was concomitantly administered with typhoid Vi polysaccharide and yellow fever vaccines *[see Adverse Reactions (6.1) and Clinical Studies (14.2, 14.7)]*. Safety and immunogenicity were similar for concomitantly administered vaccines compared to separately administered vaccines.

7.2 Use with Immune Globulin

VAQTA may be administered concomitantly with Immune Globulin, human, using separate sites and syringes. The recommended vaccination regimen for VAQTA should be followed. Consult the manufacturer's product circular for the appropriate dosage of Immune Globulin. A booster dose of VAQTA should be administered at the appropriate time as outlined in the recommended regimen for VAQTA *[see Clinical Studies (14.5)]*.

7.3 Immunosuppressive Therapy

If VAQTA is administered to a person receiving immunosuppressive therapy, an adequate immunologic response may not be obtained.

8 USE IN SPECIFIC POPULATIONS

8.1 Pregnancy

Pregnancy Category C: Animal reproduction studies have not been conducted with VAQTA. It is also not known whether VAQTA can cause fetal harm when administered to a pregnant woman or can affect reproduction capacity. VAQTA should be given to a pregnant woman only if clearly needed.

8.3 Nursing Mothers

It is not known whether VAQTA is excreted in human milk. Because many drugs are excreted in human milk, caution should be exercised when VAQTA is administered to a nursing woman.

8.4 Pediatric Use

The safety of VAQTA has been evaluated in 4374 children 12 through 23 months of age, and 2615 children/adolescents 2 through 18 years of age who received at least one 25U dose of VAQTA *[see Adverse Reactions (6) and Dosage and Administration (2)]*.

Safety and effectiveness in infants below 12 months of age have not been established.

8.5 Geriatric Use

In the post-marketing observational safety study which included 42,110 persons who received VAQTA *[see Adverse Reactions (6.2)]*, 4769 persons were 65 years of age or older and 1073 persons were 75 years of age or older. There were no adverse events judged by the investigator to be vaccine-related in the geriatric study population. In other clinical studies, 68 subjects 65 years of age or older were vaccinated with VAQTA, 10 of whom were 75 years of age or older. No overall differences in safety and immunogenicity were observed between these subjects and younger subjects; however, greater sensitivity of some older individuals cannot be ruled out. Other reported clinical experience has not identified differences in responses between the elderly and younger subjects.

8.6 Immunocompromised Individuals

Immunocompromised persons may have a diminished immune response to VAQTA and may not be protected against HAV infection.

11 DESCRIPTION

VAQTA is an inactivated whole virus vaccine derived from hepatitis A virus grown in cell culture in human MRC-5 diploid fibroblasts. It contains inactivated virus of a strain which was originally derived by further serial passage of a proven attenuated strain. The virus is grown, harvested, purified by a combination of physical and high performance liquid chromatographic techniques developed at the Merck Research Laboratories, formalin inactivated, and then adsorbed onto amorphous aluminum hydroxyphosphate sulfate.

VAQTA is a sterile suspension for intramuscular injection. One milliliter of the vaccine contains approximately 50U of hepatitis A virus antigen, which is purified and formulated without a preservative. Within the limits of current assay variability, the 50U dose of VAQTA contains less than 0.1 mcg of non-viral protein, less than 4 × 10–6 mcg of DNA, less than 10–4 mcg of bovine albumin, and less than 0.8 mcg of formaldehyde. Other process chemical residuals are less than 10 parts per billion (ppb), including neomycin.

Each 0.5-mL pediatric dose contains 25U of hepatitis A virus antigen and adsorbed onto approximately 0.225 mg of aluminum provided as amorphous aluminum hydroxyphosphate sulfate, and 35 mcg of sodium borate as a pH stabilizer, in 0.9% sodium chloride.

Each 1-mL adult dose contains 50U of hepatitis A virus antigen and adsorbed onto approximately 0.45 mg of aluminum provided as amorphous aluminum hydroxyphosphate sulfate, and 70 mcg of sodium borate as a pH stabilizer, in 0.9% sodium chloride.

12 CLINICAL PHARMACOLOGY

12.1 Mechanism of Action

VAQTA has been shown to elicit antibodies to hepatitis A as measured by ELISA.

Protection from hepatitis A disease has been shown to be related to the presence of antibody. However, the lowest titer needed to confer protection has not been determined.

13 NONCLINICAL TOXICOLOGY

13.1 Carcinogenesis, Mutagenesis, Impairment of Fertility

VAQTA has not been evaluated for its carcinogenic or mutagenic potential, or its potential to impair fertility.

14 CLINICAL STUDIES

14.1 Efficacy of VAQTA: The Monroe Clinical Study

The immunogenicity and protective efficacy of VAQTA were evaluated in a randomized, double-blind, placebo-controlled study involving 1037 susceptible healthy children and adolescents 2 through 16 years of age in a U.S. community with recurrent outbreaks of hepatitis A (The Monroe Efficacy Study). All of these children were Caucasian, and there were 51.5% male and 48.5% female. Each child received an intramuscular dose of VAQTA (25U) (N=519) or placebo (alum diluent) (N=518). Among those individuals who were initially seronegative (as measured by a modification of the HAVAB[6] radioimmunoassay [RIA]), seroconversion was achieved in >99% of vaccine recipients within 4 weeks after vaccination. The onset of seroconversion following a single dose of VAQTA was shown to parallel the onset of protection against clinical hepatitis A disease.

Table 9 Children/Adolescents from the Monroe Efficacy Study Seroconversion Rates (%) and Geometric Mean Titers (GMT) for Cohorts of Initially Seronegative Vaccinees at the Time of the Booster (25U) and 4 Weeks Later

Months Following Initial 25U Dose	Cohort* (n=960) 0 and 6 Months	Cohort* (n=35) 0 and 12 Months	Cohort* (n=39) 0 and 18 Months
	Seroconversion Rate GMT (mIU/mL) (95% CI)		
6	97% 107 (98, 117)	—	—
7	100% 10433 (9681, 11243)	—	—
12	—	91% 48 (33, 71)	—
13	—	100% 12308 (9337, 16226)	—
18	—	—	90% 50 (28, 89)
19	—	—	100% 9591 (7613, 12082)

* Blood samples were taken at prebooster and postbooster time points.

Because of the long incubation period of the disease (approximately 20 to 50 days, or longer in children), clinical efficacy was based on confirmed cases[7] of hepatitis A occurring ≥50 days after vaccination in order to exclude any children incubating the infection before vaccination. In subjects who were initially seronegative, the protective efficacy of a single dose of VAQTA was observed to be 100% with 21 cases of clinically confirmed hepatitis A occurring in the placebo group and none in the vaccine group (p<0.001). The number of clinically confirmed cases of hepatitis A ≥30 days after vaccination were also compared. In this analysis, 28 cases of clinically confirmed hepatitis A occurred in the placebo group while none occurred in the vaccine group ≥30 days after vaccination. In addition, it was observed in this trial that no cases of clinically confirmed hepatitis A occurred in the vaccine group after day 16.[8] Following demonstration of protection with a single dose and termination of the study, a booster dose was administered to a subset of vaccinees 6, 12, or 18 months after the primary dose.

No cases of clinically confirmed hepatitis A disease ≥50 days after vaccination have occurred in those vaccinees from The Monroe Efficacy Study monitored for up to 9 years.

[6] Trademark of Abbott Laboratories

[7] The clinical case definition included all of the following occurring at the same time: 1) one or more typical clinical signs or symptoms of hepatitis A (*e.g.*, jaundice, malaise, fever ≥38.3°C); 2) elevation of hepatitis A IgM antibody (HAVAB-M); 3) elevation of alanine transferase (ALT) ≥2 times the upper limit of normal.

[8] One vaccinee did not meet the pre-defined criteria for clinically confirmed hepatitis A but did have positive hepatitis A IgM and borderline liver enzyme (ALT) elevations on days 34, 50, and 58 after vaccination with mild clinical symptoms observed on days 49 and 50.

14.2 Other Clinical Studies

The efficacy of VAQTA in other age groups was based upon immunogenicity measured 4 to 6 weeks following vaccination. VAQTA was found to be immunogenic in all age groups.

Children — 12 through 23 Months of Age

In a clinical trial, children 12 through 23 months of age were randomized to receive the first dose of VAQTA with or without M-M-R II and VARIVAX (N=617) and the second dose of VAQTA with or without Tripedia and optionally either oral poliovirus vaccine (no longer licensed in the US) or IPOL (N=555). The race distribution of study subjects who received at least one dose of VAQTA was as follows: 56.7% Caucasian; 17.5% Hispanic-American; 14.3% African-American; 7.0% Native American; 3.4% other; 0.8% Oriental; 0.2% Asian; and 0.2% Indian. The distribution of subjects by gender was 53.6% male and 46.4% female. In the analysis population, there were 471 initially seronegative children 12 through 23 months of age, who received the first dose of VAQTA with (N=237) or without (N=234) M-M-R II and VARIVAX of whom 96% (95% CI: 93.7%, 97.5%) seroconverted (defined as having an anti-HAV titer ≥10 mIU/mL) post dose 1 with an anti-HAV GMT of 48 mIU/mL (95% CI: 44.7, 51.6). There were 343 children in the analysis population who received the second dose of VAQTA with (N=168) or without (N=175) Tripedia and optional oral poliovirus vaccine or IPOL of whom 100% (95% CI: 99.3%, 100%) seroconverted post dose 2 with an anti-HAV GMT of 6920 mIU/mL (95% CI: 6136, 7801). Of children who received only VAQTA at both visits, 100% (n=97) seroconverted after the second dose of VAQTA.

In a clinical trial involving 653 healthy children 12 to 15 months of age, 330 were randomized to receive VAQTA, ProQuad, and pneumococcal 7-valent conjugate vaccine concomitantly, and 323 were randomized to receive ProQuad and pneumococcal 7-valent conjugate vaccine concomitantly followed by VAQTA 6 weeks later. The race distribution of the study subjects was as follows: 60.3% Caucasian; 21.6% African-American; 9.5% Hispanic-American; 7.2% other; 1.1% Asian/Pacific; and 0.3% Native American. The distribution of subjects by gender was 50.7% male and 49.3% female. In the analysis population, the seropositivity rate for hepatitis A antibody (defined as the percent of subjects with an anti-HAV titer ≥10 mIU/mL) was 100% (n=182; 95% CI: 98.0%, 100%) post dose 2 with an anti-HAV GMT of 4977 mIU/mL (95% CI: 4068, 6089) when VAQTA was given with ProQuad and pneumococcal 7-valent conjugate vaccine and 99.4% (n=159, 95% CI: 96.5%, 100%) post dose 2 with an anti-HAV GMT of 6123 mIU/mL (95% CI: 4826, 7770) when VAQTA alone was given. These seropositivity rates were similar whether VAQTA was administered with or without ProQuad and pneumococcal 7-valent conjugate vaccine.

In an open, multicenter, randomized study involving 617 children 15 months of age, 306 were randomized to receive VAQTA with or without PedvaxHIB and INFANRIX, and 311 were randomized to receive VAQTA with or without PedvaxHIB. The race distribution of the study subjects was as follows: 63.9% Caucasian; 17.5% Hispanic-American; 14.7% Black; 2.6% other; and 1.3% Asian. The distribution of subjects by gender was 54.0% male and 46.0% female. The seropositivity rate for hepatitis A antibody (defined as the percent of subjects with an anti-HAV titer ≥ 10 mIU/mL) 4 weeks post dose 2 was 100% (n=208, 95% CI: 98.2%, 100.0%) in those who received VAQTA concomitantly with PedvaxHIB and INFANRIX or concomitantly with PedvaxHIB. In those subjects who received VAQTA alone, the seropositivity rate for hepatitis A antibody was 100% (n=183, 95% CI: 98.0%, 100.0%), regardless of baseline hepatitis A serostatus. Overall, the anti-HAV GMT in the concomitant groups was 3616.5 mIU/mL (95% CI: 3084.5, 4240.2). The anti-HAV GMT in the nonconcomitant groups was 4712.6 mIU/mL (95% CI: 3996.8, 5556.8). Comparable responses were observed in both the initially seronegative and seropositive subjects.

In three combined clinical studies 1022 initially seronegative subjects received 2 doses of VAQTA alone or concomitantly with other vaccines. Of the seronegative subjects, 99.9% achieved an anti-HAV titer ≥10 mIU/mL (95% CI: 99.5%, 100%) and an anti-HAV GMT of 5392.1 mIU/mL (95% CI: 4996.5, 5819.0) 4 weeks following dose 2 of VAQTA.

Children / Adolescents — 2 Years through 18 Years of Age

Immunogenicity data were combined from eleven randomized clinical studies in children and adolescents 2 through 18 years of age who received VAQTA (25U/0.5 mL). These included administration of VAQTA in varying doses and regimens (N=404 received 25U/0.5 mL), the Monroe Efficacy Study (N=973), and comparison studies for process and formulation changes (N=1238). The race distribution of the study subjects who received at least one dose of VAQTA in these studies was as follows: 84.8% Caucasian; 10.6% Amer-

Table 11 Seropositivity Rate, Booster Response Rate* and Geometric Mean Titer 4 Weeks Following a Booster Dose of VAQTA or HAVRIX Administered 6 to 12 Months After First Dose of HAVRIX†

First Dose	Booster Dose	Seropositivity Rate	Booster Response Rate*	Geometric Mean Titer
HAVRIX 1440 EL.U.	VAQTA 50 U	99.7% (n=313)	86.1% (n=310)	3272 (n=313)
HAVRIX 1440 EL.U.	HAVRIX 1440 EL.U.	99.3% (n=151)	80.1% (n=151)	2423 (n=151)

* Booster Response Rate is defined as greater than or equal to a tenfold rise from prebooster to postbooster titer and postbooster titer ≥100 mIU/mL.
† Study conducted in adults 18 years of age and older.

ican Indian; 2.3% African-American; 1.5% Hispanic-American; 0.6% other; 0.2% Oriental. The distribution of subjects by gender was 51.2% male and 48.8% female. The proportions of subjects who seroconverted 4 weeks after the first and second doses administered 6 months apart were 97% (n=1230; 95% CI: 96%, 98%) and 100% (n=1057; 95% CI: 99.5%, 100%) of subjects with anti-HAV GMTs of 43 mIU/mL (95% CI: 40, 45) and 10,077 mIU/mL (95% CI: 9394, 10,810), respectively.

Adults — 19 Years of Age and Older

Immunogenicity data were combined from five randomized clinical studies in adults 19 years of age and older who received VAQTA (50U/1-mL). One single-blind study evaluated doses of VAQTA with varying amounts of viral antigen and/or alum content in healthy adults ≥170 pounds and ≥30 years of age (N=208 adults administered 50U/1-mL dose). One open-label study evaluated VAQTA given with immune globulin or alone (N=164 adults who received VAQTA alone). A third study was single-blind and evaluated 3 different lots of VAQTA (N=1112). The fourth study was single-blind and evaluated doses of VAQTA with varying amounts of viral antigen in healthy adults ≥170 pounds and ≥30 years of age (N=159 adults administered the 50U/1-mL dose). The fifth study was an open-label study to evaluate various regimens for time of administration of the booster dose of VAQTA (6, 12, and 18 months post dose 1, N=354). The race distribution of the study subjects who received at least one dose of VAQTA in these studies was as follows: 93.2% Caucasian; 2.5% African-American; 2.1% Hispanic-American; 1.4% Oriental; 0.5% other; 0.3% American Indian. The distribution of subjects by gender was 44.8% male and 55.2% female. The proportion of subjects who seroconverted 4 weeks after the first and second doses administered 6 months apart was 95% (n=1411; 95% CI: 94%, 96%) and 99.9% (n=1244; 95% CI: 99.4%, 100%) with GMTs of 37 mIU/mL (95% CI: 35, 38) and 6013 mIU/mL (95% CI: 5592, 6467), respectively. Furthermore, at 2 weeks postvaccination, 69.2% (n=744; 95% CI: 65.7%, 72.5%) of adults seroconverted with an anti-HAV GMT of 16 mIU/mL after a single dose of VAQTA.

14.3 Timing of Booster Dose Administration

Children/Adolescents — 2 through 18 Years of Age

In the Monroe Efficacy Study, children were administered a second dose of VAQTA (25U/0.5 mL) 6, 12, or 18 months following the initial dose. For subjects who received both doses of VAQTA, the GMTs and proportions of subjects who seroconverted 4 weeks after the booster dose administered 6, 12, and 18 months after the first dose are presented in Table 9.
[See table 9 at top of previous page]

Adults — 19 years of age and older

Among the 5 randomized clinical studies in adults 19 years of age and older described in Section 14.2, there were additional data in which a booster dose of VAQTA (50U/1-mL) was administered 12 or 18 months after the first dose. For subjects in these studies who received both doses of VAQTA, the proportions who seroconverted 4 weeks after the booster dose administered 6, 12, and 18 months after the first dose were 100% of 1201 subjects, 98% of 91 subjects, and 100% of 84 subjects, respectively. GMTs in mIU/mL one month after the subjects received the booster dose at 6, 12, or 18 months after the primary dose were 5987 mIU/mL (95% CI: 5561, 6445), 4896 mIU/mL (95% CI: 3589, 6679), and 6043 mIU/mL (95% CI: 4687, 7793), respectively.

14.4 Duration of Immune Response

In follow-up of subjects in The Monroe Efficacy Study, in children (≥2 years of age) and adolescents who received two doses (25U) of VAQTA, detectable levels of anti-HAV antibodies (≥10 mIU/mL) were present in 100% of subjects for at least 10 years postvaccination. In subjects who received VAQTA at 0 and 6 months, the GMT was 819 mIU/mL (n=175) at 2.5 to 3.5 years and 505 mIU/mL (n=174) at 5 to 6 years, and 574 mIU/mL (n=114) at 10 years postvaccination. In subjects who received VAQTA at 0 and 12 months, the GMT was 2224 mIU/mL (n=49) at 2.5 to 3.5 years, 1191 mIU/mL (n=47) at 5 to 6 years, and 1005 mIU/mL (n=36) at 10 years postvaccination. In subjects who received VAQTA at 0 and 18 months, the GMT was 2501 mIU/mL (n=53) at 2.5 to 3.5 years, 1614 mIU/mL (n=56) at 5 to 6 years, and 1507 mIU/mL (n=41) at 10 years postvaccination.

In adults that were administered VAQTA at 0 and 6 months, the hepatitis A antibody response to date has been shown to persist at least 6 years. Detectable levels of anti-HAV antibodies (≥10 mIU/mL) were present in 100% (378/378) of subjects with a GMT of 1734 mIU/mL at 1 year, 99.2% (252/254) of subjects with a GMT of 687 mIU/mL at 2 to 3 years, 99.1% (219/221) of subjects with a GMT of 605 mIU/mL at 4 years, and 99.4% (170/171) of subjects with a GMT of 684 mIU/mL at 6 years postvaccination.

The total duration of the protective effect of VAQTA in healthy vaccinees is unknown at present.

14.5 Concomitant Administration of VAQTA and Immune Globulin

The concurrent use of VAQTA (50U) and immune globulin (IG, 0.06 mL/kg) was evaluated in an open-label, randomized clinical study involving 294 healthy adults 18 to 39 years of age. Adults were randomized to receive 2 doses of VAQTA 24 weeks apart (N=129), the first dose of VAQTA concomitant with a dose of IG followed by the second dose of VAQTA alone 24 weeks later (N=135), or IG alone (N=30). The race distribution of the study subjects who received at least one dose of VAQTA or IG in this study was as follows: 92.3% Caucasian; 4.0% Hispanic-American; 3.0% African-American; 0.3% Native American; 0.3% Asian/Pacific. The distribution of subjects by gender was 28.7% male and 71.3% female. Table 10 provides seroconversion rates and geometric mean titers (GMTs) at 4 and 24 weeks after the first dose in each treatment group and at one month after a booster dose of VAQTA (administered at 24 weeks) *[see Drug Interactions (7.2)]*.

Table 10 Seroconversion Rates (%) and Geometric Mean Titers (GMT) After Vaccination with VAQTA Plus IG, VAQTA Alone, and IG Alone

Weeks	VAQTA plus IG	VAQTA	IG
	Seroconversion Rate GMT (mIU/mL) (95% CI)		
4	100% 42 (39, 45) (n=129)	96% 38 (33, 42) (n=135)	87% 19 (15, 23) (n=30)
24	92% 83 (65, 105) (n=125)	97%* 137* (112, 169) (n=132)	0% Undetectable† (n=28)
28	100% 4872 (3716, 6388) (n=114)	100% 6498 (5111, 8261) (n=128)	N/A

N/A = Not Applicable.
* The seroconversion rate and the GMT in the group receiving VAQTA alone were significantly higher than in the group receiving VAQTA plus IG (p=0.05, p<0.001, respectively).
† Undetectable is defined as <10mIU/mL.

14.6 Interchangeability of the Booster Dose

A randomized, double-blind clinical study in 537 healthy adults, 18 to 83 years of age, evaluated the immune response to a booster dose of VAQTA and HAVRIX given at 6 or 12 months following an initial dose of HAVRIX. Subjects were randomized to receive VAQTA (50U) as a booster dose 6 months (N=232) or 12 months (N=124) following an initial dose of HAVRIX or HAVRIX (1440 EL. U) as a booster dose 6 months (N=118) or 12 months (N=63) following an initial dose of HAVRIX. The race distribution of the study subjects who received the booster dose of VAQTA or HAVRIX in this study was as follows: 87.2% Caucasian; 8.0% African-American; 1.9% Hispanic-American; 1.3% Oriental; 0.9% Asian; 0.4% Indian; 0.4% other. The distribution of subjects by gender was 44.9% male and 55.1% female. When VAQTA was given as a booster dose following HAVRIX, the vaccine produced an adequate immune response (see Table 11) *[see Dosage and Administration (2.1)]*.
[See table 11 above]

14.7 Immune Response to Concomitantly Administered Vaccines

Clinical Studies of VAQTA with M-M-R II, VARIVAX, and Tripedia

In the clinical trial in which children 12 months of age received the first dose of VAQTA concomitantly with M-M-R II and VARIVAX described in Section 14.2, rates of seroprotection to hepatitis A were similar between the two groups who received VAQTA with or without M-M-R II and VARIVAX. Measles, mumps, and rubella immune responses were tested in 241 subjects, 263 subjects, and 270 subjects, respectively. Seropositivity rates were 98.8% [95% CI: 96.4%, 99.7%] for measles, 99.6% [95% CI: 97.9%, 100%] for mumps, and 100% [95% CI: 98.6%, 100%] for rubella, which were similar to observed historical rates (seropositivity rates 99% for all three antigens, with lower bound of the 95% CI >89%) following vaccination with a first dose of M-M-R II in this age group. Data from this study were insufficient to adequately assess the immune response to VARIVAX administered concomitantly with VAQTA. In this same study, the second dose of VAQTA at 18 months of age was given with or without Tripedia (DTaP). Seropositivity rates for diphtheria and tetanus were similar to those in historical controls. However, data from this study were insufficient to assess the pertussis response of DTaP when administered with VAQTA. Rates of seroprotection to hepatitis A were similar between the two groups who received VAQTA with or without M-M-R II and VARIVAX, and between the two groups who received VAQTA with or without DTaP.

Clinical Studies of VAQTA with ProQuad and Prevnar

In the clinical trial of concomitant use of VAQTA with ProQuad and pneumococcal 7-valent conjugate vaccine in children 12 to 15 months of age described in Section 14.2, the antibody GMTs for *S. pneumoniae* types 4, 6B, 9V, 14, 18C, 19F, and 23F 6 weeks after vaccination with pneumococcal 7-valent conjugate vaccine administered concomitantly with ProQuad and VAQTA were non-inferior as compared to GMTs observed in the group given pneumococcal 7-valent conjugate vaccine with ProQuad alone (the lower bounds of the 95% CI around the fold-difference for the 7 serotypes excluded 0.5). For the varicella component of ProQuad, in subjects with baseline antibody titers <1.25 gpELISA units/mL, the proportion with a titer ≥5 gpELISA units/mL 6 weeks after their first dose of ProQuad was non-inferior (defined as -10 percentage point change) when ProQuad was administered with VAQTA and pneumococcal 7-valent conjugate vaccine as compared to the proportion with a titer ≥5 gpELISA units/mL when ProQuad was administered with pneumococcal 7-valent conjugate vaccine alone (difference in seroprotection rate -5.1% [95% CI: -9.3, -1.4%]). Hepatitis A responses were similar when compared between the two groups who received VAQTA with or without ProQuad and pneumococcal 7-valent conjugate vaccine. Seroconversion rates and antibody titers for varicella and *S. pneumoniae* types 4, 6B, 9V, 14, 18C, 19F, and 23F were similar between groups at 6 weeks postvaccination.

Clinical Studies of VAQTA with INFANRIX and PedvaxHIB

In the clinical trial of concomitant administration of VAQTA with INFANRIX and PedvaxHIB in children 15 months of age, described in Section 14.2, when the first dose of VAQTA was administered concomitantly with either INFANRIX and PedvaxHIB or PedvaxHIB, there was no interference in immune response to hepatitis A as measured by seropositivity rates after dose 2 of VAQTA compared to administration of both doses of VAQTA alone. When dose 1 of VAQTA was administered concomitantly with either PedvaxHIB and INFANRIX or PedvaxHIB, there was no interference in immune response to *Haemophilus influenzae b* (as measured by the proportion of subjects who attained an anti-polyribosylribitol phosphate antibody titer >1.0 mcg/mL at 4 weeks after vaccination), compared to subjects receiving either PedvaxHIB and INFANRIX or PedvaxHIB. When VAQTA was administered concomitantly with INFANRIX and PedvaxHIB, there was no interference in immune responses at 4 weeks after vaccination to the pertussis antigens (PT, FHA, or pertactin, as measured by GMTs) and no interference in immune responses to diphtheria toxoid or tetanus toxoid (as measured by the proportion of subjects achieving an antibody titer >0.1 IU/mL) compared to administration of INFANRIX and PedvaxHIB.

Clinical Studies of VAQTA with Typhoid Vi Polysaccharide Vaccine and Yellow Fever Vaccine, Live Attenuated

In the clinical trial of concomitant use of VAQTA with typhoid Vi polysaccharide and yellow fever vaccines in adults 18-54 years of age described in Section 6.1, the antibody response rates for typhoid Vi polysaccharide and yellow fever were adequate when typhoid Vi polysaccharide and yellow fever vaccines were administered concomitantly with

(N=80) and nonconcomitantly without VAQTA (N=80). The seropositivity rate for hepatitis A when VAQTA, typhoid Vi polysaccharide, and yellow fever vaccines were administered concomitantly was generally similar to when VAQTA was given alone *[see Drug Interactions (7.1)]*.

Data are insufficient to assess the immune response to VAQTA and poliovirus vaccine when administered concomitantly.

16 HOW SUPPLIED/STORAGE AND HANDLING

VAQTA is available in single-dose vials and prefilled Luer Lock syringes.

Pediatric/Adolescent Formulations

25U/0.5 mL in single-dose vials and prefilled Luer Lock syringes.

NDC 0006-4831-41 – box of ten 0.5-mL single dose vials.

NDC 0006-4095-09 – carton of six 0.5-mL prefilled single-dose Luer Lock syringes with tip caps.

Adult Formulations

50U/1-mL in single-dose vials and prefilled Luer Lock syringes.

NDC 0006-4841-00 – 1-mL single dose vial.

NDC 0006-4841-41 – box of ten 1-mL single dose vials.

NDC 0006-4096-09 – carton of six 1-mL prefilled single-dose Luer Lock syringes with tip caps.

Store vaccine at 2-8°C (36-46°F).

DO NOT FREEZE since freezing destroys potency.

17 PATIENT COUNSELING INFORMATION

17.1 Instructions

Information for Vaccine Recipients and Parents or Guardians

- Inform the patient, parent or guardian of the potential benefits and risks of the vaccine.
- Question the vaccine recipient, parent, or guardian about the occurrence of any symptoms and/or signs of an adverse reaction after a previous dose of hepatitis A vaccine.
- Inform the patient, parent, or guardian about the potential for adverse events that have been temporally associated with administration of VAQTA.
- Tell the patient, parent, or guardian accompanying the recipient, to report adverse events to the physician or clinic where the vaccine was administered.
- Prior to vaccination, give the patient, parent, or guardian the Vaccine Information Statements which are required by the National Childhood Vaccine Injury Act of 1986. These materials are available free of charge at the Centers for Disease Control and Prevention (CDC) website (www.cdc.gov/vaccines).
- Tell the patient, parent, or guardian that the United States Department of Health and Human Services has established a Vaccine Adverse Event Reporting System (VAERS) to accept all reports of suspected adverse events after the administration of any vaccine, including but not limited to the reporting of events required by the National Childhood Vaccine Injury Act of 1986. The VAERS toll-free number is 1-800-822-7967. Reporting forms may also be obtained at the VAERS website at (www.vaers.hhs.gov).

Manuf. and Dist. by: Merck Sharp & Dohme Corp., a subsidiary of

MERCK & CO., INC., Whitehouse Station, NJ 08889, USA

Printed in USA

USPI-I-V2511211R15

VARIVAX® ℞

[var-i-vax]

Varicella Virus Vaccine Live

Suspension for subcutaneous injection

HIGHLIGHTS OF PRESCRIBING INFORMATION

These highlights do not include all the information needed to use VARIVAX safely and effectively. See full prescribing information for VARIVAX.

VARIVAX®

Varicella Virus Vaccine Live

Suspension for subcutaneous injection

Initial U.S. Approval: 1995

RECENT MAJOR CHANGES

Warnings and Precautions (5.3, 5.6) 12/2012

INDICATIONS AND USAGE

VARIVAX is a vaccine indicated for active immunization for the prevention of varicella in individuals 12 months of age and older. (1)

DOSAGE AND ADMINISTRATION

Each dose is approximately 0.5 mL after reconstitution and is administered by subcutaneous injection. (2.1)

Children (12 months to 12 years of age)

- If a second dose is administered, there should be a minimum interval of 3 months between doses. (2.1)

Adolescents (≥13 years of age) and Adults

- Two doses, to be administered a minimum of 4 weeks apart. (2.1)

DOSAGE FORMS AND STRENGTHS

Suspension for injection (approximately 0.5-mL dose) supplied as a lyophilized vaccine to be reconstituted using the accompanying sterile diluent. (2.2, 3, 16)

CONTRAINDICATIONS

- History of severe allergic reaction to any component of the vaccine (including neomycin and gelatin) or to a previous dose of varicella vaccine. (4.1)
- Primary or acquired immunodeficiency states. (4.2)
- Any febrile illness or active infection, including untreated tuberculosis. (4.3)
- Pregnancy. (4.4, 8.1, 17)

WARNINGS AND PRECAUTIONS

- Evaluate individuals for immune competence prior to administration of VARIVAX if there is a family history of congenital or hereditary immunodeficiency. (5.2)
- Avoid contact with high-risk individuals susceptible to varicella because of possible transmission of varicella vaccine virus. (5.4)
- Defer vaccination for at least 5 months following blood or plasma transfusions, or administration of immune globulins (IG). (5.5, 7.2)
- Avoid use of salicylates for 6 weeks following administration of VARIVAX to children and adolescents. (5.6, 7.1)

ADVERSE REACTIONS

- Frequently reported (≥10%) adverse reactions in children ages 1 to 12 years include:
  - fever ≥102.0°F (38.9°C) oral: 14.7%
  - injection-site complaints: 19.3% (6.1)
- Frequently reported (≥10%) adverse reactions in adolescents and adults ages 13 years and older include:
  - fever ≥100.0°F (37.8°C) oral: 10.2%
  - injection-site complaints: 24.4% (6.1)
- Other reported adverse reactions in all age groups include:
  - varicella-like rash (injection site)
  - varicella-like rash (generalized) (6.1)

To report SUSPECTED ADVERSE REACTIONS, contact Merck Sharp & Dohme Corp., a subsidiary of Merck & Co., Inc., at 1-877-888-4231 or VAERS at 1-800-822-7967 or www.vaers.hhs.gov.

DRUG INTERACTIONS

- Reye syndrome has been reported in children and adolescents following the use of salicylates during wild-type varicella infection. (5.6, 7.1)
- Passively acquired antibodies from blood, plasma, or immunoglobulin potentially may inhibit the response to varicella vaccination. (5.5, 7.2)
- Tuberculin skin testing may be performed before VARIVAX is administered or on the same day, or six weeks following vaccination with VARIVAX. (7.3)

USE IN SPECIFIC POPULATIONS

Pregnancy: Do not administer VARIVAX to females who are pregnant; the possible effects of the vaccine on fetal development are unknown. Pregnancy should be avoided for 3 months following vaccination with VARIVAX. (4.4, 8.1, 17) Report vaccine exposure during pregnancy by calling 1-800-986-8999.

See 17 for PATIENT COUNSELING INFORMATION and FDA-approved patient labeling

Revised: 12/2012

FULL PRESCRIBING INFORMATION: CONTENTS*

*** Sections or subsections omitted from the full prescribing information are not listed**

FULL PRESCRIBING INFORMATION

1 INDICATIONS AND USAGE

VARIVAX® is a vaccine indicated for active immunization for the prevention of varicella in individuals 12 months of age and older.

2 DOSAGE AND ADMINISTRATION

Subcutaneous administration only

2.1 Recommended Dose and Schedule

VARIVAX is administered as an approximately 0.5-mL dose by subcutaneous injection into the outer aspect of the upper arm (deltoid region) or the anterolateral thigh.

Do not administer this product intravascularly or intramuscularly.

Children (12 months to 12 years of age)

If a second dose is administered, there should be a minimum interval of 3 months between doses *[see Clinical Studies (14.1)]*.

Adolescents (≥13 years of age) and Adults

Two doses of vaccine, to be administered with a minimum interval of 4 weeks between doses *[see Clinical Studies (14.1)]*.

2.2 Reconstitution Instructions

When reconstituting the vaccine, use only the sterile diluent supplied with VARIVAX. The sterile diluent does not contain preservatives or other anti-viral substances which might inactivate the vaccine virus.

Use a sterile syringe free of preservatives, antiseptics, and detergents for each reconstitution and injection of VARIVAX because these substances may inactivate the vaccine virus.

To reconstitute the vaccine, first withdraw the total volume of provided sterile diluent into a syringe. Inject all of the withdrawn diluent into the vial of lyophilized vaccine and gently agitate to mix thoroughly. Withdraw the entire contents into the syringe and inject the total volume (approximately 0.5 mL) of reconstituted vaccine subcutaneously. VARIVAX, when reconstituted, is a clear, colorless to pale yellow liquid.

Parenteral drug products should be inspected visually for particulate matter and discoloration prior to administration, whenever solution and container permit. Do not use the product if particulates are present or if it appears discolored.

To minimize loss of potency, administer VARIVAX immediately after reconstitution. Discard if reconstituted vaccine is not used within 30 minutes.

Do not freeze reconstituted vaccine.

Do not combine VARIVAX with any other vaccine through reconstitution or mixing.

3 DOSAGE FORMS AND STRENGTHS

VARIVAX is a suspension for injection supplied as a single-dose vial of lyophilized vaccine to be reconstituted using the accompanying sterile diluent *[see Dosage and Administration (2.2) and How Supplied/Storage and Handling (16)]*. A single dose after reconstitution is approximately 0.5 mL.

4 CONTRAINDICATIONS

4.1 Severe Allergic Reaction

Do not administer VARIVAX to individuals with a history of anaphylactic or severe allergic reaction to any component of the vaccine (including neomycin and gelatin) or to a previous dose of a varicella-containing vaccine.

4.2 Immunosuppression

Do not administer VARIVAX to immunosuppressed or immunodeficient individuals, including those with a history of primary or acquired immunodeficiency states, leukemia, lymphoma or other malignant neoplasms affecting the bone marrow or lymphatic system, AIDS, or other clinical manifestations of infection with human immunodeficiency virus (HIV).

Do not administer VARIVAX to individuals receiving immunosuppressive therapy, including individuals receiving immunosuppressive doses of corticosteroids.

Table 1: Fever, Local Reactions, and Rashes (%) in Children 1 to 12 Years of Age 0 to 42 Days After Receipt of a Single Dose of VARIVAX

Reaction	N	% Experiencing Reaction	Peak Occurrence During Postvaccination Days
Fever ≥102.0°F (38.9°C) Oral	8827	14.7%	0 to 42
Injection-site complaints (pain/soreness, swelling and/or erythema, rash, pruritus, hematoma, induration, stiffness)	8916	19.3%	0 to 2
Varicella-like rash (injection site) Median number of lesions	8916	3.4% 2	8 to 19
Varicella-like rash (generalized) Median number of lesions	8916	3.8% 5	5 to 26

Table 2: Fever, Local Reactions, and Rashes (%) in Adolescents and Adults 0 to 42 Days After Receipt of VARIVAX

Reaction	N	% Post Dose 1	Peak Occurrence in Postvaccination Days	N	% Post Dose 2	Peak Occurrence in Postvaccination Days
Fever ≥100.0°F (37.8°C) Oral	1584	10.2%	14 to 27	956	9.5%	0 to 42
Injection-site complaints (soreness, erythema, swelling, rash, pruritus, pyrexia, hematoma, induration, numbness)	1606	24.4%	0 to 2	955	32.5%	0 to 2
Varicella-like rash (injection site) Median number of lesions	1606	3% 2	6 to 20	955	1% 2	0 to 6
Varicella-like rash (generalized) Median number of lesions	1606	5.5% 5	7 to 21	955	0.9% 5.5	0 to 23

VARIVAX is a live, attenuated varicella-zoster vaccine (VZV) and may cause an extensive vaccine-associated rash or disseminated disease in individuals who are immunosuppressed or immunodeficient.

4.3 Concurrent Illness

Do not administer VARIVAX to individuals with any febrile illness. Do not administer VARIVAX to individuals with active, untreated tuberculosis.

4.4 Pregnancy

Do not administer VARIVAX to individuals who are pregnant because the effects of the vaccine on fetal development are unknown. Wild-type varicella (natural infection) is known to sometimes cause fetal harm. If vaccination of postpubertal females is undertaken, pregnancy should be avoided for three months following vaccination *[see Use in Specific Populations (8.1) and Patient Counseling Information (17)].*

5 WARNINGS AND PRECAUTIONS

5.1 Management of Allergic Reactions

Adequate treatment provisions, including epinephrine injection (1:1000), should be available for immediate use should anaphylaxis occur.

5.2 Family History of Immunodeficiency

Vaccination should be deferred in patients with a family history of congenital or hereditary immunodeficiency until the patient's immune status has been evaluated and the patient has been found to be immunocompetent.

5.3 Use in HIV-Infected Individuals

The Advisory Committee for Immunization Practices (ACIP) has recommendations on the use of varicella vaccine in HIV-infected individuals.

5.4 Risk of Vaccine Virus Transmission

Post-marketing experience suggests that transmission of vaccine virus may occur rarely between healthy vaccinees who develop a varicella-like rash and healthy susceptible contacts. Transmission of vaccine virus from a mother who did not develop a varicella-like rash to her newborn infant has been reported.

Due to the concern for transmission of vaccine virus, vaccine recipients should attempt to avoid whenever possible close association with susceptible high-risk individuals for up to six weeks following vaccination with VARIVAX. Susceptible high-risk individuals include:

- Immunocompromised individuals;
- Pregnant women without documented history of varicella or laboratory evidence of prior infection;
- Newborn infants of mothers without documented history of varicella or laboratory evidence of prior infection and all newborn infants born at <28 weeks gestation regardless of maternal varicella immunity.

5.5 Immune Globulins and Transfusions

Immunoglobulins should not be given concomitantly with VARIVAX. Vaccination should be deferred for at least 5 months following blood or plasma transfusions, or administration of immune globulin(s) {1}.

Following administration of VARIVAX, immune globulin(s) should not be given for 2 months thereafter unless its use outweighs the benefits of vaccination {1}. *[See Drug Interactions (7.2).]*

5.6 Salicylate Therapy

Avoid use of salicylates (aspirin) or salicylate-containing products in children and adolescents 12 months through 17 years of age for six weeks following vaccination with VARIVAX because of the association of Reye syndrome with aspirin therapy and wild-type varicella infection. *[See Drug Interactions (7.1).]*

6 ADVERSE REACTIONS

6.1 Clinical Trials Experience

Because clinical trials are conducted under widely varying conditions, adverse reaction rates observed in the clinical trials of a vaccine cannot be directly compared to rates in the clinical trials of another vaccine and may not reflect the rates observed in clinical practice. Vaccine-related adverse reactions reported during clinical trials were assessed by the study investigators to be possibly, probably, or definitely vaccine-related and are summarized below.

In clinical trials {2-9}, VARIVAX was administered to over 11,000 healthy children, adolescents, and adults.

In a double-blind, placebo-controlled study among 914 healthy children and adolescents who were serologically confirmed to be susceptible to varicella, the only adverse reactions that occurred at a significantly ($p<0.05$) greater rate in vaccine recipients than in placebo recipients were pain and redness at the injection site {2}.

Children 1 to 12 Years of Age

One-Dose Regimen in Children

In clinical trials involving healthy children monitored for up to 42 days after a single dose of VARIVAX, the frequency of fever, injection-site complaints, or rashes were reported as shown in Table 1:

[See table 1 above]

In addition, adverse events occurring a rate of ≥1% are listed in decreasing order of frequency: upper respiratory illness, cough, irritability/nervousness, fatigue, disturbed sleep, diarrhea, loss of appetite, vomiting, otitis, diaper rash/contact rash, headache, teething, malaise, abdominal pain, other rash, nausea, eye complaints, chills, lymphadenopathy, myalgia, lower respiratory illness, allergic reactions (including allergic rash, hives), stiff neck, heat rash/prickly heat, arthralgia, eczema/dry skin/dermatitis, constipation, itching.

Pneumonitis has been reported rarely (<1%) in children vaccinated with VARIVAX.

Febrile seizures have occurred at a rate of <0.1% in children vaccinated with VARIVAX.

Two-Dose Regimen in Children

Nine hundred eighty-one (981) subjects in a clinical trial received 2 doses of VARIVAX 3 months apart and were actively followed for 42 days after each dose. The 2-dose regimen of varicella vaccine had a safety profile comparable to that of the 1-dose regimen. The overall incidence of injection-site clinical complaints (primarily erythema and swelling) observed in the first 4 days following vaccination was 25.4% Postdose 2 and 21.7% Postdose 1, whereas the overall incidence of systemic clinical complaints in the 42-day follow-up period was lower Postdose 2 (66.3%) than Postdose 1 (85.8%).

Adolescents (13 Years of Age and Older) and Adults

In clinical trials involving healthy adolescents and adults, the majority of whom received two doses of VARIVAX and were monitored for up to 42 days after any dose, the frequencies of fever, injection-site complaints, or rashes are shown in Table 2.

[See table 2 below]

In addition, adverse events reported at a rate of ≥1% are listed in decreasing order of frequency: upper respiratory illness, headache, fatigue, cough, myalgia, disturbed sleep, nausea, malaise, diarrhea, stiff neck, irritability/nervousness, lymphadenopathy, chills, eye complaints, abdominal pain, loss of appetite, arthralgia, otitis, itching, vomiting, other rashes, constipation, lower respiratory illness, allergic reactions (including allergic rash, hives), contact rash, cold/canker sore.

6.2 Post-Marketing Experience

Broad use of VARIVAX could reveal adverse events not observed in clinical trials.

The following additional adverse events, regardless of causality, have been reported during post-marketing use of VARIVAX:

Body as a Whole

Anaphylaxis (including anaphylactic shock) and related phenomena such as angioneurotic edema, facial edema, and peripheral edema.

Hemic and Lymphatic System

Aplastic anemia; thrombocytopenia (including idiopathic thrombocytopenic purpura (ITP)).

Infections and Infestations

Varicella (vaccine strain).

Nervous/Psychiatric

Encephalitis; cerebrovascular accident; transverse myelitis; Guillain-Barré syndrome; Bell's palsy; ataxia; non-febrile seizures; aseptic meningitis; dizziness; paresthesia.

Respiratory

Pharyngitis; pneumonia/pneumonitis.

Skin

Stevens-Johnson syndrome; erythema multiforme; Henoch-Schönlein purpura; secondary bacterial infections of skin and soft tissue, including impetigo and cellulitis; herpes zoster.

7 DRUG INTERACTIONS

7.1 Salicylates

No cases of Reye syndrome have been observed following vaccination with VARIVAX. Vaccine recipients should avoid use of salicylates for 6 weeks after vaccination with VARIVAX, as Reye syndrome has been reported following the use of salicylates during wild-type varicella infection *[see Warnings and Precautions (5.6)].*

7.2 Immune Globulins and Transfusions

Blood, plasma, and immune globulins contain antibodies that may interfere with vaccine virus replication and decrease the immune response to VARIVAX. Vaccination should be deferred for at least 5 months following blood or plasma transfusions, or administration of immune globulin(s) {1}.

Following administration of VARIVAX, immune globulin(s) should not be given for 2 months thereafter unless its use outweighs the benefits of vaccination {1}. *[See Warnings and Precautions (5.5).]*

7.3 Tuberculin Skin Testing

Tuberculin skin testing, with tuberculin purified protein derivative (PPD), may be performed before VARIVAX is administered or on the same day, or at least 4 weeks following vaccination with VARIVAX, as other live virus vaccines may cause a temporary depression of tuberculin skin test sensitivity leading to false negative results.

8 USE IN SPECIFIC POPULATIONS

8.1 Pregnancy

Pregnancy Category: Contraindication *[see Contraindications (4.4)].* VARIVAX should not be administered to pregnant females. Pregnancy should be avoided for three months following vaccination with VARIVAX *[see Contraindications (4.4) and Patient Counseling Information (17)].*

Merck Sharp & Dohme Corp., a subsidiary of Merck & Co., Inc., maintains a Pregnancy Registry to monitor fetal outcomes of pregnant women exposed to VARIVAX. Patients and healthcare providers should report any exposure to VARIVAX during pregnancy by calling 1-800-986-8999.

8.3 Nursing Mothers

It is not known whether varicella vaccine virus is excreted in human milk. Therefore, because some viruses are excreted in human milk, caution should be exercised if VARIVAX is administered to a nursing woman. *[See Warnings and Precautions (5.4).]*

8.4 Pediatric Use

No clinical data are available on safety or efficacy of VARIVAX in children less than 12 months of age.

8.5 Geriatric Use

Clinical studies of VARIVAX did not include sufficient numbers of seronegative subjects aged 65 and over to determine whether they respond differently from younger subjects.

11 DESCRIPTION

VARIVAX [Varicella Virus Vaccine Live] is a preparation of the Oka/Merck strain of live, attenuated varicella virus. The virus was initially obtained from a child with wild-type varicella, then introduced into human embryonic lung cell cultures, adapted to and propagated in embryonic guinea pig cell cultures and finally propagated in human diploid cell cultures (WI-38). Further passage of the virus for varicella vaccine was performed at Merck Research Laboratories (MRL) in human diploid cell cultures (MRC-5) that were free of adventitious agents. This live, attenuated varicella vaccine is a lyophilized preparation containing sucrose, phosphate, glutamate, and processed gelatin as stabilizers.

VARIVAX, when reconstituted as directed, is a sterile preparation for subcutaneous injection. Each approximately 0.5-mL dose contains a minimum of 1350 plaque-forming units (PFU) of Oka/Merck varicella virus when reconstituted and stored at room temperature for a maximum of 30 minutes. Each 0.5-mL dose also contains approximately 25 mg of sucrose, 12.5 mg hydrolyzed gelatin, 3.2 mg of sodium chloride, 0.5 mg of monosodium L-glutamate, 0.45 mg of sodium phosphate dibasic, 0.08 mg of potassium phosphate monobasic, and 0.08 mg of potassium chloride. The product also contains residual components of MRC-5 cells including DNA and protein and trace quantities of sodium phosphate monobasic, EDTA, neomycin and fetal bovine serum. The product contains no preservative.

12 CLINICAL PHARMACOLOGY

12.1 Mechanism of Action

VARIVAX induces both cell-mediated and humoral immune responses to varicella-zoster virus. The relative contributions of humoral immunity and cell-mediated immunity to protection from varicella are unknown.

12.2 Pharmacodynamics

Transmission

In the placebo-controlled efficacy trial, transmission of vaccine virus was assessed in household settings (during the 8-week postvaccination period) in 416 susceptible placebo recipients who were household contacts of 445 vaccine recipients. Of the 416 placebo recipients, three developed varicella and seroconverted, nine reported a varicella-like rash and did not seroconvert, and six had no rash but seroconverted. If vaccine virus transmission occurred, it did so at a very low rate and possibly without recognizable clinical disease in contacts. These cases may represent either wild-type varicella from community contacts or a low incidence of transmission of vaccine virus from vaccinated contacts *[see Warnings and Precautions (5.4)]* {2,10}. Post-marketing experience suggests that transmission of vaccine virus may occur rarely between healthy vaccinees who develop a varicella-like rash and healthy susceptible contacts. Transmission of vaccine virus from a mother who did not develop a varicella-like rash to her newborn infant has also been reported.

Herpes Zoster

Overall, 9454 healthy children (12 months to 12 years of age) and 1648 adolescents and adults (13 years of age and older) have been vaccinated with VARIVAX in clinical trials. Eight cases of herpes zoster have been reported in children during 42,556 person-years of follow-up in clinical trials, resulting in a calculated incidence of at least 18.8 cases per 100,000 person-years. The completeness of this reporting has not been determined. One case of herpes zoster has been reported in the adolescent and adult age group during 5410 person-years of follow-up in clinical trials, resulting in a calculated incidence of 18.5 cases per 100,000 person years. All 9 cases were mild and without sequelae. Two cultures (one child and one adult) obtained from vesicles were positive for wild-type VZV as confirmed by restriction endonuclease analysis {11}. The long-term effect of VARIVAX on the incidence of herpes zoster, particularly in those vaccinees exposed to wild-type varicella, is unknown at present.

In children, the reported rate of herpes zoster in vaccine recipients appears not to exceed that previously determined in a population-based study of healthy children who had experienced wild-type varicella {12}. The incidence of herpes zoster in adults who have had wild-type varicella infection is higher than that in children.

12.4 Duration of Protection

The duration of protection of VARIVAX is unknown; however, long-term efficacy studies have demonstrated continued protection up to 10 years after vaccination {13} *[see Clinical Studies (14.1)]*. A boost in antibody levels has been observed in vaccinees following exposure to wild-type varicella which could account for the apparent long-term protection after vaccination in these studies.

14 CLINICAL STUDIES

14.1 Clinical Efficacy

The protective efficacy of VARIVAX was established by: (1) a placebo-controlled, double-blind clinical trial, (2) comparing varicella rates in vaccinees versus historical controls, and (3) assessing protection from disease following household exposure.

Clinical Data in Children

One-Dose Regimen in Children

Although no placebo-controlled trial was carried out with VARIVAX using the current vaccine, a placebo-controlled trial was conducted using a formulation containing 17,000 PFU per dose {2,14}. In this trial, a single dose of VARIVAX protected 96 to 100% of children against varicella over a two-year period. The study enrolled healthy individuals 1 to 14 years of age (n=491 vaccine, n=465 placebo). In the first year, 8.5% of placebo recipients contracted varicella, while no vaccine recipient did, for a calculated protection rate of 100% during the first varicella season. In the second year, when only a subset of individuals agreed to remain in the blinded study (n=163 vaccine, n=161 placebo), 96% protective efficacy was calculated for the vaccine group as compared to placebo.

In early clinical trials, a total of 4240 children 1 to 12 years of age received 1000 to 1625 PFU of attenuated virus per dose of VARIVAX and have been followed for up to nine years post single-dose vaccination. In this group there was considerable variation in varicella rates among studies and study sites, and much of the reported data were acquired by passive follow-up. It was observed that 0.3 to 3.8% of vaccinees per year reported varicella (called breakthrough cases). This represents an approximate 83% (95% confidence interval [CI], 82%, 84%) decrease from the age-adjusted expected incidence rates in susceptible subjects over this same period {12}. In those who developed breakthrough varicella postvaccination, the majority experienced mild disease (median of the maximum number of lesions <50). In one study, a total of 47% (27/58) of breakthrough cases had <50 lesions compared with 8% (7/92) in unvaccinated individuals, and 7% (4/58) of breakthrough cases had >300 lesions compared with 50% (46/92) in unvaccinated individuals {15}.

Among a subset of vaccinees who were actively followed in these early trials for up to nine years postvaccination, 179 individuals had household exposure to varicella. There were no reports of breakthrough varicella in 84% (150/179) of exposed children, while 16% (29/179) reported a mild form of varicella (38% [11/29] of the cases with a maximum total number of <50 lesions; no individuals with >300 lesions). This represents an 81% reduction in the expected number of varicella cases utilizing the historical attack rate of 87% following household exposure to varicella in unvaccinated individuals in the calculation of efficacy.

In later clinical trials, a total of 1114 children 1 to 12 years of age received 2900 to 9000 PFU of attenuated virus per dose of VARIVAX and have been actively followed for up to 10 years post single-dose vaccination. It was observed that 0.2% to 2.3% of vaccinees per year reported breakthrough varicella for up to 10 years post single-dose vaccination. This represents an estimated efficacy of 94% (95% CI, 93%, 96%), compared with the age-adjusted expected incidence rates in susceptible subjects over the same period {2,12,16}. In those who developed breakthrough varicella postvaccination, the majority experienced mild disease, with the median of the maximum total number of lesions <50. The severity of reported breakthrough varicella, as measured by number of lesions and maximum temperature, appeared not to increase with time since vaccination.

Among a subset of vaccinees who were actively followed in these later trials for up to 10 years postvaccination, 95 individuals were exposed to an unvaccinated individual with wild-type varicella in a household setting. There were no reports of breakthrough varicella in 92% (87/95) of exposed children, while 8% (8/95) reported a mild form of varicella (maximum total number of lesions <50; observed range, 10 to 34). This represents an estimated efficacy of 90% (95% CI, 82%, 96%) based on the historical attack rate of 87% following household exposure to varicella in unvaccinated individuals in the calculation of efficacy.

Two-Dose Regimen in Children

In a clinical trial, a total of 2216 children 12 months to 12 years of age with a negative history of varicella were randomized to receive either 1 dose of VARIVAX (n=1114) or 2 doses of VARIVAX (n=1102) given 3 months apart. Subjects were actively followed for varicella, any varicella-like illness, or herpes zoster and any exposures to varicella or herpes zoster on an annual basis for 10 years after vaccination. Persistence of VZV antibody was measured annually for 9 years. Most cases of varicella reported in recipients of 1 dose or 2 doses of vaccine were mild {13}. The estimated vaccine efficacy for the 10-year observation period was 94% for 1 dose and 98% for 2 doses ($p<0.001$). This translates to a 3.4-fold lower risk of developing varicella >42 days postvaccination during the 10-year observation period in children who received 2 doses than in those who received 1 dose (2.2% vs. 7.5%, respectively).

Clinical Data in Adolescents and Adults

Two-Dose Regimen in Adolescents and Adults

In early clinical trials, a total of 796 adolescents and adults received 905 to 1230 PFU of attenuated virus per dose of VARIVAX and have been followed for up to six years following 2-dose vaccination. A total of 50 clinical varicella cases were reported >42 days following 2-dose vaccination. Based on passive follow-up, the annual varicella breakthrough event rate ranged from <0.1 to 1.9%. The median of the maximum total number of lesions ranged from 15 to 42 per year.

Although no placebo-controlled trial was carried out in adolescents and adults, the protective efficacy of VARIVAX was determined by evaluation of protection when vaccinees received 2 doses of VARIVAX 4 or 8 weeks apart and were subsequently exposed to varicella in a household setting. Among the subset of vaccinees who were actively followed in these early trials for up to six years, 76 individuals had household exposure to varicella. There were no reports of breakthrough varicella in 83% (63/76) of exposed vaccinees, while 17% (13/76) reported a mild form of varicella. Among 13 vaccinated individuals who developed breakthrough varicella after a household exposure, 62% (8/13) of the cases reported maximum total number of lesions <50, while no individual reported >75 lesions. The attack rate of unvaccinated adults exposed to a single contact in a household has not been previously studied. Utilizing the previously reported historical attack rate of 87% for wild-type varicella following household exposure to varicella among unvaccinated children in the calculation of efficacy, this represents an approximate 80% reduction in the expected number of cases in the household setting.

In later clinical trials, a total of 220 adolescents and adults received 3315 to 9000 PFU of attenuated virus per dose of VARIVAX and have been actively followed for up to six years following 2-dose vaccination. A total of 3 clinical varicella cases were reported >42 days following 2-dose vaccination. Two cases reported <50 lesions and none reported >75. The annual varicella breakthrough event rate ranged from 0 to 1.2%. Among the subset of vaccinees who were actively followed in these later trials for up to five years, 16 individuals were exposed to an unvaccinated individual with wild-type varicella in a household setting. There were no reports of breakthrough varicella among the exposed vaccinees.

There are insufficient data to assess the rate of protective efficacy of VARIVAX against the serious complications of varicella in adults (*e.g.*, encephalitis, hepatitis, pneumonitis) and during pregnancy (congenital varicella syndrome).

14.2 Immunogenicity

In clinical trials, varicella antibodies have been evaluated following vaccination with formulations of VARIVAX containing attenuated virus ranging from 1000 to 50,000 PFU per dose in healthy individuals ranging from 12 months to 55 years of age {2,9}.

One-Dose Regimen in Children

In prelicensure efficacy studies, seroconversion was observed in 97% of vaccinees at approximately 4 to 6 weeks postvaccination in 6889 susceptible children 12 months to 12 years of age. Titers ≥5 gpELISA units/mL were induced in approximately 76% of children vaccinated with a single dose of vaccine at 1000 to 17,000 PFU per dose. Rates of breakthrough disease were significantly lower among children with VZV antibody titers ≥5 gpELISA units/mL compared with children with titers <5 gpELISA units/mL.

Two-Dose Regimen in Children

In a multicenter study, 2216 healthy children 12 months to 12 years of age received either 1 dose of VARIVAX or 2 doses administered 3 months apart. The immunogenicity results are shown in Table 3.

[See table 3 at top of next page]

The results from this study and other studies in which a second dose of VARIVAX was administered 3 to 6 years after the initial dose demonstrate significant boosting of the VZV antibodies with a second dose. VZV antibody levels after 2 doses given 3 to 6 years apart are comparable to those obtained when the 2 doses are given 3 months apart.

Two-Dose Regimen in Adolescents and Adults

In a multicenter study involving susceptible adolescents and adults 13 years of age and older, 2 doses of VARIVAX administered 4 to 8 weeks apart induced a seroconversion rate of approximately 75% in 539 individuals 4 weeks after the first dose and of 99% in 479 individuals 4 weeks after the second dose. The average antibody response in vaccinees who received the second dose 8 weeks after the first dose was higher than that in vaccinees who received the second dose 4 weeks after the first dose. In another multicenter study involving adolescents and adults, 2 doses of VARIVAX administered 8 weeks apart induced a seroconversion rate of 94% in 142 individuals 6 weeks after the first dose and 99% in 122 individuals 6 weeks after the second dose.

14.3 Persistence of Immune Response

One-Dose Regimen in Children

In clinical studies involving healthy children who received 1 dose of vaccine, detectable VZV antibodies were present in 99.0% (3886/3926) at 1 year, 99.3% (1555/1566) at 2 years, 98.6% (1106/1122) at 3 years, 99.4% (1168/1175) at 4 years, 99.2% (737/743) at 5 years, 100% (142/142) at 6 years, 97.4% (38/39) at 7 years, 100% (34/34) at 8 years, and 100% (16/16) at 10 years postvaccination.

Two-Dose Regimen in Children

In recipients of 1 dose of VARIVAX over 9 years of follow-up, the geometric mean titers (GMTs) and the percent of subjects with VZV antibody titers ≥5 gpELISA units/mL generally increased. The GMTs and percent of subjects with VZV antibody titers ≥5 gpELISA units/mL in the 2-dose recipients were higher than those in the 1-dose recipients for the first year of follow-up and generally comparable thereafter. The cumulative rate of VZV antibody persistence with both regimens remained very high at year 9 (99.0% for the 1-dose group and 98.8% for the 2-dose group).

Two-Dose Regimen in Adolescents and Adults

In clinical studies involving healthy adolescents and adults who received 2 doses of vaccine, detectable VZV antibodies were present in 97.9% (568/580) at 1 year, 97.1% (34/35) at 2 years, 100% (144/144) at 3 years, 97.0% (98/101) at 4 years, 97.4% (76/78) at 5 years, and 100% (34/34) at 6 years postvaccination.

A boost in antibody levels has been observed in vaccinees following exposure to wild-type varicella, which could account for the apparent long-term persistence of antibody levels in these studies.

14.4 Studies With Other Vaccines

Concomitant Administration with M-M-R II

In combined clinical studies involving 1080 children 12 to 36 months of age, 653 received VARIVAX and M-M-R II concomitantly at separate injection sites and 427 received the vaccines six weeks apart. Seroconversion rates and antibody levels to measles, mumps, rubella, and varicella were comparable between the two groups at approximately six weeks post-vaccination.

Concomitant Administration with Diphtheria and Tetanus Toxoids and Acellular Pertussis Vaccine Adsorbed (DTaP) and Oral Poliovirus Vaccine (OPV)

In a clinical study involving 318 children 12 months to 42 months of age, 160 received an investigational varicella-containing vaccine (a formulation combining measles, mumps, rubella, and varicella in one syringe) concomitantly with booster doses of DTaP and OPV (no longer licensed in the United States). The comparator group of 144 children received M-M-R II concomitantly with booster doses of DTaP and OPV followed by VARIVAX six weeks later. At six weeks postvaccination, seroconversion rates for measles, mumps, rubella, and VZV and the percentage of vaccinees whose titers were boosted for diphtheria, tetanus, pertussis, and polio were comparable between the two groups. Anti-VZV levels were decreased when the investigational vaccine containing varicella was administered concomitantly with DTaP {17}. No clinically significant differences were noted in adverse reactions between the two groups.

Concomitant Administration with PedvaxHIB®

In a clinical study involving 307 children 12 to 18 months of age, 150 received an investigational varicella-containing vaccine (a formulation combining measles, mumps, rubella, and varicella in one syringe) concomitantly with a booster dose of PedvaxHIB [Haemophilus b Conjugate Vaccine (Meningococcal Protein Conjugate)], while 130 received M-M-R II concomitantly with a booster dose of PedvaxHIB followed by VARIVAX 6 weeks later. At six weeks postvaccination, seroconversion rates for measles, mumps, rubella, and VZV, and GMTs for PedvaxHIB were comparable between the two groups. Anti-VZV levels were decreased when the investigational vaccine containing varicella was administered concomitantly with PedvaxHIB {18}. No clinically significant differences in adverse reactions were seen between the two groups.

Concomitant Administration with M-M-R II and COMVAX

In a clinical study involving 822 children 12 to 15 months of age, 410 received COMVAX, M-M-R II, and VARIVAX concomitantly at separate injection sites, and 412 received COMVAX followed by M-M-R II and VARIVAX given concomitantly at separate injection sites, 6 weeks later. At 6 weeks postvaccination, the immune responses for the subjects who received the concomitant doses of COMVAX, M-M-R II, and VARIVAX were similar to those of the subjects who received COMVAX followed 6 weeks later by M-M-R II and VARIVAX with respect to all antigens administered. There were no clinically important differences in reaction rates when the three vaccines were administered concomitantly versus six weeks apart.

Table 3: Summary of VZV Antibody Responses at 6 Weeks Postdose 1 and 6 Weeks Postdose 2 in Initially Seronegative Children 12 Months to 12 Years of Age (Vaccinations 3 Months Apart)

	VARIVAX 1-Dose Regimen (N=1114)	VARIVAX 2-Dose Regimen (3 months apart) (N=1102)	
	6 Weeks Postvaccination (n=892)	6 Weeks Postdose 1 (n=851)	6 Weeks Postdose 2 (n=769)
Seroconversion Rate	98.9%	99.5%	99.9%
Percent with VZV Antibody Titer ≥5 gpELISA units/mL	84.9%	87.3%	99.5%
Geometric mean titers in gpELISA units/mL (95% CI)	12.0 (11.2, 12.8)	12.8 (11.9, 13.7)	141.5 (132.3, 151.3)

N = Number of subjects vaccinated.
n = Number of subjects included in immunogenicity analysis.

15 REFERENCES

1. CDC: General Recommendations on Immunization: Recommendations of the Advisory Committee on Immunization Practices (ACIP). MMWR. 55(No. RR-15): 1-47, 2006.
2. Weibel, R.E.; et al.: Live Attenuated Varicella Virus Vaccine. Efficacy Trial in Healthy Children. N Engl J Med. 310(22): 1409-1415, 1984.
3. Arbeter, A.M.; et al.: Varicella Vaccine Trials in Healthy Children. A Summary of Comparative and Follow-up Studies. Am J Dis Child. 138: 434-438, 1984.
4. Weibel, R.E.; et al.: Live Oka/Merck Varicella Vaccine in Healthy Children. Further Clinical and Laboratory Assessment. JAMA. 254(17): 2435-2439, 1985.
5. Chartrand, D.M.; et al.: New Varicella Vaccine Production Lots in Healthy Children and Adolescents. Abstracts of the 1988 Inter-Science Conference Antimicrobial Agents and Chemotherapy: 237(Abstract #731).
6. Johnson, C.E.; et al.: Live Attenuated Varicella Vaccine in Healthy 12- to 24-Month-Old Children. Pediatrics. 81(4): 512-518, 1988.
7. Gershon, A.A.; et al.: Immunization of Healthy Adults with Live Attenuated Varicella Vaccine. J Infect Dis. 158(1): 132-137, 1988.
8. Gershon, A.A.; et al.: Live Attenuated Varicella Vaccine: Protection in Healthy Adults Compared with Leukemic Children. J Infect Dis. 161: 661-666, 1990.
9. White, C.J.; et al.: Varicella Vaccine (VARIVAX) in Healthy Children and Adolescents: Results From Clinical Trials, 1987 to 1989. Pediatrics. 87(5): 604-610, 1991.
10. Galea, S.; et al.: The Safety Profile of Varicella Vaccine: A 10-Year Review. J Infect Dis. 197(S2): 165-169, 2008.
11. Hammerschlag, M.R.; et al.: Herpes Zoster in an Adult Recipient of Live Attenuated Varicella Vaccine. J Infect Dis. 160(3): 535-537, 1989.
12. Guess, H.A.; et al.: Population-Based Studies of Varicella Complications. Pediatrics. 78(suppl): 723-727, 1986.
13. Kuter, B.J.; et al.: Ten Year Follow-up of Healthy Children who Received One or Two Injections of Varicella Vaccine. Pediatr Infect Dis J. 23: 132-37, 2004.
14. Kuter, B.J.; et al.: Oka/Merck Varicella Vaccine in Healthy Children: Final Report of a 2-Year Efficacy Study and 7-Year Follow-up Studies. Vaccine. 9: 643-647, 1991.
15. Bernstein, H.H.; et al.: Clinical Survey of Natural Varicella Compared with Breakthrough Varicella After Immunization with Live Attenuated Oka/Merck Varicella Vaccine. Pediatrics. 92(6): 833-837, 1993.
16. Wharton, M.: The Epidemiology of Varicella-zoster Virus Infections. Infect Dis Clin North Am. 10(3):571-581, 1996.
17. White, C.J. et al.: Measles, Mumps, Rubella, and Varicella Combination Vaccine: Safety and Immunogenicity Alone and in Combination with Other Vaccines Given to Children. Clin Infect Dis. 24(5): 925-931, 1997.
18. Reuman, P.D.; et al.: Safety and Immunogenicity of Concurrent Administration of Measles-Mumps-Rubella-Varicella Vaccine and PedvaxHIB® Vaccines in Healthy Children Twelve to Eighteen Months Old. Pediatr Infect Dis J. 16(7): 662-667, 1997.

16 HOW SUPPLIED/STORAGE AND HANDLING

No. 4826/4309 —VARIVAX is supplied as follows:
(1) a single-dose vial of lyophilized vaccine (package A), NDC 0006-4826-00
(2) a box of 10 vials of diluent (package B).
No. 4827/4309 —VARIVAX is supplied as follows:
(1) a box of 10 single-dose vials of lyophilized vaccine (package A), NDC 0006-4827-00
(2) a box of 10 vials of diluent (package B).

Storage

Vaccine Vial

During shipment, maintain the vaccine at a temperature between –58°F and +5°F (–50°C and –15°C). Use of dry ice may subject VARIVAX to temperatures colder than –58°F (–50°C).

Before reconstitution, store the lyophilized vaccine in a freezer at a temperature between –58°F and +5°F (–50°C and –15°C). Any freezer (*e.g.*, chest, frost-free) that reliably maintains a temperature between –58°F and +5°F (–50°C and –15°C) and has a separate sealed freezer door is acceptable for storing VARIVAX.VARIVAX may be stored at refrigerator temperature (36°F to 46°F, 2°C to 8°C) for up to 72 continuous hours prior to reconstitution. Vaccine stored at 2°C to 8°C which is not used within 72 hours of removal from +5°F (–15°C) storage should be discarded.

Before reconstitution, protect from light.

DISCARD IF RECONSTITUTED VACCINE IS NOT USED WITHIN 30 MINUTES.

Diluent Vial

The vial of diluent should be stored separately at room temperature (68°F to 77°F, 20°C to 25°C), or in the refrigerator. **For further product information, call 1-800-9-VARIVAX (1-800-982-7482).**

17 PATIENT COUNSELING INFORMATION

See FDA-Approved Patient Labeling (Patient Information).
Discuss the following with the patient:

- Question the patient, parent, or guardian about reactions to previous vaccines.
- Provide a copy of the patient information (PPI) located at the end of this insert and discuss any questions or concerns.
- Inform patient, parent, or guardian that vaccination with VARIVAX may not result in protection of all healthy, susceptible children, adolescents, and adults.
- Inform female patients to avoid pregnancy for three months following vaccination.
- Inform patient, parent, or guardian of the benefits and risks of VARIVAX.
- Instruct patient, parent, or guardian to report any adverse reactions or any symptoms of concern to their healthcare professional.

The U.S. Department of Health and Human Services has established a Vaccine Adverse Event Reporting System (VAERS) to accept all reports of suspected adverse events after the administration of any vaccine. For information or a copy of the vaccine reporting form, call the VAERS toll-free number at 1-800-822-7967, or report online at http://www.vaers.hhs.gov.

Dist. by: Merck Sharp & Dohme Corp., a subsidiary of **MERCK & CO., INC.**, Whitehouse Station, NJ 08889, USA

USPI-I-V2101212R706

Patient Information about
VARIVAX® (pronounced "VAR ih vax")
Generic name: Varicella Virus Vaccine Live

This is a summary of information about VARIVAX®. You should read it before you or your child get the vaccine. If you have any questions about the vaccine after reading this leaflet, you should ask your healthcare professional. This is a summary only. It does not take the place of talking about VARIVAX with your doctor, nurse, or other healthcare professional. Only your healthcare professional can decide if VARIVAX is right for you or your child.

What is VARIVAX and how does it work?

VARIVAX is also known as Varicella Virus Vaccine Live. It is a live virus vaccine that is given as a shot. It is meant to help prevent chickenpox. Chickenpox is sometimes called varicella (pronounced VAR ih sell a).
VARIVAX contains a weakened form of chickenpox virus.

VARIVAX works by helping the immune system protect you or your child from getting chickenpox.
VARIVAX may not protect everyone who gets it.
VARIVAX does not treat chickenpox once you or your child have it.

What do I need to know about chickenpox?

Chickenpox is an illness that occurs most often in children who are 5 to 9 years old. It can be passed to others. The illness can include headache, fever, and general discomfort. Then an itchy rash occurs, which can turn into blisters. The most common complication is that the blisters can get infected. Less common but very serious complications can occur. These include pneumonia, inflammation of the brain, Reye syndrome (which affects the liver and the brain), and death. Severe disease and serious complications are more likely to occur in adolescents and adults.

Who should not get VARIVAX?

Do not get VARIVAX if you or your child:
- are allergic to any of its ingredients. (This includes gelatin or neomycin. See the ingredient list at the end of this leaflet.)
- have a weakened immune system, such as an immune deficiency, an inherited immune disorder, leukemia, lymphoma, or HIV/AIDS.
- take high doses of steroids by mouth or in a shot.
- have active tuberculosis that is not treated.
- have a fever.
- are pregnant or plan to get pregnant within the next three months.

What should I tell my healthcare professional before getting VARIVAX?

Tell your healthcare professional if you or your child:
- have or have had any medical problems.
- have received blood or plasma transfusions or human serum globulin within the last 5 months.
- take any medicines. (This includes non-prescription medicines and dietary supplements.)
- have any allergies. (This includes allergies to neomycin or gelatin.)
- had an allergic reaction to any other vaccine.
- are pregnant or plan to become pregnant within the next three months.
- are breast-feeding.

How is VARIVAX given?

VARIVAX is given as a shot to people who are 12 months old or older. If your child is 12 months to 12 years old and your doctor gives a second dose, the second dose must be given at least 3 months after the first shot.
A second dose should be given to those who first get the vaccine when they are 13 years old or older. This second dose should be given 4 to 8 weeks after the first dose.
Your doctor or healthcare professional will use the official recommendations to decide the number of shots needed and when to get them.
If a dose is missed, your healthcare professional will let you know when you should have it.

What should you or your child avoid when getting VARIVAX?

Do not take aspirin or aspirin-containing products for 6 weeks after getting VARIVAX.
It is rare, but possible, that once you have the vaccine, you could spread the chickenpox virus to others. Whenever possible, try to avoid contact with certain groups of people for up to six weeks after receiving the vaccine. This is because the disease for these groups may be quite serious. These groups include:
- people who have a weakened immune system.
- pregnant women who have never had chickenpox.
- newborn babies whose mothers have never had chickenpox.
- newborn babies born at less than 28 weeks of pregnancy.

Tell your doctor or healthcare professional if you or your child expect to have contact with someone who falls into one of these groups.

What are the possible side effects of VARIVAX?

The most common side effects reported after taking VARIVAX are:
- Fever
- Pain, swelling, itching, or redness at the site of the shot
- Chickenpox-like rash on the body or at the site of the shot
- Irritability

Other less common side effects have also been reported.
- Tingling of the skin
- Shingles

Tell your healthcare professional if you have any of the following problems within a short time after getting VARIVAX because they may be signs of an allergic reaction:
- Shortness of breath or wheezing
- Rash or hives

Other side effects have been reported. Some of them were serious. These include bruising more easily than normal; red or purple, flat, pinhead spots under the skin; severe paleness; difficulty walking; severe skin disorders; skin infection; and chickenpox. Rarely, swelling of the brain, stroke, inflammation of the lungs (known as pneumonia or pneumonitis), and seizures with or without a fever have been reported. It is not known if these rare side effects are related to the vaccine.
Your doctor has a more complete list of side effects for VARIVAX.
Tell your doctor or healthcare professional if you or your child have any new or unusual symptoms after getting VARIVAX.
You may also report any adverse reactions to your doctor or your child's doctor or directly to the Vaccine Adverse Event Reporting System (VAERS). The VAERS toll-free number is 1-800-822-7967 or report online to www.vaers.hhs.gov.

What are the ingredients of VARIVAX?

Active Ingredient: a weakened form of chickenpox virus.
Inactive Ingredients: sucrose, hydrolyzed gelatin, sodium chloride, monosodium L-glutamate, sodium phosphate dibasic, potassium phosphate monobasic, potassium chloride, residual components of MRC-5 cells including DNA and protein, sodium phosphate monobasic, EDTA, neomycin, fetal bovine serum.

What else should I know about VARIVAX?

If you get VARIVAX while you are pregnant, please call 1-800-986-8999. Or, you can have your healthcare professional call.
This leaflet summarizes important information about VARIVAX.
If you would like more information, talk to your healthcare professional, visit the web site at www.merckvaccines.com, or call 1-800-Merck-90.

Rx Only

Dist by: Merck Sharp & Dohme Corp., a subsidiary of **MERCK & CO., INC.**, Whitehouse Station, NJ 08889, USA

USPPI-I-V2101212R706

VICTRELIS® ℞

[vĭc-TRĔL-ĭs]
(boceprevir)
Capsules for oral use

HIGHLIGHTS OF PRESCRIBING INFORMATION
These highlights do not include all the information needed to use VICTRELIS safely and effectively. See full prescribing information for VICTRELIS.
VICTRELIS® (boceprevir) Capsules for oral use
Initial U.S. Approval: 2011

RECENT MAJOR CHANGES

Indications and Usage (1)	02/2013
Dosage and Administration (2.1, 2.3)	02/2013
Contraindications (4)	11/2012
Warnings and Precautions	
Pregnancy (Use with Ribavirin and Peginterferon Alfa) (5.1)	02/2013
Anemia (Use with Ribavirin and Peginterferon Alfa) (5.2)	02/2013
Neutropenia (Use with Ribavirin and Peginterferon Alfa) (5.3)	02/2013
Hypersensitivity (5.4)	11/2012
Laboratory Tests (5.6)	02/2013

INDICATIONS AND USAGE

VICTRELIS is a hepatitis C virus (HCV) NS3/4A protease inhibitor indicated for the treatment of chronic hepatitis C (CHC) genotype 1 infection, in combination with peginterferon alfa and ribavirin, in adult patients (18 years of age or older) with compensated liver disease, including cirrhosis, who are previously untreated or who have failed previous interferon and ribavirin therapy, including prior null responders, partial responders, and relapsers. (1)
- VICTRELIS must not be used as a monotherapy and should only be used in combination with peginterferon alfa and ribavirin. (1)
- The efficacy of VICTRELIS has not been studied in patients who have previously failed therapy with a treatment regimen that includes VICTRELIS or other HCV NS3/4A protease inhibitors. (1)

DOSAGE AND ADMINISTRATION

- 800 mg administered orally three times daily (every 7 to 9 hours) with food (a meal or light snack). (2)
- VICTRELIS must be administered in combination with peginterferon alfa and ribavirin. Initiate therapy with peginterferon alfa and ribavirin for 4 weeks, then add VICTRELIS to peginterferon alfa and ribavirin regimen. The duration of treatment is based on viral response, prior response status and presence of cirrhosis. (2)
- Refer to peginterferon alfa and ribavirin Package Inserts for specific dosing instructions. (2)

DOSAGE FORMS AND STRENGTHS

Capsules: 200 mg (3)

CONTRAINDICATIONS

- **All contraindications to peginterferon alfa and ribavirin also apply since VICTRELIS must be administered with peginterferon alfa and ribavirin. (4)**
- Because ribavirin may cause birth defects and fetal death, boceprevir in combination with peginterferon alfa and ribavirin is contraindicated in pregnant women and in men whose female partners are pregnant. (4)
- Contraindicated in patients with a history of a hypersensitivity reaction to boceprevir. (4)
- Coadministration with drugs that are highly dependent on CYP3A4/5 for clearance, and for which elevated plasma concentrations are associated with serious and/or life-threatening events is contraindicated. (4)
- Coadministration with potent CYP3A4/5 inducers where significantly reduced boceprevir plasma concentrations may be associated with reduced efficacy is contraindicated. (4)

WARNINGS AND PRECAUTIONS

Use of VICTRELIS with Ribavirin and Peginterferon alfa:
- **Ribavirin may cause birth defects and fetal death; avoid pregnancy in female patients and female partners of male patients.** Patients must have a negative pregnancy test prior to therapy; use two or more forms of contraception, and have monthly pregnancy tests. (5.1)
- Anemia - The addition of VICTRELIS to peginterferon alfa and ribavirin is associated with an additional decrease in hemoglobin concentrations compared with peginterferon alfa and ribavirin alone. (5.2)
- Neutropenia - The addition of VICTRELIS to peginterferon alfa and ribavirin may result in worsening of neutropenia associated with peginterferon alfa and ribavirin therapy alone. (5.3)
- Hypersensitivity – Serious acute hypersensitivity reactions (e.g., urticaria, angioedema) have been observed during combination therapy with VICTRELIS, peginterferon alfa and ribavirin. (5.4)

ADVERSE REACTIONS

The most commonly reported adverse reactions (greater than 35% of subjects) in clinical trials in adult subjects receiving the combination of VICTRELIS with PegIntron and REBETOL were fatigue, anemia, nausea, headache and dysgeusia. (6.1)
To report SUSPECTED ADVERSE REACTIONS, contact Merck Sharp & Dohme Corp., a subsidiary of Merck & Co., Inc., at 1-877-888-4231 or FDA at 1-800-FDA-1088 or www.fda.gov/medwatch.

DRUG INTERACTIONS

- VICTRELIS is a strong inhibitor of CYP3A4/5 and is partly metabolized by CYP3A4/5. The potential for drug-drug interactions must be considered prior to and during therapy. (4, 7, 12.3)

USE IN SPECIFIC POPULATIONS

- Cirrhosis: Safety and efficacy have not been studied in patients with decompensated cirrhosis or in patients with an organ transplant. (8.7, 8.10)
- Co-infection with Human Immunodeficiency Virus (HIV): Safety and efficacy have not been established in patients co-infected with HCV and HIV. (8.8)
- Co-infection with Hepatitis B Virus (HBV): Safety and efficacy have not been studied in patients co-infected with HCV and HBV. (8.9)
- Pediatrics: Safety and efficacy have not been studied in pediatric patients. (8.4)

See 17 for PATIENT COUNSELING INFORMATION and Medication Guide

Revised: 02/2013

FULL PRESCRIBING INFORMATION: CONTENTS*

*** Sections or subsections omitted from the full prescribing information are not listed**

FULL PRESCRIBING INFORMATION

1 INDICATIONS AND USAGE

VICTRELIS® (boceprevir) is indicated for the treatment of chronic hepatitis C genotype 1 infection, in combination with peginterferon alfa and ribavirin, in adult patients (18 years and older) with compensated liver disease, including cirrhosis, who are previously untreated or who have failed previous interferon and ribavirin therapy, including prior null responders, partial responders, and relapsers *[see Clinical Studies (14)]*.

The following points should be considered when initiating VICTRELIS for treatment of chronic hepatitis C infection:

- VICTRELIS must not be used as monotherapy and should only be used in combination with peginterferon alfa and ribavirin.
- The efficacy of VICTRELIS has not been studied in patients who have previously failed therapy with a treatment regimen that includes VICTRELIS or other HCV NS3/4A protease inhibitors.
- Poorly interferon responsive patients who were treated with VICTRELIS in combination with peginterferon alfa and ribavirin have a lower likelihood of achieving a sustained virologic response (SVR), and a higher rate of detection of resistance-associated substitutions upon treatment failure, compared to patients with a greater response to peginterferon alfa and ribavirin *[see Microbiology (12.4) and Clinical Studies (14)]*.

2 DOSAGE AND ADMINISTRATION

VICTRELIS must be administered in combination with peginterferon alfa and ribavirin. The dose of VICTRELIS is 800 mg (four 200-mg capsules) three times daily (every 7 to 9 hours) with food [a meal or light snack] (see Table 1). Refer to the peginterferon alfa and ribavirin Package Inserts for instructions on dosing.

The following dosing recommendations differ for some subgroups from the dosing studied in the Phase 3 trials *[see Clinical Studies (14)]*. Response-Guided Therapy (RGT) is recommended for most individuals, but longer dosing is recommended in targeted subgroups (e.g., patients with cirrhosis).

Table 1 Duration of Therapy in Patients Without Cirrhosis Who Are Previously Untreated or Who Previously Failed Interferon and Ribavirin Therapy

	ASSESSMENT* (HCV-RNA Results†)		RECOMMENDATION
	At Treatment Week 8	At Treatment Week 24	
Previously Untreated Patients	Not Detected	Not Detected	Complete three-medicine regimen at TW28.
	Detected	Not Detected	1. Continue all three medicines and finish through TW36; and then 2. Administer peginterferon alfa and ribavirin and finish through TW48.
Previous Partial Responders or Relapsers‡	Not Detected	Not Detected	Complete three-medicine regimen at TW36.
	Detected	Not Detected	1. Continue all three medicines and finish through TW36; and then 2. Administer peginterferon alfa and ribavirin and finish through TW48.
Previous Null Responders‡	Detected or Not Detected	Not Detected	Continue all three medicines and finish through TW48.

* **TREATMENT FUTILITY**
If the patient has HCV-RNA results greater than or equal to 100 IU/mL at TW12, then discontinue three-medicine regimen.
If the patient has confirmed, detectable HCV-RNA at TW24, then discontinue three-medicine regimen.
† "Not Detected" refers to HCV-RNA assay results reported as "Target Not Detected" or "HCV-RNA Not Detected". In clinical trials, HCV-RNA in plasma was measured using a Roche COBAS® TaqMan® assay with a lower limit of quantification of 25 IU/mL and a limit of detection of 9.3 IU/mL. See Warnings and Precautions (5.6) for a description of HCV-RNA assay recommendations.
‡ *See Clinical Studies (14)* for definitions of previous response to interferon and ribavirin therapy.

Table 2 Drugs that are contraindicated with VICTRELIS

Drug Class	Drugs Within Class that are Contraindicated With VICTRELIS	Clinical Comments
Alpha 1-Adrenoreceptor antagonist	Alfuzosin	Increased alfuzosin concentrations can result in hypotension.
Anticonvulsants	Carbamazepine, phenobarbital, phenytoin	May lead to loss of virologic response to VICTRELIS
Antimycobacterial Agents	Rifampin	May lead to loss of virologic response to VICTRELIS.
Ergot Derivatives	Dihydroergotamine, ergonovine, ergotamine, methylergonovine	Potential for acute ergot toxicity characterized by peripheral vasospasm and ischemia of the extremities and other tissues.
GI Motility Agent	Cisapride	Potential for cardiac arrhythmias.
Herbal Products	St. John's Wort (hypericum perforatum)	May lead to loss of virologic response to VICTRELIS.
HMG-CoA Reductase Inhibitors	Lovastatin, simvastatin	Potential for myopathy, including rhabdomyolysis.
Oral Contraceptives	Drospirenone	Potential for hyperkalemia.
PDE5 enzyme Inhibitor	REVATIO® (sildenafil) or ADCIRCA® (tadalafil) when used for the treatment of pulmonary arterial hypertension*	Potential for PDE5 inhibitor-associated adverse events, including visual abnormalities, hypotension, prolonged erection, and syncope.
Neuroleptic	Pimozide	Potential for cardiac arrhythmias.
Sedative/Hypnotics	Triazolam; orally administered midazolam†	Prolonged or increased sedation or respiratory depression.

* See *Drug Interactions, Table 5* for coadministration of sildenafil and tadalafil when dosed for erectile dysfunction.
† See *Drug Interactions, Table 5* for parenterally administered midazolam.

2.1 VICTRELIS/Peginterferon alfa/Ribavirin Combination Therapy: Patients Without Cirrhosis Who Are Previously Untreated or Who Previously Failed Interferon and Ribavirin Therapy

- Initiate therapy with peginterferon alfa and ribavirin for 4 weeks (Treatment Weeks 1–4).
- Add VICTRELIS 800 mg (four 200-mg capsules) orally three times daily (every 7 to 9 hours) to peginterferon alfa and ribavirin regimen after 4 weeks of treatment. Based on the patient's HCV-RNA levels at Treatment Week (TW) 8, TW12 and TW24, use the following guidelines to determine duration of treatment (see Table 1).

[See table 1 above]

Consideration should be given to treating previously untreated patients who are poorly interferon responsive (as determined at TW4) with 4 weeks peginterferon alfa and ribavirin followed by 44 weeks of VICTRELIS 800 mg orally three times daily (every 7 to 9 hours) in combination with peginterferon alfa and ribavirin in order to maximize rates of SVR.

2.2 VICTRELIS/Peginterferon alfa/Ribavirin Combination Therapy: Patients with Cirrhosis

Patients with compensated cirrhosis should receive 4 weeks peginterferon alfa and ribavirin followed by 44 weeks

VICTRELIS 800 mg (four 200-mg capsules) three times daily (every 7 to 9 hours) in combination with peginterferon alfa and ribavirin.

2.3 Dose Modification

Dose reduction of VICTRELIS is not recommended.

If a patient has a serious adverse reaction potentially related to peginterferon alfa and/or ribavirin, the peginterferon alfa and/or ribavirin dose should be reduced or discontinued. Refer to the peginterferon alfa and ribavirin Package Inserts for additional information about how to reduce and/or discontinue the peginterferon alfa and/or ribavirin dose. VICTRELIS must not be administered in the absence of peginterferon alfa and ribavirin. If peginterferon alfa or ribavirin is permanently discontinued, VICTRELIS must also be discontinued.

2.4 Discontinuation of Dosing Based on Treatment Futility

Discontinuation of therapy is recommended in all patients with 1) HCV-RNA levels of greater than or equal to 100 IU per mL at TW12; or 2) confirmed detectable HCV-RNA levels at TW24.

3 DOSAGE FORMS AND STRENGTHS

VICTRELIS 200 mg Capsules, red-colored cap with the Merck logo printed in yellow ink, and a yellow-colored body with "314" printed in red ink.

4 CONTRAINDICATIONS

Contraindications to peginterferon alfa and ribavirin also apply to VICTRELIS combination treatment.

VICTRELIS in combination with peginterferon alfa and ribavirin is contraindicated in:

- Pregnant women and men whose female partners are pregnant because of the risks for birth defects and fetal death associated with ribavirin *[see Warnings and Precautions (5.1) and Use in Specific Populations (8.1)]*.
- Patients with a history of a hypersensitivity reaction to boceprevir *[see Warnings and Precautions (5.4)]*.

Coadministration with drugs that are highly dependent on CYP3A4/5 for clearance, and for which elevated plasma concentrations are associated with serious and/or life-threatening events, including those in Table 2, is contraindicated *[see also Drug Interactions (7)]*.

Coadministration with potent CYP3A4/5 inducers, where significantly reduced boceprevir plasma concentrations may be associated with reduced efficacy, including those in Table 2, is contraindicated *[see also Drug Interactions (7)]*.

[See table 2 at top of previous page]

5 WARNINGS AND PRECAUTIONS

5.1 Pregnancy (Use with Ribavirin and Peginterferon Alfa)

Ribavirin may cause birth defects and/or death of the exposed fetus. Extreme care must be taken to avoid pregnancy in female patients and in female partners of male patients. Ribavirin therapy should not be started unless a report of a negative pregnancy test has been obtained immediately prior to initiation of therapy. Women of childbearing potential and men must use at least two forms of effective contraception during treatment and for at least 6 months after treatment has concluded. One of these forms of contraception can be a combined oral contraceptive product containing at least 1 mg of norethindrone. Oral contraceptives containing lower doses of norethindrone and other forms of hormonal contraception have not been studied or are contraindicated. Routine monthly pregnancy tests must be performed during this time *[see Contraindications (4) and Drug Interactions (7)]*.

5.2 Anemia (Use with Ribavirin and Peginterferon Alfa)

Anemia has been reported with peginterferon alfa and ribavirin therapy. The addition of VICTRELIS to peginterferon alfa and ribavirin is associated with an additional decrease in hemoglobin concentrations. Complete blood counts should be obtained pretreatment, and at Treatment Weeks 2, 4, 8, and 12, and should be monitored closely at other time points, as clinically appropriate. If hemoglobin is less than 10 g per dL, a decrease in dosage or interruption of ribavirin is recommended; and if hemoglobin is less than 8.5 g per dL, discontinuation of ribavirin is recommended *[see Adverse Reactions (6.1) and Clinical Studies (14)]*. If ribavirin is permanently discontinued for management of anemia, then peginterferon alfa and VICTRELIS must also be discontinued *[see Dosage and Administration (2.3)]*.

Refer to the Package Insert for ribavirin for additional information regarding dosage reduction and/or interruption.

In clinical trials with VICTRELIS, the proportion of subjects who experienced hemoglobin values less than 10 g per dL and less than 8.5 g per dL was higher in subjects treated with the combination of VICTRELIS with PegIntron®/REBETOL® than in those treated with PegIntron/REBETOL alone (see Table 4). With the interventions used for anemia management in the clinical trials, the average additional decrease of hemoglobin was approximately 1 g per dL.

Table 3 Adverse Events Reported in ≥10% of Subjects Receiving the Combination of VICTRELIS with PegIntron/REBETOL and Reported at a Rate of ≥5% than PegIntron/REBETOL alone

Adverse Events	Previously Untreated (SPRINT-1 & SPRINT-2)		Previous Treatment Failures (RESPOND-2)	
	Percentage of Subjects Reporting Adverse Events		Percentage of Subjects Reporting Adverse Events	
Body System Organ Class	VICTRELIS + PegIntron + REBETOL (n=1225)	PegIntron + REBETOL (n=467)	VICTRELIS + PegIntron + REBETOL (n=323)	PegIntron + REBETOL (n=80)
Median Exposure (days)	**197**	**216**	**253**	**104**
Blood and Lymphatic System Disorders				
Anemia	50	30	45	20
Neutropenia	25	19	14	10
Gastrointestinal Disorders				
Nausea	46	42	43	38
Dysgeusia	35	16	44	11
Diarrhea	25	22	24	16
Vomiting	20	13	15	8
Dry Mouth	11	10	15	9
General Disorders and Administration Site Conditions				
Fatigue	58	59	55	50
Chills	34	29	33	30
Asthenia	15	18	21	16
Metabolism and Nutrition Disorders				
Decreased Appetite	25	24	26	16
Musculoskeletal and Connective Tissue Disorders				
Arthralgia	19	19	23	16
Nervous System Disorders				
Dizziness	19	16	16	10
Psychiatric Disorders				
Insomnia	34	34	30	24
Irritability	22	23	21	13
Respiratory, Thoracic, and Mediastinal Disorders				
Dyspnea Exertional	8	8	11	5
Skin and Subcutaneous Tissue Disorders				
Alopecia	27	27	22	16
Dry Skin	18	18	22	9
Rash	17	19	16	6

In clinical trials, the median time to onset of hemoglobin less than 10 g per dL from the initiation of therapy was similar among subjects treated with the combination of VICTRELIS and PegIntron/REBETOL (71 days with a range of 15-337 days), compared to those who received PegIntron/REBETOL (71 days with a range of 8-337 days). Certain adverse reactions consistent with symptoms of anemia, such as dyspnea, exertional dyspnea, dizziness and syncope were reported more frequently in subjects who received the combination of VICTRELIS with PegIntron/REBETOL than in those treated with PegIntron/REBETOL alone *[see Adverse Reactions (6.1)]*.

In clinical trials with VICTRELIS, dose modifications (generally of PegIntron/REBETOL) due to anemia occurred twice as often in subjects treated with the combination of VICTRELIS with PegIntron/REBETOL (26%) compared to PegIntron/REBETOL (13%). The proportion of subjects who discontinued study drug due to anemia was 1% in subjects treated with the combination of VICTRELIS with PegIntron/REBETOL and 1% in subjects who received PegIntron/REBETOL. The use of erythropoiesis stimulating agents (ESAs) was permitted for management of anemia, at the investigator's discretion, with or without ribavirin dose reduction in the Phase 2 and 3 clinical trials. The proportion of subjects who received an ESA was 43% in those treated with the combination of VICTRELIS with PegIntron/REBETOL compared to 24% in those treated with PegIntron/REBETOL alone. The proportion of subjects who received a transfusion for the management of anemia was 3% of subjects treated with the combination of VICTRELIS with PegIntron/REBETOL compared to less than 1% in subjects who received PegIntron/REBETOL alone.

Thromboembolic events have been associated with ESA use in other disease states; and have also been reported with peginterferon alfa use in hepatitis C patients. Thromboembolic events were reported in clinical trials with VICTRELIS among subjects receiving the combination of VICTRELIS with PegIntron/REBETOL, and among those receiving PegIntron/REBETOL alone, regardless of ESA use. No definite causality assessment or benefit risk assessment could be made for these events due to the presence of confounding factors and lack of randomization of ESA use.

A randomized, parallel-arm, open-label clinical trial was conducted in previously untreated CHC subjects with genotype 1 infection to compare use of an ESA versus ribavirin dose reduction for initial management of anemia during

Table 4 Selected Hematological Parameters

	Previously Untreated (SPRINT-1 & SPRINT-2)		Previous Treatment Failures (RESPOND-2)	
	Percentage of Subjects Reporting Selected Hematological Parameters		Percentage of Subjects Reporting Selected Hematological Parameters	
Hematological Parameters	VICTRELIS + PegIntron + REBETOL (n=1225)	PegIntron + REBETOL (n=467)	VICTRELIS + PegIntron + REBETOL (n=323)	PegIntron + REBETOL (n=80)
Hemoglobin (g/dL)				
<10	49	29	49	25
<8.5	6	3	10	1
Neutrophils ($\times 10^9$/L)				
<0.75	31	18	26	13
<0.5	8	4	7	4
Platelets ($\times 10^9$/L)				
<50	3	1	4	0
<25	<1	0	0	0

therapy with VICTRELIS in combination with peginterferon alfa-2b and ribavirin. Similar SVR rates were reported in subjects who were randomized to receive ribavirin dose reduction compared to subjects who were randomized to receive an ESA. In this trial, use of ESAs was associated with an increased risk of thromboembolic events including pulmonary embolism, acute myocardial infarction, cerebrovascular accident, and deep vein thrombosis compared to ribavirin dose reduction alone. The treatment discontinuation rate due to anemia was similar in subjects randomized to receive ribavirin dose reduction compared to subjects randomized to receive ESA (2% in each group). The transfusion rate was 4% in subjects randomized to receive ribavirin dose reduction and 2% in subjects randomized to receive ESA.

Ribavirin dose reduction is recommended for the initial management of anemia.

5.3 Neutropenia (Use with Ribavirin and Peginterferon Alfa)

In Phase 2 and 3 clinical trials, seven percent of subjects receiving the combination of VICTRELIS with PegIntron/REBETOL had neutrophil counts of less than 0.5×10^9 per L compared to 4% of subjects receiving PegIntron/REBETOL alone (see Table 4). Three subjects experienced severe or life-threatening infections associated with neutropenia, and two subjects experienced life-threatening neutropenia while receiving the combination of VICTRELIS with PegIntron/REBETOL. Complete blood count (with white blood cell differential counts) must be conducted in all patients prior to initiating VICTRELIS/peginterferon alfa/ribavirin combination therapy. Complete blood counts should be obtained at Treatment Weeks 4, 8, and 12, and should be monitored closely at other time points, as clinically appropriate. Decreases in neutrophil counts may require dose reduction or discontinuation of peginterferon alfa and ribavirin. If peginterferon alfa and ribavirin are permanently discontinued, then VICTRELIS must also be discontinued *[see Dosage and Administration (2.3)]*.

Refer to Package Inserts for peginterferon alfa and ribavirin for additional information regarding dose reduction or discontinuation for peginterferon alfa and ribavirin.

5.4 Hypersensitivity

Serious acute hypersensitivity reactions (e.g., urticaria, angioedema) have been observed during combination therapy with VICTRELIS, peginterferon alfa and ribavirin. If such an acute reaction occurs, combination therapy should be discontinued and appropriate medical therapy immediately instituted *[see Contraindications (4) and Adverse Reactions (6.2)]*.

5.5 Drug Interactions

See Table 2 for a listing of drugs that are contraindicated for use with VICTRELIS due to potentially life-threatening adverse events, significant drug interactions or loss of virologic activity *[see Contraindications (4)]*. Please refer to Table 5 for established and other potentially significant drug interactions *[see Drug Interactions (7.3)]*.

5.6 Laboratory Tests

HCV-RNA levels should be monitored at Treatment Weeks 4, 8, 12, and 24, at the end of treatment, during treatment follow-up, and for other time points as clinically indicated. Use of a sensitive real-time reverse-transcription polymerase chain reaction (RT-PCR) assay for monitoring HCV-RNA levels during treatment is recommended. The assay should have a lower limit of HCV-RNA quantification of equal to or less than 25 IU per mL, and a limit of HCV-RNA detection of approximately 10 to 15 IU per mL. For the purposes of assessing Response-Guided Therapy milestones, a confirmed "detectable but below limit of quantification" HCV-RNA result should not be considered equivalent to an "undetectable" HCV-RNA result (reported as "Target Not Detected" or "HCV-RNA Not Detected").

Complete blood count (with white blood cell differential counts) must be conducted in all patients prior to initiating VICTRELIS/peginterferon alfa/ribavirin combination therapy. Complete blood counts should be obtained at Treatment Weeks 2, 4, 8, and 12, and should be monitored closely at other time points, as clinically appropriate.

Refer to the Package Inserts for peginterferon alfa and ribavirin, including pregnancy testing requirements.

6 ADVERSE REACTIONS

See peginterferon alfa and ribavirin Package Inserts for description of adverse reactions associated with their use.

6.1 Clinical Trials Experience

Because clinical trials are conducted under widely varying conditions, adverse reaction rates observed in clinical trials of VICTRELIS cannot be directly compared to rates in the clinical trials of another drug and may not reflect the rates observed in practice.

The following serious and otherwise important adverse drug reactions (ADRs) are discussed in detail in another section of the labeling:

- Anemia *[see Warnings and Precautions (5.2) and Patient Counseling Information (17.2)]*
- Neutropenia *[see Warnings and Precautions (5.3) and Patient Counseling Information (17.3)]*
- Hypersensitivity *[see Contraindications (4), Warnings and Precautions (5.4) and Patient Counseling Information (17.4)]*

The most commonly reported adverse reactions (more than 35% of subjects regardless of investigator's causality assessment) in adult subjects were fatigue, anemia, nausea, headache, and dysgeusia when VICTRELIS was used in combination with PegIntron and REBETOL.

The safety of the combination of VICTRELIS 800 mg three times daily with PegIntron/REBETOL was assessed in 2095 subjects with chronic hepatitis C in one Phase 2, open-label trial and two Phase 3, randomized, double-blind, placebo-controlled clinical trials. SPRINT-1 (subjects who were previously untreated) evaluated the use of VICTRELIS in combination with PegIntron/REBETOL with or without a four-week lead-in period with PegIntron/REBETOL compared to PegIntron/REBETOL alone. SPRINT-2 (subjects who were previously untreated) and RESPOND-2 (subjects who had failed previous therapy) evaluated the use of VICTRELIS 800 mg three times daily in combination with PegIntron/REBETOL with a four-week lead-in period with PegIntron/REBETOL compared to PegIntron/REBETOL alone *[see Clinical Studies (14)]*. The population studied had a mean age of 49 years (3% of subjects were older than 65 years of age), 39% were female, 82% were white and 15% were black.

During the four week lead-in period with PegIntron/REBETOL in subjects treated with the combination of VICTRELIS with PegIntron/REBETOL, 28/1263 (2%) subjects experienced adverse reactions leading to discontinuation of treatment. During the entire course of treatment, the proportion of subjects who discontinued treatment due to adverse reactions was 13% for subjects receiving the combination of VICTRELIS with PegIntron/REBETOL and 12% for subjects receiving PegIntron/REBETOL alone. Events resulting in discontinuation were similar to those seen in previous studies with PegIntron/REBETOL. Only anemia and fatigue were reported as events that led to discontinuation in more than 1% of subjects in any arm.

Adverse reactions that led to dose modifications of any drug (primarily PegIntron and REBETOL) occurred in 39% of subjects receiving the combination of VICTRELIS with PegIntron/REBETOL compared to 24% of subjects receiving PegIntron/REBETOL alone. The most common reason for dose reduction was anemia, which occurred more frequently in subjects receiving the combination of VICTRELIS with PegIntron/REBETOL than in subjects receiving PegIntron/REBETOL alone.

Serious adverse events were reported in 11% of subjects receiving the combination of VICTRELIS with PegIntron/REBETOL and in 8% of subjects receiving PegIntron/REBETOL.

Adverse events (regardless of investigator's causality assessment) reported in greater than or equal to 10% of subjects receiving the combination of VICTRELIS with PegIntron/REBETOL and reported at a rate of greater than or equal to 5% than PegIntron/REBETOL alone in SPRINT-1, SPRINT-2, and RESPOND-2 are presented in Table 3.

[See table 3 at top of previous page]

Other Important Adverse Reactions Reported in Clinical Trials

Among subjects (previously untreated subjects or those who failed previous therapy) who received VICTRELIS in combination with peginterferon alfa and ribavirin, the following adverse drug reactions were reported. These events are notable because of their seriousness, severity, or increased frequency in subjects who received VICTRELIS in combination with peginterferon alfa and ribavirin compared with subjects who received only peginterferon alfa and ribavirin.

Gastrointestinal Disorders

Dysgeusia (alteration of taste) was an adverse event reported at an increased frequency in subjects receiving VICTRELIS in combination with peginterferon alfa and ribavirin compared with subjects receiving peginterferon alfa and ribavirin alone (Table 3). Adverse events such as dry mouth, nausea, vomiting and diarrhea were also reported at an increased frequency in subjects receiving VICTRELIS in combination with peginterferon alfa and ribavirin.

Laboratory Values

Changes in selected hematological parameters during treatment of adult subjects with the combination of VICTRELIS with PegIntron and REBETOL are described in Table 4.

Hemoglobin

Decreases in hemoglobin may require a decrease in dosage/interruption or discontinuation of ribavirin *[see Warnings and Precautions (5.2) and Clinical Studies (14); see Package Insert for ribavirin]*. If ribavirin is permanently discontinued, then peginterferon alfa and VICTRELIS must also be discontinued *[see Dosage and Administration (2.3)]*.

Neutrophils and Platelets

The proportion of subjects with decreased neutrophil and platelet counts was higher in subjects treated with VICTRELIS in combination with PegIntron/REBETOL compared to subjects receiving PegIntron/REBETOL alone. Three percent of subjects receiving the combination of VICTRELIS with PegIntron/REBETOL had platelet counts of less than 50×10^9 per L compared to 1% of subjects receiving PegIntron/REBETOL alone. Decreases in neutrophils or platelets may require a decrease in dosage or interruption of peginterferon alfa, or discontinuation of therapy *[see Package Inserts for peginterferon alfa and ribavirin]*. If peginterferon alfa is permanently discontinued, then ribavirin and VICTRELIS must also be discontinued *[see Dosage and Administration (2.3)]*.

[See table 4 above]

6.2 Postmarketing Experience

The following adverse reactions have been identified during post-approval use of VICTRELIS in combination with peginterferon alfa and ribavirin. Because these reactions are reported voluntarily from a population of uncertain size, it is not always possible to reliably estimate their frequency or establish a causal relationship to drug exposure.

Gastrointestinal Disorders: mouth ulceration, stomatitis

Skin and Subcutaneous Tissue Disorders: angioedema, urticaria *[see Warnings and Precautions (5.4)]*; drug rash with eosinophilia and systemic symptoms (DRESS) syndrome, exfoliative rash, exfoliative dermatitis, Stevens-Johnson syndrome, toxic skin eruption, toxicoderma

Table 5 Established and Other Potentially Significant Drug Interactions

Concomitant Drug Class: Drug Name	Effect on Concentration of Boceprevir or Concomitant Drug	Recommendations
Antiarrhythmics: amiodarone, bepridil, propafenone, quinidine	↑ antiarrhythmics	Coadministration with VICTRELIS has the potential to produce serious and/or life-threatening adverse events and has not been studied. Caution is warranted and therapeutic concentration monitoring of these drugs is recommended if they are used concomitantly with VICTRELIS.
digoxin	↑ digoxin	Digoxin concentrations increased when administered with VICTRELIS *[see Clinical Pharmacology (12.3)]*. Measure serum digoxin concentrations before initiating VICTRELIS. Continue monitoring digoxin concentrations; consult the digoxin prescribing information for information on titrating the digoxin dose.
Anticoagulant: warfarin	↑ or ↓ warfarin	Concentrations of warfarin may be altered when co-administered with VICTRELIS. Monitor INR closely.
Antidepressants: trazodone, desipramine	↑ trazodone ↑ desipramine	Plasma concentrations of trazodone and desipramine may increase when administered with VICTRELIS, resulting in adverse events such as dizziness, hypotension and syncope. Use with caution and consider a lower dose of trazodone or desipramine.
escitalopram	↓escitalopram	Exposure of escitalopram was slightly decreased when coadministered with VICTRELIS. Selective serotonin reuptake inhibitors such as escitalopram have a wide therapeutic index, but doses may need to be adjusted when combined with VICTRELIS.
Antifungals: ketoconazole*, itraconazole, posaconazole, voriconazole	↑ boceprevir ↑ itraconazole ↑ ketoconazole ↑ posaconazole ↑ voriconazole	Plasma concentrations of ketoconazole, itraconazole, voriconazole or posaconazole may be increased with VICTRELIS. When coadministration is required, doses of ketoconazole and itraconazole should not exceed 200 mg/day.
Anti-gout: colchicine	↑ colchicine	Significant increases in colchicine levels are expected; fatal colchicine toxicity has been reported with other strong CYP3A4 inhibitors. Patients with renal or hepatic impairment should not be given colchicine with VICTRELIS. Treatment of gout flares (during treatment with VICTRELIS): 0.6 mg (1 tablet) × 1 dose, followed by 0.3 mg (half tablet) 1 hour later. Dose to be repeated no earlier than 3 days. Prophylaxis of gout flares (during treatment with VICTRELIS): If the original regimen was 0.6 mg twice a day, reduce dose to 0.3 mg once a day. If the original regimen was 0.6 mg once a day, reduce the dose to 0.3 mg once every other day. Treatment of familial Mediterranean fever (FMF) (during treatment with VICTRELIS): Maximum daily dose of 0.6 mg (may be given as 0.3 mg twice a day).
Anti-infective: clarithromycin	↑ clarithromycin	Concentrations of clarithromycin may be increased with VICTRELIS; however, no dosage adjustment is necessary for patients with normal renal function.
Antimycobacterial: rifabutin	↓ boceprevir ↑ rifabutin	Increases in rifabutin exposure are anticipated, while exposure of boceprevir may be decreased. Doses have not been established for the 2 drugs when used in combination. Concomitant use is not recommended.
Calcium Channel Blockers, dihydropyridine: felodipine, nifedipine, nicardipine	↑ dihydropyridine calcium channel blockers	Plasma concentrations of dihydropyridine calcium channel blockers may increase when administered with VICTRELIS. Caution is warranted and clinical monitoring is recommended.
Corticosteroid, systemic: dexamethasone	↓ boceprevir	Coadministration of VICTRELIS with CYP3A4/5 inducers may decrease plasma concentrations of boceprevir, which may result in loss of therapeutic effect. Therefore, this combination should be avoided if possible and used with caution if necessary.
prednisone*	↑ prednisone	Concentrations of prednisone and its active metabolite, prednisolone, increased when administered with VICTRELIS *[see Clinical Pharmacology (12.3)]*. No dose adjustment of prednisone is necessary when co-administered with VICTRELIS. Patients receiving prednisone and VICTRELIS should be monitored appropriately.

(Table continued on next page)

7 DRUG INTERACTIONS

See also *Contraindications (4), Warnings and Precautions (5.5),* and *Clinical Pharmacology (12.3).*

7.1 Potential for VICTRELIS to Affect Other Drugs

Boceprevir is a strong inhibitor of CYP3A4/5. Drugs metabolized primarily by CYP3A4/5 may have increased exposure when administered with VICTRELIS, which could increase or prolong their therapeutic and adverse effects. Boceprevir does not inhibit CYP1A2, CYP2A6, CYP2B6, CYP2C8, CYP2C9, CYP2C19, CYP2D6 or CYP2E1 *in vitro*. In addition, boceprevir does not induce CYP1A2, CYP2B6, CYP2C8, CYP2C9, CYP2C19 or CYP3A4/5 *in vitro*.

Boceprevir is a potential inhibitor of p-glycoprotein (P-gp) based on *in vitro* studies. In a drug interaction trial conducted with digoxin, VICTRELIS had limited p-glycoprotein inhibitory potential at clinically relevant concentrations.

7.2 Potential for Other Drugs to Affect VICTRELIS

Boceprevir is primarily metabolized by aldo-ketoreductase (AKR). In drug interaction trials conducted with AKR inhibitors diflunisal and ibuprofen, boceprevir exposure did not increase to a clinically significant extent. VICTRELIS may be coadministered with AKR inhibitors.

Boceprevir is partly metabolized by CYP3A4/5. It is also a substrate for p-glycoprotein. Coadministration of VICTRELIS with drugs that induce or inhibit CYP3A4/5 could decrease or increase exposure to boceprevir.

7.3 Established and Other Potential Significant Drug Interactions

Table 5 provides recommendations based on established or potentially clinically significant drug interactions. VICTRELIS is contraindicated with drugs that are potent inducers of CYP3A4/5 and drugs that are highly dependent on CYP3A4/5 for clearance, and for which elevated plasma concentrations are associated with serious and/or life-threatening events *[see Contraindications (4)]*.

[See table 5 above and on pages 1824 and 1825]

8 USE IN SPECIFIC POPULATIONS

8.1 Pregnancy

VICTRELIS must be administered in combination with peginterferon alfa and ribavirin *[see Dosage and Administration (2)]*.

Pregnancy Category X: Use with Ribavirin and Peginterferon Alfa

Significant teratogenic and/or embryocidal effects have been demonstrated in all animal species exposed to ribavirin; and therefore ribavirin is contraindicated in women who are pregnant and in the male partners of women who are pregnant *[see Contraindications (4), Warnings and Precautions (5.1) and ribavirin Package Inserts]*. Interferons have abortifacient effects in animals and should be assumed to have abortifacient potential in humans *[see peginterferon alfa Package Inserts]*.

Extreme caution must be taken to avoid pregnancy in female patients and female partners of male patients while taking this combination. Women of childbearing potential and their male partners should not receive ribavirin unless they are using effective contraception (two reliable forms) during treatment with ribavirin and for 6 months after treatment. One of these reliable forms of contraception can be a combined oral contraceptive product containing at least 1 mg of norethindrone. Oral contraceptives containing lower doses of norethindrone and other forms of hormonal contraception have not been studied or are contraindicated *[see Contraindications (4) and Warnings and Precautions (5.1)]*. **In case of exposure during pregnancy, a Ribavirin Pregnancy Registry has been established to monitor maternal-fetal outcomes of pregnancies in female patients and female partners of male patients exposed to ribavirin during treatment and for 6 months following cessation of treatment. Physicians and patients are encouraged to report such cases by calling 1-800-593-2214.**

Pregnancy Category B: VICTRELIS

VICTRELIS must not be used as a monotherapy *[see Indications and Usage (1)]*. There are no adequate and well-controlled studies with VICTRELIS in pregnant women.

No effects on fetal development have been observed in rats and rabbits at boceprevir AUC exposures approximately 11.8- and 2.0-fold higher, respectively, than those in humans at the recommended dose of 800 mg three times daily *[see Nonclinical Toxicology (13.1)]*.

8.3 Nursing Mothers

It is not known whether VICTRELIS is excreted into human breast milk. Levels of boceprevir and/or metabolites in the milk of lactating rats were slightly higher than levels observed in maternal blood. Peak blood concentrations of boceprevir and/or metabolites in nursing pups were less than 1% of those of maternal blood concentrations. Because of the potential for adverse reactions from the drug in nursing infants, a decision must be made whether to discontinue nursing or discontinue treatment with VICTRELIS, taking into account the importance of the therapy to the mother.

8.4 Pediatric Use

The safety, efficacy, and pharmacokinetic profile of VICTRELIS in pediatric patients have not been studied.

8.5 Geriatric Use

Clinical studies of VICTRELIS did not include sufficient numbers of subjects aged 65 and over to determine whether they respond differently from younger subjects. In general, caution should be exercised in the administration and monitoring of VICTRELIS in geriatric patients due to the greater frequency of decreased hepatic function, concomitant diseases and other drug therapy *[see Clinical Pharmacology (12.3)]*.

8.6 Renal Impairment

No dosage adjustment of VICTRELIS is required for patients with any degree of renal impairment *[see Clinical Pharmacology (12.3)]*.

Table 5 *(cont.)* Established and Other Potentially Significant Drug Interactions

Concomitant Drug Class: Drug Name	Effect on Concentration of Boceprevir or Concomitant Drug	Recommendations
Corticosteroid, inhaled: budesonide, fluticasone	↑ budesonide ↑ fluticasone	Concomitant use of inhaled budesonide or fluticasone with VICTRELIS may result in increased plasma concentrations of budesonide or fluticasone, resulting in significantly reduced serum cortisol concentrations. Avoid coadministration if possible, particularly for extended durations.
Endothelin Receptor Antagonist: bosentan	↑ bosentan	Concentrations of bosentan may be increased when coadministered with VICTRELIS. Use with caution and monitor closely.
HIV Integrase Inhibitor: raltegravir*	↔ raltegravir	No dose adjustment required for VICTRELIS or raltegravir.
HIV Non-Nucleoside Reverse Transcriptase Inhibitors: efavirenz*	↓ boceprevir	Plasma trough concentrations of boceprevir were decreased when VICTRELIS was coadministered with efavirenz, which may result in loss of therapeutic effect. Avoid combination.
etravirine*	↓ etravirine	Concentrations of etravirine decreased when coadministered with VICTRELIS. The clinical significance of the reductions in etravirine pharmacokinetic parameters has not been directly assessed.
HIV Protease Inhibitors: atazanavir/ritonavir*	↓ atazanavir ↓ ritonavir	Concomitant administration of boceprevir and atazanavir/ritonavir resulted in reduced steady-state exposures to atazanavir and ritonavir. Coadministration of atazanavir/ritonavir and boceprevir is not recommended.
darunavir/ritonavir*	↓ darunavir ↓ ritonavir ↓ boceprevir	Concomitant administration of boceprevir and darunavir/ritonavir resulted in reduced steady-state exposures to boceprevir, darunavir and ritonavir. Coadministration of darunavir/ritonavir and boceprevir is not recommended.
lopinavir/ritonavir*	↓ lopinavir ↓ ritonavir ↓ boceprevir	Concomitant administration of boceprevir and lopinavir/ritonavir resulted in reduced steady-state exposures to boceprevir, lopinavir and ritonavir. Coadministration of lopinavir/ritonavir and boceprevir is not recommended.
ritonavir*	↓ boceprevir	When boceprevir is administered with ritonavir alone, boceprevir concentrations are decreased.
HMG-CoA Reductase Inhibitors: atorvastatin*	↑ atorvastatin	Exposure to atorvastatin was increased when administered with VICTRELIS. Use the lowest effective dose of atorvastatin, but do not exceed a daily dose of 40 mg when coadministered with VICTRELIS.
pravastatin*	↑ pravastatin	Concomitant administration of pravastatin with VICTRELIS increased exposure to pravastatin. Treatment with pravastatin can be initiated at the recommended dose when coadministered with VICTRELIS. Close clinical monitoring is warranted.
Immunosuppressants: cyclosporine* tacrolimus* sirolimus	↑cyclosporine	Dose adjustments of cyclosporine should be anticipated when administered with VICTRELIS and should be guided by close monitoring of cyclosporine blood concentrations, and frequent assessments of renal function and cyclosporine-related side effects.
	↑tacrolimus	Concomitant administration of VICTRELIS with tacrolimus requires significant dose reduction and prolongation of the dosing interval for tacrolimus, with close monitoring of tacrolimus blood concentrations and frequent assessments of renal function and tacrolimus-related side effects.
	↑sirolimus	Blood concentrations of sirolimus are expected to increase significantly when administered with VICTRELIS. Close monitoring of sirolimus blood levels is recommended.
Inhaled beta-agonist: salmeterol	↑ salmeterol	Concurrent use of inhaled salmeterol and VICTRELIS is not recommended due to the risk of cardiovascular events associated with salmeterol.

(Table continued on next page)

8.7 Hepatic Impairment

No dose adjustment of VICTRELIS is required for patients with mild, moderate or severe hepatic impairment *[see Clinical Pharmacology (12.3)]*. Safety and efficacy of VICTRELIS have not been studied in patients with decompensated cirrhosis. See Package Inserts for peginterferon alfa for contraindication in hepatic decompensation.

8.8 Human Immunodeficiency Virus (HIV) Co-Infection

The safety and efficacy of VICTRELIS alone or in combination with peginterferon alfa and ribavirin for the treatment of chronic hepatitis C genotype 1 infection have not been established in patients co-infected with HIV and HCV. For data regarding drug-drug interactions with antiretroviral agents in healthy subjects, *[see Drug Interactions (7.3)* and *Clinical Pharmacology (12.3)]*.

8.9 Hepatitis B Virus (HBV) Co-Infection

The safety and efficacy of VICTRELIS alone or in combination with peginterferon alfa and ribavirin for the treatment of chronic hepatitis C genotype 1 infection in patients co-infected with HBV and HCV have not been studied.

8.10 Organ Transplantation

The safety and efficacy of VICTRELIS alone or in combination with peginterferon alfa and ribavirin for the treatment of chronic hepatitis C genotype 1 infection in liver or other organ transplant recipients have not been studied. For data regarding drug-drug interactions with immunosuppressants, see *Drug Interactions (7.3)* and *Clinical Pharmacology (12.3)*.

10 OVERDOSAGE

Daily doses of 3600 mg have been taken by healthy volunteers for 5 days without untoward symptomatic effects. There is no specific antidote for overdose with VICTRELIS. Treatment of overdosage with VICTRELIS should consist of general supportive measures, including monitoring of vital signs, and observation of the patient's clinical status.

11 DESCRIPTION

VICTRELIS (boceprevir) is an inhibitor of the hepatitis C virus (HCV) non-structural protein 3 (NS3) serine protease. Boceprevir has the following chemical name: (1R,5S)-N-[3-Amino-1-(cyclobutylmethyl)-2,3-dioxopropyl]-3-[2(S)-[[[(1,1-dimethylethyl)amino]carbonyl]amino]-3,3-dimethyl-1-oxobutyl]-6,6-dimethyl-3-azabicyclo[3.1.0]hexan-2(S)-carboxamide. The molecular formula is $C_{27}H_{45}N_5O_5$ and its molecular weight is 519.7. Boceprevir has the following structural formula:

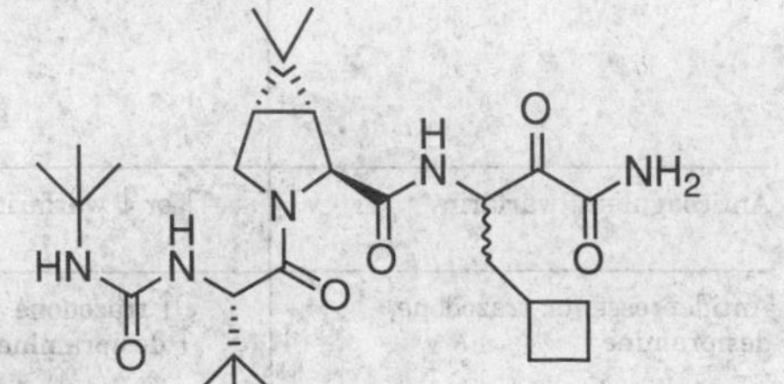

Boceprevir is manufactured as an approximately equal mixture of two diastereomers. Boceprevir is a white to off-white amorphous powder. It is freely soluble in methanol, ethanol and isopropanol and slightly soluble in water.

VICTRELIS 200 mg capsules are available as hard gelatin capsules for oral administration. Each capsule contains 200 mg of boceprevir and the following inactive ingredients: sodium lauryl sulfate, microcrystalline cellulose, lactose monohydrate, croscarmellose sodium, pre-gelatinized starch, and magnesium stearate. The red capsule cap consists of gelatin, titanium dioxide, D&C Yellow #10, FD&C Blue #1, and FD&C Red #40. The yellow capsule body contains gelatin, titanium dioxide, D&C Yellow #10, FD&C Red #40, and FD&C Yellow #6. The capsule is printed with red and yellow ink. The red ink contains shellac and red iron oxide, while the yellow ink consists of shellac, titanium dioxide, povidone and D&C Yellow #10 Aluminum Lake.

12 CLINICAL PHARMACOLOGY

12.1 Mechanism of Action

VICTRELIS is a direct acting antiviral drug against the hepatitis C virus *[see Microbiology (12.4)]*.

12.2 Pharmacodynamics

Evaluation of Effect of VICTRELIS on QTc Interval

The effect of boceprevir 800 mg and 1200 mg on QTc interval was evaluated in a randomized, multiple-dose, placebo-, and active-controlled (moxifloxacin 400 mg) 4-way crossover thorough QT study in 36 healthy subjects. In the study with demonstrated ability to detect small effects, the upper bound of the one-sided 95% confidence interval for the largest placebo-adjusted, baseline-corrected QTc based on individual correction method (QTcI) was below 10 ms, the threshold for regulatory concern. The dose of 1200 mg yields a boceprevir maximum exposure increase of approximately 15% which may not cover exposures due to coadministration with strong CYP3A4 inhibitors or use in patients with severe hepatic impairment. However, at the doses studied in the thorough QT study, no apparent concentration-QT relationship was identified. Thus, there is no expectation of a QTc effect under a higher exposure scenario.

12.3 Pharmacokinetics

VICTRELIS capsules contain a 1:1 mixture of two diastereomers, SCH534128 and SCH534129. In plasma the diastereomer ratio changes to 2:1, favoring the active diastereomer, SCH534128. Plasma concentrations of boceprevir described below consist of both diastereomers SCH534128 and SCH534129, unless otherwise specified.

In healthy subjects who received 800 mg three times daily alone, boceprevir drug exposure was characterized by AUC(τ) of 5408 ng × hr per mL (n=71), C_{max} of 1723 ng per mL (n=71), and C_{min} of 88 ng per mL (n=71). Pharmacokinetic results were similar between healthy subjects and HCV-infected subjects.

Absorption

Boceprevir was absorbed following oral administration with a median T_{max} of 2 hours. Steady state AUC, C_{max}, and C_{min} increased in a less-than-dose-proportional manner and individual exposures overlapped substantially at 800 mg and 1200 mg, suggesting diminished absorption at higher doses. Accumulation is minimal (0.8- to 1.5-fold) and pharmacokinetic steady state is achieved after approximately 1 day of three times daily dosing.

The absolute bioavailability of boceprevir has not been studied.

Effects of Food on Oral Absorption

VICTRELIS should be administered with food. Food enhanced the exposure of boceprevir by up to 65% at the

800 mg three times daily dose, relative to the fasting state. The bioavailability of boceprevir was similar regardless of meal type (e.g., high-fat vs. low-fat) or whether taken 5 minutes prior to eating, during a meal, or immediately following completion of the meal. Therefore, VICTRELIS may be taken without regard to either meal type or timing of the meal.

Distribution

Boceprevir has a mean apparent volume of distribution (Vd/F) of approximately 772 L at steady state in healthy subjects. Human plasma protein binding is approximately 75% following a single dose of boceprevir 800 mg. Boceprevir is administered as an approximately equal mixture of two diastereomers, SCH534128 and SCH534129, which rapidly interconvert in plasma. The predominant diastereomer, SCH534128, is pharmacologically active and the other diastereomer is inactive.

Metabolism

Studies *in vitro* indicate that boceprevir primarily undergoes metabolism through the aldo-ketoreductase (AKR)-mediated pathway to ketone-reduced metabolites that are inactive against HCV. After a single 800-mg oral dose of ^{14}C-boceprevir, the most abundant circulating metabolites were a diasteriomeric mixture of ketone-reduced metabolites with a mean exposure approximately 4-fold greater than that of boceprevir. Boceprevir also undergoes, to a lesser extent, oxidative metabolism mediated by CYP3A4/5.

Drug Interactions

Drug interaction studies were performed with boceprevir and drugs likely to be coadministered or drugs commonly used as probes for pharmacokinetic interactions. The effects of coadministration of boceprevir on AUC, C_{max} and C_{min} are summarized in Table 6 (effects of coadministered drugs on boceprevir) and Table 7 (effects of boceprevir on coadministered drugs).

[See table 6 at top of next page]
[See table 7 on pages 1827 and 1828]

Elimination

Boceprevir is eliminated with a mean plasma half-life (t½) of approximately 3.4 hours. Boceprevir has a mean total body clearance (CL/F) of approximately 161 L per hr. Following a single 800 mg oral dose of ^{14}C-boceprevir, approximately 79% and 9% of the dose was excreted in feces and urine, respectively, with approximately 8% and 3% of the dosed radiocarbon eliminated as boceprevir in feces and urine. The data indicate that boceprevir is eliminated primarily by the liver.

Special Populations

Hepatic Impairment

The pharmacokinetics of boceprevir was studied in adult non-HCV infected subjects with normal, mild (Child-Pugh score 5 to 6), moderate (Child-Pugh score 7 to 9), and severe (Child-Pugh score 10 to 12) hepatic impairment following a single 400 mg dose of VICTRELIS. The mean AUC of the active diastereomer of boceprevir (SCH534128) was 32% and 45% higher in subjects with moderate and severe hepatic impairment, respectively, relative to subjects with normal hepatic function. Mean C_{max} values for SCH534128 were 28% and 62% higher in moderate and severe hepatic impairment, respectively. Subjects with mild hepatic impairment had similar SCH534128 exposure as subjects with normal hepatic function. A similar magnitude of effect is anticipated for boceprevir. No dosage adjustment of VICTRELIS is recommended for patients with hepatic impairment *[see Use in Specific Populations (8.7)]*. See peginterferon alfa Package Insert for contraindication in patients with hepatic decompensation.

Renal Impairment

The pharmacokinetics of boceprevir was studied in non-HCV-infected subjects with end-stage renal disease (ESRD) requiring hemodialysis following a single 800 mg dose of VICTRELIS. The mean AUC of boceprevir was 10% lower in subjects with ESRD requiring hemodialysis relative to subjects with normal renal function. Hemodialysis removed less than 1% of the boceprevir dose. No dosage adjustment of VICTRELIS is required in patients with any degree of renal impairment.

Gender

Population pharmacokinetic analysis of VICTRELIS indicated that gender had no apparent effect on exposure.

Race

Population pharmacokinetic analysis of VICTRELIS indicated that race had no apparent effect on exposure.

Age

Population pharmacokinetic analysis of VICTRELIS showed that boceprevir exposure was not different across subjects 19 to 65 years old.

12.4 Microbiology

Mechanism of Action

Boceprevir is an inhibitor of the HCV NS3/4A protease that is necessary for the proteolytic cleavage of the HCV encoded polyprotein into mature forms of the NS4A, NS4B, NS5A and NS5B proteins. Boceprevir covalently, yet reversibly, binds to the NS3 protease active site serine (S139) through an (alpha)-ketoamide functional group to inhibit viral replication in HCV-infected host cells. In a biochemical assay, boceprevir inhibited the activity of recombinant HCV genotype 1a and 1b NS3/4A protease enzymes, with K_i values of 14 nM for each subtype.

Activity in Cell Culture

The EC_{50} and EC_{90} values for boceprevir against an HCV replicon constructed from a single genotype 1b isolate were approximately 200 nM and 400 nM, respectively, in a 72-hour cell culture assay. Boceprevir cell culture anti-HCV activity was approximately 2-fold lower for an HCV replicon derived from a single genotype 1a isolate, relative to the 1b isolate-derived replicon. In replicon assays, boceprevir had approximately 2-fold reduced activity against a genotype 2a isolate relative to genotype 1a and 1b replicon isolates. In a biochemical assay, boceprevir had approximately 3- and 2-fold reduced activity against NS3/4A proteases derived from single isolates representative of HCV genotypes 2 and 3a, respectively, relative to a genotype 1b-derived NS3/4A protease. The presence of 50% human serum reduced the cell culture anti-HCV activity of boceprevir by approximately 3-fold.

Evaluation of varying combinations of boceprevir and interferon alfa-2b that produced 90% suppression of replicon RNA in cell culture showed additivity of effect without evidence of antagonism.

Resistance

In HCV Replicon Cell Culture and Biochemical Studies

The activity of boceprevir against the HCV genotype 1a replicon was reduced (2- to 6-fold) by the following amino acid substitutions in the NS3 protease domain: V36A/L/M, Q41R, T54A/S, V55A, R155K and V158I. A greater than 10-fold reduction in boceprevir susceptibility was conferred by the amino acid substitutions R155T and A156S. The V55I and D168N single substitutions did not reduce sensitivity to boceprevir. The following double amino acid substitutions conferred more than 10-fold reduced sensitivity to boceprevir: V55A+I170V, T54S+R155K, R155K+D168N, R155T+D168N and V36M+R155K.

The activity of boceprevir against the HCV genotype 1b replicon was reduced (2- to 8- fold) by the following amino acid substitutions in the NS3 protease domain: V36A/M, Q41R, F43S, T54A/G/S, V55A/I, R155K, V158I, V170M and M175L. A greater than 10-fold reduction in boceprevir susceptibility was conferred by the amino acid substitutions A156S/T/V, V170A and V36M+R155K. The D168V single substitution did not reduce sensitivity to boceprevir.

Additional NS3 protease domain substitutions that have not been evaluated in the HCV replicon but have been shown to reduce boceprevir activity against the HCV NS3/4A protease in a biochemical assay include F43C and R155G/I/M/Q.

Resistance-associated amino acid substitutions for HCV genotype 1a and 1b observed in clinical trials are presented in Table 8.

In Clinical Studies

An as-treated, pooled genotypic resistance analysis was conducted for subjects who received four weeks of PegIntron/REBETOL followed by VICTRELIS 800 mg three times daily in combination with PegIntron/REBETOL in two

Table 5 *(cont.)* Established and Other Potentially Significant Drug Interactions

Concomitant Drug Class: Drug Name	Effect on Concentration of Boceprevir or Concomitant Drug	Recommendations
Narcotic Analgesic/Opioid Dependence: methadone*	↓ R-methadone	Plasma concentrations of *R*-methadone decreased when coadministered with VICTRELIS *[see Clinical Pharmacology (12.3)]*. The observed changes are not considered clinically relevant. No dose adjustment of methadone or VICTRELIS is recommended. Individual patients may require additional titration of their methadone dosage when VICTRELIS is started or stopped to ensure clinical effect of methadone.
buprenorphine/naloxone*	↑ buprenorphine/ naloxone	Plasma concentrations of buprenorphine and naloxone increased when coadministered with VICTRELIS *[see Clinical Pharmacology (12.3)]*. The observed changes are not considered clinically relevant. No dose adjustment of buprenorphine/naloxone or VICTRELIS is recommended.
Oral hormonal contraceptives: drospirenone/ethinyl estradiol*	↑ drospirenone ↓ ethinyl estradiol	Concentrations of drospirenone increased in the presence of boceprevir. Thus, the use of drospirenone-containing products is contraindicated during treatment with VICTRELIS due to potential for hyperkalemia *[see Contraindications (4)]*.
norethindrone/ethinyl estradiol*	↓ ethinyl estradiol ↔ norethindrone	Concentrations of ethinyl estradiol decreased in the presence of boceprevir. Norethindrone C_{max} decreased 17% in the presence of boceprevir *[see Clinical Pharmacology (12.3)]*. Coadministration of VICTRELIS with a combined oral contraceptive containing ethinyl estradiol and at least 1 mg of norethindrone is not likely to alter the effectiveness of this combined oral contraceptive *[see Use in Specific Populations (8.1)]*. Patients using estrogens as hormone replacement therapy should be clinically monitored for signs of estrogen deficiency.
PDE5 inhibitors: sildenafil, tadalafil, vardenafil	↑ sildenafil ↑ tadalafil ↑ vardenafil	Increases in PDE5 inhibitor concentrations are expected, and may result in an increase in adverse events, including hypotension, syncope, visual disturbances, and priapism. Use of REVATIO® (sildenafil) or ADCIRCA® (tadalafil) for the treatment of pulmonary arterial hypertension (PAH) is contraindicated with VICTRELIS *[see Contraindications (4)]*. Use of PDE5 inhibitors for erectile dysfunction: Use with caution in combination with VICTRELIS with increased monitoring for PDE5 inhibitor-associated adverse events. Do not exceed the following doses: Sildenafil: 25 mg every 48 hours Tadalafil: 10 mg every 72 hours Vardenafil: 2.5 mg every 24 hours
Proton Pump Inhibitor: omeprazole*	↔ omeprazole	No dose adjustment of omeprazole or VICTRELIS is recommended.
Sedative/hypnotics: alprazolam; IV midazolam	↑ midazolam ↑ alprazolam	Close clinical monitoring for respiratory depression and/or prolonged sedation should be exercised during coadministration of VICTRELIS. A lower dose of IV midazolam or alprazolam should be considered.

* These combinations have been studied; see *Clinical Pharmacology (12.3)* for magnitude of interaction.

Table 6 Summary of the Effect of Co-administered Drugs on Boceprevir in Healthy Subjects or HCV Positive Genotype-1 Subjects

Co-administered Drug	Co-administered Drug Dose/ Schedule	Boceprevir Dose/ Schedule	Ratio Estimate of Boceprevir Pharmacokinetic Parameters (in Combination vs. Alone) (90% CI of the Ratio Estimate) *		
			Change in mean C_{max}	Change in mean AUC	Change in mean C_{min}
Atazanavir/Ritonavir	300 mg/100 mg daily × 22 days	800 mg three times daily × 6 days	0.93 (0.80-1.08)	0.95 (0.87-1.05)	0.82 (0.68-0.98)
Atorvastatin	40 mg single dose	800 mg three times daily × 7 days	1.04 (0.89-1.21)	0.95 (0.90-1.01)	N/A
Buprenorphine/ Naloxone	Buprenorphine: 8-24 mg + Naloxone: 2-6 mg daily × 6 days	800 mg three times daily × 6 days	0.82 (0.71-0.94)	0.88 (0.76-1.02)	0.95 (0.70-1.28)
Cyclosporine	100 mg single dose	800 mg single dose	1.08 (0.97-1.20)	1.16 (1.06-1.26)	N/A
Darunavir/Ritonavir	600 mg/100 mg two times daily × 22 days	800 mg three times daily × 6 days	0.75 (0.67-0.85)	0.68 (0.65-0.72)	0.65 (0.56-0.76)
Diflunisal	250 mg two times daily × 7 days	800 mg three times daily × 12 days	0.86 (0.56-1.32)	0.96 (0.79-1.17)	1.31 (1.04-1.65)
Efavirenz	600 mg daily × 16 days	800 mg three times daily × 6 days	0.92 (0.78-1.08)	0.81 (0.75-0.89)	0.56 (0.42-0.74)
Escitalopram	10 mg single dose	800 mg three times daily × 11 days	0.91 (0.81-1.02)	1.02 (0.96-1.08)	N/A
Etravirine	200 mg two times daily × 11-14 days	800 mg three times daily × 11-14 days	1.10 (0.94-1.29)	1.10 (0.94-1.28)	0.88† (0.66-1.17)
Ibuprofen	600 mg three times daily × 6 days	400 mg single oral dose	0.94 (0.67-1.32)	1.04 (0.90-1.20)	N/A
Ketoconazole	400 mg two times daily × 6 days	400 mg single oral dose	1.41 (1.00-1.97)	2.31 (2.00-2.67)	N/A
Lopinavir/Ritonavir	400 mg/100 mg two times daily × 22 days	800 mg three times daily × 6 days	0.50 (0.45-0.55)	0.55 (0.49-0.61)	0.43 (0.36-0.53)
Methadone	20-150 mg daily × 6 days	800 mg three times daily × 6 days	0.62 (0.53-0.72)	0.80 (0.69-0.93)	1.03 (0.75-1.42)
Omeprazole	40 mg daily × 5 days	800 mg three times daily × 5 days	0.94 (0.86-1.02)	0.92 (0.87-0.97)	1.17† (0.97-1.42)
Peginterferon alfa-2b	1.5 mcg/kg subcutaneous weekly × 2 weeks	400 mg three times daily × 1 week	0.88 (0.66-1.18)	1.00* (0.89-1.13)	N/A
Pravastatin	40 mg single dose	800 mg three times daily × 6 days	0.93 (0.83-1.04)	0.94 (0.88-1.01)	N/A
Ritonavir	100 mg daily × 12 days	400 mg three times daily × 15 days	0.73 (0.57-0.93)	0.81 (0.73-0.91)	1.04 (0.62-1.75)
Tacrolimus	0.5 mg single dose	800 mg single dose	0.97 (0.84-1.13)	1.00* (0.95-1.06)	N/A
Tenofovir	300 mg daily × 7 days	800 mg three times daily × 7 days	1.05 (0.98-1.12)	1.08 (1.02-1.14)	1.08 (0.97-1.20)

N/A = not available
* No effect = 1.00
† $C_{8\ hours}$

Phase 3 studies, SPRINT-2 and RESPOND-2. Among subjects treated with VICTRELIS who did not achieve a sustained virologic response, and for whom samples were analyzed, 53% had one or more specific post-baseline, treatment-emergent NS3 protease domain amino acid substitutions detected by a population-based sequencing assay (Table 8). Similar patterns of treatment-emergent substitutions were observed in P06086, a Phase 3 clinical trial in previously untreated CHC subjects with genotype 1 infection comparing the use of ESA to ribavirin dose reduction for initial management of anemia during therapy with VICTRELIS in combination with PegIntron/REBETOL. Nearly all of these substitutions have been shown to reduce boceprevir anti-HCV activity in cell culture or biochemical assays. Among subjects treated with VICTRELIS in SPRINT-2 and RESPOND-2 who did not achieve SVR and for whom post-baseline samples were analyzed, 31% of PegIntron/REBETOL-responsive subjects, as defined by greater than or equal to 1-$\log_{10}$ decline in viral load at Treatment Week 4 (end of 4-week PegIntron/REBETOL lead-in period), had detectable treatment-emergent substitutions, compared to 68% of subjects with less than 1-$\log_{10}$ decline in viral load at Treatment Week 4. Clear patterns of boceprevir treatment-emergent substitutions in the NS3 helicase domain or NS4A coding regions of the HCV genome were not observed.

Table 8 Treatment-Emergent NS3 Protease Domain Amino Acid Substitutions Detected Among Subjects treated with VICTRELIS in SPRINT-2, RESPOND-2 and P06086 Who Did Not Achieve a Sustained Virologic Response (SVR)

	Subjects Infected with HCV Genotype 1a	Subjects Infected with HCV Genotype 1b
>10% of subjects treated with VICTRELIS who did not achieve SVR	V36M, T54S, R155K	T54A, T54S, V55A, A156S, V170A
<1% to 10% of subjects treated with VICTRELIS who did not achieve SVR	V36A, T54A, V55A, V55I, V107I, R155T, A156S, A156T, V158I, D168N, I170F, I170T, I170V	V36A, V36M, T54C, T54G, V107I, R155C, R155K, A156T, A156V, V158I, I/V170T, M175L

Persistence of Resistance-Associated Substitutions

Data from an ongoing, long-term follow-up study of subjects who did not achieve SVR in Phase 2 trials with VICTRELIS, with a median duration of follow-up of approximately 2 years, indicate that HCV populations harboring certain post-baseline, treatment-emergent substitutions may decline in relative abundance over time. However, among those subjects with available data, one or more treatment-emergent substitutions remained detectable with a population-based sequencing assay in 25% of subjects after 2.5 years of follow-up. The most common NS3 substitutions detected after 2.5 years of follow-up were T54S and R155K. The lack of detection of a substitution based on a population-based assay does not necessarily indicate that viral populations carrying that substitution have declined to a background level that may have existed prior to treatment. The long-term clinical impact of the emergence or persistence of boceprevir-resistance-associated substitutions is unknown. No data are available regarding the efficacy of VICTRELIS among subjects who were previously exposed to VICTRELIS, or who previously failed treatment with a regimen containing VICTRELIS.

Effect of Baseline HCV Polymorphisms on Treatment Response

A pooled analysis was conducted to explore the association between the detection of baseline NS3/4A amino acid polymorphisms and treatment outcome in the two Phase 3 studies, SPRINT-2 and RESPOND-2.

Baseline resistance associated polymorphisms were detected in 7% of subjects by a population-based sequencing method. Overall, the presence of these polymorphisms alone did not impact SVR rates in subjects treated with VICTRELIS. However, among subjects with a relatively poor response to PegIntron/REBETOL during the 4-week lead-in period, the efficacy of VICTRELIS appeared to be reduced for those who had V36M, T54A, T54S, V55A or R155K detected at baseline. Subjects with these baseline polymorphisms and reduced response to PegIntron/REBETOL represented approximately 1% of the total number of subjects treated with VICTRELIS.

Cross-Resistance

Many of the treatment-emergent NS3 amino acid substitutions detected in subjects treated with VICTRELIS who did not achieve SVR in the Phase 3 clinical trials have been demonstrated to reduce the anti-HCV activity of other HCV NS3/4A protease inhibitors. The impact of prior exposure to VICTRELIS or treatment failure on the efficacy of other HCV NS3/4A protease inhibitors has not been studied. The efficacy of VICTRELIS has not been established for patients with a history of exposure to other NS3/4A protease inhibitors. Cross-resistance is not expected between VICTRELIS and interferons, or VICTRELIS and ribavirin.

Table 7 Summary of the Effect of Boceprevir on Co-administered Drugs in Healthy Subjects or HCV Positive Genotype-1 Subjects

Co-administered Drug	Co-administered Drug Dose/ Schedule	Boceprevir Dose/ Schedule	Ratio Estimate of Co-administered Pharmacokinetic Parameters (in Combination vs. Alone) (90% CI of the Ratio Estimate) *		
			Change in mean C_{max}	Change in mean AUC(τ)	Change in mean C_{min}
Atazanavir/Ritonavir	300 mg/100 mg daily × 22 days	800 mg three times daily × 6 days	Atazanavir: 0.75 (0.64-0.88) Ritonavir: 0.73 (0.64-0.83)	Atazanavir: 0.65† (0.55-0.78) Ritonavir: 0.64 (0.58-0.72)	Atazanavir: 0.51 (0.44-0.61) Ritonavir: 0.55 (0.45-0.67)
Atorvastatin	40 mg single dose	800 mg three times daily × 7 days	2.66 (1.81-3.90)	2.30‡ (1.84-2.88)	N/A
Buprenorphine/ Naloxone	Buprenorphine: 8-24 mg + Naloxone: 2-6 mg daily × 6 days	800 mg three times daily × 6 days	Buprenorphine: 1.18 (0.93-1.50) Naloxone: 1.09 (0.79-1.51)	Buprenorphine: 1.19 (0.91-1.57) Naloxone: 1.33 (0.90-1.98)	Buprenorphine: 1.31 (0.95-1.79) Naloxone: N/A
Cyclosporine	100 mg single dose	800 mg three times daily × 7 days	2.01 (1.69-2.40)	2.68‡ (2.38-3.03)	N/A
Darunavir/Ritonavir	600 mg/100 mg two times daily × 22 days	800 mg three times daily × 6 days	Darunavir: 0.64 (0.58-0.71) Ritonavir: 0.87 (0.76-1.00)	Darunavir: 0.56† (0.51-0.61) Ritonavir: 0.73 (0.68-0.79)	Darunavir: 0.41 (0.38-0.45) Ritonavir: 0.55 (0.52-0.59)
Digoxin	0.25 mg single dose	800 mg three times daily × 10 days	1.18 (1.07-1.31)	1.19‡ (1.12-1.27)	N/A
Drospirenone/ Ethinyl estradiol	Drospirenone: 3 mg + Ethinyl estradiol : 0.02 mg daily × 14 days	800 mg three times daily × 7 days	Drospirenone: 1.57 (1.46-1.70) Ethinyl estradiol: 1.00 (0.91-1.10)	Drospirenone: 1.99 (1.87-2.11) Ethinyl estradiol: 0.76 (0.73-0.79)	N/A
Efavirenz	600 mg daily × 16 days	800 mg three times daily × 6 days	1.11 (1.02-1.20)	1.20 (1.15-1.26)	N/A
Escitalopram	10 mg single dose	800 mg three times daily × 11 days	0.81 (0.76-0.87)	0.79‡ (0.71-0.87)	N/A
Etravirine	200 mg two times daily × 11-14 days	800 mg three times daily × 11-14 days	0.76 (0.68-0.85)	0.77 (0.66-0.91)	0.71 (0.54-0.95)
Lopinavir/Ritonavir	400 mg/100 mg two times daily × 22 days	800 mg three times daily × 6 days	Lopinavir: 0.70 (0.65-0.77) Ritonavir: 0.88 (0.72-1.07)	Lopinavir: 0.66† (0.60-0.72) Ritonavir: 0.78 (0.71-0.87)	Lopinavir: 0.57 (0.49-0.65) Ritonavir: 0.58 (0.52-0.65)
Methadone	20-150 mg daily × 6 days	800 mg three times daily × 6 days	*R*-methadone: 0.90 (0.71-1.13) *S*-methadone: 0.83 (0.64-1.09)	*R*-methadone: 0.85 (0.74-0.96) *S*-methadone: 0.78 (0.66-0.93)	*R*-methadone: 0.81 (0.66-1.00) *S*-methadone: 0.74 (0.58-0.95)
Midazolam	4 mg single oral dose	800 mg three times daily × 6 days	2.77 (2.36-3.25)	5.30 (4.66-6.03)	N/A
Norethindrone/ Ethinyl estradiol	Norethindrone: 1 mg + Ethinyl estradiol : 0.035 mg daily × 21 days	800 mg three times daily × 28 days	Norethindrone: 0.83 (0.76-0.90) Ethinyl estradiol: 0.79 (0.75 -0.84)	Norethindrone: 0.96 (0.87-1.06) Ethinyl estradiol: 0.74 (0.68-0.80)	N/A
Omeprazole	40 mg daily × 5 days	800 mg three times daily × 5 days	1.03 (0.85-1.26)	1.06 (0.90-1.25)	1.12 § (0.75-1.67)

(Table continued on next page)

12.5 Pharmacogenomics

A genetic variant near the gene encoding interferon-lambda-3 (*IL28B rs12979860*, a C to T change) is a strong predictor of response to PegIntron/REBETOL. *IL28B rs12979860* was genotyped in 653 of 1048 (62%) subjects in SPRINT-2 (previously untreated) and 259 of 394 (66%) subjects in RESPOND-2 (previous partial responders and relapsers) *[see Clinical Studies (14) for trial descriptions]*. Among subjects that received at least one dose of placebo or VICTRELIS (Modified-Intent-to-Treat population), SVR rates tended to be lower in subjects with the C/T and T/T genotypes compared to those with the C/C genotype, particularly among previously untreated subjects receiving 48 weeks of PegIntron and REBETOL (see Table 9). Among previous treatment failures, subjects of all genotypes appeared to have higher SVR rates with regimens containing VICTRELIS. The results of this retrospective subgroup analysis should be viewed with caution because of the small sample size and potential differences in demographic or clinical characteristics of the substudy population relative to the overall trial population.

[See table 9 at top of next page]

13 NONCLINICAL TOXICOLOGY

13.1 Carcinogenesis, Mutagenesis, Impairment of Fertility

Carcinogenesis and Mutagenesis

Use with Ribavirin and Peginterferon alfa: Ribavirin is genotoxic in *in vitro* and *in vivo* assays. Ribavirin was not oncogenic in mouse and rat carcinogenicity studies at doses less than the maximum recommended daily human dose. Please refer to ribavirin Package Inserts for additional information.

Two-year carcinogenicity studies in mice and rats were conducted with boceprevir. Mice were administered doses of up to 500 mg per kg in males and 650 mg per kg in females, and rats were administered doses of up to 125 mg per kg in males and 100 mg per kg in females. In mice, no significant increases in the incidence of drug-related neoplasms were observed at the highest doses tested resulting in boceprevir AUC exposures approximately 2.3- and 6.0-fold higher in males and females, respectively, than those in humans at the recommended dose of 800 mg three times daily. In rats, no increases in the incidence of drug-related neoplasms were observed at the highest doses tested resulting in boceprevir AUC exposures similar to those in humans at the recommended dose of 800 mg three times daily.

Boceprevir was not genotoxic in a battery of *in vitro* or *in vivo* assays, including bacterial mutagenicity, chromosomal aberration in human peripheral blood lymphocytes and mouse micronucleus assays.

Impairment of Fertility

Use with Ribavirin and Peginterferon alfa: In fertility studies in male animals, ribavirin induced reversible testicular toxicity; while peginterferon alfa may impair fertility in females. Please refer to Package Inserts for ribavirin and peginterferon alfa for additional information.

Boceprevir-induced reversible effects on fertility and early embryonic development in female rats, with no effects observed at a 75 mg per kg dose level. At this dose, boceprevir AUC exposures are approximately 1.3-fold higher than those in humans at the recommended dose of 800 mg three times daily. Decreased fertility was also observed in male rats, most likely as a consequence of testicular degeneration. No testicular degeneration was observed at a 15 mg per kg dose level resulting in boceprevir AUC exposures of less than those in humans at the recommended dose of 800 mg three times daily. Testicular degeneration was not observed in mice or monkeys administered boceprevir for 3 months at doses of up to 900 or 1000 mg per kg, respectively. At these doses, boceprevir AUC exposures are approximately 6.8- and 4.4-fold higher in mice and monkeys, respectively, than those in humans at the recommended dose of 800 mg three times daily. Additionally, limited clinical monitoring has revealed no evidence of testicular toxicity in human subjects.

14 CLINICAL STUDIES

The efficacy of VICTRELIS as a treatment for chronic hepatitis C (genotype 1) infection was assessed in approximately 1500 adult subjects who were previously untreated (SPRINT-2) or who had failed previous peginterferon alfa and ribavirin therapy (RESPOND-2) in Phase 3 clinical studies.

Previously Untreated Subjects

SPRINT-2 was a randomized, double-blind, placebo-controlled study comparing two therapeutic regimens of VICTRELIS 800 mg orally three times daily in combination with PR [PegIntron 1.5 micrograms per kg per week subcutaneously and weight-based dosing with REBETOL (600–1400 mg per day orally divided twice daily)] to PR alone in adult subjects who had chronic hepatitis C (HCV genotype 1) infection with detectable levels of HCV-RNA and were not previously treated with interferon alfa therapy. Subjects were randomized in a 1:1:1 ratio within two separate cohorts (Cohort 1/non-Black and Cohort 2/Black) and were stratified by HCV genotype (1a or 1b) and by HCV-RNA viral load (less than or equal to 400,000 IU per mL vs. more than 400,000 IU per mL) to one of the following three treatment arms:

- PegIntron + REBETOL for 48 weeks (PR48).
- PegIntron + REBETOL for four weeks followed by VICTRELIS 800 mg three times daily + PegIntron + REBETOL for 24 weeks. The subjects were then continued on different regimens based on Treatment Week (TW) 8 through TW24 response-guided therapy (boceprevir-RGT). All subjects in this treatment arm were limited to 24 weeks of therapy with VICTRELIS.
  - Subjects with undetectable HCV-RNA (Target Not Detected) at TW8 (early responders) and remained undetectable through TW24 discontinued therapy and entered follow-up at the TW28 visit.

Table 7 *(cont.)* Summary of the Effect of Boceprevir on Co-administered Drugs in Healthy Subjects or HCV Positive Genotype-1 Subjects

Co-administered Drug	Co-administered Drug Dose/ Schedule	Boceprevir Dose/ Schedule	Ratio Estimate of Co-administered Pharmacokinetic Parameters (in Combination vs. Alone) (90% CI of the Ratio Estimate) *		
			Change in mean C_{max}	Change in mean AUC(τ)	Change in mean C_{min}
Peginterferon alfa-2b	1.5 mcg/kg subcutaneous weekly × 2 weeks	200 mg or 400 mg three times daily × 1 week	N/A	0.99[¶,#] (0.83-1.17)	N/A
Pravastatin	40 mg single dose	800 mg three times daily × 6 days	1.49 (1.03-2.14)	1.63[‡] (1.01-2.62)	N/A
Prednisone	40 mg single dose	800 mg three times daily × 6 days	Prednisone: 0.99 (0.94-1.04) Prednisolone: 1.16 (1.09-1.24)	Prednisone: 1.22 (1.16-1.28) Prednisolone: 1.37 (1.31-1.44)	Prednisone: N/A Prednisolone: N/A
Raltegravir	400 mg single dose	800 mg three times daily × 10 days	1.11 (0.91-1.36)	1.04 (0.88-1.22)	0.75[Þ] (0.45-1.23)
Tacrolimus	0.5 mg single dose	800 mg three times daily × 11 days	9.90 (7.96-12.3)	17.1[‡] (14.0-20.8)	N/A
Tenofovir	300 mg daily × 7 days	800 mg three times daily × 7 days	1.32 (1.19-1.45)	1.05 (1.01-1.09)	N/A

N/A = not available
* No effect = 1.00
† $AUC_{0\text{-}last}$
‡ $AUC_{0\text{-}inf}$
§ $C_{8\ hours}$
¶ 0-168 hours
\# Reported AUC is 200 mg and 400 mg cohorts combined.
Þ $C_{12\ hours}$

Table 9 Sustained Virologic Response (SVR) Rates by IL28B rs12979860 Genotype

Clinical Study	*IL28B rs12979860* Genotype	SVR, % (n/N)		
		PR48*	Boceprevir-RGT*	Boceprevir-PR48*
SPRINT-2 (Previously Untreated Subjects)				
	C/C	78 (50/64)	82 (63/77)	80 (44/55)
	C/T	28 (33/116)	65 (67/103)	71 (82/115)
	T/T	27 (10/37)	55 (23/42)	59 (26/44)
RESPOND-2 (Previous Partial Responders and Relapsers)				
	C/C	46 (6/13)	79 (22/28)	77 (17/22)
	C/T	17 (5/29)	61 (38/62)	73 (48/66)
	T/T	50 (5/10)	55 (6/11)	72 (13/18)

* For description of each treatment arm, see *Clinical Studies (14)*.

- ◦ Subjects with detectable HCV-RNA at TW8 or any subsequent treatment week but subsequently achieving undetectable HCV-RNA (Target Not Detected) at TW24 (late responders) were changed in a blinded fashion to placebo at the TW28 visit and continued therapy with PegIntron + REBETOL for an additional 20 weeks, for a total treatment duration of 48 weeks.
- PegIntron + REBETOL for four weeks followed by VICTRELIS 800 mg three times daily + PegIntron + REBETOL for 44 weeks (boceprevir-PR48).

All subjects with detectable HCV-RNA in plasma at TW24 were discontinued from treatment. Sustained Virologic Response (SVR) was defined as plasma HCV-RNA less than 25 IU/mL at Follow-up Week 24. Plasma HCV-RNA results at Follow-up Week 12 were used if plasma HCV-RNA results at Follow-up Week 24 were missing.

Mean age of subjects randomized was 49 years. The racial distribution of subjects was as follows: 82% White, 14% Black, and 4% others. The distribution of subjects by gender was 60% men and 40% women.

The addition of VICTRELIS to PegIntron and REBETOL significantly increased the SVR rates compared to PegIntron and REBETOL alone in the combined cohort (63% to 66% in arms containing VICTRELIS vs. 38% PR48 control) for randomized subjects who received at least one dose of any study medication (Full-Analysis-Set population). SVR rates for Blacks who received the combination of VICTRELIS with PegIntron and REBETOL were 42% to 53% in a predefined analysis (see Table 10).

[See table 10 at top of next page]

In subjects with cirrhosis at baseline, sustained virologic response was higher in those who received treatment with the combination of VICTRELIS with PegIntron and REBETOL for 44 weeks after lead-in therapy with PegIntron and REBETOL (10/24, 42%) compared to those who received RGT (5/16, 31%).

Sustained Virologic Response (SVR) Based on TW8 HCV-RNA Results

Table 11 presents sustained virologic response based on TW8 HCV-RNA results in previously untreated subjects. Fifty-seven percent (208/368) of subjects in the boceprevir-RGT arm and 56% (204/366) of subjects in the boceprevir-PR48 arm had undetectable HCV-RNA (Target Not Detected) at TW8 (early responders) compared with 17% (60/363) of subjects in the PR48 arm.

[See table 11 at top of next page]

Among subjects with detectable HCV-RNA at TW8 who had attained undetectable HCV-RNA (Target Not Detected) at TW24 and completed at least 28 weeks of treatment, the SVR rates were 66% (45/68) in boceprevir-RGT arm (4 weeks of PegIntron and REBETOL then 24 weeks of VICTRELIS with PegIntron and REBETOL followed by 20 weeks of PegIntron and REBETOL alone) and 75% (55/73) in boceprevir-PR48 arms (4 weeks of PegIntron and REBETOL then 44 weeks of VICTRELIS with PegIntron and REBETOL).

Previous Partial Responders and Relapsers to Interferon and Ribavirin Therapy

RESPOND-2 was a randomized, parallel-group, double-blind study comparing two therapeutic regimens of VICTRELIS 800 mg orally three times daily in combination with PR [PegIntron 1.5 micrograms per kg per week subcutaneously and weight-based ribavirin (600–1400 mg per day orally divided twice daily)] compared to PR alone in adult subjects with chronic hepatitis C (HCV genotype 1) infection with demonstrated interferon responsiveness (as defined historically by a decrease in HCV-RNA viral load greater than or equal to $2\text{-}\log_{10}$ by Week 12, but never achieved SVR [partial responders] or undetectable HCV-RNA at end of prior treatment with a subsequent detectable HCV-RNA in plasma [relapsers]). Subjects with less than $2\text{-}\log_{10}$ decrease in HCV-RNA by week 12 of previous treatment (prior null responders) were not eligible for enrollment in this trial. Subjects were randomized in a 1:2:2 ratio and stratified based on response to their previous qualifying regimen (relapsers vs. partial responders) and by HCV subtype (1a vs. 1b) to one of the following treatment arms:

- PegIntron + REBETOL for 48 weeks (PR48)
- PegIntron + REBETOL for 4 weeks followed by VICTRELIS 800 mg three times daily + PegIntron + REBETOL for 32 weeks. The subjects were then continued on different treatment regimens based on TW8 and TW12 response-guided therapy (boceprevir-RGT). All subjects in this treatment arm were limited to 32 weeks of VICTRELIS.
  - ◦ Subjects with undetectable HCV-RNA (Target Not Detected) at TW8 (early responders) and TW12 completed therapy at TW36 visit.
  - ◦ Subjects with a detectable HCV-RNA at TW8 but subsequently undetectable (Target Not Detected) at TW12 (late responders) were changed in a blinded fashion to placebo at the TW36 visit and continued treatment with PegIntron + REBETOL for an additional 12 weeks, for a total treatment duration of 48 weeks.
- PegIntron + REBETOL for 4 weeks followed by VICTRELIS 800 mg three times daily + PegIntron + REBETOL for 44 weeks (boceprevir-PR48).

All subjects with detectable HCV-RNA in plasma at TW12 were discontinued from treatment. Sustained Virologic Response (SVR) was defined as plasma HCV-RNA less than 25 IU/mL at Follow-up Week 24. Plasma HCV-RNA results at Follow-up Week 12 were used if plasma HCV-RNA results at Follow-up Week 24 were missing.

Mean age of subjects randomized was 53 years. The racial distribution of subjects was as follows: 85% White, 12% Black, and 3% others. The distribution of subjects by gender was 67% men and 33% women.

The addition of VICTRELIS to the PegIntron and REBETOL therapy significantly increased the SVR rates compared to PegIntron/REBETOL alone (59% to 66% in arms containing VICTRELIS vs. 23% PR48 control) for randomized subjects who received at least one dose of any study medication (Full-Analysis-Set population) (see Table 12).

[See table 12 at top of page 1830]

In subjects with cirrhosis at baseline, sustained virologic response was higher in those who received treatment with the combination of VICTRELIS with PegIntron and REBETOL for 44 weeks after 4 weeks of lead-in therapy with PegIntron and REBETOL (17/22, 77%) compared to those who received RGT (6/17, 35%).

Sustained Virologic Response (SVR) Based on TW8 HCV-RNA Results

Table 13 presents sustained virologic response based on TW8 HCV-RNA results in subjects who were relapsers or partial responders to previous interferon and ribavirin therapy. Forty-six percent (74/162) of subjects in the boceprevir-RGT arm and 52% (84/161) in the boceprevir-PR48 had undetectable HCV-RNA (Target Not Detected) at TW8 (early responders) compared with 9% (7/80) in the PR48 arm.

[See table 13 at top of page 1830]

Among subjects with detectable HCV-RNA at TW8 who attained an undetectable HCV-RNA (Target Not Detected) at TW12 and completed at least 36 weeks of treatment, the SVR rates were 79% (27/34) in boceprevir-RGT arm (4 weeks of PegIntron and REBETOL then 32 weeks of VICTRELIS with PegIntron and REBETOL followed by 12 weeks of PegIntron and REBETOL alone) and 72% (29/40) in boceprevir-PR48 arm (4 weeks of PegIntron and REBETOL then 44 weeks of VICTRELIS with PegIntron and REBETOL).

Interferon Responsiveness during Lead-In Therapy with Peginterferon alfa and Ribavirin

Previously Untreated Subjects

In previously untreated subjects evaluated in SPRINT-2, interferon-responsiveness (defined as greater than or equal to 1-log_{10} decline in viral load at TW4) was predictive of SVR. Subjects treated with VICTRELIS who demonstrated interferon responsiveness at TW4 achieved SVR rates of 81% (203/252) in boceprevir-RGT arm and 79% (200/254) in boceprevir-PR48 arm, compared to 52% (134/260) in subjects treated with PegIntron/REBETOL.

Subjects treated with VICTRELIS who demonstrated poor interferon responsiveness (defined as less than 1-log_{10} decline in viral load at TW4), achieved SVR rates of 28% (27/97) in boceprevir-RGT arm and 38% (36/95) in boceprevir-PR48 arm, compared to 4% (3/83) in subjects treated with PegIntron/REBETOL. Subjects with less than a 0.5-log_{10} decline in viral load at TW4 achieved SVR rates of 28% (13/47) in boceprevir-RGT arm and 30% (11/37) in boceprevir-PR48 arm, compared to 0% (0/25) in subjects treated with PegIntron/REBETOL. Subjects with less than a 0.5-log_{10} decline in viral load at TW4 with peginterferon alfa plus ribavirin therapy alone are predicted to have a null response (less than 2-log_{10} viral load decline at TW12) to peginterferon alfa and ribavirin.

Previous Partial Responders and Relapsers to Interferon and Ribavirin Therapy

In subjects who were previous relapsers and partial responders evaluated in RESPOND-2, interferon-responsiveness (defined as greater than or equal to 1-log_{10} decline in viral load at TW4) was predictive of SVR. Subjects treated with VICTRELIS who demonstrated interferon responsiveness at TW4 achieved SVR rates of 74% (81/110) in boceprevir-RGT arm and 79% (90/114) in boceprevir-PR48 arm, compared to 27% (18/67) in subjects treated with PegIntron/REBETOL. Subjects treated with VICTRELIS who demonstrated poor interferon responsiveness (defined as less than 1-log_{10} decline in viral load at TW4) achieved SVR rates of 33% (15/46) in boceprevir-RGT arm and 34% (15/44) in boceprevir-PR48 arm, compared to 0% (0/12) in subjects treated with PegIntron/REBETOL.

Prior Null Responders to Interferon and Ribavirin Therapy

PROVIDE is an ongoing, open-label, single-arm study of VICTRELIS 800 mg orally three times daily in combination with peginterferon alfa-2b 1.5 micrograms per kg per week subcutaneously and weight-based ribavirin (600 – 1,400 mg per day orally divided twice daily) in adult subjects with chronic hepatitis C (HCV) genotype 1 infection who did not achieve SVR while in the peginterferon alfa/ribavirin control arms of previous Phase 2 and 3 studies of combination therapy with VICTRELIS. Subjects who enrolled in PROVIDE within 2 weeks after the last dose of peginterferon alfa/ribavirin in the parent study received VICTRELIS 800 mg three times daily + peginterferon alfa-2b + ribavirin for 44 weeks. Subjects who were not able to enroll in this study within 2 weeks received PegIntron/REBETOL lead-in for 4 weeks followed by VICTRELIS 800 mg three times daily + peginterferon alfa-2b + ribavirin for 44 weeks.

Among the subjects who were null responders in the peginterferon alfa/ribavirin control arm of the parent study that received the 4-week PegIntron/REBETOL lead-in treatment followed by VICTRELIS 800 mg three times daily + PegIntron/REBETOL for 44 weeks, 38% (20/52) achieved SVR, and the relapse rate was 14% (3/22).

Use of Ribavirin Dose Reduction versus Erythropoiesis Stimulating Agent (ESA) in the Management of Anemia in Previously Untreated Subjects

A randomized, parallel-arm, open-label study was conducted to compare two strategies for the management of anemia (use of ESA versus ribavirin dose reduction) in 687 subjects with previously untreated CHC genotype 1 infection who became anemic during therapy with VICTRELIS 800 mg orally three times daily plus peginterferon alfa-2b 1.5 micrograms per kg per week subcutaneously and weight-based ribavirin (600 – 1,400 mg per day orally divided twice daily). The study enrolled subjects with serum hemoglobin concentrations of less than 15 g per dL. Subjects were treated for 4 weeks with peginterferon alfa-2b and ribavirin followed by up to 44 weeks of VICTRELIS plus peginterferon alfa-2b and ribavirin. If a subject became anemic (serum hemoglobin of approximately less than or equal to 10 g per dL within the treatment period), the subject was randomized in a 1:1 ratio to either ribavirin dose reduction (N=249) or use of erythropoietin 40,000 units subcutaneously once weekly for the management of the anemia (N=251). If serum hemoglobin concentrations continued to decrease to less than or equal to 8.5 g per dL, subjects could be treated with additional anemia interventions, including the addition of erythropoietin (18% of those in the ribavirin dose reduction arm) or ribavirin dose reduction (37% of those in the ESA arm).

Mean age of subjects randomized was 49 years. The racial distribution of subjects was as follows: 77% White, 19% Black, and 4% other. The distribution of subjects by gender was 37% men and 63% women.

Table 10 Sustained Virologic Response (SVR)*, † and Relapse Rates‡ for Previously Untreated Subjects

Study Cohorts	Boceprevir-RGT	Boceprevir-PR48	PR48
Cohort 1 Plus Cohort 2 (all subjects)	n=368	n=366	n=363
SVR† %	63	66	38
Relapse‡ % (n/N)	9 (24/257)	9 (24/265)	22 (39/176)
Cohort 1 Plus Cohort 2 (subjects without cirrhosis)			
SVR†,§ % (n/N)	65 (228/352)	68 (232/342)	38 (132/350)
Cohort 1 (non-Black)	n=316	n=311	n=311
SVR† %	67	68	40
Relapse‡ % (n/N)	9 (21/232)	8 (18/230)	23 (37/162)
Cohort 2 (Black)	n=52	n=55	n=52
SVR† %	42	53	23
Relapse‡ % (n/N)	12 (3/25)	17 (6/35)	14 (2/14)

* The Full Analysis Set (FAS) consisted of all randomized subjects (N=1097) who received at least one dose of any study medication (PegIntron, REBETOL, or VICTRELIS).

† Sustained Virologic Response (SVR): reported as plasma HCV-RNA <25 IU/mL at follow-up week (FW) 24. The last available HCV-RNA value in the period at or after FW24 was used. If HCV-RNA value at FW24 was missing, the FW12 value was carried forward.

‡ Relapse rate was the proportion of subjects with undetectable HCV-RNA (Target Not Detected) at End of Treatment (EOT) and HCV-RNA ≥25 IU/mL at End of Follow-up (EOF) among subjects who were undetectable at EOT and not missing End of Follow-up (EOF) data.

§ Includes subjects with missing baseline data regarding cirrhosis as diagnosed by liver biopsy.

Table 11 Sustained Virologic Response (SVR) by HCV-RNA Detectability at TW8 in Previously Untreated Subjects in the Combined Cohort

	Boceprevir-RGT	Boceprevir-PR48	PR48
SVR by TW8 Detectability, % (n/N)*	N=337	N=335	N=331
Undetectable (Target Not Detected)	88 (184/208)	90 (184/204)	85 (51/60)
Detectable	36 (46/129)	40 (52/131)	30 (82/271)

* Denominator included only subjects with HCV-RNA results at TW8.

The overall intent-to-treat SVR rate for all enrolled subjects (including those subjects who were not randomized to RBV dose reduction or ESA for the management of anemia) was 63% (431/687). The SVR rate in subjects randomized who received ribavirin dose reduction was 71% (178/249), similar to the SVR rate of 71% (178/251) in subjects randomized to receive an ESA. The relapse rates in subjects randomized to receive ribavirin dose reduction or an ESA were 10% (19/196) and 10% (19/197), respectively.

16 HOW SUPPLIED/STORAGE AND HANDLING

16.1 How Supplied

VICTRELIS 200 mg capsules are comprised of a red-colored cap with the Merck logo printed in yellow ink, and a yellow-colored body with "314" printed in red ink. The capsules are packaged into a carton with 28 bottles containing 12 capsules (NDC 0085-0314-02).

16.2 Storage and Handling

VICTRELIS Capsules should be refrigerated at 2–8°C (36–46°F) until dispensed. Avoid exposure to excessive heat. For patient use, refrigerated capsules of VICTRELIS can remain stable until the expiration date printed on the label. VICTRELIS can also be stored at room temperature up to 25°C (77°F) for 3 months. Keep container tightly closed.

17 PATIENT COUNSELING INFORMATION

• See FDA-approved patient labeling (Medication Guide)

VICTRELIS must be used in combination with peginterferon alfa and ribavirin, and thus all contraindications and warnings for peginterferon alfa and ribavirin also apply. If peginterferon alfa or ribavirin is permanently discontinued, VICTRELIS must also be discontinued *[see Dosage and Administration (2.3)]*.

17.1 Pregnancy

Ribavirin must not be used by women who are pregnant or by men whose female partners are pregnant. Ribavirin therapy should not be initiated until a report of a negative pregnancy test has been obtained immediately before starting therapy. Female patients of childbearing potential and male patients with female partners of childbearing potential must be advised of the teratogenic/embryocidal risks of ribavirin and must be instructed to practice effective contraception during therapy and for 6 months post-therapy. Patients should be advised to notify the healthcare provider immediately in the event of a pregnancy *[see Contraindications (4) and Warnings and Precautions (5.1)]*.

Women of childbearing potential and men must use at least two forms of effective contraception during treatment and for at least 6 months after treatment has been stopped; routine monthly pregnancy tests must be performed during this time. One of these reliable forms of contraception can be a combined oral contraceptive product containing at least 1 mg of norethindrone. Oral contraceptives containing lower doses of norethindrone and other forms of hormonal contraception have not been studied or are contraindicated *[see Contraindications (4) and Warnings and Precautions (5.1)]*.

To monitor maternal and fetal outcomes of pregnant women exposed to ribavirin, the Ribavirin Pregnancy Registry has been established. Patients should be encouraged to register by calling 1-800-593-2214.

17.2 Anemia

Patients should be informed that anemia may be increased when VICTRELIS is administered with peginterferon alfa and ribavirin *[see Warnings and Precautions (5.2) and Adverse Reactions (6.1)]*. Patients should be advised that laboratory evaluations are required prior to starting therapy and periodically thereafter *[see Warnings and Precautions (5.6)]*.

17.3 Neutropenia

Patients should be informed that neutropenia may be increased when VICTRELIS is administered with peginterferon alfa and ribavirin *[see Warnings and Precautions (5.3) and Adverse Reactions (6.1)]*. Patients should be advised that laboratory evaluations are required prior to starting therapy and periodically thereafter *[see Warnings and Precautions (5.6)]*.

Table 12 Sustained Virologic Response (SVR)*, † and Relapse‡ Rates for Subjects Who have Failed Previous Therapy with Peginterferon Alfa and Ribavirin (Previous Partial Responders and Relapsers)

		Boceprevir-RGT	Boceprevir-PR48	PR48
		N=162	N=161	N=80
SVR† %		59	66	23
Relapse‡ % (n/N)		14 (16/111)	12 (14/121)	28 (7/25)
SVR (subjects without cirrhosis) § (n/N)		62 (90/145)	65 (90/139)	26 (18/70)
SVR by Response to Previous Peginterferon and Ribavirin Therapy				
Previous Response	Relapser, % (n/N)	70 (73/105)	75 (77/103)	31 (16/51)
	Partial responder, % (n/N)	40 (23/57)	52 (30/58)	7 (2/29)

Previous Partial Responder = subject who failed to achieve SVR after at least 12 weeks of previous treatment with peginterferon alfa and ribavirin, but demonstrated a ≥2-$\log_{10}$ reduction in HCV-RNA by Week 12.

Previous Relapser = subject who failed to achieve SVR after at least 12 weeks of previous treatment with peginterferon alfa and ribavirin, but had undetectable HCV-RNA at the end of treatment.

* The Full Analysis Set (FAS) consisted of all randomized subjects (N=403) who received at least one dose of any study medication (PegIntron, REBETOL, or VICTRELIS).

† Sustained Virologic Response (SVR): reported as plasma HCV-RNA <25 IU/mL at follow-up week (FW) 24. The last available HCV-RNA value in the period at or after FW24 was used. If HCV-RNA value at FW24 was missing, the FW12 value was carried forward.

‡ Relapse rate was the proportion of subjects with undetectable HCV-RNA (Target Not Detected) at End of Treatment (EOT) and HCV-RNA ≥25 IU/mL at End of Follow-up (EOF) among subjects who were undetectable at EOT and not missing End of Follow-up (EOF) data.

§ Includes subjects with missing baseline data regarding cirrhosis as diagnosed by liver biopsy.

Table 13 Sustained Virologic Response (SVR) by HCV-RNA Detectability at TW8 in Subjects Who Have Failed Previous Therapy (Previous Partial Responders and Relapsers)

	Boceprevir-RGT	Boceprevir-PR48	PR48
SVR by TW8 Detectability, % (n/N)*	N=146	N=154	N=72
Undetectable (Target Not Detected)	88 (65/74)	88 (74/84)	100 (7/7)
Detectable	40 (29/72)	43 (30/70)	14 (9/65)

* Denominator included only subjects with HCV-RNA results at TW8.

17.4 Hypersensitivity

Patients should be informed that serious acute hypersensitivity reactions have been observed during combination therapy with VICTRELIS, peginterferon alfa, and ribavirin therapy *[see Contraindications (4) and Warnings and Precautions (5.4)]*. If symptoms of acute hypersensitivity reactions (e.g., itching; hives; swelling of the face, eyes, lips, tongue, or throat; trouble breathing or swallowing) occur, patients should seek medical advice promptly.

17.5 Usage Safeguards

Patients should be advised that VICTRELIS must not be used alone due to the high probability of resistance without combination anti-HCV therapies *[see Indications and Usage (1)]*. See peginterferon alfa and ribavirin Package Inserts for additional patient counseling information on the use of these drugs in combination with VICTRELIS.

Patients should be informed of the potential for serious drug interactions with VICTRELIS, and that some drugs should not be taken with VICTRELIS *[see Contraindications (4), Warnings and Precautions (5.5), Drug Interactions (7), and Clinical Pharmacology (12.3)]*.

Patients should be advised that the total daily dose of VICTRELIS is packaged into a single bottle containing 12-capsules and the patient should take four capsules three times daily with food.

17.6 Missed VICTRELIS Doses

If a patient misses a dose and it is less than 2 hours before the next dose is due, the missed dose should be skipped. If a patient misses a dose and it is 2 or more hours before the next dose is due, the patient should take the missed dose with food and resume the normal dosing schedule.

17.7 Hepatitis C Virus Transmission

Patients should be informed that the effect of treatment of hepatitis C infection on transmission is not known, and that appropriate precautions to prevent transmission of the hepatitis C virus should be taken.

Merck Sharp & Dohme Corp., a subsidiary of **Merck & Co., Inc.**, Whitehouse Station, NJ 08889, USA

U.S. Patent Nos. 7,012,066; 7,244,721

Trademarks depicted herein are the property of their respective owners.

503034-BCV-CP-USPI.62

MEDICATION GUIDE

VICTRELIS® (vic-TREL-is)

(boceprevir)

Capsules

Read this Medication Guide before you start taking VICTRELIS and each time you get a refill. There may be new information. This information does not take the place of talking with your healthcare provider about your medical condition or treatment.

VICTRELIS is taken along with peginterferon alfa and ribavirin. You should also read those Medication Guides.

What is the most important information I should know about VICTRELIS?

VICTRELIS, in combination with peginterferon alfa and ribavirin, may cause birth defects or death of your unborn baby. If you are pregnant or your sexual partner is pregnant or plans to become pregnant, do not take these medicines. You or your sexual partner should not become pregnant while taking VICTRELIS, peginterferon alfa, and ribavirin combination therapy and for 6 months after treatment is over.

- **Females and males must use 2 effective forms of birth control during treatment and for 6 months after treatment with VICTRELIS, peginterferon alfa, and ribavirin combination therapy.** Hormonal forms of birth control such as implants, injections, vaginal rings, and some birth control pills may not work during treatment with VICTRELIS. The use of certain types of birth control pills may be acceptable. Talk to your healthcare provider about forms of birth control that may be used during this time.
- Females must have a pregnancy test before starting treatment with VICTRELIS, peginterferon alfa, and ribavirin combination therapy, every month while being treated, and every month for 6 months after treatment with VICTRELIS, peginterferon alfa, and ribavirin combination therapy is over.
- If you or your female sexual partner becomes pregnant while taking VICTRELIS, peginterferon alfa, and ribavirin combination therapy or within 6 months after you stop taking these medicines, tell your healthcare provider right away. You or your healthcare provider should contact the Ribavirin Pregnancy Registry by calling 1-800-593-2214. The Ribavirin Pregnancy Registry collects information about what happens to mothers and their babies if the mother takes ribavirin while she is pregnant.

- **Do not take VICTRELIS alone to treat chronic hepatitis C infection.** VICTRELIS must be used with peginterferon alfa and ribavirin to treat chronic hepatitis C infection.

What is VICTRELIS?

VICTRELIS is a prescription medicine used with the medicines peginterferon alfa and ribavirin to treat long-lasting (chronic) hepatitis C genotype 1 infection in adults with stable (compensated) liver disease who have not been treated before or who have failed previous treatment.

It is not known if VICTRELIS is safe and effective in children under 18 years of age.

Who should not take VICTRELIS?

See "What is the most important information I should know about VICTRELIS?"

Do not take VICTRELIS if you:

- have had an allergic reaction to boceprevir or any of the ingredients in VICTRELIS. See the end of this Medication Guide for a complete list of ingredients in VICTRELIS.
- take certain medicines. **VICTRELIS may cause serious side effects when taken with certain medicines.** Read the section **"What should I tell my healthcare provider before taking VICTRELIS?"**

Talk to your healthcare provider before taking VICTRELIS if you have any of the conditions listed below.

What should I tell my healthcare provider before taking VICTRELIS?

Before you take VICTRELIS, tell your healthcare provider if you:

- have certain blood disorders such as low red blood cell count (anemia) or a certain type of low white blood cell count (neutropenia)
- have liver problems other than hepatitis C infection
- have human immunodeficiency virus (HIV) or any other immunity problems
- have had an organ transplant
- plan to have surgery
- have any other medical condition
- are breastfeeding. It is not known if VICTRELIS passes into breast milk. You and your healthcare provider should decide if you will take VICTRELIS or breastfeed. You should not do both.

Tell your healthcare provider about all the medicines you take, including prescription and non-prescription medicines, vitamins, and herbal supplements.

VICTRELIS and other medicines may affect each other. This can cause you to have too much or not enough VICTRELIS or your other medicines in your body, affecting the way VICTRELIS and your other medicines work, or causing side effects that can be serious or life-threatening. Do not start taking a new medicine without telling your healthcare provider or pharmacist.

Do not take VICTRELIS if you take a medicine that contains:

- alfuzosin hydrochloride (UROXATRAL®)
- anti-seizure medicines:
  - carbamazepine (CARBATROL®, EPITOL®, EQUETRO®, TEGRETOL®, TEGRETOL® XR, TERIL™)
  - phenobarbital
  - phenytoin (DILANTIN®)
- cisapride (PROPULSID®)
- drospirenone-containing birth control medicines, including:
  - YAZ®, YASMIN®, ZARAH®, OCELLA®, GIANVI®, BEYAZ®, ANGELIQ®, LORYNA™, SYEDA™, SAFYRAL™
- ergot-containing medicines, including:
  - dihydroergotamine mesylate (D.H.E. 45®, MIGRANAL®)
  - ergonovine and methylergonovine (ERGOTRATE®, METHERGINE®)
  - ergotamine tartrate (CAFERGOT®, MIGERGOT®, ERGOMAR®, ERGOSTAT, MEDIHALER ERGOTAMINE, WIGRAINE, WIGRETTES)
- lovastatin (ADVICOR®, ALTOPREV®, MEVACOR®)
- midazolam, when taken by mouth
- pimozide (ORAP®)
- rifampin (RIFADIN®, RIFAMATE®, RIFATER®, RIMACTANE)
- sildenafil (REVATIO®), when used for treating lung problems
- simvastatin (SIMCOR®, VYTORIN®, JUVISYNC™, ZOCOR®)
- St. John's Wort (Hypericum perforatum) or products containing St. John's Wort

- tadalafil (ADCIRCA®), when used for treating lung problems
- triazolam (HALCION®)

Tell your healthcare provider if you are taking or starting to take any of these medicines:

- atazanavir (REYATAZ®)
- clarithromycin (BIAXIN®, BIAXIN® XL, PREVPAC®)
- darunavir (PREZISTA®)
- dexamethasone
- efavirenz (SUSTIVA®, ATRIPLA®)
- etravirine (INTELENCE®)
- itraconazole (ONMEL™, SPORANOX®)
- ketoconazole (NIZORAL®)
- lopinavir (KALETRA®)
- posaconazole (NOXAFIL®)
- rifabutin (MYCOBUTIN®)
- ritonavir (NORVIR®, KALETRA®)
- voriconazole (VFEND®)

Your healthcare provider may need to monitor your therapy more closely if you take VICTRELIS with the following medicines. Talk to your doctor if you are taking or starting to take these medicines:

- alprazolam (XANAX®)
- amiodarone (CORDARONE®, NEXTERONE®, PACERONE®)
- atorvastatin (LIPITOR®)
- bepridil (VASCOR)
- bosentan (TRACLEER®)
- budesonide (PULMICORT®, PULMICORT FLEXIHALER®, RHINOCORT®, PULMICORT RESPULES®, SYMBICORT®)
- buprenorphine (BUTRANS®, BUPRENEX®, SUBOXONE®, SUBUTEX®)
- cyclosporine (GENGRAF ®, NEORAL®, SANDIMMUNE®)
- desipramine (NORPRAMIN®)
- digoxin (LANOXIN®)
- escitalopram (LEXAPRO®)
- felodipine (PLENDIL®)
- fluticasone (VERAMYST®, FLOVENT® HFA, FLOVENT® DISKUS, ADVAIR® HFA, ADVAIR DISKUS®)
- hormonal forms of birth control, including birth control pills, vaginal rings, implants and injections
- hormone replacement therapy
- methadone (METHADOSE®,DOLOPHINE®)
- naloxone
- nifedipine (PROCARDIA®, ADALAT® CC, PROCARDIA XL®, AFEDITAB® CR)
- nicardipine (CARDENE® SR, CARDENE®)
- omeprazole
- prednisone
- oral and IV prednisolone
- pravastatin (PRAVACHOL®)
- propafenone (RHYTHMOL, RHYTHMOL SR®)
- quinidine
- raltegravir (ISENTRESS®)
- salmeterol (ADVAIR® HFA, ADVAIR DISKUS®, SEREVENT®)
- sildenafil (VIAGRA®), when used for treating erectile dysfunction
- sirolimus (RAPAMUNE®)
- tacrolimus (PROGRAF®)
- tadalafil (CIALIS®), when used for treating erectile dysfunction
- colchicine (COLCRYS®, Probenecid and Colchicine, COL-Probenecid)
- trazodone (OLEPTRO ®)
- vardenafil (STAXYN®, LEVITRA®), when used for treating erectile dysfunction
- warfarin (COUMADIN®, JANTOVEN®)

Know the medicines you take. Keep a list of them to show your healthcare provider and pharmacist when you get a new medicine.

How should I take VICTRELIS?

- Take VICTRELIS exactly as your healthcare provider tells you to take it.
- Your healthcare provider will tell you how much to take and when to take it.
- Take VICTRELIS with food (a meal or light snack).
- VICTRELIS is packaged into single daily-use bottles. Each bottle has your entire day's worth of medicine. Make sure you are taking the correct amount of medicine each time.
- If you miss a dose of VICTRELIS and it is less than 2 hours before the next dose, the missed dose should be skipped.
- If you miss a dose of VICTRELIS and it is 2 or more hours before the next dose, take the missed dose with food. Take your next dose at your normal time and continue the normal dosing schedule.
- Do not double the next dose. If you have questions about what to do, call your healthcare provider.
- Your healthcare provider should do blood tests before you start treatment, at weeks 4, 8, 12, and 24, and at other times as needed during treatment, to see how well the medicines are working and to check for side effects.
- If you take too much VICTRELIS, call your healthcare provider or go to the nearest hospital emergency room right away.

What are the possible side effects of VICTRELIS?

VICTRELIS may cause serious side effects, including:

See "What is the most important information I should know about VICTRELIS?"

Serious allergic reactions. Serious allergic reactions can happen and may become severe requiring treatment in a hospital. Tell your healthcare provider right away if you have any of these symptoms:

- itching
- hives
- swelling of your face, eyes, lips, tongue, or throat
- trouble breathing or swallowing

Blood problems. VICTRELIS can affect your bone marrow and cause low red blood cell, and low white blood cell, counts. In some people, these blood counts may fall to dangerously low levels. If your blood cell counts become very low, you can get anemia or infections.

The most common side effects of VICTRELIS in combination with peginterferon alfa and ribavirin include:

- tiredness
- nausea
- headache
- change in taste

Additionally, while the medicine has been on the market, serious skin reactions, including blistering or peeling of the skin, have been reported. Tell your healthcare provider about any side effect that bothers you or that does not go away.

These are not all the possible side effects of VICTRELIS. For more information, ask your healthcare provider or pharmacist.

Call your doctor for medical advice about side effects. You may report side effects to FDA at 1-800-FDA-1088.

How should I store VICTRELIS?

- Store VICTRELIS capsules in a refrigerator at 36 to 46°F (2 to 8°C). Safely throw away refrigerated VICTRELIS after the expiration date.
- VICTRELIS capsules may also be stored at room temperature up to 77°F (25°C) for 3 months.
- Keep VICTRELIS in a tightly closed container and away from heat.

Keep VICTRELIS and all medicines out of the reach of children.

General information about the safe and effective use of VICTRELIS.

It is not known if treatment with VICTRELIS will prevent you from infecting another person with the hepatitis C virus during your treatment. Talk with your healthcare provider about ways to prevent spreading the hepatitis C virus.

Medicines are sometimes prescribed for purposes other than those listed in a Medication Guide.

Do not use VICTRELIS for a condition for which it was not prescribed. Do not give VICTRELIS to other people, even if they have the same symptoms that you have. It may harm them.

This Medication Guide summarizes the most important information about VICTRELIS. If you would like more information, talk with your healthcare provider. You can ask your pharmacist or healthcare provider for information about VICTRELIS that is written for health professionals. For more information, go to www.victrelis.com or call 1-877-888-4231.

What are the ingredients in VICTRELIS?

Active ingredients: boceprevir

Inactive ingredients: sodium lauryl sulfate, microcrystalline cellulose, lactose monohydrate, croscarmellose sodium, pre-gelatinized starch, and magnesium stearate.

Red capsule shell: gelatin, titanium dioxide, D&C Yellow #10, FD&C Blue #1, FD&C Red #40.

Yellow capsule shell: gelatin, titanium dioxide, D&C Yellow #10, FD&C Red #40, FD&C Yellow #6.

Red printing ink: shellac, red iron oxide. **Yellow printing ink:** shellac, titanium dioxide, povidone, D&C Yellow #10 Aluminum Lake.

This Medication Guide has been approved by the U.S. Food and Drug Administration.

Merck Sharp & Dohme Corp., a subsidiary of **Merck & Co., Inc.**, Whitehouse Station, NJ 08889, USA

Revised: 02/2013

503034-BCV-CP-MG.34

Shown in Product Identification Guide, page 309

VYTORIN® ℞

[*vī-tŏr-in*]

(ezetimibe/simvastatin)

Tablets

HIGHLIGHTS OF PRESCRIBING INFORMATION

These highlights do not include all the information needed to use VYTORIN safely and effectively. See full prescribing information for VYTORIN.

VYTORIN® (ezetimibe/simvastatin) Tablets

Initial U.S. Approval: 2004

RECENT MAJOR CHANGES

Dosage and Administration
Coadministration with Other Drugs (2.3) 10/2012
Contraindications (4) 10/2012
Warnings and Precautions
Myopathy/Rhabdomyolysis (5.1) 10/2012

INDICATIONS AND USAGE

VYTORIN, which contains a cholesterol absorption inhibitor and an HMG-CoA reductase inhibitor (statin), is indicated as adjunctive therapy to diet to:

- reduce elevated total-C, LDL-C, Apo B, TG, and non-HDL-C, and to increase HDL-C in patients with primary (heterozygous familial and non-familial) hyperlipidemia or mixed hyperlipidemia. (1.1)
- reduce elevated total-C and LDL-C in patients with homozygous familial hypercholesterolemia (HoFH), as an adjunct to other lipid-lowering treatments. (1.2)

Limitations of Use (1.3)

- No incremental benefit of VYTORIN on cardiovascular morbidity and mortality over and above that demonstrated for simvastatin has been established.
- VYTORIN has not been studied in Fredrickson Type I, III, IV, and V dyslipidemias.

DOSAGE AND ADMINISTRATION

- Dose range is 10/10 mg/day to 10/40 mg/day. (2.1)
- Recommended usual starting dose is 10/10 or 10/20 mg/day. (2.1)
- Due to the increased risk of myopathy, including rhabdomyolysis, use of the 10/80-mg dose of VYTORIN should be restricted to patients who have been taking VYTORIN 10/80 mg chronically (e.g., for 12 months or more) without evidence of muscle toxicity. (2.2)
- Patients who are currently tolerating the 10/80-mg dose of VYTORIN who need to be initiated on an interacting drug that is contraindicated or is associated with a dose cap for simvastatin should be switched to an alternative statin or statin-based regimen with less potential for the drug-drug interaction. (2.2)
- Due to the increased risk of myopathy, including rhabdomyolysis, associated with the 10/80-mg dose of VYTORIN, patients unable to achieve their LDL-C goal utilizing the 10/40-mg dose of VYTORIN should not be titrated to the 10/80-mg dose, but should be placed on alternative LDL-C-lowering treatment(s) that provides greater LDL-C lowering. (2.2)
- Dosing of VYTORIN should occur either ≥2 hours before or ≥4 hours after administration of a bile acid sequestrant. (2.3, 7.5)

DOSAGE FORMS AND STRENGTHS

- Tablets (ezetimibe mg/simvastatin mg): 10/10, 10/20, 10/40, 10/80 (3)

CONTRAINDICATIONS

- Concomitant administration of strong CYP3A4 inhibitors. (4, 5.1)
- Concomitant administration of gemfibrozil, cyclosporine, or danazol. (4, 5.1)
- Hypersensitivity to any component of this medication (4, 6.2)
- Active liver disease or unexplained persistent elevations of hepatic transaminase levels (4, 5.2)
- Women who are pregnant or may become pregnant (4, 8.1)
- Nursing mothers (4, 8.3)

WARNINGS AND PRECAUTIONS

- **Patients should be advised of the increased risk of myopathy, including rhabdomyolysis, with the 10/80-mg dose. (5.1)**
- Patients should be advised to report promptly any unexplained and/or persistent muscle pain, tenderness, or weakness. VYTORIN should be discontinued immediately if myopathy is diagnosed or suspected. (5.1)
- Skeletal muscle effects (e.g., myopathy and rhabdomyolysis): Risks increase with higher doses and concomitant use of certain medicines. Predisposing factors include advanced age (≥65), female gender, uncontrolled hypothyroidism, and renal impairment. (4, 5.1, 8.5, 8.6)
- Liver enzyme abnormalities: Persistent elevations in hepatic transaminases can occur. Check liver enzyme tests before initiating therapy and as clinically indicated thereafter. (5.2)

- VYTORIN is not recommended in patients with moderate or severe hepatic impairment. (5.3, 12.3)

ADVERSE REACTIONS

- Common (incidence ≥2% and greater than placebo) adverse reactions in clinical trials: headache, increased ALT, myalgia, upper respiratory tract infection, and diarrhea. (6.1)

To report SUSPECTED ADVERSE REACTIONS, contact Merck Sharp & Dohme Corp., a subsidiary of Merck & Co., Inc., at 1-877-888-4231 or FDA at 1-800-FDA-1088 or www.fda.gov/medwatch.

DRUG INTERACTIONS

Drug Interactions Associated with Increased Risk of Myopathy/Rhabdomyolysis (2.3, 4, 5.1, 7.1, 7.2, 7.3, 7.6, 7.8, 12.3)

Interacting Agents	Prescribing Recommendations
Strong CYP3A4 Inhibitors, (e.g., itraconazole, ketoconazole, posaconazole, voriconazole, erythromycin, clarithromycin, telithromycin, HIV protease inhibitors, boceprevir, telaprevir, nefazodone), gemfibrozil, cyclosporine, danazol	Contraindicated with VYTORIN
Verapamil, diltiazem, dronedarone	Do not exceed 10/10 mg VYTORIN daily
Amiodarone, amlodipine, ranolazine	Do not exceed 10/20 mg VYTORIN daily
Grapefruit juice	Avoid grapefruit juice

- Coumarin anticoagulants: simvastatin prolongs INR. Achieve stable INR prior to starting VYTORIN. Monitor INR frequently until stable upon initiation or alteration of VYTORIN therapy. (7.8)
- Cholestyramine: Combination decreases exposure of ezetimibe. (2.3, 7.5)
- Other Lipid-lowering Medications: Use with other fibrate products or lipid-modifying doses (≥1 g/day) of niacin increases the risk of adverse skeletal muscle effects. Caution should be used when prescribing with VYTORIN. (5.1, 7.2, 7.4).

USE IN SPECIFIC POPULATIONS

- Moderate to severe renal impairment: Doses exceeding 10/20 mg/day should be used with caution and close monitoring (2.6, 8.6).

See 17 for PATIENT COUNSELING INFORMATION and FDA-approved patient labeling

Revised: 02/2013

FULL PRESCRIBING INFORMATION: CONTENTS*

*** Sections or subsections omitted from the full prescribing information are not listed**

FULL PRESCRIBING INFORMATION

1 INDICATIONS AND USAGE

Therapy with lipid-altering agents should be only one component of multiple risk factor intervention in individuals at significantly increased risk for atherosclerotic vascular disease due to hypercholesterolemia. Drug therapy is indicated as an adjunct to diet when the response to a diet restricted in saturated fat and cholesterol and other nonpharmacologic measures alone has been inadequate.

1.1 Primary Hyperlipidemia

VYTORIN® is indicated for the reduction of elevated total cholesterol (total-C), low-density lipoprotein cholesterol (LDL-C), apolipoprotein B (Apo B), triglycerides (TG), and non-high-density lipoprotein cholesterol (non-HDL-C), and to increase high-density lipoprotein cholesterol (HDL-C) in patients with primary (heterozygous familial and non-familial) hyperlipidemia or mixed hyperlipidemia.

1.2 Homozygous Familial Hypercholesterolemia (HoFH)

VYTORIN is indicated for the reduction of elevated total-C and LDL-C in patients with homozygous familial hypercholesterolemia, as an adjunct to other lipid-lowering treatments (e.g., LDL apheresis) or if such treatments are unavailable.

1.3 Limitations of Use

No incremental benefit of VYTORIN on cardiovascular morbidity and mortality over and above that demonstrated for simvastatin has been established.

VYTORIN has not been studied in Fredrickson type I, III, IV, and V dyslipidemias.

2 DOSAGE AND ADMINISTRATION

2.1 Recommended Dosing

The usual dosage range is 10/10 mg/day to 10/40 mg/day. The recommended usual starting dose is 10/10 mg/day or 10/20 mg/day. VYTORIN should be taken as a single daily dose in the evening, with or without food. Patients who require a larger reduction in LDL-C (greater than 55%) may be started at 10/40 mg/day in the absence of moderate to severe renal impairment (estimated glomerular filtration rate <60 mL/min/1.73 m^2). After initiation or titration of VYTORIN, lipid levels may be analyzed after 2 or more weeks and dosage adjusted, if needed.

2.2 Restricted Dosing for 10/80 mg

Due to the increased risk of myopathy, including rhabdomyolysis, particularly during the first year of treatment, use of the 10/80-mg dose of VYTORIN should be restricted to patients who have been taking VYTORIN 10/80 mg chronically (e.g., for 12 months or more) without evidence of muscle toxicity *[see Warnings and Precautions (5.1)]*.

Patients who are currently tolerating the 10/80-mg dose of VYTORIN who need to be initiated on an interacting drug that is contraindicated or is associated with a dose cap for simvastatin should be switched to an alternative statin or statin-based regimen with less potential for the drug-drug interaction.

Due to the increased risk of myopathy, including rhabdomyolysis, associated with the 10/80-mg dose of VYTORIN, patients unable to achieve their LDL-C goal utilizing the 10/40-mg dose of VYTORIN should not be titrated to the 10/80-mg dose, but should be placed on alternative LDL-C-lowering treatment(s) that provides greater LDL-C lowering.

2.3 Coadministration with Other Drugs

Patients taking Verapamil, Diltiazem, or Dronedarone

- The dose of VYTORIN should not exceed 10/10 mg/day *[see Warnings and Precautions (5.1), Drug Interactions (7.3), and Clinical Pharmacology (12.3)]*.

Patients taking Amiodarone, Amlodipine or Ranolazine

- The dose of VYTORIN should not exceed 10/20 mg/day *[see Warnings and Precautions (5.1), Drug Interactions (7.3), and Clinical Pharmacology (12.3)]*.

Patients taking Bile Acid Sequestrants

- Dosing of VYTORIN should occur either ≥2 hours before or ≥4 hours after administration of a bile acid sequestrant *[see Drug Interactions (7.5)]*.

2.4 Patients with Homozygous Familial Hypercholesterolemia

The recommended dosage for patients with homozygous familial hypercholesterolemia is VYTORIN 10/40 mg/day in the evening *[see Dosage and Administration, Restricted Dosing for 10/80 mg (2.2)]*. VYTORIN should be used as an adjunct to other lipid-lowering treatments (e.g., LDL apheresis) in these patients or if such treatments are unavailable.

2.5 Patients with Hepatic Impairment

No dosage adjustment is necessary in patients with mild hepatic impairment *[see Warnings and Precautions (5.3)]*.

2.6 Patients with Renal Impairment/Chronic Kidney Disease

In patients with mild renal impairment (estimated GFR ≥60 mL/min/1.73 m^2), no dosage adjustment is necessary. In patients with chronic kidney disease and estimated glomerular filtration rate <60 mL/min/1.73 m^2, the dose of VYTORIN is 10/20 mg/day in the evening. In such patients, higher doses should be used with caution and close monitoring *[see Warnings and Precautions (5.1); Clinical Pharmacology (12.3)]*.

2.7 Geriatric Patients

No dosage adjustment is necessary in geriatric patients *[see Clinical Pharmacology (12.3)]*.

2.8 Chinese Patients Taking Lipid-Modifying Doses (≥1 g/day Niacin) of Niacin-Containing Products

Because of an increased risk for myopathy in Chinese patients taking simvastatin 40 mg coadministered with lipid-modifying doses (≥1 g/day niacin) of niacin-containing products, caution should be used when treating Chinese patients with VYTORIN doses exceeding 10/20 mg/day coadministered with lipid-modifying doses (≥1 g/day niacin) of niacin-containing products. Because the risk for myopathy is dose-related, Chinese patients should not receive VYTORIN 10/80 mg coadministered with lipid-modifying doses of niacin-containing products. The cause of the increased risk of myopathy is not known. It is also unknown if the risk for myopathy with coadministration of simvastatin with lipid-modifying doses of niacin-containing products observed in Chinese patients applies to other Asian patients. *[See Warnings and Precautions (5.1).]*

3 DOSAGE FORMS AND STRENGTHS

- VYTORIN® 10/10, (ezetimibe 10 mg/simvastatin 10 mg tablets) are white to off-white capsule-shaped tablets with code "311" on one side.
- VYTORIN® 10/20, (ezetimibe 10 mg/simvastatin 20 mg tablets) are white to off-white capsule-shaped tablets with code "312" on one side.
- VYTORIN® 10/40, (ezetimibe 10 mg/simvastatin 40 mg tablets) are white to off-white capsule-shaped tablets with code "313" on one side.
- VYTORIN® 10/80, (ezetimibe 10 mg/simvastatin 80 mg tablets) are white to off-white capsule-shaped tablets with code "315" on one side.

4 CONTRAINDICATIONS

VYTORIN is contraindicated in the following conditions:

- Concomitant administration of strong CYP3A4 inhibitors (e.g., itraconazole, ketoconazole, posaconazole, voriconazole, HIV protease inhibitors, boceprevir, telaprevir, erythromycin, clarithromycin, telithromycin and nefazodone) *[see Warnings and Precautions (5.1)]*.
- Concomitant administration of gemfibrozil, cyclosporine, or danazol *[see Warnings and Precautions (5.1)]*.
- Hypersensitivity to any component of this medication *[see Adverse Reactions (6.2)]*.
- Active liver disease or unexplained persistent elevations in hepatic transaminase levels *[see Warnings and Precautions (5.2)]*.
- Women who are pregnant or may become pregnant. Serum cholesterol and triglycerides increase during normal pregnancy, and cholesterol or cholesterol derivatives are essential for fetal development. Because HMG-CoA reductase

inhibitors (statins), such as simvastatin, decrease cholesterol synthesis and possibly the synthesis of other biologically active substances derived from cholesterol, VYTORIN may cause fetal harm when administered to a pregnant woman. Atherosclerosis is a chronic process and the discontinuation of lipid-lowering drugs during pregnancy should have little impact on the outcome of long-term therapy of primary hypercholesterolemia. There are no adequate and well-controlled studies of VYTORIN use during pregnancy; however, in rare reports congenital anomalies were observed following intrauterine exposure to statins. In rat and rabbit animal reproduction studies, simvastatin revealed no evidence of teratogenicity. **VYTORIN should be administered to women of childbearing age only when such patients are highly unlikely to conceive.** If the patient becomes pregnant while taking this drug, VYTORIN should be discontinued immediately and the patient should be apprised of the potential hazard to the fetus *[see Use in Specific Populations (8.1)]*.

- Nursing mothers. It is not known whether simvastatin is excreted into human milk; however, a small amount of another drug in this class does pass into breast milk. Because statins have the potential for serious adverse reactions in nursing infants, women who require VYTORIN treatment should not breast-feed their infants *[see Use in Specific Populations (8.3)]*.

5 WARNINGS AND PRECAUTIONS

5.1 Myopathy/Rhabdomyolysis

Simvastatin occasionally causes myopathy manifested as muscle pain, tenderness or weakness with creatine kinase above ten times the upper limit of normal (ULN). Myopathy sometimes takes the form of rhabdomyolysis with or without acute renal failure secondary to myoglobinuria, and rare fatalities have occurred. The risk of myopathy is increased by high levels of statin activity in plasma. Predisposing factors for myopathy include advanced age (≥65 years), female gender, uncontrolled hypothyroidism, and renal impairment.

The risk of myopathy, including rhabdomyolysis, is dose related. In a clinical trial database in which 41,413 patients were treated with simvastatin, 24,747 (approximately 60%) of whom were enrolled in studies with a median follow-up of at least 4 years, the incidence of myopathy was approximately 0.03% and 0.08% at 20 and 40 mg/day, respectively. The incidence of myopathy with 80 mg (0.61%) was disproportionately higher than that observed at the lower doses. In these trials, patients were carefully monitored and some interacting medicinal products were excluded.

In a clinical trial in which 12,064 patients with a history of myocardial infarction were treated with simvastatin (mean follow-up 6.7 years), the incidence of myopathy (defined as unexplained muscle weakness or pain with a serum creatine kinase [CK] >10 times upper limit of normal [ULN]) in patients on 80 mg/day was approximately 0.9% compared with 0.02% for patients on 20 mg/day. The incidence of rhabdomyolysis (defined as myopathy with a CK >40 times ULN) in patients on 80 mg/day was approximately 0.4% compared with 0% for patients on 20 mg/day. The incidence of myopathy, including rhabdomyolysis, was highest during the first year and then notably decreased during the subsequent years of treatment. In this trial, patients were carefully monitored and some interacting medicinal products were excluded.

The risk of myopathy, including rhabdomyolysis, is greater in patients on simvastatin 80 mg compared with other statin therapies with similar or greater LDL-C-lowering efficacy and compared with lower doses of simvastatin. Therefore, the 10/80-mg dose of VYTORIN should be used only in patients who have been taking VYTORIN 10/80 mg chronically (e.g., for 12 months or more) without evidence of muscle toxicity *[see Dosage and Administration, Restricted Dosing for 10/80 mg (2.2)]*. If, however, a patient who is currently tolerating the 10/80-mg dose of VYTORIN needs to be initiated on an interacting drug that is contraindicated or is associated with a dose cap for simvastatin, that patient should be switched to an alternative statin or statin-based regimen with less potential for the drug-drug interaction. Patients should be advised of the increased risk of myopathy, including rhabdomyolysis, and to report promptly any unexplained muscle pain, tenderness or weakness. If symptoms occur, treatment should be discontinued immediately *[see Warnings and Precautions (5.2)]*.

In the Study of Heart and Renal Protection (SHARP), 9270 patients with chronic kidney disease were allocated to receive VYTORIN 10/20 mg daily (n=4650) or placebo (n=4620). During a median follow-up period of 4.9 years, the incidence of myopathy (defined as unexplained muscle weakness or pain with a serum creatine kinase [CK] >10 times upper limit of normal [ULN]) was 0.2% for VYTORIN and 0.1% for placebo: the incidence of rhabdomyolysis (defined as myopathy with a CK > 40 times ULN) was 0.09% for VYTORIN and 0.02% for placebo.

In post-marketing experience with ezetimibe, cases of myopathy and rhabdomyolysis have been reported. Most patients who developed rhabdomyolysis were taking a statin prior to initiating ezetimibe. However, rhabdomyolysis has been reported very rarely with ezetimibe monotherapy and very rarely with the addition of ezetimibe to agents known to be associated with increased risk of rhabdomyolysis, such as fibrates.

There have been rare reports of immune-mediated necrotizing myopathy (IMNM), an autoimmune myopathy, associated with statin use. IMNM is characterized by: proximal muscle weakness and elevated serum creatine kinase, which persist despite discontinuation of statin treatment; muscle biopsy showing necrotizing myopathy without significant inflammation; improvement with immunosuppressive agents.

All patients starting therapy with VYTORIN or whose dose of VYTORIN is being increased should be advised of the risk of myopathy, including rhabdomyolysis, and told to report promptly any unexplained muscle pain, tenderness or weakness particularly if accompanied by malaise or fever or if muscle signs and symptoms persist after discontinuing VYTORIN. VYTORIN therapy should be discontinued immediately if myopathy is diagnosed or suspected. In most cases, muscle symptoms and CK increases resolved when simvastatin treatment was promptly discontinued. Periodic CK determinations may be considered in patients starting therapy with VYTORIN or whose dose is being increased, but there is no assurance that such monitoring will prevent myopathy.

Many of the patients who have developed rhabdomyolysis on therapy with simvastatin have had complicated medical histories, including renal insufficiency usually as a consequence of long-standing diabetes mellitus. Such patients taking VYTORIN merit closer monitoring.

VYTORIN therapy should be discontinued if markedly elevated CPK levels occur or myopathy is diagnosed or suspected. VYTORIN therapy should also be temporarily withheld in any patient experiencing an acute or serious condition predisposing to the development of renal failure secondary to rhabdomyolysis, e.g., sepsis; hypotension; major surgery; trauma; severe metabolic, endocrine, or electrolyte disorders; or uncontrolled epilepsy.

Drug Interactions

The risk of myopathy and rhabdomyolysis is increased by high levels of statin activity in plasma. Simvastatin is metabolized by the cytochrome P450 isoform 3A4. Certain drugs that inhibit this metabolic pathway can raise the plasma levels of simvastatin and may increase the risk of myopathy. These include itraconazole, ketoconazole, posaconazole, and voriconazole, the macrolide antibiotics erythromycin and clarithromycin, and the ketolide antibiotic telithromycin, HIV protease inhibitors, boceprevir, telaprevir, the antidepressant nefazodone, or grapefruit juice. *[See Clinical Pharmacology (12.3).]* Combination of these drugs with VYTORIN is contraindicated. If short-term treatment with strong CYP3A4 inhibitors is unavoidable, therapy with VYTORIN must be suspended during the course of treatment. *[See Contraindications (4) and Drug Interactions (7).]*

The combined use of VYTORIN with gemfibrozil, cyclosporine, or danazol is contraindicated *[see Contraindications (4) and Drug Interactions (7.1 and 7.2)]*.

Caution should be used when prescribing other fibrates with VYTORIN, as these agents can cause myopathy when given alone and the risk is increased when they are co-administered *[see Drug Interactions (7.2, 7.7)]*.

Cases of myopathy, including rhabdomyolysis, have been reported with simvastatin coadministered with colchicine, and caution should be exercised when prescribing VYTORIN with colchicine *[see Drug Interactions (7.9)]*.

The benefits of the combined use of VYTORIN with the following drugs should be carefully weighed against the potential risks of combinations: other lipid-lowering drugs (other fibrates or ≥1 g/day of niacin), amiodarone, dronedarone, verapamil, diltiazem, amlodipine, or ranolazine *[see Drug Interactions (7.3) and Table 6 in Clinical Pharmacology (12.3)]*.

Cases of myopathy, including rhabdomyolysis, have been observed with simvastatin coadministered with lipid-modifying doses (≥1 g/day niacin) of niacin-containing products. In an ongoing, double-blind, randomized cardiovascular outcomes trial, an independent safety monitoring committee identified that the incidence of myopathy is higher in Chinese compared with non-Chinese patients taking simvastatin 40 mg or ezetimibe/simvastatin 10/40 mg coadministered with lipid-modifying doses of a niacin-containing product. Caution should be used when treating Chinese patients with VYTORIN in doses exceeding 10/20 mg/day coadministered with lipid-modifying doses of niacin-containing products. Because the risk for myopathy is dose-related, Chinese patients should not receive VYTORIN 10/80 mg coadministered with lipid-modifying doses of niacin-containing products. It is unknown if the risk for myopathy with coadministration of simvastatin with lipid-modifying doses of niacin-containing products observed in Chinese patients applies to other Asian patients *[see Drug Interactions (7.4)]*.

Prescribing recommendations for interacting agents are summarized in Table 1 *[see also Dosage and Administration (2.3), Drug Interactions (7), and Clinical Pharmacology (12.3)]*.

Table 1: Drug Interactions Associated with Increased Risk of Myopathy/Rhabdomyolysis

Interacting Agents	Prescribing Recommendations
Strong CYP3A4 Inhibitors, e.g.: Itraconazole Ketoconazole Posaconazole Voriconazole Erythromycin Clarithromycin Telithromycin HIV protease inhibitors Boceprevir Telaprevir Nefazodone Gemfibrozil Cyclosporine Danazol	Contraindicated with VYTORIN
Verapamil Diltiazem Dronedarone	Do not exceed 10/10 mg VYTORIN daily
Amiodarone Amlodipine Ranolazine	Do not exceed 10/20 mg VYTORIN daily
Grapefruit juice	Avoid grapefruit juice

5.2 Liver Enzymes

In three placebo-controlled, 12-week trials, the incidence of consecutive elevations (≥3 × ULN) in serum transaminases was 1.7% overall for patients treated with VYTORIN and appeared to be dose-related with an incidence of 2.6% for patients treated with VYTORIN 10/80. In controlled long-term (48-week) extensions, which included both newly-treated and previously-treated patients, the incidence of consecutive elevations (≥3 × ULN) in serum transaminases was 1.8% overall and 3.6% for patients treated with VYTORIN 10/80. These elevations in transaminases were generally asymptomatic, not associated with cholestasis, and returned to baseline after discontinuation of therapy or with continued treatment.

In SHARP, 9270 patients with chronic kidney disease were allocated to receive VYTORIN 10/20 mg daily (n=4650), or placebo (n=4620). During a median follow-up period of 4.9 years, the incidence of consecutive elevations of transaminases (>3 × ULN) was 0.7% for VYTORIN and 0.6% for placebo.

It is recommended that liver function tests be performed before the initiation of treatment with VYTORIN, and thereafter when clinically indicated. There have been rare post-marketing reports of fatal and non-fatal hepatic failure in patients taking statins, including simvastatin. If serious liver injury with clinical symptoms and/or hyperbilirubinemia or jaundice occurs during treatment with VYTORIN, promptly interrupt therapy. If an alternate etiology is not found do not restart VYTORIN. Note that ALT may emanate from muscle, therefore ALT rising with CK may indicate myopathy *[see Warnings and Precautions (5.1)]*.

VYTORIN should be used with caution in patients who consume substantial quantities of alcohol and/or have a past history of liver disease. Active liver diseases or unexplained persistent transaminase elevations are contraindications to the use of VYTORIN.

5.3 Hepatic Impairment

Due to the unknown effects of the increased exposure to ezetimibe in patients with moderate or severe hepatic impairment, VYTORIN is not recommended in these patients. *[See Clinical Pharmacology (12.3).]*

5.4 Endocrine Function

Increases in HbA1c and fasting serum glucose levels have been reported with HMG-CoA reductase inhibitors, including simvastatin.

6 ADVERSE REACTIONS

The following serious adverse reactions are discussed in greater detail in other sections of the label:

- Rhabdomyolysis and myopathy *[see Warnings and Precautions (5.1)]*
- Liver enzyme abnormalities *[see Warnings and Precautions (5.2)]*

Table 2*: Clinical Adverse Reactions Occurring in ≥2% of Patients Treated with VYTORIN and at an Incidence Greater than Placebo, Regardless of Causality

Body System/Organ Class Adverse Reaction	Placebo (%) n=371	Ezetimibe 10 mg (%) n=302	Simvastatin† (%) n=1234	VYTORIN† (%) n=1420
Body as a whole – general disorders				
Headache	5.4	6.0	5.9	5.8
Gastrointestinal system disorders				
Diarrhea	2.2	5.0	3.7	2.8
Infections and infestations				
Influenza	0.8	1.0	1.9	2.3
Upper respiratory tract infection	2.7	5.0	5.0	3.6
Musculoskeletal and connective tissue disorders				
Myalgia	2.4	2.3	2.6	3.6
Pain in extremity	1.3	3.0	2.0	2.3

* Includes two placebo-controlled combination studies in which the active ingredients equivalent to VYTORIN were coadministered and two placebo-controlled studies in which VYTORIN was administered.
† All doses.

6.1 Clinical Trials Experience

VYTORIN

Because clinical studies are conducted under widely varying conditions, adverse reaction rates observed in the clinical studies of a drug cannot be directly compared to rates in the clinical studies of another drug and may not reflect the rates observed in practice.

In the VYTORIN (ezetimibe/simvastatin) placebo-controlled clinical trials database of 1420 patients (age range 20-83 years, 52% women, 87% Caucasians, 3% Blacks, 5% Hispanics, 3% Asians) with a median treatment duration of 27 weeks, 5% of patients on VYTORIN and 2.2% of patients on placebo discontinued due to adverse reactions.

The most common adverse reactions in the group treated with VYTORIN that led to treatment discontinuation and occurred at a rate greater than placebo were:

- Increased ALT (0.9%)
- Myalgia (0.6%)
- Increased AST (0.4%)
- Back pain (0.4%)

The most commonly reported adverse reactions (incidence ≥2% and greater than placebo) in controlled clinical trials were: headache (5.8%), increased ALT (3.7%), myalgia (3.6%), upper respiratory tract infection (3.6%), and diarrhea (2.8%).

VYTORIN has been evaluated for safety in more than 10,189 patients in clinical trials.

Table 2 summarizes the frequency of clinical adverse reactions reported in ≥2% of patients treated with VYTORIN (n=1420) and at an incidence greater than placebo, regardless of causality assessment, from four placebo-controlled trials.

[See table 2 above]

Study of Heart and Renal Protection

In SHARP, 9270 patients were allocated to VYTORIN 10/20 mg daily (n=4650) or placebo (n=4620) for a median follow-up period of 4.9 years. The proportion of patients who permanently discontinued study treatment as a result of either an adverse event or abnormal safety blood result was 10.4% vs. 9.8% among patients allocated to VYTORIN and placebo, respectively. Comparing those allocated to VYTORIN vs. placebo, the incidence of myopathy (defined as unexplained muscle weakness or pain with a serum CK >10 times ULN) was 0.2% vs. 0.1% and the incidence of rhabdomyolysis (defined as myopathy with a CK >40 times ULN) was 0.09% vs. 0.02%, respectively. Consecutive elevations of transaminases (>3 × ULN) occurred in 0.7% vs. 0.6%, respectively. Patients were asked about the occurrence of unexplained muscle pain or weakness at each study visit: 21.5% vs. 20.9% patients ever reported muscle symptoms in the VYTORIN and placebo groups, respectively. Cancer was diagnosed during the trial in 9.4% vs. 9.5% of patients assigned to VYTORIN and placebo, respectively.

Ezetimibe

Other adverse reactions reported with ezetimibe in placebo-controlled studies, regardless of causality assessment: *Musculoskeletal system disorders:* arthralgia; *Infections and infestations:* sinusitis; *Body as a whole – general disorders:* fatigue.

Simvastatin

In a clinical trial in which 12,064 patients with a history of myocardial infarction were treated with simvastatin (mean follow-up 6.7 years), the incidence of myopathy (defined as unexplained muscle weakness or pain with a serum creatine kinase [CK] >10 times upper limit of normal [ULN]) in patients on 80 mg/day was approximately 0.9% compared with 0.02% for patients on 20 mg/day. The incidence of rhabdomyolysis (defined as myopathy with a CK >40 times ULN) in patients on 80 mg/day was approximately 0.4% compared with 0% for patients on 20 mg/day. The incidence of myopathy, including rhabdomyolysis, was highest during the first year and then notably decreased during the subsequent years of treatment. In this trial, patients were carefully monitored and some interacting medicinal products were excluded.

Other adverse reactions reported with simvastatin in placebo-controlled clinical studies, regardless of causality assessment: *Cardiac disorders:* atrial fibrillation; *Ear and labyrinth disorders:* vertigo; *Gastrointestinal disorders:* abdominal pain, constipation, dyspepsia, flatulence, gastritis; *Skin and subcutaneous tissue disorders:* eczema, rash; *Endocrine disorders:* diabetes mellitus; *Infections and infestations:* bronchitis, sinusitis, urinary tract infections; *Body as a whole – general disorders:* asthenia, edema/swelling; *Psychiatric disorders:* insomnia.

Laboratory Tests

Marked persistent increases of hepatic serum transaminases have been noted *[see Warnings and Precautions (5.2)]*. Elevated alkaline phosphatase and γ-glutamyl transpeptidase have been reported. About 5% of patients taking simvastatin had elevations of CK levels of 3 or more times the normal value on one or more occasions. This was attributable to the noncardiac fraction of CK *[see Warnings and Precautions (5.1)]*.

6.2 Post-Marketing Experience

Because the below reactions are reported voluntarily from a population of uncertain size, it is generally not possible to reliably estimate their frequency or establish a causal relationship to drug exposure.

The following adverse reactions have been reported in post-marketing experience for VYTORIN or ezetimibe or simvastatin: pruritus; alopecia; erythema multiforme; a variety of skin changes (e.g., nodules, discoloration, dryness of skin/mucous membranes, changes to hair/nails); dizziness; muscle cramps; myalgia; arthralgia; pancreatitis; paresthesia; peripheral neuropathy; vomiting; nausea; anemia; erectile dysfunction; interstitial lung disease; myopathy/rhabdomyolysis *[see Warnings and Precautions (5.1)]*; hepatitis/jaundice; fatal and non-fatal hepatic failure; depression; cholelithiasis; cholecystitis; thrombocytopenia; elevations in liver transaminases; elevated creatine phosphokinase.

There have been rare reports of immune-mediated necrotizing myopathy associated with statin use. *[see Warnings and Precautions (5.1)]*.

Hypersensitivity reactions, including anaphylaxis, angioedema, rash, and urticaria have been reported.

In addition, an apparent hypersensitivity syndrome has been reported rarely that has included one or more of the following features: anaphylaxis, angioedema, lupus erythematous-like syndrome, polymyalgia rheumatica, dermatomyositis, vasculitis, purpura, thrombocytopenia, leukopenia, hemolytic anemia, positive ANA, ESR increase, eosinophilia, arthritis, arthralgia, urticaria, asthenia, photosensitivity, fever, chills, flushing, malaise, dyspnea, toxic epidermal necrolysis, erythema multiforme, including Stevens-Johnson syndrome.

There have been rare postmarketing reports of cognitive impairment (e.g., memory loss, forgetfulness, amnesia, memory impairment, confusion) associated with statin use. These cognitive issues have been reported for all statins. The reports are generally nonserious, and reversible upon statin discontinuation, with variable times to symptom onset (1 day to years) and symptom resolution (median of 3 weeks).

7 DRUG INTERACTIONS

[See Clinical Pharmacology (12.3).]

VYTORIN

7.1 Strong CYP3A4 Inhibitors, cyclosporine, or danazol

Strong CYP3A4 inhibitors: The risk of myopathy is increased by reducing the elimination of the simvastatin component of VYTORIN. Hence when VYTORIN is used with an inhibitor of CYP3A4 (e.g., as listed below), elevated plasma levels of HMG-CoA reductase inhibitory activity increases the risk of myopathy and rhabdomyolysis, particularly with higher doses of VYTORIN. *[See Warnings and Precautions (5.1) and Clinical Pharmacology (12.3).]* Concomitant use of drugs labeled as having a strong inhibitory effect on CYP3A4 is contraindicated *[see Contraindications (4)]*. If treatment with itraconazole, ketoconazole, posaconazole, voriconazole, erythromycin, clarithromycin or telithromycin is unavoidable, therapy with VYTORIN must be suspended during the course of treatment.

Cyclosporine or Danazol: The risk of myopathy, including rhabdomyolysis is increased by concomitant administration of cyclosporine or danazol. Therefore, concomitant use of these drugs is contraindicated *[see Contraindications (4)*, Warnings and Precautions (5.1) and Clinical Pharmacology (12.3)].

7.2 Lipid-Lowering Drugs That Can Cause Myopathy When Given Alone

Gemfibrozil: Contraindicated with VYTORIN *[see Contraindications (4)* and *Warnings and Precautions (5.1)]*.

Other fibrates: Caution should be used when prescribing with VYTORIN *[see Warnings and Precautions (5.1)]*.

7.3 Amiodarone, Dronedarone, Ranolazine, or Calcium Channel Blockers

The risk of myopathy, including rhabdomyolysis, is increased by concomitant administration of amiodarone, dronedarone, ranolazine, or calcium channel blockers such as verapamil, diltiazem or amlodipine *[see Dosage and Administration (2.3) and Warnings and Precautions (5.1) and Table 6 in Clinical Pharmacology (12.3)]*.

7.4 Niacin

Cases of myopathy/rhabdomyolysis have been observed with simvastatin coadministered with lipid-modifying doses (≥1 g/day niacin) of niacin-containing products. The benefits of the combined use of VYTORIN with niacin should be carefully weighed against the potential risks of myopathy/rhabdomyolysis. In particular, caution should be used when treating Chinese patients with VYTORIN doses exceeding 10/20 mg/day coadministered with lipid-modifying doses of niacin-containing products. Because the risk for myopathy is dose-related, Chinese patients should not receive VYTORIN 10/80 mg coadministered with lipid-modifying doses of niacin-containing products. *[See Warnings and Precautions (5.1).]*

7.5 Cholestyramine

Concomitant cholestyramine administration decreased the mean AUC of total ezetimibe approximately 55%. The incremental LDL-C reduction due to adding VYTORIN to cholestyramine may be reduced by this interaction.

7.6 Digoxin

In one study, concomitant administration of digoxin with simvastatin resulted in a slight elevation in plasma digoxin concentrations. Patients taking digoxin should be monitored appropriately when VYTORIN is initiated.

7.7 Fibrates

The safety and effectiveness of VYTORIN administered with fibrates have not been established. Because it is known that the risk of myopathy during treatment with HMG-CoA reductase inhibitors is increased with concurrent administration of fibrates, VYTORIN should be administered with caution when used concomitantly with fibrates (other than gemfibrozil, which is contraindicated) *[see Contraindications (4) and Warnings and Precautions (5.1)]*.

Fibrates may increase cholesterol excretion into the bile, leading to cholelithiasis. In a preclinical study in dogs, ezetimibe increased cholesterol in the gallbladder bile *[see Animal Toxicology and/or Pharmacology (13.2)]*.

7.8 Coumarin Anticoagulants

Simvastatin 20-40 mg/day modestly potentiated the effect of coumarin anticoagulants: the prothrombin time, reported as International Normalized Ratio (INR), increased from a baseline of 1.7 to 1.8 and from 2.6 to 3.4 in a normal volunteer study and in a hypercholesterolemic patient study, respectively. With other statins, clinically evident bleeding and/or increased prothrombin time has been reported in a few patients taking coumarin anticoagulants concomitantly. In such patients, prothrombin time should be determined before starting VYTORIN and frequently enough during early therapy to ensure that no significant alteration of prothrombin time occurs. Once a stable prothrombin time has been documented, prothrombin times can be monitored at the intervals usually recommended for patients on coumarin anticoagulants. If the dose of VYTORIN is changed or discontinued, the same procedure should be repeated.

Simvastatin therapy has not been associated with bleeding or with changes in prothrombin time in patients not taking anticoagulants.

Concomitant administration of ezetimibe (10 mg once daily) had no significant effect on bioavailability of warfarin and prothrombin time in a study of twelve healthy adult males. There have been post-marketing reports of increased INR in patients who had ezetimibe added to warfarin. Most of these patients were also on other medications.

The effect of VYTORIN on the prothrombin time has not been studied.

7.9 Colchicine

Cases of myopathy, including rhabdomyolysis, have been reported with simvastatin coadministered with colchicine, and caution should be exercised when prescribing VYTORIN with colchicine.

8 USE IN SPECIFIC POPULATIONS

8.1 Pregnancy

Pregnancy Category X.

[See Contraindications (4).]

VYTORIN

VYTORIN is contraindicated in women who are or may become pregnant. Lipid-lowering drugs offer no benefit during pregnancy, because cholesterol and cholesterol derivatives are needed for normal fetal development. Atherosclerosis is a chronic process, and discontinuation of lipid-lowering drugs during pregnancy should have little impact on long-term outcomes of primary hypercholesterolemia therapy. There are no adequate and well-controlled studies of VYTORIN use during pregnancy; however, there are rare reports of congenital anomalies in infants exposed to statins *in utero*. Animal reproduction studies of simvastatin in rats and rabbits showed no evidence of teratogenicity. Serum cholesterol and triglycerides increase during normal pregnancy, and cholesterol or cholesterol derivatives are essential for fetal development. Because statins, such as simvastatin, decrease cholesterol synthesis and possibly the synthesis of other biologically active substances derived from cholesterol, VYTORIN may cause fetal harm when administered to a pregnant woman. If VYTORIN is used during pregnancy or if the patient becomes pregnant while taking this drug, the patient should be apprised of the potential hazard to the fetus.

Women of childbearing potential, who require VYTORIN treatment for a lipid disorder, should be advised to use effective contraception. For women trying to conceive, discontinuation of VYTORIN should be considered. If pregnancy occurs, VYTORIN should be immediately discontinued.

Ezetimibe

In oral (gavage) embryo-fetal development studies of ezetimibe conducted in rats and rabbits during organogenesis, there was no evidence of embryolethal effects at the doses tested (250, 500, 1000 mg/kg/day). In rats, increased incidences of common fetal skeletal findings (extra pair of thoracic ribs, unossified cervical vertebral centra, shortened ribs) were observed at 1000 mg/kg/day (~10 times the human exposure at 10 mg daily based on $AUC_{0\text{-}24hr}$ for total ezetimibe). In rabbits treated with ezetimibe, an increased incidence of extra thoracic ribs was observed at 1000 mg/kg/day (150 times the human exposure at 10 mg daily based on $AUC_{0\text{-}24hr}$ for total ezetimibe). Ezetimibe crossed the placenta when pregnant rats and rabbits were given multiple oral doses.

Multiple-dose studies of ezetimibe coadministered with statins in rats and rabbits during organogenesis result in higher ezetimibe and statin exposures. Reproductive findings occur at lower doses in coadministration therapy compared to monotherapy.

Simvastatin

Simvastatin was not teratogenic in rats or rabbits at doses (25, 10 mg/kg/day, respectively) that resulted in 3 times the human exposure based on mg/m^2 surface area. However, in studies with another structurally-related statin, skeletal malformations were observed in rats and mice.

There are rare reports of congenital anomalies following intrauterine exposure to statins. In a review[1] of approximately 100 prospectively followed pregnancies in women exposed to simvastatin or another structurally-related statin, the incidences of congenital anomalies, spontaneous abortions and fetal deaths/stillbirths did not exceed what would be expected in the general population. The number of cases is adequate only to exclude a 3- to 4-fold increase in congenital anomalies over the background incidence. In 89% of the prospectively followed pregnancies, drug treatment was initiated prior to pregnancy and was discontinued at some point in the first trimester when pregnancy was identified.

[1] Manson, J.M., Freyssinges, C., Ducrocq, M.B., Stephenson, W.P., Postmarketing Surveillance of Lovastatin and Simvastatin Exposure During Pregnancy, *Reproductive Toxicology*, 10(6):439-446, 1996.

8.3 Nursing Mothers

It is not known whether simvastatin is excreted in human milk. Because a small amount of another drug in this class is excreted in human milk and because of the potential for serious adverse reactions in nursing infants, women taking simvastatin should not nurse their infants. A decision should be made whether to discontinue nursing or discontinue drug, taking into account the importance of the drug to the mother *[see Contraindications (4)]*.

In rat studies, exposure to ezetimibe in nursing pups was up to half of that observed in maternal plasma. It is not known whether ezetimibe or simvastatin are excreted into human breast milk. Because a small amount of another drug in the same class as simvastatin is excreted in human milk and because of the potential for serious adverse reactions in nursing infants, women who are nursing should not take VYTORIN *[see Contraindications (4)]*.

8.4 Pediatric Use

The effects of ezetimibe coadministered with simvastatin (n=126) compared to simvastatin monotherapy (n=122) have been evaluated in adolescent boys and girls with heterozygous familial hypercholesterolemia (HeFH). In a multicenter, double-blind, controlled study followed by an open-label phase, 142 boys and 106 postmenarchal girls, 10 to 17 years of age (mean age 14.2 years, 43% females, 82% Caucasians, 4% Asian, 2% Blacks, 13% multiracial) with HeFH were randomized to receive either ezetimibe coadministered with simvastatin or simvastatin monotherapy. Inclusion in the study required 1) a baseline LDL-C level between 160 and 400 mg/dL and 2) a medical history and clinical presentation consistent with HeFH. The mean baseline LDL-C value was 225 mg/dL (range: 161-351 mg/dL) in the ezetimibe coadministered with simvastatin group compared to 219 mg/dL (range: 149-336 mg/dL) in the simvastatin monotherapy group. The patients received coadministered ezetimibe and simvastatin (10 mg, 20 mg, or 40 mg) or simvastatin monotherapy (10 mg, 20 mg, or 40 mg) for 6 weeks, coadministered ezetimibe and 40 mg simvastatin or 40 mg simvastatin monotherapy for the next 27 weeks, and open-label coadministered ezetimibe and simvastatin (10 mg, 20 mg, or 40 mg) for 20 weeks thereafter.

The results of the study at Week 6 are summarized in Table 3. Results at Week 33 were consistent with those at Week 6.

[See table 3 above]

Table 3: Mean Percent Difference at Week 6 Between the Pooled Ezetimibe Coadministered with Simvastatin Group and the Pooled Simvastatin Monotherapy Group in Adolescent Patients with Heterozygous Familial Hypercholesterolemia

	Total-C	LDL-C	Apo B	Non-HDL-C	TG*	HDL-C
Mean percent difference between treatment groups	-12%	-15%	-12%	-14%	-2%	+0.1%
95% Confidence Interval	(-15%, -9%)	(-18%, -12%)	(-15%, -9%)	(-17%, -11%)	(-9, +4)	(-3, +3)

* For triglycerides, median % change from baseline.

From the start of the trial to the end of Week 33, discontinuations due to an adverse reaction occurred in 7 (6%) patients in the ezetimibe coadministered with simvastatin group and in 2 (2%) patients in the simvastatin monotherapy group.

During the trial, hepatic transaminase elevations (two consecutive measurements for ALT and/or AST ≥3 × ULN) occurred in four (3%) individuals in the ezetimibe coadministered with simvastatin group and in two (2%) individuals in the simvastatin monotherapy group. Elevations of CPK (≥10 × ULN) occurred in two (2%) individuals in the ezetimibe coadministered with simvastatin group and in zero individuals in the simvastatin monotherapy group.

In this limited controlled study, there was no significant effect on growth or sexual maturation in the adolescent boys or girls, or on menstrual cycle length in girls.

Coadministration of ezetimibe with simvastatin at doses greater than 40 mg/day has not been studied in adolescents. Also, VYTORIN has not been studied in patients younger than 10 years of age or in pre-menarchal girls.

Ezetimibe

Based on total ezetimibe (ezetimibe + ezetimibe-glucuronide) there are no pharmacokinetic differences between adolescents and adults. Pharmacokinetic data in the pediatric population <10 years of age are not available.

Simvastatin

The pharmacokinetics of simvastatin has not been studied in the pediatric population.

8.5 Geriatric Use

Of the 10,189 patients who received VYTORIN in clinical studies, 3242 (32%) were 65 and older (this included 844 (8%) who were 75 and older). No overall differences in safety or effectiveness were observed between these subjects and younger subjects, and other reported clinical experience has not identified differences in responses between the elderly and younger patients but greater sensitivity of some older individuals cannot be ruled out. Since advanced age (≥65 years) is a predisposing factor for myopathy, VYTORIN should be prescribed with caution in the elderly. *[See Clinical Pharmacology (12.3).]*

Because advanced age (≥65 years) is a predisposing factor for myopathy, including rhabdomyolysis, VYTORIN should be prescribed with caution in the elderly. In a clinical trial of patients treated with simvastatin 80 mg/day, patients ≥65 years of age had an increased risk of myopathy, including rhabdomyolysis, compared to patients <65 years of age. *[See Warnings and Precautions (5.1) and Clinical Pharmacology (12.3).]*

8.6 Renal Impairment

In the SHARP trial of 9270 patients with moderate to severe renal impairment (6247 non-dialysis patients with median serum creatinine 2.5 mg/dL and median estimated glomerular filtration rate 25.6 mL/min/1.73 m^2, and 3023 dialysis patients), the incidence of serious adverse events, adverse events leading to discontinuation of study treatment, or adverse events of special interest (musculoskeletal adverse events, liver enzyme abnormalities, incident cancer) was similar between patients ever assigned to VYTORIN 10/20 mg (n=4650) or placebo (n=4620) during a median follow-up of 4.9 years. However, because renal impairment is a risk factor for statin-associated myopathy, doses of VYTORIN exceeding 10/20 mg should be used with caution and close monitoring in patients with moderate to severe renal impairment. *[See Dosage and Administration (2.6), Adverse Reactions (6.1), and Clinical Studies (14.3).]*

8.7 Hepatic Impairment

VYTORIN is contraindicated in patients with active liver disease or unexplained persistent elevations of hepatic transaminases. VYTORIN is not recommended in patients with moderate to severe hepatic impairment. *[See Contraindications (4) and Warnings and Precautions (5.2).]*

10 OVERDOSAGE

VYTORIN

No specific treatment of overdosage with VYTORIN can be recommended. In the event of an overdose, symptomatic and supportive measures should be employed.

Ezetimibe

In clinical studies, administration of ezetimibe, 50 mg/day to 15 healthy subjects for up to 14 days, or 40 mg/day to 18 patients with primary hyperlipidemia for up to 56 days, was generally well tolerated.

A few cases of overdosage have been reported; most have not been associated with adverse experiences. Reported adverse experiences have not been serious.

Simvastatin

Significant lethality was observed in mice after a single oral dose of 9 g/m^2. No evidence of lethality was observed in rats or dogs treated with doses of 30 and 100 g/m^2, respectively. No specific diagnostic signs were observed in rodents. At these doses the only signs seen in dogs were emesis and mucoid stools.

A few cases of overdosage with simvastatin have been reported; the maximum dose taken was 3.6 g. All patients recovered without sequelae.

The dialyzability of simvastatin and its metabolites in man is not known at present.

11 DESCRIPTION

VYTORIN contains ezetimibe, a selective inhibitor of intestinal cholesterol and related phytosterol absorption, and simvastatin, an HMG-CoA reductase inhibitor.

The chemical name of ezetimibe is 1-(4-fluorophenyl)-3(R)-[3-(4-fluorophenyl)-3(S)-hydroxypropyl]-4(S)-(4-hydroxyphenyl)-2-azetidinone. The empirical formula is $C_{24}H_{21}F_2NO_3$ and its molecular weight is 409.4.

Ezetimibe is a white, crystalline powder that is freely to very soluble in ethanol, methanol, and acetone and practically insoluble in water. Its structural formula is:

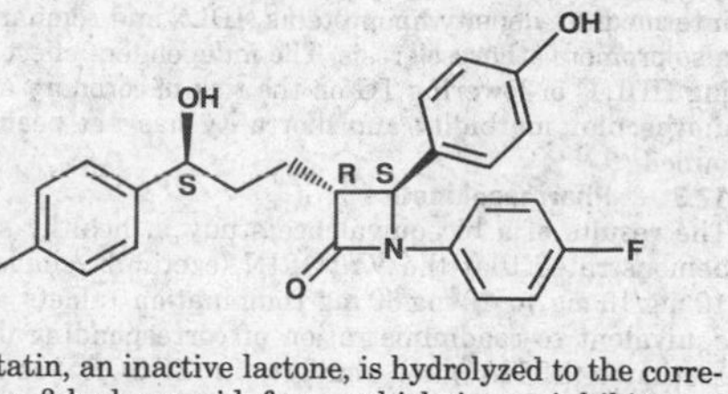

Simvastatin, an inactive lactone, is hydrolyzed to the corresponding β-hydroxyacid form, which is an inhibitor of

HMG-CoA reductase. Simvastatin is butanoic acid, 2,2-dimethyl-,1,2,3,7,8,8a-hexahydro-3,7-dimethyl-8-[2-(tetrahydro-4-hydroxy-6-oxo-2*H*-pyran-2-yl)-ethyl]-1-naphthalenyl ester, [1*S*-[1α,3α,7β,8β(2*S**,4*S**),-8aβ]]. The empirical formula of simvastatin is $C_{25}H_{38}O_5$ and its molecular weight is 418.57.

Simvastatin is a white to off-white, nonhygroscopic, crystalline powder that is practically insoluble in water and freely soluble in chloroform, methanol and ethanol. Its structural formula is:

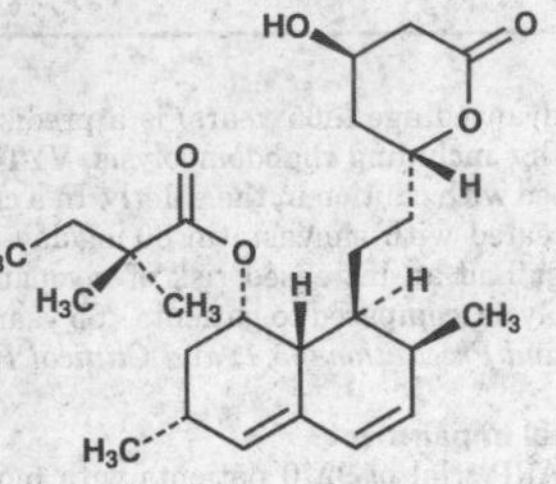

VYTORIN is available for oral use as tablets containing 10 mg of ezetimibe, and 10 mg of simvastatin (VYTORIN 10/10), 20 mg of simvastatin (VYTORIN 10/20), 40 mg of simvastatin (VYTORIN 10/40), or 80 mg of simvastatin (VYTORIN 10/80). Each tablet contains the following inactive ingredients: butylated hydroxyanisole NF, citric acid monohydrate USP, croscarmellose sodium NF, hypromellose USP, lactose monohydrate NF, magnesium stearate NF, microcrystalline cellulose NF, and propyl gallate NF.

12 CLINICAL PHARMACOLOGY

12.1 Mechanism of Action

VYTORIN

Plasma cholesterol is derived from intestinal absorption and endogenous synthesis. VYTORIN contains ezetimibe and simvastatin, two lipid-lowering compounds with complementary mechanisms of action. VYTORIN reduces elevated total-C, LDL-C, Apo B, TG, and non-HDL-C, and increases HDL-C through dual inhibition of cholesterol absorption and synthesis.

Ezetimibe

Ezetimibe reduces blood cholesterol by inhibiting the absorption of cholesterol by the small intestine. The molecular target of ezetimibe has been shown to be the sterol transporter, Niemann-Pick C1-Like 1 (NPC1L1), which is involved in the intestinal uptake of cholesterol and phytosterols. In a 2-week clinical study in 18 hypercholesterolemic patients, ezetimibe inhibited intestinal cholesterol absorption by 54%, compared with placebo. Ezetimibe had no clinically meaningful effect on the plasma concentrations of the fat-soluble vitamins A, D, and E and did not impair adrenocortical steroid hormone production.

Ezetimibe localizes at the brush border of the small intestine and inhibits the absorption of cholesterol, leading to a decrease in the delivery of intestinal cholesterol to the liver. This causes a reduction of hepatic cholesterol stores and an increase in clearance of cholesterol from the blood; this distinct mechanism is complementary to that of statins *[see Clinical Studies (14)]*.

Simvastatin

Simvastatin is a prodrug and is hydrolyzed to its active β-hydroxyacid form, simvastatin acid, after administration. Simvastatin is a specific inhibitor of 3-hydroxy-3-methylglutaryl-coenzyme A (HMG-CoA) reductase, the enzyme that catalyzes the conversion of HMG-CoA to mevalonate, an early and rate limiting step in the biosynthetic pathway for cholesterol. In addition, simvastatin reduces very-low-density lipoproteins (VLDL) and TG and increases HDL-C.

12.2 Pharmacodynamics

Clinical studies have demonstrated that elevated levels of total-C, LDL-C and Apo B, the major protein constituent of LDL, promote human atherosclerosis. In addition, decreased levels of HDL-C are associated with the development of atherosclerosis. Epidemiologic studies have established that cardiovascular morbidity and mortality vary directly with the level of total-C and LDL-C and inversely with the level of HDL-C. Like LDL, cholesterol-enriched triglyceride-rich lipoproteins, including VLDL, intermediate-density lipoproteins (IDL), and remnants, can also promote atherosclerosis. The independent effect of raising HDL-C or lowering TG on the risk of coronary and cardiovascular morbidity and mortality has not been determined.

12.3 Pharmacokinetics

The results of a bioequivalence study in healthy subjects demonstrated that the VYTORIN (ezetimibe/simvastatin) 10 mg/10 mg to 10 mg/80 mg combination tablets are bioequivalent to coadministration of corresponding doses of ezetimibe (ZETIA®) and simvastatin (ZOCOR®) as individual tablets.

Table 4: Effect of Coadministered Drugs on Total Ezetimibe

Coadministered Drug and Dosing Regimen	Total Ezetimibe* Change in AUC	Total Ezetimibe* Change in C_{max}
Cyclosporine-stable dose required (75-150 mg BID)†,‡	↑240%	↑290%
Fenofibrate, 200 mg QD, 14 days‡	↑48%	↑64%
Gemfibrozil, 600 mg BID, 7 days‡	↑64%	↑91%
Cholestyramine, 4 g BID, 14 days‡	↓55%	↓4%
Aluminum & magnesium hydroxide combination antacid, single dose§	↓4%	↓30%
Cimetidine, 400 mg BID, 7 days	↑6%	↑22%
Glipizide, 10 mg, single dose	↑4%	↓8%
Statins		
Lovastatin 20 mg QD, 7 days	↑9%	↑3%
Pravastatin 20 mg QD, 14 days	↑7%	↑23%
Atorvastatin 10 mg QD, 14 days	↓2%	↑12%
Rosuvastatin 10 mg QD, 14 days	↑13%	↑18%
Fluvastatin 20 mg QD, 14 days	↓19%	↑7%

* Based on 10 mg-dose of ezetimibe.
† Post-renal transplant patients with mild impaired or normal renal function. In a different study, a renal transplant patient with severe renal insufficiency (creatinine clearance of 13.2 mL/min/1.73 m^2) who was receiving multiple medications, including cyclosporine, demonstrated a 12-fold greater exposure to total ezetimibe compared to healthy subjects.
‡ See 7. Drug Interactions.
§ Supralox, 20 mL.

Absorption

Ezetimibe

After oral administration, ezetimibe is absorbed and extensively conjugated to a pharmacologically active phenolic glucuronide (ezetimibe-glucuronide).

Simvastatin

The availability of the β-hydroxyacid to the systemic circulation following an oral dose of simvastatin was found to be less than 5% of the dose, consistent with extensive hepatic first-pass extraction.

Effect of Food on Oral Absorption

Ezetimibe

Concomitant food administration (high-fat or non-fat meals) had no effect on the extent of absorption of ezetimibe when administered as 10-mg tablets. The C_{max} value of ezetimibe was increased by 38% with consumption of high-fat meals.

Simvastatin

Relative to the fasting state, the plasma profiles of both active and total inhibitors of HMG-CoA reductase were not affected when simvastatin was administered immediately before an American Heart Association recommended low-fat meal.

Distribution

Ezetimibe

Ezetimibe and ezetimibe-glucuronide are highly bound (>90%) to human plasma proteins.

Simvastatin

Both simvastatin and its β-hydroxyacid metabolite are highly bound (approximately 95%) to human plasma proteins. When radiolabeled simvastatin was administered to rats, simvastatin-derived radioactivity crossed the blood-brain barrier.

Metabolism and Excretion

Ezetimibe

Ezetimibe is primarily metabolized in the small intestine and liver via glucuronide conjugation with subsequent biliary and renal excretion. Minimal oxidative metabolism has been observed in all species evaluated.

In humans, ezetimibe is rapidly metabolized to ezetimibe-glucuronide. Ezetimibe and ezetimibe-glucuronide are the major drug-derived compounds detected in plasma, constituting approximately 10 to 20% and 80 to 90% of the total drug in plasma, respectively. Both ezetimibe and ezetimibe-glucuronide are eliminated from plasma with a half-life of approximately 22 hours for both ezetimibe and ezetimibe-glucuronide. Plasma concentration-time profiles exhibit multiple peaks, suggesting enterohepatic recycling.

Following oral administration of ^{14}C-ezetimibe (20 mg) to human subjects, total ezetimibe (ezetimibe + ezetimibe-glucuronide) accounted for approximately 93% of the total radioactivity in plasma. After 48 hours, there were no detectable levels of radioactivity in the plasma.

Approximately 78% and 11% of the administered radioactivity were recovered in the feces and urine, respectively, over a 10-day collection period. Ezetimibe was the major component in feces and accounted for 69% of the administered dose, while ezetimibe-glucuronide was the major component in urine and accounted for 9% of the administered dose.

Simvastatin

Simvastatin is a lactone that is readily hydrolyzed *in vivo* to the corresponding β-hydroxyacid, a potent inhibitor of HMG-CoA reductase. Inhibition of HMG-CoA reductase is a basis for an assay in pharmacokinetic studies of the β-hydroxyacid metabolites (active inhibitors) and, following base hydrolysis, active plus latent inhibitors (total inhibitors) in plasma following administration of simvastatin. The major active metabolites of simvastatin present in human plasma are the β-hydroxyacid of simvastatin and its 6′-hydroxy, 6′-hydroxymethyl, and 6′-exomethylene derivatives.

Following an oral dose of ^{14}C-labeled simvastatin in man, 13% of the dose was excreted in urine and 60% in feces. Plasma concentrations of total radioactivity (simvastatin plus ^{14}C-metabolites) peaked at 4 hours and declined rapidly to about 10% of peak by 12 hours postdose.

Specific Populations

Geriatric Patients

Ezetimibe

In a multiple-dose study with ezetimibe given 10 mg once daily for 10 days, plasma concentrations for total ezetimibe were about 2-fold higher in older (≥65 years) healthy subjects compared to younger subjects.

Simvastatin

In a study including 16 elderly patients between 70 and 78 years of age who received simvastatin 40 mg/day, the mean plasma level of HMG-CoA reductase inhibitory activity was increased approximately 45% compared with 18 patients between 18-30 years of age.

***Pediatric Patients:** [See Pediatric Use (8.4).]*

Gender

Ezetimibe

In a multiple-dose study with ezetimibe given 10 mg once daily for 10 days, plasma concentrations for total ezetimibe were slightly higher (<20%) in women than in men.

Race

Ezetimibe

Based on a meta-analysis of multiple-dose pharmacokinetic studies, there were no pharmacokinetic differences between Black and Caucasian subjects. Studies in Asian subjects indicated that the pharmacokinetics of ezetimibe was similar to those seen in Caucasian subjects.

Hepatic Impairment

Ezetimibe

After a single 10-mg dose of ezetimibe, the mean exposure (based on area under the curve [AUC]) to total ezetimibe was increased approximately 1.7-fold in patients with mild hepatic impairment (Child-Pugh score 5 to 6), compared to healthy subjects. The mean AUC values for total ezetimibe and ezetimibe increased approximately 3- to 4-fold and 5- to 6-fold, respectively, in patients with moderate (Child-Pugh score 7 to 9) or severe hepatic impairment (Child-Pugh score 10 to 15). In a 14-day, multiple-dose study (10 mg daily) in patients with moderate hepatic impairment, the mean AUC for total ezetimibe and ezetimibe increased approximately 4-fold compared to healthy subjects.

Renal Impairment

Ezetimibe

After a single 10-mg dose of ezetimibe in patients with severe renal disease (n=8; mean CrCl ≤30 mL/min/1.73 m^2), the mean AUC for total ezetimibe and ezetimibe increased approximately 1.5-fold, compared to healthy subjects (n=9).

Simvastatin

Pharmacokinetic studies with another statin having a similar principal route of elimination to that of simvastatin have suggested that for a given dose level higher systemic exposure may be achieved in patients with severe renal impairment (as measured by creatinine clearance).

Drug Interactions [See also Drug Interactions (7).]

No clinically significant pharmacokinetic interaction was seen when ezetimibe was coadministered with simvastatin. No specific pharmacokinetic drug interaction studies with VYTORIN have been conducted other than the following study with NIASPAN (Niacin extended-release tablets).

Niacin: The effect of VYTORIN (10/20 mg daily for 7 days) on the pharmacokinetics of NIASPAN extended-release tablets (1000 mg for 2 days and 2000 mg for 5 days following a low-fat breakfast) was studied in healthy subjects. The mean C_{max} and AUC of niacin increased 9% and 22%, respectively. The mean C_{max} and AUC of nicotinuric acid increased 10% and 19%, respectively (N=13). In the same study, the effect of NIASPAN on the pharmacokinetics of VYTORIN was evaluated (N=15). While concomitant NIASPAN decreased the mean C_{max} of total ezetimibe (1%), and simvastatin (2%), it increased the mean C_{max} of simvastatin acid (18%). In addition, concomitant NIASPAN increased the mean AUC of total ezetimibe (26%), simvastatin (20%), and simvastatin acid (35%).

Cases of myopathy/rhabdomyolysis have been observed with simvastatin coadministered with lipid-modifying doses (≥1 g/day niacin) of niacin-containing products. *[See Warnings and Precautions (5.1) and Drug Interactions (7.4).]*

Cytochrome P450: Ezetimibe had no significant effect on a series of probe drugs (caffeine, dextromethorphan, tolbutamide, and IV midazolam) known to be metabolized by cytochrome P450 (1A2, 2D6, 2C8/9 and 3A4) in a "cocktail" study of twelve healthy adult males. This indicates that ezetimibe is neither an inhibitor nor an inducer of these cytochrome P450 isozymes, and it is unlikely that ezetimibe will affect the metabolism of drugs that are metabolized by these enzymes.

In a study of 12 healthy volunteers, simvastatin at the 80-mg dose had no effect on the metabolism of the probe cytochrome P450 isoform 3A4 (CYP3A4) substrates midazolam and erythromycin. This indicates that simvastatin is not an inhibitor of CYP3A4 and, therefore, is not expected to affect the plasma levels of other drugs metabolized by CYP3A4.

Although the mechanism is not fully understood, cyclosporine has been shown to increase the AUC of statins. The increase in AUC for simvastatin acid is presumably due, in part, to inhibition of CYP3A4.

Simvastatin is a substrate for CYP3A4. Inhibitors of CYP3A4 can raise the plasma levels of HMG-CoA reductase inhibitory activity and increase the risk of myopathy. *[See Warnings and Precautions (5.1); Drug Interactions (7.1).]*

Ezetimibe

[See table 4 at top of previous page]

[See table 5 above]

Simvastatin

[See table 6 at top of next page]

Table 5: Effect of Ezetimibe Coadministration on Systemic Exposure to Other Drugs

Coadministered Drug and its Dosage Regimen	Ezetimibe Dosage Regimen	Change in AUC of Coadministered Drug	Change in C_{max} of Coadministered Drug
Warfarin, 25 mg single dose on Day 7	10 mg QD, 11 days	↓2% (R-warfarin) ↓4% (S-warfarin)	↑3% (R-warfarin) ↑1% (S-warfarin)
Digoxin, 0.5 mg single dose	10 mg QD, 8 days	↑2%	↓7%
Gemfibrozil, 600 mg BID, 7 days*	10 mg QD, 7 days	↓1%	↓11%
Ethinyl estradiol & Levonorgestrel, QD, 21 days	10 mg QD, Days 8-14 of 21 day oral contraceptive cycle	Ethinyl estradiol 0% Levonorgestrel 0%	Ethinyl estradiol ↓9% Levonorgestrel ↓5%
Glipizide, 10 mg on Days 1 and 9	10 mg QD, Days 2-9	↓3%	↓5%
Fenofibrate, 200 mg QD, 14 days*	10 mg QD, 14 days	↑11%	↑7%
Cyclosporine, 100 mg single dose Day 7*	20 mg QD, 8 days	↑15%	↑10%
Statins			
Lovastatin 20 mg QD, 7 days	10 mg QD, 7 days	↑19%	↑3%
Pravastatin 20 mg QD, 14 days	10 mg QD, 14 days	↓20%	↓24%
Atorvastatin 10 mg QD, 14 days	10 mg QD, 14 days	↓4%	↑7%
Rosuvastatin 10 mg QD, 14 days	10 mg QD, 14 days	↑19%	↑17%
Fluvastatin 20 mg QD, 14 days	10 mg QD, 14 days	↓39%	↓27%

* See 7. Drug Interactions.

13 NONCLINICAL TOXICOLOGY

13.1 Carcinogenesis, Mutagenesis, Impairment of Fertility

VYTORIN

No animal carcinogenicity or fertility studies have been conducted with the combination of ezetimibe and simvastatin. The combination of ezetimibe with simvastatin did not show evidence of mutagenicity *in vitro* in a microbial mutagenicity (Ames) test with *Salmonella typhimurium* and *Escherichia coli* with or without metabolic activation. No evidence of clastogenicity was observed *in vitro* in a chromosomal aberration assay in human peripheral blood lymphocytes with ezetimibe and simvastatin with or without metabolic activation. There was no evidence of genotoxicity at doses up to 600 mg/kg with the combination of ezetimibe and simvastatin (1:1) in the *in vivo* mouse micronucleus test.

Ezetimibe

A 104-week dietary carcinogenicity study with ezetimibe was conducted in rats at doses up to 1500 mg/kg/day (males) and 500 mg/kg/day (females) (~20 times the human exposure at 10 mg daily based on AUC_{0-24hr} for total ezetimibe). A 104-week dietary carcinogenicity study with ezetimibe was also conducted in mice at doses up to 500 mg/kg/day (>150 times the human exposure at 10 mg daily based on AUC_{0-24hr} for total ezetimibe). There were no statistically significant increases in tumor incidences in drug-treated rats or mice.

No evidence of mutagenicity was observed *in vitro* in a microbial mutagenicity (Ames) test with *Salmonella typhimurium* and *Escherichia coli* with or without metabolic activation. No evidence of clastogenicity was observed *in vitro* in a chromosomal aberration assay in human peripheral blood lymphocytes with or without metabolic activation. In addition, there was no evidence of genotoxicity in the *in vivo* mouse micronucleus test.

In oral (gavage) fertility studies of ezetimibe conducted in rats, there was no evidence of reproductive toxicity at doses up to 1000 mg/kg/day in male or female rats (~7 times the human exposure at 10 mg daily based on AUC_{0-24hr} for total ezetimibe).

Simvastatin

In a 72-week carcinogenicity study, mice were administered daily doses of simvastatin of 25, 100, and 400 mg/kg body weight, which resulted in mean plasma drug levels approximately 1, 4, and 8 times higher than the mean human plasma drug level, respectively, (as total inhibitory activity based on AUC) after an 80-mg oral dose. Liver carcinomas were significantly increased in high-dose females and mid- and high-dose males with a maximum incidence of 90% in males. The incidence of adenomas of the liver was significantly increased in mid- and high-dose females. Drug treatment also significantly increased the incidence of lung adenomas in mid- and high-dose males and females. Adenomas of the Harderian gland (a gland of the eye of rodents) were significantly higher in high-dose mice than in controls. No evidence of a tumorigenic effect was observed at 25 mg/kg/day.

In a separate 92-week carcinogenicity study in mice at doses up to 25 mg/kg/day, no evidence of a tumorigenic effect was observed (mean plasma drug levels were 1 times higher than humans given 80 mg simvastatin as measured by AUC).

In a two-year study in rats at 25 mg/kg/day, there was a statistically significant increase in the incidence of thyroid follicular adenomas in female rats exposed to approximately 11 times higher levels of simvastatin than in humans given 80 mg simvastatin (as measured by AUC).

A second two-year rat carcinogenicity study with doses of 50 and 100 mg/kg/day produced hepatocellular adenomas and carcinomas (in female rats at both doses and in males at 100 mg/kg/day). Thyroid follicular cell adenomas were increased in males and females at both doses; thyroid follicular cell carcinomas were increased in females at 100 mg/kg/day. The increased incidence of thyroid neoplasms appears to be consistent with findings from other statins. These treatment levels represented plasma drug levels (AUC) of approximately 7 and 15 times (males) and 22 and 25 times (females) the mean human plasma drug exposure after an 80-mg daily dose.

No evidence of mutagenicity was observed in a microbial mutagenicity (Ames) test with or without rat or mouse liver metabolic activation. In addition, no evidence of damage to genetic material was noted in an *in vitro* alkaline elution assay using rat hepatocytes, a V-79 mammalian cell forward mutation study, an *in vitro* chromosome aberration study in CHO cells, or an *in vivo* chromosomal aberration assay in mouse bone marrow.

There was decreased fertility in male rats treated with simvastatin for 34 weeks at 25 mg/kg body weight (4 times the maximum human exposure level, based on AUC, in patients receiving 80 mg/day); however, this effect was not observed during a subsequent fertility study in which simvastatin was administered at this same dose level to male rats for 11 weeks (the entire cycle of spermatogenesis including epididymal maturation). No microscopic changes were observed in the testes of rats from either study. At 180 mg/kg/day (which produces exposure levels 22 times higher than those in humans taking 80 mg/day based on surface area, mg/m^2), seminiferous tubule degeneration (necrosis and loss of spermatogenic epithelium) was observed. In dogs, there was drug-related testicular atrophy, decreased spermatogenesis, spermatocytic degeneration and giant cell formation at 10 mg/kg/day (approximately 2 times the human exposure, based on AUC, at 80 mg/day). The clinical significance of these findings is unclear.

13.2 Animal Toxicology and/or Pharmacology

CNS Toxicity

Optic nerve degeneration was seen in clinically normal dogs treated with simvastatin for 14 weeks at 180 mg/kg/day, a dose that produced mean plasma drug levels about 12 times higher than the mean plasma drug level in humans taking 80 mg/day.

A chemically similar drug in this class also produced optic nerve degeneration (Wallerian degeneration of retinogeniculate fibers) in clinically normal dogs in a dose-dependent fashion starting at 60 mg/kg/day, a dose that produced mean plasma drug levels about 30 times higher than the mean plasma drug level in humans taking the highest recommended dose (as measured by total enzyme inhibitory activity). This same drug also produced vestibulocochlear Wallerian-like degeneration and retinal ganglion cell chromatolysis in dogs treated for 14 weeks at 180 mg/kg/day, a dose that resulted in a mean plasma drug level similar to that seen with the 60 mg/kg/day dose.

CNS vascular lesions, characterized by perivascular hemorrhage and edema, mononuclear cell infiltration of perivascular spaces, perivascular fibrin deposits and necrosis of small vessels, were seen in dogs treated with simvastatin at a dose of 360 mg/kg/day, a dose that produced mean plasma drug levels that were about 14 times higher than the mean plasma drug levels in humans taking 80 mg/day. Similar CNS vascular lesions have been observed with several other drugs of this class.

There were cataracts in female rats after two years of treatment with 50 and 100 mg/kg/day (22 and 25 times the hu-

Table 6: Effect of Coadministered Drugs or Grapefruit Juice on Simvastatin Systemic Exposure

Coadministered Drug or Grapefruit Juice	Dosing of Coadministered Drug or Grapefruit Juice	Dosing of Simvastatin	Geometric Mean Ratio (Ratio* with / without coadministered drug) No Effect = 1.00		
				AUC	C_{max}
Contraindicated with VYTORIN *[see Contraindications (4) and Warnings and Precautions (5.1)]*					
Telithromycin†	200 mg QD for 4 days	80 mg	simvastatin acid‡ simvastatin	12 8.9	15 5.3
Nelfinavir†	1250 mg BID for 14 days	20 mg QD for 28 days	simvastatin acid‡ simvastatin	 6	 6.2
Itraconazole†	200 mg QD for 4 days	80 mg	simvastatin acid‡ simvastatin		13.1 13.1
Posaconazole	100 mg (oral suspension) QD for 13 days 200 mg (oral suspension) QD for 13 days	40 mg 40 mg	simvastatin acid‡ simvastatin simvastatin acid‡ simvastatin	7.3 10.3 8.5 10.6	9.2 9.4 9.5 11.4
Gemfibrozil	600 mg BID for 3 days	40 mg	simvastatin acid‡ simvastatin	2.85 1.35	2.18 0.91
Avoid grapefruit juice with VYTORIN *[see Warnings and Precautions (5.1)]*					
Grapefruit Juice§ (high dose)	200 mL of double-strength TID¶	60 mg single dose	simvastatin acid simvastatin	7 16	
Grapefruit Juice§ (low dose)	8 oz (about 237 mL) of single-strength#	20 mg single dose	simvastatin acid simvastatin	1.3 1.9	
Avoid taking with >10/10 mg VYTORIN, based on clinical and/or post-marketing simvastatin experience *[see Warnings and Precautions (5.1)]*					
Verapamil SR	240 mg QD Days 1-7 then 240 mg BID on Days 8-10	80 mg on Day 10	simvastatin acid simvastatin	2.3 2.5	2.4 2.1
Diltiazem	120 mg BID for 10 days	80 mg on Day 10	simvastatin acid simvastatin	2.69 3.10	2.69 2.88
Diltiazem	120 mg BID for 14 days	20 mg on Day 14	simvastatin	4.6	3.6
Dronedarone	400 mg BID for 14 days	40 mg QD for 14 days	simvastatin acid simvastatin	1.96 3.90	2.14 3.75
Avoid taking with >10/20 mg VYTORIN, based on clinical and/or post-marketing simvastatin experience *[see Warnings and Precautions (5.1)]*					
Amiodarone	400 mg QD for 3 days	40 mg on Day 3	simvastatin acid simvastatin	1.75 1.76	1.72 1.79
Amlodipine	10 mg QD for 10 days	80 mg on Day 10	simvastatin acid simvastatin	1.58 1.77	1.56 1.47
Ranolazine SR	1000 mg BID for 7 days	80 mg on Day 1 and Days 6-9	simvastatin acid simvastatin	2.26 1.86	2.28 1.75
No dosing adjustments required for the following:					
Fenofibrate	160 mg QD for 14 days	80 mg QD on Days 8-14	simvastatin acid simvastatin	0.64 0.89	0.89 0.83
Propranolol	80 mg single dose	80 mg single dose	total inhibitor active inhibitor	0.79 0.79	↓ from 33.6 to 21.1 ng·eq/mL ↓ from 7.0 to 4.7 ng·eq/mL

* Results based on a chemical assay except results with propranolol as indicated.
† Results could be representative of the following CYP3A4 inhibitors: ketoconazole, erythromycin, clarithromycin, HIV protease inhibitors, and nefazodone.
‡ Simvastatin acid refers to the β-hydroxyacid of simvastatin.
§ The effect of amounts of grapefruit juice between those used in these two studies on simvastatin pharmacokinetics has not been studied.
¶ Double-strength: one can of frozen concentrate diluted with one can of water. Grapefruit juice was administered TID for 2 days, and 200 mL together with single dose simvastatin and 30 and 90 minutes following single dose simvastatin on Day 3.
\# Single-strength: one can of frozen concentrate diluted with 3 cans of water. Grapefruit juice was administered with breakfast for 3 days, and simvastatin was administered in the evening on Day 3.

man AUC at 80 mg/day, respectively) and in dogs after three months at 90 mg/kg/day (19 times) and at two years at 50 mg/kg/day (5 times).

Ezetimibe

The hypocholesterolemic effect of ezetimibe was evaluated in cholesterol-fed Rhesus monkeys, dogs, rats, and mouse models of human cholesterol metabolism. Ezetimibe was found to have an ED_{50} value of 0.5 μg/kg/day for inhibiting the rise in plasma cholesterol levels in monkeys. The ED_{50} values in dogs, rats, and mice were 7, 30, and 700 μg/kg/day, respectively. These results are consistent with ezetimibe being a potent cholesterol absorption inhibitor.

In a rat model, where the glucuronide metabolite of ezetimibe (ezetimibe-glucuronide) was administered intraduodenally, the metabolite was as potent as ezetimibe in inhibiting the absorption of cholesterol, suggesting that the glucuronide metabolite had activity similar to the parent drug.

In 1-month studies in dogs given ezetimibe (0.03 to 300 mg/kg/day), the concentration of cholesterol in gallbladder bile increased ~2- to 4-fold. However, a dose of 300 mg/kg/day administered to dogs for one year did not result in gallstone formation or any other adverse hepatobiliary effects. In a 14-day study in mice given ezetimibe (0.3 to 5 mg/kg/day) and fed a low-fat or cholesterol-rich diet, the concentration of cholesterol in gallbladder bile was either unaffected or reduced to normal levels, respectively.

A series of acute preclinical studies was performed to determine the selectivity of ezetimibe for inhibiting cholesterol absorption. Ezetimibe inhibited the absorption of ^{14}C-cholesterol with no effect on the absorption of triglycerides, fatty acids, bile acids, progesterone, ethinyl estradiol, or the fat-soluble vitamins A and D.

In 4- to 12-week toxicity studies in mice, ezetimibe did not induce cytochrome P450 drug-metabolizing enzymes. In toxicity studies, a pharmacokinetic interaction of ezetimibe with statins (parents or their active hydroxy acid metabolites) was seen in rats, dogs, and rabbits.

14 CLINICAL STUDIES

14.1 Primary Hyperlipidemia

VYTORIN

VYTORIN reduces total-C, LDL-C, Apo B, TG, and non-HDL-C, and increases HDL-C in patients with hyperlipidemia. Maximal to near maximal response is generally achieved within 2 weeks and maintained during chronic therapy.

VYTORIN is effective in men and women with hyperlipidemia. Experience in non-Caucasians is limited and does not permit a precise estimate of the magnitude of the effects of VYTORIN.

Five multicenter, double-blind studies conducted with either VYTORIN or coadministered ezetimibe and simvastatin equivalent to VYTORIN in patients with primary hyperlipidemia are reported: two were comparisons with simvastatin, two were comparisons with atorvastatin, and one was a comparison with rosuvastatin.

In a multicenter, double-blind, placebo-controlled, 12-week trial, 1528 hyperlipidemic patients were randomized to one of ten treatment groups: placebo, ezetimibe (10 mg), simvastatin (10 mg, 20 mg, 40 mg, or 80 mg), or VYTORIN (10/10, 10/20, 10/40, or 10/80).

When patients receiving VYTORIN were compared to those receiving all doses of simvastatin, VYTORIN significantly lowered total-C, LDL-C, Apo B, TG, and non-HDL-C. The effects of VYTORIN on HDL-C were similar to the effects seen with simvastatin. Further analysis showed VYTORIN significantly increased HDL-C compared with placebo. (See Table 7.) The lipid response to VYTORIN was similar in patients with TG levels greater than or less than 200 mg/dL.

[See table 7 at top of next page]

In a multicenter, double-blind, controlled, 23-week study, 710 patients with known CHD or CHD risk equivalents, as defined by the NCEP ATP III guidelines, and an LDL-C ≥130 mg/dL were randomized to one of four treatment groups: coadministered ezetimibe and simvastatin equivalent to VYTORIN (10/10, 10/20, and 10/40) or simvastatin 20 mg. Patients not reaching an LDL-C <100 mg/dL had their simvastatin dose titrated at 6-week intervals to a maximal dose of 80 mg.

At Week 5, the LDL-C reductions with VYTORIN 10/10, 10/20, or 10/40 were significantly larger than with simvastatin 20 mg (see Table 8).

[See table 8 at top of next page]

In a multicenter, double-blind, 6-week study, 1902 patients with primary hyperlipidemia, who had not met their NCEP ATP III target LDL-C goal, were randomized to one of eight treatment groups: VYTORIN (10/10, 10/20, 10/40, or 10/80) or atorvastatin (10 mg, 20 mg, 40 mg, or 80 mg).

Across the dosage range, when patients receiving VYTORIN were compared to those receiving milligram-equivalent statin doses of atorvastatin, VYTORIN lowered total-C, LDL-C, Apo B, and non-HDL-C significantly more than atorvastatin. Only the 10/40 mg and 10/80 mg VYTORIN doses increased HDL-C significantly more than the corresponding milligram-equivalent statin dose of atorvastatin. The effects of VYTORIN on TG were similar to the effects seen with atorvastatin. (See Table 9.)

[See table 9 at top of page 1840]

In a multicenter, double-blind, 24-week, forced-titration study, 788 patients with primary hyperlipidemia, who had not met their NCEP ATP III target LDL-C goal, were randomized to receive coadministered ezetimibe and simvastatin equivalent to VYTORIN (10/10 and 10/20) or atorvastatin 10 mg. For all three treatment groups, the dose of the statin was titrated at 6-week intervals to 80 mg. At each pre-specified dose comparison, VYTORIN lowered LDL-C to a greater degree than atorvastatin (see Table 10).

[See table 10 at top of page 1840]

In a multicenter, double-blind, 6-week study, 2959 patients with primary hyperlipidemia, who had not met their NCEP

ATP III target LDL-C goal, were randomized to one of six treatment groups: VYTORIN (10/20, 10/40, or 10/80) or rosuvastatin (10 mg, 20 mg, or 40 mg).

The effects of VYTORIN and rosuvastatin on total-C, LDL-C, Apo B, TG, non-HDL-C and HDL-C are shown in Table 11.

[See table 11 at top of page 1841]

In a multicenter, double-blind, 24-week trial, 214 patients with type 2 diabetes mellitus treated with thiazolidinediones (rosiglitazone or pioglitazone) for a minimum of 3 months and simvastatin 20 mg for a minimum of 6 weeks were randomized to receive either simvastatin 40 mg or the coadministered active ingredients equivalent to VYTORIN 10/20. The median LDL-C and HbA1c levels at baseline were 89 mg/dL and 7.1%, respectively.

VYTORIN 10/20 was significantly more effective than doubling the dose of simvastatin to 40 mg. The median percent changes from baseline for VYTORIN vs. simvastatin were: LDL-C -25% and -5%; total-C -16% and -5%; Apo B -19% and -5%; and non-HDL-C -23% and -5%. Results for HDL-C and TG between the two treatment groups were not significantly different.

Ezetimibe

In two multicenter, double-blind, placebo-controlled, 12-week studies in 1719 patients with primary hyperlipidemia, ezetimibe significantly lowered total-C (-13%), LDL-C (-19%), Apo B (-14%), and TG (-8%), and increased HDL-C (+3%) compared to placebo. Reduction in LDL-C was consistent across age, sex, and baseline LDL-C.

Simvastatin

In two large, placebo-controlled clinical trials, the Scandinavian Simvastatin Survival Study (N=4,444 patients) and the Heart Protection Study (N=20,536 patients), the effects of treatment with simvastatin were assessed in patients at high risk of coronary events because of existing coronary heart disease, diabetes, peripheral vessel disease, history of stroke or other cerebrovascular disease. Simvastatin was proven to reduce: the risk of total mortality by reducing CHD deaths; the risk of non-fatal myocardial infarction and stroke; and the need for coronary and non-coronary revascularization procedures.

No incremental benefit of VYTORIN on cardiovascular morbidity and mortality over and above that demonstrated for simvastatin has been established.

14.2 Homozygous Familial Hypercholesterolemia (HoFH)

A double-blind, randomized, 12-week study was performed in patients with a clinical and/or genotypic diagnosis of HoFH. Data were analyzed from a subgroup of patients (n=14) receiving simvastatin 40 mg at baseline. Increasing the dose of simvastatin from 40 to 80 mg (n=5) produced a reduction of LDL-C of 13% from baseline on simvastatin 40 mg. Coadministered ezetimibe and simvastatin equivalent to VYTORIN (10/40 and 10/80 pooled, n=9), produced a reduction of LDL-C of 23% from baseline on simvastatin 40 mg. In those patients coadministered ezetimibe and simvastatin equivalent to VYTORIN (10/80, n=5), a reduction of LDL-C of 29% from baseline on simvastatin 40 mg was produced.

14.3 Chronic Kidney Disease (CKD)

The Study of Heart and Renal Protection (SHARP) was a multinational, randomized, placebo-controlled, double-blind trial that investigated the effect of VYTORIN on the time to a first major vascular event (MVE) among 9438 patients with moderate to severe chronic kidney disease (approximately one-third on dialysis at baseline) who did not have a history of myocardial infarction or coronary revascularization. An MVE was defined as nonfatal MI, cardiac death, stroke, or any revascularization procedure. Patients were allocated to treatment using a method that took into account the distribution of 8 important baseline characteristics of patients already enrolled and minimized the imbalance of those characteristics across the groups.

For the first year, 9438 patients were allocated 4:4:1, to VYTORIN 10/20, placebo, or simvastatin 20 mg daily, respectively. The 1-year simvastatin arm enabled the comparison of VYTORIN to simvastatin with regard to safety and effect on lipid levels. At 1 year the simvastatin-only arm was re-allocated 1:1 to VYTORIN 10/20 or placebo. A total of 9270 patients were ever allocated to VYTORIN 10/20 (n=4650) or placebo (n=4620) during the trial. The median follow-up duration was 4.9 years. Patients had a mean age of 61 years; 63% were male, 72% were Caucasian, and 23% were diabetic; and, for those not on dialysis at baseline, the median serum creatinine was 2.5 mg/dL and the median estimated glomerular filtration rate (eGFR) was 25.6 mL/min/1.73 m^2, with 94% of patients having an eGFR < 45 mL/min/1.73m^2. Eligibility did not depend on lipid levels. Mean LDL-C at baseline was 108 mg/dL. At 1 year, the mean LDL-C was 26% lower in the simvastatin arm and 38% lower in the VYTORIN arm relative to placebo. At the midpoint of the study (2.5 years), the mean LDL-C was 32% lower for VYTORIN relative to placebo. Patients no longer taking study medication were included in all lipid measurements.

Table 7: Response to VYTORIN in Patients with Primary Hyperlipidemia (Mean* % Change from Untreated Baseline†)

Treatment (Daily Dose)	N	Total-C	LDL-C	Apo B	HDL-C	TG*	Non-HDL-C
Pooled data (All VYTORIN doses)‡	609	-38	-53	-42	+7	-24	-49
Pooled data (All simvastatin doses)‡	622	-28	-39	-32	+7	-21	-36
Ezetimibe 10 mg	149	-13	-19	-15	+5	-11	-18
Placebo	148	-1	-2	0	0	-2	-2
VYTORIN by dose							
10/10	152	-31	-45	-35	+8	-23	-41
10/20	156	-36	-52	-41	+10	-24	-47
10/40	147	-39	-55	-44	+6	-23	-51
10/80	154	-43	-60	-49	+6	-31	-56
Simvastatin by dose							
10 mg	158	-23	-33	-26	+5	-17	-30
20 mg	150	-24	-34	-28	+7	-18	-32
40 mg	156	-29	-41	-33	+8	-21	-38
80 mg	158	-35	-49	-39	+7	-27	-45

* For triglycerides, median % change from baseline.
† Baseline - on no lipid-lowering drug.
‡ VYTORIN doses pooled (10/10-10/80) significantly reduced total-C, LDL-C, Apo B, TG, and non-HDL-C compared to simvastatin and significantly increased HDL-C compared to placebo.

Table 8: Response to VYTORIN after 5 Weeks in Patients with CHD or CHD Risk Equivalents and an LDL-C ≥130 mg/dL

	Simvastatin 20 mg	VYTORIN 10/10	VYTORIN 10/20	VYTORIN 10/40
N	253	251	109	97
Mean baseline LDL-C	174	165	167	171
Percent change LDL-C	-38	-47	-53	-59

In the primary intent-to-treat analysis, 639 (15.2%) of 4193 patients initially allocated to VYTORIN and 749 (17.9%) of 4191 patients initially allocated to placebo experienced an MVE. This corresponded to a relative risk reduction of 16% (p=0.001) (see Figure 1). Similarly, 526 (11.3%) of 4650 patients ever allocated to VYTORIN and 619 (13.4%) of 4620 patients ever allocated to placebo experienced a major atherosclerotic event (MAE; a subset of the MVE composite that excluded non-coronary cardiac deaths and hemorrhagic stroke), corresponding to a relative risk reduction of 17% (p=0.002). The trial demonstrated that treatment with VYTORIN 10/20 mg versus placebo reduced the risk for MVE and MAE in this CKD population. The study design precluded drawing conclusions regarding the independent contribution of either ezetimibe or simvastatin to the observed effect.

The treatment effect of VYTORIN on MVE was attenuated among patients on dialysis at baseline compared with those not on dialysis at baseline. Among 3023 patients on dialysis at baseline, VYTORIN reduced the risk of MVE by 6% (RR 0.94: 95% CI 0.80-1.09) compared with 22% (RR 0.78: 95% CI 0.69-0.89) among 6247 patients not on dialysis at baseline (interaction P=0.08).

Figure 1: Effect of VYTORIN on the Primary Endpoint of Risk of Major Vascular Events

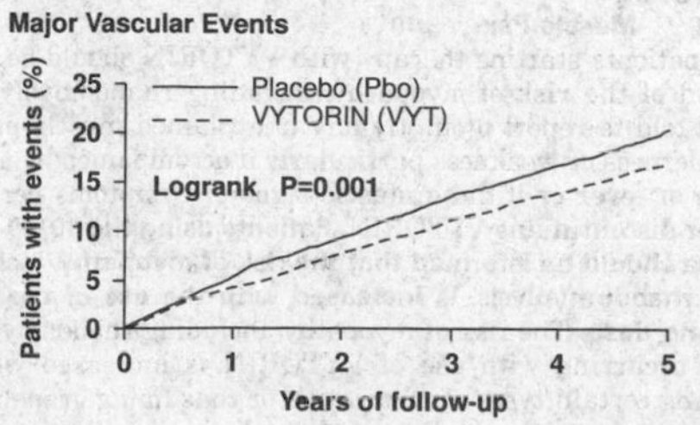

At risk						
Pbo	4191	3807	3495	3177	2419	1239
VYT	4193	3868	3567	3273	2501	1232

The individual components of MVE in all patients ever allocated to VYTORIN or placebo are presented in Table 12.

[See table 12 at top of page 1841]

Among patients not on dialysis at baseline, VYTORIN did not reduce the risk of progressing to end-stage renal disease compared with placebo (RR 0.97: 95% CI 0.89-1.05).

16 HOW SUPPLIED/STORAGE AND HANDLING

No. 3873 — Tablets VYTORIN 10/10 are white to off-white capsule-shaped tablets with code "311" on one side.
They are supplied as follows:
NDC 66582-311-31 bottles of 30
NDC 66582-311-54 bottles of 90
NDC 66582-311-82 bottles of 1000 (If repackaged in blisters, then opaque or light-resistant blisters should be used.)
NDC 66582-311-87 bottles of 10,000 (If repackaged in blisters, then opaque or light-resistant blisters should be used.)
NDC 66582-311-28 unit dose packages of 100.

No. 3874 — Tablets VYTORIN 10/20 are white to off-white capsule-shaped tablets with code "312" on one side.
They are supplied as follows:
NDC 66582-312-31 bottles of 30
NDC 66582-312-54 bottles of 90
NDC 66582-312-82 bottles of 1000 (If repackaged in blisters, then opaque or light-resistant blisters should be used.)
NDC 66582-312-87 bottles of 10,000 (If repackaged in blisters, then opaque or light-resistant blisters should be used.)
NDC 66582-312-28 unit dose packages of 100.

No. 3875 — Tablets VYTORIN 10/40 are white to off-white capsule-shaped tablets with code "313" on one side.
They are supplied as follows:
NDC 66582-313-31 bottles of 30
NDC 66582-313-54 bottles of 90
NDC 66582-313-74 bottles of 500 (If repackaged in blisters, then opaque or light-resistant blisters should be used.)
NDC 66582-313-86 bottles of 5000 (If repackaged in blisters, then opaque or light-resistant blisters should be used.)
NDC 66582-313-52 unit dose packages of 50.

No. 3876 — Tablets VYTORIN 10/80 are white to off-white capsule-shaped tablets with code "315" on one side.
They are supplied as follows:
NDC 66582-315-31 bottles of 30
NDC 66582-315-54 bottles of 90
NDC 66582-315-74 bottles of 500 (If repackaged in blisters, then opaque or light-resistant blisters should be used.)

Table 9: Response to VYTORIN and Atorvastatin in Patients with Primary Hyperlipidemia (Mean* % Change from Untreated Baseline[†])

Treatment (Daily Dose)	N	Total-C[‡]	LDL-C[‡]	Apo B[‡]	HDL-C	TG*	Non-HDL-C[‡]
VYTORIN by dose							
10/10	230	-34[§]	-47[§]	-37[§]	+8	-26	-43[§]
10/20	233	-37[§]	-51[§]	-40[§]	+7	-25	-46[§]
10/40	236	-41[§]	-57[§]	-46[§]	+9[§]	-27	-52[§]
10/80	224	-43[§]	-59[§]	-48[§]	+8[§]	-31	-54[§]
Atorvastatin by dose							
10 mg	235	-27	-36	-31	+7	-21	-34
20 mg	230	-32	-44	-37	+5	-25	-41
40 mg	232	-36	-48	-40	+4	-24	-45
80 mg	230	-40	-53	-44	+1	-32	-50

* For triglycerides, median % change from baseline.
† Baseline - on no lipid-lowering drug.
‡ VYTORIN doses pooled (10/10-10/80) provided significantly greater reductions in total-C, LDL-C, Apo B, and non-HDL-C compared to atorvastatin doses pooled (10-80).
§ $p<0.05$ for difference with atorvastatin at equal mg doses of the simvastatin component.

Table 10: Response to VYTORIN and Atorvastatin in Patients with Primary Hyperlipidemia (Mean* % Change from Untreated Baseline[†])

Treatment	N	Total-C	LDL-C	Apo B	HDL-C	TG*	Non-HDL-C
Week 6							
Atorvastatin 10 mg[‡]	262	-28	-37	-32	+5	-23	-35
VYTORIN 10/10[§]	263	-34[¶]	-46[¶]	-38[¶]	+8[¶]	-26	-43[¶]
VYTORIN 10/20[#]	263	-36[¶]	-50[¶]	-41[¶]	+10[¶]	-25	-46[¶]
Week 12							
Atorvastatin 20 mg	246	-33	-44	-38	+7	-28	-42
VYTORIN 10/20	250	-37[¶]	-50[¶]	-41[¶]	+9	-28	-46[¶]
VYTORIN 10/40	252	-39[¶]	-54[¶]	-45[¶]	+12[¶]	-31	-50[¶]
Week 18							
Atorvastatin 40 mg	237	-37	-49	-42	+8	-31	-47
VYTORIN 10/40[Þ]	482	-40[¶]	-56[¶]	-45[¶]	+11[¶]	-32	-52[¶]
Week 24							
Atorvastatin 80 mg	228	-40	-53	-45	+6	-35	-50
VYTORIN 10/80[Þ]	459	-43[¶]	-59[¶]	-49[¶]	+12[¶]	-35	-55[¶]

* For triglycerides, median % change from baseline.
† Baseline - on no lipid-lowering drug.
‡ Atorvastatin: 10 mg start dose titrated to 20 mg, 40 mg, and 80 mg through Weeks 6, 12, 18, and 24.
§ VYTORIN: 10/10 start dose titrated to 10/20, 10/40, and 10/80 through Weeks 6, 12, 18, and 24.
¶ $p \leq 0.05$ for difference with atorvastatin in the specified week.
\# VYTORIN: 10/20 start dose titrated to 10/40, 10/40, and 10/80 through Weeks 6, 12, 18, and 24.
Þ Data pooled for common doses of VYTORIN at Weeks 18 and 24.

NDC 66582-315-66 bottles of 2500 (If repackaged in blisters, then opaque or light-resistant blisters should be used.)
NDC 66582-315-52 unit dose packages of 50.

Storage

Store at 20-25°C (68-77°F). [See USP Controlled Room Temperature.] Keep container tightly closed.

Storage of 10,000, 5000, and 2500 count bottles

Store bottle of 10,000 VYTORIN 10/10 and 10/20, 5000 VYTORIN 10/40, and 2500 VYTORIN 10/80 capsule-shaped tablets at 20-25°C (68-77°F). [See USP Controlled Room Temperature.] Store in original container until time of use. When product container is subdivided, repackage into a tightly-closed, light-resistant container. Entire contents must be repackaged immediately upon opening.

17 PATIENT COUNSELING INFORMATION

See FDA-Approved Patient Labeling (Patient Information).
Patients should be advised to adhere to their National Cholesterol Education Program (NCEP)-recommended diet, a regular exercise program, and periodic testing of a fasting lipid panel.
Patients should be advised about substances they should not take concomitantly with VYTORIN *[see Contraindications (4)* and *Warnings and Precautions (5.1)]*. Patients should also be advised to inform other healthcare professionals prescribing a new medication or increasing the dose of an existing medication that they are taking VYTORIN.

17.1 Muscle Pain

All patients starting therapy with VYTORIN should be advised of the risk of myopathy, including rhabdomyolysis, and told to report promptly any unexplained muscle pain, tenderness or weakness particularly if accompanied by malaise or fever or if these muscle signs or symptoms persist after discontinuing VYTORIN. **Patients using the 10/80-mg dose should be informed that the risk of myopathy, including rhabdomyolysis, is increased with the use of the 10/80-mg dose.** The risk of myopathy, including rhabdomyolysis, occurring with use of VYTORIN is increased when taking certain types of medication or consuming grapefruit juice. Patients should discuss all medication, both prescription and over the counter, with their healthcare professional.

17.2 Liver Enzymes

It is recommended that liver function tests be performed before the initiation of VYTORIN, and thereafter when clinically indicated. All patients treated with VYTORIN should be advised to report promptly any symptoms that may indicate liver injury, including fatigue, anorexia, right upper abdominal discomfort, dark urine or jaundice.

17.3 Pregnancy

Women of childbearing age should be advised to use an effective method of birth control to prevent pregnancy while using VYTORIN. Discuss future pregnancy plans with your patients, and discuss when to stop taking VYTORIN if they are trying to conceive. Patients should be advised that if they become pregnant they should stop taking VYTORIN and call their healthcare professional.

17.4 Breast-feeding

Women who are breast-feeding should be advised to not use VYTORIN. Patients who have a lipid disorder and are breast-feeding should be advised to discuss the options with their healthcare professional.

Manufactured for: Merck Sharp & Dohme Corp., a subsidiary of
MERCK & CO., INC., Whitehouse Station, NJ 08889, USA
Manufactured by:
MSD International GmbH (Singapore Branch)
Singapore 637766
Or
Merck Sharp & Dohme (Italia) S.p.A.
Via Emilia 21,
Pavia 27100, Italy
Or
Merck Sharp & Dohme Ltd.
Cramlington, Northumberland NE23 3JU, UK
Or
Jointly manufactured by:
Merck Sharp & Dohme (Italia) S.p.A.
Via Emilia 21,
Pavia 27100, Italy
and
MSD International GmbH (Singapore Branch)
Singapore 637766
U.S. Patent Nos. 5,846,966 and RE42,461

Revised: 02/2013
USPI-T-0653A1302R026

VYTORIN® (ezetimibe/simvastatin) Tablets
Patient Information about VYTORIN (VI-tor-in)

Generic name: ezetimibe/simvastatin tablets

Read this information carefully before you start taking VYTORIN®. Review this information each time you refill your prescription for VYTORIN as there may be new information. This information does not take the place of talking with your doctor about your medical condition or your treatment. If you have any questions about VYTORIN, ask your doctor. Only your doctor can determine if VYTORIN is right for you.

What is VYTORIN?

VYTORIN contains two cholesterol-lowering medications, ezetimibe and simvastatin. VYTORIN is a prescription medicine used to lower levels of total cholesterol, LDL (bad) cholesterol, and fatty substances called triglycerides in the blood. In addition, VYTORIN raises levels of HDL (good) cholesterol. VYTORIN is for patients who cannot control their cholesterol levels by diet and exercise alone. You should stay on a cholesterol-lowering diet while taking this medicine.

VYTORIN works to reduce your cholesterol in two ways. It reduces the cholesterol absorbed in your digestive tract, as well as the cholesterol your body makes by itself. VYTORIN does not help you lose weight.

VYTORIN has not been shown to reduce heart attacks or strokes more than simvastatin alone.

The usual dose of VYTORIN is 10/10 mg to 10/40 mg 1 time each day.

VYTORIN 10/80 mg increases your chance of developing muscle damage. The 10/80 mg dose should only be used by people who:

- have been taking VYTORIN 10/80 mg chronically (such as 12 months or more) without having muscle damage
- do not need to take certain other medicines with VYTORIN that would increase your chance of getting muscle damage.

If you are unable to reach your LDL-cholesterol goal using VYTORIN 10/40 mg, your doctor should switch you to another cholesterol-lowering medicine.

For more information about cholesterol, see the section called "What should I know about high cholesterol?"

Who should not take VYTORIN?

Do not take VYTORIN if you take:

- Certain anti-fungal medicines including:
  - itraconazole
  - ketoconazole
  - posaconazole
  - voriconazole
- HIV protease inhibitors (indinavir, nelfinavir, ritonavir, saquinavir, tipranavir, or atazanavir)

- Certain hepatitis C virus protease inhibitors (such as boceprevir or telaprevir)
- Certain antibiotics, including:
  - ◦ erythromycin
  - ◦ clarithromycin
  - ◦ telithromycin
- nefazodone
- A fibric acid medicine for lowering cholesterol called gemfibrozil
- cyclosporine
- danazol

Ask your doctor if you are not sure if your medicine is listed above.

Also do not take VYTORIN:

- If you are allergic to ezetimibe or simvastatin, the active ingredients in VYTORIN, or to the inactive ingredients. For a list of inactive ingredients, see the "Inactive ingredients" section at the end of this information sheet.
- If you have active liver disease or repeated blood tests indicating possible liver problems.
- If you are pregnant, or think you may be pregnant, or planning to become pregnant or breast-feeding.
- If you are a woman of childbearing age, you should use an effective method of birth control to prevent pregnancy while using VYTORIN.

VYTORIN has not been studied in children under 10 years of age.

What should I tell my doctor before and while taking VYTORIN?

Tell your doctor right away if you have unexplained muscle pain, tenderness, or weakness especially with fever while you take VYTORIN. Muscle problems, including muscle breakdown, can be serious in some people and rarely cause kidney damage that can lead to death.

The risk of muscle breakdown is greater at higher doses of VYTORIN, particularly the 10/80 mg dose.

The risk of muscle breakdown is greater in people 65 years of age and older, females, and people with kidney or thyroid problems.

If you have muscle problems that do not go away even after your doctor has advised you to stop taking VYTORIN, notify your doctor. Your doctor may do further tests to diagnose the cause of your muscle problems.

Taking VYTORIN with certain substances can increase the risk of muscle problems. It is especially important to tell your doctor if you take:

- fibric acid derivatives (such as fenofibrate)
- amiodarone or dronedarone (drugs used to treat an irregular heartbeat)
- verapamil, diltiazem, amlodipine, or ranolazine (drugs used to treat high blood pressure, chest pain associated with heart disease, or other heart conditions)
- grapefruit juice (which should be avoided while taking VYTORIN)
- colchicine (a medicine used to treat gout)
- large doses of niacin or nicotinic acid

Tell your doctor if you are taking niacin or a niacin-containing product, as this may increase your risk of muscle problems, especially if you are Chinese.

It is also important to tell your doctor if you are taking coumarin anticoagulants (drugs that prevent blood clots, such as warfarin).

Tell your doctor about all the medicines you take, including any prescription and nonprescription medicines, vitamins, and herbal supplements.

If you have more than 1 doctor, tell all of your doctors that you take VYTORIN. This is especially important when they prescribe a new medicine or increase the dose of your other medicines.

Tell your doctor about all your medical conditions including allergies.

Tell your doctor if you:

- drink substantial quantities of alcohol or ever had liver problems. VYTORIN may not be right for you.
- are pregnant or plan to become pregnant. Do not use VYTORIN if you are pregnant, trying to become pregnant or suspect that you are pregnant. If you become pregnant while taking VYTORIN, stop taking it and contact your doctor immediately.
- are breast-feeding. Do not use VYTORIN if you are breast-feeding.

Tell other doctors prescribing a new medication that you are taking VYTORIN.

How should I take VYTORIN?

- Take VYTORIN exactly as your doctor tells you to take it.
- Take VYTORIN once a day, in the evening, with or without food.
- If you miss a dose, do not take an extra dose. Just resume your usual schedule.
- Continue to follow a cholesterol-lowering diet while taking VYTORIN. Ask your doctor if you need diet information.
- Keep taking VYTORIN unless your doctor tells you to stop. If you stop taking VYTORIN, your cholesterol may rise again.

Table 11: Response to VYTORIN and Rosuvastatin in Patients with Primary Hyperlipidemia (Mean* % Change from Untreated Baseline†)

Treatment (Daily Dose)	N	Total-C‡	LDL-C‡	Apo B‡	HDL-C	TG*	Non-HDL-C‡
VYTORIN by dose							
10/20	476	-37§	-52§	-42§	+7	-23§	-47§
10/40	477	-39¶	-55¶	-44¶	+8	-27	-50¶
10/80	474	-44#	-61#	-50#	+8	-30#	-56#
Rosuvastatin by dose							
10 mg	475	-32	-46	-37	+7	-20	-42
20 mg	478	-37	-52	-43	+8	-26	-48
40 mg	475	-41	-57	-47	+8	-28	-52

* For triglycerides, median % change from baseline.
† Baseline - on no lipid-lowering drug.
‡ VYTORIN doses pooled (10/20-10/80) provided significantly greater reductions in total-C, LDL-C, Apo B, and non-HDL-C compared to rosuvastatin doses pooled (10-40 mg).
§ $p<0.05$ vs. rosuvastatin 10 mg.
¶ $p<0.05$ vs. rosuvastatin 20 mg.
# $p<0.05$ vs. rosuvastatin 40 mg.

Table 12: Number of First Events for Each Component of the Major Vascular Event Composite Endpoint in SHARP*

Outcome	VYTORIN 10/20 (N=4650)	Placebo (N=4620)	Risk Ratio (95% CI)	P-value
Major Vascular Events	701 (15.1%)	814 (17.6%)	0.85 (0.77-0.94)	0.001
Nonfatal MI	134 (2.9%)	159 (3.4%)	0.84 (0.66-1.05)	0.12
Cardiac Death	253 (5.4%)	272 (5.9%)	0.93 (0.78-1.10)	0.38
Any Stroke	171 (3.7%)	210 (4.5%)	0.81 (0.66-0.99)	0.038
Non-hemorrhagic Stroke	131 (2.8%)	174 (3.8%)	0.75 (0.60-0.94)	0.011
Hemorrhagic Stroke	45 (1.0%)	37 (0.8%)	1.21 (0.78-1.86)	0.40
Any Revascularization	284 (6.1%)	352 (7.6%)	0.79 (0.68-0.93)	0.004

* Intention-to-treat analysis on all SHARP patients ever allocated to VYTORIN or placebo.

What should I do in case of an overdose?

Contact your doctor immediately.

What are the possible side effects of VYTORIN?

See your doctor regularly to check your cholesterol level and to check for side effects. Your doctor should do blood tests to check your liver before you start taking VYTORIN and if you have any symptoms of liver problems while you take VYTORIN. Call your doctor right away if you have the following symptoms of liver problems:

- feel tired or weak
- loss of appetite
- upper belly pain
- dark urine
- yellowing of your skin or the whites of your eyes

In clinical studies patients reported the following common side effects while taking VYTORIN: headache, muscle pain, and diarrhea (see What should I tell my doctor before and while taking VYTORIN?).

The following side effects have been reported in general use with VYTORIN or with ezetimibe or simvastatin tablets (tablets that contain the active ingredients of VYTORIN):

- allergic reactions including swelling of the face, lips, tongue, and/or throat that may cause difficulty in breathing or swallowing (which may require treatment right away), rash, hives; raised red rash, sometimes with target-shaped lesions; joint pain; muscle pain, tenderness, or weakness; alterations in some laboratory blood tests; liver problems (sometimes serious); inflammation of the pancreas; nausea; dizziness; tingling sensation; depression; gallstones; inflammation of the gallbladder; trouble sleeping; poor memory; memory loss; confusion; erectile dysfunction; breathing problems including persistent cough and/or shortness of breath or fever.

Tell your doctor if you are having these or any other medical problems while on VYTORIN. This is not a complete list of side effects. For a complete list, ask your doctor or pharmacist.

What should I know about high cholesterol?

Cholesterol is a type of fat found in your blood. Cholesterol comes from two sources. It is produced by your body and it comes from the food you eat. Your total cholesterol is made up of both LDL and HDL cholesterol.

LDL cholesterol is called "bad" cholesterol because it can build up in the wall of your arteries and form plaque. Over time, plaque build-up can cause a narrowing of the arteries. This narrowing can slow or block blood flow to your heart, brain, and other organs. High LDL cholesterol is a major cause of heart disease and one of the causes for stroke.

HDL cholesterol is called "good" cholesterol because it keeps the bad cholesterol from building up in the arteries.

Triglycerides also are fats found in your body.

General Information about VYTORIN

Medicines are sometimes prescribed for conditions that are not mentioned in patient information leaflets. Do not use VYTORIN for a condition for which it was not prescribed. Do not give VYTORIN to other people, even if they have the same condition you have. It may harm them.

This summarizes the most important information about VYTORIN. If you would like more information, talk with your doctor. You can ask your pharmacist or doctor for information about VYTORIN that is written for health professionals. For additional information, visit the following web site: vytorin.com.

Inactive ingredients:

Butylated hydroxyanisole NF, citric acid monohydrate USP, croscarmellose sodium NF, hypromellose USP, lactose monohydrate NF, magnesium stearate NF, microcrystalline cellulose NF, and propyl gallate NF.

Manufactured for: Merck Sharp & Dohme Corp., a subsidiary of

MERCK & CO., INC., Whitehouse Station, NJ 08889, USA

This patient information has been approved by the U.S. Food and Drug Administration

Revised: 10/2012
USPPI-T-0653A1210R025

Shown in Product Identification Guide, page 309

ZEMURON® ℞
(rocuronium bromide)
Injection

HIGHLIGHTS OF PRESCRIBING INFORMATION
These highlights do not include all the information needed to use ZEMURON safely and effectively. See full prescribing information for ZEMURON.
ZEMURON® (rocuronium bromide) injection solution for intravenous use
Initial U.S. Approval: 1994

INDICATIONS AND USAGE

ZEMURON is a nondepolarizing neuromuscular blocking agent indicated as an adjunct to general anesthesia to facilitate both rapid sequence and routine tracheal intubation, and to provide skeletal muscle relaxation during surgery or mechanical ventilation. (1)

DOSAGE AND ADMINISTRATION

To be administered only by experienced clinicians or adequately trained individuals supervised by an experienced clinician familiar with the use, actions, characteristics, and complications of neuromuscular blocking agents. (2)
- Individualize the dose for each patient. (2)
- Peripheral nerve stimulator recommended for determination of drug response and need for additional doses, and to evaluate recovery. (2)
- Tracheal intubation: Recommended initial dose is 0.6 mg/kg. (2.1)
- Rapid sequence intubation: 0.6 to 1.2 mg/kg. (2.2)
- Maintenance doses: Guided by response to prior dose, not administered until recovery is evident. (2.3)
- Continuous infusion: Initial rate of 10 to 12 mcg/kg/min. Start only after early evidence of spontaneous recovery from an intubating dose. (2.4)

DOSAGE FORMS AND STRENGTHS

- 5 mL multiple dose vials containing 50 mg rocuronium bromide injection (10 mg/mL). (3)
- 10 mL multiple dose vials containing 100 mg rocuronium bromide injection (10 mg/mL). (3)

CONTRAINDICATIONS

- Hypersensitivity (e.g., anaphylaxis) to rocuronium bromide or other neuromuscular blocking agents. (4)

WARNINGS AND PRECAUTIONS

- Appropriate Administration and Monitoring: Use only if facilities for intubation, mechanical ventilation, oxygen therapy, and an antagonist are immediately available. (5.1)
- Anaphylaxis: Severe anaphylaxis has been reported. Consider cross-reactivity among neuromuscular blocking agents. (5.2)
- Need for Adequate Anesthesia: Must be accompanied by adequate anesthesia or sedation. (5.3)
- Residual Paralysis: Consider using a reversal agent in cases where residual paralysis is more likely to occur. (5.4)

ADVERSE REACTIONS

Most common adverse reactions (2%) are transient hypotension and hypertension. (6.1)

To report SUSPECTED ADVERSE REACTIONS, contact Merck Sharp & Dohme Corp., a subsidiary of Merck & Co., Inc., at 1-877-888-4231 or FDA at 1-800-FDA-1088 or www.fda.gov/medwatch.

DRUG INTERACTIONS

- Succinylcholine: Use before succinylcholine has not been studied. (7.11)
- Nondepolarizing muscle relaxants: Interactions have been observed. (7.7)
- Enhanced ZEMURON activity possible: Inhalation anesthetics (7.3), certain antibiotics (7.1), quinidine (7.10), magnesium (7.6), lithium (7.4), local anesthetics (7.5), procainamide (7.8)
- Reduced ZEMURON activity possible: Anticonvulsants. (7.2)

USE IN SPECIFIC POPULATIONS

- Labor and Delivery: Not recommended for rapid sequence induction in patients undergoing Cesarean section. (8.2)
- Pediatric Use: Onset time and duration will vary with dose, age, and anesthetic technique. Not recommended for rapid sequence intubation in pediatric patients. (8.4)

See 17 for PATIENT COUNSELING INFORMATION
Revised: 08/2012

FULL PRESCRIBING INFORMATION: CONTENTS*

*** Sections or subsections omitted from the full prescribing information are not listed**

Table 1: Infusion Rates Using ZEMURON Injection (0.5 mg/mL)*

Patient Weight		Drug Delivery Rate (mcg/kg/min)									
		4	5	6	7	8	9	10	12	14	16
(kg)	(lbs)	Infusion Delivery Rate (mL/hr)									
10	22	4.8	6	7.2	8.4	9.6	10.8	12	14.4	16.8	19.2
15	33	7.2	9	10.8	12.6	14.4	16.2	18	21.6	25.2	28.8
20	44	9.6	12	14.4	16.8	19.2	21.6	24	28.8	33.6	38.4
25	55	12	15	18	21	24	27	30	36	42	48
35	77	16.8	21	25.2	29.4	33.6	37.8	42	50.4	58.8	67.2
50	110	24	30	36	42	48	54	60	72	84	96
60	132	28.8	36	43.2	50.4	57.6	64.8	72	86.4	100.8	115.2
70	154	33.6	42	50.4	58.8	67.2	75.6	84	100.8	117.6	134.4
80	176	38.4	48	57.6	67.2	76.8	86.4	96	115.2	134.4	153.6
90	198	43.2	54	64.8	75.6	86.4	97.2	108	129.6	151.2	172.8
100	220	48	60	72	84	96	108	120	144	168	192

* 50 mg ZEMURON in 100 mL solution.

FULL PRESCRIBING INFORMATION

1 INDICATIONS AND USAGE

ZEMURON® (rocuronium bromide) Injection is indicated for inpatients and outpatients as an adjunct to general anesthesia to facilitate both rapid sequence and routine tracheal intubation, and to provide skeletal muscle relaxation during surgery or mechanical ventilation.

2 DOSAGE AND ADMINISTRATION

ZEMURON is for intravenous use only. **This drug should only be administered by experienced clinicians or trained individuals supervised by an experienced clinician familiar with the use, actions, characteristics, and complications of neuromuscular blocking agents. Doses of ZEMURON injection should be individualized and a peripheral nerve stimulator should be used to monitor drug effect, need for additional doses, adequacy of spontaneous recovery or antagonism, and to decrease the complications of overdosage if additional doses are administered.**

The dosage information which follows is derived from studies based upon units of drug per unit of body weight. It is intended to serve as an initial guide to clinicians familiar with other neuromuscular blocking agents to acquire experience with ZEMURON.

In patients in whom potentiation of, or resistance to, neuromuscular block is anticipated, a dose adjustment should be considered *[see Dosage and Administration (2.5), Warnings and Precautions (5.9, 5.12), Drug Interactions (7.2, 7.3, 7.4, 7.5, 7.6, 7.8, 7.10), and Use in Specific Populations (8.6)]*.

2.1 Dose for Tracheal Intubation

The recommended initial dose of ZEMURON, regardless of anesthetic technique, is 0.6 mg/kg. Neuromuscular block sufficient for intubation (80% block or greater) is attained in a median (range) time of 1 (0.4-6) minute(s) and most patients have intubation completed within 2 minutes. Maximum blockade is achieved in most patients in less than 3 minutes. This dose may be expected to provide 31 (15-85) minutes of clinical relaxation under opioid/nitrous oxide/oxygen anesthesia. Under halothane, isoflurane, and enflurane anesthesia, some extension of the period of clinical relaxation should be expected *[see Drug Interactions (7.3)]*.

A lower dose of ZEMURON (0.45 mg/kg) may be used. Neuromuscular block sufficient for intubation (80% block or greater) is attained in a median (range) time of 1.3 (0.8-6.2) minute(s), and most patients have intubation completed within 2 minutes. Maximum blockade is achieved in most patients in less than 4 minutes. This dose may be expected to provide 22 (12-31) minutes of clinical relaxation under opioid/nitrous oxide/oxygen anesthesia. Patients receiving this low dose of 0.45 mg/kg who achieve less than 90% block (about 16% of these patients) may have a more rapid time to 25% recovery, 12 to 15 minutes.

A large bolus dose of 0.9 or 1.2 mg/kg can be administered under opioid/nitrous oxide/oxygen anesthesia without adverse effects to the cardiovascular system *[see Clinical Pharmacology (12.2)]*.

2.2 Rapid Sequence Intubation

In appropriately premedicated and adequately anesthetized patients, ZEMURON 0.6 to 1.2 mg/kg will provide excellent or good intubating conditions in most patients in less than 2 minutes *[see Clinical Studies (14.1)]*.

2.3 Maintenance Dosing

Maintenance doses of 0.1, 0.15, and 0.2 mg/kg ZEMURON, administered at 25% recovery of control T_1 (defined as 3 twitches of train-of-four), provide a median (range) of 12 (2-31), 17 (6-50), and 24 (7-69) minutes of clinical duration under opioid/nitrous oxide/oxygen anesthesia *[see Clinical Pharmacology (12.2)]*. In all cases, dosing should be guided based on the clinical duration following initial dose or prior maintenance dose and not administered until recovery of neuromuscular function is evident. A clinically insignificant cumulation of effect with repetitive maintenance dosing has been observed *[see Clinical Pharmacology (12.2)]*.

2.4 Use by Continuous Infusion

Infusion at an initial rate of 10 to 12 mcg/kg/min of ZEMURON should be initiated only after early evidence of spontaneous recovery from an intubating dose. Due to rapid redistribution *[see Clinical Pharmacology (12.3)]* and the associated rapid spontaneous recovery, initiation of the infusion after substantial return of neuromuscular function (more than 10% of control T_1) may necessitate additional bolus doses to maintain adequate block for surgery.

Upon reaching the desired level of neuromuscular block, the infusion of ZEMURON must be individualized for each patient. The rate of administration should be adjusted according to the patient's twitch response as monitored with the use of a peripheral nerve stimulator. In clinical trials, infusion rates have ranged from 4 to 16 mcg/kg/min.

Inhalation anesthetics, particularly enflurane and isoflurane, may enhance the neuromuscular blocking action of nondepolarizing muscle relaxants. In the presence of steady-state concentrations of enflurane or isoflurane, it may be necessary to reduce the rate of infusion by 30% to 50%, at 45 to 60 minutes after the intubating dose.

Spontaneous recovery and reversal of neuromuscular blockade following discontinuation of ZEMURON infusion may be expected to proceed at rates comparable to that following comparable total doses administered by repetitive bolus injections *[see Clinical Pharmacology (12.2)]*.

Infusion solutions of ZEMURON can be prepared by mixing ZEMURON with an appropriate infusion solution such as 5% glucose in water or lactated Ringers *[see Dosage and Administration (2.6)]*. These infusion solutions should be used within 24 hours of mixing. Unused portions of infusion solutions should be discarded.

Infusion rates of ZEMURON can be individualized for each patient using the following tables for 3 different concentrations of ZEMURON solution as guidelines:

[See table 1 at top of previous page]

[See table 2 above]

[See table 3 above]

Table 2: Infusion Rates Using ZEMURON Injection (1 mg/mL)*

Patient Weight		Drug Delivery Rate (mcg/kg/min)									
		4	5	6	7	8	9	10	12	14	16
(kg)	(lbs)	Infusion Delivery Rate (mL/hr)									
10	22	2.4	3	3.6	4.2	4.8	5.4	6	7.2	8.4	9.6
15	33	3.6	4.5	5.4	6.3	7.2	8.1	9	10.8	12.6	14.4
20	44	4.8	6	7.2	8.4	9.6	10.8	12	14.4	16.8	19.2
25	55	6	7.5	9	10.5	12	13.5	15	18	21	24
35	77	8.4	10.5	12.6	14.7	16.8	18.9	21	25.2	29.4	33.6
50	110	12	15	18	21	24	27	30	36	42	48
60	132	14.4	18	21.6	25.2	28.8	32.4	36	43.2	50.4	57.6
70	154	16.8	21	25.2	29.4	33.6	37.8	42	50.4	58.8	67.2
80	176	19.2	24	28.8	33.6	38.4	43.2	48	57.6	67.2	76.8
90	198	21.6	27	32.4	37.8	43.2	48.6	54	64.8	75.6	86.4
100	220	24	30	36	42	48	54	60	72	84	96

* 100 mg ZEMURON in 100 mL solution.

Table 3: Infusion Rates Using ZEMURON Injection (5 mg/mL)*

Patient Weight		Drug Delivery Rate (mcg/kg/min)									
		4	5	6	7	8	9	10	12	14	16
(kg)	(lbs)	Infusion Delivery Rate (mL/hr)									
10	22	0.5	0.6	0.7	0.8	1	1.1	1.2	1.4	1.7	1.9
15	33	0.7	0.9	1.1	1.3	1.4	1.6	1.8	2.2	2.5	2.9
20	44	1	1.2	1.4	1.7	1.9	2.2	2.4	2.9	3.4	3.8
25	55	1.2	1.5	1.8	2.1	2.4	2.7	3	3.6	4.2	4.8
35	77	1.7	2.1	2.5	2.9	3.4	3.8	4.2	5	5.9	6.7
50	110	2.4	3	3.6	4.2	4.8	5.4	6	7.2	8.4	9.6
60	132	2.9	3.6	4.3	5	5.8	6.5	7.2	8.6	10.1	11.5
70	154	3.4	4.2	5	5.9	6.7	7.6	8.4	10.1	11.8	13.4
80	176	3.8	4.8	5.8	6.7	7.7	8.6	9.6	11.5	13.4	15.4
90	198	4.3	5.4	6.5	7.6	8.6	9.7	10.8	13	15.1	17.3
100	220	4.8	6	7.2	8.4	9.6	10.8	12	14.4	16.8	19.2

* 500 mg ZEMURON in 100 mL solution.

2.5 Dosage in Specific Populations

Pediatric Patients: The recommended initial intubation dose of ZEMURON is 0.6 mg/kg; however, a lower dose of 0.45 mg/kg may be used depending on anesthetic technique and the age of the patient.

For sevoflurane (induction) ZEMURON doses of 0.45 mg/kg and 0.6 mg/kg in general produce excellent to good intubating conditions within 75 seconds. When halothane is used, a 0.6 mg/kg dose of ZEMURON resulted in excellent to good intubating conditions within 60 seconds.

The time to maximum block for an intubating dose was shortest in infants (28 days up to 3 months) and longest in neonates (birth to less than 28 days). The duration of clinical relaxation following an intubating dose is shortest in children (greater than 2 years up to 11 years) and longest in infants.

When sevoflurane is used for induction and isoflurane/nitrous oxide for maintenance of general anesthesia, maintenance dosing of ZEMURON can be administered as bolus doses of 0.15 mg/kg at reappearance of T_3 in all pediatric age groups. Maintenance dosing can also be administered at the reappearance of T_2 at a rate of 7 to 10 mcg/kg/min, with the lowest dose requirement for neonates (birth to less than 28 days) and the highest dose requirement for children (greater than 2 years up to 11 years).

When halothane is used for general anesthesia, patients ranging from 3 months old through adolescence can be administered ZEMURON maintenance doses of 0.075 to 0.125 mg/kg upon return of T_1 to 0.25% to provide clinical relaxation for 7 to 10 minutes. Alternatively, a continuous infusion of ZEMURON initiated at a rate of 12 mcg/kg/min upon return of T_1 to 10% (one twitch present in train-of-four) may also be used to maintain neuromuscular blockade in pediatric patients.

Additional information for administration to pediatric patients of all age groups is presented elsewhere in the label *[see Clinical Pharmacology (12.2)]*.

The infusion of ZEMURON must be individualized for each patient. The rate of administration should be adjusted according to the patient's twitch response as monitored with the use of a peripheral nerve stimulator. Spontaneous recovery and reversal of neuromuscular blockade following discontinuation of ZEMURON infusion may be expected to proceed at rates comparable to that following similar total exposure to single bolus doses *[see Clinical Pharmacology (12.2)]*.

ZEMURON is not recommended for rapid sequence intubation in pediatric patients.

Geriatric Patients: Geriatric patients (65 years or older) exhibited a slightly prolonged median (range) clinical duration of 46 (22-73), 62 (49-75), and 94 (64-138) minutes under opioid/nitrous oxide/oxygen anesthesia following doses of 0.6, 0.9, and 1.2 mg/kg, respectively. No differences in duration of neuromuscular blockade following maintenance doses of ZEMURON were observed between these subjects and younger subjects, and other reported clinical experience has not identified differences in response between elderly and younger patients, but greater sensitivity of some older individuals cannot be ruled out *[see Clinical Pharmacology (12.2, 12.3)]*.

Patients with Renal or Hepatic Impairment: No differences from patients with normal hepatic and kidney function were observed for onset time at a dose of 0.6 mg/kg ZEMURON. When compared to patients with normal renal and hepatic function, the mean clinical duration is similar in patients with end-stage renal disease undergoing renal transplant, and is about 1.5 times longer in patients with hepatic disease. Patients with renal failure may have a greater variation in duration of effect *[see Use in Specific Populations (8.6, 8.7) and Clinical Pharmacology (12.3)]*.

Obese Patients: In obese patients, the initial dose of ZEMURON 0.6 mg/kg should be based upon the patient's actual body weight *[see Clinical Studies (14.1)]*.

An analysis across all US controlled clinical studies indicates that the pharmacodynamics of ZEMURON are not different between obese and nonobese patients when dosed based upon their actual body weight.

Patients with Reduced Plasma Cholinesterase Activity: Rocuronium metabolism does not depend on plasma cholinesterase so dosing adjustments are not needed in patients with reduced plasma cholinesterase activity.

Patients with Prolonged Circulation Time: Because higher doses of ZEMURON produce a longer duration of action, the initial dosage should usually not be increased in these patients to reduce onset time; instead, in these situations, when feasible, more time should be allowed for the drug to achieve onset of effect *[see Warnings and Precautions (5.7)]*.

Patients with Drugs or Conditions Causing Potentiation of Neuromuscular Block: The neuromuscular blocking action of ZEMURON is potentiated by isoflurane and enflurane anesthesia. Potentiation is minimal when administration of the recommended dose of ZEMURON occurs prior to the administration of these potent inhalation agents. The median clinical duration of a dose of 0.57 to 0.85 mg/kg was 34, 38, and 42 minutes under opioid/nitrous oxide/oxygen, enflurane and isoflurane maintenance anesthesia, respectively. During 1 to 2 hours of infusion, the infusion rate of ZEMURON required to maintain about 95% block was decreased by as much as 40% under enflurane and isoflurane anesthesia *[see Drug Interactions (7.3)]*.

2.6 Preparation for Administration of ZEMURON

Diluent Compatibility: ZEMURON is compatible in solution with:

0.9% NaCl solution	sterile water for injection
5% glucose in water	lactated Ringers
5% glucose in saline	

ZEMURON is compatible in the above solutions at concentrations up to 5 mg/mL for 24 hours at room temperature in plastic bags, glass bottles, and plastic syringe pumps.

Drug Admixture Incompatibility: ZEMURON is physically incompatible when mixed with the following drugs:

amphotericin	hydrocortisone sodium succinate
amoxicillin	insulin
azathioprine	Intralipid
cefazolin	ketorolac
cloxacillin	lorazepam
dexamethasone	methohexital
diazepam	methylprednisolone
erythromycin	thiopental
famotidine	trimethoprim
furosemide	vancomycin

If ZEMURON is administered via the same infusion line that is also used for other drugs, it is important that this infusion line is adequately flushed between administration of ZEMURON and drugs for which incompatibility with ZEMURON has been demonstrated or for which compatibility with ZEMURON has not been established.

Infusion solutions should be used within 24 hours of mixing. Unused portions of infusion solutions should be discarded. ZEMURON should not be mixed with alkaline solutions *[see Warnings and Precautions (5.10)]*.

Visual Inspection: Parenteral drug products should be inspected visually for particulate matter and clarity prior to administration whenever solution and container permit. Do not use solution if particulate matter is present.

3 DOSAGE FORMS AND STRENGTHS

ZEMURON (rocuronium bromide) injection is available as

- 5 mL multiple dose vials containing 50 mg rocuronium bromide injection (10 mg/mL)
- 10 mL multiple dose vials containing 100 mg rocuronium bromide injection (10 mg/mL)

4 CONTRAINDICATIONS

ZEMURON is contraindicated in patients known to have hypersensitivity (e.g., anaphylaxis) to rocuronium bromide or other neuromuscular blocking agents *[see Warnings and Precautions (5.2)]*.

5 WARNINGS AND PRECAUTIONS

5.1 Appropriate Administration and Monitoring

ZEMURON should be administered in carefully adjusted dosages by or under the supervision of experienced clinicians who are familiar with the drug's actions and the possible complications of its use. The drug should not be administered unless facilities for intubation, mechanical ventilation, oxygen therapy, and an antagonist are immediately available. It is recommended that clinicians administering neuromuscular blocking agents such as ZEMURON employ a peripheral nerve stimulator to monitor drug effect, need for additional doses, adequacy of spontaneous recovery or antagonism, and to decrease the complications of overdosage if additional doses are administered.

5.2 Anaphylaxis

Severe anaphylactic reactions to neuromuscular blocking agents, including ZEMURON, have been reported. These reactions have, in some cases (including cases with ZEMURON), been life threatening and fatal. Due to the potential severity of these reactions, the necessary precautions, such as the immediate availability of appropriate emergency treatment, should be taken. Precautions should also be taken in those patients who have had previous anaphylactic reactions to other neuromuscular blocking agents, since cross-reactivity between neuromuscular blocking agents, both depolarizing and nondepolarizing, has been reported.

5.3 Need for Adequate Anesthesia

ZEMURON has no known effect on consciousness, pain threshold, or cerebration. Therefore, its administration must be accompanied by adequate anesthesia or sedation.

5.4 Residual Paralysis

In order to prevent complications resulting from residual paralysis, it is recommended to extubate only after the patient has recovered sufficiently from neuromuscular block. Other factors which could cause residual paralysis after extubation in the post-operative phase (such as drug interactions or patient condition) should also be considered. If not used as part of standard clinical practice the use of a reversal agent should be considered, especially in those cases where residual paralysis is more likely to occur.

5.5 Long-Term Use in an Intensive Care Unit

ZEMURON has not been studied for long-term use in the intensive care unit (ICU). As with other nondepolarizing neuromuscular blocking drugs, apparent tolerance to ZEMURON may develop during chronic administration in the ICU. While the mechanism for development of this resistance is not known, receptor up-regulation may be a contributing factor. **It is strongly recommended that neuromuscular transmission be monitored continuously during administration and recovery with the help of a nerve stimulator. Additional doses of ZEMURON or any other neuromuscular blocking agent should not be given until there is a definite response (one twitch of the train-of-four) to nerve stimulation.** Prolonged paralysis and/or skeletal muscle weakness may be noted during initial attempts to wean from the ventilator patients who have chronically received neuromuscular blocking drugs in the ICU.

Myopathy after long-term administration of other nondepolarizing neuromuscular blocking agents in the ICU alone or in combination with corticosteroid therapy has been reported. Therefore, for patients receiving both neuromuscular blocking agents and corticosteroids, the period of use of the neuromuscular blocking agent should be limited as much as possible and only used in the setting where in the opinion of the prescribing physician, the specific advantages of the drug outweigh the risk.

5.6 Malignant Hyperthermia (MH)

ZEMURON has not been studied in MH-susceptible patients. Because ZEMURON is always used with other agents, and the occurrence of malignant hyperthermia during anesthesia is possible even in the absence of known triggering agents, clinicians should be familiar with early signs, confirmatory diagnosis, and treatment of malignant hyperthermia prior to the start of any anesthetic.

In an animal study in MH-susceptible swine, the administration of ZEMURON Injection did not appear to trigger malignant hyperthermia.

5.7 Prolonged Circulation Time

Conditions associated with an increased circulatory delayed time, e.g., cardiovascular disease or advanced age, may be associated with a delay in onset time *[see Dosage and Administration (2.5)]*.

5.8 QT Interval Prolongation

The overall analysis of ECG data in pediatric patients indicates that the concomitant use of ZEMURON with general anesthetic agents can prolong the QTc interval *[see Clinical Studies (14.3)]*.

5.9 Conditions/Drugs Causing Potentiation of, or Resistance to, Neuromuscular Block

Potentiation: Nondepolarizing neuromuscular blocking agents have been found to exhibit profound neuromuscular blocking effects in cachectic or debilitated patients, patients with neuromuscular diseases, and patients with carcinomatosis.

Certain inhalation anesthetics, particularly enflurane and isoflurane, antibiotics, magnesium salts, lithium, local anesthetics, procainamide, and quinidine have been shown to increase the duration of neuromuscular block and decrease infusion requirements of neuromuscular blocking agents *[see Drug Interactions (7.3)]*.

In these or other patients in whom potentiation of neuromuscular block or difficulty with reversal may be anticipated, a decrease from the recommended initial dose of ZEMURON should be considered *[see Dosage and Administration (2.5)]*.

Resistance: Resistance to nondepolarizing agents, consistent with up-regulation of skeletal muscle acetylcholine receptors, is associated with burns, disuse atrophy, denervation, and direct muscle trauma. Receptor up-regulation may also contribute to the resistance to nondepolarizing muscle relaxants which sometimes develops in patients with cerebral palsy, patients chronically receiving anticonvulsant agents such as carbamazepine or phenytoin, or with chronic exposure to nondepolarizing agents. When ZEMURON is administered to these patients, shorter durations of neuromuscular block may occur, and infusion rates may be higher due to the development of resistance to nondepolarizing muscle relaxants.

Potentiation or Resistance: Severe acid-base and/or electrolyte abnormalities may potentiate or cause resistance to the neuromuscular blocking action of ZEMURON. No data are available in such patients and no dosing recommendations can be made.

ZEMURON-induced neuromuscular blockade was modified by alkalosis and acidosis in experimental pigs. Both respiratory and metabolic acidosis prolonged the recovery time. The potency of ZEMURON was significantly enhanced in metabolic acidosis and alkalosis, but was reduced in respiratory alkalosis. In addition, experience with other drugs has suggested that acute (e.g., diarrhea) or chronic (e.g., adrenocortical insufficiency) electrolyte imbalance may alter neuromuscular blockade. Since electrolyte imbalance and acid-base imbalance are usually mixed, either enhancement or inhibition may occur.

5.10 Incompatibility with Alkaline Solutions

ZEMURON, which has an acid pH, should not be mixed with alkaline solutions (e.g., barbiturate solutions) in the same syringe or administered simultaneously during intravenous infusion through the same needle.

5.11 Increase in Pulmonary Vascular Resistance

ZEMURON may be associated with increased pulmonary vascular resistance, so caution is appropriate in patients with pulmonary hypertension or valvular heart disease *[see Clinical Studies (14.1)]*.

5.12 Use In Patients with Myasthenia

In patients with myasthenia gravis or myasthenic (Eaton-Lambert) syndrome, small doses of nondepolarizing neuromuscular blocking agents may have profound effects. In such patients, a peripheral nerve stimulator and use of a small test dose may be of value in monitoring the response to administration of muscle relaxants.

5.13 Extravasation

If extravasation occurs, it may be associated with signs or symptoms of local irritation. The injection or infusion should be terminated immediately and restarted in another vein.

6 ADVERSE REACTIONS

In clinical trials, the most common adverse reactions (2%) are transient hypotension and hypertension.

The following adverse reactions are described, or described in greater detail, in other sections:

- Anaphylaxis *[see Warnings and Precautions (5.2)]*
- Residual paralysis *[see Warnings and Precautions (5.4)]*
- Myopathy *[see Warnings and Precautions (5.5)]*
- Increased pulmonary vascular resistance *[see Warnings and Precautions (5.11)]*

6.1 Clinical Trials Experience

Because clinical trials are conducted under widely varying conditions, adverse reaction rates observed in the clinical trials of a drug cannot be directly compared to rates in the clinical trials of another drug and may not reflect the rates observed in practice.

Clinical studies in the US (n=1137) and Europe (n=1394) totaled 2531 patients. The patients exposed in the US clinical studies provide the basis for calculation of adverse reaction rates. The following adverse reactions were reported in patients administered ZEMURON (all events judged by investigators during the clinical trials to have a possible causal relationship):

Adverse reactions in greater than 1% of patients: None

Adverse reactions in less than 1% of patients (probably related or relationship unknown):

Cardiovascular: arrhythmia, abnormal electrocardiogram, tachycardia

Digestive: nausea, vomiting

Respiratory: asthma (bronchospasm, wheezing, or rhonchi), hiccup

Skin and Appendages: rash, injection site edema, pruritus

In the European studies, the most commonly reported reactions were transient hypotension (2%) and hypertension (2%); these are in greater frequency than the US studies (0.1% and 0.1%). Changes in heart rate and blood pressure were defined differently from in the US studies in which changes in cardiovascular parameters were not considered as adverse events unless judged by the investigator as unexpected, clinically significant, or thought to be histamine related.

In a clinical study in patients with clinically significant cardiovascular disease undergoing coronary artery bypass graft, hypertension and tachycardia were reported in some patients, but these occurrences were less frequent in patients receiving beta or calcium channel-blocking drugs. In some patients, ZEMURON was associated with transient increases (30% or greater) in pulmonary vascular resistance. In another clinical study of patients undergoing abdominal aortic surgery, transient increases (30% or greater) in pulmonary vascular resistance were observed in about 24% of patients receiving ZEMURON 0.6 or 0.9 mg/kg.

In pediatric patient studies worldwide (n=704), tachycardia occurred at an incidence of 5.3% (n=37), and it was judged by the investigator as related in 10 cases (1.4%).

6.2 Postmarketing Experience

In clinical practice, there have been reports of severe allergic reactions (anaphylactic and anaphylactoid reactions and shock) with ZEMURON, including some that have been life-threatening and fatal *[see Warnings and Precautions (5.2)]*. Because these reactions were reported voluntarily from a population of uncertain size, it is not possible to reliably estimate their frequency.

7 DRUG INTERACTIONS

7.1 Antibiotics

Drugs which may enhance the neuromuscular blocking action of nondepolarizing agents such as ZEMURON include certain antibiotics (e.g., aminoglycosides; vancomycin; tetracyclines; bacitracin; polymyxins; colistin; and sodium colistimethate). If these antibiotics are used in conjunction with ZEMURON, prolongation of neuromuscular block may occur.

7.2 Anticonvulsants
In 2 of 4 patients receiving chronic anticonvulsant therapy, apparent resistance to the effects of ZEMURON was observed in the form of diminished magnitude of neuromuscular block, or shortened clinical duration. As with other nondepolarizing neuromuscular blocking drugs, if ZEMURON is administered to patients chronically receiving anticonvulsant agents such as carbamazepine or phenytoin, shorter durations of neuromuscular block may occur and infusion rates may be higher due to the development of resistance to nondepolarizing muscle relaxants. While the mechanism for development of this resistance is not known, receptor upregulation may be a contributing factor *[see Warnings and Precautions (5.9)]*.

7.3 Inhalation Anesthetics
Use of inhalation anesthetics has been shown to enhance the activity of other neuromuscular blocking agents (enflurane > isoflurane > halothane).
Isoflurane and enflurane may also prolong the duration of action of initial and maintenance doses of ZEMURON and decrease the average infusion requirement of ZEMURON by 40% compared to opioid/nitrous oxide/oxygen anesthesia. No definite interaction between ZEMURON and halothane has been demonstrated. In one study, use of enflurane in 10 patients resulted in a 20% increase in mean clinical duration of the initial intubating dose, and a 37% increase in the duration of subsequent maintenance doses, when compared in the same study to 10 patients under opioid/nitrous oxide/oxygen anesthesia. The clinical duration of initial doses of ZEMURON of 0.57 to 0.85 mg/kg under enflurane or isoflurane anesthesia, as used clinically, was increased by 11% and 23%, respectively. The duration of maintenance doses was affected to a greater extent, increasing by 30% to 50% under either enflurane or isoflurane anesthesia.
Potentiation by these agents is also observed with respect to the infusion rates of ZEMURON required to maintain approximately 95% neuromuscular block. Under isoflurane and enflurane anesthesia, the infusion rates are decreased by approximately 40% compared to opioid/nitrous oxide/oxygen anesthesia. The median spontaneous recovery time (from 25% to 75% of control T_1) is not affected by halothane, but is prolonged by enflurane (15% longer) and isoflurane (62% longer). Reversal-induced recovery of ZEMURON neuromuscular block is minimally affected by anesthetic technique *[see Dosage and Administration (2.5) and Warnings and Precautions (5.9)]*.

7.4 Lithium Carbonate
Lithium has been shown to increase the duration of neuromuscular block and decrease infusion requirements of neuromuscular blocking agents *[see Warnings and Precautions (5.9)]*.

7.5 Local Anesthetics
Local anesthetics have been shown to increase the duration of neuromuscular block and decrease infusion requirements of neuromuscular blocking agents *[see Warnings and Precautions (5.9)]*.

7.6 Magnesium
Magnesium salts administered for the management of toxemia of pregnancy may enhance neuromuscular blockade *[see Warnings and Precautions (5.9)]*.

7.7 Nondepolarizing Muscle Relaxants
There are no controlled studies documenting the use of ZEMURON before or after other nondepolarizing muscle relaxants. Interactions have been observed when other nondepolarizing muscle relaxants have been administered in succession.

7.8 Procainamide
Procainamide has been shown to increase the duration of neuromuscular block and decrease infusion requirements of neuromuscular blocking agents *[see Warnings and Precautions (5.9)]*.

7.9 Propofol
The use of propofol for induction and maintenance of anesthesia does not alter the clinical duration or recovery characteristics following recommended doses of ZEMURON.

7.10 Quinidine
Injection of quinidine during recovery from use of muscle relaxants is associated with recurrent paralysis. This possibility must also be considered for ZEMURON *[see Warnings and Precautions (5.9)]*.

7.11 Succinylcholine
The use of ZEMURON before succinylcholine, for the purpose of attenuating some of the side effects of succinylcholine, has not been studied.
If ZEMURON is administered following administration of succinylcholine, it should not be given until recovery from succinylcholine has been observed. The median duration of action of ZEMURON 0.6 mg/kg administered after a 1 mg/kg dose of succinylcholine when T_1 returned to 75% of control was 36 minutes (range: 14-57, n=12) vs. 28 minutes (range: 17-51, n=12) without succinylcholine.

8 USE IN SPECIFIC POPULATIONS

8.1 Pregnancy
Pregnancy Category C: Developmental toxicology studies have been performed with rocuronium bromide in pregnant, conscious, nonventilated rabbits and rats. Inhibition of neuromuscular function was the endpoint for high-dose selection. The maximum tolerated dose served as the high dose and was administered intravenously 3 times a day to rats (0.3 mg/kg, 15%-30% of human intubation dose of 0.6-1.2 mg/kg based on the body surface unit of mg/m^2) from Day 6 to 17 and to rabbits (0.02 mg/kg, 25% human dose) from Day 6 to 18 of pregnancy. High-dose treatment caused acute symptoms of respiratory dysfunction due to the pharmacological activity of the drug. Teratogenicity was not observed in these animal species. The incidence of late embryonic death was increased at the high dose in rats, most likely due to oxygen deficiency. Therefore, this finding probably has no relevance for humans because immediate mechanical ventilation of the intubated patient will effectively prevent embryo-fetal hypoxia. However, there are no adequate and well-controlled studies in pregnant women. ZEMURON should be used during pregnancy only if the potential benefit justifies the potential risk to the fetus.

8.2 Labor and Delivery
The use of ZEMURON in Cesarean section has been studied in a limited number of patients *[see Clinical Studies (14.1)]*. ZEMURON is not recommended for rapid sequence induction in Cesarean section patients.

8.4 Pediatric Use
The use of ZEMURON has been studied in pediatric patients 3 months to 14 years of age under halothane anesthesia. Of the pediatric patients anesthetized with halothane who did not receive atropine for induction, about 80% experienced a transient increase (30% or greater) in heart rate after intubation. One of the 19 infants anesthetized with halothane and fentanyl who received atropine for induction experienced this magnitude of change *[see Dosage and Administration (2.5) and Clinical Studies (14.3)]*.
ZEMURON was also studied in pediatric patients up to 17 years of age, including neonates, under sevoflurane (induction) and isoflurane/nitrous oxide (maintenance) anesthesia. Onset time and clinical duration varied with dose, the age of the patient, and anesthetic technique. The overall analysis of ECG data in pediatric patients indicates that the concomitant use of ZEMURON with general anesthetic agents can prolong the QTc interval. The data also suggest that ZEMURON may increase heart rate. However, it was not possible to conclusively identify an effect of ZEMURON independent of that of anesthesia and other factors. Additionally, when examining plasma levels of ZEMURON in correlation to QTc interval prolongation, no relationship was observed *[see Dosage and Administration (2.5), Warnings and Precautions (5.8), and Clinical Studies (14.3)]*.
ZEMURON is not recommended for rapid sequence intubation in pediatric patients. Recommendations for use in pediatric patients are discussed in other sections *[see Dosage and Administration (2.5) and Clinical Pharmacology (12.2)]*.

8.5 Geriatric Use
ZEMURON was administered to 140 geriatric patients (65 years or greater) in US clinical trials and 128 geriatric patients in European clinical trials. The observed pharmacokinetic profile for geriatric patients (n=20) was similar to that for other adult surgical patients *[see Clinical Pharmacology (12.3)]*. Onset time and duration of action were slightly longer for geriatric patients (n=43) in clinical trials. Clinical experiences and recommendations for use in geriatric patients are discussed in other sections *[see Dosage and Administration (2.5), Clinical Pharmacology (12.2), and Clinical Studies (14.2)]*.

8.6 Patients with Hepatic Impairment
Since ZEMURON is primarily excreted by the liver, it should be used with caution in patients with clinically significant hepatic impairment. ZEMURON 0.6 mg/kg has been studied in a limited number of patients (n=9) with clinically significant hepatic impairment under steady-state isoflurane anesthesia. After ZEMURON 0.6 mg/kg, the median (range) clinical duration of 60 (35-166) minutes was moderately prolonged compared to 42 minutes in patients with normal hepatic function. The median recovery time of 53 minutes was also prolonged in patients with cirrhosis compared to 20 minutes in patients with normal hepatic function. Four of 8 patients with cirrhosis, who received ZEMURON 0.6 mg/kg under opioid/nitrous oxide/oxygen anesthesia, did not achieve complete block. These findings are consistent with the increase in volume of distribution at steady state observed in patients with significant hepatic impairment *[see Clinical Pharmacology (12.3)]*. If used for rapid sequence induction in patients with ascites, an increased initial dosage may be necessary to assure complete block. Duration will be prolonged in these cases. The use of doses higher than 0.6 mg/kg has not been studied *[see Dosage and Administration (2.5)]*.

8.7 Patients with Renal Impairment
Due to the limited role of the kidney in the excretion of ZEMURON, usual dosing guidelines should be followed. In patients with renal dysfunction, the duration of neuromuscular blockade was not prolonged; however, there was substantial individual variability (range: 22-90 minutes) *[see Clinical Pharmacology (12.3)]*.

10 OVERDOSAGE

Overdosage with neuromuscular blocking agents may result in neuromuscular block beyond the time needed for surgery and anesthesia. The primary treatment is maintenance of a patent airway, controlled ventilation, and adequate sedation until recovery of normal neuromuscular function is assured. Once evidence of recovery from neuromuscular block is observed, further recovery may be facilitated by administration of an anticholinesterase agent in conjunction with an appropriate anticholinergic agent.
Reversal of Neuromuscular Blockade: **Anticholinesterase agents should not be administered prior to the demonstration of some spontaneous recovery from neuromuscular blockade. The use of a nerve stimulator to document recovery is recommended.**
Patients should be evaluated for adequate clinical evidence of neuromuscular recovery, e.g., 5-second head lift, adequate phonation, ventilation, and upper airway patency. Ventilation must be supported while patients exhibit any signs of muscle weakness.
Recovery may be delayed in the presence of debilitation, carcinomatosis, and concomitant use of certain drugs which enhance neuromuscular blockade or separately cause respiratory depression. Under such circumstances the management is the same as that of prolonged neuromuscular blockade.

11 DESCRIPTION

ZEMURON (rocuronium bromide) injection is a nondepolarizing neuromuscular blocking agent with a rapid to intermediate onset depending on dose and intermediate duration. Rocuronium bromide is chemically designated as 1-[17β-(acetyloxy)-3α-hydroxy-2β-(4-morpholinyl)-5α-androstan-16β-yl]-1-(2-propenyl)pyrrolidinium bromide.
The structural formula is:

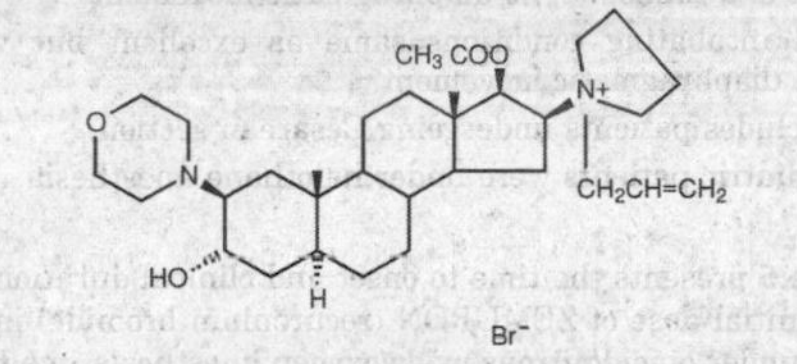

The chemical formula is $C_{32}H_{53}BrN_2O_4$ with a molecular weight of 609.70. The partition coefficient of rocuronium bromide in n-octanol/water is 0.5 at 20°C.
ZEMURON is supplied as a sterile, nonpyrogenic, isotonic solution that is clear, colorless to yellow/orange, for intravenous injection only. Each mL contains 10 mg rocuronium bromide and 2 mg sodium acetate. The aqueous solution is adjusted to isotonicity with sodium chloride and to a pH of 4 with acetic acid and/or sodium hydroxide.

12 CLINICAL PHARMACOLOGY

12.1 Mechanism of Action
ZEMURON is a nondepolarizing neuromuscular blocking agent with a rapid to intermediate onset depending on dose and intermediate duration. It acts by competing for cholinergic receptors at the motor end-plate. This action is antagonized by acetylcholinesterase inhibitors, such as neostigmine and edrophonium.

12.2 Pharmacodynamics
The ED_{95} (dose required to produce 95% suppression of the first [T_1] mechanomyographic [MMG] response of the adductor pollicis muscle [thumb] to indirect supramaximal train-of-four stimulation of the ulnar nerve) during opioid/nitrous oxide/oxygen anesthesia is approximately 0.3 mg/kg. Patient variability around the ED_{95} dose suggests that 50% of patients will exhibit T_1 depression of 91% to 97%.
Table 4 presents intubating conditions in patients with intubation initiated at 60 to 70 seconds.

Table 4: Percent of Excellent or Good Intubating Conditions and Median (Range) Time to Completion of Intubation in Patients with Intubation Initiated at 60 to 70 Seconds

ZEMURON Dose (mg/kg) Administered Over 5 sec	Percent of Patients with Excellent or Good Intubating Conditions	Time to Completion of Intubation (min)
Adults* 18 to 64 yrs		
0.45 (n=43)	86%	1.6 (1.0-7.0)
0.6 (n=51)	96%	1.6 (1.0-3.2)
Infants† 3 mo to 1 yr		
0.6 (n=18)	100%	1.0 (1.0-1.5)

Table 5: Median (Range) Time to Onset and Clinical Duration Following Initial (Intubating) Dose During Opioid/Nitrous Oxide/Oxygen Anesthesia (Adults) and Halothane Anesthesia (Pediatric Patients)

ZEMURON Dose (mg/kg) Administered Over 5 sec	Time to ≥80% Block (min)	Time to Maximum Block (min)	Clinical Duration (min)
Adults 18 to 64 yrs			
0.45 (n=50)	1.3 (0.8-6.2)	3.0 (1.3-8.2)	22 (12-31)
0.6 (n=142)	1.0 (0.4-6.0)	1.8 (0.6-13.0)	31 (15-85)
0.9 (n=20)	1.1 (0.3-3.8)	1.4 (0.8-6.2)	58 (27-111)
1.2 (n=18)	0.7 (0.4-1.7)	1.0 (0.6-4.7)	67 (38-160)
Geriatric ≥65 yrs			
0.6 (n=31)	2.3 (1.0-8.3)	3.7 (1.3-11.3)	46 (22-73)
0.9 (n=5)	2.0 (1.0-3.0)	2.5 (1.2-5.0)	62 (49-75)
1.2 (n=7)	1.0 (0.8-3.5)	1.3 (1.2-4.7)	94 (64-138)
Infants 3 mo to 1 yr			
0.6 (n=17)	—	0.8 (0.3-3.0)	41 (24-68)
0.8 (n=9)	—	0.7 (0.5-0.8)	40 (27-70)
Pediatric 1 to 12 yrs			
0.6 (n=27)	0.8 (0.4-2.0)	1.0 (0.5-3.3)	26 (17-39)
0.8 (n=18)	—	0.5 (0.3-1.0)	30 (17-56)

n=the number of patients who had time to maximum block recorded.
Clinical duration=time until return to 25% of control T_1. Patients receiving doses of 0.45 mg/kg who achieved less than 90% block (16% of these patients) had about 12 to 15 minutes to 25% recovery.

Pediatric† 1 to 12 yrs		
0.6 (n=12)	100%	1.0 (0.5-2.3)

Excellent intubating conditions=jaw relaxed, vocal cords apart and immobile, no diaphragmatic movement.

Good intubating conditions=same as excellent but with some diaphragmatic movement.

* Excludes patients undergoing Cesarean section.

† Pediatric patients were under halothane anesthesia.

Table 5 presents the time to onset and clinical duration for the initial dose of ZEMURON (rocuronium bromide) injection under opioid/nitrous oxide/oxygen anesthesia in adults and geriatric patients, and under halothane anesthesia in pediatric patients.

[See table 5 above]

Table 6 presents the time to onset and clinical duration for the initial dose of ZEMURON (rocuronium bromide) Injection under sevoflurane (induction) and isoflurane/nitrous oxide (maintenance) anesthesia in pediatric patients.

Table 6: Median (Range) Time to Onset and Clinical Duration Following Initial (Intubating) Dose During Sevoflurane (induction) and Isoflurane/Nitrous Oxide (maintenance) Anesthesia (Pediatric Patients)

ZEMURON Dose (mg/kg) Administered Over 5 sec	Time to Maximum Block (min)	Time to Reappearance T_3 (min)
Neonates birth to <28 days		
0.45 (n=5)	1.1 (0.6-2.2)	40.3 (32.5-62.6)
0.6 (n=10)	1.0 (0.2-2.1)	49.7 (16.6-119.0)
1 (n=6)	0.6 (0.3-1.8)	114.4 (92.6-136.3)
Infants 28 days to ≤3 mo		
0.45 (n=9)	0.5 (0.4-1.3)	49.1 (13.5-79.9)
0.6 (n=11)	0.4 (0.2-0.8)	59.8 (32.3-87.8)
1 (n=5)	0.3 (0.2-0.7)	103.3 (90.8-155.4)
Toddlers >3 mo to ≤2 yrs		
0.45 (n=17)	0.8 (0.3-1.9)	39.2 (16.9-59.4)
0.6 (n=29)	0.6 (0.2-1.6)	44.2 (18.9-68.8)
1 (n=15)	0.5 (0.2-1.5)	72.0 (36.2-128.2)
Children >2 yrs to ≤11 yrs		
0.45 (n=14)	0.9 (0.4-1.9)	21.5 (17.5-38.0)
0.6 (n=37)	0.8 (0.3-1.7)	36.7 (20.1-65.9)
1 (n=16)	0.7 (0.4-1.2)	53.1 (31.2-89.9)
Adolescents >11 to ≤17 yrs		
0.45 (n=18)	1.0 (0.5-1.7)	37.5 (18.3-65.7)
0.6 (n=31)	0.9 (0.2-2.1)	41.4 (16.3-91.2)
1 (n=14)	0.7 (0.5-1.2)	67.1 (25.6-93.8)

n=the number of patients with the highest number of observations for time to maximum block or reappearance T_3.

The time to 80% or greater block and clinical duration as a function of dose are presented in **Figures 1** and **2**.

Figure 1: Time to 80% or Greater Block vs. Initial Dose of ZEMURON by Age Group (Median, 25th and 75th Percentile, and Individual Values)

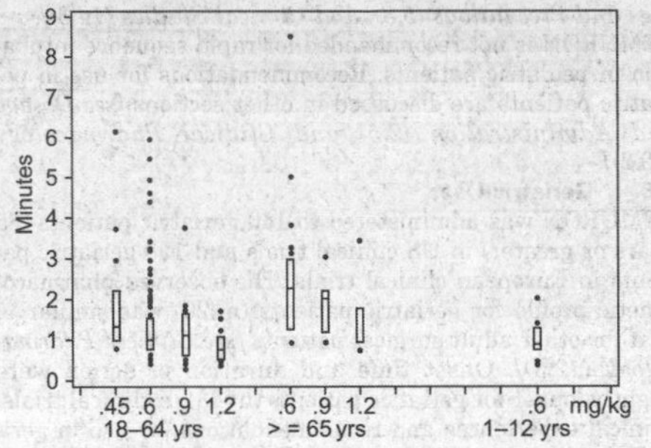

Figure 2: Duration of Clinical Effect vs. Initial Dose of ZEMURON by Age Group (Median, 25th and 75th Percentile, and Individual Values)

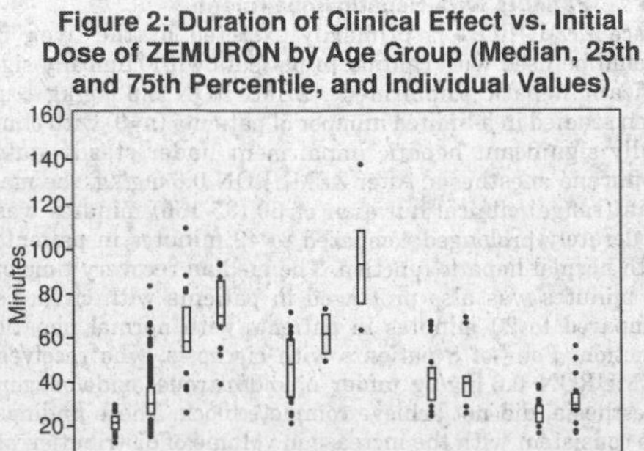

The clinical durations for the first 5 maintenance doses, in patients receiving 5 or more maintenance doses are represented in **Figure 3** *[see Dosage and Administration (2.3)]*.

[See figure 3 at top of next column]

Figure 3: Duration of Clinical Effect vs. Number of ZEMURON Maintenance Doses, by Dose

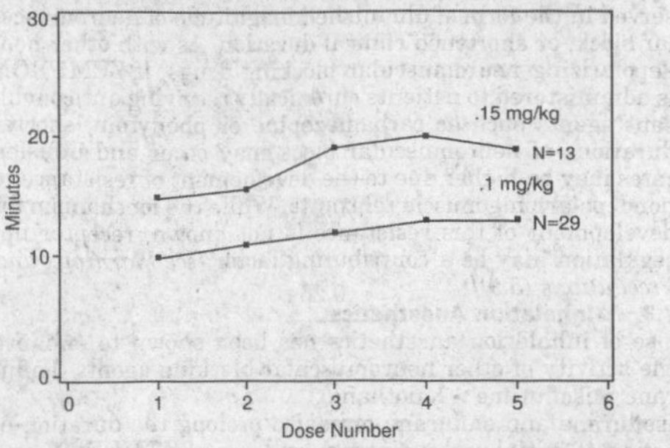

Once spontaneous recovery has reached 25% of control T_1, the neuromuscular block produced by ZEMURON is readily reversed with anticholinesterase agents, e.g., edrophonium or neostigmine.

The median spontaneous recovery from 25% to 75% T_1 was 13 minutes in adult patients. When neuromuscular block was reversed in 36 adults at a T_1 of 22% to 27%, recovery to a T_1 of 89 (50-132)% and T_4/T_1 of 69 (38-92)% was achieved within 5 minutes. Only 5 of 320 adults reversed received an additional dose of reversal agent. The median (range) dose of neostigmine was 0.04 (0.01-0.09) mg/kg and the median (range) dose of edrophonium was 0.5 (0.3-1.0) mg/kg.

In geriatric patients (n=51) reversed with neostigmine, the median T_4/T_1 increased from 40% to 88% in 5 minutes.

In clinical trials with halothane, pediatric patients (n=27) who received 0.5 mg/kg edrophonium had increases in the median T_4/T_1 from 37% at reversal to 93% after 2 minutes. Pediatric patients (n=58) who received 1 mg/kg edrophonium had increases in the median T_4/T_1 from 72% at reversal to 100% after 2 minutes. Infants (n=10) who were reversed with 0.03 mg/kg neostigmine recovered from 25% to 75% T_1 within 4 minutes.

There were no reports of less than satisfactory clinical recovery of neuromuscular function.

The neuromuscular blocking action of ZEMURON may be enhanced in the presence of potent inhalation anesthetics *[see Drug Interactions (7.3)]*.

Hemodynamics: There were no dose-related effects on the incidence of changes from baseline (30% or greater) in mean arterial blood pressure (MAP) or heart rate associated with ZEMURON administration over the dose range of 0.12 to 1.2 mg/kg ($4 \times ED_{95}$) within 5 minutes after ZEMURON administration and prior to intubation. Increases or decreases in MAP were observed in 2% to 5% of geriatric and other adult patients, and in about 1% of pediatric patients. Heart rate changes (30% or greater) occurred in 0% to 2% of geriatric and other adult patients. Tachycardia (30% or greater) occurred in 12 of 127 pediatric patients. Most of the pediatric patients developing tachycardia were from a single study where the patients were anesthetized with halothane and who did not receive atropine for induction *[see Clinical Studies (14.3)]*. In US studies, laryngoscopy and tracheal intubation following ZEMURON administration were accompanied by transient tachycardia (30% or greater increases) in about one-third of adult patients under opioid/nitrous oxide/oxygen anesthesia. Animal studies have indicated that the ratio of vagal:neuromuscular block following ZEMURON administration is less than vecuronium but greater than pancuronium. The tachycardia observed in some patients may result from this vagal blocking activity.

Histamine Release: In studies of histamine release, clinically significant concentrations of plasma histamine occurred in 1 of 88 patients. Clinical signs of histamine release (flushing, rash, or bronchospasm) associated with the administration of ZEMURON were assessed in clinical trials and reported in 9 of 1137 (0.8%) patients.

12.3 Pharmacokinetics

Adult and Geriatric Patients: In an effort to maximize the information gathered in the *in vivo* pharmacokinetic studies, the data from the studies was used to develop population estimates of the parameters for the subpopulations represented (e.g., geriatric, pediatric, renal, and hepatic impairment). These population-based estimates and a measure of the estimate variability are contained in the following section.

Following intravenous administration of ZEMURON, plasma levels of rocuronium follow a three-compartment open model. The rapid distribution half-life is 1 to 2 minutes and the slower distribution half-life is 14 to 18 minutes. Rocuronium is approximately 30% bound to human plasma proteins. In geriatric and other adult surgical patients undergoing either opioid/nitrous oxide/oxygen or inhalational anesthesia, the observed pharmacokinetic profile was essentially unchanged.

Table 7: Mean (SD) Pharmacokinetic Parameters in Adults (n=22; ages 27 to 58 yrs) and Geriatric (n=20; 65 yrs or greater) During Opioid/Nitrous Oxide/Oxygen Anesthesia

PK Parameters	Adults (Ages 27-58 yrs)	Geriatrics (≥65 yrs)
Clearance (L/kg/hr)	0.25 (0.08)	0.21 (0.06)
Volume of Distribution at Steady State (L/kg)	0.25 (0.04)	0.22 (0.03)
$t_{1/2}$ β Elimination (hr)	1.4 (0.4)	1.5 (0.4)

In general, studies with normal adult subjects did not reveal any differences in the pharmacokinetics of rocuronium due to gender.

Studies of distribution, metabolism, and excretion in cats and dogs indicate that rocuronium is eliminated primarily by the liver. The rocuronium analog 17-desacetyl-rocuronium, a metabolite, has been rarely observed in the plasma or urine of humans administered single doses of 0.5 to 1 mg/kg with or without a subsequent infusion (for up to 12 hr) of rocuronium. In the cat, 17-desacetyl-rocuronium has approximately one-twentieth the neuromuscular blocking potency of rocuronium. The effects of renal failure and hepatic disease on the pharmacokinetics and pharmacodynamics of rocuronium in humans are consistent with these findings.

In general, patients undergoing cadaver kidney transplant have a small reduction in clearance which is offset pharmacokinetically by a corresponding increase in volume, such that the net effect is an unchanged plasma half-life. Patients with demonstrated liver cirrhosis have a marked increase in their volume of distribution resulting in a plasma half-life approximately twice that of patients with normal hepatic function. **Table 8** shows the pharmacokinetic parameters in subjects with either impaired renal or hepatic function.

[See table 8 above]

Table 8: Mean (SD) Pharmacokinetic Parameters in Adults with Normal Renal and Hepatic Function (n=10, ages 23 to 65), Renal Transplant Patients (n=10, ages 21 to 45), and Hepatic Dysfunction Patients (n=9, ages 31 to 67) During Isoflurane Anesthesia

PK Parameters	Normal Renal and Hepatic Function	Renal Transplant Patients	Hepatic Dysfunction Patients
Clearance (L/kg/hr)	0.16 (0.05)*	0.13 (0.04)	0.13 (0.06)
Volume of Distribution at Steady State (L/kg)	0.26 (0.03)	0.34 (0.11)	0.53 (0.14)
$t_{1/2}$ β Elimination (hr)	2.4 (0.8)*	2.4 (1.1)	4.3 (2.6)

* Differences in the calculated $t_{1/2}$ β and Cl between this study and the study in young adults vs. geriatrics (≥65 years) is related to the different sample populations and anesthetic techniques.

The net result of these findings is that subjects with renal failure have clinical durations that are similar to but somewhat more variable than the duration that one would expect in subjects with normal renal function. Hepatically impaired patients, due to the large increase in volume, may demonstrate clinical durations approaching 1.5 times that of subjects with normal hepatic function. In both populations the clinician should individualize the dose to the needs of the patient *[see Dosage and Administration (2.5)]*.

Tissue redistribution accounts for most (about 80%) of the initial amount of rocuronium administered. As tissue compartments fill with continued dosing (4-8 hours), less drug is redistributed away from the site of action and, for an infusion-only dose, the rate to maintain neuromuscular blockade falls to about 20% of the initial infusion rate. The use of a loading dose and a smaller infusion rate reduces the need for adjustment of dose.

Pediatric Patients: Under halothane anesthesia, the clinical duration of effects of ZEMURON did not vary with age in patients 4 months to 8 years of age. The terminal half-life and other pharmacokinetic parameters of rocuronium in these pediatric patients are presented in **Table 9.**

Table 9: Mean (SD) Pharmacokinetic Parameters of Rocuronium in Pediatric Patients (ages 3 to less than 12 mos, n=6; 1 to less than 3 yrs, n=5; 3 to less than 8 yrs, n=7) During Halothane Anesthesia

PK Parameters	Patient Age Range: 3 to <12 mos	1 to <3 yrs	3 to <8 yrs
Clearance (L/kg/hr)	0.35 (0.08)	0.32 (0.07)	0.44 (0.16)
Volume of Distribution at Steady State (L/kg)	0.30 (0.04)	0.26 (0.06)	0.21 (0.03)
$t_{1/2}$ β Elimination (hr)	1.3 (0.5)	1.1 (0.7)	0.8 (0.3)

Pharmacokinetics of ZEMURON were evaluated using a population analysis of the pooled pharmacokinetic datasets from 2 trials under sevoflurane (induction) and isoflurane/nitrous oxide (maintenance) anesthesia. All pharmacokinetic parameters were found to be linearly proportional to body weight. In patients under the age of 18 years clearance (CL) and volume of distribution (Vss) increase with body-weight (kg) and age (years). As a result the terminal half-life of ZEMURON decreases with increasing age from 1.1 hour to 0.7-0.8 hour. **Table 10** presents the pharmacokinetic parameters in the different age groups in the studies with sevoflurane (induction) and isoflurane/nitrous oxide (maintenance) anesthesia.

[See table 10 above]

Table 10: Mean (SD) Pharmacokinetic Parameters of Rocuronium in Pediatric Patients During Sevoflurane (induction) and Isoflurane/Nitrous Oxide (maintenance) Anesthesia

PK Parameters	Patient Age Range: Birth to <28 days	28 days to ≤3 mos	3 mos to ≤2 yrs	2 to ≤11 yrs	11 to ≤17 yrs
CL (L/kg/hr)	0.31 (0.07)	0.30 (0.08)	0.33 (0.10)	0.35 (0.09)	0.29 (0.14)
Volume of Distribution (L/kg)	0.42 (0.06)	0.31 (0.03)	0.23 (0.03)	0.18 (0.02)	0.18 (0.01)
$t_{1/2}$ β (hr)	1.1 (0.2)	0.9 (0.3)	0.8 (0.2)	0.7 (0.2)	0.8 (0.3)

13 NONCLINICAL TOXICOLOGY

13.1 Carcinogenesis, Mutagenesis, Impairment of Fertility

Studies in animals have not been performed with rocuronium bromide to evaluate carcinogenic potential or impairment of fertility. Mutagenicity studies (Ames test, analysis of chromosomal aberrations in mammalian cells, and micronucleus test) conducted with rocuronium bromide did not suggest mutagenic potential.

14 CLINICAL STUDIES

In US clinical studies, a total of 1137 patients received ZEMURON, including 176 pediatric, 140 geriatric, 55 obstetric, and 766 other adults. Most patients (90%) were ASA physical status I or II, about 9% were ASA III, and 10 patients (undergoing coronary artery bypass grafting or valvular surgery) were ASA IV. In European clinical studies, a total of 1394 patients received ZEMURON, including 52 pediatric, 128 geriatric (65 years or greater), and 1214 other adults.

14.1 Adult Patients

Intubation using doses of ZEMURON 0.6 to 0.85 mg/kg was evaluated in 203 adults in 11 clinical studies. Excellent to good intubating conditions were generally achieved within 2 minutes and maximum block occurred within 3 minutes in most patients. Doses within this range provide clinical relaxation for a median (range) time of 33 (14-85) minutes under opioid/nitrous oxide/oxygen anesthesia. Larger doses (0.9 and 1.2 mg/kg) were evaluated in 2 studies with 19 and 16 patients under opioid/nitrous oxide/oxygen anesthesia and provided 58 (27-111) and 67 (38-160) minutes of clinical relaxation, respectively.

Cardiovascular Disease: In 1 clinical study, 10 patients with clinically significant cardiovascular disease undergoing coronary artery bypass graft received an initial dose of 0.6 mg/kg ZEMURON. Neuromuscular block was maintained during surgery with bolus maintenance doses of 0.3 mg/kg. Following induction, continuous 8 mcg/kg/min infusion of ZEMURON produced relaxation sufficient to support mechanical ventilation for 6 to 12 hours in the surgical intensive care unit (SICU) while the patients were recovering from surgery.

Rapid Sequence Intubation: Intubating conditions were assessed in 230 patients in 6 clinical studies where anesthesia was induced with either thiopental (3-6 mg/kg) or propofol (1.5-2.5 mg/kg) in combination with either fentanyl (2-5 mcg/kg) or alfentanil (1 mg). Most of the patients also received a premedication such as midazolam or temazepam. Most patients had intubation attempted within 60 to 90 seconds of administration of ZEMURON 0.6 mg/kg or succinylcholine 1 to 1.5 mg/kg. Excellent or good intubating conditions were achieved in 119/120 (99% [95% confidence interval: 95%-99.9%]) patients receiving ZEMURON and in 108/110 (98% [94%-99.8%]) patients receiving succinylcholine. The duration of action of ZEMURON 0.6 mg/kg is longer than succinylcholine and at this dose is approximately equivalent to the duration of other intermediate-acting neuromuscular blocking drugs.

Obese Patients: ZEMURON was dosed according to actual body weight (ABW) in most clinical studies. The administration of ZEMURON in the 47 of 330 (14%) patients who were at least 30% or more above their ideal body weight (IBW) was not associated with clinically significant differences in the onset, duration, recovery, or reversal of ZEMURON-induced neuromuscular block.

In 1 clinical study in obese patients, ZEMURON 0.6 mg/kg was dosed according to ABW (n=12) or IBW (n=11). Obese patients dosed according to IBW had a longer time to maximum block, a shorter median (range) clinical duration of 25 (14-29) minutes, and did not achieve intubating conditions comparable to those dosed based on ABW. These results support the recommendation that obese patients be dosed based on actual body weight *[see Dosage and Administration (2.5)]*.

Obstetric Patients: ZEMURON 0.6 mg/kg was administered with thiopental, 3 to 4 mg/kg (n=13) or 4 to 6 mg/kg (n=42), for rapid sequence induction of anesthesia for Cesarean section. No neonate had APGAR scores greater than 7 at 5 minutes. The umbilical venous plasma concentrations were 18% of maternal concentrations at delivery. Intubating conditions were poor or inadequate in 5 of 13 women receiving 3 to 4 mg/kg thiopental when intubation was attempted 60 seconds after drug injection. Therefore, ZEMURON is not recommended for rapid sequence induction in Cesarean section patients.

14.2 Geriatric Patients

ZEMURON was evaluated in 55 geriatric patients (ages 65-80 years) in 6 clinical studies. Doses of 0.6 mg/kg provided excellent to good intubating conditions in a median (range) time of 2.3 (1-8) minutes. Recovery times from 25% to 75% after these doses were not prolonged in geriatric patients compared to other adult patients *[see Dosage and Administration (2.5) and Use in Specific Populations (8.5)]*.

14.3 Pediatric Patients

ZEMURON 0.45, 0.6, or 1 mg/kg was evaluated under sevoflurane (induction) and isoflurane/nitrous oxide (maintenance) anesthesia for intubation in 326 patients in 2 studies. In 1 of these studies maintenance bolus and infusion requirements were evaluated in 137 patients. In all age groups, doses of 0.6 mg/kg provided time to maximum block in about 1 minute. Across all age groups, median (range) time to reappearance of T_3 for doses of 0.6 mg/kg was shortest in the children [36.7 (20.1-65.9) minutes] and longest in infants [59.8 (32.3-87.8) minutes]. For pediatric patients older than 3 months, the time to recovery was shorter after stopping infusion maintenance when compared with bolus maintenance *[see Dosage and Administration (2.5) and Use in Specific Populations (8.4)]*.

ZEMURON 0.6 or 0.8 mg/kg was evaluated for intubation in 75 pediatric patients (n=28; age 3-12 months, n=47; age 1-12 years) in 3 studies using halothane (1%-5%) and nitrous oxide (60%-70%) in oxygen. Doses of 0.6 mg/kg provided a median (range) time to maximum block of 1 (0.5-3.3) minute(s). This dose provided a median (range) time of clinical relaxation of 41 (24-68) minutes in 3-month to 1-year-old infants and 26 (17-39) minutes in 1- to 12-year-old pediatric patients *[see Dosage and Administration (2.5) and Use in Specific Populations (8.4)]*.

16 HOW SUPPLIED/STORAGE AND HANDLING

ZEMURON (rocuronium bromide) injection is available in the following:

- ZEMURON 5 mL multiple dose vials containing 50 mg rocuronium bromide injection (10 mg/mL)
  Box of 10 NDC 0052-0450-15
- ZEMURON 10 mL multiple dose vials containing 100 mg rocuronium bromide injection (10 mg/mL)
  Box of 10 NDC 0052-0450-16

The packaging of this product contains **no** natural rubber (latex).

ZEMURON should be stored in a refrigerator, 2-8°C (36-46°F). DO NOT FREEZE. Upon removal from refrigeration to room temperature storage conditions (25°C/77°F), use ZEMURON within 60 days. Use opened vials of ZEMURON within 30 days.

Safety and Handling: There is no specific work exposure limit for ZEMURON. In case of eye contact, flush with water for at least 10 minutes.

17 PATIENT COUNSELING INFORMATION

Obtain information about your patient's medical history, current medications, any history of hypersensitivity to rocuronium bromide or other neuromuscular blocking agents. If applicable, inform your patients that certain medical conditions and medications might influence how ZEMURON works.

In addition, inform your patient that severe anaphylactic reactions to neuromuscular blocking agents, including ZEMURON, have been reported. Since allergic cross-reactivity has been reported in this class, request information from your patients about previous anaphylactic reactions to other neuromuscular blocking agents.

Manuf. for: Merck Sharp & Dohme Corp., a subsidiary of **MERCK & CO., INC.,** Whitehouse Station, NJ 08889, USA

Manufactured by: Organon (Ireland) Ltd., Swords, Co. Dublin, Ireland, a subsidiary of **Merck & Co., Inc.**, Whitehouse Station, NJ 08889, USA.

Revised: 09/2012
900085-ROC-SOi-USPI.3

Shown in Product Identification Guide, page 309

ZETIA® ℞

[zĕt'-ē-ă]
(ezetimibe)
Tablets

HIGHLIGHTS OF PRESCRIBING INFORMATION

These highlights do not include all the information needed to use ZETIA safely and effectively. See full prescribing information for ZETIA.

ZETIA® (ezetimibe) Tablets
Initial U.S. Approval: 2002

INDICATIONS AND USAGE

ZETIA is an inhibitor of intestinal cholesterol (and related phytosterol) absorption indicated as an adjunct to diet to:

- Reduce elevated total-C, LDL-C, Apo B, and non-HDL-C in patients with primary hyperlipidemia, alone or in combination with an HMG-CoA reductase inhibitor (statin) (1.1)
- Reduce elevated total-C, LDL-C, Apo B, and non-HDL-C in patients with mixed hyperlipidemia in combination with fenofibrate (1.1)
- Reduce elevated total-C and LDL-C in patients with homozygous familial hypercholesterolemia (HoFH), in combination with atorvastatin or simvastatin (1.2)
- Reduce elevated sitosterol and campesterol in patients with homozygous sitosterolemia (phytosterolemia) (1.3)

Limitations of Use (1.4)

- The effect of ZETIA on cardiovascular morbidity and mortality has not been determined.
- ZETIA has not been studied in Fredrickson Type I, III, IV, and V dyslipidemias.

DOSAGE AND ADMINISTRATION

- One 10-mg tablet once daily, with or without food (2.1)
- Dosing of ZETIA should occur either ≥2 hours before or ≥4 hours after administration of a bile acid sequestrant. (2.3, 7.4)

DOSAGE FORMS AND STRENGTHS

- Tablets: 10 mg (3)

CONTRAINDICATIONS

- Statin contraindications apply when ZETIA is used with a statin:
  - Active liver disease, which may include unexplained persistent elevations in hepatic transaminase levels (4, 5.2)
  - Women who are pregnant or may become pregnant (4, 8.1)
  - Nursing mothers (4, 8.3)
- Known hypersensitivity to product components (4, 6.2)

WARNINGS AND PRECAUTIONS

- ZETIA is not recommended in patients with moderate or severe hepatic impairment. (5.4, 8.7, 12.3)
- Liver enzyme abnormalities and monitoring: Persistent elevations in hepatic transaminase can occur when ZETIA is added to a statin. Therefore, when ZETIA is added to statin therapy, monitor hepatic transaminase levels before and during treatment according to the recommendations for the individual statin used. (5.2)
- Skeletal muscle effects (e.g., myopathy and rhabdomyolysis):
  - Cases of myopathy and rhabdomyolysis have been reported in patients treated with ZETIA co-administered with a statin and with ZETIA administered alone. Risk for skeletal muscle toxicity increases with higher doses of statin, advanced age (>65), hypothyroidism, renal impairment, and depending on the statin used, concomitant use of other drugs. (5.3, 6.2)

ADVERSE REACTIONS

- Common adverse reactions in clinical trials:
  - ZETIA co-administered with a statin (incidence ≥2% and greater than statin alone):
    - nasopharyngitis, myalgia, upper respiratory tract infection, arthralgia, and diarrhea (6)
  - ZETIA administered alone (incidence ≥2% and greater than placebo):
    - upper respiratory tract infection, diarrhea, arthralgia, sinusitis, and pain in extremity (6)

To report SUSPECTED ADVERSE REACTIONS, contact Merck Sharp & Dohme Corp., a subsidiary of Merck & Co., Inc., at 1-877-888-4231 or FDA at 1-800-FDA-1088 or www.fda.gov/medwatch.

DRUG INTERACTIONS

- Cyclosporine: Combination increases exposure of ZETIA and cyclosporine. Cyclosporine concentrations should be monitored in patients taking ZETIA concomitantly. (7.1, 12.3)
- Fenofibrate: Combination increases exposure of ZETIA. If cholelithiasis is suspected in a patient receiving ZETIA and fenofibrate, gallbladder studies are indicated and alternative lipid-lowering therapy should be considered. (6.1, 7.3)
- Fibrates: Co-administration of ZETIA with fibrates other than fenofibrate is not recommended until use in patients is adequately studied. (7.2)
- Cholestyramine: Combination decreases exposure of ZETIA. (2.3, 7.4, 12.3)

See 17 for PATIENT COUNSELING INFORMATION and FDA-approved patient labeling

Revised: 02/2013

FULL PRESCRIBING INFORMATION: CONTENTS*

*** Sections or subsections omitted from the full prescribing information are not listed**

FULL PRESCRIBING INFORMATION

1 INDICATIONS AND USAGE

Therapy with lipid-altering agents should be only one component of multiple risk factor intervention in individuals at significantly increased risk for atherosclerotic vascular disease due to hypercholesterolemia. Drug therapy is indicated as an adjunct to diet when the response to a diet restricted in saturated fat and cholesterol and other nonpharmacologic measures alone has been inadequate.

1.1 Primary Hyperlipidemia

Monotherapy

ZETIA®, administered alone, is indicated as adjunctive therapy to diet for the reduction of elevated total cholesterol (total-C), low-density lipoprotein cholesterol (LDL-C), apolipoprotein B (Apo B), and non-high-density lipoprotein cholesterol (non-HDL-C) in patients with primary (heterozygous familial and non-familial) hyperlipidemia.

Combination Therapy with HMG-CoA Reductase Inhibitors (Statins)

ZETIA, administered in combination with a 3-hydroxy-3-methylglutaryl-coenzyme A (HMG-CoA) reductase inhibitor (statin), is indicated as adjunctive therapy to diet for the reduction of elevated total-C, LDL-C, Apo B, and non-HDL-C in patients with primary (heterozygous familial and non-familial) hyperlipidemia.

Combination Therapy with Fenofibrate

ZETIA, administered in combination with fenofibrate, is indicated as adjunctive therapy to diet for the reduction of elevated total-C, LDL-C, Apo B, and non-HDL-C in adult patients with mixed hyperlipidemia.

1.2 Homozygous Familial Hypercholesterolemia (HoFH)

The combination of ZETIA and atorvastatin or simvastatin is indicated for the reduction of elevated total-C and LDL-C levels in patients with HoFH, as an adjunct to other lipid-lowering treatments (e.g., LDL apheresis) or if such treatments are unavailable.

1.3 Homozygous Sitosterolemia

ZETIA is indicated as adjunctive therapy to diet for the reduction of elevated sitosterol and campesterol levels in patients with homozygous familial sitosterolemia.

1.4 Limitations of Use

The effect of ZETIA on cardiovascular morbidity and mortality has not been determined.

ZETIA has not been studied in Fredrickson Type I, III, IV, and V dyslipidemias.

2 DOSAGE AND ADMINISTRATION

2.1 General Dosing Information

The recommended dose of ZETIA is 10 mg once daily.

ZETIA can be administered with or without food.

2.2 Concomitant Lipid-Lowering Therapy

ZETIA may be administered with a statin (in patients with primary hyperlipidemia) or with fenofibrate (in patients with mixed hyperlipidemia) for incremental effect. For convenience, the daily dose of ZETIA may be taken at the same time as the statin or fenofibrate, according to the dosing recommendations for the respective medications.

2.3 Co-Administration with Bile Acid Sequestrants

Dosing of ZETIA should occur either ≥2 hours before or ≥4 hours after administration of a bile acid sequestrant *[see Drug Interactions (7.4)]*.

2.4 Patients with Hepatic Impairment

No dosage adjustment is necessary in patients with mild hepatic impairment *[see Warnings and Precautions (5.4)]*.

2.5 Patients with Renal Impairment

No dosage adjustment is necessary in patients with renal impairment *[see Clinical Pharmacology (12.3)]*. When given with simvastatin in patients with moderate to severe renal impairment (estimated glomerular filtration rate <60 mL/min/1.73 m^2), doses of simvastatin exceeding 20 mg should be used with caution and close monitoring *[see Use in Specific Populations (8.6)]*.

2.6 Geriatric Patients

No dosage adjustment is necessary in geriatric patients *[see Clinical Pharmacology (12.3)]*.

3 DOSAGE FORMS AND STRENGTHS

10-mg tablets are white to off-white, capsule-shaped tablets debossed with "414" on one side.

4 CONTRAINDICATIONS

ZETIA is contraindicated in the following conditions:

- The combination of ZETIA with a statin is contraindicated in patients with active liver disease or unexplained persistent elevations in hepatic transaminase levels.
- Women who are pregnant or may become pregnant. Because statins decrease cholesterol synthesis and possibly the synthesis of other biologically active substances derived from cholesterol, ZETIA in combination with a statin may cause fetal harm when administered to pregnant women. Additionally, there is no apparent benefit to therapy during pregnancy, and safety in pregnant women has not been established. If the patient becomes pregnant while taking this drug, the patient should be apprised of the potential hazard to the fetus and the lack of known clinical benefit with continued use during pregnancy. *[See Use in Specific Populations (8.1).]*
- Nursing mothers. Because statins may pass into breast milk, and because statins have the potential to cause serious adverse reactions in nursing infants, women who require ZETIA treatment in combination with a statin should be advised not to nurse their infants *[see Use in Specific Populations (8.3)]*.
- Patients with a known hypersensitivity to any component of this product. Hypersensitivity reactions including anaphylaxis, angioedema, rash and urticaria have been reported with ZETIA *[see Adverse Reactions (6.2)]*.

5 WARNINGS AND PRECAUTIONS

5.1 Use with Statins or Fenofibrate

Concurrent administration of ZETIA with a specific statin or fenofibrate should be in accordance with the product labeling for that medication.

5.2 Liver Enzymes

In controlled clinical monotherapy studies, the incidence of consecutive elevations (≥3 × the upper limit of normal [ULN]) in hepatic transaminase levels was similar between ZETIA (0.5%) and placebo (0.3%).

In controlled clinical combination studies of ZETIA initiated concurrently with a statin, the incidence of consecutive elevations (≥3 × ULN) in hepatic transaminase levels was 1.3% for patients treated with ZETIA administered with statins and 0.4% for patients treated with statins alone. These elevations in transaminases were generally asymptomatic, not associated with cholestasis, and returned to baseline after discontinuation of therapy or with continued treatment. When ZETIA is co-administered with a statin, liver tests should be performed at initiation of therapy and according to the recommendations of the statin. Should an increase in ALT or AST ≥3 × ULN persist, consider withdrawal of ZETIA and/or the statin.

5.3 Myopathy/Rhabdomyolysis

In clinical trials, there was no excess of myopathy or rhabdomyolysis associated with ZETIA compared with the relevant control arm (placebo or statin alone). However, myopathy and rhabdomyolysis are known adverse reactions to statins and other lipid-lowering drugs. In clinical trials, the incidence of creatine phosphokinase (CPK) >10 × ULN was 0.2% for ZETIA vs. 0.1% for placebo, and 0.1% for ZETIA co-administered with a statin vs. 0.4% for statins alone. Risk for skeletal muscle toxicity increases with higher doses of statin, advanced age (>65), hypothyroidism, renal impairment, and depending on the statin used, concomitant use of other drugs.

In post-marketing experience with ZETIA, cases of myopathy and rhabdomyolysis have been reported. Most patients who developed rhabdomyolysis were taking a statin prior to initiating ZETIA. However, rhabdomyolysis has been reported with ZETIA monotherapy and with the addition of ZETIA to agents known to be associated with increased risk of rhabdomyolysis, such as fibrates. ZETIA and any statin or fibrate that the patient is taking concomitantly should be immediately discontinued if myopathy is diagnosed or suspected. The presence of muscle symptoms and a CPK level >10 × the ULN indicates myopathy.

5.4 Hepatic Impairment

Due to the unknown effects of the increased exposure to ezetimibe in patients with moderate to severe hepatic impairment, ZETIA is not recommended in these patients. *[See Clinical Pharmacology (12.3).]*

6 ADVERSE REACTIONS

The following serious adverse reactions are discussed in greater detail in other sections of the label:

- Liver enzyme abnormalities *[see Warnings and Precautions (5.2)]*
- Rhabdomyolysis and myopathy *[see Warnings and Precautions (5.3)]*

Monotherapy Studies: In the ZETIA controlled clinical trials database (placebo-controlled) of 2396 patients with a median treatment duration of 12 weeks (range 0 to 39 weeks), 3.3% of patients on ZETIA and 2.9% of patients on placebo discontinued due to adverse reactions. The most common adverse reactions in the group of patients treated with ZETIA that led to treatment discontinuation and occurred at a rate greater than placebo were:

- Arthralgia (0.3%)
- Dizziness (0.2%)
- Gamma-glutamyltransferase increased (0.2%)

The most commonly reported adverse reactions (incidence ≥2% and greater than placebo) in the ZETIA monotherapy controlled clinical trial database of 2396 patients were: upper respiratory tract infection (4.3%), diarrhea (4.1%), arthralgia (3.0%), sinusitis (2.8%), and pain in extremity (2.7%).

Statin Co-Administration Studies: In the ZETIA + statin controlled clinical trials database of 11,308 patients with a median treatment duration of 8 weeks (range 0 to 112 weeks), 4.0% of patients on ZETIA + statin and 3.3% of patients on statin alone discontinued due to adverse reactions. The most common adverse reactions in the group of patients treated with ZETIA + statin that led to treatment discontinuation and occurred at a rate greater than statin alone were:

- Alanine aminotransferase increased (0.6%)
- Myalgia (0.5%)
- Fatigue, aspartate aminotransferase increased, headache, and pain in extremity (each at 0.2%)

The most commonly reported adverse reactions (incidence ≥2% and greater than statin alone) in the ZETIA + statin controlled clinical trial database of 11,308 patients were: nasopharyngitis (3.7%), myalgia (3.2%), upper respiratory tract infection (2.9%), arthralgia (2.6%) and diarrhea (2.5%).

6.1 Clinical Trials Experience

Because clinical studies are conducted under widely varying conditions, adverse reaction rates observed in the clinical studies of a drug cannot be directly compared to rates in the clinical studies of another drug and may not reflect the rates observed in clinical practice.

Monotherapy

In 10 double-blind, placebo-controlled clinical trials, 2396 patients with primary hyperlipidemia (age range 9–86 years, 50% women, 90% Caucasians, 5% Blacks, 3% Hispanics, 2% Asians) and elevated LDL-C were treated with ZETIA 10 mg/day for a median treatment duration of 12 weeks (range 0 to 39 weeks).

Adverse reactions reported in ≥2% of patients treated with ZETIA and at an incidence greater than placebo in placebo-controlled studies of ZETIA, regardless of causality assessment, are shown in **Table 1**.

TABLE 1: Clinical Adverse Reactions Occurring in ≥2% of Patients Treated with ZETIA and at an Incidence Greater than Placebo, Regardless of Causality

Body System/Organ Class Adverse Reaction	ZETIA 10 mg (%) n = 2396	Placebo (%) n = 1159
Gastrointestinal disorders		
Diarrhea	4.1	3.7
General disorders and administration site conditions		
Fatigue	2.4	1.5
Infections and infestations		
Influenza	2.0	1.5
Sinusitis	2.8	2.2
Upper respiratory tract infection	4.3	2.5
Musculoskeletal and connective tissue disorders		
Arthralgia	3.0	2.2
Pain in extremity	2.7	2.5

The frequency of less common adverse reactions was comparable between ZETIA and placebo.

Combination with a Statin

In 28 double-blind, controlled (placebo or active-controlled) clinical trials, 11,308 patients with primary hyperlipidemia (age range 10–93 years, 48% women, 85% Caucasians, 7% Blacks, 4% Hispanics, 3% Asians) and elevated LDL-C were treated with ZETIA 10 mg/day concurrently with or added to on-going statin therapy for a median treatment duration of 8 weeks (range 0 to 112 weeks).

The incidence of consecutive increased transaminases (≥3 × ULN) was higher in patients receiving ZETIA administered with statins (1.3%) than in patients treated with statins alone (0.4%). *[See Warnings and Precautions (5.2).]*

Clinical adverse reactions reported in ≥2% of patients treated with ZETIA + statin and at an incidence greater than statin, regardless of causality assessment, are shown in **Table 2**.

TABLE 2: Clinical Adverse Reactions Occurring in ≥2% of Patients Treated with ZETIA Co-Administered with a Statin and at an Incidence Greater than Statin, Regardless of Causality

Body System/Organ Class Adverse Reaction	All Statins* (%) n = 9361	ZETIA + All Statins* (%) n = 11,308
Gastrointestinal disorders		
Diarrhea	2.2	2.5
General disorders and administration site conditions		
Fatigue	1.6	2.0
Infections and infestations		
Influenza	2.1	2.2
Nasopharyngitis	3.3	3.7
Upper respiratory tract infection	2.8	2.9
Musculoskeletal and connective tissue disorders		
Arthralgia	2.4	2.6
Back pain	2.3	2.4
Myalgia	2.7	3.2
Pain in extremity	1.9	2.1

* All Statins = all doses of all statins

Combination with Fenofibrate

This clinical study involving 625 patients with mixed dyslipidemia (age range 20–76 years, 44% women, 79% Caucasians, 0.1% Blacks, 11% Hispanics, 5% Asians) treated for up to 12 weeks and 576 patients treated for up to an additional 48 weeks evaluated co-administration of ZETIA and fenofibrate. This study was not designed to compare treatment groups for infrequent events. Incidence rates (95% CI) for clinically important elevations (≥3 × ULN, consecutive) in hepatic transaminase levels were 4.5% (1.9, 8.8) and 2.7% (1.2, 5.4) for fenofibrate monotherapy (n=188) and ZETIA co-administered with fenofibrate (n=183), respectively, adjusted for treatment exposure. Corresponding incidence rates for cholecystectomy were 0.6% (95% CI: 0.0%, 3.1%) and 1.7% (95% CI: 0.6%, 4.0%) for fenofibrate monotherapy and ZETIA co-administered with fenofibrate, respectively *[see Drug Interactions (7.3)]*. The numbers of patients exposed to co-administration therapy as well as fenofibrate and ezetimibe monotherapy were inadequate to assess gallbladder disease risk. There were no CPK elevations >10 × ULN in any of the treatment groups.

6.2 Post-Marketing Experience

Because the reactions below are reported voluntarily from a population of uncertain size, it is generally not possible to reliably estimate their frequency or establish a causal relationship to drug exposure.

The following additional adverse reactions have been identified during post-approval use of ZETIA:

Hypersensitivity reactions, including anaphylaxis, angioedema, rash, and urticaria; erythema multiforme; arthralgia; myalgia; elevated creatine phosphokinase; myopathy/rhabdomyolysis *[see Warnings and Precautions (5.3)]*; elevations in liver transaminases; hepatitis; abdominal pain; thrombocytopenia; pancreatitis; nausea; dizziness; paresthesia; depression; headache; cholelithiasis; cholecystitis.

7 DRUG INTERACTIONS

[See Clinical Pharmacology (12.3).]

7.1 Cyclosporine

Caution should be exercised when using ZETIA and cyclosporine concomitantly due to increased exposure to both ezetimibe and cyclosporine. Cyclosporine concentrations should be monitored in patients receiving ZETIA and cyclosporine.

The degree of increase in ezetimibe exposure may be greater in patients with severe renal insufficiency. In patients treated with cyclosporine, the potential effects of the increased exposure to ezetimibe from concomitant use should be carefully weighed against the benefits of alterations in lipid levels provided by ezetimibe.

TABLE 3: Mean Percent Difference at Week 6 Between the Pooled ZETIA Co-Administered with Simvastatin Group and the Pooled Simvastatin Monotherapy Group in Adolescent Patients with Heterozygous Familial Hypercholesterolemia

	Total-C	LDL-C	Apo B	Non-HDL-C	TG*	HDL-C
Mean percent difference between treatment groups	-12%	-15%	-12%	-14%	-2%	+0.1%
95% Confidence Interval	(-15%, -9%)	(-18%, -12%)	(-15%, -9%)	(-17%, -11%)	(-9%, +4%)	(-3%, +3%)

* For triglycerides, median % change from baseline.

7.2 Fibrates
The efficacy and safety of co-administration of ezetimibe with fibrates other than fenofibrate have not been studied. Fibrates may increase cholesterol excretion into the bile, leading to cholelithiasis. In a preclinical study in dogs, ezetimibe increased cholesterol in the gallbladder bile *[see Nonclinical Toxicology (13.2)]*. Co-administration of ZETIA with fibrates other than fenofibrate is not recommended until use in patients is adequately studied.

7.3 Fenofibrate
If cholelithiasis is suspected in a patient receiving ZETIA and fenofibrate, gallbladder studies are indicated and alternative lipid-lowering therapy should be considered *[see Adverse Reactions (6.1) and the product labeling for fenofibrate]*.

7.4 Cholestyramine
Concomitant cholestyramine administration decreased the mean area under the curve (AUC) of total ezetimibe approximately 55%. The incremental LDL-C reduction due to adding ezetimibe to cholestyramine may be reduced by this interaction.

7.5 Coumarin Anticoagulants
If ezetimibe is added to warfarin, a coumarin anticoagulant, the International Normalized Ratio (INR) should be appropriately monitored.

8 USE IN SPECIFIC POPULATIONS

8.1 Pregnancy
Pregnancy Category C:
There are no adequate and well-controlled studies of ezetimibe in pregnant women. Ezetimibe should be used during pregnancy only if the potential benefit justifies the risk to the fetus.
In oral (gavage) embryo-fetal development studies of ezetimibe conducted in rats and rabbits during organogenesis, there was no evidence of embryolethal effects at the doses tested (250, 500, 1000 mg/kg/day). In rats, increased incidences of common fetal skeletal findings (extra pair of thoracic ribs, unossified cervical vertebral centra, shortened ribs) were observed at 1000 mg/kg/day (~10 × the human exposure at 10 mg daily based on AUC_{0-24hr} for total ezetimibe). In rabbits treated with ezetimibe, an increased incidence of extra thoracic ribs was observed at 1000 mg/kg/day (150 × the human exposure at 10 mg daily based on AUC_{0-24hr} for total ezetimibe). Ezetimibe crossed the placenta when pregnant rats and rabbits were given multiple oral doses.
Multiple-dose studies of ezetimibe given in combination with statins in rats and rabbits during organogenesis result in higher ezetimibe and statin exposures. Reproductive findings occur at lower doses in combination therapy compared to monotherapy.
All statins are contraindicated in pregnant and nursing women. When ZETIA is administered with a statin in a woman of childbearing potential, refer to the pregnancy category and product labeling for the statin. *[See Contraindications (4).]*

8.3 Nursing Mothers
It is not known whether ezetimibe is excreted into human breast milk. In rat studies, exposure to total ezetimibe in nursing pups was up to half of that observed in maternal plasma. Because many drugs are excreted in human milk, caution should be exercised when ZETIA is administered to a nursing woman. ZETIA should not be used in nursing mothers unless the potential benefit justifies the potential risk to the infant.

8.4 Pediatric Use
The effects of ZETIA co-administered with simvastatin (n=126) compared to simvastatin monotherapy (n=122) have been evaluated in adolescent boys and girls with heterozygous familial hypercholesterolemia (HeFH). In a multicenter, double-blind, controlled study followed by an open-label phase, 142 boys and 106 postmenarchal girls, 10 to 17 years of age (mean age 14.2 years, 43% females, 82% Caucasians, 4% Asian, 2% Blacks, 13% multi-racial) with HeFH were randomized to receive either ZETIA co-administered with simvastatin or simvastatin monotherapy. Inclusion in the study required 1) a baseline LDL-C level between 160 and 400 mg/dL and 2) a medical history and clinical presentation consistent with HeFH. The mean baseline LDL-C value was 225 mg/dL (range: 161–351 mg/dL) in the ZETIA co-administered with simvastatin group compared to 219 mg/dL (range: 149–336 mg/dL) in the simvastatin monotherapy group. The patients received co-administered ZETIA and simvastatin (10 mg, 20 mg, or 40 mg) or simvastatin monotherapy (10 mg, 20 mg, or 40 mg) for 6 weeks, co-administered ZETIA and 40-mg simvastatin or 40-mg simvastatin monotherapy for the next 27 weeks, and open-label co-administered ZETIA and simvastatin (10 mg, 20 mg, or 40 mg) for 20 weeks thereafter.
The results of the study at Week 6 are summarized in **Table 3**. Results at Week 33 were consistent with those at Week 6. [See table 3 above]
From the start of the trial to the end of Week 33, discontinuations due to an adverse reaction occurred in 7 (6%) patients in the ZETIA co-administered with simvastatin group and in 2 (2%) patients in the simvastatin monotherapy group.
During the trial, hepatic transaminase elevations (two consecutive measurements for ALT and/or AST ≥3 × ULN) occurred in four (3%) individuals in the ZETIA co-administered with simvastatin group and in two (2%) individuals in the simvastatin monotherapy group. Elevations of CPK (≥10 × ULN) occurred in two (2%) individuals in the ZETIA co-administered with simvastatin group and in zero individuals in the simvastatin monotherapy group.
In this limited controlled study, there was no significant effect on growth or sexual maturation in the adolescent boys or girls, or on menstrual cycle length in girls.
Co-administration of ZETIA with simvastatin at doses greater than 40 mg/day has not been studied in adolescents. Also, ZETIA has not been studied in patients younger than 10 years of age or in pre-menarchal girls.
Based on total ezetimibe (ezetimibe + ezetimibe-glucuronide), there are no pharmacokinetic differences between adolescents and adults. Pharmacokinetic data in the pediatric population <10 years of age are not available.

8.5 Geriatric Use
Monotherapy Studies
Of the 2396 patients who received ZETIA in clinical studies, 669 (28%) were 65 and older, and 111 (5%) were 75 and older.
Statin Co-Administration Studies
Of the 11,308 patients who received ZETIA + statin in clinical studies, 3587 (32%) were 65 and older, and 924 (8%) were 75 and older.
No overall differences in safety and effectiveness were observed between these patients and younger patients, and other reported clinical experience has not identified differences in responses between the elderly and younger patients, but greater sensitivity of some older individuals cannot be ruled out *[see Clinical Pharmacology (12.3)]*.

8.6 Renal Impairment
When used as monotherapy, no dosage adjustment of ZETIA is necessary.
In the Study of Heart and Renal Protection (SHARP) trial of 9270 patients with moderate to severe renal impairment (6247 non-dialysis patients with median serum creatinine 2.5 mg/dL and median estimated glomerular filtration rate 25.6 mL/min/1.73 m^2, and 3023 dialysis patients), the incidence of serious adverse events, adverse events leading to discontinuation of study treatment, or adverse events of special interest (musculoskeletal adverse events, liver enzyme abnormalities, incident cancer) was similar between patients ever assigned to ezetimibe 10 mg plus simvastatin 20 mg (n=4650) or placebo (n=4620) during a median follow-up of 4.9 years. However, because renal impairment is a risk factor for statin-associated myopathy, doses of simvastatin exceeding 20 mg should be used with caution and close monitoring when administered concomitantly with ZETIA in patients with moderate to severe renal impairment.

8.7 Hepatic Impairment
ZETIA is not recommended in patients with moderate to severe hepatic impairment *[see Warnings and Precautions (5.4)* and *Clinical Pharmacology (12.3)]*.
ZETIA given concomitantly with a statin is contraindicated in patients with active liver disease or unexplained persistent elevations of hepatic transaminase levels *[see Contraindications (4); Warnings and Precautions (5.2) and Clinical Pharmacology (12.3)]*.

10 OVERDOSAGE

In clinical studies, administration of ezetimibe, 50 mg/day to 15 healthy subjects for up to 14 days, 40 mg/day to 18 patients with primary hyperlipidemia for up to 56 days, and 40 mg/day to 27 patients with homozygous sitosterolemia for 26 weeks was generally well tolerated. One female patient with homozygous sitosterolemia took an accidental overdose of ezetimibe 120 mg/day for 28 days with no reported clinical or laboratory adverse events.
In the event of an overdose, symptomatic and supportive measures should be employed.

11 DESCRIPTION

ZETIA (ezetimibe) is in a class of lipid-lowering compounds that selectively inhibits the intestinal absorption of cholesterol and related phytosterols. The chemical name of ezetimibe is 1-(4-fluorophenyl)-3(R)-[3-(4-fluorophenyl)-3(S)-hydroxypropyl]-4(S)-(4-hydroxyphenyl)-2-azetidinone. The empirical formula is $C_{24}H_{21}F_2NO_3$. Its molecular weight is 409.4 and its structural formula is:

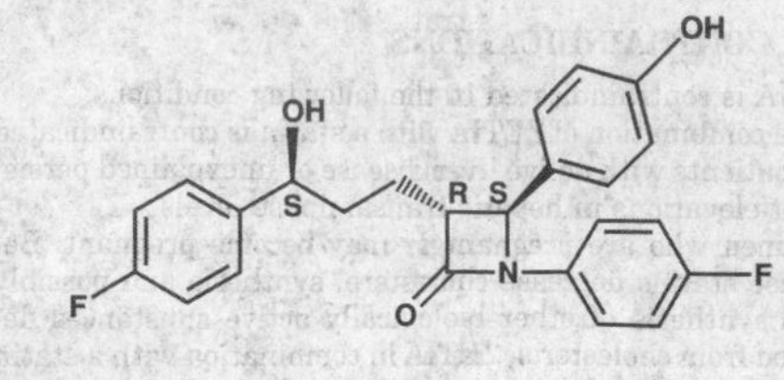

Ezetimibe is a white, crystalline powder that is freely to very soluble in ethanol, methanol, and acetone and practically insoluble in water. Ezetimibe has a melting point of about 163°C and is stable at ambient temperature. ZETIA is available as a tablet for oral administration containing 10 mg of ezetimibe and the following inactive ingredients: croscarmellose sodium NF, lactose monohydrate NF, magnesium stearate NF, microcrystalline cellulose NF, povidone USP, and sodium lauryl sulfate NF.

12 CLINICAL PHARMACOLOGY

12.1 Mechanism of Action
Ezetimibe reduces blood cholesterol by inhibiting the absorption of cholesterol by the small intestine. In a 2-week clinical study in 18 hypercholesterolemic patients, ZETIA inhibited intestinal cholesterol absorption by 54%, compared with placebo. ZETIA had no clinically meaningful effect on the plasma concentrations of the fat-soluble vitamins A, D, and E (in a study of 113 patients), and did not impair adrenocortical steroid hormone production (in a study of 118 patients).
The cholesterol content of the liver is derived predominantly from three sources. The liver can synthesize cholesterol, take up cholesterol from the blood from circulating lipoproteins, or take up cholesterol absorbed by the small intestine. Intestinal cholesterol is derived primarily from cholesterol secreted in the bile and from dietary cholesterol.
Ezetimibe has a mechanism of action that differs from those of other classes of cholesterol-reducing compounds (statins, bile acid sequestrants [resins], fibric acid derivatives, and plant stanols). The molecular target of ezetimibe has been shown to be the sterol transporter, Niemann-Pick C1-Like 1 (NPC1L1), which is involved in the intestinal uptake of cholesterol and phytosterols.
Ezetimibe does not inhibit cholesterol synthesis in the liver, or increase bile acid excretion. Instead, ezetimibe localizes at the brush border of the small intestine and inhibits the absorption of cholesterol, leading to a decrease in the delivery of intestinal cholesterol to the liver. This causes a reduction of hepatic cholesterol stores and an increase in clearance of cholesterol from the blood; this distinct mechanism is complementary to that of statins and of fenofibrate *[see Clinical Studies (14.1)]*.

12.2 Pharmacodynamics
Clinical studies have demonstrated that elevated levels of total-C, LDL-C and Apo B, the major protein constituent of LDL, promote human atherosclerosis. In addition, decreased levels of HDL-C are associated with the development of atherosclerosis. Epidemiologic studies have established that cardiovascular morbidity and mortality vary directly with the level of total-C and LDL-C and inversely with the level of HDL-C. Like LDL, cholesterol-enriched triglyceride-rich lipoproteins, including very-low-density lipoproteins (VLDL), intermediate-density lipoproteins (IDL), and remnants, can also promote atherosclerosis. The independent effect of raising HDL-C or lowering TG on the risk of coronary and cardiovascular morbidity and mortality has not been determined.
ZETIA reduces total-C, LDL-C, Apo B, non-HDL-C, and TG, and increases HDL-C in patients with hyperlipidemia. Administration of ZETIA with a statin is effective in improving serum total-C, LDL-C, Apo B, non-HDL-C, TG, and HDL-C beyond either treatment alone. Administration of ZETIA with fenofibrate is effective in improving serum total-C, LDL-C, Apo B, and non-HDL-C in patients with mixed hyperlipidemia as compared to either treatment alone. The ef-

fects of ezetimibe given either alone or in addition to a statin or fenofibrate on cardiovascular morbidity and mortality have not been established.

12.3 Pharmacokinetics

Absorption

After oral administration, ezetimibe is absorbed and extensively conjugated to a pharmacologically active phenolic glucuronide (ezetimibe-glucuronide). After a single 10-mg dose of ZETIA to fasted adults, mean ezetimibe peak plasma concentrations (C_{max}) of 3.4 to 5.5 ng/mL were attained within 4 to 12 hours (T_{max}). Ezetimibe-glucuronide mean C_{max} values of 45 to 71 ng/mL were achieved between 1 and 2 hours (T_{max}). There was no substantial deviation from dose proportionality between 5 and 20 mg. The absolute bioavailability of ezetimibe cannot be determined, as the compound is virtually insoluble in aqueous media suitable for injection.

Effect of Food on Oral Absorption

Concomitant food administration (high-fat or non-fat meals) had no effect on the extent of absorption of ezetimibe when administered as ZETIA 10-mg tablets. The C_{max} value of ezetimibe was increased by 38% with consumption of high-fat meals. ZETIA can be administered with or without food.

Distribution

Ezetimibe and ezetimibe-glucuronide are highly bound (>90%) to human plasma proteins.

Metabolism and Excretion

Ezetimibe is primarily metabolized in the small intestine and liver via glucuronide conjugation (a phase II reaction) with subsequent biliary and renal excretion. Minimal oxidative metabolism (a phase I reaction) has been observed in all species evaluated.

In humans, ezetimibe is rapidly metabolized to ezetimibe-glucuronide. Ezetimibe and ezetimibe-glucuronide are the major drug-derived compounds detected in plasma, constituting approximately 10 to 20% and 80 to 90% of the total drug in plasma, respectively. Both ezetimibe and ezetimibe-glucuronide are eliminated from plasma with a half-life of approximately 22 hours for both ezetimibe and ezetimibe-glucuronide. Plasma concentration-time profiles exhibit multiple peaks, suggesting enterohepatic recycling.

Following oral administration of ^{14}C-ezetimibe (20 mg) to human subjects, total ezetimibe (ezetimibe + ezetimibe-glucuronide) accounted for approximately 93% of the total radioactivity in plasma. After 48 hours, there were no detectable levels of radioactivity in the plasma.

Approximately 78% and 11% of the administered radioactivity were recovered in the feces and urine, respectively, over a 10-day collection period. Ezetimibe was the major component in feces and accounted for 69% of the administered dose, while ezetimibe-glucuronide was the major component in urine and accounted for 9% of the administered dose.

Specific Populations

Geriatric Patients: In a multiple-dose study with ezetimibe given 10 mg once daily for 10 days, plasma concentrations for total ezetimibe were about 2-fold higher in older (≥65 years) healthy subjects compared to younger subjects.

Pediatric Patients: *[See Use in Specific Populations (8.4).]*

Gender: In a multiple-dose study with ezetimibe given 10 mg once daily for 10 days, plasma concentrations for total ezetimibe were slightly higher (<20%) in women than in men.

Race: Based on a meta-analysis of multiple-dose pharmacokinetic studies, there were no pharmacokinetic differences between Black and Caucasian subjects. Studies in Asian subjects indicated that the pharmacokinetics of ezetimibe were similar to those seen in Caucasian subjects.

Hepatic Impairment: After a single 10-mg dose of ezetimibe, the mean AUC for total ezetimibe was increased approximately 1.7-fold in patients with mild hepatic impairment (Child-Pugh score 5 to 6), compared to healthy subjects. The mean AUC values for total ezetimibe and ezetimibe were increased approximately 3- to 4-fold and 5- to 6-fold, respectively, in patients with moderate (Child-Pugh score 7 to 9) or severe hepatic impairment (Child-Pugh score 10 to 15). In a 14-day, multiple-dose study (10 mg daily) in patients with moderate hepatic impairment, the mean AUC values for total ezetimibe and ezetimibe were increased approximately 4-fold on Day 1 and Day 14 compared to healthy subjects. Due to the unknown effects of the increased exposure to ezetimibe in patients with moderate or severe hepatic impairment, ZETIA is not recommended in these patients *[see Warnings and Precautions (5.4)]*.

Renal Impairment: After a single 10-mg dose of ezetimibe in patients with severe renal disease (n=8; mean CrCl ≤30 mL/min/1.73 m²), the mean AUC values for total ezetimibe, ezetimibe-glucuronide, and ezetimibe were increased approximately 1.5-fold, compared to healthy subjects (n=9).

Drug Interactions [See also Drug Interactions (7)]

ZETIA had no significant effect on a series of probe drugs (caffeine, dextromethorphan, tolbutamide, and IV midazolam) known to be metabolized by cytochrome P450 (1A2, 2D6, 2C8/9 and 3A4) in a "cocktail" study of twelve healthy adult males. This indicates that ezetimibe is neither an inhibitor nor an inducer of these cytochrome P450 isozymes, and it is unlikely that ezetimibe will affect the metabolism of drugs that are metabolized by these enzymes.

[See table 4 above]

[See table 5 above]

TABLE 4: Effect of Co-Administered Drugs on Total Ezetimibe

Co-Administered Drug and Dosing Regimen	Total Ezetimibe* Change in AUC	Total Ezetimibe* Change in C_{max}
Cyclosporine-stable dose required (75–150 mg BID)†,‡	↑240%	↑290%
Fenofibrate, 200 mg QD, 14 days‡	↑48%	↑64%
Gemfibrozil, 600 mg BID, 7 days‡	↑64%	↑91%
Cholestyramine, 4 g BID, 14 days‡	↓55%	↓4%
Aluminum & magnesium hydroxide combination antacid, single dose§	↓4%	↓30%
Cimetidine, 400 mg BID, 7 days	↑6%	↑22%
Glipizide, 10 mg, single dose	↑4%	↓8%
Statins		
Lovastatin 20 mg QD, 7 days	↑9%	↑3%
Pravastatin 20 mg QD, 14 days	↑7%	↑23%
Atorvastatin 10 mg QD, 14 days	↓2%	↑12%
Rosuvastatin 10 mg QD, 14 days	↑13%	↑18%
Fluvastatin 20 mg QD, 14 days	↓19%	↑7%

* Based on 10-mg dose of ezetimibe.

† Post-renal transplant patients with mild impaired or normal renal function. In a different study, a renal transplant patient with severe renal insufficiency (creatinine clearance of 13.2 mL/min/1.73 m²) who was receiving multiple medications, including cyclosporine, demonstrated a 12-fold greater exposure to total ezetimibe compared to healthy subjects.

‡ See Drug Interactions (7).

§ Supralox, 20 mL.

TABLE 5: Effect of Ezetimibe Co-Administration on Systemic Exposure to Other Drugs

Co-Administered Drug and its Dosage Regimen	Ezetimibe Dosage Regimen	Change in AUC of Co-Administered Drug	Change in C_{max} of Co-Administered Drug
Warfarin, 25-mg single dose on Day 7	10 mg QD, 11 days	↓2% (R-warfarin) ↓4% (S-warfarin)	↑3% (R-warfarin) ↑1% (S-warfarin)
Digoxin, 0.5-mg single dose	10 mg QD, 8 days	↑2%	↓7%
Gemfibrozil, 600 mg BID, 7 days*	10 mg QD, 7 days	↓1%	↓11%
Ethinyl estradiol & Levonorgestrel, QD, 21 days	10 mg QD, days 8–14 of 21d oral contraceptive cycle	Ethinyl estradiol 0% Levonorgestrel 0%	Ethinyl estradiol ↓9% Levonorgestrel ↓5%
Glipizide, 10-mg on Days 1 and 9	10 mg QD, days 2–9	↓3%	↓5%
Fenofibrate, 200 mg QD, 14 days*	10 mg QD, 14 days	↑11%	↑7%
Cyclosporine, 100-mg single dose Day 7*	20 mg QD, 8 days	↑15%	↑10%
Statins			
Lovastatin 20 mg QD, 7 days	10 mg QD, 7 days	↑19%	↑3%
Pravastatin 20 mg QD, 14 days	10 mg QD, 14 days	↓20%	↓24%
Atorvastatin 10 mg QD, 14 days	10 mg QD, 14 days	↓4%	↑7%
Rosuvastatin 10 mg QD, 14 days	10 mg QD, 14 days	↑19%	↑17%
Fluvastatin 20 mg QD, 14 days	10 mg QD, 14 days	↓39%	↓27%

* See Drug Interactions (7).

13 NONCLINICAL TOXICOLOGY

13.1 Carcinogenesis, Mutagenesis, Impairment of Fertility

A 104-week dietary carcinogenicity study with ezetimibe was conducted in rats at doses up to 1500 mg/kg/day (males) and 500 mg/kg/day (females) (~20 × the human exposure at 10 mg daily based on AUC_{0-24hr} for total ezetimibe). A 104-week dietary carcinogenicity study with ezetimibe was also conducted in mice at doses up to 500 mg/kg/day (>150 × the human exposure at 10 mg daily based on AUC_{0-24hr} for total ezetimibe). There were no statistically significant increases in tumor incidences in drug-treated rats or mice.

No evidence of mutagenicity was observed *in vitro* in a microbial mutagenicity (Ames) test with *Salmonella typhimurium* and *Escherichia coli* with or without metabolic activation. No evidence of clastogenicity was observed *in vitro* in a chromosomal aberration assay in human peripheral blood lymphocytes with or without metabolic activation. In addition, there was no evidence of genotoxicity in the *in vivo* mouse micronucleus test.

In oral (gavage) fertility studies of ezetimibe conducted in rats, there was no evidence of reproductive toxicity at doses

TABLE 6: Response to ZETIA in Patients with Primary Hyperlipidemia (Mean* % Change from Untreated Baseline†)

	Treatment Group	N	Total-C	LDL-C	Apo B	Non-HDL-C	TG*	HDL-C
Study 1‡	Placebo	205	+1	+1	-1	+1	-1	-1
	Ezetimibe	622	-12	-18	-15	-16	-7	+1
Study 2‡	Placebo	226	+1	+1	-1	+2	+2	-2
	Ezetimibe	666	-12	-18	-16	-16	-9	+1
Pooled Data‡ (Studies 1 & 2)	Placebo	431	0	+1	-2	+1	0	-2
	Ezetimibe	1288	-13	-18	-16	-16	-8	+1

* For triglycerides, median % change from baseline.
† Baseline - on no lipid-lowering drug.
‡ ZETIA significantly reduced total-C, LDL-C, Apo B, non-HDL-C, and TG, and increased HDL-C compared to placebo.

TABLE 7: Response to Addition of ZETIA to On-Going Statin Therapy* in Patients with Hyperlipidemia (Mean† % Change from Treated Baseline‡)

Treatment (Daily Dose)	N	Total-C	LDL-C	Apo B	Non-HDL-C	TG†	HDL-C
On-going Statin + Placebo§	390	-2	-4	-3	-3	-3	+1
On-going Statin + ZETIA§	379	-17	-25	-19	-23	-14	+3

* Patients receiving each statin: 40% atorvastatin, 31% simvastatin, 29% others (pravastatin, fluvastatin, cerivastatin, lovastatin).
† For triglycerides, median % change from baseline.
‡ Baseline - on a statin alone.
§ ZETIA + statin significantly reduced total-C, LDL-C, Apo B, non-HDL-C, and TG, and increased HDL-C compared to statin alone.

TABLE 8: Response to ZETIA and Atorvastatin Initiated Concurrently in Patients with Primary Hyperlipidemia (Mean* % Change from Untreated Baseline†)

Treatment (Daily Dose)	N	Total-C	LDL-C	Apo B	Non-HDL-C	TG*	HDL-C
Placebo	60	+4	+4	+3	+4	-6	+4
ZETIA	65	-14	-20	-15	-18	-5	+4
Atorvastatin 10 mg	60	-26	-37	-28	-34	-21	+6
ZETIA + Atorvastatin 10 mg	65	-38	-53	-43	-49	-31	+9
Atorvastatin 20 mg	60	-30	-42	-34	-39	-23	+4
ZETIA + Atorvastatin 20 mg	62	-39	-54	-44	-50	-30	+9
Atorvastatin 40 mg	66	-32	-45	-37	-41	-24	+4
ZETIA + Atorvastatin 40 mg	65	-42	-56	-45	-52	-34	+5
Atorvastatin 80 mg	62	-40	-54	-46	-51	-31	+3
ZETIA + Atorvastatin 80 mg	63	-46	-61	-50	-58	-40	+7
Pooled data (All Atorvastatin Doses)‡	248	-32	-44	-36	-41	-24	+4
Pooled data (All ZETIA + Atorvastatin Doses)‡	255	-41	-56	-45	-52	-33	+7

* For triglycerides, median % change from baseline.
† Baseline - on no lipid-lowering drug.
‡ ZETIA + all doses of atorvastatin pooled (10–80 mg) significantly reduced total-C, LDL-C, Apo B, non-HDL-C, and TG, and increased HDL-C compared to all doses of atorvastatin pooled (10–80 mg).

up to 1000 mg/kg/day in male or female rats (~7 × the human exposure at 10 mg daily based on AUC_{0-24hr} for total ezetimibe).

13.2 Animal Toxicology and/or Pharmacology

The hypocholesterolemic effect of ezetimibe was evaluated in cholesterol-fed Rhesus monkeys, dogs, rats, and mouse models of human cholesterol metabolism. Ezetimibe was found to have an ED_{50} value of 0.5 μg/kg/day for inhibiting the rise in plasma cholesterol levels in monkeys. The ED_{50} values in dogs, rats, and mice were 7, 30, and 700 μg/kg/day, respectively. These results are consistent with ZETIA being a potent cholesterol absorption inhibitor.

In a rat model, where the glucuronide metabolite of ezetimibe (SCH 60663) was administered intraduodenally, the metabolite was as potent as the parent compound (SCH 58235) in inhibiting the absorption of cholesterol, suggesting that the glucuronide metabolite had activity similar to the parent drug.

In 1-month studies in dogs given ezetimibe (0.03 to 300 mg/kg/day), the concentration of cholesterol in gallbladder bile increased ~2- to 4-fold. However, a dose of 300 mg/kg/day administered to dogs for one year did not result in gallstone formation or any other adverse hepatobiliary effects. In a 14-day study in mice given ezetimibe (0.3 to 5 mg/kg/day) and fed a low-fat or cholesterol-rich diet, the concentration of cholesterol in gallbladder bile was either unaffected or reduced to normal levels, respectively.

A series of acute preclinical studies was performed to determine the selectivity of ZETIA for inhibiting cholesterol absorption. Ezetimibe inhibited the absorption of ^{14}C-cholesterol with no effect on the absorption of triglycerides, fatty acids, bile acids, progesterone, ethinyl estradiol, or the fat-soluble vitamins A and D.

In 4- to 12-week toxicity studies in mice, ezetimibe did not induce cytochrome P450 drug metabolizing enzymes. In toxicity studies, a pharmacokinetic interaction of ezetimibe with statins (parents or their active hydroxy acid metabolites) was seen in rats, dogs, and rabbits.

14 CLINICAL STUDIES

14.1 Primary Hyperlipidemia

ZETIA reduces total-C, LDL-C, Apo B, non-HDL-C, and TG, and increases HDL-C in patients with hyperlipidemia. Maximal to near maximal response is generally achieved within 2 weeks and maintained during chronic therapy.

Monotherapy

In two multicenter, double-blind, placebo-controlled, 12-week studies in 1719 patients with primary hyperlipidemia, ZETIA significantly lowered total-C, LDL-C, Apo B, non-HDL-C, and TG, and increased HDL-C compared to placebo (see **Table 6**). Reduction in LDL-C was consistent across age, sex, and baseline LDL-C.

[See table 6 above]

Combination with Statins

ZETIA Added to On-going Statin Therapy

In a multicenter, double-blind, placebo-controlled, 8-week study, 769 patients with primary hyperlipidemia, known coronary heart disease or multiple cardiovascular risk factors who were already receiving statin monotherapy, but who had not met their NCEP ATP II target LDL-C goal were randomized to receive either ZETIA or placebo in addition to their on-going statin.

ZETIA, added to on-going statin therapy, significantly lowered total-C, LDL-C, Apo B, non-HDL-C, and TG, and increased HDL-C compared with a statin administered alone (see **Table 7**). LDL-C reductions induced by ZETIA were generally consistent across all statins.

[See table 7 above]

ZETIA Initiated Concurrently with a Statin

In four multicenter, double-blind, placebo-controlled, 12-week trials, in 2382 hyperlipidemic patients, ZETIA or placebo was administered alone or with various doses of atorvastatin, simvastatin, pravastatin, or lovastatin.

When all patients receiving ZETIA with a statin were compared to all those receiving the corresponding statin alone, ZETIA significantly lowered total-C, LDL-C, Apo B, non-HDL-C, and TG, and, with the exception of pravastatin, increased HDL-C compared to the statin administered alone. LDL-C reductions induced by ZETIA were generally consistent across all statins. (See footnote ‡, **Tables 8** to **11**.)

[See table 8 above]
[See table 9 at top of next page]
[See table 10 at top of next page]
[See table 11 at top of page 1854]

Combination with Fenofibrate

In a multicenter, double-blind, placebo-controlled, clinical study in patients with mixed hyperlipidemia, 625 patients were treated for up to 12 weeks and 576 for up to an additional 48 weeks. Patients were randomized to receive placebo, ZETIA alone, 160-mg fenofibrate alone, or ZETIA and 160-mg fenofibrate in the 12-week study. After completing the 12-week study, eligible patients were assigned to ZETIA co-administered with fenofibrate or fenofibrate monotherapy for an additional 48 weeks.

ZETIA co-administered with fenofibrate significantly lowered total-C, LDL-C, Apo B, and non-HDL-C compared to fenofibrate administered alone. The percent decrease in TG and percent increase in HDL-C for ZETIA co-administered with fenofibrate were comparable to those for fenofibrate administered alone (see **Table 12**).

[See table 12 at top of page 1854]

The changes in lipid endpoints after an additional 48 weeks of treatment with ZETIA co-administered with fenofibrate or with fenofibrate alone were consistent with the 12-week data displayed above.

14.2 Homozygous Familial Hypercholesterolemia (HoFH)

A study was conducted to assess the efficacy of ZETIA in the treatment of HoFH. This double-blind, randomized, 12-week study enrolled 50 patients with a clinical and/or genotypic diagnosis of HoFH, with or without concomitant LDL apheresis, already receiving atorvastatin or simvastatin (40 mg). Patients were randomized to one of three treatment groups, atorvastatin or simvastatin (80 mg), ZETIA administered with atorvastatin or simvastatin (40 mg), or ZETIA administered with atorvastatin or simvastatin (80 mg). Due to decreased bioavailability of ezetimibe in patients concomitantly receiving cholestyramine *[see Drug Interactions (7.4)]*, ezetimibe was dosed at least 4 hours before or after administration of resins. Mean baseline LDL-C was 341 mg/dL in those patients randomized to atorvastatin 80 mg or simvastatin 80 mg alone and 316 mg/dL in the group randomized to ZETIA plus atorvastatin 40 or 80 mg or simvastatin 40 or 80 mg. ZETIA, administered with atorvastatin or simvastatin (40- and 80-mg statin groups, pooled), significantly reduced LDL-C (21%) compared with increasing the dose of simvastatin or atorvastatin monotherapy from 40 to 80 mg (7%). In those treated with ZETIA plus 80-mg atorvastatin or with ZETIA plus 80-mg simvastatin, LDL-C was reduced by 27%.

14.3 Homozygous Sitosterolemia (Phytosterolemia)

A study was conducted to assess the efficacy of ZETIA in the treatment of homozygous sitosterolemia. In this multicenter, double-blind, placebo-controlled, 8-week trial, 37 patients with homozygous sitosterolemia with elevated plasma sitosterol levels (>5 mg/dL) on their current therapeutic regimen (diet, bile-acid-binding resins, statins, ileal bypass surgery and/or LDL apheresis), were randomized to receive ZETIA (n=30) or placebo (n=7). Due to decreased bioavailability of ezetimibe in patients concomitantly receiving cholestyramine *[see Drug Interactions (7.4)]*, ezetimibe was dosed at least 2 hours before or 4 hours after resins were administered. Excluding the one subject receiving LDL apheresis, ZETIA significantly lowered plasma sitosterol and campesterol, by 21% and 24% from baseline, respectively. In contrast, patients who received placebo had increases in sitosterol and campesterol of 4% and 3% from baseline, respectively. For patients treated with ZETIA, mean plasma levels of plant sterols were reduced progressively over the course of the study. The effects of reducing plasma sitosterol and campesterol on reducing the risks of cardiovascular morbidity and mortality have not been established.

Reductions in sitosterol and campesterol were consistent between patients taking ZETIA concomitantly with bile acid sequestrants (n=8) and patients not on concomitant bile acid sequestrant therapy (n=21).

Limitations of Use

The effect of ZETIA on cardiovascular morbidity and mortality has not been determined.

TABLE 9: Response to ZETIA and Simvastatin Initiated Concurrently in Patients with Primary Hyperlipidemia (Mean* % Change from Untreated Baseline†)

Treatment (Daily Dose)	N	Total-C	LDL-C	Apo B	Non-HDL-C	TG*	HDL-C
Placebo	70	-1	-1	0	-1	+2	+1
ZETIA	61	-13	-19	-14	-17	-11	+5
Simvastatin 10 mg	70	-18	-27	-21	-25	-14	+8
ZETIA + Simvastatin 10 mg	67	-32	-46	-35	-42	-26	+9
Simvastatin 20 mg	61	-26	-36	-29	-33	-18	+6
ZETIA + Simvastatin 20 mg	69	-33	-46	-36	-42	-25	+9
Simvastatin 40 mg	65	-27	-38	-32	-35	-24	+6
ZETIA + Simvastatin 40 mg	73	-40	-56	-45	-51	-32	+11
Simvastatin 80 mg	67	-32	-45	-37	-41	-23	+8
ZETIA + Simvastatin 80 mg	65	-41	-58	-47	-53	-31	+8
Pooled data (All Simvastatin Doses)‡	263	-26	-36	-30	-34	-20	+7
Pooled data (All ZETIA + Simvastatin Doses)‡	274	-37	-51	-41	-47	-29	+9

* For triglycerides, median % change from baseline.
† Baseline - on no lipid-lowering drug.
‡ ZETIA + all doses of simvastatin pooled (10–80 mg) significantly reduced total-C, LDL-C, Apo B, non-HDL-C, and TG, and increased HDL-C compared to all doses of simvastatin pooled (10–80 mg).

TABLE 10: Response to ZETIA and Pravastatin Initiated Concurrently in Patients with Primary Hyperlipidemia (Mean* % Change from Untreated Baseline†)

Treatment (Daily Dose)	N	Total-C	LDL-C	Apo B	Non-HDL-C	TG*	HDL-C
Placebo	65	0	-1	-2	0	-1	+2
ZETIA	64	-13	-20	-15	-17	-5	+4
Pravastatin 10 mg	66	-15	-21	-16	-20	-14	+6
ZETIA + Pravastatin 10 mg	71	-24	-34	-27	-32	-23	+8
Pravastatin 20 mg	69	-15	-23	-18	-20	-8	+8
ZETIA + Pravastatin 20 mg	66	-27	-40	-31	-36	-21	+8
Pravastatin 40 mg	70	-22	-31	-26	-28	-19	+6
ZETIA + Pravastatin 40 mg	67	-30	-42	-32	-39	-21	+8
Pooled data (All Pravastatin Doses)‡	205	-17	-25	-20	-23	-14	+7
Pooled data (All ZETIA + Pravastatin Doses)‡	204	-27	-39	-30	-36	-21	+8

* For triglycerides, median % change from baseline.
† Baseline - on no lipid-lowering drug.
‡ ZETIA + all doses of pravastatin pooled (10–40 mg) significantly reduced total-C, LDL-C, Apo B, non-HDL-C, and TG compared to all doses of pravastatin pooled (10–40 mg).

16 HOW SUPPLIED/STORAGE AND HANDLING

No. 3861 — Tablets ZETIA, 10 mg, are white to off-white, capsule-shaped tablets debossed with "414" on one side. They are supplied as follows:

NDC 66582-414-31 bottles of 30
NDC 66582-414-54 bottles of 90
NDC 66582-414-74 bottles of 500
NDC 66582-414-76 bottles of 5000
NDC 66582-414-28 unit dose packages of 100.

Storage

Store at 25°C (77°F); excursions permitted to 15–30°C (59–86°F). [See USP Controlled Room Temperature.] Protect from moisture.

17 PATIENT COUNSELING INFORMATION

See FDA-Approved Patient Labeling (Patient Information). Patients should be advised to adhere to their National Cholesterol Education Program (NCEP)-recommended diet, a regular exercise program, and periodic testing of a fasting lipid panel.

17.1 Muscle Pain

All patients starting therapy with ezetimibe should be advised of the risk of myopathy and told to report promptly any unexplained muscle pain, tenderness or weakness. The risk of this occurring is increased when taking certain types of medication. Patients should discuss all medication, both prescription and over-the-counter, with their physician.

17.2 Liver Enzymes

Liver tests should be performed when ZETIA is added to statin therapy and according to statin recommendations.

17.3 Pregnancy

Women of childbearing age should be advised to use an effective method of birth control to prevent pregnancy while using ZETIA added to statin therapy. Discuss future pregnancy plans with your patients, and discuss when to stop combination ZETIA and statin therapy if they are trying to conceive. Patients should be advised that if they become pregnant they should stop taking combination ZETIA and statin therapy and call their healthcare professional.

17.4 Breastfeeding

Women who are breastfeeding should be advised to not use ZETIA added to statin therapy. Patients who have a lipid disorder and are breastfeeding should be advised to discuss the options with their healthcare professionals.

Merck Sharp & Dohme Corp., a subsidiary of
MERCK & CO., INC., Whitehouse Station, NJ 08889, USA
U.S. Patent Nos. 5,846,966; 7,030,106 and RE 42,461.

Revised: 02/2013
USPI-T-06531302R025

ZETIA® (ezetimibe) Tablets

Patient Information about ZETIA (zĕt´-ē-ä)

Generic name: ezetimibe (ĕ-zĕt´-ĕ-mīb)

Read this information carefully before you start taking ZETIA® and each time you get more ZETIA. There may be new information. This information does not take the place of talking with your doctor about your medical condition or your treatment. If you have any questions about ZETIA, ask your doctor. Only your doctor can determine if ZETIA is right for you.

What is ZETIA?

ZETIA is a medicine used to lower levels of total cholesterol and LDL (bad) cholesterol in the blood. ZETIA is for patients who cannot control their cholesterol levels by diet and exercise alone. It can be used by itself or with other medicines to treat high cholesterol. You should stay on a cholesterol-lowering diet while taking this medicine.

ZETIA works to reduce the amount of cholesterol your body absorbs. ZETIA does not help you lose weight. ZETIA has not been shown to prevent heart disease or heart attacks.

For more information about cholesterol, see the "What should I know about high cholesterol?" section that follows.

Who should not take ZETIA?

- Do not take ZETIA if you are allergic to ezetimibe, the active ingredient in ZETIA, or to the inactive ingredients. For a list of inactive ingredients, see the "Inactive ingredients" section that follows.
- If you have active liver disease, do not take ZETIA while taking cholesterol-lowering medicines called statins.
- If you are pregnant or breastfeeding, do not take ZETIA while taking a statin.
- If you are a woman of childbearing age, you should use an effective method of birth control to prevent pregnancy while using ZETIA added to statin therapy.

ZETIA has not been studied in children under age 10.

What should I tell my doctor before and while taking ZETIA?

Tell your doctor about any prescription and nonprescription medicines you are taking or plan to take, including natural or herbal remedies.

Tell your doctor about all your medical conditions including allergies.

Tell your doctor if you:

- ever had liver problems. ZETIA may not be right for you.
- are pregnant or plan to become pregnant. Your doctor will discuss with you whether ZETIA is right for you.
- are breastfeeding. We do not know if ZETIA can pass to your baby through your milk. Your doctor will discuss with you whether ZETIA is right for you.
- experience unexplained muscle pain, tenderness, or weakness.

How should I take ZETIA?

- Take ZETIA once a day, with or without food. It may be easier to remember to take your dose if you do it at the same time every day, such as with breakfast, dinner, or at bedtime. If you also take another medicine to reduce your cholesterol, ask your doctor if you can take them at the same time.
- If you forget to take ZETIA, take it as soon as you remember. However, do not take more than one dose of ZETIA a day.

TABLE 11: Response to ZETIA and Lovastatin Initiated Concurrently in Patients with Primary Hyperlipidemia (Mean* % Change from Untreated Baseline†)

Treatment (Daily Dose)	N	Total-C	LDL-C	Apo B	Non-HDL-C	TG*	HDL-C
Placebo	64	+1	0	+1	+1	+6	0
ZETIA	72	-13	-19	-14	-16	-5	+3
Lovastatin 10 mg	73	-15	-20	-17	-19	-11	+5
ZETIA + Lovastatin 10 mg	65	-24	-34	-27	-31	-19	+8
Lovastatin 20 mg	74	-19	-26	-21	-24	-12	+3
ZETIA + Lovastatin 20 mg	62	-29	-41	-34	-39	-27	+9
Lovastatin 40 mg	73	-21	-30	-25	-27	-15	+5
ZETIA + Lovastatin 40 mg	65	-33	-46	-38	-43	-27	+9
Pooled data (All Lovastatin Doses)‡	220	-18	-25	-21	-23	-12	+4
Pooled data (All ZETIA + Lovastatin Doses)‡	192	-29	-40	-33	-38	-25	+9

* For triglycerides, median % change from baseline.
† Baseline - on no lipid-lowering drug.
‡ ZETIA + all doses of lovastatin pooled (10–40 mg) significantly reduced total-C, LDL-C, Apo B, non-HDL-C, and TG, and increased HDL-C compared to all doses of lovastatin pooled (10–40 mg).

TABLE 12: Response to ZETIA and Fenofibrate Initiated Concurrently in Patients with Mixed Hyperlipidemia (Mean* % Change from Untreated Baseline† at 12 weeks)

Treatment (Daily Dose)	N	Total-C	LDL-C	Apo B	TG*	HDL-C	Non-HDL-C
Placebo	63	0	0	-1	-9	+3	0
ZETIA	185	-12	-13	-11	-11	+4	-15
Fenofibrate 160 mg	188	-11	-6	-15	-43	+19	-16
ZETIA + Fenofibrate 160 mg	183	-22	-20	-26	-44	+19	-30

* For triglycerides, median % change from baseline.
† Baseline - on no lipid-lowering drug.

- Continue to follow a cholesterol-lowering diet while taking ZETIA. Ask your doctor if you need diet information.
- Keep taking ZETIA unless your doctor tells you to stop. It is important that you keep taking ZETIA even if you do not feel sick.

See your doctor regularly to check your cholesterol level and to check for side effects. Your doctor may do blood tests to check your liver before you start taking ZETIA with a statin and during treatment.

What are the possible side effects of ZETIA?

In clinical studies patients reported few side effects while taking ZETIA. These included diarrhea, joint pains, and feeling tired.

Patients have experienced severe muscle problems while taking ZETIA, usually when ZETIA was added to a statin drug. If you experience unexplained muscle pain, tenderness, or weakness while taking ZETIA, contact your doctor immediately. You need to do this promptly, because on rare occasions, these muscle problems can be serious, with muscle breakdown resulting in kidney damage.

Additionally, the following side effects have been reported in general use: allergic reactions (which may require treatment right away) including swelling of the face, lips, tongue, and/or throat that may cause difficulty in breathing or swallowing, rash, and hives; raised red rash, sometimes with target-shaped lesions; joint pain; muscle aches; alterations in some laboratory blood tests; liver problems; stomach pain; inflammation of the pancreas; nausea; dizziness; tingling sensation; depression; headache; gallstones; inflammation of the gallbladder.

Tell your doctor if you are having these or any other medical problems while on ZETIA. For a complete list of side effects, ask your doctor or pharmacist.

What should I know about high cholesterol?

Cholesterol is a type of fat found in your blood. Your total cholesterol is made up of LDL and HDL cholesterol.

LDL cholesterol is called "bad" cholesterol because it can build up in the wall of your arteries and form plaque. Over time, plaque build-up can cause a narrowing of the arteries. This narrowing can slow or block blood flow to your heart, brain, and other organs. High LDL cholesterol is a major cause of heart disease and one of the causes for stroke.

HDL cholesterol is called "good" cholesterol because it keeps the bad cholesterol from building up in the arteries.

Triglycerides also are fats found in your blood.

General information about ZETIA

Medicines are sometimes prescribed for conditions that are not mentioned in patient information leaflets. Do not use ZETIA for a condition for which it was not prescribed. Do not give ZETIA to other people, even if they have the same condition you have. It may harm them.

This summarizes the most important information about ZETIA. If you would like more information, talk with your doctor. You can ask your pharmacist or doctor for information about ZETIA that is written for health professionals.

Inactive ingredients:

Croscarmellose sodium, lactose monohydrate, magnesium stearate, microcrystalline cellulose, povidone, and sodium lauryl sulfate.

Merck Sharp & Dohme Corp., a subsidiary of
MERCK & CO., INC., Whitehouse Station, NJ 08889, USA
U.S. Patent Nos. 5,846,966; 7,030,106 and RE 42,461.

Revised: 02/2013
USPPI-T-06531302R025

Shown in Product Identification Guide, page 309

ZIOPTAN™ ℞
(tafluprost ophthalmic solution) 0.0015%

HIGHLIGHTS OF PRESCRIBING INFORMATION

These highlights do not include all the information needed to use ZIOPTAN (tafluprost ophthalmic solution) 0.0015% safely and effectively. See full prescribing information for ZIOPTAN.

ZIOPTAN™ (tafluprost ophthalmic solution) 0.0015%
Initial U.S. Approval: 2012

INDICATIONS AND USAGE

- ZIOPTAN (tafluprost ophthalmic solution) 0.0015% is a prostaglandin analog indicated for reducing elevated intraocular pressure in patients with open-angle glaucoma or ocular hypertension. (1)

DOSAGE AND ADMINISTRATION

- One drop in the affected eye(s) once daily in the evening. (2)

DOSAGE FORMS AND STRENGTHS

- Ophthalmic solution containing tafluprost 0.015 mg/mL. (3)

CONTRAINDICATIONS

- None. (4)

WARNINGS AND PRECAUTIONS

- Pigmentation

Pigmentation of the iris, periorbital tissue (eyelid) and eyelashes can occur. Iris pigmentation is likely to be permanent. (5.1)

- Eyelash Changes

Gradual changes to eyelashes including increased length, thickness and number of lashes. Usually reversible. (5.2)

ADVERSE REACTIONS

- Most common ocular adverse reaction is conjunctival hyperemia (range 4% – 20%). (6.1)

To report SUSPECTED ADVERSE REACTIONS, contact Merck Sharp & Dohme Corp., a subsidiary of Merck & Co., Inc., at 1-877-888-4231 or FDA at 1-800-FDA-1088 or www.fda.gov/medwatch.

USE IN SPECIFIC POPULATIONS

- Use in pediatric patients is not recommended because of potential safety concerns related to increased pigmentation following long-term chronic use. (8.4)

See 17 for PATIENT COUNSELING INFORMATION and FDA-approved patient labeling

Revised: 08/2013

FULL PRESCRIBING INFORMATION: CONTENTS*

*** Sections or subsections omitted from the full prescribing information are not listed**

FULL PRESCRIBING INFORMATION

1 INDICATIONS AND USAGE

ZIOPTAN™ (tafluprost ophthalmic solution) 0.0015% is indicated for reducing elevated intraocular pressure in patients with open-angle glaucoma or ocular hypertension.

2 DOSAGE AND ADMINISTRATION

The recommended dose is one drop of ZIOPTAN in the conjunctival sac of the affected eye(s) once daily in the evening. The dose should not exceed once daily since it has been shown that more frequent administration of prostaglandin analogs may lessen the intraocular pressure lowering effect.

Reduction of the intraocular pressure starts approximately 2 to 4 hours after the first administration with the maximum effect reached after 12 hours.

ZIOPTAN may be used concomitantly with other topical ophthalmic drug products to lower intraocular pressure. If more than one topical ophthalmic product is being used, each one should be administered at least 5 minutes apart.

The solution from one individual unit is to be used immediately after opening for administration to one or both eyes. Since sterility cannot be maintained after the individual unit is opened, the remaining contents should be discarded immediately after administration.

3 DOSAGE FORMS AND STRENGTHS

Ophthalmic solution containing tafluprost 0.015 mg/mL.

4 CONTRAINDICATIONS

None.

5 WARNINGS AND PRECAUTIONS

5.1 Pigmentation

Tafluprost ophthalmic solution has been reported to cause changes to pigmented tissues. The most frequently reported changes have been increased pigmentation of the iris, periorbital tissue (eyelid) and eyelashes. Pigmentation is expected to increase as long as tafluprost is administered. The pigmentation change is due to increased melanin content in the melanocytes rather than to an increase in the number of melanocytes. After discontinuation of tafluprost, pigmentation of the iris is likely to be permanent, while pigmentation of the periorbital tissue and eyelash changes have been reported to be reversible in some patients. Patients who receive treatment should be informed of the possibility of increased pigmentation. The long term effects of increased pigmentation are not known.

Iris color change may not be noticeable for several months to years. Typically, the brown pigmentation around the pupil spreads concentrically towards the periphery of the iris and the entire iris or parts of the iris become more brownish. Neither nevi nor freckles of the iris appear to be affected by treatment. While treatment with ZIOPTAN can be continued in patients who develop noticeably increased iris pigmentation, these patients should be examined regularly. *[See Patient Counseling Information (17.3).]*

5.2 Eyelash Changes

ZIOPTAN may gradually change eyelashes and vellus hair in the treated eye. These changes include increased length, color, thickness, shape and number of lashes. Eyelash changes are usually reversible upon discontinuation of treatment.

5.3 Intraocular Inflammation

ZIOPTAN should be used with caution in patients with active intraocular inflammation (e.g., iritis/uveitis) because the inflammation may be exacerbated.

5.4 Macular Edema

Macular edema, including cystoid macular edema, has been reported during treatment with prostaglandin F2α analogs. ZIOPTAN should be used with caution in aphakic patients, in pseudophakic patients with a torn posterior lens capsule, or in patients with known risk factors for macular edema.

6 ADVERSE REACTIONS

6.1 Clinical Studies Experience

Because clinical studies are conducted under widely varying conditions, adverse reaction rates observed in the clinical studies of a drug cannot be directly compared to rates in the clinical studies of another drug and may not reflect the rates observed in practice.

Preservative-containing or preservative-free tafluprost 0.0015% was evaluated in 905 patients in five controlled clinical studies of up to 24-months duration. The most common adverse reaction observed in patients treated with tafluprost was conjunctival hyperemia which was reported in a range of 4% – 20% of patients. Approximately 1% of patients discontinued therapy due to ocular adverse reactions.

Ocular adverse reactions reported at an incidence of ≥2% in these clinical studies included ocular stinging/irritation (7%), ocular pruritus including allergic conjunctivitis (5%), cataract (3%), dry eye (3%), ocular pain (3%), eyelash darkening (2%), growth of eyelashes (2%) and vision blurred (2%).

Nonocular adverse reactions reported at an incidence of 2% – 6% in these clinical studies in patients treated with tafluprost 0.0015% were headache (6%), common cold (4%), cough (3%) and urinary tract infection (2%).

6.2 Postmarketing Experience

The following adverse reactions have been identified during postapproval use of tafluprost. Because postapproval adverse reactions are reported voluntarily from a population of uncertain size, it is not always possible to reliably estimate their frequency or establish a causal relationship to drug exposure.

Respiratory disorders: exacerbation of asthma, dyspnea
Eye disorders: iritis/uveitis

In postmarketing use with prostaglandin analogs, periorbital and lid changes including deepening of the eyelid sulcus have been observed.

8 USE IN SPECIFIC POPULATIONS

8.1 Pregnancy

Pregnancy Category C.

Teratogenic effects: In embryo-fetal development studies in rats and rabbits, tafluprost administered intravenously was teratogenic. Tafluprost caused increases in post-implantation losses in rats and rabbits and reductions in fetal body weights in rats. Tafluprost also increased the incidence of vertebral skeletal abnormalities in rats and the incidence of skull, brain and spine malformations in rabbits. In rats, there were no adverse effects on embryo-fetal development at a dose of 3 mcg/kg/day corresponding to maternal plasma levels of tafluprost acid that were 343 times the maximum clinical exposure based on C_{max}. In rabbits, effects were seen at a tafluprost dose of 0.03 mcg/kg/day corresponding to maternal plasma levels of tafluprost acid during organogenesis that were approximately 5 times higher than the clinical exposure based on C_{max}. At the no-effect dose in rabbits (0.01 mcg/kg/day), maternal plasma levels of tafluprost acid were below the lower level of quantification (20 pg/mL).

In a pre- and postnatal development study in rats, increased mortality of newborns, decreased body weights and delayed pinna unfolding were observed in offsprings. The no observed adverse effect level was at a tafluprost intravenous dose of 0.3 mcg/kg/day which is greater than 3 times the maximum recommended clinical dose based on body surface area comparison.

There are no adequate and well-controlled studies in pregnant woman. Although animal reproduction studies are not always predictive of human response, ZIOPTAN should not be used during pregnancy unless the potential benefit justifies the potential risk to the fetus.

Women of childbearing age/potential should have adequate contraceptive measures in place.

8.3 Nursing Mothers

A study in lactating rats demonstrated that radio-labeled tafluprost and/or its metabolites were excreted in milk. It is not known whether this drug or its metabolites are excreted in human milk. Because many drugs are excreted in human milk, caution should be exercised when ZIOPTAN is administered to a nursing woman.

8.4 Pediatric Use

Use in pediatric patients is not recommended because of potential safety concerns related to increased pigmentation following long-term chronic use.

8.5 Geriatric Use

No overall clinical differences in safety or effectiveness have been observed between elderly and other adult patients.

11 DESCRIPTION

Tafluprost is a fluorinated analog of prostaglandin F2α. The chemical name for tafluprost is 1-methylethyl (*5Z*)-7-{(*1R*, *2R*, *3R*, *5S*)-2-[(*1E*)-3,3-difluoro-4-phenoxy-1-butenyl]-3,5-dihydroxycyclopentyl]-5-heptenoate. The molecular formula of tafluprost is $C_{25}H_{34}F_2O_5$ and its molecular weight is 452.53.

Its structural formula is:

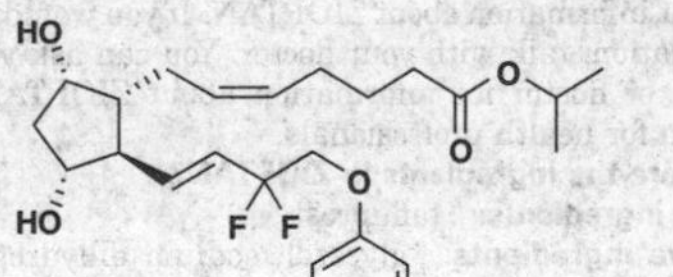

Tafluprost is a colorless to light yellow viscous liquid that is practically insoluble in water.

ZIOPTAN (tafluprost ophthalmic solution) 0.0015% is supplied as a sterile solution of tafluprost with a pH range of 5.5 – 6.7 and an Osmolality range of 260 – 300 mOsmol/kg. ZIOPTAN contains Active: tafluprost 0.015 mg/mL; Inactives: glycerol, sodium dihydrogen phosphate dihydrate, disodium edetate, polysorbate 80, hydrochloric acid and/or sodium hydroxide (to adjust pH) and Water for Injection. ZIOPTAN does not contain a preservative.

12 CLINICAL PHARMACOLOGY

12.1 Mechanism of Action

Tafluprost acid, a prostaglandin analog is a selective FP prostanoid receptor agonist which is believed to reduce intraocular pressure by increasing uveoscleral outflow. The exact mechanism of action is unknown at this time.

12.3 Pharmacokinetics

Absorption

Following instillation, tafluprost is absorbed through the cornea and is hydrolyzed to the biologically active acid metabolite, tafluprost acid. Following instillation of one drop of the 0.0015% solution once daily into each eye of healthy volunteers, the plasma concentrations of tafluprost acid peaked at a median time of 10 minutes on both Days 1 and 8. The mean plasma C_{max} of tafluprost acid were 26 pg/mL and 27 pg/mL on Day 1, and Day 8, respectively. The mean plasma AUC estimates of tafluprost acid were 394 pg*min/mL and 432 pg*min/mL on Day 1 and 8, respectively.

Metabolism

Tafluprost, an ester prodrug, is hydrolyzed to its biologically active acid metabolite in the eye. The acid metabolite is further metabolized via fatty acid β-oxidation and phase II conjugation.

Elimination

Mean plasma tafluprost acid concentrations were below the limit of quantification of the bioanalytical assay (10 pg/mL) at 30 minutes following topical ocular administration of tafluprost 0.0015% ophthalmic solution.

13 NONCLINICAL TOXICOLOGY

13.1 Carcinogenesis, Mutagenesis, Impairment of Fertility

Tafluprost was not carcinogenic when administered subcutaneously daily for 24 months at doses up to 30 mcg/kg/day in rats and for 18 months at doses up to 100 mcg/kg/day in mice (over 1600 and 1300 times, respectively, the maximum clinical exposure based on plasma AUC).

Tafluprost was not mutagenic or clastogenic in a battery of genetic toxicology studies, including an *in vitro* microbial mutagenesis assay, an *in vitro* chromosomal aberration assay in Chinese hamster lung cells, and an *in vivo* mouse micronucleus assay in bone marrow.

In rats, no adverse effects on mating performance or fertility were observed with intravenous dosing of tafluprost at a dose of 100 mcg/kg/day (over 14000 times the maximum clinical exposure based on plasma C_{max} or over 3600 times based on plasma AUC).

14 CLINICAL STUDIES

In clinical studies up to 24 months in duration, patients with open-angle glaucoma or ocular hypertension and baseline pressure of 23–26 mm Hg who were treated with ZIOPTAN dosed once daily in the evening demonstrated reductions in intraocular pressure at 3 and 6 months of 6–8 mmHg and 5–8 mmHg, respectively.

16 HOW SUPPLIED/STORAGE AND HANDLING

ZIOPTAN (tafluprost ophthalmic solution) 0.0015% is supplied as a sterile solution in translucent low density polyethylene single-use containers packaged in foil pouches (10 single-use containers per pouch). Each single-use container has 0.3 mL solution corresponding to 0.0045 mg tafluprost.
NDC 0006-3931-30; Unit-of-Use Carton of 30.
NDC 0006-3931-54; Unit-of-Use Carton of 90.

Storage:

Store refrigerated at 2–8°C (36–46°F). Store in the original pouch. After the pouch is opened, the single-use containers may be stored in the opened foil pouch for up to 28 days at room temperature: 20–25°C (68–77°F). Protect from moisture. Write down the date you open the foil pouch in the space provided on the pouch. Discard any unused containers 28 days after first opening the pouch.

17 PATIENT COUNSELING INFORMATION

See FDA-Approved Patient Labeling (Patient Information).

17.1 Nightly Application

Advise patients to not exceed once daily dosing since more frequent administration may decrease the intraocular pressure lowering effect of ZIOPTAN.

17.2 Handling the Single-Use Container

Advise patients that ZIOPTAN is a sterile solution that does not contain a preservative. The solution from one individual unit is to be used immediately after opening for administration to one or both eyes. Since sterility cannot be maintained after the individual unit is opened, the remaining contents should be discarded immediately after administration.

17.3 Potential for Pigmentation

Advise patients about the potential for increased brown pigmentation of the iris, which may be permanent. Also inform patients about the possibility of eyelid skin darkening, which may be reversible after discontinuation of ZIOPTAN.

17.4 Potential for Eyelash Changes

Inform patients of the possibility of eyelash and vellus hair changes in the treated eye during treatment with ZIOPTAN. These changes may result in a disparity between eyes in length, thickness, pigmentation, number of eyelashes or vellus hairs, and/or direction of eyelash growth. Eyelash changes are usually reversible upon discontinuation of treatment.

17.5 When to Seek Physician Advice

Advise patients that if they develop a new ocular condition (e.g., trauma or infection), experience a sudden decrease in visual acuity, have ocular surgery, or develop any ocular reactions, particularly conjunctivitis and eyelid reactions, they should immediately seek their physician's advice concerning the continued use of ZIOPTAN.

17.6 Use with Other Ophthalmic Drugs

If more than one topical ophthalmic drug is being used, the drugs should be administered at least five (5) minutes between applications.

17.7 Storage Information

Instruct patients on proper storage of cartons, unopened foil pouches, and opened foil pouches *[see How Supplied/Stor-*

age and Handling (16)]. Recommended storage for cartons and unopened foil pouches is to store refrigerated at 2–8°C (36–46°F). After the pouch is opened, the single-use containers may be stored in the opened foil pouch for up to 28 days at room temperature: 20–25°C (68–77°F). Protect from moisture.

Manufactured for: Merck Sharp & Dohme Corp., a subsidiary of
MERCK & CO., INC., Whitehouse Station, NJ 08889, USA
Manufactured by:
Laboratoire Unither
ZI de la Guerie
F-50211 COUTANCES Cedex
France
For patent information: www.merck.com/product/patent/home.html

USPI-PF-24521308R005

PATIENT INFORMATION
ZIOPTAN™ (zye OP tan)
(tafluprost ophthalmic solution) 0.0015%

Read this Patient Information before you start using ZIOPTAN™ and each time you get a refill. There may be new information. This information does not take the place of talking to your doctor about your medical condition or your treatment.

What is ZIOPTAN?
ZIOPTAN is a prescription sterile eye drop solution. ZIOPTAN is used to lower the pressure in the eye (intraocular pressure) in people with open-angle glaucoma or ocular hypertension when their eye pressure is too high. ZIOPTAN belongs to a group of medicines called prostaglandin analogs.
ZIOPTAN is not for use in children.

What should I tell my doctor before using ZIOPTAN?
Before you use ZIOPTAN, tell your doctor if you:
- have or have had eye problems including any surgery on your eye or eyes
- are using any other eye medicines
- have any other medical problems
- are pregnant or plan to become pregnant. It is not known if ZIOPTAN will harm your unborn baby. You should use an effective method of birth control while you use ZIOPTAN. If you become pregnant while using ZIOPTAN talk to your doctor right away.
- are breastfeeding or plan to breastfeed. It is not known if ZIOPTAN passes into your breast milk. Talk to your doctor about the best way to feed your baby if you use ZIOPTAN.

Tell your doctor about all the medicines you take, including prescription and non-prescription medicines, vitamins, and herbal supplements.
Know the medicines you take. Keep a list of them to show your doctor and pharmacist when you get a new medicine.

How should I take ZIOPTAN?
Read the Instructions for Use at the end of this Patient Information leaflet for additional instructions about the right way to use ZIOPTAN.
- **Use 1 drop of ZIOPTAN in your eye (or eyes) each evening.** Talk to your doctor or pharmacist if you are not sure how to use ZIOPTAN.
- Your ZIOPTAN may not work as well if you use it more than 1 time each evening.
- If you use other medicines in your eye, wait at least 5 minutes between using ZIOPTAN and your other eye medicines.
- Use your ZIOPTAN right away after opening. Each ZIOPTAN single-use container is sterile and is to be used 1 time then thrown away. Do not save any ZIOPTAN that may be left over after you use your medicine. Using ZIOPTAN that is not sterile may cause other eye problems.

What are the possible side effects of ZIOPTAN?
ZIOPTAN may cause serious side effects including:
- **changes in the color of your eye (iris).** Your iris may become more brown in color while using ZIOPTAN. This color change may not go away when you stop using ZIOPTAN. If ZIOPTAN is used in 1 eye only, the color of that eye may always be a different color from the color of your other eye.
- **darkening of the color of the skin around your eye (eyelid).** These skin changes usually go away when you stop using ZIOPTAN.
- **increasing the length, thickness, color, or number of your eyelashes.** These eyelash changes usually go away when you stop using ZIOPTAN.
- **hair growth on your eyelids.** This hair growth usually goes away when you stop using ZIOPTAN.

The most common side effects of ZIOPTAN include:
- redness, stinging or itching of your eye
- cataract formation
- dry eye
- eye pain
- blurred vision
- headache
- common cold
- cough
- urinary tract infection

Tell your doctor if you have any new eye problems while using ZIOPTAN including:
- an eye injury
- an eye infection
- a sudden loss of vision
- eye surgery
- swelling and redness of and around your eye (conjunctivitis)
- problems with your eyelids

Additionally, the following side effects have been reported in general use:
- worsening of asthma
- shortness of breath

Tell your doctor if you have any other side effects that bother you.
These are not all the possible side effects of ZIOPTAN. For more information, ask your doctor or pharmacist.
Call your doctor for medical advice about side effects. You may report side effects to FDA at 1-800-FDA-1088.

How should I store ZIOPTAN?
Keep the foil pouches and ZIOPTAN single-use containers dry.
Before opening the foil pouches:
- Store the unopened foil pouches in a refrigerator between 36°F to 46°F (2°C to 8°C).
- Do not open the pouch containing ZIOPTAN until you are ready to use the eye drops.

After opening the foil pouch:
- Store the opened foil pouch at room temperature, between 68°F to 77°F (20°C to 25°C), for up to 28 days.
- Throw away all unused ZIOPTAN single-use containers in the opened foil pouch after 28 days.
- Keep the ZIOPTAN single-use containers in their original foil pouch.
- After opening the foil pouch, refrigeration is not required.

Keep ZIOPTAN and all medicines out of the reach of children.

General information about the safe and effective use of ZIOPTAN.
Do not use ZIOPTAN for a condition for which it was not prescribed. Do not give ZIOPTAN to other people, even if they have the same symptoms that you have. It may harm them.
This Patient Information leaflet summarizes the most important information about ZIOPTAN. If you would like more information, talk with your doctor. You can ask your pharmacist or doctor for information about ZIOPTAN that is written for health professionals.

What are the ingredients in ZIOPTAN?
Active ingredients: tafluprost
Inactive ingredients: glycerol, sodium dihydrogen phosphate dihydrate, disodium edetate, and polysorbate 80, hydrochloric acid and/or sodium hydroxide, and water

Instructions for Use
Read these Instructions for Use before using your ZIOPTAN and each time you get a refill. There may be new information. This leaflet does not take the place of talking with your doctor about your medical condition or your treatment.

Important:
- **ZIOPTAN is for the eye only. Do not swallow ZIOPTAN.**
- ZIOPTAN single-use containers are packaged in a foil pouch.
- **Do not** use the ZIOPTAN single-use containers if the foil pouch is opened.
- Write down the date you open the foil pouch in the space provided on the pouch.

Every time you use ZIOPTAN:

Step 1.	Wash your hands.
Step 2.	Take the strip of single-use containers from the foil pouch.
Step 3.	Pull off one single-use container from the strip.
Step 4.	Put the remaining strip of single-use containers back in the foil pouch and fold the edge to close the pouch.

Step 5.	Hold the single-use container upright. Make sure that your ZIOPTAN medicine is in the bottom part of the single-use container. **See Figure A.**	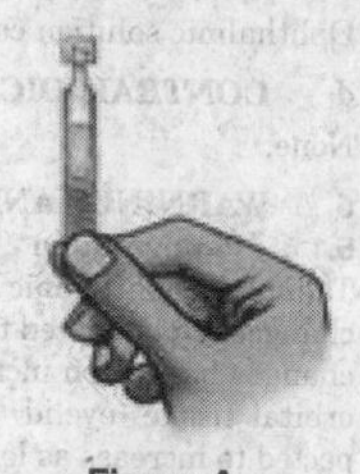 **Figure A**
Step 6.	Open the single-use container by twisting off the tab. **See Figure B.**	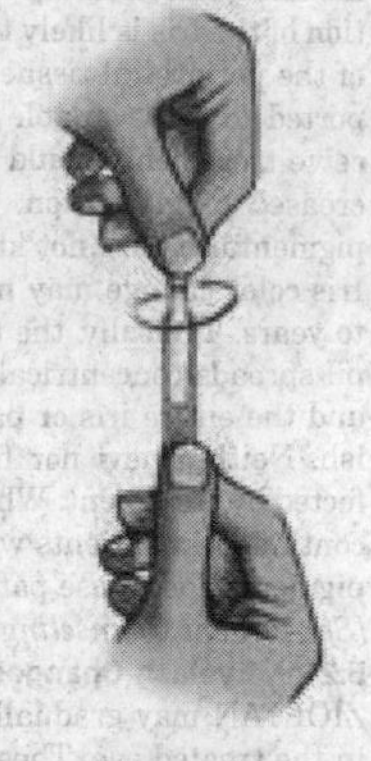 **Figure B**
Step 7.	Tilt your head backwards. If you are unable to tilt your head, lie down.	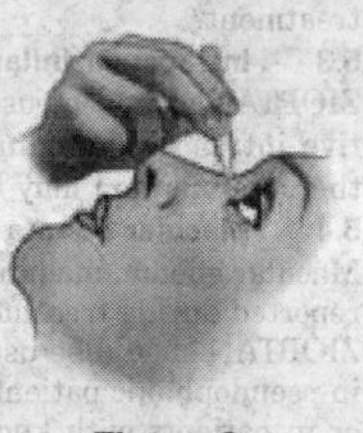 **Figure C**
Step 8.	Place the tip of the single-use container close to your eye. Be careful not to touch your eye with the tip of the single-use container. **See Figure C.**	
Step 9.	Pull your lower eyelid downwards and look up.	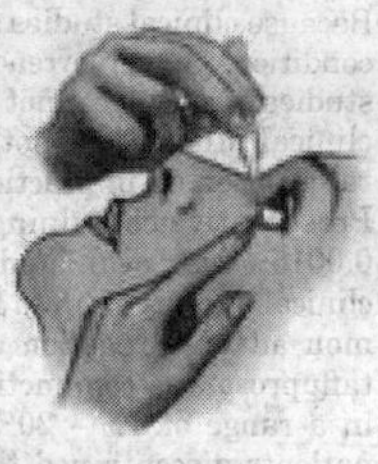 **Figure D**
Step 10.	Gently squeeze the container and let 1 drop of ZIOPTAN fall into the space between your lower eyelid and your eye. If a drop misses your eye, try again. **See Figure D.**	

- If your doctor has told you to use ZIOPTAN drops in both eyes, repeat Steps 7 to 10 for your other eye.
- There is enough ZIOPTAN in one single-use container for both of your eyes.
- **Throw away the opened single-use container with any remaining ZIOPTAN right away.**

This Patient Information and Instructions for Use have been approved by the U.S. Food and Drug Administration.
Rx only
Manufactured for: Merck Sharp & Dohme Corp., a subsidiary of
MERCK & CO., INC., Whitehouse Station, NJ 08889, USA
Manufactured by:
Laboratoire Unither
ZI de la Guerie
F-50211 COUTANCES Cedex
France
For patent information: www.merck.com/product/patent/home.html

Revised: 08/2013
USPPI-PF-24521308R005

Shown in Product Identification Guide, page 309

ZOCOR ℞
(simvastatin)
Tablets

HIGHLIGHTS OF PRESCRIBING INFORMATION
These highlights do not include all the information needed to use ZOCOR safely and effectively. See full prescribing information for ZOCOR.
ZOCOR (simvastatin) Tablets
Initial U.S. Approval: 1991

RECENT MAJOR CHANGES

Dosage and Administration
Coadministration with Other Drugs (2.3) 10/2012
Contraindications (4) 10/2012
Warnings and Precautions
Myopathy/Rhabdomyolysis (5.1) 10/2012

INDICATIONS AND USAGE

ZOCOR® is an HMG-CoA reductase inhibitor (statin) indicated as an adjunctive therapy to diet to:
- Reduce the risk of total mortality by reducing CHD deaths and reduce the risk of non-fatal myocardial infarction, stroke, and the need for revascularization procedures in patients at high risk of coronary events. (1.1)
- Reduce elevated total-C, LDL-C, Apo B, TG and increase HDL-C in patients with primary hyperlipidemia (heterozygous familial and nonfamilial) and mixed dyslipidemia. (1.2)
- Reduce elevated TG in patients with hypertriglyceridemia and reduce TG and VLDL-C in patients with primary dysbeta-lipoproteinemia. (1.2)
- Reduce total-C and LDL-C in adult patients with homozygous familial hypercholesterolemia. (1.2)
- Reduce elevated total-C, LDL-C, and Apo B in boys and postmenarchal girls, 10 to 17 years of age with heterozygous familial hypercholesterolemia after failing an adequate trial of diet therapy. (1.2, 1.3)

Limitations of Use
ZOCOR has not been studied in Fredrickson Types I and V dyslipidemias. (1.4)

DOSAGE AND ADMINISTRATION

- Dose range is 5 to 40 mg/day. (2.1)
- Recommended usual starting dose is 10 or 20 mg once a day in the evening. (2.1)
- Recommended starting dose for patients at high risk of CHD is 40 mg/day. (2.1)
- Due to the increased risk of myopathy, including rhabdomyolysis, use of the 80-mg dose of ZOCOR should be restricted to patients who have been taking simvastatin 80 mg chronically (e.g., for 12 months or more) without evidence of muscle toxicity. (2.2)
- Patients who are currently tolerating the 80-mg dose of ZOCOR who need to be initiated on an interacting drug that is contraindicated or is associated with a dose cap for simvastatin should be switched to an alternative statin with less potential for the drug-drug interaction. (2.2)
- Due to the increased risk of myopathy, including rhabdomyolysis, associated with the 80-mg dose of ZOCOR, patients unable to achieve their LDL-C goal utilizing the 40-mg dose of ZOCOR should not be titrated to the 80-mg dose, but should be placed on alternative LDL-C-lowering treatment(s) that provides greater LDL-C lowering. (2.2)
- Adolescents (10-17 years of age) with HeFH: starting dose is 10 mg/day; maximum recommended dose is 40 mg/day. (2.5)

DOSAGE FORMS AND STRENGTHS

Tablets: 5 mg; 10 mg; 20 mg; 40 mg; 80 mg (3)

CONTRAINDICATIONS

- Concomitant administration of strong CYP3A4 inhibitors. (4, 5.1)
- Concomitant administration of gemfibrozil, cyclosporine, or danazol. (4, 5.1)
- Hypersensitivity to any component of this medication. (4, 6.2)
- Active liver disease, which may include unexplained persistent elevations in hepatic transaminase levels. (4, 5.2)
- Women who are pregnant or may become pregnant. (4, 8.1)
- Nursing mothers. (4, 8.3)

WARNINGS AND PRECAUTIONS

- **Patients should be advised of the increased risk of myopathy including rhabdomyolysis with the 80-mg dose. (5.1)**
- Skeletal muscle effects (e.g., myopathy and rhabdomyolysis): Risks increase with higher doses and concomitant use of certain medicines. Predisposing factors include advanced age (≥65), female gender, uncontrolled hypothyroidism, and renal impairment. (4, 5.1, 8.5, 8.6)
- Patients should be advised to report promptly any unexplained and/or persistent muscle pain, tenderness, or weakness. ZOCOR therapy should be discontinued immediately if myopathy is diagnosed or suspected. See Drug Interaction table. (5.1)
- Liver enzyme abnormalities: Persistent elevations in hepatic transaminases can occur. Check liver enzyme tests before initiating therapy and as clinically indicated thereafter. (5.2)

ADVERSE REACTIONS

Most common adverse reactions (incidence ≥5.0%) are: upper respiratory infection, headache, abdominal pain, constipation, and nausea. (6.1)
To report SUSPECTED ADVERSE REACTIONS, contact Merck Sharp & Dohme Corp., a subsidiary of Merck & Co., Inc., at 1-877-888-4231 or FDA at 1-800-FDA-1088 or www.fda.gov/medwatch.

DRUG INTERACTIONS

Drug Interactions Associated with Increased Risk of Myopathy/Rhabdomyolysis (2.3, 4, 5.1, 7.1, 7.2, 7.3, 12.3)

Interacting Agents	Prescribing Recommendations
Strong CYP3A4 inhibitors (e.g., itraconazole, ketoconazole, posaconazole, voriconazole, erythromycin, clarithromycin, telithromycin, HIV protease inhibitors, boceprevir, telaprevir, nefazodone), gemfibrozil, cyclosporine, danazol	Contraindicated with simvastatin
Verapamil, diltiazem, dronedarone	Do not exceed 10 mg simvastatin daily
Amiodarone, amlodipine, ranolazine	Do not exceed 20 mg simvastatin daily
Grapefruit juice	Avoid grapefruit juice

- Other Lipid-lowering Medications: Use with other fibrate products or lipid-modifying doses (≥1 g/day) of niacin increases the risk of adverse skeletal muscle effects. Caution should be used when prescribing with simvastatin. (5.1, 7.2, 7.4)
- Coumarin anticoagulants: Concomitant use with ZOCOR prolongs INR. Achieve stable INR prior to starting ZOCOR. Monitor INR frequently until stable upon initiation or alteration of ZOCOR therapy. (7.6)

USE IN SPECIFIC POPULATIONS

- Severe renal impairment: patients should be started at 5 mg/day and be closely monitored. (2.6, 8.6)

See 17 for PATIENT COUNSELING INFORMATION
Revised: 10/2012

FULL PRESCRIBING INFORMATION: CONTENTS*

*** Sections or subsections omitted from the full prescribing information are not listed**

FULL PRESCRIBING INFORMATION

1 INDICATIONS AND USAGE

Therapy with lipid-altering agents should be only one component of multiple risk factor intervention in individuals at significantly increased risk for atherosclerotic vascular disease due to hypercholesterolemia. Drug therapy is indicated as an adjunct to diet when the response to a diet restricted in saturated fat and cholesterol and other nonpharmacologic measures alone has been inadequate. In patients with coronary heart disease (CHD) or at high risk of CHD, ZOCOR[1] can be started simultaneously with diet.

[1]Registered trademark of Merck Sharp & Dohme Corp., a subsidiary of **Merck & Co., Inc.**

1.1 Reductions in Risk of CHD Mortality and Cardiovascular Events

In patients at high risk of coronary events because of existing coronary heart disease, diabetes, peripheral vessel disease, history of stroke or other cerebrovascular disease, ZOCOR is indicated to:
- Reduce the risk of total mortality by reducing CHD deaths.
- Reduce the risk of non-fatal myocardial infarction and stroke.
- Reduce the need for coronary and non-coronary revascularization procedures.

1.2 Hyperlipidemia

ZOCOR is indicated to:
- Reduce elevated total cholesterol (total-C), low-density lipoprotein cholesterol (LDL-C), apolipoprotein B (Apo B), and triglycerides (TG), and to increase high-density lipoprotein cholesterol (HDL-C) in patients with primary hyperlipidemia (Fredrickson type IIa, heterozygous familial and nonfamilial) or mixed dyslipidemia (Fredrickson type IIb).
- Reduce elevated TG in patients with hypertriglyceridemia (Fredrickson type IV hyperlipidemia).
- Reduce elevated TG and VLDL-C in patients with primary dysbetalipoproteinemia (Fredrickson type III hyperlipidemia).
- Reduce total-C and LDL-C in patients with homozygous familial hypercholesterolemia as an adjunct to other lipid-lowering treatments (e.g., LDL apheresis) or if such treatments are unavailable.

1.3 Adolescent Patients with Heterozygous Familial Hypercholesterolemia (HeFH)

ZOCOR is indicated as an adjunct to diet to reduce total-C, LDL-C, and Apo B levels in adolescent boys and girls who are at least one year post-menarche, 10-17 years of age, with HeFH, if after an adequate trial of diet therapy the following findings are present:
1. LDL cholesterol remains ≥190 mg/dL; or
2. LDL cholesterol remains ≥160 mg/dL and
- There is a positive family history of premature cardiovascular disease (CVD) or
- Two or more other CVD risk factors are present in the adolescent patient.

The minimum goal of treatment in pediatric and adolescent patients is to achieve a mean LDL-C <130 mg/dL. The optimal age at which to initiate lipid-lowering therapy to decrease the risk of symptomatic adulthood CAD has not been determined.

1.4 Limitations of Use

ZOCOR has not been studied in conditions where the major abnormality is elevation of chylomicrons (i.e., hyperlipidemia Fredrickson types I and V).

2 DOSAGE AND ADMINISTRATION

2.1 Recommended Dosing

The usual dosage range is 5 to 40 mg/day. In patients with CHD or at high risk of CHD, ZOCOR can be started simultaneously with diet. The recommended usual starting dose is 10 or 20 mg once a day in the evening. For patients at high risk for a CHD event due to existing CHD, diabetes, peripheral vessel disease, history of stroke or other cerebrovascular disease, the recommended starting dose is 40 mg/day. Lipid determinations should be performed after 4 weeks of therapy and periodically thereafter.

2.2 Restricted Dosing for 80 mg

Due to the increased risk of myopathy, including rhabdomyolysis, particularly during the first year of treatment, use of the 80-mg dose of ZOCOR should be restricted to patients who have been taking simvastatin 80 mg chronically (e.g., for 12 months or more) without evidence of muscle toxicity *[see Warnings and Precautions (5.1)].*

Patients who are currently tolerating the 80-mg dose of ZOCOR who need to be initiated on an interacting drug that is contraindicated or is associated with a dose cap for simvastatin should be switched to an alternative statin with less potential for the drug-drug interaction.

Due to the increased risk of myopathy, including rhabdomyolysis, associated with the 80-mg dose of ZOCOR, patients unable to achieve their LDL-C goal utilizing the 40-mg dose of ZOCOR should not be titrated to the 80-mg dose, but should be placed on alternative LDL-C-lowering treatment(s) that provides greater LDL-C lowering.

2.3 Coadministration with Other Drugs

Patients taking Verapamil, Diltiazem, or Dronedarone

- The dose of ZOCOR should not exceed 10 mg/day *[see Warnings and Precautions (5.1), Drug Interactions (7.3), and Clinical Pharmacology (12.3)].*

Patients taking Amiodarone, Amlodipine or Ranolazine

- The dose of ZOCOR should not exceed 20 mg/day *[see Warnings and Precautions (5.1), Drug Interactions (7.3), and Clinical Pharmacology (12.3)].*

2.4 Patients with Homozygous Familial Hypercholesterolemia

The recommended dosage is 40 mg/day in the evening *[see Dosage and Administration, Restricted Dosing for 80 mg (2.2)].* ZOCOR should be used as an adjunct to other lipid-lowering treatments (e.g., LDL apheresis) in these patients or if such treatments are unavailable.

2.5 Adolescents (10-17 years of age) with Heterozygous Familial Hypercholesterolemia

The recommended usual starting dose is 10 mg once a day in the evening. The recommended dosing range is 10 to 40 mg/day; the maximum recommended dose is 40 mg/day. Doses should be individualized according to the recommended goal of therapy [see NCEP Pediatric Panel Guidelines[2] and *Clinical Studies (14.2)*]. Adjustments should be made at intervals of 4 weeks or more.

[2] National Cholesterol Education Program (NCEP): Highlights of the Report of the Expert Panel on Blood Cholesterol Levels in Children and Adolescents. *Pediatrics.* 89(3):495-501. 1992.

2.6 Patients with Renal Impairment

Because ZOCOR does not undergo significant renal excretion, modification of dosage should not be necessary in patients with mild to moderate renal impairment. However, caution should be exercised when ZOCOR is administered to patients with severe renal impairment; such patients should be started at 5 mg/day and be closely monitored *[see Warnings and Precautions (5.1) and Clinical Pharmacology (12.3)].*

2.7 Chinese Patients Taking Lipid-Modifying Doses (≥1 g/day Niacin) of Niacin-Containing Products

Because of an increased risk for myopathy in Chinese patients taking simvastatin 40 mg coadministered with lipid-modifying doses (≥1 g/day niacin) of niacin-containing products, caution should be used when treating Chinese patients with simvastatin doses exceeding 20 mg/day coadministered with lipid-modifying doses of niacin-containing products. Because the risk for myopathy is dose-related, Chinese patients should not receive simvastatin 80 mg coadministered with lipid-modifying doses of niacin-containing products. The cause of the increased risk of myopathy is not known. It is also unknown if the risk for myopathy with coadministration of simvastatin with lipid-modifying doses of niacin-containing products observed in Chinese patients applies to other Asian patients. *[See Warnings and Precautions (5.1).]*

3 DOSAGE FORMS AND STRENGTHS

- Tablets ZOCOR 5 mg are buff, oval, film-coated tablets, coded MSD 726 on one side and ZOCOR 5 on the other.
- Tablets ZOCOR 10 mg are peach, oval, film-coated tablets, coded MSD 735 on one side and plain on the other.
- Tablets ZOCOR 20 mg are tan, oval, film-coated tablets, coded MSD 740 on one side and plain on the other.
- Tablets ZOCOR 40 mg are brick red, oval, film-coated tablets, coded MSD 749 on one side and plain on the other.
- Tablets ZOCOR 80 mg are brick red, capsule-shaped, film-coated tablets, coded 543 on one side and 80 on the other.

4 CONTRAINDICATIONS

ZOCOR is contraindicated in the following conditions:

- Concomitant administration of strong CYP3A4 inhibitors (e.g., itraconazole, ketoconazole, posaconazole, voriconazole, HIV protease inhibitors, boceprevir, telaprevir, erythromycin, clarithromycin, telithromycin and nefazodone) *[see Warnings and Precautions (5.1)].*
- Concomitant administration of gemfibrozil, cyclosporine, or danazol *[see Warnings and Precautions (5.1)].*
- Hypersensitivity to any component of this medication *[see Adverse Reactions (6.2)].*
- Active liver disease, which may include unexplained persistent elevations in hepatic transaminase levels *[see Warnings and Precautions (5.2)].*
- Women who are pregnant or may become pregnant. Serum cholesterol and triglycerides increase during normal pregnancy, and cholesterol or cholesterol derivatives are essential for fetal development. Because HMG-CoA reductase inhibitors (statins) decrease cholesterol synthesis and possibly the synthesis of other biologically active substances derived from cholesterol, ZOCOR may cause fetal harm when administered to a pregnant woman. Atherosclerosis is a chronic process and the discontinuation of lipid-lowering drugs during pregnancy should have little impact on the outcome of long-term therapy of primary hypercholesterolemia. There are no adequate and well-controlled studies of use with ZOCOR during pregnancy; however, in rare reports congenital anomalies were observed following intrauterine exposure to statins. In rat and rabbit animal reproduction studies, simvastatin revealed no evidence of teratogenicity. **ZOCOR should be administered to women of childbearing age only when such patients are highly unlikely to conceive.** If the patient becomes pregnant while taking this drug, ZOCOR should be discontinued immediately and the patient should be apprised of the potential hazard to the fetus *[see Use in Specific Populations (8.1)].*
- Nursing mothers. It is not known whether simvastatin is excreted into human milk; however, a small amount of another drug in this class does pass into breast milk. Because statins have the potential for serious adverse reactions in nursing infants, women who require treatment with ZOCOR should not breastfeed their infants *[see Use in Specific Populations (8.3)].*

5 WARNINGS AND PRECAUTIONS

5.1 Myopathy/Rhabdomyolysis

Simvastatin occasionally causes myopathy manifested as muscle pain, tenderness or weakness with creatine kinase (CK) above ten times the upper limit of normal (ULN). Myopathy sometimes takes the form of rhabdomyolysis with or without acute renal failure secondary to myoglobinuria, and rare fatalities have occurred. The risk of myopathy is increased by high levels of statin activity in plasma. Predisposing factors for myopathy include advanced age (≥65 years), female gender, uncontrolled hypothyroidism, and renal impairment.

The risk of myopathy, including rhabdomyolysis, is dose related. In a clinical trial database in which 41,413 patients were treated with ZOCOR, 24,747 (approximately 60%) of whom were enrolled in studies with a median follow-up of at least 4 years, the incidence of myopathy was approximately 0.03% and 0.08% at 20 and 40 mg/day, respectively. The incidence of myopathy with 80 mg (0.61%) was disproportionately higher than that observed at the lower doses. In these trials, patients were carefully monitored and some interacting medicinal products were excluded.

In a clinical trial in which 12,064 patients with a history of myocardial infarction were treated with ZOCOR (mean follow-up 6.7 years), the incidence of myopathy (defined as unexplained muscle weakness or pain with a serum creatine kinase [CK] >10 times upper limit of normal [ULN]) in patients on 80 mg/day was approximately 0.9% compared with 0.02% for patients on 20 mg/day. The incidence of rhabdomyolysis (defined as myopathy with a CK >40 times ULN) in patients on 80 mg/day was approximately 0.4% compared with 0% for patients on 20 mg/day. The incidence of myopathy, including rhabdomyolysis, was highest during the first year and then notably decreased during the subsequent years of treatment. In this trial, patients were carefully monitored and some interacting medicinal products were excluded.

The risk of myopathy, including rhabdomyolysis, is greater in patients on simvastatin 80 mg compared with other statin therapies with similar or greater LDL-C-lowering efficacy and compared with lower doses of simvastatin. Therefore, the 80-mg dose of ZOCOR should be used only in patients who have been taking simvastatin 80 mg chronically (e.g., for 12 months or more) without evidence of muscle toxicity *[see Dosage and Administration, Restricted Dosing for 80 mg (2.2)].* If, however, a patient who is currently tolerating the 80-mg dose of ZOCOR needs to be initiated on an interacting drug that is contraindicated or is associated with a dose cap for simvastatin, that patient should be switched to an alternative statin with less potential for the drug-drug interaction. Patients should be advised of the increased risk of myopathy, including rhabdomyolysis, and to report promptly any unexplained muscle pain, tenderness or weakness. If symptoms occur, treatment should be discontinued immediately. *[See Warnings and Precautions (5.2).]*

There have been rare reports of immune-mediated necrotizing myopathy (IMNM), an autoimmune myopathy, associated with statin use. IMNM is characterized by: proximal muscle weakness and elevated serum creatine kinase, which persist despite discontinuation of statin treatment; muscle biopsy showing necrotizing myopathy without significant inflammation; improvement with immunosuppressive agents.

All patients starting therapy with ZOCOR, or whose dose of ZOCOR is being increased, should be advised of the risk of myopathy, including rhabdomyolysis, and told to report promptly any unexplained muscle pain, tenderness or weakness particularly if accompanied by malaise or fever or if muscle signs and symptoms persist after discontinuing ZOCOR. ZOCOR therapy should be discontinued immediately if myopathy is diagnosed or suspected. In most cases, muscle symptoms and CK increases resolved when treatment was promptly discontinued. Periodic CK determinations may be considered in patients starting therapy with ZOCOR or whose dose is being increased, but there is no assurance that such monitoring will prevent myopathy.

Many of the patients who have developed rhabdomyolysis on therapy with simvastatin have had complicated medical histories, including renal insufficiency usually as a consequence of long-standing diabetes mellitus. Such patients merit closer monitoring. ZOCOR therapy should be discontinued if markedly elevated CPK levels occur or myopathy is diagnosed or suspected. ZOCOR therapy should also be temporarily withheld in any patient experiencing an acute or serious condition predisposing to the development of renal failure secondary to rhabdomyolysis, e.g., sepsis; hypotension; major surgery; trauma; severe metabolic, endocrine, or electrolyte disorders; or uncontrolled epilepsy.

Drug Interactions

The risk of myopathy and rhabdomyolysis is increased by high levels of statin activity in plasma. Simvastatin is metabolized by the cytochrome P450 isoform 3A4. Certain drugs which inhibit this metabolic pathway can raise the plasma levels of simvastatin and may increase the risk of myopathy. These include itraconazole, ketoconazole, posaconazole, voriconazole, the macrolide antibiotics erythromycin and clarithromycin, and the ketolide antibiotic telithromycin, HIV protease inhibitors, boceprevir, telaprevir, the antidepressant nefazodone, or grapefruit juice *[see Clinical Pharmacology (12.3)].* Combination of these drugs with simvastatin is contraindicated. If short-term treatment with strong CYP3A4 inhibitors is unavoidable, therapy with simvastatin must be suspended during the course of treatment. *[See Contraindications (4) and Drug Interactions (7.1).]*

The combined use of simvastatin with gemfibrozil, cyclosporine, or danazol is contraindicated *[see Contraindications (4) and Drug Interactions (7.1 and 7.2)].*

Caution should be used when prescribing other fibrates with simvastatin, as these agents can cause myopathy when given alone and the risk is increased when they are coadministered *[see Drug Interactions (7.2)].*

Cases of myopathy, including rhabdomyolysis, have been reported with simvastatin coadministered with colchicine, and caution should be exercised when prescribing simvastatin with colchicine *[see Drug Interactions (7.7)].*

The benefits of the combined use of simvastatin with the following drugs should be carefully weighed against the potential risks of combinations: other lipid-lowering drugs (other fibrates or ≥1 g/day of niacin), amiodarone, dronedarone, verapamil, diltiazem, amlodipine, or ranolazine *[see Drug Interactions (7.3) and Table 3 in Clinical Pharmacology (12.3)].*

Cases of myopathy, including rhabdomyolysis, have been observed with simvastatin coadministered with lipid-modifying doses (≥1 g/day niacin) of niacin-containing products. In an ongoing, double-blind, randomized cardiovascular outcomes trial, an independent safety monitoring committee identified that the incidence of myopathy is higher in Chinese compared with non-Chinese patients taking simvastatin 40 mg coadministered with lipid-modifying doses of a niacin-containing product. Caution should be used when treating Chinese patients with simvastatin in doses exceeding 20 mg/day coadministered with lipid-modifying doses of niacin-containing products. Because the risk for myopathy is dose-related, Chinese patients should not receive simvastatin 80 mg coadministered with lipid-modifying doses of niacin-containing products. It is unknown if the risk for myopathy with coadministration of simvastatin with lipid-modifying doses of niacin-containing products observed in Chinese patients applies to other Asian patients *[see Drug Interactions (7.4)]*.

Prescribing recommendations for interacting agents are summarized in Table 1 *[see also Dosage and Administration (2.3), Drug Interactions (7), Clinical Pharmacology (12.3)]*.

TABLE 1: Drug Interactions Associated with Increased Risk of Myopathy/Rhabdomyolysis

Interacting Agents	Prescribing Recommendations
Strong CYP3A4 Inhibitors, e.g.: Itraconazole, Ketoconazole, Posaconazole, Voriconazole, Erythromycin, Clarithromycin, Telithromycin, HIV protease inhibitors, Boceprevir, Telaprevir, Nefazodone; Gemfibrozil; Cyclosporine; Danazol	Contraindicated with simvastatin
Verapamil; Diltiazem; Dronedarone	Do not exceed 10 mg simvastatin daily
Amiodarone; Amlodipine; Ranolazine	Do not exceed 20 mg simvastatin daily
Grapefruit juice	Avoid grapefruit juice

5.2 Liver Dysfunction

Persistent increases (to more than 3× the ULN) in serum transaminases have occurred in approximately 1% of patients who received simvastatin in clinical studies. When drug treatment was interrupted or discontinued in these patients, the transaminase levels usually fell slowly to pretreatment levels. The increases were not associated with jaundice or other clinical signs or symptoms. There was no evidence of hypersensitivity.

In the Scandinavian Simvastatin Survival Study (4S) *[see Clinical Studies (14.1)]*, the number of patients with more than one transaminase elevation to >3× ULN, over the course of the study, was not significantly different between the simvastatin and placebo groups (14 [0.7%] vs. 12 [0.6%]). Elevated transaminases resulted in the discontinuation of 8 patients from therapy in the simvastatin group (n=2,221) and 5 in the placebo group (n=2,223). Of the 1,986 simvastatin treated patients in 4S with normal liver function tests (LFTs) at baseline, 8 (0.4%) developed consecutive LFT elevations to >3× ULN and/or were discontinued due to transaminase elevations during the 5.4 years (median follow-up) of the study. Among these 8 patients, 5 initially developed these abnormalities within the first year. All of the patients in this study received a starting dose of 20 mg of simvastatin; 37% were titrated to 40 mg.

In 2 controlled clinical studies in 1,105 patients, the 12-month incidence of persistent hepatic transaminase elevation without regard to drug relationship was 0.9% and 2.1% at the 40- and 80-mg dose, respectively. No patients developed persistent liver function abnormalities following the initial 6 months of treatment at a given dose.

It is recommended that liver function tests be performed before the initiation of treatment, and thereafter when clinically indicated. There have been rare postmarketing reports of fatal and non-fatal hepatic failure in patients taking statins, including simvastatin. If serious liver injury with clinical symptoms and/or hyperbilirubinemia or jaundice occurs during treatment with ZOCOR, promptly interrupt therapy. If an alternate etiology is not found do not restart ZOCOR. Note that ALT may emanate from muscle, therefore ALT rising with CK may indicate myopathy *[see Warnings and Precautions (5.1)]*.

The drug should be used with caution in patients who consume substantial quantities of alcohol and/or have a past history of liver disease. Active liver diseases or unexplained transaminase elevations are contraindications to the use of simvastatin.

As with other lipid-lowering agents, moderate (less than 3× ULN) elevations of serum transaminases have been reported following therapy with simvastatin. These changes appeared soon after initiation of therapy with simvastatin, were often transient, were not accompanied by any symptoms and did not require interruption of treatment.

5.3 Endocrine Function

Increases in HbA1c and fasting serum glucose levels have been reported with HMG-CoA reductase inhibitors, including ZOCOR.

6 ADVERSE REACTIONS

6.1 Clinical Trials Experience

Because clinical studies are conducted under widely varying conditions, adverse reaction rates observed in the clinical studies of a drug cannot be directly compared to rates in the clinical studies of another drug and may not reflect the rates observed in practice.

In the pre-marketing controlled clinical studies and their open extensions (2,423 patients with median duration of follow-up of approximately 18 months), 1.4% of patients were discontinued due to adverse reactions. The most common adverse reactions that led to treatment discontinuation were: gastrointestinal disorders (0.5%), myalgia (0.1%), and arthralgia (0.1%). The most commonly reported adverse reactions (incidence ≥5%) in simvastatin controlled clinical trials were: upper respiratory infections (9.0%), headache (7.4%), abdominal pain (7.3%), constipation (6.6%), and nausea (5.4%).

Scandinavian Simvastatin Survival Study

In 4S involving 4,444 (age range 35-71 years, 19% women, 100% Caucasians) treated with 20-40 mg/day of ZOCOR (n=2,221) or placebo (n=2,223) over a median of 5.4 years, adverse reactions reported in ≥2% of patients and at a rate greater than placebo are shown in Table 2.

TABLE 2: Adverse Reactions Reported Regardless of Causality by ≥2% of Patients Treated with ZOCOR and Greater than Placebo in 4S

	ZOCOR (N = 2,221) %	Placebo (N = 2,223) %
Body as a Whole		
Edema/swelling	2.7	2.3
Abdominal pain	5.9	5.8
Cardiovascular System Disorders		
Atrial fibrillation	5.7	5.1
Digestive System Disorders		
Constipation	2.2	1.6
Gastritis	4.9	3.9
Endocrine Disorders		
Diabetes mellitus	4.2	3.6
Musculoskeletal Disorders		
Myalgia	3.7	3.2
Nervous System / Psychiatric Disorders		
Headache	2.5	2.1
Insomnia	4.0	3.8
Vertigo	4.5	4.2
Respiratory System Disorders		
Bronchitis	6.6	6.3
Sinusitis	2.3	1.8
Skin / Skin Appendage Disorders		
Eczema	4.5	3.0
Urogenital System Disorders		
Infection, urinary tract	3.2	3.1

Heart Protection Study

In the Heart Protection Study (HPS), involving 20,536 patients (age range 40-80 years, 25% women, 97% Caucasians, 3% other races) treated with ZOCOR 40 mg/day (n=10,269) or placebo (n=10,267) over a mean of 5 years, only serious adverse reactions and discontinuations due to any adverse reactions were recorded. Discontinuation rates due to adverse reactions were 4.8% in patients treated with ZOCOR compared with 5.1% in patients treated with placebo. The incidence of myopathy/rhabdomyolysis was <0.1% in patients treated with ZOCOR.

Other Clinical Studies

In a clinical trial in which 12,064 patients with a history of myocardial infarction were treated with ZOCOR (mean follow-up 6.7 years), the incidence of myopathy (defined as unexplained muscle weakness or pain with a serum creatine kinase [CK] >10 times upper limit of normal [ULN]) in patients on 80 mg/day was approximately 0.9% compared with 0.02% for patients on 20 mg/day. The incidence of rhabdomyolysis (defined as myopathy with a CK >40 times ULN) in patients on 80 mg/day was approximately 0.4% compared with 0% for patients on 20 mg/day. The incidence of myopathy, including rhabdomyolysis, was highest during the first year and then notably decreased during the subsequent years of treatment. In this trial, patients were carefully monitored and some interacting medicinal products were excluded.

Other adverse reactions reported in clinical trials were: diarrhea, rash, dyspepsia, flatulence, and asthenia.

Laboratory Tests

Marked persistent increases of hepatic transaminases have been noted *[see Warnings and Precautions (5.2)]*. Elevated alkaline phosphatase and γ-glutamyl transpeptidase have also been reported. About 5% of patients had elevations of CK levels of 3 or more times the normal value on one or more occasions. This was attributable to the noncardiac fraction of CK. *[See Warnings and Precautions (5.1).]*

Adolescent Patients (ages 10-17 years)

In a 48-week, controlled study in adolescent boys and girls who were at least 1 year post-menarche, 10-17 years of age (43.4% female, 97.7% Caucasians, 1.7% Hispanics, 0.6% Multiracial) with heterozygous familial hypercholesterolemia (n=175), treated with placebo or ZOCOR (10-40 mg daily), the most common adverse reactions observed in both groups were upper respiratory infection, headache, abdominal pain, and nausea *[see Use in Specific Populations (8.4) and Clinical Studies (14.2)]*.

6.2 Post-Marketing Experience

Because the below reactions are reported voluntarily from a population of uncertain size, it is generally not possible to reliably estimate their frequency or establish a causal relationship to drug exposure. The following additional adverse reactions have been identified during postapproval use of simvastatin: pruritus, alopecia, a variety of skin changes (e.g., nodules, discoloration, dryness of skin/mucous membranes, changes to hair/nails), dizziness, muscle cramps, myalgia, pancreatitis, paresthesia, peripheral neuropathy, vomiting, anemia, erectile dysfunction, interstitial lung disease, rhabdomyolysis, hepatitis/jaundice, fatal and non-fatal hepatic failure, and depression.

There have been rare reports of immune-mediated necrotizing myopathy associated with statin use *[see Warnings and Precautions (5.1)]*.

An apparent hypersensitivity syndrome has been reported rarely which has included some of the following features: anaphylaxis, angioedema, lupus erythematous-like syndrome, polymyalgia rheumatica, dermatomyositis, vasculitis, purpura, thrombocytopenia, leukopenia, hemolytic anemia, positive ANA, ESR increase, eosinophilia, arthritis, arthralgia, urticaria, asthenia, photosensitivity, fever, chills, flushing, malaise, dyspnea, toxic epidermal necrolysis, erythema multiforme, including Stevens-Johnson syndrome.

There have been rare postmarketing reports of cognitive impairment (e.g., memory loss, forgetfulness, amnesia, memory impairment, confusion) associated with statin use. These cognitive issues have been reported for all statins. The reports are generally nonserious, and reversible upon statin discontinuation, with variable times to symptom onset (1 day to years) and symptom resolution (median of 3 weeks).

7 DRUG INTERACTIONS

7.1 Strong CYP3A4 Inhibitors, cyclosporine, or danazol

Strong CYP3A4 inhibitors: Simvastatin, like several other inhibitors of HMG-CoA reductase, is a substrate of CYP3A4. Simvastatin is metabolized by CYP3A4 but has no CYP3A4 inhibitory activity; therefore it is not expected to affect the plasma concentrations of other drugs metabolized by CYP3A4.

Elevated plasma levels of HMG-CoA reductase inhibitory activity increases the risk of myopathy and rhabdomyolysis, particularly with higher doses of simvastatin. *[See Warnings and Precautions (5.1) and Clinical Pharmacology (12.3).]* Concomitant use of drugs labeled as having a strong inhibitory effect on CYP3A4 is contraindicated *[see Contraindications (4)]*. If treatment with itraconazole, ketoconazole, posaconazole, voriconazole, erythromycin, clarithromycin or telithromycin is unavoidable, therapy with simvastatin must be suspended during the course of treatment.

Cyclosporine or Danazol: The risk of myopathy, including rhabdomyolysis is increased by concomitant administration of cyclosporine or danazol. Therefore, concomitant use of these drugs is contraindicated. *[see Contraindications (4), Warnings and Precautions (5.1) and Clinical Pharmacology (12.3)]*.

7.2 Lipid-Lowering Drugs That Can Cause Myopathy When Given Alone

Gemfibrozil: Contraindicated with simvastatin *[see Contraindications (4) and Warnings and Precautions (5.1)]*.

Other fibrates: Caution should be used when prescribing with simvastatin *[see Warnings and Precautions (5.1)]*.

7.3 Amiodarone, Dronedarone, Ranolazine, or Calcium Channel Blockers

The risk of myopathy, including rhabdomyolysis, is increased by concomitant administration of amiodarone, dronedarone, ranolazine, or calcium channel blockers such as verapamil, diltiazem, or amlodipine *[see Dosage and Administration (2.3) and Warnings and Precautions (5.1), and Table 3 in Clinical Pharmacology (12.3)]*.

7.4 Niacin
Cases of myopathy/rhabdomyolysis have been observed with simvastatin coadministered with lipid-modifying doses (≥1 g/day niacin) of niacin-containing products. In particular, caution should be used when treating Chinese patients with simvastatin doses exceeding 20 mg/day coadministered with lipid-modifying doses of niacin-containing products. Because the risk for myopathy is dose-related, Chinese patients should not receive simvastatin 80 mg coadministered with lipid-modifying doses of niacin-containing products. *[See Warnings and Precautions (5.1) and Clinical Pharmacology (12.3).]*

7.5 Digoxin
In one study, concomitant administration of digoxin with simvastatin resulted in a slight elevation in digoxin concentrations in plasma. Patients taking digoxin should be monitored appropriately when simvastatin is initiated *[see Clinical Pharmacology (12.3)]*.

7.6 Coumarin Anticoagulants
In two clinical studies, one in normal volunteers and the other in hypercholesterolemic patients, simvastatin 20-40 mg/day modestly potentiated the effect of coumarin anticoagulants: the prothrombin time, reported as International Normalized Ratio (INR), increased from a baseline of 1.7 to 1.8 and from 2.6 to 3.4 in the volunteer and patient studies, respectively. With other statins, clinically evident bleeding and/or increased prothrombin time has been reported in a few patients taking coumarin anticoagulants concomitantly. In such patients, prothrombin time should be determined before starting simvastatin and frequently enough during early therapy to ensure that no significant alteration of prothrombin time occurs. Once a stable prothrombin time has been documented, prothrombin times can be monitored at the intervals usually recommended for patients on coumarin anticoagulants. If the dose of simvastatin is changed or discontinued, the same procedure should be repeated. Simvastatin therapy has not been associated with bleeding or with changes in prothrombin time in patients not taking anticoagulants.

7.7 Colchicine
Cases of myopathy, including rhabdomyolysis, have been reported with simvastatin coadministered with colchicine, and caution should be exercised when prescribing simvastatin with colchicine.

8 USE IN SPECIFIC POPULATIONS

8.1 Pregnancy
Pregnancy Category X [See Contraindications (4).]
ZOCOR is contraindicated in women who are or may become pregnant. Lipid lowering drugs offer no benefit during pregnancy, because cholesterol and cholesterol derivatives are needed for normal fetal development. Atherosclerosis is a chronic process, and discontinuation of lipid-lowering drugs during pregnancy should have little impact on long-term outcomes of primary hypercholesterolemia therapy. There are no adequate and well-controlled studies of use with ZOCOR during pregnancy; however, there are rare reports of congenital anomalies in infants exposed to statins *in utero*. Animal reproduction studies of simvastatin in rats and rabbits showed no evidence of teratogenicity. Serum cholesterol and triglycerides increase during normal pregnancy, and cholesterol or cholesterol derivatives are essential for fetal development. Because statins decrease cholesterol synthesis and possibly the synthesis of other biologically active substances derived from cholesterol, ZOCOR may cause fetal harm when administered to a pregnant woman. If ZOCOR is used during pregnancy or if the patient becomes pregnant while taking this drug, the patient should be apprised of the potential hazard to the fetus.
There are rare reports of congenital anomalies following intrauterine exposure to statins. In a review[3] of approximately 100 prospectively followed pregnancies in women exposed to simvastatin or another structurally-related statin, the incidences of congenital anomalies, spontaneous abortions, and fetal deaths/stillbirths did not exceed those expected in the general population. However, the study was only able to exclude a 3- to 4-fold increased risk of congenital anomalies over the background rate. In 89% of these cases, drug treatment was initiated prior to pregnancy and was discontinued during the first trimester when pregnancy was identified.
Simvastatin was not teratogenic in rats or rabbits at doses (25, 10 mg/kg/day, respectively) that resulted in 3 times the human exposure based on mg/m^2 surface area. However, in studies with another structurally-related statin, skeletal malformations were observed in rats and mice.
Women of childbearing potential, who require treatment with ZOCOR for a lipid disorder, should be advised to use effective contraception. For women trying to conceive, discontinuation of ZOCOR should be considered. If pregnancy occurs, ZOCOR should be immediately discontinued.

[3]Manson, J.M., Freyssinges, C., Ducrocq, M.B., Stephenson, W.P., Postmarketing Surveillance of Lovastatin and Simvastatin Exposure During Pregnancy, *Reproductive Toxicology*, 10(6):439-446, 1996.

8.3 Nursing Mothers
It is not known whether simvastatin is excreted in human milk. Because a small amount of another drug in this class is excreted in human milk and because of the potential for serious adverse reactions in nursing infants, women taking simvastatin should not nurse their infants. A decision should be made whether to discontinue nursing or discontinue drug, taking into account the importance of the drug to the mother *[see Contraindications (4)]*.

8.4 Pediatric Use
Safety and effectiveness of simvastatin in patients 10-17 years of age with heterozygous familial hypercholesterolemia have been evaluated in a controlled clinical trial in adolescent boys and in girls who were at least 1 year post-menarche. Patients treated with simvastatin had an adverse reaction profile similar to that of patients treated with placebo. **Doses greater than 40 mg have not been studied in this population.** In this limited controlled study, there was no significant effect on growth or sexual maturation in the adolescent boys or girls, or on menstrual cycle length in girls. *[See Dosage and Administration (2.5), Adverse Reactions (6.1), Clinical Studies (14.2).]* Adolescent females should be counseled on appropriate contraceptive methods while on simvastatin therapy *[see Contraindications (4) and Use in Specific Populations (8.1)]*. Simvastatin has not been studied in patients younger than 10 years of age, nor in pre-menarchal girls.

8.5 Geriatric Use
Of the 2,423 patients who received ZOCOR in Phase III clinical studies and the 10,269 patients in the Heart Protection Study who received ZOCOR, 363 (15%) and 5,366 (52%), respectively were ≥65 years old. In HPS, 615 (6%) were ≥75 years old. No overall differences in safety or effectiveness were observed between these subjects and younger subjects, and other reported clinical experience has not identified differences in responses between the elderly and younger patients, but greater sensitivity of some older individuals cannot be ruled out. Since advanced age (≥65 years) is a predisposing factor for myopathy, ZOCOR should be prescribed with caution in the elderly. *[See Clinical Pharmacology (12.3).]*
A pharmacokinetic study with simvastatin showed the mean plasma level of statin activity to be approximately 45% higher in elderly patients between 70-78 years of age compared with patients between 18-30 years of age. In 4S, 1,021 (23%) of 4,444 patients were 65 or older. Lipid-lowering efficacy was at least as great in elderly patients compared with younger patients, and ZOCOR significantly reduced total mortality and CHD mortality in elderly patients with a history of CHD. In HPS, 52% of patients were elderly (4,891 patients 65-69 years and 5,806 patients 70 years or older). The relative risk reductions of CHD death, non-fatal MI, coronary and non-coronary revascularization procedures, and stroke were similar in older and younger patients *[see Clinical Studies (14.1)]*. In HPS, among 32,145 patients entering the active run-in period, there were 2 cases of myopathy/rhabdomyolysis; these patients were aged 67 and 73. Of the 7 cases of myopathy/rhabdomyolysis among 10,269 patients allocated to simvastatin, 4 were aged 65 or more (at baseline), of whom one was over 75. There were no overall differences in safety between older and younger patients in either 4S or HPS.
Because advanced age (≥65 years) is a predisposing factor for myopathy, including rhabdomyolysis, ZOCOR should be prescribed with caution in the elderly. In a clinical trial of patients treated with simvastatin 80 mg/day, patients ≥65 years of age had an increased risk of myopathy, including rhabdomyolysis, compared to patients <65 years of age. *[See Warnings and Precautions (5.1) and Clinical Pharmacology (12.3).]*

8.6 Renal Impairment
Caution should be exercised when ZOCOR is administered to patients with severe renal impairment. *[See Dosage and Administration (2.6).]*

8.7 Hepatic Impairment
ZOCOR is contraindicated in patients with active liver disease which may include unexplained persistent elevations in hepatic transaminase levels *[see Contraindications (4) and Warnings and Precautions (5.2)]*.

10 OVERDOSAGE

Significant lethality was observed in mice after a single oral dose of 9 g/m^2. No evidence of lethality was observed in rats or dogs treated with doses of 30 and 100 g/m^2, respectively. No specific diagnostic signs were observed in rodents. At these doses the only signs seen in dogs were emesis and mucoid stools.
A few cases of overdosage with ZOCOR have been reported; the maximum dose taken was 3.6 g. All patients recovered without sequelae. Supportive measures should be taken in the event of an overdose. The dialyzability of simvastatin and its metabolites in man is not known at present.

11 DESCRIPTION

ZOCOR (simvastatin) is a lipid-lowering agent that is derived synthetically from a fermentation product of *Aspergillus terreus*. After oral ingestion, simvastatin, which is an inactive lactone, is hydrolyzed to the corresponding β-hydroxyacid form. This is an inhibitor of 3-hydroxy-3-methylglutaryl-coenzyme A (HMG-CoA) reductase. This enzyme catalyzes the conversion of HMG-CoA to mevalonate, which is an early and rate-limiting step in the biosynthesis of cholesterol.
Simvastatin is butanoic acid, 2,2-dimethyl-,1,2,3,7,8,8a-hexahydro-3,7-dimethyl-8-[2-(tetrahydro-4-hydroxy-6-oxo-2*H*-pyran-2-yl)-ethyl]-1-naphthalenyl ester, [1*S*-[1α,3α,7β, 8β(2*S**,4*S**),-8aβ]]. The empirical formula of simvastatin is $C_{25}H_{38}O_5$ and its molecular weight is 418.57. Its structural formula is:

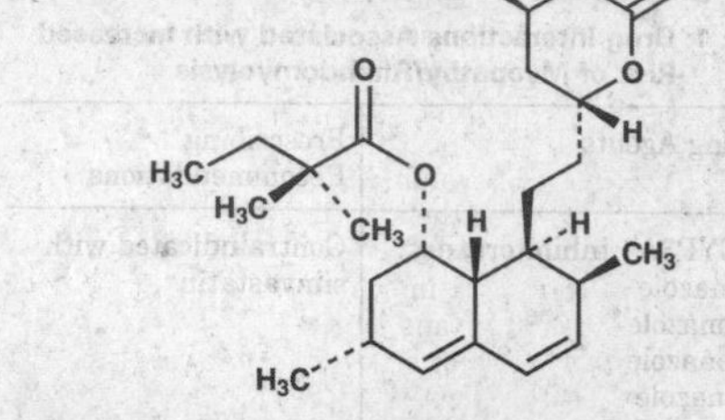

Simvastatin is a white to off-white, nonhygroscopic, crystalline powder that is practically insoluble in water, and freely soluble in chloroform, methanol and ethanol.
Tablets ZOCOR for oral administration contain either 5 mg, 10 mg, 20 mg, 40 mg or 80 mg of simvastatin and the following inactive ingredients: ascorbic acid, citric acid, hydroxypropyl cellulose, hypromellose, iron oxides, lactose, magnesium stearate, microcrystalline cellulose, starch, talc, and titanium dioxide. Butylated hydroxyanisole is added as a preservative.

12 CLINICAL PHARMACOLOGY

12.1 Mechanism of Action
Simvastatin is a prodrug and is hydrolyzed to its active β-hydroxyacid form, simvastatin acid, after administration. Simvastatin is a specific inhibitor of 3-hydroxy-3-methylglutaryl-coenzyme A (HMG-CoA) reductase, the enzyme that catalyzes the conversion of HMG-CoA to mevalonate, an early and rate limiting step in the biosynthetic pathway for cholesterol. In addition, simvastatin reduces VLDL and TG and increases HDL-C.

12.2 Pharmacodynamics
Epidemiological studies have demonstrated that elevated levels of total-C, LDL-C, as well as decreased levels of HDL-C are associated with the development of atherosclerosis and increased cardiovascular risk. Lowering LDL-C decreases this risk. However, the independent effect of raising HDL-C or lowering TG on the risk of coronary and cardiovascular morbidity and mortality has not been determined.

12.3 Pharmacokinetics
Simvastatin is a lactone that is readily hydrolyzed *in vivo* to the corresponding β-hydroxyacid, a potent inhibitor of HMG-CoA reductase. Inhibition of HMG-CoA reductase is the basis for an assay in pharmacokinetic studies of the β-hydroxyacid metabolites (active inhibitors) and, following base hydrolysis, active plus latent inhibitors (total inhibitors) in plasma following administration of simvastatin.
Following an oral dose of ^{14}C-labeled simvastatin in man, 13% of the dose was excreted in urine and 60% in feces. Plasma concentrations of total radioactivity (simvastatin plus ^{14}C-metabolites) peaked at 4 hours and declined rapidly to about 10% of peak by 12 hours postdose. Since simvastatin undergoes extensive first-pass extraction in the liver, the availability of the drug to the general circulation is low (<5%).
Both simvastatin and its β-hydroxyacid metabolite are highly bound (approximately 95%) to human plasma proteins. Rat studies indicate that when radiolabeled simvastatin was administered, simvastatin-derived radioactivity crossed the blood-brain barrier.
The major active metabolites of simvastatin present in human plasma are the β-hydroxyacid of simvastatin and its 6′-hydroxy, 6′-hydroxymethyl, and 6′-exomethylene derivatives. Peak plasma concentrations of both active and total inhibitors were attained within 1.3 to 2.4 hours postdose. While the recommended therapeutic dose range is 5 to 40 mg/day, there was no substantial deviation from linearity of AUC of inhibitors in the general circulation with an increase in dose to as high as 120 mg. Relative to the fasting state, the plasma profile of inhibitors was not affected when simvastatin was administered immediately before an American Heart Association recommended low-fat meal.
In a study including 16 elderly patients between 70 and 78 years of age who received ZOCOR 40 mg/day, the mean plasma level of HMG-CoA reductase inhibitory activity was increased approximately 45% compared with 18 patients between 18-30 years of age. Clinical study experience in the

elderly (n=1522), suggests that there were no overall differences in safety between elderly and younger patients *[see Use in Specific Populations (8.5)]*.

Kinetic studies with another statin, having a similar principal route of elimination, have suggested that for a given dose level higher systemic exposure may be achieved in patients with severe renal insufficiency (as measured by creatinine clearance).

Although the mechanism is not fully understood, cyclosporine has been shown to increase the AUC of statins. The increase in AUC for simvastatin acid is presumably due, in part, to inhibition of CYP3A4.

The risk of myopathy is increased by high levels of HMG-CoA reductase inhibitory activity in plasma. Inhibitors of CYP3A4 can raise the plasma levels of HMG-CoA reductase inhibitory activity and increase the risk of myopathy *[see Warnings and Precautions (5.1) and Drug Interactions (7.1)]*.

[See table 3 above]

In a study of 12 healthy volunteers, simvastatin at the 80-mg dose had no effect on the metabolism of the probe cytochrome P450 isoform 3A4 (CYP3A4) substrates midazolam and erythromycin. This indicates that simvastatin is not an inhibitor of CYP3A4, and, therefore, is not expected to affect the plasma levels of other drugs metabolized by CYP3A4.

Coadministration of simvastatin (40 mg QD for 10 days) resulted in an increase in the maximum mean levels of cardioactive digoxin (given as a single 0.4 mg dose on day 10) by approximately 0.3 ng/mL.

13 NONCLINICAL TOXICOLOGY

13.1 Carcinogenesis, Mutagenesis, Impairment of Fertility

In a 72-week carcinogenicity study, mice were administered daily doses of simvastatin of 25, 100, and 400 mg/kg body weight, which resulted in mean plasma drug levels approximately 1, 4, and 8 times higher than the mean human plasma drug level, respectively (as total inhibitory activity based on AUC) after an 80-mg oral dose. Liver carcinomas were significantly increased in high-dose females and mid- and high-dose males with a maximum incidence of 90% in males. The incidence of adenomas of the liver was significantly increased in mid- and high-dose females. Drug treatment also significantly increased the incidence of lung adenomas in mid- and high-dose males and females. Adenomas of the Harderian gland (a gland of the eye of rodents) were significantly higher in high-dose mice than in controls. No evidence of a tumorigenic effect was observed at 25 mg/kg/day.

In a separate 92-week carcinogenicity study in mice at doses up to 25 mg/kg/day, no evidence of a tumorigenic effect was observed (mean plasma drug levels were 1 times higher than humans given 80 mg simvastatin as measured by AUC).

In a two-year study in rats at 25 mg/kg/day, there was a statistically significant increase in the incidence of thyroid follicular adenomas in female rats exposed to approximately 11 times higher levels of simvastatin than in humans given 80 mg simvastatin (as measured by AUC).

A second two-year rat carcinogenicity study with doses of 50 and 100 mg/kg/day produced hepatocellular adenomas and carcinomas (in female rats at both doses and in males at 100 mg/kg/day). Thyroid follicular cell adenomas were increased in males and females at both doses; thyroid follicular cell carcinomas were increased in females at 100 mg/kg/day. The increased incidence of thyroid neoplasms appears to be consistent with findings from other statins. These treatment levels represented plasma drug levels (AUC) of approximately 7 and 15 times (males) and 22 and 25 times (females) the mean human plasma drug exposure after an 80 milligram daily dose.

No evidence of mutagenicity was observed in a microbial mutagenicity (Ames) test with or without rat or mouse liver metabolic activation. In addition, no evidence of damage to genetic material was noted in an *in vitro* alkaline elution assay using rat hepatocytes, a V-79 mammalian cell forward mutation study, an *in vitro* chromosome aberration study in CHO cells, or an *in vivo* chromosomal aberration assay in mouse bone marrow.

There was decreased fertility in male rats treated with simvastatin for 34 weeks at 25 mg/kg body weight (4 times the maximum human exposure level, based on AUC, in patients receiving 80 mg/day); however, this effect was not observed during a subsequent fertility study in which simvastatin was administered at this same dose level to male rats for 11 weeks (the entire cycle of spermatogenesis including epididymal maturation). No microscopic changes were observed in the testes of rats from either study. At 180 mg/kg/day, (which produces exposure levels 22 times higher than those in humans taking 80 mg/day based on surface area, mg/m^2), seminiferous tubule degeneration (necrosis and loss of spermatogenic epithelium) was observed. In dogs, there was drug-related testicular atrophy, de-

TABLE 3: Effect of Coadministered Drugs or Grapefruit Juice on Simvastatin Systemic Exposure

Coadministered Drug or Grapefruit Juice	Dosing of Coadministered Drug or Grapefruit Juice	Dosing of Simvastatin	Geometric Mean Ratio (Ratio* with / without coadministered drug) No Effect = 1.00		
				AUC	C_{max}
Contraindicated with simvastatin *[see Contraindications (4) and Warnings and Precautions (5.1)]*					
Telithromycin†	200 mg QD for 4 days	80 mg	simvastatin acid‡ simvastatin	12 8.9	15 5.3
Nelfinavir†	1250 mg BID for 14 days	20 mg QD for 28 days	simvastatin acid‡ simvastatin	 6	 6.2
Itraconazole†	200 mg QD for 4 days	80 mg	simvastatin acid‡ simvastatin		13.1 13.1
Posaconazole	100 mg (oral suspension) QD for 13 days	40 mg	simvastatin acid simvastatin	7.3 10.3	9.2 9.4
	200 mg (oral suspension) QD for 13 days	40 mg	simvastatin acid simvastatin	8.5 10.6	9.5 11.4
Gemfibrozil	600 mg BID for 3 days	40 mg	simvastatin acid simvastatin	2.85 1.35	2.18 0.91
Avoid grapefruit juice with simvastatin *[see Warnings and Precautions (5.1)]*					
Grapefruit Juice§ (high dose)	200 mL of double-strength TID¶	60 mg single dose	simvastatin acid simvastatin	7 16	
Grapefruit Juice§ (low dose)	8 oz (about 237mL) of single-strength#	20 mg single dose	simvastatin acid simvastatin	1.3 1.9	
Avoid taking with >10 mg simvastatin, based on clinical and/or post-marketing experience *[see Warnings and Precautions (5.1)]*					
Verapamil SR	240 mg QD Days 1-7 then 240 mg BID on Days 8-10	80 mg on Day 10	simvastatin acid simvastatin	2.3 2.5	2.4 2.1
Diltiazem	120 mg BID for 10 days	80 mg on Day 10	simvastatin acid simvastatin	2.69 3.10	2.69 2.88
Diltiazem	120 mg BID for 14 days	20 mg on Day 14	simvastatin	4.6	3.6
Dronedarone	400 mg BID for 14 days	40 mg QD for 14 days	simvastatin acid simvastatin	1.96 3.90	2.14 3.75
Avoid taking with >20 mg simvastatin, based on clinical and/or post-marketing experience *[see Warnings and Precautions (5.1)]*					
Amiodarone	400 mg QD for 3 days	40 mg on Day 3	simvastatin acid simvastatin	1.75 1.76	1.72 1.79
Amlodipine	10 mg QD × 10 days	80 mg on Day 10	simvastatin acid simvastatin	1.58 1.77	1.56 1.47
Ranolazine SR	1000 mg BID for 7 days	80 mg on Day 1 and Days 6-9	simvastatin acid simvastatin	2.26 1.86	2.28 1.75
No dosing adjustments required for the following:					
Fenofibrate	160 mg QD × 14 days	80 mg QD on Days 8-14	simvastatin acid simvastatin	0.64 0.89	0.89 0.83
Niacin extended-releaseÞ	2 g single dose	20 mg single dose	simvastatin acid simvastatin	1.6 1.4	1.84 1.08
Propranolol	80 mg single dose	80 mg single dose	total inhibitor active inhibitor	0.79 0.79	↓ from 33.6 to 21.1 ng•eq/mL ↓ from 7.0 to 4.7 ng•eq/mL

* Results based on a chemical assay except results with propranolol as indicated.
† Results could be representative of the following CYP3A4 inhibitors: ketoconazole, erythromycin, clarithromycin, HIV protease inhibitors, and nefazodone.
‡ Simvastatin acid refers to the β-hydroxyacid of simvastatin.
§ The effect of amounts of grapefruit juice between those used in these two studies on simvastatin pharmacokinetics has not been studied.
¶ Double-strength: one can of frozen concentrate diluted with one can of water. Grapefruit juice was administered TID for 2 days, and 200 mL together with single dose simvastatin and 30 and 90 minutes following single dose simvastatin on Day 3.
\# Single-strength: one can of frozen concentrate diluted with 3 cans of water. Grapefruit juice was administered with breakfast for 3 days, and simvastatin was administered in the evening on Day 3.
Þ Because Chinese patients have an increased risk for myopathy with simvastatin coadministered with lipid-modifying doses (≥ 1 gram/day niacin) of niacin-containing products, and the risk is dose-related, Chinese patients should not receive simvastatin 80 mg coadministered with lipid-modifying doses of niacin-containing products *[see Warnings and Precautions (5.1) and Drug Interactions (7.4)]*.

TABLE 4: Summary of Heart Protection Study Results

Endpoint	ZOCOR (N=10,269) n (%)*	Placebo (N=10,267) n (%)*	Risk Reduction (%) (95% CI)	p-Value
Primary				
Mortality	1,328 (12.9)	1,507 (14.7)	13 (6-19)	p=0.0003
CHD mortality	587 (5.7)	707 (6.9)	18 (8-26)	p=0.0005
Secondary				
Non-fatal MI	357 (3.5)	574 (5.6)	38 (30-46)	p<0.0001
Stroke	444 (4.3)	585 (5.7)	25 (15-34)	p<0.0001
Tertiary				
Coronary revascularization	513 (5)	725 (7.1)	30 (22-38)	p<0.0001
Peripheral and other non-coronary revascularization	450 (4.4)	532 (5.2)	16 (5-26)	p=0.006

* n = number of patients with indicated event

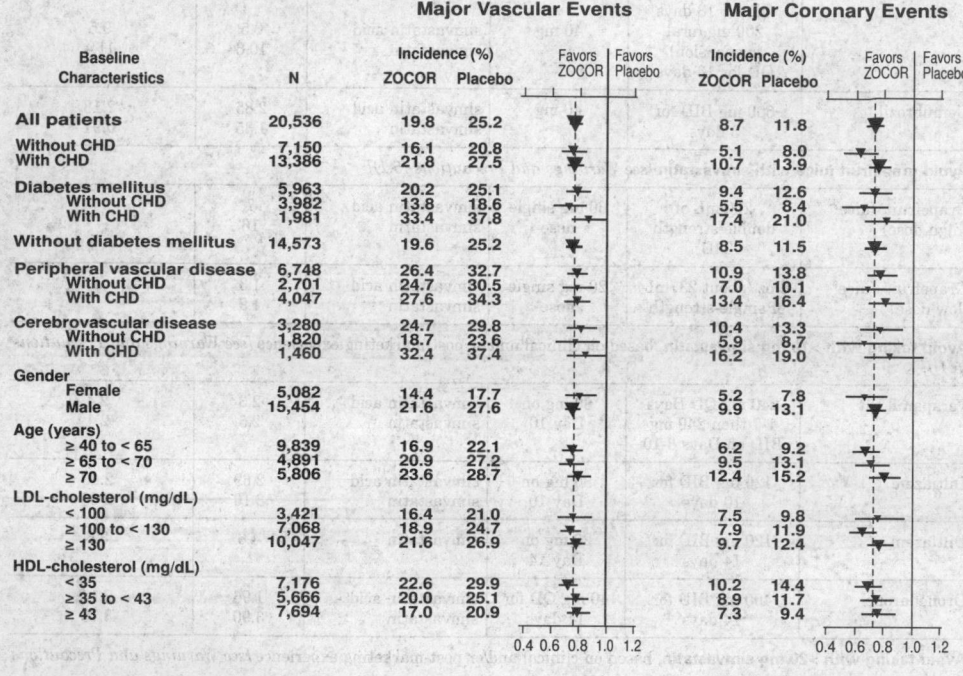

Baseline Characteristics	N	Major Vascular Events: Incidence (%) ZOCOR	Major Vascular Events: Incidence (%) Placebo	Major Coronary Events: Incidence (%) ZOCOR	Major Coronary Events: Incidence (%) Placebo
All patients	20,536	19.8	25.2	8.7	11.8
Without CHD	7,150	16.1	20.8	5.1	8.0
With CHD	13,386	21.8	27.5	10.7	13.9
Diabetes mellitus	5,963	20.2	25.1	9.4	12.6
Without CHD	3,982	13.8	18.6	5.5	8.4
With CHD	1,981	33.4	37.8	17.4	21.0
Without diabetes mellitus	14,573	19.6	25.2	8.5	11.5
Peripheral vascular disease	6,748	26.4	32.7	10.9	13.8
Without CHD	2,701	24.7	30.5	7.0	10.1
With CHD	4,047	27.6	34.3	13.4	16.4
Cerebrovascular disease	3,280	24.7	29.8	10.4	13.3
Without CHD	1,820	18.7	23.6	5.9	8.7
With CHD	1,460	32.4	37.4	16.2	19.0
Gender					
Female	5,082	14.4	17.7	5.2	7.8
Male	15,454	21.6	27.6	9.9	13.1
Age (years)					
≥ 40 to < 65	9,839	16.9	22.1	6.2	9.2
≥ 65 to < 70	4,891	20.9	27.2	9.5	13.1
≥ 70	5,806	23.6	28.7	12.4	15.2
LDL-cholesterol (mg/dL)					
< 100	3,421	16.4	21.0	7.5	9.8
≥ 100 to < 130	7,068	18.9	24.7	7.9	11.9
≥ 130	10,047	21.6	26.9	9.7	12.4
HDL-cholesterol (mg/dL)					
< 35	7,176	22.6	29.9	10.2	14.4
≥ 35 to < 43	5,666	20.0	25.1	8.9	11.7
≥ 43	7,694	17.0	20.9	7.3	9.4

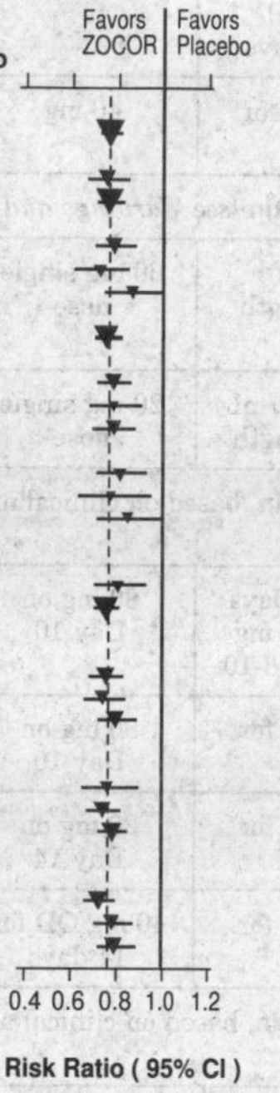

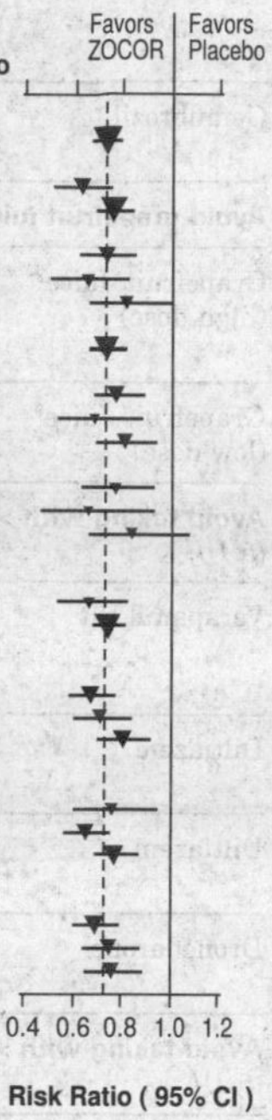

N = number of patients in each subgroup. The inverted triangles are point estimates of the relative risk, with their 95% confidence intervals represented as a line. The area of a triangle is proportional to the number of patients with MVE or MCE in the subgroup relative to the number with MVE or MCE, respectively, in the entire study population. The vertical solid line represents a relative risk of one. The vertical dashed line represents the point estimate of relative risk in the entire study population.

Figure 1: The Effects of Treatment with ZOCOR on Major Vascular Events and Major Coronary Events in HPS

creased spermatogenesis, spermatocytic degeneration and giant cell formation at 10 mg/kg/day, (approximately 2 times the human exposure, based on AUC, at 80 mg/day). The clinical significance of these findings is unclear.

13.2 Animal Toxicology and/or Pharmacology

CNS Toxicity

Optic nerve degeneration was seen in clinically normal dogs treated with simvastatin for 14 weeks at 180 mg/kg/day, a dose that produced mean plasma drug levels about 12 times higher than the mean plasma drug level in humans taking 80 mg/day.

A chemically similar drug in this class also produced optic nerve degeneration (Wallerian degeneration of retinogeniculate fibers) in clinically normal dogs in a dose-dependent fashion starting at 60 mg/kg/day, a dose that produced mean plasma drug levels about 30 times higher than the mean plasma drug level in humans taking the highest recommended dose (as measured by total enzyme inhibitory activity). This same drug also produced vestibulocochlear Wallerian-like degeneration and retinal ganglion cell chromatolysis in dogs treated for 14 weeks at 180 mg/kg/day, a dose that resulted in a mean plasma drug level similar to that seen with the 60 mg/kg/day dose.

CNS vascular lesions, characterized by perivascular hemorrhage and edema, mononuclear cell infiltration of perivascular spaces, perivascular fibrin deposits and necrosis of small vessels were seen in dogs treated with simvastatin at a dose of 360 mg/kg/day, a dose that produced mean plasma drug levels that were about 14 times higher than the mean plasma drug levels in humans taking 80 mg/day. Similar CNS vascular lesions have been observed with several other drugs of this class.

There were cataracts in female rats after two years of treatment with 50 and 100 mg/kg/day (22 and 25 times the human AUC at 80 mg/day, respectively) and in dogs after three months at 90 mg/kg/day (19 times) and at two years at 50 mg/kg/day (5 times).

14 CLINICAL STUDIES

14.1 Clinical Studies in Adults

Reductions in Risk of CHD Mortality and Cardiovascular Events

In 4S, the effect of therapy with ZOCOR on total mortality was assessed in 4,444 patients with CHD and baseline total cholesterol 212-309 mg/dL (5.5-8.0 mmol/L). In this multicenter, randomized, double-blind, placebo-controlled study, patients were treated with standard care, including diet, and either ZOCOR 20-40 mg/day (n=2,221) or placebo (n=2,223) for a median duration of 5.4 years. Over the course of the study, treatment with ZOCOR led to mean reductions in total-C, LDL-C and TG of 25%, 35%, and 10%, respectively, and a mean increase in HDL-C of 8%. ZOCOR significantly reduced the risk of mortality by 30% (p=0.0003, 182 deaths in the ZOCOR group vs 256 deaths in the placebo group). The risk of CHD mortality was significantly reduced by 42% (p=0.00001, 111 vs 189 deaths). There was no statistically significant difference between groups in non-cardiovascular mortality. ZOCOR significantly decreased the risk of having major coronary events (CHD mortality plus hospital-verified and silent non-fatal myocardial infarction [MI]) by 34% (p<0.00001, 431 vs 622 patients with one or more events). The risk of having a hospital-verified non-fatal MI was reduced by 37%. ZOCOR significantly reduced the risk for undergoing myocardial revascularization procedures (coronary artery bypass grafting or percutaneous transluminal coronary angioplasty) by 37% (p<0.00001, 252 vs 383 patients). ZOCOR significantly reduced the risk of fatal plus non-fatal cerebrovascular events (combined stroke and transient ischemic attacks) by 28% (p=0.033, 75 vs 102 patients). ZOCOR reduced the risk of major coronary events to a similar extent across the range of baseline total and LDL cholesterol levels. Because there were only 53 female deaths, the effect of ZOCOR on mortality in women could not be adequately assessed. However, ZOCOR significantly lessened the risk of having major coronary events by 34% (60 vs 91 women with one or more event). The randomization was stratified by angina alone (21% of each treatment group) or a previous MI. Because there were only 57 deaths among the patients with angina alone at baseline, the effect of ZOCOR on mortality in this subgroup could not be adequately assessed. However, trends in reduced coronary mortality, major coronary events and revascularization procedures were consistent between this group and the total study cohort. Additionally, ZOCOR resulted in similar decreases in relative risk for total mortality, CHD mortality, and major coronary events in elderly patients (≥65 years), compared with younger patients.

The Heart Protection Study (HPS) was a large, multicenter, placebo-controlled, double-blind study with a mean duration of 5 years conducted in 20,536 patients (10,269 on ZOCOR 40 mg and 10,267 on placebo). Patients were allocated to treatment using a covariate adaptive method[4] which took into account the distribution of 10 important baseline characteristics of patients already enrolled and minimized the imbalance of those characteristics across the groups. Patients had a mean age of 64 years (range 40-80 years), were 97% Caucasian and were at high risk of developing a major coronary event because of existing CHD (65%), diabetes (Type 2, 26%; Type 1, 3%), history of stroke or other cerebrovascular disease (16%), peripheral vessel disease (33%), or hypertension in males ≥65 years (6%). At baseline, 3,421 patients (17%) had LDL-C levels below 100 mg/dL, of whom 953 (5%) had LDL-C levels below 80 mg/dL; 7,068 patients (34%) had levels between 100 and 130 mg/dL; and 10,047 patients (49%) had levels greater than 130 mg/dL.

The HPS results showed that ZOCOR 40 mg/day significantly reduced: total and CHD mortality; non-fatal MI, stroke, and revascularization procedures (coronary and non-coronary) (see Table 4).

[See table 4 above]

Two composite endpoints were defined in order to have sufficient events to assess relative risk reductions across a range of baseline characteristics (see Figure 1). A composite of major coronary events (MCE) was comprised of CHD mortality and non-fatal MI (analyzed by time-to-first event; 898 patients treated with ZOCOR had events and 1,212 patients on placebo had events). A composite of major vascular events (MVE) was comprised of MCE, stroke and revascularization procedures including coronary, peripheral and other non-coronary procedures (analyzed by time-to-first event; 2,033 patients treated with ZOCOR had events and 2,585 patients on placebo had events). Significant relative risk reductions were observed for both composite endpoints (27% for MCE and 24% for MVE, p<0.0001). Treatment with ZOCOR produced significant relative risk reductions for all components of the composite endpoints. The risk reductions produced by ZOCOR in both MCE and MVE were evident and consistent regardless of cardiovascular disease related medical history at study entry (i.e., CHD alone; or peripheral vascular disease, cerebrovascular disease, diabetes or treated hypertension, with or without CHD), gender, age, creatinine levels up to the entry limit of 2.3 mg/dL, baseline levels of LDL-C, HDL-C, apolipoprotein B and A-1, baseline concomitant cardiovascular medications (i.e., aspirin, beta blockers, or calcium channel blockers), smoking status, alcohol intake, or obesity. Diabetics showed risk reductions for MCE and MVE due to ZOCOR treatment regardless of baseline HbA1c levels or obesity with the greatest effects seen for diabetics without CHD.

[See figure 1 above]

Angiographic Studies

In the Multicenter Anti-Atheroma Study, the effect of simvastatin on atherosclerosis was assessed by quantitative coronary angiography in hypercholesterolemic patients with CHD. In this randomized, double-blind, controlled study, patients were treated with simvastatin 20 mg/day or placebo. Angiograms were evaluated at baseline, two and four years. The co-primary study endpoints were mean change per-patient in minimum and mean lumen diameters, indicating focal and diffuse disease, respectively.

ZOCOR significantly slowed the progression of lesions as measured in the Year 4 angiogram by both parameters, as well as by change in percent diameter stenosis. In addition, simvastatin significantly decreased the proportion of patients with new lesions and with new total occlusions.

Modifications of Lipid Profiles

Primary Hyperlipidemia (Fredrickson type IIa and IIb)

ZOCOR has been shown to be effective in reducing total-C and LDL-C in heterozygous familial and non-familial forms of hyperlipidemia and in mixed hyperlipidemia. Maximal to near maximal response is generally achieved within 4-6 weeks and maintained during chronic therapy. ZOCOR consistently and significantly decreased total-C, LDL-C, total-C/HDL-C ratio, and LDL-C/HDL-C ratio; ZOCOR also decreased TG and increased HDL-C (see Table 5).

[See table 5 above]

Hypertriglyceridemia (Fredrickson type IV)

The results of a subgroup analysis in 74 patients with type IV hyperlipidemia from a 130-patient, double-blind, placebo-controlled, 3-period crossover study are presented in Table 6.

[See table 6 below]

Dysbetalipoproteinemia (Fredrickson type III)

The results of a subgroup analysis in 7 patients with type III hyperlipidemia (dysbetalipoproteinemia) (apo E2/2) (VLDL-C/TG>0.25) from a 130-patient, double-blind, placebo-controlled, 3-period crossover study are presented in Table 7.

[See table 7 below]

Homozygous Familial Hypercholesterolemia

In a controlled clinical study, 12 patients 15-39 years of age with homozygous familial hypercholesterolemia received simvastatin 40 mg/day in a single dose or in 3 divided doses, or 80 mg/day in 3 divided doses. In 11 patients with reductions in LDL-C, the mean LDL-C changes for the 40- and 80-mg doses were 14% (range 8% to 23%, median 12%) and 30% (range 14% to 46%, median 29%), respectively. One patient had an increase of 15% in LDL-C. Another patient with absent LDL-C receptor function had an LDL-C reduction of 41% with the 80-mg dose.

Endocrine Function

In clinical studies, simvastatin did not impair adrenal reserve or significantly reduce basal plasma cortisol concentration. Small reductions from baseline in basal plasma testosterone in men were observed in clinical studies with simvastatin, an effect also observed with other statins and the bile acid sequestrant cholestyramine. There was no effect on plasma gonadotropin levels. In a placebo-controlled, 12-week study there was no significant effect of simvastatin 80 mg on the plasma testosterone response to human chorionic gonadotropin. In another 24-week study, simvastatin 20-40 mg had no detectable effect on spermatogenesis. In 4S, in which 4,444 patients were randomized to simvastatin 20-40 mg/day or placebo for a median duration of 5.4 years, the incidence of male sexual adverse events in the two treatment groups was not significantly different. Because of these factors, the small changes in plasma testosterone are unlikely to be clinically significant. The effects, if any, on the pituitary-gonadal axis in pre-menopausal women are unknown.

---

[4]D.R. Taves, Minimization: a new method of assigning patients to treatment and control groups. Clin. Pharmacol. Ther. 15 (1974), pp. 443-453

14.2 Clinical Studies in Adolescents

In a double-blind, placebo-controlled study, 175 patients (99 adolescent boys and 76 post-menarchal girls) 10-17 years of age (mean age 14.1 years) with heterozygous familial hypercholesterolemia (HeFH) were randomized to simvastatin (n=106) or placebo (n=67) for 24 weeks (base study). Inclusion in the study required a baseline LDL-C level between 160 and 400 mg/dL and at least one parent with an LDL-C level >189 mg/dL. The dosage of simvastatin (once daily in the evening) was 10 mg for the first 8 weeks, 20 mg for the second 8 weeks, and 40 mg thereafter. In a 24-week extension, 144 patients elected to continue therapy with simvastatin 40 mg or placebo.

ZOCOR significantly decreased plasma levels of total-C, LDL-C, and Apo B (see Table 8). Results from the extension at 48 weeks were comparable to those observed in the base study.

[See table 8 above]

After 24 weeks of treatment, the mean achieved LDL-C value was 124.9 mg/dL (range: 64.0-289.0 mg/dL) in the ZOCOR 40 mg group compared to 207.8 mg/dL (range: 128.0-334.0 mg/dL) in the placebo group.

The safety and efficacy of doses above 40 mg daily have not been studied in children with HeFH. The long-term efficacy of simvastatin therapy in childhood to reduce morbidity and mortality in adulthood has not been established.

16 HOW SUPPLIED/STORAGE AND HANDLING

No. 8360 — Tablets ZOCOR 5 mg are buff, oval, film-coated tablets, coded MSD 726 on one side and ZOCOR 5 on the other. They are supplied as follows:

NDC 0006-0726-31 unit of use bottles of 30.

No. 8146 — Tablets ZOCOR 10 mg are peach, oval, film-coated tablets, coded MSD 735 on one side and plain on the other. They are supplied as follows:

TABLE 5: Mean Response in Patients with Primary Hyperlipidemia and Combined (mixed) Hyperlipidemia (Mean Percent Change from Baseline After 6 to 24 Weeks)

TREATMENT	N	TOTAL-C	LDL-C	HDL-C	TG*
Lower Dose Comparative Study† (Mean % Change at Week 6)					
ZOCOR 5 mg q.p.m.	109	-19	-26	10	-12
ZOCOR 10 mg q.p.m.	110	-23	-30	12	-15
Scandinavian Simvastatin Survival Study‡ (Mean % Change at Week 6)					
Placebo	2223	-1	-1	0	-2
ZOCOR 20 mg q.p.m.	2221	-28	-38	8	-19
Upper Dose Comparative Study§ (Mean % Change Averaged at Weeks 18 and 24)					
ZOCOR 40 mg q.p.m.	433	-31	-41	9	-18
ZOCOR 80 mg q.p.m.¶	664	-36	-47	8	-24
Multi-Center Combined Hyperlipidemia Study# (Mean % Change at Week 6)					
Placebo	125	1	2	3	-4
ZOCOR 40 mg q.p.m.	123	-25	-29	13	-28
ZOCOR 80 mg q.p.m.	124	-31	-36	16	-33

* median percent change
† mean baseline LDL-C 244 mg/dL and median baseline TG 168 mg/dL
‡ mean baseline LDL-C 188 mg/dL and median baseline TG 128 mg/dL
§ mean baseline LDL-C 226 mg/dL and median baseline TG 156 mg/dL
¶ 21% and 36% median reduction in TG in patients with TG ≤200 mg/dL and TG >200 mg/dL, respectively. Patients with TG >350 mg/dL were excluded
\# mean baseline LDL-C 156 mg/dL and median baseline TG 391 mg/dL.

TABLE 6: Six-week, Lipid-lowering Effects of Simvastatin in Type IV Hyperlipidemia Median Percent Change (25th and 75th percentile) from Baseline*

TREATMENT	N	Total-C	LDL-C	HDL-C	TG	VLDL-C	Non-HDL-C
Placebo	74	+2 (-7, +7)	+1 (-8, +14)	+3 (-3, +10)	-9 (-25, +13)	-7 (-25, +11)	+1 (-9, +8)
ZOCOR 40 mg/day	74	-25 (-34, -19)	-28 (-40, -17)	+11 (+5, +23)	-29 (-43, -16)	-37 (-54, -23)	-32 (-42, -23)
ZOCOR 80 mg/day	74	-32 (-38, -24)	-37 (-46, -26)	+15 (+5, +23)	-34 (-45, -18)	-41 (-57, -28)	-38 (-49, -32)

* The median baseline values (mg/dL) for the patients in this study were: total-C = 254, LDL-C = 135, HDL-C = 36, TG = 404, VLDL-C = 83, and non-HDL-C = 215.

TABLE 7: Six-week, Lipid-lowering Effects of Simvastatin in Type III Hyperlipidemia Median Percent Change (min, max) from Baseline*

TREATMENT	N	Total-C	LDL-C + IDL	HDL-C	TG	VLDL-C+IDL	Non-HDL-C
Placebo	7	-8 (-24, +34)	-8 (-27, +23)	-2 (-21, +16)	+4 (-22, +90)	-4 (-28, +78)	-8 (-26, -39)
ZOCOR 40 mg/day	7	-50 (-66, -39)	-50 (-60, -31)	+7 (-8, +23)	-41 (-74, -16)	-58 (-90, -37)	-57 (-72, -44)
ZOCOR 80 mg/day	7	-52 (-55, -41)	-51 (-57, -28)	+7 (-5, +29)	-38 (-58, +2)	-60 (-72, -39)	-59 (-61, -46)

* The median baseline values (mg/dL) were: total-C = 324, LDL-C = 121, HDL-C = 31, TG = 411, VLDL-C = 170, and non-HDL-C = 291.

TABLE 8: Lipid-Lowering Effects of Simvastatin in Adolescent Patients with Heterozygous Familial Hypercholesterolemia (Mean Percent Change from Baseline)

Dosage	Duration	N		Total-C	LDL-C	HDL-C	TG*	Apo B
Placebo	24 Weeks	67	% Change from Baseline (95% CI)	1.6 (-2.2, 5.3)	1.1 (-3.4, 5.5)	3.6 (-0.7, 8.0)	-3.2 (-11.8, 5.4)	-0.5 (-4.7, 3.6)
			Mean baseline, mg/dL (SD)	278.6 (51.8)	211.9 (49.0)	46.9 (11.9)	90.0 (50.7)	186.3 (38.1)
ZOCOR	24 Weeks	106	% Change from Baseline (95% CI)	-26.5 (-29.6, -23.3)	-36.8 (-40.5, -33.0)	8.3 (4.6, 11.9)	-7.9 (-15.8, 0.0)	-32.4 (-35.9, -29.0)
			Mean baseline, mg/dL (SD)	270.2 (44.0)	203.8 (41.5)	47.7 (9.0)	78.3 (46.0)	179.9 (33.8)

* median percent change

NDC 0006-0735-31 unit of use bottles of 30
NDC 0006-0735-54 unit of use bottles of 90.

No. 8147 — Tablets ZOCOR 20 mg are tan, oval, film-coated tablets, coded MSD 740 on one side and plain on the other. They are supplied as follows:

NDC 0006-0740-31 unit of use bottles of 30
NDC 0006-0740-54 unit of use bottles of 90.

No. 8148 — Tablets ZOCOR 40 mg are brick red, oval, film-coated tablets, coded MSD 749 on one side and plain on the other. They are supplied as follows:

NDC 0006-0749-31 unit of use bottles of 30
NDC 0006-0749-54 unit of use bottles of 90.
No. 6577 — Tablets ZOCOR 80 mg are brick red, capsule-shaped, film-coated tablets, coded 543 on one side and 80 on the other. They are supplied as follows:
NDC 0006-0543-31 unit of use bottles of 30
NDC 0006-0543-54 unit of use bottles of 90.
Storage
Store between 5-30°C (41-86°F).

17 PATIENT COUNSELING INFORMATION

Patients should be advised to adhere to their National Cholesterol Education Program (NCEP)-recommended diet, a regular exercise program, and periodic testing of a fasting lipid panel.

Patients should be advised about substances they should not take concomitantly with simvastatin *[see Contraindications (4) and Warnings and Precautions (5.1)]*. Patients should also be advised to inform other healthcare professionals prescribing a new medication or increasing the dose of an existing medication that they are taking ZOCOR.

17.1 Muscle Pain

All patients starting therapy with ZOCOR should be advised of the risk of myopathy, including rhabdomyolysis, and told to report promptly any unexplained muscle pain, tenderness or weakness particularly if accompanied by malaise or fever or if these muscle signs or symptoms persist after discontinuing ZOCOR. **Patients using the 80-mg dose should be informed that the risk of myopathy, including rhabdomyolysis, is increased with use of the 80-mg dose.** The risk of myopathy, including rhabdomyolysis, occurring with use of ZOCOR is increased when taking certain types of medication or consuming grapefruit juice. Patients should discuss all medication, both prescription and over the counter, with their healthcare professional.

17.2 Liver Enzymes

It is recommended that liver function tests be performed before the initiation of ZOCOR, and thereafter when clinically indicated. All patients treated with ZOCOR should be advised to report promptly any symptoms that may indicate liver injury, including fatigue, anorexia, right upper abdominal discomfort, dark urine or jaundice.

17.3 Pregnancy

Women of childbearing age should be advised to use an effective method of birth control to prevent pregnancy while using ZOCOR. Discuss future pregnancy plans with your patients, and discuss when to stop taking ZOCOR if they are trying to conceive. Patients should be advised that if they become pregnant they should stop taking ZOCOR and call their healthcare professional.

17.4 Breastfeeding

Women who are breastfeeding should not use ZOCOR. Patients who have a lipid disorder and are breastfeeding should be advised to discuss the options with their healthcare professional.

Manuf. for: Merck Sharp & Dohme Corp., a subsidiary of **MERCK & CO., INC.**, Whitehouse Station, NJ 08889, USA
By:
MERCK SHARP & DOHME LTD.
Cramlington, Northumberland, UK NE23 3JU
Revised: 10/2012
USPI-T-07331210R060

Shown in Product Identification Guide, page 309

ZOLINZA® ℞
[zō-linz'-a]
(vorinostat)
Capsules

HIGHLIGHTS OF PRESCRIBING INFORMATION
These highlights do not include all the information needed to use ZOLINZA safely and effectively. See full prescribing information for ZOLINZA.
ZOLINZA® (vorinostat) Capsules
Initial U.S. Approval: 2006

RECENT MAJOR CHANGES

Dosage and Administration
Dose Modifications (2.2) 04/2013

INDICATIONS AND USAGE

ZOLINZA is a histone deacetylase (HDAC) inhibitor indicated for the treatment of cutaneous manifestations in patients with cutaneous T-cell lymphoma (CTCL) who have progressive, persistent or recurrent disease on or following two systemic therapies. (1)

DOSAGE AND ADMINISTRATION

- 400 mg orally once daily with food. (2.1)
- If patient is intolerant to therapy, reduce the dose to 300 mg orally once daily with food. If necessary, reduce the dose further to 300 mg once daily with food for 5 consecutive days each week. (2.2, 5)
- Reduce dose in patients with mild or moderate hepatic impairment. (2.2)

DOSAGE FORMS AND STRENGTHS

- Capsules: 100 mg (3)

CONTRAINDICATIONS

- None (4)

WARNINGS AND PRECAUTIONS

- Pulmonary embolism and deep vein thrombosis: Monitor for pertinent signs and symptoms. (5.1)
- Thrombocytopenia and anemia: May require dose modification or discontinuation. Monitor blood counts every 2 weeks during the first 2 months of therapy and monthly thereafter. (2.2, 5.2, 6)
- Gastrointestinal Toxicity: Nausea, vomiting and diarrhea; patients may require antiemetics, antidiarrheals, and fluid and electrolyte replacement to prevent dehydration. (5.3, 6, 17.1)
- Hyperglycemia: Monitor blood glucose every 2 weeks during the first 2 months of therapy and monthly thereafter. (5.4)
- Clinical chemistry abnormalities: Measure and correct abnormal electrolytes, creatinine, magnesium and calcium at baseline. Monitor every 2 weeks during the first 2 months of therapy and at least monthly during treatment. (5.5)
- Severe thrombocytopenia with gastrointestinal bleeding has been reported with concomitant use of ZOLINZA and other HDAC inhibitors (e.g., valproic acid). Monitor platelet counts more frequently. (5.6, 7.2)
- Fetal harm can occur when administered to a pregnant woman. Women should be apprised of the potential harm to the fetus. (5.7)

ADVERSE REACTIONS

- The most common adverse reactions (incidence ≥20%) are diarrhea, fatigue, nausea, thrombocytopenia, anorexia and dysgeusia. (6)

To report SUSPECTED ADVERSE REACTIONS, contact Merck Sharp & Dohme Corp., a subsidiary of Merck & Co., Inc., at 1-877-888-4231 or FDA at 1-800-FDA-1088 or www.fda.gov/medwatch.

DRUG INTERACTIONS

- Coumarin-derivative anticoagulants: Prolongation of prothrombin time and International Normalized Ratio (INR) have been observed with concomitant use. Monitor INR frequently. (7.1)

See 17 for PATIENT COUNSELING INFORMATION and FDA-approved patient labeling

Revised: 04/2013

FULL PRESCRIBING INFORMATION: CONTENTS*

*** Sections or subsections omitted from the full prescribing information are not listed**

FULL PRESCRIBING INFORMATION

1 INDICATIONS AND USAGE

ZOLINZA® is indicated for the treatment of cutaneous manifestations in patients with cutaneous T-cell lymphoma who have progressive, persistent or recurrent disease on or following two systemic therapies.

2 DOSAGE AND ADMINISTRATION

2.1 Dosing Information

The recommended dose is 400 mg orally once daily with food.

Treatment may be continued as long as there is no evidence of progressive disease or unacceptable toxicity.

ZOLINZA capsules should not be opened or crushed *[see How Supplied/Storage and Handling (16)]*.

2.2 Dose Modifications

If a patient is intolerant to therapy, the dose may be reduced to 300 mg orally once daily with food. The dose may be further reduced to 300 mg once daily with food for 5 consecutive days each week, as necessary.

Hepatic Impairment

Reduce the starting dose to 300 mg orally once daily with food in patients with mild to moderate hepatic impairment (bilirubin 1 to 3 × ULN or AST > ULN). There is insufficient evidence to recommend a starting dose for patients with severe hepatic impairment (bilirubin > 3 × ULN). *[see Use in Specific Populations (8.6) and Clinical Pharmacology (12.3)]*.

3 DOSAGE FORMS AND STRENGTHS

100 mg white, opaque, hard gelatin capsules with "568" over "100 mg" printed within radial bar in black ink on the capsule body.

4 CONTRAINDICATIONS

None.

5 WARNINGS AND PRECAUTIONS

5.1 Thromboembolism

Pulmonary embolism occurred in 5% (4/86) of patients receiving ZOLINZA, and deep vein thrombosis has also been reported. Monitor for signs and symptoms of these events, particularly in patients with a prior history of thromboembolic events *[see Adverse Reactions (6)]*.

5.2 Myelosuppression

Treatment with ZOLINZA can cause dose-related thrombocytopenia and anemia. Monitor blood counts every 2 weeks during the first 2 months of therapy and monthly thereafter. Adjust dosage or discontinue treatment with ZOLINZA as clinically appropriate. *[See Dosage and Administration (2.2), Warnings and Precautions (5.6) and Adverse Reactions (6).]*

5.3 Gastrointestinal Toxicity

Gastrointestinal disturbances, including nausea, vomiting and diarrhea, have been reported *[see Adverse Reactions (6)]* and may require the use of antiemetic and antidiarrheal medications. Fluid and electrolytes should be replaced to prevent dehydration *[see Adverse Reactions (6.1)]*. Pre-existing nausea, vomiting, and diarrhea should be adequately controlled before beginning therapy with ZOLINZA.

5.4 Hyperglycemia

Hyperglycemia has been observed in patients receiving ZOLINZA and was severe in 5% (4/86) of patients *[see Adverse Reactions (6.1)]*. Monitor serum glucose every 2 weeks during the first 2 months of therapy and monthly thereafter.

5.5 Clinical Chemistry Abnormalities

Obtain chemistry tests, including serum electrolytes, creatinine, magnesium, and calcium, every 2 weeks during the first 2 months of therapy and monthly thereafter. Correct hypokalemia and hypomagnesemia prior to administration of ZOLINZA. Monitor potassium and magnesium more frequently in symptomatic patients (e.g., patients with nausea, vomiting, diarrhea, fluid imbalance or cardiac symptoms).

5.6 Severe thrombocytopenia when combined with other Histone Deacetylase (HDAC) Inhibitors

Severe thrombocytopenia leading to gastrointestinal bleeding has been reported with concomitant use of ZOLINZA and other HDAC inhibitors (e.g., valproic acid). Monitor platelet counts more frequently. *[See Drug Interactions (7.2)]*.

5.7 Pregnancy

Pregnancy Category D

ZOLINZA can cause fetal harm when administered to a pregnant woman. There are no adequate and well-controlled studies of ZOLINZA in pregnant women. Results of animal studies indicate that vorinostat crosses the placenta and is found in fetal plasma at levels up to 50% of maternal concentrations. Doses up to 50 and 150 mg/kg/day were tested in rats and rabbits, respectively (~0.5 times the human exposure based on $AUC_{0\text{-}24\ hours}$). Treatment-related, developmental effects including decreased mean live fetal weights, incomplete ossifications of the skull, thoracic vertebra, sternebra, and skeletal variations (cervical ribs, supernumerary ribs, vertebral count and sacral arch variations) in rats at the highest dose of vorinostat tested. Reductions in mean live fetal weight and an elevated incidence of incomplete ossification of the metacarpals were seen in rabbits dosed at 150 mg/kg/day. The no observed effect levels (NOELs) for these findings were 15 and 50 mg/kg/day (<0.1 times the human exposure based on AUC) in rats and rabbits, respectively. A dose-related increase in the incidence of malformations of the gall bladder was noted in all drug treatment groups in rabbits versus the concurrent control. If this drug is used during pregnancy, or if the patient becomes pregnant while taking this drug, the patient should be apprised of the potential hazard to the fetus.

6 ADVERSE REACTIONS

The following serious adverse reactions have been associated with ZOLINZA in clinical trials and are discussed in greater detail in other sections of the label [*see Warnings and Precautions (5)*].

Thromboembolism [*see Warnings and Precautions (5.1)*]
Myelosuppression [*see Warnings and Precautions (5.2)*]
Gastrointestinal Toxicity [*see Warnings and Precautions (5.3)*]
Hyperglycemia [*see Warnings and Precautions (5.4)*]
Clinical Chemistry Abnormalities [*see Warnings and Precautions (5.5)*]
Severe thrombocytopenia when combined with other Histone Deacetylase (HDAC) Inhibitors [*see Warnings and Precautions (5.6)*]

The most common drug-related adverse reactions can be classified into 4 symptom complexes: gastrointestinal symptoms (diarrhea, nausea, anorexia, weight decrease, vomiting, constipation), constitutional symptoms (fatigue, chills), hematologic abnormalities (thrombocytopenia, anemia), and taste disorders (dysgeusia, dry mouth). The most common serious drug-related adverse reactions were pulmonary embolism and anemia.

6.1 Clinical Trials Experience

Because clinical trials are conducted under widely varying conditions, adverse reaction rates observed in the clinical trials of a drug cannot be directly compared to rates in the clinical trials of another drug and may not reflect the rates observed in practice.

The safety of ZOLINZA was evaluated in 107 CTCL patients in two single arm clinical studies in which 86 patients received 400 mg once daily.

The data described below reflect exposure to ZOLINZA 400 mg once daily in the 86 patients for a median number of 97.5 days on therapy (range 2 to 480+ days). Seventeen (19.8%) patients were exposed beyond 24 weeks and 8 (9.3%) patients were exposed beyond 1 year. The population of CTCL patients studied was 37 to 83 years of age, 47.7% female, 52.3% male, and 81.4% white, 16.3% black, and 1.2% Asian or multi-racial.

Common Adverse Reactions

Table 1 summarizes the frequency of CTCL patients with specific adverse reactions, using the National Cancer Institute-Common Terminology Criteria for Adverse Events (NCI-CTCAE, version 3.0).

Table 1: Clinical or Laboratory Adverse Reactions Occurring in CTCL Patients (Incidence ≥10% of patients)

	ZOLINZA 400 mg once daily (N=86)			
Adverse Reactions	**All Grades**		**Grades 3-5***	
	n	**%**	**n**	**%**
Fatigue	45	52.3	3	3.5
Diarrhea	45	52.3	0	0.0
Nausea	35	40.7	3	3.5
Dysgeusia	24	27.9	0	0.0
Thrombocytopenia	22	25.6	5	5.8
Anorexia	21	24.4	2	2.3
Weight Decreased	18	20.9	1	1.2
Muscle Spasms	17	19.8	2	2.3
Alopecia	16	18.6	0	0.0
Dry Mouth	14	16.3	0	0.0
Blood Creatinine Increased	14	16.3	0	0.0
Chills	14	16.3	1	1.2
Vomiting	13	15.1	1	1.2
Constipation	13	15.1	0	0.0
Dizziness	13	15.1	1	1.2
Anemia	12	14.0	2	2.3
Decreased Appetite	12	14.0	1	1.2
Peripheral Edema	11	12.8	0	0.0
Headache	10	11.6	0	0.0
Pruritus	10	11.6	1	1.2
Cough	9	10.5	0	0.0
Upper Respiratory Infection	9	10.5	0	0.0
Pyrexia	9	10.5	1	1.2

* No Grade 5 reactions were reported.

The frequencies of more severe thrombocytopenia, anemia [*see Warnings and Precautions (5.2)*] and fatigue were increased at doses higher than 400 mg once daily of ZOLINZA.

Serious Adverse Reactions

The most common serious adverse reactions in the 86 CTCL patients in two clinical trials were pulmonary embolism reported in 4.7% (4/86) of patients, squamous cell carcinoma reported in 3.5% (3/86) of patients and anemia reported in 2.3% (2/86) of patients. There were single events of cholecystitis, death (of unknown cause), deep vein thrombosis, enterococcal infection, exfoliative dermatitis, gastrointestinal hemorrhage, infection, lobar pneumonia, myocardial infarction, ischemic stroke, pelviureteric obstruction, sepsis, spinal cord injury, streptococcal bacteremia, syncope, T-cell lymphoma, thrombocytopenia and ureteric obstruction.

Discontinuations

Of the CTCL patients who received the 400-mg once daily dose, 9.3% (8/86) of patients discontinued ZOLINZA due to adverse reactions. These adverse reactions, regardless of causality, included anemia, angioneurotic edema, asthenia, chest pain, exfoliative dermatitis, death, deep vein thrombosis, ischemic stroke, lethargy, pulmonary embolism, and spinal cord injury.

Dose Modifications

Of the CTCL patients who received the 400-mg once daily dose, 10.5% (9/86) of patients required a dose modification of ZOLINZA due to adverse reactions. These adverse reactions included increased serum creatinine, decreased appetite, hypokalemia, leukopenia, nausea, neutropenia, thrombocytopenia and vomiting. The median time to the first adverse reactions resulting in dose reduction was 42 days (range 17 to 263 days).

Laboratory Abnormalities

Laboratory abnormalities were reported in all of the 86 CTCL patients who received the 400-mg once-daily dose.

Increased serum glucose was reported as a laboratory abnormality in 69% (59/86) of CTCL patients who received the 400-mg once daily dose; only 4 of these abnormalities were severe (Grade 3). Increased serum glucose was reported as an adverse reaction in 8.1% (7/86) of CTCL patients who received the 400-mg once daily dose. [*See Warnings and Precautions (5.4).*]

Transient increases in serum creatinine were detected in 46.5% (40/86) of CTCL patients who received the 400-mg once daily dose. Of these laboratory abnormalities, 34 were NCI CTCAE Grade 1, 5 were Grade 2, and 1 was Grade 3. Proteinuria was detected as a laboratory abnormality (51.4%) in 38 of 74 patients tested. The clinical significance of this finding is unknown.

Dehydration

Based on reports of dehydration as a serious drug-related adverse reaction in clinical trials, patients were instructed to drink at least 2 L/day of fluids for adequate hydration. [*See Warnings and Precautions (5.3, 5.5).*]

Adverse Reactions in Non-CTCL Patients

The frequencies of individual adverse reactions were substantially higher in the non-CTCL population. Drug-related serious adverse reactions reported in the non-CTCL population which were not observed in the CTCL population included single events of blurred vision, asthenia, hyponatremia, tumor hemorrhage, Guillain-Barré syndrome, renal failure, urinary retention, cough, hemoptysis, hypertension, and vasculitis.

In patients recovering from bowel surgery and treated perioperatively with ZOLINZA, anastomotic healing complications including fistulas, perforations, and abscess formation have occurred.

7 DRUG INTERACTIONS

7.1 Coumarin-Derivative Anticoagulants

Prolongation of prothrombin time (PT) and International Normalized Ratio (INR) were observed in patients receiving ZOLINZA concomitantly with coumarin-derivative anticoagulants. Physicians should monitor PT and INR more frequently in patients concurrently administered ZOLINZA and coumarin derivatives.

7.2 Other HDAC Inhibitors

Severe thrombocytopenia and gastrointestinal bleeding have been reported with concomitant use of ZOLINZA and other HDAC inhibitors (e.g., valproic acid). Monitor platelet count every 2 weeks for the first 2 months. [*See Warnings and Precautions (5.6).*]

8 USE IN SPECIFIC POPULATIONS

8.1 Pregnancy

Pregnancy Category D [See Warnings and Precautions (5.7)]

8.3 Nursing Mothers

It is not known whether this drug is excreted in human milk. Because many drugs are excreted in human milk and because of the potential for serious adverse reactions in nursing infants from ZOLINZA, a decision should be made whether to discontinue nursing or discontinue the drug, taking into account the importance of the drug to the mother.

8.4 Pediatric Use

The safety and effectiveness of ZOLINZA in pediatric patients have not been established.

8.5 Geriatric Use

Of the total number of patients with CTCL in trials (N=107), 46 % were 65 years of age and over, while 15 % were 75 years of age and over. No overall differences in safety or effectiveness were observed between these subjects and younger subjects, and other reported clinical experience has not identified differences in responses between the elderly and younger patients, but greater sensitivity of some older individuals should be considered, reflecting the greater frequency of decreased hepatic, renal, or cardiac function, and of concomitant disease or other drug therapy.

8.6 Use in Patients with Hepatic Impairment

ZOLINZA was studied in 42 patients with non-CTCL cancer and varying degrees of hepatic impairment after single and multiple-dose administration. Compared to patients with normal liver function, AUC increases of 50 to 66% were observed in patients with hepatic impairment. The incidence of Grade 3 or 4 thrombocytopenia increased in patients with mild (bilirubin of 1 to 1.5 × ULN and AST < ULN, or bilirubin ≤ ULN and AST > ULN) and moderate (bilirubin 1.5 to ≤ 3 × ULN) hepatic impairment treated daily at doses of 300 and 200 mg respectively.

Patients with severe hepatic impairment (bilirubin > 3 × ULN) have not been treated at doses greater than 200 mg a day. Reduce the initial dose of ZOLINZA in patients with bilirubin 1 to 3 × ULN or AST > ULN. [*See Dosage and Administration (2.2) and Clinical Pharmacology (12.3).*]

8.7 Use in Patients with Renal Impairment

Vorinostat was not evaluated in patients with renal impairment. However, renal excretion does not play a role in the elimination of vorinostat. Patients with pre-existing renal impairment should be treated with caution. [*See Clinical Pharmacology (12.3).*]

10 OVERDOSAGE

No specific information is available on the treatment of overdosage of ZOLINZA.

In the event of overdose, it is reasonable to employ the usual supportive measures, e.g., remove unabsorbed material from the gastrointestinal tract, employ clinical monitoring, and institute supportive therapy, if required. It is not known if vorinostat is dialyzable.

11 DESCRIPTION

ZOLINZA contains vorinostat, which is described chemically as *N*-hydroxy-*N'*-phenyloctanediamide.

The empirical formula is $C_{14}H_{20}N_2O_3$. The molecular weight is 264.32 and the structural formula is:

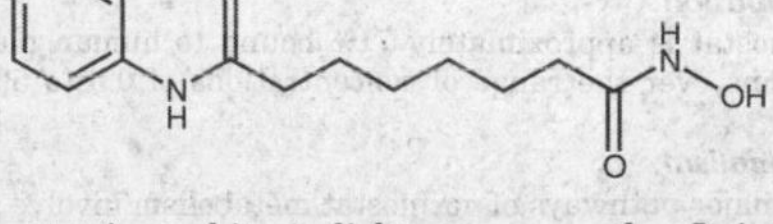

Vorinostat is a white to light orange powder. It is very slightly soluble in water, slightly soluble in ethanol, isopropanol and acetone, freely soluble in dimethyl sulfoxide and insoluble in methylene chloride. It has no chiral centers and is non-hygroscopic. The differential scanning calorimetry ranged from 161.7 (endotherm) to 163.9°C. The pH of saturated water solutions of vorinostat drug substance was 6.6. The pKa of vorinostat was determined to be 9.2.

Each 100 mg ZOLINZA capsule for oral administration contains 100 mg vorinostat and the following inactive ingredients: microcrystalline cellulose, sodium croscarmellose and magnesium stearate. The capsule shell excipients are titanium dioxide, gelatin and sodium lauryl sulfate.

12 CLINICAL PHARMACOLOGY

12.1 Mechanism of Action

Vorinostat inhibits the enzymatic activity of histone deacetylases HDAC1, HDAC2 and HDAC3 (Class I) and HDAC6 (Class II) at nanomolar concentrations (IC_{50}<86 nM). These enzymes catalyze the removal of acetyl groups from the lysine residues of proteins, including histones and transcription factors. In some cancer cells, there is an overexpression of HDACs, or an aberrant recruitment of HDACs to oncogenic transcription factors causing hypoacetylation of core nucleosomal histones. Hypoacetylation of histones is associated with a condensed chromatin structure and repression of gene transcription. Inhibition of HDAC activity allows for the accumulation of acetyl groups on the histone lysine residues resulting in an open chromatin structure and transcriptional activation. *In vitro*, vorinostat causes the accumulation of acetylated histones and induces cell cycle arrest and/or apoptosis of some transformed cells. The mechanism of the antineoplastic effect of vorinostat has not been fully characterized.

12.2 Pharmacodynamics

Cardiac Electrophysiology

A randomized, partially-blind, placebo-controlled, 2-period crossover study was performed to assess the effects of a single 800-mg dose of vorinostat on the QTc interval in 24 patients with advanced cancer. This study was conducted to assess the impact of vorinostat on ventricular repolarization. The upper bound of the 90% confidence interval of the placebo-adjusted mean QTc interval change-from-baseline was less than 10 msec at every time point through 24 hours. Based on these study results, administration of a single supratherapeutic 800-mg dose of vorinostat does not appear to prolong the QTc interval in patients with advanced cancer; however the study did not include a positive control to demonstrate assay sensitivity. In the fasted state, oral administration of a single 800-mg dose of vorinostat resulted in a mean AUC and C_{max} and median T_{max} of 8.6±5.7 μM•hr and 1.7±0.67 μM and 2.1 (0.5-6) hours, respectively.

In clinical studies in patients with CTCL, three of 86 CTCL patients exposed to 400 mg once daily had Grade 1 (>450-470 msec) or 2 (>470-500 msec or increase of >60 msec above baseline) clinical adverse reactions of QTc prolongation. In a retrospective analysis of three Phase 1 and two Phase 2 studies, 116 patients had a baseline and at least one follow-up ECG. Four patients had Grade 2 (>470-500 msec or increase of >60 msec above baseline) and 1 patient had Grade 3 (>500 msec) QTc prolongation. In 49 non-CTCL patients from 3 clinical trials who had complete evaluation of QT interval, 2 had QTc measurements of >500 msec and 1 had a QTc prolongation of >60 msec.

12.3 Pharmacokinetics

Absorption

The pharmacokinetics of vorinostat were evaluated in 23 patients with relapsed or refractory advanced cancer. After oral administration of a single 400-mg dose of vorinostat with a high-fat meal, the mean ± standard deviation area under the curve (AUC) and peak serum concentration (C_{max}) and the median (range) time to maximum concentration (T_{max}) were 5.5±1.8 μM•hr, 1.2±0.62 μM and 4 (2-10) hours, respectively.

In the fasted state, oral administration of a single 400-mg dose of vorinostat resulted in a mean AUC and C_{max} and median T_{max} of 4.2±1.9 μM•hr and 1.2±0.35 μM and 1.5 (0.5-10) hours, respectively. Therefore, oral administration of vorinostat with a high-fat meal resulted in an increase (33%) in the extent of absorption and a modest decrease in the rate of absorption (T_{max} delayed 2.5 hours) compared to the fasted state. However, these small effects are not expected to be clinically meaningful. In clinical trials of patients with CTCL, vorinostat was taken with food.

At steady state in the fed-state, oral administration of multiple 400-mg doses of vorinostat resulted in a mean AUC and C_{max} and a median T_{max} of 6.0±2.0 μM•hr, 1.2±0.53 μM and 4 (0.5-14) hours, respectively.

Distribution

Vorinostat is approximately 71% bound to human plasma proteins over the range of concentrations of 0.5 to 50 μg/mL.

Metabolism

The major pathways of vorinostat metabolism involve glucuronidation and hydrolysis followed by β-oxidation. Human serum levels of two metabolites, *O*-glucuronide of vorinostat and 4-anilino-4-oxobutanoic acid were measured. Both metabolites are pharmacologically inactive. Compared to vorinostat, the mean steady state serum exposures in humans of the *O*-glucuronide of vorinostat and 4-anilino-4-oxobutanoic acid were 4-fold and 13-fold higher, respectively.

In vitro studies using human liver microsomes indicate negligible biotransformation by cytochromes P450 (CYP).

Excretion

Vorinostat is eliminated predominantly through metabolism with less than 1% of the dose recovered as unchanged drug in urine, indicating that renal excretion does not play a role in the elimination of vorinostat. The mean urinary recovery of two pharmacologically inactive metabolites at steady state was 16±5.8% of vorinostat dose as the *O*-glucuronide of vorinostat, and 36±8.6% of vorinostat dose as 4-anilino-4-oxobutanoic acid. Total urinary recovery of vorinostat and these two metabolites averaged 52±13.3% of vorinostat dose. The mean terminal half-life ($t_{1/2}$) was ~2.0 hours for both vorinostat and the *O*-glucuronide metabolite, while that of the 4-anilino-4-oxobutanoic acid metabolite was 11 hours.

Specific Populations

Gender, Race & Age

Based upon an exploratory analysis of limited data, gender, race and age do not appear to have meaningful effects on the pharmacokinetics of vorinostat.

Pediatric

Vorinostat was not evaluated in patients <18 years of age.

Hepatic Impairment

The single dose pharmacokinetics of a 400 mg ZOLINZA dose was evaluated in patients with non-CTCL cancers with varying degrees of hepatic impairment. The mean AUC of vorinostat in patients with mild (bilirubin > 1 to 1.5 × ULN or AST > ULN but bilirubin ≤ ULN) and moderate (bilirubin 1.5 to ≤ 3 × ULN) hepatic impairment increased by 50% compared to the AUC of vorinostat in patients with normal hepatic function. The mean vorinostat AUC in patients with severe hepatic impairment (bilirubin > 3 × ULN) increased by 66% compared to the AUC of patients with normal hepatic function.

The safety of multiple daily doses of ZOLINZA was also evaluated in patients with non-CTCL cancers with varying degrees of hepatic impairment. The highest dose studied in mild, moderate and severe hepatic impairment was 400, 300 and 200 mg daily respectively. The incidence of Grade 3 or 4 adverse reactions was similar among the hepatic function groups. The most common Grade 3 or 4 adverse reaction was thrombocytopenia.

Reduce the dose in patients with mild to moderate hepatic impairment. There is not enough data in patients with severe hepatic impairment to recommend a dose modification. *[See Dosage and Administration (2.2) and Use in Specific Populations (8.6).]*

Renal Insufficiency

Vorinostat was not evaluated in patients with renal impairment. However, renal excretion does not play a role in the elimination of vorinostat. *[See Use in Specific Populations (8.7).]*

Pharmacokinetic effects of vorinostat with other agents

Vorinostat is not an inhibitor of CYP drug metabolizing enzymes in human liver microsomes at steady state C_{max} of the 400 mg dose (C_{max} of 1.2 μM vs IC_{50} of >75 μM). Gene expression studies in human hepatocytes detected some potential for suppression of CYP2C9 and CYP3A4 activities by vorinostat at concentrations higher (≥10 μM) than pharmacologically relevant. Thus, vorinostat is not expected to affect the pharmacokinetics of other agents. As vorinostat is not eliminated via the CYP pathways, it is anticipated that vorinostat will not be subject to drug-drug interactions when co-administered with drugs that are known CYP inhibitors or inducers. However, no formal clinical studies have been conducted to evaluate drug interactions with vorinostat.

In vitro studies indicate that vorinostat is not a substrate of human P-glycoprotein (P-gp). In addition, vorinostat has no inhibitory effect on human P-gp-mediated transport of vinblastine (a marker P-gp substrate) at concentrations of up to 100 μM. Thus, vorinostat is not likely to inhibit P-gp at the pharmacologically relevant serum concentration of 2 μM (C_{max}) in humans.

13 NONCLINICAL TOXICOLOGY

13.1 Carcinogenesis, Mutagenesis, Impairment of Fertility

Carcinogenicity studies have not been performed with vorinostat.

Vorinostat was mutagenic *in vitro* in the bacterial reverse mutation assays (Ames test), caused chromosomal aberrations *in vitro* in Chinese hamster ovary (CHO) cells and increased the incidence of micro-nucleated erythrocytes when administered to mice (Mouse Micronucleus Assay).

Effects on the female reproductive system were identified in the oral fertility study when females were dosed for 14 days prior to mating through gestational day 7. Doses of 15, 50 and 150 mg/kg/day to rats resulted in approximate exposures of 0.15, 0.36 and 0.70 times the expected clinical exposure based on AUC. Dose dependent increases in corpora lutea were noted at ≥15 mg/kg/day, which resulted in increased peri-implantation losses were noted at ≥50 mg/kg/day. At 150 mg/kg/day, there were increases in the incidences of dead fetuses and in resorptions.

No effects on reproductive performance were observed in male rats dosed (20, 50, 150 mg/kg/day; approximate exposures of 0.15, 0.36 and 0.70 times the expected clinical exposure based on AUC), for 70 days prior to mating with untreated females. *[See Warnings and Precautions (5.7).]*

14 CLINICAL STUDIES

Cutaneous T-cell Lymphoma

In two open-label clinical studies, patients with refractory CTCL have been evaluated to determine their response rate to oral ZOLINZA. One study was a single-arm clinical study and the other assessed several dosing regimens. In both studies, patients were treated until disease progression or intolerable toxicity.

Study 1

In an open-label, single-arm, multicenter non-randomized study, 74 patients with advanced CTCL were treated with ZOLINZA at a dose of 400 mg once daily. The primary endpoint was response rate to oral ZOLINZA in the treatment of skin disease in patients with advanced CTCL (Stage IIB and higher) who had progressive, persistent, or recurrent disease on or following two systemic therapies. Enrolled patients should have received, been intolerant to or not a candidate for bexarotene. Extent of skin disease was quantitatively assessed by investigators using a modified Severity Weighted Assessment Tool (SWAT). The investigator measured the percentage total body surface area (%TBSA) involvement separately for patches, plaques, and tumors within 12 body regions using the patient's palm as a "ruler". The total %TBSA for each lesion type was multiplied by a severity weighting factor (1=patch, 2=plaque and 4=tumor) and summed to derive the SWAT score. Efficacy was measured as either a Complete Clinical Response (CCR) defined as no evidence of disease, or Partial Response (PR) defined as a ≥50% decrease in SWAT skin assessment score compared to baseline. Both CCR and PR had to be maintained for at least 4 weeks.

Secondary efficacy endpoints included response duration, time to progression, and time to objective response.

The population had been exposed to a median of three prior therapies (range 1 to 12).

Table 2 summarizes the demographic and disease characteristics of the Study 1 population.

Table 2: Baseline Patient Characteristics (All Patients As Treated)

Characteristics	Vorinostat (N=74)
Age (year)	
Mean (SD)	61.2 (11.3)
Median (Range)	60.0 (39.0, 83.0)
Gender, n (%)	
Male	38 (51.4%)
Female	36 (48.6%)
CTCL stage, n (%)	
IB	11 (14.9%)
IIA	2 (2.7%)
IIB	19 (25.7%)
III	22 (29.7%)
IVA	16 (21.6%)
IVB	4 (5.4%)
Racial Origin, n (%)	
Asian	1 (1.4%)
Black	11 (14.9%)
Other	1 (1.4%)
White	61 (82.4%)
Time from Initial CTCL Diagnosis (year)	
Median (Range)	2.6 (0.0, 27.3)
Clinical Characteristics	
Number of prior systemic treatments, median (range)	3.0 (1.0, 12.0)

The overall objective response rate was 29.7% (22/74, 95% CI [19.7 to 41.5%]) in all patients treated with ZOLINZA. In patients with Stage IIB and higher CTCL, the overall objective response rate was 29.5% (18/61). One patient with Stage IIB CTCL achieved a CCR. Median times to response were 55 and 56 days (range 28 to 171 days), respectively in the overall population and in patients with Stage IIB and higher CTCL. However, in rare cases it took up to 6 months for patients to achieve an objective response to ZOLINZA.

The median response duration was not reached since the majority of responses continued at the time of analysis, but was estimated to exceed 6 months for both the overall population and in patients with Stage IIB and higher CTCL. When end of response was defined as a 50% increase in SWAT score from the nadir, the estimated median response duration was 168 days and the median time to tumor progression was 202 days.

Using a 25% increase in SWAT score from the nadir as criterion for tumor progression, the estimated median time-to-progression was 148 days for the overall population and 169 days in the 61 patients with Stage IIB and higher CTCL.

Response to any previous systemic therapy does not appear to be predictive of response to ZOLINZA.

Study 2

In an open-label, non-randomized study, ZOLINZA was evaluated to determine the response rate for patients with CTCL who were refractory or intolerant to at least one treatment. In this study, 33 patients were assigned to one of 3 cohorts: Cohort 1, 400 mg once daily; Cohort 2, 300 mg twice daily 3 days/week; or Cohort 3, 300 mg twice daily for 14 days followed by a 7-day rest (induction). In Cohort 3, if at least a partial response was not observed then patients were dosed with a maintenance regimen of 200 mg twice daily. The primary efficacy endpoint, objective response, was measured by the 7-point Physician's Global Assessment (PGA) scale. The investigator assessed improvement or worsening in overall disease compared to baseline based on overall clinical impression. Index and non-index cutaneous lesions as well as cutaneous tumors, lymph nodes and all other disease manifestations were also assessed and included in the overall clinical impression. CCR required 100% clearing of all findings, and PR required at least 50% improvement in disease findings.

The median age was 67.0 years (range 26.0 to 82.0). Fifty-five percent of patients were male, and 45% of patients were female. Fifteen percent of patients had Stage IA, IB, or IIA CTCL and 85% of patients had Stage IIB, III, IVA, or IVB CTCL. The median number of prior systemic therapies was 4 (range 0.0 to 11.0).

In all patients treated, the objective response was 24.2% (8/33) in the overall population, 25% (7/28) in patients with Stage IIB or higher disease and 36.4% (4/11) in patients with Sezary syndrome. The overall response rates were 30.8%, 9.1% and 33.3% in Cohort 1, Cohort 2 and Cohort 3, respectively. The 300 mg twice daily regimen had higher toxicity with no additional clinical benefit over the 400 mg once daily regimen. No CCR was observed.

Among the 8 patients who responded to study treatment, the median time to response was 83.5 days (range 25 to 153 days). The median response duration was 106 days (range 66 to 136 days). Median time to progression was 211.5 days (range 94 to 255 days).

15 REFERENCES

1. OSHA Hazardous Drugs. *OSHA*. [http://www.osha.gov/SLTC/hazardousdrugs/index.html]

16 HOW SUPPLIED/STORAGE AND HANDLING

ZOLINZA capsules, 100 mg, are white, opaque hard gelatin capsules with "568" over "100 mg" printed within the radial bar in black ink on the capsule body. They are supplied as follows:

NDC 0006-0568-40.

Each bottle contains 120 capsules.

Storage and Handling

Store at 20-25°C (68-77°F), excursions permitted between 15-30°C (59-86°F). [See USP Controlled Room Temperature.]

Procedures for proper handling and disposal of anticancer drugs should be considered. Several guidelines on this subject have been published.[1] There is no general agreement that all of the procedures recommended in the guidelines are necessary or appropriate.

ZOLINZA (vorinostat) capsules should not be opened or crushed. Direct contact of the powder in ZOLINZA capsules with the skin or mucous membranes should be avoided. If such contact occurs, wash thoroughly as outlined in the references. Personnel should avoid exposure to crushed and/or broken capsules *[see Nonclinical Toxicology (13.1)]*.

17 PATIENT COUNSELING INFORMATION

See FDA-Approved Patient Labeling (Patient Information)

17.1 Instructions

Patients should be instructed to drink at least 2 L/day of fluid to prevent dehydration and should promptly report excessive vomiting or diarrhea to their physician. Patients should be instructed about the signs of deep vein thrombosis and should consult their physician should any evidence of deep vein thrombosis develop. Patients receiving ZOLINZA should seek immediate medical attention if unusual bleeding occurs. ZOLINZA capsules should not be opened or crushed.

Patients should be instructed to read the patient insert carefully.

Manuf. for: Merck Sharp & Dohme Corp., a subsidiary of **MERCK & CO., INC.**, Whitehouse Station, NJ 08889, USA

Manufactured by:
Patheon, Inc.
Mississauga, Ontario, Canada L5N 7K9
U.S. Patent Nos. RE 38,506 E; 6,087,367

Revised: 04/2013
USPI-C-0683-1304R006

Patient Information
ZOLINZA® (zo LINZ ah)
(vorinostat)
Capsules

Read the patient information that comes with ZOLINZA before you start taking it and each time you get a refill. There may be new information. This leaflet is a summary of the information for patients. Your doctor or pharmacist can give you additional information. This leaflet does not take the place of talking with your doctor about your medical condition or your treatment.

What is ZOLINZA?

ZOLINZA is a prescription medicine used to treat a type of cancer called cutaneous T-cell lymphoma (CTCL) in patients when the CTCL gets worse, does not go away, or comes back after treatment with other medicines.

ZOLINZA has not been studied in children under the age of 18.

What should I tell my doctor before taking ZOLINZA?

Tell your doctor about all of your medical conditions, including if you:

- Have any allergies
- Have had a blood clot in your lung (pulmonary embolus)
- Have had a blood clot in a vein (a blood vessel) anywhere in your body (deep vein thrombosis)
- Have nausea, vomiting, or diarrhea
- Have liver disease
- Have high blood sugar or diabetes
- Are pregnant or plan to become pregnant. ZOLINZA may harm your unborn baby. ZOLINZA has not been studied in pregnant women. If you use ZOLINZA during pregnancy, tell your doctor immediately.
- Are breastfeeding or plan to breastfeed. It is not known if ZOLINZA will pass into your breast milk. Talk to your doctor about the best way to feed your baby while you are taking ZOLINZA.

Tell your doctor about all of the medicines you take, including prescription and non-prescription medicines, vitamins and herbal supplements. Some medicines may affect how ZOLINZA works, or ZOLINZA may affect how your other medicines work. **Especially tell your doctor if you take:**

- **Valproic acid:** a medicine used to treat seizures. Your doctor will decide if you should continue to take valproic acid and may want to test your blood more frequently.
- **COUMADIN®: (warfarin) or any other blood thinner.** Ask your doctor if you are not sure if you are taking a blood thinner. Your doctor may want to test your blood more frequently.

Know the medicines you take. Keep a list of your medicines and show it to your doctor and pharmacist when you get a new medicine.

How should I take ZOLINZA?

- Take ZOLINZA exactly as your doctor tells you to.
- Your doctor will tell you how many ZOLINZA capsules to take and when to take them.
- Swallow each capsule whole. Do not chew or break open the capsule. If you can't swallow ZOLINZA capsules whole, tell your doctor. You may need a different medicine.
- Take ZOLINZA with food.
- If ZOLINZA capsules are accidentally opened or crushed, do not touch the capsules or the powder contents of the capsules. If the powder from an open or crushed capsule gets on your skin or in your eyes, wash the contacted area well with plenty of plain water. Call your doctor.
- **Drink at least eight 8-ounce glasses of liquids every day while taking ZOLINZA.** Drinking enough fluids may help to decrease the chances of losing too much fluid from your body (dehydration) especially if you are having symptoms such as nausea, vomiting or diarrhea while taking ZOLINZA.
- If you miss a dose, take it as soon as you remember. If you do not remember until it is almost time for your next dose, just skip the missed dose. Just take the next dose at your regular time. Do not take two doses of ZOLINZA at the same time.
- If you take too much ZOLINZA, call your doctor, local emergency room, or poison control center right away.
- Your doctor will check your blood cell counts, blood sugar, blood electrolytes, and other chemistries every two weeks for the first two months of your treatment with ZOLINZA and then monthly. Your doctor may decide to do other tests to check your health as needed.
- If you have high blood sugar (hyperglycemia) or diabetes, continue to monitor your blood sugar as your doctor tells you to. Your doctor may need to change your diet or medicine to help control your blood sugar while you take ZOLINZA. Be sure to tell your doctor if you are unable to eat or drink normally due to nausea, vomiting or diarrhea.

What are the possible side effects of ZOLINZA?

ZOLINZA may cause **serious side effects.** Tell your doctor right away if you have any of the following symptoms:

- **Blood clots in the legs (deep vein thrombosis)**
  - sudden swelling in a leg
  - pain or tenderness in the leg. The pain may only be felt when standing or walking.
  - increased warmth in the area where the swelling is.
  - skin redness or change in skin color
- **Blood clots that travel to the lungs (pulmonary embolus)**
  - sudden sharp chest pain
  - rapid pulse
  - shortness of breath
  - fainting
  - cough with bloody secretions
  - feeling anxious
  - sweating
- **Dehydration** (loss of too much fluid from the body). This can happen if you are having nausea, vomiting or diarrhea and can not drink fluids well.
- **Changes in blood tests:** Your doctor will periodically do blood tests to check your blood counts and electrolytes.
  - **Low red blood cells.** Low red blood cells may make you feel tired and get tired easily. You may look pale, and feel short of breath.
  - **Low platelets.** Low platelets can cause unusual bleeding or bruising under the skin. Talk to your doctor right away if this happens.
- **High blood sugar** (blood glucose). If you have high blood sugar or diabetes, monitor your blood sugar frequently as directed by your doctor. Tell your doctor right away if your blood sugar is higher than normal.

In addition, the most common side effects with ZOLINZA include:

- **Stomach and intestinal problems,** including diarrhea, nausea, vomiting, loss of appetite, constipation and weight loss
- **Tiredness**
- **Dizziness**
- **Headache**
- **Changes in the way things taste and dry mouth**
- **Muscle aches**
- **Hair loss**
- **Chills**
- **Fever**
- **Upper respiratory infection**
- **Cough**
- **Increase in blood creatinine**
- **Swelling in the foot, ankle, and leg**
- **Itching**

Tell your doctor if you have any side effect that bothers you or that does not go away.

These are not all the possible side effects of ZOLINZA. For more information, ask your doctor or pharmacist.

General information about ZOLINZA

Medicines are sometimes prescribed for conditions that are not mentioned in patient information leaflets. Do not use ZOLINZA for a condition for which it was not prescribed. Do not give ZOLINZA to other people, even if they have the same symptoms you have. It may harm them.

Keep ZOLINZA and all medicines out of the reach of children.

This leaflet summarizes the most important information about ZOLINZA. If you would like to know more information, talk to your doctor. You can ask your doctor or pharmacist for information about ZOLINZA that is written for health professionals.

What are the ingredients in ZOLINZA?

Active ingredient: vorinostat

Inactive ingredients: microcrystalline cellulose, sodium croscarmellose and magnesium stearate. The inactive ingredients in the capsule shell are titanium dioxide, gelatin, and sodium lauryl sulfate.

How should I store ZOLINZA?

Store ZOLINZA at room temperature, 68°F-77°F (20°C-25°C).

Merck Sharp & Dohme Corp., a subsidiary of
MERCK & CO., INC., Whitehouse Station, NJ 08889, USA

Manufactured by:
Patheon, Inc.
Mississauga, Ontario, Canada L5N 7K9
U.S. Patent Nos. RE 38,506 E; 6,087,367

Revised: 04/2013
USPPI-C-0683-1304R006

Shown in Product Identification Guide, page 309

ZOSTAVAX® ℞
[ZOS tah vax]
(Zoster Vaccine Live)
Suspension for subcutaneous injection

HIGHLIGHTS OF PRESCRIBING INFORMATION

These highlights do not include all the information needed to use ZOSTAVAX safely and effectively. See full prescribing information for ZOSTAVAX.

ZOSTAVAX® (Zoster Vaccine Live)
Suspension for subcutaneous injection
Initial U.S. Approval: 2006

INDICATIONS AND USAGE

ZOSTAVAX is a live attenuated virus vaccine indicated for prevention of herpes zoster (shingles) in individuals 50 years of age and older. (1)

Limitations of Use of ZOSTAVAX:
- ZOSTAVAX is not indicated for the treatment of zoster or postherpetic neuralgia (PHN) (1)
- ZOSTAVAX is not indicated for prevention of primary varicella infection (Chickenpox) (1)

DOSAGE AND ADMINISTRATION

Single 0.65 mL subcutaneous injection (2.1)

DOSAGE FORMS AND STRENGTHS

Single dose vials with not less than 19,400 plaque-forming units [PFU] per 0.65 mL dose when reconstituted to a suspension. (2.1, 3, 16)

CONTRAINDICATIONS

- History of anaphylactic/anaphylactoid reaction to gelatin, neomycin, or any other component of the vaccine. (4.1)
- Immunosuppression or Immunodeficiency. (4.2)
- Pregnancy. (4.3, 8.1)

WARNINGS AND PRECAUTIONS

- Hypersensitivity reactions including anaphylaxis have occurred with ZOSTAVAX (5.1)
- Transmission of vaccine virus may occur between vaccinees and susceptible contacts (5.2)
- Avoid pregnancy for 3 months following vaccination with ZOSTAVAX (8.1)
- Deferral should be considered in acute illness (for example, in the presence of fever) or in patients with active untreated tuberculosis (5.3)

ADVERSE REACTIONS

The most frequent adverse reactions, reported in ≥1% of subjects vaccinated with ZOSTAVAX, were headache and injection-site reactions. (6)

To report SUSPECTED ADVERSE REACTIONS, contact Merck Sharp & Dohme Corp., a subsidiary of Merck & Co., Inc., at 1-877-888-4231 or VAERS at 1-800-822-7967 or www.vaers.hhs.gov.

DRUG INTERACTIONS

In a randomized clinical study, a reduced immune response to ZOSTAVAX as measured by gpELISA was observed in individuals who received concurrent administration of PNEUMOVAX® 23 and ZOSTAVAX compared with individuals who received these vaccines 4 weeks apart. Consider administration of the two vaccines separated by at least 4 weeks (7.1, 14.3).

USE IN SPECIFIC POPULATIONS

Pregnancy: Do not administer ZOSTAVAX to females who are pregnant. Animal reproduction studies have not been conducted. It is not known whether ZOSTAVAX can cause fetal harm. (4.3, 8.1) Pregnancy Registry Available - call 1-800-986-8999.

See 17 for PATIENT COUNSELING INFORMATION and FDA-approved patient labeling

Revised: 04/2013

FULL PRESCRIBING INFORMATION: CONTENTS*

*** Sections or subsections omitted from the full prescribing information are not listed**

FULL PRESCRIBING INFORMATION

1 INDICATIONS AND USAGE

ZOSTAVAX is a live attenuated virus vaccine indicated for prevention of herpes zoster (shingles) in individuals 50 years of age and older.

Limitations of Use of ZOSTAVAX:
- ZOSTAVAX is not indicated for the treatment of zoster or postherpetic neuralgia (PHN).
- ZOSTAVAX is not indicated for prevention of primary varicella infection (Chickenpox).

2 DOSAGE AND ADMINISTRATION

Subcutaneous administration only. Do not inject intravascularly or intramuscularly.

2.1 Recommended Dose and Schedule

Administer ZOSTAVAX as a single 0.65-mL dose subcutaneously in the deltoid region of the upper arm.

2.2 Preparation for Administration

Use only sterile syringes free of preservatives, antiseptics, and detergents for each injection and/or reconstitution of ZOSTAVAX. Preservatives, antiseptics and detergents may inactivate the vaccine virus.

ZOSTAVAX is stored frozen and should be reconstituted immediately upon removal from the freezer.

When reconstituted, ZOSTAVAX is a semi-hazy to translucent, off-white to pale yellow liquid.

Reconstitution:
- Use only the diluent supplied.
- Withdraw the entire contents of the diluent into a syringe.
- To avoid excessive foaming, slowly inject all of the diluent in the syringe into the vial of lyophilized vaccine and gently agitate to mix thoroughly.
- Withdraw the entire contents of reconstituted vaccine into a syringe and inject the total volume subcutaneously.
- **ADMINISTER IMMEDIATELY AFTER RECONSTITUTION** to minimize loss of potency. Discard reconstituted vaccine if not used within 30 minutes. Do not freeze reconstituted vaccine.

3 DOSAGE FORMS AND STRENGTHS

ZOSTAVAX is a lyophilized preparation of live, attenuated varicella-zoster virus (Oka/Merck) to be reconstituted with sterile diluent to give a single dose suspension with a minimum of 19,400 PFU (plaque forming units) when stored at room temperature for up to 30 minutes.

4 CONTRAINDICATIONS

4.1 Hypersensitivity

Do not administer ZOSTAVAX to individuals with a history of anaphylactic/anaphylactoid reaction to gelatin, neomycin or any other component of the vaccine. Neomycin allergy manifested as contact dermatitis is not a contraindication to receiving this vaccine.[1]

4.2 Immunosuppression

ZOSTAVAX is a live, attenuated varicella-zoster vaccine and administration may result in disseminated disease in individuals who are immunosuppressed or immunodeficient. Do not administer ZOSTAVAX to immunosuppressed or immunodeficient individuals including those with a history of primary or acquired immunodeficiency states, leukemia, lymphoma or other malignant neoplasms affecting the bone marrow or lymphatic system, AIDS or other clinical manifestations of infection with human immunodeficiency viruses, and those on immunosuppressive therapy.

4.3 Pregnancy

Do not administer ZOSTAVAX to pregnant women. It is not known whether ZOSTAVAX can cause fetal harm when administered to a pregnant woman or can affect reproduction capacity. However, naturally occurring VZV infection is known to sometimes cause fetal harm. Therefore, ZOSTAVAX should not be administered to pregnant women, and pregnancy should be avoided for 3 months following administration of ZOSTAVAX.

5 WARNINGS AND PRECAUTIONS

5.1 Hypersensitivity Reactions

Serious adverse reactions, including anaphylaxis, have occurred with ZOSTAVAX. Adequate treatment provisions, including epinephrine injection (1:1,000), should be available for immediate use should an anaphylactic/anaphylactoid reaction occur.

5.2 Transmission of Vaccine Virus

Transmission of vaccine virus may occur between vaccinees and susceptible contacts.

5.3 Concurrent Illness

Deferral should be considered in acute illness (for example, in the presence of fever) or in patients with active untreated tuberculosis.

5.4 Limitations of Vaccine Effectiveness

Vaccination with ZOSTAVAX does not result in protection of all vaccine recipients.

The duration of protection beyond 4 years after vaccination with ZOSTAVAX is unknown. The need for revaccination has not been defined.

6 ADVERSE REACTIONS

The most frequent adverse reactions, reported in ≥1% of subjects vaccinated with ZOSTAVAX, were headache and injection-site reactions.

6.1 Clinical Trials Experience

Because clinical trials are conducted under widely varying conditions, rates of adverse reactions observed in the clinical trials of a vaccine cannot be directly compared to rates in the clinical trials of another vaccine and may not reflect the rates observed in practice.

ZOSTAVAX Efficacy and Safety Trial (ZEST) in Subjects 50 to 59 Years of Age

In the ZEST study, subjects received a single dose of either ZOSTAVAX (N=11,184) or placebo (N=11,212). The racial distribution across both vaccination groups was similar: White (94.4%); Black (4.2%); Hispanic (3.3%) and Other (1.4%) in both vaccination groups. The gender distribution was 38% male and 62% female in both vaccination groups. The age distribution of subjects enrolled, 50 to 59 years, was similar in both vaccination groups. All subjects received a vaccination report card (VRC) to record adverse events occurring from Days 1 to 42 postvaccination.

In the ZEST study, serious adverse events occurred at a similar rate in subjects vaccinated with ZOSTAVAX (0.6%) or placebo (0.5%) from Days 1 to 42 postvaccination.

In the ZEST study, all subjects were monitored for adverse reactions. An anaphylactic reaction was reported for one subject vaccinated with ZOSTAVAX.

Most Common Adverse Reactions and Experiences in the ZEST Study

The overall incidence of vaccine-related injection-site adverse reactions within 5 days post-vaccination was greater for subjects vaccinated with ZOSTAVAX as compared to subjects who received placebo (63.6% for ZOSTAVAX and 14.0% for placebo). Injection-site adverse reactions occurring at an incidence ≥1% within 5 days post-vaccination are shown in Table 1.

Table 1
Injection-Site Adverse Reactions Reported in ≥1% of Adults Who Received ZOSTAVAX or Placebo Within 5 Days Post-Vaccination in the ZOSTAVAX Efficacy and Safety Trial

Injection-Site Adverse Reaction	ZOSTAVAX (N = 11094) %	Placebo (N = 11116) %
*Solicited**		
Pain	53.9	9.0
Erythema	48.1	4.3
Swelling	40.4	2.8
Unsolicited		
Pruritis	11.3	0.7
Warmth	3.7	0.2
Hematoma	1.6	1.6
Induration	1.1	0.0

* Solicited on the Vaccination Report Card

Systemic adverse reactions and experiences reported during Days 1-42 at an incidence of ≥1% in either vaccination group were headache (ZOSTAVAX 9.4%, placebo 8.2%) and pain in the extremity (ZOSTAVAX 1.3%, placebo 0.8%), respectively.

The overall incidence of systemic adverse experiences reported during Days 1-42 was higher for ZOSTAVAX (35.4%) than for placebo (33.5%).

Shingles Prevention Study (SPS) in Subjects 60 Years of Age and Older

In the SPS, the largest clinical trial of ZOSTAVAX, subjects received a single dose of either ZOSTAVAX (n=19,270) or placebo (n=19,276). The racial distribution across both vaccination groups was similar: White (95%); Black (2.0%); Hispanic (1.0%) and Other (1.0%) in both vaccination groups. The gender distribution was 59% male and 41% female in

Table 2: Number of Subjects with ≥1 Serious Adverse Events (0-42 Days Postvaccination) in the Shingles Prevention Study

Cohort	ZOSTAVAX n/N %	Placebo n/N %	Relative Risk (95% CI)
Overall Study Cohort (60 years of age and older)	255/18671 1.4%	254/18717 1.4%	1.01 (0.85, 1.20)
60-69 years old	113/10100 1.1%	101/10095 1.0%	1.12 (0.86, 1.46)
70-79 years old	115/7351 1.6%	132/7333 1.8%	0.87 (0.68, 1.11)
≥80 years old	27/1220 2.2%	21/1289 1.6%	1.36 (0.78, 2.37)
AE Monitoring Substudy Cohort (60 years of age and older)	64/3326 1.9%	41/3249 1.3%	1.53 (1.04, 2.25)
60-69 years old	22/1726 1.3%	18/1709 1.1%	1.21 (0.66, 2.23)
70-79 years old	31/1383 2.2%	19/1367 1.4%	1.61 (0.92, 2.82)
≥80 years old	11/217 5.1%	4/173 2.3%	2.19 (0.75, 6.45)

N=number of subjects in cohort with safety follow-up
n=number of subjects reporting an SAE 0-42 Days postvaccination

both vaccination groups. The age distribution of subjects enrolled, 59-99 years, was similar in both vaccination groups. The Adverse Event Monitoring Substudy of the SPS, designed to provide detailed data on the safety profile of the zoster vaccine (n=3,345 received ZOSTAVAX and n=3,271 received placebo) used vaccination report cards (VRC) to record adverse events occurring from Days 0 to 42 postvaccination (97% of subjects completed VRC in both vaccination groups). In addition, monthly surveillance for hospitalization was conducted through the end of the study, 2 to 5 years postvaccination.

The remainder of subjects in the SPS (n=15,925 received ZOSTAVAX and n=16,005 received placebo) were actively followed for safety outcomes through Day 42 postvaccination and passively followed for safety after Day 42.

Serious Adverse Events Occurring 0-42 Days Postvaccination

In the overall SPS study population, serious adverse events occurred at a similar rate (1.4%) in subjects vaccinated with ZOSTAVAX or placebo.

In the AE Monitoring Substudy, the rate of SAEs was increased in the group of subjects who received ZOSTAVAX as compared to the group of subjects who received placebo (Table 2).

[See table 2 above]

Among reported serious adverse events in the SPS (Days 0 to 42 postvaccination), serious cardiovascular events occurred more frequently in subjects who received ZOSTAVAX (20 [0.6%]) than in subjects who received placebo (12 [0.4%]) in the AE Monitoring Substudy. The frequencies of serious cardiovascular events were similar in subjects who received ZOSTAVAX (81 [0.4%]) and in subjects who received placebo (72 [0.4%]) in the entire study cohort (Days 0 to 42 postvaccination).

Serious Adverse Events Occurring Over the Entire Course of the Study

Rates of hospitalization were similar among subjects who received ZOSTAVAX and subjects who received placebo in the AE Monitoring Substudy, throughout the entire study.

Fifty-one individuals (1.5%) receiving ZOSTAVAX were reported to have congestive heart failure (CHF) or pulmonary edema compared to 39 individuals (1.2%) receiving placebo in the AE Monitoring Substudy; 58 individuals (0.3%) receiving ZOSTAVAX were reported to have congestive heart failure (CHF) or pulmonary edema compared to 45 (0.2%) individuals receiving placebo in the overall study.

In the SPS, all subjects were monitored for vaccine-related SAEs. Investigator-determined, vaccine-related serious adverse experiences were reported for 2 subjects vaccinated with ZOSTAVAX (asthma exacerbation and polymyalgia rheumatica) and 3 subjects who received placebo (Goodpasture's syndrome, anaphylactic reaction, and polymyalgia rheumatica).

Deaths

The incidence of death was similar in the groups receiving ZOSTAVAX or placebo during the Days 0-42 postvaccination period; 14 deaths occurred in the group of subjects who received ZOSTAVAX and 16 deaths occurred in the group of subjects who received placebo. The most common reported cause of death was cardiovascular disease (10 in the group of subjects who received ZOSTAVAX, 8 in the group of subjects who received placebo). The overall incidence of death occurring at any time during the study was similar between vaccination groups: 793 deaths (4.1%) occurred in subjects who received ZOSTAVAX and 795 deaths (4.1%) in subjects who received placebo.

Most Common Adverse Reactions and Experiences in the AE Monitoring Substudy of the SPS

Injection-site adverse reactions reported at an incidence ≥1% are shown in Table 3. Most of these adverse reactions were reported as mild in intensity. The overall incidence of vaccine-related injection-site adverse reactions was significantly greater for subjects vaccinated with ZOSTAVAX versus subjects who received placebo (48% for ZOSTAVAX and 17% for placebo).

Table 3: Injection-Site Adverse Reactions* in ≥1% of Adults Who Received ZOSTAVAX or Placebo Within 5 Days Postvaccination from the AE Monitoring Substudy of the Shingles Prevention Study

Adverse Reaction	ZOSTAVAX (N = 3345) %	Placebo (N = 3271) %
Solicited†		
Erythema	35.6	6.9
Pain/Tenderness	34.3	8.3
Swelling	26.1	4.5
Unsolicited		
Hematoma	1.6	1.4
Pruritis	6.9	1.0
Warmth	1.6	0.3

* Patients instructed to report adverse experiences on a Vaccination Report Card
† Solicited on the Vaccination Report Card

Headache was the only systemic adverse reaction reported on the vaccine report card between Days 0-42 by ≥1% of subjects in the AE Monitoring Substudy in either vaccination group (ZOSTAVAX 1.4%, placebo 0.8%).

The numbers of subjects with elevated temperature (≥38.3°C [≥101.0°F]) within 42 days postvaccination were similar in the ZOSTAVAX and the placebo vaccination groups [27 (0.8%) vs. 27 (0.9%), respectively].

The following adverse experiences in the AE Monitoring Substudy of the SPS (Days 0 to 42 postvaccination) were reported at an incidence ≥1% and greater in subjects who received ZOSTAVAX than in subjects who received placebo, respectively: respiratory infection (65 [1.9%] vs. 55 [1.7%]), fever (59 [1.8%] vs. 53 [1.6%]), flu syndrome (57 [1.7%] vs. 52 [1.6%]), diarrhea (51 [1.5%] vs. 41 [1.3%]), rhinitis (46 [1.4%] vs. 36 [1.1%]), skin disorder (35 [1.1%] vs. 31 [1.0%]), respiratory disorder (35 [1.1%] vs. 27 [0.8%]), asthenia (32 [1.0%] vs. 14 [0.4%]).

6.2 VZV Rashes Following Vaccination

Within the 42-day postvaccination reporting period in the ZEST, noninjection-site zoster-like rashes were reported by 34 subjects (19 for ZOSTAVAX and 15 for placebo). Of 24 specimens that were adequate for Polymerase Chain Reaction (PCR) testing, wild-type VZV was detected in 10 (3 for ZOSTAVAX, 7 for placebo) of these specimens. The Oka/Merck strain of VZV was not detected from any of these specimens. Of reported varicella-like rashes (n=124, 69 for ZOSTAVAX and 55 for placebo), 23 had specimens that were available and adequate for PCR testing. VZV was detected in one of these specimens in the ZOSTAVAX group; however, the virus strain (wild-type or Oka/Merck strain) could not be determined.

Within the 42-day postvaccination reporting period in the SPS, noninjection-site zoster-like rashes were reported by 53 subjects (17 for ZOSTAVAX and 36 for placebo). Of 41 specimens that were adequate for Polymerase Chain Reaction (PCR) testing, wild-type VZV was detected in 25 (5 for ZOSTAVAX, 20 for placebo) of these specimens. The Oka/Merck strain of VZV was not detected from any of these specimens.

Of reported varicella-like rashes (n=59), 10 had specimens that were available and adequate for PCR testing. VZV was not detected in any of these specimens.

In clinical trials in support of the initial licensure of the frozen formulation of ZOSTAVAX, the reported rates of noninjection-site zoster-like and varicella-like rashes within 42 days postvaccination were also low in both zoster vaccine and placebo recipients. Of 17 reported varicella-like rashes and non-injection site zoster-like rashes, 10 specimens were available and adequate for PCR testing, and 2 subjects had varicella (onset Day 8 and 17) confirmed to be Oka/Merck strain.

6.3 Postmarketing Experience

The following additional adverse reactions have been identified during postmarketing use of ZOSTAVAX. Because these reactions are reported voluntarily from a population of uncertain size, it is generally not possible to reliably estimate their frequency or establish a causal relationship to the vaccine.

Gastrointestinal disorders: nausea

Skin and subcutaneous tissue disorders: rash

Musculoskeletal and connective tissue disorders: arthralgia; myalgia

General disorders and administration site conditions: injection-site rash; pyrexia; injection-site urticaria; transient injection-site lymphadenopathy

Immune system disorders: hypersensitivity reactions including anaphylactic reactions

Reporting Adverse Events

The U.S. Department of Health and Human Services has established a Vaccine Adverse Event Reporting System (VAERS) to accept all reports of suspected adverse events after the administration of any vaccine. For information or a copy of the vaccine reporting form, call the VAERS toll-free number at 1-800-822-7967 or report online to www.vaers.hhs.gov.[2]

7 DRUG INTERACTIONS

7.1 Concomitant Administration with Other Vaccines

In a randomized clinical study, a reduced immune response to ZOSTAVAX as measured by gpELISA was observed in individuals who received concurrent administration of PNEUMOVAX® 23 and ZOSTAVAX compared with individuals who received these vaccines 4 weeks apart. Consider administration of the two vaccines separated by at least 4 weeks *[see Clinical Studies (14.3)]*.

For concomitant administration of ZOSTAVAX with trivalent inactivated influenza vaccine, *[see Clinical Studies (14.3)]*.

7.2 Antiviral Medications

Concurrent administration of ZOSTAVAX and antiviral medications known to be effective against VZV has not been evaluated.

8 USE IN SPECIFIC POPULATIONS

8.1 Pregnancy

Pregnancy Category: Contraindication *[see Contraindications (4.3)]*.

Vaccinees and health care providers are encouraged to report any exposure to ZOSTAVAX during pregnancy by calling 1-800-986-8999.

8.3 Nursing Mothers

ZOSTAVAX is not indicated in women who are nursing. It is not known whether VZV is secreted in human milk. Therefore, because some viruses are secreted in human milk, caution should be exercised if ZOSTAVAX is administered to a nursing woman.

8.4 Pediatric Use

ZOSTAVAX is not indicated for prevention of primary varicella infection (Chickenpox) and should not be used in children and adolescents.

8.5 Geriatric Use

The median age of subjects enrolled in the largest (N=38,546) clinical study of ZOSTAVAX was 69 years (range 59-99 years). Of the 19,270 subjects who received ZOSTAVAX, 10,378 were 60-69 years of age, 7,629 were 70-79 years of age, and 1,263 were 80 years of age or older.

Table 4: Efficacy of ZOSTAVAX on HZ Incidence Compared with Placebo in the ZOSTAVAX Efficacy and Safety Trial*

Age group (yrs.)	ZOSTAVAX			Placebo			Vaccine Efficacy (95% CI)
	# subjects	# HZ cases	Incidence rate of HZ per 1000 person-yrs.	# subjects	# HZ cases	Incidence rate of HZ per 1000 person-yrs.	
50-59	11211	30	1.994	11228	99	6.596	69.8% (54.1%, 80.6%)

* The analysis was performed on the intent-to-treat (ITT) population that included all subjects randomized in the ZEST study.

Table 5: Efficacy of ZOSTAVAX on HZ Incidence Compared with Placebo in the Shingles Prevention Study*

Age group† (yrs.)	ZOSTAVAX			Placebo			Vaccine Efficacy (95% CI)
	# subjects	# HZ cases	Incidence rate of HZ per 1000 person-yrs.	# subjects	# HZ cases	Incidence rate of HZ per 1000 person-yrs.	
Overall	19254	315	5.4	19247	642	11.1	51% (44%, 58%)
60-69	10370	122	3.9	10356	334	10.8	64% (56%, 71%)
70-79	7621	156	6.7	7559	261	11.4	41% (28%, 52%)
≥80	1263	37	9.9	1332	47	12.2	18% (-29%, 48%)

* The analysis was performed on the Modified Intent-To-Treat (MITT) population that included all subjects randomized in the study who were followed for at least 30 days postvaccination and did not develop an evaluable case of HZ within the first 30 days postvaccination.

† Age strata at randomization were 60-69 and ≥70 years of age.

11 DESCRIPTION

ZOSTAVAX is a lyophilized preparation of the Oka/Merck strain of live, attenuated varicella-zoster virus (VZV). ZOSTAVAX, when reconstituted as directed, is a sterile suspension for subcutaneous administration. Each 0.65-mL dose contains a minimum of 19,400 PFU (plaque-forming units) of Oka/Merck strain of VZV when reconstituted and stored at room temperature for up to 30 minutes.

Each dose contains 31.16 mg of sucrose, 15.58 mg of hydrolyzed porcine gelatin, 3.99 mg of sodium chloride, 0.62 mg of monosodium L-glutamate, 0.57 mg of sodium phosphate dibasic, 0.10 mg of potassium phosphate monobasic, 0.10 mg of potassium chloride; residual components of MRC-5 cells including DNA and protein; and trace quantities of neomycin and bovine calf serum. The product contains no preservatives.

12 CLINICAL PHARMACOLOGY

12.1 Mechanism of Action

The risk of developing zoster appears to be related to a decline in VZV-specific immunity. ZOSTAVAX was shown to boost VZV-specific immunity, which is thought to be the mechanism by which it protects against zoster and its complications. *[See Clinical Studies (14).]*

Herpes zoster (HZ), commonly known as shingles or zoster, is a manifestation of the reactivation of varicella zoster virus (VZV), which, as a primary infection, produces chickenpox (varicella). Following initial infection, the virus remains latent in the dorsal root or cranial sensory ganglia until it reactivates, producing zoster. Zoster is characterized by a unilateral, painful, vesicular cutaneous eruption with a dermatomal distribution.

Pain associated with zoster may occur during the prodrome, the acute eruptive phase, and the postherpetic phase of the infection. Pain occurring in the postherpetic phase of infection is commonly referred to as postherpetic neuralgia (PHN).

Serious complications, such as PHN, scarring, bacterial superinfection, allodynia, cranial and motor neuron palsies, pneumonia, encephalitis, visual impairment, hearing loss, and death can occur as the result of zoster.

13 NONCLINICAL TOXICOLOGY

13.1 Carcinogenesis, Mutagenesis, Impairment of Fertility

ZOSTAVAX has not been evaluated for its carcinogenic or mutagenic potential, or its potential to impair fertility.

14 CLINICAL STUDIES

In two large clinical trials (ZEST and SPS), ZOSTAVAX significantly reduced the risk of developing zoster when compared with placebo (see Table 4 and Table 5).

14.1 ZOSTAVAX Efficacy and Safety Trial (ZEST) in Subjects 50 to 59 Years of Age

Efficacy of ZOSTAVAX was evaluated in the ZOSTAVAX Efficacy and Safety Trial (ZEST), a placebo-controlled, double-blind clinical trial in which 22,439 subjects 50 to 59 years of age were randomized to receive a single dose of either ZOSTAVAX (n=11,211) or placebo (n=11,228). Subjects were followed for the development of zoster for a median of 1.3 years (range 0 to 2 years). Confirmed zoster cases were determined by Polymerase Chain Reaction (PCR) [86%] or, in the absence of virus detection, by a Clinical Evaluation Committee [14%]. The primary efficacy analysis included all subjects randomized in the study (intent-to-treat [ITT] analysis).

Compared with placebo, ZOSTAVAX significantly reduced the risk of developing zoster by 69.8% (95% CI [54.1, 80.6%]) in subjects 50 to 59 years of age (Table 4).

[See table 4 above]

Immune responses to vaccination were evaluated in a random 10% subcohort (n=1,136 for ZOSTAVAX and n=1,133 for placebo) of the subjects enrolled in the ZEST study. VZV antibody levels (Geometric Mean Titers, GMT), as measured by glycoprotein enzyme-linked immunosorbent assay (gpELISA) 6 weeks postvaccination, were increased 2.3-fold [95% CI (2.2, 2.4)] in the group of subjects who received ZOSTAVAX compared to subjects who received placebo; the specific antibody level that correlates with protection from zoster has not been established.

14.2 Shingles Prevention Study (SPS) in Subjects 60 Years of Age and Older

Efficacy of ZOSTAVAX was evaluated in the Shingles Prevention Study (SPS), a placebo-controlled, double-blind clinical trial in which 38,546 subjects 60 years of age or older were randomized to receive a single dose of either ZOSTAVAX (n=19,270) or placebo (n=19,276). Subjects were followed for the development of zoster for a median of 3.1 years (range 31 days to 4.90 years). The study excluded people who were immunocompromised or using corticosteroids on a regular basis, anyone with a previous history of HZ, and those with conditions that might interfere with study evaluations, including people with cognitive impairment, severe hearing loss, those who were non-ambulatory, and those whose survival was not considered to be at least 5 years. Randomization was stratified by age, 60-69 and ≥70 years of age. Suspected zoster cases were confirmed by Polymerase Chain Reaction (PCR) [93%], viral culture [1%], or in the absence of virus detection, as determined by a Clinical Evaluation Committee [6%]. Individuals in both vaccination groups who developed zoster were given famciclovir, and, as necessary, pain medications. The primary efficacy analysis included all subjects randomized in the study who were followed for at least 30 days postvaccination and did not develop an evaluable case of HZ within the first 30 days postvaccination (Modified Intent-To-Treat [MITT] analysis). ZOSTAVAX significantly reduced the risk of developing zoster when compared with placebo (Table 5). In the SPS, vaccine efficacy for the prevention of HZ was highest for those subjects 60-69 years of age and declined with increasing age.

[See table 5 above]

Forty-five subjects were excluded from the MITT analysis (16 in the group of subjects who received ZOSTAVAX and 29 in the group of subjects who received placebo), including 24 subjects with evaluable HZ cases that occurred in the first 30 days postvaccination (6 evaluable HZ cases in the group of subjects who received ZOSTAVAX and 18 evaluable HZ cases in the group of subjects who received placebo).

Suspected HZ cases were followed prospectively for the development of HZ-related complications. Table 6 compares the rates of PHN defined as HZ-associated pain (rated as 3 or greater on a 10-point scale by the study subject and occurring or persisting at least 90 days) following the onset of rash in evaluable cases of HZ.

[See table 6 below]

Table 6: Postherpetic Neuralgia (PHN)* in the Shingles Prevention Study†

Age group (yrs.)‡	ZOSTAVAX					Placebo					Vaccine efficacy against PHN in subjects who develop HZ postvaccination (95% CI)
	# subjects	# HZ cases	# PHN cases	Incidence rate of PHN per 1,000 person-yrs.	% HZ cases with PHN	# subjects	# HZ cases	# PHN cases	Incidence rate of PHN per 1,000 person-yrs.	% HZ cases with PHN	
Overall	19254	315	27	0.5	8.6%	19247	642	80	1.4	12.5%	39%§ (7%, 59%)
60-69	10370	122	8	0.3	6.6%	10356	334	23	0.7	6.9%	5% (-107%, 56%)
70-79	7621	156	12	0.5	7.7%	7559	261	45	2.0	17.2%	55% (18%, 76%)
≥80	1263	37	7	1.9	18.9%	1332	47	12	3.1	25.5%	26% (-69%, 68%)

* PHN was defined as HZ-associated pain rated as ≥3 (on a 0-10 scale), persisting or appearing more than 90 days after onset of HZ rash using Zoster Brief Pain Inventory (ZBPI)[3].

† The table is based on the Modified Intent-To-Treat (MITT) population that included all subjects randomized in the study who were followed for at least 30 days postvaccination and did not develop an evaluable case of HZ within the first 30 days postvaccination.

‡ Age strata at randomization were 60-69 and ≥70 years of age.

§ Age-adjusted estimate based on the age strata (60-69 and ≥70 years of age) at randomization.

The median duration of clinically significant pain (defined as ≥3 on a 0-10 point scale) among HZ cases in the group of subjects who received ZOSTAVAX as compared to the group of subjects who received placebo was 20 days vs. 22 days based on the confirmed HZ cases.

Overall, the benefit of ZOSTAVAX in the prevention of PHN can be primarily attributed to the effect of the vaccine on the prevention of herpes zoster. Vaccination with ZOSTAVAX in the SPS reduced the incidence of PHN in individuals 70 years of age and older who developed zoster postvaccination. Other prespecified zoster-related complications were reported less frequently in subjects who received ZOSTAVAX compared to subjects who received placebo. Among HZ cases, zoster-related complications were reported at similar rates in both vaccination groups (Table 7). [See table 7 above]

Table 7: Specific complications* of zoster among HZ cases in the Shingles Prevention Study

Complication	ZOSTAVAX (N = 19,270)		Placebo (N = 19,276)	
	(n = 321)	% Among Zoster Cases	(n = 659)	% Among Zoster Cases
Allodynia	135	42.1	310	47.0
Bacterial Superinfection	3	0.9	7	1.1
Dissemination	5	1.6	11	1.7
Impaired Vision	2	0.6	9	1.4
Ophthalmic Zoster	35	10.9	69	10.5
Peripheral Nerve Palsies (motor)	5	1.6	12	1.8
Ptosis	2	0.6	9	1.4
Scarring	24	7.5	57	8.6
Sensory Loss	7	2.2	12	1.8

N=number of subjects randomized
n=number of zoster cases, including those cases occurring within 30 days postvaccination, with these data available
* Complications reported at a frequency of ≥1% in at least one vaccination group among subjects with zoster

Visceral complications reported by fewer than 1% of subjects with zoster included 3 cases of pneumonitis and 1 case of hepatitis in the placebo group, and 1 case of meningoencephalitis in the vaccine group.

Immune responses to vaccination were evaluated in a subset of subjects enrolled in the Shingles Prevention Study (N=1,395). VZV antibody levels (Geometric Mean Titers, GMT), as measured by glycoprotein enzyme-linked immunosorbent assay (gpELISA) 6 weeks postvaccination, were increased 1.7-fold (95% CI: [1.6 to 1.8]) in the group of subjects who received ZOSTAVAX compared to subjects who received placebo; the specific antibody level that correlates with protection from zoster has not been established.

14.3 Concomitant Use Studies

In a double-blind, controlled substudy, 374 adults in the US, 60 years of age and older (median age = 66 years), were randomized to receive trivalent inactivated influenza vaccine (TIV) and ZOSTAVAX concurrently (N=188), or TIV alone followed 4 weeks later by ZOSTAVAX alone (N=186). The antibody responses to both vaccines at 4 weeks postvaccination were similar in both groups.

In a double-blind, controlled clinical trial, 473 adults, 60 years of age or older, were randomized to receive ZOSTAVAX and PNEUMOVAX 23 concomitantly (N=237), or PNEUMOVAX 23 alone followed 4 weeks later by ZOSTAVAX alone (N=236). At 4 weeks postvaccination, the VZV antibody levels following concomitant use were significantly lower than the VZV antibody levels following nonconcomitant administration (GMTs of 338 vs. 484 gpELISA units/mL, respectively; GMT ratio = 0.70 (95% CI: [0.61, 0.80])).

15 REFERENCES

1. Reitschel RL, Bernier R. Neomycin sensitivity and the MMR vaccine. JAMA 1981;245(6):571.
2. Atkinson WL, Pickering LK, Schwartz B, Weniger BG, Iskander JK, Watson JC. General recommendations on immunization: Recommendations of the Advisory Committee on Immunization Practices (ACIP) and the American Academy of Family Physicians (AAFP). MMWR 2002;51(RR02):1-36.
3. Coplan PM, Schmader K, Nikas A, Chan ISF, Choo P, Levin MJ, et al. Development of a measure of the burden of pain due to herpes zoster and postherpetic neuralgia for prevention trials: Adaptation of the brief pain inventory. J Pain 2004;5(6):344-56.

16 HOW SUPPLIED/STORAGE AND HANDLING

No. 4963-00 — ZOSTAVAX is supplied as follows: (1) a package of 1 single-dose vial of lyophilized vaccine, **NDC** 0006-4963-00 (package A); and (2) a separate package of 10 vials of diluent (package B).

No. 4963-41 — ZOSTAVAX is supplied as follows: (1) a package of 10 single-dose vials of lyophilized vaccine, **NDC** 0006-4963-41 (package A); and (2) a separate package of 10 vials of diluent (package B).

Storage

To maintain potency, ZOSTAVAX must be stored frozen between -58°F and +5°F (-50°C and -15°C). Use of dry ice may subject ZOSTAVAX to temperatures colder than -58°F (-50°C).

Before reconstitution, ZOSTAVAX SHOULD BE STORED FROZEN at a temperature between -58°F and +5°F (-50°C and -15°C) until it is reconstituted for injection. Any freezer, including frost-free, that has a separate sealed freezer door and reliably maintains a temperature between -58°F and +5°F (-50°C and -15°C) is acceptable for storing ZOSTAVAX.

ZOSTAVAX may be stored and/or transported at refrigerator temperature between 36°F and 46°F (2°C to 8°C) for up to 72 continuous hours prior to reconstitution. Vaccine stored between 36°F and 46°F (2°C to 8°C) that is not used within 72 hours of removal from +5°F (-15°C) storage should be discarded. ZOSTAVAX should be reconstituted immediately upon removal from the freezer. The diluent should be stored separately at room temperature (68°F to 77°F, 20°C to 25°C), or in the refrigerator (36°F to 46°F, 2°C to 8°C).

For further product information call 1-800-MERCK-90.

Before reconstitution, protect from light.

DO NOT FREEZE RECONSTITUTED VACCINE.

17 PATIENT COUNSELING INFORMATION

[See FDA-Approved Patient Labeling.]

- Question the patient about reactions to previous vaccines.
- Provide a copy of the patient information (PPI) located at the end of this insert and discuss any questions or concerns.
- Inform patient of the benefits and risks of ZOSTAVAX, including the potential risk of transmitting the vaccine virus to susceptible individuals, such as immunosuppressed or immunodeficient individuals or pregnant women who have not had chickenpox.
- Instruct patient to report any adverse reactions or any symptoms of concern to their healthcare professional.

Dist. by: Merck Sharp & Dohme Corp., a subsidiary of
MERCK & CO., INC., Whitehouse Station, NJ 08889, USA
Revised: 04/2013
Printed in USA
USPI-I-V2111304R016

Patient Information about

ZOSTAVAX® (pronounced "ZOS tah vax")

Generic name: Zoster Vaccine Live

You should read this summary of information about ZOSTAVAX before you are vaccinated. If you have any questions about ZOSTAVAX after reading this leaflet, you should ask your health care provider. This information does not take the place of talking about ZOSTAVAX with your doctor, nurse, or other health care provider. Only your health care provider can decide if ZOSTAVAX is right for you.

What is ZOSTAVAX and how does it work?

ZOSTAVAX is a vaccine that is used for adults 50 years of age or older to prevent shingles (also known as zoster).

ZOSTAVAX contains a weakened chickenpox virus (varicella-zoster virus).

ZOSTAVAX works by helping your immune system protect you from getting shingles.

If you do get shingles even though you have been vaccinated, ZOSTAVAX may help prevent the nerve pain that can follow shingles in some people. ZOSTAVAX does not protect everyone, so some people who get the vaccine may still get shingles.

ZOSTAVAX cannot be used to treat shingles, or the nerve pain that may follow shingles, once you have it.

What do I need to know about shingles and the virus that causes it?

Shingles is caused by the same virus that causes chickenpox. Once you have had chickenpox, the virus can stay in your nervous system for many years. For reasons that are not fully understood, the virus may become active again and give you shingles. Age and problems with the immune system may increase your chances of getting shingles.

Shingles is a rash that is usually on one side of the body. The rash begins as a cluster of small red spots that often blister. The rash can be painful. Shingles rashes usually last up to 30 days and, for most people, the pain associated with the rash lessens as it heals.

Who should not get ZOSTAVAX?

You should not get ZOSTAVAX if you:

- are allergic to any of its ingredients.
- are allergic to gelatin or neomycin.
- have a weakened immune system (for example, an immune deficiency, leukemia, lymphoma, or HIV/AIDS).
- take high doses of steroids by injection or by mouth.
- are pregnant or plan to get pregnant.

You should not get ZOSTAVAX to prevent chickenpox.

Children should not get ZOSTAVAX.

How is ZOSTAVAX given?

ZOSTAVAX is given as a single dose by injection under the skin.

What should I tell my health care provider before I get ZOSTAVAX?

You should tell your health care provider if you:

- have or have had any medical problems.
- take any medicines, including non-prescription medicines, and dietary supplements.
- have any allergies, including allergies to neomycin or gelatin.
- had an allergic reaction to another vaccine.
- are pregnant or plan to become pregnant.
- are breast-feeding.

Tell your health care provider if you expect to be in close contact (including household contact) with newborn infants, someone who may be pregnant and has not had chickenpox or been vaccinated against chickenpox, or someone who has problems with their immune system. Your health care provider can tell you what situations you may need to avoid.

Can I get ZOSTAVAX with other vaccines?

Talk to your health care provider if you plan to get ZOSTAVAX at the same time as the flu vaccine.

Talk to your health care provider if you plan to get ZOSTAVAX at the same time as PNEUMOVAX® 23 because it may be better to get these vaccines at least 4 weeks apart.

What are the possible side effects of ZOSTAVAX?

The most common side effects that people in the clinical studies reported after receiving the vaccine include:

- redness, pain, itching, swelling, hard lump, warmth, or bruising where the shot was given.
- headache

The following additional side effects have been reported with ZOSTAVAX:

- allergic reactions, which may be serious and may include difficulty in breathing or swallowing. If you have an allergic reaction, call your doctor right away.
- chickenpox
- fever
- hives at the injection site
- joint pain
- muscle pain
- nausea
- rash
- rash at the injection site
- swollen glands near the injection site (that may last a few days to a few weeks)

Tell your healthcare provider if you have any new or unusual symptoms after you receive ZOSTAVAX. For a complete list of side effects, ask your health care provider.

Call 1-800-986-8999 to report any exposure to ZOSTAVAX during pregnancy.

What are the ingredients of ZOSTAVAX?

Active Ingredient: a weakened form of the varicella-zoster virus.

Inactive Ingredients: sucrose, hydrolyzed porcine gelatin, sodium chloride, monosodium L-glutamate, sodium phosphate dibasic, potassium phosphate monobasic, potassium chloride.

This leaflet summarizes important information about ZOSTAVAX. If you would like more information, talk to your health care provider or visit the website at www.ZOSTAVAX.com or call 1-800-622-4477.

Rx Only

Issued June 2011
9989115

Dist. by: Merck Sharp & Dohme Corp., a subsidiary of **MERCK & CO., INC.**, Whitehouse Station, NJ 08889, USA

Merck Sharp & Dohme Corp.,

for product information, please see Merck

Mission Pharmacal Company

10999 IH 10 WEST, SUITE 1000
SAN ANTONIO, TX 78230-1355

Direct All Inquiries to:
PO Box 786099
San Antonio, TX 78278–6099
TOLL FREE: (800) 292-7364
Customer Service (M–W 7A–5:30P Central Time
Th 7:30A–5P Central Time)
(210) 696-8400; FAX: (210) 696-6010

AVAR™-e Emollient Cream ℞

(sodium sulfacetamide 10% and sulfur 5%)

Rx Only
FOR EXTERNAL USE ONLY.
NOT FOR OPHTHALMIC USE.

DESCRIPTION:

Each gram of AVAR™-*e* Emollient Cream (sodium sulfacetamide 10% w/w and sulfur 5% w/w) contains 100 mg of sodium sulfacetamide and 50 mg of colloidal sulfur in an emollient cream vehicle containing isostearyl palmitate, glyceryl stearate (and) PEG-100 stearate, emulsifying wax, cetyl alcohol, dimethicone, purified water, sodium thiosulfate, glycerine, sodium lactate, disodium EDTA, nicotinamide, benzyl alcohol, phenoxyethanol, zinc oxide and fragrance.

Sodium sulfacetamide is a sulfonamide with antibacterial activity while sulfur acts as a keratolytic agent. Sodium sulfacetamide is $C_8H_9N_2NaO_3S{\cdot}H_2O$ with molecular weight of 254.24. Chemically, it is N-[(4-aminophenyl)sulfonyl]-acetamide, monosodium salt, monohydrate. The structural formula is:

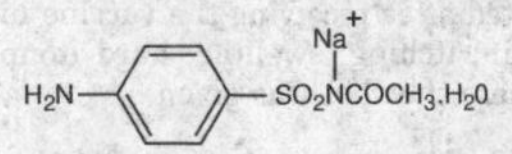

CLINICAL PHARMACOLOGY:

The most widely accepted mechanism of action of sulfonamides is the Woods-Fildes theory, which is based on the fact that sulfonamides act as competitive antagonists to para-aminobenzoic acid (PABA), an essential component for bacterial growth. While absorption through intact skin has not been determined, sodium sulfacetamide is readily absorbed from the gastrointestinal tract when taken orally and excreted in the urine, largely unchanged. The biological half-life has variously been reported as 7 to 12.8 hours.

The exact mode of action of sulfur in the treatment of acne is unknown, but it has been reported that it inhibits the growth of *Propionibacterium acnes* and the formation of free fatty acids.

INDICATIONS:

AVAR™-*e* Emollient Cream is indicated for use in the topical control of acne vulgaris, acne rosacea and seborrheic dermatitis.

CONTRAINDICATIONS:

AVAR™-*e* Emollient Cream is contraindicated for use by patients having known hypersensitivity to sulfonamides, sulfur or any other component of this preparation. AVAR™-*e* Emollient Cream is not to be used by patients with kidney disease.

WARNINGS:

Although rare, sensitivity to sodium sulfacetamide may occur. Therefore, caution and careful supervision should be observed when prescribing this drug for patients who may be prone to hypersensitivity to topical sulfonamides. Systemic toxic reactions such as agranulocytosis, acute hemolytic anemia, purpura hemorrhagica, drug fever, jaundice and contact dermatitis indicate hypersensitivity to sulfonamides. Particular caution should be employed if areas of denuded or abraded skin are involved.

Sulfonamides are known to cause Stevens-Johnson syndrome in hypersensitive individuals. Stevens-Johnson syndrome also has been reported following the use of sodium sulfacetamide topically. Cases of drug induced systemic lupus erythematosus from topical sulfacetamide also have been reported. In one of these cases, there was a fatal outcome. **KEEP OUT OF REACH OF CHILDREN.**

PRECAUTIONS: FOR EXTERNAL USE ONLY. NOT FOR OPHTHALMIC USE.

General: If irritation develops, use of the product should be discontinued and appropriate therapy instituted. Patients should be carefully observed for possible local irritation or sensitization during long-term therapy. The object of this therapy is to achieve desquamation without irritation, but sodium sulfacetamide and sulfur can cause reddening and scaling of the epidermis. These side effects are not unusual in the treatment of acne vulgaris, but patients should be cautioned about the possibility.

Carcinogenesis, Mutagenesis and Impairment of Fertility:
Long-term studies in animals have not been performed to evaluate carcinogenic potential.

Pregnancy:
Category C. Animal reproduction studies have not been conducted with AVAR™-*e* Emollient Cream. It is also not known whether AVAR™-*e* Emollient Cream can cause fetal harm when administered to a pregnant woman or can affect reproduction capacity. AVAR™-*e* Emollient Cream should be given to a pregnant woman only if clearly needed.

Nursing Mothers:
It is not known whether sodium sulfacetamide is excreted in human milk following topical use of AVAR™-*e* Emollient Cream. However, small amounts of orally administered sulfonamides have been reported to be excreted in human milk. In view of this and because many drugs are excreted in human milk, caution should be exercised when AVAR™-*e* Emollient Cream is administered to a nursing woman.

Pediatric Use:
Safety and effectiveness in children under the age of 12 has not been established.

ADVERSE REACTIONS:

Although rare, sodium sulfacetamide may cause local irritation.

Call your doctor for medical advice about side effects. To report SUSPECTED ADVERSE REACTIONS, contact the FDA at 1-800-FDA-1088 or www.fda.gov/medwatch.

DOSAGE AND ADMINISTRATION:

Wash hands. Cleanse affected area. Apply a thin layer 1 to 3 times daily or as directed by a physician. Massage the cream completely and uniformly into the skin.

HOW SUPPLIED:

AVAR™-*e* Emollient Cream is supplied in a 45 g (1.6 oz.) tube, NDC 0178-0470-45, and in 5 g sample packets, NDC 0178-0470-05.

Store at 25°C (77°F); excursions permitted to 15° to 30°C (59° to 86°F).

See USP Controlled Room Temperature.

Note: Protect from freezing and excessive heat. The product may tend to darken slightly on storage. Slight discoloration does not impair the efficacy or safety of the product. Keep container or packet tightly closed.

Occasionally, a slight yellowish discoloration may occur when an excessive amount of the product is used and comes in contact with white fabrics. This discoloration, however, presents no problem, as it is readily removed by ordinary laundering without bleaches.

Distributed by:
Mission Pharmacal Company
San Antonio, TX 78230-1355
Patent Pending
Rev 0911

AVAR™-e LS Emollient Cream ℞

(sodium sulfacetamide 10% and sulfur 2%)

Rx Only
FOR EXTERNAL USE ONLY.
NOT FOR OPHTHALMIC USE.

DESCRIPTION:

Each gram of AVAR™-*e* LS Emollient Cream (sodium sulfacetamide 10% w/w and sulfur 2% w/w) contains 100 mg of sodium sulfacetamide and 20 mg of colloidal sulfur in an emollient cream vehicle containing isostearyl palmitate, glyceryl stearate (and) PEG-100 stearate, emulsifying wax, cetyl alcohol, dimethicone, purified water, sodium thiosulfate, gum arabica, glycerine, sodium lactate, disodium EDTA, nicotinamide, benzyl alcohol, phenoxyethanol, zinc oxide and fragrance.

Sodium sulfacetamide is a sulfonamide with antibacterial activity while sulfur acts as a keratolytic agent. Sodium sulfacetamide is $C_8H_9N_2NaO_3S{\cdot}H_2O$ with molecular weight of 254.24. Chemically, it is N-[(4-aminophenyl)sulfonyl]-acetamide, monosodium salt, monohydrate. The structural formula is:

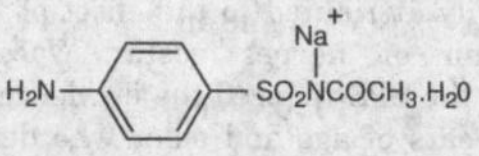

CLINICAL PHARMACOLOGY:

The most widely accepted mechanism of action of sulfonamides is the Woods-Fildes theory, which is based on the fact that sulfonamides act as competitive antagonists to para-aminobenzoic acid (PABA), an essential component for bacterial growth. While absorption through intact skin has not been determined, sodium sulfacetamide is readily absorbed from the gastrointestinal tract when taken orally and excreted in the urine, largely unchanged. The biological half-life has variously been reported as 7 to 12.8 hours.

The exact mode of action of sulfur in the treatment of acne is unknown, but it has been reported that it inhibits the growth of *Propionibacterium acnes* and the formation of free fatty acids.

INDICATIONS:

AVAR™-*e* LS Emollient Cream is indicated for use in the topical control of acne vulgaris, acne rosacea and seborrheic dermatitis.

CONTRAINDICATIONS:

AVAR™-*e* LS Emollient Cream is contraindicated for use by patients having known hypersensitivity to sulfonamides, sulfur or any other component of this preparation. AVAR™-*e* LS Emollient Cream is not to be used by patients with kidney disease.

WARNINGS:

Although rare, sensitivity to sodium sulfacetamide may occur. Therefore, caution and careful supervision should be observed when prescribing this drug for patients who may be prone to hypersensitivity to topical sulfonamides. Systemic toxic reactions such as agranulocytosis, acute hemolytic anemia, purpura hemorrhagica, drug fever, jaundice and contact dermatitis indicate hypersensitivity to sulfonamides. Particular caution should be employed if areas of denuded or abraded skin are involved.

Sulfonamides are known to cause Stevens-Johnson syndrome in hypersensitive individuals. Stevens-Johnson syndrome also has been reported following the use of sodium sulfacetamide topically. Cases of drug induced systemic lupus erythematosus from topical sulfacetamide also have been reported. In one of these cases, there was a fatal outcome. **KEEP OUT OF REACH OF CHILDREN.**

PRECAUTIONS: FOR EXTERNAL USE ONLY. NOT FOR OPHTHALMIC USE.

General: If irritation develops, use of the product should be discontinued and appropriate therapy instituted. Patients should be carefully observed for possible local irritation or sensitization during long-term therapy. The object of this therapy is to achieve desquamation without irritation, but sodium sulfacetamide and sulfur can cause reddening and scaling of the epidermis. These side effects are not unusual in the treatment of acne vulgaris, but patients should be cautioned about the possibility.

Carcinogenesis, Mutagenesis and Impairment of Fertility:
Long-term studies in animals have not been performed to evaluate carcinogenic potential.

Pregnancy:
Category C. Animal reproduction studies have not been conducted with AVAR™-*e* LS Emollient Cream. It is also not known whether AVAR™-*e* LS Emollient Cream can cause fetal harm when administered to a pregnant woman or can affect reproduction capacity. AVAR™-*e* LS Emollient Cream should be given to a pregnant woman only if clearly needed.

Nursing Mothers:
It is not known whether sodium sulfacetamide is excreted in human milk following topical use of AVAR™-*e* LS Emollient Cream. However, small amounts of orally administered sulfonamides have been reported to be excreted in human milk. In view of this and because many drugs are excreted in human milk, caution should be exercised when AVAR™-*e* LS Emollient Cream is administered to a nursing woman.

Pediatric Use:
Safety and effectiveness in children under the age of 12 has not been established.

ADVERSE REACTIONS:

Although rare, sodium sulfacetamide may cause local irritation.

Call your doctor for medical advice about side effects. To report SUSPECTED ADVERSE REACTIONS, contact the FDA at 1-800-FDA-1088 or www.fda.gov/medwatch.

DOSAGE AND ADMINISTRATION:
Wash hands. Cleanse affected area. Apply a thin layer 1 to 3 times daily or as directed by a physician. Massage the cream completely and uniformly into the skin.

HOW SUPPLIED:
AVAR™-*e* LS Emollient Cream is supplied in a 45 g (1.6 oz.) tube, NDC 0178-0465-45, and in 5 g sample packets, NDC 0178-0465-05.
Store at 25°C (77°F); excursions permitted to 15° to 30°C (59° to 86°F).
See USP Controlled Room Temperature.
Note: Protect from freezing and excessive heat. The product may tend to darken slightly on storage. Slight discoloration does not impair the efficacy or safety of the product. Keep tube or packet tightly closed.
Occasionally, a slight yellowish discoloration may occur when an excessive amount of the product is used and comes in contact with white fabrics. This discoloration, however, presents no problem, as it is readily removed by ordinary laundering without bleaches.
Distributed by:
Mission Pharmacal Company
San Antonio, TX 78230-1355
Patent Pending
Rev 0911

AVAR™ CLEANSER ℞

(sodium sulfacetamide 10% and sulfur 5%)
Rx Only
FOR EXTERNAL USE ONLY.
NOT FOR OPHTHALMIC USE.

DESCRIPTION
Each gram of AVAR™ Cleanser (sodium sulfacetamide 10% w/w and sulfur 5% w/w) contains 100 mg of sodium sulfacetamide and 50 mg of colloidal sulfur in a mild aqueous based cleansing vehicle containing benzyl alcohol, cetyl alcohol, gum arabic, fragrance, phenoxyethanol, propylene glycol, purified water, sodium lauryl sulfate, sodium magnesium silicate, sodium thiosulfate and stearyl alcohol.
Sodium sulfacetamide is a sulfonamide with antibacterial activity while sulfur acts as a keratolytic agent. Sodium sulfacetamide is $C_8H_9N_2NaO_3S \bullet H_2O$ with molecular weight of 254.24. Chemically, it is N-[(4-aminophenyl)sulfonyl]-acetamide, monosodium salt, monohydrate. The structural formula is:

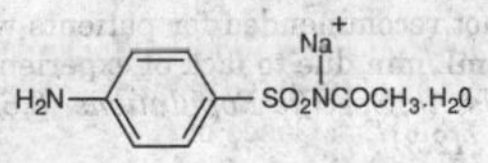

CLINICAL PHARMACOLOGY
The most widely accepted mechanism of action of sulfonamides is the Woods-Fildes theory, which is based on the fact that sulfonamides act as competitive antagonists to para-aminobenzoic acid (PABA), an essential component for bacterial growth. While absorption through intact skin has not been determined, sodium sulfacetamide is readily absorbed from the gastrointestinal tract when taken orally and excreted in the urine, largely unchanged. The biological half-life has variously been reported as 7 to 12.8 hours.
The exact mode of action of sulfur in the treatment of acne is unknown, but it has been reported that it inhibits the growth of *Propionibacterium acnes* and the formation of free fatty acids.

INDICATIONS
AVAR™ Cleanser is indicated for use in the topical control of acne vulgaris, acne rosacea and seborrheic dermatitis.

CONTRAINDICATIONS
AVAR™ Cleanser is contraindicated for use by patients having known hypersensitivity to sulfonamides, sulfur or any other component of this preparation. AVAR™ Cleanser is not to be used by patients with kidney disease.

WARNINGS
Although rare, sensitivity to sodium sulfacetamide may occur. Therefore, caution and careful supervision should be observed when prescribing this drug for patients who may be prone to hypersensitivity to topical sulfonamides. Systemic toxic reactions such as agranulocytosis, acute hemolytic anemia, purpura hemorrhagica, drug fever, jaundice and contact dermatitis indicate hypersensitivity to sulfonamides. Particular caution should be employed if areas of denuded or abraded skin are involved.
Sulfonamides are known to cause Stevens-Johnson syndrome in hypersensitive individuals. Stevens-Johnson syndrome also has been reported following the use of sodium sulfacetamide topically. Cases of drug induced systemic lupus erythematosus from topical sulfacetamide also have been reported. In one of these cases, there was a fatal outcome. **KEEP OUT OF REACH OF CHILDREN.**

PRECAUTIONS
FOR EXTERNAL USE ONLY. NOT FOR OPHTHALMIC USE.
General: If irritation develops, use of the product should be discontinued and appropriate therapy instituted. Patients should be carefully observed for possible local irritation or sensitization during long-term therapy. The object of this therapy is to achieve desquamation without irritation, but sodium sulfacetamide and sulfur can cause reddening and scaling of the epidermis. These side effects are not unusual in the treatment of acne vulgaris, but patients should be cautioned about the possibility.
Carcinogenesis, Mutagenesis and Impairment of Fertility: Long-term studies in animals have not been performed to evaluate carcinogenic potential.
Pregnancy:
Category C. Animal reproduction studies have not been conducted with AVAR™ Cleanser. It is also not known whether AVAR™ Cleanser can cause fetal harm when administered to a pregnant woman or can affect reproduction capacity. AVAR™ Cleanser should be given to a pregnant woman only if clearly needed.
Nursing Mothers:
It is not known whether sodium sulfacetamide is excreted in human milk following topical use of AVAR™ Cleanser. However, small amounts of orally administered sulfonamides have been reported to be excreted in human milk. In view of this and because many drugs are excreted in human milk, caution should be exercised when AVAR™ Cleanser is administered to a nursing woman.
Pediatric Use:
Safety and effectiveness in children under the age of 12 has not been established.

ADVERSE REACTIONS
Although rare, sodium sulfacetamide may cause local irritation.
Call your doctor for medical advice about side effects. To report SUSPECTED ADVERSE REACTIONS, contact the FDA at 1-800-FDA-1088 or www.fda.gov/medwatch.

DOSAGE AND ADMINISTRATION
Wash affected areas with AVAR™ Cleanser 1 to 2 times daily or as directed by a physician. Avoid contact with eyes or mucous membranes. Wet skin and liberally apply to areas to be cleansed, massage gently into skin for 10 to 20 seconds working into a full lather, rinse thoroughly and pat dry. If drying occurs, it may be controlled by rinsing cleanser off sooner or using cleanser less often.

HOW SUPPLIED
AVAR™ Cleanser is supplied in an 8 oz. (227 g) bottle, NDC 0178-0480-08, and in 5 g sample packets, NDC 0178-0480-05.
Store at 25°C (77°F); excursions permitted to 15° to 30°C (59° to 86°F). See USP Controlled Room Temperature.
Note: Protect from freezing and excessive heat. The product may tend to darken slightly on storage. Slight discoloration does not impair the efficacy or safety of the product. Keep container or packet tightly closed.
Occasionally, a slight yellowish discoloration may occur when an excessive amount of the product is used and comes in contact with white fabrics. This discoloration, however, presents no problem, as it is readily removed by ordinary laundering without bleaches.
Distributed by:
Mission Pharmacal Company
San Antonio, TX 78230-1355
Patent Pending
Rev 0911

AVAR™ LS CLEANSER ℞

(sodium sulfacetamide 10% and sulfur 2%)
Rx Only
FOR EXTERNAL USE ONLY.
NOT FOR OPHTHALMIC USE.

DESCRIPTION
Each gram of AVAR™ LS Cleanser (sodium sulfacetamide 10% w/w and sulfur 2% w/w) contains 100 mg of sodium sulfacetamide and 20 mg of colloidal sulfur in a mild aqueous based cleansing vehicle containing purified water, propylene glycol, stearyl alcohol, cetyl alcohol, sodium magnesium silicate, sodium lauryl sulfate, phenoxyethanol, benzyl alcohol, gum arabic, sodium thiosulfate and fragrance.
Sodium sulfacetamide is a sulfonamide with antibacterial activity while sulfur acts as a keratolytic agent. Sodium sulfacetamide is $C_8H_9N_2NaO_3S \bullet H_2O$ with molecular weight of 254.24. Chemically, it is N-[(4-aminophenyl)sulfonyl]-acetamide, monosodium salt, monohydrate. The structural formula is:

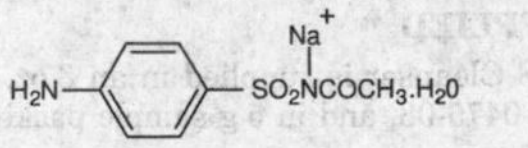

CLINICAL PHARMACOLOGY
The most widely accepted mechanism of action of sulfonamides is the Woods-Fildes theory, which is based on the fact that sulfonamides act as competitive antagonists to para-aminobenzoic acid (PABA), an essential component for bacterial growth. While absorption through intact skin has not been determined, sodium sulfacetamide is readily absorbed from the gastrointestinal tract when taken orally and excreted in the urine, largely unchanged. The biological half-life has variously been reported as 7 to 12.8 hours.
The exact mode of action of sulfur in the treatment of acne is unknown, but it has been reported that it inhibits the growth of *Propionibacterium acnes* and the formation of free fatty acids.

INDICATIONS
AVAR™ LS Cleanser is indicated for use in the topical control of acne vulgaris, acne rosacea and seborrheic dermatitis.

CONTRAINDICATIONS
AVAR™ LS Cleanser is contraindicated for use by patients having known hypersensitivity to sulfonamides, sulfur or any other component of this preparation. AVAR™ LS Cleanser is not to be used by patients with kidney disease.

WARNINGS
Although rare, sensitivity to sodium sulfacetamide may occur. Therefore, caution and careful supervision should be observed when prescribing this drug for patients who may be prone to hypersensitivity to topical sulfonamides. Systemic toxic reactions such as agranulocytosis, acute hemolytic anemia, purpura hemorrhagica, drug fever, jaundice and contact dermatitis indicate hypersensitivity to sulfonamides. Particular caution should be employed if areas of denuded or abraded skin are involved.
Sulfonamides are known to cause Stevens-Johnson syndrome in hypersensitive individuals. Stevens-Johnson syndrome also has been reported following the use of sodium sulfacetamide topically. Cases of drug induced systemic lupus erythematosus from topical sulfacetamide also have been reported. In one of these cases, there was a fatal outcome. **KEEP OUT OF REACH OF CHILDREN.**

PRECAUTIONS
FOR EXTERNAL USE ONLY. NOT FOR OPHTHALMIC USE.
General: If irritation develops, use of the product should be discontinued and appropriate therapy instituted. Patients should be carefully observed for possible local irritation or sensitization during long-term therapy. The object of this therapy is to achieve desquamation without irritation, but sodium sulfacetamide and sulfur can cause reddening and scaling of the epidermis. These side effects are not unusual in the treatment of acne vulgaris, but patients should be cautioned about the possibility.
Carcinogenesis, Mutagenesis and Impairment of Fertility: Long-term studies in animals have not been performed to evaluate carcinogenic potential.
Pregnancy:
Category C. Animal reproduction studies have not been conducted with AVAR™ LS Cleanser. It is also not known whether AVAR™ LS Cleanser can cause fetal harm when administered to a pregnant woman or can affect reproduction capacity. AVAR™ LS Cleanser should be given to a pregnant woman only if clearly needed.
Nursing Mothers:
It is not known whether sodium sulfacetamide is excreted in human milk following topical use of AVAR™ LS Cleanser. However, small amounts of orally administered sulfonamides have been reported to be excreted in human milk. In view of this and because many drugs are excreted in human milk, caution should be exercised when AVAR™ LS Cleanser is administered to a nursing woman.
Pediatric Use:
Safety and effectiveness in children under the age of 12 has not been established.

ADVERSE REACTIONS
Although rare, sodium sulfacetamide may cause local irritation.
Call your doctor for medical advice about side effects. To report SUSPECTED ADVERSE REACTIONS, contact the FDA at 1-800-FDA-1088 or www.fda.gov/medwatch.

DOSAGE AND ADMINISTRATION
Wash affected areas with AVAR™ LS Cleanser 1 to 2 times daily or as directed by a physician. Avoid contact with eyes or mucous membranes. Wet skin and liberally apply to areas to be cleansed, massage gently into skin for 10 to 20 seconds working into a full lather, rinse thoroughly and pat dry. If drying occurs, it may be controlled by rinsing cleanser off sooner or using cleanser less often.

HOW SUPPLIED

AVAR™ LS Cleanser is supplied in an 8 oz. (227 g) bottle, NDC 0178-0475-08, and in 5 g sample packets, NDC 0178-0475-05.

Store at 25°C (77°F); excursions permitted to 15° to 30°C (59° to 86°F). See USP Controlled Room Temperature.

Note: Protect from freezing and excessive heat. The product may tend to darken slightly on storage. Slight discoloration does not impair the efficacy or safety of the product. Keep container or packet tightly closed.

Occasionally, a slight yellowish discoloration may occur when an excessive amount of the product is used and comes in contact with white fabrics. This discoloration, however, presents no problem, as it is readily removed by ordinary laundering without bleaches.

Distributed by:
Mission Pharmacal Company
San Antonio, TX 78230-1355
Patent Pending
Rev 0911

BINOSTO ℞

(alendronate sodium)
effervescent tablets for oral solution

HIGHLIGHTS OF PRESCRIBING INFORMATION

These highlights do not include all the information needed to use BINOSTO™ safely and effectively. See full prescribing information for BINOSTO. BINOSTO (alendronate sodium) effervescent tablets for oral solution. Initial U.S. Approval 1995

INDICATIONS AND USAGE

BINOSTO is a bisphosphonate indicated for:
- Treatment of osteoporosis in postmenopausal women (1.1)
- Treatment to increase bone mass in men with osteoporosis (1.2)

Important limitation of use: The optimal duration of use has not been determined. Patients should have the need for continued therapy re-evaluated on a periodic basis. (1.3)

DOSAGE AND ADMINISTRATION

- 70 mg BINOSTO effervescent tablet once weekly. (2.1, 2.2)
- Dissolve one tablet of BINOSTO in approximately half a glass of plain room temperature water (4 oz). Wait at least 5 minutes after the effervescence stops, stir the solution for approximately 10 seconds and consume contents. (2.3)
- Must be taken *at least* **30** minutes before the first food, beverage, or medication of the day. (2.3)
- Do not lie down for at least 30 minutes after taking BINOSTO and until after the first food of the day. (2.3)

DOSAGE FORMS AND STRENGTHS

Effervescent tablets, 70 mg (3)

CONTRAINDICATIONS

- Abnormalities of the esophagus which delay emptying such as stricture or achalasia (4, 5.1)
- Inability to stand/sit upright for at least 30 minutes (4, 5.1)
- Increased risk of aspiration. (4)
- Hypocalcemia (4, 5.2)
- Hypersensitivity to any component of this product (4, 6.2)

WARNINGS AND PRECAUTIONS

- Severe irritation of upper gastrointestinal mucosa can occur. Follow dosing instructions. Use caution in patients with active upper GI disease. Discontinue if new or worsening symptoms occur. (5.1)
- Hypocalcemia can worsen and must be corrected prior to use. (5.2)
- Severe bone, joint, muscle pain may occur. Discontinue use if severe symptoms develop. (5.3)
- Osteonecrosis of the jaw has been reported. (5.4)
- Atypical femur fractures have been reported. Evaluate new thigh or groin pain to rule out an incomplete femoral fracture. (5.5)
- Each tablet contains 650 mg sodium, equivalent to 1650 mg NaCl. Use caution in patients on sodium restriction. (5.7)

ADVERSE REACTIONS

The most common adverse reactions (incidence ≥3%) are abdominal pain, acid regurgitation, constipation, diarrhea, dyspepsia, musculoskeletal pain, and nausea. (6.1)

To report SUSPECTED ADVERSE REACTIONS, contact Mission Pharmacal Company at 1-855-778-0177or FDA at 1-800-FDA-1088 or www.fda.gov/medwatch

DRUG INTERACTIONS

- Calcium supplements, antacids or oral medications containing multivalent cations interfere with absorption of alendronate. (7.1)
- Aspirin and nonsteroidal anti-inflammatory drug use may worsen GI irritation; caution should be used. (7.2, 7.3)

USE IN SPECIFIC POPULATIONS

- BINOSTO is not indicated for use in pediatric patients. (8.4)
- BINOSTO is not recommended in patients with renal impairment (creatinine clearance <35 mL/min). (2.5, 5.6, 8.6)

See 17 for PATIENT COUNSELING INFORMATION and Medication Guide

Revised: 06/2012

FULL PRESCRIBING INFORMATION: CONTENTS*

*** Sections or subsections omitted from the full prescribing information are not listed**

FULL PRESCRIBING INFORMATION

1 INDICATIONS AND USAGE

1.1 Treatment of Osteoporosis in Postmenopausal Women

BINOSTO effervescent tablet 70 mg is indicated for the treatment of osteoporosis in postmenopausal women. For the treatment of osteoporosis, alendronate sodium increases bone mass and reduces the incidence of fractures, including those of the hip and spine (vertebral compression fractures). *[See Clinical Studies (14.1)]*

1.2 Treatment to Increase Bone Mass in Men With Osteoporosis

BINOSTO is indicated for treatment to increase bone mass in men with osteoporosis *[see Clinical Studies (14.2)]*.

1.3 Important Limitations of Use

The safety and effectiveness of BINOSTO for the treatment of osteoporosis are based on clinical data of four years duration. The optimal duration of use has not been determined. All patients on bisphosphonate therapy should have the need for continued therapy re-evaluated on a periodic basis.

2 DOSAGE AND ADMINISTRATION

2.1 Treatment of Osteoporosis in Postmenopausal Women

The recommended dosage is one 70 mg effervescent tablet once weekly.

2.2 Treatment to Increase Bone Mass in Men With Osteoporosis

The recommended dosage is one 70 mg effervescent tablet once weekly.

2.3 Dosing Instructions

To assure adequate drug absorption and to decrease the risk of esophageal adverse reactions, dosing instructions should be followed:

- BINOSTO should only be taken upon arising for the day and must be taken at least 30 minutes before the first food, beverage, or medication of the day.
- Dissolve the effervescent tablet in 4 ounces room temperature plain water only (not mineral water or flavored water).
- After the effervescence stops, wait at least 5 minutes and then stir the solution for approximately 10 seconds and ingest.
- Patients should not lie down for at least 30 minutes after taking BINOSTO and until after their first food of the day.
- BINOSTO should not be taken at bedtime or before arising for the day.
- Waiting less than 30 minutes, or taking BINOSTO with food, beverages (other than plain water) or other medications will lessen the effect of BINOSTO by decreasing its absorption into the body *[see Drug Interactions (7.1)]*.
- Failure to follow these instructions may increase the risk of esophageal adverse reactions *[see Warnings and Precautions (5.1)]*.

2.4 Recommendations for Calcium and Vitamin D Supplementation

Patients should receive supplemental calcium and vitamin D, if dietary intake is inadequate *[see Warnings and Precautions (5.2)]*. Patients at increased risk for vitamin D insufficiency (e.g., over the age of 70 years, nursing home-bound, or chronically ill) may need vitamin D supplementation. Patients with gastrointestinal malabsorption syndromes may require higher doses of vitamin D supplementation and measurement of 25-hydroxyvitamin D should be considered.

2.5 Dosing in Severe Renal Impairment

BINOSTO is not recommended for patients with creatinine clearance <35 mL/min due to lack of experience in this population. *[see Use in Specific Populations (8.6) and Clinical Pharmacology (12.3)]*.

3 DOSAGE FORMS AND STRENGTHS

BINOSTO effervescent tablets are round, flat-faced, white to off-white tablets, 25 mm in diameter, with beveled edges, with "M" debossed on one side, containing 91.37 mg of alendronate sodium, which is equivalent to 70 mg of free alendronic acid.

4 CONTRAINDICATIONS

- Abnormalities of the esophagus which delay esophageal emptying such as stricture or achalasia *[see Warnings and Precautions (5.1)]*
- Inability to stand or sit upright for at least 30 minutes *[see Dosage and Administration (2.3); Warnings and Precautions (5.1)]*
- Do not administer BINOSTO to patients at increased risk of aspiration
- Hypocalcemia *[see Warnings and Precautions (5.2)]*
- Hypersensitivity to any component of this product. Hypersensitivity reactions including urticaria and angioedema have been reported *[see Adverse Reactions (6.2)]*.

5 WARNINGS AND PRECAUTIONS

5.1 Upper Gastrointestinal Adverse Reactions

BINOSTO, like other bisphosphonates administered orally, may cause local irritation of the upper gastrointestinal mucosa. Because of these possible irritant effects and a potential for worsening of the underlying disease, caution should be used when BINOSTO is given to patients with active upper gastrointestinal problems (such as known Barrett's esophagus, dysphagia, other esophageal diseases, gastritis, duodenitis, or ulcers).

Esophageal adverse experiences, such as esophagitis, esophageal ulcers and esophageal erosions, occasionally with bleeding and rarely followed by esophageal stricture or perforation, have been reported in patients receiving treatment with oral bisphosphonates including alendronate sodium. In some cases these have been severe and required hospitalization. Physicians should therefore be alert to any signs or symptoms signaling a possible esophageal reaction and patients should be instructed to discontinue BINOSTO and seek medical attention if they develop dysphagia, odynophagia, retrosternal pain or new or worsening heartburn.

The risk of severe esophageal adverse experiences appears to be greater in patients who lie down after taking oral bisphosphonates including alendronate sodium, and/or who continue to take oral bisphosphonates including alendronate sodium after developing symptoms suggestive of esophageal irritation. Therefore, it is very important that the full dosing instructions are provided to, and understood by, the patient *[see Dosage and Administration (2.3)]*. In patients who cannot comply with dosing instructions due to mental disability, therapy with BINOSTO should be used under appropriate supervision.

There have been post-marketing reports of gastric and duodenal ulcers with oral bisphosphonate use, some severe and with complications, although no increased risk was observed in controlled clinical trials *[see Adverse Reactions (6.2)]*.

5.2 Mineral Metabolism

Hypocalcemia must be corrected before initiating therapy with BINOSTO *[see Contraindications (4)]*. Other disorders affecting mineral metabolism (such as vitamin D deficiency) should also be effectively treated. In patients with these conditions, serum calcium and symptoms of hypocalcemia should be monitored during therapy with BINOSTO.

Presumably due to the effects of BINOSTO on increasing bone mineral, small, asymptomatic decreases in serum calcium and phosphate may occur. Patients should receive adequate calcium and vitamin D intake.

5.3 Musculoskeletal Pain

In post marketing experience, severe and occasionally incapacitating bone, joint, and/or muscle pain has been reported in patients taking bisphosphonates that are approved for the treatment of osteoporosis *[see Adverse Reactions (6.2)]*. This category of drugs includes BINOSTO. Most of the patients were postmenopausal women. The time to onset of symptoms varied from one day to several months after starting the drug. Discontinue use if severe symptoms develop. Most patients had relief of symptoms after stopping. A subset had recurrence of symptoms when rechallenged with the same drug or another bisphosphonate.

In placebo-controlled clinical studies of alendronate sodium, the percentages of patients with these symptoms were similar in the alendronate sodium and placebo groups.

5.4 Osteonecrosis of the Jaw

Osteonecrosis of the jaw (ONJ), which can occur spontaneously, is generally associated with tooth extraction and/or local infection with delayed healing, and has been reported in patients taking bisphosphonates, including alendronate sodium. Known risk factors for osteonecrosis of the jaw include invasive dental procedures (e.g., tooth extraction, dental implants, boney surgery), diagnosis of cancer, concomitant therapies (e.g., chemotherapy, corticosteroids), poor oral hygiene, and co-morbid disorders (e.g., periodontal and/or other pre-existing dental disease, anemia, coagulopathy, infection, ill-fitting dentures).

For patients requiring invasive dental procedures, discontinuation of bisphosphonate treatment may reduce the risk for ONJ. Clinical judgment of the treating physician and/or oral surgeon should guide the management plan of each patient based on individual benefit/risk assessment.

Patients who develop osteonecrosis of the jaw while on bisphosphonate therapy should receive care by an oral surgeon. In these patients, extensive dental surgery to treat ONJ may exacerbate the condition. Discontinuation of bisphosphonate therapy should be considered based on individual benefit/risk assessment.

5.5 Atypical Subtrochanteric and Diaphyseal Femoral Fractures

Atypical, low-energy, or low trauma fractures of the femoral shaft have been reported in bisphosphonate-treated patients. These fractures can occur anywhere in the femoral shaft from just below the lesser trochanter to above the supracondylar flare and are transverse or short oblique in orientation without evidence of comminution. Causality has not been established as these fractures also occur in osteoporotic patients who have not been treated with bisphosphonates.

Atypical femur fractures most commonly occur with minimal or no trauma to the affected area. They may be bilateral and many patients report prodromal pain in the affected area, usually presenting as dull, aching thigh pain, weeks to months before a complete fracture occurs. A number of reports note that patients were also receiving treatment with glucocorticoids (e.g., prednisone) at the time of fracture.

Any patient with a history of bisphosphonate exposure who presents with thigh or groin pain should be suspected of having an atypical fracture and should be evaluated to rule out an incomplete femur fracture. Patients presenting with an atypical fracture should also be assessed for symptoms and signs of fracture in the contralateral limb. Interruption of bisphosphonate therapy should be considered, pending a risk/benefit assessment, on an individual basis.

5.6 Renal Impairment

BINOSTO is not recommended for patients with creatinine clearance <35 mL/min *[see Dosage and Administration (2.5)]*.

Table 1 Osteoporosis Treatment Studies in Postmenopausal Women
Adverse Reactions Considered Possibly, Probably, or Definitely Drug Related by the Investigators and Reported in ≥1% of Patients

	United States/Multinational Studies		Fracture Intervention Trial	
	Alendronate Sodium* % (N=196)	Placebo % (N=397)	Alendronate Sodium** % (N=3236)	Placebo % (N=3223)
Gastrointestinal				
Abdominal pain	6.6	4.8	1.5	1.5
Nausea	3.6	4.0	1.1	1.5
Dyspepsia	3.6	3.5	1.1	1.2
Constipation	3.1	1.8	0.0	0.2
Diarrhea	3.1	1.8	0.6	0.3
Flatulence	2.6	0.5	0.2	0.3
Acid regurgitation	2.0	4.3	1.1	0.9
Esophageal ulcer	1.5	0.0	0.1	0.1
Vomiting	1.0	1.5	0.2	0.3
Dysphagia	1.0	0.0	0.1	0.1
Abdominal distention	1.0	0.8	0.0	0.0
Gastritis	0.5	1.3	0.6	0.7
Musculoskeletal				
Musculoskeletal (bone, muscle or joint) pain	4.1	2.5	0.4	0.3
Muscle cramp	0.0	1.0	0.2	0.1
Nervous system/psychiatric				
Headache	2.6	1.5	0.2	0.2
Dizziness	0.0	1.0	0.0	0.1
Special senses				
Taste perversion	0.5	1.0	0.1	0.0

* 10 mg/day for three years
** 5 mg/day for 2 years and 10 mg/day for either 1 or 2 additional years

5.7 Patients Sensitive to High Sodium Intake

Each BINOSTO effervescent tablet contains 650 mg of sodium, equivalent to approximately 1650 mg of salt (NaCl). Use caution in patients who must restrict their sodium intake, including some patients with a history of heart failure, hypertension, or other cardiovascular diseases *[see Patient Counseling Information (17.3)]*.

6 ADVERSE REACTIONS

6.1 Clinical Trials Experience

Because clinical trials are conducted under widely varying conditions, adverse reaction rates observed in the clinical trials of a drug cannot be directly compared to rates in the clinical trials of another drug and may not reflect the rates observed in clinical practice.

The safety of BINOSTO (alendronate sodium) effervescent tablet 70 mg is based on clinical trial data of alendronate sodium 10 mg daily and alendronate sodium 70 mg weekly.

Treatment of Osteoporosis in Postmenopausal Women

Daily Dosing

The safety of alendronate sodium 10 mg daily in the treatment of postmenopausal osteoporosis was assessed in four clinical trials that enrolled 7453 women aged 44-84 years. Study 1 and Study 2 were identically designed, three-year, placebo-controlled, double-blind, multicenter studies (United States and Multinational n=994); Study 3 was the three year vertebral fracture cohort of the Fracture Intervention Trial [FIT] (n=2027) and Study 4 was the four-year clinical fracture cohort of FIT (n=4432). Overall, 3620 patients were exposed to placebo and 3432 patients exposed to alendronate. Patients with pre-existing gastrointestinal disease and concomitant use of non-steroidal anti-inflammatory drugs were included in these clinical trials. In Study 1 and Study 2 all women received 500 mg elemental calcium as carbonate. In Study 3 and Study 4 all women with dietary calcium intake less than 1000 mg per day received 500 mg calcium and 250 IU Vitamin D per day.

Among patients treated with alendronate 10 mg or placebo in Study 1 and Study 2, and all patients in Study 3 and Study 4, the incidence of all-cause mortality was 1.8% in the placebo group and 1.8% in the alendronate group. The incidence of serious adverse events was 30.7% in the placebo group and 30.9% in the alendronate group. The percentage of patients who discontinued the study due to any clinical adverse event was 9.5% in the placebo group and 8.9% in the alendronate group. Adverse reactions from these studies considered by the investigators as possibly, probably, or definitely drug related in ≥1% of patients treated with either alendronate or placebo are presented in Table 1.

[See table 1 above]

Rarely, rash and erythema have occurred.

Gastrointestinal Adverse Reactions: One patient treated with alendronate sodium (10 mg/day), who had a history of peptic ulcer disease and gastrectomy and who was taking concomitant aspirin developed an anastomotic ulcer with mild hemorrhage, which was considered drug related. Aspirin and alendronate sodium were discontinued and the patient recovered. In the Study 1 and Study 2 populations, 49-54% had a history of gastrointestinal disorders at baseline and 54-89% used nonsteroidal anti-inflammatory drugs or aspirin at some time during the studies *[see Warnings and Precautions (5.1)]*.

Laboratory Test Findings: In double-blind, multicenter, controlled studies, asymptomatic, mild, and transient decreases in serum calcium and phosphate were observed in approximately 18% and 10%, respectively, of patients taking alendronate versus approximately 12% and 3% of those taking placebo. However, the incidences of decreases in serum calcium to <8.0 mg/dL (2.0 mM) and serum phosphate to ≤2.0 mg/dL (0.65 mM) were similar in both treatment groups.

Weekly Dosing

The safety of alendronate sodium 70 mg once weekly for the treatment of postmenopausal osteoporosis was assessed in a one-year, double-blind, multicenter study comparing alendronate 70 mg once weekly and alendronate 10 mg daily. The overall safety and tolerability profiles of once weekly alendronate 70 mg and alendronate 10 mg daily were similar. The adverse reactions considered by the investigators as possibly, probably, or definitely drug related in ≥1% of patients in either treatment group are presented in Table 2.

Table 2 Osteoporosis Treatment Studies in Postmenopausal Women
Adverse Reactions Considered Possibly, Probably, or Definitely Drug Related by the Investigators and Reported in ≥1% of Patients

	Once Weekly Alendronate Sodium 70 mg % (N=519)	Once Daily Alendronate Sodium 10 mg % (N=370)
Gastrointestinal		
Abdominal pain	3.7	3.0
Dyspepsia	2.7	2.2
Acid regurgitation	1.9	2.4
Nausea	1.9	2.4
Abdominal distention	1.0	1.4
Constipation	0.8	1.6
Flatulence	0.4	1.6
Gastritis	0.2	1.1
Gastric ulcer	0.0	1.1
Musculoskeletal		
Musculoskeletal (bone, muscle, joint) pain	2.9	3.2
Muscle cramp	0.2	1.1

Osteoporosis in Men

In two placebo-controlled, double-blind, multicenter studies in men (a two-year study of alendronate sodium 10 mg/day and a one-year study of once weekly alendronate sodium 70 mg) the rates of discontinuation of therapy due to any

Table 3 Osteoporosis Studies in Men
Adverse Reactions Considered Possibly, Probably, or Definitely Drug Related by the Investigators and Reported in ≥2% of Patients

	Two-Year Study Once Daily Alendronate Sodium 10 mg % (N=146)	Two-Year Study Placebo % (N=95)	One-Year Study Once Weekly Alendronate Sodium 70 mg % (N=109)	One-Year Study Placebo % (N=58)
Gastrointestinal				
Acid regurgitation	4.1	3.2	0.0	0.0
Flatulence	4.1	1.1	0.0	0.0
Gastroesophageal reflux disease	0.7	3.2	2.8	0.0
Dyspepsia	3.4	0.0	2.8	1.7
Diarrhea	1.4	1.1	2.8	0.0
Abdominal pain	2.1	1.1	0.9	3.4
Nausea	2.1	0.0	0.0	0.0

clinical adverse event were 2.7% for alendronate 10 mg/day vs. 10.5% for placebo, and 6.4% for once weekly alendronate 70 mg vs. 8.6% for placebo. The adverse reactions considered by the investigators as possibly, probably, or definitely drug related in ≥2% of patients treated with either alendronate or placebo are presented in the following table. [See table 3 above]

6.2 Post-Marketing Experience

The following adverse reactions have been identified during post-approval use of alendronate sodium. Because these reactions are reported voluntarily from a population of uncertain size, it is not always possible to reliably estimate their frequency or establish a causal relationship to drug exposure.

Body as a Whole: hypersensitivity reactions including urticaria and rarely angioedema. Transient symptoms of myalgia, malaise, asthenia and rarely, fever have been reported with alendronate, typically in association with initiation of treatment. Rarely, symptomatic hypocalcemia has occurred, generally in association with predisposing conditions. Rarely, peripheral edema.

Gastrointestinal: esophagitis, esophageal erosions, esophageal ulcers, rarely esophageal stricture or perforation, and oropharyngeal ulceration. Gastric or duodenal ulcers, some severe and with complications have also been reported *[see Dosage and Administration (2.3); Warnings and Precautions (5.1)]*.

Dental: Localized osteonecrosis of the jaw, generally associated with tooth extraction and/or local infection with delayed healing, has been reported rarely *[see Warnings and Precautions (5.4)]*.

Musculoskeletal: bone, joint, and/or muscle pain, occasionally severe, and rarely incapacitating *[see Warnings and Precautions (5.3)]* ; joint swelling; low-energy femoral shaft and subtrochanteric fractures *[see Warnings and Precautions (5.5)]*.

Nervous system: dizziness and vertigo.

Skin: rash (occasionally with photosensitivity), pruritus, alopecia, rarely severe skin reactions, including Stevens-Johnson syndrome and toxic epidermal necrolysis.

Special Senses: rarely uveitis, scleritis or episcleritis.

7 DRUG INTERACTIONS

7.1 Calcium Supplements/Antacids

Co-administration of BINOSTO and calcium, antacids, or oral medications containing multivalent cations will interfere with absorption of BINOSTO. Therefore, patients must wait at least one-half hour after taking BINOSTO before taking any other oral medications.

7.2 Aspirin

In clinical studies, the incidence of upper gastrointestinal adverse events was increased in patients receiving concomitant therapy with daily doses of alendronate sodium greater than 10 mg and aspirin-containing products.

7.3 Nonsteroidal Anti-inflammatory Drugs (NSAIDs)

BINOSTO may be administered to patients taking NSAIDs. In a 3-year, controlled, clinical study (n=2027) during which a majority of patients received concomitant NSAIDs, the incidence of upper gastrointestinal adverse events was similar in patients taking alendronate sodium 5 or 10 mg/day compared to those taking placebo. However, since NSAID use is associated with gastrointestinal irritation, caution should be used during concomitant use with BINOSTO.

8 USE IN SPECIFIC POPULATIONS

8.1 Pregnancy

Pregnancy Category C:

There are no studies in pregnant women. BINOSTO should be used during pregnancy only if the potential benefit justifies the potential risk to the mother and fetus.

Bisphosphonates are incorporated into the bone matrix, from which they are gradually released over a period of years. The amount of bisphosphonate incorporated into adult bone, and hence, the amount available for release back into the systemic circulation, is directly related to the dose and duration of bisphosphonate use. There are no data on fetal risk in humans. However, there is a theoretical risk of fetal harm, predominantly skeletal, if a woman becomes pregnant after completing a course of bisphosphonate therapy. The impact of variables such as time between cessation of bisphosphonate therapy to conception, the particular bisphosphonate used, and the route of administration (intravenous versus oral) on the risk has not been studied.

Reproduction studies in rats showed decreased postimplantation survival and decreased body weight gain in normal pups at doses less than half of the recommended clinical dose. Sites of incomplete fetal ossification were statistically significantly increased in rats beginning at approximately 3 times the clinical dose in vertebral (cervical, thoracic, and lumbar), skull, and sternebral bones. No similar fetal effects were seen when pregnant rabbits were treated with doses approximately 10 times the clinical dose.

Both total and ionized calcium decreased in pregnant rats at approximately 4 times the clinical dose resulting in delays and failures of delivery. Protracted parturition due to maternal hypocalcemia occurred in rats at doses as low as one tenth the clinical dose when rats were treated from before mating through gestation. Maternotoxicity (late pregnancy deaths) also occurred in the female rats treated at approximately 4 times the clinical dose for varying periods of time ranging from treatment only during pre-mating to treatment only during early, middle, or late gestation; these deaths were lessened but not eliminated by cessation of treatment. Calcium supplementation either in the drinking water or by minipump could not ameliorate the hypocalcemia or prevent maternal and neonatal deaths due to delays in delivery; intravenous calcium supplementation prevented maternal, but not fetal deaths.

Exposure multiples based on surface area, mg/m^2, were calculated using a 40-mg human daily dose. Animal dose ranged between 1 and 15 mg/kg/day in rats and up to 40 mg/kg/day in rabbits.

8.3 Nursing Mothers

It is not known whether alendronate is excreted in human milk. Because many drugs are excreted in human milk, caution should be exercised when BINOSTO is administered to nursing women.

8.4 Pediatric Use

BINOSTO is not indicated for use in pediatric patients.

The safety and efficacy of alendronate sodium were examined in a randomized, double-blind, placebo-controlled two-year study of 139 pediatric patients, aged 4-18 years, with severe osteogenesis imperfecta (OI). One-hundred-and-nine patients were randomized to 5 mg alendronate sodium daily (weight <40 kg) or 10 mg alendronate sodium daily (weight ≥40 kg) and 30 patients to placebo. The mean baseline lumbar spine BMD Z-score of the patients was -4.5. The mean change in lumbar spine BMD Z-score from baseline to Month 24 was 1.3 in the alendronate-treated patients and 0.1 in the placebo-treated patients. Treatment with alendronate sodium did not reduce the risk of fracture. Sixteen percent of the alendronate-treated patients who sustained a radiologically-confirmed fracture by Month 12 of the study had delayed fracture healing (callus remodeling) or fracture non-union when assessed radiographically at Month 24 compared with 9% of the placebo-treated patients. In alendronate-treated patients, bone histomorphometry data obtained at Month 24 demonstrated decreased bone turnover and delayed mineralization time; however, there were no mineralization defects. There were no statistically significant differences between the alendronate sodium and placebo groups in reduction of bone pain. The oral bioavailability in children was similar to that observed in adults.

The overall safety profile of alendronate sodium in OI patients treated for up to 24 months was generally similar to that of adults with osteoporosis treated with alendronate sodium. However, there was an increased occurrence of vomiting in OI patients treated with alendronate sodium compared to placebo. During the 24-month treatment period, vomiting was observed in 32 of 109 (29.4%) patients treated with alendronate sodium and 3 of 30 (10%) patients treated with placebo.

In a pharmacokinetic study, 6 of 24 pediatric OI patients who received a single oral dose of alendronate sodium 35 or 70 mg developed fever, flu-like symptoms, and/or mild lymphocytopenia within 24 to 48 hours after administration. These events, lasting no more than 2 to 3 days and responding to acetaminophen, are consistent with an acute-phase response that has been reported in patients receiving bisphosphonates, including alendronate sodium. *[See Adverse Reactions (6.2).]*

8.5 Geriatric Use

Of the patients receiving alendronate sodium in the Fracture Intervention Trial (FIT), 71% (n=2302) were ≥65 years of age and 17% (n=550) were ≥75 years of age. Of the patients receiving alendronate sodium in the United States and Multinational osteoporosis treatment studies in women and osteoporosis studies in men, *[see Clinical Studies (14.1), (14.2)]*, 45% and 54%, respectively, were 65 years of age or over. No overall differences in efficacy or safety were observed between these patients and younger patients, but greater sensitivity of some older individuals cannot be ruled out.

8.6 Renal Impairment

BINOSTO is not recommended for patients with creatinine clearance <35 mL/min. No dosage adjustment is necessary in patients with creatinine clearance values between 35-60 mL/min *[see Dosage and Administration (2.5) and Clinical Pharmacology (12.3)]*.

8.7 Hepatic Impairment

As there is evidence that alendronate is not metabolized or excreted in the bile, no studies were conducted in patients with hepatic impairment. No dosage adjustment is necessary *[see Clinical Pharmacology (12.3)]*.

10 OVERDOSAGE

Significant lethality after single oral doses was seen in female rats and mice at 552 mg/kg (3256 mg/m^2) and 966 mg/kg (2898 mg/m^2), respectively. In males, these values were slightly higher, 626 and 1280 mg/kg, respectively. There was no lethality in dogs at oral doses up to 200 mg/kg (4000 mg/m^2).

No specific information is available on the treatment of overdosage with BINOSTO. Hypocalcemia, hypophosphatemia, and upper gastrointestinal adverse events, such as upset stomach, heartburn, esophagitis, gastritis, or ulcer, may result from oral overdosage. Milk or antacids should be given to bind alendronate. Due to the risk of esophageal irritation, vomiting should not be induced and the patient should remain fully upright.

Dialysis would not be beneficial.

11 DESCRIPTION

BINOSTO (alendronate sodium) is a bisphosphonate that acts as a specific inhibitor of osteoclast-mediated bone resorption. Bisphosphonates are synthetic analogs of pyrophosphate that bind to the hydroxyapatite found in bone.

Alendronate sodium is chemically described as (4 amino-1-hydroxybutylidene) bisphosphonic acid, monosodium salt, trihydrate. The molecular formula of alendronate sodium is $C_4H_{12}NNaO_7P_2 \bullet 3H_2O$ and its molecular weight is 325.12. The structural formula of alendronate sodium is

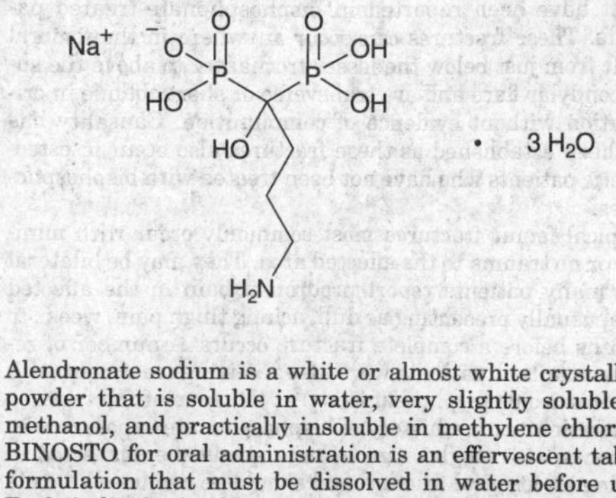

Alendronate sodium is a white or almost white crystalline powder that is soluble in water, very slightly soluble in methanol, and practically insoluble in methylene chloride.

BINOSTO for oral administration is an effervescent tablet formulation that must be dissolved in water before use. Each individual tablet contains 91.37 mg of alendronate sodium, which is equivalent to 70 mg of free alendronic acid. Each tablet also contains the following inactive ingredients: monosodium citrate anhydrous, citric acid anhdydrous, sodium hydrogen carbonate, and sodium carbonate anhydrous as buffering agents, strawberry flavor, acesulfame potassium, and sucralose.

Once the effervescent tablet is dissolved in water, the alendronate sodium is present in a citrate-buffered solution.

12 CLINICAL PHARMACOLOGY

12.1 Mechanism of Action

Animal studies have indicated the following mode of action. At the cellular level, alendronate shows preferential localization to sites of bone resorption, specifically under osteoclasts. The osteoclasts adhere normally to the bone surface but lack the ruffled border that is indicative of active resorption. Alendronate does not interfere with osteoclast recruitment or attachment, but it does inhibit osteoclast activity. Studies in mice on the localization of radioactive [^{3}H]alendronate in bone showed about 10-fold higher uptake on osteoclast surfaces than on osteoblast surfaces. Bones examined 6 and 49 days after [^{3}H]alendronate administration in rats and mice, respectively, showed that normal bone was formed on top of the alendronate, which was incorporated inside the matrix. While incorporated in bone matrix, alendronate is not pharmacologically active. Thus, alendronate must be continuously administered to suppress osteoclasts on newly formed resorption surfaces. Histomorphometry in baboons and rats showed that alendronate treatment reduces bone turnover (i.e., the number of sites at which bone is remodeled). In addition, bone formation exceeds bone resorption at these remodeling sites, leading to progressive gains in bone mass.

12.2 Pharmacodynamics

Alendronate is a bisphosphonate that binds to bone hydroxyapatite and specifically inhibits the activity of osteoclasts, the bone-resorbing cells. Alendronate reduces bone resorption with no direct effect on bone formation, although the latter process is ultimately reduced because bone resorption and formation are coupled during bone turnover.

Osteoporosis in Postmenopausal Women

Osteoporosis is characterized by low bone mass that leads to an increased risk of fracture. The diagnosis can be confirmed by the finding of low bone mass, evidence of fracture on x-ray, a history of osteoporotic fracture, or height loss or kyphosis, indicative of vertebral (spinal) fracture. Osteoporosis occurs in both males and females but is most common among women following the menopause, when bone turnover increases and the rate of bone resorption exceeds that of bone formation. These changes result in progressive bone loss and lead to osteoporosis in a significant proportion of women over age 50. Fractures, usually of the spine, hip, and wrist, are the common consequences. From age 50 to age 90, the risk of hip fracture in white women increases 50-fold and the risk of vertebral fracture 15- to 30-fold. It is estimated that approximately 40% of 50-year-old women will sustain one or more osteoporosis-related fractures of the spine, hip, or wrist during their remaining lifetimes. Hip fractures, in particular, are associated with substantial morbidity, disability, and mortality.

Daily oral doses of alendronate sodium (5, 20, and 40 mg for six weeks) in postmenopausal women produced biochemical changes indicative of dose-dependent inhibition of bone resorption, including decreases in urinary calcium and urinary markers of bone collagen degradation (such as deoxypyridinoline and cross-linked N-telopeptides of type I collagen). These biochemical changes tended to return toward baseline values as early as 3 weeks following the discontinuation of therapy with alendronate and did not differ from placebo after 7 months.

Long-term treatment of osteoporosis with alendronate sodium 10 mg/day (for up to five years) reduced urinary excretion of markers of bone resorption, deoxypyridinoline and cross-linked N-telopeptides of type I collagen, by approximately 50% and 70%, respectively, to reach levels similar to those seen in healthy premenopausal women. Similar decreases were seen in patients in osteoporosis prevention studies who received alendronate sodium 5 mg/day. The decrease in the rate of bone resorption indicated by these markers was evident as early as 1 month and at 3 to 6 months reached a plateau that was maintained for the entire duration of treatment with alendronate sodium. In osteoporosis treatment studies alendronate sodium 10 mg/day decreased the markers of bone formation, osteocalcin and bone specific alkaline phosphatase by approximately 50%, and total serum alkaline phosphatase by approximately 25 to 30% to reach a plateau after 6 to 12 months. In osteoporosis prevention studies alendronate sodium 5 mg/day decreased osteocalcin and total serum alkaline phosphatase by approximately 40% and 15%, respectively. Similar reductions in the rate of bone turnover were observed in postmenopausal women during one-year studies with once weekly alendronate sodium 70 mg for the treatment of osteoporosis and once weekly alendronate sodium 35 mg for the prevention of osteoporosis. These data indicate that the rate of bone turnover reached a new steady state, despite the progressive increase in the total amount of alendronate deposited within bone.

As a result of inhibition of bone resorption, asymptomatic reductions in serum calcium and phosphate concentrations were also observed following treatment with alendronate sodium. In the long-term studies, reductions from baseline in serum calcium (approximately 2%) and phosphate (approximately 4 to 6%) were evident the first month after the initiation of alendronate sodium 10 mg. No further decreases in serum calcium were observed for the five-year duration of treatment; however, serum phosphate returned toward prestudy levels during years three through five. Similar reductions were observed with alendronate sodium 5 mg/day. In one-year studies with once weekly alendronate sodium 35 and 70 mg, similar reductions were observed at 6 and 12 months. The reduction in serum phosphate may reflect not only the positive bone mineral balance due to alendronate sodium but also a decrease in renal phosphate reabsorption.

Osteoporosis in Men

Treatment of men with osteoporosis with alendronate sodium 10 mg/day for two years reduced urinary excretion of cross-linked N-telopeptides of type I collagen by approximately 60% and bone-specific alkaline phosphatase by approximately 40%. Similar reductions were observed in a one-year study in men with osteoporosis receiving once weekly alendronate sodium 70 mg.

12.3 Pharmacokinetics

Absorption

Relative to an intravenous (IV) reference dose, the mean oral bioavailability of alendronate in women was 0.64% for doses ranging from 5 to 70 mg when administered after an overnight fast and two hours before a standardized breakfast. Oral bioavailability of the 10 mg tablet in men (0.59%) was similar to that in women when administered after an overnight fast and 2 hours before breakfast.

BINOSTO 70 mg effervescent tablet and alendronate sodium 70 mg tablet are bioequivalent.

A study evaluating the effect of food on the bioavailability of BINOSTO was performed in 119 healthy women. Bioavailability was decreased (by approximately 50%) when 70 mg alendronate sodium was administered 15 minutes before a standardized breakfast, when compared to dosing 4 hours before eating.

In studies of treatment and prevention of osteoporosis, alendronate was effective when administered at least 30 minutes before breakfast.

Bioavailability was negligible whether alendronate sodium was administered with or up to 2 hours after a standardized breakfast. Concomitant administration of alendronate with coffee or orange juice reduced bioavailability by approximately 60%.

Distribution

Preclinical studies (in male rats) show that alendronate sodium transiently distributes to soft tissues following 1 mg/kg IV administration but is then rapidly redistributed to bone or excreted in the urine. The mean steady-state volume of distribution, exclusive of bone, is at least 28 L in humans. Concentrations of drug in plasma following therapeutic oral doses are too low (less than 5 ng/mL) for analytical detection. Protein binding in human plasma is approximately 78%.

Metabolism

There is no evidence that alendronate sodium is metabolized in animals or humans.

Excretion

Following a single IV dose of [^{14}C]alendronate, approximately 50% of the radioactivity was excreted in the urine within 72 hours and little or no radioactivity was recovered in the feces. Following a single 10 mg IV dose, the renal clearance of alendronate was 71 mL/min (64, 78; 90% confidence interval [CI]), and systemic clearance did not exceed 200 mL/min. Plasma concentrations fell by more than 95% within 6 hours following IV administration. The terminal half-life in humans is estimated to exceed 10 years, probably reflecting release of alendronate from the skeleton. Based on the above, it is estimated that after 10 years of oral treatment with alendronate sodium (10 mg daily) the amount of alendronate released daily from the skeleton is approximately 25% of that absorbed from the gastrointestinal tract.

Specific Populations

Gender: Bioavailability and the fraction of an intravenous dose excreted in urine were similar in men and women.

Geriatric: Bioavailability and disposition (urinary excretion) were similar in elderly and younger patients. No dosage adjustment is necessary in elderly patients.

Race: Pharmacokinetic differences due to race have not been studied.

Renal Impairment: Preclinical studies show that, in rats with kidney failure, increasing amounts of drug are present in plasma, kidney, spleen, and tibia. In healthy controls, drug that is not deposited in bone is rapidly excreted in the urine. No evidence of saturation of bone uptake was found after 3 weeks dosing with cumulative intravenous doses of 35 mg/kg in young male rats. Although no formal renal impairment pharmacokinetic study has been conducted in patients, it is likely that, as in animals, elimination of alendronate via the kidney will be reduced in patients with impaired renal function. Therefore, somewhat greater accumulation of alendronate in bone might be expected in patients with impaired renal function.

No dosage adjustment is necessary for patients with creatinine clearance 35 to 60 mL/min. BINOSTO is not recommended for patients with creatinine clearance <35 mL/min due to lack of experience with alendronate in renal failure.

Drug Interactions

Intravenous ranitidine was shown to double the bioavailability of oral alendronate. The clinical significance of this increased bioavailability and whether similar increases will occur in patients given oral H_2-antagonists is unknown.

In healthy subjects, oral prednisone (20 mg three times daily for five days) did not produce a clinically meaningful change in the oral bioavailability of alendronate (a mean increase ranging from 20 to 44%).

Products containing calcium and other multivalent cations are likely to interfere with absorption of alendronate

13 NONCLINICAL TOXICOLOGY

13.1 Carcinogenesis, Mutagenesis, Impairment of Fertility

Harderian gland (a retro-orbital gland not present in humans) adenomas were increased in high-dose female mice (p=0.003) in a 92-week oral carcinogenicity study at doses of alendronate of 1, 3, and 10 mg/kg/day (males) or 1, 2, and 5 mg/kg/day (females). These doses are equivalent to 0.12 to 1.2 times a maximum recommended daily dose of 40 mg, based on surface area, mg/m^2. The relevance of this finding to humans is unknown.

Parafollicular cell (thyroid) adenomas were increased in high-dose male rats (p=0.003) in a 2-year oral carcinogenicity study at doses of 1 and 3.75 mg/kg body weight. These doses are equivalent to 0.26 and 1 times a 40 mg human daily dose based on surface area, mg/m^2. The relevance of this finding to humans is unknown.

Alendronate sodium was not genotoxic in the in vitro microbial mutagenesis assay with and without metabolic activation, in an in vitro mammalian cell mutagenesis assay, in an in vitro alkaline elution assay in rat hepatocytes, and in an in vivo chromosomal aberration assay in mice. In an in vitro chromosomal aberration assay in Chinese hamster ovary cells, however, alendronate gave equivocal results.

Alendronate sodium had no effect on fertility (male or female) in rats at oral doses up to 5 mg/kg/day (1.3 times a 40 mg human daily dose based on surface area, mg/m^2).

13.2 Animal Toxicology and/or Pharmacology

The relative inhibitory activities on bone resorption and mineralization of alendronate and etidronate were compared in the Schenk assay, which is based on histological examination of the epiphyses of growing rats. In this assay, the lowest dose of alendronate that interfered with bone mineralization (leading to osteomalacia) was 6000-fold the antiresorptive dose. The corresponding ratio for etidronate was one to one. These data suggest that alendronate administered in therapeutic doses is highly unlikely to induce osteomalacia.

14 CLINICAL STUDIES

14.1 Treatment of Osteoporosis in Postmenopausal Women

BINOSTO (alendronate sodium) effervescent tablet 70 mg is bioequivalent to alendronate sodium tablet 70 mg. The fracture reduction efficacy and bone mineral density changes attributed to BINOSTO are based on clinical trial data of alendronate sodium 10 mg daily and alendronate sodium 70 mg weekly.

Daily Dosing

The efficacy of alendronate sodium 10 mg daily was assessed in four clinical trials. Study 1, a three-year, multicenter double-blind, placebo-controlled, US clinical study enrolled 478 patients with a BMD T-score at or below minus 2.5 with or without a prior vertebral fracture; Study 2, a three-year, multicenter double blind placebo controlled Multinational clinical study enrolled 516 patients with a BMD T-score at or below minus 2.5 with or without a prior vertebral fracture; Study 3, the Three-Year Study of the Fracture Intervention Trial (FIT) a study which enrolled 2027 postmenopausal patients with at least one baseline vertebral fracture; and Study 4, the Four-Year Study of FIT: a study which enrolled 4432 postmenopausal patients with low bone mass but without a baseline vertebral fracture.

Effect on Fracture Incidence

To assess the effects of alendronate sodium on the incidence of vertebral fractures (detected by digitized radiography; approximately one third of these were clinically symptomatic), the U.S. and Multinational studies were combined in an analysis that compared placebo to the pooled dosage groups of alendronate sodium (5 or 10 mg for three years or 20 mg for two years followed by 5 mg for one year). There was a statistically significant reduction in the proportion of patients treated with alendronate experiencing one or more new vertebral fractures relative to those treated with placebo (3.2% vs. 6.2%; a 48% relative risk reduction). A reduction in the total number of new vertebral fractures (4.2 vs. 11.3 per 100 patients) was also observed. In the pooled analysis, patients who received alendronate had a loss in stature that was statistically significantly less than was observed in those who received placebo (-3.0 mm vs. -4.6 mm).

Table 4 Effect of Alendronate Sodium on Fracture Incidence in the Three-Year Study of FIT (Patients With Vertebral Fracture at Baseline)

	Percent of Patients			
	Alendronate Sodium (N=1022)	Placebo (N=1005)	Absolute Reduction in Fracture Incidence	Relative Reduction in Fracture Risk %
Patients with:				
Vertebral fractures (diagnosed by X-ray)*				
≥1 new vertebral fracture	7.9	15.0	7.1	47†
≥2 new vertebral fractures	0.5	4.9	4.4	90†
Clinical (symptomatic) fractures				
Any clinical (symptomatic) fracture	13.8	18.1	4.3	26‡
≥1 clinical (symptomatic) vertebral fracture	2.3	5.0	2.7	54§
Hip fracture	1.1	2.2	1.1	51¶
Wrist (forearm) fracture	2.2	4.1	1.9	48¶

*Number evaluable for vertebral fractures: alendronate, n=984; placebo, n=966
†p<0.001, ‡p=0.007, §p<0.01, ¶p<0.05

Table 5 Effect of Alendronate on Fracture Incidence in Osteoporotic* Patients in the Four-Year Study of FIT (Patients Without Vertebral Fracture at Baseline)

	Percent of Patients			
	Alendronate Sodium (n=1545)	Placebo (n=1521)	Absolute Reduction in Fracture Incidence	Relative Reduction in Fracture Risk (%)
Patients with:				
Vertebral fractures (diagnosed by X-ray)†				
≥1 new vertebral fracture	2.5	4.8	2.3	48‡
≥2 new vertebral fractures	0.1	0.6	0.5	78§
Clinical (symptomatic) fractures				
Any clinical (symptomatic) fracture	12.9	16.2	3.3	22¶
≥1 clinical (symptomatic) vertebral fracture	1.0	1.6	0.6	41 (NS)#
Hip fracture	1.0	1.4	0.4	29 (NS)#
Wrist (forearm) fracture	3.9	3.8	-0.1	NS#

*Baseline femoral neck BMD at least 2 SD below the mean for young adult women
†Number evaluable for vertebral fractures: alendronate, n=1426; placebo, n=1428
‡p<0.001, §p=0.035, ¶p=0.01
#Not significant. This study was not powered to detect differences at these sites.

Figure 3 Osteoporosis Treatment in Studies in Postmenopausal Women Time Course Effect of Alendronate Sodium 10 mg/day Versus Placebo: Lumbar Spine BMD Percent Change From Baseline

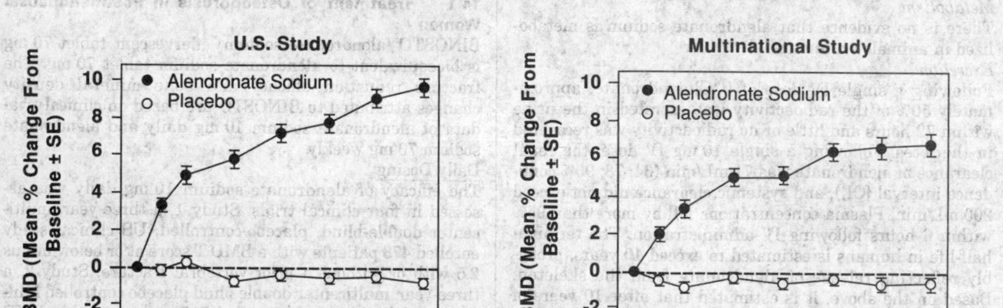

The Fracture Intervention Trial (FIT) consisted of two studies in postmenopausal women: the Three-Year Study of patients who had at least one baseline radiographic vertebral fracture and the Four-Year Study of patients with low bone mass but without a baseline vertebral fracture. In both studies of FIT, 96% of randomized patients completed the studies (i.e., had a closeout visit at the scheduled end of the study); approximately 80% of patients were still taking study medication upon completion.

Fracture Intervention Trial: Three-Year Study (patients with at least one baseline radiographic vertebral fracture)

This randomized, double-blind, placebo-controlled, 2027-patient study (alendronate, n=1022; placebo, n=1005) demonstrated that treatment with alendronate sodium resulted in statistically significant reductions in fracture incidence at three years as shown in Table 4.

[See table 4 above]

Furthermore, in this population of patients with baseline vertebral fracture, treatment with alendronate sodium significantly reduced the incidence of hospitalizations (25.0% vs. 30.7%).

In the Three-Year Study of FIT, fractures of the hip occurred in 22 (2.2%) of 1005 patients on placebo and 11 (1.1%) of 1022 patients on alendronate sodium, p=0.047. Figure 1 displays the cumulative incidence of hip fractures in this study.

[See figure 1 at top of next column]

Fracture Intervention Trial: Four-Year Study (patients with low bone mass but without a baseline radiographic vertebral fracture)

This randomized, double-blind, placebo-controlled, 4432-patient study (alendronate, n=2214; placebo, n=2218) further investigated the reduction in fracture incidence due to alendronate sodium. The intent of the study was to recruit women with osteoporosis, defined as a baseline femoral

Figure 1 Cumulative Incidence of Hip Fractures in the Three-Year Study of FIT (Patients With Radiographic Vertebral Fracture at Baseline)

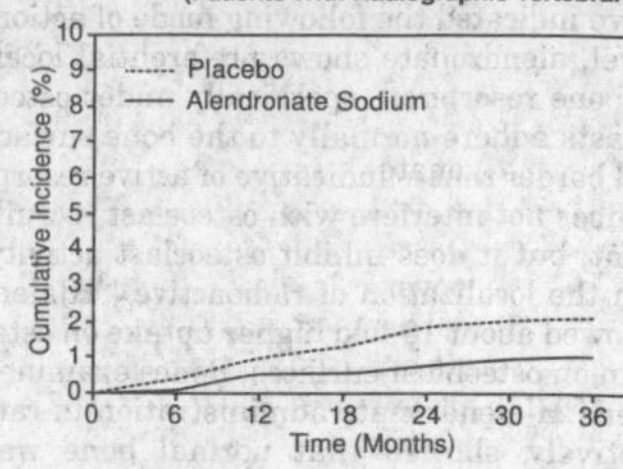

neck BMD at least two standard deviations below the mean for young adult women. However, due to subsequent revisions to the normative values for femoral neck BMD, 31% of patients were found not to meet this entry criterion and thus this study included both osteoporotic and non-osteoporotic women. The results are shown in Table 5 for the patients with osteoporosis.

[See table 5 at left]

Fracture Results Across Studies

In the Three-Year Study of FIT, alendronate sodium reduced the percentage of women experiencing at least one new radiographic vertebral fracture from 15.0% to 7.9% (47% relative risk reduction, p<0.001); in the Four-Year Study of FIT, the percentage was reduced from 3.8% to 2.1% (44% relative risk reduction, p=0.001); and in the combined U.S./Multinational studies, from 6.2% to 3.2% (48% relative risk reduction, p=0.034).

Alendronate sodium reduced the percentage of women experiencing multiple (two or more) new vertebral fractures from 4.2% to 0.6% (87% relative risk reduction, p<0.001) in the combined U.S./Multinational studies and from 4.9% to 0.5% (90% relative risk reduction, p<0.001) in the Three-Year Study of FIT. In the Four-Year Study of FIT, alendronate sodium reduced the percentage of osteoporotic women experiencing multiple vertebral fractures from 0.6% to 0.1% (78% relative risk reduction, p=0.035).

Thus, alendronate sodium reduced the incidence of radiographic vertebral fractures in osteoporotic women whether or not they had a previous radiographic vertebral fracture.

Effect on Bone Mineral Density

The bone mineral density efficacy of alendronate sodium 10 mg once daily in postmenopausal women, 44 to 84 years of age, with osteoporosis (lumbar spine bone mineral density [BMD] of at least 2 standard deviations below the premenopausal mean) was demonstrated in 4 double-blind, placebo-controlled clinical studies of 2 or 3 years' duration. Figure 2 shows the mean increases in BMD of the lumbar spine, femoral neck, and trochanter in patients receiving alendronate sodium 10 mg/day relative to placebo-treated patients at three years for each of these studies.

Figure 2 Osteoporosis Treatment Studies in Postmenopausal Women Increase in BMD Alendronate Sodium 10 mg/day at Three Years

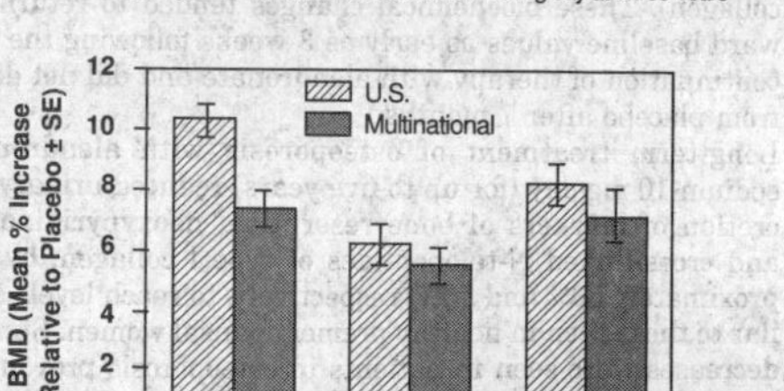

At 3 years significant increases in BMD, relative both to baseline and placebo, were seen at each measurement site in each study in patients who received alendronate 10 mg/day. Total body BMD also increased significantly in each study, suggesting that the increases in bone mass of the spine and hip did not occur at the expense of other skeletal sites. Increases in BMD were evident as early as 3 months and continued throughout the 3 years of treatment. (*See figures below* for lumbar spine results.) In the 2-year extension of these studies, treatment of 147 patients with alendronate sodium 10 mg/day resulted in continued increases in BMD at the lumbar spine and trochanter (absolute additional increases between years 3 and 5: lumbar spine, 0.94%; trochanter, 0.88%). BMD at the femoral neck, forearm and total body were maintained. Alendronate sodium was similarly effective regardless of age, race, baseline rate of bone turnover, and baseline BMD in the range studied (at least 2 standard deviations below the premenopausal mean).

[See figure 3 above]

In patients with postmenopausal osteoporosis treated with alendronate sodium 10 mg/day for one or two years, the effects of treatment withdrawal were assessed. Following discontinuation, there were no further increases in bone mass and the rates of bone loss were similar to those of the placebo groups.

Bone Histology

Bone histology in 270 postmenopausal patients with osteoporosis treated with alendronate sodium at doses ranging from 1 to 20 mg/day for one, two, or three years revealed normal mineralization and structure, as well as the expected decrease in bone turnover relative to placebo. These data, together with the normal bone histology and increased bone strength observed in rats and baboons exposed to long-term alendronate treatment, support the conclusion that bone formed during therapy with alendronate sodium is of normal quality.

Effect on height

Alendronate sodium, over a three- or four-year period, was associated with statistically significant reductions in loss of height vs. placebo in patients with and without baseline radiographic vertebral fractures. At the end of the FIT studies the between-treatment group differences were 3.2 mm in the Three-Year Study and 1.3 mm in the Four-Year Study.

Weekly dosing

The therapeutic equivalence of once weekly alendronate sodium 70 mg (n=519) and alendronate sodium 10 mg daily (n=370) was demonstrated in a one-year, double-blind, multicenter study of postmenopausal women with osteoporosis. In the primary analysis of completers, the mean increases from baseline in lumbar spine BMD at 1 year were 5.1% (4.8, 5.4%; 95% CI) in the 70 mg once-weekly group (n=440) and 5.4% (5.0, 5.8%; 95% CI) in the 10 mg daily group (n=330). The 2 treatment groups were also similar with regard to BMD increases at other skeletal sites. The results of the intention-to-treat analysis were consistent with the primary analysis of completers.

14.2 Treatment to Increase Bone Mass in Men with Osteoporosis

The efficacy of alendronate sodium in men with hypogonadal or idiopathic osteoporosis was demonstrated in two clinical studies.

Daily Dosing

A two-year, double-blind, placebo-controlled, multicenter study of alendronate sodium 10 mg once daily enrolled a total of 241 men between the ages of 31 and 87 (mean, 63). All patients in the trial had either: 1) a BMD T-score ≤-2 at the femoral neck and ≤-1 at the lumbar spine, or 2) a baseline osteoporotic fracture and a BMD T-score ≤-1 at the femoral neck. At two years, the mean increases relative to placebo in BMD in men receiving alendronate sodium 10 mg/day were significant at the following sites: lumbar spine, 5.3%; femoral neck, 2.6%; trochanter, 3.1%; and total body, 1.6%. Treatment with alendronate sodium also reduced height loss (alendronate, -0.6 mm vs. placebo, -2.4 mm).

Weekly dosing

A one-year, double-blind, placebo-controlled, multicenter study of once weekly alendronate sodium 70 mg enrolled a total of 167 men between the ages of 38 and 91 (mean, 66). Patients in the study had either: 1) a BMD T-score ≤ -2 at the femoral neck and ≤-1 at the lumbar spine, 2) a BMD T-score ≤-2 at the lumbar spine and ≤-1 at the femoral neck, or 3) a baseline osteoporotic fracture and a BMD Tscore ≤-1 at the femoral neck. At one year, the mean increases relative to placebo in BMD in men receiving alendronate sodium 70 mg once weekly were significant at the following sites: lumbar spine, 2.8%; femoral neck, 1.9%; trochanter, 2.0%; and total body, 1.2%. These increases in BMD were similar to those seen at one year in the alendronate sodium 10 mg once-daily study.

In both studies, BMD responses were similar regardless of age (≥65 years vs. <65 years), gonadal function (baseline testosterone <9 ng/dL vs. ≥9 ng/dL), or baseline BMD (femoral neck and lumbar spine T-score ≤-2.5 vs. >-2.5).

16 HOW SUPPLIED/STORAGE AND HANDLING

BINOSTO effervescent tablets are round, flat faced, white to off-white tablets with beveled edges and "M" debossed on one side. BINOSTO effervescent tablets, 70 mg are provided in blisters made of aluminum foil composite, as follows:

NDC 0178–0101–02 carton containing 4 units of use blisters

NDC 0178–0101–03 carton containing 12 units of use blisters

Store at 20°C to 25°C (68°F to 77°F), excursions permitted to 15°C to 30°C (59°F to 86°F), [See USP Controlled Room Temperature.] Protect from moisture. Store tablets in original blister package until use.

17 PATIENT COUNSELING INFORMATION

See FDA-approved patient labeling (Medication Guide).

Physicians should instruct their patients to read the Medication Guide before starting therapy with BINOSTO and to reread it each time the prescription is renewed.

17.1 Osteoporosis Recommendations, Including Calcium and Vitamin D Supplementation

Patients should be instructed to take supplemental calcium and vitamin D, if daily dietary intake is inadequate. Weight-bearing exercise should be considered along with the modification of certain behavioral factors, such as cigarette smoking and/or excessive alcohol consumption, if these factors exist.

17.2 Dosing Instructions

Patients should be instructed that it is necessary to follow all dosing instructions for BINOSTO:

- BINOSTO should only be taken upon arising for the day and must be taken at least 30 minutes before the first food, beverage, or medication of the day.
- Patients should not attempt to swallow, chew, or suck on the tablet because of a potential for oropharyngeal ulceration.
- Patients should be instructed to dissolve the effervescent tablet in 4 ounces room temperature plain water only (not mineral water or flavored water).
- Patients should be instructed to wait at least 5 minutes after the effervescence stops and then stir the solution for approximately 10 seconds and then consume the contents.
- Patients should be instructed not to lie down for at least 30 minutes after taking BINOSTO and until after their first food of the day.
- Patients should be specifically instructed not to take BINOSTO at bedtime or before arising for the day.
- Patients should be instructed that waiting less than 30 minutes, or taking BINOSTO with food, beverages (other than plain water) or other medications will lessen the effect of BINOSTO by decreasing its absorption into the body *[see Drug Interactions (7.1)]*. Even dosing with orange juice or coffee has been shown to markedly reduce the absorption of BINOSTO *[see Clinical Pharmacology (12.3)]*.
- Patients should be informed that failure to follow these instructions may increase their risk of esophageal problems. *[see Warnings and Precautions (5.1)]*.

Patients should be instructed that if they develop symptoms of esophageal disease (such as difficulty or pain upon swallowing, retrosternal pain or new or worsening heartburn) they should stop taking BINOSTO and consult their physician. *[see Warnings and Precautions (5.1)]*.

Patients should be instructed that if they miss a dose of once weekly BINOSTO, they should take one dose on the morning after they remember. They should not take 2 doses on the same day but should return to taking one dose once a week, as originally scheduled on their chosen day.

17.3 Patients on Sodium Restriction

Patients who are prescribed sodium restricted diets should be informed that BINOSTO contains 650 mg of sodium which is equivalent to approximately 1650 mg NaCl per tablet.

Manufactured for: Mission Pharmacal Company, San Antonio, TX 78230

Medication Guide

BINOSTO™ (BIN-oss-tow)

(alendronate sodium)

Effervescent Tablets

Read the Medication Guide that comes with BINOSTO™ before you start taking it and each time you get a refill. There may be new information. This Medication Guide does not take the place of talking with your doctor about your medical condition or treatment.

What is the most important information I should know about BINOSTO Effervescent Tablet?

BINOSTO Effervescent Tablet can cause serious side effects, including:

1. Esophagus problems
2. Low calcium levels in your blood (hypocalcemia)
3. Bone, joint, or muscle pain
4. Severe jaw bone problems (osteonecrosis)
5. Unusual thigh bone fractures

1. **Esophagus problems.**
   Some people who take BINOSTO may develop problems in the esophagus (the tube that connects the mouth and the stomach).
   These problems include irritation, inflammation, or ulcers of the esophagus which may sometimes bleed.
   - **It is important that you take BINOSTO exactly as prescribed to help lower your chance of getting esophagus problems. (See the section "How should I take BINOSTO?")**
   - **Stop taking BINOSTO and call your doctor right away if you get chest pain, new or worsening heartburn, or have trouble or pain when you swallow.**
2. **Low calcium levels in your blood (hypocalcemia).**
   BINOSTO may lower the calcium levels in your blood. If you have low blood calcium before you start taking BINOSTO, it may get worse during treatment. Your low blood calcium must be treated before you take BINOSTO. Most people with low blood calcium levels do not have symptoms, but some people may have symptoms. Call your doctor right away if you have symptoms of low blood calcium such as:
   - Spasms, twitches, or cramps in your muscles
   - Numbness or tingling in your fingers, toes, or around your mouth

   Your doctor may prescribe calcium and vitamin D to help prevent low calcium levels in your blood, while you take BINOSTO. Take calcium and vitamin D as your doctor tells you to.
3. **Bone, joint, or muscle pain.**
   Some people who take BINOSTO develop severe bone, joint, or muscle pain.
4. **Severe jaw bone problems (osteonecrosis).**
   Severe jaw bone problems may happen when you take BINOSTO. Your doctor should examine your mouth before you start BINOSTO. Your doctor may tell you to see your dentist before you start BINOSTO. It is important for you to practice good mouth care during treatment with BINOSTO.
5. **Unusual thigh bone fractures.**
   Some people have developed unusual fractures in their thigh bone. Symptoms of a fracture may include new or unusual pain in your hip, groin, or thigh.

Call your doctor right away if you have any of these side effects.

What is BINOSTO Effervescent Tablet?

BINOSTO is a prescription medicine used to:

- Treat thinning of your bones (osteoporosis) in women after menopause. BINOSTO helps reduce the chance of having a hip or spinal fracture (break).
- Increase bone mass in men who have osteoporosis.

It is not known how long BINOSTO works for the treatment of osteoporosis. You should see your doctor regularly to determine if BINOSTO is still right for you.

BINOSTO is not for use in children.

Who should not take BINOSTO Effervescent Tablet?

Do not take BINOSTO if you:

- Have certain problems with your esophagus, the tube that connects your mouth with your stomach
- Cannot stand or sit upright for at least 30 minutes
- Have trouble swallowing liquids
- Have low levels of calcium in your blood
- Are allergic to BINOSTO or any of its ingredients. See the end of this leaflet for a complete list of ingredients in BINOSTO.

What should I tell my doctor before taking BINOSTO Effervescent Tablet?

Before you start taking BINOSTO, tell your doctor about all of your medical conditions, including if you:

- Have problems with swallowing
- Have stomach or digestive problems
- Have low blood calcium
- Plan to have dental surgery or teeth removed
- Have kidney problems
- Have been told you have trouble absorbing minerals in your stomach or intestines (malabsorption syndrome)
- Have been told to lower your salt intake
- Are pregnant or planning to become pregnant. It is not known if BINOSTO can harm your unborn baby.
- Are breastfeeding or plan to breastfeed. It is not known if BINOSTO passes into your milk and may harm your baby.

Tell your doctor about all medicines you take, including prescription and non-prescription medicines, vitamins, and herbal supplements.

Especially tell your doctor if you take:

- calcium
- antacids
- aspirin
- Nonsteroidal Anti-Inflammatory (NSAID) medicines

Know the medicines you take. Keep a list of them and show it to your doctor and pharmacist each time you get a new medicine.

How should I take BINOSTO Effervescent Tablet?

- Take BINOSTO exactly as your doctor tells you.
- BINOSTO is taken 1 time each week. Choose the day of the week that best fits your schedule, then take BINOSTO on the same day every week.
- **BINOSTO works only if you take it on an empty stomach.**
- Take BINOSTO **after** you get up for the day and **30 minutes before** taking your first food, drink, or other medicine.
- Take BINOSTO while you are sitting or standing.
- **Do not swallow, chew or suck on a BINOSTO tablet.**
- **Do not dissolve BINOSTO in:**
  - mineral or flavored water
  - coffee
  - tea
  - soda
  - juice
- **You must dissolve your BINOSTO effervescent tablet in plain water at room temperature before you take it. To prepare your BINOSTO liquid medicine:**

  Step 1. Place the BINOSTO tablet in about a half glass (4 ounces) of plain water. The water should **not** be cold or hot, and should be at room temperature.

  Step 2. Wait at least 5 minutes after the bubbling (effervescence) stops for the BINOSTO tablet to completely dissolve in the water.

Step 3. Stir the liquid medicine for about 10 seconds.
Step 4. Drink all of the BINOSTO liquid medicine in the glass.

After you take BINOSTO, wait at least 30 minutes before you:
- lie down. You may sit, stand or walk, and do normal activities like reading.
- take your first food or drink, except for plain water.
- take other medicines, including antacids, calcium, and other supplements and vitamins.

Do not lie down until after you eat your first food of the day.
- If you miss a dose of BINOSTO, do not take it later in the day. Take your missed dose on the next morning after you remember and then return to your normal schedule. Do not take 2 doses on the same day.
- If you think you took more than your prescribed dose of BINOSTO, drink a full glass of milk and call your doctor right away. Do not try to vomit. Do not lie down.

What should I avoid while taking BINOSTO Effervescent Tablet?
BINOSTO contains a high amount of salt in each tablet. Avoid eating foods with a high amount of salt if your doctor has told you to limit how much salt you eat.

What are the possible side effects of BINOSTO Effervescent Tablet?
BINOSTO may cause serious side effects.
- See **"What is the most important information I should know about BINOSTO?"**

The most common side effects of BINOSTO are:
- Stomach area (abdominal) pain
- Heartburn
- Constipation
- Diarrhea
- Upset stomach
- Pain in your bones, joints, or muscles
- Nausea

You may get allergic reactions, such as hives or, in rare cases, swelling of your face, lips, tongue, or throat.
Tell your doctor about any side effect that bothers you or that does not go away.
These are not all the side effects with BINOSTO. Ask your doctor or pharmacist for more information.
Call your doctor for medical advice about side effects. You may report side effects to FDA at 1-800-FDA-1088.

How should I store BINOSTO Effervescent Tablet?
- Store BINOSTO at room temperature between 68°F to 77°F (20°C to 25°C).
- Keep BINOSTO tablets in their original blister pack until you use them.
- Protect BINOSTO from moisture.

Keep BINOSTO and all medicines out of the reach of children.

General information about the safe and effective use of BINOSTO Effervescent Tablet
Medicines are sometimes prescribed for purposes other than those listed in a Medication Guide. Do not use BINOSTO for a condition for which it was not prescribed. Do not give BINOSTO to other people, even if they have the same symptoms you have. It may harm them.
This Medication Guide summarizes the most important information about BINOSTO. If you would like more information, talk with your doctor. You can ask your doctor or pharmacist for information about BINOSTO that is written for health professionals.
For more information, go to www.BINOSTO.com, or call 1-855-778-0177.

What are the ingredients in BINOSTO Effervescent Tablet?
Active ingredient: alendronate sodium
Inactive ingredients: monosodium citrate anhydrous, citric acid anhydrous, sodium hydrogen carbonate, sodium carbonate anhydrous, strawberry flavor, acesulfame potassium, and sucralose.
This Medication Guide has been approved by the U.S. Food and Drug Administration.
Manufactured for:
Mission Pharmacal Company
San Antonio, TX 78230
Issued: July 2012

CITRANATAL ASSURE® ℞
Rx Prenatal Vitamin Tablet and 300 mg DHA capsule

DESCRIPTION
CitraNatal Assure® is a prescription prenatal/postnatal multivitamin/mineral tablet with FERR-EASE®, a patented dual-iron delivery comprising both a quick release and slow release iron, and a capsule of an essential fatty acid. The prenatal vitamin is a white, coated, oval multivitamin/mineral tablet. The tablet is debossed "0893" on one side and is blank on the other. The essential fatty acid DHA capsule is caramel colored and contains a light yellow to orange semi-solid mixture.

Each prenatal tablet contains:	
Vitamin C (Ascorbic acid)	120 mg
Calcium (Calcium citrate)	125 mg
Iron (Carbonyl iron, ferrous gluconate)	35 mg
Vitamin D_3 (Cholecalciferol)	400 IU
Vitamin E (dl-alpha tocopheryl acetate)	30 IU
Thiamin (Vitamin B_1)	3 mg
Riboflavin (Vitamin B_2)	3.4 mg
Niacinamide (Vitamin B_3)	20 mg
Vitamin B_6 (Pyridoxine HCl)	25 mg
Folic Acid	1 mg
Iodine (Potassium iodide)	150 mcg
Zinc (Zinc oxide)	25 mg
Copper (Cupric oxide)	2 mg
Docusate Sodium	50 mg
Each DHA gelatin capsule contains:	
Docosahexaenoic Acid (DHA, 40% from 750 mg Algal Oil)	300 mg
Eicosapentaenoic Acid (EPA)	Not more than 0.750 mg

Other ingredients in DHA gelatin capsule: High Oleic Sunflower Oil, Sunflower Lecithin, Rosemary Extract, Tocopherols, Ascorbyl Palmitate.

INDICATIONS
CitraNatal Assure® is a multivitamin/mineral prescription drug indicated for use in improving the nutritional status of women prior to conception, throughout pregnancy, and in the postnatal period for both lactating and nonlactating mothers.

CONTRAINDICATIONS
This product is contraindicated in patients with a known hypersensitivity to any of the ingredients.

> **WARNING:** Accidental overdose of **iron-containing** products is a leading cause of fatal poisoning in children under 6. KEEP THIS PRODUCT OUT OF THE REACH OF CHILDREN. In case of accidental overdose, call a doctor or poison control center immediately.

WARNING
Ingestion of more than 3 grams of omega-3 fatty acids per day has been shown to have potential antithrombotic effects, including an increased bleeding time and INR. Administration of omega-3 fatty acids should be avoided in patients on anticoagulants and in those known to have an inherited or acquired bleeding diathesis.

WARNING
Folic acid alone is improper therapy in the treatment of pernicious anemia and other megaloblastic anemias where vitamin B_{12} is deficient.

PRECAUTIONS
Folic acid in doses above 0.1 mg daily may obscure pernicious anemia in that hematologic remission can occur while neurological manifestations progress.

ADVERSE REACTIONS
Allergic sensitization has been reported following both oral and parenteral administration of folic acid.

DOSAGE AND ADMINISTRATION
One tablet and one capsule daily or as directed by a physician.
STORAGE: Store at 20-25°C (68-77°F)
NOTICE: Contact with moisture can discolor or erode the tablet.

HOW SUPPLIED
Six child-resistant blister packs of 5 tablets and 5 capsules each - **NDC** 0178-0893-30
To report a serious adverse event or obtain product information, call (210) 696-8400.
Please consult your health care provider with any dietary concerns.
Rev 0113

CITRANATAL B-CALM® ℞
Rx Prenatal Vitamin and two 25 mg each Vitamin B_6 tablets

A prescription prenatal supplement with 1 mg folic acid and a high level of vitamin B_6 which may act as an antiemetic.

DESCRIPTION
CitraNatal B-Calm® is a prescription prenatal multivitamin/mineral tablet with B_6, along with two vitamin B_6 tablets. The prenatal tablet contains FERR-EASE®, a patented dual-iron delivery comprising both a quick release and slow release iron. The prenatal tablet is white, coated, modified oval, and is debossed with "0832" on one side and is blank on the other. The B_6 25 mg tablets are white to off-white, uncoated, round, and are debossed with "B" on one side and "6" on the other.

Each prenatal tablet contains:	
Vitamin C (Ascorbic acid)	120 mg
Calcium (Calcium citrate)	120 mg
Iron (Carbonyl iron, ferrous gluconate)	20 mg
Vitamin D_3 (Cholecalciferol)	400 IU
Vitamin B_6 (Pyridoxine HCI)	25 mg
Folic Acid	1 mg
Each vitamin B_6 tablet contains:	
Vitamin B_6 (Pyridoxine HCl)	25 mg

INDICATIONS
CitraNatal B-Calm® is a multivitamin/mineral prescription drug indicated for use in improving the nutritional status of women prior to conception, throughout pregnancy, and in the postnatal period for both lactating and nonlactating mothers. CitraNatal B-Calm® may be used in conjunction with a physician prescribed regimen to help minimize pregnancy related nausea and vomiting.

CONTRAINDICATIONS
This product is contraindicated in patients with a known hypersensitivity to any of the ingredients.

> **WARNING:** Accidental overdose of **iron-containing** products is a leading cause of fatal poisoning in children under 6. KEEP THIS AND ALL DRUGS OUT OF THE REACH OF CHILDREN. In case of accidental overdose, call a doctor or poison control center immediately.

WARNING
Folic acid alone is improper therapy in the treatment of pernicious anemia and other megaloblastic anemias where vitamin B_{12} is deficient.

PRECAUTION
Folic acid in doses above 0.1 mg daily may obscure pernicious anemia, in that hematologic remission can occur while neurological manifestations remain progressive.

ADVERSE REACTIONS
Allergic sensitization has been reported following both oral and parenteral administration of folic acid.

DOSAGE AND ADMINISTRATION
One tablet every eight hours, beginning with "Tablet 1", or as directed by a physician.
STORAGE
Store at 20-25°C (68-77°F)
NOTICE: Contact with moisture can discolor or erode tablets.

HOW SUPPLIED
Six child-resistant blister packs of 5 multivitamin/multimineral tablets and 10 vitamin B_6 tablets each - **NDC** 0178-0832-30.
To report a serious adverse event or obtain product information, call (210) 696-8400.
Please consult your health care provider with any dietary concerns.
Rev. 0113

CITRANATAL® 90 DHA ℞
Rx Prenatal Vitamin Tablet and 300 mg DHA Capsule

DESCRIPTION
CitraNatal® 90 DHA is a prescription prenatal/postnatal multivitamin/mineral tablet with FERR-EASE®, a patented dual-iron delivery comprising both a quick release and slow release iron, and a capsule of an essential fatty acid. The prenatal vitamin is a scored, white, oval multivitamin/mineral tablet. The tablet is debossed "CN 90" on one side and "08" bisect "29"; on the other. The essential fatty acid DHA capsule is caramel colored and contains a light yellow to orange semi-solid mixture.

Each prenatal tablet contains:	
Vitamin C (Ascorbic acid)	120 mg
Calcium (Calcium citrate)	160 mg
Iron (Carbonyl iron, ferrous gluconate)	90 mg
Vitamin D_3 (Cholecalciferol)	400 IU

Vitamin E (dl-alpha tocopheryl acetate)	30 IU
Thiamin (Vitamin B_1)	3 mg
Riboflavin (Vitamin B_2)	3.4 mg
Niacinamide (Vitamin B_3)	20 mg
Vitamin B_6 (Pyridoxine HCl)	20 mg
Folic Acid	1 mg
Iodine (Potassium iodide)	150 mcg
Zinc (Zinc oxide)	25 mg
Copper (Cupric oxide)	2 mg
Docusate Sodium	50 mg

Each DHA gelatin capsule contains:

Docosahexaenoic Acid (DHA, 40% from 750 mg Algal Oil)	300 mg
Eicosapentaenoic Acid (EPA)	Not more than 0.750 mg

Other ingredients in DHA gelatin capsule: High Oleic Sunflower Oil, Sunflower Lecithin, Rosemary Extract, Tocopherols, Ascorbyl Palmitate.

INDICATIONS

CitraNatal® 90 DHA is a multivitamin/mineral prescription drug indicated for use in improving the nutritional status of women prior to conception, throughout pregnancy, and in the postnatal period for both lactating and nonlactating mothers.

CONTRAINDICATIONS

This product is contraindicated in patients with a known hypersensitivity to any of the ingredients.

> **WARNING**
> Accidental overdose of **iron-containing** products is a leading cause of fatal poisoning in children under 6. KEEP THIS PRODUCT OUT OF THE REACH OF CHILDREN. In case of accidental overdose, call a doctor or poison control center immediately.

WARNING

Ingestion of more than 3 grams of omega-3 fatty acids per day has been shown to have potential antithrombotic effects, including an increased bleeding time and INR. Administration of omega-3 fatty acids should be avoided in patients on anticoagulants and in those known to have an inherited or acquired bleeding diathesis.

WARNING

Folic acid alone is improper therapy in the treatment of pernicious anemia and other megaloblastic anemias where vitamin B_{12} is deficient.

PRECAUTIONS

Folic acid in doses above 0.1 mg daily may obscure pernicious anemia in that hematologic remission can occur while neurological manifestations progress.

ADVERSE REACTIONS

Allergic sensitization has been reported following both oral and parenteral administration of folic acid.

DOSAGE AND ADMINISTRATION

One tablet and one capsule daily or as directed by a physician.
STORAGE: Store at 20-25°C (68-77°F)

NOTICE

Contact with moisture can discolor or erode the tablet.

HOW SUPPLIED

Six child-resistant blister packs of 5 tablets and 5 capsules each - **NDC** 0178-0829-30
To report a serious adverse event or obtain product information, call (210) 696-8400.
Please consult your health care provider with any dietary concerns.
Rev 0113

CITRANATAL HARMONY® ℞

Rx Prenatal Vitamin Gel Cap

DESCRIPTION

CitraNatal Harmony® is a prescription prenatal/postnatal multivitamin/mineral soft gelatin capsule. The prenatal vitamin is a purple, opaque soft gelatin capsule containing a greenish-gray liquid to semi-solid fill. The capsule is printed "0797" in white ink.

Each prenatal capsule contains:

Calcium (Calcium citrate)	104 mg
Iron (Carbonyl iron)	29 mg
Vitamin D_3 (Cholecalciferol)	400 IU
Vitamin E (dl-alpha tocopheryl acetate)	30 IU
Vitamin B_6 (Pyridoxine HCl)	25 mg
Folic Acid	1 mg
Docusate Sodium	50 mg
Docosahexaenoic Acid (DHA 40% from 650 mg Algal Oil)	265 mg

INDICATIONS

CitraNatal Harmony® is a multivitamin/mineral prescription drug indicated for use in improving the nutritional status of women prior to conception, throughout pregnancy, and in the postnatal period for both lactating and nonlactating mothers.

CONTRAINDICATIONS

This product is contraindicated in patients with a known hypersensitivity to any of the ingredients.

> **WARNING**
> Accidental overdose of **iron-containing** products is a leading cause of fatal poisoning in children under 6. KEEP THIS PRODUCT OUT OF THE REACH OF CHILDREN. In case of accidental overdose, call a doctor or poison control center immediately.

WARNING

Ingestion of more than 3 grams of omega-3 fatty acids per day has been shown to have potential antithrombotic effects, including an increased bleeding time and INR. Administration of omega-3 fatty acids should be avoided in patients on anticoagulants and in those known to have an inherited or acquired bleeding diathesis.

WARNING

Folic acid alone is improper therapy in the treatment of pernicious anemia and other megaloblastic anemias where vitamin B_{12} is deficient.

PRECAUTIONS

Folic acid in doses above 0.1 mg daily may obscure pernicious anemia in that hematologic remission can occur while neurological manifestations progress.

ADVERSE REACTIONS

Allergic sensitization has been reported following both oral and parenteral administration of folic acid.
CAUTION: Exercise caution to ensure that the prescribed dosage of DHA does not exceed 1 gram (1000 mg) per day.

DOSAGE AND ADMINISTRATION

One capsule daily or as directed by a physician.
Store at controlled room temperature.
NOTICE: Contact with moisture can discolor or erode the capsule.

HOW SUPPLIED

Bottles of 30 capsules each—**NDC** 0178-0797-30.
To report a serious adverse event or obtain product information, call (210) 696-8400.
Please consult your health care provider with any dietary concerns.
Rev 1112

Eletone® Cream ℞

Nonsteroidal Dermatitis Therapy with Hydrolipid Technology™

Rx Only
For topical dermatological use only.

PRODUCT DESCRIPTION: Eletone® Cream is a nonsteroidal, lipid-rich, fragrance free emulsion formulated with Hydrolipid Technology™ for the management and relief of burning, itching, and redness associated with various types of dermatoses. There are no restrictions on age or duration of use and the product has a low potential for irritation.

INDICATIONS FOR USE: Eletone® Cream is indicated for the management and relief of burning, itching, and redness associated with various types of dermatoses, including atopic dermatitis, allergic contact dermatitis, and radiation dermatitis (post-radiation treatment).

CONTRAINDICATIONS: THIS PRODUCT SHOULD NOT BE USED DURING THE PERIOD OF TIME WHEN RADIATION TREATMENT IS OCCURRING BECAUSE OF THE INCREASED RISK OF SKIN TOXICITY WHEN RADIATING THROUGH PETROLATUM AND OIL. Eletone® Cream is contraindicated in patients with a known hypersensitivity to any of the components of the formulation.

PRECAUTIONS: Eletone® Cream is for external use only. Eletone® Cream does not contain a sunscreen and should always be used in conjunction with a sunscreen in sun exposed areas.

INSTRUCTIONS FOR USE: Apply liberally to the affected areas three times daily or as needed. If skin is broken, cover Eletone® Cream with a dressing of choice.

INGREDIENTS: Eletone® Cream contains petrolatum, purified water, mineral oil, cetostearyl alcohol, ceteth-20, citric acid, sodium citrate, propylparaben, and butylparaben.

HOW SUPPLIED: Eletone® Cream is available in a 100 gram tube **NHRIC** 0178-0368-01.
Store at 25°C (77°F); excursions permitted to 15-30°C (59-86°F) [see USP Controlled Room Temperature].
CAUTION: Rx only. Federal law restricts this device to sale by or on the order of a physician.
Protected under U.S. Patent No. 5,635,497
Eletone® is a medical device registered with the United States Food and Drug Administration
Rev 0412

FERRALET® 90 ℞

Carbonyl Iron/ferrous gluconate tablet

DESCRIPTION

Each green film-coated tablet for oral administration contains:

Iron (Carbonyl iron, ferrous gluconate)	90 mg
Folic Acid	1 mg
Vitamin B_{12} (Cyanocobalamin)	12 mcg
Vitamin C (Ascorbic acid)	120 mg
Docusate sodium	50 mg

Inactive Ingredients: Povidone, croscarmellose sodium, acrylic resin, color added, magnesium stearate, FD&C Yellow No. 5, magnesium silicate, FD&C Blue No. 1, polyethylene glycol, vitamin A palmitate, ethyl vanillin.

CLINICAL PHARMACOLOGY

Oral iron is absorbed most efficiently when administered between meals. Iron is critical for normal hemoglobin synthesis to maintain oxygen transport for energy production and proper function of cells. Adequate amounts of iron are necessary for effective erythropoiesis. Iron also serves as a cofactor of several essential enzymes, including cytochromes, which are involved in electron transport.
Folic acid is required for nucleoprotein synthesis and the maintenance of normal erythropoiesis. Folic acid is the precursor of tetrahydrofolic acid, which is involved as a cofactor for transformylation reactions in the biosynthesis of purines and thymidylates of nucleic acids. Deficiency of folic acid may account for the defective deoxyribonucleic acid (DNA) synthesis that leads to megaloblast formation and megaloblastic macrocytic anemias. Vitamin B_{12} is essential to growth, cell reproduction, hematopoiesis, nucleic acid, and myelin synthesis. Deficiency may result in megaloblastic anemia or pernicious anemia.

INDICATIONS AND USAGE

Ferralet® 90 is indicated for the treatment of all anemias that are responsive to oral iron therapy. These include: hypochromic anemia associated with pregnancy, chronic and/or acute blood loss, metabolic disease, post-surgical convalescence, and dietary needs.

CONTRAINDICATIONS

Hypersensitivity to any of the ingredients. Hemolytic anemia, hemochromatosis, and hemosiderosis are contraindications to iron therapy.

WARNING

Folic acid alone is improper therapy in the treatment of pernicious anemia and other megaloblastic anemias where vitamin B_{12} is deficient.

> **WARNING:** Accidental overdose of **iron-containing** products is a leading cause of fatal poisoning in children under 6. KEEP THIS PRODUCT OUT OF REACH OF CHILDREN. In case of accidental overdose, call a doctor or poison control center immediately.

PRECAUTIONS

General: Take 2 hours after meals. Do not exceed recommended dose. Discontinue use if symptoms of intolerance appear. The type of anemia and underlying cause or causes should be determined before starting therapy with Ferralet® 90 tablets. Ensure Hgb, Hct, and reticulocyte counts are determined before starting therapy and periodically thereafter during prolonged treatment. Periodically review therapy to determine if it needs to be continued without change or if a dose change is indicated. This product contains FD&C Yellow No. 5 (tartrazine) which may cause allergic-type reactions (including bronchial asthma) in certain susceptible persons. Although the overall incidence of FD&C Yellow No. 5 (tartrazine) sensitivity in the general population is low, it is frequently seen in patients who also have aspirin hypersensitivity.
Folic Acid: Folic acid in doses above 0.1 mg daily may obscure pernicious anemia in that hematologic remission can occur while neurological manifestations remain progressive.

Pernicious anemia should be excluded before using these products since folic acid may mask the symptoms of pernicious anemia.

Pediatric Use: Safety and effectiveness in pediatric patients have not been established.

Geriatric Use: Dosing for elderly patients should be administered with caution. Due to the greater frequency of decreased hepatic, renal, or cardiac function, and of concomitant disease or other drug therapy, dosing should start at the lower end of the dosing range.

ADVERSE REACTIONS

Adverse reactions with iron therapy may include GI irritation, constipation, diarrhea, nausea, vomiting, and dark stools. Adverse reactions with iron therapy are usually transient. Allergic sensitization has been reported following both oral and parenteral administration of folic acid.

DRUG INTERACTIONS: Prescriber should be aware of a number of iron/drug interactions, including antacids, tetracyclines, or fluoroquinolones.

OVERDOSAGE

Symptoms: abdominal pain, metabolic acidosis, anuria, CNS damage, coma, convulsions, death, dehydration, diffuse vascular congestion, hepatic cirrhosis, hypotension, hypothermia, lethargy, nausea, vomiting, diarrhea, tarry stools, melena, hematemesis, tachycardia, hyperglycemia, drowsiness, pallor, cyanosis, lassitude, seizures, and shock.

DOSAGE AND ADMINISTRATION

One tablet daily or as directed by a physician. Do not chew tablet.

STORAGE:

Store at 25° C (77° F). Excursions permitted to 15°-30° C (59°-86° F). (See USP Controlled Room Temperature.)

NOTICE: Contact with moisture can discolor or erode the tablet.

HOW SUPPLIED

Ferralet® 90 (NDC 0178-0089-90) is a green, modified rectangle shaped, film-coated tablet, debossed with "F6" on one side and blank on the other, and packaged in bottles of 90.

To report a serious adverse event or obtain product information, call (210) 696-8400.

Rev 0112

LITHOSTAT® ℞

(Acetohydroxamic Acid)
Tablets

DESCRIPTION: Acetohydroxamic acid (AHA) is a stable, synthetic compound derived from hydroxylamine and ethyl acetate. Its molecular structure is similar to urea:

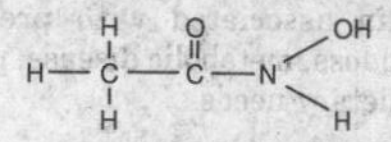

ACETOHYDROXAMIC ACID

AHA is weakly acidic, highly soluble in water, and chelates metals - notably iron. The molecular weight is 75.068. AHA has a pKa of 9.32 and a melting point of 89-91° C. AHA is a urease inhibitor. Available as 250 mg tablets.

CLINICAL PHARMACOLOGY: AHA reversibly inhibits the bacterial enzyme urease, thereby inhibiting the hydrolysis of urea and production of ammonia in urine infected with urea-splitting organisms. The reduced ammonia levels and decreased pH enhance the effectiveness of antimicrobial agents and allow an increased cure rate of these infections.

AHA is well absorbed from the gastrointestinal tract after oral administration; peak blood levels occur from 0.25 to 1 hour after dosing. The compound is distributed throughout body water, and there is no known binding to any tissue. AHA chelates with dietary iron within the gut. This reaction may interfere with absorption of AHA and with iron. Concomitant hypochromic anemia should be treated with intramuscular iron.

In rodents, the metabolic fate of AHA is well known; 55% is excreted unchanged in urine, 25% is excreted as acetamide or acetate and 7% is excreted by the lungs as carbon dioxide. Less than 1% is excreted in the feces. Approximately 5% of the administered dose is unaccounted for. In rodents, AHA shows a dose-related change in pharmacokinetics; with increasing dose, there is an increase in the half-life and an increase in the percent of the administered dose recovered in urine as unchanged AHA.

Pharmacokinetics in man are generally similar to rodents including the dose-related increase in half-life, but they are not as well characterized as in the rodent. Thirty-six to sixty-five percent (36-65%) of the oral dosage is excreted unchanged in the urine. It is unaltered AHA in the urine that provides the therapeutic effect, but the precise concentration of AHA in urine that is necessary to inhibit urease is incompletely delineated. Therapeutic benefit may be obtained from concentrations as low as 8 mcg/ml; higher concentrations (i.e., 30 mcg/ml) are expected to provide more complete inhibition of urease. The plasma half-life of AHA is approximately 5-10 hours in subjects with normal renal function and is prolonged in patients with reduced renal function.

Acetohydroxamic acid has been evaluated clinically in patients with urea-splitting urinary infections, often accompanied by struvite stone disease, that were recalcitrant to other forms of medical and surgical management. In these clinical trials, AHA reduced the pathologically elevated urinary ammonia and pH levels that result from the hydrolysis of urea by the enzyme, urease.

AHA does not acidify urine directly nor does it have a direct antibacterial effect. The usefulness of reducing ammonia levels and decreasing urinary pH is suggested by single (not yet replicated) clinical trials in which urease inhibition 1) allowed successful antibiotic treatment of urea-splitting Proteus infections after surgical removal of struvite stones in patients not cured by 3 months of antibacterial treatment alone, and 2) reduced the rate of stone growth in patients who were not candidates for surgical removal of stones.

INDICATIONS AND USAGE: Acetohydroxamic acid is indicated as adjunctive therapy in patients with chronic urea-splitting urinary infection. AHA is intended to decrease urinary ammonia and alkalinity, but it should not be used in lieu of curative surgical treatment (for patients with stones) or antimicrobial treatment. Long-term treatment with AHA may be warranted to maintain urease inhibition as long as urea-splitting infection is present. Experience with AHA does not go beyond 7 years. A patient package insert should be distributed to each patient who receives AHA.

CONTRAINDICATIONS: Acetohydroxamic acid should not be used in:

a. patients whose physical state and disease are amenable to definitive surgery and appropriate antimicrobial agents
b. patients whose urine is infected by non-urease producing organisms
c. patients whose urinary infections can be controlled by culture-specific oral antimicrobial agents
d. patients whose renal function is poor (i.e., serum creatinine more than 2.5 mg/dl and/or creatinine clearance less than 20 ml/min)
e. female patients who do not evidence a satisfactory method of contraception
f. patients who are pregnant

Acetohydroxamic acid may cause fetal harm when administered to a pregnant woman. AHA was teratogenic (retarded and/or clubbed rear leg at 750 mg/kg and above and exencephaly and encephalocele at 1,500 mg/kg) when given intraperitoneally to rats. AHA is contraindicated in women who are or may become pregnant. If this drug is used during pregnancy, or if the patient becomes pregnant while taking this drug, the patient should be informed of the potential hazard to the fetus.

WARNINGS: A Coombs negative hemolytic anemia has occurred in patients receiving AHA. Gastrointestinal upset characterized by nausea, vomiting, anorexia and generalized malaise have accompanied the most severe forms of hemolytic anemia. Approximately 15% of patients receiving AHA have had only laboratory findings of an anemia. However, most patients developed a mild reticulocytosis. The untoward reactions have reverted to normal following cessation of treatment. A complete blood count, including a reticulocyte count, is recommended after two weeks of treatment. If the reticulocyte count exceeds 6%, a reduced dosage should be entertained. A CBC and reticulocyte count are recommended at 3-month intervals for the duration of treatment.

PRECAUTIONS: GENERAL: Hematologic Effects: Bone marrow depression (leukopenia, anemia, and thrombocytopenia) has occurred in experimental animals receiving large doses of AHA, but has not been seen in man to date. AHA is a known inhibitor of DNA synthesis and also chelates metals - notably iron. Its bone marrow suppressant effect is probably related to its ability to inhibit DNA synthesis, but anemia could also be related to depletion of iron stores. To date, the only clinical effect noted has been hemolysis, with a decrease in the circulating red blood cells, hemoglobin and hematocrit. Abnormalities in platelet or white blood cell count have not been noted. However, clinical monitoring of the platelet and white cell count is recommended.

Monitoring Liver Function: Abnormalities of liver function have not been reported to date. However, a chlorobenzene derivative of acetohydroxamic acid caused significant liver dysfunction in an unrelated study. Therefore, close monitoring of liver function is recommended. (See Carcinogenesis for discussion of possible hepatic carcinogenesis.)

Use In Patients With Renal Impairment: Since AHA is eliminated primarily by the kidneys, patients with significantly impaired renal function should be closely monitored, and a reduction of daily dose may be needed to avoid excessive drug accumulation. (See Dosage and Administration.)

DRUG INTERACTIONS: AHA has been used concomitantly with insulin, oral and parenteral antibiotics, and progestational agents. No clinically significant interactions have been noted, but until wider clinical experience is obtained, AHA should be used with caution in patients receiving other therapeutic agents.

AHA taken in association with alcoholic beverages has resulted in a rash. (See Adverse Reactions.)

AHA chelates heavy metals-notably iron. The absorption of iron and AHA from the intestinal lumen may be reduced when both drugs are taken concomitantly. When iron administration is indicated, intramuscular iron is probably the product of choice.

CARCINOGENESIS, MUTAGENESIS, IMPAIRMENT OF FERTILITY: Well controlled, long-term animal studies that identify the carcinogenic potential of AHA treatment have not been conducted. Acetamide, a metabolite of AHA, has been shown to cause hepatocellular carcinoma in rats at oral doses 1,500 times the human dose. AHA is cytotoxic and was positive for mutagenicity in the Ames test.

PREGNANCY: Pregnancy Category X. (See Contraindications.)

NURSING MOTHERS: It is not known whether AHA is secreted in human milk. Because many drugs are excreted in human milk, and because of the potential for serious adverse reactions in nursing infants from AHA, a decision should be made to discontinue nursing or the drug, taking into account the significance of the drug to the mother's well being.

PEDIATRIC USE: Children with chronic, recalcitrant, urea-splitting urinary infection may benefit from treatment with AHA. However, detailed studies involving dosage and dose intervals in children have not been established. Children have tolerated a dose of 10 mg/kg/day, taken in two or three divided doses, satisfactorily for periods up to one year. Close monitoring of such patients is mandatory.

ADVERSE REACTIONS: Experience with AHA is limited. About 150 patients have been treated, most for periods of more than a year.

Adverse reactions have occurred in up to thirty percent (30%) of the patients receiving AHA. In some instances the reactions were symptomatic; in others only changes in laboratory parameters were noted. Adverse reactions seem to be more prevalent in patients with preexisting thrombophlebitis or phlebothrombosis and/or in patients with advanced degrees of renal insufficiency. The risk of adverse reactions is highest during the first year of treatment. Chronic treatment does not seem to increase the risk nor the severity of adverse reactions.

The following reactions have been reported:

NEUROLOGICAL: Mild headaches are commonly reported (about 30%) during the first 48 hours of treatment. These headaches are mild, responsive to oral salicylate-type analgesics, and usually disappear spontaneously. The headaches have not been associated with vertigo, tinnitus, or visual or auditory abnormalities. Tremulousness and nervousness have also been reported.

GASTROINTESTINAL: Gastrointestinal symptoms, nausea, vomiting, anorexia, and malaise have occurred in 20-25% of patients. In most patients the symptoms were mild, transitory, and did not result in interruption of treatment. Approximately 3% of patients developed a hemolytic anemia of sufficient magnitude to warrant interruption in treatment; several of these patients also had symptoms of gastrointestinal upset.

HEMATOLOGICAL: Approximately 15% of patients have had laboratory findings characteristic of a hemolytic anemia. A mild reticulocytosis (5- 6%) without anemia, is even more prevalent. The laboratory findings are occasionally accompanied by systemic symptoms such as malaise, lethargy and fatigue, and gastrointestinal symptoms. Symptoms and laboratory findings have invariably improved following cessation of treatment with AHA. The hematological abnormalities are more prevalent in patients with advanced renal failure.

DERMATOLOGICAL: A nonpruritic, macular skin rash has occurred in the upper extremities and on the face of several patients taking AHA on a long-term basis, usually when AHA has been taken concomitantly with alcoholic beverages, but in a few patients in the absence of alcohol consumption. The rash commonly appears 30-45 minutes after ingestion of alcoholic beverages; it characteristically disappears spontaneously in 30-60 minutes. The rash may be associated with a general sensation of warmth. In some patients the rash is sufficiently severe to warrant discontinuation of treatment, but most patients have continued treatment, avoiding alcohol or using smaller quantities of it. Alopecia has also been reported in patients taking AHA.

CARDIOVASCULAR: Superficial phlebitis involving the lower extremities has occurred in several patients on AHA during the early (Phase II) clinical trials. Several of the affected patients had had phlebitic episodes prior to treatment. One patient developed deep vein thrombosis of the lower extremities. The patient with phlebothrombosis had an associated traumatic injury to the groin. It is unclear whether the phlebitis was related to or exacerbated by treatment with AHA. No patient in the three (3) year controlled (Phase III) clinical trial developed phlebitis. In all instances these vascular abnormalities returned to normal following appropriate medical therapy. Embolic phenomena have been reported in three patients taking AHA in the Phase II trial. The phlebitis and emboli resolved following discontinuation of AHA and implementation of appropriate medical therapy. Several patients have resumed treatment with AHA without ill effect. Palpitations have also been reported in patients taking AHA.

RESPIRATORY: No symptoms have been reported. Radiographic evidence of small pulmonary emboli has been seen in three patients with phlebitis in their lower legs.

PSYCHIATRIC: Depression, anxiety, nervousness, and tremulousness have been observed in approximately 20% of patients taking AHA. In most patients the symptoms were mild and transitory, but in about 6% of patients the symptoms were sufficiently distressing to warrant interruption or discontinuation of treatment.

OVERDOSAGE: Acute deliberate overdosage in man has not occurred, but would be expected to induce the following symptoms: anorexia, malaise, lethargy, diminished sense of well being, tremulousness, anxiety, nausea and vomiting. Laboratory findings are likely to include an elevated reticulocyte count and a severe hemolytic reaction requiring hospitalization, symptomatic treatment, and possibly blood transfusions. Concomitant reduction in platelets and/or white blood cells should be anticipated.

Milder overdosages resulting in hemolysis have occurred in an occasional patient with reduced renal function after several weeks or months of continuous treatment.

The acute LD 50 of AHA in animals (rats) is 4.8 gm/kg.

Recommended treatment for an overdosage reaction consists of (1) cessation of treatment, (2) close monitoring of hematologic status, (3) symptomatic treatment, and (4) blood transfusions as required by the clinical circumstances. The drug is probably dialyzable, but this property has not been tested clinically.

DOSAGE AND ADMINISTRATION: AHA should be administered orally, one tablet 3-4 times a day in a total daily dose of 10-15 mg/kg/day. The recommended starting dose is 12 mg/kg/day, administered at 6-8 hour intervals at a time when the stomach is empty. The maximum daily dose should be no more than 1.5 grams, regardless of body weight.

The dosage should be reduced in patients with reduced renal function. Patients whose serum creatinine is greater than 1.8 mg/dl should take no more than 1.0 gm/day; such patients should be dosed at q-12-h intervals. Further reductions in dosage to prevent the accumulation of toxic concentrations in the blood may also be desirable. Insufficient data exists to accurately characterize the optimum dose and/or dose interval in patients with moderate degrees of renal insufficiency.

Patients with advanced renal insufficiency (i.e., serum creatinine more than 2.5 mg/dl) should not be treated with AHA. The risk of accumulation of toxic blood levels of AHA seems to be greater than the chances for a beneficial effect in such patients.

In children an initial dose of 10 mg/kg/day is recommended. Close monitoring of the patient's clinical condition and hematologic status is recommended. Titration of the dose to higher or lower levels may be required to obtain an optimum therapeutic effect and/or to reduce the risk of side effects.

HOW SUPPLIED: LITHOSTAT®, NDC 0178-0500-01, is available for oral administration as 250 mg white, round tablets, in unit of use packages of 100 tablets. Each Lithostat® tablet is debossed MPC 500 on one side and blank on the other side. LITHOSTAT® should be stored in a dry place at room temperature, 15° - 30°C (59° - 86°F). Container should be closed tightly.

C08 Rev 010060

PATIENT INFORMATION

PLEASE READ THIS INFORMATION BEFORE USING THIS DRUG.

GENERAL INFORMATION: It has been known for many years that urinary infection may cause the formation of urinary stones. As these stones form, bacteria are trapped within the stones. The trapped bacteria cause the stones to grow, and the stones protect the bacteria from antibiotics. Surgical removal of the stone attempts to break this vicious cycle - many times successfully. However, if infection persists or if a small stone fragment persists, then there is an increased risk of stone recurrence. Multiple operations to remove kidney stones may result in damage and scarring of the kidney. In some situations removal of the kidney may be necessary.

In some instances stones may form initially as a result of non-infectious (i.e., metabolic) causes. If a metabolic stone becomes infected, then an "infection stone" may grow onto the "metabolic stone." Stone analysis and/or biochemical tests will usually determine which factors are present.

Experimental investigations have identified an enzyme called urease which is made by some (but not all) bacteria. Urease reacts with urine to make ammonia. Ammonia changes the acidity of the urine and the change in acidity encourages stone formation. LITHOSTAT® (acetohydroxamic acid) inhibits urease and thereby reduces urinary ammonia. In some instances, LITHOSTAT® enhances the effectiveness of antibiotics and thereby makes urinary infection easier to control.

WHAT IS LITHOSTAT®? LITHOSTAT® is a drug which prevents the excessive buildup of ammonia in your urine, which controls the acidity and alkalinity (pH) of your urine. The cause of excessive ammonia and alkalinity in your urine is a bacterial infection.

WHAT CAN LITHOSTAT® DO? Treatment with LITHOSTAT® is prescribed to decrease urinary ammonia. This may increase the chance of controlling your infection with antibiotics and may help the treatment of your kidney stones. Dissolution of existing stones is unlikely.

LITHOSTAT® should not be used in place of surgical treatment. Surgical removal of all stones and elimination of all infection with antibiotics offers the possibility of curative treatment. LITHOSTAT® is likely to be more effective after large stones or obstructing stones have been removed.

WHAT ARE THE PROBLEMS OR SIDE EFFECTS WITH LITHOSTAT®? The complete spectrum of side effects induced by LITHOSTAT® (acetohydroxamic acid) is unknown. However, some side effects which have been reported to date have been headaches, abdominal discomfort, nausea, loss of hair, shakiness, and anemia. Lifethreatening problems (blood clot in the legs) occurred in several patients with advanced disease in early investigation. In more extensive later investigations, this problem has not occurred. No patient has died as a consequence of taking LITHOSTAT®. The most serious side effects seem to occur in patients with poor kidney function and/or in patients with a previous history of these conditions.

Problems related to LITHOSTAT® have disappeared following cessation of the drug and initiation of appropriate medical treatment. Most patients have resumed treatment without ill effect.

A flushing skin reaction (i.e., redness, warmth, and tingling) has occurred in several patients who consumed alcohol during treatment with LITHOSTAT®. The reaction persisted approximately 30 minutes and disappeared without treatment. The cause and significance of this reaction are unknown. Consequently, patients are encouraged to abstain from consumption of alcoholic beverages while being treated with LITHOSTAT®.

In animal studies doses of LITHOSTAT® about 20 times the maximum human dose have caused fetal abnormalities (birth defects) indicating a potential for such an adverse effect in an exposed human fetus. Therefore, LITHOSTAT® should not be given to pregnant women or to any sexually active woman of child-baring age, not using a highly effective method of contraception (oral contraceptive or IUD).

An acceptable long-term study of the cancer causing potential of LITHOSTAT® has not been conducted, but a known metabolite of LITHOSTAT®, acetamide, is carcinogenic (cancer-causing) to the liver in rats at doses about 80 times the maximum human dose of LITHOSTAT®. LITHOSTAT® thus must be considered a potential human carcinogen. LITHOSTAT® kills tissue cells grown in tissue culture and alters genetic material in cells grown in culture.

LITHOSTAT® may induce other adverse reactions which have not yet been recognized.

Unusual symptoms should be reported to your physician. Mild symptoms usually do not warrant discontinuation of treatment. Severe symptoms may necessitate temporary cessation of treatment and/or alteration of dosage.

WHAT ABOUT TAKING OTHER DRUGS WITH LITHOSTAT®? Only take those drugs prescribed by your physician. Do not take prescription drugs or over the counter preparations without your physician' s specific prescription or recommendation. Drugs that contain iron should not be taken at the same time as LITHOSTAT®, (acetohydroxamic acid).

LITHOSTAT® reacts with iron, and may not be absorbed into the bloodstream. Both the iron you take and the LITHOSTAT® you take may be ineffective if both drugs are taken together.

HOW IMPORTANT IS MY DAILY DOSAGE OF LITHOSTAT®? If you fail to follow your daily dosage schedule with LITHOSTAT® you will probably suffer a setback in treatment effectiveness and new kidney stone formation is likely. LITHOSTAT® plus antibiotic therapy must be taken exactly as your physician prescribes it for optimum effectiveness.

IN CONCLUSION: Your daily dosage of LITHOSTAT® (acetohydroxamic acid) is important to the proper treatment of your condition. Any unusual side effects should be reported to your physician at once.

Rx only.

Rev 1006

OVACE® PLUS SHAMPOO ℞

(sodium sulfacetamide 10%)

Rx Only

FOR EXTERNAL USE ONLY. NOT FOR OPHTHALMIC USE.

DESCRIPTION

Each gram of OVACE® Plus Shampoo (sodium sulfacetamide 10% w/w) contains 100 mg of sodium sulfacetamide in a vehicle consisting of cetearyl alcohol (and) PEG-3 distearoylamidoethylmonium methosulfate (and) polysorbate 60, citric acid anhydrous, cocamide MEA, cocamidopropyl betaine, ethylene glycol distearate, Flamenco Super Blue, fragrance, magnesium aluminum silicate, methylparaben, PEG-150 distearate, propylparaben, purified water, sodium chloride and sodium laureth sulfate. Sodium sulfacetamide is $C_8H_9N_2NaO_3S \cdot H_2O$ with molecular weight of 254.24. Chemically, it is N-[(4-aminophenyl)sulfonyl]-acetamide, monosodium salt, monohydrate. The structural formula is:

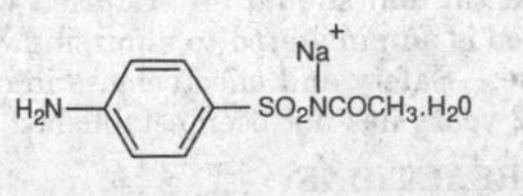

Sodium sulfacetamide is an odorless, white, crystalline powder with a bitter taste. It is freely soluble in water, sparingly soluble in alcohol, while practically insoluble in benzene, in chloroform and in ether.

CLINICAL PHARMACOLOGY

Sodium sulfacetamide exerts a bacteriostatic effect against sulfonamide sensitive Gram-positive and Gram-negative microorganisms commonly isolated from secondary cutaneous pyogenic infections. It acts by restricting the synthesis of folic acid required by bacteria for growth, by its competition with para-aminobenzoic acid. There is no clinical data available on the degree and rate of systemic absorption of OVACE® Plus Shampoo when applied to the skin or scalp. However, significant absorption of sodium sulfacetamide through the skin has been reported.

The following in vitro data is available but the clinical significance is unknown. Organisms that show susceptibility to sodium sulfacetamide are: Streptococci, Staphylococci, E. coli, Klebsiella pneumoniae, Pseudomonas pyocyanea, Salmonella species, Proteus vulgaris, Nocardia and Actinomyces.

INDICATIONS AND USAGE

OVACE® Plus Shampoo is intended for topical application in the following scaling dermatoses: seborrheic dermatitis and seborrhea sicca (dandruff). Shake well before using.

CONTRAINDICATIONS

OVACE® Plus Shampoo is contraindicated in persons with known or suspected hypersensitivity to sulfonamides or to any of the ingredients of the product.

WARNINGS

Sulfonamides are known to cause Stevens-Johnson syndrome in hypersensitive individuals. Stevens-Johnson syndrome also has been reported following the use of sodium sulfacetamide topically. Cases of drug-induced systemic lupus erythematosus from topical sulfacetamide also have been reported. In one of these cases, there was a fatal outcome. **KEEP OUT OF THE REACH OF CHILDREN.**

PRECAUTIONS

FOR EXTERNAL USE ONLY. NOT FOR OPHTHALMIC USE.

General: Nonsusceptible organisms, including fungi, may proliferate with the use of this preparation. Hypersensitivity reactions may recur when a sulfonamide is readministered, irrespective of the route of administration, and cross hypersensitivity between different sulfonamides may occur. If OVACE® Plus Shampoo produces signs of hypersensitivity or other untoward reactions, discontinue use of the preparation. Systemic absorption of topical sulfonamides is greater following application to large, infected, abraded, denuded or severely burned areas. Under these circumstances, any of the adverse effects produced by the systemic administration of these agents could potentially occur and appropriate observations and laboratory determinations should be performed.

Information for Patients: Patients should discontinue OVACE® Plus Shampoo if the condition becomes worse, or if a rash develops in the area being treated or elsewhere. OVACE® Plus Shampoo also should be discontinued promptly and the physician notified if any arthritis, fever or sores in the mouth develop.

Drug Interactions: OVACE® Plus Shampoo is incompatible with silver preparations.

Pharmacology: OVACE® Plus Shampoo has a bacteriostatic effect against Gram-positive and Gram-negative microorganisms commonly isolated from secondary cutaneous pyogenic infections.

Carcinogenesis, Mutagenesis and Impairment of Fertility: Long-term animal studies for carcinogenic potential have not been performed on OVACE® Plus Shampoo to date. Studies on reproduction and fertility also have not been performed. Chromosomal nondisjunction has been reported in the yeast, Saccharomyces cerevisiae, following application of sodium sulfacetamide. The significance of this finding to the topical use of sodium sulfacetamide in the human is unknown.

Pregnancy: Category C. Animal reproduction studies have not been conducted with OVACE® Plus Shampoo. It is also not known whether OVACE® Plus Shampoo can affect reproduction capacity or cause fetal harm when administered to a pregnant woman. OVACE® Plus Shampoo should be used by a pregnant woman only if clearly needed or when potential benefits outweigh potential hazards to the fetus.

Nursing Mothers: It is not known whether this drug is excreted in human milk. Because many drugs are excreted in human milk, caution should be exercised when OVACE® Plus Shampoo is administered to a nursing woman.

Pediatric Use: Safety and effectiveness in children under the age of 12 years has not been established.

ADVERSE REACTIONS

Reports of irritation and hypersensitivity to sodium sulfacetamide are uncommon. The following adverse reactions, reported after administration of sterile ophthalmic sodium sulfacetamide, are noteworthy: instances of Stevens-Johnson syndrome and instances of local hypersensitivity which progressed to a syndrome resembling systemic lupus erythematosus; in one case a fatal outcome was reported (see WARNINGS). **You should call your doctor for medical advice about side effects. To report a serious adverse event, call 1-800-298-1087.**

OVERDOSAGE

The oral LD_{50} of sulfacetamide in mice is 16.5 g/kg. In the event of overdosage, emergency treatment should be started immediately.

Manifestations: Overdosage may cause nausea and vomiting. Large oral overdosage may cause hematuria, crystalluria and renal shutdown due to the precipitation of sulfa crystals in the renal tubules and the urinary tract. For treatment, contact your local Poison Control Center or your doctor.

DOSAGE AND ADMINISTRATION

Apply to wet hair and massage vigorously into scalp. Rinse thoroughly. For best results, use at least twice a week or as directed by a doctor. Avoid contact with eyes or mucous membranes. Do not use on an infant less than 2 months of age.

HOW SUPPLIED

OVACE® Plus Shampoo is available in an 8 fl. oz. (237 mL) bottle, NDC 0178-0485-08 and 5 g sample packets, NDC 0178-0485-05.

Store at 20°C to 25°C (68°F to 77°F), excursions permitted between 15°C and 30°C (between 59°F and 86°F). Brief exposure to temperatures up to 40°C (104°F) may be tolerated provided the mean kinetic temperature does not exceed 25°C (77°F); however, such exposure should be minimized.

Note: Protect from freezing and excessive heat. The product may tend to darken slightly on storage. Slight discoloration does not impair the efficacy or safety of the product. Keep container or packet tightly closed.

Occasionally, a slight yellowish discoloration may occur when an excessive amount of the product is used and comes in contact with white fabrics. This discoloration, however, presents no problem as it is readily removed by ordinary laundering without bleaches.

Distributed by:
Mission Pharmacal Company
San Antonio, TX 78230-1355
Patent Pending
v1 Rev. 02/2012

OVACE® PLUS WASH ℞

(sodium sulfacetamide 10%)
Cleansing Gel
Rx Only
FOR EXTERNAL USE ONLY. NOT FOR OPHTHALMIC USE.

DESCRIPTION

Each gram of OVACE® Plus Wash (sodium sulfacetamide 10% w/w) contains 100 mg of sodium sulfacetamide incorporated into a specially formulated oil and water emulsion (OIW™), delivered in a gel vehicle consisting of cocamidopropyl betaine, sodium thiosulfate, emulsifying wax, glyceryl stearate SE, cetearyl alcohol (and) PEG-3 distearoylamidoethylmonium methosulfate (and) polysorbate 60, PEG-150 pentaerythrityl tetrastearate (and) aqua (and) PEG-6 caprylic/capric glycerides, methylparaben, purified water, sodium laureth ether sulfate, disodium EDTA dihydrate, xanthan gum and fragrance.

Sodium sulfacetamide is $C_8H_9N_2NaO_3S \bullet H_2O$ with molecular weight of 254.24. Chemically, it is N-[(4-aminophenyl)sulfonyl]-acetamide, monosodium salt, monohydrate. The structural formula is:

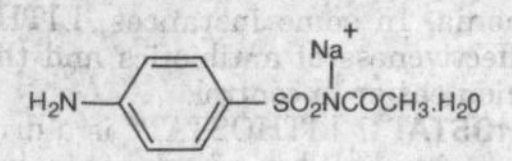

Sodium sulfacetamide is an odorless, white, crystalline powder with a bitter taste. It is freely soluble in water, sparingly soluble in alcohol, while practically insoluble in benzene, in chloroform and in ether.

This OIW™ formulation has been shown to provide gradual and prolonged release of the active ingredient into the skin.

CLINICAL PHARMACOLOGY

Sodium sulfacetamide exerts a bacteriostatic effect against sulfonamide sensitive Gram-positive and Gram-negative microorganisms commonly isolated from secondary cutaneous pyogenic infections. It acts by restricting the synthesis of folic acid required by bacteria for growth, by its competition with para-aminobenzoic acid. There is no clinical data available on the degree and rate of systemic absorption of OVACE® Plus Wash when applied to the skin or scalp. However, significant absorption of sodium sulfacetamide through the skin has been reported.

The following in vitro data is available but the clinical significance is unknown. Organisms that show susceptibility to sodium sulfacetamide are: Streptococci, Staphylococci, E. coli, Klebsiella pneumoniae, Pseudomonas pyocyanea, Salmonella species, Proteus vulgaris, Nocardia and Actinomyces.

INDICATIONS AND USAGE

OVACE® Plus Wash is intended for topical application in the following scaling dermatoses: seborrheic dermatitis and seborrhea sicca (dandruff). It also is indicated for the treatment of secondary bacterial infections of the skin due to organisms susceptible to sulfonamides.

CONTRAINDICATIONS

OVACE® Plus Wash is contraindicated in persons with known or suspected hypersensitivity to sulfonamides or to any of the ingredients of the product.

WARNINGS

Sulfonamides are known to cause Stevens-Johnson syndrome in hypersensitive individuals. Stevens-Johnson syndrome also has been reported following the use of sodium sulfacetamide topically. Cases of drug-induced systemic lupus erythematosus from topical sulfacetamide also have been reported. In one of these cases, there was a fatal outcome. **KEEP OUT OF THE REACH OF CHILDREN.**

PRECAUTIONS

FOR EXTERNAL USE ONLY. NOT FOR OPHTHALMIC USE.

General: Nonsusceptible organisms, including fungi, may proliferate with the use of this preparation. Hypersensitivity reactions may recur when a sulfonamide is readministered, irrespective of the route of administration, and cross hypersensitivity between different sulfonamides may occur. If OVACE® Plus Wash produces signs of hypersensitivity or other untoward reactions, discontinue use of the preparation. Systemic absorption of topical sulfonamides is greater following application to large, infected, abraded, denuded or severely burned areas. Under these circumstances, any of the adverse effects produced by the systemic administration of these agents could potentially occur, and appropriate observations and laboratory determinations should be performed.

Information for Patients: Patients should discontinue OVACE® Plus Wash if the condition becomes worse, or if a rash develops in the area being treated or elsewhere. OVACE® Plus Wash also should be discontinued promptly and the physician notified if any arthritis, fever or sores in the mouth develop.

Drug Interactions: OVACE® Plus Wash is incompatible with silver preparations.

Pharmacology: OVACE® Plus Wash has a bacteriostatic effect against Gram-positive and Gram-negative microorganisms commonly isolated from secondary cutaneous pyogenic infections.

Carcinogenesis, Mutagenesis and Impairment of Fertility: Long-term animal studies for carcinogenic potential have not been performed on OVACE® Plus Wash to date. Studies on reproduction and fertility also have not been performed. Chromosomal nondisjunction has been reported in the yeast, Saccharomyces cerevisiae, following application of sodium sulfacetamide. The significance of this finding to the topical use of sodium sulfacetamide in the human is unknown.

Pregnancy: Category C. Animal reproduction studies have not been conducted with OVACE® Plus Wash. It is also not known whether OVACE® Plus Wash can affect reproduction capacity or cause fetal harm when administered to a pregnant woman. OVACE® Plus Wash should be used by a pregnant woman only if clearly needed or when potential benefits outweigh potential hazards to the fetus.

Nursing Mothers: It is not known whether this drug is excreted in human milk. Because many drugs are excreted in human milk, caution should be exercised when OVACE® Plus Wash is administered to a nursing woman.

Pediatric Use: Safety and effectiveness in children under the age of 12 years has not been established.

ADVERSE REACTIONS

Reports of irritation and hypersensitivity to sodium sulfacetamide are uncommon. The following adverse reactions, reported after administration of sterile ophthalmic sodium sulfacetamide, are noteworthy: instances of Stevens-Johnson syndrome and instances of local hypersensitivity which progressed to a syndrome resembling systemic lupus erythematosus; in one case a fatal outcome was reported (see WARNINGS). **Call your doctor for medical advice about side effects. To report SUSPECTED ADVERSE REACTIONS, contact the FDA at 1-800-FDA-1088 or www.fda.gov/medwatch.**

OVERDOSAGE

The oral LD_{50} of sulfacetamide in mice is 16.5 g/kg. In the event of overdosage, emergency treatment should be started immediately.

Manifestations: Overdosage may cause nausea and vomiting. Large oral overdosage may cause hematuria, crystalluria and renal shutdown due to the precipitation of sulfa crystals in the renal tubules and the urinary tract. For treatment, contact your local Poison Control Center or your doctor.

DOSAGE AND ADMINISTRATION

Seborrheic dermatitis including seborrhea sicca - Wash affected areas twice daily (morning and evening), or as directed by your physician. Avoid contact with eyes or mucous membranes. Wet skin and liberally apply to areas to be cleansed, massage gently into skin working into a full lather, rinse thoroughly, pat dry and repeat after 10 to 20 seconds. Rinsing with plain water will remove any excess medication. Repeat application as described for 8 to 10 days. If skin dryness occurs it may be controlled by rinsing cleanser off sooner or using less frequently. Regular shampooing following OVACE® Plus Wash is not necessary, but the hair should be shampooed at least once a week. As the condition subsides, the interval between applications may be lengthened. Applications once or twice weekly or every other week may prevent recurrence. Should the condition recur after stopping therapy, the application of OVACE® Plus Wash should be reinitiated as at the beginning of treatment.

Secondary cutaneous bacterial infections - Wet skin and liberally apply to areas to be cleansed, massage gently into skin for 10 to 20 seconds working into a full lather, rinse thoroughly and pat dry. Rinsing with plain water will remove any excess medication. Repeat application as described for 8 to 10 days. If skin dryness occurs it may be controlled by rinsing cleanser off sooner or using less often.

HOW SUPPLIED

OVACE® Plus Wash is available in a 12 fl. oz. (355 mL) bottle, NDC 0178-0490-12, and 5 g sample packets, NDC 0178-0490-05.

Store at 25°C (77°F); excursions permitted to 15°C to 30°C (59°F to 86°F). See USP Controlled Room Temperature.

Note: Protect from freezing and excessive heat. The product may tend to darken slightly on storage. Slight discoloration does not impair the efficacy or safety of the product. Keep container or packet tightly closed.

Occasionally, a slight yellowish discoloration may occur when an excessive amount of the product is used and comes in contact with white fabrics. This discoloration, however, presents no problem, as it is readily removed by ordinary laundering without bleaches.

Distributed by:
Mission Pharmacal Company
San Antonio, TX 78230-1355
Patent Pending
Rev 0911

THIOLA® ℞

(Tiopronin)
Tablets

DESCRIPTION

THIOLA® (Tiopronin) is a reducing and complexing thiol compound. Tiopronin is N-(2-Mercaptopropionyl) glycine and has the following structure:

$$CH_3\text{-}\underset{\displaystyle SH}{\underset{|}{CH}}\text{-}CONHCH_2\text{-}COOH$$

Tiopronin has the empirical formula $C_5H_9NO_3S$ and a molecular weight of 163.20. In this drug product tiopronin exists as a dl racemic mixture.

Tiopronin is a white crystalline powder which is freely soluble in water.

THIOLA® tablets are white, sugar coated tablets, each containing 100 mg. of Tiopronin and are taken orally.

Inactive ingredients: Calcium carbonate, carnauba wax, ethyl cellulose, Eudragit E 100, hydroxy-propyl cellulose, lactose, magnesium stearate, povidone, sugar, talc, titanium dioxide.

CLINICAL PHARMACOLOGY

THIOLA® is an active reducing agent which undergoes thiol-disulfide exchange with cystine to form a mixed disulfide of Thiola-cysteine.

$$2R\text{-}SH + R'\text{-}S\text{-}S\text{-}R' \rightleftharpoons 2R\text{-}S\text{-}S\text{-}R' + 2H^+$$

Thiola Cystine ⇌ Thiola-cysteine

From this reaction, a water-soluble mixed disulfide is formed and the amount of sparingly soluble cystine is reduced. When THIOLA® is given orally, up to 48% of dose appears in urine during the first 4 hours and up to 78% by 72 hours. Thus, in patients with cystinuria, sufficient amount of THIOLA® or its active metabolites could appear in urine to react with cystine, lowering cystine excretion.

The decrement in urinary cystine produced by THIOLA® is generally proportional to the dose. A reduction in urinary cystine of 250-350 mg/day at a THIOLA® dosage of 1 g/day, and a decline of approximately 500 mg/day at a dosage of 2 g/day, might be expected. THIOLA® causes a sustained reduction in cystine excretion without apparent loss of effectiveness. THIOLA® has a rapid onset and offset of action, showing a fall in cystine excretion on the first day of administration and a rise on the first day of drug withdrawal.

INDICATIONS AND USAGE

THIOLA® is indicated for the prevention of cystine (kidney) stone formation in patients with severe homozygous cystinuria with urinary cystine greater than 500 mg/day, who are resistant to treatment with conservative measures of high fluid intake, alkali and diet modification, or who have adverse reactions to d-penicillamine.

Cystine stones typically occur in approximately 10,000 persons in the United States who are homozygous for cystinuria. These persons excrete abnormal amounts of cystine in urine of over 250 mg/g creatinine, as well as excessive amounts of other dibasic amino acids (lysine, arginine and ornithine). In addition, they show varying intestinal transport defects for these same amino acids. The stone formation is the result of poor aqueous solubility of cystine.

Since there are no known inhibitors of the crystallization of cystine, the stone formation is determined primarily by the urinary supersaturation of cystine. Thus, cystine stones could theoretically form whenever urinary cystine concentration exceeds the solubility limit. Cystine solubility in urine is pH-dependent, and ranges from 170-300 mg/liter at pH 5, 190-400 mg/liter at pH 7 and 220-500 mg/liter at pH 7.5.

The goal of therapy is to reduce urinary cystine concentration below its solubility limit. It may be accomplished by dietary means aimed at reducing cystine synthesis and by a high fluid intake in order to increase urine volume and thereby lower cystine concentration.

Unfortunately, the above conservative measures alone may be ineffective in controlling cystine stone formation in some homozygous patients with severe cystinuria (urinary cystine exceeding 500 mg/day). In such patients, d-penicillamine has been used as an additional therapy. Like THIOLA™, dpenicillamine undergoes thiol-disulfide exchange with cystine, thereby lowering the amount of sparingly soluble cystine in urine.

However, d-penicillamine treatment is frequently accompanied by adverse reactions, such as dermatologic complications, hypersensitivity reactions, hematologic abnormalities and renal disturbances. THIOLA® may have a particular therapeutic role in such patients.

CONTRAINDICATIONS

The use of THIOLA® during pregnancy is contraindicated, except in those with severe cystinuria where the anticipated benefit of inhibited stone formation clearly outweighs possible hazards of treatment (see PRECAUTIONS).

THIOLA® should not be begun again in patients with a prior history of developing agranulocytosis, aplastic anemia or thrombocytopenia on this medication.

Mothers maintained on THIOLA® treatment should not nurse their infants.

WARNINGS

Despite apparent lower toxicity of THIOLA™, THIOLA® may potentially cause all the serious adverse reactions reported for d-penicillamine. Thus, although no death has been reported to result directly from THIOLA® treatment, a fatal outcome from THIOLA® is possible, as has been reported with d-penicillamine therapy from such complications as aplastic anemia, agranulocytosis, thrombocytopenia, Goodpasture's syndrome or myasthenia gravis.

Leukopenia of the granulocytic series may develop without eosinophilia. Thrombocytopenia may be immunologic in origin or occur on an idiosyncratic basis. The reduction in peripheral blood white count to less than 3500/cubic mm or in platelet count to below 100,000 cubic mm mandates cessation of therapy. Patients should be instructed to report promptly the occurrence of any symptom or sign of these hematological abnormalities, such as fever, sore throat, chills, bleeding or easy bruisability.

Proteinuria, sometimes sufficiently severe to cause nephrotic syndrome, may develop from membranous glomerulopathy. A close observation of affected patients is mandatory.

The following complications, though rare, have been reported during d-penicillamine therapy and could occur during THIOLA® treatment. When there are abnormal urinary findings associated with hemoptysis and pulmonary infiltrates suggestive of Goodpasture's syndrome, THIOLA® treatment should be stopped. Appearance of myasthenic syndrome or myasthenia gravis requires cessation of treatment. When pemphigus-type reactions develop, THIOLA® therapy should be stopped. Steroid treatment may be necessary.

PRECAUTIONS

Patients should be advised of the potential development of complications and to report promptly the occurrence of any symptom or sign of them.

To help monitor potential complications, the following tests are recommended: peripheral blood counts, direct platelet count, hemoglobin, serum albumin, liver function tests, 24-hour urinary protein and routine urinalysis at 3-6 month intervals during treatment. In order to assess effect on stone disease, urinary cystine analysis should be monitored frequently during the first 6 months when the optimum dose schedule is being determined, and at 6-month intervals thereafter. Abdominal roentogenogram (KUB) is advised on a yearly basis to monitor the size and appearance/disappearance of stone(s).

CARCINOGENESIS, MUTAGENESIS, IMPAIRMENT OF FERTILITY: Long-term carcino-genicity studies in animals have not been performed. High doses of THIOLA® in experimental animals have been shown to interfere with maintenance of pregnancy and viability of the fetus.

USE IN PREGNANCY: Pregnancy category C. D-penicillamine has been shown to cause skeletal defects and cleft palates in the fetus when given to pregnant rats at 10 times the dose recommended for human use. A similar teratogenicity might be expected for THIOLA® although no such findings could be related to the drug in studies in mice and rats at doses up to 10 times the highest recommended human dose.

There are no adequate and well-controlled studies in pregnant women. THIOLA® should be used during pregnancy only if the potential benefit justifies potential risk to the fetus.

NURSING MOTHERS: Because THIOLA® may be excreted in milk and because of the potential serious adverse reactions of nursing infants from THIOLA®, mothers taking THIOLA® should not nurse their infants.

PEDIATRIC USE: Safety and effectiveness below the age of 9 have not been established.

ADVERSE REACTIONS

Some patients may develop drug fever, usually during the first month of therapy. THIOLA® treatment should be discontinued until the fever subsides. It may be reinstated at a small dose, with a gradual increase in dosage until the desired level is achieved.

A generalized rash (erythematous, maculopapular or morbilliform) accompanied by pruritis may develop during the first few months of treatment. It may be controlled by antihistamine therapy, typically recedes when THIOLA® treatment is discontinued, and seldom recurs when THIOLA® treatment is restarted at a lower dosage. Less commonly, rash may appear late in the course of treatment (of more than 6 months). Located usually in the trunk, the late rash is associated with intense pruritis, recedes slowly after discontinuing treatment, and usually recurs upon resumption of treatment.

A drug reaction simulating lupus erythematous, manifested by fever, arthralgia and lymphadenopathy may develop. It may be associated with a positive antinuclear antibody test, but not necessarily with nephropathy. It may require discontinuance of THIOLA® treatment.

A reduction in taste perception may develop. It is believed to be the result of chelation of trace metals by THIOLA™. Hypogeusia is often self-limiting.

Unlike during d-penicillamine therapy, vitamin B_6 deficiency is uncommonly associated with THIOLA® treatment.

Some patients may complain of wrinkling and friability of skin. This complication usually occurs after long-term treatment, and is believed to result from the effect of THIOLA® on collagen.

A multiclinic trial involving 66 cystinuric patients in the United States indicated that THIOLA® is associated with fewer or less severe adverse reactions than d-penicillamine. Among those who had to stop taking d-penicillamine due to toxicity, 64.7% could take THIOLA®. In those without prior history of d-penicillamine treatment, only 5.9% developed reactions of sufficient severity to require THIOLA® withdrawal. A review of available literature supports the findings from this trial.

Despite this apparent reduced toxicity to THIOLA® relative to d-penicillamine, THIOLA® treatment may potentially be associated with all the adverse reactions reported with d-penicillamine. They include:

Gastrointestinal side-effects (nausea, emesis, diarrhea or softstools, anorexia, abdominal pain, bloating or flatus) in about 1 in 6 patients;

Impairment in taste and smell in about 1 in 25 patients;

Dermatologic complications (pharyngitis, oral ulcers, rash, ecchymosis, prurites, uritcaria, warts, skin wrinkling, pemphigus, elastosis perforans serpiginosa) in about 1 in 6 patients;

Hypersensitivity reactions (laryngeal edema, dyspnea, respiratory distress, fever, chills, arthralgia, weakness, fatigue, myalgia, adenopathy) in about 1 in 25 patients;

Hematologic abnormalities (increased bleeding, anemia, leukopenia, thrombocytopenia, eosinophilia) in about 1 in 25 patients;

Renal complications (proteinuria, nephrotic syndrome, hematuria) in about 1 in 20 patients;

Pulmonary manifestations (bronchiolitis, hemoptysis, pulmonary infiltrates, dyspnea) in about 1 in 50 patients;

Neurologic complications (myasthenic syndrome) in about 1 in 50 patients.

These reactions are more likely to develop during THIOLA® therapy among patients who had previously shown toxicity to d-penicillamine.

In patients who had previously manifested adverse reactions to d-penicillamine, adverse reactions to THIOLA® are more likely to occur than in patients who took THIOLA® for the first time. A close supervision with a careful monitoring of potential side effects is mandatory during THIOLA® treatment. Patients should be told to report promptly any symptoms suggesting toxicity. The treatment with THIOLA® should be stopped if severe toxicity develops.

Jaundice and abnormal liver function tests have been reported during THIOLA® therapy for non-cystinuric conditions. A direct cause and effect relationship, based upon these foreign reports, has not been established. Although such complications were not encountered in the small multicenter trials in the United States, patients should be carefully monitored and if any abnormalities are noted, the drug should be discontinued and the patient treated by appropriate measures.

DOSAGE AND ADMINISTRATION

It is recommended that a conservative treatment program should be attempted first. At least 3 liters of fluid (10-10 oz. glassfuls) should be provided, including two glasses with each meal and at bedtime. The patients should be expected to awake at night to urinate; they should drink two more glasses of fluids before returning to bed. Additional fluids should be consumed if there is excessive sweating or intestinal fluid loss. A minimum urine output of 2 liters/day on a consistent basis should be sought. A modest amount of alkali should be provided in order to maintain urinary pH at a high normal range (6.5-7.0). Potassium alkali are advantageous over sodium alkali, because they do not cause hypercalciuria and are less likely to cause the complication of calcium stones.

Excessive alkali therapy is not advisable. When urinary pH increases above 7.0 with alkali therapy, the complication of calcium phosphate nephrolithiasis may ensue because of the enhanced urinary supersaturation of hydroxyapatite in an alkaline environment.

In patients who continue to form cystine stones on the above conservative program, THIOLA® may be added to the treatment program. THIOLA® may also be substituted for d-penicillamine in patients who have developed toxicity to the latter drug. In both situations, the conservative treatment program should be continued.

The dose of THIOLA® should not be arbitrary but should be based on that amount required to reduce urinary cystine concentration to below its solubility limit (generally <250 mg/liter). The extent of the decline in cystine excretion is generally dependent on the THIOLA® dosage.

THIOLA® may be begun at a dosage of 800 mg/day in adult patients with cystine stones. In a multiclinic trial, average dose of THIOLA® was about 1000 mg/day. However, some patients require a smaller dose. In children, initial dosage may be based on 15 mg/kg/day. Urinary cystine should be measured at 1 month after THIOLA® treatment, and every 3 months thereafter. THIOLA® dosage should be readjusted depending on the urinary cystine value. Whenever possible, THIOLA® should be given in divided doses 3 times/day at least one hour before or 2 hours after meals.

In patients who had shown severe toxicity to d-penicillamine, THIOLA® might be begun at a lower dosage.

HOW SUPPLIED

THIOLA® (NDC 0178-0900-01), is available for oral administration as 100 mg. round, white, sugar coated tablets in bottles of 100 tablets each. Each tablet is imprinted in red with "M" on one side and blank on the other side. Store at 25°C (77°F); excursions permitted to 15-30°C (59-86°F) [see USP Controlled Room Temperature].

Rx only.

Rev 1006

TINDAMAX® ℞

[tin-da-max]

(tinidazole)

HIGHLIGHTS OF PRESCRIBING INFORMATION

These highlights do not include all the information needed to use Tindamax® safely and effectively. See full prescribing information for Tindamax®.

Tindamax® (tinidazole) tablets for oral use

Initial U.S. Approval: 2004

To reduce the development of drug-resistant bacteria and maintain the effectiveness of Tindamax and other antibacterial drugs, Tindamax should be used only to treat or prevent infections that are proven or strongly suspected to be caused by bacteria.

WARNING: POTENTIAL RISK FOR CARCINOGENICITY

See full prescribing information for complete boxed warning.

Carcinogenicity has been seen in mice and rats treated chronically with metronidazole, another nitroimidazole agent *(13.1)*. Although such data have not been reported for tinidazole, the two drugs are structurally related and have similar biologic effects. Use should be limited to approved indications only.

RECENT MAJOR CHANGES

Indications and Usage, Bacterial Vaginosis *(1.4)* 5/2007

Dosage and Administration, Bacterial Vaginosis *(2.6)* 5/2007

INDICATIONS AND USAGE

Tindamax is a nitroimidazole antimicrobial indicated for:
- Trichomoniasis *(1.1)*
- Giardiasis: in patients age 3 and older *(1.2)*
- Amebiasis: in patients age 3 and older *(1.3)*
- Bacterial Vaginosis: in non-pregnant, adult women *(1.4, 8.1)*

DOSAGE AND ADMINISTRATION

- Trichomoniasis: a single 2 g oral dose taken with food. Treat sexual partners with the same dose and at the same time *(2.3)*
- Giardiasis: Adults: a single 2 g dose taken with food. Pediatric patients older than three years of age: a single dose of 50 mg/kg (up to 2 g) with food *(2.4)*
- Amebiasis, *Intestinal:* Adults: 2 g per day for 3 days with food. Pediatric patients older than three years of age: 50 mg/kg/day (up to 2 g per day) for 3 days with food *(2.5)*.
Amebic liver abscess: Adults: 2 g per day for 3-5 days with food. Pediatric patients older than three years of age: 50 mg/kg/day (up to 2 g per day) for 3-5 days with food *(2.5)*
- Bacterial vaginosis: Non-pregnant, adult women: 2 g once daily for 2 days taken with food, or 1 g once daily for 5 days taken with food *(2.6)*

DOSAGE FORMS AND STRENGTHS

Tablets: 250 mg and 500 mg *(3)*

CONTRAINDICATIONS

- Prior history of hypersensitivity to tinidazole or other nitroimidazole derivatives *(4, 6.1, 6.2)*
- First trimester of pregnancy *(4, 8.1)*
- Nursing mothers, unless breast-feeding is interrupted during tinidazole therapy and for 3 days following the last dose *(4, 8.3)*

WARNINGS AND PRECAUTIONS

- Seizures and neuropathy have been reported. Discontinue Tindamax if abnormal neurologic signs develop *(5.1)*
- Vaginal candidiasis may develop with Tindamax and require treatment with an antifungal agent *(5.2)*
- Use Tindamax with caution in patients with blood dyscrasias. Tindamax may produce transient leukopenia and neutropenia *(5.3, 7.3)*

ADVERSE REACTIONS

Most common adverse reactions for a single 2 g dose of tinidazole (incidence >1%) are metallic/bitter taste, nausea, weakness/fatigue/malaise, dyspepsia/ cramps/epigastric discomfort, vomiting, anorexia, headache, dizziness and constipation *(6.1)*

To report SUSPECTED ADVERSE REACTIONS, contact Mission Pharmacal Company at 1-800-298-1087 or FDA at 1-800-FDA-1088 or www.fda.gov/medwatch

DRUG INTERACTIONS

The following drug interactions were reported for metronidazole, a chemically-related nitroimidazole and may therefore occur with tinidazole:
- Warfarin and other oral coumarin anticoagulants: Anticoagulant dosage may need adjustment during and up to 8 days after tinidazole therapy *(7.1)*
- Alcohol-containing beverages/preparations: Avoid during and up to 3 days after tinidazole therapy *(7.1)*
- Lithium: Monitor serum lithium concentrations *(7.1)*
- Cyclosporine, tacrolimus: Monitor for toxicities of these immunosuppressive drugs *(7.1)*
- Fluorouracil: Monitor for fluorouracil-associated toxicities *(7.1)*
- Phenytoin, fosphenytoin: Adjustment of anticonvulsant and/or tinidazole dose(s) may be needed *(7.1, 7.2)*
- CYP3A4 inducers/inhibitors: Monitor for decreased tinidazole effect or increased adverse reactions *(7.2)*

USE IN SPECIFIC POPULATIONS

- Pediatric Use: Data on tinidazole use in children is limited to treatment of giardiasis and amebiasis in patients age 3 and older *(8.4)*
- Hemodialysis patients: If tinidazole is administered the same day and prior to hemodialysis, administer an additional ½ dose after end of hemodialysis *(8.6, 12.3)*

See 17 for PATIENT COUNSELING INFORMATION

Revised: 08/2007

FULL PRESCRIBING INFORMATION: CONTENTS*

*** Sections or subsections omitted from the full prescribing information are not listed**

FULL PRESCRIBING INFORMATION

WARNING: POTENTIAL RISK FOR CARCINOGENICITY

Carcinogenicity has been seen in mice and rats treated chronically with metronidazole, another nitroimidazole agent *(13.1)*. Although such data have not been reported for tinidazole, the two drugs are structurally related and have similar biologic effects. **Its use should be reserved for the conditions described in INDICATIONS AND USAGE *(1)*.**

1 INDICATIONS AND USAGE

1.1 Trichomoniasis

Tinidazole is indicated for the treatment of trichomoniasis caused by *Trichomonas vaginalis*. The organism should be identified by appropriate diagnostic procedures. Because trichomoniasis is a sexually transmitted disease with potentially serious sequelae, partners of infected patients should be treated simultaneously in order to prevent re-infection *[see Clinical Studies (14.1)]*.

1.2 Giardiasis

Tinidazole is indicated for the treatment of giardiasis caused by *Giardia duodenalis* (also termed *G. lamblia*) in both adults and pediatric patients older than three years of age *[see Clinical Studies (14.2)]*.

1.3 Amebiasis

Tinidazole is indicated for the treatment of intestinal amebiasis and amebic liver abscess caused by *Entamoeba histolytica* in both adults and pediatric patients older than three years of age. It is not indicated in the treatment of asymptomatic cyst passage *[see Clinical Studies (14.3, 14.4)]*.

1.4 Bacterial Vaginosis

Tinidazole is indicated for the treatment of bacterial vaginosis (formerly referred to as *Haemophilus* vaginitis, *Gardnerella* vaginitis, nonspecific vaginitis, or anaerobic vaginosis) in non-pregnant women *[see Use in Specific Populations (8.1) and Clinical Studies (14.5)]*.

Other pathogens commonly associated with vulvovaginitis such as *Trichomonas vaginalis, Chlamydia trachomatis, Neisseria gonorrhoeae, Candida albicans* and *Herpes simplex* virus should be ruled out.

To reduce the development of drug-resistant bacteria and maintain the effectiveness of Tindamax and other antibacterial drugs, Tindamax should be used only to treat or prevent infections that are proven or strongly suspected to be caused by susceptible bacteria. When culture and susceptibility information are available, they should be considered in selecting or modifying antibacterial therapy. In the absence of such data, local epidemiology and susceptibility patterns may contribute to the empiric selection of therapy.

2 DOSAGE AND ADMINISTRATION

2.1 Dosing Instructions

It is advisable to take tinidazole with food to minimize the incidence of epigastric discomfort and other gastrointestinal side-effects. Food does not affect the oral bioavailability of tinidazole *[see Clinical Pharmacology (12.3)]*.

Alcoholic beverages should be avoided when taking tinidazole and for 3 days afterwards *[see Drug Interactions (7.1)]*.

2.2 Compounding of the Oral Suspension

For those unable to swallow tablets, tinidazole tablets may be crushed in artificial cherry syrup to be taken with food.

Procedure for Extemporaneous Pharmacy Compounding of the Oral Suspension: Pulverize four 500 mg oral tablets with a mortar and pestle. Add approximately 10 mL of cherry syrup to the powder and mix until smooth. Transfer the suspension to a graduated amber container. Use several small rinses of cherry syrup to transfer any remaining drug in the mortar to the final suspension for a final volume of 30 mL. The suspension of crushed tablets in artificial cherry syrup is stable for 7 days at room temperature. When this suspension is used, it should be shaken well before each administration.

2.3 Trichomoniasis

The recommended dose in both females and males is a single 2 g oral dose taken with food. Since trichomoniasis is a sexually transmitted disease, sexual partners should be treated with the same dose and at the same time.

2.4 Giardiasis

The recommended dose in adults is a single 2 g dose taken with food. In pediatric patients older than three years of age, the recommended dose is a single dose of 50 mg/kg (up to 2 g) with food.

2.5 Amebiasis

Intestinal: The recommended dose in adults is a 2 g dose per day for 3 days taken with food. In pediatric patients older than three years of age, the recommended dose is 50 mg/kg/day (up to 2 g per day) for 3 days with food.

Amebic Liver Abscess: The recommended dose in adults is a 2 g dose per day for 3-5 days taken with food. In pediatric patients older than three years of age, the recommended dose is 50 mg/kg/day (up to 2 g per day) for 3-5 days with food. There are limited pediatric data on durations of therapy exceeding 3 days, although a small number of children were treated for 5 days without additional reported adverse reactions. Children should be closely monitored when treatment durations exceed 3 days.

2.6 Bacterial Vaginosis

The recommended dose in non-pregnant females is a 2 g oral dose once daily for 2 days taken with food or a 1 g oral dose once daily for 5 days taken with food. The use of tinidazole in pregnant patients has not been studied for bacterial vaginosis.

3 DOSAGE FORMS AND STRENGTHS

- 250 mg tablets are pink, round, scored tablets, with TM debossed on one side and 250 on the other
- 500 mg tablets are pink, oval, scored tablets, with TM debossed on one side and 500 on the other

4 CONTRAINDICATIONS

The use of tinidazole is contraindicated:

- In patients with a previous history of hypersensitivity to tinidazole or other nitroimidazole derivatives. Reported reactions have ranged in severity from urticaria to Stevens-Johnson syndrome *[see Adverse Reactions (6.1, 6.2)]*.
- During first trimester of pregnancy *[see Use in Specific Populations (8.1)]*.
- In nursing mothers: Interruption of breast-feeding is recommended during tinidazole therapy and for 3 days following the last dose *[see Use in Specific Populations (8.3)]*.

5 WARNINGS AND PRECAUTIONS

5.1 Neurological Adverse Reactions

Convulsive seizures and peripheral neuropathy, the latter characterized mainly by numbness or paresthesia of an extremity, have been reported in patients treated with tinidazole. The appearance of abnormal neurologic signs demands the prompt discontinuation of tinidazole therapy.

5.2 Vaginal Candidiasis

The use of tinidazole may result in *Candida* vaginitis. In a clinical study of 235 women who received tinidazole for bacterial vaginosis, a vaginal fungal infection developed in 11 (4.7%) of all study subjects *[see Clinical Studies (14.5)]*.

5.3 Blood Dyscrasia

Tinidazole should be used with caution in patients with evidence of or history of blood dyscrasia *[see Drug Interactions (7.3)]*.

5.4 Drug Resistance

Prescribing Tindamax in the absence of a proven or strongly suspected bacterial infection or a prophylactic indication is unlikely to provide benefit to the patient and increases the risk of the development of drug-resistant bacteria.

6 ADVERSE REACTIONS

6.1 Clinical Studies Experience

Because clinical trials are conducted under widely varying conditions, adverse reaction rates observed in the clinical trials of a drug cannot be directly compared to rates in the clinical trials of another drug and may not reflect the rates observed in practice.

Among 3669 patients treated with a single 2 g dose of tinidazole, in both controlled and uncontrolled trichomoniasis and giardiasis clinical studies, adverse reactions were reported by 11.0% of patients. For multi-day dosing in controlled and uncontrolled amebiasis studies, adverse reactions were reported by 13.8% of 1765 patients. Common (≥ 1% incidence) adverse reactions reported by body system are as follows. (Note. Data described in Table 1 below are pooled from studies with variable designs and safety evaluations.)

Table 1. Adverse Reactions Summary of Published Reports

	2 g single dose	Multi-day dose
GI: Metallic/bitter taste	3.7%	6.3%
Nausea	3.2%	4.5%
Anorexia	1.5%	2.5%
Dyspepsia/cramps/epigastric discomfort	1.8%	1.4%
Vomiting	1.5%	0.9%
Constipation	0.4%	1.4%
CNS: Weakness/fatigue/malaise	2.1%	1.1%
Dizziness	1.1%	0.5%
Other: Headache	1.3%	0.7%
Total patients with adverse reactions	11.0% (403/3669)	13.8% (244/1765)

Other adverse reactions reported with tinidazole include:

Central Nervous System: Two serious adverse reactions reported include convulsions and transient peripheral neuropathy including numbness and paresthesia *[see Warnings and Precautions (5.1)]*. Other CNS reports include vertigo, ataxia, giddiness, insomnia, drowsiness.

Gastrointestinal: tongue discoloration, stomatitis, diarrhea

Hypersensitivity: urticaria, pruritis, rash, flushing, sweating, dryness of mouth, fever, burning sensation, thirst, salivation, angioedema

Renal: darkened urine

Cardiovascular: palpitations

Hematopoietic: transient neutropenia, transient leukopenia

Other: *Candida* overgrowth, increased vaginal discharge, oral candidiasis, hepatic abnormalities including raised transaminase level, arthralgias, myalgias, and arthritis.

[See table 1 above]

Rare reported adverse reactions include bronchospasm, dyspnea, coma, confusion, depression, furry tongue, pharyngitis and reversible thrombocytopenia.

Adverse Reactions in Pediatric Patients: In pooled pediatric studies, adverse reactions reported in pediatric patients taking tinidazole were similar in nature and frequency to adult findings including nausea, vomiting, diarrhea, taste change, anorexia, and abdominal pain.

Bacterial vaginosis: The most common adverse reactions in treated patients (incidence >2%), which were not identified in the trichomoniasis, giardiasis and amebiasis studies, are gastrointestinal: decreased appetite, and flatulence; renal: urinary tract infection, painful urination, and urine abnormality; and other reactions including pelvic pain, vulvo-vaginal discomfort, vaginal odor, menorrhagia, and upper respiratory tract infection *[See Clinical Studies (14.5)]*.

6.2 Postmarketing Experience

The following adverse reactions have been identified and reported during post-approval use of Tindamax. Because the reports of these reactions are voluntary and the population is of uncertain size, it is not always possible to reliably estimate the frequency of the reaction or establish a causal relationship to drug exposure.

Severe acute hypersensitivity reactions have been reported on initial or subsequent exposure to tinidazole. Hypersensitivity reactions may include urticaria, pruritis, angioedema, Stevens-Johnson syndrome and erythema multiforme.

7 DRUG INTERACTIONS

Although not specifically identified in studies with tinidazole, the following drug interactions were reported for metronidazole, a chemically-related nitroimidazole. Therefore, these drug interactions may occur with tinidazole.

7.1 Potential Effects of Tinidazole on Other Drugs

Warfarin and Other Oral Coumarin Anticoagulants: As with metronidazole, tinidazole may enhance the effect of warfarin and other coumarin anticoagulants, resulting in a prolongation of prothrombin time. The dosage of oral anticoagulants may need to be adjusted during tinidazole co-administration and up to 8 days after discontinuation.

Alcohols, Disulfiram: Alcoholic beverages and preparations containing ethanol or propylene glycol should be avoided during tinidazole therapy and for 3 days afterward because abdominal cramps, nausea, vomiting, headaches, and flushing may occur. Psychotic reactions have been reported in alcoholic patients using metronidazole and disulfiram concurrently. Though no similar reactions have been reported with tinidazole, tinidazole should not be given to patients who have taken disulfiram within the last two weeks.

Lithium: Metronidazole has been reported to elevate serum lithium levels. It is not known if tinidazole shares this property with metronidazole, but consideration should be given to measuring serum lithium and creatinine levels after several days of simultaneous lithium and tinidazole treatment to detect potential lithium intoxication.

Phenytoin, Fosphenytoin: Concomitant administration of oral metronidazole and intravenous phenytoin was reported to result in prolongation of the half-life and reduction in the clearance of phenytoin. Metronidazole did not significantly affect the pharmacokinetics of orally-administered phenytoin.

Cyclosporine, Tacrolimus: There are several case reports suggesting that metronidazole has the potential to increase the levels of cyclosporine and tacrolimus. During tinidazole co-administration with either of these drugs, the patient should be monitored for signs of calcineurin-inhibitor associated toxicities.

Fluorouracil: Metronidazole was shown to decrease the clearance of fluorouracil, resulting in an increase in side-effects without an increase in therapeutic benefits. If the concomitant use of tinidazole and fluorouracil cannot be avoided, the patient should be monitored for fluorouracil-associated toxicities.

7.2 Potential Effects of Other Drugs on Tinidazole

CYP3A4 Inducers and Inhibitors: Simultaneous administration of tinidazole with drugs that induce liver microsomal enzymes, i.e., CYP3A4 inducers such as *phenobarbital, rifampin, phenytoin,* and *fosphenytoin* (a pro-drug of phenytoin), may accelerate the elimination of tinidazole, decreasing the plasma level of tinidazole. Simultaneous administration of drugs that inhibit the activity of liver microsomal enzymes, i.e., CYP3A4 inhibitors such as *cimetidine* and *ketoconazole*, may prolong the half-life and decrease the plasma clearance of tinidazole, increasing the plasma concentrations of tinidazole.

Cholestyramine: Cholestyramine was shown to decrease the oral bioavailability of metronidazole by 21%. Thus, it is advisable to separate dosing of cholestyramine and tinidazole to minimize any potential effect on the oral bioavailability of tinidazole.

Oxytetracycline: Oxytetracycline was reported to antagonize the therapeutic effect of metronidazole.

7.3 Laboratory Test Interactions

Tinidazole, like metronidazole, may interfere with certain types of determinations of serum chemistry values, such as aspartate aminotransferase (AST, SGOT), alanine aminotransferase (ALT, SGPT), lactate dehydrogenase (LDH), triglycerides, and hexokinase glucose. Values of zero may be observed. All of the assays in which interference has been reported involve enzymatic coupling of the assay to oxidation-reduction of nicotinamide adenine dinucleotide ($NAD^+ \leftrightarrow NADH$). Potential interference is due to the similarity of absorbance peaks of NADH and tinidazole.

Tinidazole, like metronidazole, may produce transient leukopenia and neutropenia; however, no persistent hematological abnormalities attributable to tinidazole have been observed in clinical studies. Total and differential leukocyte counts are recommended if re-treatment is necessary.

8 USE IN SPECIFIC POPULATIONS

8.1 Pregnancy

Teratogenic effects: Pregnancy Category C

The use of tinidazole in pregnant patients has not been studied. Since tinidazole crosses the placental barrier and enters fetal circulation it should not be administered to pregnant patients in the first trimester.

Embryo-fetal developmental toxicity studies in pregnant mice indicated no embryo-fetal toxicity or malformations at the highest dose level of 2,500 mg/kg (approximately 6.3-fold the highest human therapeutic dose based upon body surface area conversions). In a study with pregnant rats a slightly higher incidence of fetal mortality was observed at a maternal dose of 500 mg/kg (2.5-fold the highest human therapeutic dose based upon body surface area conversions). No biologically relevant neonatal developmental effects were observed in rat neonates following maternal doses as high as 600 mg/kg (3-fold the highest human therapeutic dose based upon body surface area conversions). Although there is some evidence of mutagenic potential and animal reproduction studies are not always predictive of human response, the use of tinidazole after the first trimester of pregnancy requires that the potential benefits of the drug be weighed against the possible risks to both the mother and the fetus.

8.3 Nursing Mothers

Tinidazole is excreted in breast milk in concentrations similar to those seen in serum. Tinidazole can be detected in breast milk for up to 72 hours following administration. Interruption of breast-feeding is recommended during tinidazole therapy and for 3 days following the last dose.

8.4 Pediatric Use

Other than for use in the treatment of giardiasis and amebiasis in pediatric patients older than three years of age, safety and effectiveness of tinidazole in pediatric patients have not been established.

Pediatric Administration: For those unable to swallow tablets, tinidazole tablets may be crushed in artificial cherry syrup, to be taken with food *[see Dosage and Administration (2.2)]*.

8.5 Geriatric Use

Clinical studies of tinidazole did not include sufficient numbers of subjects aged 65 and over to determine whether they respond differently from younger subjects. In general, dose selection for an elderly patient should be cautious, reflecting the greater frequency of decreased hepatic, renal, or cardiac function, and of concomitant disease or other drug therapy.

8.6 Renal Impairment

Because the pharmacokinetics of tinidazole in patients with severe renal impairment (CrCL < 22 mL/min) are not significantly different from those in healthy subjects, no dose adjustments are necessary in these patients.

Patients undergoing hemodialysis: If tinidazole is administered on the same day as and prior to hemodialysis, it is recommended that an additional dose of tinidazole equivalent to one-half of the recommended dose be administered after the end of the hemodialysis *[see Clinical Pharmacology (12.3)]*.

8.7 Hepatic Impairment

There are no data on tinidazole pharmacokinetics in patients with impaired hepatic function. Reduced elimination of metronidazole, a chemically-related nitroimidazole, has been reported in this population. Usual recommended doses of tinidazole should be administered cautiously in patients with hepatic dysfunction *[see Clinical Pharmacology (12.3)]*.

10 OVERDOSAGE

There are no reported overdoses with tinidazole in humans.

Treatment of Overdosage: There is no specific antidote for the treatment of overdosage with tinidazole; therefore, treatment should be symptomatic and supportive. Gastric lavage may be helpful. Hemodialysis can be considered because approximately 43% of the amount present in the body is eliminated during a 6-hour hemodialysis session.

11 DESCRIPTION

Tinidazole is a synthetic antiprotozoal and antibacterial agent. It is 1-(2-ethylsulfonylethyl)-2-methyl-5-nitroimidazole, a second-generation 2-methyl-5-nitroimidazole, which has the following chemical structure:

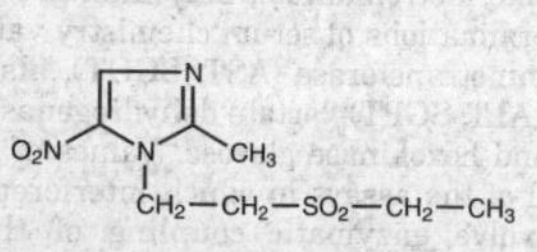

Tindamax pink oral tablets contain 250 mg or 500 mg of tinidazole. Inactive ingredients include croscarmellose sodium, FD&C Red 40 lake, FD&C Yellow 6 lake, hypromellose, magnesium stearate, microcrystalline cellulose, polydextrose, polyethylene glycol, pregelatinized corn starch, titanium dioxide, and triacetin.

12 CLINICAL PHARMACOLOGY

12.1 Mechanism of Action

Tinidazole is an antiprotozoal, antibacterial agent. *[See Clinical Pharmacology (12.4)]*.

12.3 Pharmacokinetics

Absorption: After oral administration, tinidazole is rapidly and completely absorbed. A bioavailability study of Tindamax tablets was conducted in adult healthy volunteers. All subjects received a single oral dose of 2 g (four 500 mg tablets) of Tindamax following an overnight fast. Oral administration of four 500 mg tablets of Tindamax under fasted conditions produced a mean peak plasma concentration (C_{max}) of 47.7 (±7.5) µg/mL with a mean time to peak concentration (T_{max}) of 1.6 (±0.7) hours, and a mean area under the plasma concentration-time curve (AUC, 0-∞) of 901.6 (± 126.5) µg.hr/mL at 72 hours. The elimination half-life ($T_{1/2}$) was 13.2 (±1.4) hours. Mean plasma levels decreased to 14.3 µg/mL at 24 hours, 3.8 µg/mL at 48 hours and 0.8 µg/mL at 72 hours following administration. Steady-state conditions are reached in 2½-3 days of multi-day dosing.

Administration of Tindamax tablets with food resulted in a delay in T_{max} of approximately 2 hours and a decline in C_{max} of approximately 10%, compared to fasted conditions. However, administration of Tindamax with food did not affect AUC or $T_{1/2}$ in this study.

In healthy volunteers, administration of crushed Tindamax tablets in artificial cherry syrup, [prepared as described in *Dosage and Administration (2.2)*] after an overnight fast had no effect on any pharmacokinetic parameter as compared to tablets swallowed whole under fasted conditions.

Distribution: Tinidazole is distributed into virtually all tissues and body fluids and also crosses the blood-brain barrier. The apparent volume of distribution is about 50 liters. Plasma protein binding of tinidazole is 12%. Tinidazole crosses the placental barrier and is secreted in breast milk.

Metabolism: Tinidazole is significantly metabolized in humans prior to excretion. Tinidazole is partly metabolized by oxidation, hydroxylation, and conjugation. Tinidazole is the major drug-related constituent in plasma after human treatment, along with a small amount of the 2-hydroxymethyl metabolite.

Tinidazole is biotransformed mainly by CYP3A4. In an *in vitro* metabolic drug interaction study, tinidazole concentrations of up to 75 µg/mL did not inhibit the enzyme activities of CYP1A2, CYP2B6, CYP2C9, CYP2D6, CYP2E1, and CYP3A4.

The potential of tinidazole to induce the metabolism of other drugs has not been evaluated.

Elimination: The plasma half-life of tinidazole is approximately 12-14 hours. Tinidazole is excreted by the liver and the kidneys. Tinidazole is excreted in the urine mainly as unchanged drug (approximately 20-25% of the administered dose). Approximately 12% of the drug is excreted in the feces.

Patients with impaired renal function: The pharmacokinetics of tinidazole in patients with severe renal impairment (CrCL < 22 mL/min) are not significantly different from the pharmacokinetics seen in healthy subjects. However, during hemodialysis, clearance of tinidazole is significantly increased; the half-life is reduced from 12.0 hours to 4.9 hours. Approximately 43% of the amount present in the body is eliminated during a 6-hour hemodialysis session *[see Use in Specific Populations (8.6)]*. The pharmacokinetics of tinidazole in patients undergoing routine continuous peritoneal dialysis have not been investigated.

Patients with impaired hepatic function: There are no data on tinidazole pharmacokinetics in patients with impaired hepatic function. Reduction of metabolic elimination of metronidazole, a chemically-related nitroimidazole, in patients with hepatic dysfunction has been reported in several studies *[see Use in Specific Populations (8.7)]*.

12.4 Microbiology

Mechanism of Action: Tinidazole is an antiprotozoal, antibacterial agent. The nitro-group of tinidazole is reduced by cell extracts of *Trichomonas*. The free nitro-radical generated as a result of this reduction may be responsible for the antiprotozoal activity. Chemically reduced tinidazole was shown to release nitrites and cause damage to purified bacterial DNA *in vitro*. Additionally, the drug caused DNA base changes in bacterial cells and DNA strand breakage in mammalian cells. The mechanism by which tinidazole exhibits activity against *Giardia* and *Entamoeba* species is not known.

Antibacterial: Culture and sensitivity testing of bacteria are not routinely performed to establish the diagnosis of bacterial vaginosis *[see Indications and Usage (1.4)]*; standard methodology for the susceptibility testing of potential bacterial pathogens, *Gardnerella vaginalis, Mobiluncus spp.* or *Mycoplasma hominis*, has not been defined. The following *in vitro* data are available, but their clinical significance is unknown. Tinidazole is active *in vitro* against most strains of the following organisms that have been reported to be associated with bacterial vaginosis:

- *Bacteroides spp.*
- *Gardnerella vaginalis*
- *Prevotella spp.*

Tinidazole does not appear to have activity against most strains of vaginal lactobacilli.

Antiprotozoal: Tinidazole demonstrates activity both *in vitro* and in clinical infections against the following protozoa: *Trichomonas vaginalis; Giardia duodenalis* (also termed *G. lamblia*); and *Entamoeba histolytica*.

For protozoal parasites, standardized susceptibility tests do not exist for use in clinical microbiology laboratories.

Drug Resistance: The development of resistance to tinidazole by *G. duodenalis, E. histolytica*, or bacteria associated with bacterial vaginosis has not been examined.

Cross-resistance: Approximately 38% of *T. vaginalis* isolates exhibiting reduced susceptibility to metronidazole also show reduced susceptibility to tinidazole *in vitro*. The clinical significance of such an effect is not known.

13 NONCLINICAL TOXICOLOGY

13.1 Carcinogenesis, Mutagenesis, Impairment of Fertility

Metronidazole, a chemically-related nitroimidazole, has been reported to be carcinogenic in mice and rats but not hamsters. In several studies metronidazole showed evidence of pulmonary, hepatic, and lymphatic tumorigenesis in mice and mammary and hepatic tumors in female rats. Tinidazole carcinogenicity studies in rats, mice or hamsters have not been reported.

Tinidazole was mutagenic in the TA 100, *S. typhimurium* tester strain both with and without the metabolic activation system and was negative for mutagenicity in the TA 98 strain. Mutagenicity results were mixed (positive and negative) in the TA 1535, 1537, and 1538 strains. Tinidazole was also mutagenic in a tester strain of *Klebsiella pneumonia*. Tinidazole was negative for mutagenicity in a mammalian cell culture system utilizing Chinese hamster lung V79 cells (HGPRT test system) and negative for genotoxicity in the Chinese hamster ovary (CHO) sister chromatid exchange assay. Tinidazole was positive for *in vivo* genotoxicity in the mouse micronucleus assay.

In a 60-day fertility study, tinidazole reduced fertility and produced testicular histopathology in male rats at a 600 mg/kg/day dose level (approximately 3-fold the highest human therapeutic dose based upon body surface area conversions). Spermatogenic effects resulted from 300 and 600 mg/kg/day dose levels. The no observed adverse reaction level for testicular and spermatogenic effects was 100 mg/kg/day (approximately 0.5-fold the highest human therapeutic dose based upon body surface area conversions). This effect is characteristic of agents in the 5-nitroimidazole class.

13.2 Animal Toxicology and/or Pharmacology

In acute studies with mice and rats, the LD_{50} for mice was generally > 3,600 mg/kg for oral administration and was > 2,300 mg/kg for intraperitoneal administration. In rats, the LD_{50} was > 2,000 mg/kg for both oral and intraperitoneal administration.

A repeated-dose toxicology study has been performed in beagle dogs using oral dosing of tinidazole at 100 mg/kg/day, 300 mg/kg/day, and 1000 mg/kg/day for 28-days. On Day 18 of the study, the highest dose was lowered to 600 mg/kg/day due to severe clinical symptoms. The two compound-related effects observed in the dogs treated with tinidazole were increased atrophy of the thymus in both sexes at the middle and high doses, and atrophy of the prostate at all doses in the males. A no-adverse-effect level (NOAEL) of 100 mg/kg/day for females was determined. There was no NOAEL identified for males because of minimal atrophy of the prostate at 100 mg/kg/day (approximately 0.9-fold the highest human dose based upon plasma AUC comparisons).

14 CLINICAL STUDIES

14.1 Trichomoniasis

Tinidazole (2 g single oral dose) use in trichomoniasis has been well documented in 34 published reports from the world literature involving over 2,800 patients treated with tinidazole. In four published, blinded, randomized, comparative studies of the 2 g tinidazole single oral dose where efficacy was assessed by culture at time points post-treatment ranging from one week to one month, reported cure rates ranged from 92% (37/40) to 100% (65/65) (n=172 total subjects). In four published, blinded, randomized, comparative studies where efficacy was assessed by wet mount between 7-14 days post-treatment, reported cure rates ranged from 80% (8/10) to 100% (16/16) (n=116 total subjects). In these studies, tinidazole was superior to placebo and comparable to other anti-trichomonal drugs. The single oral 2 g tinidazole dose was also assessed in four open-label trials in men (one comparative to metronidazole and 3 single-arm studies). Parasitological evaluation of the urine was performed both pre- and post-treatment and reported cure rates ranged from 83% (25/30) to 100% (80/80) (n=142 total subjects).

14.2 Giardiasis

Tinidazole (2 g single dose) use in giardiasis has been documented in 19 published reports from the world literature involving over 1,600 patients (adults and pediatric patients). In eight controlled studies involving a total of 619 subjects of whom 299 were given the 2 g × 1 day (50 mg/kg × 1 day in pediatric patients) oral dose of tinidazole, reported cure rates ranged from 80% (40/50) to 100% (15/15). In three of these trials where the comparator was 2 to 3 days of various doses of metronidazole, reported cure rates for metronidazole were 76% (19/25) to 93% (14/15). Data comparing a single 2 g dose of tinidazole to usually recommended 5-7 days of metronidazole are limited.

14.3 Intestinal Amebiasis

Tinidazole use in intestinal amebiasis has been documented in 26 published reports from the world literature involving over 1,400 patients. Most reports utilized tinidazole 2 g/day × 3 days. In four published, randomized, controlled studies (1 investigator single- blind, 3 open-label) of the 2 g/day × 3 days oral dose of tinidazole, reported cure rates after 3 days of therapy among a total of 220 subjects ranged from 86% (25/29) to 93% (25/27).

Table 2. Efficacy of Tindamax in the Treatment of Bacterial Vaginosis in a Randomized, Double-Blind, Double-Dummy, Placebo-Controlled Trial: Modified Intent-to-Treat Population[1] (n=227)

Outcome	Tindamax 1 g × 5 days (n=76)	Tindamax 2 g × 2 days (n=73)	Placebo (n=78)
	% Cure	% Cure	% Cure
Therapeutic Cure	36.8	27.4	5.1
Difference[2]	31.7	22.3	
97.5% CI[3]	(16.8, 46.6)	(8.0, 36.6)	
Clinical Cure	51.3	35.6	11.5
Difference[2]	39.8	24.1	
97.5% CI[3]	(23.3, 56.3)	(7.8, 40.3)	
Nugent Score Cure	38.2	27.4	5.1
Difference[2]	33.1	22.3	
97.5% CI[3]	(18.1, 48.0)	(8.0, 36.6)	

[1] Modified Intent-to-Treat defined as all patients randomized with a baseline Nugent score of at least 4
[2] Difference in cure rates (Tindamax-placebo)
[3] CI: confidence interval
p-values for both Tindamax regimens vs. placebo for therapeutic, clinical and Nugent score cure rates for both 2 and 5 days <0.001

14.4 Amebic Liver Abscess

Tinidazole use in amebic liver abscess has been documented in 18 published reports from the world literature involving over 470 patients. Most reports utilized tinidazole 2 g/day × 2-5 days. In seven published, randomized, controlled studies (1 double-blind, 1 single-blind, 5 open-label) of the 2 g/day × 2-5 days oral dose of tinidazole accompanied by aspiration of the liver abscess when clinically necessary, reported cure rates among 133 subjects ranged from 81% (17/21) to 100% (16/16). Four of these studies utilized at least 3 days of tinidazole.

14.5 Bacterial Vaginosis

A randomized, double-blind, placebo-controlled clinical trial in 235 non-pregnant women was conducted to evaluate the efficacy of tinidazole for the treatment of bacterial vaginosis. A clinical diagnosis of bacterial vaginosis was based on Amsel's criteria and defined by the presence of an abnormal homogeneous vaginal discharge that (a) has a pH of greater than 4.5, (b) emits a "fishy" amine odor when mixed with a 10% KOH solution, and (c) contains ≥20% clue cells on microscopic examination. Clinical cure required a return to normal vaginal discharge and resolution of all Amsel's criteria. A microbiologic diagnosis of bacterial vaginosis was based on Gram stain of the vaginal smear demonstrating (a) markedly reduced or absent *Lactobacillus* morphology, (b) predominance of *Gardnerella* morphotype, and (c) absent or few white blood cells, with quantification of these bacterial morphotypes to determine the Nugent score, where a score ≥4 was required for study inclusion and a score of 0-3 considered a microbiologic cure. Therapeutic cure was a composite endpoint, consisting of both a clinical cure and microbiologic cure. In patients with all four Amsel's criteria and with a baseline Nugent score ≥4, tinidazole oral tablets given as either 2 g once daily for 2 days or 1 g once daily for 5 days demonstrated superior efficacy over placebo tablets as measured by therapeutic cure, clinical cure, and a microbiologic cure.

[See table 2 above]

The therapeutic cure rates reported in this clinical study conducted with Tindamax were based on resolution of 4 out of 4 Amsel's criteria and a Nugent score of <4. The cure rates for previous clinical studies with other products approved for bacterial vaginosis were based on resolution of either 2 or 3 out of 4 Amsel's criteria. At the time of approval for other products for bacterial vaginosis, there was no requirement for a Nugent score on Gram stain, resulting in higher reported rates of cure for bacterial vaginosis for those products than for those reported here for tinidazole.

16 HOW SUPPLIED/STORAGE AND HANDLING

Tindamax 250 mg tablets are pink, round, scored tablets, with TM debossed on one side and 250 on the other, supplied in bottles with child-resistant caps as:

NDC 0178-8250-40 Bottle of 40

Tindamax 500 mg tablets are pink, oval, scored tablets, with TM debossed on one side and 500 on the other, supplied in bottles with child-resistant caps as:

NDC 0178-8500-60 Bottle of 60
NDC 0178-8500-20 Bottle of 20

Professional Samples:

NDC 0178-8500-02 Bottle of 2

Storage: Store at controlled room temperature 20-25° C (68-77° F); excursions permitted to 15-30° C (59-86° F) [see USP]. Protect contents from light.

17 PATIENT COUNSELING INFORMATION

17.1 Administration of Drug

Patients should be told to take Tindamax with food to minimize the incidence of epigastric discomfort and other gastrointestinal side-effects. Food does not affect the oral bioavailability of tinidazole.

17.2 Alcohol Avoidance

Patients should be told to avoid alcoholic beverages and preparations containing ethanol or propylene glycol during Tindamax therapy and for 3 days afterward because abdominal cramps, nausea, vomiting, headaches, and flushing may occur.

17.3 Drug Resistance

Patients should be counseled that antibacterial drugs including Tindamax should only be used to treat bacterial infections. They do not treat viral infections (e.g., the common cold). When Tindamax is prescribed to treat a bacterial infection, patients should be told that although it is common to feel better early in the course of therapy, the medication should be taken exactly as directed. Skipping doses or not completing the full course of therapy may (1) decrease the effectiveness of the immediate treatment and (2) increase the likelihood that bacteria will develop resistance and will not be treatable by Tindamax or other antibacterial drugs in the future.

Rev 0907

URIBEL ℞

Rx Only

DESCRIPTION

Uribel® capsules for oral administration.

Each capsule contains:

Methenamine	118 mg
Sodium Phosphate Monobasic	40.8 mg
Phenyl Salicylate	36 mg
Methylene Blue	10 mg
Hyoscyamine Sulfate	0.12 mg

HYOSCYAMINE SULFATE. [620-61-1] [3(S)-endo]-α-(Hydroxymethyl)-benzeneacetic acid 8-methyl-8-azabicyclo[3.2.1]oct-3-yl ester sulfate(2:1)(salt); 1αH,5αH-tropan-3α-ol(-)-tropate (ester) sulfate(2:1)(salt); 3α-tropanyl S-(-)-tropate; I-tropic acid ester with tropine; I-tropine tropate. $C_{34}H_{48}N_2O_{10}S$. Hyoscyamine Sulfate is an alkaloid of belladonna. Exists as a white crystalline powder. Its solutions are alkaline to litmus. Affected by light, it is slightly soluble in water; freely soluble in alcohol; sparingly soluble in ether.

METHENAMINE. [100-97-0] 1,3,5,7-Tetraazatricyclo [3.3.1.-$1^{3,7}$] decane; hexamethylenetetramine; HMT; HMTA; hexamine; 1,3,5,7-tetraazaadamantane hexamethylenemine; Uritone; Urotropin. $C_6H_{12}N_4$; mol wt 140.19; C 51.40%, H 8.63%, N 39.96%. Methenamine (hexamethylenetetramine) exists as colorless, lustrous crystals or white crystalline powder. Its solutions are alkaline to litmus. Freely soluble in water, soluble in alcohol and in chloroform.

METHYLENE BLUE. [61-73-4] 3,7-Bis(dimethylamino) phenothiazin-5-ium chloride; C.I. Basic Blue 9; methylthionium chloride; tetramethylthionine chloride; 3,7-bis(dimethylamino) phenazathionium chloride. $C_{16}H_{18}ClN_3S$; mol wt 319.85, C 60.08%, H 5.67%, Cl 11.08%, N 13.14%, S 10.03%. Methylene Blue (Methylthionine chloride) exists as dark green crystals. It is soluble in water and in chloroform; sparingly soluble in alcohol.

PHENYL SALICYLATE. [118-55-8] 2-Hydroxybenzoic acid phenyl ester; Salol. $C_{13}H_{10}O_3$; mol wt 214.22, C 72.89%, H 4.71%, O 22.41%. Made by the action of phosphorus oxychloride on a mixture of phenol and salicylic acid. Phenyl Salicylate exists as white crystals with a melting point of 41°-43° C. It is very slightly soluble in water and freely soluble in alcohol.

SODIUM PHOSPHATE MONOBASIC. [7558-80-7] Phosphoric acid sodium salt (1:1); Sodium biphosphate; sodium dihydrogen phosphate; acid sodium phosphate; monosodium orthophosphate; primary sodium phosphate; H_2NaO_4P; mol wt 119.98, H 1.68%, Na 19.16%, O 53.34%, P 25.82%. Monohydrate, white, odorless slightly deliquesce crystals or granules. At 100° C loses all its water; when ignited it converts to metaphosphate. It is freely soluble in water and practically insoluble in alcohol. The aqueous solution is acid. pH of 0.1 molar aqueous solution at 25° C: 4.5.

Uribel® capsules contain inactive ingredients: Dicalcium Phosphate, FD&C Blue #1, FD&C Red #3, Gelatin, Magnesium Stearate, Microcrystalline Cellulose, Povidone, Propylene Glycol, Shellac, Silicon Dioxide, Sodium Hydroxide, Stearic Acid, and Titanium Dioxide.

CLINICAL PHARMACOLOGY

HYOSCYAMINE SULFATE is a parasympatholytic which relaxes smooth muscles and thus produces an antispasmodic effect. It is well absorbed from the gastrointestinal tract and is rapidly distributed throughout the body tissues. Most is excreted in the urine within 12 hours, 13% to 50% being unchanged. Its biotransformation is hepatic. Its protein binding is moderate.

METHENAMINE degrades in an acidic environment releasing formaldehyde which provides bactericidal or bacteriostatic action. It is well absorbed from the gastrointestinal tract. 70% - 90% reaches the urine unchanged at which point it is hydrolyzed if the urine is acidic. Within 24 hours it is almost completely (90%) excreted; of this at a pH of 5, approximately 20% is formaldehyde. Protein binding- some formaldehyde is bound to substances in the urine and surrounding tissues. Methenamine is freely distributed to body tissue and fluids but is not clinically significant as it does not hydrolyze at pH greater than 6.8.

METHYLENE BLUE possesses weak antiseptic properties. It is well absorbed by the gastrointestinal tract and rapidly reduced to leukomethylene blue which is stabilized in some combination form in the urine. 75% is excreted unchanged.

PHENYL SALICYLATE releases salicylate, a mild analgesic for pain.

SODIUM PHOSPHATE MONOBASIC an acidifier, helps to maintain an acid pH in the urine necessary for the degradation of methenamine.

INDICATIONS AND USAGE

Uribel® capsules are indicated for the treatment of symptoms of irritative voiding. Indicated for the relief of local symptoms, such as inflammation, hypermotility, and pain, which accompany lower urinary tract infections. Indicated for the relief of urinary tract symptoms caused by diagnostic procedures.

CONTRAINDICATIONS

Hypersensitivity to any of the ingredients is possible. Risk benefits should be carefully considered when the following medical problems exist: cardiac disease (especially cardiac arrhythmias, congestive heart failure, coronary heart disease, and mitral stenosis); gastrointestinal tract obstructive disease; glaucoma; myasthenia gravis, acute urinary retention may be precipitated in obstructive uropathy (such as bladder neck obstruction due to prostatic hypertrophy).

WARNINGS

Do not exceed recommended dosage. If rapid pulse, dizziness or blurring of vision occurs discontinue use immediately.

PRECAUTIONS

Cross sensitivity and/or related problems

Patients intolerant of belladona alkaloids or salicylates may be intolerant of this medication also. Delay in gastric emptying could complicate the management of gastric ulcers.

Pregnancy/Reproduction (FDA Pregnancy Category C)

Hyoscyamine and methenamine cross the placenta. Studies concerning the effect of hyoscyamine and methenamine on pregnancy and reproduction have not been done in animals or humans. Thus it is not known whether **Uribel®** capsules cause fetal harm when administered to a pregnant woman or can effect reproduction capacity. **Uribel®** capsules should be given to a pregnant woman only if clearly needed.

Breast feeding

Problems in humans have not been demonstrated; however, methenamine and traces of hyoscyamine are excreted in breast milk. Accordingly, **Uribel® capsules** should be given to a nursing mother with caution and only if clearly needed.

Prolonged use
There have been no studies to establish the safety of prolonged use in humans. No known long-term animal studies have been performed to evaluate carcinogenic potential.
Pediatric use
Infants and young children are especially susceptible to the toxic effect of the belladona alkaloids.
Geriatric use
Use with caution in elderly patients as they may respond to usual doses of hyoscyamine with excitement, agitation, drowsiness or confusion.

ADVERSE REACTION

Cardiovascular: rapid heartbeat, flushing
Central Nervous System: blurred vision, dizziness, drowsiness
Genitourinary: difficult micturition, acute urinary retention
Gastrointestinal: dry mouth, nausea and vomiting
Respiratory: shortness of breath or trouble breathing
Serious allergic reactions to this drug are rare. Seek immediate medical attention if you notice symptoms of a serious allergic reaction, including itching, rash, severe dizziness, swelling or trouble breathing.
This medication can cause urine and sometimes stools to turn blue to blue-green. This effect is harmless and will subside after medication is stopped.
Call your doctor or physician for medical advice about side effects. To report SUSPECTED ADVERSE REACTIONS, contact Star Pharmaceuticals, LLC at 1-800-845-7827 or FDA at 1-800-FDA-1088, www.fda.gov/medwatch.
Drug interactions
Because of this product's effect on gastrointestinal motility and gastric emptying, it may decrease the absorption of other oral medications during concurrent use such as: urinary alkalizers; thiazide diuretics (may cause the urine to become alkaline reducing the effectiveness of methenamine by inhibiting its conversion to formaldehyde); antimuscarinics (concurrent use may intensify antimuscarinic effects of hyoscyamine because of secondary antimuscarinic activities of these medications); antacids/antidiarrheals (may reduce absorption of hyoscyamine, concurrent use with antacids may cause urine to become alkaline, reducing effectiveness of methenamine by inhibiting its conversion to formaldehyde). Doses of these medications should be spaced 1 hour apart from doses of hyoscyamine; antimyasthenics (concurrent use with hyoscyamine may further reduce intestinal motility); ketoconazole (patients should be advised to take this combination at least 2 hours after ketoconazole); monoamine oxidase (MAO) inhibitors (concurrent use may intensify antimuscarinic side effects), opioid (narcotic analgesics may result in increased risk of severe constipation); sulfonamides (these drugs may precipitate with formaldehyde in the urine, increasing the danger of crystalluria). Patients should be advised that the urine may become blue to blue-green and the feces may be discolored as a result of the excretion of the methylene blue.

DRUG ABUSE AND DEPENDENCE

A dependence on the use of **Uribel® capsules** has not been reported and due to the nature of its ingredients, abuse of **Uribel® capsules** is not expected.

OVERDOSAGE

Emesis or gastric lavage. Slow intravenous administration of physostigmine in doses of 1 to 4 mg (0.5 to 1 mg in children), repeated as needed in one to two hours to reverse severe antimuscarinic symptoms.
Administration of small doses of diazepam to control excitement and seizures. Artificial respiration with oxygen if needed for respiratory depression. Adequate hydration. Symptomatic treatment as necessary.
If overdose is suspected, contact your local poison center or emergency room immediately. US residents can contact the US National Poison Hotline at 1-800-222-1222.

DOSAGE AND ADMINISTRATION

Adults
One capsule orally 4 times per day followed by liberal fluid intake.
Older Children
Dosage must be individualized by physician. Not recommended for use in children six years of age or younger.

HOW SUPPLIED

Uribel® capsules are purple/purple capsules imprinted "S 111". NDC 0076-0111-01, Bottle of 100 Capsules and NDC 0076-0111-02, Carton of 20 individually pouched capsules.
STORAGE
Dispense in a tight, light-resistant container as defined in the USP/NF with a child resistant closure.
Store at controlled room temperature 20°-25° C (68°-77° F)
Keep in a cool dry place.
Keep container tightly closed.

WARNING: Keep this and all drugs out of the reach of children.
Rx Only

COMPANIES

Rx Only
Uribel® is a registered trademark of Star Pharmaceuticals, LLC
Distributed by:
MISSION PHARMACAL COMPANY
San Antonio, TX 78230
Manufactured for:
STAR PHARMACEUTICALS, LLC
Ft. Lauderdale, FL 33306
Rev 04/10

UROCIT®-K ℞
[yu 'ro-cit kay]
(Potassium Citrate)
Extended-release tablets for oral use

HIGHLIGHTS OF PRESCRIBING INFORMATION
These highlights do not include all the information needed to use Urocit®-K safely and effectively. See full prescribing information for Urocit®-K.
Urocit®-K (Potassium Citrate) Extended-release tablets for oral use
Initial U.S. Approval: 1985

RECENT MAJOR CHANGES

Dosage and Administration, Urocit®-K 15 mEq *(2.2, 2.3)* 12/2009
Dosage Forms and Strengths, Urocit®-K 15 mEq *(3)* 12/2009
Description, Urocit®-K 15 mEq *(11)* 12/2009
Clinical Studies *(14)* 12/2009
How Supplied/Storage and Handling, Urocit®-K 15 mEq *(16)* 12/2009

INDICATIONS AND USAGE

Urocit®-K is a citrate salt of potassium indicated for the management of:
- Renal tubular acidosis (RTA) with calcium stones *(1.1)*
- Hypocitraturic calcium oxalate nephrolithiasis of any etiology *(1.2)*
- Uric acid lithiasis with or without calcium stones *(1.3)*

DOSAGE AND ADMINISTRATION

Objective: To restore normal urinary citrate (greater than 320 mg/day and as close to the normal mean of 640 mg/day as possible), and to increase urinary pH to a level of 6.0 to 7.0.
- Severe hypocitraturia (urinary citrate < 150 mg/day): therapy should be initiated at 60 mEq per day; a dose of 30 mEq two times per day or 20 mEq three times per day with meals or within 30 minutes after meals or bedtime snack *(2.2)*
- Mild to moderate hypocitraturia (urinary citrate >150 mg/day): therapy should be initiated at 30 mEq per day; a dose of 15 mEq two times per day or 10 mEq three times per day with meals or within 30 minutes after meals or bedtime snack *(2.3)*

DOSAGE FORMS AND STRENGTHS

Tablets: 5 mEq, 10 mEq and 15 mEq *(3)*

CONTRAINDICATIONS

- Patients with hyperkalemia (or who have conditions predisposing them to hyperkalemia). Such conditions include chronic renal failure, uncontrolled diabetes mellitus, acute dehydration, strenuous physical exercise in unconditioned individuals, adrenal insufficiency, extensive tissue breakdown *(4)*
- Patients for whom there is cause for arrest or delay in tablet passage through the gastrointestinal tract such as those suffering from delayed gastric emptying, esophageal compression, intestinal obstruction or stricture *(4)*
- Patients with peptic ulcer disease *(4)*
- Patients with active urinary tract infection *(4)*
- Patients with renal insufficiency (glomerular filtration rate of less than 0.7 ml/kg/min) *(4)*

WARNINGS AND PRECAUTIONS

- Hyperkalemia: In patients with impaired mechanisms for excreting potassium, Urocit®-K administration can produce hyperkalemia and cardiac arrest. Potentially fatal hyperkalemia can develop rapidly and be asymptomatic. The use of Urocit®-K in patients with chronic renal failure, or any other condition which impairs potassium excretion such as severe myocardial damage or heart failure, should be avoided *(5.1)*
- Gastrointestinal lesions: if there is severe vomiting, abdominal pain or gastrointestinal bleeding, Urocit®-K should be discontinued immediately and the possibility of bowel perforation or obstruction investigated *(5.2)*

ADVERSE REACTIONS

Some patients may develop minor gastrointestinal complaints such as abdominal discomfort, vomiting, diarrhea, loose bowel movements or nausea. These may be alleviated by taking the dose with meals or snacks or by reducing the dosage *(6.1)*
To report SUSPECTED ADVERSE REACTIONS, contact Mission Pharmacal Company at 1-800-298-1087 or FDA at 1-800-FDA-1088 or *www.fda.gov/medwatch*

DRUG INTERACTIONS

The following drug interactions may occur with potassium citrate:
- Potassium-sparing diuretics: concomitant administration should be avoided since the simultaneous administration of these agents can produce severe hyperkalemia *(7.1)*
- Drugs that slow gastrointestinal transit time: These agents (such as anticholinergics) can be expected to increase the gastrointestinal irritation produced by potassium salts *(7.2)*

USE IN SPECIFIC POPULATIONS

- Pregnant women: Pregnancy Category C; animal reproduction studies have not been conducted. It is not known whether Urocit®-K can cause fetal harm when administered to a pregnant woman or can affect reproduction capacity. Urocit®-K should be given to a pregnant woman only if clearly needed *(8.1)*
- Nursing mothers: The normal potassium ion content of human milk is about 13 mEq/L. It is not known if Urocit®-K has an effect on this content. Urocit®-K should be given to a woman who is breast feeding only if clearly needed *(8.3)*
- Pediatric Use: Safety and effectiveness in children have not been established *(8.4)*

See 17 for PATIENT COUNSELING INFORMATION
Revised: 04/2010

FULL PRESCRIBING INFORMATION: CONTENTS*

*** Sections or subsections omitted from the full prescribing information are not listed**

FULL PRESCRIBING INFORMATION

1 INDICATIONS AND USAGE

1.1 Renal tubular acidosis (RTA) with calcium stones
Potassium citrate is indicated for the management of renal tubular acidosis *[see Clinical Studies (14.1)]*.

1.2 Hypocitraturic calcium oxalate nephrolithiasis of any etiology
Potassium citrate is indicated for the management of Hypocitraturic calcium oxalate nephrolithiasis *[see Clinical Studies (14.2)]*.

1.3 Uric acid lithiasis with or without calcium stones

Potassium citrate is indicated for the management of Uric acid lithiasis with or without calcium stones *[see Clinical Studies (14.3)]*.

2 DOSAGE AND ADMINISTRATION

2.1 Dosing Instructions

Treatment with extended release potassium citrate should be added to a regimen that limits salt intake (avoidance of foods with high salt content and of added salt at the table) and encourages high fluid intake (urine volume should be at least two liters per day). The objective of treatment with Urocit®-K is to provide Urocit®-K in sufficient dosage to restore normal urinary citrate (greater than 320 mg/day and as close to the normal mean of 640 mg/day as possible), and to increase urinary pH to a level of 6.0 or 7.0.

Monitor serum electrolytes (sodium, potassium, chloride and carbon dioxide), serum creatinine and complete blood counts every four months and more frequently in patients with cardiac disease, renal disease or acidosis. Perform electrocardiograms periodically. Treatment should be discontinued if there is hyperkalemia, a significant rise in serum creatinine or a significant fall in blood hemocrit or hemoglobin.

2.2 Severe Hypocitraturia

In patients with severe hypocitraturia (urinary citrate < 150 mg/day), therapy should be initiated at a dosage of 60 mEq/day (30 mEq two times/day or 20 mEq three times/day with meals or within 30 minutes after meals or bedtime snack). Twenty-four hour urinary citrate and/or urinary pH measurements should be used to determine the adequacy of the initial dosage and to evaluate the effectiveness of any dosage change. In addition, urinary citrate and/or pH should be measured every four months. Doses of Urocit®-K greater than 100 mEq/day have not been studied and should be avoided.

2.3 Mild to Moderate Hypocitraturia

In patients with mild to moderate hypocitraturia (urinary citrate > 150 mg/day) therapy should be initiated at 30 mEq/day (15 mEq two times/day or 10 mEq three times/day within 30 minutes after meals or bedtime snack). Twenty-four hour urinary citrate and/or urinary pH measurements should be used to determine the adequacy of the initial dosage and to evaluate the effectiveness of any dosage change. Doses of Urocit®-K greater than 100 mEq/day have not been studied and should be avoided.

3 DOSAGE FORMS AND STRENGTHS

- 5 mEq tablets are uncoated, tan to yellowish in color, modified ball shaped, with MPC 600 debossed on one side and blank on the other
- 10 mEq tablets are uncoated, tan to yellowish in color, elliptical shaped, with 610 debossed on one side and MISSION on the other
- 15 mEq tablets are uncoated, tan to yellowish in color, modified rectangle shaped, with M15 debossed on one side and blank on the other

4 CONTRAINDICATIONS

Urocit®-K is contraindicated:

- In patients with hyperkalemia (or who have conditions pre-disposing them to hyperkalemia), as a further rise in serum potassium concentration may produce cardiac arrest. Such conditions include: chronic renal failure, uncontrolled diabetes mellitus, acute dehydration, strenuous physical exercise in unconditioned individuals, adrenal insufficiency, extensive tissue breakdown or the administration of a potassium-sparing agent (such as triamterene, spironolactone or amiloride).
- In patients in whom there is cause for arrest or delay in tablet passage through the gastrointestinal tract, such as those suffering from delayed gastric emptying, esophageal compression, intestinal obstruction or stricture, or those taking anticholinergic medication.
- In patients with peptic ulcer disease because of its ulcerogenic potential.
- In patients with active urinary tract infection (with either urea-splitting or other organisms, in association with either calcium or struvite stones). The ability of Urocit®-K to increase urinary citrate may be attenuated by bacterial enzymatic degradation of citrate. Moreover, the rise in urinary pH resulting from Urocit®-K therapy might promote further bacterial growth.
- In patients with renal insufficiency (glomerular filtration rate of less than 0.7 ml/kg/min), because of the danger of soft tissue calcification and increased risk for the development of hyperkalemia.

5 WARNINGS AND PRECAUTIONS

5.1 Hyperkalemia

In patients with impaired mechanisms for excreting potassium, Urocit®-K administration can produce hyperkalemia and cardiac arrest. Potentially fatal hyperkalemia can develop rapidly and be asymptomatic. The use of Urocit®-K in patients with chronic renal failure, or any other condition which impairs potassium excretion such as severe myocardial damage or heart failure, should be avoided. Closely monitor for signs of hyperkalemia with periodic blood tests and ECGs.

5.2 Gastrointestinal Lesions

Because of reports of upper gastrointestinal mucosal lesions following administration of potassium chloride (wax-matrix), an endoscopic examination of the upper gastrointestinal mucosa was performed in 30 normal volunteers after they had taken glycopyrrolate 2 mg p.o. t.i.d., Urocit®-K 95 mEq/day, wax-matrix potassium chloride 96 mEq/day or wax-matrix placebo, in thrice daily schedule in the fasting state for one week. Urocit®-K and the wax-matrix formulation of potassium chloride were indistinguishable but both were significantly more irritating than the wax-matrix placebo. In a subsequent, similar study, lesions were less severe when glycopyrrolate was omitted.

Solid dosage forms of potassium chlorides have produced stenotic and/or ulcerative lesions of the small bowel and deaths. These lesions are caused by a high local concentration of potassium ions in the region of the dissolving tablets, which injured the bowel. In addition, perhaps because wax-matrix preparations are not enteric-coated and release some of their potassium content in the stomach, there have been reports of upper gastrointestinal bleeding associated with these products. The frequency of gastrointestinal lesions with wax-matrix potassium chloride products is estimated at one per 100,000 patient-years. Experience with Urocit®-K is limited, but a similar frequency of gastrointestinal lesions should be anticipated.

If there is severe vomiting, abdominal pain or gastrointestinal bleeding, Urocit®-K should be discontinued immediately and the possibility of bowel perforation or obstruction investigated.

6 ADVERSE REACTIONS

6.1 Postmarketing Experience

Some patients may develop minor gastrointestinal complaints during Urocit®-K therapy, such as abdominal discomfort, vomiting, diarrhea, loose bowel movements or nausea. These symptoms are due to the irritation of the gastrointestinal tract, and may be alleviated by taking the dose with meals or snacks, or by reducing the dosage. Patients may find intact matrices in their feces.

7 DRUG INTERACTIONS

7.1 Potential Effects of Potassium citrate on Other Drugs

Potassium-sparing Diuretics: Concomitant administration of Urocit®-K and a potassium-sparing diuretic (such as triamterene, spironolactone or amiloride) should be avoided since the simultaneous administration of these agents can produce severe hyperkalemia.

7.2 Potential Effects of Other Drugs on Potassium citrate

Drugs that slow gastrointestinal transit time: These agents (such as anticholinergics) can be expected to increase the gastrointestinal irritation produced by potassium salts.

8 USE IN SPECIFIC POPULATIONS

8.1 Pregnancy

Pregnancy Category C

Animal reproduction studies have not been conducted. It is also not known whether Urocit®-K can cause fetal harm when administered to a pregnant woman or can affect reproduction capacity. Urocit®-K should be given to a pregnant woman only if clearly needed.

8.3 Nursing Mothers

The normal potassium ion content of human milk is about 13 mEq/L. It is not known if Urocit®-K has an effect on this content. Urocit®-K should be given to a woman who is breast feeding only if clearly needed.

8.4 Pediatric Use

Safety and effectiveness in children have not been established.

10 OVERDOSAGE

Treatment of Overdosage: The administration of potassium salts to persons without predisposing conditions for hyperkalemia rarely causes serious hyperkalemia at recommended dosages. It is important to recognize that hyperkalemia is usually asymptomatic and may be manifested only by an increased serum potassium concentration and characteristic electrocardiographic changes (peaking of T-wave, loss of P-wave, depression of S-T segment and prolongation of the QT interval). Late manifestations include muscle paralysis and cardiovascular collapse from cardiac arrest.

Treatment measures for hyperkalemia include the following:

1. Patients should be closely monitored for arrhythmias and electrolyte changes.
2. Elimination of medications containing potassium and of agents with potassium-sparing properties such as potassium-sparing diuretics, ARBs, ACE inhibitors, NSAIDs, certain nutritional supplements and many others.
3. Elimination of foods containing high levels of potassium such as almonds, apricots, bananas, beans (lima, pinto, white), cantaloupe, carrot juice (canned), figs, grapefruit juice, halibut, milk, oat bran, potato (with skin), salmon, spinach, tuna and many others.
4. Intravenous calcium gluconate if the patient is at no risk or low risk of developing digitalis toxicity.
5. Intravenous administration of 300-500 mL/hr of 10% dextrose solution containing 10-20 units of crystalline insulin per 1,000 mL.
6. Correction of acidosis, if present, with intravenous sodium bicarbonate.
7. Hemodialysis or peritoneal dialysis.
8. Exchange resins may be used. However, this measure alone is not sufficient for the acute treatment of hyperkalemia.

Lowering potassium levels too rapidly in patients taking digitalis can produce digitalis toxicity.

11 DESCRIPTION

Urocit®-K is a citrate salt of potassium. Its empirical formula is $K_3C_6H_5O_7 \bullet H_2O$, and it has the following chemical structure:

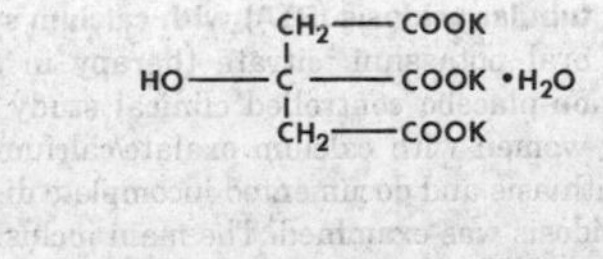

Urocit®-K yellowish to tan, oral wax-matrix tablets, contain 5 mEq (540 mg) potassium citrate, 10 mEq (1080 mg) potassium citrate and 15 mEq (1620 mg) potassium citrate each. Inactive ingredients include carnauba wax and magnesium stearate.

12 CLINICAL PHARMACOLOGY

12.1 Mechanism of Action

When Urocit®-K is given orally, the metabolism of absorbed citrate produces an alkaline load. The induced alkaline load in turn increases urinary pH and raises urinary citrate by augmenting citrate clearance without measurably altering ultrafilterable serum citrate. Thus, Urocit®-K therapy appears to increase urinary citrate principally by modifying the renal handling of citrate, rather than by increasing the filtered load of citrate. The increased filtered load of citrate may play some role, however, as in small comparisons of oral citrate and oral bicarbonate, citrate had a greater effect on urinary citrate.

In addition to raising urinary pH and citrate, Urocit®-K increases urinary potassium by approximately the amount contained in the medication. In some patients, Urocit®-K causes a transient reduction in urinary calcium.

The changes induced by Urocit®-K produce urine that is less conducive to the crystallization of stone-forming salts (calcium oxalate, calcium phosphate and uric acid). Increased citrate in the urine, by complexing with calcium, decreases calcium ion activity and thus the saturation of calcium oxalate. Citrate also inhibits the spontaneous nucleation of calcium oxalate and calcium phosphate (brushite).

The increase in urinary pH also decreases calcium ion activity by increasing calcium complexation to dissociated anions. The rise in urinary pH also increases the ionization of uric acid to the more soluble urate ion.

Urocit®-K therapy does not alter the urinary saturation of calcium phosphate, since the effect of increased citrate complexation of calcium is opposed by the rise in pH-dependent dissociation of phosphate. Calcium phosphate stones are more stable in alkaline urine.

In the setting of normal renal function, the rise in urinary citrate following a single dose begins by the first hour and lasts for 12 hours. With multiple doses the rise in citrate excretion reaches its peak by the third day and averts the normally wide circadian fluctuation in urinary citrate, thus maintaining urinary citrate at a higher, more constant level throughout the day. When the treatment is withdrawn, urinary citrate begins to decline toward the pre-treatment level on the first day.

The rise in citrate excretion is directly dependent on the Urocit®-K dosage. Following long-term treatment, Urocit®-K at a dosage of 60 mEq/day raises urinary citrate by approximately 400 mg/day and increases urinary pH by approximately 0.7 units.

In patients with severe renal tubular acidosis or chronic diarrheal syndrome where urinary citrate may be very low (<100 mg/day), Urocit®-K may be relatively ineffective in raising urinary citrate. A higher dose of Urocit®-K may therefore be required to produce a satisfactory citraturic response. In patients with renal tubular acidosis in whom urinary pH may be high, Urocit®-K produces a relatively small rise in urinary pH.

Table 1. Effect of Urocit®-K In Patients With Calcium Oxalate Nephrolithiasis.

	Stones Formed Per Year			
Group	**Baseline**	**On Treatment**	**Remission***	**Any Decrease**
I (n=19)	12 ± 30	0.9 ± 1.3	58%	95%
II (n=37)	1.2 ± 2	0.4 ± 1.5	89%	97%
III (n=15)	4.2 ± 7	0.7 ± 2	67%	100%
IV (n=18)	3.4 ± 8	0.5 ± 2	94%	100%
Total (n=89)	4.3 ±15	0.6 ± 2	80%	98%

*Remission defined as "the percentage of patients remaining free of newly formed stones during treatment".

14 CLINICAL STUDIES

The pivotal Urocit®-K trials were non-randomized and non-placebo controlled where dietary management may have changed coincidentally with pharmacological treatment. Therefore, the results as presented in the following sections may overstate the effectiveness of the product.

14.1 Renal tubular acidosis (RTA) with calcium stones

The effect of oral potassium citrate therapy in a non-randomized, non-placebo controlled clinical study of five men and four women with calcium oxalate/calcium phosphate nephrolithiasis and documented incomplete distal renal tubular acidosis was examined. The main inclusion criterion was a history of stone passage or surgical removal of stones during the 3 years prior to initiation of potassium citrate therapy. All patients began alkali treatment with 60-80 mEq potassium citrate daily in 3 or 4 divided doses. Throughout treatment, patients were instructed to stay on a sodium restricted diet (100 mEq/day) and to reduce oxalate intake (limited intake of nuts, dark roughage, chocolate and tea). A moderate calcium restriction (400-800 mg/day) was imposed on patients with hypercalciuria.

X-rays of the urinary tract, available in all patients, were reviewed to determine presence of pre-existing stones, appearance of new stones, or change in the number of stones. Potassium citrate therapy was associated with inhibition of new stone formation in patients with distal tubular acidosis. Three of the nine patients continued to pass stones during the on-treatment phase. While it is likely that these patients passed pre-existing stones during therapy, the most conservative assumption is that the passed stones were newly formed. Using this assumption, the stone-passage remission rate was 67%. All patients had a reduced stone formation rate. Over the first 2 years of treatment, the on-treatment stone formation rate was reduced from 13±27 to 1±2 per year.

14.2 Hypocitraturic calcium oxalate nephrolithiasis of any etiology

Eighty-nine patients with hypocitraturic calcium nephrolithiasis or uric acid lithiasis with or without calcium nephrolithiasis participated in this non-randomized, non-placebo controlled clinical study. Four groups of patients were treated with potassium citrate: Group 1 was comprised of 19 patients, 10 with renal tubular acidosis and 9 with chronic diarrheal syndrome, Group 2 was comprised of 37 patients, 5 with uric acid stones alone, 6 with uric acid lithiasis and calcium stones, 3 with type 1 absorptive hypercalciuria, 9 with type 2 absorptive hypercalciuria and 14 with hypocitraturia. Group 3 was comprised of 15 patients with history of relapse on other therapy and Group 4 was comprised of 18 patients, 9 with type 1 absorptive hypercalciuria and calcium stones, 1 with type 2 absorptive hypercalciuria and calcium stones, 2 with hyperuricosuric calcium oxalate nephrolithiasis, 4 with uric acid lithiasis accompanied by calcium stones and 2 with hypocitraturia and hyperuricemia accompanied by calcium stones. The dose of potassium citrate ranged from 30 to 100 mEq per day, and usually was 20 mEq administered orally 3 times daily. Patients were followed in an outpatient setting every 4 months during treatment and were studied over a period from 1 to 4.33 years. A three-year retrospective pre-study history for stone passage or removal was obtained and corroborated by medical records. Concomitant therapy (with thiazide or allopurinol) was allowed if patients had hypercalciuria, hyperuricosuria or hyperuricemia. Group 2 was treated with potassium citrate alone.

In all groups, treatment that included potassium citrate was associated with a sustained increase in urinary citrate excretion from subnormal values to normal values (400 to 700 mg/day), and a sustained increase in urinary pH from 5.6-6.0 to approximately 6.5. The stone formation rate was reduced in all groups as shown in **Table 1**.

[See table 1 above]

14.3 Uric acid lithiasis with or without calcium stones

A long-term non-randomized, non-placebo controlled clinical trial with eighteen adult patients with uric acid lithiasis participated in the study. Six patients formed only uric acid stones, and the remaining 12 patients formed mixed stones containing both uric acid and calcium salts or formed both uric acid stones (without calcium salts) and calcium stones (without uric acid) on separate occasions.

Eleven of the 18 patients received potassium citrate alone. Six of the 7 other patients also received allopurinol for hyperuricemia with gouty arthritis, symptomatic hyperuricemia, or hyperuricosuria. One patient also received hydrochlorothiazide because of unclassified hypercalciuria. The main inclusion criterion was a history of stone passage or surgical removal of stones during the 3 years prior to initiation of potassium citrate therapy. All patients received potassium citrate at a dosage of 30-80 mEq/day in three-to-four divided doses and were followed every four months for up to 5 years.

While on potassium citrate treatment, urinary pH rose significantly from a low value of 5.3 ± 0.3 to within normal limits (6.2 to 6.5). Urinary citrate which was low before treatment rose to the high normal range and only one stone was formed in the entire group of 18 patients.

15 REFERENCES

1. Pak, C. (1987). Citrate and Renal Calculi. *Mineral and Electrolyte Metabolism* 13, 257-266.
2. Pak, C. (1985). Long-Term Treatment of Calcium Nephrolithiasis with Potassium Citrate. *The Journal of Urology* 134, 11-19.
3. Preminger, G.M., K. Sakhaee, C. Skurla and C.Y.C. Pak. (1985). Prevention of Recurrent Calcium Stone Formation with Potassium Citrate Therapy in Patients with Distal Renal Tubular Acidosis. *The Journal of Urology* 134, 20-23.
4. Pak, C.Y.C., K. Sakhaee and C. Fuller. (1986). Successful Management of Uric Acid Nephrolithiasis with Potassium Citrate. *Kidney International* 30, 422-428.
5. Hollander-Rodriguez, J et al. (2006). Hyperkalemia, *American Family Physician*, Vol. 73/No. 2.
6. Greenberg, A et al. (1998). Hyperkalemia: treatment options. *Semen Nephrol*. Jan; 18 (1): 46-57.

16 HOW SUPPLIED/STORAGE AND HANDLING

Urocit®-K 5 mEq tablets are uncoated, tan to yellowish in color, modified ball shaped, with MPC 600 debossed on one side and blank on the other, supplied in bottles as:
NDC 0178-0600-01 Bottle of 100

Urocit®-K 10 mEq tablets are uncoated, tan to yellowish in color, elliptical shaped, with 610 debossed on one side and MISSION on the other, supplied in bottles as:
NDC 0178-0610-01 Bottle of 100

Urocit®-K 15 mEq tablets are uncoated, tan to yellowish in color, modified rectangle shaped, with M15 debossed on one side and blank on the other, supplied in bottles as:
NDC 0178-0615-01 Bottle of 100

Storage: Store in a tight container.

17 PATIENT COUNSELING INFORMATION

17.1 Administration of Drug

Tell patients to take each dose without crushing, chewing or sucking the tablet.

Tell patients to take this medicine only as directed. This is especially important if the patient is also taking both diuretics and digitalis preparations.

Tell patients to check with the doctor if there is trouble swallowing tablets or if the tablet seems to stick in the throat.

Tell patients to check with the doctor at once if tarry stools or other evidence of gastrointestinal bleeding is noticed.

Tell patients that their doctor will perform regular blood tests and electrocardiograms to ensure safety.

Rev 0410

MSD International GmbH,

for product information, please see Merck

MSD Oss B.V.,

for product information, please see Merck

NeoPharm, Co. Ltd.

#928, TAMNIP-DONG, YUSEONG-GU, DAEJEON, SOUTH KOREA (ZIP: 305-510)

ATOPALM — OTC

Moisturizing Hydrocortisone Cream

Active Ingredient

Hydrocortisone 1%

Purpose

Anti-itch

Uses for the temporary relief of itching associated with minor skin irritation, inflammation and rashes due to:
- eczema
- insect bites
- poison ivy, poison oak, or poison sumac
- soaps
- detergents
- jewelry
- seborrheic dermatitis
- psoriasis
- external genital and anal itching

Other uses of this product should be only under the advice and supervision of a doctor.

Warnings

For external use only.

Do not use
- for the treatment of diaper rash. Consult a doctor
- for external genital itching if you have a vaginal discharge. Consult a doctor.

When using this product
- avoid contact with the eyes
- do not begin the use of any other hydrocortisone product unless you have consulted a doctor
- for external anal itching do not exceed the recommended daily dosage unless directed by a doctor. In case of bleeding, consult a doctor promptly.
- Do not put this product in rectum by using fingers or any mechanical devise for application.

Stop use and ask a doctor if
- condition worsens or if symptoms persist for more than 7 days or clean up and then occur again within a few days. Stop use and do not begin use of any other hydrocortisone products unless you have consulted a doctor. Do not exceed recommended daily dosage unless directed by a doctor.

Ask a doctor or a pharmacist before use if you are using any other hydrocortisone product.

Keep out of reach of children. If swallowed, get medical help or contact a Poison Control Center immediately.

Directions

Adults and children 2 years of age and older
- apply to affected area not more than 3 to 4 times daily

Children under 2 years of age
- Do not use. Consult a doctor.

For external anal itching
- adults: when practical, cleanse the affected area with mild soap and warm water and rinse thoroughly. Gently dry by patting or blotting with toilet tissue or a soft cloth before application of this product.
- children under 12 years of age with external anal itching, consult a doctor.

Other Information
- store at room temperature
- see end of carton or tube crimp for lot number and expiration date

Inactive Ingredients Water, Butylene glycol, Cetyl alcohol, PEG-15 glyceryl stearate, Olive oil, Stearic acid, Glyceryl stearate, Squalane, PEG-10 glyceryl stearate, Cholesterol, BHT, Myristoyl/Palmitoyl Oxostearamide/Arachamide MEA, Methylparaben, Propylparaben

Questions? Call 1-855-ATOPALM

US Patent # US 6221371B1

Shown in Product Identification Guide, page 309

PSORIAPALM **OTC**
Non-Greasy Psoriasis Lotion

Drug Facts

Active ingredient
Salicylic Acid 2%

Purpose
Psoriasis and Seborrheic Dermatitis

Uses
relieves and helps prevent recurrence of skin:
- itching
- irritation
- redness
- flaking
- scaling

due to psoriasis and seborrheic dermatitis

Warnings
For external use only
Ask a doctor before use if condition covers a large area of the body.
When using this product avoid contact with the eyes. If contact occurs, rinse the eyes thoroughly with water.
Stop use and ask a doctor if condition worsens or does not improve after regular use as directed
Keep out of reach of children. If swallowed, get medical help or contact a Poison Control Center immediately.

Directions
Apply to affected areas one to four times daily or as directed by a doctor

Other Information
Store at room temperature 15° - 30°C (59° - 86°F). Keep out of direct sunlight.

Inactive ingredients
WATER, BUTYLENE GLYCOL, CETYL ALCOHOL, ISOPROPYL MYRISTATE, POLYSORBATE 60, STEARIC ACID, DIMETHICONE, GLYCERYL STEARATE, OCTYLDODECANOL, MYRISTOYL/PALMITOYL OXOSTEARAMIDE/ARACHAMIDE MEA, PANTHENOL, TOCOPHERYL ACETATE, CHOLESTEROL, XANTHAN GUM, METHYLBENZYL METHYLBENZIMIDAZOLE PIPERIDINYLMETHANONE, POLYACRYLAMIDE, C13-14 ISOPARAFFIN, LAURETH-7, SODIUM HYDROXIDE, METHYLPARABEN, PROPYLPARABEN

Questions?
Visit our website at www.psoriapalm.com
Shown in Product Identification Guide, page 309

Novartis Pharmaceuticals Corporation

ONE HEALTH PLAZA
EAST HANOVER, NJ 07936
(for branded products)

For Information Contact (branded products):
Customer Interaction Center
(888) NOW-NOVA [888-669-6682]
www.pharma.us.novartis.com

AFINITOR ℞
[a-fin-it-or]
(everolimus)
tablets for oral administration

AFINITOR DISPERZ
(everolimus tablets for oral suspension)

The following prescribing information is based on official labeling in effect July 2013.

HIGHLIGHTS OF PRESCRIBING INFORMATION
These highlights do not include all the information needed to use AFINITOR safely and effectively. See full prescribing information for AFINITOR.
AFINITOR (everolimus) tablets for oral administration
AFINITOR DISPERZ (everolimus tablets for oral suspension)
Initial U.S. Approval: 2009

RECENT MAJOR CHANGES

Indications and Usage (1)	08/2012
Dosage and Administration (2)	08/2012
Warnings and Precautions (5)	08/2012

INDICATIONS AND USAGE

AFINITOR is a kinase inhibitor indicated for the treatment of:
- postmenopausal women with advanced hormone receptor-positive, HER2-negative breast cancer (advanced HR+ BC) in combination with exemestane after failure of treatment with letrozole or anastrozole. (1.1)
- adults with progressive neuroendocrine tumors of pancreatic origin (PNET) that are unresectable, locally advanced or metastatic. The safety and effectiveness of AFINITOR in the treatment of patients with carcinoid tumors have not been established. (1.2)
- adults with advanced renal cell carcinoma (RCC) after failure of treatment with sunitinib or sorafenib. (1.3)
- adults with renal angiomyolipoma and tuberous sclerosis complex (TSC), not requiring immediate surgery. The effectiveness of AFINITOR in the treatment of renal angiomyolipoma is based on an analysis of durable objective responses in patients treated for a median of 8.3 months. Further follow-up of patients is required to determine long-term outcomes. (1.4)

AFINITOR and AFINITOR DISPERZ are kinase inhibitors indicated for the treatment of:
- pediatric and adult patients with tuberous sclerosis complex (TSC) who have subependymal giant cell astrocytoma (SEGA) that requires therapeutic intervention but cannot be curatively resected. The effectiveness is based on demonstration of durable objective response, as evidenced by reduction in SEGA tumor volume. Improvement in disease-related symptoms and overall survival in patients with SEGA and TSC has not been demonstrated. (1.5)

DOSAGE AND ADMINISTRATION

Advanced HR+ BC, advanced PNET, advanced RCC, or renal angiomyolipoma with TSC:
- 10 mg once daily with or without food. (2.1)
- For patients with hepatic impairment, reduce the AFINITOR dose. (2.2)
- If moderate inhibitors of CYP3A4 and/or P-glycoprotein (PgP) are required, reduce the AFINITOR dose to 2.5 mg once daily; if tolerated, consider increasing to 5 mg once daily. (2.2)
- If strong inducers of CYP3A4 are required, increase AFINITOR dose in 5 mg increments to a maximum of 20 mg once daily. (2.2)

SEGA with TSC:
- 4.5 mg/m^2 once daily; adjust dose to attain trough concentrations of 5-15 ng/mL. (2.3)
- Assess trough concentrations approximately 2 weeks after initiation of treatment, a change in dose, a change in co-administration of CYP3A4 and/or PgP inducers or inhibitors, a change in hepatic function, or a change in dosage form between AFINITOR Tablets and AFINITOR DISPERZ. (2.3, 2.4)
- For patients with severe hepatic impairment reduce the starting dose of AFINITOR Tablets or AFINITOR DISPERZ. (2.3, 2.5)
- If concomitant use of moderate inhibitors of CYP3A4 and/or PgP is required, reduce the dose of AFINITOR Tablets or AFINITOR DISPERZ by 50%. (2.3, 2.5)
- If concomitant use of strong inducers of CYP3A4 is required, double the dose of AFINITOR Tablets or AFINITOR DISPERZ. (2.3, 2.5)

DOSAGE FORMS AND STRENGTHS

AFINITOR Tablets: 2.5 mg, 5 mg, 7.5 mg, and 10 mg tablets with no score (3.1)
AFINITOR DISPERZ (everolimus tablets for oral suspension): 2 mg, 3 mg, and 5 mg tablets for oral suspension with no score (3.2)

CONTRAINDICATIONS

Hypersensitivity to everolimus, to other rapamycin derivatives, or to any of the excipients (4)

WARNINGS AND PRECAUTIONS

- Non-infectious pneumonitis: Monitor for clinical symptoms or radiological changes; fatal cases have occurred. Manage by dose reduction or discontinuation until symptoms resolve, and consider use of corticosteroids. (5.1)
- Infections: Increased risk of infections, some fatal. Monitor for signs and symptoms, and treat promptly. (5.2)
- Oral ulceration: Mouth ulcers, stomatitis, and oral mucositis are common. Management includes mouthwashes and topical treatments. (5.3)
- Renal failure: Cases of renal failure (including acute renal failure), some with a fatal outcome, have been observed. (5.4)
- Laboratory test alterations: Elevations of serum creatinine, blood glucose, and lipids may occur. Decreases in hemoglobin, neutrophils, and platelets may also occur. Monitor renal function, blood glucose, lipids, and hematologic parameters prior to treatment and periodically thereafter. (5.6)
- Vaccinations: Avoid live vaccines and close contact with those who have received live vaccines. (5.9)
- Embryo-fetal toxicity: Fetal harm can occur when administered to a pregnant woman. Apprise women of potential harm to the fetus. (5.10, 8.1)

ADVERSE REACTIONS

Advanced HR+ BC, advanced PNET, advanced RCC: Most common adverse reactions (incidence ≥30%) include stomatitis, infections, rash, fatigue, diarrhea, edema, abdominal pain, nausea, fever, asthenia, cough, headache and decreased appetite. (6.1, 6.2, 6.3)
Renal angiomyolipoma with TSC: Most common adverse reaction (incidence ≥ 30%) is stomatitis. (6.4)
SEGA with TSC: Most common adverse reactions (incidence ≥ 30%) are stomatitis and respiratory tract infection. (6.5)

To report SUSPECTED ADVERSE REACTIONS, contact Novartis Pharmaceuticals Corporation at 1-888-669-6682 or FDA at 1-800-FDA-1088 or www.fda.gov/medwatch.

DRUG INTERACTIONS

- Strong CYP3A4 inhibitors: Avoid concomitant use. (2.2, 2.5, 5.7, 7.1)
- Moderate CYP3A4 and/or PgP inhibitors: If combination is required, use caution and reduce dose of AFINITOR. (2.2, 2.3, 2.5, 5.7, 7.1)
- Strong CYP3A4 inducers: Avoid concomitant use. If combination cannot be avoided, increase dose of AFINITOR. (2.2, 2.3, 2.5, 5.7, 7.2)

USE IN SPECIFIC POPULATIONS

- Nursing mothers: Discontinue drug or nursing, taking into consideration the importance of drug to the mother. (8.3)
- Hepatic impairment: For advanced HR+ BC, advanced PNET, advanced RCC, or renal angiomyolipoma with TSC patients with hepatic impairment, reduce AFINITOR dose. For SEGA patients with severe hepatic impairment, reduce the starting dose of AFINITOR Tablets or AFINITOR DISPERZ. (2.2, 2.3, 2.5, 5.8, 8.7)

See 17 for PATIENT COUNSELING INFORMATION and FDA-approved patient labeling

Revised: 08/2012

FULL PRESCRIBING INFORMATION: CONTENTS*

*** Sections or subsections omitted from the full prescribing information are not listed**

FULL PRESCRIBING INFORMATION

1 INDICATIONS AND USAGE

1.1 Advanced Hormone Receptor-Positive, HER2-Negative Breast Cancer (Advanced HR+ BC)

AFINITOR® is indicated for the treatment of postmenopausal women with advanced hormone receptor-positive, HER2-negative breast cancer (advanced HR+ BC) in combination with exemestane, after failure of treatment with letrozole or anastrozole.

1.2 Advanced Neuroendocrine Tumors of Pancreatic Origin (PNET)

AFINITOR® is indicated for the treatment of adult patients with progressive neuroendocrine tumors of pancreatic origin (PNET) with unresectable, locally advanced or metastatic disease.

The safety and effectiveness of AFINITOR® in the treatment of patients with carcinoid tumors have not been established.

1.3 Advanced Renal Cell Carcinoma (RCC)

AFINITOR® is indicated for the treatment of adult patients with advanced renal cell carcinoma (RCC) after failure of treatment with sunitinib or sorafenib.

1.4 Renal Angiomyolipoma with Tuberous Sclerosis Complex (TSC)

AFINITOR® is indicated for the treatment of adult patients with renal angiomyolipoma and tuberous sclerosis complex (TSC), not requiring immediate surgery.

The effectiveness of AFINITOR in the treatment of renal angiomyolipoma is based on an analysis of durable objective responses in patients treated for a median of 8.3 months. Further follow-up of patients is required to determine long-term outcomes.

1.5 Subependymal Giant Cell Astrocytoma (SEGA) with Tuberous Sclerosis Complex (TSC)

AFINITOR® Tablets and AFINITOR® DISPERZ are indicated in pediatric and adult patients with tuberous sclerosis complex (TSC) for the treatment of subependymal giant cell astrocytoma (SEGA) that requires therapeutic intervention but cannot be curatively resected.

The effectiveness of AFINITOR Tablets and AFINITOR DISPERZ is based on demonstration of durable objective response, as evidenced by reduction in SEGA tumor volume. Improvement in disease-related symptoms and overall survival in patients with SEGA and TSC have not been demonstrated *[see Clinical Studies (14.5)]*.

2 DOSAGE AND ADMINISTRATION

AFINITOR is available in two dosage forms: tablets (AFINITOR Tablets) and tablets for oral suspension (AFINITOR DISPERZ). AFINITOR DISPERZ is recommended only for the treatment of patients with subependymal giant cell astrocytoma (SEGA) and tuberous sclerosis complex (TSC) in conjunction with therapeutic drug monitoring *[see Clinical Pharmacology (12.3)]*.

2.1 Recommended Dose in Advanced Hormone Receptor-Positive, HER2-Negative Breast Cancer, Advanced PNET, Advanced RCC, and Renal Angiomyolipoma with TSC

The recommended dose of AFINITOR Tablets is 10 mg, to be taken once daily at the same time every day. Administer either consistently with food or consistently without food [see Clinical Pharmacology (12.3)]. AFINITOR Tablets should be swallowed whole with a glass of water. Do not break or crush tablets.

Continue treatment until disease progression or unacceptable toxicity occurs.

2.2 Dose Modifications in Advanced Hormone Receptor-Positive, HER2-Negative Breast Cancer, Advanced PNET, Advanced RCC, and Renal Angiomyolipoma with TSC

Adverse Reactions

Management of severe or intolerable adverse reactions may require temporary dose reduction and/or interruption of AFINITOR therapy. If dose reduction is required, the suggested dose is approximately 50% lower than the daily dose previously administered *[see Warnings and Precautions (5)]*.

Table 1 summarizes recommendations for dose reduction, interruption or discontinuation of AFINITOR in the management of adverse reactions. General management recommendations are also provided as applicable. Clinical judgment of the treating physician should guide the management plan of each patient based on individual benefit/risk assessment.

[See table 1 at top of next page]

Hepatic Impairment

Hepatic impairment will increase the exposure to everolimus *[see Warnings and Precautions (5.8) and Use in Specific Populations (8.7)]*. Dose adjustments are recommended:

- Mild hepatic impairment (Child-Pugh class A) – The recommended dose is 7.5 mg daily; the dose may be decreased to 5 mg if not well tolerated.
- Moderate hepatic impairment (Child-Pugh class B) – The recommended dose is 5 mg daily; the dose may be decreased to 2.5 mg if not well tolerated.
- Severe hepatic impairment (Child-Pugh class C) – If the desired benefit outweighs the risk, a dose of 2.5 mg daily may be used but must not be exceeded.

Dose adjustments should be made if a patient's hepatic (Child-Pugh) status changes during treatment.

CYP3A4 and/or P-glycoprotein (PgP) Inhibitors

Avoid the use of strong CYP3A4 inhibitors (e.g., ketoconazole, itraconazole, clarithromycin, atazanavir, nefazodone, saquinavir, telithromycin, ritonavir, indinavir, nelfinavir, voriconazole) *[see Warnings and Precautions (5.7) and Drug Interactions (7.1)]*.

Use caution when co-administered with moderate CYP3A4 and/or PgP inhibitors (e.g., amprenavir, fosamprenavir, aprepitant, erythromycin, fluconazole, verapamil, diltiazem). If patients require co-administration of a moderate CYP3A4 and/or PgP inhibitor, reduce the AFINITOR dose to 2.5 mg daily. The reduced dose of AFINITOR is predicted to adjust the area under the curve (AUC) to the range observed without inhibitors. An AFINITOR dose increase from 2.5 mg to 5 mg may be considered based on patient tolerance. If the moderate inhibitor is discontinued, a washout period of approximately 2 to 3 days should be allowed before the AFINITOR dose is increased. If the moderate inhibitor is discontinued, the AFINITOR dose should be returned to the dose used prior to initiation of the moderate CYP3A4 and/or PgP inhibitor.

Grapefruit, grapefruit juice, and other foods that are known to inhibit cytochrome P450 and PgP activity may increase everolimus exposures and should be avoided during treatment.

Strong CYP3A4 Inducers

Avoid the use of concomitant strong CYP3A4 inducers (e.g., phenytoin, carbamazepine, rifampin, rifabutin, rifapentine, phenobarbital). If patients require co-administration of a strong CYP3A4 inducer, consider increasing the AFINITOR dose from 10 mg daily up to 20 mg daily, using 5 mg increments. This dose of AFINITOR is predicted, based on pharmacokinetic data, to adjust the AUC to the range observed without inducers. However, there are no clinical data with this dose adjustment in patients receiving strong CYP3A4 inducers. If the strong inducer is discontinued, the AFINITOR dose should be returned to the dose used prior to initiation of the strong CYP3A4 inducer *[see Warnings and Precautions (5.7) and Drug Interactions (7.2)]*.

St. John's Wort (*Hypericum perforatum*) may decrease everolimus exposure unpredictably and should be avoided.

2.3 Recommended Dose in SEGA with TSC

The recommended starting dose is 4.5 mg/m^2, once daily. The recommended starting dose for patients with severe hepatic impairment (Child-Pugh class C) or requiring moderate CYP3A4 and/or PgP inhibitors is 2.5 mg/m^2, once daily *[see Dosage and Administration (2.5)]*. The recommended starting dose for patients requiring a concomitant strong CYP3A4 inducer is 9 mg/m^2, once daily *[see Dosage and Administration (2.5)]*. Round dose to the nearest strength of either AFINITOR Tablets or AFINITOR DISPERZ.

Use therapeutic drug monitoring to guide subsequent dosing *[see Dosage and Administration (2.4)]*. Adjust dose at two week intervals as needed to achieve and maintain trough concentrations of 5 to 15 ng/mL *[see Dosage and Administration (2.4, 2.5)]*.

Continue treatment until disease progression or unacceptable toxicity occurs. The optimal duration of therapy is unknown.

2.4 Therapeutic Drug Monitoring in SEGA with TSC

Monitor everolimus whole blood trough levels routinely in all patients. When possible, use the same assay and laboratory for therapeutic drug monitoring throughout treatment.

Assess trough concentrations approximately two weeks after initiation of treatment, a change in dose, a change in co-administration of CYP3A4 and/or PgP inducers or inhibitors, a change in hepatic function, or a change in dosage form between AFINITOR Tablets and AFINITOR DISPERZ. Once a stable dose is attained, monitor trough concentrations every 3 to 6 months in patients with changing body surface area or every 6 to 12 months in patients with stable body surface area for the duration of treatment.

Titrate the dose to attain trough concentrations of 5 to 15 ng/mL.

- For trough concentrations less than 5 ng/mL, increase the daily dose by 2.5 mg (in patients taking AFINITOR Tablets) or 2 mg (in patients taking AFINITOR DISPERZ).
- For trough concentrations greater than 15 ng/mL, reduce the daily dose by 2.5 mg (in patients taking AFINITOR Tablets) or 2 mg (in patients taking AFINITOR DISPERZ).
- If dose reduction is required for patients receiving the lowest available strength, administer every other day.

2.5 Dose Modifications in SEGA with TSC

Adverse Reactions

Reduce dose or withhold AFINITOR Tablets or AFINITOR DISPERZ for severe or intolerable adverse reactions *[see Warnings and Precautions (5)]*. Reduce the dose of AFINITOR Tablets or AFINITOR DISPERZ by approximately 50%. If dose reduction is required for patients receiving the lowest available strength, administer every other day *[see Table 1 in Dosage and Administration (2.2)]*.

Hepatic Impairment

- Reduce the starting dose of AFINITOR Tablets or AFINITOR DISPERZ by approximately 50% in patients with SEGA who have severe hepatic impairment (Child-Pugh class C) *[see Dosage and Administration (2.3)]*. Adjustment to the starting dose for patients with SEGA who have mild (Child-Pugh class A) or moderate (Child-Pugh class B) hepatic impairment may not be needed. Subsequent dosing should be based on therapeutic drug monitoring.
- Assess everolimus trough concentrations approximately two weeks after commencing treatment, a change in dose, or any change in hepatic function *[see Dosage and Administration (2.3, 2.4)]*.

CYP3A4 and/or P-glycoprotein (PgP) Inhibitors

Avoid the use of concomitant strong CYP3A4 inhibitors (e.g., ketoconazole, itraconazole, clarithromycin, atazanavir, nefazodone, saquinavir, telithromycin, ritonavir, indinavir, nelfinavir, voriconazole) in patients receiving AFINITOR Tablets or AFINITOR DISPERZ *[see Warnings and Precautions (5.7) and Drug Interactions (7.1)]*.

For patients who require treatment with moderate CYP3A4 and/or PgP inhibitors (e.g., amprenavir, fosamprenavir, aprepitant, erythromycin, fluconazole, verapamil, diltiazem):

- Reduce the AFINITOR Tablets or AFINITOR DISPERZ dose by approximately 50%. Administer every other day if dose reduction is required for patients receiving the lowest available strength *[see Dosage and Administration (2.3)]*.
- Assess everolimus trough concentrations approximately two weeks after dose reduction *[see Dosage and Administration (2.3, 2.4)]*.
- Resume the dose that was used prior to initiating the CYP3A4 and/or PgP inhibitor 2 to 3 days after discontinu-

ation of a moderate inhibitor. Assess the everolimus trough concentration approximately two weeks later *[see Dosage and Administration (2.3, 2.4)]*.

Do not ingest foods or nutritional supplements (e.g., grapefruit, grapefruit juice) that are known to inhibit cytochrome P450 or PgP activity.

Strong CYP3A4 Inducers

Avoid the use of concomitant strong CYP3A4 inducers (e.g., phenytoin, carbamazepine, rifampin, rifabutin, rifapentine, phenobarbital) if alternative therapy is available *[see Warnings and Precautions (5.7) and Drug Interactions (7.2)]*. For patients who require treatment with a strong CYP3A4 inducer:

- Double the dose of AFINITOR Tablets or AFINITOR DISPERZ *[see Dosage and Administration (2.3)]*.
- Assess the everolimus trough concentration two weeks after doubling the dose and adjust the dose if necessary to maintain a trough concentration of 5 to 15 ng/mL *[see Dosage and Administration (2.3, 2.4)]*.
- Return the AFINITOR Tablets or AFINITOR DISPERZ dose to that used prior to initiating the strong CYP3A4 inducer if the strong inducer is discontinued, and assess the everolimus trough concentrations approximately two weeks later *[see Dosage and Administration (2.3, 2.4)]*.

Do not ingest foods or nutritional supplements (e.g., St. John's Wort (*Hypericum perforatum*)) that are known to induce cytochrome P450 activity.

2.6 Administration of AFINITOR Tablets in SEGA with TSC

Do not combine the two dosage forms (AFINITOR Tablets and AFINITOR DISPERZ) to achieve the desired dose. Use one dosage form or the other.

Administer AFINITOR Tablets orally once daily at the same time every day. Administer either consistently with food or consistently without food *[see Clinical Pharmacology (12.3)]*.

AFINITOR Tablets should be swallowed whole with a glass of water. Do not break or crush tablets.

2.7 Administration and Preparation of AFINITOR DISPERZ in SEGA with TSC

Do not combine the two dosage forms (AFINITOR Tablets and AFINITOR DISPERZ) to achieve the desired dose. Use one dosage form or the other.

Administer AFINITOR DISPERZ (everolimus tablets for oral suspension) as a suspension only.

Administer AFINITOR DISPERZ orally once daily at the same time every day. Administer either consistently with food or consistently without food *[see Clinical Pharmacology (12.3)]*.

Administer suspension immediately after preparation. Discard suspension if not administered within 60 minutes after preparation.

Prepare suspension in water only.

Using an oral syringe:

- Place the prescribed dose of AFINITOR DISPERZ into a 10-mL syringe. Do not exceed a total of 10 mg per syringe. If higher doses are required, prepare an additional syringe. Do not break or crush tablets.
- Draw approximately 5 mL of water and 4 mL of air into the syringe.
- Place the filled syringe into a container (tip up) for 3 minutes, until the AFINITOR DISPERZ tablets are in suspension.
- Gently invert the syringe 5 times immediately prior to administration.
- After administration of the prepared suspension, draw approximately 5 mL of water and 4 mL of air into the same syringe, and swirl the contents to suspend remaining particles. Administer the entire contents of the syringe.

Using a small drinking glass:

- Place the prescribed dose of AFINITOR DISPERZ into a small drinking glass (maximum size 100 mL) containing approximately 25 mL of water. Do not exceed a total of 10 mg of AFINITOR DISPERZ per glass. If higher doses are required, prepare an additional glass. Do not break or crush tablets.
- Allow 3 minutes for suspension to occur.
- Stir the contents gently with a spoon, immediately prior to drinking.
- After administration of the prepared suspension, add 25 mL of water and stir with the same spoon to re-suspend remaining particles. Administer the entire contents of the glass.

Table 1: AFINITOR Dose Adjustment and Management Recommendation for Adverse Reactions

Adverse Drug Reaction	Severity[a]	AFINITOR Dose Adjustment[b] and Management Recommendations
Non-infectious pneumonitis	Grade 1 Asymptomatic, radiographic findings only	No dose adjustment required. Initiate appropriate monitoring.
	Grade 2 Symptomatic, not interfering with ADL[c]	Consider interruption of therapy, rule out infection and consider treatment with corticosteroids until symptoms improve to ≤ grade 1. Re-initiate AFINITOR at a lower dose. Discontinue treatment if failure to recover within 4 wks.
	Grade 3 Symptomatic, interfering with ADL[c]; O2 indicated	Interrupt AFINITOR until symptoms resolve to ≤ grade 1. Rule out infection, and consider treatment with corticosteroids. Consider re-initiating AFINITOR at a lower dose. If toxicity recurs at grade 3, consider discontinuation.
	Grade 4 Life-threatening, ventilatory support indicated	Discontinue AFINITOR, rule out infection, and consider treatment with corticosteroids.
Stomatitis	Grade 1 Minimal symptoms, normal diet	No dose adjustment required. Manage with non-alcoholic or salt water (0.9%) mouth wash several times a day.
	Grade 2 Symptomatic but can eat and swallow modified diet	Temporary dose interruption until recovery to grade ≤1. Re-initiate AFINITOR at the same dose. If stomatitis recurs at grade 2, interrupt dose until recovery to grade ≤1. Re-initiate AFINITOR at a lower dose. Manage with topical analgesic mouth treatments (e.g. benzocaine, butyl aminobenzoate, tetracaine hydrochloride, menthol or phenol) with or without topical corticosteroids (i.e. triamcinolone oral paste).[d]
	Grade 3 Symptomatic and unable to adequately aliment or hydrate orally	Temporary dose interruption until recovery to grade ≤1. Re-initiate AFINITOR at a lower dose. Manage with topical analgesic mouth treatments (i.e. benzocaine, butyl aminobenzoate, tetracaine hydrochloride, menthol or phenol) with or without topical corticosteroids (i.e. triamcinolone oral paste).[d]
	Grade 4 Symptoms associated with life-threatening consequences	Discontinue AFINITOR and treat with appropriate medical therapy.
Other non-hematologic toxicities (excluding metabolic events)	Grade 1	If toxicity is tolerable, no dose adjustment required. Initiate appropriate medical therapy and monitor.
	Grade 2	If toxicity is tolerable, no dose adjustment required. Initiate appropriate medical therapy and monitor. If toxicity becomes intolerable, temporary dose interruption until recovery to grade ≤1. Re-initiate AFINITOR at the same dose. If toxicity recurs at grade 2, interrupt AFINITOR until recovery to grade ≤1. Re-initiate AFINITOR at a lower dose.
	Grade 3	Temporary dose interruption until recovery to grade ≤1. Initiate appropriate medical therapy and monitor. Consider re-initiating AFINITOR at a lower dose. If toxicity recurs at grade 3, consider discontinuation.
	Grade 4	Discontinue AFINITOR and treat with appropriate medical therapy.
Metabolic events (e.g. hyperglycemia, dyslipidemia)	Grade 1	No dose adjustment required. Initiate appropriate medical therapy and monitor.
	Grade 2	No dose adjustment required. Manage with appropriate medical therapy and monitor.
	Grade 3	Temporary dose interruption. Re-initiate Afinitor at a lower dose. Manage with appropriate medical therapy and monitor.
	Grade 4	Discontinue AFINITOR and treat with appropriate medical therapy.

[a] Severity grade description: 1 = mild symptoms; 2 = moderate symptoms; 3 = severe symptoms; 4 = life-threatening symptoms.
[b] If dose reduction is required, the suggested dose is approximately 50% lower than the dose previously administered.
[c] Activities of daily living (ADL)
[d] Avoid using agents containing alcohol, hydrogen peroxide, iodine, and thyme derivatives in management of stomatitis as they may worsen mouth ulcers.

3 DOSAGE FORMS AND STRENGTHS

3.1 AFINITOR (everolimus) Tablets

2.5 mg tablet
White to slightly yellow, elongated tablets with a bevelled edge and no score, engraved with "LCL" on one side and "NVR" on the other.

5 mg tablet
White to slightly yellow, elongated tablets with a bevelled edge and no score, engraved with "5" on one side and "NVR" on the other.

7.5 mg tablet
White to slightly yellow, elongated tablets with a bevelled edge and no score, engraved with "7P5" on one side and "NVR" on the other.

10 mg tablet
White to slightly yellow, elongated tablets with a bevelled edge and no score, engraved with "UHE" on one side and "NVR" on the other.

Table 2: Adverse Reactions Reported ≥ 10% of Patients with Advanced HR+ BC*

	AFINITOR (10 mg/day) + exemestane[a] N=482			Placebo + exemestane[a] N=238		
	All grades %	Grade 3 %	Grade 4 %	All grades %	Grade 3 %	Grade 4 %
Any adverse reaction	**100**	**41**	**9**	**90**	**22**	**5**
Gastrointestinal disorders						
Stomatitis[b]	67	8	0	11	0.8	0
Diarrhea	33	2	0.2	18	0.8	0
Nausea	29	0.2	0.2	28	1	0
Vomiting	17	0.8	0.2	12	0.8	0
Constipation	14	0.4	0	13	0.4	0
Dry mouth	11	0	0	7	0	0
General disorders and administration site conditions						
Fatigue	36	4	0.4	27	1	0
Edema peripheral	19	1	0	6	0.4	0
Pyrexia	15	0.2	0	7	0.4	0
Asthenia	13	2	0.2	4	0	0
Infections and infestations						
Infections[c]	50	4	1	25	2	0
Investigations						
Weight decreased	25	1	0	6	0	0
Metabolism and nutrition disorders						
Decreased appetite	30	1	0	12	0.4	0
Hyperglycemia	14	5	0.4	2	0.4	0
Musculoskeletal and connective tissue disorders						
Arthralgia	20	0.8	0	17	0	0
Back pain	14	0.2	0	10	0.8	0
Pain in extremity	9	0.4	0	11	2	0
Nervous system disorders						
Dysgeusia	22	0.2	0	6	0	0
Headache	21	0.4	0	14	0	0
Psychiatric disorders						
Insomnia	13	0.2	0	8	0	0
Respiratory, thoracic and mediastinal disorders						
Cough	24	0.6	0	12	0	0
Dyspnea	21	4	0.2	11	0.8	0.4
Epistaxis	17	0	0	1	0	0
Pneumonitis[d]	19	4	0.2	0.4	0	0
Skin and subcutaneous tissue disorders						
Rash	39	1	0	6	0	0
Pruritus	13	0.2	0	5	0	0
Alopecia	10	0	0	5	0	0
Vascular disorders						
Hot flush	6	0	0	14	0	0
Median duration of treatment[e]		**23.9 weeks**			**13.4 weeks**	

CTCAE Version 3.0
[*] 160 patients (33.2%) were exposed to AFINITOR therapy for a period of ≥ 32 weeks)
[a] Exemestane (25 mg/day)
[b] Includes stomatitis, mouth ulceration, aphthous stomatitis, glossodynia, gingival pain, glossitis and lip ulceration
[c] Includes all preferred terms within the 'infections and infestations' system organ class, the most common being nasopharyngitis (10%), urinary tract infection (10%), upper respiratory tract infection (5%), pneumonia (4%), bronchitis (4%), cystitis (3%), sinusitis (3%), and also including candidiasis (<1%), and sepsis (<1%), and hepatitis C (<1%).
[d] Includes pneumonitis, interstitial lung disease, lung infiltration, and pulmonary fibrosis
[e] Exposure to AFINITOR or placebo

3.2 AFINITOR DISPERZ (everolimus tablets for oral suspension)

2 mg tablet for oral suspension
White to slightly yellowish, round, flat tablets with a bevelled edge and no score, engraved with "D2" on one side and "NVR" on the other.
3 mg tablet for oral suspension
White to slightly yellowish, round, flat tablets with a bevelled edge and no score, engraved with "D3" on one side and "NVR" on the other.
5 mg tablet for oral suspension
White to slightly yellowish, round, flat tablets with a bevelled edge and no score, engraved with "D5" on one side and "NVR" on the other.

4 CONTRAINDICATIONS

AFINITOR is contraindicated in patients with hypersensitivity to the active substance, to other rapamycin derivatives, or to any of the excipients. Hypersensitivity reactions manifested by symptoms including, but not limited to, anaphylaxis, dyspnea, flushing, chest pain, or angioedema (e.g., swelling of the airways or tongue, with or without respiratory impairment) have been observed with everolimus and other rapamycin derivatives.

5 WARNINGS AND PRECAUTIONS

5.1 Non-infectious Pneumonitis

Non-infectious pneumonitis is a class effect of rapamycin derivatives, including AFINITOR. Non-infectious pneumonitis was reported in up to 19% of patients treated with AFINITOR in clinical trials. The incidence of Common Terminology Criteria (CTC) grade 3 and 4 non-infectious pneumonitis was up to 4.0% and up to 0.2%, respectively *[see Adverse Reactions (6.1, 6.2, 6.3, 6.4, 6.5)]*. Fatal outcomes have been observed.

Consider a diagnosis of non-infectious pneumonitis in patients presenting with non-specific respiratory signs and symptoms such as hypoxia, pleural effusion, cough, or dyspnea, and in whom infectious, neoplastic, and other causes have been excluded by means of appropriate investigations. Advise patients to report promptly any new or worsening respiratory symptoms.

Patients who develop radiological changes suggestive of non-infectious pneumonitis and have few or no symptoms may continue AFINITOR therapy without dose alteration. Imaging appears to overestimate the incidence of clinical pneumonitis.

If symptoms are moderate, consider interrupting therapy until symptoms improve. The use of corticosteroids may be indicated. AFINITOR may be reintroduced at a daily dose approximately 50% lower than the dose previously administered *[see Table 1 in Dosage and Administration (2.2)]*.

For cases of grade 4 non-infectious pneumonitis, discontinue AFINITOR. Corticosteroids may be indicated until clinical symptoms resolve. For cases of grade 3 non-infectious pneumonitis interrupt AFINITOR until resolution to less than or equal to grade 1. AFINITOR may be re-introduced at a daily dose approximately 50% lower than the dose previously administered depending on the individual clinical circumstances *[see Table 1 in Dosage and Administration (2.2)]*. If toxicity recurs at grade 3, consider discontinuation of AFINITOR. The development of pneumonitis has been reported even at a reduced dose.

5.2 Infections

AFINITOR has immunosuppressive properties and may predispose patients to bacterial, fungal, viral, or protozoal infections, including infections with opportunistic pathogens *[see Adverse Reactions (6.1, 6.2, 6.3, 6.4, 6.5)]*. Localized and systemic infections, including pneumonia, mycobacterial infections, other bacterial infections, invasive fungal infections, such as aspergillosis or candidiasis, and viral infections including reactivation of hepatitis B virus have occurred in patients taking AFINITOR. Some of these infections have been severe (e.g., leading to respiratory or hepatic failure) or fatal. Physicians and patients should be aware of the increased risk of infection with AFINITOR. Complete treatment of pre-existing invasive fungal infections prior to starting treatment with AFINITOR. While taking AFINITOR, be vigilant for signs and symptoms of infection; if a diagnosis of an infection is made, institute appropriate treatment promptly and consider interruption or discontinuation of AFINITOR. If a diagnosis of invasive systemic fungal infection is made, discontinue AFINITOR and treat with appropriate antifungal therapy.

5.3 Oral Ulceration

Mouth ulcers, stomatitis, and oral mucositis have occurred in patients treated with AFINITOR at an incidence ranging from 44-86% across the clinical trial experience. Grade 3 or 4 stomatitis was reported in 4-9% of patients *[see Adverse Reactions (6.1, 6.2, 6.3, 6.4, 6.5)]*. In such cases, topical treatments are recommended, but alcohol-, peroxide-, iodine-, or thyme- containing mouthwashes should be avoided as they may exacerbate the condition. Antifungal agents should not be used unless fungal infection has been diagnosed *[see Drug Interactions (7.1)]*.

5.4 Renal Failure

Cases of renal failure (including acute renal failure), some with a fatal outcome, have been observed in patients treated with AFINITOR *[see Laboratory Tests and Monitoring (5.6)]*.

5.5 Geriatric Patients

In the randomized advanced hormone receptor-positive, HER2-negative breast cancer study, the incidence of deaths due to any cause within 28 days of the last AFINITOR dose was 6% in patients ≥ 65 years of age compared to 2% in patients < 65 years of age. Adverse reactions leading to permanent treatment discontinuation occurred in 33% of patients ≥ 65 years of age compared to 17% in patients < 65 years of age. Careful monitoring and appropriate dose adjustments for adverse reactions are recommended *[see Dosage and Administration (2.2), Use in Specific Populations (8.5)]*.

5.6 Laboratory Tests and Monitoring

Renal Function
Elevations of serum creatinine and proteinuria have been reported in clinical trials *[see Adverse Reactions (6.1, 6.2, 6.3, 6.4, 6.5)]*. Monitoring of renal function, including measurement of blood urea nitrogen (BUN), urinary protein, or serum creatinine, is recommended prior to the start of AFINITOR therapy and periodically thereafter.

Blood Glucose and Lipids
Hyperglycemia, hyperlipidemia, and hypertriglyceridemia have been reported in clinical trials *[see Adverse Reactions (6.1, 6.2, 6.3, 6.4, 6.5)]*. Monitoring of fasting serum glucose and lipid profile is recommended prior to the start of AFINITOR therapy and periodically thereafter. When possible, optimal glucose and lipid control should be achieved before starting a patient on AFINITOR.

Hematologic Parameters
Decreased hemoglobin, lymphocytes, neutrophils, and platelets have been reported in clinical trials *[see Adverse Reactions (6.1, 6.2, 6.3, 6.4, 6.5)]*. Monitoring of complete blood count is recommended prior to the start of AFINITOR therapy and periodically thereafter.

5.7 Drug-drug Interactions

Due to significant increases in exposure of everolimus, co-administration with strong CYP3A4 inhibitors should be avoided *[see Dosage and Administration (2.2, 2.5) and Drug Interactions (7.1)]*.

A reduction of the AFINITOR dose is recommended when co-administered with a moderate CYP3A4 and/or PgP inhibitor *[see Dosage and Administration (2.2, 2.5) and Drug Interactions (7.1)]*.

An increase in the AFINITOR dose is recommended when co-administered with a strong CYP3A4 inducer *[see Dosage and Administration (2.2, 2.5) and Drug Interactions (7.2)]*.

5.8 Hepatic Impairment

Exposure to everolimus was increased in patients with hepatic impairment *[see Clinical Pharmacology (12.3)]*.

For advanced HR+ BC, advanced PNET, advanced RCC, and renal angiomyolipoma with TSC patients with severe hepatic impairment (Child-Pugh class C), AFINITOR may be used at a reduced dose if the desired benefit outweighs the risk. For patients with mild (Child-Pugh class A) or moderate (Child-Pugh class B) hepatic impairment, a dose reduction is recommended *[see Dosage and Administration (2.2) and Clinical Pharmacology (12.3)]*.

For patients with SEGA and mild or moderate hepatic impairment, adjust the dose of AFINITOR Tablets or AFINITOR DISPERZ based on therapeutic drug monitoring. For patients with SEGA and severe hepatic impairment, reduce the starting dose of AFINITOR Tablets or AFINITOR DISPERZ by approximately 50% and adjust subsequent doses based on therapeutic drug monitoring *[see Dosage and Administration (2.4, 2.5)]*.

5.9 Vaccinations

During AFINITOR treatment, avoid the use of live vaccines and avoid close contact with individuals who have received live vaccines (e.g., intranasal influenza, measles, mumps, rubella, oral polio, BCG, yellow fever, varicella, and TY21a typhoid vaccines).

For pediatric patients with SEGA that do not require immediate treatment, complete the recommended childhood series of live virus vaccinations according to American Council on Immunization Practices (ACIP) guidelines prior to the start of therapy. An accelerated vaccination schedule may be appropriate.

5.10 Embryo-fetal Toxicity

There are no adequate and well-controlled studies of AFINITOR in pregnant women; however, based on the mechanism of action, AFINITOR can cause fetal harm. Everolimus caused embryo-fetal toxicities in animals at maternal exposures that were lower than human exposures. If this drug is used during pregnancy or if the patient becomes pregnant while taking this drug, the patient should be apprised of the potential hazard to a fetus. Women of childbearing potential should be advised to use a highly effective method of contraception while using AFINITOR and for up to 8 weeks after ending treatment *[see Use in Specific Populations (8.1)]*.

6 ADVERSE REACTIONS

The following serious adverse reactions are discussed in greater detail in another section of the label *[see Warnings and Precautions (5)]*:

- Non-infectious pneumonitis *[see Warnings and Precautions (5.1)]*.
- Infections *[see Warnings and Precautions (5.2)]*.
- Oral ulcers *[see Warnings and Precautions (5.3)]*.
- Renal failure *[see Warnings and Precautions (5.4)]*.

Because clinical trials are conducted under widely varying conditions, the adverse reaction rates observed cannot be directly compared to rates in other trials and may not reflect the rates observed in clinical practice.

6.1 Clinical Study Experience in Advanced Hormone Receptor-Positive, HER2-Negative Breast Cancer

The efficacy and safety of AFINITOR (10 mg/day) plus exemestane (25 mg/day) (n=485) versus placebo plus exemestane (25 mg/day) (n=239) was evaluated in a randomized, controlled trial in patients with advanced or metastatic hormone receptor-positive, HER2-negative breast cancer. The median age of patients was 61 years (range 28-93), and 75% were Caucasian. Safety results are based on a median follow-up of approximately 13 months.

The most common adverse reactions (incidence ≥ 30%) were stomatitis, infections, rash, fatigue, diarrhea, and decreased appetite. The most common grade 3/4 adverse reactions (incidence ≥ 2%) were stomatitis, infections, hyperglycemia, fatigue, dyspnea, pneumonitis, and diarrhea. The most common laboratory abnormalities (incidence ≥ 50%) were hypercholesterolemia, hyperglycemia, increased AST, anemia, leukopenia, thrombocytopenia, lymphopenia, increased ALT, and hypertriglyceridemia. The most common grade 3/4 laboratory abnormalities (incidence ≥ 3%) were lymphopenia, hyperglycemia, anemia, decreased potassium, increased AST, increased ALT, and thrombocytopenia.

Fatal adverse reactions occurred more frequently in patients who received AFINITOR plus exemestane (2%) compared to patients on the placebo plus exemestane arm (0.4%). The rates of treatment-emergent adverse events resulting in permanent discontinuation were 24% and 5% for the AFINITOR plus exemestane and placebo plus exemestane treatment groups, respectively. Dose adjustments (interruptions or reductions) were more frequent among patients in the AFINITOR plus exemestane arm than in the placebo plus exemestane arm (63% versus 14%).

Table 2 compares the incidence of treatment-emergent adverse reactions reported with an incidence of ≥10% for patients receiving AFINITOR 10 mg daily versus placebo.

[See table 2 at top of previous page]

Key observed laboratory abnormalities are presented in Table 3.

[See table 3 above]

Table 3: Key Laboratory Abnormalities Reported in ≥ 10% of Patients with Advanced HR+ BC

Laboratory parameter	AFINITOR (10 mg/day) + exemestane[a] N=482 All grades %	Grade 3 %	Grade 4 %	Placebo + exemestane[a] N=238 All grades %	Grade 3 %	Grade 4 %
Hematology[b]						
Hemoglobin decreased	68	6	0.6	40	0.8	0.4
WBC decreased	58	1	0	28	5	0.8
Platelets decreased	54	3	0.2	5	0	0.4
Lymphocytes decreased	54	11	0.6	37	5	0.8
Neutrophils decreased	31	2	0	11	0.8	0.8
Clinical chemistry						
Glucose increased	69	9	0.4	44	0.8	0.4
Cholesterol increased	70	0.6	0.2	38	0.8	0.8
Aspartate transaminase (AST) increased	69	4	0.2	45	3	0.4
Alanine transaminase (ALT) increased	51	4	0.2	29	5	0
Triglycerides increased	50	0.8	0	26	0	0
Albumin decreased	33	0.8	0	16	0.8	0
Potassium decreased	29	4	0.2	7	1	0
Creatinine increased	24	2	0.2	13	0	0

CTCAE Version 3.0

[a] Exemestane (25 mg/day)

[b] Reflects corresponding adverse drug reaction reports of anemia, leukopenia, lymphopenia, neutropenia, and thrombocytopenia (collectively as pancytopenia), which occurred at lower frequency.

6.2 Clinical Study Experience in Advanced Pancreatic Neuroendocrine Tumors

In a randomized, controlled trial of AFINITOR (n=204) versus placebo (n=203) in patients with advanced PNET the median age of patients was 58 years (range 20-87), 79% were Caucasian, and 55% were male. Patients on the placebo arm could cross over to open-label AFINITOR upon disease progression.

The most common adverse reactions (incidence ≥ 30%) were stomatitis, rash, diarrhea, fatigue, edema, abdominal pain, nausea, fever, and headache. The most common grade 3-4 adverse reactions (incidence ≥ 5%) were stomatitis and diarrhea. The most common laboratory abnormalities (incidence ≥ 50%) were decreased hemoglobin, hyperglycemia, alkaline phosphatase increased, hypercholesterolemia, bicarbonate decreased, and increased aspartate transaminase (AST). The most common grade 3-4 laboratory abnormalities (incidence ≥ 3%) were hyperglycemia, lymphopenia, decreased hemoglobin, hypophosphatemia, increased alkaline phosphatase, neutropenia, increased aspartate transaminase (AST), potassium decreased, and thrombocytopenia. Deaths during double-blind treatment where an adverse event was the primary cause occurred in 7 patients on AFINITOR and 1 patient on placebo. Causes of death on the AFINITOR arm included one case of each of the following: acute renal failure, acute respiratory distress, cardiac arrest, death (cause unknown), hepatic failure, pneumonia, and sepsis. There was 1 death due to pulmonary embolism on the placebo arm. After cross-over to open-label AFINITOR, there were 3 additional deaths, one due to hypoglycemia and cardiac arrest in a patient with insulinoma, one due to MI with CHF, and the other due to sudden death.

The rates of treatment-emergent adverse events resulting in permanent discontinuation were 20% and 6% for the AFINITOR and placebo treatment groups, respectively. Dose delay or reduction was necessary in 61% of everolimus patients and 29% of placebo patients. grade 3-4 renal failure occurred in 6 patients in the everolimus arm and 3 patients in the placebo arm. Thrombotic events included 5 patients with pulmonary embolus in the everolimus arm and 1 in the placebo arm as well as 3 patients with thrombosis in the everolimus arm and 2 in the placebo arm.

Table 4 compares the incidence of treatment-emergent adverse reactions reported with an incidence of ≥ 10% for patients receiving AFINITOR 10 mg daily versus placebo.

[See table 4 at top of next page]

Key observed laboratory abnormalities are presented in Table 5.

[See table 5 at top of page 1899]

6.3 Clinical Study Experience in Advanced Renal Cell Carcinoma

The data described below reflect exposure to AFINITOR (n=274) and placebo (n=137) in a randomized, controlled trial in patients with metastatic renal cell carcinoma who received prior treatment with sunitinib and/or sorafenib. The median age of patients was 61 years (range 27-85), 88% were Caucasian, and 78% were male. The median duration of blinded study treatment was 141 days (range 19-451) for patients receiving AFINITOR and 60 days (range 21-295) for those receiving placebo.

The most common adverse reactions (incidence ≥ 30%) were stomatitis, infections, asthenia, fatigue, cough, and diarrhea. The most common grade 3-4 adverse reactions (incidence ≥ 3%) were infections, dyspnea, fatigue, stomatitis, dehydration, pneumonitis, abdominal pain, and asthenia. The most common laboratory abnormalities (incidence ≥ 50%) were anemia, hypercholesterolemia, hypertriglyceridemia, hyperglycemia, lymphopenia, and increased creatinine. The most common grade 3-4 laboratory abnormalities (incidence ≥ 3%) were lymphopenia, hyperglycemia, anemia, hypophosphatemia, and hypercholesterolemia. Deaths due to acute respiratory failure (0.7%), infection (0.7%), and acute renal failure (0.4%) were observed on the AFINITOR arm but none on the placebo arm. The rates of treatment-emergent adverse events (irrespective of causality) resulting in permanent discontinuation were 14% and 3% for the AFINITOR and placebo treatment groups, respectively. The most common adverse reactions (irrespective of causality) leading to treatment discontinuation were pneumonitis and dyspnea. Infections, stomatitis, and pneumonitis were the most common reasons for treatment delay or dose reduction. The most common medical interventions required during AFINITOR treatment were for infections, anemia, and stomatitis.

Table 6 compares the incidence of treatment-emergent adverse reactions reported with an incidence of ≥ 10% for patients receiving AFINITOR 10 mg daily versus placebo. Within each MedDRA system organ class, the adverse reactions are presented in order of decreasing frequency.

[See table 6 at top of page 1899]

Other notable adverse reactions occurring more frequently with AFINITOR than with placebo, but with an incidence of < 10% include:

Gastrointestinal disorders: Abdominal pain (9%), dry mouth (8%), hemorrhoids (5%), dysphagia (4%)

General disorders and administration site conditions: Weight decreased (9%), chest pain (5%), chills (4%), impaired wound healing (< 1%)

Respiratory, thoracic and mediastinal disorders: Pleural effusion (7%), pharyngolaryngeal pain (4%), rhinorrhea (3%)

Skin and subcutaneous tissue disorders: Hand-foot syndrome (reported as palmar-plantar erythrodysesthesia syndrome) (5%), nail disorder (5%), erythema (4%), onychoclasis (4%), skin lesion (4%), acneiform dermatitis (3%)

Metabolism and nutrition disorders: Exacerbation of preexisting diabetes mellitus (2%), new onset of diabetes mellitus (< 1%)

Psychiatric disorders: Insomnia (9%)

Nervous system disorders: Dizziness (7%), paresthesia (5%)

Eye disorders: Eyelid edema (4%), conjunctivitis (2%)

Vascular disorders: Hypertension (4%), deep vein thrombosis (< 1%)

Renal and urinary disorders: Renal failure (3%)

Cardiac disorders: Tachycardia (3%), congestive cardiac failure (1%)

Musculoskeletal and connective tissue disorders: Jaw pain (3%)

Hematologic disorders: Hemorrhage (3%)

Key laboratory abnormalities are presented in Table 7.

[See table 7 at top of page 1900]

6.4 Clinical Study Experience in Renal Angiomyolipoma with Tuberous Sclerosis Complex

The data described below are based on a randomized (2:1), double-blind, placebo-controlled trial of AFINITOR in 118 patients with renal angiomyolipoma as a feature of TSC (n=113) or sporadic lymphangioleiomyomatosis (n=5). The median age of patients was 31 years (range 18 to 61 years), 89% were Caucasian, and 34% were male. The median du-

Table 4: Adverse Reactions Reported ≥ 10% of Patients with Advanced PNET

	AFINITOR N=204			Placebo N=203		
	All grades %	Grade 3 %	Grade 4 %	All grades %	Grade 3 %	Grade 4 %
Any adverse reaction	**100**	**49**	**13**	**98**	**32**	**8**
Gastrointestinal disorders						
Stomatitis[a]	70	7	0	20	0	0
Diarrhea[b]	50	5	0.5	25	3	0
Abdominal pain	36	4	0	32	6	1
Nausea	32	2	0	33	2	0
Vomiting	29	1	0	21	2	0
Constipation	14	0	0	13	0.5	0
Dry mouth	11	0	0	4	0	0
General disorders and administration site conditions						
Fatigue/malaise	45	3	0.5	27	2	0.5
Edema (general and peripheral)	39	1	0.5	12	1	0
Fever	31	0.5	0.5	13	0.5	0
Asthenia	19	3	0	20	3	0
Infections and infestations						
Nasopharyngitis/rhinitis/URI	25	0	0	13	0	0
Urinary tract infection	16	0	0	6	0.5	0
Investigations						
Weight decreased	28	0.5	0	11	0	0
Metabolism and nutrition disorders						
Decreased appetite	30	1	0	18	1	0
Diabetes mellitus	10	2	0	0.5	0	0
Musculoskeletal and connective tissue disorders						
Arthralgia	15	1	0.5	7	0.5	0
Back pain	15	1	0	11	1	0
Pain in extremity	14	0.5	0	6	1	0
Muscle spasms	10	0	0	4	0	0
Nervous system disorders						
Headache/migraine	30	0.5	0	15	1	0
Dysgeusia	19	0	0	5	0	0
Dizziness	12	0.5	0	7	0	0
Psychiatric disorders						
Insomnia	14	0	0	8	0	0
Respiratory, thoracic and mediastinal disorders						
Cough/productive cough	25	0.5	0	13	0	0
Epistaxis	22	0	0	1	0	0
Dyspnea/dyspnea exertional	20	2	0.5	7	0.5	0
Pneumonitis[c]	17	3	0.5	0	0	0
Oropharyngeal pain	11	0	0	6	0	0
Skin and subcutaneous disorders						
Rash	59	0.5	0	19	0	0
Nail disorders	22	0.5	0	2	0	0
Pruritus/pruritus generalized	21	0	0	13	0	0
Dry skin/xeroderma	13	0	0	6	0	0
Vascular disorders						
Hypertension	13	1	0	6	1	0
Median duration of treatment (wks)		**37**			**16**	

CTCAE Version 3.0

[a] Includes stomatitis, aphthous stomatitis, gingival pain/swelling/ulceration, glossitis, glossodynia, lip ulceration, mouth ulceration, tongue ulceration, and mucosal inflammation.

[b] Includes diarrhea, enteritis, enterocolitis, colitis, defecation urgency, and steatorrhea.

[c] Includes pneumonitis, interstitial lung disease, pulmonary fibrosis and restrictive pulmonary disease.

ration of blinded study treatment was 48 weeks (range 2 to 115 weeks) for patients receiving AFINITOR and 45 weeks (range 9 to 115 weeks) for those receiving placebo.

The most common adverse reaction reported for AFINITOR (incidence ≥ 30%) was stomatitis. The most common Grade 3-4 adverse reactions (incidence ≥ 2%) were stomatitis and amenorrhea. The most common laboratory abnormalities (incidence ≥ 50%) were hypercholesterolemia, hypertriglyceridemia, and anemia. The most common Grade 3-4 laboratory abnormality (incidence ≥ 3%) was hypophosphatemia.

The rate of adverse reactions resulting in permanent discontinuation was 3.8% in the AFINITOR-treated patients. Adverse reactions leading to permanent discontinuation in the AFINITOR arm were hypersensitivity/angioedema/bronchospasm, convulsion, and hypophosphatemia. Dose adjustments (interruptions or reductions) due to adverse reactions occurred in 52% of AFINITOR-treated patients. The most common adverse reaction leading to AFINITOR dose adjustment was stomatitis.

Table 8 compares the incidence of adverse reactions reported with an incidence of ≥ 10% for patients receiving AFINITOR and occurring more frequently with AFINITOR than with placebo. Laboratory abnormalities are described separately in Table 9.

[See table 8 at top of page 1900]

Amenorrhea occurred in 15% of AFINITOR-treated females (8 of 52) and 4% (1 of 26) of females in the placebo group. Other adverse reactions involving the female reproductive system were menorrhagia (10%), menstrual irregularities (10%), and vaginal hemorrhage (8%).

The following additional adverse reactions occurred: epistaxis (9%), decreased appetite (6%), otitis media (6%), depression (5%), abnormal taste (5%), hypersensitivity (3%), and pneumonitis (1%).

[See table 9 at top of page 1900]

6.5 Clinical Study Experience in Subependymal Giant Cell Astrocytoma with Tuberous Sclerosis Complex

The data described below are based on a randomized (2:1), double-blind, placebo-controlled trial (Study 1) of AFINITOR in 117 patients with subependymal giant cell astrocytoma (SEGA) and tuberous sclerosis complex (TSC). The median age of patients was 9.5 years (range 0.8 to 26 years), 93% were Caucasian, and 57% were male. The median duration of blinded study treatment was 52 weeks (range 24 to 89 weeks) for patients receiving AFINITOR and 47 weeks (range 14 to 88 weeks) for those receiving placebo.

The most common adverse reactions reported for AFINITOR (incidence ≥ 30%) were stomatitis and respiratory tract infection. The most common Grade 3-4 adverse reactions (incidence ≥ 2%) were stomatitis, pyrexia, pneumonia, gastroenteritis, aggression, agitation, and amenorrhea. The most common key laboratory abnormalities (incidence ≥ 50%) were hypercholesterolemia and elevated partial thromboplastin time. The most common Grade 3-4 laboratory abnormality (incidence ≥ 3%) was neutropenia.

There were no adverse reactions resulting in permanent discontinuation. Dose adjustments (interruptions or reductions) due to adverse reactions occurred in 55% of AFINITOR-treated patients. The most common adverse reaction leading to AFINITOR dose adjustment was stomatitis.

Table 10 compares the incidence of adverse reactions reported with an incidence of ≥ 10% for patients receiving AFINITOR and occurring more frequently with AFINITOR than with placebo. Laboratory abnormalities are described separately in Table 11.

[See table 10 at top of page 1901]

Amenorrhea occurred in 17% of AFINITOR-treated females aged 10 to 55 years (3 of 18) and none of the females in the placebo group. For this same group of AFINITOR-treated females, the following menstrual abnormalities were reported: dysmenorrhea (6%), menorrhagia (6%), metrorrhagia (6%), and unspecified menstrual irregularity (6%).

The following additional adverse reactions occurred in AFINITOR-treated patients: nausea (8%), pain in extremity (8%), insomnia (6%), pneumonia (6%), epistaxis (5%), hypersensitivity (3%), and pneumonitis (1%).

[See table 11 at top of page 1901]

Longer-term follow-up of 34.2 months (range 4.7 to 47.1 months) from a non-randomized, open-label, 28-patient trial resulted in the following additional notable adverse reactions and key laboratory abnormalities: cellulitis (29%), hyperglycemia (25%), and elevated creatinine (14%).

7 DRUG INTERACTIONS

Everolimus is a substrate of CYP3A4, and also a substrate and moderate inhibitor of the multidrug efflux pump PgP. *In vitro*, everolimus is a competitive inhibitor of CYP3A4 and a mixed inhibitor of CYP2D6.

7.1 Agents That May Increase Everolimus Blood Concentrations

CYP3A4 Inhibitors and PgP Inhibitors

In healthy subjects, compared to AFINITOR treatment alone there were significant increases in everolimus exposure when AFINITOR was coadministered with:

- ketoconazole (a strong CYP3A4 inhibitor and a PgP inhibitor) - C_{max} and AUC increased by 3.9- and 15.0-fold, respectively.
- erythromycin (a moderate CYP3A4 inhibitor and a PgP inhibitor) - C_{max} and AUC increased by 2.0- and 4.4-fold, respectively.
- verapamil (a moderate CYP3A4 inhibitor and a PgP inhibitor) - C_{max} and AUC increased by 2.3- and 3.5-fold, respectively.

Concomitant strong inhibitors of CYP3A4 should not be used *[see Dosage and Administration (2.2, 2.5) and Warnings and Precautions (5.7)]*.

Use caution when AFINITOR is used in combination with moderate CYP3A4 and/or PgP inhibitors. If alternative treatment cannot be administered reduce the AFINITOR dose *[see Dosage and Administration (2.2, 2.5) and Warnings and Precautions (5.7)]*.

7.2 Agents That May Decrease Everolimus Blood Concentrations

CYP3A4 Inducers

In healthy subjects, co-administration of AFINITOR with rifampin, a strong inducer of CYP3A4, decreased everolimus AUC and C_{max} by 63% and 58% respectively, compared to everolimus treatment alone. Consider a dose increase of AFINITOR when co-administered with strong CYP3A4 inducers if alternative treatment cannot be administered. St. John's Wort may decrease everolimus exposure unpredictably and should be avoided *[see Dosage and Administration (2.2, 2.5)]*.

7.3 Drugs That May Have Their Plasma Concentrations Altered by Everolimus

Studies in healthy subjects indicate that there are no clinically significant pharmacokinetic interactions between AFINITOR and the HMG-CoA reductase inhibitors atorvastatin (a CYP3A4 substrate) and pravastatin (a non-CYP3A4 substrate) and population pharmacokinetic analyses also detected no influence of simvastatin (a CYP3A4 substrate) on the clearance of AFINITOR.

A study in healthy subjects demonstrated that co-administration of an oral dose of midazolam (sensitive CYP3A4 substrate) with everolimus resulted in a 25% increase in midazolam C_{max} and a 30% increase in midazolam $AUC_{(0-inf)}$.

Coadministration of everolimus and exemestane increased exemestane C_{min} by 45% and C_{2h} by 64%. However, the corresponding estradiol levels at steady state (4 weeks) were not different between the two treatment arms. No increase in adverse events related to exemestane was observed in patients with hormone receptor-positive, HER2-negative advanced breast cancer receiving the combination.

Coadministration of everolimus and depot octreotide increased octreotide Cmin by approximately 50%.

8 USE IN SPECIFIC POPULATIONS

8.1 Pregnancy

Pregnancy Category D *[see Warnings and Precautions (5.10)]*.

There are no adequate and well-controlled studies of AFINITOR in pregnant women; however, based on the mechanism of action, AFINITOR can cause fetal harm when administered to a pregnant woman. Everolimus caused embryo-fetal toxicities in animals at maternal exposures that were lower than human exposures. If this drug is used during pregnancy or if the patient becomes pregnant while taking the drug, the patient should be apprised of the potential hazard to the fetus. Women of childbearing potential should be advised to use a highly effective method of contraception while receiving AFINITOR and for up to 8 weeks after ending treatment.

In animal reproductive studies, oral administration of everolimus to female rats before mating and through organogenesis induced embryo-fetal toxicities, including increased resorption, pre-implantation and post-implantation loss, decreased numbers of live fetuses, malformation (e.g., sternal cleft), and retarded skeletal development. These effects occurred in the absence of maternal toxicities. Embryo-fetal toxicities in rats occurred at doses ≥ 0.1 mg/kg (0.6 mg/m^2) with resulting exposures of approximately 4% of the exposure (AUC_{0-24h}) achieved in patients receiving the 10 mg daily dose of everolimus. In rabbits, embryotoxicity evident as an increase in resorptions occurred at an oral dose of 0.8 mg/kg (9.6 mg/m^2), approximately 1.6 times either the 10 mg daily dose or the median dose administered to SEGA patients on a body surface area basis. The effect in rabbits occurred in the presence of maternal toxicities.

In a pre- and post-natal development study in rats, animals were dosed from implantation through lactation. At the dose of 0.1 mg/kg (0.6 mg/m^2), there were no adverse effects on delivery and lactation or signs of maternal toxicity; however, there were reductions in body weight (up to 9% reduction from the control) and in survival of offspring (~5% died or missing). There were no drug-related effects on the developmental parameters (morphological development, motor activity, learning, or fertility assessment) in the offspring.

8.3 Nursing Mothers

It is not known whether everolimus is excreted in human milk. Everolimus and/or its metabolites passed into the milk of lactating rats at a concentration 3.5 times higher than in maternal serum. Because many drugs are excreted in human milk and because of the potential for serious adverse reactions in nursing infants from everolimus, a decision should be made whether to discontinue nursing or to discontinue the drug, taking into account the importance of the drug to the mother.

8.4 Pediatric Use

Pediatric use of AFINITOR Tablets and AFINITOR DISPERZ is recommended for patients 1 year of age and older with TSC for the treatment of SEGA that requires therapeutic intervention but cannot be curatively resected. The safety and effectiveness of AFINITOR Tablets and AFINITOR DISPERZ have not been established in pediatric patients with renal angiomyolipoma with TSC in the absence of SEGA.

The effectiveness of AFINITOR in pediatric patients with SEGA was demonstrated in two clinical trials based on demonstration of durable objective response, as evidenced by reduction in SEGA tumor volume *[see Clinical Studies (14.5)]*. Improvement in disease-related symptoms and overall survival in pediatric patients with SEGA has not been demonstrated. The long term effects of AFINITOR on growth and pubertal development are unknown.

Study 1 was a randomized, double-blind, multicenter trial comparing AFINITOR (n=78) to placebo (n=39) in pediatric and adult patients. The median age was 9.5 years (range 0.8 to 26 years). At the time of randomization, a total of 20 patients were < 3 years of age, 54 patients were 3 to < 12 years of age, 27 patients were 12 to < 18 years of age, and 16 patients were ≥ 18 years of age. The overall nature, type, and frequency of adverse reactions across the age groups evaluated were similar, with the exception of a higher per patient incidence of infectious serious adverse events in patients < 3 years of age. A total of 6 of 13 patients (46%) < 3 years of age had at least one serious adverse event due to infection, compared to 2 of 7 patients (29%) treated with placebo. No patient in any age group discontinued AFINITOR due to infection *[see Adverse Reactions (6.5)]*. Subgroup analyses showed reduction in SEGA volume with AFINITOR treatment in all pediatric age subgroups.

Study 2 was an open-label, single-arm, single-center trial of AFINITOR (N=28) in patients aged ≥ 3 years; median age was 11 years (range 3 to 34 years). A total of 16 patients were 3 to < 12 years, 6 patients were 12 to < 18 years, and 6 patients were ≥ 18 years. The frequency of adverse reactions across the age groups was generally similar *[see Adverse Reactions (6.5)]*. Subgroup analyses showed reductions in SEGA volume with AFINITOR treatment in all pediatric age subgroups.

Everolimus clearance normalized to body surface area was higher in pediatric patients than in adults with SEGA *[see Clinical Pharmacology (12.3)]*.The recommended starting dose and subsequent requirement for therapeutic drug monitoring to achieve and maintain trough concentrations of 5 to 15 ng/mL are the same for adult and pediatric patients with SEGA *[see Dosage and Administration (2.3, 2.4)]*.

Table 5: Key Laboratory Abnormalities Reported in ≥ 10% of Patients with Advanced PNET

Laboratory parameter	AFINITOR N=204		Placebo N=203	
	All grades %	Grade 3-4 %	All grades %	Grade 3-4 %
Hematology				
Hemoglobin decreased	86	15	63	1
Lymphocytes decreased	45	16	22	4
Platelets decreased	45	3	11	0
WBC decreased	43	2	13	0
Neutrophils decreased	30	4	17	2
Clinical chemistry				
Alkaline phosphatase increased	74	8	66	8
Glucose (fasting) increased	75	17	53	6
Cholesterol increased	66	0.5	22	0
Bicarbonate decreased	56	0	40	0
Aspartate transaminase (AST) increased	56	4	41	4
Alanine transaminase (ALT) increased	48	2	35	2
Phosphate decreased	40	10	14	3
Triglycerides increased	39	0	10	0
Calcium decreased	37	0.5	12	0
Potassium decreased	23	4	5	0
Creatinine increased	19	2	14	0
Sodium decreased	16	1	16	1
Albumin decreased	13	1	8	0
Bilirubin increased	10	1	14	2
Potassium increased	7	0	10	0.5

CTCAE Version 3.0

Table 6: Adverse Reactions Reported in at least 10% of Patients with RCC and at a Higher Rate in the AFINITOR Arm than in the Placebo Arm

	AFINITOR 10 mg/day N=274			Placebo N=137		
	All grades %	Grade 3 %	Grade 4 %	All grades %	Grade 3 %	Grade 4 %
Any adverse reaction	97	52	13	93	23	5
Gastrointestinal disorders						
Stomatitis[a]	44	4	<1	8	0	0
Diarrhea	30	1	0	7	0	0
Nausea	26	1	0	19	0	0
Vomiting	20	2	0	12	0	0
Infections and infestations[b]	37	7	3	18	1	0
General disorders and administration site conditions						
Asthenia	33	3	<1	23	4	0
Fatigue	31	5	0	27	3	<1
Edema peripheral	25	<1	0	8	<1	0
Pyrexia	20	<1	0	9	0	0
Mucosal inflammation	19	1	0	1	0	0
Respiratory, thoracic and mediastinal disorders						
Cough	30	<1	0	16	0	0
Dyspnea	24	6	1	15	3	0
Epistaxis	18	0	0	0	0	0
Pneumonitis[c]	14	4	0	0	0	0
Skin and subcutaneous tissue disorders						
Rash	29	1	0	7	0	0
Pruritus	14	<1	0	7	0	0
Dry skin	13	<1	0	5	0	0
Metabolism and nutrition disorders						
Anorexia	25	1	0	14	<1	0
Nervous system disorders						
Headache	19	<1	<1	9	<1	0
Dysgeusia	10	0	0	2	0	0
Musculoskeletal and connective tissue disorders						
Pain in extremity	10	1	0	7	0	0
Median duration of treatment (d)		141			60	

CTCAE Version 3.0

[a] Stomatitis (including aphthous stomatitis), and mouth and tongue ulceration.

[b] Includes all preferred terms within the 'infections and infestations' system organ class, the most common being nasopharyngitis (6%), pneumonia (6%), urinary tract infection (5%), bronchitis (4%), and sinusitis (3%), and also including aspergillosis (<1%), candidiasis (<1%), and sepsis (<1%).

[c] Includes pneumonitis, interstitial lung disease, lung infiltration, pulmonary alveolar hemorrhage, pulmonary toxicity, and alveolitis.

8.5 Geriatric Use

In the randomized advanced hormone receptor positive, HER2-negative breast cancer study, 40% of AFINITOR-treated patients were ≥ 65 years of age, while 15% were 75 and over. No overall differences in effectiveness were observed between elderly and younger subjects. The incidence of deaths due to any cause within 28 days of the last AFINITOR dose was 6% in patients ≥ 65 years of age compared to 2% in patients < 65 years of age. Adverse reactions leading to permanent treatment discontinuation occurred in 33% of patients ≥ 65 years of age compared to 17% in patients < 65 years of age *[see Warnings and Precautions (5.5)]*.

In two other randomized trials (advanced renal cell carcinoma and advanced neuroendocrine tumors of pancreatic origin), no overall differences in safety or effectiveness were observed between elderly and younger subjects. In the randomized advanced RCC study, 41% of AFINITOR treated patients were ≥ 65 years of age, while 7% were 75 and over. In the randomized advanced PNET study, 30% of

Table 7: Key Laboratory Abnormalities Reported in Patients with RCC at a Higher Rate in the AFINITOR Arm than the Placebo Arm

Laboratory parameter	AFINITOR 10 mg/day N=274			Placebo N=137		
	All grades %	Grade 3 %	Grade 4 %	All grades %	Grade 3 %	Grade 4 %
Hematology[a]						
Hemoglobin decreased	92	12	1	79	5	<1
Lymphocytes decreased	51	16	2	28	5	0
Platelets decreased	23	1	0	2	0	<1
Neutrophils decreased	14	0	<1	4	0	0
Clinical chemistry						
Cholesterol increased	77	4	0	35	0	0
Triglycerides increased	73	<1	0	34	0	0
Glucose increased	57	15	<1	25	1	0
Creatinine increased	50	1	0	34	0	0
Phosphate decreased	37	6	0	8	0	0
Aspartate transaminase (AST) increased	25	<1	<1	7	0	0
Alanine transaminase (ALT) increased	21	1	0	4	0	0
Bilirubin increased	3	<1	<1	2	0	0

CTCAE Version 3.0
[a] Reflects corresponding adverse drug reaction reports of anemia, leukopenia, lymphopenia, neutropenia, and thrombocytopenia (collectively pancytopenia), which occurred at lower frequency.

Table 8: Adverse Reactions Reported in ≥ 10% of AFINITOR-treated Patients with Renal Angiomyolipoma

	AFINITOR N=79			Placebo N=39		
	All grades %	Grade 3 %	Grade 4 %	All grades %	Grade 3 %	Grade 4 %
Any adverse reaction	**100**	**25**	**5**	**97**	**8**	**5**
Gastrointestinal disorders						
Stomatitis[a]	78	6	0	23	0	0
Vomiting	15	0	0	5	0	0
Diarrhea	14	0	0	5	0	0
General disorders and administration site conditions						
Peripheral edema	13	0	0	8	0	0
Infections and infestations						
Upper respiratory tract infection	11	0	0	5	0	0
Musculoskeletal and connective tissue disorders						
Arthralgia	13	0	0	5	0	0
Respiratory, thoracic and mediastinal disorders						
Cough	20	0	0	13	0	0
Skin and subcutaneous tissue disorders						
Acne	22	0	0	5	0	0

Grading according to CTCAE Version 3.0
[a] Includes stomatitis, aphthous stomatitis, mouth ulceration, gingival pain, glossitis, and glossodynia.

Table 9: Key Laboratory Abnormalities Reported in AFINITOR-treated Patients with Renal Angiomyolipoma

	AFINITOR N=79			Placebo N=39		
	All grades %	Grade 3 %	Grade 4 %	All grades %	Grade 3 %	Grade 4 %
Hematology						
Anemia	61	0	0	49	0	0
Leucopenia	37	0	0	21	0	0
Neutropenia	25	0	1	26	0	0
Lymphopenia	20	1	0	8	0	0
Thrombocytopenia	19	0	0	3	0	0
Clinical chemistry						
Hypercholesterolemia	85	1	0	46	0	0
Hypertriglyceridemia	52	0	0	10	0	0
Hypophosphatemia	49	5	0	15	0	0
Alkaline phosphatase increased	32	1	0	10	0	0
Elevated aspartate transaminase (AST)	23	1	0	8	0	0
Elevated alanine transaminase (ALT)	20	1	0	15	0	0
Fasting hyperglycemia	14	0	0	8	0	0

Grading according to CTCAE Version 3.0

AFINITOR-treated patients were ≥ 65 years of age, while 7% were 75 and over.

Other reported clinical experience has not identified differences in response between the elderly and younger patients, but greater sensitivity of some older individuals cannot be ruled out *[see Clinical Pharmacology (12.3)]*.

No dosage adjustment in initial dosing is required in elderly patients, but close monitoring and appropriate dose adjustments for adverse reactions is recommended *[see Dosage and Administration (2.2), Clinical Pharmacology (12.3)]*.

8.6 Renal Impairment

No clinical studies were conducted with AFINITOR in patients with decreased renal function. Renal impairment is not expected to influence drug exposure and no dosage adjustment of everolimus is recommended in patients with renal impairment *[see Clinical Pharmacology (12.3)]*.

8.7 Hepatic Impairment

The safety, tolerability and pharmacokinetics of AFINITOR were evaluated in a 34 subject single oral dose study of everolimus in subjects with impaired hepatic function relative to subjects with normal hepatic function. Exposure was increased in patients with mild (Child-Pugh class A), moderate (Child-Pugh class B), and severe (Child-Pugh class C) hepatic impairment *[see Clinical Pharmacology (12.3)]*.

For advanced HR+ BC, advanced PNET, advanced RCC, and renal angiomyolipoma with TSC patients with severe hepatic impairment, AFINITOR may be used at a reduced dose if the desired benefit outweighs the risk. For patients with mild (Child-Pugh class A) or moderate (Child-Pugh class B) hepatic impairment, a dose reduction is recommended *[see Dosage and Administration (2.2)]*.

For patients with SEGA who have severe hepatic impairment (Child-Pugh class C), reduce the starting dose of AFINITOR Tablets or AFINITOR DISPERZ by approximately 50%. For patients with SEGA who have mild (Child-Pugh class A) or moderate (Child-Pugh class B) hepatic impairment, adjustment to the starting dose may not be needed. Subsequent dosing should be based on therapeutic drug monitoring *[see Dosage and Administration (2.4, 2.5)]*.

10 OVERDOSAGE

In animal studies, everolimus showed a low acute toxic potential. No lethality or severe toxicity was observed in either mice or rats given single oral doses of 2000 mg/kg (limit test).

Reported experience with overdose in humans is very limited. Single doses of up to 70 mg have been administered. The acute toxicity profile observed with the 70 mg dose was consistent with that for the 10 mg dose.

11 DESCRIPTION

AFINITOR (everolimus), an inhibitor of mTOR, is an antineoplastic agent.

The chemical name of everolimus is (1R,9S,12S,15R,16E,18R,19R,21R,23S,24E,26E,28E,30S,32S,35R)-1,18- dihydroxy-12-[(1R)-2-[(1S,3R,4R)-4-(2-hydroxyethoxy)-3-methoxycyclohexyl]-1-methylethyl]-19,30-dimethoxy-15,17,21,23,29,35-hexamethyl-11,36-dioxa-4-aza-tricyclo[30.3.1.$0^{4,9}$]hexatriaconta-16,24,26,28-tetraene-2,3,10,14,20-pentaone.

The molecular formula is $C_{53}H_{83}NO_{14}$ and the molecular weight is 958.2. The structural formula is:

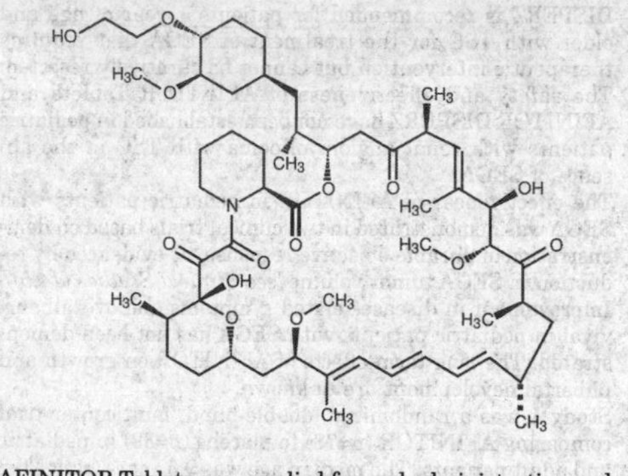

AFINITOR Tablets are supplied for oral administration and contain 2.5 mg, 5 mg, 7.5 mg, or 10 mg of everolimus. The tablets also contain anhydrous lactose, butylated hydroxytoluene, crospovidone, hypromellose, lactose monohydrate, and magnesium stearate as inactive ingredients.

AFINITOR DISPERZ (everolimus tablets for oral suspension) is supplied for oral administration and contains 2 mg, 3 mg, or 5 mg of everolimus. The tablets for oral suspension also contain butylated hydroxytoluene, colloidal silicon dioxide, crospovidone, hypromellose, lactose monohydrate, magnesium stearate, mannitol, and microcrystalline cellulose as inactive ingredients.

12 CLINICAL PHARMACOLOGY

12.1 Mechanism of Action

Everolimus is an inhibitor of mammalian target of rapamycin (mTOR), a serine-threonine kinase, downstream of the PI3K/AKT pathway. The mTOR pathway is dysregulated in several human cancers. Everolimus binds to an intracellular protein, FKBP-12, resulting in an inhibitory complex formation with mTOR complex 1 (mTORC1) and thus inhibition of mTOR kinase activity. Everolimus reduced the activity of S6 ribosomal protein kinase (S6K1) and eukaryotic elongation factor 4E-binding protein (4E-BP1), downstream effectors of mTOR, involved in protein synthesis. S6K1 is a substrate of mTORC1 and phosphorylates the activation domain 1 of the estrogen receptor which results in ligand-independent activation of the receptor. In addition, everolimus inhibited the expression of hypoxia-inducible factor (e.g., HIF-1) and reduced the expression of vascular endothelial growth factor (VEGF). Inhibition of mTOR by everolimus has been shown to reduce cell proliferation, angiogenesis, and glucose uptake in *in vitro* and/or *in vivo* studies.

Constitutive activation of the PI3K/Akt/mTOR pathway can contribute to endocrine resistance in breast cancer. *In vitro* studies show that estrogen-dependent and HER2+ breast cancer cells are sensitive to the inhibitory effects of everolimus, and that combination treatment with everolimus and Akt, HER2, or aromatase inhibitors enhances the anti-tumor activity of everolimus in a synergistic manner.

Two regulators of mTORC1 signaling are the oncogene suppressors tuberin-sclerosis complexes 1 and 2 (*TSC1, TSC2*). Loss or inactivation of either *TSC1* or *TSC2* leads to activation of downstream signaling. In TSC, a genetic disorder, inactivating mutations in either the *TSC1* or the *TSC2* gene lead to hamartoma formation throughout the body.

12.2 Pharmacodynamics

Exposure Response Relationships

Markers of protein synthesis show that inhibition of mTOR is complete after a 10 mg daily dose.

In patients with SEGA, higher everolimus trough concentrations appear to be associated with larger reductions in SEGA volume. However, as responses have been observed at trough concentrations as low as 5 ng/mL, once acceptable efficacy has been achieved, additional dose increase may not be necessary.

12.3 Pharmacokinetics

Absorption

In patients with advanced solid tumors, peak everolimus concentrations are reached 1 to 2 hours after administration of oral doses ranging from 5 mg to 70 mg. Following single doses, C_{max} is dose-proportional between 5 mg and 10 mg. At doses of 20 mg and higher, the increase in C_{max} is less than dose-proportional, however AUC shows dose-proportionality over the 5 mg to 70 mg dose range. Steady-state was achieved within 2 weeks following once-daily dosing.

Dose Proportionality in Patients with SEGA and TSC: In patients with SEGA and TSC, everolimus C_{min} was approximately dose-proportional within the dose range from 1.35 mg/m^2 to 14.4 mg/m^2.

Food effect: In healthy subjects, high fat meals reduced systemic exposure to AFINITOR 10 mg tablet (as measured by AUC) by 22% and the peak blood concentration C_{max} by 54%. Light fat meals reduced AUC by 32% and C_{max} by 42%. Food, however, had no apparent effect on the post absorption phase concentration-time profile.

Relative bioavailability of AFINITOR DISPERZ (everolimus tablets for oral suspension): The $AUC_{0-\infty}$ of AFINITOR DISPERZ was equivalent to that of AFINITOR Tablets; the C_{max} of this dosage form was 20-36% lower than that of AFINITOR Tablets. The predicted trough concentrations at steady-state were similar after daily administration.

Distribution

The blood-to-plasma ratio of everolimus, which is concentration-dependent over the range of 5 to 5000 ng/mL, is 17% to 73%. The amount of everolimus confined to the plasma is approximately 20% at blood concentrations observed in cancer patients given AFINITOR 10 mg/day. Plasma protein binding is approximately 74% both in healthy subjects and in patients with moderate hepatic impairment.

Metabolism

Everolimus is a substrate of CYP3A4 and PgP. Following oral administration, everolimus is the main circulating component in human blood. Six main metabolites of everolimus have been detected in human blood, including three monohydroxylated metabolites, two hydrolytic ring-opened products, and a phosphatidylcholine conjugate of everolimus. These metabolites were also identified in animal species used in toxicity studies, and showed approximately 100-times less activity than everolimus itself.

In vitro, everolimus competitively inhibited the metabolism of CYP3A4 and was a mixed inhibitor of the CYP2D6 substrate dextromethorphan.

Excretion

No specific excretion studies have been undertaken in cancer patients. Following the administration of a 3 mg single dose of radiolabeled everolimus in patients who were receiving cyclosporine, 80% of the radioactivity was recovered from the feces, while 5% was excreted in the urine. The parent substance was not detected in urine or feces. The mean elimination half-life of everolimus is approximately 30 hours.

Patients with Renal Impairment

Approximately 5% of total radioactivity was excreted in the urine following a 3 mg dose of [^{14}C]-labeled everolimus. In a population pharmacokinetic analysis which included 170 patients with advanced cancer, no significant influence of creatinine clearance (25–178 mL/min) was detected on oral clearance (CL/F) of everolimus *[see Use in Specific Populations (8.6)]*.

Table 10: Adverse Reactions Reported in ≥10% of AFINITOR-treated Patients with SEGA in Study 1

	AFINITOR N=78			Placebo N=39		
	All grades %	Grade 3 %	Grade 4 %	All grades %	Grade 3 %	Grade 4 %
Any adverse reaction	**97**	**36**	**3**	**92**	**23**	**3**
Gastrointestinal disorders						
Stomatitis[a]	62	9	0	26	3	0
Vomiting	22	1	0	13	0	0
Diarrhea	17	0	0	5	0	0
Constipation	10	0	0	3	0	0
Infections and infestations						
Respiratory tract infection[b]	31	1	1	23	0	0
Gastroenteritis[c]	10	4	1	3	0	0
Pharyngitis streptococcal	10	0	0	3	0	0
General disorders and administration site conditions						
Pyrexia	23	6	0	18	3	0
Fatigue	14	0	0	3	0	0
Psychiatric disorders						
Anxiety, aggression or other behavioral disturbance[d]	21	5	0	3	0	0
Skin and subcutaneous tissue disorders						
Rash[e]	21	0	0	8	0	0
Acne	10	0	0	5	0	0

Grading according to CTCAE Version 3.0

[a] Includes mouth ulceration, stomatitis, and lip ulceration

[b] Includes respiratory tract infection, upper respiratory tract infection, and respiratory tract infection viral

[c] Includes gastroenteritis, gastroenteritis viral, and gastrointestinal infection

[d] Includes agitation, anxiety, panic attack, aggression, abnormal behavior, and obsessive compulsive disorder

[e] Includes rash, rash generalized, rash macular, rash maculo-papular, rash papular, dermatitis allergic, and urticaria

Table 11: Key Laboratory Abnormalities Reported in AFINITOR-treated Patients with SEGA in Study 1

	AFINITOR N=78			Placebo N=39		
	All grades %	Grade 3 %	Grade 4 %	All grades %	Grade 3 %	Grade 4 %
Hematology						
Elevated partial thromboplastin time	72	3	0	44	5	0
Neutropenia	46	9	0	41	3	0
Anemia	41	0	0	21	0	0
Clinical chemistry						
Hypercholesterolemia	81	0	0	39	0	0
Elevated aspartate transaminase (AST)	33	0	0	0	0	0
Hypertriglyceridemia	27	0	0	15	0	0
Elevated alanine transaminase (ALT)	18	0	0	3	0	0
Hypophosphatemia	9	1	0	3	0	0

Grading according to CTCAE Version 3.0

Patients with Hepatic Impairment

The safety, tolerability and pharmacokinetics of AFINITOR were evaluated in a single oral dose study of everolimus in subjects with impaired hepatic function relative to subjects with normal hepatic function. Compared to normal subjects (N=13), there was a 1.8-fold, 3.2-fold, and 3.6-fold increase in exposure (i.e. AUC) for subjects with mild (Child-Pugh class A, N=6), moderate (Child-Pugh class B, N=9), and severe (Child-Pugh class C, N=6) hepatic impairment, respectively. In another study, the average AUC of everolimus in eight subjects with moderate hepatic impairment (Child-Pugh class B) was twice that found in eight subjects with normal hepatic function.

For advanced HR+ BC, advanced PNET, advanced RCC, and renal angiomyolipoma with TSC patients with severe hepatic impairment, AFINITOR may be used at a reduced dose if the desired benefit outweighs the risk. For patients with moderate or mild hepatic impairment, a dose reduction is recommended *[see Dosage and Administration (2.2)]*.

For patients with SEGA and mild or moderate hepatic impairment, adjust the dose of AFINITOR Tablets or AFINITOR DISPERZ based on therapeutic drug monitoring. For patients with SEGA and severe hepatic impairment, reduce the starting dose of AFINITOR Tablets or AFINITOR DISPERZ by approximately 50% and adjust subsequent doses based on therapeutic drug monitoring *[see Dosage and Administration (2.4, 2.5)]*.

Effects of Age and Gender

In a population pharmacokinetic evaluation in cancer patients, no relationship was apparent between oral clearance and patient age or gender.

In patients with SEGA, the geometric mean C_{min} values normalized to mg/m^2 dose in patients aged < 10 years and 10 to 18 years were lower by 54% and 40%, respectively, than those observed in adults (> 18 years of age), suggesting that everolimus clearance normalized to body surface area was higher in pediatric patients as compared to adults.

Ethnicity

Based on a cross-study comparison, Japanese patients (n=6) had on average exposures that were higher than non-Japanese patients receiving the same dose.

Based on analysis of population pharmacokinetics, oral clearance (CL/F) is on average 20% higher in Black patients than in Caucasians.

The significance of these differences on the safety and efficacy of everolimus in Japanese or Black patients has not been established.

12.6 QT/QTc Prolongation Potential

In a randomized, placebo-controlled, crossover study, 59 healthy subjects were administered a single oral dose of AFINITOR (20 mg and 50 mg) and placebo. There is no indication of a QT/QTc prolonging effect of AFINITOR in single doses up to 50 mg.

13 NONCLINICAL TOXICOLOGY

13.1 Carcinogenesis, Mutagenesis, Impairment of Fertility

Administration of everolimus for up to 2 years did not indicate oncogenic potential in mice and rats up to the highest doses tested (0.9 mg/kg) corresponding respectively to 3.9 and 0.2 times the estimated clinical exposure (AUC_{0-24h}) at the 10 mg daily human dose.

Everolimus was not genotoxic in a battery of *in vitro* assays (Ames mutation test in *Salmonella*, mutation test in L5178Y mouse lymphoma cells, and chromosome aberration assay in V79 Chinese hamster cells). Everolimus was not genotoxic in an *in vivo* mouse bone marrow micronucleus test at doses up to 500 mg/kg/day (1500 mg/m^2/day, approximately 255-fold the 10 mg daily human dose, and 103-fold the maximum dose administered to patients with SEGA, based on the body surface area), administered as two doses, 24 hours apart.

Based on non-clinical findings, male fertility may be compromised by treatment with AFINITOR. In a 13-week male

Table 12: Progression-free Survival Results

Analysis	AFINITOR + exemestane[a] N = 485	Placebo + exemestane[a] N = 239	Hazard ratio	P-value
Median progression-free survival (months, 95% CI)				
Investigator radiological review	7.8 (6.9 to 8.5)	3.2 (2.8 to 4.1)	0.45[b] (0.38 to 0.54)	<0.0001[c]
Independent radiological review	11.0 (9.7 to 15.0)	4.1 (2.9 to 5.6)	0.38[b] (0.3 to 0.5)	<0.0001[c]
Best overall response (%, 95% CI)				
Objective response rate (ORR)[d]	12.6% (9.8 to 15.9)	1.7% (0.5 to 4.2)	n/a[e]	

[a] Exemestane (25 mg/day)
[b] Hazard ratio is obtained from the stratified Cox proportional-hazards model by sensitivity to prior hormonal therapy and presence of visceral metastasis
[c] p-value is obtained from the one-sided log-rank test stratified by sensitivity to prior hormonal therapy and presence of visceral metastasis
[d] Objective response rate = proportion of patients with CR or PR
[e] not applicable

Table 13: Progression-free Survival Results

Analysis	N	AFINITOR N=207	Placebo N=203	Hazard Ratio (95%CI)	p-value
	410	Median progression-free survival (months) (95% CI)			
Investigator radiological review		11.0 (8.4 to 13.9)	4.6 (3.1 to 5.4)	0.35 (0.27 to 0.45)	<0.001
Central radiological review		13.7 (11.2 to 18.8)	5.7 (5.4 to 8.3)	0.38 (0.28 to 0.51)	<0.001
Adjudicated radiological review[a]		11.4 (10.8 to 14.8)	5.4 (4.3 to 5.6)	0.34 (0.26 to 0.44)	<0.001

[a] includes adjudication for discrepant assessments between investigator radiological review and central radiological review

fertility study in rats, testicular morphology was affected at 0.5 mg/kg and above. Sperm motility, sperm count, and plasma testosterone levels were diminished in rats treated with 5 mg/kg. These doses result in exposures which are within the range of therapeutic exposure (52 ng.hr/mL and 414 ng.hr/mL respectively compared to 560 ng.hr/mL human exposure at 10 mg/day), and resulted in infertility in the rats at 5 mg/kg. Effects on male fertility occurred at the $AUC_{0\text{-}24h}$ values below that of therapeutic exposure (approximately 10%-81% of the $AUC_{0\text{-}24h}$ in patients receiving the 10 mg daily dose). After a 10-13 week non-treatment period, the fertility index increased from zero (infertility) to 60% (12/20 mated females were pregnant).

Oral doses of everolimus in female rats at ≥0.1 mg/kg (approximately 4% the $AUC_{0\text{-}24h}$ in patients receiving the 10 mg daily dose) resulted in increases in pre-implantation loss, suggesting that the drug may reduce female fertility. Everolimus crossed the placenta and was toxic to the conceptus *[see Use in Specific Populations (8.1)]*.

13.2 Animal Toxicology and/or Pharmacology

In juvenile rat toxicity studies, dose-related delayed attainment of developmental landmarks including delayed eye-opening, delayed reproductive development in males and females and increased latency time during the learning and memory phases were observed at doses as low as 0.15 mg/kg/day.

14 CLINICAL STUDIES

14.1 Advanced Hormone Receptor-Positive, HER2-Negative Breast Cancer

A randomized, double-blind, multicenter study of AFINITOR plus exemestane versus placebo plus exemestane was conducted in 724 postmenopausal women with estrogen receptor-positive, HER 2/neu-negative advanced breast cancer with recurrence or progression following prior therapy with letrozole or anastrozole. Randomization was stratified by documented sensitivity to prior hormonal therapy (yes vs. no) and by the presence of visceral metastasis (yes vs. no). Sensitivity to prior hormonal therapy was defined as either (1) documented clinical benefit (complete response [CR], partial response [PR], stable disease ≥ 24 weeks) to at least one prior hormonal therapy in the advanced setting or (2) at least 24 months of adjuvant hormonal therapy prior to recurrence. Patients were permitted to have received 0-1 prior lines of chemotherapy for advanced disease.

The primary endpoint for the trial was progression-free survival (PFS) evaluated by RECIST (Response Evaluation Criteria in Solid Tumors), based on investigator (local radiology) assessment. Other endpoints included overall survival (OS), objective response rate (ORR), and safety.

Patients were randomly allocated in a 2:1 ratio to AFINITOR 10 mg/day plus exemestane 25 mg/day (n = 485) or to placebo plus exemestane 25 mg/day (n = 239). The two treatment groups were generally balanced with respect to baseline demographics and disease characteristics. Patients were not permitted to cross over to AFINITOR at the time of disease progression.

The median progression-free survival by investigator assessment at the time of the final PFS analysis was 7.8 and 3.2 months in the AFINITOR and placebo arms, respectively [HR = 0.45 (95% CI: 0.38, 0.54), one-sided log-rank p < 0.0001] (see Table 12 and Figure 1). The results of the PFS analysis based on independent central radiological assessment were consistent with the investigator assessment. PFS results were also consistent across the subgroups of age, race, presence and extent of visceral metastases, and sensitivity to prior hormonal therapy.

Objective response rate was 12.6% (95% CI: 9.8, 15.9) in the AFINITOR plus exemestane arm vs. 1.7% (95% CI: 0.5, 4.2) in the placebo plus exemestane arm. There were 3 complete responses (0.6%) and 58 partial responses (12.0%) in the AFINITOR plus exemestane arm. There were no complete responses and 4 partial responses (1.7%) in the placebo plus exemestane arm.

The overall survival results were not mature at the time of the interim analysis, and no statistically significant treatment-related difference in OS was noted [HR=0.77 (95% CI: 0.57, 1.04)].

[See table 12 above]

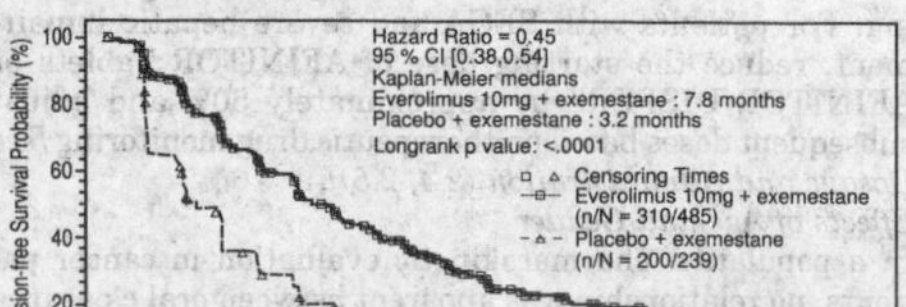

Figure 1: Kaplan-Meier Progression-free Survival Curves (Investigator Radiological Review)

14.2 Advanced Neuroendocrine Tumors

Locally Advanced or Metastatic Advanced Pancreatic Neuroendocrine Tumors (PNET)

A randomized, double-blind, multi-center trial of AFINITOR plus best supportive care (BSC) versus placebo plus BSC was conducted in patients with locally advanced or metastatic advanced pancreatic neuroendocrine tumors (PNET) and disease progression within the prior 12 months. Patients were stratified by prior cytotoxic chemotherapy (yes/no) and by WHO performance status (0 vs. 1 and 2). Treatment with somatostatin analogs was allowed as part of BSC. The primary endpoint for the trial was progression-free survival (PFS) evaluated by RECIST (Response Evaluation Criteria in Solid Tumors). After documented radiological progression, patients could be unblinded by the investigator; those randomized to placebo were then able to receive open-label AFINITOR. Other endpoints included safety, objective response rate [ORR (complete response (CR) or partial response (PR)], response duration, and overall survival.

Patients were randomized 1:1 to receive either AFINITOR 10 mg/day (n=207) or placebo (n=203). Demographics were well balanced (median age 58 years, 55% male, 79% Caucasian). Crossover from placebo to open-label AFINITOR occurred in 73% (148/203) of patients.

The trial demonstrated a statistically significant improvement in PFS (median 11.0 months versus 4.6 months), resulting in a 65% risk reduction in investigator-determined PFS (HR 0.35; 95%CI: 0.27 to 0.45; p<0.001) (see Table 13 and Figure 2). PFS improvement was observed across all patient subgroups, irrespective of prior somatostatin analog use. The PFS results by investigator radiological review, central radiological review and adjudicated radiological review are shown below in Table 13.

[See table 13 above]

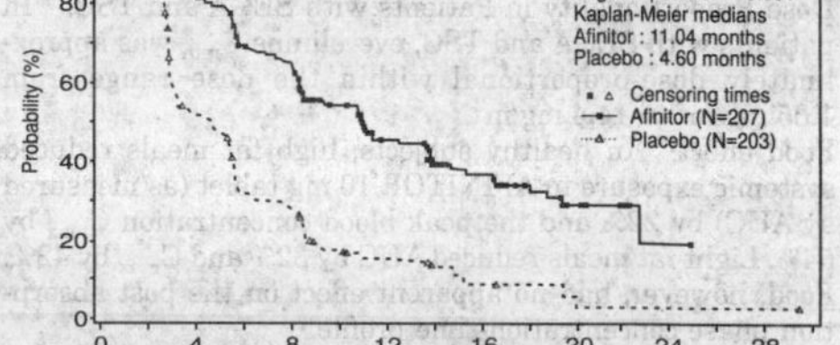

Figure 2: Kaplan-Meier Investigator-Determined Progression-free Survival Curves

Investigator-determined response rate was low (4.8%) in the AFINITOR arm and there were no complete responses. The overall survival results are not yet mature and no statistically significant treatment-related difference in OS was noted [HR=1.05 (95% CI: 0.71 to 1.55)].

Locally Advanced or Metastatic Carcinoid Tumors

In a randomized, double-blind, multi-center trial in 429 patients with carcinoid tumors, AFINITOR plus depot octreotide (Sandostatin LAR®) was compared to placebo plus depot octreotide. After documented radiological progression, patients could be unblinded by the investigator: those randomized to placebo were then able to receive open-label AFINITOR plus depot octreotide. The study did not meet the primary efficacy endpoint (PFS) and the OS interim analysis numerically favored the placebo plus depot octreotide arm. Therefore, the use of AFINITOR in patients with carcinoid tumors remains investigational.

14.3 Advanced Renal Cell Carcinoma

An international, multi-center, randomized, double-blind trial comparing AFINITOR 10 mg daily and placebo, both in conjunction with best supportive care, was conducted in patients with metastatic RCC whose disease had progressed despite prior treatment with sunitinib, sorafenib, or both sequentially. Prior therapy with bevacizumab, interleukin 2, or interferon-α was also permitted. Randomization was stratified according to prognostic score and prior anticancer therapy *[see References (15)]*.

Progression-free survival (PFS), documented using Response Evaluation Criteria in Solid Tumors (RECIST) was assessed via a blinded, independent, central radiologic review. After documented radiological progression, patients could be unblinded by the investigator: those randomized to placebo were then able to receive open-label AFINITOR 10 mg daily.

In total, 416 patients were randomized 2:1 to receive AFINITOR (n=277) or placebo (n=139). Demographics were well balanced between the two arms (median age 61 years; 77% male, 88% Caucasian, 74% received prior sunitinib or sorafenib, and 26% received both sequentially).

AFINITOR was superior to placebo for PFS (see Table 14 and Figure 3). The treatment effect was similar across prog-

nostic scores and prior sorafenib and/or sunitinib. Final overall survival (OS) results yield a hazard ratio of 0.90 (95% CI: 0.71 to 1.14), with no statistically significant difference between the two treatment groups. Planned crossover from placebo due to disease progression to open label AFINITOR occurred in 111 of the 139 patients (79.9%) and may have confounded the OS benefit.
[See table 14 above]

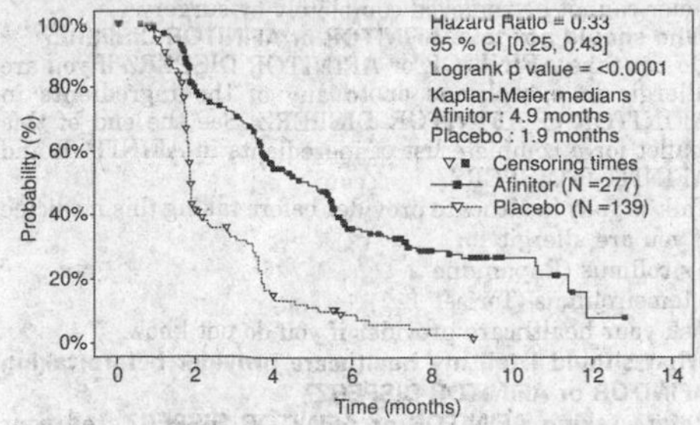

Figure 3: Kaplan-Meier Progression-free Survival Curves

Table 14: Efficacy Results by Central Radiologic Review

	AFINITOR N=277	Placebo N=139	Hazard Ratio (95% CI)	p-value [a]
Median Progression-free Survival (95% CI)	4.9 months (4.0 to 5.5)	1.9 months (1.8 to 1.9)	0.33 (0.25 to 0.43)	<0.0001
Objective Response Rate	2%	0%	n/a [b]	n/a [b]

[a] Log-rank test stratified by prognostic score.
[b] Not applicable.

14.4 Renal Angiomyolipoma with Tuberous Sclerosis Complex

A randomized (2:1), double-blind, placebo-controlled trial of AFINITOR was conducted in 118 patients with renal angiomyolipoma as a feature of TSC (n=113) or sporadic lymphangioleiomyomatosis (n=5).

The key eligibility requirements for this trial were at least one angiomyolipoma of ≥ 3 cm in longest diameter on CT/MRI based on local radiology assessment, no immediate indication for surgery, and age ≥ 18 years. Patients received daily oral AFINITOR 10 mg or matching placebo until disease progression or unacceptable toxicity. CT or MRI scans for disease assessment were obtained at baseline, 12, 24, and 48 weeks and annually thereafter. Clinical and photographic assessment of skin lesions were conducted at baseline and every 12 weeks thereafter until treatment discontinuation. The major efficacy outcome measure was angiomyolipoma response rate based on independent central radiology review, which was defined as a ≥ 50% reduction in angiomyolipoma volume, absence of new angiomyolipoma lesion ≥ 1 cm, absence of kidney volume increase ≥ 20%, and no angiomyolipoma related bleeding of ≥ grade 2. Key supportive efficacy outcome measures were time to angiomyolipoma progression and skin lesion response rate. Analyses of efficacy outcome measures were limited to the blinded treatment period which ended 6 months after the last patient was randomized. The comparative angiomyolipoma response rate analysis was stratified by use of enzyme-inducing antiepileptic drugs (EIAEDs) at randomization (yes/no).

Of the 118 patients enrolled, 79 were randomized to AFINITOR and 39 to placebo. The median age was 31 years (range 18 to 61 years), 34% were male, and 89% were Caucasian. At baseline, 17% of patients were receiving EIAEDs. On central radiology review at baseline, 92% of patients had at least one angiomyolipoma of ≥ 3 cm in longest diameter, 29% had angiomyolipomas ≥ 8 cm, 78% had bilateral angiomyolipomas, and 97% had skin lesions. The median values for the sum of all target renal angiomyolipoma lesions at baseline were 85 cm^3 (range 9 to 1612 cm^3) and 120 cm^3 (range 3 to 4520 cm^3) in the AFINITOR and placebo arms respectively. Forty-six (39%) patients had prior renal embolization or nephrectomy. The median duration of follow-up was 8.3 months (range 0.7 to 24.8 months).

The renal angiomyolipoma response rate was statistically significantly higher in AFINITOR-treated patients; there were 33 (41.8%) patients with angiomyolipoma responses in the AFINITOR arm as compared to none in the placebo arm. Results are displayed in Table 15. The median response duration is 5.3+ months (range 2.3+ to 19.6+ months).

Table 15: Angiomyolipoma Response

	AFINITOR N=79	Placebo N=39	p-value
Primary analysis			
Angiomyolipoma response rate[a] - %	**41.8**	**0**	**<0.0001**
95% CI	(30.8, 53.4)	(0.0, 9.0)	

[a] Per independent central radiology review

There were 3 patients in the AFINITOR arm and 8 patients in the placebo arm with documented angiomyolipoma progression by central radiologic review. The time to angiomyolipoma progression was statistically significantly longer in the AFINITOR arm (HR 0.08 [95% CI: 0.02, 0.37]; p <0.0001).

Skin lesion response rates were assessed by local investigators in 77 patients in the AFINITOR arm and 37 patients in the placebo arm with skin lesions at study entry. The skin lesion response rate was statistically significantly higher in the AFINITOR arm (26% vs. 0, p=0.0011); all skin lesion responses were partial responses, defined as visual improvement in 50%-99% skin lesions, considering all skin lesions, durable for at least eight weeks (Physician's Global Assessment of Clinical Condition).

14.5 Subependymal Giant Cell Astrocytoma with Tuberous Sclerosis Complex

Study 1 was a randomized (2:1), double-blind, placebo-controlled trial of AFINITOR Tablets conducted in 117 pediatric and adult patients with subependymal giant cell astrocytoma (SEGA) and tuberous sclerosis complex (TSC). Eligible patients had at least one SEGA lesion ≥ 1.0 cm in longest diameter on MRI based on local radiology assessment and one or more of the following: serial radiological evidence of SEGA growth, a new SEGA lesion ≥ 1 cm in longest diameter, or new or worsening hydrocephalus. Patients randomized to the treatment arm received AFINITOR Tablets at a starting dose of 4.5 mg/m^2 daily, with subsequent dose adjustments as needed to achieve and maintain everolimus trough concentrations of 5 to 15 ng/mL as tolerated. AFINITOR/matched placebo treatment continued until disease progression or unacceptable toxicity. MRI scans for disease assessment were obtained at baseline, 12, 24, and 48 weeks, and annually thereafter.

The main efficacy outcome measure was SEGA response rate based on independent central radiology review. SEGA response was defined as a ≥ 50% reduction in the sum of SEGA volume relative to baseline, in the absence of unequivocal worsening of non-target SEGA lesions, a new SEGA lesion ≥ 1 cm, and new or worsening hydrocephalus. Analysis of SEGA response rate was limited to the blinded treatment period which ended 6 months after the last patient was randomized. The analysis of SEGA response rate was stratified by use of enzyme-inducing antiepileptic drugs (EIAEDs) at randomization (yes/no).

Of the 117 patients enrolled, 78 were randomized to AFINITOR and 39 to placebo. The median age was 9.5 years (range 0.8 to 26 years; 69% were 3 to < 18 years at enrollment; 17% were < 3 years at enrollment), 57% were male, and 93% were Caucasian. At baseline, 18% of patients were receiving EIAEDs. Based on central radiology review at baseline, 98% of patients had at least one SEGA lesion ≥ 1.0 cm in longest diameter, 79% had bilateral SEGAs, 43% had ≥ 2 target SEGA lesions, 26% had growth in or into the inferior surface of the ventricle, 9% had evidence of growth beyond the subependymal tissue adjacent to the ventricle, and 7% had radiographic evidence of hydrocephalus. The median values for the sum of all target SEGA lesions at baseline were 1.63 cm^3 (range 0.18 to 25.15 cm^3) and 1.30 cm^3 (range 0.32 to 9.75 cm^3) in the AFINITOR and placebo arms respectively. Eight (7%) patients had prior SEGA-related surgery. The median duration of follow-up was 8.4 months (range 4.6 to 17.2 months).

The SEGA response rate was statistically significantly higher in AFINITOR-treated patients. There were 27 (35%) patients with SEGA responses in the AFINITOR arm and no SEGA responses in the placebo arm. Results are displayed in Table 16. At the time of the final analysis, all SEGA responses were ongoing and the median duration of response was 5.3 months (range 2.1 to 8.4 months). No patient in either treatment arm required surgical intervention during the course of Study 1.

Table 16: SEGA response

	AFINITOR N=78	Placebo N=39	p-value
Final analysis			
SEGA response rate[a] - (%)	**35**	**0**	**<0.0001**
95% CI	24, 46	0, 9	

[a] Per independent central radiology review

With a median follow-up of 8.4 months, SEGA progression was detected in 6 of 39 (15.4%) patients randomized to receive placebo and none of the 78 patients randomized to receive AFINITOR.

Study 2 was an open-label, single-arm trial conducted to evaluate the safety and efficacy of AFINITOR in patients with SEGA and TSC. Serial radiological evidence of SEGA growth was required for entry. Change in SEGA volume at the end of the core 6-month treatment phase was assessed via independent central radiology review. In total, 28 patients received treatment with AFINITOR; median age was 11 years (range 3-34), 61% male, 86% Caucasian. Four patients had surgical resection of their SEGA lesions with subsequent re-growth prior to receiving AFINITOR treatment. After the core treatment phase, patients could continue to receive AFINITOR treatment as part of an extension treatment phase where SEGA volume was assessed every 6 months. The median duration of treatment was 34.2 months (range 4.7-47.1 months).

At 6 months, 9 out of 28 patients (32%, 95% CI: 16% to 52%) had a ≥ 50% reduction in the tumor volume of their largest SEGA lesion. The median duration of response for these 9 patients was 11.8 months (range 3.2 to 39.1 months). Seven of these 9 patients had an ongoing volumetric reduction of ≥ 50% at the data cutoff.

Three of 4 patients who had prior surgery experienced a ≥ 50% reduction in the tumor volume of their largest SEGA lesion. One of these three patients responded by month 6. No patient developed new lesions.

15 REFERENCES

- Motzer RJ, Bacik J, Schwartz LH, et al. Prognostic factors for survival in previously treated patients with metastatic renal cell cancer. J Clin Oncol (2004) 22:454-63.
- NIOSH Alert: Preventing occupational exposures to antineoplastic and other hazardous drugs in healthcare settings. 2004. U.S. Department of Health and Human Services, Public Health Service, Centers for Disease Control and Prevention, National Institute for Occupational Safety and Health, DHHS (NIOSH) Publication No. 2004-165.
- OSHA Technical Manual, TED 1-0.15A, Section VI: Chapter 2. Controlling Occupational Exposure to Hazardous Drugs. OSHA, 1999. http://www.osha.gov/dts/osta/otm/otm_vi/otm_vi_2.html
- American Society of Health-System Pharmacists. ASHP guidelines on handling hazardous drugs. Am J Health-Syst Pharm. (2006) 63:1172-93.
- Polovich, M., White, J. M., & Kelleher, L.O. (eds.) 2005. Chemotherapy and biotherapy guidelines and recommendations for practice (2nd. ed.) Pittsburgh, PA: Oncology Nursing Society.

16 HOW SUPPLIED/STORAGE AND HANDLING

AFINITOR (everolimus) Tablets

2.5 mg tablets

White to slightly yellow, elongated tablets with a bevelled edge and no score, engraved with "LCL" on one side and "NVR" on the other; available in:

Blisters of 28 tablets .... NDC 0078-0594-51

Each carton contains 4 blister cards of 7 tablets each

5 mg tablets

White to slightly yellow, elongated tablets with a bevelled edge and no score, engraved with "5" on one side and "NVR" on the other; available in:

Blisters of 28 tablets .... NDC 0078-0566-51

Each carton contains 4 blister cards of 7 tablets each

7.5 mg tablets

White to slightly yellow, elongated tablets with a bevelled edge and no score, engraved with "7P5" on one side and "NVR" on the other; available in:

Blisters of 28 tablets .... NDC 0078-0620-51

Each carton contains 4 blister cards of 7 tablets each

10 mg tablets

White to slightly yellow, elongated tablets with a bevelled edge and no score, engraved with "UHE" on one side and "NVR" on the other; available in:

Blisters of 28 tablets .... NDC 0078-0567-51

Each carton contains 4 blister cards of 7 tablets each

AFINITOR DISPERZ (everolimus tablets for oral suspension)
2 mg tablets for oral suspension
White to slightly yellowish, round, flat tablets with a bevelled edge and no score, engraved with "D2" on one side and "NVR" on the other; available in:
Blisters of 28 tablets .... NDC 0078-0626-51
Each carton contains 4 blister cards of 7 tablets each
3 mg tablets for oral suspension
White to slightly yellowish, round, flat tablets with a bevelled edge and no score, engraved with "D3" on one side and "NVR" on the other; available in:
Blisters of 28 tablets .... NDC 0078-0627-51
Each carton contains 4 blister cards of 7 tablets each
5 mg tablets for oral suspension
White to slightly yellowish, round, flat tablets with a bevelled edge and no score, engraved with "D5" on one side and "NVR" on the other; available in:
Blisters of 28 tablets .... NDC 0078-0628-51
Each carton contains 4 blister cards of 7 tablets each
Store AFINITOR (everolimus) Tablets and AFINITOR DISPERZ (everolimus tablets for oral suspension) at 25°C (77°F); excursions permitted between 15°–30°C (59°–86°F). See USP Controlled Room Temperature. Store in the original container, protect from light and moisture. Keep this and all drugs out of the reach of children.
Procedures for proper handling and disposal of anticancer drugs should be considered. Several guidelines on this subject have been published *[see References (15)]*.
AFINITOR tablets should not be crushed. Do not take tablets which are crushed or broken.

17 PATIENT COUNSELING INFORMATION

17.1 Non-infectious Pneumonitis
Warn patients of the possibility of developing non-infectious pneumonitis. In clinical studies, some non-infectious pneumonitis cases have been severe and occasionally fatal. Advise patients to report promptly any new or worsening respiratory symptoms *[see Warnings and Precautions (5.1)]*.
17.2 Infections
Inform patients that they are more susceptible to infections while being treated with AFINITOR and that cases of hepatitis B reactivation have been associated with AFINITOR treatment. In clinical studies, some of these infections have been severe (e.g., leading to respiratory or hepatic failure) and occasionally fatal. Patients should be aware of the signs and symptoms of infection and should report any such signs or symptoms promptly to their physician *[see Warnings and Precautions (5.2)]*.
17.3 Oral Ulceration
Inform patients of the possibility of developing mouth ulcers, stomatitis, and oral mucositis. In such cases, mouthwashes and/or topical treatments are recommended, but these should not contain alcohol, peroxide, iodine, or thyme *[see Warnings and Precautions (5.3)]*.
17.4 Renal Failure
Inform patients of the possibility of developing kidney failure. In some cases kidney failure has been severe and occasionally fatal. Inform patients of the need for the healthcare provider to monitor kidney function, especially in patients with risk factors that may impair kidney function *[see Warnings and Precautions (5.4)]*.
17.5 Laboratory Tests and Monitoring
Inform patients of the need to monitor blood chemistry and hematology prior to the start of AFINITOR therapy and periodically thereafter *[see Warnings and Precautions (5.6)]*.
17.6 Drug-drug Interactions
Advise patients to inform their healthcare providers of all concomitant medications, including over-the-counter medications and dietary supplements. Inform the patients to avoid concomitant administration of strong CYP3A4 inhibitors or inducers while on AFINITOR treatment *[see Dosage and Administration (2.2, 2.5), Warnings and Precautions (5.7), Drug Interactions (7.1, 7.2)]*.
17.7 Vaccinations
Advise patients to avoid the use of live vaccines and close contact with those who have received live vaccines *[see Warnings and Precautions (5.9)]*.
17.8 Embryo-fetal Toxicity
Advise female patients of childbearing potential that AFINITOR may cause fetal harm and that a highly effective method of contraception should be used during therapy with AFINITOR and for 8 weeks after ending treatment *[see Warnings and Precautions (5.10)]*.
17.9 Safe Handling Practices for AFINITOR DISPERZ
Advise patients and their caregivers to read and carefully follow the FDA approved AFINITOR DISPERZ "Instructions for Use" to minimize unintended exposure to AFINITOR.
17.10 Dosing Instructions
Advise patients that AFINITOR is available in two dosage forms: tablets (AFINITOR Tablets) and tablets for oral suspension (AFINITOR DISPERZ). AFINITOR DISPERZ is recommended only for the treatment of patients with SEGA and TSC in conjunction with therapeutic drug monitoring *[see Dosage and Administration (2) and Clinical Pharmacology (12.3)]*.
Inform patients to take AFINITOR Tablets orally once daily at the same time every day, either consistently with food or consistently without food. Inform patients that AFINITOR Tablets should be swallowed whole with a glass of water.
Inform patients that AFINITOR DISPERZ should be taken as a suspension only and should not be swallowed whole. The suspension should be taken orally once daily at the same time every day, either consistently with food or consistently without food. Review the procedures for preparation of the AFINITOR DISPERZ suspension with patients *[see Dosage and Administration (2.7)]*. Refer patients to the "Instructions for Use" pamphlet for additional information regarding these procedures.
Instruct patients that if they miss a dose of AFINITOR, they may still take it up to 6 hours after the time they would normally take it. If more than 6 hours have elapsed, they should be instructed to skip the dose for that day. The next day, they should take AFINITOR at the usual time. Warn patients to not take 2 doses to make up for the one that they missed.

PATIENT INFORMATION
AFINITOR® (a-fin-it-or)
(everolimus)
Tablets
AFINITOR® DISPERZ (a-fin-it-or dis-perz)
(everolimus tablets for oral suspension)
Read this Patient Information leaflet that comes with AFINITOR or AFINITOR DISPERZ before you start taking it and each time you get a refill. There may be new information. This information does not take the place of talking to your healthcare provider about your medical condition or treatment.
What is the most important information I should know about AFINITOR and AFINITOR DISPERZ?
AFINITOR and AFINITOR DISPERZ can cause serious side effects. These serious side effects include:
1. **You may develop lung or breathing problems.** In some people lung or breathing problems may be severe, and can even lead to death. Tell your healthcare provider right away if you have any of these symptoms:
- New or worsening cough
- Shortness of breath
- Chest pain
- Difficulty breathing or wheezing

2. **You may be more likely to develop an infection,** such as pneumonia, or a bacterial, fungal or viral infection. Viral infections may include active hepatitis B in people who have had hepatitis B in the past (reactivation). In some people these infections may be severe, and can even lead to death. You may need to be treated as soon as possible.
Tell your healthcare provider right away if you have a temperature of 100.5°F or above, chills, or do not feel well.
Symptoms of hepatitis B or infection may include the following:
- Fever
- Chills
- Skin rash
- Joint pain and inflammation
- Tiredness
- Loss of appetite
- Nausea
- Pale stools or dark urine
- Yellowing of the skin
- Pain in the upper right side of the stomach

3. **You may develop kidney failure.** In some people this may be severe and can even lead to death. Your healthcare provider should do tests to check your kidney function before and during your treatment with AFINITOR or AFINITOR DISPERZ.

If you have any of the serious side effects listed above, you may need to stop taking AFINITOR or AFINITOR DISPERZ for a while or use a lower dose. Follow your healthcare provider's instructions.
What is AFINITOR?
AFINITOR is a prescription medicine used to treat:
- advanced hormone receptor-positive, HER2-negative breast cancer, along with the medicine exemestane, in postmenopausal women who have already received certain other medicines for their cancer.
- adults with a type of pancreatic cancer known as pancreatic neuroendocrine tumor (PNET), that has progressed and cannot be treated with surgery.
  It is not known if AFINITOR is safe and effective in people with carcinoid tumors.
- adults with advanced kidney cancer (renal cell carcinoma or RCC) when certain other medicines have not worked.
- people with the following types of tumors that are seen with a genetic condition called tuberous sclerosis complex (TSC):
  - adults with a kidney tumor called angiomyolipoma, when their kidney tumor does not require surgery right away.
  - adults and children with a brain tumor called subependymal giant cell astrocytoma (SEGA) when the tumor cannot be removed completely by surgery.

What is AFINITOR DISPERZ?
AFINITOR DISPERZ is a prescription medicine used to treat:
- adults and children with a genetic condition called tuberous sclerosis complex (TSC) who have a brain tumor called subependymal giant cell astrocytoma (SEGA) when the tumor cannot be removed completely by surgery.

Who should not take AFINITOR or AFINITOR DISPERZ?
Do not take AFINITOR or AFINITOR DISPERZ if you are allergic to everolimus or to any of the ingredients in AFINITOR or AFINITOR DISPERZ. See the end of this leaflet for a complete list of ingredients in AFINITOR and AFINITOR DISPERZ.
Talk to your healthcare provider before taking this medicine if you are allergic to:
- sirolimus (Rapamune®)
- temsirolimus (Torisel®)

Ask your healthcare provider if you do not know.
What should I tell my healthcare provider before taking AFINITOR or AFINITOR DISPERZ?
Before taking AFINITOR or AFINITOR DISPERZ, tell your healthcare provider about all of your medical conditions, including if you:
- Have or have had kidney problems
- Have or have had liver problems
- Have diabetes or high blood sugar
- Have high blood cholesterol levels
- Have any infections
- Previously had hepatitis B
- Are scheduled to receive any vaccinations. You should not receive a "live vaccine" or be around people who have recently received a "live vaccine" during your treatment with AFINITOR or AFINITOR DISPERZ. If you are not sure about the type of immunization or vaccine, ask your healthcare provider.
- Have other medical conditions.
- Are pregnant, or could become pregnant. AFINITOR or AFINITOR DISPERZ can cause harm to your unborn baby. You should use effective birth control while using AFINITOR or AFINITOR DISPERZ and for 8 weeks after stopping treatment.
- Are breastfeeding or plan to breastfeed. It is not known if AFINITOR or AFINITOR DISPERZ passes into your breast milk. You and your healthcare provider should decide if you will take AFINITOR or AFINITOR DISPERZ, or breastfeed. You should not do both.

Tell your healthcare provider about all of the medicines you take, including prescription and non-prescription medicines, vitamins, and herbal supplements.
AFINITOR or AFINITOR DISPERZ may affect the way other medicines work, and other medicines can affect how AFINITOR or AFINITOR DISPERZ work. Using AFINITOR or AFINITOR DISPERZ with other medicines can cause serious side effects.
Know the medicines you take. Keep a list of them and show it to your healthcare provider and pharmacist when you get a new medicine. Especially tell your healthcare provider if you take:
- St. John's Wort (Hypericum perforatum)
- Medicine for:
  - Fungal infections
  - Bacterial infections
  - Tuberculosis
  - Seizures
  - HIV-AIDS
  - Heart conditions or high blood pressure
- Medicines that weaken your immune system (your body's ability to fight infections and other problems)

Ask your healthcare provider or pharmacist if you are not sure if your medicine is one of those taken for the conditions listed above. If you are taking any medicines for the conditions listed above, your healthcare provider might need to prescribe a different medicine or your dose of AFINITOR or AFINITOR DISPERZ may need to be changed. You should also tell your healthcare provider before you start taking any new medicine.
How should I take AFINITOR or AFINITOR DISPERZ?
- Your healthcare provider will prescribe the dose of AFINITOR or AFINITOR DISPERZ that is right for you.
- Take AFINITOR or AFINITOR DISPERZ exactly as your healthcare provider tells you to.
- Your healthcare provider may change your dose of AFINITOR or AFINITOR DISPERZ if needed.
- Use scissors to open the blister pack.

AFINITOR:
- Swallow AFINITOR tablets whole with a glass of water. Do not take any tablet that is broken or crushed.

AFINITOR DISPERZ:
- If your healthcare provider prescribes AFINITOR DISPERZ for you, see the "Instructions for Use" that come with your medicine for instructions on how to prepare and take your dose.

- Each dose of AFINITOR DISPERZ must be prepared as a suspension before it is given.
- AFINITOR DISPERZ can cause harm to an unborn baby. When possible, the suspension should be prepared by an adult who is not pregnant or planning to become pregnant.
- Anyone who prepares suspensions of AFINITOR DISPERZ for another person should wear gloves to avoid possible contact with the medicine.
- Take AFINITOR or AFINITOR DISPERZ one time each day at about the same time.
- Take AFINITOR or AFINITOR DISPERZ the same way each time, either with food or without food.
- If you take too much AFINITOR or AFINITOR DISPERZ contact your healthcare provider or go to the nearest hospital emergency department right away. Take the pack of AFINITOR or AFINITOR DISPERZ with you.
- If you miss a dose of AFINITOR or AFINITOR DISPERZ, you may still take it up to 6 hours after the time you normally take it. If it is more than 6 hours after you normally take your AFINITOR or AFINITOR DISPERZ, skip the dose for that day. The next day, take AFINITOR or AFINITOR DISPERZ at your usual time. Do not take 2 doses to make up for the one that you missed. If you are not sure about what to do, call your healthcare provider.
- You should have blood tests before you start AFINITOR or AFINITOR DISPERZ and as needed during your treatment. These will include tests to check your blood cell count, kidney and liver function, cholesterol, and blood sugar levels.
- If you take AFINITOR or AFINITOR DISPERZ to treat SEGA, you will also need to have blood tests regularly to measure how much medicine is in your blood. This will help your healthcare provider decide how much AFINITOR or AFINITOR DISPERZ you need to take.

What should I avoid while taking AFINITOR or AFINITOR DISPERZ?

You should not drink grapefruit juice or eat grapefruit during your treatment with AFINITOR or AFINITOR DISPERZ. It may make the amount of AFINITOR in your blood increase to a harmful level.

What are the possible side effects of AFINITOR or AFINITOR DISPERZ?

AFINITOR and AFINITOR DISPERZ can cause serious side effects.

- **See "What is the most important information I should know about AFINITOR and AFINITOR DISPERZ?" for more information.**

Common side effects of AFINITOR in people with advanced hormone receptor-positive, HER 2-negative breast cancer, advanced pancreatic neuroendocrine tumors, and advanced kidney cancer include:

- Mouth ulcers. AFINITOR can cause mouth ulcers and sores. Tell your healthcare provider if you have pain, discomfort, or open sores in your mouth. Your healthcare provider may tell you to use a special mouthwash or mouth gel that does not contain alcohol, peroxide, iodine, or thyme.
- Infections
- Feeling weak or tired
- Cough, shortness of breath
- Diarrhea and constipation
- Rash, dry skin, and itching
- Nausea and vomiting
- Fever
- Loss of appetite, weight loss
- Swelling of arms, hands, feet, ankles, face or other parts of the body
- Abnormal taste
- Dry mouth
- Inflammation of lining of the digestive system
- Headache
- Nose bleeds
- Pain in arms and legs, mouth and throat, back or joints
- High blood glucose
- High blood pressure
- Difficulty sleeping
- Hair loss
- Muscle spasms
- Feeling dizzy
- Nail disorders

Common side effects of AFINITOR and AFINITOR DISPERZ in people who have SEGA or renal angiomyolipoma with TSC include:

- Mouth ulcers. AFINITOR can cause mouth ulcers and sores. Tell your healthcare provider if you have pain, discomfort, or open sores in your mouth. Your healthcare provider may tell you to use a special mouthwash or mouth gel that does not contain alcohol, peroxide iodine, or thyme.
- Infections
- Nausea and vomiting
- Diarrhea and constipation
- Swelling of your hands, arms, legs, and feet
- Joint pain
- Cough
- Skin problems (such as rash, acne, or dry skin)
- Fever
- Feeling tired
- Anxiety, aggression, and other abnormal behaviors
- Absence of menstrual periods (menstruation). You may miss one or more menstrual periods. Tell your healthcare provider if this happens.
- Low red blood cells, white blood cells or platelets
- Increased blood cholesterol level and certain other blood tests
- Increased blood sugar levels
- Decreased blood phosphate levels

Tell your healthcare provider if you have any side effect that bothers you or does not go away.

These are not all the possible side effects of AFINITOR and AFINITOR DISPERZ. For more information, ask your healthcare provider or pharmacist.

Call your doctor for medical advice about side effects. You may report side effects to FDA at 1-800-FDA-1088.

How should I store AFINITOR or AFINITOR DISPERZ?

- Store AFINITOR or AFINITOR DISPERZ at room temperature, between 68°F to 77°F (20°C to 25°C).
- Keep AFINITOR or AFINITOR DISPERZ in the pack it comes in.
- Open the blister pack just before taking AFINITOR or AFINITOR DISPERZ.
- Keep AFINITOR or AFINITOR DISPERZ dry and away from light.
- Do not use AFINITOR or AFINITOR DISPERZ that is out of date or no longer needed.

Keep AFINITOR or AFINITOR DISPERZ and all medicines out of the reach of children.

General information about AFINITOR and AFINITOR DISPERZ

Medicines are sometimes prescribed for purposes other than those listed in a Patient Information leaflet. Do not use AFINITOR or AFINITOR DISPERZ for a condition for which it was not prescribed. Do not give AFINITOR or AFINITOR DISPERZ to other people, even if they have the same problem you have. It may harm them.

This leaflet summarizes the most important information about AFINITOR and AFINITOR DISPERZ. If you would like more information, talk with your healthcare provider. You can ask your healthcare provider or pharmacist for information written for healthcare professionals.

For more information call 1-888-423-4648 or go to www.AFINITOR.com.

What are the ingredients in AFINITOR?

Active ingredient: everolimus.

Inactive ingredients: anhydrous lactose, butylated hydroxytoluene, crospovidone, hypromellose, lactose monohydrate, and magnesium stearate.

What are the ingredients in AFINITOR DISPERZ?

Active ingredient: everolimus.

Inactive ingredients: butylated hydroxytoluene, colloidal silicon dioxide, crospovidone, hypromellose, lactose monohydrate, magnesium stearate, mannitol, and microcrystalline cellulose.

This Patient Information has been approved by the U.S. Food and Drug Administration.

Manufactured by:
Novartis Pharma Stein AG
Stein, Switzerland

Distributed by:
Novartis Pharmaceuticals Corporation
East Hanover, New Jersey 07936

The brands listed are the trademarks or register marks of their respective owners and are not trademarks or register marks of Novartis.

T2012-153/T2012-154
August 2012/August 2012

Shown in Product Identification Guide, page 309

AMTURNIDE ℞

(aliskiren, amlodipine and hydrochlorothiazide) tablets, for oral use

The following prescribing information is based on official labeling in effect July 2013.

HIGHLIGHTS OF PRESCRIBING INFORMATION

These highlights do not include all the information needed to use AMTURNIDE safely and effectively. See full prescribing information for AMTURNIDE.

Amturnide (aliskiren, amlodipine and hydrochlorothiazide) tablets, for oral use

Initial U.S. Approval: 2010

WARNING: FETAL TOXICITY

See full prescribing information for complete boxed warning.

- **When pregnancy is detected, discontinue Amturnide as soon as possible. (5.1)**
- **Drugs that act directly on the renin-angiotensin system can cause injury and death to the developing fetus. (5.1)**

RECENT MAJOR CHANGES

Boxed Warning: Fetal Toxicity	02/2012
Contraindications: Concomitant use with ARBs or ACEIs in diabetes (4)	03/2012
Contraindications (4)	09/2012
Warnings and Precautions (5.1, 5.13)	02/2012
Warnings and Precautions (5.2, 5.4, 5.6, 5.10)	03/2012
Warnings and Precautions (5.3)	09/2012
Warnings and Precautions (5.4, 5.5)	09/2012

INDICATIONS AND USAGE

Amturnide is a combination of aliskiren, a renin inhibitor, amlodipine besylate, a dihydropyridine calcium channel blocker, and hydrochlorothiazide (HCTZ), a thiazide diuretic. Amturnide is indicated for the treatment of hypertension, to lower blood pressure. Lowering blood pressure reduces the risk of fatal and nonfatal cardiovascular events, primarily strokes and myocardial infarctions:

- Not indicated for initial therapy. (1)

DOSAGE AND ADMINISTRATION

- Dose once-daily. Titrate as needed up to a maximum dose of 300/10/25 mg.
- Amturnide may be used as add-on/switch therapy for patients not adequately controlled on any two of the following: aliskiren, dihydropyridine calcium channel blockers, and thiazide diuretics. (2.2)
- Amturnide may be substituted for its individually titrated aliskiren, amlodipine and HCTZ. (2.3)

DOSAGE FORMS AND STRENGTHS

Tablets (aliskiren/ amlodipine/ HCTZ): 150/5/12.5, 300/5/12.5, 300/5/25, 300/10/12.5, 300/10/25 mg. (3)

CONTRAINDICATIONS

- Do not use with angiotensin receptor blockers (ARBs) or ACE inhibitors (ACEI) in patients with diabetes (4)
- Anuria (4)
- Hypersensitivity to sulfonamide-derived drugs or to any of the components (4)

WARNINGS AND PRECAUTIONS

- Avoid concomitant use with ARBs or ACEIs in patients with renal impairment (GFR<60 mL/min) (5.2)
- Anaphylactic Reactions and Head and Neck Angioedema: Discontinue Amturnide and monitor until signs and symptoms resolve. (5.3)
- Hypotension: Correct volume depletion prior to initiation. (5.4)
- Increased angina or myocardial infarction may occur upon dosage initiation or increase in amlodipine. (5.5)
- Impaired renal function: Monitor serum creatinine periodically (5.6)
- HCTZ may exacerbate or activate systemic lupus erythematosus. (5.8)
- Hyperkalemia: Monitor potassium levels periodically. (5.10)
- Acute myopia and secondary angle closure glaucoma: Discontinue HCTZ. (5.12)
- Hypersensitivity Reactions: May occur from HCTZ component. (5.7)

ADVERSE REACTIONS

The most common adverse events (incidence ≥2%) are: peripheral edema, dizziness, headache and nasopharyngitis. (6.1)

To report SUSPECTED ADVERSE REACTIONS, contact Novartis Pharmaceuticals Corporation at 1-888-669-6682 or FDA at 1-800-FDA-1088 or www.fda.gov/medwatch.

DRUG INTERACTIONS

- Cyclosporine: Avoid concomitant use (7, 12.3)
- Itraconazole: Avoid concomitant use (7, 12.3)
- NSAIDs use may lead to increased risk of renal impairment and loss of antihypertensive effect (7)
- If simvastatin is co-administered with amlodipine, do not exceed doses greater than 20 mg daily of simvastatin (7)
- Antidiabetic Drugs: Antidiabetic dosage adjustment may be required. (7)
- Cholestyramine and Colestipol: Reduce absorption of thiazides. (7)
- Lithium: Increased risk of lithium toxicity when used with diuretics. Monitor serum lithium concentrations during concurrent use. (7)

USE IN SPECIFIC POPULATIONS

Nursing Mothers: Discontinue drug or nursing. (8.3)

See 17 for PATIENT COUNSELING INFORMATION and FDA-approved patient labeling

Revised: 09/2012

FULL PRESCRIBING INFORMATION: CONTENTS*

*** Sections or subsections omitted from the full prescribing information are not listed**

FULL PRESCRIBING INFORMATION

WARNING: FETAL TOXICITY
- **When pregnancy is detected, discontinue Amturnide as soon as possible. (5.1)**
- **Drugs that act directly on the renin-angiotensin system can cause injury and death to the developing fetus. (5.1)**

1 INDICATIONS AND USAGE

Amturnide is indicated for the treatment of hypertension, to lower blood pressure. Lowering blood pressure reduces the risk of fatal and nonfatal cardiovascular events, primarily strokes and myocardial infarctions. These benefits have been seen in controlled trials of antihypertensive drugs from a wide variety of pharmacologic classes, including amlodipine and hydrochlorothiazide. There are no controlled trials demonstrating risk reduction with Amturnide. Control of high blood pressure should be part of comprehensive cardiovascular risk management, including, as appropriate, lipid control, diabetes management, antithrombotic therapy, smoking cessation, exercise, and limited sodium intake. Many patients will require more than one drug to achieve blood pressure goals. For specific advice on goals and management, see published guidelines, such as those of the National High Blood Pressure Education Program's Joint National Committee on Prevention, Detection, Evaluation, and Treatment of High Blood Pressure (JNC).

Numerous antihypertensive drugs, from a variety of pharmacologic classes and with different mechanisms of action, have been shown in randomized controlled trials to reduce cardiovascular morbidity and mortality, and it can be concluded that it is blood pressure reduction, and not some other pharmacologic property of the drugs, that is largely responsible for those benefits. The largest and most consistent cardiovascular outcome benefit has been a reduction in the risk of stroke, but reductions in myocardial infarction and cardiovascular mortality also have been seen regularly. Elevated systolic or diastolic pressure causes increased cardiovascular risk, and the absolute risk increase per mmHg is greater at higher blood pressures, so that even modest reductions of severe hypertension can provide substantial benefit. Relative risk reduction from blood pressure reduction is similar across populations with varying absolute risk, so the absolute benefit is greater in patients who are at higher risk independent of their hypertension (for example, patients with diabetes or hyperlipidemia), and such patients would be expected to benefit from more aggressive treatment to a lower blood pressure goal.

Some antihypertensive drugs have smaller blood pressure effects (as monotherapy) in black patients, and many antihypertensive drugs have additional approved indications and effects (e.g., on angina, heart failure, or diabetic kidney disease). These considerations may guide selection of therapy.

This fixed combination drug is not indicated for initial therapy of hypertension.

2 DOSAGE AND ADMINISTRATION

2.1 General Considerations

Dose once-daily. The dosage may be increased after 2 weeks of therapy. The maximum recommended dose of Amturnide is 300/10/25 mg.

2.2 Add-on/Switch Therapy

Use Amturnide for patients not adequately controlled with any two of the following: aliskiren, dihydropyridine calcium channel blockers, and thiazide diuretics.

Switch a patient who experiences dose-limiting adverse reactions attributed to an individual component—while on any dual combination of the components of Amturnide—to Amturnide at a lower dose of that component to achieve similar blood pressure reductions.

2.3 Replacement Therapy

For patients receiving aliskiren, amlodipine and HCTZ from separate tablets, substitute Amturnide containing the same component doses.

2.4 Relationship to Meals

Patients should establish a routine pattern for taking Amturnide, either with or without a meal. High-fat meals decrease absorption of aliskiren substantially *[see Clinical Pharmacology (12.3)]*.

3 DOSAGE FORMS AND STRENGTHS

Tablets are convex ovaloid with a beveled edge, film-coated, and unscored, in the following strengths:

Aliskiren/ Amlodipine/HCTZ (mg)	Color	Embossing Side 1/side 2
150/5/12.5	Violet white	YIY/NVR
300/5/12.5	Light pink	LIL/NVR
300/5/25	Pale orange brown	OIO/NVR
300/10/12.5	Light red	UIU/NVR
300/10/25	Brown	VIV/NVR

4 CONTRAINDICATIONS

Do not use aliskiren with ARBs or ACEIs in patients with diabetes *[see Warnings and Precautions (5.2), Clinical Studies (14.2)]*.

Amturnide is contraindicated in patients with anuria or hypersensitivity to sulfonamide-derived drugs like HCTZ or to any of the components *[see Warnings and Precautions (5.8) and Adverse Reactions (6.1)]*. Hypersensitivity reactions may range from urticaria to anaphylaxis.

5 WARNINGS AND PRECAUTIONS

5.1 Fetal Toxicity

Pregnancy Category D

Use of drugs that act on the renin-angiotensin system during the second and third trimesters of pregnancy reduces fetal renal function and increases fetal and neonatal morbidity and death. Resulting oligohydramnios can be associated with fetal lung hypoplasia and skeletal deformations. Potential neonatal adverse effects include skull hypoplasia, anuria, hypotension, renal failure, and death. When pregnancy is detected, discontinue Amturnide as soon as possible *[see Use in Specific Populations (8.1)]*.

5.2 Renal Impairment/Hyperkalemia/Hypotension when Amturnide is given in combination with ARBs or ACEIs

Amturnide is contraindicated in patients with diabetes who are receiving ARBs or ACEIs because of the increased risk of renal impairment, hyperkalemia, and hypotension *[see Contraindications (4) and Clinical Studies (14.2)]*.

Avoid use of Amturnide with ARBs or ACEI in patients with moderate renal impairment (GFR <60 ml/min).

5.3 Anaphylactic Reactions and Head and Neck Angioedema

Aliskiren

Hypersensitivity reactions such as anaphylactic reactions and angioedema of the face, extremities, lips, tongue, glottis and/or larynx have been reported in patients treated with aliskiren and has necessitated hospitalization and intubation. This may occur at any time during treatment and has occurred in patients with and without a history of angioedema with ACE inhibitors or angiotensin receptor antagonists. Anaphylactic reactions have been reported from postmarketing experience with unknown frequency. If angioedema involves the throat, tongue, glottis or larynx, or if the patient has a history of upper respiratory surgery, airway obstruction may occur and be fatal. Patients who experience these effects, even without respiratory distress, require prolonged observation and appropriate monitoring measures since treatment with antihistamines and corticosteroids may not be sufficient to prevent respiratory involvement. Prompt administration of subcutaneous epinephrine solution 1:1000 (0.3 to 0.5 mL) and measures to ensure a patent airway may be necessary.

Discontinue Amturnide immediately in patients who develop anaphylactic reactions or angioedema, and do not re-administer.

5.4 Hypotension

In patients with an activated renin-angiotensin-aldosterone system, such as volume- and/or salt-depleted patients receiving high doses of diuretics, symptomatic hypotension may occur in patients receiving renin-angiotensin-aldosterone system (RAAS) blockers. Correct these conditions prior to administration of Amturnide, or start the treatment under close medical supervision.

A transient hypotensive response is not a contraindication to further treatment, which usually can be continued without difficulty once the blood pressure has stabilized.

Amlodipine besylate

Symptomatic hypotension is possible, particularly in patients with severe aortic stenosis. Because of the gradual onset of action, acute hypotension is unlikely.

5.5 Risk of Myocardial Infarction or Increased Angina

Worsening angina and acute myocardial infarction can develop after starting or increasing the dose of amlodipine, particularly with severe obstructive coronary artery disease.

5.6 Impaired Renal Function

Monitor renal function periodically in patients treated with Amturnide. Changes in renal function, including acute renal failure, can be caused by drugs that affect the renin-angiotensin system and by diuretics. Patients whose renal function may depend in part on the activity of the renin-angiotensin system (e.g., patients with renal artery stenosis, severe heart failure, post-myocardial infarction or volume depletion) or patients receiving ARB, ACEI or nonsteroidal anti-inflammatory (NSAID) therapy may be at particular risk of developing acute renal failure on Amturnide *[see Contraindications (4), Warnings and Precautions (5.2), Clinical Studies (14.2)]*. Consider withholding or discontinuing therapy in patients who develop a clinically significant decrease in renal function on Amturnide.

5.7 Hypersensitivity Reactions

Hydrochlorothiazide

Hypersensitivity reactions to HCTZ may occur in patients with or without a history of allergy or bronchial asthma, but are more likely in patients with such a history.

5.8 Systemic Lupus Erythematosus

Thiazide diuretics have been reported to cause exacerbation or activation of systemic lupus erythematosus.

5.9 Lithium Interaction

Lithium generally should not be given with thiazides *[see Drug Interactions (7)]*.

5.10 Serum Electrolyte Abnormalities

Amturnide

In a short-term controlled trial the incidence of patients with hypertension not concomitantly treated with an ARB or ACEI who developed hypokalemia (serum potassium <3.5 mEq/L) was 11.0% of Amturnide-treated patients compared to 19.0% of amlodipine/HCTZ patients, 4.4% of aliskiren/HCTZ patients, and 2.1% of aliskiren/amlodipine patients; the incidence of hyperkalemia (serum potassium >5.5 mEq/L) was 3.0% compared to 2.0% of amlodipine/HCTZ patients, 0.7% of aliskiren/HCTZ patients, and 0.7% of aliskiren/amlodipine patients. No Amturnide-treated patients discontinued due to increase or decrease of serum potassium.

Aliskiren

Monitor serum potassium periodically in patients receiving aliskiren. Drugs that affect the renin-angiotensin system can cause hyperkalemia. Risk factors for the development of hyperkalemia include renal insufficiency, diabetes, combination use with ARBs or ACEI *[see Contraindications (4),*

Warnings and Precautions (5.2), and Clinical Studies (14.2)], NSAIDs, or potassium supplements or potassium sparing diuretics.

Hydrochlorothiazide

Hydrochlorothiazide can cause hypokalemia and hyponatremia. Hypomagnesemia can result in hypokalemia which appears difficult to treat despite potassium repletion.

If hypokalemia is accompanied by clinical signs (e.g., muscular weakness, paresis, or ECG alterations), Amturnide should be discontinued. Correction of hypokalemia and any coexisting hypomagnesemia is recommended prior to the initiation of thiazides.

5.11 Cyclosporine or Itraconazole

When aliskiren was given with cyclosporine or itraconazole, the blood concentrations of aliskiren were significantly increased. Avoid concomitant use of Amturnide with cyclosporine or itraconazole *[see Drug Interactions (7)]*.

5.12 Acute Myopia and Secondary Angle-Closure Glaucoma

Hydrochlorothiazide, a sulfonamide, can cause an idiosyncratic reaction, resulting in transient myopia and acute angle-closure glaucoma. Symptoms include acute onset of decreased visual acuity or ocular pain and typically occur within hours to weeks of drug initiation. Untreated acute angle-closure glaucoma can lead to permanent vision loss. The primary treatment is to discontinue hydrochlorothiazide as rapidly as possible. Prompt medical or surgical treatments may need to be considered if the intraocular pressure remains uncontrolled. Risk factors for developing acute angle-closure glaucoma may include a history of sulfonamide or penicillin allergy.

5.13 Metabolic Disturbances

Hydrochlorothiazide

Hydrochlorothiazide may alter glucose tolerance and raise serum levels of cholesterol and triglycerides.

Hydrochlorothiazide may raise the serum uric acid level due to reduced clearance of uric acid and may cause or exacerbate hyperuricemia and precipitate gout in susceptible patients.

Hydrochlorothiazide decreases urinary calcium excretion and may cause elevation of serum calcium. Monitor calcium levels in patients with hypercalcemia receiving Amturnide.

6 ADVERSE REACTIONS

6.1 Clinical Studies Experience

The following serious adverse reactions are discussed in greater detail in other sections of the label:

- Risk of fetal/neonatal morbidity and mortality *[see Warnings and Precautions (5.1)]*
- Head and neck angioedema *[see Warnings and Precautions (5.3)]*
- Hypotension *[see Warnings and Precautions (5.4)]*

Because clinical trials are conducted under widely varying conditions, adverse reaction rates observed in the clinical trials of a drug cannot be directly compared to rates in clinical trials of another drug and may not reflect the rates observed in practice.

Amturnide

Amturnide has been evaluated for safety in 1155 patients treated with Amturnide, including 182 patients for over 1 year.

In a short-term controlled trial, there were 60.5% males, 84.1% Caucasians, 10% Blacks, 6.4% Hispanics, and 19.1% who were ≥ 65 years of age. In this study, the overall incidence of adverse events on therapy with Amturnide was similar to that observed with the individual components. The overall frequency of adverse events was similar between men and women and Black and White patients. Discontinuation of therapy because of a clinical adverse event in this study occurred in 3.6% of patients treated with Amturnide versus 2.4% in aliskiren/amlodipine, 0.7% in aliskiren/HCTZ, and 2.7% in amlodipine/HCTZ.

Table 1. Adverse events in a short-term controlled trial that occurred in at least 2% of patients treated with Amturnide

	Amturnide	Ali/ amlo	Ali/ HCTZ	Amlo/ HCTZ
Edema peripheral	7.1%	8.0%	2.0%	4.1%
Dizziness	3.6%	2.4%	3.4%	1.7%
Headache	3.6%	3.1%	4.0%	5.1%
Nasopharyngitis	2.6%	0.7%	2.0%	3.4%

In a long-term safety trial, the safety profile was similar to that seen in the short-term controlled trial.

Aliskiren

Aliskiren has been evaluated for safety in 6460 patients, including 1740 treated for longer than 6 months, and 1250 for longer than 1 year. In placebo-controlled clinical trials, discontinuation of therapy because of a clinical adverse event, including uncontrolled hypertension, occurred in 2.2% of patients treated with aliskiren, versus 3.5% of patients given placebo. These data do not include information from the ALTITUDE study which evaluated the use of aliskiren in combination with ARBs or ACEI *[see Contraindications (4), Warnings and Precautions (5.2), and Clinical Studies (14.2)]*.

Two cases of angioedema with respiratory symptoms were reported with aliskiren use in the clinical studies. Two other cases of periorbital edema without respiratory symptoms were reported as possible angioedema and resulted in discontinuation. The rate of these angioedema cases in the completed studies was 0.06%.

In addition, 26 other cases of edema involving the face, hands, or whole body were reported with aliskiren use, including 4 leading to discontinuation.

In the placebo-controlled studies, however, the incidence of edema involving the face, hands, or whole body was 0.4% with aliskiren compared with 0.5% with placebo. In a long-term active-controlled study with aliskiren and HCTZ arms, the incidence of edema involving the face, hands, or whole body was 0.4% in both treatment arms.

Aliskiren produces dose-related gastrointestinal (GI) adverse reactions. Diarrhea was reported by 2.3% of patients at 300 mg, compared to 1.2% in placebo patients. In women and the elderly (age ≥65) increases in diarrhea rates were evident starting at a dose of 150 mg daily, with rates for these subgroups at 150 mg similar to those seen at 300 mg for men or younger patients (all rates about 2%). Other GI symptoms included abdominal pain, dyspepsia, and gastroesophageal reflux, although increased rates for abdominal pain and dyspepsia were distinguished from placebo only at 600 mg daily. Diarrhea and other GI symptoms were typically mild and rarely led to discontinuation.

Aliskiren was associated with a slight increase in cough in the placebo-controlled studies (1.1% for any aliskiren use versus 0.6% for placebo). In active-controlled trials with ACE inhibitor (ramipril, lisinopril) arms, the rates of cough for the aliskiren arms were about one-third to one-half the rates in the ACE inhibitor arms.

Other adverse reactions with increased rates for aliskiren compared to placebo included rash (1% versus 0.3%), and renal stones (0.2% versus 0%).

Single episodes of tonic-clonic seizures with loss of consciousness were reported in 2 patients treated with aliskiren in the clinical trials. One patient had predisposing causes for seizures and had a negative electroencephalogram (EEG) and cerebral imaging following the seizures; for the other patient, EEG and imaging results were not reported. Aliskiren was discontinued and there was no rechallenge in either case.

No clinically meaningful changes in vital signs or in ECG (including QTc interval) were observed in patients treated with aliskiren.

Amlodipine

Amlodipine (Norvasc®) has been evaluated for safety in more than 11,000 patients in U.S. and foreign clinical trials. Other adverse events that have been reported at <1% but >0.1% of patients in controlled clinical trials or under conditions of open trials or marketing experience where a causal relationship is uncertain were:

Cardiovascular: arrhythmia (including ventricular tachycardia and atrial fibrillation), bradycardia, chest pain, peripheral ischemia, syncope, postural hypotension, vasculitis

Central and Peripheral Nervous System: neuropathy peripheral, paresthesia, tremor, vertigo

Gastrointestinal: anorexia, constipation, dyspepsia,** dysphagia, diarrhea, flatulence, pancreatitis, vomiting, gingival hyperplasia

General: allergic reaction, asthenia,** back pain, hot flushes, malaise, pain, rigors, weight gain, weight decrease

Musculoskeletal System: arthralgia, arthrosis, muscle cramps,** myalgia

Psychiatric: sexual dysfunction (male** and female), insomnia, nervousness, depression, abnormal dreams, anxiety, depersonalization

Respiratory System: dyspnea, epistaxis

Skin and Appendages: angioedema, erythema multiforme, pruritus,** rash,** rash erythematous, rash maculopapular

**These events occurred in less than 1% in placebo-controlled trials, but the incidence of these side effects was between 1% and 2% in all multiple dose studies.

Special Senses: abnormal vision, conjunctivitis, diplopia, eye pain, tinnitus

Urinary System: micturition frequency, micturition disorder, nocturia

Autonomic Nervous System: dry mouth, sweating increased

Metabolic and Nutritional: hyperglycemia, thirst

Hemopoietic: leukopenia, purpura, thrombocytopenia

Other events reported with amlodipine at a frequency of ≤0.1% of patients include: cardiac failure, pulse irregularity, extrasystoles, skin discoloration, urticaria, skin dryness, alopecia, dermatitis, muscle weakness, twitching, ataxia, hypertonia, migraine, cold and clammy skin, apathy, agitation, amnesia, gastritis, increased appetite, loose stools, rhinitis, dysuria, polyuria, parosmia, taste perversion, abnormal visual accommodation, and xerophthalmia. Other reactions occurred sporadically and cannot be distinguished from medications or concurrent disease states such as myocardial infarction and angina.

HCTZ

Other adverse reactions not listed above that have been reported with HCTZ, without regard to causality, are listed below:

Body as a Whole: weakness

Digestive: pancreatitis, jaundice (intrahepatic cholestatic jaundice), sialadenitis, cramping, gastric irritation

Hematologic: aplastic anemia, agranulocytosis, hemolytic anemia

Hypersensitivity: photosensitivity, urticaria, necrotizing angiitis (vasculitis and cutaneous vasculitis), fever, respiratory distress including pneumonitis and pulmonary edema, anaphylactic reactions

Musculoskeletal: muscle spasm

Nervous System/Psychiatric: restlessness

Renal: renal failure, renal dysfunction, interstitial nephritis

Skin: erythema multiforme including Stevens-Johnson syndrome, exfoliative dermatitis including toxic epidermal necrolysis

Special Senses: transient blurred vision, xanthopsia

Clinical Laboratory Test Abnormalities

Clinical laboratory findings for Amturnide in patients with hypertension not concomitantly treated with an ARB or ACEI were obtained in a controlled trial of Amturnide administered at the maximal dose of 300/10/25 mg compared to maximal doses of dual therapies, i.e., aliskiren/amlodipine 300/10 mg, aliskiren/HCTZ 300/25 mg and amlodipine/HCTZ 10/25 mg.

RBC Count, Hemoglobin and Hematocrit

Small mean changes from baseline were seen in RBC count, hemoglobin and hematocrit in patients treated with Amturnide. This effect is also seen with other agents acting on the renin angiotensin system. In aliskiren monotherapy trials these decreases led to slight increases in rates of anemia compared to placebo (0.1% for any aliskiren use, 0.3% for aliskiren 600 mg daily, versus 0% for placebo). No patients discontinued Amturnide because of anemia.

Blood Urea Nitrogen (BUN)/Creatinine

No patients with hypertension not concomitantly treated with an ARB or ACEI treated with Amturnide had elevations in BUN >40 mg/dL or creatinine >2.0 mg/dL.

Liver Function Tests

Occasional elevations (greater than 150% from baseline) in ALT (SGPT) were observed in 2.7% of patients treated with Amturnide, compared with 1.7-2.7% in patients treated with the dual combinations. No patients were discontinued due to abnormal liver function tests.

6.2 Postmarketing Experience

The following adverse reactions have been identified during post-approval use of either aliskiren, amlodipine or hydrochlorothiazide. Because these reactions are reported voluntarily from a population of uncertain size, it is not always possible to estimate their frequency or establish a causal relationship to drug exposure:

Aliskiren:

Hypersensitivity: anaphylactic reactions and angioedema requiring airway management and hospitalization.

Peripheral edema, severe cutaneous adverse reactions, including Stevens-Johnson syndrome and toxic epidermal necrolysis.

Amlodipine: The following postmarketing event has been reported infrequently where a causal relationship is uncertain: gynecomastia. In postmarketing experience, jaundice and hepatic enzyme elevations (mostly consistent with cholestasis or hepatitis), in some cases severe enough to require hospitalization, have been reported in association with use of amlodipine.

Hydrochlorothiazide:

Acute renal failure, renal disorder, aplastic anemia, erythema multiforme, pyrexia, muscle spasm, asthenia, acute angle-closure glaucoma, bone marrow failure, worsening of diabetes control, hypokalemia, blood lipids increased, hyponatremia, hypomagnesemia, hypercalcemia, hyperchloremic alkalosis, impotence, visual impairment.

Pathological changes in the parathyroid gland of patients with hypercalcemia and hypophosphatemia have been observed in a few patients on prolonged thiazide therapy. If hypercalcemia occurs, further diagnostic evaluation is necessary.

7 DRUG INTERACTIONS

No drug interaction studies have been conducted between Amturnide and other drugs. In a phase III sub-study, there was no clinically relevant change in the exposure of aliskiren, amlodipine, and HCTZ observed with Amturnide compared to the dual combinations of aliskiren and amlodipine, amlodipine and HCTZ, and aliskiren and HCTZ. Studies with the individual aliskiren, amlodipine, and HCTZ components are described below.

Aliskiren

Cyclosporine: Avoid co-administration of cyclosporine with aliskiren.

Itraconazole: Avoid co-administration of itraconazole with aliskiren *[see Clinical Pharmacology (12.3)]*.

Non-Steroidal Anti-Inflammatory Agents (NSAIDs) including selective Cyclooxygenase-2 inhibitors (COX-2 inhibitors): In patients who are elderly, volume-depleted (including those on diuretic therapy), or with compromised renal function, co-administration of NSAIDs, including selective COX-2 inhibitors with agents that affect the renin-angiotensin system, including aliskiren, may result in deterioration of renal function, including possible acute renal failure. These effects are usually reversible. Monitor renal function periodically in patients receiving aliskiren and NSAID therapy.

The antihypertensive effect of aliskiren may be attenuated by NSAIDs.

Amlodipine

Simvastatin: Co-administration of simvastatin with amlodipine increases the systemic exposure of simvastatin. Limit the dose of simvastatin in patients on amlodipine to 20 mg daily.

CYP3A4 Inhibitors: Co-administration with CYP3A inhibitors (moderate and strong) result in increased systemic exposure to amlodipine warranting dose reduction. Monitor for symptoms of hypotension and edema when amlodipine is co-administered with CYP3A4 inhibitors to determine the need for dose adjustment.

CYP3A4 Inducers: No information is available on the quantitative effects of CYP3A4 inducers on amlodipine. Blood pressure should be monitored when amlodipine is co-administered with CYP3A4 inducers.

HCTZ

When administered concurrently, the following drugs may interact with thiazide diuretics.

Antidiabetic drugs (oral agents and insulin): Dosage adjustment of the antidiabetic drug may be required.

Lithium: Diuretic agents increase the risk of lithium toxicity. Refer to the package insert for lithium before use of such preparation with Amturnide. Monitoring of serum lithium concentrations is recommended during concurrent use.

Nonsteroidal anti-inflammatory drugs (NSAIDs) and COX-2 selective agents: When Amturnide and nonsteroidal anti-inflammatory agents are used concomitantly, observe the patient to determine if the desired effect of the diuretic is obtained.

Ion exchange resins: Staggering the dosage of hydrochlorothiazide and resin (e.g., cholestyramine, colestipol) such that hydrochlorothiazide is administered at least 4 hours before or 4-6 hours after the administration of resins would potentially minimize the interaction *[see Clinical Pharmacology (12.3)]*.

8 USE IN SPECIFIC POPULATIONS

8.1 Pregnancy

Pregnancy Category D

Use of drugs that act on the renin-angiotensin system during the second and third trimesters of pregnancy reduces fetal renal function and increases fetal and neonatal morbidity and death. Resulting oligohydramnios can be associated with fetal lung hypoplasia and skeletal deformations. Potential neonatal adverse effects include skull hypoplasia, anuria, hypotension, renal failure, and death. When pregnancy is detected, discontinue Amturnide as soon as possible. These adverse outcomes are usually associated with use of drugs in the second and third trimesters of pregnancy. Most epidemiologic studies examining fetal abnormalities after exposure to antihypertensive use in the first trimester have not distinguished drugs affecting the renin-angiotensin system from other antihypertensive agents. Appropriate management of maternal hypertension during pregnancy is important to optimize outcomes for both mother and fetus. In the unusual case that there is no appropriate alternative to therapy with drugs affecting the renin-angiotensin system for a particular patient, apprise the mother of the potential risk to the fetus. Perform serial ultrasound examinations to assess the intra-amniotic environment. If oligohydramnios is observed, discontinue Amturnide, unless it is considered lifesaving for the mother. Fetal testing may be appropriate, based on the week of pregnancy. Patients and physicians should be aware, however, that oligohydramnios may not appear until after the fetus has sustained irreversible injury. Closely observe infants with histories of in utero exposure to Amturnide for hypotension, oliguria, and hyperkalemia [*see use in Specific Populations (8.4)*].

Animal Data

No reproductive toxicity studies have been conducted with the combination of aliskiren, amlodipine besylate and HCTZ. However, these studies have been conducted for aliskiren, amlodipine besylate and HCTZ alone.

Aliskiren

In developmental toxicity studies, pregnant rats and rabbits received oral aliskiren hemifumarate during organogenesis at doses up to 20 and 7 times the maximum recommended human dose (MRHD) based on body surface area (mg/m^2), respectively, in rats and rabbits. (Actual animal doses were up to 600 mg/kg/day in rats and up to 100 mg/kg/day in rabbits.) No teratogenicity was observed; however, fetal birth weight was decreased in rabbits at doses 3.2 times the MRHD based on body surface area (mg/m^2). Aliskiren was present in placentas, amniotic fluid and fetuses of pregnant rabbits.

Amlodipine

No evidence of teratogenicity or embryo/fetal toxicity was found when pregnant rats and rabbits were treated orally with amlodipine maleate at doses up to 10 mg amlodipine/kg/day during their respective periods of major organogenesis. However, litter size was significantly decreased (by about 50%) and the number of intrauterine deaths was significantly increased (about 5-fold). Amlodipine has been shown to prolong both the gestation period and the duration of labor in rats at this dose.

HCTZ

When pregnant mice and rats were given HCTZ at doses up to 3000 and 1000 mg/kg/day, respectively (about 600 and 400 times the MRHD), during their respective periods of major organogenesis, there was no evidence of fetal harm. Thiazides can cross the placenta, and concentrations reached in the umbilical vein approach those in the maternal plasma. Hydrochlorothiazide, like other diuretics, can cause placental hypoperfusion. It accumulates in the amniotic fluid, with reported concentrations up to 19 times higher than in umbilical vein plasma. Use of thiazides during pregnancy is associated with a risk of fetal or neonatal jaundice or thrombocytopenia. Since they do not prevent or alter the course of EPH (Edema, Proteinuria, Hypertension) gestosis (pre eclampsia), these drugs should not be used to treat hypertension in pregnant women. The use of hydrochlorothiazide for other indications (e.g. heart disease) in pregnancy should be avoided.

8.3 Nursing Mothers

It is not known whether aliskiren or amlodipine is excreted in human milk, but thiazides are excreted in human milk. Both aliskiren and amlodipine are secreted in the milk of lactating rats. Because of the potential for serious adverse reactions in human milk-fed infants from Amturnide, a decision should be made whether to discontinue nursing or discontinue Amturnide, taking into account the importance of the drug to the mother.

8.4 Pediatric Use

Safety and effectiveness of Amturnide in pediatric patients have not been established.

Neonates with a history of in utero exposure to Amturnide:

If oliguria or hypotension occurs, direct attention towards support of blood pressure and renal perfusion. Exchange transfusions or dialysis may be required as a means of reversing hypotension and/or substituting for disordered renal function.

8.5 Geriatric Use

As individual components, exposure to aliskiren, amlodipine and hydrochlorothiazide is increased in elderly patients, thus consider lower initial doses of Amturnide *[see Clinical Pharmacology (12.3)]*.

In the short-term controlled clinical trial of Amturnide, 19% of patients treated with Amturnide were ≥ 65 years. No overall differences in safety or effectiveness were observed between these subjects and younger subjects. Other reported clinical experience has not identified differences in responses between the elderly and younger patients, but greater sensitivity of some older individuals cannot be ruled out.

8.6 Hepatic Impairment

Exposure to amlodipine is increased in patients with hepatic insufficiency, thus consider using lower doses of Amturnide *[see Clinical Pharmacology (12.3)]*.

Hydrochlorothiazide

Minor alterations of fluid and electrolyte balance may precipitate hepatic coma in patients with impaired hepatic function or progressive liver disease.

8.7 Renal Impairment

Exposure to hydrochlorothiazide increases in patients with renal insufficiency, thus consider using lower doses of Amturnide *[see Clinical Pharmacology (12.3)]*.

Safety and effectiveness of Amturnide in patients with severe renal impairment (creatinine clearance <30 mL/min) have not been established as these patients were excluded in clinical trials *[see Warnings and Precautions (5.6), Clinical Pharmacology (12.3) and Clinical Studies (14)]*.

10 OVERDOSAGE

Aliskiren

Limited data are available related to overdosage in humans. The most likely manifestation of overdosage would be hypotension. If symptomatic hypotension occurs, provide supportive treatment.

Aliskiren is poorly dialyzed. Therefore, hemodialysis is not adequate to treat aliskiren overexposure *[see Clinical Pharmacology (12.3)]*.

Amlodipine

Overdosage might be expected to cause excessive peripheral vasodilation with marked hypotension and possibly a reflex tachycardia. Marked and potentially prolonged systemic hypotension up to and including shock with fatal outcome have been reported. In humans, experience with intentional overdosage of amlodipine is limited.

Single oral doses of amlodipine maleate equivalent to 40 mg amlodipine/kg and 100 mg amlodipine/kg in mice and rats, respectively, caused deaths. Single oral amlodipine maleate doses equivalent to 4 or more mg amlodipine/kg or higher in dogs (11 or more times the maximum recommended human dose on a mg/m2 basis) caused a marked peripheral vasodilation and hypotension.

If massive overdose occurs, initiate active cardiac and respiratory monitoring. Frequent blood pressure measurements are essential. If hypotension occurs, provide cardiovascular support including elevation of the extremities and the judicious administration of fluids. If hypotension remains unresponsive to these conservative measures, consider administration of vasopressors (such as phenylephrine), with attention to circulating volume and urine output. As amlodipine is highly protein bound, hemodialysis is not likely to be of benefit. Administration of activated charcoal to healthy volunteers immediately or up to two hours after ingestion of amlodipine has been shown to significantly decrease amlodipine absorption.

HCTZ

The most common signs and symptoms of overdose observed in humans are those caused by electrolyte depletion (hypokalemia, hypochloremia, hyponatremia) and dehydration resulting from excessive diuresis. If digitalis has also been administered, hypokalemia may accentuate cardiac arrhythmias. The degree to which HCTZ is removed by hemodialysis has not been established. The oral LD_{50} of HCTZ is greater than 10 g/kg in both mice and rats. These doses are 1946 and 3892 times, respectively, the MRHD of 25 mg/day, when based on a mg/m^2 basis of a 60-kg individual.

11 DESCRIPTION

Amturnide is a single tablet for oral administration of aliskiren hemifumarate (an orally active, nonpeptide, potent direct renin inhibitor), amlodipine besylate (a dihydropyridine calcium channel blocker) and HCTZ (a diuretic).

Aliskiren hemifumarate

Aliskiren hemifumarate is chemically described as (2S,4S,5S,7S)-N-(2-carbamoyl-2-methylpropyl)-5-amino-4-hydroxy-2,7-diisopropyl-8-[4-methoxy-3-(3-methoxypropoxy)-phenyl]-octanamide hemifumarate, and its structural formula is

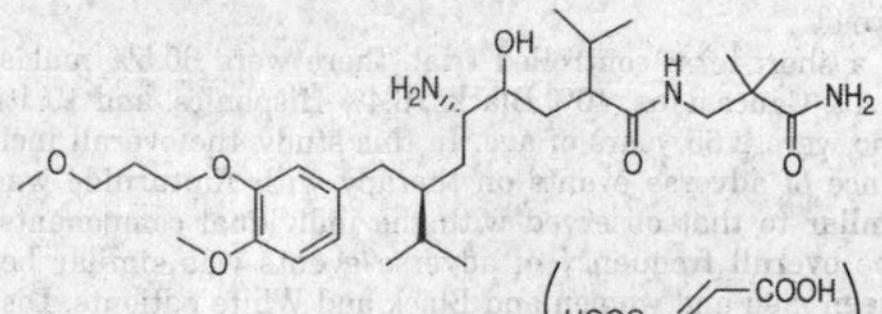

Molecular formula: $C_{30}H_{53}N_3O_6 \cdot 0.5\ C_4H_4O_4$

Aliskiren hemifumarate is a white to slightly yellowish powder with a molecular weight of 609.8 (free base- 551.8). It is highly soluble in water, and freely soluble in methanol, ethanol and isopropanol.

Amlodipine

Amlodipine besylate, USP is chemically described as 3-ethyl 5-methyl (±)-2-[(2-aminoethoxy)methyl]-4-(*o*-chlorophenyl)-1,4-dihydro-6-methyl-3,5-pyridinedicarboxylate, monobenzenesulfonate and its structural formula is

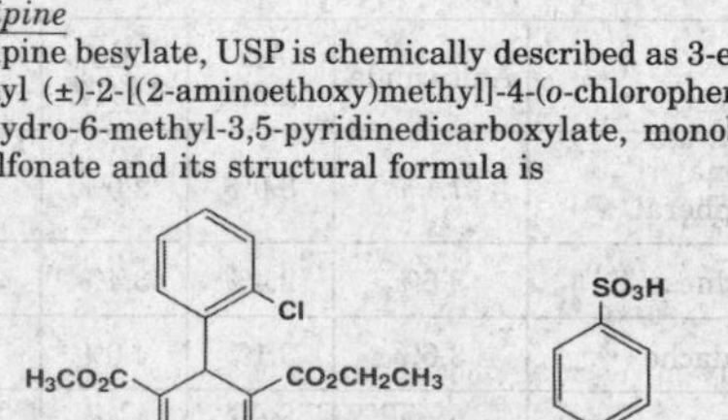

Molecular formula: $C_{20}H_{25}ClN_2O_5 \cdot C_6H_6O_3S$

Amlodipine besylate is a white to pale yellow crystalline powder with a molecular weight of 567.1. It is slightly soluble in water and sparingly soluble in ethanol.

HCTZ

HCTZ, USP is a white, or practically white, practically odorless, crystalline powder. It is slightly soluble in water; freely soluble in sodium hydroxide solution, in *n*-butylamine, and in dimethylformamide; sparingly soluble in methanol; and insoluble in ether, in chloroform, and in dilute mineral acids. HCTZ is chemically described as 6-chloro-3,4-dihydro-2*H*-1,2,4-benzothiadiazine-7-sulfonamide 1,1-dioxide.

HCTZ is a thiazide diuretic. Its empirical formula is $C_7H_8ClN_3O_4S_2$, its molecular weight is 297.73, and its structural formula is

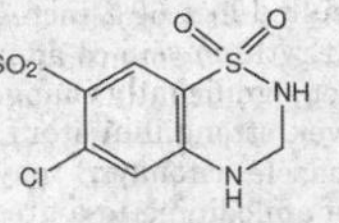

The inactive ingredients for all strengths of the tablets may contain colloidal silicon dioxide, crospovidone, hypromellose, iron oxide red, iron oxide yellow, iron oxide black, magnesium stearate, microcrystalline cellulose, polyethylene glycol, povidone, talc, and titanium dioxide.

12 CLINICAL PHARMACOLOGY

12.1 Mechanism of Action

Amturnide

The effects of combined treatment of aliskiren, amlodipine and HCTZ arise from the actions of these three agents on different but complementary mechanisms that regulate blood pressure. Together, inhibition of the renin-angiotensin-aldosterone system (RAAS), inhibition of calcium channel-mediated vasoconstriction, and increase of sodium chloride excretion lowers blood pressure to a greater degree than the individual components.

Aliskiren

Renin is secreted by the kidney in response to decreases in blood volume and renal perfusion. Renin cleaves angiotensinogen to form the inactive decapeptide angiotensin I (Ang I). Ang I is converted to the active octapeptide angiotensin II (Ang II) by angiotensin-converting enzyme (ACE) and non-ACE pathways. Ang II is a powerful vasoconstrictor and leads to the release of catecholamines from the adrenal medulla and prejunctional nerve endings. It also promotes aldosterone secretion and sodium reabsorption. Together, these effects increase blood pressure. Ang II also inhibits renin release, thus providing a negative feedback to the system. This cycle, from renin through angiotensin to aldosterone and its associated negative feedback loop, is known as the renin-angiotensin-aldosterone system (RAAS). Aliskiren is a direct renin inhibitor, decreasing plasma renin activity (PRA) and inhibiting the conversion of angiotensinogen to Ang I. Whether aliskiren affects other RAAS components, e.g., ACE or non-ACE pathways, is not known.

All agents that inhibit the RAAS, including renin inhibitors, suppress the negative feedback loop, leading to a compensatory rise in plasma renin concentration. When this rise occurs during treatment with ACE inhibitors and ARBs, the result is increased levels of PRA. During treatment with aliskiren, however, the effect of increased renin levels is blocked, so that PRA, Ang I and Ang II are all reduced, whether aliskiren is used as monotherapy or in combination with other antihypertensive agents.

Amlodipine

Amlodipine is a dihydropyridine calcium channel blocker that inhibits the transmembrane influx of calcium ions into vascular smooth muscle and cardiac muscle. Experimental data suggest that amlodipine binds to both dihydropyridine and nondihydropyridine binding sites. The contractile processes of cardiac muscle and vascular smooth muscle are dependent upon the movement of extracellular calcium ions into these cells through specific ion channels. Amlodipine inhibits calcium ion influx across cell membranes selectively, with a greater effect on vascular smooth muscle cells than on cardiac muscle cells. Negative inotropic effects can be detected *in vitro* but such effects have not been seen in intact animals at therapeutic doses. Serum calcium concentration is not affected by amlodipine. Within the physiologic pH range, amlodipine is an ionized compound (pKa=8.6), and its kinetic interaction with the calcium channel receptor is characterized by a gradual rate of association and dissociation with the receptor binding site, resulting in a gradual onset of effect.

Amlodipine is a peripheral arterial vasodilator that acts directly on vascular smooth muscle to cause a reduction in peripheral vascular resistance and reduction in blood pressure.

HCTZ

The mechanism of action of the antihypertensive effect of thiazides is unknown.

HCTZ is a thiazide diuretic. Thiazides affect the renal tubular mechanisms of electrolyte reabsorption, directly increasing excretion of sodium and chloride in approximately equivalent amounts. Indirectly, the diuretic action of HCTZ reduces plasma volume, with consequent increases in plasma renin activity, increases in aldosterone secretion, increases in urinary potassium loss, and decreases in serum potassium. The renin-aldosterone link is mediated by angiotensin II, so coadministration of agents that block the production or function of angiotensin II tends to reverse the potassium loss associated with these diuretics.

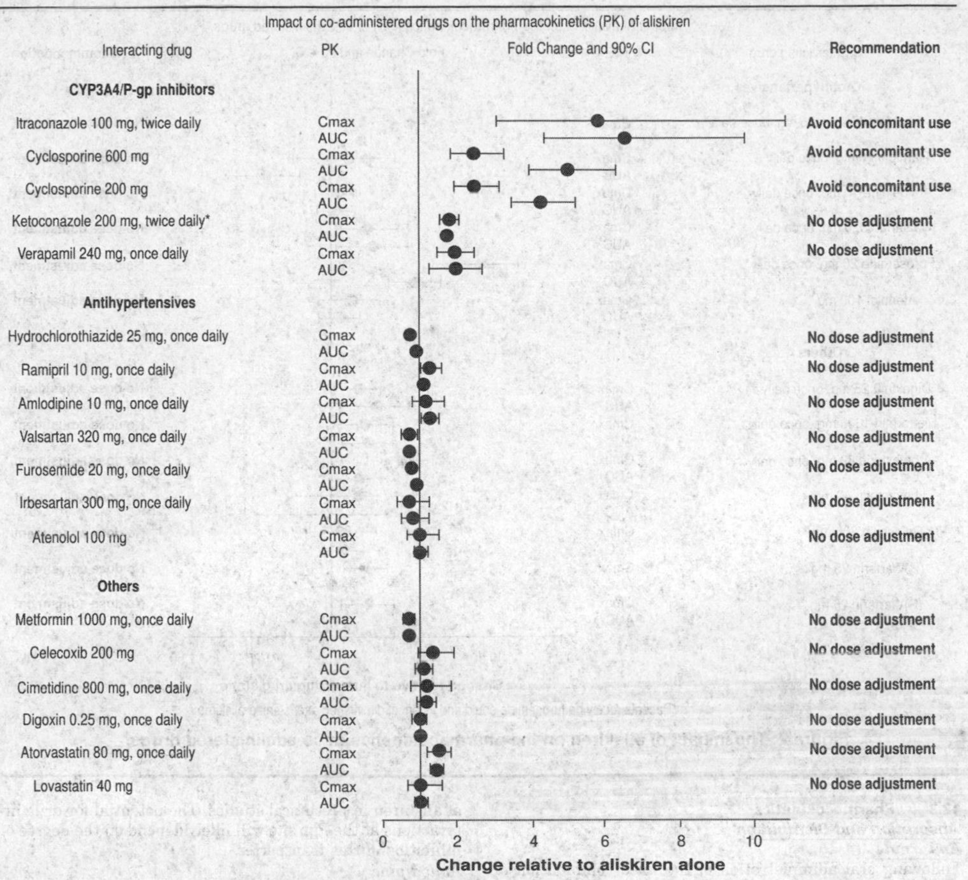

*A 400 mg once daily dose was not studied, but would be expected to increase aliskiren blood levels further.

Figure 1: The impact of co-administered drugs on the pharmacokinetics of aliskiren.

12.2 Pharmacodynamics

Amturnide

In an active-controlled trial which established the clinical efficacy of Amturnide in hypertensive patients, Amturnide was associated with a 34% reduction in PRA compared to a 63% reduction with aliskiren/amlodipine, 64% reduction with aliskiren/HCTZ and a 170% elevation with amlodipine/HCTZ.

Aliskiren

PRA reductions in clinical trials ranged from approximately 50% to 80%, were not dose-related and did not correlate with blood pressure reductions. The clinical implications of the differences in effect on PRA are not known.

Amlodipine

Following administration of therapeutic doses to patients with hypertension, amlodipine produces vasodilation resulting in a reduction of supine and standing blood pressures. These decreases in blood pressure are not accompanied by a significant change in heart rate or plasma catecholamine levels with chronic dosing. Although the acute intravenous administration of amlodipine decreases arterial blood pressure and increases heart rate in hemodynamic studies of patients with chronic stable angina, chronic oral administration of amlodipine in clinical trials did not lead to clinically significant changes in heart rate or blood pressures in normotensive patients with angina.

With chronic once-daily administration, antihypertensive effectiveness is maintained for at least 24 hours. Plasma concentrations correlate with effect in both young and elderly patients. The magnitude of reduction in blood pressure with amlodipine is also correlated with the height of pretreatment elevation; thus, individuals with moderate hypertension (diastolic pressure 105-114 mmHg) had about 50% greater response than patients with mild hypertension (diastolic pressure 90-104 mmHg). Normotensive subjects experienced no clinically significant change in blood pressure (+1/-2 mmHg).

In hypertensive patients with normal renal function, therapeutic doses of amlodipine resulted in a decrease in renal vascular resistance and an increase in glomerular filtration rate and effective renal plasma flow without change in filtration fraction or proteinuria.

As with other calcium channel blockers, hemodynamic measurements of cardiac function at rest and during exercise (or pacing) in patients with normal ventricular function treated with amlodipine have generally demonstrated a small increase in cardiac index without significant influence on dP/dt or on left ventricular end diastolic pressure or volume. In hemodynamic studies, amlodipine has not been associated with a negative inotropic effect when administered in therapeutic dose range to intact animals and man, even when co-administered with beta-blockers to man. Similar findings, however, have been observed in normal or well-compensated patients with heart failure with agents possessing significant negative inotropic effects.

Amlodipine does not change sinoatrial nodal function or atrioventricular conduction in intact animals or man. In patients with chronic stable angina, intravenous administration of 10 mg did not significantly alter A-H and H-V conduction and sinus node recovery time after pacing. Similar results were obtained in patients receiving amlodipine and concomitant beta-blockers. In clinical studies in which amlodipine was administered in combination with beta-blockers to patients with either hypertension or angina, no adverse effects of electrocardiographic parameters were observed. In clinical trials with angina patients alone, amlodipine therapy did not alter electrocardiographic intervals or produce higher degrees of AV blocks.

Amlodipine has indications other than hypertension, which can be found in the Norvasc® package insert.

HCTZ

After oral administration of HCTZ, diuresis begins within 2 hours, peaks in about 4 hours, and lasts about 6 to 12 hours.

Drug Interactions

Hydrochlorothiazide

Alcohol, barbiturates, or narcotics: Potentiation of orthostatic hypotension may occur.

Skeletal muscle relaxants: Possible increased responsiveness to muscle relaxants such as curare derivatives.

Digitalis glycosides: Thiazide-induced hypokalemia or hypomagnesemia may predispose the patient to digoxin toxicity.

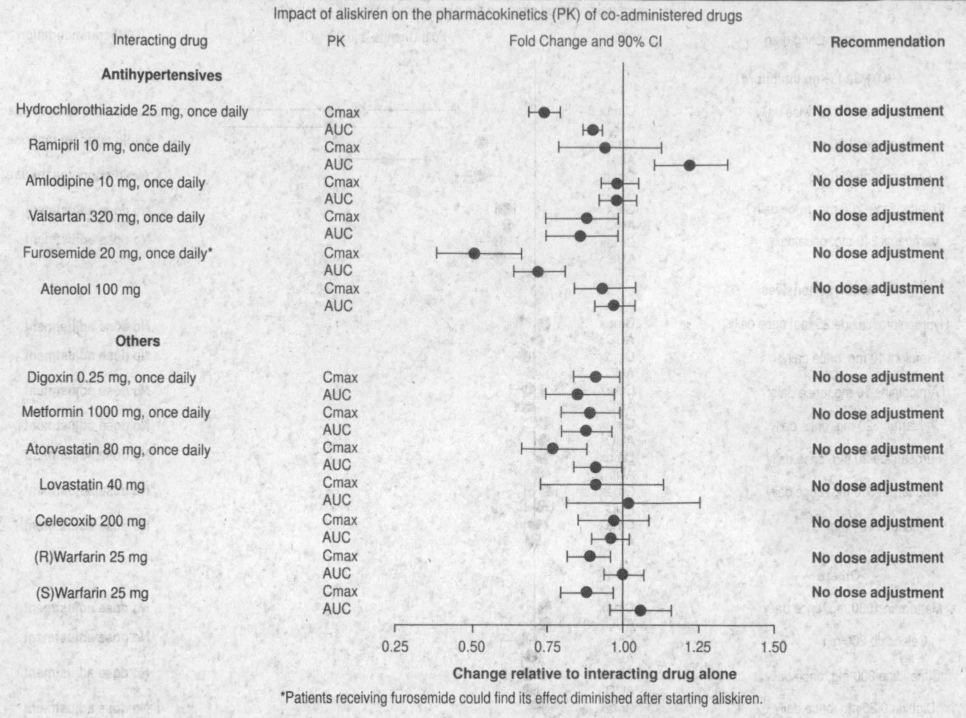

Figure 2: The impact of aliskiren on the pharmacokinetics of co-administered drugs.

12.3 Pharmacokinetics

Absorption and Distribution

Amturnide

Following oral administration of the fixed combination of aliskiren, amlodipine, and HCTZ, peak concentrations were achieved within 1-2 hours, 6-12 hours, and 1-4 hours for aliskiren, amlodipine and HCTZ, respectively. The rate and extent of absorption of aliskiren, amlodipine, and HCTZ following administration of the fixed combination are similar to when they are administered as individual dosage forms. When Amturnide is taken with food, mean AUC and C_{max} of aliskiren are decreased by 78% and 89%, respectively. There is no impact of food on the exposures of amlodipine and HCTZ.

Aliskiren

Aliskiren is poorly absorbed (bioavailability about 2.5%). Following oral administration, peak plasma concentrations of aliskiren are reached within 1 to 3 hours. When taken with a high fat meal, mean AUC and C_{max} of aliskiren are decreased by 71% and 85% respectively. In the clinical trials of aliskiren, it was administered without requiring a fixed relation of administration to meals.

Amlodipine

Peak plasma concentrations of amlodipine are reached 6-12 hours after an oral administration of amlodipine. Absolute bioavailability has been estimated to be between 64% and 90%. The bioavailability of amlodipine is not altered by the presence of food.

The apparent volume of distribution of amlodipine is about 21 L/kg. Approximately 93% of circulating amlodipine is bound to plasma proteins in hypertensive patients.

HCTZ

The estimated absolute bioavailability of hydrochlorothiazide after oral administration is about 70%. Peak plasma hydrochlorothiazide concentrations (C_{max}) are reached within 2 to 5 hours after oral administration. There is no clinically significant effect of food on the bioavailability of hydrochlorothiazide.

Hydrochlorothiazide binds to albumin (40 to 70%) and distributes into erythrocytes. Following oral administration, plasma hydrochlorothiazide concentrations decline bi-exponentially, with a mean distribution half-life of about 2 hours and an elimination half-life of about 10 hours.

Metabolism and Elimination

Aliskiren

The effective half-life for aliskiren is 24 hours. Steady state blood levels are reached in about 7 – 8 days. About one-fourth of the absorbed dose appears in the urine as parent drug. How much of the absorbed dose is metabolized is unknown. Based on the *in vitro* studies, the major enzyme responsible for aliskiren metabolism appears to be CYP 3A4. Aliskiren does not inhibit the CYP450 isoenzymes (CYP 1A2, 2C8, 2C9, 2C19, 2D6, 2E1, and 3A) or induce CYP 3A4.

Transporters: Pgp (MDR1/Mdr1a/1b) was found to be the major efflux system involved in absorption and disposition of aliskiren in preclinical studies. The potential for drug interactions at the Pgp site will likely depend on the degree of inhibition of this transporter.

Amlodipine

Amlodipine is extensively (about 90%) converted to inactive metabolites via hepatic metabolism, with 10% of the parent compound and 60% of the metabolites excreted in the urine. Elimination of amlodipine from the plasma is biphasic, with a terminal elimination half-life of about 30-50 hours. Steady state plasma levels are reached after once-daily dosing for 7-8 days.

HCTZ

About 70% of an orally administered dose of hydrochlorothiazide is eliminated in the urine as unchanged drug.

Drug interactions:

Aliskiren

The effects of co-administered drugs on the pharmacokinetics of aliskiren, and vice versa, were studied in several single and multiple dose studies. Pharmacokinetic measures indicating the magnitude of these interactions are presented in Figure 1 (impact of co-administered drugs on aliskiren) and Figure 2 (impact on co-administered drugs).

[See figure 1 at top of previous page]

Warfarin: There was no clinically significant effect of a single dose of warfarin 25 mg on the pharmacokinetics of aliskiren.

[See figure 2 above]

Amlodipine

In vitro data in human plasma indicate that amlodipine has no effect on the protein binding of digoxin, phenytoin, warfarin, and indomethacin.

Cimetidine: Co-administration of amlodipine with cimetidine did not alter the pharmacokinetics of amlodipine.

Grapefruit juice: Co-administration of 240 mL of grapefruit juice with a single oral dose of amlodipine 10 mg in 20 healthy volunteers had no significant effect on the pharmacokinetics of amlodipine.

Maalox® (antacid): Co-administration of the antacid Maalox with a single dose of amlodipine had no significant effect on the pharmacokinetics of amlodipine.

Sildenafil: A single 100 mg dose of sildenafil in subjects with essential hypertension had no effect on the pharmacokinetic parameters of amlodipine. When amlodipine and sildenafil were used in combination, each agent independently exerted its own blood pressure lowering effect.

Atorvastatin: Co-administration of multiple 10 mg doses of amlodipine with 80 mg of atorvastatin resulted in no significant change in the steady-state pharmacokinetic parameters of atorvastatin.

Digoxin: Co-administration of amlodipine with digoxin did not change serum digoxin levels or digoxin renal clearance in normal volunteers.

Ethanol (alcohol): Single and multiple 10 mg doses of amlodipine had no significant effect on the pharmacokinetics of ethanol.

Warfarin: Co-administration of amlodipine with warfarin did not change the warfarin prothrombin response time.

Simvastatin: Co-administration of multiple doses of 10 mg of amlodipine with 80 mg simvastatin resulted in a 77% increase in exposure to simvastatin compared to simvastatin alone.

CYP3A inhibitors: Co-administration of a 180 mg daily dose of diltiazem with 5 mg amlodipine in elderly hypertensive patients resulted in a 60% increase in amlodipine systemic exposure. Erythromycin co-administration in healthy volunteers did not significantly change amlodipine systemic exposure. However, strong inhibitors of CYP3A4 (e.g. ketoconazole, itraconazole, ritonavir) may increase the plasma concentrations of amlodipine to a greater extent.

Hydrochlorothiazide

Drugs that alter gastrointestinal motility: The bioavailability of thiazide-type diuretics may be increased by anticholinergic agents (e.g. atropine, biperiden), apparently due to a decrease in gastrointestinal motility and the stomach emptying rate. Conversely, pro-kinetic drugs may decrease the bioavailability of thiazide diuretics.

Cholestyramine: In a dedicated drug interaction study, administration of cholestyramine 2 hours before hydrochlorothiazide resulted in a 70% reduction in exposure to hydrochlorothiazide. Further, administration of hydrochlorothiazide 2 hours before cholestyramine, resulted in 35% reduction in exposure to hydrochlorothiazide.

Antineoplastic agents (e.g. cyclophosphamide, methotrexate): Concomitant use of thiazide diuretics may reduce renal excretion of cytotoxic agents and enhance their myelosuppressive effects.

Special Populations

Pediatric Patients

The pharmacokinetics of Amturnide have not been investigated in patients <18 years of age.

Geriatric Patients

Impact of aging on aliskiren pharmacokinetics has been assessed. When compared to young adults (18-40 years), aliskiren mean AUC and C_{max} in elderly subjects (> 65 years) are increased by 57% and 28%, respectively. In the elderly, clearance of amlodipine is decreased with resulting increases in peak plasma levels, elimination half-life and area-under-the-plasma-concentration curve. Limited data suggest that the systemic clearance of hydrochlorothiazide is reduced in both healthy and hypertensive elderly subjects compared to young healthy volunteers *[see Use in Specific Populations (8.5)]*.

Race

With Amturnide, pharmacokinetic differences due to race have not been studied. The pharmacokinetic differences among Blacks, Caucasians, and Japanese are minimal with aliskiren therapy.

Hepatic Impairment

The pharmacokinetics of aliskiren is not significantly affected in patients with mild-to-severe liver disease. Patients with hepatic insufficiency have decreased clearance of amlodipine with resulting increase in AUC of approximately 40%-60% *[see Warnings and Precautions (5.6) and Use in Specific Populations (8.6)]*.

Renal Impairment

The pharmacokinetics of aliskiren were evaluated in patients with varying degrees of renal impairment. Rate and extent of exposure (AUC and C_{max}) of aliskiren in subjects with renal impairment did not show a consistent correlation with the severity of renal impairment.

The pharmacokinetics of aliskiren following administration of a single oral dose of 300 mg was evaluated in patients with End Stage Renal Disease (ESRD) undergoing hemodialysis. When compared to matched healthy subjects, changes in the rate and extent of aliskiren exposure (C_{max} and AUC) in ESRD patients undergoing hemodialysis was not clinically significant. Timing of hemodialysis did not significantly alter the pharmacokinetics of aliskiren in ESRD patients.

The pharmacokinetics of amlodipine is not significantly influenced by renal impairment.

In a study in individuals with impaired renal function, the mean elimination half-life of hydrochlorothiazide was doubled in individuals with mild/moderate renal impairment (30 < CLcr < 90 mL/min) and tripled in severe renal impairment (≤ 30 mL/min), compared to individuals with normal renal function (CLcr > 90 mL/min) *[see Warnings and Precautions (5.7) and Use in Specific Populations (8.7)]*.

13 NONCLINICAL TOXICOLOGY

13.1 Carcinogenesis, Mutagenesis, Impairment of Fertility

Studies with Aliskiren hemifumarate, Amlodipine besylate and HCTZ

No carcinogenicity, mutagenicity or fertility studies have been conducted with the combination of aliskiren hemifumarate, amlodipine besylate and HCTZ. However, these studies have been conducted for aliskiren hemifumarate, amlodipine besylate and HCTZ alone.

Studies with Aliskiren hemifumarate

Carcinogenic potential was assessed in a 2-year rat study and a 6-month transgenic (rasH2) mouse study with aliskiren hemifumarate at oral doses of up to 1500 mg aliskiren/kg/day. Although there were no statistically significant increases in tumor incidence associated with exposure to aliskiren, mucosal epithelial hyperplasia (with or without erosion/ulceration) was observed in the lower gastrointestinal tract at doses of 750 or more mg/kg/day in both species, with a colonic adenoma identified in one rat and a cecal adenocarcinoma identified in another, rare tumors in the strain of rat studied. On a systemic exposure (AUC_{0-24h}) basis, 1500 mg/kg/day in the rat is about 4 times and in the mouse about 1.5 times the maximum recommended human dose (300 mg aliskiren/day). Mucosal hyperplasia in the cecum or colon of rats was also observed at doses of 250 mg/kg/day (the lowest tested dose) as well as at higher doses in 4- and 13-week studies.

Aliskiren hemifumarate was devoid of genotoxic potential in the Ames reverse mutation assay with *S. typhimurium* and *E. coli*, the *in vitro* Chinese hamster ovary cell chromosomal aberration assay, the *in vitro* Chinese hamster V79 cell gene mutation test and the *in vivo* rat bone marrow micronucleus assay.

Fertility of male and female rats was unaffected at doses of up to aliskiren 250 mg/kg/day (8 times the maximum recommended human dose of aliskiren 300 mg/60 kg on a mg/m^2 basis).

Studies with Amlodipine besylate

Rats and mice treated with amlodipine maleate in the diet for up to two years, at concentrations calculated to provide daily dosage levels of 0.5, 1.25, and 2.5 mg amlodipine/kg/day, showed no evidence of a carcinogenic effect of the drug. For the mouse, the highest dose was, on mg/m^2 basis, similar to the maximum recommended human dose (MRHD) of 10 mg amlodipine/day. For the rat, the highest dose was, on a mg/m^2 basis, about twice the MRHD.

Mutagenicity studies conducted with amlodipine maleate revealed no drug-related effects at either the gene or chromosome level.

There was no effect on the fertility of rats treated orally with amlodipine maleate (males for 64 days and females for 14 days prior to mating) at doses of up to 10 mg amlodipine/kg/day (about 8 times the MRHD of 10 mg/day on a mg/m^2 basis).

Studies with HCTZ

Two-year feeding studies in mice and rats conducted under the auspices of the National Toxicology Program (NTP) uncovered no evidence of a carcinogenic potential of HCTZ in female mice (at doses of up to approximately 600 mg/kg/day) or in male and female rats (at doses of up to approximately 100 mg/kg/day). These doses in mice and rats are about 117 and 39 times, respectively, the MRHD of 25 mg/day, when based on a mg/m^2 basis of a 60 kg individual. The NTP, however, found equivocal evidence for hepatocarcinogenicity in male mice.

HCTZ was not genotoxic *in vitro* in the Ames mutagenicity assay of *S. typhimurium* strains TA 98, TA 100, TA 1535, TA 1537, and TA 1538 and in the Chinese Hamster Ovary (CHO) test for chromosomal aberrations, or *in vivo* in assays using mouse germinal cell chromosomes, Chinese hamster bone marrow chromosomes, and the Drosophila sex-linked recessive lethal trait gene. Positive test results were obtained only in the *in vitro* CHO Sister Chromatid Exchange (clastogenicity) and in the Mouse Lymphoma Cell (mutagenicity) assays, using concentrations of HCTZ from 43 to 1300 mcg/mL, and in the *Aspergillus Nidulans* nondisjunction assay at an unspecified concentration.

HCTZ was not teratogenic and had no adverse effects on the fertility of mice and rats of either sex in studies wherein these species were exposed, via their diet, to doses of up to 100 and 4 mg/kg, respectively, prior to mating and throughout gestation. These doses of HCTZ in mice and rats represent 19 and 1.5 times, respectively, the maximum recommended human dose on a mg/m^2 basis. (Calculations assume an oral dose of 25 mg/day and a 60-kg patient.)

13.2 Animal Toxicology and/or Pharmacology

Reproductive Toxicology Studies

[See Use in Specific Populations (8.1).]

14 CLINICAL STUDIES

14.1 Amturnide

Amturnide was studied in a double-blind, active-controlled study in 1181 treated hypertensive patients, of whom 773 were classified as moderately hypertensive (SBP 160-180 mmHg) and 408 as severely hypertensive (SBP 180-200 mmHg) at baseline. The mean baseline systolic/diastolic blood pressure for all randomized patients was approximately 173/105 mmHg. A total of 61% of patients were male, 19% were 65 years or older, 84% were Caucasian, and 10% were Black.

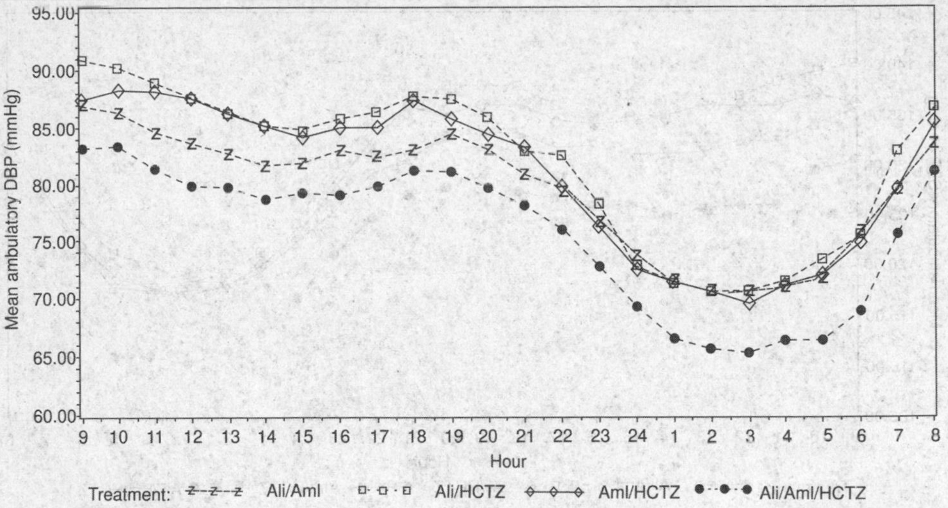

Figure 5. Mean Ambulatory Diastolic Blood Pressure at Endpoint by Treatment and Clock Hour

At study initiation, patients assigned to the dual combination treatments received lower doses of their treatment combination (aliskiren 150 mg plus amlodipine 5 mg, aliskiren 150 mg plus HCTZ 12.5 mg, or amlodipine 5 mg plus HCTZ 12.5 mg), while patients assigned to the Amturnide arm received aliskiren/HCTZ 150/12.5 mg. After 3 days, Amturnide patients were titrated to aliskiren/amlodipine/HCTZ 150/5/12.5 mg, while all other patients continued receiving their initial doses. After 4 weeks, all patients were titrated to their full target doses of aliskiren/amlodipine/HCTZ 300/10/25 mg, aliskiren/amlodipine 300/10, aliskiren/HCTZ 300/25 mg, or amlodipine/HCTZ 10/25 mg.

Amturnide produced greater reductions in blood pressure than did any of the 3 dual combination treatments ($p<0.001$ for both diastolic and systolic blood pressure reductions). The reductions in systolic/diastolic blood pressure with Amturnide were 9.9/6.3 mmHg greater than with aliskiren/HCTZ, 7.2/3.6 mmHg greater than with amlodipine/HCTZ, and 6.6/2.6 mmHg greater than with aliskiren/amlodipine. In the severe hypertensive patients, Amturnide produced greater reductions in blood pressure than each of the 3 dual combination treatments ($p<0.001$ for both diastolic and systolic blood pressure reductions). The reductions in systolic/diastolic blood pressure with Amturnide were 16.3/8.2 mmHg greater than with aliskiren/HCTZ, 9.6/4.8 mmHg greater than with amlodipine/HCTZ, and 11.4/4.9 mmHg greater than with aliskiren/amlodipine.

The distribution of reductions in blood pressure on each treatment are shown in Figure 3 for diastolic blood pressure and in Figure 4 for systolic blood pressure. For example, Figure 3 shows that 50% of patients on Amturnide had more than 20.2 mmHg reduction in diastolic blood pressure compared to 18.7 mmHg on aliskiren/amlodipine combination, 12.7 mmHg on aliskiren/HCTZ combination, and 15.3 mmHg on amlodipine/HCTZ combination. Similarly, Figure 4 shows that 50% of patients on Amturnide had more than 36.3 mmHg reduction in systolic blood pressure compared to 30.8 mmHg on aliskiren/amlodipine combination, 28.3 mmHg on aliskiren/HCTZ combination, and 31.0 mmHg on amlodipine/HCTZ combination. The time course over which blood pressure effects developed is shown in Figures 5 and 6. As the trial had no placebo control, the treatment effects shown in Figures 3-6 include a placebo effect of unknown size.

The antihypertensive effect of Amturnide was similar in patients with and without diabetes, obese and non-obese patients, in patients ≥65 years of age and <65 years of age, and in women and men.

[See figure 3 at top of next column]

[See figure 4 at top of next column]

[See figure 5 above]

[See figure 6 at top of next page]

There are no trials of the Amturnide triple combination tablet demonstrating reductions in cardiovascular risk in patients with hypertension, but two of the components, amlodipine and hydrochlorothiazide, have demonstrated such benefits.

14.2 Aliskiren in Patients with Diabetes treated with ARB or ACEI (ALTITUDE study)

Patients with diabetes with renal disease (defined either by the presence of albuminuria or reduced GFR) were randomized to aliskiren 300 mg daily (n=4283) or placebo (n=4296). All patients were receiving background therapy with an

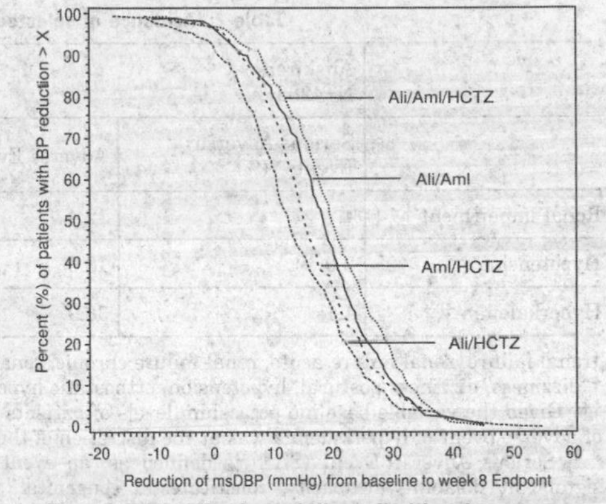

Figure 3. Distribution of diastolic blood pressure responses on Amturnide and combinations of two drugs.

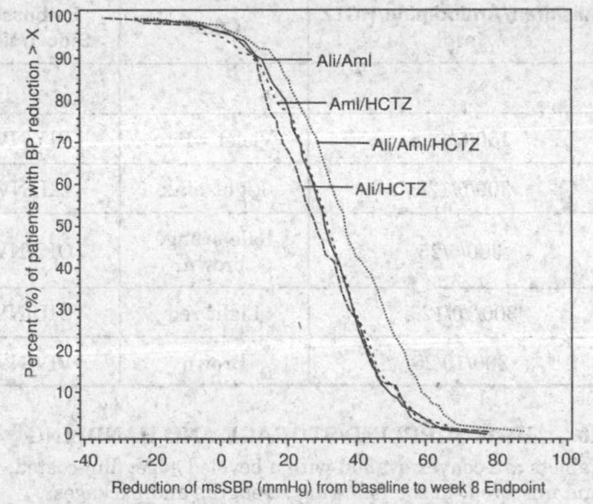

Figure 4. Distribution of systolic blood pressure responses on Amturnide and combinations of two drugs.

ARB or ACEI. The primary efficacy outcome was the time to the first event of the primary composite endpoint consisting of cardiovascular death, resuscitated sudden death, non-fatal myocardial infarction, non-fatal stroke, unplanned hospitalization for heart failure, onset of end stage renal disease, renal death, and doubling of serum creatinine concentration from baseline sustained for at least one month. After a median follow up of about 27 months, the trial was terminated early for lack of efficacy. Higher risk of renal impairment, hypotension and hyperkalemia was observed in aliskiren compared to placebo treated patients, as shown in the table below.

[See table 2 at top of next page]

The risk of stroke (2.7% aliskiren vs 2.0% placebo) and death (6.9% aliskiren vs. 6.4% placebo) were also numerically higher in aliskiren treated patients.

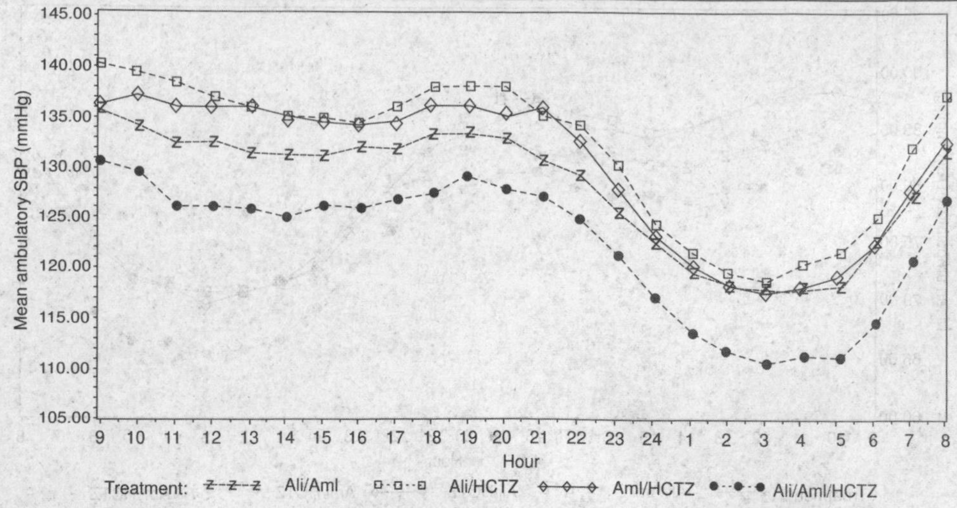

Figure 6. Mean Ambulatory Systolic Blood Pressure at Endpoint by Treatment and Clock Hour

Table 2: Incidence of selected adverse events in ALTITUDE

	Aliskiren N=4283		Placebo N=4296	
	Serious Adverse Events* (%)	Adverse Events (%)	Serious Adverse Events* (%)	Adverse Events (%)
Renal impairment †	4.7	12.4	3.3	10.4
Hypotension ††	2.0	18.6	1.7	14.8
Hyperkalemia †††	1.1	36.9	0.3	27.1

†renal failure, renal failure acute, renal failure chronic, renal impairment

††dizziness, dizziness postural, hypotension, orthostatic hypotension, presyncope, syncope

††† Given the variable baseline potassium levels of patients with renal insufficiency on dual RAAS therapy, the reporting of adverse event of hyperkalemia was at the discretion of the investigator.

* A Serious Adverse Event (SAE) is defined as: an event which is fatal or life-threatening, results in persistent or significant disability/incapacity, constitutes a congenital anomaly/birth defect, requires inpatient hospitalization or prolongation of existing hospitalization, or is medically significant (i.e. defined as an event that jeopardizes the patient or may require medical or surgical intervention to prevent one of the outcomes previously listed).

Aliskiren/Amlodipine/HCTZ (mg)	Color	Embossing Side 1/side 2	NDC 0078-XXXX-XX		
			Bottle/30	Bottle/90	Blister/100
150/5/12.5	Violet white	YIY/NVR	0610-15	0610-34	0610-35
300/5/12.5	Light pink	LIL/NVR	0611-15	0611-34	0611-35
300/5/25	Pale orange brown	OIO/NVR	0612-15	0612-34	0612-35
300/10/12.5	Light red	UIU/NVR	0613-15	0613-34	0613-35
300/10/25	Brown	VIV/NVR	0614-15	0614-34	0614-35

16 HOW SUPPLIED/STORAGE AND HANDLING

Tablets are convex ovaloid with a beveled edge, film-coated, and unscored, in the following strengths and packages:
[See third table above]

Storage

Store at 25°C (77°F); excursions permitted to 15-30°C (59-86°F) in original container.

Protect from heat and moisture.

Dispense in original container.

17 PATIENT COUNSELING INFORMATION

See FDA-Approved Patient Labeling (Patient Information)

Instruct patients to read the Patient Package Insert before starting Amturnide and to reread each time the prescription is renewed. Instruct patients to inform their doctor or pharmacist if they develop any unusual symptom, or if any known symptom persists or worsens.

Pregnancy

Female patients of childbearing age should be told about the consequences of exposure to Amturnide during pregnancy. Discuss treatment options with women planning to become pregnant. Patients should be asked to report pregnancies to their physicians as soon as possible.

Symptomatic Hypotension

Caution patients receiving Amturnide that lightheadedness can occur, especially during the first days of therapy, and that it should be reported to the prescribing physician. Tell patients that if syncope occurs, discontinue Amturnide until the physician has been consulted.

Caution all patients that inadequate fluid intake, excessive perspiration, diarrhea, or vomiting can lead to an excessive fall in blood pressure, with the same consequences of lightheadedness and possible syncope.

Anaphylactic Reactions and Angioedema

Advise patients to report immediately any signs or symptoms suggesting a severe allergic reaction (difficulty breathing or swallowing, tightness of the chest, hives, general rash, swelling, itching, dizziness, vomiting, or abdominal pain) or angioedema (swelling of face, extremities, eyes, lips, tongue, difficulty in swallowing or breathing) and to take no more drug until they have consulted with the prescribing physician. Angioedema, including laryngeal edema, may occur at any time during treatment with Amturnide.

Potassium Supplements

Tell patients receiving Amturnide not to use potassium supplements or salt substitutes containing potassium without consulting the prescribing physician.

Relationship to Meals

Patient should establish a routine pattern for taking Amturnide either with or without a meal. High-fat meals decrease absorption substantially.

T2012-177
September 2012

FDA-Approved Patient Labeling
Patient Information
Amturnide™ *(AM-turn-ide)*
Amturnide
(aliskiren, amlodipine and hydrochlorothiazide)
Tablets

Read the Patient Information leaflet that comes with Amturnide before you start taking it and each time you get a refill. There may be new information. This leaflet does not take the place of talking with your doctor about your medical condition and treatment. If you have any questions about Amturnide, ask your doctor or pharmacist.

What is the most important information I should know about Amturnide?

Amturnide can cause harm or death to an unborn baby. Talk to your doctor about other ways to lower your blood pressure if you plan to become pregnant. If you get pregnant while taking Amturnide, tell your doctor right away.

What is Amturnide?

Amturnide is a prescription medicine used to lower blood pressure (hypertension). Amturnide is not for use as the first medicine to treat your high blood pressure.

Amturnide contains 3 different prescription medicines:
- aliskiren, a direct renin inhibitor (DRI)
- amlodipine, a calcium channel blocker (CCB) and
- hydrochlorothiazide (HCTZ), a diuretic (water pill)

It is not known if Amturnide is safe and works in children under 18 years of age.

Who should not take Amturnide?

Do not take Amturnide if you:
- If you get pregnant, stop taking Amturnide and call your doctor right away. If you plan to become pregnant, talk to your doctor about other treatment options for your high blood pressure.
- have diabetes and are taking a kind of medicine called an angiotensin-receptor-blocker or angiotensin-converting-enzyme-inhibitor.
- have low or no urine output
- are allergic to any ingredients in Amturnide or other medicines that contain sulfonamide. See the end of this leaflet for a complete list of ingredients in Amturnide.

What should I tell my doctor before taking Amturnide?

Before taking Amturnide, tell your doctor if you:
- have kidney problems
- have liver problems
- have lupus
- have had an allergic reaction to another blood pressure medicine. Symptoms may include: swelling of the face, lips, tongue, throat, arms and legs, and trouble breathing.
- suffer from heart disorders or if you experienced a heart attack
- have any other medical problems
- are pregnant or planning to become pregnant. **See "What is the most important information I should know about Amturnide?"**
- are breast-feeding. It is not known if Amturnide passes into your breast milk and if it can harm your baby. You and your doctor should decide if you will take Amturnide or breastfeed. You should not do both.

Tell your doctor about all the medicines you take including prescription and nonprescription medicines, vitamins and herbal supplements. Amturnide and certain other medicines may affect each other and cause side effects.

Especially tell your doctor if you are taking:
- a kind of medicine called angiotensin receptor blocker or angiotensin converting enzyme inhibitor
- water pills (also called "diuretics")
- medicines for treating fungus or fungal infections
- cyclosporine (Gengraf®, Neoral, Sandimmune), a medicine used to suppress the immune system
- potassium-containing medicines, potassium supplements, or salt substitutes containing potassium
- cholesterol lowering medicines
  - simvastatin (Zocor®) oratorvastatin (Lipitor®)
  - cholestyramine (Questran, Questran Light, Cholestyramine Light, Locholest Light, Locholest, Prevalite)
  - colestipol (Colestipol hydrochloride, Colestid, Flavored Colestid)
- medicines used to treat diabetes, including insulin
- lithium, a medicine used to treat some types of depression. You should not take Amturnide if you are taking lithium.
- nonsteroidal anti-inflammatory (NSAIDs) medicines. Ask your doctor if you are not sure if you are taking one of these medicines.
- sleeping pills and anti-seizure medicines called barbiturates
- medicines used to treat AIDS or HIV infections (such as ritonavir, indinavir)
- narcotic pain medicines.

Ask your doctor if you are not sure whether you are taking one of the medicines listed above.
Know the medicines you take. Keep a list of them to show your doctor or pharmacist when you get a new medicine. Your doctor or pharmacist will know what medicines are safe to take together.

How should I take Amturnide?

- Take Amturnide exactly as prescribed by your doctor. It is important to take Amturnide every day to control your blood pressure.
- Take Amturnide one time a day, at about the same time each day.
- Take Amturnide the same way every day, either with or without a meal.
- Your doctor may change your dose of Amturnide if needed. Do not change the amount of Amturnide you take without talking to your doctor.
- If you miss a dose of Amturnide, take it as soon as you remember. If it is close to your next dose, do not take the missed dose. Just take the next dose at your regular time.
- If you take too much Amturnide, call your doctor or a Poison Control Center, or go to the nearest hospital emergency room.

What should I avoid while taking Amturnide?

Drinking alcohol. Drinking alcohol during treatment with Amturnide can cause you to have low blood pressure. **See "What are the possible side effects of Amturnide?"**

What are the possible side effects of Amturnide?

Amturnide may cause serious side effects, including:

- **Harm to an unborn baby causing injury or death. See "What is the most important information I should know about Amturnide?"**
- **Severe Allergic Reactions and Angioedema.** Aliskiren, one of the medicines in Amturnide, can cause difficulty breathing or swallowing, tightness of the chest, hives, general rash, swelling, itching, dizziness, vomiting, or abdominal pain (signs of a severe allergic reaction). Aliskiren can also cause swelling of your face, lips, tongue, throat, arms and legs, or the whole body (signs of angioedema). Get medical help right away and tell your doctor if you get any one or more of these symptoms. Serious allergic reactions can happen at any time while you are taking Amturnide.
- **Low blood pressure (hypotension).** Your blood pressure may get too low if you also take water pills, are on a low-salt diet, get dialysis treatments, have heart problems, or get sick with vomiting or diarrhea. Drinking alcohol and taking certain medicines (barbiturates or narcotics) can cause low blood pressure to get worse. Lie down if you feel faint or dizzy, and call your doctor right away.
- **Worsening chest pain or heart attack.** When you first start taking Amturnide or increase your dose, you may have a heart attack or your angina may get worse. If that happens, call your doctor right away or go directly to the nearest hospital emergency room.
- **Allergic reactions.** Hydrochlorothiazide, one of the medicines in Amturnide, can cause allergic reactions.
- **Worsening of lupus.** One of the medicines in Amturnide may cause your lupus to become active or get worse. Tell your doctor if your lupus gets worse or becomes active while taking Amturnide.
- **Low potassium level (hypokalemia).** Your doctor will do blood tests to check your potassium levels.
- **Eye problems.** One of the medicines in Amturnide can cause eye problems that may lead to vision loss. Symptoms of eye problems can happen within hours to weeks of starting Amturnide. Tell your doctor right away if you have:
  - decrease in vision
  - eye pain

The most common side effects of Amturnide include:

- swelling of your ankles, feet, and hands
- dizziness
- headache
- stuffy or runny nose and sore throat

Common side effects of Amturnide include:

- diarrhea
- cough
- tiredness
- high levels of potassium in the blood (hyperkalemia)

Tell your doctor if you have any side effect that bothers you or that does not go away. These are not all of the possible side effects of Amturnide. For more information ask your doctor or pharmacist.
Call your doctor for medical advice about side effects. You may report side effects to FDA at 1-800-FDA-1088.

How should I store Amturnide?

- Store Amturnide tablets at room temperature between 59°F to 86°F (15°C to 30°C).
- Keep Amturnide in the original container.
- Protect Amturnide from heat and moisture.

Keep Amturnide and all medicines out of the reach of children.

General information about Amturnide

Medicines are sometimes prescribed for conditions not listed in the patient information leaflet. Do not take Amturnide for a condition for which it was not prescribed. Do not give Amturnide to other people, even if they have the same condition or symptoms you have. It may harm them. This leaflet summarizes the most important information about Amturnide. If you have questions about Amturnide, talk with your doctor. You can ask your doctor or pharmacist for information that is written for healthcare professionals.
For more information about Amturnide, visit www.Amturnide.com, or call 1-888-NOW-NOVA (1-888-669-6682).

What are the ingredients in Amturnide?

Active ingredients: Aliskiren hemifumarate, amlodipine besylate, and HCTZ.
Inactive ingredients: colloidal silicon dioxide, crospovidone, hypromellose, iron oxide red, iron oxide yellow, iron oxide black, magnesium stearate, microcrystalline cellulose, polyethylene glycol, povidone, talc, and titanium dioxide.

What is high blood pressure (hypertension)?

Blood pressure is the force of blood in your blood vessels when your heart beats and when your heart rests. You have high blood pressure when the force is too much.
High blood pressure makes the heart work harder to pump blood through the body and causes damage to blood vessels. Amturnide can help your blood vessels relax so your blood pressure is lower. Medicines that lower your blood pressure may lower your chance of having a stroke or heart attack.
Distributed by:
Novartis Pharmaceuticals Corporation
East Hanover, New Jersey 07936
© Novartis
T2012-178
September 2012

Shown in Product Identification Guide, page 309

ARCAPTA™ NEOHALER™ ℞

[ar-CAP-ta]
(indacaterol inhalation powder)

The following prescribing information is based on official labeling in effect July 2013.

HIGHLIGHTS OF PRESCRIBING INFORMATION

These highlights do not include all the information needed to use ARCAPTA NEOHALER safely and effectively. See full prescribing information for ARCAPTA NEOHALER.
ARCAPTA™ NEOHALER™ (indacaterol inhalation powder)
Initial U.S. Approval: 2011

WARNING: ASTHMA-RELATED DEATH
See full prescribing information for complete boxed warning

- **Long-acting $beta_2$-adrenergic agonists (LABA) increase the risk of asthma-related death (5.1).**
- **A placebo-controlled study with another long-acting $beta_2$-adrenergic agonist (salmeterol) showed an increase in asthma-related deaths in patients receiving salmeterol. (5.1)**
- **This finding of an increased risk of asthma-related death with salmeterol is considered a class effect of LABA, including indacaterol, the active ingredient in ARCAPTA NEOHALER. The safety and efficacy of ARCAPTA NEOHALER in patients with asthma have not been established. ARCAPTA NEOHALER is not indicated for the treatment of asthma. (4, 5.1)**

RECENT MAJOR CHANGES

Contraindications (4) 09/2012
Warnings and Precautions, Immediate Hypersensitivity Reactions (5.4) 09/2012

INDICATIONS AND USAGE

ARCAPTA NEOHALER is a long-acting $beta_2$-adrenergic agonist indicated for:
The long term, once-daily maintenance bronchodilator treatment of airflow obstruction in patients with chronic obstructive pulmonary disease (COPD), including chronic bronchitis and/or emphysema. (1.1)
Important limitations:

- ARCAPTA NEOHALER is NOT indicated to treat acute deteriorations of chronic obstructive pulmonary disease. (1.2)
- ARCAPTA NEOHALER is NOT indicated for asthma. (1.2)

DOSAGE AND ADMINISTRATION

For oral inhalation only. DO NOT swallow ARCAPTA capsule. ARCAPTA capsules should **always** be used with the NEOHALER inhaler **only**.
75 mcg inhaled every day (once-daily). (2)

DOSAGE FORMS AND STRENGTHS

Inhalation powder hard capsules: 75 mcg. (3)

CONTRAINDICATIONS

- All LABA are contraindicated in patients with asthma without use of a long-term asthma control medication. (4) ARCAPTA NEOHALER is not indicated for the treatment of asthma.
- ARCAPTA NEOHALER is contraindicated in patients with a history of hypersensitivity to indacaterol or to any of the ingredients. (4)

WARNINGS AND PRECAUTIONS

- Do not initiate in acutely deteriorating COPD patients (5.2)
- Do not use for relief of acute symptoms. Concomitant short-acting $beta_2$-agonists can be used as needed for acute relief (5.2)
- Do not exceed the recommended dose. Excessive use or use in conjunction with other medications containing LABA can result in clinically significant cardiovascular effects and may be fatal (5.3)
- Immediate hypersensitivity reactions may occur. Discontinue immediately. (5.4)
- Life-threatening paradoxical bronchospasm can occur. Discontinue immediately. (5.5)
- Use with caution in patients with cardiovascular or convulsive disorders, thyrotoxicosis or sensitivity to sympathomimetic drugs. (5.6, 5.7)

ADVERSE REACTIONS

Most common adverse reactions (>2% and more common than placebo) are cough, oropharyngeal pain, nasopharyngitis, headache and nausea. (6)
To report SUSPECTED ADVERSE REACTIONS, contact Novartis Pharmaceuticals Corporation at 1-888-669-6682 or FDA at 1-800-FDA-1088 or www.fda.gov/medwatch.

DRUG INTERACTIONS

- Other adrenergic drugs may potentiate effect: Use with caution. (5.3, 7.1)
- Xanthine derivatives, steroids, diuretics or non-potassium sparing diuretics may potentiate hypokalemia or ECG changes. Use with caution. (7.2, 7.3)
- MAO inhibitors, tricyclic antidepressants, and drugs that prolong QTc interval may potentiate effect on cardiovascular system. Use with extreme caution. (7.4)
- Beta-blockers may decrease effectiveness: Use with caution and only when medically necessary. (7.5)

See 17 for PATIENT COUNSELING INFORMATION and Medication Guide

Revised: 09/2012

FULL PRESCRIBING INFORMATION: CONTENTS*

*** Sections or subsections omitted from the full prescribing information are not listed**

FULL PRESCRIBING INFORMATION

WARNING: ASTHMA-RELATED DEATH

Long-acting beta$_2$-adrenergic agonists (LABA) increase the risk of asthma-related death. Data from a large placebo-controlled US study that compared the safety of another long-acting beta$_2$-adrenergic agonist (salmeterol) or placebo added to usual asthma therapy showed an increase in asthma-related deaths in patients receiving salmeterol. This finding with salmeterol is considered a class effect of LABA, including indacaterol, the active ingredient in ARCAPTA NEOHALER. The safety and efficacy of ARCAPTA NEOHALER in patients with asthma have not been established. ARCAPTA NEOHALER is not indicated for the treatment of asthma. [See *Contraindications (4), Warnings and Precautions (5.1)*].

1 INDICATIONS AND USAGE

1.1 Maintenance Treatment of COPD

ARCAPTA NEOHALER is a long-acting beta$_2$-agonist indicated for long-term, once-daily maintenance bronchodilator treatment of airflow obstruction in patients with chronic obstructive pulmonary disease (COPD), including chronic bronchitis and/or emphysema.

1.2 Important Limitations of Use

ARCAPTA NEOHALER is not indicated to treat acute deteriorations of chronic obstructive pulmonary disease [*see Warnings and Precautions (5.2)*].

ARCAPTA NEOHALER is not indicated to treat asthma. The safety and effectiveness of ARCAPTA NEOHALER in asthma have not been established.

2 DOSAGE AND ADMINISTRATION

DO NOT SWALLOW ARCAPTA CAPSULES
FOR USE WITH NEOHALER DEVICE ONLY
FOR ORAL INHALATION ONLY

ARCAPTA capsules must not be swallowed as the intended effects on the lungs will not be obtained. The contents of ARCAPTA capsules are only for oral inhalation and should only be used with the NEOHALER device.

The recommended dosage of ARCAPTA NEOHALER is the once-daily inhalation of the contents of one 75 mcg ARCAPTA capsule using the NEOHALER inhaler.

ARCAPTA NEOHALER should be administered once daily every day at the same time of the day by the orally inhaled route only. If a dose is missed, the next dose should be taken as soon as it is remembered. Do not use ARCAPTA NEOHALER more than one time every 24 hours.

ARCAPTA capsules must always be stored in the blister, and only removed IMMEDIATELY BEFORE USE.

No dosage adjustment is required for geriatric patients, patients with mild and moderate hepatic impairment, or renally impaired patients. No data are available for subjects with severe hepatic impairment [*see Clinical Pharmacology (12.3)*].

3 DOSAGE FORMS AND STRENGTHS

Inhalation powder:

75 mcg: hard gelatin capsule with black product code "IDL 75" above a bar printed on one side of the capsule and the logo " " printed on the other side

4 CONTRAINDICATIONS

All LABA are contraindicated in patients with asthma without use of a long-term asthma control medication. [*see Warnings and Precautions (5.1)*]. ARCAPTA NEOHALER is not indicated for the treatment of asthma.

ARCAPTA NEOHALER is contraindicated in patients with a history of hypersensitivity to indacaterol or to any of the ingredients. [*see Warnings and Precautions (5.4)*].

5 WARNINGS AND PRECAUTIONS

5.1 Asthma-Related Death [*See Boxed Warning*]

- **Data from a large placebo-controlled study in asthma patients showed that long-acting beta$_2$-adrenergic agonists may increase the risk of asthma-related death. Data are not available to determine whether the rate of death in patients with COPD is increased by long-acting beta$_2$-adrenergic agonists.**
- **A 28-week, placebo-controlled US study comparing the safety of another long-acting beta$_2$-adrenergic agonist (salmeterol) with placebo, each added to usual asthma therapy, showed an increase in asthma-related deaths in patients receiving salmeterol (13/13,176 in patients treated with salmeterol vs. 3/13,179 in patients treated with placebo; RR 4.37, 95% CI 1.25, 15.34). The increased risk of asthma-related death is considered a class effect of the long-acting beta$_2$-adrenergic agonists, including ARCAPTA NEOHALER. No study adequate to determine whether the rate of asthma-related death is increased in patients treated with ARCAPTA NEOHALER has been conducted. The safety and efficacy of ARCAPTA NEOHALER in patients with asthma have not been established. ARCAPTA NEOHALER is not indicated for the treatment of asthma. [*see Contraindications (4)*].**
- **Serious asthma-related events, including death, were reported in clinical studies with ARCAPTA NEOHALER. The sizes of these studies were not adequate to precisely quantify the differences in serious asthma exacerbation rates between treatment groups. [*see Adverse Reactions (6.2)*].**

5.2 Deterioration of Disease and Acute Episodes

ARCAPTA NEOHALER should not be initiated in patients with acutely deteriorating COPD, which may be a life-threatening condition. ARCAPTA NEOHALER has not been studied in patients with acutely deteriorating COPD. The use of ARCAPTA NEOHALER in this setting is inappropriate.

ARCAPTA NEOHALER should not be used for the relief of acute symptoms, i.e. as rescue therapy for the treatment of acute episodes of bronchospasm. ARCAPTA NEOHALER has not been studied in the relief of acute symptoms and extra doses should not be used for that purpose. Acute symptoms should be treated with an inhaled short-acting beta$_2$-agonist.

When beginning ARCAPTA NEOHALER, patients who have been taking inhaled, short-acting beta$_2$-agonists on a regular basis (e.g., four times a day) should be instructed to discontinue the regular use of these drugs and use them only for symptomatic relief of acute respiratory symptoms. When prescribing ARCAPTA NEOHALER, the healthcare provider should also prescribe an inhaled, short-acting beta$_2$-agonist and instruct the patient on how it should be used. Increasing inhaled beta$_2$-agonist use is a signal of deteriorating disease for which prompt medical attention is indicated.

COPD may deteriorate acutely over a period of hours or chronically over several days or longer. If ARCAPTA NEOHALER no longer controls the symptoms of bronchoconstriction, or the patient's inhaled, short-acting beta$_2$-agonist becomes less effective or the patient needs more inhalation of short-acting beta$_2$-agonist than usual, these may be markers of deterioration of disease. In this setting, a re-evaluation of the patient and the COPD treatment regimen should be undertaken at once. Increasing the daily dosage of ARCAPTA NEOHALER beyond the recommended dose is not appropriate in this situation.

5.3 Excessive Use of ARCAPTA NEOHALER and Use with Other Long-Acting Beta$_2$-Agonists

As with other inhaled beta$_2$-adrenergic drugs, ARCAPTA NEOHALER should not be used more often, at higher doses than recommended, or in conjunction with other medications containing long-acting beta$_2$-agonists, as an overdose may result. Clinically significant cardiovascular effects and fatalities have been reported in association with excessive use of inhaled sympathomimetic drugs.

5.4 Immediate Hypersensitivity Reactions

Immediate hypersensitivity reactions may occur after administration of ARCAPTA NEOHALER. If signs suggesting allergic reactions (in particular, difficulties in breathing or swallowing, swelling of tongue, lips and face, urticaria, skin rash) occur, ARCAPTA NEOHALER should be discontinued immediately and alternative therapy instituted.

5.5 Paradoxical Bronchospasm

As with other inhaled beta$_2$-agonists, ARCAPTA NEOHALER may produce paradoxical bronchospasm that may be life-threatening. If paradoxical bronchospasm occurs, ARCAPTA NEOHALER should be discontinued immediately and alternative therapy instituted.

5.6 Cardiovascular Effects

ARCAPTA NEOHALER, like other beta$_2$-agonists, can produce a clinically significant cardiovascular effect in some patients as measured by increases in pulse rate, systolic or diastolic blood pressure, or symptoms. If such effects occur, ARCAPTA NEOHALER may need to be discontinued. In addition, beta-agonists have been reported to produce ECG changes, such as flattening of the T wave, prolongation of the QTc interval, and ST segment depression, although the clinical significance of these findings is unknown. Therefore, ARCAPTA NEOHALER, like other sympathomimetic amines, should be used with caution in patients with cardiovascular disorders, especially coronary insufficiency, cardiac arrhythmias, and hypertension.

5.7 Coexisting Conditions

ARCAPTA NEOHALER, like other sympathomimetic amines, should be used with caution in patients with convulsive disorders or thyrotoxicosis, and in patients who are unusually responsive to sympathomimetic amines. Doses of the related beta$_2$-agonist albuterol, when administered intravenously, have been reported to aggravate pre-existing diabetes mellitus and ketoacidosis.

5.8 Hypokalemia and Hyperglycemia

Beta$_2$-agonist medications may produce significant hypokalemia in some patients, possibly through intracellular shunting, which has the potential to produce adverse cardiovascular effects [*see Clinical Pharmacology (12.2)*]. The decrease in serum potassium is usually transient, not requiring supplementation. Inhalation of high doses of beta$_2$-adrenergic agonists may produce increases in plasma glucose.

Clinically notable decreases in serum potassium or changes in blood glucose were infrequent during clinical studies with long-term administration of ARCAPTA NEOHALER with the rates similar to those for placebo controls. ARCAPTA NEOHALER has not been investigated in patients whose diabetes mellitus is not well controlled.

6 ADVERSE REACTIONS

Long-acting beta$_2$-adrenergic agonists, such as ARCAPTA NEOHALER, increase the risk of asthma-related death. ARCAPTA NEOHALER is not indicated for the treatment of asthma [See *Boxed Warning* and *Warning and Precautions (5.1)*].

6.1 Clinical Trials Experience in Chronic Obstructive Pulmonary Disease

Because clinical trials are conducted under widely varying conditions, adverse reaction rates observed in the clinical trials of a drug cannot be directly compared to rates in the clinical trials of another drug and may not reflect the rates observed in practice.

The ARCAPTA NEOHALER safety database reflects exposure of 2516 patients to ARCAPTA NEOHALER at doses of 75 mcg or greater for at least 12 weeks in six confirmatory randomized, double-blind, placebo and active-controlled clinical trials (see Section 14). In these trials, 449 patients were exposed to the recommended dose of 75 mcg for up to 3 months, and 144, 583 and 425 COPD patients were exposed to a dose of 150, 300 or 600 mcg for one year, respectively. Overall, patients had a mean pre-bronchodilator forced expiratory volume in one second (FEV$_1$) percent predicted of 54%. The mean age of patients was 64 years, with 47% of patients aged 65 years or older, and the majority (88%) was Caucasian.

In these six clinical trials, 48% of patients treated with any dose of ARCAPTA NEOHALER reported an adverse reaction compared with 43% of patients treated with placebo. The proportion of patients who discontinued treatment due to adverse reaction was 5% for ARCAPTA NEOHALER-treated patients and 5% for placebo-treated patients. The most common adverse reactions that lead to discontinuation of ARCAPTA NEOHALER were COPD and dyspnea.

The most common serious adverse reactions were COPD exacerbation, pneumonia, angina pectoris, and atrial fibrillation, which occurred at similar rates across treatment groups.

Table 1 displays adverse drug reactions reported by at least 2% of patients (and higher than placebo) during a 3 month exposure at the recommended 75 mcg once daily dose. Adverse drug reactions are listed according to MedDRA (version 13.0) system organ class and sorted in descending order of frequency.

Table 1: Number and frequency of adverse drug reactions greater than 2% (and higher than placebo) in COPD patients exposed to ARCAPTA NEOHALER 75 mcg for up to 3 months in multiple dose, controlled trials

	Indacaterol 75 mcg once daily	Placebo
	n=449	n=445
	n (%)	n (%)
Respiratory, thoracic and mediastinal disorders		
- Cough	29 (6.5)	20 (4.5)
- Oropharyngeal pain	10 (2.2)	3 (0.7)

Infections and infestations		
- Nasopharyngitis	24 (5.3)	12 (2.7)
Nervous system disorders		
- Headache	23 (5.1)	11 (2.5)
Gastrointestinal disorders		
- Nausea	11 (2.4)	4 (0.9)

In these trials the overall frequency of all cardiovascular adverse reactions was 2.5% for ARCAPTA NEOHALER 75 mcg and 1.6% for placebo during a 3 month exposure. There were no frequently occurring specific cardiovascular adverse reactions for ARCAPTA NEOHALER 75 mcg (frequency at least 1% and greater than placebo).

Additional adverse drug reactions reported in greater than 2% (and higher than on placebo) in patients dosed with 150, 300 or 600 mcg for up to 12 months were as follows:

- Musculoskeletal and connective tissue disorders: muscle spasm, musculoskeletal pain
- General disorders and administration site conditions: edema peripheral
- Metabolism and nutrition disorder: diabetes mellitus, hyperglycemia
- Infections and infestations: sinusitis, upper respiratory tract infection

Cough experienced post-inhalation

In the clinical trials, health care providers observed during clinic visits that an average of 24% of patients experienced a cough on at least 20% of visits following inhalation of the recommended 75 mcg dose of ARCAPTA NEOHALER compared to 7% of patients receiving placebo. The cough usually occurred within 15 seconds following inhalation and lasted for no more than 15 seconds. Cough following inhalation in clinical trials was not associated with bronchospasm, exacerbations, deteriorations of disease or loss of efficacy.

6.2 Clinical Trials Experience in Asthma

In a 6-month randomized, active controlled asthma safety trial, 805 adult patients with moderate to severe persistent asthma were treated with ARCAPTA NEOHALER 300 mcg (n=268), ARCAPTA NEOHALER 600 mcg (n=268), and salmeterol (n=269), all concomitant with inhaled corticosteroids, which were not co-randomized. Of these patients, there were 2 respiratory-related deaths in the ARCAPTA NEOHALER 300 mcg dose group. There were no deaths in the ARCAPTA NEOHALER 600 mcg dose group or in the salmeterol active control group. Serious adverse reactions related to asthma exacerbation were reported for 2 patients in the indacaterol 300 mcg group, 3 patients in the indacaterol 600 mcg group, and no patients in the salmeterol active control group.

In addition, a two-week dose-ranging trial was conducted in 511 adult patients with mild persistent asthma taking inhaled corticosteroids. No deaths, intubations, or serious adverse reactions related to asthma exacerbation were reported in this trial.

6.3 Postmarketing Experience

The following adverse reactions have been identified during worldwide post-approval use of indacaterol, the active ingredient in ARCAPTA NEOHALER. Because these reactions are reported voluntarily from a population of uncertain size, it is not always possible to reliably estimate their frequency or establish a causal relationship to drug exposure. These adverse reactions are: hypersensitivity reactions, paradoxical bronchospasm, tachycardia/heart rate increase/palpitations, pruritus/rash and dizziness.

7 DRUG INTERACTIONS

7.1 Adrenergic Drugs

If additional adrenergic drugs are to be administered by any route, they should be used with caution because the sympathetic effects of ARCAPTA NEOHALER may be potentiated [*see Warnings and Precautions (5.3, 5.6, 5.7, 5.8)*].

7.2 Xanthine Derivatives, Steroids, or Diuretics

Concomitant treatment with xanthine derivatives, steroids, or diuretics may potentiate any hypokalemic effect of ARCAPTA NEOHALER [*see Warnings and Precautions (5.8)*].

7.3 Non-Potassium Sparing Diuretics

The ECG changes or hypokalemia that may result from the administration of non-potassium sparing diuretics (such as loop or thiazide diuretics) can be acutely worsened by beta-agonists, especially when the recommended dose of the beta-agonist is exceeded. Although the clinical relevance of these effects is not known, caution is advised in the co-administration of ARCAPTA NEOHALER with non-potassium-sparing diuretics.

7.4 Monoamine Oxidase Inhibitors, Tricyclic Antidepressants, QTc Prolonging Drugs

Indacaterol, as with other beta$_2$-agonists, should be administered with extreme caution to patients being treated with monoamine oxidase inhibitors, tricyclic antidepressants, or other drugs known to prolong the QTc interval because the action of adrenergic agonists on the cardiovascular system may be potentiated by these agents. Drugs that are known to prolong the QTc interval may have an increased risk of ventricular arrhythmias.

7.5 Beta-Blockers

Beta-adrenergic receptor antagonists (beta-blockers) and ARCAPTA NEOHALER may interfere with the effect of each other when administered concurrently. Beta-blockers not only block the therapeutic effects of beta-agonists, but may produce severe bronchospasm in COPD patients. Therefore, patients with COPD should not normally be treated with beta-blockers. However, under certain circumstances, e.g. as prophylaxis after myocardial infarction, there may be no acceptable alternatives to the use of beta-blockers in patients with COPD. In this setting, cardioselective beta-blockers could be considered, although they should be administered with caution.

7.6 Inhibitors of Cytochrome P450 3A4 and P-gp Efflux Transporter

Drug interaction studies were carried out using potent and specific inhibitors of CYP3A4 and P-gp (i.e., ketoconazole, erythromycin, verapamil and ritonavir). The data suggest that systemic clearance is influenced by modulation of both P-gp and CYP3A4 activities and that the 1.9-fold $AUC_{0\text{-}24}$ increase caused by the strong dual inhibitor ketoconazole reflects the impact of maximal combined inhibition. ARCAPTA NEOHALER was evaluated in clinical trials for up to one year at doses up to 600 mcg. No dose adjustment is warranted at the 75 mcg dose. [*See Drug-drug Interaction (12.3)*]

8 USE IN SPECIFIC POPULATIONS

8.1 Pregnancy

Teratogenic Effects: Pregnancy Category C.

There are no adequate and well-controlled studies with ARCAPTA NEOHALER in pregnant women. ARCAPTA NEOHALER should be used during pregnancy only if the potential benefit justifies the potential risk to the fetus.

Indacaterol was not teratogenic following subcutaneous administration to rats and rabbits at doses up to 1 mg/kg, approximately 130 and 260 times, respectively, the 75 mcg dose on a mg/m^2 basis.

8.2 Labor and Delivery

There are no adequate and well-controlled human studies that have investigated effects of ARCAPTA NEOHALER on preterm labor or labor at term. Because of the potential for beta-agonist interference with uterine contractility, use of ARCAPTA NEOHALER during labor should be restricted to those patients in whom the benefits clearly outweigh the risks.

8.3 Nursing Mothers

It is not known that the active component of ARCAPTA NEOHALER, indacaterol, is excreted in human milk. Because many drugs are excreted in human milk and because indacaterol has been detected in the milk of lactating rats, caution should be exercised when ARCAPTA NEOHALER is administered to nursing women.

8.4 Pediatric Use

ARCAPTA NEOHALER is not indicated for use in children. The safety and effectiveness of ARCAPTA NEOHALER in pediatric patients have not been established.

8.5 Geriatric Use

Based on available data, no adjustment of ARCAPTA NEOHALER dosage in geriatric patients is warranted. Of the total number of patients who received ARCAPTA NEOHALER at the recommended dose of 75 mcg once daily in the clinical studies from the pooled 3-month database, 239 were <65 years, 153 were 65–74 years and 57 were ≥75 years of age.

No overall differences in effectiveness were observed, and in the 3-month pooled data, the adverse drug reaction profile was similar in the older population compared to the patient population overall. When treated at higher doses (300 mcg and 600 mcg) over the course of a year, the adverse drug reaction profiles for patients >65 years was similar to that of the general patient population.

8.6 Hepatic Impairment

Patients with mild and moderate hepatic impairment showed no relevant changes in C_{max} or AUC, nor did protein binding differ between mild and moderate hepatically impaired subjects and their healthy controls. Studies in subjects with severe hepatic impairment were not performed.

8.7 Renal Impairment

Due to the very low contribution of the urinary pathway to total body elimination, a study in renally impaired subjects was not performed.

10 OVERDOSAGE

10.1 Human Experience

In COPD patients single doses of 40 times the 75 mcg dose were associated with moderate increases in pulse rate, systolic blood pressure and QTc interval.

The expected signs and symptoms associated with overdosage of ARCAPTA NEOHALER are those of excessive beta-adrenergic stimulation and occurrence or exaggeration of any of the signs and symptoms, e.g., angina, hypertension or hypotension, tachycardia, with rates up to 200 bpm, arrhythmias, nervousness, headache, tremor, dry mouth, palpitation, muscle cramps, nausea, dizziness, fatigue, malaise, hypokalemia, hyperglycemia, metabolic acidosis and insomnia. As with all inhaled sympathomimetic medications, cardiac arrest and even death may be associated with an overdose of ARCAPTA NEOHALER.

Treatment of overdosage consists of discontinuation of ARCAPTA NEOHALER together with institution of appropriate symptomatic and supportive therapy. The judicious use of a cardioselective beta-receptor blocker may be considered, bearing in mind that such medication can produce bronchospasm. There is insufficient evidence to determine if dialysis is beneficial for overdosage of ARCAPTA NEOHALER. Cardiac monitoring is recommended in cases of overdosage.

11 DESCRIPTION

ARCAPTA NEOHALER consists of a dry powder formulation of indacaterol maleate for oral inhalation only with the NEOHALER inhaler. The inhalation powder is packaged in clear gelatin capsules.

Each clear, hard gelatin capsule contains a dry powder blend of 75 mcg of indacaterol (equivalent to 97 mcg of indacaterol maleate) with approximately 25 mg of lactose monohydrate (which contains trace levels of milk protein) as the carrier.

The active component of ARCAPTA NEOHALER is indacaterol maleate, a (R) enantiomer. Indacaterol maleate is a selective beta$_2$-adrenergic agonist. Its chemical name is (R)-5-[2-(5,6-Diethylindan-2-ylamino)-1-hydroxyethyl]-8-hydroxy-1H-quinolin-2-one maleate; its structural formula is

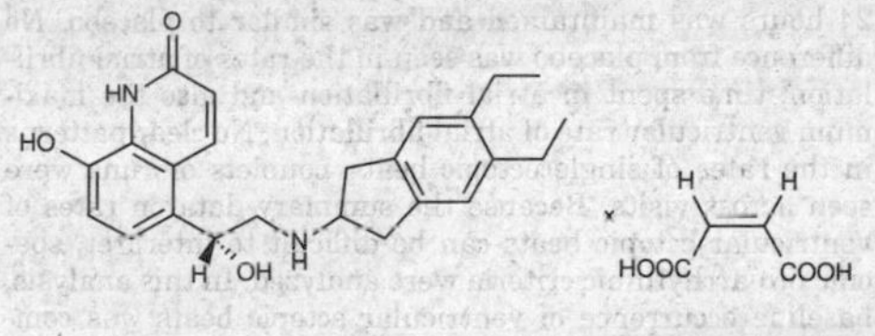

Indacaterol maleate has a molecular weight of 508.56, and its empirical formula is $C_{24}H_{28}N_2O_3 \bullet C_4H_4O_4$. Indacaterol maleate is a white to very slightly grayish or very slightly yellowish powder. Indacaterol maleate is freely soluble in N-methylpyrrolidone and dimethylformamide, slightly soluble in methanol, ethanol, propylene glycol and polyethylene glycol 400, very slightly soluble in water, isopropyl alcohol and practically insoluble in 0.9% sodium chloride in water, ethyl acetate and n-octanol.

The NEOHALER inhaler is a plastic device used for inhaling ARCAPTA. The amount of drug delivered to the lung will depend on patient factors, such as inspiratory flow rate and inspiratory time. Under standardized *in vitro* testing at a fixed flow rate of 60 L/min for 2 seconds, the NEOHALER inhaler delivered 57 mcg for the 75 mcg dose strength (equivalent to 73.9 mcg of indacaterol maleate) from the mouthpiece. Peak inspiratory flow rates (PIFR) achievable through the NEOHALER inhaler were evaluated in 26 adult patients with COPD of varying severity. Mean PIFR was 95 L/min (range 52-133 L/min) for adult patients. Approximately ninety-five percent of the population studied generated a PIFR through the device exceeding 60 L/min.

12 CLINICAL PHARMACOLOGY

12.1 Mechanism of Action

Indacaterol is a long-acting beta$_2$-adrenergic agonist.

When inhaled, indacaterol acts locally in the lung as a bronchodilator. Although beta$_2$-receptors are the predominant adrenergic receptors in bronchial smooth muscle and beta$_1$-receptors are the predominant receptors in the heart, there are also beta$_2$-adrenergic receptors in the human heart comprising 10%-50% of the total adrenergic receptors. The precise function of these receptors is not known, but their presence raises the possibility that even highly selective beta$_2$-adrenergic agonists may have cardiac effects.

The pharmacological effects of beta$_2$-adrenoceptor agonist drugs, including indacaterol, are at least in part attributable to stimulation of intracellular adenyl cyclase, the enzyme that catalyzes the conversion of adenosine triphosphate (ATP) to cyclic-3′, 5′-adenosine monophosphate (cyclic monophosphate). Increased cyclic AMP levels cause relaxation of bronchial smooth muscle. *In vitro* studies have shown that indacaterol has more than 24-fold greater agonist activity at beta$_2$-receptors compared to beta$_1$-receptors and 20-fold greater agonist activity compared to beta$_3$-receptors. This selectivity profile is similar to formoterol. The clinical significance of these findings is unknown.

12.2 Pharmacodynamics

Systemic Safety

The major adverse effects of inhaled beta$_2$-adrenergic agonists occur as a result of excessive activation of systemic beta-adrenergic receptors. The most common adverse effects in adults include skeletal muscle tremor and cramps, insomnia, tachycardia, decreases in serum potassium and increases in plasma glucose.

Changes in serum potassium and plasma glucose were evaluated in COPD patients in double-blind Phase III studies. In pooled data, at the recommended 75 mcg dose, at 1 hour post-dose at week 12, there was no change compared to placebo in serum potassium, and change in mean plasma glucose was 0.07 mmol/L.

Electrophysiology

The effect of ARCAPTA NEOHALER on the QT interval was evaluated in a double-blind, placebo- and active (moxifloxacin)-controlled study following multiple doses of indacaterol 150 mcg, 300 mcg or 600 mcg once-daily for 2 weeks in 404 healthy volunteers. Fridericia's method for heart rate correction was employed to derive the corrected QT interval (QTcF). Maximum mean prolongation of QTcF intervals were <5 ms, and the upper limit of the 90% confidence interval was below 10 ms for all time-matched comparisons versus placebo. During these studies, there were no clinically meaningful QT-interval prolongations. There was no evidence of a clinically relevant concentration-delta QTc relationship in the range of doses evaluated.

The effect of 150 mcg and 300 mcg once daily of ARCAPTA NEOHALER on heart rate and rhythm was assessed using continuous 24-hour ECG recording (Holter monitoring) in a subset of 605 patients with COPD from a 26-week, double-blind, placebo-controlled Phase III study. Holter monitoring occurred once at baseline and up to 3 times during the 26-week treatment period (at weeks 2, 12 and 26). A comparison of the mean heart rate over 24 hours showed no increase from baseline. The hourly heart rate analysis was similar compared to placebo. The pattern of diurnal variation over 24 hours was maintained and was similar to placebo. No difference from placebo was seen in the rates of atrial fibrillation, time spent in atrial fibrillation and also the maximum ventricular rate of atrial fibrillation. No clear patterns in the rates of single ectopic beats, couplets or runs were seen across visits. Because the summary data on rates of ventricular ectopic beats can be difficult to interpret, specific pro-arrhythmic criteria were analyzed. In this analysis, baseline occurrence of ventricular ectopic beats was compared to change from baseline, setting certain parameters for the change to describe the pro-arrhythmic response. The number of patients with a documented pro-arrhythmic response was very similar compared to placebo. Overall, there was no clinically relevant difference in the development of arrhythmic events in patients receiving indacaterol treatment over those patients who received placebo.

Tachyphylaxis/Tolerance

Tolerance to the effects of inhaled beta-agonists can occur with regularly-scheduled, chronic use. In two 12-week clinical efficacy trials in 323 and 318 adult patients with COPD, ARCAPTA NEOHALER improvement in lung function (as measured by the forced expiratory volume in one second, FEV$_1$) observed at Week 4 with ARCAPTA NEOHALER was consistently maintained over the 12-week treatment period in both trials.

12.3 Pharmacokinetics

Absorption

The median time to reach peak serum concentrations of indacaterol was approximately 15 minutes after single or repeated inhaled doses. Systemic exposure to indacaterol increased with increasing dose (150 mcg to 600 mcg) in a dose proportional manner, and was about dose-proportional in the dose range of 75 mcg to 150 mcg. Absolute bioavailability of indacaterol after an inhaled dose was on average 43-45%. Systemic exposure results from a composite of pulmonary and intestinal absorption.

Indacaterol serum concentrations increased with repeated once-daily administration. Steady-state was achieved within 12 to 15 days. The mean accumulation ratio of indacaterol, i.e. AUC over the 24-hour dosing interval on day 14 or day 15 compared to day 1, was in the range of 2.9 to 3.8 for once-daily inhaled doses between 75 mcg and 600 mcg.

Distribution

After intravenous infusion the volume of distribution (Vz) of indacaterol was 2,361 L to 2,557 L indicating an extensive distribution. The *in vitro* human serum and plasma protein binding was 94.1-95.3% and 95.1-96.2%, respectively.

Metabolism

After oral administration of radiolabeled indacaterol in the human ADME (absorption, distribution, metabolism, excretion) study unchanged indacaterol was the main component in serum, accounting for about one third of total drug-related AUC over 24 hours. A hydroxylated derivative was the most prominent metabolite in serum. Phenolic O-glucuronides of indacaterol and hydroxylated indacaterol were further prominent metabolites. A diastereomer of the hydroxylated derivative, a N-glucuronide of indacaterol, and C- and N-dealkylated products were further metabolites identified.

In vitro investigations indicated that UGT1A1 was the only UGT isoform that metabolized indacaterol to the phenolic O-glucuronide. The oxidative metabolites were found in incubations with recombinant CYP1A1, CYP2D6, and CYP3A4. CYP3A4 is concluded to be the predominant isoenzyme responsible for hydroxylation of indacaterol.

In vitro investigations indicated that indacaterol is a low affinity substrate for the efflux pump P-gp.

In vitro investigations indicated that indacaterol has negligible potential to cause metabolic interactions with medications (by inhibition or induction of cytochrome P450 enzymes, or induction of UGT1A1) at the systemic exposure levels achieved in clinical practice. *In vitro* investigation furthermore indicated that, *in vivo*, indacaterol is unlikely to significantly inhibit transporter proteins such as P-gp, MRP2, BCRP, the cationic substrate transporters hOCT1 and hOCT2, and the human multidrug and toxin extrusion transporters hMATE1 and hMATE2K, and that indacaterol has negligible potential to induce P-gp or MRP2.

Elimination

In clinical studies which included urine collection the amount of indacaterol excreted unchanged *via* urine was generally lower than 2% of the dose. Renal clearance of indacaterol was, on average, between 0.46 and 1.2 L/h. When compared with the serum clearance of indacaterol of 18.8 L/h to 23.3 L/h, it is evident that renal clearance plays a minor role (about 2 to 6% of systemic clearance) in the elimination of systemically available indacaterol.

In a human ADME study where indacaterol was given orally, the fecal route of excretion was dominant over the urinary route. Indacaterol was excreted into human feces primarily as unchanged parent drug (54% of the dose) and, to a lesser extent, hydroxylated indacaterol metabolites (23% of the dose). Mass balance was complete with ≥90% of the dose recovered in the excreta.

Indacaterol serum concentrations declined in a multi-phasic manner with an average terminal half-life ranging from 45.5 to 126 hours. The effective half-life, calculated from the accumulation of indacaterol after repeated dosing with once daily doses between 75 mcg and 600 mcg ranged from 40 to 56 hours which is consistent with the observed time-to-steady state of approximately 12-15 days.

Special Populations

A population pharmacokinetic analysis was performed for indacaterol utilizing data from 3 controlled clinical trials that included 1,844 patients with COPD aged 40 to 88 years who received treatment with ARCAPTA NEOHALER.

The population analysis showed that no dose adjustment is warranted based on the effect of age, gender and weight on systemic exposure in COPD patients after inhalation of ARCAPTA NEOHALER. The population pharmacokinetic analysis did not suggest any difference between ethnic subgroups in this population.

Hepatic Impairment

Patients with mild and moderate hepatic impairment showed no relevant changes in C_{max} or AUC of indacaterol, nor did protein binding differ between mild and moderate hepatically impaired subjects and their healthy controls. Studies in subjects with severe hepatic impairment were not performed.

Renal Impairment

Due to the very low contribution of the urinary pathway to total body elimination, a study in renally impaired subjects was not performed.

Drug-drug Interaction

Drug interaction studies were carried out using potent and specific inhibitors of CYP3A4 and P-gp (i.e., ketoconazole, erythromycin, verapamil and ritonavir).

Verapamil: Co-administration of indacaterol 300 mcg (single dose) with verapamil (80 mg t.i.d for 4 days) showed 2-fold increase in indacaterol $AUC_{0\text{-}24}$, and 1.5-fold increase in indacaterol C_{max}.

Erythromycin: Co-administration of indacaterol inhalation powder 300 mcg (single dose) with erythromycin (400 mg q.i.d for 7 days) showed a 1.4-fold increase in indacaterol $AUC_{0\text{-}24}$, and 1.2-fold increase in indacaterol C_{max}

Ketoconazole: Co-administration of indacaterol inhalation powder 300 mcg (single dose) with ketoconazole (200 mg b.i.d for 7 days) caused a 1.9-fold increase in indacaterol $AUC_{0\text{-}24}$, and 1.3-fold increase in indacaterol C_{max}

Ritonavir: Co-administration of indacaterol 300 mcg (single dose) with ritonavir (300 mg b.i.d for 7.5 days) resulted in a 1.7-fold increase in indacaterol $AUC_{0\text{-}24}$ whereas indacaterol C_{max} was unaffected. *[See Drug Interactions (7.6)].*

12.4 Pharmacogenomics

The pharmacokinetics of indacaterol were prospectively investigated in subjects with the *UGT1A1* $(TA)_7/(TA)_7$ genotype (low UGT1A1 expression; also referred to as *28) and the $(TA)_6$, $(TA)_6$ genotype. Steady-state AUC and C_{max} of indacaterol were 1.2-fold higher in the $[(TA)_7, (TA)_7]$ genotype, suggesting no relevant effect of UGT1A1 genotype of indacaterol exposure.

13 NONCLINICAL TOXICOLOGY

13.1 Carcinogenesis, Mutagenesis, Impairment of Fertility

Long-term studies were conducted in transgenic mice using oral administration and in rats using inhalation administration to evaluate the carcinogenic potential of indacaterol maleate. Indacaterol did not show a statistically significant increase in tumor formation in mice or rats.

Lifetime treatment of rats resulted in increased incidences of benign ovarian leiomyoma and focal hyperplasia of ovarian smooth muscle in females at doses approximately 270-times the dose of 75 mcg once-daily for humans (on a mg/m^2 basis).

A 26-week oral (gavage) study in CB6F1/TgrasH2 hemizygous mice with indacaterol did not show any evidence of tumorigenicity at doses approximately 39,000-times the dose of 75 mcg once-daily for humans (on a mg/m^2 basis).

Increases in leiomyomas of the female rat genital tract have been similarly demonstrated with other beta$_2$-adrenergic agonist drugs. The relevance of these findings to human use is unknown.

Indacaterol was not mutagenic or clastogenic in Ames test, chromosome aberration test in V79 Chinese hamster cells, and bone marrow micronucleus test in rats.

Indacaterol did not impair fertility of rats in reproduction studies.

14 CLINICAL STUDIES

The ARCAPTA NEOHALER COPD clinical development program included three dose-ranging trials and six confirmatory trials (Trial 3, a 26-week seamless adaptive design trial that included an initial 2 week dose ranging phase; Trials 4, 5, and 6, 12-week trials; Trial 7, a 26-week trial; and Trial 8, a 52 week trial).

Dose-ranging trials:

Dose selection for ARCAPTA NEOHALER for COPD was based on three dose-ranging trials (Trial 1, a 2-week dose-ranging trial in an asthma population; Trial 2, a 2-week dose-ranging trial in a COPD population; and Trial 3, a 26-week adaptive seamless design trial that included an initial 2-week dose ranging phase). Although ARCAPTA NEOHALER is not indicated for asthma, dose selection was primarily based upon the results from the dose-ranging trial in asthma patients (Trial 1) as an asthma population is the most responsive to beta-agonist bronchodilation and is most likely to demonstrate a dose response. Dose-ranging in COPD patients (Trials 2 and 3) provided supportive information.

Dose-ranging in asthma

ARCAPTA NEOHALER is not indicated for asthma.

Trial 1 was a 2-week, randomized, double-blinded, placebo-controlled design that enrolled 511 patients with persistent asthma 18 years of age and older. All enrolled patients were required to be taking inhaled corticosteroids, had a forced expiratory volume in one second (FEV$_1$) of ≥ 50% and ≤ 90% predicted, and FEV$_1$ reversibility after albuterol of at least 12% and at least 200 mL. Trial 1 included ARCAPTA NEOHALER doses of 18.75, 37.5, 75, and 150 mcg once daily, a salmeterol active control group, and placebo. The trial showed that the effect on FEV$_1$ in patients treated with ARCAPTA NEOHALER 18.75 and 37.5 mcg doses was lower compared to patients treated with other ARCAPTA NEOHALER doses, particularly after the first dose. The effect did not clearly differ between the 75 and 150 mcg doses. Results of the ARCAPTA NEOHALER and placebo treatment arms are as follows. After the first dose (Day 1), the peak (4 hour) FEV$_1$ was 2.58L in the placebo group, with a treatment difference of 0.04L (95% CI -0.01, 0.09) in the 18.75 mcg ARCAPTA NEOHALER group, 0.04L (-0.01, 0.09) in the 37.5 mcg group, 0.12L (0.07, 0.17) in the 75 mcg group, and 0.15L (0.10, 0.20) in the 150 mcg group. The Day 2 trough FEV$_1$ was 2.45L in the placebo group, with a treatment difference of 0.02L (95% CI -0.05, 0.08), 0.08L (0.01, 0.15), 0.09L (0.03, 0.16) and 0.16L (0.09, 0.22) in the ARCAPTA NEOHALER groups, respectively. At Day 14, the peak (4 hour) FEV$_1$ was 2.55L in the placebo group, with a treatment difference of 0.12L (95% CI 0.05, 0.20) in the 18.75 mcg ARCAPTA NEOHALER group, 0.14L (0.06, 0.21) in the 37.5 mcg group, 0.23L (0.15, 0.30) in the 75 mcg group, and 0.20L (0.13, 0.27) in the 150 mcg group. The Day 15 FEV$_1$ (primary endpoint) was 2.42L in the placebo group, with a treatment difference of 0.09L (95% CI 0.00, 0.17), 0.11L (0.02, 0.19), 0.17L (0.08, 0.26), and 0.12L (0.04, 0.21) in the ARCAPTA NEOHALER groups, respectively.

Dose-ranging in COPD

Trial 2 was a 2-week, randomized, double-blinded, placebo-controlled design that enrolled 552 patients with a clinical diagnosis of COPD, who were 40 years or older, had a smoking history of at least 10 pack years, had a postbronchodilator FEV_1 less than 80% and at least 30% of the predicted normal value and a post-bronchodilator ratio of FEV_1 over forced vital capacity (FEV_1/FVC) of less than 70%. Trial 2 included ARCAPTA NEOHALER doses of 18.75, 37.5, 75 and 150 mcg once daily, a salmeterol active control group, and placebo. Results of the ARCAPTA NEOHALER and placebo arms are shown in Figure 1. The trial showed that the effect on FEV_1 in patients treated with ARCAPTA NEOHALER 18.75 mcg dose was lower compared to patients treated with other ARCAPTA NEOHALER doses. Although a dose-response relationship was observed at Day 1, the effect did not clearly differ among the 37.5, 75 and 150 mcg doses by Day 15.

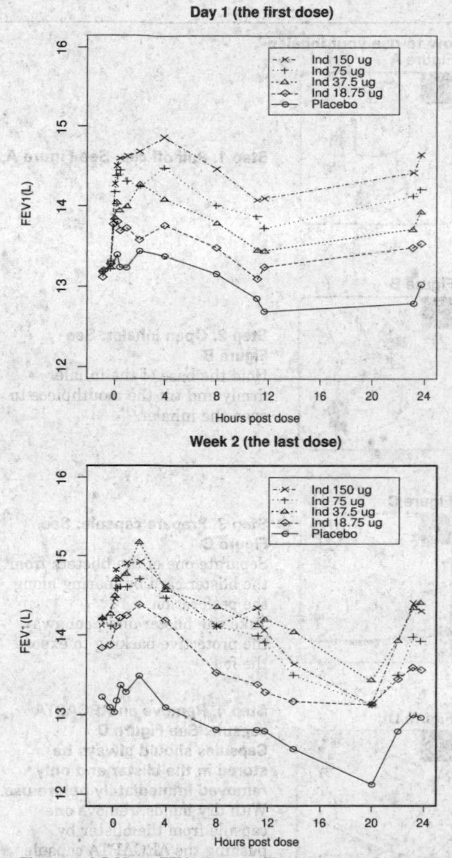

Figure 1: LS Mean FEV1 time profile curve over 24 hours after ARCAPTA NEOHALER Day 1 and Week 2 in Trial 2 (COPD dose ranging)

The 2-week dose ranging phase of Trial 3 included ARCAPTA NEOHALER doses of 75, 150, 300, and 600 mcg once daily, placebo, and two active comparators. Although a dose-response relationship was observed at week 2, the effect did not clearly differ among the ARCAPTA NEOHALER doses.

Confirmatory Trials:

The ARCAPTA NEOHALER COPD development program included six confirmatory trials that were randomized, double-blinded placebo and active-controlled in design (Trial 3, a 26-week seamless adaptive design trial that included an initial 2 week dose-ranging phase; Trials 4, 5, and 6, 12-week trials; Trial 7, a 26-week trial; and Trial 8, a 52 week trial). After the initial 2-week dose-ranging portion of the design, Trial 3 was conducted with ARCAPTA NEOHALER doses of 150 mcg and 300 mcg once daily, placebo, and an active comparator. Trials 4 and 5 were conducted with ARCAPTA NEOHALER dose of 75 mcg once daily, and placebo. Trial 6 was conducted with ARCAPTA NEOHALER dose of 150 mcg once daily and placebo. Trial 7 was conducted with ARCAPTA NEOHALER dose of 150 mcg once daily, an active comparator, and placebo. Trial 8 was conducted with ARCAPTA NEOHALER doses of 300 mcg and 600 mcg once daily, an active comparator, and placebo.

As Trials 3, 6, 7, and 8 were conducted with doses of ARCAPTA NEOHALER higher than 75 mcg, the results of Trials 4 and 5, which included ARCAPTA NEOHALER 75 mcg are the focus of this section.

These six trials enrolled 5474 patients with a clinical diagnosis of COPD, who were 40 years or older, had a smoking history of at least 10 pack years, had a post-bronchodilator FEV_1 less than 80% and at least 30% of the predicted normal value and a post-bronchodilator ratio of FEV_1 over FVC of less than 70%.

Assessment of efficacy in these six COPD trials was based on FEV_1. The primary efficacy endpoint was 24-hour post-dose trough FEV_1 (defined as the average of two FEV_1 measurements taken after 23 hours 10 minutes and 23 hours and 45 minutes after the previous dose) after 12 weeks of treatment in all 6 trials. Other efficacy variables included other FEV_1 and FVC time points, rescue medication use, symptoms, and health-related quality of life measured using the St. George's Respiratory Questionnaire (SGRQ).

In all six confirmatory COPD trials, all doses of ARCAPTA NEOHALER tested (75 mcg, 150 mcg, 300 mcg, and 600 mcg) showed significantly greater 24-hour post-dose trough FEV_1 compared to placebo at 12 weeks. Results of Trials 4 and 5, which compared ARCAPTA NEOHALER at the dose of 75 mcg once daily to placebo are shown in Table 2.

Table 2: LS Mean for trough FEV_1 at 12 weeks

Treatment	Trough FEV_1 at Week 12 (liters)	Treatment Difference LS Mean (95% CI)
Trial 4 (N=323)		
Indacaterol 75 mcg	1.38	0.12 (0.08, 0.15)
Placebo	1.26	
Trial 5 (N=318)		
Indacaterol 75 mcg	1.49	0.14 (0.10, 0.18)
Placebo	1.35	

In addition, serial FEV_1 measurements in patients treated with ARCAPTA NEOHALER demonstrated a bronchodilatory treatment effect after the first dose compared to placebo at 5 minutes post dose of 0.09 L (Trial 4) and 0.10 L (Trial 5). The mean peak improvement relative to baseline within the first 4 hours after the first dose (Day 1) was 0.19 L (Trial 4) and 0.22 L (Trial 5) and was 0.24 L (Trial 4) and 0.27 L (Trial 5) after 12 weeks. Improvement in lung function observed at week 4 was consistently maintained over the 12-week treatment period in both trials. In Trial 5, 24-hour spirometry was assessed in a subset of 239 patients. See Figure 2.

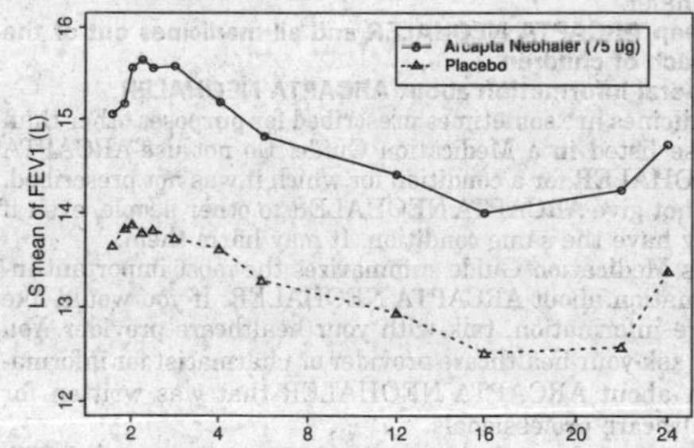

Figure 2: LS Mean FEV1 time profile curve over 24 hours at Week 12 in Trial 5

In both COPD clinical trials including the 75 mcg dose (Trials 4 and 5), patients treated with ARCAPTA NEOHALER used less daily rescue albuterol during the trial compared to patients treated with placebo.

Health-related quality of life was measured using the St. George's Respiratory Questionnaire (SGRQ) in all six confirmatory COPD clinical trials. SGRQ is a disease-specific patient reported instrument which measures symptoms, activities, and its impact on daily life. At week 12, pooled data from these trials demonstrated an improvement over placebo in SGRQ total score of -3.8 with a 95% CI of (-5.3, -2.3) for the ARCAPTA NEOHALER 75 mcg dose, -4.6 with a 95% CI of (-5.5, -3.6) for 150 mcg, and -3.8 with a 95% CI of (-4.9, -2.8) for 300 mcg. The confidence intervals for this change are widely overlapping with no dose ordering. Results from individual studies were variable, but are generally consistent with the pooled data results.

16 HOW SUPPLIED/STORAGE AND HANDLING

16.1 How Supplied

75 mcg ARCAPTA NEOHALER contains ARCAPTA (indacaterol inhalation powder) capsules packaged in aluminum blister cards, one NEOHALER inhaler, and an FDA approved Medication Guide.

Unit Dose (blister pack), Box of 30 (5 blister cards with 6 capsules each) NDC 0078-0619-15

The NEOHALER inhaler consists of a white protective cap and a base with mouthpiece, capsule chamber and two translucent red push buttons.

16.2 Storage and Handling

Store in a dry place at 25°C (77°F); excursions permitted to 15-30°C (59-86° F) [*see USP Controlled Room Temperature*].

75 mcg: Protect capsule from light and moisture.

- ARCAPTA capsules should be used with the NEOHALER inhaler only. The NEOHALER inhaler should not be used with any other capsules.
- Capsules should always be stored in the blister and only removed from the blister immediately before use.
- Always use the new NEOHALER inhaler provided with each new prescription.

Keep out of the reach of children.

17 PATIENT COUNSELING INFORMATION

See FDA-approved patient labeling (Medication Guide)

17.1 Asthma-Related Death

Patients should be informed that LABA, such as ARCAPTA NEOHALER, increase the risk of asthma-related death. ARCAPTA NEOHALER is not indicated for the treatment of asthma.

17.2 Instructions for Administering ARCAPTA NEOHALER

It is important for patients to understand how to correctly administer ARCAPTA capsules using the NEOHALER device [*see Instructions for Use at the end of the Medication Guide*]. Patients should be instructed that ARCAPTA capsules should only be administered via the NEOHALER device and the NEOHALER device should not be used for administering other medications. **The contents of ARCAPTA capsules are for oral inhalation only and must not be swallowed.**

ARCAPTA capsules should always be stored in sealed blisters. Only one ARCAPTA capsule should be removed immediately before use, or its effectiveness may be reduced. Additional ARCAPTA capsules that are exposed to air (i.e. not intended for immediate use) should be discarded.

17.3 Not for Acute Symptoms

ARCAPTA NEOHALER is not meant to relieve acute symptoms or exacerbations of COPD and extra doses should not be used for that purpose. Acute symptoms should be treated with an inhaled, short-acting beta$_2$-agonist such as albuterol. (The healthcare provider should provide the patient with such medication and instruct the patient in how it should be used.)

Patients should be instructed to notify their physician immediately if they experience any of the following:

- Worsening of symptoms
- Decreasing effectiveness of inhaled, short-acting beta$_2$-agonists
- Need for more inhalations than usual of inhaled, short-acting beta$_2$-agonists
- Significant decrease in lung function as outlined by the physician.

Patients should not stop therapy with ARCAPTA NEOHALER without physician/provider guidance since symptoms may recur after discontinuation.

17.4 Do Not Use Additional Long-Acting Beta$_2$-Agonists

Patients who have been taking inhaled, short-acting beta$_2$-agonists on a regular basis should be instructed to discontinue the regular use of these products and use them only for the symptomatic relief of acute symptoms.

When patients are prescribed ARCAPTA NEOHALER, other inhaled medications containing long-acting beta2-agonists should not be used. Patients should not use more than the recommended once daily dose of ARCAPTA NEOHALER. Excessive use of sympathomimetics may cause significant cardiovascular effects, and may be fatal.

17.5 Risks Associated With Beta-Agonist Therapy

Patients should be informed of adverse effects associated with beta$_2$-agonists, such as palpitations, chest pain, rapid heart rate, tremor, or nervousness.

T2012-174

September 2012

Medication Guide

ARCAPTA™ (ar CAP-ta) NEOHALER™

(indacaterol inhalation powder)

> **Important: Do not swallow ARCAPTA capsules. ARCAPTA capsules are used only with the NEOHALER inhaler that comes with ARCAPTA NEOHALER. Never place a capsule in the mouthpiece of the NEOHALER inhaler.**

Read the Medication Guide that comes with ARCAPTA NEOHALER before you start using it and each time you get a refill. There may be new information. This Medication Guide does not take the place of talking to your health care provider about your medical condition or treatment.

What is the most important information I should know about ARCAPTA NEOHALER?

ARCAPTA NEOHALER has been approved for COPD only. Therefore, ARCAPTA NEOHALER is NOT to be used in asthma.

ARCAPTA NEOHALER can cause serious side effects, including:
- **People with asthma who take long-acting beta$_2$ adrenergic-agonist (LABA) medicines, such as ARCAPTA NEOHALER, have an increased risk of death from asthma problems.**
- **It is not known if LABA medicines, such as ARCAPTA NEOHALER, increase the risk of death in people with chronic obstructive pulmonary disease (COPD).**
- Get emergency medical care if:
  - breathing problems worsen quickly
  - you use your rescue inhaler medicine, but it does not relieve your breathing problems.

What is ARCAPTA NEOHALER?
ARCAPTA NEOHALER is used long term, 1 time each day, in controlling symptoms of chronic obstructive pulmonary disease (COPD) in adults with COPD.
LABA medicines such as ARCAPTA NEOHALER help the muscles around the airways in your lungs stay relaxed to prevent symptoms, such as wheezing, cough, chest tightness and shortness of breath.
ARCAPTA NEOHALER is not for use to treat sudden symptoms of COPD. Always have a short-acting beta$_2$-agonist medicine with you to treat sudden symptoms. If you do not have an inhaled, short-acting bronchodilator, contact your healthcare provider to have one prescribed for you.
It is not known if ARCAPTA NEOHALER is safe and effective in people with asthma.
ARCAPTA NEOHALER should not be used in children. It is not known if ARCAPTA NEOHALER is safe and effective in children.

Who should not use ARCAPTA NEOHALER?
Do not use ARCAPTA NEOHALER if you:
- **have asthma.**
- **have had an allergic reaction to indacaterol or any of the ingredients in ARCAPTA NEOHALER. Ask your healthcare provider if you are not sure. See the end of the Medication Guide for a list of ingredients in ARCAPTA NEOHALER.**

What should I tell my healthcare provider before using ARCAPTA NEOHALER?
Tell your healthcare provider about all of your health conditions, including if you:
- have heart problems
- have high blood pressure
- have seizures
- have thyroid problems
- have diabetes
- are pregnant or planning to become pregnant. It is not known if ARCAPTA NEOHALER can harm your unborn baby.
- are breastfeeding. It is not known if ARCAPTA NEOHALER passes into your milk and if it can harm your baby.
- are allergic to ARCAPTA NEOHALER or any of its ingredients, any other medicines, or food products.

ARCAPTA NEOHALER contains lactose (milk sugar) and a small amount of milk proteins. It is possible that allergic reactions may happen in patients who have a severe milk protein allergy.
Tell your doctor about all the medicines you take, including prescription and non-prescription medicines, vitamins, and herbal supplements. ARCAPTA NEOHALER and certain other medicines may interact with each other. This may cause serious side effects.
Know the medicines you take. Keep a list of your medicines with you to show your healthcare provider and pharmacist each time you get a new medicine.

How should I use ARCAPTA NEOHALER?
- **Read the step-by-step instructions for using ARCAPTA NEOHALER at the end of this Medication Guide.**
- **Use ARCAPTA NEOHALER 1 time each day at the same time of the day.**
- If you miss a dose of ARCAPTA NEOHALER, take it as soon as you remember. Do not take more than one dose in 24 hours.
- **Do not swallow ARCAPTA capsules.** ARCAPTA capsules should always be used with the NEOHALER inhaler only.
- Always use the new NEOHALER inhaler that is provided with each new prescription.
- **ARCAPTA NEOHALER does not relieve sudden symptoms of COPD.** Always have a rescue inhaler medicine with you to treat sudden symptoms. If you do not have a rescue inhaler medicine, call your healthcare provider to have one prescribed for you.
- Do not stop using ARCAPTA NEOHALER or other medicines to control or treat your COPD unless told to do so by your healthcare provider because your symptoms might get worse. Your healthcare provider will change your medicines as needed.
- **Do not use ARCAPTA NEOHALER:**
  - more often than prescribed
  - more medicine than prescribed for you, or
  - with other LABA medicines
- **Call your health care provider or get emergency medical care right away if:**
  - your breathing problems worsen with ARCAPTA NEOHALER
  - you need to use your rescue medicine more often than usual
  - your rescue inhaler medicine does not work as well for you at relieving your symptoms

What are the possible side effects with ARCAPTA NEOHALER?
ARCAPTA NEOHALER can cause serious side effects, including:
- **See "What is the most important information I should know about ARCAPTA NEOHALER?"**
- If your COPD symptoms worsen over time do not increase your dose of ARCAPTA NEOHALER, instead call your healthcare provider.
- serious allergic reactions including rash, hives, swelling of the tongue, lips and face, difficulties in breathing or swallowing. Call your healthcare provider or get emergency medical care if you get any symptoms of a serious allergic reaction.
- sudden shortness of breath that may be life-threatening
- fast or irregular heartbeat (palpitations)
- increased blood pressure
- chest pain
- low blood potassium (which may cause symptoms of muscle spasm, muscle weakness or abnormal heart rhythm)
- high blood sugar

Common side effects of ARCAPTA NEOHALER include:
- runny nose
- cough
- sore throat
- headache
- nausea

Tell your healthcare provider about any side effect that bothers you or that does not go away.
These are not all the side effects with ARCAPTA NEOHALER. Ask your healthcare provider or pharmacist for more information.
Call your doctor for medical advice about side effects. You may report side effects to FDA at 1-800-FDA-1088.

How should I store ARCAPTA NEOHALER?
- Store ARCAPTA NEOHALER (inhaler and blister-packaged capsules) in a dry place 59° F to 86° F (15°C to 30°C). Protect ARCAPTA NEOHALER (inhaler and blister-packaged capsules) from moisture.
- Do not remove ARCAPTA capsules from their foil package until just before use.
- Keep ARCAPTA capsules out of the light.
- Do not store ARCAPTA capsules in the NEOHALER inhaler.
- **Keep ARCAPTA NEOHALER and all medicines out of the reach of children.**

General Information about ARCAPTA NEOHALER
Medicines are sometimes prescribed for purposes other than those listed in a Medication Guide. Do not use ARCAPTA NEOHALER for a condition for which it was not prescribed. Do not give ARCAPTA NEOHALER to other people, even if they have the same condition. It may harm them.
This Medication Guide summarizes the most important information about ARCAPTA NEOHALER. If you would like more information, talk with your healthcare provider. You can ask your healthcare provider or pharmacist for information about ARCAPTA NEOHALER that was written for healthcare professionals.
For more information, go to www.arcapta.com or call 1-888-669-6682.
Active ingredient: indacaterol
Inactive ingredients: lactose monohydrate (contains trace levels of milk protein)
T2012-175
Revised September 2012

Instructions for Use
ARCAPTA™ (ar-CAP-ta) NEOHALER™ (indacaterol inhalation powder)
Do not swallow ARCAPTA capsules.
Follow the instructions below for using ARCAPTA NEOHALER. You will breathe-in (inhale) the medicine in the ARCAPTA capsules from the NEOHALER inhaler. If you have any questions, ask your healthcare provider or pharmacist.

ARCAPTA NEOHALER

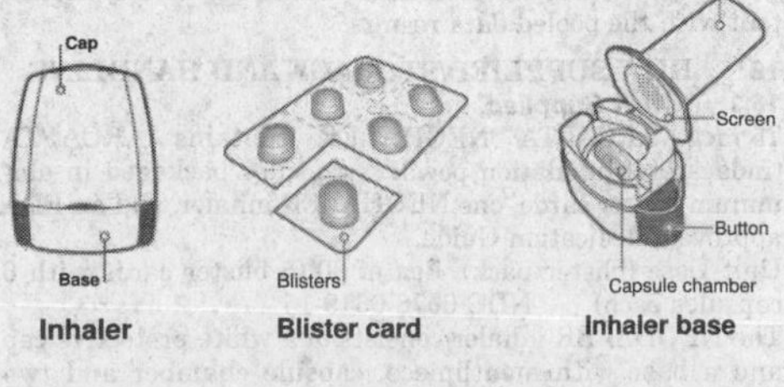

Inhaler **Blister card** **Inhaler base**

ARCAPTA NEOHALER consists of both the inhaler and the blister-packaged capsules. Each package contains ARCAPTA capsules and a NEOHALER inhaler.
- ARCAPTA capsules come in blister cards (see figure above).
- NEOHALER inhaler consists of a cap and a base (see figure above).

Your inhaler is made to give you the medicine contained in the capsules.
Do not use ARCAPTA capsules with any other capsule inhaler, and **do not** use NEOHALER inhaler to take any other capsule medicine.

How to use your inhaler

Figure A

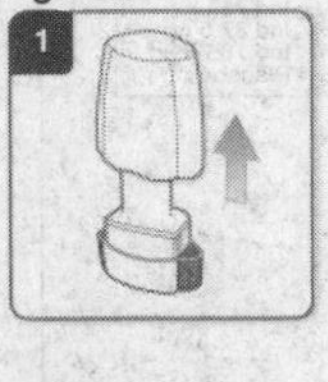

Step 1. Pull off cap. See Figure A.

Figure B

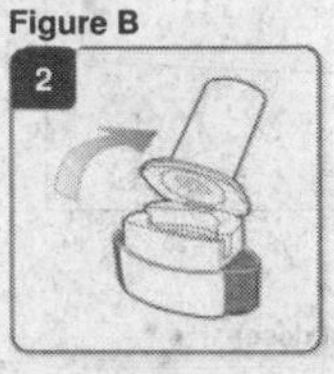

Step 2. Open inhaler: See Figure B
Hold the base of the inhaler firmly and tilt the mouthpiece to open the inhaler.

Figure C

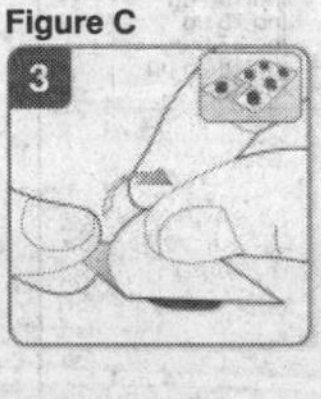

Step 3. Prepare capsule: See Figure C
Separate one of the blisters from the blister card by tearing along the perforation.
Take one blister and peel away the protective backing to expose the foil.

Figure D

Step 4. Remove an ARCAPTA capsule: See Figure D
Capsules should always be stored in the blister and only removed immediately before use.
With dry hands, remove one capsule from the blister by pushing the ARCAPTA capsule through the foil.
Do not swallow ARCAPTA capsule.

Figure E

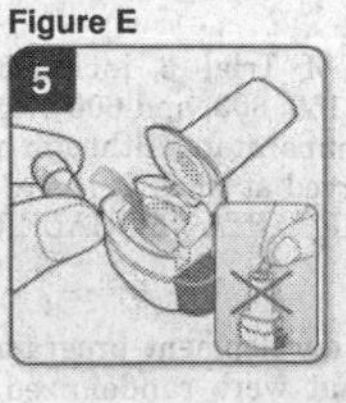

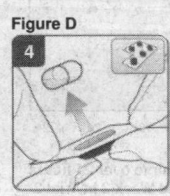

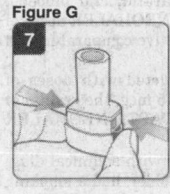

Step 5. Insert capsule: See Figure E
Place the capsule into the capsule chamber.
Do not place a capsule directly into the mouthpiece.

Figure F

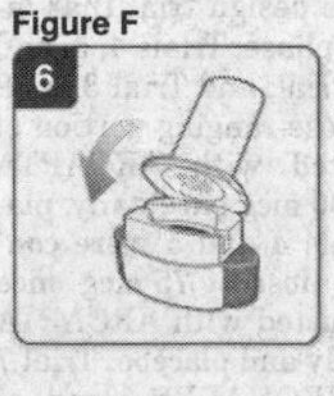

Step 6. Close the inhaler: See Figure F
Close the inhaler fully. You should hear a '**click**' as it fully closes.

Figure G

Step 7. Pierce the capsule: See Figure G
Hold the inhaler upright.
Press both buttons fully one time. You should hear a '**click**' as the capsule is being pierced.
Do not press the piercing buttons more than one time.

Figure H

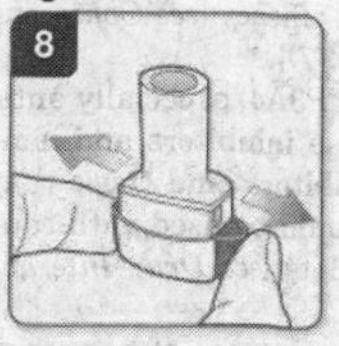

Step 8. Release the buttons fully. See Figure H

Figure I

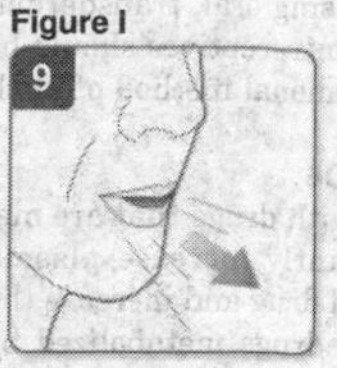

Step 9. Breathe out: See Figure I
Before placing the mouthpiece in your mouth, breathe out fully. **Never blow into the mouthpiece.**

Figure J

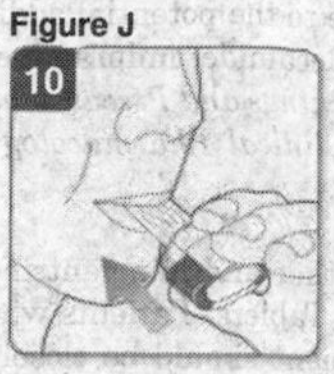

Step 10. Inhale the medicine: See Figure J
Before breathing in, place the mouthpiece in your mouth and close your lips around the mouthpiece. Hold the inhaler with the buttons to the left and right (not up and down).
Breathe in rapidly and steadily, as deeply as you can. **Do not press the piercing buttons.**
Note: See Figure K

Figure K

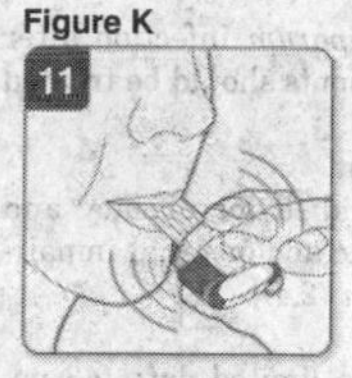

As you breathe in through the inhaler, the capsule spins around in the chamber and you should hear a whirring noise.
If you do not hear a whirring noise, the capsule may be stuck in the capsule cavity. If this occurs, open the inhaler and carefully loosen the capsule by tapping the base of the device. Do not press the piercing buttons to loosen the capsule. **(Repeat steps 9 and 10 if needed).**

Figure L

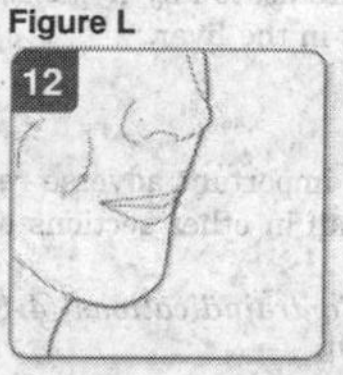

Step 11. Hold breath: See Figure L
Continue to hold your breath as long as comfortably possible while removing the inhaler from your mouth. Then breathe out.
Open the inhaler to see if any powder is left in the capsule. **If there is powder left in the capsule, close the inhaler and repeat steps 9 to 12.** Most people are able to empty the capsule in one or two inhalations.
Some people may cough soon after inhaling the medicine. If you do, don't worry, as long as the capsule is empty, you have received the full dose.

Figure M

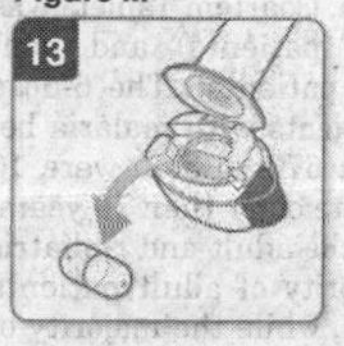

Step 12. Remove capsule: See Figure M
After you have finished taking your daily dose of the ARCAPTA NEOHALER, open the mouthpiece again, remove the empty capsule by tipping it out, and discard it. Close the inhaler and replace the cap.
Do not store the capsules in the NEOHALER device.

Additional Information
Occasionally, very small pieces of the capsule can get past the screen and enter your mouth. If this happens, you may be able to feel these pieces on your tongue. It is not harmful if these pieces are swallowed or inhaled. **The chances of the capsule shattering will be increased if the capsule is pierced more than once (Step 7).** Therefore it is recommended that you follow the storage directions, remove the capsule from the blister immediately before use and pierce each capsule only once.
How to clean your inhaler
Cleaning the device is not necessary, however, if desired, a clean, dry lint-free cloth, or a clean, dry soft brush may be used to wipe the inhaler between uses.
Remember:
- ARCAPTA capsules should be stored in the blister, and only removed immediately before use.
- Do not breathe into the NEOHALER inhaler.
- Do not place the ARCAPTA capsule directly into the mouthpiece of the NEOHALER inhaler.
- Do not store the ARCAPTA capsule in the NEOHALER inhaler chamber.
- Always release the push buttons prior to inhalation
- Do not wash the NEOHALER inhaler. **Keep it dry.**
- Always keep the NEOHALER inhaler and ARCAPTA capsules in a dry place.
- Always use the new NEOHALER inhaler that comes with your refill.
- Do not use ARCAPTA capsules with inhalers from other medicines.
- Keep this and all drugs out of the reach of children.

This Medication Guide has been approved by the U.S. Food and Drug Administration.
Manufactured by:
Novartis Pharma Stein AG
Stein, Switzerland
Distributed by:
Novartis Pharmaceuticals Corporation
East Hanover, New Jersey 07936
© Novartis
T2012-179
Revised September 2012

Shown in Product Identification Guide, page 309

COARTEM ℞
[co-AR-tem]
(artemether/lumefantrine)
Tablets

The following prescribing information is based on official labeling in effect July 2013.

HIGHLIGHTS OF PRESCRIBING INFORMATION
These highlights do not include all the information needed to use Coartem Tablets safely and effectively. See full prescribing information for Coartem Tablets.
Coartem (artemether/lumefantrine) Tablets
Initial U.S. Approval: 2009

RECENT MAJOR CHANGES

Contraindications (4.2)	08/2012
Warnings and Precautions (5.1)	04/2013
Warnings and Precautions (5.2)	04/2013
Warnings and Precautions (5.3)	08/2012

INDICATIONS AND USAGE

- Coartem (artemether and lumefantrine) Tablets are indicated for treatment of acute, uncomplicated malaria infections due to *Plasmodium falciparum* in patients of 5 kg bodyweight and above. (1)
- Coartem Tablets have been shown to be effective in geographical regions where resistance to chloroquine has been reported. (1)
- Coartem Tablets should not be used to treat severe malaria or to prevent malaria. (1)

DOSAGE AND ADMINISTRATION

- Coartem Tablets should be taken with food. (2.1, 5.2)
- Tablets may be crushed and mixed with one to two teaspoons of water immediately prior to administration to patients, including children. (2.1)
- Coartem Tablets should be administered over 3-days for a total of 6 doses: an initial dose, second dose after 8 hours and then twice daily (morning and evening) for the following two days. (2.2, 2.3)
- The adult dosage for patients with bodyweight of 35 kg and above is 4 tablets per dose for a total of 6 doses. (2.2)
- The number of tablets per dose for children is determined by bodyweight, as shown in the chart below. (2.3)

Tablets per dose by bodyweight; total of 6 doses over 3 days

5 to <15 kg	1 tablet
15 to <25 kg	2 tablets
25 to <35 kg	3 tablets
35 kg and over	4 tablets

DOSAGE FORMS AND STRENGTHS

Tablets are scored and contain 20 mg artemether and 120 mg lumefantrine. (3)

CONTRAINDICATIONS

- Known hypersensitivity to artemether, lumefantrine, or to any of the excipients. (4.1)
- Co-administration of strong inducers of CYP3A4 such as rifampin, carbamazepine, phenytoin and St. John's wort with Coartem Tablets. (4.2, 7.1, 12.3)

WARNINGS AND PRECAUTIONS

- Avoid use in patients with known QT prolongation, those with hypokalemia or hypomagnesemia, and those taking other drugs that prolong the QT interval. (5.1, 12.6)
- Halofantrine and Coartem Tablets should not be administered within one month of each other due to potential additive effects on the QT interval. (5.1, 5.2, 12.3)
- Antimalarials should not be given concomitantly, unless there is no other treatment option, due to limited safety data. (5.2)
- QT prolonging drugs, including quinine and quinidine, should be used cautiously following Coartem Tablets. (5.1, 5.2, 7.7, 12.3)
- Substrates, inhibitors, or inducers of CYP3A4, including antiretroviral medications, should be used cautiously with Coartem Tablets, due to a potential loss of efficacy of the concomitant drug or additive QT prolongation. (5.3, 7.2, 7.3)

ADVERSE REACTIONS

The most common adverse reactions in adults (>30%) are headache, anorexia, dizziness, asthenia, arthralgia and myalgia. The most common adverse reactions in children (>12%) are pyrexia, cough, vomiting, anorexia and headache. (6.2)

To report SUSPECTED ADVERSE REACTIONS, contact Novartis Pharmaceuticals Corporation at 1-888-669-6682 or FDA at 1-800-FDA-1088 or www.fda.gov/medwatch

DRUG INTERACTIONS

- CYP3A4 Inducers: Potential for loss of antimalarial efficacy. (4.2, 5.3, 7.1, 12.3)
- CYP3A4 Inhibitors: Use cautiously due to potential for QT prolongation. (5.3, 7.2, 12.3)
- Antiretrovirals: Use cautiously due to potential for QT prolongation, loss of antiviral efficacy, or loss of antimalarial efficacy of Coartem Tablets. (5.3, 7.3, 12.3)
- Mefloquine: If used immediately before treatment, monitor for decreased efficacy of Coartem Tablets and encourage food consumption. (2.1, 7.4, 12.3)
- Hormonal Contraceptives: Effectiveness may be reduced; use an additional method of birth control. (5.3, 7.5, 12.3)
- CYP2D6 Substrates: Monitor for adverse reactions and potential QT prolongation. (5.1, 5.4, 7.6)

USE IN SPECIFIC POPULATIONS

- Pregnancy: Based on animal data, may increase fetal loss. (8.1)
- Nursing Mothers: Use caution when administering to a nursing woman. (8.3)
- Pediatric Use: Studied in children 2 months of age and older with a bodyweight of 5 kg and greater. (8.4)
- Geriatric Use: Not studied in geriatric patients. (8.5)

See 17 for PATIENT COUNSELING INFORMATION and FDA-approved patient labeling

Revised: 04/2013

FULL PRESCRIBING INFORMATION: CONTENTS*

*** Sections or subsections omitted from the full prescribing information are not listed**

FULL PRESCRIBING INFORMATION

1 INDICATIONS AND USAGE

Coartem (artemether/lumefantrine) Tablets are indicated for treatment of acute, uncomplicated malaria infections due to *Plasmodium falciparum* in patients of 5 kg bodyweight and above. Coartem Tablets have been shown to be effective in geographical regions where resistance to chloroquine has been reported [*see Clinical Studies (14.1)*].

Limitations of Use:
- Coartem Tablets are not approved for patients with severe or complicated *P. falciparum* malaria.
- Coartem Tablets are not approved for the prevention of malaria.

2 DOSAGE AND ADMINISTRATION

2.1 Administration Instructions

Coartem Tablets should be taken with food. Patients with acute malaria are frequently averse to food. Patients should be encouraged to resume normal eating as soon as food can be tolerated since this improves absorption of artemether and lumefantrine.

For patients who are unable to swallow the tablets such as infants and children, Coartem Tablets may be crushed and mixed with a small amount of water (one to two teaspoons) in a clean container for administration immediately prior to use. The container can be rinsed with more water and the contents swallowed by the patient. The crushed tablet preparation should be followed whenever possible by food/drink (e.g., milk, formula, pudding, broth, and porridge).

In the event of vomiting within 1 to 2 hours of administration, a repeat dose should be taken. If the repeat dose is vomited, the patient should be given an alternative antimalarial for treatment.

2.2 Dosage in Adult Patients (>16 years of age)

A 3-day treatment schedule with a total of 6 doses is recommended for adult patients with a bodyweight of 35 kg and above:

Four tablets as a single initial dose, 4 tablets again after 8 hours and then 4 tablets twice daily (morning and evening) for the following two days (total course of 24 tablets).

For patients weighing less than 35 kg, *see* Dosage in Pediatric Patients (2.3).

2.3 Dosage in Pediatric Patients

A 3-day treatment schedule with a total of 6 doses is recommended as below:

5 kg to less than 15 kg bodyweight: One tablet as an initial dose, 1 tablet again after 8 hours and then 1 tablet twice daily (morning and evening) for the following two days (total course of 6 tablets).

15 kg to less than 25 kg bodyweight: Two tablets as an initial dose, 2 tablets again after 8 hours and then 2 tablets twice daily (morning and evening) for the following two days (total course of 12 tablets).

25 kg to less than 35 kg bodyweight: Three tablets as an initial dose, 3 tablets again after 8 hours and then 3 tablets twice daily (morning and evening) for the following two days (total course of 18 tablets).

35 kg bodyweight and above: Four tablets as a single initial dose, 4 tablets again after 8 hours and then 4 tablets twice daily (morning and evening) for the following two days (total course of 24 tablets).

2.4 Dosage in Patients with Hepatic or Renal Impairment

No specific pharmacokinetic studies have been carried out in patients with hepatic or renal impairment. Most patients with acute malaria present with some degree of related hepatic and/or renal impairment. In clinical studies, the adverse event profile did not differ in patients with mild or moderate hepatic impairment compared to patients with normal hepatic function. No specific dose adjustments are needed for patients with mild or moderate hepatic impairment.

In clinical studies, the adverse event profile did not differ in patients with mild or moderate renal impairment compared to patients with normal renal function. There were few patients with severe renal impairment in clinical studies. There is no significant renal excretion of lumefantrine, artemether and dihydroartemisinin (DHA) in healthy volunteers and while clinical experience in this population is limited, no dose adjustment is recommended.

Caution should be exercised when administering Coartem Tablets in patients with severe hepatic or renal impairment [*see Warnings and Precautions (5.6)*].

3 DOSAGE FORMS AND STRENGTHS

Coartem Tablets contain 20 mg of artemether and 120 mg of lumefantrine. Coartem Tablets are supplied as yellow, round, flat tablets with beveled edges and scored on one side. Tablets are imprinted with N/C on one side and CG on the other side.

4 CONTRAINDICATIONS

4.1 Hypersensitivity

- Known hypersensitivity to artemether, lumefantrine, or to any of the excipients of Coartem Tablets [*see Adverse Reactions (6.3)*].

4.2 Strong CYP3A4 Inducers

- Co-administration of strong inducers of CYP3A4 such as rifampin, carbamazepine, phenytoin and St. John's wort with Coartem Tablets can result in decreased concentrations of artemether and/or lumefantrine and loss of antimalarial efficacy [*see Warnings and Precautions (5.3), Drug Interactions (7.1),* and *Clinical Pharmacology (12.3)*].

5 WARNINGS AND PRECAUTIONS

5.1 Prolongation of the QT Interval

Some antimalarials (e.g., halofantrine, quinine, quinidine) including Coartem Tablets have been associated with prolongation of the QT interval on the electrocardiogram.

Coartem Tablets should be avoided in patients:
- with congenital prolongation of the QT interval (e.g., long QT syndrome) or any other clinical condition known to prolong the QTc interval such as patients with a history of symptomatic cardiac arrhythmias, with clinically relevant bradycardia or with severe cardiac disease.
- with a family history of congenital prolongation of the QT interval or sudden death.
- with known disturbances of electrolyte balance, e.g., hypokalemia or hypomagnesemia.
- receiving other medications that prolong the QT interval, such as class IA (quinidine, procainamide, disopyramide), or class III (amiodarone, sotalol) antiarrhythmic agents; antipsychotics (pimozide, ziprasidone); antidepressants; certain antibiotics (macrolide antibiotics, fluoroquinolone antibiotics, imidazole, and triazole antifungal agents) [*see Clinical Pharmacology (12.6)*].
- receiving medications that are metabolized by the cytochrome enzyme CYP2D6 which also have cardiac effects (e.g., flecainide, imipramine, amitriptyline, clomipramine) [*see Warnings and Precautions (5.4), Drug Interactions (7.6),* and *Clinical Pharmacology (12.3)*].

5.2 Use of QT Prolonging Drugs and Other Antimalarials

Halofantrine and Coartem Tablets should not be administered within one month of each other due to the long elimination half-life of lumefantrine (3-6 days) and potential additive effects on the QT interval [*see Warnings and Precautions (5.1)* and *Clinical Pharmacology (12.3)*].

Antimalarials should not be given concomitantly with Coartem Tablets, unless there is no other treatment option, due to limited safety data.

Drugs that prolong the QT interval, including antimalarials such as quinine and quinidine, should be used cautiously following Coartem Tablets, due to the long elimination half-life of lumefantrine (3-6 days) and the potential for additive effects on the QT interval; ECG monitoring is advised if use of drugs that prolong the QT interval is medically required [*see Warnings and Precautions (5.1), Drug Interactions (7.7),* and *Clinical Pharmacology (12.3)*].

If mefloquine is administered immediately prior to Coartem Tablets there may be a decreased exposure to lumefantrine, possibly due to a mefloquine-induced decrease in bile production. Therefore, patients should be monitored for decreased efficacy and food consumption should be encouraged while taking Coartem Tablets [*see Dosage and Administration (2.1), Drug Interactions (7.4),* and *Clinical Pharmacology (12.3)*].

5.3 Drug Interactions with CYP3A4

When Coartem Tablets are co-administered with substrates of CYP3A4 it may result in decreased concentrations of the substrate and potential loss of substrate efficacy. When Coartem Tablets are co-administered with an inhibitor of CYP3A4, including grapefruit juice it may result in increased concentrations of artemether and/or lumefantrine and potentiate QT prolongation. When Coartem Tablets are co-administered with inducers of CYP3A4 it may result in decreased concentrations of artemether and/or lumefantrine and loss of antimalarial efficacy [*see Contraindications (4.2)* and *Drug Interactions (7)*].

Drugs that have a mixed effect on CYP3A4, especially antiretroviral drugs such as HIV protease inhibitors and non-nucleoside reverse transcriptase inhibitors, and those that have an effect on the QT interval should be used with caution in patients taking Coartem Tablets [*see Drug Interactions (7.3, 7.7)*].

Coartem Tablets may reduce the effectiveness of hormonal contraceptives. Therefore, patients using oral, transdermal patch, or other systemic hormonal contraceptives should be advised to use an additional non-hormonal method of birth control [*see Drug Interactions (7.5)*].

5.4 Drug Interactions with CYP2D6

Administration of Coartem Tablets with drugs that are metabolized by CYP2D6 may significantly increase plasma concentrations of the co-administered drug and increase the risk of adverse effects. Many of the drugs metabolized by CYP2D6 can prolong the QT interval and should not be administered with Coartem Tablets due to the potential additive effect on the QT interval (e.g., flecainide, imipramine, amitriptyline, clomipramine) [*see Warnings and Precautions (5.1), Drug Interactions (7.6),* and *Clinical Pharmacology (12.3)*].

5.5 Recrudescence

Food enhances absorption of artemether and lumefantrine following administration of Coartem Tablets. Patients who remain averse to food during treatment should be closely monitored as the risk of recrudescence may be greater [*see Dosage and Administration (2.1)*].

In the event of recrudescent *P. falciparum* infection after treatment with Coartem Tablets, patients should be treated with a different antimalarial drug.

5.6 Hepatic and Renal Impairment

Coartem Tablets have not been studied for efficacy and safety in patients with severe hepatic and/or renal impairment [*see Dosage and Administration (2.4)*].

5.7 *Plasmodium vivax* Infection

Coartem Tablets have been shown in limited data (43 patients) to be effective in treating the erythrocytic stage of *P. vivax* infection. However, relapsing malaria caused by *P. vivax* requires additional treatment with other antimalarial agents to achieve radical cure i.e., eradicate any hypnozoites forms that may remain dormant in the liver.

6 ADVERSE REACTIONS

6.1 Serious Adverse Reactions

The following serious and otherwise important adverse reactions are discussed in greater detail in other sections of labeling:
- Hypersensitivity Reactions [*see Contraindications (4.1)* and *Postmarketing Experience (6.3)*].

6.2 Clinical Studies Experience

Because clinical trials are conducted under widely varying conditions, adverse reaction rates observed in the clinical trials of a drug cannot be directly compared to rates in the clinical trials of another drug and may not reflect the rate observed in practice.

The data described below reflect exposure to a 6-dose regimen of Coartem Tablets in 1,979 patients including 647 adults (older than 16 years) and 1,332 children (16 years and younger). For the 6-dose regimen, Coartem Tablets was studied in active-controlled (366 patients) and non-controlled, open-label trials (1,613 patients). The 6-dose Coartem Tablets population was patients with malaria between ages 2 months and 71 years: 67% (1,332) were 16 years and younger and 33% (647) were older than 16 years. Males represented 73% and 53% of the adult and pediatric populations, respectively. The majority of adult patients were enrolled in studies in Thailand, while the majority of pediatric patients were enrolled in Africa.

Tables 1 and 2 show the most frequently reported adverse reactions (≥3%) in adults and children respectively who received the 6-dose regimen of Coartem Tablets. Adverse reactions collected in clinical trials included signs and symptoms at baseline but only treatment emergent adverse events, defined as events that appeared or worsened after the start of treatment, are presented below. In adults, the most frequently reported adverse reactions were headache, anorexia, dizziness, and asthenia. In children, the adverse reactions were pyrexia, cough, vomiting, anorexia, and headache. Most adverse reactions were mild, did not lead to discontinuation of study medication, and resolved.

In limited comparative studies, the adverse reaction profile of Coartem Tablets appeared similar to that of another antimalarial regimen.

Discontinuation of Coartem Tablets due to adverse drug reactions occurred in 1.1% of patients treated with the 6-dose regimen overall: 0.2% (1/647) in adults and 1.6% (21/1,332) in children.

[See table 1 at right]
[See table 2 below]
Clinically significant adverse reactions reported in adults and/or children treated with the 6-dose regimen of Coartem Tablets which occurred in clinical studies at <3% regardless of causality are listed below:

Blood and lymphatic system disorders: eosinophilia
Ear and labyrinth disorders: tinnitus
Eye disorders: conjunctivitis
Gastrointestinal disorders: constipation, dyspepsia, dysphagia, peptic ulcer
General disorders: gait disturbance
Infections and infestations: abscess, acrodermatitis, bronchitis, ear infection, gastroenteritis, helminthic infection, hookworm infection, impetigo, influenza, lower respiratory tract infection, malaria, nasopharyngitis, oral herpes, pneumonia, respiratory tract infection, subcutaneous abscess, upper respiratory tract infection, urinary tract infection
Investigations: alanine aminotransferase increased, aspartate aminotransferase increased, hematocrit decreased, lymphocyte morphology abnormal, platelet count decreased, platelet count increased, white blood cell count decreased, white blood cell count increased
Metabolism and nutrition disorders: hypokalemia
Musculoskeletal and connective tissue disorders: back pain
Nervous system disorders: ataxia, clonus, fine motor delay, hyperreflexia, hypoaesthesia, nystagmus, tremor
Psychiatric disorders: agitation, mood swings
Renal and urinary disorders: hematuria, proteinuria
Respiratory, thoracic and mediastinal disorders: asthma, pharyngo-laryngeal pain
Skin and subcutaneous tissue disorders: urticaria

6.3 Postmarketing Experience
The following adverse reactions have been identified during post-approval use of Coartem Tablets. Because these events are reported voluntarily from a population of uncertain size, it is not always possible to reliably estimate their frequency or establish a causal relationship to drug exposure.

- Hypersensitivity reactions including urticaria and angioedema. Serious skin reactions (bullous eruption) have been rarely reported.

7 DRUG INTERACTIONS

7.1 Rifampin
Oral administration of rifampin, a strong CYP3A4 inducer, with Coartem Tablets resulted in significant decreases in exposure to artemether, dihydroartemisinin (DHA, metabolite of artemether) and lumefantrine by 89%, 85% and 68%, respectively, when compared to exposure values after Coartem Tablets alone. Concomitant use of strong inducers of CYP3A4 such as rifampin, carbamazepine, phenytoin and St. John's wort is contraindicated with Coartem Tablets [*see Contraindications (4.2)* and *Clinical Pharmacology (12.3)*].

7.2 Ketoconazole
Concurrent oral administration of ketoconazole, a potent CYP3A4 inhibitor, with a single dose of Coartem Tablets resulted in a moderate increase in exposure to artemether, DHA, and lumefantrine in a study of 15 healthy subjects. No dose adjustment of Coartem Tablets is necessary when administered with ketoconazole or other potent CYP3A4 inhibitors. However, due to the potential for increased concentrations of lumefantrine which could lead to QT prolongation, Coartem Tablets should be used cautiously with drugs that inhibit CYP3A4 [*see Warnings and Precautions (5.1, 5.3)* and *Clinical Pharmacology (12.3)*].

7.3 Antiretroviral Drugs
Both artemether and lumefantrine are metabolized by CYP3A4. Antiretroviral drugs, such as protease inhibitors and non-nucleoside reverse transcriptase inhibitors, are known to have variable patterns of inhibition, induction or competition for CYP3A4. Therefore, the effects of antiretroviral drugs on the exposure to artemether, DHA, and lumefantrine are also variable [*see Clinical Pharmacology (12.3)*]. Coartem Tablets should be used cautiously in patients on antiretroviral drugs because decreased artemether, DHA, and/or lumefantrine concentrations may result in a decrease of antimalarial efficacy of Coartem Tablets, and increased lumefantrine concentrations may cause QT prolongation [*see Warnings and Precautions (5.3)*].

7.4 Prior Use of Mefloquine
Administration of three doses of mefloquine followed 12 hours later by a 6-dose regimen of Coartem Tablets in 14 healthy volunteers demonstrated no effect of mefloquine on plasma concentrations of artemether or the artemether/DHA ratio. However, exposure to lumefantrine was reduced, possibly due to lower absorption secondary to a mefloquine-induced decrease in bile production. Patients should be monitored for decreased efficacy and food consumption should be encouraged with administration of Coartem Tablets [*see Warnings and Precautions (5.2)* and *Clinical Pharmacology (12.3)*].

7.5 Hormonal Contraceptives
In vitro, the metabolism of ethinyl estradiol and levonorgestrel was not induced by artemether, DHA, or lumefantrine. However, artemether has been reported to weakly induce, in humans, the activity of CYP2C19, CYP2B6, and CYP3A. Therefore, Coartem Tablets may potentially reduce the effectiveness of hormonal contraceptives. Patients using oral, transdermal patch, or other systemic hormonal contraceptives should be advised to use an additional non-hormonal method of birth control [*see Warnings and Precautions (5.3)* and *Clinical Pharmacology (12.3)*].

Table 1: Adverse Reactions Occurring in 3% or More of Adult Patients Treated in Clinical Trials with the 6-dose Regimen of Coartem Tablets

System Organ Class	Preferred Term	Adults* N=647 (%)
Nervous system disorders	Headache	360 (56)
	Dizziness	253 (39)
Metabolism and nutrition disorders	Anorexia	260 (40)
General disorders and administration site conditions	Asthenia	243 (38)
	Pyrexia	159 (25)
	Chills	147 (23)
	Fatigue	111 (17)
	Malaise	20 (3)
Musculoskeletal and connective tissue disorders	Arthralgia	219 (34)
	Myalgia	206 (32)
Gastrointestinal disorders	Nausea	169 (26)
	Vomiting	113 (17)
	Abdominal pain	112 (17)
	Diarrhea	46 (7)
Psychiatric disorders	Sleep disorder	144 (22)
	Insomnia	32 (5)
Cardiac disorders	Palpitations	115 (18)
Hepatobiliary disorders	Hepatomegaly	59 (9)
Blood and lymphatic system disorders	Splenomegaly	57 (9)
	Anemia	23 (4)
Respiratory, thoracic and mediastinal disorders	Cough	37 (6)
Skin and subcutaneous tissue disorders	Pruritus	24 (4)
	Rash	21 (3)
Ear and labyrinth disorders	Vertigo	21 (3)
Infections and infestations	Malaria	18 (3)
	Nasopharyngitis	17 (3)

* Adult patients defined as >16 years of age

Table 2: Adverse Reactions Occurring in 3% or More of Pediatric Patients Treated in Clinical Trials with the 6-dose Regimen of Coartem Tablets

System Organ Class	Preferred Term	Children* N=1,332 (%)
General disorders and administration site conditions	Pyrexia	381 (29)
	Chills	72 (5)
	Asthenia	63 (5)
	Fatigue	46 (3)
Respiratory, thoracic and mediastinal disorders	Cough	302 (23)
Gastrointestinal disorders	Vomiting	242 (18)
	Abdominal pain	112 (8)
	Diarrhea	100 (8)
	Nausea	61 (5)
Infections and infestations	*Plasmodium falciparum* infection	224 (17)
	Rhinitis	51 (4)
Metabolism and nutrition disorders	Anorexia	175 (13)
Nervous system disorders	Headache	168 (13)
	Dizziness	56 (4)
Blood and lymphatic system disorders	Splenomegaly	124 (9)
	Anemia	115 (9)
Hepatobiliary disorders	Hepatomegaly	75 (6)
Investigations	Aspartate aminotransferase increased	51 (4)
Musculoskeletal and connective tissue disorders	Arthralgia	39 (3)
	Myalgia	39 (3)
Skin and subcutaneous tissue disorders	Rash	38 (3)

* Children defined as patients ≤16 years of age

7.6 CYP2D6 Substrates

Lumefantrine inhibits CYP2D6 *in vitro*. Administration of Coartem Tablets with drugs that are metabolized by CYP2D6 may significantly increase plasma concentrations of the co-administered drug and increase the risk of adverse effects. Many of the drugs metabolized by CYP2D6 can prolong the QT interval and should not be administered with Coartem Tablets due to the potential additive effect on the QT interval (e.g., flecainide, imipramine, amitriptyline, clomipramine) [*see Warnings and Precautions (5.1, 5.4)* and *Clinical Pharmacology (12.3)*].

7.7 Sequential Use of Quinine

A single dose of intravenous quinine (10 mg/kg bodyweight) concurrent with the final dose of a 6-dose regimen of Coartem Tablets demonstrated no effect of intravenous quinine on the systemic exposure of DHA or lumefantrine. Quinine exposure was also not altered. Exposure to artemether was decreased. This decrease in artemether exposure is not thought to be clinically significant. However, quinine and other drugs that prolong the QT interval should be used cautiously following treatment with Coartem Tablets due to the long elimination half-life of lumefantrine and the potential for additive QT effects; ECG monitoring is advised if use of drugs that prolong the QT interval is medically required [*see Warnings and Precautions (5.2)* and *Clinical Pharmacology (12.3)*].

7.8 Interaction with Drugs that are Known to Prolong the QT Interval

Coartem is to be used with caution when co-administered with drugs that may cause prolonged QT interval such as antiarrhythmics of classes IA and III, neuroleptics and antidepressant agents, certain antibiotics including some agents of the following classes: macrolides, fluoroquinolones, imidazole, and triazole antifungal agents [*see Warnings and Precautions (5.1, 5.2)*].

8 USE IN SPECIFIC POPULATIONS

8.1 Pregnancy

Pregnancy Category C

Safety data from an observational pregnancy study of approximately 500 pregnant women who were exposed to Coartem Tablets (including a third of patients who were exposed in the first trimester), and published data of over 1,000 pregnant patients who were exposed to artemisinin derivatives, did not show an increase in adverse pregnancy outcomes or teratogenic effects over background rate.

The efficacy of Coartem Tablets in the treatment of acute, uncomplicated malaria in pregnant women has not been established.

Coartem Tablets should be used during pregnancy only if the potential benefit justifies the potential risk to the fetus.

Pregnant rats dosed during the period of organogenesis at or higher than a dose of about half the highest clinical dose of 1120 mg artemether-lumefantrine per day (based on body surface area comparisons), showed increases in fetal loss, early resorptions and post implantation loss. No adverse effects were observed in animals dosed at about one-third the highest clinical dose. Similarly, dosing in pregnant rabbits at about three times the clinical dose (based on body surface area comparisons) resulted in abortions, preimplantation loss, post implantation loss and decreases in the number of live fetuses. No adverse reproductive effects were detected in rabbits at two times the clinical dose. Embryo-fetal loss is a significant reproductive toxicity. Other artemisinins are known to be embryotoxic in animals. However, because metabolic profiles in animals and humans are dissimilar, artemether exposures in animals may not be predictive of human exposures [*see Nonclinical Toxicology (13.2)*]. These data cannot rule out an increased risk for early pregnancy loss or fetal defects in humans.

8.3 Nursing Mothers

It is not known whether artemether or lumefantrine is excreted in human milk. Because many drugs are excreted in human milk, caution should be exercised when Coartem Tablets are administered to a nursing woman. Animal data suggest both artemether and lumefantrine are excreted into breast milk. The benefits of breastfeeding to mother and infant should be weighed against potential risk from infant exposure to artemether and lumefantrine through breast milk.

8.4 Pediatric Use

The safety and effectiveness of Coartem Tablets have been established for the treatment of acute, uncomplicated malaria in studies involving pediatric patients weighing 5 kg or more [*see Clinical Studies (14.1)*]. The safety and efficacy have not been established in pediatric patients who weigh less than 5 kg. Children from non-endemic countries were not included in clinical trials.

8.5 Geriatric Use

Clinical studies of Coartem Tablets did not include sufficient numbers of subjects aged 65 years and over to determine they respond differently from younger subjects. In general, the greater frequency of decreased hepatic, renal, or cardiac function, and of concomitant disease or other drug therapy in elderly patients should be considered when prescribing Coartem Tablets.

8.6 Hepatic and Renal Impairment

No specific pharmacokinetic studies have been performed in patients with either hepatic or renal impairment. Coartem Tablets have not been studied for efficacy and safety in patients with severe hepatic and/or renal impairment. Based on the pharmacokinetic data in 16 healthy subjects showing no or insignificant renal excretion of lumefantrine, artemether and DHA, no dose adjustment for the use of Coartem in patients with renal impairment is advised. No dosage adjustment is necessary in patients with mild to moderate hepatic impairment [*see Dosage and Administration (2.4)* and *Warnings and Precautions (5.6)*].

10 OVERDOSAGE

There is no information on overdoses of Coartem Tablets higher than the doses recommended for treatment.

In cases of suspected overdosage, symptomatic and supportive therapy, which would include ECG and blood electrolyte monitoring, should be given as appropriate.

11 DESCRIPTION

Coartem Tablets contain a fixed combination of two antimalarial active ingredients, artemether, an artemisinin derivative, and lumefantrine. Both components are blood schizontocides. The chemical name of artemether is (3*R*,5a*S*,6*R*,8a*S*,9*R*,10*S*,12*R*,12a*R*)-10-methoxy-3,6,9-trimethyldecahydro-3,12-epoxypyrano[4,3-*j*]-1,2-benzodioxepine. Artemether is a white, crystalline powder that is freely soluble in acetone, soluble in methanol and ethanol, and practically insoluble in water. It has the empirical formula $C_{16}H_{26}O_5$ with a molecular weight of 298.4, and the following structural formula:

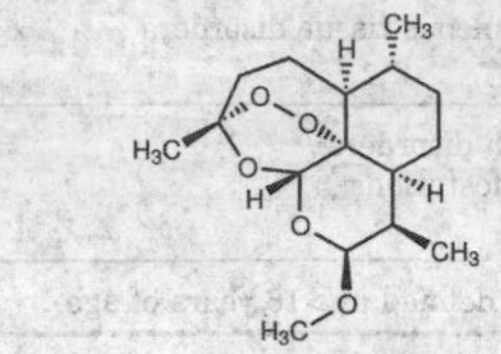

The chemical name of lumefantrine is (1*RS*)-2-(dibutylamino)-1-[(9Z)-2,7-dichloro-9-[(4-chlorophenyl) methylene]-*9H*-fluorene-4-yl]ethanol. Lumefantrine is a yellow, crystalline powder that is freely soluble in N,N-dimethylformamide, chloroform, and ethyl acetate; soluble in dichloromethane; slightly soluble in ethanol and methanol; and insoluble in water. It has the empirical formula $C_{30}H_{32}Cl_3NO$ with a molecular weight of 528.9, and the following structural formula:

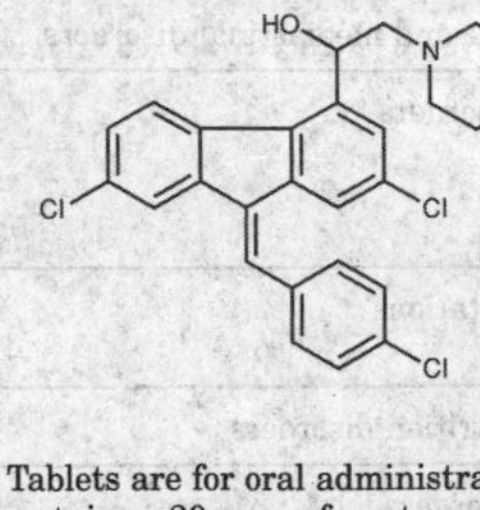

Coartem Tablets are for oral administration. Each Coartem Tablet contains 20 mg of artemether and 120 mg lumefantrine. The inactive ingredients are colloidal silicon dioxide, croscarmellose sodium, hypromellose, magnesium stearate, microcrystalline cellulose, and polysorbate 80.

12 CLINICAL PHARMACOLOGY

12.1 Mechanism of Action

Coartem Tablets, a fixed dose combination of artemether and lumefantrine in the ratio of 1:6, is an antimalarial agent [*see Clinical Pharmacology (12.4)*].

12.3 Pharmacokinetics

Absorption

Following administration of Coartem Tablets to healthy volunteers and patients with malaria, artemether is absorbed with peak plasma concentrations reached about 2 hours after dosing. Absorption of lumefantrine, a highly lipophilic compound, starts after a lag-time of up to 2 hours, with peak plasma concentrations about 6 to 8 hours after administration. The single dose (4 tablets) pharmacokinetic parameters for artemether, dihydroartemisinin (DHA), an active antimalarial metabolite of artemether, and lumefantrine in adult Caucasian healthy volunteers are given in Table 3. Multiple dose data after the 6-dose regimen of Coartem Tablets in adult malaria patients are given in Table 4.

Table 3: Single Dose Pharmacokinetic Parameters[a] for Artemether, Dihydroartemisinin (DHA), and Lumefantrine under Fed Conditions

	Study 2102 (n=50)	Study 2104 (n=48)
Artemether		
C_{max} (ng/mL)	60.0 ± 32.5	83.8 ± 59.7
t_{max} (h)	1.50	2.00
AUC_{last} (ng•h/mL)	146 ± 72.2	259 ± 150
$t_{1/2}$ (h)	1.6 ± 0.7	2.2 ± 1.9
DHA		
C_{max} (ng/mL)	104 ± 35.3	90.4 ± 48.9
t_{max} (h)	1.76	2.00
AUC_{last} (ng•h/mL)	284 ± 83.8	285 ± 98.0
$t_{1/2}$ (h)	1.6 ± 0.6	2.2 ± 1.5
Lumefantrine		
C_{max} (µg/mL)	7.38 ± 3.19	9.80 ± 4.20
t_{max} (h)	6.01	8.00
AUC_{last} (µg•h/mL)	158 ± 70.1	243 ± 117
$t_{1/2}$ (h)	101 ± 35.6	119 ± 51.0

[a]Mean ± SD C_{max}, AUC_{last}, $t_{1/2}$ and Median t_{max}

Food enhances the absorption of both artemether and lumefantrine. In healthy volunteers, the relative bioavailability of artemether was increased between two- to three-fold, and that of lumefantrine sixteen-fold when Coartem Tablets were taken after a high-fat meal compared under fasted conditions. Patients should be encouraged to take Coartem Tablets with a meal as soon as food can be tolerated [*see Dosage and Administration (2.1)*].

Distribution

Artemether and lumefantrine are both highly bound to human serum proteins *in vitro* (95.4% and 99.7%, respectively). Dihydroartemisinin is also bound to human serum proteins (47% to 76%). Protein binding to human plasma proteins is linear.

Biotransformation

In human liver microsomes and recombinant CYP450 enzymes, the metabolism of artemether was catalyzed predominantly by CYP3A4/5. Dihydroartemisinin (DHA) is an active metabolite of artemether. The metabolism of artemether was also catalyzed to a lesser extent by CYP2B6, CYP2C9 and CYP2C19. *In vitro* studies with artemether at therapeutic concentrations revealed no significant inhibition of the metabolic activities of CYP1A2, CYP2A6, CYP2C9, CYP2C19, CYP2D6, CYP2E1, CYP3A4/5, and CYP4A9/11. *In vitro* studies with artemether, DHA, and lumefantrine at therapeutic concentrations revealed no significant induction of the metabolic activities of CYP1A1, CYP1A2, CYP2B6, CYP2C8, CYP2C9, CYP2C19, CYP3A4, or CYP3A5.

During repeated administration of Coartem Tablets, systemic exposure of artemether decreased significantly, while concentrations of DHA increased, although not to a statistically significant degree. The artemether/DHA AUC ratio is 1.2 after a single dose and 0.3 after 6 doses given over 3 days. This suggests that there was induction of enzymes responsible for the metabolism of artemether.

In human liver microsomes and in recombinant CYP450 enzymes, lumefantrine was metabolized mainly by CYP3A4 to desbutyl-lumefantrine. The systemic exposure to the metabolite desbutyl-lumefantrine was less than 1% of the exposure to the parent compound. *In vitro*, lumefantrine significantly inhibits the activity of CYP2D6 at therapeutic plasma concentrations.

Caution is recommended when combining Coartem Tablets with substrates, inhibitors, or inducers of CYP3A4, especially antiretroviral drugs and those that prolong the QT interval (e.g., macrolide antibiotics, pimozide) [*see Contraindications (4.2), Warnings and Precautions (5.1, 5.2, 5.3),* and *Drug Interactions (7)*].

Co-administration of Coartem Tablets with CYP2D6 substrates may result in increased plasma concentrations of the CYP2D6 substrate and increase the risk of adverse reactions. In addition, many of the drugs metabolized by CYP2D6 can prolong the QT interval and should not be administered with Coartem Tablets due to the potential additive effect on the QT interval (e.g., flecainide, imipramine, amitriptyline, clomipramine) [*see Warnings and Precautions (5.1, 5.4)* and *Drug Interactions (7.6)*].

Elimination

Artemether and DHA are cleared from plasma with an elimination half-life of about 2 hours. Lumefantrine is eliminated more slowly, with an elimination half-life of 3-6 days in healthy volunteers and in patients with *falciparum* malaria. Demographic characteristics such as sex and weight appear to have no clinically relevant effects on the pharmacokinetics of artemether and lumefantrine.

In 16 healthy volunteers, neither lumefantrine nor artemether was found in the urine after administration of Coartem, and urinary excretion of DHA amounted to less than 0.01% of the artemether dose.

Hepatic and Renal Impairment

No specific pharmacokinetic studies have been performed in patients with either hepatic or renal impairment. There is no significant renal excretion of lumefantrine, artemether and DHA in healthy volunteers and while clinical experience in this population is limited, no dose adjustment in renal impairment is recommended [*see Dosage and Administration (2.4)*].

Pediatric Patients

The PK of artemether, DHA, and lumefantrine were obtained in two pediatric studies by sparse sampling using a population based approach. PK estimates derived from a composite plasma concentration profile for artemether, DHA, and lumefantrine are provided in Table 4.

Systemic exposure to artemether, DHA, and lumefantrine, when dosed on a mg/kg body weight basis in pediatric patients (≥5 to <35 kg body weight), is comparable to that of the recommended dosing regimen in adult patients.

[See table 4 above]

Geriatric Patients

No specific pharmacokinetic studies have been performed in patients older than 65 years of age.

Drug Interactions

Rifampin (strong CYP3A4 inducer)

Oral administration of rifampin (600 mg daily), a strong CYP3A4 inducer, with Coartem Tablets (6-dose regimen over 3 days) in six HIV-1 and tuberculosis co-infected adults without malaria resulted in significant decreases in exposure, in terms of AUC, to artemether, DHA and lumefantrine by 89%, 85% and 68%, respectively, when compared to exposure values after Coartem Tablets alone. Concomitant use of strong inducers of CYP3A4 such as rifampin, carbamazepine, phenytoin and St. John's wort is contraindicated with Coartem Tablets [*see Contraindications (4.2)*].

Ketoconazole (potent CYP3A4 inhibitor)

Concurrent oral administration of ketoconazole (400 mg on Day 1 followed by 200 mg on days 2, 3, 4 and 5) with Coartem Tablets (single dose of 4 tablets of 20 mg artemether/120 mg lumefantrine per tablet) with a meal led to an increase in exposure, in terms of area under the curve (AUC), of artemether (2.3-fold), DHA (1.5-fold), and lumefantrine (1.6-fold) in 13 healthy subjects. The pharmacokinetics of ketoconazole were not evaluated. Based on this study, dose adjustment of Coartem Tablets is considered unnecessary when administered with ketoconazole or other CYP3A4 inhibitors. However, due to the potential for increased concentrations of lumefantrine which could lead to QT prolongation, Coartem Tablets should be used cautiously with other drugs that inhibit CYP3A4 (e.g., antiretroviral drugs, macrolide antibiotics, antidepressants, imidazole antifungal agents) [*see Warnings and Precautions (5.1, 5.3)*].

Antimalarials

The oral administration of mefloquine in 14 healthy volunteers administered as three doses of 500 mg, 250 mg and 250 mg, followed 12 hours later by Coartem Tablets (6 doses of 4 tablets of 20 mg artemether/120 mg lumefantrine per tablet), had no effect on plasma concentrations of artemether or the artemether/DHA ratio. In the same study, there was a 30% reduction in C_{max} and 40% reduction in AUC of lumefantrine, possibly due to lower absorption secondary to a mefloquine-induced decrease in bile production.

Intravenous administration of a single dose of quinine (10 mg/kg bodyweight) concurrent with the last dose of a 6-dose regimen of Coartem Tablets had no effect on systemic exposure of DHA, lumefantrine or quinine in 14 healthy volunteers. Mean AUC of artemether were 46% lower when administered with quinine compared to Coartem Tablets alone. This decrease in artemether exposure is not thought to be clinically significant. However, quinine should be used cautiously in patients following treatment with Coartem Tablets due to the long elimination half-life of lumefantrine and the potential for additive effects on the QT interval; ECG monitoring is advised if use of quinine is medically required [*see Warnings and Precautions (5.2)*].

Antiretroviral Drugs

The oral administration of lopinavir/ritonavir (400 mg/100 mg twice daily for 26 days) in 10 healthy volunteers co-administered with Coartem Tablets (6-dose regimen over 3 days), resulted in a decrease in systemic exposures, in terms of AUC, to artemether and DHA by approximately 40%, but an increase in exposure to lumefantrine by approximately 2.3-fold. The oral administration of efavirenz (600 mg once daily for 26 days) in 12 healthy volunteers co-administered with Coartem Tablets (6-dose regimen over 3 days), resulted in a decrease in exposures to artemether, DHA, and lumefantrine by approximately 50%, 45%, and 20%, respectively. Exposures to lopinavir/ritonavir and efavirenz were not significantly affected by concomitant use of Coartem Tablets. Coartem Tablets should be used cautiously in patients on antiretroviral drugs such as HIV protease inhibitors and non-nucleoside reverse transcriptase inhibitors because decreased artemether, DHA, and/or lumefantrine concentrations may result in a decrease of antimalarial efficacy of Coartem Tablets, and increased lumefantrine concentrations may cause QT prolongation [*see Warnings and Precautions (5.3)* and *Drug Interactions (7.3)*].

Table 4: Summary of Pharmacokinetic Parameters for Lumefantrine, Artemether and DHA in Pediatric and Adult Patients with Malaria Following Administration of a 6-dose Regimen of Coartem Tablets

Drug	Adults[1]	Pediatric patients (body weight, kg)[2] 5 - <15	15 - <25	25 - <35
Lumefantrine				
Mean C_{max}, range (μg/mL)	5.60 - 9.0	4.71 – 12.6		Not Available
Mean AUC_{last}, range (μg•h/mL)	410 - 561	372 – 699		Not Available
Artemether				
Mean C_{max} ± SD (ng/mL)	186 ± 125	223 ± 309	198 ± 179	174 ± 145
Dihydroartemisinin				
Mean C_{max} ± SD (ng/mL)	101 ± 58	54.7 ± 58.9	79.8 ± 80.5	65.3 ± 23.6

[1] There are a total of 181 adults for lumefantrine pharmacokinetic parameters and a total of 25 adults for artemether and dihydroartemisinin pharmacokinetic parameters.

[2] There are 477 children for the lumefantrine pharmacokinetic parameters; for artemether and dihydroartemisinin pharmacokinetic parameters there are 55, 29, and 8 children for the 5 to <15, 15 to <25 and the 25 to <35 kg groups, respectively.

Table 5: Clinical Efficacy of Coartem Tablets versus Components (mITT Population)[1]

Study No. Region/patient ages	28-day cure rate[2] n/N (%) patients	Median FCT[3] [25th,75th percentile]	Median PCT [25th,75th percentile]
Study 1			
China, ages 13 - 57 years			
Coartem Tablets	50/51 (98.0)	24 hours [9, 48]	30 hours [24, 36]
Artemether[4]	24/52 (46.2)	21 hours [12, 30]	30 hours [24, 33]
Lumefantrine[5]	47/52 (90.4)	60 hours [36, 78]	54 hours [45, 66]
Study 2			
China, ages 12 - 65 years			
Coartem Tablets	50/52 (96.2)	21 hours [6, 33]	30 hours [24, 36]
Lumefantrine[6]	45/51 (88.2)	36 hours [12, 60]	48 hours [42, 60]

[1]In mITT analysis, patients whose status was uncertain were classified as treatment failures.

[2]Efficacy cure rate based on blood smear microscopy.

[3]For patients who had a body temperature >37.5°C at baseline only

[4]95% CI (Coartem Tablets – artemether) on 28-day cure rate: 37.8%, 66.0%

[5]P-value comparing Coartem Tablets to lumefantrine on parasite clearance time (PCT) and fever clearance time (FCT): <0.001

[6]P-value comparing Coartem Tablets to lumefantrine on parasite clearance time (PCT): <0.001 and on fever clearance time (FCT): <0.05

Hormonal Contraceptives

No clinical drug-drug interaction studies between Coartem Tablets and hormonal contraceptives have been performed. *In vitro* studies revealed that the metabolism of ethinyl estradiol and levonorgestrel was not induced by artemether, DHA or lumefantrine. However, artemether has been reported to weakly induce, in humans, the activity of CYP2C19, CYP2B6, and CYP3A. Therefore, co-administration of Coartem Tablets may potentially reduce the effectiveness of hormonal contraceptives [*see Warnings and Precautions (5.3)* and *Drug Interactions (7.5)*].

12.4 Microbiology

Mechanism of Action

Coartem Tablets, a fixed ratio of 1:6 parts of artemether and lumefantrine, respectively, is an antimalarial agent. Artemether is rapidly metabolized into an active metabolite dihydroartemisinin (DHA). The antimalarial activity of artemether and DHA has been attributed to endoperoxide moiety. The exact mechanism by which lumefantrine, exerts its antimalarial effect is not well defined. Available data suggest lumefantrine inhibits the formation of β-hematin by forming a complex with hemin. Both artemether and lumefantrine were shown to inhibit nucleic acid and protein synthesis.

Activity In Vitro and In Vivo

Artemether and lumefantrine are active against the erythrocytic stages of *Plasmodium falciparum*.

Drug Resistance

Strains of *P. falciparum* with a moderate decrease in susceptibility to artemether or lumefantrine alone can be selected *in vitro* or *in vivo*, but not maintained in the case of artemether. The clinical relevance of such an effect is not known.

12.6 Effects on the Electrocardiogram

In a healthy adult volunteer parallel group study including a placebo and moxifloxacin control group (n=42 per group), the administration of the 6-dose regimen of Coartem Tablets was associated with prolongation of QTcF (Fridericia). Following administration of a 6-dose regimen of Coartem Tablets consisting of 4 tablets per dose (total of 4 tablets of 80 mg artemether/480 mg lumefantrine) taken with food, the maximum mean change from baseline and placebo adjusted QTcF was 7.5 msec (1-sided 95% Upper CI: 11 msec). There was a concentration-dependent increase in QTcF for lumefantrine.

In clinical trials conducted in children, no patient had QTcF >500 msec. Over 5% of patients had an increase in QTcF of over 60 msec.

In clinical trials conducted in adults, QTcF prolongation of >500 msec was reported in 3 (0.3%) of patients. Over 6% of adults had a QTcF increase of over 60 msec from baseline.

13 NONCLINICAL TOXICOLOGY

13.1 Carcinogenesis, Mutagenesis, Impairment of Fertility

Carcinogenesis

Carcinogenicity studies were not conducted.

Mutagenesis

No evidence of mutagenicity was detected. The artemether: lumefantrine combination was evaluated using the *Salmonella* and *Escherichia*/mammalian-microsome mutagenicity test, the gene mutation test with Chinese hamster cells V79, the cytogenetic test on Chinese hamster cells *in vitro*, and the rat micronucleus test, *in vivo*.

Impairment of Fertility

Pregnancy rates were reduced by about one half in female rats dosed for 2 to 4 weeks with the artemether-lumefantrine combination at 1000 mg/kg (about 9 times the clinical dose based on body surface area comparisons). Male rats dosed for 70 days showed increases in abnormal sperm (87% abnormal) and increased testes weights at 30 mg/kg doses (about one third the clinical dose). Higher doses (about 9 times the clinical dose) resulted in decreased sperm motility and 100% abnormal sperm cells.

13.2 Animal Toxicology and/or Pharmacology

Neonatal rats (7-21 days old) were more sensitive to the toxic effects of artemether (a component of Coartem) than older juvenile rats or adults. Mortality and severe clinical signs were observed in neonatal rats at doses which were well tolerated in pups above 22 days old.

14 CLINICAL STUDIES

14.1 Treatment of Acute, Uncomplicated *P. falciparum* Malaria

The efficacy of Coartem Tablets was evaluated for the treatment of acute, uncomplicated malaria caused by *P. falciparum* in HIV negative patients in 8 clinical studies. Uncom-

Table 6: Clinical Efficacy of 6-dose Regimen of Coartem Tablets

Study No. Region/ages	28-day cure rate[1] n/N (%) patients mITT[3]	28-day cure rate[1] n/N (%) patients Evaluable	Median FCT[2] [25th, 75th percentile]	Median PCT [25th, 75th percentile]
Study 3 Thailand, ages 3 – 62 years	96/118 (81.4)	93/96 (96.9)	35 hours [20, 46]	44 hours [22, 47]
Early failure[4]	0	0		
Late failure[5]	4 (3.4)	3 (3.1)		
Lost to follow up	18 (15.3)			
Other[6]	0			
Study 4 Thailand, ages 2 – 63 years	130/149 (87.2)	130/134 (97.0)	22 hours [19, 44]	NA
Early failure[4]	0	0		
Late failure[5]	4 (2.7)	4 (3.0)		
Lost to follow up	13 (8.7)			
Other[6]	2 (1.3)			
Study 5 Thailand, ages 12 – 71 years	148/164 (90.2)	148/155 (95.5)	29 hours [8, 51]	29 hours [18, 40]
Early failure[4]	0	0		
Late failure[5]	7 (4.3)	7 (4.5)		
Lost to follow up	9 (5.5)			
Other[6]	0			
Study 6 Europe/Columbia, ages 16 – 66 years	120/162 (74.1)	119/124 (96.0)	37 hours [18, 44]	42 hours [34, 63]
Early failure[4]	6 (3.7)	1 (0.8)		
Late failure[5]	3 (1.9)	3 (2.4)		
Lost to follow up	17 (10.5)			
Other[6]	16 (9.9)	1 (0.8)		
Study 7 Africa, ages 2 months – 9 years	268/310 (86.5)	267/300 (89.0)	8 hours [8, 24]	24 hours [24, 36]
Early failure[4]	2 (0.6)	0		
Late failure[5]	34 (11.0)	33 (11.0)		
Lost to follow up	2 (0.6)			
Other[6]	4 (1.3)			
Study 8 Africa, ages 3 months – 12 years	374/452 (82.7)	370/419 (88.3)	8 hours [8, 23]	35 hours [24, 36]
Early failure[4]	13 (2.9)	0		
Late failure[5]	49 (10.8)	49 (11.7)		
Lost to follow up	6 (1.3)			
Other[6]	10 (2.2)			

[1] Efficacy cure rate based on blood smear microscopy
[2] For patients who had a body temperature >37.5°C at baseline only
[3] In mITT analysis, patients whose status was uncertain were classified as treatment failures.
[4] Early failures were usually defined as patients withdrawn for unsatisfactory therapeutic effect within the first 7 days or because they received another antimalarial medication within the first 7 days
[5] Late failures were defined as patients achieving parasite clearance within 7 days but having parasite reappearance including recrudescence or new infection during the 28 day follow-up period
[6] Other includes withdrawn due to protocol violation or non-compliance, received additional medication after day 7, withdrew consent, missing day 7 or 28 assessment

Table 7: Clinical Efficacy by Weight for Pediatric Studies

Study No. Age category	Coartem Tablets 6-dose Regimen mITT population[1] Median PCT [25th,75th percentile]	mITT population[1] 28-day cure rate[2] n/N (%) patients	Evaluable population 28-day cure rate[2] n/N (%) patients
Study 7			
5 - <10 kg	24 [24, 36]	133/154 (86.4)	133/149 (89.3)
10 - <15 kg	35 [24, 36]	94/110 (85.5)	94/107 (87.9)
15 -25 kg	24 [24, 36]	41/46 (89.1)	40/44 (90.9)
Study 8[3]			
5 - <10 kg	36 [24, 36]	61/83 (73.5)	61/69 (88.4)
10 - <15 kg	35 [24, 36]	160/190 (84.2)	157/179 (87.7)
15 - <25 kg	35 [24, 36]	123/145 (84.8)	123/140 (87.9)
25 - <35 kg	26 [24, 36]	30/34 (88.2)	29/31 (93.5)

[1] In mITT analysis, patients whose status was uncertain were classified as treatment failures.
[2] Efficacy cure rate based on blood smear microscopy
[3] Coartem Tablets administered as crushed tablets

plicated malaria was defined as symptomatic *P. falciparum* malaria without signs and symptoms of severe malaria or evidence of vital organ dysfunction. Baseline parasite density ranged from 500/μL - 200,000/μL (0.01% to 4% parasitemia) in the majority of patients. Studies were conducted in partially immune and non-immune adults and children (≥5kg body weight) with uncomplicated malaria in China, Thailand, sub-Saharan Africa, Europe, and South America. Patients who had clinical features of severe malaria, severe cardiac, renal, or hepatic impairment were excluded.

The studies include two 4-dose studies assessing the efficacy of the components of the regimen, a study comparing a 4-dose versus a 6-dose regimen, and 5 additional 6-dose regimen studies.

Coartem Tablets were administered at 0, 8, 24, and 48 hours in the 4-dose regimen, and at 0, 8, 24, 36, 48, and 60 hours in the 6-dose regimen. Efficacy endpoints consisted of:

- 28 day cure rate, defined as clearance of asexual parasites (the erythrocytic stage) within 7 days without recrudescence by day 28
- parasite clearance time (PCT), defined as time from first dose until first total and continued disappearance of asexual parasite which continues for a further 48 hours
- fever clearance time (FCT), defined as time from first dose until the first time body temperature fell below 37.5°C and remained below 37.5°C for at least a further 48 hours (only for patients with temperature >37.5°C at baseline)

The modified intent to treat (mITT) population includes all patients with malaria diagnosis confirmation who received at least one dose of study drug. Evaluable patients generally are all patients who had a day 7 and a day 28 parasitological assessment or experienced treatment failure by day 28.

Studies 1 and 2: The two studies which assessed the efficacy of Coartem Tablets (4 doses of 4 tablets of 20 mg artemether/120 mg lumefantrine) compared to each component alone were randomized, double-blind, comparative, single center, conducted in China. The efficacy results (Table 5) support that the combination of artemether and lumefantrine in Coartem Tablets had a significantly higher 28-day cure rate compared to artemether and had a significantly faster parasite clearance time (PCT) and fever clearance time (FCT) compared to lumefantrine.

[See table 5 at top of previous page]

Results of 4-dose studies conducted in areas with high resistance such as Thailand during 1995-96 showed lower efficacy results than the above studies. Therefore, Study 3 was conducted.

Study 3: Study 3 was a randomized, double-blind, two-center study conducted in Thailand in adults and children (aged ≥2 years), which compared the 4-dose regimen (administered over 48 hours) of Coartem Tablets to a 6-dose regimen (administered over 60 hours). Twenty-eight day cure rate in mITT subjects was 81% (96/118) for the Coartem Tablets 6-dose arm as compared to 71% (85/120) in the 4-dose arm.

Studies 4, 5, 6, 7, and 8: In these studies, Coartem Tablets were administered as the 6-dose regimen.

In study 4, a total of 150 adults and children aged ≥2 years received Coartem Tablets. In study 5, a total 164 adults and children ≥12 years received Coartem Tablets. Both studies were conducted in Thailand.

Study 6 was a study of 165 non-immune adults residing in regions non-endemic for malaria (Europe and Colombia) who contracted acute uncomplicated *falciparum* malaria when traveling in endemic regions.

Study 7 was conducted in Africa in 310 infants and children aged 2 months to 9 years, weighing 5 kg to 25 kg, with an axillary temperature ≥37.5°C.

Study 8 was conducted in Africa in 452 infants and children, aged 3 months to 12 years, weighing 5 kg to <35 kg, with fever (≥37.5°C axillary or ≥38°C rectally) or history of fever in the preceding 24 hours.

Results of 28-day cure rate, median parasite clearance time (PCT), and fever clearance time (FCT) for Studies 3 to 8 are reported in Table 6.

[See table 6 above]

In all studies, patients' signs and symptoms of malaria resolved when parasites were cleared.

In studies conducted in areas with high transmission rates, such as Africa, reappearance of *P. falciparum* parasites may be due to recrudescence or a new infection.

The efficacy by body weight category for studies 7 and 8 is summarized in Table 7.

[See table 7 above]

The efficacy of Coartem Tablets for the treatment *P. falciparum* infections mixed with *P. vivax* was assessed in a small number of patients. Coartem Tablets are only active against the erythrocytic phase of *P. vivax* malaria. Of the 43 patients with mixed infections at baseline, all cleared their parasitemia within 48 hours. However, parasite relapse occurred commonly (14/43; 33%). Relapsing malaria caused by *P. vivax* requires additional treatment with other antimalarial agents to achieve radical cure i.e., eradicate any hypnozoite forms that may remain dormant in the liver.

16 HOW SUPPLIED/STORAGE AND HANDLING

Coartem (artemether/lumefantrine) Tablets

20 mg/120 mg Tablets - yellow, round flat tablets with beveled edges and scored on one side. Tablets are imprinted with N/C on one side and CG on the other.

Bottle of 24 NDC 0078-0568-45

Store at 25°C (77°F); excursions permitted to 15-30°C (59-86°F) [*see USP Controlled Room Temperature*].

Dispense in tight container (USP).

17 PATIENT COUNSELING INFORMATION

See FDA-Approved Patient Labeling.
Information for Safe Use

- Instruct patients to take Coartem Tablets with food. Patients who do not have an adequate intake of food are at risk for recrudescence of malaria.
- Patients with known hypersensitivity to artemether, lumefantrine, or to any of the excipients should not receive Coartem Tablets.
- Instruct patients to inform their physician of any personal or family history of QT prolongation or proarrhythmic conditions such as hypokalemia, bradycardia, or recent myocardial ischemia.
- Instruct patients to inform their physician if they are taking any other medications that prolong the QT interval, such as class IA (quinidine, procainamide, disopyramide), or class III (amiodarone, sotalol) antiarrhythmic agents; antipsychotics (pimozide, ziprasidone); antidepressants; certain antibiotics (macrolide antibiotics, fluoroquinolone antibiotics, imidazole, and triazole antifungal agents).
- Instruct patients to notify their physicians if they have any symptoms of prolongation of the QT interval, including prolonged heart palpitations or a loss of consciousness.
- Instruct patients to avoid medications that are metabolized by the cytochrome enzyme CYP2D6 while receiving Coartem Tablets since these drugs also have cardiac effects (e.g., flecainide, imipramine, amitriptyline, clomipramine).
- Inform patients that based on animal data, Coartem Tablets administered during pregnancy may result in fetal loss. Fetal defects have been reported when artemisinins are administered to animals.
- Halofantrine and Coartem Tablets should not be administered within one month of each other due to potential additive effects on the QT interval.
- Antimalarials should not be given concomitantly with Coartem Tablets, unless there is no other treatment option, due to limited safety data.
- QT prolonging drugs, including quinine and quinidine, should be used cautiously following Coartem Tablets due to the long elimination half-life of lumefantrine and the potential for additive effects on the QT interval. ECG monitoring is advised if use of drugs that prolong the QT interval is medically required.
- Closely monitor food intake in patients who received mefloquine immediately prior to treatment with Coartem Tablets.
- Use Coartem Tablets cautiously in patients receiving other drugs that are substrates, inhibitors or inducers of CYP3A4, including grapefruit juice, especially those that prolong the QT interval or are antiretroviral drugs.
- Co-administration of strong inducers of CYP3A4 such as rifampin, carbamazepine, phenytoin and St. John's wort is contraindicated with Coartem Tablets.
- Coartem Tablets may reduce the effectiveness of hormonal contraceptives. Therefore, patients using oral, transdermal patch, or other systemic hormonal contraceptives should be advised to use an additional non-hormonal method of birth control.
- Inform patients that Coartem Tablets can cause hypersensitivity reactions. Instruct patients to discontinue the drug at the first sign of a skin rash, hives or other skin reactions, a rapid heartbeat, difficulty in swallowing or breathing, any swelling suggesting angioedema (e.g., swelling of the lips, tongue, face, tightness of the throat, hoarseness), or other symptoms of an allergic reaction.

T2013-42
April 2013

FDA-APPROVED PATIENT LABELING
Patient Information
Coartem®
(co-AR-tem)
(artemether and lumefantrine)
Tablets

Read this patient information before you start taking Coartem. There may be new information. This information does not take the place of talking to your healthcare provider about your medical condition or your treatment.

What is Coartem?

Coartem is a prescription medicine used to treat uncomplicated malaria in adults and children who weigh at least 11 pounds (5 kg).

Who should not take Coartem?

Do not take Coartem if you are allergic to any of the ingredients. See the end of this leaflet for a complete list of ingredients in Coartem.

Do not take Coartem if you are taking rifampin (medicine to treat leprosy or tuberculosis), certain medicines used to treat epilepsy (such as carbamazepine, phenytoin), or St. John's wort (*Hypericum perforatum*, a medicinal plant or extract of this medicinal plant).

What should I tell my healthcare provider before taking Coartem?

Before you take Coartem, tell your healthcare provider about all your medical conditions including if you have:

- heart disease or a family history of heart problems or heart disease
- liver or kidney problems
- recently taken other medicines used to treat malaria
- if you are pregnant or are planning to become pregnant. Coartem may increase your risk for loss of pregnancy. Fetal defects have been reported when artemisinins are administered to animals. Talk to your healthcare provider before taking Coartem.
- if you are breast-feeding. It is not known if Coartem passes into your breast milk. You and your doctor will decide the best way to feed your baby if you take Coartem.

Tell your doctor about all the medicines you take, including prescription and non-prescription medicines, vitamins, and herbal supplements. Coartem and other medicines may affect each other causing side effects. Coartem may affect the way other medicines work and other medicines may affect how Coartem works.

Especially tell your doctor if you take:

- any other medicines to treat or prevent malaria
- medicines for your heart
- antipsychotic medicines
- antidepressants
- medicines for seizures or trigeminal neuralgia (facial nerve pain)
- antibiotics (including medicines to treat tuberculosis)
- medicines to treat HIV-infection
- hormonal methods of birth control (for example, birth control pills or patch). If you are taking a hormonal birth control medicine, you should also use an additional method of birth control.

Ask your healthcare provider if you are not sure if your medicine is one that is listed above. Know the medicines you take. Keep a list of your medicines with you to show your healthcare providers when you get a new medicine.

How should I take Coartem?

- Take Coartem exactly as prescribed.
- If you weigh 77 pounds (35 kg) or more, one dose of Coartem is 4 tablets.
- If you weigh less than 77 pounds (35 kg), your healthcare provider will tell you how many tablets to take for each dose.
- A full course of treatment is 6 doses of Coartem taken over 3 days:

Day 1: take 1 dose; 8 hours later take 1 dose
Day 2: take 1 dose in the morning, 1 dose in the evening
Day 3: take 1 dose in the morning, 1 dose in the evening

Take Coartem for 3 days even if you are feeling better.

- Every dose of Coartem should be taken with food, such as milk, infant formula, pudding, porridge, or broth. It is important for you to eat as soon as you can so that your malaria will go away and not get worse.
- Do not drink grapefruit juice while you take Coartem. Drinking grapefruit juice during treatment with Coartem can cause you to have too much medicine in your blood.
- Coartem may be crushed and mixed with one to two teaspoons of water in a clean container.
- If you vomit within 1 hour of taking Coartem you should take another dose of Coartem. If you vomit the second dose, tell your healthcare provider. A different medicine may need to be prescribed for you.

Tell your healthcare provider right away if:

- your malaria does not get better
- you vomited any of your doses of Coartem
- you are not able to eat
- you get flu-like symptoms (chills, fever, muscle pains, or headaches) again after you have finished your treatment with Coartem.
- you have any change in the way your heart beats or a loss of consciousness (fainting).

What are the possible side effects of Coartem?

Coartem can cause serious side effects including:

- **A heart problem called QT prolongation** that can cause an abnormal heartbeat can happen in people who take Coartem. The chance of this happening is higher in people with a family history of prolonged QT interval, low potassium (hypokalemia), and in people who take medicines to control heartbeats.
- **Allergic reactions.** Symptoms of an allergic reaction include: rash, hives, fast heartbeat, trouble swallowing or breathing, swelling of lips, tongue, face, tightness of the throat, or trouble speaking. If you have a serious allergic reaction, stop taking Coartem and get emergency medical help right away.

The most common side effects in adults are:

- headache
- feeling dizzy
- feeling weak
- loss of appetite
- muscle and joint pain or stiffness
- feeling tired
- chills
- fever

The most common side effects in children are:

- fever
- cough
- vomiting
- headache
- loss of appetite

These are not all the possible side effects of Coartem. For more information, ask your doctor or pharmacist. Call your doctor for medical advice about side effects. You may report side effects to FDA at 1-800-FDA-1088.

How should I store Coartem?

Store Coartem between 59°F to 86°F (15°C to 30°C).

Keep Coartem and all medicines out of the reach of children.

General information about the safe and effective use of Coartem.

Medicines are sometimes prescribed for purposes other than those listed in patient information leaflets. Do not use Coartem for a condition for which it was not prescribed. Do not give Coartem to other people, even if they have the same symptoms that you have. It may harm them.

This patient information leaflet summarizes the most important information about Coartem. If you would like more information about Coartem talk with your healthcare provider. You can ask your healthcare provider or pharmacist for information about Coartem that is written for health professionals. For more information call 1-888-294-6287.

What are the ingredients in Coartem?

Active ingredients include: artemether, lumefantrine
Inactive ingredients include: colloidal silicon dioxide, croscarmellose sodium, hypromellose, magnesium stearate, microcrystalline cellulose, polysorbate 80

Distributed by:
Novartis Pharmaceuticals Corporation
East Hanover, New Jersey 07936
© Novartis
T2013-43
April 2013

Shown in Product Identification Guide, page 309

DIOVAN ℞

[*DYE'-o-van*]
(valsartan)
Tablets

The following prescribing information is based on official labeling in effect July 2013.

HIGHLIGHTS OF PRESCRIBING INFORMATION
These highlights do not include all the information needed to use Diovan safely and effectively. See full prescribing information for Diovan.
Diovan (valsartan) Tablets
Initial U.S. Approval: 1996

WARNING: FETAL TOXICITY
See full prescribing information for complete boxed warning.
- **When pregnancy is detected, discontinue Diovan as soon as possible. (5.1)**
- **Drugs that act directly on the renin-angiotensin system can cause injury and death to the developing fetus. (5.1)**

RECENT MAJOR CHANGES

Boxed Warning: Fetal Toxicity	01/2012
Indications and Usage: Benefits of lowering blood pressure (1)	12/2011
Dosage and Administration: Pediatric Hypertension 6-16 years of age (2.2)	02/2012
Contraindications: Known hypersensitivity (4)	07/2012
Contraindications: Dual RAS Blockade in Diabetics (4)	10/2012
Warnings and Precautions: Fetal Toxicity (5.1)	01/2012
Drug Interactions: Dual Blockade of the Renin-Angiotensin System (7)	10/2012

INDICATIONS AND USAGE

Diovan is an angiotensin II receptor blocker (ARB) indicated for:

- Treatment of **hypertension**, to lower blood pressure. Lowering blood pressure reduces the risk of fatal and nonfatal cardiovascular events, primarily strokes and myocardial infarctions (1.1)
- Treatment of **heart failure** (NYHA class II-IV); Diovan significantly reduced hospitalization for heart failure (1.2)
- Reduction of cardiovascular mortality in clinically stable patients with left ventricular failure or left ventricular dysfunction **following myocardial infarction** (1.3)

Indication	Starting Dose	Dose Range	Target Maintenance Dose*
Adult Hypertension (2.1)	80 or 160 mg once daily	80-320 mg once daily	---
Pediatric Hypertension (6-16 years) (2.2)	1.3 mg/kg once daily (up to 40 mg total)	1.3-2.7 mg/kg once daily (up to 40-160 mg total)	---
Heart Failure (2.3)	40 mg twice daily	40-160 mg twice daily	160 mg twice daily
Post-Myocardial Infarction (2.4)	20 mg twice daily	20-160 mg twice daily	160 mg twice daily

* as tolerated by patient

DOSAGE AND ADMINISTRATION

[See table above]

DOSAGE FORMS AND STRENGTHS

Tablets (mg): 40 (scored), 80, 160, 320 (3)

CONTRAINDICATIONS

Known hypersensitivity to any component; Do not coadminister aliskiren with Diovan in patients with diabetes (4)

WARNINGS AND PRECAUTIONS

- Observe for signs and symptoms of hypotension (5.2)
- Monitor renal function and potassium in susceptible patients (5.3, 5.4)

ADVERSE REACTIONS

Hypertension: Most common adverse reactions are headache, dizziness, viral infection, fatigue and abdominal pain (6.1)

Heart Failure: Most common adverse reactions are dizziness, hypotension, diarrhea, arthralgia, back pain, fatigue and hyperkalemia (6.1)

Post-Myocardial Infarction: Most common adverse reactions which caused patients to discontinue therapy are hypotension, cough and increased blood creatinine (6.1)

To report SUSPECTED ADVERSE REACTIONS, contact Novartis Pharmaceuticals Corporation at 1-888-669-6682 or FDA at 1-800-FDA-1088 or www.fda.gov/medwatch.

DRUG INTERACTIONS

- Potassium sparing diuretics, potassium supplements or salt substitutes may lead to increases in serum potassium, and in heart failure patients, increases in serum creatinine (7)
- NSAID use may lead to increased risk of renal impairment and loss of antihypertensive effect (7)
- Dual inhibition of the renin-angiotensin system: Increased risk of renal impairment, hypotension, and hyperkalemia (7)

USE IN SPECIFIC POPULATIONS

Nursing Mothers: Nursing or drug should be discontinued (8.3); **Pediatrics**: Efficacy and safety data support use in 6-16 year old patients; use is not recommended in patients <6 years old (6.1, 8.4)

See 17 for PATIENT COUNSELING INFORMATION and FDA-approved patient labeling

Revised: 10/2012

FULL PRESCRIBING INFORMATION: CONTENTS*

*** Sections or subsections omitted from the full prescribing information are not listed**

FULL PRESCRIBING INFORMATION

WARNING: FETAL TOXICITY
- **When pregnancy is detected, discontinue Diovan as soon as possible. (5.1)**
- **Drugs that act directly on the renin-angiotensin system can cause injury and death to the developing fetus. (5.1)**

1 INDICATIONS AND USAGE

1.1 Hypertension

Diovan® (valsartan) is indicated for the treatment of hypertension, to lower blood pressure. Lowering blood pressure reduces the risk of fatal and nonfatal cardiovascular events, primarily strokes and myocardial infarctions. These benefits have been seen in controlled trials of antihypertensive drugs from a wide variety of pharmacologic classes including the class to which valsartan principally belongs. There are no controlled trials in hypertensive patients demonstrating risk reduction with Diovan.

Control of high blood pressure should be part of comprehensive cardiovascular risk management, including, as appropriate, lipid control, diabetes management, antithrombotic therapy, smoking cessation, exercise, and limited sodium intake. Many patients will require more than one drug to achieve blood pressure goals. For specific advice on goals and management, see published guidelines, such as those of the National High Blood Pressure Education Program's Joint National Committee on Prevention, Detection, Evaluation, and Treatment of High Blood Pressure (JNC).

Numerous antihypertensive drugs, from a variety of pharmacologic classes and with different mechanisms of action, have been shown in randomized controlled trials to reduce cardiovascular morbidity and mortality, and it can be concluded that it is blood pressure reduction, and not some other pharmacologic property of the drugs, that is largely responsible for those benefits. The largest and most consistent cardiovascular outcome benefit has been a reduction in the risk of stroke, but reductions in myocardial infarction and cardiovascular mortality also have been seen regularly.

Elevated systolic or diastolic pressure causes increased cardiovascular risk, and the absolute risk increase per mmHg is greater at higher blood pressures, so that even modest reductions of severe hypertension can provide substantial benefit. Relative risk reduction from blood pressure reduction is similar across populations with varying absolute risk, so the absolute benefit is greater in patients who are at higher risk independent of their hypertension (for example, patients with diabetes or hyperlipidemia), and such patients would be expected to benefit from more aggressive treatment to a lower blood pressure goal.

Some antihypertensive drugs have smaller blood pressure effects (as monotherapy) in black patients, and many antihypertensive drugs have additional approved indications and effects (e.g., on angina, heart failure, or diabetic kidney disease). These considerations may guide selection of therapy.

Diovan may be used alone or in combination with other antihypertensive agents.

1.2 Heart Failure

Diovan is indicated for the treatment of heart failure (NYHA class II-IV). In a controlled clinical trial, Diovan significantly reduced hospitalizations for heart failure. There is no evidence that Diovan provides added benefits when it is used with an adequate dose of an ACE inhibitor. *[See Clinical Studies (14.2)]*

1.3 Post-Myocardial Infarction

In clinically stable patients with left ventricular failure or left ventricular dysfunction following myocardial infarction, Diovan is indicated to reduce cardiovascular mortality. *[See Clinical Studies (14.3)]*

2 DOSAGE AND ADMINISTRATION

2.1 Adult Hypertension

The recommended starting dose of Diovan (valsartan) is 80 mg or 160 mg once daily when used as monotherapy in patients who are not volume-depleted. Patients requiring greater reductions may be started at the higher dose. Diovan may be used over a dose range of 80 mg to 320 mg daily, administered once a day.

The antihypertensive effect is substantially present within 2 weeks and maximal reduction is generally attained after 4 weeks. If additional antihypertensive effect is required over the starting dose range, the dose may be increased to a maximum of 320 mg or a diuretic may be added. Addition of a diuretic has a greater effect than dose increases beyond 80 mg.

No initial dosage adjustment is required for elderly patients, for patients with mild or moderate renal impairment, or for patients with mild or moderate liver insufficiency. Care should be exercised with dosing of Diovan in patients with hepatic or severe renal impairment.

Diovan may be administered with other antihypertensive agents.

Diovan may be administered with or without food.

2.2 Pediatric Hypertension 6-16 years of age

For children who can swallow tablets, the usual recommended starting dose is 1.3 mg/kg once daily (up to 40 mg total). The dosage should be adjusted according to blood pressure response. Doses higher than 2.7 mg/kg (up to 160 mg) once daily have not been studied in pediatric patients 6 to 16 years old.

For children who cannot swallow tablets, or children for whom the calculated dosage (mg/kg) does not correspond to the available tablet strengths of Diovan, the use of a suspension is recommended. Follow the suspension preparation instructions below (see **Preparation of Suspension**) to administer valsartan as a suspension. When the suspension is replaced by a tablet, the dose of valsartan may have to be increased. The exposure to valsartan with the suspension is 1.6 times greater than with the tablet.

No data are available in pediatric patients either undergoing dialysis or with a glomerular filtration rate <30 mL/min/1.73 m^2. *[See Pediatric Use (8.4)]*

Diovan is not recommended for patients <6 years old. *[See Adverse Reactions (6.1), Clinical Studies (14.1)]*

Preparation of Suspension (for 160 mL of a 4 mg/mL suspension)

Add 80 mL of Ora-Plus®* oral suspending vehicle to an amber glass bottle containing 8 Diovan 80 mg tablets, and shake for a minimum of 2 minutes. Allow the suspension to stand for a minimum of 1 hour. After the standing time, shake the suspension for a minimum of 1 additional minute. Add 80 mL of Ora-Sweet SF®* oral sweetening vehicle to the bottle and shake the suspension for at least 10 seconds to disperse the ingredients. The suspension is homogenous and can be stored for either up to 30 days at room temperature (below 30°C/86°F) or up to 75 days at refrigerated conditions (2-8°C/35-46°F) in the glass bottle with a child-resistant screw-cap closure. Shake the bottle well (at least 10 seconds) prior to dispensing the suspension.

*Ora-Sweet SF® and Ora-Plus® are registered trademarks of Paddock Laboratories, Inc.

2.3 Heart Failure

The recommended starting dose of Diovan is 40 mg twice daily. Uptitration to 80 mg and 160 mg twice daily should be done to the highest dose, as tolerated by the patient. Consideration should be given to reducing the dose of concomitant diuretics. The maximum daily dose administered in clinical trials is 320 mg in divided doses.

2.4 Post-Myocardial Infarction

Diovan may be initiated as early as 12 hours after a myocardial infarction. The recommended starting dose of Diovan is 20 mg twice daily. Patients may be uptitrated within 7 days to 40 mg twice daily, with subsequent titrations to a target maintenance dose of 160 mg twice daily, as tolerated by the patient. If symptomatic hypotension or renal dysfunction occurs, consideration should be given to a dosage reduction. Diovan may be given with other standard post-myocardial infarction treatment, including thrombolytics, aspirin, beta-blockers, and statins.

3 DOSAGE FORMS AND STRENGTHS

40 mg are scored yellow ovaloid tablets with beveled edges, imprinted NVR/DO (Side 1/Side 2)
80 mg are pale red almond-shaped tablets with beveled edges, imprinted NVR/DV
160 mg are grey-orange almond-shaped tablets with beveled edges, imprinted NVR/DX
320 mg are dark grey-violet almond-shaped tablets with beveled edges, imprinted NVR/DXL

4 CONTRAINDICATIONS

Do not use in patients with known hypersensitivity to any component.
Do not coadminister aliskiren with Diovan in patients with diabetes [*See Drug Interactions (7)*].

5 WARNINGS AND PRECAUTIONS

5.1 Fetal Toxicity

Pregnancy Category D

Use of drugs that act on the renin-angiotensin system during the second and third trimesters of pregnancy reduces fetal renal function and increases fetal and neonatal morbidity and death. Resulting oligohydramnios can be associated with fetal lung hypoplasia and skeletal deformations. Potential neonatal adverse effects include skull hypoplasia, anuria, hypotension, renal failure, and death. When pregnancy is detected, discontinue Diovan as soon as possible. [*see Use in Specific Populations (8.1)*].

5.2 Hypotension

Excessive hypotension was rarely seen (0.1%) in patients with uncomplicated hypertension treated with Diovan alone. In patients with an activated renin-angiotensin system, such as volume- and/or salt-depleted patients receiving high doses of diuretics, symptomatic hypotension may occur. This condition should be corrected prior to administration of Diovan, or the treatment should start under close medical supervision.

Caution should be observed when initiating therapy in patients with heart failure or post-myocardial infarction patients. Patients with heart failure or post-myocardial infarction patients given Diovan commonly have some reduction in blood pressure, but discontinuation of therapy because of continuing symptomatic hypotension usually is not necessary when dosing instructions are followed. In controlled trials in heart failure patients, the incidence of hypotension in valsartan-treated patients was 5.5% compared to 1.8% in placebo-treated patients. In the Valsartan in Acute Myocardial Infarction Trial (VALIANT), hypotension in post-myocardial infarction patients led to permanent discontinuation of therapy in 1.4% of valsartan-treated patients and 0.8% of captopril-treated patients.

If excessive hypotension occurs, the patient should be placed in the supine position and, if necessary, given an intravenous infusion of normal saline. A transient hypotensive response is not a contraindication to further treatment, which usually can be continued without difficulty once the blood pressure has stabilized.

5.3 Impaired Renal Function

Changes in renal function including acute renal failure can be caused by drugs that inhibit the renin-angiotensin system and by diuretics. Patients whose renal function may depend in part on the activity of the renin-angiotensin system (e.g. patients with renal artery stenosis, chronic kidney disease, severe congestive heart failure, or volume depletion) may be at particular risk of developing acute renal failure on Diovan. Monitor renal function periodically in these patients. Consider withholding or discontinuing therapy in patients who develop a clinically significant decrease in renal function on Diovan [*See Drug Interactions (7)*].

5.4 Hyperkalemia

Some patients with heart failure have developed increases in potassium. These effects are usually minor and transient, and they are more likely to occur in patients with pre-existing renal impairment. Dosage reduction and/or discontinuation of Diovan may be required. [*see Adverse Reactions (6.1)*]

6 ADVERSE REACTIONS

6.1 Clinical Studies Experience

Because clinical studies are conducted under widely varying conditions, adverse reaction rates observed in the clinical studies of a drug cannot be directly compared to rates in the clinical studies of another drug and may not reflect the rates observed in practice.

Adult Hypertension

Diovan (valsartan) has been evaluated for safety in more than 4,000 patients, including over 400 treated for over 6 months, and more than 160 for over 1 year. Adverse reactions have generally been mild and transient in nature and have only infrequently required discontinuation of therapy. The overall incidence of adverse reactions with Diovan was similar to placebo.

The overall frequency of adverse reactions was neither dose-related nor related to gender, age, race, or regimen. Discontinuation of therapy due to side effects was required in 2.3% of valsartan patients and 2.0% of placebo patients. The most common reasons for discontinuation of therapy with Diovan were headache and dizziness.

The adverse reactions that occurred in placebo-controlled clinical trials in at least 1% of patients treated with Diovan and at a higher incidence in valsartan (n=2,316) than placebo (n=888) patients included viral infection (3% vs. 2%), fatigue (2% vs. 1%), and abdominal pain (2% vs. 1%).

Headache, dizziness, upper respiratory infection, cough, diarrhea, rhinitis, sinusitis, nausea, pharyngitis, edema, and arthralgia occurred at a more than 1% rate but at about the same incidence in placebo and valsartan patients.

In trials in which valsartan was compared to an ACE inhibitor with or without placebo, the incidence of dry cough was significantly greater in the ACE-inhibitor group (7.9%) than in the groups who received valsartan (2.6%) or placebo (1.5%). In a 129-patient trial limited to patients who had had dry cough when they had previously received ACE inhibitors, the incidences of cough in patients who received valsartan, HCTZ, or lisinopril were 20%, 19%, and 69% respectively ($p < 0.001$).

Dose-related orthostatic effects were seen in less than 1% of patients. An increase in the incidence of dizziness was observed in patients treated with Diovan 320 mg (8%) compared to 10 to 160 mg (2% to 4%).

Diovan has been used concomitantly with hydrochlorothiazide without evidence of clinically important adverse interactions.

Other adverse reactions that occurred in controlled clinical trials of patients treated with Diovan (>0.2% of valsartan patients) are listed below. It cannot be determined whether these events were causally related to Diovan.

Body as a Whole: Allergic reaction and asthenia
Cardiovascular: Palpitations
Dermatologic: Pruritus and rash
Digestive: Constipation, dry mouth, dyspepsia, and flatulence
Musculoskeletal: Back pain, muscle cramps, and myalgia
Neurologic and Psychiatric: Anxiety, insomnia, paresthesia, and somnolence
Respiratory: Dyspnea
Special Senses: Vertigo
Urogenital: Impotence

Other reported events seen less frequently in clinical trials included chest pain, syncope, anorexia, vomiting, and angioedema.

Pediatric Hypertension

Diovan has been evaluated for safety in over 400 pediatric patients aged 6 to 17 years and more than 160 pediatric patients aged 6 months to 5 years. No relevant differences were identified between the adverse experience profile for pediatric patients aged 6-16 years and that previously reported for adult patients. Headache and hyperkalemia were the most common adverse events suspected to be study drug-related in older children (6 to 17 years old) and younger children (6 months to 5 years old), respectively. Hyperkalemia was mainly observed in children with underlying renal disease. Neurocognitive and developmental assessment of pediatric patients aged 6 to 16 years revealed no overall clinically relevant adverse impact after treatment with Diovan for up to 1 year.

Diovan is not recommended for pediatric patients under 6 years of age. In a study (n=90) of pediatric patients (1-5 years), two deaths and three cases of on-treatment transaminase elevations were seen in the one-year open-label extension phase. These 5 events occurred in a study population in which patients frequently had significant comorbidities. A causal relationship to Diovan has not been established. In a second study in which 75 children aged 1 to 6 years were randomized, no deaths and one case of marked liver transaminase elevations occurred during a 1 year open-label extension.

Heart Failure

The adverse experience profile of Diovan in heart failure patients was consistent with the pharmacology of the drug and the health status of the patients. In the Valsartan Heart Failure Trial, comparing valsartan in total daily doses up to 320 mg (n=2,506) to placebo (n=2,494), 10% of valsartan patients discontinued for adverse reactions vs. 7% of placebo patients.

The table shows adverse reactions in double-blind short-term heart failure trials, including the first 4 months of the Valsartan Heart Failure Trial, with an incidence of at least 2% that were more frequent in valsartan-treated patients than in placebo-treated patients. All patients received standard drug therapy for heart failure, frequently as multiple medications, which could include diuretics, digitalis, beta-blockers. About 93% of patients received concomitant ACE inhibitors.

	Valsartan (n=3,282)	Placebo (n=2,740)
Dizziness	17%	9%
Hypotension	7%	2%
Diarrhea	5%	4%
Arthralgia	3%	2%
Fatigue	3%	2%
Back Pain	3%	2%
Dizziness, postural	2%	1%
Hyperkalemia	2%	1%
Hypotension, postural	2%	1%

Discontinuations occurred in 0.5% of valsartan-treated patients and 0.1% of placebo patients for each of the following: elevations in creatinine and elevations in potassium.

Other adverse reactions with an incidence greater than 1% and greater than placebo included headache NOS, nausea, renal impairment NOS, syncope, blurred vision, upper abdominal pain and vertigo. (NOS = not otherwise specified).

From the long-term data in the Valsartan Heart Failure Trial, there did not appear to be any significant adverse reactions not previously identified.

Post-Myocardial Infarction

The safety profile of Diovan was consistent with the pharmacology of the drug and the background diseases, cardiovascular risk factors, and clinical course of patients treated in the post-myocardial infarction setting. The table shows the percent of patients discontinued in the valsartan and captopril-treated groups in the Valsartan in Acute Myocardial Infarction Trial (VALIANT) with a rate of at least 0.5% in either of the treatment groups.

Discontinuations due to renal dysfunction occurred in 1.1% of valsartan-treated patients and 0.8% of captopril-treated patients.

	Valsartan (n=4,885)	Captopril (n=4,879)
Discontinuation for adverse reaction	5.8%	7.7%
Adverse reactions		
Hypotension NOS	1.4%	0.8%
Cough	0.6%	2.5%
Blood creatinine increased	0.6%	0.4%
Rash NOS	0.2%	0.6%

6.2 Post-Marketing Experience

The following additional adverse reactions have been reported in post-marketing experience:

Hypersensitivity: There are rare reports of angioedema. Some of these patients previously experienced angioedema with other drugs including ACE inhibitors. Diovan should not be re-administered to patients who have had angioedema.
Digestive: Elevated liver enzymes and very rare reports of hepatitis
Renal: Impaired renal function, renal failure
Clinical Laboratory Tests: Hyperkalemia
Dermatologic: Alopecia
Blood and Lymphatic: There are very rare reports of thrombocytopenia
Vascular: Vasculitis

Rare cases of rhabdomyolysis have been reported in patients receiving angiotensin II receptor blockers.

Because these reactions are reported voluntarily from a population of uncertain size, it is not always possible to reliably estimate their frequency or establish a causal relationship to drug exposure.

7 DRUG INTERACTIONS

No clinically significant pharmacokinetic interactions were observed when Diovan (valsartan) was coadministered with amlodipine, atenolol, cimetidine, digoxin, furosemide, glyburide, hydrochlorothiazide, or indomethacin. The valsartan-atenolol combination was more antihypertensive than either component, but it did not lower the heart rate more than atenolol alone.

Coadministration of valsartan and warfarin did not change the pharmacokinetics of valsartan or the time-course of the anticoagulant properties of warfarin.

CYP 450 Interactions: *In vitro* metabolism studies indicate that CYP 450 mediated drug interactions between valsartan and coadministered drugs are unlikely because of the low extent of metabolism *[see Clinical Pharmacology (12.3)]*.

Transporters: The results from an *in vitro* study with human liver tissue indicate that valsartan is a substrate of the hepatic uptake transporter OATP1B1 and the hepatic efflux transporter MRP2. Coadministration of inhibitors of the uptake transporter (rifampin, cyclosporine) or efflux transporter (ritonavir) may increase the systemic exposure to valsartan.

Potassium: Concomitant use of valsartan with other agents that block the renin-angiotensin system, potassium sparing diuretics (e.g. spironolactone, triamterene, amiloride), potassium supplements, or salt substitutes containing potassium may lead to increases in serum potassium and in heart failure patients to increases in serum creatinine. If co-medication is considered necessary, monitoring of serum potassium is advisable.

Non-Steroidal Anti-Inflammatory Agents including Selective Cyclooxygenase-2 Inhibitors (COX-2 Inhibitors): In patients who are elderly, volume-depleted (including those on diuretic therapy), or with compromised renal function, coadministration of NSAIDs, including selective COX-2 inhibitors, with angiotensin II receptor antagonists, including valsartan, may result in deterioration of renal function, including possible acute renal failure. These effects are usually reversible. Monitor renal function periodically in patients receiving valsartan and NSAID therapy.

The antihypertensive effect of angiotensin II receptor antagonists, including valsartan may be attenuated by NSAIDs including selective COX-2 inhibitors.

Dual Blockade of the Renin-Angiotensin System (RAS): Dual blockade of the RAS with angiotensin receptor blockers, ACE inhibitors, or aliskiren is associated with increased risks of hypotension, hyperkalemia, and changes in renal function (including acute renal failure) compared to monotherapy. Closely monitor blood pressure, renal function and electrolytes in patients on Diovan and other agents that affect the RAS.

Do not coadminister aliskiren with Diovan in patients with diabetes. Avoid use of aliskiren with Diovan in patients with renal impairment (GFR <60 mL/min).

7.1 Clinical Laboratory Test Findings

In controlled clinical trials, clinically important changes in standard laboratory parameters were rarely associated with administration of Diovan.

Creatinine: Minor elevations in creatinine occurred in 0.8% of patients taking Diovan and 0.6% given placebo in controlled clinical trials of hypertensive patients. In heart failure trials, greater than 50% increases in creatinine were observed in 3.9% of Diovan-treated patients compared to 0.9% of placebo-treated patients. In post-myocardial infarction patients, doubling of serum creatinine was observed in 4.2% of valsartan-treated patients and 3.4% of captopril-treated patients.

Hemoglobin and Hematocrit: Greater than 20% decreases in hemoglobin and hematocrit were observed in 0.4% and 0.8%, respectively, of Diovan patients, compared with 0.1% and 0.1% in placebo-treated patients. One valsartan patient discontinued treatment for microcytic anemia.

Liver Function Tests: Occasional elevations (greater than 150%) of liver chemistries occurred in Diovan-treated patients. Three patients (< 0.1%) treated with valsartan discontinued treatment for elevated liver chemistries.

Neutropenia: Neutropenia was observed in 1.9% of patients treated with Diovan and 0.8% of patients treated with placebo.

Serum Potassium: In hypertensive patients, greater than 20% increases in serum potassium were observed in 4.4% of Diovan-treated patients compared to 2.9% of placebo-treated patients. In heart failure patients, greater than 20% increases in serum potassium were observed in 10.0% of Diovan-treated patients compared to 5.1% of placebo-treated patients.

Blood Urea Nitrogen (BUN): In heart failure trials, greater than 50% increases in BUN were observed in 16.6% of Diovan-treated patients compared to 6.3% of placebo-treated patients.

8 USE IN SPECIFIC POPULATIONS

8.1 Pregnancy

Pregnancy Category D

Use of drugs that act on the renin-angiotensin system during the second and third trimesters of pregnancy reduces fetal renal function and increases fetal and neonatal morbidity and death. Resulting oligohydramnios can be associated with fetal lung hypoplasia and skeletal deformations. Potential neonatal adverse effects include skull hypoplasia, anuria, hypotension, renal failure, and death. When pregnancy is detected, discontinue Diovan as soon as possible. These adverse outcomes are usually associated with use of these drugs in the second and third trimesters of pregnancy. Most epidemiologic studies examining fetal abnormalities after exposure to antihypertensive use in the first trimester have not distinguished drugs affecting the renin-angiotensin system from other antihypertensive agents. Appropriate management of maternal hypertension during pregnancy is important to optimize outcomes for both mother and fetus.

In the unusual case that there is no appropriate alternative to therapy with drugs affecting the renin-angiotensin system for a particular patient, apprise the mother of the potential risk to the fetus. Perform serial ultrasound examinations to assess the intra-amniotic environment. If oligohydramnios is observed, discontinue Diovan, unless it is considered lifesaving for the mother. Fetal testing may be appropriate, based on the week of pregnancy. Patients and physicians should be aware, however, that oligohydramnios may not appear until after the fetus has sustained irreversible injury. Closely observe infants with histories of in utero exposure to Diovan for hypotension, oliguria, and hyperkalemia. *[see Use in Specific Populations (8.4)]*

8.3 Nursing Mothers

It is not known whether Diovan is excreted in human milk. Diovan was excreted in the milk of lactating rats; however, animal breast milk drug levels may not accurately reflect human breast milk levels. Because many drugs are excreted into human milk and because of the potential for adverse reactions in nursing infants from Diovan, a decision should be made whether to discontinue nursing or discontinue the drug, taking into account the importance of the drug to the mother.

8.4 Pediatric Use

The antihypertensive effects of Diovan have been evaluated in two randomized, double-blind clinical studies in pediatric patients from 1-5 and 6-16 years of age *[see Clinical Studies (14.1)]*. The pharmacokinetics of Diovan have been evaluated in pediatric patients 1 to 16 years of age *[see Pharmacokinetics, Special Populations, Pediatric (12.3)]*. Diovan was generally well tolerated in children 6-16 years and the adverse experience profile was similar to that described for adults.

In children and adolescents with hypertension where underlying renal abnormalities may be more common, renal function and serum potassium should be closely monitored as clinically indicated.

Diovan is not recommended for pediatric patients under 6 years of age due to safety findings for which a relationship to treatment could not be excluded *[see Adverse Reactions, Pediatric Hypertension (6.1)]*.

No data are available in pediatric patients either undergoing dialysis or with a glomerular filtration rate <30 mL/min/1.73 m^2.

There is limited clinical experience with Diovan in pediatric patients with mild to moderate hepatic impairment *[See Warnings and Precautions (5.3)]*.

Daily oral dosing of neonatal/juvenile rats with valsartan at doses as low as 1 mg/kg/day (about 10% of the maximum recommended pediatric dose on a mg/m^2 basis) from postnatal day 7 to postnatal day 70 produced persistent, irreversible kidney damage. These kidney effects in neonatal rats represent expected exaggerated pharmacological effects that are observed if rats are treated during the first 13 days of life. Since this period coincides with up to 44 weeks after conception in humans, it is not considered to point toward an increased safety concern in 6 to 16 year old children.

Neonates with a history of in utero exposure to Diovan:

If oliguria or hypotension occurs, direct attention toward support of blood pressure and renal perfusion. Exchange transfusions or dialysis may be required as a means of reversing hypotension and/or substituting for disordered renal function.

8.5 Geriatric Use

In the controlled clinical trials of valsartan, 1,214 (36.2%) hypertensive patients treated with valsartan were ≥65 years and 265 (7.9%) were ≥75 years. No overall difference in the efficacy or safety of valsartan was observed in this patient population, but greater sensitivity of some older individuals cannot be ruled out.

Of the 2,511 patients with heart failure randomized to valsartan in the Valsartan Heart Failure Trial, 45% (1,141) were 65 years of age or older. In the Valsartan in Acute Myocardial Infarction Trial (VALIANT), 53% (2,596) of the 4,909 patients treated with valsartan and 51% (2,515) of the 4,885 patients treated with valsartan + captopril were 65 years of age or older. There were no notable differences in efficacy or safety between older and younger patients in either trial.

8.6 Renal Impairment

Safety and effectiveness of Diovan in patients with severe renal impairment (CrCl ≤ 30 mL/min) have not been established. No dose adjustment is required in patients with mild (CrCl 60-90 mL/min) or moderate (CrCl 30-60) renal impairment.

8.7 Hepatic Impairment

No dose adjustment is necessary for patients with mild-to-moderate liver disease. No dosing recommendations can be provided for patients with severe liver disease.

10 OVERDOSAGE

Limited data are available related to overdosage in humans. The most likely manifestations of overdosage would be hypotension and tachycardia; bradycardia could occur from parasympathetic (vagal) stimulation. Depressed level of consciousness, circulatory collapse and shock have been reported. If symptomatic hypotension should occur, supportive treatment should be instituted.

Diovan (valsartan) is not removed from the plasma by hemodialysis.

Valsartan was without grossly observable adverse effects at single oral doses up to 2000 mg/kg in rats and up to 1000 mg/kg in marmosets, except for salivation and diarrhea in the rat and vomiting in the marmoset at the highest dose (60 and 31 times, respectively, the maximum recommended human dose on a mg/m^2 basis). (Calculations assume an oral dose of 320 mg/day and a 60-kg patient.)

11 DESCRIPTION

Diovan (valsartan) is a nonpeptide, orally active, and specific angiotensin II receptor blocker acting on the AT_1 receptor subtype.

Valsartan is chemically described as *N*-(1-oxopentyl)-*N*-[[2'-(1*H*-tetrazol-5-yl) [1,1'-biphenyl]-4-yl]methyl]-L-valine. Its empirical formula is $C_{24}H_{29}N_5O_3$, its molecular weight is 435.5, and its structural formula is

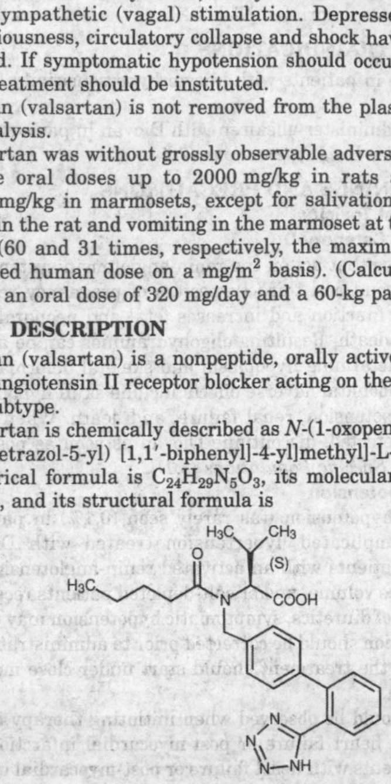

Valsartan is a white to practically white fine powder. It is soluble in ethanol and methanol and slightly soluble in water.

Diovan is available as tablets for oral administration, containing 40 mg, 80 mg, 160 mg or 320 mg of valsartan. The inactive ingredients of the tablets are colloidal silicon dioxide, crospovidone, hydroxypropyl methylcellulose, iron oxides (yellow, black and/or red), magnesium stearate, microcrystalline cellulose, polyethylene glycol 8000, and titanium dioxide.

12 CLINICAL PHARMACOLOGY

12.1 Mechanism of Action

Angiotensin II is formed from angiotensin I in a reaction catalyzed by angiotensin-converting enzyme (ACE, kininase II). Angiotensin II is the principal pressor agent of the renin-angiotensin system, with effects that include vasoconstriction, stimulation of synthesis and release of aldosterone, cardiac stimulation, and renal reabsorption of sodium. Diovan (valsartan) blocks the vasoconstrictor and aldosterone-secreting effects of angiotensin II by selectively blocking the binding of angiotensin II to the AT_1 receptor in many tissues, such as vascular smooth muscle and the adrenal gland. Its action is therefore independent of the pathways for angiotensin II synthesis.

There is also an AT_2 receptor found in many tissues, but AT_2 is not known to be associated with cardiovascular homeostasis. Valsartan has much greater affinity (about 20,000-fold) for the AT_1 receptor than for the AT_2 receptor. The increased plasma levels of angiotensin II following AT_1 receptor blockade with valsartan may stimulate the unblocked AT_2 receptor. The primary metabolite of valsartan is essentially inactive with an affinity for the AT_1 receptor about one-200th that of valsartan itself.

Blockade of the renin-angiotensin system with ACE inhibitors, which inhibit the biosynthesis of angiotensin II from angiotensin I, is widely used in the treatment of hypertension. ACE inhibitors also inhibit the degradation of bradykinin, a reaction also catalyzed by ACE. Because valsartan does not inhibit ACE (kininase II), it does not affect the response to bradykinin. Whether this difference has clinical relevance is not yet known. Valsartan does not bind to or block other hormone receptors or ion channels known to be important in cardiovascular regulation.

Blockade of the angiotensin II receptor inhibits the negative regulatory feedback of angiotensin II on renin secretion, but the resulting increased plasma renin activity and angiotensin II circulating levels do not overcome the effect of valsartan on blood pressure.

12.2 Pharmacodynamics

Valsartan inhibits the pressor effect of angiotensin II infusions. An oral dose of 80 mg inhibits the pressor effect by about 80% at peak with approximately 30% inhibition persisting for 24 hours. No information on the effect of larger doses is available.

Removal of the negative feedback of angiotensin II causes a 2- to 3-fold rise in plasma renin and consequent rise in angiotensin II plasma concentration in hypertensive patients. Minimal decreases in plasma aldosterone were observed after administration of valsartan; very little effect on serum potassium was observed.

In multiple-dose studies in hypertensive patients with stable renal insufficiency and patients with renovascular hypertension, valsartan had no clinically significant effects on glomerular filtration rate, filtration fraction, creatinine clearance, or renal plasma flow.

In multiple-dose studies in hypertensive patients, valsartan had no notable effects on total cholesterol, fasting triglycerides, fasting serum glucose, or uric acid.

12.3 Pharmacokinetics

Valsartan peak plasma concentration is reached 2 to 4 hours after dosing. Valsartan shows bi-exponential decay kinetics following intravenous administration, with an average elimination half-life of about 6 hours. Absolute bioavailability for Diovan is about 25% (range 10%-35%). The bioavailability of the suspension *[see Dosage and Administration; Pediatric Hypertension (2.2)]* is 1.6 times greater than with the tablet. With the tablet, food decreases the exposure (as measured by AUC) to valsartan by about 40% and peak plasma concentration (C_{max}) by about 50%. AUC and C_{max} values of valsartan increase approximately linearly with increasing dose over the clinical dosing range. Valsartan does not accumulate appreciably in plasma following repeated administration.

Metabolism and Elimination: Valsartan, when administered as an oral solution, is primarily recovered in feces (about 83% of dose) and urine (about 13% of dose). The recovery is mainly as unchanged drug, with only about 20% of dose recovered as metabolites. The primary metabolite, accounting for about 9% of dose, is valeryl 4-hydroxy valsartan. *In vitro* metabolism studies involving recombinant CYP 450 enzymes indicated that the CYP 2C9 isoenzyme is responsible for the formation of valeryl-4-hydroxy valsartan. Valsartan does not inhibit CYP 450 isozymes at clinically relevant concentrations. CYP 450 mediated drug interaction between valsartan and coadministered drugs are unlikely because of the low extent of metabolism.

Following intravenous administration, plasma clearance of valsartan is about 2 L/h and its renal clearance is 0.62 L/h (about 30% of total clearance).

Distribution: The steady state volume of distribution of valsartan after intravenous administration is small (17 L), indicating that valsartan does not distribute into tissues extensively. Valsartan is highly bound to serum proteins (95%), mainly serum albumin.

Special Populations:

Pediatric: In a study of pediatric hypertensive patients (n=26, 1-16 years of age) given single doses of a suspension of Diovan (mean: 0.9 to 2 mg/kg), the clearance (L/h/kg) of valsartan for children was similar to that of adults receiving the same formulation.

Geriatric: Exposure (measured by AUC) to valsartan is higher by 70% and the half-life is longer by 35% in the elderly than in the young. No dosage adjustment is necessary *[see Dosage and Administration (2.1)]*.

Gender: Pharmacokinetics of valsartan does not differ significantly between males and females.

Heart Failure: The average time to peak concentration and elimination half-life of valsartan in heart failure patients are similar to those observed in healthy volunteers. AUC and C_{max} values of valsartan increase linearly and are almost proportional with increasing dose over the clinical dosing range (40 to 160 mg twice a day). The average accumulation factor is about 1.7. The apparent clearance of valsartan following oral administration is approximately 4.5 L/h. Age does not affect the apparent clearance in heart failure patients.

Renal Insufficiency: There is no apparent correlation between renal function (measured by creatinine clearance) and exposure (measured by AUC) to valsartan in patients with different degrees of renal impairment. Consequently, dose adjustment is not required in patients with mild-to-moderate renal dysfunction. No studies have been performed in patients with severe impairment of renal function (creatinine clearance <10 mL/min). Valsartan is not removed from the plasma by hemodialysis. In the case of severe renal disease, exercise care with dosing of valsartan *[see Dosage and Administration (2.1)]*.

Hepatic Insufficiency: On average, patients with mild-to-moderate chronic liver disease have twice the exposure (measured by AUC values) to valsartan of healthy volunteers (matched by age, sex and weight). In general, no dosage adjustment is needed in patients with mild-to-moderate liver disease. Care should be exercised in patients with liver disease *[see Dosage and Administration (2.1)]*.

	Placebo (N=2,499)	Valsartan (N=2,511)	Hazard Ratio (95% CI*)	Nominal p-value
All-cause mortality	484 (19.4%)	495 (19.7%)	1.02 (0.90-1.15)	0.8
HF morbidity	801 (32.1%)	723 (28.8%)	0.87 (0.79-0.97)	0.009

* CI = Confidence Interval

	Without ACE Inhibitor		With ACE Inhibitor	
	Placebo (N=181)	Valsartan (N=185)	Placebo (N=2,318)	Valsartan (N=2,326)
Events (%)	77 (42.5%)	46 (24.9%)	724 (31.2%)	677 (29.1%)
Hazard ratio (95% CI)	0.51 (0.35, 0.73)		0.92 (0.82, 1.02)	
p-value	0.0002		0.0965	

13 NONCLINICAL TOXICOLOGY

13.1 Carcinogenesis, Mutagenesis, Impairment of Fertility

There was no evidence of carcinogenicity when valsartan was administered in the diet to mice and rats for up to 2 years at doses up to 160 and 200 mg/kg/day, respectively. These doses in mice and rats are about 2.6 and 6 times, respectively, the maximum recommended human dose on a mg/m^2 basis. (Calculations assume an oral dose of 320 mg/day and a 60-kg patient.)

Mutagenicity assays did not reveal any valsartan-related effects at either the gene or chromosome level. These assays included bacterial mutagenicity tests with *Salmonella* (Ames) and *E coli*; a gene mutation test with Chinese hamster V79 cells; a cytogenetic test with Chinese hamster ovary cells; and a rat micronucleus test.

Valsartan had no adverse effects on the reproductive performance of male or female rats at oral doses up to 200 mg/kg/day. This dose is 6 times the maximum recommended human dose on a mg/m^2 basis. (Calculations assume an oral dose of 320 mg/day and a 60-kg patient.)

13.2 Animal Toxicology and/or Pharmacology

Reproductive Toxicology Studies

No teratogenic effects were observed when valsartan was administered to pregnant mice and rats at oral doses up to 600 mg/kg/day and to pregnant rabbits at oral doses up to 10 mg/kg/day. However, significant decreases in fetal weight, pup birth weight, pup survival rate, and slight delays in developmental milestones were observed in studies in which parental rats were treated with valsartan at oral, maternally toxic (reduction in body weight gain and food consumption) doses of 600 mg/kg/day during organogenesis or late gestation and lactation. In rabbits, fetotoxicity (i.e., resorptions, litter loss, abortions, and low body weight) associated with maternal toxicity (mortality) was observed at doses of 5 and 10 mg/kg/day. The no observed adverse effect doses of 600, 200 and 2 mg/kg/day in mice, rats and rabbits represent 9, 6, and 0.1 times, respectively, the maximum recommended human dose on a mg/m^2 basis. Calculations assume an oral dose of 320 mg/day and a 60-kg patient.

14 CLINICAL STUDIES

14.1 Hypertension

Adult Hypertension

The antihypertensive effects of Diovan (valsartan) were demonstrated principally in 7 placebo-controlled, 4- to 12-week trials (one in patients over 65) of dosages from 10 to 320 mg/day in patients with baseline diastolic blood pressures of 95-115. The studies allowed comparison of once-daily and twice-daily regimens of 160 mg/day; comparison of peak and trough effects; comparison (in pooled data) of response by gender, age, and race; and evaluation of incremental effects of hydrochlorothiazide.

Administration of valsartan to patients with essential hypertension results in a significant reduction of sitting, supine, and standing systolic and diastolic blood pressure, usually with little or no orthostatic change.

In most patients, after administration of a single oral dose, onset of antihypertensive activity occurs at approximately 2 hours, and maximum reduction of blood pressure is achieved within 6 hours. The antihypertensive effect persists for 24 hours after dosing, but there is a decrease from peak effect at lower doses (40 mg) presumably reflecting loss of inhibition of angiotensin II. At higher doses, however (160 mg), there is little difference in peak and trough effect. During repeated dosing, the reduction in blood pressure with any dose is substantially present within 2 weeks, and maximal reduction is generally attained after 4 weeks. In long-term follow-up studies (without placebo control), the effect of valsartan appeared to be maintained for up to 2 years. The antihypertensive effect is independent of age, gender or race. The latter finding regarding race is based on pooled data and should be viewed with caution, because antihypertensive drugs that affect the renin-angiotensin system (that is, ACE inhibitors and angiotensin-II blockers) have generally been found to be less effective in low-renin hypertensives (frequently blacks) than in high-renin hypertensives (frequently whites). In pooled, randomized, controlled trials of Diovan that included a total of 140 blacks and 830 whites, valsartan and an ACE-inhibitor control were generally at least as effective in blacks as whites. The explanation for this difference from previous findings is unclear.

Abrupt withdrawal of valsartan has not been associated with a rapid increase in blood pressure.

The blood pressure lowering effect of valsartan and thiazide-type diuretics are approximately additive.

The 7 studies of valsartan monotherapy included over 2,000 patients randomized to various doses of valsartan and about 800 patients randomized to placebo. Doses below 80 mg were not consistently distinguished from those of placebo at trough, but doses of 80, 160 and 320 mg produced dose-related decreases in systolic and diastolic blood pressure, with the difference from placebo of approximately 6-9/3-5 mmHg at 80-160 mg and 9/6 mmHg at 320 mg. In a controlled trial the addition of HCTZ to valsartan 80 mg resulted in additional lowering of systolic and diastolic blood pressure by approximately 6/3 and 12/5 mmHg for 12.5 and 25 mg of HCTZ, respectively, compared to valsartan 80 mg alone.

Patients with an inadequate response to 80 mg once daily were titrated to either 160 mg once daily or 80 mg twice daily, which resulted in a comparable response in both groups.

In controlled trials, the antihypertensive effect of once-daily valsartan 80 mg was similar to that of once-daily enalapril 20 mg or once-daily lisinopril 10 mg.

There are no trials of Diovan demonstrating reductions in cardiovascular risk in patients with hypertension, but at least one pharmacologically similar drug has demonstrated such benefits.

There was essentially no change in heart rate in valsartan-treated patients in controlled trials.

Pediatric Hypertension

The antihypertensive effects of Diovan were evaluated in two randomized, double-blind clinical studies.

In a clinical study involving 261 hypertensive pediatric patients 6 to 16 years of age, patients who weighed < 35 kg received 10, 40 or 80 mg of valsartan daily (low, medium and high doses), and patients who weighed ≥ 35 kg received 20, 80, and 160 mg of valsartan daily (low, medium and high doses). Renal and urinary disorders, and essential hypertension with or without obesity were the most common underlying causes of hypertension in children enrolled in this study. At the end of 2 weeks, valsartan reduced both systolic and diastolic blood pressure in a dose-dependent manner. Overall, the three dose levels of valsartan (low, medium and high) significantly reduced systolic blood pressure by -8, -10, -12 mm Hg from the baseline, respectively. Patients were re-randomized to either continue receiving the same dose of valsartan or were switched to placebo. In patients who continued to receive the medium and high doses of valsartan, systolic blood pressure at trough was -4 and -7 mm Hg lower than patients who received the placebo treatment. In patients receiving the low dose of valsartan, systolic blood pressure at trough was similar to that of patients who received the placebo treatment. Overall, the dose-dependent antihypertensive effect of valsartan was consistent across all the demographic subgroups.

	Placebo (N=181)	Valsartan (N=185)	Hazard Ratio (95% CI)
Components of HF morbidity			
All-cause mortality	49 (27.1%)	32 (17.3%)	0.59 (0.37, 0.91)
Sudden death with resuscitation	2 (1.1%)	1 (0.5%)	0.47 (0.04, 5.20)
CHF therapy	1 (0.6%)	0 (0.0%)	–
CHF hospitalization	48 (26.5%)	24 (13.0%)	0.43 (0.27, 0.71)
Cardiovascular mortality	40 (22.1%)	29 (15.7%)	0.65 (0.40, 1.05)
Non-fatal morbidity	49 (27.1%)	24 (13.0%)	0.42 (0.26, 0.69)

	Valsartan vs. Captopril (N=4,909) (N=4,909)			Valsartan + Captopril vs. Captopril (N=4,885) (N=4,909)		
	No. of Deaths Valsartan/Captopril	Hazard Ratio CI	p-value	No. of Deaths Comb/Captopril	Hazard Ratio CI	p-value
All-cause mortality	979 (19.9%)/ 958 (19.5%)	1.001 (0.902, 1.111)	0.98	941 (19.3%)/ 958 (19.5%)	0.984 (0.886, 1.093)	0.73
CV mortality	827 (16.8%)/ 830 (16.9%)	0.976 (0.875, 1.090)				
CV mortality, hospitalization for HF, and recurrent non-fatal MI	1,529 (31.1%)/ 1,567 (31.9%)	0.955 (0.881, 1.035)				

Tablet	Color	Deboss		NDC 0078-####-##					
		Side 1	Side 2	Bottle of					Blister
				30	90	3500	7000	14000	Packages of 100
40 mg	Yellow	NVR	DO	0423-15	–	–	–	–	0423-06
80 mg	Pale red	NVR	DV	–	0358-34	–	–	0358-33	0358-06
160 mg	Grey-orange	NVR	DX	–	0359-34	–	0359-17	–	0359-06
320 mg	Dark grey-violet	NVR	DXL	–	0360-34	0360-11	–	–	0360-06

In a clinical study involving 90 hypertensive pediatric patients 1 to 5 years of age with a similar study design, there was some evidence of effectiveness, but safety findings for which a relationship to treatment could not be excluded mitigate against recommending use in this age group. *[see Adverse Reactions (6.1)].*

14.2 Heart Failure

The Valsartan Heart Failure Trial (Val-HeFT) was a multinational, double-blind study in which 5,010 patients with NYHA class II (62%) to IV (2%) heart failure and LVEF <40%, on baseline therapy chosen by their physicians, were randomized to placebo or valsartan (titrated from 40 mg twice daily to the highest tolerated dose or 160 mg twice daily) and followed for a mean of about 2 years. Although Val-HeFT's primary goal was to examine the effect of valsartan when added to an ACE inhibitor, about 7% were not receiving an ACE inhibitor. Other background therapy included diuretics (86%), digoxin (67%), and beta-blockers (36%). The population studied was 80% male, 46% 65 years or older and 89% Caucasian. At the end of the trial, patients in the valsartan group had a blood pressure that was 4 mmHg systolic and 2 mmHg diastolic lower than the placebo group. There were two primary end points, both assessed as time to first event: all-cause mortality and heart failure morbidity, the latter defined as all-cause mortality, sudden death with resuscitation, hospitalization for heart failure, and the need for intravenous inotropic or vasodilatory drugs for at least 4 hours. These results are summarized in the table below.

[See first table at top of previous page]

Although the overall morbidity result favored valsartan, this result was largely driven by the 7% of patients not receiving an ACE inhibitor, as shown in the following table.

[See second table at top of previous page]

The modest favorable trend in the group receiving an ACE inhibitor was largely driven by the patients receiving less than the recommended dose of ACE inhibitor. Thus, there is little evidence of further clinical benefit when valsartan is added to an adequate dose of ACE inhibitor.

Secondary end points in the subgroup not receiving ACE inhibitors were as follows.

[See first table above]

In patients not receiving an ACE inhibitor, valsartan-treated patients had an increase in ejection fraction and reduction in left ventricular internal diastolic diameter (LVIDD).

Effects were generally consistent across subgroups defined by age and gender for the population of patients not receiving an ACE inhibitor. The number of black patients was small and does not permit a meaningful assessment in this subset of patients.

14.3 Post-Myocardial Infarction

The VALsartan In Acute myocardial iNfarcTion trial (VALIANT) was a randomized, controlled, multinational, double-blind study in 14,703 patients with acute myocardial infarction and either heart failure (signs, symptoms or radiological evidence) or left ventricular systolic dysfunction (ejection fraction ≤40% by radionuclide ventriculography or ≤35% by echocardiography or ventricular contrast angiography). Patients were randomized within 12 hours to 10 days after the onset of myocardial infarction symptoms to one of three treatment groups: valsartan (titrated from 20 or 40 mg twice daily to the highest tolerated dose up to a maximum of 160 mg twice daily), the ACE inhibitor, captopril (titrated from 6.25 mg three times daily to the highest tolerated dose up to a maximum of 50 mg three times daily), or the combination of valsartan plus captopril. In the combination group, the dose of valsartan was titrated from 20 mg twice daily to the highest tolerated dose up to a maximum of 80 mg twice daily; the dose of captopril was the same as for monotherapy. The population studied was 69% male, 94% Caucasian, and 53% were 65 years of age or older. Baseline therapy included aspirin (91%), beta-blockers (70%), ACE inhibitors (40%), thrombolytics (35%) and statins (34%). The mean treatment duration was 2 years. The mean daily dose of Diovan in the monotherapy group was 217 mg.

The primary endpoint was time to all-cause mortality. Secondary endpoints included (1) time to cardiovascular (CV) mortality, and (2) time to the first event of cardiovascular mortality, reinfarction, or hospitalization for heart failure. The results are summarized in the table below:

[See second table above]

There was no difference in overall mortality among the three treatment groups. There was thus no evidence that combining the ACE inhibitor captopril and the angiotensin II blocker valsartan was of value.

The data were assessed to see whether the effectiveness of valsartan could be demonstrated by showing in a non-inferiority analysis that it preserved a fraction of the effect of captopril, a drug with a demonstrated survival effect in this setting. A conservative estimate of the effect of captopril (based on a pooled analysis of 3 post-infarction studies of captopril and 2 other ACE inhibitors) was a 14-16% reduction in mortality compared to placebo. Valsartan would be considered effective if it preserved a meaningful fraction of that effect and unequivocally preserved some of that effect. As shown in the table, the upper bound of the CI for the hazard ratio (valsartan/captopril) for overall or CV mortality is 1.09-1.11, a difference of about 9-11%, thus making it unlikely that valsartan has less than about half of the estimated effect of captopril and clearly demonstrating an effect of valsartan. The other secondary endpoints were consistent with this conclusion.

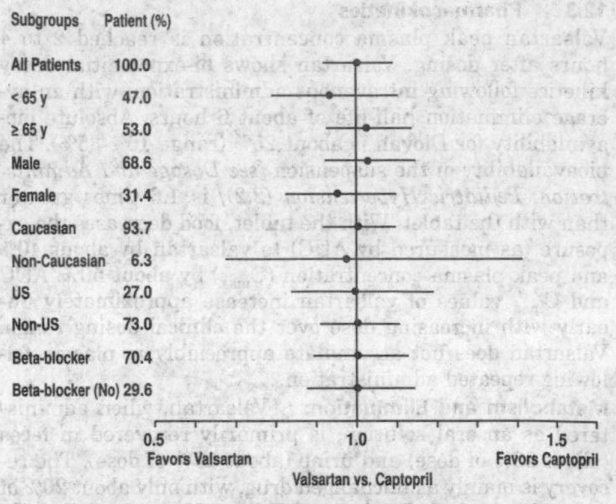

Effects on Mortality Amongst Subgroups in VALIANT

There were no clear differences in all-cause mortality based on age, gender, race, or baseline therapies, as shown in the figure above.

16 HOW SUPPLIED/STORAGE AND HANDLING

Diovan (valsartan) is available as tablets containing valsartan 40 mg, 80 mg, 160 mg, or 320 mg. All strengths are packaged in bottles and unit dose blister packages (10 strips of 10 tablets) as described below.

40 mg tablets are scored on one side and ovaloid with bevelled edges. 80 mg, 160 mg, and 320 mg tablets are unscored and almond-shaped with bevelled edges.

[See third table above]

Store at 25°C (77°F); excursions permitted to 15-30°C (59 - 86°F) [see USP Controlled Room Temperature].

Protect from moisture.

Dispense in tight container (USP).

17 PATIENT COUNSELING INFORMATION

Information for Patients

Pregnancy: Female patients of childbearing age should be told about the consequences of exposure to Diovan during pregnancy. Discuss treatment options with women planning to become pregnant. Patients should be asked to report pregnancies to their physicians as soon as possible.

T2012-184
October 2012

DIOVAN (DYE'-o-van)
(valsartan) Tablets

Read the Patient Information that comes with DIOVAN before you take it and each time you get a refill. There may be new information. This leaflet does not take the place of talking with your doctor about your medical condition or treatment. If you have any questions about DIOVAN, ask your doctor or pharmacist.

What is the most important information I should know about DIOVAN?

DIOVAN can cause harm or death to an unborn baby. Talk to your doctor about other ways to lower your blood pressure if you plan to become pregnant. If you get pregnant while taking DIOVAN, tell your doctor right away.

What is DIOVAN?

DIOVAN is a prescription medicine called an angiotensin receptor blocker (ARB). It is used in adults to:

- lower high blood pressure (hypertension) in adults and children, 6 to 16 years of age.
- treat heart failure in adults. In these patients, DIOVAN may lower the need for hospitalization that happens from heart failure.
- improve the chance of living longer after a heart attack (myocardial infarction) in adults.

DIOVAN is not for children under 6 years of age or children with certain kidney problems.

High Blood Pressure (Hypertension). Blood pressure is the force in your blood vessels when your heart beats and when your heart rests. You have high blood pressure when the force is too much. DIOVAN can help your blood vessels relax so your blood pressure is lower. Medicines that lower your blood pressure lower your chance of having a stroke or heart attack.

High blood pressure makes the heart work harder to pump blood throughout the body and causes damage to the blood vessels. If high blood pressure is not treated, it can lead to stroke, heart attack, heart failure, kidney failure and vision problems.

Heart Failure occurs when the heart is weak and cannot pump enough blood to your lungs and the rest of your body. Just walking or moving can make you short of breath, so you may have to rest a lot.

Heart Attack (Myocardial Infarction): A heart attack is caused by a blocked artery that results in damage to the heart muscle.

What should I tell my doctor before taking DIOVAN?

Tell your doctor about all your medical conditions including whether you:

- have any allergies. See the end of this leaflet for a complete list of ingredients in DIOVAN.
- have a heart condition
- have liver problems
- have kidney problems
- **are pregnant or planning to become pregnant.** See "What is the most important information I should know about DIOVAN?"
- are breast-feeding. It is not known if DIOVAN passes into your breast milk. You and your doctor should decide if you will take DIOVAN or breast-feed, but not both. Talk with your doctor about the best way to feed your baby if you take DIOVAN.
- have ever had a reaction called angioedema, to another blood pressure medicine. Angioedema causes swelling of the face, lips, tongue and/or throat, and may cause difficulty breathing.

Tell your doctor about all the medicines you take including prescription and nonprescription medicines, vitamins and herbal supplements. Especially tell your doctor if you take:

- other medicines for high blood pressure or a heart problem
- water pills (also called "diuretics")
- potassium supplements. Your doctor may check the amount of potassium in your blood periodically
- a salt substitute. Your doctor may check the amount of potassium in your blood periodically
- Nonsteroidal anti-inflammatory drugs (like ibuprofen or naproxen)
- certain antibiotics (rifamycin group), a drug used to protect against transplant rejection (cyclosporin) or an antiretroviral drug used to treat HIV/AIDS infection (ritonavir). These drugs may increase the effect of valsartan.

Know the medicines you take. Keep a list of your medicines with you to show to your doctor and pharmacist when a new medicine is prescribed. Talk to your doctor or pharmacist before you start taking any new medicine. Your doctor or pharmacist will know what medicines are safe to take together.

How should I take DIOVAN?

- Take DIOVAN exactly as prescribed by your doctor.
- For treatment of high blood pressure, take DIOVAN one time each day, at the same time each day.
- If your child cannot swallow tablets, or if tablets are not available in the prescribed strength, your pharmacist will mix DIOVAN as a liquid suspension for your child. If your child switches between taking the tablet and the suspension, your doctor will adjust the dose as needed. Shake the bottle of suspension well for at least 10 seconds before pouring the dose of medicine to give to your child.
- For adult patients with heart failure or who have had a heart attack, take DIOVAN two times each day, at the same time each day. Your doctor may start you on a low dose of DIOVAN and may increase the dose during your treatment.
- DIOVAN can be taken with or without food.
- If you miss a dose, take it as soon as you remember. If it is close to your next dose, do not take the missed dose. Take the next dose at your regular time.
- If you take too much DIOVAN, call your doctor or Poison Control Center, or go to the nearest hospital emergency room.

What are the possible side effects of DIOVAN?

DIOVAN may cause the following serious side effects:

Injury or death to an unborn baby. See "What is the most important information I should know about DIOVAN?"

Low Blood Pressure (Hypotension). Low blood pressure is most likely to happen if you also take water pills, are on a low-salt diet, get dialysis treatments, have heart problems, or get sick with vomiting or diarrhea. Lie down, if you feel faint or dizzy. Call your doctor right away.

Kidney problems. Kidney problems may get worse if you already have kidney disease. Some patients will have changes on blood tests for kidney function and may need a lower dose of DIOVAN. Call your doctor if you get swelling in your feet, ankles, or hands, or unexplained weight gain. If you have heart failure, your doctor should check your kidney function before prescribing DIOVAN.

The most common side effects of DIOVAN used to treat people with high blood pressure include:

- headache
- dizziness
- flu symptoms
- tiredness
- stomach (abdominal) pain

Side effects were generally mild and brief. They generally have not caused patients to stop taking DIOVAN.

The most common side effects of DIOVAN used to treat people with heart failure include:

- dizziness
- low blood pressure
- diarrhea
- joint and back pain
- tiredness
- high blood potassium

Common side effects of DIOVAN used to treat people after a heart attack which caused them to stop taking the drug include:

- low blood pressure
- cough
- high blood creatinine (decreased kidney function)
- rash

Tell your doctor if you get any side effect that bothers you or that does not go away.

These are not all the possible side effects of DIOVAN. For a complete list, ask your doctor or pharmacist.

How do I store DIOVAN?

- Store DIOVAN tablets at room temperature between 59° to 86°F (15°C - 30°C).
- Keep DIOVAN tablets in a closed container in a dry place.
- Store bottles of DIOVAN suspension at room temperature less than 86°F (30°C) for up to 30 days, or refrigerate between 35°F - 46°F (2°C - 8°C) for up to 75 days.
- Keep DIOVAN and all medicines out of the reach of children.

General information about DIOVAN

Medicines are sometimes prescribed for conditions that are not mentioned in patient information leaflets. Do not use DIOVAN for a condition for which it was not prescribed. Do not give DIOVAN to other people, even if they have the same symptoms you have. It may harm them.

This leaflet summarizes the most important information about DIOVAN. If you would like more information, talk with your doctor. You can ask your doctor or pharmacist for information about DIOVAN that is written for health professionals.

For more information about DIOVAN, ask your pharmacist or doctor, visit www.DIOVAN.com on the Internet, or call **1-866-404-6361.**

What are the ingredients in DIOVAN?

Active ingredient: valsartan

Inactive ingredients: colloidal silicon dioxide, crospovidone, hydroxypropyl methylcellulose, iron oxides (yellow, black and/or red), magnesium stearate, microcrystalline cellulose, polyethylene glycol 8000, and titanium dioxide

Distributed by:
Novartis Pharmaceuticals Corp.
East Hanover, NJ 07936

T2012-137
July 2012

Shown in Product Identification Guide, page 309

DIOVAN HCT® ℞

[DYE'-o-van HCT]
(valsartan and hydrochlorothiazide USP)
Tablets

The following prescribing information is based on official labeling in effect July 2013.

HIGHLIGHTS OF PRESCRIBING INFORMATION

These highlights do not include all the information needed to use Diovan HCT safely and effectively. See full prescribing information for Diovan HCT.

Diovan HCT® (valsartan and hydrochlorothiazide USP)
Tablets
Initial U.S. Approval: 1998

WARNING: FETAL TOXICITY

See full prescribing information for complete boxed warning.

- **When pregnancy is detected, discontinue Diovan HCT as soon as possible. (5.1)**
- **Drugs that act directly on the renin-angiotensin system can cause injury and death to the developing fetus. (5.1)**

RECENT MAJOR CHANGES

Boxed Warning: Fetal Toxicity	01/2012
Indications and Usage: Benefits of lowering blood pressure (1)	12/2011
Contraindications: Dual RAS Blockade in Diabetics (4)	10/2012
Warnings and Precautions: Fetal Toxicity (5.1)	01/2012
Warnings and Precautions: Potassium Abnormalities (5.7)	07/2012
Drug Interactions: Dual Blockade of the Renin-Angiotensin System (7)	10/2012

INDICATIONS AND USAGE

Diovan HCT is the combination tablet of valsartan (Diovan), an angiotensin II receptor blocker (ARB) and hydrochlorothiazide (HCTZ), a diuretic. Diovan HCT is indicated for the treatment of hypertension, to lower blood pressure:

- In patients not adequately controlled with monotherapy (1)
- As initial therapy in patients likely to need multiple drugs to achieve their blood pressure goals (1)

Lowering blood pressure reduces the risk of fatal and nonfatal cardiovascular events, primarily strokes and myocardial infarctions.

DOSAGE AND ADMINISTRATION

- Dose once daily. Titrate as needed to a maximum dose of 320/25mg (2)
- May be used as add-on/switch therapy for patients not adequately controlled on any of the components (valsartan or HCTZ) (2)
- May be substituted for titrated components (2.3)

DOSAGE FORMS AND STRENGTHS

Tablets (valsartan/HCTZ mg): 80/12.5, 160/12.5, 160/25, 320/12.5, 320/25 (3)

CONTRAINDICATIONS

Anuria; Hypersensitivity to any sulfonamide-derived drugs or any component; Do not coadminister aliskiren with Diovan HCT in patients with diabetes (4)

WARNINGS AND PRECAUTIONS

- Hypotension: Correct volume depletion prior to initiation (5.2)
- Observe for signs of fluid or electrolyte imbalance (5.9)
- Monitor renal function and potassium in susceptible patients (5.3, 5.7)
- Exacerbation or activation of systemic lupus erythematosus (5.5)
- Acute angle-closure glaucoma (5.8)

ADVERSE REACTIONS

The most common reasons for discontinuation of therapy with Diovan HCT were headache and dizziness. The only adverse experience that occurred in ≥2% of patients treated with Diovan HCT and at a higher incidence than placebo was nasopharyngitis (2.4% vs. 1.9%). (6.1)

To report SUSPECTED ADVERSE REACTIONS, contact Novartis Pharmaceuticals Corporation at 1-888-669-6682 or FDA at 1-800-FDA-1088 or www.fda.gov/medwatch.

DRUG INTERACTIONS

- Antidiabetic drugs: Dosage adjustment of antidiabetic may be required (7)
- Cholestyramine and colestipol: Reduced absorption of thiazides (12.3)
- Lithium: Diuretics increase risk of lithium toxicity. Monitor serum lithium concentrations during concurrent use. (7)
- Non-Steroidal Anti-Inflammatory Drugs (NSAIDs): May increase risk of renal impairment. Can reduce diuretic, natriuretic and antihypertensive effects of diuretics. (7)
- Dual inhibition of the renin-angiotensin system: Increased risk of renal impairment, hypotension, and hyperkalemia (7)

USE IN SPECIFIC POPULATIONS

Nursing Mothers: Nursing or drug should be discontinued (8.3)

See 17 for PATIENT COUNSELING INFORMATION and FDA-approved patient labeling

Revised: 10/2012

FULL PRESCRIBING INFORMATION: CONTENTS*

*** Sections or subsections omitted from the full prescribing information are not listed**

FULL PRESCRIBING INFORMATION

> **WARNING: FETAL TOXICITY**
> - **When pregnancy is detected, discontinue Diovan HCT as soon as possible. (5.1)**
> - **Drugs that act directly on the renin-angiotensin system can cause injury and death to the developing fetus. (5.1)**

1 INDICATIONS AND USAGE

Diovan HCT (valsartan and hydrochlorothiazide, USP) is indicated for the treatment of hypertension, to lower blood pressure. Lowering blood pressure reduces the risk of fatal and nonfatal cardiovascular events, primarily strokes and myocardial infarctions. These benefits have been seen in controlled trials of antihypertensive drugs from a wide variety of pharmacologic classes, including hydrochlorothiazide and the ARB class to which valsartan principally belongs. There are no controlled trials demonstrating risk reduction with Diovan HCT.

Control of high blood pressure should be part of comprehensive cardiovascular risk management, including, as appropriate, lipid control, diabetes management, antithrombotic therapy, smoking cessation, exercise, and limited sodium intake. Many patients will require more than 1 drug to achieve blood pressure goals. For specific advice on goals and management, see published guidelines, such as those of the National High Blood Pressure Education Program's Joint National Committee on Prevention, Detection, Evaluation, and Treatment of High Blood Pressure (JNC).

Numerous antihypertensive drugs, from a variety of pharmacologic classes and with different mechanisms of action, have been shown in randomized controlled trials to reduce cardiovascular morbidity and mortality, and it can be concluded that it is blood pressure reduction, and not some other pharmacologic property of the drugs, that is largely responsible for those benefits. The largest and most consistent cardiovascular outcome benefit has been a reduction in the risk of stroke, but reductions in myocardial infarction and cardiovascular mortality have also been seen regularly.

Elevated systolic or diastolic pressure causes increased cardiovascular risk, and the absolute risk increase per mmHg is greater at higher blood pressures, so that even modest reductions of severe hypertension can provide substantial benefit. Relative risk reduction from blood pressure reduction is similar across populations with varying absolute risk, so the absolute benefit is greater in patients who are at higher risk independent of their hypertension (for example, patients with diabetes or hyperlipidemia), and such patients would be expected to benefit from more aggressive treatment to a lower blood pressure goal.

Some antihypertensive drugs have smaller blood pressure effects (as monotherapy) in black patients, and many antihypertensive drugs have additional approved indications and effects (e.g., on angina, heart failure, or diabetic kidney disease). These considerations may guide selection of therapy.

Add-On Therapy

Diovan HCT may be used in patients whose blood pressure is not adequately controlled on monotherapy.

Replacement Therapy

Diovan HCT may be substituted for the titrated components.

Initial Therapy

Diovan HCT may be used as initial therapy in patients who are likely to need multiple drugs to achieve blood pressure goals.

The choice of Diovan HCT as initial therapy for hypertension should be based on an assessment of potential benefits and risks.

Patients with stage 2 hypertension are at a relatively high risk for cardiovascular events (such as strokes, heart attacks, and heart failure), kidney failure, and vision problems, so prompt treatment is clinically relevant. The decision to use a combination as initial therapy should be individualized and should be shaped by considerations such as baseline blood pressure, the target goal, and the incremental likelihood of achieving goal with a combination compared to monotherapy. Individual blood pressure goals may vary based upon the patient's risk.

Data from the high dose multifactorial trial [*see Clinical Studies (14.1)*] provides estimates of the probability of reaching a target blood pressure with Diovan HCT compared to valsartan or hydrochlorothiazide monotherapy. The figures below provide estimates of the likelihood of achieving systolic or diastolic blood pressure control with Diovan HCT 320/25 mg, based upon baseline systolic or diastolic blood pressure. The curve of each treatment group was estimated by logistic regression modeling. The estimated likelihood at the right tail of each curve is less reliable due to small numbers of subjects with high baseline blood pressures.

[See figures 1 through 4 above]

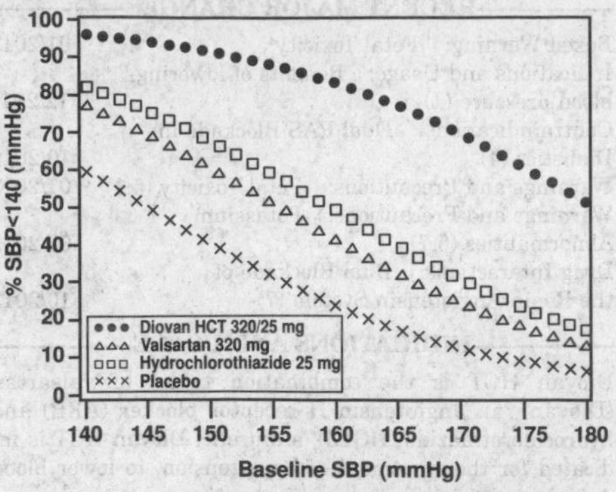

Figure 1: Probability of Achieving Systolic Blood Pressure <140 mmHg at Week 8

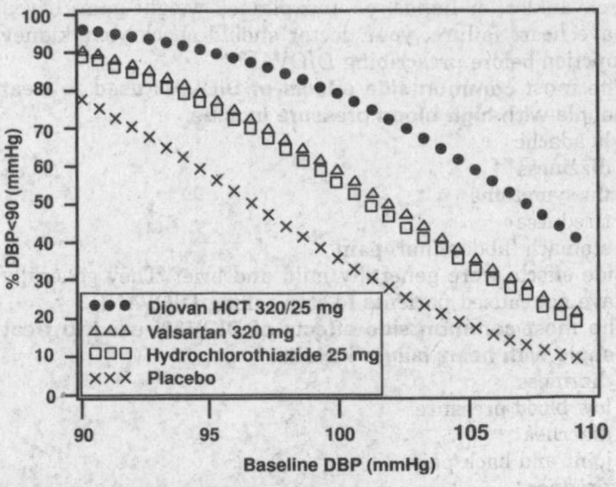

Figure 2: Probability of Achieving Diastolic Blood Pressure <90 mmHg at Week 8

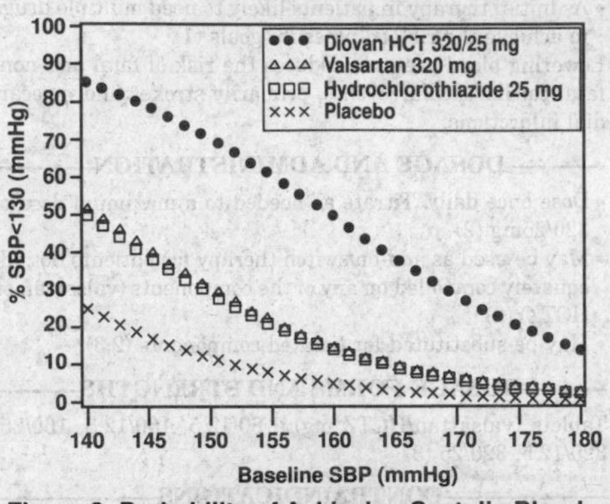

Figure 3: Probability of Achieving Systolic Blood Pressure <130 mmHg at Week 8

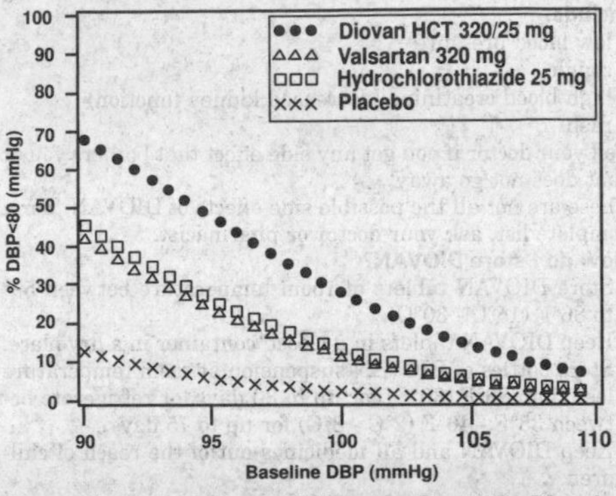

Figure 4: Probability of Achieving Diastolic Blood Pressure <80 mmHg at Week 8

For example, a patient with a baseline blood pressure of 160/100 mmHg has about a 41% likelihood of achieving a goal of <140 mmHg (systolic) and 60% likelihood of achieving <90 mmHg (diastolic) on valsartan alone and the likelihood of achieving these goals on HCTZ alone is about 50% (systolic) or 57% (diastolic). The likelihood of achieving these goals on Diovan HCT rises to about 84% (systolic) or 80% (diastolic). The likelihood of achieving these goals on placebo is about 23% (systolic) or 36% (diastolic).

2 DOSAGE AND ADMINISTRATION

2.1 General Considerations

The usual starting dose is Diovan HCT 160/12.5 mg once daily. The dosage can be increased after 1 to 2 weeks of therapy to a maximum of one 320/25 tablet once daily as needed to control blood pressure [*see Clinical Studies (14.2)*]. Maximum antihypertensive effects are attained within 2 to 4 weeks after a change in dose.

2.2 Add-On Therapy

A patient whose blood pressure is not adequately controlled with valsartan (or another ARB) alone or hydrochlorothiazide alone may be switched to combination therapy with Diovan HCT.

A patient who experiences dose-limiting adverse reactions on either component alone may be switched to Diovan HCT containing a lower dose of that component in combination with the other to achieve similar blood pressure reductions. The clinical response to Diovan HCT should be subsequently evaluated and if blood pressure remains uncontrolled after 3 to 4 weeks of therapy, the dose may be titrated up to a maximum of 320/25 mg.

2.3 Replacement Therapy

Diovan HCT may be substituted for the titrated components.

2.4 Initial Therapy

Diovan HCT is not recommended as initial therapy in patients with intravascular volume depletion [*see Warnings and Precautions (5.2)*].

2.5 Use with Other Antihypertensive Drugs

Diovan HCT may be administered with other antihypertensive agents.

3 DOSAGE FORMS AND STRENGTHS

80/12.5 mg tablets, imprinted CG/HGH (Side 1/Side 2)
160/12.5 mg tablets, imprinted CG/HHH
160/25 mg tablets, imprinted NVR/HXH
320/12.5 mg tablets, imprinted NVR/HIL
320/25 mg tablets, imprinted NVR/CTI

4 CONTRAINDICATIONS

Diovan HCT (valsartan and hydrochlorothiazide, USP) is contraindicated in patients who are hypersensitive to any component of this product.

Because of the hydrochlorothiazide component, this product is contraindicated in patients with anuria or hypersensitivity to other sulfonamide-derived drugs.
Do not coadminister aliskiren with Diovan HCT in patients with diabetes [*see Drug Interactions (7)*].

5 WARNINGS AND PRECAUTIONS

5.1 Fetal Toxicity

Pregnancy Category D

Use of drugs that act on the renin-angiotensin system during the second and third trimesters of pregnancy reduces fetal renal function and increases fetal and neonatal morbidity and death. Resulting oligohydramnios can be associated with fetal lung hypoplasia and skeletal deformations. Potential neonatal adverse effects include skull hypoplasia, anuria, hypotension, renal failure, and death. When pregnancy is detected, discontinue Diovan HCT as soon as possible [*see Use in Specific Populations (8.1)*].
Intrauterine exposure to thiazide diuretics is associated with fetal or neonatal jaundice, thrombocytopenia, and possibly other adverse reactions that have occurred in adults.

5.2 Hypotension in Volume- and/or Salt-Depleted Patients

Excessive reduction of blood pressure was rarely seen (0.7%) in patients with uncomplicated hypertension treated with Diovan HCT in controlled trials. In patients with an activated renin-angiotensin system, such as volume- and/or salt-depleted patients receiving high doses of diuretics, symptomatic hypotension may occur. This condition should be corrected prior to administration of Diovan HCT, or the treatment should start under close medical supervision.
If hypotension occurs, the patient should be placed in the supine position and, if necessary, given an intravenous infusion of normal saline. A transient hypotensive response is not a contraindication to further treatment, which usually can be continued without difficulty once the blood pressure has stabilized.

5.3 Impaired Renal Function

Changes in renal function including acute renal failure can be caused by drugs that inhibit the renin-angiotensin system and by diuretics. Patients whose renal function may depend in part on the activity of the renin-angiotensin system (e.g., patients with renal artery stenosis, chronic kidney disease, severe congestive heart failure, or volume depletion) may be at particular risk of developing acute renal failure on Diovan HCT. Monitor renal function periodically in these patients. Consider withholding or discontinuing therapy in patients who develop a clinically significant decrease in renal function on Diovan HCT [*see Drug Interactions (7)*].

5.4 Hypersensitivity Reaction

Hydrochlorothiazide: Hypersensitivity reactions to hydrochlorothiazide may occur in patients with or without a history of allergy or bronchial asthma, but are more likely in patients with such a history.

5.5 Systemic Lupus Erythematosus

Hydrochlorothiazide: Thiazide diuretics have been reported to cause exacerbation or activation of systemic lupus erythematosus.

5.6 Lithium Interaction

Hydrochlorothiazide: Lithium generally should not be given with thiazides [*see Drug Interactions (7)*].

5.7 Potassium Abnormalities

Valsartan – Hydrochlorothiazide: In the controlled trials of various doses of Diovan HCT the incidence of hypertensive patients who developed hypokalemia (serum potassium <3.5 mEq/L) was 3.0%; the incidence of hyperkalemia (serum potassium >5.7 mEq/L) was 0.4%.
Hydrochlorothiazide can cause hypokalemia and hyponatremia. Hypomagnesemia can result in hypokalemia which appears difficult to treat despite potassium repletion. Drugs that inhibit the renin-angiotensin system can cause hyperkalemia. Monitor serum electrolytes periodically.
If hypokalemia is accompanied by clinical signs (e.g. muscular weakness, paresis, or ECG alterations), Diovan HCT should be discontinued. Correction of hypokalemia and any coexisting hypomagnesemia is recommended prior to the initiation of thiazides.
Some patients with heart failure have developed increases in potassium with Diovan therapy. These effects are usually minor and transient, and they are more likely to occur in patients with pre-existing renal impairment. Dosage reduction and/or discontinuation of the diuretic and/or Diovan may be required [*see Adverse Reactions (6.1)*].

5.8 Acute Myopia and Secondary Angle-Closure Glaucoma

Hydrochlorothiazide, a sulfonamide, can cause an idiosyncratic reaction, resulting in acute transient myopia and acute angle-closure glaucoma. Symptoms include acute onset of decreased visual acuity or ocular pain and typically occur within hours to weeks of drug initiation. Untreated acute angle-closure glaucoma can lead to permanent vision loss. The primary treatment is to discontinue hydrochlorothiazide as rapidly as possible. Prompt medical or surgical treatments may need to be considered if the intraocular pressure remains uncontrolled. Risk factors for developing acute angle-closure glaucoma may include a history of sulfonamide or penicillin allergy.

5.9 Metabolic Disturbances

Hydrochlorothiazide

Hydrochlorothiazide may alter glucose tolerance and raise serum levels of cholesterol and triglycerides.
Hydrochlorothiazide may raise the serum uric acid level due to reduced clearance of uric acid and may cause or exacerbate hyperuricemia and precipitate gout in susceptible patients.
Hydrochlorothiazide decreases urinary calcium excretion and may cause elevations of serum calcium. Monitor calcium levels in patients with hypercalcemia receiving Diovan HCT.

6 ADVERSE REACTIONS

6.1 Clinical Trials Experience

Because clinical studies are conducted under widely varying conditions, adverse reactions rates observed in the clinical studies of a drug cannot be directly compared to rates in the clinical studies of another drug and may not reflect the rates observed in practice. The adverse reaction information from clinical trials does, however, provide a basis for identifying the adverse events that appear to be related to drug use and for approximating rates.

Hypertension

Diovan HCT (valsartan and hydrochlorothiazide, USP) has been evaluated for safety in more than 5700 patients, including over 990 treated for over 6 months, and over 370 for over 1 year. Adverse experiences have generally been mild and transient in nature and have only infrequently required discontinuation of therapy. The overall incidence of adverse reactions with Diovan HCT was comparable to placebo.
The overall frequency of adverse reactions was neither dose-related nor related to gender, age, or race. In controlled clinical trials, discontinuation of therapy due to side effects was required in 2.3% of valsartan-hydrochlorothiazide patients and 3.1% of placebo patients. The most common reasons for discontinuation of therapy with Diovan HCT were headache and dizziness.
The only adverse reaction that occurred in controlled clinical trials in at least 2% of patients treated with Diovan HCT and at a higher incidence in valsartan-hydrochlorothiazide (n=4372) than placebo (n=262) patients was nasopharyngitis (2.4% vs. 1.9%).
Dose-related orthostatic effects were seen in fewer than 1% of patients. In individual trials, a dose-related increase in the incidence of dizziness was observed in patients treated with Diovan HCT.
Other adverse reactions that have been reported with valsartan-hydrochlorothiazide (>0.2% of valsartan-hydrochlorothiazide patients in controlled clinical trials) without regard to causality, are listed below:
Cardiovascular: Palpitations and tachycardia
Ear and Labyrinth: Tinnitus and vertigo
Gastrointestinal: Dyspepsia, diarrhea, flatulence, dry mouth, nausea, abdominal pain, abdominal pain upper, and vomiting
General and Administration Site Conditions: Asthenia, chest pain, fatigue, peripheral edema and pyrexia
Infections and Infestations: Bronchitis, bronchitis acute, influenza, gastroenteritis, sinusitis, upper respiratory tract infection, and urinary tract infection
Investigations: Blood urea increased
Musculoskeletal: Arthralgia, back pain, muscle cramps, myalgia, and pain in extremity
Nervous System: Dizziness postural, paresthesia, and somnolence
Psychiatric: Anxiety and insomnia
Renal and Urinary: Pollakiuria
Reproductive System: Erectile dysfunction
Respiratory, Thoracic and Mediastinal: Dyspnea, cough, nasal congestion, pharyngolaryngeal pain, and sinus congestion
Skin and Subcutaneous Tissue: Hyperhidrosis and rash
Vascular: Hypotension
Other reported reactions seen less frequently in clinical trials included abnormal vision, anaphylaxis, bronchospasm, constipation, depression, dehydration, decreased libido, dysuria, epistaxis, flushing, gout, increased appetite, muscle weakness, pharyngitis, pruritus, sunburn, syncope, and viral infection.

Initial Therapy - Hypertension

In a clinical study in patients with severe hypertension (diastolic blood pressure ≥110 mmHg and systolic blood pressure ≥140 mmHg), the overall pattern of adverse reactions reported through 6 weeks of follow-up was similar in patients treated with Diovan HCT as initial therapy and in patients treated with valsartan as initial therapy. Comparing the groups treated with Diovan HCT (force-titrated to 320/25 mg) and valsartan (force-titrated to 320 mg), dizziness was observed in 6% and 2% of patients, respectively. Hypotension was observed in 1% of those patients receiving Diovan HCT and 0% of patients receiving valsartan. There were no reported cases of syncope in either treatment group. Laboratory changes with Diovan HCT as initial therapy in patients with severe hypertension were similar to those reported with Diovan HCT in patients with less severe hypertension [*see Clinical Studies (14.2) and Drug Interactions (7)*].
Valsartan: In trials in which valsartan was compared to an ACE inhibitor with or without placebo, the incidence of dry cough was significantly greater in the ACE inhibitor group (7.9%) than in the groups who received valsartan (2.6%) or placebo (1.5%). In a 129-patient trial limited to patients who had had dry cough when they had previously received ACE inhibitors, the incidences of cough in patients who received valsartan, hydrochlorothiazide, or lisinopril were 20%, 19%, 69% respectively (p <0.001).
Other reported reactions seen less frequently in clinical trials included chest pain, syncope, anorexia, vomiting, and angioedema.
Hydrochlorothiazide: Other adverse reactions not listed above that have been reported with hydrochlorothiazide, without regard to causality, are listed below:
Body As A Whole: weakness
Digestive: pancreatitis, jaundice (intrahepatic cholestatic jaundice), sialadenitis, cramping, gastric irritation
Hematologic: aplastic anemia, agranulocytosis, leukopenia, hemolytic anemia, thrombocytopenia
Hypersensitivity: purpura, photosensitivity, urticaria, necrotizing angiitis (vasculitis and cutaneous vasculitis), fever, respiratory distress including pneumonitis and pulmonary edema, anaphylactic reactions
Metabolic: hyperglycemia, glycosuria, hyperuricemia
Musculoskeletal: muscle spasm
Nervous System/Psychiatric: restlessness
Renal: renal failure, renal dysfunction, interstitial nephritis
Skin: erythema multiforme including Stevens-Johnson syndrome, exfoliative dermatitis including toxic epidermal necrolysis
Special Senses: transient blurred vision, xanthopsia

Clinical Laboratory Test Findings

In controlled clinical trials, clinically important changes in standard laboratory parameters were rarely associated with administration of Diovan HCT.
Creatinine/Blood Urea Nitrogen (BUN): Minor elevations in creatinine and BUN occurred in 2% and 15% respectively, of patients taking Diovan HCT and 0.4% and 6% respectively, given placebo in controlled clinical trials
Hemoglobin and Hematocrit: Greater than 20% decreases in hemoglobin and hematocrit were observed in less than 0.1% of Diovan HCT patients, compared with 0% in placebo-treated patients
Liver Function Tests: Occasional elevations (greater than 150%) of liver chemistries occurred in Diovan HCT-treated patients
Neutropenia: Neutropenia was observed in 0.1% of patients treated with Diovan HCT and 0.4% of patients treated with placebo

6.2 Postmarketing Experience

The following additional adverse reactions have been reported in valsartan or valsartan/hydrochlorothiazide postmarketing experience. Because these reactions are reported voluntarily from a population of uncertain size, it is not always possible to reliably estimate their frequency or establish a causal relationship to drug exposure.
Hypersensitivity: There are rare reports of angioedema. Some of these patients previously experienced angioedema with other drugs including ACE inhibitors. Diovan HCT should not be re-administered to patients who have had angioedema.
Digestive: Elevated liver enzymes and very rare reports of hepatitis
Renal: Impaired renal function
Clinical Laboratory Tests: Hyperkalemia
Dermatologic: Alopecia
Vascular: Vasculitis
Nervous System: Syncope
Rare cases of rhabdomyolysis have been reported in patients receiving angiotensin II receptor blockers.

Hydrochlorothiazide:

The following additional adverse reactions have been reported in post-marketing experience with hydrochlorothiazide:
Acute renal failure, renal disorder, aplastic anemia, erythema multiforme, pyrexia, muscle spasm, asthenia, acute angle-closure glaucoma, bone marrow failure, worsening of diabetes control, hypokalemia, blood lipids increased, hyponatremia, hypomagnesemia, hypercalcemia, hypochloremic alkalosis, impotence, and visual impairment.
Pathological changes in the parathyroid gland of patients with hypercalcemia and hypophosphatemia have been observed in a few patients on prolonged thiazide therapy. If hypercalcemia occurs, further diagnostic evaluation is necessary.

7 DRUG INTERACTIONS

Valsartan: No clinically significant pharmacokinetic interactions were observed when valsartan was coadministered with amlodipine, atenolol, cimetidine, digoxin, furosemide, glyburide, hydrochlorothiazide, or indomethacin. The valsartan-atenolol combination was more antihypertensive than either component, but it did not lower the heart rate more than atenolol alone.

Coadministration of valsartan and warfarin did not change the pharmacokinetics of valsartan or the time-course of the anticoagulant properties of warfarin.

CYP 450 Interactions: In vitro metabolism studies indicate that CYP 450 mediated drug interactions between valsartan and co-administered drugs are unlikely because of the low extent of metabolism [*see Clinical Pharmacology (12.3)*].

Transporters: The results from an *in vitro* study with human liver tissue indicate that valsartan is a substrate of the hepatic uptake transporter OATP1B1 and the hepatic efflux transporter MRP2. Coadministration of inhibitors of the uptake transporter (rifampin, cyclosporine) or efflux transporter (ritonavir) may increase the systemic exposure to valsartan.

Non-Steroidal Anti-Inflammatory Agents including Selective Cyclooxygenase-2 Inhibitors (COX-2 Inhibitors): In patients who are elderly, volume-depleted (including those on diuretic therapy), or with compromised renal function, coadministration of NSAIDs, including selective COX-2 inhibitors, with angiotensin II receptor antagonists, including valsartan, may result in deterioration of renal function, including possible acute renal failure. These effects are usually reversible. Monitor renal function periodically in patients receiving valsartan and NSAID therapy.

The antihypertensive effect of angiotensin II receptor antagonists, including valsartan may be attenuated by NSAIDs including selective COX-2 inhibitors.

Potassium: Concomitant use of valsartan with other agents that block the renin-angiotensin system, potassium sparing diuretics (e.g. spironolactone, triamterene, amiloride), potassium supplements, or salt substitutes containing potassium may lead to increases in serum potassium and in heart failure patients to increases in serum creatinine. If co-medication is considered necessary, monitoring of serum potassium is advisable.

Dual Blockade of the Renin-Angiotensin System (RAS): Dual blockade of the RAS with angiotensin receptor blockers, ACE inhibitors, or aliskiren is associated with increased risks of hypotension, hyperkalemia, and changes in renal function (including acute renal failure) compared to monotherapy. Closely monitor blood pressure, renal function, and electrolytes in patients on Diovan HCT and other agents that affect the RAS.

Do not coadminister aliskiren with Diovan HCT in patients with diabetes. Avoid use of aliskiren with Diovan HCT in patients with renal impairment (GFR <60 mL/min).

Hydrochlorothiazide: When administered concurrently, the following drugs may interact with thiazide diuretics:

Antidiabetic Drugs (oral agents and insulin) - Dosage adjustment of the antidiabetic drug may be required.

Lithium - Diuretic agents increase the risk of lithium toxicity. Refer to the package insert for lithium preparations before use of such preparations with Diovan HCT. Monitoring of serum lithium concentrations is recommended during concurrent use.

Nonsteroidal Anti-inflammatory Drugs (NSAIDs and COX-2 selective inhibitors) - When Diovan HCT and nonsteroidal anti-inflammatory agents are used concomitantly, the patient should be observed closely to determine if the desired effect of the diuretic is obtained.

Carbamazepine – May lead to symptomatic hyponatremia.

Ion exchange resins: Staggering the dosage of hydrochlorothiazide and ion exchange resins (e.g., cholestyramine, colestipol) such that hydrochlorothiazide is administered at least 4 hours before or 4-6 hours after the administration of resins would potentially minimize the interaction [*see Clinical Pharmacology (12.3)*].

Cyclosporine: Concomitant treatment with cyclosporine may increase the risk of hyperuricemia and gout-type complications.

8 USE IN SPECIFIC POPULATIONS

8.1 Pregnancy

Pregnancy Category D

Use of drugs that act on the renin-angiotensin system during the second and third trimesters of pregnancy reduces fetal renal function and increases fetal and neonatal morbidity and death. Resulting oligohydramnios can be associated with fetal lung hypoplasia and skeletal deformations. Potential neonatal adverse effects include skull hypoplasia, anuria, hypotension, renal failure, and death. When pregnancy is detected, discontinue Diovan HCT as soon as possible. These adverse outcomes are usually associated with use of these drugs in the second and third trimester of pregnancy. Most epidemiologic studies examining fetal abnormalities after exposure to antihypertensive use in the first trimester have not distinguished drugs affecting the renin-angiotensin system from other antihypertensive agents. Appropriate management of maternal hypertension during pregnancy is important to optimize outcomes for both mother and fetus.

In the unusual case that there is no appropriate alternative to therapy with drugs affecting the renin-angiotensin system for a particular patient, apprise the mother of the potential risk to the fetus. Perform serial ultrasound examinations to assess the intra-amniotic environment. If oligohydramnios is observed, discontinue Diovan HCT, unless it is considered lifesaving for the mother. Fetal testing may be appropriate, based on the week of pregnancy. Patients and physicians should be aware, however, that oligohydramnios may not appear until after the fetus has sustained irreversible injury. Closely observe infants with histories of in utero exposure to Diovan HCT for hypotension, oliguria, and hyperkalemia [*see Use in Specific Populations (8.4)*].

Hydrochlorothiazide

Thiazides can cross the placenta, and concentrations reached in the umbilical vein approach those in the maternal plasma. Hydrochlorothiazide, like other diuretics, can cause placental hypoperfusion. It accumulates in the amniotic fluid, with reported concentrations up to 19 times higher than in umbilical vein plasma. Use of thiazides during pregnancy is associated with a risk of fetal or neonatal jaundice or thrombocytopenia. Since they do not prevent or alter the course of EPH (Edema, Proteinuria, Hypertension) gestosis (pre-eclampsia), these drugs should not be used to treat hypertension in pregnant women. The use of hydrochlorothiazide for other indications (e.g., heart disease) in pregnancy should be avoided.

8.3 Nursing Mothers

It is not known whether valsartan is excreted in human milk. Valsartan was excreted into the milk of lactating rats; however, animal breast milk drug levels may not accurately reflect human breast milk levels. Hydrochlorothiazide is excreted in human breast milk. Because many drugs are excreted into human milk and because of the potential for adverse reactions in nursing infants from Diovan HCT, a decision should be made whether to discontinue nursing or discontinue the drug, taking into account the importance of the drug to the mother.

8.4 Pediatric Use

Safety and effectiveness of Diovan HCT in pediatric patients have not been established.

Neonates with a history of in utero exposure to Diovan HCT:

If oliguria or hypotension occurs, direct attention toward support of blood pressure and renal perfusion. Exchange transfusions or dialysis may be required as a means of reversing hypotension and/or substituting for disordered renal function.

8.5 Geriatric Use

In the controlled clinical trials of Diovan HCT, 764 (17.5%) patients treated with valsartan-hydrochlorothiazide were ≥65 years and 118 (2.7%) were ≥75 years. No overall difference in the efficacy or safety of valsartan-hydrochlorothiazide was observed between these patients and younger patients, but greater sensitivity of some older individuals cannot be ruled out.

8.6 Renal Impairment

Safety and effectiveness of Diovan HCT in patients with severe renal impairment (CrCl ≤ 30 mL/min) have not been established. No dose adjustment is required in patients with mild (CrCl 60-90 mL/min) or moderate (CrCl 30-60) renal impairment.

8.7 Hepatic Impairment

Valsartan

No dose adjustment is necessary for patients with mild-to-moderate liver disease. No dosing recommendations can be provided for patients with severe liver disease.

Hydrochlorothiazide

Minor alterations of fluid and electrolyte balance may precipitate hepatic coma in patients with impaired hepatic function or progressive liver disease.

10 OVERDOSAGE

Valsartan - Hydrochlorothiazide: Limited data are available related to overdosage in humans. The most likely manifestations of overdosage would be hypotension and tachycardia; bradycardia could occur from parasympathetic (vagal) stimulation. Depressed level of consciousness, circulatory collapse and shock have been reported. If symptomatic hypotension should occur, supportive treatment should be instituted.

Valsartan is not removed from the plasma by dialysis.

The degree to which hydrochlorothiazide is removed by hemodialysis has not been established. The most common signs and symptoms observed in patients are those caused by electrolyte depletion (hypokalemia, hypochloremia, hyponatremia) and dehydration resulting from excessive diuresis. If digitalis has also been administered, hypokalemia may accentuate cardiac arrhythmias.

In rats and marmosets, single oral doses of valsartan up to 1524 and 762 mg/kg in combination with hydrochlorothiazide at doses up to 476 and 238 mg/kg, respectively, were very well tolerated without any treatment-related effects. These no adverse effect doses in rats and marmosets, respectively, represent 46.5 and 23 times the maximum recommended human dose (MRHD) of valsartan and 188 and 113 times the MRHD of hydrochlorothiazide on a mg/m^2 basis. (Calculations assume an oral dose of 320 mg/day valsartan in combination with 25 mg/day hydrochlorothiazide and a 60-kg patient.)

Valsartan: Valsartan was without grossly observable adverse effects at single oral doses up to 2000 mg/kg in rats and up to 1000 mg/kg in marmosets, except for salivation and diarrhea in the rat and vomiting in the marmoset at the highest dose (60 and 31 times, respectively, the MRHD on a mg/m^2 basis). (Calculations assume an oral dose of 320 mg/day and a 60-kg patient.)

Hydrochlorothiazide: The oral LD_{50} of hydrochlorothiazide is greater than 10 g/kg in both mice and rats, which represents 2027 and 4054 times, respectively, the MRHD on a mg/m^2 basis. (Calculations assume an oral dose of 25 mg/day and a 60-kg patient.)

11 DESCRIPTION

Diovan HCT (valsartan and hydrochlorothiazide, USP) is a combination of valsartan, an orally active, specific angiotensin II receptor blocker (ARB) acting on the AT_1 receptor subtype, and hydrochlorothiazide, a diuretic.

Valsartan, a nonpeptide molecule, is chemically described as *N*-(1-oxopentyl)-*N*-[[2′-(1*H*-tetrazol-5-yl)[1,1′-biphenyl]-4-yl]methyl]-L-Valine. Its empirical formula is $C_{24}H_{29}N_5O_3$, its molecular weight is 435.5, and its structural formula is

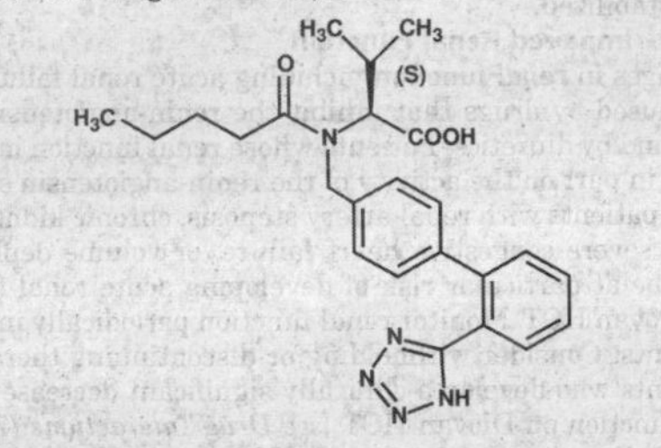

Valsartan is a white to practically white fine powder. It is soluble in ethanol and methanol and slightly soluble in water.

Hydrochlorothiazide USP is a white, or practically white, practically odorless, crystalline powder. It is slightly soluble in water; freely soluble in sodium hydroxide solution, in *n*-butylamine, and in dimethylformamide; sparingly soluble in methanol; and insoluble in ether, in chloroform, and in dilute mineral acids. Hydrochlorothiazide is chemically described as 6-chloro-3,4-dihydro-2*H*-1,2,4-benzothiadiazine-7-sulfonamide 1,1-dioxide.

Hydrochlorothiazide is a thiazide diuretic. Its empirical formula is $C_7H_8ClN_3O_4S_2$, its molecular weight is 297.73, and its structural formula is

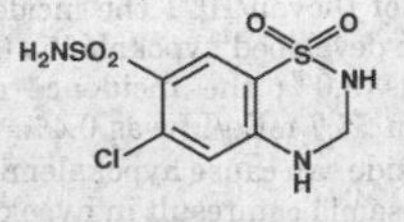

Diovan HCT tablets are formulated for oral administration to contain valsartan and hydrochlorothiazide, USP 80/12.5 mg, 160/12.5 mg, 160/25 mg, 320/12.5 mg, and 320/25 mg. The inactive ingredients of the tablets are colloidal silicon dioxide, crospovidone, hydroxypropyl methylcellulose, iron oxides, magnesium stearate, microcrystalline cellulose, polyethylene glycol, talc, and titanium dioxide.

12 CLINICAL PHARMACOLOGY

12.1 Mechanism of Action

Angiotensin II is formed from angiotensin I in a reaction catalyzed by angiotensin-converting enzyme (ACE, kininase II). Angiotensin II is the principal pressor agent of the renin-angiotensin system, with effects that include vasoconstriction, stimulation of synthesis and release of aldosterone, cardiac stimulation, and renal reabsorption of sodium. Valsartan blocks the vasoconstrictor and aldosterone-secreting effects of angiotensin II by selectively blocking the binding of angiotensin II to the AT_1 receptor in many tissues, such as vascular smooth muscle and the adrenal gland. Its action is therefore independent of the pathways for angiotensin II synthesis.

There is also an AT_2 receptor found in many tissues, but AT_2 is not known to be associated with cardiovascular homeostasis. Valsartan has much greater affinity (about 20000-fold) for the AT_1 receptor than for the AT_2 receptor. The primary metabolite of valsartan is essentially inactive with an affinity for the AT_1 receptor about one 200th that of valsartan itself.

Blockade of the renin-angiotensin system with ACE inhibitors, which inhibit the biosynthesis of angiotensin II from angiotensin I, is widely used in the treatment of hypertension. ACE inhibitors also inhibit the degradation of bradykinin, a reaction also catalyzed by ACE. Because valsartan does not inhibit ACE (kininase II) it does not affect the response to bradykinin. Whether this difference has clinical relevance is not yet known. Valsartan does not bind to or block other hormone receptors or ion channels known to be important in cardiovascular regulation.

Blockade of the angiotensin II receptor inhibits the negative regulatory feedback of angiotensin II on renin secretion, but the resulting increased plasma renin activity and angiotensin II circulating levels do not overcome the effect of valsartan on blood pressure.

Hydrochlorothiazide is a thiazide diuretic. Thiazides affect the renal tubular mechanisms of electrolyte reabsorption, directly increasing excretion of sodium and chloride in approximately equivalent amounts. Indirectly, the diuretic action of hydrochlorothiazide reduces plasma volume, with consequent increases in plasma renin activity, increases in aldosterone secretion, increases in urinary potassium loss, and decreases in serum potassium. The renin-aldosterone link is mediated by angiotensin II, so coadministration of an angiotensin II receptor antagonist tends to reverse the potassium loss associated with these diuretics.

The mechanism of the antihypertensive effect of thiazides is unknown.

12.2 Pharmacodynamics

Valsartan: Valsartan inhibits the pressor effect of angiotensin II infusions. An oral dose of 80 mg inhibits the pressor effect by about 80% at peak with approximately 30% inhibition persisting for 24 hours. No information on the effect of larger doses is available.

Removal of the negative feedback of angiotensin II causes a 2- to 3-fold rise in plasma renin and consequent rise in angiotensin II plasma concentration in hypertensive patients. Minimal decreases in plasma aldosterone were observed after administration of valsartan; very little effect on serum potassium was observed.

Hydrochlorothiazide: After oral administration of hydrochlorothiazide, diuresis begins within 2 hours, peaks in about 4 hours and lasts about 6 to 12 hours.

Drug Interactions

Hydrochlorothiazide:

Alcohol, barbiturates, or narcotics: Potentiation of orthostatic hypotension may occur.

Skeletal muscle relaxants: Possible increased responsiveness to muscle relaxants such as curare derivatives.

Digitalis glycosides: Thiazide-induced hypokalemia or hypomagnesemia may predispose the patient to digoxin toxicity.

12.3 Pharmacokinetics

Valsartan: Valsartan peak plasma concentration is reached 2 to 4 hours after dosing. Valsartan shows bi-exponential decay kinetics following intravenous administration, with an average elimination half-life of about 6 hours. Absolute bioavailability for the capsule formulation is about 25% (range 10%-35%). Food decreases the exposure (as measured by AUC) to valsartan by about 40% and peak plasma concentration (C_{max}) by about 50%. AUC and C_{max} values of valsartan increase approximately linearly with increasing dose over the clinical dosing range. Valsartan does not accumulate appreciably in plasma following repeated administration.

Hydrochlorothiazide: The estimated absolute bioavailability of hydrochlorothiazide after oral administration is about 70%. Peak plasma hydrochlorothiazide concentrations (C_{max}) are reached within 2 to 5 hours after oral administration. There is no clinically significant effect of food on the bioavailability of hydrochlorothiazide.

Hydrochlorothiazide binds to albumin (40 to 70%) and distributes into erythrocytes. Following oral administration, plasma hydrochlorothiazide concentrations decline bi-exponentially, with a mean distribution half-life of about 2 hours and an elimination half-life of about 10 hours.

Diovan HCT: Diovan HCT may be administered with or without food.

Distribution

Valsartan: The steady state volume of distribution of valsartan after intravenous administration is small (17 L), indicating that valsartan does not distribute into tissues extensively. Valsartan is highly bound to serum proteins (95%), mainly serum albumin.

Metabolism

Valsartan: The primary metabolite, accounting for about 9% of dose, is valeryl 4-hydroxy valsartan. *In vitro* metabolism studies involving recombinant CYP 450 enzymes indicated that the CYP 2C9 isoenzyme is responsible for the formation of valeryl-4-hydroxy valsartan. Valsartan does not inhibit CYP 450 isozymes at clinically relevant concentrations. CYP 450 mediated drug interaction between valsartan and coadministered drugs are unlikely because of the low extent of metabolism.

Hydrochlorothiazide: Is not metabolized.

Excretion

Valsartan: Valsartan, when administered as an oral solution, is primarily recovered in feces (about 83% of dose) and urine (about 13% of dose). The recovery is mainly as unchanged drug, with only about 20% of dose recovered as metabolites.

Following intravenous administration, plasma clearance of valsartan is about 2 L/h and its renal clearance is 0.62 L/h (about 30% of total clearance).

Hydrochlorothiazide: About 70% of an orally administered dose of hydrochlorothiazide is eliminated in the urine as unchanged drug.

Special Populations

Geriatric: Exposure (measured by AUC) to valsartan is higher by 70% and the half-life is longer by 35% in the elderly than in the young. A limited amount of data suggest that the systemic clearance of hydrochlorothiazide is reduced in both healthy and hypertensive elderly subjects compared to young healthy volunteers.

Gender: Pharmacokinetics of valsartan do not differ significantly between males and females.

Race: Pharmacokinetic differences due to race have not been studied.

Renal Insufficiency: There is no apparent correlation between renal function (measured by creatinine clearance) and exposure (measured by AUC) to valsartan in patients with different degrees of renal impairment. Valsartan has not been studied in patients with severe impairment of renal function (creatinine clearance <10 mL/min). Valsartan is not removed from the plasma by hemodialysis.

In a study in individuals with impaired renal function, the mean elimination half-life of hydrochlorothiazide was doubled in individuals with mild/moderate renal impairment (30 < CrCl < 90 mL/min) and tripled in severe renal impairment (≤ 30 mL/min), compared to individuals with normal renal function (CrCl > 90 mL/min) [*see Use in Specific Populations (8.6)*].

Hepatic Insufficiency: On average, patients with mild-to-moderate chronic liver disease have twice the exposure (measured by AUC values) to valsartan of healthy volunteers (matched by age, sex, and weight) *[see Use in Specific Populations (8.7)]*.

Drug Interactions

Hydrochlorothiazide:

Drugs that alter gastrointestinal motility: The bioavailability of thiazide-type diuretics may be increased by anticholinergic agents (e.g., atropine, biperiden), apparently due to a decrease in gastrointestinal motility and the stomach emptying rate. Conversely, pro-kinetic drugs may decrease the bioavailability of thiazide diuretics.

Cholestyramine: In a dedicated drug interaction study, administration of cholestyramine 2 hours before hydrochlorothiazide resulted in a 70% reduction in exposure to hydrochlorothiazide. Further, administration of hydrochlorothiazide 2 hours before cholestyramine resulted in 35% reduction in exposure to hydrochlorothiazide.

Antineoplastic agents (e.g., cyclophosphamide, methotrexate): Concomitant use of thiazide diuretics may reduce renal excretion of cytotoxic agents and enhance their myelosuppressive effects.

13 NONCLINICAL TOXICOLOGY

13.1 Carcinogenesis, Mutagenesis, Impairment of Fertility

Valsartan-Hydrochlorothiazide: No carcinogenicity, mutagenicity, or fertility studies have been conducted with the combination of valsartan and hydrochlorothiazide. However, these studies have been conducted for valsartan as well as hydrochlorothiazide alone. Based on the preclinical safety and human pharmacokinetic studies, there is no indication of any adverse interaction between valsartan and hydrochlorothiazide.

Valsartan: There was no evidence of carcinogenicity when valsartan was administered in the diet to mice and rats for up to 2 years at doses up to 160 and 200 mg/kg/day, respectively. These doses in mice and rats are about 2.6 and 6 times, respectively, the MRHD on a mg/m^2 basis. (Calculations assume an oral dose of 320 mg/day and a 60-kg patient.)

Mutagenicity assays did not reveal any valsartan-related effects at either the gene or chromosome level. These assays included bacterial mutagenicity tests with *Salmonella* (Ames) and *E. coli*; a gene mutation test with Chinese hamster V79 cells; a cytogenetic test with Chinese hamster ovary cells; and a rat micronucleus test.

Valsartan had no adverse effects on the reproductive performance of male or female rats at oral doses up to 200 mg/kg/day. This dose is about 6 times the MRHD on a mg/m^2 basis. (Calculations assume an oral dose of 320 mg/day and a 60-kg patient.)

Hydrochlorothiazide: Two-year feeding studies in mice and rats conducted under the auspices of the National Toxicology Program (NTP) uncovered no evidence of a carcinogenic potential of hydrochlorothiazide in female mice (at doses of up to approximately 600 mg/kg/day) or in male and female rats (at doses of up to approximately 100 mg/kg/day). The NTP, however, found equivocal evidence for hepatocarcinogenicity in male mice.

Hydrochlorothiazide was not genotoxic *in vitro* in the Ames mutagenicity assay of *Salmonella Typhimurium* strains TA 98, TA 100, TA 1535, TA 1537, and TA 1538 and in the Chinese Hamster Ovary (CHO) test for chromosomal aberrations, or *in vivo* in assays using mouse germinal cell chromosomes, Chinese hamster bone marrow chromosomes, and the Drosophila sex-linked recessive lethal trait gene. Positive test results were obtained only in the *in vitro* CHO Sister Chromatid Exchange (clastogenicity) and in the Mouse Lymphoma Cell (mutagenicity) assays, using concentrations of hydrochlorothiazide from 43 to 1300 mcgm/mL, and in the Aspergillus Nidulans non-disjunction assay at an unspecified concentration.

Hydrochlorothiazide had no adverse effects on the fertility of mice and rats of either sex in studies wherein these species were exposed, via their diet, to doses of up to 100 and 4 mg/kg, respectively, prior to mating and throughout gestation. These doses of hydrochlorothiazide in mice and rats represent 19 and 1.5 times, respectively, the MRHD on a mg/m^2 basis. (Calculations assume an oral dose of 25 mg/day and a 60-kg patient.)

13.3 Developmental Toxicity Studies

Valsartan-Hydrochlorothiazide: There was no evidence of teratogenicity in mice, rats, or rabbits treated orally with valsartan at doses up to 600, 100, and 10 mg/kg/day, respectively, in combination with hydrochlorothiazide at doses up to 188, 31, and 3 mg/kg/day. These non-teratogenic doses in mice, rats and rabbits, respectively, represent 9, 3.5, and 0.5 times the MRHD of valsartan and 38, 13, and 2 times the MRHD of hydrochlorothiazide on a mg/m^2 basis. (Calculations assume an oral dose of 320 mg/day valsartan in combination with 25 mg/day hydrochlorothiazide and a 60-kg patient.)

Fetotoxicity was observed in association with maternal toxicity in rats and rabbits at valsartan doses of ≥200 and 10 mg/kg/day, respectively, in combination with hydrochlorothiazide doses of ≥63 and 3 mg/kg/day. Fetotoxicity in rats was considered to be related to decreased fetal weights and included fetal variations of sternebrae, vertebrae, ribs and/or renal papillae. Fetotoxicity in rabbits included increased numbers of late resorptions with resultant increases in total resorptions, postimplantation losses, and decreased number of live fetuses. The no observed adverse effect doses in mice, rats and rabbits for valsartan were 600, 100, and 3 mg/kg/day, respectively, in combination with hydrochlorothiazide doses of 188, 31, and 1 mg/kg/day. These no adverse effect doses in mice, rats, and rabbits, respectively, represent 9, 3, and 0.18 times the MRHD of valsartan and 38, 13, and 0.5 times the MRHD of hydrochlorothiazide on a mg/m^2 basis. (Calculations assume an oral dose of 320 mg/day valsartan in combination with 25 mg/day hydrochlorothiazide and a 60-kg patient.)

Valsartan: No teratogenic effects were observed when valsartan was administered to pregnant mice and rats at oral doses up to 600 mg/kg/day and to pregnant rabbits at oral doses up to 10 mg/kg/day. However, significant decreases in fetal weight, pup birth weight, pup survival rate, and slight delays in developmental milestones were observed in studies in which parental rats were treated with valsartan at oral, maternally toxic (reduction in body weight gain and food consumption) doses of 600 mg/kg/day during organogenesis or late gestation and lactation. In rabbits, fetotoxicity (i.e., resorptions, litter loss, abortions, and low body weight) associated with maternal toxicity (mortality) was observed at doses of 5 and 10 mg/kg/day. The no observed adverse effect doses of 600, 200, and 2 mg/kg/day in mice, rats, and rabbits represent 9, 6, and 0.1 times, respectively, the MRHD on a mg/m^2 basis. (Calculations assume an oral dose of 320 mg/day and a 60-kg patient.)

Hydrochlorothiazide: Under the auspices of the National Toxicology Program, pregnant mice and rats that received hydrochlorothiazide via gavage at doses up to 3000 and 1000 mg/kg/day, respectively, on gestation days 6 through 15 showed no evidence of teratogenicity. These doses of hydrochlorothiazide in mice and rats represent 608 and 405 times, respectively, the MRHD on a mg/m^2 basis. (Calculations assume an oral dose of 25 mg/day and a 60-kg patient.)

14 CLINICAL STUDIES

14.1 Hypertension

Valsartan-Hydrochlorothiazide: In controlled clinical trials including over 7600 patients, 4372 patients were exposed to valsartan (80, 160, and 320 mg) and concomitant hydrochlorothiazide (12.5 and 25 mg). Two factorial trials compared various combinations of 80/12.5 mg, 80/25 mg, 160/12.5 mg, 160/25 mg, 320/12.5 mg, and 320/25 mg with their respective components and placebo. The combination of valsartan and hydrochlorothiazide resulted in additive placebo-adjusted decreases in systolic and diastolic blood pressure at trough of 14-21/8-11 mmHg at 80/12.5 mg to 320/25 mg, compared to 7-10/4-5 mmHg for valsartan 80 mg to 320 mg, and 5-11/2-5 mmHg for hydrochlorothiazide 12.5 mg to 25 mg alone.

Three other controlled trials investigated the addition of hydrochlorothiazide to patients who did not respond adequately to valsartan 80 mg to valsartan 320 mg, resulted in the additional lowering of systolic and diastolic blood pressure by approximately 4-12/2-5 mmHg.

The maximal antihypertensive effect was attained 4 weeks after the initiation of therapy, the first time point at which blood pressure was measured in these trials.

In long-term follow-up studies (without placebo control) the effect of the combination of valsartan and hydrochlorothiazide appeared to be maintained for up to 2 years. The antihypertensive effect is independent of age or gender. The overall response to the combination was similar for black and non-black patients.

There was essentially no change in heart rate in patients treated with the combination of valsartan and hydrochlorothiazide in controlled trials.

There are no trials of the Diovan HCT combination tablet demonstrating reductions in cardiovascular risk in patients with hypertension, but the hydrochlorothiazide component and several ARBs, which are the same pharmacological class as the valsartan component, have demonstrated such benefits.

Valsartan: The antihypertensive effects of valsartan were demonstrated principally in 7 placebo-controlled, 4- to 12-week trials (1 in patients over 65) of dosages from 10 to 320 mg/day in patients with baseline diastolic blood pressures of 95-115. The studies allowed comparison of once-daily and twice-daily regimens of 160 mg/day; comparison of peak and trough effects; comparison (in pooled data) of response by gender, age, and race; and evaluation of incremental effects of hydrochlorothiazide.

Administration of valsartan to patients with essential hypertension results in a significant reduction of sitting, supine, and standing systolic and diastolic blood pressure, usually with little or no orthostatic change.

In most patients, after administration of a single oral dose, onset of antihypertensive activity occurs at approximately 2 hours, and maximum reduction of blood pressure is achieved within 6 hours. The antihypertensive effect persists for 24 hours after dosing, but there is a decrease from peak effect at lower doses (40 mg) presumably reflecting loss of inhibition of angiotensin II. At higher doses, however (160 mg), there is little difference in peak and trough effect. During repeated dosing, the reduction in blood pressure with any dose is substantially present within 2 weeks, and maximal reduction is generally attained after 4 weeks. In long-term follow-up studies (without placebo control) the effect of valsartan appeared to be maintained for up to 2 years. The antihypertensive effect is independent of age, gender or race. The latter finding regarding race is based on pooled data and should be viewed with caution, because antihypertensive drugs that affect the renin-angiotensin system (that is, ACE inhibitors and angiotensin II blockers) have generally been found to be less effective in low-renin hypertensives (frequently blacks) than in high-renin hypertensives (frequently whites). In pooled, randomized, controlled trials of Diovan that included a total of 140 blacks and 830 whites, valsartan and an ACE-inhibitor control were generally at least as effective in blacks as whites. The explanation for this difference from previous findings is unclear.

Abrupt withdrawal of valsartan has not been associated with a rapid increase in blood pressure.

The 7 studies of valsartan monotherapy included over 2000 patients randomized to various doses of valsartan and about 800 patients randomized to placebo. Doses below 80 mg were not consistently distinguished from those of placebo at trough, but doses of 80, 160 and 320 mg produced dose-related decreases in systolic and diastolic blood pressure, with the difference from placebo of approximately 6-9/3-5 mmHg at 80-160 mg and 9/6 mmHg at 320 mg.

Patients with an inadequate response to 80 mg once daily were titrated to either 160 mg once daily or 80 mg twice daily, which resulted in a comparable response in both groups.

In another 4-week study, 1876 patients randomized to valsartan 320 mg once daily had an incremental blood pressure reduction 3/1 mmHg lower than did 1900 patients randomized to valsartan 160 mg once daily.

In controlled trials, the antihypertensive effect of once daily valsartan 80 mg was similar to that of once daily enalapril 20 mg or once daily lisinopril 10 mg.

There was essentially no change in heart rate in valsartan-treated patients in controlled trials.

14.2 Initial Therapy - Hypertension

The safety and efficacy of Diovan HCT as initial therapy for patients with severe hypertension (defined as a sitting diastolic blood pressure ≥110 mmHg and systolic blood pressure ≥140 mmHg off all antihypertensive therapy) was studied in a 6-week multicenter, randomized, double-blind study. Patients were randomized to either Diovan HCT (valsartan and hydrochlorothiazide 160/12.5 mg once daily) or to valsartan (160 mg once daily) and followed for blood pressure response. Patients were force-titrated at 2-week intervals. Patients on combination therapy were subsequently titrated to 160/25 mg followed by 320/25 mg valsartan/hydrochlorothiazide. Patients on monotherapy were subsequently titrated to 320 mg valsartan followed by a titration to 320 mg valsartan to maintain the blind.

The study randomized 608 patients, including 261 (43%) females, 147 (24%) blacks, and 75 (12%) ≥65 years of age. The mean blood pressure at baseline for the total population was 168/112 mmHg. The mean age was 52 years. After 4 weeks of therapy, reductions in systolic and diastolic blood pressure were 9/5 mmHg greater in the group treated with Diovan HCT compared to valsartan. Similar trends were seen when the patients were grouped according to gender, race, or age.

16 HOW SUPPLIED/STORAGE AND HANDLING

Diovan HCT (valsartan and hydrochlorothiazide, USP) is available as non-scored tablets containing valsartan/hydrochlorothiazide 80/12.5 mg, 160/12.5 mg, 160/25 mg, 320/12.5 mg, and 320/25 mg. Strengths are available as follows.

80/12.5 mg Tablet - Light orange, ovaloid, with slightly convex faces debossed CG on 1 side and HGH on the other side.
Bottles of 90 NDC 0078-0314-34
Bottles of 14,000 NDC 0078-0314-33
Unit Dose (blister pack) NDC 0078-0314-06
Box of 100 (strips of 10)

160/12.5 mg Tablet - Dark red, ovaloid, with slightly convex faces debossed CG on 1 side and HHH on the other side.
Bottles of 90 NDC 0078-0315-34
Bottles of 7,000 NDC 0078-0315-17
Unit Dose (blister pack) NDC 0078-0315-06
Box of 100 (strips of 10)
Unit Dose (blister pack of 30) NDC 0078-0315-15

160/25 mg Tablet - Brown orange, ovaloid, with slightly convex faces debossed NVR on 1 side and HXH on the other side.
Bottles of 90 NDC 0078-0383-34
Bottles of 7,000 NDC 0078-0383-17
Unit Dose (blister pack) NDC 0078-0383-06
Box of 100 (strips of 10)
Unit Dose (blister pack of 30) NDC 0078-0383-15

320/12.5 mg Tablet - Pink, ovaloid, with beveled edge, debossed NVR on 1 side and HIL on the other side.
Bottles of 90 NDC 0078-0471-34
Bottles of 3,500 NDC 0078-0471-11
Unit Dose (blister pack) NDC 0078-0471-06
Box of 100 (strips of 10)
Unit Dose (blister pack of 30) NDC 0078-0471-15

320/25 mg Tablet - Yellow, ovaloid, with beveled edge, debossed NVR on 1 side and CTI on the other side.
Bottles of 90 NDC 0078-0472-34
Bottles of 3,500 NDC 0078-0472-11
Unit Dose (blister pack) NDC 0078-0472-06
Box of 100 (strips of 10)
Unit Dose (blister pack of 30) NDC 0078-0472-15

Store at 25°C (77°F); excursions permitted to 15-30°C (59-86°F) [see USP Controlled Room Temperature].
Protect from moisture.
Dispense in tight container (USP).

17 PATIENT COUNSELING INFORMATION

Information for Patients

Pregnancy: Female patients of childbearing age should be told about the consequences of exposure to Diovan HCT during pregnancy. Discuss treatment options with women planning to become pregnant. Patients should be asked to report pregnancies to their physicians as soon as possible.

Symptomatic Hypotension: A patient receiving Diovan HCT should be cautioned that lightheadedness can occur, especially during the first days of therapy, and that it should be reported to the prescribing physician. The patients should be told that if syncope occurs, Diovan HCT should be discontinued until the physician has been consulted.

All patients should be cautioned that inadequate fluid intake, excessive perspiration, diarrhea, or vomiting can lead to an excessive fall in blood pressure, with the same consequences of lightheadedness and possible syncope.

Potassium Supplements: A patient receiving Diovan HCT should be told not to use potassium supplements or salt substitutes containing potassium without consulting the prescribing physician.

T2012-186
October 2012

FDA-Approved Patient Labeling
PATIENT INFORMATION
DIOVAN HCT (DYE'-o-van HCT)
(valsartan and hydrochlorothiazide)
Tablets

Read the Patient Information that comes with DIOVAN HCT before you start taking it and each time you get a refill. There may be new information. This leaflet does not take the place of talking with your doctor about your condition and treatment. If you have any questions about DIOVAN HCT, ask your doctor or pharmacist.

What is the most important information I should know about DIOVAN HCT?
Diovan HCT can cause harm or death to an unborn baby. Talk to your doctor about other ways to lower your blood pressure if you plan to become pregnant. If you get pregnant while taking Diovan HCT, tell your doctor right away.

What is DIOVAN HCT?
DIOVAN HCT contains 2 prescription medicines:
1. valsartan, an angiotensin receptor blocker (ARB)
2. hydrochlorothiazide (HCTZ), a water pill (diuretic)

DIOVAN HCT may be used to lower high blood pressure (hypertension) in adults-
- when 1 medicine to lower your high blood pressure is not enough.
- as the first medicine to lower high blood pressure if your doctor decides you are likely to need more than 1 medicine.

DIOVAN HCT has not been studied in children under 18 years of age.

Who should not take DIOVAN HCT?
Do not take DIOVAN HCT if you:
- **are allergic to any of the ingredients in DIOVAN HCT.** See the end of this leaflet for a complete list of ingredients in DIOVAN HCT.
- make less urine due to kidney problems.
- are allergic to medicines that contain sulfonamides.

What should I tell my doctor before taking DIOVAN HCT?
Tell your doctor about all your medical conditions including if you:
- **are pregnant or plan to become pregnant.** See "What is the most important information I should know about DIOVAN HCT?"
- **are breastfeeding.** DIOVAN HCT passes into breast milk. You should choose either to take DIOVAN HCT or breastfeed, but not both.
- **have liver problems**
- **have kidney problems**
- **have or had gallstones**
- **have Lupus**
- **have low levels of potassium** (with or without symptoms such as muscle weakness, muscle spasms, abnormal heart rhythm) or magnesium in your blood
- **have high levels of calcium in your blood** (with or without symptoms such as nausea, vomiting, constipation, stomach pain, frequent urination, thirst, muscle weakness and twitching).
- **have high levels of uric acid in the blood.**
- **have ever had a reaction called angioedema, to another blood pressure medication. Angioedema causes swelling of the face, lips, tongue, throat and may cause difficulty breathing.**

Tell your doctor about all the medicines you take including prescription and nonprescription medicines, vitamins and herbal supplements. Some of your other medicines and DIOVAN HCT could affect each other, causing serious side effects. Especially, tell your doctor if you take:
- other medicines for high blood pressure or a heart problem
- water pills (diuretics)
- potassium supplements. Your doctor may check the amount of potassium in your blood periodically.
- a salt substitute. Your doctor may check the amount of potassium in your blood periodically.
- antidiabetic medicines including insulin
- narcotic pain medicines
- sleeping pills
- lithium, a medicine used in some types of depression (Eskalith®, Lithobid®, Lithium Carbonate, Lithium Citrate)
- aspirin or other medicines called Non-Steroidal Anti-Inflammatory Drugs (NSAIDs), like ibuprofen or naproxen
- digoxin or other digitalis glycosides (a heart medicine)
- muscle relaxants (medicines used during operations)
- certain cancer medicines, like cyclophosphamide or methotrexate
- certain antibiotics (rifamycin group), a drug used to protect against transplant rejection (cyclosporin) or an anti-retroviral drug used to treat HIV/AIDS infection (ritonavir). These drugs may increase the effect of valsartan.

Ask your doctor if you are not sure if you are taking 1 of these medicines.

Know the medicines you take. Keep a list of your medicines with you to show to your doctor and pharmacist when a new medicine is prescribed. Talk to your doctor or pharmacist before you start taking any new medicine. Your doctor or pharmacist will know what medicines are safe to take together.

How should I take DIOVAN HCT?

- Take DIOVAN HCT exactly as prescribed by your doctor. Your doctor may change your dose if needed.
- Take DIOVAN HCT once each day.
- DIOVAN HCT can be taken with or without food.
- If you miss a dose, take it as soon as you remember. If it is close to your next dose, do not take the missed dose. Just take the next dose at your regular time.
- If you take too much DIOVAN HCT, call your doctor or Poison Control Center, or go to the nearest hospital emergency room.

What should I avoid while taking DIOVAN HCT?

You should not take DIOVAN HCT during pregnancy. See "What is the most important information I should know about DIOVAN HCT?"

What are the possible side effects of DIOVAN HCT?

DIOVAN HCT may cause serious side effects including:

- **Harm to an unborn baby causing injury and even death.** See "What is the most important information I should know about DIOVAN HCT?"
- **Low blood pressure (hypotension).** Low blood pressure is most likely to happen if you:
  - take water pills
  - are on a low salt diet
  - get dialysis treatments
  - have heart problems
  - get sick with vomiting or diarrhea
  - drink alcohol

Lie down if you feel faint or dizzy. Call your doctor right away.

- **Allergic reactions.** People with and without allergy problems or asthma who take DIOVAN HCT may get allergic reactions.
- **Worsening of Lupus.** Hydrochlorothiazide, 1 of the medicines in DIOVAN HCT may cause Lupus to become active or worse.
- **Fluid and electrolyte (salt) problems.** Tell your doctor about any of the following signs and symptoms of fluid and electrolyte problems:

• dry mouth	• drowsiness	• muscle fatigue
• thirst	• restlessness	• very low urine output
• lack of energy (lethargic)	• confusion	• fast heartbeat
• weakness	• seizures	• nausea and vomiting
	• muscle pain or cramps	

- **Kidney problems.** Kidney problems may become worse in people that already have kidney disease. Some people will have changes on blood tests for kidney function and may need a lower dose of DIOVAN HCT. Call your doctor if you get swelling in your feet, ankles, or hands, or unexplained weight gain. If you have heart failure, your doctor should check your kidney function before prescribing DIOVAN HCT.
- **Skin rash.** Call your doctor right away if you have an unusual skin rash.
- **Eye Problems.** One of the medicines in DIOVAN HCT can cause eye problems that may lead to vision loss. Symptoms of eye problems can happen within hours to weeks of starting DIOVAN HCT. Tell your doctor right away if you have:
  - decrease in vision
  - eye pain

Other side effects were generally mild and brief. They generally have not caused patients to stop taking DIOVAN HCT.

Tell your doctor if you have any side effect that bothers you or that does not go away.

These are not all the possible side effects of DIOVAN HCT. For a complete list, ask your doctor or pharmacist.

Call your doctor for medical advice about side effects. You may report side effects to FDA at 1-800-FDA-1088.

How do I store DIOVAN HCT?

- Store DIOVAN HCT tablets at room temperature between 59°F to 86°F (15°C to 30°C).
- Keep DIOVAN HCT in a closed container in a dry place.

Keep DIOVAN HCT and all medicines out of the reach of children.

General information about DIOVAN HCT

Medicines are sometimes prescribed for conditions that are not mentioned in patient information leaflets. Do not use DIOVAN HCT for a condition for which it was not prescribed. Do not give DIOVAN HCT to other people, even if they have the same symptoms you have. It may harm them. This leaflet summarizes the most important information about DIOVAN HCT. If you would like more information, talk with your doctor. You can ask your doctor or pharmacist for information about DIOVAN HCT that is written for health professionals. For more information about DIOVAN HCT, go to www.DIOVAN.com or call 1-866-404-6359.

What are the ingredients in DIOVAN HCT?

Active ingredients: Valsartan and hydrochlorothiazide

Inactive ingredients: colloidal silicon dioxide, crospovidone, hydroxypropyl methylcellulose, iron oxides, magnesium stearate, microcrystalline cellulose, polyethylene glycol, talc, and titanium dioxide.

What is high blood pressure (hypertension)?

Blood pressure is the force in your blood vessels when your heart beats and when your heart rests. You have high blood pressure when the force is too much. DIOVAN HCT can help your blood vessels relax and reduce the amount of water in your body so your blood pressure is lower. Medicines that lower blood pressure lower your risk of having a stroke or heart attack.

High blood pressure makes the heart work harder to pump blood throughout the body and causes damage to the blood vessels. If high blood pressure is not treated, it can lead to stroke, heart attack, heart failure, kidney failure, and vision problems.

Eskalith® and Lithobid® are registered trademarks of Noven Pharmaceuticals, Inc.

Distributed by:
Novartis Pharmaceuticals Corporation
East Hanover, New Jersey 07936

T2012-187
October 2012

Shown in Product Identification Guide, page 309

EXELON® PATCH ℞

[ĕx′ə-lŏn]

(rivastigmine transdermal system)

The following prescribing information is based on official labeling in effect July 2013.

HIGHLIGHTS OF PRESCRIBING INFORMATION

These highlights do not include all the information needed to use EXELON PATCH safely and effectively. See full prescribing information for EXELON PATCH.

EXELON® PATCH (rivastigmine transdermal system)

Initial U.S. Approval: 2000

RECENT MAJOR CHANGES

Indications and Usage (1.1) 06/2013
Dosage and Administration (2.1, 2.2) 06/2013
Contraindications (4) 06/2013
Warnings and Precautions (5.3) 06/2013

INDICATIONS AND USAGE

Exelon Patch is an acetylcholinesterase inhibitor indicated for treatment of:

- Mild, moderate, and severe dementia of the Alzheimer's type (1.1)
- Mild to moderate dementia associated with Parkinson's disease (1.2)

DOSAGE AND ADMINISTRATION

- Apply patch on intact skin for a 24-hour period; replace with a new patch every 24 hours (2.1, 2.4)
- **Initiate treatment with 4.6 mg/24 hours Exelon Patch (2.1)**
- **After a minimum of 4 weeks, if tolerated, increase dose to 9.5 mg/24 hours, which is the minimum effective dose (2.1)**
- **Following a minimum additional 4 weeks, may increase dosage to maximum dosage of 13.3 mg/24 hours (2.1)**
- **Mild to Moderate Alzheimer's Disease and Parkinson's Disease Dementia:** Exelon Patch 9.5 mg/24 hours or 13.3 mg/24 hours once daily (2.1)
- **Severe Alzheimer's Disease:** Exelon Patch 13.3 mg/24 hours once daily (2.1)
- For treatment interruption longer than 3 days, retitrate dosage starting at 4.6 mg/24 hours (2.1)
- Consider dose adjustments in patients with (2.2):
  - Mild to moderate hepatic impairment (8.7)
  - Low (<50 kg) body weight (8.8)

DOSAGE FORMS AND STRENGTHS

Exelon Patch: 4.6 mg/24 hours or 9.5 mg/24 hours or 13.3 mg/24 hours (3)

CONTRAINDICATIONS

Patients with known hypersensitivity to rivastigmine, other carbamate derivatives, or other components of the formulation or previous history of application site reactions with rivastigmine transdermal patch suggestive of allergic contact dermatitis (4, 6.2)

WARNINGS AND PRECAUTIONS

- *Overdose from medication errors:* Hospitalization and, rarely, death have been reported due to application of multiple patches at same time. Ensure patients or caregivers receive instruction on proper dosing and administration. (5.1)
- *Gastrointestinal adverse reactions:* May include significant nausea, vomiting, diarrhea, anorexia/decreased appetite, and weight loss, and may necessitate treatment interruption. Dehydration may result from prolonged vomiting or diarrhea and can be associated with serious outcomes. (5.2)
- *Skin reactions:* Application site reactions may occur with the patch form of rivastigmine. Discontinue treatment if application site reactions spread beyond the patch size, if there is evidence of a more intense local reaction (e.g., increasing erythema, edema, papules, vesicles), and if symptoms do not significantly improve within 48 hours after patch removal. (5.3)

ADVERSE REACTIONS

Most commonly observed adverse reactions (>5% and higher than with placebo): Nausea, vomiting, and diarrhea (6.1)

To report SUSPECTED ADVERSE REACTIONS, contact Novartis Pharmaceuticals Corporation at 1-888-669-6682 or FDA at 1-800-FDA-1088 or www.fda.gov/medwatch.

DRUG INTERACTIONS

Cholinomimetic and anticholinergic drugs: Avoid concomitant use unless clinically necessary (7.1)

See 17 for PATIENT COUNSELING INFORMATION and FDA-approved patient labeling

Revised: 07/2013

FULL PRESCRIBING INFORMATION: CONTENTS*

*** Sections or subsections omitted from the full prescribing information are not listed**

FULL PRESCRIBING INFORMATION

1 INDICATIONS AND USAGE

1.1 Alzheimer's Disease

Exelon Patch is indicated for the treatment of dementia of the Alzheimer's type (AD). Efficacy has been demonstrated in patients with mild, moderate, and severe Alzheimer's disease.

1.2 Parkinson's Disease Dementia

Exelon Patch is indicated for the treatment of mild to moderate dementia associated with Parkinson's disease (PDD).

2 DOSAGE AND ADMINISTRATION

2.1 Recommended Dosing

Initial Dose

Initiate treatment with one 4.6 mg/24 hours Exelon Patch applied to the skin once daily *[see Dosage and Administration (2.4)]*.

Dose Titration

Increase the dose only after a minimum of 4 weeks at the previous dose, and only if the previous dose has been well tolerated. For mild to moderate AD and PDD patients continue the recommended effective dose of 9.5 mg/24 hours for as long as therapeutic benefit persists. Patients can then be increased to the maximum effective dose of 13.3 mg/24 hours dose. For patients with severe AD, 13.3 mg/24 hours is the recommended effective dose. Doses higher than 13.3 mg/24 hours confer no appreciable additional benefit, and are associated with an increase in the incidence of adverse reactions *[see Warnings and Precautions (5.2), Adverse Reactions (6.1)]*.

Mild to Moderate Alzheimer's Disease and Mild to Moderate Parkinson's Disease Dementia

The effective dosage of Exelon Patch is 9.5 mg/24 hours or 13.3 mg/24 hours administered once per day; replace with a new patch every 24 hours.

Severe Alzheimer's Disease

The effective dosage of Exelon Patch in patients with severe Alzheimer's disease is 13.3 mg/24 hours administered once per day; replace with a new patch every 24 hours.

Interruption of Treatment

If dosing is interrupted for 3 days or fewer, restart treatment with the same or lower strength Exelon Patch. If dosing is interrupted for more than 3 days, restart treatment with the 4.6 mg/24 hours Exelon Patch and titrate as described above.

2.2 Dosing in Specific Populations

Dosing Modifications in Patients with Hepatic Impairment

Consider using the 4.6 mg/24 hours Exelon Patch as both the initial and maintenance dose in patients with mild (Child-Pugh score 5 to 6) to moderate (Child-Pugh score 7 to 9) hepatic impairment *[see Use in Specific Populations (8.7), Clinical Pharmacology (12.3)]*.

Dosing Modifications in Patients with Low Body Weight

Because rivastigmine blood levels vary with weight [see Use in Specific Populations (8.8), Clinical Pharmacology (12.3)], carefully titrate and monitor patients with low body weight (<50kg) for toxicities (e.g., excessive nausea, vomiting) and consider reducing the maintenance dose to the 4.6 mg/24 hours Exelon Patch if such toxicities develop.

2.3 Switching to Exelon Patch from Exelon Capsules or Exelon Oral Solution

Patients treated with Exelon Capsules or Oral Solution may be switched to Exelon Patch as follows:

- A patient who is on a total daily dose of <6 mg of oral rivastigmine can be switched to the 4.6 mg/24 hours Exelon Patch.
- A patient who is on a total daily dose of 6 mg to 12 mg of oral rivastigmine can be switched to the 9.5 mg/24 hours Exelon Patch.

Instruct patients or caregivers to apply the first patch on the day following the last oral dose.

2.4 Important Administration Instructions

Exelon Patch is for transdermal use on intact skin.

(a) Do not use the patch if the pouch seal is broken or the patch is cut, damaged, or changed in any way.

(b) Apply the Exelon Patch once a day

- Press down firmly for 30 seconds until the edges stick well when applying to clean, dry, hairless, intact healthy skin in a place that will not be rubbed against by tight clothing.
- Use the upper or lower back as the site of application because the patch is less likely to be removed by the patient. If sites on the back are not accessible, apply the patch to the upper arm or chest.
- Do not apply to a skin area where cream, lotion, or powder has recently been applied.

(c) Do not apply to skin that is red, irritated, or cut.

(d) Replace the Exelon Patch with a new patch every 24 hours. Instruct patients to only wear 1 patch at a time (remove the previous day's patch before applying a new patch) *[see Warnings and Precautions (5.1) and Overdosage (10)]*. If a patch falls off or if a dose is missed, apply a new patch immediately and then replace this patch the following day at the usual application time.

(e) Change the site of patch application daily to minimize potential irritation, although a new patch can be applied to the same general anatomic site (e.g., another spot on the upper back) on consecutive days. Do not apply a new patch to the same location for at least 14 days.

(f) May wear the patch during bathing and in hot weather. But avoid long exposure to external heat sources (excessive sunlight, saunas, solariums).

(g) Place used patches in the previously saved pouch and discard in the trash, away from pets or children.

3 DOSAGE FORMS AND STRENGTHS

Exelon Patch is available in 3 strengths. Each patch has a beige backing layer labeled as either:

- EXELON® PATCH 4.6 mg/24 hours, AMCX
- EXELON® PATCH 9.5 mg/24 hours, BHDI
- EXELON® PATCH 13.3 mg/24 hours, CNFU

4 CONTRAINDICATIONS

Exelon Patch (rivastigmine transdermal system) is contraindicated in patients with:

- known hypersensitivity to rivastigmine, other carbamate derivatives, or other components of the formulation *[see Description (11)]*.
- previous history of application site reactions with rivastigmine transdermal patch suggestive of allergic contact dermatitis *[see Warnings and Precautions (5.3)]*.

Isolated cases of generalized skin reactions have been described in postmarketing experience *[see Adverse Reactions (6.2)]*.

5 WARNINGS AND PRECAUTIONS

5.1 Medication Errors Resulting in Overdose

Medication errors with Exelon Patch have resulted in serious adverse reactions; some cases have required hospitalization, and rarely, led to death. The majority of medication errors have involved not removing the old patch when putting on a new one and the use of multiple patches at one time. Instruct patients and their caregivers on important administration instructions for Exelon Patch. *[see Dosage and Administration (2.4)]*.

5.2 Gastrointestinal Adverse Reactions

Exelon Patch can cause gastrointestinal adverse reactions, including significant nausea, vomiting, diarrhea, anorexia/decreased appetite, and weight loss. Dehydration may result from prolonged vomiting or diarrhea and can be associated with serious outcomes. The incidence and severity of these reactions are dose-related *[see Adverse Reactions (6.1)]*. For this reason, initiate treatment with Exelon Patch at a dose of 4.6 mg/24 hours and titrate to a dose of 9.5 mg/24 hours and then to a dose of 13.3 mg/24 hours, if appropriate *[see Dosage and Administration (2.1)]*.

If treatment is interrupted for more than 3 days because of intolerance, reinitiate Exelon Patch with the 4.6 mg/24 hours dose to reduce the possibility of severe vomiting and its potentially serious sequelae. A postmarketing report described a case of severe vomiting with esophageal rupture following inappropriate reinitiation of treatment of an oral formulation of rivastigmine without retitration after 8 weeks of treatment interruption.

Inform caregivers to monitor for gastrointestinal adverse reactions and to inform the physician if they occur. It is critical to inform caregivers that if therapy has been interrupted for more than 3 days because of intolerance, the next dose should not be administered without contacting the physician regarding proper retitration.

5.3 Skin Reactions

Skin application site reactions may occur with Exelon Patch and are usually mild or moderate in intensity. These reactions are not in themselves an indication of sensitization. However, use of rivastigmine patch may lead to allergic contact dermatitis.

Allergic contact dermatitis should be suspected if application site reactions spread beyond the patch size, if there is evidence of a more intense local reaction (e.g. increasing erythema, edema, papules, vesicles) and if symptoms do not significantly improve within 48 hours after patch removal. In these cases, treatment should be discontinued *[see Contraindications (4)]*.

In patients who develop application site reactions to Exelon Patch suggestive of allergic contact dermatitis and who still require rivastigmine, treatment should be switched to oral rivastigmine only after negative allergy testing and under close medical supervision. It is possible that some patients sensitized to rivastigmine by exposure to rivastigmine patch may not be able to take rivastigmine in any form.

There have been isolated postmarketing reports of patients experiencing disseminated hypersensitivity reactions of the skin when administered rivastigmine irrespective of the route of administration (oral or transdermal). In these cases, treatment should be discontinued *[see Contraindications (4)]*. Patients and caregivers should be instructed accordingly.

5.4 Other Adverse Reactions from Increased Cholinergic Activity

Neurologic Effects

Extrapyramidal Symptoms: Cholinomimetics, including rivastigmine may exacerbate or induce extrapyramidal symptoms. Worsening of parkinsonian symptoms, particularly tremor, has been observed in patients with dementia associated with Parkinson's disease who were treated with Exelon Capsules.

Seizures: Drugs that increase cholinergic activity are believed to have some potential for causing seizures. However, seizure activity also may be a manifestation of Alzheimer's disease.

Peptic Ulcers/Gastrointestinal Bleeding

Cholinesterase inhibitors, including rivastigmine, may increase gastric acid secretion due to increased cholinergic activity. Monitor patients using Exelon Patch for symptoms of active or occult gastrointestinal bleeding, especially those at increased risk for developing ulcers, e.g., those with a history of ulcer disease or those receiving concurrent nonsteroidal anti-inflammatory drugs (NSAIDs). Clinical studies of rivastigmine have shown no significant increase, relative to placebo, in the incidence of either peptic ulcer disease or gastrointestinal bleeding.

Use with Anesthesia

Rivastigmine, as a cholinesterase inhibitor, is likely to exaggerate succinylcholine-type muscle relaxation during anesthesia.

Cardiac Conduction Effects

Because rivastigmine increases cholinergic activity, use of the Exelon Patch may have vagotonic effects on heart rate (e.g., bradycardia). The potential for this action may be particularly important in patients with sick sinus syndrome or other supraventricular cardiac conduction conditions. In clinical trials, rivastigmine was not associated with any increased incidence of cardiovascular adverse events, heart rate or blood pressure changes, or ECG abnormalities.

Genitourinary Effects

Although not observed in clinical trials of rivastigmine, drugs that increase cholinergic activity may cause urinary obstruction.

Pulmonary Effects

Drugs that increase cholinergic activity, including Exelon Patch should be used with care in patients with a history of asthma or obstructive pulmonary disease.

5.5 Impairment in Driving or Use of Machinery

Dementia may cause gradual impairment of driving performance or compromise the ability to use machinery. The administration of rivastigmine may also result in adverse reactions that are detrimental to these functions. During treatment with the Exelon Patch, routinely evaluate the patient's ability to continue driving or operating machinery.

6 ADVERSE REACTIONS

Significant gastrointestinal adverse reactions including nausea, vomiting, anorexia, and weight loss are described below and elsewhere in the labeling *[see Warnings and Precautions (5.2)]*.

6.1 Clinical Trials Experience

Because clinical trials are conducted under widely varying conditions, adverse reaction rates observed in the clinical trials of a drug cannot be directly compared to rates in the clinical trials of another drug and may not reflect the rates observed in practice.

Exelon Patch has been administered to 2348 patients with Alzheimer's disease during clinical trials worldwide. Of these, 1954 patients have been treated for at least 12 weeks, 1643 patients have been treated for at least 24 weeks, and 847 patients have been treated for at least 48 weeks.

Mild to Moderate Alzheimer's Disease

24-Week International Placebo-Controlled Trial (Study 1)

Most Commonly Observed Adverse Reactions

The most commonly observed adverse reactions in patients administered Exelon Patch in Study 1 [see Clinical Studies (14)], defined as those occurring at a frequency of at least 5% in the 9.5 mg/24 hours Exelon Patch arm and at a frequency at higher than in the placebo group, were nausea, vomiting, and diarrhea. These reactions were dose-related, with each being more common in patients using the 17.4 mg/24 hours Exelon Patch than in those using the 9.5 mg/24 hours Exelon Patch.

Discontinuation Rates

In Study 1, which randomized a total of 1195 patients, the proportions of patients in the Exelon Patch 9.5 mg/24 hours, Exelon Capsules 6 mg twice daily, and placebo groups who discontinued treatment due to adverse events were 9.6%, 8.1%, and 5.0%, respectively.

The most common adverse reactions in the Exelon Patch-treated groups that led to treatment discontinuation in this study were nausea and vomiting. The proportions of patients who discontinued treatment due to nausea were 0.7%, 1.7%, and 1.3% in the Exelon Patch 9.5 mg/24 hours, Exelon Capsules 6 mg twice daily, and placebo groups, respectively. The proportions of patients who discontinued treatment due to vomiting were 0%, 2.0%, and 0.3% in the Exelon Patch 9.5 mg/24 hours, Exelon Capsules 6 mg twice daily, and placebo groups, respectively.

Adverse Reactions Observed at an Incidence of ≥2%

Table 1 lists adverse reactions seen at an incidence of ≥2% in either Exelon Patch-treated group in Study 1 and for which the rate of occurrence was greater for patients treated with that dose of Exelon Patch than for those treated with placebo. The unapproved 17.4 mg/24 hours Exelon Patch arm is included to demonstrate the increased rates of gastrointestinal adverse reactions over those seen with the 9.5 mg/24 hours Exelon Patch.

[See table 1 above]

Table 1: Proportion of Adverse Reactions Observed with a Frequency of ≥2% and Occurring at a Rate Greater Than Placebo in Study 1

	Exelon Patch 9.5 mg/24 hours	Exelon Patch 17.4 mg/24 hours	Exelon Capsule 6 mg twice daily	Placebo
Total Patients Studied	291	303	294	302
Total Percentage of Patients with ARs (%)	51	66	63	46
Nausea	7	21	23	5
Vomiting*	6	19	17	3
Diarrhea	6	10	5	3
Depression	4	4	4	1
Headache	3	4	6	2
Anxiety	3	3	2	1
Anorexia/Decreased Appetite	3	9	9	2
Weight Decreased**	3	8	5	1
Dizziness	2	7	7	2
Abdominal Pain	2	4	1	1
Urinary Tract Infection	2	2	1	1
Asthenia	2	3	6	1
Fatigue	2	2	1	1
Insomnia	1	4	2	2
Abdominal Pain Upper	1	3	2	2
Vertigo	0	2	1	1

*Vomiting was severe in 0% of patients who received Exelon Patch 9.5 mg/24 hours, 1% of patients who received Exelon Patch 17.4 mg/24 hours, 1% of patients who received the Exelon Capsule at doses up to 6 mg BID, and 0% of those who received placebo.

**Weight Decreased as presented in Table 1 is based upon clinical observations and/or adverse events reported by patients or caregivers. Body weight was also monitored at prespecified time points throughout the course of the clinical study. The proportion of patients who had weight loss equal to or greater than 7% of their baseline weight was 8% of those treated with Exelon Patch 9.5 mg/24 hours, 12% of those treated with Exelon Patch 17.4 mg/24 hours, 11% of patients who received the Exelon Capsule at doses up to 6 mg BID and 6% of those who received placebo. It is not clear how much of the weight loss was associated with anorexia, nausea, vomiting, and the diarrhea associated with the drug.

48-Week International Active Comparator-Controlled Trial (Study 2)

Most Commonly Observed Adverse Reactions

In Study 2 *[see Clinical Studies (14)]* of the commonly observed adverse reactions (≥3% in any treatment group) the most frequent event in the Exelon Patch 13.3 mg/24 hours group was nausea, followed by vomiting, fall, weight decreased, application site erythema, decreased appetite, diarrhea and urinary tract infection (Table 3). The percentage of patients with these events was higher in the Exelon Patch 13.3 mg/24 hours group than in the Exelon Patch 9.5 mg/24 hours group. Patients with nausea, vomiting, diarrhea and decreased appetite experienced these reactions more often during the first 4 weeks of the double-blind treatment phase. These reactions decreased over time in each treatment group. Weight decreased was reported to have increased over time in each treatment group.

Discontinuation Rates

Table 2 displays the most common adverse reactions leading to discontinuation during the 48-week, double-blind treatment phase in Study 2.

Table 2: Proportion of Most Common Adverse Reactions (>1% at Any Dose) Leading to Discontinuation During 48-week Double-Blind Treatment Phase in Study 2

	Exelon Patch 13.3 mg/ 24 hours	Exelon Patch 9.5 mg/ 24 hours	Total
Total Patients Studied	280	283	563
Total Percentage of Patients with ARs Leading to Discontinuation (%)	9.6	12.7	11.2
Vomiting	1.4	0.4	0.9
Application site pruritus	1.1	1.1	1.1
Aggression	0.4	1.1	0.7

Most Commonly Observed Adverse Reactions ≥3%

Other adverse reactions of interest which occurred less frequently, but which were observed in a markedly higher percentage of patients in the Exelon Patch 13.3 mg/24 hours group than in the Exelon Patch 9.5 mg/24 hours group in Study 2, included dizziness and upper abdominal pain. The percentage of patients with these reactions decreased over time in each treatment group (Table 3). The majority of patients reported adverse events of mild to moderate severity. The adverse event severity profile was generally similar for both the Exelon Patch 13.3 mg/24 hours and 9.5 mg/24 hours groups.

[See table 3 above]

Table 3: Proportion of Adverse Reactions Over Time in the 48-week Double-Blind (DB) Treatment Phase (at Least 3% in any Treatment Group) in Study 2

	Cumulative Week 0 to 48 (DB Phase)		Week 0 to 24 (DB Phase)		Week >24 to 48 (DB Phase)	
Preferred Term	Exelon Patch 13.3 mg/ 24 hours	Exelon Patch 9.5 mg/ 24 hours	Exelon Patch 13.3 mg/ 24 hours	Exelon Patch 9.5 mg/ 24 hours	Exelon Patch 13.3 mg/ 24 hours	Exelon Patch 9.5 mg/ 24 hours
Total Patients Studied	280	283	280	283	241	246
Total Percentage of Patients with ARs (%)	75	68	65	55	42	40
Nausea	12	5	10	4	4	2
Vomiting	10	5	9	3	3	2
Fall	8	6	4	4	4	3
Weight decreased*	7	3	3	1	5	2
Application site erythema	6	6	6	5	1	2
Decreased appetite	6	3	5	2	2	<1
Diarrhea	6	5	5	4	2	<1
Urinary tract infection	5	4	3	3	3	2
Agitation	5	5	4	3	1	2
Depression	5	5	3	3	3	2
Dizziness	4	1	3	<1	2	<1
Application site pruritus	4	4	4	3	<1	1
Headache	4	4	4	4	<1	<1
Insomnia	4	3	2	1	3	2
Abdominal pain upper	4	1	3	1	1	<1
Anxiety	4	3	2	2	2	1
Hypertension	3	3	3	2	1	1
Urinary incontinence	3	2	2	1	1	<1
Psychomotor hyperactivity	3	3	2	3	2	1
Aggression	2	3	1	3	1	1

*Decreased Weight as presented in Table 3 is based upon clinical observations and/or adverse events reported by patients or caregivers. Body weight was monitored as a vital sign at pre-specified time points throughout the course of the clinical study. The proportion of patients who had weight loss equal to or greater than 7% of their baseline weight was 15.2% of those treated with Exelon Patch 9.5 mg/24 hours and 18.6% of those treated with Exelon Patch 13.3 mg/24 hours during the 48-week double-blind treatment period.

Severe Alzheimer's Disease

24-Week US Controlled Trial (Study 3)

Most Commonly Observed Adverse Reactions

The most commonly observed adverse reactions in patients administered Exelon Patch in the controlled clinical trial, defined as those occurring at a frequency of at least 5% in the 13.3 mg/24 hours Exelon Patch arm and at a frequency higher than in the 4.6 mg/24 hours Exelon Patch were application site erythema, fall, insomnia, vomiting, diarrhea, weight decreased, and nausea (Table 4). Patients in the lower dose group reported more events of agitation, urinary tract infection, and hallucinations than patients in the higher dose group.

Discontinuation Rates

In Study 3 *[see Clinical Studies (14)]*, the proportions of patients in the Exelon Patch 13.3 mg/24 hours (n=355) and Exelon Patch 4.6 mg/24 hours (n=359), who discontinued treatment due to adverse reactions were 20.5% and 14.2%, respectively.

The most frequent adverse reaction leading to discontinuation in the 13.3 mg/24 hours treatment group versus the 4.6 mg/24 hours treatment group was agitation (2.8% versus 2.2%), followed by vomiting (2.5% and 1.1%), nausea (1.7% and 1.1%), decreased appetite (1.7% and 0%), aggression (1.1% and 0.3%), fall (1.1% and 0.3%) and syncope (1.1% and 0.3%). Otherwise, all AEs leading to discontinuation were reported in <1% of patients.

Most Commonly Observed Adverse Reactions ≥5%

Other adverse reactions of interest which were observed in a higher percentage of patients in the Exelon Patch 13.3 mg/24 hours group than in the Exelon Patch 4.6 mg/24 hours group, included application site erythema, fall, insomnia, vomiting, diarrhea, weight decreased, and nausea (Table 4). Overall, the majority of patients in this study experienced adverse reactions that were mild (30.7%) or moderate (32.1%) in severity. Slightly more patients in the 4.6 mg/24 hours patch group reported mild events than in the 13.3 mg/24 hours patch group, while the numbers of patients reporting moderate events were comparable between groups. Severe adverse reactions were reported at a slightly higher percentage at the higher dose (12.4%) than at the lower dose (10%) treatment groups. With the exception of severe adverse reactions of agitation (13.3 mg: 1.1%; 4.6 mg: 1.4%), fall (13.3 mg: 1.1%) and urinary tract infection (4.6 mg: 1.1%), all adverse reactions reported as severe occurred in less than 1% of patients in either treatment group.

Table 4: Proportion of Adverse Reactions in the 24-week Double-Blind (DB) Treatment Phase (at Least 5% in Any Treatment Group) in Study 3

Preferred term	Exelon Patch 13.3 mg/ 24 hours	Exelon Patch 4.6 mg/ 24 hours
Total number of patients studied	355	359
Total percentage of patients with ARs (%)	75	73
Application site erythema	13	12
Agitation	12	14
Urinary tract infection	8	10
Fall	8	6
Insomnia	7	4
Vomiting	7	3
Diarrhea	7	5
Weight decreased*	7	3
Nausea	6	3
Depression	5	4
Decreased appetite	5	1
Anxiety	5	5
Hallucination	2	5

*Weight Decreased as presented in Table 4 is based upon clinical observations and/or adverse events reported by patients or caregivers. Body weight was monitored as a vital sign at prespecified time points throughout the course of the clinical study. The proportion of patients who had weight loss equal to or greater than 7% of their baseline weight was 11% of those treated with Exelon Patch 4.6 mg/24 hours and 14.1% of those treated with Exelon Patch 13.3 mg/24 hours during the 24-week double-blind treatment.

Application Site Reactions in Studies 1, 2, and 3

A direct comparison of the rates of application site reactions reported in the placebo-controlled and active comparator controlled clinical trials cannot be made due to differences in the method of data collection employed in each of the trials.

In Study 1, cases of skin irritation were captured separately on an investigator-rated skin irritation scale and not as adverse events unless they fulfilled the criteria for a serious adverse event. Among the skin reactions reported were the following: application site reactions, application site dermatitis, and application site irritation.

In Study 2, cases of application site reactions were captured as patient or caregiver reported adverse events. The most commonly reported skin irritation events for both treatment groups were application site erythema and application site pruritus. These events occurred more frequently during the first 24 weeks of the double-blind period and decreased over time in each treatment group after 24 weeks (Table 3). The most common reason for discontinuation due to application site reactions was application site pruritus which occurred in 1.1% of the patients in each treatment group (Table 2).

In Study 3, cases of application site reactions were captured as patient or caregiver reported adverse events. The most commonly reported skin irritation events during the 24 weeks of the study were application site erythema and application site pruritus (Table 4). The most common reason for discontinuation due to application site reactions were application site erythema and application site pruritus which occurred in less than 1% of patients in each treatment group.

Other Adverse Events Observed During Clinical Trials

The frequencies represent the proportion of 2348 patients from 3 controlled and 4 open-label trials in North America, Europe, Latin America, Asia, and Japan who experienced that event while receiving Exelon Patch. All patch doses are pooled.

All adverse events occurring in approximately 0.1% of patients are included, except for those already listed elsewhere in labeling, too general to be informative, or relatively minor events.

Events are classified by system organ class and listed using the following definitions: *Frequent*–those occurring in at least 1/100 patients; *Infrequent*–those occurring in 1/100 to 1/1000 patients. These adverse events are not necessarily related to Exelon Patch treatment and in most cases were observed at a similar frequency in placebo-treated patients in the controlled studies.

Cardiac Disorders: *Infrequent*: Bradycardia, atrial fibrillation, atrioventricular block, arrhythmia, supraventricular extrasystole.

Ear and Labyrinth Disorders: *Infrequent*: Tinnitus.

Eye Disorders: *Infrequent*: Vision blurred.

Gastrointestinal System: *Frequent*: Constipation, gastritis. *Infrequent*: Gastroesophageal reflux disease, hematochezia, hematemesis, pancreatitis, salivary hypersecretion.

General Disorders and Administration Site Conditions: *Infrequent*: Chest pain.

Injury, Poisoning and Procedural Complications: *Infrequent*: Hip fracture.

Investigations: *Infrequent*: Blood creatine phosphokinase increased, lipase increased, blood amylase increased, electrocardiogram QT prolonged.

Metabolic and Nutritional Disorders: *Frequent*: Dehydration. *Infrequent*: Hypokalemia, hyponatremia.

Nervous System Disorders: *Infrequent*: Migraine.

Psychiatric Disorders: *Infrequent*: Delirium.

Respiratory, Thoracic, and Mediastinal Disorders: *Infrequent*: Dyspnea, bronchospasm.

Skin and Subcutaneous Tissue Disorders: *Frequent*: Pruritus. *Infrequent*: Erythema, eczema, dermatitis, rash erythematous, skin ulcer.

Vascular Disorders: *Infrequent*: Hypotension, cerebrovascular accident.

Other Adverse Reactions Observed with Exelon Capsules or Oral Solution

The following additional adverse reactions have been observed with Exelon Capsules/Oral Solution:

Confusion, duodenal ulcers, angina pectoris, myocardial infarction, tremor

Parkinson's Disease Dementia

76-week International Open-Label Trial (Study 4)

Exelon Patch has been administered to 288 patients with mild to moderate Parkinson's Disease Dementia in a single, 76-week, open-label, active-comparator safety study. Of these, 256 have been treated for at least 12 weeks, 232 for at least 24 weeks, and 196 for at least 52 weeks.

Treatment with Exelon Patch was initiated at 4.6 mg/24 hours and if well tolerated the dose was increased after 4 weeks to 9.5 mg/24 hours. Exelon Capsule (target maintenance dose of 12 mg/day) served as the active comparator and was administered to 294 patients. Treatment emergent adverse reactions are presented in Table 5.

Table 5: Proportion of Adverse Reactions Reported at a Rate ≥2% During the Initial 24-Week Period in Study 4

Adverse drug reactions	Exelon Patch
Total patients studied	288
	Percentage (%)
Psychiatric disorders	
Insomnia	6
Depression	6
Anxiety	5
Agitation	3
Nervous system disorders	
Tremor	7
Dizziness	6
Somnolence	4
Hypokinesia	4
Bradykinesia	4
Cogwheel rigidity	3
Dyskinesia	3
Gastrointestinal disorders	
Abdominal pain	2
Vascular disorders	
Hypertension	3
General disorders and administration site conditions	
Fall	12
Application site erythema	11
Application site irritation, pruritus, rash	3; 5; 2
Fatigue	4
Asthenia	2
Gait disturbance	4

Additional adverse reactions observed during the 76-week prospective, open-label study in patients with dementia associated with Parkinson's disease treated with Exelon transdermal patches: Frequent (those occurring in at least 1/100 patients): dehydration, weight decreased, aggression, hallucination visual.

In patients with dementia associated with Parkinson's disease the following adverse drug reactions have only been observed in clinical trials with Exelon Capsules: Frequent: nausea, vomiting, decreased appetite, restlessness, worsening of Parkinson's disease, bradycardia, diarrhea, dyspepsia, salivary hypersecretion, sweating increased; Infrequent (those occurring between 1/100 to 1/1000 patients): dystonia, atrial fibrillation, atrioventricular block.

6.2 Postmarketing Experience

The following additional adverse reactions have been identified based on postmarketing spontaneous reports and are not listed above. Because these reactions are reported voluntarily from a population of uncertain size, it is not always possible to reliably estimate their frequency or establish a causal relationship to drug exposure.

Hypertension, application site hypersensitivity, urticaria, blister, allergic dermatitis, seizure, worsening of Parkinson's disease in patients with Parkinson's disease who were treated with Exelon Patch, tachycardia, abnormal liver function tests, disseminated cutaneous hypersensitivity reactions.

7 DRUG INTERACTIONS

7.1 Cholinomimetic and Anticholinergic Drugs

Rivastigmine may increase the cholinergic effects of other cholinomimetic drugs. Rivastigmine may also interfere with the activity of anticholinergic medications. Avoid concomitant use of rivastigmine with drugs having these pharmacologic effects unless deemed clinically necessary.

8 USE IN SPECIFIC POPULATIONS

8.1 Pregnancy

Pregnancy Category B

There are no adequate and well-controlled studies in pregnant women. No dermal reproduction studies in animals have been conducted. Oral reproduction studies conducted in pregnant rats and rabbits revealed no evidence of teratogenicity. Studies in rats showed slightly decreased fetal/pup weight, usually at doses causing some maternal toxicity. Because animal reproduction studies are not always predictive of human response, this drug should be used during pregnancy only if clearly needed.

8.3 Nursing Mothers

Rivastigmine and its metabolites are excreted in rat milk following oral administration of rivastigmine; levels of rivastigmine plus metabolites in rat milk are approximately 2 times that in maternal plasma. It is not known whether rivastigmine is excreted in human milk. Because many drugs are excreted in human milk and because of the potential for serious adverse reactions in nursing infants from Exelon Patch, a decision should be made whether to discontinue nursing or to discontinue the drug, taking into account the importance of the drug to the mother.

8.4 Pediatric Use

Safety and effectiveness in pediatric patients have not been established. Use of Exelon Patch in children and adolescents (below 18 years of age) is not recommended.

8.5 Geriatric Use

Of the total number of subjects in clinical studies of Exelon Patch, 88% were 65 years and over, while 55% were 75 years and over. No overall differences in safety or effectiveness were observed between these subjects and younger subjects, and other reported clinical experience has not identified differences in responses between the elderly and younger patients, but greater sensitivity of some older individuals cannot be ruled out.

8.6 Renal Impairment

No dose adjustment is necessary for patients with renal impairment *[see Clinical Pharmacology (12.3)]*.

8.7 Hepatic Impairment

In patients with mild or moderate hepatic impairment (Child-Pugh score 5 to 9), clearance of oral rivastigmine was reduced *[see Clinical Pharmacology (12.3)]*. In these patients, consider using the lowest dose Exelon Patch (4.6 mg/24 hours) for both initial and maintenance therapy. No data are available on the use of rivastigmine in patients with severe hepatic impairment.

8.8 Low or High Body Weight

Because rivastigmine blood levels vary with weight [see Clinical Pharmacology (12.3)], careful titration and monitoring should be performed in patients with low or high body weights. In patients with low body weight (<50 kg), monitor closely for toxicities (e.g., excessive nausea, vomiting), and consider reducing the maintenance dose to the 4.6 mg/24 hour Exelon Patch if such toxicities develop. In patients with body weight >100 kg, consider the use of doses higher than 9.5 mg/24 hours.

10 OVERDOSAGE

Overdose with Exelon Patch has been reported in the postmarketing setting *[see Warnings and Precautions (5.1)]*. Overdoses have occurred from application of more than one patch at one time and not removing the previous day's patch before applying a new patch. The symptoms reported in these overdose cases are similar to those seen in cases of overdose associated with rivastigmine oral formulations.

Because strategies for the management of overdose are continually evolving, it is advisable to contact a Poison Control Center to determine the latest recommendations for the management of an overdose of any drug. As rivastigmine has a plasma half-life of about 3.4 hours after patch administration and a duration of acetylcholinesterase inhibition of about 9 hours, it is recommended that in cases of asymptomatic overdose the patch should be immediately removed and no further patch should be applied for the next 24 hours.

As in any case of overdose, general supportive measures should be utilized. Overdosage with cholinesterase inhibitors can result in cholinergic crisis characterized by severe nausea, vomiting, salivation, sweating, bradycardia, hypotension, respiratory depression, and convulsions. Increasing muscle weakness is a possibility and may result in death if respiratory muscles are involved. Atypical responses in blood pressure and heart rate have been reported with other drugs that increase cholinergic activity when coadministered with quaternary anticholinergics such as glycopyrrolate. Due to the short plasma elimination half-life of rivastigmine after patch administration, dialysis (hemodialysis, peritoneal dialysis, or hemofiltration) would not be clinically indicated in the event of an overdose.
In overdose accompanied by severe nausea and vomiting, the use of antiemetics should be considered.

11 DESCRIPTION

Exelon Patch (rivastigmine transdermal system) contains rivastigmine, a reversible cholinesterase inhibitor known chemically as (S)-3-[1-(dimethylamino) ethyl]phenyl ethylmethylcarbamate. It has an empirical formula of $C_{14}H_{22}N_2O_2$ as the base and a molecular weight of 250.34 (as the base). Rivastigmine is a viscous, clear, and colorless to yellow to very slightly brown liquid that is sparingly soluble in water and very soluble in ethanol, acetonitrile, n-octanol and ethyl acetate.
The distribution coefficient at 37°C in n-octanol/phosphate buffer solution pH 7 is 4.27.

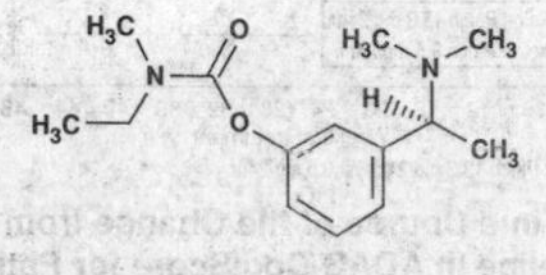

Exelon Patch is for transdermal administration. The patch is a 4-layer laminate containing the backing layer, drug matrix, adhesive matrix and overlapping release liner (see Figure 1). The release liner is removed and discarded prior to use.

Figure 1: Cross Section of the Exelon Patch

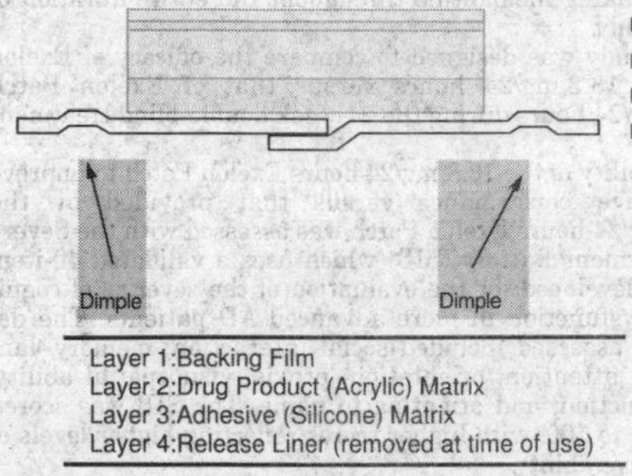

Excipients within the formulation include acrylic copolymer, poly(butylmethacrylate, methylmethacrylate), silicone adhesive applied to a flexible polymer backing film, silicone oil, and vitamin E.

12 CLINICAL PHARMACOLOGY

12.1 Mechanism of Action

Although the precise mechanism of action of rivastigmine is unknown, it is thought to exert its therapeutic effect by enhancing cholinergic function. This is accomplished by increasing the concentration of acetylcholine through reversible inhibition of its hydrolysis by cholinesterase. The effect of rivastigmine may lessen as the disease process advances and fewer cholinergic neurons remain functionally intact. There is no evidence that rivastigmine alters the course of the underlying dementing process.

12.2 Pharmacodynamics

After a 6-mg oral dose of rivastigmine in humans, anticholinesterase activity is present in cerebrospinal fluid for about 10 hours, with a maximum inhibition of about 60% 5 hours after dosing.
In vitro and *in vivo* studies demonstrate that the inhibition of cholinesterase by rivastigmine is not affected by the concomitant administration of memantine, an N-methyl-D-aspartate receptor antagonist.

12.3 Pharmacokinetics

Absorption
After the initial application of Exelon Patch, there is a lag time of 0.5 to 1 hour in the absorption of rivastigmine. Concentrations then rise slowly typically reaching a maximum after 8 hours, although maximum values (C_{max}) can also occur later (at 10 to 16 hours). After the peak, plasma concentrations slowly decrease over the remainder of the 24-hour period of application. At steady state, trough levels are approximately 60 to 80% of peak levels.
Exelon Patch 9.5 mg/24 hours gave exposure approximately the same as that provided by an oral dose of 6 mg twice daily (i.e., 12 mg/day). Inter-subject variability in exposure was lower (43% to 49%) for the Exelon Patch formulation as compared with the oral formulations (73% to 103%). Fluctuation (between C_{max} and C_{min}) is less for Exelon Patch than for the oral formulation of rivastigmine.
Figure 2 displays rivastigmine plasma concentrations over 24 hours for the 3 available patch strengths.

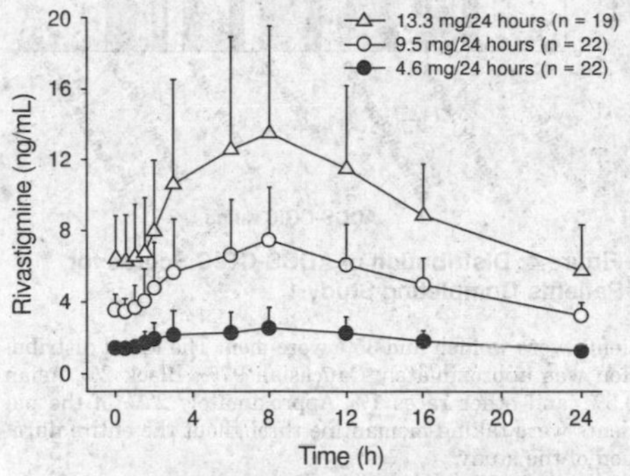

Figure 2: Rivastigmine Plasma Concentrations Following Dermal 24-Hour Patch Application

Over a 24-hour dermal application, approximately 50% of the drug content of the patch is released from the system. Exposure (AUC_{∞}) to rivastigmine (and metabolite NAP266-90) was highest when the patch was applied to the upper back, chest, or upper arm. Two other sites (abdomen and thigh) could be used if none of the 3 other sites is available, but the practitioner should be aware that the rivastigmine plasma exposure associated with these sites was approximately 20% to 30% lower.
There was no relevant accumulation of rivastigmine or the metabolite NAP226-90 in plasma in patients with Alzheimer's disease with daily dosing.
The pharmacokinetic profile of rivastigmine transdermal patches was comparable in patients with Alzheimer's disease and in patients with dementia associated with Parkinson's disease.

Distribution
Rivastigmine is weakly bound to plasma proteins (approximately 40%) over the therapeutic range. It readily crosses the blood-brain barrier, reaching CSF peak concentrations in 1.4 to 2.6 hours. It has an apparent volume of distribution in the range of 1.8 to 2.7 L/kg.

Metabolism
Rivastigmine is extensively metabolized primarily via cholinesterase-mediated hydrolysis to the decarbamylated metabolite NAP226-90. *In vitro*, this metabolite shows minimal inhibition of acetylcholinesterase (<10%). Based on evidence from *in vitro* and animal studies, the major cytochrome P450 isoenzymes are minimally involved in rivastigmine metabolism.
The metabolite-to-parent AUC_{∞} ratio was about 0.7 after Exelon Patch application versus 3.5 after oral administration, indicating that much less metabolism occurred after dermal treatment. Less NAP226-90 is formed following patch application, presumably because of the lack of presystemic (hepatic first pass) metabolism. Based on *in vitro* studies, no unique metabolic routes were detected in human skin.

Elimination
Renal excretion of the metabolites is the major route of elimination. Unchanged rivastigmine is found in trace amounts in the urine. Following administration of ^{14}C-rivastigmine, renal elimination was rapid and essentially complete (>90%) within 24 hours. Less than 1% of the administered dose is excreted in the feces. The apparent elimination half-life in plasma is approximately 3 hours after patch removal. Renal clearance was approximately 2.1 to 2.8 L/hr.

Renal Impairment
No study was conducted with Exelon Patch in subjects with renal impairment. Based on population analysis creatinine clearance did not show any clear effect on steady state concentrations of rivastigmine or its metabolite. No dosage adjustment is necessary in patients with renal impairment.

Hepatic Impairment
No pharmacokinetic study was conducted with Exelon Patch in subjects with hepatic impairment. After multiple 6-mg twice daily oral dosing, the mean clearance of rivastigmine was 65% lower in mild (n=7, Child-Pugh score 5 to 6) and moderate (n=3, Child-Pugh score 7 to 9) hepatically impaired patients (biopsy proven, liver cirrhosis) than in healthy subjects (n=10) *[see Dosage and Administration (2.2), Specific Population (8.7)]*.

Body Weight
A relationship between drug exposure at steady state (rivastigmine and metabolite NAP226-90) and body weight was observed in Alzheimer's dementia patients. Rivastigmine exposure is higher in subjects with low body weight. Compared to a patient with a body weight of 65 kg, the rivastigmine steady-state concentrations in a patient with a body weight of 35 kg would be approximately doubled, while for a patient with a body weight of 100 kg the concentrations would be approximately halved *[see Dosage and Administration (2.2)]*.

Age
Age had no impact on the exposure to rivastigmine in Alzheimer's disease patients treated with Exelon Patch.

Gender or Race
No specific pharmacokinetic study was conducted to investigate the effect of gender and race on the disposition of Exelon Patch. A population pharmacokinetic analysis of oral rivastigmine indicated that neither gender (n=277 males and 348 females) nor race (n=575 Caucasian, 34 Black, 4 Asian, and 12 Other) affected clearance of the drug. Similar results were seen with analyses of pharmacokinetic data obtained after the administration of Exelon Patch.

Smoking
Population pharmacokinetic analysis showed that nicotine use increased the oral clearance of rivastigmine by 23% (n=75 smokers and 549 nonsmokers).

Drug Interaction Studies
No specific interaction studies have been conducted with Exelon Patch. Information presented below is from studies with oral rivastigmine.

Effect of Rivastigmine on the Metabolism of Other Drugs
Rivastigmine is primarily metabolized through hydrolysis by esterases. Minimal metabolism occurs via the major cytochrome P450 isoenzymes. Based on *in vitro* studies, no pharmacokinetic drug interactions with drugs metabolized by the following isoenzyme systems are expected: CYP1A2, CYP2D6, CYP3A4/5, CYP2E1, CYP2C9, CYP2C8, CYP2C19, or CYP2B6.
No pharmacokinetic interaction was observed between rivastigmine taken orally and digoxin, warfarin, diazepam or fluoxetine in studies in healthy volunteers. The increase in prothrombin time induced by warfarin is not affected by administration of rivastigmine.

Effect of Other Drugs on the Metabolism of Rivastigmine
Drugs that induce or inhibit CYP450 metabolism are not expected to alter the metabolism of rivastigmine.
Population pharmacokinetic analysis with a database of 625 patients showed that the pharmacokinetics of rivastigmine taken orally were not influenced by commonly prescribed medications such as antacids (n=77), antihypertensives (n=72), ß-blockers (n=42), calcium channel blockers (n=75), antidiabetics (n=21), nonsteroidal anti-inflammatory drugs (n=79), estrogens (n=70), salicylate analgesics (n=177), antianginals (n=35), and antihistamines (n=15).

13 NONCLINICAL TOXICOLOGY

13.1 Carcinogenesis, Mutagenesis, Impairment of Fertility

Carcinogenesis
In oral carcinogenicity studies conducted at doses up to 1.1 mg base/kg/day in rats and 1.6 mg base/kg/day in mice, rivastigmine was not carcinogenic.
In a dermal carcinogenicity study conducted at doses up to 0.75 mg base/kg/day in mice, rivastigmine was not carcinogenic. The mean rivastigmine plasma exposure (AUC) at this dose was less than that in humans at the maximum recommended human dose (13.3 mg/24 hours).
Mutagenesis
Rivastigmine was clastogenic in *in vitro* chromosomal aberration assays in mammalian cells in the presence, but not the absence, of metabolic activation. Rivastigmine was negative in an *in vitro* bacterial reverse mutation (Ames) assay, an *in vitro* HGPRT assay, and in an *in vivo* mouse micronucleus test.
Impairment of Fertility
No fertility or reproduction studies of dermal rivastigmine have been conducted in animals. Rivastigmine had no effect on fertility or reproductive performance in rats at oral doses up to 1.1 mg base/kg/day.

14 CLINICAL STUDIES

The effectiveness of the Exelon Patch in dementia of the Alzheimer's type and dementia associated with Parkinson's disease was based on the results of 3 controlled trials of Exelon Patch in patients with Alzheimer's disease (Studies 1, 2, and 3) (see below); 3 controlled trials of oral rivastigmine in patients with dementia of the Alzheimer's type; and 1 controlled trial of oral rivastigmine in patients with dementia associated with Parkinson's disease. See the prescribing information for oral rivastigmine for details of the four studies of oral rivastigmine.

Mild to Moderate Alzheimer's Disease

International 24-Week Study of Exelon Patch in Dementia of the Alzheimer's Type (Study 1)

This study was a randomized double-blind, double dummy clinical investigation in patients with Alzheimer's disease [diagnosed by NINCDS-ADRDA and DSM-IV criteria, Mini-Mental Status Examination (MMSE) score ≥10 and ≤20] (Study 1). The mean age of patients participating in this trial was 74 years with a range of 50 to 90 years. Approximately 67% of patients were women, and 33% were men. The racial distribution was Caucasian 75%, Black 1%, Asian 9%, and other races 15%.

The effectiveness of the Exelon Patch was evaluated in Study 1 using a dual outcome assessment strategy, evaluating for changes in both cognitive performance and overall clinical effect.

The ability of the Exelon Patch to improve cognitive performance was assessed with the cognitive subscale of the Alzheimer's Disease Assessment Scale (ADAS-Cog), a multi-item instrument that has been extensively validated in longitudinal cohorts of Alzheimer's disease patients. The ADAS-Cog examines selected aspects of cognitive performance including elements of memory, orientation, attention, reasoning, language, and praxis. The ADAS-Cog scoring range is from 0 to 70, with higher scores indicating greater cognitive impairment. Elderly normal adults may score as low as 0 or 1, but it is not unusual for non-demented adults to score slightly higher.

The ability of the Exelon Patch to produce an overall clinical effect was assessed using the Alzheimer's Disease Cooperative Study-Clinical Global Impression of Change (ADCS-CGIC). The ADCS-CGIC is a more standardized form of the Clinician's Interview-Based Impression Of Change-Plus (CIBIC-Plus) and is also scored as a 7-point categorical rating; scores range from 1, indicating "markedly improved," to 4, indicating "no change," to 7, indicating "marked worsening."

In Study 1, 1195 patients were randomized to 1 of the following 4 treatments: Exelon Patch 9.5 mg/24 hours, Exelon Patch 17.4 mg/24 hours, Exelon Capsules in a dose of 6 mg twice daily, or placebo. This 24-week study was divided into a 16-week titration phase followed by an 8-week maintenance phase. In the active treatment arms of this study, doses below the target dose were permitted during the maintenance phase in the event of poor tolerability.

Figure 3 illustrates the time course for the change from baseline in ADAS-Cog scores for all 4 treatment groups over the 24-week study. At 24 weeks, the mean differences in the ADAS-Cog change scores for the Exelon-treated patients compared to the patients on placebo, were 1.8, 2.9, and 1.8 units for the Exelon Patch 9.5 mg/24 hours, Exelon Patch 17.4 mg/24 hours, and Exelon Capsule 6 mg twice daily groups, respectively. The difference between each of these groups and placebo was statistically significant. Although a slight improvement was observed with the 17.4 mg/24 hours patch compared to the 9.5 mg/24 hours patch on this outcome measure, no meaningful difference between the two was seen on the global evaluation (see Figure 4).

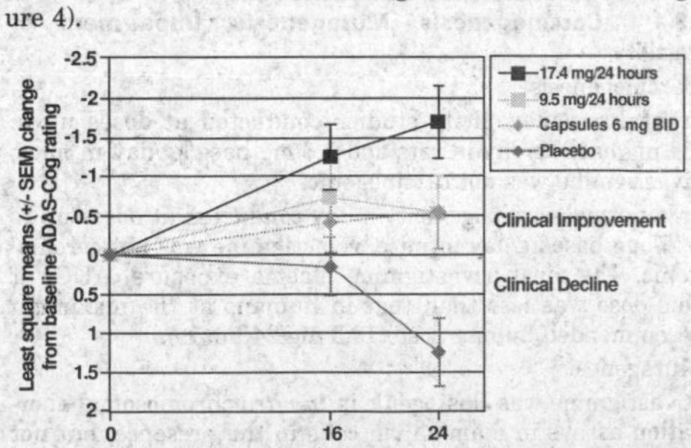

Figure 3: Time Course of the Change from Baseline in ADAS-Cog Score for Patients Observed at Each Time Point in Study 1

Figure 4 presents the distribution of patients' scores on the ADCS-CGIC for all 4 treatment groups. At 24 weeks, the mean difference in the ADCS-CGIC scores for the comparison of patients in each of the Exelon-treated groups with the patients on placebo was 0.2 units. The difference between each of these groups and placebo was statistically significant.

[See figure 4 at top of next column]

International 48-Week Study of Exelon Patch in Dementia of the Alzheimer's Type (Study 2)

This study was a randomized double-blind clinical investigation in patients with Alzheimer's disease [diagnosed by NINCDS-ADRDA and DSM-IV criteria, Mini-Mental State Examination (MMSE) score ≥10 and ≤24] (Study 2). The mean age of patients participating in this trial was 76 years with a range of 50 to 85 years. Approximately 65% of patients were women and 35% were men. The racial distribution was approximately Caucasian 97%, Black 2%, Asian 0.5%, and other races 1%. Approximately 27% of the patients were taking memantine throughout the entire duration of the study.

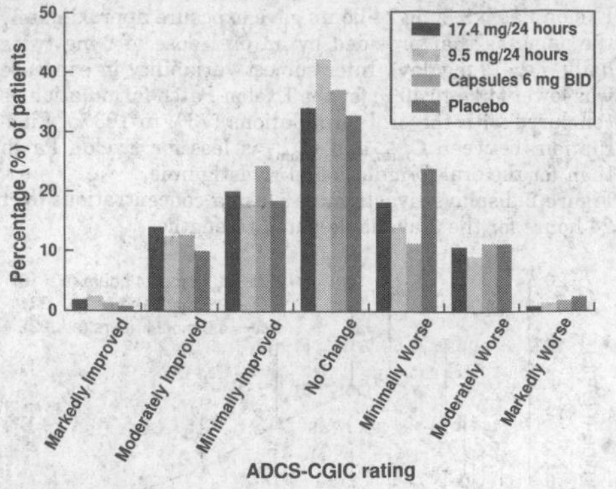

Figure 4: Distribution of ADCS-CGIC Scores for Patients Completing Study 1

Alzheimer's disease patients who received 24 to 48 weeks open-label treatment with Exelon Patch 9.5mg/24 hours and who demonstrated functional and cognitive decline were randomized into treatment with either Exelon Patch 9.5 mg/24 hours or Exelon Patch 13.3 mg/24 hours in a 48-week, double-blind treatment phase. Functional decline was assessed by the investigator and cognitive decline was defined as a decrease in the MMSE score of ≥2 points from the previous visit or a decrease of ≥3 points from baseline.

Study 2 was designed to compare the efficacy of Exelon Patch 13.3 mg/24 hours versus that of Exelon Patch 9.5 mg/24 hours during the 48-week, double-blind treatment phase.

The ability of the Exelon Patch 13.3 mg/24 hours to improve cognitive performance over that provided by the Exelon Patch 9.5 mg/24 hours was assessed by the cognitive subscale of the Alzheimer's Disease Assessment Scale (ADAS-Cog) *[see Clinical Studies, International 24-Week Study (14)]*.

The ability of the Exelon Patch 13.3 mg/24 hours to improve overall function versus that provided by Exelon Patch 9.5 mg/24 hours was assessed by the instrumental subscale of the Alzheimer's Disease Cooperative Study Activities of Daily Living (ADCS-IADL). The ADCS-IADL subscale is composed of items 7 to 23 of the caregiver-based ADCS-ADL scale. The ADCS-IADL assesses activities such as those necessary for communicating and interacting with other people, maintaining a household, and conducting hobbies and interests. A sum score is calculated by adding the scores of the individual items and can range from 0 to 56, with higher scores indicating less impairment.

Out of a total of 1584 patients enrolled in the initial open-label phase of the study, 567 patients were classified as decliners and were randomized into the 48-week double-blind treatment phase of the study. Two hundred eighty-seven (287) patients entered the 9.5 mg/24 hours Exelon Patch treatment group and 280 patients entered the 13.3 mg/24 hours Exelon Patch treatment group.

Figure 5 illustrates the time course for the mean change from double-blind baseline in ADCS-IADL scores for each treatment group over the course of the 48-week treatment phase of the study. Decline in the mean ADCS-IADL score from the double-blind baseline for the Intent to Treat–Last Observation Carried Forward (ITT-LOCF) analysis was less at each timepoint in the 13.3 mg/24 hour Exelon Patch treatment group than in the 9.5 mg/24 hours Exelon Patch treatment group. The 13.3 mg/24 hours dose was statistically significantly superior to the 9.5mg/24 hours dose at weeks 16, 24, 32, and 48 (primary endpoint).

Figure 6 illustrates the time course for the mean change from double-blind baseline in ADAS-Cog scores for both treatment groups over the 48-week treatment phase. The between-treatment group difference for Exelon Patch 13.3 mg/24 hours versus Exelon Patch 9.5 mg/24 hours was nominally statistically significant at week 24 (p=0.027), but not at week 48 (p=0.227), which was the primary endpoint.

[See figure 5 at top of next column]
[See figure 6 at top of next column]

Severe Alzheimer's Disease

24-Week United States Study with Exelon Patch in Severe Alzheimer's Disease (Study 3)

This was a 24-week randomized double-blind, clinical investigation in patients with severe Alzheimer's disease [diagnosed by NINCDS-ADRDA and DSM-IV criteria, Mini-Mental State Examination (MMSE) score ≥3 and ≤12]. The mean age of patients participating in this trial was 78 years with a range of 51 to 96 years with 62% aged >75 years.

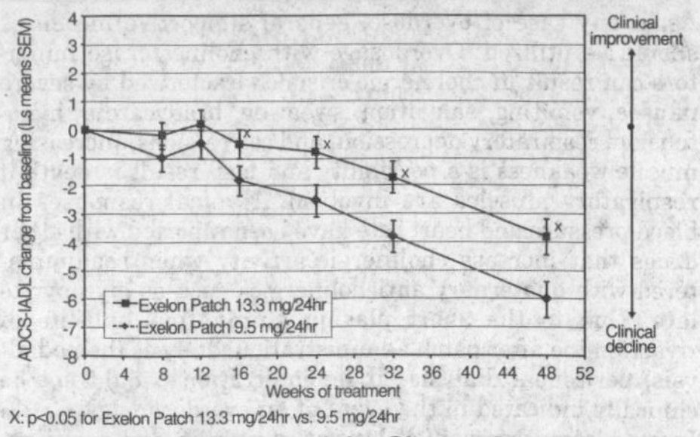

Figure 5: Time Course of the Change from Double-Blind Baseline in ADCS-IADL Score for Patients Observed at Each Time Point in Study 2

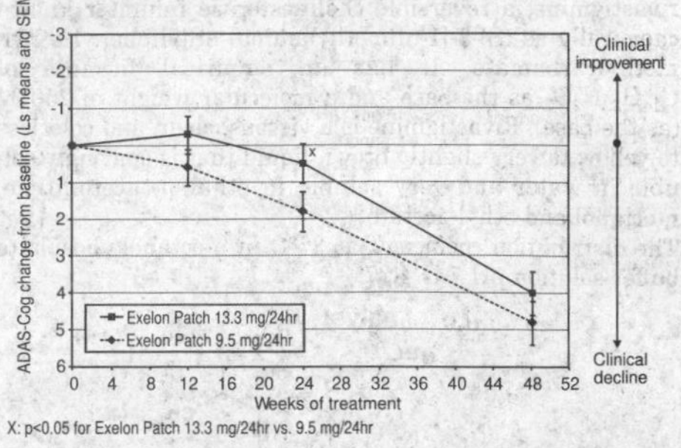

Figure 6: Time Course of the Change from Double-Blind Baseline in ADAS-Cog Score for Patients Observed at Each Time Point in Study 2

Approximately 65% of patients were women and 35% were men. The racial distribution was approximately Caucasian 87%, Black 7%, Asian 1%, and other races 5%. Patients on a stable dose of memantine were permitted to enter the study. Approximately 61% of the patients in each treatment group were taking memantine throughout the entire duration of the study.

The study was designed to compare the efficacy of Exelon Patch 13.3 mg/24 hours versus that of Exelon Patch 4.6 mg/24 hours during the 24-week double-blind treatment phase.

The ability of the 13.3 mg/24 hours Exelon Patch to improve cognitive performance versus that provided by the 4.6 mg/24 hours Exelon Patch was assessed with the Severe Impairment Battery (SIB) which uses a validated 40-item scale developed for the evaluation of the severity of cognitive dysfunction in more advanced AD patients. The domains assessed included social interaction, memory, language, attention, orientation, praxis, visuospatial ability, construction, and orienting to name. The SIB was scored from 0 to 100, with higher scores reflecting higher levels of cognitive ability.

The ability of the 13.3 mg/24 hours Exelon Patch to improve overall function versus that provided by the 4.6 mg/24 hours Exelon Patch was assessed with the Alzheimer's Disease Cooperative Study-Activities of Daily Living-Severe Impairment Version (ADCS-ADL-SIV) which is a caregiver-based ADL scale composed of 19 items developed for use in clinical studies of dementia. It is designed to assess the patient's performance of both basic and instrumental activities of daily living such as those necessary for personal care, communicating and interacting with other people, maintaining a household, conducting hobbies and interests, and making judgments and decisions. A sum score is calculated by adding the scores of the individual items and can range from 0 to 54, with higher scores indicating less functional impairment.

In this study, 716 patients were randomized into one of the following treatments: Exelon Patch 13.3 mg/24 hours or Exelon Patch 4.6 mg/24 hours in a 1:1 ratio. This 24-week study was divided into an 8-week titration phase followed by a 16-week maintenance phase. In the active treatment arms of this study, temporary dose adjustments below the target dose were permitted during the titration and maintenance phase in the event of poor tolerability.

Figure 7 illustrates the time course for the mean change from baseline SIB scores for each treatment group over the course of the 24-week treatment phase of the study. Decline in the mean SIB score from the baseline for the Modified Full Analysis Set (MFAS)-Last Observation Carried Forward (LOCF) analysis was less at each timepoint in the 13.3 mg/24 hour Exelon Patch treatment group than in the 4.6 mg/24 hours Exelon Patch treatment group. The 13.3 mg/24 hours dose was statistically significantly superior to the 4.6 mg/24 hours dose at weeks 16 and 24 (primary endpoint).

Figure 8 illustrates the time course for the mean change from baseline in ADCS-ADL-SIV scores for each treatment group over the course of the 24-week treatment phase of the study. Decline in the mean ADCS-ADL-SIV score from baseline for the MFAS-LOCF analysis was less at each timepoint in the 13.3 mg/24 hour Exelon Patch treatment group than in the 4.6 mg/24 hours Exelon Patch treatment group. The 13.3 mg/24 hours dose was statistically significantly superior to the 4.6 mg/24 hours dose at weeks 16 and 24 (primary endpoint).

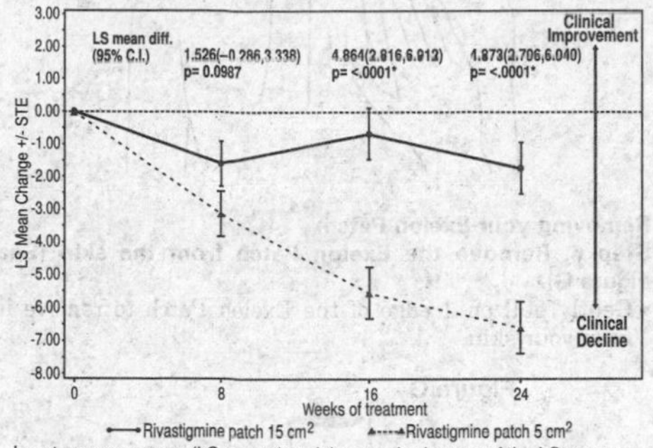

Least squares means (LS means) and the standard errors of the LS means (STE) are based on an analysis of covariance model adjusted for pooled center and baseline.
* indicating statistical significance at a level of 0.05

Figure 7: Time Course of the Change from Baseline in SIB Score for Patients Observed at Each Time Point (Modified Full Analysis Set-LOCF)

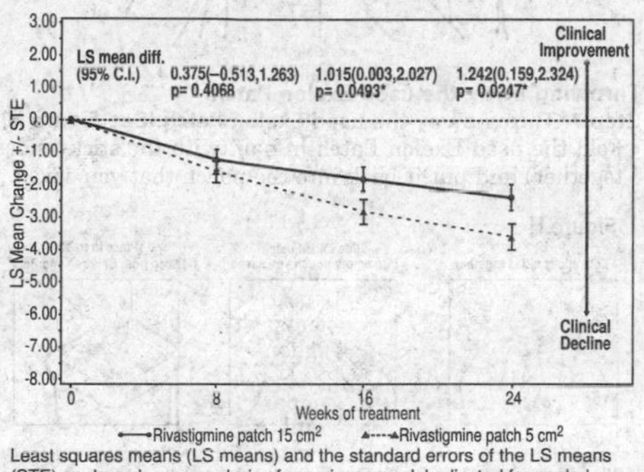

Least squares means (LS means) and the standard errors of the LS means (STE) are based on an analysis of covariance model adjusted for pooled center and baseline.
* indicating statistical significance at a level of 0.05

Figure 8: Time Course of the Change from Baseline in ADCS-ADL-SIV Score for Patients Observed at Each Time Point (Modified Full Analysis Set-LOCF)

16 HOW SUPPLIED/STORAGE AND HANDLING

Exelon Patch: 4.6 mg/24 hours
Each patch of 5 cm^2 contains 9 mg rivastigmine base with *in vivo* release rate of 4.6 mg/24 hours.

Carton of 30 ....NDC 0078-0501-15

Exelon Patch: 9.5 mg/24 hours
Each patch of 10 cm^2 contains 18 mg rivastigmine base with *in vivo* release rate of 9.5 mg/24 hours.

Carton of 30 ....NDC 0078-0502-15

Exelon Patch: 13.3 mg/24 hours
Each patch of 15 cm^2 contains 27 mg rivastigmine base with *in vivo* release rate of 13.3 mg/24 hours.

Carton of 30 ....NDC 0078-0503-15

Store at 25°C (77°F); excursions permitted to 15°C to 30°C (59°F to 86°F) [see USP Controlled Room Temperature]. Keep Exelon Patch in the individual sealed pouch until use. Each pouch contains 1 patch. Used systems should be folded, with the adhesive surfaces pressed together, and discarded safely.

17 PATIENT COUNSELING INFORMATION

See FDA-approved patient labeling (Patient Information).

Importance of Correct Usage
Inform patients or caregivers of the importance of applying the correct dose on the correct part of the body. They should be instructed to rotate the application site in order to minimize skin irritation. The same site should not be used within 14 days. The previous day's patch must be removed before applying a new patch to a different skin location. Exelon Patch should be replaced every 24 hours and the time of day should be consistent. It may be helpful for this to be part of a daily routine, such as the daily bath or shower. Only 1 patch should be worn at a time.

Instruct patients or caregivers to avoid exposure of the patch to external heat sources (excessive sunlight, saunas, solariums) for long periods of time.

Instruct patients who have missed a dose to apply a new patch immediately. They may apply the next patch at the usual time the next day. Instruct patients to not apply 2 patches to make up for 1 missed.

Inform the patient or caregiver to contact the physician for retitration instructions if treatment has been interrupted.

Discarding Used Patches
Instruct patients or caregivers to fold the patch in half after use, return the used patch to its original pouch, and discard it out of the reach and sight of children and pets. They should also be informed that drug still remains in the patch after 24-hour usage. They should be instructed to avoid eye contact and to wash their hands after handling the patch. In case of accidental contact with the eyes, or if their eyes become red after handling the patch, they should be instructed to rinse immediately with plenty of water and to seek medical advice if symptoms do not resolve.

Gastrointestinal Adverse Reactions
Inform patients or caregivers of the potential gastrointestinal adverse reactions such as nausea, vomiting, and diarrhea, including the possibility of dehydration due to these symptoms. Explain that Exelon Patch may affect the patient's appetite and/or the patient's weight. Patients and caregivers should be instructed to look for these adverse reactions, in particular when treatment is initiated or the dose is increased. Instruct patients and caregivers to inform a physician if these adverse reactions persist.

Skin Reactions
Inform patients or caregivers about the potential for allergic contact dermatitis reactions to occur. Patients or caregivers should be instructed to inform a physician if application site reactions spread beyond the patch size, if there is evidence of a more intense local reaction (e.g., increasing erythema, edema, papules, vesicles) and if symptoms do not significantly improve within 48 hours after patch removal.

Concomitant Use of Drugs with Cholinergic Action
Inform patients or caregivers that while wearing Exelon Patch, patients should not be taking Exelon Capsules or Exelon Oral Solution or other drugs with cholinergic effects.

T2013-66
July 2013

Patient Information
Exelon (ECS-'el-on) Patch
(rivastigmine transdermal system)
Exelon Patch is for skin use only.

What is Exelon Patch?
Exelon Patch is a prescription medicine used to treat:
- Mild, moderate, and severe memory problems (dementia) associated with Alzheimer's disease.
- Mild to moderate memory problems (dementia) associated with Parkinson's disease.

Based on clinical trials conducted over 6 to 12 months Exelon Patch was shown to help with cognition which includes (memory, understanding communication, reasoning) and with doing daily tasks. Exelon Patch does not work the same in all people. Some people treated with Exelon Patch may:
- Seem much better
- Get better in small ways or stay the same
- Get worse but slower than expected
- Not change and then get worse as expected

Some patients will not benefit from treatment with Exelon Patch. Exelon Patch does not cure Alzheimer's disease. All patients with Alzheimer's disease get worse over time.

Exelon Patch comes as a transdermal system that delivers rivastigmine (the medicine in Exelon Patch) through the skin.

It is not known if Exelon Patch is safe or effective in children under 18 years of age.

Who should not use Exelon Patch?
Do not use Exelon Patch if you:
- are allergic to rivastigmine, carbamate derivatives, or any of the ingredients in Exelon Patch. See the end of this leaflet for a complete list of ingredients in Exelon Patch.
- have had a skin reaction that:
  - spread beyond the Exelon Patch size
  - had blisters, increased skin redness, or swelling
  - did not get better within 48 hours after you removed the Exelon Patch

Ask your healthcare provider if you are not sure if you should use Exelon Patch.

What should I tell my healthcare provider before using Exelon Patch?
Before you use Exelon Patch, tell your healthcare provider if you:
- have or have had a stomach ulcer
- are planning to have surgery
- have or have had problems with your heart
- have problems passing urine
- have or have had seizures
- have problems with movement (tremors)
- have asthma or breathing problems
- have a loss of appetite or are losing weight
- have had a skin reaction to rivastigmine (the medicine in Exelon Patch) in the past.
- have any other medical conditions
- are pregnant or plan to become pregnant. It is not known if the medicine in Exelon Patch will harm your unborn baby. Talk to your healthcare provider if you are pregnant or plan to become pregnant.
- are breastfeeding or plan to breastfeed. It is not known if the medicine in Exelon Patch passes into your breast milk. You and your healthcare provider should decide if you will use Exelon Patch or breastfeed. You should not do both.

Tell your healthcare provider about all the medicines you take, including prescription and over-the counter medicines, vitamins, and herbal supplements.

Especially tell your healthcare provider if you take:
- a medicine used to treat inflammation [nonsteroidal anti-inflammatory drugs (NSAIDs)]
- other medicines used to treat Alzheimer's or Parkinson's disease
- an anticholinergic medicine, such as an allergy or cold medicine, a medicine to treat bladder or bowel spasms, or certain asthma medicines, or certain medicines to prevent motion or travel sickness

Ask your healthcare provider if you are not sure if your medicine is one listed above.

Know the medicines you take. Keep a list of them to show to your healthcare provider and pharmacist when you get a new medicine.

How should I use Exelon Patch?
- Use Exelon Patch exactly as your healthcare provider tells you to use it.
- Exelon Patches come in 3 different dosage strengths.
- Your healthcare provider may change your dose as needed.
- Wear only 1 Exelon Patch at a time.
- Exelon Patch is for skin use only.
- Only apply Exelon Patch to healthy skin that is clean, dry, hairless, and free of redness, irritation, burns or cuts.
- Avoid applying Exelon Patch to areas on your body that will be rubbed against tight clothing.
- Do not apply Exelon Patch to skin that has cream, lotion, or powder on it.
- Change your Exelon Patch every 24 hours at the same time of day. You may write the date and time you put on the Exelon Patch with a ballpoint pen before applying the patch to help you remember when to remove it.
- Change your application site every day to avoid skin irritation. You can use the same area, but do not use the exact same spot for at least 14 days after your last application.
- Check to see if the Exelon Patch has become loose when you are bathing, swimming, or showering.
- Exelon Patch is designed to deliver medication during the time it is worn. If your Exelon Patch falls off before its usual replacement time, put on a new Exelon Patch right away. Replace the new patch the next day at the same time as usual. Do not use overlays, bandages, or tape to secure an Exelon Patch that has become loose or try to reapply an Exelon Patch that has fallen off.
- If you miss a dose or forget to change your Exelon Patch apply your next Exelon Patch as soon as you remember. Do not apply 2 Exelon Patches to make up for the missed dose.
- If you miss more than 3 doses of applying Exelon Patch, call your healthcare provider before putting on a new Exelon Patch. You may need to restart Exelon Patch at a lower dose.
- Always remove the old Exelon Patch from the previous day before you apply a new one.
- **Having more than 1 Exelon Patch on your body at the same time can cause you to get too much medicine.** If you accidentally use more than 1 Exelon Patch at a time, call your healthcare provider right away. If you are unable to reach your healthcare provider, call your local Poison Control Center at 1-800-222-1222 or go to the nearest hospital emergency room right away.

What should I avoid while using Exelon Patch?
- Do not touch your eyes after you touch the Exelon Patch. In case of accidental contact with your eyes or if your eyes become red after handling the patch, rinse immediately with plenty of water and seek medical advice if symptoms do not resolve.
- Exelon Patch can cause drowsiness, dizziness, weakness, or fainting. Do not drive, operate heavy machinery, or do other dangerous activities until you know how Exelon Patch affects you.
- Avoid exposure to heat sources such as excessive sunlight, saunas, or sun-rooms for long periods of time.

What are the possible side effects of Exelon Patch?
Exelon Patch may cause serious side effects, including:
- **Medication overdose.** Hospitalization and rarely death may happen when people accidently wear more than 1 patch at the same time. It is important that the old Exelon Patch be removed before you apply a new one. Do not wear more than 1 Exelon Patch at a time.
- **Stomach or bowel (intestinal) problems, including:**
  - nausea
  - vomiting
  - diarrhea

∘ dehydration
∘ loss of appetite
∘ weight loss
∘ bleeding in your stomach (ulcers)

- **Skin reactions.** Some people have had a serious skin reaction called allergic contact dermatitis (ACD) when using Exelon Patch. Stop using Exelon Patch and call your healthcare provider right away if you experience reactions that spread beyond the patch size, are intense in nature and do not improve within 48 hours after the patch is removed. Symptoms of ACD may be intense and include:
  ∘ itching, redness, swelling, warmth or tenderness of the skin
  ∘ peeling or blistering of the skin that may ooze, drain or crust over
- **heart problems**
- **seizures**
- **problems with movement (tremors)**

The most common side effects of Exelon Patch include:

- depression
- headache
- anxiety
- dizziness
- stomach pain
- urinary tract infections
- muscle weakness
- tiredness
- trouble sleeping

Tell your healthcare provider if you have any side effect that bothers you or that does not go away.

These are not all the possible side effects of Exelon Patch. For more information, ask your healthcare provider or pharmacist.

Call your doctor for medical advice about side effects. You may report side effects to the FDA at 1-800-FDA-1088.

How should I store Exelon Patch?

- Store Exelon Patch between 68°F to 77°F (20°C to 25°C).
- Keep Exelon Patch in the sealed pouch until ready to use.

Keep Exelon Patch and all medicines out of the reach of children.

General information about the safe and effective use of Exelon Patch.

Medicines are sometimes prescribed for purposes other than those listed in the Patient Information leaflet. Do not use Exelon Patch for a condition for which it was not prescribed. Do not give Exelon Patch to other people, even if they have the same symptoms you have. It may harm them.

This Patient Information leaflet summarizes the most important information about Exelon Patch. If you would like more information, talk with your healthcare provider. You can ask your pharmacist or healthcare provider for information about Exelon Patch that is written for health professionals.

For more information, go to www.EXELONPATCH.com or call 1-888-669-6682.

What are the ingredients of Exelon Patch?

Active ingredient: rivastigmine

Excipients include: acrylic copolymer, poly (butylmethacrylate, methylmethacrylate), silicone adhesive applied to a flexible polymer backing film, silicone oil, and vitamin E

T2013-67
July 2013

Instructions for Use

Exelon (ECS-'el-on) Patch

(rivastigmine transdermal system)

You will need the following supplies (See Figure A):

Exelon Patch is supplied in cartons containing 30 patches (see Figure A)

Figure A

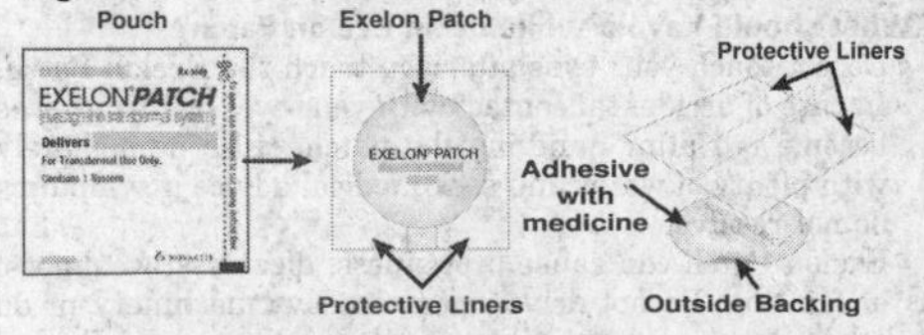

- Exelon Patch is a thin, beige, plastic patch that sticks to the skin. Each Exelon Patch is sealed in a pouch that protects it until you are ready to put it on (See Figure A).
- **Only 1 Exelon Patch should be worn at a time. Do not apply more than 1 Exelon Patch at a time to the body.**
- Do not open the pouch or remove the Exelon Patch until you are ready to apply it.

Using Exelon Patch:

Step 1. Choose an area to apply the Exelon Patch (See Figure B).

- **Instructions for Caregivers:** Apply Exelon Patch to the upper or lower back if it is likely that the patient will remove it. If this is not a concern, the Exelon Patch can be applied **instead** to the upper arm **or** chest. Do not apply the Exelon Patch to areas where it can be rubbed off by tight clothing or belts.
- Only apply the Exelon Patch to healthy skin that is clean, dry, hairless, and free of redness, irritation, burns or cuts.

Figure B

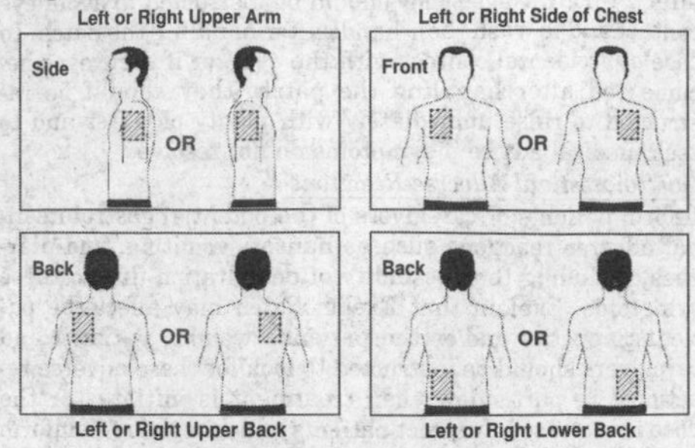

The diagram represents areas on the body where Exelon Patch may be applied. Only 1 patch should be worn at a time. Do not apply multiple patches to the body.

Step 2. Remove the Exelon Patch from the pouch (See Figure C).

Carefully cut the pouch along the dotted line to open and remove the Exelon Patch. Save the pouch for later use.

Figure C

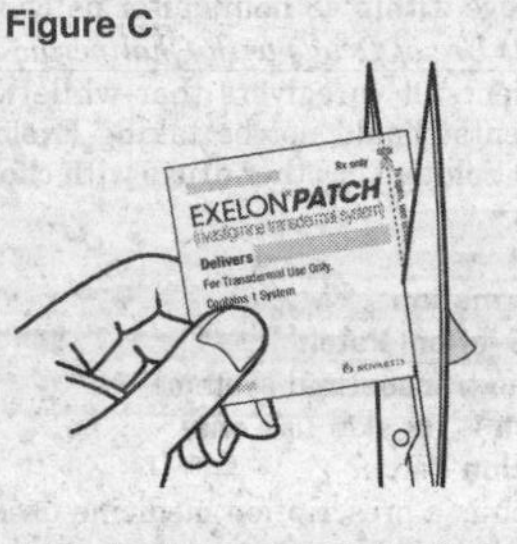

- **Do not cut or fold the Exelon Patch itself.**

Step 3. Remove 1 side of the adhesive liner (See Figure D).

- A protective liner covers the sticky (adhesive) side of the Exelon Patch. Peel off 1 side of the protective cover. Do not touch the sticky part of the Exelon Patch with your fingers.

Figure D

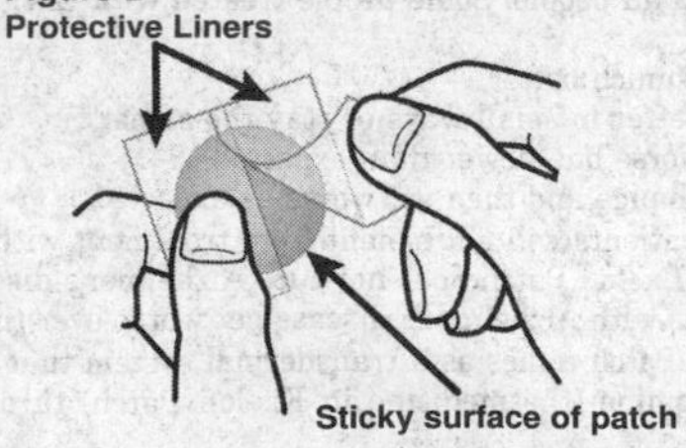

Step 4. Apply the Exelon Patch to your skin (See Figure E).

- Apply the sticky (adhesive) side of the Exelon Patch to your chosen area of skin **and** then peel off the other side of the protective cover.

Figure E

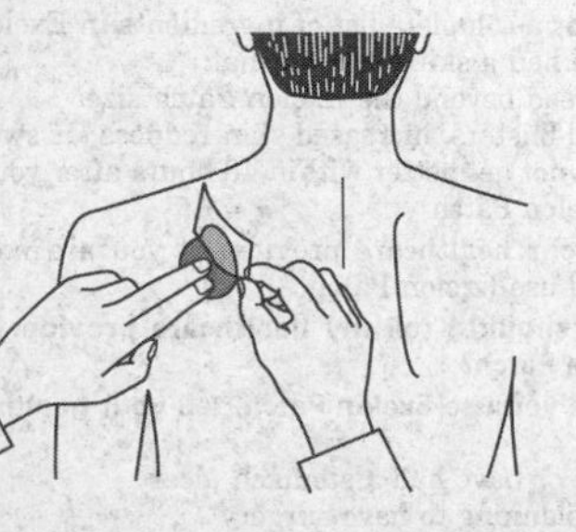

- **Press down on the Exelon Patch firmly for 30 seconds to make sure that the edges stick to your skin (See Figure F).**

[See figure F at top of next column]

Step 5: Wash your hands with soap and water right away.

Note:

- If your Exelon Patch falls off, select a new area, and repeat Steps 2 to 5 to apply a new Exelon Patch.
- Be sure to replace the new Exelon Patch the next day at the same time as usual.

Figure F

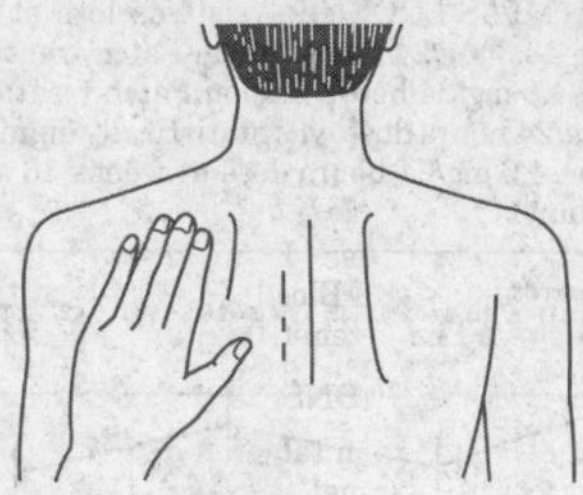

Removing your Exelon Patch:

Step 6. Remove the Exelon Patch from the skin (See Figure G).

- Gently pull on 1 edge of the Exelon Patch to remove it from your skin.

Figure G

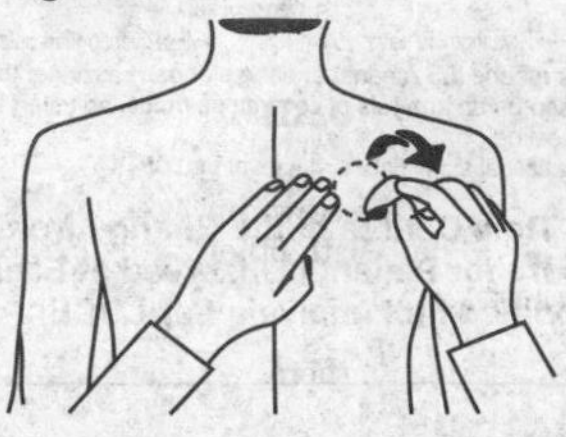

Throwing away the used Exelon Patch:

Step 7. Throw away the used Exelon Patch (See Figure H).

- Fold the used Exelon Patch in half (with the sticky sides together) and put it back into the pouch that you saved.

Figure H

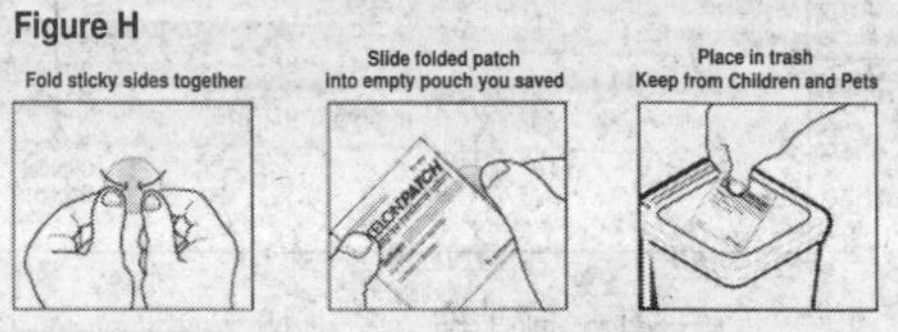

Fold sticky sides together
Slide folded patch into empty pouch you saved
Place in trash Keep from Children and Pets

- Throw away the used Exelon Patch safely and out of the reach of children and pets.
- Some medicine stays in the patch for 24 hours after you use it and should be folded together (sticky side together) and safely thrown away. Do not try to re-use Exelon Patches.

Step 8: Wash your hands with soap and water right away.

- After you remove the Exelon Patch, if any adhesive remains on your skin, you can use soap and water or an oil-based substance (such as baby oil) to remove the adhesive. Alcohol or other dissolving liquids (such as nail polish) should not be used.

This Patient Information and Instructions for Use have been approved by the U.S. Food and Drug Administration.

Distributed by:
Novartis Pharmaceuticals Corporation
East Hanover, New Jersey 07936
©Novartis
T2013-68
July 2013

Shown in Product Identification Guide, page 310

EXFORGE ℞

[X-phorj]

(amlodipine and valsartan)

Tablets

The following prescribing information is based on official labeling in effect July 2013.

HIGHLIGHTS OF PRESCRIBING INFORMATION

These highlights do not include all the information needed to use Exforge safely and effectively. See full prescribing information for Exforge.

Exforge (amlodipine and valsartan) Tablets

Initial U.S. Approval: 2007

WARNING: FETAL TOXICITY

See full prescribing information for complete boxed warning.

- **When pregnancy is detected, discontinue Exforge as soon as possible. (5.1)**
- **Drugs that act directly on the renin-angiotensin system can cause injury and death to the developing fetus. (5.1)**

RECENT MAJOR CHANGES

Boxed Warning: Fetal Toxicity	01/2012
Indications and Usage: Benefits of lowering blood pressure (1)	12/2011
Contraindications: Known hypersensitivity (4)	09/2012
Contraindications: Dual RAS Blockade in Diabetics (4)	11/2012
Warnings and Precautions: Fetal Toxicity (5.1)	01/2012
Drug Interactions: Dual Blockade of the Renin-Angiotensin System (7)	11/2012

INDICATIONS AND USAGE

Exforge is the combination tablet of amlodipine, a dihydropyridine calcium channel blocker (DHP CCB), and valsartan, an angiotensin II receptor blocker (ARB). Exforge is indicated for the treatment of hypertension, to lower blood pressure:

- In patients not adequately controlled on monotherapy (1)
- As initial therapy in patients likely to need multiple drugs to achieve their blood pressure goals (1).

Lowering blood pressure reduces the risk of fatal and nonfatal cardiovascular events, primarily strokes and myocardial infarctions.

DOSAGE AND ADMINISTRATION

General Considerations:

- Majority of effect attained within 2 weeks (2.1)
- May be administered with other antihypertensive agents (2.1)

Hypertension:

- May be used as add-on therapy for patients not controlled on monotherapy (2.2)
- Patients who experience dose-limiting adverse reactions on monotherapy may be switched to Exforge containing a lower dose of that component (2.2)
- May be substituted for titrated components (2.3)
- When used as initial therapy: Initiate with 5/160 mg, then titrate upwards as necessary to a maximum of 10/320 mg once daily (2.4)

DOSAGE FORMS AND STRENGTHS

Tablets (amlodipine/valsartan mg): 5/160, 10/160, 5/320, 10/320 (3)

CONTRAINDICATIONS

Known hypersensitivity to any component;
Do not coadminister aliskiren with Exforge in patients with diabetes (4)

WARNINGS AND PRECAUTIONS

- Hypotension: Correct volume depletion prior to initiation (5.2)
- Increased angina and/or myocardial infarction (5.3)
- Monitor renal function and potassium in susceptible patients (5.4, 5.5)

ADVERSE REACTIONS

In placebo-controlled clinical trials, discontinuation due to side effects occurred in 1.8% of patients in the Exforge-treated patients and 2.1% in the placebo-treated group. The most common reasons for discontinuation of therapy with Exforge were peripheral edema and vertigo. The adverse experiences that occurred in clinical trials (≥2% of patients) at a higher incidence than placebo included peripheral edema, nasopharyngitis, upper respiratory tract infection, and dizziness. (6.1)

To report SUSPECTED ADVERSE REACTIONS, contact Novartis Pharmaceuticals Corporation at 1-888-669-6682 or FDA at 1-800-FDA-1088 or www.fda.gov/medwatch.

DRUG INTERACTIONS

- If simvastatin is coadministered with amlodipine, do not exceed doses greater than 20 mg daily of simvastatin (7)
- NSAID use may lead to increased risk of renal impairment and loss of anti-hypertensive effect (7)
- Dual inhibition of the renin-angiotensin system: Increased risk of renal impairment, hypotension, and hyperkalemia (7)

USE IN SPECIFIC POPULATIONS

Start amlodipine or add amlodipine at 2.5 mg in patients ≥75 years old or in patients with hepatic impairment. (8.5, 8.7)

Nursing Mothers: Avoid use while nursing – discontinue either nursing or drug (8.3)

See 17 for PATIENT COUNSELING INFORMATION and FDA-approved patient labeling

Revised: 11/2012

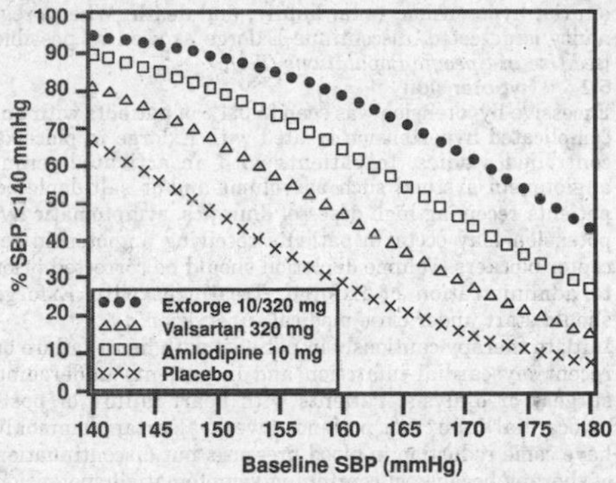

Figure 1: Probability of Achieving Systolic Blood Pressure <140 mmHg at Week 8

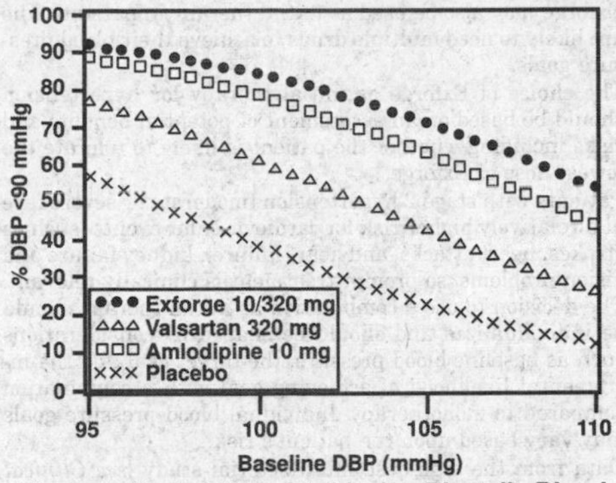

Figure 2: Probability of Achieving Diastolic Blood Pressure <90 mmHg at Week 8

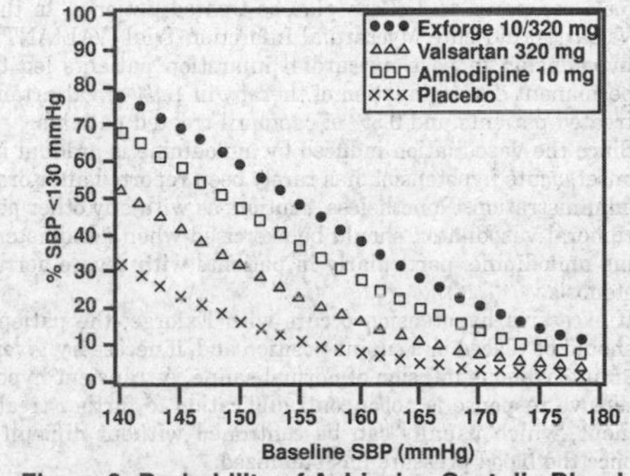

Figure 3: Probability of Achieving Systolic Blood Pressure <130 mmHg at Week 8

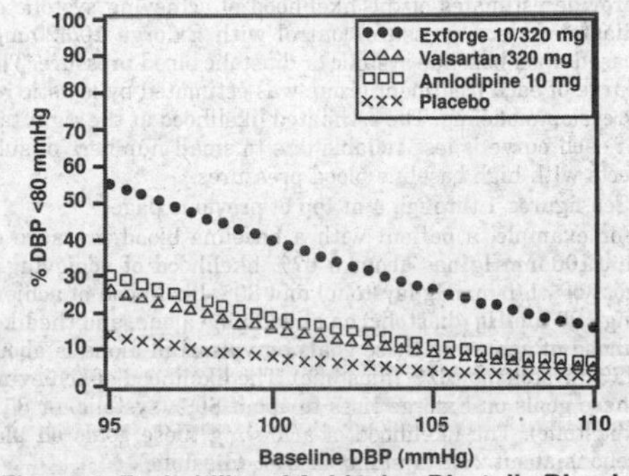

Figure 4: Probability of Achieving Diastolic Blood Pressure <80 mmHg at Week 8

FULL PRESCRIBING INFORMATION: CONTENTS*

*** Sections or subsections omitted from the full prescribing information are not listed**

FULL PRESCRIBING INFORMATION

WARNING: FETAL TOXICITY

- **When pregnancy is detected, discontinue Exforge as soon as possible. (5.1)**
- **Drugs that act directly on the renin-angiotensin system can cause injury and death to the developing fetus. (5.1)**

1 INDICATIONS AND USAGE

1.1 Hypertension

Exforge (amlodipine and valsartan) is indicated for the treatment of hypertension, to lower blood pressure. Lowering blood pressure reduces the risk of fatal and nonfatal cardiovascular events, primarily strokes and myocardial infarctions. These benefits have been seen in controlled trials of antihypertensive drugs from a wide variety of pharmacologic classes, including amlodipine and the ARB class to which valsartan principally belongs. There are no controlled trials demonstrating risk reduction with Exforge.

Control of high blood pressure should be part of comprehensive cardiovascular risk management, including, as appropriate, lipid control, diabetes management, antithrombotic therapy, smoking cessation, exercise, and limited sodium intake. Many patients will require more than 1 drug to achieve blood pressure goals. For specific advice on goals and management, see published guidelines, such as those of the National High Blood Pressure Education Program's Joint National Committee on Prevention, Detection, Evaluation, and Treatment of High Blood Pressure (JNC).

Numerous antihypertensive drugs, from a variety of pharmacologic classes and with different mechanisms of action, have been shown in randomized controlled trials to reduce cardiovascular morbidity and mortality, and it can be concluded that it is blood pressure reduction, and not some other pharmacologic property of the drugs, that is largely responsible for those benefits. The largest and most consistent cardiovascular outcome benefit has been a reduction in the risk of stroke, but reductions in myocardial infarction and cardiovascular mortality also have been seen regularly.

Elevated systolic or diastolic pressure causes increased cardiovascular risk, and the absolute risk increase per mmHg is greater at higher blood pressures, so that even modest reductions of severe hypertension can provide substantial benefit. Relative risk reduction from blood pressure reduction is similar across populations with varying absolute risk, so the absolute benefit is greater in patients who are at higher risk independent of their hypertension (for example, patients with diabetes or hyperlipidemia), and such patients would be expected to benefit from more aggressive treatment to a lower blood pressure goal.

Some antihypertensive drugs have smaller blood pressure effects (as monotherapy) in black patients, and many antihypertensive drugs have additional approved indications and effects (e.g., on angina, heart failure, or diabetic kidney disease). These considerations may guide selection of therapy. Exforge (amlodipine and valsartan) is indicated for the treatment of hypertension.

Exforge may be used in patients whose blood pressure is not adequately controlled on either monotherapy.

Exforge may also be used as initial therapy in patients who are likely to need multiple drugs to achieve their blood pressure goals.

The choice of Exforge as initial therapy for hypertension should be based on an assessment of potential benefits and risks including whether the patient is likely to tolerate the lowest dose of Exforge.

Patients with stage 2 hypertension (moderate or severe) are at a relatively higher risk for cardiovascular events (such as strokes, heart attacks, and heart failure), kidney failure and vision problems, so prompt treatment is clinically relevant. The decision to use a combination as initial therapy should be individualized and should be shaped by considerations such as baseline blood pressure, the target goal and the incremental likelihood of achieving goal with a combination compared to monotherapy. Individual blood pressure goals may vary based upon the patient's risk.

Data from the high-dose multifactorial study [*see Clinical Studies (14)*] provide estimates of the probability of reaching a blood pressure goal with Exforge compared to amlodipine or valsartan monotherapy. The figures below provide estimates of the likelihood of achieving systolic or diastolic blood pressure control with Exforge 10/320 mg, based upon baseline systolic or diastolic blood pressure. The curve of each treatment group was estimated by logistic regression modeling. The estimated likelihood at the right tail of each curve is less reliable due to small numbers of subjects with high baseline blood pressures.

[See figures 1 through 4 at top of previous page]

For example, a patient with a baseline blood pressure of 160/100 mmHg has about a 67% likelihood of achieving a goal of <140 mmHg (systolic) and 80% likelihood of achieving <90 mmHg (diastolic) on amlodipine alone, and the likelihood of achieving these goals on valsartan alone is about 47% (systolic) or 62% (diastolic). The likelihood of achieving these goals on Exforge rises to about 80% (systolic) or 85% (diastolic). The likelihood of achieving these goals on placebo is about 28% (systolic) or 37% (diastolic).

2 DOSAGE AND ADMINISTRATION

2.1 General Considerations

Dose once daily. The dosage can be increased after 1 to 2 weeks of therapy to a maximum of one 10/320mg tablet once daily as needed to control blood pressure. The majority of the antihypertensive effect is attained within 2 weeks after initiation of therapy or a change in dose.

Exforge may be administered with or without food.

Exforge may be administered with other antihypertensive agents.

2.2 Add-on Therapy

A patient whose blood pressure is not adequately controlled with amlodipine (or another dihydropyridine calcium-channel blocker) alone or with valsartan (or another angiotensin II receptor blocker) alone may be switched to combination therapy with Exforge.

A patient who experiences dose-limiting adverse reactions on either component alone may be switched to Exforge containing a lower dose of that component in combination with the other to achieve similar blood pressure reductions. The clinical response to Exforge should be subsequently evaluated and if blood pressure remains uncontrolled after 3 to 4 weeks of therapy, the dose may be titrated up to a maximum of 10/320 mg.

2.3 Replacement Therapy

For convenience, patients receiving amlodipine and valsartan from separate tablets may instead wish to receive tablets of Exforge containing the same component doses.

2.4 Initial Therapy

A patient may be initiated on Exforge if it is unlikely that control of blood pressure would be achieved with a single agent. The usual starting dose is Exforge 5/160 mg once daily in patients who are not volume-depleted.

3 DOSAGE FORMS AND STRENGTHS

5/160 mg tablets, debossed with NVR/ECE (side 1/side 2)
10/160 mg tablets, debossed with NVR/UIC
5/320 mg tablets, debossed with NVR/CSF
10/320 mg tablets, debossed with NVR/LUF

4 CONTRAINDICATIONS

Do not use in patients with known hypersensitivity to any component.

Do not coadminister aliskiren with Exforge in patients with diabetes *[see Drug Interactions (7)]*.

5 WARNINGS AND PRECAUTIONS

5.1 Fetal Toxicity

Pregnancy Category D

Use of drugs that act on the renin-angiotensin system during the second and third trimesters of pregnancy reduces fetal renal function and increases fetal and neonatal morbidity and death. Resulting oligohydramnios can be associated with fetal lung hypoplasia and skeletal deformations. Potential neonatal adverse effects include skull hypoplasia, anuria, hypotension, renal failure, and death. When pregnancy is detected, discontinue Exforge as soon as possible [*see Use in Specific Populations (8.1)*].

5.2 Hypotension

Excessive hypotension was seen in 0.4% of patients with uncomplicated hypertension treated with Exforge in placebo-controlled studies. In patients with an activated renin-angiotensin system, such as volume-and/or salt-depleted patients receiving high doses of diuretics, symptomatic hypotension may occur in patients receiving angiotensin receptor blockers. Volume depletion should be corrected prior to administration of Exforge. Treatment with Exforge should start under close medical supervision.

Initiate therapy cautiously in patients with heart failure or recent myocardial infarction and in patients undergoing surgery or dialysis. Patients with heart failure or post-myocardial infarction patients given valsartan commonly have some reduction in blood pressure, but discontinuation of therapy because of continuing symptomatic hypotension usually is not necessary when dosing instructions are followed. In controlled trials in heart failure patients, the incidence of hypotension in valsartan-treated patients was 5.5% compared to 1.8% in placebo-treated patients. In the Valsartan in Acute Myocardial Infarction Trial (VALIANT), hypotension in post-myocardial infarction patients led to permanent discontinuation of therapy in 1.4% of valsartan-treated patients and 0.8% of captopril-treated patients.

Since the vasodilation induced by amlodipine is gradual in onset, acute hypotension has rarely been reported after oral administration. Nonetheless, caution, as with any other peripheral vasodilator, should be exercised when administering amlodipine, particularly in patients with severe aortic stenosis.

If excessive hypotension occurs with Exforge, the patient should be placed in a supine position and, if necessary, given an intravenous infusion of normal saline. A transient hypotensive response is not a contraindication to further treatment, which usually can be continued without difficulty once the blood pressure has stabilized.

5.3 Risk of Myocardial Infarction or Increased Angina

Worsening angina and acute myocardial infarction can develop after starting or increasing the dose of amlodipine, particularly in patients with severe obstructive coronary artery disease.

5.4 Impaired Renal Function

Changes in renal function including acute renal failure can be caused by drugs that inhibit the renin-angiotensin system and by diuretics. Patients whose renal function may depend in part on the activity of the renin-angiotensin system (e.g. patients with renal artery stenosis, chronic kidney disease, severe congestive heart failure, or volume depletion) may be at particular risk of developing acute renal failure on Exforge. Monitor renal function periodically in these patients. Consider withholding or discontinuing therapy in patients who develop a clinically significant decrease in renal function on Exforge *[see Drug Interactions (7)]*.

5.5 Hyperkalemia

Drugs that inhibit the renin-angiotensin system can cause hyperkalemia. Monitor serum electrolytes periodically.

Some patients with heart failure have developed increases in potassium with valsartan therapy. These effects are usually minor and transient, and they are more likely to occur in patients with pre-existing renal impairment. Dosage reduction and/or discontinuation of Exforge may be required [*see Adverse Reactions (6.1)*].

6 ADVERSE REACTIONS

6.1 Clinical Trials Experience

Because clinical trials are conducted under widely varying conditions, adverse reaction rates observed in the clinical trials of a drug cannot be directly compared to rates in the clinical trials of another drug and may not reflect the rates observed in practice. The adverse reaction information from clinical trials does, however, provide a basis for identifying the adverse events that appear to be related to drug use and for approximating rates.

Studies with Exforge:

Exforge has been evaluated for safety in over 2600 patients with hypertension; over 1440 of these patients were treated for at least 6 months and over 540 of these patients were treated for at least 1 year. Adverse reactions have generally been mild and transient in nature and have only infrequently required discontinuation of therapy.

The hazards [*see Warnings and Precautions (5)*] of valsartan are generally independent of dose; those of amlodipine are a mixture of dose-dependent phenomena (primarily peripheral edema) and dose-independent phenomena, the former much more common than the latter.

The overall frequency of adverse reactions was neither dose-related nor related to gender, age, or race. In placebo-controlled clinical trials, discontinuation due to side effects occurred in 1.8% of patients in the Exforge-treated patients and 2.1% in the placebo-treated group. The most common reasons for discontinuation of therapy with Exforge were peripheral edema (0.4%), and vertigo (0.2%).

The adverse reactions that occurred in placebo-controlled clinical trials in at least 2% of patients treated with Exforge but at a higher incidence in amlodipine/valsartan patients (n=1437) than placebo (n=337) included peripheral edema (5.4% vs. 3.0%), nasopharyngitis (4.3% vs. 1.8%), upper respiratory tract infection (2.9% vs 2.1%) and dizziness (2.1% vs 0.9%).

Orthostatic events (orthostatic hypotension and postural dizziness) were seen in less than 1% of patients.

Other adverse reactions that occurred in placebo-controlled clinical trials with Exforge (≥0.2%) are listed below. It cannot be determined whether these events were causally related to Exforge.

Blood and Lymphatic System Disorders: Lymphadenopathy

Cardiac Disorders: Palpitations, tachycardia

Ear and Labyrinth Disorders: Ear pain

Gastrointestinal Disorders: Diarrhea, nausea, constipation, dyspepsia, abdominal pain, abdominal pain upper, gastritis, vomiting, abdominal discomfort, abdominal distention, dry mouth, colitis

General Disorders and Administration Site Conditions: Fatigue, chest pain, asthenia, pitting edema, pyrexia, edema

Immune System Disorders: Seasonal allergies

Infections and Infestations: Nasopharyngitis, sinusitis, bronchitis, pharyngitis, gastroenteritis, pharyngotonsillitis, bronchitis acute, tonsillitis

Injury and Poisoning: Epicondylitis, joint sprain, limb injury

Metabolism and Nutrition Disorders: Gout, non-insulin-dependent diabetes mellitus, hypercholesterolemia

Musculoskeletal and Connective Tissue Disorders: Arthralgia, back pain, muscle spasms, pain in extremity, myalgia, osteoarthritis, joint swelling, musculoskeletal chest pain

Nervous System Disorders: Headache, sciatica, paresthesia, cervicobrachial syndrome, carpal tunnel syndrome, hypoesthesia, sinus headache, somnolence

Psychiatric Disorders: Insomnia, anxiety, depression

Renal and Urinary Disorders: Hematuria, nephrolithiasis, pollakiuria

Reproductive System and Breast Disorders: Erectile dysfunction

Respiratory, Thoracic and Mediastinal Disorders: Cough, pharyngolaryngeal pain, sinus congestion, dyspnea, epistaxis, productive cough, dysphonia, nasal congestion

Skin and Subcutaneous Tissue Disorders: Pruritus, rash, hyperhidrosis, eczema, erythema

Vascular Disorders: Flushing, hot flush

Isolated cases of the following clinically notable adverse reactions were also observed in clinical trials: exanthema, syncope, visual disturbance, hypersensitivity, tinnitus, and hypotension.

Studies with Amlodipine:

Norvasc®* has been evaluated for safety in more than 11000 patients in U.S. and foreign clinical trials. Other adverse events that have been reported <1% but >0.1% of patients in controlled clinical trials or under conditions of open trials or marketing experience where a causal relationship is uncertain were:

Cardiovascular: arrhythmia (including ventricular tachycardia and atrial fibrillation), bradycardia, chest pain, peripheral ischemia, syncope, postural hypotension, vasculitis

Central and Peripheral Nervous System: neuropathy peripheral, tremor

Gastrointestinal: anorexia, dysphagia, pancreatitis, gingival hyperplasia

General: allergic reaction, hot flushes, malaise, rigors, weight gain, weight loss

Musculoskeletal System: arthrosis, muscle cramps

Psychiatric: sexual dysfunction (male and female), nervousness, abnormal dreams, depersonalization

Respiratory System: dyspnea

Skin and Appendages: angioedema, erythema multiforme, rash erythematous, rash maculopapular

Special Senses: abnormal vision, conjunctivitis, diplopia, eye pain, tinnitus

Urinary System: micturition frequency, micturition disorder, nocturia

Autonomic Nervous System: sweating increased

Metabolic and Nutritional: hyperglycemia, thirst

Hemopoietic: leukopenia, purpura, thrombocytopenia

Other events reported with amlodipine at a frequency of ≤0.1% of patients include: cardiac failure, pulse irregularity, extrasystoles, skin discoloration, urticaria, skin dryness, alopecia, dermatitis, muscle weakness, twitching, ataxia, hypertonia, migraine, cold and clammy skin, apathy, agitation, amnesia, gastritis, increased appetite, loose stools, rhinitis, dysuria, polyuria, parosmia, taste perversion, abnormal visual accommodation, and xerophthalmia. Other reactions occurred sporadically and cannot be distinguished from medications or concurrent disease states such as myocardial infarction and angina.

Adverse reactions reported for amlodipine for indications other than hypertension may be found in the prescribing information for Norvasc.

Studies with Valsartan:

Diovan® has been evaluated for safety in more than 4000 hypertensive patients in clinical trials. In trials in which valsartan was compared to an ACE inhibitor with or without placebo, the incidence of dry cough was significantly greater in the ACE inhibitor group (7.9%) than in the groups who received valsartan (2.6%) or placebo (1.5%). In a 129-patient trial limited to patients who had had dry cough when they had previously received ACE inhibitors, the incidences of cough in patients who received valsartan, HCTZ, or lisinopril were 20%, 19%, and 69% respectively (p<0.001).

Other adverse reactions, not listed above, occurring in >0.2% of patients in controlled clinical trials with valsartan are:

Body as a Whole: allergic reaction, asthenia

Musculoskeletal: muscle cramps

Neurologic and Psychiatric: paresthesia

Respiratory: sinusitis, pharyngitis

Urogenital: impotence

Other reported events seen less frequently in clinical trials were: angioedema.

Adverse reactions reported for valsartan for indications other than hypertension may be found in the prescribing information for Diovan.

Clinical Lab Test Findings:

Creatinine: In hypertensive patients, greater than 50% increases in creatinine occurred in 0.4% of patients receiving Exforge and 0.6% receiving placebo. In heart failure patients, greater than 50% increases in creatinine were observed in 3.9% of valsartan-treated patients compared to 0.9% of placebo-treated patients. In post-myocardial infarction patients, doubling of serum creatinine was observed in 4.2% of valsartan-treated patients and 3.4% of captopril-treated patients.

Liver Function Tests: Occasional elevations (greater than 150%) of liver chemistries occurred in Exforge-treated patients.

Serum Potassium: In hypertensive patients, greater than 20% increases in serum potassium were observed in 2.8% of Exforge-treated patients compared to 3.4% of placebo-treated patients. In heart failure patients, greater than 20% increases in serum potassium were observed in 10% of valsartan-treated patients compared to 5.1% of placebo-treated patients.

Blood Urea Nitrogen (BUN): In hypertensive patients, greater than 50% increases in BUN were observed in 5.5% of Exforge-treated patients compared to 4.7% of placebo-treated patients. In heart failure patients, greater than 50% increases in BUN were observed in 16.6% of valsartan-treated patients compared to 6.3% of placebo-treated patients.

Neutropenia: Neutropenia was observed in 1.9% of patients treated with Diovan and 0.8% of patients treated with placebo.

6.2 Postmarketing Experience

Amlodipine: Gynecomastia has been reported infrequently and a causal relationship is uncertain. Jaundice and hepatic enzyme elevations (mostly consistent with cholestasis or hepatitis), in some cases severe enough to require hospitalization, have been reported in association with use of amlodipine.

Valsartan: The following additional adverse reactions have been reported in postmarketing experience with valsartan:

Blood and Lymphatic: Decrease in hemoglobin, decrease in hematocrit, neutropenia,

Hypersensitivity: There are rare reports of angioedema. Some of these patients previously experienced angioedema with other drugs including ACE inhibitors. Exforge should not be re-administered to patients who have had angioedema.

Digestive: Elevated liver enzymes and very rare reports of hepatitis

Renal: Impaired renal function, renal failure

Clinical Laboratory Tests: Hyperkalemia

Dermatologic: Alopecia

Vascular: Vasculitis

Rare cases of rhabdomyolysis have been reported in patients receiving angiotensin II receptor blockers.

7 DRUG INTERACTIONS

No drug interaction studies have been conducted with Exforge and other drugs, although studies have been conducted with the individual amlodipine and valsartan components.

Studies with Amlodipine

Simvastatin: Coadministration of simvastatin with amlodipine increases the systemic exposure of simvastatin. Limit the dose of simvastatin in patients on amlodipine to 20 mg daily.

CYP3A4 Inhibitors: Coadministration with CYP3A4 inhibitors (moderate and strong) result in increased systemic exposure to amlodipine warranting dose reduction. Monitor for symptoms of hypotension and edema when amlodipine is coadministered with CYP3A4 inhibitors to determine the need for dose adjustment.

CYP3A4 Inducers: No information is available on the quantitative effects of CYP3A4 inducers on amlodipine. Blood pressure should be monitored when amlodipine is coadministered with CYP3A4 inducers.

Studies with Valsartan

No clinically significant pharmacokinetic interactions were observed when valsartan was coadministered with amlodipine, atenolol, cimetidine, digoxin, furosemide, glyburide, hydrochlorothiazide, or indomethacin. The valsartan-atenolol combination was more antihypertensive than either component, but it did not lower the heart rate more than atenolol alone.

Warfarin: Coadministration of valsartan and warfarin did not change the pharmacokinetics of valsartan or the time-course of the anticoagulant properties of warfarin.

Non-Steroidal Anti-Inflammatory Agents including Selective Cyclooxygenase-2 Inhibitors (COX-2 Inhibitors): In patients who are elderly, volume-depleted (including those on diuretic therapy), or with compromised renal function, coadministration of NSAIDs, including selective COX-2 inhibitors, with angiotensin II receptor antagonists, including valsartan, may result in deterioration of renal function, including possible acute renal failure. These effects are usually reversible. Monitor renal function periodically in patients receiving valsartan and NSAID therapy.

The antihypertensive effect of angiotensin II receptor antagonists, including valsartan may be attenuated by NSAIDs including selective COX-2 inhibitors.

Potassium: Concomitant use of valsartan with other agents that block the renin-angiotensin system, potassium sparing diuretics (e.g., spironolactone, triamterene, amiloride), potassium supplements, or salt substitutes containing potassium may lead to increases in serum potassium and in heart failure patients to increases in serum creatinine. If co-medication is considered necessary, monitoring of serum potassium is advisable.

CYP 450 Interactions: In vitro metabolism studies indicate that CYP 450 mediated drug interactions between valsartan and coadministered drugs are unlikely because of low extent of metabolism [see Pharmacokinetics, Valsartan (12.3)].

Transporters: The results from an in vitro study with human liver tissue indicate that valsartan is a substrate of the hepatic uptake transporter OATP1B1 and the hepatic efflux transporter MRP2. Coadministration of inhibitors of the uptake transporter (rifampin, cyclosporine) or efflux transporter (ritonavir) may increase the systemic exposure to valsartan.

Dual Blockade of the Renin-Angiotensin System (RAS): Dual blockade of the RAS with angiotensin receptor blockers, ACE inhibitors, or aliskiren is associated with increased risks of hypotension, hyperkalemia, and changes in renal function (including acute renal failure) compared to monotherapy. Closely monitor blood pressure, renal function, and electrolytes in patients on Exforge and other agents that affect the RAS.

Do not coadminister aliskiren with Exforge in patients with diabetes. Avoid use of aliskiren with Exforge in patients with renal impairment (GFR <60 mL/min).

8 USE IN SPECIFIC POPULATIONS

8.1 Pregnancy

Pregnancy Category D

Use of drugs that act on the renin-angiotensin system during the second and third trimesters of pregnancy reduces fetal renal function and increases fetal and neonatal morbidity and death. Resulting oligohydramnios can be associated with fetal lung hypoplasia and skeletal deformations. Potential neonatal adverse effects include skull hypoplasia, anuria, hypotension, renal failure, and death. When pregnancy is detected, discontinue Exforge as soon as possible. These adverse outcomes are usually associated with use of these drugs in the second and third trimester of pregnancy. Most epidemiologic studies examining fetal abnormalities after exposure to antihypertensive use in the first trimester have not distinguished drugs affecting the renin-angiotensin system from other antihypertensive agents. Appropriate management of maternal hypertension during pregnancy is important to optimize outcomes for both mother and fetus.

In the unusual case that there is no appropriate alternative to therapy with drugs affecting the renin-angiotensin system for a particular patient, apprise the mother of the potential risk to the fetus. Perform serial ultrasound examinations to assess the intra-amniotic environment. If oligohydramnios is observed, discontinue Exforge, unless it is considered lifesaving for the mother. Fetal testing may be appropriate, based on the week of pregnancy. Patients and physicians should be aware, however, that oligohydramnios may not appear until after the fetus has sustained irreversible injury.

Closely observe infants with histories of in utero exposure to Exforge for hypotension, oliguria, and hyperkalemia [*see Use in Specific Populations (8.4)*].

8.2 Labor and Delivery

The effect of Exforge on labor and delivery has not been studied.

8.3 Nursing Mothers

It is not known whether amlodipine is excreted in human milk. In the absence of this information, it is recommended that nursing be discontinued while amlodipine is administered.

It is not known whether valsartan is excreted in human milk. Valsartan was excreted into the milk of lactating rats; however, animal breast milk drug levels may not accurately reflect human breast milk levels. Because many drugs are excreted into human milk and because of the potential for adverse reactions in nursing infants from Exforge, a decision should be made whether to discontinue nursing or discontinue the drug, taking into account the importance of the drug to the mother.

8.4 Pediatric Use

Safety and effectiveness of Exforge in pediatric patients have not been established.

Neonates with a history of in utero exposure to Exforge:

If oliguria or hypotension occurs, direct attention toward support of blood pressure and renal perfusion. Exchange transfusions or dialysis may be required as a means of reversing hypotension and/or substituting for disordered renal function.

8.5 Geriatric Use

In controlled clinical trials, 323 (22.5%) hypertensive patients treated with Exforge were ≥65 years and 79 (5.5%) were ≥75 years. No overall differences in the efficacy or safety of Exforge was observed in this patient population, but greater sensitivity of some older individuals cannot be ruled out.

Amlodipine: Clinical studies of amlodipine besylate tablets did not include sufficient numbers of subjects aged 65 and over to determine whether they respond differently from younger subjects. Other reported clinical experience has not identified differences in responses between the elderly and younger patients. In general, dose selection for an elderly patient should be cautious, usually starting at the low end of the dosing range, reflecting the greater frequency of decreased hepatic, renal or cardiac function, and of concomitant disease or other drug therapy. Elderly patients have decreased clearance of amlodipine with a resulting increase of AUC of approximately 40-60%, and a lower initial dose may be required.

Valsartan: In the controlled clinical trials of valsartan, 1214 (36.2%) of hypertensive patients treated with valsartan were ≥65 years and 265 (7.9%) were ≥75 years. No overall difference in the efficacy or safety of valsartan was observed in this patient population, but greater sensitivity of some older individuals cannot be ruled out.

8.6 Renal Impairment

Safety and effectiveness of Exforge in patients with severe renal impairment (CrCl< 30 mL/min) have not been established. No dose adjustment is required in patients with mild (60-90 mL/min) or moderate (CrCl 30-60) renal impairment.

8.7 Hepatic Impairment

Amlodipine

Exposure to amlodipine is increased in patients with hepatic insufficiency, thus consider using lower doses of Exforge [*see Clinical Pharmacology (12.3)*].

Valsartan

No dose adjustment is necessary for patients with mild-to-moderate disease. No dosing recommendations can be provided for patients with severe liver disease.

10 OVERDOSAGE

Information on Amlodipine

Single oral doses of amlodipine maleate equivalent to 40 mg/kg and 100 mg/kg amlodipine in mice and rats, respectively, caused deaths. Single oral doses equivalent to 4 or more mg/kg amlodipine in dogs (11 or more times the maximum recommended human dose on a mg/m^2 basis) caused a marked peripheral vasodilation and hypotension.

Overdosage might be expected to cause excessive peripheral vasodilation with marked hypotension. In humans, experience with intentional overdosage of amlodipine is limited. Marked and potentially prolonged systemic hypotension up to and including shock with fatal outcome have been reported.

If massive overdose should occur, initiate active cardiac and respiratory monitoring. Frequent blood pressure measurements are essential. Should hypotension occur, cardiovascular support including elevation of the extremities and the judicious administration of fluids should be initiated. If hypotension remains unresponsive to these conservative measures, consider administration of vasopressors (such as phenylephrine) with attention to circulating volume and urine output. As amlodipine is highly protein bound, hemodialysis is not likely to be of benefit. Administration of activated charcoal to healthy volunteers immediately or up to two hours after ingestion of amlodipine has been shown to significantly decrease amlodipine absorption.

Information on Valsartan

Limited data are available related to overdosage in humans. The most likely effect of overdose with valsartan would be peripheral vasodilation, hypotension, and tachycardia; bradycardia could occur from parasympathetic (vagal) stimulation. Depressed level of consciousness, circulatory collapse, and shock have been reported. If symptomatic hypotension should occur, supportive treatment should be instituted.

Valsartan is not removed from the plasma by hemodialysis. Valsartan was without grossly observable adverse effects at single oral doses up to 2000 mg/kg in rats and up to 1000 mg/kg in marmosets, except for the salivation and diarrhea in the rat and vomiting in the marmoset at the highest dose (60 and 37 times, respectively, the maximum recommended human dose (MRHD) on a mg/m^2 basis). (Calculations assume an oral dose of 320 mg/day and a 60-kg patient.)

11 DESCRIPTION

Exforge is a fixed combination of amlodipine and valsartan. Exforge contains the besylate salt of amlodipine, a dihydropyridine calcium-channel blocker (CCB). Amlodipine besylate is a white to pale yellow crystalline powder, slightly soluble in water and sparingly soluble in ethanol. Amlodipine besylate's chemical name is 3-Ethyl-5-methyl(4RS)-2-[(2-aminoethoxy)methyl]-4-(2-chlorophenyl)-6-methyl-1,4-dihydropyridine-3,5-dicarboxylate benzenesulphonate; its structural formula is

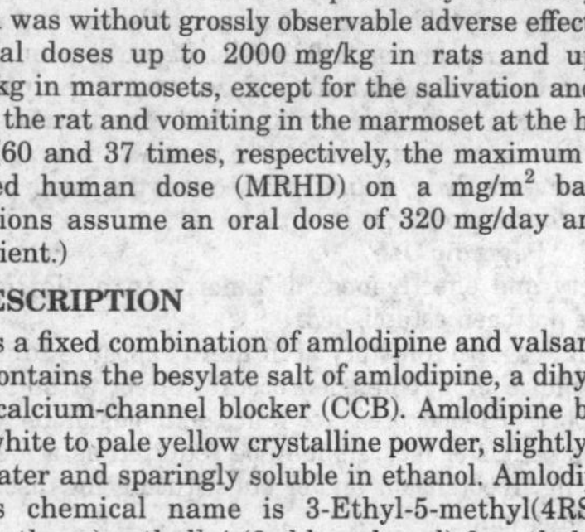

Its empirical formula is $C_{20}H_{25}ClN_2O_5 \bullet C_6H_6O_3S$ and its molecular weight is 567.1.

Valsartan is a nonpeptide, orally active, and specific angiotensin II antagonist acting on the AT_1 receptor subtype. Valsartan is a white to practically white fine powder, soluble in ethanol and methanol and slightly soluble in water. Valsartan's chemical name is N-(1-oxopentyl)-N-[[2′-(1H-tetrazol-5-yl) [1,1′-biphenyl]-4-yl]methyl]-L-valine; its structural formula is

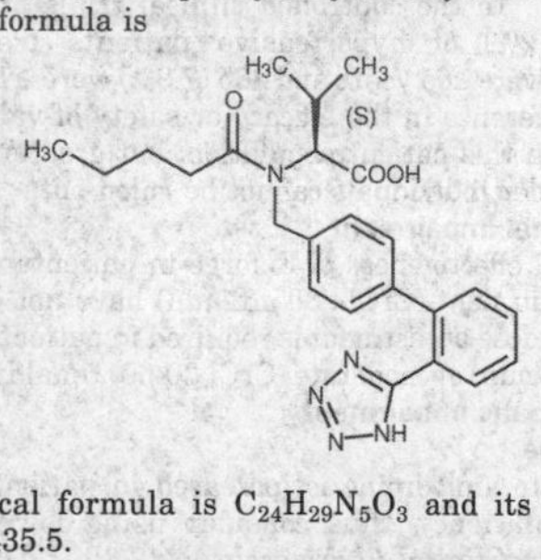

Its empirical formula is $C_{24}H_{29}N_5O_3$ and its molecular weight is 435.5.

Exforge tablets are formulated in 4 strengths for oral administration with a combination of amlodipine besylate, equivalent to 5 mg or 10 mg of amlodipine free-base, with 160 mg, or 320 mg of valsartan providing for the following available combinations: 5/160 mg, 10/160 mg, 5/320 mg, and 10/320 mg.

The inactive ingredients for all strengths of the tablets are colloidal silicon dioxide, crospovidone, magnesium stearate, and microcrystalline cellulose. Additionally the 5/320 mg and 10/320 mg strengths contain iron oxide yellow and sodium starch glycolate. The film coating contains hypromellose, iron oxides, polyethylene glycol, talc, and titanium dioxide.

12 CLINICAL PHARMACOLOGY

12.1 Mechanism of Action

Amlodipine

Amlodipine is a dihydropyridine calcium channel blocker that inhibits the transmembrane influx of calcium ions into vascular smooth muscle and cardiac muscle. Experimental data suggest that amlodipine binds to both dihydropyridine and nondihydropyridine binding sites. The contractile processes of cardiac muscle and vascular smooth muscle are dependent upon the movement of extracellular calcium ions into these cells through specific ion channels. Amlodipine inhibits calcium ion influx across cell membranes selectively, with a greater effect on vascular smooth muscle cells than on cardiac muscle cells. Negative inotropic effects can be detected *in vitro* but such effects have not been seen in intact animals at therapeutic doses. Serum calcium concentration is not affected by amlodipine. Within the physiologic pH range, amlodipine is an ionized compound (pKa=8.6), and its kinetic interaction with the calcium channel receptor is characterized by a gradual rate of association and dissociation with the receptor binding site, resulting in a gradual onset of effect.

Amlodipine is a peripheral arterial vasodilator that acts directly on vascular smooth muscle to cause a reduction in peripheral vascular resistance and reduction in blood pressure.

Valsartan

Angiotensin II is formed from angiotensin I in a reaction catalyzed by angiotensin-converting enzyme (ACE, kininase II). Angiotensin II is the principal pressor agent of the renin-angiotensin system, with effects that include vasoconstriction, stimulation of synthesis and release of aldosterone, cardiac stimulation, and renal reabsorption of sodium. Valsartan blocks the vasoconstrictor and aldosterone-secreting effects of angiotensin II by selectively blocking the binding of angiotensin II to the AT_1 receptor in many tissues, such as vascular smooth muscle and the adrenal gland. Its action is therefore independent of the pathways for angiotensin II synthesis.

There is also an AT_2 receptor found in many tissues, but AT_2 is not known to be associated with cardiovascular homeostasis. Valsartan has much greater affinity (about 20,000-fold) for the AT_1 receptor than for the AT_2 receptor. The increased plasma levels of angiotensin following AT_1 receptor blockade with valsartan may stimulate the unblocked AT_2 receptor. The primary metabolite of valsartan is essentially inactive with an affinity for the AT_1 receptor about one-200th that of valsartan itself.

Blockade of the renin-angiotensin system with ACE inhibitors, which inhibit the biosynthesis of angiotensin II from angiotensin I, is widely used in the treatment of hypertension. ACE inhibitors also inhibit the degradation of bradykinin, a reaction also catalyzed by ACE. Because valsartan does not inhibit ACE (kininase II), it does not affect the response to bradykinin. Whether this difference has clinical relevance is not yet known. Valsartan does not bind to or block other hormone receptors or ion channels known to be important in cardiovascular regulation.

Blockade of the angiotensin II receptor inhibits the negative regulatory feedback of angiotensin II on renin secretion, but the resulting increased plasma renin activity and angiotensin II circulating levels do not overcome the effect of valsartan on blood pressure.

12.2 Pharmacodynamics

Amlodipine

Following administration of therapeutic doses to patients with hypertension, amlodipine produces vasodilation resulting in a reduction of supine and standing blood pressures. These decreases in blood pressure are not accompanied by a significant change in heart rate or plasma catecholamine levels with chronic dosing. Although the acute intravenous administration of amlodipine decreases arterial blood pressure and increases heart rate in hemodynamic studies of patients with chronic stable angina, chronic oral administration of amlodipine in clinical trials did not lead to clinically significant changes in heart rate or blood pressures in normotensive patients with angina.

With chronic, once-daily administration, antihypertensive effectiveness is maintained for at least 24 hours. Plasma concentrations correlate with effect in both young and elderly patients. The magnitude of reduction in blood pressure with amlodipine is also correlated with the height of pretreatment elevation; thus, individuals with moderate hypertension (diastolic pressure 105-114 mmHg) had about a 50% greater response than patients with mild hypertension (diastolic pressure 90-104 mmHg). Normotensive subjects experienced no clinically significant change in blood pressure (+1/-2 mmHg).

In hypertensive patients with normal renal function, therapeutic doses of amlodipine resulted in a decrease in renal vascular resistance and an increase in glomerular filtration rate and effective renal plasma flow without change in filtration fraction or proteinuria.

As with other calcium channel blockers, hemodynamic measurements of cardiac function at rest and during exercise (or pacing) in patients with normal ventricular function treated with amlodipine have generally demonstrated a small increase in cardiac index without significant influence on dP/dt or on left ventricular end diastolic pressure or volume. In hemodynamic studies, amlodipine has not been associated with a negative inotropic effect when administered in the therapeutic dose range to intact animals and man, even when coadministered with beta-blockers to man. Similar findings, however, have been observed in normals or well-compensated patients with heart failure with agents possessing significant negative inotropic effects.

Amlodipine does not change sinoatrial nodal function or atrioventricular (AV) conduction in intact animals or man. In patients with chronic stable angina, intravenous administration of 10 mg did not significantly alter A-H and H-V conduction and sinus node recovery time after pacing. Similar results were obtained in patients receiving amlodipine and concomitant beta-blockers. In clinical studies in which amlodipine was administered in combination with beta-blockers to patients with either hypertension or angina, no adverse effects of electrocardiographic (ECG) parameters were observed. In clinical trials with angina patients alone, amlodipine therapy did not alter electrocardiographic intervals or produce higher degrees of AV blocks.

Amlodipine has indications other than hypertension which can be found in the Norvasc* package insert.

Valsartan

Valsartan inhibits the pressor effect of angiotensin II infusions. An oral dose of 80 mg inhibits the pressor effect by about 80% at peak with approximately 30% inhibition persisting for 24 hours. No information on the effect of larger doses is available.

Removal of the negative feedback of angiotensin II causes a 2- to 3-fold rise in plasma renin and consequent rise in angiotensin II plasma concentration in hypertensive patients. Minimal decreases in plasma aldosterone were observed after administration of valsartan; very little effect on serum potassium was observed.

In multiple dose studies in hypertensive patients with stable renal insufficiency and patients with renovascular hypertension, valsartan had no clinically significant effects on glomerular filtration rate, filtration fraction, creatinine clearance, or renal plasma flow.

Administration of valsartan to patients with essential hypertension results in a significant reduction of sitting, supine, and standing systolic blood pressure, usually with little or no orthostatic change. Valsartan has indications other than hypertension which can be found in the Diovan package insert.

Exforge

Exforge has been shown to be effective in lowering blood pressure. Both amlodipine and valsartan lower blood pressure by reducing peripheral resistance, but calcium influx blockade and reduction of angiotensin II vasoconstriction are complementary mechanisms.

12.3 Pharmacokinetics

Amlodipine

Peak plasma concentrations of amlodipine are reached 6-12 hours after administration of amlodipine alone. Absolute bioavailability has been estimated to be between 64% and 90%. The bioavailability of amlodipine is not altered by the presence of food.

The apparent volume of distribution of amlodipine is 21 L/kg. Approximately 93% of circulating amlodipine is bound to plasma proteins in hypertensive patients.

Amlodipine is extensively (about 90%) converted to inactive metabolites via hepatic metabolism with 10% of the parent compound and 60% of the metabolites excreted in the urine. Elimination of amlodipine from the plasma is biphasic with a terminal elimination half-life of about 30-50 hours. Steady state plasma levels of amlodipine are reached after 7-8 days of consecutive daily dosing.

Valsartan

Following oral administration of valsartan alone peak plasma concentrations of valsartan are reached in 2-4 hours. Absolute bioavailability is about 25% (range 10%-35%). Food decreases the exposure (as measured by AUC) to valsartan by about 40% and peak plasma concentration (C_{max}) by about 50%.

The steady state volume of distribution of valsartan after intravenous administration is 17 L indicating that valsartan does not distribute into tissues extensively. Valsartan is highly bound to serum proteins (95%), mainly serum albumin.

Valsartan shows biexponential decay kinetics following intravenous administration with an average elimination half-life of about 6 hours. The recovery is mainly as unchanged drug, with only about 20% of dose recovered as metabolites. The primary metabolite, accounting for about 9% of dose, is valeryl 4-hydroxy valsartan. In vitro metabolism studies involving recombinant CYP 450 enzymes indicated that the CYP 2C9 isoenzyme is responsible for the formation of valeryl-4-hydroxy valsartan. Valsartan does not inhibit CYP 450 isozymes at clinically relevant concentrations. CYP 450 mediated drug interaction between valsartan and coadministered drugs are unlikely because of the low extent of metabolism.

Valsartan, when administered as an oral solution, is primarily recovered in feces (about 83% of dose) and urine (about 13% of dose). Following intravenous administration, plasma clearance of valsartan is about 2 L/h and its renal clearance is 0.62 L/h (about 30% of total clearance).

Exforge

Following oral administration of Exforge in normal healthy adults, peak plasma concentrations of valsartan and amlodipine are reached in 3 and 6-8 hours, respectively. The rate and extent of absorption of valsartan and amlodipine from Exforge are the same as when administered as individual tablets. The bioavailabilities of amlodipine and valsartan are not altered by the coadministration of food.

Special Populations

Geriatric

Studies with Amlodipine: Elderly patients have decreased clearance of amlodipine with a resulting increase in peak plasma levels, elimination half-life and AUC.

Studies with Valsartan: Exposure (measured by AUC) to valsartan is higher by 70% and the half-life is longer by 35% in the elderly than in the young. No dosage adjustment is necessary.

Gender

Studies with Valsartan: Pharmacokinetics of valsartan does not differ significantly between males and females.

Renal Insufficiency

Studies with Amlodipine: The pharmacokinetics of amlodipine is not significantly influenced by renal impairment.

Studies with Valsartan: There is no apparent correlation between renal function (measured by creatinine clearance) and exposure (measured by AUC) to valsartan in patients with different degrees of renal impairment. Consequently, dose adjustment is not required in patients with mild-to-moderate renal dysfunction. No studies have been performed in patients with severe impairment of renal function (creatinine clearance <10 mL/min). Valsartan is not removed from the plasma by hemodialysis. In the case of severe renal disease, exercise care with dosing of valsartan.

Hepatic Insufficiency

Studies with Amlodipine: Patients with hepatic insufficiency have decreased clearance of amlodipine with resulting increase in AUC of approximately 40%-60%.

Studies with Valsartan: On average, patients with mild-to-moderate chronic liver disease have twice the exposure (measured by AUC values) to valsartan of healthy volunteers (matched by age, sex and weight). In general, no dosage adjustment is needed in patients with mild-to-moderate liver disease. Care should be exercised in patients with liver disease.

Drug Interactions

In vitro data in human plasma indicate that amlodipine has no effect on the protein binding of digoxin, phenytoin, warfarin and indomethacin.

Cimetidine: Coadministration of amlodipine with cimetidine did not alter the pharmacokinetics of amlodipine.

Grapefruit juice: Coadministration of 240 mL of grapefruit juice with a single oral dose of amlodipine 10 mg in 20 healthy volunteers had no significant effect on the pharmacokinetics of amlodipine.

Maalox® (antacid): Coadministration of the antacid Maalox with a single dose of amlodipine had no significant effect on the pharmacokinetics of amlodipine.

Sildenafil: A single 100 mg dose of sildenafil (Viagra®**) in subjects with essential hypertension had no effect on the pharmacokinetic parameters of amlodipine. When amlodipine and sildenafil were used in combination, each agent independently exerted its own blood pressure lowering effect.

Atorvastatin: Coadministration of multiple 10 mg doses of amlodipine with 80 mg of atorvastatin resulted in no significant change in the steady state pharmacokinetic parameters of atorvastatin.

Digoxin: Coadministration of amlodipine with digoxin did not change serum digoxin levels or digoxin renal clearance in normal volunteers.

Warfarin: Coadministration of amlodipine with warfarin did not change the warfarin prothrombin response time.

Simvastatin: Coadministration of multiple doses of 10 mg of amlodipine with 80 mg simvastatin resulted in a 77% increase in exposure to simvastatin compared to simvastatin alone. Limit the dose of simvastatin in patients on amlodipine to 20 mg daily.

CYP3A4 Inhibitors: Coadministration of a 180 mg daily dose of diltiazem with 5 mg amlodpidine in elderly hypertensives patients resulted in a 60% increase in amlodipine systemic exposure. Erythromycin coadministration in healthy volunteers did not significantly change amlodipine systemic exposure. However, strong inhbitors of CYP3A4 (i.e., ketoconazole, itraconazole, ritonavir) may increase the plasma concentrations of amlodipine to a greater extent.

Table 1: Effect of Exforge on Sitting Diastolic Blood Pressure

Amlodipine dosage	Valsartan dosage							
	0 mg		80 mg		160 mg		320 mg	
	Mean Change*	Placebo-subtracted	Mean Change*	Placebo-subtracted	Mean Change*	Placebo-subtracted	Mean Change*	Placebo-subtracted
0 mg	-6.4	---	-9.5	-3.1	-10.9	-4.5	-13.2	-6.7
5 mg	-11.1	-4.7	-14.2	-7.8	-14.0	-7.6	-15.7	-9.3

*Mean Change and Placebo-Subtracted Mean Change from Baseline (mmHg) at Week 8 in Sitting Diastolic Blood Pressure. Mean baseline diastolic BP was 99.3 mmHg.

Table 2: Effect of Exforge on Sitting Systolic Blood Pressure

Amlodipine dosage	Valsartan dosage							
	0 mg		80 mg		160 mg		320 mg	
	Mean Change*	Placebo-subtracted	Mean Change*	Placebo-subtracted	Mean Change*	Placebo-subtracted	Mean Change*	Placebo-subtracted
0 mg	-6.2	---	-12.9	-6.8	-14.3	-8.2	-16.3	-10.1
5 mg	-14.8	-8.6	-20.7	-14.5	-19.4	-13.2	-22.4	-16.2

*Mean Change and Placebo-Subtracted Mean Change from Baseline (mmHg) at Week 8 in Sitting Systolic Blood Pressure. Mean baseline systolic BP was 152.8 mmHg.

Table 3: Effect of Exforge on Sitting Diastolic Blood Pressure

Amlodipine dosage	Valsartan dosage					
	0 mg		160 mg		320 mg	
	Mean Change*	Placebo-subtracted	Mean Change*	Placebo-subtracted	Mean Change*	Placebo-subtracted
0 mg	-8.2	---	-12.8	- 4.5	-12.8	-4.5
10 mg	-15.0	-6.7	- 17.2	- 9.0	-18.1	-9.9

*Mean Change and Placebo-Subtracted Mean Change from Baseline (mmHg) at Week 8 in Sitting Diastolic Blood Pressure. Mean baseline diastolic BP was 99.1 mmHg.

13 NONCLINICAL TOXICOLOGY

13.1 Carcinogenesis, Mutagenesis, Impairment of Fertility

Studies with Amlodipine

Rats and mice treated with amlodipine maleate in the diet for up to 2 years, at concentrations calculated to provide daily dosage levels of 0.5, 1.25, and 2.5 mg amlodipine/kg/day, showed no evidence of a carcinogenic effect of the drug. For the mouse, the highest dose was, on mg/m^2 basis, similar to the MRHD of 10 mg amlodipine/day. For the rat, the highest dose was, on a mg/m^2 basis, about 2.5 the MRHD. (Calculations based on a 60-kg patient.)

Mutagenicity studies conducted with amlodipine maleate revealed no drug-related effects at either the gene or chromosome level.

There was no effect on the fertility of rats treated orally with amlodipine maleate (males for 64 days and females for 14 days prior to mating) at doses of up to 10 mg amlodipine/kg/day (about 10 times the MRHD of 10 mg/day on a mg/m^2 basis).

Studies with Valsartan

There was no evidence of carcinogenicity when valsartan was administered in the diet to mice and rats for up to 2 years at concentrations calculated to provide doses of up to 160 and 200 mg/kg/day, respectively. These doses in mice and rats are about 2.4 and 6 times, respectively, the MRHD of 320 mg/day on a mg/m^2 basis. (Calculations based on a 60 kg patient.)

Mutagenicity assays did not reveal any valsartan-related effects at either the gene or chromosome level. These assays included bacterial mutagenicity tests with Salmonella and E. coli, a gene mutation test with Chinese hamster V79 cells, a cytogenetic test with Chinese hamster ovary cells, and a rat micronucleus test.

Valsartan had no adverse effects on the reproductive performance of male or female rats at oral doses of up to 200 mg/kg/day. This dose is about 6 times the MRHD on a mg/m^2 basis.

13.3 Developmental Toxicity Studies

Studies with Amlodipine

No evidence of teratogenicity or other embryo/fetal toxicity was found when pregnant rats and rabbits were treated orally with amlodipine maleate at doses of up to 10 mg amlodipine/kg/day (respectively, about 10 and 20 times the MRHD of 10 mg amlodipine on a mg/m^2 basis) during their respective periods of major organogenesis. (Calculations based on a patient weight of 60 kg.) However, litter size was significantly decreased (by about 50%) and the number of intrauterine deaths was significantly increased (about 5-fold) for rats receiving amlodipine maleate at a dose equivalent to 10 mg amlodipine/kg/day for 14 days before mating and throughout mating and gestation. Amlodipine maleate has been shown to prolong both the gestation period and the duration of labor in rats at this dose. There are no adequate and well-controlled studies in pregnant women. Amlodipine should be used during pregnancy only if the potential benefit justifies the potential risk to the fetus.

Studies with Valsartan

No teratogenic effects were observed when valsartan was administered to pregnant mice and rats at oral doses of up to 600 mg/kg/day and to pregnant rabbits at oral doses of up to 10 mg/kg/day. However, significant decreases in fetal weight, pup birth weight, pup survival rate, and slight delays in developmental milestones were observed in studies in which parental rats were treated with valsartan at oral, maternally toxic (reduction in body weight gain and food consumption) doses of 600 mg/kg/day during organogenesis or late gestation and lactation. In rabbits, fetotoxicity (i.e., resorptions, litter loss, abortions, and low body weight) associated with maternal toxicity (mortality) was observed at doses of 5 and 10 mg/kg/day. The no observed adverse effect doses of 600, 200, and 2 mg/kg/day in mice, rats and rabbits, respectively, are about 9, 6, and 0.1 times the MRHD of 320 mg/day on a mg/m^2 basis. (Calculations based on a patient weight of 60 kg.)

Studies with Amlodipine Besylate and Valsartan

In the oral embryofetal development study in rats using amlodipine besylate plus valsartan at doses equivalent to 5 mg/kg/day amlodipine plus 80 mg/kg/day valsartan, 10 mg/kg/day amlodipine plus 160 mg/kg/day valsartan, and 20 mg/kg/day amlodipine plus 320 mg/kg/day valsartan, treatment-related maternal and fetal effects (developmental delays and alterations noted in the presence of significant maternal toxicity) were noted with the high dose combination. The no-observed-adverse-effect level (NOAEL) for embryofetal effects was 10 mg/kg/day amlodipine plus 160 mg/kg/day valsartan. On a systemic exposure [$AUC_{(0-\infty)}$] basis, these doses are, respectively, 4.3, and 2.7 times the systemic exposure [$AUC_{(0-\infty)}$] in humans receiving the MRHD (10/320 mg/60 kg).

Table 4: Effect of Exforge on Sitting Systolic Blood Pressure

Amlodipine dosage	Valsartan dosage					
	0 mg		160 mg		320 mg	
	Mean Change*	Placebo-subtracted	Mean Change*	Placebo-subtracted	Mean Change*	Placebo-subtracted
0 mg	-11.0	---	-18.1	-7.0	-18.5	-7.5
10 mg	-22.2	-11.2	-26.6	-15.5	-26.9	-15.9

*Mean Change and Placebo-Subtracted Mean Change from Baseline (mmHg) at Week 8 in Sitting Systolic Blood Pressure. Mean baseline systolic BP was 156.7 mmHg.

Table 5: Effect of Exforge on Sitting Diastolic/Systolic Blood Pressure

Treatment Group	Diastolic BP		Systolic BP	
	Mean change*	Treatment Difference**	Mean change*	Treatment Difference**
Exforge 10/160 mg	-11.4	-4.8	-13.9	-5.7
Exforge 5/160 mg	-9.6	-3.1	-12.0	-3.9
Valsartan 160 mg	-6.6	---	-8.2	---

*Mean Change from Baseline at Week 8 in Sitting Diastolic/Systolic Blood Pressure. Mean baseline BP was 149.5/96.5 (systolic/diastolic) mmHg
**Treatment Difference = difference in mean BP reduction between Exforge and the control group (Valsartan 160 mg)

Table 6: Effect of Exforge on Sitting Diastolic/Systolic Blood Pressure

Treatment Group	Diastolic BP		Systolic BP	
	Mean change*	Treatment Difference**	Mean change*	Treatment Difference**
Exforge 10/160 mg	-11.8	-1.8	-12.7	-1.9
Amlodipine 10 mg	-10.0	---	-10.8	---

*Mean Change from Baseline at Week 8 in Sitting Diastolic/Systolic Blood Pressure. Mean baseline BP was 147.0/95.1 (systolic/diastolic) mmHg
**Treatment Difference = difference in mean BP reduction between Exforge and the control group (Amlodipine 10 mg)

14 CLINICAL STUDIES

Exforge was studied in 2 placebo-controlled and 4 active-controlled trials in hypertensive patients. In a double-blind, placebo-controlled study, a total of 1012 patients with mild-to-moderate hypertension received treatments of 3 combinations of amlodipine and valsartan (5/80, 5/160, 5/320 mg) or amlodipine alone (5 mg), valsartan alone (80, 160, or 320 mg) or placebo. All doses with the exception of the 5/320 mg dose were initiated at the randomized dose. The high dose was titrated to that dose after a week at a dose of 5/160 mg. At week 8, the combination treatments were statistically significantly superior to their monotherapy components in reduction of diastolic and systolic blood pressures.

[See table 1 at top of previous page]

[See table 2 at top of previous page]

In a double-blind, placebo controlled study, a total of 1246 patients with mild to moderate hypertension received treatments of 2 combinations of amlodipine and valsartan (10/160, 10/320 mg), or amlodipine alone (10 mg), valsartan alone (160 or 320 mg) or placebo. With the exception of the 10/320 mg dose, treatment was initiated at the randomized dose. The high dose was initiated at a dose of 5/160 mg and titrated to the randomized dose after 1 week. At week 8, the combination treatments were statistically significantly superior to their monotherapy components in reduction of diastolic and systolic blood pressures.

[See table 3 at top of previous page]

[See table 4 above]

In a double-blind, active-controlled study, a total of 947 patients with mild to moderate hypertension who were not adequately controlled on valsartan 160 mg received treatments of 2 combinations of amlodipine and valsartan (10/160, 5/160 mg) or valsartan alone (160 mg). At week 8, the combination treatments were statistically significantly superior to the monotherapy component in reduction of diastolic and systolic blood pressures.

[See table 5 above]

In a double-blind, active-controlled study, a total of 944 patients with mild to moderate hypertension who were not adequately controlled on amlodipine 10 mg received a combination of amlodipine and valsartan (10/160 mg) or amlodipine alone (10 mg). At week 8, the combination treatment was statistically significantly superior to the monotherapy component in reduction of diastolic and systolic blood pressures.

[See table 6 above]

Exforge was also evaluated for safety in a 6-week, double-blind, active-controlled trial of 130 hypertensive patients with severe hypertension (mean baseline BP of 171/113 mmHg). Adverse events were similar in patients with severe hypertension and mild/moderate hypertension treated with Exforge.

A wide age range of the adult population, including the elderly was studied (range 19-92 years, mean 54.7 years). Women comprised almost half of the studied population (47.3%). Of the patients in the studied Exforge group, 87.6% were Caucasian. Black and Asian patients each represented approximately 4% of the population in the studied Exforge group.

Two additional double-blind, active-controlled studies were conducted in which Exforge was administered as initial therapy. In 1 study, a total of 572 black patients with moderate to severe hypertension were randomized to receive either combination amlodipine/valsartan or amlodipine monotherapy for 12 weeks. The initial dose of amlodipine/valsartan was 5/160 mg for 2 weeks with forced titration to 10/160 mg for 2 weeks, followed by optional titration to 10/320 mg for 4 weeks and optional addition of HCTZ 12.5 mg for 4 weeks. The initial dose of amlodipine was 5 mg for 2 weeks with forced titration to 10 mg for 2 weeks, followed by optional titration to 10 mg for 4 weeks and optional addition of HCTZ 12.5 mg for 4 weeks. At the primary endpoint of 8 weeks, the treatment difference between amlodipine/valsartan and amlodipine was 6.7/2.8 mmHg.

In the other study of similar design, a total of 646 patients with moderate to severe hypertension (MSSBP of ≥160 mmHg and <200 mmHg) were randomized to receive either combination amlodipine/valsartan or amlodipine monotherapy for 8 weeks. The initial dose of amlodipine/valsartan was 5/160 mg for 2 weeks with forced titration to 10/160 mg for 2 weeks, followed by the optional addition of HCTZ 12.5 mg for 4 weeks. The initial dose of amlodipine was 5 mg for 2 weeks with forced titration to 10 mg for 2 weeks, followed by the optional addition of HCTZ 12.5 mg for 4 weeks. At the primary endpoint of 4 weeks, the treatment difference between amlodipine/valsartan and amlodipine was 6.6/3.9 mmHg.

There are no trials of the Exforge combination tablet demonstrating reductions in cardiovascular risk in patients with hypertension, but the amlodipine component and several ARBs, which are the same pharmacological class as the valsartan component, have demonstrated such benefits.

16 HOW SUPPLIED/STORAGE AND HANDLING

Exforge is available as non-scored tablets containing amlodipine besylate equivalent to 5 mg, or 10 mg of amlodipine free-base with valsartan 160 mg or 320 mg, providing for the following available combinations: 5/160 mg, 10/160 mg, 5/320 mg, and 10/320 mg.

All strengths are packaged in bottles of 30 and 90 count.

5/160 mg Tablets - dark yellow, ovaloid shaped, film-coated tablet with beveled edge, debossed with "NVR" on one side and "ECE" on the other side.

Bottles of 30 NDC # 0078-0488-15
Bottles of 90 NDC # 0078-0488-34

10/160 mg Tablets - light yellow, ovaloid shaped, film-coated tablet with beveled edge, debossed with "NVR" on one side and "UIC" on the other side.

Bottles of 30 NDC # 0078-0489-15
Bottles of 90 NDC # 0078-0489-34

5/320 mg Tablets - very dark yellow, ovaloid shaped, film-coated tablet with beveled edge, debossed with "NVR" on one side and "CSF" on the other side.

Bottles of 30 NDC # 0078-0490-15
Bottles of 90 NDC # 0078-0490-34

10/320 mg Tablets - dark yellow, ovaloid shaped, film-coated tablet with beveled edge, debossed with "NVR" on one side and "LUF" on the other side.

Bottles of 30 NDC # 0078-0491-15
Bottles of 90 NDC # 0078-0491-34

Store at 25°C (77°F); excursions permitted to 15-30°C (59-86°F). [See USP Controlled Room Temperature.] Protect from moisture.

17 PATIENT COUNSELING INFORMATION

Information for Patients

Pregnancy: Female patients of childbearing age should be told about the consequences of exposure to Exforge during pregnancy. Discuss treatment options with women planning to become pregnant. Patients should be asked to report pregnancies to their physicians as soon as possible.

T2012-215
November 2012

FDA-APPROVED PATIENT LABELING

PATIENT INFORMATION
EXFORGE (X-phorj)
(amlodipine and valsartan)
Tablets

Read the Patient Information that comes with EXFORGE before you start taking it and each time you get a refill. There may be new information. This leaflet does not take the place of talking with your doctor about your medical condition or treatment. If you have any questions about EXFORGE, ask your doctor or pharmacist.

What is the most important information I should know about EXFORGE?

- EXFORGE can cause harm or death to an unborn baby.
- Talk to your doctor about other ways to lower your blood pressure if you plan to become pregnant.
- If you get pregnant while taking EXFORGE, tell your doctor right away.

What is EXFORGE?

EXFORGE contains 2 prescription medicines:
1. amlodipine, a calcium channel blocker
2. valsartan, an angiotensin receptor blocker (ARB).

EXFORGE may be used to lower high blood pressure (hypertension) in adults

- when 1 medicine to lower your high blood pressure is not enough
- as the first medicine to lower high blood pressure if your doctor decides you are likely to need more than 1 medicine.

EXFORGE has not been studied in children under 18 years of age.

What should I tell my doctor before taking EXFORGE?

Tell your doctor about all of your medical conditions, including if you:

- **are pregnant or plan to become pregnant.** See "What is the most important information I should know about EXFORGE?"

- **are breastfeeding or plan to breastfeed.** EXFORGE may pass into your milk. Do not breastfeed while you are taking EXFORGE.
- have heart problems
- have liver problems
- have kidney problems
- are vomiting or having a lot of diarrhea
- have ever had a reaction called angioedema, to another blood pressure medicine. Angioedema causes swelling of the face, lips, tongue, throat, and may cause difficulty breathing.

Tell your doctor about all the medicines you take, including prescription and nonprescription medicines, vitamins, and herbal supplements. Some of your other medicines and EXFORGE could affect each other, causing serious side effects.

Especially tell your doctor if you take:

- simvastatin or other cholesterol lowering medicine
- other medicines for high blood pressure or a heart problem
- water pills (diuretics)
- potassium supplements. Your doctor may check the amount of potassium in your blood periodically.
- a salt substitute. Your doctor may check the amount of potassium in your blood periodically.
- nonsteroidal anti-inflammatory drugs (like ibuprofen or naproxen)
- medicines used to prevent and treat fungal skin infections (such as Ketoconazole, itraconazole)
- medicines used to treat bacterial infections (such as clarithromycin, telithromycin)
- certain antibiotics (rifamycin group), a drug used to protect against transplant rejection (cyclosporin) or an antiretroviral drug used to treat HIV/AIDS infection (ritonavir). These drugs may increase the effect of valsartan.

Know the medicines you take. Keep a list of your medicines and show it to your doctor or pharmacist when you get a new medicine. Talk to your doctor or pharmacist before you start taking any new medicine. Your doctor or pharmacist will know what medicines are safe to take together.

How should I take EXFORGE?

- Take EXFORGE exactly as your doctor tells you.
- Take EXFORGE once each day.
- EXFORGE can be taken with or without food.
- If you miss a dose, take it as soon as you remember. If it is close to your next dose, do not take the missed dose. Just take the next dose at your regular time.
- If you take too much EXFORGE, call your doctor or Poison Control Center, or go to the emergency room.
- Tell all your doctors or dentist you are taking EXFORGE if you:
  - are going to have surgery
  - go for kidney dialysis

What should I avoid while taking EXFORGE?

You should not take EXFORGE during pregnancy. See "What is the most important information I should know about EXFORGE?"

What are the possible side effects of EXFORGE?

EXFORGE may cause **serious side effects** including:

- **harm to an unborn baby causing injury and even death.** See "What is the most important information I should know about EXFORGE?"
- **low blood pressure (hypotension).** Low blood pressure is most likely to happen if you:
  - take water pills
  - are on a low-salt diet
  - get dialysis treatments
  - have heart problems
  - get sick with vomiting or diarrhea
  - drink alcohol

Lie down if you feel faint or dizzy. Call your doctor right away.

- **more heart attacks and chest pain (angina)** in people that already have severe heart problems. This may happen when you start EXFORGE or when there is an increase in your dose of EXFORGE. Get emergency help if you get worse chest pain or chest pain that does not go away.
- **kidney problems.** Kidney problems may become worse in people that already have kidney disease. Some people will have changes in blood tests for kidney function and may need a lower dose of EXFORGE. Call your doctor if you have swelling in your feet, ankles, or hands or unexplained weight gain. If you have heart failure, your doctor should check your kidney function before prescribing EXFORGE.
- **laboratory blood test changes in people with heart failure.** Some people with heart failure who take valsartan, 1 of the medicines in EXFORGE, have changes in blood tests including increased potassium and decreased kidney function.

The most common side effects of EXFORGE include:

- swelling (edema) of the hands, ankles, or feet
- nasal congestion, sore throat, and discomfort when swallowing
- upper respiratory tract infection (head or chest cold)
- dizziness

Tell your doctor if you have any side effect that bothers you or that does not go away.

These are not all the possible side effects of EXFORGE. For more information, ask your doctor or pharmacist.

Call your doctor for medical advice about side effects. You may report side effects to FDA at 1-800-FDA-1088.

How should I store EXFORGE?

- Store EXFORGE at room temperature between 59°F to 86°F (15°C to 30°C).
- Keep EXFORGE dry (protect it from moisture).

Keep EXFORGE and all medicines out of the reach of children.

General Information about EXFORGE

Medicines are sometimes prescribed for conditions that are not mentioned in the patient information leaflet. Do not use EXFORGE for a condition for which it was not prescribed. Do not give EXFORGE to other people, even if they have the same symptoms that you have. It may harm them.

This patient information leaflet summarizes the most important information about EXFORGE. If you would like more information about EXFORGE, talk with your doctor. You can ask your doctor or pharmacist for information about EXFORGE that is written for health professionals. For more information go to www.EXFORGE.com or call 1-888-839-3674.

What are the ingredients in EXFORGE?

Active ingredients: Amlodipine besylate and valsartan

The inactive ingredients of all strengths of the tablets are colloidal silicon dioxide, crospovidone, magnesium stearate, and microcrystalline cellulose. Additionally, the 5/320 mg and 10/320 mg strengths contain iron oxide yellow and sodium starch glycolate. The film coating contains hypromellose, iron oxides, polyethylene glycol, talc, and titanium dioxide.

What is high blood pressure (hypertension)?

Blood pressure is the force of blood in your blood vessels when your heart beats and when your heart rests. You have high blood pressure when the force is too much. EXFORGE can help your blood vessels relax so your blood pressure is lower. Medicines that lower blood pressure lower your chance of having a stroke or heart attack.

High blood pressure makes the heart work harder to pump blood throughout the body and causes damage to blood vessels. If high blood pressure is not treated, it can lead to stroke, heart attack, heart failure, kidney failure, and vision problems.

*Norvasc® is a registered trademark of Pfizer, Inc.
**Viagra® is a registered trademark of Pfizer, Inc.

Distributed by:
Novartis Pharmaceuticals Corporation
East Hanover, New Jersey 07936
©Novartis
T2012-189
September 2012

Shown in Product Identification Guide, page 310

EXFORGE HCT® ℞

[X-phorj HCT]
(amlodipine, valsartan, hydrochlorothiazide)
Tablets

The following prescribing information is based on official labeling in effect July 2013.

HIGHLIGHTS OF PRESCRIBING INFORMATION

These highlights do not include all the information needed to use Exforge HCT safely and effectively. See full prescribing information for Exforge HCT.

Exforge HCT® (amlodipine, valsartan, hydrochlorothiazide) Tablets

Initial U.S. Approval: 2009

> **WARNING: FETAL TOXICITY**
>
> ***See full prescribing information for complete boxed warning.***
>
> - **When pregnancy is detected, discontinue Exforge HCT as soon as possible. (5.1)**
> - **Drugs that act directly on the renin-angiotensin system can cause injury and death to the developing fetus. (5.1)**

RECENT MAJOR CHANGES

Boxed Warning: Fetal Toxicity	01/2012
Indications and Usage: Benefits of lowering blood pressure (1)	12/2011
Contraindications: Known hypersensitivity (4)	09/2012
Contraindications: Dual RAS Blockade in Diabetics (4)	11/2012
Warnings and Precautions: Fetal Toxicity (5.1)	01/2012
Drug Interactions: Dual Blockade of the Renin-Angiotensin System (7)	11/2012

INDICATIONS AND USAGE

- Exforge HCT is a combination tablet of amlodipine, a dihydropyridine calcium channel blocker (DHP CCB), valsartan, an angiotensin II receptor blocker (ARB), and hydrochlorothiazide, a thiazide diuretic. Exforge HCT is indicated for the treatment of hypertension to lower blood pressure. Lowering blood pressure reduces the risk of fatal and nonfatal cardiovascular events, primarily strokes, and myocardial infarctions. (1)
- Not indicated for initial therapy

DOSAGE AND ADMINISTRATION

- Dose once-daily. Titrate up to a maximum dose of 10/320/25 mg
- Exforge HCT may be used as add-on/switch therapy for patients not adequately controlled on any two of the following antihypertensive classes: calcium channel blockers, angiotensin receptor blockers, and diuretics.
- Exforge HCT may be substituted for its individually titrated components (2).

DOSAGE FORMS AND STRENGTHS

Tablets: (amlodipine/valsartan/hydrochlorothiazide mg) 5/160/12.5, 10/160/12.5, 5/160/25, 10/160/25, 10/320/25 (3)

CONTRAINDICATIONS

- Anuria (4)
- Hypersensitivity to sulfonamide-derived drugs (4)
- Known hypersensitivity to any component (4)
- Do not coadminister aliskiren with Exforge HCT in patients with diabetes (4)

WARNINGS AND PRECAUTIONS

- Hypotension: Correct volume depletion prior to initiation (5.2)
- Increased angina and/or myocardial infarction (5.3)
- Monitor renal function and potassium in susceptible patients (5.4, 5.5)
- Exacerbation or activation of systemic lupus erythematosus (5.7)
- Observe for signs of fluid or electrolyte imbalance (5.9)
- Acute angle-closure glaucoma (5.10)

ADVERSE REACTIONS

Most common adverse events (≥2% incidence) are dizziness, peripheral edema, headache, dyspepsia, fatigue, muscle spasms, back pain, nausea and nasopharyngitis. (6.1)

To report SUSPECTED ADVERSE REACTIONS, contact Novartis Pharmaceuticals Corporation at 1-888-669-6682 or FDA at 1-800-FDA-1088 or www.fda.gov/medwatch.

DRUG INTERACTIONS

- If simvastatin is coadministered with amlodipine, do not exceed doses greater than 20 mg daily of simvastatin (7)
- Antidiabetic drugs: Dosage adjustment of antidiabetic may be required (7)
- Cholestyramine and colestipol: Reduced absorption of thiazides (12.3)
- Lithium: Diuretics increase risk of lithium toxicity. Monitor serum lithium concentrations during concurrent use. (7)
- NSAID use may lead to increased risk of renal impairment and loss of anti-hypertensive effect (7)
- Dual inhibition of the renin-angiotensin system: Increased risk of renal impairment, hypotension, and hyperkalemia (7)

USE IN SPECIFIC POPULATIONS

Nursing Mothers: Avoid use while nursing – discontinue either nursing or drug (8.3)

See 17 for PATIENT COUNSELING INFORMATION and FDA-approved patient labeling

Revised: 11/2012

FULL PRESCRIBING INFORMATION: CONTENTS*

*** Sections or subsections omitted from the full prescribing information are not listed**

FULL PRESCRIBING INFORMATION

WARNING: FETAL TOXICITY
- **When pregnancy is detected, discontinue Exforge HCT as soon as possible. (5.1)**
- **Drugs that act directly on the renin-angiotensin system can cause injury and death to the developing fetus. (5.1)**

1 INDICATIONS AND USAGE

Exforge HCT (amlodipine, valsartan, hydrochlorothiazide) is indicated for the treatment of hypertension, to lower blood pressure. Lowering blood pressure reduces the risk of fatal and nonfatal cardiovascular events, primarily strokes and myocardial infarctions. These benefits have been seen in controlled trials of antihypertensive drugs from a wide variety of pharmacologic classes, including amlodipine, hydrochlorothiazide, and the ARB class to which valsartan principally belongs. There are no controlled trials demonstrating risk reduction with Exforge HCT.

Control of high blood pressure should be part of comprehensive cardiovascular risk management, including, as appropriate, lipid control, diabetes management, antithrombotic therapy, smoking cessation, exercise, and limited sodium intake. Many patients will require more than 1 drug to achieve blood pressure goals. For specific advice on goals and management, see published guidelines, such as those of the National High Blood Pressure Education Program's Joint National Committee on Prevention, Detection, Evaluation, and Treatment of High Blood Pressure (JNC).

Numerous antihypertensive drugs, from a variety of pharmacologic classes and with different mechanisms of action, have been shown in randomized controlled trials to reduce cardiovascular morbidity and mortality, and it can be concluded that it is blood pressure reduction, and not some other pharmacologic property of the drugs, that is largely responsible for those benefits. The largest and most consistent cardiovascular outcome benefit has been a reduction in the risk of stroke, but reductions in myocardial infarction and cardiovascular mortality also have been seen regularly.

Elevated systolic or diastolic pressure causes increased cardiovascular risk, and the absolute risk increase per mmHg is greater at higher blood pressures, so that even modest reductions of severe hypertension can provide substantial benefit. Relative risk reduction from blood pressure reduction is similar across populations with varying absolute risk, so the absolute benefit is greater in patients who are at higher risk independent of their hypertension (for example, patients with diabetes or hyperlipidemia), and such patients would be expected to benefit from more aggressive treatment to a lower blood pressure goal.

Some antihypertensive drugs have smaller blood pressure effects (as monotherapy) in black patients, and many antihypertensive drugs have additional approved indications and effects (e.g., on angina, heart failure, or diabetic kidney disease). These considerations may guide selection of therapy.

This fixed combination drug is not indicated for the initial therapy of hypertension [see *Dosage and Administration* (2)].

2 DOSAGE AND ADMINISTRATION

2.1 General Considerations

Dose once-daily. The dosage may be increased after 2 weeks of therapy. The full blood pressure lowering effect was achieved 2 weeks after being on the maximal dose of Exforge HCT. The maximum recommended dose of Exforge HCT is 10/320/25 mg.

2.2 Add-on / Switch Therapy

Exforge HCT may be used for patients not adequately controlled on any 2 of the following antihypertensive classes: calcium channel blockers, angiotensin receptor blockers, and diuretics.

A patient who experiences dose-limiting adverse reactions to an individual component while on any dual combination of the components of Exforge HCT may be switched to Exforge HCT containing a lower dose of that component to achieve similar blood pressure reductions.

2.3 Replacement Therapy

Exforge HCT may be substituted for the individually titrated components.

2.4 Use with Other Antihypertensive Drugs

Exforge HCT may be administered with other antihypertensive agents.

3 DOSAGE FORMS AND STRENGTHS

- 5 mg amlodipine /160 mg valsartan /12.5 mg hydrochlorothiazide Tablets – White, non-scored, film-coated tablet, ovaloid, biconvex with beveled edge with debossing "NVR" on one side and "VCL" on the other side.
- 10 mg amlodipine /160 mg valsartan /12.5 mg hydrochlorothiazide Tablets – Pale yellow, non-scored, film-coated tablet, ovaloid, biconvex with beveled edge with debossing "NVR" on one side and "VDL" on the other side.
- 5 mg amlodipine /160 mg valsartan /25 mg hydrochlorothiazide Tablets – Yellow, non-scored, film-coated tablet, ovaloid, biconvex with beveled edge with debossing "NVR" on one side and "VEL" on the other side.
- 10 mg amlodipine /160 mg valsartan /25 mg hydrochlorothiazide Tablets – Brown-yellow, non-scored, film-coated tablet, ovaloid, biconvex with beveled edge with debossing "NVR" on one side and "VHL" on the other side.
- 10 mg amlodipine /320 mg valsartan /25 mg hydrochlorothiazide Tablets – Brown-yellow, non-scored, film-coated tablet, ovaloid, biconvex with beveled edge with debossing "NVR" on one side and "VFL" on the other side.

4 CONTRAINDICATIONS

Do not use in patients with anuria, hypersensitivity to other sulfonamide-derived drugs, or hypersensitivity to any component of this product.

Do not coadminister aliskiren with Exforge HCT in patients with diabetes *[see Drug Interactions (7)]*.

5 WARNINGS AND PRECAUTIONS

5.1 Fetal Toxicity

Pregnancy Category D

Use of drugs that act on the renin-angiotensin system during the second and third trimesters of pregnancy reduces fetal renal function and increases fetal and neonatal morbidity and death. Resulting oligohydramnios can be associated with fetal lung hypoplasia and skeletal deformations. Potential neonatal adverse effects include skull hypoplasia, anuria, hypotension, renal failure, and death. When pregnancy is detected, discontinue Exforge HCT as soon as possible *[see Use in Specific Populations (8.1)]*.

5.2 Hypotension in Volume- or Salt-Depleted Patients

Excessive hypotension, including orthostatic hypotension, was seen in 1.7% of patients treated with the maximum dose of Exforge HCT (10/320/25 mg) compared to 1.8% of valsartan/HCTZ (320/25 mg) patients, 0.4% of amlodipine/valsartan (10/320 mg) patients, and 0.2% of HCTZ/amlodipine (25/10 mg) patients in a controlled trial in patients with moderate to severe uncomplicated hypertension. In patients with an activated renin-angiotensin system, such as volume- or salt-depleted patients receiving high doses of diuretics, symptomatic hypotension may occur in patients receiving angiotensin receptor blockers. Correct this condition prior to administration of Exforge HCT.

Exforge HCT has not been studied in patients with heart failure, recent myocardial infarction, or in patients undergoing surgery or dialysis. Patients with heart failure or post-myocardial infarction patients given valsartan commonly have some reduction in blood pressure, but discontinuation of therapy because of continuing symptomatic hypotension usually is not necessary when dosing instructions are followed. In controlled trials in heart failure patients, the incidence of hypotension in valsartan-treated patients was 5.5% compared to 1.8% in placebo-treated patients. In the Valsartan in Acute Myocardial Infarction Trial (VALIANT), hypotension in post-myocardial infarction patients led to permanent discontinuation of therapy in 1.4% of valsartan-treated patients and 0.8% of captopril-treated patients.

Since the vasodilation induced by amlodipine is gradual in onset, acute hypotension has rarely been reported after oral administration. Do not initiate treatment with Exforge HCT in patients with aortic or mitral stenosis or obstructive hypertrophic cardiomyopathy.

If excessive hypotension occurs with Exforge HCT, the patient should be placed in a supine position and, if necessary, given an intravenous infusion of normal saline. A transient hypotensive response is not a contraindication to further treatment, which usually can be continued without difficulty once the blood pressure has stabilized.

5.3 Increased Angina and/or Myocardial Infarction

Worsening angina and acute myocardial infarction can develop after starting or increasing the dose of amlodipine, particularly in patients with severe obstructive coronary artery disease.

5.4 Impaired Renal Function

Changes in renal function including acute renal failure can be caused by drugs that inhibit the renin-angiotensin system and by diuretics. Patients whose renal function may depend in part on the activity of the renin-angiotensin system (e.g., patients with renal artery stenosis, chronic kidney disease, severe congestive heart failure, or volume depletion) may be at particular risk of developing acute renal failure on Exforge HCT. Monitor renal function periodically in these patients. Consider withholding or discontinuing therapy in patients who develop a clinically significant decrease in renal function on Exforge HCT *[see Drug Interactions (7)]*.

5.5 Potassium Abnormalities

In the controlled trial of Exforge HCT in moderate to severe hypertensive patients, the incidence of hypokalemia (serum potassium <3.5 mEq/L) at any time post-baseline with the maximum dose of Exforge HCT (10/320/25 mg) was 10% compared to 25% with HCTZ/amlodipine (25/10 mg), 7% with valsartan/HCTZ (320/25 mg), and 3% with amlodipine/valsartan (10/320 mg). One patient (0.2%) discontinued therapy due to an adverse event of hypokalemia in each of the Exforge HCT and HCTZ/amlodipine groups. The incidence of hyperkalemia (serum potassium >5.7 mEq/L) was 0.4% with Exforge HCT compared to 0.2-0.7% with the dual therapies.

Some patients with heart failure have developed increases in potassium on valsartan. These effects are usually minor and transient, and they are more likely to occur in patients with pre-existing renal impairment. Dosage reduction and/or discontinuation of the diuretic and/or valsartan may be required.

Hydrochlorothiazide can cause hypokalemia and hyponatremia. Hypomagnesemia can result in hypokalemia which appears difficult to treat despite potassium repletion. Drugs that inhibit the renin-angiotensin system can cause hyperkalemia. Monitor serum electrolytes periodically.

If hypokalemia is accompanied by clinical signs (e.g., muscular weakness, paresis, or ECG alterations), Exforge HCT should be discontinued. Correction of hypokalemia and any coexisting hypomagnesmia is recommended prior to the initiation of thiazides.

5.6 Hypersensitivity Reaction

Hypersensitivity reactions to hydrochlorothiazide may occur in patients with or without a history of allergy or bronchial asthma, but are more likely in patients with such a history.

5.7 Systemic Lupus Erythematosus

Thiazide diuretics have been reported to cause exacerbation or activation of systemic lupus erythematosus.

5.8 Lithium Interaction

Lithium generally should not be given with thiazides [see *Drug Interactions, Hydrochlorothiazide, Lithium* (7)].

5.9 Metabolic Imbalances

Hydrochlorothiazide may alter glucose tolerance and raise serum levels of cholesterol and triglycerides.

Hydrochlorothiazide may raise the serum uric acid level due to reduced clearance of uric acid and may cause or exacerbate hyperuricemia and precipitate gout in susceptible patients.

Hydrochlorothiazide decreases urinary calcium excretion and may cause elevations of serum calcium. Monitor calcium levels in patients with hypercalcemia receiving Exforge HCT.

5.10 Acute Myopia and Secondary Angle-Closure Glaucoma

Hydrochlorothiazide, a sulfonamide, can cause an idiosyncratic reaction, resulting in acute transient myopia and acute angle-closure glaucoma. Symptoms include acute onset of decreased visual acuity or ocular pain and typically occur within hours to weeks of drug initiation. Untreated acute angle-closure glaucoma can lead to permanent vision loss. The primary treatment is to discontinue hydrochlorothiazide as rapidly as possible. Prompt medical or surgical treatments may need to be considered if the intraocular pressure remains uncontrolled. Risk factors for developing acute angle-closure glaucoma may include a history of sulfonamide or penicillin allergy.

6 ADVERSE REACTIONS

6.1 Clinical Trials Experience

Because clinical studies are conducted under widely varying conditions, adverse reaction rates observed in the clinical studies of a drug cannot be directly compared to rates in the clinical studies of another drug and may not reflect the rates observed in clinical practice.

In the controlled trial of Exforge HCT, where only the maximum dose (10/320/25 mg) was evaluated, safety data were obtained in 582 patients with hypertension. Adverse reactions have generally been mild and transient in nature and have only infrequently required discontinuation of therapy. The overall frequency of adverse reactions was similar between men and women, younger (<65 years) and older (≥65 years) patients, and black and white patients. In the active controlled clinical trial, discontinuation because of adverse events occurred in 4.0% of patients treated with Exforge HCT 10/320/25 mg compared to 2.9% of patients treated with valsartan/HCTZ 320/25 mg, 1.6% of patients treated with amlodipine/valsartan 10/320 mg, and 3.4% of patients treated with HCTZ/amlodipine 25/10 mg. The most common reasons for discontinuation of therapy with Exforge HCT were dizziness (1.0%) and hypotension (0.7%).

The most frequent adverse events that occurred in the active controlled clinical trial in at least 2% of patients treated with Exforge HCT are presented in the table below:

[See table above]

Preferred Term	Aml/Val/HCTZ 10/320/25 mg N=582 n (%)	Val/HCTZ 320/25 mg N=559 n (%)	Aml/Val 10/320 mg N=566 n (%)	HCTZ/Aml 25/10 mg N=561 n (%)
Dizziness	48 (8.2)	40 (7.2)	14 (2.5)	23 (4.1)
Edema	38 (6.5)	8 (1.4)	65 (11.5)	63 (11.2)
Headache	30 (5.2)	31 (5.5)	30 (5.3)	40 (7.1)
Dyspepsia	13 (2.2)	5 (0.9)	6 (1.1)	2 (0.4)
Fatigue	13 (2.2)	15 (2.7)	12 (2.1)	8 (1.4)
Muscle spasms	13 (2.2)	7 (1.3)	7 (1.2)	5 (0.9)
Back pain	12 (2.1)	13 (2.3)	5 (0.9)	12 (2.1)
Nausea	12 (2.1)	7 (1.3)	10 (1.8)	12 (2.1)
Nasopharyngitis	12 (2.1)	13 (2.3)	13 (2.3)	12 (2.1)

Orthostatic events (orthostatic hypotension and postural dizziness) were seen in 0.5% of patients. Other adverse reactions that occurred in clinical trials with Exforge HCT (>0.2%) are listed below. It cannot be determined whether these events were causally related to Exforge HCT.

Cardiac Disorders: tachycardia

Ear and Labyrinth Disorders: vertigo, tinnitus

Eye Disorders: vision blurred

Gastrointestinal Disorders: diarrhea, abdominal pain upper, vomiting, abdominal pain, toothache, dry mouth, gastritis, hemorrhoids

General Disorders and Administration Site Conditions: asthenia, noncardiac chest pain, chills, malaise

Infections and Infestations: upper respiratory tract infection, bronchitis, influenza, pharyngitis, tooth abscess, gastroenteritis viral, respiratory tract infection, rhinitis, urinary tract infection

Injury, Poisoning and Procedural Complications: back injury, contusion, joint sprain, procedural pain

Investigations: blood uric acid increased, blood creatine phosphokinase increased, weight decreased

Metabolism and Nutrition Disorders: hypokalemia, diabetes mellitus, hyperlipidemia, hyponatremia

Musculoskeletal and Connective Tissue Disorders: pain in extremity, arthralgia, musculoskeletal pain, muscular weakness, musculoskeletal weakness, musculoskeletal stiffness, joint swelling, neck pain, osteoarthritis, tendonitis

Nervous System Disorders: paresthesia, somnolence, syncope, carpal tunnel syndrome, disturbance in attention, dizziness postural, dysgeusia, head discomfort, lethargy, sinus headache, tremor

Psychiatric Disorders: anxiety, depression, insomnia

Renal and Urinary Disorders: pollakiuria

Reproductive System and Breast Disorders: erectile dysfunction

Respiratory, Thoracic and Mediastinal Disorders: dyspnea, nasal congestion, cough, pharyngolaryngeal pain

Skin and Subcutaneous Tissue Disorders: pruritus, hyperhidrosis, night sweats, rash

Vascular Disorders: hypotension

Isolated cases of the following clinically notable adverse reactions were also observed in clinical trials: anorexia, constipation, dehydration, dysuria, increased appetite, viral infection.

Amlodipine

Amlodipine has been evaluated for safety in more than 11000 patients in US and foreign clinical trials. Other adverse reactions not listed above that have been reported in <1% but >0.1% of patients in controlled clinical trials or under conditions of open trials or marketing experience where a causal relationship is uncertain were:

Cardiovascular: arrhythmia (including ventricular tachycardia and atrial fibrillation), bradycardia, chest pain, peripheral ischemia, syncope, postural hypotension, vasculitis

Central and Peripheral Nervous System: neuropathy peripheral, tremor

Gastrointestinal: anorexia, dysphagia, pancreatitis, gingival hyperplasia

General: allergic reaction, hot flushes, malaise, rigors, weight gain

Musculoskeletal System: arthrosis, muscle cramps

Psychiatric: sexual dysfunction (male and female), nervousness, abnormal dreams, depersonalization

Skin and Appendages: angioedema, erythema multiforme, rash erythematous, rash maculopapular

Special Senses: abnormal vision, conjunctivitis, diplopia, eye pain, tinnitus

Urinary System: micturition frequency, micturition disorder, nocturia

Autonomic Nervous System: sweating increased

Metabolic and Nutritional: hyperglycemia, thirst

Hemopoietic: leukopenia, purpura, thrombocytopenia

Other adverse reactions reported with amlodipine at a frequency of ≤0.1% of patients include: cardiac failure, pulse irregularity, extrasystoles, skin discoloration, urticaria, skin dryness, alopecia, dermatitis, muscle weakness, twitching, ataxia, hypertonia, migraine, cold and clammy skin, apathy, agitation, amnesia, gastritis, increased appetite, loose stools, rhinitis, dysuria, polyuria, parosmia, taste perversion, abnormal visual accommodation, and xerophthalmia. Other reactions occurred sporadically and cannot be distinguished from medications or concurrent disease states such as myocardial infarction and angina.

Adverse reactions reported for amlodipine for indications other than hypertension may be found in its full prescribing information.

Valsartan

Valsartan has been evaluated for safety in more than 4000 hypertensive patients in clinical trials. In trials in which valsartan was compared to an ACE inhibitor with or without placebo, the incidence of dry cough was significantly greater in the ACE inhibitor group (7.9%) than in the groups who received valsartan (2.6%) or placebo (1.5%). In a 129-patient trial limited to patients who had dry cough when they had previously received ACE inhibitors, the incidences of cough in patients who received valsartan, HCTZ, or lisinopril were 20%, 19%, and 69% respectively (p<0.001).

Other adverse reactions, not listed above, occurring in >0.2% of patients in controlled clinical trials with valsartan are:

Digestive: flatulence

Respiratory: sinusitis, pharyngitis

Urogenital: impotence

Adverse reactions reported for valsartan for indications other than hypertension may be found in the prescribing information for Diovan.

Hydrochlorothiazide

Other adverse reactions not listed above that have been reported with hydrochlorothiazide, without regard to causality, are listed below:

Body as a Whole: weakness

Digestive: pancreatitis, jaundice (intrahepatic cholestatic jaundice), sialadenitis, cramping, gastric irritation

Hematologic: aplastic anemia, agranulocytosis, hemolytic anemia

Hypersensitivity: photosensitivity, urticaria, necrotizing angiitis (vasculitis and cutaneous vasculitis), fever, respiratory distress including pneumonitis and pulmonary edema, anaphylactic reactions

Metabolic: glycosuria, hyperuricemia

Nervous System/Psychiatric: restlessness

Renal: renal failure, renal dysfunction, interstitial nephritis

Skin: erythema multiforme including Stevens-Johnson syndrome, exfoliative dermatitis including toxic epidermal necrolysis

Special Senses: transient blurred vision, xanthopsia.

Clinical Laboratory Test Findings

Clinical laboratory test findings for Exforge HCT were obtained in a controlled trial of Exforge HCT administered at the maximal dose of 10/320/25 mg compared to maximal doses of dual therapies, i.e., valsartan/HCTZ 320/25 mg, amlodipine/valsartan 10/320 mg, and HCTZ/amlodipine 25/10 mg. Findings for the components of Exforge HCT were obtained from other trials.

Creatinine: In hypertensive patients, greater than 50% increases in creatinine occurred in 2.1% of Exforge HCT patients compared to 2.4% of valsartan/HCTZ patients, 0.7% of amlodipine/valsartan patients, and 1.8% of HCTZ/amlodipine patients.

In heart failure patients, greater than 50% increases in creatinine were observed in 3.9% of valsartan-treated patients compared to 0.9% of placebo-treated patients. In post-myocardial infarction patients, doubling of serum creatinine was observed in 4.2% of valsartan-treated patients and 3.4% of captopril-treated patients.

Liver Function Tests: Occasional elevations (greater than 150%) of liver chemistries occurred in Exforge HCT-treated patients.

Blood Urea Nitrogen (BUN): In hypertensive patients, greater than 50% increases in BUN were observed in 30% of Exforge HCT-treated patients compared to 29% of valsartan/HCTZ patients, 15.8% of amlodipine/valsartan patients, and 18.5% of HCTZ/amlodipine patients. The majority of BUN values remained within normal limits.

In heart failure patients, greater than 50% increases in BUN were observed in 17% of valsartan-treated patients compared to 6% of placebo-treated patients.

Serum Electrolytes (Potassium): In hypertensive patients, greater than 20% decreases in serum potassium were observed in 6.5% of Exforge HCT-treated patients compared to 3.3% of valsartan/HCTZ patients, 0.4% of amlodipine/valsartan patients, and 19.3% of HCTZ/amlodipine patients. Greater than 20% increases in potassium were observed in 3.5% of Exforge HCT-treated patients compared to 2.4% of valsartan/HCTZ patients, 6.2% of amlodipine/valsartan patients, and 2.2% of HCTZ/amlodipine patients. In heart failure patients, greater than 20% increases in serum potassium were observed in 10% of valsartan-treated patients compared to 5.1% of placebo-treated patients [*see Warnings and Precautions (5.5)*].

Neutropenia: Neutropenia (<1500/L) was observed in 1.9% of patients treated with valsartan and 0.8% of patients treated with placebo.

6.2 Postmarketing Experience

The following additional adverse reactions have been reported in postmarketing experience. Because these reactions are reported voluntarily from a population of uncertain size, it is not always possible to reliably estimate their frequency or establish a causal relationship to drug exposure.

Amlodipine

With amlodipine, gynecomastia has been reported infrequently and a causal relationship is uncertain. Jaundice and hepatic enzyme elevations (mostly consistent with cholestasis or hepatitis), in some cases severe enough to require hospitalization, have been reported in association with use of amlodipine.

Valsartan

The following additional adverse reactions have been reported in postmarketing experience with valsartan or valsartan/hydrochlorothiazide:

Blood and Lymphatic: Decrease in hemoglobin, decrease in hematocrit, neutropenia

Hypersensitivity: There are rare reports of angioedema. Some of these patients previously experienced angioedema with other drugs including ACE inhibitors. Exforge HCT should not be re-administered to patients who have had angioedema.

Digestive: Elevated liver enzymes and very rare reports of hepatitis

Renal: Impaired renal function, renal failure

Clinical Laboratory Tests: Hyperkalemia

Dermatologic: Alopecia

Vascular: Vasculitis

Nervous System: Syncope

Rare cases of rhabdomyolysis have been reported in patients receiving angiotensin II receptor blockers.

Hydrochlorothiazide

The following additional adverse reactions have been reported in post-marketing experience with hydrochlorothiazide:

Acute renal failure, renal disorder, aplastic anemia, erythema multiforme, pyrexia, muscle spasm, asthenia, acute angle-closure glaucoma, bone marrow failure, worsening of diabetes control, hypokalemia, blood lipids increased, hyponatremia, hypomagnesemia, hypercalcemia, hypochloremic alkalosis, impotence, visual impairment.

Pathological changes in the parathyroid gland of patients with hypercalcemia and hypophosphatemia have been observed in a few patients on prolonged thiazide therapy. If hypercalcemia occurs, further diagnostic evaluation is necessary.

7 DRUG INTERACTIONS

No drug interaction studies have been conducted with Exforge HCT and other drugs, although studies have been conducted with the individual components. A pharmacokinetic drug-drug interaction study has been conducted to address the potential for pharmacokinetic interaction between the triple combination, Exforge HCT, and the corresponding 3 double combinations. No clinically relevant interaction was observed.

Amlodipine

Simvastatin: Coadministration of simvastatin with amlodipine increases the systemic exposure of simvastatin. Limit the dose of simvastatin in patients on amlodipine to 20 mg daily.

CYP3A4 Inhibitors: Coadministration with CYP3A inhibitors (moderate and strong) result in increased systemic exposure to amlodipine warranting dose reduction. Monitor for symptoms of hypotension and edema when amlodipine is coadministered with CYP3A4 inhibitors to determine the need for dose adjustment.

CYP3A4 Inducers: No information is available on the quantitative effects of CYP3A4 inducers on amlodipine. Blood pressure should be monitored when amlodipine is coadministered with CYP3A4 inducers.

Valsartan

No clinically significant pharmacokinetic interactions were observed when valsartan was coadministered with amlodipine, atenolol, cimetidine, digoxin, furosemide, glyburide, hydrochlorothiazide, or indomethacin. The valsartan-atenolol combination was more antihypertensive than either component, but it did not lower the heart rate more than atenolol alone.

In vitro metabolism studies have indicated that CYP450 mediated drug interaction between valsartan and coadministered drugs are unlikely because of the low extent of metabolism [see *Pharmacokinetics – Valsartan*, (12.3)].

Coadministration of valsartan and warfarin did not change the pharmacokinetics of valsartan or the time-course of the anticoagulant properties of warfarin.

Potassium: Concomitant use of valsartan with other agents that block the renin-angiotensin system, potassium-sparing diuretics (e.g., spironolactone, triamterene, amiloride), potassium supplements, or salt substitutes containing potassium may lead to increases in serum potassium and in heart failure patients to increases in serum creatinine. If co-medication is considered necessary, monitoring of serum potassium is advisable.

Non-Steroidal Anti-Inflammatory Agents including Selective Cyclooxygenase-2 Inhibitors (COX-2 Inhibitors): In patients who are elderly, volume-depleted (including those on diuretic therapy), or with compromised renal function, coadministration of NSAIDs, including selective COX-2 inhibitors, with angiotensin II receptor antagonists, including valsartan, may result in deterioration of renal function, including possible acute renal failure. These effects are usually reversible. Monitor renal function periodically in patients receiving valsartan and NSAID therapy.

The antihypertensive effect of angiotensin II receptor antagonists, including valsartan may be attenuated by NSAIDs including selective COX-2 inhibitors.

Dual Blockade of the Renin-Angiotensin System (RAS): Dual blockade of the RAS with angiotensin receptor blockers, ACE inhibitors, or aliskiren is associated with increased risks of hypotension, hyperkalemia, and changes in renal function (including acute renal failure) compared to monotherapy. Closely monitor blood pressure, renal function, and electrolytes in patients on Exforge HCT and other agents that affect the RAS.

Do not coadminister aliskiren with Exforge HCT in patients with diabetes. Avoid use of aliskiren with Exforge HCT in patients with renal impairment (GFR <60 mL/min).

Hydrochlorothiazide

When administered concurrently the following drugs may interact with thiazide diuretics:

Antidiabetic drugs (oral agents and insulin): Dosage adjustment of the antidiabetic drug may be required.

Lithium: Diuretic agents increase the risk of lithium toxicity. Refer to the package insert for lithium preparations before use of such preparations with Exforge HCT. Monitoring of serum lithium concentrations is recommended during concurrent use.

Non-steroidal anti-inflammatory drugs (NSAIDs and COX-2 selective inhibitors): When Exforge HCT and nonsteroidal anti-inflammatory agents are used concomitantly, the patient should be observed closely to determine if the desired effect of diuretic is obtained.

Carbamazepine: May lead to symptomatic hyponatremia.

Ion exchange resins: Staggering the dosage of hydrochlorothiazide and ion exchange resins (e.g., cholestyramine, colestipol) such that hydrochlorothiazide is administered at least 4 hours before or 4-6 hours after the administration of resins would potentially minimize the interaction. *[see Clinical Pharmacology (12.3)]*

Cyclosporine: Concomitant treatment with cyclosporine may increase the risk of hyperuricemia and gout-type complications.

8 USE IN SPECIFIC POPULATIONS

8.1 Pregnancy

Pregnancy Category D

Use of drugs that act on the renin-angiotensin system during the second and third trimesters of pregnancy reduces fetal renal function and increases fetal and neonatal morbidity and death. Resulting oligohydramnios can be associated with fetal lung hypoplasia and skeletal deformations. Potential neonatal adverse effects include skull hypoplasia, anuria, hypotension, renal failure, and death. When pregnancy is detected, discontinue Exforge HCT as soon as possible. These adverse outcomes are usually associated with use of these drugs in the second and third trimester of pregnancy. Most epidemiologic studies examining fetal abnormalities after exposure to antihypertensive use in the first trimester have not distinguished drugs affecting the renin-angiotensin system from other antihypertensive agents. Appropriate management of maternal hypertension during pregnancy is important to optimize outcomes for both mother and fetus.

In the unusual case that there is no appropriate alternative to therapy with drugs affecting the renin-angiotensin system for a particular patient, apprise the mother of the potential risk to the fetus. Perform serial ultrasound examinations to assess the intra-amniotic environment. If oligohydramnios is observed, discontinue Exforge HCT, unless it is considered lifesaving for the mother. Fetal testing may be appropriate, based on the week of pregnancy. Patients and physicians should be aware, however, that oligohydramnios may not appear until after the fetus has sustained irreversible injury. Closely observe infants with histories of in utero exposure to Exforge HCT for hypotension, oliguria, and hyperkalemia. *[see Use in Specific Populations (8.4)]*

Hydrochlorothiazide

Thiazides can cross the placenta, and concentrations reached in the umbilical vein approach those in the maternal plasma. Hydrochlorothiazide, like other diuretics, can cause placental hypoperfusion. It accumulates in the amniotic fluid, with required concentrations up to 19 times higher than in umbilical vein plasma. Use of thiazides during pregnancy is associated with a risk of fetal or neonatal jaundice of thrombocytopenia. Since they do not prevent or alter the course of EPH (Edema, Proteinuria, Hypertension) gestosis (pre-eclampsia), these drugs should not be used to treat hypertension in pregnant women. The use of hydrochlorothiazide for other indications (e.g., heart disease) in pregnancy should be avoided.

8.3 Nursing Mothers

It is not known whether amlodipine and valsartan are excreted in human milk, but thiazides are excreted in human milk and valsartan is excreted in rat milk. Because of the potential for adverse effects on the nursing infant, a decision should be made whether to discontinue nursing or discontinue the drug, taking into account the importance of the drug to the mother.

8.4 Pediatric Use

The safety and effectiveness of Exforge HCT in pediatric patients have not been established.

Neonates with a history of in utero exposure to Exforge HCT: If oliguria or hypotension occurs, direct attention toward support of blood pressure and renal perfusion. Exchange transfusions or dialysis may be required as a means of reversing hypotension and/or substituting for disordered renal function.

8.5 Geriatric Use

Exposure to amlodipine is increased in elderly patients, thus consider lower initial doses of Exforge HCT *[see Clinical Pharmacology (12.3)]*.

In controlled clinical trials, 82 hypertensive patients treated with Exforge HCT were ≥65 years and 13 were ≥75 years. No overall differences in the efficacy or safety of Exforge HCT were observed in this patient population, but greater sensitivity of some older individuals cannot be ruled out.

8.6 Renal Impairment

Safety and effectiveness of Exforge HCT in patients with severe renal impairment (CrCl< 30 mL/min) have not been established. No dose adjustment is required in patients with mild (60-90 mL/min) or moderate (CrCl 30-60) renal impairment.

8.7 Hepatic Impairment

Amlodipine

Exposure to amlodipine is increased in patients with hepatic insufficiency, thus consider using lower doses of Exforge HCT [*see Clinical Pharmacology (12.3)*].

Valsartan

No dose adjustment is necessary for patients with mild-to-moderate disease. No dosing recommendations can be provided for patients with severe liver disease.

Hydrochlorothiazide

Minor alterations of fluid and electrolyte balance may precipitate hepatic coma in patients with impaired hepatic function or progressive liver disease.

10 OVERDOSAGE

Limited data are available related to overdosage in humans. The most likely manifestations of overdosage would be hypotension and tachycardia; bradycardia could occur from parasympathetic (vagal) stimulation. If symptomatic hypotension should occur, supportive treatment should be instituted.

Amlodipine

Single oral doses of amlodipine maleate equivalent to 40 mg/kg and 100 mg/kg amlodipine in mice and rats, respectively, caused deaths. Single oral doses equivalent to 4 or more mg/kg amlodipine in dogs (11 or more times the maximum recommended human dose on a mg/m^2 basis) caused a marked peripheral vasodilation and hypotension. Overdosage might be expected to cause excessive peripheral vasodilation with marked hypotension. In humans, experience with intentional overdosage of amlodipine is limited. Marked and potentially prolonged systemic hypotension up to and including shock with fatal outcome have been reported.

If massive overdose should occur, initiate active cardiac and respiratory monitoring. Frequent blood pressure measurements are essential. Should hypotension occur, initiate cardiovascular support including elevation of the extremities and the judicious administration of fluids. If hypotension remains unresponsive to these conservative measures, consider administration of vasopressors (such as phenylephrine) with attention to circulating volume and urine output. As amlodipine is highly protein bound, hemodialysis is not likely to be of benefit. Administration of activated charcoal to healthy volunteers immediately or up to two hours after ingestion of amlodipine has been shown to significantly decrease amlodipine absorption.

Valsartan

Depressed level of consciousness, circulatory collapse, and shock have been reported.

Valsartan is not removed from the plasma by hemodialysis. Valsartan was without grossly observable adverse effects at single oral doses up to 2000 mg/kg in rats and up to 1000 mg/kg in marmosets, except for salivation and diarrhea in the rat and vomiting in the marmoset at the highest dose (60 and 31 times, respectively, the maximum recommended human dose (MHRD) on a mg/m^2 basis). (Calculations assume an oral dose of 320 mg/day and a 60-kg patient.)

Hydrochlorothiazide

The degree to which hydrochlorothiazide is removed by hemodialysis has not been established. The most common signs and symptoms observed in patients are those caused by electrolyte depletion (hypokalemia, hypochloremia, hyponatremia) and dehydration resulting from excessive diuresis. If digitalis has also been administered, hypokalemia may accentuate cardiac arrhythmias.

The oral LD_{50} of hydrochlorothiazide is greater than 10 g/kg in both mice and rats, 2000 and 4000 times, respectively, the MHRD on a mg/m^2 basis. (Calculations assume an oral dose of 25 mg/day and a 60-kg patient.)

Valsartan and Hydrochlorothiazide

In rats and marmosets, single oral doses of valsartan up to 1524 and 762 mg/kg in combination with hydrochlorothiazide at doses up to 476 and 238 mg/kg, respectively, were very well tolerated without any treatment-related effects. These no adverse effect doses in rats and marmosets, respectively, represent 46.5 and 23 times the MRHD of valsartan and 188 and 113 times the MRHD of hydrochlorothiazide on a mg/m^2 basis. (Calculations assume an oral dose of 320 mg/day valsartan in combination with 25 mg/day hydrochlorothiazide and a 60-kg patient.)

11 DESCRIPTION

Exforge HCT is a fixed combination of amlodipine, valsartan, and hydrochlorothiazide.

Exforge HCT contains the besylate salt of amlodipine, a dihydropyridine calcium channel blocker (CCB). Amlodipine besylate, USP is a white to pale yellow crystalline powder, slightly soluble in water and sparingly soluble in ethanol. Amlodipine besylate's chemical name is 3-Ethyl 5-methyl (±)-2-[(2-aminoethoxy)methyl]-4-(*o*-chlorophenyl)-1,4-dihydro-6-methyl-3,5-pyridinedicarboxylate, monobenzenesulfonate ; its structural formula is

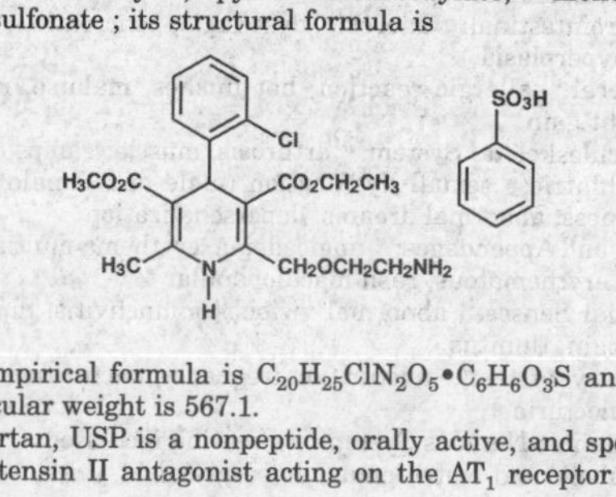

Its empirical formula is $C_{20}H_{25}ClN_2O_5 \cdot C_6H_6O_3S$ and its molecular weight is 567.1.

Valsartan, USP is a nonpeptide, orally active, and specific angiotensin II antagonist acting on the AT_1 receptor subtype. Valsartan is a white to practically white fine powder, soluble in ethanol and methanol and slightly soluble in water. Valsartan's chemical name is N-(1-oxopentyl)-N-[[2'-(1*H*-tetrazol-5-yl) [1,1'-biphenyl]-4-yl]methyl]-L-valine; its structural formula is

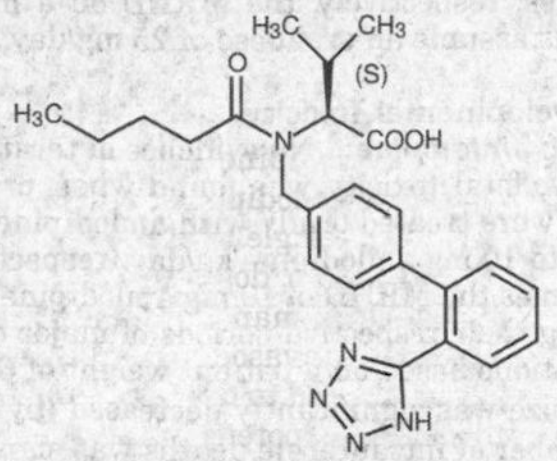

Its empirical formula is $C_{24}H_{29}N_5O_3$ and its molecular weight is 435.5.

Hydrochlorothiazide, USP is a white, or practically white, practically odorless, crystalline powder. It is slightly soluble in water; freely soluble in sodium hydroxide solution, in *n*-butylamine, and in dimethylformamide; sparingly soluble in methanol; and insoluble in ether, in chloroform, and in dilute mineral acids. Hydrochlorothiazide is chemically described as 6-chloro-3,4-dihydro-2*H*-1,2,4-benzothiadiazine-7- sulfonamide 1,1-dioxide.

Hydrochlorothiazide is a thiazide diuretic. Its empirical formula is $C_7H_8ClN_3O_4S_2$, its molecular weight is 297.73, and its structural formula is

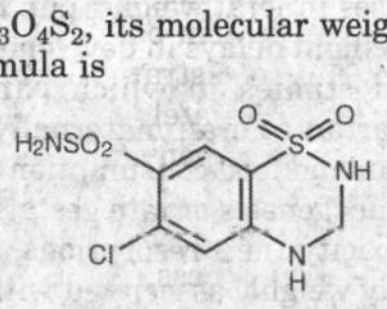

Exforge HCT film-coated tablets are formulated in 5 strengths for oral administration with a combination of amlodipine besylate, valsartan, and hydrochlorothiazide, providing for the following available combinations: 5/160/12.5 mg, 10/160/12.5 mg, 5/160/25 mg, 10/160/25 mg, and 10/320/25 mg amlodipine besylate/valsartan/hydrochlorothiazide. The inactive ingredients for all strengths of the tablets include microcrystalline cellulose; crospovidone; colloidal anhydrous silica; magnesium stearate; hypromellose, macrogol 4000, and talc. Additionally, the 5/160/12.5 mg strength contains titanium dioxide; the 10/160/12.5 mg strength contains titanium dioxide and yellow and red iron oxides; the 5/160/25 mg strength contains titanium dioxide and yellow iron oxide, and the 10/160/25 mg and 10/320/25 mg strengths both contain yellow iron oxide.

12 CLINICAL PHARMACOLOGY

12.1 Mechanism of Action

The active ingredients of Exforge HCT target 3 separate mechanisms involved in blood pressure regulation. Specifically, amlodipine blocks the contractile effects of calcium on cardiac and vascular smooth muscle cells; valsartan blocks the vasoconstriction and sodium retaining effects of angiotensin II on cardiac, vascular smooth muscle, adrenal and renal cells; and hydrochlorothiazide directly promotes the excretion of sodium and chloride in the kidney leading to reductions in intravascular volume. A more detailed description of the mechanism of action of each individual component follows.

Amlodipine

Amlodipine is a dihydropyridine calcium channel blocker that inhibits the transmembrane influx of calcium ions into vascular smooth muscle and cardiac muscle. Experimental data suggest that amlodipine binds to both dihydropyridine and nondihydropyridine binding sites. The contractile processes of cardiac muscle and vascular smooth muscle are dependent upon the movement of extracellular calcium ions into these cells through specific ion channels. Amlodipine inhibits calcium ion influx across cell membranes selectively, with a greater effect on vascular smooth muscle cells than on cardiac muscle cells. Negative inotropic effects can be detected in vitro but such effects have not been seen in intact animals at therapeutic doses. Serum calcium concentration is not affected by amlodipine. Within the physiologic pH range, amlodipine is an ionized compound (pKa=8.6), and its kinetic interaction with the calcium channel receptor is characterized by a gradual rate of association and dissociation with the receptor binding site, resulting in a gradual onset of effect.

Amlodipine is a peripheral arterial vasodilator that acts directly on vascular smooth muscle to cause a reduction in peripheral vascular resistance and reduction in blood pressure.

Valsartan

Angiotensin II is formed from angiotensin I in a reaction catalyzed by angiotensin-converting enzyme (ACE, kininase II). Angiotensin II is the principal pressor agent of the renin-angiotensin system, with effects that include vasoconstriction, stimulation of synthesis and release of aldosterone, cardiac stimulation, and renal reabsorption of sodium. Valsartan blocks the vasoconstrictor and aldosterone-secreting effects of angiotensin II by selectively blocking the binding of angiotensin II to the AT_1 receptor in many tissues, such as vascular smooth muscle and the adrenal gland. Its action is therefore independent of the pathways for angiotensin II synthesis.

There is also an AT_2 receptor found in many tissues, but AT_2 is not known to be associated with cardiovascular homeostasis. Valsartan has much greater affinity (about 20000-fold) for the AT_1 receptor than for the AT_2 receptor. The increased plasma levels of angiotensin following AT_1 receptor blockade with valsartan may stimulate the unblocked AT_2 receptor. The primary metabolite of valsartan is essentially inactive with an affinity for the AT_1 receptor about one-200th that of valsartan itself.

Blockade of the renin-angiotensin system with ACE inhibitors, which inhibit the biosynthesis of angiotensin II from angiotensin I, is widely used in the treatment of hypertension. ACE inhibitors also inhibit the degradation of bradykinin, a reaction also catalyzed by ACE. Because valsartan does not inhibit ACE (kininase II), it does not affect the response to bradykinin. Whether this difference has clinical relevance is not yet known. Valsartan does not bind to or block other hormone receptors or ion channels known to be important in cardiovascular regulation.

Blockade of the angiotensin II receptor inhibits the negative regulatory feedback of angiotensin II on renin secretion, but the resulting increased plasma renin activity and angiotensin II circulating levels do not overcome the effect of valsartan on blood pressure.

Hydrochlorothiazide

Hydrochlorothiazide is a thiazide diuretic. Thiazides affect the renal tubular mechanisms of electrolyte reabsorption, directly increasing excretion of sodium and chloride in approximately equivalent amounts. Indirectly, the diuretic action of hydrochlorothiazide reduces plasma volume, with consequent increases in plasma renin activity, increases in aldosterone secretion, increases in urinary potassium loss, and decreases in serum potassium. The renin-aldosterone link is mediated by angiotensin II, so coadministration of an angiotensin II receptor antagonist tends to reverse the potassium loss associated with these diuretics.

The mechanism of the antihypertensive effect of thiazides is unknown.

12.2 Pharmacodynamics

Exforge HCT has been shown to be effective in lowering blood pressure. The 3 components of Exforge HCT (amlodipine, valsartan, hydrochlorothiazide) lower the blood pressure through complementary mechanisms, each working at a separate site and blocking different effector pathways. The pharmacodynamics of each individual component are described below.

Exforge HCT has not been studied in indications other than hypertension.

Amlodipine

Following administration of therapeutic doses to patients with hypertension, amlodipine produces vasodilation resulting in a reduction of supine and standing blood pressures. These decreases in blood pressure are not accompanied by a significant change in heart rate or plasma catecholamine levels with chronic dosing. Although the acute intravenous administration of amlodipine decreases arterial blood pressure and increases heart rate in hemodynamic studies of patients with chronic stable angina, chronic oral administration of amlodipine in clinical trials did not lead to clinically significant changes in heart rate or blood pressures in normotensive patients with angina.

With chronic, once-daily administration, antihypertensive effectiveness is maintained for at least 24 hours. Plasma concentrations correlate with effect in both young and elderly patients. The magnitude of reduction in blood pressure with amlodipine is also correlated with the height of pretreatment elevation; thus, individuals with moderate hypertension (diastolic pressure 105-114 mmHg) had about a 50% greater response than patients with mild hypertension (diastolic pressure 90-104 mmHg). Normotensive subjects experienced no clinically significant change in blood pressure (+1/-2 mmHg).

In hypertensive patients with normal renal function, therapeutic doses of amlodipine resulted in a decrease in renal vascular resistance and an increase in glomerular filtration rate and effective renal plasma flow without change in filtration fraction or proteinuria.

As with other calcium channel blockers, hemodynamic measurements of cardiac function at rest and during exercise (or pacing) in patients with normal ventricular function treated with amlodipine have generally demonstrated a small increase in cardiac index without significant influence on dP/dt or on left ventricular end diastolic pressure or volume. In hemodynamic studies, amlodipine has not been associated with a negative inotropic effect when administered in the therapeutic dose range to intact animals and man, even when coadministered with beta-blockers to man. Similar findings, however, have been observed in normals or well-compensated patients with heart failure with agents possessing significant negative inotropic effects.

Amlodipine does not change sinoatrial nodal function or atrioventricular conduction in intact animals or man. In patients with chronic stable angina, intravenous administration of 10 mg did not significantly alter A-H and H-V conduction and sinus node recovery time after pacing. Similar results were obtained in patients receiving amlodipine and concomitant beta-blockers. In clinical studies in which amlodipine was administered in combination with beta-blockers to patients with either hypertension or angina, no adverse effects of electrocardiographic (ECG) parameters were observed. In clinical trials with angina patients alone, amlodipine therapy did not alter ECG intervals or produce higher degrees of AV blocks.

Amlodipine has indications other than hypertension which are described in its full prescribing information.

Valsartan

Valsartan inhibits the pressor effect of angiotensin II infusions. An oral dose of 80 mg inhibits the pressor effect by about 80% at peak with approximately 30% inhibition persisting for 24 hours. No information on the effect of larger doses is available.

Removal of the negative feedback of angiotensin II causes a 2- to 3-fold rise in plasma renin and consequent rise in angiotensin II plasma concentration in hypertensive patients. Minimal decreases in plasma aldosterone were observed after administration of valsartan; very little effect on serum potassium was observed.

Administration of valsartan to patients with essential hypertension results in a significant reduction of sitting, supine, and standing systolic blood pressure, usually with little or no orthostatic change.

Valsartan has indications other than hypertension which are described in its full prescribing information.

Hydrochlorothiazide

After oral administration of hydrochlorothiazide, diuresis begins within 2 hours, peaks in about 4 hours and lasts about 6 to 12 hours.

12.3 Pharmacokinetics

Exforge HCT

Following oral administration of Exforge HCT in normal healthy adults, peak plasma concentrations of amlodipine, valsartan and HCTZ are reached in about 6 hours, 3 hours, and 2 hours, respectively. The rate and extent of absorption of amlodipine, valsartan and HCTZ from Exforge HCT are the same as when administered as individual dosage forms. The bioavailability of amlodipine, valsartan, and HCTZ were not altered when Exforge HCT was administered with food. Exforge HCT may be administered with or without food.

Amlodipine

Peak plasma concentrations of amlodipine are reached 6-12 hours after administration of amlodipine alone. Absolute bioavailability has been estimated to be between 64% and 90%. The apparent volume of distribution of amlodipine is 21 L/kg. Approximately 93% of circulating amlodipine is bound to plasma proteins in hypertensive patients.

Amlodipine is extensively (about 90%) converted to inactive metabolites via hepatic metabolism with 10% of the parent compound and 60% of the metabolites excreted in the urine.

Elimination of amlodipine from the plasma is biphasic with a terminal elimination half-life of about 30-50 hours. Steady state plasma levels of amlodipine are reached after 7 to 8 days of consecutive daily dosing.

Valsartan

Following oral administration of valsartan alone peak plasma concentrations of valsartan are reached in 2 to 4 hours. Absolute bioavailability is about 25% (range 10%-35%).

The steady state volume of distribution of valsartan after intravenous administration is 17 L indicating that valsartan does not distribute into tissues extensively. Valsartan is highly bound to serum proteins (95%), mainly serum albumin.

Valsartan shows biexponential decay kinetics following intravenous administration with an average elimination half-life of about 6 hours. The recovery is mainly as unchanged drug, with only about 20% of dose recovered as metabolites. The primary metabolite, accounting for about 9% of dose, is valeryl 4-hydroxy valsartan. In vitro metabolism studies involving recombinant CYP450 enzymes indicated that the CYP2C9 isoenzyme is responsible for the formation of valeryl-4-hydroxy valsartan. Valsartan does not inhibit CYP450 isozymes at clinically relevant concentrations. CYP450 mediated drug interaction between valsartan and coadministered drugs are unlikely because of the low extent of metabolism.

Valsartan, when administered as an oral solution, is primarily recovered in feces (about 83% of dose) and urine (about 13% of dose). Following intravenous administration, plasma clearance of valsartan is about 2 L/h and its renal clearance is 0.62 L/h (about 30% of total clearance).

Hydrochlorothiazide

The estimated absolute bioavailability of hydrochlorothiazide after oral administration is about 70%. Peak plasma hydrochlorothiazide concentrations (C_{max}) are reached within 2 to 5 hours after oral administration. There is no clinically significant effect of food on the bioavailability of hydrochlorothiazide.

Hydrochlorothiazide binds to albumin (40% to 70%) and distributes into erythrocytes. Following oral administration, plasma hydrochlorothiazide concentrations decline biexponentially, with a mean distribution half-life of about 2 hours and an elimination half-life of about 10 hours.

About 70% of an orally administered dose of hydrochlorothiazide is eliminated in the urine as unchanged drug.

Special Populations

Geriatric: Elderly patients have decreased clearance of amlodipine with a resulting increase in peak plasma levels, elimination half-life, and AUC. Exposure (measured by AUC) to valsartan is higher by 70% and the half-life is longer by 35% in the elderly than in the young. Limited amount of data suggest that the systemic clearance of hydrochlorothiazide is reduced in both healthy and hypertensive elderly subjects compared to young healthy volunteers.

Gender: Pharmacokinetics of valsartan do not differ significantly between males and females.

Race: Pharmacokinetic differences due to race have not been studied.

Renal Insufficiency: The pharmacokinetics of amlodipine are not significantly influenced by renal impairment. There is no apparent correlation between renal function (measured by creatinine clearance) and exposure (measured by AUC) to valsartan in patients with different degrees of renal impairment. Valsartan has not been studied in patients with severe impairment of renal function (creatinine clearance <10 mL/min). Valsartan is not removed from the plasma by hemodialysis.

In a study in individuals with impaired renal function, the mean elimination half-life of hydrochlorothiazide was doubled in individuals with mild/moderate renal impairment (30 < CrCl < 90 mL/min) and tripled in severe renal impairment (≤ 30 mL/min), compared to individuals with normal renal function (CrCl > 90 mL/min). *[see Use in Special Populations (8.6)]*

Hepatic Insufficiency: Patients with hepatic insufficiency have decreased clearance of amlodipine with resulting increase in AUC of approximately 40%-60%. On average, patients with mild-to-moderate chronic liver disease have twice the exposure (measured by AUC values) to valsartan of healthy volunteers (matched by age, sex, and weight). *[see Use in Special Populations (8.7)]*

Drug Interactions

Amlodipine:

In vitro data in human plasma indicate that amlodipine has no effect on the protein binding of digoxin, phenytoin, warfarin, and indomethacin.

Cimetidine: Coadministration of amlodipine with cimetidine did not alter the pharmacokinetics of amlodipine.

Grapefruit juice: Coadministration of 240 mL of grapefruit juice with a single oral dose of amlodipine 10 mg in 20 healthy volunteers had no significant effect on the pharmacokinetics of amlodipine.

Maalox® (antacid): Coadministration of the antacid Maalox with a single dose of amlodipine had no significant effect on the pharmacokinetics of amlodipine.

Sildenafil: A single 100 mg dose of sildenafil in subjects with essential hypertension had no effect on the pharmacokinetic parameters of amlodipine. When amlodipine and sildenafil were used in combination, each agent independently exerted its own blood pressure lowering effect.

Atorvastatin: Coadministration of multiple 10 mg doses of amlodipine with 80 mg of atorvastatin resulted in no significant change in the steady state pharmacokinetic parameters of atorvastatin.

Digoxin: Coadministration of amlodipine with digoxin did not change serum digoxin levels or digoxin renal clearance in normal volunteers.

Ethanol (alcohol): Single and multiple 10 mg doses of amlodipine had no significant effect on the pharmacokinetics of ethanol.

Warfarin: Coadministration of amlodipine with warfarin did not change the warfarin prothrombin response time.

Simvastatin: Coadministration of multiple doses of 10 mg of amlodipine with 80 mg simvastatin resulted in a 77% increase in exposure to simvastatin compared to simvastatin alone. Limit the dose of simvastatin in patients on amlodipine to 20 mg daily.

CYP3A4 Inhibitors: Coadministration of a 180 mg daily dose of diltiazem with 5 mg amlodipine in elderly hypertensive patients resulted in a 60% increase in amlodipine systemic exposure. Erythromycin coadministration in healthy volunteers did not significantly change amlodipine systemic exposure. However, strong inhibitors of CYP3A4 (e.g., ketoconazole, itraconazole, ritonavir) may increase the plasma concentrations of amlodipine to a greater extent.

Hydrochlorothiazide:

Drugs that alter gastrointestinal motility: The bioavailability of thiazide-type diuretics may be increased by anticholinergic agents (e.g., atropine, biperiden), apparently due to a decrease in gastrointestinal motility and the stomach emptying rate. Conversely, pro-kinetic drugs may decrease the bioavailability of thiazide diuretics.

Cholestyramine: In a dedicated drug interaction study, administration of cholestyramine 2 hours before hydrochlorothiazide resulted in a 70% reduction in exposure to hydrochlorothiazide. Further, administration of hydrochlorothiazide 2 hours before cholestyramine resulted in 35% reduction in exposure to hydrochlorothiazide.

Antineoplastic agents (e.g. cyclophosphamide, methotrexate): Concomitant use of thiazide diuretics may reduce renal excretion of cytotoxic agents and enhance their myelosuppressive effects.

Alcohol, barbiturates, or narcotics: Potentiation of orthostatic hypotension may occur.

Skeletal muscle relaxants: Possible increased responsiveness to muscle relaxants such as curare derivatives.

Digitalis glycosides: Thiazide-induced hypokalemia or hypomagnesemia may predispose the patient to digoxin toxicity.

13 NONCLINICAL TOXICOLOGY

13.1 Carcinogenesis, Mutagenesis, Impairment of Fertility

Studies with amlodipine/valsartan/hydrochlorothiazide: No carcinogenicity, mutagenicity, or fertility studies have been conducted with this combination. However, these studies have been conducted for amlodipine, valsartan and hydrochlorothiazide alone. Based on the preclinical safety and human pharmacokinetic studies, there is no indication of any toxicologically significant adverse interaction between these components.

Studies with amlodipine: Rats and mice treated with amlodipine maleate in the diet for up to two years, at concentrations calculated to provide daily dosage levels of 0.5, 1.25, and 2.5 mg amlodipine/kg/day, showed no evidence of a carcinogenic effect of the drug. For the mouse, the highest dose was, on mg/m^2 basis, similar to the MRHD of 10 mg amlodipine/day. For the rat, the highest dose was, on a mg/m^2 basis, about 2.5 times the MRHD. (Calculations based on a 60-kg patient.)

Mutagenicity studies conducted with amlodipine maleate revealed no drug-related effects at either the gene or chromosome level.

There was no effect on the fertility of rats treated orally with amlodipine maleate (males for 64 days and females for 14 days prior to mating) at doses of up to 10 mg amlodipine/kg/day (about 10 times the MRHD of 10 mg/day on a mg/m^2 basis).

Studies with valsartan: There was no evidence of carcinogenicity when valsartan was administered in the diet to mice and rats for up to 2 years at concentrations calculated to provide doses of up to 160 and 200 mg/kg/day, respectively. These doses in mice and rats are about 2.4 and 6 times, respectively, the MRHD of 320 mg/day on a mg/m^2 basis. (Calculations based on a 60 kg patient.)

Mutagenicity assays did not reveal any valsartan-related effects at either the gene or chromosome level. These assays included bacterial mutagenicity tests with Salmonella and E. coli, a gene mutation test with Chinese hamster V79 cells, a cytogenetic test with Chinese hamster ovary cells, and a rat micronucleus test.

Valsartan had no adverse effects on the reproductive performance of male or female rats at oral doses of up to 200 mg/kg/day. This dose is about 6 times the MRHD on a mg/m^2 basis.

Studies with hydrochlorothiazide: Two-year feeding studies in mice and rats conducted under the auspices of the National Toxicology Program (NTP) uncovered no evidence of a carcinogenic potential of hydrochlorothiazide in female mice (at doses of up to approximately 600 mg/kg/day) or in male and female rats (at doses of up to approximately 100 mg/kg/day). The NTP, however, found equivocal evidence for hepatocarcinogenicity in male mice.

Hydrochlorothiazide was not genotoxic *in vitro* in the Ames mutagenicity assay of Salmonella Typhimurium strains TA 98, TA 100, TA 1535, TA 1537, and TA 1538 and in the Chinese Hamster Ovary (CHO) test for chromosomal aberrations, or *in vivo* in assays using mouse germinal cell chromosomes, Chinese hamster bone marrow chromosomes, and the Drosophila sex-linked recessive lethal trait gene. Positive test results were obtained in the *in vitro* CHO Sister Chromatid Exchange (clastogenicity) and Mouse Lymphoma Cell (mutagenicity) assays and in the Aspergillus Nidulans non-disjunction assay.

Hydrochlorothiazide had no adverse effects on the fertility of mice and rats of either sex in studies wherein these species were exposed via diet at doses of up to 100 and 4 mg/kg, respectively, prior to mating and throughout gestation. These doses of hydrochlorothiazide in mice and rats are 19 and 1.5 times, respectively, the MRHD on a mg/m^2 basis. (Calculations assume an oral dose of 25 mg/day and a 60-kg patient.)

13.3 Developmental Toxicity

Studies with amlodipine: No evidence of teratogenicity or other embryo/fetal toxicity was found when pregnant rats and rabbits were treated orally with amlodipine maleate at doses of up to 10 mg amlodipine/kg/day (respectively, about 10 and 20 times the MRHD of 10 mg amlodipine on a mg/m^2 basis) during their respective periods of major organogenesis. (Calculations based on a patient weight of 60 kg.) However, litter size was significantly decreased (by about 50%) and the number of intrauterine deaths was significantly increased (about 5-fold) for rats receiving amlodipine maleate at a dose equivalent to 10 mg amlodipine/kg/day for 14 days before mating and throughout mating and gestation. Amlodipine maleate has been shown to prolong both the gestation period and the duration of labor in rats at this dose. There are no adequate and well controlled studies in pregnant women.

Studies with valsartan: No teratogenic effects were observed when valsartan was administered to pregnant mice and rats at oral doses of up to 600 mg/kg/day and to pregnant rabbits at oral doses of up to 10 mg/kg/day. However, significant decreases in fetal weight, pup birth weight, pup survival rate, and slight delays in developmental milestones were observed in studies in which parental rats were treated with valsartan at oral, maternally toxic (reduction in body weight gain and food consumption) doses of 600 mg/kg/day during organogenesis or late gestation and lactation. In rabbits, fetotoxicity (i.e., resorptions, litter loss, abortions, and low body weight) associated with maternal toxicity (mortality) was observed at doses of 5 and 10 mg/kg/day. The no observed adverse effect doses of 600, 200 and 2 mg/kg/day in mice, rats and rabbits, respectively, are about 9, 6 and 0.1 times the MRHD of 320 mg/day on a mg/m^2 basis. (Calculations based on a patient weight of 60 kg.)

Studies with hydrochlorothiazide: Under the auspices of the National Toxicology Program, pregnant mice and rats that received hydrochlorothiazide via gavage at doses up to 3000 and 1000 mg/kg/day, respectively, on gestation days 6 through 15 showed no evidence of teratogenicity. These doses of hydrochlorothiazide in mice and rats are 608 and 405 times, respectively, the MRHD on a mg/m^2 basis. (Calculations assume an oral dose of 25 mg/day and a 60-kg patient.)

Studies with amlodipine and valsartan: In the oral embryofetal development study in rats using amlodipine besylate plus valsartan at doses equivalent to 5 mg/kg/day amlodipine plus 80 mg/kg/day valsartan, 10 mg/kg/day amlodipine plus 160 mg/kg/day valsartan, and 20 mg/kg/day amlodipine plus 320 mg/kg/day valsartan, treatment-related maternal and fetal effects (developmental delays and alterations noted in the presence of significant maternal toxicity) were noted with the high dose combination. The no-observed-adverse-effect level (NOAEL) for embryo-fetal effects was 10 mg/kg/day amlodipine plus 160 mg/kg/day valsartan. On a systemic exposure [$AUC_{(0-\infty)}$] basis, these doses are, respectively, 4.3 and 2.7 times the systemic exposure [$AUC_{(0-\infty)}$] in humans receiving the MRHD (10/320 mg/60 kg).

Studies with valsartan and hydrochlorothiazide: There was no evidence of teratogenicity in mice, rats, or rabbits treated orally with valsartan at doses up to 600, 100, and 10 mg/kg/day, respectively, in combination with hydrochlorothiazide at doses up to 188, 31, and 3 mg/kg/day. These non-teratogenic doses in mice, rats and rabbits are, respectively, 9, 3.5, and 0.5 times the MRHD of valsartan and 38, 13 and 2 times the MRHD of hydrochlorothiazide on a mg/m^2 basis. (Calculations assume an oral dose of 320 mg/day valsartan in combination with 25 mg/day hydrochlorothiazide in a 60-kg patient.)

Fetotoxicity was observed in association with maternal toxicity in rats at valsartan/hydrochlorothiazide doses ≥200/63 mg/kg/day and in rabbits at valsartan/hydrochlorothiazide doses of 10/3 mg/kg/day. Evidence of fetotoxicity in rats consisted of decreased fetal weight and fetal variations of sternebrae, vertebrae, ribs, and/or renal papillae. Evidence of fetotoxicity in rabbits included increased numbers of late resorptions with resultant increases in total resorptions, postimplantation losses, and decreased number of live fetuses. The no observed adverse effect doses of the valsartan/hydrochlorothiazide combination in mice, rats and rabbits were 600/188, 100/31 and 3/1 mg/kg/day, respectively. These doses in mice, rats and rabbits are, respectively, 9, 3 and 0.18 times the MRHD of valsartan and 38, 13, and 0.5 times the MRHD of hydrochlorothiazide on a mg/m^2 basis. (Calculations assume an oral dose of 320 mg/day valsartan in combination with 25 mg/day hydrochlorothiazide in a 60-kg patient.)

14 CLINICAL STUDIES

Exforge HCT was studied in a double-blind, active controlled study in hypertensive patients. A total of 2271 patients with moderate to severe hypertension (mean baseline systolic/diastolic blood pressure was 170/107 mmHg) received treatments of amlodipine/valsartan/HCTZ 10/320/25 mg, valsartan/HCTZ 320/25 mg, amlodipine/valsartan 10/320 mg, or HCTZ/amlodipine 25/10 mg. At study initiation patients assigned to the 2-component arms received lower doses of their treatment combination while patients assigned to the Exforge HCT arm received 160/12.5 mg valsartan/hydrochlorothiazide. After 1 week, Exforge HCT patients were titrated to 5/160/12.5 mg amlodipine/valsartan/hydrochlorothiazide, while all other patients continued receiving their initial doses. After 2 weeks, all patients were titrated to their full treatment dose. A total of 55% of patients were male, 14% were 65 years or older, 72% were Caucasian, and 17% were black.

At week 8, the triple combination therapy produced greater reductions in blood pressure than each of the 3 dual combination treatments ($p<0.0001$ for both diastolic and systolic blood pressures reductions). The reductions in systolic/diastolic blood pressure with Exforge HCT were 7.6/5.0 mmHg greater than with valsartan/HCTZ, 6.2/3.3 mmHg greater than with amlodipine/valsartan, and 8.2/5.3 mmHg greater than with amlodipine/HCTZ (see Figure 1). The full blood pressure lowering effect was achieved 2 weeks after being on the maximal dose of Exforge HCT (see Figure 2 and Figure 3). As the pivotal study was an active-controlled trial, the treatment effects shown in Figure 1, 2, and 3 include a placebo effect of unknown size.

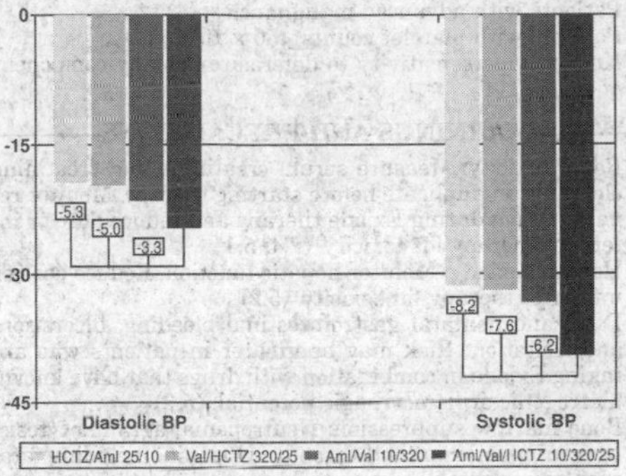

Figure 1: Reduction in Mean Blood Pressure at Endpoint

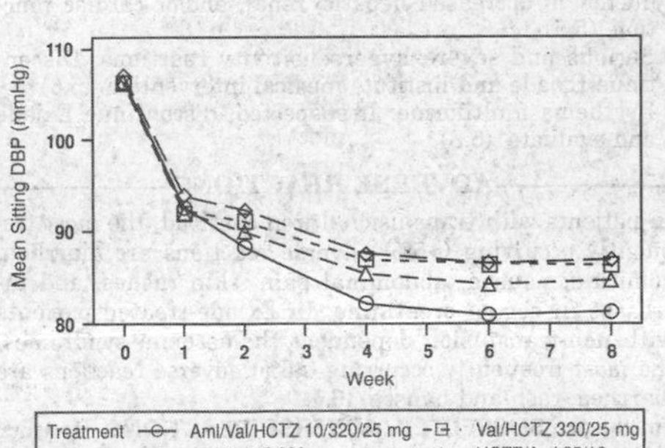

Figure 2: Mean Sitting Diastolic Blood Pressure by Treatment and Week

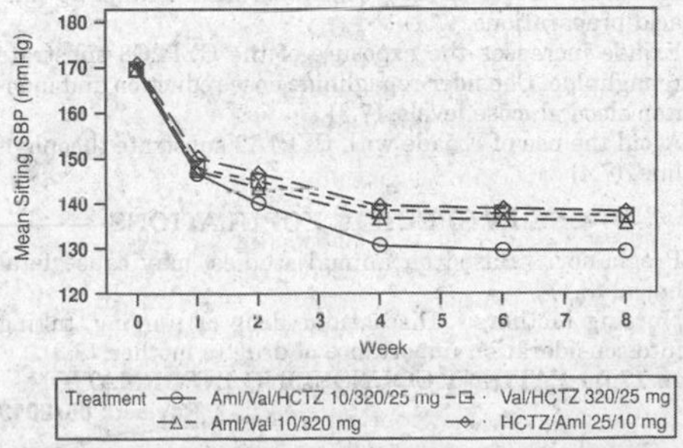

Figure 3: Mean Sitting Systolic Blood Pressure by Treatment and Week

A subgroup of 283 patients was studied with ambulatory blood pressure monitoring. The blood pressure lowering effect in the triple therapy group was maintained throughout the 24-hour period (see Figure 4 and Figure 5).

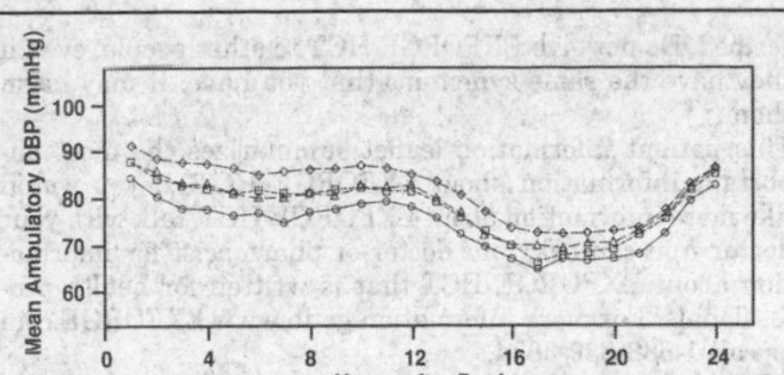

Figure 4: Mean Ambulatory Diastolic Blood Pressure at Endpoint by Treatment and Hour

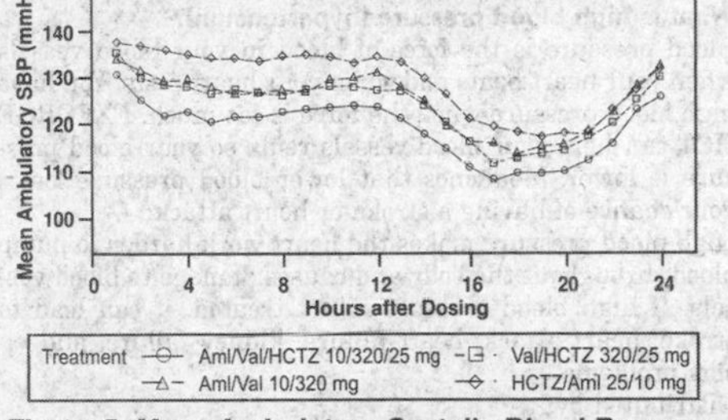

Figure 5: Mean Ambulatory Systolic Blood Pressure at Endpoint by Treatment and Hour

There are no trials of the Exforge HCT combination tablet demonstrating reductions in cardiovascular risk in patients with hypertension, but both the amlodipine and hydrochlorothiazide components and several ARBs, which are the same pharmacological class as the valsartan component, have demonstrated such benefits.

16 HOW SUPPLIED/STORAGE AND HANDLING

Exforge HCT (amlodipine, valsartan, hydrochlorothiazide) is available as film-coated tablets containing amlodipine besylate equivalent to 5 mg or 10 mg of amlodipine free-base with valsartan 160 mg or 320 mg, and hydrochlorothiazide 12.5 mg or 25 mg, providing for the following available combinations: 5/160/12.5 mg, 10/160/12.5 mg, 5/160/25 mg, 10/160/25 mg, and 10/320/25 mg. All strengths are packaged in bottles of 30 and 90 tablets.

5 mg amlodipine /160 mg valsartan /12.5 mg hydrochlorothiazide Tablets – White, non-scored, film-coated tablet, ovaloid, biconvex with beveled edge with debossing "NVR" on one side and "VCL" on the other side.

Bottles of 30	NDC 0078-0559-15
Bottles of 90	NDC 0078-0559-34

10 mg amlodipine /160 mg valsartan /12.5 mg hydrochlorothiazide Tablets – Pale yellow, non-scored, film-coated tablet, ovaloid, biconvex with beveled edge with debossing "NVR" on one side and "VDL" on the other side.

Bottles of 30	NDC 0078-0561-15
Bottles of 90	NDC 0078-0561-34

5 mg amlodipine /160 mg valsartan /25 mg hydrochlorothiazide Tablets – Yellow, non-scored, film-coated tablet, ovaloid, biconvex with beveled edge with debossing "NVR" on one side and "VEL" on the other side.

Bottles of 30	NDC 0078-0560-15
Bottles of 90	NDC 0078-0560-34

10 mg amlodipine /160 mg valsartan /25 mg hydrochlorothiazide Tablets – Brown-yellow, non-scored, film-coated tablet, ovaloid, biconvex with beveled edge with debossing "NVR" on one side and "VHL" on the other side.

Bottles of 30	NDC 0078-0562-15
Bottles of 90	NDC 0078-0562-34

10 mg amlodipine /320 mg valsartan /25 mg hydrochlorothiazide Tablets – Brown-yellow, non-scored, film-coated tablet, ovaloid, biconvex with beveled edge with debossing "NVR" on one side and "VFL" on the other side.

Bottles of 30	NDC 0078-0563-15
Bottles of 90	NDC 0078-0563-34

Store at 25°C (77°F); excursions permitted to 15-30°C (59-86°F), [see USP controlled room temperature.]

Protect from moisture.

Dispense in tight container (USP).

17 PATIENT COUNSELING INFORMATION

Pregnancy: Female patients of childbearing age should be told about the consequences of exposure to Exforge HCT during pregnancy. Discuss treatment options with women planning to become pregnant. Patients should be asked to report pregnancies to their physicians as soon as possible.

Symptomatic Hypotension: A patient receiving Exforge HCT should be cautioned that lightheadedness can occur, especially during the first days of therapy, and that it should be reported to the prescribing physician. The patients should be told that if syncope occurs, Exforge HCT should be discontinued until the physician has been consulted.

All patients should be cautioned that inadequate fluid intake, excessive perspiration, diarrhea, or vomiting can lead to an excessive fall in blood pressure, with the same consequences of lightheadedness and possible syncope.

Potassium Supplements: A patient receiving Exforge HCT should be told not to use potassium supplements or salt substitutes containing potassium without consulting the prescribing physician.

T2012-214

November 2012

Information for Patients

Patient Information

Exforge HCT (X-phorj HCT)

(amlodipine and valsartan and hydrochlorothiazide) Tablets

Read the Patient Information that comes with EXFORGE HCT before you start taking it and each time you get a refill. There may be new information. This leaflet does not take the place of talking with your doctor about your medical condition or treatment.

What is the most important information I should know about EXFORGE HCT?

- EXFORGE HCT can cause harm or death to an unborn baby.
- Talk to your doctor about other ways to lower your blood pressure if you plan to become pregnant.
- If you get pregnant while taking EXFORGE HCT, tell your doctor right away.

What is EXFORGE HCT?

EXFORGE HCT contains 3 prescription medicines:

1. amlodipine, a calcium channel blocker
2. valsartan, an angiotensin receptor blocker, and
3. hydrochlorothiazide, a diuretic (water pill)

EXFORGE HCT may be used to lower blood pressure in adults when 2 medicines to lower your high blood pressure are not enough.

EXFORGE HCT has not been studied in children under 18 years of age.

Who should not take EXFORGE HCT?

Do not take EXFORGE HCT if you have low or no urine output (anuria).

What should I tell my doctor before taking EXFORGE HCT?

Tell your doctor about all of your medical conditions, including if you:

- **are pregnant or plan to become pregnant.** See "What is the most important information I should know about EXFORGE HCT?"
- **are breastfeeding or plan to breastfeed.** EXFORGE HCT may pass into your milk. Do not breastfeed while you are taking EXFORGE HCT.
- are allergic to any of the ingredients in EXFORGE HCT. See the end of this leaflet for a list of the ingredients in EXFORGE HCT.
- have heart problems
- have liver problems
- have kidney problems
- are vomiting or having a lot of diarrhea
- have or had gallstones
- have Lupus
- have low levels of potassium (with or without symptoms such as muscle weakness, muscle spasms, abnormal heart rhythm) or magnesium in your blood
- have high levels of calcium in your blood (with or without symptoms such as nausea, vomiting, constipation, stomach pain, frequent urination, thirst, muscle weakness, and twitching).
- have high levels of uric acid in the blood.
- have ever had a reaction called angioedema, to another blood pressure medicine. Angioedema causes swelling of the face, lips, tongue, and may cause difficulty breathing.

Tell your doctor about all the medicines you take, including prescription and nonprescription medicines, vitamins, and herbal supplements. Some of your other medicines and EXFORGE HCT could affect each other, causing serious side effects.

Especially tell your doctor if you take:

- simvastatin or other cholesterol lowering medicine
- other medicines for high blood pressure or a heart problem
- water pills ("diuretics")
- potassium supplements. Your doctor may check the amount of potassium in your blood periodically.
- salt substitute containing potassium. Your doctor may check the amount of potassium in your blood periodically.
- diabetes medicine including insulin
- narcotic pain medicines
- sleeping pills and antiseizure medicines called barbiturates
- lithium, a medicine used to treat some types of depression
- aspirin or other medicines called nonsteroidal anti-inflammatory drugs (NSAIDs), like ibuprofen or naproxen
- steroids
- alcohol

- digoxin or other digitalis glycosides (a heart medicine)
- muscle relaxants (medicines used during operations)
- certain cancer medicines, like cyclophosphamide or methotrexate
- medicines used to prevent and treat fungal infections (such as ketoconazole, intraconazole).
- medicines used to treat bacterial infections (such as clarithromycin, telithromycin).
- certain antibiotics (rifamycin group), a drug used to protect against transplant rejection (cyclosporin) or an antiretroviral drug used to treat HIV/AIDS infection (ritonavir). These drugs may increase the effect of valsartan.

Know the medicines you take. Keep a list of your medicines and show it to your doctor or pharmacist when you get a new medicine.

How should I take EXFORGE HCT?

- Take EXFORGE HCT exactly as your doctor tells you.
- Take EXFORGE HCT one time each day.
- EXFORGE HCT can be taken with or without food.
- If you miss a dose, take it as soon as you remember. If it is close to your next dose, do not take the missed dose. Just take the next dose at the regular time.
- If you take too much EXFORGE HCT, call your doctor or Poison Control Center, or go to the emergency room.
- Tell all your doctors and dentist you are taking EXFORGE HCT. This is especially important if you:
  - are going to have surgery
  - go for kidney dialysis

What are the possible side effects of EXFORGE HCT?

EXFORGE HCT may cause **serious side effects** including:

- **harm to an unborn baby causing injury or death. See "What is the most important information I should know about EXFORGE HCT?"**
- **low blood pressure** (hypotension). Low blood pressure is most likely to happen if you:
  - take water pills
  - are on a low salt diet
  - have heart problems
  - get dialysis treatments
  - get sick with vomiting or diarrhea
  - drink alcohol.

Lie down if you feel faint or dizzy. If you faint (lose consciousness), stop taking EXFORGE HCT. Call your doctor right away.

- Get emergency help if you get worse chest pain or chest pain that does not go away.
- **kidney problems.** Kidney problems may become worse in people that already have kidney disease. Some people will have changes in blood tests for kidney function and may need a lower dose of EXFORGE HCT. Call your doctor if you have swelling in your feet, ankles, or hands, or unexplained weight gain. If you have heart failure, your doctor should check your kidney function before prescribing EXFORGE HCT.
- **laboratory blood test changes in people with heart failure.** Some people with heart failure who take valsartan, one of the medicines in EXFORGE HCT, have changes in blood tests including increased potassium and decreased kidney function.
- **allergic reactions**
- **skin rash.** Call your doctor right away if you get an unusual skin rash.
- **eye problems.** One of the medicines in EXFORGE HCT can cause eye problems that may lead to vision loss. Symptoms of eye problems can happen within hours to weeks of starting EXFORGE HCT. Tell your doctor right away if you have:
  - decrease in vision
  - eye pain

The **most common** side effects of EXFORGE HCT include:

- dizziness
- swelling (edema) of the hands, ankles, or feet
- headache
- indigestion
- tiredness
- muscle spasms
- back pain
- nausea.

Tell your doctor if you have any side effect that bothers you or that does not go away.

These are not all the possible side effects of EXFORGE HCT. For more information, ask your doctor or pharmacist. Call your doctor for medical advice about side effects. You may report side effects to FDA at 1-800-FDA-1088.

How should I store EXFORGE HCT?

- Store EXFORGE HCT at room temperature between 59°F to 86°F (15°C to 30°C).
- Keep EXFORGE HCT dry (protect it from moisture).

Keep EXFORGE HCT and all medicines out of the reach of children.

General Information about EXFORGE HCT

Medicines are sometimes prescribed for conditions that are not mentioned in the patient information leaflet. Do not use EXFORGE HCT for a condition for which it was not prescribed. Do not give EXFORGE HCT to other people, even if they have the same symptoms that you have. It may harm them.

This patient information leaflet summarizes the most important information about EXFORGE HCT. If you would like more information about EXFORGE HCT, talk with your doctor. You can ask your doctor or pharmacist for information about EXFORGE HCT that is written for health professionals. For more information go to www.EXFORGE.com or call 1-888-839-3674.

What are the ingredients in EXFORGE HCT?

Active ingredients: amlodipine besylate, valsartan, and hydrochlorothiazide

The inactive ingredients of all strengths of the tablets are crospovidone, magnesium stearate, microcrystalline cellulose, and colloidal anhydrous silica. The film coating contains hypromellose, talc, macrogol 4000, and may contain titanium dioxide or yellow and red iron oxides.

What is high blood pressure (hypertension)?

Blood pressure is the force of blood in your blood vessels when your heart beats and when your heart rests. You have high blood pressure when the force is too much. EXFORGE HCT can help your blood vessels relax so your blood pressure is lower. Medicines that lower blood pressure lower your chance of having a stroke or heart attack.

High blood pressure makes the heart work harder to pump blood throughout the body and causes damage to blood vessels. If high blood pressure is not treated, it can lead to stroke, heart attack, heart failure, kidney failure, and vision problems.

Distributed by:
Novartis Pharmaceuticals Corporation
East Hanover, New Jersey 07936
© Novartis
T2012-191
September 2012

Shown in Product Identification Guide, page 310

EXJADE® ℞

[x-jāde]
(deferasirox)
tablets, for oral suspension

The following prescribing information is based on official labeling in effect July 2013.

HIGHLIGHTS OF PRESCRIBING INFORMATION

These highlights do not include all the information needed to use EXJADE safely and effectively. See full prescribing information for EXJADE.

EXJADE® (deferasirox) tablets, for oral suspension
Initial U.S. Approval: 2005

> **WARNING: RENAL FAILURE, HEPATIC FAILURE, AND GASTROINTESTINAL HEMORRHAGE**
> ***See full prescribing information for complete boxed warning***
> **Exjade may cause:**
> - **renal toxicity, including failure (5.1)**
> - **hepatic toxicity, including failure (5.2)**
> - **gastrointestinal hemorrhage (5.3)**
>
> **Exjade therapy requires close patient monitoring, including laboratory tests of renal and hepatic function. (5)**

RECENT MAJOR CHANGES

Boxed Warning	09/2012
Indications and Usage (1)	05/2013
Dosage and Administration (2)	05/2013
Warnings and Precautions (5)	01/2013

INDICATIONS AND USAGE

Exjade is an iron chelator indicated for the treatment of chronic iron overload due to blood transfusions in patients 2 years of age and older. This indication is based on reduction in serum ferritin and liver iron concentration. An improvement in survival or disease-related symptoms has not been established. (1.1)

Exjade is indicated for the treatment of chronic iron overload in patients 10 years of age and older with non-transfusion dependent thalassemia syndromes and with a liver iron (Fe) concentration (LIC) of at least 5 mg Fe per gram of dry weight and a serum ferritin greater than 300 mcg/L. This indication is based on achievement of an LIC less than 5 mg Fe/g dw. An improvement in survival or disease-related symptoms has not been established. (1.2)

Limitation of Use

Controlled clinical trials of Exjade in patients with myelodysplastic syndromes (MDS) and chronic iron overload due to blood transfusion have not been performed. (1.3)

The safety and efficacy of Exjade when administered with other iron chelation therapy have not been established. (1.3)

DOSAGE AND ADMINISTRATION

- In patients with transfusional iron overload, the recommended initial daily dose is 20 mg per kg body weight once daily, as oral suspension. Calculate dose to the nearest whole tablet. (2.1)
- In patients with non-transfusion-dependent thalassemia syndromes, the recommended initial daily dose is 10 mg per kg body weight once daily, as oral suspension. Calculate dose to the nearest whole tablet. (2.2)
- Monitor serum ferritin monthly and adjust dose accordingly. (2.1, 2.2)
- Monitor LIC every 6 months and adjust dose accordingly. (2.2)
- Do not chew or swallow tablets whole. (2.3)
- Take on an empty stomach at least 30 minutes before food. Disperse tablets by stirring in an appropriate amount of water, orange juice, or apple juice. (2.3)
- Reduce the starting dose in patients with moderate (Child-Pugh B) hepatic impairment by 50%. Avoid the use of Exjade in patients with severe (Child-Pugh C) hepatic impairment. (2.4)
- Reduce the starting dose by 50% in patients with renal impairment (ClCr 40-60 mL/min). (2.4)

DOSAGE FORMS AND STRENGTHS

Tablets for oral suspension: 125 mg, 250 mg, 500 mg. (3)

CONTRAINDICATIONS

- Serum creatinine greater than 2 times the age-appropriate upper limit of normal or creatinine clearance less than 40 mL/min. (4)
- Patients with poor performance status. (4)
- Patients with high-risk myelodysplastic syndromes (MDS). (4)
- Patients with advanced malignancies. (4)
- Patients with platelet counts $<50 \times 10^9$/L. (4)
- Known hypersensitivity to deferasirox or any component of Exjade. (4)

WARNINGS AND PRECAUTIONS

- Renal toxicity: Measure serum creatinine and creatinine clearance in duplicate before starting therapy. Monitor renal function during Exjade therapy and reduce dose or interrupt therapy for toxicity. (2.4, 5.1)
- Hepatic toxicity: Monitor hepatic function. Reduce dose or interrupt therapy for toxicity. (5.2)
- Fatal and nonfatal gastrointestinal bleeding, ulceration, and irritation: Risk may be greater in patients who are taking Exjade in combination with drugs that have known ulcerogenic or hemorrhagic potential. (5.3)
- Bone marrow suppression: Neutropenia, agranulocytosis, worsening anemia, and thrombocytopenia, including fatal events; monitor blood counts during Exjade therapy. Interrupt therapy for toxicity. (5.4)
- Elderly: Monitor closely for toxicity due to the greater frequency of decreased hepatic, renal, and/or cardiac function. (5.5)
- Serious and severe hypersensitivity reactions: Discontinue Exjade and institute medical intervention. (5.6)
- Erythema multiforme: If suspected, discontinue Exjade and evaluate. (5.8)

ADVERSE REACTIONS

In patients with transfusional iron overload, the most frequently occurring (>5%) adverse reactions are diarrhea, vomiting, nausea, abdominal pain, skin rashes, and increases in serum creatinine. In Exjade-treated patients with non-transfusion dependent thalassemia syndromes, the most frequently occurring (>5%) adverse reactions are diarrhea, rash and nausea. (6.1)

To report SUSPECTED ADVERSE REACTIONS, contact Novartis Pharmaceuticals Corporation at 1-888-669-6682 or FDA at 1-800-FDA-1088 or www.fda.gov/medwatch.

DRUG INTERACTIONS

- Avoid the use of Exjade with aluminum-containing antacid preparations. (7.1)
- Exjade increases the exposure of the CYP2C8 substrate repaglinide. Consider repaglinide dose reduction and monitor blood glucose levels. (7.3)
- Avoid the use of Exjade with CYP1A2 substrate theophylline. (7.4)

USE IN SPECIFIC POPULATIONS

- Pregnancy: Based on animal studies, may cause fetal harm. (8.1)
- Nursing Mothers: Discontinue drug or nursing, taking into consideration importance of drug to mother. (8.3)

See 17 for PATIENT COUNSELING INFORMATION

Revised: 05/2013

FULL PRESCRIBING INFORMATION: CONTENTS*

*** Sections or subsections omitted from the full prescribing information are not listed**

FULL PRESCRIBING INFORMATION

WARNING: RENAL FAILURE, HEPATIC FAILURE, AND GASTROINTESTINAL HEMORRHAGE

Renal Failure

- **Exjade can cause acute renal failure and death, particularly in patients with comorbidities and those who are in the advanced stages of their hematologic disorders.**
- **Measure serum creatinine and determine creatinine clearance in duplicate prior to initiation of therapy and monitor renal function at least monthly thereafter. For patients with baseline renal impairment or increased risk of acute renal failure, monitor creatinine weekly for the first month, then at least monthly. Consider dose reduction, interruption, or discontinuation based on increases in serum creatinine *[see Dosage and Administration (2.4, 2.5) and Warnings and Precautions (5.1)]*.**

Hepatic Failure

- **Exjade can cause hepatic injury including hepatic failure and death.**
- **Measure serum transaminases and bilirubin in all patients prior to initiating treatment, every 2 weeks during the first month, and at least monthly thereafter.**
- **Avoid use of Exjade in patients with severe (Child-Pugh C) hepatic impairment and reduce the dose in patients with moderate (Child Pugh B) hepatic impairment *[see Dosage and Administration (2.4) and Warnings and Precautions (5.2)]*.**

Gastrointestinal Hemorrhage

- **Exjade can cause gastrointestinal (GI) hemorrhages, which may be fatal, especially in elderly patients who have advanced hematologic malignancies and/or low platelet counts.**
- **Monitor patients and discontinue Exjade for suspected GI ulceration or hemorrhage *[see Warnings and Precautions (5.3)]*.**

1 INDICATIONS AND USAGE

1.1 Treatment of Chronic Iron Overload Due to Blood Transfusions (Transfusional Iron Overload)

Exjade is indicated for the treatment of chronic iron overload due to blood transfusions (transfusional hemosiderosis) in patients 2 years of age and older. This indication is based on a reduction of liver iron concentrations and serum ferritin levels *[see Clinical Studies (14)]*. An improvement in survival or disease-related symptoms has not been established *[see Indications and Usage (1.3)]*.

1.2 Treatment of Chronic Iron Overload in Non-Transfusion Dependent Thalassemia Syndromes

Exjade is indicated for the treatment of chronic iron overload in patients 10 years of age and older with non-transfusion dependent thalassemia syndromes and with a liver iron concentration (LIC) of at least 5 milligrams of iron per gram of liver dry weight (mg Fe/g dw) and a serum ferritin greater than 300 mcg/L. This indication is based on achievement of an LIC less than 5 mg Fe/g dw *[see Clinical Studies (14)]*. An improvement in survival or disease-related symptoms has not been established.

1.3 Limitation of Use

Controlled clinical trials of Exjade with myelodysplastic syndromes (MDS) and chronic iron overload due to blood transfusions have not been performed *[see Clinical Studies (14)]*.

The safety and efficacy of Exjade when administered with other iron chelation therapy have not been established.

2 DOSAGE AND ADMINISTRATION

2.1 Transfusional Iron Overload

Exjade therapy should only be considered when a patient has evidence of chronic transfusional iron overload. The evidence should include the transfusion of at least 100 mL/kg of packed red blood cells (e.g., at least 20 units of packed red blood cells for a 40-kg person or more in individuals weighing more than 40 kg), and a serum ferritin consistently greater than 1000 mcg/L.

Prior to starting therapy, obtain:

- serum ferritin level
- baseline serum creatinine in duplicate (due to variations in measurements) and determine the creatinine clearance (Cockcroft-Gault method) *[see Dosage and Administration (2.4) and Warnings and Precautions (5.1)]*
- serum transaminases and bilirubin *[see Dosage and Administration (2.4) and Warnings and Precautions (5.2)]*
- baseline auditory and ophthalmic examinations *[see Warnings and Precautions (5.9)]*

The recommended initial dose of Exjade for patients 2 years of age and older is 20 mg per kg body weight orally, once daily. Calculate doses (mg per kg per day) to the nearest whole tablet.

After commencing therapy, monitor serum ferritin monthly and adjust the dose of Exjade, if necessary, every 3-6 months based on serum ferritin trends. Make dose adjustments in steps of 5 or 10 mg per kg and tailor adjustments to the individual patient's response and therapeutic goals. In patients not adequately controlled with doses of 30 mg per kg (e.g., serum ferritin levels persistently above 2500 mcg/L and not showing a decreasing trend over time), doses of up to 40 mg per kg may be considered. Doses above 40 mg per kg are not recommended.

If the serum ferritin falls consistently below 500 mcg/L, consider temporarily interrupting therapy with Exjade *[see Warnings and Precautions (5.10)]*.

2.2 Iron Overload in Non-Transfusion Dependent Thalassemia Syndromes

Exjade therapy should only be considered when a patient with a non-transfusion dependent thalassemia syndrome has an LIC of at least 5 mg Fe/g dw and a serum ferritin greater than 300 mcg/L.

Prior to starting therapy, obtain:

- LIC by liver biopsy or by an FDA cleared or approved method for identifying patients for treatment with deferasirox therapy
- Serum ferritin level on at least 2 measurements 1 month apart *[see Clinical Studies (14)]*
- Baseline serum creatinine in duplicate (due to variations in measurements) and determine the creatinine clearance (Cockcroft-Gault method) *[see Dosage and Administration (2.4) and Warnings and Precautions (5.1)]*
- Serum transaminases and bilirubin *[see Dosage and Administration (2.4) and Warnings and Precautions (5.2)]*
- Baseline auditory and ophthalmic examinations *[see Warnings and Precautions (5.9)]*

Initiating therapy:

- The recommended initial dose of Exjade is 10 mg per kg body weight orally once daily. Calculate doses (mg per kg per day) to the nearest whole tablet.
- If the baseline LIC is greater than 15 mg Fe/g dw, consider increasing the dose to 20 mg/kg/day after 4 weeks.

During therapy:

- Monitor serum ferritin monthly. Interrupt treatment when serum ferritin is less than 300 mcg/L and obtain an LIC to determine whether the LIC has fallen to less than 3 mg Fe/g dw.
- Monitor LIC every 6 months.
- After 6 months of therapy, if the LIC remains greater than 7 mg Fe/g dw, increase the dose of deferasirox to a maximum of 20 mg/kg/day. Do not exceed a maximum of 20 mg/kg/day.
- If after 6 months of therapy, the LIC is 3-7 mg Fe/g dw, continue treatment with deferasirox at no more than 10 mg/kg/day.
- When the LIC is less than 3 mg Fe/g dw, interrupt treatment with deferasirox and continue to monitor the LIC.
- Monitor blood counts, hepatic function, and renal function *[see Warnings and Precautions (5.1, 5.2, 5.4)]*.

Restart treatment when the LIC rises again to more than 5 mg Fe/g dw.

2.3 Administration

Do not chew tablets or swallow them whole.

Take Exjade once daily on an empty stomach at least 30 minutes before food, preferably at the same time each day. Completely disperse tablets by stirring in water, orange juice, or apple juice until a fine suspension is obtained. Disperse doses of less than 1 g in 3.5 ounces of liquid and doses of 1 g or greater in 7 ounces of liquid. After swallowing the suspension, resuspend any residue in a small volume of liquid and swallow. Do not take Exjade with aluminum-containing antacid products *[see Drug Interactions (7.1)]*.

2.4 Use in Patients with Baseline Hepatic or Renal Impairment

Patients with Baseline Hepatic Impairment

Mild (Child-Pugh A) hepatic impairment: No dose adjustment is necessary.

Moderate (Child-Pugh B) hepatic impairment: Reduce the starting dose by 50%.

Severe (Child-Pugh C) hepatic impairment: Avoid Exjade *[see Warnings and Precautions (5.2) and Use in Specific Populations (8.7)]*.

Patients with Baseline Renal Impairment

For patients with renal impairment (ClCr 40-60 mL/min), reduce the starting dose by 50% *[see Use in Specific Populations (8.6)]*. Do not use Exjade in patients with serum creatinine greater than 2 times the upper limit of normal or creatinine clearance less than 40 mL/min *[see Contraindications (4)]*.

2.5 Dose Modifications for Increases in Serum Creatinine on Exjade

For serum creatinine increases while receiving Exjade *[see Warnings and Precautions (5.1)]* modify the dose as follows:

Transfusional Iron Overload

Adults and Adolescents (ages 16 and older):

- If the serum creatinine increases by 33% or more above the average baseline measurement, repeat the serum creatinine within 1 week, and if still elevated by 33% or more, reduce the dose by 10 mg per kg.

Pediatric Patients (ages 2-15 years):

- Reduce the dose by 10 mg per kg if serum creatinine increases to greater than 33% above the average baseline measurement and greater than the age appropriate upper limit of normal.

All Patients (regardless of age):

- Discontinue therapy for serum creatinine greater than 2 times the age-appropriate upper limit of normal or for creatinine clearance <40 mL/min. *[see Contraindications (4)]*

Non-Transfusion Dependent Thalassemia Syndromes

Adults and Adolescents (ages 16 and older):

- If the serum creatinine increases by 33% or more above the average baseline measurement, repeat the serum creatinine within 1 week, and if still elevated by 33% or more, interrupt therapy if the dose is 5 mg per kg, or reduce by 50% if the dose is 10 or 20 mg per kg.

Pediatric Patients (ages 10-15 years):

- Reduce the dose by 5 mg per kg if serum creatinine increases to greater than 33% above the average baseline measurement and greater than the age appropriate upper limit of normal.

All Patients (regardless of age):

- Discontinue therapy for serum creatinine greater than 2 times the age-appropriate upper limit of normal or for creatinine clearance <40 mL/min *[see Contraindications (4)]*.

2.6 Dose Modifications Based on Concomitant Medications

UDP-glucuronosyltransferases (UGT) Inducers

Concomitant use of UGT inducers decreases Exjade systemic exposure. Avoid the concomitant use of potent UGT inducers (e.g., rifampicin, phenytoin, phenobarbital, ritonavir) with Exjade. If you must administer Exjade with 1 of these agents, consider increasing the initial dose of Exjade by 50%, and monitor serum ferritin levels and clinical responses for further dose modification *[see Dosage and Administration (2.1, 2.2) and Drug Interactions (7.5)]*.

Bile Acid Sequestrants

Concomitant use of bile acid sequestrants decreases Exjade systemic exposure. Avoid the concomitant use of bile acid sequestrants (e.g., cholestyramine, colesevelam, colestipol) with Exjade. If you must administer Exjade with one of these agents, consider increasing the initial dose of Exjade by 50%, and monitor serum ferritin levels and clinical responses for further dose modification *[see Dosage and Administration (2.1, 2.2) and Drug Interactions (7.6)]*.

3 DOSAGE FORMS AND STRENGTHS

- 125 mg tablets
  Off-white, round, flat tablet with beveled edge and imprinted with "J" and "125" on one side and "NVR" on the other.
- 250 mg tablets
  Off-white, round, flat tablet with beveled edge and imprinted with "J" and "250" on one side and "NVR" on the other.
- 500 mg tablets
  Off-white, round, flat tablet with beveled edge and imprinted with "J" and "500" on one side and "NVR" on the other.

4 CONTRAINDICATIONS

Exjade is contraindicated in patients with:

- Serum creatinine greater than 2 times the age-appropriate upper limit of normal or creatinine clearance less than 40 mL/min *[see Warning and Precautions (5.1)]*;
- Poor performance status;
- High-risk myelodysplastic syndromes;
- Advanced malignancies;
- Platelet counts $<50 \times 10^9$/L;
- Known hypersensitivity to deferasirox or any component of Exjade *[see Warnings and Precautions (5.6) and Adverse Reactions (6.2)]*.

5 WARNINGS AND PRECAUTIONS

5.1 Renal Toxicity, Renal Failure, and Proteinuria

Exjade can cause acute renal failure, fatal in some patients and requiring dialysis in others. Postmarketing experience showed that most fatalities occurred in patients with multiple comorbidities and who were in advanced stages of their hematological disorders. In the clinical trials, Exjade-treated patients experienced dose-dependent increases in serum creatinine. In patients with transfusional iron overload, these increases in creatinine occurred at a greater frequency compared to deferoxamine-treated patients (38% versus 14%, respectively, in Study 1 and 36% versus 22%, respectively, in Study 3) *[see Adverse Reactions (6.1) and (6.2)]*.

Measure serum creatinine in duplicate (due to variations in measurements) and determine the creatinine clearance (estimated by the Cockcroft-Gault method) before initiating therapy in all patients in order to establish a reliable pretreatment baseline. Monitor serum creatinine weekly during the first month after initiation or modification of therapy and at least monthly thereafter. Monitor serum creatinine and/or creatinine clearance more frequently if creatinine levels are increasing. Dose reduction, interruption, or discontinuation based on increases in serum creatinine may be necessary *[see Dosage and Administration (2.5)]*.

Exjade is contraindicated in patients with creatinine clearance less than 40 mL/minute or serum creatinine greater than 2 times the age appropriate upper limit of normal.

Renal tubular damage, including Fanconi's Syndrome, has been reported in patients treated with Exjade, most commonly in children and adolescents with β-thalassemia and serum ferritin levels <1500 mcg/L.

Intermittent proteinuria (urine protein/creatinine ratio >0.6 mg/mg) occurred in 18.6% of Exjade-treated patients compared to 7.2% of deferoxamine-treated patients in Study 1. In clinical trials in patients with transfusional iron overload, Exjade was temporarily withheld until the urine protein/creatinine ratio fell below 0.6 mg/mg. Monthly monitoring for proteinuria is recommended. The mechanism and clinical significance of the proteinuria are uncertain *[see Adverse Reactions (6.1)]*.

5.2 Hepatic Toxicity and Failure

Exjade can cause hepatic injury, fatal in some patients. In Study 1, 4 patients (1.3%) discontinued Exjade because of hepatic toxicity (drug-induced hepatitis in 2 patients and increased serum transaminases in 2 additional patients). Hepatic toxicity appears to be more common in patients greater than 55 years of age. Hepatic failure was more common in patients with significant comorbidities, including liver cirrhosis and multiorgan failure *[see Adverse Reactions (6.1)]*.

Measure transaminases (AST and ALT) and bilirubin in all patients before the initiation of treatment and every 2 weeks during the first month and at least monthly thereafter. Consider dose modifications or interruption of treatment for severe or persistent elevations.

Avoid the use of Exjade in patients with severe (Child-Pugh C) hepatic impairment. Reduce the starting dose in patients with moderate (Child-Pugh B) hepatic impairment *[see Dosage and Administration (2.4), and Use in Specific Populations (8.7)]*. Patients with mild (Child-Pugh A) or moderate (Child-Pugh B) hepatic impairment may be at higher risk for hepatic toxicity.

5.3 Gastrointestinal (GI) Hemorrhage

GI hemorrhage, including deaths, has been reported, especially in elderly patients who had advanced hematologic malignancies and/or low platelet counts. Nonfatal upper GI irritation, ulceration and hemorrhage have been reported in patients, including children and adolescents, receiving Exjade *[see Adverse Reactions (6.1)]*. Monitor for signs and symptoms of GI ulceration and hemorrhage during Exjade therapy and promptly initiate additional evaluation and treatment if a serious GI adverse event is suspected. The risk of gastrointestinal hemorrhage may be increased when administering Exjade in combination with drugs that have ulcerogenic or hemorrhagic potential, such as nonsteroidal anti-inflammatory drugs (NSAIDs), corticosteroids, oral bisphosphonates, or anticoagulants.

5.4 Bone Marrow Suppression

Neutropenia, agranulocytosis, worsening anemia, and thrombocytopenia, including fatal events, have been reported in patients treated with Exjade. Preexisting hematologic disorders may increase this risk. Monitor blood counts in all patients. Interrupt treatment with Exjade in patients who develop cytopenias until the cause of the cytopenia has been determined. Exjade is contraindicated in patients with platelet counts below 50×10^9/L.

5.5 Increased Risk of Toxicity in the Elderly

Exjade has been associated with serious and fatal adverse reactions in the postmarketing setting, predominantly in elderly patients. Monitor elderly patients treated with Exjade more frequently for toxicity *[see Use in Specific Populations (8.5)]*.

5.6 Hypersensitivity

Exjade may cause serious hypersensitivity reactions (such as anaphylaxis and angioedema), with the onset of the reaction usually occurring within the first month of treatment *[see Adverse Reactions (6.2)]*. If reactions are severe, discontinue Exjade and institute appropriate medical intervention. Exjade is contraindicated in patients with known hypersensitivity to Exjade.

5.7 Skin Rash

Rashes may occur during Exjade treatment *[see Adverse Reactions (6.1)]*. For rashes of mild to moderate severity, Exjade may be continued without dose adjustment, since the rash often resolves spontaneously. In severe cases, interrupt treatment with Exjade. Reintroduction at a lower dose with escalation may be considered in combination with a short period of oral steroid administration.

5.8 Erythema Multiforme

Erythema multiforme has been reported during Exjade therapy. If erythema multiforme is suspected, discontinue Exjade and evaluate.

5.9 Auditory and Ocular Abnormalities

Auditory disturbances (high frequency hearing loss, decreased hearing), and ocular disturbances (lens opacities, cataracts, elevations in intraocular pressure, and retinal disorders) were reported at a frequency of <1% with Exjade therapy in the clinical studies. Perform auditory and ophthalmic testing (including slit lamp examinations and dilated fundoscopy) before starting Exjade treatment and thereafter at regular intervals (every 12 months). If disturbances are noted, monitor more frequently. Consider dose reduction or interruption.

5.10 Overchelation

For patients with transfusional iron overload, measure serum ferritin monthly to assess for possible overchelation of iron. If the serum ferritin falls below 500 mcg/L, consider interrupting therapy with Exjade, since overchelation may increase Exjade toxicity *[see Dosage and Administration (2.1)]*.

For patients with non-transfusion dependent thalassemia, measure LIC by liver biopsy or by using an FDA-cleared or approved method for monitoring patients receiving deferasirox therapy every 6 months on treatment. Interrupt Exjade administration when the LIC is less than 3 mg Fe/g dw. Measure serum ferritin monthly, and if the serum ferritin falls below 300 mcg/L, interrupt Exjade and obtain a confirmatory LIC *[see Clinical Studies (14)]*.

6 ADVERSE REACTIONS

6.1 Clinical Trials Experience

The following adverse reactions are also discussed in other sections of the labeling:

- Renal Toxicity, Renal Failure, and Proteinuria *[see Warnings and Precautions (5.1)]*
- Hepatic Toxicity and Failure *[see Warnings and Precautions (5.2)]*
- Gastrointestinal (GI) Hemorrhage *[see Warnings and Precautions (5.3)]*
- Bone Marrow Suppression *[see Warnings and Precautions (5.4)]*
- Skin Rash *[see Warnings and Precautions (5.7)]*
- Auditory and Ocular Abnormalities *[see Warnings and Precautions (5.9]*

Because clinical trials are conducted under widely varying conditions, adverse reaction rates observed in the clinical trials of a drug cannot be directly compared to rates in the clinical trials of another drug and may not reflect the rates observed in practice.

Transfusional Iron Overload

A total of 700 adult and pediatric patients were treated with Exjade (deferasirox) for 48 weeks in premarketing studies. These included 469 patients with ß-thalassemia, 99 with rare anemias, and 132 with sickle cell disease. Of these patients, 45% were male, 70% were Caucasian and 292 patients were <16 years of age. In the sickle cell disease population, 89% of patients were black. Median treatment duration among the sickle cell patients was 51 weeks. Of the 700 patients treated, 469 (403 ß-thalassemia and 66 rare anemias) were entered into extensions of the original clinical protocols. In ongoing extension studies, median durations of treatment were 88-205 weeks.

Six hundred twenty-seven patients with MDS were enrolled across 5 uncontrolled trials. These studies varied in duration from 1 to 5 years. The discontinuation rate across studies in the first year was 46% (AEs 20%, withdrawal of consent 10%, death 8%, other 4%, lab abnormalities 3%, and lack of efficacy 1%). Among 47 patients enrolled in the study of 5-year duration, 10 remained on Exjade at the completion of the study.

Table 1 displays adverse reactions occurring in >5% of Exjade-treated β-thalassemia patients (Study 1), sickle cell disease patients (Study 3), and patients with MDS (MDS pool). Abdominal pain, nausea, vomiting, diarrhea, skin rashes, and increases in serum creatinine were the most frequent adverse reactions reported with a suspected relationship to Exjade. Gastrointestinal symptoms, increases in serum creatinine, and skin rash were dose related.

[See table 1 below]

Table 1. Adverse Reactions* Occurring in >5% of Exjade-treated Patients in Study 1, Study 3, and MDS Pool

	Study 1 (β-Thalassemia)		Study 3 (Sickle Cell Disease)		MDS Pool
Preferred Term	EXJADE N=296 n (%)	Deferoxamine N=290 n (%)	EXJADE N=132 n (%)	Deferoxamine N=63 n (%)	EXJADE N=627 n (%)
Abdominal Pain**	63 (21)	41 (14)	37 (28)	9 (14)	145 (23)
Diarrhea	35 (12)	21 (7)	26 (20)	3 (5)	297 (47)
Creatinine Increased***	33 (11)	0 (0)	9 (7)	0	89 (14)
Nausea	31 (11)	14 (5)	30 (23)	7 (11)	161 (26)
Vomiting	30 (10)	28 (10)	28 (21)	10 (16)	83 (13)
Rash	25 (8)	9 (3)	14 (11)	3 (5)	83 (13)

* Adverse reaction frequencies are based on adverse events reported regardless of relationship to study drug.
** Includes 'abdominal pain', 'abdominal pain lower', and 'abdominal pain upper' which were reported as adverse events.
*** Includes 'blood creatinine increased' and 'blood creatinine abnormal' which were reported as adverse events. Also see Table 2.

In Study 1, a total of 113 (38%) patients treated with Exjade had increases in serum creatinine >33% above baseline on 2 separate occasions (Table 2) and 25 (8%) patients required dose reductions. Increases in serum creatinine appeared to be dose related *[see Warnings and Precautions (5.1)]*. In this study, 17 (6%) patients treated with Exjade developed elevations in SGPT/ALT levels >5 times the upper limit of normal at 2 consecutive visits. Of these, 2 patients had liver biopsy proven drug-induced hepatitis and both discontinued Exjade therapy *[see Warnings and Precautions (5.2)]*. An additional 2 patients, who did not have elevations in SGPT/ALT >5 times the upper limit of normal, discontinued Exjade because of increased SGPT/ALT. Increases in transaminases did not appear to be dose related. Adverse reactions that led to discontinuations included abnormal liver function tests (2 patients) and drug-induced hepatitis (2 patients), skin rash, glycosuria/proteinuria, Henoch Schönlein purpura, hyperactivity/insomnia, drug fever, and cataract (1 patient each).

In Study 3, a total of 48 (36%) patients treated with Exjade had increases in serum creatinine >33% above baseline on 2 separate occasions (Table 2) *[see Warnings and Precautions (5.1)]*. Of the patients who experienced creatinine increases in Study 3, 8 Exjade-treated patients required dose reductions. In this study, 5 patients in the Exjade group developed elevations in SGPT/ALT levels >5 times the upper limit of normal at 2 consecutive visits and 1 patient subsequently had Exjade permanently discontinued. Four additional patients discontinued Exjade due to adverse reactions with a suspected relationship to study drug, including diarrhea, pancreatitis associated with gallstones, atypical tuberculosis, and skin rash.

In the MDS pool, in the first year, a total of 229 (37%) patients treated with Exjade had increases in serum creatinine >33% above baseline on 2 consecutive occasions (Table 2) and 8 (3.5%) patients permanently discontinued *[see Warnings and Precautions (5.1)]*. A total of 5 (0.8%) patients developed SGPT/ALT levels >5 times the upper limit of normal at 2 consecutive visits. The most frequent adverse reactions that led to discontinuation included increases in serum creatinine, diarrhea, nausea, rash, and vomiting. Death was reported in the first year in 52 (8%) of patients *[see Clinical Studies (14)]*.

[See table 2 above]

Non-Transfusion Dependent Thalassemia Syndromes

In Study 4, 110 patients with NTDT received 1 year of treatment with Exjade 5 or 10 mg/kg/day and 56 patients received placebo in a double-blind, randomized trial. In Study 5, 130 of the patients who completed Study 4 were treated with open-label Exjade at 5, 10, or 20 mg/kg/day (depending on the baseline LIC) for 1 year *[see Clinical Studies (14)]*. Table 3 displays adverse reactions occurring in >5% in any group. The most frequent adverse reactions with a suspected relationship to study drug were nausea, rash, and diarrhea.

Table 3. Adverse Reactions Occurring in >5% in NTDT Patients

	Study 4		Study 5
	EXJADE N=110 n (%)	Placebo N=56 n (%)	EXJADE N=130 n (%)
Any adverse reaction	**31 (28)**	**9 (16)**	**27 (21)**
Nausea	7 (6)	4 (7)	2 (2)
Rash	7 (6)	1 (2)	2 (2)
Diarrhea	5 (5)	1 (2)	7 (5)

In Study 4, 1 patient in the placebo 10 mg/kg/day group experienced an ALT increase to >5 times ULN and >2 times baseline (Table 4). Three Exjade-treated patients (all in the 10 mg/kg/day group) had 2 consecutive serum creatinine level increases >33% from baseline and >ULN. Serum creatinine returned to normal in all 3 patients (in 1 spontaneously and in the other 2 after drug interruption). Two additional cases of ALT increase and 2 additional cases of serum creatinine increase were observed in the 1-year extension of Study 4.

Table 4. Number (%) of NTDT Patients with Increases in Serum Creatinine or SGPT/ALT

	Study 4		Study 5
Laboratory Parameter	**EXJADE N=110 n (%)**	**Placebo N=56 n (%)**	**EXJADE N=130 n (%)**
Serum creatinine (>33% increase from baseline and >ULN at ≥2 consecutive postbaseline values)	3 (3%)	0	2 (2%)
SGPT/ALT (>5 × ULN and >2 × baseline)	1 (1%)	1 (2%)	2 (2%)

Table 2. Number (%) of Patients with Increases in Serum Creatinine or SGPT/ALT in Study 1, Study 3, and MDS Pool

	Study 1 (β-Thalassemia)		Study 3 (Sickle Cell Disease)		MDS Pool
Laboratory Parameter	**EXJADE N=296 n (%)**	**Deferoxamine N=290 n (%)**	**EXJADE N=132 n (%)**	**Deferoxamine N=63 n (%)**	**EXJADE N=627 n (%)**
Serum Creatinine					
Creatinine increase >33% at 2 consecutive postbaseline visits	113 (38)	41 (14)	48 (36)	14 (22)	229 (37)
Creatinine increase >33% and <ULN at 2 consecutive postbaseline visits	7 (2)	1 (0)	3 (2)	2 (3)	126 (20)
SGPT/ALT					
SGPT/ALT >5 × ULN at 2 postbaseline visits	25 (8)	7 (2)	2 (2)	0	9 (1)
SGPT/ALT >5 × ULN at 2 consecutive postbaseline visits	17 (6)	5 (2)	5 (4)	0	5 (1)

Proteinuria

In clinical studies, urine protein was measured monthly. Intermittent proteinuria (urine protein/creatinine ratio >0.6 mg/mg) occurred in 18.6% of Exjade-treated patients compared to 7.2% of deferoxamine-treated patients in Study 1 *[see Warnings and Precautions (5.1)]*.

Other Adverse Reactions

In the population of more than 5,000 patients with transfusional iron overload who have been treated with Exjade during clinical trials, adverse reactions occurring in 0.1% to 1% of patients included gastritis, edema, sleep disorder, pigmentation disorder, dizziness, anxiety, maculopathy, cholelithiasis, pyrexia, fatigue, pharyngolaryngeal pain, early cataract, hearing loss, gastrointestinal hemorrhage, gastric ulcer (including multiple ulcers), duodenal ulcer, and renal tubulopathy (Fanconi's Syndrome). Adverse reactions occurring in 0.01% to 0.1% of patients included optic neuritis, esophagitis, and erythema multiforme. Adverse reactions which most frequently led to dose interruption or dose adjustment during clinical trials were rash, gastrointestinal disorders, infections, increased serum creatinine, and increased serum transaminases.

6.2 Postmarketing Experience

The following adverse reactions have been spontaneously reported during post-approval use of Exjade in the transfusional iron overload setting. Because these reactions are reported voluntarily from a population of uncertain size, in which patients may have received concomitant medication, it is not always possible to reliably estimate frequency or establish a causal relationship to drug exposure.

Skin and subcutaneous tissue disorders: leukocytoclastic vasculitis, urticaria, alopecia

Immune system disorders: hypersensitivity reactions (including anaphylaxis and angioedema)

Renal and urinary disorders: acute renal failure, tubulointerstitial nephritis

Hepatobiliary disorders: hepatic failure

Gastrointestinal disorders: gastrointestinal hemorrhage

Blood and lymphatic system disorders: worsening anemia

7 DRUG INTERACTIONS

7.1 Aluminum Containing Antacid Preparations

The concomitant administration of Exjade and aluminum-containing antacid preparations has not been formally studied. Although deferasirox has a lower affinity for aluminum than for iron, avoid use of Exjade with aluminum-containing antacid preparations due to the mechanism of action of Exjade.

7.2 Agents Metabolized by CYP3A4

Deferasirox may induce CYP3A4 resulting in a decrease in CYP3A4 substrate concentration when these drugs are coadministered. Closely monitor patients for signs of reduced effectiveness when deferasirox is administered with drugs metabolized by CYP3A4 (e.g., alfentanil, aprepitant, budesonide, buspirone, conivaptan, cyclosporine, darifenacin, darunavir, dasatinib, dihydroergotamine, dronedarone, eletriptan, eplerenone, ergotamine, everolimus, felodipine, fentanyl, hormonal contraceptive agents, indinavir, fluticasone, lopinavir, lovastatin, lurasidone, maraviroc, midazolam, nisoldipine, pimozide, quetiapine, quinidine, saquinavir, sildenafil, simvastatin, sirolimus, tacrolimus, tolvaptan, tipranavir, triazolam, ticagrelor, and vardenafil) *[see Clinical Pharmacology (12.3)]*.

7.3 Agents Metabolized by CYP2C8

Deferasirox inhibits CYP2C8 resulting in an increase in CYP2C8 substrate (e.g., repaglinide and paclitaxel) concentration when these drugs are coadministered. If Exjade and repaglinide are used concomitantly, consider decreasing the dose of repaglinide and perform careful monitoring of blood glucose levels. Closely monitor patients for signs of exposure related toxicity when Exjade is coadministered with other CYP2C8 substrates *[see Clinical Pharmacology (12.3)]*.

7.4 Agents Metabolized by CYP1A2

Deferasirox inhibits CYP1A2 resulting in an increase in CYP1A2 substrate (e.g., alosetron, caffeine, duloxetine, melatonin, ramelteon, tacrine, theophylline, tizanidine) concentration when these drugs are coadministered. An increase in theophylline plasma concentrations could lead to clinically significant theophylline induced CNS or other adverse reactions. Avoid the concomitant use of theophylline or other CYP1A2 substrates with a narrow therapeutic index (e.g., tizanidine) with Exjade. Monitor theophylline concentrations and consider theophylline dose modification if you must coadminister theophylline with Exjade. Closely monitor patients for signs of exposure related toxicity when Exjade is coadministered with other drugs metabolized by CYP1A2 [see Clinical Pharmacology (12.3)].

7.5 Agents Inducing UDP-glucuronosyltransferase (UGT) Metabolism

Deferasirox is a substrate of UGT1A1 and to a lesser extent UGT1A3. The concomitant use of Exjade with potent UGT inducers (e.g., rifampicin, phenytoin, phenobarbital, ritonavir) may result in a decrease in Exjade efficacy due to a possible decrease in deferasirox concentration. Avoid the concomitant use of potent UGT inducers with Exjade. Consider increasing the initial dose of Exjade if you must coadminister these agents together *[see Dosage and Administration (2.5) and Clinical Pharmacology (12.3)]*.

7.6 Bile Acid Sequestrants

Avoid the concomitant use of bile acid sequestrants (e.g., cholestyramine, colesevelam, colestipol) with Exjade due to a possible decrease in deferasirox concentration. If you must coadminister these agents together, consider increasing the initial dose of Exjade *[see Dosage and Administration (2.5) and Clinical Pharmacology (12.3)]*.

8 USE IN SPECIFIC POPULATIONS

8.1 Pregnancy

Pregnancy Category C

There are no adequate and well-controlled studies with Exjade in pregnant women. Administration of deferasirox to animals during pregnancy and lactation resulted in decreased offspring viability and an increase in renal anomalies in male offspring at exposures that were less than the recommended human exposure. Exjade should be used during pregnancy only if the potential benefit justifies the potential risk to the fetus.

In embryofetal developmental studies, pregnant rats and rabbits received oral deferasirox during the period of organogenesis at doses up to (100 mg per kg/day in rats and 50 mg per kg/day in rabbits) 0.8 times the Maximum Recommended Human Dose (MRHD) on a mg/m^2 basis. These doses resulted in maternal toxicity but no fetal harm was observed.

In a prenatal and postnatal developmental study, pregnant rats received oral deferasirox daily from organogenesis through lactation day 20 at doses (10, 30, and 90 mg per kg/day) 0.08, 0.2, and 0.7 times the MRHD on a mg/m^2 basis. Maternal toxicity, loss of litters, and decreased offspring viability occurred at 0.7 times the MRHD on a mg/m^2 basis, and increases in renal anomalies in male offspring occurred at 0.2 times the MRHD on a mg/m^2 basis.

8.3 Nursing Mothers

It is not known whether Exjade is excreted in human milk. Deferasirox and its metabolites were excreted in rat milk. Because many drugs are excreted in human milk and because of the potential for serious adverse reactions in nursing infants from deferasirox and its metabolites, a decision should be made whether to discontinue nursing or to discontinue the drug, taking into account the importance of the drug to the mother.

8.4 Pediatric Use

Of the 700 patients with transfusional iron overload who received Exjade during clinical studies, 292 were pediatric patients 2 - <16 years of age with various congenital and acquired anemias, including 52 patients age 2 - <6 years, 121 patients age 6 - <12 years and 119 patients age 12 - <16 years. Seventy percent of these patients had β-thalassemia. Children between the ages of 2 - <6 years have a systemic exposure to Exjade approximately 50% of that of adults [*see Clinical Pharmacology (12.3)*]. However, the safety and efficacy of Exjade in pediatric patients was similar to that of adult patients, and younger pediatric patients responded similarly to older pediatric patients. The recommended starting dose and dosing modification are the same for children and adults [*see Clinical Studies (14), Indications and Usage (1), and Dosage and Administration (2.1)*].

Growth and development in patients with chronic iron overload due to blood transfusions were within normal limits in children followed for up to 5 years in clinical trials.

Sixteen pediatric patients (10 to <16 years of age) with chronic iron overload and non-transfusional-dependent thalassemia were treated with Exjade in clinical studies. The safety and efficacy of Exjade in these children was similar to that seen in the adults. The recommended starting dose and dosing modification are the same for children and adults with chronic iron overload in non-transfusional-dependent thalassemia [*see Clinical Studies (14), Indications and Usage (1.2), and Dosage and Administration (2.2)*].

Safety and effectiveness have not been established in pediatric patients with chronic iron overload due to blood transfusions who are less than 2 years of age or pediatric patients with chronic iron overload and non-transfusional-dependent thalassemia who are less than 10 years of age.

8.5 Geriatric Use

Four hundred thirty-one (431) patients ≥65 years of age were studied in clinical trials of Exjade in the transfusional iron overload setting. The majority of these patients had myelodysplastic syndrome (MDS) (n=393). In these trials, elderly patients experienced a higher frequency of adverse reactions than younger patients. Monitor elderly patients for early signs or symptoms of adverse reactions that may require a dose adjustment. Elderly patients are at increased risk for toxicity due to the greater frequency of decreased hepatic, renal, or cardiac function, and of concomitant disease or other drug therapy. Dose selection for an elderly patient should be cautious, usually starting at the low end of the dosing range.

8.6 Renal Impairment

For patients with renal impairment (ClCr 40-60 mL/min), reduce the starting dose by 50% [*see Dosage and Administration (2.4) and Clinical Pharmacology (12.3)*]. Exjade is contraindicated in patients with a creatinine clearance <40 mL/min or serum creatinine >2 times the age-appropriate upper limit of normal [*see Contraindications (4)*].

Exjade can cause renal failure. Monitor serum creatinine and calculate creatinine clearance (using Cockcroft-Gault method) during treatment in all patients. Reduce, interrupt or discontinue Exjade dosing based on increases in serum creatinine [*see Dosage and Administration (2.4, 2.5) and Warnings and Precautions (5.1)*].

8.7 Hepatic Impairment

In a single dose (20 mg/kg) study in patients with varying degrees of hepatic impairment, deferasirox exposure was increased compared to patients with normal hepatic function. The average total (free and bound) AUC of deferasirox increased 16% in 6 patients with mild (Child-Pugh A) hepatic impairment, and 76% in 6 patients with moderate (Child-Pugh B) hepatic impairment compared to 6 patients with normal hepatic function. The impact of severe (Child-Pugh C) hepatic impairment was assessed in only 1 patient.

Avoid the use of Exjade in patients with severe (Child-Pugh C) hepatic impairment. For patients with moderate (Child-Pugh B) hepatic impairment, the starting dose should be reduced by 50%. Closely monitor patients with mild (Child-Pugh A) or moderate (Child-Pugh B) hepatic impairment for efficacy and adverse reactions that may require dose titration [*see Dosage and Administration (2.4), and Warnings and Precautions (5.2)*].

10 OVERDOSAGE

Cases of overdose (2-3 times the prescribed dose for several weeks) have been reported. In 1 case, this resulted in hepatitis which resolved without long-term consequences after a dose interruption. Single doses up to 80 mg per kg per day in iron overloaded β-thalassemic patients have been tolerated with nausea and diarrhea noted. In healthy volunteers, single doses of up to 40 mg per kg per day were tolerated. There is no specific antidote for Exjade. In case of overdose, induce vomiting and employ gastric lavage.

11 DESCRIPTION

Exjade (deferasirox) is an iron chelating agent. Exjade tablets for oral suspension contain 125 mg, 250 mg, or 500 mg deferasirox. Deferasirox is designated chemically as 4-[3,5-Bis (2-hydroxyphenyl)-1H-1,2,4-triazol-1-yl]-benzoic acid and its structural formula is:

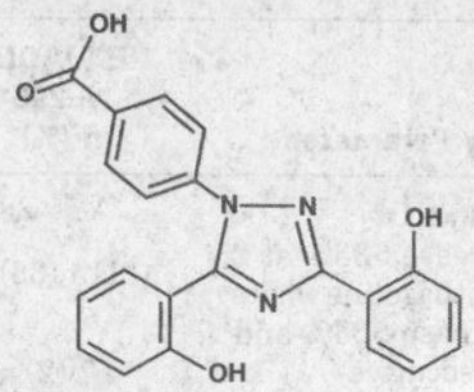

Deferasirox is a white to slightly yellow powder. Its molecular formula is $C_{21}H_{15}N_3O_4$ and its molecular weight is 373.4.

Inactive Ingredients: Lactose monohydrate (NF), crospovidone (NF), povidone (K30) (NF), sodium lauryl sulphate (NF), microcrystalline cellulose (NF), silicon dioxide (NF), and magnesium stearate (NF).

12 CLINICAL PHARMACOLOGY

12.1 Mechanism of Action

Exjade (deferasirox) is an orally active chelator that is selective for iron (as Fe^{3+}). It is a tridentate ligand that binds iron with high affinity in a 2:1 ratio. Although deferasirox has very low affinity for zinc and copper there are variable decreases in the serum concentration of these trace metals after the administration of deferasirox. The clinical significance of these decreases is uncertain.

12.2 Pharmacodynamics

Pharmacodynamic effects tested in an iron balance metabolic study showed that deferasirox (10, 20, and 40 mg per kg per day) was able to induce a mean net iron excretion (0.119, 0.329, and 0.445 mg Fe/kg body weight per day, respectively) within the clinically relevant range (0.1-0.5 mg per kg per day). Iron excretion was predominantly fecal.

12.3 Pharmacokinetics

Absorption

Exjade is absorbed following oral administration with median times to maximum plasma concentration (t_{max}) of about 1.5-4 hours. The C_{max} and AUC of deferasirox increase approximately linearly with dose after both single administration and under steady-state conditions. Exposure to deferasirox increased by an accumulation factor of 1.3-2.3 after multiple doses. The absolute bioavailability (AUC) of deferasirox tablets for oral suspension is 70% compared to an intravenous dose. The bioavailability (AUC) of deferasirox was variably increased when taken with a meal.

Distribution

Deferasirox is highly (~99%) protein bound almost exclusively to serum albumin. The percentage of deferasirox confined to the blood cells was 5% in humans. The volume of distribution at steady state (V_{ss}) of deferasirox is 14.37 ± 2.69 L in adults.

Metabolism

Glucuronidation is the main metabolic pathway for deferasirox, with subsequent biliary excretion. Deconjugation of glucuronidates in the intestine and subsequent reabsorption (enterohepatic recycling) is likely to occur. Deferasirox is mainly glucuronidated by UGT1A1 and to a lesser extent UGT1A3. CYP450-catalyzed (oxidative) metabolism of deferasirox appears to be minor in humans (about 8%). Deconjugation of glucuronide metabolites in the intestine and subsequent reabsorption (enterohepatic recycling) was confirmed in a healthy volunteer study in which the administration of cholestyramine 12 g twice daily (strongly binds to deferasirox and its conjugates) 4 and 10 hours after a single dose of deferasirox resulted in a 45% decrease in deferasirox exposure (AUC) by interfering with the enterohepatic recycling of deferasirox.

Excretion

Deferasirox and metabolites are primarily (84% of the dose) excreted in the feces. Renal excretion of deferasirox and metabolites is minimal (8% of the administered dose). The mean elimination half-life ($t_{1/2}$) ranged from 8-16 hours following oral administration.

Drug Interactions

Midazolam: In healthy volunteers, the concomitant administration of Exjade and midazolam (a CYP3A4 probe substrate) resulted in a decrease of midazolam peak concentration by 23% and exposure by 17%. In the clinical setting, this effect may be more pronounced. The study was not adequately designed to conclusively assess the potential induction of CYP3A4 by deferasirox [*see Drug Interactions (7.2)*].

Repaglinide: In a healthy volunteer study, the concomitant administration of Exjade (30 mg per kg/day for 4 days) and the CYP2C8 probe substrate repaglinide (single dose of 0.5 mg) resulted in an increase in repaglinide systemic exposure (AUC) to 2.3-fold of control and an increase in C_{max} of 62% [*see Drug Interactions (7.3)*].

Theophylline: In a healthy volunteer study, the concomitant administration of Exjade (repeated dose of 30 mg per kg/day) and the CYP1A2 substrate theophylline (single dose of 120 mg) resulted in an approximate doubling of the theophylline AUC and elimination half-life. The single dose C_{max} was not affected, but an increase in theophylline C_{max} is expected to occur with chronic dosing [*see Drug Interactions (7.4)*].

Rifampicin: In a healthy volunteer study, the concomitant administration of Exjade (single dose of 30 mg per kg) and the potent UDP-glucuronosyltransferase (UGT) inducer rifampicin (600 mg/day for 9 days) resulted in a decrease of deferasirox systemic exposure (AUC) by 44% [*see Drug Interactions (7.5)*].

Cholesytramine: The concomitant use of Exjade with bile acid sequestrants may result in a decrease in Exjade efficacy. In healthy volunteers, the administration of cholesytramine after a single dose of deferasirox resulted in a 45% decrease in deferasirox exposure (AUC) [*see Drug Interactions (7.6)*].

In vitro studies:

- Cytochrome P450 Enzymes: Deferasirox inhibits human CYP3A4, CYP2C8, CYP1A2, CYP2A6, CYP2D6, and CYP2C19 *in vitro*.
- Transporter Systems: The addition of cyclosporin A (PgP/MRP1/MRP2 inhibitor) or verapamil (PgP/MRP1 inhibitor) did not influence ICL670 permeability *in vitro*.

Pharmacokinetics in Specific Populations

Pediatric: Following oral administration of single or multiple doses, systemic exposure of adolescents and children to deferasirox was less than in adult patients. In children <6 years of age, systemic exposure was about 50% lower than in adults.

Geriatric: The pharmacokinetics of deferasirox have not been studied in elderly patients (65 years of age or older).

Gender: Females have a moderately lower apparent clearance (by 17.5%) for deferasirox compared to males.

Renal Impairment: Compared to patients with MDS and ClCr >60 mL/min, patients with MDS and ClCr 40 to 60 mL/min (n=34) had approximately 50% higher mean deferasirox trough plasma concentrations.

12.6 QT Prolongation

The effect of 20 and 40 mg per kg per day of deferasirox on the QT interval was evaluated in a single-dose, double-blind, randomized, placebo- and active-controlled (moxifloxacin 400 mg), parallel group study in 182 healthy male and female volunteers age 18-65 years. No evidence of prolongation of the QTc interval was observed in this study.

13 NONCLINICAL TOXICOLOGY

13.1 Carcinogenesis, Mutagenesis, Impairment of Fertility

A 104-week oral carcinogenicity study in Wistar rats showed no evidence of carcinogenicity from deferasirox at doses up to 60 mg per kg per day (0.48 times the MRHD on a mg/m^2 basis). A 26-week oral carcinogenicity study in p53 (+/-) transgenic mice has shown no evidence of carcinogenicity from deferasirox at doses up to 200 mg per kg per day (0.81 times the MRHD on a mg/m^2 basis) in males and 300 mg per kg per day (1.21 times the MRHD on a mg/m^2 basis) in females.

Deferasirox was negative in the Ames test and chromosome aberration test with human peripheral blood lymphocytes. It was positive in 1 of 3 *in vivo* oral rat micronucleus tests.

Deferasirox at oral doses up to 75 mg per kg per day (0.6 times the MRHD on a mg/m^2 basis) was found to have no adverse effect on fertility and reproductive performance of male and female rats.

14 CLINICAL STUDIES

Transfusional Iron Overload

The primary efficacy study, Study 1, was a multicenter, open-label, randomized, active comparator control study to compare Exjade (deferasirox) and deferoxamine in patients with β-thalassemia and transfusional hemosiderosis. Patients ≥2 years of age were randomized in a 1:1 ratio to receive either oral Exjade at starting doses of 5, 10, 20, or 30 mg per kg once daily or subcutaneous Desferal (deferoxamine) at starting doses of 20 to 60 mg per kg for at least 5 days per week based on LIC (liver iron concentration) at baseline (2-3, >3-7, >7-14 and >14 mg Fe/g dry weight). Patients randomized to deferoxamine who had LIC values <7 mg Fe/g dry weight were permitted to continue on their prior deferoxamine dose, even though the dose may have been higher than specified in the protocol.

Patients were to have a liver biopsy at baseline and end of study (after 12 months) for LIC. The primary efficacy endpoint was defined as a reduction in LIC of ≥3 mg Fe/g dry weight for baseline values ≥10 mg Fe/g dry weight, reduction of baseline values between 7 and <10 to <7 mg Fe/g dry weight, or maintenance or reduction for baseline values <7 mg Fe/g dry weight.

A total of 586 patients were randomized and treated, 296 with Exjade and 290 with deferoxamine. The mean age was 17.1 years (range, 2-53 years); 52% were females and 88% were Caucasian. The primary efficacy population consisted of 553 patients (Exjade n=276; deferoxamine n=277) who had LIC evaluated at baseline and 12 months or discontinued due to an adverse event. The percentage of patients achieving the primary endpoint was 52.9% for Exjade and 66.4% for deferoxamine. The relative efficacy of Exjade to deferoxamine cannot be determined from this study.

In patients who had an LIC at baseline and at end of study, the mean change in LIC was -2.4 mg Fe/g dry weight in patients treated with Exjade and -2.9 mg Fe/g dry weight in patients treated with deferoxamine.

Reduction of LIC and serum ferritin was observed with Exjade doses of 20 to 30 mg per kg per day. Exjade doses below 20 mg per kg per day failed to provide consistent lowering of LIC and serum ferritin levels (Figure 1). Therefore, a starting dose of 20 mg per kg per day is recommended [*see Dosage and Administration (2.1)*].

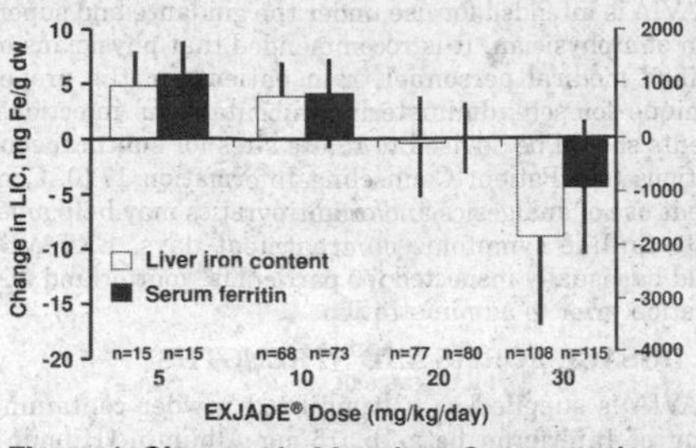

Figure 1. Changes in Liver Iron Concentration and Serum Ferritin Following EXJADE (5-30 mg/kg per day) in Study 1

Study 2 was an open-label, noncomparative trial of efficacy and safety of Exjade given for 1 year to patients with chronic anemias and transfusional hemosiderosis. Similar to Study 1, patients received 5, 10, 20, or 30 mg per kg per day of Exjade based on baseline LIC.

A total of 184 patients were treated in this study: 85 patients with β-thalassemia and 99 patients with other congenital or acquired anemias (myelodysplastic syndromes, n=47; Diamond-Blackfan syndrome, n=30; other, n=22). 19% of patients were <16 years of age and 16% were ≥65 years of age. There was a reduction in the absolute LIC from baseline to end of study (-4.2 mg Fe/g dry weight).

Study 3 was a multicenter, open-label, randomized trial of the safety and efficacy of Exjade relative to deferoxamine given for 1 year in patients with sickle cell disease and transfusional hemosiderosis. Patients were randomized to Exjade at doses of 5, 10, 20, or 30 mg per kg per day or subcutaneous deferoxamine at doses of 20-60 mg per kg per day for 5 days per week according to baseline LIC.

A total of 195 patients were treated in this study: 132 with Exjade and 63 with deferoxamine. 44% of patients were <16 years of age and 91% were black. At end of study, the mean change in LIC (as measured by magnetic susceptometry by a superconducting quantum interference device) in the per protocol-1 (PP-1) population, which consisted of patients who had at least 1 post-baseline LIC assessment, was -1.3 mg Fe/g dry weight for patients receiving Exjade (n=113) and -0.7 mg Fe/g dry weight for patients receiving deferoxamine (n=54).

One-hundred five (105) patients with thalassemia major and cardiac iron overload were enrolled in a study assessing the change in cardiac MRI T2* value (measured in milliseconds, ms) before and after treatment with deferasirox. Cardiac T2* values at baseline ranged from 5 to <20 ms. The geometric mean of cardiac T2* in the 68 patients who completed 3 years of Exjade therapy increased from 11.98 ms at baseline to 17.12 ms at 3 years. Cardiac T2* values improved in patients with severe cardiac iron overload (<10 ms) and in those with mild to moderate cardiac iron overload (≥10 to <20 ms). The clinical significance of these observations is unknown.

Six hundred twenty-seven patients with MDS were enrolled across 5 uncontrolled trials. Two hundred thirty-nine of the 627 patients were enrolled in trials that limited enrollment to patients with IPSS Low or Intermediate 1 risk MDS and the remaining 388 patients were enrolled in trials that did not specify MDS risk stratification but required a life expectancy of greater than 1 year. Planned duration of treatment in these trials ranged from 1 year (365 patients) to 5 years (47 patients). These trials evaluated the effects of Exjade therapy on parameters of iron overload, including LIC (125 patients) and serum ferritin (627 patients). Percent of patients completing planned duration of treatment was 51% in the largest 1 year study, 52% in the 3-year study and 22% in the 5 year study. The major causes for treatment discontinuation were withdrawal of consent, adverse reaction, and death. Over one year of follow-up across these pooled studies, mean change in serum ferritin was -332.8 (±2615.59) mcg/L (n=593) and mean change in LIC was -5.9 (±8.32) mg Fe/g dw (n=68). Results of these pooled studies in 627 patients with MDS suggest a progressive decrease in serum ferritin and LIC beyond one year in those patients who are able to continue Exjade. No controlled trials have been performed to demonstrate that these reductions improve morbidity or mortality in patients with MDS. Adverse reactions with Exjade therapy occur more frequently in older patients [*see Use in Specific Populations (8.5)*]. In elderly patients, including those with MDS, individualize the decision to remove accumulated iron based on clinical circumstances and the anticipated clinical benefit and risks of Exjade therapy.

Table 5. Absolute Change in LIC at Week 52 in NTDT Patients

	Starting Dose[1]			
	Placebo	**EXJADE 5 mg/kg/day**	**EXJADE 10 mg/kg/day**	**EXJADE 20 mg/kg/day**
Study 4[2]				
Number of Patients	n=54	n=51	n=54	-
Mean LIC at Baseline (mg Fe/g dw)	16.1	13.4	14.4	-
Mean Change (mg Fe/g dw)	+0.4	-2.0	-3.8	-
(95% Confidence Interval)	(-0.6, +1.3)	(-2.9, -1.0)	(-4.8, -2.9)	-
Study 5				
Number of Patients	-	n=8	n=77	n=43
Mean LIC at Baseline (mg Fe/g dw)	-	5.6	8.8	23.5
Mean Change (mg Fe/g dw)	-	-1.5	-2.8	-9.1
(95% Confidence Interval)	-	(-3.7, +0.7)	(-3.4, -2.2)	(-11.0, -7.3)

[1]Randomized dose in Study 4 or assigned starting dose in Study 5
[2]Least square mean change for Study 4

Non-Transfusion Dependent Thalassemia

Study 4 was a randomized, double-blind, placebo-controlled trial of treatment with Exjade for patients 10 years of age or older with non-transfusion-dependent thalassemia syndromes and iron overload. Eligible patients had an LIC of at least 5 mg Fe/g dw measured by R2 MRI and a serum ferritin exceeding 300 mcg/L at screening (2 consecutive values at least 14 days apart from each other). A total of 166 patients were randomized, 55 to the Exjade 5 mg/kg/day dose group, 55 to the Exjade 10 mg/kg/day dose group, and 56 to placebo (28 to each matching placebo group). Doses could be increased after 6 months if the LIC exceeded 7 mg Fe/g dw and the LIC reduction from baseline was less than 15%. The patients enrolled included 89 males and 77 females. The underlying disease was beta-thalassemia intermedia in 95 (57%) patients, HbE beta-thalassemia in 49 (30%) patients, and alpha-thalassemia in 22 (13%) patients. There were 17 pediatric patients in the study. Caucasians comprised 57% of the study population and Asians comprised 42%. The median baseline LIC (range) for all patients was 12.1 (2.6-49.1) mg Fe/g dw. Follow-up was for 1 year. The primary efficacy endpoint of change in LIC from baseline to Week 52 was statistically significant in favor of both Exjade dose groups compared with placebo (p ≤0.001) (Table 5). Furthermore, a statistically significant dose effect of Exjade was observed in favor of the 10 mg/kg/day dose group (10 versus 5 mg/kg/day, p=0.009). In a descriptive analysis, the target LIC (less than 5 mg Fe/g dw) was reached by 15 (27%) of 55 patients in the 10 mg/kg/day arm, 8 (15%) of 55 patients in the 5 mg/kg/day arm and 2 (4%) of 56 patients in the combined placebo groups.

[See table 5 above]

Study 5 was an open-label trial of Exjade for the treatment of patients previously enrolled on Study 4, including crossover to active treatment for those previously treated with placebo. The starting dose of Exjade in Study 5 was assigned based on the patient's LIC at completion of Study 4, being 20 mg/kg/day for an LIC exceeding 15 mg Fe/g dw, 10 mg/kg/day for LIC 3-15 mg Fe/g dw, and observation if the LIC was less than 3 mg Fe/g dw. Patients could continue on 5 mg/kg/day if they had previously exhibited at least a 30% reduction in LIC. Doses could be increased to a maximum of 20 mg/kg/day after 6 months if the LIC was more than 7 mg Fe/g dw and the LIC reduction from baseline was less than 15%. The primary efficacy endpoint in Study 5 was the proportion of patients achieving an LIC less than 5 mg Fe/g dw. A total of 133 patients were enrolled. Twenty patients began Study 5 with an LIC less than 5 mg Fe/g dw. Of the 113 patients with a baseline LIC of at least 5 mg Fe/g dw in Study 5, the target LIC (less than 5 mg Fe/g dw) was reached by 39 (35%). The responders included 4 (10%) of 39 patients treated at 20 mg/kg/day for a baseline LIC exceeding 15 mg Fe/g dw, and 31 (51%) of 61 patients treated at 10 mg/kg/day for a baseline LIC between 5 and 15 mg Fe/g dw. The absolute change in LIC at Week 52 by starting dose is shown in Table 5 above.

16 HOW SUPPLIED/STORAGE AND HANDLING

Exjade is provided as 125 mg, 250 mg, and 500 mg tablets for oral suspension.

125 mg
Off-white, round, flat tablet with beveled edge and imprinted with "J" and "125" on one side and "NVR" on the other.
Bottles of 30 tablets..............................(NDC 0078-0468-15)

250 mg
Off-white, round, flat tablet with beveled edge and imprinted with "J" and "250" on one side and "NVR" on the other.
Bottles of 30 tablets..............................(NDC 0078-0469-15)

500 mg
Off-white, round, flat tablet with beveled edge and imprinted with "J" and "500" on one side and "NVR" on the other.
Bottles of 30 tablets..............................(NDC 0078-0470-15)

Store Exjade tablets at 25°C (77°F); excursions are permitted to 15–30°C (59–86°F) [see USP Controlled Room Temperature]. Protect from moisture.

17 PATIENT COUNSELING INFORMATION

- Advise patients to take Exjade once daily on an empty stomach at least 30 minutes prior to food, preferably at the same time every day. Instruct patients to completely disperse the tablets in water, orange juice, or apple juice, and drink the resulting suspension immediately. After the suspension has been swallowed, resuspend any residue in a small volume of the liquid and swallow [*see Dosage and Administration (2.3)*].
- Advise patients not to chew tablets or swallow them whole [*see Dosage and Administration (2.3)*].
- Caution patients not to take aluminum-containing antacids and Exjade simultaneously [*see Drug Interactions (7.1)*].
- Because auditory and ocular disturbances have been reported with Exjade, conduct auditory testing and ophthalmic testing before starting Exjade treatment and thereafter at regular intervals [*see Warnings and Precautions (5.9)*].
- Caution patients experiencing dizziness to avoid driving or operating machinery [*see Adverse Reactions (6.1)*].
- Caution patients about the potential for the development of GI ulcers or bleeding when taking Exjade in combination with drugs that have ulcerogenic or hemorrhagic potential, such as NSAIDs, corticosteroids, oral bisphosphonates, or anticoagulants [*see Warnings and Precautions (5.3)*].
- Caution patients about potential loss of effectiveness of drugs metabolized by CYP3A4 (e.g., cyclosporine, simvastatin, hormonal contraceptive agents) when Exjade is administered with these drugs [*see Drug Interactions (7.2)*].
- Caution patients about potential loss of effectiveness of Exjade when administered with drugs that are potent UGT inducers (e.g., rifampicin, phenytoin, phenobarbital, ritonavir). Based on serum ferritin levels and clinical response, consider increases in the dose of Exjade when concomitantly used with potent UGT inducers [*see Drug Interactions (7.5)*].
- Caution patients about potential loss of effectiveness of Exjade when administered with drugs that are bile acid sequestrants (e.g., cholestyramine, colesevelam, colestipol). Based on serum ferritin levels and clinical response, consider increases in the dose of Exjade when concomitantly used with bile acid sequestrants [*see Drug Interactions (7.6)*].
- Perform careful monitoring of glucose levels when repaglinide is used concomitantly with Exjade. An interaction between Exjade and other CYP2C8 substrates like paclitaxel cannot be excluded [*see Drug Interactions (7.3)*].
- Advise patients that blood tests will be performed because Exjade may affect your kidneys, liver, or blood cells. The blood tests will be performed every month or more frequently if you are at increased risk of complications (e.g., preexisting kidney condition, are elderly, have multiple

medical conditions, or are taking medicine that affects your organs). There have been reports of severe kidney and liver problems, blood disorders, stomach hemorrhage and death in patients taking Exjade *[see Warnings and Precautions (5.1, 5.2, 5.3, 5.4, and 5.5)]*.

- Skin rashes may occur during Exjade treatment and if severe, interrupt treatment. Serious allergic reactions (which include swelling of the throat) have been reported in patients taking Exjade, usually within the first month of treatment. If reactions are severe, advise patients to stop taking Exjade and contact their doctor immediately *[see Warnings and Precautions (5.6, 5.7, and 5.8)]*.

Manufactured by:
Novartis Pharma Stein AG
Stein, Switzerland
Distributed by:
Novartis Pharmaceuticals Corporation
East Hanover, New Jersey 07936
© Novartis
T2013-41
May 2013

Shown in Product Identification Guide, page 310

EXTAVIA® ℞

(Interferon beta-1b)
Kit for subcutaneous use

The following prescribing information is based on official labeling in effect July 2013.

HIGHLIGHTS OF PRESCRIBING INFORMATION

These highlights do not include all the information needed to use Extavia safely and effectively. See full prescribing information for Extavia.

Extavia (Interferon beta-1b) Kit for subcutaneous use
Initial U.S. Approval: 1993

INDICATIONS AND USAGE

Extavia is an interferon beta indicated for the treatment of relapsing forms of multiple sclerosis to reduce the frequency of clinical exacerbations. Patients with multiple sclerosis in whom efficacy has been demonstrated include patients who have experienced a first clinical episode and have MRI features consistent with multiple sclerosis. (1)

DOSAGE AND ADMINISTRATION

- For subcutaneous use only. (2)
- The recommended dose is 0.25 mg injected subcutaneously every other day. Generally, start at 0.0625 mg (0.25 mL) subcutaneously every other day, and increase over a six week period to 0.25 mg (1 mL) every other day. (2)
- Instruct patients in the use of aseptic technique when administering Extavia. (17.6)

DOSAGE FORMS AND STRENGTHS

Lyophilized powder containing 0.3 mg of Interferon beta-1b, 15 mg Albumin (Human), USP, and 15 mg Mannitol, USP. (3).

CONTRAINDICATIONS

History of hypersensitivity to natural or recombinant interferon beta, Albumin (Human), USP, or any other component of the formulation. (4)

WARNINGS AND PRECAUTIONS

- Depression and suicide: advise patients to immediately report any symptom of depression and/or suicidal ideation; consider discontinuation of Extavia if depression occurs. (5.1)
- Injection site necrosis: do not administer Extavia into affected area until it is fully healed; if multiple lesions occur, therapy should be discontinued until healing occurs. (5.2)
- Injection site reactions. (5.3)
- Anaphylaxis and other allergic reactions. (5.4)
- Flu-Like Symptom Complex. (5.5)
- Leukopenia: monitor CBC. (5.6, 5.8)
- Liver enzymes abnormalities: monitor liver function tests. (5.7, 5.8)
- Monitor thyroid function tests every 6 months in patients with history of thyroid dysfunction. (5.8)

ADVERSE REACTIONS

In controlled studies with interferon beta-1b, the most common adverse reactions (at least 2% more than placebo) were: Lymphopenia, neutropenia, leukopenia, lymphadenopathy, headache, insomnia, incoordination, hypertension, dyspnea, abdominal pain, increased liver enzymes, rash, skin disorder, hypertonia, myalgia, urinary urgency, metrorrhagia, impotence, injection site reaction, asthenia, flu-like symptom complex, pain, fever, chills, peripheral edema, chest pain, malaise, and injection site necrosis (6.1)

To report SUSPECTED ADVERSE REACTIONS, contact Novartis Pharmaceuticals Corporation at 1-888-669-6682 or FDA at 1-800-FDA-1088 or www.fda.gov/medwatch.

DRUG INTERACTIONS

No formal drug interaction studies have been conducted. (7)

USE IN SPECIFIC POPULATIONS

- Pregnancy: Based on animal data, may cause fetal harm. (8.1)
- Nursing Mothers: use EXTAVIA with caution. (8.3)
- Pediatric Use: Safety and efficacy not established in patients under 18 years of age. (8.3)
- Geriatric Use: Safety and efficacy not established in patients age 65 years or older. (8.4)

See 17 for PATIENT COUNSELING INFORMATION and Medication Guide

Revised: 03/2012

FULL PRESCRIBING INFORMATION: CONTENTS*

*** Sections or subsections omitted from the full prescribing information are not listed**

FULL PRESCRIBING INFORMATION

1 INDICATIONS AND USAGE

EXTAVIA (Interferon beta-1b) is indicated for the treatment of relapsing forms of multiple sclerosis to reduce the frequency of clinical exacerbations. Patients with multiple sclerosis in whom efficacy has been demonstrated include patients who have experienced a first clinical episode and have MRI features consistent with multiple sclerosis.

2 DOSAGE AND ADMINISTRATION

The recommended dose of EXTAVIA is 0.25 mg injected subcutaneously every other day.

Generally, patients should be started at 0.0625 mg (0.25 mL) subcutaneously every other day, and increased over a six week period to 0.25 mg (1 mL) every other day (see Table 1).

Table 1. Schedule for Dose Titration

	Recommended Titration	EXTAVIA Dose	Volume
Weeks 1-2	25%	0.0625 mg	0.25 mL
Weeks 3-4	50%	0.125 mg	0.5 mL
Weeks 5-6	75%	0.1875 mg	0.75 mL
Week 7+	100%	0.25 mg	1 mL

To reconstitute lyophilized EXTAVIA for injection, attach the prefilled syringe containing the diluent (Sodium Chloride, 0.54% Solution) to the EXTAVIA vial using the vial adapter. Slowly inject 1.2 mL of diluent into the EXTAVIA vial. Gently swirl the vial to dissolve the drug completely; do not shake. Foaming may occur during reconstitution or if the vial is swirled or shaken too vigorously. If foaming occurs, allow the vial to sit undisturbed until the foam settles. Visually inspect the reconstituted product before use; discard the product if it contains particulate matter or is discolored. Keeping the syringe and vial adapter in place, turn the assembly over so that the vial is on top. Withdraw the appropriate dose of EXTAVIA solution. Remove the vial from the vial adapter before injecting EXTAVIA. One mL of reconstituted EXTAVIA solution contains 0.25 mg of Interferon beta-1b/mL.

EXTAVIA is intended for use under the guidance and supervision of a physician. It is recommended that physicians or qualified medical personnel train patients in the proper technique for self-administering subcutaneous injections. Patients should be advised to rotate sites for subcutaneous injections (see Patient Counseling Information 17.6). Concurrent use of analgesics and/or antipyretics may help ameliorate flu-like symptoms on treatment days. EXTAVIA should be visually inspected for particulate matter and discoloration prior to administration.

3 DOSAGE FORMS AND STRENGTHS

EXTAVIA is supplied as a lyophilized powder containing 0.3 mg of Interferon beta-1b, 15 mg Albumin (Human), USP, and 15 mg Mannitol, USP. Drug is packaged in a clear glass, single-use vial (3 mL capacity). A pre-filled single-use syringe containing 1.2 mL of diluent (Sodium Chloride, 0.54% solution), two alcohol prep pads, and one vial adapter with attached 27 gauge needle are included for each vial of drug. EXTAVIA and the diluent are for single-use only. Unused portions should be discarded. Store at room temperature.

4 CONTRAINDICATIONS

EXTAVIA is contraindicated in patients with a history of hypersensitivity to natural or recombinant interferon beta, Albumin (Human), USP, or any other component of the formulation.

5 WARNINGS AND PRECAUTIONS

5.1 Depression and Suicide

EXTAVIA (Interferon beta-1b) should be used with caution in patients with depression, a condition that is common in people with multiple sclerosis. Depression and suicide have been reported to occur with increased frequency in patients receiving interferon compounds, including Interferon beta-1b. Patients treated with EXTAVIA should be advised to report immediately any symptoms of depression and/or suicidal ideation to their prescribing physicians. If a patient develops depression, cessation of EXTAVIA therapy should be considered.

In the four randomized controlled studies there were three suicides and eight suicide attempts among the 1532 patients in the Interferon beta-1b treated groups compared to one suicide and four suicide attempts among the 965 patients in the placebo groups.

5.2 Injection Site Necrosis

Injection site necrosis (ISN) has been reported in 4% of patients in controlled clinical trials *[see Adverse Reactions (6.1)]*. Typically, injection site necrosis occurs within the first four months of therapy, although post-marketing reports have been received of ISN occurring over one year after initiation of therapy. Necrosis may occur at a single or multiple injection sites. The necrotic lesions are typically three cm or less in diameter, but larger areas have been reported. Generally the necrosis has extended only to subcutaneous fat. However, there are also reports of necrosis extending to and including fascia overlying muscle. In some lesions where biopsy results are available, vasculitis has been reported. For some lesions debridement and, infrequently, skin grafting have been required.

As with any open lesion, it is important to avoid infection and, if it occurs, to treat the infection. Time to healing was varied depending on the severity of the necrosis at the time treatment was begun. In most cases healing was associated with scarring.

Some patients have experienced healing of necrotic skin lesions while Interferon beta-1b therapy continued; others have not. Whether to discontinue therapy following a single site of necrosis is dependent on the extent of necrosis. For patients who continue therapy with EXTAVIA after injection site necrosis has occurred, EXTAVIA should not be administered into the affected area until it is fully healed. If multiple lesions occur, therapy should be discontinued until healing occurs.

Patient understanding and use of aseptic self-injection techniques and procedures should be periodically reevaluated, particularly if injection site necrosis has occurred.

5.3 Injection Site Reactions

In controlled clinical trials, injection site reactions occurred in 78% of patients receiving Interferon beta-1b with injection site necrosis in 4%. Injection site inflammation (42%), injection site pain (16%), injection site hypersensitivity (4%), injection site necrosis (4%), injection site mass (2%), injection site edema (2%) and non-specific reactions were significantly associated with Interferon beta-1b treatment. The incidence of injection site reactions tended to decrease over time. Approximately 69% of patients experienced the event during the first three months of treatment, compared to approximately 40% at the end of the studies.

5.4 Anaphylaxis

Anaphylaxis has been reported as a rare complication of Interferon beta-1b use. Other allergic reactions have included dyspnea, bronchospasm, tongue edema, skin rash and urticaria *[see Adverse Reactions (6.1)]*.

5.5 Flu-Like Symptom Complex

In controlled clinical trials, the rate of flu-like symptom complex was approximately 57%. The incidence decreased over time, with only 10% of patients reporting flu-like symptom complex at the end of the studies. The median duration of flu-like symptom complex in Study 1 was 7.5 days *[see Clinical Studies (14)]*.

5.6 Leukopenia

In controlled clinical trials, leukopenia was reported in 18% of patients receiving Interferon beta-1b, leading to a reduction of the dose of Interferon beta-1b in some patients [see Adverse Reactions (6.1)]. Monitoring of complete blood and differential white blood cell counts is recommended *[see Warnings and Precautions (5.8)]*.

5.7 Hepatic enzymes elevations

In controlled clinical trials, elevations of SGPT to greater than five times baseline value were reported in 12% of patients receiving Interferon beta-1b, and increase of SGOT to greater than five times baseline value were reported in 4% of patients receiving Interferon beta-1b, leading to dose-reduction or discontinuation of treatment in some patients *[see Adverse Reactions (6.1)]*. Monitoring of liver function tests is recommended *[see Warnings and Precautions (5.8)]*.

5.8 Laboratory Tests

In addition to those laboratory tests normally required for monitoring patients with multiple sclerosis, complete blood and differential white blood cell counts, platelet counts and blood chemistries, including liver function tests, are recommended at regular intervals (one, three, and six months) following introduction of EXTAVIA therapy, and then periodically thereafter in the absence of clinical symptoms. Thyroid function tests are recommended every six months in patients with a history of thyroid dysfunction or as clinically indicated. Patients with myelosuppression may require more intensive monitoring of complete blood cell counts, with differential and platelet counts.

5.9 Albumin (Human), USP

This product contains albumin, a derivative of human blood. Based on effective donor screening and product manufacturing processes, it carries an extremely remote risk for transmission of viral diseases. A theoretical risk for transmission of Creutzfeldt-Jakob disease (CJD) also is considered extremely remote. No cases of transmission of viral diseases or CJD have ever been identified for albumin.

6 ADVERSE REACTIONS

6.1 Clinical Studies Experience

In all studies, the most serious adverse reactions with Interferon beta-1b were depression, suicidal ideation and injection site necrosis (*see Warnings and Precautions*). The incidence of depression of any severity was approximately 30% in both Interferon beta-1b-treated patients and placebo-treated patients. Anaphylaxis and other allergic reactions have been reported in patients using Interferon beta-1b [*see Warnings and Precautions (5.4)]*. The most commonly reported adverse reactions were lymphopenia (lymphocytes<1500/mm^3), injection site reaction, asthenia, flu-like symptom complex, headache, and pain. The most frequently reported adverse reactions resulting in clinical intervention (e.g., discontinuation of Interferon beta 1b, adjustment in dosage, or the need for concomitant medication to treat an adverse reaction symptom) were depression, flu-like symptom complex, injection site reactions, leukopenia, increased liver enzymes, asthenia, hypertonia, and myasthenia.

Because clinical trials are conducted under widely varying conditions and over varying lengths of time, adverse reaction rates observed in the clinical trials of Interferon beta-1b cannot be directly compared to rates in clinical trials of other drugs, and may not reflect the rates observed in practice. The adverse reaction information from clinical trials does, however, provide a basis for identifying the adverse events that appear to be related to drug use and for approximating rates.

The data described below reflect exposure to Interferon beta-1b in the four placebo controlled trials of 1407 patients with MS treated with 0.25 mg or 0.16 mg/m^2, including 1261 exposed for greater than one year. The population encompassed an age range from 18 – 65 years. Sixty-four percent (64%) of the patients were female. The percentages of Caucasian, Black, Asian, and Hispanic patients were 94.8%, 3.5%, 0.1%, and 0.7%, respectively.

The safety profiles for Interferon beta-1b-treated patients with SPMS and RRMS were similar. Clinical experience with Interferon beta-1b in other populations (patients with cancer, HIV positive patients, etc.) provides additional data regarding adverse reactions; however, experience in non-MS populations may not be fully applicable to the MS population.

Table 2 enumerates adverse events and laboratory abnormalities that occurred among all patients treated with 0.25 mg or 0.16 mg/m^2 Interferon beta-1b every other day for periods of up to three years in the four placebo controlled trials (Study 1-4) at an incidence that was at least 2.0% more than that observed in the placebo patients (System Organ Class, MedDRA v. 8.0).

Table 2. Adverse Reactions and Laboratory Abnormalities

System Organ Class MedDRA v. 8.0 [#] Adverse Reaction	Placebo (n=965)	Interferon beta-1b (n=1407)
Blood and lymphatic system disorders		
Lymphocytes count decreased (< 1500/mm^3) [x]	66%	86%
Absolute neutrophil count decreased (< 1500/mm^3) [x]	5%	13%
White blood cell count decreased (< 3000/mm^3) [x]	4%	13%
Lymphadenopathy	3%	6%
Nervous system disorders		
Headache	43%	50%
Insomnia	16%	21%
Incoordination	15%	17%
Vascular disorders		
Hypertension	4%	6%
Respiratory, thoracic and mediastinal disorders		
Dyspnea	3%	6%
Gastrointestinal disorders		
Abdominal pain	11%	16%
Hepatobiliary disorders		
Alanine aminotransferase increased(SGPT > 5 times baseline)[x]	4%	12%
Aspartate aminotransferase increased(SGOT > 5 times baseline)[x]	1%	4%
Skin and subcutaneous tissue disorders		
Rash	15%	21%
Skin disorder	8%	10%
Musculoskeletal and connective tissue disorders		
Hypertonia	33%	40%
Myalgia	14%	23%
Renal and urinary disorders		
Urinary urgency	8%	11%
Reproductive system and breast disorders		
Metrorrhagia*	7%	9%
Impotence**	6%	8%
General disorders and administration site conditions		
Injection site reaction (various kinds) [o]	26%	78%
Asthenia	48%	53%
Flu-like symptoms (complex)[§]	37%	57%
Pain	35%	42%
Fever	19%	31%
Chills	9%	21%
Peripheral edema	10%	12%
Chest pain	6%	9%
Malaise	3%	6%
Injection site necrosis	0%	4%

[#] except for "injection site reaction (various kinds)[o]" and "flu-like symptom complex[§]" the most appropriate MedDRA term is used to describe a certain reaction and its synonyms and related conditions.

[x] laboratory abnormality

* pre-menopausal women

** men

[o] "Injection site reaction (various kinds)" comprises all adverse events occurring at the injection site (except injection site necrosis), i.e., the following terms: injection site reaction, injection site hemorrhage, injection site hypersensitivity, injection site inflammation, injection site mass, injection site pain, injection site edema and injection site atrophy.

[§] "Flu-like symptom complex" denotes flu syndrome and/or a combination of at least two AEs from fever, chills, myalgia, malaise, sweating.

Laboratory Abnormalities

In the four clinical trials, leukopenia was reported in 18% and 6% of patients in Interferon beta-1b- and placebo-treated groups, respectively. No patients were withdrawn or dose reduced for neutropenia in Study 1. Three percent (3%) of patients in Studies 2 and 3 experienced leukopenia and were dose-reduced. Monitoring of complete blood and differential white blood cell counts is recommended *[see Warnings and Precautions (5.6, 5.8)]*.

Other abnormalities included increase of SGPT to greater than five times baseline value (12%), and increase of SGOT to greater than five times baseline value (4%). In Study 1, two patients were dose reduced for increased hepatic enzymes; one continued on treatment and one was ultimately withdrawn. In Studies 2 and 3, 1.5% of Interferon beta-1b patients were dose-reduced or interrupted treatment for increased hepatic enzymes. In Study 4, 1.7% of patients were withdrawn from treatment due to increased hepatic enzymes, two of them after a dose reduction. In Studies 1-4, nine (0.6%) patients were withdrawn from treatment with Interferon beta-1b for any laboratory abnormality, including four (0.3%) patients following dose reduction. Monitoring of liver function tests is recommended *[see Warnings and Precautions (5.7, 5.8)]*.

6.2 Postmarketing Experience

The following adverse events have been observed during postmarketing experience with Interferon beta-1b and are classified within body system categories:

Blood and lymphatic system disorders: Anemia, Thrombocytopenia

Endocrine disorders: Hypothyroidism, Hyperthyroidism, Thyroid dysfunction

Metabolism and nutrition disorders: Hypocalcemia, Hyperuricemia, Triglyceride increased, Anorexia, Weight decrease

Psychiatric disorders: Confusion, Depersonalization, Emotional lability

Nervous system disorders: Ataxia, Convulsion, Paresthesia, Psychotic symptoms

Cardiac disorders: Cardiomyopathy

Vascular disorders: Deep vein thrombosis, Pulmonary embolism

Respiratory, thoracic and mediastinal disorders: Bronchospasm, Pneumonia

Gastrointestinal disorders: Pancreatitis, Vomiting

Hepatobiliary disorders: Hepatitis, Gamma GT increased

Skin and subcutaneous tissue disorders: Pruritus, Skin discoloration, Urticaria

Renal and urinary disorders: Urinary tract infection, Urosepsis

General disorders and administration site conditions: Fatal capillary leak syndrome[1]

[1]The administration of cytokines to patients with a pre-existing monoclonal gammopathy has been associated with the development of this syndrome.

6.3 Immunogenicity

As with all therapeutic proteins, there is a potential for immunogenicity. Serum samples were monitored for the development of antibodies to Interferon beta-1b during Study 1 *[see Clinical Studies (14)]*. In patients receiving 0.25 mg every other day 56/124 (45%) were found to have serum neutralizing activity at one or more of the time points tested. In Study 4 *[see Clinical Studies (14)]*, neutralizing activity was measured every 6 months and at end of study. At individual visits after start of therapy, activity was observed in 16.5% up to 25.2% of the Interferon beta-1b treated patients. Such neutralizing activity was measured at least once in 75 (29.9%) out of 251 Interferon beta-1b patients who provided samples during treatment phase; of these, 17 (22.7%) converted to negative status later in the study.

Based on all the available evidence, the relationship between antibody formation and clinical safety or efficacy is not known.

These data reflect the percentage of patients whose test results were considered positive for antibodies to Interferon beta-1b using a biological neutralization assay that measures the ability of immune sera to inhibit the production of the interferon-inducible protein, MxA. Neutralization assays are highly dependent on the sensitivity and specificity of the assay. Additionally, the observed incidence of neutralizing activity in an assay may be influenced by several factors including sample handling, timing of sample collection, concomitant medications, and underlying disease. For these reasons, comparison of the incidence of antibodies to Interferon beta-1b with the incidence of antibodies to other products may be misleading.

Anaphylactic reactions have rarely been reported with the use of Interferon beta-1b *[see Warnings and Precautions (5.4)]*.

Table 3. Two Year RRMS Study Results. Primary and Secondary Clinical Outcomes

Efficacy Parameters	Treatment Groups			Statistical Comparisons p-value		
Primary End Points	Placebo N=123	0.05 mg N=125	0.25 mg N=124	Placebo vs 0.05 mg	0.05 mg vs 0.25 mg	Placebo vs 0.25 mg
Annual exacerbation rate	1.31	1.14	0.90	0.005	0.113	**0.0001**
Proportion of exacerbation-free patients†	16%	18%	25%	0.609	0.288	**0.094**
Exacerbation frequency per patient: 0† 1 2 3 4 ≥5	20 32 20 15 15 21	22 31 28 15 7 16	29 39 17 14 9 8	0.151	0.077	**0.001**
Secondary Endpoints ††						
Median number of months to first on-study exacerbation	5	6	9	0.299	0.097	**0.010**
Rate of moderate or severe exacerbations per year	0.47	0.29	0.23	0.020	0.257	**0.001**
Mean number of moderate or severe exacerbation days per patient	44.1	33.2	19.5	0.229	0.064	**0.001**
Mean change in EDSS score‡ at endpoint	0.21	0.21	-0.07	0.995	0.108	**0.144**
Mean change in Scripps score‡‡ at endpoint	-0.53	-0.50	0.66	0.641	0.051	**0.126**
Median duration in days per exacerbation	36	33	35.5	ND	ND	**ND**
% change in mean MRI lesion area at endpoint	21.4%	9.8%	-0.9%	0.015	0.019	**0.0001**

ND Not done

† 14 exacerbation free patients (0 from placebo, six from 0.05 mg, and eight from 0.25 mg) dropped out of the study before completing six months of therapy. These patients are excluded from this analysis.

†† Sequelae and Functional Neurologic Status, both required by protocol, were not analyzed individually but are included as a function of the EDSS.

‡ EDSS scores range from 1-10, with higher scores reflecting greater disability

‡‡ Scripps neurologic rating scores range from 0-100, with smaller scores reflecting greater disability.

7 DRUG INTERACTIONS

No formal drug interaction studies have been conducted with Interferon beta-1b. In the placebo controlled studies in MS, corticosteroids or ACTH were administered for treatment of relapses for periods of up to 28 days in patients (N=664) receiving Interferon beta-1b.

8 USE IN SPECIFIC POPULATIONS

8.1 Pregnancy

Pregnancy Category C: There are no adequate and well-controlled studies of Interferon beta-1b in pregnant women; however, spontaneous abortions while on treatment were reported in four patients participating in the Interferon beta-1b RRMS clinical trial. Interferon beta-1b should be used during pregnancy only if the potential benefit justifies the potential risk to the fetus.

When Interferon beta-1b (doses ranging from 0.028 to 0.42 mg/kg) was administered to pregnant rhesus monkeys throughout the period of organogenesis (gestation days 20 to 70), a dose-related abortifacient effect was observed. The low effect dose is approximately 3 times the recommended human dose of 0.25 mg on a body surface are (mg/m^2) basis. A no-effect dose for embryo-fetal developmental toxicity in rhesus monkeys was not established.

8.3 Nursing Mothers

It is not known whether Interferon beta-1b is excreted in human milk. Because many drugs are excreted in human milk and because of the potential for serious adverse reactions in nursing infants from Interferon beta-1b, a decision should be made to either discontinue nursing or discontinue the drug, taking into account the importance of drug to the mother.

8.4 Pediatric Use

Safety and efficacy in pediatric patients have not been established.

8.5 Geriatric Use

Clinical studies of Interferon beta-1b did not include sufficient numbers of patients aged 65 and over to determine whether they respond differently than younger patients.

10 OVERDOSAGE

Safety of doses higher than 0.25 mg every other day has not been adequately evaluated. The maximum amount of Interferon beta-1b that can be safely administered has not been determined.

11 DESCRIPTION

EXTAVIA® (Interferon beta-lb) is a purified, sterile, lyophilized protein product produced by recombinant DNA techniques. Interferon beta-1b is manufactured by bacterial fermentation of a strain of Escherichia coli that bears a genetically engineered plasmid containing the gene for human interferon beta$_{ser17}$. The native gene was obtained from human fibroblasts and altered in a way that substitutes serine for the cysteine residue found at position 17. Interferon beta-1b has 165 amino acids and an approximate molecular weight of 18,500 daltons. It does not include the carbohydrate side chains found in the natural material. EXTAVIA contains the same active ingredients as other Interferon beta-1b products. For this reason, these products should not be given concomitantly.

The specific activity of EXTAVIA is approximately 32 million international units (IU)/mg Interferon beta-lb. Each vial contains 0.3 mg of Interferon beta-lb. The unit measurement is derived by comparing the antiviral activity of the product to the World Health Organization (WHO) reference standard of recombinant human interferon beta. Mannitol, USP and Albumin (Human), USP (15 mg each/ vial) are added as stabilizers.

Lyophilized EXTAVIA is a sterile, white to off-white powder, for subcutaneous injection after reconstitution with the diluent supplied (Sodium Chloride, 0.54% Solution).

12 CLINICAL PHARMACOLOGY

12.1 Mechanism of Action

The mechanism of action of Interferon beta-1b in patients with multiple sclerosis is unknown.

12.2 Pharmacodynamics

Interferons (IFNs) are a family of naturally occurring proteins, produced by eukaryotic cells in response to viral infection and other biologic agents. Four major groups of interferons have been distinguished: alpha, beta, gamma and lambda. Interferons-alpha and -beta comprise the Type I interferons, interferon-gamma is the sole Type II interferon, and interferon-lambda is designated as Type III interferon. Type I interferons have considerably overlapping but also distinct biologic activities. The bioactivities of IFNs are mediated by their interactions with specific receptors found on the surfaces of human cells. Differences in bioactivites induced by IFNs likely reflect divergences in the signal transduction process induced by IFN-receptor binding.

Interferon beta-1b receptor binding induces the expression of proteins that are responsible for the pleiotropic bioactivities of Interferon beta-1b. A number of these proteins (including neopterin, β_2-microglobulin, MxA protein, and IL-10) have been measured in blood fractions from Interferon beta-1b-treated patients and Interferon beta-1b-treated healthy volunteers. Immunomodulatory effects of Interferon beta-1b include the enhancement of suppressor T cell activity, reduction of pro-inflammatory cytokine production, down-regulation of antigen presentation, and inhibition of lymphocyte trafficking into the central nervous system. It is not known if these effects play an important role in the observed clinical activity of Interferon beta-1b in multiple sclerosis (MS).

12.3 Pharmacokinetics

Because serum concentrations of Interferon beta-1b are low or not detectable following subcutaneous administration of 0.25 mg or less of Interferon beta-1b, pharmacokinetic information in patients with MS receiving the recommended dose of Interferon beta-1b is not available. Following single and multiple daily subcutaneous administrations of 0.5 mg Interferon beta-1b to healthy volunteers (N=12), serum Interferon beta-1b concentrations were generally below 100 IU/mL. Peak serum Interferon beta-1b concentrations occurred between one to eight hours, with a mean peak serum interferon concentration of 40 IU/mL. Bioavailability, based on a total dose of 0.5 mg Interferon beta-1b given as two subcutaneous injections at different sites, was approximately 50%.

After intravenous administration of Interferon beta-1b (0.006 mg to 2.0 mg), similar pharmacokinetic profiles were obtained from healthy volunteers (N=12) and from patients with diseases other than MS (N=142). In patients receiving single intravenous doses up to 2.0 mg, increases in serum concentrations were dose proportional. Mean serum clearance values ranged from 9.4 mL/min•kg $^{-1}$ to 28.9 mL/ min•kg^{-1} and were independent of dose. Mean terminal elimination half-life values ranged from 8.0 minutes to 4.3 hours and mean steady-state volume of distribution values ranged from 0.25 L/kg to 2.88 L/kg. Three-times-a-week intravenous dosing for two weeks resulted in no accumulation of Interferon beta-1b in sera of patients. Pharmacokinetic parameters after single and multiple intravenous doses of Interferon beta-1b were comparable.

Following every other day subcutaneous administration of 0.25 mg Interferon beta-1b in healthy volunteers, biologic response marker levels (neopterin, β_2- microglobulin, MxA protein, and the immunosuppressive cytokine, IL-10) increased significantly above baseline six-twelve hours after the first Interferon beta-1b dose. Biologic response marker levels peaked between 40 and 124 hours and remained elevated above baseline throughout the seven-day (168-hour) study. The relationship between serum Interferon beta-1b levels or induced biologic response marker levels and the clinical effects of Interferon beta-1b in multiple sclerosis is unknown.

13 NONCLINICAL TOXICOLOGY

13.1 Carcinogenesis, Mutagenesis, Impairment of Fertility

Carcinogenesis: Interferon beta-1b has not been tested for its carcinogenic potential in animals.

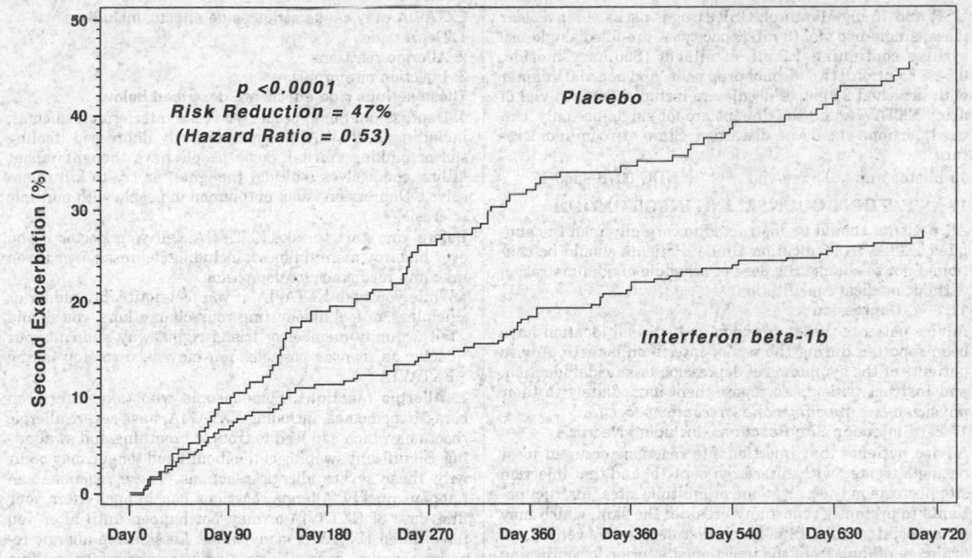

Interferon beta-1b	n=292	287	249	237	223	210	206	200	47
Placebo	n=176	158	139	126	115	111	101	96	34

Figure 2 – Onset of Second Exacerbation by Time on Study (Kaplan-Meier Methodology)

Figure 1

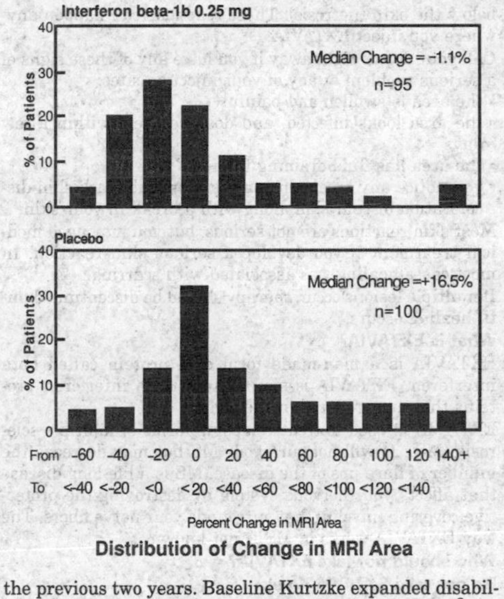

Distribution of Change in MRI Area

Mutagenesis: Interferon beta-1b was not genotoxic in the *in vitro* Ames bacterial test or the *in vitro* chromosomal aberration assay in human peripheral blood lymphocytes. Interferon beta-1b treatment of mouse BALBc-3T3 cells did not result in increased transformation frequency in an *in vitro* model of tumor transformation.

Impairment of fertility: Administration of Interferon beta-1b (doses of up to 0.33 mg/kg) to normally cycling female rhesus monkeys had no apparent adverse effects on either menstrual cycle duration or associated hormonal profiles (progesterone and estradiol) when administered over three consecutive menstrual cycles. The highest dose tested is approximately 30 times the recommended human dose of 0.25 mg on a body surface area (mg/m^2) basis. The potential for other effects on fertility or reproductive performance was not evaluated.

14 CLINICAL STUDIES

The clinical effects of Interferon beta-1b were studied in four randomized, multicenter, double-blind, placebo-controlled studies in patients with multiple sclerosis.

The effectiveness of Interferon beta-1b in relapsing-remitting MS (Study 1) was evaluated in a double blind, multiclinic, randomized, parallel, placebo controlled clinical investigation of two years' duration. The study enrolled MS patients, aged 18 to 50, who were ambulatory (EDSS of ≤ 5.5), exhibited a relapsing-remitting clinical course, met Poser's criteria[1] for clinically definite and/or laboratory supported definite MS and had experienced at least two exacerbations over two years preceding the trial without exacerbation in the preceding month. Patients who had received prior immunosuppressant therapy were excluded.

An exacerbation was defined as the appearance of a new clinical sign/symptom or the clinical worsening of a previous sign/symptom (one that had been stable for at least 30 days) that persisted for a minimum of 24 hours.

Patients selected for study were randomized to treatment with either placebo (N=123), 0.05 mg of Interferon beta-1b (N=125), or 0.25 mg of Interferon beta-1b (N=124) self-administered subcutaneously every other day. Outcome based on the 372 randomized patients was evaluated after two years.

Patients who required more than three 28-day courses of corticosteroids were removed from the study. Minor analgesics (acetaminophen, codeine), antidepressants, and oral baclofen were allowed ad libitum, but chronic nonsteroidal anti-inflammatory drug (NSAID) use was not allowed.

The primary protocol-defined outcome measures were 1) frequency of exacerbations per patient and 2) proportion of exacerbation free patients. A number of secondary clinical and magnetic resonance imaging (MRI) measures were also employed. All patients underwent annual T2 MRI imaging and a subset of 52 patients at one site had MRIs performed every six weeks for assessment of new or expanding lesions.

The study results are shown in **Table 3**.

[See table 3 at top of previous page]

Of the 372 RRMS patients randomized, 72 (19%) failed to complete two full years on their assigned treatments.

Over the two-year period, there were 25 MS-related hospitalizations in the 0.25 mg Interferon beta-1b-treated group compared to 48 hospitalizations in the placebo group. In comparison, non-MS hospitalizations were evenly distributed among the groups, with 16 in the 0.25 mg Interferon beta-1b group and 15 in the placebo group. The average number of days of MS-related steroid use was 41 days in the 0.25 mg Interferon beta-1b group and 55 days in the placebo group (p=0.004).

MRI data were also analyzed for patients in this study. A frequency distribution of the observed percent changes in MRI area at the end of two years was obtained by grouping the percentages in successive intervals of equal width. Figure 1 displays a histogram of the proportions of patients, which fell into each of these intervals. The median percent change in MRI area for the 0.25 mg group was -1.1%, which was significantly smaller than the 16.5% observed for the placebo group (p=0.0001).

[See figure 1 at top of next column]

In an evaluation of frequent MRI scans (every six weeks) on 52 patients at one site, the percent of scans with new or expanding lesions was 29% in the placebo group and 6% in the 0.25 mg treatment group (p=0.006).

The exact relationship between MRI findings and clinical status of patients is unknown. Changes in lesion area often do not correlate with changes in disability progression. The prognostic significance of the MRI findings in this study has not been evaluated.

Studies 2 and 3 were multicenter, randomized, double-blind, placebo controlled trials conducted to assess the effect of Interferon beta-1b in patients with SPMS. Study 2 was conducted in Europe and Study 3 was conducted in North America. Both studies enrolled patients with clinically definite or laboratory-supported MS in the secondary progressive phase, and who had evidence of disability progression (both Study 2 and 3) or two relapses (Study 2 only) within the previous two years. Baseline Kurtzke expanded disability status scale (EDSS) scores ranged from 3.0 to 6.5. [2] Patients in Study 2 were randomized to receive Interferon beta-1b 0.25 mg (n=360) or placebo (n=358). Patients in Study 3 were randomized to Interferon beta-1b 0.25 mg (n=317), Interferon beta-1b 0.16 mg/m^2 of body surface area (n=314, mean assigned dose 0.30 mg), or placebo (n=308). Test agents were administered subcutaneously, every other day for three years.

The primary outcome measure was progression of disability, defined as a 1.0 point increase in the EDSS score, or a 0.5 point increase for patients with baseline EDSS ≥ 6.0. In Study 2, time to progression in EDSS was longer in the Interferon beta-1b treatment group (p=0.005), with estimated annualized rates of progression of 16% and 19% in the Interferon beta-1b and placebo groups, respectively. In Study 3, the rates of progression did not differ significantly between treatment groups, with estimated annualized rates of progression of 12%, 14%, and 12% in the Interferon beta-1b fixed dose, surface area-adjusted dose, and placebo groups, respectively.

Multiple analyses, including covariate and subset analyses based on sex, age, disease duration, clinical disease activity prior to study enrollment, MRI measures at baseline and early changes in MRI following treatment were evaluated in order to interpret the discordant study results. No demographic or disease-related factors enabled identification of a patient subset where Interferon beta-1b treatment was predictably associated with delayed progression of disability.

In Studies 2 and 3, like Study 1, a statistically significant decrease in the incidence of relapses associated with Interferon beta-1b treatment was demonstrated. In Study 2, the mean annual relapse rates were 0.42 and 0.63 in the Interferon beta-1b and placebo groups, respectively (p<0.001). In Study 3, the mean annual relapse rates were 0.16, 0.20, and 0.28, for the fixed dose, surface area-adjusted dose, and placebo groups, respectively (p<0.02).

MRI endpoints in both Study 2 and Study 3 showed lesser increases in T2 MRI lesion area and decreased number of active MRI lesions in patients in the Interferon beta-1b groups. The exact relationship between MRI findings and the clinical status of patients is unknown. Changes in MRI findings often do not correlate with changes in disability progression. The prognostic significance of the MRI findings in these studies is not known.

In Study 4, 468 patients who had recently (within 60 days) experienced an isolated demyelinating event, and who had lesions typical of multiple sclerosis on brain MRI were randomized to receive either 0.25 mg Interferon beta-1b (n = 292) or placebo (n= 176) subcutaneously every other day (ratio 5:3). The primary outcome measure was time to development of a second exacerbation with involvement of at least two distinct anatomical regions. Secondary outcomes were brain MRI measures, including the cumulative number of newly active lesions, and the absolute change in T2 lesion volume. Patients were followed for up to two years or until they fulfilled the primary endpoint.

Eight percent of subjects on Interferon beta-1b and 6% of subjects on placebo withdrew from the study for a reason other than the development of a second exacerbation. Time to development of a second exacerbation was significantly delayed in patients treated with Interferon beta-1b compared to placebo (p<0.0001). The Kaplan-Meier estimates of the percentage of patients developing an exacerbation within 24 months were 45% in the placebo group and 28% of the Interferon beta-1b group (Figure 2). The risk for developing a second exacerbation in the Interferon beta-1b group was 53% of the risk in the placebo group (Hazard ratio= 0.53; 95% confidence interval 0.39 to 0.73).

[See figure 2 above]

Patients treated with Interferon beta-1b demonstrated a lower number of newly active lesions during the course of the study. A significant difference between Interferon beta-1b and placebo was not seen in the absolute change in T2 lesion volume during the course of the study.

Safety and efficacy of treatment with Interferon beta-1b beyond three years are not known.

15 REFERENCES

1. Poser CM, et al. Ann Neurol 1983; 13(3): 227-231.
2. Kurtzke JF. Neurology 1983; 33(11): 1444-1452.

16 HOW SUPPLIED/STORAGE AND HANDLING

The reconstituted product contains no preservative. Before reconstitution with diluent, store EXTAVIA at room temperature 25°C (77°F). Excursions of 15° to 30°C (59° to 86°F) are permitted. After reconstitution, if not used immediately, the product should be refrigerated and used within three hours. Do not freeze.

EXTAVIA is supplied as a lyophilized powder containing 0.3 mg of Interferon beta-1b, 15 mg Albumin (Human),

USP, and 15 mg Mannitol, USP. Drug is packaged in a clear glass, single-use vial (3 mL capacity). A pre-filled single-use syringe containing 1.2 mL of diluent (Sodium Chloride, 0.54% solution), two alcohol prep pads, and one vial adapter with attached 27 gauge needle are included for each vial of drug. EXTAVIA and the diluent are for single-use only. Unused portions should be discarded. Store at room temperature.

15 blister units, 0.3 mg/vial NDC 0078-0569-12

17 PATIENT COUNSELING INFORMATION

All patients should be instructed to carefully read the supplied EXTAVIA Medication Guide. Patients should be cautioned not to change the dose or schedule of administration without medical consultation.

17.1 Depression

Advise patients that depression and suicidal ideation have been reported during the use of Interferon beta-1b. Advise patients of the symptoms of depression or suicidal ideation, and instruct patients to report them immediately to their physician *[see Warnings and Precautions (5.1)]*.

17.2 Injection Site Reactions, Including Necrosis

Advise patients that injection site reactions occur in most patients treated with Interferon beta-1b, and that injection site necrosis may occur at one or multiple sites. Instruct patients to promptly report any break in the skin, which may be associated with blue-black discoloration, swelling, or drainage of fluid from the injection site, prior to continuing their EXTAVIA therapy *[see Warnings and Precautions (5.2, 5.3)]*.

17.3 Allergic Reactions and Anaphylaxis

Advise patients of the symptoms of allergic reactions and anaphylaxis, and instruct patients to seek immediate medical attention if these symptoms occur *[see Warnings and Precautions (5.4)]*.

17.4 Flu-like Symptoms

Patients should be informed that flu-like symptoms are common following initiation of therapy with Interferon beta-1b. In controlled clinical trials, antipyretics and analgesics were permitted for relief of these symptoms. In addition, gradual dose titration during initiation of Interferon beta-1b treatment may reduce flu-like symptoms *[see Warnings and Precautions (5.5) and Dosage And Administration (2)]*.

17.5 Pregnancy

Advise patients that EXTAVIA should not be used during pregnancy unless the potential benefit justifies the potential risk to the fetus *[see Use in Special Population (8.1)]*.

17.6 Instruction on Self-injection Technique and Procedures

Patients should be instructed in the use of aseptic technique when administering EXTAVIA. Appropriate instruction for reconstitution of EXTAVIA and methods of self-injection should be provided, including careful review of the EXTAVIA Medication Guide. The first injection should be performed under the supervision of an appropriately qualified health care professional.

Patients should be cautioned against the re-use of needles or syringes and instructed in safe disposal procedures. A puncture resistant container for disposal of used needles and syringes should be supplied to the patient along with instructions for safe disposal of full containers.

Patients should be advised of the importance of rotating areas of injection with each dose, to minimize the likelihood of severe injection site reactions, including necrosis or localized infection, (see Choose an Injection Site section of the Medication Guide).

Manufactured by:
Bayer HealthCare Pharmaceuticals Inc.
Montville, NJ 07045
Distributed by:
Novartis Pharmaceuticals Corporation
East Hanover, NJ 07936
For
Novartis Pharmaceuticals Corporation
East Hanover, NJ 07936
U.S. License No. 1244

MEDICATION GUIDE

EXTAVIA ***(ex tā vee uh)*** Interferon beta-1b

Read the Medication Guide that comes with EXTAVIA before you start taking it and each time you get a refill. There may be new information. This Medication Guide does not take the place of talking with your doctor about your medical condition or your treatment.

What is the most important information I should know about EXTAVIA?

EXTAVIA and other Interferon beta-1b medicines will not cure multiple sclerosis (MS) but have been shown to decrease the number of flare-ups of the disease. Interferon beta-1b medicines, including EXTAVIA, can cause serious side effects. Before you start to take EXTAVIA, you should talk to your doctor about the possible risks and benefits of EXTAVIA.

EXTAVIA may cause serious side effects, including:

1. Depression
2. Allergic reactions
3. Injection site problems

These serious side effects are described below.

1. Depression. Some people who take interferon medicines, including EXTAVIA, become seriously depressed (feeling sad or sinking spirits). Some people have thoughts about killing themselves (suicidal thoughts) or try to kill themselves. Depression is not uncommon in people with multiple sclerosis.

Before you start to take EXTAVIA, tell your doctor if you ever had any mental illness, including depression, or if you take any medicines for depression.

- While you take EXTAVIA, if you feel noticeably sadder or helpless, or feel like hurting yourself or others, you should tell a family member or friend right away and call your doctor as soon as possible. You may need to stop taking EXTAVIA.

2. Allergic reactions. Some people who take Interferon beta-1b medicines, including EXTAVIA, have severe allergic reactions which can lead to trouble breathing and swallowing. Significant swelling of the mouth and tongue may occur with these severe allergic reactions. These reactions can happen quickly. Allergic reactions can happen after your first dose of EXTAVIA or may not happen until after you have taken EXTAVIA many times. Less severe allergic reactions such as rash, itching, skin bumps or minor swelling of the mouth and tongue can also happen. If you think you are having an allergic reaction, stop taking EXTAVIA right away and call your doctor.

3. Injection site problems. Interferon beta-1b medicines, including EXTAVIA, may cause redness, pain or swelling at the place where an injection was given (injection site). Serious skin reactions can happen in some people, including skin infections or areas of severe damage to skin and tissue below the skin (necrosis). These reactions can happen anywhere you inject EXTAVIA.

Call your doctor right away if you have any of these signs of a serious problem at any of your injection sites:

- the area is swollen and painful
- the area looks infected, and does not heal within a few days
- the area has fluid draining from it
- you notice any breaks in your skin or blue-black skin discoloration of your skin along with a break in your skin.

Most skin reactions are not serious, but you may need medical treatment if you develop a serious skin reaction. In most cases healing was associated with scarring.

If multiple lesions occur, therapy should be discontinued until healing occurs.

What is EXTAVIA?

EXTAVIA is a man-made form of a protein called beta interferon. EXTAVIA is similar to certain interferon proteins that are produced in the body.

EXTAVIA is used to treat relapsing forms of multiple sclerosis (MS). It will not cure your MS but may decrease the number of flare-ups of the disease. MS is a life-long disease that affects your nervous system by destroying the protective covering (myelin) that surrounds your nerve fibers. The way EXTAVIA works in MS is not known.

Who should not take EXTAVIA?

Do not take EXTAVIA if you:

- have had an allergic reaction such as trouble breathing, skin flushing, or hives, with another interferon beta product, or to human albumin.
- are allergic to any of the ingredients in EXTAVIA. See the end of this Medication Guide for a list of the ingredients in EXTAVIA.

What should I tell my doctor before taking EXTAVIA?

Tell your doctor about all your medical conditions, including if you have:

- or had depression, anxiety (feeling uneasy, nervous, or fearful), or trouble sleeping
- liver problems
- thyroid problems
- blood problems, such as bleeding or bruising easily, and low red blood cells (anemia) or low white blood cells
- are pregnant or plan to become pregnant. If you become pregnant while you take EXTAVIA, stop taking EXTAVIA and call your doctor right away. Interferon beta-1b medicines, including EXTAVIA, may cause you to lose your pregnancy (miscarriage) or may cause harm to your unborn child. You and your doctor will need to decide whether the possible benefit of taking EXTAVIA is more important than the possible risks to your unborn child.
- are breastfeeding or plan to breastfeed. It is not known if EXTAVIA passes into your milk. You and your doctor should decide if you will breastfeed or take EXTAVIA. You should not do both without talking with your doctor.

Tell your doctor about all the medicines you take, including prescription and non-prescription medicines, vitamins, and herbal supplements.

Know the medicines you take. Keep a list of them and show it to your doctor and pharmacist when you get a new medicine.

How should I take EXTAVIA?

- Take EXTAVIA exactly as prescribed by your doctor. Do not change your dose unless told to by your doctor.
- If your doctor decides that you or a caregiver may be able to give your injections of EXTAVIA at home, your doctor or nurse should instruct you on the right way to prepare and inject EXTAVIA. Do not try to inject EXTAVIA yourself until you have been instructed by your doctor or nurse the right way to prepare and give the injections.
- EXTAVIA is given by injection under the skin (subcutaneous injection) every other day.
- If you miss a dose of EXTAVIA, take your next dose as soon as you remember or are able to take it. Take your next injection about 2 days after that dose. If you are not sure when you should take your next dose, call your doctor.
- **Do not take EXTAVIA two days in a row (consecutive days).**
- Call your doctor right away if you take more than your prescribed dose of EXTAVIA, or take it two days in a row.
- **Always use a new, unopened, vial of EXTAVIA and syringe for each injection. Throw away any unused medicine. Do not reuse any vials, syringes, or needles.**
- It is important for you to change your injection site each time you inject EXTAVIA. This will lessen the chance of you having a serious skin reaction at the site where you inject EXTAVIA.
- Avoid injecting EXTAVIA into an area of skin that is sore, red, infected or has other problems.
- See the end of this Medication Guide for detailed Patient Instructions for Use for information about how to mix and inject EXTAVIA the right way.

What are the possible side effects of EXTAVIA?

EXTAVIA can cause serious side effects. See "What is the most important information I should know about EXTAVIA?".

Common side effects of EXTAVIA include:

- **Flu-like symptoms.** Most people have flu-like symptoms (fever, chills, sweating, muscle aches and tiredness) when taking EXTAVIA. These symptoms may lessen or go away over time. Talk to your doctor about whether you should take a non-prescription medicine for pain, or to lower fever before or after you take your dose of EXTAVIA.
- **Liver problems.** EXTAVIA may affect your liver function. Your doctor will do blood tests to check for these problems while you take EXTAVIA. Tell your doctor if you have any of these symptoms of a liver problem:
  - yellowing of the skin and whites of the eyes
  - easy bruising
  - right-sided stomach area (abdominal) pain
- **Blood problems.** You may have a decrease in the amount of certain blood cells, including white blood cells (blood cells that fight infection), red blood cells (blood cells that carry oxygen to body tissues), or platelets (blood cells that help you form blood clots). If this decrease is severe, your body may be less able to fight infections, you may feel tired or sluggish, or you may bruise or bleed easily.
- **Thyroid problems.** Your thyroid function may change. Symptoms of changes in the function of your thyroid include feeling cold or hot much of the time, or change in your weight (gain or loss) without a change in your diet or amount of exercise you are getting.
- **Asthenia.** You may feel excessively or unusually fatigued. Talk to your doctor about your fatigue if it is persistent and bothersome to you.
- **Headache.** You may develop headaches. You should tell your doctor if you experience headaches while taking EXTAVIA, and you should make a plan with your doctor for monitoring your headaches. Talk to your doctor about whether you should take an additional medicine for the headaches.
- **Pain.** You may experience pain while taking EXTAVIA. Talk to your doctor about whether you should take a non-prescription medicine for pain and keep your doctor informed about any changes in the pain you experience.

You should discuss with your doctor the need for blood testing to monitor for these problems. Your doctor will arrange for testing your blood at regular intervals to help detect blood, thyroid, liver, or other problems that may develop. These blood tests will be needed even if you do not have any symptoms.

Tell your doctor if you have any side effect that bothers you or that does not go away. These are not all the possible side effects of EXTAVIA. For more information ask your doctor or pharmacist.

Call your doctor for medical advice about side effects. You may report side effects to FDA at 1-800-FDA-1088.

How should I store EXTAVIA?

- Before mixing, store EXTAVIA at room temperature 25°C (77°F). Storage at temperatures between 15° to 30°C (59° to 86°F) for brief periods of time are acceptable.

- After mixing, if you can not inject EXTAVIA right away, refrigerate the medicine and inject it **within 3 hours.** If you can not inject the mixed medicine within 3 hours, do not use it. Follow the information in the Patient Instructions for Use section "Dispose of used needles, syringes, and vials" for the right way to throw away the syringe with the unused medicine, and needle.
- Do not freeze EXTAVIA.

Keep EXTAVIA and all medicines out of the reach of children.

General information about EXTAVIA

Medicines are sometimes prescribed for purposes other than those listed in a Medication Guide. Do not use EXTAVIA for a condition for which it has not been prescribed. Do not give EXTAVIA to other people even if they have the same symptoms that you have. It may harm them.

This Medication Guide summarizes the most important information about EXTAVIA. If you would like more information, talk with your doctor. You can ask your doctor or pharmacist for information about EXTAVIA that is written for health professionals. For more information go to the web site www.EXTAVIA.com or call the EXTAVIA toll-free medical information line at 1-888-669-6682.

What are the ingredients in EXTAVIA?

Active ingredient: interferon beta-1b

Inactive ingredients: mannitol, albumin (human).

The diluent contains sodium chloride solution.

EXTAVIA Patient Instructions for Use

If your doctor decides that you or a caregiver may be able to give your injections of EXTAVIA at home, your doctor or nurse should instruct you on the right way to prepare and inject EXTAVIA. To lower your risk of infection, it is important that you follow the technique that your doctor or nurse discussed with you to prepare and inject EXTAVIA. Do not try to inject EXTAVIA yourself until you have been shown by your doctor or nurse the right way to prepare and give the injections.

It is important for you to read, understand, and follow these instructions. Call your doctor if you or your caregiver has any questions about the right way to prepare or inject EXTAVIA.

Important safety information

- Do not leave the blister pack containing EXTAVIA where others might tamper with it.
- Keep the blister pack containing EXTAVIA out of the reach of children.
- Do not open the blister pack or take out any of the items until right before you are ready to use them.
- Do not use EXTAVIA if the seal on the vial is broken. If the seal is broken, the product may not be safe for you to use.
- Do not use EXTAVIA after the expiration date shown on the blister pack label or box (Figure 1). If it has expired, return the entire pack to the pharmacy.

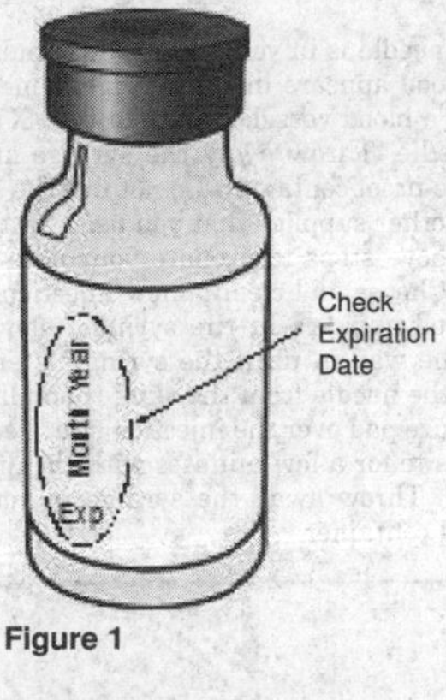

Figure 1

- Do not use any of the items in the blister pack more than one time. See the section at the end of this leaflet, "Dispose of used syringes, needles, and vials". Throw away any open and unused medicine.

Gather your supplies.

You will need the following supplies to get ready to give your injection of EXTAVIA:

- **A blister pack containing the following items (Figure 2)**
- a vial of EXTAVIA
- a prefilled syringe of diluent (Sodium Chloride, 0.54% solution)
- a vial adapter with a 27-gauge needle attached (in its own container)
- two (2) alcohol wipes

[See figure 2 above]

- a dry cotton ball and gauze
- a sharps disposal container (Figure 3). See the section "Dispose of used syringes, needles, and vials."

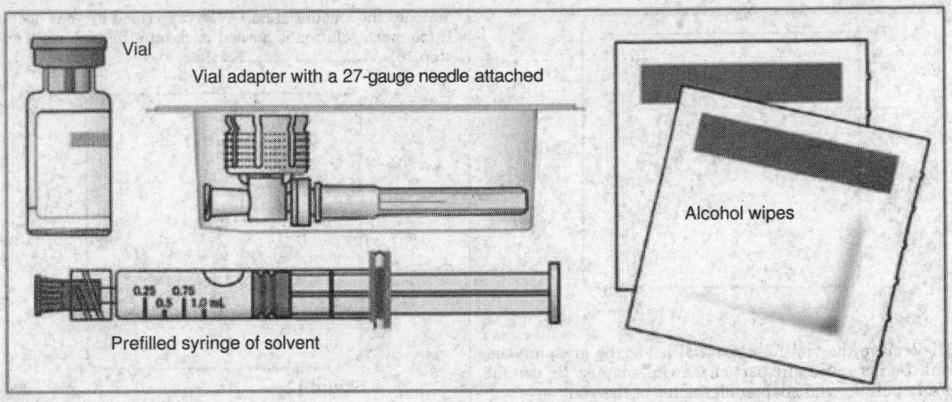

Figure 2

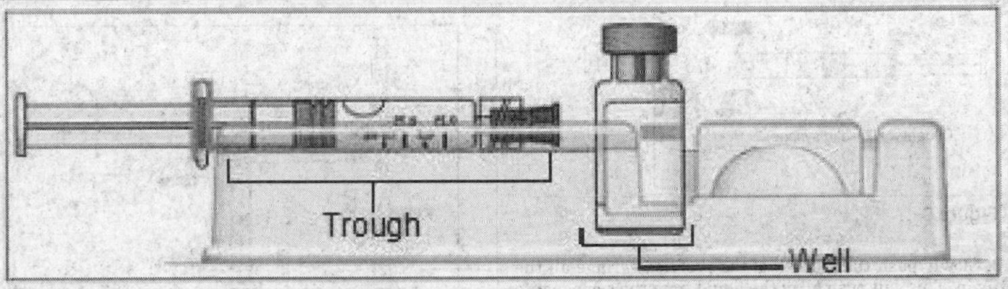

Figure 4

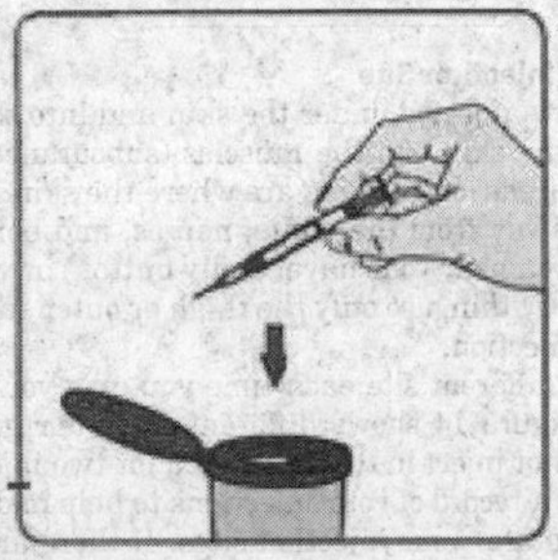

Figure 3

Prepare for self-injection

1. Wash your hands well with soap and water.
2. Open the blister pack by peeling off the label and take out all the items. Make sure the blister pack containing the vial adapter is sealed. Check to make sure the rubber cap on the diluent syringe is firmly attached.
3. Turn the blister pack over, and place the vial in the well (vial holder) and place the prefilled syringe in the U-shaped trough (Figure 4).

[See figure 4 above]

Mix EXTAVIA

4. Remove the EXTAVIA vial from the well and take the cap off the vial (Figure 5).

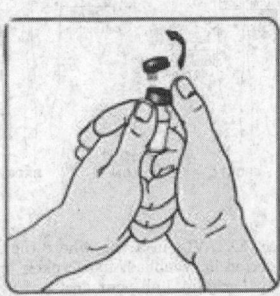

Figure 5

5. Place the vial back in the vial holder.
6. Use an alcohol wipe to clean the top of the vial (Figure 6). Wipe in one direction only.

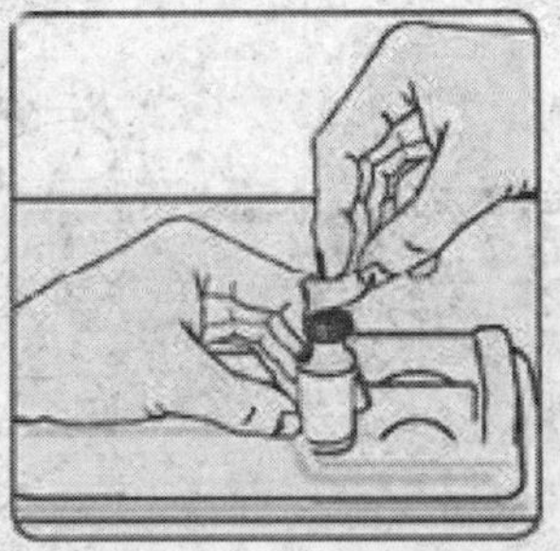

Figure 6

7. Leave the alcohol wipe on top of the vial until step 9 below.
8. Peel the label off the container with the vial adapter in it, but do not remove the vial adapter. The vial adapter is sterile, so do not touch it.
9. Remove the alcohol wipe from the top of the vial. Pick up the container that holds the vial adapter. Turn over the container keeping the vial adaptor inside. Put the adapter on top of the vial. Push down on the adapter until it pierces the rubber top of the vial and snaps in place (Figure 7). Lift the container off the vial adapter.

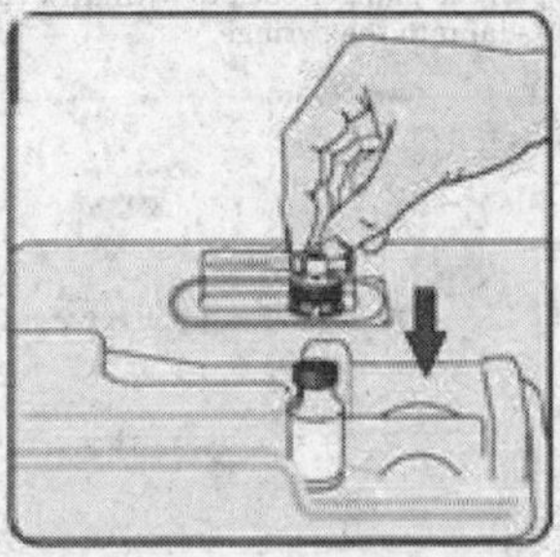

Figure 7

10. Remove the rubber cap from the prefilled syringe using a twist and pull motion (Figure 8). Throw away the rubber cap.

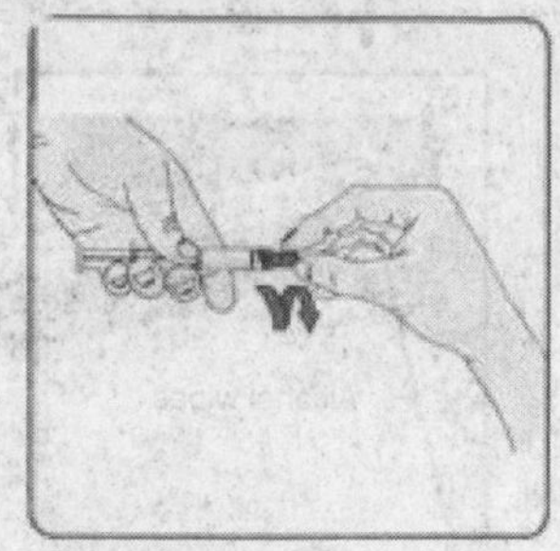
Figure 8

11. Remove the vial from the vial holder by grasping the vial. Do not touch any part of the vial adapter. Be careful not to pull the vial adapter off the top of the vial.
12. Connect the prefilled syringe of diluent to the vial adapter by turning clockwise and tighten carefully (Figure 9).

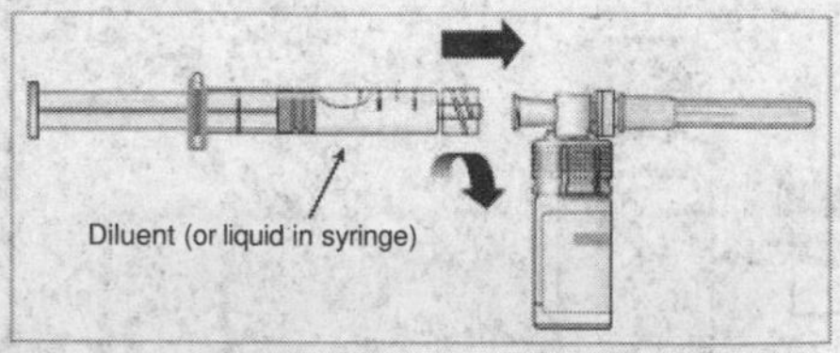

Figure 9

13. Slowly push the plunger of the prefilled syringe all the way in. This will push all of the liquid from the syringe into the vial (Figure 10). Continue to hold the plunger while you mix EXTAVIA with the liquid from the syringe. If you do not hold the plunger in it may return to its original position after you let go.

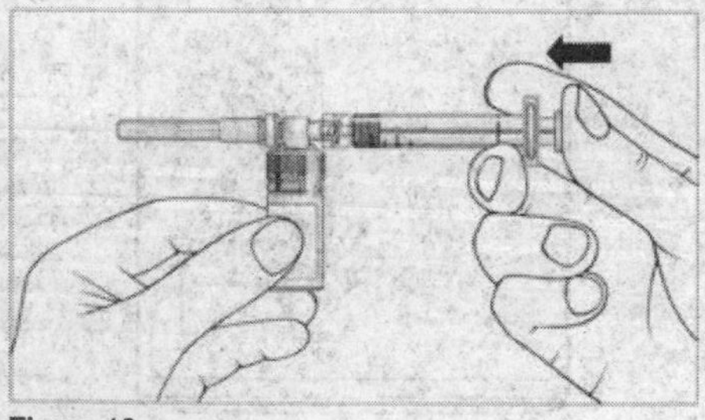
Figure 10

14. Gently swirl the vial to completely dissolve the white powder (EXTAVIA). **Do not shake.** Shaking and even gentle mixing can cause foaming of the medicine. If there is foam, let the vial sit until the foam settles.
15. After the powder dissolves, look closely at the solution in the vial. Do not use the solution if it is not clear or colorless, or if it contains particles.
The injection should be given right away after you mix EXTAVIA and let any foam in the solution settle. If you must wait for any reason before giving yourself the injection, you may refrigerate the medicine after you mix it. But you should use it within three hours.
16. With your thumb still pushing the plunger, turn the syringe and vial, so that the vial is on top (Figure 11).
17. Slowly pull the plunger back to withdraw the entire contents of the vial into the syringe.

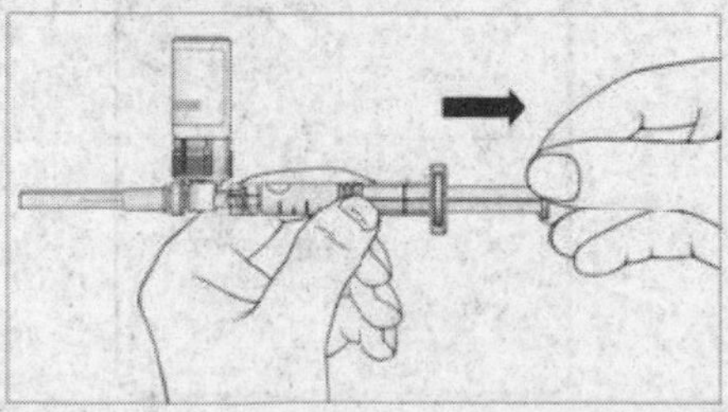
Figure 11

18. Turn the syringe so that the needle end is pointing up. Remove any air bubbles by tapping the outside of the syringe with your fingers (Figure 12). Slowly push the plunger to the 1 mL mark on the syringe or to the mark that matches the amount of EXTAVIA prescribed by your doctor. If too much solution is pushed back into the vial, return to step 16.

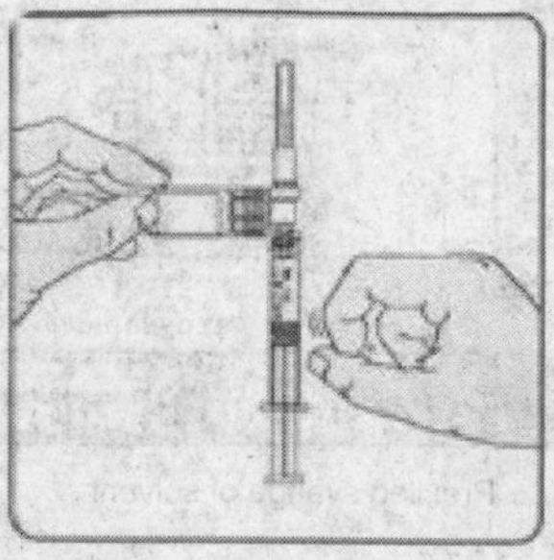
Figure 12

19. Remove the vial adapter and the vial from the syringe by twisting the vial adapter (Figure 13).

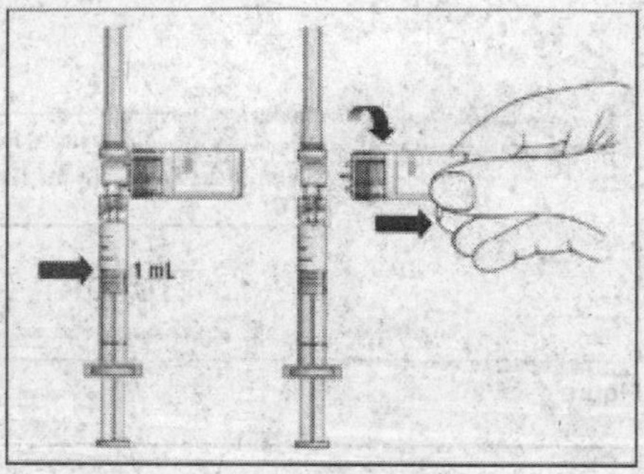

Figure 13

Choose an Injection Site
- EXTAVIA is injected under the skin and into the fat layer between the skin and the muscles (subcutaneous tissue). The best areas for injection are where the skin is loose and soft and away from the joints, nerves, and bones. Do not use the area near your navel (belly button) or waistline. If you are very thin, use only the thigh or outer surface of the arm for injection.
- Choose a different site each time you give yourself an injection. Figure 14 shows different areas for giving injections. Do not inject in the same area for two injections in a row. Keep a record of your injections to help make sure you change (rotate) your injection sites. If there are any sites that are difficult for you to reach, you can ask someone who has been trained to give the injection to you.

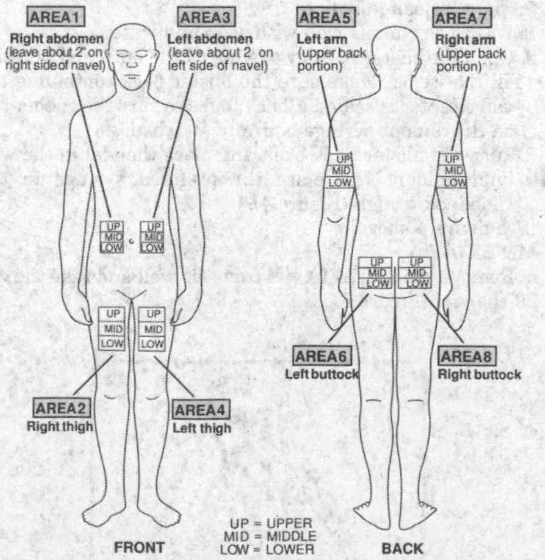

Figure 14

- Do not inject EXTAVIA in a site where the skin is red, bruised, infected, or scabbed, has broken open, or has lumps, bumps, or pain. Tell your doctor if you find skin conditions like the ones mentioned here or any other unusual looking areas where you have been given injections.

Injecting EXTAVIA
20. Using a circular motion, clean the injection site with an alcohol wipe, starting at the injection site and moving outward (Figure 15). Let the skin area air dry.

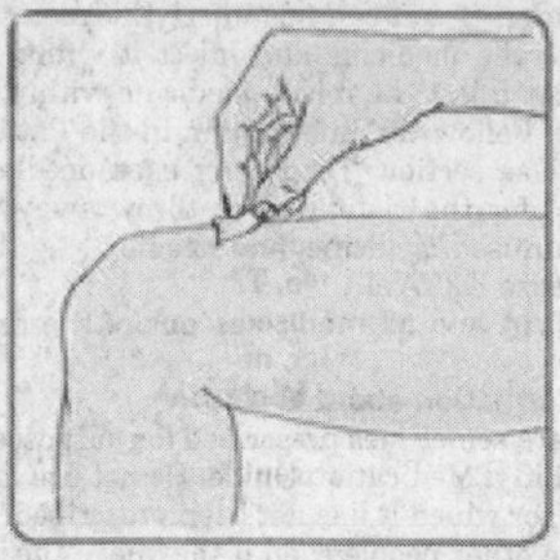
Figure 15

21. Remove the cap from the needle (Figure 16).

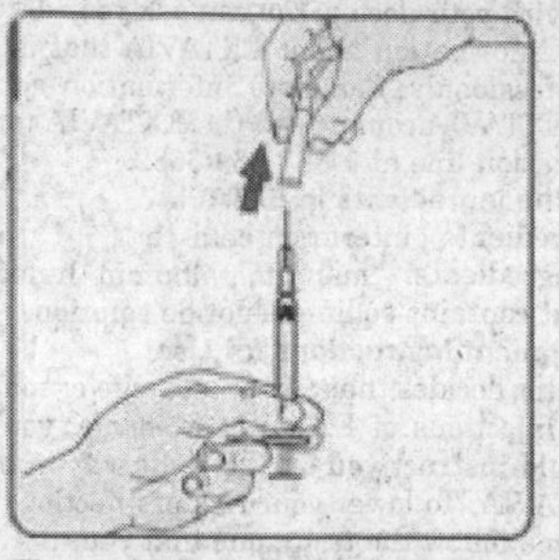
Figure 16

22. Gently pinch the skin around the site with your thumb and forefinger of the other hand (Figure 17). Insert the needle straight up and down into your skin at a 90° angle with a quick, dart-like motion.

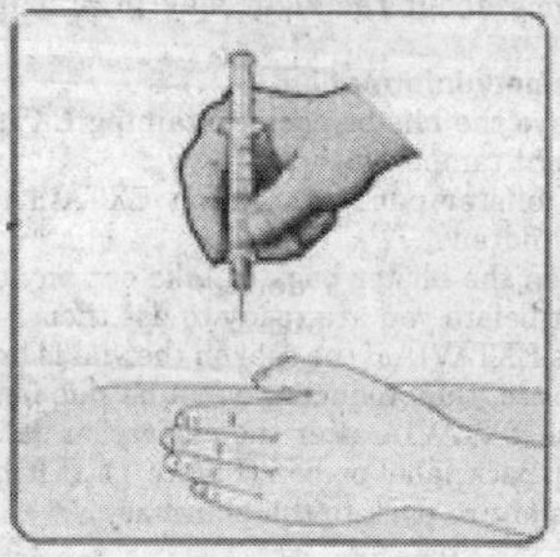
Figure 17

23. Once the needle is in your skin, slowly pull back on the plunger. If blood appears in the syringe it means that you have entered a blood vessel. Do not inject EXTAVIA. Withdraw the needle. Throw away the syringe and needle in your puncture-proof container. Do not use the same syringe or any of the other supplies that you used for this injection. Repeat the above steps to prepare your dose using a new blister pack. Choose and clean a new injection site.
24. If no blood appears in the syringe, slowly push the plunger all the way in until the syringe is empty (Figure 18). Remove the needle from the skin; then place a dry cotton ball or gauze pad over the injection site. Gently massage the injection site for a few minutes with the dry cotton ball or gauze pad. Throw away the syringe in your puncture-proof disposal container.

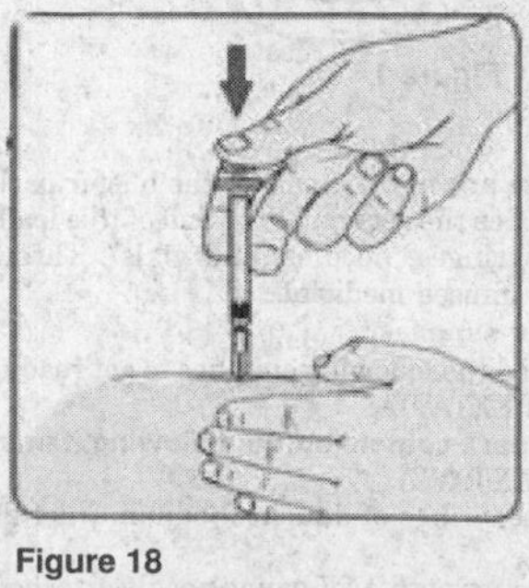
Figure 18

Dispose of used syringes, needles, and vials
- To prevent needle-stick injury and spread of infection, do not try to re-cap the needle.
- Place used needles, syringes, and vials in a closeable, puncture-resistant container. You may use a sharps container (such as a red biohazard container), a hard plastic

container (such as a detergent bottle), or a metal container (such as an empty coffee can). Do not use glass or clear plastic containers. Ask your doctor for instructions on the right way to throw away (dispose of) the container. There may be state and local laws about how you should throw away used needles and syringes.

- **Do not throw used needles, syringes, or vials in your household trash or recycle.** Throw away any unused medicine. Do not save any unused EXTAVIA for a future dose.

Keep the disposal container, needles, syringes, and vials of EXTAVIA out of the reach of children.

Manufactured by:
Bayer HealthCare Pharmaceuticals Inc.
Montville, NJ 07045
Distributed by:
Novartis Pharmaceuticals Corporation
East Hanover, NJ 07936
For
Novartis Pharmaceuticals Corporation
East Hanover, NJ 07936
U.S. License No. 1244
This Medication Guide has been approved by the U.S. Food and Drug Administration

T2012-69/T2012-70
March 2012/March 2012

FANAPT® ℞
[fan-apt]
(iloperidone)
tablets

The following prescribing information is based on official labeling in effect July 2013.

HIGHLIGHTS OF PRESCRIBING INFORMATION
These highlights do not include all the information needed to use FANAPT safely and effectively. See full prescribing information for FANAPT.
FANAPT® (iloperidone) tablets
Initial U.S. Approval: 2009

> **WARNING: INCREASED MORTALITY IN ELDERLY PATIENTS WITH DEMENTIA-RELATED PSYCHOSIS**
> ***See full prescribing information for complete boxed warning.***
> **Elderly patients with dementia-related psychosis treated with antipsychotic drugs are at an increased risk of death. FANAPT is not approved for use in patients with dementia-related psychosis. (5.1)**

RECENT MAJOR CHANGES
Warnings and Precautions, Metabolic Changes (5.5) 01/2012

INDICATIONS AND USAGE
FANAPT is an atypical antipsychotic agent indicated for the treatment of schizophrenia in adults. (1) Efficacy was established in two short-term (4- and 6-week) placebo- and active-controlled studies of adult patients with schizophrenia. (14) In choosing among treatments, prescribers should consider the ability of FANAPT to prolong the QT interval and the use of other drugs first. Prescribers should also consider the need to titrate FANAPT slowly to avoid orthostatic hypotension, which may lead to delayed effectiveness compared to some other drugs that do not require similar titration.

DOSAGE AND ADMINISTRATION
The recommended target dosage of FANAPT tablets is 12 to 24 mg/day administered twice daily. This target dosage range is achieved by daily dosage adjustments, alerting patients to symptoms of orthostatic hypotension, starting at a dose of 1 mg twice daily, then moving to 2 mg, 4 mg, 6 mg, 8 mg, 10 mg, and 12 mg twice daily on days 2, 3, 4, 5, 6, and 7 respectively, to reach the 12 mg/day to 24 mg/day dose range. FANAPT can be administered without regard to meals. (2.1)

DOSAGE FORMS AND STRENGTHS
1 mg, 2 mg, 4 mg, 6 mg, 8 mg, 10 mg and 12 mg tablets. (3)

CONTRAINDICATIONS
Known hypersensitivity to FANAPT or to any components in the formulation. (4)

WARNINGS AND PRECAUTIONS
- *Elderly patients with dementia-related psychosis* who are treated with atypical antipsychotic drugs are at an increased risk of death and cerebrovascular-related adverse events, including stroke. (5.1)
- *QT prolongation:* Prolongs QT interval and may be associated with arrhythmia and sudden death-consider using other antipsychotics first. Avoid use of FANAPT in combination with other drugs that are known to prolong QTc; use caution and consider dose modification when prescribing FANAPT with other drugs that inhibit FANAPT metabolism. Monitor serum potassium and magnesium in patients at risk for electrolyte disturbances. (1, 5.2, 7.1, 7.3, 12.3)
- *Neuroleptic Malignant Syndrome:* Manage with immediate discontinuation of drug and close monitoring. (5.3)
- *Tardive dyskinesia:* Discontinue if clinically appropriate. (5.4)
- *Metabolic Changes:* Atypical antipsychotic drugs have been associated with metabolic changes that may increase cardiovascular/cerebrovascular risk. These metabolic changes include hyperglycemia, dyslipidemia, and weight gain. (5.5)
  - *Hyperglycemia and diabetes mellitus:* Monitor patients for symptoms of hyperglycemia including polydipsia, polyuria, polyphagia, and weakness. Monitor glucose regularly in patients at risk for diabetes. (5.5)
  - *Dyslipidemia:* Undesirable alterations have been observed in patients treated with atypical antipsychotics. (5.5)
  - *Weight Gain:* Weight gain has been reported. Monitor weight. (5.5)
- *Seizures:* Use cautiously in patients with a history of seizures or with conditions that lower seizure threshold. (5.6)
- *Orthostatic hypotension:* Dizziness, tachycardia, and syncope can occur with standing. (5.7)
- *Leukopenia, Neutropenia, and Agranulocytosis* have been reported with antipsychotics. Patients with a pre-existing low white blood cell count (WBC) or a history of leukopenia/neutropenia should have their complete blood count (CBC) monitored frequently during the first few months of therapy and should discontinue FANAPT at the first sign of a decline in WBC in the absence of other causative factors. (5.8)
- *Suicide:* Close supervision of high risk patients. (5.12)
- *Priapism:* Cases have been reported in association with FANAPT treatment. (5.13)
- *Potential for cognitive and motor impairment:* Use caution when operating machinery. (5.14)
- See Full Prescribing Information for additional *WARNINGS and PRECAUTIONS.*

ADVERSE REACTIONS
Commonly observed adverse reactions (incidence >5% and two-fold greater than placebo) were: dizziness, dry mouth, fatigue, nasal congestion, orthostatic hypotension, somnolence, tachycardia, and weight increased. (6.1)

To report SUSPECTED ADVERSE REACTIONS, contact Novartis Pharmaceuticals Corporation at 1-888-669-6682 or FDA at 1-800-FDA-1088 or www.fda.gov/medwatch.

DRUG INTERACTIONS
- The dose of FANAPT should be reduced in patients coadministered a strong CYP2D6 or CYP3A4 inhibitor. (2.2, 7.1)

USE IN SPECIFIC POPULATIONS
- Pregnancy: No human or animal data. Use only if clearly needed. (8.1)
- Nursing Mothers: Should not breast feed. (8.3)
- Pediatric Use: Safety and effectiveness not established in children and adolescents. (8.4)
- Hepatic Impairment: Not recommended for patients with hepatic impairment. (8.7)
- The dose of FANAPT should be reduced in patients who are poor metabolizers of CYP2D6. (12.3)

See 17 for PATIENT COUNSELING INFORMATION
Revised: 01/2013

FULL PRESCRIBING INFORMATION: CONTENTS*

*** Sections or subsections omitted from the full prescribing information are not listed**

FULL PRESCRIBING INFORMATION

> **WARNING: INCREASED MORTALITY IN ELDERLY PATIENTS WITH DEMENTIA-RELATED PSYCHOSIS**
> **Elderly patients with dementia-related psychosis treated with antipsychotic drugs are at an increased risk of death. Analysis of seventeen placebo-controlled trials (modal duration 10 weeks), largely in patients taking atypical antipsychotic drugs, revealed a risk of death in the drug-treated patients of between 1.6 to 1.7 times the risk of death in placebo-treated patients. Over the course of a typical 10-week controlled trial, the rate of death in drug-treated patients was about 4.5%, compared to a rate of about 2.6% in the placebo group. Although the causes of death were varied, most of the deaths appeared to be either cardiovascular (e.g., heart failure, sudden death) or infectious (e.g., pneumonia) in nature.**
> **Observational studies suggest that, similar to atypical antipsychotic drugs, treatment with conventional antipsychotic drugs may increase mortality. The extent to which the findings of increased mortality in observational studies may be attributed to the antipsychotic drug as opposed to some characteristic(s) of the patients is not clear. FANAPT is not approved for the treatment of patients with Dementia-Related Psychosis. [see Warnings and Precautions (5.1)]**

1 INDICATIONS AND USAGE
FANAPT® tablets are indicated for the treatment of adults with schizophrenia. Efficacy was established in two short-term (4- and 6-week) placebo- and active-controlled studies of adult patients with schizophrenia *[see Clinical Studies (14)]*.

When deciding among the alternative treatments available for this condition, the prescriber should consider the finding that FANAPT is associated with prolongation of the QTc interval *[see Warnings and Precautions (5.2)]*. Prolongation of the QTc interval is associated in some other drugs with the ability to cause torsade de pointes-type arrhythmia, a potentially fatal polymorphic ventricular tachycardia which can result in sudden death. In many cases this would lead to the conclusion that other drugs should be tried first. Whether FANAPT will cause torsade de pointes or increase the rate of sudden death is not yet known.

Patients must be titrated to an effective dose of FANAPT. Thus, control of symptoms may be delayed during the first 1 to 2 weeks of treatment compared to some other antipsychotic drugs that do not require a similar titration. Prescribers should be mindful of this delay when selecting an antipsychotic drug for the treatment of schizophrenia *[see Dosage and Administration (2.1) and Clinical Studies (14)]*.

The effectiveness of FANAPT in long-term use, that is, for more than 6 weeks, has not been systematically evaluated in controlled trials. Therefore, the physician who elects to use FANAPT for extended periods should periodically re-evaluate the long-term usefulness of the drug for the individual patient *[see Dosage and Administration (2.3)]*.

2 DOSAGE AND ADMINISTRATION

2.1 Usual Dose

FANAPT must be titrated slowly from a low starting dose to avoid orthostatic hypotension due to its alpha-adrenergic blocking properties. The recommended starting dose for FANAPT tablets is 1 mg twice daily. Dose increases to reach the target range of 6-12 mg twice daily (12-24 mg/day) may be made with daily dosage adjustments not to exceed 2 mg twice daily (4 mg/day). The maximum recommended dose is 12 mg twice daily (24 mg/day). FANAPT doses above 24 mg/day have not been systematically evaluated in the clinical trials. Efficacy was demonstrated with FANAPT in a dose range of 6 to 12 mg twice daily. Prescribers should be mindful of the fact that patients need to be titrated to an effective dose of FANAPT. Thus, control of symptoms may be delayed during the first 1 to 2 weeks of treatment compared to some other antipsychotic drugs that do not require similar titration. Prescribers should also be aware that some adverse effects associated with FANAPT use are dose related.

FANAPT can be administered without regard to meals.

2.2 Dosage in Special Populations

Dosage adjustments are not routinely indicated on the basis of age, gender, race, or renal impairment status *[see Use in Specific Populations (8.6, 8.7)]*.

Dosage adjustment for patients taking FANAPT concomitantly with potential CYP2D6 inhibitors: FANAPT dose should be reduced by one-half when administered concomitantly with strong CYP2D6 inhibitors such as fluoxetine or paroxetine. When the CYP2D6 inhibitor is withdrawn from the combination therapy, FANAPT dose should then be increased to where it was before *[see Drug Interactions (7.1)]*.

Dosage adjustment for patients taking FANAPT concomitantly with potential CYP3A4 inhibitors: FANAPT dose should be reduced by one-half when administered concomitantly with strong CYP3A4 inhibitors such as ketoconazole or clarithromycin. When the CYP3A4 inhibitor is withdrawn from the combination therapy, FANAPT dose should be increased to where it was before *[see Drug Interactions (7.1)]*.

Dosage adjustment for patients taking FANAPT who are poor metabolizers of CYP2D6: FANAPT dose should be reduced by one-half for poor metabolizers of CYP2D6 *[see Pharmacokinetics (12.3)]*.

Hepatic Impairment: FANAPT is not recommended for patients with hepatic impairment.

2.3 Maintenance Treatment

Although there is no body of evidence available to answer the question of how long the patient treated with FANAPT should be maintained, it is generally recommended that responding patients be continued beyond the acute response. Patients should be periodically reassessed to determine the need for maintenance treatment.

2.4 Reinitiation of Treatment in Patients Previously Discontinued

Although there are no data to specifically address reinitiation of treatment, it is recommended that the initiation titration schedule be followed whenever patients have had an interval off FANAPT of more than 3 days.

2.5 Switching from Other Antipsychotics

There are no specific data to address how patients with schizophrenia can be switched from other antipsychotics to FANAPT or how FANAPT can be used concomitantly with other antipsychotics. Although immediate discontinuation of the previous antipsychotic treatment may be acceptable for some patients with schizophrenia, more gradual discontinuation may be most appropriate for others. In all cases, the period of overlapping antipsychotic administration should be minimized.

3 DOSAGE FORMS AND STRENGTHS

FANAPT tablets are available in the following strengths: 1 mg, 2 mg, 4 mg, 6 mg, 8 mg, 10 mg and 12 mg. The tablets are white, round, flat, beveled-edged and identified with a logo debossed on one side and tablet strength "1", "2", "4", "6", "8", "10", or "12" debossed on the other side.

Table 1: Change in Fasting Glucose

	Placebo	FANAPT® 24 mg/day
	Mean Change from Baseline (mg/dL)	
	n=114	n=228
Serum Glucose Change from Baseline	-0.5	6.6
	Proportion of Patients with Shifts	
Serum Glucose Normal to High (<100 mg/dL to ≥126 mg/dL)	2.5% (2/80)	10.7% (18/169)

4 CONTRAINDICATIONS

FANAPT is contraindicated in individuals with a known hypersensitivity reaction to the product. Reactions have included pruritus and urticaria.

5 WARNINGS AND PRECAUTIONS

5.1 Increased Risks in Elderly Patients with Dementia-Related Psychosis

Increased Mortality

Elderly patients with dementia-related psychosis treated with atypical antipsychotic drugs are at an increased risk of death compared to placebo. FANAPT is not approved for the treatment of patients with dementia-related psychosis *[see Boxed Warning]*.

Cerebrovascular Adverse Events, Including Stroke

In placebo-controlled trials with risperidone, aripiprazole, and olanzapine in elderly patients with dementia, there was a higher incidence of cerebrovascular adverse events (cerebrovascular accidents and transient ischemic attacks) including fatalities compared to placebo-treated patients. FANAPT is not approved for the treatment of patients with dementia-related psychosis *[see Boxed Warning]*.

5.2 QT Prolongation

In an open-label QTc study in patients with schizophrenia or schizoaffective disorder (n=160), FANAPT was associated with QTc prolongation of 9 msec at an iloperidone dose of 12 mg twice daily. The effect of FANAPT on the QT interval was augmented by the presence of CYP450 2D6 or 3A4 metabolic inhibition (paroxetine 20 mg once daily and ketoconazole 200 mg twice daily, respectively). Under conditions of metabolic inhibition for both 2D6 and 3A4, FANAPT 12 mg twice daily was associated with a mean QTcF increase from baseline of about 19 msec.

No cases of torsade de pointes or other severe cardiac arrhythmias were observed during the pre-marketing clinical program.

The use of FANAPT should be avoided in combination with other drugs that are known to prolong QTc including Class 1A (e.g., quinidine, procainamide) or Class III (e.g., amiodarone, sotalol) antiarrhythmic medications, antipsychotic medications (e.g., chlorpromazine, thioridazine), antibiotics (e.g., gatifloxacin, moxifloxacin), or any other class of medications known to prolong the QTc interval (e.g., pentamidine, levomethadyl acetate, methadone). FANAPT should also be avoided in patients with congenital long QT syndrome and in patients with a history of cardiac arrhythmias.

Certain circumstances may increase the risk of torsade de pointes and/or sudden death in association with the use of drugs that prolong the QTc interval, including (1) bradycardia; (2) hypokalemia or hypomagnesemia; (3) concomitant use of other drugs that prolong the QTc interval; and (4) presence of congenital prolongation of the QT interval; (5) recent acute myocardial infarction; and/or (6) uncompensated heart failure.

Caution is warranted when prescribing FANAPT with drugs that inhibit FANAPT metabolism *[see Drug Interactions (7.1)]*, and in patients with reduced activity of CYP2D6 *[see Clinical Pharmacology (12.3)]*.

It is recommended that patients being considered for FANAPT treatment who are at risk for significant electrolyte disturbances have baseline serum potassium and magnesium measurements with periodic monitoring. Hypokalemia (and/or hypomagnesemia) may increase the risk of QT prolongation and arrhythmia. FANAPT should be avoided in patients with histories of significant cardiovascular illness, e.g., QT prolongation, recent acute myocardial infarction, uncompensated heart failure, or cardiac arrhythmia. FANAPT should be discontinued in patients who are found to have persistent QTc measurements >500 ms.

If patients taking FANAPT experience symptoms that could indicate the occurrence of cardiac arrhythmias, e.g., dizziness, palpitations, or syncope, the prescriber should initiate further evaluation, including cardiac monitoring.

5.3 Neuroleptic Malignant Syndrome (NMS)

A potentially fatal symptom complex sometimes referred to as Neuroleptic Malignant Syndrome (NMS) has been reported in association with administration of antipsychotic drugs, including FANAPT. Clinical manifestations include hyperpyrexia, muscle rigidity, altered mental status (including catatonic signs) and evidence of autonomic instability (irregular pulse or blood pressure, tachycardia, diaphoresis, and cardiac dysrhythmia). Additional signs may include elevated creatine phosphokinase, myoglobinuria (rhabdomyolysis), and acute renal failure.

The diagnostic evaluation of patients with this syndrome is complicated. In arriving at a diagnosis, it is important to identify cases in which the clinical presentation includes both serious medical illness (e.g., pneumonia, systemic infection, etc.) and untreated or inadequately treated extrapyramidal signs and symptoms (EPS). Other important considerations in the differential diagnosis include central anticholinergic toxicity, heat stroke, drug fever, and primary central nervous system (CNS) pathology.

The management of this syndrome should include: (1) immediate discontinuation of the antipsychotic drugs and other drugs not essential to concurrent therapy, (2) intensive symptomatic treatment and medical monitoring, and (3) treatment of any concomitant serious medical problems for which specific treatments are available. There is no general agreement about specific pharmacological treatment regimens for NMS.

If a patient requires antipsychotic drug treatment after recovery from NMS, the potential reintroduction of drug therapy should be carefully considered. The patient should be carefully monitored, since recurrences of NMS have been reported.

5.4 Tardive Dyskinesia

Tardive dyskinesia is a syndrome consisting of potentially irreversible, involuntary, dyskinetic movements, which may develop in patients treated with antipsychotic drugs. Although the prevalence of the syndrome appears to be highest among the elderly, especially elderly women, it is impossible to rely on prevalence estimates to predict, at the inception of antipsychotic treatment, which patients are likely to develop the syndrome. Whether antipsychotic drug products differ in their potential to cause tardive dyskinesia is unknown.

The risk of developing tardive dyskinesia and the likelihood that it will become irreversible are believed to increase as the duration of treatment and the total cumulative dose of antipsychotic administered increases. However, the syndrome can develop, although much less commonly, after relatively brief treatment periods at low doses.

There is no known treatment for established cases of tardive dyskinesia, although the syndrome may remit, partially or completely, if antipsychotic treatment is withdrawn. Antipsychotic treatment itself, however, may suppress (or partially suppress) the signs and symptoms of the syndrome and thereby may possibly mask the underlying process. The effect that symptomatic suppression has upon the long-term course of the syndrome is unknown.

Given these considerations, FANAPT should be prescribed in a manner that is most likely to minimize the occurrence of tardive dyskinesia. Chronic antipsychotic treatment should generally be reserved for patients who suffer from a chronic illness that (1) is known to respond to antipsychotic drugs, and (2) for whom alternative, equally effective, but potentially less harmful treatments are not available or appropriate. In patients who do require chronic treatment, the smallest dose and the shortest duration of treatment producing a satisfactory clinical response should be sought. The need for continued treatment should be reassessed periodically.

If signs and symptoms of tardive dyskinesia appear in a patient on FANAPT, drug discontinuation should be considered. However, some patients may require treatment with FANAPT despite the presence of the syndrome.

5.5 Metabolic Changes

Atypical antipsychotic drugs have been associated with metabolic changes that may increase cardiovascular/cerebrovascular risk. These metabolic changes include hyperglycemia, dyslipidemia, and body weight gain *[see Patient Counseling Information (17.3)]*. While all atypical antipsychotic drugs have been shown to produce some metabolic changes, each drug in the class has its own specific risk profile.

Hyperglycemia and Diabetes Mellitus

Hyperglycemia, in some cases extreme and associated with ketoacidosis or hyperosmolar coma or death, has been reported in patients treated with atypical antipsychotics including FANAPT. Assessment of the relationship between atypical antipsychotic use and glucose abnormalities is complicated by the possibility of an increased background risk of diabetes mellitus in patients with schizophrenia and the increasing incidence of diabetes mellitus in the general population. Given these confounders, the relationship between atypical antipsychotic use and hyperglycemia-related adverse events is not completely understood. However, epidemiological studies suggest an increased risk of treatment-emergent hyperglycemia-related adverse events in patients treated with the atypical antipsychotics included in these studies. Because FANAPT was not marketed at the time these studies were performed, it is not known if FANAPT is associated with this increased risk.

Patients with an established diagnosis of diabetes mellitus who are started on atypical antipsychotics should be monitored regularly for worsening of glucose control. Patients with risk factors for diabetes mellitus (e.g., obesity, family history of diabetes) who are starting treatment with atypical antipsychotics should undergo fasting blood glucose testing at the beginning of treatment and periodically during treatment. Any patient treated with atypical antipsychotics should be monitored for symptoms of hyperglycemia including polydipsia, polyuria, polyphagia, and weakness. Patients who develop symptoms of hyperglycemia during treatment with atypical antipsychotics should undergo fasting blood glucose testing. In some cases, hyperglycemia has resolved when the atypical antipsychotic was discontinued; however, some patients required continuation of antidiabetic treatment despite discontinuation of the suspect drug.

Data from a 4- week, fixed-dose study in adult subjects with schizophrenia, in which fasting blood samples were drawn, are presented in Table 1.

[See table 1 at top of previous page]

Pooled analyses of glucose data from clinical studies including longer term trials are shown in Table 2.

Table 2: Change in Glucose

Mean Change from Baseline (mg/dL)	3-6 months	6-12 months	>12 months
FANAPT 10-16 mg/day	1.8 (N=773)	5.4 (N=723)	5.4 (N=425)
FANAPT 20-24 mg/day	-3.6 (N=34)	-9.0 (N=31)	-18.0 (N=20)

Dyslipidemia

Undesirable alterations in lipids have been observed in patients treated with atypical antipsychotics.

Data from a placebo-controlled, 4-week, fixed-dose study, in which fasting blood samples were drawn, in adult subjects with schizophrenia are presented in Table 3.

Table 3: Change in Fasting Lipids

	Placebo	FANAPT® 24 mg/day
	Mean Change from Baseline (mg/dL)	
Cholesterol	**n=114**	**n=228**
Change from baseline	-2.17	8.18
LDL	**n=109**	**n=217**
Change from baseline	-1.41	9.03
HDL	**n=114**	**n=228**
Change from baseline	-3.35	0.55
Triglycerides	**n=114**	**n=228**
Change from baseline	16.47	-0.83
	Proportion of Patients with Shifts	
Cholesterol		
Normal to High (<200 mg/dL to ≥240 mg/dL)	1.4% (1/72)	3.6% (5/141)
LDL		
Normal to High (<100 mg/dL to ≥160 mg/dL)	2.4% (1/42)	1.1% (1/90)
HDL		
Normal to Low (≥40 mg/dL to <40 mg/dL)	23.8% (19/80)	12.1% (20/166)
Triglycerides		
Normal to High (<150 mg/dL to ≥200 mg/dL)	8.3% (6/72)	10.1% (15/148)

Pooled analyses of cholesterol and triglyceride data from clinical studies including longer term trials are shown in Tables 4 and 5.

Table 4: Change in Cholesterol

Mean Change from Baseline (mg/dL)	3-6 months	6-12 months	>12 months
FANAPT 10-16 mg/day	-3.9 (N=783)	-3.9 (N=726)	-7.7 (N=428)
FANAPT 20-24 mg/day	-19.4 (N=34)	-23.2 (N=31)	-19.4 (N=20)

Table 5: Change in Triglycerides

Mean Change from Baseline (mg/dL)	3-6 months	6-12 months	>12 months
FANAPT 10-16 mg/day	-8.9 (N=783)	-8.9 (N=726)	-17.7 (N=428)
FANAPT 20-24 mg/day	-26.6 (N=34)	-35.4 (N=31)	-17.7 (N=20)

Weight Gain

Weight gain has been observed with atypical antipsychotic use. Clinical monitoring of weight is recommended.

Across all short- and long-term studies, the overall mean change from baseline at endpoint was 2.1 kg.

Changes in body weight (kg) and the proportion of subjects with ≥7% gain in body weight from four placebo-controlled, 4- or 6-week, fixed- or flexible-dose studies in adult subjects are presented in Table 6.

Table 6: Change in Body Weight

	Placebo n=576	FANAPT 10-16 mg/day n=481	FANAPT 20-24 mg/day n=391
Weight (kg) Change from Baseline	-0.1	2.0	2.7
Weight Gain ≥7% increase from Baseline	4%	12%	18%

5.6 Seizures

In short-term placebo-controlled trials (4- to 6-weeks), seizures occurred in 0.1% (1/1344) of patients treated with FANAPT compared to 0.3% (2/587) on placebo. As with other antipsychotics, FANAPT should be used cautiously in patients with a history of seizures or with conditions that potentially lower the seizure threshold, e.g., Alzheimer's dementia. Conditions that lower the seizure threshold may be more prevalent in a population of 65 years or older.

5.7 Orthostatic Hypotension and Syncope

FANAPT can induce orthostatic hypotension associated with dizziness, tachycardia, and syncope. This reflects its alpha1-adrenergic antagonist properties. In double-blind placebo-controlled short-term studies, where the dose was increased slowly, as recommended above, syncope was reported in 0.4% (5/1344) of patients treated with FANAPT, compared with 0.2% (1/587) on placebo. Orthostatic hypotension was reported in 5% of patients given 20-24 mg/day, 3% of patients given 10-16 mg/day, and 1% of patients given placebo. More rapid titration would be expected to increase the rate of orthostatic hypotension and syncope.

FANAPT should be used with caution in patients with known cardiovascular disease (e.g., heart failure, history of myocardial infarction, ischemia, or conduction abnormalities), cerebrovascular disease, or conditions that predispose the patient to hypotension (dehydration, hypovolemia, and treatment with antihypertensive medications). Monitoring of orthostatic vital signs should be considered in patients who are vulnerable to hypotension.

5.8 Leukopenia, Neutropenia and Agranulocytosis

In clinical trial and postmarketing experience, events of leukopenia/neutropenia have been reported temporally related to antipsychotic agents. Agranulocytosis (including fatal cases) has also been reported.

Possible risk factors for leukopenia/neutropenia include preexisting low white blood cell count (WBC) and history of drug induced leukopenia/neutropenia. Patients with a preexisting low WBC or a history of drug induced leukopenia/neutropenia should have their complete blood count (CBC) monitored frequently during the first few months of therapy and should discontinue FANAPT at the first sign of a decline in WBC in the absence of other causative factors.

Patients with neutropenia should be carefully monitored for fever or other symptoms or signs of infection and treated promptly if such symptoms or signs occur. Patients with severe neutropenia (absolute neutrophil count <1000/mm^3) should discontinue FANAPT and have their WBC followed until recovery.

5.9 Hyperprolactinemia

As with other drugs that antagonize dopamine D2 receptors, FANAPT elevates prolactin levels.

Hyperprolactinemia may suppress hypothalamic GnRH, resulting in reduced pituitary gonadotropin secretion. This, in turn, may inhibit reproductive function by impairing gonadalsteroidogenesis in both female and male patients. Galactorrhea, amenorrhea, gynecomastia, and impotence have been reported with prolactin-elevating compounds. Long-standing hyperprolactinemia when associated with hypogonadism may lead to decreased bone density in both female and male patients.

Tissue culture experiments indicate that approximately one-third of human breast cancers are prolactin-dependent *in vitro*, a factor of potential importance if the prescription of these drugs is contemplated in a patient with previously detected breast cancer. Mammary gland proliferative changes and increases in serum prolactin were seen in mice and rats treated with FANAPT *[see Nonclinical Toxicology (13.1)]*. Neither clinical studies nor epidemiologic studies conducted to date have shown an association between chronic administration of this class of drugs and tumorigenesis in humans; the available evidence is considered too limited to be conclusive at this time.

In a short-term placebo-controlled trial (4-weeks), the mean change from baseline to endpoint in plasma prolactin levels for the FANAPT 24 mg/day-treated group was an increase of 2.6 ng/mL compared to a decrease of 6.3 ng/mL in the placebo-group. In this trial, elevated plasma prolactin levels were observed in 26% of adults treated with FANAPT compared to 12% in the placebo group. In the short-term trials, FANAPT was associated with modest levels of prolactin elevation compared to greater prolactin elevations observed with some other antipsychotic agents. In pooled analysis from clinical studies including longer term trials, in 3210 adults treated with iloperidone, gynecomastia was reported in 2 male subjects (0.1%) compared to 0% in placebo-treated patients, and galactorrhea was reported in 8 female subjects (0.2%) compared to 3 female subjects (0.5%) in placebo-treated patients.

5.10 Body Temperature Regulation

Disruption of the body's ability to reduce core body temperature has been attributed to antipsychotic agents. Appropriate care is advised when prescribing FANAPT for patients who will be experiencing conditions which may contribute to an elevation in core body temperature, e.g., exercising strenuously, exposure to extreme heat, receiving concomitant medication with anticholinergic activity, or being subject to dehydration.

5.11 Dysphagia

Esophageal dysmotility and aspiration have been associated with antipsychotic drug use. Aspiration pneumonia is a common cause of morbidity and mortality in elderly patients, in particular those with advanced Alzheimer's dementia. FANAPT and other antipsychotic drugs should be used cautiously in patients at risk for aspiration pneumonia *[see Boxed Warning]*.

5.12 Suicide

The possibility of a suicide attempt is inherent in psychotic illness, and close supervision of high-risk patients should accompany drug therapy. Prescriptions for FANAPT should be written for the smallest quantity of tablets consistent with good patient management in order to reduce the risk of overdose.

5.13 Priapism

Three cases of priapism were reported in the pre-marketing FANAPT program. Drugs with alpha-adrenergic blocking effects have been reported to induce priapism. FANAPT shares this pharmacologic activity. Severe priapism may require surgical intervention.

5.14 Potential for Cognitive and Motor Impairment

FANAPT, like other antipsychotics, has the potential to impair judgment, thinking or motor skills. In short-term, placebo-controlled trials, somnolence (including sedation) was reported in 11.9% (104/874) of adult patients treated with FANAPT at doses of 10 mg/day or greater versus 5.3% (31/587) treated with placebo. Patients should be cautioned about operating hazardous machinery, including automobiles, until they are reasonably certain that therapy with FANAPT does not affect them adversely.

6 ADVERSE REACTIONS

6.1 Clinical Studies Experience

Because clinical trials are conducted under widely varying conditions, adverse reaction rates observed in the clinical trial of a drug cannot be directly compared to rates in the clinical trials of another drug and may not reflect the rates observed in clinical practice. The information below is derived from a clinical trial database for FANAPT consisting of 2070 patients exposed to FANAPT at doses of 10 mg/day or greater, for the treatment of schizophrenia. Of these, 806 received FANAPT for at least 6 months, with 463 exposed to FANAPT for at least 12 months. All of these patients who received FANAPT were participating in multiple-dose clin-

Table 7: Treatment-Emergent Adverse Reactions in Short-Term, Fixed- or Flexible-Dose, Placebo-Controlled Trials in Adult Patients*

Body System or Organ Class / Dictionary-derived Term	Placebo (N=587)	Percentage of Patients Reporting Reaction FANAPT 10-16 mg/day (N=483)	FANAPT 20-24 mg/day (N=391)
Body as a Whole			
Arthralgia	2	3	3
Fatigue	3	4	6
Musculoskeletal Stiffness	1	1	3
Weight Increased	1	1	9
Cardiac Disorders			
Tachycardia	1	3	12
Eye Disorders			
Vision Blurred	2	3	1
Gastrointestinal Disorders			
Nausea	8	7	10
Dry Mouth	1	8	10
Diarrhea	4	5	7
Abdominal Discomfort	1	1	3
Infections			
Nasopharyngitis	3	4	3
Upper Respiratory Tract Infection	1	2	3
Nervous System Disorders			
Dizziness	7	10	20
Somnolence	5	9	15
Extrapyramidal Disorder	4	5	4
Tremor	2	3	3
Lethargy	1	3	1
Reproductive System			
Ejaculation Failure	<1	2	2
Respiratory			
Nasal Congestion	2	5	8
Dyspnea	<1	2	2
Skin			
Rash	2	3	2
Vascular Disorders			
Orthostatic Hypotension	1	3	5
Hypotension	<1	<1	3

*Table includes adverse reactions that were reported in 2% or more of patients in any of the FANAPT dose groups and which occurred at greater incidence than in the placebo group. Figures rounded to the nearest integer.

ical trials. The conditions and duration of treatment with FANAPT varied greatly and included (in overlapping categories), open-label and double-blind phases of studies, inpatients and outpatients, fixed-dose and flexible-dose studies, and short-term and longer-term exposure.

Adverse reactions during exposure were obtained by general inquiry and recorded by clinical investigators using their own terminology. Consequently, to provide a meaningful estimate of the proportion of individuals experiencing adverse reactions, reactions were grouped in standardized categories using MedDRA terminology.

The stated frequencies of adverse reactions represent the proportions of individuals who experienced a treatment-emergent adverse reaction of the type listed. A reaction was considered treatment emergent if it occurred for the first time or worsened while receiving therapy following baseline evaluation.

The information presented in these sections was derived from pooled data from four placebo-controlled, 4- or 6-week, fixed- or flexible-dose studies in patients who received FANAPT at daily doses within a range of 10 to 24 mg (n=874).

Adverse Reactions Occurring at an Incidence of 2% or More among FANAPT-Treated Patients and More Frequent than Placebo

Table 7 enumerates the pooled incidences of treatment-emergent adverse reactions that were spontaneously reported in four placebo-controlled, 4- or 6-week, fixed- or flexible-dose studies, listing those reactions that occurred in 2% or more of patients treated with FANAPT in any of the dose groups, and for which the incidence in FANAPT-treated patients in any dose group was greater than the incidence in patients treated with placebo.

[See table 7 above]

Dose-Related Adverse Reactions in Clinical Trials

Based on the pooled data from four placebo-controlled, 4- or 6-week, fixed- or flexible-dose studies, adverse reactions that occurred with a greater than 2% incidence in the patients treated with FANAPT, and for which the incidence in patients treated with FANAPT 20-24 mg/day were twice than the incidence in patients treated with FANAPT 10-16 mg/day were: abdominal discomfort, dizziness, hypotension, musculoskeletal stiffness, tachycardia, and weight increased.

Common and Drug-Related Adverse Reactions in Clinical Trials

Based on the pooled data from four placebo-controlled, 4- or 6-week, fixed- or flexible-dose studies, the following adverse reactions occurred in ≥5% incidence in the patients treated with FANAPT and at least twice the placebo rate for at least one dose: dizziness, dry mouth, fatigue, nasal congestion, somnolence, tachycardia, orthostatic hypotension, and weight increased. Dizziness, tachycardia, and weight increased were at least twice as common on 20-24 mg/day as on 10-16 mg/day.

Extrapyramidal Symptoms (EPS) in Clinical Trials

Pooled data from the four placebo-controlled, 4- or 6-week, fixed- or flexible-dose studies provided information regarding treatment-emergent EPS. Adverse event data collected from those trials showed the following rates of EPS-related adverse events as shown in Table 8.

Table 8: Percentage of EPS Compared to Placebo

Adverse Event Term	Placebo (%) (N=587)	FANAPT 10-16 mg/day (%) (N=483)	FANAPT 20-24 mg/day (%) (N=391)
All EPS events	**11.6**	**13.5**	**15.1**
Akathisia	2.7	1.7	2.3
Bradykinesia	0	0.6	0.5
Dyskinesia	1.5	1.7	1.0
Dystonia	0.7	1.0	0.8
Parkinsonism	0	0.2	0.3
Tremor	1.9	2.5	3.1

Adverse Reactions Associated with Discontinuation of Treatment in Clinical Trials

Based on the pooled data from four placebo-controlled, 4- or 6-week, fixed- or flexible-dose studies, there was no difference in the incidence of discontinuation due to adverse events between FANAPT-treated (5%) and placebo-treated (5%) patients. The types of adverse events that led to discontinuation were similar for the FANAPT- and placebo-treated patients.

Demographic Differences in Adverse Reactions in Clinical Trials

An examination of population subgroups in the four placebo-controlled, 4- or 6-week, fixed- or flexible-dose studies did not reveal any evidence of differences in safety on the basis of age, gender or race *[see Warnings and Precautions (5.1)]*.

Laboratory Test Abnormalities in Clinical Trials

There were no differences between FANAPT and placebo in the incidence of discontinuation due to changes in hematology, urinalysis, or serum chemistry.

In short-term placebo-controlled trials (4- to 6-weeks), there were 1.0% (13/1342) iloperidone-treated patients with hematocrit at least one time below the extended normal range during post-randomization treatment, compared to 0.3% (2/585) on placebo. The extended normal range for lowered hematocrit was defined in each of these trials as the value 15% below the normal range for the centralized laboratory that was used in the trial.

Other Reactions During the Pre-marketing Evaluation of FANAPT

The following is a list of MedDRA terms that reflect treatment-emergent adverse reactions in patients treated with FANAPT at multiple doses ≥ 4 mg/day during any phase of a trial with the database of 3210 FANAPT-treated patients. All reported reactions are included except those already listed in Table 7, or other parts of the *Adverse Reactions (6)* section, those considered in the *Warnings and Precautions (5)*, those reaction terms which were so general as to be uninformative, reactions reported in fewer than 3 patients and which were neither serious nor life-threatening, reactions that are otherwise common as background reactions, and reactions considered unlikely to be drug related. It is important to emphasize that, although the reactions reported occurred during treatment with FANAPT, they were not necessarily caused by it.

Reactions are further categorized by MedDRA system organ class and listed in order of decreasing frequency according to the following definitions: frequent adverse events are those occurring in at least 1/100 patients (only those not listed in Table 7 appear in this listing); infrequent adverse reactions are those occurring in 1/100 to 1/1000 patients; rare events are those occurring in fewer than 1/1000 patients.

Blood and Lymphatic Disorders: Infrequent – anemia, iron deficiency anemia; *Rare* – leukopenia

Cardiac Disorders: Frequent – palpitations; *Rare* – arrhythmia, atrioventricular block first degree, cardiac failure (including congestive and acute)

Ear and Labyrinth Disorders: Infrequent – vertigo, tinnitus

Endocrine Disorders: Infrequent – hypothyroidism

Eye Disorders: Frequent - conjunctivitis (including allergic); *Infrequent* – dry eye, blepharitis, eyelid edema, eye swelling, lenticular opacities, cataract, hyperemia (including conjunctival)

Gastrointestinal Disorders: Infrequent – gastritis, salivary hypersecretion, fecal incontinence, mouth ulceration; *Rare* - aphthous stomatitis, duodenal ulcer, hiatus hernia, hyperchlorhydria, lip ulceration, reflux esophagitis, stomatitis

General Disorders and Administrative Site Conditions: Infrequent – edema (general, pitting, due to cardiac disease), difficulty in walking, thirst; *Rare* - hyperthermia

Hepatobiliary Disorders: Infrequent – cholelithiasis

Investigations: Frequent: weight decreased; *Infrequent* – hemoglobin decreased, neutrophil count increased, hematocrit decreased

Metabolism and Nutrition Disorders: Infrequent – increased appetite, dehydration, hypokalemia, fluid retention

Musculoskeletal and Connective Tissue Disorders: Frequent – myalgia, muscle spasms; *Rare* – torticollis

Nervous System Disorders: Infrequent – paresthesia, psychomotor hyperactivity, restlessness, amnesia, nystagmus; *Rare* – restless legs syndrome

Psychiatric Disorders: Frequent – restlessness, aggression, delusion; *Infrequent* – hostility, libido decreased, paranoia, anorgasmia, confusional state, mania, catatonia, mood swings, panic attack, obsessive-compulsive disorder, bulimia nervosa, delirium, polydipsia psychogenic, impulse-control disorder, major depression

Renal and Urinary Disorders: Frequent – urinary incontinence; *Infrequent* – dysuria, pollakiuria, enuresis, nephrolithiasis; *Rare* – urinary retention, renal failure acute

Reproductive System and Breast Disorders: Frequent – erectile dysfunction; *Infrequent* – testicular pain, amenorrhea, breast pain; *Rare* – menstruation irregular, gynecomastia, menorrhagia, metrorrhagia, postmenopausal hemorrhage, prostatitis.

Respiratory, Thoracic and Mediastinal Disorders: Infrequent – epistaxis, asthma, rhinorrhea, sinus congestion, nasal dryness; *Rare* – dry throat, sleep apnea syndrome, dyspnea exertional

6.2 Postmarketing Experience

The following adverse reactions have been identified during postapproval use of Fanapt: retrograde ejaculation. Because these reactions were reported voluntarily from a population of uncertain size, it is not possible to reliably estimate their frequency or establish a causal relationship to drug exposure.

7 DRUG INTERACTIONS

Given the primary CNS effects of FANAPT, caution should be used when it is taken in combination with other centrally acting drugs and alcohol. Due to its α1-adrenergic receptor antagonism, FANAPT has the potential to enhance the effect of certain antihypertensive agents.

7.1 Potential for Other Drugs to Affect FANAPT

Iloperidone is not a substrate for CYP1A1, CYP1A2, CYP2A6, CYP2B6, CYP2C8, CYP2C9, CYP2C19, or CYP2E1 enzymes. This suggests that an interaction of iloperidone with inhibitors or inducers of these enzymes, or other factors, like smoking, is unlikely.

Both CYP3A4 and CYP2D6 are responsible for iloperidone metabolism. Inhibitors of CYP3A4 (e.g., ketoconazole) or CYP2D6 (e.g., fluoxetine, paroxetine) can inhibit iloperidone elimination and cause increased blood levels.

Ketoconazole: Co-administration of ketoconazole (200 mg twice daily for 4 days), a potent inhibitor of CYP3A4, with a 3 mg single dose of iloperidone to 19 healthy volunteers, ages 18-45, increased the AUC of iloperidone and its metabolites P88 and P95 by 57%, 55% and 35%, respectively. Iloperidone doses should be reduced by about one-half when administered with ketoconazole or other strong inhibitors of CYP3A4 (e.g., itraconazole). Weaker inhibitors (e.g., erythromycin, grapefruit juice) have not been studied. When the CYP3A4 inhibitor is withdrawn from the combination therapy, the iloperidone dose should be returned to the previous level.

***Fluoxetine*:** Co-administration of fluoxetine (20 mg twice daily for 21 days), a potent inhibitor of CYP2D6, with a single 3 mg dose of iloperidone to 23 healthy volunteers, ages 29-44, who were classified as CYP2D6 extensive metabolizers, increased the AUC of iloperidone and its metabolite P88, by about 2-3 fold, and decreased the AUC of its metabolite P95 by one-half. Iloperidone doses should be reduced by one-half when administered with fluoxetine. When fluoxetine is withdrawn from the combination therapy, the iloperidone dose should be returned to the previous level. Other strong inhibitors of CYP2D6 would be expected to have similar effects and would need appropriate dose reductions. When the CYP2D6 inhibitor is withdrawn from the combination therapy, iloperidone dose could then be increased to the previous level.

Paroxetine: Co-administration of paroxetine (20 mg/day for 5-8 days), a potent inhibitor of CYP2D6, with multiple doses of iloperidone (8 or 12 mg twice daily) to patients with schizophrenia ages 18-65 resulted in increased mean steady-state peak concentrations of iloperidone and its metabolite P88, by about 1.6 fold, and decreased mean steady-state peak concentrations of its metabolite P95 by one-half. Iloperidone doses should be reduced by one-half when administered with paroxetine. When paroxetine is withdrawn from the combination therapy, the iloperidone dose should be returned to the previous level. Other strong inhibitors of CYP2D6 would be expected to have similar effects and would need appropriate dose reductions. When the CYP2D6 inhibitor is withdrawn from the combination therapy, iloperidone dose could then be increased to previous levels.

Paroxetine and Ketoconazole: Co-administration of paroxetine (20 mg once daily for 10 days), a CYP2D6 inhibitor, and ketoconazole (200 mg twice daily) with multiple doses of iloperidone (8 or 12 mg twice daily) to patients with schizophrenia ages 18-65 resulted in a 1.4 fold increase in steady-state concentrations of iloperidone and its metabolite P88 and a 1.4 fold decrease in the P95 in the presence of paroxetine. So giving iloperidone with inhibitors of both of its metabolic pathways did not add to the effect of either inhibitor given alone. Iloperidone doses should therefore be reduced by about one-half if administered concomitantly with both a CYP2D6 and CYP3A4 inhibitor.

7.2 Potential for FANAPT to Affect Other Drugs

In vitro studies in human liver microsomes showed that iloperidone does not substantially inhibit the metabolism of drugs metabolized by the following cytochrome P450 isozymes: CYP1A1, CYP1A2, CYP2A6, CYP2B6, CYP2C8, CYP2C9, or CYP2E1. Based on *in vitro* studies, iloperidone is a time-dependent inhibitor of CYP3A at therapeutic exposure levels. Co-administration of iloperidone may lead to an increase in plasma levels of drugs that are predominantly eliminated by CYP3A4. Furthermore, *in vitro* studies in human liver microsomes showed that iloperidone does not have enzyme inducing properties, specifically for the following cytochrome P450 isozymes: CYP1A2, CYP2C8, CYP2C9, CYP2C19, CYP3A4 and CYP3A5.

Dextromethorphan: A study in healthy volunteers showed that changes in the pharmacokinetics of dextromethorphan (80 mg dose) when a 3 mg dose of iloperidone was co-administered resulted in a 17% increase in total exposure and a 26% increase in C_{max} of dextromethorphan. Thus, an interaction between iloperidone and other CYP2D6 substrates is unlikely.

Fluoxetine: A single 3 mg dose of iloperidone had no effect on the pharmacokinetics of fluoxetine (20 mg twice daily).

7.3 Drugs that Prolong the QT Interval

FANAPT should not be used with any other drugs that prolong the QT interval *[see Warnings and Precautions (5.2)]*.

8 USE IN SPECIFIC POPULATIONS

8.1 Pregnancy

Pregnancy Category C

FANAPT caused developmental toxicity, but was not teratogenic, in rats and rabbits.

In an embryo-fetal development study, pregnant rats were given 4, 16, or 64 mg/kg/day (1.6, 6.5, and 26 times the maximum recommended human dose [MRHD] of 24 mg/day on a mg/m^2 basis) of iloperidone orally during the period of organogenesis. The highest dose caused increased early intrauterine deaths, decreased fetal weight and length, decreased fetal skeletal ossification, and an increased incidence of minor fetal skeletal anomalies and variations; this dose also caused decreased maternal food consumption and weight gain.

In an embryo-fetal development study, pregnant rabbits were given 4, 10, or 25 mg/kg/day (3, 8, and 20 times the MRHD on a mg/m^2 basis) of iloperidone during the period of organogenesis. The highest dose caused increased early intrauterine deaths and decreased fetal viability at term; this dose also caused maternal toxicity.

In additional studies in which rats were given iloperidone at doses similar to the above beginning from either preconception or from day 17 of gestation and continuing through weaning, adverse reproductive effects included prolonged pregnancy and parturition, increased stillbirth rates, increased incidence of fetal visceral variations, decreased fetal and pup weights, and decreased post-partum pup survival. There were no drug effects on the neurobehavioral or reproductive development of the surviving pups. No-effect doses ranged from 4 to 12 mg/kg except for the increase in stillbirth rates which occurred at the lowest dose tested of 4 mg/kg, which is 1.6 times the MRHD on a mg/m^2 basis. Maternal toxicity was seen at the higher doses in these studies.

The iloperidone metabolite P95, which is a major circulating metabolite of iloperidone in humans but is not present in significant amounts in rats, was given to pregnant rats during the period of organogenesis at oral doses of 20, 80, or 200 mg/kg/day. No teratogenic effects were seen. Delayed skeletal ossification occurred at all doses. No significant maternal toxicity was produced. Plasma levels of P95 (AUC) at the highest dose tested were 2 times those in humans receiving the MRHD of iloperidone.

There are no adequate and well-controlled studies in pregnant women.

Non-Teratogenic Effects

Neonates exposed to antipsychotic drugs, during the third trimester of pregnancy are at risk for extrapyramidal and/or withdrawal symptoms following delivery. There have been reports of agitation, hypertonia, hypotonia, tremor, somnolence, respiratory distress and feeding disorder in these neonates. These complications have varied in severity; while in some cases symptoms have been self-limited, in other cases neonates have required intensive care unit support and prolonged hospitalization.

FANAPT should be used during pregnancy only if the potential benefit justifies the potential risk to the fetus.

8.2 Labor and Delivery

The effect of FANAPT on labor and delivery in humans is unknown.

8.3 Nursing Mothers

FANAPT was excreted in milk of rats during lactation. It is not known whether FANAPT or its metabolites are excreted in human milk. It is recommended that women receiving FANAPT should not breast feed.

8.4 Pediatric Use

Safety and effectiveness in pediatric and adolescent patients have not been established.

8.5 Geriatric Use

Clinical Studies of FANAPT in the treatment of schizophrenia did not include sufficient numbers of patients aged 65 years and over to determine whether or not they respond differently than younger adult patients. Of the 3210 patients treated with FANAPT in pre-marketing trials, 25 (0.5%) were ≥65 years old and there were no patients ≥75 years old.

Studies of elderly patients with psychosis associated with Alzheimer's disease have suggested that there may be a different tolerability profile (i.e., increased risk in mortality and cerebrovascular events including stroke) in this population compared to younger patients with schizophrenia *[see Boxed Warning and Warnings and Precautions (5.1)]*. The safety and efficacy of FANAPT in the treatment of patients with psychosis associated with Alzheimer's disease has not been established. If the prescriber elects to treat such patients with FANAPT, vigilance should be exercised.

8.6 Renal Impairment

Because FANAPT is highly metabolized, with less than 1% of the drug excreted unchanged, renal impairment alone is unlikely to have a significant impact on the pharmacokinetics of FANAPT. Renal impairment (creatinine clearance <30 mL/min) had minimal effect on maximum plasma concentrations (C_{max}) of iloperidone (given in a single dose of 3 mg) and its metabolites P88 and P95 in any of the three analytes measured. $AUC_{0-\infty}$ was increased by 24%, decreased by 6%, and increased by 52% for iloperidone, P88 and P95, respectively, in subjects with renal impairment.

8.7 Hepatic Impairment

A study in mild and moderate liver impairment has not been conducted. FANAPT is not recommended for patients with hepatic impairment.

8.8 Smoking Status

Based on *in vitro* studies utilizing human liver enzymes, FANAPT is not a substrate for CYP1A2; smoking should therefore not have an effect on the pharmacokinetics of FANAPT.

9 DRUG ABUSE AND DEPENDENCE

9.1 Controlled Substance

FANAPT is not a controlled substance.

9.2 Abuse

FANAPT has not been systematically studied in animals or humans for its potential for abuse, tolerance, or physical dependence. While the clinical trials did not reveal any tendency for drug-seeking behavior, these observations were not systematic and it is not possible to predict on the basis of this experience the extent to which a CNS active drug, FANAPT, will be misused, diverted, and/or abused once marketed. Consequently, patients should be evaluated carefully for a history of drug abuse, and such patients should be observed closely for signs of FANAPT misuse or abuse (e.g. development of tolerance, increases in dose, drug-seeking behavior).

10 OVERDOSAGE

10.1 Human Experience

In pre-marketing trials involving over 3210 patients, accidental or intentional overdose of FANAPT was documented in eight patients ranging from 48 mg to 576 mg taken at once and 292 mg taken over a three-day period. No fatalities were reported from these cases. The largest confirmed single ingestion of FANAPT was 576 mg; no adverse physical effects were noted for this patient. The next largest confirmed ingestion of FANAPT was 438 mg over a four-day period; extrapyramidal symptoms and a QTc interval of 507 msec were reported for this patient with no cardiac sequelae. This patient resumed FANAPT treatment for an additional 11 months. In general, reported signs and symptoms were those resulting from an exaggeration of the known pharmacological effects (e.g., drowsiness and sedation, tachycardia and hypotension) of FANAPT.

10.2 Management of Overdose

There is no specific antidote for FANAPT. Therefore appropriate supportive measures should be instituted. In case of acute overdose, the physician should establish and maintain an airway and ensure adequate oxygenation and ventilation. Gastric lavage (after intubation, if patient is unconscious) and administration of activated charcoal together with a laxative should be considered. The possibility of obtundation, seizures or dystonic reaction of the head and neck following overdose may create a risk of aspiration with induced emesis. Cardiovascular monitoring should commence immediately and should include continuous ECG monitoring to detect possible arrhythmias. If antiarrhythmic therapy is administered, disopyramide, procainamide and quinidine should not be used, as they have the potential for QT-prolonging effects that might be additive to those of FANAPT. Similarly, it is reasonable to expect that the alpha-blocking properties of bretylium might be additive to those of FANAPT, resulting in problematic hypotension. Hypotension and circulatory collapse should be treated with appropriate measures such as intravenous fluids or sympathomimetic agents (epinephrine and dopamine should not be used, since beta stimulation may worsen hypotension in the setting of FANAPT-induced alpha blockade). In cases of severe extrapyramidal symptoms, anticholinergic medication should be administered. Close medical supervision should continue until the patient recovers.

11 DESCRIPTION

FANAPT is a psychotropic agent belonging to the chemical class of piperidinyl-benzisoxazole derivatives. Its chemical name is 4′-[3-[4-(6-Fluoro-1,2-benzisoxazol-3-yl)piperidino] propoxy]-3′-methoxyacetophenone. Its molecular formula is $C_{24}H_{27}FN_2O_4$ and its molecular weight is 426.48. The structural formula is:

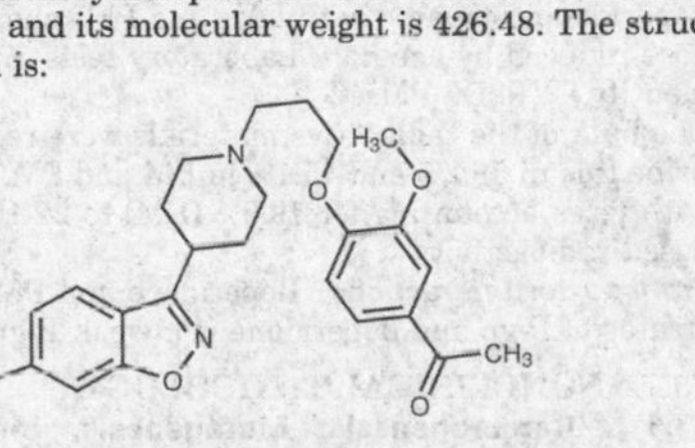

Iloperidone is a white to off-white finely crystalline powder. It is practically insoluble in water, very slightly soluble in 0.1 N HCl and freely soluble in chloroform, ethanol, methanol, and acetonitrile.

FANAPT tablets are intended for oral administration only. Each round, uncoated tablet contains 1 mg, 2 mg, 4 mg, 6 mg, 8 mg, 10 mg, or 12 mg of iloperidone. Inactive ingredients are: lactose monohydrate, microcrystalline cellulose, hydroxypropylmethylcellulose, crospovidone, magnesium stearate, colloidal silicon dioxide, and purified water (removed during processing). The tablets are white, round, flat, beveled-edged and identified with a logo debossed on one side and tablet strength "1", "2", "4", "6", "8", "10", or "12" debossed on the other side.

12 CLINICAL PHARMACOLOGY

12.1 Mechanism of Action

The mechanism of action of FANAPT, as with other drugs having efficacy in schizophrenia, is unknown. However it is proposed that the efficacy of FANAPT is mediated through a combination of dopamine type 2 (D_2) and serotonin type 2 (5-HT_2) antagonisms.

12.2 Pharmacodynamics

FANAPT exhibits high (nM) affinity binding to serotonin 5-HT_{2A}dopamine D_2 and D_3 receptors, and norepinephrine NEα1 receptors (K_i values of 5.6, 6.3, 7.1, and 0.36 nM, respectively). FANAPT has moderate affinity for dopamine D_4, and serotonin 5-HT_6 and 5-HT_7 receptors (K_i values of 25, 43, and 22, nM respectively), and low affinity for the serotonin 5-HT_{1A}, dopamine D_1, and histamine H_1 receptors (K_i values of 168, 216 and 437 nM, respectively). FANAPT has no appreciable affinity (K_i>1000 nM) for cholinergic muscarinic receptors. FANAPT functions as an antagonist at the dopamine D_2, D_3, serotonin 5-HT_{1A} and norepinephrine α_1/α_{2C} receptors. The affinity of the FANAPT metabolite P88 is generally equal or less than that of the parent compound. In contrast, the metabolite P95 only shows affinity for 5-HT_{2A} (K_i value of 3.91) and the $NE_{\alpha 1A}$, $NE_{\alpha 1B}$, $NE_{\alpha 1D}$, and $NE_{\alpha 2C}$ receptors (K_i values of 4.7, 2.7, 8.8 and 4.7 nM respectively).

12.3 Pharmacokinetics

The observed mean elimination half-lives for iloperidone, P88 and P95 in CYP2D6 extensive metabolizers (EM) are 18, 26 and 23 hours, respectively, and in poor metabolizers (PM) are 33, 37 and 31 hours, respectively. Steady-state concentrations are attained within 3-4 days of dosing. Iloperidone accumulation is predictable from single-dose pharmacokinetics. The pharmacokinetics of iloperidone is more than dose proportional. Elimination of iloperidone is mainly through hepatic metabolism involving two P450 isozymes, CYP2D6 and CYP3A4.

Absorption: Iloperidone is well absorbed after administration of the tablet with peak plasma concentrations occurring within 2 to 4 hours; while the relative bioavailability of the tablet formulation compared to oral solution is 96%. Administration of iloperidone with a standard high-fat meal did not significantly affect the C_{max} or AUC of iloperidone, P88, or P95, but delayed T_{max} by 1 hour for iloperidone, 2 hours for P88 and 6 hours for P95. FANAPT can be administered without regard to meals.

Distribution: Iloperidone has an apparent clearance (clearance / bioavailability) of 47 to 102 L/h, with an apparent volume of distribution of 1340-2800 L. At therapeutic concentrations, iloperidone and its metabolites are ~95% bound to serum proteins.

Metabolism and Elimination: Iloperidone is metabolized primarily by three biotransformation pathways: carbonyl reduction, hydroxylation (mediated by CYP2D6) and *O*-demethylation (mediated by CYP3A4). There are two predominant iloperidone metabolites, P95 and P88. The iloperidone metabolite P95 represents 47.9% of the AUC of iloperidone and its metabolites in plasma at steady-state for extensive metabolizers (EM) and 25% for poor metabolizers (PM). The active metabolite P88 accounts for 19.5% and 34.0% of total plasma exposure in EM and PM, respectively. Approximately 7-10% of Caucasians and 3-8% of Black/African Americans lack the capacity to metabolize CYP2D6 substrates and are classified as poor metabolizers (PM), whereas the rest are intermediate, extensive or ultrarapid metabolizers. Co-administration of FANAPT with known strong inhibitors of CYP2D6 like fluoxetine results in a 2.3 fold increase in iloperidone plasma exposure, and therefore one-half of the FANAPT dose should be administered.

Similarly, PMs of CYP2D6 have higher exposure to iloperidone compared with EMs and PMs should have their dose reduced by one-half. Laboratory tests are available to identify CYP2D6 PMs.

The bulk of the radioactive materials were recovered in the urine (mean 58.2% and 45.1% in EM and PM, respectively), with feces accounting for 19.9% (EM) to 22.1% (PM) of the dosed radioactivity.

Transporter Interaction: Iloperidone and P88 are not substrates of P-gp and iloperidone is a weak P-gp inhibitor.

13 NONCLINICAL TOXICOLOGY

13.1 Carcinogenesis, Mutagenesis, Impairment of Fertility

Carcinogenesis: Lifetime carcinogenicity studies were conducted in CD-1 mice and Sprague Dawley rats. Iloperidone was administered orally at doses of 2.5, 5.0 and 10 mg/kg/day to CD-1 mice and 4, 8 and 16 mg/kg/day to Sprague Dawley rats (0.5, 1.0 and 2.0 times and 1.6, 3.2 and 6.5 times, respectively, the maximum recommended human dose [MRHD] of 24 mg/day on a mg/m^2 basis). There was an increased incidence of malignant mammary gland tumors in female mice treated with the lowest dose (2.5 mg/kg/day) only. There were no treatment-related increases in neoplasia in rats.

The carcinogenic potential of the iloperidone metabolite P95, which is a major circulating metabolite of iloperidone in humans but is not present at significant amounts in mice or rats, was assessed in a lifetime carcinogenicity study in Wistar rats at oral doses of 25, 75 and 200 mg/kg/day in males and 50, 150 and 250 (reduced from 400) mg/kg/day in females.

Drug-related neoplastic changes occurred in males, in the pituitary gland (pars distalis adenoma) at all doses and in the pancreas (islet cell adenoma) at the high dose. Plasma levels of P95 (AUC) in males at the tested doses (25, 75, and 200 mg/kg/day) were approximately 0.4, 3, and 23 times, respectively, the human exposure to P95 at the MRHD of iloperidone.

An increase in mammary, pituitary and endocrine pancreas neoplasms has been found in rodents after chronic administration of other antipsychotic drugs and is considered to be mediated by prolonged dopamine D2 antagonism and hyperprolactinemia. Increases in serum prolactin were seen in mice and rats treated with iloperidone. The relevance of these tumor findings in rodents in terms of human risk is unknown.

Mutagenesis: Iloperidone was negative in the Ames test and in the *in vivo* mouse bone marrow and rat liver micronucleus tests. Iloperidone induced chromosomal aberrations in Chinese Hamster Ovary (CHO) cells *in vitro* at concentrations which also caused some cytotoxicity.

The iloperidone metabolite P95 was negative in the Ames test, the V79 chromosome aberration test, and an *in vivo* mouse bone marrow micronucleus test.

Impairment of Fertility: Iloperidone decreased fertility at 12 and 36 mg/kg in a study in which both male and female rats were treated. The no-effect dose was 4 mg/kg, which is 1.6 times the maximum recommended human dose of 24 mg/day on a mg/m^2 basis.

14 CLINICAL STUDIES

The efficacy of FANAPT in the treatment of schizophrenia was supported by two placebo- and active-controlled short-term (4- and 6-week) trials. Both trials enrolled patients who met the DSM-III/IV criteria for schizophrenia.

Two instruments were used for assessing psychiatric signs and symptoms in these studies. The Positive and Negative Syndrome Scale (PANSS) and Brief Psychiatric Rating Scale (BPRS) are both multi-item inventories of general psychopathology usually used to evaluate the effects of drug treatment in schizophrenia.

A 6-week, placebo-controlled trial (n=706) involved two flexible dose ranges of FANAPT (12-16 mg/day or 20-24 mg/day) compared to placebo and an active control (risperidone). For the 12-16 mg/day group, the titration schedule of FANAPT was 1 mg twice daily on days 1 and 2, 2 mg twice daily on days 3 and 4, 4 mg twice daily on days 5 and 6, and 6 mg twice daily on day 7. For the 20-24 mg/day group, the titration schedule of FANAPT was 1 mg twice daily on day 1, 2 mg twice daily on day 2, 4 mg twice daily on day 3, 6 mg twice daily on days 4 and 5, 8 mg twice daily on day 6, and 10 mg twice daily on day 7. The primary endpoint was change from baseline on the BPRS total score at the end of treatment (Day 42). Both the 12-16 mg/day and the 20-24 mg/day dose ranges of FANAPT were superior to placebo on the BPRS total score. The active control antipsychotic drug appeared to be superior to FANAPT in this trial within the first 2 weeks, a finding that may in part be explained by the more rapid titration that was possible for that drug. In patients in this study who remained on treatment for at least two weeks, iloperidone appeared to have had comparable efficacy to the active control.

A 4-week, placebo-controlled trial (n=604) involved one fixed dose of FANAPT (24 mg/day) compared to placebo and an active control (ziprasidone). The titration schedule for this study was similar to that for the 6-week study. This study involved titration of FANAPT starting at 1 mg twice daily on day 1 and increasing to 2, 4, 6, 8, 10 and 12 mg twice daily on days 2, 3, 4, 5, 6, and 7. The primary endpoint was change from baseline on the PANSS total score at the end of treatment (Day 28). The 24 mg/day FANAPT dose was superior to placebo in the PANSS total score. FANAPT appeared to have similar efficacy to the active control drug which also needed a slow titration to the target dose.

16 HOW SUPPLIED/STORAGE AND HANDLING

FANAPT tablets are white, round and identified with a logo debossed on one side and tablet strength "1", "2", "4", "6", "8", "10", or "12" debossed on the other side. Tablets are supplied in the following strengths and package configurations:

Package Configuration	Tablet Strength (mg)	NDC Code
Bottles of 60	1 mg	0078-0595-20
Bottles of 60	2 mg	0078-0596-20
Bottles of 60	4 mg	0078-0597-20
Bottles of 60	6 mg	0078-0598-20
Bottles of 60	8 mg	0078-0599-20
Bottles of 60	10 mg	0078-0600-20
Bottles of 60	12 mg	0078-0601-20
Titration Pack	2×1 mg, 2×2 mg, 2×4 mg, 2×6 mg (Total of 8 tablets)	0078-0602-08

Storage

Store FANAPT tablets at controlled room temperature, 25°C (77°F); excursions permitted to 15° - 30 °C (59° - 86°F) [See USP Controlled Room Temperature]. Protect FANAPT tablets from exposure to light and moisture.

17 PATIENT COUNSELING INFORMATION

Physicians are advised to discuss the following issues with patients for whom they prescribe FANAPT:

17.1 QT Interval Prolongation

Patients should be advised to consult their physician immediately if they feel faint, lose consciousness or have heart palpitations. Patients should be counseled not to take FANAPT with other drugs that cause QT interval prolongation *[see Warnings and Precautions (5.2)]*. Patients should be told to inform physicians that they are taking FANAPT before any new drug is taken.

17.2 Neuroleptic Malignant Syndrome

Patients and caregivers should be counseled that a potentially fatal symptom complex sometimes referred to as NMS has been reported in association with administration of antipsychotic drugs, including FANAPT. Signs and symptoms of NMS include hyperpyrexia, muscle rigidity, altered mental status, and evidence of autonomic instability (irregular pulse or blood pressure, tachycardia, diaphoresis, and cardiac dysrhythmia) *[see Warnings and Precautions (5.3)]*.

17.3 Metabolic Changes

Patients should be aware of the symptoms of hyperglycemia (high blood sugar) and diabetes mellitus. Patients who are diagnosed with diabetes, those with risk factors for diabetes, or those who develop these symptoms during treatment should have their blood glucose monitored at the beginning of and periodically during treatment. Patients should be counseled that weight gain has occurred during treatment with FANAPT. Clinical monitoring of weight is recommended. *[see Warnings and Precautions (5.5)]*.

17.4 Orthostatic Hypotension

Patients should be advised of the risk of orthostatic hypotension, particularly at the time of initiating treatment, reinitiating treatment, or increasing the dose *[see Warnings and Precautions (5.7)]*.

17.5 Interference with Cognitive and Motor Performance

Because FANAPT may have the potential to impair judgment, thinking, or motor skills, patients should be cautioned about operating hazardous machinery, including automobiles, until they are reasonably certain that FANAPT therapy does not affect them adversely *[see Warnings and Precautions (5.14)]*.

17.6 Pregnancy

Patients should be advised to notify their physician if they become pregnant or intend to become pregnant during therapy with FANAPT *[see Use in Specific Populations (8.1)]*.

17.7 Nursing

Patients should be advised not to breast-feed an infant if they are taking FANAPT *[see Use in Specific Populations (8.3)]*.

17.8 Concomitant Medication

Patients should be advised to inform their physicians if they are taking, or plan to take, any prescription or over-the-counter drugs, since there is a potential for interactions *[see Drug Interactions (7)]*.

17.9 Alcohol

Patients should be advised to avoid alcohol while taking FANAPT.

17.10 Heat Exposure and Dehydration

Patients should be advised regarding appropriate care in avoiding overheating and dehydration.

Fanapt® is a registered trademark of Vanda Pharmaceuticals Inc. and is used by Novartis Pharmaceuticals Corporation under license.

Distributed by:
Novartis Pharmaceuticals Corporation
East Hanover, NJ 07936
T2013-07
January 2013

Shown in Product Identification Guide, page 310

FEMARA ℞
[fĕm-ara]
(letrozole)
tablets

The following prescribing information is based on official labeling in effect July 2013.

HIGHLIGHTS OF PRESCRIBING INFORMATION
These highlights do not include all the information needed to use Femara safely and effectively. See full prescribing information for Femara.
Femara (letrozole) tablets
Initial U.S. Approval: 1997

INDICATIONS AND USAGE

Femara is an aromatase inhibitor indicated for:
- Adjuvant treatment of postmenopausal women with hormone receptor positive early breast cancer (1.1)
- Extended adjuvant treatment of postmenopausal women with early breast cancer who have received prior standard adjuvant tamoxifen therapy (1.2)
- First and second-line treatment of postmenopausal women with hormone receptor positive or unknown advanced breast cancer (1.3)

DOSAGE AND ADMINISTRATION

Femara tablets are taken orally without regard to meals (2):
- Recommended dose: 2.5 mg once daily (2.1)
- Patients with cirrhosis or severe hepatic impairment: 2.5 mg every other day (2.5, 5.3)

DOSAGE FORMS AND STRENGTHS

2.5 milligram tablets (3)

CONTRAINDICATIONS

Women of premenopausal endocrine status, including pregnant women (4)

WARNINGS AND PRECAUTIONS

- Decreases in bone mineral density may occur. Consider bone mineral density monitoring (5.1)
- Increases in total cholesterol may occur. Consider cholesterol monitoring. (5.2)
- Fatigue, dizziness and somnolence may occur. Exercise caution when operating machinery (5.4)

ADVERSE REACTIONS

The most common adverse reactions (>20%) were hot flashes, arthralgia (6.1); flushing, asthenia, edema, arthralgia, headache, dizziness, hypercholesterolemia, sweating increased, bone pain (6.2, 6.3); and musculoskeletal (6.4).

To report SUSPECTED ADVERSE REACTIONS, contact Novartis Pharmaceuticals Corporation at 1-888-669-6682 or FDA at 1-800-FDA-1088 or www.fda.gov/medwatch.

See 17 for PATIENT COUNSELING INFORMATION

Revised: 12/2011

FULL PRESCRIBING INFORMATION: CONTENTS*

*** Sections or subsections omitted from the full prescribing information are not listed**

FULL PRESCRIBING INFORMATION

1 INDICATIONS AND USAGE

1.1 Adjuvant Treatment of Early Breast Cancer

Femara (letrozole) is indicated for the adjuvant treatment of postmenopausal women with hormone receptor positive early breast cancer.

1.2 Extended Adjuvant Treatment of Early Breast Cancer

Femara is indicated for the extended adjuvant treatment of early breast cancer in postmenopausal women, who have received 5 years of adjuvant tamoxifen therapy. The effectiveness of Femara in extended adjuvant treatment of early breast cancer is based on an analysis of disease-free survival in patients treated with Femara for a median of 60 months *[see Clinical Studies (14.2, 14.3)]*.

1.3 First and Second-Line Treatment of Advanced Breast Cancer

Femara is indicated for first-line treatment of postmenopausal women with hormone receptor positive or unknown, locally advanced or metastatic breast cancer. Femara is also indicated for the treatment of advanced breast cancer in postmenopausal women with disease progression following antiestrogen therapy *[see Clinical Studies (14.4, 14.5)]*.

2 DOSAGE AND ADMINISTRATION

2.1 Recommended Dose

The recommended dose of Femara is one 2.5 mg tablet administered once a day, without regard to meals.

2.2 Use in Adjuvant Treatment of Early Breast Cancer

In the adjuvant setting, the optimal duration of treatment with letrozole is unknown. The planned duration of treatment in the study was 5 years with 73% of the patients having completed adjuvant therapy. Treatment should be discontinued at relapse *[see Clinical Studies (14.1)]*.

2.3 Use in Extended Adjuvant Treatment of Early Breast Cancer

In the extended adjuvant setting, the optimal treatment duration with Femara is not known. The planned duration of treatment in the study was 5 years. In the final updated analysis, conducted at a median follow-up of 62 months, the median treatment duration was 60 months. Seventy-one percent of patients were treated for at least 3 years and 58% of patients completed least 4.5 years of extended adjuvant treatment. The treatment should be discontinued at tumor relapse *[see Clinical Studies (14.2)]*.

2.4 Use in First and Second-Line Treatment of Advanced Breast Cancer

In patients with advanced disease, treatment with Femara should continue until tumor progression is evident. *[see Clinical Studies (14.4, 14.5)]*

2.5 Use in Hepatic Impairment

No dosage adjustment is recommended for patients with mild to moderate hepatic impairment, although Femara blood concentrations were modestly increased in subjects with moderate hepatic impairment due to cirrhosis. The dose of Femara in patients with cirrhosis and severe hepatic dysfunction should be reduced by 50% *[see Warnings and Precautions (5.3)]*. The recommended dose of Femara for such patients is 2.5 mg administered every other day. The effect of hepatic impairment on Femara exposure in noncirrhotic cancer patients with elevated bilirubin levels has not been determined.

2.6 Use in Renal Impairment

No dosage adjustment is required for patients with renal impairment if creatinine clearance is ≥10 mL/min. *[see Clinical Pharmacology (12.3)]*.

3 DOSAGE FORMS AND STRENGTHS

2.5 mg tablets: dark yellow, film-coated, round, slightly biconvex, with beveled edges (imprinted with the letters FV on one side and CG on the other side).

4 CONTRAINDICATIONS

Femara may cause fetal harm when administered to a pregnant woman and the clinical benefit to premenopausal women with breast cancer has not been demonstrated. Femara is contraindicated in women who are or may become pregnant. If Femara is used during pregnancy, or if the patient becomes pregnant while taking this drug, the patient should be apprised of the potential hazard to a fetus. *[see Use in Specific Populations (8.1)]*

5 WARNINGS AND PRECAUTIONS

5.1 Bone Effects

Use of Femara may cause decreases in bone mineral density (BMD). Consideration should be given to monitoring BMD. Results of a substudy to evaluate safety in the adjuvant setting comparing the effect on lumbar spine (L2-L4) bone mineral density (BMD) of adjuvant treatment with letrozole to that with tamoxifen showed at 24 months a median decrease in lumbar spine BMD of 4.1% in the letrozole arm compared to a median increase of 0.3% in the tamoxifen arm (difference = 4.4%) (P<0.0001) *[See Adverse reactions (6.1)]*. Updated results from the BMD sub-study in the extended adjuvant setting demonstrated that at 2 years patients receiving letrozole had a median decrease from baseline of 3.8% in hip BMD compared to a median decrease of 2.0% in the placebo group. The changes from baseline in lumbar spine BMD in letrozole and placebo treated groups were not significantly different *[see Adverse Reactions (6.2)]*. In the adjuvant trial the incidence of bone fractures at any time after randomization was 13.8% for letrozole and 10.5% for tamoxifen. The incidence of osteoporosis was 5.1% for letrozole and 2.7% for tamoxifen *[See Adverse Reactions (6.1)]*. In the extended adjuvant trial the incidence of bone fractures at any time after randomization was 13.3% for letrozole and 7.8% for placebo. The incidence of new osteoporosis was 14.5% for letrozole and 7.8% for placebo *[see Adverse Reactions (6.3)]*.

5.2 Cholesterol

Consideration should be given to monitoring serum cholesterol. In the adjuvant trial hypercholesterolemia was reported in 52.3% of letrozole patients and 28.6% of tamoxifen patients. CTC grade 3-4 hypercholesterolemia was reported in 0.4% of letrozole patients and 0.1% of tamoxifen patients. Also in the adjuvant setting, an increase of ≥1.5 × ULN in total cholesterol (generally non-fasting) was observed in patients on monotherapy who had baseline total serum cholesterol within the normal range (i.e., <=1.5 × ULN) in 151/1843 (8.2%) on letrozole vs 57/1840 (3.2%). Lipid lowering medications were required for 25% of patients on letrozole and 16% on tamoxifen *[see Adverse Reactions (6.1)]*.

5.3 Hepatic Impairment

Subjects with cirrhosis and severe hepatic impairment who were dosed with 2.5 mg of Femara experienced approximately twice the exposure to Femara as healthy volunteers with normal liver function. Therefore, a dose reduction is recommended for this patient population. The effect of hepatic impairment on Femara exposure in cancer patients with elevated bilirubin levels has not been determined. *[see Dosage and Administration (2.5)]*

5.4 Fatigue and Dizziness

Because fatigue, dizziness, and somnolence have been reported with the use of Femara, caution is advised when driving or using machinery until it is known how the patient reacts to Femara use.

5.5 Laboratory Test Abnormalities

No dose-related effect of Femara on any hematologic or clinical chemistry parameter was evident. Moderate decreases in lymphocyte counts, of uncertain clinical significance, were observed in some patients receiving Femara 2.5 mg. This depression was transient in about half of those affected. Two patients on Femara developed thrombocytopenia; relationship to the study drug was unclear. Patient withdrawal due to laboratory abnormalities, whether related to study treatment or not, was infrequent.

Table 1: Patients with Adverse Reactions (CTC Grades 1-4, Irrespective of Relationship to Study Drug) in the Adjuvant Study – Monotherapy Arms Analysis (Median Follow-up 73 Months; Median Treatment 60 Months)

	Grades 1-4				Grades 3-4			
Adverse Reaction	Femara N=2448 n (%)		tamoxifen N=2447 n (%)		Femara N=2448 n (%)		tamoxifen N=2447 n (%)	
Pts with any adverse event	2310	(94.4)	2214	(90.5)	635	(25.9)	604	(24.7)
Hypercholesterolemia	1280	(52.3)	700	(28.6)	11	(0.4)	6	(0.2)
Hot Flashes/Flushes	821	(33.5)	929	(38.0)	0	-	0	-
Arthralgia/Arthritis	618	(25.2)	501	(20.4)	85	(3.5)	50	(2.0)
Night Sweats	357	(14.6)	426	(17.4)	0	-	0	-
Bone Fractures[2]	338	(13.8)	257	(10.5)	-	-	-	-
Weight Increase	317	(12.9)	378	(15.4)	27	(1.1)	39	(1.6)
Nausea	283	(11.6)	277	(11.3)	6	(0.2)	9	(0.4)
Bone Fractures[1]	247	(10.1)	174	(7.1)	-	-	-	-
Fatigue (Lethargy, Malaise, Asthenia)	235	(9.6)	250	(10.2)	6	(0.2)	7	(0.3)
Myalgia	217	(8.9)	212	(8.7)	18	(0.7)	14	(0.6)
Edema	164	(6.7)	160	(6.5)	3	(0.1)	1	(<0.1)
Weight Decrease	140	(5.7)	129	(5.3)	8	(0.3)	5	(0.2)
Vaginal Bleeding	128	(5.2)	320	(13.1)	1	(<0.1)	8	(0.3)
Back Pain	125	(5.1)	136	(5.6)	7	(0.3)	11	(0.4)
Osteoporosis NOS	124	(5.1)	66	(2.7)	10	(0.4)	5	(0.2)
Bone pain	123	(5.0)	109	(4.5)	6	(0.2)	4	(0.2)
Depression	119	(4.9)	114	(4.7)	16	(0.7)	14	(0.6)
Vaginal Irritation	111	(4.5)	77	(3.1)	2	(<0.1)	2	(<0.1)
Headache	105	(4.3)	94	(3.8)	9	(0.4)	5	(0.2)
Pain in extremity	103	(4.2)	79	(3.2)	6	(0.2)	4	(0.2)
Osteopenia	87	(3.6)	74	(3.0)	0	-	2	(<0.1)
Dizziness/Light-Headedness	84	(3.4)	84	(3.4)	1	(<0.1)	6	(0.2)
Alopecia	83	(3.4)	84	(3.4)	0	-	0	-
Vomiting	80	(3.3)	80	(3.3)	3	(0.1)	5	(0.2)
Cataract	49	(2.0)	54	(2.2)	16	(0.7)	17	(0.7)
Constipation	49	(2.0)	71	(2.9)	3	(0.1)	1	(<0.1)
Breast pain	37	(1.5)	43	(1.8)	1	(<0.1)	0	-
Anorexia	20	(0.8)	20	(0.8)	1	(<0.1)	1	(<0.1)
Endometrial Hyperplasia/Cancer[2,3]	11/1909	(0.6)	70/1943	(3.6)	-	-	-	-
Endometrial Proliferation Disorders	10	(0.3)	71	(1.8)	0	-	14	(0.6)
Endometrial Hyperplasia/Cancer[1,3]	6/1909	(0.3)	57/1943	(2.9)	-	-	-	-
Other Endometrial Disorders	2	(<0.1)	3	(0.1)	0	-	0	-
Myocardial Infarction[1]	24	(1.0)	12	(0.5)	-	-	-	-
Myocardial Infarction[2]	37	(1.5)	25	(1.0)	-	-	-	-
Myocardial Ischemia	6	(0.2)	9	(0.4)	-	-	-	-
Cerebrovascular Accident[1]	52	(2.1)	46	(1.9)	-	-	-	-
Cerebrovascular Accident[2]	70	(2.9)	63	(2.6)	-	-	-	-
Angina[1]	26	(1.1)	24	(1.0)	-	-	-	-
Angina[2]	32	(1.3)	31	(1.3)	-	-	-	-
Thromboembolic Event[1]	51	(2.1)	89	(3.6)	-	-	-	-
Thromboembolic Event[2]	71	(2.9)	111	(4.5)	-	-	-	-
Other Cardiovascular[1]	260	(10.6)	256	(10.5)	-	-	-	-
Other Cardiovascular[2]	312	(12.7)	337	(13.8)	-	-	-	-
Second Malignancies[1]	53	(2.2)	78	(3.2)	-	-	-	-
Second Malignancies[2]	102	(4.2)	119	(4.9)	-	-	-	-

[1] During study treatment, based on Safety Monotherapy population
[2] Any time after randomization, including post treatment follow-up
[3] Excluding women who had undergone hysterectomy before study entry

6 ADVERSE REACTIONS

The most serious adverse reactions from the use of Femara are:

- Bone effects *[see Warnings and Precautions (5.1)]*
- Increases in cholesterol *[see Warnings and Precautions (5.2)]*

Because clinical trials are conducted under widely varying conditions, adverse reactions rates observed in the clinical trials of a drug cannot be directly compared to rates in the clinical trials of another drug and may not reflect the rates observed in practice.

6.1 Adjuvant Treatment of Early Breast Cancer

The median treatment duration of adjuvant treatment was 60 months and the median duration of follow-up for safety was 73 months for patients receiving Femara and tamoxifen.

Certain adverse reactions were prospectively specified for analysis, based on the known pharmacologic properties and side effect profiles of the two drugs.

Adverse reactions were analyzed irrespective of whether a symptom was present or absent at baseline. Most adverse reactions reported (approximately 75% of patients reporting 1 or more AE) were Grade 1 or Grade 2 applying the Common Toxicity Criteria Version 2.0/ Common Terminology Criteria for Adverse Events, version 3.0. Table 1 describes adverse reactions (Grades 1-4) irrespective of relationship to study treatment in the adjuvant trial for the monotherapy arms analysis (safety population).

[See table 1 above]

Note: Cardiovascular (including cerebrovascular and thromboembolic), skeletal and urogenital/endometrial events and second malignancies were collected life-long. All of these events were assumed to be of CTC grade 3-5 and were not individually graded.

When considering all grades during study treatment, a higher incidence of events was seen for Femara regarding fractures (10.1% vs 7.1%), myocardial infarctions (1.0% vs 0.5%), and arthralgia (25.2% vs 20.4%) (Femara vs tamoxifen respectively). A higher incidence was seen for tamoxifen regarding thromboembolic events (2.1% vs 3.6%), endometrial hyperplasia/cancer (0.3% vs 2.9%), and endometrial proliferation disorders (0.3% vs 1.8%) (Femara vs tamoxifen respectively).

At a median follow up of 73 months, a higher incidence of events was seen for Femara (13.8%) than for tamoxifen (10.5%) regarding fractures. A higher incidence was seen for tamoxifen compared to Femara regarding thromboembolic events (4.5% vs 2.9%), and endometrial hyperplasia or cancer (2.9% vs 0.4%) (tamoxifen vs Femara, respectively).

Bone Study: Results of a phase 3 safety trial in 262 post menopausal women with resected receptor positive early breast cancer in the adjuvant setting comparing the effect on lumbar spine (L2-L4) bone mineral density (BMD) of adjuvant treatment with letrozole to that with tamoxifen showed at 24 months a median decrease in lumbar spine BMD of 4.1% in the letrozole arm compared to a median increase of 0.3% in the tamoxifen arm (difference = 4.4%) ($P<0.0001$). No patients with a normal BMD at baseline became osteoporotic over the 2 years and only 1 patient with osteopenia at baseline (T score of -1.9) developed osteoporosis during the treatment period (assessment by central review). The results for total hip BMD were similar, although the differences between the two treatments were less pronounced. During the 2 year period, fractures were reported by 4 of 103 patients (4%) in the letrozole arm, and 6 of 97 patients (6%) in the tamoxifen arm.

Lipid Study: In a phase 3 safety trial in 262 post menopausal women with resected receptor positive early breast cancer at 24 months comparing the effects on lipid profiles of adjuvant letrozole to tamoxifen, 12% of patients on letrozole had at least one total cholesterol value of a higher CTCAE grade than at baseline compared with 4% of patients on tamoxifen.

6.2 Extended Adjuvant Treatment of Early Breast Cancer, Median Treatment Duration of 24 Months

The median duration of extended adjuvant treatment was 24 months and the median duration of follow-up for safety was 28 months for patients receiving Femara and placebo.

Table 2 describes the adverse reactions occurring at a frequency of at least 5% in any treatment group during treatment. Most adverse reactions reported were Grade 1 and Grade 2 based on the Common Toxicity Criteria Version 2.0. In the extended adjuvant setting, the reported drug-related adverse reactions that were significantly different from placebo were hot flashes, arthralgia/arthritis, and myalgia.

[See table 2 at top of next page]

Based on a median follow-up of patients for 28 months,the incidence of clinical fractures from the core randomized study in patients who received Femara was 5.9% (152) and placebo was 5.5% (142). The incidence of self-reported osteoporosis was higher in patients who received Femara 6.9% (176) than in patients who received placebo 5.5% (141). Bisphosphonates were administered to 21.1% of the patients who received Femara and 18.7% of the patients who received placebo.

The incidence of cardiovascular ischemic events from the core randomized study was comparable between patients who received Femara 6.8% (175) and placebo 6.5% (167).

A patient-reported measure that captures treatment impact on important symptoms associated with estrogen deficiency demonstrated a difference in favor of placebo for vasomotor and sexual symptom domains.

Bone Sub-study: *[see Warnings and Precautions (5.1)].*

Lipid Sub-study: In the extended adjuvant setting, based on a median duration of follow-up of 62 months, there was no significant difference between Femara and placebo in total cholesterol or in any lipid fraction at any time over 5 years. Use of lipid lowering drugs or dietary management of elevated lipids was allowed. *[see Warnings and Precautions (5.2)].*

6.3 Updated Analysis, Extended Adjuvant Treatment of Early Breast Cancer, Median Treatment Duration of 60 Months

The extended adjuvant treatment trial was unblinded early [*see Adverse Reactions* (6.2)]. At the updated (final analysis), overall the side effects seen were consistent to those seen at a median treatment duration of 24 months.

During treatment or within 30 days of stopping treatment (median duration of treatment 60 months) a higher rate of fractures was observed for Femara (10.4%) compared to placebo (5.8%), as also a higher rate of osteoporosis (Femara 12.2% vs placebo 6.4%).

Based on 62 months median duration of follow-up in the randomized letrozole arm in the Safety population the incidence of new fractures at any time after randomization was 13.3% for letrozole and 7.8% for placebo. The incidence of new osteoporosis was 14.5% for letrozole and 7.8% for placebo.

During treatment or within 30 days of stopping treatment (median duration of treatment 60 months) the incidence of cardiovascular events was 9.8% for Femara and 7.0% for placebo.

Based on 62 months median duration of follow-up in the randomized letrozole arm in the Safety population the incidence of cardiovascular disease at any time after randomization was 14.4% for letrozole and 9.8% for placebo.

Lipid sub-study: In the extended adjuvant setting, based on a median duration of follow-up of 62 months, there was no significant difference between Femara and placebo in total cholesterol or in any lipid fraction over 5 years. Use of lipid lowering drugs or dietary management of elevated lipids was allowed. *[see Warnings and Precautions(5.2)]*

6.4 First-Line Treatment of Advanced Breast Cancer

A total of 455 patients were treated for a median time of exposure of 11 months. The incidence of adverse reactions was similar for Femara and tamoxifen. The most frequently reported adverse reactions were bone pain, hot flushes, back pain, nausea, arthralgia and dyspnea. Discontinuations for adverse reactions other than progression of tumor occurred in 10/455 (2%) of patients on Femara and in 15/455 (3%) of patients on tamoxifen.

Adverse reactions, regardless of relationship to study drug, that were reported in at least 5% of the patients treated with Femara 2.5 mg or tamoxifen 20 mg in the first-line treatment study are shown in Table 3.

Table 3: Percentage (%) of Patients with Adverse Reactions

Adverse Reaction	Femara 2.5 mg (N=455) %	tamoxifen 20 mg (N=455) %
General Disorders		
Fatigue	13	13
Chest Pain	8	9
Edema Peripheral	5	6
Pain NOS	5	7
Weakness	6	4
Investigations		
Weight Decreased	7	5
Vascular Disorders		
Hot Flushes	19	16
Hypertension	8	4
Gastrointestinal Disorders		
Nausea	17	17
Constipation	10	11
Diarrhea	8	4
Vomiting	7	8
Infections/Infestations		
Influenza	6	4
Urinary Tract Infection NOS	6	3
Injury, Poisoning and Procedural Complications		
Post-Mastectomy Lymphedema	7	7
Metabolism and Nutrition Disorders		
Anorexia	4	6
Musculoskeletal and Connective Tissue Disorders		
Bone Pain	22	21
Back Pain	18	19
Arthralgia	16	15
Pain in Limb	10	8
Nervous System Disorders		
Headache NOS	8	7
Psychiatric Disorders		
Insomnia	7	4
Reproductive System and Breast Disorders		
Breast Pain	7	7
Respiratory, Thoracic and Mediastinal Disorders		
Dyspnea	18	17
Cough	13	13
Chest Wall Pain	6	6

Other less frequent (≤2%) adverse reactions considered consequential for both treatment groups, included peripheral thromboembolic events, cardiovascular events, and cerebrovascular events. Peripheral thromboembolic events included venous thrombosis, thrombophlebitis, portal vein thrombosis and pulmonary embolism. Cardiovascular events included angina, myocardial infarction, myocardial ischemia, and coronary heart disease. Cerebrovascular events included transient ischemic attacks, thrombotic or hemorrhagic strokes and development of hemiparesis.

6.5 Second- Line Treatment of Advanced Breast Cancer

Study discontinuations in the megestrol acetate comparison study for adverse reactions other than progression of tumor were 5/188 (2.7%) on Femara 0.5 mg, in 4/174 (2.3%) on Femara 2.5 mg, and in 15/190 (7.9%) on megestrol acetate. There were fewer thromboembolic events at both Femara doses than on the megestrol acetate arm (0.6% vs 4.7%). There was also less vaginal bleeding (0.3% vs 3.2%) on Femara than on megestrol acetate. In the aminoglutethimide comparison study, discontinuations for reasons other than progression occurred in 6/193 (3.1%) on 0.5 mg Femara, 7/185 (3.8%) on 2.5 mg Femara, and 7/178 (3.9%) of patients on aminoglutethimide.

Comparisons of the incidence of adverse reactions revealed no significant differences between the high and low dose Femara groups in either study. Most of the adverse reactions observed in all treatment groups were mild to moderate in severity and it was generally not possible to distinguish adverse reactions due to treatment from the consequences of the patient's metastatic breast cancer, the effects of estrogen deprivation, or intercurrent illness.

Adverse reactions, regardless of relationship to study drug, that were reported in at least 5% of the patients treated with Femara 0.5 mg, Femara 2.5 mg, megestrol acetate, or aminoglutethimide in the two controlled trials are shown in Table 4.

[See table 4 above]

Other less frequent (<5%) adverse reactions considered consequential and reported in at least 3 patients treated with Femara, included hypercalcemia, fracture, depression, anxiety, pleural effusion, alopecia, increased sweating and vertigo.

Table 2: Percentage of Patients with Adverse Reactions

	Number (%) of Patients with Grade 1-4 Adverse Reaction		Number (%) of Patients with Grade 3-4 Adverse Reaction	
	Femara N=2563	Placebo N=2573	Femara N=2563	Placebo N=2573
Any Adverse Reaction	2232 (87.1)	2174 (84.5)	419 (16.3)	389 (15.1)
Vascular Disorders	1375 (53.6)	1230 (47.8)	59 (2.3)	74 (2.9)
Flushing	1273 (49.7)	1114 (43.3)	3 (0.1)	0 -
General Disorders	1154 (45)	1090 (42.4)	30 (1.2)	28 (1.1)
Asthenia	862 (33.6)	826 (32.1)	16 (0.6)	7 (0.3)
Edema NOS	471 (18.4)	416 (16.2)	4 (0.2)	3 (0.1)
Musculoskeletal Disorders	978 (38.2)	836 (32.5)	71 (2.8)	50 (1.9)
Arthralgia	565 (22)	465 (18.1)	25 (1)	20 (0.8)
Arthritis NOS	173 (6.7)	124 (4.8)	10 (0.4)	5 (0.2)
Myalgia	171 (6.7)	122 (4.7)	8 (0.3)	6 (0.2)
Back Pain	129 (5)	112 (4.4)	8 (0.3)	7 (0.3)
Nervous System Disorders	863 (33.7)	819 (31.8)	65 (2.5)	58 (2.3)
Headache	516 (20.1)	508 (19.7)	18 (0.7)	17 (0.7)
Dizziness	363 (14.2)	342 (13.3)	9 (0.4)	6 (0.2)
Skin Disorders	830 (32.4)	787 (30.6)	17 (0.7)	16 (0.6)
Sweating Increased	619 (24.2)	577 (22.4)	1 (<0.1)	0 -
Gastrointestinal Disorders	725 (28.3)	731 (28.4)	43 (1.7)	42 (1.6)
Constipation	290 (11.3)	304 (11.8)	6 (0.2)	2 (<0.1)
Nausea	221 (8.6)	212 (8.2)	3 (0.1)	10 (0.4)
Diarrhea NOS	128 (5)	143 (5.6)	12 (0.5)	8 (0.3)
Metabolic Disorders	551 (21.5)	537 (20.9)	24 (0.9)	32 (1.2)
Hypercholesterolemia	401 (15.6)	398 (15.5)	2 (<0.1)	5 (0.2)
Reproductive Disorders	303 (11.8)	357 (13.9)	9 (0.4)	8 (0.3)
Vaginal Hemorrhage	123 (4.8)	171 (6.6)	2 (<0.1)	5 (0.2)
Vulvovaginal Dryness	137 (5.3)	127 (4.9)	0 -	0 -
Psychiatric Disorders	320 (12.5)	276 (10.7)	21 (0.8)	16 (0.6)
Insomnia	149 (5.8)	120 (4.7)	2 (<0.1)	2 (<0.1)
Respiratory Disorders	279 (10.9)	260 (10.1)	30 (1.2)	28 (1.1)
Dyspnea	140 (5.5)	137 (5.3)	21 (0.8)	18 (0.7)
Investigations	184 (7.2)	147 (5.7)	13 (0.5)	13 (0.5)
Infections and Infestations	166 (6.5)	163 (6.3)	40 (1.6)	33 (1.3)
Renal Disorders	130 (5.1)	100 (3.9)	12 (0.5)	6 (0.2)

Table 4: Percentage (%) of Patients with Adverse Reactions

Adverse Reaction	Pooled Femara 2.5 mg (N=359) %	Pooled Femara 0.5 mg (N=380) %	megestrol acetate 160 mg (N=189) %	aminoglutethimide 500 mg (N=178) %
Body as a Whole				
Fatigue	8	6	11	3
Chest Pain	6	3	7	3
Peripheral Edema[1]	5	5	8	3
Asthenia	4	5	4	5
Weight Increase	2	2	9	3
Cardiovascular				
Hypertension	5	7	5	6
Digestive System				
Nausea	13	15	9	14
Vomiting	7	7	5	9
Constipation	6	7	9	7
Diarrhea	6	5	3	4
Pain-Abdominal	6	5	9	8
Anorexia	5	3	5	5
Dyspepsia	3	4	6	5
Infections/Infestations				
Viral Infection	6	5	6	3
Lab Abnormality				
Hypercholesterolemia	3	3	0	6
Musculoskeletal System				
Musculoskeletal[2]	21	22	30	14
Arthralgia	8	8	8	3
Nervous System				
Headache	9	12	9	7
Somnolence	3	2	2	9
Dizziness	3	5	7	3
Respiratory System				
Dyspnea	7	9	16	5
Coughing	6	5	7	5
Skin and Appendages				
Hot Flushes	6	5	4	3
Rash[3]	5	4	3	12
Pruritus	1	2	5	3

[1] Includes peripheral edema, leg edema, dependent edema, edema
[2] Includes musculoskeletal pain, skeletal pain, back pain, arm pain, leg pain
[3] Includes rash, erythematous rash, maculopapular rash, psoriasiform rash, vesicular rash

6.6 First and Second-Line Treatment of Advanced Breast Cancer

In the combined analysis of the first- and second-line metastatic trials and post-marketing experiences other adverse reactions that were reported were cataract, eye irritation, palpitations, cardiac failure, tachycardia, dysesthesia (including hypesthesia/paresthesia), arterial thrombosis, memory impairment, irritability, nervousness, urticaria, increased urinary frequency, leukopenia, stomatitis cancer pain, pyrexia, vaginal discharge, appetite increase, dryness of skin and mucosa (including dry mouth), and disturbances of taste and thirst.

6.7 Postmarketing Experience

Cases of blurred vision, increased hepatic enzymes, angioedema, anaphylactic reactions, toxic epidermal necrolysis, erythema multiforme, and hepatitis have been reported. Cases of carpal tunnel syndrome and trigger finger have been identified during post approval use of Femara.

7 DRUG INTERACTIONS

Tamoxifen

Coadministration of Femara and tamoxifen 20 mg daily resulted in a reduction of letrozole plasma levels of 38% on average. Clinical experience in the second-line breast cancer trials indicates that the therapeutic effect of Femara therapy is not impaired if Femara is administered immediately after tamoxifen.

Cimetidine

A pharmacokinetic interaction study with cimetidine showed no clinically significant effect on letrozole pharmacokinetics.

Warfarin

An interaction study with warfarin showed no clinically significant effect of letrozole on warfarin pharmacokinetics.

Other anticancer agents

There is no clinical experience to date on the use of Femara in combination with other anticancer agents.

8 USE IN SPECIFIC POPULATIONS

8.1 Pregnancy

Pregnancy Category X *[see Contraindications (4)].* Femara may cause fetal harm when administered to a pregnant woman and the clinical benefit to premenopausal women with breast cancer has not been demonstrated. Femara is contraindicated in women who are or may become pregnant. If this drug is used during pregnancy, or if the patient becomes pregnant while taking this drug, the patient should be apprised of the potential hazard to a fetus.

Femara caused adverse pregnancy outcomes, including congenital malformations, in rats and rabbits at doses much smaller than the daily maximum recommended human dose (MRHD) on a mg/m^2 basis. Effects included increased post-implantation pregnancy loss and resorptions, fewer live fetuses, and fetal malformations affecting the renal and skeletal systems. Animal data and letrozole's mechanism of action raise concerns that letrozole could be a human teratogen as well.

Reproduction studies in rats showed embryo and fetal toxicity at letrozole doses during organogenesis equal to or greater than 1/100 the daily maximum recommended human dose (MHRD) (mg/m^2 basis). Adverse effects included: intrauterine mortality; increased resorptions and postimplantation loss; decreased numbers of live fetuses; and fetal anomalies including absence and shortening of renal papilla, dilation of ureter, edema and incomplete ossification of frontal skull and metatarsals. Letrozole doses 1/10 the daily MHRD (mg/m^2 basis) caused fetal domed head and cervical/centrum vertebral fusion. In rabbits, letrozole caused embryo and fetal toxicity at doses about 1/100,000 and 1/10,000 the daily MHRD respectively (mg/m^2 basis). Fetal anomalies included incomplete ossification of the skull, sternebrae, and fore- and hind legs. *[see Nonclinical Toxicology (13.2)].*

Physicians should discuss the need for adequate contraception with women who are recently menopausal. Contraception should be used until postmenopausal status is clinically well established.

8.3 Nursing Mothers

It is not known if letrozole is excreted in human milk. Because many drugs are excreted in human milk and because of the potential for serious adverse reactions in nursing infants from letrozole, a decision should be made whether to discontinue nursing or to discontinue the drug, taking into account the importance of the drug to the mother.

8.4 Pediatric Use

The safety and effectiveness in pediatric patients have not been established.

8.5 Geriatric Use

The median age of patients in all studies of first-line and second-line treatment of metastatic breast cancer was 64-65 years. About 1/3 of the patients were ≥70 years old. In the first-line study, patients ≥70 years of age experienced longer time to tumor progression and higher response rates than patients <70.

For the extended adjuvant setting, more than 5,100 postmenopausal women were enrolled in the clinical study. In total, 41% of patients were aged 65 years or older at enrollment, while 12% were 75 or older. In the extended adjuvant setting, no overall differences in safety or efficacy were observed between these older patients and younger patients, and other reported clinical experience has not identified differences in responses between the elderly and younger patients, but greater sensitivity of some older individuals cannot be ruled out.

In the adjuvant setting, more than 8,000 postmenopausal women were enrolled in the clinical study. In total, 36 % of patients were aged 65 years or older at enrollment, while 12% were 75 or older. More adverse reactions were generally reported in elderly patients irrespective of study treatment allocation. However, in comparison to tamoxifen, no overall differences with regards to the safety and efficacy profiles were observed between elderly patients and younger patients.

10 OVERDOSAGE

Isolated cases of Femara overdose have been reported. In these instances, the highest single dose ingested was 62.5 mg or 25 tablets. While no serious adverse reactions were reported in these cases, because of the limited data available, no firm recommendations for treatment can be made. However, emesis could be induced if the patient is alert. In general, supportive care and frequent monitoring of vital signs are also appropriate. In single-dose studies, the highest dose used was 30 mg, which was well tolerated; in multiple-dose trials, the largest dose of 10 mg was well tolerated.

Lethality was observed in mice and rats following single oral doses that were equal to or greater than 2,000 mg/kg (about 4,000 to 8,000 times the daily maximum recommended human dose on a mg/m^2 basis); death was associated with reduced motor activity, ataxia and dyspnea. Lethality was observed in cats following single IV doses that were equal to or greater than 10 mg/kg (about 50 times the daily maximum recommended human dose on a mg/m^2 basis); death was preceded by depressed blood pressure and arrhythmias.

11 DESCRIPTION

Femara tablets for oral administration contains 2.5 mg of letrozole, a nonsteroidal aromatase inhibitor (inhibitor of estrogen synthesis). It is chemically described as 4,4'-(1H-1,2,4-Triazol-1-ylmethylene)dibenzonitrile, and its structural formula is

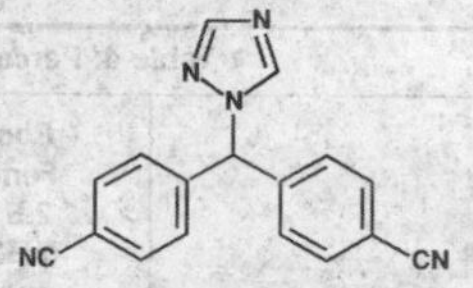

Letrozole is a white to yellowish crystalline powder, practically odorless, freely soluble in dichloromethane, slightly soluble in ethanol, and practically insoluble in water. It has a molecular weight of 285.31, empirical formula $C_{17}H_{11}N_5$, and a melting range of 184°C-185°C.

Femara is available as 2.5 mg tablets for oral administration.

Inactive Ingredients: Colloidal silicon dioxide, ferric oxide, hydroxypropyl methylcellulose, lactose monohydrate, magnesium stearate, maize starch, microcrystalline cellulose, polyethylene glycol, sodium starch glycolate, talc, and titanium dioxide.

12 CLINICAL PHARMACOLOGY

12.1 Mechanism of Action

The growth of some cancers of the breast is stimulated or maintained by estrogens. Treatment of breast cancer thought to be hormonally responsive (i.e., estrogen and/or progesterone receptor positive or receptor unknown) has included a variety of efforts to decrease estrogen levels (ovariectomy, adrenalectomy, hypophysectomy) or inhibit estrogen effects (antiestrogens and progestational agents). These interventions lead to decreased tumor mass or delayed progression of tumor growth in some women.

In postmenopausal women, estrogens are mainly derived from the action of the aromatase enzyme, which converts adrenal androgens (primarily androstenedione and testosterone) to estrone and estradiol. The suppression of estrogen biosynthesis in peripheral tissues and in the cancer tissue itself can therefore be achieved by specifically inhibiting the aromatase enzyme.

Letrozole is a nonsteroidal competitive inhibitor of the aromatase enzyme system; it inhibits the conversion of androgens to estrogens. In adult nontumor- and tumor-bearing female animals, letrozole is as effective as ovariectomy in reducing uterine weight, elevating serum LH, and causing the regression of estrogen-dependent tumors. In contrast to ovariectomy, treatment with letrozole does not lead to an increase in serum FSH. Letrozole selectively inhibits gonadal steroidogenesis but has no significant effect on adrenal mineralocorticoid or glucocorticoid synthesis.

Letrozole inhibits the aromatase enzyme by competitively binding to the heme of the cytochrome P450 subunit of the enzyme, resulting in a reduction of estrogen biosynthesis in all tissues. Treatment of women with letrozole significantly lowers serum estrone, estradiol and estrone sulfate and has not been shown to significantly affect adrenal corticosteroid synthesis, aldosterone synthesis, or synthesis of thyroid hormones.

12.2 Pharmacodynamics

In postmenopausal patients with advanced breast cancer, daily doses of 0.1 mg to 5 mg Femara (letrozole) suppress plasma concentrations of estradiol, estrone, and estrone sulfate by 75%-95% from baseline with maximal suppression achieved within two-three days. Suppression is dose-related, with doses of 0.5 mg and higher giving many values of estrone and estrone sulfate that were below the limit of detection in the assays. Estrogen suppression was maintained throughout treatment in all patients treated at 0.5 mg or higher.

Letrozole is highly specific in inhibiting aromatase activity. There is no impairment of adrenal steroidogenesis. No clinically-relevant changes were found in the plasma concentrations of cortisol, aldosterone, 11-deoxycortisol, 17-hydroxy-progesterone, ACTH or in plasma renin activity among postmenopausal patients treated with a daily dose of Femara 0.1 mg to 5 mg. The ACTH stimulation test performed after 6 and 12 weeks of treatment with daily doses of 0.1, 0.25, 0.5, 1, 2.5, and 5 mg did not indicate any attenuation of aldosterone or cortisol production. Glucocorticoid or mineralocorticoid supplementation is, therefore, not necessary.

No changes were noted in plasma concentrations of androgens (androstenedione and testosterone) among healthy postmenopausal women after 0.1, 0.5, and 2.5 mg single doses of Femara or in plasma concentrations of androstenedione among postmenopausal patients treated with daily doses of 0.1 mg to 5 mg. This indicates that the blockade of estrogen biosynthesis does not lead to accumulation of androgenic precursors. Plasma levels of LH and FSH were not affected by letrozole in patients, nor was thyroid function as evaluated by TSH levels, T3 uptake, and T4 levels.

12.3 Pharmacokinetics

Absorption and Distribution: Letrozole is rapidly and completely absorbed from the gastrointestinal tract and absorption is not affected by food. It is metabolized slowly to an inactive metabolite whose glucuronide conjugate is excreted renally, representing the major clearance pathway. About 90% of radiolabeled letrozole is recovered in urine. Letrozole's terminal elimination half-life is about 2 days and steady-state plasma concentration after daily 2.5 mg dosing is reached in 2-6 weeks. Plasma concentrations at steady state are 1.5 to 2 times higher than predicted from the concentrations measured after a single dose, indicating a slight non-linearity in the pharmacokinetics of letrozole upon daily administration of 2.5 mg. These steady-state levels are maintained over extended periods, however, and continuous accumulation of letrozole does not occur. Letrozole is weakly protein bound and has a large volume of distribution (approximately 1.9 L/kg).

Metabolism and Excretion: Metabolism to a pharmacologically-inactive carbinol metabolite (4,4'-methanol-bisbenzonitrile) and renal excretion of the glucuronide conjugate of this metabolite is the major pathway of letrozole clearance. Of the radiolabel recovered in urine, at least 75% was the glucuronide of the carbinol metabolite, about 9% was two unidentified metabolites, and 6% was unchanged letrozole.

In human microsomes with specific CYP isozyme activity, CYP3A4 metabolized letrozole to the carbinol metabolite while CYP2A6 formed both this metabolite and its ketone analog. In human liver microsomes, letrozole strongly inhibited CYP2A6 and moderately inhibited CYP2C19.

Pediatric, Geriatric and Race: In the study populations (adults ranging in age from 35 to >80 years), no change in pharmacokinetic parameters was observed with increasing age. Differences in letrozole pharmacokinetics between adult and pediatric populations have not been studied. Differences in letrozole pharmacokinetics due to race have not been studied.

Renal Impairment: In a study of volunteers with varying renal function (24-hour creatinine clearance: 9-116 mL/min), no effect of renal function on the pharmacokinetics of single doses of 2.5 mg of Femara was found. In addition, in a study of 347 patients with advanced breast cancer, about half of whom received 2.5 mg Femara and half 0.5 mg Femara, renal impairment (calculated creatinine clearance: 20-50 mL/min) did not affect steady-state plasma letrozole concentrations.

Hepatic Impairment: In a study of subjects with mild to moderate non-metastatic hepatic dysfunction (e.g., cirrhosis, Child-Pugh classification A and B), the mean AUC values of the volunteers with moderate hepatic impairment were 37% higher than in normal subjects, but still within the range seen in subjects without impaired function.

In a pharmacokinetic study, subjects with liver cirrhosis and severe hepatic impairment (Child-Pugh classification C, which included bilirubins about 2-11 times ULN with minimal to severe ascites) had two-fold increase in exposure

Table 5: Adjuvant Study - Patient and Disease Characteristics (ITT Population)

Characteristic	Primary Core Analysis (PCA) Femara N=4003 n (%)	Primary Core Analysis (PCA) tamoxifen N=4007 n (%)	Monotherapy Arms Analysis (MAA) Femara N=2463 n (%)	Monotherapy Arms Analysis (MAA) tamoxifen N=2459 n (%)
Age (median, years)	61	61	61	61
Age range (years)	38-89	39-90	38-88	39-90
Hormone receptor status (%)				
ER+ and/or PgR+	99.7	99.7	99.7	99.7
Both unknown	0.3	0.3	0.3	0.3
Nodal status (%)				
Node negative	52	52	50	52
Node positive	41	41	43	41
Nodal status unknown	7	7	7	7
Prior adjuvant chemotherapy (%)	24	24	24	24

Table 6: Updated Adjuvant Study Results - Monotherapy Arms Analysis (Median Follow-up 73 Months)

		Femara N=2463		tamoxifen N=2459		Hazard ratio	
		Events (%)	5-year rate	Events (%)	5-year rate	(95% CI)	*P*
Disease-free survival[1]	ITT	445 (18.1)	87.4	500 (20.3)	84.7	0.87 (0.76, 0.99)	0.03
	Censor	445	87.4	483	84.2	0.84 (0.73, 0.95)	
0 positive nodes	ITT	165	92.2	189	90.3	0.88 (0.72, 1.09)	
1-3 positive nodes	ITT	151	85.6	163	83.0	0.85 (0.68, 1.06)	
>=4 positive nodes	ITT	123	71.2	142	62.6	0.81 (0.64, 1.03)	
Adjuvant chemotherapy	ITT	119	86.4	150	80.6	0.77 (0.60, 0.98)	
No chemotherapy	ITT	326	87.8	350	86.1	0.91 (0.78, 1.06)	
Systemic DFS[2]	ITT	401	88.5	446	86.6	0.88 (0.77,1.01)	
Time to distant metastasis[3]	ITT	257	92.4	298	90.1	0.85 (0.72, 1.00)	
Adjuvant chemotherapy	ITT	84	-	109	-	0.75 (0.56-1.00)	
No chemotherapy	ITT	173	-	189	-	0.90 (0.73,1.11)	
Distant DFS[4]	ITT	385	89.0	432	87.1	0.87 (0.76,1.00)	
Contralateral breast cancer	ITT	34	99.2	44	98.6	0.76 (0.49, 1.19)	
Overall survival	ITT	303	91.8	343	90.9	0.87 (0.75, 1.02)	
	Censor	303	91.8	338	90.1	0.82 (0.70, 0.96)	
0 positive nodes	ITT	107	95.2	121	94.8	0.90 (0.69.1.16)	
1-3 positive nodes	ITT	99	90.8	114	90.6	0.81(0.62,1.06)	
>=4 positive nodes	ITT	92	80.2	104	73.6	0.86 (0.65, 1.14)	
Adjuvant chemotherapy	ITT	76	91.5	96	88.4	0.79 (0.58, 1.06)	
No chemotherapy	ITT	227	91.9	247	91.8	0.91 (0.76, 1.08)	

Definition of:

[1] Disease-free survival: Interval from randomization to earliest event of invasive loco-regional recurrence, distant metastasis, invasive contralateral breast cancer, or death without a prior event

[2] Systemic disease-free survival: Interval from randomization to invasive regional recurrence, distant metastasis, or death without a prior cancer event

[3] Time to distant metastasis: Interval from randomization to distant metastasis

[4] Distant disease-free survival: Interval from randomization to earlier event of relapse in a distant site or death from any cause

ITT analysis ignores selective crossover in tamoxifen arms

Censored analysis censors follow-up at the date of selective crossover in 632 patients who crossed to Femara or another aromatase inhibitor after the tamoxifen arms were unblinded in 2005

Table 8: Extended Adjuvant Study Results

	Femara N = 2582	Placebo N = 2586	Hazard Ratio (95% CI)	*P*-Value
Disease Free Survival (DFS)[1] Events	122 (4.7%)	193 (7.5%)	0.62 (0.49, 0.78)[2]	0.00003
Local Breast Recurrence	9	22		
Local Chest Wall Recurrence	2	8		
Regional Recurrence	7	4		
Distant Recurrence	55	92	0.61 (0.44 - 0.84)	0.003
Contralateral Breast Cancer	19	29		
Deaths Without Recurrence or Contralateral Breast Cancer	30	38		

CI = confidence interval for hazard ratio. Hazard ratio of less than 1.0 indicates difference in favor of Femara (lesser risk of recurrence); hazard ratio greater than 1.0 indicates difference in favor of placebo (higher risk of recurrence with Femara).

[1] First event of loco-regional recurrence, distant relapse, contralateral breast cancer or death from any cause

[2] Analysis stratified by receptor status, nodal status and prior adjuvant chemotherapy (stratification factors as at randomization). *P*-value based on stratified logrank test.

(AUC) and 47% reduction in systemic clearance. Breast cancer patients with severe hepatic impairment are thus expected to be exposed to higher levels of letrozole than patients with normal liver function receiving similar doses of this drug. *[see Dosage and Administration (2.5)]*

13 NONCLINICAL TOXICOLOGY

13.1 Carcinogenesis, Mutagenesis, Impairment of Fertility

A conventional carcinogenesis study in mice at doses of 0.6 to 60 mg/kg/day (about 1 to 100 times the daily maximum recommended human dose on a mg/m^2 basis) administered by oral gavage for up to 2 years revealed a dose-related increase in the incidence of benign ovarian stromal tumors. The incidence of combined hepatocellular adenoma and carcinoma showed a significant trend in females when the high dose group was excluded due to low survival. In a separate study, plasma $AUC_{0\text{-}12hr}$ levels in mice at 60 mg/kg/day were 55 times higher than the $AUC_{0\text{-}24hr}$ level in breast cancer patients at the recommended dose. The carcinogenicity study in rats at oral doses of 0.1 to 10 mg/kg/day (about 0.4 to 40 times the daily maximum recommended human dose on a mg/m^2 basis) for up to 2 years also produced an increase in the incidence of benign ovarian stromal tumors at 10 mg/kg/day. Ovarian hyperplasia was observed in females at doses equal to or greater than 0.1 mg/kg/day. At 10 mg/kg/day, plasma $AUC_{0\text{-}24hr}$ levels in rats were 80 times higher than the level in breast cancer patients at the recommended dose.

Femara (letrozole) was not mutagenic in *in vitro* tests (Ames and E.coli bacterial tests) but was observed to be a potential clastogen in *in vitro* assays (CHO K1 and CCL 61 Chinese hamster ovary cells). Letrozole was not clastogenic *in vivo* (micronucleus test in rats).

Studies to investigate the effect of letrozole on fertility have not been conducted; however, repeated dosing caused sexual inactivity in females and atrophy of the reproductive tract in males and females at doses of 0.6, 0.1 and 0.03 mg/kg in mice, rats and dogs, respectively (about one, 0.4 and 0.4 the daily maximum recommended human dose on a mg/m^2 basis, respectively).

Letrozole administered to young (postnatal day 7) rats for 12 weeks duration at 0.003, 0.03, 0.3 mg/kg/day by oral gavage, resulted in adverse skeletal/growth effects (bone maturation, bone mineral density) and neuroendocrine and reproductive developmental perturbations of the hypothalamic-pituitary axis at exposures less than exposure anticipated at the clinical dose of 2.5 mg/day. Decreased fertility was accompanied by hypertrophy of the hypophysis and testicular changes that included degeneration of the seminiferous tubular epithelium and atrophy of the female reproductive tract. Young rats in this study were allowed to recover following discontinuation of letrozole treatment for 42 days. Histopathological changes were not reversible at clinically relevant exposures.

13.2 Animal Toxicology and/or Pharmacology

Reproductive Toxicology: Reproduction studies in rats at letrozole doses equal to or greater than 0.003 mg/kg (about 1/100 the daily maximum recommended human dose on a mg/m^2 basis) administered during the period of organogenesis, have shown that letrozole is embryotoxic and fetotoxic, as indicated by intrauterine mortality, increased resorption, increased postimplantation loss, decreased numbers of live fetuses and fetal anomalies including absence and shortening of renal papilla, dilation of ureter, edema and incomplete ossification of frontal skull and metatarsals. Letrozole was teratogenic in rats. A 0.03 mg/kg dose (about 1/10 the daily maximum recommended human dose on a mg/m^2 basis) caused fetal domed head and cervical/centrum vertebral fusion.

Letrozole is embryotoxic at doses equal to or greater than 0.002 mg/kg and fetotoxic when administered to rabbits at 0.02 mg/kg (about 1/100,000 and 1/10,000 the daily maximum recommended human dose on a mg/m^2 basis, respectively). Fetal anomalies included incomplete ossification of the skull, sternebrae, and fore- and hind legs.

14 CLINICAL STUDIES

14.1 Updated Adjuvant Treatment of Early Breast Cancer

In a multicenter study enrolling over 8,000 postmenopausal women with resected, receptor-positive early breast cancer, one of the following treatments was randomized in a double-blind manner:

Option 1:

A. tamoxifen for 5 years

B. Femara for 5 years

C. tamoxifen for 2 years followed by Femara for 3 years

D. Femara for 2 years followed by tamoxifen for 3 years

Option 2:

A. tamoxifen for 5 years

B. Femara for 5 years

The study in the adjuvant setting, BIG 1-98 was designed to answer two primary questions: whether Femara for 5 years was superior to tamoxifen for 5 years (Primary Core Analysis) and whether switching endocrine treatments at 2 years was superior to continuing the same agent for a total of 5 years (Sequential Treatments Analysis). Selected baseline characteristics for the study population are shown in Table 5.

The primary endpoint of this trial was disease-free survival (DFS) (i.e., interval between randomization and earliest occurrence of a local, regional, or distant recurrence, or invasive contralateral breast cancer, or death from any cause). The secondary endpoints were overall survival (OS), systemic disease-free survival (SDFS), invasive contralateral breast cancer, time to breast cancer recurrence (TBR) and time to distant metastasis (TDM).

The Primary Core Analysis (PCA) included all patients and all follow-up in the monotherapy arms in both randomization options, but follow-up in the two sequential treatments arms was truncated 30 days after switching treatments. The PCA was conducted at a median treatment duration of 24 months and a median follow-up of 26 months. Femara was superior to tamoxifen in all endpoints except overall survival and contralateral breast cancer [e.g., DFS: hazard ratio, HR 0.79; 95% CI (0.68, 0.92); *P*=0.002; SDFS: HR 0.83; 95% CI (0.70, 0.97); TDM: HR 0.73; 95% CI (0.60, 0.88); OS: HR 0.86; 95% CI (0.70, 1.06).

In 2005, based on recommendations by the independent Data Monitoring Committee, the tamoxifen arms were un-

Table 9: Update of Extended Adjuvant Study Results

	Femara N = 2582 (%)	Placebo N = 2586 (%)	Hazard Ratio[1] (95% CI)	*P*-Value[2]
Disease Free Survival (DFS) events[3]	344 (13.3)	402 (15.5)	0.89 (0.77, 1.03)	0.12
Breast cancer recurrence (Protocol definition of DFS events[4])	209	286	0.75 (0.63, 0.89)	0.001
Local Breast Recurrence	15	44		
Local Chest Wall Recurrence	6	14		
Regional Recurrence	10	8		
Distant Recurrence	140	167		
Distant recurrence (first or subsequent events)	142	169	0.88 (0.70,1.10)	0.246
Contralateral Breast Cancer	37	53		
Deaths Without Recurrence or Contralateral Breast Cancer	135	116		

[1] Adjusted by receptor status, nodal status and prior chemotherapy
[2] Stratified logrank test, stratified by receptor status, nodal status and prior chemotherapy
[3] DFS events defined as earliest of loco-regional recurrence, distant metastasis, contralateral breast cancer or death from any cause, and ignoring switches to Femara in 60% of the placebo arm.
[4] Protocol definition does not include deaths from any cause

Table 11: Results of First-Line Treatment of Advanced Breast Cancer

	Femara 2.5 mg N=453	tamoxifen 20 mg N=454	Hazard or Odds Ratio (95% CI) *P*-Value (2-Sided)
Median Time to Progression	9.4 months	6.0 months	0.72 (0.62, 0.83)[1] $P<0.0001$
Objective Response Rate			
(CR + PR)	145 (32%)	95 (21%)	1.77 (1.31, 2.39)[2] $P=0.0002$
(CR)	42 (9%)	15 (3%)	2.99 (1.63, 5.47)[2] $P=0.0004$
Duration of Objective Response			
Median	18 months (N=145)	16 months (N=95)	
Overall Survival	35 months (N=458)	32 months (N=458)	$P=0.5136$[3]

[1] Hazard ratio
[2] Odds ratio
[3] Overall logrank test

blinded and patients were allowed to complete initial adjuvant therapy with Femara (if they had received tamoxifen for at least 2 years) or to start extended adjuvant treatment with Femara (if they had received tamoxifen for at least 4.5 years) if they remained alive and disease-free. In total, 632 patients crossed to Femara or another aromatase inhibitor. Approximately 70% (448) of these 632 patients crossed to Femara to complete initial adjuvant therapy and most of these crossed in years 3 to 4. All of these patients were in Option 1. A total of 184 patients started extended adjuvant therapy with Femara (172 patients) or with another aromatase inhibitor (12 patients). To explore the impact of this selective crossover, results from analyses censoring follow-up at the date of the selective crossover (in the tamoxifen arm) are presented for the Monotherapy Arms Analysis (MAA).

The PCA allowed the results of Femara for 5 years compared with tamoxifen for 5 years to be reported in 2005 after a median follow-up of only 26 months. The design of the PCA is not optimal to evaluate the effect of Femara after a longer time (because follow-up was truncated in two arms at around 25 months). The Monotherapy Arms Analysis (ignoring the two sequential treatment arms) provided follow-up equally as long in each treatment and did not overemphasize early recurrences as the PCA did. The MAA thus provides the clinically appropriate updated efficacy results in answer to the first primary question, despite the confounding of the tamoxifen reference arm by the selective crossover to Femara. The updated results for the MAA are summarized in Table 6. Median follow-up for this analysis is 73 months.

The Sequential Treatments Analysis (STA) addresses the second primary question of the study. The primary analysis for the Sequential Treatments Analysis (STA) was from switch (or equivalent time-point in monotherapy arms) + 30 days (STA-S) with a two-sided test applied to each pair-wise comparison at the 2.5% level. Additional analyses were conducted from randomization (STA-R) but these comparisons (added in light of changing medical practice) were underpowered for efficacy.

[See table 5 at top of previous page]
[See table 6 at top of previous page]

Figure 1 shows the Kaplan-Meier curves for Disease-Free Survival Monotherapy Analysis

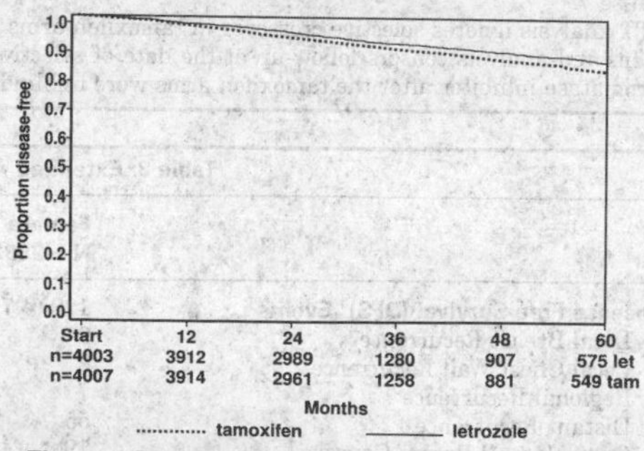

Figure 1 Disease-Free Survival (Median follow-up 73 months, ITT Approach)

DFS events defined as loco-regional recurrence, distant metastasis, invasive contralateral breast cancer, or death from any cause (i.e., definition excludes second non-breast primary cancers).

The medians of overall survival for both arms were not reached for the Monotherapy Arms Analysis (MAA). There was no statistically significant difference in overall survival. The hazard ratio for survival in the Femara arm compared to the tamoxifen arm was 0.87, with 95% CI (0.75, 1.02) (see Table 6).

There were no significant differences in DFS, OS, SDFS, and Distant DFS from switch in the Sequential Treatments Analysis with respect to either monotherapy (e.g., [Tamoxifen 2 years followed by] Femara 3 years versus tamoxifen beyond 2 years, DFS HR 0.89; 97.5% CI 0.68, 1.15 and [Femara 2 years followed by] tamoxifen 3 years versus Femara beyond 2 years, DFS HR 0.93; 97.5% CI 0.71, 1.22). There were no significant differences in DFS, OS, SDFS, and Distant DFS from randomization in the Sequential Treatments Analyses.

14.2 Extended Adjuvant Treatment of Early Breast Cancer, Median Treatment Duration of 24 Months

A double-blind, randomized, placebo-controlled trial of Femara was performed in over 5,100 postmenopausal women with receptor-positive or unknown primary breast cancer who were disease free after 5 years of adjuvant treatment with tamoxifen.

The planned duration of treatment for patients in the study was 5 years, but the trial was terminated early because of an interim analysis showing a favorable Femara effect on time without recurrence or contralateral breast cancer. At the time of unblinding, women had been followed for a median of 28 months, 30% of patients had completed 3 or more years of follow-up and less than 1% of patients had completed 5 years of follow-up.

Selected baseline characteristics for the study population are shown in Table 7.

Table 7: Selected Study Population Demographics (Modified ITT Population)

Baseline Status	Femara N=2582	Placebo N=2586
Hormone Receptor Status (%)		
ER+ and/or PgR+	98	98
Both Unknown	2	2
Nodal Status (%)		
Node Negative	50	50
Node Positive	46	46
Nodal Status Unknown	4	4
Chemotherapy	46	46

Table 8 shows the study results. Disease-free survival was measured as the time from randomization to the earliest event of loco-regional or distant recurrence of the primary disease or development of contralateral breast cancer or death. DFS by hormone receptor status, nodal status and adjuvant chemotherapy were similar to the overall results. Data were premature for an analysis of survival.

[See table 8 at top of previous page]

14.3 Updated Analyses of Extended Adjuvant Treatment of Early Breast Cancer, Median Treatment Duration of 60 Months

[See table 9 above]

Updated analyses were conducted at a median follow-up of 62 months. In the Femara arm, 71% of the patients were treated for a least 3 years and 58% of patients completed at least 4.5 years of extended adjuvant treatment. After the unblinding of the study at a median follow-up of 28 months, approximately 60% of the selected patients in the placebo arm opted to switch to Femara.

In this updated analysis shown in Table 9, Femara significantly reduced the risk of breast cancer recurrence or contralateral breast cancer compared with placebo (HR 0.75; 95% CI 0.63, 0.89; $P=0.001$). However, in the updated DFS analysis (interval between randomization and earliest event of loco-regional recurrence, distant metastasis, contralateral breast cancer, or death from any cause) the treatment difference was heavily diluted by 60% of the patients in the placebo arm switching to Femara and accounting for 64% of the total placebo patient- years of follow-up. Ignoring these switches, the risk of DFS event was reduced by a non-significant 11% (HR 0.89; 95% CI 0.77, 1.03). There was no significant difference in distant disease-free survival or overall survival.

14.4 First-Line Treatment of Advanced Breast Cancer

A randomized, double-blind, multinational trial compared Femara 2.5 mg with tamoxifen 20 mg in 916 postmenopausal patients with locally advanced (Stage IIIB or loco-regional recurrence not amenable to treatment with surgery or radiation) or metastatic breast cancer. Time to progression (TTP) was the primary endpoint of the trial. Selected baseline characteristics for this study are shown in Table 10.

Table 10: Selected Study Population Demographics

Baseline Status	Femara N=458	tamoxifen N=458
Stage of Disease		
IIIB	6%	7%
IV	93%	92%
Receptor Status		
ER and PgR Positive	38%	41%
ER or PgR Positive	26%	26%
Both Unknown	34%	33%
ER[-] or PgR[-]/Other Unknown	<1%	0
Previous Antiestrogen Therapy		
Adjuvant	19%	18%
None	81%	82%
Dominant Site of Disease		
Soft Tissue	25%	25%

Bone	32%	29%
Viscera	43%	46%

Femara was superior to tamoxifen in TTP and rate of objective tumor response (see Table 11).
Table 11 summarizes the results of the trial, with a total median follow-up of approximately 32 months. (All analyses are unadjusted and use 2-sided *P*-values.)
[See table 11 at top of previous page]
Figure 2 shows the Kaplan-Meier curves for TTP.

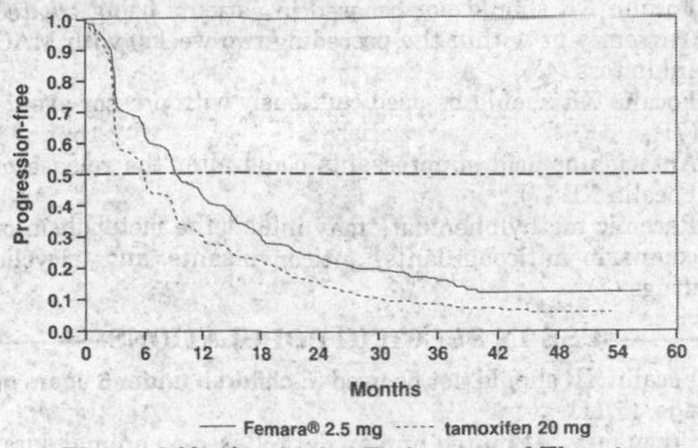

Figure 2 Kaplan-Meier Estimates of Time to Progression (Tamoxifen Study)

Table 12 shows results in the subgroup of women who had received prior antiestrogen adjuvant therapy, Table 13, results by disease site and Table 14, the results by receptor status.

Table 12: Efficacy in Patients Who Received Prior Antiestrogen Therapy

Variable	Femara 2.5 mg N=84	tamoxifen 20 mg N=83
Median Time to Progression (95% CI)	8.9 months (6.2, 12.5)	5.9 months (3.2, 6.2)
Hazard Ratio for TTP (95% CI)	0.60 (0.43, 0.84)	
Objective Response Rate (CR + PR)	22 (26%)	7 (8%)
Odds Ratio for Response (95% CI)	3.85 (1.50, 9.60)	

Hazard ratio less than 1 or odds ratio greater than 1 favors Femara; hazard ratio greater than 1 or odds ratio less than 1 favors tamoxifen.

Table 13: Efficacy by Disease Site

	Femara 2.5 mg	tamoxifen 20 mg
Dominant Disease Site		
Soft Tissue:	N=113	N=115
Median TTP	12.1 months	6.4 months
Objective Response Rate	50%	34%
Bone:	N=145	N=131
Median TTP	9.5 months	6.3 months
Objective Response Rate	23%	15%
Viscera:	N=195	N=208
Median TTP	8.3 months	4.6 months
Objective Response Rate	28%	17%

[See table 14 above]
Hazard ratio less than 1 or odds ratio greater than 1 favors Femara; hazard ratio greater than 1 or odds ratio less than 1 favors tamoxifen.
Figure 3 shows the Kaplan-Meier curves for survival.

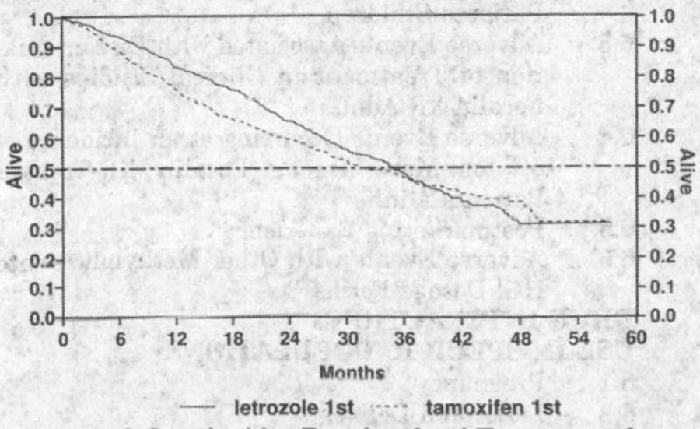

Figure 3 Survival by Randomized Treatment Arm

Legend: Randomized Femara: n=458, events 57%, median overall survival 35 months (95% CI 32 to 38 months) Randomized tamoxifen: n=458, events 57%, median overall survival 32 months (95% CI 28 to 37 months)

Table 14: Efficacy by Receptor Status

Variable	Femara 2.5 mg	tamoxifen 20 mg
Receptor Positive	N=294	N=305
Median Time to Progression (95% CI)	9.4 months (8.9, 11.8)	6.0 months (5.1, 8.5)
Hazard Ratio for TTP (95% CI)	0.69 (0.58, 0.83)	
Objective Response Rate (CR+PR)	97 (33%)	66 (22%)
Odds Ratio for Response 95% CI)	1.78 (1.20, 2.60)	
Receptor Unknown	N=159	N=149
Median Time to Progression (95% CI)	9.2 months (6.1, 12.3)	6.0 months (4.1, 6.4)
Hazard Ratio for TTP (95% CI)	0.77 (0.60, 0.99)	
Objective Response Rate (CR+PR)	48 (30%)	29 (20%)
Odds Ratio for Response (95% CI)	1.79 (1.10, 3.00)	

Table 16: Megestrol Acetate Study Results

	Femara 0.5 mg N=188	Femara 2.5 mg N=174	megestrol acetate N=190
Objective Response (CR + PR)	22 (11.7%)	41 (23.6%)	31 (16.3%)
Median Duration of Response	552 days	(Not reached)	561 days
Median Time to Progression	154 days	170 days	168 days
Median Survival	633 days	730 days	659 days
Odds Ratio for Response	Femara 2.5: Femara 0.5=2.33 (95% CI: 1.32, 4.17); *P*=0.004*		Femara 2.5: megestrol=1.58 (95% CI: 0.94, 2.66); *P*=0.08*
Relative Risk of Progression	Femara 2.5: Femara 0.5=0.81 (95% CI: 0.63, 1.03); *P*=0.09		Femara 2.5: megestrol=0.77 (95% CI: 0.60, 0.98); *P*=0.03*

* two-sided *P*-value

Overall logrank *P*=0.5136 (i.e., there was no significant difference between treatment arms in overall survival).
The median overall survival was 35 months for the Femara group and 32 months for the tamoxifen group, with a *P*-value 0.5136. Study design allowed patients to cross over upon progression to the other therapy. Approximately 50% of patients crossed over to the opposite treatment arm and almost all patients who crossed over had done so by 36 months. The median time to crossover was 17 months (Femara to tamoxifen) and 13 months (tamoxifen to Femara). In patients who did not cross over to the opposite treatment arm, median survival was 35 months with Femara (n=219, 95% Cl 29 to 43 months) vs 20 months with tamoxifen (n=229, 95% Cl 16 to 26 months).

14.5 Second-Line Treatment of Advanced Breast Cancer
Femara was initially studied at doses of 0.1 mg to 5.0 mg daily in six non-comparative Phase I/II trials in 181 postmenopausal estrogen/progesterone receptor positive or unknown advanced breast cancer patients previously treated with at least antiestrogen therapy. Patients had received other hormonal therapies and also may have received cytotoxic therapy. Eight (20%) of forty patients treated with Femara 2.5 mg daily in Phase I/II trials achieved an objective tumor response (complete or partial response).
Two large randomized, controlled, multinational (predominantly European) trials were conducted in patients with advanced breast cancer who had progressed despite antiestrogen therapy. Patients were randomized to Femara 0.5 mg daily, Femara 2.5 mg daily, or a comparator (megestrol acetate 160 mg daily in one study; and aminoglutethimide 250 mg b.i.d. with corticosteroid supplementation in the other study). In each study over 60% of the patients had received therapeutic antiestrogens, and about one-fifth of these patients had an objective response. The megestrol acetate controlled study was double-blind; the other study was open label. Selected baseline characteristics for each study are shown in Table 15.

Table 15: Selected Study Population Demographics

Parameter	megestrol acetate study	aminoglutethimide study
No. of Participants	552	557
Receptor Status		
ER/PR Positive	57%	56%
ER/PR Unknown	43%	44%
Previous Therapy		
Adjuvant Only	33%	38%
Therapeutic +/- Adj.	66%	62%
Sites of Disease		
Soft Tissue	56%	50%
Bone	50%	55%
Viscera	40%	44%

Confirmed objective tumor response (complete response plus partial response) was the primary endpoint of the trials. Responses were measured according to the Union Internationale Contre le Cancer (UICC) criteria and verified by independent, blinded review. All responses were confirmed by a second evaluation 4-12 weeks after the documentation of the initial response.
Table 16 shows the results for the first trial, with a minimum follow-up of 15 months, that compared Femara 0.5 mg, Femara 2.5 mg, and megestrol acetate 160 mg daily. (All analyses are unadjusted.)
[See table 16 above]
The Kaplan-Meier curves for progression for the megestrol acetate study are shown in Figure 4.

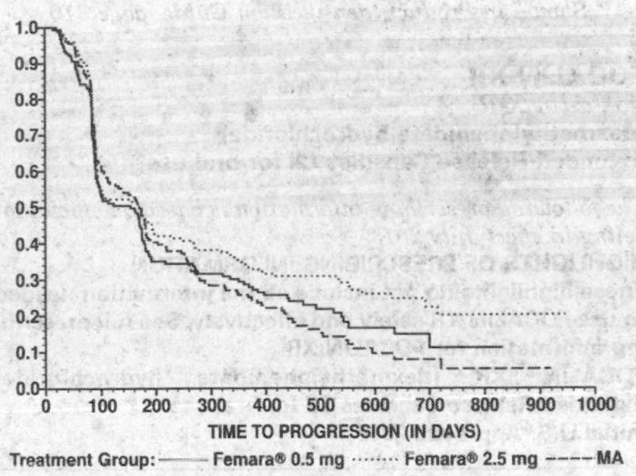

Figure 4 Kaplan-Meier Estimates of Time to Progression (Megestrol Acetate Study)

The results for the study comparing Femara to aminoglutethimide, with a minimum follow-up of 9 months, are shown in Table 17. (Unadjusted analyses are used.)
[See table 17 at top of next page]
The Kaplan-Meier curves for progression for the aminoglutethimide study is shown in Figure 5.

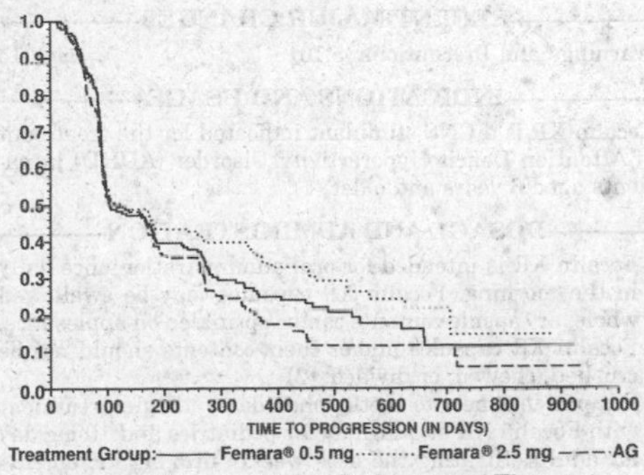

Figure 5 Kaplan-Meier Estimates of Time to Progression (Aminoglutethimide Study)

Table 17: Aminoglutethimide Study Results

	Femara 0.5 mg N=193	Femara 2.5 mg N=185	aminoglutethimide N=179
Objective Response (CR + PR)	34 (17.6%)	34 (18.4%)	22 (12.3%)
Median Duration of Response	619 days	706 days	450 days
Median Time to Progression	103 days	123 days	112 days
Median Survival	636 days	792 days	592 days
Odds Ratio for Response	Femara 2.5: Femara 0.5=1.05 (95% CI: 0.62, 1.79); P=0.85*		Femara 2.5: aminoglutethimide=1.61 (95% CI: 0.90, 2.87); P=0.11*
Relative Risk of Progression	Femara 2.5: Femara 0.5=0.86 (95% CI: 0.68, 1.11); P=0.25*		Femara 2.5: aminoglutethimide=0.74 (95% CI: 0.57, 0.94); P=0.02*

* two-sided P-value

16 HOW SUPPLIED/STORAGE AND HANDLING

Packaged in HDPE bottles with a safety screw cap.
2.5 milligram tablets
Bottles of 30 tablets.................................NDC 0078-0249-15
Store at 25°C (77°F); excursions permitted to 15-30°C (59-86°F) [see USP Controlled Room Temperature].

17 PATIENT COUNSELING INFORMATION

Information for Patients

Pregnancy: Femara is contraindicated in women of pre-menopausal endocrine status. The physician needs to discuss the necessity of adequate contraception with women who have the potential to become pregnant including women who are perimenopausal or who recently became postmenopausal, until their postmenopausal status is fully established.

Fatigue and Dizziness: Since fatigue and dizziness have been observed with the use of Femara and somnolence was uncommonly reported, caution is advised when driving or using machinery.

Bone Effects: Consideration should be given to monitoring bone mineral density.

Novartis Pharmaceuticals Corporation
East Hanover, New Jersey, 07936

T2012-10
December 2011

Shown in Product Identification Guide, page 310

FOCALIN XR Ⓒ

[fōk'ă-lĭn X-R]
(dexmethylphenidate hydrochloride)
Extended-Release Capsules CII for oral use

The following prescribing information is based on official labeling in effect July 2013.

HIGHLIGHTS OF PRESCRIBING INFORMATION

These highlights do not include all the information needed to use FOCALIN XR safely and effectively. See full prescribing information for FOCALIN XR.

FOCALIN XR (dexmethylphenidate hydrochloride) Extended-Release Capsules CII for oral use
Initial U.S. Approval: 2005

> **WARNING: DRUG DEPENDENCE**
> ***See full prescribing information for complete boxed warning***
> **Focalin XR should be given cautiously to patients with a history of drug dependence or alcoholism. Chronic abusive use can lead to marked tolerance and psychological dependence, with varying degrees of abnormal behavior.**

RECENT MAJOR CHANGES

Warnings and Precautions (5.10) 06/2013

INDICATIONS AND USAGE

Focalin XR is a CNS stimulant indicated for the treatment of Attention Deficit Hyperactivity Disorder (ADHD) in patients aged 6 years and older (1)

DOSAGE AND ADMINISTRATION

- Focalin XR is intended for oral administration once daily in the morning. Focalin XR capsules may be swallowed whole, or capsule contents can be sprinkled on applesauce. Focalin XR capsules and/or their contents should not be crushed, chewed, or divided. (2)
- For patients new to methylphenidate: Begin treatment with Focalin XR at 5 mg/day for pediatrics and 10 mg/day for adults, titrating the dose weekly in 5 mg increments for pediatrics and in 10 mg increments for adults. Doses above 30 mg/day in children and 40 mg/day in adults have not been studied. (2.1)
- For patients already using methylphenidate: Initiate Focalin XR therapy with half (1/2) the current total daily dose of methylphenidate. (2.2)
- Patients already using Focalin (dexmethylphenidate) immediate release: switch to the same daily dose of Focalin XR. (2.2)

DOSAGE FORMS AND STRENGTHS

Extended-release capsules: 5, 10, 15, 20, 25, 30, 35, and 40 mg (3)

CONTRAINDICATIONS

- Agitation, marked anxiety, and tension (4.1)
- Known hypersensitivity to methylphenidate or product components (4.2)
- Glaucoma (4.3)
- History of motor tics or a family history or diagnosis of Tourette's syndrome (4.4)
- During, or within a minimum of 14 days following discontinuation of treatment with a monoamine oxidase inhibitor (MAOI) (4.5)

WARNINGS AND PRECAUTIONS

- Serious Cardiovascular Events: Sudden death has been reported in association with CNS stimulant treatment at usual doses in children and adolescents with structural cardiac abnormalities or other serious heart problems. Sudden death, stroke, and myocardial infarction have been reported in adults taking stimulant drugs at usual doses for ADHD. Stimulant products generally should not be used in patients with known structural cardiac abnormalities, cardiomyopathy, serious heart rhythm abnormalities, coronary artery disease, or other serious heart problems. (5.1)
- Increased Blood Pressure and Heart Rate: have been reported. Monitor patients for changes in blood pressure and heart rate. Caution should be exercised in treating patients whose underlying medical conditions might be compromised by increases in blood pressure or heart rate. (5.2)
- Assess Cardiovascular Status: prior to stimulant treatment, assess for cardiac disease with history and exam and, if suggested by findings, conduct further cardiac evaluation. Patients with emerging symptoms suggestive of cardiac disease should undergo a prompt cardiac evaluation. (5.3)
- Psychotic Symptoms: may be exacerbated in patients with psychotic disorders. (5.4)
- Bipolar Disorder: Use with particular care in ADHD patients with comorbid Bipolar Disorder. Before initiating stimulant therapy, obtain a detailed psychiatric history for patients with comorbid depressive symptoms, in order to determine risk for Bipolar Disorder. (5.5)
- Emergence of New Psychotic or Manic Symptoms: Treatment-emergent psychotic or manic symptoms without a prior history can be caused by stimulants at usual doses. Discontinuation of stimulant therapy may be indicated. (5.6)
- Aggression: Monitor for appearance of or worsening of aggressive behavior or hostility. (5.7)
- Long-Term Suppression of Growth: monitor height and weight in pediatric patients at appropriate intervals. Patients who are not growing or gaining weight as expected may need to have their treatment interrupted. (5.8)
- Seizures: The threshold for seizures may be lowered. In the presence of seizure, discontinue treatment. (5.9)
- Peripheral Vasculopathy, including Raynaud's phenomenon: Stimulants used to treat ADHD are associated with peripheral vasculopathy, including Raynaud's phenomenon. Careful observation for digital changes is necessary during treatment with ADHD stimulants. (5.10)
- Visual Disturbance: difficulties with accommodation and blurring of vision have been reported with stimulant treatment. (5.11)
- Hematologic Monitoring: periodic monitoring of CBC with differential is advised during prolonged therapy. (5.13)

ADVERSE REACTIONS

Most common adverse reactions (at least 5% and twice the incidence among placebo-treated patients) are dyspepsia, decreased appetite, headache, and anxiety for pediatric patients and dry mouth, dyspepsia, headache, and anxiety for adult patients (6).

To report SUSPECTED ADVERSE REACTIONS, contact Novartis Pharmaceuticals Corporation at 1-888-669-6682 or FDA at 1-800-FDA-1088 or www.fda.gov/medwatch.

DRUG INTERACTIONS

- Focalin XR should not be used in patients being treated (currently or within the preceding two weeks) with MAO Inhibitors (4.5)
- Focalin XR should be used cautiously with pressor agents (7)
- Antacids or acid suppressants could alter the release of Focalin XR (7)
- Racemic methylphenidate may inhibit the metabolism of coumarin anticoagulants, anticonvulsants, and tricyclic drugs (7)

USE IN SPECIFIC POPULATIONS

- Focalin XR should not be used in **children under 6 years of age.** (5.11)
- Pregnancy: Limited human data. Based on animal data, may cause fetal harm. (8.1)
- Nursing Mothers: Caution should be exercised when administered to a nursing woman. (8.3)

See 17 for PATIENT COUNSELING INFORMATION and Medication Guide

Revised: 06/2013

FULL PRESCRIBING INFORMATION: CONTENTS*

*** Sections or subsections omitted from the full prescribing information are not listed**

FULL PRESCRIBING INFORMATION

WARNING: DRUG DEPENDENCE

Focalin XR should be given cautiously to patients with a history of drug dependence or alcoholism. Chronic abusive use can lead to marked tolerance and psychological dependence with varying degrees of abnormal behavior. Frank psychotic episodes can occur, especially with parenteral abuse. Careful supervision is required during withdrawal from abusive use, since severe depression may occur. Withdrawal following chronic therapeutic use may unmask symptoms of the underlying disorder that may require follow-up.

1 INDICATIONS AND USAGE

Focalin XR is indicated for the treatment of Attention Deficit Hyperactivity Disorder (ADHD) in patients aged 6 years and older.

The effectiveness of Focalin XR in the treatment of ADHD in patients aged 6 years and older was established in 2 placebo-controlled studies in patients meeting DSM-IV criteria for ADHD [*see Clinical Studies (14)*].

A diagnosis of Attention Deficit Hyperactivity Disorder (ADHD; DSM-IV) implies the presence of hyperactive-impulsive or inattentive symptoms that caused impairment and were present before age 7 years. The symptoms must cause clinically significant impairment, e.g., in social, academic, or occupational functioning, and be present in 2 or more settings, e.g., school (or work) and at home. The symptoms must not be better accounted for by another mental disorder. For the Inattentive Type, at least 6 of the following symptoms must have persisted for at least 6 months: lack of attention to details/careless mistakes; lack of sustained attention; poor listener; failure to follow through on tasks; poor organization; avoids tasks requiring sustained mental effort; loses things; easily distracted; forgetful. For the Hyperactive-Impulsive Type, at least 6 of the following symptoms must have persisted for at least 6 months: fidgeting/squirming; leaving seat; inappropriate running/climbing; difficulty with quiet activities; "on the go"; excessive talking; blurting answers; can't wait turn; intrusive. The Combined Types requires both inattentive and hyperactive-impulsive criteria to be met.

Special Diagnostic Considerations

Specific etiology of this syndrome is unknown, and there is no single diagnostic test. Adequate diagnosis requires the use not only of medical but of special psychological, educational, and social resources. Learning may or may not be impaired. The diagnosis must be based upon a complete history and evaluation of the child and not solely on the presence of the required number of DSM-IV characteristics.

Need for Comprehensive Treatment Program

Focalin XR is indicated as an integral part of a total treatment program for ADHD that may include other measures (psychological, educational, social) for patients with this syndrome. Drug treatment may not be indicated for all children with this syndrome. Stimulants are not intended for use in the child who exhibits symptoms secondary to environmental factors and/or other primary psychiatric disorders, including psychosis. Appropriate educational placement is essential and psychosocial intervention is often helpful. When remedial measures alone are insufficient, the decision to prescribe stimulant medication will depend upon the physician's assessment of the chronicity and severity of the child's symptoms.

Long-Term Use

The effectiveness of Focalin XR for long-term use, i.e., for more than 7 weeks, has not been systematically evaluated in controlled trials. Therefore, the physician who elects to use Focalin XR for extended periods should periodically reevaluate the long-term usefulness of the drug for the individual patient [*see Dosage and Administration (2.3)*].

2 DOSAGE AND ADMINISTRATION

Focalin XR is for oral administration once daily in the morning.

Focalin XR may be swallowed as whole capsules or alternatively may be administered by sprinkling the capsule contents on a small amount of applesauce (see specific instructions below). Focalin XR capsules and/or their contents should not be crushed, chewed, or divided.

The capsules may be carefully opened and the beads sprinkled over a spoonful of applesauce. The mixture of drug and applesauce should be consumed immediately in its entirety. The drug and applesauce mixture should not be stored for future use.

Dosage should be individualized according to the needs and responses of the patient.

2.1 Patients New to Methylphenidate

The recommended starting dose of Focalin XR for patients who are not currently taking dexmethylphenidate or racemic methylphenidate, or for patients who are on stimulants other than methylphenidate, is 5 mg/day for pediatric patients and 10 mg/day for adult patients.

Dosage may be adjusted in 5 mg increments for pediatric patients and in 10 mg increments for adult patients. In general, dosage adjustments may proceed at approximately weekly intervals. The patient should be observed for a sufficient duration at a given dose to ensure that a maximal benefit has been achieved before a dose increase is considered. In dose-response (fixed-dose) studies (pediatric from 10 to 30 mg/day and adult from 20 to 40 mg/day), all doses were effective vs. placebo. There was no clear finding, however, of greater average benefits for the higher doses compared to the lower doses. Adverse events and discontinuations, however, were dose-related. Doses above 30 mg/day in pediatrics and 40 mg/day in adults have not been studied and are not recommended.

2.2 Patients Currently Using Methylphenidate

For patients currently using methylphenidate, the recommended starting dose of Focalin XR is half the total daily dose of racemic methylphenidate. Patients currently using Focalin (dexmethylphenidate) may be switched to the same daily dose of Focalin XR.

2.3 Maintenance/Extended Treatment

There is no body of evidence available from controlled trials to indicate how long the patient with ADHD should be treated with Focalin XR. It is generally agreed, however, that pharmacological treatment of ADHD may be needed for extended periods. Nevertheless, the physician who elects to use Focalin XR for extended periods in patients with ADHD should periodically reevaluate the long-term usefulness of the drug for the individual patient with periods off medication to assess the patient's functioning without pharmacotherapy. Improvement may be sustained when the drug is either temporarily or permanently discontinued.

2.4 Dose Reduction and Discontinuation

If paradoxical aggravation of symptoms or other adverse events occur, the dosage should be reduced, or, if necessary, the drug should be discontinued.

If improvement is not observed after appropriate dosage adjustment over a 1-month period, the drug should be discontinued.

3 DOSAGE FORMS AND STRENGTHS

5 mg extended-release capsules
10 mg extended-release capsules
15 mg extended-release capsules
20 mg extended-release capsules
25 mg extended-release capsules
30 mg extended-release capsules
35 mg extended-release capsules
40 mg extended-release capsules

4 CONTRAINDICATIONS

4.1 Agitation

Focalin XR is contraindicated in patients with marked anxiety, tension, and agitation, since the drug may aggravate these symptoms.

4.2 Hypersensitivity to Methylphenidate

Focalin XR is contraindicated in patients known to be hypersensitive to methylphenidate, or other components of the product. Hypersensitivity reactions, including angioedema and anaphylactic reactions, have been observed in patients treated with methylphenidate [*see Adverse Reactions (6.5, 6.6)*].

4.3 Glaucoma

Focalin XR is contraindicated in patients with glaucoma.

4.4 Tics

Focalin XR is contraindicated in patients with motor tics or with a family history or diagnosis of Tourette's syndrome [*see Adverse Reactions (6.1)*].

4.5 Monoamine Oxidase Inhibitors

Focalin XR is contraindicated during treatment with monoamine oxidase inhibitors, and also within a minimum of 14 days following discontinuation of treatment with a monoamine oxidase inhibitor (hypertensive crises may result).

5 WARNINGS AND PRECAUTIONS

5.1 Sudden Death and Preexisting Structural Cardiac Abnormalities or Other Serious Heart Problems

Children and Adolescents

Sudden death has been reported in association with CNS stimulant treatment at usual doses in children and adolescents with structural cardiac abnormalities or other serious heart problems. Although some serious heart problems alone carry an increased risk of sudden death, stimulant products generally should not be used in children or adolescents with known serious structural cardiac abnormalities, cardiomyopathy, serious heart rhythm abnormalities, or other serious cardiac problems that may place them at increased vulnerability to the sympathomimetic effects of a stimulant drug.

Adults

Sudden death, stroke, and myocardial infarction have been reported in adults taking stimulant drugs at usual doses for ADHD. Although the role of stimulants in these adult cases is also unknown, adults have a greater likelihood than children of having serious structural cardiac abnormalities, cardiomyopathy, serious heart rhythm abnormalities, coronary artery disease, or other serious cardiac problems. Adults with such abnormalities should also generally not be treated with stimulant drugs.

5.2 Hypertension and Other Cardiovascular Conditions

Stimulant medications cause a modest increase in average blood pressure (about 2-4 mmHg) and average heart rate (about 3-6 bpm), and individuals may have larger increases. While the mean changes alone would not be expected to have short-term consequences, all patients should be monitored for larger changes in heart rate and blood pressure. Caution is indicated in treating patients whose underlying medical conditions might be compromised by increases in blood pressure or heart rate, e.g., those with preexisting hypertension, heart failure, recent myocardial infarction, or ventricular arrhythmia.

5.3 Assessing Cardiovascular Status in Patients being Treated with Stimulant Medications

Children, adolescents, or adults who are being considered for treatment with stimulant medications should have a careful history (including assessment for a family history of sudden death or ventricular arrhythmia) and physical exam to assess for the presence of cardiac disease, and should receive further cardiac evaluation if findings suggest such disease (e.g., electrocardiogram and echocardiogram). Patients who develop symptoms such as exertional chest pain, unexplained syncope, or other symptoms suggestive of cardiac disease during stimulant treatment should undergo a prompt cardiac evaluation.

5.4 Preexisting Psychosis

Administration of stimulants may exacerbate symptoms of behavior disturbance and thought disorder in patients with a preexisting psychotic disorder.

5.5 Bipolar Illness

Particular care should be taken in using stimulants to treat ADHD in patients with comorbid bipolar disorder because of concern for possible induction of a mixed/manic episode in such patients. Prior to initiating treatment with a stimulant, patients with comorbid depressive symptoms should be adequately screened to determine if they are at risk for bipolar disorder; such screening should include a detailed psychiatric history, including a family history of suicide, bipolar disorder, and depression.

5.6 Emergence of New Psychotic or Manic Symptoms

Treatment emergent psychotic or manic symptoms, e.g., hallucinations, delusional thinking, or mania in children and adolescents without a prior history of psychotic illness or mania can be caused by stimulants at usual doses. If such symptoms occur, consideration should be given to a possible causal role of the stimulant, and discontinuation of treatment may be appropriate. In a pooled analysis of multiple short-term, placebo-controlled studies, such symptoms occurred in about 0.1% (4 patients with events out of 3,482 exposed to methylphenidate or amphetamine for several weeks at usual doses) of stimulant-treated patients compared to 0 in placebo-treated patients.

5.7 Aggression

Aggressive behavior or hostility is often observed in children and adolescents with ADHD, and has been reported in clinical trials and the post marketing experience of some medications indicated for the treatment of ADHD. Although there is no systematic evidence that stimulants cause aggressive behavior or hostility, patients beginning treatment for ADHD should be monitored for the appearance of or worsening of aggressive behavior or hostility.

5.8 Long-Term Suppression of Growth

Careful follow-up of weight and height in children ages 7 to 10 years who were randomized to either methylphenidate or

Table 2. Dose-related Adverse Events from a Fixed-dose Study of Double-Blind Treatment in Pediatric Patients by Organ-System and Preferred Term

ADVERSE EVENT	Focalin XR 10 mg/d N=64	Focalin XR 20 mg/d N=60	Focalin XR 30 mg/d N=58	Placebo N=63
Gastrointestinal Disorders	22%	23%	29%	24%
Vomiting	2%	8%	9%	0
Metabolism and Nutritional Disorders	16%	17%	22%	5%
Anorexia	5%	5%	7%	0
Psychiatric Disorders	19%	20%	38%	8%
Insomnia	5%	8%	17%	3%
Depression	0	0	3%	0
Mood Swings	0	0	3%	2%
Other Adverse Events				
Irritability	0	2%	5%	0
Nasal Congestion	0	0	5%	0
Pruritus	0	0	3%	0

Table 3. Treatment-Emergent Adverse Events[1] Occurring During Double-Blind Treatment–Adults

	Focalin XR 20 mg N=57	Focalin XR 30 mg N=54	Focalin XR 40 mg N=54	Placebo N=53
No. of Patients with AEs				
Total	84%	94%	85%	68%
Primary System Organ Class/ Adverse Event Preferred Term				
Gastrointestinal Disorders	28%	32%	44%	19%
Dry Mouth	7%	20%	20%	4%
Dyspepsia	5%	9%	9%	2%
Nervous System Disorders	37%	39%	50%	28%
Headache	26%	30%	39%	19%
Psychiatric Disorders	40%	43%	46%	30%
Anxiety	5%	11%	11%	2%
Respiratory, Thoracic and Mediastinal Disorders	16%	9%	15%	8%
Pharyngolaryngeal Pain	4%	4%	7%	2%

[1]Events, regardless of causality, for which the incidence was at least 5% in a Focalin XR group and which appeared to increase with randomized dose. Incidence has been rounded to the nearest whole number.

nonmedication treatment groups over 14 months, as well as in naturalistic subgroups of newly methylphenidate-treated and nonmedication treated children over 36 months (to the ages of 10 to 13 years), suggests that consistently medicated children (i.e., treatment for 7 days per week throughout the year) have a temporary slowing in growth rate (on average, a total of about 2 cm less growth in height and 2.7 kg less growth in weight over 3 years), without evidence of growth rebound during this period of development. In the 7-week, double-blind, placebo-controlled study of Focalin XR, the mean weight gain was greater for patients receiving placebo (+0.4 kg) than for patients receiving Focalin XR (-0.5 kg). Published data are inadequate to determine whether chronic use of amphetamines may cause a similar suppression of growth, however, it is anticipated that they likely have this effect as well. Therefore, growth should be monitored during treatment with stimulants, and patients who are not growing or gaining height or weight as expected may need to have their treatment interrupted.

5.9 Seizures

There is some clinical evidence that stimulants may lower the convulsive threshold in patients with prior history of seizures, in patients with prior EEG abnormalities in absence of seizures, and, very rarely, in patients without a history of seizures and no prior EEG evidence of seizures. In the presence of seizures, the drug should be discontinued.

5.10 Peripheral Vasculopathy, Including Raynaud's Phenomenon

Stimulants, including Focalin XR, used to treat ADHD are associated with peripheral vasculopathy, including Raynaud's phenomenon. Signs and symptoms are usually intermittent and mild; however, very rare sequelae include digital ulceration and/or soft tissue breakdown. Effects of peripheral vasculopathy, including Raynaud's phenomenon, were observed in postmarketing reports at different times and at therapeutic doses in all age groups throughout the course of treatment. Signs and symptoms generally improve after reduction in dose or discontinuation of drug. Careful observation for digital changes is necessary during treating with ADHD stimulants. Further clinical evaluation (e.g., rheumatology referral) may be appropriate for certain patients.

5.11 Visual Disturbance

Difficulties with accommodation and blurring of vision have been reported with stimulant treatment.

5.12 Use in Children Under Six Years of Age

Focalin XR should not be used in children under 6 years of age, since safety and efficacy in this age group have not been established.

5.13 Hematologic Monitoring

Periodic CBC, differential, and platelet counts are advised during prolonged therapy.

6 ADVERSE REACTIONS

Focalin XR was administered to 46 children and 7 adolescents with ADHD for up to 7 weeks and 206 adults with ADHD in clinical studies. During the clinical studies, 101 adult patients were treated for at least 6 months.

Adverse events during exposure were obtained primarily by general inquiry and recorded by clinical investigators using terminology of their own choosing. Consequently, it is not possible to provide a meaningful estimate of the proportion of individuals experiencing adverse events without first grouping similar types of events into a smaller number of standardized event categories. In the tables and listings that follow, MedDRA terminology has been used to classify reported adverse events. The stated frequencies of adverse events represent the proportion of individuals who experienced, at least once, a treatment-emergent adverse event of the type listed. An event was considered treatment emergent if it occurred for the first time or worsened while receiving therapy following baseline evaluation.

6.1 Adverse Events Associated with Discontinuation of Treatment in Acute Clinical Studies with Focalin XR-Children

Overall, 50 of 684 children treated with Focalin immediate-release formulation (7.3%) experienced an adverse event that resulted in discontinuation. The most common reasons for discontinuation were twitching (described as motor or vocal tics), anorexia, insomnia, and tachycardia (approximately 1% each). None of the 53 Focalin XR-treated pediatric patients discontinued treatment due to adverse events in the 7-week, placebo-controlled study.

6.2 Adverse Events Occurring at an Incidence of 5% or More Among Focalin XR-Treated Patients-Children

Table 1 enumerates treatment-emergent adverse events for the placebo-controlled, parallel-group study in children and adolescents with ADHD at flexible Focalin XR doses of 5-30 mg/day. The table includes only those events that occurred in 5% or more of patients treated with Focalin XR and for which the incidence in patients treated with Focalin XR was at least twice the incidence in placebo-treated patients. The prescriber should be aware that these figures cannot be used to predict the incidence of adverse events in the course of usual medical practice where patient characteristics and other factors differ from those which prevailed in the clinical trials. Similarly, the cited frequencies cannot be compared with figures obtained from other clinical investigations involving different treatments, uses, and investigators. The cited figures, however, do provide the prescribing physician with some basis for estimating the relative contribution of drug and nondrug factors to the adverse event incidence rate in the population studied.

Table 1.Treatment-Emergent Adverse Events[1] Occurring During Double-Blind Treatment–Pediatric Patients

	Focalin XR N=53	Placebo N=47
No. of Patients with AEs		
Total	76%	57%
Primary System Organ Class/ Adverse Event Preferred Term		
Gastrointestinal Disorders	38%	19%
Dyspepsia	8%	4%
Metabolism and Nutrition Disorders	34%	11%
Decreased Appetite	30%	9%
Nervous System Disorders	30%	13%
Headache	25%	11%
Psychiatric Disorders	26%	15%
Anxiety	6%	0%

[1]Events, regardless of causality, for which the incidence for patients treated with Focalin XR was at least 5% and twice the incidence among placebo-treated patients. Incidence has been rounded to the nearest whole number.

Table 2 below enumerates the incidence of dose-related adverse events that occurred during a fixed-dose, double-blind, placebo-controlled trial of Focalin XR up to 30mg/day versus placebo in children and adolescents with ADHD.

[See table 2 above]

6.3 Adverse Events Associated with Discontinuation of Treatment in Clinical Studies with Focalin XR-Adults

In the adult placebo-controlled study, 10.7% of the Focalin XR-treated patients and 7.5% of the placebo-treated patients discontinued for adverse events. Among Focalin XR-treated patients, insomnia (1.8%, n=3), feeling jittery (1.8%, n=3), anorexia (1.2%, n=2), and anxiety (1.2%, n=2) were the reasons for discontinuation reported by more than 1 patient.

6.4 Adverse Events Occurring at an Incidence of 5% or More Among Focalin XR-Treated Patients-Adults

Table 3 enumerates treatment-emergent adverse events for the placebo-controlled, parallel-group study in adults with ADHD at fixed Focalin XR doses of 20, 30, and 40 mg/day. The table includes only those events that occurred in 5% or more of patients in a Focalin XR dose group and for which the incidences in patients treated with Focalin XR appeared to increase with dose. The prescriber should be aware that these figures cannot be used to predict the incidence of adverse events in the course of usual medical practice where patient characteristics and other factors differ from those which prevailed in the clinical trials. Similarly, the cited frequencies cannot be compared with figures obtained from other clinical investigations involving different treatments, uses, and investigators. The cited figures, however, do provide the prescribing physician with some basis for estimating the relative contribution of drug and non-drug factors to the adverse event incidence rate in the population studied.

[See table 3 above]

Two other adverse reactions occurring in clinical trials with Focalin XR at a frequency greater than placebo, but which were not dose related were: feeling jittery (12% and 2%, respectively) and dizziness (6% and 2%, respectively).

Table 4 summarizes changes in vital signs and weight that were recorded in the adult study (N=218) of Focalin XR in the treatment of ADHD.

[See table 4 at top of next page]

6.5 Postmarketing Experience

The following additional adverse reactions have been identified during postapproval use of Focalin XR. Because these reactions are reported voluntarily from a population of uncertain size, it is not always possible to reliably estimate their frequency:

Immune System Disorders: hypersensitivity reactions, including angioedema and anaphylaxis

6.6 Adverse Events with Other Methylphenidate HCl Dosage Forms

Nervousness and insomnia are the most common adverse reactions reported with other methylphenidate products. In children, loss of appetite, abdominal pain, weight loss during prolonged therapy, insomnia, and tachycardia may occur more frequently; however, any of the other adverse reactions listed below may also occur.

Other reactions include:

Cardiac: angina, arrhythmia, palpitations, pulse increased or decreased, tachycardia

Gastrointestinal: abdominal pain, nausea

Immune: hypersensitivity reactions including skin rash, urticaria, fever, arthralgia, exfoliative dermatitis, erythema multiforme with histopathological findings of necrotizing vasculitis, and thrombocytopenic purpura
Metabolism/Nutrition: anorexia, weight loss during prolonged therapy
Nervous System: dizziness, drowsiness, dyskinesia, headache, rare reports of Tourette's syndrome, toxic psychosis
Vascular: blood pressure increased or decreased, cerebral arteritis and/or occlusion

Although a definite causal relationship has not been established, the following have been reported in patients taking methylphenidate:
Blood/Lymphatic: leukopenia and/or anemia
Hepatobiliary: abnormal liver function, ranging from transaminase elevation to hepatic coma
Psychiatric: transient depressed mood, aggressive behavior
Skin/Subcutaneous: scalp hair loss

Very rare reports of neuroleptic malignant syndrome (NMS) have been received, and, in most of these, patients were concurrently receiving therapies associated with NMS. In a single report, a 10-year-old boy who had been taking methylphenidate for approximately 18 months experienced an NMS-like event within 45 minutes of ingesting his first dose of venlafaxine. It is uncertain whether this case represented a drug-drug interaction, a response to either drug alone, or some other cause.

7 DRUG INTERACTIONS

Focalin XR should not be used in patients being treated (currently or within the preceding 2 weeks) with MAO Inhibitors [*see Contraindications (4.5)*].

Because of possible effects on blood pressure, Focalin XR should be used cautiously with pressor agents.

Methylphenidate may decrease the effectiveness of drugs used to treat hypertension.

Dexmethylphenidate is metabolized primarily to *d*-ritalinic acid by de-esterification and not through oxidative pathways.

The effects of gastrointestinal pH alterations on the absorption of dexmethylphenidate from Focalin XR have not been studied. Since the modified release characteristics of Focalin XR are pH dependent, the coadministration of antacids or acid suppressants could alter the release of dexmethylphenidate.

Human pharmacologic studies have shown that racemic methylphenidate may inhibit the metabolism of coumarin anticoagulants, anticonvulsants (e.g., phenobarbital, phenytoin, primidone), and tricyclic drugs (e.g., imipramine, clomipramine, desipramine). Downward dose adjustments of these drugs may be required when given concomitantly with methylphenidate. It may be necessary to adjust the dosage and monitor plasma drug concentration (or, in the case of coumarin, coagulation times), when initiating or discontinuing methylphenidate.

8 USE IN SPECIFIC POPULATIONS

8.1 Pregnancy

Pregnancy Category C

There are no adequate and well controlled studies of Focalin in pregnant women. Dexmethylphenidate did not cause major malformations in rats or rabbits; however, it did cause delayed skeletal ossification and decreased postweaning weight gain in rats. Focalin XR should be used during pregnancy only if the potential benefit justifies the potential risk to the fetus.

In studies conducted in rats and rabbits, dexmethylphenidate was administered orally at doses of up to 20 and 100 mg/kg/day, respectively, during the period of organogenesis. No evidence of teratogenic activity was found in either the rat or rabbit study; however, delayed fetal skeletal ossification was observed at the highest dose level in rats. When dexmethylphenidate was administered to rats throughout pregnancy and lactation at doses of up to 20 mg/kg/day, postweaning body weight gain was decreased in male offspring at the highest dose, but no other effects on postnatal development were observed. At the highest doses tested, plasma levels (AUCs) of dexmethylphenidate in pregnant rats and rabbits were approximately 5 and 1 times, respectively, those in adults dosed with 20 mg/day.

Racemic methylphenidate has been shown to have teratogenic effects in rabbits when given in doses of 200 mg/kg/day throughout organogenesis.

8.2 Labor and Delivery

Focalin XR has not been studied in labor and delivery.

8.3 Nursing Mothers

It is not known whether dexmethylphenidate is excreted in human milk. Because many drugs are excreted in human milk, caution should be exercised if Focalin XR is administered to a nursing woman. Information from 4 published case reports on the use of racemic methylphenidate during breastfeeding suggest that at maternal doses of 35-80 mg/day, milk concentrations of methylphenidate range from undetectable to 15.4 ng/mL. Based on these limited data, the calculated infant daily dose for an exclusively breastfed infant would be about 0.4-2.9 μg/kg/day or about 0.2-0.7% of the maternal weight adjusted dose.

Table 4. Changes (Mean ± SD) in Vital Signs and Weight by Randomized Dose During Double-Blind Treatment-Adults

	Focalin XR 20 mg (N=57)	Focalin XR 30 mg (N=54)	Focalin XR 40 mg (N=54)	Placebo (N=53)
Pulse (bpm)	3.1 ± 11.1	4.3 ± 11.7	6.0 ± 10.1	-1.4 ± 9.3
Diastolic BP (mmHg)	-0.2 ± 8.2	1.2 ± 8.9	2.1 ± 8.0	0.3 ± 7.8
Weight (kg)	-1.4 ± 2.0	-1.2 ± 1.9	-1.7 ± 2.3	-0.1 ± 3.9

8.4 Pediatric Use

The safety and efficacy of Focalin XR in children under 6 years old have not been established. Long-term effects of Focalin in children have not been well established [*see Warnings and Precautions (5.11)*].

In a study conducted in young rats, racemic methylphenidate was administered orally at doses of up to 100 mg/kg/day for 9 weeks, starting early in the postnatal period (Postnatal Day 7) and continuing through sexual maturity (Postnatal Week 10). When these animals were tested as adults (Postnatal Weeks 13-14), decreased spontaneous locomotor activity was observed in males and females previously treated with 50 mg/kg/day (approximately 6 times the maximum recommended human dose [MRHD] of racemic methylphenidate on a mg/m^2 basis) or greater, and a deficit in the acquisition of a specific learning task was seen in females exposed to the highest dose (12 times the racemic MRHD on a mg/m^2 basis). The no effect level for juvenile neurobehavioral development in rats was 5 mg/kg/day (half the racemic MRHD on a mg/m^2 basis). The clinical significance of the long-term behavioral effects observed in rats is unknown.

8.5 Geriatric Use

Focalin XR has not been studied in the geriatric population.

9 DRUG ABUSE AND DEPENDENCE

9.1 Controlled Substance Class

Focalin XR, like other methylphenidate products, is classified as a Schedule II controlled substance by Federal regulation.

9.2 Abuse, Dependence, Tolerance

See the complete boxed warning for drug abuse and dependence information at the beginning of *Full Prescribing Information.*

10 OVERDOSAGE

10.1 Signs and Symptoms

Signs and symptoms of acute methylphenidate overdosage, resulting principally from overstimulation of the CNS and from excessive sympathomimetic effects, may include the following: vomiting, agitation, tremors, hyperreflexia, muscle twitching, convulsions (may be followed by coma), euphoria, confusion, hallucinations, delirium, sweating, flushing, headache, hyperpyrexia, tachycardia, palpitations, cardiac arrhythmias, hypertension, mydriasis, and dryness of mucous membranes.

10.2 Poison Control Center

The physician may wish to consider contacting a poison control center for up-to-date information on the management of overdosage with methylphenidate.

10.3 Recommended Treatment

As with the management of all overdosage, the possibility of multiple drug ingestion should be considered.

When treating overdose, practitioners should bear in mind that there is a prolonged release of dexmethylphenidate from Focalin XR.

Treatment consists of appropriate supportive measures. The patient must be protected against self-injury and against external stimuli that would aggravate overstimulation already present. Gastric contents may be evacuated by gastric lavage as indicated. Before performing gastric lavage, control agitation and seizures if present and protect the airway. Other measures to detoxify the gut include administration of activated charcoal and a cathartic. Intensive care must be provided to maintain adequate circulation and respiratory exchange; external cooling procedures may be required for hyperpyrexia.

Efficacy of peritoneal dialysis for Focalin overdosage has not been established.

11 DESCRIPTION

Focalin XR is an extended-release formulation of dexmethylphenidate with a bi-modal release profile. Focalin XR uses the proprietary SODAS® (Spheroidal Oral Drug Absorption System) technology. Each bead-filled Focalin XR capsule contains half the dose as immediate-release beads and half as enteric-coated, delayed-release beads, thus providing an immediate release of dexmethylphenidate and a second delayed release of dexmethylphenidate. Focalin XR is available as 5, 10, 15, 20, 25, 30, 35, and 40 mg extended-release capsules. Focalin XR 5, 10, 15, 20, 25, 30, 35, and 40 mg extended-release capsules provide in a single dose the same amount of dexmethylphenidate as dosages of 2.5, 5, 7.5, 10, 12.5, 15, 17.5, or 20 mg of Focalin given b.i.d. as tablets.

Dexmethylphenidate hydrochloride, the *d-threo* enantiomer of racemic methylphenidate hydrochloride, is a central nervous system (CNS) stimulant.

Dexmethylphenidate hydrochloride is methyl α-phenyl-2-piperidineacetate hydrochloride, (R,R')-(+)-. Its empirical formula is $C_{14}H_{19}NO_2 \bullet HCl$. Its molecular weight is 269.77 and its structural formula is:

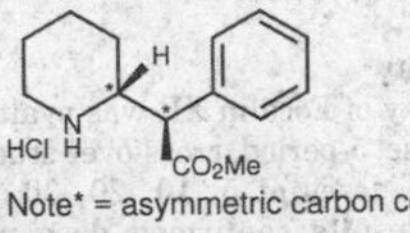

Note* = asymmetric carbon center

Dexmethylphenidate hydrochloride is a white to off white powder. Its solutions are acid to litmus. It is freely soluble in water and in methanol, soluble in alcohol, and slightly soluble in chloroform and in acetone.

Inactive ingredients: ammonio methacrylate copolymer, FD&C Blue #2 (5 mg, 15 mg, 25 mg, 35 mg, and 40 mg strengths), FDA/E172 yellow iron oxide (10 mg, 15 mg, 30 mg, 35 mg, and 40 mg strengths), gelatin, ink Tan SW-8010, methacrylic acid copolymer, polyethylene glycol, sugar spheres, talc, titanium dioxide, and triethyl citrate.

12 CLINICAL PHARMACOLOGY

12.1 Mechanism of Action

Dexmethylphenidate hydrochloride, the active ingredient in Focalin XR, is a central nervous system stimulant. Dexmethylphenidate, the more pharmacologically active *d*-enantiomer of racemic methylphenidate, is thought to block the reuptake of norepinephrine and dopamine into the presynaptic neuron and increase the release of these monoamines into the extraneuronal space. The mode of therapeutic action in Attention Deficit Hyperactivity Disorder (ADHD) is not known.

12.2 Pharmacodynamics

Effects on QT Interval

The effect of Focalin XR on the QT interval was evaluated in a double-blind, placebo- and open-label active (moxifloxacin)-controlled study following single doses of Focalin XR 40mg in 75 healthy volunteers. ECGs were collected up to 12 hours postdose. Frederica's method for heart rate correction was employed to derive the corrected QT interval (QTcF). The maximum mean prolongation of QTcF intervals was <5 ms, and the upper limit of the 90% confidence interval was below 10 ms for all time matched comparisons versus placebo. This was below the threshold of clinical concern and there was no evident-exposure response relationship.

12.3 Pharmacokinetics

Absorption

Focalin XR produces a bi-modal plasma concentration-time profile (i.e., 2 distinct peaks approximately 4 hours apart) when orally administered to healthy adults. The initial rate of absorption for Focalin XR is similar to that of Focalin tablets as shown by the similar rate parameters between the 2 formulations, i.e., first peak concentration (C_{max1}), and time to the first peak (t_{max1}), which is reached in 1.5 hours (typical range 1-4 hours). The mean time to the interpeak minimum (t_{minip}) is slightly shorter, and time to the second peak (t_{max2}) is slightly longer for Focalin XR given once daily (about 6.5 hours, range 4.5-7 hours) compared to Focalin tablets given in 2 doses 4 hours apart (see Figure 1), although the ranges observed are greater for Focalin XR.

Focalin XR given once daily exhibits a lower second peak concentration (C_{max2}), higher interpeak minimum concentrations (C_{minip}), and fewer peak and trough fluctuations than Focalin tablets given in 2 doses given 4 hours apart. This is due to an earlier onset and more prolonged absorption from the delayed-release beads (see Figure 1).

The AUC (exposure) after administration of Focalin XR given once daily is equivalent to the same total dose of Focalin tablets given in 2 doses 4 hours apart. The variability in C_{max}, C_{min}, and AUC is similar between Focalin XR and Focalin IR with approximately a 3-fold range in each.

Radiolabeled racemic methylphenidate is well absorbed after oral administration with approximately 90% of the radioactivity recovered in urine. However, due to first pass metabolism the mean absolute bioavailability of dexmethylphenidate when administered in various formulations was 22%-25%.

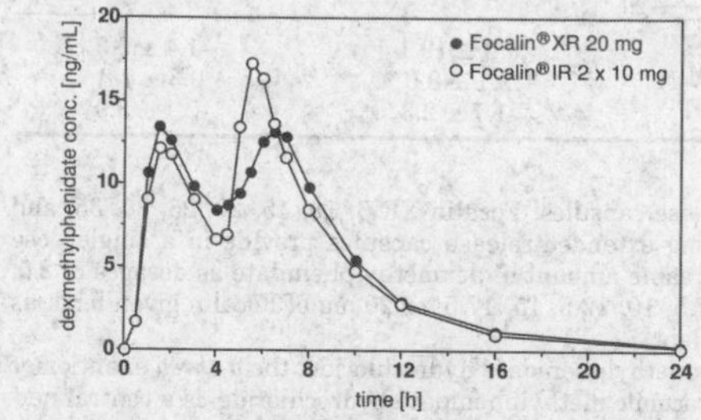

Figure 1. Mean Dexmethylphenidate Plasma Concentration-Time Profiles After Administration of 1 x 20 mg Focalin XR (n=24) Capsules and 2 x 10 mg Focalin Immediate-Release Tablets (n=25)

Dose Proportionality

Dose proportionality of Focalin XR was evaluated in a randomized, single-dose, 5-period, cross-over study with administration of single doses of 5, 10, 20, 30, and 40 mg to healthy adults. Results confirmed dose proportionality within this dose range.

Food Effects

Administration times relative to meals and meal composition may need to be individually titrated.

No food effect study was performed with Focalin XR. However, the effect of food has been studied in adults with racemic methylphenidate in the same type of extended-release formulation. The findings of that study are considered applicable to Focalin XR. After a high fat breakfast, there was a longer lag time until absorption began and variable delays in the time until the first peak concentration, the time until the interpeak minimum, and the time until the second peak. The first peak concentration and the extent of absorption were unchanged after food relative to the fasting state, although the second peak was approximately 25% lower. The effect of a high fat lunch was not examined. There is no evidence of dose dumping in the presence or absence of food. There were no differences in the plasma concentration-time profile, when administered with applesauce, compared to administration in the fasting condition. The results are expected not to differ for Focalin XR.

For patients unable to swallow the capsule, the contents may be sprinkled on applesauce and administered [*see Dosage and Administration (2)*].

Distribution

The plasma protein binding of dexmethylphenidate is not known; racemic methylphenidate is bound to plasma proteins by 12%-15%, independent of concentration. Dexmethylphenidate shows a volume of distribution of 2.65±1.11 L/kg. Plasma dexmethylphenidate concentrations decline monophasically following oral administration of Focalin XR.

Metabolism and Excretion

In humans, dexmethylphenidate is metabolized primarily to *d*-α-phenyl-piperidine acetic acid (also known as *d*-ritalinic acid) by de-esterification. This metabolite has little or no pharmacological activity. There is no *in vivo* interconversion to the *l-threo*-enantiomer, based on a finding of no levels of *l-threo*-methylphenidate being detectable after administration of up to 40 mg dexmethylphenidate in adults. After oral dosing of radiolabeled racemic methylphenidate in humans, about 90% of the radioactivity was recovered in urine. The main urinary metabolite of racemic (*d,l*-) methylphenidate was *d,l*-ritalinic acid, accountable for approximately 80% of the dose. Urinary excretion of parent compound accounted for 0.5% of an intravenous dose.

In vitro studies showed that dexmethylphenidate did not inhibit cytochrome P450 isoenzymes at concentrations observed after therapeutic doses.

Intravenous dexmethylphenidate was eliminated with a mean clearance of 0.40±0.12 $L/kg.h^{-1}$ corresponding to 0.56±0.18 L/min. The mean terminal elimination half-life of dexmethylphenidate was just over 3 hours in healthy adults and typically varied between 2 and 4.5 hours with an occasional subject exhibiting a terminal half-life between 5 and 7 hours. Children tend to have slightly shorter half-lives with means of 2–3 hours.

Special Populations

Gender

After administration of Focalin XR the first peak, (C_{max1}), was on average 45% higher in women. The interpeak minimum and the second peak also tended to be slightly higher in women although the difference was not statistically significant, and these patterns remained even after weight normalization. Pharmacokinetic parameters for dexmethylphenidate after Focalin immediate-release tablets were similar for boys and girls.

Race

There is insufficient experience with the use of Focalin XR to detect ethnic variations in pharmacokinetics.

Age

The pharmacokinetics of dexmethylphenidate after Focalin XR administration have not been studied in children less than 18 years of age. When a similar formulation of racemic methylphenidate was examined in 15 children between 10 and 12 years of age and 3 children with ADHD between 7 and 9 years of age, the time to the first peak was similar, although the time until the between peak minimum, and the time until the second peak were delayed and more variable in children compared to adults. After administration of the same dose to children and adults, concentrations in children were approximately twice the concentrations observed in adults. This higher exposure is almost completely due to smaller body size as no relevant age-related differences in dexmethylphenidate pharmacokinetic parameters (i.e., clearance and volume of distribution) are observed after normalization to dose and weight.

Renal Insufficiency

There is no experience with the use of Focalin XR in patients with renal insufficiency. After oral administration of radiolabeled racemic methylphenidate in humans, methylphenidate was extensively metabolized and approximately 80% of the radioactivity was excreted in the urine in the form of racemic ritalinic acid which is pharmacologically inactive. Very little unchanged drug is excreted in the urine, thus renal insufficiency is expected to have little effect on the pharmacokinetics of Focalin XR.

Hepatic Insufficiency

There is no experience with the use of Focalin XR in patients with hepatic insufficiency [*see Drug Interactions (7)*].

13 NONCLINICAL TOXICOLOGY

13.1 Carcinogenesis, Mutagenesis, and Impairment of Fertility

Carcinogenesis

Lifetime carcinogenicity studies have not been carried out with dexmethylphenidate. In a lifetime carcinogenicity study carried out in B6C3F1 mice, racemic methylphenidate caused an increase in hepatocellular adenomas, and in males only, an increase in hepatoblastomas at a daily dose of approximately 60 mg/kg/day. Hepatoblastoma is a relatively rare rodent malignant tumor type. There was no increase in total malignant hepatic tumors. The mouse strain used is sensitive to the development of hepatic tumors, and the significance of these results to humans is unknown.

Racemic methylphenidate did not cause any increase in tumors in a lifetime carcinogenicity study carried out in F344 rats; the highest dose used was approximately 45 mg/kg/day.

In a 24-week study of racemic methylphenidate in the transgenic mouse strain p53+/-, which is sensitive to genotoxic carcinogens, there was no evidence of carcinogenicity. Mice were fed diets containing the same concentrations as in the lifetime carcinogenicity study; the high-dose group was exposed to 60-74 mg/kg/day of racemic methylphenidate.

Mutagenesis

Dexmethylphenidate was not mutagenic in the *in vitro* Ames reverse mutation assay, the *in vitro* mouse lymphoma cell forward mutation assay, or the *in vivo* mouse bone marrow micronucleus test.

Racemic methylphenidate was not mutagenic in the *in vitro* Ames reverse mutation assay or the *in vitro* mouse lymphoma cell forward mutation assay, and was negative *in vivo* in the mouse bone marrow micronucleus assay. However, sister chromatid exchanges and chromosome aberrations were increased, indicative of a weak clastogenic response, in an *in vitro* assay of racemic methylphenidate in cultured Chinese Hamster Ovary (CHO) cells.

Impairment of Fertility

Racemic methylphenidate did not impair fertility in male or female mice that were fed diets containing the drug in an 18-week Continuous Breeding study. The study was conducted at doses of up to 160 mg/kg/day.

14 CLINICAL STUDIES

The effectiveness of Focalin XR in the treatment of ADHD was established in randomized, double-blind, placebo-controlled studies in children and adolescents and in adults who met Diagnostic and Statistical Manual 4th edition (DSM-IV) criteria for ADHD [*see Indications and Usage (1)*].

14.1 Children and Adolescents

The effectiveness of Focalin XR was established in a randomized, double-blind, placebo-controlled, parallel-group study in 103 pediatric patients (ages 6 to 12, n=86; ages 13 to 17, n=17) who met DSM-IV criteria for ADHD. Patients were randomized to receive either a flexible dose of Focalin XR (5 to 30 mg/day) or placebo once daily for 7 weeks. During the first 5 weeks of treatment patients were titrated to their optimal dose and in the last 2 weeks of the study patients remained on their optimal dose without dose changes or interruption.

Signs and symptoms of ADHD were evaluated by comparing the mean change from baseline to endpoint for Focalin XR– and placebo-treated patients using an intent-to-treat analysis of the primary efficacy outcome measure, the DSM-IV total subscale score of the Conners ADHD/DSM-IV Scales for teachers (CADS-T).

There was a statistically significant treatment effect in favor of Focalin XR. There were insufficient adolescents enrolled in this study to assess the efficacy for Focalin XR in the adolescent population. However, pharmacokinetic considerations and evidence of effectiveness of immediate-release Focalin in adolescents support the effectiveness of Focalin XR in this population.

In 2 additional studies in pediatric patients aged 6-12 years who received 20 mg Focalin XR or placebo in a cross-over design, Focalin XR was found to have a statistically significant treatment effect versus placebo on the Swanson, Kotkin, Agler, M-Flynn & Pelham (SKAMP) rating scale combined score at all time points after dosing in each study (0.5, 1, 3, 4, 5, 7, 9, 10, 11, and 12 hours in one study and 1, 2, 4, 6, 8, 9, 10, 11, and 12 hours in the other study). A treatment effect was also observed 0.5 hours after administration of Focalin XR 20 mg in an additional study of ADHD patients aged 6-12 years. The SKAMP is a reliable and validated scale that assesses specific classroom behaviors related to attention (e.g., getting started, sticking with activities, completing work, and stopping for transition) and deportment or behavior (e.g., remaining quiet, remaining seated, interacting with other students, and interacting with the teacher.) Each item is rated on a 7-point impairment scale, and an average rating per item is calculated for the subscales of Attention and Deportment.

14.2 Adults

The effectiveness of Focalin XR was established in a randomized, double-blind, placebo-controlled, parallel-group study in 221 adult patients (ages 18 to 60) who met DSM-IV criteria for ADHD. Patients were randomized to receive either a fixed dose of Focalin XR (20, 30, or 40 mg/day) or placebo once daily for 5 weeks. Patients randomized to Focalin XR were initiated on a 10 mg/day starting dose and titrated in increments of 10 mg/week to the randomly assigned fixed dose. Patients were maintained on their fixed dose (20, 30, or 40 mg/day) for a minimum of 2 weeks.

Signs and symptoms of ADHD were evaluated by comparing the mean change from baseline to endpoint for Focalin XR– and placebo-treated patients using an intent-to-treat analysis of the primary efficacy outcome measure, the investigator-administered DSM-IV Attention-Deficit/Hyperactivity Disorder Rating Scale (DSM-IV ADHD RS).

All three Focalin XR doses were statistically significantly superior to placebo. There was no obvious increase in effectiveness with increasing dose.

15 REFERENCES

American Psychiatric Association. Diagnosis and Statistical Manual of Mental Disorders. 4th ed. Washington DC: American Psychiatric Association 1994.

16 HOW SUPPLIED/STORAGE AND HANDLING

5 mg Extended-Release Capsules (NDC 0078-0430-05) light-blue, (imprinted NVR D5) supplied in bottles of 100

10 mg Extended-Release Capsules (NDC 0078-0431-05) light caramel (imprinted NVR D10) supplied in bottles of 100

15 mg Extended-Release Capsules (NDC 0078-0493-05) green (imprinted NVR D15) supplied in bottles of 100

20 mg Extended-Release Capsules (NDC 0078-0432-05) white (imprinted NVR D20) supplied in bottles of 100

25 mg Extended-Release Capsules (NDC 0078-0608-05) light-blue and white (imprinted NVR D25) supplied in bottles of 100

30 mg Extended-Release Capsules (NDC 0078-0433-05) light caramel and white (imprinted NVR D30) supplied in bottles of 100

35 mg Extended-Release Capsules (NDC 0078-0609-05) light-blue and light caramel (imprinted NVR D35) supplied in bottles of 100

40 mg Extended-Release Capsules (NDC 0078-0434-05) green and white (imprinted NVR D40) supplied in bottles of 100

Store FOCALIN XR at 25°C (77°F), excursions permitted 15°-30°C (59°-86°F). [See USP Controlled Room Temperature.]

Dispense in tight container (USP).

17 PATIENT COUNSELING INFORMATION

17.1 Information for Patients

Prescribers or other health professionals should inform patients, their families, and their caregivers about the benefits and risks associated with treatment with dexmethylphenidate and should counsel them in its appropriate use. A patient Medication Guide is available for Focalin XR. The prescriber or health professional should instruct patients, their families, and their caregivers to read the Medication Guide and should assist them in understanding its contents. Patients should be given the opportunity to discuss the contents of the Medication Guide and to obtain answers to any questions they may have. The complete text of the Medication Guide is reprinted at the end of this document.

Circulation problems in fingers and toes [Peripheral vasculopathy, including Raynaud's phenomenon]

- Instruct patients beginning treatment with Focalin XR about the risk of peripheral vasculopathy, including Raynaud's Phenomenon, and associated signs and symptoms: fingers or toes may feel numb, cool, painful, and/or may change color from pale, to blue, to red.
- Instruct patients to report to their physician any new numbness, pain, skin color change, or sensitivity to temperature in fingers or toes.
- **Instruct patients to call their physician immediately with any signs of unexplained wounds appearing on fingers or toes while taking Focalin XR.**
- Further clinical evaluation (e.g., rheumatology referral) may be appropriate for certain patients.

T2013-55
June 2013

MEDICATION GUIDE
FOCALIN XR
(dexmethylphenidate hydrochloride) extended-release capsules CII

Read the Medication Guide that comes with FOCALIN XR before you or your child starts taking it and each time you get a refill. There may be new information. This Medication Guide does not take the place of talking to your doctor about your or your child's treatment with FOCALIN XR.

What is the most important information I should know about FOCALIN XR?

The following have been reported with use of dexmethylphenidate hydrochloride and other stimulant medicines.

1. Heart-related problems:

- **sudden death in patients who have heart problems or heart defects**
- **stroke and heart attack in adults**
- **increased blood pressure and heart rate**

Tell your doctor if you or your child have any heart problems, heart defects, high blood pressure, or a family history of these problems.

Your doctor should check you or your child carefully for heart problems before starting FOCALIN XR.

Your doctor should check your or your child's blood pressure and heart rate regularly during treatment with FOCALIN XR.

Call your doctor right away if you or your child has any signs of heart problems such as chest pain, shortness of breath, or fainting while taking FOCALIN XR.

2. Mental (Psychiatric) problems:

All Patients

- **new or worse behavior and thought problems**
- **new or worse bipolar illness**
- **new or worse aggressive behavior or hostility**

Children and Teenagers

- **new psychotic symptoms (such as hearing voices, believing things that are not true, are suspicious) or new manic symptoms**

Tell your doctor about any mental problems you or your child have, or about a family history of suicide, bipolar illness, or depression.

Call your doctor right away if you or your child have any new or worsening mental symptoms or problems while taking FOCALIN XR, especially seeing or hearing things that are not real, believing things that are not real, or are suspicious.

3. Circulation problems in fingers and toes [Peripheral vasculopathy, including Raynaud's phenomenon]: fingers or toes may feel numb, cool, painful, and/or may change color from pale, to blue, to red.

- Tell your doctor if you have or your child has numbness, pain, skin color change, or sensitivity to temperature in the fingers or toes.
- **Call your doctor right away if you have or your child has any signs of unexplained wounds appearing on fingers or toes while taking FOCALIN XR.**

What Is FOCALIN XR?

FOCALIN XR is a central nervous system stimulant prescription medicine. **It is used for the treatment of attention deficit and hyperactivity disorder (ADHD).** FOCALIN XR may help increase attention and decrease impulsiveness and hyperactivity in patients with ADHD.

FOCALIN XR should be used as a part of a total treatment program for ADHD that may include counseling or other therapies.

FOCALIN XR is a federally controlled substance (CII) because it can be abused or lead to dependence. Keep FOCALIN XR in a safe place to prevent misuse and abuse. Selling or giving away FOCALIN XR may harm others, and is against the law.

Tell your doctor if you or your child have (or have a family history of) ever abused or been dependent on alcohol, prescription medicines or street drugs.

Who should not take FOCALIN XR?

FOCALIN XR should not be taken if you or your child:

- are very anxious, tense, or agitated.
- have an eye problem called glaucoma.
- have tics or Tourette's syndrome, or a family history of Tourette's syndrome. Tics are hard-to-control repeated movements or sounds.
- are taking or have taken within the past 14 days an anti-depression medicine called a monoamine oxidase inhibitor or MAOI.
- are allergic to anything in FOCALIN XR. See the end of this Medication Guide for a complete list of ingredients.

FOCALIN XR should not be used in children less than 6 years old because it has not been studied in this age group.

FOCALIN XR may not be right for you or your child. Before starting FOCALIN XR tell your or your child's doctor about all health conditions (or a family history of) including:

- heart problems, heart defects, high blood pressure
- mental problems including psychosis, mania, bipolar illness, or depression
- tics or Tourette's syndrome
- seizures or have had an abnormal brain wave test (EEG)
- circulation problems in fingers or toes

Tell your doctor if you or your child is pregnant, planning to become pregnant, or breastfeeding.

Can FOCALIN XR be taken with other medicines?

Tell your doctor about all of the medicines that you or your child takes including prescription and nonprescription medicines, vitamins, and herbal supplements. FOCALIN XR and some medicines may interact with each other and cause serious side effects. Sometimes the doses of other medicines will need to be adjusted while taking FOCALIN XR.

Your doctor will decide whether FOCALIN XR can be taken with other medicines.

Especially tell your doctor if you or your child takes:

- anti-depression medicines including MAOIs
- seizure medicines
- blood thinner medicines
- blood pressure medicines
- antacids
- cold or allergy medicines that contain decongestants

Know the medicines that you or your child takes. Keep a list of your medicines with you to show your doctor and pharmacist.

Do not start any new medicine while taking FOCALIN XR without talking to your doctor first.

How should FOCALIN XR be taken?

- **Take FOCALIN XR exactly as prescribed.** Your doctor may adjust the dose until it is right for you or your child.
- Take FOCALIN XR once each day in the morning. FOCALIN XR is an extended-release capsule. It releases medicine into your body throughout the day.
- FOCALIN XR can be taken with or without food. Taking FOCALIN XR with food may slow the time it takes for the medicine to start working.
- Swallow FOCALIN XR capsules whole with water or other liquids. **Do not chew, crush, or divide the capsules or the beads in the capsule.** If you or your child cannot swallow the capsule, open it and sprinkle the small beads of medicine over a spoonful of applesauce and swallow it right away without chewing.
- From time to time, your doctor may stop FOCALIN XR treatment for a while to check ADHD symptoms.
- Your doctor may do regular checks of the blood, heart, and blood pressure while taking FOCALIN XR. Children should have their height and weight checked often while taking FOCALIN XR. FOCALIN XR treatment may be stopped if a problem is found during these check-ups.
- **If you or your child takes too much FOCALIN XR or overdoses, call your doctor or poison control center right away, or get emergency treatment.**

What are possible side effects of FOCALIN XR?

See **"What is the most important information I should know about FOCALIN XR?"** for information on reported heart and mental problems.

Other serious side effects include:

- Serious allergic reactions (symptoms can be difficulty breathing, swelling of the face, neck and throat, rashes and hives, fever)
- slowing of growth (height and weight) in children
- seizures, mainly in patients with a history of seizures
- eyesight changes or blurred vision

Common side effects include:

• headache	• decreased appetite
• upset stomach	• dry mouth
• trouble sleeping	• dizziness
• anxiety	• nervousness

Talk to your doctor if you or your child has side effects that are bothersome or do not go away.

This is not a complete list of possible side effects. Ask your doctor or pharmacist for more information.

How should I store FOCALIN XR?

- Store FOCALIN XR in a safe place at room temperature, 59°F to 86°F (15°C to 30°C).
- **Keep FOCALIN XR and all medicines out of the reach of children.**

General information about FOCALIN XR.

Medicines are sometimes prescribed for purposes other than those listed in a Medication Guide. Do not use FOCALIN XR for a condition for which it was not prescribed. Do not give FOCALIN XR to other people, even if they have the same condition. It may harm them and it is against the law.

This Medication Guide summarizes the most important information about FOCALIN XR. If you would like more information, talk with your doctor. You can ask your doctor or pharmacist for information about FOCALIN XR that was written for healthcare professionals. For more information about FOCALIN XR call 1-888-669-6682.

What are the ingredients in FOCALIN XR?

Active Ingredient: dexmethylphenidate hydrochloride

Inactive Ingredients: ammonio methacrylate copolymer, FD&C Blue #2 (5 mg, 15 mg, 25 mg, 35 mg, and 40 mg strengths), FDA/E172 yellow iron oxide (10 mg, 15 mg, 30 mg, 35 mg, and 40 mg strengths), gelatin, ink Tan SW-8010, methacrylic acid copolymer, polyethylene glycol, sugar spheres, talc, titanium dioxide, and triethyl citrate.

This Medication Guide has been approved by the U.S. Food and Drug Administration.

Focalin XR is a trademark of Novartis AG
SODAS® is a registered trademark of Alkermes Pharma Ireland Limited
This product is covered by US patents including 5,837,284, 5,908,850, 6,228,398, 6,355,656, and 6,635,284.
Manufactured for
Novartis Pharmaceuticals Corporation
East Hanover, New Jersey 07936
By Alkermes Gainesville LLC
Gainesville, GA 30504
© Novartis
T2013-56
June 2013

Shown in Product Identification Guide, page 310

GILENYA™ ℞

[je-LEN-yah]
(fingolimod)
capsules

The following prescribing information is based on official labeling in effect July 2013.

HIGHLIGHTS OF PRESCRIBING INFORMATION

These highlights do not include all the information needed to use GILENYA™ safely and effectively. See full prescribing information for GILENYA.

GILENYA (fingolimod) capsules
Initial U.S. Approval: 2010

RECENT MAJOR CHANGES

Dosage and Administration (2)	04/2012
Contraindications (4)	04/2012
Warnings and Precautions (5.1, 5.7)	04/2012

INDICATIONS AND USAGE

GILENYA is a sphingosine 1-phosphate receptor modulator indicated for the treatment of patients with relapsing forms of multiple sclerosis to reduce the frequency of clinical exacerbations and to delay the accumulation of physical disability. (1)

DOSAGE AND ADMINISTRATION

- Recommended dose: 0.5 mg orally once daily, with or without food (2)
- First Dose Monitoring:
  - Observe all patients for signs and symptoms of bradycardia for at least 6 hours after first dose with hourly pulse and blood pressure measurement. Obtain ECG prior to dosing and at the end of the observation period.
  - Patients who develop a heart rate <45 bpm, or a new onset 2nd degree or higher atrioventricular block should be

monitored until resolution of the finding. Patients at lowest post-dose heart rate at the end of the observation period should be monitored until heart rate increases.

- In patients experiencing symptomatic bradycardia, begin continuous ECG monitoring until the symptoms have resolved; if pharmacological intervention is required to treat bradycardia, continuous ECG monitoring should continue overnight in a medical facility, and first-dose monitoring procedures should be repeated for the second dose.
- Patients at higher risk of symptomatic bradycardia or heart block because of a coexisting medical condition or certain concomitant medications should be observed overnight with continuous ECG monitoring (2).
- Patients with prolonged QTc interval at baseline or during the observation period, or taking drugs with known risk of torsades de pointes should be observed overnight with continuous ECG monitoring (2).

DOSAGE FORMS AND STRENGTHS

0.5 mg hard capsules. (3)

CONTRAINDICATIONS

- Recent (within the last 6 months) occurrence of: myocardial infarction, unstable angina, stroke, transient ischemic attack, decompensated heart failure requiring hospitalization, or Class III/IV heart failure (4)
- History or presence of Mobitz Type II 2nd degree or 3rd degree AV block or sick sinus syndrome, unless patient has a pacemaker (4)
- Baseline QTc interval ≥500 ms (4)
- Treatment with Class Ia or Class III anti-arrhythmic drugs (4)

WARNINGS AND PRECAUTIONS

- Decrease in heart rate and/or atrioventricular conduction after first dose of GILENYA: Monitor patients (2, 5.1)
- Infections: GILENYA may increase the risk of infections. A recent CBC should be available before initiating treatment with GILENYA. Monitor for signs and symptoms of infection during treatment and for two months after discontinuation. Do not start GILENYA treatment in patients with active acute or chronic infections. (5.2)
- Macular edema: Can occur with or without visual symptoms. An ophthalmologic evaluation should be performed before starting GILENYA and at 3-4 months after treatment initiation. Monitor visual acuity at baseline and during routine evaluations of patients. Patients with diabetes mellitus or a history of uveitis are at increased risk and should have regular ophthalmologic evaluations. (5.3)
- Decrease in pulmonary function tests with GILENYA: Obtain spirometry and diffusion lung capacity for carbon monoxide (DLCO) when clinically indicated. (5.4)
- Hepatic effects: GILENYA may increase liver transaminases. Recent liver enzyme results should be available before starting GILENYA. Assess liver enzymes if hepatic injury is suspected. Discontinue GILENYA if significant liver injury occurs (5.5)
- Fetal risk: Women of childbearing potential should use effective contraception during and for 2 months after stopping GILENYA (5.6)

ADVERSE REACTIONS

Most common adverse reactions (incidence ≥10% and > placebo): Headache, influenza, diarrhea, back pain, liver transaminase elevations and cough. (6.1)

To report SUSPECTED ADVERSE REACTIONS, contact Novartis Pharmaceuticals Corporation at 1-888-669-6682 or FDA at 1-800-FDA-1088 or www.fda.gov/medwatch.

DRUG INTERACTIONS

- Ketoconazole: Monitor patients closely, as GILENYA exposure is increased by 70% during concomitant use with systemic ketoconazole, and risk of adverse reactions is greater. (7, 12,3)
- Vaccines: Avoid live attenuated vaccines during, and for 2 months after stopping GILENYA treatment, due to risk of infection. (5.2, 7)

USE IN SPECIFIC POPULATIONS

- Pregnancy: Based on animal data, may cause fetal harm. Pregnancy registry available. (8.1)
- Pediatric patients: Safety and effectiveness not established. (8.4)
- Hepatic impairment: Monitor patients with severe hepatic impairment closely, as GILENYA exposure is doubled, and risk of adverse reactions is greater. (5.5, 8.6, 12.3)

See 17 for PATIENT COUNSELING INFORMATION and Medication Guide

Revised: 05/2012

FULL PRESCRIBING INFORMATION: CONTENTS*

*** Sections or subsections omitted from the full prescribing information are not listed**

FULL PRESCRIBING INFORMATION

1 INDICATIONS AND USAGE

GILENYA is indicated for the treatment of patients with relapsing forms of multiple sclerosis (MS) to reduce the frequency of clinical exacerbations and to delay the accumulation of physical disability.

2 DOSAGE AND ADMINISTRATION

Recommended Dose

The recommended dose of GILENYA is 0.5 mg orally once daily. Fingolimod doses higher than 0.5 mg are associated with a greater incidence of adverse reactions without additional benefit. GILENYA can be taken with or without food.

First Dose Monitoring

Initiation of GILENYA treatment results in a decrease in heart rate [*see Warnings and Precautions (5.1) and Clinical Pharmacology (12.2)*]. After the first dose of GILENYA, the heart rate decrease starts within an hour and the Day 1 nadir generally occurs within approximately 6 hours, although the nadir can be observed up to 24 hours after the first dose in some patients.

The first dose of GILENYA should be administered in a setting in which resources to appropriately manage symptomatic bradycardia are available. In order to assess patient response to the first dose of fingolimod, observe all patients for 6 hours for signs and symptoms of bradycardia with hourly pulse and blood pressure measurement. Obtain in all patients an electrocardiogram prior to dosing, and at the end of the observation period.

Additional observation should be instituted until the finding has resolved in the following situations:

- The heart rate 6 hours post-dose is <45 bpm
- The heart rate 6 hours post-dose is at the lowest value post-dose (suggesting that the maximum pharmacodynamic effect on the heart may not have occurred)
- The ECG 6-hours post-dose shows new onset second degree or higher AV block

Should post-dose symptomatic bradycardia occur, initiate appropriate management, begin continuous ECG monitoring, and continue observation until the symptoms have resolved.

Should a patient require pharmacologic intervention for symptomatic bradycardia, continuous overnight ECG monitoring in a medical facility should be instituted, and the first dose monitoring strategy should be repeated after the second dose of GILENYA.

Patients with some pre-existing conditions (e.g., ischemic heart disease, history of myocardial infarction, congestive heart failure, history of cardiac arrest, cerebrovascular disease, history of symptomatic bradycardia, history of recurrent syncope, severe untreated sleep apnea, AV block, sino-atrial heart block) may poorly tolerate the GILENYA-induced bradycardia, or experience serious rhythm disturbances after the first dose of GILENYA. Prior to treatment with GILENYA, these patients should have a cardiac evaluation by a physician appropriately trained to conduct such evaluation, and, if treated with GILENYA, should be monitored overnight with continuous ECG in a medical facility after the first dose. GILENYA is contraindicated in patients who in the last 6 months experienced myocardial infarction, unstable angina, stroke, transient ischemic attack (TIA), decompensated heart failure requiring hospitalization or Class III/IV heart failure) [*see Contraindications (4)*].

Since initiation of GILENYA treatment results in decreased heart rate and may prolong the QT interval, patients with a prolonged QTc interval (>450 msec males, >470 msec females) before dosing or during 6 hour observation, or at additional risk for QT prolongation (e.g., hypokalemia, hypomagnesemia, congenital long-QT syndrome), or on concurrent therapy with QT prolonging drugs with a known risk of torsades de pointes (e.g., citalopram, chlorpromazine, haloperidol, methadone, erythromycin) should be monitored overnight with continuous ECG in a medical facility [*see Drug Interactions (7)*].

Experience with GILENYA is limited in patients receiving concurrent therapy with drugs that slow heart rate or atrioventricular conduction (e.g., beta blockers, heart-rate lowering calcium channel blockers such as diltiazem or verapamil, or digoxin). Because the initiation of GILENYA treatment is also associated with slowing of the heart rate, concomitant use of these drugs during GILENYA initiation may be associated with severe bradycardia or heart block. The possibility to switch to drugs that do not slow the heart rate or atrioventricular conduction should be evaluated by the physician prescribing these drugs before initiating GILENYA. In patients who cannot switch, overnight continuous ECG monitoring after the first dose is recommended [*see Drug Interactions (7)*].

Clinical data indicate effects of GILENYA on heart rate are maximal after the first dose although milder effects on heart rate may persist for, on average, 2-4 weeks after initiation of therapy at which time heart rate generally returns to baseline. Physicians should continue to be alert to patient reports of cardiac symptoms.

Re-initiation of Therapy Following Discontinuation

If GILENYA therapy is discontinued for more than 14 days, after the first month of treatment, the effects on heart rate and AV conduction may recur on reintroduction of GILENYA treatment and the same precautions (first dose monitoring) as for initial dosing should apply. Within the first 2 weeks of treatment, first dose procedures are recommended after interruption of one day or more, during week 3 and 4 of treatment first dose procedures are recommended after treatment interruption of more than 7 days.

3 DOSAGE FORMS AND STRENGTHS

GILENYA is available as 0.5 mg hard capsules with a white opaque body and bright yellow cap imprinted with "FTY 0.5 mg" on the cap and two radial bands imprinted on the capsule body with yellow ink.

4 CONTRAINDICATIONS

Patients who in the last 6 months experienced myocardial infarction, unstable angina, stroke, TIA, decompensated heart failure requiring hospitalization or Class III/IV heart failure

History or presence of Mobitz Type II second-degree or third-degree atrioventricular (AV) block or sick sinus syndrome, unless patient has a functioning pacemaker

Baseline QTc interval ≥500 ms

Treatment with Class Ia or Class III anti-arrhythmic drugs

5 WARNINGS AND PRECAUTIONS

5.1 Bradyarrhythmia and Atrioventricular Blocks

Because of a risk for bradyarrhythmia and atrioventricular (AV) blocks, patients should be monitored during GILENYA treatment initiation [*see Dosage and Administration (2)*].

Reduction in heart rate

After the first dose of GILENYA, the heart rate decrease starts within an hour. On Day 1, the maximal decline in heart rate generally occurs within 6 hours and recovers, although not to baseline levels, by 8-10 hours post dose. Because of physiological diurnal variation, there is a second period of heart rate decrease within 24 hours after the first dose. In some patients, heart rate decrease during the second period is more pronounced than the decrease observed in the first 6 hours. Heart rates below 40 beats per minute were rarely observed. Adverse reactions of symptomatic bradycardia following the first dose were reported in 0.5% of patients receiving GILENYA 0.5 mg, but in no patient on placebo. Patients who experienced bradycardia were generally asymptomatic, but some patients experienced hypotension, dizziness, fatigue, palpitations, and chest pain that usually resolved within the first 24 hours on treatment.

Following the second dose, a further decrease in heart rate may occur when compared to the heart rate prior to the second dose, but this change is of a smaller magnitude than that observed following the first dose. With continued dosing, the heart rate returns to baseline within one month of chronic treatment.

Atrioventricular blocks

Initiation of GILENYA treatment has resulted in transient AV conduction delays. In controlled clinical trials, adverse reactions of first-degree AV block (prolonged PR interval on ECG) following the first dose were reported in 0.1% of patients receiving GILENYA 0.5 mg, but in no patient on placebo. Second-degree AV blocks following the first dose were also identified in 0.1% of patients receiving GILENYA 0.5 mg, but in no patient on placebo. In a study of 698 patients with available 24-hour Holter monitoring data after their first dose (N=351 on GILENYA 0.5 mg and N=347 on placebo), second-degree AV blocks, Mobitz types I (Wenckebach) and/or II, were reported in 3.7% (N=13) of patients receiving GILENYA 0.5 mg and 2% (N=7) of patients on placebo. The conduction abnormalities were usually transient and asymptomatic, and resolved within the first 24 hours on treatment, but they occasionally required treatment with atropine or isoproterenol.

Post-marketing experience

In the post-marketing setting, third degree AV block and AV block with junctional escape have been observed during the first-dose six-hour observation period with GILENYA. Isolated delayed onset events, including transient asystole and unexplained death, have occurred within 24 hours of the first dose. These events were confounded by concomitant medications and/or pre-existing disease, and the relationship to GILENYA is uncertain. Cases of syncope were also reported after the first dose of GILENYA.

5.2 Infections

Risk of infections

GILENYA causes a dose-dependent reduction in peripheral lymphocyte count to 20 - 30% of baseline values because of reversible sequestration of lymphocytes in lymphoid tissues. GILENYA may therefore increase the risk of infections, some serious in nature [see *Clinical Pharmacology* (12.2)].

Before initiating treatment with GILENYA, a recent CBC (i.e. within 6 months) should be available. Consider suspending treatment with GILENYA if a patient develops a serious infection, and reassess the benefits and risks prior to re-initiation of therapy. Because the elimination of fingolimod after discontinuation may take up to two months, continue monitoring for infections throughout this period. Instruct patients receiving GILENYA to report symptoms of infections to a physician. Patients with active acute or chronic infections should not start treatment until the infection(s) is resolved.

Two patients died of herpetic infections during GILENYA controlled studies in the premarketing database (one disseminated primary herpes zoster and one herpes simplex encephalitis). In both cases, the patients were receiving a fingolimod dose (1.25 mg) higher than recommended for the treatment of MS (0.5 mg), and had received high dose corticosteroid therapy for suspected MS relapse. No deaths due to viral infections occurred in patients treated with GILENYA 0.5 mg in the premarketing database.

In MS controlled studies, the overall rate of infections (72%) and serious infections (2%) with GILENYA 0.5 mg was similar to placebo. However, bronchitis and, to a lesser extent, pneumonia were more common in GILENYA-treated patients.

Concomitant use with antineoplastic, immunosuppressive or immune modulating therapies

GILENYA has not been administered concomitantly with antineoplastic, immunosuppressive or immune modulating therapies used for treatment of MS. Concomitant use of GILENYA with any of these therapies would be expected to increase the risk of immunosuppression [see Drug Interactions (7)].

Varicella zoster virus antibody testing/vaccination

As for any immune modulating drug, before initiating GILENYA therapy, patients without a history of chickenpox or without vaccination against varicella zoster virus (VZV) should be tested for antibodies to VZV. VZV vaccination of antibody-negative patients should be considered prior to commencing treatment with GILENYA, following which initiation of treatment with GILENYA should be postponed for 1 month to allow the full effect of vaccination to occur.

5.3 Macular Edema

In patients receiving GILENYA 0.5 mg, macular edema occurred in 0.4% of patients. An adequate ophthalmologic evaluation should be performed at baseline and 3-4 months after treatment initiation. If patients report visual disturbances at any time while on GILENYA therapy, additional ophthalmologic evaluation should be undertaken.

In MS controlled studies involving 1204 patients treated with GILENYA 0.5 mg and 861 patients treated with placebo, macular edema with or without visual symptoms was reported in 0.4% of patients treated with GILENYA 0.5 mg and 0.1% of patients treated with placebo; it occurred predominantly in the first 3-4 months of therapy. Some patients presented with blurred vision or decreased visual acuity, but others were asymptomatic and diagnosed on routine ophthalmologic examination. Macular edema generally improved or resolved with or without treatment after drug discontinuation, but some patients had residual visual acuity loss even after resolution of macular edema.

Continuation of GILENYA in patients who develop macular edema has not been evaluated. A decision on whether or not to discontinue GILENYA therapy should include an assessment of the potential benefits and risks for the individual patient. The risk of recurrence after rechallenge has not been evaluated.

Macular edema in patients with history of uveitis or diabetes mellitus

Patients with a history of uveitis and patients with diabetes mellitus are at increased risk of macular edema during GILENYA therapy. The incidence of macular edema is also increased in MS patients with a history of uveitis. The rate was approximately 20% in patients with a history of uveitis vs. 0.6% in those without a history of uveitis, in the combined experience with all doses of fingolimod. MS patients with diabetes mellitus or a history of uveitis should undergo an ophthalmologic evaluation prior to initiating GILENYA therapy and have regular follow-up ophthalmologic evaluations while receiving GILENYA therapy. GILENYA has not been tested in MS patients with diabetes mellitus.

5.4 Respiratory Effects

Dose-dependent reductions in forced expiratory volume over 1 second (FEV1) and diffusion lung capacity for carbon monoxide (DLCO) were observed in patients treated with GILENYA as early as 1 month after treatment initiation. At Month 24, the reduction from baseline in the percent of predicted values for FEV1 was 3.1% for GILENYA 0.5 mg and 2% for placebo. For DLCO, the reductions from baseline in percent of predicted values at Month 24 were 3.8% for GILENYA 0.5 mg and 2.7% for placebo. The changes in FEV1 appear to be reversible after treatment discontinuation. There is insufficient information to determine the reversibility of the decrease of DLCO after drug discontinuation. In MS controlled trials, dyspnea was reported in 5% of patients receiving GILENYA 0.5 mg and 4% of patients receiving placebo. Several patients discontinued GILENYA because of unexplained dyspnea during the extension (uncontrolled) studies. GILENYA has not been tested in MS patients with compromised respiratory function.

Spirometric evaluation of respiratory function and evaluation of DLCO should be performed during therapy with GILENYA if clinically indicated.

5.5 Hepatic Effects

Elevations of liver enzymes may occur in patients receiving GILENYA. Recent (i.e. within last 6 months) transaminase and bilirubin levels should be available before initiation of GILENYA therapy.

During clinical trials, 3-fold the upper limit of normal (ULN) or greater elevation in liver transaminases occurred in 8% of patients treated with GILENYA 0.5 mg, as compared to 2% of patients on placebo. Elevations 5-fold the ULN occurred in 2% of patients on GILENYA and 1% of patients on placebo. In clinical trials, GILENYA was discontinued if the elevation exceeded 5 times the ULN. Recurrence of liver transaminase elevations occurred with rechallenge in some patients, supporting a relationship to drug. The majority of elevations occurred within 6-9 months. Serum transaminase levels returned to normal within approximately 2 months after discontinuation of GILENYA.

Liver enzymes should be monitored in patients who develop symptoms suggestive of hepatic dysfunction, such as unexplained nausea, vomiting, abdominal pain, fatigue, anorexia, or jaundice and/or dark urine. GILENYA should be discontinued if significant liver injury is confirmed. Patients with pre-existing liver disease may be at increased risk of developing elevated liver enzymes when taking GILENYA.

Because GILENYA exposure is doubled in patients with severe hepatic impairment, these patients should be closely monitored, as the risk of adverse reactions is greater [see *Use in Specific Populations* (8.6) and *Clinical Pharmacology* (12.3)].

5.6 Fetal Risk

Based on animal studies, GILENYA may cause fetal harm. Because it takes approximately 2 months to eliminate GILENYA from the body, women of childbearing potential should use effective contraception to avoid pregnancy during and for 2 months after stopping GILENYA treatment.

5.7 Blood Pressure Effects

In MS clinical trials, patients treated with GILENYA 0.5 mg had an average increase of approximately 2 mmHg in systolic pressure, and approximately 1 mmHg in diastolic pressure, first detected after approximately 1 month of treatment initiation, and persisting with continued treatment. In controlled studies involving 854 MS patients on GILENYA 0.5 mg and 511 MS patients on placebo, hypertension was reported as an adverse reaction in 5% of patients on GILENYA 0.5 mg and in 3% of patients on placebo. Blood pressure should be monitored during treatment with GILENYA.

5.8 Immune System Effects Following GILENYA Discontinuation

Fingolimod remains in the blood and has pharmacodynamic effects, including decreased lymphocyte counts, for up to 2 months following the last dose of GILENYA. Lymphocyte counts generally return to the normal range within 1-2 months of stopping therapy [see *Clinical Pharmacology* (12.2)]. Because of the continuing pharmacodynamic effects of fingolimod, initiating other drugs during this period warrants the same considerations needed for concomitant administration (e.g., risk of additive immunosuppressant effects) [see *Drug Interactions* (7)].

6 ADVERSE REACTIONS

The following serious adverse reactions are described elsewhere in labeling:

- Bradyarrhythmia and atrioventricular blocks [see *Warnings and Precautions* (5.1)]
- Infections [see *Warnings and Precautions* (5.2)]
- Macular edema [see *Warnings and Precautions* (5.3)]
- Respiratory effects [see *Warnings and Precautions* (5.4)]
- Hepatic effects [see *Warnings and Precautions* (5.5)]

The most frequent adverse reactions (incidence ≥10% and > placebo) for GILENYA 0.5 mg were headache, influenza, diarrhea, back pain, liver enzyme elevations, and cough. The only adverse event leading to treatment interruption reported at an incidence >1% for GILENYA 0.5 mg was serum transaminase elevations (3.8%).

6.1 Clinical Trials Experience

A total of 1703 patients on GILENYA (0.5 or 1.25 mg once daily) constituted the safety population in the 2 controlled studies in patients with relapsing remitting MS (RRMS) [*see Clinical Studies (14)*].

Study 1 was a 2-year placebo-controlled clinical study in 1272 MS patients treated with GILENYA 0.5 mg (n=425), GILENYA 1.25 mg (n=429) or placebo (n= 418).

Table 1 Adverse Reactions in Study 1 (occurring in ≥1% of patients, and reported for GILENYA 0.5 mg at ≥1% higher rate than for placebo)

Primary System Organ Class Preferred Term	GILENYA 0.5 mg N=425 %	Placebo N=418 %
Infections		
Influenza viral infections	13	10
Herpes viral infections	9	8
Bronchitis	8	4
Sinusitis	7	5
Gastroenteritis	5	3
Tinea infections	4	1
Cardiac Disorders		
Bradycardia	4	1
Nervous system disorders		
Headache	25	23
Dizziness	7	6
Paresthesia	5	4
Migraine	5	1
Gastrointestinal disorders		
Diarrhea	12	7
General disorders and administration site conditions		
Asthenia	3	1
Musculoskeletal and connective tissue disorders		
Back pain	12	7
Skin and subcutaneous tissue disorders		
Alopecia	4	2
Eczema	3	2
Pruritus	3	1
Investigations		
ALT/AST increased	14	5
GGT increased	5	1
Weight decreased	5	3
Blood triglycerides increased	3	1
Respiratory, thoracic and mediastinal disorders		
Cough	10	8
Dyspnea	8	5
Psychiatric disorders		
Depression	8	7
Eye disorders		
Vision blurred	4	1
Eye pain	3	1
Vascular disorders		
Hypertension	6	4

Blood and lymphatic system disorders		
Lymphopenia	4	1
Leukopenia	3	<1

Adverse reactions in Study 2, a 1-year active-controlled (vs. interferon beta-1a, n=431) study including 849 patients with MS treated with fingolimod, were generally similar to those in Study 1.

Vascular Events

Vascular events, including ischemic and hemorrhagic strokes, peripheral arterial occlusive disease and posterior reversible encephalopathy syndrome were reported in premarketing clinical trials in patients who received GILENYA doses (1.25-5 mg) higher than recommended for use in MS. No vascular events were observed with GILENYA 0.5 mg in the premarketing database.

Lymphomas

Cases of lymphoma (cutaneous T-cell lymphoproliferative disorders or diffuse B-cell lymphoma) were reported in premarketing clinical trials in MS patients receiving GILENYA at, or above, the recommended dose of 0.5 mg. Based on the small number of cases and short duration of exposure, the relationship to GILENYA remains uncertain.

7 DRUG INTERACTIONS

QT prolonging drugs

GILENYA has not been studied in patients treated with drugs that prolong the QT interval. Drugs that prolong the QT interval have been associated with cases of torsades de pointes in patients with bradycardia. Since initiation of GILENYA treatment results in decreased heart rate and may prolong the QT interval, patients on QT prolonging drugs with a known risk of torsades de pointes (e.g., citalopram, chlorpromazine, haloperidol, methadone, erythromycin) should be monitored overnight with continuous ECG in a medical facility [*see Dosage and Administration (2) and Warnings and Precautions (5.1)*].

Ketoconazole

The blood levels of fingolimod and fingolimod-phosphate are increased by 1.7-fold when used concomitantly with ketoconazole. Patients who use GILENYA and systemic ketoconazole concomitantly should be closely monitored, as the risk of adverse reactions is greater.

Vaccines

Vaccination may be less effective during and for up to 2 months after discontinuation of treatment with GILENYA [*see Clinical Pharmacology* (12.2)]. The use of live attenuated vaccines should be avoided during and for 2 months after treatment with GILENYA because of the risk of infection.

Antineoplastic, immunosuppressive or immunomodulating therapies

Antineoplastic, immunosuppressive or immune modulating therapies are expected to increase the risk of immunosuppression. Use caution when switching patients from long-acting therapies with immune effects such as natalizumab or mitoxantrone.

Drugs that slow heart rate or atrioventricular conduction (e.g., beta blockers or diltiazem)

Experience with GILENYA in patients receiving concurrent therapy with drugs that slow the heart rate or atrioventricular conduction (e.g., beta blockers, digoxin, or heart-rate slowing calcium channel blockers such as diltiazem or verapamil) is limited. Because initiation of GILENYA treatment may result in an additional decrease in heart rate, concomitant use of these drugs during GILENYA initiation may be associated with severe bradycardia or heart block. Seek advice from the prescribing physician regarding the possibility to switch to drugs that do not slow the heart rate or atrioventricular conduction before initiating GILENYA. In patients who cannot switch, consider extended monitoring, including overnight, after the first dose [*see Dosage and Administration (2) and Warnings and Precautions (5.1)*].

Laboratory test interaction

Because GILENYA reduces blood lymphocyte counts via redistribution in secondary lymphoid organs, peripheral blood lymphocyte counts cannot be utilized to evaluate the lymphocyte subset status of a patient treated with GILENYA. A recent CBC should be available before initiating treatment with GILENYA.

8 USE IN SPECIFIC POPULATIONS

8.1 Pregnancy

Pregnancy Category C

There are no adequate and well-controlled studies in pregnant women. In oral studies conducted in rats and rabbits, fingolimod demonstrated developmental toxicity, including teratogenicity (rats) and embryolethality, when given to pregnant animals. In rats, the highest no-effect dose was less than the recommended human dose (RHD) of 0.5 mg/day on a body surface area (mg/m^2) basis. The most common fetal visceral malformations in rats included persistent truncus arteriosus and ventricular septal defect. The receptor affected by fingolimod (sphingosine 1-phosphate receptor) is known to be involved in vascular formation during embryogenesis. Because it takes approximately 2 months to eliminate fingolimod from the body, potential risks to the fetus may persist after treatment ends [see *Warnings and Precautions* (5.7, 5.8)]. GILENYA should be used during pregnancy only if the potential benefit justifies the potential risk to the fetus.

Pregnancy Registry

A pregnancy registry has been established to collect information about the effect of GILENYA use during pregnancy. Physicians are encouraged to enroll pregnant patients, or pregnant women may register themselves in the GILENYA pregnancy registry by calling 1-877-598-7237 or visiting www.gilenyapregnancyregistry.com.

Animal Data

When fingolimod was orally administered to pregnant rats during the period of organogenesis (0, 0.03, 0.1, and 0.3 mg/kg/day or 0, 1, 3, and 10 mg/kg/day), increased incidences of fetal malformations and embryo-fetal deaths were observed at all but the lowest dose tested (0.03 mg/kg/day), which is less than the RHD on a mg/m^2 basis. Oral administration to pregnant rabbits during organogenesis (0, 0.5, 1.5, and 5 mg/kg/day) resulted in increased incidences of embryo-fetal mortality and fetal growth retardation at the mid and high doses. The no-effect dose for these effects in rabbits (0.5 mg/kg/day) is approximately 20 times the RHD on a mg/m^2 basis.

When fingolimod was orally administered to female rats during pregnancy and lactation (0, 0.05, 0.15, and 0.5 mg/kg/day), pup survival was decreased at all doses and a neurobehavioral (learning) deficit was seen in offspring at the high dose. The low-effect dose of 0.05 mg/kg/day is similar to the RHD on a mg/m^2 basis.

8.2 Labor and Delivery

The effects of GILENYA on labor and delivery are unknown.

8.3 Nursing Mothers

Fingolimod is excreted in the milk of treated rats. It is not known whether this drug is excreted in human milk. Because many drugs are excreted in human milk and because of the potential for serious adverse reactions in nursing infants from GILENYA, a decision should be made whether to discontinue nursing or to discontinue the drug, taking into account the importance of the drug to the mother.

8.4 Pediatric Use

The safety and effectiveness of GILENYA in pediatric patients with MS below the age of 18 have not been established.

8.5 Geriatric Use

Clinical MS studies of GILENYA did not include sufficient numbers of patients aged 65 years and over to determine whether they respond differently than younger patients. GILENYA should be used with caution in patients aged 65 years and over, reflecting the greater frequency of decreased hepatic, or renal, function and of concomitant disease or other drug therapy.

8.6 Hepatic Impairment

Because fingolimod, but not fingolimod-phosphate, exposure is doubled in patients with severe hepatic impairment, patients with severe hepatic impairment should be closely monitored, as the risk of adverse reactions may be greater [See *Warnings and Precautions (5.5)* and *Clinical Pharmacology* (12.3)].

No dose adjustment is needed in patients with mild or moderate hepatic impairment.

8.7 Renal Impairment

The blood level of some GILENYA metabolites is increased (up to 13-fold) in patients with severe renal impairment [see *Clinical Pharmacology* (12.3)]. The toxicity of these metabolites has not been fully explored. The blood level of these metabolites has not been assessed in patients with mild or moderate renal impairment.

10 OVERDOSAGE

GILENYA can induce bradycardia as well as AV conduction blocks (including complete AV block). The decline in heart rate usually starts within one hour of the first dose and is maximal within 6 hours in most patients *[see Warnings and Precautions (5.1)]*. In case of GILENYA overdosage, observe patients overnight with continuous ECG monitoring in a medical facility, and obtain regular measurements of blood pressure *[see Dosage and Administration (2)]*.

Neither dialysis nor plasma exchange results in removal of fingolimod from the body.

11 DESCRIPTION

Fingolimod is a sphingosine 1-phosphate receptor modulator.

Chemically, fingolimod is 2-amino-2-[2-(4-octylphenyl)-ethyl]propan-1,3-diol hydrochloride. Its structure is shown below:

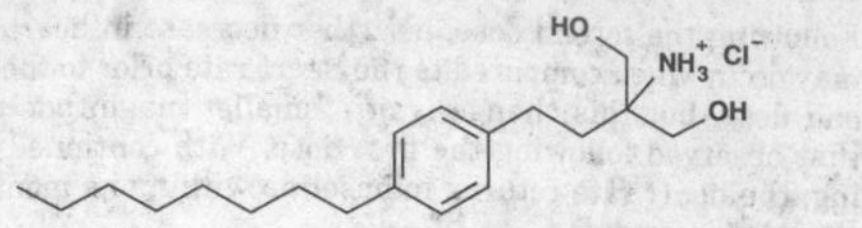

Fingolimod hydrochloride is a white to practically white powder that is freely soluble in water and alcohol and soluble in propylene glycol. It has a molecular weight of 343.93. GILENYA is provided as 0.5 mg hard gelatin capsules for oral use. Each capsule contains 0.56 mg of fingolimod hydrochloride, equivalent to 0.5 mg of fingolimod.

Each GILENYA 0.5 mg capsule contains the following inactive ingredients: gelatin, magnesium stearate, mannitol, titanium dioxide, yellow iron oxide.

12 CLINICAL PHARMACOLOGY

12.1 Mechanism of Action

Fingolimod is metabolized by sphingosine kinase to the active metabolite, fingolimod-phosphate. Fingolimod-phosphate is a sphingosine 1-phosphate receptor modulator, and binds with high affinity to sphingosine 1-phosphate receptors 1, 3, 4, and 5. Fingolimod-phosphate blocks the capacity of lymphocytes to egress from lymph nodes, reducing the number of lymphocytes in peripheral blood. The mechanism by which fingolimod exerts therapeutic effects in multiple sclerosis is unknown, but may involve reduction of lymphocyte migration into the central nervous system.

12.2 Pharmacodynamics

Heart rate and rhythm

Fingolimod causes a transient reduction in heart rate and AV conduction at treatment initiation [*see Warnings and Precautions (5.1)*].

Heart rate progressively increases after the first day, returning to baseline values within 1 month of the start of chronic treatment.

Autonomic responses of the heart, including diurnal variation of heart rate and response to exercise, are not affected by fingolimod treatment.

Fingolimod treatment is not associated with a decrease in cardiac output.

Potential to prolong the QT interval

In a thorough QT interval study of doses of 1.25 or 2.5 mg fingolimod at steady-state, when a negative chronotropic effect of fingolimod was still present, fingolimod treatment resulted in a prolongation of QTc, with the upper bound of the 90% confidence interval (CI) of 14.0 ms. There is no consistent signal of increased incidence of QTc outliers, either absolute or change from baseline, associated with fingolimod treatment. In MS studies, there was no clinically relevant prolongation of QT interval, but patients at risk for QT prolongation were not included in clinical studies.

Immune system

Effects on immune cell numbers in the blood

In a study in which 12 subjects received GILENYA 0.5 mg daily, the lymphocyte count decreased to approximately 60% of baseline within 4-6 hours after the first dose. With continued daily dosing, the lymphocyte count continued to decrease over a 2-week period, reaching a nadir count of approximately 500 cells/μL or approximately 30% of baseline. In a placebo-controlled study in 1272 MS patients (of whom 425 received fingolimod 0.5 mg daily and 418 received placebo), 18% (N=78) of patients on fingolimod 0.5 mg reached a nadir of < 200 cells/μL on at least one occasion. No patient on placebo reached a nadir of < 200 cells/μL. Low lymphocyte counts are maintained with chronic daily dosing of GILENYA 0.5 mg daily.

Chronic fingolimod dosing leads to a mild decrease in the neutrophil count to approximately 80% of baseline. Monocytes are unaffected by fingolimod.

Peripheral lymphocyte count increases are evident within days of stopping fingolimod treatment and typically normal counts are reached within 1 to 2 months.

Effect on antibody response

The immunogenicity of keyhole limpet Hemocyanin (KLH) and pneumococcal polysaccharide vaccine (PPV-23) immunization were assessed by IgM and IgG titers in a steady-state, randomized, placebo-controlled study in healthy volunteers. Compared to placebo, antigen-specific IgM titers were decreased by 91% and 25% in response to KLH and PPV, respectively, in subjects on GILENYA 0.5 mg. Similarly, IgG titers were decreased by 45% and 50%, in response to KLH and PPV, respectively, in subjects on GILENYA 0.5 mg daily compared to placebo. The responder rate for GILENYA 0.5 mg as measured by the number of subjects with a >4-fold increase in KLH IgG was comparable to placebo and 25% lower for PPV-23 IgG, while the number of subjects with a >4 fold increase in KLH and PPV-23 IgM was 75% and 40% lower, respectively, compared to placebo. The capacity to mount a skin delayed-type hypersensitivity reaction to *Candida* and tetanus toxoid was decreased by approximately 30% in subjects on GILENYA 0.5 mg daily, compared to placebo. Immunologic responses were further decreased with fingolimod 1.25 mg (a dose higher than recommended in MS) [see *Warnings and Precautions* (5.2)].

Pulmonary function

Single fingolimod doses ≥5 mg (10-fold the recommended dose) are associated with a dose-dependent increase in airway resistance. In a 14-day study of 0.5, 1.25, or 5 mg/day, fingolimod was not associated with impaired oxygenation or oxygen desaturation with exercise or an increase in airway responsiveness to methacholine. Subjects on fingolimod treatment had a normal bronchodilator response to inhaled beta-agonists.

In a 14-day placebo-controlled study of patients with moderate asthma, no effect was seen for GILENYA 0.5mg (recommended dose in MS). A 10% reduction in mean FEV1 at 6 hour after dosing was observed in patients receiving fingolimod 1.25 mg (a dose higher than recommended for use in MS) on Day 10 of treatment. Fingolimod 1.25 mg was associated with a 5-fold increase in the use of rescue short acting beta-agonists.

12.3 Pharmacokinetics

Absorption

The T_{max} of fingolimod is 12-16 hours. The apparent absolute oral bioavailability is 93%.

Food intake does not alter C_{max} or exposure (AUC) of fingolimod or fingolimod-phosphate. Therefore GILENYA may be taken without regard to meals.

Steady-state blood concentrations are reached within 1 to 2 months following once-daily administration and steady-state levels are approximately 10-fold greater than with the initial dose.

Distribution

Fingolimod highly (86%) distributes in red blood cells. Fingolimod-phosphate has a smaller uptake in blood cells of <17%. Fingolimod and fingolimod-phosphate are >99.7% protein bound. Fingolimod and fingolimod-phosphate protein binding is not altered by renal or hepatic impairment. Fingolimod is extensively distributed to body tissues with a volume of distribution of about 1200±260 L.

Metabolism

The biotransformation of fingolimod in humans occurs by three main pathways: by reversible stereoselective phosphorylation to the pharmacologically active (*S*)-enantiomer of fingolimod-phosphate, by oxidative biotransformation mainly via the cytochrome P450 4F2 isoenzyme and subsequent fatty acid-like degradation to inactive metabolites, and by formation of pharmacologically inactive non-polar ceramide analogs of fingolimod.

Fingolimod is primarily metabolized via human CYP4F2 with a minor contribution of CYP2D6, 2E1, 3A4, and 4F12. Inhibitors or inducers of these isozymes might alter the exposure of fingolimod or fingolimod-phosphate. The involvement of multiple CYP isoenzymes in the oxidation of fingolimod suggests that the metabolism of fingolimod will not be subject to substantial inhibition in the presence of an inhibitor of a single specific CYP isozyme.

Following single oral administration of [^{14}C] fingolimod, the major fingolimod-related components in blood, as judged from their contribution to the AUC up to 816 hours post-dose of total radiolabeled components, are fingolimod itself (23.3%), fingolimod-phosphate (10.3%), and inactive metabolites [M3 carboxylic acid metabolite (8.3%), M29 ceramide metabolite (8.9%), and M30 ceramide metabolite (7.3%)].

Elimination

Fingolimod blood clearance is 6.3±2.3 L/h, and the average apparent terminal half-life ($t_{1/2}$) is 6-9 days. Blood levels of fingolimod-phosphate decline in parallel with those of fingolimod in the terminal phase, yielding similar half-lives for both.

After oral administration, about 81% of the dose is slowly excreted in the urine as inactive metabolites. Fingolimod and fingolimod-phosphate are not excreted intact in urine but are the major components in the feces with amounts of each representing less than 2.5% of the dose.

Special Populations

Renal Impairment

In patients with severe renal impairment, fingolimod C_{max} and AUC are increased by 32% and 43%, respectively, and fingolimod-phosphate C_{max} and AUC are increased by 25% and 14%, respectively, with no change in apparent elimination half-life. Based on these findings, the GILENYA 0.5 mg dose is appropriate for use in patients with renal impairment. The systemic exposure of two metabolites (M2 and M3) is increased by 3- and 13-fold, respectively. The toxicity of these metabolites has not been fully characterized.

A study in patients with mild or moderate renal impairment has not been conducted.

Hepatic Impairment

In subjects with mild, moderate, or severe hepatic impairment, no change in fingolimod C_{max} was observed, but fingolimod AUC was increased respectively by 12%, 44%, and 103%. In patients with severe hepatic impairment, fingolimod-phosphate C_{max} was decreased by 22% and AUC was not substantially changed. The pharmacokinetics of fingolimod-phosphate were not evaluated in patients with mild or moderate hepatic impairment. The apparent elimination half-life of fingolimod is unchanged in subjects with mild hepatic impairment, but is prolonged by about 50% in patients with moderate or severe hepatic impairment.

Patients with severe hepatic impairment should be closely monitored, as the risk of adverse reactions is greater [See *Warnings and Precautions* (5.5)].

No dose adjustment is needed in patients with mild or moderate hepatic impairment.

Race

The effects of race on fingolimod and fingolimod-phosphate pharmacokinetics cannot be adequately assessed due to a low number of non-white patients in the clinical program.

Gender

Gender has no clinically significant influence on fingolimod and fingolimod-phosphate pharmacokinetics.

Geriatric patients

The mechanism for elimination and results from population pharmacokinetics suggest that dose adjustment would not be necessary in elderly patients. However, clinical experience in patients aged above 65 years is limited.

Pharmacokinetic interactions

Ketoconazole

The coadministration of ketoconazole (a potent inhibitor of CYP3A and CYP4F) 200 mg twice daily at steady-state and a single dose of fingolimod 5 mg led to a 70% increase in AUC of fingolimod and fingolimod-phosphate. Patients who use GILENYA and systemic ketoconazole concomitantly should be closely monitored, as the risk of adverse reactions is greater. [See *Drug Interactions (7)*].

Potential of fingolimod and fingolimod-phosphate to inhibit the metabolism of co-medications

In vitro inhibition studies in pooled human liver microsomes and specific metabolic probe substrates demonstrate that fingolimod has little or no capacity to inhibit the activity of the following CYP450 enzymes: CYP1A2, CYP2A6, CYP2B6, CYP2C9, CYP2C19, CYP2D6, CYP2E1, CYP3A4/5, or CYP4A9/11, and similarly fingolimod-phosphate has little or no capacity to inhibit the activity of CYP1A2, CYP2A6, CYP2C8, CYP2C9, CYP2C19, CYP2D6, CYP2E1, or CYP3A4 at concentrations up to three orders of magnitude of therapeutic concentrations. Therefore, fingolimod and fingolimod-phosphate are unlikely to reduce the clearance of drugs that are mainly cleared through metabolism by the major cytochrome P450 isoenzymes described above. The potential of fingolimod to inhibit CYP2C8 and fingolimod-phosphate to inhibit CYP2B6 is unknown.

Potential of fingolimod and fingolimod-phosphate to induce its own and/or the metabolism of co-medications

Fingolimod was examined for its potential to induce human CYP3A4, CYP1A2, CYP4F2, and MDR1 (P-glycoprotein) mRNA and CYP3A, CYP1A2, CYP2B6, CYP2C8, CYP2C9, CYP2C19, and CYP4F2 activity in primary human hepatocytes. Fingolimod did not induce mRNA or activity of the different CYP450 enzymes and MDR1 with respect to the vehicle control; therefore, no clinically relevant induction of the tested CYP450 enzymes or MDR1 by fingolimod are expected at therapeutic concentrations. The potential of fingolimod-phosphate to induce CYP450 isoenzymes is unknown.

Transporters

Fingolimod as well as fingolimod-phosphate are not expected to inhibit the uptake of co-medications and/or biologics transported by OATP1B1, OATP1B3, or NTCP. Similarly, they are not expected to inhibit the efflux of co-medications and/or biologics transported by the breast cancer resistant protein (MXR), the bile salt export pump (BSEP), the multidrug resistance-associated protein 2 (MRP2), and MDR1-mediated transport at therapeutic concentrations.

Cyclosporine

The pharmacokinetics of single-dose fingolimod were not altered during coadministration with cyclosporine at steady-state, nor was cyclosporine steady-state pharmacokinetics altered by fingolimod. These data indicate that GILENYA is unlikely to reduce the clearance of drugs mainly cleared by CYP3A4 and show that the potent inhibition of transporters MDR1, MRP2, and OATP-C does not influence fingolimod disposition.

Isoproterenol, atropine, atenolol, and diltiazem

Single-dose fingolimod and fingolimod-phosphate exposure was not altered by coadministered isoproterenol or atropine. Likewise, the single-dose pharmacokinetics of fingolimod and fingolimod-phosphate and the steady-state pharmacokinetics of both atenolol and diltiazem were unchanged during the coadministration of the latter two drugs individually with fingolimod.

Population pharmacokinetics analysis

A population pharmacokinetics evaluation performed in MS patients did not provide evidence for a significant effect of fluoxetine and paroxetine (strong CYP2D6 inhibitors) and carbamazepine (potent enzyme inducer) on fingolimod or fingolimod-phosphate pre-dose concentrations. In addition, the following commonly co-prescribed substances had no clinically relevant effect (<20%) on fingolimod or fingolimod-phosphate pre-dose concentrations: baclofen, gabapentin, oxybutynin, amantadine, modafinil, amitriptyline, pregabalin, and corticosteroids.

13 NONCLINICAL TOXICOLOGY

13.1 Carcinogenesis, Mutagenesis, Impairment of Fertility

Oral carcinogenicity studies of fingolimod were conducted in mice and rats. In mice, fingolimod was administered at oral doses of 0, 0.025, 0.25, and 2.5 mg/kg/day for up to 2 years. The incidence of malignant lymphoma was increased in males and females at the mid and high dose. The lowest dose tested (0.025 mg/kg/day) is less than the recommended human dose (RHD) of 0.5 mg/day on a body surface area (mg/m^2) basis. In rats, fingolimod was administered at oral doses of 0, 0.05, 0.15, 0.5, and 2.5 mg/kg/day. No increase in tumors was observed. The highest dose tested (2.5 mg/kg/day) is approximately 50 times the RHD on a mg/m^2 basis.

Fingolimod was negative in a battery of *in vitro* (Ames, mouse lymphoma thymidine kinase, chromosomal aberration in mammalian cells) and *in vivo* (micronucleus in mouse and rat) assays.

When fingolimod was administered orally (0, 1, 3, and 10 mg/kg/day) to male and female rats prior to and during mating, and continuing to Day 7 of gestation in females, no effect on fertility was observed up to the highest dose tested (10 mg/kg), which is approximately 200 times the RHD on a mg/m^2 basis.

13.2 Animal Toxicology and/or Pharmacology

Lung toxicity was observed in two different strains of rat and in dog and monkey. The primary findings included increase in lung weight, associated with smooth muscle hypertrophy, hyperdistension of the alveoli, and/or increased collagen. Insufficient or lack of pulmonary collapse at necropsy, generally correlated with microscopic changes, was observed in all species. In rat and monkey, lung toxicity was observed at all oral doses tested in chronic studies. The lowest doses tested in rat (0.05 mg/kg/day in the 2-year carcinogenicity study) and monkey (0.5 mg/kg/day in the 39-week toxicity study) are similar to and approximately 20 times the RHD on a mg/m^2 basis, respectively.

In the 52-week oral study in monkey, respiratory distress associated with ketamine administration was observed at doses of 3 and 10 mg/kg/day; the most affected animal became hypoxic and required oxygenation. As ketamine is not generally associated with respiratory depression, this effect was attributed to fingolimod. In a subsequent study in rat, ketamine was shown to potentiate the bronchoconstrictive effects of fingolimod. The relevance of these findings to humans is unknown.

Table 2 Clinical and MRI Results of Study 1

	GILENYA 0.5 mg N=425	Placebo N=418	p-value
Clinical Endpoints			
Annualized relapse rate (primary endpoint)	0.18	0.40	<0.001
Percentage of patients without relapse	70%	46%	<0.001
Hazard ratio‡ of disability progression (95% CI)	0.70 (0.52, 0.96)		0.02
MRI Endpoint			
Mean (median) number of new or newly enlarging T2 lesions over 24 months	2.5(0)	9.8 (5.0)	<0.001
Mean (median) number of T1 Gd-enhancing lesions at Month 24	0.2(0)	1.1 (0)	<0.001

All analyses of clinical endpoints were intent-to-treat. MRI analysis used evaluable dataset.
‡ Hazard ratio is an estimate of the relative risk of having the event of disability progression on GILENYA as compared to placebo.

Table 3 Clinical and MRI Results of Study 2

	GILENYA 0.5 mg N=429	Interferon beta-1a IM 30 µg N=431	p-value
Clinical Endpoints			
Annualized relapse rate (primary endpoint)	0.16	0.33	<0.001
Percentage of patients without relapse	83%	70%	<0.001
Hazard ratio‡ of disability progression (95% CI)	0.71 (0.42, 1.21)		0.21
MRI Endpoint			
Mean (median) number of new or newly enlarging T2 lesions over 12 months	1.6 (0)	2.6 (1.0)	0.002
Mean (median) number of T1 Gd-enhancing lesions at Month 12	0.2 (0)	0.5 (0)	<0.001

All analyses of clinical endpoints were intent-to–treat. MRI analysis used evaluable dataset.
‡ Hazard ratio is an estimate of the relative risk of having the event of disability progression on GILENYA as compared to control.

14 CLINICAL STUDIES

The efficacy of GILENYA was demonstrated in 2 studies that evaluated once-daily doses of GILENYA 0.5 mg and 1.25 mg in patients with relapsing remitting MS (RRMS). Both studies included patients who had experienced at least 2 clinical relapses during the 2 years prior to randomization or at least 1 clinical relapse during the 1 year prior to randomization, and had an Expanded Disability Status Scale (EDSS) score from 0 to 5.5. Study 1 was a 2-year randomized, double-blind, placebo-controlled study in patients with RRMS who had not received any interferon-beta or glatiramer acetate for at least the previous 3 months and had not received any natalizumab for at least the previous 6 months. Neurological evaluations were performed at screening, every 3 months and at time of suspected relapse. MRI evaluations were performed at screening, month 6, month 12, and month 24. The primary endpoint was the annualized relapse rate.

Median age was 37 years, median disease duration was 6.7 years and median EDSS score at baseline was 2.0. Patients were randomized to receive GILENYA 0.5 mg (n=425), 1.25 mg (n=429), or placebo (n=418) for up to 24 months. Median time on study drug was 717 days on 0.5 mg, 715 days on 1.25 mg and 719 days on placebo.

The annualized relapse rate was significantly lower in patients treated with GILENYA than in patients who received placebo. The secondary endpoint was the time to 3-month confirmed disability progression as measured by at least a 1-point increase from baseline in EDSS (0.5 point increase for patients with baseline EDSS of 5.5) sustained for 3 months. Time to onset of 3-month confirmed disability progression was significantly delayed with GILENYA treatment compared to placebo. The 1.25 mg dose resulted in no additional benefit over the GILENYA 0.5 mg dose. The results for this study are shown in Table 2 and Figure 1.

[See table 2 at top of previous page]

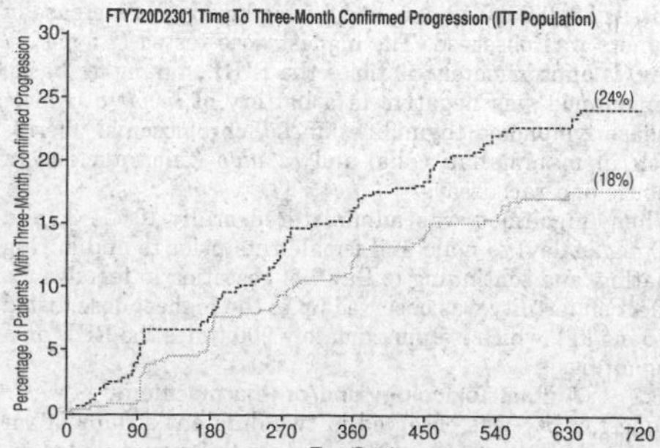

Figure 1 Time to 3-month Confirmed Disability Progression – Study 1 (ITT population)

Study 2 was a 1-year randomized, double-blind, double-dummy, active-controlled study in patients with RRMS who had not received any natalizumab in the previous 6 months. Prior therapy with interferon-beta or glatiramer acetate up to the time of randomization was permitted.

Neurological evaluations were performed at screening, every 3 months, and at the time of suspected relapses. MRI evaluations were performed at screening and at month 12. The primary endpoint was the annualized relapse rate.

Median age was 36 years, median disease duration was 5.9 years, and median EDSS score at baseline was 2.0. Patients were randomized to receive GILENYA 0.5 mg (n=431), 1.25 mg (n=426), or interferon beta-1a, 30 micrograms via the intramuscular route (IM) once weekly (n=435) for up to 12 months. Median time on study drug was 365 days on GILENYA 0.5 mg, 354 days on 1.25 mg, and 361 days on interferon beta-1a IM.

The annualized relapse rate was significantly lower in patients treated with GILENYA 0.5 mg than in patients who received interferon beta-1a IM. The key secondary endpoints were number of new and newly enlarging T2 lesions and time to onset of 3-month confirmed disability progression as measured by at least a 1-point increase from baseline in EDSS (0.5 point increase for those with baseline EDSS of 5.5) sustained for 3 months. The number of new and newly enlarging T2 lesions was significantly lower in patients treated with GILENYA than in patients who received interferon beta-1a IM. There was no significant difference in the time to 3-month confirmed disability progression between GILENYA and interferon beta-1a-treated patients at 1 year. The 1.25 mg dose resulted in no additional benefit over the GILENYA 0.5 mg dose. The results for this study are shown in Table 3.

[See table 3 above]

Pooled results of study 1 and study 2 showed a consistent and statistically significant reduction of annualized relapse rate compared to comparator in subgroups defined by gender, age, prior MS therapy, and disease activity.

16 HOW SUPPLIED/STORAGE AND HANDLING

0.5 mg GILENYA capsules are hard gelatin capsules with a white opaque body and bright yellow cap imprinted with "FTY 0.5 mg" on the cap and two radial bands imprinted on the capsule body with yellow ink.

GILENYA capsules are supplied in blister packs.

Carton of 28 capsules containing 2 folded blister cards of 14 capsules per blister card NDC 0078-0607-51

Carton of 7 capsules containing 1 blister card of 7 capsules per blister card NDC 0078-0607-89

GILENYA capsules should be stored at 25°C (77°F); excursions permitted to 15-30°C (59-86°F). Protect from moisture.

17 PATIENT COUNSELING INFORMATION

See Medication Guide.

A Medication Guide is required for distribution with GILENYA. Encourage patients to read the GILENYA Medication Guide. The complete text of the Medication Guide is reprinted at the end of this document.

17.1 Benefits and Risks

Summarize for patients the benefits and potential risks of treatment with GILENYA. Tell patients to take GILENYA once daily as prescribed. Tell patients not to discontinue GILENYA without first discussing this with the prescribing physician.

17.2 Cardiac Effects

Advise patients that initiation of GILENYA treatment results in a transient decrease in heart rate. Inform patients that they will need to be observed in the doctor's office or other facility for at least 6 hours after the first dose. Advise patients that if GILENYA is discontinued for more than 14 days, effects similar to those observed on treatment initiation may be seen and observation for at least 6 hours will be needed on treatment re-initiation, and that the same precautions will be taken if treatment is interrupted for more than one day within the first 2 weeks of treatment, or for more than 7 days during week 3 and 4 of treatment.

17.3 Risk of Infections

Inform patients that they may be more likely to get infections when taking GILENYA, and that they should contact their physician if they develop symptoms of infection. Advise patients that the use of some vaccines should be avoided during treatment with GILENYA and for 2 months after discontinuation. Advise patients who have not had chickenpox or vaccination to consider VZV vaccination prior to commencing treatment with GILENYA.

17.4 Macular Edema

Advise patients that GILENYA may cause macular edema, and that they should contact their physician if they experience any changes in their vision. Inform patients with diabetes mellitus or a history of uveitis that their risk of macular edema is increased.

17.5 Respiratory Effects

Advise patients that they should contact their physician if they experience new onset or worsening of dyspnea.

17.6 Hepatic Effects

Inform patients that GILENYA may increase liver enzymes. Advise patients that they should contact their physician if they have any unexplained nausea, vomiting, abdominal pain, fatigue, anorexia, or jaundice and/or dark urine.

17.7 Fetal Risk

Inform patients that, based on animal studies, GILENYA may cause fetal harm. Discuss with women of childbearing age whether they are pregnant, might be pregnant or are trying to become pregnant. Advise women of childbearing age of the need for effective contraception during GILENYA treatment and for two months after stopping GILENYA. Advise the patient that if she should nevertheless become pregnant, she should immediately inform her physician.

17.8 Persistence of GILENYA effects after drug discontinuation

Advise patients that GILENYA remains in the blood and continues to have effects, including decreased blood lymphocyte counts, for up to two months following the last dose.

MEDICATION GUIDE

GILENYA™ (je-LEN-yah)
(fingolimod)
capsules

Read this Medication Guide before you start using GILENYA and each time you get a refill. There may be new information. This information does not take the place of talking with your doctor about your medical condition or your treatment.

What is the most important information I should know about GILENYA?

GILENYA may cause serious side effects, including:

1. Slow heart rate (bradycardia or bradyarrhythmia) when you start taking GILENYA. GILENYA can cause your heart rate to slow down, especially after you take your first dose. You will have a test to check the electrical activity of your heart (ECG) before you take your first dose of GILENYA.

You should stay in a medical facility for at least 6 hours after you take your first dose of GILENYA.

After you take your first dose of GILENYA:

- Your pulse and blood pressure should be checked every hour.
- You should be watched by a healthcare professional to see if you have any serious side effects. If your heart rate slows down too much, you may have symptoms such as:
  - dizziness
  - tiredness
  - feeling like your heart is beating slowly or skipping beats
- If you have any of the symptoms of slow heart rate, they will usually happen during the first 6 hours after your first dose of GILENYA. Symptoms can happen up to 24 hours after you take your first GILENYA dose.
- 6 hours after you take your first dose of GILENYA you will have another ECG. If your ECG shows any heart problems or if your heart rate is still too low or continues to decrease, you will continue to be watched.
- If you have any serious side effects after your first dose of GILENYA, especially those that require treatment with other medicines, you will stay in the medical facility to be watched overnight. You will also be watched for any serious side effects for at least 6 hours after you take your second dose of GILENYA the next day.
- If you have certain types of heart problems, or if you are taking certain types of medicines that can affect your heart, you will be watched overnight after you take your first dose of GILENYA.

Your slow heart rate will usually return to normal within 1 month after you start taking GILENYA.

Call your doctor or go to the nearest emergency room right away if you have any symptoms of slow heart rate.

2. Infections. GILENYA can increase your risk of serious infections. GILENYA lowers the number of white blood cells (lymphocytes) in your blood. This will usually go back to normal within 2 months of stopping treatment. Your doctor may do a blood test before you start taking GILENYA. Call your doctor right away if you have any of these symptoms of an infection:

- fever
- tiredness
- body aches
- chills
- nausea
- vomiting

3. A problem with your vision called macular edema. Macular edema can cause some of the same vision symptoms as an MS attack (optic neuritis). You may not notice any symptoms with macular edema. Macular edema usually starts in the first 3 to 4 months after you start taking GILENYA. Your doctor should test your vision before you start taking GILENYA and 3 to 4 months after you start taking GILENYA, or any time you notice vision changes during treatment with GILENYA. Your risk of macular edema may be higher if you have diabetes or have had an inflammation of your eye called uveitis.

Call your doctor right away if you have any of the following:
- blurriness or shadows in the center of your vision
- a blind spot in the center of your vision
- sensitivity to light
- unusually colored (tinted) vision

What is GILENYA?

GILENYA is a prescription medicine used to treat relapsing forms of multiple sclerosis (MS) in adults. GILENYA can decrease the number of MS flare-ups (relapses). GILENYA does not cure MS, but it can help slow down the physical problems that MS causes.

It is not known if GILENYA is safe and effective in children under age 18.

Who should not take GILENYA?

Do not take GILENYA if you:
- have had a heart attack, unstable angina, stroke or warning stroke or certain types of heart failure in the last 6 months
- have certain types of irregular or abnormal heartbeat (arrhythmia), including patients in whom a heart finding called prolonged QT is seen on ECG before starting GILENYA
- are taking certain medicines that change your heart rhythm

If any of the above situations apply to you, tell your doctor.

What should I tell my doctor before taking GILENYA?

Before you take GILENYA, tell your doctor about all your medical conditions, including if you had or now have:
- an irregular or abnormal heartbeat (arrhythmia)
- a history of stroke or warning stroke
- heart problems, including heart attack or angina
- a history of repeated fainting (syncope)
- a fever or infection, or you are unable to fight infections. Tell your doctor if you have had chicken pox or have received the vaccine for chicken pox. Your doctor may do a blood test for chicken pox virus. You may need to get the vaccine for chicken pox and then wait 1 month before you start taking GILENYA.
- eye problems, especially an inflammation of the eye called uveitis.
- diabetes
- breathing problems, including during your sleep
- liver problems
- high blood pressure
- Are pregnant or plan to become pregnant. GILENYA may harm your unborn baby. Talk to your doctor if you are pregnant or are planning to become pregnant.
  - Tell your doctor right away if you become pregnant while taking GILENYA or if you become pregnant within 2 months after you stop taking GILENYA.
  - If you are a female who can become pregnant, you should use effective birth control during your treatment with GILENYA and for at least 2 months after you stop taking GILENYA.

Pregnancy Registry: There is a registry for women who become pregnant during treatment with GILENYA. If you become pregnant while taking GILENYA, talk to your doctor about registering with the GILENYA Pregnancy Registry. The purpose of this registry is to collect information about your health and your baby's health.

For more information, you can call the GILENYA Pregnancy Registry at 1-877-598-7237 or visit www.gilenyapregnancyregistry.com.
- Are breastfeeding or plan to breastfeed. It is not known if GILENYA passes into your breast milk. You and your doctor should decide if you will take GILENYA or breastfeed. You should not do both.

Tell your doctor about all the medicines you take, including prescription and non-prescription medicines, vitamins, and herbal supplements.

Know the medicines you take. Keep a list of your medicines with you to show your doctor and pharmacist when you get a new medicine.

Using GILENYA and other medicines together may affect each other causing serious side effects.

Especially tell your doctor if you take:
- Medicines for:
  - heart problems or
  - high blood pressure or
  - other medicines that may lower your heart rate or change your heart rhythm
- Vaccines. Tell your doctor if you have been vaccinated within 1 month before you start taking GILENYA. You should not get certain vaccines while you take GILENYA and for at least 2 months after you stop taking GILENYA. If you take certain vaccines, you may get the infection the vaccine should have prevented. Vaccines may not work as well when given during GILENYA treatment.
- Medicines that could raise your chance of getting infections, such as medicines to treat cancer or to control your immune system.
- ketoconazole (an antifungal drug) by mouth

Ask your doctor or pharmacist for a list of these medicines if you are not sure.

How should I take GILENYA?
- Your first dose of GILENYA will be given in a medical facility where you will be watched for at least 6 hours after your first dose of GILENYA. See **"What is the most important information I should know about GILENYA?"**
- Take GILENYA exactly as your doctor tells you to take it.
- Take GILENYA 1 time each day.
- Take GILENYA with or without food.
- Do not stop taking GILENYA without talking with your doctor first.
- If you start GILENYA again after stopping for 2 weeks or more, you will start taking GILENYA again in your doctor's office or clinic.

What are possible side effects of GILENYA?

GILENYA can cause serious side effects.

See **"What is the most important information I should know about GILENYA?"**

Serious side effects include:
- **Breathing Problems.** Some people who take GILENYA have shortness of breath. Call your doctor right away if you have trouble breathing.
- **Liver problems.** GILENYA may cause liver problems. Your doctor should do blood tests to check your liver before you start taking GILENYA. Call your doctor right away if you have any of the following symptoms of liver problems:
  - nausea
  - vomiting
  - stomach pain
  - loss of appetite
  - tiredness
  - your skin or the whites of your eyes turn yellow
  - dark urine

The most common side effects of GILENYA include:
- headache
- flu
- diarrhea
- back pain
- abnormal liver tests
- cough

Tell your doctor if you have any side effect that bothers you or that does not go away.

These are not all of the possible side effects of GILENYA. For more information, ask your doctor or pharmacist. Call your doctor for medical advice about side effects. You may report side effects to FDA at 1-800-FDA-1088.

How do I store GILENYA?
- Store GILENYA in the original blister pack in a dry place.
- Store GILENYA at room temperature between 59°F to 86°F (15°C to 30°C).
- Keep GILENYA and all medicines out of the reach of children.

General information about GILENYA

Medicines are sometimes prescribed for purposes other than those listed in a Medication Guide. Do not use GILENYA for a condition for which it was not prescribed. Do not give GILENYA to other people, even if they have the same symptoms you have. It may harm them.

This Medication Guide summarizes the most important information about GILENYA. If you would like more information, talk with your doctor. You can ask your doctor or pharmacist for information about GILENYA that is written for healthcare professionals.

For more information, go to www.pharma.US.Novartis.com or call 1-888-669-6682.

What are the ingredients in GILENYA?

Active ingredient: fingolimod

Inactive ingredients: gelatin, magnesium stearate, mannitol, titanium dioxide, yellow iron oxide.

This Medication Guide has been approved by the U.S. Food and Drug Administration.

GILENYA is a trademark of Novartis AG.

Manufactured by:
Novartis Pharma Stein AG
Stein, Switzerland

Distributed by:
Novartis Pharmaceuticals Corporation
East Hanover, New Jersey 07936

T2012-108/T2012-109
May 2012/May 2012

Shown in Product Identification Guide, page 310

GLEEVEC ℞

[glē-vĕk]
(imatinib mesylate)
tablets for oral use

The following prescribing information is based on official labeling in effect July 2013.

HIGHLIGHTS OF PRESCRIBING INFORMATION

These highlights do not include all the information needed to use Gleevec safely and effectively. See full prescribing information for Gleevec.

GLEEVEC (imatinib mesylate) tablets for oral use
Initial U.S. Approval: 2001

RECENT MAJOR CHANGES

Indications and Usage, Newly Diagnosed Pediatric Ph+ ALL (1.4) 01/2013

INDICATIONS AND USAGE

Gleevec is a kinase inhibitor indicated for the treatment of:
- Newly diagnosed adult and pediatric patients with Philadelphia chromosome positive chronic myeloid leukemia (Ph+ CML) in chronic phase (1.1)
- Patients with Philadelphia chromosome positive chronic myeloid leukemia (Ph+ CML) in blast crisis (BC), accelerated phase (AP), or in chronic phase (CP) after failure of interferon-alpha therapy (1.2)
- Adult patients with relapsed or refractory Philadelphia chromosome positive acute lymphoblastic leukemia (Ph+ ALL) (1.3)
- Pediatric patients with newly diagnosed Philadelphia chromosome positive acute lymphoblastic leukemia (Ph+ ALL) in combination with chemotherapy (1.4)
- Adult patients with myelodysplastic/ myeloproliferative diseases (MDS/MPD) associated with PDGFR (platelet-derived growth factor receptor) gene re-arrangements (1.5)
- Adult patients with aggressive systemic mastocytosis (ASM) without the D816V c-Kit mutation or with c-Kit mutational status unknown (1.6)
- Adult patients with hypereosinophilic syndrome (HES) and/or chronic eosinophilic leukemia (CEL) who have the FIP1L1-PDGFRα fusion kinase (mutational analysis or FISH demonstration of CHIC2 allele deletion) and for patients with HES and/or CEL who are FIP1L1-PDGFRα fusion kinase negative or unknown (1.7)
- Adult patients with unresectable, recurrent and/or metastatic dermatofibrosarcoma protuberans (DFSP) (1.8)
- Patients with Kit (CD117) positive unresectable and/or metastatic malignant gastrointestinal stromal tumors (GIST) (1.9)
- Adjuvant treatment of adult patients following resection of Kit (CD117) positive GIST (1.10)

DOSAGE AND ADMINISTRATION

- Adults with Ph+ CML CP (2.1): 400 mg/day
- Adults with Ph+ CML AP or BC (2.1): 600 mg/day
- Pediatrics with Ph+ CML CP (2.2): 340 mg/m²/day
- Adults with Ph+ ALL (2.3): 600 mg/day
- Pediatrics with Ph+ ALL (2.4): 340 mg/m²/day
- Adults with MDS/MPD (2.5): 400 mg/day
- Adults with ASM (2.6): 100 mg/day or 400 mg/day
- Adults with HES/CEL (2.7): 100 mg/day or 400 mg/day
- Adults with DFSP (2.8): 800 mg/day
- Adults with metastatic and/or unresectable GIST (2.9): 400 mg/day
- Adjuvant treatment of adults with GIST (2.10): 400 mg/day
- Patients with mild to moderate hepatic impairment (2.11): 400 mg/day
- Patients with severe hepatic impairment (2.11): 300 mg/day

All doses of Gleevec should be taken with a meal and a large glass of water. Doses of 400 mg or 600 mg should be administered once daily, whereas a dose of 800 mg should be administered as 400 mg twice a day. Gleevec can be dissolved in water or apple juice for patients having difficulty swallowing. Daily dosing of 800 mg and above should be accomplished using the 400 mg tablet to reduce exposure to iron.

DOSAGE FORMS AND STRENGTHS

Tablets (scored): 100 mg and 400 mg (3)

CONTRAINDICATIONS

None (4)

WARNINGS AND PRECAUTIONS

- Edema and severe fluid retention have occurred. Weigh patients regularly and manage unexpected rapid weight gain by drug interruption and diuretics (5.1, 6.1, 6.11)
- Cytopenias, particularly anemia, neutropenia, and thrombocytopenia, have occurred. Manage with dose reduction or dose interruption and in rare cases discontinuation of treatment. Perform complete blood counts weekly for the first month, biweekly for the second month, and periodically thereafter (5.2)

- Severe congestive heart failure and left ventricular dysfunction have been reported, particularly in patients with comorbidities and risk factors. Patients with cardiac disease or risk factors for cardiac failure should be monitored and treated (5.3)
- Severe hepatotoxicity including fatalities may occur. Assess liver function before initiation of treatment and monthly thereafter or as clinically indicated. Monitor liver function when combined with chemotherapy known to be associated with liver dysfunction (5.4)
- Grade 3/4 hemorrhage has been reported in clinical studies in patients with newly diagnosed CML and with GIST. GI tumor sites may be the source of GI bleeds in GIST (5.5)
- Gastrointestinal perforations, some fatal, have been reported (5.6)
- Cardiogenic shock/left ventricular dysfunction has been associated with the initiation of Gleevec in patients with conditions associated with high eosinophil levels (e.g., HES, MDS/MPD and ASM) (5.7)
- Bullous dermatologic reactions (e.g., erythema multiforme and Stevens-Johnson syndrome) have been reported with the use of Gleevec (5.8)
- Hypothyroidism has been reported in thyroidectomy patients undergoing levothyroxine replacement. Closely monitor TSH levels in such patients (5.9)
- Consider potential toxicities, specifically, liver, kidney, and cardiac toxicity, and immunosuppression from long-term use (5.10)
- Fetal harm can occur when administered to a pregnant woman. Women should be apprised of the potential harm to the fetus (5.11, 8.1)
- Growth retardation occurring in children and preadolescents receiving Gleevec has been reported. Close monitoring of growth in children under Gleevec treatment is recommended (5.12, 6.13)
- Tumor lysis syndrome. Close monitoring is recommended (5.13)
- Reports of motor vehicle accidents have been received in patients receiving Gleevec. Caution patients about driving a car or operating machinery (5.14)

ADVERSE REACTIONS

The most frequently reported adverse reactions (≥30%) were edema, nausea, vomiting, muscle cramps, musculoskeletal pain, diarrhea, rash, fatigue and abdominal pain (6.1, 6.11)

To report SUSPECTED ADVERSE REACTIONS, contact Novartis Pharmaceuticals Corporation at 1-888-669-6682 or FDA at 1-800-FDA-1088 or www.fda.gov/medwatch.

DRUG INTERACTIONS

- CYP3A4 inducers may decrease Gleevec C_{max} and AUC (2.11, 7.1)
- CYP3A4 inhibitors may increase Gleevec C_{max} and AUC (7.2)
- Gleevec is an inhibitor of CYP3A4 and CYP2D6 which may increase the C_{max} and AUC of other drugs (7.3, 7.4)
- Patients who require anticoagulation should receive low-molecular weight or standard heparin and not warfarin (7.3)

USE IN SPECIFIC POPULATIONS

- There is no experience in children less than 1 year of age (8.4)
- Pregnancy: Sexually active female patients should use highly effective contraception during treatment (5.11)

See 17 for PATIENT COUNSELING INFORMATION

Revised: 02/2013

Table 1 Dose Adjustments for Neutropenia and Thrombocytopenia

ASM associated with eosinophilia (starting dose 100 mg)	ANC <1.0 × 10^9/L and/or platelets <50 × 10^9/L	1. Stop Gleevec until ANC ≥1.5 × 10^9/L and platelets ≥75 × 10^9/L 2. Resume treatment with Gleevec at previous dose (i.e., dose before severe adverse reaction)
HES/CEL with FIP1L1-PDGFRα fusion kinase (starting dose 100 mg)	ANC <1.0 × 10^9/L and/or platelets <50 × 10^9/L	1. Stop Gleevec until ANC ≥1.5 × 10^9/L and platelets ≥75 × 10^9/L 2. Resume treatment with Gleevec at previous dose (i.e., dose before severe adverse reaction)
Chronic Phase CML (starting dose 400 mg) MDS/MPD, ASM and HES/CEL (starting dose 400 mg) GIST (starting dose 400 mg)	ANC <1.0 × 10^9/L and/or platelets <50 × 10^9/L	1. Stop Gleevec until ANC ≥1.5 × 10^9/L and platelets ≥75 × 10^9/L 2. Resume treatment with Gleevec at the original starting dose of 400 mg 3. If recurrence of ANC <1.0 × 10^9/L and/or platelets <50 × 10^9/L, repeat step 1 and resume Gleevec at a reduced dose of 300 mg
Ph+ CML : Accelerated Phase and Blast Crisis (starting dose 600 mg) Ph+ ALL (starting dose 600 mg)	ANC <0.5 × 10^9/L and/or platelets <10 × 10^9/L	1. Check if cytopenia is related to leukemia (marrow aspirate or biopsy) 2. If cytopenia is unrelated to leukemia, reduce dose of Gleevec to 400 mg 3. If cytopenia persists 2 weeks, reduce further to 300 mg 4. If cytopenia persists 4 weeks and is still unrelated to leukemia, stop Gleevec until ANC ≥1 × 10^9/L and platelets ≥20 × 10^9/L and then resume treatment at 300 mg
DFSP (starting dose 800 mg)	ANC <1.0 × 10^9/L and/or platelets <50 × 10^9/L	1. Stop Gleevec until ANC ≥1.5 × 10^9/L and platelets ≥75 × 10^9/L 2. Resume treatment with Gleevec at 600 mg 3. In the event of recurrence of ANC <1.0 × 10^9/L and/or platelets <50 × 10^9/L, repeat step 1 and resume Gleevec at reduced dose of 400 mg
Pediatric newly diagnosed chronic phase CML (starting dose 340 mg/m^2)	ANC <1.0 × 10^9/L and/or platelets <50 × 10^9/L	1. Stop Gleevec until ANC ≥1.5 × 10^9/L and platelets ≥75 × 10^9/L 2. Resume treatment with Gleevec at previous dose (i.e., dose before severe adverse reaction) 3. In the event of recurrence of ANC <1.0 × 10^9/L and/or platelets <50 × 10^9/L, repeat step 1 and resume Gleevec at reduced dose of 260 mg/m^2

FULL PRESCRIBING INFORMATION: CONTENTS*

*** Sections or subsections omitted from the full prescribing information are not listed**

FULL PRESCRIBING INFORMATION

1 INDICATIONS AND USAGE

1.1 Newly Diagnosed Philadelphia Positive Chronic Myeloid Leukemia (Ph+ CML)

Newly diagnosed adult and pediatric patients with Philadelphia chromosome positive chronic myeloid leukemia in chronic phase.

1.2 Ph+ CML in Blast Crisis (BC), Accelerated Phase (AP) or Chronic Phase (CP) After Interferon-alpha (IFN) Therapy

Patients with Philadelphia chromosome positive chronic myeloid leukemia in blast crisis, accelerated phase, or in chronic phase after failure of interferon-alpha therapy.

1.3 Adult patients with Ph+ Acute Lymphoblastic Leukemia (ALL)

Adult patients with relapsed or refractory Philadelphia chromosome positive acute lymphoblastic leukemia.

1.4 Pediatric patients with Ph+ Acute Lymphoblastic Leukemia (ALL)

Pediatric patients with newly diagnosed Philadelphia chromosome positive acute lymphoblastic leukemia (Ph+ ALL) in combination with chemotherapy.

1.5 Myelodysplastic/Myeloproliferative Diseases (MDS/MPD)

Adult patients with myelodysplastic/ myeloproliferative diseases associated with PDGFR (platelet-derived growth factor receptor) gene re-arrangements.

1.6 Aggressive Systemic Mastocytosis (ASM)

Adult patients with aggressive systemic mastocytosis without the D816V c-Kit mutation or with c-Kit mutational status unknown.

1.7 Hypereosinophilic Syndrome (HES) and/or Chronic Eosinophilic Leukemia (CEL)

Adult patients with hypereosinophilic syndrome and/or chronic eosinophilic leukemia who have the FIP1L1-PDGFRα fusion kinase (mutational analysis or FISH demonstration of CHIC2 allele deletion) and for patients with HES and/or CEL who are FIP1L1-PDGFRα fusion kinase negative or unknown.

1.8 Dermatofibrosarcoma Protuberans (DFSP)

Adult patients with unresectable, recurrent and/or metastatic dermatofibrosarcoma protuberans.

1.9 Kit+ Gastrointestinal Stromal Tumors (GIST)

Patients with Kit (CD117) positive unresectable and/or metastatic malignant gastrointestinal stromal tumors.

1.10 Adjuvant Treatment of GIST

Adjuvant treatment of adult patients following complete gross resection of Kit (CD117) positive GIST.

2 DOSAGE AND ADMINISTRATION

Therapy should be initiated by a physician experienced in the treatment of patients with hematological malignancies or malignant sarcomas, as appropriate. The prescribed dose should be administered orally, with a meal and a large glass of water. Doses of 400 mg or 600 mg should be administered once daily, whereas a dose of 800 mg should be administered as 400 mg twice a day.

In children, Gleevec treatment can be given as a once-daily dose in CML and Ph+ ALL. Alternatively, in children with CML the daily dose may be split into two - one portion dosed in the morning and one portion in the evening. There is no experience with Gleevec treatment in children under 1 year of age.

For patients unable to swallow the film-coated tablets, the tablets may be dispersed in a glass of water or apple juice. The required number of tablets should be placed in the appropriate volume of beverage (approximately 50 mL for a 100 mg tablet, and 200 mL for a 400 mg tablet) and stirred with a spoon. The suspension should be administered immediately after complete disintegration of the tablet(s).

For daily dosing of 800 mg and above, dosing should be accomplished using the 400 mg tablet to reduce exposure to iron.

Treatment may be continued as long as there is no evidence of progressive disease or unacceptable toxicity.

2.1 Adult Patients with Ph+ CML CP, AP, and BC

The recommended dose of Gleevec is 400 mg/day for adult patients in chronic phase CML and 600 mg/day for adult patients in accelerated phase or blast crisis.

In CML, a dose increase from 400 mg to 600 mg in adult patients with chronic phase disease, or from 600 mg to 800 mg (given as 400 mg twice daily) in adult patients in accelerated phase or blast crisis may be considered in the absence of severe adverse drug reaction and severe non-leukemia related neutropenia or thrombocytopenia in the following circumstances: disease progression (at any time), failure to achieve a satisfactory hematologic response after at least 3 months of treatment, failure to achieve a cytogenetic response after 6-12 months of treatment, or loss of a previously achieved hematologic or cytogenetic response.

2.2 Pediatric Patients with Ph+ CML CP

The recommended dose of Gleevec for children with newly diagnosed Ph+ CML is 340 mg/m^2/day (not to exceed 600 mg).

Table 2 Adverse Reactions Regardless of Relationship to Study Drug Reported in Newly Diagnosed CML Clinical Trial (≥10% of Gleevec Treated Patients)[(1)]

	All Grades		CTC Grades 3/4	
Preferred Term	Gleevec N=551 (%)	IFN+Ara–C N=533 (%)	Gleevec N=551 (%)	IFN+Ara–C N=533 (%)
Fluid Retention	61.7	11.1	2.5	0.9
– Superficial Edema	59.9	9.6	1.5	0.4
– Other Fluid Retention Reactions[2]	6.9	1.9	1.3	0.6
Nausea	49.5	61.5	1.3	5.1
Muscle Cramps	49.2	11.8	2.2	0.2
Musculoskeletal Pain	47.0	44.8	5.4	8.6
Diarrhea	45.4	43.3	3.3	3.2
Rash and Related Terms	40.1	26.1	2.9	2.4
Fatigue	38.8	67.0	1.8	25.1
Headache	37.0	43.3	0.5	3.8
Joint Pain	31.4	38.1	2.5	7.7
Abdominal Pain	36.5	25.9	4.2	3.9
Nasopharyngitis	30.5	8.8	0	0.4
Hemorrhage	28.9	21.2	1.8	1.7
- GI Hemorrhage	1.6	1.1	0.5	0.2
- CNS Hemorrhage	0.2	0.4	0	0.4
Myalgia	24.1	38.8	1.5	8.3
Vomiting	22.5	27.8	2.0	3.4
Dyspepsia	18.9	8.3	0	0.8
Cough	20.0	23.1	0.2	0.6
Pharyngolaryngeal Pain	18.1	11.4	0.2	0
Upper Respiratory Tract Infection	21.2	8.4	0.2	0.4
Dizziness	19.4	24.4	0.9	3.8
Pyrexia	17.8	42.6	0.9	3.0
Weight Increased	15.6	2.6	2.0	0.4
Insomnia	14.7	18.6	0	2.3
Depression	14.9	35.8	0.5	13.1
Influenza	13.8	6.2	0.2	0.2
Bone Pain	11.3	15.6	1.6	3.4
Constipation	11.4	14.4	0.7	0.2
Sinusitis	11.4	6.0	0.2	0.2

[(1)]All adverse reactions occurring in ≥10% of Gleevec treated patients are listed regardless of suspected relationship to treatment.

[(2)]Other fluid retention reactions include pleural effusion, ascites, pulmonary edema, pericardial effusion, anasarca, edema aggravated, and fluid retention not otherwise specified.

2.3 Adults Patients with Ph+ ALL

The recommended dose of Gleevec is 600 mg/day for adult patients with relapsed/refractory Ph+ ALL.

2.4 Pediatric Patients with Ph+ ALL

The recommended dose of Gleevec to be given in combination with chemotherapy to children with newly diagnosed Ph+ ALL is 340mg/m^2/day (not to exceed 600mg).

2.5 MDS/MPD

The recommended dose of Gleevec is 400 mg/day for adult patients with MDS/MPD.

2.6 ASM

The recommended dose of Gleevec is 400 mg/day for adult patients with ASM without the D816V c-Kit mutation. If c-Kit mutational status is not known or unavailable, treatment with Gleevec 400 mg/day may be considered for patients with ASM not responding satisfactorily to other therapies. For patients with ASM associated with eosinophilia, a clonal hematological disease related to the fusion kinase FIP1L1-PDGFRα, a starting dose of 100 mg/day is recommended. Dose increase from 100 mg to 400 mg for these patients may be considered in the absence of adverse drug reactions if assessments demonstrate an insufficient response to therapy.

2.7 HES/CEL

The recommended dose of Gleevec is 400 mg/day for adult patients with HES/CEL. For HES/CEL patients with demonstrated FIP1L1-PDGFRα fusion kinase, a starting dose of 100 mg/day is recommended. Dose increase from 100 mg to 400 mg for these patients may be considered in the absence of adverse drug reactions if assessments demonstrate an insufficient response to therapy.

2.8 DFSP

The recommended dose of Gleevec is 800 mg/day for adult patients with DFSP.

2.9 Metastatic or Unresectable GIST

The recommended dose of Gleevec is 400 mg/day for adult patients with unresectable and/or metastatic, malignant GIST. A dose increase up to 800 mg daily (given as 400 mg twice daily) may be considered, as clinically indicated, in patients showing clear signs or symptoms of disease progression at a lower dose and in the absence of severe adverse drug reactions.

2.10 Adjuvant GIST

The recommended dose of Gleevec is 400 mg/day for the adjuvant treatment of adult patients following complete gross resection of GIST. In clinical trials one year of Gleevec and three years of Gleevec were studied. In the patient population defined in Study 2, three years of Gleevec is recommended [*see Clinical Studies (14.8)*]. The optimal treatment duration with Gleevec is not known.

2.11 Dose Modification Guidelines

Concomitant Strong CYP3A4 inducers: The use of concomitant strong CYP3A4 inducers should be avoided (e.g., dexamethasone, phenytoin, carbamazepine, rifampin, rifabutin, rifampacin, phenobarbital). If patients must be co-administered a strong CYP3A4 inducer, based on pharmacokinetic studies, the dosage of Gleevec should be increased by at least 50%, and clinical response should be carefully monitored [*see Drug Interactions (7.1)*].

Hepatic Impairment: Patients with mild and moderate hepatic impairment do not require a dose adjustment and should be treated per the recommended dose. A 25% decrease in the recommended dose should be used for patients with severe hepatic impairment [*see Use in Specific Populations (8.6)*].

Renal Impairment: Patients with moderate renal impairment (CrCL=20-39 mL/min) should receive a 50% decrease in the recommended starting dose and future doses can be increased as tolerated. Doses greater than 600 mg are not recommended in patients with mild renal impairment (CrCL=40-59 mL/min). For patients with moderate renal impairment doses greater than 400 mg are not recommended.

Imatinib should be used with caution in patients with severe renal impairment. A dose of 100 mg/day was tolerated in two patients with severe renal impairment [*See Warnings and Precautions (5.3), Use in Specific Populations (8.7)*].

2.12 Dose Adjustment for Hepatotoxicity and Non-Hematologic Adverse Reactions

If elevations in bilirubin >3 × institutional upper limit of normal (IULN) or in liver transaminases >5 × IULN occur, Gleevec should be withheld until bilirubin levels have returned to a <1.5 × IULN and transaminase levels to <2.5 × IULN. In adults, treatment with Gleevec may then be continued at a reduced daily dose (i.e., 400 mg to 300 mg, 600 mg to 400 mg or 800 mg to 600 mg). In children, daily doses can be reduced under the same circumstances from 340 mg/m^2/day to 260 mg/m^2/day.

If a severe non-hematologic adverse reaction develops (such as severe hepatotoxicity or severe fluid retention), Gleevec should be withheld until the event has resolved. Thereafter, treatment can be resumed as appropriate depending on the initial severity of the event.

Table 3 Adverse Reactions Regardless of Relationship to Study Drug Reported in Other CML Clinical Trials (≥10% of All Patients in any Trial)[(1)]

	Myeloid Blast Crisis (n=260) %		Accelerated Phase (n=235) %		Chronic Phase, IFN Failure (n=532) %	
Preferred Term	**All Grades**	**Grade 3/4**	**All Grades**	**Grade 3/4**	**All Grades**	**Grade 3/4**
Fluid Retention	72	11	76	6	69	4
-Superficial Edema	66	6	74	3	67	2
-Other Fluid Retention Reactions [(2)]	22	6	15	4	7	2
Nausea	71	5	73	5	63	3
Muscle Cramps	28	1	47	0.4	62	2
Vomiting	54	4	58	3	36	2
Diarrhea	43	4	57	5	48	3
Hemorrhage	53	19	49	11	30	2
- CNS Hemorrhage	9	7	3	3	2	1
- GI Hemorrhage	8	4	6	5	2	0.4
Musculoskeletal Pain	42	9	49	9	38	2
Fatigue	30	4	46	4	48	1
Skin Rash	36	5	47	5	47	3
Pyrexia	41	7	41	8	21	2
Arthralgia	25	5	34	6	40	1
Headache	27	5	32	2	36	0.6
Abdominal Pain	30	6	33	4	32	1
Weight Increased	5	1	17	5	32	7
Cough	14	0.8	27	0.9	20	0
Dyspepsia	12	0	22	0	27	0
Myalgia	9	0	24	2	27	0.2
Nasopharyngitis	10	0	17	0	22	0.2
Asthenia	18	5	21	5	15	0.2
Dyspnea	15	4	21	7	12	0.9
Upper Respiratory Tract Infection	3	0	12	0.4	19	0
Anorexia	14	2	17	2	7	0
Night Sweats	13	0.8	17	1	14	0.2
Constipation	16	2	16	0.9	9	0.4
Dizziness	12	0.4	13	0	16	0.2
Pharyngitis	10	0	12	0	15	0
Insomnia	10	0	14	0	14	0.2
Pruritus	8	1	14	0.9	14	0.8
Hypokalemia	13	4	9	2	6	0.8
Pneumonia	13	7	10	7	4	1
Anxiety	8	0.8	12	0	8	0.4
Liver Toxicity	10	5	12	6	6	3
Rigors	10	0	12	0.4	10	0
Chest Pain	7	2	10	0.4	11	0.8
Influenza	0.8	0.4	6	0	11	0.2
Sinusitis	4	0.4	11	0.4	9	0.4

(1) All adverse reactions occurring in ≥10% of patients are listed regardless of suspected relationship to treatment.
(2) Other fluid retention reactions include pleural effusion, ascites, pulmonary edema, pericardial effusion, anasarca, edema aggravated, and fluid retention not otherwise specified.

Table 4 Lab Abnormalities in Newly Diagnosed CML Clinical Trial

	Gleevec N=551 %		IFN+Ara–C N=533 %	
CTC Grades	**Grade 3**	**Grade 4**	**Grade 3**	**Grade 4**
Hematology Parameters*				
– Neutropenia*	13.1	3.6	20.8	4.5
– Thrombocytopenia*	8.5	0.4	15.9	0.6
– Anemia	3.3	1.1	4.1	0.2
Biochemistry Parameters				
– Elevated Creatinine	0	0	0.4	0
– Elevated Bilirubin	0.9	0.2	0.2	0
– Elevated Alkaline Phosphatase	0.2	0	0.8	0
– Elevated SGOT /SGPT	4.7	0.5	7.1	0.4

*p<0.001 (difference in Grade 3 plus 4 abnormalities between the two treatment groups)

2.13 Dose Adjustment for Hematologic Adverse Reactions

Dose reduction or treatment interruptions for severe neutropenia and thrombocytopenia are recommended as indicated in Table 1.

[See table 1 at top of page 1996]

3 DOSAGE FORMS AND STRENGTHS

100 mg film coated tablets

Very dark yellow to brownish orange, film-coated tablets, round, biconvex with bevelled edges, debossed with "NVR" on one side, and "SA" with score on the other side

400 mg film coated tablets

Very dark yellow to brownish orange, film-coated tablets, ovaloid, biconvex with bevelled edges, debossed with "400" on one side with score on the other side, and "SL" on each side of the score

4 CONTRAINDICATIONS

None

5 WARNINGS AND PRECAUTIONS

5.1 Fluid Retention and Edema

Gleevec is often associated with edema and occasionally serious fluid retention [*see Adverse Reactions (6.1)*]. Patients should be weighed and monitored regularly for signs and symptoms of fluid retention. An unexpected rapid weight gain should be carefully investigated and appropriate treatment provided. The probability of edema was increased with higher Gleevec dose and age >65 years in the CML studies. Severe superficial edema was reported in 1.5% of newly diagnosed CML patients taking Gleevec, and in 2%-6% of other adult CML patients taking Gleevec. In addition, other severe fluid retention (e.g., pleural effusion, pericardial effusion, pulmonary edema, and ascites) reactions were reported in 1.3% of newly diagnosed CML patients taking Gleevec, and in 2%-6% of other adult CML patients taking Gleevec. Severe fluid retention was reported in 9% to 13.1% of patients taking Gleevec for GIST [*see Adverse Reactions (6.11)*].

5.2 Hematologic Toxicity

Treatment with Gleevec is associated with anemia, neutropenia, and thrombocytopenia. Complete blood counts should be performed weekly for the first month, biweekly for the second month, and periodically thereafter as clinically indicated (for example, every 2-3 months). In CML, the occurrence of these cytopenias is dependent on the stage of disease and is more frequent in patients with accelerated phase CML or blast crisis than in patients with chronic phase CML. In pediatric CML patients the most frequent toxicities observed were Grade 3 or 4 cytopenias including neutropenia, thrombocytopenia and anemia. These generally occur within the first several months of therapy [*see Dosage and Administration (2.12)*].

5.3 Severe Congestive Heart Failure and Left Ventricular Dysfunction

Severe congestive heart failure and left ventricular dysfunction have been reported in patients taking Gleevec. Most of the patients with reported cardiac reactions have had other co-morbidities and risk factors, including advanced age and previous medical history of cardiac disease. In an international randomized phase 3 study in 1,106 patients with newly diagnosed Ph+ CML in chronic phase, severe cardiac failure and left ventricular dysfunction were observed in 0.7% of patients taking Gleevec compared to 0.9% of patients taking IFN + Ara-C. Patients with cardiac disease or risk factors for cardiac or history of renal failure should be monitored carefully and any patient with signs or symptoms consistent with cardiac or renal failure should be evaluated and treated.

5.4 Hepatotoxicity

Hepatotoxicity, occasionally severe, may occur with Gleevec [*see Adverse Reactions (6.3)*]. Cases of fatal liver failure and severe liver injury requiring liver transplants have been reported with both short-term and long-term use of Gleevec. Liver function (transaminases, bilirubin, and alkaline phosphatase) should be monitored before initiation of treatment and monthly, or as clinically indicated. Laboratory abnormalities should be managed with Gleevec interruption and/or dose reduction [*see Dosage and Administration (2.12)*].

When Gleevec is combined with chemotherapy, liver toxicity in the form of transaminase elevation and hyperbilirubinemia has been observed. Additionally, there have been reports of acute liver failure. Monitoring of hepatic function is recommended.

5.5 Hemorrhage

In the newly diagnosed CML trial, 1.8% of patients had Grade 3/4 hemorrhage. In the Phase 3 unresectable or metastatic GIST studies 211 patients (12.9%) reported Grade 3/4 hemorrhage at any site. In the Phase 2 unresectable or metastatic GIST study 7 patients (5%) had a total of 8 CTC Grade 3/4 hemorrhages; gastrointestinal (GI) (3 patients), intra-tumoral (3 patients) or both (1 patient). Gastrointestinal tumor sites may have been the source of GI hemorrhages. Patients should therefore be monitored for gastrointestinal symptoms at the start of therapy.

5.6 Gastrointestinal Disorders

Gleevec is sometimes associated with GI irritation. Gleevec should be taken with food and a large glass of water to minimize this problem. There have been rare reports, including fatalities, of gastrointestinal perforation.

5.7 Hypereosinophilic Cardiac Toxicity

In patients with hypereosinophilic syndrome with occult infiltration of HES cells within the myocardium, cases of cardiogenic shock/left ventricular dysfunction have been associated with HES cell degranulation upon the initiation of Gleevec therapy. The condition was reported to be reversible with the administration of systemic steroids, circulatory support measures and temporarily withholding Gleevec. Myelodysplastic/ myeloproliferative disease and systemic mastocytosis may be associated with high eosinophil levels. Performance of an echocardiogram and determination of serum troponin should therefore be considered in patients with HES/CEL, and in patients with MDS/MPD or ASM associated with high eosinophil levels. If either is abnormal, the prophylactic use of systemic steroids (1-2 mg/kg) for one to two weeks concomitantly with Gleevec should be considered at the initiation of therapy.

5.8 Dermatologic Toxicities

Bullous dermatologic reactions, including erythema multiforme and Stevens-Johnson syndrome, have been reported with use of Gleevec. In some cases of bullous dermatologic reactions, including erythema multiforme and Stevens-Johnson syndrome reported during postmarketing surveillance, a recurrent dermatologic reaction was observed upon re-challenge. Several foreign post-marketing reports have described cases in which patients tolerated the reintroduction of Gleevec therapy after resolution or improvement of the bullous reaction. In these instances, Gleevec was resumed at a dose lower than that at which the reaction occurred and some patients also received concomitant treatment with corticosteroids or antihistamines.

5.9 Hypothyroidism

Clinical cases of hypothyroidism have been reported in thyroidectomy patients undergoing levothyroxine replacement during treatment with Gleevec. TSH levels should be closely monitored in such patients.

5.10 Toxicities from Long-Term Use

It is important to consider potential toxicities suggested by animal studies, specifically, *liver, kidney, and cardiac toxicity and immunosuppression*. Severe liver toxicity was observed in dogs treated for 2 weeks, with elevated liver enzymes, hepatocellular necrosis, bile duct necrosis, and bile duct hyperplasia. Renal toxicity was observed in monkeys treated for 2 weeks, with focal mineralization and dilation of the renal tubules and tubular nephrosis. Increased BUN and creatinine were observed in several of these animals. An increased rate of opportunistic infections was observed with chronic imatinib treatment in laboratory animal studies. In a 39-week monkey study, treatment with imatinib resulted in worsening of normally suppressed malarial infections in these animals. Lymphopenia was observed in animals (as in humans). Additional long-term toxicities were identified in a 2-year rat study. Histopathological examination of the treated rats that died on study revealed cardiomyopathy (both sexes), chronic progressive nephropathy (females) and preputial gland papilloma as principal causes of death or reasons for sacrifice. Non-neoplastic lesions seen in this 2-year study which were not identified in earlier preclinical studies were the cardiovascular system, pancreas, endocrine organs and teeth. The most important changes included cardiac hypertrophy and dilatation, leading to signs of cardiac insufficiency in some animals.

5.11 Use in Pregnancy

Pregnancy Category D

Gleevec can cause fetal harm when administered to a pregnant woman. Imatinib mesylate was teratogenic in rats when administered during organogenesis at doses approximately equal to the maximum human dose of 800 mg/day based on body surface area. Significant post-implantation loss was seen in female rats administered imatinib mesylate at doses approximately one-half the maximum human dose of 800 mg/day based on body surface area. Sexually active female patients of reproductive potential taking Gleevec should use highly effective contraception. If this drug is used during pregnancy or if the patient becomes pregnant while taking this drug, the patient should be apprised of the potential hazard to a fetus [*see Use in Specific Populations (8.1)*].

5.12 Children and Adolescents

Growth retardation has been reported in children and preadolescents receiving Gleevec. The long term effects of prolonged treatment with Gleevec on growth in children are unknown. Therefore, close monitoring of growth in children under Gleevec treatment is recommended [*see Adverse Reactions (6.13)*].

5.13 Tumor Lysis Syndrome

Cases of Tumor Lysis Syndrome (TLS), including fatal cases, have been reported in patients with CML, GIST, ALL and eosinophilic leukemia receiving Gleevec. The patients at risk of TLS are those with tumors having a high proliferative rate or high tumor burden prior to treatment. These patients should be monitored closely and appropriate precautions taken. Due to possible occurrence of TLS, correction of clinically significant dehydration and treatment of high uric acid levels are recommended prior to initiation of Gleevec.

5.14 Driving and Using Machinery

Reports of motor vehicle accidents have been received in patients receiving Gleevec. While most of these reports are not suspected to be caused by Gleevec, patients should be advised that they may experience undesirable effects such as dizziness, blurred vision or somnolence during treatment with Gleevec. Therefore, caution should be recommended when driving a car or operating machinery.

6 ADVERSE REACTIONS

Because clinical trials are conducted under widely varying conditions, the adverse reaction rates observed cannot be directly compared to rates on other clinical trials and may not reflect the rates observed in clinical practice.

6.1 Chronic Myeloid Leukemia

The majority of Gleevec-treated patients experienced adverse reactions at some time. Most reactions were of mild-to-moderate grade, but drug was discontinued for drug-related adverse reactions in 2.4% of newly diagnosed patients, 4% of patients in chronic phase after failure of interferon-alpha therapy, 4% in accelerated phase and 5% in blast crisis.

The most frequently reported drug-related adverse reactions were edema, nausea and vomiting, muscle cramps, musculoskeletal pain, diarrhea and rash (Table 2 for newly diagnosed CML, Table 3 for other CML patients). Edema was most frequently periorbital or in lower limbs and was managed with diuretics, other supportive measures, or by reducing the dose of Gleevec [*see Dosage and Administration (2.12)*]. The frequency of severe superficial edema was 1.5%-6%.

Table 5 Lab Abnormalities in Other CML Clinical Trials

	Myeloid Blast Crisis (n=260) 600 mg n=223 400 mg n=37 %		Accelerated Phase (n=235) 600 mg n=158 400 mg n=77 %		Chronic Phase, IFN Failure (n=532) 400 mg %	
CTC Grades[1]	Grade 3	Grade 4	Grade 3	Grade 4	Grade 3	Grade 4
Hematology Parameters						
– Neutropenia	16	48	23	36	27	9
– Thrombocytopenia	30	33	31	13	21	<1
– Anemia	42	11	34	7	6	1
Biochemistry Parameters						
– Elevated Creatinine	1.5	0	1.3	0	0.2	0
– Elevated Bilirubin	3.8	0	2.1	0	0.6	0
– Elevated Alkaline Phosphatase	4.6	0	5.5	0.4	0.2	0
– Elevated SGOT (AST)	1.9	0	3.0	0	2.3	0
– Elevated SGPT (ALT)	2.3	0.4	4.3	0	2.1	0

[1]CTC Grades: neutropenia (Grade 3 ≥0.5-1.0 × 10^9/L, Grade 4 <0.5 × 10^9/L), thrombocytopenia (Grade 3 ≥10-50 × 10^9/L, Grade 4 <10 × 10^9/L), anemia (hemoglobin ≥65-80 g/L, Grade 4 <65 g/L), elevated creatinine (Grade 3 >3-6 × upper limit normal range [ULN], Grade 4 >6 × ULN), elevated bilirubin (Grade 3 >3-10 × ULN, Grade 4 >10 × ULN), elevated alkaline phosphatase (Grade 3 >5-20 × ULN, Grade 4 >20 × ULN), elevated SGOT or SGPT (Grade 3 >5-20 × ULN, Grade 4 >20 × ULN)

Table 6 Adverse Reactions Reported More Frequently in Patients Treated with Study Drug (>5%) or in Cycles with Study Drug (>1%)

Adverse Event	Per Patient Incidence Ph+ALL With Gleevec N = 92	Per Patient Incidence Ph- ALL No Gleevec N = 65	Per Patient Per Cycle Incidence With Gleevec* N = 778	Per Patient Per Cycle Incidence No Gleevec** N = 647
Grade 3 and 4 Adverse Events				
Nausea and/or Vomiting	15 (16%)	6 (9%)	28 (4%)	8 (1%)
Hypokalemia	31 (34%)	16 (25%)	72 (9%)	32(5%)
Pneumonitis	7 (8%)	1 (1%)	7(1%)	1(<1%)
Pleural effusion	6 (7%)	0	6 (1%)	0
Abdominal Pain	8 (9%)	2 (3%)	9 (1%)	3(<1%)
Anorexia	10 (11%)	3 (5%)	19 (2%)	4 (1%)
Hemorrhage	11 (12%)	4 (6%)	17 (2%)	8 (1%)
Hypoxia	8 (9%)	2 (3%)	12 (2%)	2 (<1%)
Myalgia	5 (5%)	0	4 (1%)	1 (<1%)
Stomatitis	15 (16%)	8 (12%)	22 (3%)	14 (2%)
Diarrhea	8 (9%)	3 (5%)	12 (2%)	3 (<1%)
Rash / Skin Disorder	4 (4%)	0	5 (1%)	0
Infection	49 (53%)	32 (49%)	131 (17%)	92 (14%)
Hepatic (transaminase and/or bilirubin)	52 (57%)	38 (58%)	172 (22%)	113 (17%)
Hypotension	10 (11%)	5 (8%)	16 (2%)	6 (1%)
Myelosuppression				
Neutropenia (<750/µL)	92 (100%)	63 (97%)	556 (71%)	218 (34%)
Thrombocytopenia (<75,000/µL)	90 (92%)	63 (97%)	431 (55%)	329 (51%)

* Defined as the frequency of AEs per patient per treatment cycles that included Gleevec (includes patients with Ph+ ALL that received cycles with Gleevec

** Defined as the frequency of AEs per patient per treatment cycles that did not include Gleevec (includes patients with Ph+ALL that received cycles without Gleevec as well as all patients with Ph- ALL who did not receive Gleevec in any treatment cycle)

A variety of adverse reactions represent local or general fluid retention including pleural effusion, ascites, pulmonary edema and rapid weight gain with or without superficial edema. These reactions appear to be dose related, were more common in the blast crisis and accelerated phase studies (where the dose was 600 mg/day), and are more common in the elderly. These reactions were usually managed by interrupting Gleevec treatment and using diuretics or other appropriate supportive care measures. A few of these reactions may be serious or life threatening, and one patient with blast crisis died with pleural effusion, congestive heart failure, and renal failure.

Adverse reactions, regardless of relationship to study drug, that were reported in at least 10% of the Gleevec treated patients are shown in Tables 2 and 3.

[See table 2 at top of page 1997]

[See table 3 at top of previous page]

6.2 Hematologic Toxicity

Cytopenias, and particularly neutropenia and thrombocytopenia, were a consistent finding in all studies, with a higher frequency at doses ≥750 mg (Phase 1 study). The occurrence of cytopenias in CML patients was also dependent on the stage of the disease.

In patients with newly diagnosed CML, cytopenias were less frequent than in the other CML patients (see Tables 4 and 5). The frequency of Grade 3 or 4 neutropenia and thrombocytopenia was between 2- and 3-fold higher in blast crisis and accelerated phase compared to chronic phase (see Tables 4 and 5). The median duration of the neutropenic and thrombocytopenic episodes varied from 2 to 3 weeks, and from 2 to 4 weeks, respectively.

These reactions can usually be managed with either a reduction of the dose or an interruption of treatment with Gleevec, but in rare cases require permanent discontinuation of treatment.

[See table 4 at top of previous page]

[See table 5 above]

6.3 Hepatotoxicity

Severe elevation of transaminases or bilirubin occurred in approximately 5% of CML patients (see Tables 4 and 5) and were usually managed with dose reduction or interruption (the median duration of these episodes was approximately 1 week). Treatment was discontinued permanently because of liver laboratory abnormalities in less than 1.0% of CML patients. One patient, who was taking acetaminophen regularly for fever, died of acute liver failure. In the Phase 2 GIST trial, Grade 3 or 4 SGPT (ALT) elevations were observed in 6.8% of patients and Grade 3 or 4 SGOT (AST) elevations were observed in 4.8% of patients. Bilirubin elevation was observed in 2.7% of patients.

6.4 Adverse Reactions in Pediatric Population

Single agent therapy

The overall safety profile of pediatric patients treated with Gleevec in 93 children studied was similar to that found in studies with adult patients, except that musculoskeletal pain was less frequent (20.5%) and peripheral edema was not reported. Nausea and vomiting were the most commonly reported individual adverse reactions with an incidence similar to that seen in adult patients. Although most patients experienced adverse reactions at some time during the study, the incidence of Grade 3/4 adverse reactions was low.

In combination with multi-agent chemotherapy

Pediatric and young adult patients with very high risk ALL, defined as those with an expected 5 year event-free survival (EFS) less than 45%, were enrolled after induction therapy on a multicenter, non-randomized cooperative group pilot protocol. The study population included patients with a median age of 10 years (1 to 21 years), 61% of whom were male, 75% were white, 7% were black and 6% were Asian/Pacific Islander. Patients with Ph+ ALL (n=92) were assigned to receive Gleevec and treated in 5 successive cohorts. Gleevec exposure was systematically increased in successive cohorts by earlier introduction and more prolonged duration.

The safety of Gleevec given in combination with intensive chemotherapy was evaluated by comparing the incidence of grade 3 and 4 adverse events, neutropenia (<750/µL) and thrombocytopenia (<75,000/ µL) in the 92 patients with Ph+ ALL compared to 65 patients with Ph- ALL enrolled on the trial who did not receive Gleevec. The safety was also evaluated comparing the incidence of adverse events in cycles of therapy administered with or without Gleevec. The protocol included up to 18 cycles of therapy. Patients were exposed to a cumulative total of 1425 cycles of therapy, 778 with Gleevec and 647 without Gleevec. The adverse events that were reported with a 5% or greater incidence in patients with Ph+ ALL compared to Ph- ALL or with a 1% or greater incidence in cycles of therapy that included Gleevec are presented in Table 6.

[See table 6 at top of previous page]

6.5 Adverse Reactions in Other Subpopulations

In older patients (≥65 years old), with the exception of edema, where it was more frequent, there was no evidence of an increase in the incidence or severity of adverse reactions. In women there was an increase in the frequency of neutropenia, as well as Grade 1/2 superficial edema, headache, nausea, rigors, vomiting, rash, and fatigue. No differences were seen that were related to race but the subsets were too small for proper evaluation.

6.6 Acute Lymphoblastic Leukemia

The adverse reactions were similar for Ph+ ALL as for Ph+ CML. The most frequently reported drug-related adverse reactions reported in the Ph+ ALL studies were mild nausea and vomiting, diarrhea, myalgia, muscle cramps and rash, which were easily manageable. Superficial edema was a common finding in all studies and were described primarily as periorbital or lower limb edemas. These edemas were rarely severe and may be managed with diuretics, other supportive measures, or in some patients by reducing the dose of Gleevec.

6.7 Myelodysplastic/Myeloproliferative Diseases

Adverse reactions, regardless of relationship to study drug, that were reported in at least 10% of the patients treated with Gleevec for MDS/MPD in the phase 2 study, are shown in Table 7.

Table 7 Adverse Reactions Regardless of Relationship to Study Drug Reported (More than One Patient) in MPD Patients in the Phase 2 Study (≥10% All Patients) All Grades

Preferred Term	N=7 n (%)
Nausea	4 (57.1)
Diarrhea	3 (42.9)
Anemia	2 (28.6)
Fatigue	2 (28.6)
Muscle Cramp	3 (42.9)
Arthralgia	2 (28.6)
Periorbital Edema	2 (28.6)

6.8 Aggressive Systemic Mastocytosis

All ASM patients experienced at least one adverse reaction at some time. The most frequently reported adverse reactions were diarrhea, nausea, ascites, muscle cramps, dyspnea, fatigue, peripheral edema, anemia, pruritus, rash and lower respiratory tract infection. None of the 5 patients in the phase 2 study with ASM discontinued Gleevec due to drug-related adverse reactions or abnormal laboratory values.

6.9 Hypereosinophilic Syndrome and Chronic Eosinophilic Leukemia

The safety profile in the HES/CEL patient population does not appear to be different from the safety profile of Gleevec observed in other hematologic malignancy populations, such as Ph+ CML. All patients experienced at least one adverse reaction, the most common being gastrointestinal, cutaneous and musculoskeletal disorders. Hematological abnormalities were also frequent, with instances of CTC Grade 3 leukopenia, neutropenia, lymphopenia, and anemia.

6.10 Dermatofibrosarcoma Protuberans

Adverse reactions, regardless of relationship to study drug, that were reported in at least 10% of the 12 patients treated with Gleevec for DFSP in the phase 2 study are shown in Table 8.

Table 8 Adverse Reactions Regardless of Relationship to Study Drug Reported in DFSP Patients in the Phase 2 Study (≥10% All Patients) All Grades

Preferred term	N=12 n (%)
Nausea	5 (41.7)
Diarrhea	3 (25.0)
Vomiting	3 (25.0)
Periorbital Edema	4 (33.3)
Face Edema	2 (16.7)
Rash	3 (25.0)
Fatigue	5 (41.7)
Edema Peripheral	4 (33.3)
Pyrexia	2 (16.7)
Eye Edema	4 (33.3)
Lacrimation Increased	3 (25.0)
Dyspnea Exertional	2 (16.7)
Anemia	3 (25.0)
Rhinitis	2 (16.7)
Anorexia	2 (16.7)

Clinically relevant or severe laboratory abnormalities in the 12 patients treated with Gleevec for DFSP in the phase 2 study are presented in Table 9.

Table 9 Laboratory Abnormalities Reported in DFSP Patients in the Phase 2 Study

CTC Grades[1]	N=12 Grade 3	Grade 4
Hematology Parameters		
- Anemia	17 %	0 %
- Thrombocytopenia	17 %	0 %
- Neutropenia	0 %	8 %
Biochemistry Parameters		
- Elevated Creatinine	0 %	8 %

[1]CTC Grades: neutropenia (Grade 3 ≥0.5-1.0 × 10^9/L, Grade 4 <0.5 × 10^9/L), thrombocytopenia (Grade 3 ≥10 - 50 × 10^9/L, Grade 4 <10 × 10^9/L), anemia (Grade 3 ≥65-80 g/L, Grade 4 <65 g/L), elevated creatinine (Grade 3 >3-6 × upper limit normal range [ULN], Grade 4 >6 × ULN),

Table 10 Number (%) of Patients with Adverse Reactions Regardless of Relationship to Study Drug where Frequency is ≥10% in any One Group (Full Analysis Set) in the Phase 3 Unresectable and/or Malignant Metastatic GIST Clinical Trials

Reported or Specified Term	Imatinib 400 mg N=818 All Grades %	Imatinib 400 mg N=818 Grades 3/4/5 %	Imatinib 800 mg[1] N=822 All Grades %	Imatinib 800 mg[1] N=822 Grades 3/4/5 %
Edema	76.7	9.0	86.1	13.1
Fatigue/lethargy, malaise, asthenia	69.3	11.7	74.9	12.2
Nausea	58.1	9.0	64.5	7.8
Abdominal pain/cramping	57.2	13.8	55.2	11.8
Diarrhea	56.2	8.1	58.2	8.6
Rash/desquamation	38.1	7.6	49.8	8.9
Vomiting	37.4	9.2	40.6	7.5
Myalgia	32.2	5.6	30.2	3.8
Anemia	32.0	4.9	34.8	6.4
Anorexia	31.1	6.6	35.8	4.7
Other GI toxicity	25.2	8.1	28.1	6.6
Headache	22.0	5.7	19.7	3.6
Other pain (excluding tumor related pain)	20.4	5.9	20.8	5.0
Other dermatology /skin toxicity	17.6	5.9	20.1	5.7
Leukopenia	17.0	0.7	19.6	1.6
Other constitutional symptoms	16.7	6.4	15.2	4.4
Cough	16.1	4.5	14.5	3.2
Infection (without neutropenia)	15.5	6.6	16.5	5.6
Pruritus	15.4	5.4	18.9	4.3
Other neurological toxicity	15.0	6.4	15.2	4.9
Constipation	14.8	5.1	14.4	4.1
Other renal/genitourinary toxicity	14.2	6.5	13.6	5.2
Arthralgia (joint pain)	13.6	4.8	12.3	3.0
Dyspnea (shortness of breath)	13.6	6.8	14.2	5.6
Fever in absence of neutropenia (ANC<1.0 × 10^9/L)	13.2	4.9	12.9	3.4
Sweating	12.7	4.6	8.5	2.8
Other hemorrhage	12.3	6.7	13.3	6.1
Weight gain	12.0	1.0	10.6	0.6
Alopecia	11.9	4.3	14.8	3.2
Dyspepsia/heartburn	11.5	0.6	10.9	0.5
Neutropenia/ granulocytopenia	11.5	3.1	16.1	4.1
Rigors/chills	11.0	4.6	10.2	3.0
Dizziness/ lightheadedness	11.0	4.8	10.0	2.8
Creatinine increase	10.8	0.4	10.1	0.6
Flatulence	10.0	0.2	10.1	0.1
Stomatitis/pharyngitis (oral/pharyngeal mucositis)	9.2	5.4	10.0	4.3
Lymphopenia	6.0	0.7	10.1	1.9

6.11 Gastrointestinal Stromal Tumors

Unresectable and/or Malignant Metastatic GIST

In the Phase 3 trials the majority of Gleevec-treated patients experienced adverse reactions at some time. The most frequently reported adverse reactions were edema, fatigue, nausea, abdominal pain, diarrhea, rash, vomiting, myalgia, anemia, and anorexia. Drug was discontinued for adverse reactions in a total of 89 patients (5.4%). Superficial edema, most frequently periorbital or lower extremity edema was managed with diuretics, other supportive measures, or by reducing the dose of Gleevec [*see Dosage and Administration (2.12)*]. Severe (CTC Grade 3/4) edema was observed in 182 patients (11.1%).

Adverse reactions, regardless of relationship to study drug, that were reported in at least 10% of the patients treated with Gleevec are shown in Table 10.

Overall the incidence of all grades of adverse reactions and the incidence of severe adverse reactions (CTC Grade 3 and above) were similar between the two treatment arms except for edema, which was reported more frequently in the 800 mg group.

[See table 10 above]

Clinically relevant or severe abnormalities of routine hematologic or biochemistry laboratory values were not reported or evaluated in the Phase 3 GIST trials. Severe abnormal laboratory values reported in the Phase 2 GIST trial are presented in Table 11.

[See table 11 at top of next page]

Adjuvant Treatment of GIST

In Study 1, the majority of both Gleevec and placebo treated patients experienced at least one adverse reaction at some time. The most frequently reported adverse reactions were similar to those reported in other clinical studies in other patient populations and include diarrhea, fatigue, nausea, edema, decreased hemoglobin, rash, vomiting, and abdominal pain. No new adverse reactions were reported in the adjuvant GIST treatment setting that had not been previously reported in other patient populations including patients with unresectable and/or malignant metastatic GIST. Drug was discontinued for adverse reactions in 57 patients (17%) and 11 patients (3%) of the Gleevec and placebo treated pa-

Table 11 Laboratory Abnormalities in the Phase 2 Unresectable and/or Malignant Metastatic GIST Trial

	400 mg (n=73) %		600 mg (n=74) %	
CTC Grades[1]	**Grade 3**	**Grade 4**	**Grade 3**	**Grade 4**
Hematology Parameters				
– Anemia	3	0	8	1
– Thrombocytopenia	0	0	1	0
– Neutropenia	7	3	8	3
Biochemistry Parameters				
– Elevated Creatinine	0	0	3	0
– Reduced Albumin	3	0	4	0
– Elevated Bilirubin	1	0	1	3
– Elevated Alkaline Phosphatase	0	0	3	0
– Elevated SGOT (AST)	4	0	3	3
– Elevated SGPT (ALT)	6	0	7	1

[1]CTC Grades: neutropenia (Grade 3 ≥0.5-1.0 × 10^9/L, Grade 4 <0.5 × 10^9/L), thrombocytopenia (Grade 3 ≥10 - 50 × 10^9/L, Grade 4 <10 × 10^9/L), anemia (Grade 3 ≥65-80 g/L, Grade 4 <65 g/L), elevated creatinine (Grade 3 >3-6 × upper limit normal range [ULN], Grade 4 >6 × ULN), elevated bilirubin (Grade 3 >3-10 × ULN, Grade 4 >10 × ULN), elevated alkaline phosphatase, SGOT or SGPT (Grade 3 >5-20 × ULN, Grade 4 >20 × ULN), albumin (Grade 3 <20 g/L)

Table 12: Adverse Reactions Regardless of Relationship to Study Drug Reported in Study 1 (≥5% of Gleevec Treated Patients)[(1)]

	All CTC Grades		CTC Grade 3 and above	
	Gleevec (n=337)	**Placebo (n=345)**	**Gleevec (n=337)**	**Placebo (n=345)**
Preferred Term	**%**	**%**	**%**	**%**
Diarrhea	59.3	29.3	3.0	1.4
Fatigue	57.0	40.9	2.1	1.2
Nausea	53.1	27.8	2.4	1.2
Periorbital Edema	47.2	14.5	1.2	0
Hemoglobin Decreased	46.9	27.0	0.6	0
Peripheral Edema	26.7	14.8	0.3	0
Rash (Exfoliative)	26.1	12.8	2.7	0
Vomiting	25.5	13.9	2.4	0.6
Abdominal Pain	21.1	22.3	3.0	1.4
Headache	19.3	20.3	0.6	0
Dyspepsia	17.2	13.0	0.9	0
Anorexia	16.9	8.7	0.3	0
Weight Increased	16.9	11.6	0.3	0
Liver enzymes (ALT) Increased	16.6	13.0	2.7	0
Muscle spasms	16.3	3.3	0	0
Neutrophil Count Decreased	16.0	6.1	3.3	0.9
Arthralgia	15.1	14.5	0	0.3
White Blood Cell Count Decreased	14.5	4.3	0.6	0.3
Constipation	12.8	17.7	0	0.3
Dizziness	12.5	10.7	0	0.3
Liver Enzymes (AST) Increased	12.2	7.5	2.1	0
Myalgia	12.2	11.6	0	0.3
Blood Creatinine Increased	11.6	5.8	0	0.3
Cough	11.0	11.3	0	0
Pruritus	11.0	7.8	0.9	0
Weight Decreased	10.1	5.2	0	0
Hyperglycemia	9.8	11.3	0.6	1.7
Insomnia	9.8	7.2	0.9	0
Lacrimation Increased	9.8	3.8	0	0
Alopecia	9.5	6.7	0	0
Flatulence	8.9	9.6	0	0
Rash	8.9	5.2	0.9	0
Abdominal Distension	7.4	6.4	0.3	0.3
Back Pain	7.4	8.1	0.6	0
Pain in Extremity	7.4	7.2	0.3	0
Hypokalemia	7.1	2.0	0.9	0.6
Depression	6.8	6.4	0.9	0.6
Facial Edema	6.8	1.2	0.3	0
Blood Alkaline Phosphatase Increased	6.5	7.5	0	0
Dry skin	6.5	5.2	0	0
Dysgeusia	6.5	2.9	0	0
Abdominal Pain Upper	6.2	6.4	0.3	0
Neuropathy Peripheral	5.9	6.4	0	0
Hypocalcemia	5.6	1.7	0.3	0
Leukopenia	5.0	2.6	0.3	0
Platelet Count Decreased	5.0	3.5	0	0
Stomatitis	5.0	1.7	0.6	0
Upper Respiratory Tract Infection	5.0	3.5	0	0
Vision Blurred	5.0	2.3	0	0

[(1)]All adverse reactions occurring in ≥5% of patients are listed regardless of suspected relationship to treatment. A patient with multiple occurrences of an adverse reaction is counted only once in the adverse reaction category.

tients respectively. Edema, gastrointestinal disturbances (nausea, vomiting, abdominal distention and diarrhea), fatigue, low hemoglobin, and rash were the most frequently reported adverse reactions at the time of discontinuation.

In Study 2, discontinuation of therapy due to adverse reactions occurred in 15 patients (8%) and 27 patients (14%) of the Gleevec 12-month and 36-month treatment arms, respectively. As in previous trials the most common adverse reactions were diarrhea, fatigue, nausea, edema, decreased hemoglobin, rash, vomiting, and abdominal pain.

Adverse reactions, regardless of relationship to study drug, that were reported in at least 5% of the patients treated with Gleevec are shown in Table 12 (Study 1) and Table 13 (Study 2). There were no deaths attributable to Gleevec treatment in either trial.

[See table 12 below]
[See table 13 at top of next page]

6.12 Additional Data from Multiple Clinical Trials

The following adverse reactions have been reported during clinical trials of Gleevec.

Cardiac Disorders:
Estimated 0.1%-1%: congestive cardiac failure, tachycardia, palpitations, pulmonary edema
Estimated 0.01%-0.1%: arrhythmia, atrial fibrillation, cardiac arrest, myocardial infarction, angina pectoris, pericardial effusion

Vascular Disorders:
Estimated 1%-10%: flushing, hemorrhage
Estimated 0.1%-1%: hypertension, hypotension, peripheral coldness, Raynauds phenomenon, hematoma, subdural hematoma

Clinical Laboratory Tests:
Estimated 0.1%-1%: blood CPK increased, blood LDH increased
Estimated 0.01%-0.1%: blood amylase increased

Dermatologic:
Estimated 1%-10%: dry skin, alopecia, face edema, erythema, photosensitivity reaction
Estimated 0.1%-1%: exfoliative dermatitis, bullous eruption, nail disorder, purpura, psoriasis, rash pustular, contusion, sweating increased, urticaria, ecchymosis, increased tendency to bruise, hypotrichosis, skin hypopigmentation, skin hyperpigmentation, onychoclasis, folliculitis, petechiae
Estimated 0.01%-0.1%: vesicular rash, Stevens-Johnson syndrome, acute generalized exanthematous pustulosis, acute febrile neutrophilic dermatosis (Sweet's syndrome), nail discoloration, angioneurotic edema, erythema multiforme, leucocytoclastic vasculitis

Digestive:
Estimated 1%-10%: abdominal distention, gastroesophageal reflux, dry mouth, gastritis
Estimated 0.1%-1%: gastric ulcer, stomatitis, mouth ulceration, eructation, melena, esophagitis, ascites, hematemesis, chelitis, dysphagia, pancreatitis
Estimated 0.01%-0.1%: colitis, ileus, inflammatory bowel disease

General Disorders and Administration Site Conditions:
Estimated 1%-10%: weakness, anasarca, chills
Estimated 0.1%-1%: malaise

Hematologic:
Estimated 1%-10%: pancytopenia, febrile neutropenia
Estimated 0.1%-1%: thrombocythemia, lymphopenia, bone marrow depression, eosinophilia, lymphadenopathy
Estimated 0.01%-0.1%: hemolytic anemia, aplastic anemia

Hepatobiliary:
Estimated 0.1%-1%: hepatitis, jaundice
Estimated 0.01%-0.1%: hepatic failure and hepatic necrosis[1]

Hypersensitivity:
Estimated 0.01%-0.1%: angioedema

Infections:
Estimated 0.1%-1%: sepsis, herpes simplex, herpes zoster, cellulitis, urinary tract infection, gastroenteritis
Estimated 0.01%-0.1%: fungal infection

Metabolic and Nutritional:
Estimated 1%-10%: weight decreased
Estimated 0.1%-1%: hypophosphatemia, dehydration, gout, increased appetite, decreased appetite, hyperuricemia, hypercalcemia, hyperglycemia, hyponatremia
Estimated 0.01%-0.1%: hyperkalemia, hypomagnesemia

Musculoskeletal:
Estimated 1%-10%: joint swelling
Estimated 0.1%-1%: joint and muscle stiffness
Estimated 0.01%-0.1%: muscular weakness, arthritis

Nervous System/Psychiatric:
Estimated 1%-10%: paresthesia, hypesthesia
Estimated 0.1%-1%: syncope, peripheral neuropathy, somnolence, migraine, memory impairment, libido decreased, sciatica, restless leg syndrome, tremor
Estimated 0.01%-0.1%: increased intracranial pressure[1], confusional state, convulsions, optic neuritis

Renal:
Estimated 0.1%-1%: renal failure acute, urinary frequency increased, hematuria, renal pain

Reproductive:
Estimated 0.1%-1%: breast enlargement, menorrhagia, sexual dysfunction, gynecomastia, erectile dysfunction, menstruation irregular, nipple pain, scrotal edema

Table 13: Adverse Reactions Regardless of Relationship to Study Drug by Preferred Term All Grades and 3/4 Grades (≥5% of Gleevec Treated Patients) Study 2[(1)]

Preferred Term	All CTC Grades		CTC Grades 3 and above	
	Gleevec 12 Months (N=194) %	Gleevec 36 Months (N=198) %	Gleevec 12 Months (N=194) %	Gleevec 36 Months (N=198) %
Patients with at least one AE	99.0	100.0	20.1	32.8
Hemoglobin decreased	72.2	80.3	0.5	0.5
Periorbital edema	59.3	74.2	0.5	1.0
Blood lactate dehydrogenase increased	43.3	60.1	0	0
Diarrhea	43.8	54.0	0.5	2.0
Nausea	44.8	51.0	1.5	0.5
Muscle spasms	30.9	49.0	0.5	1.0
Fatigue	48.5	48.5	1.0	0.5
White blood cell count decreased	34.5	47.0	2.1	3.0
Pain	25.8	45.5	1.0	3.0
Blood creatinine increased	30.4	44.4	0	0
Edema peripheral	33.0	40.9	0.5	1.0
Dermatitis	29.4	38.9	2.1	1.5
Aspartate aminotransferase increased	30.9	37.9	1.5	3.0
Alanine aminotransferase increased	28.9	34.3	2.1	3.0
Neutrophil count decreased	24.2	33.3	4.6	5.1
Hypoproteinemia	23.7	31.8	0	0
Infection	13.9	27.8	1.5	2.5
Weight increased	13.4	26.8	0	0.5
Pruritus	12.9	25.8	0	0
Flatulence	19.1	24.7	1.0	0.5
Vomiting	10.8	22.2	0.5	1.0
Dyspepsia	17.5	21.7	0.5	1.0
Hypoalbuminemia	11.9	21.2	0	0
Edema	10.8	19.7	0	0.5
Abdominal distension	11.9	19.2	0.5	0
Headache	8.2	18.2	0	0
Lacrimation increased	18.0	17.7	0	0
Arthralgia	8.8	17.2	0	1.0
Blood alkaline phosphatase increased	10.8	16.7	0	0.5
Dyspnea	6.2	16.2	0.5	1.5
Myalgia	9.3	15.2	0	1.0
Platelet count decreased	11.3	14.1	0	0
Blood bilirubin increased	11.3	13.1	0	0
Dysgeusia	9.3	12.6	0	0
Paresthesia	5.2	12.1	0	0.5
Vision blurred	10.8	11.1	1.0	0.5
Alopecia	11.3	10.6	0	0
Decreased appetite	9.8	10.1	0	0
Constipation	8.8	9.6	0	0
Pyrexia	6.2	9.6	0	0
Depression	3.1	8.1	0	0
Abdominal pain	2.6	7.6	0	0
Conjunctivitis	5.2	7.6	0	0
Photosensitivity reaction	3.6	7.1	0	0
Dizziness	4.6	6.6	0.5	0
Hemorrhage	3.1	6.6	0	0
Dry skin	6.7	6.1	0.5	0
Nasopharyngitis	1.0	6.1	0	0.5
Palpitations	5.2	5.1	0	0

[(1)]All adverse reactions occurring in ≥5% of patients are listed regardless of suspected relationship to treatment.
A patient with multiple occurrences of an adverse reaction is counted only once in the adverse reaction category.

Respiratory:
Estimated 1%-10%: epistaxis
Estimated 0.1%-1%: pleural effusion
Estimated 0.01%-0.1%: interstitial pneumonitis, pulmonary fibrosis, pleuritic pain, pulmonary hypertension, pulmonary hemorrhage

Special Senses:
Estimated 1%-10%: conjunctivitis, vision blurred, eyelid edema, conjunctival hemorrhage, dry eye
Estimated 0.1%-1%: vertigo, tinnitus, eye irritation, eye pain, orbital edema, scleral hemorrhage, retinal hemorrhage, blepharitis, macular edema, hearing loss
Estimated 0.01%-0.1%: papilledema[1], glaucoma, cataract
[1]Including some fatalities

6.13 Postmarketing Experience

The following additional adverse reactions have been identified during post approval use of Gleevec. Because these reactions are reported voluntarily from a population of uncertain size, it is not always possible to reliably estimate their frequency or establish a causal relationship to drug exposure.

Nervous system disorders: cerebral edema[1]
Eye disorders: vitreous hemorrhage
Cardiac disorders: pericarditis, cardiac tamponade[1]
Vascular disorders: thrombosis/embolism, anaphylactic shock
Respiratory, thoracic and mediastinal disorders: acute respiratory failure[1], interstitial lung disease
Gastrointestinal disorders: ileus/intestinal obstruction, tumor hemorrhage/tumor necrosis, gastrointestinal perforation[1] [*see Warnings and Precautions (5.6)*], diverticulitis
Skin and subcutaneous tissue disorders: lichenoid keratosis, lichen planus, toxic epidermal necrolysis, palmar-plantar erythrodysesthesia syndrome
Musculoskeletal and connective tissue disorders: avascular necrosis/hip osteonecrosis, rhabdomyolysis/myopathy, growth retardation in children
Reproduction disorders: hemorrhagic corpus luteum/ hemorrhagic ovarian cyst
[1]Including some fatalities

7 DRUG INTERACTIONS

7.1 Agents Inducing CYP3A Metabolism

Pretreatment of healthy volunteers with multiple doses of rifampin followed by a single dose of Gleevec, increased Gleevec oral-dose clearance by 3.8-fold, which significantly ($p<0.05$) decreased mean C_{max} and AUC.

Similar findings were observed in patients receiving 400-1200 mg/day Gleevec concomitantly with enzyme-inducing anti-epileptic drugs (EIAED) (e.g., carbamazepine, oxcarbamazepine, phenytoin, fosphenytoin, phenobarbital, and primidone). The mean dose normalized AUC for imatinib in the patients receiving EIAED's decreased by 73% compared to patients not receiving EIAED.

Concomitant administration of Gleevec and St. John's Wort led to a 30% reduction in the AUC of imatinib.

Consider alternative therapeutic agents with less enzyme induction potential in patients when rifampin or other CYP3A4 inducers are indicated. Gleevec doses up to 1200 mg/day (600 mg BID) have been given to patients receiving concomitant strong CYP3A4 inducers [*see Dosage and Administration (2.11)*].

7.2 Agents Inhibiting CYP3A Metabolism

There was a significant increase in exposure to imatinib (mean C_{max} and AUC increased by 26% and 40%, respectively) in healthy subjects when Gleevec was co-administered with a single dose of ketoconazole (a CYP3A4 inhibitor). Caution is recommended when administering Gleevec with strong CYP3A4 inhibitors (e.g., ketoconazole, itraconazole, clarithromycin, atazanavir, indinavir, nefazodone, nelfinavir, ritonavir, saquinavir, telithromycin, and voriconazole). Grapefruit juice may also increase plasma concentrations of imatinib and should be avoided. Substances that inhibit the cytochrome P450 isoenzyme (CYP3A4) activity may decrease metabolism and increase imatinib concentrations.

7.3 Interactions with Drugs Metabolized by CYP3A4

Gleevec increases the mean C_{max} and AUC of simvastatin (CYP3A4 substrate) 2- and 3.5-fold, respectively, suggesting an inhibition of the CYP3A4 by Gleevec. Particular caution is recommended when administering Gleevec with CYP3A4 substrates that have a narrow therapeutic window (e.g., alfentanil, cyclosporine, diergotamine, ergotamine, fentanyl, pimozide, quinidine, sirolimus or tacrolimus).

Gleevec will increase plasma concentration of other CYP3A4 metabolized drugs (e.g., triazolo-benzodiazepines, dihydropyridine calcium channel blockers, certain HMG-CoA reductase inhibitors, etc.).

Because warfarin is metabolized by CYP2C9 and CYP3A4, patients who require anticoagulation should receive low-molecular weight or standard heparin instead of warfarin.

7.4 Interactions with Drugs Metabolized by CYP2D6

Gleevec increased the mean C_{max} and AUC of metoprolol by approximately 23% suggesting that Gleevec has a weak inhibitory effect on CYP2D6-mediated metabolism. No dose adjustment is necessary, however, caution is recommended when administering Gleevec with CYP2D6 substrates that have a narrow therapeutic window.

7.5 Interaction with Acetaminophen

In vitro, Gleevec inhibits the acetaminophen O-glucuronidate pathway (K_i 58.5 µM). Co-administration of Gleevec (400 mg/day for eight days) with acetaminophen (1000 mg single dose on day eight) in patients with CML did not result in any changes in the pharmacokinetics of acetaminophen. Gleevec pharmacokinetics were not altered in the presence of single-dose acetaminophen. There is no pharmacokinetic or safety data on the concomitant use of Gleevec at doses >400 mg/day or the chronic use of concomitant acetaminophen and Gleevec.

8 USE IN SPECIFIC POPULATIONS

8.1 Pregnancy

Pregnancy Category D [*see Warnings and Precautions (5.11)*].

Gleevec can cause fetal harm when administered to a pregnant woman. There have been post-market reports of spontaneous abortions and infant congenital anomalies from women who have taken Gleevec. Imatinib mesylate was teratogenic in rats when administered during organogenesis at doses ≥100 mg/kg (approximately equal to the maximum human dose of 800 mg/day based on body surface area). Teratogenic effects included exencephaly or encephalocele, absent/reduced frontal and absent parietal bones. Female rats administered doses ≥45 mg/kg (approximately one-half the maximum human dose of 800 mg/day based on body surface area) also experienced significant post-implantation loss as evidenced by either early fetal resorption or stillbirths, non-viable pups and early pup mortality between postpartum Days 0 and 4. At doses higher than 100 mg/kg, total fetal loss was noted in all animals. Fetal loss was not seen at doses ≤30 mg/kg (one-third the maximum human dose of 800 mg).

There are no adequate and well-controlled studies with Gleevec in pregnant women. Women should be advised not to become pregnant when taking Gleevec. If this drug is used during pregnancy, or if the patient becomes pregnant while taking this drug, the patient should be apprised of the potential hazard to the fetus.

8.3 Nursing Mothers

Imatinib and its active metabolite are excreted into human milk. Based on data from three breastfeeding women taking Gleevec, the milk:plasma ratio is about 0.5 for imatinib and about 0.9 for the active metabolite. Considering the combined concentration of imatinib and active metabolite, a breastfed infant could receive up to 10% of the maternal therapeutic dose based on body weight. Because of the potential for serious adverse reactions in nursing infants from Gleevec, a decision should be made whether to discontinue nursing or to discontinue the drug, taking into account the importance of the drug to the mother.

8.4 Pediatric Use

Gleevec safety and efficacy have been demonstrated in children with newly diagnosed Ph+ chronic phase CML and Ph+ ALL. There are no data in children under 1 year of age. As in adult patients, imatinib was rapidly absorbed after oral administration in pediatric patients, with a C_{max} of 2-4 hours. Apparent oral clearance was similar to adult values (11.0 L/hr/m^2 in children vs. 10.0 L/hr/m^2 in adults), as was the half-life (14.8 hours in children vs. 17.1 hours in adults). Dosing in children at both 260 mg/m^2 and 340 mg/m^2 achieved an AUC similar to the 400 mg dose in adults. The comparison of AUC on Day 8 vs. Day 1 at 260 mg/m^2 and 340 mg/m^2 dose levels revealed a 1.5- and 2.2-fold drug accumulation, respectively, after repeated once-daily dosing. Mean imatinib AUC did not increase proportionally with increasing dose.

Based on pooled population pharmacokinetic analysis in pediatric patients with hematological disorders (CML, Ph+ ALL, or other hematological disorders treated with imatinib), clearance of imatinib increases with increasing body surface area (BSA). After correcting for the BSA effect, other demographics such as age, body weight and body mass index did not have clinically significant effects on the exposure of imatinib. The analysis confirmed that exposure of imatinib in pediatric patients receiving 260 mg/m^2 once daily (not exceeding 400 mg once daily) or 340 mg/m^2 once daily (not exceeding 600 mg once daily) were similar to those in adult patients who received imatinib 400 mg or 600 mg once daily.

8.5 Geriatric Use

In the CML clinical studies, approximately 20% of patients were older than 65 years. In the study of patients with newly diagnosed CML, 6% of patients were older than 65 years. No difference was observed in the safety profile in patients older than 65 years as compared to younger patients, with the exception of a higher frequency of edema [*see Warnings and Precautions (5.1)*]. The efficacy of Gleevec was similar in older and younger patients.

In the unresectable or metastatic GIST study, 16% of patients were older than 65 years. No obvious differences in the safety or efficacy profile were noted in patients older than 65 years as compared to younger patients, but the small number of patients does not allow a formal analysis. In the adjuvant GIST study, 221 patients (31%) were older than 65 years. No difference was observed in the safety profile in patients older than 65 years as compared to younger patients, with the exception of a higher frequency of edema. The efficacy of Gleevec was similar in patients older than 65 years and younger patients.

8.6 Hepatic Impairment

The effect of hepatic impairment on the pharmacokinetics of both imatinib and its major metabolite, CGP74588, was assessed in 84 cancer patients with varying degrees of hepatic impairment (Table 14) at imatinib doses ranging from 100-800 mg. Exposure to both imatinib and CGP74588 was comparable between each of the mildly and moderately hepatically-impaired groups and the normal group. Patients with severe hepatic impairment tend to have higher exposure to both imatinib and its metabolite than patients with normal hepatic function. At steady state, the mean C_{max}/dose and AUC/dose for imatinib increased by about 63% and 45%, respectively, in patients with severe hepatic impairment compared to patients with normal hepatic function. The mean C_{max}/dose and AUC/dose for CGP74588 increased by about 56% and 55%, respectively, in patients with severe hepatic impairment compared to patients with normal hepatic function [*see Dosage and Administration (2.11)*].

[See table 14 above]

8.7 Renal Impairment

The effect of renal impairment on the pharmacokinetics of imatinib was assessed in 59 cancer patients with varying degrees of renal impairment (Table 15) at single and steady state imatinib doses ranging from 100 to 800 mg/day. The mean exposure to imatinib (dose normalized AUC) in patients with mild and moderate renal impairment increased 1.5- to 2-fold compared to patients with normal renal function. The AUCs did not increase for doses greater than 600 mg in patients with mild renal impairment. The AUCs did not increase for doses greater than 400 mg in patients with moderate renal impairment. Two patients with severe renal impairment were dosed with 100 mg/day and their exposures were similar to those seen in patients with normal renal function receiving 400 mg/day. Dose reductions are necessary for patients with moderate and severe renal impairment [*See Dosage and Administration (2.11)*].

Table 15 Renal Function Classification

Renal Dysfunction	Renal Function Tests
Mild	CrCL = 40-59 mL/min
Moderate	CrCL = 20-39 mL/min
Severe	CrCL = <20 mL/min

CrCL = Creatinine Clearance

10 OVERDOSAGE

Experience with doses greater than 800 mg is limited. Isolated cases of Gleevec overdose have been reported. In the event of overdosage, the patient should be observed and appropriate supportive treatment given.

Table 14 Liver Function Classification

Liver Function Test	Normal (n=14)	Mild (n=30)	Moderate (n=20)	Severe (n=20)
Total Bilirubin	≤ULN	>1.0-1.5x ULN	>1.5-3x ULN	>3-10x ULN
SGOT	≤ULN	>ULN (can be normal if Total Bilirubin is >ULN)	Any	Any

ULN=upper limit of normal for the institution

Adult Overdose

1,200 to 1,600 mg (duration varying between 1 to 10 days): Nausea, vomiting, diarrhea, rash erythema, edema, swelling, fatigue, muscle spasms, thrombocytopenia, pancytopenia, abdominal pain, headache, decreased appetite.

1,800 to 3,200 mg (as high as 3,200 mg daily for 6 days): Weakness, myalgia, increased CPK, increased bilirubin, gastrointestinal pain.

6,400 mg (single dose): One case in the literature reported one patient who experienced nausea, vomiting, abdominal pain, pyrexia, facial swelling, neutrophil count decreased, increase transaminases.

8 to 10 g (single dose): Vomiting and gastrointestinal pain have been reported.

A patient with myeloid blast crisis experienced Grade 1 elevations of serum creatinine, Grade 2 ascites and elevated liver transaminase levels, and Grade 3 elevations of bilirubin after inadvertently taking 1,200 mg of Gleevec daily for 6 days. Therapy was temporarily interrupted and complete reversal of all abnormalities occurred within 1 week. Treatment was resumed at a dose of 400 mg daily without recurrence of adverse reactions. Another patient developed severe muscle cramps after taking 1,600 mg of Gleevec daily for 6 days. Complete resolution of muscle cramps occurred following interruption of therapy and treatment was subsequently resumed. Another patient that was prescribed 400 mg daily, took 800 mg of Gleevec on Day 1 and 1,200 mg on Day 2. Therapy was interrupted, no adverse reactions occurred and the patient resumed therapy.

Pediatric Overdose

One 3 year-old male exposed to a single dose of 400 mg experienced vomiting, diarrhea and anorexia and another 3 year-old male exposed to a single dose of 980 mg experienced decreased white blood cell count and diarrhea.

11 DESCRIPTION

Imatinib is a small molecule kinase inhibitor. Gleevec film-coated tablets contain imatinib mesylate equivalent to 100 mg or 400 mg of imatinib free base. Imatinib mesylate is designated chemically as 4-[(4-Methyl-1-piperazinyl)-methyl]-N-[4-methyl-3-[[4-(3-pyridinyl)-2-pyrimidinyl]amino]-phenyl]benzamide methanesulfonate and its structural formula is

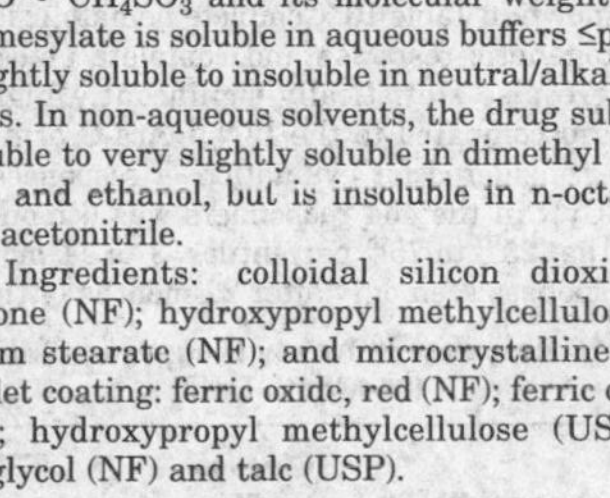

Imatinib mesylate is a white to off-white to brownish or yellowish tinged crystalline powder. Its molecular formula is $C_{29}H_{31}N_7O \bullet CH_4SO_3$ and its molecular weight is 589.7. Imatinib mesylate is soluble in aqueous buffers ≤pH 5.5 but is very slightly soluble to insoluble in neutral/alkaline aqueous buffers. In non-aqueous solvents, the drug substance is freely soluble to very slightly soluble in dimethyl sulfoxide, methanol, and ethanol, but is insoluble in n-octanol, acetone, and acetonitrile.

Inactive Ingredients: colloidal silicon dioxide (NF); crospovidone (NF); hydroxypropyl methylcellulose (USP); magnesium stearate (NF); and microcrystalline cellulose (NF). Tablet coating: ferric oxide, red (NF); ferric oxide, yellow (NF); hydroxypropyl methylcellulose (USP); polyethylene glycol (NF) and talc (USP).

12 CLINICAL PHARMACOLOGY

12.1 Mechanism of Action

Imatinib mesylate is a protein-tyrosine kinase inhibitor that inhibits the bcr-abl tyrosine kinase, the constitutive abnormal tyrosine kinase created by the Philadelphia chromosome abnormality in CML. Imatinib inhibits proliferation and induces apoptosis in bcr-abl positive cell lines as well as fresh leukemic cells from Philadelphia chromosome positive chronic myeloid leukemia. Imatinib inhibits colony formation in assays using *ex vivo* peripheral blood and bone marrow samples from CML patients.

In vivo, imatinib inhibits tumor growth of bcr-abl transfected murine myeloid cells as well as bcr-abl positive leukemia lines derived from CML patients in blast crisis.

Imatinib is also an inhibitor of the receptor tyrosine kinases for platelet-derived growth factor (PDGF) and stem cell factor (SCF), c-kit, and inhibits PDGF- and SCF-mediated cellular events. *In vitro*, imatinib inhibits proliferation and induces apoptosis in GIST cells, which express an activating c-kit mutation.

12.3 Pharmacokinetics

The pharmacokinetics of Gleevec have been evaluated in studies in healthy subjects and in population pharmacokinetic studies in over 900 patients. The pharmacokinetics of Gleevec are similar in CML and GIST patients. Imatinib is well absorbed after oral administration with C_{max} achieved within 2-4 hours post-dose. Mean absolute bioavailability is 98%. Following oral administration in healthy volunteers, the elimination half-lives of imatinib and its major active metabolite, the N-demethyl derivative (CGP74588), are approximately 18 and 40 hours, respectively. Mean imatinib AUC increases proportionally with increasing doses ranging from 25 mg-1,000 mg. There is no significant change in the pharmacokinetics of imatinib on repeated dosing, and accumulation is 1.5- to 2.5-fold at steady state when Gleevec is dosed once daily. At clinically relevant concentrations of imatinib, binding to plasma proteins in *in vitro* experiments is approximately 95%, mostly to albumin and α1-acid glycoprotein.

CYP3A4 is the major enzyme responsible for metabolism of imatinib. Other cytochrome P450 enzymes, such as CYP1A2, CYP2D6, CYP2C9, and CYP2C19, play a minor role in its metabolism. The main circulating active metabolite in humans is the N-demethylated piperazine derivative, formed predominantly by CYP3A4. It shows *in vitro* potency similar to the parent imatinib. The plasma AUC for this metabolite is about 15% of the AUC for imatinib. The plasma protein binding of N-demethylated metabolite CGP74588 is similar to that of the parent compound. Human liver microsome studies demonstrated that Gleevec is a potent competitive inhibitor of CYP2C9, CYP2D6, and CYP3A4/5 with Ki values of 27, 7.5, and 8 μM, respectively.

Imatinib elimination is predominately in the feces, mostly as metabolites. Based on the recovery of compound(s) after an oral ^{14}C-labeled dose of imatinib, approximately 81% of the dose was eliminated within 7 days, in feces (68% of dose) and urine (13% of dose). Unchanged imatinib accounted for 25% of the dose (5% urine, 20% feces), the remainder being metabolites.

Typically, clearance of imatinib in a 50-year-old patient weighing 50 kg is expected to be 8 L/h, while for a 50-year-old patient weighing 100 kg the clearance will increase to 14 L/h. The inter-patient variability of 40% in clearance does not warrant initial dose adjustment based on body weight and/or age but indicates the need for close monitoring for treatment-related toxicity.

13 NONCLINICAL TOXICOLOGY

13.1 Carcinogenesis, Mutagenesis, Impairment of Fertility

In the 2-year rat carcinogenicity study administration of imatinib at 15, 30, and 60 mg/kg/day resulted in a statistically significant reduction in the longevity of males at 60 mg/kg/day and females at ≥30 mg/kg/day. Target organs for neoplastic changes were the kidneys (renal tubule and renal pelvis), urinary bladder, urethra, preputial and clitoral gland, small intestine, parathyroid glands, adrenal glands and non-glandular stomach. Neoplastic lesions were not seen at: 30 mg/kg/day for the kidneys, urinary bladder, urethra, small intestine, parathyroid glands, adrenal glands and non-glandular stomach, and 15 mg/kg/day for the preputial and clitoral gland. The papilloma/carcinoma of the preputial/clitoral gland were noted at 30 and 60 mg/kg/day, representing approximately 0.5 to 4 or 0.3 to 2.4 times the human daily exposure (based on AUC) at 400 mg/day or 800 mg/day, respectively, and 0.4 to 3.0 times the daily exposure in children (based on AUC) at 340 mg/m^2. The renal tubule adenoma/carcinoma, renal pelvis transitional cell neoplasms, the urinary bladder and urethra transitional cell papillomas, the small intestine adenocarcinomas, the parathyroid glands adenomas, the benign and malignant medullary tumors of the adrenal glands and the non-glandular stomach papillomas/carcinomas were noted at 60 mg/kg/day. The relevance of these findings in the rat carcinogenicity study for humans is not known.

Positive genotoxic effects were obtained for imatinib in an *in vitro* mammalian cell assay (Chinese hamster ovary) for clastogenicity (chromosome aberrations) in the presence of metabolic activation. Two intermediates of the manufacturing process, which are also present in the final product, are positive for mutagenesis in the Ames assay. One of these intermediates was also positive in the mouse lymphoma assay. Imatinib was not genotoxic when tested in an *in vitro* bacterial cell assay (Ames test), an *in vitro* mammalian cell assay (mouse lymphoma) and an *in vivo* rat micronucleus assay.

In a study of fertility, male rats were dosed for 70 days prior to mating and female rats were dosed 14 days prior to mating and through to gestational Day 6. Testicular and epididymal weights and percent motile sperm were decreased at 60 mg/kg, approximately three-fourths the maximum clinical dose of 800 mg/day based on body surface area. This was not seen at doses ≤20 mg/kg (one-fourth the maximum human dose of 800 mg). The fertility of male and female rats was not affected.

In a pre- and post-natal development study in female rats dosed with imatinib mesylate at 45 mg/kg (approximately one-half the maximum human dose of 800 mg/day, based on body surface area) from gestational Day 6 until the end of lactation, red vaginal discharge was noted on either gestational Day 14 or 15. In the first generation offspring at this same dose level, mean body weights were reduced from birth until terminal sacrifice. First generation offspring fertility was not affected but reproductive effects were noted at 45 mg/kg/day including an increased number of resorptions and a decreased number of viable fetuses.

Fertility was not affected in the preclinical fertility and early embryonic development study although lower testes and epididymal weights as well as a reduced number of motile sperm were observed in the high dose males rats. In the preclinical pre- and postnatal study in rats, fertility in the first generation was also not affected by Gleevec.

Human studies on male patients receiving Gleevec and its affect on male fertility and spermatogenesis have not been performed. Male patients concerned about their fertility on Gleevec treatment should consult with their physician.

14 CLINICAL STUDIES

14.1 Chronic Myeloid Leukemia

Chronic Phase, Newly Diagnosed: An open-label, multicenter, international randomized Phase 3 study has been conducted in patients with newly diagnosed Philadelphia chromosome positive (Ph+) chronic myeloid leukemia (CML) in chronic phase. This study compared treatment with either single-agent Gleevec or a combination of interferon-alpha (IFN) plus cytarabine (Ara-C). Patients were allowed to cross over to the alternative treatment arm if they failed to show a complete hematologic response (CHR) at 6 months, a major cytogenetic response (MCyR) at 12 months, or if they lost a CHR or MCyR. Patients with increasing WBC or severe intolerance to treatment were also allowed to cross over to the alternative treatment arm with the permission of the study monitoring committee (SMC). In the Gleevec arm, patients were treated initially with 400 mg daily. Dose escalations were allowed from 400 mg daily to 600 mg daily, then from 600 mg daily to 800 mg daily. In the IFN arm, patients were treated with a target dose of IFN of 5 MIU/m^2/day subcutaneously in combination with subcutaneous Ara-C 20 mg/m^2/day for 10 days/month.

A total of 1,106 patients were randomized from 177 centers in 16 countries, 553 to each arm. Baseline characteristics were well balanced between the two arms. Median age was 51 years (range 18-70 years), with 21.9% of patients ≥60 years of age. There were 59% males and 41% females; 89.9% Caucasian and 4.7% Black patients. At the cut-off for this analysis (7 years after last patient had been recruited), the median duration of first-line treatment was 82 and 8 months in the Gleevec and IFN arm, respectively. The median duration of second-line treatment with Gleevec was 64 months. Sixty percent of patients randomized to Gleevec are still receiving first-line treatment. In these patients, the average dose of Gleevec was 403 mg ± 57 mg. Overall, in patients receiving first line Gleevec, the average daily dose delivered was 406 mg ± 76 mg. Due to discontinuations and cross-overs, only 2% of patients randomized to IFN were still on first-line treatment. In the IFN arm, withdrawal of consent (14%) was the most frequent reason for discontinuation of first-line therapy, and the most frequent reason for cross over to the Gleevec arm was severe intolerance to treatment (26%) and progression (14%).

The primary efficacy endpoint of the study was progression-free survival (PFS). Progression was defined as any of the following events: progression to accelerated phase or blast crisis (AP/BC), death, loss of CHR or MCyR, or in patients not achieving a CHR an increasing WBC despite appropriate therapeutic management. The protocol specified that the progression analysis would compare the intent to treat (ITT) population: patients randomized to receive Gleevec were compared with patients randomized to receive IFN. Patients that crossed over prior to progression were not censored at the time of cross-over, and events that occurred in these patients following cross-over were attributed to the original randomized treatment. The estimated rate of progression-free survival at 84 months in the ITT population was 81.2 % [95% CI: 78, 85] in the Gleevec arm and 60.6 % [56, 65] in the IFN arm (p<0.0001, log-rank test), (Figure 1). With 7 years follow up there were 93 (16.8%) progression events in the Gleevec arm: 37(6.7%) progression to AP/BC, 31(5.6%) loss of MCyR, 15 (2.7%) loss of CHR or increase in WBC and 10 (1.8%) CML unrelated deaths. In contrast, there were 165 (29.8%) events in the IFN+Ara-C arm of which 130 occurred during first-line treatment with IFN-Ara-C. The estimated rate of patients free of progression to accelerated phase (AP) or blast crisis (BC) at 84 months was 92.5%[90, 95] in the Gleevec arm compared to the 85.1%, [82, 89] (p≤0.001) in the IFN arm, (Figure 2). The annual rates of any progression events have decreased with time on therapy. The probability of remaining progression free at 60 months was 95% for patients who were in complete cytogenetic response (CCyR) with molecular response (≥3 log reduction in Bcr-Abl transcripts as measured by quantitative reverse transcriptase polymerase chain reaction) at 12 months, compared to 89% for patients in complete cytogenetic response but without a major molecular response and 70% in patients who were not in complete cytogenetic response at this time point (p<0.001).

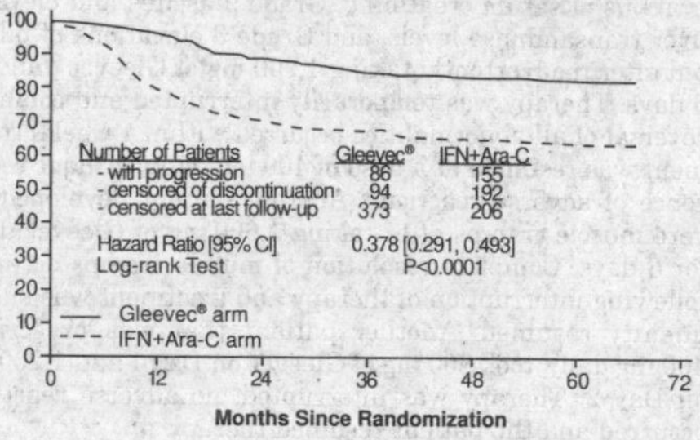

Figure 1 Progression Free Survival (ITT Principle)

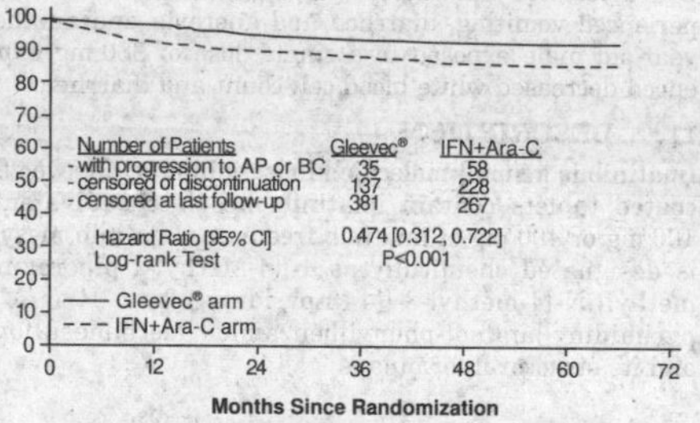

Figure 2 Time to Progression to AP or BC (ITT Principle)

A total of 71 (12.8%) and 85 (15.4%) patients died in the Gleevec and IFN+Ara-C group, respectively. At 84 months the estimated overall survival is 86.4% (83, 90) vs. 83.3% (80, 87) in the randomized Gleevec and the IFN+Ara-C group, respectively (p=0.073 log-rank test). The hazard ratio is 0.750 with 95% CI 0.547-1.028. This time-to-event endpoint may be affected by the high crossover rate from IFN+Ara-C to Gleevec. Major cytogenetic response, hematologic response, evaluation of minimal residual disease (molecular response), time to accelerated phase or blast crisis and survival were main secondary endpoints. Response data are shown in Table 16. Complete hematologic response, major cytogenetic response and complete cytogenetic response were also statistically significantly higher in the Gleevec arm compared to the IFN + Ara-C arm (no crossover data considered for evaluation of responses). Median time to CCyR in the 454 responders was 6 months (range 2-64 months, 25th to 75th percentiles=3 to 11 months) with 10% of responses seen only after 22 months of therapy).

Table 16 Response in Newly Diagnosed CML Study (84-Month Data)

(Best Response Rate)	Gleevec n=553	IFN+Ara–C n=553
Hematologic Response[1]		
CHR Rate n (%)	534 (96.6%)*	313 (56.6%)*
[95% CI]	[94.7%, 97.9%]	[52.4%, 60.8%]
Cytogenetic Response[2]		
Major Cytogenetic Response n (%)	472 (85.4 %)*	93 (16.8%)*
[95% CI]	[82.1%, 88.2%]	[13.8%, 20.2%]
Unconfirmed[3]	88.6%*	23.3%*
Complete Cytogenetic Response n (%)	413 (74.7%)*	36 (6.5%)*
[95% CI]	[70.8, 78.3]	[4.6, 8.9]
Unconfirmed[3]	82.5%*	11.6%*

*p<0.001, Fischer's exact test

[1]**Hematologic response criteria** (all responses to be confirmed after ≥4 weeks):
WBC<10 × 10^9/L, platelet <450 × 10^9/L, myelocyte + metamyelocyte <5% in blood, no blasts and promyelocytes in blood, no extramedullary involvement.

[2]**Cytogenetic response criteria** (confirmed after ≥4 weeks): complete (0% Ph+ metaphases) or partial (1%-35%). A major response (0%-35%) combines both complete and partial responses.

[3]**Unconfirmed cytogenetic response** is based on a single bone marrow cytogenetic evaluation, therefore unconfirmed complete or partial cytogenetic responses might have had a lesser cytogenetic response on a subsequent bone marrow evaluation.

Molecular response was defined as follows: in the peripheral blood, after 12 months of therapy, reduction of ≥3 logarithms in the amount of bcr-abl transcripts (measured by real-time quantitative reverse transcriptase PCR assay) over a standardized baseline. Molecular response was only evaluated in a subset of patients who had a complete cytogenetic response by 12 months or later (N=333). The molecular response rate in patients who had a complete cytogenetic response in the Gleevec arm was 59% at 12 months and 72% at 24 months.

Physical, functional, and treatment-specific biologic response modifier scales from the FACT-BRM (Functional Assessment of Cancer Therapy - Biologic Response Modifier) instrument were used to assess patient-reported general effects of interferon toxicity in 1,067 patients with CML in chronic phase. After one month of therapy to six months of therapy, there was a 13%-21% decrease in median index from baseline in patients treated with IFN, consistent with increased symptoms of IFN toxicity. There was no apparent change from baseline in median index for patients treated with Gleevec.

Late Chronic Phase CML and Advanced Stage CML: Three international, open-label, single-arm phase 2 studies were conducted to determine the safety and efficacy of Gleevec in patients with Ph+ CML: 1) in the chronic phase after failure of IFN therapy, 2) in accelerated phase disease, or 3) in myeloid blast crisis. About 45% of patients were women and 6% were Black. In clinical studies 38%-40% of patients were ≥60 years of age and 10%-12% of patients were ≥70 years of age.

Chronic Phase, Prior Interferon-Alpha Treatment: 532 patients were treated at a starting dose of 400 mg; dose escalation to 600 mg was allowed. The patients were distributed in three main categories according to their response to prior interferon: failure to achieve (within 6 months), or loss of a complete hematologic response (29%), failure to achieve (within 1 year) or loss of a major cytogenetic response (35%), or intolerance to interferon (36%). Patients had received a median of 14 months of prior IFN therapy at doses ≥25 × 10^6 IU/week and were all in late chronic phase, with a median time from diagnosis of 32 months. Effectiveness was evaluated on the basis of the rate of hematologic response and by bone marrow exams to assess the rate of major cytogenetic response (up to 35% Ph+ metaphases) or complete cytogenetic response (0% Ph+ metaphases). Median duration of treatment was 29 months with 81% of patients treated for ≥24 months (maximum = 31.5 months). Efficacy results are reported in Table 16. Confirmed major cytogenetic response rates were higher in patients with IFN intolerance (66%) and cytogenetic failure (64%), than in patients with hematologic failure (47%). Hematologic response was achieved in 98% of patients with cytogenetic failure, 94% of patients with hematologic failure, and 92% of IFN-intolerant patients.

Accelerated Phase: 235 patients with accelerated phase disease were enrolled. These patients met one or more of the following criteria: ≥15%-<30% blasts in PB or BM; ≥30% blasts + promyelocytes in PB or BM; ≥20% basophils in PB; and <100 × 10^9/L platelets. The first 77 patients were started at 400 mg, with the remaining 158 patients starting at 600 mg.

Effectiveness was evaluated primarily on the basis of the rate of hematologic response, reported as either complete hematologic response, no evidence of leukemia (i.e., clearance of blasts from the marrow and the blood, but without a full peripheral blood recovery as for complete responses), or return to chronic phase CML. Cytogenetic responses were also evaluated. Median duration of treatment was 18 months with 45% of patients treated for ≥24 months (maximum=35 months). Efficacy results are reported in Table 17.

Response rates in accelerated phase CML were higher for the 600 mg dose group than for the 400 mg group: hematologic response (75% vs. 64%), confirmed and unconfirmed major cytogenetic response (31% vs. 19%).

Myeloid Blast Crisis: 260 patients with myeloid blast crisis were enrolled. These patients had ≥30% blasts in PB or BM and/or extramedullary involvement other than spleen or liver; 95 (37%) had received prior chemotherapy for treatment of either accelerated phase or blast crisis ("pretreated patients") whereas 165 (63%) had not ("untreated patients"). The first 37 patients were started at 400 mg; the remaining 223 patients were started at 600 mg.

Effectiveness was evaluated primarily on the basis of rate of hematologic response, reported as either complete hematologic response, no evidence of leukemia, or return to chronic phase CML using the same criteria as for the study in accelerated phase. Cytogenetic responses were also assessed. Median duration of treatment was 4 months with 21% of patients treated for ≥12 months and 10% for ≥24 months (maximum=35 months). Efficacy results are reported in Table 17. The hematologic response rate was higher in untreated patients than in treated patients (36% vs. 22%, respectively) and in the group receiving an initial dose of 600 mg rather than 400 mg (33% vs. 16%). The confirmed and unconfirmed major cytogenetic response rate was also higher for the 600 mg dose group than for the 400 mg dose group (17% vs. 8%).

[See table 17 above]

The median time to hematologic response was 1 month. In late chronic phase CML, with a median time from diagnosis of 32 months, an estimated 87.8% of patients who achieved MCyR maintained their response 2 years after achieving their initial response. After 2 years of treatment, an estimated 85.4% of patients were free of progression to AP or BC, and estimated overall survival was 90.8% [88.3, 93.2]. In accelerated phase, median duration of hematologic response was 28.8 months for patients with an initial dose of 600 mg (16.5 months for 400 mg). An estimated 63.8% of patients who achieved MCyR were still in response 2 years after achieving initial response. The median survival was 20.9 [13.1, 34.4] months for the 400 mg group and was not yet reached for the 600 mg group (p=0.0097). An estimated 46.2% [34.7, 57.7] vs. 65.8% [58.4, 73.3] of patients were still alive after 2 years of treatment in the 400 mg vs. 600 mg dose groups, respectively. In blast crisis, the estimated median duration of hematologic response is 10 months. An estimated 27.2% [16.8, 37.7] of hematologic responders maintained their response 2 years after achieving their initial response. Median survival was 6.9 [5.8, 8.6] months, and an estimated 18.3% [13.4, 23.3] of all patients with blast crisis were alive 2 years after start of study.

Efficacy results were similar in men and women and in patients younger and older than age 65. Responses were seen in Black patients, but there were too few Black patients to allow a quantitative comparison.

Table 17 Response in CML Studies

	Chronic Phase IFN Failure (n=532) 400 mg	Accelerated Phase (n=235) 600 mg n=158 400 mg n=77	Myeloid Blast Crisis (n=260) 600 mg n=223 400 mg n=37
		% of patients [CI $_{95\%}$]	
Hematologic Response[1]	95% [92.3–96.3]	71% [64.8–76.8]	31% [25.2–36.8]
Complete Hematologic Response (CHR)	95%	38%	7%
No Evidence of Leukemia (NEL)	Not applicable	13%	5%
Return to Chronic Phase (RTC)	Not applicable	20%	18%
Major Cytogenetic Response[2]	60% [55.3–63.8]	21% [16.2–27.1]	7% [4.5–11.2]
(Unconfirmed[3])	(65%)	(27%)	(15%)
Complete[4] (Unconfirmed[3])	39% (47%)	16% (20%)	2% (7%)

[1] **Hematologic response criteria** (all responses to be confirmed after ≥4 weeks):
CHR:Chronic phase study [WBC <10 × 10^9/L, platelet <450 × 10^9/L, myelocytes + metamyelocytes <5% in blood, no blasts and promyelocytes in blood, basophils <20%, no extramedullary involvement] and in the accelerated and blast crisis studies [ANC ≥1.5 × 10^9/L, platelets ≥100 × 10^9/L, no blood blasts, BM blasts <5% and no extramedullary disease]
NEL: Same criteria as for CHR but ANC ≥1 × 10^9/L and platelets ≥20 × 10^9/L (accelerated and blast crisis studies)
RTC: <15% blasts BM and PB, <30% blasts + promyelocytes in BM and PB, <20% basophils in PB, no extramedullary disease other than spleen and liver (accelerated and blast crisis studies).
BM=bone marrow, PB=peripheral blood

[2] **Cytogenetic response criteria** (confirmed after ≥4 weeks): complete (0% Ph+ metaphases) or partial (1%-35%). A major response (0%-35%) combines both complete and partial responses.

[3] **Unconfirmed cytogenetic response** is based on a single bone marrow cytogenetic evaluation, therefore unconfirmed complete or partial cytogenetic responses might have had a lesser cytogenetic response on a subsequent bone marrow evaluation.

[4] **Complete cytogenetic response** confirmed by a second bone marrow cytogenetic evaluation performed at least 1 month after the initial bone marrow study.

14.2 Pediatric CML

A total of 51 pediatric patients with newly diagnosed and untreated CML in chronic phase were enrolled in an open-label, multicenter, single arm phase 2 trial. Patients were treated with Gleevec 340 mg/m²/day, with no interruptions in the absence of dose limiting toxicity. Complete hematologic response (CHR) was observed in 78% of patients after 8 weeks of therapy. The complete cytogenetic response rate (CCyR) was 65%, comparable to the results observed in adults. Additionally, partial cytogenetic response (PCyR) was observed in 16%. The majority of patients who achieved a CCyR developed the CCyR between months 3 and 10 with a median time to response based on the Kaplan-Meier estimate of 6.74 months. Patients were allowed to be removed from protocol therapy to undergo alternative therapy including hematopoietic stem cell transplantation. Thirty one children received stem cell transplantation. Of the 31 children, 5 were transplanted after disease progression on study and 1 withdrew from study during first week treatment and received transplant approximately 4 months after withdrawal. Twenty five children withdrew from protocol therapy to undergo stem cell transplant after receiving a median of 9 twenty-eight day courses (range 4 to 24). Of the 25 patients 13 (52%) had CCyR and 5 (20%) had PCyR at the end of protocol therapy.

One open-label, single-arm study enrolled 14 pediatric patients with Ph+ chronic phase CML recurrent after stem cell transplant or resistant to interferon-alpha therapy. These patients had not previously received Gleevec and ranged in age from 3-20 years old; 3 were 3-11 years old, 9 were 12-18 years old, and 2 were >18 years old. Patients were treated at doses of 260 mg/m²/day (n=3), 340 mg/m²/day (n=4), 440 mg/m²/day (n=5) and 570 mg/m²/day (n=2). In the 13 patients for whom cytogenetic data are available, 4 achieved a major cytogenetic response, 7 achieved a complete cytogenetic response, and 2 had a minimal cytogenetic response.

In a second study, 2 of 3 patients with Ph+ chronic phase CML resistant to interferon-alpha therapy achieved a complete cytogenetic response at doses of 242 and 257 mg/m²/day.

14.3 Acute Lymphoblastic Leukemia

A total of 48 Philadelphia chromosome positive acute lymphoblastic leukemia (Ph+ ALL) patients with relapsed/refractory disease were studied, 43 of whom received the recommended Gleevec dose of 600 mg/day. In addition 2 patients with relapsed/refractory Ph+ ALL received Gleevec 600 mg/day in a phase 1 study.

Confirmed and unconfirmed hematologic and cytogenetic response rates for the 43 relapsed/refractory Ph+ALL phase 2 study patients and for the 2 phase 1 patients are shown in Table 18. The median duration of hematologic response was 3.4 months and the median duration of MCyR was 2.3 months.

Table 18 Effect of Gleevec on Relapsed/Refractory Ph+ ALL.

	Phase 2 Study (N=43)	Phase 1 Study (N=2)
CHR	8 (19%)	2 (100%)
NEL	5 (12%)	
RTC/PHR	11 (26%)	
MCyR	15 (35%)	
CCyR	9 (21%)	
PCyR	6 (14%)	

14.4 Pediatric ALL

Pediatric and young adult patients with very high risk ALL, defined as those with an expected 5 year event-free survival (EFS) less than 45%, were enrolled after induction therapy on a multicenter, non-randomized cooperative group pilot protocol.

The safety and effectiveness of Gleevec (340 mg/m²/day) in combination with intensive chemotherapy was evaluated in a subgroup of patients with Ph+ ALL. The protocol included intensive chemotherapy and hematopoietic stem cell transplant after 2 courses of chemotherapy for patients with an appropriate HLA-matched family donor. There were 92 eligible patients with Ph+ ALL enrolled. The median age was 9.5 years (1 to 21 years), 64% were male, 75% were white, 9% were Asian/Pacific Islander, and 5% were black. In 5 successive cohorts of patients, Gleevec exposure was systematically increased by earlier introduction and prolonged duration. Cohort 1 received the lowest intensity and cohort 5 received the highest intensity of Gleevec exposure.

There were 50 patients with Ph+ ALL assigned to cohort 5 all of whom received Gleevec plus chemotherapy; 30 were treated exclusively with chemotherapy and Gleevec and 20 received chemotherapy plus Gleevec and then underwent hematopoietic stem cell transplant, followed by further Gleevec treatment. Patients in cohort 5 treated with chemotherapy received continuous daily exposure to Gleevec beginning in the first course of post induction chemotherapy continuing through maintenance cycles 1 through 4 chemotherapy. During maintenance cycles 5 through 12 Gleevec was administered 28 days out of the 56 day cycle. Patients who underwent hematopoietic stem cell transplant received 42 days of Gleevec prior to HSCT, and 28 weeks (196 days) of Gleevec after the immediate post transplant period. The estimated 4-year EFS of patients in cohort 5 was 70% (95% CI: 54, 81). The median follow-up time for EFS at data cutoff in cohort 5 was 40.5 months.

14.5 Myelodysplastic/Myeloproliferative Diseases

An open label, multicenter, phase 2 clinical trial was conducted testing Gleevec in diverse populations of patients suffering from life-threatening diseases associated with Abl, Kit or PDGFR protein tyrosine kinases. This study included 7 patients with MDS/MPD. These patients were treated with Gleevec 400 mg daily. The ages of the enrolled patients ranged from 20 to 86 years. A further 24 patients with MDS/MPD aged 2 to 79 years were reported in 12 published case reports and a clinical study. These patients also received Gleevec at a dose of 400 mg daily with the exception of three patients who received lower doses. Of the total population of 31 patients treated for MDS/MPD, 14 (45%) achieved a complete hematological response and 12 (39%) a major cytogenetic response (including 10 with a complete cytogenetic response). Sixteen patients had a translocation, involving chromosome 5q33 or 4q12, resulting in a PDGFR gene re-arrangement. All of these patients responded hematologically (13 completely). Cytogenetic response was evaluated in 12 out of 14 patients, all of whom responded (10 patients completely). Only 1(7%) out of the 14 patients without a translocation associated with PDGFR gene re-arrangement achieved a complete hematological response and none achieved a major cytogenetic response. A further patient with a PDGFR gene re-arrangement in molecular relapse after bone marrow transplant responded molecularly. Median duration of therapy was 12.9 months (0.8-26.7) in the 7 patients treated within the phase 2 study and ranged between 1 week and more than 18 months in responding patients in the published literature. Results are provided in Table 19. Response durations of phase 2 study patients ranged from 141+ days to 457+ days.

Table 19 Response in MDS/MPD

	N	Complete Hematologic Response N (%)	Major Cytogenetic Response N (%)
Overall Population	31	14 (45)	12 (39)
Chromosome 5 Translocation	14	11 (79)	11 (79)
Chromosome 4 Translocation	2	2 (100)	1 (50)
Others / no Translocation	14	1 (7)	0 (0)
Molecular Relapse	1	NE[1]	NE[1]

[1] NE: Not Evaluable

14.6 Aggressive Systemic Mastocytosis

One open-label, multicenter, phase 2 study was conducted testing Gleevec in diverse populations of patients with life-threatening diseases associated with Abl, Kit or PDGFR protein tyrosine kinases. This study included 5 patients with aggressive systemic mastocytosis (ASM) treated with

Table 20 Response in ASM

Cytogenetic Abnormality	Number of Patients	Complete Hematologic Response N (%)	Partial Hematologic Response N (%)
FIP1L1-PDGFRα Fusion Kinase (or CHIC2 Deletion)	7	7(100%)	0%
Juxtamembrane Mutation	2	0 (0%)	2 (100%)
Unknown or No Cytogenetic Abnormality Detected	15	0(0%)	7 (44%)
D816V Mutation	4	1* (25%)	0%
Total	28	8 (29%)	9 (32%)

* Patient had concomitant CML and ASM

Table 21 Response in HES/CEL

Cytogenetic Abnormality	Number of Patients	Complete Hematological Response N (%)	Partial Hematological Response N (%)
Positive FIP1L1-PDGFRα Fusion Kinase	61	61 (100%)	0%
Negative FIP1L1-PDGFRα Fusion Kinase	56	12 (21%)	9 (16%)
Unknown Cytogenetic Abnormality	59	34 (58%)	7 (12%)
Total	176	107 (61%)	23 (13%)

100 mg to 400 mg of Gleevec daily. These 5 patients ranged from 49 to 74 years of age. In addition to these 5 patients, 10 published case reports and case series describe the use of Gleevec in 23 additional patients with ASM aged 26 to 85 years who also received 100 mg to 400 mg of Gleevec daily. Cytogenetic abnormalities were evaluated in 20 of the 28 ASM patients treated with Gleevec from the published reports and in the phase 2 study. Seven of these 20 patients had the FIP1L1-PDGFRα fusion kinase (or CHIC2 deletion). Patients with this cytogenetic abnormality were predominantly males and had eosinophilia associated with their systemic mast cell disease. Two patients had a Kit mutation in the juxtamembrane region (one Phe522Cys and one K509I) and four patients had a D816V c-Kit mutation (not considered sensitive to Gleevec), one with concomitant CML.

Of the 28 patients treated for ASM, 8 (29%) achieved a complete hematologic response and 9 (32%) a partial hematologic response (61% overall response rate). Median duration of Gleevec therapy for the 5 ASM patients in the phase 2 study was 13 months (range 1.4-22.3 months) and between 1 month and more than 30 months in the responding patients described in the published medical literature. A summary of the response rates to Gleevec in ASM is provided in Table 20. Response durations of literature patients ranged from 1+ to 30+ months.

[See table 20 above]

Gleevec has not been shown to be effective in patients with less aggressive forms of systemic mastocytosis (SM). Gleevec is therefore not recommended for use in patients with cutaneous mastocytosis, indolent systemic mastocytosis (smoldering SM or isolated bone marrow mastocytosis), SM with an associated clonal hematological non-mast cell lineage disease, mast cell leukemia, mast cell sarcoma or extracutaneous mastocytoma. Patients that harbor the D816V mutation of c-Kit are not sensitive to Gleevec and should not receive Gleevec.

14.7 Hypereosinophilic Syndrome/Chronic Eosinophilic Leukemia

One open-label, multicenter, phase 2 study was conducted testing Gleevec in diverse populations of patients with life-threatening diseases associated with Abl, Kit or PDGFR protein tyrosine kinases. This study included 14 patients with Hypereosinophilic Syndrome/Chronic Eosinophilic Leukemia (HES/CEL). HES patients were treated with 100 mg to 1000 mg of Gleevec daily. The ages of these patients ranged from 16 to 64 years. A further 162 patients with HES/CEL aged 11 to 78 years were reported in 35 published case reports and case series. These patients received Gleevec at doses of 75 mg to 800 mg daily. Hematologic response rates are summarized in Table 21. Response durations for literature patients ranged from 6+ weeks to 44 months.

[See table 21 above]

14.8 Dermatofibrosarcoma Protuberans

Dermatofibrosarcoma Protuberans (DFSP) is a cutaneous soft tissue sarcoma. It is characterized by a translocation of chromosomes 17 and 22 that results in the fusion of the collagen type 1 alpha 1 gene and the PDGF B gene.

An open-label, multicenter, phase 2 study was conducted testing Gleevec in a diverse population of patients with life-threatening diseases associated with Abl, Kit or PDGFR protein tyrosine kinases. This study included 12 patients with DFSP who were treated with Gleevec 800 mg daily (age range 23 to 75 years). DFSP was metastatic, locally recurrent following initial surgical resection and not considered amenable to further surgery at the time of study entry. A further 6 DFSP patients treated with Gleevec are reported in 5 published case reports, their ages ranging from 18 months to 49 years. The total population treated for DFSP therefore comprises 18 patients, 8 of them with metastatic disease. The adult patients reported in the published literature were treated with either 400 mg (4 cases) or 800 mg (1 case) Gleevec daily. A single pediatric patient received 400 mg/m^2/daily, subsequently increased to 520 mg/m^2/daily. Ten patients had the PDGF B gene rearrangement, 5 had no available cytogenetics and 3 had complex cytogenetic abnormalities. Responses to treatment are described in Table 22.

Table 22 Response in DFSP

	Number of Patients (n=18)	%
Complete Response	7	39
Partial Response *	8	44
Total Responders	15	83

* 5 patients made disease free by surgery

Twelve of these 18 patients either achieved a complete response (7 patients) or were made disease free by surgery after a partial response (5 patients, including one child) for a total complete response rate of 67%. A further 3 patients achieved a partial response, for an overall response rate of 83%. Of the 8 patients with metastatic disease, five responded (62%), three of them completely (37%). For the 10 study patients with the PDGF B gene rearrangement there were 4 complete and 6 partial responses. The median duration of response in the phase 2 study was 6.2 months, with a maximum duration of 24.3 months, while in the published literature it ranged between 4 weeks and more than 20 months.

14.9 Gastrointestinal Stromal Tumors

Unresectable and/or Malignant Metastatic GIST

Two open-label, randomized, multinational Phase 3 studies were conducted in patients with unresectable or metastatic malignant gastrointestinal stromal tumors (GIST). The two study designs were similar allowing a predefined combined analysis of safety and efficacy. A total of 1640 patients were enrolled into the two studies and randomized 1:1 to receive either 400 mg or 800 mg orally daily continuously until disease progression or unacceptable toxicity. Patients in the 400 mg daily treatment group who experienced disease progression were permitted to crossover to receive treatment with 800 mg daily. The studies were designed to compare response rates, progression-free survival and overall survival between the dose groups. Median age at patient entry was 60 years. Males comprised 58% of the patients enrolled. All patients had a pathologic diagnosis of CD117 positive unresectable and/or metastatic malignant GIST.

The primary objective of the two studies was to evaluate either progression-free survival (PFS) with a secondary objective of overall survival (OS) in one study or overall survival with a secondary objective of PFS in the other study. A planned analysis of both OS and PFS from the combined datasets from these two studies was conducted. Results from this combined analysis are shown in Table 23.

Table 23 Overall Survival, Progression-Free Survival and Tumor Response Rates in the Phase 3 GIST Trials

	Gleevec 400 mg N=818	Gleevec 800 mg N=822
Progression-Free Survival (months)	18.9	23.2
Median		
95% CI	17.4-21.2	20.8-24.9
Overall Survival (months)	49.0	48.7
95% CI	45.3-60.0	45.3-51.6
Best Overall Tumor Response		
Response	43 (5.3%)	41 (5.0%)
Complete Response (CR)	377 (46.1%)	402 (48.9%)
Partial Response (PR)		

Median follow up for the combined studies was 37.5 months. There were no observed differences in overall survival between the treatment groups (p=0.98). Patients who crossed over following disease progression from the 400 mg/day treatment group to the 800 mg/day treatment group (n=347) had a 3.4 month median and a 7.7 month mean exposure to Gleevec following crossover.

One open-label, multinational Phase 2 study was conducted in patients with Kit (CD117) positive unresectable or metastatic malignant GIST. In this study, 147 patients were enrolled and randomized to receive either 400 mg or 600 mg orally q.d. for up to 36 months. The primary outcome of the study was objective response rate. Tumors were required to be measurable at entry in at least one site of disease, and response characterization was based on Southwestern Oncology Group (SWOG) criteria. There were no differences in response rates between the 2 dose groups. The response rate was 68.5% for the 400 mg group and 67.6% for the 600 mg group. The median time to response was 12 weeks (range was 3-98 weeks) and the estimated median duration of response is 118 weeks (95% CI: 86, not reached).

Adjuvant Treatment of GIST

In the adjuvant setting, Gleevec was investigated in a multicenter, double-blind, placebo-controlled, randomized trial involving 713 patients (Study 1). Patients were randomized one to one to Gleevec at 400 mg/day or matching placebo for 12 months. The ages of these patients ranged from 18 to 91 years. Patients were included who had a histologic diagnosis of primary GIST, expressing KIT protein by immunochemistry and a tumor size ≥3 cm in maximum dimension with complete gross resection of primary GIST within 14 to 70 days prior to registration.

Recurrence-free survival (RFS) was defined as the time from date of randomization to the date of recurrence or death from any cause. In a planned interim analysis, the median follow up was 15 months in patients without a RFS event; there were 30 RFS events in the 12-month Gleevec arm compared to 70 RFS events in the placebo arm with a hazard ratio of 0.398 (95% CI: 0.259, 0.610), p<0.0001. After the interim analysis of RFS, 79 of the 354 patients initially randomized to the placebo arm were eligible to cross over to the 12-month Gleevec arm. Seventy-two of these 79 patients subsequently crossed over to Gleevec therapy. In an updated analysis, the median follow-up for patients without a RFS event was 50 months. There were 74 (21%) RFS events in the 12-month Gleevec arm compared to 98 (28%) events in the placebo arm with a hazard ratio of 0.718 (95% CI: 0.531-0.971) (Figure 3). The median follow-up for OS in patients still living was 61 months. There were 26 (7%) and 33 (9%) deaths in the 12-month Gleevec and placebo arms, respectively with a hazard ratio of 0.816 (95% CI: 0.488-1.365).

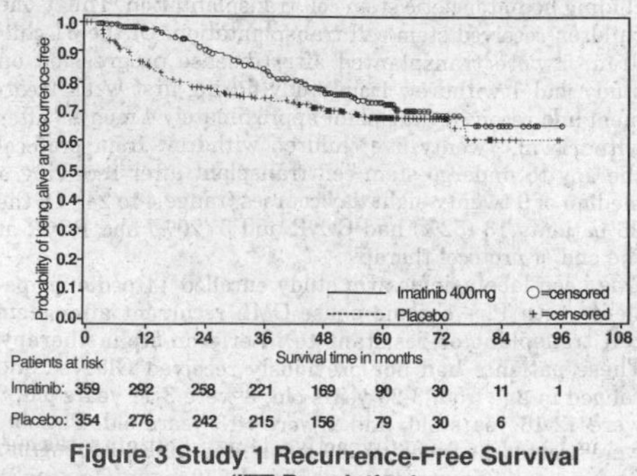

Figure 3 Study 1 Recurrence-Free Survival (ITT Population)

A second randomized, multicenter, open label, phase 3 trial in the adjuvant setting (Study 2) compared 12 months of Gleevec treatment to 36 months of Gleevec treatment at 400 mg/day in adult patients with KIT (CD117) positive GIST after surgical resection with one of the following: tumor diameter >5 cm and mitotic count >5/50 high power fields (HPF), or tumor diameter >10 cm and any mitotic count, or tumor of any size with mitotic count >10/50 HPF, or tumors ruptured into the peritoneal cavity. There were a total of 397 patients randomized in the trial with 199 patients on the 12-month treatment arm and 198 patients on the 36-month treatment arm. The median age was 61 years (range 22 to 84 years).

RFS was defined as the time from date of randomization to the date of recurrence or death from any cause. The median follow-up for patients without a RFS event was 42 months. There were 84 (42%) RFS events in the 12-month treatment arm and 50 (25%) RFS events in the 36 month treatment arm. Thirty-six months of Gleevec treatment significantly prolonged RFS compared to 12 months of Gleevec treatment with a hazard ratio of 0.46 (95% CI: 0.32, 0.65), p<0.0001 (Figure 4).

The median follow-up for overall survival (OS) in patients still living was 48 months. There were 25 (13%) deaths in the 12-month treatment arm and 12 (6%) deaths in the 36-month treatment arm. Thirty-six months of Gleevec treatment significantly prolonged OS compared to 12 months of Gleevec treatment with a hazard ratio of 0.45 (95% CI: 0.22, 0.89), p=0.0187 (Figure 5).

[See figure 4 above]

[See figure 5 below]

15 REFERENCES

1. Preventing Occupational Exposures to Antineoplastic and Other Hazardous Drugs in Health Care Settings. NIOSH Alert 2004-165.
2. OSHA Technical Manual, TED 1-0.15A, Section VI: Chapter 2. Controlling Occupational Exposure to Hazardous Drugs. OSHA, 1999. http://www.osha.gov/dts/osta/otm/otm_vi/otm_vi_2.html
3. American Society of Health-System Pharmacists. ASHP guidelines on handling hazardous drugs. *Am J Health-Syst Pharm.* 2006;63:1172-1193.
4. Polovich, M., White, J. M., & Kelleher, L.O. (eds.) 2005. Chemotherapy and biotherapy guidelines and recommendations for practice (2nd. ed.) Pittsburgh, PA: Oncology Nursing Society

16 HOW SUPPLIED/STORAGE AND HANDLING

Each film-coated tablet contains 100 mg or 400 mg of imatinib free base.

100 mg Tablets

Very dark yellow to brownish orange, film-coated tablets, round, biconvex with bevelled edges, debossed with "NVR" on one side, and "SA" with score on the other side.

Bottles of 90 tablets NDC 0078-0401-34

400 mg Tablets

Very dark yellow to brownish orange, film-coated tablets, ovaloid, biconvex with bevelled edges, debossed with "400" on one side with score on the other side, and "SL" on each side of the score.

Bottles of 30 tablets NDC 0078-0438-15

Storage and Handling

Store at 25°C (77°F); excursions permitted to 15-30°C (59-86°F) [see USP Controlled Room Temperature]. Protect from moisture.

Dispense in a tight container, USP.

Procedures for proper handling and disposal of anticancer drugs should be considered. Several guidelines on this subject have been published.[1-4]

Gleevec tablets should not be crushed. Direct contact of crushed tablets with the skin or mucous membranes should be avoided. If such contact occurs, wash thoroughly as outlined in the references. Personnel should avoid exposure to crushed tablets [*see Nonclinical Toxicology (13.1)*].

17 PATIENT COUNSELING INFORMATION

17.1 Dosing and Administration

Patients should be informed to take Gleevec exactly as prescribed, not to change their dose or to stop taking Gleevec unless they are told to do so by their doctor. If patients miss a dose they should be advised to take their dose as soon as possible unless it is almost time for their next dose in which case the missed dose should not be taken. A double dose should not be taken to make up for any missed dose. Patients should be advised to take Gleevec with a meal and a large glass of water.

17.2 Pregnancy and Breast-Feeding

Patients should be advised to inform their doctor if they are or think they may be pregnant. Women of reproductive potential should be advised to avoid becoming pregnant while taking Gleevec. Sexually active female patients taking Gleevec should use highly effective contraception. Patients should also be advised not to breast feed while taking Gleevec.

17.3 Adverse Reactions

Patients should be advised to tell their doctor if they experience side effects during Gleevec therapy including fever, shortness of breath, blood in their stools, jaundice, sudden weight gain, symptoms of cardiac failure, or if they have a history of cardiac disease or risk factors for cardiac failure.

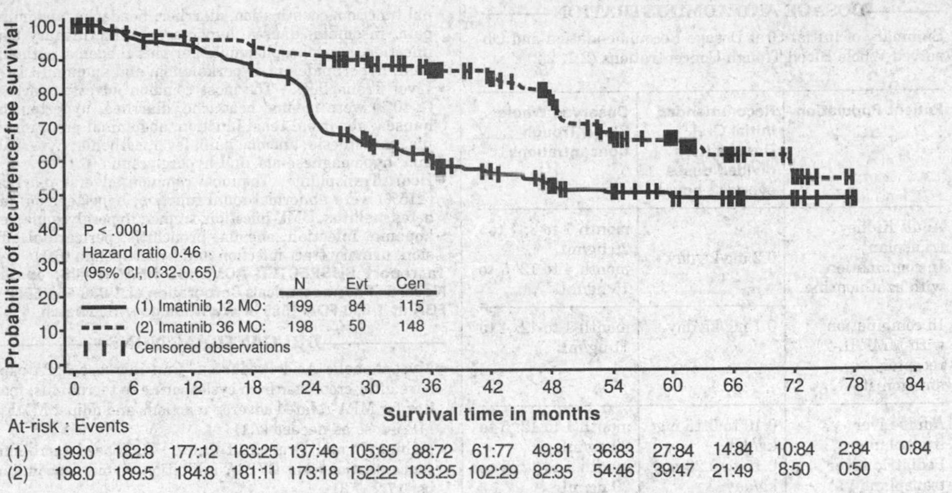

Figure 4 Study 2 Recurrence-Free Survival (ITT Population)

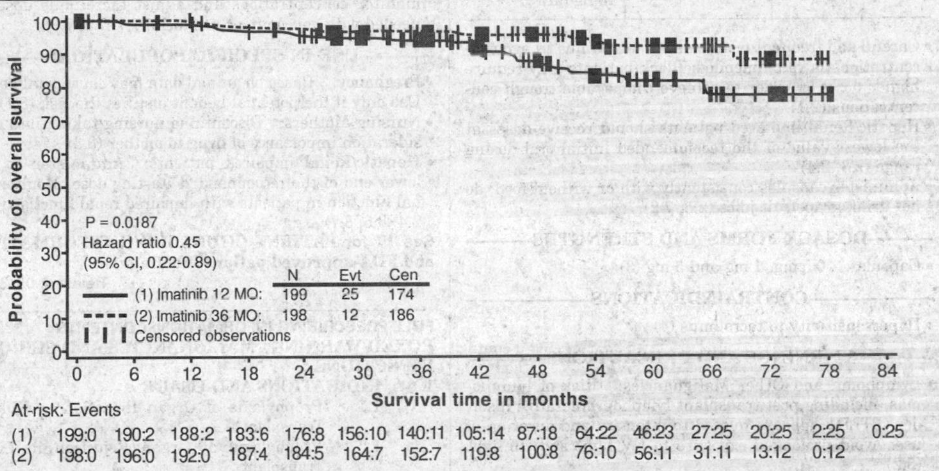

Figure 5 Study 2 Overall Survival (ITT Population)

17.4 Drug Interactions

Patients should be advised not to take any other medications, including over-the-counter medications such as herbal products without talking to their doctor or pharmacist first. Examples of other medications that should not be taken with Gleevec are warfarin, erythromycin, and phenytoin. Patients should also be advised to tell their doctor if they are taking or plan to take iron supplements. Patients should also avoid grapefruit juice and other foods known to inhibit CYP3A4 while taking Gleevec.

17.5 Pediatric

Patients should be advised that growth retardation has been reported in children and pre-adolescents receiving Gleevec. The long term effects of prolonged treatment with Gleevec on growth in children are unknown. Therefore, close monitoring of growth in children under Gleevec treatment is recommended.

17.6 Driving and Using Machines

Patients should be advised that they may experience undesirable effects such as dizziness, blurred vision or somnolence during treatment with Gleevec. Therefore, caution patients about driving a car or operating machinery.

Distributed by:
Novartis Pharmaceuticals Corporation
East Hanover, New Jersey 07936
© Novartis
T2013-17
February 2013

Shown in Product Identification Guide, page 310

HECORIA™ ℞
(tacrolimus capsules, USP)

The following prescribing information is based on official labeling in effect July 2013.

HIGHLIGHTS OF PRESCRIBING INFORMATION

These highlights do not include all the information needed to use Hecoria safely and effectively. See full prescribing information for Hecoria.

Hecoria™ (tacrolimus capsules, USP)
Initial U.S. Approval: 1994

WARNING: MALIGNANCIES AND SERIOUS INFECTIONS

See full prescribing information for complete boxed warning

- **Increased risk of development of lymphoma and other malignancies, particularly of the skin, due to immunosuppression (5.2)**
- **Increased susceptibility to bacterial, viral, fungal, and protozoal infections, including opportunistic infections (5.3, 5.4, 5.5)**
- **Only physicians experienced in immunosuppressive therapy and management of organ transplant patients should prescribe Hecoria (tacrolimus) capsules (5.1)**

RECENT MAJOR CHANGES

Warnings and Precautions, Use with CYP3A4 Inhibitors and Inducers Including Those That Prolong QT (5.13) 07/2012

INDICATIONS AND USAGE

Hecoria (tacrolimus capsules, USP) is a calcineurin-inhibitor immunosuppressant indicated for (1)

- Prophylaxis of organ rejection in patients receiving allogeneic liver, kidney, or heart transplants (1.1, 1.2, 1.3)
- Use concomitantly with adrenal corticosteroids; in kidney and heart transplant, use in conjunction with azathioprine or mycophenolate mofetil (MMF) (1.1, 1.2, 1.3)
- Limitations of Use (1.4):
  - Do not use simultaneously with cyclosporine
  - Intravenous use reserved for patients who cannot tolerate capsules orally
  - Use with sirolimus is not recommended in liver and heart transplant; use with sirolimus in kidney transplant has not been established

DOSAGE AND ADMINISTRATION

Summary of Initial Oral Dosage Recommendation and Observed Whole Blood Trough Concentrations (2.1, 2.2).

Patient Population	Recommended Initial Oral Dosage (two divided doses every 12 hours)	Observed Whole Blood Trough Concentrations
Adult Kidney transplant In combination with azathioprine	0.2 mg/kg/day	month 1 to 3: 7 to 20 ng/mL month 4 to 12: 5 to 15 ng/mL
In combination with MMF/IL-2 receptor antagonist	0.1 mg/kg/day	month 1 to 12: 4 to 11 ng/mL
Adult Liver transplant Pediatric Liver transplant	0.10 to 0.15 mg/kg/day 0.15 to 0.20 mg/kg/day	month 1 to 12: 5 to 20 ng/mL month 1 to 12: 5 to 20 ng/mL
Adult Heart transplant	0.075 mg/kg/day	month 1 to 3: 10 to 20 ng/mL month ≥4: 5 to 15 ng/mL

- Careful and frequent monitoring of tacrolimus trough concentrations is recommended; Black patients may require higher doses in order to achieve comparable trough concentrations (2.1)
- Hepatic/Renal impaired patients should receive doses at the lowest value of the recommended initial oral dosing range (2.3, 2.4)
- Administer capsules consistently with or without food; do not drink grapefruit juice (2.5, 7.2)

DOSAGE FORMS AND STRENGTHS

- Capsules: 0.5 mg, 1 mg and 5 mg (3)

CONTRAINDICATIONS

- Hypersensitivity to tacrolimus (4)

WARNINGS AND PRECAUTIONS

- Lymphoma and Other Malignancies: Risk of lymphomas, including post transplant lymphoproliferative disorder (PTLD); appears related to intensity and duration of use. Avoid prolonged exposure to UV light and sunlight (5.2)
- Serious infections: Increased risk of bacterial, viral, fungal and protozoal infections, including opportunistic infections: combination immunosuppression should be used with caution (5.3)
- Polyoma Virus Infections: Serious, sometimes fatal outcomes, including polyoma virus-associated nephropathy (PVAN), mostly due to BK virus, and JC virus-associated progressive multifocal leukoencephalopathy (PML); consider reducing immunosuppression (5.4)
- Cytomegalovirus (CMV) Infections: Increased risk of CMV viremia and disease; consider reducing immunosuppression (5.5)
- New Onset Diabetes After Transplant: Monitor blood glucose (5.6)
- Nephrotoxicity: Acute and/or chronic; reduce the dose; use caution with other nephrotoxic drugs (5.7)
- Neurotoxicity: Risk of Posterior Reversible Encephalopathy Syndrome, monitor for neurologic abnormalities; reduce or discontinue tacrolimus and other immunosuppressants (5.8)
- Hyperkalemia: Monitor serum potassium levels. Careful consideration should be given prior to use of other agents also associated with hyperkalemia (5.9)
- Hypertension: May require antihypertensive therapy. Monitor relevant drug-drug interactions (5.10)
- Anaphylactic Reactions with IV formulation: Observe patients receiving tacrolimus injection for signs and symptoms of anaphylaxis (5.11)
- Use with Sirolimus: Not recommended in liver and heart transplant due to increased risk of serious adverse reactions (5.12)
- Myocardial Hypertrophy: Consider dosage reduction or discontinuation (5.14)
- Immunizations: Use of live vaccines should be avoided (5.15)
- Pure Red Cell Aplasia: Discontinuation should be considered (5.16)

ADVERSE REACTIONS

- Kidney Transplant: The most common adverse reactions (≥ 30%) were infection, tremor, hypertension, abnormal renal function, constipation, diarrhea, headache, abdominal pain, insomnia, nausea, hypomagnesemia, urinary tract infection, hypophosphatemia, peripheral edema, asthenia, pain, hyperlipidemia, hyperkalemia, and anemia (6.1)
- Liver Transplant: The most common adverse reactions (≥ 40%) were tremor, headache, diarrhea, hypertension, nausea, abnormal renal function, abdominal pain, insomnia, paresthesia, anemia, pain, fever, asthenia, hyperkalemia, hypomagnesemia, and hyperglycemia (6.1)
- Heart Transplant: The most common adverse reactions (≥15%) were abnormal renal function, hypertension, diabetes mellitus, CMV infection, tremor, hyperglycemia, leukopenia, infection, anemia, bronchitis, pericardial effusion, urinary tract infection and hyperlipemia (6.1)

To report SUSPECTED ADVERSE REACTIONS, contact Novartis Pharmaceuticals Corporation at 1-888-669-6682 or FDA at 1-800-FDA-1088 or www.fda.gov/medwatch

DRUG INTERACTIONS

- Mycophenolic Acid Products: Can increase MPA exposure after crossover from cyclosporine to tacrolimus; monitor for MPA-related adverse reactions and adjust MMF or MPA-dose as needed (7.1)
- Nelfinavir and Grapefruit Juice: Increased tacrolimus concentrations via CYP3A inhibition; avoid concomitant use (7.2, 7.3)
- CYP3A Inhibitors: Increased tacrolimus concentrations; monitor concentrations and adjust tacrolimus dose as needed with concomitant use (5.13, 7.3, 7.4, 7.5, 7.6)
- CYP3A4 Inducers: Decreased tacrolimus concentrations; monitor concentrations and adjust tacrolimus dose as needed with concomitant use (5.13, 7.7, 7.8, 7.9)

USE IN SPECIFIC POPULATIONS

- Pregnancy: Based on animal data may cause fetal harm. Use only if the potential benefit justifies the risk (8.1)
- Nursing Mothers: Discontinue nursing taking into consideration importance of drug to mother (8.3)
- Hepatic/Renal impaired patients: Administer at the lower end of the recommended starting dose. Monitor renal function in patients with impaired renal function (2.3, 2.4, 8.6, 8.7)

See 17 for PATIENT COUNSELING INFORMATION and FDA-approved patient labeling

Revised: 03/2013

FULL PRESCRIBING INFORMATION: CONTENTS*

*** Sections or subsections omitted from the full prescribing information are not listed**

FULL PRESCRIBING INFORMATION

BOXED WARNING - MALIGNANCIES AND SERIOUS INFECTIONS

- **Increased risk of development of lymphoma and other malignancies, particularly of the skin, due to immunosuppression [see WARNINGS AND PRECAUTIONS (5.2)].**
- **Increased susceptibility to bacterial, viral, fungal, and protozoal infections, including opportunistic infections [see WARNINGS AND PRECAUTIONS (5.3, 5.4, 5.5)].**
- **Only physicians experienced in immunosuppressive therapy and management of organ transplant patients should prescribe Hecoria (tacrolimus) capsules. Patients receiving the drug should be managed in facilities equipped and staffed with adequate laboratory and supportive medical resources. The physician responsible for maintenance therapy should have complete information requisite for the follow-up of the patient [see WARNINGS AND PRECAUTIONS (5.1)]**

1 INDICATIONS AND USAGE

1.1 Prophylaxis of Organ Rejection in Kidney Transplant

Hecoria (tacrolimus capsules, USP) is indicated for the prophylaxis of organ rejection in patients receiving allogeneic kidney transplants. It is recommended that Hecoria be used concomitantly with azathioprine or mycophenolate mofetil (MMF) and adrenal corticosteroids [see **CLINICAL STUDIES (14.1)**]. Therapeutic drug monitoring is recommended for all patients receiving Hecoria [see **DOSAGE AND ADMINISTRATION (2.6)**].

1.2 Prophylaxis of Organ Rejection in Liver Transplant

Hecoria (tacrolimus capsules, USP) is indicated for the prophylaxis of organ rejection in patients receiving allogeneic liver transplants. It is recommended that Hecoria be used concomitantly with adrenal corticosteroids [see **CLINICAL STUDIES (14.2)**]. Therapeutic drug monitoring is recommended for all patients receiving Hecoria [see **DOSAGE AND ADMINISTRATION (2.6)**].

1.3 Prophylaxis of Organ Rejection in Heart Transplant

Hecoria (tacrolimus capsules, USP) is indicated for the prophylaxis of organ rejection in patients receiving allogeneic heart transplants. It is recommended that Hecoria be used concomitantly with azathioprine or mycophenolate mofetil (MMF) and adrenal corticosteroids [see **CLINICAL STUDIES (14.3)**]. Therapeutic drug monitoring is recommended for all patients receiving Hecoria [see **DOSAGE AND ADMINISTRATION (2.6)**].

1.4 Limitations of Use

Hecoria (tacrolimus capsules, USP) should not be used simultaneously with cyclosporine [see **DOSAGE AND ADMINISTRATION (2.5)**].

Tacrolimus injection should be reserved for patients unable to take Hecoria orally [see **DOSAGE AND ADMINISTRATION (2.1)** and **WARNINGS AND PRECAUTIONS (5.11)**].

Use with sirolimus is not recommended in liver and heart transplant. The safety and efficacy of Hecoria with sirolimus has not been established in kidney transplant [see **WARNINGS AND PRECAUTIONS (5.12)**].

2 DOSAGE AND ADMINISTRATION

2.1 Dosage in Adult Kidney, Liver, or Heart Transplant Patients

The initial oral dosage recommendations for adult patients with kidney, liver, or heart transplants along with recommendations for whole blood trough concentrations are shown in **Table 1**. The initial dose of Hecoria (tacrolimus capsules, USP) should be administered no sooner than 6 hours after transplantation in the liver and heart transplant patients. In kidney transplant patients, the initial dose of Hecoria may be administered within 24 hours of transplantation, but should be delayed until renal function has recovered. For blood concentration monitoring details see **DOSAGE AND ADMINISTRATION (2.6)**.

Table 1. Summary of Initial Oral Dosage Recommendations and Observed Whole Blood Trough Concentrations in Adults

Patient Population	Recommended Hecoria Initial Oral Dosage Note: daily doses should be administered as two divided doses, every 12 hours	Observed Tacrolimus Whole Blood Trough Concentrations
Adult kidney transplant patients In combination with azathioprine	0.2 mg/kg/day	month 1 to 3: 7 to 20 ng/mL month 4 to 12: 5 to 15 ng/mL
In combination with MMF/IL-2 receptor antagonist[a]	0.1 mg/kg/day	month 1 to 12: 4 to 11 ng/mL
Adult liver transplant patients	0.10 to 0.15 mg/kg/day	month 1 to 12: 5 to 20 ng/mL
Adult heart transplant patients	0.075 mg/kg/day	month 1 to 3: 10 to 20 ng/mL month ≥4: 5 to 15 ng/mL

[a]In a second smaller trial, the initial dose of tacrolimus was 0.15 to 0.2 mg/kg/day and observed tacrolimus concentrations were 6 to 16 ng/mL during months 1 to 3 and 5 to 12 ng/mL during months 4 to 12 [see **CLINICAL STUDIES (14.1)**].

Dosing should be titrated based on clinical assessments of rejection and tolerability. Lower Hecoria dosages than the recommended initial dosage may be sufficient as maintenance therapy. Adjunct therapy with adrenal corticosteroids is recommended early post-transplant.

The data in kidney transplant patients indicate that the Black patients required a higher dose to attain comparable trough concentrations compared to Caucasian patients (**Table 2**).

[See table 2 above]

Table 2. Comparative Dose and Trough Concentrations Based on Race

Time After Transplant	Caucasian n=114		Black n=56	
	Dose (mg/kg)	Trough Concentrations (ng/mL)	Dose (mg/kg)	Trough Concentrations (ng/mL)
Day 7	0.18	12	0.23	10.9
Month 1	0.17	12.8	0.26	12.9
Month 6	0.14	11.8	0.24	11.5
Month 12	0.13	10.1	0.19	11

Initial Dose – Injection

Tacrolimus injection should be used only as a continuous IV infusion and when the patient cannot tolerate oral administration of Hecoria (tacrolimus capsules, USP). Tacrolimus injection should be discontinued as soon as the patient can tolerate oral administration of Hecoria, usually within 2 to 3 days. In a patient receiving an IV infusion, the first dose of oral therapy should be given 8 to 12 hours after discontinuing the IV infusion.

The observed trough concentrations described above pertain to oral administration of Hecoria only; while monitoring Hecoria concentrations in patients receiving tacrolimus injection as a continuous IV infusion may have some utility, the observed concentrations will not represent comparable exposures to those estimated by the trough concentrations observed in patients on oral therapy.

The recommended starting dose of tacrolimus injection is 0.03 to 0.05 mg/kg/day in kidney and liver transplant and 0.01 mg/kg/day in heart transplant given as a continuous IV infusion. Adult patients should receive doses at the lower end of the dosing range. Concomitant adrenal corticosteroid therapy is recommended early post-transplantation.

Anaphylactic reactions have occurred with injectables containing castor oil derivatives, such as tacrolimus injection [see **WARNINGS AND PRECAUTIONS (5.11)**].

2.2 Dosage in Pediatric Liver Transplant Patients

The initial oral dosage recommendations for pediatric patients with liver transplants along with recommendations for whole blood trough concentrations are shown in **Table 3**. For blood concentration monitoring details see **DOSAGE AND ADMINISTRATION (2.6)**. If necessary, pediatric patients may start on an IV dose of 0.03 to 0.05 mg/kg/day.

Table 3. Summary of Initial Oral Dosage Recommendations and Observed Whole Blood Trough Concentrations in Children

Patient Population	Recommended Hecoria Initial Oral Dosage Note: daily doses should be administered as two divided doses, every 12 hours	Observed Tacrolimus Whole Blood Trough Concentrations
Pediatric liver transplant patients	0.15 to 0.20 mg/kg/day	Month 1 to 12: 5 to 20 ng/mL

Pediatric liver transplantation patients without pre-existing renal or hepatic dysfunction have required and tolerated higher doses than adults to achieve similar blood concentrations.

Experience in pediatric kidney and heart transplantation patients is limited.

2.3 Dosage Adjustment in Patients with Renal Impairment

Due to its potential for nephrotoxicity, consideration should be given to dosing Hecoria (tacrolimus capsules, USP) at the lower end of the therapeutic dosing range in patients who have received a liver or heart transplant and have pre-existing renal impairment. Further reductions in dose below the targeted range may be required.

In kidney transplant patients with post-operative oliguria, the initial dose of Hecoria should be administered no sooner than 6 hours and within 24 hours of transplantation, but may be delayed until renal function shows evidence of recovery.

2.4 Dosage Adjustments in Patients with Hepatic Impairment

Due to the reduced clearance and prolonged half-life, patients with severe hepatic impairment (Child Pugh ≥ 10) may require lower doses of Hecoria (tacrolimus capsules, USP). Close monitoring of blood concentrations is warranted.

The use of Hecoria in liver transplant recipients experiencing post-transplant hepatic impairment may be associated with increased risk of developing renal insufficiency related to high whole-blood concentrations of tacrolimus. These patients should be monitored closely and dosage adjustments should be considered. Some evidence suggests that lower doses should be used in these patients [see **DOSAGE AND ADMINISTRATION (2.1), USE IN SPECIFIC POPULATIONS (8.7)** and **CLINICAL PHARMACOLOGY (12.3)**].

2.5 Administration Instructions

It is recommended that patients initiate oral therapy with Hecoria (tacrolimus capsules, USP) if possible.

Initial dosage and observed tacrolimus whole blood trough concentrations for adults are shown in **Table 1** and for pediatrics in **Table 3** [see **DOSAGE AND ADMINISTRATION (2.1, 2.2)**]; for blood concentration monitoring details in kidney transplant patients [see **DOSAGE AND ADMINISTRATION (2.1)**].

It is important to take Hecoria consistently every day either with or without food because the presence and composition of food decreases the bioavailability of Hecoria [see **CLINICAL PHARMACOLOGY (12.3)**].

Patients should not eat grapefruit or drink grapefruit juice in combination with Hecoria [see **DRUG INTERACTIONS (7.2)**].

Hecoria should not be used simultaneously with cyclosporine. Hecoria or cyclosporine should be discontinued at least 24 hours before initiating the other. In the presence of elevated Hecoria or cyclosporine concentrations, dosing with the other drug usually should be further delayed.

In patients unable to take oral Hecoria (tacrolimus capsules, USP), therapy may be initiated with tacrolimus injection as a continuous IV infusion. If IV therapy is necessary, conversion from IV to oral tacrolimus is recommended as soon as oral therapy can be tolerated. This usually occurs within 2 to 3 days. In patients receiving an IV infusion, the first dose of oral therapy should be given 8 to 12 hours after discontinuing the IV infusion.

2.6 Therapeutic Drug Monitoring

Monitoring of tacrolimus blood concentrations in conjunction with other laboratory and clinical parameters is considered an essential aid to patient management for the evaluation of rejection, toxicity, dose adjustments and compliance. Observed whole blood trough concentrations can be found in **Table 1**. Factors influencing frequency of monitoring include but are not limited to hepatic or renal dysfunction, the addition or discontinuation of potentially interacting drugs and the post-transplant time. Blood concentration monitoring is not a replacement for renal and liver function monitoring and tissue biopsies. Data from clinical trials show that tacrolimus whole blood concentrations were most variable during the first week post-transplantation.

The relative risks of toxicity and efficacy failure are related to tacrolimus whole blood trough concentrations. Therefore, monitoring of whole blood trough concentrations is recommended to assist in the clinical evaluation of toxicity and efficacy failure.

Methods commonly used for the assay of tacrolimus include high performance liquid chromatography with tandem mass spectrometric detection (HPLC/MS/MS) and immunoassays. Immunoassays may react with metabolites as well as parent compound. Therefore assay results obtained with immunoassays may have a positive bias relative to results of HPLC/MS. The bias may depend upon the specific assay and laboratory. Comparison of the concentrations in published literature to patient concentrations using the current assays must be made with detailed knowledge of the assay methods and biological matrices employed. Whole blood is the matrix of choice and specimens should be collected into tubes containing ethylene diamine tetraacetic acid (EDTA) anti-coagulant. Heparin anti-coagulation is not recommended because of the tendency to form clots on storage. Samples which are not analyzed immediately should be stored at room temperature or in a refrigerator and assayed within 7 days; see assay instructions for specifics. If samples are to be kept longer they should be deep frozen at -20° C. One study showed drug recovery >90% for samples stored at -20° C for 6 months, with reduced recovery observed after 6 months.

3 DOSAGE FORMS AND STRENGTHS

Hecoria (tacrolimus capsules, USP) is available in 0.5 mg, 1 mg, and 5 mg strengths.

Hecoria (tacrolimus capsules, USP) containing white to off white powder equivalent to 0.5 mg of anhydrous tacrolimus, are hard gelatin capsules with white opaque body and ivory cap. The body is imprinted "0.5 mg" and cap is imprinted "HECORIA" in black ink.

Hecoria (tacrolimus capsules, USP) containing white to off white powder equivalent to 1 mg of anhydrous tacrolimus, are hard gelatin capsules with white opaque body and brown cap. The body is imprinted "1 mg" and cap is imprinted "HECORIA" in black ink.

Hecoria (tacrolimus capsules, USP) containing white to off white powder equivalent to 5 mg of anhydrous tacrolimus, are hard gelatin capsules with white opaque body and orange cap. The body is imprinted "5 mg" and cap is imprinted "HECORIA" in black ink.

4 CONTRAINDICATIONS

Hecoria (tacrolimus) capsules are contraindicated in patients with a hypersensitivity to tacrolimus. Hypersensitivity symptoms reported include dyspnea, rash, pruritus, and acute respiratory distress syndrome [see **ADVERSE REACTIONS (6)**].

5 WARNINGS AND PRECAUTIONS

5.1 Management of Immunosuppression

Only physicians experienced in immunosuppressive therapy and management of organ transplant patients should use Hecoria (tacrolimus) capsules. Patients receiving the drug should be managed in facilities equipped and staffed with adequate laboratory and supportive medical resources. The physicians responsible for maintenance therapy should have complete information requisite for the follow up of the patient [see **BOXED WARNING**].

5.2 Lymphoma and Other Malignancies

Patients receiving immunosuppressants, including Hecoria (tacrolimus) capsules, are at increased risk of developing lymphomas and other malignancies, particularly of the skin [see **BOXED WARNING**]. The risk appears to be related to the intensity and duration of immunosuppression rather than to the use of any specific agent.

As usual for patients with increased risk for skin cancer, exposure to sunlight and UV light should be limited by wearing protective clothing and using a sunscreen with a high protection factor.

Post transplant lymphoproliferative disorder (PTLD) has been reported in immunosuppressed organ transplant recipients. The majority of PTLD events appear related to Epstein Barr Virus (EBV) infection. The risk of PTLD appears greatest in those individuals who are EBV seronegative, a population which includes many young children.

5.3 Serious Infections

Patients receiving immunosuppressants, including Hecoria (tacrolimus) capsules, are at increased risk of developing bacterial, viral, fungal, and protozoal infections, including opportunistic infections [see **BOXED WARNING** and **WARNINGS AND PRECAUTIONS (5.4, 5.5)**]. These infections may lead to serious, including fatal, outcomes. Because of the danger of oversuppression of the immune system which can increase susceptibility to infection, combination immunosuppressant therapy should be used with caution.

5.4 Polyoma Virus Infections

Patients receiving immunosuppressants, including Hecoria (tacrolimus) capsules, are at increased risk for opportunistic infections, including polyoma virus infections. Polyoma virus infections in transplant patients may have serious, and sometimes fatal, outcomes. These include polyoma virus-associated nephropathy (PVAN), mostly due to BK virus infection, and JC virus-associated progressive multifocal leukoencephalopathy (PML) which have been observed in patients receiving tacrolimus [see **ADVERSE REACTIONS (6.2)**].

PVAN is associated with serious outcomes, including deteriorating renal function and kidney graft loss [see **ADVERSE REACTIONS (6.2)**]. Patient monitoring may help detect patients at risk for PVAN.

Cases of PML have been reported in patients treated with Hecoria. PML, which is sometimes fatal, commonly presents with hemiparesis, apathy, confusion, cognitive deficiencies and ataxia. Risk factors for PML include treatment with immunosuppressant therapies and impairment of immune function. In immunosuppressed patients, physicians should consider PML in the differential diagnosis in patients reporting neurological symptoms and consultation with a neurologist should be considered as clinically indicated.

Reductions in immunosuppression should be considered for patients who develop evidence of PVAN or PML. Physicians should also consider the risk that reduced immunosuppression represents to the functioning allograft.

5.5 Cytomegalovirus (CMV) Infections

Patients receiving immunosuppressants, including Hecoria (tacrolimus) capsules, are at increased risk of developing CMV viremia and CMV disease. The risk of CMV disease is highest among transplant recipients seronegative for CMV at time of transplant who receive a graft from a CMV seropositive donor. Therapeutic approaches to limiting CMV disease exist and should be routinely provided. Patient monitoring may help detect patients at risk for CMV disease. Consideration should be given to reducing the amount of immunosuppression in patients who develop CMV viremia and/or CMV disease.

5.6 New Onset Diabetes After Transplant

Tacrolimus was shown to cause new onset diabetes mellitus in clinical trials of kidney, liver, and heart transplantation. New onset diabetes after transplantation may be reversible in some patients. Black and Hispanic kidney transplant patients are at an increased risk. Blood glucose concentrations should be monitored closely in patients using Hecoria (tacrolimus) capsules [see **ADVERSE REACTIONS (6.1)**].

5.7 Nephrotoxicity

Hecoria (tacrolimus) capsules, like other calcineurin-inhibitors, can cause acute or chronic nephrotoxicity, particularly when used in high doses. Acute nephrotoxicity is most often related to vasoconstriction of the afferent renal arteriole, is characterized by increasing serum creatinine, hyperkalemia, and/or a decrease in urine output, and is typically reversible. Chronic calcineurin-inhibitor nephrotoxicity is associated with increased serum creatinine, decreased kidney graft life, and characteristic histologic changes observed on renal biopsy; the changes associated with chronic calcineurin-inhibitor nephrotoxicity are typically progressive. Patients with impaired renal function should be monitored closely as the dosage of tacrolimus may need to be reduced. In patients with persistent elevations of serum creatinine who are unresponsive to dosage adjustments, consideration should be given to changing to another immunosuppressive therapy.

Based on reported adverse reactions terms related to decreased renal function, nephrotoxicity was reported in approximately 52% of kidney transplantation patients and in 40% and 36% of liver transplantation patients receiving tacrolimus in the U.S. and European randomized trials, respectively, and in 59% of heart transplantation patients in a European randomized trial [see **ADVERSE REACTIONS (6.1)**].

Due to the potential for additive or synergistic impairment of renal function, care should be taken when administering Hecoria with drugs that may be associated with renal dysfunction. These include, but are not limited to, aminoglycosides, ganciclovir, amphotericin B, cisplatin, nucleotide reverse transcriptase inhibitors (e.g., tenofovir) and protease inhibitors (e.g., ritonavir, indinavir). Similarly, care should be exercised when administering with CYP3A4 inhibitors such as antifungal drugs (e.g., ketoconazole), calcium channel blockers (e.g., diltiazem, verapamil), and macrolide antibiotics (e.g., clarithromycin, erythromycin, troleandomycin) which will result in increased tacrolimus whole blood concentrations due to inhibition of tacrolimus metabolism [see **DRUG INTERACTIONS (7.3, 7.4, 7.5, 7.6)**].

5.8 Neurotoxicity

Hecoria (tacrolimus) capsules may cause a spectrum of neurotoxicities, particularly when used in high doses. The most severe neurotoxicities include posterior reversible encephalopathy syndrome (PRES), delirium, and coma. Patients treated with tacrolimus have been reported to develop PRES. Symptoms indicating PRES include headache, altered mental status, seizures, visual disturbances and hypertension. Diagnosis may be confirmed by radiological procedure. If PRES is suspected or diagnosed, blood pressure control should be maintained and immediate reduction of immunosuppression is advised. This syndrome is characterized by reversal of symptoms upon reduction or discontinuation of immunosuppression.

Coma and delirium, in the absence of PRES, have also been associated with high plasma concentrations of tacrolimus. Seizures have occurred in adult and pediatric patients receiving Hecoria [see **ADVERSE REACTIONS (6.1)**].

Less severe neurotoxicities, include tremors, parathesias, headache, and other changes in motor function, mental status, and sensory function [see **ADVERSE REACTIONS (6.1)**] . Tremor and headache have been associated with high whole-blood concentrations of tacrolimus and may respond to dosage adjustment.

5.9 Hyperkalemia

Hyperkalemia has been reported with Hecoria (tacrolimus) capsule use. Serum potassium levels should be monitored. Careful consideration should be given prior to use of other agents also associated with hyperkalemia (e.g., potassium-sparing diuretics, ACE inhibitors, angiotensin receptor blockers) during Hecoria therapy [see **ADVERSE REACTIONS (6.1)**].

5.10 Hypertension

Hypertension is a common adverse effect of Hecoria (tacrolimus) capsules therapy and may require antihypertensive therapy [see **ADVERSE REACTIONS (6.1)**]. The control of blood pressure can be accomplished with any of the common antihypertensive agents, though careful consideration should be given prior to use of antihypertensive agents associated with hyperkalemia (e.g., potassium-sparing diuretics, ACE inhibitors, angiotensin receptor blockers) [see **WARNINGS AND PRECAUTIONS (5.9)**]. Calcium-channel blocking agents may increase tacrolimus blood concentrations and therefore require dosage reduction of Hecoria [see **DRUG INTERACTIONS (7.5)**].

5.11 Anaphylactic Reactions with Tacrolimus Injection

Anaphylactic reactions have occurred with injectables containing castor oil derivatives, including tacrolimus, in a small percentage of patients (0.6%). The exact cause of these reactions is not known. Tacrolimus injection should be reserved for patients who are unable to take tacrolimus capsules [see **INDICATIONS AND USAGE (1.4)**].

Patients receiving tacrolimus injection should be under continuous observation for at least the first 30 minutes following the start of the infusion and at frequent intervals thereafter. If signs or symptoms of anaphylaxis occur, the infusion should be stopped. An aqueous solution of epinephrine should be available at the bedside as well as a source of oxygen.

5.12 Use with Sirolimus

The safety and efficacy of Hecoria (tacrolimus) capsules with sirolimus has not been established in kidney transplant patients.

Use of sirolimus with tacrolimus in studies of de novo liver transplant patients was associated with an excess mortality, graft loss, and hepatic artery thrombosis (HAT) and is not recommended [see **INDICATIONS AND USAGE (1.4)**].

Use of sirolimus (2 mg per day) with tacrolimus in heart transplant patients in a U.S. trial was associated with increased risk of renal function impairment, wound healing complications, and insulin-dependent post–transplant diabetes mellitus, and is not recommended [see **CLINICAL STUDIES (14.3)**].

5.13 Use with CYP3A4 Inhibitors and Inducers Including Those That Prolong QT

Coadministration with strong CYP3A4-inhibitors (e.g., telaprevir, boceprevir, ritonavir, ketoconazole, itraconazole, voriconazole, clarithromycin) and strong inducers (e.g., rifampin, rifabutin) is not recommended without adjustments in the dosing regimen of tacrolimus and subsequent close monitoring of tacrolimus whole blood trough concentrations and tacrolimus-associated adverse reactions [see **DRUG INTERACTIONS (7)**].

When coadministering tacrolimus with other substrates and/or inhibitors of CYP3A4 that also have the potential to prolong the QT interval, a reduction in tacrolimus dose, close monitoring of tacrolimus whole blood concentrations, and monitoring for QT prolongation is recommended. Use of tacrolimus with amiodarone has been reported to result in increased tacrolimus whole blood concentrations with or without concurrent QT prolongation.

5.14 Myocardial Hypertrophy

Myocardial hypertrophy has been reported in infants, children, and adults, particularly those with high tacrolimus trough concentrations, and is generally manifested by echocardiographically demonstrated concentric increases in left ventricular posterior wall and interventricular septum thickness. This condition appears reversible in most cases following dose reduction or discontinuance of therapy. In patients who develop renal failure or clinical manifestations of ventricular dysfunction while receiving tacrolimus therapy, echocardiographic evaluation should be considered. If myocardial hypertrophy is diagnosed, dosage reduction or discontinuation of Hecoria (tacrolimus) capsules should be considered [see **ADVERSE REACTIONS (6.2)**].

5.15 Immunizations

The use of live vaccines should be avoided during treatment with tacrolimus; examples include (not limited to) the following: intranasal influenza, measles, mumps, rubella, oral polio, BCG, yellow fever, varicella, and TY21a typhoid vaccines.

5.16 Pure Red Cell Aplasia

Cases of pure red cell aplasia (PRCA) have been reported in patients treated with tacrolimus. A mechanism for tacrolimus-induced PRCA has not been elucidated. All patients reported risk factors for PRCA such as parvovirus B19 infection, underlying disease, or concomitant medications associated with PRCA. If PRCA is diagnosed, discontinuation of Hecoria (tacrolimus) capsules should be considered [see **ADVERSE REACTIONS (6.2)**].

6 ADVERSE REACTIONS

The following serious and otherwise important adverse drug reactions are discussed in greater detail in other sections of labeling:

- Lymphoma and Other Malignancies [see **BOXED WARNING, WARNINGS AND PRECAUTIONS (5.2)**]
- Serious Infections [see **BOXED WARNING, WARNINGS AND PRECAUTIONS (5.3)**]
- Polyoma Virus Infections [see **BOXED WARNING, WARNINGS AND PRECAUTIONS (5.4)**]
- CMV Infections [see **BOXED WARNING, WARNINGS AND PRECAUTIONS (5.5)**]
- New Onset Diabetes After Transplant [see **WARNINGS AND PRECAUTIONS (5.6)**]
- Nephrotoxicity [see **WARNINGS AND PRECAUTIONS (5.7)**]
- Neurotoxicity [see **WARNINGS AND PRECAUTIONS (5.8)**]
- Hyperkalemia [see **WARNINGS AND PRECAUTIONS (5.9)**]
- Hypertension [see **WARNINGS AND PRECAUTIONS (5.10)**]
- Anaphylaxis with Tacrolimus Injection [see **WARNINGS AND PRECAUTIONS (5.11)**]
- Myocardial Hypertrophy [see **WARNINGS AND PRECAUTIONS (5.14)**]
- Pure Red Cell Aplasia [see **WARNINGS AND PRECAUTIONS (5.16)**]

6.1 Clinical Studies Experience

Because clinical trials are conducted under widely varying conditions, adverse reaction rates observed in the clinical trials of a drug cannot be directly compared to rates in the clinical trials of another drug and may not reflect the rates observed in practice. In addition, the clinical trials were not designed to establish comparative differences across study arms with regards to the adverse reactions discussed below.

Table 5. Kidney Transplantation: Adverse Reactions Occurring in ≥ 10% of Patients Treated with Tacrolimus in Conjunction with MMF (Study 1)

	Tacrolimus (Group C)	Cyclosporine (Group A)	Cyclosporine (Group B)
	(N=403)	(N=384)	(N=408)
Diarrhea	25%	16%	13%
Urinary Tract Infection	24%	28%	24%
Anemia	17%	19%	17%
Hypertension	13%	14%	12%
Leukopenia	13%	10%	10%
Edema Peripheral	11%	12%	13%
Hyperlipidemia	10%	15%	13%

Key: Group A = CsA/MMF/CS, B = CsA/MMF/CS/Daclizumab, C = Tac/MMF/CS/Daclizumab
CsA = Cyclosporine, CS = Corticosteroids, Tac = Tacrolimus, MMF = mycophenolate mofetil

Kidney Transplant

The incidence of adverse reactions was determined in three randomized kidney transplant trials. One of the trials used azathioprine (AZA) and corticosteroids and two of the trials used mycophenolate mofetil (MMF) and corticosteroids concomitantly for maintenance immunosuppression.

Tacrolimus-based immunosuppression in conjunction with azathioprine and corticosteroids following kidney transplantation was assessed in trial where 205 patients received tacrolimus based immunosuppression and 207 patients received cyclosporine based immunosuppression. The trial population had a mean age of 43 years (mean±sd was 43±13 years on tacrolimus and 44±12 years on cyclosporine arm), the distribution was 61% male, and the composition was White (58%), Black (25%), Hispanic (12%) and Other (5%). The 12 month post-transplant information from this trial is presented below.

The most common adverse reactions (≥ 30%) observed in tacrolimus-treated kidney transplant patients are: infection, tremor, hypertension, abnormal renal function, constipation, diarrhea, headache, abdominal pain, insomnia, nausea, hypomagnesemia, urinary tract infection, hypophosphatemia, peripheral edema, asthenia, pain, hyperlipidemia, hyperkalemia and anemia.

Adverse reactions that occurred in ≥ 15% of kidney transplant patients treated with tacrolimus in conjunction with azathioprine are presented below:

Table 4. Kidney Transplantation: Adverse Reactions Occurring in ≥ 15% of Patients Treated with Tacrolimus in Conjunction with Azathioprine (AZA)

	Tacrolimus/ AZA (N=205)	Cyclosporine/ AZA (N=207)
Nervous System		
Tremor	54%	34%
Headache	44%	38%
Insomnia	32%	30%
Paresthesia	23%	16%
Dizziness	19%	16%
Gastrointestinal		
Diarrhea	44%	41%
Nausea	38%	36%
Constipation	35%	43%
Vomiting	29%	23%
Dyspepsia	28%	20%
Cardiovascular		
Hypertension	50%	52%
Chest Pain	19%	13%
Urogenital		
Creatinine Increased	45%	42%
Urinary Tract Infection	34%	35%
Metabolic and Nutritional		
Hypophosphatemia	49%	53%
Hypomagnesemia	34%	17%
Hyperlipemia	31%	38%
Hyperkalemia	31%	32%
Diabetes Mellitus	24%	9%
Hypokalemia	22%	25%
Hyperglycemia	22%	16%
Edema	18%	19%
Hemic and Lymphatic		
Anemia	30%	24%
Leukopenia	15%	17%
Miscellaneous		
Infection	45%	49%
Peripheral Edema	36%	48%
Asthenia	34%	30%
Abdominal Pain	33%	31%
Pain	32%	30%
Fever	29%	29%
Back Pain	24%	20%
Respiratory System		
Dyspnea	22%	18%
Cough Increased	18%	15%
Musculoskeletal		
Arthralgia	25%	24%
Skin		
Rash	17%	12%
Pruritus	15%	7%

Two trials were conducted for tacrolimus-based immunosuppression in conjunction with MMF and corticosteroids. In the non-US trial (Study 1), the incidence of adverse reactions was based on 1195 kidney transplant patients that received tacrolimus (Group C, n=403), or one of two cyclosporine (CsA) regimens (Group A, n=384 and Group B, n=408) in combination with MMF and corticosteroids; all patients, except those in one of the two cyclosporine groups, also received induction with daclizumab. The trial population had a mean age of 46 years (range 17 to 76), the distribution was 65% male, and the composition was 93% Caucasian. The 12 month post-transplant information from this trial is presented below.

Adverse reactions that occurred in ≥ 10% of kidney transplant patients treated with tacrolimus in conjunction with MMF in Study 1 [Note: This trial was conducted entirely outside of the United States. Such trials often report a lower incidence of adverse reactions in comparison to U.S. trials] are presented below:

[See table 5 above]

In the U.S. trial (Study 2) with tacrolimus-based immunosuppression in conjunction with MMF and corticosteroids, 424 kidney transplant patients received tacrolimus (n=212) or cyclosporine (n=212) in combination with MMF 1 gram twice daily, basiliximab induction, and corticosteroids. The trial population had a mean age of 48 years (range 17 to 77), the distribution was 63% male, and the composition was White (74%), Black (20%), Asian (3%) and other (3%). The 12 month post-transplant information from this trial is presented below.

Adverse reactions that occurred in ≥15% of kidney transplant patients treated with tacrolimus in conjunction with MMF in Study 2 are presented below:

Table 6. Kidney Transplantation: Adverse Reactions Occurring in ≥ 15% of Patients Treated with Tacrolimus in Conjunction with MMF (Study 2)

	Tacrolimus/ MMF (N=212)	Cyclosporine/ MMF (N=212)
Gastrointestinal Disorders		
Diarrhea	44%	26%
Nausea	39%	47%
Constipation	36%	41%
Vomiting	26%	25%
Dyspepsia	18%	15%
Injury, Poisoning, and Procedural Complications		
Post-Procedural Pain	29%	27%
Incision Site Complication	28%	23%
Graft Dysfunction	24%	18%
Metabolism and Nutrition Disorders		
Hypomagnesemia	28%	22%
Hypophosphatemia	28%	21%
Hyperkalemia	26%	19%
Hyperglycemia	21%	15%
Hyperlipidemia	18%	25%
Hypokalemia	16%	18%
Nervous System Disorders		
Tremor	34%	20%
Headache	24%	25%
Blood and Lymphatic System Disorders		
Anemia	30%	28%
Leukopenia	16%	12%
Miscellaneous		
Edema Peripheral	35%	46%
Hypertension	32%	35%
Insomnia	30%	21%
Urinary Tract Infection	26%	22%
Blood Creatinine Increased	23%	23%

Less frequently observed adverse reactions in both liver transplantation and kidney transplantation patients are described under the subsection *Less Frequently Reported Adverse Reactions.*

Liver Transplantation

There were two randomized comparative liver transplant trials. In the U.S. trial, 263 adult and pediatric patients re-

Table 7. Liver Transplantation: Adverse Reactions Occurring in ≥ 15% of Patients Treated with Tacrolimus

	U.S. TRIAL		EUROPEAN TRIAL	
	Tacrolimus (N=250)	Cyclosporine/AZA (N=250)	Tacrolimus (N=264)	Cyclosporine/AZA (N=265)
Nervous System				
Headache	64%	60%	37%	26%
Insomnia	64%	68%	32%	23%
Tremor	56%	46%	48%	32%
Paresthesia	40%	30%	17%	17%
Gastrointestinal				
Diarrhea	72%	47%	37%	27%
Nausea	46%	37%	32%	27%
LFT Abnormal	36%	30%	6%	5%
Anorexia	34%	24%	7%	5%
Vomiting	27%	15%	14%	11%
Constipation	24%	27%	23%	21%
Cardiovascular				
Hypertension	47%	56%	38%	43%
Urogenital				
Kidney Function Abnormal	40%	27%	36%	23%
Creatinine Increased	39%	25%	24%	19%
BUN Increased	30%	22%	12%	9%
Oliguria	18%	15%	19%	12%
Urinary Tract Infection	16%	18%	21%	19%
Metabolic and Nutritional				
Hypomagnesemia	48%	45%	16%	9%
Hyperglycemia	47%	38%	33%	22%
Hyperkalemia	45%	26%	13%	9%
Hypokalemia	29%	34%	13%	16%
Hemic and Lymphatic				
Anemia	47%	38%	5%	1%
Leukocytosis	32%	26%	8%	8%
Thrombocytopenia	24%	20%	14%	19%
Miscellaneous				
Pain	63%	57%	24%	22%
Abdominal Pain	59%	54%	29%	22%
Asthenia	52%	48%	11%	7%
Fever	48%	56%	19%	22%
Back Pain	30%	29%	17%	17%
Ascites	27%	22%	7%	8%
Peripheral Edema	26%	26%	12%	14%
Respiratory System				
Pleural Effusion	30%	32%	36%	35%
Dyspnea	29%	23%	5%	4%
Atelectasis	28%	30%	5%	4%
Skin and Appendages				
Pruritus	36%	20%	15%	7%
Rash	24%	19%	10%	4%

ceived tacrolimus and steroids and 266 patients received cyclosporine-based immunosuppressive regimen (CsA/AZA). The trial population had a mean age of 44 years (range 0.4 to 70), the distribution was 52% male, and the composition was White (78%), Black (5%), Asian (2%), Hispanic (13%) and Other (2%). In the European trial, 270 patients received tacrolimus and steroids and 275 patients received CsA/AZA. The trial population had a mean age of 46 years (range 15 to 68), the distribution was 59% male, and the composition was White (95.4%), Black (1%), Asian (2%) and Other (2%). The proportion of patients reporting more than one adverse event was > 99% in both the tacrolimus group and the CsA/AZA group. Precautions must be taken when comparing the incidence of adverse reactions in the U.S. trial to that in the European trial. The 12-month post-transplant information from the U.S. trial and from the European trial is presented below. The two trials also included different patient populations and patients were treated with immunosuppressive regimens of differing intensities. Adverse reactions reported in ≥15% in tacrolimus patients (combined trial results) are presented below for the two controlled trials in liver transplantation.

The most common adverse reactions (≥ 40%) observed in tacrolimus-treated liver transplant patients are: tremor, headache, diarrhea, hypertension, nausea, abnormal renal function, abdominal pain, insomnia, paresthesia, anemia, pain, fever, asthenia, hyperkalemia, hypomagnesemia, and hyperglycemia. These all occur with oral administration of tacrolimus and some may respond to a reduction in dosing (e.g., tremor, headache, paresthesia, hypertension). Diarrhea was sometimes associated with other gastrointestinal complaints such as nausea and vomiting.

[See table 7 above]

Less frequently observed adverse reactions in both liver transplantation and kidney transplantation patients are described under the subsection *Less Frequently Reported Adverse Reactions*.

Heart Transplantation

The incidence of adverse reactions was determined based on two trials in primary orthotopic heart transplantation. In a trial conducted in Europe, 314 patients received a regimen of antibody induction, corticosteroids and azathioprine (AZA) in combination with tacrolimus (n=157) or cyclosporine (n=157) for 18 months. The trial population had a mean age of 51 years (range 18 to 65), the distribution was 82% male, and the composition was White (96%), Black (3%) and other (1%).

The most common adverse reactions (≥15%) observed in tacrolimus-treated heart transplant patients are: abnormal renal function, hypertension, diabetes mellitus, CMV infection, tremor, hyperglycemia, leukopenia, infection, anemia, bronchitis, pericardial effusion, urinary tract infection and hyperlipemia.

Adverse reactions in heart transplant patients in the European trial are presented below:

Table 8. Heart Transplantation: Adverse Reactions Occurring in ≥15% of Patients Treated with Tacrolimus in Conjunction with Azathioprine (AZA)

	Tacrolimus/ AZA	Cyclosporine/ AZA
	(n=157)	(n=157)
Cardiovascular System		
Hypertension	62%	59%
Pericardial Effusion	15%	14%
Body as a Whole		
CMV Infection	32%	30%
Infection	24%	21%
Metabolism and Nutrition Disorders		
Diabetes Mellitus	26%	16%
Hyperglycemia	23%	17%
Hyperlipemia	18%	27%
Hemic and Lymphatic System		
Anemia	50%	36%
Leukopenia	48%	39%
Urogenital System		
Kidney Function Abnormal	56%	57%
Urinary Tract Infection	16%	12%

Respiratory System		
Bronchitis	17%	18%
Nervous System		
Tremor	15%	6%

In the European trial, the cyclosporine trough concentrations were above the pre-defined target range (i.e., 100 to 200 ng/mL) at Day 122 and beyond in 32 to 68% of the patients in the cyclosporine treatment arm, whereas the tacrolimus trough concentrations were within the pre-defined target range (i.e., 5 to 15 ng/mL) in 74 to 86% of the patients in the tacrolimus treatment arm.

In the U.S. trial, the incidence of adverse reactions was based on 331 heart transplant patients that received corticosteroids and tacrolimus in combination with sirolimus (n=109), tacrolimus in combination with MMF (n=107) or cyclosporine modified in combination with MMF (n=115) for 1 year. The trial population had a mean age of 53 years (range 18 to 75), the distribution was 78% male, and the composition was White (83%), Black (13%) and other (4%). Only selected targeted treatment-emergent adverse reactions were collected in the U.S. heart transplantation trial. Those reactions that were reported at a rate of 15% or greater in patients treated with tacrolimus and MMF include the following: any target adverse reactions (99%), hypertension (89%), hyperglycemia requiring antihyperglycemic therapy (70%), hypertriglyceridemia (65%), anemia (hemoglobin <10 g/dL) (65%), fasting blood glucose >140 mg/dL (on two separate occasions) (61%), hypercholesterolemia (57%), hyperlipidemia (34%), WBCs <3000 cells/mcL (34%), serious bacterial infections (30%), magnesium <1.2 mEq/L (24%), platelet count <75,000 cells/mcL (19%), and other opportunistic infections (15%).

Other targeted treatment-emergent adverse reactions in tacrolimus-treated patients occurred at a rate of less than 15%, and include the following: Cushingoid features, impaired wound healing, hyperkalemia, *Candida* infection, and CMV infection/syndrome.

New Onset Diabetes After Transplant

Kidney Transplant

New Onset Diabetes After Transplant (NODAT) is defined as a composite of fasting plasma glucose ≥126 mg/dL, HbA_{1C} ≥ 6%, insulin use ≥ 30 days or oral hypoglycemic use. In a trial in kidney transplant patients (Study 2), NODAT was observed in 75% in the tacrolimus-treated and 61% in the Neoral-treated patients without pre-transplant history of diabetes mellitus (Table 9) [see **CLINICAL STUDIES (14.1)**].

Table 9. Incidence of New Onset Diabetes After Transplant at 1 Year in Kidney Transplant Recipients in a Phase 3 Trial (Study 2)

Parameter	Treatment Group	
	Tacrolimus/MMF (n = 212)	Neoral/MMF (n = 212)
NODAT	112/150 (75%)	93/152 (61%)
Fasting Plasma Glucose ≥ 126 mg/dL	96/150 (64%)	80/152 (53%)
HbA_{1C} ≥ 6%	59/150 (39%)	28/152 (18%)
Insulin Use ≥ 30 days	9/150 (6%)	4/152 (3%)
Oral Hypoglycemic Use	15/150 (10%)	5/152 (3%)

In early trials of tacrolimus, Post-Transplant Diabetes Mellitus (PTDM) was evaluated with a more limited criteria of "use of insulin for 30 or more consecutive days with < 5 day gap" in patients without a prior history of insulin-dependent diabetes mellitus or non-insulin dependent diabetes mellitus. Data are presented in **Tables 10 to 13**. PTDM was reported in 20% of tacrolimus/Azathioprine (AZA)-treated kidney transplant patients without pre-transplant history of diabetes mellitus in a Phase 3 trial (**Table 10**). The median time to onset of PTDM was 68 days. Insulin dependence was reversible in 15% of these PTDM patients at one year and in 50% at 2 years post-transplant. Black and Hispanic kidney transplant patients were at an increased risk of development of PTDM (**Table 11**).

Table 10. Incidence of Post-Transplant Diabetes Mellitus and Insulin Use at 2 Years in Kidney Transplant Recipients in a Phase 3 Trial using Azathioprine (AZA)

Status of PTDM[a]	Tacrolimus/AZA	CsA/AZA
Patients without pre-transplant history of diabetes mellitus	151	151
New onset PTDM[a], 1st Year	30/151 (20%)	6/151 (4%)
Still insulin-dependent at one year in those without prior history of diabetes	25/151 (17%)	5/151 (3%)
New onset PTDM[a] post 1 year	1	0
Patients with PTDM[a] at 2 years	16/151 (11%)	5/151 (3%)

[a] Use of insulin for 30 or more consecutive days, with < 5 day gap, without a prior history of insulin-dependent diabetes mellitus or non-insulin dependent diabetes mellitus.

Table 11. Development of Post-Transplant Diabetes Mellitus by Race or Ethnicity and by Treatment Group During First Year Post Kidney Transplantation in a Phase 3 Trial

Patient Race	Patients Who Developed PTDM[a]	
	Tacrolimus	Cyclosporine
Black	15/41 (37%)	3 (8%)
Hispanic	5/17 (29%)	1 (6%)
Caucasian	10/82 (12%)	1 (1%)
Other	0/11 (0%)	1 (10%)
Total	30/151 (20%)	6 (4%)

[a] Use of insulin for 30 or more consecutive days, with < 5 day gap, without a prior history of insulin-dependent diabetes mellitus or non-insulin dependent diabetes mellitus.

Liver Transplant

Insulin-dependent PTDM was reported in 18% and 11% of tacrolimus-treated liver transplant patients and was reversible in 45% and 31% of these patients at 1 year post-transplant, in the U.S. and European randomized trials, respectively (**Table 12**). Hyperglycemia was associated with the use of tacrolimus in 47% and 33% of liver transplant recipients in the U.S. and European randomized trials, respectively, and may require treatment [see **ADVERSE REACTIONS (6.1)**].

[See table 12 above]

Table 12. Incidence of Post-Transplant Diabetes Mellitus and Insulin Use at 1 Year in Liver Transplant Recipients

Status of PTDM[a]	US Trial		European Trial	
	Tacrolimus	Cyclosporine	Tacrolimus	Cyclosporine
Patients at risk[b]	239	236	239	249
New Onset PTDM[a]	42 (18%)	30 (13%)	26 (11%)	12 (5%)
Patients still on insulin at 1 year	23 (10%)	19 (8%)	18 (8%)	6 (2%)

[a] Use of insulin for 30 or more consecutive days, with < 5 day gap, without a prior history of insulin-dependent diabetes mellitus or non-insulin dependent diabetes mellitus.
[b] Patients without pre-transplant history of diabetes mellitus.

Heart Transplant

Insulin-dependent PTDM was reported in 13% and 22% of tacrolimus-treated heart transplant patients receiving mycophenolate mofetil (MMF) or azathioprine (AZA) and was reversible in 30% and 17% of these patients at one year post-transplant, in the U.S. and European randomized trials, respectively (Table 13). Hyperglycemia defined as two fasting plasma glucose levels ≥126 mg/dL was reported with the use of tacrolimus plus MMF or AZA in 32% and 35% of heart transplant recipients in the U.S. and European randomized trials, respectively, and may require treatment [see **ADVERSE REACTIONS (6.1)**].

[See table 13 above]

Table 13. Incidence of Post-Transplant Diabetes Mellitus and Insulin Use at 1 Year in Heart Transplant Recipients

Status of PTDM[a]	US Trial		European Trial	
	Tacrolimus/MMF	Cyclosporine/MMF	Tacrolimus/AZA	Cyclosporine/AZA
Patients at risk[b]	75	83	132	138
New Onset PTDM[a]	10 (13%)	6 (7%)	29 (22%)	5 (4%)
Patients still on insulin at 1 year[c]	7 (9%)	1 (1%)	24 (18%)	4 (3%)

[a] Use of insulin for 30 or more consecutive days without a prior history of insulin-dependent diabetes mellitus or non-insulin dependent diabetes mellitus.
[b] Patients without pre-transplant history of diabetes mellitus.
[c] 7 to 12 months for the U.S. trial.

Less Frequently Reported Adverse Reactions (>3% and <15%)

The following adverse reactions were reported in either liver, kidney, and/or heart transplant recipients who were treated with tacrolimus in clinical trials.

Nervous System [see **WARNINGS AND PRECAUTIONS (5.8)**]

Abnormal dreams, agitation, amnesia, anxiety, confusion, convulsion, crying, depression, elevated mood, emotional lability, encephalopathy, haemorrhagic stroke, hallucinations, hypertonia, incoordination, monoparesis, myoclonus, nerve compression, nervousness, neuralgia, neuropathy, paralysis flaccid, psychomotor skills impaired, psychosis, quadriparesis, somnolence, thinking abnormal, vertigo, writing impaired

Special Senses

Abnormal vision, amblyopia, ear pain, otitis media, tinnitus

Gastrointestinal

Cholangitis, cholestatic jaundice, duodenitis, dysphagia, esophagitis, flatulence, gastritis, gastroesophagitis, gastrointestinal hemorrhage, GGT increase, GI disorder, GI perforation, hepatitis, hepatitis granulomatous, ileus, increased appetite, jaundice, liver damage, oesophagitis ulcerative, oral moniliasis, pancreatic pseudocyst, rectal disorder, stomatitis

Cardiovascular

Abnormal ECG, angina pectoris, arrhythmia, atrial fibrillation, atrial flutter, bradycardia, cardiac fibrillation, cardiopulmonary failure, cardiovascular disorder, congestive heart failure, deep thrombophlebitis, echocardiogram abnormal, electrocardiogram QRS complex abnormal, electrocardiogram ST segment abnormal, heart failure, heart rate decreased, hemorrhage, hypotension, peripheral vascular disorder, phlebitis, postural hypotension, syncope, tachycardia, thrombosis, vasodilatation

Urogenital

Acute kidney failure [see **WARNINGS AND PRECAUTIONS (5.7)**], albuminuria, BK nephropathy, bladder spasm, cystitis, dysuria, hematuria, hydronephrosis, kidney failure, kidney tubular necrosis, nocturia, pyuria, toxic nephropathy, urge incontinence, urinary frequency, urinary incontinence, urinary retention, vaginitis

Metabolic/Nutritional

Acidosis, alkaline phosphatase increased, alkalosis, ALT (SGPT) increased, AST (SGOT) increased, bicarbonate decreased, bilirubinemia, dehydration, GGT increased, gout, healing abnormal, hypercalcemia, hypercholesterolemia, hyperphosphatemia, hyperuricemia, hypervolemia, hypocalcemia, hypoglycemia, hyponatremia, hypoproteinemia, lactic dehydrogenase increase, weight gain

Endocrine
Cushing's syndrome
Hemic / Lymphatic
Coagulation disorder, ecchymosis, haematocrit increased, haemoglobin abnormal, hypochromic anemia, leukocytosis, polycythemia, prothrombin decreased, serum iron decreased
Miscellaneous
Abdomen enlarged, abscess, accidental injury, allergic reaction, cellulitis, chills, fall, feeling abnormal, flu syndrome, generalized edema, hernia, mobility decreased, peritonitis, photosensitivity reaction, sepsis, temperature intolerance, ulcer
Musculoskeletal
Arthralgia, cramps, generalized spasm, joint disorder, leg cramps, myalgia, myasthenia, osteoporosis
Respiratory
Asthma, emphysema, hiccups, lung disorder, lung function decreased, pharyngitis, pneumonia, pneumothorax, pulmonary edema, respiratory disorder, rhinitis, sinusitis, voice alteration
Skin
Acne, alopecia, exfoliative dermatitis, fungal dermatitis, herpes simplex, herpes zoster, hirsutism, neoplasm skin benign, skin discoloration, skin disorder, skin ulcer, sweating

6.2 Postmarketing Adverse Reactions

The following adverse reactions have been reported from worldwide marketing experience with tacrolimus. Because these reactions are reported voluntarily from a population of uncertain size it is not always possible to reliably estimate their frequency or establish a causal relationship to drug exposure. Decisions to include these reactions in labeling are typically based on one or more of the following factors: (1) seriousness of the reaction, (2) frequency of the reporting, or (3) strength of causal connection to the drug.
Other reactions include:

Cardiovascular
Atrial fibrillation, atrial flutter, cardiac arrhythmia, cardiac arrest, electrocardiogram T wave abnormal, flushing, myocardial infarction, myocardial ischaemia, pericardial effusion, QT prolongation, Torsade de Pointes, venous thrombosis deep limb, ventricular extrasystoles, ventricular fibrillation, myocardial hypertrophy [see **WARNINGS AND PRECAUTIONS (5.14)**].
Gastrointestinal
Bile duct stenosis, colitis, enterocolitis, gastroenteritis, gastroesophageal reflux disease, hepatic cytolysis, hepatic necrosis, hepatotoxicity, impaired gastric emptying, liver fatty, mouth ulceration, pancreatitis haemorrhagic, pancreatitis necrotizing, stomach ulcer, venoocclusive liver disease
Hemic/Lymphatic
Agranulocytosis, disseminated intravascular coagulation, hemolytic anemia, neutropenia, pancytopenia, thrombocytopenic purpura, thrombotic thrombocytopenic purpura, pure red cell aplasia [see **WARNINGS AND PRECAUTIONS (5.16)**]
Infections
Cases of progressive multifocal leukoencephalopathy (PML), sometimes fatal; polyoma virus-associated nephropathy, (PVAN) including graft loss [see **WARNINGS AND PRECAUTIONS (5.4)**]
Metabolic/Nutritional
Glycosuria, increased amylase including pancreatitis, weight decreased
Miscellaneous
Feeling hot and cold, feeling jittery, hot flushes, multi-organ failure, primary graft dysfunction
Nervous System
Carpal tunnel syndrome, cerebral infarction, hemiparesis, leukoencephalopathy, mental disorder, mutism, posterior reversible encephalopathy syndrome (PRES) [see **WARNINGS AND PRECAUTIONS (5.8)**], progressive multifocal leukoencephalopathy (PML) [see **WARNINGS AND PRECAUTIONS (5.4)**], quadriplegia, speech disorder, syncope
Respiratory
Acute respiratory distress syndrome, interstitial lung disease, lung infiltration, respiratory distress, respiratory failure
Skin
Stevens-Johnson syndrome, toxic epidermal necrolysis
Special Senses
Blindness, blindness cortical, hearing loss including deafness, photophobia
Urogenital
Acute renal failure, cystitis haemorrhagic, hemolytic-uremic syndrome, micturition disorder

7 DRUG INTERACTIONS

Since tacrolimus is metabolized mainly by CYP3A enzymes, drugs or substances known to inhibit these enzymes may increase tacrolimus whole blood concentrations. Drugs known to induce CYP3A enzymes may decrease tacrolimus whole blood concentrations [see **WARNINGS AND PRECAUTIONS (5.13)** and **CLINICAL PHARMACOLOGY (12.3)**].

7.1 Mycophenolic Acid Products

With a given dose of mycophenolic acid (MPA) products, exposure to MPA is higher with tacrolimus co-administration than with cyclosporine co-administration because cyclosporine interrupts the enterohepatic recirculation of MPA while tacrolimus does not. Clinicians should be aware that there is also a potential for increased MPA exposure after crossover from cyclosporine to Hecoria (tacrolimus) capsules in patients concomitantly receiving MPA-containing products.

7.2 Grapefruit Juice

Grapefruit juice inhibits CYP3A-enzymes resulting in increased tacrolimus whole blood trough concentrations, and patients should avoid eating grapefruit or drinking grapefruit juice with tacrolimus [see **DOSAGE AND ADMINISTRATION (2.5)**].

7.3 Protease Inhibitors

Most protease inhibitors inhibit CYP3A enzymes and may increase tacrolimus whole blood concentrations. It is recommended to avoid concomitant use of tacrolimus with nelfinavir unless the benefits outweigh the risks [see **CLINICAL PHARMACOLOGY (12.3)**]. Whole blood concentrations of tacrolimus are markedly increased when coadministered with telaprevir or with boceprevir [see **CLINICAL PHARMACOLOGY (12.3)**]. Monitoring of tacrolimus whole blood concentrations and tacrolimus-associated adverse reactions, and appropriate adjustments in the dosing regimen of tacrolimus are recommended when tacrolimus and protease inhibitors (e.g., ritonavir, telaprevir, boceprevir) are used concomitantly.

7.4 Antifungal Agents

Frequent monitoring of whole blood concentrations and appropriate dosage adjustments of tacrolimus are recommended when concomitant use of the following antifungal drugs with tacrolimus is initiated or discontinued [see **CLINICAL PHARMACOLOGY (12.3)**].
Azoles: Voriconazole, posaconazole, itraconazole, ketoconazole, fluconazole and clotrimazole inhibit CYP3A metabolism of tacrolimus and increase tacrolimus whole blood concentrations. When initiating therapy with voriconazole or posaconazole in patients already receiving tacrolimus, it is recommended that the tacrolimus dose be initially reduced to one-third of the original dose and the subsequent tacrolimus doses be adjusted based on the tacrolimus whole blood concentrations.
Caspofungin is an inducer of CYP3A and decreases whole blood concentrations of tacrolimus.

7.5 Calcium Channel Blockers

Verapamil, diltiazem, nifedipine, and nicardipine inhibit CYP3A metabolism of tacrolimus and may increase tacrolimus whole blood concentrations. Monitoring of whole blood concentrations and appropriate dosage adjustments of tacrolimus are recommended when these calcium channel blocking drugs and tacrolimus are used concomitantly.

7.6 Antibacterials

Erythromycin, clarithromycin, troleandomycin and chloramphenicol inhibit CYP3A metabolism of tacrolimus and may increase tacrolimus whole blood concentrations. Monitoring of blood concentrations and appropriate dosage adjustments of tacrolimus are recommended when these drugs and tacrolimus are used concomitantly.

7.7 Antimycobacterials

Rifampin [see **CLINICAL PHARMACOLOGY (12.3)**] and rifabutin are inducers of CYP3A enzymes and may decrease tacrolimus whole blood concentrations. Monitoring of whole blood concentrations and appropriate dosage adjustments of tacrolimus are recommended when these antimycobacterial drugs and tacrolimus are used concomitantly.

7.8 Anticonvulsants

Phenytoin, carbamazepine and phenobarbital induce CYP3A enzymes and may decrease tacrolimus whole blood concentrations. Monitoring of whole blood concentrations and appropriate dosage adjustments of tacrolimus are recommended when these drugs and tacrolimus are used concomitantly.
Concomitant administration of phenytoin with tacrolimus may also increase phenytoin plasma concentrations. Thus, frequent monitoring phenytoin plasma concentrations and adjusting the phenytoin dose as needed are recommended when tacrolimus and phenytoin are administered concomitantly.

7.9 St. John's Wort (*Hypericum perforatum*)

St. John's Wort induces CYP3A enzymes and may decrease tacrolimus whole blood concentrations. Monitoring of whole blood concentrations and appropriate dosage adjustments of tacrolimus are recommended when St. John's Wort and tacrolimus are coadministered.

7.10 Gastric Acid Suppressors/Neutralizers

Lansoprazole and omeprazole, as CYP2C19 and CYP3A4 substrates, may potentially inhibit the CYP3A4 metabolism of tacrolimus and thereby substantially increase tacrolimus whole blood concentrations, especially in transplant patients who are intermediate or poor CYP2C19 metabolizers, as compared to those patients who are efficient CYP2C19 metabolizers.
Cimetidine may also inhibit the CYP3A4 metabolism of tacrolimus and thereby substantially increase tacrolimus whole blood concentrations.
Coadministration with magnesium and aluminum hydroxide antacids increase tacrolimus whole blood concentrations [see **CLINICAL PHARMACOLOGY (12.3)**]. Monitoring of whole blood concentrations and appropriate dosage adjustments of tacrolimus are recommended when these drugs and tacrolimus are used concomitantly.

7.11 Others

Bromocriptine, nefazodone, metoclopramide, danazol, ethinyl estradiol, amiodarone and methylprednisolone may inhibit CYP3A metabolism of tacrolimus and increase tacrolimus whole blood concentrations. Monitoring of blood concentrations and appropriate dosage adjustments of tacrolimus are recommended when these drugs and tacrolimus are coadministered.

8 USE IN SPECIFIC POPULATIONS

8.1 Pregnancy

Pregnancy Category C - There are no adequate and well-controlled studies in pregnant women. Tacrolimus is transferred across the placenta. The use of tacrolimus during pregnancy in humans has been associated with neonatal hyperkalemia and renal dysfunction. Tacrolimus given orally to pregnant rabbits at 0.5 to 4.3 times the clinical dose and pregnant rats at 0.8 to 6.9 times the clinical dose was associated with an increased incidence of fetal death *in utero*, fetal malformations (cardiovascular, skeletal, omphalocele, and gallbladder agenesis) and maternal toxicity. Hecoria (tacrolimus) capsules should be used during pregnancy only if the potential benefit to the mother justifies the potential risk to the fetus.
In pregnant rabbits, tacrolimus at oral doses of 0.32 and 1 mg/kg, 0.5 to 4.3 times the clinical dose range (0.075 to 0.2 mg/kg) based on body surface area, was associated with maternal toxicity as well as an increased incidence of abortions. At the 1 mg/kg dose, fetal rabbits showed an increased incidence of malformations (ventricular hypoplasia, interventricular septal defect, bulbous aortic arch, stenosis of ductus arteriosis, interrupted ossification of vertebral arch, vertebral and rib malformations, omphalocele, and gallbladder agenesis) and developmental variations. In pregnant rats, tacrolimus at oral doses of 3.2 mg/kg, 2.6 to 6.9 times the clinical dose range was associated with maternal toxicity, an increase in late resorptions, decreased numbers of live births, and decreased pup weight and viability. Tacrolimus, given orally to pregnant rats after organogenesis and during lactation at 1 and 3.2 mg/kg, 0.8 to 6.9 times the recommended clinical dose range was associated with reduced pup weights and pup viability (3.2 mg/kg only); among the high dose pups that died early, an increased incidence of kidney hydronephrosis was observed.

8.3 Nursing Mothers

Tacrolimus is excreted in human milk. As the effect of chronic exposure to tacrolimus in healthy infants is not established, patients maintained on Hecoria (tacrolimus) capsules should discontinue nursing taking into consideration importance of drug to the mother.

8.4 Pediatric Use

The safety and efficacy of Hecoria (tacrolimus) capsules in pediatric kidney and heart transplant patients have not been established. Successful liver transplants have been performed in pediatric patients (ages up to 16 years) using tacrolimus. Two randomized active-controlled trials of tacrolimus in primary liver transplantation included 56 pediatric patients. Thirty-one patients were randomized to tacrolimus-based and 25 to cyclosporine-based therapies. Additionally, a minimum of 122 pediatric patients were studied in an uncontrolled trial of tacrolimus in living related donor liver transplantation. Pediatric patients generally required higher doses of tacrolimus to maintain blood trough concentrations of tacrolimus similar to adult patients [see **DOSAGE AND ADMINISTRATION (2.2)**].

8.5 Geriatric Use

Clinical trials of tacrolimus did not include sufficient numbers of subjects aged 65 and over to determine whether they respond differently from younger subjects. Other reported clinical experience has not identified differences in responses between the elderly and younger patients. In general, dose selection for an elderly patient should be cautious, usually starting at the low end of the dosing range, reflecting the greater frequency of decreased hepatic, renal, or cardiac function, and of concomitant disease or other drug therapy.

8.6 Use in Renal Impairment

The pharmacokinetics of tacrolimus in patients with renal impairment was similar to that in healthy volunteers with normal renal function. However, consideration should be given to dosing Hecoria (tacrolimus) capsules at the lower end of the therapeutic dosing range in patients who have received a liver or heart transplant and have pre-existing renal impairment. Further reductions in dose below the targeted range may be required [see **DOSAGE AND ADMINISTRATION (2.3)** and **CLINICAL PHARMACOLOGY (12.3)**].

8.7 Use in Hepatic Impairment

The mean clearance of tacrolimus was substantially lower in patients with severe hepatic impairment (mean Child-Pugh score: >10) compared to healthy volunteers with normal hepatic function. Close monitoring of tacrolimus trough concentrations is warranted in patients with hepatic impairment [see **CLINICAL PHARMACOLOGY (12.3)**].

The use of Hecoria (tacrolimus) capsules in liver transplant recipients experiencing post-transplant hepatic impairment may be associated with increased risk of developing renal insufficiency related to high whole-blood trough concentrations of tacrolimus. These patients should be monitored closely and dosage adjustments should be considered. Some evidence suggests that lower doses should be used in these patients [see **DOSAGE AND ADMINISTRATION (2.3)** and **CLINICAL PHARMACOLOGY (12.3)**].

10 OVERDOSAGE

Limited overdosage experience is available. Acute overdosages of up to 30 times the intended dose have been reported. Almost all cases have been asymptomatic and all patients recovered with no sequelae. Acute overdosage was sometimes followed by adverse reactions consistent with those listed in **ADVERSE REACTIONS (6)** (including tremors, abnormal renal function, hypertension, and peripheral edema); in one case of acute overdosage, transient urticaria and lethargy were observed. Based on the poor aqueous solubility and extensive erythrocyte and plasma protein binding, it is anticipated that tacrolimus is not dialyzable to any significant extent; there is no experience with charcoal hemoperfusion. The oral use of activated charcoal has been reported in treating acute overdoses, but experience has not been sufficient to warrant recommending its use. General supportive measures and treatment of specific symptoms should be followed in all cases of overdosage.

In acute oral and IV toxicity studies, mortalities were seen at or above the following doses: in adult rats, 52 times the recommended human oral dose; in immature rats, 16 times the recommended oral dose; and in adult rats, 16 times the recommended human IV dose (all based on body surface area corrections).

11 DESCRIPTION

Hecoria is available for oral administration as capsules (tacrolimus capsules) containing the equivalent of 0.5 mg, 1 mg or 5 mg of anhydrous tacrolimus. In addition, each capsule contains the following inactive ingredients: croscarmellose sodium, hypromellose, lactose monohydrate, and magnesium stearate.

The Hecoria (tacrolimus) capsule shell for 0.5 mg strength consists of gelatin, titanium dioxide and yellow iron oxide.

The Hecoria (tacrolimus) capsule shell for 1 mg strength consists of black iron oxide, gelatin, red iron oxide, titanium dioxide, and yellow iron oxide.

The Hecoria (tacrolimus) capsule shell for 5 mg strength consists of red iron oxide, gelatin, and titanium dioxide.

Hecoria (tacrolimus capsules, USP) 0.5 mg, 1 mg and 5 mg are printed with edible black ink. The black ink is comprised of ammonia, black iron oxide, butyl alcohol, potassium hydroxide, propylene glycol, and shellac.

Tacrolimus, previously known as FK506, is the active ingredient in Hecoria (tacrolimus capsules, USP). Tacrolimus is a macrolide immunosuppressant produced by *Streptomyces tsukubaensis*. Chemically, tacrolimus is designated as [3S-[3R*[E(1S*,3S*,4S*)],4S*,5R*,8S*,9E,12R,14R*, 15S*, 16R*,18S*,19S*,26aR*]] 5,6,8,11,12,13,14,15,16,17,18, 19, 24,25,26,26a-hexadecahydro-5,19-dihydroxy-3-[2-(4-hydroxy-3-methoxycyclohexyl)-1-methylethenyl]-14,16-dimethoxy-4,10,12,18-tetramethyl-8-(2-propenyl)-15,19-epoxy-3H-pyrido[2,1-c][1,4] oxaazacyclotricosine-1,7,20,21(4H, 23H)-tetrone, monohydrate.

The chemical structure of tacrolimus is:

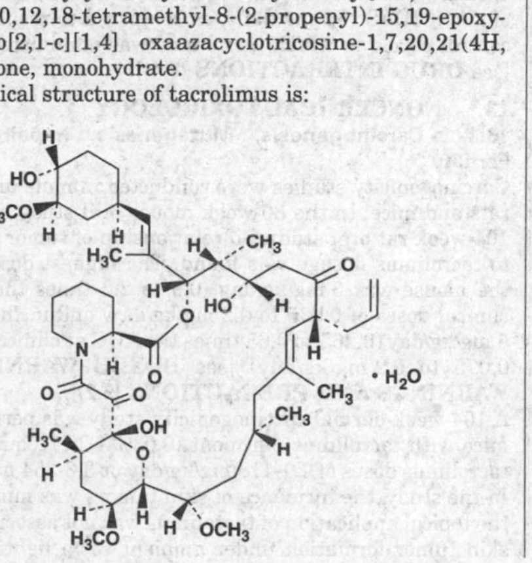

Table 14. Pharmacokinetics Parameters (mean±S.D.) of Tacrolimus in Healthy Volunteers and Patients

Population	N	Route (Dose)	C_{max} (ng/mL)	T_{max} (hr)	AUC (ng•hr/mL)	$t_{1/2}$ (hr)	Cl (L/hr/kg)	V (L/kg)
Healthy Volunteers	8	IV (0.025 mg/kg/4hr)	a	a	598[b] ± 125	34.2 ± 7.7	0.040 ± 0.009	1.91 ± 0.31
	16	PO (5 mg)	29.7 ± 7.2	1.6 ± 0.7	243[c] ± 73	34.8 ± 11.4	0.041[d] ± 0.008	1.94[d] ± 0.53
Kidney Transplant Patients	26	IV (0.02 mg/kg/12 hr)	a	a	294[e] ± 262	18.8 ± 16.7	0.083 ± 0.050	1.41 ± 0.66
		PO (0.2 mg/kg/day)	19.2 ± 10.3	3	203[e] ± 42	f	f	f
		PO (0.3 mg/kg/day)	24.2 ± 15.8	1.5	288[e] ± 93	f	f	f
Liver Transplant Patients	17	IV (0.05 mg/kg/12 hr)	a	a	3300[e] ± 2130	11.7 ± 3.9	0.053 ± 0.017	0.85 ± 0.30
		PO (0.3 mg/kg/day)	68.5 ± 30	2.3 ± 1.5	519[e] ± 179	f	f	f
Heart Transplant Patients	11	IV (0.01 mg/kg/day as a continuous infusion)	a	a	954[g] ± 334	23.6 ± 9.22	23.6 ± 0.015	
	11	PO (0.75 mg/kg/day)[h]	14.7 ± 7.79	2.1 [0.5-6][i]	82.7[j] ± 63.2	a	f	f
	14	PO (0.15 mg/kg/day)[h]	24.5 ± 13.7	1.5 [0.4-4][i]	142[j] ± 116	a	f	f

[a]not applicable
[b]AUC_{0-120}
[c]AUC_{0-72}
[d]Corrected for individual bioavailability
[e]AUC_{0-inf}
[f]not available
[g]AUC_{0-t}
[h]Determined after the first dose
[i]Median [range]
[j]AUC0-12

Tacrolimus has a molecular formula of $C_{44}H_{69}NO_{12}•H_2O$ and a formula weight of 822.03. Tacrolimus appears as white crystals or crystalline powder. It is practically insoluble in water, freely soluble in ethanol, and very soluble in methanol and chloroform.

USP Dissolution test 2 and Organic Impurities procedure 2 used.

12 CLINICAL PHARMACOLOGY

12.1 Mechanism of Action

Tacrolimus inhibits T-lymphocyte activation, although the exact mechanism of action is not known. Experimental evidence suggests that tacrolimus binds to an intracellular protein, FKBP-12. A complex of tacrolimus-FKBP-12, calcium, calmodulin, and calcineurin is then formed and the phosphatase activity of calcineurin inhibited. This effect may prevent the dephosphorylation and translocation of nuclear factor of activated T-cells (NF-AT), a nuclear component thought to initiate gene transcription for the formation of lymphokines (such as interleukin-2, gamma interferon). The net result is the inhibition of T-lymphocyte activation (i.e., immunosuppression).

Tacrolimus prolongs the survival of the host and transplanted graft in animal transplant models of liver, kidney, heart, bone marrow, small bowel and pancreas, lung and trachea, skin, cornea, and limb.

In animals, tacrolimus has been demonstrated to suppress some humoral immunity and, to a greater extent, cell-mediated reactions such as allograft rejection, delayed type hypersensitivity, collagen-induced arthritis, experimental allergic encephalomyelitis, and graft versus host disease.

12.3 Pharmacokinetics

Tacrolimus activity is primarily due to the parent drug. The pharmacokinetic parameters (mean±S.D.) of tacrolimus have been determined following intravenous (IV) and/or oral (PO) administration in healthy volunteers, and in kidney transplant, liver transplant, and heart transplant patients (**Table 14**).

[See table 14 above]

Due to intersubject variability in tacrolimus pharmacokinetics, individualization of dosing regimen is necessary for optimal therapy [see **DOSAGE AND ADMINISTRATION (2.6)**]. Pharmacokinetic data indicate that whole blood concentrations rather than plasma concentrations serve as the more appropriate sampling compartment to describe tacrolimus pharmacokinetics.

Absorption

Absorption of tacrolimus from the gastrointestinal tract after oral administration is incomplete and variable. The absolute bioavailability of tacrolimus was 17±10% in adult kidney transplant patients (N=26), 22±6% in adult liver transplant patients (N=17), 23±9% in adult heart transplant patients (N=11) and 18±5% in healthy volunteers (N=16).

A single dose trial conducted in 32 healthy volunteers established the bioequivalence of the 1 mg and 5 mg capsules. Another single dose trial in 32 healthy volunteers established the bioequivalence of the 0.5 mg and 1 mg capsules. Tacrolimus maximum blood concentrations (C_{max}) and area under the curve (AUC) appeared to increase in a dose-proportional fashion in 18 fasted healthy volunteers receiving a single oral dose of 3, 7, and 10 mg.

In 18 kidney transplant patients, tacrolimus trough concentrations from 3 to 30 ng/mL measured at 10 to 12 hours post-dose (C_{min}) correlated well with the AUC (correlation coefficient 0.93). In 24 liver transplant patients over a concentration range of 10 to 60 ng/mL, the correlation coefficient was 0.94. In 25 heart transplant patients over a concentration range of 2 to 24 ng/mL, the correlation coefficient was 0.89 after an oral dose of 0.075 or 0.15 mg/kg/day at steady-state.

Food Effects

The rate and extent of tacrolimus absorption were greatest under fasted conditions. The presence and composition of food decreased both the rate and extent of tacrolimus absorption when administered to 15 healthy volunteers.

The effect was most pronounced with a high-fat meal (848 kcal, 46% fat): mean AUC and C_{max} were decreased 37% and 77%, respectively; T_{max} was lengthened 5-fold. A high-carbohydrate meal (668 kcal, 85% carbohydrate) decreased mean AUC and mean C_{max} by 28% and 65%, respectively.

In healthy volunteers (N=16), the time of the meal also affected tacrolimus bioavailability. When given immediately following the meal, mean C_{max} was reduced 71%, and mean AUC was reduced 39%, relative to the fasted condition.

Table 15. Pharmacokinetic In Renal and Hepatic Impaired Patients

Population (No. of Patients)	Dose	$AUC_{0\text{-}t}$ (ng•hr/mL)	$t_{1/2}$ (hr)	V (L/kg)	Cl (L/hr/kg)
Renal Impairment (n=12)	0.02 mg/kg/4hr IV	393±123 (t=60 hr)	26.3±9.2	1.07 ±0.20	0.038 ±0.014
Mild Hepatic Impairment (n=6)	0.02 mg/kg/4hr IV	367±107 (t=72 hr)	60.6±43.8 Range: 27.8 to 141	3.1±1.6	0.042 ±0.02
	7.7 mg PO	488±320 (t=72 hr)	66.1±44.8 Range: 29.5 to 138	3.7±4.7[a]	0.034 ±0.019[a]
Severe Hepatic Impairment (n=6, IV)	0.02 mg/kg/4hr IV (n=2) 0.01 mg/kg/8hr IV (n=4)	762±204 (t=120 hr) 289±117 (t=144 hr)	198±158 Range: 81 to 436	3.9±1	0.017 ±0.013
(n=5, PO)[b]	8 mg PO (n=1) 5 mg PO (n=4) 4 mg PO (n=1)	658 (t=120 hr) 533±156 (t=144 hr)	119±35 Range: 85 to 178	3.1±3.4[a]	0.016 ±0.011[a]

[a] corrected for bioavailability
[b] 1 patient did not receive the PO dose

When administered 1.5 hours following the meal, mean C_{max} was reduced 63%, and mean AUC was reduced 39%, relative to the fasted condition.

In 11 liver transplant patients, tacrolimus administered 15 minutes after a high fat (400 kcal, 34% fat) breakfast, resulted in decreased AUC (27±18%) and C_{max} (50±19%), as compared to a fasted state.

Hecoria (tacrolimus) capsules should be taken consistently every day either with or without food because the presence and composition of food decreases the bioavailability of Hecoria [see **DOSAGE AND ADMINISTRATION (2.5)**].

Distribution

The plasma protein binding of tacrolimus is approximately 99% and is independent of concentration over a range of 5 to 50 ng/mL. Tacrolimus is bound mainly to albumin and alpha-1-acid glycoprotein, and has a high level of association with erythrocytes. The distribution of tacrolimus between whole blood and plasma depends on several factors, such as hematocrit, temperature at the time of plasma separation, drug concentration, and plasma protein concentration. In a U.S. trial, the ratio of whole blood concentration to plasma concentration averaged 35 (range 12 to 67).

Metabolism

Tacrolimus is extensively metabolized by the mixed-function oxidase system, primarily the cytochrome P-450 system (CYP3A). A metabolic pathway leading to the formation of 8 possible metabolites has been proposed. Demethylation and hydroxylation were identified as the primary mechanisms of biotransformation *in vitro*. The major metabolite identified in incubations with human liver microsomes is 13-demethyl tacrolimus. In *in vitro* studies, a 31-demethyl metabolite has been reported to have the same activity as tacrolimus.

Excretion

The mean clearance following IV administration of tacrolimus is 0.040, 0.083, 0.053, and 0.051 L/hr/kg in healthy volunteers, adult kidney transplant patients, adult liver transplant patients, and adult heart transplant patients, respectively. In man, less than 1% of the dose administered is excreted unchanged in urine.

In a mass balance study of IV administered radiolabeled tacrolimus to 6 healthy volunteers, the mean recovery of radiolabel was 77.8±12.7%. Fecal elimination accounted for 92.4±1% and the elimination half-life based on radioactivity was 48.1±15.9 hours whereas it was 43.5±11.6 hours based on tacrolimus concentrations. The mean clearance of radiolabel was 0.029±0.015 L/hr/kg and clearance of tacrolimus was 0.029±0.009 L/hr/kg. When administered PO, the mean recovery of the radiolabel was 94.9±30.7%. Fecal elimination accounted for 92.6±30.7%, urinary elimination accounted for 2.3±1.1% and the elimination half-life based on radioactivity was 31.9±10.5 hours whereas it was 48.4±12.3 hours based on tacrolimus concentrations. The mean clearance of radiolabel was 0.226±0.116 L/hr/kg and clearance of tacrolimus 0.172±0.088 L/hr/kg.

Specific Populations

Pediatric

Pharmacokinetics of tacrolimus have been studied in liver transplantation patients, 0.7 to 13.2 years of age. Following oral administration to 9 patients, mean AUC and C_{max} were 337±167 ng•hr/mL and 48.4±27.9 ng/mL, respectively. The absolute bioavailability was 31±24%.

Whole blood trough concentrations from 31 patients less than 12 years old showed that pediatric patients needed higher doses than adults to achieve similar tacrolimus trough concentrations [see **DOSAGE AND ADMINISTRATION (2.2)**].

Pharmacokinetics of tacrolimus have also been studied in kidney transplantation patients, 8.2±2.4 years of age. Following oral administration, mean AUC and C_{max} were 181±65 (range 81 to 300) ng•hr/mL and 30±11 (range 14 to 49) ng/mL, respectively. The absolute bioavailability was 19±14 (range 5.2 to 56) %.

Renal and Hepatic Impairment

The mean pharmacokinetic parameters for tacrolimus following single administrations to patients with renal and hepatic impairment are given in **Table 15**.

[See table 15 above]

Renal Impairment: Tacrolimus pharmacokinetics following a single IV administration were determined in 12 patients (7 not on dialysis and 5 on dialysis, serum creatinine of 3.9±1.6 and 12±2.4 mg/dL, respectively) prior to their kidney transplant. The pharmacokinetic parameters obtained were similar for both groups. The mean clearance of tacrolimus in patients with renal dysfunction was similar to that in normal volunteers (**Table 15**) [see **DOSAGE AND ADMINISTRATION (2.3)** and **USE IN SPECIFIC POPULATIONS (8.6)**].

Hepatic Impairment: Tacrolimus pharmacokinetics have been determined in six patients with mild hepatic dysfunction (mean Pugh score: 6.2) following oral administrations. The mean clearance of tacrolimus in patients with mild hepatic dysfunction was not substantially different from that in normal volunteers (see previous table). Tacrolimus pharmacokinetics were studied in 6 patients with severe hepatic dysfunction (mean Pugh score: >10). The mean clearance was substantially lower in patients with severe hepatic dysfunction, irrespective of the route of administration [see **DOSAGE AND ADMINISTRATION (2.4)** and **USE IN SPECIFIC POPULATIONS (8.7)**].

Race

The pharmacokinetics of tacrolimus have been studied following single IV and oral administration of tacrolimus to 10 African-American, 12 Latino-American, and 12 Caucasian healthy volunteers. There were no significant pharmacokinetic differences among the three ethnic groups following a 4-hour IV infusion of 0.015 mg/kg. However, after single oral administration of 5 mg, mean (±SD) tacrolimus C_{max} in African-Americans (23.6±12.1 ng/mL) was significantly lower than in Caucasians (40.2±12.6 ng/mL) and the Latino-Americans (36.2±15.8 ng/mL) (p<0.01). Mean $AUC_{0\text{-}inf}$ tended to be lower in African-Americans (203±115 ng•hr/mL) than Caucasians (344±186 ng•hr/mL) and Latino-Americans (274±150 ng•hr/mL). The mean (±SD) absolute oral bioavailability (F) in African-Americans (12±4.5%) and Latino-Americans (14±7.4%) was significantly lower than in Caucasians (19±5.8%, p=0.011). There was no significant difference in mean terminal $T_{1/2}$ among the three ethnic groups (range from approximately 25 to 30 hours). A retrospective comparison of African-American and Caucasian kidney transplant patients indicated that African-American patients required higher tacrolimus doses to attain similar trough concentrations [see **DOSAGE AND ADMINISTRATION (2.1)**].

Gender

A formal trial to evaluate the effect of gender on tacrolimus pharmacokinetics has not been conducted, however, there was no difference in dosing by gender in the kidney transplant trial. A retrospective comparison of pharmacokinetics in healthy volunteers, and in kidney, liver, and heart transplant patients indicated no gender-based differences.

Drug Interactions

Frequent monitoring of whole blood concentrations and appropriate dosage adjustments of tacrolimus are recommended when concomitant use of the following drugs with tacrolimus is initiated or discontinued [see **DRUG INTERACTIONS (7)**].

Telaprevir: In a single dose study in 9 healthy volunteers, coadministration of tacrolimus (0.5 mg single dose) with telaprevir (750 mg three times daily for 13 days) increased the tacrolimus dose normalized Cmax by 9.3-fold and AUC by 70-fold compared to tacrolimus alone [see **DRUG INTERACTIONS (7.3)**].

Boceprevir: In a single dose study in 12 subjects, coadministration of tacrolimus (0.5 mg single dose) with boceprevir (800 mg three times daily for 11 days) increased tacrolimus C_{max} by 9.9-fold and AUC by 17-fold compared to tacrolimus alone [see **DRUG INTERACTIONS (7.3)**].

Nelfinavir: Based on a clinical study of 5 liver transplant recipients, co-administration of tacrolimus with nelfinavir increased blood concentrations of tacrolimus significantly and, as a result, a reduction in the tacrolimus dose by an average of 16-fold was needed to maintain mean trough tacrolimus blood concentrations of 9.7 ng/mL. It is recommended to avoid concomitant use of Hecoria (tacrolimus) capsules and nelfinavir unless the benefits outweigh the risks [see **DRUG INTERACTIONS (7.3)**].

Rifampin: In a study of 6 normal volunteers, a significant decrease in tacrolimus oral bioavailability (14±6% vs. 7±3%) was observed with concomitant rifampin administration (600 mg). In addition, there was a significant increase in tacrolimus clearance (0.036±0.008 L/hr/kg vs. 0.053±0.010 L/hr/kg) with concomitant rifampin administration [see **DRUG INTERACTIONS (7.7)**].

Magnesium-aluminum-hydroxide: In a single-dose crossover study in healthy volunteers, coadministration of tacrolimus and magnesium-aluminum-hydroxide resulted in a 21% increase in the mean tacrolimus AUC and a 10% decrease in the mean tacrolimus C_{max} relative to tacrolimus administration alone [see **DRUG INTERACTIONS (7.10)**].

Ketoconazole: In a study of 6 normal volunteers, a significant increase in tacrolimus oral bioavailability (14±5% vs. 30±8%) was observed with concomitant ketoconazole administration (200 mg). The apparent oral clearance of tacrolimus during ketoconazole administration was significantly decreased compared to tacrolimus alone (0.430±0.129 L/hr/kg vs. 0.148±0.043 L/hr/kg). Overall, IV clearance of tacrolimus was not significantly changed by ketoconazole co-administration, although it was highly variable between patients [see **DRUG INTERACTIONS (7.4)**].

Voriconazole (see complete prescribing information for Voriconazole): Repeat oral dose administration of voriconazole (400 mg every 12 hours for one day, then 200 mg every 12 hours for 6 days) increased tacrolimus (0.1 mg/kg single dose) C_{max} and AUCτ in healthy subjects by an average of 2-fold (90% CI: 1.9, 2.5) and 3-fold (90% CI: 2.7, 3.8), respectively [see **DRUG INTERACTIONS (7.4)**].

Posaconazole (see complete prescribing information for Noxafil®): Repeat oral administration of posaconazole (400 mg twice daily for 7 days) increased tacrolimus (0.05 mg/kg single dose) C_{max} and AUC in healthy subjects by an average of 2-fold (90% CI: 2.01, 2.42) and 4.5-fold (90% CI: 4.03, 5.19), respectively [see **DRUG INTERACTIONS (7.4)**].

Caspofungin (see complete prescribing information for CANCIDAS®): Caspofungin reduced the blood $AUC_{0\text{-}12}$ of tacrolimus by approximately 20%, peak blood concentration (C_{max}) by 16%, and 12-hour blood concentration (C12hr) by 26% in healthy adult subjects when tacrolimus (2 doses of 0.1 mg/kg 12 hours apart) was administered on the 10th day of CANCIDAS® 70 mg daily, as compared to results from a control period in which tacrolimus was administered alone [see **DRUG INTERACTIONS (7.4)**].

13 NONCLINICAL TOXICOLOGY

13.1 Carcinogenesis, Mutagenesis, Impairment of Fertility

Carcinogenicity studies were conducted in male and female rats and mice. In the 80-week mouse oral study and in the 104-week rat oral study, no relationship of tumor incidence to tacrolimus dosage was found. The highest dose used in the mouse was 3 mg/kg/day (0.9 to 2.2 times the AUC at clinical doses of 0.075 to 0.2 mg/kg/day) and in the rat was 5 mg/kg/day (0.265 to 0.65 times the AUC at clinical doses of 0.075 to 0.2 mg/kg/day) [see **BOXED WARNING** and **WARNINGS AND PRECAUTIONS (5.2)**].

A 104-week dermal carcinogenicity study was performed in mice with tacrolimus ointment (0.03% - 3%), equivalent to tacrolimus doses of 1.1-118 mg/kg/day or 3.3-354 mg/m²/day. In the study, the incidence of skin tumors was minimal and the topical application of tacrolimus was not associated with skin tumor formation under ambient room lighting. However, a statistically significant elevation in the incidence of pleomorphic lymphoma in high dose male (25/50) and female animals (27/50) and in the incidence of undifferentiated lymphoma in high dose female animals (13/50) was noted in the mouse dermal carcinogenicity study. Lymphomas were noted in the mouse dermal carcinogenicity study at a daily dose of 3.5 mg/kg (0.1% tacrolimus ointment). No drug-related tumors were noted in the mouse dermal carcinogenicity study at a daily dose of 1.1 mg/kg (0.03% tacrolimus ointment). The relevance of topical administration of tacrolimus in the setting of systemic tacrolimus use is unknown.

The implications of these carcinogenicity studies to the human condition are limited; doses of tacrolimus were administered that likely induced immunosuppression in these animals impairing their immune system's ability to inhibit unrelated carcinogenesis.

No evidence of genotoxicity was seen in bacterial (*Salmonella* and *E. coli*) or mammalian (Chinese hamster lung-derived cells) *in vitro* assays of mutagenicity, the *in vitro* CHO/HGPRT assay of mutagenicity, or *in vivo* clastogenicity assays performed in mice; tacrolimus did not cause unscheduled DNA synthesis in rodent hepatocytes.

Tacrolimus given orally at 1 mg/kg (0.8 to 2.2 times the clinical dose range of 0.075 to 0.2 mg/kg/day based on body surface area) to male and female rats, prior to and during mating, as well as to dams during gestation and lactation, was associated with embryolethality and adverse effects on female reproduction. Effects on female reproductive function (parturition) and embryolethal effects were indicated by a higher rate of pre-implantation loss and increased numbers of undelivered and nonviable pups. When given at 3.2 mg/kg (2.6 to 6.9 times the clinical dose range based on body surface area), tacrolimus was associated with maternal and paternal toxicity as well as reproductive toxicity including marked adverse effects on estrus cycles, parturition, pup viability, and pup malformations.

14 CLINICAL STUDIES

14.1 Kidney Transplantation

Tacrolimus/azathioprine (AZA)

Tacrolimus-based immunosuppression in conjunction with azathioprine and corticosteroids following kidney transplantation was assessed in a randomized, multicenter, non-blinded, prospective trial. There were 412 kidney transplant patients enrolled at 19 clinical sites in the United States. Study therapy was initiated when renal function was stable as indicated by a serum creatinine ≤ 4 mg/dL (median of 4 days after transplantation, range 1 to 14 days). Patients less than 6 years of age were excluded.

There were 205 patients randomized to tacrolimus-based immunosuppression and 207 patients were randomized to cyclosporine-based immunosuppression. All patients received prophylactic induction therapy consisting of an antilymphocyte antibody preparation, corticosteroids and azathioprine. Overall 1 year patient and graft survival was 96.1% and 89.6%, respectively.

Data from this trial of tacrolimus in conjunction with azathioprine indicate that during the first three months of that trial, 80% of the patients maintained trough concentrations between 7 to 20 ng/mL, and then between 5 to 15 ng/mL, through 1 year.

Tacrolimus/mycophenolate mofetil (MMF)

Tacrolimus-based immunosuppression in conjunction with MMF, corticosteroids, and induction has been studied. In a randomized, open-label, multi-center trial (Study 1), 1589 kidney transplant patients received tacrolimus (Group C, n=401), sirolimus (Group D, n=399), or one of two cyclosporine (CsA) regimens (Group A, n=390 and Group B, n=399) in combination with MMF and corticosteroids; all patients, except those in one of the two cyclosporine groups, also received induction with daclizumab. The trial was conducted outside the United States; the trial population was 93% Caucasian. In this trial, mortality at 12 months in patients receiving tacrolimus/MMF was similar (3%) compared to patients receiving cyclosporine/MMF (3% and 2%) or sirolimus/MMF (3%). Patients in the tacrolimus group exhibited higher estimated creatinine clearance rates (eCL_{cr}) using the Cockcroft-Gault formula (**Table 16**) and experienced fewer efficacy failures, defined as biopsy proven acute rejection (BPAR), graft loss, death, and/or lost to follow-up (**Table 17**) in comparison to each of the other three groups. Patients randomized to tacrolimus/MMF were more likely to develop diarrhea and diabetes after the transplantation and experienced similar rates of infections compared to patients randomized to either cyclosporine/MMF regimen [see **ADVERSE REACTIONS (6.1)**].

[See table 16 above]
[See table 17 above]

Table 16. Estimated Creatinine Clearance at 12 Months (Study 1)

Group	eCL_{cr} [mL/min] at Month 12[a]				
	N	MEAN	SD	MEDIAN	Treatment Difference with Group C (99.2% CI[b])
(A) CsA/MMF/CS	390	56.5	25.8	56.9	-8.6 (-13.7, -3.7)
(B) CsA/MMF/CS/Daclizumab	399	58.9	25.6	60.9	-6.2 (-11.2, -1.2)
(C) Tac/MMF/CS/Daclizumab	401	65.1	27.4	66.2	-
(D) Siro/MMF/CS/Daclizumab	399	56.2	27.4	57.3	-8.9 (-14.1, -3.9)
Total	1589	59.2	26.8	60.5	

Key: CsA =Cyclosporine, CS=Corticosteroids, Tac=Tacrolimus, Siro=Sirolimus

[a] All death/graft loss (n=41, 27, 23 and 42 in Groups A, B, C and D) and patients whose last recorded creatinine values were prior to month 3 visit (n=10, 9, 7 and 9 in Groups A, B, C and D, respectively) were inputed with Glomerular Filtration Rate (GFR) of 10 mL/min; a subject's last observed creatinine value from month 3 on was used for the remainder of subjects with missing creatinine at month 12 (n=11, 12, 15 and 19 for Groups A, B, C and D, respectively). Weight was also imputed in the calculation of estimated GFR, if missing.

[b] Adjusted for multiple (6) pairwise comparisons using Bonferroni corrections.

Table 17. Incidence of BPAR, Graft Loss, Death or Loss to Follow-up at 12 Months (Study 1)

	Group A N=390	Group B N=399	Group C N=401	Group D N=399
Overall Failure	141 (36.2%)	126 (31.6%)	82 (20.4%)	185 (46.4%)
Components of efficacy failure				
BPAR	113 (29%)	106 (26.6%)	60 (15%)	152 (38.1%)
Graft loss excluding death	28 (7.2%)	20 (5%)	12 (3%)	30 (7.5%)
Mortality	13 (3.3%)	7 (1.8%)	11 (2.7%)	12 (3%)
Lost to follow-up	5 (1.3%)	7 (1.8%)	5 (1.3%)	6 (1.5%)
Treatment Difference of efficacy failure compared to Group C (99.2% CI[a])	15.8% (7.1%, 24.3%)	11.2% (2.7%, 19.5%)	-	26% (17.2%, 34.7%)

Key: Group A=CsA/MMF/CS, B=CsA/MMF/CS/Daclizumab, C=Tac/MMF/CS/Daclizumab, and D=Siro/MMF/CS/Daclizumab

[a] Adjusted for multiple (6) pairwise comparisons using Bonferroni corrections.

The protocol-specified target tacrolimus trough concentrations ($C_{trough,Tac}$) were 3 to 7 ng/mL; however, the observed median $C_{troughs,Tac}$ approximated 7 ng/mL throughout the 12-month trial (**Table 18**). Approximately 80% of patients maintained tacrolimus whole blood concentrations between 4 to 11 ng/mL through 1 year post-transplant.

Table 18. Tacrolimus Whole Blood Trough Concentrations (Study 1)

Time	Median (P10-P90[a]) tacrolimus whole blood trough concentrations (ng/mL)
Day 30 (N=366)	6.9 (4.4 to 11.3)
Day 90 (N=351)	6.8 (4.1 to 10.7)
Day 180 (N=355)	6.5 (4 to 9.6)
Day 365 (N=346)	6.5 (3.8 to 10)

[a] 10 to the 90th Percentile: range of $C_{trough,Tac}$ that excludes lowest 10% and highest 10% of $C_{trough,Tac}$

The protocol-specified target cyclosporine trough concentrations ($C_{trough,CsA}$) for Group B were 50 to 100 ng/mL; however, the observed median $C_{troughs,CsA}$ approximated 100 ng/mL throughout the 12-month trial. The protocol-specified target $C_{troughs,CsA}$ for Group A were 150 to 300 ng/mL for the first 3 months and 100 to 200 ng/mL from month 4 to month 12; the observed median $C_{troughs,CsA}$ approximated 225 ng/mL for the first 3 months and 140 ng/mL from month 4 to month 12.

While patients in all groups started MMF at 1 gram twice daily, the MMF dose was reduced to less than 2 g per day in 63% of patients in the tacrolimus treatment arm by month 12 (**Table 19**); approximately 50% of these MMF dose reductions were due to adverse reactions. By comparison, the MMF dose was reduced to less than 2 g per day in 49% and 45% of patients in the two cyclosporine arms (Group A and Group B, respectively), by month 12 and approximately 40% of MMF dose reductions were due to adverse reactions.

Table 19. MMF Dose Over Time in Tacrolimus/MMF (Group C) (Study 1)

Time period (Days)	Time-averaged MMF dose (grams per day)[a]		
	Less than 2	2	Greater than 2
0 to 30 (N=364)	37%	60%	2%
0 to 90 (N=373)	47%	51%	2%
0 to 180 (N=377)	56%	42%	2%
0 to 365 (N=380)	63%	36%	1%

Key: Time-averaged MMF dose = (total MMF dose)/(duration of treatment)

[a] Percentage of patients for each time-averaged MMF dose range during various treatment periods.
Administration of 2 g per day of time-averaged MMF dose means that MMF dose was not reduced in those patients during the treatment periods.

In a second randomized, open-label, multi-center trial (Study 2), 424 kidney transplant patients received tacrolimus (N=212) or cyclosporine (N=212) in combination with MMF 1 gram twice daily, basiliximab induction, and corticosteroids. In this trial, the rate for the combined endpoint of BPAR, graft failure, death, and/or lost to follow-up at 12 months in the tacrolimus/MMF group was similar to the rate in the cyclosporine/MMF group. There was, however, an imbalance in mortality at 12 months in those patients receiving tacrolimus/MMF (4%) compared to those receiving cyclosporine/MMF (2%), including cases attributed to overimmunosuppression (**Table 20**).

Table 20. Incidence of BPAR, Graft Loss, Death or Loss to Follow-up at 12 Months (Study 2)

	Tacrolimus/MMF	Cyclosporine/MMF
	(N=212)	(N=212)
Overall Failure	32 (15.1%)	36 (17%)
Components of efficacy failure		
BPAR	16 (7.5%)	29 (13.7%)
Graft loss excluding death	6 (2.8%)	4 (1.9%)
Mortality	9 (4.2%)	5 (2.4%)
Lost to follow-up	4 (1.9%)	1 (0.5%)
Treatment Difference of efficacy failure compared to tacrolimus/MMF group (95% CI[a])		1.9% (-5.2%, 9%)

[a] 95% confidence interval calculated using Fisher's Exact Test

The protocol-specified target tacrolimus whole blood trough concentrations ($C_{trough,Tac}$) in Study 2 were 7 to 16 ng/mL for the first three months and 5 to 15 ng/mL thereafter. The observed median $C_{troughs,Tac}$ approximated 10 ng/mL during the first three months and 8 ng/mL from month 4 to month 12 (**Table 21**). Approximately 80% of patients maintained tacrolimus whole trough blood concentrations between 6 to 16 ng/mL during months 1 through 3 and, then, between 5 to 12 ng/mL from month 4 through 1 year.

Table 21. Tacrolimus Whole Blood Trough Concentrations (Study 2)

Time	Median (P10-P90[a]) tacrolimus whole blood trough concentrations (ng/mL)
Day 30 (N=174)	10.5 (6.3 to 16.8)
Day 60 (N=179)	9.2 (5.9 to 15.3)
Day 120 (N=176)	8.3 (4.6 to 13.3)
Day 180 (N=171)	7.8 (5.5 to 13.2)
Day 365 (N=178)	7.1 (4.2 to 12.4)

[a] 10 to 90th Percentile: range of $C_{trough,Tac}$ that excludes lowest 10% and highest 10% of $C_{trough,Tac}$

The protocol-specified target cyclosporine whole blood concentrations ($C_{trough,CsA}$) were 125 to 400 ng/mL for the first three months, and 100 to 300 ng/mL thereafter. The observed median $C_{troughs,CsA}$ approximated 280 ng/mL during the first three months and 190 ng/mL from month 4 to month 12.

Patients in both groups started MMF at 1 gram twice daily. The MMF dose was reduced to less than 2 grams per day by month 12 in 62% of patients in the tacrolimus/MMF group (**Table 22**) and in 47% of patients in the cyclosporine/MMF group. Approximately 63% and 55% of these MMF dose reductions were because of adverse reactions in the tacrolimus/MMF group and the cyclosporine/MMF group, respectively [see **ADVERSE REACTIONS (6.1)**].

Table 22. MMF Dose Over Time in the Tacrolimus/MMF Group (Study 2)

Time period (Days)	Time-averaged MMF dose (grams per day)[a]		
	Less than 2	2	Greater than 2
0 to 30 (N=212)	25%	69%	6%
0 to 90 (N=212)	41%	53%	6%
0 to 180 (N=212)	52%	41%	7%
0 to 365 (N=212)	62%	34%	4%

Key: Time-averaged MMF dose=(total MMF dose)/(duration of treatment)

[a] Percentage of patients for each time-averaged MMF dose range during various treatment periods. Two grams per day of time-averaged MMF dose means that MMF dose was not reduced in those patients during the treatment periods.

14.2 Liver Transplantation

The safety and efficacy of tacrolimus-based immunosuppression following orthotopic liver transplantation were assessed in two prospective, randomized, non-blinded multicenter trials. The active control groups were treated with a cyclosporine-based immunosuppressive regimen (CsA/AZA). Both trials used concomitant adrenal corticosteroids as part of the immunosuppressive regimens. These trials compared patient and graft survival rates at 12 months following transplantation.

In one trial, 529 patients were enrolled at 12 clinical sites in the United States; prior to surgery, 263 were randomized to the tacrolimus-based immunosuppressive regimen and 266 to the CsA/AZA. In 10 of the 12 sites, the same CsA/AZA protocol was used, while 2 sites used different control protocols. This trial excluded patients with renal dysfunction, fulminant hepatic failure with Stage IV encephalopathy, and cancers; pediatric patients (≤ 12 years old) were allowed.

In the second trial, 545 patients were enrolled at 8 clinical sites in Europe; prior to surgery, 270 were randomized to the tacrolimus-based immunosuppressive regimen and 275 to CsA/AZA. In this trial, each center used its local standard CsA/AZA protocol in the active-control arm. This trial excluded pediatric patients, but did allow enrollment of subjects with renal dysfunction, fulminant hepatic failure in Stage IV encephalopathy, and cancers other than primary hepatic with metastases.

One-year patient survival and graft survival in the tacrolimus-based treatment groups were similar to those in the CsA/AZA treatment groups in both trials. The overall 1-year patient survival (CsA/AZA and tacrolimus-based treatment groups combined) was 88% in the U.S. trial and 78% in the European trial. The overall 1-year graft survival (CsA/AZA and tacrolimus-based treatment groups combined) was 81% in the U.S. trial and 73% in the European trial. In both trials, the median time to convert from IV to oral tacrolimus dosing was 2 days.

Although there is a lack of direct correlation between tacrolimus concentrations and drug efficacy, data from clinical trials of liver transplant patients have shown an increasing incidence of adverse reactions with increasing trough blood concentrations. Most patients are stable when trough whole blood concentrations are maintained between 5 to 20 ng/mL. Long-term post-transplant patients often are maintained at the low end of this target range.

Data from the U.S. clinical trial show that the median trough blood concentrations, measured at intervals from the second week to one year post-transplantation ranged from 9.8 ng/mL to 19.4 ng/mL.

14.3 Heart Transplantation

Two open-label, randomized, comparative trials evaluated the safety and efficacy of tacrolimus-based and cyclosporine-based immunosuppression in primary orthotopic heart transplantation. In a trial conducted in Europe, 314 patients received a regimen of antibody induction, corticosteroids and azathioprine in combination with tacrolimus or cyclosporine modified for 18 months. In a 3-arm trial conducted in the US, 331 patients received corticosteroids and tacrolimus plus sirolimus, tacrolimus plus mycophenolate mofetil (MMF) or cyclosporine modified plus MMF for 1 year.

In the European trial, patient/graft survival at 18 months post-transplant was similar between treatment arms, 92% in the tacrolimus group and 90% in the cyclosporine group. In the U.S. trial, patient and graft survival at 12 months was similar with 93% survival in the tacrolimus plus MMF group and 86% survival in the cyclosporine modified plus MMF group. In the European trial, the cyclosporine trough concentrations were above the pre-defined target range (i.e., 100 to 200 ng/mL) at Day 122 and beyond in 32 to 68% of the patients in the cyclosporine treatment arm, whereas the tacrolimus trough concentrations were within the pre-defined target range (i.e., 5 to 15 ng/mL) in 74 to 86% of the patients in the tacrolimus treatment arm. Data from this European trial indicate that from 1 week to 3 months post-transplant, approximately 80% of patients maintained trough concentrations between 8 to 20 ng/mL and, from 3 months through 18 months post-transplant, approximately 80% of patients maintained trough concentrations between 6 to 18 ng/mL.

The U.S. trial contained a third arm of a combination regimen of sirolimus, 2 mg per day, and full-dose tacrolimus; however, this regimen was associated with increased risk of wound healing complications, renal function impairment, and insulin-dependent post-transplant diabetes mellitus, and is not recommended [see **WARNINGS AND PRECAUTIONS (5.12)**].

16 HOW SUPPLIED/STORAGE AND HANDLING

Hecoria (tacrolimus capsules, USP) containing white to off-white powder equivalent to 0.5 mg of anhydrous tacrolimus, are hard gelatin capsules with white opaque body and ivory cap. The body is imprinted "0.5 mg" and cap is imprinted "HECORIA" in black ink.

They are supplied as follows:

NDC 0078-0616-05, bottle of 100 capsules with child-resistant closure

Hecoria (tacrolimus capsules, USP) containing white to off-white powder equivalent to 1 mg of anhydrous tacrolimus, are hard gelatin capsules with white opaque body and brown cap. The body is imprinted "1 mg" and cap is imprinted "HECORIA" in black ink.

They are supplied as follows:

NDC 0078-0617-05, bottle of 100 capsules with child-resistant closure

Hecoria (tacrolimus capsules, USP) containing white to off-white powder equivalent to 5 mg of anhydrous tacrolimus, are hard gelatin capsules with white opaque body and orange cap. The body is imprinted "5 mg" and cap is imprinted "HECORIA" in black ink.

They are supplied as follows:

NDC 0078-0618-05, bottle of 100 capsules with child-resistant closure.

Hecoria capsules should be stored at 20° to 25°C (68° to 77°F) [see USP Controlled Room Temperature].

17 PATIENT COUNSELING INFORMATION

17.1 Administration

Advise patients to:

- Take Hecoria (tacrolimus) capsules at the same 12-hour intervals every day to achieve consistent blood concentrations.
- Take Hecoria consistently either with or without food because the presence and composition of food decreases the bioavailability of Hecoria.
- Not to eat grapefruit or drink grapefruit juice in combination with Hecoria [see **DRUG INTERACTIONS (7.2)**].

17.2 Development of Lymphoma and Other Malignancies

Inform patients they are at increased risk of developing lymphomas and other malignancies, particularly of the skin, due to immunosuppression. Advise patients to limit exposure to sunlight and ultraviolet (UV) light by wearing protective clothing and use a sunscreen with a high protection factor [see **WARNINGS AND PRECAUTIONS (5.2)**].

17.3 Increased Risk of Infection

Inform patients they are at increased risk of developing a variety of infections, including opportunistic infections, due to immunosuppression and to contact their physician if they develop any symptoms of infection [see **WARNINGS AND PRECAUTIONS (5.3, 5.4, 5.5)**].

17.4 New Onset Diabetes After Transplant

Inform patients that Hecoria (tacrolimus) capsules can cause diabetes mellitus and should be advised to contact their physician if they develop frequent urination, increased thirst or hunger [see **WARNINGS AND PRECAUTIONS (5.6)**].

17.5 Nephrotoxicity

Inform patients that Hecoria (tacrolimus) capsules can have toxic effects on the kidney that should be monitored. Advise patients to attend all visits and complete all blood tests ordered by their medical team [see **WARNINGS AND PRECAUTIONS (5.7)**].

17.6 Neurotoxicity

Inform patients that they are at risk of developing adverse neurologic effects including seizure, altered mental status, and tremor. Advise patients to contact their physician should they develop vision changes, deliriums, or tremors [see **WARNINGS AND PRECAUTIONS (5.8)**].

17.7 Hyperkalemia

Inform patients that Hecoria (tacrolimus) capsules can cause hyperkalemia. Monitoring of potassium levels may be necessary, especially with concomitant use of other drugs known to cause hyperkalemia [see **WARNINGS AND PRECAUTIONS (5.9)**].

17.8 Hypertension

Inform patients that Hecoria (tacrolimus) capsules can cause high blood pressure which may require treatment with anti-hypertensive therapy [see **WARNINGS AND PRECAUTIONS (5.10)**].

17.9 Drug Interactions

Instruct patients to tell their health care providers when they start or stop taking all the medicines, including prescription medicines and non-prescription medicines, natural or herbal remedies, nutritional supplements and vitamins [see **DRUG INTERACTIONS (7)**].

17.10 Pregnant Women and Nursing Mothers

Instruct patients to tell their healthcare providers if they plan to become pregnant or breast-feed their infant [see **USE IN SPECIFIC POPULATIONS (8.1, 8.3)**]

17.11 Immunizations

Inform patients that Hecoria (tacrolimus) capsules can interfere with the usual response to immunizations and that they should avoid live vaccines [see **WARNINGS AND PRECAUTIONS (5.15)**].

T2013-13
March 2013

PATIENT INFORMATION

Hecoria™ (tacrolimus capsules, USP)

Read this Patient Information before you start taking Hecoria (tacrolimus) capsules and each time you get a refill. There may be new information. This information does not take the place of talking with your doctor about your medical condition or your treatment.

What is the most important information I should know about Hecoria (tacrolimus) capsules?

Hecoria (tacrolimus) capsules can cause serious side effects, including:

1. Increased risk of cancer. People who take Hecoria have an increased risk of getting some kinds of cancer, including skin and lymph gland cancer (lymphoma).

2. Increased risk of infection. Hecoria is a medicine that affects your immune system. Hecoria can lower the ability of your immune system to fight infections. Serious infections can happen in people receiving Hecoria that can cause death. **Call your doctor right away if you have symptoms of an infection such as:**

- fever
- sweats or chills
- cough or flu-like symptoms
- muscle aches
- warm, red, or painful areas on your skin

What are Hecoria (tacrolimus) capsules?

Hecoria is a prescription medicine used with other medicines to help prevent organ rejection in people who have had a kidney, liver, or heart transplant and Hecoria is not for use with medicines called cyclosporines (Gengraf®, Neoral®, and Sandimmune®).

Hecoria is not for use with a medicine called sirolimus (Rapamune®) in people who have had a liver or heart transplant.

It is not known if Hecoria is safe and effective when used with sirolimus in people who have had kidney transplants.

It is not known if Hecoria is safe and effective in children who have had a kidney or heart transplant.

Who should not take Hecoria (tacrolimus) capsules?

Do not take Hecoria if you are allergic to tacrolimus or any of the ingredients in Hecoria. See the end of this leaflet for a complete list of ingredients in Hecoria.

What should I tell my doctor before taking Hecoria (tacrolimus) capsules?

Before you take Hecoria, tell your doctor if you:

- plan to receive any live vaccines
- have or have had liver, kidney or heart problems
- are pregnant or plan to become pregnant. Hecoria may harm your unborn baby. Talk to your doctor if you are pregnant or plan to become pregnant.
- Are breastfeeding or plan to breastfeed. Hecoria can pass into your breast milk. You and your doctor should decide if you will take Hecoria or breastfeed. You should not do both.

Tell your doctor about all the medicines you take, including prescription and non-prescription medicines, vitamins, and herbal supplements.

Especially tell your doctor if you take:

- cyclosporine (Gengraf®, Neoral®, and Sandimmune®)
- sirolimus (Rapamune®)
- nelfinavir (Viracept®)
- telaprevir (Incivek™)
- boceprevir (Victrelis™)
- amiodarone (Cordarone™, Nexterone™, Pacerone™)

Ask your doctor or pharmacist if you are not sure if you take any of the medicines listed above.

Hecoria may affect the way other medicines work, and other medicines may affect how Hecoria works.

Know the medicines you take. Keep a list of your medicines and show it to your doctor and pharmacist when you get a new medicine.

How should I take Hecoria (tacrolimus) capsules?

- Take Hecoria exactly as your doctor tells you to take it.
- Your doctor will tell you how many Hecoria capsules to take and when to take them.
- Your doctor may change your Hecoria dose if needed. Do not stop taking or change your dose of Hecoria without talking to your doctor.
- Take Hecoria with or without food.
- Take Hecoria the same way every day. For example, if you choose to take Hecoria with food, you should always take Hecoria with food.
- Take Hecoria at the same time each day, 12 hours apart. For example, if you take your first dose at 7:00 a.m. you should take your second dose at 7:00 p.m.
  - Taking Hecoria at the same time each day helps to keep enough medicine in your body to give your transplanted organ the around-the-clock medicine it needs.
- **Do not** eat grapefruit or drink grapefruit juice while taking Hecoria.
- If you take too much Hecoria, call your doctor or go to the nearest hospital emergency room right away.

What should I avoid while taking Hecoria (tacrolimus) capsules?

- While you take Hecoria you should not receive any live vaccines such as:
  - flu vaccine through your nose
  - measles
  - mumps
  - rubella
  - polio by mouth
  - BCG (TB vaccine)
  - yellow fever
  - chicken pox (varicella)
  - typhoid
- Avoid exposure to sunlight and UV light such as tanning machines. Wear protective clothing and use a sunscreen.

What are the possible side effects of Hecoria (tacrolimus) capsules?

Hecoria may cause serious side effects, including:

- See **"What is the most important information I should know about Hecoria?"**
- **high blood sugar (diabetes).** Your doctor may do certain tests to check for diabetes while you take Hecoria. Call your doctor right away if you have:
  - frequent urination
  - increased thirst or hunger
  - blurred vision
  - confusion
  - drowsiness
  - loss of appetite
  - fruity smell on your breath
  - nausea, vomiting, or stomach pain
- **kidney problems.** Your doctor may do certain tests to check your kidney function while you take Hecoria.
- **nervous system problems.** Call your doctor right away if you get any of these symptoms while taking Hecoria. These could be signs of a serious nervous system problem:
  - confusion
  - coma
  - muscle tremors
  - numbness and tingling
  - headache
  - seizures
  - vision changes
- **high levels of potassium in your blood.** Your doctor may do certain tests to check your potassium level while you take Hecoria.
- **high blood pressure.** Your doctor will monitor your blood pressure while you take Hecoria.
- **heart problems (myocardial hypertrophy).** Tell your doctor right away if you get any of these symptoms of heart problems while taking Hecoria:
  - shortness of breath
  - chest pain
  - feel lightheaded
  - feel faint

The most common side effects of Hecoria (tacrolimus) capsules in people receiving kidney transplant are:

- infection
- tremors (shaking of the body)
- high blood pressure
- kidney problems
- constipation
- diarrhea
- headache
- stomach pain
- trouble sleeping
- nausea
- low levels of phosphate in your blood
- swelling of the hands, ankles, or legs
- weakness
- pain
- high levels of fat in your blood
- high levels of potassium in your blood
- low red blood cell count (anemia)

The most common side effects of Hecoria (tacrolimus) capsules in people receiving liver transplants are:

- shaking of the body tremors
- headache
- diarrhea
- high blood pressure
- nausea
- kidney problems
- stomach pain
- trouble sleeping
- numbness or tingling in your hands or feet
- anemia
- pain
- fever
- weakness
- high levels of potassium in the blood
- low levels of magnesium in the blood

The most common side effects of Hecoria (tacrolimus) capsules for heart transplant patients are:

- kidney problems
- high blood pressure

Tell your doctor if you have any side effect that bothers you or that does not go away.

These are not all the possible side effects of Hecoria. For more information, ask your doctor or pharmacist.

Call your doctor for medical advice about side effects. You may report side effects to FDA at 1-800-FDA-1088.

How should I store Hecoria (tacrolimus) capsules?

- Store Hecoria at 20° to 25°C (68° to 77° F).
- Safely throw away medicine that is out of date or no longer needed.

Keep Hecoria and all medicines out of reach of children.

General information about the safe and effective use of Hecoria (tacrolimus) capsules

Medicines are sometimes prescribed for purposes other than those listed in a Patient Information leaflet. Do not use Hecoria for a condition for which it was not prescribed. Do not give Hecoria to other people, even if they have the same symptoms that you have. It may harm them.

How do Hecoria (tacrolimus) capsules protect my new organ?

The body's immune system protects the body against any thing that it does not recognize as part of the body. For example, when the immune system detects a virus or bacteria it tries to get rid of it to prevent infection. When a person has a liver, kidney, or heart transplant, the immune system does not recognize the new organ as a part of the body and tries to get rid of it, too. This is called "rejection". Hecoria protects your new organ by slowing down the body's immune system.

This Patient Information leaflet summarizes the most important information about Hecoria. If you would like more information, talk with your doctor. You can ask your pharmacist or doctor for information about Hecoria that is written for health professionals.

For more information contact Novartis Pharmaceuticals Corporation at 1-888-669-6682.

What are the ingredients in Hecoria (tacrolimus) capsules?

Active ingredient: tacrolimus

Inactive ingredients: croscarmellose sodium, hypromellose, lactose monohydrate, and magnesium stearate.

The Hecoria capsule shell for 0.5 mg strength consists of gelatin, titanium dioxide and yellow iron oxide.

The Hecoria capsule shell for 1 mg strength consists of black iron oxide, gelatin, red iron oxide, titanium dioxide, and yellow iron oxide.

The Hecoria capsule shell for 5 mg strength consists of red iron oxide, gelatin, and titanium dioxide.

Hecoria capsules 0.5 mg, 1 mg and 5 mg are printed with edible black ink. The black ink is comprised of ammonia, black iron oxide, butyl alcohol, potassium hydroxide, propylene glycol, and shellac.

This Patient Information has been approved by the U.S. Food and Drug Administration.

Manufactured in India by Sandoz Private Limited
Distributed by: Novartis Pharmaceuticals Corporation
East Hanover, NJ 07936

T2013-14
March 2013

Shown in Product Identification Guide, page 310

ILARIS ℞
(canakinumab)
injection for subcutaneous use

The following prescribing information is based on official labeling in effect July 2013.

HIGHLIGHTS OF PRESCRIBING INFORMATION

These highlights do not include all the information needed to use ILARIS safely and effectively. See full prescribing information for ILARIS

ILARIS (canakinumab) injection for subcutaneous use
Initial U.S. Approval: 2009

RECENT MAJOR CHANGES

Indications and Usage, Systemic Juvenile Idiopathic Arthritis (SJIA) (1.2)	05/2013
Dosage and Administration, Systemic Juvenile Idiopathic Arthritis (SJIA) (2.3)	05/2013
Warnings and Precautions, Macrophage Activation Syndrome (SJIA) (5.5)	05/2013

INDICATIONS AND USAGE

ILARIS is an interleukin-1β blocker indicated for the treatment of:

Cryopyrin-Associated Periodic Syndromes (CAPS), in adults and children 4 years of age and older including:
- Familial Cold Autoinflammatory Syndrome (FCAS) (1.1)
- Muckle-Wells Syndrome (MWS) (1.1)

Active Systemic Juvenile Idiopathic Arthritis (SJIA) in patients aged 2 years and older (1.2)

DOSAGE AND ADMINISTRATION

Cryopyrin-Associated Periodic Syndromes
150 mg for CAPS patients with body weight greater than 40 kg and 2 mg/kg for CAPS patients with body weight greater than or equal to 15 kg and less than or equal to 40 kg. For children 15 to 40 kg with an inadequate response, the dose can be increased to 3 mg/kg. Administer subcutaneously every 8 weeks. (2.2)

Systemic Juvenile Idiopathic Arthritis (SJIA)
4 mg/kg (with a maximum of 300mg) for patients with a body weight greater than or equal to 7.5kg. Administer subcutaneously every 4 weeks. (2.3)

DOSAGE FORMS AND STRENGTHS

Sterile, single-use, glass vial containing 180 mg of ILARIS as a lyophilized powder for reconstitution. (3)

CONTRAINDICATIONS

Confirmed hypersensitivity to the active substance or to any of the excipients. (4)

WARNINGS AND PRECAUTIONS

- Interleukin-1 blockade may interfere with immune response to infections. Treatment with medications that work through inhibition of IL-1 has been associated with an increased risk of serious infections. ILARIS has been associated with an increased incidence of serious infections. Physicians should exercise caution when administering ILARIS to patients with infections, a history of recurring infections or underlying conditions which may predispose them to infections. Discontinue treatment with ILARIS if a patient develops a serious infection. Do not administer ILARIS to patients during an active infection requiring medical intervention. (5.1)
- Live vaccines should not be given concurrently with ILARIS. Prior to initiation of therapy with ILARIS, patients should receive all recommended vaccinations. (5.4)

ADVERSE REACTIONS

CAPS: The most common adverse reactions greater than 10% reported by patients with CAPS treated with ILARIS are nasopharyngitis, diarrhea, influenza, headache and nausea. (6)

SJIA: The most common adverse drug reactions greater than 10% reported by patients with SJIA treated with ILARIS are infections (nasopharyngitis and upper respiratory tract infections), abdominal pain and injection site reactions. (6)

To report SUSPECTED ADVERSE REACTIONS, contact Novartis Pharmaceuticals Corporation at 1-888-669-6682 or FDA at 1-800-FDA-1088 or www.fda.gov/medwatch

DRUG INTERACTIONS

No formal drug interaction studies have been conducted with ILARIS. (7)

USE IN SPECIFIC POPULATIONS

- Pregnancy: No Human data. Because animal reproduction studies are not always predictive of human response, this drug should be used during pregnancy only if clearly needed. (8.1)
- Nursing Mothers: Caution should be exercised when administered to a nursing woman. (8.3)

See 17 for PATIENT COUNSELING INFORMATION and Medication Guide

Revised: 05/2013

FULL PRESCRIBING INFORMATION: CONTENTS*

*** Sections or subsections omitted from the full prescribing information are not listed**

FULL PRESCRIBING INFORMATION

1 INDICATIONS AND USAGE

1.1 Cryopyrin-Associated Periodic Syndromes (CAPS)

ILARIS (canakinumab) is an interleukin-1β blocker indicated for the treatment of Cryopyrin-Associated Periodic Syndromes (CAPS), in adults and children 4 years of age and older including:
- Familial Cold Autoinflammatory Syndrome (FCAS)
- Muckle-Wells Syndrome (MWS)

1.2 Systemic Juvenile Idiopathic Arthritis (SJIA)

ILARIS is indicated for the treatment of active Systemic Juvenile Idiopathic Arthritis (SJIA) in patients aged 2 years and older.

2 DOSAGE AND ADMINISTRATION

2.1 General Dosing Information

INJECTION FOR SUBCUTANEOUS USE ONLY.

2.2 Cryopyrin-Associated Periodic Syndromes (CAPS)

The recommended dose of ILARIS is 150 mg for CAPS patients with body weight greater than 40 kg. For CAPS patients with body weight greater than or equal to 15 kg and less than or equal to 40 kg, the recommended dose is 2 mg/kg. For children 15 to 40 kg with an inadequate response, the dose can be increased to 3 mg/kg.

ILARIS is administered every eight weeks as a single dose via subcutaneous injection.

2.3 Systemic Juvenile Idiopathic Arthritis (SJIA)

The recommended dose of ILARIS for SJIA patients with a body weight greater than or equal to 7.5kg is 4mg/kg (with a maximum of 300mg) administered every four weeks via subcutaneous injection.

2.4 Four Steps for Preparation and Administration

STEP 1: Using aseptic technique, reconstitute each vial of ILARIS by slowly injecting 1 mL of preservative-free Sterile Water for Injection with a 1 mL syringe and an 18 gauge × 2" needle.

STEP 2: Swirl the vial slowly at an angle of about 45° for approximately 1 minute and allow to stand for 5 minutes. Do not shake. Then gently turn the vial upside down and back again ten times. Avoid touching the rubber stopper with your fingers.

STEP 3: Allow to stand for about 15 minutes at room temperature to obtain a clear solution. The reconstituted solution has a final concentration of 150mg/mL. Do not shake. Do not use if particulate matter is present in the solution. Tap the side of the vial to remove any residual liquid from the stopper. The reconstituted solution should be essentially free from particulates, and clear to opalescent. The solution should be colorless or may have a slight brownish-yellow tint. If the solution has a distinctly brown discoloration it should not be used. If not used within 60 minutes of reconstitution, the solution should be stored in the refrigerator at 2 to 8° C (36 to 46° F) and used within 4 hours. Slight foaming of the product upon reconstitution is not unusual.

STEP 4: Using a sterile syringe and needle carefully withdraw the required volume depending on the dose to be administered (0.2 mL to 1 mL) and subcutaneously inject using a 27 gauge × 0.5" needle.

Injection into scar tissue should be avoided as this may result in insufficient exposure to ILARIS.

ILARIS 180-mg powder for solution for injection is supplied in a single-use vial. Any unused product or waste material should be disposed of in accordance with local requirements.

3 DOSAGE FORMS AND STRENGTHS

ILARIS is supplied as a 180 mg white lyophilized powder for solution for subcutaneous injection. Reconstitution with 1 mL of preservative-free Sterile Water for Injection is required prior to subcutaneous administration of the drug, resulting in a total volume of 1.2 mL reconstituted solution. The reconstituted ILARIS is a clear to slightly opalescent, colorless to a slight brownish yellow tint, essentially free from particulates, 150 mg/mL solution.

4 CONTRAINDICATIONS

Confirmed hypersensitivity to the active substance or to any of the excipients *[see Warnings and Precautions (5.3) and Adverse Reactions (6.2)]*.

5 WARNINGS AND PRECAUTIONS

5.1 Serious Infections

ILARIS has been associated with an increased risk of serious infections. Physicians should exercise caution when administering ILARIS to patients with infections, a history of recurring infections or underlying conditions which may predispose them to infections. ILARIS should not be administered to patients during an active infection requiring medical intervention. Administration of ILARIS should be discontinued if a patient develops a serious infection.

Infections, predominantly of the upper respiratory tract, in some instances serious, have been reported with ILARIS. Generally, the observed infections responded to standard therapy. Isolated cases of unusual or opportunistic infections were reported during ILARIS treatment. In clinical trials, ILARIS has not been administered concomitantly with tumor necrosis factor (TNF) inhibitors. An increased incidence of serious infections has been associated with administration of another IL-1 blocker in combination with TNF inhibitors. Co-administration of ILARIS with TNF inhibitors is not recommended because this may increase the risk of serious infections *[see Drug Interactions (7.1)]*.

Drugs that affect the immune system by blocking TNF have been associated with an increased risk of new tuberculosis and reactivation of latent tuberculosis (TB). It is possible that use of IL-1 inhibitors such as ILARIS increases the risk of reactivation of tuberculosis or of opportunistic infections. Prior to initiating immunomodulatory therapies, including ILARIS, patients should be evaluated for active and latent tuberculosis infection. Appropriate screening tests should be performed in all patients. ILARIS has not been studied in patients with a positive tuberculosis screen, and the safety of ILARIS in individuals with latent tuberculosis infection is unknown. Patients testing positive in tuberculosis screening should be treated according to standard medical practice prior to therapy with ILARIS. All patients should be instructed to seek medical advice if signs, symptoms, or high risk exposure suggestive of tuberculosis (e.g. persistent cough, weight loss, subfebrile temperature) appear during or after ILARIS therapy.

Healthcare providers should follow current CDC guidelines both to evaluate for and to treat possible latent tuberculosis infections before initiating therapy with ILARIS.

5.2 Immunosuppression

The impact of treatment with anti-interleukin-1 (IL-1) therapy on the development of malignancies is not known. However, treatment with immunosuppressants, including ILARIS, may result in an increase in the risk of malignancies.

5.3 Hypersensitivity

Hypersensitivity reactions have been reported with ILARIS therapy. During clinical trials, no anaphylactic reactions have been reported. It should be recognized that symptoms of the underlying disease being treated may be similar to symptoms of hypersensitivity. ILARIS should not be administered to any patients with known clinical hypersensitivity to ILARIS *[see Contraindications (4) and Adverse Reactions (6.2)]*.

5.4 Immunizations

Live vaccines should not be given concurrently with ILARIS *[see Drug Interactions (7.2)]*. Since no data are available on either the efficacy or on the risks of secondary transmission of infection by live vaccines in patients receiving ILARIS, live vaccines should not be given concurrently with ILARIS. In addition, because ILARIS may interfere with normal immune response to new antigens, vaccinations may not be effective in patients receiving ILARIS. No data are available on the effectiveness of vaccinations with inactivated (killed) antigens in patients receiving ILARIS. *[see Drug Interactions (7.2)]*.

Because IL-1 blockade may interfere with immune response to infections, it is recommended that prior to initiation of therapy with ILARIS, adult and pediatric patients receive all recommended vaccinations, as appropriate, including pneumococcal vaccine and inactivated influenza vaccine. (See current recommended immunization schedules at the website of the Centers for Disease Control, http://www.cdc.gov/vaccines/recs/schedules/).

5.5 Macrophage Activation Syndrome

Macrophage activation syndrome (MAS) is a known, life-threatening disorder that may develop in patients with rheumatic conditions, in particular SJIA, and should be aggressively treated. Physicians should be attentive to symptoms of infection or worsening of SJIA, as these are known triggers for MAS. Eleven cases of MAS were observed in 201 SJIA patients treated with canakinumab in clinical trials. Based on the clinical trial experience, ILARIS does not appear to increase the incidence of MAS in SJIA patients, but no definitive conclusion can be made.

6 ADVERSE REACTIONS

395 patients, including approximately 250 children (aged 2 to 17 years) have been treated with ILARIS in interventional trials in CAPS or SJIA. The most frequently reported adverse drug reactions were infections predominantly of the upper respiratory tract. The majority of the events were mild to moderate although serious infections were observed. The type and frequency of adverse drug reactions appeared to be consistent over time.

6.1 Clinical Trial Experience

Because clinical trials are conducted under widely varying conditions, adverse reaction rates observed in the clinical trials of a drug cannot be directly compared to rates in the clinical trials of another drug and may not reflect the rates observed in practice.

Treatment of CAPS

The data described herein reflect exposure to ILARIS in 104 adult and pediatric CAPS patients, (including 20 FCAS, 72 MWS, 10 MWS/NOMID (Neonatal Onset Multisystem Inflammatory Disorder) overlap, 1 non-FCAS non-MWS, and 1 mis-diagnosed in placebo-controlled (35 patients) and uncontrolled trials. Sixty-two patients were exposed to ILARIS for at least 6 months, 56 for at least 1 year and 4 for at least 3 years. A total of 9 serious adverse reactions were reported for CAPS patients. Among these were vertigo (2 patients), infections (3 patients), including intra-abdominal abscess following appendectomy (1 patient). The most commonly reported adverse reactions associated with ILARIS treatment in the CAPS patients were nasopharyngitis, diarrhea, influenza, headache, and nausea. One patient discontinued treatment due to potential infection.

CAPS Study 1 investigated the safety of ILARIS in an 8-week, open-label period (Part 1), followed by a 24-week, randomized withdrawal period (Part 2), followed by a 16-week, open-label period (Part 3). All patients were treated with ILARIS 150 mg subcutaneously or 2 mg/kg if body weight was greater than or equal to 15 kg and less than or equal to 40 kg (see Table 1).

Since all CAPS patients received ILARIS in Part 1, there are no controlled data on adverse events (AEs). Data in Table 1 are for all AEs for all CAPS patients receiving canakinumab. In CAPS Study 1, no pattern was observed for any type or frequency of adverse events throughout the three study periods.

Table 1 Number (%) of Patients with AEs by Preferred Terms, in > 10% of Patients in Parts 1 to 3 of the Phase 3 Trial for CAPS Patients

Preferred Term	ILARIS N=35 n (%)
n % of Patients with Adverse Events	35 (100)
Nasopharyngitis	12 (34)
Diarrhea	7 (20)
Influenza	6 (17)
Rhinitis	6 (17)
Nausea	5 (14)
Headache	5 (14)
Bronchitis	4 (11)
Gastroenteritis	4 (11)
Pharyngitis	4 (11)
Weight increased	4 (11)
Musculoskeletal pain	4(11)
Vertigo	4(11)

Vertigo

Vertigo has been reported in 9 to 14% of patients in CAPS studies, exclusively in MWS patients, and reported as a serious adverse event in two cases. All events resolved with continued treatment with ILARIS.

Injection Site Reactions

In CAPS Study 1, subcutaneous injection site reactions were observed in 9% of patients in Part 1 with mild tolerability reactions; in Part 2, one patient each (7%) had a mild or a moderate tolerability reaction and, in Part 3, one patient had a mild local tolerability reaction. No severe injection-site reactions were reported and none led to discontinuation of treatment.

Table 2 Tabulated summary of adverse drug reactions from pivotal SJIA clinical trials

	SJIA Study 2			SJIA Study 1	
	Part I	Part II			
	ILARIS N=177 n (%) (IR)^	ILARIS N=50 n (%) (IR)	Placebo N=50 n (%) (IR)	ILARIS N=43 n (%) (IR)	Placebo N=41 n (%) (IR)
Infections and infestations					
Infection (e.g. nasopharyngitis, (viral) upper respiratory tract infection, pneumonia, rhinitis, pharyngitis, tonsillitis, sinusitis, urinary tract infection, gastroenteritis, viral infection)	97 (54.8%) (0.91)	27 (54%) (0.59)	19 (38%) (0.63)	13 (30.2%) (1.26)	5 (12.2%) (1.37)
Gastrointestinal disorders					
Abdominal pain (upper)	25 (14.1%) (0.16)	8 (16%) (0.15)	6 (12%) (0.08)	3 (7%) (0.25)	1 (2.4%) (0.23)
Skin and subcutaneous tissue disorders					
Injection site reaction*					
mild	19 (10.7%)	6 (12.0%)	2 (4.0%)	0	3 (7.3%)
moderate	2 (1.1%)	1 (2.0%)	0	0	0

n= number of patients

^ IR=Exposure adjusted incidence rate per 100 patient-days

* No injection site reaction led to study discontinuation

Treatment of SJIA

A total of 201 SJIA patients aged 2 to less than 20 years have received ILARIS in clinical trials. The safety of ILARIS compared to placebo was investigated in two phase 3 studies *[see Clinical Studies (14.2)]*. Patients in SJIA Study 1 received a single dose of ILARIS 4mg/kg (n=43) or placebo (n=41) via subcutaneous injection and were assessed at Day 15 for the efficacy endpoints and had a safety analysis up to Day 29. SJIA Study 2 was a two-part study with an open-label, single-arm active treatment period (Part I) followed by a randomized, double-blind, placebo-controlled, event-driven withdrawal design (Part II). Overall, 177 patients were enrolled into the study and received ILARIS 4 mg/kg (up to 300 mg maximum) in Part I, and 100 patients received ILARIS 4mg/kg (up to 300mg maximum) every 4 weeks or placebo in Part II. Adverse drug reactions listed in Table 2 showed higher rates than placebo from both trials. The adverse drug reactions associated with ILARIS treatment in SJIA patients were infections, abdominal pain, and injection site reactions.

Adverse reactions are listed according to MedDRA version 15.0 system organ class.

[See table 2 above]

6.2 Hypersensitivity

During clinical trials, no anaphylactic reactions have been reported. In CAPS trials one patient discontinued and in SJIA trials no patients discontinued due to hypersensitivity reactions. ILARIS should not be administered to any patients with known clinical hypersensitivity to ILARIS *[see Contraindications (4) and Warnings and Precautions (5.3)]*.

6.3 Immunogenicity

A biosensor binding assay or a bridging immunoassay was used to detect antibodies directed against canakinumab in patients who received ILARIS. Antibodies against ILARIS were observed in approximately 1.5% and 3.1% of the patients treated with ILARIS for CAPS and SJIA, respectively. No neutralizing antibodies were detected. No apparent correlation of antibody development to clinical response or adverse events was observed. The CAPS clinical studies employed the biosensor binding assay, and most of the SJIA clinical studies employed the bridging assay. The data obtained in an assay are highly dependent on several factors including assay sensitivity and specificity, assay methodology, sample handling, timing of sample collection, concomitant medications, underlying disease, and the number of patients tested. For these reasons, comparison of the incidence of antibodies to canakinumab between the CAPS and SJIA clinical studies or with the incidence of antibodies to other products may be misleading.

6.4 Laboratory Findings

Hematology

During clinical trials with ILARIS, mean values decreased for white blood cells, neutrophils and platelets.

In the randomized, placebo-controlled portion of SJIA Study 2 decreased white blood cell counts (WBC) less than or equal to 0.8× lower limit of normal (LLN) were reported in 5 patients (10.4%)in the ILARIS group compared to 2 (4.0%) in the placebo group. Transient decreases in absolute neutrophil counts (ANC) to less than 1×109/L were reported in 3 patients (6.0%) in the ILARIS group compared to1 patient (2.0%) in the placebo group. One case of ANC counts less than 0.5x109/L was observed in the ILARIS group and none in the placebo group.

Mild (less than LLN and greater than 75×109/L) and transient decreases in platelet counts were observed in 3 (6.3%) ILARIS treated patients versus 1 (2.0%) placebo-treated patient.

Hepatic transaminases

Elevations of transaminases have been observed in patients treated with ILARIS.

In the randomized, placebo-controlled portion of SJIA Study 2, high ALT and/or AST greater than or equal to 3× upper limit of normal (ULN) were reported in 2 (4.1%) ILARIS-treated patients and 1 (2.0%) placebo patient. All patients had normal values at the next visit.

Bilirubin

Asymptomatic and mild elevations of serum bilirubin have been observed in patients treated with ILARIS without concomitant elevations of transaminases.

7 DRUG INTERACTIONS

Interactions between ILARIS and other medicinal products have not been investigated in formal studies.

7.1 TNF-Blocker and IL-1 Blocking Agent

An increased incidence of serious infections and an increased risk of neutropenia have been associated with administration of another IL-1 blocker in combination with TNF inhibitors in another patient population. Use of ILARIS with TNF inhibitors may also result in similar toxicities and is not recommended because this may increase the risk of serious infections *[see Warnings and Precautions (5.1)]*.

The concomitant administration of ILARIS with other drugs that block IL-1 has not been studied. Based upon the potential for pharmacological interactions between ILARIS and a recombinant IL-1ra, concomitant administration of ILARIS and other agents that block IL-1 or its receptors is not recommended.

7.2 Immunization

No data are available on either the effects of live vaccination or the secondary transmission of infection by live vaccines in patients receiving ILARIS. Therefore, live vaccines should not be given concurrently with ILARIS. It is recommended that, if possible, pediatric and adult patients should complete all immunizations in accordance with current immunization guidelines prior to initiating ILARIS therapy *[see Warnings and Precautions (5.4)]*.

7.3 Cytochrome P450 Substrates

The formation of CYP450 enzymes is suppressed by increased levels of cytokines (e.g., IL-1) during chronic inflammation. Thus it is expected that for a molecule that binds to IL-1, such as canakinumab, the formation of CYP450 enzymes could be normalized. This is clinically relevant for CYP450 substrates with a narrow therapeutic index, where the dose is individually adjusted (e.g., warfarin). Upon initiation of canakinumab, in patients being treated with these types of medicinal products, therapeutic monitoring of the effect or drug concentration should be performed and the individual dose of the medicinal product may need to be adjusted as needed.

8 USE IN SPECIFIC POPULATIONS

8.1 Pregnancy

Pregnancy Category C

Canakinumab has been shown to produce delays in fetal skeletal development when evaluated in marmoset monkeys using doses 11-fold the maximum recommended human dose (MRHD) and greater (based on a plasma area under the time-concentration curve [AUC] comparison). Doses producing exposures within the clinical exposure range at the MRHD were not evaluated. Similar delays in fetal skeletal development were observed in mice administered a murine analog of canakinumab. There are no adequate and well-controlled studies of ILARIS in pregnant women. Because animal reproduction studies are not always predictive of human response, this drug should be used during pregnancy only if clearly needed.

Embryofetal developmental toxicity studies were performed in marmoset monkeys and mice. Pregnant marmoset monkeys were administered canakinumab subcutaneously twice weekly at doses of 15, 50 or 150 mg/kg (representing 11 to 110-fold the human dose based on a plasma AUC comparison at the MRHD) from gestation days 25 to 109 which revealed no evidence of embryotoxicity or fetal malformations. There were increases in the incidence of incomplete ossification of the terminal caudal vertebra and misaligned and/or bipartite vertebra in fetuses at all dose levels when compared to concurrent controls suggestive of delay in skeletal development in the marmoset. Since canakinumab does not cross-react with mouse or rat IL-1, pregnant mice were subcutaneously administered a murine analog of canakinumab at doses of 15, 50, or 150 mg/kg on gestation days 6, 11 and 17. The incidence of incomplete ossification of the parietal and frontal skull bones of fetuses was increased in a dose-dependent manner at all dose levels tested.

8.3 Nursing Mothers

It is not known whether canakinumab is excreted in human milk. Because many drugs are excreted in human milk, caution should be exercised when ILARIS is administered to a nursing woman.

8.4 Pediatric Use

The CAPS trials with ILARIS included a total of 23 pediatric patients with an age range from 4 years to 17 years (11 adolescents were treated subcutaneously with 150 mg , and 12 children were treated with 2 mg/kg based on body weight greater than or equal to 15 kg and less than or equal to 40 kg). The majority of patients achieved improvement in clinical symptoms and objective markers of inflammation (e.g., Serum Amyloid A and C-Reactive Protein). Overall, the efficacy and safety of ILARIS in pediatric and adult patients were comparable. Infections of the upper respiratory tract were the most frequently reported infection. The safety and effectiveness of ILARIS in CAPS patients under 4 years of age has not been established *[see Pharmacokinetics (12.3)]*.

The safety and efficacy of ILARIS in SJIA patients under 2 years of age have not been established *[see Pharmacokinetics (12.3)]*.

8.5 Geriatric Use

Clinical studies of ILARIS did not include sufficient numbers of subjects aged 65 and over to determine whether they respond differently from younger subjects.

8.6 Patients with Renal Impairment

No formal studies have been conducted to examine the pharmacokinetics of ILARIS administered subcutaneously in patients with renal impairment.

8.7 Patients with Hepatic Impairment

No formal studies have been conducted to examine the pharmacokinetics of ILARIS administered subcutaneously in patients with hepatic impairment.

10 OVERDOSAGE

No confirmed case of overdose has been reported. In the case of overdose, it is recommended that the subject be monitored for any signs and symptoms of adverse reactions or effects, and appropriate symptomatic treatment be instituted immediately.

11 DESCRIPTION

Canakinumab is a recombinant, human anti-human-IL-1β monoclonal antibody that belongs to the IgG1/κ isotype subclass. It is expressed in a murine Sp2/0-Ag14 cell line and comprised of two 447- (or 448-) residue heavy chains and two 214-residue light chains, with a molecular mass of 145157 Daltons when deglycosylated. Both heavy chains of canakinumab contain oligosaccharide chains linked to the protein backbone at asparagine 298 (Asn 298).

The biological activity of canakinumab is measured by comparing its inhibition of IL-1β-dependent expression of the reporter gene luciferase to that of a canakinumab internal reference standard, using a stably transfected cell line.

ILARIS is supplied in a sterile, single-use, colorless, 6 mL glass vial with coated stopper and aluminum flip-off cap. Each vial contains 180 mg of canakinumab as a white, preservative-free, lyophilized powder. Reconstitution with 1 mL of preservative-free Sterile Water for Injection is required prior to subcutaneous administration of the drug. The reconstituted canakinumab is a 150 mg/mL solution essentially free of particulates, clear to slightly opalescent, and is colorless or may have a slightly brownish-yellow tint. A volume of up to 1 mL can be withdrawn for delivery of 150 mg/mL canakinumab for subcutaneous administration. Each reconstituted vial contains 180 mg canakinumab, sucrose, L-histidine, L-histidine HCl monohydrate, polysorbate 80 and Sterile Water for Injection. No preservatives are present.

12 CLINICAL PHARMACOLOGY

12.1 Mechanism of Action

Canakinumab is a human monoclonal anti-human IL-1β antibody of the IgG1/κ isotype. Canakinumab binds to human IL-1β and neutralizes its activity by blocking its interaction with IL-1 receptors, but it does not bind IL-1α or IL-1 receptor antagonist (IL-1ra).

CAPS refer to rare genetic syndromes generally caused by mutations in the NLRP-3 [nucleotide-binding domain, leucine rich family (NLR), pyrin domain containing 3] gene (also known as Cold-Induced Auto-inflammatory Syndrome-1 [CIAS1]). CAPS disorders are inherited in an autosomal dominant pattern with male and female offspring equally affected. Features common to all disorders include fever, urticaria-like rash, arthralgia, myalgia, fatigue, and conjunctivitis.

The NLRP-3 gene encodes the protein cryopyrin, an important component of the inflammasome. Cryopyrin regulates the protease caspase-1 and controls the activation of interleukin-1 beta (IL-1β). Mutations in NLRP-3 result in an overactive inflammasome resulting in excessive release of activated IL-1β that drives inflammation. Systemic juvenile idiopathic arthritis (SJIA) is a severe autoinflammatory disease, driven by innate immunity by means of pro-inflammatory cytokines such as interleukin 1β (IL-1β).

12.2 Pharmacodynamics

C-reactive protein and Serum Amyloid A (SAA) are indicators of inflammatory disease activity that are elevated in patients with CAPS. Elevated SAA has been associated with the development of systemic amyloidosis in patients with CAPS. Following ILARIS treatment, CRP and SAA levels normalize within 8 days. In SJIA the median percent reduction in CRP from baseline to Day 15 was 91%. Improvement in pharmacodynamic markers may not be representative of clinical response.

12.3 Pharmacokinetics

Absorption

The peak serum canakinumab concentration (Cmax) of 16 ± 3.5 μg/mL occurred approximately 7 days after subcutaneous administration of a single, 150-mg dose subcutaneously to adult CAPS patients. The mean terminal half-life was 26 days. The absolute bioavailability of subcutaneous canakinumab was estimated to be 66%. Exposure parameters (such as AUC and Cmax) increased in proportion to dose over the dose range of 0.30 to 10 mg/kg given as intravenous infusion or from 150 to 300 mg as subcutaneous injection.

Distribution

Canakinumab binds to serum IL-1β. Canakinumab volume of distribution (Vss) varied according to body weight and was estimated to be 6.01 liters in a typical CAPS patient weighing 70 kg, and 3.2 liters in a SJIA patient weighing 33 kg. The expected accumulation ratio was 1.3-fold for CAPS patients and 1.6-fold for SJIA patients following 6 months of subcutaneous dosing of 150 mg ILARIS every 8 weeks and 4mg/kg every 4 weeks, respectively.

Elimination

Clearance (CL) of canakinumab varied according to body weight and was estimated to be 0.174 L/day in a typical CAPS patient weighing 70 kg and 0.11 L/day in a SJIA patient weighing 33 kg. There was no indication of accelerated clearance or time-dependent change in the pharmacokinetic properties of canakinumab following repeated administration. No gender- or age-related pharmacokinetic differences were observed after correction for body weight.

Pediatrics

Pharmacokinetic properties are similar in CAPS and SJIA pediatric populations.

In CAPS patients, peak concentrations of canakinumab occurred between 2 to 7 days following single subcutaneous administration of ILARIS 150 mg or 2 mg/kg in pediatric patients. The terminal half-life ranged from 22.9 to 25.7 days, similar to the pharmacokinetic properties observed in adults.

In SJIA, exposure parameters (such as AUC and Cmax) were comparable across age groups from 2 years of age and above following subcutaneous administration of canakinumab 4 mg/kg every 4 weeks.

13 NONCLINICAL TOXICOLOGY

13.1 Carcinogenesis, Mutagenesis, Impairment of Fertility

Long-term animal studies have not been performed to evaluate the carcinogenic potential of canakinumab.

The mutagenic potential of canakinumab was not evaluated.

As canakinumab does not cross-react with rodent IL-1β, male and female fertility was evaluated in a mouse model using a murine analog of canakinumab. Male mice were treated weekly beginning 4 weeks prior to mating and continuing through 3 weeks after mating. Female mice were treated weekly for 2 weeks prior to mating through gestation day 3 or 4. The murine analog of canakinumab did not alter either male or female fertility parameters at subcutaneous doses up to 150 mg/kg.

14 CLINICAL STUDIES

14.1 Treatment of CAPS

The efficacy and safety of ILARIS for the treatment of CAPS was demonstrated in CAPS Study 1, a 3-part trial in patients 9 to 74 years of age with the MWS phenotype of CAPS. Throughout the trial, patients weighing more than 40 kg received ILARIS 150 mg and patients weighing 15 to 40 kg received 2 mg/kg. Part 1 was an 8-week open-label, single-dose period where all patients received ILARIS. Patients who achieved a complete clinical response and did not relapse by Week 8 were randomized into Part 2, a 24-week randomized, double-blind, placebo-controlled withdrawal period. Patients who completed Part 2 or experienced a disease flare entered Part 3, a 16-week open-label active treatment phase. A complete response was defined as ratings of minimal or better for physician's assessment of disease activity (PHY) and assessment of skin disease (SKD) and had serum levels of C-Reactive Protein (CRP) and Serum Amyloid A (SAA) less than 10 mg/L. A disease flare was defined as a CRP and/or SAA values greater than 30 mg/L and either a score of mild or worse for PHY or a score of minimal or worse for PHY and SKD.

In Part 1, a complete clinical response was observed in 71% of patients one week following initiation of treatment and in 97% of patients by Week 8 (see Figure 1 and Table 2). In the randomized withdrawal period, a total of 81% of the patients randomized to placebo flared as compared to none (0%) of the patients randomized to ILARIS. The 95% confidence interval for treatment difference in the proportion of flares was 53% to 96%. At the end of Part 2, all 15 patients treated with ILARIS had absent or minimal disease activity and skin disease (see Table 3).

In a second trial, patients 4 to 74 years of age with both MWS and FCAS phenotypes of CAPS were treated in an open-label manner. Treatment with ILARIS resulted in clinically significant improvement of signs and symptoms and in normalization of high CRP and SAA in a majority of patients within 1 week.

[See table 3 at top of next page]

Markers of inflammation CRP and SAA normalized within 8 days of treatment in the majority of patients. Normal mean CRP (Figure 1) and SAA values were sustained throughout CAPS Study 1 in patients continuously treated with canakinumab. After withdrawal of canakinumab in Part 2 CRP (figure 1) and SAA values again returned to abnormal values and subsequently normalized after reintroduction of canakinumab in Part 3. The pattern of normalization of CRP and SAA was similar.

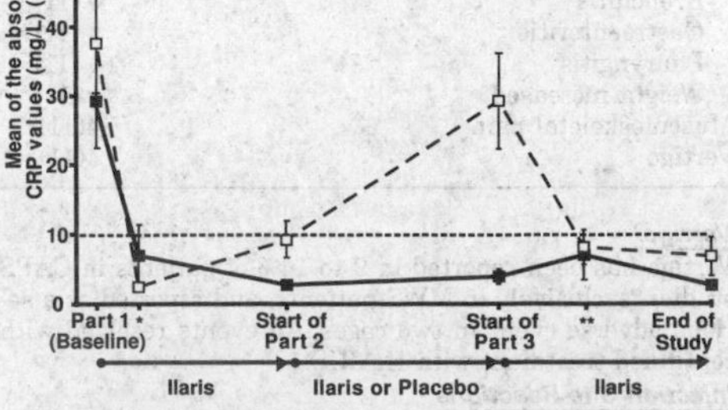

*1 week after the start of Part 1; **8 weeks after the start of Part 3

Figure 1. Mean C-Reactive Protein Levels at the End of Parts 1, 2 and 3 of CAPS Study 1

14.2 Treatment of SJIA

The efficacy of ILARIS for the treatment of active SJIA was assessed in two phase 3 studies (SJIA Study 1 and SJIA Study 2). Patients enrolled were aged 2 to less than 20 years (mean age at baseline: 8.5 years) with a confirmed diagnosis of SJIA at least 2 months before enrollment (mean disease duration at baseline: 3.5 years). Patients had active disease defined as greater than or equal to 2 joints with active arthritis (mean number of active joints at baseline: 15.4), documented spiking, intermittent fever (body temperature greater than 38°C) for at least 1 day within 1 week before study drug administration, and CRP greater than 30 mg/L (normal range less than 10 mg/L)(mean CRP at baseline: 200.5 mg/L). Patients were allowed to continue their stable dose of methotrexate, corticosteroids, and/or NSAIDs without change, except for tapering of the corticosteroid dose as per study design in SJIA Study 2 (see below).

SJIA Study 1 was a randomized, double-blind, placebo-controlled, single-dose 4-week study assessing the short term efficacy of ILARIS in 84 patients randomized to receive a single subcutaneous dose of 4 mg/kg ILARIS or placebo (43 patients received ILARIS and 41 patients received placebo). The primary objective of this study was to demonstrate the superiority of ILARIS versus placebo in the proportion of patients who achieved at least 30% improvement in an adapted pediatric American College of Rheumatology (ACR) response criterion which included both the pediatric ACR core set (ACR30 response) and absence of fever (temperature less than or equal to 38°C in the preceding 7 days) at Day 15.

Pediatric ACR responses are defined by achieving levels of percentage improvement (30%, 50%, and 70%) from baseline in at least 3 of the 6 core outcome variables, with worsening of greater than or equal to 30% in no more than one of the remaining variables. Core outcome variables included a physician global assessment of disease activity, parent or patient global assessment of wellbeing, number of joints with active arthritis, number of joints with limited range of motion, CRP, and functional ability (Childhood Health Assessment Questionnaire - CHAQ).

Percentages of patients by pediatric ACR response are presented in Table 4.

[See table 4 above]

Results for the components of the pediatric ACR core set were consistent with the overall ACR response results, for systemic and arthritic components including the reduction in the total number of active joints and joints with limited range of motion. Among the patients who returned for a Day 15 visit, the mean change in patient pain score (0-100 mm visual analogue scale) was -50.0 mm on ILARIS (N=43), as compared to +4.5 mm on placebo (N=25). The mean change in pain score among ILARIS treated patients was consistent through Day 29. All patients treated with ILARIS had no fever at Day 3 compared to 87% of patients treated with placebo.

SJIA Study 2 was a randomized, double-blind, placebo controlled, withdrawal study of flare prevention by ILARIS in patients with active SJIA. Flare was defined by worsening of greater than or equal to 30% in at least 3 of the 6 core Pediatric ACR response variables combined with improvement of greater than or equal to 30% in no more than 1 of the 6 variables, or reappearance of fever not due to infection for at least 2 consecutive days. The study consisted of two major parts. 177 patients were enrolled in the study and received 4mg/kg ILARIS subcutaneously every 4 weeks in Part I and 100 of these patients continued into Part II to receive either ILARIS 4mg/kg or placebo subcutaneously every 4 weeks.

Corticosteroid dose tapering

Of the total 128 patients who entered the open-label portion of Study 2 taking corticosteroids, 92 attempted corticosteroid tapering. Fifty-seven (62%) of the 92 patients who attempted to taper were able to successfully taper their corticosteroid dose and 42 (46%) discontinued corticosteroids

Time to Flare

Part II was a randomized withdrawal design to demonstrate that the time to flare was longer with ILARIS than with placebo. Follow-up stopped when 37 events had been observed resulting in patients being followed for different lengths of time. The probability of experiencing a flare over time in Part II was statistically lower for the ILARIS treatment group than for the placebo group (Figure 2). This corresponded to a 64% relative reduction in the risk of flare for patients in the ILARIS group as compared to those in the placebo group (hazard ratio of 0.36; 95% CI: 0.17 to 0.75).

[See figure 2 above]

Table 3 Physician's Global Assessment of Auto-Inflammatory Disease Activity and Assessment of Skin Disease: Frequency Table and Treatment Comparison in Part 2 (Using LOCF, ITT Population)

	ILARIS N= 15			Placebo N= 16	
	Baseline	Start of Part 2 (Week 8)	End of Part 2	Start of Part 2 (Week 8)	End of Part 2
Physician's Global Assessment of Auto-Inflammatory Disease Activity - n (%)					
Absent	0/31 (0)	9/15 (60)	8/15 (53)	8/16 (50)	0/16 (0)
Minimal	1/31 (3)	4/15 (27)	7/15 (47)	8/16 (50)	4/16 (25)
Mild	7/31 (23)	2/15 (13)	0/15 (0)	0/16 (0)	8/16 (50)
Moderate	19/31 (61)	0/15 (0)	0/15 (0)	0/16 (0)	4/16 (25)
Severe	4/31 (13)	0/15 (0)	0/15 (0)	0/16 (0)	0/16 (0)
Assessment of Skin Disease – n (%)					
Absent	3/31 (10)	13/15 (87)	14/15 (93)	13/16 (81)	5/16 (31)
Minimal	6/31 (19)	2/15 (13)	1/15 (7)	3/16 (19)	3/16 (19)
Mild	9/31 (29)	0/15 (0)	0/15 (0)	0/16 (0)	5/16 (31)
Moderate	12/31 (39)	0/15 (0)	0/15 (0)	0/16 (0)	3/16 (19)
Severe	1/32 (3)	0/15 (0)	0/15 (0)	0/16 (0)	0/16 (0)

Table 4 Pediatric ACR response at Days 15 and 29

	Day 15			Day 29		
	ILARIS N=43	**Placebo N=41**	**Weighted Difference[1] (95% CI)[2]**	**ILARIS N=43**	**Placebo N=41**	**Weighted Difference[1] (95% CI)[2]**
ACR30	84%	10%	70% (56%, 84%)	81%	10%	70% (56%, 84%)
ACR50	67%	5%	65% (50%, 80%)	79%	5%	76% (63%, 88%)
ACR70	60%	2%	64% (49%, 79%)	67%	2%	67% (52%, 81%)

[1]Weighted difference is the difference between the ILARIS and placebo response rates, adjusted for the stratification factors (number of active joints, previous response to anakinra, and level of oral corticosteroid use)
[2]CI: confidence interval for the weighted difference

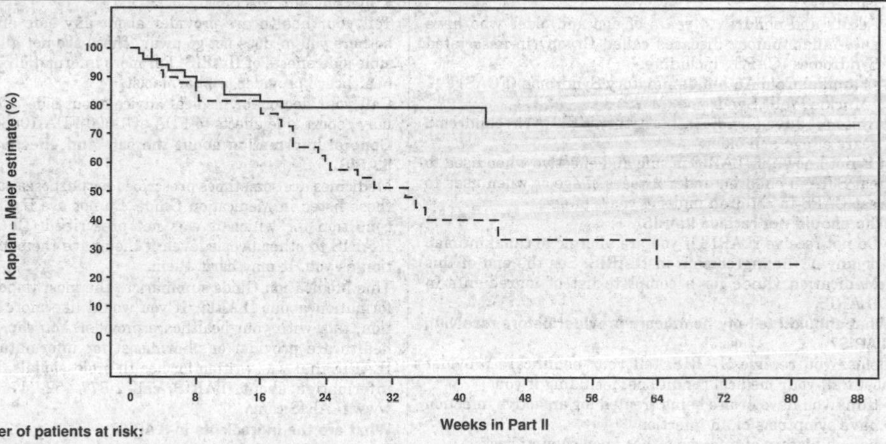

Number of patients at risk:	0	8	16	24	32	40	48	56	64	72	80	88
——— ACZ885	50	45	37	32	25	17	11	9	6	3	2	1
– – – Placebo	50	41	36	23	16	8	5	4	4	1	1	

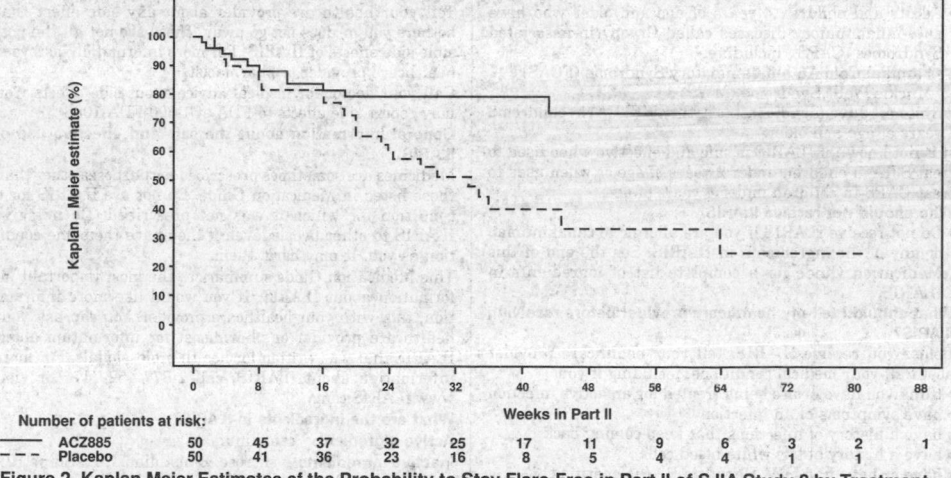

Figure 2. Kaplan Meier Estimates of the Probability to Stay Flare-Free in Part II of SJIA Study 2 by Treatment

*Very few patients were followed for more than 48 weeks

16 HOW SUPPLIED/STORAGE AND HANDLING

Carton of 1 vial NDC 0078-0582-61

Each single-use vial of ILARIS contains a sterile, preservative free, white lyophilized powder containing 180 mg of canakinumab. Each vial is to be reconstituted with 1 mL of preservative-free Sterile Water for Injection resulting in a final concentration of 150 mg/mL.

Special Precautions for Storage

The unopened vial must be stored refrigerated at 2 to 8° C (36 to 46° F). Do not freeze. Store in the original carton to protect from light. Do not use beyond the date stamped on the label. After reconstitution, ILARIS should be kept from light, and can be kept at room temperature if used within 60 minutes of reconstitution. Otherwise, it should be refrigerated at 2 to 8° C (36 to 46° F) and used within 4 hours of reconstitution. ILARIS does not contain preservatives. Unused portions of ILARIS should be discarded.

Keep this and all drugs out of the reach of children.

17 PATIENT COUNSELING INFORMATION

See FDA-approved patient labeling (Medication Guide)

Patients should be advised of the potential benefits and risks of ILARIS. Physicians should instruct their patients to read the Medication Guide before starting ILARIS therapy.

Drug Administration

Patients should be advised that healthcare providers should perform administration of ILARIS, by the subcutaneous injection route.

Infections

Patients should be cautioned that ILARIS use has been associated with serious infections. Patients should be counseled to contact their healthcare professional immediately if they develop an infection after starting ILARIS. Treatment with ILARIS should be discontinued if a patient develops a serious infection. Patients should be counseled not to take any IL-1 blocking drug, including ILARIS, if they are also taking a drug that blocks TNF such as etanercept, infliximab, or adalimumab. Use of ILARIS with other IL-1 blocking agents, such as rilonacept and anakinra is not recommended. Patients should be cautioned not to receive ILARIS if they have a chronic or active infection, including HIV, Hepatitis B or Hepatitis C.

Vaccinations

Prior to initiation of therapy with ILARIS, physicians should review with adult and pediatric patients their vaccination history relative to current medical guidelines for vaccine use, including taking into account the potential of increased risk of infection during treatment with ILARIS.

Injection-site Reactions

Physicians should explain to patients that a very small number of patients in the clinical trials experienced a reaction at the subcutaneous injection site. Injection-site reactions may include pain, erythema, swelling, pruritus, bruising, mass, inflammation, dermatitis, edema, urticaria, vesicles, warmth, and hemorrhage. Healthcare providers should be cautioned to avoid injecting into an area that is already swollen or red. Any persistent reaction should be brought to the attention of the prescribing physician.

Hypersensitivity

Patients should be counseled to contact their healthcare provider immediately if they develop signs of allergic reaction such as difficulty breathing or swallowing, nausea, dizziness, skin rash, itching, hives, palpitations or low blood pressure.

Manufactured by:
Novartis Pharma Stein AG
Stein, Switzerland
Distributed by:
Novartis Pharmaceuticals Corporation
East Hanover, New Jersey 07936
© Novartis
T2013-33
May 2013

Medication Guide

ILARIS® (i-LAHR-us)
(canakinumab)
injection for subcutaneous use

What is the most important information I should know about ILARIS?

ILARIS can cause serious side effects, including:

- **Increased risk of serious infections.** ILARIS can lower the ability of your immune system to fight infections. Your healthcare provider should:
  - test you for tuberculosis (TB) before you receive ILARIS
  - monitor you closely for symptoms of TB during treatment with ILARIS
  - check you for symptoms of any type of infection before, during, and after your treatment with ILARIS

Tell your healthcare provider right away if you have any symptoms of an infection such as fever, sweats or chills, cough, flu-like symptoms, weight loss, shortness of breath, blood in your phlegm, sores on your body, warm or painful areas on your body, diarrhea or stomach pain, or feeling very tired.

What is ILARIS?

ILARIS is a prescription medicine injected by your healthcare provider just below the skin (subcutaneous) used to treat:

- Adults and children 4 years of age and older who have auto-inflammatory diseases called Cryopyrin-Associated Syndromes (CAPS), including:
  - Familial Cold Auto-inflammatory Syndrome (FCAS)
  - Muckle-Wells Syndrome (MWS)
- Systemic Juvenile Idiopathic Arthritis (SJIA) in children 2 years of age and older.

It is not known if ILARIS is safe and effective when used to treat SJIA in children under 2 years of age or when used to treat CAPS in children under 4 years of age.

Who should not receive ILARIS?

- Do not receive ILARIS if you are allergic to canakinumab or any of the ingredients in ILARIS. See the end of this Medication Guide for a complete list of ingredients in ILARIS.

What should I tell my healthcare provider before receiving ILARIS?

Before you receive ILARIS, tell your healthcare provider about all your medical conditions, including if you:

- think you have or are being treated for an active infection
- have symptoms of an infection
- have a history of infections that keep coming back
- have a history of low white blood cells
- have or have had HIV, Hepatitis B, or Hepatitis C
- are scheduled to receive any immunizations (vaccines). You should not get 'live vaccines' if you are receiving ILARIS.
- are pregnant or planning to become pregnant. It is not known if ILARIS will harm your unborn baby. Tell your healthcare provider right away if you become pregnant while receiving ILARIS.
- are breastfeeding or planning to breastfeed. It is not known if ILARIS passes into your breast milk. You and your healthcare provider should decide if you will receive ILARIS or breastfeed. You should not do both.

Tell your healthcare provider about all the medicines you take, including prescription and nonprescription medicines, vitamins, and herbal supplements. Especially tell your healthcare provider if you take:

- Medicines that affect your immune system
- Medicines called IL-1 blocking agents such as Kineret® (anakinra), Arcalyst® (rilonacept)
- Medicines called Tumor Necrosis Factor (TNF) inhibitors such as Enbrel® (etanercept), Humira® (adalimumab), Remicade® (infliximab), Simponi® (golimumab), or Cimzia® (certolizumab pegol)
- Medicines that effect enzyme metabolism

Ask your healthcare provider if you are not sure.

How will I receive ILARIS?

- ILARIS is given by your healthcare provider every 8 weeks for CAPS and every 4 weeks for SJIA.

What are the possible side effects of ILARIS?

ILARIS can cause serious side effects, including:

- See "What is the most important information I should know about ILARIS?"
- **decreased ability of your body to fight infections (immunosuppression).** For people treated with medicines that cause immunosuppression like ILARIS, the chances of getting cancer may increase.
- **allergic reactions.** Allergic reactions can happen while you are receiving ILARIS. Call your healthcare provider right away if you have any of these symptoms of an allergic reaction:
  - rash
  - itching and hives
  - difficulty breathing or swallowing
  - dizziness or feeling faint
- **risk of infection with live vaccines.** You should not get live vaccines if you are receiving ILARIS. Tell your healthcare provider if you are scheduled to receive any vaccines.

The most common side effects of ILARIS include:

When ILARIS is used for the treatment of CAPS:

- cold symptoms
- diarrhea
- flu (influenza)
- runny nose
- nausea
- headache
- cough
- weight gain
- body aches
- feeling like you are spinning (vertigo)
- injection site reactions (such as redness, swelling, warmth, or itching)

When ILARIS is used for treatment of the SJIA:

- cold symptoms
- upper respiratory tract infection
- pneumonia
- runny nose
- sore throat
- urinary tract infection
- nausea, vomiting, and diarrhea (gastroenteritis)
- stomach pain
- injection site reactions

Tell your healthcare provider about any side effect that bothers you or does not go away. These are not all the possible side effects of ILARIS. For more information, ask your healthcare provider or pharmacist.

Call your doctor for medical advice about side effects. You may report side effects to FDA at 1-800-FDA-1088

General information about the safe and effective use of ILARIS.

Medicines are sometimes prescribed for purposes other than those listed in Medication Guide. Do not use ILARIS for a condition for which it was not prescribed. Do not give ILARIS to other people, even if they have the same condition as you. It may harm them.

This Medication Guide summarizes the most important information about ILARIS. If you would like more information, talk with your healthcare provider. You can ask your healthcare provider or pharmacist for information about ILARIS that was written for health professionals. For more information about ILARIS, call 1-877-452-7471 or visit www.ILARIS.com.

What are the ingredients in ILARIS?

Active ingredient: canakinumab

Inactive ingredients: sucrose, L-histidine, L-histidine HCl monohydrate, polysorbate 80, preservative-free sterile water for injection

What are CAPS?

CAPS are a group of illnesses that run in families where patients make too much IL-1β. The IL-1β triggers inflammation. This leads to symptoms such as rash, fever/chills, joint pain, fatigue, and eye pain and redness.

What is SJIA?

SJIA is an autoinflammatory disorder which can be caused by having too much or being too sensitive to certain proteins, including interleukin-1β (IL-1β), and can lead to symptoms such as fever, rash, headache, fatigue, or painful joints and muscles.

What is Macrophage Activation Syndrome (MAS)?

MAS is a syndrome associated with SJIA that can lead to death. Tell your healthcare provider right away if your SJIA symptoms get worse or if you have any of these symptoms of an infection:

- a fever lasting longer than 3 days
- a cough that does not go away
- redness in one part of your body
- warm feeling or swelling of your skin

This Medication Guide has been approved by the U.S. Food and Drug Administration.

Manufactured by:
Novartis Pharma Stein AG
Stein, Switzerland
Distributed by:
Novartis Pharmaceuticals Corporation
East Hanover, New Jersey 07936
© Novartis

Kineret®, Arcalyst®, Enbrel®, Humira®, Remicade®, Simponi®, and Cimzia® are trademarks of Amgen, Regeneron, Immunex Corporation, Abbott Laboratories, Centocor Ortho Biotech Inc., Janssen Biotech Inc., and the UCB Group of companies, respectively.

T2013-34
Revised: May 2013

Shown in Product Identification Guide, page 310

MYFORTIC® ℞

[mi-for-tic]
(mycophenolic acid)
delayed-release tablets, for oral use

The following prescribing information is based on official labeling in effect July 2013.

HIGHLIGHTS OF PRESCRIBING INFORMATION

These highlights do not include all the information needed to use MYFORTIC safely and effectively. See full prescribing information for MYFORTIC.

MYFORTIC® (mycophenolic acid) delayed-release tablets, for oral use

Initial U.S. Approval: 2004

> **WARNING: EMBRYOFETAL TOXICITY, MALIGNANCIES, AND SERIOUS INFECTIONS**
>
> ***See full prescribing information for complete boxed warning***
>
> - **Use during pregnancy is associated with increased risks of pregnancy loss and congenital malformations. Females of reproductive potential must be counseled regarding pregnancy prevention and planning. (5.1, 8.1, 8.6)**
> - **Increased risk of development of lymphoma and other malignancies, particularly of the skin, due to immunosuppression. (5.4)**
> - **Increased susceptibility to bacterial, viral, fungal, and protozoal infections, including opportunistic infections. (5.5, 5.6, 5.7)**
> - **Only physicians experienced in immunosuppressive therapy and management of organ transplant patients should prescribe Myfortic. (5.3)**

RECENT MAJOR CHANGES

Warnings and Precautions, Embryofetal Toxicity (5.1) 06/2012

INDICATIONS AND USAGE

- Myfortic is an antimetabolite immunosuppressant indicated for prophylaxis of organ rejection in adult patients receiving kidney transplants and in pediatric patients at least 5 years of age and older who are at least 6 months post kidney transplant. (1.1)
- Use in combination with cyclosporine and corticosteroids. (1.1)

Limitations of Use:

- Myfortic delayed release tablets and mycophenolate mofetil tablets and capsules should not be used interchangeably. (1.2)

DOSAGE AND ADMINISTRATION

- In adults: 720 mg by mouth, twice daily (1440 mg total daily dose) on an empty stomach, 1 hour before or 2 hours after food intake. (2.1)
- In children: 5 years of age and older (who are at least 6 months post kidney transplant), 400 mg/m^2 by mouth, twice daily (up to a maximum of 720 mg twice daily). (2.2)
- Do not crush, chew, or cut tablet prior to ingestion. (2.3)

DOSAGE FORMS AND STRENGTHS

Myfortic is available as 180 mg and 360 mg tablets. (3)

CONTRAINDICATIONS

Known hypersensitivity to mycophenolate sodium, mycophenolic acid, mycophenolate mofetil, or to any of its excipients. (4.1)

WARNINGS AND PRECAUTIONS

- Cytomegalovirus (CMV) Infections, including viremia and disease: Consider reducing immunosuppression. (5.7)
- Blood Dyscrasias including Pure Red Cell Aplasia (PRCA): Monitor for neutropenia or anemia; consider treatment interruption or dose reduction. (5.8)
- Serious GI Tract Complications (gastrointestinal bleeding, perforations and ulcers): Administer with caution to patients with active digestive system disease. (5.9)
- Immunizations: Avoid live vaccines. (5.10)

• Patients with Hereditary Deficiency of Hypoxanthine-guanine Phosphoribosyl-transferase (HGPRT): May cause exacerbation of disease symptoms; avoid use. (5.11)

ADVERSE REACTIONS

Most common adverse reactions (≥20%): anemia, leukopenia, constipation, nausea, diarrhea, vomiting, dyspepsia, urinary tract infection, CMV infection, insomnia, and postoperative pain. (6.2)

To report SUSPECTED ADVERSE REACTIONS, contact Novartis Pharmaceuticals Corporation at 1-888-669-6682 or FDA at 1-800-FDA-1088 or www.fda.gov/medwatch.

DRUG INTERACTIONS

• Antacids with Magnesium and Aluminum Hydroxides: Decreases concentrations of mycophenolic acid (MPA); concomitant use is not recommended. (7.1)
• Azathioprine: Competition for purine metabolism; concomitant administration is not recommended. (7.2)
• Cholestyramine, Bile Acid Sequestrates, Oral Activated Charcoal, and Other Drugs that Interfere with Enterohepatic Recirculation: May decrease MPA concentrations; concomitant use is not recommended. (7.3)
• Sevelamer: May decrease MPA concentrations; concomitant use is not recommended. (7.4)
• Cyclosporine: May decrease MPA concentrations; exercise caution when switching from cyclosporine to other drugs or from other drugs to cyclosporine. (7.5)
• Norfloxacin and Metronidazole: May decrease MPA concentrations; concomitant use with both drugs is not recommended. (7.6)
• Rifampin: May decrease MPA concentrations; concomitant use is not recommended unless the benefit outweighs the risk. (7.7)
• Hormonal contraceptives: Additional barrier contraceptive methods must be used. (5.2, 7.8)
• Acyclovir, Valacyclovir, Ganciclovir, Valganciclovir, and Other Drugs that Undergo Renal Tubular Secretion: May increase concentrations of mycophenolic acid glucuronide (MPAG) and coadministered drug; monitor blood cell counts. (7.9)

USE IN SPECIFIC POPULATIONS

• Pregnancy: Can cause fetal harm. (5.1, 8.1)
• Nursing mothers: Discontinue drug or discontinue nursing while on treatment or within 6 weeks after stopping therapy, taking into consideration the importance of the drug to the mother. (8.3)
• Females of reproductive potential must be counseled regarding pregnancy prevention and planning. (5.2, 8.6)

See 17 for PATIENT COUNSELING INFORMATION and Medication Guide

Revised: 05/2013

FULL PRESCRIBING INFORMATION: CONTENTS*

*** Sections or subsections omitted from the full prescribing information are not listed**

FULL PRESCRIBING INFORMATION

WARNING: EMBRYOFETAL TOXICITY, MALIGNANCIES, AND SERIOUS INFECTIONS

- **Use during pregnancy is associated with increased risks of pregnancy loss and congenital malformations. Females of reproductive potential must be counseled regarding pregnancy prevention and planning [*see Warnings and Precautions (5.1) and Use in Specific Populations (8.1, 8.6)*].**
- **Increased risk of development of lymphoma and other malignancies, particularly of the skin, due to immunosuppression [*see Warnings and Precautions (5.4)*].**
- **Increased susceptibility to bacterial, viral, fungal, and protozoal infections, including opportunistic infections [*see Warnings and Precautions (5.5, 5.6, and 5.7)*].**
- **Only physicians experienced in immunosuppressive therapy and management of organ transplant patients should prescribe Myfortic. Patients receiving Myfortic should be managed in facilities equipped and staffed with adequate laboratory and supportive medical resources. The physician responsible for maintenance therapy should have complete information requisite for the follow-up of the patient [*see Warnings and Precautions (5.3)*].**

1 INDICATIONS AND USAGE

1.1 Prophylaxis of Organ Rejection in Kidney Transplant

Myfortic® (mycophenolic acid) is indicated for the prophylaxis of organ rejection in adult patients receiving a kidney transplant.

Myfortic is indicated for the prophylaxis of organ rejection in pediatric patients 5 years of age and older who are at least 6 months post kidney transplant.

Myfortic is to be used in combination with cyclosporine and corticosteroids.

1.2 Limitations of Use

Myfortic delayed-release tablets and mycophenolate mofetil (MMF) tablets and capsules should not be used interchangeably without physician supervision because the rate of absorption following the administration of these two products is not equivalent.

2 DOSAGE AND ADMINISTRATION

2.1 Dosage in Adult Kidney Transplant Patients

The recommended dose of Myfortic is 720 mg administered twice daily (1440 mg total daily dose).

2.2 Dosage in Pediatric Kidney Transplant Patients

The recommended dose of Myfortic in conversion (at least 6 months post-transplant) pediatric patients age 5 years and older is 400 mg/m^2 body surface area (BSA) administered twice daily (up to a maximum dose of 720 mg administered twice daily).

2.3 Administration

Myfortic tablets should be taken on an empty stomach, 1 hour before or 2 hours after food intake [**see Clinical Pharmacology (12.3)**].

Myfortic tablets should not be crushed, chewed, or cut prior to ingesting. The tablets should be swallowed whole in order to maintain the integrity of the enteric coating.

Pediatric patients with a BSA of 1.19 to 1.58 m^2 may be dosed either with three Myfortic 180 mg tablets, or one 180 mg tablet plus one 360 mg tablet twice daily (1080 mg daily dose). Patients with a BSA of >1.58 m^2 may be dosed either with four Myfortic 180 mg tablets, or two Myfortic 360 mg tablets twice daily (1440 mg daily dose). Pediatric doses for patients with BSA <1.19 m^2 cannot be accurately administered using currently available formulations of Myfortic tablets.

3 DOSAGE FORMS AND STRENGTHS

Myfortic is available as 360 mg and 180 mg tablets.

Table 1: Description of Myfortic (mycophenolic acid) Delayed-Release Tablets

Dosage Strength	360 mg	180 mg
Active ingredient	mycophenolic acid as mycophenolate sodium	mycophenolic acid as mycophenolate sodium
Appearance	Pale orange-red film-coated ovaloid tablet	Lime green film-coated round tablet with bevelled edges
Imprint	"CT" on one side	"C" on one side

4 CONTRAINDICATIONS

4.1 Hypersensitivity Reactions

Myfortic is contraindicated in patients with a hypersensitivity to mycophenolate sodium, mycophenolic acid, mycophenolate mofetil, or to any of its excipients. Reactions like rash, pruritus, hypotension, and chest pain have been observed in clinical trials and post marketing reports [*see Adverse Reactions (6)*].

5 WARNINGS AND PRECAUTIONS

5.1 Embryofetal Toxicity

Use of Myfortic during pregnancy is associated with an increased risk of first trimester pregnancy loss and an increased risk of congenital malformations, especially external ear and other facial abnormalities including cleft lip and palate, and anomalies of the distal limbs, heart, esophagus, and kidney [*see Use in Specific Populations (8.1)*].

5.2 Pregnancy Exposure Prevention and Planning

Females of reproductive potential must be aware of the increased risk of first trimester pregnancy loss and congenital malformations and must be counseled regarding pregnancy prevention and planning. For recommended pregnancy testing and contraception methods see *Use in Specific Populations (8.6)*.

5.3 Management of Immunosuppression

Only physicians experienced in immunosuppressive therapy and management of organ transplant patients should prescribe Myfortic. Patients receiving the drug should be managed in facilities equipped and staffed with adequate laboratory and supportive medical resources. The physicians responsible for maintenance therapy should have complete information requisite for the follow up of the patient. [*see Boxed Warning*]

5.4 Lymphoma and Other Malignancies

Patients receiving immunosuppressants, including Myfortic, are at increased risk of developing lymphomas and other malignancies, particularly of the skin [*see Adverse Reactions (6)*]. The risk appears to be related to the intensity and duration of immunosuppression rather than to the use of any specific agent.

As usual for patients with increased risk for skin cancer, exposure to sunlight and UV light should be limited by wearing protective clothing and using a sunscreen with a high protection factor.

Post-transplant lymphoproliferative disorder (PTLD) has been reported in immunosuppressed organ transplant recipients. The majority of PTLD events appear related to Epstein Barr Virus (EBV) infection. The risk of PTLD appears greatest in those individuals who are EBV seronegative, a population which includes many young children.

5.5 Serious Infections

Patients receiving immunosuppressants, including Myfortic, are at increased risk of developing bacterial, viral, fungal, and protozoal infections, including opportunistic infections [*see Boxed Warning and Warnings and Precautions (5.6, 5.7)*]. These infections may lead to serious, including fatal outcomes. Because of the danger of over suppression of the immune system which can increase susceptibility to infection, combination immunosuppressant therapy should be used with caution.

5.6 Polyomavirus Infections

Patients receiving immunosuppressants, including Myfortic, are at increased risk for opportunistic infections,

Table 2: Adverse Reactions (%) Reported in ≥10% of de novo Kidney Transplant Patients in Either Treatment Group

System organ class Adverse drug reactions	*de novo* Renal Trial Myfortic 1.44 grams per day (n=213)	 mycophenolate mofetil (MMF) 2 grams per day (n=210)
Blood and Lymphatic System Disorders		
Anemia	22	22
Leukopenia	19	21
Gastrointestinal System Disorders		
Constipation	38	40
Nausea	29	27
Diarrhea	24	25
Vomiting	23	20
Dyspepsia	23	19
Abdominal pain upper	14	14
Flatulence	10	13
General and Administrative Site Disorders		
Edema	17	18
Edema lower limb	16	17
Pyrexia	13	19
Investigations		
Increased blood creatinine	15	10
Infections and Infestations		
Urinary Tract Infection	29	33
CMV Infection	20	18
Metabolism and Nutrition Disorders		
Hypocalcemia	11	15
Hyperuricemia	13	13
Hyperlipidemia	12	10
Hypokalemia	13	9
Hypophosphatemia	11	9
Musculoskeletal, Connective Tissue and Bone Disorders		
Back pain	12	6
Arthralgia	7	11
Nervous System Disorder		
Insomnia	24	24
Tremor	12	14
Headache	13	11
Vascular Disorders		
Hypertension	18	18

**The trial was not designed to support comparative claims for Myfortic for the adverse reactions reported in this table

including polyomavirus infections. Polyomavirus infections in transplant patients may have serious, and sometimes fatal outcomes. These include cases of JC virus associated progressive multifocal leukoencephalopathy (PML) and polyomavirus associated nephropathy (PVAN) especially due to BK virus infection which have been observed in patients receiving Myfortic.

PVAN, especially due to BK virus infection, is associated with serious outcomes, including deteriorating renal function and renal graft loss. Patient monitoring may help detect patients at risk for PVAN.

Cases of PML, have been reported in patients treated with mycophenolic acid (MPA) derivatives which include MMF and mycophenolate sodium. PML, which is sometimes fatal, commonly presents with hemiparesis, apathy, confusion, cognitive deficiencies, and ataxia. Risk factors for PML include treatment with immunosuppressant therapies and impairment of immune function. In immunosuppressed patients, physicians should consider PML in the differential diagnosis in patients reporting neurological symptoms and consultation with a neurologist should be considered as clinically indicated.

Reduction in immunosuppression should be considered for patients who develop evidence of PML or PVAN. Physicians should also consider the risk that reduced immunosuppression represents to the functioning allograft.

5.7 Cytomegalovirus (CMV) Infections

Patients receiving immunosuppressants, including Myfortic, are at increased risk of developing CMV viremia and CMV disease. The risk of CMV disease is highest among transplant recipients seronegative for CMV at time of transplant who receive a graft from a CMV seropositive donor. Therapeutic approaches to limiting CMV disease exist and should be routinely provided. Patient monitoring may help detect patients at risk for CMV disease. Consideration should be given to reducing the amount of immunosuppression in patients who develop CMV viremia and/or CMV disease [see Adverse Reactions (6.1)].

5.8 Blood Dyscrasias Including Pure Red Cell Aplasia

Cases of pure red cell aplasia (PRCA) have been reported in patients treated with MPA derivatives in combination with other immunosuppressive agents. The mechanism for MPA derivatives induced PRCA is unknown; the relative contribution of other immunosuppressants and their combinations in an immunosuppressive regimen is also unknown. In some cases PRCA was found to be reversible with dose reduction or cessation of therapy with MPA derivatives. In transplant patients, however, reduced immunosuppression may place the graft at risk. Changes to Myfortic therapy should only be undertaken under appropriate supervision in transplant recipients in order to minimize the risk of graft rejection.

Patients receiving Myfortic should be monitored for blood dyscrasias (e.g., neutropenia or anemia). The development of neutropenia may be related to Myfortic itself, concomitant medications, viral infections, or some combination of these reactions. Complete blood count should be performed weekly during the first month, twice monthly for the second and the third month of treatment, then monthly through the first year. If blood dyscrasias occur [neutropenia develops (ANC $<1.3 \times 10^3/\mu L$) or anemia], dosing with Myfortic should be interrupted or the dose reduced, appropriate tests performed, and the patient managed accordingly.

5.9 Serious GI Tract Complications

Gastrointestinal bleeding (requiring hospitalization), intestinal perforations, gastric ulcers, and duodenal ulcers have been reported in patients treated with Myfortic. Myfortic should be administered with caution in patients with active serious digestive system disease.

5.10 Immunizations

The use of live attenuated vaccines should be avoided during treatment with Myfortic; examples include (but not limited to) the following: intranasal influenza, measles, mumps, rubella, oral polio, BCG, yellow fever, varicella, and TY21a typhoid vaccines.

5.11 Rare Hereditary Deficiencies

Myfortic is an inosine monophosphate dehydrogenase inhibitor (IMPDH Inhibitor). Myfortic should be avoided in patients with rare hereditary deficiency of hypoxanthine-guanine phosphoribosyl-transferase (HGPRT) such as Lesch-Nyhan and Kelley-Seegmiller syndromes because it may cause an exacerbation of disease symptoms characterized by the overproduction and accumulation of uric acid leading to symptoms associated with gout such as acute arthritis, tophi, nephrolithiasis or urolithiasis and renal disease including renal failure.

6 ADVERSE REACTIONS

The following adverse reactions are discussed in greater detail in other sections of the label.

- Embryofetal toxicity [*see Boxed Warning, Warnings and Precautions (5.1)*]
- Lymphomas and other malignancies [*see Boxed Warning, Warnings and Precautions (5.4)*]
- Serious infections [*see Boxed Warning, Warnings and Precautions (5.5)*]
- Polyomavirus infections including PML [*see Boxed Warning, Warnings and Precautions (5.6)*]
- Cytomegalovirus (CMV) infections [*see Boxed Warning, Warnings and Precautions (5.7)*]
- Blood dyscrasias including pure red cell aplasia [*see Warnings and Precautions (5.8)*]
- Serious GI tract complications [*see Warnings and Precautions (5.9)*]
- Rare hereditary deficiencies [*see Warnings and Precautions (5.11)*]

6.1 Clinical Studies Experience

Because clinical trials are conducted under widely varying conditions, adverse reaction rates observed in the clinical trials of a drug cannot be directly compared to rates in the clinical trials of another drug and may not reflect the rates observed in practice.

The data described below derive from two randomized, comparative, active-controlled, double-blind, double-dummy trials in prevention of acute rejection in *de novo* and converted stable kidney transplant patients.

In the *de novo* trial, patients were administered either Myfortic 1.44 grams per day (N=213) or MMF 2 grams per day (N=210) within 48 hours post-transplant for 12 months in combination with cyclosporine, USP MODIFIED and corticosteroids. Forty-one percent of patients also received antibody therapy as induction treatment. In the conversion trial, renal transplant patients who were at least 6 months post-transplant and receiving 2 grams per day MMF in combination with cyclosporine USP MODIFIED, with or without corticosteroids for at least two weeks prior to entry in the trial were randomized to Myfortic 1.44 grams per day (N=159) or MMF 2 grams per day (N=163) for 12 months.

The average age of patients in both studies was 47 years and 48 years (*de novo* study and conversion study, respectively), ranging from 22 to 75 years. Approximately 66% of patients were male; 82% were white, 12% were black, and 6% other races. About 40% of patients were from the United States and 60% from other countries.

In the *de novo* trial, the overall incidence of discontinuation due to adverse reactions was 18% (39/213) and 17% (35/210) in the Myfortic and MMF arms, respectively. The most common adverse reactions leading to discontinuation in the Myfortic arm were graft loss (2%), diarrhea (2%), vomiting (1%), renal impairment (1%), CMV infection (1%), and leukopenia (1%). The overall incidence of patients reporting dose reduction at least once during the 0-12 month study period was 59% and 60% in the Myfortic and MMF arms, respectively. The most frequent reasons for dose reduction in the Myfortic arm were adverse reactions (44%), dose reductions according to protocol guidelines (17%), dosing errors (11%) and missing data (2%).

The most common adverse reactions (≥20%) associated with the administration of Myfortic were anemia, leukopenia, constipation, nausea, diarrhea, vomiting, dyspepsia, urinary tract infection, CMV infection, insomnia and postoperative pain.

The adverse reactions reported in ≥10% of patients in the *de novo* trial are presented in the Table 2 below.

[See table 2 above]

Table 3 summarizes the incidence of opportunistic infections in *de novo* transplant patients.

Table 3: Viral and Fungal Infections (%) Reported Over 0–12 Months

	de novo Renal Trial Myfortic 1.44 grams per day (n=213) (%)	 mycophenolate mofetil (MMF) 2 grams per day (n=210) (%)
Any Cytomegalovirus	22	21
- Cytomegalovirus Disease	5	4
Herpes Simplex	8	6
Herpes Zoster	5	4
Any Fungal Infection	11	12
- Candida NOS	6	6
- Candida albicans	2	4

Lymphoma developed in 2 *de novo* patients (1%), (1 diagnosed 9 days after treatment initiation) and in 2 conversion patients (1%) receiving Myfortic with other immunosuppressive agents in the 12-month controlled clinical trials. Nonmelanoma skin carcinoma occurred in 1% *de novo* and 12% conversion patients. Other types of malignancy occurred in 1% de novo and 1% conversion patients [*see Warnings and Precautions (5.4)*].

The adverse reactions reported in <10% of *de novo* or conversion patients treated with Myfortic in combination with cyclosporine and corticosteroids are listed in Table 4.

Table 4: Adverse Reactions Reported in <10% of Patients Treated with Myfortic in Combination with Cyclosporine* and Corticosteroids

Blood and Lymphatic Disorders	Lymphocele, thrombocytopenia
Cardiac Disorder	Tachycardia
Eye Disorder	Vision blurred
Gastrointestinal Disorders	Abdominal pain, abdominal distension, gastroesophageal reflux disease, gingival hyperplasia
General Disorders and Administration Site Conditions	Fatigue, peripheral edema
Infections and Infestations	Nasopharyngitis, herpes simplex, upper respiratory infection, oral candidiasis, herpes zoster, sinusitis, influenza, wound infection, implant infection, pneumonia, sepsis
Investigations	Hemoglobin decrease, liver function tests abnormal
Metabolism and Nutrition Disorders	Hypercholesterolemia, hyperkalemia, hypomagnesemia, diabetes mellitus, hyperglycemia
Musculoskeletal and Connective Tissue Disorders	Arthralgia, pain in limb, peripheral swelling, muscle cramps, myalgia
Nervous System Disorders	Dizziness (excluding vertigo)
Psychiatric Disorders	Anxiety
Renal and Urinary Disorders	Renal tubular necrosis, renal impairment, hematuria, urinary retention
Respiratory, Thoracic and Mediastinal Disorders	Cough, dyspnea, dyspnea exertional
Skin and Subcutaneous Tissue Disorders	Acne, pruritus, rash
Vascular Disorders	Hypertension aggravated, hypotension

* USP MODIFIED

The following additional adverse reactions have been associated with the exposure to mycophenolic acid (MPA) when administered as a sodium salt or as mofetil ester:

Gastrointestinal: Intestinal perforation, gastrointestinal hemorrhage, gastric ulcers, duodenal ulcers [*see Warnings and Precautions (5.9)*], colitis (including CMV colitis), pancreatitis, esophagitis, and ileus.

Infections: Serious life-threatening infections such as meningitis and infectious endocarditis, tuberculosis, and atypical mycobacterial infection [*see Warnings and Precautions (5.5)*].

Respiratory: Interstitial lung disorders, including fatal pulmonary fibrosis.

6.2 Postmarketing Experience

The following adverse reactions have been identified during post-approval use of Myfortic or other MPA derivatives. Because these reactions are reported voluntarily from a population of uncertain size, it is not always possible to reliably estimate their frequency or establish a causal relationship to drug exposure.

- Congenital malformations and an increased incidence of first trimester pregnancy loss have been reported following exposure to MMF during pregnancy [*see Boxed Warning, Warnings and Precautions (5.1)*].
- Cases of progressive multifocal leukoencephalopathy (PML), sometimes fatal, have been reported in patients treated with MPA derivatives [*see Warnings and Precautions (5.6)*].
- Polyomavirus associated nephropathy (PVAN), especially due to BK virus infection, has been observed in patients receiving immunosuppressants, including Myfortic. This infection is associated with serious outcomes, including deteriorating renal function and renal graft loss [*see Warnings and Precautions (5.6)*].
- Cases of pure red cell aplasia (PRCA) have been reported in patients treated with MPA derivatives in combination with other immunosuppressive agents [*see Warnings and Precautions (5.8)*].

The following additional adverse reactions have been identified during postapproval use of Myfortic: agranulocytosis, asthenia, osteomyelitis, lymphadenopathy, lymphopenia, wheezing, dry mouth, gastritis, peritonitis, anorexia, alopecia, pulmonary edema, Kaposi's sarcoma.

7 DRUG INTERACTIONS

7.1 Antacids with Magnesium and Aluminum Hydroxides

Concomitant use of Myfortic and antacids decreased plasma concentrations of mycophenolic acid (MPA). It is recommended that Myfortic and antacids not be administered simultaneously [*see Clinical Pharmacology (12.3)*].

7.2 Azathioprine

Given that azathioprine and MMF inhibit purine metabolism, it is recommended that Myfortic not be administered concomitantly with azathioprine or MMF.

7.3 Cholestyramine, Bile Acid Sequestrates, Oral Activated Charcoal and Other Drugs that Interfere with Enterohepatic Recirculation

Drugs that interrupt enterohepatic recirculation may decrease MPA plasma concentrations when coadministered with MMF. Therefore, do not administer Myfortic with cholestyramine or other agents that may interfere with enterohepatic recirculation or drugs that may bind bile acids, e.g., bile acid sequestrates or oral activated charcoal, because of the potential to reduce the efficacy of Myfortic [*see Clinical Pharmacology (12.3)*].

7.4 Sevelamer

Concomitant administration of sevelamer and MMF may decrease MPA plasma concentrations. Sevelamer and other calcium free phosphate binders should not be administered simultaneously with Myfortic [*see Clinical Pharmacology (12.3)*].

7.5 Cyclosporine

Cyclosporine inhibits the enterohepatic recirculation of MPA, and therefore, MPA plasma concentrations may be decreased when Myfortic is coadministered with cyclosporine. Clinicians should be aware that there is also a potential change of MPA plasma concentrations after switching from cyclosporine to other immunosuppressive drugs or from other immunosuppressive drugs to cyclosporine in patients concomitantly receiving Myfortic [*see Clinical Pharmacology (12.3)*].

7.6 Norfloxacin and Metronidazole

MPA plasma concentrations may be decreased when MMF is administrated with norfloxacin and metronidazole. Therefore, Myfortic is not recommended to be given with the combination of norfloxacin and metronidazole. Although there will be no effect on MPA plasma concentrations when Myfortic is concomitantly administered with norfloxacin or metronidazole when given separately [*see Clinical Pharmacology (12.3)*].

7.7 Rifampin

The concomitant administration of MMF and rifampin may decrease MPA plasma concentrations. Therefore, Myfortic is not recommended to be given with rifampin concomitantly unless the benefit outweighs the risk [*see Clinical Pharmacology (12.3)*].

7.8 Hormonal Contraceptives

In a drug interaction study, mean levonorgestrel AUC was decreased by 15% when coadministered with MMF. Although Myfortic may not have any influence on the ovulation-suppressing action of oral contraceptives, it is recommended to coadminister Myfortic with hormonal contraceptives (e.g., birth control pill, transdermal patch, vaginal ring, injection, and implant) with caution, and additional barrier contraceptive methods must be used [*see Warnings and Precautions (5.2), Use in Specific Populations (8.6), and Clinical Pharmacology (12.3)*].

7.9 Acyclovir (Valacyclovir), Ganciclovir (Valganciclovir), and Other Drugs that Undergo Renal Tubular Secretion

The coadministration of MMF and acyclovir or ganciclovir may increase plasma concentrations of mycophenolic acid glucuronide (MPAG) and acyclovir/valacyclovir/ganciclovir/valganciclovir as their coexistence competes for tubular secretion. Both acyclovir/valacyclovir/ganciclovir/valganciclovir and MPAG concentrations will be also increased in the presence of renal impairment.

Acyclovir/valacyclovir/ganciclovir/valganciclovir may be taken with Myfortic; however, during the period of treatment, physicians should monitor blood cell counts [*see Clinical Pharmacology (12.3)*].

7.10 Ciprofloxacin, Amoxicillin plus Clavulanic Acid and Other Drugs that Alter the Gastrointestinal Flora

Drugs that alter the gastrointestinal flora such as ciprofloxacin or amoxicillin plus clavulanic acid may interact with MMF by disrupting enterohepatic recirculation. Interference of MPAG hydrolysis may lead to less MPA available for absorption when Myfortic is concomitantly administered with ciprofloxacin or amoxicillin plus clavulanic acid. The clinical relevance of this interaction is unclear; however, no dose adjustment of Myfortic is needed when coadministered with these drugs [*see Clinical Pharmacology (12.3)*].

7.11 Pantoprazole

Administration of a pantoprazole at a dose of 40 mg twice daily for 4 days to healthy volunteers did not alter the pharmacokinetics of a single dose of Myfortic [*see Clinical Pharmacology (12.3)*].

8 USE IN SPECIFIC POPULATIONS

8.1 Pregnancy

Pregnancy Category D [*See Warnings and Precautions (5.1)*]

For those females using Myfortic at any time during pregnancy and those becoming pregnant within 6 weeks of discontinuing therapy, the healthcare practitioner should report the pregnancy to the Mycophenolate Pregnancy Registry (1-800-617-8191). The healthcare practitioner should strongly encourage the patient to enroll in the pregnancy registry. The information provided to the registry will help the Health Care Community to better understand the effects of mycophenolate in pregnancy.

Risk Summary

Following oral or intravenous (IV) administration, MMF is metabolized to mycophenolic acid (MPA), the active ingredient in Myfortic and the active form of the drug. Use of MMF during pregnancy is associated with an increased risk of first trimester pregnancy loss and an increased risk of congenital malformations, especially external ear and other facial abnormalities including cleft lip and palate, and anomalies of the distal limbs, heart, esophagus, and kidney. In animal studies, congenital malformations and pregnancy loss occurred when pregnant rats and rabbits received mycophenolic acid at dose multiples similar to and less than clinical doses.

Risks and benefits of Myfortic should be discussed with the patient. When appropriate, consider alternative immunosuppressants with less potential for embryofetal toxicity. In certain situations, the patient and her healthcare practitioner may decide that the maternal benefits outweigh the risks to the fetus. If this drug is used during pregnancy, or if the patient becomes pregnant while taking this drug, the patient should be apprised of the potential hazard to the fetus.

Data

Human Data

In the National Transplantation Pregnancy Registry (NTPR), there were data on 33 MMF-exposed pregnancies in 24 transplant patients; there were 15 spontaneous abortions (45%) and 18 live-born infants. Four of these 18 infants had structural malformations (22%). In postmarketing data (collected from 1995 to 2007) on 77 women exposed to systemic MMF during pregnancy, 25 had spontaneous abortions and 14 had a malformed infant or fetus. Six of 14 malformed offspring had ear abnormalities. Because these postmarketing data are reported voluntarily, it is not always possible to reliably estimate the frequency of particular adverse outcomes. These malformations are similar to findings in animal reproductive toxicology studies. For comparison, the background rate for congenital anomalies in the United States is about 3%, and NTPR data show a rate of 4–5% among babies born to organ transplant patients using other immunosuppressive drugs. There are no relevant qualitative or quantitative differences in the teratogenic potential of mycophenolate sodium and MMF.

Animal Data

In a teratology study performed with mycophenolate sodium in rats, at a dose as low as 1 mg per kg, malformations in the offspring were observed, including anophthalmia, exencephaly, and umbilical hernia. The systemic exposure at this dose represents 0.05 times the clinical exposure at the dose of 1440 mg per day Myfortic. In teratology studies in rabbits, fetal resorptions and malformations occurred at doses equal to or greater than 80 mg per kg per day, in the absence of maternal toxicity (which corresponds to about 1.1 times the recommended clinical dose, based on body surface area).

8.3 Nursing Mothers

It is not known whether MPA is excreted in human milk. Because many drugs are excreted in human milk and because of the potential for serious adverse reactions in nursing infants from Myfortic, a decision should be made whether to discontinue nursing or discontinue the drug, taking into account the importance of the drug to the mother.

8.4 Pediatric Use

The safety and effectiveness of Myfortic have been established in pediatric kidney transplant patients 5 to 16 years of age who were initiated on Myfortic at least 6 months post-transplant. Use of Myfortic in this age group is supported by evidence from adequate and well-controlled studies of Myfortic in a similar population of adult kidney transplant patients with additional pharmacokinetic data in pediatric kidney transplant patients [*see Dosage and Administration (2.2, 2.3) and Clinical Pharmacology (12.3)*]. Pediatric doses for patients with BSA <1.19 m^2 cannot be accurately administered using currently available formulations of Myfortic tablets.

The safety and effectiveness of Myfortic in de novo pediatric kidney transplant patients and in pediatric kidney transplant patients below the age of 5 years have not been established.

8.5 Geriatric Use

Clinical studies of Myfortic did not include sufficient numbers of subjects aged 65 and over to determine whether they respond differently from younger subjects. Of the 372 patients treated with Myfortic in the clinical trials, 6% (N=21) were 65 years of age and older and 0.3% (N=1) were 75 years of age and older. Other reported clinical experience has not identified differences in responses between the elderly and younger patients. In general, dose selection for an elderly patient should be cautious, reflecting the greater frequency of decreased hepatic, renal, or cardiac function, and of concomitant disease or other drug therapy.

8.6 Females of Reproductive Potential

Pregnancy Exposure Prevention and Planning

Females of reproductive potential must be made aware of the increased risk of first trimester pregnancy loss and congenital malformations and must be counseled regarding pregnancy prevention and planning.

Females of reproductive potential include girls who have entered puberty and all women who have a uterus and have not passed through menopause. Menopause is the permanent end of menstruation and fertility. Menopause should be clinically confirmed by a patient's healthcare practitioner. Some commonly used diagnostic criteria include 1) 12 months of spontaneous amenorrhea (not amenorrhea induced by a medical condition or medical therapy), or 2) post-surgical from a bilateral oophorectomy.

Pregnancy Testing

To prevent unplanned exposure during pregnancy, females of reproductive potential should have a serum or urine pregnancy test with a sensitivity of at least 25 mIU/mL immediately before starting Myfortic. Another pregnancy test with the same sensitivity should be done 8 to 10 days later. Repeat pregnancy tests should be performed during routine follow-up visits. Results of all pregnancy tests should be discussed with the patient.

In the event of a positive pregnancy test, females should be counseled with regard to whether the maternal benefits of mycophenolate treatment may outweigh the risks to the fetus in certain situations.

Contraception

Females of reproductive potential taking Myfortic must receive contraceptive counseling and use acceptable contraception (see Table 5 for Acceptable Contraception Methods). Patients must use acceptable birth control during entire Myfortic therapy, and for 6 weeks after stopping Myfortic, unless the patient chooses abstinence (she chooses to avoid heterosexual intercourse completely).

Patients should be aware that Myfortic reduces blood levels of the hormones in the oral contraceptive pill and could theoretically reduce its effectiveness [*see Patient Counseling Information (17) and Drug Interactions (7.8)*].

Table 5: Acceptable Contraception Methods for Females of Reproductive Potential

Pick from the following birth control options:

Option 1

Methods to Use Alone	Intrauterine devices (IUDs) Tubal sterilization Patient's partner had a vasectomy

OR

Option 2	**Hormone Methods** choose 1		**Barrier Methods** choose 1
Choose One Hormone Method *AND* **One Barrier Method**	**Estrogen and Progesterone** Oral Contraceptive Pill Transdermal patch Vaginal ring **Progesterone-only** Injection	*AND*	Diaphragm with spermicide Cervical cap with spermicide Contraceptive sponge Male condom Female condom

OR

Option 3	**Barrier Methods** choose 1		**Barrier Methods** choose 1
Choose One Barrier Method from each column *(must choose two methods)*	Diaphragm with spermicide Cervical cap with spermicide Contraceptive sponge	*AND*	Male condom Female condom

Pregnancy Planning

For patients who are considering pregnancy, consider alternative immunosuppressants with less potential for embryofetal toxicity. Risks and benefits of Myfortic should be discussed with the patient.

10 OVERDOSAGE

Signs and Symptoms

There have been anecdotal reports of deliberate or accidental overdoses with Myfortic, whereas not all patients experienced related adverse reactions.

In those overdose cases in which adverse reactions were reported, the reactions fall within the known safety profile of the class. Accordingly an overdose of Myfortic could possibly result in oversuppression of the immune system and may increase the susceptibility to infection including opportunistic infections, fatal infections and sepsis. If blood dyscrasias occur (e.g., neutropenia with absolute neutrophil count $< 1.5 \times 10^3/\mu L$ or anemia), it may be appropriate to interrupt or discontinue Myfortic.

Possible signs and symptoms of acute overdose could include the following: hematological abnormalities such as leukopenia and neutropenia, and gastrointestinal symptoms such as abdominal pain, diarrhea, nausea and vomiting, and dyspepsia.

Treatment and Management

General supportive measures and symptomatic treatment should be followed in all cases of overdosage. Although dialysis may be used to remove the inactive metabolite mycophenolic acid glucuronide (MPAG), it would not be expected to remove clinically significant amounts of the active moiety, mycophenolic acid, due to the 98% plasma protein binding of mycophenolic acid. By interfering with enterohepatic circulation of mycophenolic acid, activated charcoal or bile sequestrates, such as cholestyramine, may reduce the systemic mycophenolic acid exposure.

11 DESCRIPTION

Myfortic® (mycophenolic acid) delayed-release tablets are an enteric formulation of mycophenolate sodium that delivers the active moiety mycophenolic acid (MPA). Myfortic is an immunosuppressive agent. As the sodium salt, MPA is chemically designated as (E)-6-(4-hydroxy-6-methoxy-7-methyl-3-oxo-1,3-dihydroisobenzofuran-5-yl)-4-methylhex-4-enoic acid sodium salt.

Its empirical formula is $C_{17}H_{19}O_6Na$. The molecular weight is 342.32 and the structural formula is

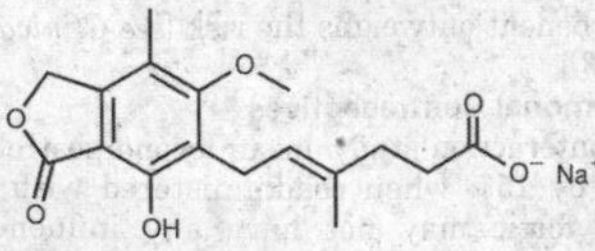

Myfortic, as the sodium salt, is a white to off-white, crystalline powder and is highly soluble in aqueous media at physiological pH and practically insoluble in 0.1 N hydrochloric acid.

Myfortic is available for oral use as delayed-release tablets containing either 180 mg or 360 mg of mycophenolic acid. Inactive ingredients include colloidal silicon dioxide, crospovidone, lactose anhydrous, magnesium stearate, povidone (K-30), and starch. The enteric coating of the tablet consists of hypromellose phthalate, titanium dioxide, iron oxide yellow, and indigotine (180 mg) or iron oxide red (360 mg).

12 CLINICAL PHARMACOLOGY

12.1 Mechanism of Action

Mycophenolic acid (MPA), an immunosuppressant, is an uncompetitive and reversible inhibitor of inosine monophosphate dehydrogenase (IMPDH), and therefore inhibits the de novo pathway of guanosine nucleotide synthesis without incorporation to DNA. T- and B-lymphocytes are critically dependent for their proliferation on de novo synthesis of purines, whereas other cell types can utilize salvage pathways. MPA has cytostatic effects on lymphocytes.

Mycophenolate sodium has been shown to prevent the occurrence of acute rejection in rat models of kidney and heart allotransplantation. Mycophenolate sodium also decreases antibody production in mice.

12.3 Pharmacokinetics

Myfortic exhibits linear and dose-proportional pharmacokinetics over the dose-range (360–2160 mg) evaluated. The absolute bioavailability of Myfortic in stable renal transplant patients on cyclosporine was 72%. MPA is highly protein bound (>98% bound to albumin). The predominant metabolite of MPA is the phenolic glucuronide (MPAG) which is pharmacologically inactive. A minor metabolite AcMPAG which is an acyl glucuronide of MPAG is also formed and has pharmacological activity comparable to MPA. MPAG undergoes renal elimination. A fraction of MPAG also undergoes biliary excretion, followed by deconjugation by gut flora and subsequent reabsorption as MPA. The mean elimination half-lives of MPA and MPAG ranged between 8 and 16 hours, and 13 and 17 hours, respectively.

Absorption

In vitro studies demonstrated that the enteric-coated Myfortic tablet does not release MPA under acidic conditions (pH <5) as in the stomach but is highly soluble in neutral pH conditions as in the intestine. Following Myfortic oral administration without food in several pharmacokinetic studies conducted in renal transplant patients, consistent with its enteric-coated formulation, the median delay (T_{lag}) in the rise of MPA concentration ranged between 0.25 and 1.25 hours and the median time to maximum concentration (T_{max}) of MPA ranged between 1.5 and 2.75 hours. In comparison, following the administration of MMF, the median T_{max} ranged between 0.5 and 1.0 hours. In stable renal transplant patients on cyclosporine, USP MODIFIED based immunosuppression, gastrointestinal absorption and absolute bioavailability of MPA following the administration of Myfortic delayed-release tablet was 93% and 72%, respectively. Myfortic pharmacokinetics is dose proportional over the dose range of 360 to 2160 mg.

Distribution

The mean (± SD) volume of distribution at steady state and elimination phase for MPA is 54 (± 25) L and 112 (± 48) L, respectively. MPA is highly protein bound to albumin, >98%. The protein binding of mycophenolic acid glucuronide (MPAG) is 82%. The free MPA concentration may increase under conditions of decreased protein binding (uremia, hepatic failure, and hypoalbuminemia).

Metabolism

MPA is metabolized principally by glucuronyl transferase to glucuronidated metabolites. The phenolic glucuronide of MPA, mycophenolic acid glucuronide (MPAG), is the predominant metabolite of MPA and does not manifest pharmacological activity. The acyl glucuronide is a minor metabolite and has comparable pharmacological activity to MPA. In stable renal transplant patients on cyclosporine, USP MODIFIED based immunosuppression, approximately 28% of the oral Myfortic dose was converted to MPAG by presystemic metabolism. The AUC ratio of MPA:MPAG:acyl glucuronide is approximately 1:24:0.28 at steady state. The mean clearance of MPA was 140 (± 30) mL/min.

Elimination

The majority of MPA dose administered is eliminated in the urine primarily as MPAG (>60%) and approximately 3% as unchanged MPA following Myfortic administration to stable renal transplant patients. The mean renal clearance of MPAG was 15.5 (± 5.9) mL/min. MPAG is also secreted in the bile and available for deconjugation by gut flora. MPA resulting from the deconjugation may then be reabsorbed and produce a second peak of MPA approximately 6-8 hours after Myfortic dosing. The mean elimination half-life of MPA and MPAG ranged between 8 and 16 hours, and 13 and 17 hours, respectively.

Food Effect

Compared to the fasting state, administration of Myfortic 720 mg with a high-fat meal (55 g fat, 1000 calories) had no effect on the systemic exposure (AUC) of MPA. However, there was a 33% decrease in the maximal concentration (C_{max}), a 3.5-hour delay in the T_{lag} (range, -6 to 18 hours), and 5.0-hour delay in the T_{max} (range, -9 to 20 hours) of MPA. To avoid the variability in MPA absorption between doses, Myfortic should be taken on an empty stomach [*see Dosage and Administration (2.3)*].

Pharmacokinetics in Renal Transplant Patients

The mean pharmacokinetic parameters for MPA following the administration of Myfortic in renal transplant patients on cyclosporine, USP MODIFIED based immunosuppression are shown in Table 6. Single-dose Myfortic pharmacokinetics predicts multiple-dose pharmacokinetics. However, in the early post-transplant period, mean MPA AUC and C_{max} were approximately one-half of those measured 6 months post-transplant.

After near equimolar dosing of Myfortic 720 mg twice daily and MMF 1000 mg twice daily (739 mg as MPA) in both the single- and multiple-dose cross-over trials, mean systemic MPA exposure (AUC) was similar.

Table 6: Mean ± SD Pharmacokinetic Parameters for MPA Following the Oral Administration of Myfortic® to Renal Transplant Patients on Cyclosporine, USP MODIFIED Based Immunosuppression

Patient	Myfortic Dosing	N	Dose (mg)	T_{max}* (hr)	C_{max} (μg/mL)	$AUC_{0\text{-}12hr}$ (μg*hr/mL)
Adult	Single	24	720	2 (0.8 – 8)	26.1 ± 12.0	66.5 ± 22.6**
Pediatric***	Single	10	450/m^2	2.5 (1.5 –24)	36.3 ± 20.9	74.3 ± 22.5**
Adult	Multiple x6 days, twice daily	10	720	2 (1.5 – 3.0)	37.0 + 13.3	67.9 ± 20.3
Adult	Multiple x28 days, twice daily	36	720	2.5 (1.5 – 8)	31.2 ± 18.1	71.2 ± 26.3
Adult	Chronic, multiple dose, twice daily					
	2 weeks post-transplant	12	720	1.8 (1.0 – 5.3)	15.0 ± 10.7	28.6 ± 11.5
	3 months post-transplant	12	720	2 (0.5 – 2.5)	26.2 ± 12.7	52.3 ± 17.4
	6 months post-transplant	12	720	2 (0 – 3)	24.1 ± 9.6	57.2 ± 15.3
Adult	Chronic, multiple dose, twice daily	18	720	1.5 (0 – 6)	18.9 ± 7.9	57.4 ± 15.0

*median (range), ** $AUC_{0\text{-}\infty}$, *** age range of 5-16 years

[See table 6 at right]

Specific Populations

Renal Insufficiency: No specific pharmacokinetic studies in individuals with renal impairment were conducted with Myfortic. However, based on studies of renal impairment with MMF, MPA exposure is not expected to be appreciably increased over the range of normal to severely impaired renal function following Myfortic administration. In contrast, MPAG exposure would be increased markedly with decreased renal function; MPAG exposure being approximately 8-fold higher in the setting of anuria. Although dialysis may be used to remove the inactive metabolite MPAG, it would not be expected to remove clinically significant amounts of the active moiety MPA. This is in large part due to the high plasma protein binding of MPA.

Hepatic Insufficiency: No specific pharmacokinetic studies in individuals with hepatic impairment were conducted with Myfortic. In a single dose (MMF 1000 mg) trial of 18 volunteers with alcoholic cirrhosis and 6 healthy volunteers, hepatic MPA glucuronidation processes appeared to be relatively unaffected by hepatic parenchymal disease when the pharmacokinetic parameters of healthy volunteers and alcoholic cirrhosis patients within this trial were compared. However, it should be noted that for unexplained reasons, the healthy volunteers in this trial had about a 50% lower AUC compared to healthy volunteers in other studies, thus making comparison between volunteers with alcoholic cirrhosis and healthy volunteers difficult. Effects of hepatic disease on this process probably depend on the particular disease. Hepatic disease, such as primary biliary cirrhosis, with other etiologies may show a different effect.

Pediatrics: Limited data are available on the use of Myfortic at a dose of 450 mg/m^2 body surface area in children. The mean MPA pharmacokinetic parameters for stable pediatric renal transplant patients, 5 to 16 years, on cyclosporine, USP MODIFIED are shown in Table 6. At the same dose administered based on body surface area, the respective mean C_{max} and AUC of MPA determined in children were higher by 33% and 18% than those determined for adults. The clinical impact of the increase in MPA exposure is not known [*see Dosage and Administration (2.2, 2.3)*].

Gender: There are no significant gender differences in Myfortic pharmacokinetics.

Elderly: Pharmacokinetics in the elderly have not been formally studied.

Ethnicity: Following a single dose administration of 720 mg of Myfortic to 18 Japanese and 18 Caucasian healthy subjects, the exposure (AUC_{inf}) for MPA and MPAG were 15% and 22% lower in Japanese subjects compared to Caucasians. The peak concentrations (C_{max}) for MPAG were similar between the two populations, however, Japanese subjects had 9.6% higher C_{max} for MPA.These results do not suggest any clinically relevant differences.

Drug Interactions:

Antacids with Magnesium and Aluminum Hydroxides:

Absorption of a single dose of Myfortic was decreased when administered to 12 stable kidney transplant patients also taking magnesium-aluminum-containing antacids (30 mL): the mean C_{max} and $AUC_{(0\text{-}t)}$ values for MPA were 25% and 37% lower, respectively, than when Myfortic was administered alone under fasting conditions [*see Drug Interactions (7.1)*].

Pantoprazole:

In a trial conducted in 12 healthy volunteers, the pharmacokinetics of MPA were observed to be similar when a single dose of 720 mg of Myfortic was administered alone and following concomitant administration of Myfortic and pantoprazole, which was administered at a dose of 40 mg twice daily for 4 days [*see Drug Interactions (7.11)*].

The following drug interaction studies were conducted following the administration of MMF:

Cholestyramine:

Following single-dose oral administration of 1.5 grams MMF to 12 healthy volunteers pretreated with 4 grams three times daily of cholestyramine for 4 days, MPA AUC decreased approximately 40%. This decrease is consistent with interruption of enterohepatic recirculation which may be due to binding of recirculating MPAG with cholestyramine in the intestine [*see Drug Interactions (7.3)*].

Sevelamer:

Concomitant administration of sevelamer and MMF in stable adult and pediatric kidney transplant patients decreased the mean MPA C_{max} and $AUC_{(0\text{-}12h)}$ by 36% and 26% respectively [*see Drug Interactions (7.4)*].

Cyclosporine:

Cyclosporine (Sandimmune®) pharmacokinetics (at doses of 275 to 415 mg/day) were unaffected by single and multiple doses of 1.5 grams twice daily of MMF in 10 stable kidney transplant patients. The mean (±SD) AUC (0-12h) and C_{max} of cyclosporine after 14 days of multiple doses of MMF were 3290 (±822) ng•h/mL and 753 (±161) ng/mL, respectively, compared to 3245 (±1088) ng•h/mL and 700 (±246) ng/mL, respectively, 1 week before administration of MMF.

A total of 73 *de novo* kidney allograft recipients on MMF therapy received either low dose cyclosporine withdrawal by 6 months post-transplant (50 to 100 ng/mL for up to 3 months post-transplant followed by complete withdrawal at month 6 post-transplant) or standard dose cyclosporine (150 to 300 ng/mL from baseline through to month 4 post-transplant and 100 to 200 ng/mL thereafter). At month 12 post-transplant, the mean MPA ($AUC_{(0\text{-}12h)}$) in the cyclosporine withdrawal group was approximately 40% higher, than that of the standard dose cyclosporine group.

Cyclosporine inhibits multidrug-resistance-associated protein 2 (MRP-2) transporter in the biliary tract, thereby preventing the excretion of MPAG into the bile that would lead to enterohepatic recirculation of MPA [*see Drug Interactions (7.5)*].

Norfloxacin and Metronidazole:

Following single-dose administration of MMF (1 g) to 11 healthy volunteers on day 4 of a 5 day course of a combination of norfloxacin and metronidazole, the mean MPA $AUC_{(0\text{-}48h)}$ was reduced by 33% compared to the administration of MMF alone (p<0.05). There was no significant effect on mean MPA $AUC_{(0\text{-}48h)}$ when MMF was concomitantly administered with norfloxacin or metronidazole separately. The mean (±SD) MPA $AUC_{(0\text{-}48h)}$ after coadministration of MMF with norfloxacin or metronidazole separately was 48.3 (±24) μg•h/mL and 42.7 (±23) μg•h/mL, respectively, compared with 56.2 (±24) μg•h/mL after administration of MMF alone [*see Drug Interactions (7.6)*].

Rifampin:

In a single heart-lung transplant patient on MMF therapy (1 gram twice daily), a 67% decrease in MPA exposure ($AUC_{(0\text{-}12h)}$) was observed with concomitant administration of MMF and 600 mg rifampin daily.

In 8 kidney transplant patients on stable MMF therapy (1 gram twice daily), administration of 300 mg rifampin twice daily resulted in a 17.5% decrease in MPA $AUC_{(0\text{-}12h)}$ due to inhibition of enterohepatic recirculation of MPAG by rifampin. Rifampin coadministration also resulted in a 22.4% increase in MPAG $AUC_{(0\text{-}12h)}$ [*see Drug Interactions (7.7)*].

Oral Contraceptives:

In a drug-drug interaction trial, mean AUCs were similar for ethinyl estradiol and norethindrone, when coadministered with MMF as compared to administration of the oral contraceptives alone [*see Drug Interactions (7.8)*].

Acyclovir:

Coadministration of MMF (1 gram) and acyclovir (800 mg) to 12 healthy volunteers resulted in no significant change in MPA AUC and C_{max}. However, MPAG and acyclovir plasma mean $AUC_{(0\text{-}24h)}$ were increased 10% and 18%, respectively. Because MPAG plasma concentrations are increased in the presence of kidney impairment, as are acyclovir concentrations, the potential exists for mycophenolate and acyclovir or its prodrug (e.g., valacyclovir) to compete for tubular secretion, further increasing the concentrations of both drugs [*see Drug Interactions (7.9)*].

Ganciclovir:

Following single-dose administration to 12 stable kidney transplant patients, no pharmacokinetic interaction was observed between MMF (1.5 grams) and intravenous ganciclovir (5 mg per kg). Mean (±SD) ganciclovir AUC and C_{max} (n=10) were 54.3 (±19.0) μg•h/mL and 11.5 (±1.8) μg/mL, respectively, after coadministration of the two drugs, compared to 51.0 (±17.0) μg•h/mL and 10.6 (±2.0) μg/mL, respectively, after administration of intravenous ganciclovir alone. The mean (±SD) AUC and C_{max} of MPA (n=12) after coadministration were 80.9 (±21.6) μg•h/mL and 27.8 (±13.9) μg/mL, respectively, compared to values of 80.3 (±16.4) μg•h/mL and 30.9 (±11.2) μg/mL, respectively, after administration of MMF alone.

Because MPAG plasma concentrations are increased in the presence of renal impairment, as are ganciclovir concentrations, the two drugs will compete for tubular secretion and thus further increases in concentrations of both drugs may occur. In patients with renal impairment in which MMF and ganciclovir or its prodrug (e.g., valganciclovir) are coadministered, patients should be monitored carefully [*see Drug Interactions (7.9)*].

Ciprofloxacin and Amoxicillin plus Clavulanic Acid:

A total of 64 MMF treated kidney transplant recipients received either oral ciprofloxacin 500 mg twice daily or amoxicillin plus clavulanic acid 375 mg three times daily for 7 or at least 14 days. Approximately 50% reductions in median trough MPA concentrations (predose) from baseline (MMF alone) were observed in 3 days following commencement of oral ciprofloxacin or amoxicillin plus clavulanic acid. These reductions in trough MPA concentrations tended to diminish within 14 days of antibiotic therapy and ceased within 3 days after discontinuation of antibiotics. The postulated mechanism for this interaction is an antibiotic-induced reduction in glucuronidase-possessing enteric organisms leading to a decrease in enterohepatic recirculation of MPA. The change in trough level may not accurately represent changes in overall MPA exposure; therefore, clinical relevance of these observations is unclear [*see Drug Interactions (7.10)*].

13 NONCLINICAL TOXICOLOGY

13.1 Carcinogenesis, Mutagenesis, Impairment of Fertility

In a 104-week oral carcinogenicity study in rats, mycophenolate sodium was not tumorigenic at daily doses up to 9 mg per kg, the highest dose tested. This dose resulted in approximately 0.6-1.2 times the systemic exposure (based on plasma AUC) observed in renal transplant patients at the recommended dose of 1440 mg per day. Similar results were observed in a parallel study in rats performed with MMF. In a 104-week oral carcinogenicity study in mice, MMF was not tumorigenic at a daily dose level as high as 180 mg per kg (which corresponds to 0.6 times the recommended mycophenolate sodium therapeutic dose, based on body surface area).

The genotoxic potential of mycophenolate sodium was determined in five assays. Mycophenolate sodium was genotoxic in the mouse lymphoma/thymidine kinase assay, the micronucleus test in V79 Chinese hamster cells, and the in vivo mouse micronucleus assay. Mycophenolate sodium was not genotoxic in the bacterial mutation assay (*Salmonella typhimurium* TA 1535, 97a, 98, 100, and 102) or the chromosomal aberration assay in human lymphocytes.

Mycophenolate mofetil generated similar genotoxic activity. The genotoxic activity of mycophenolic acid (MPA) is probably due to the depletion of the nucleotide pool required for DNA synthesis as a result of the pharmacodynamic mode of action of MPA (inhibition of nucleotide synthesis).

Mycophenolate sodium had no effect on male rat fertility at daily oral doses as high as 18 mg per kg and exhibited no testicular or spermatogenic effects at daily oral doses of 20 mg per kg for 13 weeks (approximately 2 times the systemic exposure of MPA at the recommended therapeutic dose). No effects on female fertility were seen up to a daily dose of 20 mg per kg (approximately 3 times the systemic exposure of MPA at the recommended therapeutic dose).

14 CLINICAL STUDIES

14.1 Prophylaxis of Organ Rejection in Patients Receiving Allogeneic Renal Transplants

The safety and efficacy of Myfortic in combination with cyclosporine, USP MODIFIED and corticosteroids for the prevention of organ rejection was assessed in two multicenter, randomized, double-blind active controlled trials in *de novo* and conversion renal transplant patients compared to MMF. The *de novo* trial was conducted in 423 renal transplant patients (ages 18–75 years) in Austria, Canada, Germany, Hungary, Italy, Norway, Spain, UK, and USA. Eighty-four

Table 7: Treatment Failure in de novo Renal Transplant Patients (Percent of Patients) at 6 and 12 Months of Treatment when Administered in Combination with Cyclosporine* and Corticosteroids

	Myfortic 1.44 grams per day (n=213)	mycophenolate mofetil (MMF) 2 grams per day (n=210)
6 Months	n (%)	n (%)
Treatment failure#	55 (25.8)	55 (26.2)
Biopsy-proven acute rejection	46 (21.6)	48 (22.9)
Graft loss	7 (3.3)	9 (4.3)
Death	1 (0.5)	2 (1.0)
Lost to follow-up**	3 (1.4)	0
12 Months	**n (%)**	**n (%)**
Graft loss or death or lost to follow-up***	20 (9.4)	18 (8.6)
Treatment failure##	61 (28.6)	59 (28.1)
Biopsy-proven acute rejection	48 (22.5)	51 (24.3)
Graft loss	9 (4.2)	9 (4.3)
Death	2 (0.9)	5 (2.4)
Lost to follow-up**	5 (2.3)	0

*USP MODIFIED
**Lost to follow-up indicates patients who were lost to follow-up without prior biopsy-proven acute rejection, graft loss or death
***Lost to follow-up indicates patients who were lost to follow-up without prior graft loss or death (9 Myfortic patients and 4 MMF patients)
#95% confidence interval of the difference in treatment failure at 6 months (Myfortic–MMF) is (-8.7%, 8.0%).
##95% confidence interval of the difference in treatment failure at 12 months (Myfortic–MMF) is (-8.0%, 9.1%).

Table 8: Treatment Failure in Conversion Transplant Patients (Percent of Patients) at 6 and 12 Months of Treatment when Administered in Combination with Cyclosporine* and with or without Corticosteroids

	Myfortic 1.44 grams per day (n = 159)	mycophenolate mofetil (MMF) 2 grams per day (n = 163)
6 Months	**n (%)**	**n (%)**
Treatment failure#	7 (4.4)	11 (6.7)
Biopsy-proven acute rejection	2 (1.3)	2 (1.2)
Graft loss	0	1 (0.6)
Death	0	1 (0.6)
Lost to follow-up**	5 (3.1)	7 (4.3)
12 Months	**n (%)**	**n (%)**
Graft loss or death or lost to follow-up***	10 (6.3)	17 (10.4)
Treatment failure##	12 (7.5)	20 (12.3)
Biopsy-proven acute rejection	2 (1.3)	5 (3.1)
Graft loss	0	1 (0.6)
Death	2 (1.3)	4 (2.5)
Lost to follow-up**	8 (5.0)	10 (6.1)

*USP MODIFIED
**Lost to follow-up indicates patients who were lost to follow-up without prior biopsy-proven acute rejection, graft loss, or death
***Lost to follow-up indicates patients who were lost to follow-up without prior graft loss or death (8 Myfortic patients and 12 mycophenolate mofetil patients)
#95% confidence interval of the difference in treatment failure at 6 months (Myfortic – mycophenolate mofetil) is (-7.4%, 2.7%).
##95% confidence interval of the difference in treatment failure at 12 months (Myfortic–MMF) is (-11.2%, 1.8%).

percent of randomized patients received kidneys from deceased donors. Patients were excluded if they had second or multi-organ (e.g., kidney and pancreas) transplants, or previous transplant with any other organs; kidneys from non-heart beating donors; panel reactive antibodies (PRA) of >50% at last assessment prior to transplantation, and presence of severe diarrhea, active peptic ulcer disease, or uncontrolled diabetes mellitus. Patients were administered either Myfortic 1.44 grams per day or MMF 2 grams per day within 48 hours post-transplant for 12 months in combination with cyclosporine, USP MODIFIED and corticosteroids. Forty-one percent of patients received antibody therapy as induction treatment. Treatment failure was defined as the first occurrence of biopsy proven acute rejection, graft loss, death or lost to follow-up at 6 months.

The incidence of treatment failure was similar in Myfortic- and MMF-treated patients at 6 and 12 months (Table 7). The cumulative incidence of graft loss, death and lost to follow-up at 12 months is also shown in Table 7.

[See table 7 above]

The conversion trial was conducted in 322 renal transplant patients (ages 18–75 years), who were at least 6 months post-transplant and had undergone primary or secondary, deceased donor, living related, or unrelated donor kidney transplant, stable graft function (serum creatinine <2.3 mg/mL), no change in immunosuppressive regimen due to graft malfunction, and no known clinically significant physical and/or laboratory changes for at least 2 months prior to enrollment. Patients were excluded if they had 3 or more kidney transplants, multi-organ transplants (e.g., kidney and pancreas), previous organ transplants, evidence of graft rejection or who had been treated for acute rejection within 2 months prior to screening, clinically significant infections requiring continued therapy, presence of severe diarrhea, active peptic ulcer disease, or uncontrolled diabetes mellitus.

Patients received 2 grams per day MMF in combination with cyclosporine USP MODIFIED, with or without corticosteroids for at least two weeks prior to entry in the trial. Patients were randomized to Myfortic 1.44 grams per day or MMF 2 grams per day for 12 months. The trial was conducted in Austria, Belgium, Canada, Germany, Italy, Spain, and USA. Treatment failure was defined as the first occurrence of biopsy-proven acute rejection, graft loss, death, or lost to follow-up at 6 and 12 months.

The incidences of treatment failure at 6 and 12 months were similar between Myfortic- and MMF-treated patients (Table 8). The cumulative incidence of graft loss, death and lost to follow-up at 12 months is also shown in Table 8.

[See table 8 above]

16 HOW SUPPLIED/STORAGE AND HANDLING

360 mg tablet: Pale orange-red film-coated ovaloid tablet with imprint (debossing) "CT" on one side, containing 360 mg mycophenolic acid (MPA) as mycophenolate sodium.

Bottles of 120.................................. NDC 0078-0386-66

180 mg tablet: Lime green film-coated round tablet with bevelled edges and the imprint (debossing) "C" on one side, containing 180 mg mycophenolic acid (MPA) as mycophenolate sodium.

Bottles of 120.................................. NDC 0078-0385-66

Storage

Store at 25°C (77°F); excursions permitted to 15-30°C (59-86°F) [see USP Controlled Room Temperature]. Protect from moisture. **Dispense in a tight container (USP).**

Handling

Keep out of reach and sight of children. Myfortic tablets should not be crushed or cut in order to maintain the integrity of the enteric coating [*see Dosage and Administration (2.3)*].

Teratogenic effects have been observed with mycophenolate sodium [*see Warnings and Precautions (5.1)*]. If for any reason, the Myfortic tablets must be crushed, avoid inhalation of the powder, or direct contact of the powder, with skin or mucous membranes.

17 PATIENT COUNSELING INFORMATION

See FDA-approved patient labeling (Medication Guide)

Embryofetal Toxicity

- Inform pregnant women and females of reproductive potential that use of Myfortic in pregnancy is associated with an increased risk of first trimester pregnancy loss and an increased risk of congenital malformations. [*see Use in Specific Populations (8.1)*]
- In the event of a positive pregnancy test, discuss the risks and benefits of Myfortic with the patient. Encourage her to enroll in the pregnancy registry. (1-800-617-8191). [*see Use in Specific Populations (8.1)*].

Pregnancy Exposure Prevention and Planning

- Discuss pregnancy testing, pregnancy prevention and planning with female of reproductive potential [*see Females of Reproductive Potential (8.6)*].
- Inform females of reproductive potential must use acceptable birth control during entire Myfortic therapy and for 6 weeks after stopping Myfortic, unless the patient chooses to avoid heterosexual sexual intercourse completely (abstinence) [*see Warnings and Precautions (5.2) and Females of Reproductive Potential (8.6)*].
- For patients who are considering pregnancy, discuss appropriate alternative immunosuppressants with less potential for embryofetal toxicity. Risks and benefits of Myfortic should be discussed with the patient [*see Females of Reproductive Potential (8.6)*].

Nursing Mothers

Advise patients that they should not breastfeed during Myfortic therapy [*see Nursing Mothers (8.3)*].

Development of Lymphoma and Other Malignancies

- Inform patients they are at increased risk of developing lymphomas and other malignancies, particularly of the skin, due to immunosuppression.
- Advise patients to limit exposure to sunlight and ultraviolet (UV) light by wearing protective clothing and use a sunscreen with a high protection factor.

Increased Risk of Infection

Inform patients they are at increased risk of developing a variety of infections, including opportunistic infections, due to immunosuppression and to contact their physician if they develop any symptoms of infection [*see Warnings and Precautions (5.5, 5.6, 5.7)*].

Blood Dyscrasias

Inform patients they are at increased risk for developing blood dyscrasias (e.g., neutropenia or anemia) and to immediately contact their healthcare provider if they experience any evidence of infection, unexpected bruising, bleeding, or any other manifestation of bone marrow suppression [*see Warnings and Precautions (5.8)*].

Gastrointestinal Tract Complications

Inform patients that Myfortic can cause gastrointestinal tract complications including bleeding, intestinal perforations, and gastric or duodenal ulcers. Advise the patient to contact their healthcare provider if they have symptoms of gastrointestinal bleeding or sudden onset or persistent abdominal pain.

Immunizations

Inform patients that Myfortic can interfere with the usual response to immunizations and that they should avoid live vaccines.

Administration Instructions

Advise patients to swallow Myfortic tablets whole, and not crush, chew, or cut the tablets. Inform patients to take Myfortic on an empty stomach, 1 hour before or 2 hours after food intake.

Drug Interactions

Patients should be advised to report to their doctor the use of any other medications while taking Myfortic. The simultaneous administration of any of the following drugs with Myfortic may result in clinically significant adverse reactions:

Antacids with magnesium and aluminum hydroxides

Azathioprine

Cholestyramine

Hormonal Contraceptives (e.g., birth control pill, transdermal patch, vaginal ring, injection, and implant)

Manufactured by:
Novartis Pharma Stein AG
Stein, Switzerland
Distributed by:
Novartis Pharmaceuticals Corporation
East Hanover, New Jersey 07936
T2013-35
May 2013

MEDICATION GUIDE

MYFORTIC® (my-for-tic)
(mycophenolic acid)
delayed-release tablets

Read the Medication Guide that comes with Myfortic before you start taking it and each time you get a refill. There may be new information. This Medication Guide does not take the place of talking with your healthcare provider about your medical condition or treatment. If you have any questions about Myfortic, ask your doctor.

What is the most important information I should know about Myfortic?

Myfortic can cause serious side effects including:

- **Increased risk of loss of pregnancy (miscarriage) and higher risk of birth defects.** Females who take Myfortic during pregnancy, have a higher risk of miscarriage during the first 3 months (first trimester), and a higher risk that their baby will be born with birth defects.
  If you are a female who can become pregnant:
- your doctor must talk with you about acceptable birth control methods (contraceptive counseling) while taking Myfortic.
- you should have a pregnancy test immediately before starting Myfortic and another pregnancy test 8 to 10 days later. Pregnancy tests should be repeated during routine follow-up visits with your doctor. Talk to your doctor about the results of all of your pregnancy tests.
- you must use acceptable birth control during your entire Myfortic therapy and for 6 weeks after stopping Myfortic, unless at any time you choose to avoid sexual intercourse (abstinence) with a man completely. Myfortic decreases blood levels of the hormones in birth control pills that you take by mouth. Birth control pills may not work as well while you take Myfortic and you could become pregnant. If you decide to take birth control pills while using Myfortic, you must also use another form of birth control. Talk to your doctor about other birth control methods that can be used while taking Myfortic.

If you plan to become pregnant, talk with your doctor. Your doctor will decide if other medicines to prevent rejection may be right for you.

- **If you become pregnant while taking Myfortic, do not stop taking Myfortic. Call your doctor right away.** In certain situations, you and your doctor may decide that taking Myfortic is more important to your health than the possible risks to your unborn baby.
- You and your doctor should report your pregnancy to
  - Mycophenolate Pregnancy Registry (1-800-617-8191)
  The purpose of this registry is to gather information about the health of your baby.
- **Increased risk of getting serious infections.** Myfortic weakens the body's immune system and affects your ability to fight infections. Serious infections can happen with Myfortic and can lead to death. Types of infections can include:
  - **Viral infections.** Certain viruses can live in your body and cause active infections when your immune system is weak. Viral infections that can happen with Myfortic include:
    - Shingles, other herpes infections, and cytomegalovirus (CMV). CMV can cause serious tissue and blood infections.
    - BK virus. BK virus can affect how your kidneys works and cause your transplanted kidney to fail.
  - **A brain infection called Progressive Multifocal Leukoencephalopathy (PML).** In some patients Myfortic may cause an infection of the brain that may cause death. You are at risk for this brain infection because you have a weakened immune system. You should tell your healthcare provider right away if you have any of the following symptoms:
    - Weakness on one side of the body
    - You do not care about things that you usually care about (apathy)
    - You are confused or have problems thinking
    - You cannot control your muscles
  - **Fungal infections.** Yeast and other types of fungal infections can happen with Myfortic and cause serious tissue and blood infections. **See "What are the possible side effects of Myfortic?"**

Call your doctor right away if you have any of these signs and symptoms of infection:

- Temperature of 100.5°F or greater
- Cold symptoms, such as a runny nose or sore throat
- Flu symptoms, such as an upset stomach, stomach pain, vomiting, or diarrhea
- Earache or headache
- Pain during urination or you need to urinate often
- White patches in the mouth or throat
- Unexpected bruising or bleeding
- Cuts, scrapes, or incisions that are red, warm, and oozing pus

- **Increased risk of getting certain cancers.** People who take Myfortic have a higher risk of getting lymphoma, and other cancers, especially skin cancer. Tell your doctor if you have:
  - unexplained fever, tiredness that does not go away, weight loss, or lymph node swelling
  - a brown or black skin lesion with uneven borders, or one part of the lesion does not look like other parts
  - a change in the size or color of a mole
  - a new skin lesion or bump
  - any other changes to your health

See the section "What are the possible side effects of Myfortic?" for other serious side effects.

What is Myfortic?

Myfortic is a prescription medicine given to prevent rejection (antirejection medicine) in people who have received a kidney transplant. Rejection is when the body's immune system senses the new organ as "foreign" and attacks it.

Myfortic is used with other medicines containing cyclosporine (Sandimmune®, Gengraf®, and Neoral®) and corticosteroids.

Myfortic can be used to prevent rejection in children who are 5 years or older and are stable after having a kidney transplant. It is not known if Myfortic is safe and works in children younger than 5 years. It is not known how Myfortic works in children who have just received a new kidney transplant.

Who should not take Myfortic?

Do not take Myfortic if you are allergic to mycophenolic acid, mycophenolate sodium, mycophenolate mofetil, or any of the ingredients in Myfortic. See the end of this Medication Guide for a complete list of ingredients in Myfortic.

What should I tell my doctor before I start taking Myfortic?

Tell your healthcare provider about all of your medical conditions, including if you:

- **have any digestive problems, such as ulcers**
- **plan to receive any vaccines.** You should not receive live vaccines while you take Myfortic. Some vaccines may not work as well during treatment with Myfortic.
- **have Lesch-Nyhan or Kelley-Seegmiller syndrome or another rare inherited deficiency of hypoxanthine-guanine phosphoribosyl-transferase (HGPRT).** You should not take Myfortic if you have one of these disorders.
- **are pregnant or planning to become pregnant. See "What is the most important information I should know about Myfortic"**
- **are breastfeeding or plan to breastfeed.** It is not known if Myfortic passes into breast milk. You and your doctor will decide if you will take Myfortic or breastfeed.

Tell your doctor about all the medicines you take, including prescription and nonprescription medicines, vitamins, and herbal supplements.

Some medicines may affect the way Myfortic works and Myfortic may affect how some medicines work. Especially tell your doctor if you take:

- birth control pills (oral contraceptives). **See "What is the most important information I should know about Myfortic?"**
- antacids that contain aluminum or magnesium. Myfortic and antacids should not be taken at the same time.
- acyclovir (Zovirax®), Ganciclovir (Cytovene® IV, Valcyte®)
- azathioprine (Azasan®, Imuran®)
- cholestyramine (Questran® Light, Questran®, Locholest Light, Prevalite®)

Know the medicines you take. Keep a list of your medicines with you to show your healthcare provider and pharmacist when you get a new medicine. Do not take any new medicine without talking to your doctor.

How should I take Myfortic?

- Take Myfortic exactly as prescribed. Your healthcare provider will tell you how much Myfortic to take.
- Do not stop taking or change your dose of Myfortic without talking to your healthcare provider.
- Take Myfortic on an empty stomach, either 1 hour before or 2 hours after a meal.
- Swallow Myfortic whole. Do not crush, chew, or cut Myfortic. The Myfortic tablets have a coating so that the medicine will pass through your stomach and dissolve in your intestine.
  - **If you forget to take Myfortic,** take it as soon as you remember and then take your next dose at its regular time. If it is almost time for your next dose, skip the missed dose. Do not take two doses at the same time. Call your doctor or pharmacist if you are not sure what to do.
  - **If you take more than the prescribed dose of Myfortic,** call your doctor right away.
  - **Do not change (substitute) between using Myfortic delayed-release tablets and mycophenolate mofetil tablets, capsules, or oral suspension for one another unless your healthcare provider tells you to.** These medicines are absorbed differently. This may affect the amount of medicine in your blood.
  - Be sure to keep all appointments at your transplant clinic. During these visits, your doctor may perform regular blood tests.

What should I avoid while taking Myfortic?

Avoid pregnancy. See "What is the most important information I should know about Myfortic?"

- Limit the amount of time you spend in sunlight. Avoid using tanning beds and sunlamps. People who take Myfortic have a higher risk of getting skin cancer. **See "What is the most important information I should know about Myfortic?"** Wear protective clothing when you are in the sun and use a sunscreen with a high sun protection factor (SPF 30 and above). This is especially important if your skin is fair (light colored) or you have a family history of skin cancer.
- Elderly patients 65 years of age or older may have more side effects with Myfortic because of a weaker immune system.

What are the possible side effects of Myfortic?

Myfortic can cause serious side effects.

See "What is the most important information I should know about Myfortic?"

Stomach and intestinal bleeding can happen in people who take Myfortic. Bleeding can be severe and you may have to be hospitalized for treatment.

The most common side effects of taking Myfortic include:

In people with a new transplant:

- low blood cell counts
  - red blood cells
  - white blood cells
  - platelets
- constipation
- nausea
- diarrhea
- vomiting
- urinary tract infections
- stomach upset

In people who take Myfortic for a long time (long-term) after transplant:

- low blood cell counts
  - red blood cells
  - white blood cells
- nausea
- diarrhea
- sore throat

Your healthcare provider will do blood tests before you start taking Myfortic and during treatment with Myfortic to check your blood cell counts. Tell your healthcare provider right away if you have any signs of infection **(see "What is the most important information I should know about Myfortic?")**, or any unexpected bruising or bleeding. Also, tell your healthcare provider if you have unusual tiredness, dizziness, or fainting.

These are not all the possible side effects of Myfortic. Your healthcare provider may be able to help you manage these side effects.

Call your doctor for medical advice about side effects.

You may report side effects to

- FDA MedWatch at 1-800-FDA-1088 or
- Novartis Drug Safety at 888-NOW-NOVA (1-888-669-6682).

How should I store Myfortic?

- Store Myfortic tablets at room temperature, 59° to 86°F (15° to 30°C). Myfortic does not need to be refrigerated.
- Keep the container tightly closed. Store Myfortic in a dry place.
- **Keep Myfortic and all medicines out of the reach of children.**

General information about Myfortic

Medicines are sometimes prescribed for purposes other than those listed in a Medication Guide. Do not use Myfortic for a condition for which it was not prescribed. Do not give Myfortic to other people, even if they have the same symptoms you have. It may harm them.

This Medication Guide summarizes the most important information about Myfortic. If you would like more information, talk with your doctor. You can ask your doctor or pharmacist for information about Myfortic that is written for healthcare professionals. You can also call 1-888-669-6682 or visit the Myfortic website at www.myfortic.com.

What are the ingredients in Myfortic?

Active ingredient: mycophenolic acid (as mycophenolate sodium)

Inactive ingredients: colloidal silicon dioxide, crospovidone, lactose anhydrous, magnesium stearate, povidone (K-30), and starch. The enteric coating of the tablet consists of hypromellose phthalate, titanium dioxide, iron oxide yellow, and indigotine (for the 180-mg tablet) or iron oxide red (for the 360-mg tablet)

This Medication Guide has been approved by the U.S. Food and Drug Administration.

Manufactured by:
Novartis Pharma Stein AG Stein, Switzerland
Distributed by:
Novartis Pharmaceuticals Corporation
East Hanover, New Jersey 07936
© Novartis
T2013-36
May 2013

Shown in Product Identification Guide, page 310

NEOVAL® SOFT GELATIN CAPSULES ℞

[*neō'ral*]
(cyclosporine capsules, USP)
MODIFIED

NEORAL® ORAL SOLUTION

(cyclosporine oral solution, USP)
MODIFIED
Rx only
Prescribing Information

The following prescribing information is based on official labeling in effect July 2013.

WARNING

Only physicians experienced in management of systemic immunosuppressive therapy for the indicated disease should prescribe Neoral®. At doses used in solid organ transplantation, only physicians experienced in immunosuppressive therapy and management of organ transplant recipients should prescribe Neoral®. Patients receiving the drug should be managed in facilities equipped and staffed with adequate laboratory and supportive medical resources. The physician responsible for maintenance therapy should have complete information requisite for the follow-up of the patient.

Neoral®, a systemic immunosuppressant, may increase the susceptibility to infection and the development of neoplasia. In kidney, liver, and heart transplant patients Neoral® may be administered with other immunosuppressive agents. Increased susceptibility to infection and the possible development of lymphoma and other neoplasms may result from the increase in the degree of immunosuppression in transplant patients.

Neoral® Soft Gelatin Capsules (cyclosporine capsules, USP) MODIFIED and Neoral® Oral Solution (cyclosporine oral solution, USP) MODIFIED have increased bioavailability in comparison to Sandimmune® Soft Gelatin Capsules (cyclosporine capsules, USP) and Sandimmune® Oral Solution (cyclosporine oral solution, USP). Neoral® and Sandimmune® are not bioequivalent and cannot be used interchangeably without physician supervision. For a given trough concentration, cyclosporine exposure will be greater with Neoral® than with Sandimmune®. If a patient who is receiving exceptionally high doses of Sandimmune® is converted to Neoral®, particular caution should be exercised. Cyclosporine blood concentrations should be monitored in transplant and rheumatoid arthritis patients taking Neoral® to avoid toxicity due to high concentrations. Dose adjustments should be made in transplant patients to minimize possible organ rejection due to low concentrations. Comparison of blood concentrations in the published literature with blood concentrations obtained using current assays must be done with detailed knowledge of the assay methods employed.

For Psoriasis Patients *(See also BOXED WARNING above)*

Psoriasis patients previously treated with PUVA and to a lesser extent, methotrexate or other immunosuppressive agents, UVB, coal tar, or radiation therapy, are at an increased risk of developing skin malignancies when taking Neoral®.

Cyclosporine, the active ingredient in Neoral®, in recommended dosages, can cause systemic hypertension and nephrotoxicity. The risk increases with increasing dose and duration of cyclosporine therapy. Renal dysfunction, including structural kidney damage, is a potential consequence of cyclosporine, and therefore, renal function must be monitored during therapy.

DESCRIPTION

Neoral® is an oral formulation of cyclosporine that immediately forms a microemulsion in an aqueous environment.

Cyclosporine, the active principle in Neoral®, is a cyclic polypeptide immunosuppressant agent consisting of 11 amino acids. It is produced as a metabolite by the fungus species *Beauveria nivea*.

Chemically, cyclosporine is designated as [*R*-[*R**,*R**-(*E*)]]-cyclic-(L-alanyl-D-alanyl-*N*-methyl-L-leucyl-*N*-methyl-L-leucyl-*N*-methyl-L-valyl-3-hydroxy-*N*,4-dimethyl-L-2-amino-6-octenoyl-L-α -amino-butyryl-*N*-methylglycyl-*N*-methyl-L-leucyl-L-valyl-*N*-methyl-L-leucyl).

Neoral® Soft Gelatin Capsules

(cyclosporine capsules, USP) MODIFIED are available in 25 mg and 100 mg strengths.

Each 25 mg capsule contains:

cyclosporine	25 mg
alcohol, USP dehydrated	11.9% v/v (9.5% wt/vol.)

Each 100 mg capsule contains:

cyclosporine	100 mg
alcohol, USP dehydrated	11.9% v/v (9.5% wt/vol.)

Inactive Ingredients: Corn oil-mono-di-triglycerides, polyoxyl 40 hydrogenated castor oil NF, DL-α-tocopherol USP, gelatin NF, glycerol, iron oxide black, propylene glycol USP, titanium dioxide USP, carmine, and other ingredients.

Neoral® Oral Solution

(cyclosporine oral solution, USP) MODIFIED is available in 50 mL bottles.

Each mL contains:

cyclosporine	100 mg/mL
alcohol, USP dehydrated	11.9% v/v (9.5% wt/vol.)

Inactive Ingredients: Corn oil-mono-di-triglycerides, polyoxyl 40 hydrogenated castor oil NF, DL-α -tocopherol USP, propylene glycol USP.

The chemical structure of cyclosporine (also known as cyclosporin A) is:

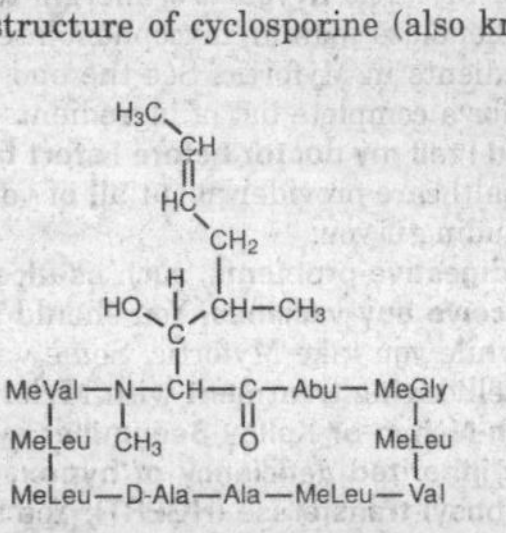

$C_{62}H_{111}N_{11}O_{12}$ Mol. Wt. 1202.63

CLINICAL PHARMACOLOGY

Cyclosporine is a potent immunosuppressive agent that in animals prolongs survival of allogeneic transplants involving skin, kidney, liver, heart, pancreas, bone marrow, small intestine, and lung. Cyclosporine has been demonstrated to suppress some humoral immunity and to a greater extent, cell-mediated immune reactions such as allograft rejection, delayed hypersensitivity, experimental allergic encephalomyelitis, Freund's adjuvant arthritis, and graft vs. host disease in many animal species for a variety of organs.

The effectiveness of cyclosporine results from specific and reversible inhibition of immunocompetent lymphocytes in the G_0- and G_1-phase of the cell cycle. T-lymphocytes are preferentially inhibited. The T-helper cell is the main target, although the T-suppressor cell may also be suppressed. Cyclosporine also inhibits lymphokine production and release including interleukin-2.

No effects on phagocytic function (changes in enzyme secretions, chemotactic migration of granulocytes, macrophage migration, carbon clearance *in vivo*) have been detected in animals. Cyclosporine does not cause bone marrow suppression in animal models or man.

Pharmacokinetics

The immunosuppressive activity of cyclosporine is primarily due to parent drug. Following oral administration, absorption of cyclosporine is incomplete. The extent of absorption of cyclosporine is dependent on the individual patient, the patient population, and the formulation. Elimination of cyclosporine is primarily biliary with only 6% of the dose (parent drug and metabolites) excreted in urine. The disposition of cyclosporine from blood is generally biphasic, with a terminal half-life of approximately 8.4 hours (range 5-18 hours). Following intravenous administration, the blood clearance of cyclosporine (assay: HPLC) is approximately 5-7 mL/min/kg in adult recipients of renal or liver allografts. Blood cyclosporine clearance appears to be slightly slower in cardiac transplant patients.

The Neoral® Soft Gelatin Capsules (cyclosporine capsules, USP) MODIFIED and Neoral® Oral Solution (cyclosporine oral solution, USP) MODIFIED are bioequivalent. Neoral® Oral Solution diluted with orange juice or apple juice is bioequivalent to Neoral Oral Solution diluted with water. The effect of milk on the bioavailability of cyclosporine when administered as Neoral Oral Solution has not been evaluated.

The relationship between administered dose and exposure (area under the concentration versus time curve, AUC) is linear within the therapeutic dose range. The intersubject variability (total, %CV) of cyclosporine exposure (AUC) when Neoral® or Sandimmune® is administered ranges from approximately 20% to 50% in renal transplant patients. This intersubject variability contributes to the need for individualization of the dosing regimen for optimal therapy *(See DOSAGE AND ADMINISTRATION)*. Intrasubject variability of AUC in renal transplant recipients (%CV) was 9%-21% for Neoral® and 19%-26% for Sandimmune®. In the same studies, intrasubject variability of trough concentrations (%CV) was 17%-30% for Neoral® and 16%-38% for Sandimmune®.

Absorption

Neoral® has increased bioavailability compared to Sandimmune®. The absolute bioavailability of cyclosporine administered as Sandimmune® is dependent on the patient population, estimated to be less than 10% in liver transplant patients and as great as 89% in some renal transplant patients. The absolute bioavailability of cyclosporine administered as Neoral® has not been determined in adults. In studies of renal transplant, rheumatoid arthritis and psoriasis patients, the mean cyclosporine AUC was approximately 20% to 50% greater and the peak blood cyclosporine concentration (C_{max}) was approximately 40% to 106% greater following administration of Neoral® compared to following administration of Sandimmune®. The dose normalized AUC in *de novo* liver transplant patients administered Neoral® 28 days after transplantation was 50% greater and C_{max} was 90% greater than in those patients administered Sandimmune®. AUC and C_{max} are also increased (Neoral® relative to Sandimmune®) in heart transplant patients, but data are very limited. Although the AUC and C_{max} values are higher on Neoral® relative to Sandimmune®, the predose trough concentrations (dose-normalized) are similar for the two formulations.

Following oral administration of Neoral®, the time to peak blood cyclosporine concentrations (T_{max}) ranged from 1.5-2.0 hours. The administration of food with Neoral® decreases the cyclosporine AUC and C_{max}. A high fat meal (669 kcal, 45 grams fat) consumed within one-half hour before Neoral® administration decreased the AUC by 13% and C_{max} by 33%. The effects of a low fat meal (667 kcal, 15 grams fat) were similar.

The effect of T-tube diversion of bile on the absorption of cyclosporine from Neoral® was investigated in eleven *de novo* liver transplant patients. When the patients were administered Neoral® with and without T-tube diversion of bile, very little difference in absorption was observed, as measured by the change in maximal cyclosporine blood concentrations from pre-dose values with the T-tube closed relative to when it was open: 6.9±41% (range -55% to 68%).

[See first table at top of next page]

Distribution

Cyclosporine is distributed largely outside the blood volume. The steady state volume of distribution during intravenous dosing has been reported as 3-5 L/kg in solid organ transplant recipients. In blood, the distribution is concentration dependent. Approximately 33%-47% is in plasma, 4%-9% in lymphocytes, 5%-12% in granulocytes, and 41%-58% in erythrocytes. At high concentrations, the binding capacity of leukocytes and erythrocytes becomes saturated. In plasma, approximately 90% is bound to proteins, primarily lipoproteins. Cyclosporine is excreted in human milk. *(See PRECAUTIONS, Nursing Mothers)*

Metabolism

Cyclosporine is extensively metabolized by the cytochrome P-450 3A enzyme system in the liver, and to a lesser degree in the gastrointestinal tract, and the kidney. The metabolism of cyclosporine can be altered by the coadministration of a variety of agents. *(See PRECAUTIONS, Drug Interactions)* At least 25 metabolites have been identified from human bile, feces, blood, and urine. The biological activity of the metabolites and their contributions to toxicity are considerably less than those of the parent compound. The major metabolites (M1, M9, and M4N) result from oxidation at the 1-beta, 9-gamma, and 4-N-demethylated positions, respectively. At steady state following the oral administration of Sandimmune®, the mean AUCs for blood concentrations of M1, M9, and M4N are about 70%, 21%, and 7.5% of the AUC for blood cyclosporine concentrations, respectively. Based on blood concentration data from stable renal transplant patients (13 patients administered Neoral® and Sandimmune® in a crossover study), and bile concentration data from *de novo* liver transplant patients (4 administered Neoral®, 3 administered Sandimmune®), the percentage of dose present as M1, M9, and M4N metabolites is similar when either Neoral® or Sandimmune® is administered.

Excretion

Only 0.1% of a cyclosporine dose is excreted unchanged in the urine. Elimination is primarily biliary with only 6% of the dose (parent drug and metabolites) excreted in the urine. Neither dialysis nor renal failure alters cyclosporine clearance significantly.

Drug Interactions

(See PRECAUTIONS, Drug Interactions) When diclofenac or methotrexate was coadministered with cyclosporine in rheumatoid arthritis patients, the AUC of diclofenac and methotrexate, each was significantly increased. *(See PRECAUTIONS, Drug Interactions)* No clinically significant pharmacokinetic interactions occurred between cyclosporine and aspirin, ketoprofen, piroxicam, or indomethacin.

Specific Populations

Renal Impairment

In a study performed in 4 subjects with end-stage renal disease (creatinine clearance <5 mL/min), an intravenous infusion of 3.5 mg/kg of cyclosporine over 4 hours administered at the end of a hemodialysis session resulted in a mean volume of distribution (Vdss) of 3.49 L/kg and systemic clearance (CL) of 0.369 L/hr/kg. This systemic CL (0.369 L/hr/kg) was approximately two thirds of the mean systemic CL (0.56 L/hr/kg) of cyclosporine in historical control subjects with normal renal function. In 5 liver transplant patients, the mean clearance of cyclosporine on and off hemodialysis was 463 mL/min and 398 mL/min, respectively. Less than 1% of the dose of cyclosporine was recovered in the dialysate.

Hepatic Impairment

Cyclosporine is extensively metabolized by the liver. Since severe hepatic impairment may result in significantly increased cyclosporine exposures, the dosage of cyclosporine may need to be reduced in these patients.

Pediatric Population

Pharmacokinetic data from pediatric patients administered Neoral® or Sandimmune® are very limited. In 15 renal transplant patients aged 3-16 years, cyclosporine whole blood clearance after IV administration of Sandimmune® was 10.6±3.7 mL/min/kg (assay: Cyclo-trac specific RIA). In a study of 7 renal transplant patients aged 2-16, the cyclosporine clearance ranged from 9.8-15.5 mL/min/kg. In 9 liver transplant patients aged 0.6-5.6 years, clearance was 9.3±5.4 mL/min/kg (assay: HPLC).

In the pediatric population, Neoral® also demonstrates an increased bioavailability as compared to Sandimmune®. In 7 liver *de novo* transplant patients aged 1.4-10 years, the absolute bioavailability of Neoral® was 43% (range 30%-68%) and for Sandimmune® in the same individuals absolute bioavailability was 28% (range 17%-42%).

[See second table above]

Geriatric Population

Comparison of single dose data from both normal elderly volunteers (N=18, mean age 69 years) and elderly rheumatoid arthritis patients (N=16, mean age 68 years) to single dose data in young adult volunteers (N=16, mean age 26 years) showed no significant difference in the pharmacokinetic parameters.

CLINICAL TRIALS

Rheumatoid Arthritis

The effectiveness of Sandimmune® and Neoral® in the treatment of severe rheumatoid arthritis was evaluated in 5 clinical studies involving a total of 728 cyclosporine treated patients and 273 placebo treated patients.

A summary of the results is presented for the "responder" rates per treatment group, with a responder being defined as a patient having *completed* the trial with a 20% improvement in the tender and the swollen joint count and a 20% improvement in 2 of 4 of investigator global, patient global, disability, and erythrocyte sedimentation rates (ESR) for the Studies 651 and 652 and 3 of 5 of investigator global, patient global, disability, visual analog pain, and ESR for Studies 2008, 654 and 302.

Study 651 enrolled 264 patients with active rheumatoid arthritis with at least 20 involved joints, who had failed at least one major RA drug, using a 3:3:2 randomization to one of the following three groups: (1) cyclosporine dosed at 2.5-5 mg/kg/day, (2) methotrexate at 7.5-15 mg/week, or (3) placebo. Treatment duration was 24 weeks. The mean cyclosporine dose at the last visit was 3.1 mg/kg/day. See Graph below.

Study 652 enrolled 250 patients with active RA with >6 active painful or tender joints who had failed at least one major RA drug. Patients were randomized using a 3:3:2 randomization to 1 of 3 treatment arms: (1) 1.5-5 mg/kg/day of cyclosporine, (2) 2.5-5 mg/kg/day of cyclosporine, and (3) placebo. Treatment duration was 16 weeks. The mean cyclosporine dose for group 2 at the last visit was 2.92 mg/kg/day. See Graph below.

Study 2008 enrolled 144 patients with active RA and >6 active joints who had unsuccessful treatment courses of aspirin and gold or Penicillamine. Patients were randomized to 1 of 2 treatment groups (1) cyclosporine 2.5-5 mg/kg/day with adjustments after the first month to achieve a target trough level and (2) placebo. Treatment duration was 24 weeks. The mean cyclosporine dose at the last visit was 3.63 mg/kg/day. See Graph below.

Study 654 enrolled 148 patients who remained with active joint counts of 6 or more despite treatment with maximally

Patient Population	Dose/day[1] (mg/d)	Dose/weight (mg/kg/d)	AUC[2] (ng·hr/mL)	C_{max} (ng/mL)	Trough[3] (ng/mL)	CL/F (mL/min)	CL/F (mL/min/kg)
	Pharmacokinetic Parameters (mean±SD)						
De novo renal transplant[4] Week 4 (N=37)	597±174	7.95±2.81	8772±2089	1802±428	361±129	593±204	7.8±2.9
Stable renal transplant[4] (N=55)	344±122	4.10±1.58	6035±2194	1333±469	251±116	492±140	5.9±2.1
De novo liver transplant[5] Week 4 (N=18)	458±190	6.89±3.68	7187±2816	1555±740	268±101	577±309	8.6±5.7
De novo rheumatoid arthritis[6] (N=23)	182±55.6	2.37±0.36	2641±877	728±263	96.4±37.7	613±196	8.3±2.8
De novo psoriasis[6] Week 4 (N=18)	189±69.8	2.48±0.65	2324±1048	655±186	74.9±46.7	723±186	10.2±3.9

[1]Total daily dose was divided into two doses administered every 12 hours
[2]AUC was measured over one dosing interval
[3]Trough concentration was measured just prior to the morning Neoral® dose, approximately 12 hours after the previous dose
[4]Assay: TDx specific monoclonal fluorescence polarization immunoassay
[5]Assay: Cyclo-trac specific monoclonal radioimmunoassay
[6]Assay: INCSTAR specific monoclonal radioimmunoassay

Patient Population	Dose/day (mg/d)	Dose/weight (mg/kg/d)	AUC[1] (ng·hr/mL)	C_{max} (ng/mL)	CL/F (mL/min)	CL/F (mL/min/kg)
	Pediatric Pharmacokinetic Parameters (mean±SD)					
Stable liver transplant[2]						
Age 2-8, Dosed TID (N=9)	101±25	5.95±1.32	2163±801	629±219	285±94	16.6±4.3
Age 8-15, Dosed BID (N=8)	188±55	4.96±2.09	4272±1462	975±281	378±80	10.2±4.0
Stable liver transplant[3]						
Age 3, Dosed BID (N=1)	120	8.33	5832	1050	171	11.9
Age 8-15, Dosed BID (N=5)	158±55	5.51±1.91	4452±2475	1013±635	328±121	11.0±1.9
Stable renal transplant[3]						
Age 7-15, Dosed BID (N=5)	328±83	7.37±4.11	6922±1988	1827±487	418±143	8.7±2.9

[1]AUC was measured over one dosing interval
[2]Assay: Cyclo-trac specific monoclonal radioimmunoassay
[3]Assay: TDx specific monoclonal fluorescence polarization immunoassay

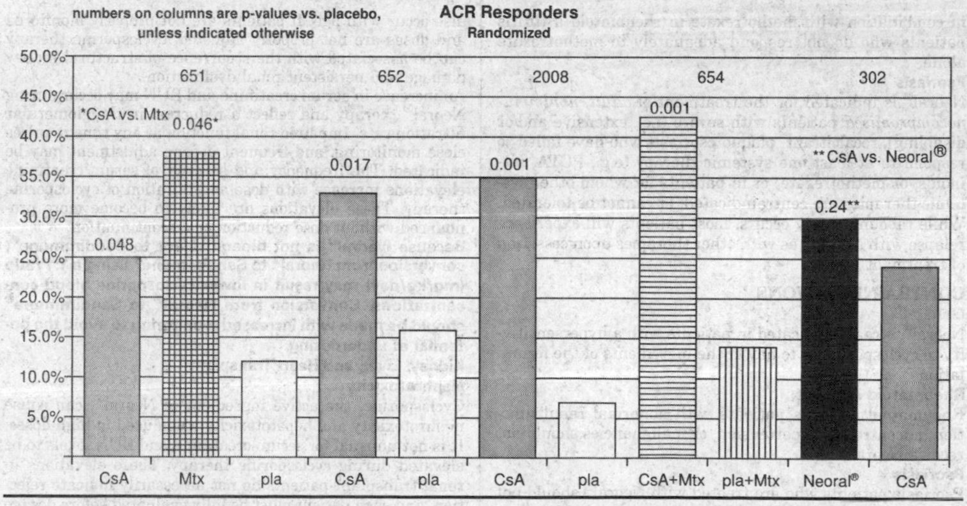

tolerated methotrexate doses for at least three months. Patients continued to take their current dose of methotrexate and were randomized to receive, in addition, one of the following medications: (1) cyclosporine 2.5 mg/kg/day with dose increases of 0.5 mg/kg/day at weeks 2 and 4 if there was no evidence of toxicity and further increases of 0.5 mg/kg/day at weeks 8 and 16 if a <30% decrease in active joint count occurred without any significant toxicity; dose decreases could be made at any time for toxicity or (2) placebo. Treatment duration was 24 weeks. The mean cyclosporine dose at the last visit was 2.8 mg/kg/day (range: 1.3-4.1). See Graph below.

Study 302 enrolled 299 patients with severe active RA, 99% of whom were unresponsive or intolerant to at least one prior major RA drug. Patients were randomized to 1 of 2 treatment groups (1) Neoral® and (2) cyclosporine, both of which were started at 2.5 mg/kg/day and increased after 4 weeks for inefficacy in increments of 0.5 mg/kg/day to a maximum of 5 mg/kg/day and decreased at any time for toxicity. Treatment duration was 24 weeks. The mean cyclosporine dose at the last visit was 2.91 mg/kg/day (range: 0.72-5.17) for Neoral® and 3.27 mg/kg/day (range: 0.73-5.68) for cyclosporine. See Graph below.

[See figure above]

INDICATIONS AND USAGE

Kidney, Liver, and Heart Transplantation

Neoral® is indicated for the prophylaxis of organ rejection in kidney, liver, and heart allogeneic transplants. Neoral® has been used in combination with azathioprine and corticosteroids.

Rheumatoid Arthritis

Neoral® is indicated for the treatment of patients with severe active, rheumatoid arthritis where the disease has not adequately responded to methotrexate. Neoral® can be used

Nephrotoxicity vs. Rejection

Parameter	Nephrotoxicity	Rejection
History	Donor >50 years old or hypotensive Prolonged kidney preservation Prolonged anastomosis time Concomitant nephrotoxic drugs	Anti-donor immune response Retransplant patient
Clinical	Often >6 weeks postop[b] Prolonged initial nonfunction (acute tubular necrosis)	Often < 4 weeks postop[b] Fever > 37.5°C Weight gain > 0.5 kg Graft swelling and tenderness Decrease in daily urine volume > 500 mL (or 50%)
Laboratory	CyA serum trough level > 200 ng/mL Gradual rise in Cr (< 0.15 mg/dl/day)[a] Cr plateau < 25% above baseline BUN/Cr ≥ 20	CyA serum trough level < 150 ng/mL Rapid rise in Cr (> 0.3 mg/dl/day)[a] Cr > 25% above baseline BUN/Cr < 20
Biopsy	Arteriolopathy (medial hypertrophy [a], hyalinosis, nodular deposits, intimal thickening, endothelial vacuolization, progressive scarring) Tubular atrophy, isometric vacuolization, isolated calcifications Minimal edema Mild focal infiltrates[c] Diffuse interstitial fibrosis, often striped form	Endovasculitis[c] (proliferation[a], intimal arteritis[b], necrosis, sclerosis) Tubulitis with RBC[b] and WBC[b] casts, some irregular vacuolization Interstitial edema[c] and hemorrhage[b] Diffuse moderate to severe mononuclear infiltrates[d] Glomerulitis (mononuclear cells)[c]
Aspiration Cytology	CyA deposits in tubular and endothelial cells Fine isometric vacuolization of tubular cells	Inflammatory infiltrate with mononuclear phagocytes, macrophages, lymphoblastoid cells, and activated T-cells These strongly express HLA-DR antigens
Urine Cytology	Tubular cells with vacuolization and granularization	Degenerative tubular cells, plasma cells, and lymphocyturia > 20% of sediment
Manometry	Intracapsular pressure < 40 mm Hg[b]	Intracapsular pressure > 40 mm Hg[b]
Ultrasonography	Unchanged graft cross sectional area	Increase in graft cross sectional area AP diameter ≥ Transverse diameter
Magnetic Resonance Imagery	Normal appearance	Loss of distinct corticomedullary junction, swelling image intensity of parachyma approaching that of psoas, loss of hilar fat
Radionuclide Scan	Normal or generally decreased perfusion Decrease in tubular function (^{131} I-hippuran) > decrease in perfusion (^{99m} Tc DTPA)	Patchy arterial flow Decrease in perfusion > decrease in tubular function Increased uptake of Indium 111 labeled platelets or Tc-99m in colloid
Therapy	Responds to decreased cyclosporine	Responds to increased steroids or antilymphocyte globulin

[a]$p < 0.05$, [b]$p < 0.01$, [c]$p < 0.001$, [d]$p < 0.0001$

in combination with methotrexate in rheumatoid arthritis patients who do not respond adequately to methotrexate alone.

Psoriasis

Neoral® is indicated for the treatment of *adult, nonimmunocompromised* patients with severe (i.e., extensive and/or disabling), recalcitrant, plaque psoriasis who have failed to respond to at least one systemic therapy (e.g., PUVA, retinoids, or methotrexate) or in patients for whom other systemic therapies are contraindicated, or cannot be tolerated.

While rebound rarely occurs, most patients will experience relapse with Neoral® as with other therapies upon cessation of treatment.

CONTRAINDICATIONS

General

Neoral® is contraindicated in patients with a hypersensitivity to cyclosporine or to any of the ingredients of the formulation.

Rheumatoid Arthritis

Rheumatoid arthritis patients with abnormal renal function, uncontrolled hypertension, or malignancies should not receive Neoral®.

Psoriasis

Psoriasis patients who are treated with Neoral® should not receive concomitant PUVA or UVB therapy, methotrexate or other immunosuppressive agents, coal tar or radiation therapy. Psoriasis patients with abnormal renal function, uncontrolled hypertension, or malignancies should not receive Neoral®.

WARNINGS

(See also BOXED WARNING)

All Patients

Cyclosporine, the active ingredient of Neoral®, can cause nephrotoxicity and hepatotoxicity. The risk increases with increasing doses of cyclosporine. Renal dysfunction including structural kidney damage is a potential consequence of Neoral® and therefore renal function must be monitored during therapy. **Care should be taken in using cyclosporine with nephrotoxic drugs. *(See PRECAUTIONS)***

Patients receiving Neoral® require frequent monitoring of serum creatinine. *(See Special Monitoring under DOSAGE AND ADMINISTRATION)* Elderly patients should be monitored with particular care, since decreases in renal function also occur with age. If patients are not properly monitored and doses are not properly adjusted, cyclosporine therapy can be associated with the occurrence of structural kidney damage and persistent renal dysfunction.

An increase in serum creatinine and BUN may occur during Neoral® therapy and reflect a reduction in the glomerular filtration rate. Impaired renal function at any time requires close monitoring, and frequent dosage adjustment may be indicated. The frequency and severity of serum creatinine elevations increase with dose and duration of cyclosporine therapy. These elevations are likely to become more pronounced without dose reduction or discontinuation.

Because Neoral® is not bioequivalent to Sandimmune®, conversion from Neoral® to Sandimmune® using a 1:1 ratio (mg/kg/day) may result in lower cyclosporine blood concentrations. Conversion from Neoral® to Sandimmune® should be made with increased monitoring to avoid the potential of underdosing.

Kidney, Liver, and Heart Transplant

Nephrotoxicity

Cyclosporine, the active ingredient of Neoral®, can cause nephrotoxicity and hepatotoxicity when used in high doses. It is not unusual for serum creatinine and BUN levels to be elevated during cyclosporine therapy. These elevations in renal transplant patients do not necessarily indicate rejection, and each patient must be fully evaluated before dosage adjustment is initiated.

Based on the historical Sandimmune® experience with oral solution, nephrotoxicity associated with cyclosporine had been noted in 25% of cases of renal transplantation, 38% of cases of cardiac transplantation, and 37% of cases of liver transplantation. Mild nephrotoxicity was generally noted 2-3 months after renal transplant and consisted of an arrest in the fall of the pre-operative elevations of BUN and creatinine at a range of 35-45 mg/dl and 2.0-2.5 mg/dl respectively. These elevations were often responsive to cyclosporine dosage reduction.

More overt nephrotoxicity was seen early after transplantation and was characterized by a rapidly rising BUN and creatinine. Since these events are similar to renal rejection episodes, care must be taken to differentiate between them. This form of nephrotoxicity is usually responsive to cyclosporine dosage reduction.

Although specific diagnostic criteria which reliably differentiate renal graft rejection from drug toxicity have not been found, a number of parameters have been significantly associated with one or the other. It should be noted however, that up to 20% of patients may have simultaneous nephrotoxicity and rejection.

[See table above]

A form of a cyclosporine-associated nephropathy is characterized by serial deterioration in renal function and morphologic changes in the kidneys. From 5%-15% of transplant recipients who have received cyclosporine will fail to show a reduction in rising serum creatinine despite a decrease or discontinuation of cyclosporine therapy. Renal biopsies from these patients will demonstrate one or several of the following alterations: tubular vacuolization, tubular microcalcifications, peritubular capillary congestion, arteriolopathy, and a striped form of interstitial fibrosis with tubular atrophy. Though none of these morphologic changes is entirely specific, a diagnosis of cyclosporine-associated structural nephrotoxicity requires evidence of these findings.

When considering the development of cyclosporine-associated nephropathy, it is noteworthy that several authors have reported an association between the appearance of interstitial fibrosis and higher cumulative doses or persistently high circulating trough concentrations of cyclosporine. This is particularly true during the first 6 post-transplant months when the dosage tends to be highest and when, in kidney recipients, the organ appears to be most vulnerable to the toxic effects of cyclosporine. Among other contributing factors to the development of interstitial fibrosis in these patients are prolonged perfusion time, warm ischemia time, as well as episodes of acute toxicity, and acute and chronic rejection. The reversibility of interstitial fibrosis and its correlation to renal function have not yet been determined. Reversibility of arteriolopathy has been reported after stopping cyclosporine or lowering the dosage.

Impaired renal function at any time requires close monitoring, and frequent dosage adjustment may be indicated.

In the event of severe and unremitting rejection, when rescue therapy with pulse steroids and monoclonal antibodies fail to reverse the rejection episode, it may be preferable to switch to alternative immunosuppressive therapy rather than increase the Neoral® dose to excessive blood concentrations.

Due to the potential for additive or synergistic impairment of renal function, caution should be exercised when coadministering Neoral with other drugs that may impair renal function. *(See PRECAUTIONS, Drug Interactions)*

Thrombotic Microangiopathy

Occasionally patients have developed a syndrome of thrombocytopenia and microangiopathic hemolytic anemia which may result in graft failure. The vasculopathy can occur in the absence of rejection and is accompanied by avid platelet consumption within the graft as demonstrated by Indium 111 labeled platelet studies. Neither the pathogenesis nor the management of this syndrome is clear. Though resolution has occurred after reduction or discontinuation of cyclosporine and 1) administration of streptokinase and heparin or 2) plasmapheresis, this appears to depend upon early detection with Indium 111 labeled platelet scans. *(See ADVERSE REACTIONS)*

Hyperkalemia

Significant hyperkalemia (sometimes associated with hyperchloremic metabolic acidosis) and hyperuricemia have been seen occasionally in individual patients.

Hepatotoxicity

Cases of hepatotoxicity and liver injury including cholestasis, jaundice, hepatitis, and liver failure have been reported in patients treated with cyclosporine. Most reports included patients with significant co-morbidities, underlying conditions and other confounding factors including infectious complications and comedications with hepatotoxic potential. In some cases, mainly in transplant patients, fatal outcomes have been reported. *(See ADVERSE REACTIONS, Postmarketing Experience, Kidney, Liver and Heart Transplantation)*

Hepatotoxicity, usually manifested by elevations in hepatic enzymes and bilirubin, was reported in patients treated with cyclosporine in clinical trials: 4% in renal transplantation, 7% in cardiac transplantation, and 4% in liver transplantation. This was usually noted during the first month of therapy when high doses of cyclosporine were used. The chemistry elevations usually decreased with a reduction in dosage.

Malignancies

As in patients receiving other immunosuppressants, those patients receiving cyclosporine are at increased risk for development of lymphomas and other malignancies, particularly those of the skin. Patients taking cyclosporine should be warned to avoid excess ultraviolet light exposure. The increased risk appears related to the intensity and duration of immunosuppression rather than to the use of specific agents. Because of the danger of oversuppression of the immune system resulting in increased risk of infection or malignancy, a treatment regimen containing multiple immunosuppressants should be used with caution. Some malignancies may be fatal. Transplant patients receiving cyclosporine are at increased risk for serious infection with fatal outcome.

Serious Infections

Patients receiving immunosuppressants, including Neoral, are at increased risk of developing bacterial, viral, fungal, and protozoal infections, including opportunistic infections. These infections may lead to serious, including fatal, outcomes. *(See BOXED WARNING, and ADVERSE REACTIONS)*

Polyoma Virus Infections

Patients receiving immunosuppressants, including Neoral, are at increased risk for opportunistic infections, including polyoma virus infections. Polyoma virus infections in transplant patients may have serious, and sometimes, fatal outcomes. These include cases of JC virus-associated progressive multifocal leukoencephalopathy (PML), and polyoma virus-associated nephropathy (PVAN), especially due to BK virus infection, which have been observed in patients receiving cyclosporine. PVAN is associated with serious outcomes, including deteriorating renal function and renal graft loss, *(See ADVERSE REACTIONS, Postmarketing Experience, Kidney, Liver and Heart Transplantation)*. Patient monitoring may help detect patients at risk for PVAN.

Cases of PML have been reported in patients treated with Neoral. PML, which is sometimes fatal, commonly presents with hemiparesis, apathy, confusion, cognitive deficiencies and ataxia. Risk factors for PML include treatment with immunosuppressant therapies and impairment of immune function. In immunosuppressed patients, physicians should consider PML in the differential diagnosis in patients reporting neurological symptoms and consultation with a neurologist should be considered as clinically indicated.

Consideration should be given to reducing the total immunosuppression in transplant patients who develop PML or PVAN. However, reduced immunosuppression may place the graft at risk.

Neurotoxicity

There have been reports of convulsions in adult and pediatric patients receiving cyclosporine, particularly in combination with high dose methylprednisolone.

Encephalopathy, including Posterior Reversible Encephalopathy Syndrome (PRES), has been described both in postmarketing reports and in the literature. Manifestations include impaired consciousness, convulsions, visual disturbances (including blindness), loss of motor function, movement disorders and psychiatric disturbances. In many cases, changes in the white matter have been detected using imaging techniques and pathologic specimens. Predisposing factors such as hypertension, hypomagnesemia, hypocholesterolemia, high-dose corticosteroids, high cyclosporine blood concentrations, and graft-versus-host disease have been noted in many but not all of the reported cases. The changes in most cases have been reversible upon discontinuation of cyclosporine, and in some cases improvement was noted after reduction of dose. It appears that patients receiving liver transplant are more susceptible to encephalopathy than those receiving kidney transplant. Another rare manifestation of cyclosporine-induced neurotoxicity, occurring in transplant patients more frequently than in other indications, is optic disc edema including papilloedema, with possible visual impairment, secondary to benign intracranial hypertension.

Care should be taken in using cyclosporine with nephrotoxic drugs. *(See PRECAUTIONS)*

Rheumatoid Arthritis

Cyclosporine nephropathy was detected in renal biopsies of 6 out of 60 (10%) rheumatoid arthritis patients after the average treatment duration of 19 months. Only one patient, out of these 6 patients, was treated with a dose ≤4 mg/kg/day. Serum creatinine improved in all but one patient after discontinuation of cyclosporine. The "maximal creatinine increase" appears to be a factor in predicting cyclosporine nephropathy.

There is a potential, as with other immunosuppressive agents, for an increase in the occurrence of malignant lymphomas with cyclosporine. It is not clear whether the risk with cyclosporine is greater than that in rheumatoid arthritis patients or in rheumatoid arthritis patients on cytotoxic treatment for this indication. Five cases of lymphoma were detected: four in a survey of approximately 2,300 patients treated with cyclosporine for rheumatoid arthritis, and another case of lymphoma was reported in a clinical trial. Although other tumors (12 skin cancers, 24 solid tumors of diverse types, and 1 multiple myeloma) were also reported in this survey, epidemiologic analyses did not support a relationship to cyclosporine other than for malignant lymphomas.

Patients should be thoroughly evaluated before and during Neoral® treatment for the development of malignancies. Moreover, use of Neoral® therapy with other immunosuppressive agents may induce an excessive immunosuppression which is known to increase the risk of malignancy.

Psoriasis

(See also BOXED WARNING for Psoriasis)

Since cyclosporine is a potent immunosuppressive agent with a number of potentially serious side effects, the risks and benefits of using Neoral® should be considered before treatment of patients with psoriasis. Cyclosporine, the active ingredient in Neoral®, can cause nephrotoxicity and hypertension *(See PRECAUTIONS)* and the risk increases with increasing dose and duration of therapy. Patients who may be at increased risk such as those with abnormal renal function, uncontrolled hypertension or malignancies, should not receive Neoral®.

Renal dysfunction is a potential consequence of Neoral® therefore renal function must be monitored during therapy. Patients receiving Neoral® require frequent monitoring of serum creatinine. *(See Special Monitoring under DOSAGE AND ADMINISTRATION)* Elderly patients should be monitored with particular care, since decreases in renal function also occur with age. If patients are not properly monitored and doses are not properly adjusted, cyclosporine therapy can cause structural kidney damage and persistent renal dysfunction.

An increase in serum creatinine and BUN may occur during Neoral® therapy and reflects a reduction in the glomerular filtration rate.

Kidney biopsies from 86 psoriasis patients treated for a mean duration of 23 months with 1.2-7.6 mg/kg/day of cyclosporine showed evidence of cyclosporine nephropathy in 18/86 (21%) of the patients. The pathology consisted of renal tubular atrophy and interstitial fibrosis. On repeat biopsy of 13 of these patients maintained on various dosages of cyclosporine for a mean of 2 additional years, the number with cyclosporine induced nephropathy rose to 26/86 (30%). The majority of patients (19/26) were on a dose of ≥5.0 mg/kg/day (the highest recommended dose is 4 mg/kg/day). The patients were also on cyclosporine for greater than 15 months (18/26) and/or had a clinically significant increase in serum creatinine for greater than 1 month (21/26). Creatinine levels returned to normal range in 7 of 11 patients in whom cyclosporine therapy was discontinued.

There is an increased risk for the development of skin and lymphoproliferative malignancies in cyclosporine-treated psoriasis patients. The relative risk of malignancies is comparable to that observed in psoriasis patients treated with other immunosuppressive agents.

Tumors were reported in 32 (2.2%) of 1439 psoriasis patients treated with cyclosporine worldwide from clinical trials. Additional tumors have been reported in 7 patients in cyclosporine postmarketing experience. Skin malignancies were reported in 16 (1.1%) of these patients; all but 2 of them had previously received PUVA therapy. Methotrexate was received by 7 patients. UVB and coal tar had been used by 2 and 3 patients, respectively. Seven patients had either a history of previous skin cancer or a potentially predisposing lesion was present prior to cyclosporine exposure. Of the 16 patients with skin cancer, 11 patients had 18 squamous cell carcinomas and 7 patients had 10 basal cell carcinomas.

There were two lymphoproliferative malignancies; one case of non-Hodgkin's lymphoma which required chemotherapy, and one case of mycosis fungoides which regressed spontaneously upon discontinuation of cyclosporine. There were four cases of benign lymphocytic infiltration: 3 regressed spontaneously upon discontinuation of cyclosporine, while the fourth regressed despite continuation of the drug. The remainder of the malignancies, 13 cases (0.9%), involved various organs.

Patients should not be treated concurrently with cyclosporine and PUVA or UVB, other radiation therapy, or other immunosuppressive agents, because of the possibility of excessive immunosuppression and the subsequent risk of malignancies. *(See CONTRAINDICATIONS)* Patients should also be warned to protect themselves appropriately when in the sun, and to avoid excessive sun exposure. Patients should be thoroughly evaluated before and during treatment for the presence of malignancies remembering that malignant lesions may be hidden by psoriatic plaques. Skin lesions not typical of psoriasis should be biopsied before starting treatment. Patients should be treated with Neoral® only after complete resolution of suspicious lesions, and only if there are no other treatment options. *(See Special Monitoring for Psoriasis Patients)*

Special Excipients

Alcohol (ethanol)

The alcohol content *(See DESCRIPTION)* of Neoral should be taken into account when given to patients in whom alcohol intake should be avoided or minimized, e.g., pregnant or breastfeeding women, in patients presenting with liver disease or epilepsy, in alcoholic patients, or pediatric patients. For an adult weighing 70 kg, the maximum daily oral dose would deliver about 1 gram of alcohol which is approximately 6% of the amount of alcohol contained in a standard drink.

PRECAUTIONS

General

Hypertension

Cyclosporine is the active ingredient of Neoral®. Hypertension is a common side effect of cyclosporine therapy which may persist. *(See ADVERSE REACTIONS and DOSAGE AND ADMINISTRATION for monitoring recommendations)*

Mild or moderate hypertension is encountered more frequently than severe hypertension and the incidence decreases over time. In recipients of kidney, liver, and heart allografts treated with cyclosporine, antihypertensive therapy may be required. *(See Special Monitoring of Rheumatoid Arthritis and Psoriasis Patients)* However, since cyclosporine may cause hyperkalemia, potassium-sparing diuretics should not be used. While calcium antagonists can be effective agents in treating cyclosporine-associated hypertension, they can interfere with cyclosporine metabolism. *(See Drug Interactions)*

Vaccination

During treatment with cyclosporine, vaccination may be less effective; and the use of live attenuated vaccines should be avoided.

Special Monitoring of Rheumatoid Arthritis Patients

Before initiating treatment, a careful physical examination, including blood pressure measurements (on at least two occasions) and two creatinine levels to estimate baseline should be performed. Blood pressure and serum creatinine should be evaluated every 2 weeks during the initial 3 months and then monthly if the patient is stable. It is advisable to monitor serum creatinine and blood pressure always after an increase of the dose of nonsteroidal anti-inflammatory drugs and after initiation of new nonsteroidal anti-inflammatory drug therapy during Neoral® treatment. If coadministered with methotrexate, CBC and liver function tests are recommended to be monitored monthly. *(See also PRECAUTIONS, General, Hypertension)*

In patients who are receiving cyclosporine, the dose of Neoral® should be decreased by 25%-50% if hypertension occurs. If hypertension persists, the dose of Neoral® should be further reduced or blood pressure should be controlled with antihypertensive agents. In most cases, blood pressure has returned to baseline when cyclosporine was discontinued.

In placebo-controlled trials of rheumatoid arthritis patients, systolic hypertension (defined as an occurrence of two systolic blood pressure readings >140 mmHg) and diastolic hypertension (defined as two diastolic blood pressure readings >90 mmHg) occurred in 33% and 19% of patients treated with cyclosporine, respectively. The corresponding placebo rates were 22% and 8%.

Special Monitoring for Psoriasis Patients

Before initiating treatment, a careful dermatological and physical examination, including blood pressure measurements (on at least two occasions) should be performed. Since Neoral® is an immunosuppressive agent, patients should be evaluated for the presence of occult infection on their first physical examination and for the presence of tumors initially, and throughout treatment with Neoral®. Skin lesions not typical for psoriasis should be biopsied before starting Neoral®. Patients with malignant or premalignant changes of the skin should be treated with Neoral® only after appropriate treatment of such lesions and if no other treatment option exists.

Baseline laboratories should include serum creatinine (on two occasions), BUN, CBC, serum magnesium, potassium, uric acid, and lipids.

The risk of cyclosporine nephropathy is reduced when the starting dose is low (2.5 mg/kg/day), the maximum dose does not exceed 4.0 mg/kg/day, serum creatinine is monitored regularly while cyclosporine is administered, and the dose of Neoral® is decreased when the rise in creatinine is greater than or equal to 25% above the patient's pretreatment level. The increase in creatinine is generally reversible upon timely decrease of the dose of Neoral® or its discontinuation.

Serum creatinine and BUN should be evaluated every 2 weeks during the initial 3 months of therapy and then monthly if the patient is stable. If the serum creatinine is greater than or equal to 25% above the patient's pretreatment level, serum creatinine should be repeated within two weeks. If the change in serum creatinine remains greater than or equal to 25% above baseline, Neoral® should be reduced by 25%-50%. If at **any time** the serum creatinine increases by greater than or equal to 50% above pretreatment level, Neoral® should be reduced by 25%-50%. Neoral® should be discontinued if reversibility (within 25% of baseline) of serum creatinine is not achievable after two dosage modifications. It is advisable to monitor serum creatinine after an increase of the dose of nonsteroidal anti-inflammatory drug and after initiation of new nonsteroidal anti-inflammatory therapy during Neoral® treatment.

Blood pressure should be evaluated every 2 weeks during the initial 3 months of therapy and then monthly if the patient is stable, or more frequently when dosage adjustments are made. Patients without a history of previous hypertension before initiation of treatment with Neoral®, should have the drug reduced by 25%-50% if found to have sustained hypertension. If the patient continues to be hyper-

Antibiotics	Antineoplastics	Antifungals	Anti-inflammatory Drugs	Gastrointestinal Agents	Immunosuppressives	Other Drugs
ciprofloxacin	melphalan	amphotericin B	azapropazon	cimetidine	tacrolimus	fibric acid derivatives
gentamicin		ketoconazole	colchicine	ranitidine		(e.g., bezafibrate,
tobramycin			diclofenac			fenofibrate)
vancomycin			naproxen			methotrexate
trimethoprim with			sulindac			
sulfamethoxazole						

tensive despite multiple reductions of Neoral®, then Neoral® should be discontinued. For patients with treated hypertension, before the initiation of Neoral® therapy, their medication should be adjusted to control hypertension while on Neoral®. Neoral® should be discontinued if a change in hypertension management is not effective or tolerable.

CBC, uric acid, potassium, lipids, and magnesium should also be monitored every 2 weeks for the first 3 months of therapy, and then monthly if the patient is stable or more frequently when dosage adjustments are made. Neoral® dosage should be reduced by 25%-50% for any abnormality of clinical concern.

In controlled trials of cyclosporine in psoriasis patients, cyclosporine blood concentrations did not correlate well with either improvement or with side effects such as renal dysfunction.

Information for Patients: Patients should be advised that any change of cyclosporine formulation should be made cautiously and only under physician supervision because it may result in the need for a change in dosage.

Patients should be informed of the necessity of repeated laboratory tests while they are receiving cyclosporine. Patients should be advised of the potential risks during pregnancy and informed of the increased risk of neoplasia. Patients should also be informed of the risk of hypertension and renal dysfunction.

Patients should be advised that during treatment with cyclosporine, vaccination may be less effective and the use of live attenuated vaccines should be avoided.

Patients should be given careful dosage instructions. Neoral® Oral Solution (cyclosporine oral solution, USP) MODIFIED should be diluted, preferably with orange or apple juice that is at room temperature. The combination of Neoral® Oral Solution (cyclosporine oral solution, USP) MODIFIED with milk can be unpalatable.

Patients should be advised to take Neoral® on a consistent schedule with regard to time of day and relation to meals. Grapefruit and grapefruit juice affect metabolism, increasing blood concentration of cyclosporine, thus should be avoided.

Laboratory Tests

In all patients treated with cyclosporine, renal and liver functions should be assessed repeatedly by measurement of serum creatinine, BUN, serum bilirubin, and liver enzymes. Serum lipids, magnesium, and potassium should also be monitored. Cyclosporine blood concentrations should be routinely monitored in transplant patients *(See DOSAGE AND ADMINISTRATION, Blood Concentration Monitoring in Transplant Patients)*, and periodically monitored in rheumatoid arthritis patients.

Drug Interactions

A. Effect of Drugs and Other Agents on Cyclosporine Pharmacokinetics and/or Safety

All of the individual drugs cited below are well substantiated to interact with cyclosporine. In addition, concomitant use of non-steroidal anti-inflammatory drugs with cyclosporine, particularly in the setting of dehydration, may potentiate renal dysfunction. Caution should be exercised when using other drugs which are known to impair renal function. *(See WARNINGS, Nephrotoxicity)*

Drugs That May Potentiate Renal Dysfunction

[See table above]

During the concomitant use of a drug that may exhibit additive or synergistic renal impairment with cyclosporine, close monitoring of renal function (in particular serum creatinine) should be performed. If a significant impairment of renal function occurs, the dosage of the coadministered drug should be reduced or an alternative treatment considered.

Cyclosporine is extensively metabolized by CYP 3A isoenzymes, in particular CYP3A4, and is a substrate of the multidrug efflux transporter P-glycoprotein. Various agents are known to either increase or decrease plasma or whole blood concentrations of cyclosporine usually by inhibition or induction of CYP3A4 or P-glycoprotein transporter or both. Compounds that decrease cyclosporine absorption such as orlistat should be avoided. Appropriate Neoral® dosage adjustment to achieve the desired cyclosporine concentrations is essential when drugs that significantly alter cyclosporine concentrations are used concomitantly. *(See Blood Concentration Monitoring)*

1. Drugs That Increase Cyclosporine Concentrations

[See first table below]

HIV Protease inhibitors

The HIV protease inhibitors (e.g., indinavir, nelfinavir, ritonavir, and saquinavir) are known to inhibit cytochrome P-450 3A and thus could potentially increase the concentrations of cyclosporine, however no formal studies of the interaction are available. Care should be exercised when these drugs are administered concomitantly.

Grapefruit juice

Grapefruit and grapefruit juice affect metabolism, increasing blood concentrations of cyclosporine, thus should be avoided.

2. Drugs/Dietary Supplements That Decrease Cyclosporine Concentrations

[See second table below]

Bosentan

Coadministration of bosentan (250–1000 mg every 12 hours based on tolerability) and cyclosporine (300 mg every 12 hours for 2 days then dosing to achieve a C_{min} of 200–250 ng/mL) for 7 days in healthy subjects resulted in decreases in the cyclosporine mean dose-normalized AUC, C_{max}, and trough concentration of approximately 50%, 30%, and 60%, respectively, compared to when cyclosporine was given alone *(See also Effect of Cyclosporine on the Pharmacokinetics and/or Safety of Other Drugs or Agents)*.

Boceprevir

Coadministration of boceprevir (800 mg three times daily for 7 days) and cyclosporine (100 mg single dose) in healthy subjects resulted in increases in the mean AUC and C_{max} of cyclosporine approximately 2.7-fold and 2-fold, respectively, compared to when cyclosporine was given alone.

Telaprevir

Coadministration of telaprevir (750 mg every 8 hours for 11 days) with cyclosporine (10 mg on day 8) in healthy subjects resulted in increases in the mean dose-normalized AUC and C_{max} of cyclosporine approximately 4.5-fold and 1.3-fold, respectively, compared to when cyclosporine (100 mg single dose) was given alone.

Calcium Channel Blockers	Antifungals	Antibiotics	Glucocorticoids	Other Drugs
diltiazem	fluconazole	azithromycin	methylprednisolone	Allopurinol
nicardipine	itraconazole	clarithromycin		Amiodarone
verapamil	ketoconazole	erythromycin		Bromocriptine
	voriconazole	quinupristin/		colchicine
		dalfopristin		danazol
				imatinib
				metoclopramide
				nefazodone
				oral contraceptives

Antibiotics	Anticonvulsants	Other Drugs/Dietary Supplements	
nafcillin	carbamazepine	bosentan	St. John's Wort
rifampin	oxcarbazepine	octreotide	
	phenobarbital	orlistat	
	phenytoin	sulfinpyrazone	
		terbinafine	
		ticlopidine	

St. John's Wort

There have been reports of a serious drug interaction between cyclosporine and the herbal dietary supplement St. John's Wort. This interaction has been reported to produce a marked reduction in the blood concentrations of cyclosporine, resulting in subtherapeutic levels, rejection of transplanted organs, and graft loss.

Rifabutin

Rifabutin is known to increase the metabolism of other drugs metabolized by the cytochrome P-450 system. The interaction between rifabutin and cyclosporine has not been studied. Care should be exercised when these two drugs are administered concomitantly.

B. Effect of Cyclosporine on the Pharmacokinetics and/or Safety of Other Drugs or Agents

Cyclosporine is an inhibitor of CYP3A4 and of the multidrug efflux transporter P-glycoprotein and may increase plasma concentrations of comedications that are substrates of CYP3A4 or P-glycoprotein or both.

Cyclosporine may reduce the clearance of digoxin, colchicine, prednisolone, HMG-CoA reductase inhibitors (statins), and, aliskiren, repaglinide, NSAIDs, sirolimus, etoposide, and other drugs. See the full prescribing information of the other drug for further information and specific recommendations. The decision on coadministration of cyclosporine with other drugs or agents should be made by the physician following the careful assessment of benefits and risks.

Digoxin

Severe digitalis toxicity has been seen within days of starting cyclosporine in several patients taking digoxin. If digoxin is used concurrently with cyclosporine, serum digoxin concentrations should be monitored.

Colchicine

There are reports on the potential of cyclosporine to enhance the toxic effects of colchicine such as myopathy and neuropathy, especially in patients with renal dysfunction. Concomitant administration of cyclosporine and colchicine results in significant increases in colchicine plasma concentrations. If colchicine is used concurrently with cyclosporine, a reduction in the dosage of colchicine is recommended.

HMG-CoA reductase inhibitors (statins)

Literature and postmarketing cases of myotoxicity, including muscle pain and weakness, myositis, and rhabdomyolysis, have been reported with concomitant administration of cyclosporine with lovastatin, simvastatin, atorvastatin, pravastatin, and, rarely fluvastatin. When concurrently administered with cyclosporine, the dosage of these statins should be reduced according to label recommendations. Statin therapy needs to be temporarily withheld or discontinued in patients with signs and symptoms of myopathy or those with risk factors predisposing to severe renal injury, including renal failure, secondary to rhabdomyolysis.

Repaglinide

Cyclosporine may increase the plasma concentrations of repaglinide and thereby increase the risk of hypoglycemia. In 12 healthy male subjects who received two doses of 100mg cyclosporine capsule orally 12 hours apart with a single dose of 0.25mg repaglinide tablet (one half of a 0.5mg tablet) orally 13 hours after the cyclosporine initial dose, the repaglinide mean Cmax and AUC were increased 1.8 fold (range: 0.6-3.7 fold) and 2.4 fold (range 1.2-5.3 fold), respectively. Close monitoring of blood glucose level is advisable for a patient taking cyclosporine and repaglinide concomitantly.

Ambrisentan

Coadministration of ambrisentan (5 mg daily) and cyclosporine (100–150 mg twice daily initially, then dosing to achieve C_{min} 150–200 ng/mL) for 8 days in healthy subjects resulted in mean increases in ambrisentan AUC and C_{max} of approximately 2-fold and 1.5–fold, respectively, compared to ambrisentan alone.

Anthracycline antibiotics

High doses of cyclosporine (e.g., at starting intravenous dose of 16 mg/kg/day) may increase the exposure to anthracycline antibiotics (e.g., doxorubicin, mitoxantrone, daunorubicin) in cancer patients.

Aliskiren

Cyclosporine alters the pharmacokinetics of aliskiren, a substrate of P-glycoprotein and CYP3A4. In 14 healthy subjects who received concomitantly single doses of cyclosporine (200 mg) and reduced dose aliskiren (75 mg), the mean Cmax of aliskiren was increased by approximately 2.5 fold (90% CI: 1.96-3.17) and the mean AUC by approximately 4.3 fold (90% CI: 3.52-5.21), compared to when these subjects received aliskiren alone. The concomitant administration of aliskiren with cyclosporine prolonged the median aliskiren elimination half-life (26 hours versus 43 to 45 hours) and the T_{max} (0.5 hours versus 1.5 to 2.0 hours). The mean AUC and C_{max} of cyclosporine were comparable to reported literature values. Coadministration of cyclosporine and aliskiren in these subjects also resulted in an increase in the number and/or intensity of adverse events, mainly headache, hot flush, nausea, vomiting, and somnolence. The coadministration of cyclosporine with aliskiren is not recommended.

Bosentan

In healthy subjects, coadministration of bosentan and cyclosporine resulted in mean increases in dose-normalized bosentan trough concentrations on day 1 and day 8 of approximately 21-fold and 2-fold, respectively, compared to when bosentan was given alone as a single dose on day 1. *(See also Effect of Drugs and Other Agents on Cyclosporine Pharmacokinetics and/or Safety)*

Potassium-Sparing Diuretics

Cyclosporine should not be used with potassium-sparing diuretics because hyperkalemia can occur. Caution is also required when cyclosporine is coadministered with potassium sparing drugs (e.g., angiotensin converting enzyme inhibitors, angiotensin II receptor antagonists), potassium containing drugs as well as in patients on a potassium rich diet. Control of potassium levels in these situations is advisable.

Nonsteroidal Anti-inflammatory Drug (NSAID) Interactions

Clinical status and serum creatinine should be closely monitored when cyclosporine is used with nonsteroidal anti-inflammatory agents in rheumatoid arthritis patients. *(See WARNINGS)*

Pharmacodynamic interactions have been reported to occur between cyclosporine and both naproxen and sulindac, in that concomitant use is associated with additive decreases in renal function, as determined by ^{99m}Tc-diethylenetriaminepentaacetic acid (DTPA) and (*p*-aminohippuric acid) PAH clearances. Although concomitant administration of diclofenac does not affect blood concentrations of cyclosporine, it has been associated with approximate doubling of diclofenac blood concentrations and occasional reports of reversible decreases in renal function. Consequently, the dose of diclofenac should be in the lower end of the therapeutic range.

Methotrexate Interaction

Preliminary data indicate that when methotrexate and cyclosporine were coadministered to rheumatoid arthritis patients (N=20), methotrexate concentrations (AUCs) were increased approximately 30% and the concentrations (AUCs) of its metabolite, 7-hydroxy methotrexate, were decreased by approximately 80%. The clinical significance of this interaction is not known. Cyclosporine concentrations do not appear to have been altered (N=6).

Sirolimus

Elevations in serum creatinine were observed in studies using sirolimus in combination with full-dose cyclosporine. This effect is often reversible with cyclosporine dose reduction. Simultaneous coadministration of cyclosporine significantly increases blood levels of sirolimus. To minimize increases in sirolimus concentrations, it is recommended that sirolimus be given 4 hours after cyclosporine administration.

Nifedipine

Frequent gingival hyperplasia when nifedipine is given concurrently with cyclosporine has been reported. The concomitant use of nifedipine should be avoided in patients in whom gingival hyperplasia develops as a side effect of cyclosporine.

Methylprednisolone

Convulsions when high dose methylprednisolone is given concurrently with cyclosporine have been reported.

Other Immunosuppressive Drugs and Agents

Psoriasis patients receiving other immunosuppressive agents or radiation therapy (including PUVA and UVB) should not receive concurrent cyclosporine because of the possibility of excessive immunosuppression.

C. Effect of Cyclosporine on the Efficacy of Live Vaccines

During treatment with cyclosporine, vaccination may be less effective. The use of live vaccines should be avoided.

For additional information on Cyclosporine Drug Interactions please contact Novartis Medical Affairs Department at 888-NOW-NOVA [888-669-6682].

Carcinogenesis, Mutagenesis, and Impairment of Fertility

Carcinogenicity studies were carried out in male and female rats and mice. In the 78-week mouse study, evidence of a statistically significant trend was found for lymphocytic lymphomas in females, and the incidence of hepatocellular carcinomas in mid-dose males significantly exceeded the control value. In the 24-month rat study, pancreatic islet cell adenomas significantly exceeded the control rate in the low dose level. Doses used in the mouse and rat studies were 0.01 to 0.16 times the clinical maintenance dose (6 mg/kg). The hepatocellular carcinomas and pancreatic islet cell adenomas were not dose related. Published reports indicate that co-treatment of hairless mice with UV irradiation and cyclosporine or other immunosuppressive agents shorten the time to skin tumor formation compared to UV irradiation alone.

Cyclosporine was not mutagenic in appropriate test systems. Cyclosporine has not been found to be mutagenic/genotoxic in the Ames Test, the V79-HGPRT Test, the micronucleus test in mice and Chinese hamsters, the chromosome-aberration tests in Chinese hamster bone-marrow, the mouse dominant lethal assay, and the DNA-repair test in sperm from treated mice. A recent study analyzing sister chromatid exchange (SCE) induction by cyclosporine using human lymphocytes *in vitro* gave indication of a positive effect (i.e., induction of SCE), at high concentrations in this system. In two published research studies, rabbits exposed to cyclosporine *in utero* (10 mg/kg/day subcutaneously) demonstrated reduced numbers of nephrons, renal hypertrophy, systemic hypertension and progressive renal insufficiency up to 35 weeks of age. Pregnant rats which received 12 mg/kg/day of cyclosporine intravenously (twice the recommended human intravenous dose) had fetuses with an increased incidence of ventricular septal defect. These findings have not been demonstrated in other species and their relevance for humans is unknown.

No impairment in fertility was demonstrated in studies in male and female rats.

Widely distributed papillomatosis of the skin was observed after chronic treatment of dogs with cyclosporine at 9 times the human initial psoriasis treatment dose of 2.5 mg/kg, where doses are expressed on a body surface area basis. This papillomatosis showed a spontaneous regression upon discontinuation of cyclosporine.

An increased incidence of malignancy is a recognized complication of immunosuppression in recipients of organ transplants and patients with rheumatoid arthritis and psoriasis. The most common forms of neoplasms are non-Hodgkin's lymphoma and carcinomas of the skin. The risk of malignancies in cyclosporine recipients is higher than in the normal, healthy population but similar to that in patients receiving other immunosuppressive therapies. Reduction or discontinuance of immunosuppression may cause the lesions to regress.

In psoriasis patients on cyclosporine, development of malignancies, especially those of the skin has been reported. *(See WARNINGS)* Skin lesions not typical for psoriasis should be biopsied before starting cyclosporine treatment. Patients with malignant or premalignant changes of the skin should be treated with cyclosporine only after appropriate treatment of such lesions and if no other treatment option exists.

Pregnancy

Pregnancy Category C

Animal studies have shown reproductive toxicity in rats and rabbits. Cyclosporine gave no evidence of mutagenic or teratogenic effects in the standard test systems with oral application (rats up to 17 mg/kg and rabbits up to 30 mg/kg per day orally.) Only at dose levels toxic to dams, were adverse effects seen in reproduction studies in rats. Cyclosporine has been shown to be embryo- and fetotoxic in rats and rabbits following oral administration at maternally toxic doses. Fetal toxicity was noted in rats at 0.8 and rabbits at 5.4 times the transplant doses in humans of 6.0 mg/kg, where dose corrections are based on body surface area. Cyclosporine was embryo- and fetotoxic as indicated by increased pre- and postnatal mortality and reduced fetal weight together with related skeletal retardation.

There are no adequate and well-controlled studies in pregnant women therefore, Neoral® should not be used during pregnancy unless the potential benefit to the mother justifies the potential risk to the fetus.

In pregnant transplant recipients who are being treated with immunosuppressants the risk of premature birth is increased. The following data represent the reported outcomes of 116 pregnancies in women receiving cyclosporine during pregnancy, 90% of whom were transplant patients, and most of whom received cyclosporine throughout the entire gestational period. The only consistent patterns of abnormality were premature birth (gestational period of 28 to 36 weeks) and low birth weight for gestational age. Sixteen fetal losses occurred. Most of the pregnancies (85 of 100) were complicated by disorders; including, preeclampsia, eclampsia, premature labor, abruptio placentae, oligohydramnios, Rh incompatibility, and fetoplacental dysfunction. Pre-term delivery occurred in 47%. Seven malformations were reported in 5 viable infants and in 2 cases of fetal loss. Twenty-eight percent of the infants were small for gestational age. Neonatal complications occurred in 27%. Therefore, the risks and benefits of using Neoral® during pregnancy should be carefully weighed.

A limited number of observations in children exposed to cyclosporine *in utero* are available, up to an age of approximately 7 years. Renal function and blood pressure in these children were normal.

Because of the possible disruption of maternal-fetal interaction, the risk/benefit ratio of using Neoral® in psoriasis patients during pregnancy should carefully be weighed with serious consideration for discontinuation of Neoral®.

The alcohol content of the Neoral formulations should also be taken into account in pregnant women. *(See WARNINGS, Special Excipients)*

Nursing Mothers

Cyclosporine is present in breast milk. Because of the potential for serious adverse drug reactions in nursing infants from Neoral, a decision should be made whether to discontinue nursing or to discontinue the drug, taking into account the importance of the drug to the mother. Neoral contains ethanol. Ethanol will be present in human milk at levels similar to that found in maternal serum and if present in breast milk will be orally absorbed by a nursing infant (*See WARNINGS*).

Pediatric Use

Although no adequate and well-controlled studies have been completed in children, transplant recipients as young as one year of age have received Neoral® with no unusual adverse effects. The safety and efficacy of Neoral® treatment in children with juvenile rheumatoid arthritis or psoriasis below the age of 18 have not been established.

Geriatric Use

In rheumatoid arthritis clinical trials with cyclosporine, 17.5% of patients were age 65 or older. These patients were more likely to develop systolic hypertension on therapy, and more likely to show serum creatinine rises ≥50% above the baseline after 3-4 months of therapy.

Clinical studies of Neoral® in transplant and psoriasis patients did not include a sufficient number of subjects aged 65 and over to determine whether they respond differently from younger subjects. Other reported clinical experiences have not identified differences in response between the elderly and younger patients. In general, dose selection for an elderly patient should be cautious, usually starting at the low end of the dosing range, reflecting the greater frequency of decreased hepatic, renal, or cardiac function, and of concomitant disease or other drug therapy.

ADVERSE REACTIONS

Kidney, Liver, and Heart Transplantation

The principal adverse reactions of cyclosporine therapy are renal dysfunction, tremor, hirsutism, hypertension, and gum hyperplasia.

Hypertension

Hypertension, which is usually mild to moderate, may occur in approximately 50% of patients following renal transplantation and in most cardiac transplant patients.

Glomerular Capillary Thrombosis

Glomerular capillary thrombosis has been found in patients treated with cyclosporine and may progress to graft failure. The pathologic changes resembled those seen in the hemolytic-uremic syndrome and included thrombosis of the renal microvasculature, with platelet-fibrin thrombi occluding glomerular capillaries and afferent arterioles, microangiopathic hemolytic anemia, thrombocytopenia, and decreased renal function. Similar findings have been observed when other immunosuppressives have been employed post-transplantation.

Hypomagnesemia

Hypomagnesemia has been reported in some, but not all, patients exhibiting convulsions while on cyclosporine therapy. Although magnesium-depletion studies in normal subjects suggest that hypomagnesemia is associated with neurologic disorders, multiple factors, including hypertension, high dose methylprednisolone, hypocholesterolemia, and nephrotoxicity associated with high plasma concentrations of cyclosporine appear to be related to the neurological manifestations of cyclosporine toxicity.

Clinical Studies

In controlled studies, the nature, severity, and incidence of the adverse events that were observed in 493 transplanted patients treated with Neoral® were comparable with those observed in 208 transplanted patients who received Sandimmune® in these same studies when the dosage of the two drugs was adjusted to achieve the same cyclosporine blood trough concentrations.

Based on the historical experience with Sandimmune®, the following reactions occurred in 3% or greater of 892 patients involved in clinical trials of kidney, heart, and liver transplants.

[See first table at top of next page]

Among 705 kidney transplant patients treated with cyclosporine oral solution (Sandimmune®) in clinical trials, the reason for treatment discontinuation was renal toxicity in 5.4%, infection in 0.9%, lack of efficacy in 1.4%, acute tubular necrosis in 1.0%, lymphoproliferative disorders in 0.3%, hypertension in 0.3%, and other reasons in 0.7% of the patients.

The following reactions occurred in 2% or less of cyclosporine-treated patients: allergic reactions, anemia, anorexia, confusion, conjunctivitis, edema, fever, brittle fingernails, gastritis, hearing loss, hiccups, hyperglycemia, migraine (Neoral®), muscle pain, peptic ulcer, thrombocytopenia, tinnitus.

Body System	Adverse Reactions	Randomized Kidney Patients		Cyclosporine Patients (Sandimmune®)		
		Sandimmune® (N=227)%	Azathioprine (N=228)%	Kidney (N=705)%	Heart (N=112)%	Liver (N=75)%
Genitourinary	Renal Dysfunction	32	6	25	38	37
Cardiovascular	Hypertension	26	18	13	53	27
	Cramps	4	<1	2	<1	0
Skin	Hirsutism	21	<1	21	28	45
	Acne	6	8	2	2	1
Central Nervous System	Tremor	12	0	21	31	55
	Convulsions	3	1	1	4	5
	Headache	2	<1	2	15	4
Gastrointestinal	Gum Hyperplasia	4	0	9	5	16
	Diarrhea	3	<1	3	4	8
	Nausea/Vomiting	2	<1	4	10	4
	Hepatotoxicity	<1	<1	4	7	4
	Abdominal Discomfort	<1	0	<1	7	0
Autonomic Nervous System	Paresthesia	3	0	1	2	1
	Flushing	<1	0	4	0	4
Hematopoietic	Leukopenia	2	19	<1	6	0
	Lymphoma	<1	0	1	6	1
Respiratory	Sinusitis	<1	0	4	3	7
Miscellaneous	Gynecomastia	<1	0	<1	4	3

Infectious Complications in Historical Randomized Studies in Renal Transplant Patients Using Sandimmune®

Complication	Cyclosporine Treatment (N=227) % of Complications	Azathioprine with Steroids* (N=228) % of Complications
Septicemia	5.3	4.8
Abscesses	4.4	5.3
Systemic Fungal Infection	2.2	3.9
Local Fungal Infection	7.5	9.6
Cytomegalovirus	4.8	12.3
Other Viral Infections	15.9	18.4
Urinary Tract Infections	21.1	20.2
Wound and Skin Infections	7.0	10.1
Pneumonia	6.2	9.2

*Some patients also received ALG.

The following reactions occurred rarely: anxiety, chest pain, constipation, depression, hair breaking, hematuria, joint pain, lethargy, mouth sores, myocardial infarction, night sweats, pancreatitis, pruritus, swallowing difficulty, tingling, upper GI bleeding, visual disturbance, weakness, weight loss.

Patients receiving immunosuppressive therapies, including cyclosporine and cyclosporine -containing regimens, are at increased risk of infections (viral, bacterial, fungal, parasitic). Both generalized and localized infections can occur. Pre-existing infections may also be aggravated. Fatal outcomes have been reported. *(See WARNINGS)*

[See second table above]

Postmarketing Experience, Kidney, Liver and Heart Transplantation

Hepatotoxicity

Cases of hepatotoxicity and liver injury including cholestasis, jaundice, hepatitis and liver failure; serious and/or fatal outcomes have been reported. *(See WARNINGS, Hepatotoxicity)*

Increased Risk of Infections

Cases of JC virus-associated progressive multifocal leukoencephalopathy (PML), sometimes fatal; and polyoma virus-associated nephropathy (PVAN), especially BK virus resulting in graft loss have been reported. *(See WARNINGS, Polyoma Virus Infection)*

Headache, including Migraine

Cases of migraine have been reported. In some cases, patients have been unable to continue cyclosporine, however, the final decision on treatment discontinuation should be made by the treating physician following the careful assessment of benefits versus risks.

Rheumatoid Arthritis

The principal adverse reactions associated with the use of cyclosporine in rheumatoid arthritis are renal dysfunction *(See WARNINGS)*, hypertension *(See PRECAUTIONS)*, headache, gastrointestinal disturbances, and hirsutism/hypertrichosis.

In rheumatoid arthritis patients treated in clinical trials within the recommended dose range, cyclosporine therapy was discontinued in 5.3% of the patients because of hypertension and in 7% of the patients because of increased creatinine. These changes are usually reversible with timely dose decrease or drug discontinuation. The frequency and severity of serum creatinine elevations increase with dose and duration of cyclosporine therapy. These elevations are likely to become more pronounced without dose reduction or discontinuation.

The following adverse events occurred in controlled clinical trials:

[See table on pages 2039 and 2040]

In addition, the following adverse events have been reported in 1% to <3% of the rheumatoid arthritis patients in the cyclosporine treatment group in controlled clinical trials.

Autonomic Nervous System: dry mouth, increased sweating

Body as a Whole: allergy, asthenia, hot flushes, malaise, overdose, procedure NOS*, tumor NOS*, weight decrease, weight increase

Cardiovascular: abnormal heart sounds, cardiac failure, myocardial infarction, peripheral ischemia

Central and Peripheral Nervous System: hypoesthesia, neuropathy, vertigo

Endocrine: goiter

Gastrointestinal: constipation, dysphagia, enanthema, eructation, esophagitis, gastric ulcer, gastritis, gastroenteritis, gingival bleeding, glossitis, peptic ulcer, salivary gland enlargement, tongue disorder, tooth disorder

Infection: abscess, bacterial infection, cellulitis, folliculitis, fungal infection, herpes simplex, herpes zoster, renal abscess, moniliasis, tonsillitis, viral infection

Hematologic: anemia, epistaxis, leukopenia, lymphadenopathy

Liver and Biliary System: bilirubinemia

Metabolic and Nutritional: diabetes mellitus, hyperkalemia, hyperuricemia, hypoglycemia

Musculoskeletal System: arthralgia, bone fracture, bursitis, joint dislocation, myalgia, stiffness, synovial cyst, tendon disorder

Neoplasms: breast fibroadenosis, carcinoma

Psychiatric: anxiety, confusion, decreased libido, emotional lability, impaired concentration, increased libido, nervousness, paroniria, somnolence

Reproductive (Female): breast pain, uterine hemorrhage

Respiratory System: abnormal chest sounds, bronchospasm

Skin and Appendages: abnormal pigmentation, angioedema, dermatitis, dry skin, eczema, nail disorder, pruritus, skin disorder, urticaria

Special Senses: abnormal vision, cataract, conjunctivitis, deafness, eye pain, taste perversion, tinnitus, vestibular disorder

Urinary System: abnormal urine, hematuria, increased BUN, micturition urgency, nocturia, polyuria, pyelonephritis, urinary incontinence

*NOS=Not Otherwise Specified

Psoriasis

The principal adverse reactions associated with the use of cyclosporine in patients with psoriasis are renal dysfunction, headache, hypertension, hypertriglyceridemia, hirsutism/hypertrichosis, paresthesia or hyperesthesia, influenza-like symptoms, nausea/vomiting, diarrhea, abdominal discomfort, lethargy, and musculoskeletal or joint pain.

In psoriasis patients treated in US controlled clinical studies within the recommended dose range, cyclosporine therapy was discontinued in 1.0% of the patients because of hypertension and in 5.4% of the patients because of increased creatinine. In the majority of cases, these changes were reversible after dose reduction or discontinuation of cyclosporine.

There has been one reported death associated with the use of cyclosporine in psoriasis. A 27-year-old male developed renal deterioration and was continued on cyclosporine. He had progressive renal failure leading to death.

Frequency and severity of serum creatinine increases with dose and duration of cyclosporine therapy. These elevations are likely to become more pronounced and may result in irreversible renal damage without dose reduction or discontinuation.

[See second table at top of page 2040]

The following events occurred in 1% to less than 3% of psoriasis patients treated with cyclosporine:

Body as a Whole: fever, flushes, hot flushes

Cardiovascular: chest pain

Central and Peripheral Nervous System: appetite increased, insomnia, dizziness, nervousness, vertigo

Gastrointestinal: abdominal distention, constipation, gingival bleeding

Liver and Biliary System: hyperbilirubinemia

Neoplasms: skin malignancies [squamous cell (0.9%) and basal cell (0.4%) carcinomas]

Reticuloendothelial: platelet, bleeding, and clotting disorders, red blood cell disorder

Respiratory: infection, viral and other infection

Skin and Appendages: acne, folliculitis, keratosis, pruritus, rash, dry skin

Urinary System: micturition frequency

Vision: abnormal vision

Mild hypomagnesemia and hyperkalemia may occur but are asymptomatic. Increases in uric acid may occur and attacks of gout have been rarely reported. A minor and dose related hyperbilirubinemia has been observed in the absence of hepatocellular damage. Cyclosporine therapy may be associated with a modest increase of serum triglycerides or cholesterol. Elevations of triglycerides (>750 mg/dL) occur in about 15% of psoriasis patients; elevations of cholesterol (>300 mg/dL) are observed in less than 3% of psoriasis patients. Generally these laboratory abnormalities are reversible upon dose reduction or discontinuation of cyclosporine.

Postmarketing Experience, Psoriasis

Cases of transformation to erythrodermic psoriasis or generalized pustular psoriasis upon either withdrawal or reduction of cyclosporine in patients with chronic plaque psoriasis have been reported.

OVERDOSAGE

There is a minimal experience with cyclosporine overdosage. Forced emesis and gastric lavage can be of value up to 2 hours after administration of Neoral®. Transient hepatotoxicity and nephrotoxicity may occur which should resolve following drug withdrawal. Oral doses of cyclosporine up to 10 g (about 150 mg/kg) have been tolerated with relatively minor clinical consequences, such as vomiting, drowsiness, headache, tachycardia and, in a few patients, moderately severe, reversible impairment of renal function. However, serious symptoms of intoxication have been reported following accidental parenteral overdosage with cyclosporine in premature neonates. General supportive measures and symptomatic treatment should be followed in all cases of overdosage. Cyclosporine is not dialyzable to any great extent, nor is it cleared well by charcoal hemoperfusion. The oral dosage at which half of experimental animals are estimated to die is 31 times, 39 times, and >54 times the human maintenance dose for transplant patients (6mg/kg; corrections based on body surface area) in mice, rats, and rabbits.

DOSAGE AND ADMINISTRATION

Neoral® Soft Gelatin Capsules (cyclosporine capsules, USP) MODIFIED and Neoral® Oral Solution (cyclosporine oral solution, USP) MODIFIED

Neoral® has increased bioavailability in comparison to Sandimmune®. Neoral® and Sandimmune® are not bioequivalent and cannot be used interchangeably without physician supervision.

The daily dose of Neoral® should always be given in two divided doses (BID). It is recommended that Neoral® be administered on a consistent schedule with regard to time of day and relation to meals. Grapefruit and grapefruit juice affect metabolism, increasing blood concentration of cyclosporine, thus should be avoided.

Specific Populations

Renal Impairment in Kidney, Liver, and Heart Transplantation

Cyclosporine undergoes minimal renal elimination and its pharmacokinetics do not appear to be significantly altered in patients with end-stage renal disease who receive routine hemodialysis treatments (*See CLINICAL PHARMACOLOGY*). However, due to its nephrotoxic potential (*See WARNINGS*), careful monitoring of renal function is recommended; cyclosporine dosage should be reduced if indicated. (*See WARNINGS and PRECAUTIONS*)

Renal Impairment in Rheumatoid Arthritis and Psoriasis

Patients with impaired renal function should not receive cyclosporine. (*See CONTRAINDICATIONS, WARNINGS and PRECAUTIONS*)

Hepatic Impairment

The clearance of cyclosporine may be significantly reduced in severe liver disease patients (*See CLINICAL PHARMACOLOGY*). Dose reduction may be necessary in patients with severe liver impairment to maintain blood concentrations within the recommended target range (*See WARNINGS and PRECAUTIONS*).

Newly Transplanted Patients

The initial oral dose of Neoral® can be given 4-12 hours prior to transplantation or be given postoperatively. The initial dose of Neoral® varies depending on the transplanted organ and the other immunosuppressive agents included in the immunosuppressive protocol. In newly transplanted patients, the initial oral dose of Neoral® is the same as the initial oral dose of Sandimmune®. Suggested initial doses are available from the results of a 1994 survey of the use of Sandimmune® in US transplant centers. The mean ± SD initial doses were 9±3 mg/kg/day for renal transplant patients (75 centers), 8±4 mg/kg/day for liver transplant patients (30 centers), and 7±3 mg/kg/day for heart transplant patients (24 centers). Total daily doses were divided into two equal daily doses. The Neoral® dose is subsequently adjusted to achieve a pre-defined cyclosporine blood concentration. *(See Blood Concentration Monitoring in Transplant Patients, below)* If cyclosporine trough blood concentrations are used, the target range is the same for Neoral® as for Sandimmune®. Using the same trough concentration target range for Neoral® as for Sandimmune® results in greater cyclosporine exposure when Neoral® is administered. *(See Pharmacokinetics, Absorption)* Dosing should be titrated based on clinical assessments of rejection and tolerability. Lower Neoral® doses may be sufficient as maintenance therapy.

Adjunct therapy with adrenal corticosteroids is recommended initially. Different tapering dosage schedules of prednisone appear to achieve similar results. A representative dosage schedule based on the patient's weight started with 2.0 mg/kg/day for the first 4 days tapered to 1.0 mg/kg/day by 1 week, 0.6 mg/kg/day by 2 weeks, 0.3 mg/kg/day by 1 month, and 0.15 mg/kg/day by 2 months and thereafter as a maintenance dose. Steroid doses may be further tapered on an individualized basis depending on status of patient and function of graft. Adjustments in dosage of prednisone must be made according to the clinical situation.

Conversion from Sandimmune® to Neoral® in Transplant Patients

In transplanted patients who are considered for conversion to Neoral® from Sandimmune®, Neoral® should be started with the same daily dose as was previously used with Sandimmune® (1:1 dose conversion). The Neoral® dose should subsequently be adjusted to attain the preconversion cyclosporine blood trough concentration. Using the same trough concentration target range for Neoral® as for Sandimmune® results in greater cyclosporine exposure when Neoral® is administered. *(See Pharmacokinetics, Absorption)* Patients with suspected poor absorption of Sandimmune® require different dosing strategies. *(See Transplant Patients with Poor Absorption of Sandimmune®, below)* In some patients, the increase in blood trough concentration is more pronounced and may be of clinical significance.

Until the blood trough concentration attains the preconversion value, it is strongly recommended that the cyclosporine blood trough concentration be monitored every 4 to 7 days after conversion to Neoral®. In addition, clinical safety parameters such as serum creatinine and blood pressure should be monitored every two weeks during the first two months after conversion. If the blood trough concentrations are outside the desired range and/or if the clinical safety parameters worsen, the dosage of Neoral® must be adjusted accordingly.

Transplant Patients with Poor Absorption of Sandimmune®

Patients with lower than expected cyclosporine blood trough concentrations in relation to the oral dose of Sandimmune® may have poor or inconsistent absorption of cyclosporine from Sandimmune®. After conversion to Neoral®, patients tend to have higher cyclosporine concentrations. **Due to the increase in bioavailability of cyclosporine following conversion to Neoral®, the cyclosporine blood trough concentration may exceed the target range. Particular caution should be exercised when converting patients to Neoral® at doses greater than 10 mg/kg/day.** The dose of Neoral® should be titrated individually based on cyclosporine trough concentrations, tolerability, and clinical response. In this population the cyclosporine blood trough concentration should be measured more frequently, at least twice a week (daily, if initial dose exceeds 10 mg/kg/day) until the concentration stabilizes within the desired range.

Neoral®/Sandimmune® Rheumatoid Arthritis
Percentage of Patients with Adverse Events ≥3% in any Cyclosporine Treated Group

Body System	Preferred Term	Studies 651+652+2008 Sandimmune®† (N=269)	Study 302 Sandimmune® (N=155)	Study 654 Methotrexate & Sandimmune® (N=74)	Study 654 Methotrexate & Placebo (N=73)	Study 302 Neoral® (N=143)	Studies 651+652+2008 Placebo (N=201)
Autonomic Nervous System Disorders							
	Flushing	2%	2%	3%	0%	5%	2%
Body As A Whole–General Disorders							
	Accidental Trauma	0%	1%	10%	4%	4%	0%
	Edema NOS*	5%	14%	12%	4%	10%	<1%
	Fatigue	6%	3%	8%	12%	3%	7%
	Fever	2%	3%	0%	0%	2%	4%
	Influenza-like symptoms	<1%	6%	1%	0%	3%	2%
	Pain	6%	9%	10%	15%	13%	4%
	Rigors	1%	1%	4%	0%	3%	1%
Cardiovascular Disorders							
	Arrhythmia	2%	5%	5%	6%	2%	1%
	Chest Pain	4%	5%	1%	1%	6%	1%
	Hypertension	8%	26%	16%	12%	25%	2%
Central and Peripheral Nervous System Disorders							
	Dizziness	8%	6%	7%	3%	8%	3%
	Headache	17%	23%	22%	11%	25%	9%
	Migraine	2%	3%	0%	0%	3%	1%
	Paresthesia	8%	7%	8%	4%	11%	1%
	Tremor	8%	7%	7%	3%	13%	4%
Gastrointestinal System Disorders							
	Abdominal Pain	15%	15%	15%	7%	15%	10%
	Anorexia	3%	3%	1%	0%	3%	3%
	Diarrhea	12%	12%	18%	15%	13%	8%
	Dyspepsia	12%	12%	10%	8%	8%	4%
	Flatulence	5%	5%	5%	4%	4%	1%
	Gastrointestinal Disorder NOS*	0%	2%	1%	4%	4%	0%
	Gingivitis	4%	3%	0%	0%	0%	1%
	Gum Hyperplasia	2%	4%	1%	3%	4%	1%
	Nausea	23%	14%	24%	15%	18%	14%
	Rectal Hemorrhage	0%	3%	0%	0%	1%	1%
	Stomatitis	7%	5%	16%	12%	6%	8%
	Vomiting	9%	8%	14%	7%	6%	5%
Hearing and Vestibular Disorders							
	Ear Disorder NOS*	0%	5%	0%	0%	1%	0%
Metabolic and Nutritional Disorders							
	Hypomagnesemia	0%	4%	0%	0%	6%	0%
Musculoskeletal System Disorders							
	Arthropathy	0%	5%	0%	1%	4%	0%
	Leg Cramps/ Involuntary Muscle Contractions	2%	11%	11%	3%	12%	1%
Psychiatric Disorders							
	Depression	3%	6%	3%	1%	1%	2%
	Insomnia	4%	1%	1%	0%	3%	2%
Renal							
	Creatinine elevations ≥30%	43%	39%	55%	19%	48%	13%
	Creatinine elevations ≥50%	24%	18%	26%	8%	18%	3%
Reproductive Disorders, Female							
	Leukorrhea	1%	0%	4%	0%	1%	0%
	Menstrual Disorder	3%	2%	1%	0%	1%	1%
Respiratory System Disorders							
	Bronchitis	1%	3%	1%	0%	1%	3%
	Coughing	5%	3%	5%	7%	4%	4%
	Dyspnea	5%	1%	3%	3%	1%	2%
	Infection NOS*	9%	5%	0%	7%	3%	10%
	Pharyngitis	3%	5%	5%	6%	4%	4%
	Pneumonia	1%	0%	4%	0%	1%	1%
	Rhinitis	0%	3%	11%	10%	1%	0%
	Sinusitis	4%	4%	8%	4%	3%	3%
	Upper Respiratory Tract	0%	14%	23%	15%	13%	0%

(Table continued on next page)

Neoral®/Sandimmune® Rheumatoid Arthritis *(cont.)*
Percentage of Patients with Adverse Events ≥3% in any Cyclosporine Treated Group

Body System	Preferred Term	Studies 651+652+2008 Sandimmune®† (N=269)	Study 302 Sandimmune® (N=155)	Study 654 Methotrexate & Sandimmune® (N=74)	Study 654 Methotrexate & Placebo (N=73)	Study 302 Neoral® (N=143)	Studies 651+652+2008 Placebo (N=201)
Skin and Appendages Disorders							
	Alopecia	3%	0%	1%	1%	4%	4%
	Bullous Eruption	1%	0%	4%	1%	1%	1%
	Hypertrichosis	19%	17%	12%	0%	15%	3%
	Rash	7%	12%	10%	7%	8%	10%
	Skin Ulceration	1%	1%	3%	4%	0%	2%
Urinary System Disorders							
	Dysuria	0%	0%	11%	3%	1%	2%
	Micturition Frequency	2%	4%	3%	1%	2%	2%
	NPN, Increased	0%	19%	12%	0%	18%	0%
	Urinary Tract Infection	0%	3%	5%	4%	3%	0%
Vascular (Extracardiac) Disorders							
	Purpura	3%	4%	1%	1%	2%	0%

† Includes patients in 2.5 mg/kg/day dose group only. *NOS=Not Otherwise Specified.

Adverse Events Occurring in 3% or More of Psoriasis Patients in Controlled Clinical Trials

Body System*	Preferred Term	Neoral® (N=182)	Sandimmune® (N=185)
Infection or Potential Infection		24.7%	24.3%
	Influenza-Like Symptoms	9.9%	8.1%
	Upper Respiratory Tract Infections	7.7%	11.3%
Cardiovascular System		28.0%	25.4%
	Hypertension**	27.5%	25.4%
Urinary System		24.2%	16.2%
	Increased Creatinine	19.8%	15.7%
Central and Peripheral Nervous System		26.4%	20.5%
	Headache	15.9%	14.0%
	Paresthesia	7.1%	4.8%
Musculoskeletal System		13.2%	8.7%
	Arthralgia	6.0%	1.1%
Body As a Whole–General		29.1%	22.2%
	Pain	4.4%	3.2%
Metabolic and Nutritional		9.3%	9.7%
Reproductive, Female		8.5% (4 of 47 females)	11.5% (6 of 52 females)
Resistance Mechanism		18.7%	21.1%
Skin and Appendages		17.6%	15.1%
	Hypertrichosis	6.6%	5.4%
Respiratory System		5.0%	6.5%
	Bronchospasm, Coughing, Dyspnea, Rhinitis	5.0%	4.9%
Psychiatric		5.0%	3.8%
Gastrointestinal System		19.8%	28.7%
	Abdominal Pain	2.7%	6.0%
	Diarrhea	5.0%	5.9%
	Dyspepsia	2.2%	3.2%
	Gum Hyperplasia	3.8%	6.0%
	Nausea	5.5%	5.9%
White cell and RES		4.4%	2.7%

*Total percentage of events within the system
**Newly occurring hypertension = SBP≥160 mm Hg and/or DBP≥90 mm Hg

Rheumatoid Arthritis

The initial dose of Neoral® is 2.5 mg/kg/day, taken twice daily as a divided (BID) oral dose. Salicylates, nonsteroidal anti-inflammatory agents, and oral corticosteroids may be continued. *(See WARNINGS and PRECAUTIONS, Drug Interactions)* Onset of action generally occurs between 4 and 8 weeks. If insufficient clinical benefit is seen and tolerability is good (including serum creatinine less than 30% above baseline), the dose may be increased by 0.5-0.75 mg/kg/day after 8 weeks and again after 12 weeks to a maximum of 4 mg/kg/day. If no benefit is seen by 16 weeks of therapy, Neoral® therapy should be discontinued.

Dose decreases by 25%-50% should be made at any time to control adverse events, e.g., hypertension elevations in serum creatinine (30% above patient's pretreatment level) or clinically significant laboratory abnormalities. *(See WARNINGS and PRECAUTIONS)*

If dose reduction is not effective in controlling abnormalities or if the adverse event or abnormality is severe, Neoral® should be discontinued. The same initial dose and dosage range should be used if Neoral® is combined with the recommended dose of methotrexate. Most patients can be treated with Neoral® doses of 3 mg/kg/day or below when combined with methotrexate doses of up to 15 mg/week. *(See CLINICAL PHARMACOLOGY, Clinical Trials)*

There is limited long-term treatment data. Recurrence of rheumatoid arthritis disease activity is generally apparent within 4 weeks after stopping cyclosporine.

Psoriasis

The initial dose of Neoral® should be 2.5 mg/kg/day. Neoral® should be taken twice daily, as a divided (1.25 mg/kg BID) oral dose. Patients should be kept at that dose for at least 4 weeks, barring adverse events. If significant clinical improvement has not occurred in patients by that time, the patient's dosage should be increased at 2-week intervals. Based on patient response, dose increases of approximately 0.5 mg/kg/day should be made to a maximum of 4.0 mg/kg/day.

Dose decreases by 25%-50% should be made at any time to control adverse events, e.g., hypertension, elevations in serum creatinine (≥25% above the patient's pretreatment level), or clinically significant laboratory abnormalities. If dose reduction is not effective in controlling abnormalities, or if the adverse event or abnormality is severe, Neoral® should be discontinued. *(See Special Monitoring of Psoriasis Patients)*

Patients generally show some improvement in the clinical manifestations of psoriasis in 2 weeks. Satisfactory control and stabilization of the disease may take 12-16 weeks to achieve. Results of a dose-titration clinical trial with Neoral® indicate that an improvement of psoriasis by 75% or more (based on PASI) was achieved in 51% of the patients after 8 weeks and in 79% of the patients after 16 weeks. Treatment should be discontinued if satisfactory response cannot be achieved after 6 weeks at 4 mg/kg/day or the patient's maximum tolerated dose. Once a patient is adequately controlled and appears stable the dose of Neoral® should be lowered, and the patient treated with the lowest dose that maintains an adequate response (this should not necessarily be total clearing of the patient). In clinical trials, cyclosporine doses at the lower end of the recommended dosage range were effective in maintaining a satisfactory response in 60% of the patients. Doses below 2.5 mg/kg/day may also be equally effective.

Upon stopping treatment with cyclosporine, relapse will occur in approximately 6 weeks (50% of the patients) to 16 weeks (75% of the patients). In the majority of patients rebound does not occur after cessation of treatment with cyclosporine. Thirteen cases of transformation of chronic plaque psoriasis to more severe forms of psoriasis have been reported. There were 9 cases of pustular and 4 cases of erythrodermic psoriasis. Long term experience with Neoral® in psoriasis patients is limited and continuous treatment for extended periods greater than one year is not recommended. Alternation with other forms of treatment should be considered in the long term management of patients with this life long disease.

Neoral® Oral Solution (cyclosporine oral solution, USP) MODIFIED–Recommendations for Administration

To make Neoral® Oral Solution (cyclosporine oral solution, USP) MODIFIED more palatable, it should be diluted with orange or apple juice that is at room temperature. Patients should avoid switching diluents frequently. Grapefruit juice affects metabolism of cyclosporine and should be avoided. The combination of Neoral® solution with milk can be unpalatable. The effect of milk on the bioavailability of cyclosporine when administered as Neoral Oral Solution has not been evaluated.

Take the prescribed amount of Neoral® Oral Solution (cyclosporine oral solution, USP) MODIFIED from the container using the dosing syringe supplied, after removal of the protective cover, and transfer the solution to a glass of orange or apple juice. Stir well and drink at once. Do not allow diluted oral solution to stand before drinking. Use a glass container (not plastic). Rinse the glass with more diluent to ensure that the total dose is consumed. After use, dry the outside of the dosing syringe with a clean towel and replace the protective cover. Do not rinse the dosing syringe with water or other cleaning agents. If the syringe requires cleaning, it must be completely dry before resuming use.

Blood Concentration Monitoring in Transplant Patients

Transplant centers have found blood concentration monitoring of cyclosporine to be an essential component of patient management. Of importance to blood concentration analysis are the type of assay used, the transplanted organ, and other immunosuppressant agents being administered. While no fixed relationship has been established, blood concentration monitoring may assist in the clinical evaluation of rejection and toxicity, dose adjustments, and the assessment of compliance.

Various assays have been used to measure blood concentrations of cyclosporine. Older studies using a nonspecific assay often cited concentrations that were roughly twice those of the specific assays. Therefore, comparison between concentrations in the published literature and an individual patient concentration using current assays must be made with detailed knowledge of the assay methods employed. Current assay results are also not interchangeable and their use should be guided by their approved labeling. A discussion of the different assay methods is contained in *Annals of Clinical Biochemistry* 1994;31:420-446. While several assays and assay matrices are available, there is a consensus that parent-compound-specific assays correlate best with clinical events. Of these, HPLC is the standard reference, but the monoclonal antibody RIAs and the monoclonal antibody FPIA offer sensitivity, reproducibility, and convenience. Most clinicians base their monitoring on trough cyclosporine concentrations. *Applied Pharmacokinetics, Principles of Therapeutic Drug Monitoring* (1992) contains a broad discussion of cyclosporine pharmacokinetics and drug monitoring techniques. Blood concentration monitoring is not a replacement for renal function monitoring or tissue biopsies.

HOW SUPPLIED

Neoral® Soft Gelatin Capsules (cyclosporine capsules, USP) MODIFIED

25 mg

Oval, blue-gray imprinted in red, "Neoral" over "25 mg." Packages of 30 unit-dose blisters (NDC 0078-0246-15).

100 mg

Oblong, blue-gray imprinted in red, "NEORAL" over "100 mg."

Packages of 30 unit-dose blisters (NDC 0078-0248-15).

Store and Dispense

In the original unit-dose container at controlled room temperature 68°-77°F (20°-25°C).

Neoral® Oral Solution (cyclosporine oral solution, USP) MODIFIED

A clear, yellow liquid supplied in 50 mL bottles containing 100 mg/mL (NDC 0078-0274-22).

Store and Dispense

In the original container at controlled room temperature 68°-77°F (20°-25°C). Do not store in the refrigerator. Once opened, the contents must be used within two months. At temperatures below 68°F (20°C) the solution may gel; light flocculation or the formation of a light sediment may also occur. There is no impact on product performance or dosing using the syringe provided. Allow to warm to room temperature 77°F (25°C) to reverse these changes.

Neoral® Soft Gelatin Capsules (cyclosporine capsules, USP) MODIFIED

Neoral® Oral Solution (cyclosporine oral solution, USP) MODIFIED

Distributed by:

Novartis Pharmaceuticals Corporation, East Hanover, New Jersey 07936

T2013-38

May 2013

Shown in Product Identification Guide, page 310

RECLAST® ℞

[RE-klast]

(zoledronic acid)

Injection

The following prescribing information is based on official labeling in effect July 2013.

HIGHLIGHTS OF PRESCRIBING INFORMATION

These highlights do not include all the information needed to use RECLAST safely and effectively. See full prescribing information for RECLAST.

Reclast® (zoledronic acid) Injection

Initial U.S. Approval: 2001

RECENT MAJOR CHANGES

Indications and Usage (1.6) 04/2013

INDICATIONS AND USAGE

Reclast is a bisphosphonate indicated for:

- Treatment and prevention of postmenopausal osteoporosis (1.1, 1.2)
- Treatment to increase bone mass in men with osteoporosis (1.3)
- Treatment and prevention of glucocorticoid-induced osteoporosis (1.4)
- Treatment of Paget's disease of bone in men and women (1.5)

Limitations of Use

Optimal duration of use has not been determined. For patients at low-risk for fracture, consider drug discontinuation after 3 to 5 years of use (1.6)

DOSAGE AND ADMINISTRATION

Infusion given intravenously over no less than 15 minutes:

- Treatment of postmenopausal osteoporosis (2.2); treatment to increase bone mass in men with osteoporosis (2.4): treatment and prevention of glucocorticoid-induced osteoporosis (2.5): 5 mg once a year
- Prevention of postmenopausal osteoporosis: 5 mg once every 2 years (2.3)
- Treatment of Paget's disease of bone: a single 5 mg infusion. Patients should receive 1500 mg elemental calcium and 800 international units vitamin D daily (2.6)

DOSAGE FORMS AND STRENGTHS

5 mg in a 100 mL ready-to-infuse solution (3)

CONTRAINDICATIONS

- Hypocalcemia (4)
- Patients with creatinine clearance less than 35 mL/min and in those with evidence of acute renal impairment (4, 5.3)
- Hypersensitivity to any component of Reclast (4, 6.2)

WARNINGS AND PRECAUTIONS

- *Products Containing Same Active Ingredient:* Patients receiving Zometa should not receive Reclast (5.1)
- *Hypocalcemia may worsen during treatment.* Patients must be adequately supplemented with calcium and vitamin D (5.2)
- *Renal Impairment:* A single dose should not exceed 5 mg and the duration of infusion should be no less than 15 minutes. Renal toxicity may be greater in patients with underlying renal impairment or with other risk factors, including advanced age or dehydration. Monitor creatinine clearance before each dose (2.7, 5.3)
- *Osteonecrosis of the Jaw (ONJ)* has been reported. All patients should have a routine oral exam by the prescriber prior to treatment (5.4)
- *Atypical Femur Fractures* have been reported. Patients with thigh or groin pain should be evaluated to rule out a femoral fracture (5.5)
- *Pregnancy:* Reclast can cause fetal harm. Women of childbearing potential should be advised (5.6, 8.1)
- *Severe Bone, Joint, and Muscle Pain* may occur. Withhold future doses of Reclast if severe symptoms occur (5.7)

ADVERSE REACTIONS

The most common adverse reactions (greater than 10%) were pyrexia, myalgia, headache, arthralgia, pain in extremity (6.1). Other important adverse reactions were flu-like illness, nausea, vomiting, diarrhea (6.2), and eye inflammation (6.1).

To report SUSPECTED ADVERSE REACTIONS, contact Novartis Pharmaceuticals Corporation at 1-888-669-6682 or FDA at 1-800-FDA-1088 or www.fda.gov/medwatch.

DRUG INTERACTIONS

- Aminoglycosides: May lower serum calcium for prolonged periods (7.1)
- Loop diuretics: May increase risk of hypocalcemia (7.2)
- Nephrotoxic drugs: Use with caution (7.3)
- Drugs primarily excreted by the kidney: Exposure may be increased with renal impairment. Monitor serum creatinine in patients at risk (7.4)

USE IN SPECIFIC POPULATIONS

Nursing Mothers: Reclast should not be given to nursing women (8.3)

Pediatric Use: Not indicated for use in pediatric patients (8.4)

Geriatric Use: Special care to monitor renal function (8.5)

See 17 for PATIENT COUNSELING INFORMATION and Medication Guide

Revised: 05/2013

FULL PRESCRIBING INFORMATION: CONTENTS*

*** Sections or subsections omitted from the full prescribing information are not listed**

FULL PRESCRIBING INFORMATION

1 INDICATIONS AND USAGE

1.1 Treatment of Osteoporosis in Postmenopausal Women

Reclast is indicated for treatment of osteoporosis in postmenopausal women. In postmenopausal women with osteoporosis, diagnosed by bone mineral density (BMD) or prevalent vertebral fracture, Reclast reduces the incidence of fractures (hip, vertebral and non-vertebral osteoporosis-related fractures). In patients at high risk of fracture, defined as a recent low-trauma hip fracture, Reclast reduces the incidence of new clinical fractures [*see Clinical Studies (14.1)*].

1.2 Prevention of Osteoporosis in Postmenopausal Women

Reclast is indicated for prevention of osteoporosis in postmenopausal women [*see Clinical Studies (14.2)*].

1.3 Osteoporosis in Men

Reclast is indicated for treatment to increase bone mass in men with osteoporosis [*see Clinical Studies (14.3)*].

1.4 Glucocorticoid-Induced Osteoporosis

Reclast is indicated for the treatment and prevention of glucocorticoid-induced osteoporosis in men and women who are either initiating or continuing systemic glucocorticoids in a daily dosage equivalent to 7.5 mg or greater of prednisone and who are expected to remain on glucocorticoids for at least 12 months [*see Clinical Studies (14.4)*].

1.5 Paget's Disease of Bone

Reclast is indicated for treatment of Paget's disease of bone in men and women. Treatment is indicated in patients with Paget's disease of bone with elevations in serum alkaline phosphatase of two times or higher than the upper limit of the age-specific normal reference range, or those who are symptomatic, or those at risk for complications from their disease [*see Clinical Studies (14.5)*].

1.6 Important Limitations of Use

The safety and effectiveness of Reclast for the treatment of osteoporosis is based on clinical data of three years duration. The optimal duration of use has not been determined. All patients on bisphosphonate therapy should have the need for continued therapy re-evaluated on a periodic basis. Patients at low-risk for fracture should be considered for drug discontinuation after 3 to 5 years of use. Patients who discontinue therapy should have their risk for fracture re-evaluated periodically.

2 DOSAGE AND ADMINISTRATION

2.1 Important Administration Instructions

Reclast injection must be administered as an intravenous infusion over no less than 15 minutes.

- Patients must be appropriately hydrated prior to administration of Reclast [*see Warnings and Precautions (5.3)*].
- Parenteral drug products should be inspected visually for particulate matter and discoloration prior to administration, whenever solution and container permit.
- Intravenous infusion should be followed by a 10 mL normal saline flush of the intravenous line.
- Administration of acetaminophen following Reclast administration may reduce the incidence of acute-phase reaction symptoms.

2.2 Treatment of Osteoporosis in Postmenopausal Women

The recommended regimen is a 5 mg infusion once a year given intravenously over no less than 15 minutes.

2.3 Prevention of Osteoporosis in Postmenopausal Women
The recommended regimen is a 5 mg infusion given once every 2 years intravenously over no less than 15 minutes.

2.4 Osteoporosis in Men
The recommended regimen is a 5 mg infusion once a year given intravenously over no less than 15 minutes.

2.5 Treatment and Prevention of Glucocorticoid-Induced Osteoporosis
The recommended regimen is a 5 mg infusion once a year given intravenously over no less than 15 minutes.

2.6 Treatment of Paget's Disease of Bone
The recommended dose is a 5 mg infusion. The infusion time must not be less than 15 minutes given over a constant infusion rate.

Re-treatment of Paget's Disease
After a single treatment with Reclast in Paget's disease an extended remission period is observed. Specific re-treatment data are not available. However, re-treatment with Reclast may be considered in patients who have relapsed, based on increases in serum alkaline phosphatase, or in those patients who failed to achieve normalization of their serum alkaline phosphatase, or in those patients with symptoms, as dictated by medical practice.

2.7 Laboratory Testing and Oral Examination Prior to Administration
- Prior to administration of each dose of Reclast, obtain a serum creatinine and creatinine clearance should be calculated based on actual body weight using Cockcroft-Gault formula before each Reclast dose. Reclast is contraindicated in patients with creatinine clearance less than 35 mL/min and in those with evidence of acute renal impairment. A 5 mg dose of Reclast administered intravenously is recommended for patients with creatinine clearance greater than or equal to 35 mL/min. There are no safety or efficacy data to support the adjustment of the Reclast dose based on baseline renal function. Therefore, no dose adjustment is required in patients with CrCl greater than or equal to 35 mL/min [*see Contraindications (4), Warnings and Precautions (5.3)*].
- A routine oral examination should be performed by the prescriber prior to initiation of Reclast treatment [*see Warnings and Precautions (5.4)*].

2.8 Calcium and Vitamin D Supplementation
- Instruct patients being treated for Paget's disease of bone on the importance of calcium and vitamin D supplementation in maintaining serum calcium levels, and on the symptoms of hypocalcemia. All patients should take 1500 mg elemental calcium daily in divided doses (750 mg two times a day, or 500 mg three times a day) and 800 international units vitamin D daily, particularly in the 2 weeks following Reclast administration [*see Warnings and Precautions (5.2)*].
- Instruct patients being treated for osteoporosis to take supplemental calcium and vitamin D if their dietary intake is inadequate. An average of at least 1200 mg calcium and 800-1000 international units vitamin D daily is recommended.

2.9 Method of Administration
The Reclast infusion time must not be less than 15 minutes given over a constant infusion rate.
The i.v. infusion should be followed by a 10 mL normal saline flush of the intravenous line.
Reclast solution for infusion must not be allowed to come in contact with any calcium or other divalent cation-containing solutions, and should be administered as a single intravenous solution through a separate vented infusion line.
If refrigerated, allow the refrigerated solution to reach room temperature before administration. After opening, the solution is stable for 24 hours at 2°C–8°C (36°F - 46°F) [*see How Supplied/Storage and Handling (16)*].

3 DOSAGE FORMS AND STRENGTHS

5 mg in a 100 mL ready to infuse solution.

4 CONTRAINDICATIONS

Reclast is contraindicated in patients with the following conditions:
- Hypocalcemia [*see Warnings and Precautions (5.2)*]
- Creatinine clearance less than 35 mL/min and in those with evidence of acute renal impairment due to an increased risk of renal failure [*see Warnings and Precautions (5.3)*].
- Known hypersensitivity to zoledronic acid or any components of Reclast. Hypersensitivity reactions including urticaria, angioedema, and anaphylactic reaction/shock have been reported [*see Post-Marketing Experience (6.2)*].

5 WARNINGS AND PRECAUTIONS

5.1 Drug Products with Same Active Ingredient
Reclast contains the same active ingredient found in Zometa, used for oncology indications, and a patient being treated with Zometa should not be treated with Reclast.

5.2 Hypocalcemia and Mineral Metabolism
Pre-existing hypocalcemia and disturbances of mineral metabolism (e.g., hypoparathyroidism, thyroid surgery, parathyroid surgery; malabsorption syndromes, excision of small intestine) must be effectively treated before initiating therapy with Reclast. Clinical monitoring of calcium and mineral levels (phosphorus and magnesium) is highly recommended for these patients [*see Contraindications (4)*].
Hypocalcemia following Reclast administration is a significant risk in Paget's disease. All patients should be instructed about the symptoms of hypocalcemia and the importance of calcium and vitamin D supplementation in maintaining serum calcium levels [*see Dosage and Administration (2.8), Adverse Reactions (6.1), Information for Patients (17)*].
All osteoporosis patients should be instructed on the importance of calcium and vitamin D supplementation in maintaining serum calcium levels [*see Dosage and Administration (2.8), Adverse Reactions (6.1), Information for Patients (17)*].

5.3 Renal Impairment
A single dose of Reclast should not exceed 5 mg and the duration of infusion should be no less than 15 minutes [*see Dosage and Administration (2)*].
Reclast is contraindicated in patients with creatinine clearance less than 35 mL/min and in those with evidence of acute renal impairment [*see Contraindications (4)*]. If history or physical signs suggest dehydration, Reclast therapy should be withheld until normovolemic status has been achieved [*see Post-Marketing Experience (6.2)*].
Reclast should be used with caution in patients with chronic renal impairment. Acute renal impairment, including renal failure, has been observed following the administration of zoledronic acid, especially in patients with pre-existing renal compromise, advanced age, concomitant nephrotoxic medications, concomitant diuretic therapy, or severe dehydration occurring before or after Reclast administration. Acute renal failure (ARF) has been observed in patients after a single administration. Rare reports of hospitalization and/or dialysis or fatal outcome occurred in patients with underlying moderate to severe renal impairment or with any of the risk factors described in this section [*see Post-Marketing Experience (6.2)*]. Renal impairment may lead to increased exposure of concomitant medications and/or their metabolites that are primarily renally excreted [*see Drug Interactions (7.4)*].
Creatinine clearance should be calculated based on actual body weight using Cockcroft-Gault formula before each Reclast dose. Transient increase in serum creatinine may be greater in patients with impaired renal function; interim monitoring of creatinine clearance should be performed in at-risk patients. Elderly patients and those receiving diuretic therapy are at increased risk of acute renal failure. These patients should have their fluid status assessed and be appropriately hydrated prior to administration of Reclast. Reclast should be used with caution with other nephrotoxic drugs [*see Drug Interactions (7.3)*]. Consider monitoring creatinine clearance in patients at-risk for ARF who are taking concomitant medications that are primarily excreted by the kidney [*see Drug Interactions (7.4)*].

5.4 Osteonecrosis of the Jaw
Osteonecrosis of the jaw (ONJ) has been reported in patients treated with bisphosphonates, including zoledronic acid. Most cases have been in cancer patients treated with intravenous bisphosphonates undergoing dental procedures. Some cases have occurred in patients with postmenopausal osteoporosis treated with either oral or intravenous bisphosphonates. A routine oral examination should be performed by the prescriber prior to initiation of bisphosphonate treatment. A dental examination with appropriate preventive dentistry should be considered prior to treatment with bisphosphonates in patients with a history of concomitant risk factors (e.g., cancer, chemotherapy, radiotherapy, corticosteroids, poor oral hygiene, pre-existing dental disease or infection, anemia, coagulopathy).
While on treatment, patients with concomitant risk factors should avoid invasive dental procedures if possible. For patients who develop ONJ while on bisphosphonate therapy, dental surgery may exacerbate the condition. For patients requiring dental procedures, there are no data available to suggest whether discontinuation of bisphosphonate treatment reduces the risk of ONJ. The clinical judgment of the treating physician should guide the management plan of each patient based on individual benefit/risk assessment [*see Adverse Reactions (6.1)*].

5.5 Atypical Subtrochanteric and Diaphyseal Femoral Fractures
Atypical, low-energy, or low trauma fractures of the femoral shaft have been reported in bisphosphonate-treated patients. These fractures can occur anywhere in the femoral shaft from just below the lesser trochanter to above the supracondylar flare and are transverse or short oblique in orientation without evidence of comminution. Causality has not been established as these fractures also occur in osteoporotic patients who have not been treated with bisphosphonates.
Atypical femur fractures most commonly occur with minimal or no trauma to the affected area. They may be bilateral and many patients report prodromal pain in the affected area, usually presenting as dull, aching thigh pain, weeks to months before a complete fracture occurs. A number of reports note that patients were also receiving treatment with glucocorticoids (e.g., prednisone) at the time of fracture.
Any patient with a history of bisphosphonate exposure who presents with thigh or groin pain should be suspected of having an atypical fracture and should be evaluated to rule out an incomplete femur fracture. Patients presenting with an atypical femur fracture should also be assessed for symptoms and signs of fracture in the contralateral limb. Interruption of bisphosphonate therapy should be considered, pending a risk/benefit assessment, on an individual basis.

5.6 Pregnancy
RECLAST SHOULD NOT BE USED DURING PREGNANCY. Reclast may cause fetal harm when administered to a pregnant woman. If the patient becomes pregnant while taking this drug, the patient should be apprised of the potential harm to the fetus. Women of childbearing potential should be advised to avoid becoming pregnant while on Reclast therapy [*see Use in Specific Populations (8.1)*].

5.7 Musculoskeletal Pain
In post-marketing experience, severe and occasionally incapacitating bone, joint, and/or muscle pain have been infrequently reported in patients taking bisphosphonates, including Reclast. The time to onset of symptoms varied from one day to several months after starting the drug. Consider withholding future Reclast treatment if severe symptoms develop. Most patients had relief of symptoms after stopping. A subset had recurrence of symptoms when rechallenged with the same drug or another bisphosphonate [*see Adverse Reactions (6.2)*].

5.8 Patients with Asthma
While not observed in clinical trials with Reclast, there have been reports of bronchoconstriction in aspirin-sensitive patients receiving bisphosphonates. Use Reclast with caution in aspirin-sensitive patients.

6 ADVERSE REACTIONS

6.1 Clinical Studies Experience
Because clinical trials are conducted under widely varying conditions, adverse reaction rates observed in the clinical trials of a drug cannot be directly compared to rates in the clinical trials of another drug and may not reflect the rates observed in practice.

Treatment of Osteoporosis in Postmenopausal Women
The safety of Reclast in the treatment of postmenopausal osteoporosis was assessed in Study 1, a large, randomized, double-blind, placebo-controlled, multinational study of 7736 postmenopausal women aged 65-89 years with osteoporosis, diagnosed by bone mineral density or the presence of a prevalent vertebral fracture. The duration of the trial was three years with 3862 patients exposed to Reclast and 3852 patients exposed to placebo administered once annually as a single 5 mg dose in 100 mL solution infused over at least 15 minutes, for a total of three doses. All women received 1000 to 1500 mg of elemental calcium plus 400 to 1200 international units of vitamin D supplementation per day.
The incidence of all-cause mortality was similar between groups: 3.4% in the Reclast group and 2.9% in the placebo group. The incidence of serious adverse events was 29.2% in the Reclast group and 30.1% in the placebo group. The percentage of patients who withdrew from the study due to adverse events was 5.4% and 4.8% for the Reclast and placebo groups, respectively.
The safety of Reclast in the treatment of osteoporosis patients with a recent (within 90 days) low-trauma hip fracture was assessed in Study 2, a randomized, double-blind, placebo-controlled, multinational endpoint-driven study of 2127 men and women aged 50-95 years; 1065 patients were randomized to Reclast and 1062 patients were randomized to placebo. Reclast was administered once annually as a single 5 mg dose in 100 mL solution infused over at least 15 minutes. The study continued until at least 211 patients had a confirmed clinical fracture in the study population who were followed for an average of approximately 2 years on study drug. Vitamin D levels were not routinely measured but a loading dose of vitamin D (50,000 to 125,000 international units orally or IM) was given to patients and they were started on 1000 to 1500 mg of elemental calcium plus 800 to 1200 international units of vitamin D supplementation per day for at least 14 days prior to the study drug infusions.
The incidence of all-cause mortality was 9.6% in the Reclast group and 13.3% in the placebo group. The incidence of serious adverse events was 38.3% in the Reclast group and 41.3% in the placebo group. The percentage of patients who withdrew from the study due to adverse events was 5.3% and 4.7% for the Reclast and placebo groups, respectively.

Adverse reactions reported in at least 2% of patients with osteoporosis and more frequently in the Reclast-treated patients than placebo-treated patients in either osteoporosis trial are shown below in Table 1.

[See table 1 above]

Renal Impairment

Treatment with intravenous bisphosphonates, including zoledronic acid, has been associated with renal impairment manifested as deterioration in renal function (i.e., increased serum creatinine) and in rare cases, acute renal failure. In the clinical trial for postmenopausal osteoporosis, patients with baseline creatinine clearance less than 30 mL/min (based on actual body weight), urine dipstick greater than or equal to 2+ protein or increase in serum creatinine of greater than 0.5 mg/dL during the screening visits were excluded. The change in creatinine clearance (measured annually prior to dosing) and the incidence of renal failure and impairment was comparable for both the Reclast and placebo treatment groups over 3 years, including patients with creatinine clearance between 30-60 mL/min at baseline. Overall, there was a transient increase in serum creatinine observed within 10 days of dosing in 1.8% of Reclast-treated patients versus 0.8% of placebo-treated patients which resolved without specific therapy [*see Warnings and Precautions (5.3)*].

Acute Phase Reaction

The signs and symptoms of acute phase reaction occurred in Study 1 following Reclast infusion including fever (18%), myalgia (9%), flu-like symptoms (8%), headache (7%), and arthralgia (7%). The majority of these symptoms occurred within the first 3 days following the dose of Reclast and usually resolved within 3 days of onset but resolution could take up to 7-14 days. In Study 2, patients without a contraindication to acetaminophen were provided with a standard oral dose at the time of the IV infusion and instructed to use additional acetaminophen at home for the next 72 hours as needed. Reclast was associated with fewer signs and symptoms of a transient acute phase reaction in this trial: fever (7%) and arthralgia (3%). The incidence of these symptoms decreased with subsequent doses of Reclast.

Laboratory Findings

In Study 1, in women with postmenopausal osteoporosis, approximately 0.2% of patients had notable declines of serum calcium levels (less than 7.5 mg/dL) following Reclast administration. No symptomatic cases of hypocalcemia were observed. In Study 2, following pre-treatment with vitamin D, no patients had treatment emergent serum calcium levels below 7.5 mg/dL.

Injection Site Reactions

In the osteoporosis trials, local reactions at the infusion site such as itching, redness and/or pain have been reported in 0% to 0.7% of patients following the administration of Reclast and 0% to 0.5% of patients following administration of placebo.

Osteonecrosis of the Jaw

In the postmenopausal osteoporosis trial, Study 1, in 7736 patients, after initiation of therapy, symptoms consistent with ONJ occurred in one patient treated with placebo and one patient treated with Reclast. Both cases resolved after appropriate treatment [*see Warnings and Precautions (5.4)*]. No reports of osteonecrosis of the jaw were reported in either treatment group in Study 2.

Atrial Fibrillation

In the postmenopausal osteoporosis trial, Study 1, adjudicated serious adverse events of atrial fibrillation in the zoledronic acid treatment group occurred in 1.3% of patients (50 out of 3862) compared to 0.4% (17 out of 3852) in the placebo group. The overall incidence of all atrial fibrillation adverse events in the zoledronic acid treatment group was reported in 2.5% of patients (96 out of 3862) in the Reclast group vs. 1.9% of patients (75 out of 3852) in the placebo group. Over 90% of these events in both treatment groups occurred more than a month after the infusion. In an ECG sub-study, ECG measurements were performed on a subset of 559 patients before and 9 to 11 days after treatment. There was no difference in the incidence of atrial fibrillation between treatment groups suggesting these events were not related to the acute infusions. In Study 2, adjudicated serious adverse events of atrial fibrillation in the zoledronic acid treatment group occurred in 1.0% of patients (11 out of 1054) compared to 1.2% (13 out of 1057) in the placebo group demonstrating no difference between treatment groups.

Ocular Adverse Events

Cases of iritis/uveitis/episcleritis/conjunctivitis have been reported in patients treated with bisphosphonates, including zoledronic acid. In the osteoporosis trials, 1 (less than 0.1%) to 9 (0.2%) patients treated with Reclast and 0 (0%) to 1 (less than 0.1%) patient treated with placebo developed iritis/uveitis/episcleritis.

Table 1. Adverse Reactions Occurring in greater than or equal to 2.0% of Patients with Osteoporosis and More Frequently than in Placebo-Treated Patients

System Organ Class	Study 1: 5 mg IV Reclast once per year % (N=3862)	Study 1: Placebo once per year % (N=3852)	Study 2: 5 mg IV Reclast once per year % (N=1054)	Study 2: Placebo once per year % (N=1057)
Blood and the Lymphatic System Disorders				
Anemia	4.4	3.6	5.3	5.2
Metabolism and Nutrition Disorders				
Dehydration	0.6	0.6	2.5	2.3
Anorexia	2.0	1.1	1.0	1.0
Nervous System Disorders				
Headache	12.4	8.1	3.9	2.5
Dizziness	7.6	6.7	2.0	4.0
Ear and Labyrinth Disorders				
Vertigo	4.3	4.0	1.3	1.7
Cardiac Disorders				
Atrial Fibrillation	2.4	1.9	2.8	2.6
Vascular Disorders				
Hypertension	12.7	12.4	6.8	5.4
Gastrointestinal Disorders				
Nausea	8.5	5.2	4.5	4.5
Diarrhea	6.0	5.6	5.2	4.7
Vomiting	4.6	3.2	3.4	3.4
Abdominal Pain Upper	4.6	3.1	0.9	1.5
Dyspepsia	4.3	4.0	1.7	1.6
Musculoskeletal, Connective Tissue and Bone Disorders				
Arthralgia	23.8	20.4	17.9	18.3
Myalgia	11.7	3.7	4.9	2.7
Pain in Extremity	11.3	9.9	5.9	4.8
Shoulder Pain	6.9	5.6	0.0	0.0
Bone Pain	5.8	2.3	3.2	1.0
Neck Pain	4.4	3.8	1.4	1.1
Muscle Spasms	3.7	3.4	1.5	1.7
Osteoarthritis	9.1	9.7	5.7	4.5
Musculoskeletal Pain	0.4	0.3	3.1	1.2
General Disorders and Administrative Site Conditions				
Pyrexia	17.9	4.6	8.7	3.1
Influenza-like Illness	8.8	2.7	0.8	0.4
Fatigue	5.4	3.5	2.1	1.2
Chills	5.4	1.0	1.5	0.5
Asthenia	5.3	2.9	3.2	3.0
Peripheral Edema	4.6	4.2	5.5	5.3
Pain	3.3	1.3	1.5	0.5
Malaise	2.0	1.0	1.1	0.5
Hyperthermia	0.3	<0.1	2.3	0.3
Chest Pain	1.3	1.1	2.4	1.8
Investigations				
Creatinine Renal Clearance Decreased	2.0	2.4	2.1	1.7

Prevention of Osteoporosis in Postmenopausal Women

The safety of Reclast in postmenopausal women with osteopenia (low bone mass) was assessed in a 2-year randomized, multi-center, double-blind, placebo-controlled study of 581 postmenopausal women aged greater than or equal to 45 years. Patients were randomized to one of three treatment groups: (1) Reclast given at randomization and Month 12 (n=198); (2) Reclast given at randomization and placebo at Month 12 (n=181); and (3) placebo given at randomization and Month 12 (n=202). Reclast was administered as a single 5 mg dose in 100 mL solution infused over at least 15 minutes. All women received 500 to 1200 mg elemental calcium plus 400 to 800 international units vitamin D supplementation per day.

The incidence of serious adverse events was similar for subjects given (1) Reclast at randomization and at Month 12 (10.6%), (2) Reclast at randomization and placebo given at Month 12 (9.4%), and (3) placebo at randomization and at Month 12 (11.4%). The percentages of patients who withdrew from the study due to adverse events were 7.1%, 7.2%, and 3.0% in the two Reclast groups and placebo group, respectively. Adverse reactions reported in at least 2% of patients with osteopenia and more frequently in the Reclast-treated patients than placebo-treated patients are shown in Table 2.

[See table 2 at top of next page]

Ocular Adverse Events

Cases of iritis/uveitis/episcleritis/conjunctivitis have been reported in patients treated with bisphosphonates, including zoledronic acid. In the osteoporosis prevention trial, 4 (1.1%) patients treated with Reclast and 0 (0%) patients treated with placebo developed iritis/uveitis.

Acute Phase Reaction

In patients given Reclast at randomization and placebo at Month 12, Reclast was associated with signs and symptoms of an acute phase reaction: myalgia (20.4%), fever (19.3%), chills (18.2%), pain (13.8%), headache (13.3%), fatigue (8.3%), arthralgia (6.1%), pain in extremity (3.9%), influenza-like illness (3.3%), and back pain (1.7%), which occurred within the first 3 days following the dose of Reclast. The majority of these symptoms were mild to moderate and resolved within 3 days of the event onset but resolution could take up to 7-14 days.

Osteoporosis in Men

The safety of Reclast in men with osteoporosis or osteoporosis secondary to hypogonadism was assessed in a two year randomized, multicenter, double-blind, active controlled group study of 302 men aged 25-86 years. One hundred fifty three (153) patients were exposed to Reclast administered once annually with a 5 mg dose in 100 mL infused over 15 minutes for up to a total of two doses, and 148 patients were exposed to a commercially-available oral weekly bisphosphonate (active control) for up to two years. All participants received 1000 mg of elemental calcium plus 800 to 1000 international units of vitamin D supplementation per day.

The incidence of all-cause mortality (one in each group) and serious adverse events were similar between the Reclast and active control treatment groups. The percentage of patients experiencing at least one adverse event was comparable between the Reclast and active control groups, with the exception of a higher incidence of post-dose symptoms in the Reclast group that occurred within 3 days after infusion. The overall safety and tolerability of Reclast was similar to the active control.

Adverse reactions reported in at least 2% of men with osteoporosis and more frequently in the Reclast-treated patients than the active control-treated patients and either (1) not reported in the postmenopausal osteoporosis treatment trial or (2) reported more frequently in the trial of osteoporosis in men are presented in Table 3. Therefore, Table 3 should be viewed in conjunction with Table 1.

Table 2. Adverse Reactions Occurring in greater than or equal to 2% of Patients with Osteopenia and More Frequently than in Placebo-Treated Patients

System Organ Class	5 mg IV Reclast Once Per Year % (n=198)	5 mg IV Reclast Once % (n=181)	Placebo once per year % (n=202)
Metabolism and nutrition disorders			
Anorexia	2.0	0.6	0.0
Nervous system disorders			
Headache	14.6	20.4	11.4
Dizziness	7.6	6.1	3.5
Hypoesthesia	5.6	2.2	2.0
Ear and labyrinth disorders			
Vertigo	2.0	1.7	1.0
Vascular disorders			
Hypertension	5.1	8.3	6.9
Gastrointestinal disorders			
Nausea	17.7	11.6	7.9
Diarrhea	8.1	6.6	7.9
Vomiting	7.6	5.0	4.5
Dyspepsia	7.1	6.6	5.0
Abdominal pain*	8.6	6.6	7.9
Constipation	6.6	7.2	6.9
Abdominal discomfort	2.0	1.1	0.5
Abdominal distension	2.0	0.6	0.0
Skin and subcutaneous tissue disorders			
Rash	3.0	2.2	2.5
Musculoskeletal and connective tissue disorders			
Arthralgia	27.3	18.8	19.3
Myalgia	19.2	22.7	6.9
Back pain	18.2	16.6	11.9
Pain in extremity	11.1	16.0	9.9
Muscle spasms	5.6	2.8	5.0
Musculoskeletal pain**	8.1	7.2	7.9
Bone pain	5.1	3.3	1.0
Neck pain	5.1	6.6	5.0
Arthritis	4.0	2.2	1.5
Joint stiffness	3.5	1.1	2.0
Joint swelling	3.0	0.6	0.0
Flank pain	2.0	0.6	0.0
Pain in jaw	2.0	3.9	2.5
General disorders and administration site conditions			
Pain	24.2	14.9	3.5
Pyrexia	21.7	21.0	4.5
Chills	18.2	18.2	3.0
Fatigue	14.6	9.9	4.0
Asthenia	6.1	2.8	1.0
Peripheral edema	5.6	3.9	3.5
Non-cardiac chest pain	3.5	7.7	3.0
Influenza-like illness	1.5	3.3	2.0
Malaise	1.0	2.2	0.5

* Combined abdominal pain, abdominal pain upper, and abdominal pain lower as one ADR
** Combined musculoskeletal pain and musculoskeletal chest pain as one ADR

Table 3: Adverse Reactions Occurring in greater than or equal to 2% of Men with Osteoporosis and More Frequently in the Reclast-Treated Patients than the Active Control-Treated Patients and either (1) Not Reported in the Postmenopausal Osteoporosis Treatment Trial or (2) Reported More Frequently in this Trial

System Organ Class	5 mg IV Reclast once per year % (N=153)	Active Control once weekly % (N=148)
Nervous System Disorders		
Headache	15.0	6.1
Lethargy	3.3	1.4
Eye Disorders		
Eye pain	2.0	0.0
Cardiac Disorders		
Atrial fibrillation	3.3	2.0
Palpitations	2.6	0.0
Respiratory, Thoracic and Mediastinal Disorders		
Dyspnea	6.5	4.7
Abdominal pain*	7.9	4.1
Skin and Subcutaneous Tissue Disorders		
Hyperhidrosis	2.6	2.0
Musculoskeletal, Connective Tissue and Bone Disorders		
Myalgia	19.6	6.8
Musculoskeletal pain**	12.4	10.8
Musculoskeletal stiffness	4.6	0.0
Renal and Urinary Disorders		
Blood creatinine increased	2.0	0.7
General Disorders and Administrative Site Conditions		
Fatigue	17.6	6.1
Pain	11.8	4.1
Chills	9.8	2.7
Influenza-like illness	9.2	2.0
Malaise	7.2	0.7
Acute phase reaction	3.9	0.0
Investigations		
C-reactive protein increased	4.6	1.4

* Combined abdominal pain, abdominal pain upper, and abdominal pain lower as one ADR
** Combined musculoskeletal pain and musculoskeletal chest pain as one ADR

Renal Impairment
Creatinine clearance was measured annually prior to dosing and changes in long-term renal function over 24 months were comparable in the Reclast and active control groups [*see Warnings and Precautions (5.3)*].

Acute Phase Reaction
Reclast was associated with signs and symptoms of an acute phase reaction: myalgia (17.1%), fever (15.7%), fatigue (12.4%), arthralgia (11.1%), pain (10.5%), chills (9.8%), headache (9.8%), influenza-like illness (8.5%), malaise (5.2%), and back pain (3.3%), which occurred within the first 3 days following the dose of Reclast. The majority of these symptoms were mild to moderate and resolved within 3 days of the event onset but resolution could take up to 7-14 days. The incidence of these symptoms decreased with subsequent doses of Reclast.

Atrial Fibrillation
The incidence of all atrial fibrillation adverse events in the Reclast treatment group was 3.3% (5 out of 153) compared to 2.0% (3 out of 148) in the active control group. However, there were no patients with adjudicated serious adverse events of atrial fibrillation in the Reclast treatment group.

Laboratory Findings
There were no patients who had treatment emergent serum calcium levels below 7.5 mg/dL.

Injection Site Reactions
There were 4 patients (2.6%) on Reclast vs. 2 patients (1.4%) on active control with local site reactions.

Osteonecrosis of the Jaw
In this trial there were no cases of osteonecrosis of the jaw [*see Warnings and Precautions (5.4)*].

Glucocorticoid-Induced Osteoporosis
The safety of Reclast in men and women in the treatment and prevention of glucocorticoid-induced osteoporosis was assessed in a randomized, multicenter, double-blind, active controlled, stratified study of 833 men and women aged 18-85 years treated with greater than or equal to 7.5 mg/day oral prednisone (or equivalent). Patients were stratified according to the duration of their pre-study corticosteroid therapy: less than or equal to 3 months prior to randomization (prevention subpopulation), and greater than 3 months prior to randomization (treatment subpopulation).
The duration of the trial was one year with 416 patients exposed to Reclast administered once as a single 5 mg dose in 100 mL infused over 15 minutes, and 417 patients exposed to a commercially-available oral daily bisphosphonate (active control) for one year. All participants received 1000 mg of elemental calcium plus 400 to 1000 international units of vitamin D supplementation per day.
The incidence of all–cause mortality was similar between treatment groups: 0.9% in the Reclast group and 0.7% in the active control group. The incidence of serious adverse events was similar between the Reclast treatment and prevention groups, 18.4% and 18.1%, respectively, and the active control treatment and prevention groups, 19.8% and 16.0%, respectively. The percentage of subjects who withdrew from the study due to adverse events was 2.2% in the Reclast group vs. 1.4% in the active control group. The overall safety and tolerability were similar between Reclast and active control groups with the exception of a higher incidence of post-dose symptoms in the Reclast group that occurred within 3 days after infusion. The overall safety and tolerability profile of Reclast in glucocorticoid-induced osteoporosis was similar to the adverse events reported in the Reclast postmenopausal osteoporosis clinical trial.
Adverse reactions reported in at least 2% of patients that were either not reported in the postmenopausal osteoporosis treatment trial or reported more frequently in the treatment and prevention of glucocorticoid-induced osteoporosis trial included the following: abdominal pain (Reclast 7.5%; active control 5.0%), and musculoskeletal pain (Reclast 3.1%; active control 1.7%). Other musculoskeletal events included back pain (Reclast 4.3%, active control 6.2%), bone pain (Reclast 3.1%, active control 2.2%), and pain in the extremity (Reclast 3.1%, active control 1.2%). In addition, the following adverse events occurred more frequently than in the postmenopausal osteoporosis trial: nausea (Reclast 9.6%; active control 8.4%), and dyspepsia (Reclast 5.5%; active control 4.3%).

Renal Impairment
Renal function measured prior to dosing and at the end of the 12 month study was comparable in the Reclast and active control groups [*see Warnings and Precautions (5.3)*].

Acute Phase Reaction
Reclast was associated with signs and symptoms of a transient acute phase reaction that was similar to that seen in the Reclast postmenopausal osteoporosis clinical trial.

Atrial Fibrillation
The incidence of atrial fibrillation adverse events was 0.7% (3 of 416) in the Reclast group compared to no adverse events in the active control group. All subjects had a prior history of atrial fibrillation and no cases were adjudicated as serious adverse events. One patient had atrial flutter in the active control group.

Laboratory Findings
There were no patients who had treatment emergent serum calcium levels below 7.5 mg/dL.

Injection Site Reactions
There were no local reactions at the infusion site.

Osteonecrosis of the Jaw
In this trial there were no cases of osteonecrosis of the jaw [*see Warnings and Precautions (5.4)*].

Paget's Disease of Bone
In the Paget's disease trials, two 6-month, double-blind, comparative, multinational studies of 349 men and women aged greater than 30 years with moderate to severe disease and with confirmed Paget's disease of bone, 177 patients were exposed to Reclast and 172 patients exposed to risedronate. Reclast was administered once as a single 5 mg

dose in 100 mL solution infused over at least 15 minutes. Risedronate was given as an oral daily dose of 30 mg for 2 months.

The incidence of serious adverse events was 5.1% in the Reclast group and 6.4% in the risedronate group. The percentage of patients who withdrew from the study due to adverse events was 1.7% and 1.2% for the Reclast and risedronate groups, respectively.

Adverse reactions occurring in at least 2% of the Paget's patients receiving Reclast (single 5 mg intravenous infusion) or risedronate (30 mg oral daily dose for 2 months) over a 6-month study period are listed by system organ class in Table 4.

Table 4. Adverse Reactions Reported in at Least 2% of Paget's Patients Receiving Reclast (Single 5 mg intravenous Infusion) or Risedronate (Oral 30 mg Daily for 2 Months) Over a 6-Month Follow-Up Period

System Organ Class	5 mg IV Reclast % (N = 177)	30 mg/day × 2 Months risedronate % (N = 172)
Infections and Infestations		
Influenza	7	5
Metabolism and Nutrition Disorders		
Hypocalcemia	3	1
Anorexia	2	2
Nervous System Disorders		
Headache	11	10
Dizziness	9	4
Lethargy	5	1
Paresthesia	2	0
Respiratory, Thoracic and Mediastinal Disorders		
Dyspnea	5	1
Gastrointestinal Disorders		
Nausea	9	6
Diarrhea	6	6
Constipation	6	5
Dyspepsia	5	4
Abdominal Distension	2	1
Abdominal Pain	2	2
Vomiting	2	2
Abdominal Pain Upper	1	2
Skin and Subcutaneous Tissue Disorders		
Rash	3	2
Musculoskeletal, Connective Tissue and Bone Disorders		
Arthralgia	9	11
Bone Pain	9	5
Myalgia	7	4
Back Pain	4	7
Musculoskeletal Stiffness	2	1
General Disorders and Administrative Site Conditions		
Influenza-like Illness	11	6
Pyrexia	9	2
Fatigue	8	4
Rigors	8	1
Pain	5	4
Peripheral Edema	3	1
Asthenia	2	1

Laboratory Findings

In the Paget's disease trials, early, transient decreases in serum calcium and phosphate levels were observed. Approximately 21% of patients had serum calcium levels less than 8.4 mg/dL 9-11 days following Reclast administration.

Renal Impairment

In clinical trials in Paget's disease there were no cases of renal deterioration following a single 5 mg 15-minute infusion [*see Warnings and Precautions (5.3)*].

Acute Phase Reaction

The signs and symptoms of acute phase reaction (influenza-like illness, pyrexia, myalgia, arthralgia, and bone pain) were reported in 25% of patients in the Reclast-treated group compared to 8% in the risedronate-treated group. Symptoms usually occur within the first 3 days following Reclast administration. The majority of these symptoms resolved within 4 days of onset.

Osteonecrosis of the Jaw

Osteonecrosis of the jaw has been reported with zoledronic acid [*see Warnings and Precautions (5.4)*].

6.2 Post-Marketing Experience

Because these reactions are reported voluntarily from a population of uncertain size, it is not always possible to reliably estimate their frequency or establish a causal relationship to drug exposure.

The following adverse reactions have been identified during post approval use of Reclast:

Acute Phase Reactions

Fever, headache, flu-like symptoms, nausea, vomiting, diarrhea, arthralgia, and myalgia. Symptoms may be significant and lead to dehydration.

Acute Renal Failure

Acute renal failure requiring hospitalization and/or dialysis or with a fatal outcome have been rarely reported. Increased serum creatinine was reported in patients with 1) underlying renal disease, 2) dehydration secondary to fever, sepsis, gastrointestinal losses, or diuretic therapy, or 3) other risk factors such as advanced age, or concomitant nephrotoxic drugs in the post-infusion period. Transient rise in serum creatinine can be correctable with intravenous fluids.

Allergic Reactions

Allergic reaction with intravenous zoledronic acid including anaphylactic reaction/shock, urticaria, angioedema, and bronchoconstriction have been reported.

Asthma Exacerbations

Asthma exacerbations have been reported.

Hypocalcemia

Hypocalcemia has been reported.

Osteonecrosis of the Jaw

Osteonecrosis of the jaw has been reported.

Ocular Adverse Events

Cases of the following events have been reported: conjunctivitis, iritis, iridocyclitis, uveitis, episcleritis, scleritis and orbital inflammation/edema.

Other

Hypotension in patients with underlying risk factors has been reported.

7 DRUG INTERACTIONS

No *in vivo* drug interaction studies have been performed for Reclast. *In vitro* and *ex vivo* studies showed low affinity of zoledronic acid for the cellular components of human blood. *In vitro* mean zoledronic acid protein binding in human plasma ranged from 28% at 200 ng/mL to 53% at 50 ng/mL. *In vivo* studies showed that zoledronic acid is not metabolized, and is excreted into the urine as the intact drug.

7.1 Aminoglycosides

Caution is advised when bisphosphonates, including zoledronic acid, are administered with aminoglycosides, since these agents may have an additive effect to lower serum calcium level for prolonged periods. This effect has not been reported in zoledronic acid clinical trials.

7.2 Loop Diuretics

Caution should also be exercised when Reclast is used in combination with loop diuretics due to an increased risk of hypocalcemia.

7.3 Nephrotoxic Drugs

Caution is indicated when Reclast is used with other potentially nephrotoxic drugs such as nonsteroidal anti-inflammatory drugs.

7.4 Drugs Primarily Excreted by the Kidney

Renal impairment has been observed following the administration of zoledronic acid in patients with pre-existing renal compromise or other risk factors [*see Warnings and Precautions (5.3)*]. In patients with renal impairment, the exposure to concomitant medications that are primarily renally excreted (e.g., digoxin) may increase. Consider monitoring serum creatinine in patients at risk for renal impairment who are taking concomitant medications that are primarily excreted by the kidney.

8 USE IN SPECIFIC POPULATIONS

8.1 Pregnancy

Pregnancy Category D [*see Warnings and Precautions (5.6)*].

RECLAST SHOULD NOT BE USED DURING PREGNANCY. If the patient becomes pregnant while taking this drug, the patient should be apprised of the potential harm to the fetus. Women of childbearing potential should be advised to avoid becoming pregnant while receiving Reclast.

Bisphosphonates are incorporated into the bone matrix, from where they are gradually released over periods of weeks to years. The extent of bisphosphonate incorporation into adult bone, and hence, the amount available for release back into the systemic circulation, is directly related to the total dose and duration of bisphosphonate use. Although there are no data on fetal risk in humans, bisphosphonates do cause fetal harm in animals, and animal data suggest that uptake of bisphosphonates into fetal bone is greater than into maternal bone. Therefore, there is a theoretical risk of fetal harm (e.g., skeletal and other abnormalities) if a woman becomes pregnant after completing a course of bisphosphonate therapy. The impact of variables such as time between cessation of bisphosphonate therapy to conception space, the particular bisphosphonate used, and the route of administration (intravenous versus oral) on this risk has not been established.

In female rats given daily subcutaneous doses of zoledronic acid beginning 15 days before mating and continuing through gestation, the number of stillbirths was increased and survival of neonates was decreased at approximately greater than or equal to 0.3 times the anticipated human systemic exposure following a 5 mg intravenous dose (based on an AUC comparison). Adverse maternal effects were observed in all dose groups at greater than or equal to 0.1 times the human systemic exposure following a 5 mg intravenous dose (based on an AUC comparison) and included dystocia and periparturient mortality in pregnant rats allowed to deliver. Maternal mortality was considered related to drug-induced inhibition of skeletal calcium mobilization, resulting in periparturient hypocalcemia. This appears to be a bisphosphonate class effect.

In pregnant rats given daily subcutaneous dose of zoledronic acid during gestation, adverse fetal effects were observed at about 2 and 4 times human systemic exposure following a 5 mg intravenous dose (based on an AUC comparison). These adverse effects included increases in pre- and post-implantation losses, decreases in viable fetuses, and fetal skeletal, visceral, and external malformations.

In pregnant rabbits given daily subcutaneous doses of zoledronic acid during gestation at doses less than or equal to 0.4 times the anticipated human systemic exposure following a 5 mg intravenous dose (based on a mg/m^2 comparison) no adverse fetal effects were observed. Maternal mortality and abortion occurred in all treatment groups (at doses greater than or equal to 0.04 times the human 5 mg intravenous dose, based on a mg/m^2 comparison). Adverse maternal effects were associated with, and may have been caused by, drug-induced hypocalcemia [*see Nonclinical Toxicology (13.3)*].

8.3 Nursing Mothers

It is not known whether Reclast is excreted in human milk. Because many drugs are excreted in human milk, and because Reclast binds to bone long-term, Reclast should not be administered to a nursing woman.

8.4 Pediatric Use

Reclast is not indicated for use in children.

The safety and effectiveness of zoledronic acid was studied in a one-year active controlled trial of 152 pediatric subjects (74 receiving zoledronic acid). The enrolled population was subjects with severe osteogenesis imperfecta, aged 1-17 years, 55% male, 84% Caucasian, with a mean lumbar spine BMD of 0.431 gm/cm^2, which is 2.7 standard deviations below the mean for age-matched controls (BMD Z-score of -2.7). At one year, increases in BMD were observed in the zoledronic acid treatment group. However, changes in BMD in individual patients with severe osteogenesis imperfecta did not necessarily correlate with the risk for fracture or the incidence or severity of chronic bone pain. The adverse events observed with zoledronic acid use in children did not raise any new safety findings beyond those previously seen in adults treated for Paget's disease of bone and treatment of osteoporosis including osteonecrosis of the jaw (ONJ) and renal impairment. However, adverse reactions seen more commonly in pediatric patients included pyrexia (61%), arthralgia (26%), hypocalcemia (22%) and headache (22%). These reactions, excluding arthralgia, occurred most frequently within three days after the first infusion and became less common with repeat dosing. No cases of ONJ or renal impairment were observed in this study. Because of long-term retention in bone, Reclast should only be used in children if the potential benefit outweighs the potential risk.

Plasma zoledronic acid concentration data was obtained from 10 patients with severe osteogenesis imperfecta (4 in the age group of 3-8 years and 6 in the age group of 9-17 years) infused with 0.05 mg/kg dose over 30 minutes. Mean C_{max} and $AUC_{(0\text{-}last)}$ was 167 ng/mL and 220 ng.h/mL respectively. The plasma concentration time profile of zoledronic acid in pediatric patients represent a multi-exponential decline, as observed in adult cancer patients at an approximately equivalent mg/kg dose.

8.5 Geriatric Use

The combined osteoporosis trials included 4863 Reclast-treated patients who were at least 65 years of age, while 2101 patients were at least 75 years old. No overall differences in efficacy or safety were observed between patients under 75 years of age with those at least 75 years of age, except that the acute phase reactions occurred less frequently in the older patients.

Of the patients receiving Reclast in the osteoporosis study in men, glucocorticoid-induced osteoporosis, and Paget's disease studies, 83, 116, and 132 patients, respectively were 65 years of age or over, while 24, 29, and 68 patients, respectively were at least 75 years of age.

However, because decreased renal function occurs more commonly in the elderly, special care should be taken to monitor renal function.

8.6 Renal Impairment

Reclast is contraindicated in patients with creatinine clearance less than 35 mL/min and in those with evidence of acute renal impairment. There are no safety or efficacy data to support the adjustment of the Reclast dose based on baseline renal function. Therefore, no dosage adjustment is required in patients with a creatinine clearance of greater than or equal to 35 mL/min [*see Warnings and Precautions (5.3), Clinical Pharmacology (12.3)*]. Risk of acute renal failure may increase with underlying renal disease and dehydration secondary to fever, sepsis, gastrointestinal losses, diuretic therapy, advanced age, etc. [*see Post-Marketing Experience (6.2)*].

8.7 Hepatic Impairment

Reclast is not metabolized in the liver. No clinical data are available for use of Reclast in patients with hepatic impairment.

10 OVERDOSAGE

Clinical experience with acute overdosage of zoledronic acid (Reclast) solution for intravenous infusion is limited. Patients who have received doses higher than those recommended should be carefully monitored. Overdosage may cause clinically significant renal impairment, hypocalcemia, hypophosphatemia, and hypomagnesemia. Clinically relevant reductions in serum levels of calcium, phosphorus, and magnesium should be corrected by intravenous administration of calcium gluconate, potassium or sodium phosphate, and magnesium sulfate, respectively.

Single doses of Reclast should not exceed 5 mg and the duration of the intravenous infusion should be no less than 15 minutes [*see Dosage and Administration (2)*].

11 DESCRIPTION

Reclast contains zoledronic acid, a bisphosphonic acid which is an inhibitor of osteoclastic bone resorption. Zoledronic acid is designated chemically as (1-Hydroxy-2-imidazol-1-yl-phosphonoethyl) phosphonic acid monohydrate and its structural formula is:

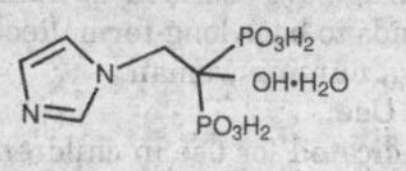

Zoledronic acid monohydrate is a white crystalline powder. Its molecular formula is $C_5H_{10}N_2O_7P_2 \bullet H_2O$ and a molar mass of 290.1 g/Mol. Zoledronic acid monohydrate is highly soluble in 0.1N sodium hydroxide solution, sparingly soluble in water and 0.1N hydrochloric acid, and practically insoluble in organic solvents. The pH of the Reclast solution for infusion is approximately 6.0 – 7.0.

Reclast Injection is available as a sterile solution in bottles for intravenous infusion. One bottle with 100 mL solution contains 5.330 mg of zoledronic acid monohydrate, equivalent to 5 mg zoledronic acid on an anhydrous basis.

Inactive Ingredients: 4950 mg of mannitol, USP; and 30 mg of sodium citrate, USP.

12 CLINICAL PHARMACOLOGY

12.1 Mechanism of Action

Reclast is a bisphosphonate and acts primarily on bone. It is an inhibitor of osteoclast-mediated bone resorption.

The selective action of bisphosphonates on bone is based on their high affinity for mineralized bone. Intravenously administered zoledronic acid rapidly partitions to bone and localizes preferentially at sites of high bone turnover. The main molecular target of zoledronic acid in the osteoclast is the enzyme farnesyl pyrophosphate synthase. The relatively long duration of action of zoledronic acid is attributable to its high binding affinity to bone mineral.

12.2 Pharmacodynamics

In the osteoporosis treatment trial, the effect of Reclast treatment on markers of bone resorption (serum beta-C-telopeptides [b-CTx]) and bone formation (bone specific alkaline phosphatase [BSAP], serum N-terminal propeptide of type I collagen [P1NP]) was evaluated in patients (subsets ranging from 517 to 1246 patients) at periodic intervals. Treatment with a 5 mg annual dose of Reclast reduces bone turnover markers to the pre-menopausal range with an approximate 55% reduction in b-CTx, a 29% reduction in BSAP and a 52% reduction in P1NP over 36 months. There was no progressive reduction of bone turnover markers with repeated annual dosing.

12.3 Pharmacokinetics

Pharmacokinetic data in patients with osteoporosis and Paget's disease of bone are not available.

Distribution: Single or multiple (q 28 days) 5-minute or 15-minute infusions of 2, 4, 8 or 16 mg zoledronic acid were given to 64 patients with cancer and bone metastases. The post-infusion decline of zoledronic acid concentrations in plasma was consistent with a triphasic process showing a rapid decrease from peak concentrations at end-of-infusion to less than 1% of C_{max} 24 hours post infusion with population half-lives of $t_{1/2\alpha}$ 0.24 hour and $t_{1/2\beta}$ 1.87 hours for the early disposition phases of the drug. The terminal elimination phase of zoledronic acid was prolonged, with very low concentrations in plasma between Days 2 and 28 post infusion, and a terminal elimination half-life $t_{1/2\gamma}$ of 146 hours. The area under the plasma concentration versus time curve ($AUC_{0\text{-}24h}$) of zoledronic acid was dose proportional from 2 to 16 mg. The accumulation of zoledronic acid measured over three cycles was low, with mean $AUC_{0\text{-}24h}$ ratios for cycles 2 and 3 versus 1 of 1.13 ± 0.30 and 1.16 ± 0.36, respectively. *In vitro* and *ex vivo* studies showed low affinity of zoledronic acid for the cellular components of human blood. *In vitro* mean zoledronic acid protein binding in human plasma ranged from 28% at 200 ng/mL to 53% at 50 ng/mL.

Metabolism: Zoledronic acid does not inhibit human P450 enzymes *in vitro*. Zoledronic acid does not undergo biotransformation *in vivo*. In animal studies, less than 3% of the administered intravenous dose was found in the feces, with the balance either recovered in the urine or taken up by bone, indicating that the drug is eliminated intact via the kidney. Following an intravenous dose of 20 nCi ^{14}C-zoledronic acid in a patient with cancer and bone metastases, only a single radioactive species with chromatographic properties identical to those of parent drug was recovered in urine, which suggests that zoledronic acid is not metabolized.

Excretion: In 64 patients with cancer and bone metastases on average (± SD) 39 ± 16% of the administered zoledronic acid dose was recovered in the urine within 24 hours, with only trace amounts of drug found in urine post Day 2. The cumulative percent of drug excreted in the urine over 0-24 hours was independent of dose. The balance of drug not recovered in urine over 0-24 hours, representing drug presumably bound to bone, is slowly released back into the systemic circulation, giving rise to the observed prolonged low plasma concentrations. The 0-24 hour renal clearance of zoledronic acid was 3.7 ± 2.0 L/h.

Zoledronic acid clearance was independent of dose but dependent upon the patient's creatinine clearance. In a study in patients with cancer and bone metastases, increasing the infusion time of a 4 mg dose of zoledronic acid from 5 minutes (n=5) to 15 minutes (n=7) resulted in a 34% decrease in the zoledronic acid concentration at the end of the infusion ([mean ± SD] 403 ± 118 ng/mL vs. 264 ± 86 ng/mL) and a 10% increase in the total AUC (378 ± 116 ng × h/mL vs. 420 ± 218 ng × h/mL). The difference between the AUC means was not statistically significant.

Specific Populations

Pediatrics: Reclast is not indicated for use in children [*see Pediatric Use (8.4)*].

Geriatrics: The pharmacokinetics of zoledronic acid was not affected by age in patients with cancer and bone metastases whose age ranged from 38 years to 84 years.

Race: The pharmacokinetics of zoledronic acid was not affected by race in patients with cancer and bone metastases.

Hepatic Impairment: No clinical studies were conducted to evaluate the effect of hepatic impairment on the pharmacokinetics of zoledronic acid.

Renal Impairment: The pharmacokinetic studies conducted in 64 cancer patients represented typical clinical populations with normal to moderately-impaired renal function. Compared to patients with creatinine clearance greater than 80 mL/min (N=37), patients with creatinine clearance = 50-80 mL/min (N=15) showed an average increase in plasma AUC of 15%, whereas patients with creatinine clearance = 30-50 mL/min (N=11) showed an average increase in plasma AUC of 43%. No dosage adjustment is required in patients with a creatinine clearance of greater than or equal to 35 mL/min. Reclast is contraindicated in patients with creatinine clearance less than 35 mL/min and in those with evidence of acute renal impairment due to an increased risk of renal failure [*see Contraindications (4), Warnings and Precautions (5.3), Use in Specific Populations (8.6)*].

13 NONCLINICAL TOXICOLOGY

13.1 Carcinogenesis, Mutagenesis, Impairment of Fertility

Carcinogenesis: Standard lifetime carcinogenicity bioassays were conducted in mice and rats. Mice were given daily oral doses of zoledronic acid of 0.1, 0.5, or 2.0 mg/kg/day. There was an increased incidence of Harderian gland adenomas in males and females in all treatment groups (at doses greater than or equal to 0.002 times the human intravenous dose of 5 mg, based on a mg/m^2 comparison). Rats were given daily oral doses of zoledronic acid of 0.1, 0.5, or 2.0 mg/kg/day. No increased incidence of tumors was observed (at doses less than or equal to 0.1 times the human intravenous dose of 5 mg, based on a mg/m^2 comparison).

Mutagenesis: Zoledronic acid was not genotoxic in the Ames bacterial mutagenicity assay, in the Chinese hamster ovary cell assay, or in the Chinese hamster gene mutation assay, with or without metabolic activation. Zoledronic acid was not genotoxic in the *in vivo* rat micronucleus assay.

Impairment of Fertility: Female rats were given daily subcutaneous doses of zoledronic acid of 0.01, 0.03, or 0.1 mg/kg beginning 15 days before mating and continuing through gestation. Effects observed in the high-dose group (equivalent to human systemic exposure following a 5 mg intravenous dose, based on an AUC comparison) included inhibition of ovulation and a decrease in the number of pregnant rats. Effects observed in both the mid-dose group and high-dose group (0.3 to 1 times human systemic exposure following a 5 mg intravenous dose, based on an AUC comparison) included an increase in pre-implantation losses and a decrease in the number of implantations and live fetuses.

13.2 Animal Pharmacology

Bone Safety Studies: Zoledronic acid is a potent inhibitor of osteoclastic bone resorption. In the ovariectomized rat, single IV doses of zoledronic acid of 4-500 μg/kg (less than 0.1 to 3.5 times human exposure at the 5 mg intravenous dose, based on a mg/m^2 comparison) suppressed bone turnover and protected against trabecular bone loss, cortical thinning and the reduction in vertebral and femoral bone strength in a dose-dependent manner. At a dose equivalent to human exposure at the 5 mg intravenous dose, the effect persisted for 8 months, which corresponds to approximately 8 remodeling cycles or 3 years in humans.

In ovariectomized rats and monkeys, weekly treatment with zoledronic acid dose-dependently suppressed bone turnover and prevented the decrease in cancellous and cortical BMD and bone strength, at yearly cumulative doses up to 3.5 times the intravenous human dose of 5 mg, based on a mg/m^2 comparison. Bone tissue was normal and there was no evidence of a mineralization defect, no accumulation of osteoid, and no woven bone.

13.3 Reproductive and Developmental Toxicology

In female rats given subcutaneous doses of zoledronic acid of 0.01, 0.03, or 0.1 mg/kg/day beginning 15 days before mating and continuing through gestation, the number of stillbirths was increased and survival of neonates was decreased in the mid- and high-dose groups (greater than or equal to 0.3 times the anticipated human systemic exposure following a 5 mg intravenous dose, based on an AUC comparison). Adverse maternal effects were observed in all dose groups (greater than or equal to 0.1 times the human systemic exposure following a 5 mg intravenous dose, based on an AUC comparison) and included dystocia and periparturient mortality in pregnant rats allowed to deliver. Maternal mortality was considered related to drug-induced inhibition of skeletal calcium mobilization, resulting in periparturient hypocalcemia. This appears to be a bisphosphonate class effect.

In pregnant rats given daily subcutaneous dose of zoledronic acid of 0.1, 0.2, or 0.4 mg/kg during gestation, adverse fetal effects were observed in the mid- and high-dose groups (about 2 and 4 times human systemic exposure following a 5 mg intravenous dose, based on an AUC comparison). These adverse effects included increases in pre- and post-implantation losses, decreases in viable fetuses, and fetal skeletal, visceral, and external malformations. Fetal skeletal effects observed in the high-dose group included unossified or incompletely ossified bones, thickened, curved or shortened bones, wavy ribs, and shortened jaw. Other adverse fetal effects observed in the high-dose group included reduced lens, rudimentary cerebellum, reduction or absence of liver lobes, reduction of lung lobes, vessel dilation, cleft palate, and edema. Skeletal variations were also observed in the low-dose group (about 1.2 times the anticipated human systemic exposure, based on an AUC comparison). Signs of maternal toxicity were observed in the high-dose group and included reduced body weights and food consumption, indicating that maximal exposure levels were achieved in this study.

In pregnant rabbits given subcutaneous doses of zoledronic acid of 0.01, 0.03, or 0.1 mg/kg/day during gestation (at doses less than or equal to 0.4 times the anticipated human systemic exposure following a 5 mg intravenous dose, based on a mg/m^2 comparison) no adverse fetal effects were observed. Maternal mortality and abortion occurred in all treatment groups (at doses greater than or equal to 0.04 times the human 5 mg intravenous dose, based on a mg/m^2 comparison). Adverse maternal effects were associated with, and may have been caused by, drug-induced hypocalcemia.

14 CLINICAL STUDIES

14.1 Treatment of Postmenopausal Osteoporosis

Study 1: The efficacy and safety of Reclast in the treatment of postmenopausal osteoporosis was demonstrated in Study 1, a randomized, double-blind, placebo-controlled, multinational study of 7736 women aged 65-89 years (mean age of 73) with either: a femoral neck BMD T-score less than or equal to -1.5 and at least two mild or one moderate existing vertebral fracture(s); or a femoral neck BMD T-score less than or equal to -2.5 with or without evidence of an existing vertebral fracture(s). Women were stratified into two groups: Stratum I: no concomitant use of osteoporosis therapy or Stratum II: baseline concomitant use of osteoporosis therapies which included calcitonin, raloxifene, tamoxifen, and hormone replacement therapy, but excluded other bisphosphonates.

Women enrolled in Stratum I (n=5661) were evaluated annually for incidence of vertebral fractures. All women

(Strata I and II) were evaluated for the incidence of hip and other clinical fractures. Reclast was administered once a year for three consecutive years, as a single 5 mg dose in 100 mL solution infused over at least 15 minutes, for a total of three doses. All women received 1000 to 1500 mg of elemental calcium plus 400 to 1200 international units of vitamin D supplementation per day.

The two primary efficacy variables were the incidence of morphometric vertebral fractures at 3 years and the incidence of hip fractures over a median duration of 3 years. The diagnosis of an incident vertebral fracture was based on both qualitative diagnosis by the radiologist and quantitative morphometric criterion. The morphometric criterion required the dual occurrence of 2 events: a relative height ratio or relative height reduction in a vertebral body of at least 20%, together with at least a 4 mm absolute decrease in height.

Effect on Vertebral Fractures

Reclast significantly decreased the incidence of new vertebral fractures at one, two, and three years as shown in Table 5.

[See table 5 above]

The reductions in vertebral fractures over three years were consistent (including new/worsening and multiple vertebral fractures) and significantly greater than placebo regardless of age, geographical region, baseline body mass index, number of baseline vertebral fractures, femoral neck BMD T-score, or prior bisphosphonate usage.

Effect on Hip Fracture over 3 years

Reclast demonstrated a 1.1% absolute reduction and 41% relative reduction in the risk of hip fractures over a median duration of follow-up of 3 years. The hip fracture event rate was 1.4% for Reclast-treated patients compared to 2.5% for placebo-treated patients.

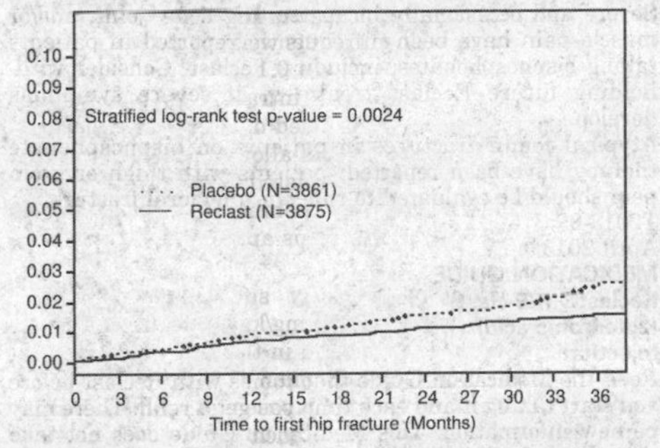

Figure 1. Cumulative Incidence of Hip Fracture Over 3 Years

The reductions in hip fractures over three years were greater for Reclast than placebo regardless of femoral neck BMD T-score.

Effect on All Clinical Fractures

Reclast demonstrated superiority to placebo in reducing the incidence of all clinical fractures, clinical (symptomatic) vertebral and non-vertebral fractures (excluding finger, toe, facial, and clinical thoracic and lumbar vertebral fractures). All clinical fractures were verified based on the radiographic and/or clinical evidence. A summary of results is presented in Table 6.

[See table 6 above]

Effect on Bone Mineral Density (BMD)

Reclast significantly increased BMD at the lumbar spine, total hip and femoral neck, relative to treatment with placebo at time points 12, 24, and 36 months. Treatment with Reclast resulted in a 6.7% increase in BMD at the lumbar spine, 6.0% at the total hip, and 5.1% at the femoral neck, over 3 years as compared to placebo.

Bone Histology

Bone biopsy specimens were obtained between Months 33 and 36 from 82 postmenopausal patients with osteoporosis treated with 3 annual doses of Reclast. Of the biopsies obtained, 81 were adequate for qualitative histomorphometry assessment, 59 were adequate for partial quantitative histomorphometry assessment, and 38 were adequate for full quantitative histomorphometry assessment. Micro CT analysis was performed on 76 specimens. Qualitative, quantitative and micro CT assessments showed bone of normal architecture and quality without mineralization defects.

Effect on Height

In the 3-year osteoporosis study, standing height was measured annually using a stadiometer. The Reclast group revealed less height loss compared to placebo (4.2 mm vs. 7.0 mm, respectively [p<0.001]).

Study 2: The efficacy and safety of Reclast in the treatment of patients with osteoporosis who suffered a recent low-trauma hip fracture was demonstrated in Study 2, a randomized, double-blind, placebo-controlled, multinational endpoint study of 2127 men and women aged 50-95 years (mean age of 74.5). Concomitant osteoporosis therapies excluding other bisphosphonates and parathyroid hormone were allowed. Reclast was administered once a year as a single 5 mg dose in 100 mL solution, infused over at least 15 minutes. The study continued until at least 211 patients had confirmed clinical fractures in the study population. Vitamin D levels were not routinely measured but a loading dose of vitamin D (50,000 to 125,000 international units orally or IM) was given to patients and they were started on 1000 to 1500 mg of elemental calcium plus 800 to 1200 international units of vitamin D supplementation per day for at least 14 days prior to the study drug infusions. The primary efficacy variable was the incidence of clinical fractures over the duration of the study.

Reclast significantly reduced the incidence of any clinical fracture by 35%. There was also a 46% reduction in the risk of a clinical vertebral fracture (Table 7).

[See table 7 above]

Effect on Bone Mineral Density (BMD)

Reclast significantly increased BMD relative to placebo at the hip and femoral neck at all timepoints (12, 24, and 36 months). Treatment with Reclast resulted in a 6.4% increase in BMD at the total hip and a 4.3% increase at the femoral neck over 36 months as compared to placebo.

14.2 Prevention of Postmenopausal Osteoporosis

The efficacy and safety of Reclast in postmenopausal women with osteopenia (low bone mass) was assessed in a 2-year randomized, multi-center, double-blind, placebo-controlled study of 581 postmenopausal women aged greater than or equal to 45 years, who were stratified by years since menopause: Stratum I women less than 5 years from menopause (n=224); Stratum II women greater than or equal to 5 years from menopause (n=357). Patients within Stratum I and II were randomized to one of three treatment groups: (1) Reclast given at randomization and at Month 12 (n=77) in Stratum I and (n=121) in Stratum II; (2) Reclast given at randomization and placebo at Month 12 (n=70) in Stratum I and (n=111) in Stratum II; and (3) Placebo given at randomization and Month 12 (n=202). Reclast was administered as a single 5 mg dose in 100 mL solution infused over at least 15 minutes. All women received 500 to 1200 mg elemental calcium plus 400 to 800 international units vitamin D supplementation per day. The primary efficacy variable was the percent change of BMD at 24 Months relative to baseline.

Effect on Bone Mineral Density (BMD)

Reclast significantly increased lumbar spine BMD relative to placebo at Month 24 across both strata. Reclast given once at randomization (and placebo given at Month 12) resulted in 4.0% increase in BMD in Stratum I patients and 4.8% increase in Stratum II patients over 24 months. Placebo given at randomization and at Month 12 resulted in 2.2% decrease in BMD in Stratum I patients and 0.7% decrease in BMD in Stratum II patients over 24 months. Therefore, Reclast given once at randomization (and placebo given at Month 12) resulted in a 6.3% increase in BMD in Stratum I patients and 5.4% increase in Stratum II patients over 24 months as compared to placebo (both p<0.0001).

Reclast also significantly increased total hip BMD relative to placebo at Month 24 across both strata. Reclast given once at randomization (and placebo given at Month 12) resulted in 2.6% increase in BMD in Stratum I patients and 2.1% in Stratum II patients over 24 months. Placebo given at randomization and at Month 12 resulted in 2.1% decrease in BMD in Stratum I patients and 1.0% decrease in BMD in Stratum II patients over 24 months. Therefore, Reclast given once at randomization (and placebo given at Month 12) resulted in a 4.7% increase in BMD in Stratum I patients and 3.2% increase in Stratum II patients over 24 months as compared to placebo (both p<0.0001).

14.3 Osteoporosis in Men

The efficacy and safety of Reclast in men with osteoporosis or significant osteoporosis secondary to hypogonadism, was

Table 5. Proportion of Patients with New Morphometric Vertebral Fractures

Outcome	Reclast (%)	Placebo (%)	Absolute Reduction in Fracture Incidence % (95% CI)	Relative Reduction in Fracture Incidence % (95% CI)
At least one new vertebral fracture (0–1 year)	1.5	3.7	2.2 (1.4, 3.1)	60 (43, 72)*
At least one new vertebral fracture (0–2 years)	2.2	7.7	5.5 (4.4, 6.6)	71 (62, 78)*
At least one new vertebral fracture (0–3 years)	3.3	10.9	7.6 (6.3, 9.0)	70 (62, 76)*

* p <0.0001

Table 6. Between–Treatment Comparisons of the Incidence of Clinical Fracture Variables Over 3 Years

Outcome	Reclast (N= 3875) Event Rate n (%)+	Placebo (N= 3861) Event Rate n (%)+	Absolute Reduction in Fracture Incidence % (95% CI)+	Relative Risk Reduction in Fracture Incidence % (95% CI)
Any clinical fracture (1)	308 (8.4)	456 (12.8)	4.4 (3.0, 5.8)	33 (23, 42)**
Clinical vertebral fracture (2)	19 (0.5)	84 (2.6)	2.1 (1.5, 2.7)	77 (63, 86)**
Non-vertebral fracture (3)	292 (8.0)	388 (10.7)	2.7 (1.4, 4.0)	25 (13, 36)*

*p-value < 0.001, **p-value <0.0001

+ Event rates based on Kaplan-Meier estimates at 36 months

(1) Excluding finger, toe, and facial fractures

(2) Includes clinical thoracic and clinical lumbar vertebral fractures

(3) Excluding finger, toe, facial, and clinical thoracic and lumbar vertebral fractures

Table 7. Between-Treatment Comparisons of the Incidence of Key Clinical Fracture Variables

Outcome	Reclast (N=1065) Event Rate n (%)+	Placebo (N=1062) Event Rate n (%)+	Absolute Reduction in Fracture Incidence % (95% CI) +	Relative Risk Reduction in Fracture Incidence % (95% CI)
Any clinical fracture (1)	92 (8.6)	139 (13.9)	5.3 (2.3, 8.3)	35 (16, 50)**
Clinical vertebral fracture (2)	21 (1.7)	39 (3.8)	2.1 (0.5, 3.7)	46 (8, 68)*

*p-value <0.05, **p-value <0.005

+ Event rates based on Kaplan-Meier estimates at 24 months

(1)Excluding finger, toe and facial fractures

(2)Including clinical thoracic and clinical lumbar vertebral fractures

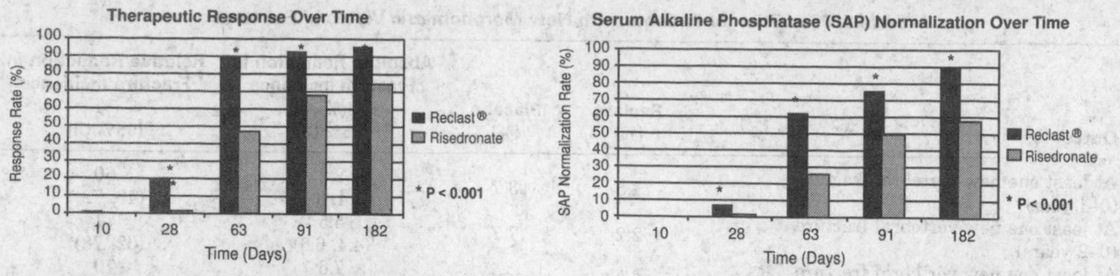

Figure 2. Therapeutic Response/Serum Alkaline Phosphatase (SAP) Normalization Over Time

assessed in a randomized, multicenter, double-blind, active controlled, study of 302 men aged 25-86 years (mean age of 64). The duration of the trial was two years. Patients were randomized to either Reclast which was administered once annually as a 5 mg dose in 100 mL infused over 15 minutes for a total of up to two doses, or to an oral weekly bisphosphonate (active control) for up to two years. All participants received 1000 mg of elemental calcium plus 800 to 1000 international units of vitamin D supplementation per day.

Effect on Bone Mineral Density (BMD)

An annual infusion of Reclast was non-inferior to the oral weekly bisphosphonate active control based on the percentage change in lumbar spine BMD at Month 24 relative to baseline (Reclast: 6.1% increase; active control: 6.2% increase).

14.4 Treatment and Prevention of Glucocorticoid-Induced Osteoporosis

The efficacy and safety of Reclast to prevent and treat glucocorticoid-induced osteoporosis (GIO) was assessed in a randomized, multicenter, double-blind, stratified, active controlled study of 833 men and women aged 18-85 years (mean age of 54.4 years) treated with greater than or equal to 7.5 mg/day oral prednisone (or equivalent). Patients were stratified according to the duration of their pre-study corticosteroid therapy: less than or equal to 3 months prior to randomization (prevention subpopulation), and greater than 3 months prior to randomization (treatment subpopulation). The duration of the trial was one year. Patients were randomized to either Reclast which was administered once as a 5 mg dose in 100 mL infused over 15 minutes, or to an oral daily bisphosphonate (active control) for one year. All participants received 1000 mg of elemental calcium plus 400 to 1000 international units of vitamin D supplementation per day.

Effect on Bone Mineral Density (BMD)

In the GIO treatment subpopulation, Reclast demonstrated a significant mean increase in lumbar spine BMD compared to the active control at one year (Reclast 4.1%, active control 2.7%) with a treatment difference of 1.4% (p<0.001). In the GIO prevention subpopulation, Reclast demonstrated a significant mean increase in lumbar spine BMD compared to active control at one year (Reclast 2.6%, active control 0.6%) with a treatment difference of 2.0% (p<0.001).

Bone Histology

Bone biopsy specimens were obtained from 23 patients (12 in the Reclast treatment group and 11 in the active control treatment group) at Month 12 treated with an annual dose of Reclast or daily oral active control. Qualitative assessments showed bone of normal architecture and quality without mineralization defects. Apparent reductions in activation frequency and remodeling rates were seen when compared with the histomorphometry results seen with Reclast in the postmenopausal osteoporosis population. The long-term consequences of this degree of suppression of bone remodeling in glucocorticoid-treated patients is unknown.

14.5 Treatment of Paget's Disease of Bone

Reclast was studied in male and female patients with moderate to severe Paget's disease of bone, defined as serum alkaline phosphatase level at least twice the upper limit of the age-specific normal reference range at the time of study entry. Diagnosis was confirmed by radiographic evidence.

The efficacy of one infusion of 5 mg Reclast vs. oral daily doses of 30 mg risedronate for 2 months was demonstrated in two identically designed 6-month randomized, double blind trials. The mean age of patients in the two trials was 70. Ninety-three percent (93%) of patients were Caucasian. Therapeutic response was defined as either normalization of serum alkaline phosphatase (SAP) or a reduction of at least 75% from baseline in total SAP excess at the end of 6 months. SAP excess was defined as the difference between the measured level and midpoint of normal range.

In both trials Reclast demonstrated a superior and more rapid therapeutic response compared with risedronate and returned more patients to normal levels of bone turnover, as evidenced by biochemical markers of formation (SAP, serum N-terminal propeptide of type I collagen [P1NP]) and resorption (serum CTx 1 [cross-linked C-telopeptides of type I collagen] and urine α-CTx).

The 6-month combined data from both trials showed that 96% (169/176) of Reclast-treated patients achieved a therapeutic response as compared with 74% (127/171) of patients treated with risedronate. Most Reclast patients achieved a therapeutic response by the Day 63 visit. In addition, at 6 months, 89% (156/176) of Reclast-treated patients achieved normalization of SAP levels, compared to 58% (99/171) of patients treated with risedronate (p<0.0001) (see Figure 2). [See figure 2 above]

The therapeutic response to Reclast was similar across demographic and disease-severity groups defined by gender, age, previous bisphosphonate use, and disease severity. At 6 months, the percentage of Reclast-treated patients who achieved therapeutic response was 97% and 95%, respectively, in each of the baseline disease severity subgroups (baseline SAP less than 3xULN, greater than or equal to 3xULN) compared to 75% and 74%, respectively, for the same disease severity subgroups of risedronate-treated patients.

In patients who had previously received treatment with oral bisphosphonates, therapeutic response rates were 96% and 55% for Reclast and risedronate, respectively. The comparatively low risedronate response was due to the low response rate (7/23, 30%) in patients previously treated with risedronate. In patients naïve to previous treatment, a greater therapeutic response was also observed with Reclast (98%) relative to risedronate (86%). In patients with symptomatic pain at screening, therapeutic response rates were 94% and 70% for Reclast and risedronate respectively. For patients without pain at screening, therapeutic response rates were 100% and 82% for Reclast and risedronate respectively.

Bone histology was evaluated in 7 patients with Paget's disease 6 months after being treated with Reclast 5 mg. Bone biopsy results showed bone of normal quality with no evidence of impaired bone remodeling and no evidence of mineralization defect.

16 HOW SUPPLIED/STORAGE AND HANDLING

Each bottle contains 5 mg/100 mL. NDC 0078-0435-61

Handling

After opening the solution, it is stable for 24 hours at 2°C–8°C (36°F-46°F).

If refrigerated, allow the refrigerated solution to reach room temperature before administration.

Storage

Store at 25°C (77°F); excursions permitted to 15°C-30°C (59°F-86°F) [see USP Controlled Room Temperature].

17 PATIENT COUNSELING INFORMATION

See FDA-Approved Medication Guide

Information for Patients

Patients should be made aware that Reclast contains the same active ingredient (zoledronic acid) found in Zometa®, and that patients being treated with Zometa should not be treated with Reclast.

Reclast is contraindicated in patients with creatinine clearance less than 35 mL/min [*see Contraindications (4)*].

Before being given Reclast, patients should tell their doctor if they have kidney problems and what medications they are taking.

Reclast should not be given if the patient is pregnant or plans to become pregnant, or if she is breast-feeding [*see Warnings and Precautions (5.6)*].

There have been reports of bronchoconstriction in aspirin-sensitive patients receiving bisphosphonates, including Reclast. Before being given Reclast, patients should tell their doctor if they are aspirin-sensitive.

If the patient had surgery to remove some or all of the parathyroid glands in their neck, or had sections of their intestine removed, or are unable to take calcium supplements they should tell their doctor.

Reclast is given as an infusion into a vein by a nurse or a doctor, and the infusion time must not be less than 15 minutes.

On the day of treatment the patient should eat and drink normally, which includes drinking at least 2 glasses of fluid such as water within a few hours prior to the infusion, as directed by their doctor, before receiving Reclast.

After getting Reclast it is strongly recommended patients with Paget's disease take calcium in divided doses (for example, 2 to 4 times a day) for a total of 1500 mg calcium a day to prevent low blood calcium levels. This is especially important for the two weeks after getting Reclast [*see Warnings and Precautions (5.2)*].

Adequate calcium and vitamin D intake is important in patients with osteoporosis and the current recommended daily intake of calcium is 1200 mg and vitamin D is 800 international units – 1000 international units daily. All patients should be instructed on the importance of calcium and vitamin D supplementation in maintaining serum calcium levels.

Patients should be aware of the most commonly associated side effects of therapy. Patients may experience one or more side effects that could include: fever, flu-like symptoms, myalgia, arthralgia, and headache. Most of these side effects occur within the first 3 days following the dose of Reclast. They usually resolve within 3 days of onset but may last for up to 7 to 14 days. Patients should consult their physician if they have questions or if these symptoms persist. The incidence of these symptoms decreased markedly with subsequent doses of Reclast.

Administration of acetaminophen following Reclast administration may reduce the incidence of these symptoms.

Physicians should inform their patients that there have been reports of persistent pain and/or a non-healing sore of the mouth or jaw, primarily in patients treated with bisphosphonates for other illnesses. If they experience these symptoms, they should inform their physician or dentist.

Severe and occasionally incapacitating bone, joint, and/or muscle pain have been infrequently reported in patients taking bisphosphonates, including Reclast. Consider withholding future Reclast treatment if severe symptoms develop.

Atypical femur fractures in patients on bisphosphonate therapy have been reported; patients with thigh or groin pain should be evaluated to rule out a femoral fracture.

T2013-39
April 2013

MEDICATION GUIDE
Reclast® (RE-clast)
(zoledronic acid)
Injection

Read the Medication Guide that comes with Reclast before you start taking it and each time you get a refill. There may be new information. This Medication Guide does not take the place of talking with your doctor about your medical condition or treatment. Talk to your doctor if you have any questions about Reclast.

What is the most important information I should know about Reclast?

You should not receive Reclast if you are already receiving Zometa. Both Reclast and Zometa contain zoledronic acid.

Reclast can cause serious side effects including:

1. Low calcium levels in your blood (hypocalcemia)
2. Severe kidney problems
3. Severe jaw bone problems (osteonecrosis)
4. Bone, joint or muscle pain
5. Unusual thigh bone fractures

1. **Low calcium levels in your blood (hypocalcemia).**

Reclast may lower the calcium levels in your blood. If you have low blood calcium before you start taking Reclast, it may get worse during treatment. Your low blood calcium must be treated before you take Reclast. Most people with low blood calcium levels do not have symptoms, but some people may have symptoms. Call your doctor right away if you have symptoms of low blood calcium such as:

- Spasms, twitches, or cramps in your muscles
- Numbness or tingling in your fingers, toes, or around your mouth

Your doctor may prescribe calcium and vitamin D to help prevent low calcium levels in your blood, while you take Reclast. Take calcium and vitamin D as your doctor tells you to.

2. **Severe kidney problems.**

Severe kidney problems may happen when you take Reclast. Severe kidney problems may lead to hospitalization or kidney dialysis and can be life-threatening. Your risk of kidney problems is higher if you:

- already have kidney problems
- take a diuretic or "water pill"
- do not have enough water in your body (dehydrated) before or after you receive Reclast
- are of advanced age since the risk increases as you get older
- take any medicines known to harm your kidneys

You should drink at least 2 glasses of fluid within a few hours before receiving Reclast to reduce the risk of kidney problems.

3. **Severe jaw bone problems (osteonecrosis).**

Severe jaw bone problems may happen when you take Reclast. Your doctor should examine your mouth before you start Reclast. Your doctor may tell you to see your dentist before you start Reclast. It is important for you to practice good mouth care during treatment with Reclast.

4. **Unusual thigh bone fractures.**

Some people have developed unusual fractures in their thigh bone. Symptoms of a fracture may include new or unusual pain in your hip, groin, or thigh.

5. **Possible harm to your unborn baby.**

Reclast should not be used if you are pregnant. Tell your doctor right away if you are pregnant or plan to become pregnant. Reclast may harm your unborn baby.

6. **Bone, joint, or muscle pain.**

Some people who take bisphosphonates develop severe bone, joint, or muscle pain.

Call your doctor right away if you have any of these side effects.

What is Reclast?

Reclast is a prescription medicine used to:

- Treat or prevent osteoporosis in women after menopause. Reclast helps reduce the chance of having a hip or spinal fracture (break).
- Increase bone mass in men with osteoporosis.
- Treat or prevent osteoporosis in either men or women who will be taking corticosteroid medicines for at least one year.
- Treat certain men and women who have Paget's disease of the bone.

It is not known how long Reclast works for the treatment and prevention of osteoporosis. You should see your doctor regularly to determine if Reclast is still right for you.

Reclast is not for use in children.

Who should not take Reclast?

Do not take Reclast if you:

- Have low levels of calcium in your blood
- Have kidney problems
- Are allergic to zoledronic acid or any of its ingredients. A list of ingredients is at the end of this leaflet.

What should I tell my doctor before taking Reclast?

Before you start Reclast, be sure to talk to your doctor if you:

- Have low blood calcium.
- Have kidney problems.
- Had parathyroid or thyroid surgery (glands in your neck).
- Have been told you have trouble absorbing minerals in your stomach or intestines (malabsorption syndrome) or have had parts of your intestine removed.
- Have asthma (wheezing) from taking aspirin.
- Plan to have dental surgery or teeth removed.
- Are pregnant, or plan to become pregnant. Reclast may harm your unborn baby. **Reclast should not be used if you are pregnant.**
- Are breastfeeding or plan to breastfeed. It is not known if Reclast passes into your milk and may harm your baby.

Tell your doctor about all the medicines you take, including prescription and non-prescription medicines, vitamins, and herbal supplements. Certain medicines may affect how Reclast works.

Especially tell your doctor if you are taking:

- An antibiotic. Certain antibiotic medicines called aminoglycosides may increase the effect of Reclast in lowering your blood calcium for a long period of time.
- A diuretic or "water pill".
- Non-steroidal anti-inflammatory medicines (NSAIDS).

Ask your doctor or pharmacist for a list of these medicines, if you are not sure.

Know the medicines you take. Keep a list of them and show it to your doctor and pharmacist each time you get a new medicine.

How will I receive Reclast?

- Your doctor will tell you how often you will receive Reclast.
- Reclast is given by infusion into your vein (intravenously). Your infusion should last at least 15 minutes.
- Before you receive Reclast, drink at least 2 glasses of fluid (such as water) within a few hours as directed by your doctor.
- You may eat before your treatment with Reclast.
- If you miss a dose of Reclast, call your doctor or healthcare provider to schedule your next dose.

What are the possible side effects of Reclast?

Reclast may cause serious side effects.

- See **"What is the most important information I should know about Reclast?"**

The most common side effects of Reclast included:

- Fever
- Pain in your bones, joints or muscles
- Pain in your arms and legs
- Headache
- Flu-like illness (fever, chills, bone, joint, or muscle pain, fatigue)
- Nausea
- Vomiting
- Diarrhea

Talk to your doctor about things you can do to help decrease some of these side effects that might happen with a Reclast infusion.

You may get allergic reactions, such as hives, swelling of your face, lips, tongue, or throat.

Tell your doctor if you have any side effect that bothers you or that does not go away.

These are not all the possible side effects of Reclast. For more information, ask your doctor or pharmacist.

Call your doctor for medical advice about side effects. You may report side effects to FDA at 1-800-FDA-1088.

General information about safe and effective use of Reclast.

Medicines are sometimes prescribed for purposes other than those listed in a Medication Guide.

This Medication Guide summarizes the most important information about Reclast. If you would like more information, talk with your doctor. You can ask your doctor or pharmacist for information about Reclast that is written for health professionals.

For more information, go to: www.RECLAST.com or call 1-866-732-5278.

What are the ingredients in Reclast?

Active ingredient: zoledronic acid monohydrate.

Inactive ingredients: mannitol and sodium citrate.

Distributed by:
Novartis Pharmaceuticals Corporation
East Hanover, New Jersey 07936

This Medication Guide has been approved by the U.S. Food and Drug Administration.

T2013-40
April 2013

Shown in Product Identification Guide, page 310

SANDIMMUNE® ℞
(cyclosporine capsules, USP)
Soft Gelatin Capsules

SANDIMMUNE®
(cyclosporine oral solution, USP)
Oral Solution

SANDIMMUNE®
(cyclosporine injection, USP)
Injection
FOR INFUSION ONLY
Rx only
Prescribing Information

The following prescribing information is based on official labeling in effect July 2013.

WARNING

Only physicians experienced in immunosuppressive therapy and management of organ transplant patients should prescribe Sandimmune® (cyclosporine). Patients receiving the drug should be managed in facilities equipped and staffed with adequate laboratory and supportive medical resources. The physician responsible for maintenance therapy should have complete information requisite for the follow-up of the patient.

Sandimmune® (cyclosporine) should be administered with adrenal corticosteroids but not with other immunosuppressive agents. Increased susceptibility to infection and the possible development of lymphoma may result from immunosuppression.

Sandimmune® Soft Gelatin Capsules (cyclosporine capsules, USP) and Sandimmune® Oral Solution (cyclosporine oral solution, USP) have decreased bioavailability in comparison to Neoral® Soft Gelatin Capsules (cyclosporine capsules, USP) MODIFIED and Neoral® Oral Solution (cyclosporine oral solution, USP) MODIFIED.

Sandimmune® and Neoral® are not bioequivalent and cannot be used interchangeably without physician supervision.

The absorption of cyclosporine during chronic administration of Sandimmune® Soft Gelatin Capsules and Oral Solution was found to be erratic. It is recommended that patients taking the soft gelatin capsules or oral solution over a period of time be monitored at repeated intervals for cyclosporine blood concentrations and subsequent dose adjustments be made in order to avoid toxicity due to high concentrations and possible organ rejection due to low absorption of cyclosporine. This is of special importance in liver transplants. Numerous assays are being developed to measure blood concentrations of cyclosporine. Comparison of concentrations in published literature to patient concentrations using current assays must be done with detailed knowledge of the assay methods employed. (See Blood Concentration Monitoring under DOSAGE AND ADMINISTRATION)

DESCRIPTION

Cyclosporine, the active principle in Sandimmune® (cyclosporine) is a cyclic polypeptide immunosuppressant agent consisting of 11 amino acids. It is produced as a metabolite by the fungus species *Beauveria nivea*.

Chemically, cyclosporine is designated as [*R*-[*R**,*R**-(*E*)]]-cyclic(L-alanyl-D-alanyl-*N*-methyl-L-leucyl-*N*-methyl-L-leucyl-*N*-methyl-L-valyl-3-hydroxy-*N*,4-dimethyl-L-2-amino-6-octenoyl-L-α-amino-butyryl-*N*-methylglycyl-*N*-methyl-L-leucyl-L-valyl-*N*-methyl-L-leucyl).

Sandimmune® Soft Gelatin Capsules (cyclosporine capsules, USP) are available in 25 mg and 100 mg strengths.

Each 25 mg capsule contains:

cyclosporine, USP	25 mg
alcohol, USP dehydrated	max 12.7% by volume

Each 100 mg capsule contains:

cyclosporine, USP	100 mg
alcohol, USP dehydrated	max 12.7% by volume

Inactive Ingredients: corn oil, gelatin, iron oxide red, linoleoyl macrogolglycerides, sorbitol, and titanium dioxide. May also contain glycerol. 100 mg capsules may contain iron oxide yellow.

Sandimmune® Oral Solution (cyclosporine oral solution, USP) is available in 50 mL bottles.

Each mL contains:

cyclosporine, USP	100 mg
alcohol, Ph. Helv.	12.5% by volume

dissolved in an olive oil, Ph. Helv./Labrafil M 1944 CS (polyoxyethylated oleic glycerides) vehicle which must be further diluted with milk, chocolate milk, or orange juice before oral administration.

Sandimmune® Injection (cyclosporine injection, USP) is available in a 5 mL sterile ampul for I.V. administration.

Each mL contains:

cyclosporine, USP	50 mg
*Cremophor® EL (polyoxyethylated castor oil)	650 mg
alcohol, Ph. Helv.	32.9% by volume
nitrogen	qs

which must be diluted further with 0.9% Sodium Chloride Injection or 5% Dextrose Injection before use.

The chemical structure of cyclosporine (also known as cyclosporin A) is

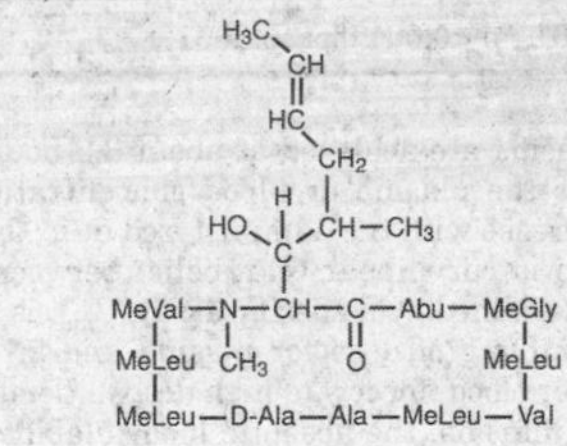

$C_{62}H_{111}N_{11}O_{12}$ Mol. Wt. 1202.63

CLINICAL PHARMACOLOGY

Sandimmune® (cyclosporine) is a potent immunosuppressive agent which in animals prolongs survival of allogeneic transplants involving skin, heart, kidney, pancreas, bone marrow, small intestine, and lung. Sandimmune® (cyclosporine) has been demonstrated to suppress some humoral immunity and to a greater extent, cell-mediated reactions such as allograft rejection, delayed hypersensitivity, experimental allergic encephalomyelitis, Freund's adjuvant arthritis, and graft vs. host disease in many animal species for a variety of organs.

Successful kidney, liver, and heart allogeneic transplants have been performed in man using Sandimmune® (cyclosporine).

The exact mechanism of action of Sandimmune® (cyclosporine) is not known. Experimental evidence suggests that the effectiveness of cyclosporine is due to specific and reversible inhibition of immunocompetent lymphocytes in the G_0- or G_1-phase of the cell cycle. T-lymphocytes are preferentially inhibited. The T-helper cell is the main target, although the T-suppressor cell may also be suppressed. Sandimmune® (cyclosporine) also inhibits lymphokine production and release including interleukin-2 or T-cell growth factor (TCGF).

No functional effects on phagocytic (changes in enzyme secretions not altered, chemotactic migration of granulocytes, macrophage migration, carbon clearance *in vivo*) or tumor cells (growth rate, metastasis) can be detected in animals. Sandimmune® (cyclosporine) does not cause bone marrow suppression in animal models or man.

The absorption of cyclosporine from the gastrointestinal tract is incomplete and variable. Peak concentrations (C_{max})

Nephrotoxicity vs. Rejection

Parameter	Nephrotoxicity	Rejection
History	Donor > 50 years old or hypotensive Prolonged kidney preservation Prolonged anastomosis time Concomitant nephrotoxic drugs	Antidonor immune response Retransplant patient
Clinical	Often > 6 weeks postop[b] Prolonged initial nonfunction (acute tubular necrosis)	Often < 4 weeks postop[b] Fever > 37.5°C Weight gain > 0.5 kg Graft swelling and tenderness Decrease in daily urine volume > 500 mL (or 50%)
Laboratory	CyA serum trough level > 200 ng/mL Gradual rise in Cr (< 0.15 mg/dl/day)[a] Cr plateau < 25% above baseline BUN/Cr ≥ 20	CyA serum trough level < 150 ng/mL Rapid rise in Cr (> 0.3 mg/dl/day)[a] Cr > 25% above baseline BUN/Cr < 20
Biopsy	Arteriolopathy (medial hypertrophy[a], hyalinosis, nodular deposits, intimal thickening, endothelial vacuolization, progressive scarring) Tubular atrophy, isometric vacuolization, isolated calcifications Minimal edema Mild focal infiltrates[c] Diffuse interstitial fibrosis, often striped form	Endovasculitis[c] (proliferation[a], intimal arteritis[b], necrosis, sclerosis) Tubulitis with RBC[b] and WBC[b] casts, some irregular vacuolization Interstitial edema[c] and hemorrhage[b] Diffuse moderate to severe mononuclear infiltrates[d] Glomerulitis (mononuclear cells)[c]
Aspiration Cytology	CyA deposits in tubular and endothelial cells Fine isometric vacuolization of tubular cells	Inflammatory infiltrate with mononuclear phagocytes, macrophages, lymphoblastoid cells, and activated T-cells These strongly express HLA-DR antigens
Urine Cytology	Tubular cells with vacuolization and granularization	Degenerative tubular cells, plasma cells, and lymphocyturia > 20% of sediment
Manometry	Intracapsular pressure < 40 mm Hg[b]	Intracapsular pressure > 40 mm Hg[b]
Ultrasonography	Unchanged graft cross-sectional area	Increase in graft cross-sectional area AP diameter ≥ Transverse diameter
Magnetic Resonance Imagery	Normal appearance	Loss of distinct corticomedullary junction, swelling, image intensity of parachyma approaching that of psoas, loss of hilar fat
Radionuclide Scan	Normal or generally decreased perfusion Decrease in tubular function (^{131} I-hippuran) > decrease in perfusion (^{99m}Tc DTPA)	Patchy arterial flow Decrease in perfusion > decrease in tubular function Increased uptake of Indium 111 labeled platelets or Tc-99m in colloid
Therapy	Responds to decreased Sandimmune® (cyclosporine)	Responds to increased steroids or antilymphocyte globulin

[a]p <0.05, [b]p <0.01, [c]p <0.001, [d]p <0.0001

in blood and plasma are achieved at about 3.5 hours. C_{max} and area under the plasma or blood concentration/time curve (AUC) increase with the administered dose; for blood, the relationship is curvilinear (parabolic) between 0 and 1400 mg. As determined by a specific assay, C_{max} is approximately 1.0 ng/mL/mg of dose for plasma and 2.7-1.4 ng/mL/mg of dose for blood (for low to high doses). Compared to an intravenous infusion, the absolute bioavailability of the oral solution is approximately 30% based upon the results in 2 patients. The bioavailability of Sandimmune® Soft Gelatin Capsules (cyclosporine capsules, USP) is equivalent to Sandimmune® Oral Solution, (cyclosporine oral solution, USP).

Cyclosporine is distributed largely outside the blood volume. In blood, the distribution is concentration dependent. Approximately 33%-47% is in plasma, 4%-9% in lymphocytes, 5%-12% in granulocytes, and 41%-58% in erythrocytes. At high concentrations, the uptake by leukocytes and erythrocytes becomes saturated. In plasma, approximately 90% is bound to proteins, primarily lipoproteins.

The disposition of cyclosporine from blood is biphasic with a terminal half-life of approximately 19 hours (range: 10-27 hours). Elimination is primarily biliary with only 6% of the dose excreted in the urine.

Cyclosporine is extensively metabolized but there is no major metabolic pathway. Only 0.1% of the dose is excreted in the urine as unchanged drug. Of 15 metabolites characterized in human urine, 9 have been assigned structures. The major pathways consist of hydroxylation of the Cγ-carbon of 2 of the leucine residues, Cη-carbon hydroxylation, and cyclic ether formation (with oxidation of the double bond) in the side chain of the amino acid 3-hydroxyl-*N*,4-dimethyl-L-2-amino-6-octenoic acid and *N*-demethylation of *N*-methyl leucine residues. Hydrolysis of the cyclic peptide chain or conjugation of the aforementioned metabolites do not appear to be important biotransformation pathways.

Specific Populations

Renal Impairment

In a study performed in 4 subjects with end-stage renal disease (creatinine clearance <5mL/min), an intravenous infusion of 3.5 mg/kg of cyclosporine over 4 hours administered at the end of a hemodialysis session resulted in a mean volume of distribution (Vdss) of 3.49 L/kg and systemic clearance (CL) of 0.369 L/hr/kg. This systemic CL (0.369 L/hr/kg) was approximately two thirds of the mean systemic CL (0.56 L/hr/kg) of cyclosporine in historical control subjects with normal renal function. In 5 liver transplant patients, the mean clearance of cyclosporine on and off hemodialysis was 463 mL/min and 398 mL/min, respectively. Less than 1% of the dose of cyclosporine was recovered in the dialysate.

Hepatic Impairment

Cyclosporine is extensively metabolized by the liver. Since severe hepatic impairment may result in significantly increased cyclosporine exposures, the dosage of cyclosporine may need to be reduced in these patients.

INDICATIONS AND USAGE

Sandimmune® (cyclosporine) is indicated for the prophylaxis of organ rejection in kidney, liver, and heart allogeneic transplants. It is always to be used with adrenal corticosteroids. The drug may also be used in the treatment of chronic rejection in patients previously treated with other immunosuppressive agents.

Because of the risk of anaphylaxis, Sandimmune® Injection (cyclosporine injection, USP) should be reserved for patients who are unable to take the soft gelatin capsules or oral solution.

CONTRAINDICATIONS

Sandimmune® Injection (cyclosporine injection, USP) is contraindicated in patients with a hypersensitivity to Sandimmune® (cyclosporine) and/or Cremophor® EL (polyoxyethylated castor oil).

WARNINGS

Kidney, Liver and Heart Transplant

(See BOXED WARNING): Sandimmune® (cyclosporine), when used in high doses, can cause hepatotoxicity and nephrotoxicity.

Nephrotoxicity

It is not unusual for serum creatinine and BUN levels to be elevated during Sandimmune® (cyclosporine) therapy. These elevations in renal transplant patients do not necessarily indicate rejection, and each patient must be fully evaluated before dosage adjustment is initiated.

Nephrotoxicity has been noted in 25% of cases of renal transplantation, 38% of cases of cardiac transplantation, and 37% of cases of liver transplantation. Mild nephrotoxicity was generally noted 2-3 months after transplant and consisted of an arrest in the fall of the preoperative elevations of BUN and creatinine at a range of 35-45 mg/dl and 2.0-2.5 mg/dl, respectively. These elevations were often responsive to dosage reduction.

More overt nephrotoxicity was seen early after transplantation and was characterized by a rapidly rising BUN and creatinine. Since these events are similar to rejection episodes, care must be taken to differentiate between them. This form of nephrotoxicity is usually responsive to Sandimmune® (cyclosporine) dosage reduction.

Although specific diagnostic criteria which reliably differentiate renal graft rejection from drug toxicity have not been found, a number of parameters have been significantly associated to one or the other. It should be noted however, that up to 20% of patients may have simultaneous nephrotoxicity and rejection.

[See table above]

A form of chronic progressive cyclosporine-associated nephrotoxicity is characterized by serial deterioration in renal function and morphologic changes in the kidneys. From 5%-15% of transplant recipients will fail to show a reduction in a rising serum creatinine despite a decrease or discontinuation of cyclosporine therapy. Renal biopsies from these patients will demonstrate an interstitial fibrosis with tubular atrophy. In addition, toxic tubulopathy, peritubular capillary congestion, arteriolopathy, and a striped form of interstitial fibrosis with tubular atrophy may be present. Though none of these morphologic changes is entirely specific, a histologic diagnosis of chronic progressive cyclosporine-associated nephrotoxicity requires evidence of these.

When considering the development of chronic nephrotoxicity it is noteworthy that several authors have reported an association between the appearance of interstitial fibrosis and higher cumulative doses or persistently high circulating trough concentrations of cyclosporine. This is particularly true during the first 6 posttransplant months when the dosage tends to be highest and when, in kidney recipients, the organ appears to be most vulnerable to the toxic effects of cyclosporine. Among other contributing factors to the development of interstitial fibrosis in these patients must be included, prolonged perfusion time, warm ischemia time, as well as episodes of acute toxicity, and acute and chronic rejection. The reversibility of interstitial fibrosis and its correlation to renal function have not yet been determined.

Impaired renal function at any time requires close monitoring, and frequent dosage adjustment may be indicated. In patients with persistent high elevations of BUN and creatinine who are unresponsive to dosage adjustments, consideration should be given to switching to other immunosuppressive therapy. In the event of severe and unremitting rejection, it is preferable to allow the kidney transplant to be rejected and removed rather than increase the Sandimmune® (cyclosporine) dosage to a very high level in an attempt to reverse the rejection.

Due to the potential for additive or synergistic impairment of renal function, caution should be exercised when coadministering Sandimmune with other drugs that may impair renal function. (See PRECAUTIONS, Drug Interactions)

Thrombotic Microangiopathy

Occasionally patients have developed a syndrome of thrombocytopenia and microangiopathic hemolytic anemia which may result in graft failure. The vasculopathy can occur in the absence of rejection and is accompanied by avid platelet consumption within the graft as demonstrated by Indium 111 labeled platelet studies. Neither the pathogenesis nor the management of this syndrome is clear. Though resolution has occurred after reduction or discontinuation of Sandimmune® (cyclosporine) and 1) administration of streptokinase and heparin or 2) plasmapheresis, this appears to depend upon early detection with Indium 111 labeled platelet scans. (See ADVERSE REACTIONS)

Hyperkalemia

Significant hyperkalemia (sometimes associated with hyperchloremic metabolic acidosis) and hyperuricemia have been seen occasionally in individual patients.

Hepatotoxicity

Cases of hepatotoxicity and liver injury including cholestasis, jaundice, hepatitis, and liver failure have been reported in patients treated with cyclosporine. Most reports included patients with significant co-morbidities, underlying conditions and other confounding factors including infectious complications and comedications with hepatotoxic potential. In some cases, mainly in transplant patients, fatal outcomes have been reported (See ADVERSE REACTIONS, Postmarketing Experience)

Hepatotoxicity, usually manifested by elevations in hepatic enzymes and bilirubin, was reported in patients treated with cyclosporine in clinical trials: 4% in renal transplantation, 7% in cardiac transplantation, and 4% in liver trans-

Drugs That May Potentiate Renal Dysfunction

Antibiotics	*Antineoplastic*	*Antifungals*	*Anti-Inflammatory Drugs*	*Gastrointestinal Agents*	*Immunosuppressives*	*Other Drugs*
ciprofloxacin	melphalan	amphotericin B	azapropazon	cimetidine	tacrolimus	fibric acid derivatives (e.g., bezafibrate, fenofibrate)
gentamicin		ketoconazole	colchicine	ranitidine		methotrexate
tobramycin			diclofenac			
trimethoprim with sulfamethoxazole			naproxen			
vancomycin			sulindac			

plantation. This was usually noted during the first month of therapy when high doses of Sandimmune® (cyclosporine) were used. The chemistry elevations usually decreased with a reduction in dosage.

Malignancies

As in patients receiving other immunosuppressants, those patients receiving Sandimmune® (cyclosporine) are at increased risk for development of lymphomas and other malignancies, particularly those of the skin. The increased risk appears related to the intensity and duration of immunosuppression rather than to the use of specific agents. Because of the danger of oversuppression of the immune system, which can also increase susceptibility to infection, Sandimmune® (cyclosporine) should not be administered with other immunosuppressive agents except adrenal corticosteroids. The efficacy and safety of cyclosporine in combination with other immunosuppressive agents have not been determined. Some malignancies may be fatal. Transplant patients receiving cyclosporine are at increased risk for serious infection with fatal outcome.

Serious Infections

Patients receiving immunosuppressants, including Sandimmune, are at increased risk of developing bacterial, viral, fungal, and protozoal infections, including opportunistic infections. These infections may lead to serious, including fatal, outcomes (See BOXED WARNING, and ADVERSE REACTIONS).

Polyoma Virus Infections

Patients receiving immunosuppressants, including Sandimmune, are at increased risk for opportunistic infections, including polyoma virus infections. Polyoma virus infections in transplant patients may have serious, and sometimes, fatal outcomes. These include cases of JC virus-associated progressive multifocal leukoencephalopathy (PML), and polyoma virus-associated nephropathy (PVAN), especially due to BK virus infection, which have been observed in patients receiving cyclosporine.

PVAN is associated with serious outcomes, including deteriorating renal function and renal graft loss, (See ADVERSE REACTIONS/Postmarketing Experience). Patient monitoring may help detect patients at risk for PVAN.

Cases of PML have been reported in patients treated with Sandimmune. PML, which is sometimes fatal, commonly presents with hemiparesis, apathy, confusion, cognitive deficiencies and ataxia. Risk factors for PML include treatment with immunosuppressant therapies and impairment of immune function. In immunosuppressed patients, physicians should consider PML in the differential diagnosis in patients reporting neurological symptoms and consultation with a neurologist should be considered as clinically indicated.

Consideration should be given to reducing the total immunosuppression in transplant patients who develop PML or PVAN. However, reduced immunosuppression may place the graft at risk.

Neurotoxicity

There have been reports of convulsions in adult and pediatric patients receiving cyclosporine, particularly in combination with high-dose methylprednisolone.

Encephalopathy, including Posterior Reversible Encephalopathy Syndrome (PRES), has been described both in postmarketing reports and in the literature. Manifestations include impaired consciousness, convulsions, visual disturbances (including blindness), loss of motor function, movement disorders and psychiatric disturbances. In many cases, changes in the white matter have been detected using imaging techniques and pathologic specimens. Predisposing factors such as hypertension, hypomagnesemia, hypocholesterolemia, high-dose corticosteroids, high cyclosporine blood concentrations, and graft-versus-host disease have been noted in many but not all of the reported cases. The changes in most cases have been reversible upon discontinuation of cyclosporine, and in some cases, improvement was noted after reduction of dose. It appears that patients receiving liver transplant are more susceptible to encephalopathy than those receiving kidney transplant. Another rare manifestation of cyclosporine-induced neurotoxicity is optic disc edema including papilloedema, with possible visual impairment, secondary to benign intracranial hypertension.

Specific Excipients

Anaphylactic Reactions

Rarely (approximately 1 in 1000), patients receiving Sandimmune® Injection (cyclosporine injection, USP) have experienced anaphylactic reactions. Although the exact cause of these reactions is unknown, it is believed to be due to the Cremophor® EL (polyoxyethylated castor oil) used as the vehicle for the I.V. formulation. These reactions can consist of flushing of the face and upper thorax, and noncardiogenic pulmonary edema, with acute respiratory distress, dyspnea, wheezing, blood pressure changes, and tachycardia. One patient died after respiratory arrest and aspiration pneumonia. In some cases, the reaction subsided after the infusion was stopped.

Patients receiving Sandimmune® Injection (cyclosporine injection, USP) should be under continuous observation for at least the first 30 minutes following the start of the infusion and at frequent intervals thereafter. If anaphylaxis occurs, the infusion should be stopped. An aqueous solution of epinephrine 1:1000 should be available at the bedside as well as a source of oxygen.

Anaphylactic reactions have not been reported with the soft gelatin capsules or oral solution which lack Cremophor® EL (polyoxyethylated castor oil). In fact, patients experiencing anaphylactic reactions have been treated subsequently with the soft gelatin capsules or oral solution without incident.

Alcohol (ethanol)

The alcohol content (See DESCRIPTION) of Sandimmune should be taken into account when given to patients in whom alcohol intake should be avoided or minimized, e.g. pregnant or breastfeeding women, in patients presenting with liver disease or epilepsy, in alcoholic patients, or pediatric patients. For an adult weighing 70 kg, the maximum daily oral dose would deliver about 1 gram of alcohol which is approximately 6% of the amount of alcohol contained in a standard drink. The daily intravenous dose would deliver approximately 15% of the amount of alcohol contained in a standard drink.

Care should be taken in using Sandimmune® (cyclosporine) with nephrotoxic drugs. (See PRECAUTIONS)

Conversion from Neoral to Sandimmune

Because Sandimmune® (cyclosporine) is not bioequivalent to Neoral®, conversion from Neoral® to Sandimmune® (cyclosporine) using a 1:1 ratio (mg/kg/day) may result in a lower cyclosporine blood concentration. Conversion from Neoral® to Sandimmune® (cyclosporine) should be made with increased blood concentration monitoring to avoid the potential of underdosing.

PRECAUTIONS

General

Patients with malabsorption may have difficulty in achieving therapeutic concentrations with Sandimmune® Soft Gelatin Capsules or Oral Solution.

Hypertension

Hypertension is a common side effect of Sandimmune® (cyclosporine) therapy. (See ADVERSE REACTIONS) Mild or moderate hypertension is more frequently encountered than severe hypertension and the incidence decreases over time. Antihypertensive therapy may be required. Control of blood pressure can be accomplished with any of the common antihypertensive agents. However, since cyclosporine may cause hyperkalemia, potassium-sparing diuretics should not be used. While calcium antagonists can be effective agents in treating cyclosporine-associated hypertension, care should be taken since interference with cyclosporine metabolism may require a dosage adjustment. (See Drug Interactions)

Vaccination

During treatment with Sandimmune® (cyclosporine), vaccination may be less effective and the use of live attenuated vaccines should be avoided.

Information for Patients

Patients should be advised that any change of cyclosporine formulation should be made cautiously and only under physician supervision because it may result in the need for a change in dosage.

Patients should be informed of the necessity of repeated laboratory tests while they are receiving the drug. They should be given careful dosage instructions, advised of the potential risks during pregnancy, and informed of the increased risk of neoplasia.

Patients using cyclosporine oral solution with its accompanying syringe for dosage measurement should be cautioned not to rinse the syringe either before or after use. Introduction of water into the product by any means will cause variation in dose.

Laboratory Tests

Renal and liver functions should be assessed repeatedly by measurement of BUN, serum creatinine, serum bilirubin, and liver enzymes.

Drug Interactions

A. Effect of Drugs and Other Agents on Cyclosporine Pharmacokinetics and/or Safety

All of the individual drugs cited below are well substantiated to interact with cyclosporine. In addition, concomitant use of nonsteroidal anti-inflammatory drugs with cyclosporine, particularly in the setting of dehydration, may potentiate renal dysfunction. Caution should be exercised when using other drugs which are known to impair renal function. (See WARNINGS, Nephrotoxicity)

[See table above]

During the concomitant use of a drug that may exhibit additive or synergistic renal impairment potential with cyclosporine, close monitoring of renal function (in particular serum creatinine) should be performed. If a significant impairment of renal function occurs, reduction in the dosage of cyclosporine and/or co-administered drug or an alternative treatment should be considered.

Cyclosporine is extensively metabolized by CYP 3A isoenzymes, in particular CYP3A4, and is a substrate of the multidrug efflux transporter P-glycoprotein. Various agents are known to either increase or decrease plasma or whole blood concentrations of cyclosporine usually by inhibition or induction of CYP3A4 or P-glycoprotein transporter or both. Compounds that decrease cyclosporine absorption such as orlistat should be avoided. Appropriate Sandimmune® (cyclosporine) dosage adjustment to achieve the desired cyclosporine concentrations is essential when drugs that significantly alter cyclosporine concentrations are used concomitantly. (See Blood Concentration Monitoring)

[See first table at top of next page]

HIV Protease inhibitors

The HIV protease inhibitors (e.g., indinavir, nelfinavir, ritonavir, and saquinavir) are known to inhibit cytochrome P-450 3A and thus could potentially increase the concentrations of cyclosporine, however no formal studies of the interaction are available. Care should be exercised when these drugs are administered concomitantly.

Grapefruit juice

Grapefruit and grapefruit juice affect metabolism, increasing blood concentrations of cyclosporine, thus should be avoided.

[See second table at top of next page]

Bosentan

Co-administration of bosentan (250-1000 mg every 12 hours based on tolerability) and cyclosporine (300 mg every 12 hours for 2 days then dosing to achieve a C_{min} of 200-250 ng/mL) for 7 days in healthy subjects resulted in decreases in the cyclosporine mean dose-normalized AUC, C_{max}, and trough concentration of approximately 50%, 30% and 60%, respectively, compared to when cyclosporine was given alone. (See also Effect of Cyclosporine on the Pharmacokinetics and/or Safety of Other Drugs or Agents)

Boceprevir

Co-administration of boceprevir (800 mg three times daily for 7 days) and cyclosporine (100 mg single dose) in healthy subjects resulted in increases in the mean AUC and C_{max} of cyclosporine approximately 2.7-fold and 2-fold, respectively, compared to when cyclosporine was given alone.

Telaprevir

Co-administration of telaprevir (750 mg every 8 hours for 11 days) with cyclosporine (10 mg on day 8) in healthy subjects resulted in increases in the mean dose-normalized AUC and C_{max} of cyclosporine approximately 4.5-fold and 1.3-fold, respectively, compared to when cyclosporine (100 mg single dose) was given alone.

1. Drugs That Increase Cyclosporine Concentrations

Calcium Channel Blockers	*Antifungals*	*Antibiotics*	*Glucocorticoids*	*Other Drugs*
diltiazem	fluconazole	azithromycin	methylprednisolone	allopurinol
nicardipine	itraconazole	clarithromycin		amiodarone
verapamil	ketoconazole	erythromycin		bromocriptine
		quinupristin/dalfopristin		colchicine
	voriconazole			danazol
				imatinib
				metoclopramide
				nefazodone
				oral contraceptives

2. Drugs/Dietary Supplements That Decrease Cyclosporine Concentrations

Antibiotics	*Anticonvulsants*	*Other Drugs / Dietary Supplements*	
nafcillin	carbamazepine	bosentan	St. John's Wort
rifampin	oxcarbazepine	octreotide	
	phenobarbital	orlistat	
	phenytoin	sulfinpyrazone	
		terbinafine	
		ticlopidine	

St. John's Wort

There have been reports of a serious drug interaction between cyclosporine and the herbal dietary supplement, St. John's Wort. This interaction has been reported to produce a marked reduction in the blood concentrations of cyclosporine, resulting in subtherapeutic levels, rejection of transplanted organs, and graft loss.

Rifabutin

Rifabutin is known to increase the metabolism of other drugs metabolized by the cytochrome P-450 system. The interaction between rifabutin and cyclosporine has not been studied. Care should be exercised when these two drugs are administered concomitantly.

B. Effect of Cyclosporine on the Pharmacokinetics and/or Safety of Other Drugs or Agents

Cyclosporine is an inhibitor of CYP3A4 and of the multidrug efflux transporter P-glycoprotein and may increase plasma concentrations of comedications that are substrates of CYP3A4 or P-glycoprotein or both.

Cyclosporine may reduce the clearance of digoxin, colchicine, prednisolone, HMG-CoA reductase inhibitors (statins) and aliskiren, repaglinide, NSAIDs, sirolimus, etoposide, and other drugs. See the full prescribing information of the other drug for further information and specific recommendations. The decision on co-administration of cyclosporine with other drugs or agents should be made by the physician following the careful assessment of benefits and risks.

Digoxin

Severe digitalis toxicity has been seen within days of starting cyclosporine in several patients taking digoxin. If digoxin is used concurrently with cyclosporine, serum digoxin concentrations should be monitored.

Colchicine

There are reports on the potential of cyclosporine to enhance the toxic effects of colchicine such as myopathy and neuropathy, especially in patients with renal dysfunction. Concomitant administration of cyclosporine and colchicine results in significant increases in colchicine plasma concentrations. If colchicine is used concurrently with cyclosporine, a reduction in the dosage of colchicine is recommended.

HMG Co-A reductase inhibitors (statins)

Literature and postmarketing cases of myotoxicity, including muscle pain and weakness, myositis, and rhabdomyolysis, have been reported with concomitant administration of cyclosporine with lovastatin, simvastatin, atorvastatin, pravastatin, and rarely, fluvastatin. When concurrently administered with cyclosporine, the dosage of these statins should be reduced according to label recommendations. Statin therapy needs to be temporarily withheld or discontinued in patients with signs and symptoms of myopathy or those with risk factors predisposing to severe renal injury, including renal failure, secondary to rhabdomyolysis.

Repaglinide

Cyclosporine may increase the plasma concentrations of repaglinide and thereby increase the risk of hypoglycemia. In 12 healthy male subjects who received two doses of 100 mg cyclosporine capsule orally 12 hours apart with a single dose of 0.25 mg repaglinide tablet (one half of a 0.5 mg tablet) orally 13 hours after the cyclosporine initial dose, the repaglinide mean C_{max} and AUC were increased 1.8 fold (range: 0.6-3.7 fold) and 2.4 fold (range 1.2-5.3 fold), respectively. Close monitoring of blood glucose level is advisable for a patient taking cyclosporine and repaglinide concomitantly.

Ambrisentan

Co-administration of ambrisentan (5 mg daily) and cyclosporine (100-150 mg twice daily initially, then dosing to achieve C_{min} 150-200 ng/mL) for 8 days in healthy subjects resulted mean increases in ambrisentan AUC and C_{max} of approximately 2-fold and 1.5-fold, respectively, compared to ambrisentan alone.

Anthracycline antibiotics

High doses of cyclosporine (e.g., at starting intravenous dose of 16 mg/kg/day) may increase the exposure to anthracycline antibiotics (e.g., doxorubicin, mitoxantrone, daunorubicin) in cancer patients.

Aliskiren

Cyclosporine alters the pharmacokinetics of aliskiren, a substrate of P-glycoprotein and CYP3A4. In 14 healthy subjects who received concomitantly single doses of cyclosporine (200 mg) and reduced dose aliskiren (75 mg), the mean C_{max} of aliskiren was increased by approximately 2.5 fold (90% CI: 1.96-3.17) and the mean AUC by approximately 4.3 fold (90% CI: 3.52-5.21), compared to when these subjects received aliskiren alone. The concomitant administration of aliskiren with cyclosporine prolonged the median aliskiren elimination half-life (26 hours versus 43 to 45 hours) and the T_{max} (0.5 hours versus 1.5 to 2.0 hours). The mean AUC and C_{max} of cyclosporine were comparable to reported literature values. Coadministration of cyclosporine and aliskiren in these subjects also resulted in an increase in the number and/or intensity of adverse events, mainly headache, hot flush, nausea, vomiting, and somnolence. The coadministration of cyclosporine with aliskiren is not recommended.

Bosentan

In healthy subjects, co-administration of bosentan and cyclosporine resulted in mean increases in dose-normalized bosentan trough concentrations on day 1 and day 8 of approximately 21-fold and 2-fold , respectively, compared to when bosentan was given alone as a single dose on day 1. (See also Effect of Drugs and Other Agents on Cyclosporine Pharmacokinetics and/or Safety)

Potassium sparing diuretics

Cyclosporine should not be used with potassium-sparing diuretics because hyperkalemia can occur. Caution is also required when cyclosporine is coadministered with potassium-sparing drugs (e.g., angiotensin-converting enzyme inhibitors, angiotensin II receptor antagonists), potassium-containing drugs as well as in patients on a potassium-rich diet. Control of potassium levels in these situations is advisable.

Nonsteroidal Anti-inflammatory Drug (NSAID) Interactions

Clinical status and serum creatinine should be closely monitored when cyclosporine is used with nonsteroidal anti-inflammatory agents in rheumatoid arthritis patients. (See WARNINGS)

Pharmacodynamic interactions have been reported to occur between cyclosporine and both naproxen and sulindac, in that concomitant use is associated with additive decreases in renal function, as determined by 99mTc-diethylenetriaminepentaacetic acid (DTPA) and (p-aminohippuric acid) PAH clearances. Although concomitant administration of diclofenac does not affect blood concentrations of cyclosporine, it has been associated with approximate doubling of diclofenac blood levels and occasional reports of reversible decreases in renal function. Consequently, the dose of diclofenac should be in the lower end of the therapeutic range.

Methotrexate Interaction

Preliminary data indicate that when methotrexate and cyclosporine were coadministered to rheumatoid arthritis patients (N=20), methotrexate concentrations (AUCs) were increased approximately 30% and the concentrations (AUCs) of its metabolite, 7-hydroxy methotrexate, were decreased by approximately 80%. The clinical significance of this interaction is not known. Cyclosporine concentrations do not appear to have been altered (N=6).

Sirolimus

Elevations in serum creatinine were observed in studies using sirolimus in combination with full-dose cyclosporine. This effect is often reversible with cyclosporine dose reduction. Simultaneous coadministration of cyclosporine significantly increases blood levels of sirolimus. To minimize increases in sirolimus blood concentrations, it is recommended that sirolimus be given 4 hours after cyclosporine administration.

Nifedipine

Frequent gingival hyperplasia when nifedipine is given concurrently with cyclosporine has been reported. The concomitant use of nifedipine should be avoided in patients in whom gingival hyperplasia develops as a side effect of cyclosporine.

Methylprednisolone

Convulsions when high dose methylprednisolone is given concomitantly with cyclosporine have been reported.

Other Immunosuppressive Drugs and Agents

Psoriasis patients receiving other immunosuppressive agents or radiation therapy (including PUVA and UVB) should not receive concurrent cyclosporine because of the possibility of excessive immunosuppression.

C. Effect of Cyclosporine on the Efficacy of Live Vaccines

During treatment with cyclosporine, vaccination may be less effective. The use of live vaccines should be avoided.

For additional information on Cyclosporine Drug Interactions please contact Novartis Medical Affairs Department at 888-NOW-NOVA (888-669-6682).

Carcinogenesis, Mutagenesis, and Impairment of Fertility

Cyclosporine gave no evidence of mutagenic or teratogenic effects in appropriate test systems. Only at dose levels toxic to dams, were adverse effects seen in reproduction studies in rats. (See Pregnancy)

Carcinogenicity studies were carried out in male and female rats and mice. In the 78-week mouse study, at doses of 1, 4, and 16 mg/kg/day, evidence of a statistically significant trend was found for lymphocytic lymphomas in females, and the incidence of hepatocellular carcinomas in mid-dose males significantly exceeded the control value. In the 24-month rat study, conducted at 0.5, 2, and 8 mg/kg/day, pancreatic islet cell adenomas significantly exceeded the control rate in the low-dose level. The hepatocellular carcinomas and pancreatic islet cell adenomas were not dose related.

No impairment in fertility was demonstrated in studies in male and female rats.

Cyclosporine has not been found mutagenic/genotoxic in the Ames Test, the V79-HGPRT Test, the micronucleus test in mice and Chinese hamsters, the chromosome-aberration tests in Chinese hamster bone marrow, the mouse dominant lethal assay, and the DNA-repair test in sperm from treated mice. A recent study analyzing sister chromatid exchange (SCE) induction by cyclosporine using human lymphocytes *in vitro* gave indication of a positive effect (i.e., induction of SCE), at high concentrations in this system. In two published research studies, rabbits exposed to cyclosporine *in utero* (10 mg/kg/day subcutaneously) demonstrated reduced numbers of nephrons, renal hypertrophy, systemic hypertension and progressive renal insufficiency up to 35 weeks of age. Pregnant rats which received 12 mg/kg/day of cyclosporine intravenously (twice the recommended human intravenous dose) had fetuses with an increased incidence of ventricular septal defect. These findings have not been demonstrated in other species and their relevance for humans is unknown.

An increased incidence of malignancy is a recognized complication of immunosuppression in recipients of organ transplants. The most common forms of neoplasms are non-Hodgkin's lymphoma and carcinomas of the skin. The risk of malignancies in cyclosporine recipients is higher than in the normal, healthy population, but similar to that in patients receiving other immunosuppressive therapies. It has been reported that reduction or discontinuance of immunosuppression may cause the lesions to regress.

Pregnancy

Pregnancy Category C

Animal studies have shown reproductive toxicity in rats and rabbits. Cyclosporine gave no evidence of mutagenic or teratogenic effects in the standard test systems with oral application (rats up to 17 mg/kg and rabbits up to 30 mg/kg per day orally). Sandimmune® Oral Solution (cyclosporine oral solution, USP) has been shown to be embryo- and fetotoxic in rats and rabbits when given in doses 2-5 times the human dose. At toxic doses (rats at 30 mg/kg/day and rab-

Body System/ Adverse Reactions	Randomized Kidney Patients Sandimmune® (N=227) %	Azathioprine (N=228) %	All Sandimmune® (cyclosporine) Patients Kidney (N=705) %	Heart (N=112) %	Liver (N=75) %
Genitourinary					
Renal Dysfunction	32	6	25	38	37
Cardiovascular					
Hypertension	26	18	13	53	27
Cramps	4	< 1	2	< 1	0
Skin					
Hirsutism	21	< 1	21	28	45
Acne	6	8	2	2	1
Central Nervous System					
Tremor	12	0	21	31	55
Convulsions	3	1	1	4	5
Headache	2	< 1	2	15	4
Gastrointestinal					
Gum Hyperplasia	4	0	9	5	16
Diarrhea	3	< 1	3	4	8
Nausea/Vomiting	2	< 1	4	10	4
Hepatotoxicity	< 1	< 1	4	7	4
Abdominal Discomfort	< 1	0	< 1	7	0
Autonomic Nervous System					
Paresthesia	3	0	1	2	1
Flushing	< 1	0	4	0	4
Hematopoietic					
Leukopenia	2	19	< 1	6	0
Lymphoma	< 1	0	1	6	1
Respiratory					
Sinusitis	< 1	0	4	3	7
Miscellaneous					
Gynecomastia	< 1	0	< 1	4	3

Renal Transplant Patients in Whom Therapy Was Discontinued

Reason for Discontinuation	Randomized Patients Sandimmune® (N=227) %	Azathioprine (N=228) %	All Sandimmune® Patients (N=705) %
Renal Toxicity	5.7	0	5.4
Infection	0	0.4	0.9
Lack of Efficacy	2.6	0.9	1.4
Acute Tubular Necrosis	2.6	0	1.0
Lymphoma/Lymphoproliferative Disease	0.4	0	0.3
Hypertension	0	0	0.3
Hematological Abnormalities	0	0.4	0
Other	0	0	0.7

Sandimmune® (cyclosporine) was discontinued on a temporary basis and then restarted in 18 additional patients.

bits at 100 mg/kg/day), Sandimmune® Oral Solution (cyclosporine oral solution, USP) was embryo- and fetotoxic as indicated by increased pre- and postnatal mortality and reduced fetal weight together with related skeletal retardations. In the well-tolerated dose range (rats at up to 17 mg/kg/day and rabbits at up to 30 mg/kg/day), Sandimmune® Oral Solution (cyclosporine oral solution, USP) proved to be without any embryolethal or teratogenic effects.

There are no adequate and well-controlled studies in pregnant women and therefore, Sandimmune® (cyclosporine) should not be used during pregnancy unless the potential benefit to the mother justifies the potential risk to the fetus.

In pregnant transplant recipients who are being treated with immunosuppressants, the risk of premature birth is increased. The following data represent the reported outcomes of 116 pregnancies in women receiving Sandimmune® (cyclosporine) during pregnancy, 90% of whom were transplant patients, and most of whom received Sandimmune® (cyclosporine) throughout the entire gestational period. Since most of the patients were not prospectively identified, the results are likely to be biased toward negative outcomes. The only consistent patterns of abnormality were premature birth (gestational period of 28 to 36 weeks) and low birth weight for gestational age. It is not possible to separate the effects of Sandimmune® (cyclosporine) on these pregnancies from the effects of the other immunosuppressants, the underlying maternal disorders, or other aspects of the transplantation milieu. Sixteen fetal losses occurred. Most of the pregnancies (85 of 100) were complicated by disorders; including, preeclampsia, eclampsia, premature labor, abruptio placentae, oligohydramnios, Rh incompatibility and fetoplacental dysfunction. Preterm delivery occurred in 47%. Seven malformations were reported in 5 viable infants and in 2 cases of fetal loss. Twenty-eight percent of the infants were small for gestational age. Neonatal complications occurred in 27%. In a report of 23 children followed up to 4 years, postnatal development was said to be normal. More information on cyclosporine use in pregnancy is available from Novartis Pharmaceuticals Corporation.

A limited number of observations in children exposed to cyclosporine *in utero* are available, up to an age of approximately 7 years. Renal function and blood pressure in these children were normal.

The alcohol content of the Sandimmune formulations should also be taken into account in pregnant women. (See WARNINGS, Special Excipients)

Nursing Mothers

Cyclosporine is present in breast milk. Because of the potential for serious adverse drug reactions in nursing infants from Sandimmune, a decision should be made whether to discontinue nursing or to discontinue the drug, taking into account the importance of the drug to the mother. Sandimmune contains ethanol. Ethanol will be present in human milk at levels similar to that found in maternal serum and if present in breast milk will be orally absorbed by a nursing infant. (See WARNINGS)

Pediatric Use

Although no adequate and well-controlled studies have been conducted in children, patients as young as 6 months of age have received the drug with no unusual adverse effects.

Geriatric Use

Clinical studies of Sandimmune® (cyclosporine) did not include sufficient numbers of subjects aged 65 and over to determine whether they respond differently from younger patients. Other reported clinical experience has not identified differences in responses between the elderly and younger patients. In general, dose selection for an elderly patient should be cautious, usually starting at the low end of the dosing range, reflecting the greater frequency of decreased hepatic, renal, or cardiac function, and of concomitant disease or other drug therapy.

ADVERSE REACTIONS

The principal adverse reactions of Sandimmune® (cyclosporine) therapy are renal dysfunction, tremor, hirsutism, hypertension, and gum hyperplasia.

Hypertension

Hypertension, which is usually mild to moderate, may occur in approximately 50% of patients following renal transplantation and in most cardiac transplant patients.

Glomerular Capillary Thrombosis

Glomerular capillary thrombosis has been found in patients treated with cyclosporine and may progress to graft failure. The pathologic changes resemble those seen in the hemolytic-uremic syndrome and include thrombosis of the renal microvasculature, with platelet-fibrin thrombi occluding glomerular capillaries and afferent arterioles, microangiopathic hemolytic anemia, thrombocytopenia, and decreased renal function. Similar findings have been observed when other immunosuppressives have been employed post-transplantation.

Hypomagnesemia

Hypomagnesemia has been reported in some, but not all, patients exhibiting convulsions while on cyclosporine therapy. Although magnesium-depletion studies in normal subjects suggest that hypomagnesemia is associated with neurologic disorders, multiple factors, including hypertension, high-dose methylprednisolone, hypocholesterolemia, and nephrotoxicity associated with high plasma concentrations of cyclosporine appear to be related to the neurological manifestations of cyclosporine toxicity.

Clinical Studies

The following reactions occurred in 3% or greater of 892 patients involved in clinical trials of kidney, heart, and liver transplants:

[See first table above]

The following reactions occurred in 2% or less of patients: allergic reactions, anemia, anorexia, confusion, conjunctivitis, edema, fever, brittle fingernails, gastritis, hearing loss, hiccups, hyperglycemia, muscle pain, peptic ulcer, thrombocytopenia, tinnitus.

The following reactions occurred rarely: anxiety, chest pain, constipation, depression, hair breaking, hematuria, joint pain, lethargy, mouth sores, myocardial infarction, night sweats, pancreatitis, pruritus, swallowing difficulty, tingling, upper GI bleeding, visual disturbance, weakness, weight loss.

[See second table above]

Patients receiving immunosuppressive therapies, including cyclosporine and cyclosporine -containing regimens, are at increased risk of infections (viral, bacterial, fungal, parasitic). Both generalized and localized infections can occur. Pre-existing infections may also be aggravated. Fatal outcomes have been reported. (see WARNINGS)

Infectious Complications in the Randomized Renal Transplant Patients

Complication	Sandimmune® Treatment (N=227) % of Complications	Standard Treatment* (N=228) % of Complications
Septicemia	5.3	4.8
Abscesses	4.4	5.3
Systemic Fungal Infection	2.2	3.9
Local Fungal Infection	7.5	9.6
Cytomegalovirus	4.8	12.3
Other Viral Infections	15.9	18.4
Urinary Tract Infections	21.1	20.2
Wound and Skin Infections	7.0	10.1
Pneumonia	6.2	9.2

*Some patients also received ALG.

Cremophor® EL (polyoxyethylated castor oil) is known to cause hyperlipemia and electrophoretic abnormalities of lipoproteins. These effects are reversible upon discontinuation of treatment but are usually not a reason to stop treatment.

Postmarketing Experience

Hepatotoxicity

Cases of hepatotoxicity and liver injury including cholestasis, jaundice, hepatitis and liver failure; serious and/or fatal outcomes have been reported. (See WARNINGS, Hepatotoxicity)

Increased Risk of Infections

Cases of JC virus-associated progressive multifocal leukoencephalopathy (PML), sometimes fatal; and polyoma virus-associated nephropathy (PVAN), especially BK virus resulting in graft loss have been reported. (See WARNINGS, Polyoma Virus Infection)

Headache, including Migraine

Cases of migraine have been reported. In some cases, patients have been unable to continue cyclosporine, however, the final decision on treatment discontinuation should be made by the treating physician following the careful assessment of benefits versus risks.

OVERDOSAGE

There is a minimal experience with overdosage. Because of the slow absorption of Sandimmune® Soft Gelatin Capsules or Oral Solution, forced emesis and gastric lavage would be of value up to 2 hours after administration. Transient hepatotoxicity and nephrotoxicity may occur which should resolve following drug withdrawal. Oral doses of cyclosporine up to 10 g (about 150 mg/kg) have been tolerated with relatively minor clinical consequences, such as vomiting, drowsiness, headache, tachycardia and, in a few patients, moderately severe, reversible impairment of renal function. However, serious symptoms of intoxication have been reported following accidental parenteral overdosage with cyclosporine in premature neonates. General supportive measures and symptomatic treatment should be followed in all cases of overdosage. Sandimmune® (cyclosporine) is not dialyzable to any great extent, nor is it cleared well by charcoal hemoperfusion. The oral LD_{50} is 2329 mg/kg in mice, 1480 mg/kg in rats, and >1000 mg/kg in rabbits. The I.V. LD_{50} is 148 mg/kg in mice, 104 mg/kg in rats, and 46 mg/kg in rabbits.

DOSAGE AND ADMINISTRATION

Sandimmune® Soft Gelatin Capsules (cyclosporine capsules, USP) and Sandimmune® Oral Solution (cyclosporine oral solution, USP)

Sandimmune® Soft Gelatin Capsules (cyclosporine capsules, USP) and Sandimmune® Oral Solution (cyclosporine oral solution, USP) have decreased bioavailability in comparison to Neoral® Soft Gelatin Capsules (cyclosporine capsules, USP) MODIFIED and Neoral® Oral Solution (cyclosporine oral solution, USP) MODIFIED. Sandimmune® and Neoral® are not bioequivalent and cannot be used interchangeably without physician supervision.

The initial oral dose of Sandimmune® (cyclosporine) should be given 4-12 hours prior to transplantation as a single dose of 15 mg/kg. Although a daily single dose of 14-18 mg/kg was used in most clinical trials, few centers continue to use the highest dose, most favoring the lower end of the scale. There is a trend towards use of even lower initial doses for renal transplantation in the ranges of 10-14 mg/kg/day. The initial single daily dose is continued postoperatively for 1-2 weeks and then tapered by 5% per week to a maintenance dose of 5-10 mg/kg/day. Some centers have successfully tapered the maintenance dose to as low as 3 mg/kg/day in selected *renal* transplant patients without an apparent rise in rejection rate.

(See Blood Concentration Monitoring, below.)

Specific Populations

Renal Impairment

Cyclosporine undergoes minimal renal elimination and its pharmacokinetics do not appear to be significantly altered in patients with end-stage renal disease who receive routine hemodialysis treatments (See CLINICAL PHARMACOLOGY). However, due to its nephrotoxic potential (See WARNINGS), careful monitoring of renal function is recommended; cyclosporine dosage should be reduced if indicated. (See WARNINGS and PRECAUTIONS)

Hepatic Impairment

The clearance of cyclosporine may be significantly reduced in severe liver disease patients (See CLINICAL PHARMACOLOGY). Dose reduction may be necessary in patients with severe liver impairment to maintain blood concentrations within the recommended target range. (See WARNINGS and PRECAUTIONS)

Pediatrics

In pediatric usage, the same dose and dosing regimen may be used as in adults although in several studies, children have required and tolerated higher doses than those used in adults.

Adjunct therapy with adrenal corticosteroids is recommended. Different tapering dosage schedules of prednisone appear to achieve similar results. A dosage schedule based on the patient's weight started with 2.0 mg/kg/day for the first 4 days tapered to 1.0 mg/kg/day by 1 week, 0.6 mg/kg/day by 2 weeks, 0.3 mg/kg/day by 1 month, and 0.15 mg/kg/day by 2 months and thereafter as a maintenance dose. Another center started with an initial dose of 200 mg tapered by 40 mg/day until reaching 20 mg/day. After 2 months at this dose, a further reduction to 10 mg/day was made. Adjustments in dosage of prednisone must be made according to the clinical situation.

To make Sandimmune® Oral Solution (cyclosporine oral solution, USP) more palatable, the oral solution may be diluted with milk, chocolate milk, or orange juice preferably at room temperature. Patients should avoid switching diluents frequently. Sandimmune® Soft Gelatin Capsules and Oral Solution should be administered on a consistent schedule with regard to time of day and relation to meals.

Take the prescribed amount of Sandimmune® (cyclosporine) from the container using the dosage syringe supplied after removal of the protective cover, and transfer the solution to a glass of milk, chocolate milk, or orange juice. Stir well and drink at once. Do not allow to stand before drinking. It is best to use a glass container and rinse it with more diluent to ensure that the total dose is taken. After use, replace the dosage syringe in the protective cover. Do not rinse the dosage syringe with water or other cleaning agents either before or after use. If the dosage syringe requires cleaning, it must be completely dry before resuming use. Introduction of water into the product by any means will cause variation in dose.

Sandimmune® Injection (cyclosporine injection, USP)
FOR INFUSION ONLY

Note: Anaphylactic reactions have occurred with Sandimmune® Injection (cyclosporine injection, USP). (See WARNINGS)

Patients unable to take Sandimmune® Soft Gelatin Capsules or Oral Solution pre- or postoperatively may be treated with the I.V. concentrate. **Sandimmune® Injection (cyclosporine injection, USP) is administered at 1/3 the oral dose.** The initial dose of Sandimmune® Injection (cyclosporine injection, USP) should be given 4-12 hours prior to transplantation as a single I.V. dose of 5-6 mg/kg/day. This daily single dose is continued postoperatively until the patient can tolerate the soft gelatin capsules or oral solution. Patients should be switched to Sandimmune® Soft Gelatin Capsules or Oral Solution as soon as possible after surgery. In pediatric usage, the same dose and dosing regimen may be used, although higher doses may be required.

Adjunct steroid therapy is to be used. (See aforementioned.)

Immediately before use, the I.V. concentrate should be diluted 1 mL Sandimmune® Injection (cyclosporine injection, USP) in 20 mL-100 mL 0.9% Sodium Chloride Injection or 5% Dextrose Injection and given in a slow intravenous infusion over approximately 2-6 hours.

Diluted infusion solutions should be discarded after 24 hours.

The Cremophor® EL (polyoxyethylated castor oil) contained in the concentrate for intravenous infusion can cause phthalate stripping from PVC.

Parenteral drug products should be inspected visually for particulate matter and discoloration prior to administration, whenever solution and container permit.

Blood Concentration Monitoring

Several study centers have found blood concentration monitoring of cyclosporine useful in patient management. While no fixed relationships have yet been established, in one series of 375 consecutive cadaveric renal transplant recipients, dosage was adjusted to achieve specific whole blood 24-hour trough concentrations of 100-200 ng/mL as determined by high-pressure liquid chromatography (HPLC).

Of major importance to blood concentration analysis is the type of assay used. The above concentrations are specific to the parent cyclosporine molecule and correlate directly to the new monoclonal specific radioimmunoassays (mRIA-sp). Nonspecific assays are also available which detect the parent compound molecule and various of its metabolites. Older studies often cited concentrations using a nonspecific assay which were roughly twice those of specific assays. Assay results are not interchangeable and their use should be guided by their approved labeling. If plasma specimens are employed, concentrations will vary with the temperature at the time of separation from whole blood. Plasma concentrations may range from 1/2-1/5 of whole blood concentrations. Refer to individual assay labeling for complete instructions. In addition, *Transplantation Proceedings* (June 1990) contains position papers and a broad consensus generated at the Cyclosporine-Therapeutic Drug Monitoring conference that year. Blood concentration monitoring is not a replacement for renal function monitoring or tissue biopsies.

HOW SUPPLIED

Sandimmune® Soft Gelatin Capsules (cyclosporine capsules, USP)

25 mg: Oblong, pink, branded "▲ 78/240". Unit dose packages of 30 capsules,

3 blister cards of 10 capsules ....NDC 0078-0240-15

100 mg: Oblong, dusty rose, branded "▲ 78/241". Unit dose packages of 30 capsules,

3 blister cards of 10 capsules ....NDC 0078-0241-15

Store and Dispense: Store at 25°C (77°F); excursions permitted to 15-30°C (59-86°F) [see USP Controlled Room Temperature].

An odor may be detected upon opening the unit dose container, which will dissipate shortly thereafter. This odor does not affect the quality of the product.

Sandimmune® Oral Solution (cyclosporine oral solution, USP)

Supplied in 50 mL bottles containing 100 mg of cyclosporine per mL NDC 0078-0110-22

A dosage syringe is provided for dispensing.

Store and Dispense: In the original container at temperatures below 30°C (86°F). Do not store in the refrigerator. Protect from freezing. Once opened, the contents must be used within 2 months.

Sandimmune® Injection (cyclosporine injection, USP)
FOR INTRAVENOUS INFUSION

Supplied as a 5 mL sterile ampul containing 50 mg of cyclosporine per mL,

in boxes of 10 ampuls ....NDC 0078-0109-01

Store and Dispense: At temperatures below 30°C (86°F). Protect from light.

FOR INFUSION ONLY

*Cremophor® is the registered trademark of BASF Aktiengesellschaft.

Distributed by:
Novartis Pharmaceuticals Corporation
East Hanover, New Jersey 07936
© Novartis
T2013-37
May 2013

SANDOSTATIN® ℞

[săn-dō-stă-tĭn]
octreotide acetate
Injection

The following prescribing information is based on official labeling in effect July 2013.

DESCRIPTION

Sandostatin® (octreotide acetate) Injection, a cyclic octapeptide prepared as a clear sterile solution of octreotide, acetate salt, in a buffered lactic acid solution for administration by deep subcutaneous (intrafat) or intravenous injection. Octreotide acetate, known chemically as L-Cysteinamide, D-phenylalanyl-L-cysteinyl-L-phenylalanyl-D-tryptophyl-L-lysyl-L-threonyl-N-[2-hydroxy-1-(hydroxymethyl)propyl]-, cyclic (2→7)-disulfide; [R-(R*, R*)] acetate salt, is a long-acting octapeptide with pharmacologic actions mimicking those of the natural hormone somatostatin.

Sandostatin Injection is available as: sterile 1-mL ampuls in 3 strengths, containing 50, 100, or 500 mcg octreotide (as acetate), and sterile 5-mL multi-dose vials in 2 strengths, containing 200 and 1000 mcg/mL of octreotide (as acetate).

Each ampul also contains:

lactic acid, USP	3.4 mg
mannitol, USP	45 mg
sodium bicarbonate, USP	qs to pH 4.2 ± 0.3
water for injection, USP	qs to 1 mL

Each mL of the multi-dose vials also contains:

lactic acid, USP	3.4 mg
mannitol, USP	45 mg
phenol, USP	5.0 mg
sodium bicarbonate, USP	qs to pH 4.2 ± 0.3
water for injection, USP	qs to 1 mL

Lactic acid and sodium bicarbonate are added to provide a buffered solution, pH to 4.2 ± 0.3.

The molecular weight of octreotide acetate is 1019.3 (free peptide, $C_{49}H_{66}N_{10}O_{10}S_2$) and its amino acid sequence is:

H-D-Phe-Cys-Phe-D-Trp-Lys-Thr-Cys-Thr-ol,
xCH_3COOH where x = 1.4 to 2.5

CLINICAL PHARMACOLOGY

Sandostatin® (octreotide acetate) exerts pharmacologic actions similar to the natural hormone, somatostatin. It is an even more potent inhibitor of growth hormone, glucagon, and insulin than somatostatin. Like somatostatin, it also suppresses LH response to GnRH, decreases splanchnic blood flow, and inhibits release of serotonin, gastrin, vasoactive intestinal peptide, secretin, motilin, and pancreatic polypeptide.

By virtue of these pharmacological actions, Sandostatin has been used to treat the symptoms associated with metastatic carcinoid tumors (flushing and diarrhea), and Vasoactive Intestinal Peptide (VIP) secreting adenomas (watery diarrhea).

Sandostatin substantially reduces growth hormone and/or IGF-I (somatomedin C) levels in patients with acromegaly.

Single doses of Sandostatin have been shown to inhibit gallbladder contractility and to decrease bile secretion in normal volunteers. In controlled clinical trials the incidence of gallstone or biliary sludge formation was markedly increased (*see WARNINGS*).

Sandostatin suppresses secretion of thyroid stimulating hormone (TSH).

Pharmacokinetics

After subcutaneous injection, octreotide is absorbed rapidly and completely from the injection site. Peak concentrations of 5.2 ng/mL (100-mcg dose) were reached 0.4 hours after dosing. Using a specific radioimmunoassay, intravenous and subcutaneous doses were found to be bioequivalent. Peak concentrations and area under the curve values were dose proportional after intravenous single doses up to 200 mcg and subcutaneous single doses up to 500 mcg and after subcutaneous multiple doses up to 500 mcg t.i.d. (1500 mcg/day).

In healthy volunteers the distribution of octreotide from plasma was rapid ($t\alpha 1/2$ = 0.2 h), the volume of distribution

(Vdss) was estimated to be 13.6 L, and the total body clearance ranged from 7 L/hr to 10 L/hr. In blood, the distribution into the erythrocytes was found to be negligible and about 65% was bound in the plasma in a concentration-independent manner. Binding was mainly to lipoprotein and, to a lesser extent, to albumin.

The elimination of octreotide from plasma had an apparent half-life of 1.7 to 1.9 hours compared with 1-3 minutes with the natural hormone. The duration of action of Sandostatin is variable but extends up to 12 hours depending upon the type of tumor. About 32% of the dose is excreted unchanged into the urine. In an elderly population, dose adjustments may be necessary due to a significant increase in the half-life (46%) and a significant decrease in the clearance (26%) of the drug.

In patients with acromegaly, the pharmacokinetics differ somewhat from those in healthy volunteers. A mean peak concentration of 2.8 ng/mL (100-mcg dose) was reached in 0.7 hours after subcutaneous dosing. The volume of distribution (Vdss) was estimated to be 21.6 ± 8.5 L and the total body clearance was increased to 18 L/h. The mean percent of the drug bound was 41.2%. The disposition and elimination half-lives were similar to normals.

In patients with renal impairment the elimination of octreotide from plasma was prolonged and total body clearance reduced. In mild renal impairment (Cl_{CR} 40-60 mL/min) octreotide $t_{1/2}$ was 2.4 hours and total body clearance was 8.8 L/hr, in moderate impairment (Cl_{CR} 10-39 mL/min) $t_{1/2}$ was 3.0 hours and total body clearance 7.3 L/hr, and in severely renally impaired patients not requiring dialysis (Cl_{CR} <10 mL/min) $t_{1/2}$ was 3.1 hours and total body clearance was 7.6 L/hr. In patients with severe renal failure requiring dialysis, total body clearance was reduced to about half that found in healthy subjects (from approximately 10 L/hr to 4.5 L/hr).

Patients with liver cirrhosis showed prolonged elimination of drug, with octreotide $t_{1/2}$ increasing to 3.7 hr and total body clearance decreasing to 5.9 L/hr, whereas patients with fatty liver disease showed $t_{1/2}$ increased to 3.4 hr and total body clearance of 8.2 L/hr.

INDICATIONS AND USAGE

Acromegaly

Sandostatin® (octreotide acetate) is indicated to reduce blood levels of growth hormone and IGF-I (somatomedin C) in acromegaly patients who have had inadequate response to or cannot be treated with surgical resection, pituitary irradiation, and bromocriptine mesylate at maximally tolerated doses. The goal is to achieve normalization of growth hormone and IGF-I (somatomedin C) levels (*see DOSAGE AND ADMINISTRATION*). In patients with acromegaly, Sandostatin reduces growth hormone to within normal ranges in 50% of patients and reduces IGF-I (somatomedin C) to within normal ranges in 50%-60% of patients. Since the effects of pituitary irradiation may not become maximal for several years, adjunctive therapy with Sandostatin to reduce blood levels of growth hormone and IGF-I (somatomedin C) offers potential benefit before the effects of irradiation are manifested.

Improvement in clinical signs and symptoms or reduction in tumor size or rate of growth were not shown in clinical trials performed with Sandostatin; these trials were not optimally designed to detect such effects.

Carcinoid Tumors

Sandostatin is indicated for the symptomatic treatment of patients with metastatic carcinoid tumors where it suppresses or inhibits the severe diarrhea and flushing episodes associated with the disease.

Sandostatin studies were not designed to show an effect on the size, rate of growth or development of metastases.

Vasoactive Intestinal Peptide Tumors (VIPomas)

Sandostatin is indicated for the treatment of the profuse watery diarrhea associated with VIP-secreting tumors. Sandostatin studies were not designed to show an effect on the size, rate of growth or development of metastases.

CONTRAINDICATIONS

Sensitivity to this drug or any of its components.

WARNINGS

Single doses of Sandostatin® (octreotide acetate) have been shown to inhibit gallbladder contractility and decrease bile secretion in normal volunteers. In clinical trials (primarily patients with acromegaly or psoriasis), the incidence of biliary tract abnormalities was 63% (27% gallstones, 24% sludge without stones, 12% biliary duct dilatation). The incidence of stones or sludge in patients who received Sandostatin for 12 months or longer was 52%. Less than 2% of patients treated with Sandostatin for 1 month or less developed gallstones. The incidence of gallstones did not appear related to age, sex or dose. Like patients without gallbladder abnormalities, the majority of patients developing gallbladder abnormalities on ultrasound had gastrointestinal symptoms. The symptoms were not specific for gallbladder disease. A few patients developed acute cholecystitis, ascending cholangitis, biliary obstruction, cholestatic hepatitis, or pancreatitis during Sandostatin therapy or following its withdrawal. One patient developed ascending cholangitis during Sandostatin therapy and died.

PRECAUTIONS

General

Sandostatin® (octreotide acetate) alters the balance between the counter-regulatory hormones, insulin, glucagon and growth hormone, which may result in hypoglycemia or hyperglycemia. Sandostatin also suppresses secretion of thyroid stimulating hormone, which may result in hypothyroidism. Cardiac conduction abnormalities have also occurred during treatment with Sandostatin. However, the incidence of these adverse events during long-term therapy was determined vigorously only in acromegaly patients who, due to their underlying disease and/or the subsequent treatment they receive, are at an increased risk for the development of diabetes mellitus, hypothyroidism, and cardiovascular disease. Although the degree to which these abnormalities are related to Sandostatin therapy is not clear, new abnormalities of glycemic control, thyroid function and ECG developed during Sandostatin therapy as described below.

Risk of Pregnancy with Normalization of IGF-1 and GH

Although acromegaly may lead to infertility, there are reports of pregnancy in acromegalic women. In women with active acromegaly who have been unable to become pregnant, normalization of GH and IGF-1 may restore fertility. Female patients of childbearing potential should be advised to use adequate contraception during treatment with octreotide.

The hypoglycemia or hyperglycemia which occurs during Sandostatin therapy is usually mild, but may result in overt diabetes mellitus or necessitate dose changes in insulin or other hypoglycemic agents. Hypoglycemia and hyperglycemia occurred on Sandostatin in 3% and 16% of acromegalic patients, respectively. Severe hyperglycemia, subsequent pneumonia, and death following initiation of Sandostatin therapy was reported in one patient with no history of hyperglycemia.

In patients with concomitant Type I diabetes mellitus, Sandostatin Injection and Sandostatin LAR® Depot (octreotide acetate for injectable suspension) are likely to affect glucose regulation, and insulin requirements may be reduced. Symptomatic hypoglycemia, which may be severe, has been reported in these patients. In non-diabetics and Type II diabetics with partially intact insulin reserves, Sandostatin Injection or Sandostatin LAR Depot administration may result in decreases in plasma insulin levels and hyperglycemia. It is therefore recommended that glucose tolerance and antidiabetic treatment be periodically monitored during therapy with these drugs.

In acromegalic patients, 12% developed biochemical hypothyroidism only, 8% developed goiter, and 4% required initiation of thyroid replacement therapy while receiving Sandostatin. Baseline and periodic assessment of thyroid function (TSH, total and/or free T_4) is recommended during chronic therapy.

In acromegalics, bradycardia (<50 bpm) developed in 25%; conduction abnormalities occurred in 10% and arrhythmias occurred in 9% of patients during Sandostatin therapy. Other EKG changes observed included QT prolongation, axis shifts, early repolarization, low voltage, R/S transition, and early R wave progression. These ECG changes are not uncommon in acromegalic patients. Dose adjustments in drugs such as beta-blockers that have bradycardia effects may be necessary. In one acromegalic patient with severe congestive heart failure, initiation of Sandostatin therapy resulted in worsening of CHF with improvement when drug was discontinued. Confirmation of a drug effect was obtained with a positive rechallenge.

Several cases of pancreatitis have been reported in patients receiving Sandostatin therapy.

Sandostatin may alter absorption of dietary fats in some patients.

In patients with severe renal failure requiring dialysis, the half-life of Sandostatin may be increased, necessitating adjustment of the maintenance dosage.

Depressed vitamin B_{12} levels and abnormal Schilling's tests have been observed in some patients receiving Sandostatin therapy, and monitoring of vitamin B_{12} levels is recommended during chronic Sandostatin therapy.

Information for Patients

Careful instruction in sterile subcutaneous injection technique should be given to the patients and to other persons who may administer Sandostatin Injection.

Laboratory Tests

Laboratory tests that may be helpful as biochemical markers in determining and following patient response depend on the specific tumor. Based on diagnosis, measurement of the following substances may be useful in monitoring the progress of therapy:

Acromegaly: Growth Hormone, IGF-I (somatomedin C)
Responsiveness to Sandostatin may be evaluated by determining growth hormone levels at 1-4 hour intervals for 8-12 hours post dose. Alternatively, a single measurement of IGF-I (somatomedin C) level may be made two weeks after drug initiation or dosage change.

Carcinoid: 5-HIAA (urinary 5-hydroxyindole acetic acid), plasma serotonin, plasma Substance P

VIPoma: VIP (plasma vasoactive intestinal peptide)

Baseline and periodic total and/or free T_4 measurements should be performed during chronic therapy (*see PRECAUTIONS – General*).

Drug Interactions

Sandostatin has been associated with alterations in nutrient absorption, so it may have an effect on absorption of orally administered drugs. Concomitant administration of Sandostatin with cyclosporine may decrease blood levels of cyclosporine and result in transplant rejection.

Patients receiving insulin, oral hypoglycemic agents, beta blockers, calcium channel blockers, or agents to control fluid and electrolyte balance, may require dose adjustments of these therapeutic agents.

Concomitant administration of octreotide and bromocriptine increases the availability of bromocriptine. Limited published data indicate that somatostatin analogs might decrease the metabolic clearance of compounds known to be metabolized by cytochrome P450 enzymes, which may be due to the suppression of growth hormones. Since it cannot be excluded that octreotide may have this effect, other drugs mainly metabolized by CYP3A4 and which have a low therapeutic index (e.g., quinidine, terfenadine) should therefore be used with caution.

Drug Laboratory Test Interactions

No known interference exists with clinical laboratory tests, including amine or peptide determinations.

Carcinogenesis/Mutagenesis/Impairment of Fertility

Studies in laboratory animals have demonstrated no mutagenic potential of Sandostatin.

No carcinogenic potential was demonstrated in mice treated subcutaneously for 85-99 weeks at doses up to 2000 mcg/kg/day (8× the human exposure based on body surface area). In a 116-week subcutaneous study in rats, a 27% and 12% incidence of injection site sarcomas or squamous cell carcinomas was observed in males and females, respectively, at the highest dose level of 1250 mcg/kg/day (10× the human exposure based on body surface area) compared to an incidence of 8%-10% in the vehicle-control groups. The increased incidence of injection site tumors was most probably caused by irritation and the high sensitivity of the rat to repeated subcutaneous injections at the same site. Rotating injection sites would prevent chronic irritation in humans. There have been no reports of injection site tumors in patients treated with Sandostatin for up to 5 years. There was also a 15% incidence of uterine adenocarcinomas in the 1250 mcg/kg/day females compared to 7% in the saline-control females and 0% in the vehicle-control females. The presence of endometritis coupled with the absence of corpora lutea, the reduction in mammary fibroadenomas, and the presence of uterine dilatation suggest that the uterine tumors were associated with estrogen dominance in the aged female rats which does not occur in humans.

Sandostatin did not impair fertility in rats at doses up to 1000 mcg/kg/day, which represents 7× the human exposure based on body surface area.

Pregnancy Category B

There are no adequate and well-controlled studies of octreotide use in pregnant women. Reproduction studies have been performed in rats and rabbits at doses up to 16 times the highest recommended human dose based on body surface area and revealed no evidence of harm to the fetus due to octreotide. However, because animal reproduction studies are not always predictive of human response, this drug should be used during pregnancy only if clearly needed.

In postmarketing data, a limited number of exposed pregnancies have been reported in patients with acromegaly. Most women were exposed to octreotide during the first trimester of pregnancy at doses ranging from 100-300 mcg/day of Sandostatin s.c. or 20-30 mg/month of Sandostatin LAR, however some women elected to continue octreotide therapy throughout pregnancy. In cases with a known outcome, no congenital malformations were reported.

Nursing Mothers

It is not known whether octreotide is excreted into human milk. Because many drugs are excreted in human milk, caution should be exercised when octreotide is administered to a nursing woman.

Pediatric Use

Safety and efficacy of Sandostatin Injection in the pediatric population have not been demonstrated.

No formal controlled clinical trials have been performed to evaluate the safety and effectiveness of Sandostatin in pediatric patients under age 6 years. In post-marketing reports, serious adverse events, including hypoxia, necrotizing enterocolitis, and death, have been reported with Sandostatin use in children, most notably in children under

2 years of age. The relationship of these events to octreotide has not been established as the majority of these pediatric patients had serious underlying co-morbid conditions.

The efficacy and safety of Sandostatin using the Sandostatin LAR Depot formulation was examined in a single randomized, double-blind, placebo-controlled, six–month pharmacokinetics study in 60 pediatric patients age 6-17 years with hypothalamic obesity resulting from cranial insult. The mean octreotide concentration after 6 doses of 40 mg Sandostatin LAR Depot administered by IM injection every four weeks was approximately 3 ng/ml. Steady-state concentrations was achieved after 3 injections of a 40 mg dose. Mean BMI increased 0.1 kg/m^2 in Sandostatin LAR Depot-treated subjects compared to 0.0 kg/m^2 in saline control-treated subjects. Efficacy was not demonstrated. Diarrhea occurred in 11 of 30 (37%) patients treated with Sandostatin LAR Depot. No unexpected adverse events were observed. However, with Sandostatin LAR Depot 40 mg once a month, the incidence of new cholelithiasis in this pediatric population (33%) was higher than that seen in other adults indications such as acromegaly (22%) or malignant carcinoid syndrome (24%), where Sandostatin LAR Depot was 10 to 30 mg once a month.

Geriatric Use

Clinical studies of Sandostatin did not include sufficient numbers of subjects aged 65 and over to determine whether they respond differently from younger subjects. Other reported clinical experience has not identified differences in responses between the elderly and younger patients. In general, dose selection for an elderly patient should be cautious, usually starting at the low end of the dosing range, reflecting the greater frequency of decreased hepatic, renal, or cardiac function, and of concomitant disease or other drug therapy.

ADVERSE REACTIONS

Gallbladder Abnormalities

Gallbladder abnormalities, especially stones and/or biliary sludge, frequently develop in patients on chronic Sandostatin® (octreotide acetate) therapy (*see WARNINGS*).

Cardiac

In acromegalics, sinus bradycardia (<50 bpm) developed in 25%; conduction abnormalities occurred in 10% and arrhythmias developed in 9% of patients during Sandostatin therapy (*see PRECAUTIONS – General*).

Gastrointestinal

Diarrhea, loose stools, nausea and abdominal discomfort were each seen in 34%-61% of acromegalic patients in U.S. studies although only 2.6% of the patients discontinued therapy due to these symptoms. These symptoms were seen in 5%-10% of patients with other disorders.

The frequency of these symptoms was not dose-related, but diarrhea and abdominal discomfort generally resolved more quickly in patients treated with 300 mcg/day than in those treated with 750 mcg/day. Vomiting, flatulence, abnormal stools, abdominal distention, and constipation were each seen in less than 10% of patients.

In rare instances, gastrointestinal side effects may resemble acute intestinal obstruction, with progressive abdominal distension, severe epigastric pain, abdominal tenderness and guarding.

Hypo/Hyperglycemia

Hypoglycemia and hyperglycemia occurred in 3% and 16% of acromegalic patients, respectively, but only in about 1.5% of other patients. Symptoms of hypoglycemia were noted in approximately 2% of patients.

Hypothyroidism

In acromegalics, biochemical hypothyroidism alone occurred in 12% while goiter occurred in 6% during Sandostatin therapy (*see PRECAUTIONS – General*). In patients without acromegaly, hypothyroidism has only been reported in several isolated patients and goiter has not been reported.

Other Adverse Events

Pain on injection was reported in 7.7%, headache in 6% and dizziness in 5%. Pancreatitis was also observed (*see WARNINGS and PRECAUTIONS*).

Other Adverse Events 1%-4%

Other events (relationship to drug not established), each observed in 1%-4% of patients, included fatigue, weakness, pruritus, joint pain, backache, urinary tract infection, cold symptoms, flu symptoms, injection site hematoma, bruise, edema, flushing, blurred vision, pollakiuria, fat malabsorption, hair loss, visual disturbance and depression.

Other Adverse Events <1%

Events reported in less than 1% of patients and for which relationship to drug is not established are listed: *Gastrointestinal:* hepatitis, jaundice, increase in liver enzymes, GI bleeding, hemorrhoids, appendicitis, gastric/peptic ulcer, gallbladder polyp; *Integumentary:* rash, cellulitis, petechiae, urticaria, basal cell carcinoma; *Musculoskeletal:* arthritis, joint effusion, muscle pain, Raynaud's phenomenon; *Cardiovascular:* chest pain, shortness of breath, thrombophlebitis, ischemia, congestive heart failure, hypertension, hypertensive reaction, palpitations, orthostatic BP decrease, tachycardia; *CNS:* anxiety, libido decrease, syncope, tremor, seizure, vertigo, Bell's Palsy, paranoia, pituitary apoplexy, increased intraocular pressure, amnesia, hearing loss, neuritis; *Respiratory:* pneumonia, pulmonary nodule, status asthmaticus; *Endocrine:* galactorrhea, hypoadrenalism, diabetes insipidus, gynecomastia, amenorrhea, polymenorrhea, oligomenorrhea, vaginitis; *Urogenital:* nephrolithiasis, hematuria; *Hematologic:* anemia, iron deficiency, epistaxis; *Miscellaneous:* otitis, allergic reaction, increased CK, weight loss.

Evaluation of 20 patients treated for at least 6 months has failed to demonstrate titers of antibodies exceeding background levels. However, antibody titers to Sandostatin were subsequently reported in three patients and resulted in prolonged duration of drug action in two patients. Anaphylactoid reactions, including anaphylactic shock, have been reported in several patients receiving Sandostatin.

Postmarketing Experience

The following adverse reactions have been identified during the postapproval use of Sandostatin. Because these reactions are reported voluntarily from a population of uncertain size, it is not always possible to reliably estimate their frequency or establish a causal relationship to drug exposure.

Gastrointestinal: intestinal obstruction
Hematologic: thrombocytopenia

OVERDOSAGE

A limited number of accidental overdoses of Sandostatin® in adults have been reported. In adults, the doses ranged from 2,400–6,000 micrograms/day administered by continuous infusion (100-250 micrograms/hour) or subcutaneously (1,500 micrograms t.i.d.). Adverse events in some patients included arrhythmia, hypotension, cardiac arrest, brain hypoxia, pancreatitis, hepatitis steatosis, hepatomegaly, lactic acidosis, flushing, diarrhea, lethargy, weakness, and weight loss.

Sandostatin Injection given in intravenous boluses of 1 mg (1000 mcg) to healthy volunteers did not result in serious ill effects, nor did doses of 30 mg (30,000 mcg) given intravenously over 20 minutes and of 120 mg (120,000 mcg) given intravenously over 8 hours to research patients.

If overdose occurs, symptomatic management is indicated. Up-to-date information about the treatment of overdose can often be obtained from the National Poison Control Center at 1-800-222-1222.

Drug Abuse and Dependence

There is no indication that Sandostatin has potential for drug abuse or dependence. Sandostatin levels in the central nervous system are negligible, even after doses up to 30,000 mcg.

DOSAGE AND ADMINISTRATION

Sandostatin® (octreotide acetate) may be administered subcutaneously or intravenously. Subcutaneous injection is the usual route of administration of Sandostatin for control of symptoms. Pain with subcutaneous administration may be reduced by using the smallest volume that will deliver the desired dose. Multiple subcutaneous injections at the same site within short periods of time should be avoided. Sites should be rotated in a systematic manner.

Parenteral drug products should be inspected visually for particulate matter and discoloration prior to administration. **Do not use if particulates and/or discoloration are observed.** Proper sterile technique should be used in the preparation of parenteral admixtures to minimize the possibility of microbial contamination. **Sandostatin is not compatible in Total Parenteral Nutrition (TPN) solutions because of the formation of a glycosyl octreotide conjugate which may decrease the efficacy of the product.**

Sandostatin is stable in sterile isotonic saline solutions or sterile solutions of dextrose 5% in water for 24 hours. It may be diluted in volumes of 50-200 mL and infused intravenously over 15-30 minutes or administered by IV push over 3 minutes. In emergency situations (e.g., carcinoid crisis) it may be given by rapid bolus.

The initial dosage is usually 50 mcg administered twice or three times daily. Upward dose titration is frequently required. Dosage information for patients with specific tumors follows.

Acromegaly

Dosage may be initiated at 50 mcg t.i.d. Beginning with this low dose may permit adaptation to adverse gastrointestinal effects for patients who will require higher doses. IGF-I (somatomedin C) levels every 2 weeks can be used to guide titration. Alternatively, multiple growth hormone levels at 0-8 hours after Sandostatin® (octreotide acetate) administration permit more rapid titration of dose. The goal is to achieve growth hormone levels less than 5 ng/mL or IGF-I (somatomedin C) levels less than 1.9 U/mL in males and less than 2.2 U/mL in females. The dose most commonly found to be effective is 100 mcg t.i.d., but some patients require up to 500 mcg t.i.d. for maximum effectiveness. Doses greater than 300 mcg/day seldom result in additional biochemical benefit, and if an increase in dose fails to provide additional benefit, the dose should be reduced. IGF-I (somatomedin C) or growth hormone levels should be reevaluated at 6-month intervals.

Sandostatin should be withdrawn yearly for approximately 4 weeks from patients who have received irradiation to assess disease activity. If growth hormone or IGF-I (somatomedin C) levels increase and signs and symptoms recur, Sandostatin therapy may be resumed.

Carcinoid Tumors

The suggested daily dosage of Sandostatin during the first 2 weeks of therapy ranges from 100-600 mcg/day in 2-4 divided doses (mean daily dosage is 300 mcg). In the clinical studies, the **median** daily maintenance dosage was approximately 450 mcg, but clinical and biochemical benefits were obtained in some patients with as little as 50 mcg, while others required doses up to 1500 mcg/day. However, experience with doses above 750 mcg/day is limited.

VIPomas

Daily dosages of 200-300 mcg in 2-4 divided doses are recommended during the initial 2 weeks of therapy (range 150-750 mcg) to control symptoms of the disease. On an individual basis, dosage may be adjusted to achieve a therapeutic response, but usually doses above 450 mcg/day are not required.

HOW SUPPLIED

Sandostatin® (octreotide acetate) Injection is available in 1-mL ampuls and 5-mL multi-dose vials as follows:

Ampuls

50 mcg/mL octreotide (as acetate)
Package of 10 ampuls NDC 0078-0180-01
100 mcg/mL octreotide (as acetate)
Package of 10 ampuls NDC 0078-0181-01
500 mcg/mL octreotide (as acetate)
Package of 10 ampuls NDC 0078-0182-01

Multi-Dose Vials

200 mcg/mL octreotide (as acetate)
Box of one NDC 0078-0183-25
1000 mcg/mL octreotide (as acetate)
Box of one NDC 0078-0184-25

Storage

For prolonged storage, Sandostatin ampuls and multi-dose vials should be stored at refrigerated temperatures 2°C-8°C (36°F-46°F) and store in outer carton in order to protect from light. At room temperature, (20°C-30°C or 70°F-86°F), Sandostatin is stable for 14 days if protected from light. The solution can be allowed to come to room temperature prior to administration. Do not warm artificially. After initial use, multiple-dose vials should be discarded within 14 days. Ampuls should be opened just prior to administration and the unused portion discarded. Dispose unused product or waste properly.

Manufactured by:
Novartis Pharma Stein AG
Stein, Switzerland
Distributed by:
Novartis Pharmaceuticals Corporation
East Hanover, NJ 07936
© Novartis
T2012-71
March 2012

Shown in Product Identification Guide, page 310

SANDOSTATIN® LAR DEPOT ℞

[*săn-dō-stă-tĭn*]
(octreotide acetate for injectable suspension)

The following prescribing information is based on official labeling in effect July 2013.

HIGHLIGHTS OF PRESCRIBING INFORMATION

These highlights do not include all the information needed to use Sandostatin LAR safely and effectively. See full prescribing information for Sandostatin LAR.

Sandostatin® LAR Depot (octreotide acetate for injectable suspension)

Initial U.S. Approval: 1988

INDICATIONS AND USAGE

Sandostatin LAR is a somatostatin analogue indicated for:
Treatment in patients who have responded to and tolerated Sandostatin Injection subcutaneous injection for:

- Acromegaly (1.1)
- Severe diarrhea/flushing episodes associated with metastatic carcinoid tumors (1.2)
- Profuse watery diarrhea associated with VIP-secreting tumors (1.3)

DOSAGE AND ADMINISTRATION

Patients not currently receiving Sandostatin Injection subcutaneously:

- Acromegaly: 50 mcg three times daily Sandostatin Injection subcutaneously for 2 weeks followed by Sandostatin LAR 20 mg intragluteally every 4 weeks for 3 months (2.1)
- Carcinoid Tumors and VIPomas: Sandostatin Injection subcutaneously 100-600 mcg/day in 2-4 divided doses for 2 weeks followed by Sandostatin LAR 20 mg every 4 weeks for 2 months (2.2)

Patients currently receiving Sandostatin Injection subcutaneously:

- Acromegaly: 20 mg every 4 weeks for 3 months (2.1)
- Carcinoid Tumors and VIPomas: 20 mg every 4 weeks for 2 months (2.2)

Renal Impairment, patients on dialysis: 10 mg every 4 weeks (2.3)

Hepatic Impairment, patients with cirrhosis: 10 mg every 4 weeks (2.4)

DOSAGE FORMS AND STRENGTHS

Vials: 10 mg per 5 mL, 20 mg per 5 mL or 30 mg per 5 mL (3)

CONTRAINDICATIONS

None (4)

WARNINGS AND PRECAUTIONS

- Gallbladder abnormalities may occur. Monitor periodically. (5.1)
- Glucose Metabolism: Hypoglycemia or hyperglycemia may occur. Glucose monitoring is recommended and antidiabetic treatment may need adjustment. (5.2)
- Thyroid Function: Hypothyroidism may occur. Monitor thyroid levels periodically. (5.3)
- Cardiac Function: Bradycardia, arrhythmia or conduction abnormalities may occur. Use with caution in at-risk patients. (5.4)

ADVERSE REACTIONS

The most common adverse reactions, occurring in ≥20% of patients are:

- Acromegaly: diarrhea, cholelithiasis, abdominal pain, flatulence (6.1)
- Carcinoid Syndrome: back pain, fatigue, headache, abdominal pain, nausea, dizziness (6.1)

To report SUSPECTED ADVERSE REACTIONS, contact Novartis Pharmaceuticals Corporation at 1-888-669-6682 or FDA at 1-800-FDA-1088 or www.fda.gov/medwatch.

DRUG INTERACTIONS

The following drugs require monitoring and possible dose adjustment when used with Sandostatin LAR: cyclosporine, insulin, oral hypoglycemic agents, beta-blockers, bromocriptine (7)

See 17 for PATIENT COUNSELING INFORMATION

Revised: 12/2011

FULL PRESCRIBING INFORMATION: CONTENTS*

*** Sections or subsections omitted from the full prescribing information are not listed**

FULL PRESCRIBING INFORMATION

1 INDICATIONS AND USAGE

Sandostatin LAR Depot 10 mg, 20 mg and 30 mg is indicated in patients in whom initial treatment with Sandostatin Injection has been shown to be effective and tolerated.

1.1 Acromegaly

Long-term maintenance therapy in acromegalic patients who have had an inadequate response to surgery and/or radiotherapy, or for whom surgery and/or radiotherapy is not an option. The goal of treatment in acromegaly is to reduce GH and IGF-1 levels to normal [*see Clinical Studies (14)* and *Dosage and Administration (2)*].

1.2 Carcinoid Tumors

Long-term treatment of the severe diarrhea and flushing episodes associated with metastatic carcinoid tumors.

1.3 Vasoactive Intestinal Peptide Tumors (VIPomas)

Long-term treatment of the profuse watery diarrhea associated with VIP-secreting tumors.

1.4 Important Limitations of Use

In patients with carcinoid syndrome and VIPomas, the effect of Sandostatin Injection and Sandostatin LAR Depot on tumor size, rate of growth and development of metastases, has not been determined.

2 DOSAGE AND ADMINISTRATION

- Sandostatin LAR Depot should be administered by a trained health care provider. It is important to closely follow the mixing instructions included in the packaging. Sandostatin LAR Depot must be administered immediately after mixing.
- **Do not directly inject diluent without preparing suspension.**
- The recommended needle size for administration of Sandostatin LAR Depot is the 1½" 19 gauge needle (supplied in the drug product kit). For patients with a greater skin to muscle depth, a 2" 19 gauge needle (not supplied) may be used.
- Sandostatin LAR Depot should be administered intramuscularly in the gluteal region at 4-week intervals. Administration of Sandostatin LAR Depot at intervals greater than 4 weeks is not recommended.
- Injection sites should be rotated in a systematic manner to avoid irritation. Deltoid injections should be avoided due to significant discomfort at the injection site when given in that area.
- **Sandostatin LAR Depot should never be administered intravenously or subcutaneously.**

The following dosage regimens are recommended.

2.1 Acromegaly

Patients Not Currently Receiving Octreotide Acetate

Patients not currently receiving octreotide acetate should begin therapy with Sandostatin Injection given subcutaneously in an initial dose of 50 mcg three times daily which may be titrated. Most patients require doses of 100 mcg to 200 mcg three times daily for maximum effect but some patients require up to 500 mcg three times daily.

Patients should be maintained on Sandostatin Injection subcutaneous for at least 2 weeks to determine tolerance to octreotide. Patients who are considered to be "responders" to the drug, based on GH and IGF-1 levels and who tolerate the drug can then be switched to Sandostatin LAR Depot in the dosage scheme described below (Patients Currently Receiving Sandostatin Injection).

Patients Currently Receiving Sandostatin Injection

Patients currently receiving Sandostatin Injection can be switched directly to Sandostatin LAR Depot in a dose of 20 mg given IM intragluteally at 4-week intervals for 3 months. After 3 months, dosage may be adjusted as follows:

- GH ≤2.5 ng/mL, IGF-1 normal and clinical symptoms controlled: maintain Sandostatin LAR Depot dosage at 20 mg every 4 weeks.
- GH >2.5 ng/mL, IGF-1 elevated, and/or clinical symptoms uncontrolled, increase Sandostatin LAR Depot dosage to 30 mg every 4 weeks.
- GH ≤1 ng/mL, IGF-1 normal and clinical symptoms controlled, reduce Sandostatin LAR Depot dosage to 10 mg every 4 weeks.
- If GH, IGF-1, or symptoms are not adequately controlled at a dose of 30 mg, the dose may be increased to 40 mg every 4 weeks. Doses higher than 40 mg are not recommended.

In patients who have received pituitary irradiation, Sandostatin LAR Depot should be withdrawn yearly for approximately 8 weeks to assess disease activity. If GH or IGF-1 levels increase and signs and symptoms recur, Sandostatin LAR Depot therapy may be resumed.

2.2 Carcinoid Tumors and VIPomas

Patients Not Currently Receiving Octreotide Acetate

Patients not currently receiving octreotide acetate should begin therapy with Sandostatin Injection given subcutaneously. The suggested daily dosage for carcinoid tumors during the first 2 weeks of therapy ranges from 100-600 mcg/day in 2-4 divided doses (mean daily dosage is 300 mcg). Some patients may require doses up to 1500 mcg/day. The suggested daily dosage for VIPomas is 200-300 mcg in 2-4 divided doses (range 150-750 mcg); dosage may be adjusted on an individual basis to control symptoms but usually doses above 450 mcg/day are not required.

Sandostatin Injection should be continued for at least 2 weeks. Thereafter, patients who are considered "responders" to octreotide acetate and who tolerate the drug may be switched to Sandostatin LAR Depot in the dosage regimen as described below (Patients Currently Receiving Sandostatin Injection).

Patients Currently Receiving Sandostatin Injection

Patients currently receiving Sandostatin Injection can be switched to Sandostatin LAR Depot in a dosage of 20 mg given IM intragluteally at 4-week intervals for 2 months. Because of the need for serum octreotide to reach therapeutically effective levels following initial injection of Sandostatin LAR Depot, carcinoid tumor and VIPoma patients should continue to receive Sandostatin Injection subcutaneously for at least 2 weeks in the same dosage they were taking before the switch. Failure to continue subcutaneous injections for this period may result in exacerbation of symptoms. (Some patients may require 3 or 4 weeks of such therapy.)

After 2 months, dosage may be adjusted as follows:

- If symptoms are adequately controlled, consider a dose reduction to 10 mg for a trial period. If symptoms recur, dosage should then be increased to 20 mg every 4 weeks. Many patients can, however, be satisfactorily maintained at a 10-mg dosage every 4 weeks.
- If symptoms are not adequately controlled, increase Sandostatin LAR Depot to 30 mg every 4 weeks if symptoms are not adequately controlled. Patients who achieve good control on a 20-mg dose may have their dose lowered to 10 mg for a trial period. If symptoms recur, dosage should then be increased to 20 mg every 4 weeks.
- Dosages higher than 30 mg are not recommended.

Despite good overall control of symptoms, patients with carcinoid tumors and VIPomas often experience periodic exacerbation of symptoms (regardless of whether they are being maintained on Sandostatin Injection or Sandostatin LAR Depot). During these periods they may be given Sandostatin Injection subcutaneously for a few days at the dosage they were receiving prior to switching to Sandostatin LAR Depot. When symptoms are again controlled, the Sandostatin Injection subcutaneous can be discontinued.

2.3 Special Populations: Renal Impairment

In patients with renal failure requiring dialysis, the starting dose should be 10 mg every 4 weeks. In other patients with renal impairment, the starting dose should be similar to a nonrenal patient (i.e., 20 mg every 4 weeks) [*see Clinical Pharmacology (12)*].

2.4 Special Populations: Hepatic Impairment – Cirrhotic Patients

In patients with established cirrhosis of the liver, the starting dose should be 10 mg every 4 weeks [*see Clinical Pharmacology (12)*].

3 DOSAGE FORMS AND STRENGTHS

Sandostatin LAR Depot is available in single-use kits containing a 5-mL vial of 10 mg, 20 mg, or 30 mg strength, a syringe containing 2.5 mL of diluent, two sterile 1½" 19 gauge needles, and two alcohol wipes. An instruction booklet for the preparation of drug suspension for injection is also included with each kit.

4 CONTRAINDICATIONS

None

5 WARNINGS AND PRECAUTIONS

5.1 Cholelithiasis and Gallbladder Sludge

Sandostatin may inhibit gallbladder contractility and decrease bile secretion, which may lead to gallbladder abnormalities or sludge. Patients should be monitored periodically [*see Adverse Reactions (6)*].

5.2 Hyperglycemia and Hypoglycemia

Octreotide alters the balance between the counter-regulatory hormones, insulin, glucagon, and growth hormone, which may result in hypoglycemia or hyperglycemia. Blood glucose levels should be monitored when Sandostatin LAR treatment is initiated, or when the dose is altered. Antidiabetic treatment should be adjusted accordingly [*see Adverse Reactions (6)*].

5.3 Thyroid Function Abnormalities

Octreotide suppresses the secretion of thyroid-stimulating hormone, which may result in hypothyroidism. Baseline and periodic assessment of thyroid function (TSH, total and/or free T_4) is recommended during chronic octreotide therapy [*see Adverse Reactions (6)*].

5.4 Cardiac Function Abnormalities

In both acromegalic and carcinoid syndrome patients, bradycardia, arrhythmias and conduction abnormalities have been reported during octreotide therapy. Other EKG changes were observed such as QT prolongation, axis shifts, early repolarization, low voltage, R/S transition, early R wave progression, and nonspecific ST-T wave changes. The relationship of these events to octreotide acetate is not established because many of these patients have underlying cardiac disease. Dose adjustments in drugs such as beta-blockers that have bradycardia effects may be necessary. In one acromegalic patient with severe congestive heart failure, initiation of Sandostatin Injection therapy resulted in worsening of CHF with improvement when drug was discontinued. Confirmation of a drug effect was obtained with a positive rechallenge [*see Adverse Reactions (6)*].

5.5 Nutrition

Octreotide may alter absorption of dietary fats.

Depressed vitamin B_{12} levels and abnormal Schilling tests have been observed in some patients receiving octreotide therapy, and monitoring of vitamin B_{12} levels is recommended during therapy with Sandostatin LAR Depot.

Octreotide has been investigated for the reduction of excessive fluid loss from the G.I. tract in patients with conditions producing such a loss. If such patients are receiving total parenteral nutrition (TPN), serum zinc may rise excessively when the fluid loss is reversed. Patients on TPN and octreotide should have periodic monitoring of zinc levels.

5.6 Monitoring: Laboratory Tests

Laboratory tests that may be helpful as biochemical markers in determining and following patient response depend on the specific tumor. Based on diagnosis, measurement of the following substances may be useful in monitoring the progress of therapy [*see Dosage and Administration (2.0)*].

Acromegaly: Growth Hormone, IGF-1 (somatomedin C)

Carcinoid: 5-HIAA (urinary 5-hydroxyindole acetic acid), plasma serotonin, plasma Substance P

VIPoma: VIP (plasma vasoactive intestinal peptide) baseline and periodic total and/or free T_4 measurements should be performed during chronic therapy

5.7 Drug Interactions

Octreotide has been associated with alterations in nutrient absorption, so it may have an effect on absorption of orally administered drugs. Concomitant administration of octreotide injection with cyclosporine may decrease blood levels of cyclosporine [*see Drug Interactions (7.2)*].

6 ADVERSE REACTIONS

6.1 Clinical Studies Experience

Because clinical trials are conducted under widely varying conditions, adverse reaction rates observed in the clinical trials of a drug cannot be directly compared to rates in the clinical trial of another drug and may not reflect the rates observed in practice.

Acromegaly

The safety of Sandostatin LAR in the treatment of acromegaly has been evaluated in three phase 3 studies in 261 patients, including 209 exposed for 48 weeks and 96 exposed for greater than 108 weeks. Sandostatin LAR was studied primarily in a double-blind, cross-over manner. Patients on subcutaneous Sandostatin Injection were switched to the LAR formulation followed by an open-label extension. The population age range was 14-81 years old and 53% were female. Approximately 35% of these acromegaly patients had not been treated with surgery and/or radiation. Most patients received a starting dose of 20 mg every 4 weeks intramuscularly. Dose was up or down titrated based on efficacy and tolerability to a final dose between 10-60 mg every 4 weeks. Table 1 below reflects adverse events from these studies regardless of presumed causality to study drug.

Table 1. Adverse Events Occurring in ≥10% of Acromegalic Patients in the Phase 3 Studies

WHO Preferred Term	Phase 3 Studies (Pooled) Number (%) of Subjects with AE's 10 mg/20 mg/30 mg (n=261) n (%)
Diarrhea	93 (35.6)
Abdominal Pain	75 (28.7)
Flatulence	66 (25.3)
Influenza-Like Symptoms	52 (19.9)
Constipation	46 (17.6)
Headache	40 (15.3)
Anemia	40 (15.3)
Injection Site Pain	36 (13.8)
Cholelithiasis	35 (13.4)
Hypertension	33 (12.6)
Dizziness	30 (11.5)
Fatigue	29 (11.1)

The safety of Sandostatin LAR in the treatment of acromegaly was also evaluated in a postmarketing randomized phase 4 study. 104 patients were randomized to either pituitary surgery or 20 mg of Sandostatin LAR. All the patients were treatment naïve ('de novo'). Crossover was allowed according to treatment response and a total of 76 patients were exposed to Sandostatin LAR. Approximately half of the patients initially randomized to Sandostatin LAR were exposed to Sandostatin LAR up to 1 year. The population age range was between 20-76 years old and 45% were female, 93% were Caucasian, and 1% Black. The majority of these patients were exposed to 30 mg every 4 weeks. Table 2 below reflects the adverse events occurring in this study regardless of presumed causality to study drug.

Table 2. Adverse Events Occurring in ≥10% of Acromegalic Patients in Phase 4 Study

WHO Preferred Term	Phase 4 Study SAS LAR N=76 n (%)	Phase 4 Study Surgery N=64 n (%)
Diarrhea	36 (47.4)	2 (3.1)
Cholelithiasis	29 (38.2)	3 (4.7)
Abdominal Pain	19 (25.0)	2 (3.1)
Nausea	12 (15.8)	5 (7.8)
Alopecia	10 (13.2)	5 (7.8)
Injection Site Pain	9 (11.8)	0
Abdominal Pain Upper	8 (10.5)	0
Headache	8 (10.5)	6 (9.4)
Epistaxis	0	7 (10.9)

Gallbladder Abnormalities

Single doses of Sandostatin Injection have been shown to inhibit gallbladder contractility and decrease bile secretion in normal volunteers. In clinical trials with Sandostatin Injection (primarily patients with acromegaly or psoriasis) in patients who had not previously received octreotide, the incidence of biliary tract abnormalities was 63% (27% gallstones, 24% sludge without stones, 12% biliary duct dilatation). The incidence of stones or sludge in patients who received Sandostatin Injection for 12 months or longer was 52%. The incidence of gallbladder abnormalities did not appear to be related to age, sex, or dose but was related to duration of exposure.

In clinical trials 52% of acromegalic patients, most of whom received Sandostatin LAR Depot for 12 months or longer, developed new biliary abnormalities including gallstones, microlithiasis, sediment, sludge, and dilatation. The incidence of new cholelithiasis was 22%, of which 7% were microstones.

Across all trials, a few patients developed acute cholecystitis, ascending cholangitis, biliary obstruction, cholestatic hepatitis, or pancreatitis during octreotide therapy or following its withdrawal. One patient developed ascending cholangitis during Sandostatin Injection therapy and died. Despite the high incidence of new gallstones in patients receiving octreotide, 1% of patients developed acute symptoms requiring cholecystectomy.

Glucose Metabolism - Hypoglycemia/Hyperglycemia

In acromegaly patients treated with either Sandostatin Injection or Sandostatin LAR Depot, hypoglycemia occurred in approximately 2% and hyperglycemia in approximately 15% of patients [*see Warnings and Precautions (5)*].

Hypothyroidism

In acromegaly patients receiving Sandostatin Injection, 12% developed biochemical hypothyroidism, 8% developed goiter, and 4% required initiation of thyroid replacement therapy while receiving Sandostatin Injection. In acromegalics treated with Sandostatin LAR Depot, hypothyroidism was reported as an adverse event in 2% and goiter in 2%. Two patients receiving Sandostatin LAR Depot required initiation of thyroid hormone replacement therapy [*see Warnings and Precautions (5)*].

Cardiac

In acromegalics, sinus bradycardia (<50 bpm) developed in 25%; conduction abnormalities occurred in 10% and arrhythmias developed in 9% of patients during Sandostatin Injection therapy. The relationship of these events to octreotide acetate is not established because many of these patients have underlying cardiac disease [*see Warnings and Precautions (5)*].

Gastrointestinal

The most common symptoms are gastrointestinal. The overall incidence of the most frequent of these symptoms in clinical trials of acromegalic patients treated for approximately 1 to 4 years is shown in Table 3.

[See table 3 below]

Only 2.6% of the patients on Sandostatin Injection in U.S. clinical trials discontinued therapy due to these symptoms. No acromegalic patient receiving Sandostatin LAR Depot discontinued therapy for a G.I. event.

In patients receiving Sandostatin LAR Depot, the incidence of diarrhea was dose related. Diarrhea, abdominal pain, and nausea developed primarily during the first month of treatment with Sandostatin LAR Depot. Thereafter, new cases of these events were uncommon. The vast majority of these events were mild-to-moderate in severity.

In rare instances, gastrointestinal adverse effects may resemble acute intestinal obstruction, with progressive abdominal distention, severe epigastric pain, abdominal tenderness, and guarding.

Dyspepsia, steatorrhea, discoloration of feces, and tenesmus were reported in 4%-6% of patients.

In a clinical trial of carcinoid syndrome, nausea, abdominal pain, and flatulence were reported in 27%-38% and constipation or vomiting in 15%-21% of patients treated with Sandostatin LAR Depot. Diarrhea was reported as an adverse event in 14% of patients but since most of the patients had diarrhea as a symptom of carcinoid syndrome, it is difficult to assess the actual incidence of drug-related diarrhea.

Pain at the Injection Site

Pain on injection, which is generally mild-to-moderate, and short-lived (usually about 1 hour) is dose related, being reported by 2%, 9%, and 11% of acromegalics receiving doses of 10 mg, 20 mg, and 30 mg, respectively, of Sandostatin LAR Depot. In carcinoid patients, where a diary was kept, pain at the injection site was reported by about 20%-25% at a 10-mg dose and about 30%-50% at the 20-mg and 30-mg dose.

Antibodies to Octreotide

Studies to date have shown that antibodies to octreotide develop in up to 25% of patients treated with octreotide acetate. These antibodies do not influence the degree of efficacy response to octreotide; however, in two acromegalic patients who received Sandostatin Injection, the duration of GH suppression following each injection was about twice as long as in patients without antibodies. It has not been determined whether octreotide antibodies will also prolong the duration of GH suppression in patients being treated with Sandostatin LAR Depot.

Carcinoid and VIPomas

The safety of Sandostatin LAR in the treatment of carcinoid tumors and VIPomas has been evaluated in one phase 3 study. Study 1 randomized 93 patients with carcinoid syndrome to Sandostatin LAR 10 mg, 20 mg, or 30 mg in a blind fashion or to open-label Sandostatin Injection subcutaneously. The population age range was between 25-78 years old and 44% were female, 95% were Caucasian and 3% Black. All the patients had symptom control on their previous Sandostatin subcutaneous treatment. 80 patients finished the initial 24 weeks of Sandostatin exposure in Study 1. In Study 1, comparable numbers of patients were randomized to each dose. Table 4 below reflects the adverse events occurring in >15% of patients regardless of presumed causality to study drug.

Table 3. Number (%) of Acromegalic Patients with Common G.I. Adverse Events

Adverse Event	Sandostatin Injection S.C. Three Times Daily n=114		Sandostatin LAR Depot Every 28 Days n=261	
	n	%	n	%
Diarrhea	66	(57.9)	95	(36.4)
Abdominal Pain or Discomfort	50	(43.9)	76	(29.1)
Nausea	34	(29.8)	27	(10.3)
Flatulence	15	(13.2)	67	(25.7)
Constipation	10	(8.8)	49	(18.8)
Vomiting	5	(4.4)	17	(6.5)

[See table 4 at right]

Gallbladder Abnormalities

In clinical trials, 62% of malignant carcinoid patients who received Sandostatin LAR Depot for up to 18 months developed new biliary abnormalities including jaundice, gallstones, sludge, and dilatation. New gallstones occurred in a total of 24% of patients.

Glucose Metabolism - Hypoglycemia/Hyperglycemia

In carcinoid patients, hypoglycemia occurred in 4% and hyperglycemia in 27% of patients treated with Sandostatin LAR Depot [*see Warnings and Precautions (5)*].

Hypothyroidism

In carcinoid patients, hypothyroidism has only been reported in isolated patients and goiter has not been reported [*see Warnings and Precautions (5)*].

Cardiac

Electrocardiograms were performed only in carcinoid patients receiving Sandostatin LAR Depot. In carcinoid syndrome patients, sinus bradycardia developed in 19%, conduction abnormalities occurred in 9%, and arrhythmias developed in 3%. The relationship of these events to octreotide acetate is not established because many of these patients have underlying cardiac disease [*see Warnings and Precautions (5)*].

Other Clinical Studies Adverse Events

Other clinically significant adverse events (relationship to drug not established) in acromegalic and/or carcinoid syndrome patients receiving Sandostatin LAR Depot were malignant hyperpyrexia, cerebral vascular disorder, rectal bleeding, ascites, pulmonary embolism, pneumonia and pleural effusion.

6.2 Postmarketing Experience

The following adverse reactions have been identified during the postapproval use of Sandostatin. Because these reactions are reported voluntarily from a population of uncertain size, it is not always possible to reliably estimate their frequency or establish a causal relationship to drug exposure.

Myocardial infarction has been observed in the postmarketing setting, mainly in patients with cardiovascular risk factors. Hypoadrenalism has been reported in some reports in patients 18 months of age and under.

Additional events reported in the postmarketing setting include anaphylactoid reactions, including anaphylactic shock, cardiac arrest, renal failure, renal insufficiency, convulsions, atrial fibrillation, aneurysm, hepatitis, increased liver enzymes, gastrointestinal hemorrhage, pancreatitis, pancytopenia, thrombocytopenia, arterial thrombosis of the arm, retinal vein thrombosis, intracranial hemorrhage, hemiparesis, paresis, deafness, visual field defect, aphasia, scotoma, status asthmaticus, pulmonary hypertension, diabetes mellitus, intestinal obstruction, peptic/gastric ulcer, appendicitis, creatinine increased, CK increased, arthritis, joint effusion, pituitary apoplexy, breast carcinoma, suicide attempt, paranoia, migraines, urticaria, facial edema, generalized edema, hematuria, orthostatic hypotension, Raynaud's syndrome, glaucoma, pulmonary nodule, pneumothorax aggravated, cellulitis, Bell's palsy, diabetes insipidus, gynecomastia, galactorrhea, gallbladder polyp, fatty liver, abdomen enlarged, libido decrease, and petechiae.

7 DRUG INTERACTIONS

7.1 Cyclosporine

Concomitant administration of octreotide injection with cyclosporine may decrease blood levels of cyclosporine and result in transplant rejection.

7.2 Insulin and Oral Hypoglycemic Drugs

Octreotide inhibits the secretion of insulin and glucagon. Therefore, blood glucose levels should be monitored when Sandostatin LAR treatment is initiated or when the dose is altered and antidiabetic treatment should be adjusted accordingly.

7.3 Bromocriptine

Concomitant administration of octreotide and bromocriptine increases the availability of bromocriptine.

7.4 Other Concomitant Drug Therapy

Concomitant administration of bradycardia-inducing drugs (e.g., beta-blockers) may have an additive effect on the reduction of heart rate associated with octreotide. Dose adjustments of concomitant medication may be necessary.

Octreotide has been associated with alterations in nutrient absorption, so it may have an effect on absorption of orally administered drugs.

7.5 Drug Metabolism Interactions

Limited published data indicate that somatostatin analogs may decrease the metabolic clearance of compounds known to be metabolized by cytochrome P450 enzymes, which may be due to the suppression of growth hormone. Since it cannot be excluded that octreotide may have this effect, other drugs mainly metabolized by CYP3A4 and which have a low therapeutic index (e.g., quinidine, terfenadine) should therefore be used with caution.

Table 4. Adverse Events Occurring in ≥15% of Carcinoid Tumor and VIPoma Patients in Study 1

	Number (%) of Subjects with AE's (n=93)			
WHO Preferred Term	**Sc N=26**	**10 mg N=22**	**20 mg N=20**	**30 mg N=25**
Abdominal Pain	8 (30.8)	8 (35.4)	2 (10.0)	5 (20.0)
Arthropathy	5 (19.2)	2 (9.1)	3 (15.0)	2 (8.0)
Back Pain	7 (26.9)	6 (27.3)	2 (10.0)	2 (8.0)
Dizziness	4 (15.4)	4 (18.2)	4 (20.0)	5 (20.0)
Fatigue	3 (11.5)	7 (31.8)	2 (10.0)	2 (8.0)
Flatulence	3 (11.5)	2 (9.1)	2 (10.0)	4 (16.0)
Generalized Pain	4 (15.4)	2 (9.1)	3 (15.0)	1 (4.0)
Headache	5 (19.2)	4 (18.2)	6 (30.0)	4 (16.0)
Musculoskeletal Pain	4 (15.4)	0	1 (5.0)	0
Myalgia	0	4 (18.2)	1 (5.0)	1 (4.0)
Nausea	8 (30.8)	9 (40.9)	6 (30.0)	6 (24.0)
Pruritus	0	4 (18.2)	0	0
Rash	1 (3.8)	0	3 (15.0)	0
Sinusitis	4 (15.4)	0	1 (5.0)	3 (12.0)
URTI	6 (23.1)	4 (18.2)	2 (10.0)	3 (12.0)
Vomiting	3 (11.5)	0	0	4 (16.0)

8 USE IN SPECIFIC POPULATIONS

8.1 Pregnancy

Pregnancy Category B

There are no adequate and well-controlled studies in pregnant women. Reproduction studies have been performed in rats and rabbits at doses up to 16× the highest recommended human dose and have revealed no evidence of harm to the fetus due to octreotide. However, because animal reproduction studies are not always predictive of human response, this drug should be used during pregnancy only if clearly needed [*see Nonclinical Toxicology (13.2)*].

8.3 Nursing Mothers

It is not known whether octreotide is excreted into human milk. Because many drugs are excreted in human milk, caution should be exercised when Sandostatin LAR Depot is administered to a nursing woman.

8.4 Pediatric Use

Safety and efficacy of Sandostatin LAR Depot in the pediatric population have not been demonstrated.

No formal controlled clinical trials have been performed to evaluate the safety and effectiveness of Sandostatin LAR Depot in pediatric patients under 6 years of age. In postmarketing reports, serious adverse events, including hypoxia, necrotizing enterocolitis, and death, have been reported with Sandostatin use in children, most notably in children under 2 years of age. The relationship of these events to octreotide has not been established as the majority of these pediatric patients had serious underlying co-morbid conditions.

The efficacy and safety of Sandostatin LAR Depot was examined in a single randomized, double-blind, placebo-controlled, six-month pharmacokinetics study in 60 pediatric patients age 6-17 years with hypothalamic obesity resulting from cranial insult. The mean octreotide concentration after 6 doses of 40 mg Sandostatin LAR Depot administered by IM injection every four weeks was approximately 3 ng/mL. Steady-state concentrations was achieved after 3 injections of a 40 mg dose. Mean BMI increased 0.1 kg/m^2 in Sandostatin LAR Depot-treated subjects compared to 0.0 kg/m^2 in saline control-treated subjects. Efficacy was not demonstrated. Diarrhea occurred in 11 of 30 (37%) patients treated with Sandostatin LAR Depot. No unexpected adverse events were observed. However, with Sandostatin LAR Depot 40 mg once a month, the incidence of new cholelithiasis in this pediatric population (33%) was higher than that seen in other adult indications such as acromegaly (22%) or malignant carcinoid syndrome (24%), where Sandostatin LAR Depot was 10 to 30 mg once a month.

8.5 Geriatric Use

Clinical studies of Sandostatin did not include sufficient numbers of subjects age 65 and over to determine whether they respond differently from younger subjects. Other reported clinical experience has not identified differences in responses between the elderly and younger patients. In general, dose selection for an elderly patient should be cautious, usually starting at the low end of the dosing range, reflecting the greater frequency of decreased hepatic, renal, or cardiac function, and of concomitant disease or other drug therapy.

8.6 Renal Impairment

In patients with renal failure requiring dialysis, the starting dose should be 10 mg. This dose should be up titrated based on clinical response and speed of response as deemed necessary by the physician. In patients with mild, moderate, or severe renal impairment there is no need to adjust the starting dose of Sandostatin. The maintenance dose should be adjusted thereafter based on clinical response and tolerability as in nonrenal patients [*see Clinical Pharmacology (12)*].

8.7 Hepatic Impairment - Cirrhotic Patients

In patients with established liver cirrhosis, the starting dose should be 10 mg. This dose should be up titrated based on clinical response and speed of response as deemed necessary by the physician. Once at a higher dose, patient should be maintained or dose adjusted based on response and tolerability as in any noncirrhotic patients [*see Clinical Pharmacology (12)*].

10 OVERDOSAGE

No frank overdose has occurred in any patient to date. Sandostatin Injection given in intravenous bolus doses of 1 mg (1000 mcg) to healthy volunteers did not result in serious ill effects, nor did doses of 30 mg (30,000 mcg) given intravenously over 20 minutes and of 120 mg (120,000 mcg) given intravenously over 8 hours to research patients. Doses of 2.5 mg (2500 mcg) of Sandostatin Injection subcutaneously have, however, caused hypoglycemia, flushing, dizziness, and nausea.

Up-to-date information about the treatment of overdose can often be obtained from a certified Regional Poison Control Center. Telephone numbers of certified Regional Poison Control Centers are listed in the Physicians' Desk Reference®**.

Mortality occurred in mice and rats given 72 mg/kg and 18 mg/kg intravenously, respectively, of octreotide.

**Trademark of PDR Network.

11 DESCRIPTION

Octreotide is the acetate salt of a cyclic octapeptide. It is a long-acting octapeptide with pharmacologic properties mimicking those of the natural hormone somatostatin. Octreotide is known chemically as L-Cysteinamide, D-phenylalanyl-L-cysteinyl-L-phenylalanyl-D-tryptophyl-L-lysyl-L-threonyl-N-[2-hydroxy-1- (hydroxy-methyl) propyl]-, cyclic (2→7)-disulfide; [R-(R*,R*)].

Sandostatin LAR Depot is available in a vial containing the sterile drug product, which when mixed with diluent, becomes a suspension that is given as a monthly intragluteal injection. The octreotide is uniformly distributed within the microspheres which are made of a biodegradable glucose star polymer, D,L-lactic and glycolic acids copolymer. Sterile mannitol is added to the microspheres to improve suspendability.

Sandostatin LAR Depot is available as: sterile 5-mL vials in 3 strengths delivering 10 mg, 20 mg, or 30 mg octreotide-free peptide. Each vial of Sandostatin LAR Depot delivers:

Name of Ingredient	10 mg	20 mg	30 mg
octreotide acetate	11.2 mg*	22.4 mg*	33.6 mg*
D, L-lactic and glycolic acids copolymer	188.8 mg	377.6 mg	566.4 mg
mannitol	41.0 mg	81.9 mg	122.9 mg

*Equivalent to 10/20/30 mg octreotide base.

Each syringe of diluent contains:

carboxymethylcellulose sodium	12.5 mg
mannitol	15.0 mg
water for injection	2.5 mL

The molecular weight of octreotide is 1019.3 (free peptide, $C_{49}H_{66}N_{10}O_{10}S_2$) and its amino acid sequence is

Table 5. Hormonal Response in Acromegalic Patients Receiving 27 to 28 Injections During[1] Treatment with Sandostatin LAR Depot

Mean Hormone Level	Sandostatin Injection S.C.		Sandostatin LAR Depot	
	n	%	n	%
GH <5.0 ng/mL	69/88	78	73/88	83
<2.5 ng/mL	44/88	50	41/88	47
<1.0 ng/mL	6/88	7	10/88	11
IGF-1 normalized	36/88	41	45/88	51
GH <5.0 ng/mL + IGF-1 normalized	36/88	41	45/88	51
<2.5 ng/mL + IGF-1 normalized	30/88	34	37/88	42
<1.0 ng/mL + IGF-1 normalized	5/88	6	10/88	11

[1]Average of monthly levels of GH and IGF-1 over the course of the trials

H-D-Phe-Cys-Phe-D-Trp-Lys-Thr-Cys-Thr-ol•xCH_3COOH
where x = 1.4 to 2.5

12 CLINICAL PHARMACOLOGY

Sandostatin LAR Depot is a long-acting dosage form consisting of microspheres of the biodegradable glucose star polymer, D,L-lactic and glycolic acids copolymer, containing octreotide. It maintains all of the clinical and pharmacological characteristics of the immediate-release dosage form Sandostatin Injection with the added feature of slow release of octreotide from the site of injection, reducing the need for frequent administration. This slow release occurs as the polymer biodegrades, primarily through hydrolysis. Sandostatin LAR Depot is designed to be injected intramuscularly (intragluteally) once every 4 weeks.

12.1 Mechanism of Action

Octreotide exerts pharmacologic actions similar to the natural hormone, somatostatin. It is an even more potent inhibitor of growth hormone, glucagon, and insulin than somatostatin. Like somatostatin, it also suppresses LH response to GnRH, decreases splanchnic blood flow, and inhibits release of serotonin, gastrin, vasoactive intestinal peptide, secretin, motilin, and pancreatic polypeptide.

By virtue of these pharmacological actions, octreotide has been used to treat the symptoms associated with metastatic carcinoid tumors (flushing and diarrhea), and Vasoactive Intestinal Peptide (VIP) secreting adenomas (watery diarrhea).

12.2 Pharmacodynamics

Octreotide substantially reduces and in many cases can normalize growth hormone and/or IGF-1 (somatomedin C) levels in patients with acromegaly.

Single doses of Sandostatin Injection given subcutaneously have been shown to inhibit gallbladder contractility and to decrease bile secretion in normal volunteers. In controlled clinical trials, the incidence of gallstone or biliary sludge formation was markedly increased [*see Warnings and Precautions (5)*].

Octreotide may cause clinically significant suppression of thyroid-stimulating hormone (TSH).

12.3 Pharmacokinetics

Sandostatin Injection

According to data obtained with the immediate-release formulation, Sandostatin Injection solution, after subcutaneous injection, octreotide is absorbed rapidly and completely from the injection site. Peak concentrations of 5.2 ng/mL (100-mcg dose) were reached 0.4 hours after dosing. Using a specific radioimmunoassay, intravenous and subcutaneous doses were found to be bioequivalent. Peak concentrations and area-under-the-curve values were dose proportional both after subcutaneous or intravenous single doses up to 400 mcg and with multiple doses of 200 mcg three times daily (600 mcg/day). Clearance was reduced by about 66% suggesting nonlinear kinetics of the drug at daily doses of 600 mcg/day compared to 150 mcg/day. The relative decrease in clearance with doses above 600 mcg/day is not defined.

In healthy volunteers, the distribution of octreotide from plasma was rapid ($t\alpha_{1/2}$ = 0.2 h), the volume of distribution (Vdss) was estimated to be 13.6 L and the total body clearance was 10 L/h.

In blood, the distribution of octreotide into the erythrocytes was found to be negligible and about 65% was bound in the plasma in a concentration-independent manner. Binding was mainly to lipoprotein and, to a lesser extent, to albumin.

The elimination of octreotide from plasma had an apparent half-life of 1.7 hours, compared with the 1-3 minutes with the natural hormone, somatostatin. The duration of action of subcutaneously administered Sandostatin Injection solution is variable but extends up to 12 hours depending upon the type of tumor, necessitating multiple daily dosing with this immediate-release dosage form. About 32% of the dose is excreted unchanged into the urine. In an elderly population, dose adjustments may be necessary due to a significant increase in the half-life (46%) and a significant decrease in the clearance (26%) of the drug.

In patients with acromegaly, the pharmacokinetics differ somewhat from those in healthy volunteers. A mean peak concentration of 2.8 ng/mL (100-mcg dose) was reached in 0.7 hours after subcutaneous dosing. The volume of distribution (Vdss) was estimated to be 21.6 ± 8.5 L and the total body clearance was increased to 18 L/h. The mean percent of the drug bound was 41.2%. The disposition and elimination half-lives were similar to normals.

The half-life in renal-impaired patients was slightly longer than normal subjects (2.4-3.1 h versus 1.9 h). The clearance in renal-impaired patients was 7.3-8.8 L/h as compared to 8.3 L/h in healthy subjects. In patients with severe renal failure requiring dialysis, clearance was reduced to about half that found in healthy subjects (from approximately 10 L/h to 4.5 L/h).

Patients with liver cirrhosis showed prolonged elimination of drug, with octreotide half-life increasing to 3.7 h and total body clearance decreasing to 5.9 L/h, whereas patients with fatty liver disease showed half-life increasing to 3.4 h and total body clearance of 8.4 L/h. In normal subjects, octreotide half-life is 1.9 h and the clearance is 8.3 L/h which is comparable with the clearance in fatty-liver patients.

Sandostatin LAR Depot

The magnitude and duration of octreotide serum concentrations after an intramuscular injection of the long-acting depot formulation Sandostatin LAR Depot reflect the release of drug from the microsphere polymer matrix. Drug release is governed by the slow biodegration of the microspheres in the muscle, but once present in the systemic circulation, octreotide distributes and is eliminated according to its known pharmacokinetic properties which are as follows.

After a single IM injection of the long-acting depot dosage form Sandostatin LAR Depot in healthy volunteer subjects, the serum octreotide concentration reached a transient initial peak of about 0.03 ng/mL/mg within 1 hour after administration progressively declining over the following 3-5 days to a nadir of <0.01 ng/mL/mg, then slowly increasing and reaching a plateau about 2-3 weeks postinjection. Plateau concentrations were maintained over a period of nearly 2-3 weeks, showing dose proportional peak concentrations of about 0.07 ng/mL/mg. After about 6 weeks postinjection, octreotide concentration slowly decreased, to <0.01 ng/mL/mg by Weeks 12 to 13, concomitant with the terminal degradation phase of the polymer matrix of the dosage form. The relative bioavailability of the long-acting release Sandostatin LAR Depot compared to immediate-release Sandostatin Injection solution given subcutaneously was 60%-63%.

In patients with acromegaly, the octreotide concentrations after single doses of 10 mg, 20 mg, and 30 mg Sandostatin LAR Depot were dose proportional. The transient Day 1 peak, amounting to 0.3 ng/mL, 0.8 ng/mL, and 1.3 ng/mL, respectively, was followed by plateau concentrations of 0.5 ng/mL, 1.3 ng/mL, and 2.0 ng/mL, respectively, achieved about 3 weeks postinjection. These plateau concentrations were maintained for nearly 2 weeks.

Following multiple doses of Sandostatin LAR Depot given every 4 weeks, steady-state octreotide serum concentrations were achieved after the third injection. Concentrations were dose proportional and higher by a factor of approximately 1.6 to 2.0 compared to the concentrations after a single dose. The steady-state octreotide concentrations were 1.2 ng/mL and 2.1 ng/mL, respectively, at trough and 1.6 ng/mL and 2.6 ng/mL, respectively, at peak with 20 mg and 30 mg Sandostatin LAR Depot given every 4 weeks. No accumulation of octreotide beyond that expected from the overlapping release profiles occurred over a duration of up to 28 monthly injections of Sandostatin LAR Depot. With the long-acting depot formulation Sandostatin LAR Depot administered IM every 4 weeks the peak-to-trough variation in octreotide concentrations ranged from 44%-68%, compared to the 163%-209% variation encountered with the daily subcutaneous three times daily regimen of Sandostatin Injection solution.

In patients with carcinoid tumors, the mean octreotide concentrations after 6 doses of 10 mg, 20 mg, and 30 mg Sandostatin LAR Depot administered by IM injection every 4 weeks were 1.2 ng/mL, 2.5 ng/mL, and 4.2 ng/mL, respectively. Concentrations were dose proportional and steady-state concentrations were reached after 2 injections of 20 mg and 30 mg and after 3 injections of 10 mg.

Sandostatin LAR Depot has not been studied in patients with renal impairment.

Sandostatin LAR Depot has not been studied in patients with hepatic impairment.

13 NONCLINICAL TOXICOLOGY

13.1 Carcinogenesis, Mutagenesis, Impairment of Fertility

Studies in laboratory animals have demonstrated no mutagenic potential of Sandostatin. No mutagenic potential of the polymeric carrier in Sandostatin LAR Depot, D,L-lactic and glycolic acids copolymer, was observed in the Ames mutagenicity test.

No carcinogenic potential was demonstrated in mice treated subcutaneously with octreotide for 85-99 weeks at doses up to 2000 mcg/kg/day (8× the human exposure based on body surface area). In a 116-week subcutaneous study in rats administered octreotide, a 27% and 12% incidence of injection site sarcomas or squamous cell carcinomas was observed in males and females, respectively, at the highest dose level of 1250 mcg/kg/day (10× the human exposure based on body surface area) compared to an incidence of 8%-10% in the vehicle-control groups. The increased incidence of injection site tumors was most probably caused by irritation and the high sensitivity of the rat to repeated subcutaneous injections at the same site. Rotating injection sites would prevent chronic irritation in humans. There have been no reports of injection site tumors in patients treated with Sandostatin Injection for at least 5 years. There was also a 15% incidence of uterine adenocarcinomas in the 1250 mcg/kg/day females compared to 7% in the saline-control females and 0% in the vehicle-control females. The presence of endometritis coupled with the absence of corpora lutea, the reduction in mammary fibroadenomas, and the presence of uterine dilatation suggest that the uterine tumors were associated with estrogen dominance in the aged female rats which does not occur in humans.

Octreotide did not impair fertility in rats at doses up to 1000 mcg/kg/day, which represents 7× the human exposure based on body surface area.

13.2 Reproductive Toxicology Studies

Reproduction studies have been performed in rats and rabbits at doses up to 16× the highest recommended human dose based on body surface area and have revealed no evidence of harm to the fetus due to octreotide.

14 CLINICAL STUDIES

14.1 Acromegaly

The clinical trials of Sandostatin LAR Depot were performed in patients who had been receiving Sandostatin Injection for a period of weeks to as long as 10 years. The acromegaly studies with Sandostatin LAR Depot described below were performed in patients who achieved GH levels of <10 ng/mL (and, in most cases <5 ng/mL) while on subcutaneous Sandostatin Injection. However, some patients enrolled were partial responders to subcutaneous Sandostatin Injection, i.e., GH levels were reduced by >50% on subcutaneous Sandostatin Injection compared to the untreated state, although not suppressed to <5 ng/mL.

Sandostatin LAR Depot was evaluated in three clinical trials in acromegalic patients.

In two of the clinical trials, a total of 101 patients were entered who had, in most cases, achieved a GH level <5 ng/mL on Sandostatin Injection given in doses of 100 mcg or 200 mcg three times daily. Most patients were switched to 20 mg or 30 mg doses of Sandostatin LAR Depot given once every 4 weeks for up to 27 to 28 injections. A few patients received doses of 10 mg and a few required doses of 40 mg. Growth hormone and IGF-1 levels were at least as well controlled with Sandostatin LAR Depot as they had been on Sandostatin Injection and this level of control remained for the entire duration of the trials.

A third trial was a 12-month study that enrolled 151 patients who had a GH level <10 ng/mL after treatment with Sandostatin Injection (most had levels <5 ng/mL). The starting dose of Sandostatin LAR Depot was 20 mg every 4 weeks for 3 doses. Thereafter, patients received 10 mg, 20 mg or 30 mg every 4 weeks, depending upon the degree of GH suppression [*see Dosage and Administration (2)*]. Growth hormone and IGF-1 were at least as well controlled on Sandostatin LAR Depot as they had been on Sandostatin Injection.

Table 5 summarizes the data on hormonal control (GH and IGF-1) for those patients in the first two clinical trials who received all 27 to 28 injections of Sandostatin LAR Depot.

[See table 5 above]

For the 88 patients in Table 5, a mean GH level of <2.5 ng/mL was observed in 47% receiving Sandostatin LAR Depot. Over the course of the trials, 42% of patients maintained mean growth hormone levels of <2.5 ng/mL and mean normal IGF-1 levels.

Table 6 summarizes the data on hormonal control (GH and IGF-1) for those patients in the third clinical trial who received all 12 injections of Sandostatin LAR Depot.

[See table 6 at top of next page]

Table 6. Hormonal Response in Acromegalic Patients Receiving 12 Injections During[1] Treatment with Sandostatin LAR Depot

Mean Hormone Level	Sandostatin Injection S.C. n	%	Sandostatin LAR Depot n	%
GH <5.0 ng/mL	116/122	95	118/122	97
<2.5 ng/mL	84/122	69	80/122	66
<1.0 ng/mL	25/122	21	28/122	23
IGF-1 normalized	82/122	67	82/122	67
GH <5.0 ng/mL + IGF-1 normalized	80/122	66	82/122	67
<2.5 ng/mL + IGF-1 normalized	65/122	53	70/122	57
<1.0 ng/mL + IGF-1 normalized	23/122	19	27/122	22

[1]Average of monthly levels of GH and IGF-1 over the course of the trial

Table 7. Average No. of Daily Stools and Flushing Episodes in Patients with Malignant Carcinoid Syndrome

Treatment	n	Daily Stools (Average No.) Baseline	Last Visit	Daily Flushing Episodes (Average No.) Baseline	Last Visit
Sandostatin Injection S.C.	26	3.7	2.6	3.0	0.5
Sandostatin LAR Depot					
10 mg	22	4.6	2.8	3.0	0.9
20 mg	20	4.0	2.1	5.9	0.6
30 mg	24	4.9	2.8	6.1	1.0

For the 122 patients in Table 6, who received all 12 injections in the third trial, a mean GH level of <2.5 ng/mL was observed in 66% receiving Sandostatin LAR Depot. Over the course of the trial, 57% of patients maintained mean growth hormone levels of <2.5 ng/mL and mean normal IGF-1 levels. In comparing the hormonal response in these trials, note that a higher percentage of patients in the third trial suppressed their mean GH to <5 ng/mL on subcutaneous Sandostatin Injection, 95%, compared to 78% across the two previous trials.

In all three trials, GH, IGF-1, and clinical symptoms were similarly controlled on Sandostatin LAR Depot as they had been on Sandostatin Injection.

Of the 25 patients who completed the trials and were partial responders to Sandostatin Injection (GH >5.0 ng/mL but reduced by >50% relative to untreated levels), 1 patient (4%) responded to Sandostatin LAR Depot with a reduction of GH to <2.5 ng/mL and 8 patients (32%) responded with a reduction of GH to <5.0 ng/mL.

Two open-label clinical studies investigated a 48-week treatment with Sandostatin LAR Depot in 143 untreated (de novo) acromegalic patients. The median reduction in tumor volume was 20.6% in Study 1 (49 patients) at 24 weeks and 24.5% in Study 2 (94 patients) at 24 weeks and 36.2% at 48 weeks.

14.2 Carcinoid Syndrome

A 6-month clinical trial of malignant carcinoid syndrome was performed in 93 patients who had previously been shown to be responsive to Sandostatin Injection. 67 patients were randomized at baseline to receive, double-blind, doses of 10 mg, 20 mg or 30 mg Sandostatin LAR Depot every 28 days and 26 patients continued, unblinded, on their previous Sandostatin Injection regimen (100-300 mcg three times daily).

In any given month after steady-state levels of octreotide were reached, approximately 35%-40% of the patients who received Sandostatin LAR Depot required supplemental subcutaneous Sandostatin Injection therapy usually for a few days, to control exacerbation of carcinoid symptoms. In any given month, the percentage of patients randomized to subcutaneous Sandostatin Injection who required supplemental treatment with an increased dose of Sandostatin Injection was similar to the percentage of patients randomized to Sandostatin LAR Depot. Over the 6-month treatment period, approximately 50%-70% of patients who completed the trial on Sandostatin LAR Depot required subcutaneous Sandostatin Injection supplemental therapy to control exacerbation of carcinoid symptoms although steady-state serum Sandostatin LAR Depot levels had been reached.

Table 7 presents the average number of daily stools and flushing episodes in malignant carcinoid patients.

[See table 7 above]

Overall, mean daily stool frequency was as well controlled on Sandostatin LAR Depot as on Sandostatin Injection (approximately 2-2.5 stools/day).

Mean daily flushing episodes were similar at all doses of Sandostatin LAR Depot and on Sandostatin Injection (approximately 0.5-1 episode/day).

In a subset of patients with variable severity of disease, median 24 hour urinary 5-HIAA (5-hydroxyindole acetic acid) levels were reduced by 38%-50% in the groups randomized to Sandostatin LAR Depot.

The reductions are within the range reported in the published literature for patients treated with octreotide (about 10%-50%).

78 patients with malignant carcinoid syndrome who had participated in this 6-month trial, subsequently participated in a 12-month extension study in which they received 12 injections of Sandostatin LAR Depot at 4-week intervals. For those who remained in the extension trial, diarrhea and flushing were as well controlled as during the 6-month trial. Because malignant carcinoid disease is progressive, as expected, a number of deaths (8 patients: 10%) occurred due to disease progression or complications from the underlying disease. An additional 22% of patients prematurely discontinued Sandostatin LAR Depot due to disease progression or worsening of carcinoid symptoms.

16 HOW SUPPLIED/STORAGE AND HANDLING

Sandostatin LAR Depot is available in single-use kits containing a 5-mL vial of 10 mg, 20 mg or 30 mg strength, a syringe containing 2.5 mL of diluent, two sterile 1½" 19 gauge needles, and two alcohol wipes. An instruction booklet for the preparation of drug suspension for injection is also included with each kit.

Drug Product Kits
10 mg kit .... NDC 0078-0340-61
20 mg kit .... NDC 0078-0341-61
30 mg kit .... NDC 0078-0342-61
Demonstration kit .... NDC 0078-9342-61

For prolonged storage, Sandostatin LAR Depot should be stored at refrigerated temperatures between 2°C-8°C (36°F-46°F) and protected from light until the time of use. Sandostatin LAR Depot drug product kit should remain at room temperature for 30-60 minutes prior to preparation of the drug suspension. However, after preparation the drug suspension must be administered immediately.

17 PATIENT COUNSELING INFORMATION

Patients with carcinoid tumors and VIPomas should be advised to adhere closely to their scheduled return visits for reinjection in order to minimize exacerbation of symptoms. Patients with acromegaly should also be urged to adhere to their return visit schedule to help assure steady control of GH and IGF-1 levels.

Sandostatin® LAR Depot vials are manufactured by:
Sandoz GmbH, Schaftenau, Austria
(Subsidiary of Novartis Pharma AG, Basle, Switzerland)
The diluent syringes are manufactured by:
Abbott Biologicals B.V.
Olst, The Netherlands
Distributed by:
Novartis Pharmaceuticals Corporation
East Hanover, New Jersey 07936
© Novartis
T2011-138

Shown in Product Identification Guide, page 311

SIMULECT® ℞

[sĭm ew lĕkt]
(basiliximab)
For Injection
Rx only

The following prescribing information is based on official labeling in effect July 2013.

Prescribing Information

WARNING

Only physicians experienced in immunosuppression therapy and management of organ transplantation patients should prescribe Simulect® (basiliximab). The physician responsible for Simulect administration should have complete information requisite for the follow-up of the patient. Patients receiving the drug should be managed in facilities equipped and staffed with adequate laboratory and supportive medical resources.

DESCRIPTION

Simulect® (basiliximab) is a chimeric (murine/human) monoclonal antibody ($IgG_{1\kappa}$), produced by recombinant DNA technology, that functions as an immunosuppressive agent, specifically binding to and blocking the interleukin-2 receptor α-chain (IL-2Rα, also known as CD25 antigen) on the surface of activated T-lymphocytes. Based on the amino acid sequence, the calculated molecular weight of the protein is 144 kilodaltons. It is a glycoprotein obtained from fermentation of an established mouse myeloma cell line genetically engineered to express plasmids containing the human heavy and light chain constant region genes and mouse heavy and light chain variable region genes encoding the RFT5 antibody that binds selectively to the IL-2Rα.

The active ingredient, basiliximab, is water soluble. The drug product, Simulect, is a sterile lyophilisate which is available in 6 mL colorless glass vials and is available in 10 mg and 20 mg strengths.

Each 10-mg vial contains 10 mg basiliximab, 3.61 mg monobasic potassium phosphate, 0.50 mg disodium hydrogen phosphate (anhydrous), 0.80 mg sodium chloride, 10 mg sucrose, 40 mg mannitol and 20 mg glycine, to be reconstituted in 2.5 mL of Sterile Water for Injection, USP. No preservatives are added.

Each 20-mg vial contains 20 mg basiliximab, 7.21 mg monobasic potassium phosphate, 0.99 mg disodium hydrogen phosphate (anhydrous), 1.61 mg sodium chloride, 20 mg sucrose, 80 mg mannitol and 40 mg glycine, to be reconstituted in 5 mL of Sterile Water for Injection, USP. No preservatives are added.

CLINICAL PHARMACOLOGY

General

Mechanism of Action: Basiliximab functions as an IL-2 receptor antagonist by binding with high affinity ($K_a = 1 \times 10^{10} M^{-1}$) to the alpha chain of the high affinity IL-2 receptor complex and inhibiting IL-2 binding. Basiliximab is specifically targeted against IL-2Rα, which is selectively expressed on the surface of activated T-lymphocytes. This specific high affinity binding of Simulect® (basiliximab) to IL-2Rα competitively inhibits IL-2-mediated activation of lymphocytes, a critical pathway in the cellular immune response involved in allograft rejection.

While in the circulation, Simulect impairs the response of the immune system to antigenic challenges. Whether the ability to respond to repeated or ongoing challenges with those antigens returns to normal after Simulect is cleared is unknown (see PRECAUTIONS).

Pharmacokinetics

Adults: Single-dose and multiple-dose pharmacokinetic studies have been conducted in patients undergoing first kidney transplantation. Cumulative doses ranged from 15 mg up to 150 mg. Peak mean ± SD serum concentration following intravenous infusion of 20 mg over 30 minutes is 7.1 ± 5.1 mg/L. There is a dose-proportional increase in C_{max} and AUC up to the highest tested single dose of 60 mg. The volume of distribution at steady state is 8.6 ± 4.1 L. The extent and degree of distribution to various body compartments have not been fully studied. The terminal half-life is 7.2 ± 3.2 days. Total body clearance is 41 ± 19 mL/h. No clinically relevant influence of body weight or gender on distribution volume or clearance has been observed in adult patients. Elimination half-life was not influenced by age (20-69 years), gender or race (see DOSAGE AND ADMINISTRATION).

Pediatric: The pharmacokinetics of Simulect have been assessed in 39 pediatric patients undergoing renal transplantation. In infants and children (1-11 years of age, n=25), the distribution volume and clearance were reduced by about 50% compared to adult renal transplantation patients. The volume of distribution at steady state was 4.8 ± 2.1 L, half-life was 9.5 ± 4.5 days and clearance was 17 ± 6 mL/h. Disposition parameters were not influenced to a clinically relevant extent by age (1-11 years of age), body weight (9-37 kg) or body surface area (0.44-1.20 m^2) in this age group. In adolescents (12-16 years of age, n=14), disposition was similar to that in adult renal transplantation patients. The volume of distribution at steady state was 7.8 ± 5.1 L, half-life was 9.1 ± 3.9 days and clearance was 31 ± 19 mL/h (see DOSAGE AND ADMINISTRATION).

Pharmacodynamics

Complete and consistent binding to IL-2Rα in adults is maintained as long as serum Simulect levels exceed 0.2 µg/mL. As concentrations fall below this threshold, the IL-2Rα sites are no longer fully bound and the number of T-cells

Table 1. Efficacy Parameters (Percentage of Patients)

	Dual-therapy Regimen (cyclosporine* and corticosteroids)					
	Study 1			Study 2		
	Placebo (N=185)	Simulect® (N=190)	p-value	Placebo (N=173)	Simulect® (N=173)	p-value
Primary endpoint						
Death, graft loss or acute rejection episode (0-6 months)	57%	42%	0.003	55%	38%	0.002
Secondary endpoints						
Death, graft loss or acute rejection episode (0-12 months)	60%	46%	0.007	58%	41%	0.001
Biopsy-confirmed rejection episode (0-6 months)	44%	30%	0.007	46%	33%	0.015
Biopsy-confirmed rejection episode (0-12 months)	46%	32%	0.005	49%	35%	0.009
Patient survival (12 months)	97%	95%	0.29	96%	97%	0.56
Patients with functioning graft (12 months)	87%	88%	0.70	93%	95%	0.50

* USP (MODIFIED)

expressing unbound IL-2Rα returns to pretherapy values within 1-2 weeks. The relationship between serum concentration and receptor saturation was assessed in 13 pediatric patients and was similar to that characterized in adult renal transplantation patients. *In vitro* studies using human tissues indicate that Simulect binds only to lymphocytes.

The duration of clinically relevant IL-2 receptor blockade after the recommended course of Simulect is not known. When basiliximab was added to a regimen of cyclosporine, USP (MODIFIED) and corticosteroids in adult patients, the duration of IL-2Rα saturation was 36 ± 14 days (mean ± SD), similar to that observed in pediatric patients (36 ± 14 days) (see DOSAGE AND ADMINISTRATION). When basiliximab was added to a triple therapy regimen consisting of cyclosporine, USP (MODIFIED), corticosteroids, and azathioprine in adults, the duration was 50 ± 20 days and when added to cyclosporine, USP (MODIFIED), corticosteroids, and mycophenolate mofetil in adults, the duration was 59 ± 17 days (see PRECAUTIONS,Drug Interactions). No significant changes to circulating lymphocyte numbers or cell phenotypes were observed by flow cytometry.

CLINICAL STUDIES

The safety and efficacy of Simulect® (basiliximab) for the prophylaxis of acute organ rejection in adults following cadaveric- or living-donor renal transplantation were assessed in four randomized, double-blind, placebo-controlled clinical studies (1,184 patients). Of these four, two studies (Study 1 [EU/CAN Study] and Study 2 [US Study]) compared two 20-mg doses of Simulect with placebo, each administered intravenously as an infusion, as part of a standard immunosuppressive regimen comprised of cyclosporine, USP (MODIFIED) and corticosteroids. The other two controlled studies compared two 20-mg doses of Simulect with placebo, each administered intravenously as a bolus injection, as part of a standard triple-immunosuppressive regimen comprised of cyclosporine, USP (MODIFIED), corticosteroids and either azathioprine or mycophenolate mofetil (Study 3 and Study 4, respectively). The first dose of Simulect or placebo was administered within 2 hours prior to transplantation surgery (Day 0) and the second dose administered on Day 4 post-transplantation. The regimen of Simulect was chosen to provide 30-45 days of IL-2Rα saturation.

729 patients were enrolled in the two studies using a dual maintenance immunosuppressive regimen comprised of cyclosporine, USP (MODIFIED) and corticosteroids, of which 363 patients were treated with Simulect and 358 patients were placebo-treated. Study 1 was conducted at 21 sites in Europe and Canada (EU/CAN Study); Study 2 was conducted at 21 sites in the USA (US Study). Patients 18-75 years of age undergoing first cadaveric- (Study 1 and Study 2) or living-donor (Study 2 only) renal transplantation, with ≥1 HLA mismatch, were enrolled.[1,2]

The primary efficacy endpoint in both studies was the incidence of death, graft loss or an episode of acute rejection during the first 6 months post-transplantation. Secondary efficacy endpoints included the primary efficacy variable measured during the first 12 months post-transplantation, the incidence of biopsy-confirmed acute rejection during the first 6 and 12 months post-transplantation, and patient survival and graft survival, each measured at 12 months post-transplantation. Table 1 summarizes the results of these studies. Figure 1 displays the Kaplan-Meier estimates of the percentage of patients by treatment group experiencing the primary efficacy endpoint during the first 12 months post-transplantation for Study 2. Patients in both studies receiving Simulect experienced a significantly lower incidence of biopsy-confirmed rejection episodes at both 6 and 12 months post-transplantation. There was no difference in the rate of delayed graft function, patient survival, or graft survival between Simulect-treated patients and placebo-treated patients in either study.

There was no evidence that the clinical benefit of Simulect was limited to specific subpopulations based on age, gender, race, donor type (cadaveric or living donor allograft) or history of diabetes mellitus.

[See table 1 above]

Figure 1
Kaplan-Meier Estimate of the Percentage of Subjects with Death, Graft Loss or First Rejection Episode (Dual Therapy)
Month: 0 –12

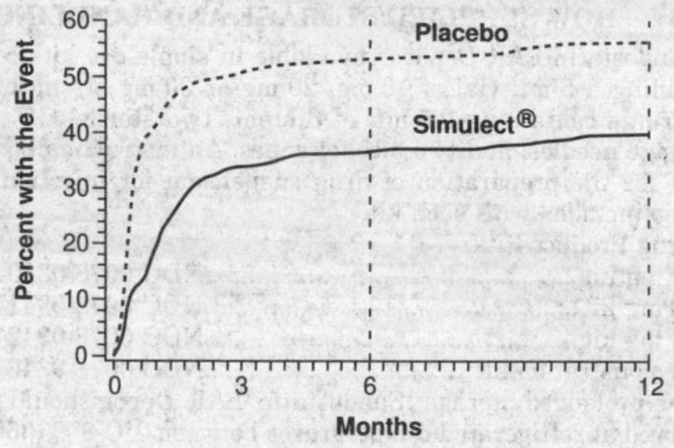

Two double-blind, randomized, placebo-controlled studies (Study 3 and Study 4) assessed the safety and efficacy of Simulect for the prophylaxis of acute renal transplant rejection in adults when used in combination with a triple immunosuppressive regimen. In Study 3, 340 patients were concomitantly treated with cyclosporine, USP (MODIFIED), corticosteroids and azathioprine (AZA), of which 168 patients were treated with Simulect and 172 patients were treated with placebo. In Study 4, 123 patients were concomitantly treated with cyclosporine, USP (MODIFIED), corticosteroids and mycophenolate mofetil (MMF), of which 59 patients were treated with Simulect and 64 patients were treated with placebo. Patients 18-70 years of age undergoing first or second cadaveric or living donor (related or unrelated) renal transplantation were enrolled in both studies. The results of Study 3 are shown in Table 2. These results are consistent with the findings from Study 1 and Study 2.

Table 2. Efficacy Parameters (Percentage of Patients)

Study 3: Triple-therapy Regimen (cyclosporine*, corticosteroids, and azathioprine)	Placebo (N=172)	Simulect® (N=168)	p-value
Primary endpoint			
Acute rejection episode (0-6 months)	35%	21%	0.005
Secondary endpoints			
Death, graft loss or acute rejection episode (0-6 months)	40%	26%	0.008
Biopsy-confirmed rejection episode (0-6 months)	29%	18%	0.023
Patient survival (12 months)	97%	98%	1.000
Patients with functioning graft (12 months)	88%	90%	0.599

*USP (MODIFIED)

In Study 4, the percentage of patients experiencing biopsy-proven acute rejection by 6 months was 15% (9 of 59 patients) in the Simulect group and 27% (17 of 64 patients) in the placebo group. Although numerically lower, the difference in acute rejection was not significant.

In a multicenter, randomized, double-blind, placebo-controlled trial of Simulect for the prevention of allograft rejection in liver transplant recipients (n=381) receiving concomitant cyclosporine, USP (MODIFIED) and steroids, the incidence of the combined endpoint of death, graft loss, or first biopsy-confirmed rejection episode at either 6 or 12 months was similar between patients randomized to receive Simulect and those randomized to receive placebo.

The efficacy of Simulect for the prophylaxis of acute rejection in recipients of a second renal allograft has not been demonstrated.

Long Term Follow-up

Five-year patient survival and graft survival data were provided by 71% and 58% of the original subjects of Study 1 and Study 2, respectively. Subjects in both studies continued to receive a dual-therapy regimen with cyclosporine, USP (MODIFIED) and corticosteroid. No difference was observed between groups in the 5-year graft survival in either Study 1 (91% Simulect group, 92% placebo group) or Study 2 (85% Simulect group, 86% placebo group). In Study 1, patient survival was lower in the Simulect-treated patients compared to the placebo-treated patients (142/163 [87%] vs. 156/164 [95%], respectively). The cause of this difference in survival is unknown. The data do not indicate an increase in malignancy- or infection-related mortality. In Study 2, patient survival in the placebo group (90%) was the same compared to Simulect group (90%).

INDICATIONS AND USAGE

Simulect® (basiliximab) is indicated for the prophylaxis of acute organ rejection in patients receiving renal transplantation when used as part of an immunosuppressive regimen that includes cyclosporine, USP (MODIFIED) and corticosteroids.

The efficacy of Simulect for the prophylaxis of acute rejection in recipients of other solid organ allografts has not been demonstrated.

CONTRAINDICATIONS

Simulect® (basiliximab) is contraindicated in patients with known hypersensitivity to basiliximab or any other component of the formulation. See composition of Simulect under DESCRIPTION.

WARNINGS. See Boxed WARNING.

General

Simulect® (basiliximab) should be administered under qualified medical supervision. Patients should be informed of the potential benefits of therapy and the risks associated with administration of immunosuppressive therapy.

While neither the incidence of lymphoproliferative disorders nor opportunistic infections was higher in Simulect-treated patients than in placebo-treated patients, patients on immunosuppressive therapy are at increased risk for developing these complications and should be monitored accordingly.

Hypersensitivity

Severe acute (onset within 24 hours) hypersensitivity reactions including anaphylaxis have been observed both on initial exposure to Simulect and/or following re-exposure after several months. These reactions may include hypotension, tachycardia, cardiac failure, dyspnea, wheezing, bronchospasm, pulmonary edema, respiratory failure, urticaria, rash, pruritus, and/or sneezing. Extreme caution should be exercised in all patients previously given Simulect when being administered a subsequent course of Simulect. A subgroup of patients may be particularly at risk of developing severe hypersensitivity reactions on re-administration. These are patients in whom concomitant immunosuppression was discontinued prematurely (e.g., due to abandoned transplantation or early loss of the graft) following the initial administration of Simulect. If a severe hypersensitivity reaction occurs, therapy with Simulect should be permanently discontinued. Medications for the treatment of severe hypersensitivity reactions including anaphylaxis should be available for immediate use.

PRECAUTIONS

General

It is not known whether Simulect® (basiliximab) use will have a long-term effect on the ability of the immune system to respond to antigens first encountered during Simulect-induced immunosuppression.

Immunogenicity

Of renal transplantation patients treated with Simulect and tested for anti-idiotype antibodies, 4/339 developed an anti-idiotype antibody response, with no deleterious clinical effect upon the patient. In none of these cases was there evidence that the presence of anti-idiotype antibody accelerated Simulect clearance or decreased the period of receptor saturation. In Study 2, the incidence of human anti-murine antibody (HAMA) in renal transplantation patients treated with Simulect was 2/138 in patients not exposed to muromonab-CD3 and 4/34 in patients who subsequently received muromonab-CD3. The available clinical data on the use of muromonab-CD3 in patients previously treated with Simulect suggest that subsequent use of muromonab-CD3 or other murine anti-lymphocytic antibody preparations is not precluded.

These data reflect the percentage of patients whose test results were considered positive for antibodies to Simulect in an ELISA assay, and are highly dependent on the sensitivity and specificity of the assay. Additionally the observed incidence of antibody positivity in an assay may be influenced by several factors including sample handling, concomitant medications, and underlying disease. For these reasons, comparison of the incidence of antibodies to Simulect with the incidence of antibodies to other products may be misleading.

Drug Interactions

No dose adjustment is necessary when Simulect is added to triple-immunosuppression regimens including cyclosporine, corticosteroids, and either azathioprine or mycophenolate mofetil. Three clinical trials have investigated Simulect use in combination with triple-therapy regimens. Pharmacokinetics were assessed in two of these trials. Total body clearance of Simulect was reduced by an average 22% and 51% when azathioprine and mycophenolate mofetil, respectively, were added to a regimen consisting of cyclosporine, USP (MODIFIED) and corticosteroids. Nonetheless, the range of individual Simulect clearance values in the presence of azathioprine (12-57 mL/h) or mycophenolate mofetil (7-54 mL/h) did not extend outside the range observed with dual therapy (10-78 mL/h). The following medications have been administered in clinical trials with Simulect with no increase in adverse reactions: ATG/ALG, azathioprine, corticosteroids, cyclosporine, mycophenolate mofetil, and muromonab-CD3.

Carcinogenesis/Mutagenesis/Impairment of Fertility

No mutagenic potential of Simulect was observed in the *in vitro* assays with Salmonella (Ames) and V79 Chinese hamster cells. No long-term or fertility studies in laboratory animals have been performed to evaluate the potential of Simulect to produce carcinogenicity or fertility impairment, respectively.

Pregnancy Category B

There are no adequate and well-controlled studies in pregnant women. No maternal toxicity, embryotoxicity, or teratogenicity was observed in cynomolgus monkeys 100 days post coitum following dosing with basiliximab during the organogenesis period; blood levels in pregnant monkeys were 13-fold higher than those seen in human patients. Immunotoxicology studies have not been performed in the offspring. Because IgG molecules are known to cross the placental barrier, because the IL-2 receptor may play an important role in development of the immune system, and because animal reproduction studies are not always predictive of human response, Simulect should only be used in pregnant women when the potential benefit justifies the potential risk to the fetus. Women of childbearing potential should use effective contraception before beginning Simulect therapy, during therapy, and for 4 months after completion of Simulect therapy.

Nursing Mothers

It is not known whether Simulect is excreted in human milk. Because many drugs including human antibodies are excreted in human milk, and because of the potential for adverse reactions, a decision should be made to discontinue nursing or to discontinue the drug, taking into account the importance of the drug to the mother.

Pediatric Use

No randomized, placebo-controlled studies have been completed in pediatric patients. In a safety and pharmacokinetic study, 41 pediatric patients (1-11 years of age [n=27], 12-16 years of age [n=14], median age 8.1 years) were treated with Simulect via intravenous bolus injection in addition to standard immunosuppressive agents including cyclosporine, USP (MODIFIED), corticosteroids, azathioprine, and mycophenolate mofetil. The acute rejection rate at 6 months was comparable to that in adults in the triple-therapy trials. The most frequently reported adverse events were hypertension, hypertrichosis, and rhinitis (49% each), urinary tract infections (46%), and fever (39%). Overall, the adverse event profile was consistent with general clinical experience in the pediatric renal transplantation population and with the profile in the controlled adult renal transplantation studies. The available pharmacokinetic data in children and adolescents are described in CLINICAL PHARMACOLOGY and DOSAGE AND ADMINISTRATION.

It is not known whether the immune response to vaccines, infection, and other antigenic stimuli administered or encountered during Simulect therapy is impaired or whether such response will remain impaired after Simulect therapy.

Geriatric Use

Controlled clinical studies of Simulect have included a small number of patients 65 years and older (Simulect 28; placebo 32). From the available data comparing Simulect and placebo-treated patients, the adverse event profile in patients ≥65 years of age is not different from patients <65 years of age and no age-related dosing adjustment is required. Caution must be used in giving immunosuppressive drugs to elderly patients.

ADVERSE REACTIONS

Because clinical trials are conducted under widely varying conditions, adverse reaction rates observed in the clinical trials of a drug cannot be directly compared to rates in the clinical trials of another drug and may not reflect the rates observed in practice. The adverse reaction information from clinical trials does, however, provide a basis for identifying the adverse events that appear to be related to drug use and for approximating rates.

The incidence of adverse events for Simulect® (basiliximab) was determined in four randomized, double-blind, placebo-controlled clinical trials for the prevention of renal allograft rejection. Two of the studies (Study 1 and Study 2), used a dual maintenance immunosuppressive regimen comprised of cyclosporine, USP (MODIFIED) and corticosteroids, whereas the other two studies (Study 3 and Study 4) used a triple-immunosuppressive regimen comprised of cyclosporine, USP (MODIFIED), corticosteroids, and either azathioprine or mycophenolate mofetil.

Simulect did not appear to add to the background of adverse events seen in organ transplantation patients as a consequence of their underlying disease and the concurrent administration of immunosuppressants and other medications. Adverse events were reported by 96% of the patients in the placebo-treated group and 96% of the patients in the Simulect-treated group. In the four placebo-controlled studies, the pattern of adverse events in 590 patients treated with the recommended dose of Simulect was similar to that in 594 patients treated with placebo. Simulect did not increase the incidence of serious adverse events observed compared with placebo.

The most frequently reported adverse events were gastrointestinal disorders, reported in 69% of Simulect-treated patients and 67% of placebo-treated patients.

The incidence and types of adverse events were similar in Simulect-treated and placebo-treated patients. The following adverse events occurred in ≥10% of Simulect-treated patients: ***Gastrointestinal System:*** constipation, nausea, abdominal pain, vomiting, diarrhea, dyspepsia; ***Body as a Whole-General:*** pain, peripheral edema, fever, viral infection; ***Metabolic and Nutritional:*** hyperkalemia, hypokalemia, hyperglycemia, hypercholesterolemia, hypophosphatemia, hyperuricemia; ***Urinary System:*** urinary tract infection; ***Respiratory System:*** dyspnea, upper respiratory tract infection; ***Skin and Appendages:*** surgical wound complications, acne; ***Cardiovascular Disorders-General:*** hypertension; ***Central and Peripheral Nervous System:*** headache, tremor; **Psychiatric:** insomnia; ***Red Blood Cell:*** anemia.

The following adverse events, not mentioned above, were reported with an incidence of ≥3% and <10% in pooled analysis of patients treated with Simulect in the four controlled clinical trials, or in an analysis of the two dual-therapy trials: ***Body as a Whole-General:*** accidental trauma, asthenia, chest pain, increased drug level, infection, face edema, fatigue, dependent edema, generalized edema, leg edema, malaise, rigors, sepsis; ***Cardiovascular:*** abnormal heart sounds, aggravated hypertension, angina pectoris, cardiac failure, chest pain, hypotension; ***Endocrine:*** increased glucocorticoids; ***Gastrointestinal:*** enlarged abdomen, esophagitis, flatulence, gastrointestinal disorder, gastroenteritis, GI hemorrhage, gum hyperplasia, melena, moniliasis, ulcerative stomatitis; ***Heart Rate and Rhythm:*** arrhythmia, atrial fibrillation, tachycardia; ***Metabolic and Nutritional:*** acidosis, dehydration, diabetes mellitus, fluid overload, hypercalcemia, hyperlipemia, hypertriglyceridemia, hypocalcemia, hypoglycemia, hypomagnesemia, hypoproteinemia, weight increase; ***Musculoskeletal:*** arthralgia, arthropathy, back pain, bone fracture, cramps, hernia, myalgia, leg pain; ***Nervous System:*** dizziness, neuropathy, paraesthesia, hypoesthesia; ***Platelet and Bleeding:*** hematoma, hemorrhage, purpura, thrombocytopenia, thrombosis; ***Psychiatric:*** agitation, anxiety, depression; ***Red Blood Cell:*** polycythemia; ***Reproductive Disorders, Male:*** genital edema, impotence; ***Respiratory:*** bronchitis, bronchospasm, abnormal chest sounds, coughing, pharyngitis, pneumonia, pulmonary disorder, pulmonary edema, rhinitis, sinusitis; ***Skin and Appendages:*** cyst, herpes simplex, herpes zoster, hypertrichosis, pruritus, rash, skin disorder, skin ulceration; ***Urinary:*** albuminuria, bladder disorder, dysuria, frequent micturition, hematuria, increased non-protein nitrogen, oliguria, abnormal renal function, renal tubular necrosis, surgery, ureteral disorder, urinary retention; ***Vascular Disorders:*** vascular disorder; ***Vision Disorders:*** cataract, conjunctivitis, abnormal vision; ***White Blood Cell:*** leucopenia. Among these events, leucopenia and hypertriglyceridemia occurred more frequently in the two triple-therapy studies using azathioprine and mycophenolate mofetil than in the dual-therapy studies.

Malignancies

The incidence of malignancies in the controlled clinical trials of renal transplant was not significantly different between groups at 1 year (9/590 Simulect-treated patients vs. 12/594 placebo-treated patients) or among patients with 5-year follow-up from Studies 1 and 2 (21/295 Simulect-treated patients vs. 21/291 placebo-treated patients). The incidence of lymphoproliferative disease was not significantly different between groups, and less than 1% in the Simulect-treated patients.

Infections

The overall incidence of cytomegalovirus infection was similar in Simulect- and placebo-treated patients (15% vs. 17%) receiving a dual- or triple-immunosuppression regimen. However, in patients receiving a triple-immunosuppression regimen, the incidence of serious cytomegalovirus infection was higher in Simulect-treated patients compared to placebo-treated patients (11% vs. 5%). The rates of infections, serious infections, and infectious organisms were similar in the Simulect- and placebo-treatment groups among dual- and triple-therapy treated patients.

Post-Marketing Experience

Severe acute hypersensitivity reactions including anaphylaxis characterized by hypotension, tachycardia, cardiac failure, dyspnea, wheezing, bronchospasm, pulmonary edema, respiratory failure, urticaria, rash, pruritus, and/or sneezing, as well as capillary leak syndrome and cytokine release syndrome, have been reported during post-marketing experience with Simulect.

OVERDOSAGE

A maximum tolerated dose of Simulect® (basiliximab) has not been determined in patients. During the course of clinical studies, Simulect has been administered to adult renal transplantation patients in single doses of up to 60 mg, or in divided doses over 3-5 days of up to 120 mg, without any associated serious adverse events. There has been one spontaneous report of a pediatric renal transplantation patient who received a single 20-mg dose (2.3 mg/kg) without adverse events.

DOSAGE AND ADMINISTRATION

Simulect® (basiliximab) is used as part of an immunosuppressive regimen that includes cyclosporine, USP (MODIFIED) and corticosteroids. Simulect is for central or peripheral intravenous administration only. Reconstituted Simulect should be given either as a bolus injection or diluted to a volume of 25 mL (10-mg vial) or 50 mL (20-mg vial) with normal saline or dextrose 5% and administered as an intravenous infusion over 20 to 30 minutes. Bolus administration may be associated with nausea, vomiting and local reactions, including pain.

Simulect should only be administered once it has been determined that the patient will receive the graft and concomitant immunosuppression. Patients previously administered Simulect should only be re-exposed to a subsequent course of therapy with extreme caution due to the potential risk of hypersensitivity (see WARNINGS).

Parenteral drug products should be inspected visually for particulate matter and discoloration before administration. After reconstitution, Simulect should be a clear-to-opalescent, colorless solution. If particulate matter is present or the solution is colored, do not use.

Care must be taken to assure sterility of the prepared solution because the drug product does not contain any antimicrobial preservatives or bacteriostatic agents.

It is recommended that after reconstitution, the solution should be used immediately. If not used immediately, it can be stored at 2°C to 8°C for 24 hours or at room temperature for 4 hours. Discard the reconstituted solution if not used within 24 hours.

No incompatibility between Simulect and polyvinyl chloride bags or infusion sets has been observed. No data are available on the compatibility of Simulect with other intravenous substances. Other drug substances should not be added or infused simultaneously through the same intravenous line.

Adults

In adult patients, the recommended regimen is two doses of 20 mg each. The first 20-mg dose should be given within 2 hours prior to transplantation surgery. The recommended second 20-mg dose should be given 4 days after transplantation. The second dose should be withheld if complications such as severe hypersensitivity reactions to Simulect or graft loss occur.

Pediatric

In pediatric patients weighing less than 35 kg, the recommended regimen is two doses of 10 mg each. In pediatric patients weighing 35 kg or more, the recommended regimen is two doses of 20 mg each. The first dose should be given within 2 hours prior to transplantation surgery. The recommended second dose should be given 4 days after transplantation. The second dose should be withheld if complications such as severe hypersensitivity reactions to Simulect or graft loss occur.

Reconstitution of 10 mg Simulect® Vial

To prepare the reconstituted solution, add 2.5 mL of Sterile Water for Injection, USP, using aseptic technique, to the vial containing the Simulect powder. Shake the vial gently to dissolve the powder.

The reconstituted solution is isotonic and may be given either as a bolus injection or diluted to a volume of 25 mL with normal saline or dextrose 5% for infusion. When mixing the solution, gently invert the bag in order to avoid foaming; DO NOT SHAKE.

Reconstitution of 20 mg Simulect® Vial

To prepare the reconstituted solution, add 5 mL of Sterile Water for Injection, USP, using aseptic technique, to the vial containing the Simulect powder. Shake the vial gently to dissolve the powder.

The reconstituted solution is isotonic and may be given either as a bolus injection or diluted to a volume of 50 mL with normal saline or dextrose 5% for infusion. When mixing the solution, gently invert the bag in order to avoid foaming; DO NOT SHAKE.

HOW SUPPLIED

Simulect® (basiliximab) is supplied in a single-use glass vial.

Each carton contains one of the following

1 Simulect 10 mg vial ....NDC 0078-0393-61

1 Simulect 20 mg vial ....NDC 0078-0331-84

Store lyophilized Simulect under refrigerated conditions (2°C to 8°C; 36°F to 46°F).

Do not use beyond the expiration date stamped on the vial.

REFERENCES

1. Kahan, B.D., Rajagopalan P.R. and Hall M., Transplantation, 67, 276-284 (1999).
2. Nashan, B., Moore R., Amlot P., Schmidt A.-G., Abeywickrama K. and Soulillou J.-P., Lancet 350, 1193-1198 (1997).

T2005-28

2027722

US License No. 1244

REV: September 2005

Novartis Pharmaceuticals Corporation

East Hanover, New Jersey 07936

Shown in Product Identification Guide, page 310

TASIGNA® ℞

[ta-sig-na]

(nilotinib)

Capsules

The following prescribing information is based on official labeling in effect July 2013.

HIGHLIGHTS OF PRESCRIBING INFORMATION

These highlights do not include all the information needed to use Tasigna safely and effectively. See full prescribing information for Tasigna.

Tasigna® (nilotinib) Capsules

Initial U.S. Approval: 2007

WARNING: QT PROLONGATION AND SUDDEN DEATHS

See full prescribing information for complete boxed warning.

- **Tasigna prolongs the QT interval. Prior to Tasigna administration and periodically, monitor for hypokalemia or hypomagnesemia and correct deficiencies (5.2). Obtain ECGs to monitor the QTc at baseline, seven days after initiation, and periodically thereafter, and following any dose adjustments (5.2, 5.3, 5.6, 5.13).**
- **Sudden deaths have been reported in patients receiving nilotinib (5.3). Do not administer Tasigna to patients with hypokalemia, hypomagnesemia, or long QT syndrome (4, 5.2).**
- **Avoid use of concomitant drugs known to prolong the QT interval and strong CYP3A4 inhibitors (5.7).**
- **Patients should avoid food 2 hours before and 1 hour after taking dose (5.8).**

INDICATIONS AND USAGE

Tasigna is a kinase inhibitor indicated for:

The treatment of newly diagnosed adult patients with Philadelphia chromosome positive chronic myeloid leukemia (Ph+ CML) in chronic phase. The study is ongoing and further data will be required to determine long-term outcome. (1.1)

The treatment of chronic phase (CP) and accelerated phase (AP) Ph+ CML in adult patients resistant to or intolerant to prior therapy that included imatinib. (1.2)

DOSAGE AND ADMINISTRATION

- Recommended Dose: Newly diagnosed Ph+ CML-CP: 300 mg orally twice daily. Resistant or intolerant Ph+ CML-CP and CML-AP: 400 mg orally twice daily. (2.1)
- Administer Tasigna approximately 12 hours apart and must not take with food. (2.1)
- Swallow the capsules whole with water. Do not consume food for at least 2 hours before the dose is taken and for at least one hour after. (2.1)
- Dose adjustment may be required for hematologic and non-hematologic toxicities, and drug interactions. (2.2)
- A lower starting dose is recommended in patients with hepatic impairment (at baseline). (2.2)

DOSAGE FORMS AND STRENGTHS

150 mg and 200 mg hard capsules (3)

CONTRAINDICATIONS

Do not use in patients with hypokalemia, hypomagnesemia, or long QT syndrome. (4)

WARNINGS AND PRECAUTIONS

- Myelosuppression: Associated with neutropenia, thrombocytopenia and anemia. CBC should be done every 2 weeks for the first 2 months, then monthly. Reversible by withholding dose. Dose reduction may be required. (5.1)
- QT Prolongation: Tasigna prolongs the QT interval. Correct hypokalemia or hypomagnesemia prior to administration and monitor periodically. (5.2) Avoid drugs known to prolong the QT interval and strong CYP3A4 inhibitors. (5.7) Use with caution in patients with hepatic impairment (5.9). Obtain ECGs at baseline, seven days after initiation, and periodically thereafter, as well as following any dose adjustments. (5.2, 5.3, 5.6, 5.13)
- Sudden deaths: Sudden deaths have been reported in patients with resistant or intolerant Ph+ CML receiving nilotinib. Ventricular repolarization abnormalities may have contributed to their occurrence.
- Pancreatitis and elevated serum lipase: Check serum lipase periodically. In case lipase elevations are accompanied by abdominal symptoms, interrupt doses and consider appropriate diagnostics to exclude pancreatitis. Caution is recommended in patients with history of pancreatitis. (5.4)
- Hepatotoxicity: Tasigna may result in elevations in bilirubin, AST/ALT, and alkaline phosphatase. Check hepatic function tests periodically. (5.5)
- Electrolyte abnormalities: Tasigna can cause hypophosphatemia, hypokalemia, hyperkalemia, hypocalcemia, and hyponatremia. Correct electrolyte abnormalities prior to initiating Tasigna and monitor periodically during therapy. (5.6, 5.13)
- Hepatic impairment: Nilotinib exposure is increased in patients with impaired hepatic function (at baseline). A dose reduction is recommended in these patients and QT interval should be monitored closely. (5.9)
- Tumor Lysis Syndrome: Cases of tumor lysis syndrome have been reported in Tasigna treated patients with resistant or intolerant CML. Due to potential for tumor lysis syndrome, maintain adequate hydration and correct uric acid levels prior to initiating therapy with Tasigna. (5.10)
- Drug interactions: Avoid concomitant use of strong inhibitors or inducers of CYP3A4. If patients must be co-administered a strong CYP3A4 inhibitor, dose reduction should be considered and the QT interval should be monitored closely. (5.7)
- Food Effects: Food increases blood levels of Tasigna.
- Avoid food 2 hours before and 1 hour after a dose. (5.8)
- Total gastrectomy: More frequent follow-up of these patients should be considered. If necessary, dose increase may be considered (5.11).
- Pregnancy: Fetal harm can occur when administered to a pregnant woman. Women should be advised not to become pregnant when taking Tasigna. (5.14, 8.1)

ADVERSE REACTIONS

The most commonly reported non-hematologic adverse reactions (≥10%) in patients with newly diagnosed Ph+ CML-CP, resistant or intolerant

Ph+ CML-CP, or resistant or intolerant Ph+ CML-AP were rash, pruritus, headache, nausea, fatigue, myalgia, nasopharyngitis, constipation, diarrhea, abdominal pain, vomiting, arthralgia, pyrexia, upper respiratory tract infection, back pain, cough, and asthenia. Hematologic adverse drug reactions include myelosuppression: thrombocytopenia, neutropenia and anemia. (6.1)

To report SUSPECTED ADVERSE REACTIONS, contact Novartis Pharmaceuticals Corporation at 1-888-669-6682 or FDA at 1-800-FDA-1088 or www.fda.gov/medwatch.

DRUG INTERACTIONS

- Tasigna is an inhibitor of CYP3A4, CYP2C8, CYP2C9, and CYP2D6. It may also induce CYP2B6, CYP2C8 and CYP2C9. Therefore, Tasigna may alter serum concentration of other drugs (7.1)
- CYP3A4 inhibitors may affect serum concentration (7.2)
- CYP3A4 inducers may affect serum concentration (7.2)

USE IN SPECIFIC POPULATIONS

- Sexually active female patients should use effective contraception during treatment (8.1)
- Should not breast-feed (8.3)
- No data to support use in pediatrics (8.4)
- A lower starting dose is recommended in patients with hepatic impairment (at baseline). (2.2, 8.7)

See 17 for PATIENT COUNSELING INFORMATION and Medication Guide

Revised: 06/2013

FULL PRESCRIBING INFORMATION: CONTENTS*

*** Sections or subsections omitted from the full prescribing information are not listed**

FULL PRESCRIBING INFORMATION

WARNING: QT PROLONGATION AND SUDDEN DEATHS

- **Tasigna prolongs the QT interval. Prior to Tasigna administration and periodically, monitor for hypokalemia or hypomagnesemia and correct deficiencies (5.2). Obtain ECGs to monitor the QTc at baseline, seven days after initiation, and periodically thereafter, and following any dose adjustments (5.2, 5.3, 5.6, 5.13).**
- **Sudden deaths have been reported in patients receiving nilotinib (5.3). Do not administer Tasigna to patients with hypokalemia, hypomagnesemia, or long QT syndrome (4, 5.2).**
- **Avoid use of concomitant drugs known to prolong the QT interval and strong CYP3A4 inhibitors (5.7).**

• Patients should avoid food 2 hours before and 1 hour after taking dose (5.8).

1 INDICATIONS AND USAGE

1.1 Newly Diagnosed Ph+ CML-CP

Tasigna (nilotinib) is indicated for the treatment of adult patients with newly diagnosed Philadelphia chromosome positive chronic myeloid leukemia (Ph+ CML) in chronic phase. The effectiveness of Tasigna is based on major molecular response and cytogenetic response rates *[see Clinical Studies (14.1)]*. The study is ongoing and further data will be required to determine long-term outcome.

1.2 Resistant or Intolerant Ph+ CML-CP and CML-AP

Tasigna is indicated for the treatment of chronic phase and accelerated phase Philadelphia chromosome positive chronic myelogenous leukemia (Ph+ CML) in adult patients resistant or intolerant to prior therapy that included imatinib. The effectiveness of Tasigna is based on hematologic and cytogenetic response rates *[see Clinical Studies (14.2)]*.

2 DOSAGE AND ADMINISTRATION

2.1 Recommended Dosing

Tasigna should be taken twice daily at approximately 12 hour intervals and must not be taken with food. The capsules should be swallowed whole with water. No food should be consumed for at least 2 hours before the dose is taken and no food should be consumed for at least one hour after the dose is taken *[see Boxed Warning, Warnings and Precautions (5.8), Clinical Pharmacology (12.3)]*.

For patients who are unable to swallow capsules, the contents of each capsule may be dispersed in one teaspoon of applesauce (puréed apple). The mixture should be taken immediately (within 15 minutes) and should not be stored for future use *[see Clinical Pharmacology (12.3)]*.

Tasigna may be given in combination with hematopoietic growth factors such as erythropoietin or G-CSF if clinically indicated. Tasigna may be given with hydroxyurea or anagrelide if clinically indicated.

Newly Diagnosed Ph+ CML-CP

The recommended dose of Tasigna is 300 mg orally twice daily *[see Clinical Pharmacology (12.3)]*.

Resistant or Intolerant Ph+ CML-CP and CML-AP

The recommended dose of Tasigna (nilotinib) is 400 mg orally twice daily *[see Clinical Pharmacology (12.3)]*.

2.2 Dose Adjustments or Modifications

QT interval prolongation:

Table 1: Dose Adjustments for QT Prolongation

ECGs with a QTc >480 msec	1. Withhold Tasigna, and perform an analysis of serum potassium and magnesium, and if below lower limit of normal, correct with supplements to within normal limits. Concomitant medication usage must be reviewed. 2. Resume within 2 weeks at prior dose if QTcF returns to <450 msec and to within 20 msec of baseline. 3. If QTcF is between 450 msec and 480 msec after 2 weeks, reduce the dose to 400 mg once daily. 4. If, following dose-reduction to 400 mg once daily, QTcF returns to >480 msec, Tasigna should be discontinued. 5. An ECG should be repeated approximately 7 days after any dose adjustment.

Myelosuppression

Tasigna may need to be withheld and/or dose reduced for hematological toxicities (neutropenia, thrombocytopenia) that are not related to underlying leukemia (Table 2).

[See table 2 above]

See Table 3 for dose adjustments for elevations of lipase, amylase, bilirubin, and/or hepatic transaminases *[see Adverse Reactions (6.1)]*.

Table 3: Dose Adjustments for Selected Non-hematologic Laboratory Abnormalities

Elevated serum lipase or amylase ≥Grade 3	1. Withhold Tasigna, and monitor serum lipase or amylase 2. Resume treatment at 400 mg once daily if serum lipase or amylase returns to ≤Grade 1
Elevated bilirubin ≥Grade 3	1. Withhold Tasigna, and monitor bilirubin 2. Resume treatment at 400 mg once daily if bilirubin returns to ≤Grade 1
Elevated hepatic transaminases ≥Grade 3	1. Withhold Tasigna, and monitor hepatic transaminases 2. Resume treatment at 400 mg once daily if hepatic transaminases returns to ≤Grade 1

Table 2: Dose Adjustments for Neutropenia and Thrombocytopenia

Newly diagnosed Ph+ CML in chronic phase at 300 mg twice daily Resistant or intolerant Ph+ CML in chronic phase or accelerated phase at 400 mg twice daily	ANC* <1.0 × 10^9/L and/or platelet counts <50 × 10^9/L	1. Stop Tasigna, and monitor blood counts 2. Resume within 2 weeks at prior dose if ANC >1.0 × 10^9/L and platelets >50 × 10^9/L 3. If blood counts remain low for >2 weeks, reduce the dose to 400 mg once daily

*ANC = absolute neutrophil count

Table 4: Dose Adjustments for Hepatic Impairment (At Baseline)

Newly diagnosed Ph+ CML in chronic phase at 300 mg twice daily	Mild, Moderate or Severe*	An initial dosing regimen of 200 mg twice daily followed by dose escalation to 300 mg twice daily based on tolerability
Resistant or intolerant Ph+ CML in chronic phase or accelerated phase at 400 mg twice daily	Mild or Moderate*	An initial dosing regimen of 300 mg twice daily followed by dose escalation to 400 mg twice daily based on tolerability
	Severe*	A starting dose of 200 mg twice daily followed by a sequential dose escalation to 300 mg twice daily and then to 400 mg twice daily based on tolerability

* Mild = mild hepatic impairment (Child-Pugh Class A); Moderate = moderate hepatic impairment (Child-Pugh Class B); Severe = severe hepatic impairment (Child-Pugh Class C) *[see Warnings and Precautions (5.9), Use in Specific Populations (8.7)]*.

Other Non-hematologic Toxicities

If other clinically significant moderate or severe non-hematologic toxicity develops, withhold dosing, and resume at 400 mg once daily when the toxicity has resolved. If clinically appropriate, escalation of the dose back to 300 mg (newly diagnosed Ph+ CML-CP) or 400 mg (resistant or intolerant Ph+ CML-CP and CML-AP) twice daily should be considered. For Grade 3 to 4 lipase elevations, dosing should be withheld, and may be resumed at 400 mg once daily. Test serum lipase levels monthly or as clinically indicated. For Grade 3 to 4 bilirubin or hepatic transaminase elevations, dosing should be withheld, and may be resumed at 400 mg once daily. Test bilirubin and hepatic transaminases levels monthly or as clinically indicated *[see Warnings and Precautions (5.4, 5.5), Use in Specific Populations (8.7)]*.

Hepatic Impairment

If possible, consider alternative therapies. If Tasigna must be administered to patients with hepatic impairment, consider the following dose reduction:

[See table 4 above]

Concomitant Strong CYP3A4 Inhibitors

Avoid the concomitant use of strong CYP3A4 inhibitors (e.g., ketoconazole, itraconazole, clarithromycin, atazanavir, indinavir, nefazodone, nelfinavir, ritonavir, saquinavir, telithromycin, voriconazole). Grapefruit products may also increase serum concentrations of nilotinib and should be avoided. Should treatment with any of these agents be required, it is recommended that therapy with Tasigna be interrupted. If patients must be co-administered a strong CYP3A4 inhibitor, based on pharmacokinetic studies, consider a dose reduction to 300 mg once daily in patients with resistant or intolerant Ph+ CML or to 200 mg once daily in patients with newly diagnosed Ph+ CML-CP. However, there are no clinical data with this dose adjustment in patients receiving strong CYP3A4 inhibitors. If the strong inhibitor is discontinued, a washout period should be allowed before the Tasigna dose is adjusted upward to the indicated dose. Close monitoring for prolongation of the QT interval is indicated for patients who cannot avoid strong CYP3A4 inhibitors *[see Boxed Warning, Warnings and Precautions (5.2, 5.7), Drug Interactions (7.2)]*.

Concomitant Strong CYP3A4 Inducers

Avoid the concomitant use of strong CYP3A4 inducers (e.g., dexamethasone, phenytoin, carbamazepine, rifampin, rifabutin, rifapentine, phenobarbital). Patients should also refrain from taking St. John's Wort. Based on the nonlinear pharmacokinetic profile of nilotinib, increasing the dose of Tasigna when co-administered with such agents is unlikely to compensate for the loss of exposure *[see Drug Interactions (7.2)]*.

3 DOSAGE FORMS AND STRENGTHS

150 mg red opaque hard gelatin capsules with black axial imprint "NVR/BCR".

200 mg light yellow opaque hard gelatin capsules with a red axial imprint "NVR/TKI".

4 CONTRAINDICATIONS

Do not use in patients with hypokalemia, hypomagnesemia, or long QT syndrome *[see Boxed Warning]*.

5 WARNINGS AND PRECAUTIONS

5.1 Myelosuppression

Treatment with Tasigna can cause Grade 3/4 thrombocytopenia, neutropenia and anemia. Perform complete blood counts every two weeks for the first 2 months and then monthly thereafter, or as clinically indicated. Myelosuppression was generally reversible and usually managed by withholding Tasigna temporarily or dose reduction *[see Dosage and Administration (2.2)]*.

5.2 QT Prolongation

Tasigna has been shown to prolong cardiac ventricular repolarization as measured by the QT interval on the surface ECG in a concentration-dependent manner *[see Adverse Reactions (6.1), Clinical Pharmacology (12.4)]*. Prolongation of the QT interval can result in a type of ventricular tachycardia called torsade de pointes, which may result in syncope, seizure, and/or death. ECGs should be performed at baseline, seven days after initiation, periodically as clinically indicated and following dose adjustments *[see Warnings and Precautions (5.13)]*.

Tasigna should not be used in patients who have hypokalemia, hypomagnesemia or long QT syndrome. Hypokalemia or hypomagnesemia must be corrected prior to initiating Tasigna and these electrolytes should be monitored periodically during therapy *[see Warnings and Precautions (5.13)]*.

Significant prolongation of the QT interval may occur when Tasigna is inappropriately taken with food and/or strong CYP3A4 inhibitors and/or medicinal products with a known potential to prolong QT. Therefore, co-administration with food must be avoided and concomitant use with strong CYP3A4 inhibitors and/or medicinal products with a known potential to prolong QT should be avoided *[see Warnings and Precautions (5.7, 5.8)]*. The presence of hypokalemia and hypomagnesemia may further enhance this effect *[see Warnings and Precautions (5.6, 5.13)]*.

5.3 Sudden Deaths

Sudden deaths have been reported in patients with CML treated with nilotinib in clinical studies (n= 5,661; 0.3%). The relative early occurrence of some of these deaths relative to the initiation of nilotinib suggests the possibility that ventricular repolarization abnormalities may have contributed to their occurrence.

5.4 Elevated Serum Lipase

The use of Tasigna can cause increases in serum lipase. Caution is recommended in patients with a previous history of pancreatitis. If lipase elevations are accompanied by abdominal symptoms, interrupt dosing and consider appropriate diagnostics to exclude pancreatitis. Test serum lipase levels monthly or as clinically indicated.

5.5 Hepatotoxicity

The use of Tasigna may result in elevations in bilirubin, AST/ALT, and alkaline phosphatase. Hepatic function tests should be checked monthly or as clinically indicated *[see Warnings and Precautions (5.13)]*.

5.6 Electrolyte Abnormalities

The use of Tasigna can cause hypophosphatemia, hypokalemia, hyperkalemia, hypocalcemia, and hyponatremia. Electrolyte abnormalities must be corrected prior to initiating Tasigna and these electrolytes should be monitored periodically during therapy *[see Warnings and Precautions (5.13)]*.

5.7 Drug Interactions

The administration of Tasigna with agents that are strong CYP3A4 inhibitors or anti-arrhythmic drugs (including, but not limited to amiodarone, disopyramide, procainamide, quinidine and sotalol) and other drugs that may prolong QT interval (including, but not limited to chloroquine, clarithromycin, haloperidol, methadone, moxifloxacin and pimozide) should be avoided. Should treatment with any of these agents be required, it is recommended that therapy with Tasigna be interrupted. If interruption of treatment with Tasigna is not possible, patients who require treatment with a drug that prolongs QT or strongly inhibits CYP3A4 should be closely monitored for prolongation of the QT interval *[see Boxed Warning, Dosage and Administration (2.2), Drug Interactions (7.2)]*.

5.8 Food Effects

The bioavailability of nilotinib is increased with food. Tasigna must not be taken with food. No food should be taken for at least 2 hours before and for at least one hour after the dose is taken. Grapefruit products and other foods that are known to inhibit CYP3A4 should be avoided *[see Boxed Warning, Drug Interactions (7.2) and Clinical Pharmacology (12.3)]*.

5.9 Hepatic Impairment

Nilotinib exposure is increased in patients with impaired hepatic function. A lower starting dose is recommended for patients with mild to severe hepatic impairment (at baseline) and QT interval should be monitored closely *[see Dosage and Administration (2.2) and Use in Specific Populations (8.7)]*.

5.10 Tumor Lysis Syndrome

Cases of tumor lysis syndrome have been reported in Tasigna treated patients with resistant or intolerant CML. Malignant disease progression, high WBC counts and/or dehydration were present in the majority of these cases. Due to potential for tumor lysis syndrome, maintain adequate hydration and correct uric acid levels prior to initiating therapy with Tasigna.

5.11 Total Gastrectomy

The exposure of nilotinib is reduced in patients with total gastrectomy. More frequent follow-up of these patients should be considered. Dose increase or alternative therapy may be considered in patients with total gastrectomy *[see Clinical Pharmacology 12.3)]*.

5.12 Lactose

Since the capsules contain lactose, Tasigna is not recommended for patients with rare hereditary problems of galactose intolerance, severe lactase deficiency with a severe degree of intolerance to lactose-containing products or of glucose-galactose malabsorption.

5.13 Monitoring Laboratory Tests

Complete blood counts should be performed every two weeks for the first two months and then monthly thereafter. Chemistry panels, including the lipid profile, should be checked periodically. ECGs should be obtained at baseline, seven days after initiation and periodically thereafter, as well as following dose adjustments *[see Warnings and Precautions (5.2)]*. Laboratory monitoring for patients receiving Tasigna may need to be performed more or less frequently at the physician's discretion.

5.14 Use in Pregnancy

There are no adequate and well controlled studies of Tasigna in pregnant women. However, Tasigna may cause fetal harm when administered to a pregnant woman. Nilotinib caused embryo-fetal toxicities in animals at maternal exposures that were lower than the expected human exposure at the recommended doses of nilotinib. If this drug is used during pregnancy, or if the patient becomes pregnant while taking this drug, the patient should be apprised of the potential hazard to the fetus. Women of child-bearing potential should avoid becoming pregnant while taking Tasigna *[see Use in Specific Populations (8.1)]*.

6 ADVERSE REACTIONS

The following serious adverse reactions can occur with Tasigna and are discussed in greater detail in other sections of the package insert *[see Boxed Warning, Warnings and Precautions (5)]*.

Myelosuppression *[see Warnings and Precautions (5.1)]*
QT prolongation *[see Boxed Warning, Warnings and Precautions (5.2)]*
Sudden deaths *[see Boxed Warning, Warnings and Precautions (5.3)]*
Elevated serum lipase *[see Warnings and Precautions (5.4)]*
Hepatotoxicity *[see Warnings and Precautions (5.5)]*
Electrolyte abnormalities *[see Boxed Warning, Warnings and Precautions (5.6)]*

6.1 Clinical Trials Experience

Because clinical trials are conducted under widely varying conditions, adverse reaction rates observed in the clinical trials of a drug cannot be directly compared to rates in the clinical trials of another drug and may not reflect the rates observed in practice.

In Patients with Newly Diagnosed Ph+ CML-CP

The data below reflect exposure to Tasigna from a randomized trial in patients with newly diagnosed Ph+ CML in chronic phase treated at the recommended dose of 300 mg twice daily (n=279). The median time on treatment in the nilotinib 300 mg twice daily group was 36.4 months (range 0.1 – 46.7 months). The median actual dose intensity was 594 mg/day in the nilotinib 300 mg twice daily group.

The most common (>10%) non-hematologic adverse drug reactions were rash, pruritus, headache, nausea, fatigue and myalgia. Upper abdominal pain, alopecia, constipation, diarrhea, dry skin, muscle spasms, arthralgia, abdominal pain, peripheral edema, vomiting, pain in extremity, dys-

Table 5: Most Frequently Reported Non-hematologic Adverse Reactions (Regardless of Relationship to Study Drug) in Patients with Newly Diagnosed Ph+ CML-CP (≥10% in Tasigna 300 mg twice daily or Imatinib 400 mg once daily groups) 36-Month Analysis[a]

		Patients with Newly Diagnosed Ph+ CML-CP			
		TASIGNA 300 mg twice daily	Imatinib 400 mg once daily	TASIGNA 300 mg twice daily	Imatinib 400 mg once daily
		N=279	N=280	N=279	N=280
Body System and Preferred Term		All Grades (%)		CTC Grades[b] 3 / 4 (%)	
Skin and subcutaneous tissue disorders	Rash	38	18	<1	2
	Pruritus	21	7	<1	0
	Alopecia	13	6	0	0
	Dry skin	10	6	0	0
Gastrointestinal disorders	Nausea	21	40	1	1
	Constipation	18	7	<1	0
	Diarrhea	16	44	<1	3
	Vomiting	14	25	0	<1
	Abdominal pain upper	17	13	1	<1
	Abdominal pain	15	11	1	<1
	Dyspepsia	8	11	0	0
Nervous system disorders	Headache	30	20	3	<1
	Dizziness	10	10	0	<1
General disorders and administration site conditions	Fatigue	22	17	1	1
	Pyrexia	13	12	<1	0
	Asthenia	13	10	<1	0
	Peripheral edema	9	20	<1	0
	Face edema	<1	13	0	<1
Musculoskeletal and connective tissue disorders	Myalgia	18	18	<1	<1
	Arthralgia	18	14	<1	<1
	Muscle spasms	12	33	0	1
	Pain in extremity	11	14	<1	<1
	Back pain	15	14	<1	1
Respiratory, thoracic and mediastinal disorders	Cough	15	11	0	0
	Oropharyngeal pain	10	6	0	0
Infections and infestations	Nasopharyngitis	24	19	0	0
	Upper respiratory tract infection	15	11	<1	0
	Influenza	11	8	0	0
Eye disorders	Eyelid edema	1	18	0	<1
	Periorbital edema	<1	15	0	0
Psychiatric disorders	Insomnia	10	9	0	0

[a] Excluding laboratory abnormalities
[b] NCI Common Terminology Criteria for Adverse Events, Version 3.0

pepsia, and asthenia were observed less commonly (≤10% and >5%) and have been of mild to moderate severity, manageable and generally did not require dose reduction. Pleural and pericardial effusions, occurred in 1% and <1% of patients, respectively. Gastrointestinal hemorrhage was reported in 2.5% of patients.

Increase in QTcF >60 msec from baseline was observed in 1 patient (0.4%) in the 300 mg twice daily treatment group. No patient had an absolute QTcF of >500 msec while on study drug.

The most common hematologic adverse drug reactions (all grades) were myelosuppression including: thrombocytopenia (18%), neutropenia (15%) and anemia (7%). See Table 7 for Grade 3/4 laboratory abnormalities.

Discontinuation due to adverse reactions, regardless of relationship to study drug, was observed in 10% of patients.

In Patients with Resistant or Intolerant Ph+ CML-CP and CML-AP

In the single open-label multicenter clinical trial, a total of 458 patients with Ph+ CML-CP and CML-AP resistant to or intolerant to at least one prior therapy including imatinib were treated (CML-CP=321; CML-AP=137) at the recommended dose of 400 mg twice daily.

The median duration of exposure in days for CML-CP and CML-AP patients is 561 (range 1-1096) and 264 (range 2-1160), respectively. The median dose intensity for patients with CML-CP and CML-AP is 789 mg/day (range 151–1110) and 780 mg/day (range 150-1149), respectively and corresponded to the planned 400 mg twice daily dosing.

The median cumulative duration in days of dose interruptions for the CML-CP patients was 20 (range 1-345), and the median duration in days of dose interruptions for the CML-AP patients was 23 (range 1–234).

In patients with CML-CP, the most commonly reported non-hematologic adverse drug reactions (≥10%) were rash, pruritus, nausea, fatigue, headache, constipation, diarrhea, vomiting and myalgia. The common serious drug-related adverse reactions (≥1% and <10%) were thrombocytopenia, neutropenia and anemia.

In patients with CML-AP, the most commonly reported non-hematologic adverse drug reactions (≥10%) were rash, pruritus and fatigue. The common serious adverse drug reactions (≥1% and <10%) were thrombocytopenia, neutropenia, febrile neutropenia, pneumonia, leukopenia, intracranial hemorrhage, elevated lipase and pyrexia.

Sudden deaths and QT prolongation were reported. The maximum mean QTcF change from baseline at steady-state was 10 msec. Increase in QTcF >60 msec from baseline was observed in 4.1% of the patients and QTcF of >500 msec was observed in 4 patients (<1%) *[see Boxed Warning, Warnings and Precautions (5.2, 5.3), Clinical Pharmacology (12.4)]*.

Discontinuation due to adverse drug reactions was observed in 16% of CML-CP and 10% of CML-AP patients.

Most Frequently Reported Adverse Reactions

Tables 5 and 6 show the percentage of patients experiencing non-hematologic adverse reactions (excluding laboratory abnormalities) regardless of relationship to study drug. Adverse reactions reported in greater than 10% of patients who received at least one dose of Tasigna are listed.

[See table 5 at top of previous page]

[See table 6 above]

Laboratory Abnormalities

Table 7 shows the percentage of patients experiencing treatment-emergent Grade 3/4 laboratory abnormalities in patients who received at least one dose of Tasigna.

[See table 7 at top of next page]

6.2 Additional Data from Clinical Trials

The following adverse drug reactions were reported in patients in the Tasigna clinical studies at the recommended doses. These adverse drug reactions are ranked under a heading of frequency, the most frequent first using the following convention: common (≥1% and <10%), uncommon (≥0.1% and <1%), and unknown frequency (single events). For laboratory abnormalities, very common events (≥10%), which were not included in Tables 5 and 6, are also reported. These adverse reactions are included based on clinical relevance and ranked in order of decreasing seriousness within each category.

Infections and Infestations: Common: folliculitis, upper respiratory tract infection (including pharyngitis, nasopharyngitis, rhinitis). Uncommon: pneumonia, bronchitis, urinary tract infection, candidiasis (including oral candidiasis), gastroenteritis. Unknown frequency: sepsis, subcutaneous abscess, anal abscess, furuncle, tinea pedis.

Neoplasms Benign, Malignant and Unspecified: Common: Skin papilloma. Unknown frequency: oral papilloma, paraproteinemia.

Blood and Lymphatic System Disorders: Common: febrile neutropenia, pancytopenia, lymphopenia. Unknown frequency: thrombocythemia, leukocytosis, eosinophilia.

Immune System Disorders: Unknown frequency: hypersensitivity.

Table 6: Most Frequently Reported Non-hematologic Adverse Reactions in Patients with Resistant or Intolerant Ph+ CML Receiving Tasigna 400 mg Twice Daily (Regardless of Relationship to Study Drug) (≥10% in any Group) 24-Month Analysis[a]

Body System and Preferred Term		CML-CP N=321 All Grades (%)	CML-CP N=321 CTC Grades[b] 3 / 4 (%)	CML-AP N=137 All Grades (%)	CML-AP N=137 CTC Grades[b] 3 / 4 (%)
Skin and subcutaneous tissue disorders	Rash	36	2	29	0
	Pruritus	32	<1	20	0
	Night sweat	12	<1	27	0
	Alopecia	11	0	12	0
Gastrointestinal disorders	Nausea	37	1	22	<1
	Constipation	26	<1	19	0
	Diarrhea	28	3	24	2
	Vomiting	29	<1	13	0
	Abdominal pain	15	2	16	3
	Abdominal pain upper	14	<1	12	<1
	Dyspepsia	10	<1	4	0
Nervous system disorders	Headache	35	2	20	1
General disorders and administration site conditions	Fatigue	32	3	23	<1
	Pyrexia	22	<1	28	2
	Asthenia	16	0	14	1
	Peripheral edema	15	<1	12	0
Musculoskeletal and connective tissue disorders	Myalgia	19	2	16	<1
	Arthralgia	26	2	16	0
	Muscle spasms	13	<1	15	0
	Bone pain	14	<1	15	2
	Pain in extremity	20	2	18	1
	Back pain	17	2	15	<1
	Musculoskeletal pain	11	<1	12	1
Respiratory, thoracic and mediastinal disorders	Cough	27	<1	18	0
	Dyspnea	15	2	9	2
	Oropharyngeal pain	11	0	7	0
Infections and infestations	Nasopharyngitis	24	<1	15	0
	Upper respiratory tract infection	12	0	10	0
Metabolism and nutrition disorders	Decreased appetite[c]	15	<1	17	<1
Psychiatric disorders	Insomnia	12	1	7	0
Vascular disorders	Hypertension	10	2	11	<1

[a] Excluding laboratory abnormalities [b] NCI Common Terminology Criteria for Adverse Events, Version 3.0 [c] Also includes preferred term anorexia

Endocrine Disorders: Uncommon: hyperthyroidism, hypothyroidism. Unknown frequency: hyperparathyroidism secondary, thyroiditis.

Metabolism and Nutrition Disorders: Very Common: hypophosphatemia. Common: electrolyte imbalance (including hypomagnesemia, hyperkalemia, hypokalemia, hyponatremia, hypocalcemia, hypercalcemia, hyperphosphatemia), diabetes mellitus, hyperglycemia, hypercholesterolemia, hyperlipidemia. Uncommon: gout, dehydration, increased appetite. Unknown frequency: hyperuricemia, hypoglycemia, dyslipidemia.

Psychiatric Disorders: Common: depression, insomnia, anxiety. Unknown frequency: disorientation, confusional state, amnesia, dysphoria.

Nervous System Disorders: Common: dizziness, peripheral neuropathy, hypoesthesia, paresthesia. Uncommon: intracranial hemorrhage, migraine, loss of consciousness (including syncope), tremor, disturbance in attention, hyperesthesia. Unknown frequency: brain edema, optic neuritis, lethargy, dysesthesia, restless legs syndrome.

Eye Disorders: Common: eye hemorrhage, periorbital edema, eye pruritus, conjunctivitis, dry eye (including xerophthalmia). Uncommon: vision impairment, vision blurred, visual acuity reduced, photopsia, hyperemia (scleral, conjunctival, ocular), eye irritation, conjunctival hemorrhage. Unknown frequency: papilloedema, diplopia, photophobia, eye swelling, blepharitis, eye pain, chorioretinopathy, conjunctivitis allergic, ocular surface disease.

Table 7: Percent Incidence of Clinically Relevant Grade 3/4* Laboratory Abnormalities

	Patient Population			
	Newly Diagnosed Ph+ CML-CP		Resistant or Intolerant Ph+	
			CML-CP	CML-AP
	TASIGNA 300 mg twice daily N=279 (%)	Imatinib 400 mg once daily N=280 (%)	TASIGNA 400 mg twice daily N=321 (%)	TASIGNA 400 mg twice daily N=137 (%)
Hematologic Parameters				
Thrombocytopenia	10	9	30[1]	42[3]
Neutropenia	12	21	31[2]	42[4]
Anemia	4	6	11	27
Biochemistry Parameters				
Elevated lipase	8	4	18	18
Hyperglycemia	6	0	12	6
Hypophosphatemia	6	9	17	15
Elevated bilirubin (total)	4	<1	7	9
Elevated SGPT (ALT)	4	3	4	4
Hyperkalemia	2	1	6	4
Hyponatremia	1	<1	7	7
Hypokalemia	<1	2	2	9
Elevated SGOT (AST)	1	1	3	2
Decreased albumin	0	<1	4	3
Hypocalcemia	<1	<1	2	5
Elevated alkaline phosphatase	0	<1	<1	1
Elevated creatinine	0	<1	<1	<1

*NCI Common Terminology Criteria for Adverse Events, version 3.0
[1]CML-CP: Thrombocytopenia: 12% were grade 3, 18% were grade 4
[2]CML-CP: Neutropenia: 16% were grade 3, 15% were grade 4
[3]CML-AP: Thrombocytopenia: 11% were grade 3, 32% were grade 4
[4]CML-AP: Neutropenia: 16% were grade 3, 26% were grade 4

Ear and Labyrinth Disorders: Common: vertigo. Unknown frequency: hearing impaired, ear pain, tinnitus.
Cardiac Disorders: Common: angina pectoris, arrhythmia (including atrioventricular block, cardiac flutter, extrasystoles, atrial fibrillation, tachycardia, bradycardia), palpitations, electrocardiogram QT prolonged. Uncommon: cardiac failure, pericardial effusion, coronary artery disease, cyanosis, cardiac murmur. Unknown frequency: myocardial infarction, ventricular dysfunction, pericarditis, ejection fraction decrease.
Vascular Disorders: Common: hypertension, flushing. Uncommon: hypertensive crisis, peripheral arterial occlusive disease, hematoma. Unknown frequency: shock hemorrhagic, hypotension, thrombosis, arteriosclerosis.
Respiratory, Thoracic and Mediastinal Disorders: Common: dyspnea, dyspnea exertional, epistaxis, cough, dysphonia. Uncommon: pulmonary edema, pleural effusion, interstitial lung disease, pleuritic pain, pleurisy, pharyngolaryngeal pain, throat irritation. Unknown frequency: pulmonary hypertension, wheezing, oropharyngeal pain.
Gastrointestinal Disorders: Common: pancreatitis, abdominal discomfort, abdominal distension, dyspepsia, dysgeusia, flatulence. Uncommon: gastrointestinal hemorrhage, melena, mouth ulceration, gastroesophageal reflux, stomatitis, esophageal pain, dry mouth, sensitivity of teeth. Unknown frequency: gastrointestinal ulcer perforation, retroperitoneal hemorrhage, hematemesis, gastric ulcer, esophagitis ulcerative, subileus, gastritis, enterocolitis, hemorrhoids, hiatus hernia, rectal hemorrhage, gingivitis.
Hepatobiliary Disorders: Very Common: hyperbilirubinemia. Common: hepatic function abnormal. Uncommon: hepatotoxicity, toxic hepatitis, jaundice. Unknown frequency: cholestasis, hepatomegaly.
Skin and Subcutaneous Tissue Disorders: Common: night sweats, eczema, urticaria, erythema, hyperhidrosis, contusion, acne, dermatitis (including allergic, exfoliative and acneiform), dry skin. Uncommon: exfoliative rash, drug eruption, pain of skin, ecchymosis, swelling of face. Unknown frequency: psoriasis, erythema multiforme, erythema nodosum, skin ulcer, palmar-plantar erythrodysesthesia syndrome, petechiae, photosensitivity, blister, dermal cyst, sebaceous hyperplasia, skin atrophy, skin discoloration, skin exfoliation, skin hyperpigmentation, skin hypertrophy, hyperkeratosis.
Musculoskeletal and Connective Tissue Disorders: Common: bone pain, musculoskeletal chest pain, musculoskeletal pain, back pain, neck pain, flank pain. Uncommon: musculoskeletal stiffness, muscular weakness, joint swelling. Unknown frequency: arthritis.
Renal and Urinary Disorders: Common: pollakiuria. Uncommon: dysuria, micturition urgency, nocturia. Unknown frequency: renal failure, hematuria, urinary incontinence, chromaturia.
Reproductive System and Breast Disorders: Uncommon: breast pain, gynecomastia, erectile dysfunction. Unknown frequency: breast induration, menorrhagia, nipple swelling.
General Disorders and Administration Site Conditions: Common: pyrexia, chest pain (including non-cardiac chest pain), pain, chest discomfort, malaise. Uncommon: face edema, gravitational edema, influenza-like illness, chills, feeling body temperature change (including feeling hot, feeling cold). Unknown frequency: localized edema.
Investigations: Very Common: alanine aminotransferase increased, aspartate aminotransferase increased, lipase increased. Common: hemoglobin decreased, blood amylase increased, gamma-glutamyltransferase increased, blood creatinine phosphokinase increased, blood alkaline phosphatase increased, weight decreased, weight increased. Uncommon: blood lactate dehydrogenase increased, blood urea increased, globulins decreased. Unknown frequency: troponin increased, blood bilirubin unconjugated increased, blood insulin increased, blood insulin decreased, insulin C-peptide decreased, lipoprotein increased (including very low density and high density), blood parathyroid hormone increased.

7 DRUG INTERACTIONS

7.1 Effects of Nilotinib on Drug Metabolizing Enzymes and Drug Transport Systems

Nilotinib is a competitive inhibitor of CYP3A4, CYP2C8, CYP2C9, CYP2D6 and UGT1A1 *in vitro*, potentially increasing the concentrations of drugs eliminated by these enzymes. *In vitro* studies also suggest that nilotinib may induce CYP2B6, CYP2C8 and CYP2C9, and decrease the concentrations of drugs which are eliminated by these enzymes.

Single-dose administration of Tasigna with midazolam (a CYP3A4 substrate) to healthy subjects increased midazolam exposure by 30%. Single-dose administration of Tasigna to healthy subjects did not change the pharmacokinetics and pharmacodynamics of warfarin (a CYP2C9 substrate). The ability of Tasigna to induce metabolism has not been determined *in vivo*. Exercise caution when co-administering Tasigna with substrates for these enzymes that have a narrow therapeutic index.

Nilotinib inhibits human P-glycoprotein (P-gp). If Tasigna is administered with drugs that are substrates of P-gp, increased concentrations of the substrate drug are likely, and caution should be exercised.

7.2 Drugs that Inhibit or Induce Cytochrome P450 3A4 Enzymes

Nilotinib undergoes metabolism by CYP3A4, and concomitant administration of strong inhibitors or inducers of CYP3A4 can increase or decrease nilotinib concentrations significantly. The administration of Tasigna with agents that are strong CYP3A4 inhibitors should be avoided *[see Boxed Warning, Dosage and Administration (2.2), Warnings and Precautions (5.2, 5.7)]*. Concomitant use of Tasigna with medicinal products and herbal preparations that are potent inducers of CYP3A4 is likely to reduce exposure to nilotinib to a clinically relevant extent. Therefore, in patients receiving Tasigna, concomitant use of alternative therapeutic agents with less potential for CYP3A4 induction should be selected.

Ketoconazole: In healthy subjects receiving ketoconazole, a CYP3A4 inhibitor, at 400 mg once daily for 6 days, systemic exposure (AUC) to nilotinib was increased approximately 3-fold.

Rifampicin: In healthy subjects receiving the CYP3A4 inducer, rifampicin, at 600 mg daily for 12 days, systemic exposure (AUC) to nilotinib was decreased approximately 80%.

7.3 Drugs that Affect Gastric pH

Nilotinib has pH-dependent solubility, with decreased solubility at higher pH. Drugs such as proton pump inhibitors that inhibit gastric acid secretion to elevate the gastric pH may decrease the solubility of nilotinib and reduce its bioavailability. In healthy subjects, co-administration of a single 400 mg dose of Tasigna with multiple doses of esomeprazole (a proton pump inhibitor) at 40 mg daily decreased the nilotinib AUC by 34%. Increasing the dose of Tasigna when co-administered with such agents is not likely to compensate for the loss of exposure. Since proton pump inhibitors affect pH of the upper GI tract for an extended period, separation of doses may not eliminate the interaction. The concomitant use of proton pump inhibitors with Tasigna is not recommended.

In healthy subjects, no significant change in nilotinib pharmacokinetics was observed when a single 400 mg dose of Tasigna was administered ten hours after and two hours before famotidine (an H2 blocker). Therefore, when the concurrent use of a H2 blocker is necessary, it may be administered approximately ten hours before and approximately two hours after the dose of Tasigna.

Administration of an antacid (aluminum hydroxide/magnesium hydroxide/simethicone) to healthy subjects, two hours before or two hours after a single 400 mg dose of Tasigna did not alter nilotinib pharmacokinetics. Therefore, if necessary, an antacid may be administered approximately two hours before or approximately two hours after the dose of Tasigna.

7.4 Drugs that Inhibit Drug Transport Systems

Nilotinib is a substrate of the efflux transporter P-glycoprotein (P-gp, ABCB1). If Tasigna is administered with drugs that inhibit P-gp, increased concentrations of nilotinib are likely, and caution should be exercised.

7.5 Drugs that May Prolong the QT Interval

The administration of Tasigna with agents that may prolong the QT interval such as anti-arrhythmic medicines should be avoided *[see Boxed Warning, Dosage and Administration (2.2), Warnings and Precautions (5.2, 5.7)]*.

8 USE IN SPECIFIC POPULATIONS

8.1 Pregnancy

Pregnancy Category D *[see Warnings and Precautions (5.14)]*.

Based on its mechanism of action and findings in animals, Tasigna may cause fetal harm when administered to a pregnant woman. There are no adequate and well controlled studies with Tasigna in pregnant women. Women should be advised to avoid becoming pregnant while on Tasigna. If this drug is used during pregnancy, or if the patient becomes pregnant while taking this drug, the patient should be apprised of the potential hazard to the fetus.

Nilotinib was studied for effects on embryo-fetal development in pregnant rats and rabbits given oral doses of 10, 30, 100 mg/kg/day, and 30, 100, 300 mg/kg/day, respectively, during organogenesis. In rats, nilotinib at doses of 100 mg/kg/day (approximately 5.7 times the AUC in patients at the dose of 400 mg twice daily) was associated with maternal toxicity (decreased gestation weight, gravid uterine weight, net weight gain, and food consumption). Nilotinib at doses ≥30 mg/kg/day (approximately 2 times the AUC in patients at the dose of 400 mg twice daily) resulted in embryo-fetal toxicity as shown by increased resorption and post-implantation loss, and at 100 mg/kg/day, a decrease in viable fetuses. In rabbits, maternal toxicity at 300 mg/kg/day (approximately one-half the human exposure based on AUC) was associated with mortality, abortion, decreased gestation weights and decreased food consumption. Embryonic toxicity (increased resorption) and minor skeletal anomalies were observed at a dose of 300 mg/kg/day. Nilotinib is not considered teratogenic.

When pregnant rats were dosed with nilotinib during organogenesis and through lactation, the adverse effects included a longer gestational period, lower pup body weights until weaning and decreased fertility indices in the pups when they reached maturity, all at a maternal dose of 360 mg/m^2 (approximately 0.7 times the clinical dose of 400 mg twice daily based on body surface area). At doses up to 120 mg/m^2 (approximately 0.25 times the clinical dose of 400 mg twice daily based on body surface area) no adverse effects were seen in the maternal animals or the pups.

8.3 Nursing Mothers

It is not known whether nilotinib is excreted in human milk. One study in lactating rats demonstrates that nilotinib is excreted into milk. Because many drugs are excreted in human milk and because of the potential for serious adverse reactions in nursing infants from Tasigna, a decision should be made whether to discontinue nursing or to discontinue the drug, taking into account the importance of the drug to the mother.

8.4 Pediatric Use

The safety and effectiveness of Tasigna in pediatric patients have not been established.

8.5 Geriatric Use

In the clinical trials of Tasigna (patients with newly diagnosed Ph+ CML-CP and resistant or intolerant Ph+ CML-CP and CML-AP), approximately 12% and 30% of patients were 65 years or over respectively.

- Patients with newly diagnosed Ph+ CML-CP: There was no difference in major molecular response between patients aged <65 years and those ≥65 years.
- Patients with resistant or intolerant CML-CP: There was no difference in major cytogenetic response rate between patients aged <65 years and those ≥65 years.
- Patients with resistant or intolerant CML-AP: The hematologic response rate was 44% in patients <65 years of age and 29% in patients ≥65 years.

No major differences for safety were observed in patients ≥65 years of age as compared to patients <65 years.

8.6 Cardiac Disorders

In the clinical trials, patients with a history of uncontrolled or significant cardiovascular disease, including recent myocardial infarction, congestive heart failure, unstable angina or clinically significant bradycardia, were excluded. Caution should be exercised in patients with relevant cardiac disorders *[see Boxed Warning, Warnings and Precautions (5.2)]*.

8.7 Hepatic Impairment

Nilotinib exposure is increased in patients with impaired hepatic function. In a study of subjects with mild to severe hepatic impairment following a single dose administration of 200 mg of Tasigna, the mean AUC values were increased on average of 35%, 35% and 56% in subjects with mild (Child-Pugh class A, score 5-6), moderate (Child-Pugh class B, score 7-9) and severe hepatic impairment (Child-Pugh class C, score 10-15), respectively, compared to a control group of subjects with normal hepatic function. Table 8 summarizes the Child-Pugh Liver Function Classification applied in this study. A lower starting dose is recommended in patients with hepatic impairment and the QT interval should be monitored closely in these patients *[see Dosage and Administration (2.2), Warnings and Precautions (5.9)]*.

Table 8: Child-Pugh Liver Function Classification

Assessment	Degree of Abnormality	Score
Encephalopathy Grade	None 1 or 2 3 or 4	1 2 3
Ascites	Absent Slight Moderate	1 2 3
Total Bilirubin (mg/dL)	<2 2 - 3 >3	1 2 3
Serum Albumin (g/dL)	>3.5 2.8 - 3.5 <2.8	1 2 3
Prothrombin Time (seconds prolonged)	<4 4 - 6 >6	1 2 3

8.8 Renal Impairment

Clinical studies have not been performed in patients with impaired renal function. Clinical studies have excluded patients with serum creatinine concentration >1.5 times the upper limit of the normal range.

Since nilotinib and its metabolites are not renally excreted, a decrease in total body clearance is not anticipated in patients with renal impairment.

10 OVERDOSAGE

Overdose with nilotinib has been reported, where an unspecified number of Tasigna capsules were ingested in combination with alcohol and other drugs. Events included neutropenia, vomiting, and drowsiness. In the event of overdose, the patient should be observed and appropriate supportive treatment given.

11 DESCRIPTION

Tasigna (nilotinib) belongs to a pharmacologic class of drugs known as kinase inhibitors.

Nilotinib drug substance, a monohydrate monohydrochloride, is a white to slightly yellowish to slightly greenish yellow powder with the anhydrous molecular formula and weight, respectively, of $C_{28}H_{22}F_3N_7O \cdot HCl \bullet H_2O$ and 584. The solubility of nilotinib in aqueous solutions decreases with increasing pH. Nilotinib is not optically active. The pK_a1 was determined to be 2.1; pK_a2 was estimated to be 5.4.

The chemical name of nilotinib is 4-methyl-N-[3-(4-methyl-1H-imidazol-1-yl)-5-(trifluoromethyl)phenyl]-3-[[4-(3-pyridinyl)-2-pyrimidinyl]amino]-benzamide, monohydrochloride, monohydrate. Its structure is shown below:

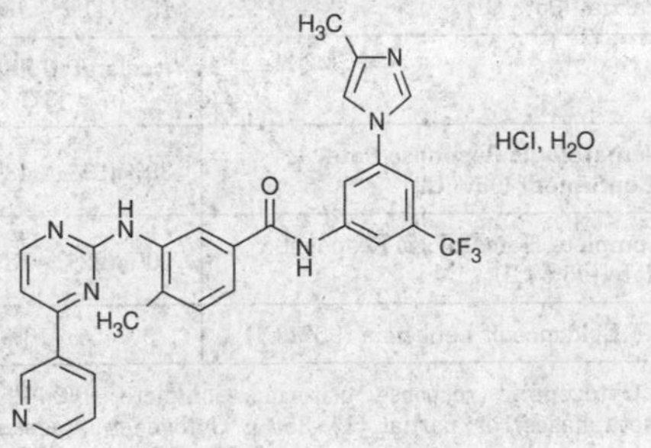

Tasigna (nilotinib) capsules, for oral use, contain 150 mg or 200 mg nilotinib base, anhydrous (as hydrochloride, monohydrate) with the following inactive ingredients: colloidal silicon dioxide, crospovidone, lactose monohydrate, magnesium stearate and polyoxamer 188. The capsules contain gelatin, iron oxide (red), iron oxide (yellow), iron oxide (black) and titanium dioxide.

12 CLINICAL PHARMACOLOGY

12.1 Mechanism of Action

Nilotinib is an inhibitor of the BCR-ABL kinase. Nilotinib binds to and stabilizes the inactive conformation of the kinase domain of ABL protein. In vitro, nilotinib inhibited BCR-ABL mediated proliferation of murine leukemic cell lines and human cell lines derived from patients with Ph+ CML. Under the conditions of the assays, nilotinib was able to overcome imatinib resistance resulting from BCR-ABL kinase mutations, in 32 out of 33 mutations tested. In vivo, nilotinib reduced the tumor size in a murine BCR-ABL xenograft model. Nilotinib inhibited the autophosphorylation of the following kinases at IC50 values as indicated: BCR-ABL (20-60 nM), PDGFR (69 nM), c-KIT (210 nM), CSF-1R (125-250 nM) and DDR1 (3.7 nM).

12.3 Pharmacokinetics

Absorption and Distribution

The absolute bioavailability of nilotinib has not been determined. As compared to an oral drink solution (pH of 1.2 to 1.3), relative bioavailability of nilotinib capsule is approximately 50%. Peak concentrations of nilotinib are reached 3 hours after oral administration.

Steady-state nilotinib exposure was dose-dependent with less than dose-proportional increases in systemic exposure at dose levels higher than 400 mg given as once daily dosing. Daily serum exposure to nilotinib following 400 mg twice daily dosing at steady state was 35% higher than with 800 mg once daily dosing. Steady state exposure (AUC) of nilotinib with 400 mg twice daily dosing was 13% higher than with 300 mg twice daily dosing. The average steady state nilotinib trough and peak concentrations did not change over 12 months. There was no relevant increase in exposure to nilotinib when the dose was increased from 400 mg twice daily to 600 mg twice daily.

The bioavailability of nilotinib was increased when given with a meal. Compared to the fasted state, the systemic exposure (AUC) increased by 82% when the dose was given 30 minutes after a high fat meal.

Single dose administration of two 200 mg nilotinib capsules each dispersed in one teaspoon of applesauce and administered within 15 minutes was shown to be bioequivalent to a single dose administration of two 200 mg intact capsules. The blood-to-serum ratio of nilotinib is 0.68. Serum protein binding is approximately 98% on the basis of *in vitro* experiments.

Median steady-state trough concentration of nilotinib was decreased by 53% in patients with total gastrectomy compared to patients who had not undergone surgeries *[see Warnings and Precautions (5.11)]*.

Pharmacokinetics, Metabolism and Excretion

The apparent elimination half-life estimated from the multiple dose pharmacokinetic studies with daily dosing was approximately 17 hours. Inter-patient variability in nilotinib AUC was 32% to 64%. Steady state conditions were achieved by Day 8. An increase in serum exposure to nilotinib between the first dose and steady state was approximately 2-fold for daily dosing and 3.8-fold for twice-daily dosing.

Main metabolic pathways identified in healthy subjects are oxidation and hydroxylation. Nilotinib is the main circulating component in the serum. None of the metabolites contribute significantly to the pharmacological activity of nilotinib.

After a single dose of radiolabeled nilotinib in healthy subjects, more than 90% of the administered dose was eliminated within 7 days: mainly in feces (93% of the dose). Parent drug accounted for 69% of the dose.

Age, body weight, gender, or ethnic origin did not significantly affect the pharmacokinetics of nilotinib.

Drug-Drug Interactions

In a Phase 1 trial of nilotinib 400 mg twice daily in combination with imatinib 400 mg daily or 400 mg twice daily, the AUC increased 30%-50% for nilotinib and approximately 20% for imatinib.

12.4 QT/QTc Prolongation

In a placebo-controlled study in healthy volunteers designed to assess the effects of Tasigna on the QT interval, administration of Tasigna was associated with concentration-dependent QT prolongation; the maximum mean placebo-adjusted QTcF change from baseline was 18 msec (1-sided 95% Upper CI: 26 msec). A positive control was not included in the QT study of healthy volunteers. Peak plasma concentrations in the QT study were 26% lower than those observed in patients enrolled in the single-arm study *[see Boxed Warning, Warnings and Precautions (5.2) and Adverse Reactions (6.1)]*.

12.5 Pharmacogenomics

Tasigna can increase bilirubin levels. A pharmacogenetic analysis of 97 patients evaluated the polymorphisms of UGT1A1 and its potential association with hyperbilirubinemia during Tasigna treatment. In this study, the (TA)7/(TA)7 genotype was associated with a statistically significant increase in the risk of hyperbilirubinemia relative to the (TA)6/(TA)6 and (TA)6/(TA)7 genotypes. However, the largest increases in bilirubin were observed in the (TA)7/(TA)7 genotype (UGT1A1*28) patients *[see Warnings and Precautions (5.5)]*.

13 NONCLINICAL TOXICOLOGY

13.1 Carcinogenesis, Mutagenesis, Impairment of Fertility

A 2-year carcinogenicity study was conducted orally in rats at nilotinib doses of 5, 15 and 40 mg/kg/day. Exposures in animals at the highest dose tested were approximately 2-3 fold the human exposure (based on AUC) at the nilotinib dose of 400 mg twice daily. The study was negative for carcinogenic findings.

Nilotinib was not mutagenic in a bacterial mutagenesis (Ames) assay, was not clastogenic in a chromosome aberration assay in human lymphocytes, did not induce DNA damage (comet assay) in L5178Y mouse lymphoma cells, nor was it clastogenic in an *in vivo* rat bone marrow micronucleus assay with two oral treatments at doses up to 2000 mg/kg/dose.

There were no effects on male or female rat and female rabbit mating or fertility at doses up to 180 mg/kg in rats (approximately 4-7 fold for males and females, respectively, the AUC in patients at the dose of 400 mg twice daily) or 300 mg/kg in rabbits (approximately one-half the AUC in patients at the dose of 400 mg twice daily). The effect of Tasigna on human fertility is unknown. In a study where male and female rats were treated with nilotinib at oral doses of 20-180 mg/kg/day (approximately 1-6.6 fold the AUC in patients at the dose of 400 mg twice daily) during the pre-mating and mating periods and then mated, and dosing of pregnant rats continued through gestation Day 6, nilotinib increased post-implantation loss and early resorption, and decreased the number of viable fetuses and litter size at all doses tested.

14 CLINICAL STUDIES

14.1 Newly Diagnosed Ph+ CML-CP

An open label, multicenter, randomized trial was conducted to determine the efficacy of Tasigna versus imatinib tablets in adult patients with cytogenetically confirmed newly diagnosed Ph+ CML-CP. Patients were within six months of diagnosis and were previously untreated for CML-CP, except for hydroxyurea and/or anagrelide. Efficacy was based on a total of 846 patients: 283 patients in the imatinib 400 mg once daily group, 282 patients in the nilotinib 300 mg twice daily group, 281 patients in the nilotinib 400 mg twice daily group.

Median age was 46 years in the imatinib group and 47 years in both nilotinib groups, with 12%, 13% and 10% of patients ≥65 years of age in imatinib 400 mg once daily, nilotinib 300 mg twice daily and nilotinib 400 mg twice daily treatment groups, respectively. There were slightly more male than female patients in all groups (56%, 56% and 62% in imatinib 400 mg once daily, nilotinib 300 mg twice daily and nilotinib 400 mg twice daily treatment groups, respectively). More than 60% of all patients were Caucasian, and 25% were Asian.

The primary data analysis was performed when all 846 patients completed 12 months of treatment (or discontinued earlier). Subsequent analyses were done when patients completed 24 and 36 months of treatment (or discontinued earlier). The median time on treatment was approximately 36 months in all three treatment groups. This study is ongoing and further data will be required to determine long-term outcome.

The primary efficacy endpoint was major molecular response (MMR) at 12 months after the start of study medication. MMR was defined as ≤0.1% BCR-ABL/ABL % by international scale measured by RQ-PCR, which corresponds to a ≥3 log reduction of BCR-ABL transcript from standardized baseline. Efficacy endpoints are summarized in Table 9 below.

Two patients in the nilotinib arm progressed to either accelerated phase or blast crisis (both within the first 6 months of treatment) while 17 patients on the imatinib arm progressed to either accelerated phase or blast crisis (8 patients within first 6 months, 4 within 6-12 months, 4 within 12-18 months and 1 within 18-24 months). Between the 24 and 36 month analyses, there were no new progressions to AP/BC in either treatment arm.

Table 9: Efficacy (MMR and CCyR) of TASIGNA Compared to Imatinib in Newly Diagnosed Ph+ CML-CP

	TASIGNA 300 mg twice daily	Imatinib 400 mg once daily
	N = 282	N = 283
MMR at 12 months (95% CI)	44% (38.4, 50.3)	22% (17.6, 27.6)
P-Value[a]	<0.0001	
CCyR[b] by 12 months (95% CI)	80% (75.0, 84.6)	65% (59.2, 70.6)
MMR at 24 months (95% CI)	62% (55.8,67.4)	38% (31.8,43.4)
CCyR[b] by 24 months (95% CI)	87% (82.4,90.6)	77% (71.7, 81.8)

[a] CMH test stratified by Sokal risk group

[b] CCyR: 0% Ph+ metaphases. Cytogenetic responses were based on the percentage of Ph-positive metaphases among ≥20 metaphase cells in each bone marrow sample.

14.2 Patients with Resistant or Intolerant Ph+ CML-CP and CML-AP

A single arm, open label, multicenter study was conducted to evaluate the efficacy and safety of Tasigna (400 mg twice daily) in patients with imatinib-resistant or -intolerant CML with separate cohorts for chronic and accelerated phase disease. The definition of imatinib resistance included failure to achieve a complete hematologic response (by 3 months), cytogenetic response (by 6 months) or major cytogenetic response (by 12 months) or progression of disease after a previous cytogenetic or hematologic response. Imatinib intolerance was defined as discontinuation of treatment due to toxicity and lack of a major cytogenetic response at time of study entry. At the time of data cut-off, 321 patients with CML-CP and 137 patients with CML-AP with a minimum follow-up of 24 months were enrolled. In this study, about 50% of CML-CP and CML-AP patients were males, over 90% (CML-CP) and 80% (CML-AP) were Caucasian, and approximately 30% were age 65 years or older.

Overall, 73% of patients were imatinib resistant while 27% were imatinib intolerant. The median time of prior imatinib treatment was approximately 32 (CML-CP) and 28 (CML-AP) months. Prior therapy included hydroxyurea in 85% of patients, interferon in 56% and stem cell or bone marrow transplant in 8%. The median highest prior imatinib dose was 600 mg/day for patients with CML-CP and CML-AP, and the highest prior imatinib dose was ≥600 mg/day in 74% of all patients with 40% of patients receiving imatinib doses ≥800 mg/day.

Median duration of nilotinib treatment was 18.4 months in patients with CML-CP and 8.7 months in patients with CML-AP.

The efficacy endpoint in CML-CP was unconfirmed major cytogenetic response (MCyR) which included complete and partial cytogenetic responses.

The efficacy endpoint in CML-AP was confirmed hematologic response (HR), defined as either a complete hematologic response (CHR) or no evidence of leukemia (NEL). The rates of response for CML-CP and CML-AP patients are reported in Table 10.

Median durations of response had not been reached at the time of data analysis.

Table 10: Efficacy of Tasigna in Resistant or Intolerant Ph+ CML-CP and CML-AP

Cytogenetic Response Rate (Unconfirmed) (%)[a]	
	Chronic Phase (n = 321)
Major (95% CI)	51% (46% - 57%)
Complete (95% CI)	37% (32% - 42%)
Partial (95% CI)	15% (11% – 19%)
	Accelerated Phase (n = 137)
Hematologic Response Rate (Confirmed) (95% CI)[b]	39% (31% - 48%)
Complete Hematologic Response Rate (95% CI)	30% (22% - 38%)
No Evidence of Leukemia (95% CI)	9% (5% -16%)

[a] Cytogenetic response criteria: Complete (0% Ph + metaphases) or partial (1%-35%). Cytogenetic responses were based on the percentage of Ph-positive metaphases among ≥20 metaphase cells in each bone marrow sample.

[b] Hematologic response = CHR + NEL (all responses confirmed after 4 weeks).

CHR (CML-CP): WBC $<10 \times 10^9$/L, platelets <450,000/mm^3, no blasts or promyelocytes in peripheral blood, <5% myelocytes + metamyelocytes in bone marrow, <20% basophils in peripheral blood, and no extramedullary involvement.

CHR (CML-AP): neutrophils $\geq 1.5 \times 10^9$/L, platelets $\geq 100 \times 10^9$/L, no myeloblasts in peripheral blood, myeloblasts <5% in bone marrow, and no extramedullary involvement.

NEL: same criteria as for CHR but neutrophils $\geq 1.0 \times 10^9$/L and platelets $\geq 20 \times 10^9$/L without transfusions or bleeding.

Patients with Chronic Phase

The MCyR rate in 321 CML-CP patients was 51%. The median time to MCyR among responders was 2.8 months (range 1 to 28 months). The median duration of MCyR cannot be estimated. The median duration of exposure on this single arm trial was 18.4 months. Among the CML-CP patients who achieved MCyR, 62% of them had MCyR lasting more than 18 months. The CCyR rate was 37%.

Patients with Accelerated Phase

The overall confirmed hematologic response rate in 137 patients with CML-AP was 39%. The median time to first hematologic response among responders was 1.0 month (range 1 to 14 months). Among the CML-AP patients who achieved HR, 44% of them had a response lasting for more than 18 months.

After imatinib failure, 24 different BCR-ABL mutations were noted in 42% of chronic phase and 54% of accelerated phase CML patients who were evaluated for mutations.

16 HOW SUPPLIED/STORAGE AND HANDLING

Tasigna (nilotinib) 150 mg capsules are red opaque hard gelatin capsules, size 1 with black axial imprint "NVR/BCR". Tasigna (nilotinib) 200 mg capsules are light yellow opaque hard gelatin capsules, size 0 with the red axial imprint "NVR/TKI." Tasigna capsules are supplied in blister packs.

150 mg

Carton of 4 blister packs of (4x28) .... NDC 0078-0592-87
Blisters of 28 capsules .... NDC 0078-0592-51

200 mg

Carton of 4 blister packs of (4x28) NDC 0078-0526-87
Blisters of 28 capsules NDC 0078-0526-51

Each blister pack contains one folded blister card of 28 capsules each, for dosing two in the morning and two in the evening at 12 hour intervals over a 7 day period.

Tasigna (nilotinib) capsules should be stored at 25°C (77°F); excursions permitted between 15°-30°C (59°-86°F) [see USP Controlled Room Temperature].

17 PATIENT COUNSELING INFORMATION

See Medication Guide

A Medication Guide is required for distribution with Tasigna. Encourage patients to read the Tasigna Medication Guide. The complete text of the Medication Guide is reprinted at the end of this document.

17.1 Taking Tasigna

Tasigna doses should be taken twice daily approximately 12 hours apart and should not be taken with food. The capsules should be swallowed whole with water.

Patients should be advised to take Tasigna on an empty stomach. Tasigna should be taken at least 2 hours after a meal. No food should be consumed for at least one hour after the dose is taken. Patients should not consume grapefruit products and other foods that are known to inhibit CYP3A4 at anytime during Tasigna treatment *[see Dosage and Administration (2.1), Warnings and Precautions (5.7, 5.8) and Medication Guide]*.

If a dose is missed, the patient should not take a make-up dose, but should resume taking the next prescribed daily dose.

Should patients be unable to swallow capsules, the contents of each capsule may be dispersed in one teaspoon of applesauce and the mixture swallowed immediately (within 15 minutes).

17.2 Drug Interactions

Tasigna and certain other medicines, including over the counter medications or herbal supplements (such as St. John's Wort), can interact with each other *[see Warnings and Precautions (5.7) and Drug Interactions (7)]*.

17.3 Pregnancy

Patients should be advised that the use of Tasigna during pregnancy may cause harm to the fetus and should not be taken during pregnancy unless necessary. Women of child-bearing potential should use highly effective contraceptives if taking Tasigna. Sexually active female patients taking Tasigna should use adequate contraception *[see Warnings and Precautions (5.14) and Use in Specific Populations (8.1)]*.

17.4 Compliance

Patients should be advised of the following:

- Continue taking Tasigna every day for as long as their doctor tells them.
- This is a long-term treatment.
- Do not change dose or stop taking Tasigna without first consulting their doctor.
- If a dose is missed, take the next dose as scheduled. Do not take a double dose to make up for the forgotten capsules.

T2013-46
June 2013

Medication Guide
TASIGNA® (ta-sig-na)
(nilotinib)
Capsules

Read this Medication Guide before you start taking Tasigna® and each time you get a refill. There may be new information. This information does not take the place of talking to your doctor about your medical condition or treatment.

What is the most important information I should know about Tasigna?

Tasigna can cause a possible life-threatening heart problem called QTc prolongation. QTc prolongation causes an irregular heartbeat, which may lead to sudden death.

Your doctor should check the electrical activity of your heart with a test called an electrocardiogram (ECG):

- before starting Tasigna
- 7 days after starting Tasigna
- with any dose changes
- regularly during Tasigna treatment

You may lower your chances for having QTc prolongation with Tasigna if you:

- Take Tasigna:
  - on an empty stomach. Do not take Tasigna with food.
  - at least 2 hours after eating any food, and
  - wait at least 1 hour before eating any food
- Avoid grapefruit, grapefruit juice, and any supplement containing grapefruit extract while taking Tasigna. Food and grapefruit products increase the amount of Tasigna in your body.
- Avoid taking other medicines or supplements with Tasigna that can also cause QTc prolongation.
- Tasigna can interact with many medicines and supplements and increase your chance for serious and life-threatening side effects.
- Do not take any other medicine while taking Tasigna unless your doctor tells you it is okay to do so.
- If you cannot swallow Tasigna capsules whole, you may open the Tasigna capsule and sprinkle the contents of each capsule in 1 teaspoon of applesauce (puréed apple). Swallow the mixture right away (within 15 minutes). For more information, see **"How should I take Tasigna?"**

Call your doctor right away if you feel lightheaded, faint or have an irregular heartbeat while taking Tasigna. These can be symptoms of QTc prolongation.

What is Tasigna?

Tasigna is a prescription medicine used to treat a type of leukemia called Philadelphia chromosome positive chronic myeloid leukemia (Ph+ CML) in adults who:

- are newly diagnosed, **or**
- are no longer benefiting from previous other treatments, including treatment with imatinib (Gleevec®), **or**
- have taken other treatments, including imatinib (Gleevec), and cannot tolerate them

It is not known if Tasigna is safe and effective in children.

Who should not take Tasigna?

Do not take if you have:

- low levels of potassium or magnesium in your blood
- long QTc syndrome

What should I tell my doctor before starting Tasigna?

Tasigna may not be right for you. Before taking Tasigna, tell your doctor about all of your medical conditions, including if you have:

- heart problems
- irregular heartbeat
- QTc prolongation or a family history of it
- liver problems
- had pancreatitis
- low blood levels of potassium or magnesium in your blood
- a severe problem with lactose (milk sugar) or other sugars. Tasigna capsules contain lactose. Most patients who have mild or moderate lactose intolerance can take Tasigna.
- had a surgical procedure involving the removal of the entire stomach (total gastrectomy)
- are pregnant or plan to become pregnant. Tasigna may harm your unborn baby. If you are able to become pregnant, you should use effective birth control during treatment with Tasigna. Talk to your doctor about the best birth control methods to prevent pregnancy while you are taking Tasigna.
- are breastfeeding or plan to breastfeed. It is not known if Tasigna passes into your breast milk. You and your doctor should decide if you will take Tasigna or breastfeed. You should not do both.

Tell your doctor about all the medicines you take, including prescription and non-prescription medicines, vitamins and herbal supplements.

If you need to take antacids (medicines to treat heartburn) do not take them at the same time that you take Tasigna. If you take:

- **a medicine to block the amount of acid produced in the stomach (H_2 blocker)**: Take these medicines **about 10 hours before** you take Tasigna, **or about 2 hours after** you take Tasigna.
- **an antacid that contains aluminum hydroxide, magnesium hydroxide and simethicone to reduce the amount of acid in the stomach**: Take these medicines **about 2 hours before or about 2 hours after** you take Tasigna.

Tasigna can interact with many medicines and supplements and increase your chance for serious and life-threatening side effects. **See "What is the most important information I should know about Tasigna?"**

Know the medicines you take. Keep a list of them and show it to your doctor and pharmacist when you get a new medicine.

How should I take Tasigna?

- Take Tasigna exactly as your doctor tells you to take it. Do not change your dose or stop taking Tasigna unless your doctor tells you.
- Tasigna is a long-term treatment.
- Your doctor will tell you how many Tasigna capsules to take and when to take them.
- **Do not take Tasigna with food. Take Tasigna at least 2 hours after you eat and at least 1 hour before you eat.**
- Swallow Tasigna capsules whole with water. If you cannot swallow Tasigna capsules whole, tell your doctor.
- **If you cannot swallow Tasigna capsules whole:**
  - Open the Tasigna capsules and sprinkle the contents in 1 teaspoon of applesauce (puréed apple).
    - Do not use more than 1 teaspoon of applesauce.
    - Only use applesauce. Do not sprinkle Tasigna onto other foods.
  - Swallow the mixture right away (within 15 minutes).
- Do not drink grapefruit juice, eat grapefruit, or take supplements containing grapefruit extract at any time during treatment. See "What is the most important information I should know about Tasigna?"
- If you miss a dose, just take your next dose as scheduled. Do not make up for a missed dose.
- If you take too much Tasigna, call your doctor or poison control center right away. Symptoms may include vomiting and drowsiness. During treatment with Tasigna your doctor will do tests to check for side effects and to see how well Tasigna is working for you. The tests will check your:
  - heart
  - blood cells (white blood cells, red blood cells, and platelets). Your blood cells should be checked every two weeks for the first two months and then monthly.
  - electrolytes (potassium, magnesium)
  - pancreas and liver function
  - bone marrow samples
- Your doctor may change your dose. Your doctor may have you stop Tasigna for some time or lower your dose if you have side effects with it.

What are the possible side effects of Tasigna?

Tasigna may cause serious side effects including:

- **See "What is the most important information I should know about Tasigna?"**
- **Low blood counts.** Low blood counts are common with Tasigna. Your doctor will check your blood counts regularly during treatment with Tasigna. Symptoms of low blood counts include:
  - unexplained bleeding or bruising
  - blood in urine or stool
  - unexplained weakness
- **Liver problems.** Symptoms include yellow skin and eyes.
- **Pancreas inflammation (pancreatitis).** Symptoms include sudden stomach area pain with nausea and vomiting.
- **Bleeding in the brain.** Symptoms include sudden headache, changes in your eyesight, not being aware of what is going on around you and becoming unconscious.
- **Tumor Lysis Syndrome (TLS).** TLS is caused by a fast breakdown of cancer cells. TLS can cause you to have:
  - kidney failure and the need for dialysis treatment
  - an abnormal heart beat

Your doctor may do blood tests to check you for TLS.

The most common side effects of Tasigna include:

• low blood count	• constipation
• rash	• muscle and joint pain
• nausea	• back pain
• fever	• muscle spasms
• headache	• weakness
• itching	• hair loss
• tiredness	• runny or stuffy nose, sneezing, sore throat
• stomach (abdominal) pain	• cough
• diarrhea	

Tell your doctor if you have any side effect that bothers you or does not go away.

These are not all of the possible side effects of Tasigna. For more information, ask your doctor or pharmacist.

Call your doctor for medical advice about side effects. You may report side effects to FDA at 1-800-FDA-1088.

How should I store Tasigna?

- Store Tasigna at room temperature between 68°F to 77°F (20°C to 25°C).
- Safely throw away medicine that is out of date or no longer needed.
- **Keep Tasigna and all medicines out of the reach of children.**

General information about Tasigna

Medicines are sometimes prescribed for purposes other than those listed in a Medication Guide. Do not use Tasigna for a condition for which it was not prescribed. Do not give Tasigna to other people, even if they have the same problem you have. It may harm them.

This Medication Guide summarizes the most important information about Tasigna. If you would like more information, talk with your doctor. You can ask your doctor or pharmacist for information about Tasigna that is written for health professionals.

For more information, go to www.us.tasigna.com or call 1-866-411-8274.

What are the ingredients in Tasigna?

Active ingredient: nilotinib

Inactive ingredients: colloidal silicon dioxide, crospovidone, lactose monohydrate, magnesium stearate and polyoxamer 188.

The capsule shell contains gelatin, iron oxide (red), iron oxide (yellow), iron oxide (black) and titanium dioxide.

This Medication Guide has been approved by the U.S. Food and Drug Administration.

Manufactured by:
Novartis Pharma Stein AG
Stein, Switzerland
Distributed by:
Novartis Pharmaceuticals Corporation
East Hanover, New Jersey 07936
Revised: June 2013

T2013-47
June 2013

Shown in Product Identification Guide, page 311

TEKAMLO ℞

[*těk'-ăm-lō*]
(aliskiren and amlodipine)
tablets, for oral use

The following prescribing information is based on official labeling in effect July 2013.

HIGHLIGHTS OF PRESCRIBING INFORMATION

These highlights do not include all the information needed to use TEKAMLO safely and effectively. See full prescribing information for TEKAMLO.

Tekamlo (aliskiren and amlodipine) tablets, for oral use

Initial U.S. Approval: 2010

> **WARNING: FETAL TOXICITY**
> ***See full prescribing information for complete boxed warning.***
> - **When pregnancy is detected, discontinue Tekamlo as soon as possible. (5.1)**
> - **Drugs that act directly on the renin-angiotensin system can cause injury and death to the developing fetus. (5.1)**

RECENT MAJOR CHANGES

Boxed Warning: Fetal Toxicity	02/2012
Contraindications: Concomitant use with ARBs or ACEIs in diabetes (4)	03/2012
Contraindications: Hypersensitivity (4)	09/2012
Warnings and Precautions: Fetal Toxicity (5.1)	02/2012
Warnings and Precautions (5.2, 5.4, 5.6, 5.8)	03/2012
Warnings and Precautions (5.3)	09/2012
Warnings and Precautions (5.4, 5.5)	09/2012

INDICATIONS AND USAGE

Tekamlo is a combination of aliskiren, a renin inhibitor, and amlodipine, a dihydropyridine calcium channel blocker, indicated for the treatment of hypertension, to lower blood pressure:

- As initial therapy in patients likely to need multiple drugs to achieve their blood pressure goals. (1)
- In patients not adequately controlled with monotherapy. (1)
- As a substitute for its titrated components. (1)

Lowering blood pressure reduces the risk of fatal and nonfatal cardiovascular events, primarily strokes and myocardial infarctions.

DOSAGE AND ADMINISTRATION

- Add-on therapy or initial therapy: Initiate with 150 mg/5 mg. Titrate as needed up to a maximum of 300 mg/10 mg. (2.1, 2.2)
- The blood pressure lowering effect is largely attained within 1-2 weeks. (2.1)
- Replacement therapy: may substitute for titrated components. (2.3)
- Administer one tablet daily with a routine pattern with regard to meals. (2.5)

DOSAGE FORMS AND STRENGTHS

Tablets (aliskiren/amlodipine): 150 mg/5 mg, 150 mg/10 mg, 300 mg/5 mg, 300 mg/10 mg. (3)

CONTRAINDICATIONS

Do not use with angiotensin receptor blockers (ARBs) or ACE inhibitors (ACEIs) in patients with diabetes (4)

Known hypersensitivity to any component (4)

WARNINGS AND PRECAUTIONS

- Avoid concomitant use with ARBs or ACEI in patients with renal impairment (GFR<60 mL/min) (5.2)
- Anaphylactic Reactions and Head and Neck Angioedema: Discontinue Tekamlo and monitor until signs and symptoms resolve. (5.3)
- Hypotension in volume- and/or salt-depleted patients: Correct imbalances before initiating therapy with Tekamlo. (5.4)

- Increased angina or myocardial infarction with calcium channel blockers may occur upon dosage initiation or increase. (5.5)
- Impaired renal function: Monitor serum creatinine periodically. (5.6)
- Hyperkalemia: Monitor potassium levels periodically. (5.8)

ADVERSE REACTIONS

The most common adverse event (incidence ≥2% and more common than with placebo) is peripheral edema. (6.1)

To report SUSPECTED ADVERSE REACTIONS, contact Novartis Pharmaceuticals Corporation at 1-888-669-6682 or FDA at 1-800-FDA-1088 or www.fda.gov/medwatch.

DRUG INTERACTIONS

- Cyclosporine: Avoid concomitant use (7, 12.3)
- Itraconazole: Avoid concomitant use (7, 12.3)
- NSAIDs use may lead to increased risk of renal impairment and loss of antihypertensive effect (7)
- If simvastatin is co-administered with amlodipine, do not exceed doses greater than 20 mg daily of simvastatin (7)

USE IN SPECIFIC POPULATIONS

Nursing Mothers: Discontinue drug or nursing. (8.3)

See 17 for PATIENT COUNSELING INFORMATION and FDA-approved patient labeling

Revised: 09/2012

FULL PRESCRIBING INFORMATION: CONTENTS*

*** Sections or subsections omitted from the full prescribing information are not listed**

FULL PRESCRIBING INFORMATION

WARNING: FETAL TOXICITY

- **When pregnancy is detected, discontinue Tekamlo as soon as possible. (5.1)**
- **Drugs that act directly on the renin-angiotensin system can cause injury and death to the developing fetus. (5.1)**

1 INDICATIONS AND USAGE

Tekamlo is indicated for the treatment of hypertension, alone or with other antihypertensive agents, to lower blood pressure. Lowering blood pressure reduces the risk of fatal and nonfatal cardiovascular events, primarily strokes and myocardial infarctions. These benefits have been seen in controlled trials of antihypertensive drugs from a wide variety of pharmacologic classes including amlodipine. There are no controlled trials demonstrating risk reduction with Tekamlo.

Control of high blood pressure should be part of comprehensive cardiovascular risk management, including, as appropriate, lipid control, diabetes management, antithrombotic therapy, smoking cessation, exercise, and limited sodium intake. Many patients will require more than one drug to achieve blood pressure goals. For specific advice on goals and management, see published guidelines, such as those of the National High Blood Pressure Education Program's Joint National Committee on Prevention, Detection, Evaluation, and Treatment of High Blood Pressure (JNC).

Numerous antihypertensive drugs, from a variety of pharmacologic classes and with different mechanisms of action, have been shown in randomized controlled trials to reduce cardiovascular morbidity and mortality, and it can be concluded that it is blood pressure reduction, and not some other pharmacologic property of the drugs, that is largely responsible for those benefits. The largest and most consistent cardiovascular outcome benefit has been a reduction in the risk of stroke, but reductions in myocardial infarction and cardiovascular mortality also have been seen regularly.

Elevated systolic or diastolic pressure causes increased cardiovascular risk, and the absolute risk increase per mmHg is greater at higher blood pressures, so that even modest reductions of severe hypertension can provide substantial benefit. Relative risk reduction from blood pressure reduction is similar across populations with varying absolute risk, so the absolute benefit is greater in patients who are at higher risk independent of their hypertension (for example, patients with diabetes or hyperlipidemia), and such patients would be expected to benefit from more aggressive treatment to a lower blood pressure goal.

Some antihypertensive drugs have smaller blood pressure effects (as monotherapy) in black patients, and many antihypertensive drugs have additional approved indications and effects (e.g., on angina, heart failure, or diabetic kidney disease). These considerations may guide selection of therapy.

Data from the high-dose multifactorial study *[see Clinical Studies (14)]* provide estimates of the probability of reaching a target blood pressure with Tekamlo compared to aliskiren or amlodipine monotherapy. The figures below provide estimates of the likelihood of achieving systolic or diastolic blood pressure control with Tekamlo 300 mg/10 mg, based upon baseline systolic or diastolic blood pressure. The curve of each treatment group was estimated by logistic regression modeling. The estimated likelihood at the right tail of each curve is less reliable because of a small number of subjects with high baseline blood pressures.

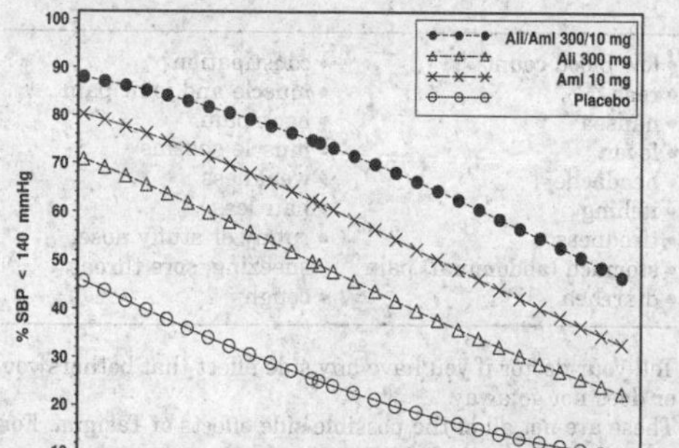

Figure 1: Probability of Achieving Systolic Blood Pressure (SBP) <140 mmHg

[See figure 2 at top of next column]
[See figure 3 at top of next column]
[See figure 4 at top of next column]

The figures above provide an approximation of the likelihood of reaching a targeted blood pressure goal (e.g. SBP<140 mmHg or <130 mmHg) for the high dose groups evaluated in the study. At all levels of baseline blood pressure, the probability of achieving any given diastolic or systolic goal is greater with the combination than for either monotherapy. For example, the mean baseline SBP/DBP for patients participating in this multifactorial study was 157/100 mmHg. A patient with a baseline blood pressure of 157/100 mmHg has about a 49% likelihood of achieving a goal of <140 mmHg (systolic) and 50% likelihood of achieving <90 mmHg (diastolic) on aliskiren alone, and the likelihood of achieving these goals on amlodipine alone is about 62% (systolic) and 69% (diastolic). The likelihood of achieving these goals on Tekamlo rises to about 74% (systolic) and 83% (diastolic). The likelihood of achieving these goals on placebo is about 25% (systolic) and 27% (diastolic) *[see Dosage and Administration (2) and Clinical Studies (14)]*.

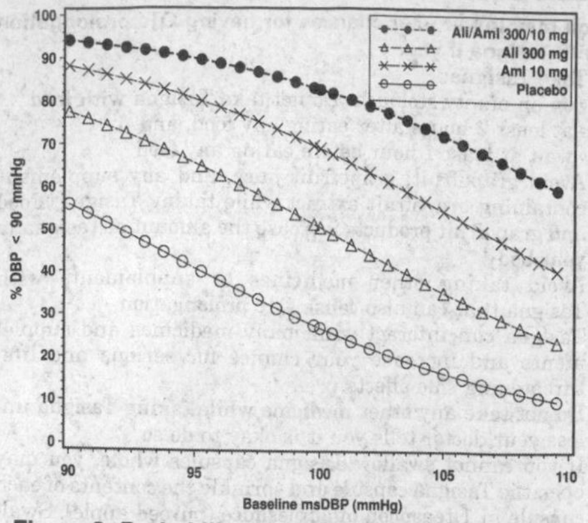

Figure 2: Probability of Achieving Diastolic Blood Pressure (DBP) <90 mmHg

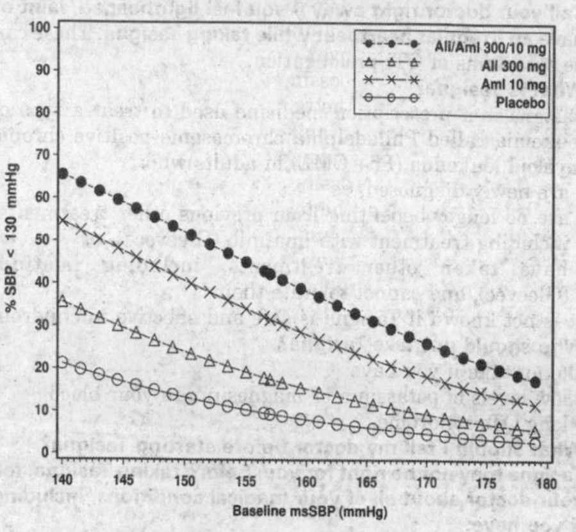

Figure 3: Probability of Achieving Systolic Blood Pressure (SBP) <130 mmHg

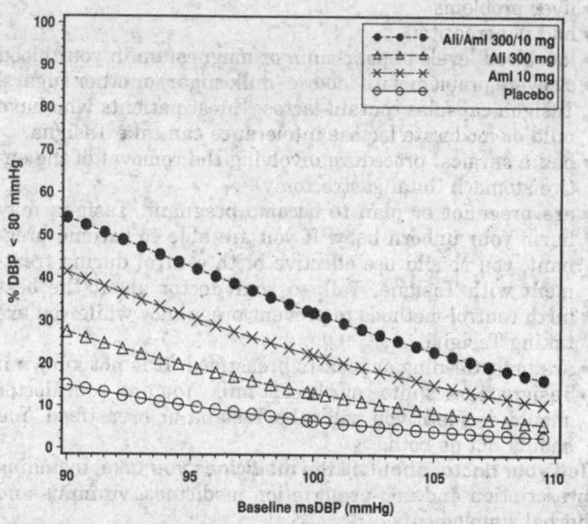

Figure 4: Probability of Achieving Diastolic Blood Pressure (DBP) <80 mmHg

2 DOSAGE AND ADMINISTRATION

2.1 General Considerations

The recommended initial once-daily dose of Tekamlo is 150 mg/5 mg. Titrate as needed to a maximum of 300 mg/10 mg.

The blood pressure lowering effects are largely attained within 1-2 weeks. If blood pressure remains uncontrolled after 2 to 4 weeks of therapy, titrate the dose to a maximum of Tekamlo 300 mg/10 mg once daily.

2.2 Add-on Therapy

Use Tekamlo for patients not adequately controlled with aliskiren alone or amlodipine besylate (or another dihydropyridine calcium channel blocker) alone.

Switch a patient who experiences dose-limiting adverse reactions on either component alone to Tekamlo containing a lower dose of that component in combination with the other to achieve similar blood pressure reductions.

2.3 Replacement Therapy

Switch patients receiving aliskiren and amlodipine besylate from separate tablets to a single tablet of Tekamlo containing the same component doses. When substituting for individual components, increase the dose of one or both of the components if blood pressure control has not been satisfactory.

2.4 Use with Other Antihypertensive Drugs

Tekamlo may be administered with some other antihypertensive agents. In diabetics, do not use in combination with angiotensin receptor blockers (ARBs) or angiotensin converting enzyme inhibitors (ACEIs) *[see Contraindications (4)]*. Concomitant use of aliskiren with an ARB or ACEI is not recommended in patients with GFR <60 ml/min *[see Warnings and Precautions (5.2)]*. It is not known whether Tekamlo decreases blood pressure further when added to maximum dosages of ACE inhibitors and beta blockers *[see Clinical Studies (14)]*.

2.5 Relationship to Meals

Advise patients to establish a routine pattern for taking Tekamlo with regard to meals. High-fat meals decrease absorption substantially *[see Clinical Pharmacology (12.3)]*.

3 DOSAGE FORMS AND STRENGTHS

- 150 mg aliskiren/5 mg amlodipine tablets: Non-scored light yellow, ovaloid convex shaped film-coated tablet with a beveled edge with debossing "T2" on one side and "NVR" on the reverse side of the tablet.
- 150 mg aliskiren/10 mg amlodipine tablets: Non-scored yellow, ovaloid convex shaped film-coated tablet with a beveled edge with debossing "T7" on one side and "NVR" on the reverse side of the tablet.
- 300 mg aliskiren/5 mg amlodipine tablets: Non-scored dark yellow, ovaloid convex shaped film-coated tablet with a beveled edge with debossing "T11" on one side and "NVR" on the reverse side of the tablet.
- 300 mg aliskiren /10 mg amlodipine tablets: Non-scored brown yellow, ovaloid convex shaped film-coated tablet with a beveled edge with debossing "T12" on one side and "NVR" on the reverse side of the tablet.

4 CONTRAINDICATIONS

Do not use aliskiren with ARBs or ACEIs in patients with diabetes *[see Warnings and Precautions (5.2), Clinical Studies (14.2)]*.

Tekamlo is contraindicated in patients with known hypersensitivity to any of the components.

5 WARNINGS AND PRECAUTIONS

5.1 Fetal Toxicity

Pregnancy Category D

Use of drugs that act on the renin-angiotensin system during the second and third trimesters of pregnancy reduces fetal renal function and increases fetal and neonatal morbidity and death. Resulting oligohydramnios can be associated with fetal lung hypoplasia and skeletal deformations. Potential neonatal adverse effects include skull hypoplasia, anuria, hypotension, renal failure, and death. When pregnancy is detected, discontinue Tekamlo as soon as possible *[see Use in Specific Populations (8.1)]*.

5.2 Renal Impairment/Hyperkalemia/Hypotension when Tekamlo is given in combination with ARBs or ACEIs

Tekamlo is contraindicated in patients with diabetes who are receiving ARBs or ACEIs because of the increased risk of renal impairment, hyperkalemia, and hypotension *[see Contraindications (4) and Clinical Studies (14.2)]*.

Avoid use of Tekamlo with ARBs or ACEIs in patients with moderate renal impairment (GFR <60 ml/min).

5.3 Anaphylactic Reactions and Head and Neck Angioedema

Aliskiren

Hypersensitivity reactions such as anaphylactic reactions and angioedema of the face, extremities, lips, tongue, glottis and/or larynx have been reported in patients treated with aliskiren and has necessitated hospitalization and intubation. This may occur at any time during treatment and has occurred in patients with and without a history of angioedema with ACE inhibitors or angiotensin receptor antagonists. Anaphylactic reactions have been reported from postmarketing experience with unknown frequency. If angioedema involves the throat, tongue, glottis or larynx, or if the patient has a history of upper respiratory surgery, airway obstruction may occur and be fatal. Patients who experience these effects, even without respiratory distress, require prolonged observation and appropriate monitoring measures since treatment with antihistamines and corticosteroids may not be sufficient to prevent respiratory involvement. Prompt administration of subcutaneous epinephrine solution 1:1000 (0.3 to 0.5 ml) and measures to ensure a patent airway may be necessary.

Discontinue Tekamlo immediately in patients who develop anaphylactic reactions or angioedema and do not readminister.

5.4 Hypotension

In patients with an activated renin-angiotensin-aldosterone system, such as volume- and/or salt-depleted patients receiving high doses of diuretics, symptomatic hypotension may occur in patients receiving renin-angiotensin-aldosterone system (RAAS) blockers. Correct these conditions prior to administration of Tekamlo, or start the treatment under close medical supervision.

A transient hypotensive response is not a contraindication to further treatment, which usually can be continued without difficulty once the blood pressure has stabilized.

Amlodipine besylate

Symptomatic hypotension is possible, particularly in patients with severe aortic stenosis. Because of the gradual onset of action, acute hypotension is unlikely.

5.5 Risk of Myocardial Infarction or Increased Angina

Worsening angina and acute myocardial infarction can develop after starting or increasing the dose of amlodipine, particularly with severe obstructive coronary artery disease.

5.6 Impaired Renal Function

Monitor renal function periodically in patients treated with Tekamlo. Changes in renal function, including acute renal failure, can be caused by drugs that affect the renin-angiotensin system. Patients whose renal function may depend in part on the activity of the renin-angiotensin system (e.g., patients with renal artery stenosis, severe heart failure, post-myocardial infarction or volume depletion) or patients receiving ARB, ACEI or non-steroidal anti-inflammatory (NSAID) therapy may be at particular risk for developing acute renal failure on Tekamlo *[see Contraindications (4), Warnings and Precautions (5.2), Clinical Studies (14.2)]*. Consider withholding or discontinuing therapy in patients who develop a clinically significant decrease in renal function.

5.7 Cyclosporine or Itraconazole

Aliskiren

When aliskiren was given with cyclosporine or itraconazole, the blood concentrations of aliskiren were significantly increased. Avoid concomitant use of aliskiren with cyclosporine or intraconazole *[see Drug Interactions (7)]*.

5.8 Hyperkalemia

Aliskiren

Monitor serum potassium periodically in patients receiving aliskiren. Drugs that affect the renin-angiotensin system can cause hyperkalemia. Risk factors for the development of hyperkalemia include renal insufficiency, diabetes, combination use with ARBs or ACEI *[see Contraindications (4), Warnings and Precautions (5.2), and Clinical Studies (14.2)]*, NSAIDs, or potassium supplements or potassium sparing diuretics.

6 ADVERSE REACTIONS

6.1 Clinical Studies Experience

The following serious adverse reactions are discussed in greater detail in other sections of the label:

- Risk of fetal/neonatal morbidity and mortality *[see Warnings and Precautions (5.1)]*
- Head and neck angioedema *[see Warnings and Precautions (5.3)]*
- Hypotension *[see Warnings and Precautions (5.4)]*

Because clinical trials are conducted under widely varying conditions, adverse reaction rates observed in the clinical trials of a drug cannot be directly compared to rates in clinical trials of another drug and may not reflect the rates observed in practice.

Tekamlo

Tekamlo has been evaluated for safety in more than 2800 patients, including 372 patients for 1 year or longer.

In a placebo-controlled study, there were 51% males, 62% Caucasians, 20% Blacks, 18% Hispanics, and 17% who were over 65 years of age. In this study, the overall incidence of adverse events on therapy with Tekamlo was similar to the individual components. Discontinuation of therapy due to a clinical adverse event in this study occurred in 1.7% of patients treated with Tekamlo (2.2% in the highest dose group) versus 1.5% of patients given placebo.

Peripheral edema is a known, dose-dependent adverse effect of amlodipine. The incidence of peripheral edema for Tekamlo in short-term double-blind placebo-controlled studies was lower than or equal to that of the corresponding amlodipine doses.

The adverse event in a placebo-controlled trial that occurred in at least 2% of patients treated with Tekamlo and at a higher incidence than placebo was peripheral edema (6.2% versus 1.0%). The incidence rate of peripheral edema at high dose was 8.9%.

In a long-term safety trial, the safety profile of adverse events was similar to that seen in the short-term controlled trials.

Aliskiren

Aliskiren has been evaluated for safety in 6460 patients, including 1740 treated for longer than 6 months, and 1250 for longer than 1 year. In placebo-controlled clinical trials, discontinuation of therapy because of a clinical adverse event, including uncontrolled hypertension, occurred in 2.2% of patients treated with aliskiren versus 3.5% of patients given placebo. These data do not include information from the ALTITUDE study which evaluated the use of aliskiren in combination with ARBs or ACEI *[see Contraindications (4), Warnings and Precautions (5.2), and Clinical Studies (14.2)]*.

Two cases of angioedema with respiratory symptoms were reported with aliskiren use in the clinical studies. Two other cases of periorbital edema without respiratory symptoms were reported as possible angioedema and resulted in discontinuation. The rate of these angioedema cases in the completed studies was 0.06%.

In addition, 26 other cases of edema involving the face, hands, or whole body were reported with aliskiren use, including 4 leading to discontinuation.

In the placebo-controlled studies, however, the incidence of edema involving the face, hands, or whole body was 0.4% with aliskiren compared with 0.5% with placebo. In a long-term active-controlled study with aliskiren and HCTZ arms, the incidence of edema involving the face, hands, or whole body was 0.4% in both treatment arms.

Aliskiren produces dose-related gastrointestinal (GI) adverse reactions. Diarrhea was reported by 2.3% of patients at 300 mg, compared to 1.2% in placebo patients. In women and the elderly (age ≥65) increases in diarrhea rates were evident starting at a dose of 150 mg daily, with rates for these subgroups at 150 mg similar to those seen at 300 mg for men or younger patients (all rates about 2%). Other GI symptoms included abdominal pain, dyspepsia, and gastroesophageal reflux, although increased rates for abdominal pain and dyspepsia were distinguished from placebo only at 600 mg daily. Diarrhea and other GI symptoms were typically mild and rarely led to discontinuation.

Aliskiren was associated with a slight increase in cough in the placebo-controlled studies (1.1% for any aliskiren use versus 0.6% for placebo). In active-controlled trials with ACE inhibitor (ramipril, lisinopril) arms, the rates of cough for the aliskiren arms were about one-third to one-half the rates in the ACE inhibitor arms.

Other adverse reactions with increased rates for aliskiren compared to placebo included rash (1% versus 0.3%), elevated uric acid (0.4% versus 0.1%), gout (0.2% versus 0.1%), and renal stones (0.2% versus 0%).

Single episodes of tonic-clonic seizures with loss of consciousness were reported in two patients treated with aliskiren in the clinical trials. One patient had predisposing causes for seizures and had a negative electroencephalogram (EEG) and cerebral imaging following the seizures; for the other patient, EEG and imaging results were not reported. Aliskiren was discontinued and there was no rechallenge in either case.

No clinically meaningful changes in vital signs or in ECG (including QTc interval) were observed in patients treated with aliskiren.

Amlodipine besylate

Amlodipine (Norvasc®) has been evaluated for safety in more than 11,000 patients in U.S. and foreign clinical trials. Other adverse events that have been reported <1% but >0.1% of patients in controlled clinical trials or under conditions of open trials or marketing experience where a causal relationship is uncertain were:

Cardiovascular: arrhythmia (including ventricular tachycardia and atrial fibrillation), bradycardia, chest pain, peripheral ischemia, syncope, postural hypotension, vasculitis

Central and Peripheral Nervous System: neuropathy peripheral, paresthesia, tremor, vertigo

Gastrointestinal: anorexia, constipation, dyspepsia,** dysphagia, diarrhea, flatulence, pancreatitis, vomiting, gingival hyperplasia

General: allergic reaction, asthenia,** back pain, hot flushes, malaise, pain, rigors, weight gain, weight decrease

Musculoskeletal System: arthralgia, arthrosis, muscle cramps,** myalgia

Psychiatric: sexual dysfunction (male** and female), insomnia, nervousness, depression, abnormal dreams, anxiety, depersonalization

Respiratory System: dyspnea, epistaxis

Skin and Appendages: angioedema, erythema multiforme, pruritus,** rash,** rash erythematous, rash maculopapular

**These events occurred in less than 1% in placebo-controlled trials, but the incidence of these side effects was between 1% and 2% in all multiple dose studies.

Special Senses: abnormal vision, conjunctivitis, diplopia, eye pain, tinnitus

Urinary System: micturition frequency, micturition disorder, nocturia

Autonomic Nervous System: dry mouth, sweating increased

Metabolic and Nutritional: hyperglycemia, thirst

Hemopoietic: leukopenia, purpura, thrombocytopenia

Other events reported with amlodipine at a frequency of ≤0.1% of patients include: cardiac failure, pulse irregularity, extrasystoles, skin discoloration, urticaria, skin dryness, alopecia, dermatitis, muscle weakness, twitching, ataxia, hypertonia, migraine, cold and clammy skin, apathy, agitation, amnesia, gastritis, increased appetite, loose stools, rhinitis, dysuria, polyuria, parosmia, taste perversion, abnormal visual accommodation, and xerophthalmia. Other reactions occurred sporadically and cannot be distinguished from medications or concurrent disease states such as myocardial infarction and angina.

Clinical Laboratory Test Abnormalities

RBC count, hemoglobin and hematocrit: Small mean changes from baseline were seen in RBC count, hemoglobin and hematocrit in patients treated with both Tekamlo and aliskiren monotherapy. This effect is also seen with other agents acting on the renin angiotensin system. In aliskiren monotherapy trials these decreases led to slight increases in rates of anemia compared to placebo (0.1% for any aliskiren use, 0.3% for aliskiren 600 mg daily, vs. 0% for placebo). No patients discontinued due to anemia.

Blood Urea Nitrogen (BUN) / Creatinine: In patients with hypertension not concomitantly treated with an ARB or ACEI, elevations in BUN (> 40 mg/dL) and creatinine (>2.0 mg/dL) in patients treated with Tekamlo were <1.0%.

Serum Potassium: In patients with hypertension not concomitantly treated with an ARB or ACEI, increases in serum potassium >5.5 mEq/L were infrequent (0.9% compared to 0.6% with placebo) *[see Contraindications (4) and Warnings and Precautions (5.10)].*

6.2 Post-marketing Experience

The following adverse reactions have been identified during postapproval use of either aliskiren or amlodipine. Because these reactions are reported voluntarily from a population of uncertain size, it is not always possible to estimate their frequency or establish a causal relationship to drug exposure:

Hypersensitivity: angioedema requiring airway management and hospitalization

Aliskiren: Peripheral edema, severe cutaneous adverse reactions, including Stevens-Johnson syndrome and toxic epidermal necrolysis

Hypersensitivity: anaphylactic reactions and angioedema requiring airway management and hospitalization

Amlodipine: The following postmarketing event has been reported infrequently where a causal relationship is uncertain: gynecomastia. In postmarketing experience, jaundice and hepatic enzyme elevations (mostly consistent with cholestasis or hepatitis), in some cases severe enough to require hospitalization, have been reported in association with use of amlodipine.

7 DRUG INTERACTIONS

No drug interaction studies have been conducted with Tekamlo and other drugs, although studies with the individual aliskiren and amlodipine besylate components are described below.

Aliskiren

Cyclosporine: Avoid co-administration of cyclosporine with aliskiren.

Itraconazole: Avoid co-administration of itraconazole with aliskiren *[see Clinical Pharmacology (12.3].*

Non-Steroidal Anti-Inflammatory Agents(NSAIDs) including selective Cyclooxygenase-2 inhibitors (COX-2 inhibitors): In patients who are elderly, volume-depleted (including those on diuretic therapy), or with compromised renal function, co-administration of NSAIDs, including selective COX-2 inhibitors with agents that affect the renin-angiotensin system, including aliskiren, may result in deterioration of renal function, including possible acute renal failure. These effects are usually reversible. Monitor renal function periodically in patients receiving aliskiren and NSAID therapy.

The antihypertensive effect of aliskiren may be attenuated by NSAIDs.

Amlodipine besylate

Simvastatin: Co-administration of simvastatin with amlodipine increases the systemic exposure of simvastatin. Limit the dose of simvastatin in patients on amlodipine to 20 mg daily.

CYP3A4 Inhibitors: Co-administration with CYP3A inhibitors (moderate and strong) result in increased systemic exposure to amlodipine warranting dose reduction. Monitor for symptoms of hypotension and edema when amlodipine is co-administered with CYP3A4 inhibitors to determine the need for dose adjustment.

CYP3A4 Inducers: No information is available on the quantitative effects of CYP3A4 inducers on amlodipine. Blood pressure should be monitored when amlodipine is co-administered with CYP3A4 inducers.

8 USE IN SPECIFIC POPULATIONS

8.1 Pregnancy

Pregnancy Category D

Use of drugs that act on the renin-angiotensin system during the second and third trimesters of pregnancy reduces fetal renal function and increases fetal and neonatal morbidity and death. Resulting oligohydramnios can be associated with fetal lung hypoplasia and skeletal deformations. Potential neonatal adverse effects include skull hypoplasia, anuria, hypotension, renal failure, and death. When pregnancy is detected, discontinue Tekamlo as soon as possible. These adverse outcomes are usually associated with use of these drugs in the second and third trimester of pregnancy. Most epidemiologic studies examining fetal abnormalities after exposure to antihypertensive use in the first trimester have not distinguished drugs affecting the renin-angiotensin system from other antihypertensive agents. Appropriate management of maternal hypertension during pregnancy is important to optimize outcomes for both mother and fetus.

In the unusual case that there is no appropriate alternative to therapy with drugs affecting the renin-angiotensin system for a particular patient, apprise the mother of the potential risk to the fetus. Perform serial ultrasound examinations to assess the intra-amniotic environment. If oligohydramnios is observed, discontinue Tekamlo, unless it is considered lifesaving for the mother. Fetal testing may be appropriate, based on the week of pregnancy. Patients and physicians should be aware, however, that oligohydramnios may not appear until after the fetus has sustained irreversible injury. Closely observe infants with histories of in utero exposure to Tekamlo for hypotension, oliguria, and hyperkalemia. *[see Use in Specific Populations (8.4)]*

Animal Data

No reproductive toxicity studies have been conducted with the combination of aliskiren and amlodipine besylate. However, these studies have been conducted for aliskiren and amlodipine besylate alone.

Aliskiren

In developmental toxicity studies, pregnant rats and rabbits received oral aliskiren hemifumarate during organogenesis at doses up to 20 and 7 times the maximum recommended human dose (MRHD) based on body surface area (mg/m^2), respectively, in rats and rabbits. (Actual animal doses were up to 600 mg/kg/day in rats and up to 100 mg/kg/day in rabbits.) No teratogenicity was observed; however, fetal birth weight was decreased in rabbits at doses 3.2 times the MRHD based on body surface area (mg/m^2). Aliskiren was present in placentas, amniotic fluid and fetuses of pregnant rabbits.

Amlodipine

No evidence of teratogenicity or embryo/fetal toxicity was found when pregnant rats and rabbits were treated orally with amlodipine maleate at doses up to 10 mg amlodipine/kg/day during their respective periods of major organogenesis. However, litter size was significantly decreased (by about 50%) and the number of intrauterine deaths was significantly increased (about 5-fold). Amlodipine has been shown to prolong both the gestation period and the duration of labor in rats at this dose.

8.3 Nursing Mothers

It is not known whether aliskiren or amlodipine is excreted in human milk. Both aliskiren and amlodipine are secreted in the milk of lactating rats. Because of the potential for serious adverse reactions in human milk-fed infants from Tekamlo, a decision should be made whether to discontinue nursing or discontinue Tekamlo, taking into account the importance of the drug to the mother.

8.4 Pediatric Use

Safety and effectiveness of Tekamlo in pediatric patients have not been established.

Neonates with a history of in utero exposure to Tekamlo:

If oliguria or hypotension occurs, direct attention toward support of blood pressure and renal perfusion. Exchange transfusions or dialysis may be required as a means of reversing hypotension and/or substituting for disordered renal function.

8.5 Geriatric Use

Exposure to aliskiren and amlodipine is increased in elderly patients, thus consider lower initial doses of Tekamlo *[see Clinical Pharmacology (12.3)].*

In the short-term controlled clinical trials of Tekamlo, 17% of patients treated with Tekamlo were ≥ 65 years. No overall differences in safety or effectiveness were observed between these subjects and younger subjects. Other reported clinical experience has not identified differences in responses between the elderly and younger patients, but greater sensitivity of some older individuals cannot be ruled out.

8.6 Hepatic Impairment

Exposure to amlodipine is increased in patients with hepatic insufficiency, thus consider using lower doses of Tekamlo *[see Clinical Pharmacology (12.3)].*

8.7 Renal Impairment

There is no impact of renal function on the pharmacokinetics of aliskiren and amlodipine. However, safety and effectiveness of Tekamlo in patients with severe renal impairment (creatinine clearance <30 mL/min) have not been established as these patients were excluded in clinical trials *[see Warnings and Precautions (5.6), Clinical Pharmacology (12.3) and Clinical Studies (14)].*

10 OVERDOSAGE

Aliskiren

Limited data are available related to overdosage in humans. The most likely manifestation of overdosage would be hypotension. If symptomatic hypotension should occur, provide supportive treatment.

Aliskiren is poorly dialyzed. Therefore, hemodialysis is not adequate to treat aliskiren overexposure *[see Clinical Pharmacology (12.3)].*

Amlodipine besylate

Overdosage might be expected to cause excessive peripheral vasodilation with marked hypotension and possibly a reflex tachycardia. Marked and potentially prolonged systemic hypotension up to and including shock with fatal outcome have been reported. In humans, experience with intentional overdosage of amlodipine is limited. Single oral doses of amlodipine maleate equivalent to 40 mg amlodipine/kg and 100 mg amlodipine/kg in mice and rats, respectively, caused deaths. Single oral amlodipine maleate doses equivalent to 4 or more mg amlodipine/kg or higher in dogs (11 or more times the maximum recommended human dose on a mg/m^2 basis) caused a marked peripheral vasodilation and hypotension.

If massive overdose should occur, initiate active cardiac and respiratory monitoring. Frequent blood pressure measurements are essential. Should hypotension occur, provide cardiovascular support including elevation of the extremities and the judicious administration of fluids. If hypotension remains unresponsive to these conservative measures, consider administration of vasopressors (such as phenylephrine) with attention to circulating volume and urine output. As amlodipine is highly protein bound, hemodialysis is not likely to be of benefit. Administration of activated charcoal to healthy volunteers immediately or up to two hours after ingestion of amlodipine has been shown to significantly decrease amlodipine absorption.

11 DESCRIPTION

Tekamlo is a single tablet for oral administration of aliskiren hemifumarate (an orally active, nonpeptide, potent direct renin inhibitor) and amlodipine besylate (a dihydropyridine calcium channel blocker).

Aliskiren hemifumarate

Aliskiren hemifumarate is chemically described as (2*S*, 4*S*,5*S*,7*S*)-N-(2-carbamoyl-2-methylpropyl)-5-amino-4-hydroxy-2,7-diisopropyl-8-[4-methoxy-3-(3-methoxypropoxy) phenyl]-octanamide hemifumarate and its structural formula is:

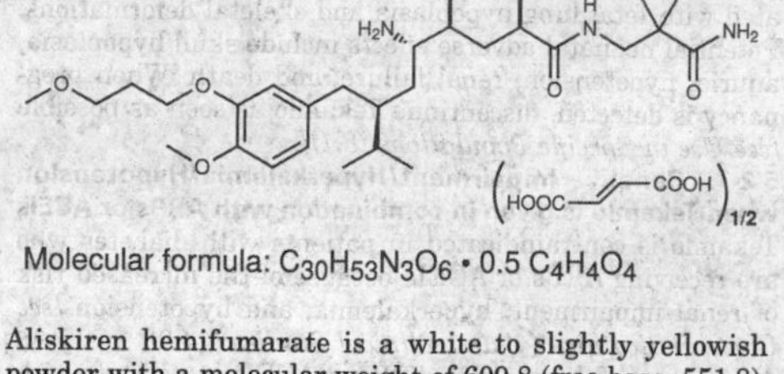

Molecular formula: $C_{30}H_{53}N_3O_6 \cdot 0.5\ C_4H_4O_4$

Aliskiren hemifumarate is a white to slightly yellowish powder with a molecular weight of 609.8 (free base- 551.8). It is highly soluble in water, and freely soluble in methanol, ethanol and isopropanol.

Amlodipine besylate

Amlodipine besylate, USP is chemically described as 3-Ethyl 5-methyl (±)-2-[(2-aminoethoxy)methyl]-4-(*o*-chlorophenyl)-1,4-dihydro-6-methyl-3,5-pyridinedicarboxylate, monobenzenesulfonate, and its structural formula is:

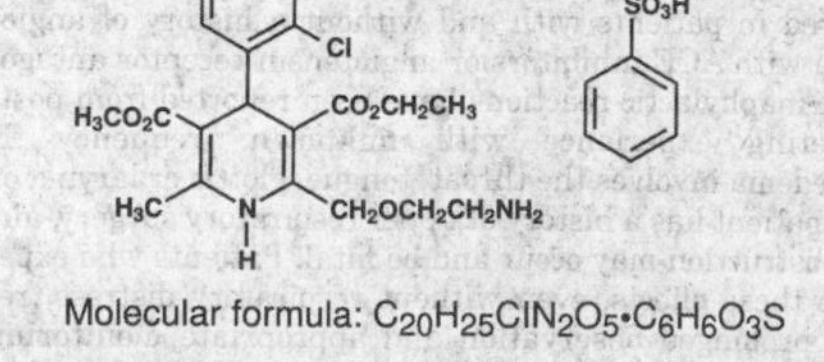

Molecular formula: $C_{20}H_{25}ClN_2O_5 \cdot C_6H_6O_3S$

Amlodipine besylate is a white to pale yellow crystalline powder with a molecular weight of 567.1. It is slightly soluble in water and sparingly soluble in ethanol.

Tekamlo tablets are formulated for oral administration to contain aliskiren hemifumarate and amlodipine besylate providing for the following available combinations: 150 mg/5 mg, 150 mg/10 mg, 300 mg/5 mg and 300 mg/10 mg aliskiren/amlodipine. The inactive ingredients for all strengths of the tablets may contain colloidal silicon dioxide, crospovidone, hypromellose, iron oxide red, iron oxide yellow, magnesium stearate, microcrystalline cellulose, polyethylene glycol, povidone, talc, and titanium dioxide.

12 CLINICAL PHARMACOLOGY

12.1 Mechanism of Action

Aliskiren

Renin is secreted by the kidney in response to decreases in blood volume and renal perfusion. Renin cleaves angiotensinogen to form the inactive decapeptide angiotensin I (Ang I). Ang I is converted to the active octapeptide angiotensin II (Ang II) by angiotensin-converting enzyme (ACE) and non ACE pathways. Ang II is a powerful vasoconstrictor and leads to the release of catecholamines from the adrenal medulla and prejunctional nerve endings. It also promotes aldosterone secretion and sodium reabsorption. Together, these effects increase blood pressure. Ang II also inhibits renin release, thus providing a negative feedback to the system. This cycle, from renin through angiotensin to aldosterone and its associated negative feedback loop, is known as the renin-angiotensin-aldosterone system (RAAS). Aliskiren is a direct renin inhibitor, decreasing plasma renin activity (PRA) and inhibiting the conversion of angiotensinogen to Ang I. Whether aliskiren affects other RAAS components, e.g., ACE or non-ACE pathways, is not known. All agents that inhibit the RAAS, including renin inhibitors, suppress the negative feedback loop, leading to a compensatory rise in plasma renin concentration. When this rise occurs during treatment with ACE inhibitors and ARBs, the result is increased levels of PRA. During treatment with aliskiren, however, the effect of increased renin levels is blocked, so that PRA, Ang I and Ang II are all reduced, whether aliskiren is used as monotherapy or in combination with other antihypertensive agents.

Amlodipine besylate

Amlodipine is a dihydropyridine calcium channel blocker that inhibits the transmembrane influx of calcium ions into vascular smooth muscle and cardiac muscle. Experimental data suggest that amlodipine binds to both dihydropyridine and nondihydropyridine binding sites. The contractile processes of cardiac muscle and vascular smooth muscle are dependent upon the movement of extracellular calcium ions into these cells through specific ion channels. Amlodipine inhibits calcium ion influx across cell membranes selectively, with a greater effect on vascular smooth muscle cells than on cardiac muscle cells. Negative inotropic effects can be detected *in vitro* but such effects have not been seen in intact animals at therapeutic doses. Serum calcium concentration is not affected by amlodipine. Within the physiologic pH range, amlodipine is an ionized compound (pKa=8.6), and its kinetic interaction with the calcium channel receptor is characterized by a gradual rate of association and dissociation with the receptor binding site, resulting in a gradual onset of effect.

Amlodipine is a peripheral arterial vasodilator that acts directly on vascular smooth muscle to cause a reduction in peripheral vascular resistance and reduction in blood pressure.

Tekamlo

The effects of combined treatment of aliskiren and amlodipine arise from the actions of these two agents on different, but complementary mechanisms that regulate blood pressure, calcium channel-mediated vasoconstriction and RAAS-mediated effects on vascular tone and sodium excretion.

12.2 Pharmacodynamics

Aliskiren

PRA reductions in clinical trials ranged from approximately 50% to 80%, were not dose-related and did not correlate with blood pressure reductions. The clinical implications of the differences in effect on PRA are not known.

Amlodipine besylate

Following administration of therapeutic doses to patients with hypertension, amlodipine produces vasodilation resulting in a reduction of supine and standing blood pressures. These decreases in blood pressure are not accompanied by a significant change in heart rate or plasma catecholamine levels with chronic dosing. Although the acute intravenous administration of amlodipine decreases arterial blood pressure and increase heart rate in hemodynamic studies of patients with chronic stable angina, chronic oral administration of amlodipine in clinical trials did not lead to clinically significant changes in heart rate or blood pressures in normotensive patients with angina.

With chronic once daily administration, antihypertensive effectiveness is maintained for at least 24 hours. Plasma concentrations correlate with effect in both young and elderly patients. The magnitude of reduction in blood pressure with amlodipine is also correlated with the height of pretreatment elevation; thus, individuals with moderate hypertension (diastolic pressure 105-114 mmHg) had about 50% greater response than patients with mild hypertension (diastolic pressure 90-104 mmHg). Normotensive subjects experienced no clinically significant change in blood pressure (+1/-2 mmHg).

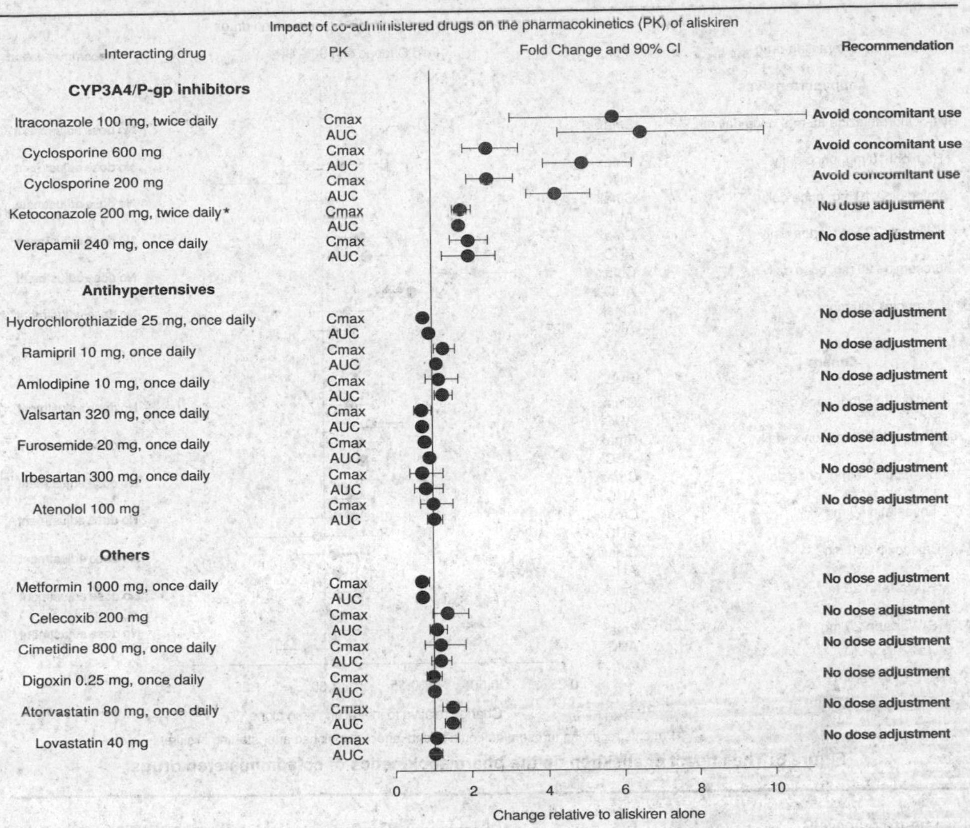

*A 400 mg once daily dose was not studied, but would be expected to increase aliskiren blood levels further.

Figure 5: The impact of co-administered drugs on the pharmacokinetics of aliskiren.

In hypertensive patients with normal renal function, therapeutic doses of amlodipine resulted in a decrease in renal vascular resistance and an increase in glomerular filtration rate and effective renal plasma flow without change in filtration fraction or proteinuria.

As with other calcium channel blockers, hemodynamic measurements of cardiac function at rest and during exercise (or pacing) in patients with normal ventricular function treated with amlodipine have generally demonstrated a small increase in cardiac index without significant influence on dP/dt or on left ventricular end diastolic pressure or volume. In hemodynamic studies, amlodipine has not been associated with a negative inotropic effect when administered in therapeutic dose range to intact animals and man, even when co-administered with beta-blockers to man. Similar findings, however, have been observed in normal or well-compensated patients with heart failure with agents possessing significant negative inotropic effects.

Amlodipine does not change sinoatrial nodal function or atrioventricular conduction in intact animals or man. In patients with chronic stable angina, intravenous administration of 10 mg did not significantly alter A-H and H-V conduction and sinus node recovery time after pacing. Similar results were obtained in patients receiving amlodipine and concomitant beta-blockers. In clinical studies in which amlodipine was administered in combination with beta-blockers to patients with either hypertension or angina, no adverse effects of electrocardiographic parameters were observed. In clinical trials with angina patients alone, amlodipine therapy did not alter electrocardiographic intervals or produce higher degrees of AV blocks.

Amlodipine has indications other than hypertension which can be found in the Norvasc® package insert.

Tekamlo

In a placebo-controlled study in hypertensive patients, amlodipine was associated with an increase in PRA (59-73% increase) whereas aliskiren monotherapy was associated with a 61-68% reduction in PRA. Aliskiren in combination with amlodipine reduced PRA (55-68% reduction).

12.3 Pharmacokinetics

Absorption and Distribution

Tekamlo

Following oral administration of the aliskiren/amlodipine combination tablets, the median peak plasma concentration times are within 3.0 hours for aliskiren and 8.0 hours for amlodipine. The rate and extent of absorption of aliskiren and amlodipine from Tekamlo are the same as when administered as individual tablets. When taken with food, mean AUC and C_{max} of aliskiren are decreased by 79% and 90%, respectively, while there is no impact of food on the AUC and C_{max} of amlodipine.

Aliskiren

Aliskiren is poorly absorbed (bioavailability about 2.5%) with an accumulation half life of about 24 hours. Steady state blood levels are reached in about 7-8 days. Following oral administration, peak plasma concentrations of aliskiren are reached within 1-3 hours. When taken with a high fat meal, mean AUC and Cmax of aliskiren are decreased by 71% and 85% respectively. In the clinical trials, aliskiren was administered without a fixed relation to meals.

Amlodipine besylate

Peak plasma concentrations of amlodipine are reached 6-12 hours after an oral administration of amlodipine. Absolute bioavailability has been estimated to be between 64% and 90%. The bioavailability of amlodipine is not altered by the presence of food.

The apparent volume of distribution of amlodipine is about 21 L/kg. Approximately 93% of circulating amlodipine is bound to plasma proteins in hypertensive patients.

Metabolism and Elimination

Aliskiren

About one-fourth of the absorbed dose appears in the urine as parent drug. How much of the absorbed dose is metabolized is unknown. Based on the in vitro studies, the major enzyme responsible for aliskiren metabolism appears to be CYP 3A4. Aliskiren does not inhibit the CYP450 isoenzymes (CYP 1A2, 2C8, 2C9, 2C19, 2D6, 2E1, and 3A) or induce CYP 3A4.

Transporters: Pgp (MDR1/Mdr1a/1b) was found to be the major efflux system involved in absorption and disposition of aliskiren in preclinical studies. The potential for drug interactions at the Pgp site will likely depend on the degree of inhibition of this transporter.

Drug interactions: The effect of co-administered drugs on the pharmacokinetics of aliskiren and vice versa, were studied in several single and multiple dose studies. Pharmacokinetic measures indicating the magnitude of these interactions are presented in Figure 5 (impact of co-administered drugs on aliskiren) and Figure 6 (impact on co-administered drugs).

[See figure 5 above]

Warfarin: There was no clinically significant effect of a single dose of warfarin 25 mg on the pharmacokinetics of aliskiren.

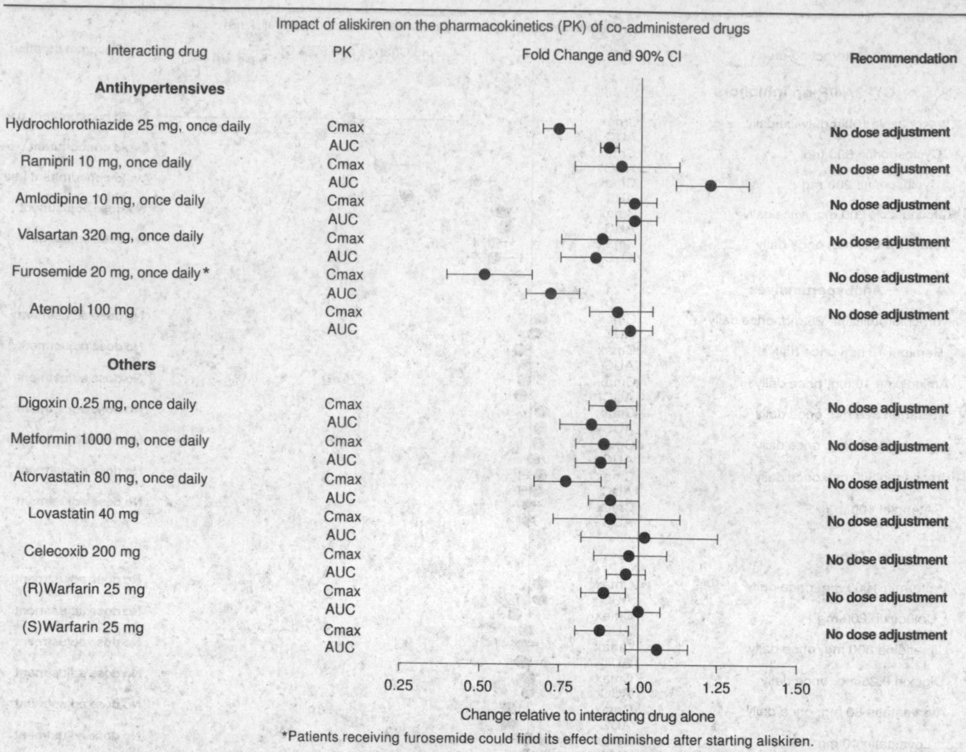

Figure 6: The impact of aliskiren on the pharmacokinetics of co-administered drugs.

[See figure 6 above]

Amlodipine besylate

Amlodipine is extensively (about 90%) converted to inactive metabolites via hepatic metabolism with 10% of the parent compound and 60% of the metabolites excreted in the urine. Elimination of amlodipine from the plasma is biphasic with a terminal elimination half-life of about 30-50 hours Steady state plasma levels are reached after once-daily dosing for 7-8 days.

<u>*Drug interactions:*</u>

Aliskiren exposure is increased slightly (AUC increased 29%) when aliskiren is co-administered with amlodipine, while amlodipine exposure remains unchanged when co-administered with aliskiren. The slight exposure increase of aliskiren in the presence of amlodipine is not clinically relevant.

In vitro data in human plasma indicate that amlodipine has no effect on the protein binding of digoxin, phenytoin, warfarin, and indomethacin.

Cimetidine: Co-administration of amlodipine with cimetidine did not alter the pharmacokinetics of amlodipine.

Grapefruit juice: Co-administration of 240 mL of grapefruit juice with a single oral dose of amlodipine 10 mg in 20 healthy volunteers had no significant effect on the pharmacokinetics of amlodipine.

Maalox® (antacid): Co-administration of the antacid Maalox with a single dose of amlodipine had no significant effect on the pharmacokinetics of amlodipine.

Sildenafil: A single 100 mg dose of sildenafil in subjects with essential hypertension had no effect on the pharmacokinetic parameters of amlodipine. When amlodipine and sildenafil were used in combination, each agent independently exerted its own blood pressure lowering effect.

Atorvastatin: Co-administration of multiple 10 mg doses of amlodipine with 80 mg of atorvastatin resulted in no significant change in the steady-state pharmacokinetic parameters of atorvastatin.

Digoxin: Co-administration of amlodipine with digoxin did not change serum digoxin levels or digoxin renal clearance in normal volunteers.

Ethanol (alcohol): Single and multiple 10 mg doses of amlodipine had no significant effect on the pharmacokinetics of ethanol.

Warfarin: Co-administration of amlodipine with warfarin did not change the warfarin prothrombin response time.

Simvastatin: Co-administration of multiple doses of 10 mg of amlodipine with 80 mg simvastatin resulted in a 77% increase in exposure to simvastatin compared to simvastatin alone.

CYP3A inhibitors: Co-administration of a 180 mg daily dose of diltiazem with 5 mg amlodipine in elderly hypertensive patients resulted in a 60% increase in amlodipine systemic exposure. Erythromycin co-administration in healthy volunteers did not significantly change amlodipine systemic exposure. However, strong inhibitors of CYP3A4 (e.g. ketoconazole, itraconazole, ritonavir) may increase the plasma concentrations of amlodipine to a greater extent.

<u>*Special Populations*</u>

Pediatric Patients

The pharmacokinetics of Tekamlo have not been investigated in patients <18 years of age.

Geriatric Patients

Impact of aging on aliskiren pharmacokinetics has been assessed. When compared to young adults (18-40 years), aliskiren mean AUC and C_{max} in elderly subjects (> 65 years) are increased by 57% and 28%, respectively. In the elderly, clearance of amlodipine is decreased with resulting increases in peak plasma levels, elimination half-life and area-under-the-plasma-concentration curve *[see Use in Specific Populations (8.5)].*

Race

With Tekamlo, pharmacokinetic differences due to race have not been studied. The pharmacokinetic differences among Blacks, Caucasians, and Japanese are minimal with aliskiren therapy.

Hepatic Impairment

The pharmacokinetics of aliskiren is not significantly affected in patients with mild-to-severe liver disease. Patients with hepatic insufficiency have decreased clearance of amlodipine with resulting increase in AUC of approximately 40%-60% *[see Use in Specific Populations (8.6)].*

Renal Impairment

The pharmacokinetics of aliskiren was evaluated in patients with varying degrees of renal impairment. Rate and extent of exposure (AUC and C_{max}) of aliskiren in subjects with renal impairment did not show a consistent correlation with the severity of renal impairment.

The pharmacokinetics of aliskiren following administration of a single oral dose of 300 mg was evaluated in patients with End Stage Renal Disease (ESRD) undergoing hemodialysis. When compared to healthy subjects, changes in the rate and extent of aliskiren exposure (Cmax and AUC) in ESRD patients undergoing hemodialysis was not clinically significant. Timing of hemodialysis did not significantly alter the pharmacokinetics of aliskiren in ESRD patients.

The pharmacokinetics of amlodipine is not significantly influenced by renal impairment *[see Warnings and Precautions (5.6) and Use in Specific Populations (8.7)].*

13 NONCLINICAL TOXICOLOGY

13.1 Carcinogenesis, Mutagenesis, Impairment of Fertility

<u>*Studies with Aliskiren hemifumarate and Amlodipine besylate*</u>

No carcinogenicity, mutagenicity or fertility studies have been conducted with the combination of aliskiren hemifumarate and amlodipine besylate. However, these studies have been conducted for aliskiren hemifumarate and amlodipine besylate alone.

<u>*Studies with Aliskiren hemifumarate*</u>

Carcinogenic potential was assessed in a 2-year rat study and a 6-month transgenic (rasH2) mouse study with aliskiren hemifumarate at oral doses of up to 1500 mg aliskiren/kg/day. Although there were no statistically significant increases in tumor incidence associated with exposure to aliskiren, mucosal epithelial hyperplasia (with or without erosion/ulceration) was observed in the lower gastrointestinal tract at doses of 750 or more mg/kg/day in both species, with a colonic adenoma identified in one rat and a cecal adenocarcinoma identified in another, rare tumors in the strain of rat studied. On a systemic exposure ($AUC_{0\text{-}24hr}$) basis, 1500 mg/kg/day in the rat is about 4 times and in the mouse about 1.5 times the maximum recommended human dose (300 mg aliskiren/day). Mucosal hyperplasia in the cecum or colon of rats was also observed at doses of 250 mg/kg/day (the lowest tested dose) as well as at higher doses in 4- and 13-week studies.

Aliskiren hemifumarate was devoid of genotoxic potential in the Ames reverse mutation assay with *S. typhimurium* and *E. coli*, the in vitro Chinese hamster ovary cell chromosomal aberration assay, the in vitro Chinese hamster V79 cell gene mutation test and the in vivo rat bone marrow micronucleus assay.

Fertility of male and female rats was unaffected at doses of up to aliskiren 250 mg/kg/day (8 times the maximum recommended human dose of aliskiren 300 mg/60 kg on a mg/m^2 basis).

<u>*Studies with Amlodipine besylate*</u>

Rats and mice treated with amlodipine maleate in the diet for up to two years, at concentrations calculated to provide daily dosage levels of 0.5, 1.25, and 2.5 mg amlodipine/kg/day, showed no evidence of a carcinogenic effect of the drug. For the mouse, the highest dose was, on mg/m^2 basis, similar to the maximum recommended human dose (MRHD) of 10 mg amlodipine/day. For the rat, the highest dose was, on a mg/m^2 basis, about twice the MRHD.

Mutagenicity studies conducted with amlodipine maleate revealed no drug-related effects at either the gene or chromosome level.

There was no effect on the fertility of rats treated orally with amlodipine maleate (males for 64 days and females for 14 days prior to mating) at doses of up to 10 mg amlodipine/kg/day (about 8 times the MRHD of 10 mg/day on a mg/m^2 basis).

13.2 Animal Toxicology and/or Pharmacology

Preclinical safety studies have demonstrated that the combination of aliskiren hemifumarate and amlodipine besylate was well tolerated in rats. The findings from the 2- and 13-week oral toxicity studies in rats were consistent with those of aliskiren hemifumarate and amlodipine besylate when both drugs were administered alone. There were no new toxicities or increased severity of the toxicities which were associated with either component.

Animal reproductive and developmental toxicology findings are described elsewhere *[see Use in Specific Populations (8.1)].*

14 CLINICAL STUDIES

14.1 Tekamlo

Tekamlo was studied in a total of 5549 patients with mild to moderate hypertension (diastolic blood pressure between 90 mmHg and 109 mmHg).

Aliskiren 150 mg and 300 mg and amlodipine besylate 5 mg and 10 mg were studied alone and in combination in an 8-week, randomized, double-blind, placebo-controlled, multifactorial study comparing the combinations 150 mg/5 mg, 150 mg/10 mg, 300 mg/5 mg and 300 mg/10 mg of aliskiren and amlodipine with their components and placebo. The combination of aliskiren and amlodipine resulted in placebo-adjusted decreases in systolic/diastolic blood pressure at trough of 14-17/9-11 mmHg compared to 4-9/3-5 mmHg for aliskiren alone and 9-14/6-8 mmHg for amlodipine alone.

Treatment with Tekamlo resulted overall in significantly greater reductions in diastolic and systolic blood pressure compared to the respective monotherapy components.

The antihypertensive effect of Tekamlo was similar in patients with and without diabetes, obese and non-obese patients, in patients ≥65 years of age and <65 years of age, and in women and men.

A subgroup of 819 patients was studied with ambulatory blood pressure monitoring. The blood pressure lowering effect in the aliskiren/amlodipine group was maintained throughout the 24-hour period (see Figure 7 and Figure 8).

[See figure 7 at top of next column]

[See figure 8 at top of next column]

Two additional double-blind, active-controlled studies of similar design were conducted in which Tekamlo was administered as initial therapy in patients with moderate to severe hypertension (SBP 160-200 mmHg). Patients were randomized to receive either combination aliskiren/amlodipine or amlodipine monotherapy. The initial dose of aliskiren/amlodipine was 150 mg/5 mg for 1 week with

Table 1: Incidence of selected adverse events in ALTITUDE

	Aliskiren N=4283		Placebo N=4296	
	Serious Adverse Events* (%)	Adverse Events (%)	Serious Adverse Events* (%)	Adverse Events (%)
Renal impairment †	4.7	12.4	3.3	10.4
Hypotension ††	2.0	18.6	1.7	14.8
Hyperkalemia †††	1.1	36.9	0.3	27.1

†renal failure, renal failure acute, renal failure chronic, renal impairment
††dizziness, dizziness postural, hypotension, orthostatic hypotension, presyncope, syncope
††† Given the variable baseline potassium levels of patients with renal insufficiency on dual RAAS therapy, the reporting of adverse event of hyperkalemia was at the discretion of the investigator.
* A Serious Adverse Event (SAE) is defined as: an event which is fatal or life-threatening, results in persistent or significant disability/incapacity, constitutes a congenital anomaly/birth defect, requires inpatient hospitalization or prolongation of existing hospitalization, or is medically significant (i.e. defined as an event that jeopardizes the patient or may require medical or surgical intervention to prevent one of the outcomes previously listed).

Table 2: Tekamlo Tablets Supply

Tablet	Color	Debossed	Debossed	NDC 0078- XXXX-XX		
Aliskiren hemifumarate/ amlodipine besylate		Side 1	Side 2	Bottle of 30	Bottle of 90	Blister Packages of 100
150 mg/5 mg	Light yellow	T2	NVR	0603-15	0603-34	0603-35
150 mg/10 mg	Yellow	T7	NVR	0604-15	0604-34	0604-35
300 mg/5 mg	Dark yellow	T11	NVR	0605-15	0605-34	0605-35
300 mg/10 mg	Brown yellow	T12	NVR	0606-15	0606-34	0606-35

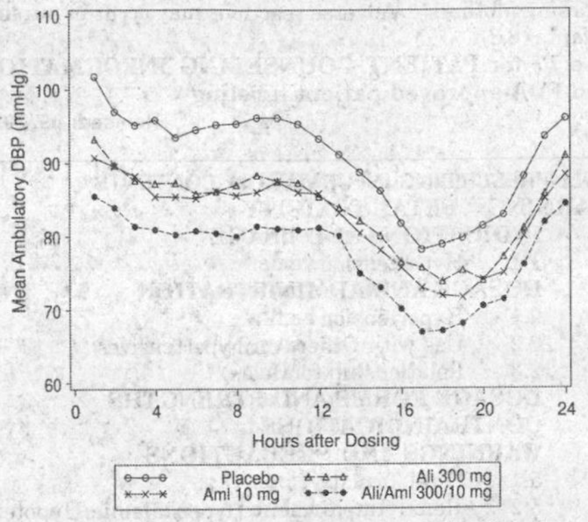

Figure 7: Mean Ambulatory Diastolic Blood Pressure at Endpoint by Treatment and Hour

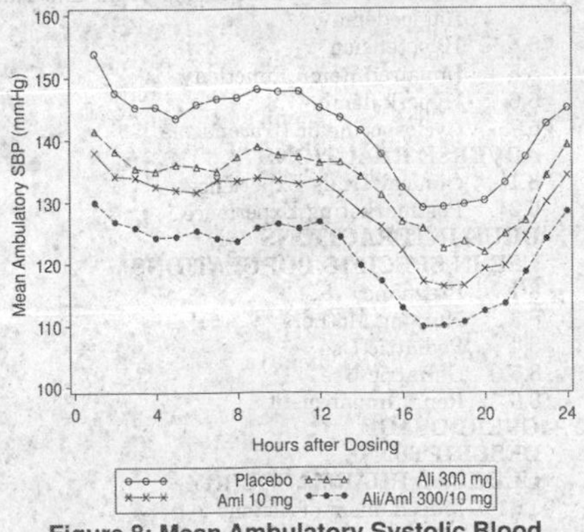

Figure 8: Mean Ambulatory Systolic Blood Pressure at Endpoint by Treatment and Hour

forced titration to 300 mg/10 mg for 7 weeks. The initial dose of amlodipine was 5 mg for 1 week with forced titration to 10 mg for 7 weeks. In one study of 443 Black patients, at the primary endpoint of 8 weeks, the treatment difference between aliskiren/amlodipine and amlodipine was 5.2/3.8 mmHg. In the other study of 484 patients, at the primary endpoint of 8 weeks, the treatment difference between aliskiren/amlodipine and amlodipine was 7.1/3.8 mmHg.
The blood pressure lowering effects of Tekamlo are largely attained within 1-2 weeks.
There are no trials of the Tekamlo combination tablet demonstrating reductions in cardiovascular risk in patients with hypertension, but the amlodipine component has demonstrated such benefits.

14.2 Aliskiren in Patients with Diabetes treated with ARB or ACEI (ALTITUDE study)

Patients with diabetes with renal disease (defined either by the presence of albuminuria or reduced GFR) were randomized to aliskiren 300 mg daily (n=4283) or placebo (n=4296). All patients were receiving background therapy with an ARB or ACEI. The primary efficacy outcome was the time to the first event of the primary composite endpoint consisting of cardiovascular death, resuscitated sudden death, nonfatal myocardial infarction, non-fatal stroke, unplanned hospitalization for heart failure, onset of end stage renal disease, renal death, and doubling of serum creatinine concentration from baseline sustained for at least one month. After a median follow up of about 27 months, the trial was terminated early for lack of efficacy. Higher risk of renal impairment, hypotension and hyperkalemia was observed in aliskiren compared to placebo treated patients, as shown in the table below.
[See table 1 above]
The risk of stroke (2.7% aliskiren vs 2.0% placebo) and death (6.9% aliskiren vs. 6.4% placebo) were also numerically higher in aliskiren treated patients.

16 HOW SUPPLIED/STORAGE AND HANDLING

Tekamlo (aliskiren and amlodipine) is supplied as follows:
150 mg aliskiren/5 mg amlodipine Tablets - Non-scored light yellow, ovaloid convex-shaped, film-coated tablet with a beveled edge with debossing "T2" on one side and "NVR" on the reverse side of the tablet. The tablet dimensions are approximately 16 × 6.3 mm.
150 mg aliskiren/10 mg amlodipine Tablets - Non-scored yellow, ovaloid convex shaped, film-coated tablet with a beveled edge with debossing "T7" on one side and "NVR" on the reverse side of the tablet. The tablet dimensions are approximately 16 × 6.3 mm.
300 mg aliskiren/5 mg amlodipine Tablets - Non-scored dark yellow, ovaloid convex-shaped, film-coated tablet with a beveled edge with debossing "T11" on one side and "NVR" on the reverse side of the tablet. The tablet dimensions are approximately 21 × 8.3 mm.
300 mg aliskiren/10 mg amlodipine Tablets - Non-scored brown yellow, ovaloid convex shaped, film-coated tablet with a beveled edge with debossing "T12" on one side and "NVR" on the reverse side of the tablet. The tablet dimensions are approximately 21 × 8.3 mm.
All strengths are packaged in bottles and unit-dose blister packages (10 strips of 10 tablets) as described below.
[See table 2 above]

Storage

Store at 25°C (77°F); excursions permitted to 15-30°C (59-86°F) in original container.
Protect from heat and moisture.
Dispense in original container.

17 PATIENT COUNSELING INFORMATION

See FDA-Approved Patient Labeling (Patient Information)
Healthcare professionals should instruct their patients to read the Patient Package Insert before starting Tekamlo and to reread each time the prescription is renewed. Patients should be instructed to inform their doctor or pharmacist if they develop any unusual symptom, or if any known symptom persists or worsens.

Pregnancy

Female patients of childbearing age should be told about the consequences of exposure to Tekamlo during pregnancy. Discuss treatment options with women planning to become pregnant. Patients should be asked to report pregnancies to their physician as soon as possible.

Symptomatic Hypotension

Caution patients receiving Tekamlo that lightheadedness can occur, especially during the first days of therapy, and that it should be reported to the prescribing physician. Tell patients that if syncope occurs, discontinue Tekamlo until the physician has been consulted.
Caution all patients that inadequate fluid intake, excessive perspiration, diarrhea, or vomiting can lead to an excessive fall in blood pressure, with the same consequences of lightheadedness and possible syncope.

Anaphylactic Reactions and Angioedema

Patients should be advised and told to report immediately any signs or symptoms suggesting a severe allergic reaction (difficulty breathing or swallowing, tightness of the chest, hives, general rash, swelling, itching, dizziness, vomiting, or abdominal pain) or angioedema (swelling of face, extremities, eyes, lips, tongue, difficulty in swallowing or breathing) and to take no more drug until they have consulted with the prescribing physician. Angioedema, including laryngeal edema, may occur at any time during treatment with Tekamlo.

Potassium Supplements

Tell patients receiving Tekamlo not to use potassium supplements or salt substitutes containing potassium without consulting the prescribing physician.

Relationship to Meals

Patients should establish a routine pattern for taking Tekamlo with regard to meals. High-fat meals decrease absorption substantially.
T2012-180
September 2012

FDA-Approved Patient Labeling
Patient Information
Tekamlo™ *(tĕk'-ăm-lō)*
Tekamlo
(aliskiren and amlodipine)
Tablets

Read the Patient Information that comes with Tekamlo before you start taking it and each time you get a refill. There may be new information. This information does not take the place of talking with your doctor about your condition and treatment. If you have any questions about Tekamlo, ask your doctor or pharmacist.

What is the most important information I should know about Tekamlo?

Tekamlo can cause harm or death to an unborn baby. Talk to your doctor about other ways to lower your blood pressure if you plan to become pregnant. If you get pregnant while taking Tekamlo, tell your doctor right away.

What is Tekamlo?

Tekamlo is a prescription medicine that may be used:
- as the first medicine to lower your high blood pressure if your doctor decides that you are likely to need more than one medicine.
- to treat your high blood pressure when one medicine to lower your high blood pressure has not worked well enough.
- if you are already taking the medicines aliskiren and amlodipine to treat your high blood pressure.

Tekamlo contains:
- aliskiren, a direct renin inhibitor (DRI)
- amlodipine, a calcium channel blocker (CCB)

Your doctor may prescribe other medicines for you to take along with Tekamlo to treat your high blood pressure.
It is not known if Tekamlo is safe and works in children under 18 years of age.

Who should not take Tekamlo?

- If you get pregnant, stop taking Tekamlo and call your doctor right away. If you plan to become pregnant, talk to your doctor about other treatment options for your high blood pressure.
- If you have diabetes and are taking a kind of medicine called an angiotensin-receptor-blocker or angiotensin-converting-enzyme-inhibitor.
- **If you are allergic** (hypersensitive) to aliskiren, amlodipine or other dihydropyridines (calcium-channel blockers, a group of medicines to lower blood pressure to which amlodipine belongs) or any of the other ingredients of Tekamlo listed at the end of this leaflet.

What should I tell my doctor before taking Tekamlo?

Before taking Tekamlo, tell your doctor if you:

- have kidney problems
- have liver problems
- have ever had an allergic reaction to another blood pressure medicine. Symptoms may include: swelling of the face, lips, tongue, throat, arms and legs, and trouble breathing.
- suffer from heart disorders or if you experienced a heart attack
- have any other medical problems
- are pregnant or planning to become pregnant. **See "What is the most important information I should know about Tekamlo?"**
- are breastfeeding. It is not known if Tekamlo passes into your breast milk and if it can harm your baby. You and your doctor should decide if you will take Tekamlo or breastfeed. You should not do both.

Tell your doctor about all the medicines you take including prescription and nonprescription medicines, vitamins and herbal supplements. Tekamlo and certain other medicines may affect each other and cause side effects.

Especially tell your doctor if you take:

- a kind of medicine called angiotensin receptor blocker or angiotensin converting enzyme inhibitor
- water pills (also called "diuretics")
- medicines for treating fungus or fungal infections
- cyclosporine (Gengraf®, Neoral, Sandimmune), a medicine used to suppress the immune system
- potassium-containing medicines, potassium supplements, or salt substitutes containing potassium
- simvastatin (Zocor®) or atorvastatin (Lipitor®)
- non-steroidal anti-inflammatory drugs (like ibuprofen or naproxen)
- medicines used to treat AIDS or HIV infections (such as ritonavir, indinavir)

Know your medicines. Keep a list of all your medicines. Show this list to your doctor or pharmacist when you get a new medicine. Your doctor or pharmacist will know what medicines are safe to take together.

How should I take Tekamlo?

- Take Tekamlo exactly as prescribed by your doctor. It is important to take Tekamlo every day to control your blood pressure.
- Take Tekamlo one time a day, about the same time each day.
- Take Tekamlo the same way every day, either with or without a meal.
- Your doctor may change your dose of Tekamlo if needed. Do not change the amount of Tekamlo you take without talking to your doctor.
- If you miss a dose of Tekamlo, take it as soon as you remember. If it is close to your next dose, do not take the missed dose. Just take the next dose at your regular time.
- If you take too much Tekamlo, call your doctor or a Poison Control Center, or go to the nearest hospital emergency room.

What are the possible side effects of Tekamlo?

Tekamlo may cause serious side effects:

- **Harm to an unborn baby, causing injury or death. See "What is the most important information I should know about Tekamlo?"**
- **Severe Allergic Reactions and Angioedema:** Aliskiren, one of the medicines in Tekamlo, can cause difficulty breathing or swallowing, tightness of the chest, hives, general rash, swelling, itching, dizziness, vomiting, or abdominal pain (signs of a severe allergic reaction). Aliskiren can also cause swelling of your face, lips, tongue, throat, arms and legs, or the whole body (signs of angioedema). Get medical help right away and tell your doctor if you get any one or more of these symptoms. Angioedema can happen at any time while you are taking Tekamlo.
- **Low blood pressure (hypotension).** Your blood pressure may get too low if you also take water pills, are on a low-salt diet, get dialysis treatments, have heart problems, or get sick with vomiting or diarrhea. Lie down if you feel faint or get dizzy. Call your doctor right away.
- **Possible increased chest pain or risk of heart attack.** It is rare, but when you first start taking Tekamlo or increase your dose, you may have a heart attack or your angina may get worse. If that happens, call your doctor right away or go directly to a hospital emergency room.

The most common side effects of Tekamlo include:

- Swelling of your lower legs

Common side effects of Tekamlo include:

- diarrhea
- cough
- dizziness
- flu-like symptoms
- tiredness
- high levels of potassium in the blood (hyperkalemia)

Tell your doctor if you have any side effect that bothers you or that does not go away.

These are not all of the possible side effects of Tekamlo. For more information, ask your doctor or pharmacist.

Call your doctor for medical advice about side effects. You may report side effects to FDA at 1-800-FDA-1088.

How do I store Tekamlo?

- Store Tekamlo tablets at room temperature between 59°F to 86°F (15°C to 30°C).
- Keep the original prescription bottle and store in a dry place.
- Protect Tekamlo from heat and moisture.

Keep Tekamlo and all medicines out of the reach of children.

General information about Tekamlo

Medicines are sometimes prescribed for conditions not listed in the patient information leaflet. Do not take Tekamlo for a condition for which it was not prescribed. Do not give Tekamlo to other people, even if they have the same condition or symptoms you have. It may harm them.

This leaflet summarizes the most important information about Tekamlo. If you have questions about Tekamlo talk with your doctor. You can ask your doctor or pharmacist for information that is written for healthcare professionals.

For more information about Tekamlo, visit www.Tekamlo.com, or call 1-888-NOW-NOVA (1-888-669-6682).

What are the ingredients in Tekamlo?

Active Ingredients: Aliskiren hemifumarate and amlodipine

Inactive ingredients: Colloidal silicon dioxide, crospovidone, hypromellose, iron oxide red, iron oxide yellow, magnesium stearate, microcrystalline cellulose, polyethylene glycol, povidone, talc, and titanium dioxide.

What is high blood pressure (hypertension)?

Blood pressure is the force of blood in your blood vessels when your heart beats and when your heart rests. You have high blood pressure when the force is too much.

High blood pressure makes the heart work harder to pump blood through the body and causes damage to blood vessels. Tekamlo can help your blood vessels relax so your blood pressure is lower. Medicines that lower your blood pressure may lower your chance of having a stroke or heart attack.

Distributed by:
Novartis Pharmaceuticals Corporation
East Hanover, New Jersey 07936
© Novartis
T2012-181
September 2012

Shown in Product Identification Guide, page 311

TEKTURNA® ℞

[tek-turn-a]
(aliskiren)
tablets, for oral use

The following prescribing information is based on official labeling in effect July 2013.

HIGHLIGHTS OF PRESCRIBING INFORMATION

These highlights do not include all the information needed to use TEKTURNA® safely and effectively. See full prescribing information for TEKTURNA®.

Tekturna® (aliskiren) tablets, for oral use
Initial U.S. Approval: 2007

WARNING: FETAL TOXICITY

See full prescribing information for complete boxed warning

- **When pregnancy is detected, discontinue Tekturna as soon as possible. (5.1)**
- **Drugs that act directly on the renin-angiotensin system can cause injury and death to the developing fetus. (5.1)**

RECENT MAJOR CHANGES

Boxed Warning: Fetal Toxicity	02/2012
Contraindications: Concomitant use with ARBs or ACEIs in diabetes (4)	03/2012
Warnings and Precautions (5.1)	02/2012
Warnings and Precautions (5.2, 5.4, 5.5, 5.6)	03/2012
Warnings and Precautions (5.3)	09/2012

INDICATIONS AND USAGE

Tekturna is a renin inhibitor (RI) indicated for:

- The treatment of hypertension, to lower blood pressure (1.1)

Lowering blood pressure reduces the risk of fatal and nonfatal cardiovascular events, primarily strokes and myocardial infarctions.

DOSAGE AND ADMINISTRATION

- Starting dose: 150 mg once daily with a routine pattern with regard to meals. If blood pressure remains uncontrolled titrate up to 300 mg daily (2.1, 2.3)
- Majority of effect of given dose attained in 2 weeks (2.1)

DOSAGE FORMS AND STRENGTHS

Tablets: 150 mg, 300 mg (3)

CONTRAINDICATIONS

Do not use with angiotensin receptor blockers (ARBs) or ACE inhibitors (ACEIs) in patients with diabetes (4)

WARNINGS AND PRECAUTIONS

- Avoid concomitant use with ARBs or ACEIs in patients with renal impairment (GFR<60 mL/min) (5.2)
- Anaphylactic Reactions and Head and Neck Angioedema: Discontinue use of Tekturna and monitor until signs and symptoms resolve (5.3)
- Hypotension in volume and/or salt depleted patients: Correct imbalances before initiating therapy with Tekturna (5.4)
- Impaired renal function: Monitor serum creatinine periodically. (5.5)
- Hyperkalemia: Monitor potassium levels periodically. (5.6)

ADVERSE REACTIONS

Most common adverse reaction: diarrhea (incidence 2.3%) (6.1)

To report SUSPECTED ADVERSE REACTIONS, contact Novartis Pharmaceuticals Corporation at 1-888-669-6682 or FDA at 1-800-FDA-1088 or www.fda.gov/medwatch.

DRUG INTERACTIONS

- Cyclosporine: Avoid concomitant use (7, 12.3)
- Itraconazole: Avoid concomitant use (7, 12.3)
- NSAIDs use may lead to increased risk of renal impairment and loss of antihypertensive effect (7)

USE IN SPECIFIC POPULATIONS

Nursing Mothers: Adverse reactions may occur in nursing infants (8.3)

See 17 for PATIENT COUNSELING INFORMATION and FDA-approved patient labeling

Revised: 09/2012

FULL PRESCRIBING INFORMATION: CONTENTS*

*** Sections or subsections omitted from the full prescribing information are not listed**

FULL PRESCRIBING INFORMATION

WARNING: FETAL TOXICITY
- **When pregnancy is detected, discontinue Tekturna as soon as possible. (5.1)**
- **Drugs that act directly on the renin-angiotensin system can cause injury and death to the developing fetus. (5.1)**

1 INDICATIONS AND USAGE

1.1 Hypertension

Tekturna is indicated for the treatment of hypertension, to lower blood pressure. Lowering blood pressure reduces the risk of fatal and nonfatal cardiovascular events, primarily strokes and myocardial infarctions. These benefits have been seen in controlled trials of antihypertensive drugs from a wide variety of pharmacologic classes. There are no controlled trials demonstrating risk reduction with Tekturna.

Control of high blood pressure should be part of comprehensive cardiovascular risk management, including, as appropriate, lipid control, diabetes management, antithrombotic therapy, smoking cessation, exercise, and limited sodium intake. Many patients will require more than one drug to achieve blood pressure goals. For specific advice on goals and management, see published guidelines, such as those of the National High Blood Pressure Education Program's Joint National Committee on Prevention, Detection, Evaluation, and Treatment of High Blood Pressure (JNC).

Numerous antihypertensive drugs, from a variety of pharmacologic classes and with different mechanisms of action, have been shown in randomized controlled trials to reduce cardiovascular morbidity and mortality, and it can be concluded that it is blood pressure reduction, and not some other pharmacologic property of the drugs, that is largely responsible for those benefits. The largest and most consistent cardiovascular outcome benefit has been a reduction in the risk of stroke, but reductions in myocardial infarction and cardiovascular mortality also have been seen regularly.

Elevated systolic or diastolic pressure causes increased cardiovascular risk, and the absolute risk increase per mmHg is greater at higher blood pressures, so that even modest reductions of severe hypertension can provide substantial benefit. Relative risk reduction from blood pressure reduction is similar across populations with varying absolute risk, so the absolute benefit is greater in patients who are at higher risk independent of their hypertension (for example, patients with diabetes or hyperlipidemia), and such patients would be expected to benefit from more aggressive treatment to a lower blood pressure goal.

Some antihypertensive drugs have smaller blood pressure effects (as monotherapy) in black patients, and many antihypertensive drugs have additional approved indications and effects (e.g., on angina, heart failure, or diabetic kidney disease). These considerations may guide selection of therapy.

2 DOSAGE AND ADMINISTRATION

2.1 Hypertension

The usual recommended starting dose of Tekturna is 150 mg once daily. In patients whose blood pressure is not adequately controlled, the daily dose may be increased to 300 mg. Doses above 300 mg did not give an increased blood pressure response but resulted in an increased rate of diarrhea. The antihypertensive effect of a given dose is substantially attained (85-90%) by 2 weeks.

2.2 Use with Other Antihypertensives

Tekturna may be administered with some other antihypertensive agents. In diabetics, do not use in combination with angiotensin receptor blockers (ARBs) or angiotensin converting enzyme inhibitors (ACEIs) *[see Contraindications (4)]*. Concomitant use of aliskiren with an ARB or ACEI is not recommended in patients with GFR <60 ml/min *[see Warnings and Precautions (5.2)]*. Most exposure to date is with diuretics, an angiotensin receptor blocker (valsartan) or a calcium channel blocker (amlodipine). Aliskiren used together with these drugs has a greater effect at their maximum recommended doses than either drug alone. It is not known whether additive effects are present when Tekturna is used with angiotensin-converting enzyme inhibitors (ACEIs) or beta blockers (BB).

2.3 Relationship to Meals

Patients should establish a routine pattern for taking Tekturna with regard to meals. High fat meals decrease absorption substantially *[see Clinical Pharmacology (12.3)]*.

3 DOSAGE FORMS AND STRENGTHS

150 mg light pink biconvex round tablet, imprinted NVR/IL (Side 1/Side 2)

300 mg light red biconvex ovaloid round tablet, imprinted NVR/IU (Side 1/Side 2)

4 CONTRAINDICATIONS

Do not use aliskiren with ARBs or ACEIs in patients with diabetes *[see Warnings and Precautions (5.2), Clinical Studies (14.3)]*.

5 WARNINGS AND PRECAUTIONS

5.1 Fetal Toxicity

Pregnancy Category D

Use of drugs that act on the renin-angiotensin system during the second and third trimesters of pregnancy reduces fetal renal function and increases fetal and neonatal morbidity and death. Resulting oligohydramnios can be associated with fetal lung hypoplasia and skeletal deformations. Potential neonatal adverse effects include skull hypoplasia, anuria, hypotension, renal failure, and death. When pregnancy is detected, discontinue Tekturna as soon as possible *[see Use in Specific Populations (8.1)]*.

5.2 Renal Impairment/Hyperkalemia/Hypotension when Tekturna is given in combination with ARBs or ACEIs

Tekturna is contraindicated in patients with diabetes who are receiving ARBs or ACEIs because of the increased risk of renal impairment, hyperkalemia, and hypotension *[see Contraindications (4) and Clinical Studies (14.3)]*.

Avoid use of Tekturna with ARBs or ACEIs in patients with moderate renal impairment (GFR <60 ml/min).

5.3 Anaphylactic Reactions and Head and Neck Angioedema

Hypersensitivity reactions such as anaphylactic reactions and angioedema of the face, extremities, lips, tongue, glottis and/or larynx have been reported in patients treated with Tekturna and has necessitated hospitalization and intubation. This may occur at any time during treatment and has occurred in patients with and without a history of angioedema with ACE inhibitors or angiotensin receptor antagonists. Anaphylactic reactions have been reported from postmarketing experience with unknown frequency. If angioedema involves the throat, tongue, glottis or larynx, or if the patient has a history of upper respiratory surgery, airway obstruction may occur and be fatal. Patients who experience these effects, even without respiratory distress, require prolonged observation and appropriate monitoring measures since treatment with antihistamines and corticosteroids may not be sufficient to prevent respiratory involvement. Prompt administration of subcutaneous epinephrine solution 1:1000 (0.3 to 0.5 ml) and measures to ensure a patent airway may be necessary.

Discontinue Tekturna immediately in patients who develop anaphylactic reactions or angioedema, and do not readminister.

5.4 Hypotension

In patients with an activated renin-angiotensin system, such as volume- and/or salt-depleted patients (e.g., those receiving high doses of diuretics), symptomatic hypotension may occur after initiation of treatment with Tekturna. This condition should be corrected prior to administration of Tekturna, or the treatment should start under close medical supervision.

A transient hypotensive response is not a contraindication to further treatment, which usually can be continued without difficulty once the blood pressure has stabilized.

5.5 Impaired Renal Function

Monitor renal function periodically in patients treated with Tekturna. Changes in renal function, including acute renal failure, can be caused by drugs that affect the renin-angiotensin system. Patients whose renal function may depend in part on the activity of the renin-angiotensin system (e.g., patients with renal artery stenosis, severe heart failure, post-myocardial infarction or volume depletion) or patients receiving ARB, ACEI or non-steroidal anti-inflammatory (NSAID) therapy may be at particular risk for developing acute renal failure on Tekturna *[see Contraindications (4), Warnings and Precautions (5.2), Clinical Studies (14.3)]*. Consider withholding or discontinuing therapy in patients who develop a clinically significant decrease in renal function.

5.6 Hyperkalemia

Monitor serum potassium periodically in patients receiving Tekturna. Drugs that affect the renin-angiotensin system can cause hyperkalemia. Risk factors for the development of hyperkalemia include renal insufficiency, diabetes, combination use with ARBs or ACEIs *[see Contraindications (4), Warnings and Precautions (5.2), and Clinical Studies (14.3)]*, NSAIDs, or potassium supplements or potassium sparing diuretics.

5.7 Cyclosporine or Itraconazole

When aliskiren was given with cyclosporine or itraconazole, the blood concentrations of aliskiren were significantly increased. Avoid concomitant use of aliskiren with cyclosporine or itraconazole *[see Drug Interactions (7)]*.

6 ADVERSE REACTIONS

6.1 Clinical Trials Experience

Because clinical trials are conducted under widely varying conditions, adverse reaction rates observed in the clinical trials of a drug cannot be directly compared to rates in clinical trials of another drug and may not reflect the rates observed in practice.

Data described below reflect the evaluation of the safety of Tekturna in more than 6,460 patients, including over 1,740 treated for longer than 6 months, and more than 1,250 patients for longer than 1 year. In placebo controlled clinical trials, discontinuation of therapy due to a clinical adverse event, including uncontrolled hypertension occurred in 2.2% of patients treated with Tekturna vs. 3.5% of patients given placebo. These data do not include information from the ALTITUDE study which evaluated the use of aliskiren in combination with ARBs or ACEIs *[see Contraindications (4), Warnings and Precautions (5.2), and Clinical Studies (14.3)]*.

Angioedema: Two cases of angioedema with respiratory symptoms were reported with Tekturna use in the clinical studies. Two other cases of periorbital edema without respiratory symptoms were reported as possible angioedema and resulted in discontinuation. The rate of these angioedema cases in the completed studies was 0.06%. In addition, 26 other cases of edema involving the face, hands, or whole body were reported with Tekturna use including 4 leading to discontinuation. In the placebo controlled studies, however, the incidence of edema involving the face, hands or whole body was 0.4% with Tekturna compared with 0.5% with placebo. In a long term active control study with Tekturna and HCTZ arms, the incidence of edema involving the face, hand or whole body was 0.4% in both treatment arms *[see Warnings and Precautions (5.2)]*.

Gastrointestinal: Tekturna produces dose-related gastrointestinal (GI) adverse reactions. Diarrhea was reported by 2.3% of patients at 300 mg, compared to 1.2% in placebo patients. In women and the elderly (age ≥ 65) increase in diarrhea rates were evident starting at a dose of 150 mg daily, with rates for these subgroups at 150 mg comparable to those seen at 300 mg for men or younger patients (all rates about 2.0-2.3%). Other GI symptoms included abdominal pain, dyspepsia, and gastroesophageal reflux, although increased rates for abdominal pain and dyspepsia were distinguished from placebo only at 600 mg daily. Diarrhea and other GI symptoms were typically mild and rarely led to discontinuation.

Cough: Tekturna was associated with a slight increase in cough in the placebo-controlled studies (1.1% for any Tekturna use vs. 0.6% for placebo). In active-controlled trials with ACE inhibitor (ramipril, lisinopril) arms, the rates of cough for the Tekturna arms were about one-third to one-half the rates in the ACE inhibitor arms.

Seizures: Single episodes of tonic-clonic seizures with loss of consciousness were reported in two patients treated with Tekturna in the clinical trials. One of these patients did have predisposing causes for seizures and had a negative electroencephalogram (EEG) and cerebral imaging following the seizures (for the other patient EEG and imaging results were not reported). Tekturna was discontinued and there was no re-challenge.

Other adverse effects with increased rates for Tekturna compared to placebo included rash (1% vs. 0.3%), elevated uric acid (0.4% vs. 0.1%), gout (0.2% vs. 0.1%) and renal stones (0.2% vs. 0%).

Aliskiren's effect on ECG intervals was studied in a randomized, double-blind, placebo and active-controlled (moxifloxacin), 7-day repeat dosing study with Holter-monitoring and 12 lead ECGs throughout the interdosing interval. No effect of aliskiren on QT interval was seen.

Clinical Laboratory Findings

In controlled clinical trials, clinically relevant changes in standard laboratory parameters were rarely associated with the administration of Tekturna in patients with hypertension not concomitantly treated with an ARB or ACEI. In multiple-dose studies in hypertensive patients, Tekturna had no clinically important effects on total cholesterol, HDL, fasting triglycerides, or fasting glucose.

Blood Urea Nitrogen, Creatinine: In patients with hypertension not concomitantly treated with an ARB or ACEI, minor increases in blood urea nitrogen (BUN) or serum creatinine were observed in less than 7% of patients treated with Tekturna alone vs. 6% on placebo *[see Warnings and Precautions (5.2)]*.

Hemoglobin and Hematocrit: Small decreases in hemoglobin and hematocrit (mean decreases of approximately 0.08 g/dL and 0.16 volume percent, respectively, for all aliskiren monotherapy) were observed. The decreases were dose-related and were 0.24 g/dL and 0.79 volume percent for 600 mg daily. This effect is also seen with other agents acting on the renin angiotensin system, such as angiotensin inhibitors and angiotensin receptor blockers and may be mediated by reduction of angiotensin II which stimulates erythropoietin production via the AT1 receptor. These decreases led to slight increases in rates of anemia with aliskiren compared to placebo were observed (0.1% for any aliskiren use, 0.3% for aliskiren 600 mg daily, vs 0% for placebo). No patients discontinued therapy due to anemia.

Serum Potassium: In patients with hypertension not concomitantly treated with an ARB or ACEI, increases in serum potassium >5.5 mEq/L were infrequent (0.9% compared to 0.6% with placebo) *[See Contraindications (4) and Warnings and Precautions (5.6)]*.

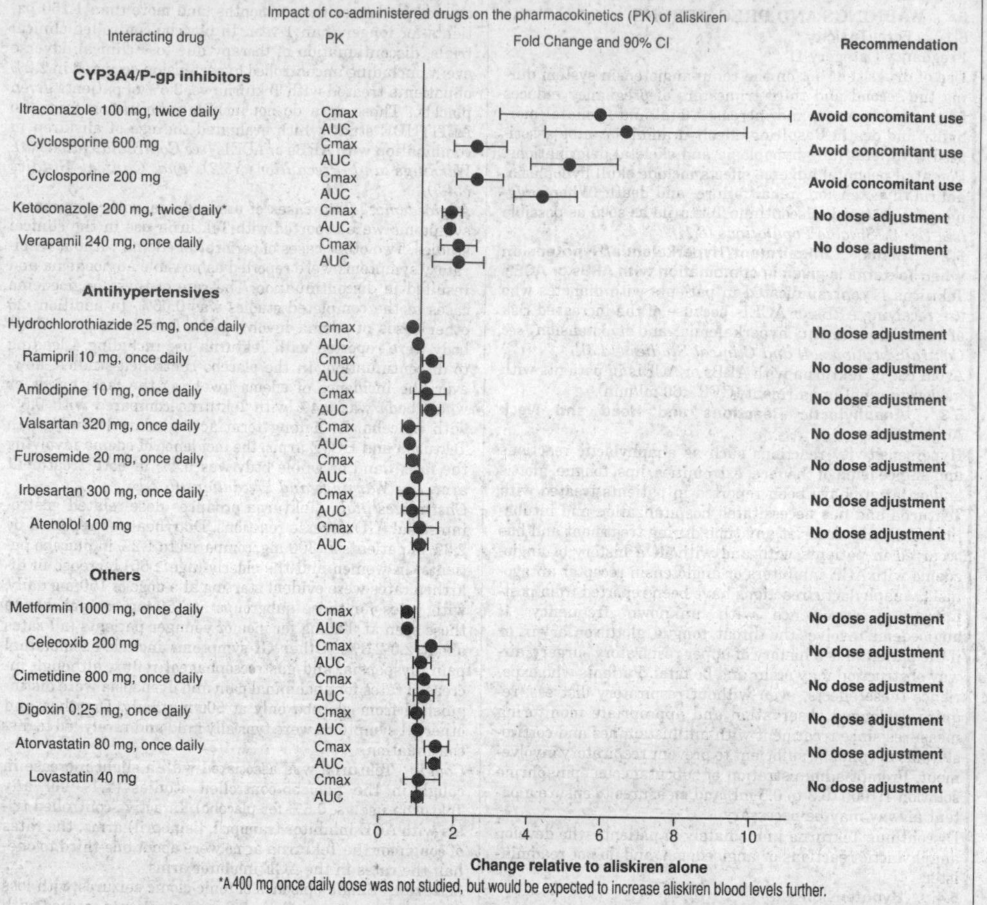

Figure 1: The impact of co-administered drugs on the pharmacokinetics of aliskiren.

Serum Uric Acid: Aliskiren monotherapy produced small median increases in serum uric acid levels (about 6 µmol/L) while HCTZ produced larger increases (about 30 µmol/L). The combination of aliskiren with HCTZ appears to be additive (about 40 µmol/L increase). The increases in uric acid appear to lead to slight increases in uric acid-related AEs: elevated uric acid (0.4% vs 0.1%), gout (0.2% vs. 0.1%), and renal stones (0.2% vs 0%).

Creatine Kinase: Increases in creatine kinase of >300% were recorded in about 1% of aliskiren monotherapy patients vs. 0.5% of placebo patients. Five cases of creatine kinase rises, three leading to discontinuation and one diagnosed as subclinical rhabdomyolysis, and another as myositis, were reported as adverse events with aliskiren use in the clinical trials. No cases were associated with renal dysfunction.

6.2 Postmarketing Experience

The following adverse reactions have been reported in aliskiren post-marketing experience. Because these reactions are reported voluntarily from a population of uncertain size, it is not always possible to estimate their frequency or establish a causal relationship to drug exposure.

Hypersensitivity: anaphylactic reactions and angioedema requiring airway management and hospitalization

Peripheral edema

Severe cutaneous adverse reactions, including Stevens-Johnson syndrome and toxic epidermal necrolysis

7 DRUG INTERACTIONS

Cyclosporine: Avoid co-administration of cyclosporine with aliskiren.

Itraconazole: Avoid co-administration of itraconazole with aliskiren *[See Clinical Pharmacology (12.3)]*.

Non-Steroidal Anti-Inflammatory Agents (NSAIDs) including selective Cyclooxygenase-2 inhibitors (COX-2 inhibitors): In patients who are elderly, volume-depleted (including those on diuretic therapy), or with compromised renal function, co-administration of NSAIDs, including selective COX-2 inhibitors with agents that affect the renin-angiotensin system, including aliskiren, may result in deterioration of renal function, including possible acute renal failure. These effects are usually reversible. Monitor renal function periodically in patients receiving aliskiren and NSAID therapy.

The antihypertensive effect of aliskiren may be attenuated by NSAIDs.

8 USE IN SPECIFIC POPULATIONS

8.1 Pregnancy

Pregnancy Category D

Use of drugs that act on the renin-angiotensin system during the second and third trimesters of pregnancy reduces fetal renal function and increases fetal and neonatal morbidity and death. Resulting oligohydramnios can be associated with fetal lung hypoplasia and skeletal deformations. Potential neonatal adverse effects include skull hypoplasia, anuria, hypotension, renal failure, and death. When pregnancy is detected, discontinue Tekturna as soon as possible. These adverse outcomes are usually associated with use of these drugs in the second and third trimester of pregnancy. Most epidemiologic studies examining fetal abnormalities after exposure to antihypertensive use in the first trimester have not distinguished drugs affecting the renin-angiotensin system from other antihypertensive agents. Appropriate management of maternal hypertension during pregnancy is important to optimize outcomes for both mother and fetus.

In the unusual case that there is no appropriate alternative to therapy with drugs affecting the renin-angiotensin system for a particular patient, apprise the mother of the potential risk to the fetus. Perform serial ultrasound examinations to assess the intra-amniotic environment. If oligohydramnios is observed, discontinue Tekturna, unless it is considered lifesaving for the mother. Fetal testing may be appropriate, based on the week of pregnancy. Patients and physicians should be aware, however, that oligohydramnios may not appear until after the fetus has sustained irreversible injury. Closely observe infants with histories of in utero exposure to Tekturna for hypotension, oliguria, and hyperkalemia. *[see Use in Specific Populations (8.4)]*

8.3 Nursing Mothers

It is not known whether aliskiren is excreted in human breast milk. Aliskiren was secreted in the milk of lactating rats. Because of the potential for adverse effects on the nursing infant, a decision should be made whether to discontinue nursing or discontinue the drug, taking into account the importance of the drug to the mother.

8.4 Pediatric Use

Safety and effectiveness of aliskiren in pediatric patients <18 years have not been established.

Neonates with a history of in utero exposure to Tekturna:
If oliguria or hypotension occurs, direct attention toward support of blood pressure and renal perfusion. Exchange transfusions or dialysis may be required as a means of reversing hypotension and/or substituting for disordered renal function.

8.5 Geriatric Use

Of the total number of patients receiving aliskiren in clinical studies, 1,275 (19%) were 65 years or older and 231 (3.4%) were 75 years or older. No overall differences in safety or effectiveness were observed between these subjects and younger subjects. Other reported clinical experience has not identified differences in responses between the elderly and younger patients, but greater sensitivity of some older individuals cannot be ruled out.

8.6 Renal Impairment

Safety and effectiveness of Tekturna in patients with severe renal impairment (CrCL <30 ml/min) have not been established as patients with eGFR <30ml/min were excluded in clinical trials *[see Clinical Studies (14)]*.

10 OVERDOSAGE

Limited data are available related to overdosage in humans. The most likely manifestation of overdosage would be hypotension. If symptomatic hypotension occurs, supportive treatment should be initiated.

Aliskiren is poorly dialyzed. Therefore, hemodialysis is not adequate to treat aliskiren overexposure *[see Clinical Pharmacology (12.3)]*.

11 DESCRIPTION

Tekturna contains aliskiren hemifumarate, a renin inhibitor, that is provided as tablets for oral administration. Aliskiren hemifumarate is chemically described as (2S, 4S,5S,7S)-N-(2-carbamoyl-2-methylpropyl)-5-amino-4-hydroxy-2,7-diisopropyl-8-[4-methoxy-3-(3-methoxypropoxy) phenyl]-octanamide hemifumarate and its structural formula is

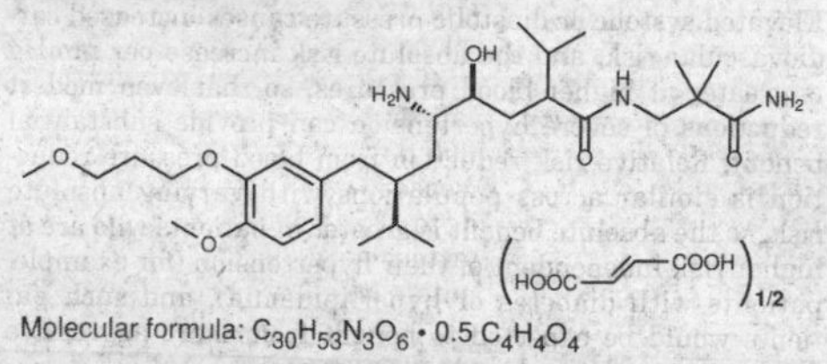

Molecular formula: $C_{30}H_{53}N_3O_6 \cdot 0.5\ C_4H_4O_4$

Aliskiren hemifumarate is a white to slightly yellowish crystalline powder with a molecular weight of 609.8 (free base- 551.8). It is soluble in phosphate buffer, n-octanol, and highly soluble in water.

12 CLINICAL PHARMACOLOGY

12.1 Mechanism of Action

Renin is secreted by the kidney in response to decreases in blood volume and renal perfusion. Renin cleaves angiotensinogen to form the inactive decapeptide angiotensin I (Ang I). Ang I is converted to the active octapeptide angiotensin II (Ang II) by angiotensin-converting enzyme (ACE) and non-ACE pathways. Ang II is a powerful vasoconstrictor and leads to the release of catecholamines from the adrenal medulla and prejunctional nerve endings. It also promotes aldosterone secretion and sodium reabsorption. Together, these effects increase blood pressure. Ang II also inhibits renin release, thus providing a negative feedback to the system. This cycle, from renin through angiotensin to aldosterone and its associated negative feedback loop, is known as the renin-angiotensin-aldosterone system (RAAS). Aliskiren is a direct renin inhibitor, decreasing plasma renin activity (PRA) and inhibiting the conversion of angiotensinogen to Ang I. Whether aliskiren affects other RAAS components, e.g., ACE or non-ACE pathways, is not known. All agents that inhibit the RAAS, including renin inhibitors, suppress the negative feedback loop, leading to a compensatory rise in plasma renin concentration. When this rise occurs during treatment with ACE inhibitors and ARBs, the result is increased levels of PRA. During treatment with aliskiren, however, the effect of increased renin levels is blocked so that PRA, Ang I and Ang II are all reduced, whether aliskiren is used as monotherapy or in combination with other antihypertensive agents.

12.2 Pharmacodynamics

In placebo controlled clinical trials, plasma renin activity (PRA) was decreased in a range of 50-80%. This reduction in PRA was not dose-related and did not correlate with blood pressure reductions. The clinical implications of the differences in effect on PRA are not known.

12.3 Pharmacokinetics

Aliskiren is poorly absorbed (bioavailability about 2.5%) with an approximate accumulation half life of 24 hours. Steady state blood levels are reached in about 7-8 days.

Absorption and Distribution

Following oral administration, peak plasma concentrations of aliskiren are reached within 1 – 3 hours. When taken with a high fat meal, mean AUC and C_{max} of aliskiren are decreased by 71% and 85% respectively. In the clinical trials of aliskiren, it was administered without requiring a fixed relation of administration to meals.

Metabolism and Elimination

About one fourth of the absorbed dose appears in the urine as parent drug. How much of the absorbed dose is metabolized is unknown. Based on the in vitro studies, the major enzyme responsible for aliskiren metabolism appears to be CYP 3A4. Aliskiren does not inhibit the CYP450 isoenzymes (CYP 1A2, 2C8, 2C9, 2C19, 2D6, 2E1, and 3A) or induce CYP 3A4.

Transporters: Pgp (MDR1/Mdr1a/1b) was found to be the major efflux system involved in absorption and disposition of aliskiren in preclinical studies. The potential for drug interactions at the Pgp site will likely depend on the degree of inhibition of this transporter.

Drug interactions

The effect of co-administered drugs on the pharmacokinetics of aliskiren and vice versa, were studied in several single and multiple dose studies. Pharmacokinetic measures indicating the magnitude of these interactions are presented in Figure 1 (impact of co-administered drugs on aliskiren) and Figure 2 (impact of aliskiren on co-administered drugs).

[See figure 1 at top of previous page]

Warfarin: There was no clinically significant effect of a single dose of warfarin 25 mg on the pharmacokinetics of aliskiren.

[See figure 2 above]

Special Populations

Renally Impaired Patients: Aliskiren was evaluated in patients with varying degrees of renal insufficiency. The rate and extent of exposure (AUC and C_{max}) of aliskiren in subjects with renal impairment did not show a consistent correlation with the severity of renal impairment. Adjustment of the starting dose is not required in these patients *[see Warnings and Precautions (5.2)]*.

The pharmacokinetics of aliskiren following administration of a single oral dose of 300 mg was evaluated in patients with End Stage Renal Disease (ESRD) undergoing hemodialysis. When compared to matched healthy subjects, changes in the rate and extent of aliskiren exposure (C_{max} and AUC) in ESRD patients undergoing hemodialysis was not clinically significant.

Timing of hemodialysis did not significantly alter the pharmacokinetics of aliskiren in ESRD patients. Therefore, no dose adjustment is warranted in ESRD patients receiving hemodialysis.

Hepatically Impaired Patients: The pharmacokinetics of aliskiren were not significantly affected in patients with mild to severe liver disease. Consequently, adjustment of the starting dose is not required in these patients.

Pediatric Patients: The pharmacokinetics of aliskiren have not been investigated in patients <18 years of age.

Geriatric Patients: Exposure (measured by AUC) is increased in elderly patients ≥65 years. Adjustment of the starting dose is not required in these patients.

Race: The pharmacokinetic differences between Blacks, Caucasians, and the Japanese are minimal.

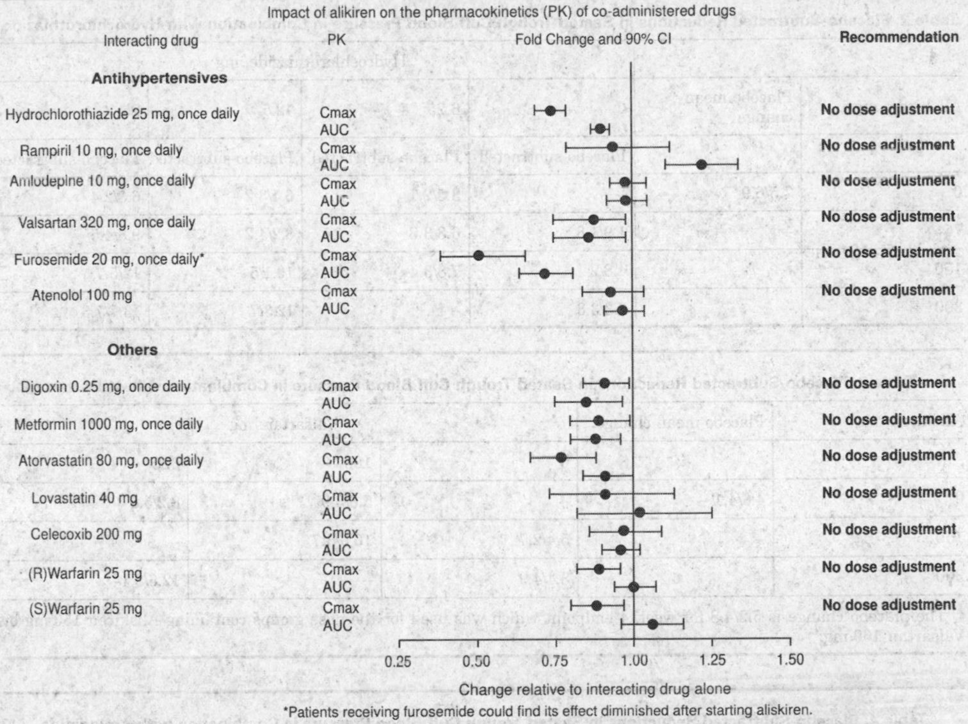

Figure 2: The impact of aliskiren on the pharmacokinetics of co-administered drugs.

Table 1: Reductions in Seated Trough Cuff Blood Pressure in the Placebo-Controlled Studies

Study	Placebo mean change	Aliskiren daily dose, mg			
		75	150	300	600
		Placebo-subtracted	Placebo-subtracted	Placebo-subtracted	Placebo-subtracted
1	2.9/3.3	5.7/4*	5.9/4.5*	11.2/7.5*	--
2	5.3/6.3	--	6.1/2.9*	10.5/5.4*	10.4/5.2*
3	10/8.6	2.2/1.7	2.1/1.7	5.1/3.7*	--
4	7.5/6.9	1.9/1.8	4.8/2*	8.3/3.3*	--
5	3.8/4.9	--	9.3/5.4*	10.9/6.2*	12.1/7.6*
6	4.6/4.1	--	--	8.4/4.9†	--

*p<0.05 vs. placebo by ANCOVA with Dunnett's procedure for multiple comparisons
†p<0.05 vs. placebo by ANCOVA for the pairwise comparison.

13 NONCLINICAL TOXICOLOGY

13.1 Carcinogenesis, Mutagenesis, Impairment of Fertility

Carcinogenic potential was assessed in a 2-year rat study and a 6-month transgenic (rasH2) mouse study with aliskiren hemifumarate at oral doses of up to 1500 mg aliskiren/kg/day. Although there were no statistically significant increases in tumor incidence associated with exposure to aliskiren, mucosal epithelial hyperplasia (with or without erosion/ulceration) was observed in the lower gastrointestinal tract at doses of ≥750 mg/kg/day in both species, with a colonic adenoma identified in one rat and a cecal adenocarcinoma identified in another, rare tumors in the strain of rat studied. On a systemic exposure (AUC_{0-24hr}) basis, 1500 mg/kg/day in the rat is about 4 times and in the mouse about 1.5 times the maximum recommended human dose (300 mg aliskiren/day). Mucosal hyperplasia in the cecum or colon of rats was also observed at doses of 250 mg/kg/day (the lowest tested dose) as well as at higher doses in 4- and 13-week studies.

Aliskiren hemifumarate was devoid of genotoxic potential in the Ames reverse mutation assay with *S. typhimurium* and *E. coli*, the in vitro Chinese hamster ovary cell chromosomal aberration assay, the in vitro Chinese hamster V79 cell gene mutation test and the in vivo mouse bone marrow micronucleus assay.

Fertility of male and female rats was unaffected at doses of up to 250 mg aliskiren/kg/day (8 times the maximum recommended human dose of 300 mg Tekturna/60 kg on a mg/m^2 basis.)

13.2 Animal Toxicology and/or Pharmacology

Reproductive Toxicology Studies: Reproductive toxicity studies of aliskiren hemifumarate did not reveal any evidence of teratogenicity at oral doses up to 600 mg aliskiren/kg/day (20 times the maximum recommended human dose (MRHD) of 300 mg/day on a mg/m^2 basis) in pregnant rats or up to 100 mg aliskiren/kg/day (7 times the MRHD on a mg/m^2 basis) in pregnant rabbits. Fetal birth weight was adversely affected in rabbits at 50 mg/kg/day (3.2 times the MRHD on a mg/m^2 basis). Aliskiren was present in placenta, amniotic fluid and fetuses of pregnant rabbits.

14 CLINICAL STUDIES

14.1 Aliskiren Monotherapy

The antihypertensive effects of Tekturna have been demonstrated in six randomized, double-blind, placebo-controlled 8 week clinical trials in patients with mild-to-moderate hypertension. The placebo response and placebo-subtracted changes from baseline in seated trough cuff blood pressure are shown in Table 1.

[See table 1 above]

The studies included approximately 2,730 patients given doses of 75-600 mg of aliskiren and 1,231 patients given placebo. As shown in Table 1, there is some increase in response with administered dose in all studies, with reasonable effects seen at 150-300 mg, and no clear further increases at 600 mg. A substantial proportion (85%-90%) of the blood pressure lowering effect was observed within 2 weeks of treatment studies with ambulatory blood pressure monitoring showed reasonable control throughout the interdosing interval; the ratios of mean daytime to mean night-time ambulatory BP range from 0.6 to 0.9.

Patients in the placebo-controlled trials continued open-label aliskiren for up to one year. A persistent blood pressure lowering effect was demonstrated by a randomized withdrawal study (patients randomized to continue drug or placebo), which showed a statistically significant difference between patients kept on aliskiren and those randomized to placebo. With cessation of treatment, blood pressure gradually returned toward baseline levels over a period of several weeks. There was no evidence of rebound hypertension after abrupt cessation of therapy.

Aliskiren lowered blood pressure in all demographic subgroups, although Black patients tended to have smaller reduction than Caucasians and Asians, as has been seen with ACE inhibitors and ARBs.

There are no studies of Tekturna or members of the direct renin inhibitors demonstrating reductions in cardiovascular risk in patients with hypertension.

14.2 Aliskiren in Combination with Other Antihypertensives

Hydrochlorothiazide

Aliskiren 75, 150, and 300 mg and hydrochlorothiazide 6.25, 12.5, and 25 mg were studied alone and in combination in an 8-week, 2,776-patient, randomized, double-blind, placebo-controlled, parallel-group, 15-arm factorial study. Blood pressure reductions with the combinations were greater than the reductions with the monotherapies as shown in Table 2.

Table 2: Placebo-Subtracted Reductions in Seated Trough Cuff Blood Pressure in Combination with Hydrochlorothiazide

		Hydrochlorothiazide, mg			
Aliskiren, mg	Placebo mean change	0	6.25	12.5	25
		Placebo-subtracted	Placebo-subtracted	Placebo-subtracted	Placebo-subtracted
0	7.5/6.9	--	3.5/2.1	6.4/3.2	6.8/2.4
75	--	1.9/1.8	6.8/3.8	8.2/4.2	9.8/4.5
150	--	4.8/2	7.8/3.4	10.1/5	12/5.7
300	--	8.3/3.3	--	12.3/7	13.7/7.3

Table 3: Placebo-Subtracted Reductions in Seated Trough Cuff Blood Pressure in Combination with Valsartan

Aliskiren, mg	Placebo mean change	Valsartan, mg		
		0	160	320
0	4.6/4.1*	--	5.6/3.9	8.2/5.6
150	--	5.4/2.7	10.0/5.7	--
300	--	8.4/4.9	--	12.6/8.1

* The placebo change is 5.2/4.8 for week 4 endpoint which was used for the dose groups containing Aliskiren 150 mg or Valsartan 160 mg.

Table 4: Placebo-Subtracted Reductions in Seated Trough Cuff Blood Pressure in Combination with Amlodipine

Aliskiren, mg	Placebo mean change	Amlodipine, mg		
		0	5	10
0	5.4/6.8	--	5.6/9.0	8.5/14.3
150	--	2.6/3.9	8.6/13.9	10.8/17.1
300	--	4.9/8.6	9.6/15.0	11.1/16.4

Table 5: Incidence of selected adverse events in ALTITUDE

	Aliskiren N=4283		Placebo N=4296	
	Serious Adverse Events* (%)	Adverse Events (%)	Serious Adverse Events* (%)	Adverse Events (%)
Renal impairment †	4.7	12.4	3.3	10.4
Hypotension ††	2.0	18.6	1.7	14.8
Hyperkalemia †††	1.1	36.9	0.3	27.1

†renal failure, renal failure acute, renal failure chronic, renal impairment
††dizziness, dizziness postural, hypotension, orthostatic hypotension, presyncope, syncope
††† Given the variable baseline potassium levels of patients with renal insufficiency on dual RAAS therapy, the reporting of adverse event of hyperkalemia was at the discretion of the investigator.
* A Serious Adverse Event (SAE) is defined as: an event which is fatal or life-threatening, results in persistent or significant disability/incapacity, constitutes a congenital anomaly/birth defect, requires inpatient hospitalization or prolongation of existing hospitalization, or is medically significant (i.e. defined as an event that jeopardizes the patient or may require medical or surgical intervention to prevent one of the outcomes previously listed).

[See table 2 above]

Valsartan

Aliskiren 150 and 300 mg and valsartan 160 and 320 mg were studied alone and in combination in an 8-week, 1,797-patient, randomized, double-blind, placebo-controlled, parallel-group, 4-arm, dose-escalation study. The dosages of aliskiren and valsartan were started at 150 and 160 mg, respectively, and increased at four weeks to 300 mg and 320 mg, respectively. Seated trough cuff blood pressure was measured at baseline, 4, and 8 weeks. Blood pressure reductions with the combinations were greater than the reductions with the monotherapies as shown in Table 3.

[See table 3 above]

Amlodipine

Aliskiren 150 mg and 300 mg and amlodipine besylate 5 mg and 10 mg were studied alone and in combination in an 8-week, 1,685-patient, randomized, double-blind, placebo-controlled, multifactorial study. Treatment with aliskiren and amlodipine resulted overall in significantly greater reductions in diastolic and systolic blood pressure compared to the respective monotherapy components as shown in Table 4.

[See table 4 above]

ACE inhibitors

Aliskiren has not been studied when added to maximal doses of ACE inhibitors to determine whether aliskiren produces additional blood pressure reduction.

14.3 Aliskiren in Patients with Diabetes treated with ARB or ACEI (ALTITUDE study)

Patients with diabetes with renal disease (defined either by the presence of albuminuria or reduced GFR) were randomized to aliskiren 300 mg daily (n=4283) or placebo (n=4296). All patients were receiving background therapy with an ARB or ACEI. The primary efficacy outcome was the time to the first event of the primary composite endpoint consisting of cardiovascular death, resuscitated sudden death, non-fatal myocardial infarction, non-fatal stroke, unplanned hospitalization for heart failure, onset of end stage renal disease, renal death, and doubling of serum creatinine concentration from baseline sustained for at least one month. After a median follow up of about 27 months, the trial was terminated early for lack of efficacy. Higher risk of renal impairment, hypotension and hyperkalemia was observed in aliskiren compared to placebo treated patients, as shown in the table below.

[See table 5 below]

The risk of stroke (2.7% aliskiren vs 2.0% placebo) and death (6.9% aliskiren vs. 6.4% placebo) were also numerically higher in aliskiren treated patients.

16 HOW SUPPLIED/STORAGE AND HANDLING

Tekturna is supplied as a light-pink, biconvex round tablet containing 150 mg of aliskiren, and as a light-red biconvex ovaloid tablet containing 300 mg of aliskiren. Tablets are imprinted with NVR on one side and IL, IU, on the other side of the 150, and 300 mg tablets, respectively.

All strengths are packaged in bottles and unit-dose blister packages (10 strips or 10 tablets) as described below in Table 6.

[See table 6 at top of next page]

Store at 25°C (77°F); excursions permitted to 15-30°C (59-86°F) [See USP Controlled Room Temperature]. Protect from moisture.

Dispense in original container.

17 PATIENT COUNSELING INFORMATION

See FDA-approved patient labeling (Patient Information)

Information for Patients

Pregnancy: Female patients of child bearing age should be told about the consequences of exposure to Tekturna during pregnancy. Discuss treatment options with women planning to become pregnant. Patients should be asked to report pregnancies to their physicians as soon as possible.

Anaphylactic Reactions and Angioedema: Patients should be advised and told to report immediately any signs or symptoms suggesting a severe allergic reaction (difficulty breathing or swallowing, tightness of the chest, hives, general rash, swelling, itching, dizziness, vomiting, or abdominal pain) or angioedema (swelling of face, extremities, eyes, lips, tongue, difficulty in swallowing or breathing) and to take no more drug until they have consulted with the prescribing physicians. Angioedema, including laryngeal edema, may occur at any time during treatment with Tekturna.

Symptomatic Hypotension: A patient receiving Tekturna should be cautioned that lightheadedness can occur, especially during the first days of therapy, and that it should be reported to the prescribing physician. The patients should be told that if syncope occurs, Tekturna should be discontinued until the physician has been consulted.

All patients should be cautioned that inadequate fluid intake, excessive perspiration, diarrhea, or vomiting can lead to an excessive fall in blood pressure, with the same consequences of lightheadedness and possible syncope.

Potassium Supplements: A patient receiving Tekturna should be told not to use potassium supplements or salt substitutes containing potassium without consulting the prescribing physician.

Relationship to Meals: Patients should establish a routine pattern for taking Tekturna with regard to meals. High-fat meals decrease absorption substantially.

T2012-172
September 2012

FDA approved patient labeling

PATIENT INFORMATION

Tekturna (pronounced tek-turn-a)
(aliskiren)
Tablets

Dosing Strengths:
150 mg tablets
300 mg tablets

Available by Prescription Only

Read the patient information that comes with Tekturna before you start taking it and each time you get a refill. There may be new information. This leaflet does not replace talking to your doctor about your condition or treatment. If you have any questions about Tekturna, ask your doctor or pharmacist.

What is the most important information I should know about Tekturna?

Tekturna can cause harm or death to an unborn baby. Talk to your doctor about other ways to lower your blood pressure if you plan to become pregnant. If you get pregnant while taking Tekturna, tell your doctor right away.

What Is Tekturna?

Tekturna can help your blood vessels relax and widen so blood pressure is lower. Tekturna is a type of prescription medicine called a direct renin inhibitor. By reducing renin, it helps to reduce blood pressure.

What Is High Blood Pressure (Hypertension)?

Blood pressure is the force that pushes the blood through your blood vessels to all the organs of your body. You have high blood pressure when the force of your blood moving through your blood vessels is too great. Renin (pronounced REE-nin) is a chemical in the body that starts a process that makes blood vessels narrow, leading to high blood pressure. Drugs that lower blood pressure lower your risk of having a stroke or heart attack.

Table 6: Tekturna Tablets Supply

Tablet	Color	Imprint	Imprint	NDC 0078-XXXX-XX		
		Side 1	Side 2	Bottle of 30	Bottle of 90	Blister Packages of 100
150 mg	Light-Pink	NVR	IL	0485-15	0485-34	0485-35
300 mg	Light-Red	NVR	IU	0486-15	0486-34	0486-35

High blood pressure makes the heart work harder to pump blood throughout the body and causes damage to the blood vessels. If high blood pressure is not treated, it can lead to stroke, heart attack, heart failure, kidney failure, and vision problems.

Who Should Not Take Tekturna?

- **If you get pregnant, stop taking Tekturna and call your doctor right away. If you plan to become pregnant, talk to your doctor about other treatment options for your high blood pressure.**
- **If you have diabetes and are taking a kind of medicine called an angiotensin-receptor-blocker or angiotensin-converting-enzyme-inhibitor.**
- **Do not take Tekturna if you are allergic to any of its ingredients. See the end of this leaflet for a complete list of the ingredients in Tekturna.**
- **Tekturna has not been studied in children under 18 years of age.**

What Should I Tell My Doctor Before Taking Tekturna?

Tell your doctor about all your medical conditions, including whether you:

- have kidney problems.
- are pregnant or planning to become pregnant, see "What is the most important information I should know about Tekturna?"
- are breast-feeding. It is not known if Tekturna passes into your breast milk. You should choose either to take Tekturna or breast-feed, but not both.
- are allergic to any of the ingredients in Tekturna, see "What are the ingredients in Tekturna?"
- have ever had a reaction called angioedema, to an ACE inhibitor medicine. Angioedema causes swelling of the face, lips, tongue, throat, arms, and legs, and may cause difficulty breathing.

Tell your doctor about all the medicines you take including prescription and nonprescription medicines, vitamins and herbal supplements. Especially tell your doctor if you are taking:

- a kind of medicine called angiotensin receptor blocker or angiotensin converting enzyme inhibitor
- Atorvastatin (medicine to lower cholesterol in your blood).
- water pills (also called "diuretics").
- medicines for treating fungus or fungal infections.
- cyclosporine (a medicine used to suppress the immune system).
- potassium-containing medicines, potassium supplements, or salt substitutes containing potassium.
- nonsteroidal anti-inflammatory drugs (like ibuprofen or naproxen)

Your doctor or pharmacist will know what medicines are safe to take together.

How Should I Take Tekturna?

- Take Tekturna once a day, at the same time each day. As with any blood pressure medication, it is important to take Tekturna on a regular daily basis exactly as prescribed by your doctor.
- Tekturna can be taken by itself or safely in combination with other medicines to lower high blood pressure. Your doctor may change your dose if needed.
- Tekturna can be taken with or without food.
- If you miss a dose, take it as soon as you remember. If it is close to your next dose, do not take the missed dose. Just take the next dose at your regular time.
- If you take too much Tekturna, call your doctor or Poison Control Center, or go to the nearest hospital emergency room.

What Are Possible Side Effects Of Tekturna?

Tekturna may cause serious side effects:

- **Injury or death to an unborn baby.** See "What is the most important information I should know about Tekturna?"
- **Low blood pressure (hypotension).** Your blood pressure may get too low if you also take water pills, are on a low-salt diet, get dialysis treatments, have heart problems, or get sick with vomiting or diarrhea. Lie down if you feel faint or dizzy. Call your doctor right away.
- **Severe Allergic Reactions and Angioedema**: Aliskiren may cause difficulty breathing or swallowing, tightness of the chest, hives, general rash, swelling, itching, dizziness, vomiting, or abdominal pain (signs of a severe allergic reaction). Aliskiren can also cause swelling of the face, lips, tongue, throat, arms and legs or the whole body (signs of angioedema). Get medical help right away and tell your doctor if you get any one or more of these symptoms. Angioedema can happen at any time while you are taking Tekturna.

Common side effects of Tekturna include:

diarrhea
cough
dizziness
headache
flu-like symptoms
back pain
tiredness
high levels of potassium in the blood (hyperkalemia)

Less common side effects include rash.

Tell your doctor if you have any side effect that bothers you or that does not go away. These are not all of the possible side effects of Tekturna. For a complete list of side effects, ask your doctor or pharmacist.

How Do I Store Tekturna?

- Store Tekturna tablets at room temperature between 59° to 86°F (15°-30°C).
- Keep Tekturna in the original prescription bottle in a dry place. Do not remove the desiccant (drying agent) from the bottle.
- Keep Tekturna and all medicines out of the reach of children.

General Information About Tekturna

Medicines are sometimes prescribed for conditions not listed in the patient information leaflet. Do not take Tekturna for a condition for which it was not prescribed. Do not give Tekturna to other people, even if they have the same condition or symptoms you have. It may harm them. This leaflet summarizes the most important information about Tekturna. If you have more questions about Tekturna talk with your doctor. You can ask your doctor or pharmacist for information that is written for healthcare professionals.

For more information about Tekturna, ask your doctor or pharmacist, visit www.Tekturna.com, or call 1-888-Tekturna (1-888-835-8876).

What are the ingredients in Tekturna?

Active Ingredients: Aliskiren (Tekturna)

Inactive Ingredients: colloidal silicone dioxide, crospovidone, hypromellose, iron oxide colorants, magnesium stearate, microcrystalline cellulose, polyethylene glycol, talc, and titanium dioxide.

Manufactured by:
Novartis Pharma AG, Stein, Switzerland
Novartis Pharma Produktions GmbH, Wehr, Germany
Distributed by:
Novartis Pharmaceuticals Corporation
East Hanover, NJ 07936
© Novartis
T2012-173
September 2012

Shown in Product Identification Guide, page 311

TEKTURNA HCT ℞

[*tek-turn-a HCT*]
(aliskiren and hydrochlorothiazide) tablets, for oral use

The following prescribing information is based on official labeling in effect July 2013.

HIGHLIGHTS OF PRESCRIBING INFORMATION

These highlights do not include all the information needed to use TEKTURNA HCT safely and effectively. See full prescribing information for TEKTURNA HCT.

Tekturna HCT (aliskiren and hydrochlorothiazide) tablets, for oral use

Initial U.S. Approval: 2008

> **WARNING: FETAL TOXICITY**
>
> ***See full prescribing information for complete boxed warning***
>
> - **When pregnancy is detected, discontinue Tekturna HCT as soon as possible. (5.1)**
> - **Drugs that act directly on the renin-angiotensin system can cause injury and death to the developing fetus. (5.1)**

RECENT MAJOR CHANGES

Boxed Warning: Fetal Toxicity	02/2012
Contraindications: Concomitant use with ARBs or ACEIs in diabetes (4)	03/2012
Warnings and Precautions (5.1)	02/2012
Warnings and Precautions (5.2, 5.4, 5.5, 5.9)	03/2012
Warnings and Precautions (5.3)	09/2012

INDICATIONS AND USAGE

Tekturna HCT is a combination of aliskiren, a renin inhibitor, and hydrochlorothiazide (HCTZ), a thiazide diuretic, indicated for the treatment of hypertension, to lower blood pressure:

- In patients not adequately controlled with monotherapy
- As initial therapy in patients likely to need multiple drugs to achieve their blood pressure goals (1)

Lowering blood pressure reduces the risk of fatal and nonfatal cardiovascular events, primarily strokes and myocardial infarction.

DOSAGE AND ADMINISTRATION

- The antihypertensive effect is largely manifested within 1 week, with maximal effects seen at around 4 weeks. If blood pressure remains uncontrolled after 2 to 4 weeks of therapy, titrate up to a maximum of 300/25 mg. (2.2)
- Order of increasing mean effect: 150/12.5 mg, 150/25 mg or 300/12.5 mg, and 300/25 mg (2.1)
- One tablet daily, with a routine pattern with regard to meals. (2.7)
- Add-on or Initial therapy: Initiate with 150/12.5mg. Titrate as needed up to a maximum of 300/25 mg. (2.3, 2.5)
- Replacement therapy: May be substituted for titrated components (2.4)

DOSAGE FORMS AND STRENGTHS

Tablets (mg aliskiren/mg HCTZ): 150/12.5, 150/25, 300/12.5, 300/25 (3)

CONTRAINDICATIONS

Do not use with angiotensin receptor blockers (ARBs) or ACE inhibitors (ACEIs) in patients with diabetes (4)
Anuria (4)
Hypersensitivity to sulfonamide-derived drugs (4)

WARNINGS AND PRECAUTIONS

- Avoid concomitant use with ARBs or ACEIs in patients with renal impairment (GFR<60 mL/min) (5.2)
- Anaphylactic Reactions and Head and Neck Angioedema: Discontinue Tekturna HCT and monitor until signs and symptoms resolve. (5.3)
- Hypotension: Correct volume depletion prior to initiation. (5.4)
- Impaired renal function: Monitor serum creatinine periodically. (5.5)
- Hypersensitivity Reactions: May occur from HCTZ component (5.6)
- Hyperkalemia: Monitor potassium levels periodically. (5.9)
- Hydrochlorothiazide has been associated with acute angle-closure glaucoma (5.11)

ADVERSE REACTIONS

The most common adverse reactions (incidence ≥1.5% and more common than with placebo) are: dizziness and diarrhea. (6.1)

To report SUSPECTED ADVERSE REACTIONS, contact Novartis Pharmaceuticals Corporation at 1-888-669-6682 or FDA at 1-800-FDA-1088 or www.fda.gov/medwatch.

DRUG INTERACTIONS

- Cyclosporine: Avoid concomitant use (7, 12.3)
- Itraconazole: Avoid concomitant use (7, 12.3)
- NSAIDs use may lead to increased risk of renal impairment and loss of antihypertensive effect (7)
- Antidiabetic Drugs: Dosage adjustment of antidiabetic may be required (7)
- Cholestyramine and Colestipol: Reduced absorption of thiazides (7)
- Lithium: Increased risk of lithium toxicity when used with diuretics. Monitor serum lithium concentrations during concurrent use. (7)

USE IN SPECIFIC POPULATIONS

Nursing Mothers: Nursing or drug should be discontinued. (8.3)

See 17 for PATIENT COUNSELING INFORMATION and FDA-approved patient labeling

Revised: 09/2012

FULL PRESCRIBING INFORMATION: CONTENTS*

*** Sections or subsections omitted from the full prescribing information are not listed**

FULL PRESCRIBING INFORMATION

WARNING: FETAL TOXICITY
- **When pregnancy is detected, discontinue Tekturna HCT as soon as possible. (5.1)**
- **Drugs that act directly on the renin-angiotensin system can cause injury and death to the developing fetus. (5.1)**

1 INDICATIONS AND USAGE

Tekturna HCT is indicated for the treatment of hypertension, to lower blood pressure. Lowering blood pressure reduces the risk of fatal and nonfatal cardiovascular events, primarily strokes and myocardial infarctions. These benefits have been seen in controlled trials of antihypertensive drugs from a wide variety of pharmacologic classes including hydrochlorothiazide. There are no controlled trials demonstrating risk reduction with Tekturna HCT.

Control of high blood pressure should be part of comprehensive cardiovascular risk management, including, as appropriate, lipid control, diabetes management, antithrombotic therapy, smoking cessation, exercise, and limited sodium intake. Many patients will require more than one drug to achieve blood pressure goals. For specific advice on goals and management, see published guidelines, such as those of the National High Blood Pressure Education Program's Joint National Committee on Prevention, Detection, Evaluation, and Treatment of High Blood Pressure (JNC).

Numerous antihypertensive drugs, from a variety of pharmacologic classes and with different mechanisms of action, have been shown in randomized controlled trials to reduce cardiovascular morbidity and mortality, and it can be concluded that it is blood pressure reduction, and not some other pharmacologic property of the drugs, that is largely responsible for those benefits. The largest and most consistent cardiovascular outcome benefit has been a reduction in the risk of stroke, but reductions in myocardial infarction and cardiovascular mortality also have been seen regularly. Elevated systolic or diastolic pressure causes increased cardiovascular risk, and the absolute risk increase per mmHg is greater at higher blood pressures, so that even modest reductions of severe hypertension can provide substantial benefit. Relative risk reduction from blood pressure reduction is similar across populations with varying absolute risk, so the absolute benefit is greater in patients who are at higher risk independent of their hypertension (for example, patients with diabetes or hyperlipidemia), and such patients would be expected to benefit from more aggressive treatment to a lower blood pressure goal.

Some antihypertensive drugs have smaller blood pressure effects (as monotherapy) in black patients, and many antihypertensive drugs have additional approved indications and effects (e.g., on angina, heart failure, or diabetic kidney disease). These considerations may guide selection of therapy.

Add-On Therapy

A patient whose blood pressure is not adequately controlled with aliskiren alone or hydrochlorothiazide alone may be switched to combination therapy with Tekturna HCT.

A patient whose blood pressure is controlled with hydrochlorothiazide alone but who experiences hypokalemia may be switched to combination therapy with Tekturna HCT.

A patient who experiences dose-limiting adverse reactions on either component alone may be switched to Tekturna HCT containing a lower dose of that component in combination with the other to achieve similar blood pressure reductions.

Replacement Therapy

Tekturna HCT may be substituted for the titrated components.

Initial Therapy

Tekturna HCT may be used as initial therapy in patients who are likely to need multiple drugs to achieve their blood pressure goals.

The choice of Tekturna HCT as initial therapy should be based on an assessment of potential benefits and risks.

Patients with Stage 2 hypertension are at a relatively high risk for cardiovascular events (such as strokes, heart attacks, and heart failure), kidney failure, and vision problems, so prompt treatment is clinically relevant. The decision to use a combination as initial therapy should be individualized and should be shaped by considerations such as baseline blood pressure, the target goal, and the incremental likelihood of achieving goal with a combination compared to monotherapy. Individual blood pressure goals may vary based upon the patient's risk.

Data from the high-dose multifactorial study *[see Clinical Studies (14)]* provide estimates of the probability of reaching a target blood pressure with Tekturna HCT compared to aliskiren or hydrochlorothiazide monotherapy. The figures below provide estimates of the likelihood of achieving systolic or diastolic blood pressure control with Tekturna HCT 300/25 mg, based upon baseline systolic or diastolic blood pressure. The curve of each treatment group was estimated by logistic regression modeling. The estimated likelihood at the right tail of each curve is less reliable because of small numbers of subjects with high baseline blood pressures.

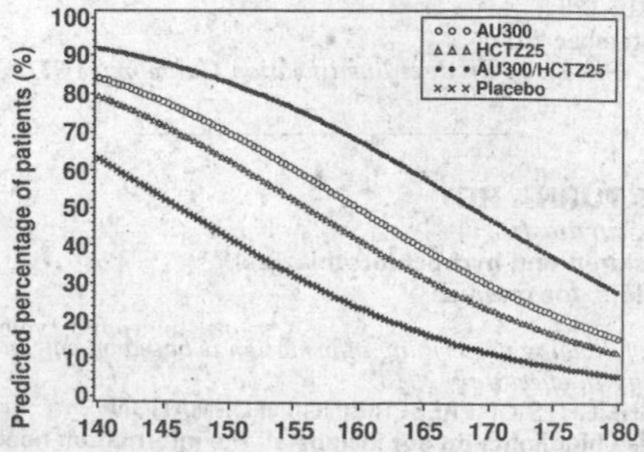

Figure 1: Probability of Achieving Systolic Blood Pressure (SBP) <140 mmHg

[See figure 2 at top of next column]
[See figure 3 at top of next column]
[See figure 4 at top of next column]

At all levels of baseline blood pressure, the probability of achieving any given diastolic or systolic goal is greater with the combination than for either monotherapy. For example, the mean baseline msSBP/msDBP for patients participating in this multifactorial study was 154/99 mmHg. A patient with a baseline blood pressure of 154/99 mmHg has about a 62% chance of achieving a goal of <140 mmHg (systolic) and 61% chance of achieving <90 mmHg (diastolic) on aliskiren alone, and the chance of achieving these goals on

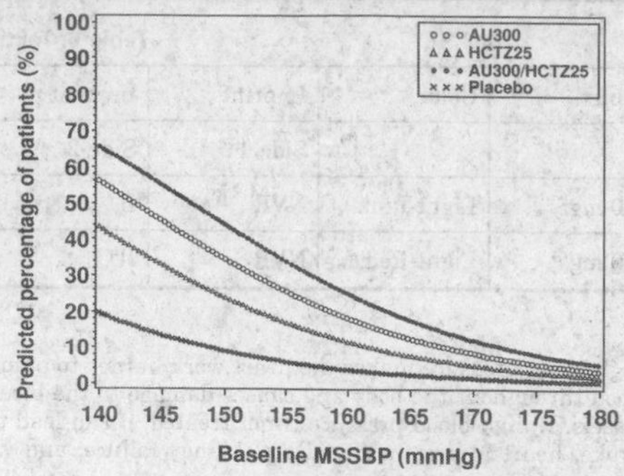

Figure 2: Probability of Achieving Systolic Blood Pressure (SBP) <130 mmHg

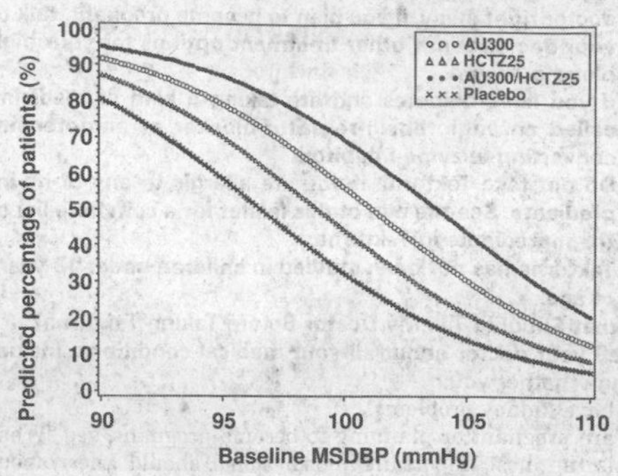

Figure 3: Probability of Achieving Diastolic Blood Pressure (DBP) <90 mmHg

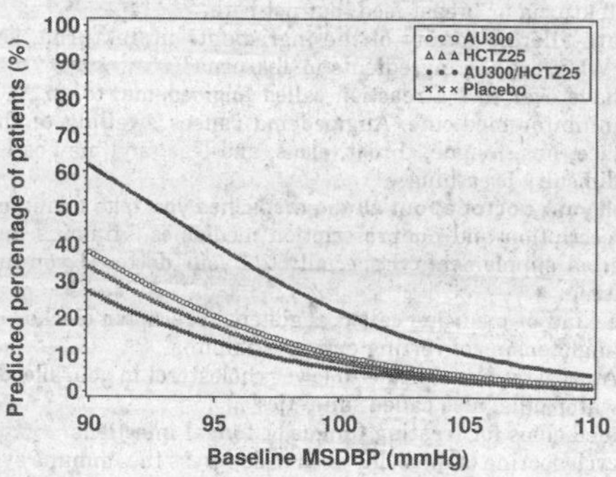

Figure 4: Probability of Achieving Diastolic Blood Pressure (DBP) <80 mmHg

hydrochlorothiazide alone is about 54% (systolic) and 49% (diastolic). The chance of achieving these goals on Tekturna HCT rises to about 77% (systolic) and 74% (diastolic). The chance of achieving these goals on placebo is about 34% (systolic) and 37% (diastolic) *[see Dosage and Administration (2) and Clinical Studies (14)]*.

2 DOSAGE AND ADMINISTRATION

2.1 Dose Selection

The recommended once-daily doses of Tekturna HCT in order of increasing mean effect are 150/12.5 mg, 150/25 mg or 300/12.5 mg, and 300/25 mg.

2.2 Dose Titration

The antihypertensive effect of Tekturna HCT is largely manifested within 1 week, with maximal effects generally seen at around 4 weeks. If blood pressure remains uncontrolled after 2 to 4 weeks of therapy, the dose may be titrated up to a maximum of aliskiren 300 mg/hydrochlorothiazide 25 mg.

2.3 Add-On Therapy

A patient whose blood pressure is not adequately controlled with aliskiren alone or hydrochlorothiazide alone may be switched to combination therapy with Tekturna HCT. The usual recommended starting dose is 150/12.5 mg once daily as needed to control blood pressure. The dose may be titrated up to a maximum of aliskiren 300 mg/hydrochlorothiazide 25 mg once daily.

2.4 Replacement Therapy

Tekturna HCT may be substituted for the individually titrated components.

2.5 Initial Therapy

The usual recommended starting dose is 150/12.5 mg once daily as needed to control blood pressure. The dose may be titrated up to a maximum of aliskiren 300 mg/hydrochlorothiazide 25 mg once daily.

Tekturna HCT is not recommended for use as initial therapy in patients with intravascular volume depletion *[see Warnings and Precautions (5.4)]*.

2.6 Use with Other Antihypertensive Drugs

Tekturna HCT may be administered with some other antihypertensive agents. In diabetics, do not use in combination with angiotensin receptor blockers (ARBs) or angiotensin converting enzyme inhibitors (ACEIs) *[see Contraindications (4)]*. Concomitant use of aliskiren with an ARB or ACEI is not recommended in patients with GFR <60 ml/min *[see Warnings and Precautions (5.2)]*. There are no data available with use of Tekturna HCT with angiotensin-converting enzyme inhibitors or beta blockers *[see Clinical Studies (14)]*.

2.7 Relationship to Meals

Patients should establish a routine pattern for taking Tekturna HCT with regard to meals. High-fat meals decrease absorption substantially *[see Clinical Pharmacology (12.3)]*.

3 DOSAGE FORMS AND STRENGTHS

- 150 mg/12.5 mg tablets: white, biconvex ovaloid, film-coated tablets imprinted with NVR/LCI
- 150 mg/25 mg tablets: pale yellow, biconvex ovaloid, film-coated tablets imprinted with NVR/CLL
- 300 mg/12.5 mg tablets: violet white, biconvex ovaloid, film-coated tablets imprinted with NVR/CVI
- 300 mg/25 mg tablets: light yellow, biconvex ovaloid, film-coated tablets imprinted with NVR/CVV

4 CONTRAINDICATIONS

Do not use aliskiren with ARBs or ACEIs in patients with diabetes *[see Warnings and Precautions (5.2), Clinical Studies (14.4)]*.

Because of the hydrochlorothiazide component, Tekturna HCT is contraindicated in patients with anuria or hypersensitivity to sulfonamide-derived drugs *[see Warnings and Precautions (5.6) and Adverse Reactions (6.1)]*. Hypersensitivity reactions may range from urticaria to anaphylaxis *[see Adverse Reactions (6.1)]*.

5 WARNINGS AND PRECAUTIONS

5.1 Fetal Toxicity

Pregnancy Category D

Use of drugs that act on the renin-angiotensin system during the second and third trimesters of pregnancy reduces fetal renal function and increases fetal and neonatal morbidity and death. Resulting oligohydramnios can be associated with fetal lung hypoplasia and skeletal deformations. Potential neonatal adverse effects include skull hypoplasia, anuria, hypotension, renal failure, and death. When pregnancy is detected, discontinue Tekturna HCT as soon as possible *[see Use in Specific Populations (8.1)]*.

Thiazides cross the placenta, and use of thiazides during pregnancy is associated with a risk of fetal or neonatal jaundice, thrombocytopenia, and possible other adverse reactions that have occurred in Tekturna HCT.

5.2 Renal Impairment/Hyperkalemia/Hypotension when Tekturna HCT is given in combination with ARBs or ACEIs

Tekturna HCT is contraindicated in patients with diabetes who are receiving ARBs or ACEIs because of the increased risk of renal impairment, hyperkalemia, and hypotension *[see Contraindications (4) and Clinical Studies (14.4)]*.

Avoid use of Tekturna HCT with ARBs or ACEIs in patients with moderate renal impairment (GFR <60 ml/min).

5.3 Anaphylactic Reactions and Head and Neck Angioedema

Aliskiren

Hypersensitivity reactions such as anaphylactic reactions and angioedema of the face, extremities, lips, tongue, glottis and/or larynx have been reported in patients treated with Tekturna and has necessitated hospitalization and intubation. This may occur at any time during treatment and has occurred in patients with and without a history of angioedema with ACE inhibitors or angiotensin receptor antagonists. Anaphylactic reactions have been reported from post-marketing experience with unknown frequency. If angioedema involves the throat, tongue, glottis or larynx, or if the patient has a history of upper respiratory surgery, airway obstruction may occur and be fatal. Patients who experience these effects, even without respiratory distress, require prolonged observation and appropriate monitoring measures since treatment with antihistamines and corticosteroids may not be sufficient to prevent respiratory involvement. Prompt administration of subcutaneous epinephrine solution 1:1000 (0.3 to 0.5 ml) and measures to ensure a patent airway may be necessary.

Discontinue Tekturna HCT immediately in patients who develop anaphylactic reactions or angioedema, and do not readminister.

5.4 Hypotension

In patients with an activated renin-angiotensin system, such as volume- and/or salt-depleted patients receiving high doses of diuretics, symptomatic hypotension may occur. Correct these conditions prior to administration of Tekturna HCT, or the treatment should start under close medical supervision.

A transient hypotensive response is not a contraindication to further treatment, which usually can be continued without difficulty once the blood pressure has stabilized.

5.5 Impaired Renal Function

Monitor renal function periodically in patients treated with Tekturna HCT. Changes in renal function, including acute renal failure, can be caused by drugs that affect the renin-angiotensin system and by diuretics. Patients whose renal function may depend in part on the activity of the renin-angiotensin system (e.g., patients with renal artery stenosis, severe heart failure, post-myocardial infarction or volume depletion) or patients receiving ARB, ACEI or non-steroidal anti-inflammatory (NSAID) therapy may be at particular risk of developing acute renal failure on Tekturna HCT *[see Contraindications (4), Warnings and Precautions (5.2), Clinical Studies (14.4)]*. Consider withholding or discontinuing therapy in patients who develop a clinically significant decrease in renal function on Tekturna HCT.

5.6 Hypersensitivity Reactions

Hydrochlorothiazide

Hypersensitivity reactions to hydrochlorothiazide may occur in patients with or without a history of allergy or bronchial asthma, but are more likely in patients with such a history.

5.7 Systemic Lupus Erythematosus

Hydrochlorothiazide

Thiazide diuretics have been reported to cause exacerbation or activation of systemic lupus erythematosus.

5.8 Lithium Interaction

Hydrochlorothiazide

Lithium generally should not be given with thiazides *[see Drug Interactions (7)]*.

5.9 Serum Electrolyte Abnormalities

Tekturna HCT

In the short-term controlled trials of various doses of Tekturna HCT, in patients with hypertension not concomitantly treated with an ARB or ACEI, the incidence of hypertensive patients who developed hypokalemia (serum potassium <3.5 mEq/L) was 2.2%; the incidence of hyperkalemia (serum potassium >5.5 mEq/L) was 0.8%. No patients discontinued due to increase or decrease of serum potassium.

Aliskiren

Monitor serum potassium periodically in patients receiving aliskiren. Drugs that affect the renin-angiotensin system can cause hyperkalemia. Risk factors for the development of hyperkalemia include renal insufficiency, diabetes, combination use with ARBs or ACEI *[see Contraindications (4), Warnings and Precautions (5.2), and Clinical Studies (14.4)]*, NSAIDs, or potassium supplements or potassium sparing diuretics.

Hydrochlorothiazide

Hydrochlorothiazide can cause hypokalemia and hyponatremia. Hypomagnesemia can result in hypokalemia which appears difficult to treat despite potassium repletion.

If hypokalemia is accompanied by clinical signs (e.g., muscular weakness, paresis, or ECG alterations), Tekturna HCT should be discontinued. Correction of hypokalemia and any coexisting hypomagnesemia is recommended prior to the initiation of thiazides.

5.10 Cyclosporine or Itraconazole

Aliskiren

When aliskiren was given with cyclosporine or itraconazole, the blood concentrations of aliskiren were significantly increased. Avoid concomitant use of aliskiren with cyclosporine or itraconazole *[see Drug Interactions (7)]*.

5.11 Acute Myopia and Secondary Angle-Closure Glaucoma

Hydrochlorothiazide, a sulfonamide, can cause an idiosyncratic reaction, resulting in acute transient myopia and acute angle-closure glaucoma. Symptoms include acute onset of decreased visual acuity or ocular pain and typically occur within hours to weeks of drug initiation. Untreated acute angle-closure glaucoma can lead to permanent vision loss. The primary treatment is to discontinue hydrochlorothiazide as rapidly as possible. Prompt medical or surgical treatments may need to be considered if the intraocular pressure remains uncontrolled. Risk factors for developing acute angle-closure glaucoma may include a history of sulfonamide or penicillin allergy.

5.12 Metabolic Disturbances

Hydrochlorothiazide

Hydrochlorothiazide may alter glucose tolerance and raise serum levels of cholesterol and triglycerides.

Hydrochlorothiazide may raise the serum uric acid level due to reduced clearance of uric acid and may cause or exacerbate hyperuricemia and precipitate gout in susceptible patients.

Hydrochlorothiazide decreases urinary calcium excretion and may cause elevations of serum calcium. Monitor calcium levels in patients with hypercalcemia receiving Tekturna HCT.

6 ADVERSE REACTIONS

6.1 Clinical Studies Experience

The following serious adverse reactions are discussed in greater detail in other sections of the label:

- Risk of fetal/neonatal morbidity and mortality *[see Warnings and Precautions (5.1)]*.
- Head and neck angioedema *[see Warnings and Precautions (5.3)]*.
- Hypotension in volume- and/or salt-depleted patients *[see Warnings and Precautions (5.4)]*.

Because clinical trials are conducted under widely varying conditions, adverse reaction rates observed in the clinical trials of a drug cannot be directly compared to rates in clinical trials of another drug and may not reflect the rates observed in practice.

Tekturna HCT

Tekturna HCT has been evaluated for safety in more than 2,700 patients, including over 700 treated for 6 months and 190 for over 1 year. In placebo-controlled clinical trials, discontinuation of therapy due to a clinical adverse event (including uncontrolled hypertension) occurred in 2.7% of patients treated with Tekturna HCT versus 3.6% of patients given placebo.

Adverse events in placebo-controlled trials that occurred in at least 1% of patients treated with Tekturna HCT and at a higher incidence than placebo included dizziness (2.3% vs. 1%), influenza (2.3% vs. 1.6%), diarrhea (1.6% vs. 0.5%), cough (1.3% vs. 0.5%), vertigo (1.2% vs. 0.5%), asthenia (1.2% vs. 0%), and arthralgia (1% vs. 0.5%).

Aliskiren

Aliskiren has been evaluated for safety in 6,460 patients, including 1,740 treated for longer than 6 months, and 1,250 for longer than 1 year. In placebo-controlled clinical trials, discontinuation of therapy due to a clinical adverse event, including uncontrolled hypertension occurred in 2.2% of patients treated with aliskiren, versus 3.5% of patients given placebo. These data do not include information from the ALTITUDE study which evaluated the use of aliskiren in combination with ARBs or ACEIs *[see Contraindications (4), Warnings and Precautions (5.2), and Clinical Studies (14.4)]*.

Two cases of angioedema with respiratory symptoms were reported with aliskiren use in the clinical studies. Two other cases of periorbital edema without respiratory symptoms were reported as possible angioedema and resulted in discontinuation. The rate of these angioedema cases in the completed studies was 0.06%.

In addition, 26 other cases of edema involving the face, hands, or whole body were reported with aliskiren use, including 4 leading to discontinuation.

In the placebo-controlled studies, however, the incidence of edema involving the face, hands, or whole body was 0.4% with aliskiren compared with 0.5% with placebo. In a long-term active-controlled study with aliskiren and HCTZ arms, the incidence of edema involving the face, hands, or whole body was 0.4% in both treatment arms.

Aliskiren produces dose-related gastrointestinal (GI) adverse reactions. Diarrhea was reported by 2.3% of patients at 300 mg, compared to 1.2% in placebo patients. In women and the elderly (age ≥65) increases in diarrhea rates were evident starting at a dose of 150 mg daily, with rates for these subgroups at 150 mg comparable to those seen at 300 mg for men or younger patients (all rates about 2% to 2.3%). Other GI symptoms included abdominal pain, dyspepsia, and gastroesophageal reflux, although increased rates for abdominal pain and dyspepsia were distinguished from placebo only at 600 mg daily. Diarrhea and other GI symptoms were typically mild and rarely led to discontinuation.

Aliskiren was associated with a slight increase in cough in the placebo-controlled studies (1.1% for any aliskiren use vs. 0.6% for placebo). In active-controlled trials with ACE inhibitor (ramipril, lisinopril) arms, the rates of cough for the aliskiren arms were about one-third to one-half the rates in the ACE inhibitor arms.

Other adverse reactions with increased rates for aliskiren compared to placebo included rash (1% vs. 0.3%) and renal stones (0.2% vs. 0%).

Single episodes of tonic-clonic seizures with loss of consciousness were reported in two patients treated with aliskiren in the clinical trials. One patient had predisposing causes for seizures and had a negative electroencephalogram (EEG) and cerebral imaging following the seizures; for the other patient, EEG and imaging results were not reported. Aliskiren was discontinued and there was no rechallenge in either case.

No clinically meaningful changes in vital signs or in ECG (including QTc interval) were observed in patients treated with aliskiren.

Hydrochlorothiazide

Other adverse reactions that have been reported with hydrochlorothiazide, without regard to causality, are listed below:

Body As A Whole: weakness

Digestive: pancreatitis, jaundice (intrahepatic cholestatic jaundice), sialadenitis, cramping, gastric irritation
Hematologic: aplastic anemia, agranulocytosis, leukopenia, hemolytic anemia, thrombocytopenia;
Hypersensitivity: purpura, photosensitivity, urticaria, necrotizing angiitis (vasculitis and cutaneous vasculitis), fever, respiratory distress including pneumonitis and pulmonary edema, anaphylactic reactions
Metabolic: hyperglycemia, glycosuria, hyperuricemia
Musculoskeletal: muscle spasm
Nervous System/Psychiatric: restlessness
Renal: renal failure, renal dysfunction, interstitial nephritis
Skin: erythema multiforme including Stevens-Johnson syndrome, exfoliative dermatitis including toxic epidermal necrolysis
Special Senses: transient blurred vision, xanthopsia

Clinical Laboratory Test Abnormalities

In controlled clinical trials, clinically important changes in standard laboratory parameters were rarely associated with administration of Tekturna HCT in patients with hypertension not concomitantly treated with an ARB or ACEI.

Blood Urea Nitrogen (BUN)/Creatinine: In patients with hypertension not concomitantly treated with an ARB or ACEI, elevations (greater than 50% increase) in BUN and creatinine occurred in 11.8% and 0.9%, respectively, of patients taking Tekturna HCT, and 7% and 1.1%, respectively, of patients given placebo in short-term controlled clinical trials. No patients were discontinued due to an increase in either BUN or creatinine.

Hemoglobin and Hematocrit: A greater than 20% decrease in hemoglobin and hematocrit were observed in <0.1% and 0.1%, respectively, of patients treated with Tekturna HCT, compared with 0% in placebo-treated patients. No patients were discontinued due to anemia.

Liver Function Tests: Occasional elevations (greater than 150%) in ALT (SGPT) were observed in 1.2% of patients treated with Tekturna HCT, compared with 0% in placebo-treated patients. No patients were discontinued due to abnormal liver function tests.

6.2 Post-Marketing Experience

The following adverse reactions have been reported in aliskiren or hydrochlorothiazide post-marketing experience. Because these reactions are reported voluntarily from a population of uncertain size, it is not always possible to estimate their frequency or establish a causal relationship to drug exposure.

Aliskiren

Hypersensitivity: anaphylactic reactions and angioedema requiring airway management and hospitalization

Peripheral edema

Severe cutaneous adverse reactions, including Stevens-Johnson syndrome and toxic epidermal necrolysis

Hydrochlorothiazide

Acute renal failure, renal disorder, aplastic anemia, erythema mutliforme, pyrexia, muscle spasm, asthenia, acute angle-closure glaucoma, bone marrow failure, worsening of diabetes control, hypokalemia, blood lipids increased, hyponatremia, hypomagnesemia, hypercalcemia, hyperchloremic alkalosis, impotence, visual impairment

Pathological changes in the parathyroid gland of patients with hypercalcemia and hypophosphatemia have been observed in a few patients on prolonged thiazide therapy. If hypercalcemia occurs, further diagnostic evaluation is necessary.

7 DRUG INTERACTIONS

No drug interaction studies have been conducted with Tekturna HCT and other drugs, although studies with the individual aliskiren and hydrochlorothiazide components are described below.

Aliskiren

Cyclosporine: Avoid co-administration of cyclosporine with aliskiren.

Itraconazole: Avoid co-administration of itraconazole with aliskiren *[See Clinical Pharmacology (12.3)]*.

Non-Steroidal Anti-Inflammatory Agents (NSAIDs) including selective Cyclooxygenase-2 inhibitors (COX-2 inhibitors): In patients who are elderly, volume-depleted (including those on diuretic therapy), or with compromised renal function, co-administration of NSAIDs, including selective COX-2 inhibitors with agents that affect the renin-angiotensin system, including aliskiren, may result in deterioration of renal function, including possible acute renal failure. These effects are usually reversible. Monitor renal function periodically in patients receiving aliskiren and NSAID therapy.

The antihypertensive effect of aliskiren may be attenuated by NSAIDs.

Hydrochlorothiazide

When administered concurrently, the following drugs may interact with thiazide diuretics.

Antidiabetic drugs (oral agents and insulin): Dosage adjustment of the antidiabetic drug may be required.

Lithium: Diuretic agents increase the risk of lithium toxicity. Refer to the package insert for lithium before use of such preparation with Tekturna HCT. Monitoring of serum lithium concentrations is recommended during concurrent use.

Nonsteroidal anti-inflammatory drugs: When Tekturna HCT and nonsteroidal anti-inflammatory agents are used concomitantly, the patient should be observed closely to determine if the desired effect of the diuretic is obtained.

Ion exchange resins: Staggering the dosage of hydrochlorothiazide and ion exchange resins (e.g., cholestyramine, colestipol) such that hydrochlorothiazide is administered at least 4 hours before or 4-6 hours after the administration of resins would potentially minimize the interaction *[see Clinical Pharmacology (12.3)]*.

8 USE IN SPECIFIC POPULATIONS

8.1 Pregnancy

Pregnancy Category D

Use of drugs that act on the renin-angiotensin system during the second and third trimesters of pregnancy reduces fetal renal function and increases fetal and neonatal morbidity and death. Resulting oligohydramnios can be associated with fetal lung hypoplasia and skeletal deformations. Potential neonatal adverse effects include skull hypoplasia, anuria, hypotension, renal failure, and death. When pregnancy is detected, discontinue Tekturna HCT as soon as possible. These adverse outcomes are usually associated with use of these drugs in the second and third trimester of pregnancy. Most epidemiologic studies examining fetal abnormalities after exposure to antihypertensive use in the first trimester have not distinguished drugs affecting the renin-angiotensin system from other antihypertensive agents. Appropriate management of maternal hypertension during pregnancy is important to optimize outcomes for both mother and fetus.

In the unusual case that there is no appropriate alternative to therapy with drugs affecting the renin-angiotensin system for a particular patient, apprise the mother of the potential risk to the fetus. Perform serial ultrasound examinations to assess the intra-amniotic environment. If oligohydramnios is observed, discontinue Tekturna HCT, unless it is considered lifesaving for the mother. Fetal testing may be appropriate, based on the week of pregnancy. Patients and physicians should be aware, however, that oligohydramnios may not appear until after the fetus has sustained irreversible injury. Closely observe infants with histories of in utero exposure to Tekturna HCT for hypotension, oliguria, and hyperkalemia. *[see Use in Specific Populations (8.4)]*

Thiazides cross the placenta, and use of thiazides during pregnancy is associated with a risk of fetal or neonatal jaundice, thrombocytopenia, and possible other adverse reactions that have occurred in adults.

Reproductive toxicity studies of aliskiren hemifumarate did not reveal any evidence of teratogenicity at oral doses up to 600 mg aliskiren/kg/day (20 times the maximum recommended human dose [MRHD] of 300 mg/day on a mg/m^2 basis) in pregnant rats or up to 100 mg aliskiren/kg/day (seven times the MRHD on a mg/m^2 basis) in pregnant rabbits. Fetal birth weight was adversely affected in rabbits at 50 mg/kg/day (3.2 times the MRHD on a mg/m^2 basis). Aliskiren was present in placenta, amniotic fluid and fetuses of pregnant rabbits.

When pregnant mice and rats were given hydrochlorothiazide at doses up to 3000 and 1000 mg/kg/day, respectively (about 600 and 400 times the MRHD) during their respective periods of major organogenesis, there was no evidence of fetal harm.

Hydrochlorothiazide

Thiazides can cross the placenta, and concentrations reached in the umbilical vein approach those in the maternal plasma. Hydrochlorothiazide, like other diuretics, can cause placental hypoperfusion. It accumulates in the amniotic fluid, with reported concentrations up to 19 times higher than in umbilical vein plasma. Use of thiazides during pregnancy is associated with a risk of fetal or neonatal jaundice or thrombocytopenia. Since they do not prevent or alter the course of EPH (Edema, Proteinuria, Hypertension) gestosis (pre eclampsia), these drugs should not be used to treat hypertension in pregnant women. The use of hydrochlorothiazide for other indications (e.g. heart disease) in pregnancy should be avoided.

8.3 Nursing Mothers

It is not known whether aliskiren is excreted in human milk, but aliskiren was secreted in the milk of lactating rats. Thiazides appear in human milk. Because of the potential for adverse effects on the nursing infant, a decision should be made whether to discontinue nursing or discontinue the drug, taking into account the importance of the drug to the mother.

8.4 Pediatric Use

Safety and effectiveness in pediatric patients have not been established.

Neonates with a history of in utero exposure to Tekturna HCT:

If oliguria or hypotension occurs, direct attention toward support of blood pressure and renal perfusion. Exchange transfusions or dialysis may be required as a means of reversing hypotension and/or substituting for disordered renal function.

8.5 Geriatric Use

In the short-term controlled clinical trials of Tekturna HCT, 325 (19.6%) patients treated with Tekturna HCT were ≥65 years and 53 (3.2%) were ≥75 years.

No overall differences in safety or effectiveness were observed between these subjects and younger subjects, and other reported clinical experience has not identified differences in responses between the elderly and younger patients, but greater sensitivity of some older individuals cannot be ruled out.

8.6 Renal Impairment

Safety and effectiveness of Tekturna HCT in patients with severe renal impairment (CrCl ≤ 30 mL/min) have not been established. No dose adjustment is required in patients with mild (CrCl 60-90 mL/min) or moderate (CrCl 30-60) renal impairment.

8.7 Hepatic Impairment

Aliskiren

No dose adjustment is necessary for patients with mild-to-severe liver disease.

Hydrochlorothiazide

Minor alterations of fluid and electrolyte balance may precipitate hepatic coma in patients with impaired hepatic function or progressive liver disease.

10 OVERDOSAGE

Aliskiren

Limited data are available related to overdosage in humans. The most likely manifestation of overdosage would be hypotension. If symptomatic hypotension should occur, supportive treatment should be initiated.

Aliskiren is poorly dialyzed. Therefore, hemodialysis is not adequate to treat aliskiren overexposure *[see Clinical Pharmacology (12.3)]*.

Hydrochlorothiazide

The most common signs and symptoms of overdose observed in humans are those caused by electrolyte depletion (hypokalemia, hypochloremia, hyponatremia) and dehydration resulting from excessive diuresis. If digitalis has also been administered, hypokalemia may accentuate cardiac arrhythmias. The degree to which hydrochlorothiazide is removed by hemodialysis has not been established. The oral LD_{50} of hydrochlorothiazide is greater than 10 g/kg in both mice and rats.

11 DESCRIPTION

Tekturna HCT is a fixed combination of aliskiren, an orally active, nonpeptide, direct renin inhibitor, and hydrochlorothiazide, a thiazide diuretic that is provided as tablets for oral administration.

Aliskiren

Aliskiren hemifumarate is chemically described as (2S, 4S,5S,7S)-N-(2-carbamoyl-2-methylpropyl)-5-amino-4-hydroxy-2,7-diisopropyl-8-[4-methoxy-3-(3-methoxypropoxy)-phenyl]-octanamide hemifumarate and its structural formula is

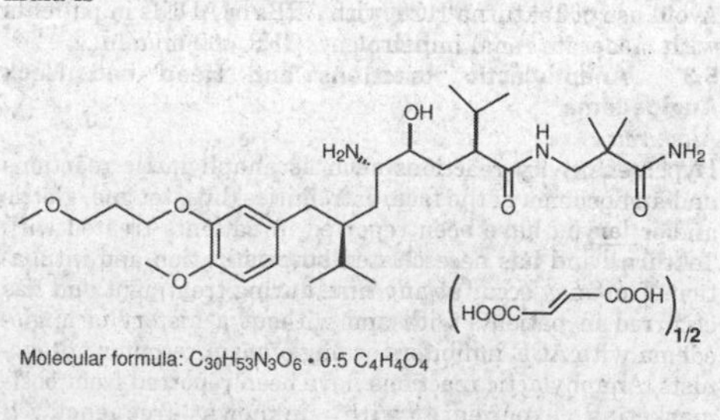

Molecular formula: $C_{30}H_{53}N_3O_6 \cdot 0.5\ C_4H_4O_4$

Aliskiren hemifumarate is a white to slightly yellowish crystalline powder with a molecular weight of 609.8 (free base- 551.8). It is soluble in phosphate buffer, n-octanol, and highly soluble in water.

Hydrochlorothiazide

Hydrochlorothiazide USP is a white, or practically white, practically odorless, crystalline powder. It is slightly soluble in water; freely soluble in sodium hydroxide solution, in *n*-butylamine, and in dimethylformamide; sparingly soluble in methanol; and insoluble in ether, in chloroform, and in dilute mineral acids. Hydrochlorothiazide is chemically described as 6-chloro-3,4-dihydro-2*H*-1,2,4-benzothiadiazine-7-sulfonamide 1,1-dioxide.

Hydrochlorothiazide is a thiazide diuretic. Its empirical formula is $C_7H_8ClN_3O_4S_2$, its molecular weight is 297.73, and its structural formula is

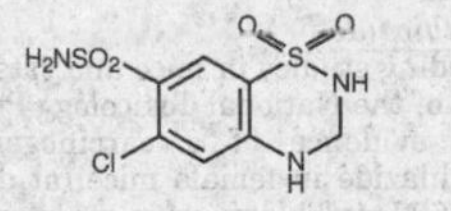

Tekturna HCT tablets are formulated for oral administration to contain aliskiren and hydrochlorothiazide, USP 150/12.5 mg, 150/25 mg, 300/12.5 mg and 300/25 mg. The inactive ingredients for all strengths of the tablets are colloidal silicon dioxide, crospovidone, hydroxypropyl methylcellulose, iron oxide colorants, lactose, magnesium stearate, microcrystalline cellulose, polyethylene glycol, povidone, talc, titanium dioxide, and wheat starch.

12 CLINICAL PHARMACOLOGY

12.1 Mechanism of Action

Aliskiren

Renin is secreted by the kidney in response to decreases in blood volume and renal perfusion. Renin cleaves angiotensinogen to form the inactive decapeptide angiotensin I (Ang I). Ang I is converted to the active octapeptide angiotensin II (Ang II) by angiotensin-converting enzyme (ACE) and non-ACE pathways. Ang II is a powerful vasoconstrictor and leads to the release of catecholamines from the adrenal medulla and prejunctional nerve endings. It also promotes aldosterone secretion and sodium reabsorption. Together, these effects increase blood pressure. Ang II also inhibits renin release, thus providing a negative feedback to the system. This cycle, from renin through angiotensin to aldosterone and its associated negative feedback loop, is known as the renin-angiotensin-aldosterone system (RAAS). Aliskiren is a direct renin inhibitor, decreasing plasma renin activity (PRA) and inhibiting the conversion of angiotensinogen to Ang I. Whether aliskiren affects other RAAS components, e.g., ACE or non-ACE pathways, is not known.

All agents that inhibit the RAAS, including renin inhibitors, suppress the negative feedback loop, leading to a compensatory rise in plasma renin concentration. When this rise occurs during treatment with ACE inhibitors and ARBs, the result is increased levels of PRA. During treatment with aliskiren, however, the effect of increased renin levels is blocked, so that PRA, Ang I and Ang II are all reduced, whether aliskiren is used as monotherapy or in combination with other antihypertensive agents.

Hydrochlorothiazide

Hydrochlorothiazide is a thiazide diuretic. Thiazides affect the renal tubular mechanisms of electrolyte reabsorption, directly increasing excretion of sodium and chloride in approximately equivalent amounts. Indirectly, the diuretic action of hydrochlorothiazide reduces plasma volume, with consequent increases in plasma renin activity, increases in aldosterone secretion, increases in urinary potassium loss, and decreases in serum potassium. The renin-aldosterone link is mediated by angiotensin II, so coadministration of agents that block the production or function of angiotensin II tends to reverse the potassium loss associated with these diuretics.

The mechanism of action of the antihypertensive effect of thiazides is unknown.

12.2 Pharmacodynamics

Tekturna HCT

In placebo-controlled clinical trials, PRA was decreased with aliskiren monotherapy (ranging from 54% to 65%) and increased with hydrochlorothiazide monotherapy (ranging from 4% to 72%). Treatment with Tekturna HCT resulted in PRA reductions ranging from approximately 46% to 63% in various doses despite the increase in PRA with hydrochlorothiazide treatment. The clinical implications of the differences in effect on PRA are not known.

Aliskiren

PRA reductions in clinical trials ranged from approximately 50% to 80%, were not dose-related and did not correlate with blood pressure reductions. The clinical implications of the differences in effect on PRA are not known.

Hydrochlorothiazide

After oral administration of hydrochlorothiazide, diuresis begins within 2 hours, peaks in about 4 hours, and lasts about 6 to 12 hours.

Drug Interactions

Hydrochlorothiazide

Alcohol, barbiturates, or narcotics: Potentiation of orthostatic hypotension may occur.

Skeletal muscle relaxants: Possible increased responsiveness to muscle relaxants such as curare derivatives.

Digitalis glycosides: Thiazide-induced hypokalemia or hypomagnesemia may predispose the patient to digoxin toxicity.

12.3 Pharmacokinetics

Absorption and Distribution

Tekturna HCT

Following oral administration of Tekturna HCT combination tablets, the median peak plasma concentration time is within 1 hour for aliskiren and 2.5 hours for hydrochlorothiazide. When taken with food, mean AUC and C_{max} of aliskiren are decreased by 60% and 82%, respectively; mean AUC and C_{max} of hydrochlorothiazide increased by 13% and 10%, respectively. As a result, patients should establish a routine pattern for taking Tekturna HCT with regard to meals.

Aliskiren

Aliskiren is poorly absorbed (bioavailability about 2.5%). Following oral administration, peak plasma concentrations of aliskiren are reached within 1 to 3 hours. When taken with a high fat meal, mean AUC and C_{max} of aliskiren are decreased by 71% and 85% respectively. In the clinical trials of aliskiren, it was administered without requiring a fixed relation of administration to meals.

Hydrochlorothiazide

The estimated absolute bioavailability of hydrochlorothiazide after oral administration is about 70%. Peak plasma hydrochlorothiazide concentrations (C_{max}) are reached within 2 to 5 hours after oral administration. There is no clinically significant effect of food on the bioavailability of hydrochlorothiazide.

Hydrochlorothiazide binds to albumin (40 to 70%) and distributes into erythrocytes. Following oral administration, plasma hydrochlorothiazide concentrations decline bi-exponentially, with a mean distribution half-life of about 2 hours and an elimination half-life of about 10 hours.

Metabolism and Elimination

Aliskiren

The effective half-life for aliskiren is 24 hours. Steady state blood levels are reached in about 7 – 8 days. About one-fourth of the absorbed dose appears in the urine as parent drug. How much of the absorbed dose is metabolized is unknown. Based on the *in vitro* studies, the major enzyme responsible for aliskiren metabolism appears to be CYP 3A4. Aliskiren does not inhibit the CYP450 isoenzymes (CYP 1A2, 2C8, 2C9, 2C19, 2D6, 2E1, and 3A) or induce CYP 3A4.

Transporters: Pgp (MDR1/Mdr1a/1b) was found to be the major efflux system involved in absorption and disposition of aliskiren in preclinical studies. The potential for drug interactions at the Pgp site will likely depend on the degree of inhibition of this transporter.

Hydrochlorothiazide

About 70% of an orally administered dose of hydrochlorothiazide is eliminated in the urine as unchanged drug.

Drug interactions:

Aliskiren

The effect of co-administered drugs on the pharmacokinetics of aliskiren and vice versa, were studied in several single and multiple dose studies. Pharmacokinetic measures indicating the magnitude of these interactions are presented in Figure 5 (impact of co-administered drugs on aliskiren) and Figure 6 (impact on co-administered drugs).

[See figure 5 above]

Warfarin: There was no clinically significant effect of a single dose of warfarin 25 mg on the pharmacokinetics of aliskiren.

[See figure 6 at top of next page]

Hydrochlorothiazide

Drugs that alter gastrointestinal motility: The bioavailability of thiazide-type diuretics may be increased by anticholinergic agents (e.g. atropine, biperiden), apparently due to a decrease in gastrointestinal motility and the stomach emptying rate. Conversely, pro-kinetic drugs may decrease the bioavailability of thiazide diuretics.

Cholestyramine: In a dedicated drug interaction study, administration of cholestyramine 2 hours before hydrochlorothiazide resulted in a 70% reduction in exposure to hydrochlorothiazide. Further, administration of hydrochlorothiazide 2 hours before cholestyramine, resulted in 35% reduction in exposure to hydrochlorothiazide.

Antineoplastic agents (e.g. cyclophosphamide, methotrexate): Concomitant use of thiazide diuretics may reduce renal excretion of cytotoxic agents and enhance their myelosuppressive effects.

Special Populations

Pediatric Patients

The pharmacokinetics of aliskiren have not been investigated in patients <18 years of age.

Geriatric Patients

Aliskiren

The pharmacokinetics of aliskiren were studied in the elderly (≥65 years). Exposure (measured by AUC) is increased in elderly patients.

Hydrochlorothiazide

A limited amount of data suggest that the systemic clearance of hydrochlorothiazide is reduced in both healthy and hypertensive elderly subjects compared to young healthy volunteers.

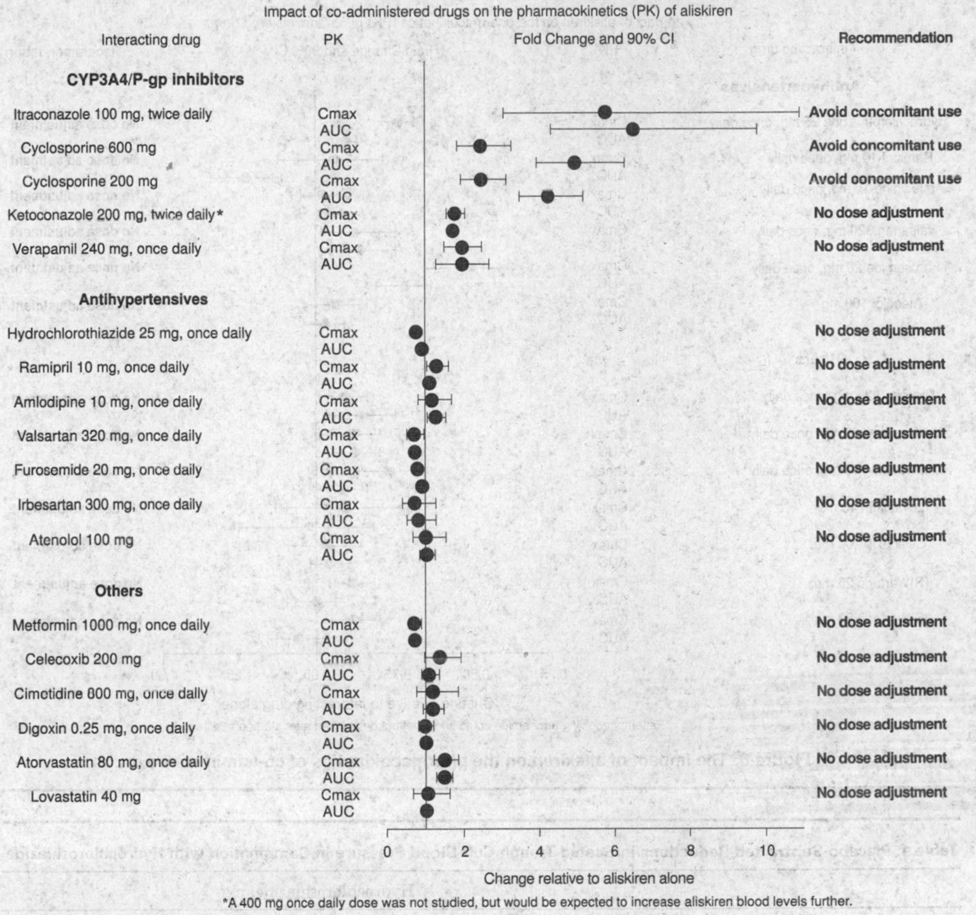

Figure 5: The impact of co-administered drugs on the pharmacokinetics of aliskiren

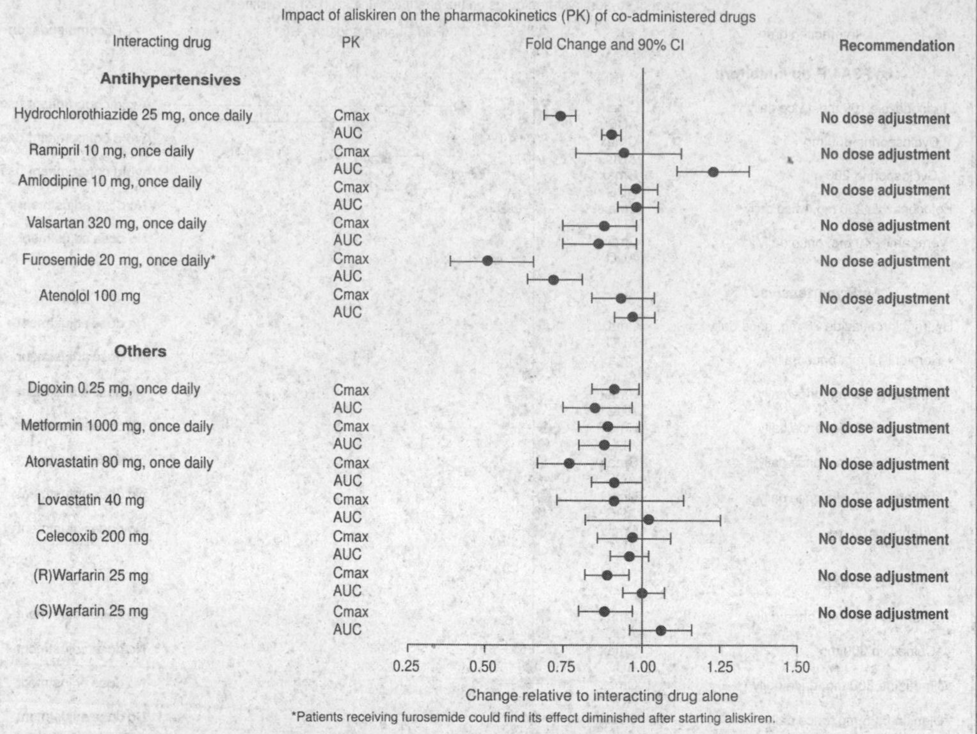

Figure 6: The impact of aliskiren on the pharmacokinetics of co-administered drugs

Table 1: Placebo-Subtracted Reductions in Seated Trough Cuff Blood Pressure in Combination with Hydrochlorothiazide

		Hydrochlorothiazide, mg			
		0	6.25	12.5	25
Aliskiren, mg	Placebo Mean Change	Placebo-subtracted	Placebo-subtracted	Placebo-subtracted	Placebo-subtracted
0	7.5/6.9	--	3.5/2.1	6.4/3.2	6.8/2.4
75	--	1.9/1.8	6.8/3.8	8.2/4.2	9.8/4.5
150	--	4.8/2	7.8/3.4	10.1/5	12/5.7
300	--	8.3/3.3	--	12.3/7	13.7/7.3

Race

Too few non-Caucasians have been studied with Tekturna HCT to assess pharmacokinetic differences among races. The pharmacokinetic differences among Blacks, Caucasians, and Japanese are minimal with aliskiren therapy.

Renal Impairment

Aliskiren

The pharmacokinetics of aliskiren were evaluated in patients with varying degrees of renal impairment. Rate and extent of exposure (AUC and C_{max}) of aliskiren in subjects with renal impairment did not show a consistent correlation with the severity of renal impairment *[see Use in Specific Populations (8.6)]*.

The pharmacokinetics of aliskiren following administration of a single oral dose of 300 mg was evaluated in patients with End Stage Renal Disease (ESRD) undergoing hemodialysis. When compared to matched healthy subjects, changes in the rate and extent of aliskiren exposure (Cmax and AUC) in ESRD patients undergoing hemodialysis were not clinically significant.

Timing of hemodialysis did not significantly alter the pharmacokinetics of aliskiren in ESRD patients. Therefore, no dose adjustment is warranted in ESRD patients receiving hemodialysis.

Hydrochlorothiazide

In a study in individuals with impaired renal function, the mean elimination half-life of hydrochlorothiazide was doubled in individuals with mild/moderate renal impairment (30 < CLcr < 90 mL/min) and tripled in severe renal impairment (≤ 30 mL/min), compared to individuals with normal renal function (CLcr > 90 mL/min) *[see Use in Specific Populations (8.6)]*.

Hepatic Impairment

Aliskiren

The pharmacokinetics of aliskiren were not significantly affected in patients with mild-to-severe liver disease *[see Use in Specific Populations (8.7)]*.

13 NONCLINICAL TOXICOLOGY

13.1 Carcinogenesis, Mutagenesis, Impairment of Fertility

Tekturna HCT

No carcinogenicity, mutagenicity or fertility studies have been conducted with Tekturna HCT. However, these studies have been conducted for aliskiren as well as hydrochlorothiazide alone.

Aliskiren

Carcinogenic potential was assessed in a 2-year rat study and a 6-month transgenic (rasH2) mouse study with aliskiren hemifumarate at oral doses of up to 1500 mg aliskiren/kg/day. Although there were no statistically significant increases in tumor incidence associated with exposure to aliskiren, mucosal epithelial hyperplasia (with or without erosion/ulceration) was observed in the lower gastrointestinal tract at doses of 750 or more mg/kg/day in both species, with a colonic adenoma identified in one rat and a cecal adenocarcinoma identified in another, rare tumors in the strain of rat studied. On a systemic exposure (AUC_{0-24hr}) basis, 1500 mg/kg/day in the rat is about 4 times and in the mouse about 1.5 times the maximum recommended human dose (300 mg aliskiren/day). Mucosal hyperplasia in the cecum or colon of rats was also observed at doses of 250 mg/kg/day (the lowest tested dose) as well as at higher doses in 4- and 13-week studies.

Aliskiren hemifumarate was devoid of genotoxic potential in the Ames reverse mutation assay with *S. typhimurium* and *E. coli*, the in vitro Chinese hamster ovary cell chromosomal aberration assay, the in vitro Chinese hamster V79 cell gene mutation test and the in vivo mouse bone marrow micronucleus assay.

Fertility of male and female rats was unaffected at doses of up to 250 mg aliskiren/kg/day (8 times the maximum recommended human dose of 300 mg Tekturna/60 kg on a mg/m^2 basis).

Hydrochlorothiazide

Two-year feeding studies in mice and rats conducted under the auspices of the National Toxicology Program (NTP) uncovered no evidence of a carcinogenic potential of hydrochlorothiazide in female mice (at doses of up to approximately 600 mg/kg/day) or in male and female rats (at doses of up to approximately 100 mg/kg/day). The NTP, however, found equivocal evidence for hepatocarcinogenicity in male mice.

Hydrochlorothiazide was not genotoxic in vitro in the Ames mutagenicity assay of *S. typhimurium* strains TA 98, TA 100, TA 1535, TA 1537, and TA 1538 and in the Chinese Hamster Ovary (CHO) test for chromosomal aberrations, or in vivo in assays using mouse germinal cell chromosomes, Chinese hamster bone marrow chromosomes, and the Drosophila sex-linked recessive lethal trait gene. Positive test results were obtained only in the in vitro CHO Sister Chromatid Exchange (clastogenicity) and in the Mouse Lymphoma Cell (mutagenicity) assays, using concentrations of hydrochlorothiazide from 43 to 1300 mcgm/mL, and in the Aspergillums Nidulans nondisjunction assay at an unspecified concentration.

Hydrochlorothiazide was not teratogenic and had no adverse effects on the fertility of mice and rats of either sex in studies wherein these species were exposed, via their diet, to doses of up to 100 and 4 mg/kg, respectively, prior to mating and throughout gestation. These doses of hydrochlorothiazide in mice and rats represent 19 and 1.5 times, respectively, the maximum recommended human dose on a mg/m^2 basis. (Calculations assume an oral dose of 25 mg/day and a 60-kg patient.)

14 CLINICAL STUDIES

14.1 Tekturna HCT

In all clinical trials including over 6,200 patients, more than 2,700 patients were exposed to combinations of aliskiren and hydrochlorothiazide. The safety and efficacy of Tekturna HCT were evaluated in patients with mild-to-moderate hypertension in an 8-week, randomized, double-blind, placebo-controlled, parallel-group, 15-arm factorial trial (n=2762). Patients were randomized to receive various combinations of aliskiren (75 mg to 300 mg) plus hydrochlorothiazide (6.25 mg to 25 mg) once daily (without titrating up from monotherapy) and followed for blood pressure response. The combination of aliskiren and hydrochlorothiazide resulted in additive placebo-adjusted decreases in systolic and diastolic blood pressure at trough of 10-14/5-7 mmHg at doses of 150-300 mg/12.5-25 mg, compared to 5-8/2-3 mmHg for aliskiren 150 mg to 300 mg and 6-7/2-3 mmHg for hydrochlorothiazide 12.5 mg to 25 mg, alone. Blood pressure reductions with the combinations were greater than the reductions with the monotherapies as shown in Table 1.

[See table 1 above]

The safety and efficacy of Tekturna HCT as initial therapy was evaluated in this trial. All patients randomized to the combination groups received the combination treatment of Tekturna HCT at assigned doses as initial therapy without titration from monotherapy. The figures *[see Indications and Usage (1)]* display the probability that a patient will achieve systolic or diastolic blood pressure goal with Tekturna HCT 300/25 mg, based upon their baseline systolic or diastolic blood pressure. At all levels of baseline blood pressure, the probability of achieving any given diastolic or systolic goal is greater with the combination than for either monotherapy.

The antihypertensive effect of Tekturna HCT was largely manifested within 1 week. The maximum antihypertensive effect was generally attained after about 4 weeks of therapy.

One active-controlled trial investigated the addition of 300 mg aliskiren in obese hypertensive patients who did not respond adequately to hydrochlorothiazide 25 mg, and showed incremental decreases of systolic and diastolic blood pressure of approximately 7/4 mmHg.

In long-term follow-up studies (without placebo control) the effect of the combination of aliskiren and hydrochlorothiazide was maintained for over 1 year.

The antihypertensive effect was independent of age and gender. There were too few non-Caucasians to assess differences in blood pressure effects by race.

14.2 Aliskiren Monotherapy

The antihypertensive effects of aliskiren have been demonstrated in six randomized, double-blind, placebo-controlled, 8-week clinical trials in patients with mild-to-moderate hypertension. The placebo response and placebo-subtracted changes from baseline in seated trough cuff blood pressure are shown in Table 2.

[See table 2 at top of next page]

The studies included approximately 2,730 patients given doses of 75 mg to 600 mg of aliskiren and 1,231 patients given placebo. As shown in Table 2, there is some increase in response with administered dose in all studies, with reasonable effects seen at 150 mg to 300 mg, and no clear further increase at 600 mg. A substantial proportion (85% to 90%) of the blood pressure lowering effect was observed within 2 weeks of treatment. Studies with ambulatory blood pressure monitoring showed reasonable control throughout the interdosing interval, e.g., the ratios of mean daytime to mean nighttime ambulatory BP ranged from 0.6 to 0.9.

Patients in the placebo-controlled trials continued open-label aliskiren for up to one year. A persistent blood pressure lowering effect was demonstrated by a randomized withdrawal study (patients randomized to continued drug or placebo), which showed a statistically significant difference between patients kept on aliskiren and those randomized to placebo. With cessation of treatment, blood pressure gradually returned toward baseline levels over a period of several weeks. There was no evidence of rebound hypertension after abrupt cessation of therapy.

The effectiveness of aliskiren was demonstrated across all demographic subgroups, although Black patients tended to have smaller reductions in blood pressure than Caucasians and Asians, as has been seen with ACE inhibitors and ARBs.

14.3 Aliskiren in Combination with Other Antihypertensives

Valsartan

Aliskiren 150 mg and 300 mg and valsartan 160 mg and 320 mg were studied alone and in combination in an 8-week, 1,797-patient, randomized, double-blind, placebo-controlled, parallel-group, 4-arm, dose-escalation study. The dosages of aliskiren and valsartan were started at 150 mg and 160 mg, respectively, and increased at four weeks to 300 mg and 320 mg, respectively. Seated trough cuff blood pressure was measured at baseline, 4, and 8 weeks. Blood pressure reductions with the combinations were greater than the reductions with the monotherapies as shown in Table 3.

Table 3: Placebo-Subtracted Reductions in Seated Trough Cuff Blood Pressure of Aliskiren in Combination with Valsartan

		Valsartan, mg		
Aliskiren, mg	Placebo Mean Change	0	160	320
0	4.6/4.1*	--	5.6/3.9	8.2/5.6
150	--	5.4/2.7	10.0/5.7	--
300	--	8.4/4.9	--	12.6/8.1

* The placebo change is 5.2/4.8 for Week 4 endpoint which was used for the dose groups containing aliskiren 150 mg or valsartan 160 mg.

Amlodipine

Aliskiren 150 mg and 300 mg and amlodipine besylate 5 mg and 10 mg were studied alone and in combination in an 8-week, 1,685-patient, randomized, double-blind, placebo-controlled, multifactorial study. Treatment with aliskiren and amlodipine resulted overall in significantly greater reductions in diastolic and systolic blood pressure compared to the respective monotherapy components as shown in Table 4.

Table 4: Placebo-Subtracted Reductions in Seated Trough Cuff Blood Pressure in Combination with Amlodipine

Aliskiren, mg	Placebo mean change	Amlodipine, mg		
		0	5	10
0	5.4/6.8	--	5.6/9.0	8.5/14.3
150	--	2.6/3.9	8.6/13.9	10.8/17.1
300	--	4.9/8.6	9.6/15.0	11.1/16.4

ACE Inhibitors

Aliskiren has not been studied when added to maximal doses of ACE inhibitors to determine whether aliskiren produces additional blood pressure reduction.

There are no trials of the Tekturna HCT combination tablet demonstrating reductions in cardiovascular risk in patients with hypertension, but the hydrochlorothiazide component has demonstrated such benefits.

14.4 Aliskiren in Patients with Diabetes treated with ARB or ACEI (ALTITUDE study)

Patients with diabetes with renal disease (defined either by the presence of albuminuria or reduced GFR) were randomized to aliskiren 300 mg daily (n=4283) or placebo (n=4296). All patients were receiving background therapy with an ARB or ACEI. The primary efficacy outcome was the time to the first event of the primary composite endpoint consisting of cardiovascular death, resuscitated sudden death, non-fatal myocardial infarction, non-fatal stroke, unplanned hospitalization for heart failure, onset of end stage renal disease, renal death, and doubling of serum creatinine concentration from baseline sustained for at least one month. After a median follow up of about 27 months, the trial was terminated early for lack of efficacy. Higher risk of renal impairment, hypotension and hyperkalemia was observed in aliskiren compared to placebo treated patients, as shown in the table below.

[See table 5 above]

The risk of stroke (2.7% aliskiren vs 2.0% placebo) and death (6.9% aliskiren vs. 6.4% placebo) were also numerically higher in aliskiren treated patients.

Table 2: Reductions in Seated Trough Cuff Blood Pressure in the Placebo-Controlled Studies of Aliskiren Monotherapy

		Aliskiren Daily Dose, mg			
		75	150	300	600
Study	Placebo Mean Change	Placebo-subtracted	Placebo-subtracted	Placebo-subtracted	Placebo-subtracted
1	2.9/3.3	5.7/4*	5.9/4.5*	11.2/7.5*	--
2	5.3/6.3	--	6.1/2.9*	10.5/5.4*	10.4/5.2*
3	10/8.6	2.2/1.7	2.1/1.7	5.1/3.7*	--
4	7.5/6.9	1.9/1.8	4.8/2*	8.3/3.3*	--
5	3.8/4.9	--	9.3/5.4*	10.9/6.2*	12.1/7.6*
6	4.6/4.1	--	--	8.4/4.9†	--

*p<0.05 vs. placebo by ANCOVA with Dunnett's procedure for multiple comparisons.
†p<0.05 vs. placebo by ANCOVA for the pairwise comparison.

Table 5: Incidence of selected adverse events in ALTITUDE

	Aliskiren N=4283		Placebo N=4296	
	Serious Adverse Events* (%)	Adverse Events (%)	Serious Adverse Events* (%)	Adverse Events (%)
Renal impairment †	4.7	12.4	3.3	10.4
Hypotension ††	2.0	18.6	1.7	14.8
Hyperkalemia †††	1.1	36.9	0.3	27.1

†renal failure, renal failure acute, renal failure chronic, renal impairment
††dizziness, dizziness postural, hypotension, orthostatic hypotension, presyncope, syncope
††† Given the variable baseline potassium levels of patients with renal insufficiency on dual RAAS therapy, the reporting of adverse event of hyperkalemia was at the discretion of the investigator.
* A Serious Adverse Event (SAE) is defined as: an event which is fatal or life-threatening, results in persistent or significant disability/incapacity, constitutes a congenital anomaly/birth defect, requires inpatient hospitalization or prolongation of existing hospitalization, or is medically significant (i.e. defined as an event that jeopardizes the patient or may require medical or surgical intervention to prevent one of the outcomes previously listed).

Table 6: Tekturna HCT Tablets Supply

Tablet	Color	Imprint	Imprint	NDC 0078- XXXX-XX		
Aliskiren/HCTZ		Side 1	Side 2	Bottle of 30	Bottle of 90	Blister Packages of 100
150 mg/12.5 mg	White	NVR	LCI	0521-15	0521-34	0521-35
150 mg/25 mg	Pale Yellow	NVR	CLL	0522-15	0522-34	0522-35
300 mg/12.5 mg	Violet White	NVR	CVI	0523-15	0523-34	0523-35
300 mg/25 mg	Light Yellow	NVR	CVV	0524-15	0524-34	0524-35

16 HOW SUPPLIED/STORAGE AND HANDLING

Tekturna HCT is supplied as biconvex, ovaloid film-coated tablets.

All strengths are packaged in bottles and unit-dose blister packages (10 strips of 10 tablets) as described below.

[See table 6 above]

Storage

Store at 25ºC (77ºF); excursions permitted to 15-30ºC (59-86ºF) *[See USP Controlled Room Temperature].*

Protect from moisture.

Dispense in original container.

17 PATIENT COUNSELING INFORMATION

See FDA-approved patient labeling (Patient Information)

Healthcare professionals should instruct their patients to read the Patient Package Insert before starting Tekturna HCT and to reread each time the prescription is renewed. Patients should be instructed to inform their doctor or pharmacist if they develop any unusual symptom, or if any known symptom persists or worsens.

Pregnancy

Female patients of childbearing age should be told about the consequences of exposure to Tekturna HCT during pregnancy. Discuss treatment options with women planning to become pregnant. Patients should be asked to report pregnancies to their physicians as soon as possible.

Symptomatic Hypotension

A patient receiving Tekturna HCT should be cautioned that lightheadedness can occur, especially during the first days of therapy, and that it should be reported to the prescribing physician. The patients should be told that if syncope occurs, Tekturna HCT should be discontinued until the physician has been consulted.

All patients should be cautioned that inadequate fluid intake, excessive perspiration, diarrhea, or vomiting can lead to an excessive fall in blood pressure, with the same consequences of lightheadedness and possible syncope.

Anaphylactic Reactions and Angioedema

Patients should be advised and told to report immediately any signs or symptoms suggesting a severe allergic reaction (difficulty breathing or swallowing, tightness of the chest, hives, general rash, swelling, itching, dizziness, vomiting, or abdominal pain) or angioedema (swelling of face, extremities, eyes, lips, tongue, difficulty in swallowing or breathing) and to take no more drug until they have consulted with the prescribing physician. Angioedema, including laryngeal edema, may occur at any time during treatment with Tekturna HCT.

Potassium Supplements

A patient receiving Tekturna HCT should be told not to use potassium supplements or salt substitutes containing potassium without consulting the prescribing physician.

Relationship to Meals

Patients should establish a routine pattern for taking Tekturna HCT with regard to meals. High-fat meals decrease absorption substantially.

T2012-182
September 2012

FDA-Approved Patient Labeling
Patient Information
Tekturna HCT® (tek-turn-a HCT)
(aliskiren and hydrochlorothiazide, USP)
Combination Tablets

Read the Patient Information that comes with Tekturna HCT before you start taking it and each time you get a refill. There may be new information. This leaflet does not take the place of talking with your doctor about your condition and treatment.

What is the most important information I should know about Tekturna HCT?

Tekturna HCT can cause harm or death to an unborn baby. Talk to your doctor about other ways to lower your blood pressure if you plan to become pregnant. If you get pregnant while taking Tekturna HCT, tell your doctor right away.

What is Tekturna HCT?

Tekturna HCT contains two prescription medicines in one tablet that work together to lower blood pressure. It contains:

- aliskiren (Tekturna), a direct renin inhibitor (DRI)
- hydrochlorothiazide, a diuretic (water pill)

Aliskiren (Tekturna) reduces the effect of renin, and the harmful process that narrows blood vessels. Aliskiren also helps blood vessels relax and widen so blood pressure is lower. Hydrochlorothiazide reduces the amount of salt and water in your body so your blood pressure is lower.

Tekturna HCT may be used to lower high blood pressure in adults

- when one medicine to lower high blood pressure is not enough
- as the first medicine to lower high blood pressure if your doctor decides that you are likely to need more than one medicine

Tekturna HCT has not been studied in children under 18 years of age.

Your doctor may prescribe other medicines for you to take, along with Tekturna HCT to treat your high blood pressure.

What is high blood pressure (hypertension)?

Blood pressure is the force that pushes the blood through your blood vessels to all the organs of your body. You have high blood pressure when the force of your blood moving through your blood vessels is too great. One cause of high blood pressure is renin, a chemical in the body that starts a process that makes blood vessels narrow, leading to high blood pressure.

Tekturna HCT reduces high blood pressure. Medicines that lower your blood pressure lower your chance of having a stroke or heart attack. High blood pressure makes the heart work harder to pump blood throughout the body and causes damage to the blood vessels. If high blood pressure is not treated, it can lead to stroke, heart attack, heart failure, kidney failure, and vision problems.

Who should not take Tekturna HCT?

- **If you get pregnant, stop taking Tekturna HCT and call your doctor right away. If you plan to become pregnant, talk to your doctor about other treatment options for your high blood pressure.**
- **If you have diabetes and are taking a kind of medicine called an angiotensin-receptor-blocker or angiotensin-converting-enzyme-inhibitor.**
- **Do not take Tekturna HCT if you make very little or no urine due to kidney problems.**
- **Do not take Tekturna HCT if you are allergic to any of its ingredients. See the end of this leaflet for a complete list of the ingredients in Tekturna HCT.**

What should I tell my doctor before taking Tekturna HCT?

Tell your doctor about all your medical conditions, including whether you:

- have kidney problems
- are pregnant or planning to become pregnant. See "What is the most important information I should know about Tekturna HCT?"
- have any allergies or asthma
- have liver problems
- have systemic lupus erythematosus (SLE). Tekturna HCT can make your SLE active or worse.
- have ever had a reaction called angioedema, to an ACE inhibitor medicine. Angioedema causes swelling of the face, lips, tongue, throat, arms and legs, and may cause difficulty breathing.
- are breast-feeding. It is not known if Tekturna HCT passes into your breast milk.

Tell your doctor about all the medicines you take including prescription and nonprescription medicines, vitamins and herbal supplements. Especially tell your doctor if you are taking:

- a kind of medicine called angiotensin receptor blocker or angiotensin converting enzyme inhibitor
- atorvastatin (medicine to lower cholesterol in your blood)
- water pills (also called "diuretics")
- medicines for treating fungus or fungal infections
- cyclosporine (a medicine used to suppress the immune system)
- potassium-containing medicines, potassium supplements, or salt substitutes containing potassium
- cholestyramine (for example; Questran, Questran Light, Cholestyramine Light, Locholest Light, Locholest, Prevalite) (medicines to lower the cholesterol in your blood)
- colestipol (for example; Colestipol hydrochloride, Colestid, Flavored Colestid) (medicines to lower the cholesterol in your blood)
- medicines to treat diabetes, including insulin
- lithium, a medicine used in some types of depression. Do not take Tekturna HCT if you are taking lithium.
- Nonsteroidal anti-inflammatory (NSAIDs) medicines. Ask your doctor if you are not sure if you are taking one of these medicines.
- blood thinners
- barbiturate or narcotic medicines. Ask your doctor if you are not sure if you are taking one of these medicines.

Your doctor or pharmacist will know what medicines are safe to take together. Know your medicines. Keep a list of your medicines and show it to your doctor or pharmacist when you get a new medicine.

How should I take Tekturna HCT?

- Take Tekturna HCT exactly as prescribed by your doctor. It is important to take Tekturna HCT every day to control your blood pressure.
- Take Tekturna HCT once each day, about the same time each day.
- Take Tekturna HCT the same way every day, either with or without a meal.
- Your doctor may change your dose of Tekturna HCT if needed.
- If you miss a dose of Tekturna HCT, take it as soon as you remember. If it is close to your next dose, do not take the missed dose. Just take the next dose at your regular time.
- If you take too much Tekturna HCT, call your doctor or a Poison Control Center, or go to the nearest hospital emergency room.

What are the possible side effects of Tekturna HCT?

Tekturna HCT may cause serious side effects:

- **Injury or death to an unborn baby.** See "What is the most important information I should know about Tekturna HCT?"
- **Low blood pressure (hypotension).** Your blood pressure may get too low if you also take water pills, are on a low-salt diet, get dialysis treatments, have heart problems, or get sick with vomiting or diarrhea. Drinking alcohol and taking certain medicines (barbiturates or narcotics) can cause low blood pressure to get worse. Lie down if you feel faint or dizzy, and call your doctor right away.
- **Severe Allergic Reactions and Angioedema.** Aliskiren, one of the medicines in Tekturna HCT, can cause difficulty breathing or swallowing, tightness of the chest, hives, general rash, swelling, itching, dizziness, vomiting, or abdominal pain (signs of a severe allergic reaction). Aliskiren can also cause swelling of the face, lips, tongue, throat, arms and legs, or the whole body (signs of angioedema). Get medical help right away and tell your doctor if you get any one or more of these symptoms. Angioedema can happen at any time while you are taking Tekturna HCT.
- **Active or worsened Systemic Lupus Erythematosus (SLE).** If you have SLE, tell your doctor right away if you get any new or worse symptoms.
- **Eye problems.** One of the medicines in Tekturna HCT can cause eye problems that may lead to vision loss. Symptoms of eye problems can happen within hours to weeks of starting Tekturna HCT. Tell your doctor right away if you have:
  - ■ Decrease in vision
  - ■ Eye pain

Common side effects of Tekturna HCT include:

- dizziness
- flu-like symptoms
- diarrhea
- cough
- tiredness
- high levels of potassium in the blood (hyperkalemia)

Other less common side effects include skin rash.

Tell your doctor if you have any side effect that bothers you or that does not go away. These are not all of the possible side effects of Tekturna HCT. For a complete list of side effects, ask your doctor or pharmacist.

How do I store Tekturna HCT?

- Store Tekturna HCT tablets at room temperature between 59°F-86°F (15°C-30°C).
- Keep Tekturna HCT in the original prescription bottle in a dry place. Do not remove the desiccant (drying agent) from the bottle.

Keep Tekturna HCT and all medicines out of the reach of children.

General information about Tekturna HCT

Medicines are sometimes prescribed for conditions not listed in the patient information leaflet. Do not take Tekturna HCT for a condition for which it was not prescribed. Do not give Tekturna HCT to other people, even if they have the same condition or symptoms you have. It may harm them.

This leaflet summarizes the most important information about Tekturna HCT. If you have questions about Tekturna HCT talk with your doctor. You can ask your doctor or pharmacist for information that is written for healthcare professionals.

For more information about Tekturna HCT, visit www.TekturnaHCT.com, or call 1-888-669-6682.

What are the ingredients in Tekturna HCT?

Active ingredients: Aliskiren and hydrochlorothiazide

Inactive ingredients: Colloidal silicon dioxide, crospovidone, hydroxypropyl methylcellulose, iron oxide colorants, lactose, magnesium stearate, microcrystalline cellulose, polyethylene glycol, povidone, talc, titanium dioxide, and wheat starch.

Call your doctor for medical advice about side effects. You may report side effects to FDA at 1-800-FDA-1088.

Manufactured by:
Novartis Pharma Produktions GmbH
Wehr, Germany
Distributed by:
Novartis Pharmaceuticals Corporation
East Hanover, New Jersey 07936
© Novartis
T2012-183
September 2012

Shown in Product Identification Guide, page 311

TOBI® ℞
[toe-bye]
(tobramycin inhalation solution, USP)
Nebulizer Solution – For Inhalation Use Only
Rx only
Prescribing Information

The following prescribing information is based on official labeling in effect July 2013.

DESCRIPTION

TOBI® is a tobramycin solution for inhalation. It is a sterile, clear, slightly yellow, non-pyrogenic, aqueous solution with the pH and salinity adjusted specifically for administration by a compressed air driven reusable nebulizer. The chemical formula for tobramycin is $C_{18}H_{37}N_5O_9$ and the molecular weight is 467.52. Tobramycin is *O*-3-amino-3-deoxy-α-D-glucopyranosyl-(1→4)-*O*-[2,6-diamino-2,3,6-trideoxy-α-D-*ribo*-hexopyranosyl-(1→6)]-2-deoxy-L-streptamine. The structural formula for tobramycin is:

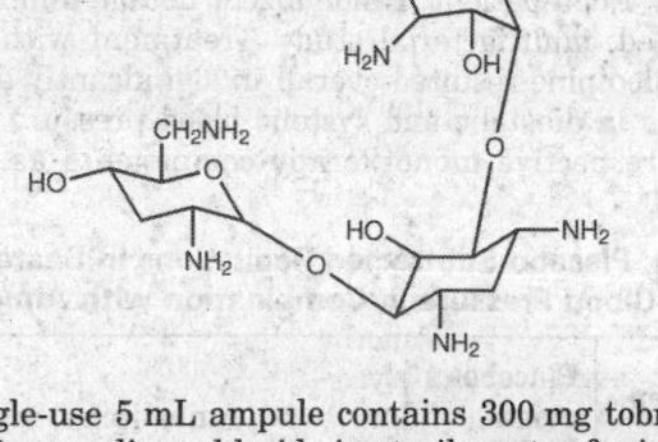

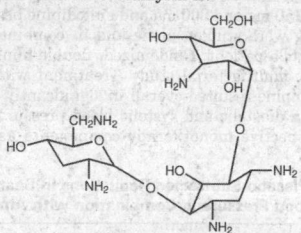

Each single-use 5 mL ampule contains 300 mg tobramycin and 11.25 mg sodium chloride in sterile water for injection. Sulfuric acid and sodium hydroxide are added to adjust the pH to 6.0. Nitrogen is used for sparging. All ingredients meet USP requirements. The formulation contains no preservatives.

CLINICAL PHARMACOLOGY

TOBI® is specifically formulated for administration by inhalation. When inhaled, tobramycin is concentrated in the airways.

Pharmacokinetics

TOBI® contains tobramycin, a cationic polar molecule that does not readily cross epithelial membranes.(1) The bioavailability of TOBI® may vary because of individual differences in nebulizer performance and airway pathology.(2) Following administration of TOBI®, tobramycin remains concentrated primarily in the airways.

Sputum Concentrations: Ten minutes after inhalation of the first 300-mg dose of TOBI®, the average concentration of tobramycin was 1237 μg/g (ranging from 35 to 7414 μg/g) in sputum. Tobramycin does not accumulate in sputum; after 20 weeks of therapy with the TOBI® regimen, the average concentration of tobramycin at ten minutes after inhalation was 1154 μg/g (ranging from 39 to 8085 μg/g) in sputum. High variability of tobramycin concentration in sputum was observed. Two hours after inhalation, sputum concentrations declined to approximately 14% of tobramycin levels at ten minutes after inhalation.

Serum Concentrations: The average serum concentration of tobramycin one hour after inhalation of a single 300-mg dose of TOBI® by cystic fibrosis patients was 0.95 µg/mL. After 20 weeks of therapy on the TOBI® regimen, the average serum tobramycin concentration one hour after dosing was 1.05 µg/mL.

Elimination: The elimination half-life of tobramycin from serum is approximately 2 hours after intravenous (IV) administration. Assuming tobramycin absorbed following inhalation behaves similarly to tobramycin following IV administration, systemically absorbed tobramycin is eliminated principally by glomerular filtration. Unabsorbed tobramycin, following TOBI® administration, is probably eliminated primarily in expectorated sputum.

Microbiology

Tobramycin is an aminoglycoside antibiotic produced by *Streptomyces tenebrarius.*[1] It acts primarily by disrupting protein synthesis, leading to altered cell membrane permeability, progressive disruption of the cell envelope, and eventual cell death.[3]

Tobramycin has *in-vitro* activity against a wide range of gram-negative organisms including *Pseudomonas aeruginosa*. It is bactericidal at concentrations equal to or slightly greater than inhibitory concentrations.

Susceptibility Testing

A single sputum sample from a cystic fibrosis patient may contain multiple morphotypes of *Pseudomonas aeruginosa* and each morphotype may have a different level of *in-vitro* susceptibility to tobramycin. Treatment for 6 months with TOBI® in two clinical studies did not affect the susceptibility of the majority of *P. aeruginosa* isolates tested; however, increased minimum inhibitory concentrations (MICs) were noted in some patients. The clinical significance of this information has not been clearly established in the treatment of *P. aeruginosa* in cystic fibrosis patients. For additional information regarding the effects of TOBI® on *P. aeruginosa* MIC values and bacterial sputum density, please refer to the CLINICAL STUDIES section.

The *in-vitro* antimicrobial susceptibility test methods used for parenteral tobramycin therapy can be used to monitor the susceptibility of *P. aeruginosa* isolated from cystic fibrosis patients. If decreased susceptibility is noted, the results should be reported to the clinician.

Susceptibility breakpoints established for parenteral administration of tobramycin do not apply to aerosolized administration of TOBI®. The relationship between *in-vitro* susceptibility test results and clinical outcome with TOBI® therapy is not clear.

INDICATIONS AND USAGE

TOBI® is indicated for the management of cystic fibrosis patients with *P. aeruginosa*.

Safety and efficacy have not been demonstrated in patients under the age of 6 years, patients with FEV_1 <25% or >75% predicted, or patients colonized with *Burkholderia cepacia* (see CLINICAL STUDIES).

CONTRAINDICATIONS

TOBI® is contraindicated in patients with a known hypersensitivity to any aminoglycoside.

WARNINGS

Caution should be exercised when prescribing TOBI® to patients with known or suspected renal, auditory, vestibular, or neuromuscular dysfunction. Patients receiving concomitant parenteral aminoglycoside therapy should be monitored as clinically appropriate.

Aminoglycosides can cause fetal harm when administered to a pregnant woman. Aminoglycosides cross the placenta, and streptomycin has been associated with several reports of total, irreversible, bilateral congenital deafness in pediatric patients exposed *in utero*. Patients who use TOBI® during pregnancy, or become pregnant while taking TOBI® should be apprised of the potential hazard to the fetus.

Ototoxicity

Ototoxicity, as measured by complaints of hearing loss or by audiometric evaluations, did not occur with TOBI® therapy during clinical studies. However, transient tinnitus occurred in eight TOBI®-treated patients versus no placebo patients in the clinical studies. Tinnitus may be a sentinel symptom of ototoxicity, and therefore the onset of this symptom warrants caution (see ADVERSE REACTIONS). Ototoxicity, manifested as both auditory and vestibular toxicity, has been reported with parenteral aminoglycosides. Vestibular toxicity may be manifested by vertigo, ataxia or dizziness.

In postmarketing experience, patients receiving TOBI® have reported hearing loss. Some of these reports occurred in patients with previous or concomitant treatment with systemic aminoglycosides. Patients with hearing loss frequently reported tinnitus.

Nephrotoxicity

Nephrotoxicity was not seen during TOBI® clinical studies but has been associated with aminoglycosides as a class. If nephrotoxicity occurs in a patient receiving TOBI®, tobramycin therapy should be discontinued until serum concentrations fall below 2 µg/mL.

Muscular Disorders

TOBI® should be used cautiously in patients with muscular disorders, such as myasthenia gravis or Parkinson's disease, since aminoglycosides may aggravate muscle weakness because of a potential curare-like effect on neuromuscular function.

Bronchospasm

Bronchospasm can occur with inhalation of TOBI®. In clinical studies of TOBI®, changes in FEV_1 measured after the inhaled dose were similar in the TOBI® and placebo groups. Bronchospasm should be treated as medically appropriate.

PRECAUTIONS

Information for Patients

NOTE: In addition to information provided below, a Patient Medication Guide providing instructions for proper use of TOBI® is contained inside the package.

Safety Information

TOBI® is in a class of antibiotics that have caused hearing loss, dizziness, kidney damage, and harm to a fetus. Ringing in the ears and hoarseness were two symptoms that were seen in more patients taking TOBI® than placebo in research studies. Patients with cystic fibrosis can have many symptoms. Some of these symptoms may be related to your medications. If you have new or worsening symptoms, you should tell your doctor.

Hearing: You should tell your doctor if you have ringing in the ears, dizziness, or any changes in hearing.

Kidney Damage: Inform your doctor if you have any history of kidney problems.

Pregnancy: If you want to become pregnant or are pregnant while on TOBI®, you should talk with your doctor about the possibility of TOBI® causing any harm.

Nursing Mothers: If you are nursing a baby, you should talk with your doctor before using TOBI®.

TOBI® Packaging

TOBI® comes in a single dose, ready-to-use ampule containing 300 mg tobramycin. Each foil pouch contains 4 ampules, for 2 days of TOBI® therapy.

Dosage

The 300 mg dose of TOBI® is the same for patients regardless of age or weight. TOBI® has not been studied in patients less than 6 years old. Doses should be inhaled as close to 12 hours apart as possible and not less than 6 hours apart.

You should not mix TOBI® with dornase alfa (PULMOZYME®, Genentech) in the nebulizer.

If you are taking several medications the recommended order is as follows: bronchodilator first, followed by chest physiotherapy, then other inhaled medications and, finally, TOBI®.

Treatment Schedule

You should take TOBI® in repeated cycles of 28 days on drug followed by 28 days off drug. You should take TOBI® twice a day during the 28-day period on drug.

How To Administer TOBI®

THIS INFORMATION IS NOT INTENDED TO REPLACE CONSULTATION WITH YOUR PHYSICIAN AND CF CARE TEAM ABOUT PROPERLY TAKING MEDICATION OR USING INHALATION EQUIPMENT.

TOBI® is specifically formulated for inhalation using a PARI LC PLUS™ Reusable Nebulizer and a DeVilbiss® Pulmo-Aide® air compressor. TOBI® can be taken at home, school, or at work. The following are instructions on how to use the DeVilbiss® Pulmo-Aide® air compressor and PARI LC PLUS™ Reusable Nebulizer to administer TOBI®.

You will need the following supplies:

- TOBI® plastic ampule (vial)
- DeVilbiss® Pulmo-Aide® air compressor
- PARI LC PLUS™ Reusable Nebulizer
- Tubing to connect the nebulizer and compressor
- Clean paper or cloth towels
- Nose clips (optional)

It is important that your nebulizer and compressor function properly before starting your TOBI® therapy.

Note: Please refer to the manufacturers' care and use instructions for important information.

Preparing Your TOBI® for Inhalation

1. Wash your hands thoroughly with soap and water.

2a. TOBI® is packaged with 4 ampules per foil pouch.

2b. Separate one ampule by gently pulling apart at the bottom tabs. Store all remaining ampules in the refrigerator as directed.

3. Lay out the contents of a PARI LC PLUS™ Reusable Nebulizer package on a clean, dry paper or cloth towel. You should have the following parts:

- Nebulizer Top and Bottom (Nebulizer Cup) Assembly
- Inspiratory Valve Cap
- Mouthpiece with Valve
- Tubing

4. Remove the Nebulizer Top from the Nebulizer Cup by twisting the Nebulizer Top counter-clockwise, and then lifting. Place the Nebulizer Top on the clean paper or cloth towel. Stand the Nebulizer Cup upright on the towel.

5. Connect one end of the tubing to the compressor air outlet. The tubing should fit snugly. Plug in your compressor to an electrical outlet.

6. Open the TOBI® ampule by holding the bottom tab with one hand and twisting off the top of the ampule with the other hand. Be careful not to squeeze the ampule until you are ready to empty its contents into the Nebulizer Cup.

7. Squeeze **all** the contents of the ampule into the Nebulizer Cup.

8. Replace the Nebulizer Top. Note: In order to insert the Nebulizer Top into the Nebulizer Cup, the semi-circle halfway down the stem of the Nebulizer Top should face the Nebulizer Outlet.

9. Attach the Mouthpiece to the Nebulizer Outlet. Then firmly push the Inspiratory Valve Cap in place on the Nebulizer Top. Note: the Inspiratory Valve Cap will fit snugly.

10. Connect the free end of the tubing to the Air Intake on the bottom of the nebulizer, making sure to keep the nebulizer upright. Press the tubing on the Air Intake firmly.

TOBI® Treatment

1. Turn on the compressor.
2. Check for a steady mist from the Mouthpiece. If there is no mist, check all tubing connections and confirm that the compressor is working properly.
3. Sit or stand in an upright position that will allow you to breathe normally.
4. Place Mouthpiece between your teeth and on top of your tongue and breathe normally only through your mouth. Nose clips may help you breathe through your mouth and not through your nose. Do not block airflow with your tongue.
5. Continue treatment until all your TOBI® is gone, and there is no longer any mist being produced. You may hear a sputtering sound when the Nebulizer Cup is empty. The entire TOBI® treatment should take approximately 15 minutes to complete. Note: if you are interrupted, need to cough or rest during your TOBI® treatment, turn off the compressor to save your medication. Turn the compressor back on when you are ready to resume your therapy.
6. Follow the nebulizer cleaning and disinfecting instructions after completing therapy.

Cleaning Your Nebulizer

To reduce the risk of infection, illness or injury from contamination, you must thoroughly clean all parts of the nebulizer as instructed after each treatment. Never use a nebulizer with a clogged nozzle. If the nozzle is clogged, no aerosol mist is produced, which will alter the effectiveness of the treatment. Replace the nebulizer if clogging occurs.

1. Remove tubing from nebulizer and disassemble nebulizer parts.
2. Wash all parts (except tubing) with warm water and liquid dish soap.
3. Rinse thoroughly with warm water and shake out water.
4. Air dry or hand dry nebulizer parts on a clean, lint-free cloth. Reassemble nebulizer when dry, and store.
5. You can also wash all parts of the nebulizer in a dishwasher (except tubing). Place the nebulizer parts in a dishwasher basket, then place on the top rack of the dishwasher. Remove and dry the parts when the cycle is complete.

Disinfecting Your Nebulizer

Your nebulizer is for your use only - Do not share your nebulizer with other people. You must regularly disinfect the nebulizer. Failure to do so could lead to serious or fatal illness.

Clean the nebulizer as described above. Every other treatment day, disinfect the nebulizer parts (except tubing) by boiling them in water for a full 10 minutes. Dry parts on a clean, lint-free cloth.

Care and Use of Your Pulmo-Aide® Compressor

Follow the manufacturer's instructions for care and use of your compressor.

Filter Change:

1. DeVilbiss® Compressor filters should be changed every six months or sooner if filter turns completely gray in color.

Compressor Cleaning:

1. With power switch in the "Off" position, unplug power cord from wall outlet.
2. Wipe outside of the compressor cabinet with a clean, damp cloth every few days to keep dust free.

Caution: Do not submerge in water; doing so will result in compressor damage.

Storage Instructions

You should store TOBI® ampules in a refrigerator (2-8°C or 36-46°F). However, when you don't have a refrigerator available (e.g., transporting your TOBI®), you may store the foil pouches (opened or unopened) at room temperature (up to 25°C/77°F) for up to 28 days.

Avoid exposing TOBI® ampules to intense light.

Unrefrigerated TOBI®, which is normally slightly yellow, may darken with age; however, the color change does not indicate any change in the quality of the product.
You should not use TOBI® if it is cloudy, if there are particles in the solution, or if it has been stored at room temperature for more than 28 days. You should not use TOBI® beyond the expiration date stamped on the ampule.

Additional Information

Nebulizer: 1-800-327-8632
Compressor: 1-800-338-1988
TOBI®: 1-888-NOW-NOVA (1-888-669-6682)

Laboratory Tests

Audiograms

Clinical studies of TOBI® did not identify hearing loss using audiometric tests which evaluated hearing up to 8000 Hz. **Physicians should consider an audiogram for patients who show any evidence of auditory dysfunction, or who are at increased risk for auditory dysfunction.** Tinnitus may be a sentinel symptom of ototoxicity, and therefore the onset of this symptom warrants caution.

Serum Concentrations

In patients with normal renal function treated with TOBI®, serum tobramycin concentrations are approximately 1 µg/mL 1 hour after dose administration and do not require routine monitoring. Serum concentrations of tobramycin in patients with renal dysfunction or patients treated with concomitant parenteral tobramycin should be monitored at the discretion of the treating physician.

Renal Function

The clinical studies of TOBI® did not reveal any imbalance in the percentage of patients in the TOBI® and placebo groups who experienced at least a 50% rise in serum creatinine from baseline (see ADVERSE REACTIONS). Laboratory tests of urine and renal function should be conducted at the discretion of the treating physician.

Drug Interactions

In clinical studies of TOBI®, patients taking TOBI® concomitantly with dornase alfa (PULMOZYME®, Genentech), ß-agonists, inhaled corticosteroids, other anti-pseudomonal antibiotics, or parenteral aminoglycosides demonstrated adverse experience profiles similar to the study population as a whole.
Concurrent and/or sequential use of TOBI® with other drugs with neurotoxic or ototoxic potential should be avoided. Some diuretics can enhance aminoglycoside toxicity by altering antibiotic concentrations in serum and tissue. TOBI® should not be administered concomitantly with ethacrynic acid, furosemide, urea, or mannitol.

Carcinogenesis, Mutagenesis, Impairment of Fertility

A two-year rat inhalation toxicology study to assess carcinogenic potential of TOBI® has been completed. Rats were exposed to TOBI® for up to 1.5 hours per day for 95 weeks. The clinical formulation of the drug was used for this carcinogenicity study. Serum levels of tobramycin of up to 35 mcg/mL were measured in rats, in contrast to the average 1 mcg/mL levels observed in cystic fibrosis patients in clinical trials. There was no drug-related increase in the incidence of any variety of tumor.
Additionally, TOBI® has been evaluated for genotoxicity in a battery of *in-vitro* and *in-vivo* tests. The Ames bacterial reversion test, conducted with 5 tester strains, failed to show a significant increase in revertants with or without metabolic activation in all strains. Tobramycin was negative in the mouse lymphoma forward mutation assay, did not induce chromosomal aberrations in Chinese hamster ovary cells, and was negative in the mouse micronucleus test.
Subcutaneous administration of up to 100 mg/kg of tobramycin did not affect mating behavior or cause impairment of fertility in male or female rats.

Pregnancy

Teratogenic Effects – Pregnancy Category D

(See WARNINGS.)
No reproduction toxicology studies have been conducted with TOBI®. However, subcutaneous administration of tobramycin at doses of 100 or 20 mg/kg/day during organogenesis was not teratogenic in rats or rabbits, respectively. Doses of tobramycin ≥40 mg/kg/day were severely maternally toxic to rabbits and precluded the evaluation of teratogenicity. Aminoglycosides can cause fetal harm (e.g., congenital deafness) when administered to a pregnant woman. Ototoxicity was not evaluated in offspring during nonclinical reproduction toxicity studies with tobramycin. If TOBI® is used during pregnancy, or if the patient becomes pregnant while taking TOBI®, the patient should be apprised of the potential hazard to the fetus.

Nursing Mothers

It is not known if TOBI® will reach sufficient concentrations after administration by inhalation to be excreted in human breast milk. Because of the potential for ototoxicity and nephrotoxicity in infants, a decision should be made whether to terminate nursing or discontinue TOBI®.

Pediatric Use

The safety and efficacy of TOBI® have not been studied in pediatric patients under 6 years of age.

ADVERSE REACTIONS

TOBI® was generally well tolerated during two clinical studies in 258 cystic fibrosis patients ranging in age from 6 to 48 years. Patients received TOBI® in alternating periods of 28 days on and 28 days off drug in addition to their standard cystic fibrosis therapy for a total of 24 weeks.
Voice alteration and tinnitus were the only adverse experiences reported by significantly more TOBI®-treated patients. Thirty-three patients (13%) treated with TOBI® complained of voice alteration compared to 17 (7%) placebo patients. Voice alteration was more common in the on-drug periods.
Eight patients from the TOBI® group (3%) reported tinnitus compared to no placebo patients. All episodes were transient, resolved without discontinuation of the TOBI® treatment regimen, and were not associated with loss of hearing in audiograms. Tinnitus is one of the sentinel symptoms of cochlear toxicity, and patients with this symptom should be carefully monitored for high frequency hearing loss. The numbers of patients reporting vestibular adverse experiences such as dizziness were similar in the TOBI® and placebo groups.
Nine (3%) patients in the TOBI® group and nine (3%) patients in the placebo group had increases in serum creatinine of at least 50% over baseline. In all nine patients in the TOBI® group, creatinine decreased at the next visit.
Table 1 lists the percent of patients with treatment-emergent adverse experiences (spontaneously reported and solicited) that occurred in >5% of TOBI® patients during the two Phase III studies.

Table 1: Percent of Patients With Treatment Emergent Adverse Experiences Occurring in >5% of TOBI® Patients

Adverse Event	TOBI® (n=258) %	Placebo (n=262) %
Cough Increased	46.1	47.3
Pharyngitis	38.0	39.3
Sputum Increased	37.6	39.7
Asthenia	35.7	39.3
Rhinitis	34.5	33.6
Dyspnea	33.7	38.5
Fever[1]	32.9	43.5
Lung Disorder	31.4	31.3
Headache	26.7	32.1
Chest Pain	26.0	29.8
Sputum Discoloration	21.3	19.8
Hemoptysis	19.4	23.7
Anorexia	18.6	27.9
Lung Function Decreased[2]	16.3	15.3
Asthma	15.9	20.2
Vomiting	14.0	22.1
Abdominal Pain	12.8	23.7
Voice Alteration	12.8	6.5
Nausea	11.2	16.0
Weight Loss	10.1	15.3
Pain	8.1	12.6
Sinusitis	8.1	9.2
Ear Pain	7.4	8.8
Back Pain	7.0	8.0
Epistaxis	7.0	6.5
Taste Perversion	6.6	6.9
Diarrhea	6.2	10.3
Malaise	6.2	5.3
Lower Respiratory Tract Infection	5.8	8.0
Dizziness	5.8	7.6
Hyperventilation	5.4	9.9
Rash	5.4	6.1

[1] Includes subjective complaints of fever.
[2] Includes reported decreases in pulmonary function tests or decreased lung volume on chest radiograph associated with intercurrent illness or study drug administration.

OVERDOSAGE

Signs and symptoms of acute toxicity from overdosage of IV tobramycin might include dizziness, tinnitus, vertigo, loss of high-tone hearing acuity, respiratory failure, and neuromuscular blockade. Administration by inhalation results in low systemic bioavailability of tobramycin. Tobramycin is not significantly absorbed following oral administration. Tobramycin serum concentrations may be helpful in monitoring overdosage.
In all cases of suspected overdosage, physicians should contact the Regional Poison Control Center for information about effective treatment. In the case of any overdosage, the possibility of drug interactions with alterations in drug disposition should be considered.

DOSAGE AND ADMINISTRATION

The recommended dosage for both adults and pediatric patients 6 years of age and older is 1 single-use ampule (300 mg) administered BID for 28 days. Dosage is not adjusted by weight. All patients should be administered 300 mg BID. The doses should be taken as close to 12 hours apart as possible; they should not be taken less than 6 hours apart.
TOBI® is inhaled while the patient is sitting or standing upright and breathing normally through the mouthpiece of the nebulizer. Nose clips may help the patient breathe through the mouth.
TOBI® is administered BID in alternating periods of 28 days. After 28 days of therapy, patients should stop TOBI® therapy for the next 28 days, and then resume therapy for the next 28 day on/28 day off cycle.
TOBI® is supplied as a single-use ampule and is administered by inhalation, using a hand-held PARI LC PLUS™ Reusable Nebulizer with a DeVilbiss® Pulmo-Aide® compressor. TOBI® is not for subcutaneous, intravenous or intrathecal administration.

Usage

TOBI® is administered by inhalation over an approximately 15-minute period, using a hand-held PARI LC PLUS™ Reusable Nebulizer with a DeVilbiss® Pulmo-Aide® compressor. TOBI® should not be diluted or mixed with dornase alfa (PULMOZYME®, Genentech) in the nebulizer.
During clinical studies, patients on multiple therapies were instructed to take them first, followed by TOBI®.

HOW SUPPLIED

TOBI® 300 mg is available as follows:
NDC 0078-0494-71
5 mL single-dose ampule (carton of 56)

Storage

TOBI® should be stored under refrigeration at 2-8°C/36-46°F. Upon removal from the refrigerator, or if refrigeration is unavailable, TOBI® pouches (opened or unopened) may be stored at room temperature (up to 25°C/77°F) for up to 28 days. TOBI® should not be used beyond the expiration date stamped on the ampule when stored under refrigeration (2-8°C/36-46°F) or beyond 28 days when stored at room temperature (25°C/77°F).
TOBI® ampules should not be exposed to intense light. The solution in the ampule is slightly yellow, but may darken with age if not stored in the refrigerator; however, the color change does not indicate any change in the quality of the product as long as it is stored within the recommended storage conditions.

Clinical Studies

Two identically designed, double-blind, randomized, placebo-controlled, parallel group, 24-week clinical studies (Study 1 and Study 2) at a total of 69 cystic fibrosis centers in the United States were conducted in cystic fibrosis patients with *P. aeruginosa*. Subjects who were less than 6 years of age, had a baseline creatinine of >2 mg/dL, or had *Burkholderia cepacia* isolated from sputum were excluded. All subjects had baseline FEV_1 % predicted between 25% and 75%. In these clinical studies, 258 patients received TOBI® therapy on an outpatient basis (see Table 2) using a hand-held PARI LC PLUS™ Reusable Nebulizer with a DeVilbiss® Pulmo-Aide® compressor.
[See table 2 at left]
All patients received either TOBI® or placebo (saline with 1.25 mg quinine for flavoring) in addition to standard treatment recommended for cystic fibrosis patients, which included oral and parenteral anti-pseudomonal therapy, β_2-agonists, cromolyn, inhaled steroids, and airway clearance techniques. In addition, approximately 77% of patients were concurrently treated with dornase alfa (PULMOZYME®, Genentech).

Table 2: Dosing Regimens in Clinical Studies

	Cycle 1		Cycle 2		Cycle 3	
	28 days	28 days	28 days	28 days	28 days	28 days
TOBI® regimen n=258	TOBI® 300 mg BID	No drug	TOBI® 300 mg BID	No drug	TOBI® 300 mg BID	No drug
Placebo regimen n=262	placebo BID	No drug	placebo BID	No drug	placebo BID	No drug

In each study, TOBI® treated patients experienced significant improvement in pulmonary function. Improvement was demonstrated in the TOBI® group in Study 1 by an average increase in FEV_1 % predicted of about 11% relative to baseline (Week 0) during 24 weeks compared to no average change in placebo patients. In Study 2, TOBI®-treated patients had an average increase of about 7% compared to an average decrease of about 1% in placebo patients. Figure 1 shows the average relative change in FEV_1% predicted over 24 weeks for both studies.

Figure 1: Relative Change From Baseline in FEV_1% Predicted

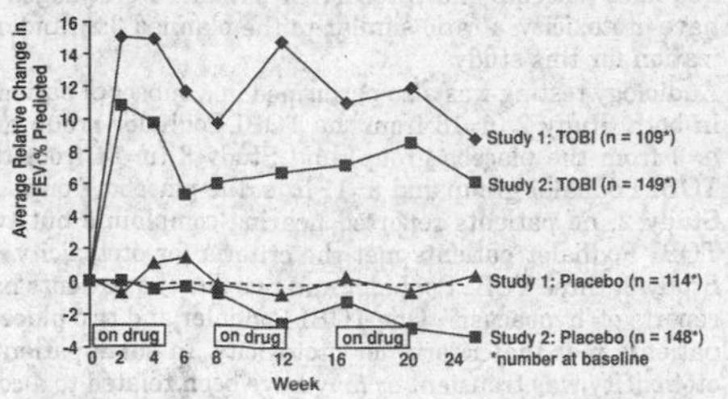

In each study, TOBI® therapy resulted in a significant reduction in the number of *P. aeruginosa* colony forming units (CFUs) in sputum during the on-drug periods. Sputum bacterial density returned to baseline during the off-drug periods. Reductions in sputum bacterial density were smaller in each successive cycle. (see Figure 2).

Figure 2: Absolute Change From Baseline in Log_{10} CFUs

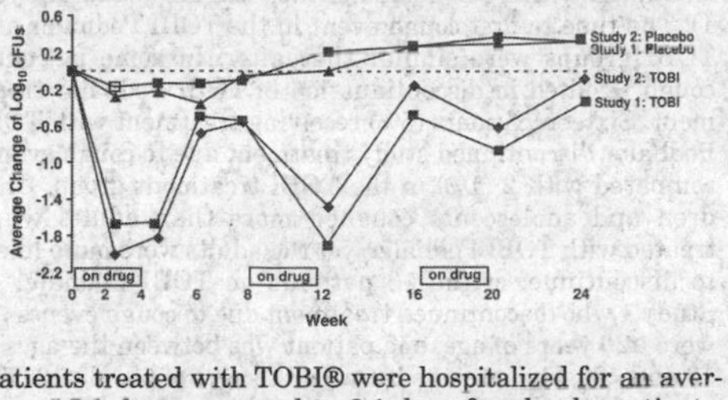

Patients treated with TOBI® were hospitalized for an average of 5.1 days compared to 8.1 days for placebo patients. Patients treated with TOBI® required an average of 9.6 days of parenteral anti-pseudomonal antibiotic treatment compared to 14.1 days for placebo patients. During the 6 months of treatment, 40% of TOBI® patients and 53% of placebo patients were treated with parenteral anti-pseudomonal antibiotics.

The relationship between *in-vitro* susceptibility test results and clinical outcome with TOBI® therapy is not clear. However, 4 TOBI® patients who began the clinical trial with *P. aeruginosa* isolates having MIC values ≥128 μg/mL did not experience an improvement in FEV_1 or a decrease in sputum bacterial density.

Treatment with TOBI® did not affect the susceptibility of the majority of *P. aeruginosa* isolates during the 6-month studies. However, some *P. aeruginosa* isolates did exhibit increased tobramycin MICs. The percentage of patients with *P. aeruginosa* isolates with tobramycin MICs ≥16 μg/mL was 13% at the beginning, and 23% at the end of 6 months of the TOBI® regimen.

REFERENCES

1. Neu HC. Tobramycin: an overview. [Review]. J Infect Dis 1976; Suppl 134:S3-19.
2. Weber A, Smith A, Williams-Warren J et al. Nebulizer delivery of tobramycin to the lower respiratory tract. Pediatr Pulmonol 1994; 17 (5):331-9.
3. Bryan LE. Aminoglycoside resistance. Bryan LE, Ed. Antimicrobial drug resistance. Orlando, FL:Academic Press, 1984: 241-77.

U.S. Patent 5,508,269; other patents pending.

Distributed by:
Novartis Pharmaceuticals Corporation
East Hanover, New Jersey 07936
REV: NOVEMBER 2009 T2009-119

Shown in Product Identification Guide, page 311

TOBI® PODHALER™ ℞
(tobramycin inhalation powder)
for oral inhalation use

The following prescribing information is based on official labeling in effect July 2013.

HIGHLIGHTS OF PRESCRIBING INFORMATION

These highlights do not include all the information needed to use TOBI Podhaler safely and effectively. See full prescribing information for TOBI Podhaler.

TOBI® PODHALER™ (tobramycin inhalation powder), for oral inhalation use
Initial U.S. Approval: 1975

INDICATIONS AND USAGE

TOBI Podhaler is an antibacterial aminoglycoside indicated for the management of cystic fibrosis patients with *Pseudomonas aeruginosa*.

Safety and efficacy have not been demonstrated in patients under the age of 6 years, patients with forced expiratory volume in 1 second (FEV_1) <25% or >80%, or patients colonized with *Burkholderia cepacia* (1).

DOSAGE AND ADMINISTRATION

- DO NOT swallow TOBI Podhaler capsules (2)
- For use with the Podhaler device only (2)
- For oral inhalation only (2)
- The recommended dosage is the inhalation of four 28 mg capsules twice-daily for 28 days (2)

DOSAGE FORMS AND STRENGTHS

Inhalation powder: 28 mg in a capsule (3)

CONTRAINDICATIONS

Known hypersensitivity to any aminoglycoside (4)

WARNINGS AND PRECAUTIONS

- Caution should be exercised when prescribing TOBI Podhaler to patients with known or suspected auditory, vestibular, renal, or neuromuscular dysfunction (5.1, 5.2, 5.3)
- Ototoxicity, as measured by complaints of hearing loss or tinnitus, was reported in clinical trials (5.1)
- Aminoglycosides may aggravate muscle weakness because of a potential curare-like effect on neuromuscular function (5.3)
- Bronchospasm can occur with inhalation of TOBI Podhaler (5.4)
- Audiograms, serum concentrations, and renal function should be monitored as appropriate (5.5)
- Fetal harm can occur when aminoglycosides are administered to a pregnant woman. Apprise women of the potential hazard to the fetus (5.6)

ADVERSE REACTIONS

The most common adverse reactions (≥10 % of TOBI Podhaler and TOBI patients in primary safety population) are cough, lung disorder, productive cough, dyspnea, pyrexia, oropharyngeal pain, dysphonia, hemoptysis, and headache (6.1)

To report SUSPECTED ADVERSE REACTIONS, contact Novartis Pharmaceuticals Corporation at 1-888-669-6682 or FDA at 1-800-FDA-1088 or www.fda.gov/medwatch.

DRUG INTERACTIONS

Concurrent and/or sequential use of TOBI Podhaler with other drugs with neurotoxic, nephrotoxic, or ototoxic potential should be avoided (7)

USE IN SPECIFIC POPULATIONS

- Aminoglycosides can cause fetal harm when administered to a pregnant woman (8.1)
- Nursing mother: discontinue drug or nursing, taking into consideration the importance of the drug to the mother (8.3)

See 17 for PATIENT COUNSELING INFORMATION and FDA-approved patient labeling

Revised: 03/2013

FULL PRESCRIBING INFORMATION: CONTENTS*

*** Sections or subsections omitted from the full prescribing information are not listed**

FULL PRESCRIBING INFORMATION

1 INDICATIONS AND USAGE

TOBI Podhaler is indicated for the management of cystic fibrosis patients with *Pseudomonas aeruginosa*.

Safety and efficacy have not been demonstrated in patients under the age of 6 years, patients with forced expiratory volume in 1 second (FEV_1) <25% or >80% predicted, or patients colonized with *Burkholderia cepacia* [see *Clinical Studies (14)*].

2 DOSAGE AND ADMINISTRATION

DO NOT SWALLOW TOBI PODHALER CAPSULES
FOR USE WITH THE PODHALER DEVICE ONLY
FOR ORAL INHALATION ONLY

TOBI Podhaler capsules must not be swallowed as the intended effects in the lungs will not be obtained. The contents of TOBI Podhaler capsules are only for oral inhalation and should only be used with the Podhaler device.

The recommended dosage of TOBI Podhaler for both adults and pediatric patients 6 years of age and older is the inhalation of the contents of four 28 mg TOBI Podhaler capsules twice-daily for 28 days using the Podhaler device.

Refer to the Instructions For Use (IFU) for full administration information.

Dosage is not adjusted by weight. Each dose of four capsules should be taken as close to 12 hours apart as possible; each dose should not be taken less than 6 hours apart.

TOBI Podhaler is administered twice-daily in alternating periods of 28 days. After 28 days of therapy, patients should stop TOBI Podhaler therapy for the next 28 days, and then resume therapy for the next 28 day on and 28 day off cycle.

TOBI Podhaler capsules should always be stored in the blister and each capsule should only be removed IMMEDIATELY BEFORE USE.

For patients taking several different inhaled medications and/or performing chest physiotherapy, the order of therapies should follow the physician's recommendation. It is recommended that TOBI Podhaler is taken last.

3 DOSAGE FORMS AND STRENGTHS

Inhalation powder:

28 mg: clear, colorless hypromellose capsule with "NVR AVCI" in blue radial imprint on one part of the capsule and the Novartis logo "ⓑ" in blue radial imprint on the other part of the capsule.

4 CONTRAINDICATIONS

TOBI Podhaler is contraindicated in patients with a known hypersensitivity to any aminoglycoside.

5 WARNINGS AND PRECAUTIONS

5.1 Ototoxicity

Caution should be exercised when prescribing TOBI Podhaler to patients with known or suspected auditory or vestibular dysfunction.

Ototoxicity, as measured by complaints of hearing loss or tinnitus, was reported by patients in the TOBI Podhaler clinical studies [see *Adverse Reactions (6.1)*]. Tinnitus may be a sentinel symptom of ototoxicity, and therefore the onset of this symptom warrants caution. Ototoxicity, manifested as both auditory (hearing loss) and vestibular toxicity, has been reported with parenteral aminoglycosides. Vestibular toxicity may be manifested by vertigo, ataxia or dizziness.

5.2 Nephrotoxicity

Caution should be exercised when prescribing TOBI Podhaler to patients with known or suspected renal dysfunction.

Nephrotoxicity was not observed during TOBI Podhaler clinical studies but has been associated with aminoglycosides as a class.

5.3 Neuromuscular Disorders

Caution should be exercised when prescribing TOBI Podhaler to patients with known or suspected neuromuscular dysfunction.

TOBI Podhaler should be used cautiously in patients with neuromuscular disorders, such as myasthenia gravis or Parkinson's disease, since aminoglycosides may aggravate muscle weakness because of a potential curare-like effect on neuromuscular function.

5.4 Bronchospasm

Bronchospasm can occur with inhalation of TOBI Podhaler [see *Adverse Reactions (6.1)*]. Bronchospasm should be treated as medically appropriate.

5.5 Laboratory Tests

Audiograms

Physicians should consider an audiogram at baseline, particularly for patients at increased risk of auditory dysfunction.

If a patient reports tinnitus or hearing loss during TOBI Podhaler therapy, the physician should refer that patient for audiological assessment.

Serum Concentrations

In patients treated with TOBI Podhaler, serum tobramycin concentrations are approximately 1 to 2 μg/mL one hour after dose administration and do not require routine monitoring. Serum concentrations of tobramycin in patients with known or suspected auditory or renal dysfunction or patients treated with a concomitant parenteral aminoglycoside (or other nephrotoxic or ototoxic medications) should be monitored at the discretion of the treating physician. If ototoxicity or nephrotoxicity occurs in a patient receiving TOBI Podhaler, tobramycin therapy should be discontinued until serum concentrations fall below 2 μg/mL.

The serum concentration of tobramycin should only be monitored through venipuncture and not finger prick blood sampling. Contamination of the skin of the fingers with tobramycin may lead to falsely increased measurements of serum levels of the drug. This contamination cannot be completely avoided by hand washing before testing.

Renal Function

Laboratory tests of urine and renal function should be conducted at the discretion of the treating physician.

5.6 Use in Pregnancy

Aminoglycosides can cause fetal harm when administered to a pregnant woman. Aminoglycosides cross the placenta, and streptomycin has been associated with several reports of total, irreversible, bilateral congenital deafness in pediatric patients exposed *in utero*. Patients who use TOBI Podhaler during pregnancy, or become pregnant while taking TOBI Podhaler should be apprised of the potential hazard to the fetus [see *Use in Specific Populations (8.1)*].

6 ADVERSE REACTIONS

6.1 Clinical Trials Experience

Because clinical trials are conducted under widely varying conditions, adverse reaction rates observed in the clinical trials of a drug cannot be directly compared to rates in the clinical trials of another drug and may not reflect the rates observed in practice.

TOBI Podhaler has been evaluated for safety in 425 cystic fibrosis patients exposed to at least one dose of TOBI Podhaler, including 273 patients who were exposed across three cycles (6 months) of treatment. Each cycle consisted of 28 days on-treatment (with 112 mg administered twice daily) and 28 days off-treatment. Patients with serum creatinine ≥ 2 mg/dL and blood urea nitrogen (BUN) ≥ 40 mg/dL were excluded from clinical studies. There were 218 males and 207 females in this population, and reflecting the cystic fibrosis population in the U.S., the vast majority of patients were Caucasian. There were 221 patients ≥ 20 years old, 121 patients ≥ 13 to < 20 years old, and 83 patients ≥ 6 to < 13 years old. There were 239 patients with screening FEV_1 % predicted ≥ 50%, 156 patients with screening FEV_1 % predicted < 50%, and 30 patients with missing FEV_1 % predicted.

The primary safety population reflects patients from Study 1, an open-label study comparing TOBI Podhaler with TOBI (tobramycin inhalation solution, USP) over three cycles of 4 weeks on treatment followed by 4 weeks off treatment. Randomization, in a planned 3:2 ratio, resulted in 308 patients treated with TOBI Podhaler and 209 patients treated with TOBI. For both the TOBI Podhaler and TOBI groups, mean exposure to medication for each cycle was 28-29 days. The mean age for both arms was between 25 and 26 years old. The mean baseline FEV_1 % predicted for both arms was 53%.

Table 1 displays adverse drug reactions reported by at least 2% of TOBI Podhaler patients in Study 1, inclusive of all cycles (on and off treatment). Adverse drug reactions are listed according to MedDRA system organ class and sorted within system organ class group in descending order of frequency.

Table 1: Adverse reactions reported in Study 1 (occurring in ≥2% of TOBI Podhaler patients)

Primary System Organ Class Preferred Term	TOBI Podhaler N=308 %	TOBI N=209 %
Respiratory, thoracic, and mediastinal disorders		
Cough	48.4	31.1
Lung disorder[1]	33.8	30.1
Productive cough	18.2	19.6
Dyspnea	15.6	12.4
Oropharyngeal pain	14.0	10.5
Dysphonia	13.6	3.8
Hemoptysis	13.0	12.4
Nasal congestion	8.1	7.2
Rales	7.1	6.2
Wheezing	6.8	6.2
Chest discomfort	6.5	2.9
Throat irritation	4.5	1.9
Gastrointestinal disorders		
Nausea	7.5	9.6
Vomiting	6.2	5.7
Diarrhea	4.2	1.9
Dysgeusia	3.9	0.5
Infections and infestations		
Upper respiratory tract infection	6.8	8.6
Investigations		
Pulmonary function test decreased	6.8	8.1
Forced expiratory volume decreased	3.9	1.0
Blood glucose increased	2.9	0.5
Vascular disorders		
Epistaxis	2.6	1.9
Nervous system disorders		
Headache	11.4	12.0
General disorders and administration site conditions		
Pyrexia	15.6	12.4
Musculoskeletal and connective tissue disorders		
Musculoskeletal chest pain	4.5	4.8
Skin and subcutaneous tissue disorders		
Rash	2.3	2.4

[1]This includes adverse events of pulmonary or cystic fibrosis exacerbations

Adverse drug reactions that occurred in <2% of patients treated with TOBI Podhaler in Study 1 were: bronchospasm (TOBI Podhaler 1.6%, TOBI 0.5%); deafness including deafness unilateral (reported as mild to moderate hearing loss or increased hearing loss) (TOBI Podhaler 1.0%, TOBI 0.5%); and tinnitus (TOBI Podhaler 1.9%, TOBI 2.4%).

Discontinuations in Study 1 were higher in the TOBI Podhaler arm compared to TOBI (27% TOBI Podhaler vs 18% TOBI). This was driven primarily by discontinuations due to adverse events (14% TOBI Podhaler vs 8% TOBI). Higher rates of discontinuation were seen in subjects ≥ 20 years old and those with baseline FEV_1 % predicted < 50%. Respiratory related hospitalizations occurred in 24% of the patients in the TOBI Podhaler arm and 22% of the patients in the TOBI arm. There was an increased new usage of antipseudomonal medication in the TOBI Podhaler arm (65% TOBI Podhaler vs 55% TOBI). This included oral antibiotics in 55% of TOBI Podhaler patients and 40% of TOBI patients and intravenous antibiotics in 35% of TOBI Podhaler patients and 33% of TOBI patients. Median time to first antipseudomonal usage was 89 days in the TOBI Podhaler arm and 112 days in the TOBI arm.

The supportive safety population reflects patients from two studies: Study 2, a double-blind, placebo-controlled design for the first treatment cycle, followed by all patients receiving TOBI Podhaler (replaced placebo) for two additional cycles, and Study 3, a double-blind, placebo-controlled trial for one treatment cycle only. Placebo in these studies was inhaled powder without the active ingredient, tobramycin. The patient population for these studies was much younger than in Study 1 (mean age 13 years old).

Adverse drug reactions reported more frequently by TOBI Podhaler patients in the placebo-controlled cycle (Cycle 1) of Study 2, which included 46 TOBI Podhaler and 49 placebo patients, were:

Respiratory, thoracic, and mediastinal disorders
Pharyngolaryngeal pain (TOBI Podhaler 10.9%, placebo 0%); dysphonia (TOBI Podhaler 4.3%, placebo 0%)
Gastrointestinal disorders
Dysgeusia (TOBI Podhaler 6.5%, placebo 2.0%)

Adverse drug reactions reported more frequently by TOBI Podhaler patients in Study 3, which included 30 TOBI Podhaler and 32 placebo patients, were:

Respiratory, thoracic, and mediastinal disorders
Cough (TOBI Podhaler 10%, placebo 0%)
Ear and labyrinth disorders
Hypoacusis (TOBI Podhaler 10%, placebo 6.3%)

Audiometric assessment

In Study 1, audiology testing was performed in a subset of approximately 25% of TOBI Podhaler (n=78) and TOBI (n=45) patients. Using the criteria for either ear of ≥ 10 dB loss at two consecutive frequencies, ≥ 20 dB loss at any frequency, or loss of response at three consecutive frequencies where responses were previously obtained, five TOBI Podhaler patients and three TOBI patients were judged to have ototoxicity, a ratio similar to the planned 3:2 randomization for this study.

Audiology testing was also performed in a subset of patients in both Study 2 (n=13 from the TOBI Podhaler group and n=9 from the placebo group) and Study 3 (n=14 from the TOBI Podhaler group and n=11 from the placebo group). In Study 2, no patients reported hearing complaints but two TOBI Podhaler patients met the criteria for ototoxicity. In Study 3, three TOBI Podhaler and two placebo patients had reports of 'hypoacusis'. One TOBI Podhaler and two placebo patients met the criteria for ototoxicity. In some patients, ototoxicity was transient or may have been related to a conductive defect.

Cough

Cough is a common symptom in cystic fibrosis, reported in 42% of the patients in Study 1 at baseline. Cough was the most frequently reported adverse event in Study 1 and was more common in the TOBI Podhaler arm (48% TOBI Podhaler vs 31 % TOBI). There was a higher rate of cough adverse event reporting during the first week of active treatment with TOBI Podhaler (i.e., the first week of Cycle 1). The time to first cough event in the TOBI Podhaler and TOBI groups were similar thereafter. In some patients, cough resulted in discontinuation of TOBI Podhaler treatment. Sixteen patients (5%) receiving treatment with TOBI Podhaler discontinued study treatment due to cough events compared with 2 (1%) in the TOBI treatment group. Children and adolescents coughed more than adults when treated with TOBI Podhaler, yet the adults were more likely to discontinue: of the 16 patients on TOBI Podhaler in Study 1 who discontinued treatment due to cough events, 14 were ≥20 years of age, one patient was between the ages of 13 and <20, and one was between the ages of 6 and <13. The rates of bronchospasm (as measured by ≥20% decrease in FEV_1 % predicted post-dose) were approximately 5% in both treatment groups, and none of these patients experienced concomitant cough.

In Study 2, cough was the most commonly reported adverse event during the first cycle of treatment (the double blind period of treatment) and occurred more frequently in placebo-treated patients (26.5%) than patients treated with TOBI Podhaler (13%). Similar percentages of patients in both treatment groups reported cough as a baseline symptom. In Study 3, cough events were reported by three patients in the TOBI Podhaler group (10%) and none in the placebo group (0%).

7 DRUG INTERACTIONS

No clinical drug interaction studies have been performed with TOBI Podhaler. In clinical studies, patients receiving TOBI Podhaler continued to take dornase alfa, bronchodilators, inhaled corticosteroids, and macrolides. No clinical signs of drug interactions with these medicines were identified.

Concurrent and/or sequential use of TOBI Podhaler with other drugs with neurotoxic, nephrotoxic, or ototoxic potential should be avoided.

Some diuretics can enhance aminoglycoside toxicity by altering antibiotic concentrations in serum and tissue. TOBI Podhaler should not be administered concomitantly with ethacrynic acid, furosemide, urea, or mannitol.

8 USE IN SPECIFIC POPULATIONS

8.1 Pregnancy

Teratogenic Effects – Pregnancy Category D [see *Warnings and Precautions (5.6)*]

No reproduction toxicology studies have been conducted with TOBI Podhaler. However, subcutaneous administration of tobramycin at doses of 100 or 20 mg/kg/day during organogenesis was not teratogenic in rats or rabbits, respectively. Doses of tobramycin ≥ 40 mg/kg/day were severely maternally toxic to rabbits and precluded the evaluation of teratogenicity. Ototoxicity was not evaluated in offspring during nonclinical reproduction toxicity studies with tobramycin.

Aminoglycosides can cause fetal harm (e.g., congenital deafness) when administered to a pregnant woman. No adequate and well-controlled studies of TOBI Podhaler in pregnant women have been conducted. If TOBI Podhaler is used during pregnancy, or if the patient becomes pregnant while taking TOBI Podhaler, the patient should be apprised of the potential hazard to the fetus.

8.3 Nursing Mothers

The amount of tobramycin excreted in human breast milk after administration by inhalation is not known. Because of the potential for ototoxicity and nephrotoxicity in infants, a decision should be made whether to terminate nursing or discontinue the drug, taking into account the importance of the drug to the mother.

8.4 Pediatric Use

Patients 6 years and older were included in the Phase 3 studies with TOBI Podhaler; 206 patients below 20 years of age received TOBI Podhaler. No dosage adjustments are needed based on age. The overall pattern of adverse events in pediatric patients was similar to the adults. Dysgeusia (taste disturbance) was more commonly reported in younger patients six to 19 years of age than in patients 20 years and older, 7.4% vs 2.7%, respectively. Safety and effectiveness in pediatric patients below the age of 6 years have not been established.

8.5 Geriatric Use

Clinical studies of TOBI Podhaler did not include sufficient numbers of subjects aged 65 years and over to determine whether they respond differently from younger subjects. Tobramycin is known to be substantially excreted by the kidney, and the risk of adverse reactions to this drug may be greater in patients with impaired renal function. Because elderly patients are more likely to have decreased renal function, it may be useful to monitor renal function [see *Warnings and Precautions (5.2, 5.5)*].

8.6 Renal Impairment

Tobramycin is primarily excreted unchanged in the urine and renal function is expected to affect the exposure to tobramycin. The risk of adverse reactions to this drug may be greater in patients with impaired renal function. Patients with serum creatinine > 2 mg/dL and blood urea nitrogen (BUN) > 40 mg/dL have not been included in clinical studies and there are no data in this population to support a recommendation regarding dose adjustment with TOBI Podhaler [see *Warnings and Precautions (5.2, 5.5)*].

8.7 Hepatic Impairment

No studies have been performed in patients with hepatic impairment. As tobramycin is not metabolized, an effect of hepatic impairment on the exposure to tobramycin is not expected.

8.8 Organ Transplantation

Adequate data do not exist for the use of TOBI Podhaler in patients after organ transplantation.

10 OVERDOSAGE

The maximum tolerated daily dose of TOBI Podhaler has not been established.

In the event of accidental oral ingestion of TOBI Podhaler capsules, systemic toxicity is unlikely as tobramycin is poorly absorbed. Tobramycin serum concentrations may be helpful in monitoring overdosage.

Acute toxicity should be treated with immediate withdrawal of TOBI Podhaler, and baseline tests of renal function should be undertaken.

Hemodialysis may be helpful in removing tobramycin from the body.

In all cases of suspected overdosage, physicians should contact the Regional Poison Control Center for information about effective treatment. In the case of any overdosage, the possibility of drug interactions with alterations in drug disposition should be considered.

11 DESCRIPTION

TOBI Podhaler consists of a dry powder formulation of tobramycin for oral inhalation only with the Podhaler device. The inhalation powder is filled into clear, colorless hypromellose capsules.

Each clear, colorless hypromellose capsule contains a spray dried powder of 28 mg of tobramycin active ingredient with 1,2-distearoyl-sn-glycero-3-phosphocholine (DSPC), calcium chloride, and sulfuric acid (for pH adjustment).

The active component of TOBI Podhaler is tobramycin. Tobramycin is an aminoglycoside antibiotic. Its chemical name is *O*-3-amino-3-deoxy-α-D-glucopyranosyl-(1→4)-*O*-[2,6-diamino-2,3,6-trideoxy-α-D-ribo-hexopyranosyl-(1→6)]-2-deoxy-L-streptamine; its structural formula is:

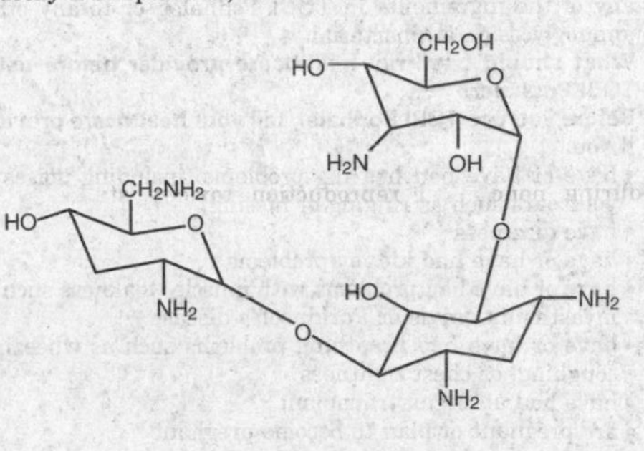

Tobramycin has a molecular weight of 467.52, and its empirical formula is $C_{18}H_{37}N_5O_9$. Tobramycin is a white to almost white powder; visually free from any foreign contaminants. Tobramycin is freely soluble in water, very slightly soluble in ethanol, and practically insoluble in chloroform and ether.

The Podhaler device is a plastic device used to inhale the dry powder contained in the TOBI Podhaler capsule. Under standardized *in vitro* testing at a fixed flow rate of 60 L/min and volume of 2 L for 2 seconds, the Podhaler device has a target delivered dose of 102 mg of tobramycin from the mouthpiece (4 capsules per dose). Peak inspiratory flow rate and inhaled volumes were explored in 96 cystic fibrosis patients aged 6 years and older. Older patients with significant disease progression and associated decreases in forced expiratory volume (FEV_1) and younger patients with inhaled volumes < 1 L were able to generate inspiratory flow rates and volumes required to receive their medication when following the instructions for use. However, no pediatric patients aged 6 to 10 years with FEV_1 less than 40% predicted were evaluated.

12 CLINICAL PHARMACOLOGY

12.1 Mechanism of Action

Tobramycin is an aminoglycoside antibiotic [see *Clinical Pharmacology (12.4)*].

12.3 Pharmacokinetics

Absorption

TOBI Podhaler contains tobramycin, a cationic polar molecule that does not readily cross epithelial membranes. TOBI Podhaler is specifically formulated for administration by oral inhalation. The systemic exposure to tobramycin after inhalation of TOBI Podhaler is expected to result from pulmonary absorption of the dose fraction delivered to the lungs as tobramycin and is not absorbed to any appreciable extent when administered via the oral route.

Serum concentrations

After inhalation of a 112 mg single dose (4 × 28 mg capsules) of TOBI Podhaler in cystic fibrosis patients, the maximum serum concentration (C_{max}) of tobramycin was 1.02 ± 0.53 μg/mL (mean ± SD) and the median time to reach the peak concentration (T_{max}) was 1 hour. In comparison, after inhalation of a single 300 mg dose of TOBI, C_{max} was 1.04 ± 0.58 μg/mL and median T_{max} was 1 hour. The extent of systemic exposure (AUC_{0-12}) was also similar: 4.6 ± 2.0 μg·h/mL following the 112 mg TOBI Podhaler dose and 4.8 ± 2.5 μg·h/mL following the 300 mg TOBI dose. At the end of a 4-week dosing cycle of TOBI Podhaler (112 mg twice daily), the maximum serum concentration of tobramycin 1 hour after dosing ranged from 1.48 ± 0.69 μg/mL to 1.99 ± 0.59 μg/mL (mean ± SD).

Sputum concentrations

After inhalation of a 112 mg single dose (4 × 28 mg capsules) of TOBI Podhaler in cystic fibrosis patients, sputum C_{max} of tobramycin was 1048 ± 1080 μg/g (mean ± SD). In comparison, after inhalation of a single 300 mg dose of TOBI, sputum C_{max} was 737 ± 1028 μg/g. The variability in pharmacokinetic parameters was higher in sputum as compared to serum.

Distribution

A population pharmacokinetic analysis for TOBI Podhaler in cystic fibrosis patients estimated the apparent volume of distribution of tobramycin in the central compartment to be 85.1 L for a typical CF patient.

Binding of tobramycin to serum proteins is negligible.

Metabolism

Tobramycin is not metabolized and is primarily excreted unchanged in the urine.

Elimination

Tobramycin is eliminated from the systemic circulation primarily by glomerular filtration of the unchanged compound. Systemically absorbed tobramycin following TOBI Podhaler administration is also expected to be eliminated principally by glomerular filtration.

The apparent terminal half-life of tobramycin in serum after inhalation of a 112 mg single dose of TOBI Podhaler was approximately 3 hours in cystic fibrosis patients and consistent with the half-life of tobramycin after TOBI inhalation.

A population pharmacokinetic analysis for TOBI Podhaler in cystic fibrosis patients aged 6 to 58 years estimated the apparent serum clearance of tobramycin to be 14.5 L/h. No clinically relevant covariates that were predictive of tobramycin clearance were identified from this analysis.

12.4 Microbiology

Mechanism of Action

Tobramycin is an aminoglycoside antimicrobial produced by *Streptomyces tenebrarius*. It acts primarily by disrupting protein synthesis leading to altered cell membrane permeability, progressive disruption of the cell envelope, and eventual cell death.

Tobramycin has *in vitro* activity against Gram-negative bacteria including *P. aeruginosa*. It is bactericidal *in vitro* at peak concentrations equal to or slightly greater than the minimum inhibitory concentration.

Susceptibility Testing

Interpretive criteria for inhaled antibacterial products are not defined. The *in vitro* antimicrobial susceptibility test methods used to determine the susceptibility for parenteral tobramycin therapy can be used to monitor the susceptibility of *P. aeruginosa* isolated from cystic fibrosis patients [1, 2, 3]. The relationship between *in vitro* susceptibility test results and clinical outcome with TOBI Podhaler therapy is not clear. A single sputum sample from a cystic fibrosis patient may contain multiple morphotypes of *P. aeruginosa* and each morphotype may require a different concentration of tobramycin to inhibit its growth *in vitro*. Patients should be monitored for changes in tobramycin susceptibility.

Development of Resistance

In clinical studies, some increases from baseline to the end of the treatment period were observed in the tobramycin MIC for *P. aeruginosa* morphotypes. In general, a higher percentage of patients treated with TOBI Podhaler had increases in tobramycin MIC compared with placebo or patients treated with TOBI inhalation solution.

The clinical significance of changes in MICs for *P. aeruginosa* has not been clearly established in the treatment of cystic fibrosis patients.

Cross-Resistance

Some emerging resistance to aztreonam, ceftazidime, ciprofloxacin, imipenem, or meropenem were observed in the TOBI Podhaler clinical trials. As other anti-pseudomonal antibiotics were concomitantly utilized in many patients in the clinical trials, the association with TOBI Podhaler is not clear.

Other

No trends were observed in the isolation of treatment-emergent bacterial respiratory pathogens (*Burkholderia cepacia, Stenotrophomonas maltophilia, Staphylococcus aureus* and *Achromobacter xylosoxidans*).

13 NONCLINICAL TOXICOLOGY

13.1 Carcinogenesis, Mutagenesis, Impairment of Fertility

Carcinogenicity studies were not conducted with TOBI Podhaler. A two-year rat inhalation toxicology study to assess carcinogenic potential of TOBI (tobramycin inhalation solution, USP) has been completed. Rats were exposed to TOBI for up to 1.5 hours per day for 95 weeks. Serum levels of tobramycin of up to 35 μg/mL were measured in rats, in contrast to the maximum 1.99 ± 0.59 μg/mL level observed in cystic fibrosis patients in TOBI Podhaler clinical trials. There was no drug-related increase in the incidence of any variety of tumor.

Additionally, tobramycin has been evaluated for genotoxicity in a battery of *in vitro* and *in vivo* tests. The Ames bacterial reversion test, conducted with 5 tester strains, failed to show a significant increase in revertants with or without metabolic activation in all strains. Tobramycin was negative in the mouse lymphoma forward mutation assay, did not induce chromosomal aberrations in Chinese hamster ovary cells, and was negative in the mouse micronucleus test.

Subcutaneous administration of up to 100 mg/kg of tobramycin did not affect mating behavior or cause impairment of fertility in male or female rats.

14 CLINICAL STUDIES

The Phase 3 clinical development program included two placebo-controlled studies (Studies 2 and 3) and one open-label study (Study 1), which randomized and dosed 157 and 517 patients, respectively, with a clinical diagnosis of cystic fibrosis, confirmed by quantitative pilocarpine iontophoresis sweat chloride test, well-characterized disease causing mutations in each CFTR gene, or abnormal nasal transepithelial potential difference characteristic of cystic fibrosis.

In the placebo-controlled studies, all patients were aged between 6 and 21 years old and had an FEV_1 at screening within the range of 25% to 80% (inclusive) of predicted normal values for their age, sex, and height based upon Knudson criteria. In addition, all patients were infected with *P. aeruginosa* as demonstrated by a positive sputum or throat culture (or bronchoalveolar lavage) within 6 months prior to screening, and also in a sputum culture taken at the screening visit. Among the 76 patients treated with TOBI Podhaler, 37% were males and 63% were females. Thirty-six patients were between 6 and 12 years of age, and 40 patients were between 13 and 21 years of age. Patients had a mean baseline FEV_1 of 56% of predicted normal value.

In both studies, >90% of patients received concomitant therapies for cystic fibrosis related indications. The most frequently used other antibacterial drugs (any route of administration) were azithromycin, ciprofloxacin, and ceftazidime. Consistent with the population of cystic fibrosis patients, the most frequently used concomitant medications included oral pancreatic enzyme preparations, mucolytics (especially dornase alfa), and selective β2-adrenoreceptor agonists.

Study 2

Study 2 was a randomized, three-cycle, two-arm trial. Each cycle comprised of 28 days on treatment followed by 28 days off treatment. The first cycle was double-blind, placebo-controlled with eligible patients randomized 1:1 to TOBI Podhaler (4 × 28 mg capsules twice daily) or placebo. Upon completion of the first cycle, patients who were randomized to the placebo treatment group received TOBI Podhaler for Cycles 2 and 3. The total treatment period was 24 weeks.

A total of 95 patients were randomized into Study 2 and received TOBI Podhaler (n=46) or placebo (n=49) in Cycle 1. All patients were less than 22 years of age (mean age 13.3 years) and had not received inhaled antipseudomonal antibiotics within four months prior to screening; 56% were female and 84% were Caucasian. This study was stopped early for demonstrated benefit and the primary analysis used the set of patients included in the interim analysis (n=79); 16 patients did not have data on the primary endpoint at that time. Of the 79 patients included in the interim analysis, 18 patients were excluded due to a failure to meet spirometry quality review criteria as determined by an external review panel. This resulted in a total of 61 patients, 29 in the TOBI Podhaler arm and 32 in the placebo arm, who were included in the primary analysis.

In the primary analysis, TOBI Podhaler significantly improved lung function compared with placebo as measured by the relative change in FEV_1 % predicted from baseline to the end of Cycle 1 dosing. This analysis adjusted for the covariates of baseline FEV_1 % predicted, age, and region, and imputed for missing data. Treatment with TOBI Podhaler and placebo resulted in relative increases in FEV_1 % predicted of 12.54% and 0.09%, respectively (LS mean difference = 12.44%; 95% CI: 4.89, 20.00; p=0.002). Analysis of absolute changes in FEV_1 % predicted showed LS means of 6.38% for TOBI Podhaler and -0.52% for placebo with a difference of 6.90% (95% CI: 2.40, 11.40). Improvements in lung function were achieved during the subsequent cycles of treatment with TOBI Podhaler, although the magnitude was reduced (Figure 1).

The percentage of patients using new antipseudomonal antibiotics in Cycle 1 was greater in the placebo treatment group (18.4%) compared with the TOBI Podhaler treatment group (13.1%). During the first cycle, 8.7% of TOBI Podhaler patients and 10.2% of placebo patients were treated with parenteral antipseudomonal antibiotics. In Cycle 1, two patients (4.4%) in the TOBI Podhaler treatment group required respiratory-related hospitalizations, compared with six patients (12.2%) in the placebo treatment group.

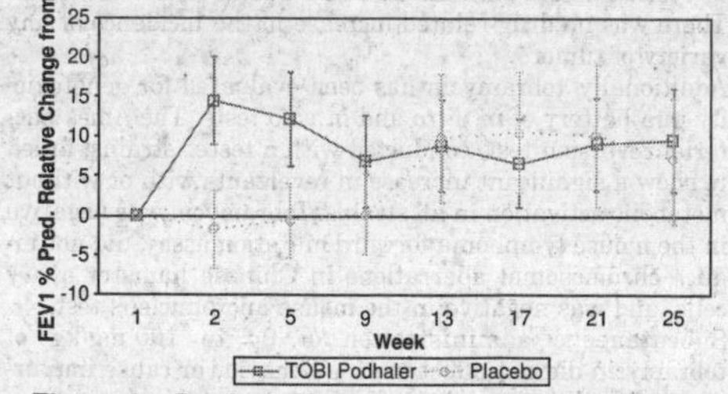

Figure 1 – Study 2: Mean relative change in FEV_1 % predicted from baseline in Cycles 1-3 by treatment group

Error bars represent the mean relative change (95% CI)

Study 3

Study 3 was a randomized, double-blind, placebo-controlled trial, similar in design to Study 2. Eligible patients were randomized 1:1 to receive TOBI Podhaler (4 × 28 mg capsules twice daily) or placebo for one cycle (28 days on-treatment and 28 days off-treatment).

A total of 62 patients were randomized into Study 3 and allocated to TOBI Podhaler (n=32) or placebo (n=30). All patients were less than 22 years of age (mean age 12.9 years) and had not received inhaled antipseudomonal antibiotics within 4 months prior to screening; 64.5% were female and 98.4% were Caucasian.

In this study, the results were not statistically significant for the primary lung function endpoint when adjusting for the covariates of age (<13 years, ≥13 years) and FEV_1 % predicted at screening (< 50%, ≥ 50%) and imputing for missing data. Improvement in lung function for TOBI Podhaler compared with placebo was evaluated using the relative change in FEV_1 % predicted from baseline to the end of Cycle 1 dosing. Treatment with TOBI Podhaler (8.19%) compared to placebo (2.27%) failed to achieve statistical significance in relative change in FEV_1 % predicted (LS mean difference = 5.91%; 95% CI: -2.54, 14.37; p=0.167). Analyses of absolute changes in FEV_1 % predicted showed LS means of 4.86% for TOBI Podhaler and 0.48% for placebo with a difference of 4.38% (95% CI:-0.17, 8.94).

Study 1

Study 1 was a randomized, open-label, active-controlled parallel arm trial. Eligible patients were randomized 3:2 to TOBI Podhaler (4 × 28 mg capsules twice daily) or TOBI (300 mg/5 mL twice daily). Treatment was administered for 28 days, followed by 28 days off therapy (one cycle) for three cycles. The total treatment period was 24 weeks. The time to administer a dose of TOBI Podhaler (10th to 90th percentiles) ranged from 2-7 minutes at the end of the dosing period for Cycle 1, and 2-6 minutes at the end of the dosing period for Cycle 3.

A total of 517 patients were randomized in Study 1 and received TOBI Podhaler (n=308) or TOBI (n=209). Patients were predominantly 20 years of age or older (mean age 25.6 years) with no inhaled antipseudomonal antibiotic use within 28 days prior to study drug administration; 45% were female and 91% were Caucasian.

The primary purpose of Study 1 was to evaluate safety. Interpretation of efficacy results in Study 1 is limited by several factors including open-label design, testing of multiple secondary endpoints, and missing values for the outcome of FEV_1 % predicted. The number (%) of patients with missing values for FEV_1 % predicted at Weeks 5 and 25 in the TOBI Podhaler treated group were 40 (13.0%) and 86 (27.9%) compared to 15 (7.2%) and 40 (19.1%) in the TOBI treated group. Using imputation of the missing data, the mean differences (TOBI Podhaler minus TOBI) in the percent relative change from baseline in FEV_1 % predicted at Weeks 5 and 25 were -0.87 (95% CI: -3.80, 2.07) and 1.62 (95% CI: -0.90, 4.14), respectively.

15 REFERENCES

1. Clinical and Laboratory Standards Institute (CLSI). Methods for Dilution Antimicrobial Susceptibility Tests for Bacteria that Grow Aerobically – Ninth Edition; Approved Standard. CLSI Document M7-A9. CLSI, 950 West Valley Rd., Suite 2500, Wayne, PA 19087, 2012.
2. CLSI. Performance Standards for Antimicrobial Disk Susceptibility Tests; Approved Standard – 11th ed. CLSI document M02-A11. CLSI, 2012.
3. CLSI. Performance Standards for Antimicrobial Susceptibility Testing; 22nd Informational Supplement. CLSI document M100-S22. CLSI, 2012

16 HOW SUPPLIED/STORAGE AND HANDLING

16.1 How Supplied

TOBI Podhaler contains aluminum blister-packaged 28 mg TOBI Podhaler (tobramycin inhalation powder) clear, colorless hypromellose capsules with "NVR AVCI" in blue radial imprint on one part of the capsule and the Novartis logo "ʋ" in blue radial imprint on the other part of the capsule, and Podhaler devices.

Each Podhaler device consists of the inhaler body, mouthpiece, capsule chamber and blue push button. The Podhaler device is provided in a case that protects the device during shipment, storage and its one week in-use period.

Unit Dose (blister pack), Box of 224 capsules contains: NDC 0078-0630-35

- 4 weekly packs, each containing:
  - 56 capsules (7 blister cards of 8 capsules)
  - 1 Podhaler device
- 1 reserve Podhaler device

16.2 Information for Patients

Store at 25°C (77°F); excursions permitted to 15-30°C (59-86°F)

Protect TOBI Podhaler from moisture.

- TOBI Podhaler capsules should be used with the Podhaler device only. The Podhaler device should not be used with any other capsules.
- Capsules should always be stored in the blister and each capsule should only be removed immediately before use.
- Always use the new Podhaler device provided with each weekly pack.

Keep this and all drugs out of the reach of children.

17 PATIENT COUNSELING INFORMATION

See *FDA-Approved Patient Labeling*

Information for Patients

Information on the long term efficacy and safety of TOBI Podhaler is limited. There is no information in patients with limited pulmonary reserve (FEV_1 <25% predicted). Decreased susceptibility of Pseudomonas aeruginosa to tobramycin has been seen with use of TOBI Podhaler. The relationship between in vitro susceptibility test results and clinical outcome with TOBI Podhaler therapy is not clear. Occurrence of decreased susceptibility on treatment should be monitored, and treatment with an alternative therapy should be considered if clinical worsening is observed.

TOBI Podhaler may not be tolerated by all patients. Patients should be instructed to consider alternative therapy if they are unable to tolerate TOBI Podhaler. Patients should be advised to complete a full 28-day course of TOBI Podhaler, even if they are feeling better. After 28 days of therapy, patients should stop TOBI Podhaler therapy for the next 28 days, and then resume therapy for the next 28 day on and 28 day off cycle.

It is important for patients to understand how to correctly administer TOBI Podhaler capsules using the Podhaler device. It is recommended that caregivers and patients be adequately trained in the proper use of the TOBI Podhaler prior to use. [See Instructions for Use at the end of the Patient Information leaflet.] Caregivers should provide assistance to children using TOBI Podhaler (including preparing the dose for inhalation) particularly for those aged 10 years or younger, and should continue to supervise them until they are able to use the Podhaler device properly without help.

For patients taking several different inhaled medications and/or performing chest physiotherapy, advise the patient regarding the order they should take the therapies. It is recommended that TOBI Podhaler be taken last.

17.1 Ototoxicity

Inform patients that ototoxicity, as measured by complaints of hearing loss or tinnitus, was reported by patients in the TOBI Podhaler clinical studies. Physicians should consider an audiogram at baseline, particularly for patients at increased risk of auditory dysfunction. If a patient reports tinnitus or hearing loss during TOBI Podhaler therapy, the physician should refer that patient for audiological assessment.

Patients should be reminded that vestibular toxicity may manifest as vertigo, ataxia, or dizziness.

17.2 Bronchospasm

Inform patients that bronchospasm can occur with inhalation of TOBI Podhaler.

17.3 Risks Associated with Aminoglycosides

Inform patients of adverse reactions associated with aminoglycosides such as nephrotoxicity and neuromuscular disorders.

17.4 Laboratory Tests

Inform patients of the need to monitor hearing, serum concentrations of tobramycin, or renal function as necessary during treatment with TOBI Podhaler.

17.5 Pregnancy

Inform patients that aminoglycosides can cause fetal harm when administered to a pregnant woman. Advise them to inform their doctor if they are pregnant, become pregnant, or plan to become pregnant.

17.6 Cough

Inform patients that cough was reported with the use of TOBI Podhaler in clinical trials. If coughing that may be experienced with TOBI Podhaler becomes bothersome or cannot be tolerated, advise patients that tobramycin inhalation solution or alternative therapeutic options may be considered.

T2013-20

March 2013

Patient Information

TOBI (TOH-bee) Podhaler (POD-hay-ler)

(tobramycin inhalation powder)

For Oral Inhalation

Important information: Do not swallow TOBI Podhaler capsules. TOBI Podhaler capsules are used only with the Podhaler device and inhaled through your mouth (oral inhalation). Never place a capsule in the mouthpiece of the Podhaler device.

Read this Patient Information before you start using TOBI Podhaler and each time you get a refill. There may be new information. This information does not take the place of talking to your healthcare provider about your medical condition or treatment.

What is TOBI Podhaler?

TOBI Podhaler is a prescription medicine used to treat people with cystic fibrosis who have a bacterial infection called Pseudomonas aeruginosa. TOBI Podhaler contains an antibacterial medicine called tobramycin (an aminoglycoside).

It is not known if TOBI Podhaler is safe and effective:

- in children under 6 years of age
- in people who have an FEV1 less than 25% predicted
- in people who are colonized with a bacterium called *Burkholderia cepacia*
- when used for more than 3 cycles

Who should not use TOBI Podhaler?

Do not use TOBI Podhaler if you are allergic to tobramycin, any of the ingredients in TOBI Podhaler, or to any other aminoglycoside antibacterial.

What should I tell my healthcare provider before using TOBI Podhaler?

Before you use TOBI Podhaler, tell your healthcare provider if you:

- have or have had hearing problems (including noises in your ears such as ringing or hissing)
- have dizziness
- have or have had kidney problems
- have or have had problems with muscle weakness such as myasthenia gravis or Parkinson's disease
- have or have had breathing problems such as wheezing, coughing, or chest tightness
- have had an organ transplant
- are pregnant or plan to become pregnant

- are breastfeeding or plan to breastfeed. It is not known if TOBI Podhaler passes into your breast milk.

Tell your healthcare provider about all the medicines you take, including prescription and non-prescription medicines, vitamins, and herbal supplements.

Using TOBI Podhaler with certain other medicines can cause serious side effects.

If you are using TOBI Podhaler, you should discuss with your healthcare provider if you should take:

- other medicines that may harm your nervous system, kidneys, or hearing
- "water pills" (diuretics) such as Edecrin (ethacrynic acid), Lasix (furosemide), or mannitol
- urea

Ask your healthcare provider or pharmacist for a list of these medicines, if you are not sure.

Know the medicines you take. Keep a list of them and show it to your healthcare provider and pharmacist when you get a new medicine.

How should I use TOBI Podhaler?

- See the step-by-step Instructions for Use at the end of this Patient Information leaflet about the right way to use TOBI Podhaler. Do not use TOBI Podhaler unless your healthcare provider has taught you how to use it the right way. Ask your healthcare provider or pharmacist if you are not sure.
- Always use TOBI Podhaler exactly as your healthcare provider tells you to use it. Ask your healthcare provider or pharmacist if you are not sure.
- The usual dose for adults and children over 6 years of age is:
  - The content of 4 TOBI Podhaler capsules inhaled by mouth in the morning using your Podhaler device and the content of 4 TOBI Podhaler capsules inhaled by mouth in the evening using your Podhaler device.
  - Check to see that each capsule is empty after inhaling. If powder remains in the capsule, repeat inhalation until the capsule is empty.
- Each dose of 4 TOBI Podhaler capsules should be taken as close to 12 hours as possible.
- You should not take your dose of 4 TOBI Podhaler capsules less than 6 hours apart.
- If you forget to take TOBI Podhaler and there are at least 6 hours to your next dose, take your dose as soon as you can. Otherwise, wait for your next dose. Do not double the dose to make up for the missed dose.
- After using TOBI Podhaler for 28 days, you should stop using it and wait 28 days. After you have stopped using TOBI Podhaler for 28 days, you should start using TOBI Podhaler again for 28 days. Complete the full 28 day course even if you are feeling better. It is important that you keep to the 28-day on, 28-day off cycle (See Figure A).

ON TOBI Podhaler	OFF TOBI Podhaler
Take TOBI Podhaler twice a day, every day for 28 days	Do not take any TOBI Podhaler for the next 28 days

Repeat cycle

(Figure A)

- If you are taking several different medicines inhaled through your mouth, your healthcare provider will tell you how to take your medicines the right way.
- If you are doing therapies for cystic fibrosis (chest physiotherapy), you should take TOBI Podhaler after your therapies are done.
- If you inhale too much TOBI Podhaler, tell your healthcare provider right away.
- If you accidentally swallow TOBI Podhaler capsules, tell your healthcare provider right away.
- Use a new Podhaler device every 7 days.
- Caregivers should help children who are 10 years of age and younger use TOBI Podhaler, and should keep watching them use their TOBI Podhaler until they are able to use it the right way without help.

What are the possible side effects of TOBI Podhaler?

TOBI Podhaler can cause serious side effects, including:

- hearing loss or ringing in the ears (ototoxicity). Tell your healthcare provider right away if you have hearing loss or you hear noises in your ears such as ringing or hissing. Tell your healthcare provider if you develop vertigo, difficulty with balance or dizziness.
- worsening kidney problems (nephrotoxicity). TOBI Podhaler is in a class of drugs which may cause worsening kidney problems, especially in people with known or suspected kidney problems. Your healthcare provider may do a blood test to check how your kidneys are working while you are using TOBI Podhaler.
- worsening muscle weakness. TOBI Podhaler is in a class of drugs which can cause muscle weakness to get worse in people who already have problems with muscle weakness (myasthenia gravis or Parkinson's disease).
- severe breathing problems (bronchospasm). Tell your healthcare provider right away if you get any of these symptoms of bronchospasm with using TOBI Podhaler:
  - shortness of breath with wheezing
  - coughing and chest tightness
- TOBI Podhaler is in a class of drugs which may cause harm to an unborn baby.

The most common side effects of TOBI Podhaler include:

- cough
- worsening of lung problems or cystic fibrosis
- productive cough
- shortness of breath
- fever
- sore throat
- changes in your voice (hoarseness)
- coughing up blood
- headache
- altered taste

Laboratory tests show reduced tobramycin activity against *Pseudomonas aeruginosa* bacteria in some patients with the use of TOBI Podhaler. The relationship between these lab results and how well TOBI Podhaler works is not clear. Let your healthcare provider know if your symptoms worsen.

Some patients may be unable to continue TOBI Podhaler and need to consider alternative therapies. Tell your healthcare provider about any side effect that bothers you enough to stop treatment or that does not go away.

These are not all of the possible side effects of TOBI Podhaler. For more information, ask your healthcare provider or pharmacist.

Call your doctor for medical advice about side effects. You may report side effects to FDA at 1-800-FDA-1088.

General information about the safe and effective use of TOBI Podhaler

Medicines are sometimes prescribed for purposes other than those listed in a patient information leaflet. Do not use TOBI Podhaler for a condition for which it was not prescribed. Do not give TOBI Podhaler to other people, even if they have the same problem you have. It may harm them.

This leaflet summarizes the most important information about TOBI Podhaler. If you would like more information, talk with your healthcare provider. You can ask your healthcare provider or pharmacist for information about TOBI Podhaler that was written for healthcare professionals.

For more information, go to www.TOBIPodhaler.com or call 1-877-999-TOBI (8624).

What are the ingredients in TOBI Podhaler?

Active ingredient: tobramycin

Inactive ingredients: 1,2-distearoyl-sn-glycero-3-phosphocholine (DSPC), calcium chloride, and sulfuric acid (for pH adjustment)

What is *Pseudomonas aeruginosa?*

It is a very common bacterium that infects the lungs of nearly everyone with cystic fibrosis at some time during their lives. Some people do not get this infection until later in their lives, while others get it very young. It is one of the most damaging bacteria for people with cystic fibrosis. If the infection is not properly managed, it will continue to damage your lungs causing further problems to your breathing.

T2013-21

March 2013

Instructions for Use

TOBI Podhaler

Follow the instructions below for using your TOBI Podhaler. You will breathe in (inhale) the medicine in the TOBI Podhaler capsules using the Podhaler device. If you have any questions, ask your healthcare provider or pharmacist.

Each TOBI Podhaler package contains (See Figure A):

- 4 weekly packs (28-day supply), each containing:
  - 56 capsules (7 blister cards of 8 capsules). Each blister card contains 8 TOBI Podhaler capsules (4 capsules for inhalation in the morning and 4 capsules for inhalation in the evening).
  - 1 Podhaler device and its storage case
- 1 reserve Podhaler device (to be used if needed) and its storage case

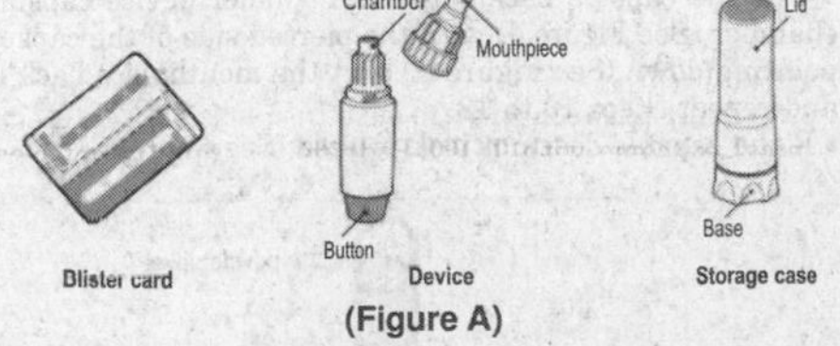

(Figure A)

Please note the following:

- **Do not** swallow TOBI Podhaler capsules. The powder in the capsule is for you to inhale using the Podhaler device.
- Only use the Podhaler device contained in this pack. **Do not** use TOBI Podhaler capsules with any other device, and **do not** use the Podhaler device to take any other medicine.
- When you start a new weekly (7 day) pack of capsules, use the new Podhaler device that is supplied in the pack and discard the used device and its case. Each Podhaler device is only used for one week (7 days).
- Always keep the TOBI Podhaler capsules in the blister card. Only remove 1 capsule at a time just before you are going to use it.
- Doses should be inhaled as close to 12 hours apart as possible and not less than 6 hours apart.
- Once in a while, very small pieces of the capsules can get into your mouth and you may be able to feel these pieces on your tongue. These small pieces will not hurt you if you swallow or inhale them.
- The reserve Podhaler device provided in the package may be used if the Podhaler device:
  - is wet, dirty, or broken
  - has been dropped
  - does not seem to be piercing the capsule properly (see Step 17)

Getting ready:

- **Wash and dry your hands completely** (See Figure B).

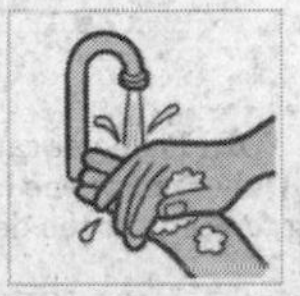

Figure B

Preparing your TOBI Podhaler dose

Step 1: Just before use, hold the base of the Podhaler device and unscrew the lid in a counter-clockwise direction (See Figure C). Set the lid aside.

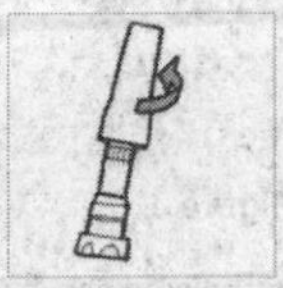

Figure C

Step 2: Stand the Podhaler device upright in the base of the case (See Figure D).

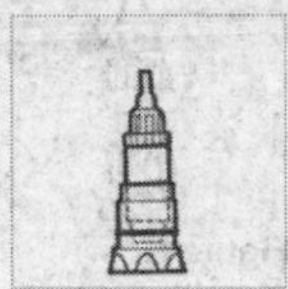

Figure D

Step 3: Hold the body of the Podhaler device and unscrew the mouthpiece in a counter-clockwise direction (See Figure E). Set the mouthpiece aside on a clean, dry surface.

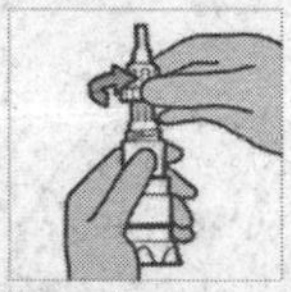

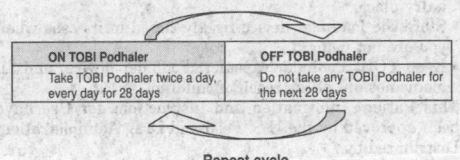

Figure E

Step 4: Take 1 blister card and tear the pre-cut lines along the length (See Figure F) then tear at the pre-cut lines along the width (See Figure G).

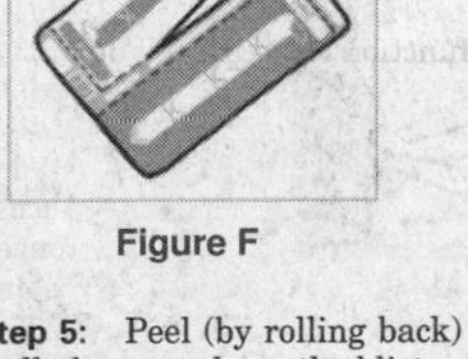

Figure F

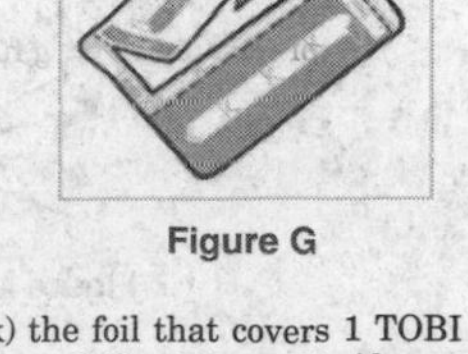

Figure G

Step 5: Peel (by rolling back) the foil that covers 1 TOBI Podhaler capsule on the blister card (See Figure H). Always hold the foil close to where you are peeling.

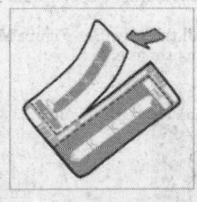

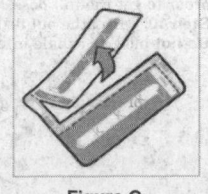

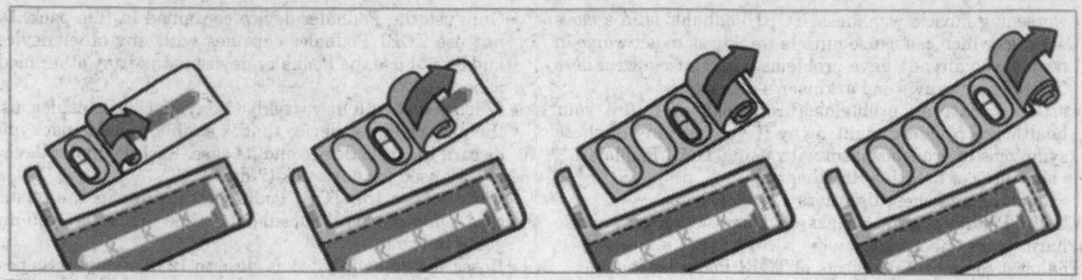
Figure I

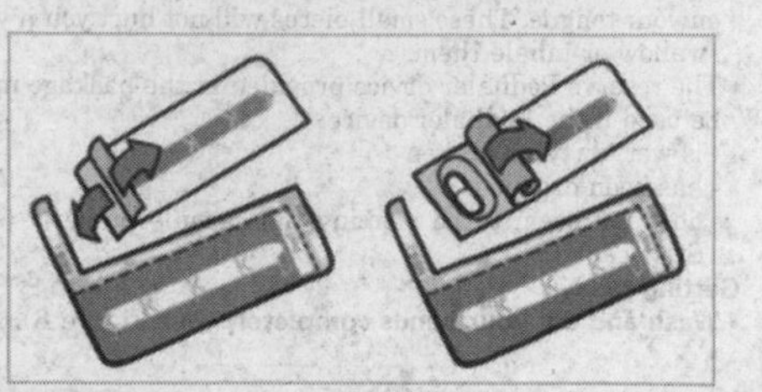
Figure H

Step 6: Take out 1 TOBI Podhaler capsule from the blister card (See Figure I). Only remove one capsule at a time just before you are going to use it in the device.
[See figure 1 above]

Step 7: Immediately, place the TOBI Podhaler capsule in the capsule chamber at the top of the Podhaler device (See Figure J). **Do not** put the capsule directly into the top of the mouthpiece.

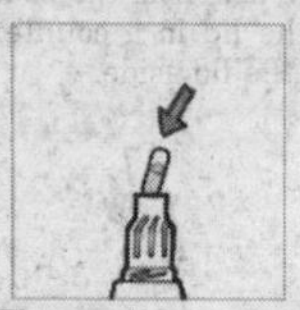
Figure J

Step 8: Put the mouthpiece back on your Podhaler device and screw the mouthpiece in a clockwise direction until it is tight (See Figure K). **Do not** overtighten.

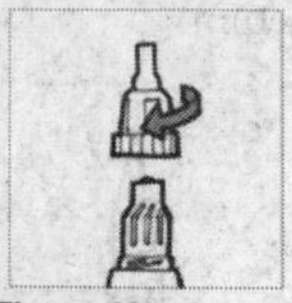
Figure K

Step 9: Hold the Podhaler device with the mouthpiece pointing down. Put your thumb on the blue button and press the blue button all the way down (See Figure L). Let go of the blue button. **Do not** press the blue button more than 1 time. The chances of the capsule breaking into pieces will be increased if the capsule is accidentally pierced more than once.

Figure L

Taking your TOBI Podhaler dose:
You will need to inhale at least twice from each capsule in order to get the full dose.

Step 10: Breathe out (exhale) all the way (See Figure M). **Do not** blow or exhale into the mouthpiece.

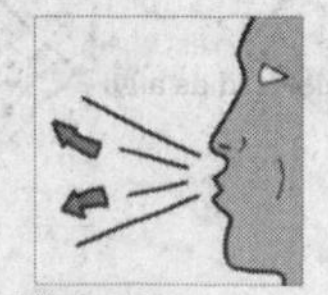
Figure M

Step 11: Place your mouth over the mouthpiece and close your lips tightly around it (See Figure N).

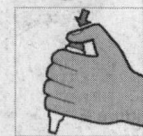

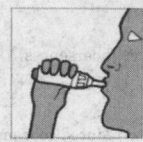
Figure N

Step 12: Inhale deeply with a single breath (See Figure O).

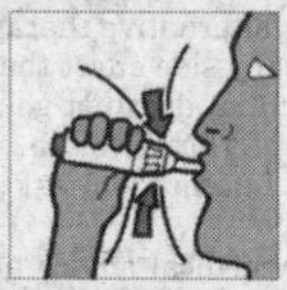
Figure O

Step 13: Remove the Podhaler device from your mouth, and hold your breath for about 5 seconds, then exhale normally away from the Podhaler device.

Step 14: Take a few normal breaths away from the Podhaler device. **Do not** blow or exhale into the mouthpiece.

Step 15: For your second inhalation, repeat steps 10 through 13 using the same capsule.

Step 16: Unscrew the mouthpiece and remove the TOBI Podhaler capsule from the capsule chamber (See Figure P).

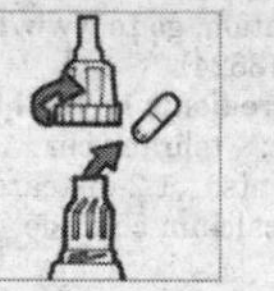

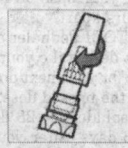
Figure P

Step 17: Look at the used capsule. It should be pierced and empty. There will be a fine coating of powder remaining on the inside of the capsule (See Figure Q). If it is pierced and empty, throw it away and go to Step 18.

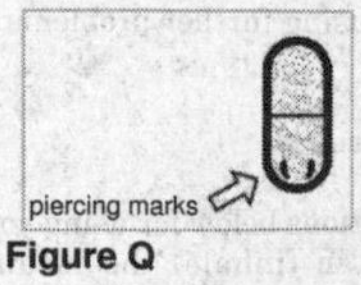

Figure Q

- If the capsule is pierced but still contains more than just a fine coating of powder (See Figure R for an example):

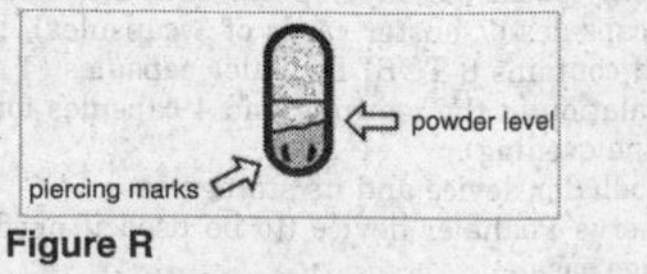

Figure R

○ Put the capsule back into the Podhaler device capsule-chamber (See Figure J) with the pierced side of the capsule pointing down (See Figure R). Put the mouthpiece back on and repeat Steps 10 to 13.

- If the capsule does not look pierced (See Figure S):

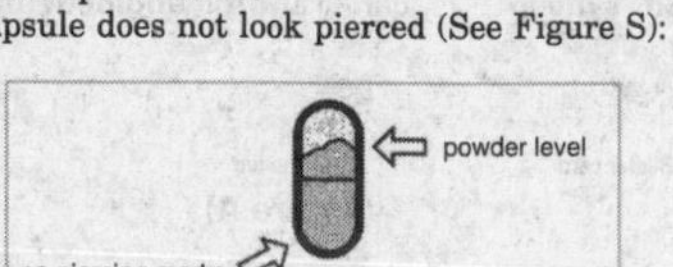

Figure S

○ Put the capsule back into the Podhaler device capsule-chamber (See Figure J). Put the mouthpiece back on and repeat Steps 9 to 17.

■ If the capsule still does not look pierced and still has some powder in it, use the reserve Podhaler device provided in the TOBI Podhaler package and repeat Steps 1 to 3, then 7 to 17.

Step 18: Repeat Steps 6 to 17 for 3 more times until your whole dose (4 capsules) has been taken (See Figure T).

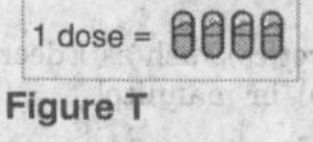

Figure T

After your TOBI Podhaler dose:

Step 19: Throw away all the empty TOBI Podhaler capsules. **Do not** store the TOBI Podhaler capsules in the Podhaler device.

Step 20: Put the mouthpiece back on to your Podhaler device and twist the mouthpiece in a clockwise direction until it is tight (See Figure K). **Do not** overtighten.

Step 21: Wipe the mouthpiece with a clean, dry cloth (See Figure U).

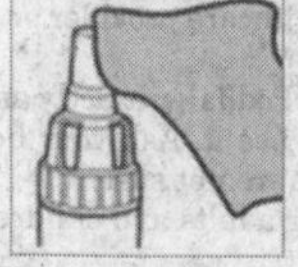
Figure U

- **Do not** wash the Podhaler device with water. Your Podhaler device needs to stay dry at all times to work the right way.

Step 22: Place your Podhaler device back in the storage case base.

Step 23: Place the lid back on the storage case base and screw the cover in a clockwise direction until it is tight (See Figure V).

Figure V

How should I store TOBI Podhaler?

- Store your Podhaler device and blister-packaged capsules at room temperature between 68°F to 77°F (20°C to 25°C).
- Keep the TOBI Podhaler capsules and Podhaler device in a dry place.
- Store the Podhaler device tightly closed in its case when you are not using it.
- Keep TOBI Podhaler capsules, Podhaler device, and all medicines out of the reach of children.

This Patient Information and Instructions for Use have been approved by the U.S. Food and Drug Administration.

Distributed by:
Novartis Pharmaceuticals Corporation
East Hanover, NJ 07936
© Novartis
T2013-22
March 2013

Shown in Product Identification Guide, page 311

XOLAIR® ℞
[zō-lər]
(omalizumab)
For injection, for subcutaneous use

The following prescribing information is based on official labeling in effect July 2013.

HIGHLIGHTS OF PRESCRIBING INFORMATION
These highlights do not include all the information needed to use Xolair safely and effectively. See full prescribing information for Xolair.
XOLAIR® [omalizumab]
For injection, for subcutaneous use
Initial U.S. Approval: 2003

WARNING: ANAPHYLAXIS
See full prescribing information for complete boxed warning
Anaphylaxis, presenting as bronchospasm, hypotension, syncope, urticaria, and/or angioedema of the throat or tongue, has been reported to occur after administration of Xolair. Anaphylaxis has occurred after the first dose of Xolair but also has occurred beyond 1 year after beginning treatment. Closely observe patients for an appropriate period of time after Xolair

administration and be prepared to manage anaphylaxis that can be life-threatening. Inform patients of the signs and symptoms of anaphylaxis and have them seek immediate medical care should symptoms occur.

RECENT MAJOR CHANGES

Indications and Usage, Pediatric Patients (Age 0 to <12) (1) 01/2010
Use in Specific Populations, Pediatric Use (Age 0 to <12) (8.4) 01/2010
Warnings and Precautions, Fever, Arthralgia, and Rash (5.6) 07/2010
Adverse Reactions, Postmarketing Experience (6.2) 07/2010

INDICATIONS AND USAGE

Xolair is indicated for:
- Moderate to severe persistent asthma in patients with a positive skin test or in vitro reactivity to a perennial aeroallergen and symptoms that are inadequately controlled with inhaled corticosteroids.

Important Limitations of use:
- Not indicated for other allergic conditions. (1)
- Not indicated for acute bronchospasm or status asthmaticus (1, 5.3)
- Not indicated for pediatric patients less than 12 years of age (1, 8.4)

DOSAGE AND ADMINISTRATION

For subcutaneous (SC) administration only.
Administer Xolair 150 to 375 mg SC every 2 or 4 weeks. (2.1)
- Determine dose (mg) and dosing frequency by serum total IgE level (IU/mL), measured before the start of treatment, and body weight (kg). See the dose determination charts (2.1)
- Divide doses of more than 150 mg among more than one injection site to limit injections to not more than 150 mg per site. (2.3)

DOSAGE FORMS AND STRENGTHS

- Lyophilized, sterile powder in a single-use 5mL vial, 150 mg (3)

CONTRAINDICATIONS

- Severe hypersensitivity reaction to Xolair or any ingredient of Xolair. (4, 5.1)

WARNINGS AND PRECAUTIONS

- Anaphylaxis—Administer only in a healthcare setting prepared to manage anaphylaxis that can be life-threatening and observe patients for an appropriate period of time after administration. (5.1)
- Malignancy— Malignancies have been observed in clinical studies. (5.2)
- Acute Asthma Symptoms—Do not use for the treatment of acute bronchospasm or status asthmaticus. (5.3)
- Corticosteroid Reductions—Do not abruptly discontinue corticosteroids upon initiation of Xolair therapy. (5.4)
- Fever, Arthralgia, and Rash— Stop Xolair if patients develop signs and symptoms similar to serum sickness (5.6)
- Eosinophilic Conditions—Be alert to eosinophilia, vasculitic rash, worsening pulmonary symptoms, cardiac complications, and/or neuropathy, especially upon reduction of oral corticosteroids. (5.5)

ADVERSE REACTIONS

In the adult and adolescent patients (≥12 years of age), the most commonly observed adverse reactions in clinical studies (≥1% more frequent in Xolair-treated patients) were arthralgia, pain (general), leg pain, fatigue, dizziness, fracture, arm pain, pruritus, dermatitis, and earache. (6.1)
To report SUSPECTED ADVERSE REACTIONS, contact Genentech at 1-888-835-2555 or FDA at 1-800-FDA-1088 or www.fda.gov/medwatch

DRUG INTERACTIONS

- No formal drug interaction studies have been performed. (7)

USE IN SPECIFIC POPULATIONS

- Pregnancy: No adequate data in humans. Xolair Pregnancy Exposure Registry available (1-866-496-5247) (8.1)

See 17 for PATIENT COUNSELING INFORMATION and Medication Guide

Revised: 07/2010

FULL PRESCRIBING INFORMATION: CONTENTS*

*** Sections or subsections omitted from the full prescribing information are not listed**

Table 1: Administration Every 4 Weeks: Xolair Doses (milligrams) Administered by Subcutaneous Injection Every 4 Weeks for Adults and Adolescents 12 Years of Age and Older

Pre-treatment Serum IgE (IU/mL)	Body Weight (kg) 30-60	> 60-70	> 70-90	> 90-150
≥ 30-100	150	150	150	300
> 100-200	300	300	300	SEE TABLE 2
> 200-300	300			
> 300-400				
> 400-500				
> 500-600				

Table 2: Administration Every 2 Weeks: Xolair Doses (milligrams) Administered by Subcutaneous Injection Every 2 Weeks for Adults and Adolescents 12 Years of Age and Older

Pre-treatment Serum IgE (IU/mL)	Body Weight (kg) 30-60	> 60-70	> 70-90	> 90-150
≥ 30-100		SEE TABLE 1		
> 100-200				225
> 200-300		225	225	300
> 300-400	225	225	300	
> 400-500	300	300	375	
> 500-600	300	375		DO NOT DOSE
> 600-700	375			

FULL PRESCRIBING INFORMATION

> WARNING: Anaphylaxis
>
> **Anaphylaxis presenting as bronchospasm, hypotension, syncope, urticaria, and/or angioedema of the throat or tongue, has been reported to occur after administration of Xolair. Anaphylaxis has occurred as early as after the first dose of Xolair, but also has occurred beyond 1 year after beginning regularly administered treatment. Because of the risk of anaphylaxis, observe patients closely for an appropriate period of time after Xolair administration. Health care providers administering Xolair should be prepared to manage anaphylaxis that can be life-threatening. Inform patients of the signs and symptoms of anaphylaxis and instruct them to seek immediate medical care should symptoms occur [*see Warnings and Precautions (5.1)*].**

1 INDICATIONS AND USAGE

Xolair (omalizumab) is indicated for adults and adolescents (12 years of age and above) with moderate to severe persistent asthma who have a positive skin test or in vitro reactivity to a perennial aeroallergen and whose symptoms are inadequately controlled with inhaled corticosteroids.
Xolair has been shown to decrease the incidence of asthma exacerbations in these patients.
Important Limitations of Use
- Xolair is not indicated for treatment of other allergic conditions.
- Xolair is not indicated for the relief of acute bronchospasm or status asthmaticus.
- Xolair is not indicated for use in pediatric patients less than 12 years of age.

2 DOSAGE AND ADMINISTRATION

2.1 Dosing

Administer Xolair (omalizumab) 150 to 375 mg by subcutaneous (SC) injection every 2 or 4 weeks. Determine doses (mg) and dosing frequency by serum total IgE level (IU/mL), measured before the start of treatment, and body weight (kg). *See the dose determination charts below (Table 1 and Table 2) for appropriate dose assignment.*
Periodically reassess the need for continued therapy based upon the patient's disease severity and level of asthma control.
[See table 1 above]
[See table 2 above]

2.2 Dosing Adjustments

Adjust doses for significant changes in body weight (see Table 1 and Table 2).
Total IgE levels are elevated during treatment and remain elevated for up to one year after the discontinuation of treatment. Therefore, re-testing of IgE levels during Xolair treatment cannot be used as a guide for dose determination.
- Interruptions lasting less than one year: Dose based on serum IgE levels obtained at the initial dose determination.
- Interruptions lasting one year or more: Re-test total serum IgE levels for dose determination.

2.3 Preparation and Administration

Prepare Xolair for subcutaneous injection using Sterile Water for Injection (SWFI), USP, ONLY. Each vial of Xolair is for single use only and contains no preservatives.

Reconstitution
The lyophilized product takes 15-20 minutes to dissolve. The fully reconstituted product will appear clear or slightly opalescent and it is acceptable if there are a few small bubbles or foam around the edge of the vial. The reconstituted product is somewhat viscous; in order to obtain the full 1.2 mL dose, ALL OF THE PRODUCT MUST BE WITHDRAWN from the vial before expelling any air or excess solution from the syringe.
Use the solution within 8 hours following reconstitution when stored in the vial at 2-8°C (36-46°F), or within 4 hours of reconstitution when stored at room temperature. Reconstituted Xolair vials should be protected from sunlight.
Preparation
STEP 1: Draw 1.4 mL of SWFI, USP into a 3 mL syringe equipped with a 1 inch, 18-gauge needle.
STEP 2: Place the vial upright on a flat surface and using standard aseptic technique, insert the needle and inject the SWFI, USP directly onto the product.
STEP 3: Keeping the vial upright, gently swirl the upright vial for approximately 1 minute to evenly wet the powder. Do not shake.
STEP 4: After completing STEP 3, gently swirl the vial for 5-10 seconds approximately every 5 minutes in order to dissolve any remaining solids. There should be no visible gel like particles in the solution. Do not use if foreign particles are present.
Note: If it takes longer than 20 minutes to dissolve completely, repeat STEP 4 until there are no visible gel-like particles in the solution. Do not use if the contents of the vial do not dissolve completely by 40 minutes.
STEP 5: Invert the vial for 15 seconds in order to allow the solution to drain toward the stopper. Using a new 3 mL syringe equipped with a 1-inch, 18-gauge needle, insert the needle into the inverted vial. Position the needle tip at the very bottom of the solution in the vial stopper when drawing the solution into the syringe. Before removing the needle from the vial, pull the plunger all the way back to the end of the syringe barrel in order to remove all of the solution from the inverted vial.
STEP 6: Replace the 18-gauge needle with a 25-gauge needle for subcutaneous injection.
STEP 7: Expel air, large bubbles, and any excess solution in order to obtain the required 1.2 mL dose. A thin layer of small bubbles may remain at the top of the solution in the syringe.
Administration
Administer Xolair by subcutaneous injection. The injection may take 5-10 seconds to administer because the solution is slightly viscous. Each vial delivers 1.2 mL (150 mg) of Xolair. Do not administer more than 150 mg per injection site. Divide doses of more than 150 mg among two or more injection sites. (Table 3).

Table 3: Number of Injections and Total Injection Volumes

Xolair Dose (mg)	Number of Injections	Total Volume Injected (mL)
150	1	1.2
225	2	1.8
300	2	2.4
375	3	3.0

3 DOSAGE FORMS AND STRENGTHS
150 mg of omalizumab as lyophilized, sterile powder in a single-use 5 mL vial.

4 CONTRAINDICATIONS
The use of Xolair is contraindicated in the following:
Severe hypersensitivity reaction to Xolair or any ingredient of Xolair [*see Warnings and Precautions (5.1)*].

5 WARNINGS AND PRECAUTIONS
5.1 Anaphylaxis
Anaphylaxis has been reported to occur after administration of Xolair in premarketing clinical trials and in postmarketing spontaneous reports. Signs and symptoms in these reported cases have included bronchospasm, hypotension, syncope, urticaria, and/or angioedema of the throat or tongue. Some of these events have been life-threatening. In premarketing clinical trials the frequency of anaphylaxis attributed to Xolair use was estimated to be 0.1%. In postmarketing spontaneous reports, the frequency of anaphylaxis attributed to Xolair use was estimated to be at least 0.2% of patients based on an estimated exposure of about 57,300 patients from June 2003 through December 2006. Anaphylaxis has occurred as early as after the first dose of Xolair, but also has occurred beyond one year after beginning regularly scheduled treatment.
Administer Xolair only in a healthcare setting by healthcare providers prepared to manage anaphylaxis that can be life-threatening. Observe patients closely for an appropriate period of time after administration of Xolair, taking into account the time to onset of anaphylaxis seen in premarketing clinical trials and postmarketing spontaneous reports [*see Adverse Reactions (6)*]. Inform patients of the signs and symptoms of anaphylaxis, and instruct them to seek immediate medical care should signs or symptoms occur.
Discontinue Xolair in patients who experience a severe hypersensitivity reaction [*see Contraindications (4)*].

5.2 Malignancy
Malignant neoplasms were observed in 20 of 4127 (0.5%) Xolair-treated patients compared with 5 of 2236 (0.2%) control patients in clinical studies of adults and adolescents (≥ 12 years of age) with asthma and other allergic disorders. The observed malignancies in Xolair-treated patients were a variety of types, with breast, non-melanoma skin, prostate, melanoma, and parotid occurring more than once, and five other types occurring once each. The majority of patients were observed for less than 1 year. The impact of longer exposure to Xolair or use in patients at higher risk for malignancy (e.g., elderly, current smokers) is not known [*see Adverse Reactions (6)*].

5.3 Acute Asthma Symptoms
Xolair has not been shown to alleviate asthma exacerbations acutely. Do not use Xolair to treat acute bronchospasm or status asthmaticus.

5.4 Corticosteroid Reduction
Do not discontinue systemic or inhaled corticosteroids abruptly upon initiation of Xolair therapy. Decrease corticosteroids gradually under the direct supervision of a physician.

5.5 Eosinophilic Conditions
In rare cases, patients with asthma on therapy with Xolair may present with serious systemic eosinophilia sometimes presenting with clinical features of vasculitis consistent with Churg-Strauss syndrome, a condition which is often treated with systemic corticosteroid therapy. These events usually, but not always, have been associated with the reduction of oral corticosteroid therapy. Physicians should be alert to eosinophilia, vasculitic rash, worsening pulmonary symptoms, cardiac complications, and/or neuropathy presenting in their patients. A causal association between Xolair and these underlying conditions has not been established.

5.6 Fever, Arthralgia, and Rash
In post-approval use, some patients have experienced a constellation of signs and symptoms including arthritis/arthralgia, rash (urticaria or other forms), fever and lymphadenopathy with an onset 1 to 5 days after the first or subsequent injections of Xolair. These signs and symptoms have recurred after additional doses in some patients. Although circulating immune complexes or a skin biopsy consistent with a Type III reaction were not seen with these cases, these signs and symptoms are similar to those seen in patients with serum sickness. Physicians should stop Xolair if a patient develops this constellation of signs and symptoms. [*see Adverse Reactions, Postmarketing Experience (6.2)*]

5.7 Parasitic (Helminth) Infection
Monitor patients at high risk of geohelminth infection while on Xolair therapy. Insufficient data are available to determine the length of monitoring required for geohelminth infections after stopping Xolair treatment.
In a one-year clinical trial conducted in Brazil in patients at high risk for geohelminthic infections (roundworm, hookworm, whipworm, threadworm), 53% (36/68) of Xolair-treated patients experienced an infection, as diagnosed by standard stool examination, compared to 42% (29/69) of placebo controls. The point estimate of the odds ratio for infection was 1.96, with a 95% confidence interval (0.88, 4.36) indicating that in this study a patient who had an infection was anywhere from 0.88 to 4.36 times as likely to have received Xolair than a patient who did not have an infection. Response to appropriate anti-geohelminth treatment of infection as measured by stool egg counts was not different between treatment groups.

5.8 Laboratory Tests
Serum total IgE levels increase following administration of Xolair due to formation of Xolair:IgE complexes [*see Clinical Pharmacology (12.2)*]. Elevated serum total IgE levels may persist for up to 1 year following discontinuation of Xolair. Do not use serum total IgE levels obtained less than 1 year following discontinuation to reassess the dosing regimen because these levels may not reflect steady state free IgE levels.

6 ADVERSE REACTIONS
Use of Xolair has been associated with:
• Anaphylaxis [*see Boxed Warning and Warnings and Precautions (5.1)*]
• Malignancies [*see Warnings and Precautions (5.2)*]
Anaphylaxis was reported in 3 of 3507 (0.1%) patients in clinical trials. Anaphylaxis occurred with the first dose of Xolair in two patients and with the fourth dose in one patient. The time to onset of anaphylaxis was 90 minutes after administration in two patients and 2 hours after administration in one patient. In clinical trials the observed incidence of malignancy among Xolair-treated patients (0.5%) was numerically higher than among patients in control groups (0.2%).

6.1 Clinical Trials Experience
Adult and Adolescent Patients 12 years of Age and Older
The data described below reflect Xolair exposure for 2076 adult and adolescent patients ages 12 and older, including 1687 patients exposed for six months and 555 exposed for one year or more, in either placebo-controlled or other controlled asthma studies. The mean age of patients receiving Xolair was 42 years, with 134 patients 65 years of age or older; 60% were women, and 85% Caucasian. Patients received Xolair 150 to 375 mg every 2 or 4 weeks or, for patients assigned to control groups, standard therapy with or without a placebo. Because clinical studies are conducted under widely varying conditions, adverse reaction rates observed in the clinical studies of one drug cannot be directly compared with rates in the clinical studies of another drug and may not reflect the rates observed in medical practice.
The adverse events most frequently resulting in clinical intervention (e.g., discontinuation of Xolair, or the need for concomitant medication to treat an adverse event) were injection site reaction (45%), viral infections (23%), upper respiratory tract infection (20%), sinusitis (16%), headache (15%), and pharyngitis (11%). These events were observed at similar rates in Xolair-treated patients and control patients.
Table 4 shows adverse reactions from four placebo-controlled asthma studies that occurred ≥ 1% and more frequently in patients receiving Xolair than in those receiving placebo. Adverse events were classified using preferred terms from the International Medical Nomenclature (IMN) dictionary. Injection site reactions were recorded separately from the reporting of other adverse events and are described following Table 4.

Table 4: Adverse Reactions ≥ 1% More Frequent in Xolair-Treated Adult or Adolescent Patients 12 years of age and older: Four placebo-controlled asthma studies

Adverse reaction	Xolair n = 738 (%)	Placebo n = 717 (%)
Body as a whole		
Pain	7	5
Fatigue	3	2
Musculoskeletal system		
Arthralgia	8	6
Fracture	2	1
Leg pain	4	2
Arm pain	2	1
Nervous system		
Dizziness	3	2
Skin and appendages		
Pruritus	2	1
Dermatitis	2	1
Special senses		
Earache	2	1

There were no differences in the incidence of adverse reactions based on age (among patients under 65), gender or race.

Injection Site Reactions
Injection site reactions of any severity occurred at a rate of 45% in Xolair-treated patients compared with 43% in placebo-treated patients. The types of injection site reactions included: bruising, redness, warmth, burning, stinging, itching, hive formation, pain, indurations, mass, and inflammation.
Severe injection site reactions occurred more frequently in Xolair-treated patients compared with patients in the placebo group (12% versus 9%).
The majority of injection site reactions occurred within 1 hour-post injection, lasted less than 8 days, and generally decreased in frequency at subsequent dosing visits.

Immunogenicity
Antibodies to Xolair were detected in approximately 1/1723 (< 0.1%) of patients treated with Xolair. The data reflect the percentage of patients whose test results were considered positive for antibodies to Xolair in an ELISA assay and are highly dependent on the sensitivity and specificity of the assay. Additionally, the observed incidence of antibody positivity in the assay may be influenced by several factors including sample handling, timing of sample collection, concomitant medications, and underlying disease. Therefore, comparison of the incidence of antibodies to Xolair with the incidence of antibodies to other products may be misleading.

6.2 Postmarketing Experience
The following adverse reactions have been identified during postapproval use of Xolair in adult and adolescent patients

12 years of age and older. Because these reactions are reported voluntarily from a population of uncertain size, it is not always possible to reliably estimate their frequency or establish a causal relationship to drug exposure.

Anaphylaxis: Based on spontaneous reports and an estimated exposure of about 57,300 patients from June 2003 through December 2006, the frequency of anaphylaxis attributed to Xolair use was estimated to be at least 0.2% of patients. Diagnostic criteria of anaphylaxis were skin or mucosal tissue involvement, and, either airway compromise, and/or reduced blood pressure with or without associated symptoms, and a temporal relationship to Xolair administration with no other identifiable cause. Signs and symptoms in these reported cases included bronchospasm, hypotension, syncope, urticaria, angioedema of the throat or tongue, dyspnea, cough, chest tightness, and/or cutaneous angioedema. Pulmonary involvement was reported in 89% of the cases. Hypotension or syncope was reported in 14% of cases. Fifteen percent of the reported cases resulted in hospitalization. A previous history of anaphylaxis unrelated to Xolair was reported in 24% of the cases.

Of the reported cases of anaphylaxis attributed to Xolair, 39% occurred with the first dose, 19% occurred with the second dose, 10% occurred with the third dose, and the rest after subsequent doses. One case occurred after 39 doses (after 19 months of continuous therapy, anaphylaxis occurred when treatment was restarted following a 3 month gap). The time to onset of anaphylaxis in these cases was up to 30 minutes in 35%, greater than 30 and up to 60 minutes in 16%, greater than 60 and up to 90 minutes in 2%, greater than 90 and up to 120 minutes in 6%, greater than 2 hours and up to 6 hours in 5%, greater than 6 hours and up to 12 hours in 14%, greater than 12 hours and up to 24 hours in 8%, and greater than 24 hours and up to 4 days in 5%. In 9% of cases the times to onset were unknown.

Twenty-three patients who experienced anaphylaxis were rechallenged with Xolair and 18 patients had a recurrence of similar symptoms of anaphylaxis. In addition, anaphylaxis occurred upon rechallenge with Xolair in 4 patients who previously experienced urticaria only.

Eosinophilic Conditions: Eosinophilic conditions have been reported [*see Warnings and Precautions (5.5)*].

Fever, Arthralgia, and Rash: A constellation of signs and symptoms including arthritis/arthralgia, rash (urticaria or other forms), fever and lymphadenopathy similar to serum sickness have been reported in postapproval use of Xolair [*see Warnings and Precautions (5.6)*]

Hematologic: Severe thrombocytopenia has been reported.

Skin: Hair loss has been reported.

7 DRUG INTERACTIONS

No formal drug interaction studies have been performed with Xolair. The concomitant use of Xolair and allergen immunotherapy has not been evaluated.

8 USE IN SPECIFIC POPULATIONS

8.1 Pregnancy

Teratogenic Effects: Pregnancy Category B

There are no adequate and well-controlled studies of Xolair in pregnant women. Reproduction studies have been performed in Cynomolgus monkeys at subcutaneous doses up to 10 times the maximum recommended human dose on a mg/kg basis and have revealed no evidence of impaired fertility or harm to the fetus due to Xolair. Because animal reproduction studies are not always predictive of human response, administer Xolair during pregnancy only if clearly needed [*see Nonclinical Toxicology (13.2)*].

Pregnancy Exposure Registry

To monitor outcomes of pregnant women exposed to Xolair, including women who are exposed to at least one dose of Xolair within 8 weeks prior to conception or any time during pregnancy, a pregnancy exposure registry has been established. Encourage patients to call 1-866-4XOLAIR (1-866-496-5247) to enroll in the Xolair Pregnancy Exposure Registry. Call this number to obtain further information about this registry.

8.3 Nursing Mothers

There are no data from controlled clinical trials on the use of Xolair by nursing mothers. It is not known whether Xolair is excreted in human breast milk. However, IgG is excreted in human breast milk and therefore it is expected that Xolair will be excreted in human breast milk. The potential for Xolair absorption or harm to the infant is unknown; therefore caution should be exercised when Xolair is administered to a nursing woman.

The excretion of omalizumab in milk was evaluated in female Cynomolgus monkeys at a subcutaneous dose approximately 10 times the maximum recommended human dose on a mg/kg basis. Neonatal plasma levels of omalizumab after in utero exposure and 28 days of nursing were between 11% and 94% of the maternal plasma level. Milk levels of omalizumab were 1.5% of maternal blood concentration [*see Nonclinical Toxicology (13.2)*].

8.4 Pediatric Use

Safety and effectiveness of Xolair were evaluated in 2 studies in 926 (Xolair 624; placebo 302) asthma patients 6 to <12 years of age. One study was a pivotal study of similar design and conduct to that of adult and adolescent studies 1 and 2 [*see Clinical Trials (14)*]. The other study was primarily a safety study and included evaluation of efficacy as a secondary outcome. In the pivotal study, Xolair-treated patients had a statistically significant reduction in the rate of exacerbations (exacerbation was defined as worsening of asthma that required treatment with systemic corticosteroids or a doubling of the baseline ICS dose), but other efficacy variables such as nocturnal symptom scores, beta-agonist use, and measures of airflow (FEV_1) were not significantly different in Xolair-treated patients compared to placebo. Considering the risk of anaphylaxis and malignancy seen in Xolair-treated patients ≥12 years old and the modest efficacy of Xolair in the pivotal pediatric study, the risk-benefit assessment does not support the use of Xolair in patients 6 to <12 years of age. Although patients treated with Xolair in these two studies did not develop anaphylaxis or malignancy, the studies are not adequate to address these concerns because patients with a history of anaphylaxis or malignancy were excluded, and the duration of exposure and sample size were not large enough to exclude these risks in patients 6 to <12 years of age. Furthermore, there is no reason to expect that younger pediatric patients would not be at risk of anaphylaxis and malignancy seen in adult and adolescent patients with Xolair. [*see Warnings and Precautions (5.1) (5.2); and Adverse Reactions (6)*].

Studies in patients 0-5 years of age were not required because of the safety concerns of anaphylaxis and malignancy associated with the use of Xolair in adults and adolescents.

8.5 Geriatric Use

In clinical trials 134 patients 65 years of age or older were treated with Xolair. Although there were no apparent age-related differences observed in these studies, the number of patients aged 65 and over is not sufficient to determine whether they respond differently from younger patients.

10 OVERDOSAGE

The maximum tolerated dose of Xolair has not been determined. Single intravenous doses of up to 4000 mg have been administered to patients without evidence of dose limiting toxicities. The highest cumulative dose administered to patients was 44,000 mg over a 20 week period, which was not associated with toxicities.

11 DESCRIPTION

Xolair (omalizumab) is a recombinant DNA-derived humanized IgG1κ monoclonal antibody that selectively binds to human immunoglobulin E (IgE). The antibody has a molecular weight of approximately 149 kiloDaltons. Xolair is produced by a Chinese hamster ovary cell suspension culture in a nutrient medium containing the antibiotic gentamicin. Gentamicin is not detectable in the final product.

Xolair is a sterile, white, preservative free, lyophilized powder contained in a single use vial that is reconstituted with Sterile Water for Injection (SWFI), USP, and administered as a subcutaneous (SC) injection. Each 202.5 mg vial of omalizumab also contains L-histidine (1.8 mg), L-histidine hydrochloride monohydrate (2.8 mg), polysorbate 20 (0.5 mg) and sucrose (145.5 mg) and is designed to deliver 150 mg of omalizumab in 1.2 mL after reconstitution with 1.4 mL SWFI, USP.

12 CLINICAL PHARMACOLOGY

12.1 Mechanism of Action

Omalizumab inhibits the binding of IgE to the high-affinity IgE receptor (FcεRI) on the surface of mast cells and basophils. Reduction in surface-bound IgE on FcεRI-bearing cells limits the degree of release of mediators of the allergic response. Treatment with Xolair also reduces the number of FcεRI receptors on basophils in atopic patients.

12.2 Pharmacodynamics

In clinical studies, serum free IgE levels were reduced in a dose dependent manner within 1 hour following the first dose and maintained between doses. Mean serum free IgE decrease was greater than 96% using recommended doses. Serum total IgE levels (i.e., bound and unbound) increased after the first dose due to the formation of omalizumab:IgE complexes, which have a slower elimination rate compared with free IgE. At 16 weeks after the first dose, average serum total IgE levels were five-fold higher compared with pre-treatment when using standard assays. After discontinuation of Xolair dosing, the Xolair-induced increase in total IgE and decrease in free IgE were reversible, with no observed rebound in IgE levels after drug washout. Total IgE levels did not return to pre-treatment levels for up to one year after discontinuation of Xolair.

12.3 Pharmacokinetics

After SC administration, omalizumab is absorbed with an average absolute bioavailability of 62%. Following a single SC dose in adult and adolescent patients with asthma, omalizumab was absorbed slowly, reaching peak serum concentrations after an average of 7-8 days. The pharmacokinetics of omalizumab are linear at doses greater than 0.5 mg/kg. Following multiple doses of Xolair, areas under the serum concentration-time curve from Day 0 to Day 14 at steady state were up to 6-fold of those after the first dose.

In vitro, omalizumab forms complexes of limited size with IgE. Precipitating complexes and complexes larger than 1 million daltons in molecular weight are not observed in vitro or in vivo. Tissue distribution studies in Cynomolgus monkeys showed no specific uptake of ^{125}I-omalizumab by any organ or tissue. The apparent volume of distribution in patients following SC administration was 78 ± 32 mL/kg.

Clearance of omalizumab involves IgG clearance processes as well as clearance via specific binding and complex formation with its target ligand, IgE. Liver elimination of IgG includes degradation in the liver reticuloendothelial system (RES) and endothelial cells. Intact IgG is also excreted in bile. In studies with mice and monkeys, omalizumab:IgE complexes were eliminated by interactions with Fcγ receptors within the RES at rates that were generally faster than IgG clearance. In asthma patients omalizumab serum elimination half-life averaged 26 days, with apparent clearance averaging 2.4 ± 1.1 mL/kg/day. In addition, doubling body weight approximately doubled apparent clearance.

Special Populations

The population pharmacokinetics of omalizumab were analyzed to evaluate the effects of demographic characteristics. Analyses of these data suggest that no dose adjustments are necessary for age (12-76 years), race, ethnicity, or gender.

13 NONCLINICAL TOXICOLOGY

13.1 Carcinogenesis, Mutagenesis, Impairment of Fertility

No long-term studies have been performed in animals to evaluate the carcinogenic potential of Xolair.

No evidence of mutagenic activity was observed in Ames tests using six different strains of bacteria with and without metabolic activation at omalizumab concentrations up to 5000 μg/mL.

There were no effects on fertility and reproductive performance in male and female Cynomolgus monkeys that received Xolair at subcutaneous doses up to 75 mg/kg/week (approximately 5 times the maximum recommended human dose on an AUC basis).

13.2 Animal Toxicology and/or Pharmacology

Reproductive Toxicology Studies:

Reproductive studies have been performed in Cynomolgus monkeys at subcutaneous doses up to 75 mg/kg (approximately 10 times the maximum recommended human dose on a mg/kg basis) and have revealed no evidence of maternal toxicity, embryotoxicity, or teratogenicity when administered throughout organogenesis and did not elicit adverse effects on fetal or neonatal growth when administered throughout late gestation, delivery and nursing. IgG molecules are known to cross the placental barrier [*see Use in Specific Populations (8.1)*].

Lactation Studies:

The excretion of omalizumab in milk was evaluated in female Cynomolgus monkeys receiving a subcutaneous dose of 75 mg/kg/week (approximately 10 times the maximum recommended human dose on a mg/kg basis). Neonatal plasma levels of omalizumab after in utero exposure and 28 days of nursing were between 11% and 94% of the maternal plasma level. Milk levels of Xolair were 1.5% of maternal blood concentration. [*see Use in Specific Population (8.3)*].

14 CLINICAL STUDIES

Adult and Adolescent Patients 12 Years of Age and Older

The safety and efficacy of Xolair were evaluated in three randomized, double-blind, placebo-controlled, multicenter trials.

The trials enrolled patients 12 to 76 years old, with moderate to severe persistent (NHLBI criteria) asthma for at least one year, and a positive skin test reaction to a perennial aeroallergen. In all trials, Xolair dosing was based on body weight and baseline serum total IgE concentration. All patients were required to have a baseline IgE between 30 and 700 IU/mL and body weight not more than 150 kg. Patients were treated according to a dosing table to administer at least 0.016 mg/kg/IU (IgE/mL) of Xolair or a matching volume of placebo over each 4-week period. The maximum Xolair dose per 4 weeks was 750 mg.

In all three studies an exacerbation was defined as a worsening of asthma that required treatment with systemic corticosteroids or a doubling of the baseline ICS dose. Most exacerbations were managed in the out-patient setting and the majority were treated with systemic steroids. Hospitalization rates were not significantly different between Xolair and placebo-treated patients; however, the overall hospitalization rate was small. Among those patients who experienced an exacerbation, the distribution of exacerbation severity was similar between treatment groups.

Table 5: Frequency of Asthma Exacerbations per Patient by Phase in Studies 1 and 2

	Stable Steroid Phase (16 wks)			
	Study 1		Study 2	
Exacerbations per patient	Xolair N = 268 (%)	Placebo N = 257 (%)	Xolair N = 274 (%)	Placebo N = 272 (%)
0	85.8	76.7	87.6	69.9
1	11.9	16.7	11.3	25.0
≥ 2	2.2	6.6	1.1	5.1
p-Value	0.005		< 0.001	
Mean number exacerbations/patient	0.2	0.3	0.1	0.4
	Steroid Reduction Phase (12 wks)			
Exacerbations per patient	Xolair N = 268 (%)	Placebo N = 257 (%)	Xolair N = 274 (%)	Placebo N = 272 (%)
0	78.7	67.7	83.9	70.2
1	19.0	28.4	14.2	26.1
≥ 2	2.2	3.9	1.8	3.7
p-Value	0.004		< 0.001	
Mean number exacerbations/patient	0.2	0.4	0.2	0.3

Table 6: Asthma Symptoms and Pulmonary Function During Stable Steroid Phase of Study 1

	Xolair N = 268*		Placebo N = 257*	
Endpoint	Mean Baseline	Median Change (Baseline to Wk 16)	Mean Baseline	Median Change (Baseline to Wk 16)
Total asthma symptom score	4.3	-1.5†	4.2	-1.1†
Nocturnal asthma score	1.2	-0.4†	1.1	-0.2†
Daytime asthma score	2.3	-0.9†	2.3	-0.6†
FEV_1 % predicted	68	3†	68	0†

Asthma symptom scale: total score from 0 (least) to 9 (most); nocturnal and daytime scores from 0 (least) to 4 (most symptoms).

*Number of patients available for analysis ranges 255-258 in the Xolair group and 238-239 in the placebo group.

†Comparison of Xolair versus placebo ($p < 0.05$).

Table 7: Percentage of Patients with Asthma Exacerbations by Subgroup and Phase in Study 3

	Stable Steroid Phase (16 wks)			
	Inhaled Only		Oral + Inhaled	
	Xolair N = 126	Placebo N = 120	Xolair N = 50	Placebo N = 45
% Patients with ≥ 1 exacerbations	15.9	15.0	32.0	22.2
Difference (95% CI)	0.9 (-9.7, 13.7)		9.8 (-10.5, 31.4)	
	Steroid Reduction Phase (16 wks)			
	Xolair N = 126	Placebo N = 120	Xolair N = 50	Placebo N = 45
% Patients with ≥ 1 exacerbations	22.2	26.7	42.0	42.2
Difference (95% CI)	-4.4 (-17.6, 7.4)		-0.2 (-22.4, 20.1)	

Studies 1 and 2

At screening, patients in Studies 1 and 2 had a forced expiratory volume in one second (FEV_1) between 40% and 80% predicted. All patients had a FEV_1 improvement of at least 12% following beta$_2$-agonist administration. All patients were symptomatic and were being treated with inhaled corticosteroids (ICS) and short acting beta$_2$-agonists. Patients receiving other concomitant controller medications were excluded, and initiation of additional controller medications while on study was prohibited. Patients currently smoking were excluded.

Each study was comprised of a run-in period to achieve a stable conversion to a common ICS (beclomethasone dipropionate), followed by randomization to Xolair or placebo. Patients received Xolair for 16 weeks with an unchanged corticosteroid dose unless an acute exacerbation necessitated an increase. Patients then entered an ICS reduction phase of 12 weeks during which ICS dose reduction was attempted in a step-wise manner.

The distribution of the number of asthma exacerbations per patient in each group during a study was analyzed separately for the stable steroid and steroid-reduction periods.

In both Studies 1 and 2 the number of exacerbations per patient was reduced in patients treated with Xolair compared with placebo (Table 5).

Measures of airflow (FEV_1) and asthma symptoms were also evaluated in these studies. The clinical relevance of the treatment-associated differences is unknown. Results from the stable steroid phase Study 1 are shown in Table 6. Results from the stable steroid phase of Study 2 and the steroid reduction phases of both Studies 1 and 2 were similar to those presented in Table 6.

[See table 5 at left]

[See table 6 below]

Study 3

In Study 3, there was no restriction on screening FEV_1, and unlike Studies 1 and 2, long-acting beta$_2$-agonists were allowed. Patients were receiving at least 1000 µg/day fluticasone propionate and a subset was also receiving oral corticosteroids. Patients receiving other concomitant controller medications were excluded, and initiation of additional controller medications while on study was prohibited. Patients currently smoking were excluded.

The study was comprised of a run-in period to achieve a stable conversion to a common ICS (fluticasone propionate), followed by randomization to Xolair or placebo. Patients were stratified by use of ICS-only or ICS with concomitant use of oral steroids. Patients received Xolair for 16 weeks with an unchanged corticosteroid dose unless an acute exacerbation necessitated an increase. Patients then entered an ICS reduction phase of 16 weeks during which ICS or oral steroid dose reduction was attempted in a step-wise manner.

The number of exacerbations in patients treated with Xolair was similar to that in placebo-treated patients (Table 7). The absence of an observed treatment effect may be related to differences in the patient population compared with Studies 1 and 2, study sample size, or other factors.

[See table 7 below]

In all three of the studies, a reduction of asthma exacerbations was not observed in the Xolair-treated patients who had FEV_1 > 80% at the time of randomization. Reductions in exacerbations were not seen in patients who required oral steroids as maintenance therapy.

Pediatric Patients 6 to < 12 Years of Age

Clinical studies with Xolair in pediatric patients 6 to 11 years of age have been conducted [*see Use in Specific Populations (8.4)*]

Pediatric Patients <6 Years of Age

Clinical studies have with Xolair in pediatric patients less than 6 years of age have not been conducted [*see Use in Specific Populations (8.4)*]

16 HOW SUPPLIED/STORAGE AND HANDLING

Xolair (omalizumab) is supplied as a lyophilized, sterile powder in a single-use, 5 mL vial without preservatives. Each vial delivers 150 mg of Xolair upon reconstitution with 1.4 mL SWFI, USP. Each carton contains one single-use vial of Xolair® (omalizumab) NDC 50242-040-62.

Xolair should be shipped at controlled ambient temperature (≤ 30°C [≤ 86°F]). Store Xolair under refrigerated conditions 2-8°C (36-46°F). Do not use beyond the expiration date stamped on carton.

Use the solution for subcutaneous administration within 8 hours following reconstitution when stored in the vial at 2-8°C (36-46°F), or within 4 hours of reconstitution when stored at room temperature.

Reconstituted Xolair vials should be protected from direct sunlight.

17 PATIENT COUNSELING INFORMATION

[*See Medication Guide*]

17.1 Information for Patients

Provide and instruct patients to read the accompanying Medication Guide before starting treatment and before each subsequent treatment. The complete text of the Medication Guide is reprinted at the end of this document.

Inform patients of the risk of life-threatening anaphylaxis with Xolair including the following points [*see Warnings and Precautions (5.1)*]:

- There have been reports of anaphylaxis up to 4 days after administration of Xolair
- Xolair should only be administered in a healthcare setting by healthcare providers.
- Patients should be closely observed following administration
- Patients should be informed of the signs and symptoms of anaphylaxis
- Patients should be instructed to seek immediate medical care should such signs or symptoms occur

Instruct patients receiving Xolair not to decrease the dose of, or stop taking any other asthma medications unless otherwise instructed by their physician. Inform patients that they may not see immediate improvement in their asthma after beginning Xolair therapy.

Pregnancy Exposure Registry

Encourage pregnant women exposed to Xolair to enroll in the Xolair Pregnancy Exposure Registry [1-866-4XOLAIR (1-866-496-5247)] (8.1)

MEDICATION GUIDE
XOLAIR®
(omalizumab)
IMPORTANT: XOLAIR SHOULD ALWAYS BE INJECTED IN YOUR DOCTOR'S OFFICE.

WHAT IS THE MOST IMPORTANT INFORMATION I SHOULD KNOW ABOUT XOLAIR?

A severe allergic reaction called anaphylaxis has happened in some patients after they received Xolair. Anaphylaxis is a life-threatening condition and can lead to death so get emergency medical treatment right away if symptoms occur.

Signs and Symptoms of anaphylaxis include:
- wheezing, shortness of breath, cough, chest tightness, or trouble breathing
- low blood pressure, dizziness, fainting, rapid or weak heartbeat, anxiety, or feeling of "impending doom"
- flushing, itching, hives, or feeling warm
- swelling of the throat or tongue, throat tightness, hoarse voice, or trouble swallowing

Get emergency medical treatment right away if you have signs or symptoms of anaphylaxis after receiving Xolair.

Anaphylaxis from Xolair can happen:
- right after receiving a Xolair injection or hours later
- after any Xolair injection. Anaphylaxis has occurred after the first Xolair injection or after many Xolair injections.

Your healthcare provider should watch you for some time in the office for signs or symptoms of anaphylaxis after injecting Xolair. If you have signs or symptoms of anaphylaxis, tell your healthcare provider right away.

Your healthcare provider should instruct you about getting emergency medical treatment and further medical care if you have signs or symptoms of anaphylaxis after leaving the doctor's office.

WHAT IS XOLAIR?

Xolair is an injectable medicine for patients 12 years of age and older with moderate to severe persistent allergic asthma whose asthma symptoms are not controlled by asthma medicines called inhaled corticosteroids. A skin or blood test is done to see if you have allergic asthma.

WHAT ELSE SHOULD I KNOW ABOUT XOLAIR?
- You should not receive Xolair if you have ever had an allergic reaction to a Xolair injection.
- Do not change or stop taking any of your other asthma medicines unless your healthcare provider tells you to do so.
- There are other possible side effects with Xolair. Talk to your doctor for more information. You can also go to www.xolair.com or call 1-866-4XOLAIR (1-866-496-5247).
- **You may report side effects to FDA at 1-800-FDA-1088.**

This Medication Guide has been approved by the U.S. Food and Drug Administration.

XOLAIR®
(omalizumab)
Manufactured by:
Genentech, Inc.
A Member of the Roche Group
1 DNA Way
South San Francisco, CA 94080-4990
Jointly marketed by:
Genentech USA, Inc.
A Member of the Roche Group
1 DNA Way
South San Francisco, CA 94080-499
Novartis Pharmaceuticals Corporation
One Health Plaza
East Hanover, NJ 07936-1080
7390209/XOL-400050
LX1331
4855302
Initial US Approval: June 2003
Revision Date: July 2010

Shown in Product Identification Guide, page 311

ZOMETA® ℞
[zō-mĕ-ta]
(zoledronic acid)
Injection
Ready-to-Use Solution for Intravenous Infusion (For Single Use)
Concentrate for Intravenous Infusion

The following prescribing information is based on official labeling in effect July 2013.

HIGHLIGHTS OF PRESCRIBING INFORMATION
These highlights do not include all the information needed to use Zometa safely and effectively. See full prescribing information for Zometa.
Zometa® (zoledronic acid) Injection
Ready-to-Use Solution for Intravenous Infusion (For Single Use)
Concentrate for Intravenous Infusion
Initial U.S. Approval: 2001

RECENT MAJOR CHANGES

Warnings and Precautions, addition of atypical subtrochanteric and diaphyseal femoral fractures (5.6) 03/2012

INDICATIONS AND USAGE

Zometa is a bisphosphonate indicated for the treatment of:
- Hypercalcemia of malignancy. (1.1)
- Patients with multiple myeloma and patients with documented bone metastases from solid tumors, in conjunction with standard antineoplastic therapy. Prostate cancer should have progressed after treatment with at least one hormonal therapy. (1.2)

Important limitation of use: The safety and efficacy of Zometa has not been established for use in hyperparathyroidism or nontumor-related hypercalcemia. (1.3)

DOSAGE AND ADMINISTRATION

Hypercalcemia of malignancy (2.1)
- 4 mg as a single-use intravenous infusion over no less than 15 minutes.
- 4 mg as retreatment after a minimum of 7 days.

Multiple myeloma and bone metastasis from solid tumors. (2.2)
- 4 mg as a single-use intravenous infusion over no less than 15 minutes every 3-4 weeks for patients with creatinine clearance of greater than 60 mL/min.
- Reduce the dose for patients with renal impairment.
- Coadminister oral calcium supplements of 500 mg and a multiple vitamin containing 400 IU of Vitamin D daily.

Administer through a separate vented infusion line and do not allow to come in contact with any calcium or divalent cation-containing solutions. (2.3)

DOSAGE FORMS AND STRENGTHS

4 mg/100 mL single-use ready-to-use bottle (3)
4 mg/5 mL single-use vial of concentrate (3)

CONTRAINDICATIONS

Hypersensitivity to any component of Zometa (4)

WARNINGS AND PRECAUTIONS
- Patients being treated with Zometa should not be treated with Reclast®. (5.1)
- Adequately rehydrate patients with hypercalcemia of malignancy prior to administration of Zometa and monitor electrolytes during treatment. (5.2)
- Renal toxicity may be greater in patients with renal impairment. Do not use doses greater than 4 mg. Treatment in patients with severe renal impairment is not recommended. Monitor serum creatinine before each dose. (5.3)
- Osteonecrosis of the jaw has been reported. Preventive dental exams should be performed before starting Zometa. Avoid invasive dental procedures. (5.4)
- Severe incapacitating bone, joint, muscle pain may occur. Discontinue Zometa if severe symptoms occur. (5.5)
- Zometa can cause fetal harm. Women of childbearing potential should be advised of the potential hazard to the fetus and to avoid becoming pregnant. (5.9, 8.1)
- Atypical subtrochanteric and diaphyseal femoral fractures have been reported in patients receiving bisphosphonate therapy. These fractures may occur after minimal or no trauma. Evaluate patients with thigh or groin pain to rule out a femoral fracture. Consider drug discontinuation in patients suspected to have an atypical femur fracture. (5.6)

ADVERSE REACTIONS

The most common adverse events (greater than 25%) were nausea, fatigue, anemia, bone pain, constipation, fever, vomiting, and dyspnea (6.1)

To report SUSPECTED ADVERSE REACTIONS, contact Novartis Pharmaceuticals Corporation at 1-888-669-6682 or FDA at 1-800-FDA-1088 or www.fda.gov/medwatch.

DRUG INTERACTIONS
- Aminoglycosides: May have an additive effect to lower serum calcium for prolonged periods. (7.1)
- Loop diuretics: Concomitant use with Zometa may increase risk of hypocalcemia. (7.2)
- Nephrotoxic drugs: Use with caution. (7.3)

USE IN SPECIFIC POPULATIONS
- Nursing Mothers: It is not known whether Zometa is excreted in human milk. (8.3)
- Pediatric Use: Not indicated for use in pediatric patients. (8.4)
- Geriatric Use: Special care to monitor renal function. (8.5)

See 17 for PATIENT COUNSELING INFORMATION
Revised: 11/2012

FULL PRESCRIBING INFORMATION: CONTENTS*

*** Sections or subsections omitted from the full prescribing information are not listed**

FULL PRESCRIBING INFORMATION

1 INDICATIONS AND USAGE

1.1 Hypercalcemia of Malignancy

Zometa is indicated for the treatment of hypercalcemia of malignancy defined as an albumin-corrected calcium (cCa) of greater than or equal to 12 mg/dL [3.0 mmol/L] using the formula: cCa in mg/dL=Ca in mg/dL + 0.8 (4.0 g/dL - patient albumin (g/dL)).

1.2 Multiple Myeloma and Bone Metastases of Solid Tumors

Zometa is indicated for the treatment of patients with multiple myeloma and patients with documented bone metastases from solid tumors, in conjunction with standard antineoplastic therapy. Prostate cancer should have progressed after treatment with at least one hormonal therapy.

1.3 Important Limitation of Use

The safety and efficacy of Zometa in the treatment of hypercalcemia associated with hyperparathyroidism or with other nontumor-related conditions have not been established.

2 DOSAGE AND ADMINISTRATION

Parenteral drug products should be inspected visually for particulate matter and discoloration prior to administration, whenever solution and container permit.

2.1 Hypercalcemia of Malignancy

The maximum recommended dose of Zometa in hypercalcemia of malignancy (albumin-corrected serum calcium greater than or equal to 12 mg/dL [3.0 mmol/L]) is 4 mg. The 4-mg dose must be given as a single-dose intravenous infusion over **no less than 15 minutes**. Patients who receive Zometa should have serum creatinine assessed prior to each treatment.

Dose adjustments of Zometa are not necessary in treating patients for hypercalcemia of malignancy presenting with mild-to-moderate renal impairment prior to initiation of therapy (serum creatinine less than 400 µmol/L or less than 4.5 mg/dL).

Patients should be adequately rehydrated prior to administration of Zometa [*see Warnings and Precautions (5.2)*].

Consideration should be given to the severity of, as well as the symptoms of, tumor-induced hypercalcemia when considering use of Zometa. Vigorous saline hydration, an integral part of hypercalcemia therapy, should be initiated promptly and an attempt should be made to restore the urine output to about 2 L/day throughout treatment. Mild or asymptomatic hypercalcemia may be treated with conservative measures (i.e., saline hydration, with or without loop diuretics). Patients should be hydrated adequately throughout the treatment, but overhydration, especially in those patients who have cardiac failure, must be avoided. Diuretic therapy should not be employed prior to correction of hypovolemia.

Retreatment with Zometa 4 mg may be considered if serum calcium does not return to normal or remain normal after initial treatment. It is recommended that a minimum of 7 days elapse before retreatment, to allow for full response to the initial dose. Renal function must be carefully monitored in all patients receiving Zometa and serum creatinine must be assessed prior to retreatment with Zometa [*see Warnings and Precautions (5.2)*].

2.2 Multiple Myeloma and Metastatic Bone Lesions of Solid Tumors

The recommended dose of Zometa in patients with multiple myeloma and metastatic bone lesions from solid tumors for patients with creatinine clearance greater than 60 mL/min is 4 mg infused over **no less than 15 minutes** every 3-4 weeks. The optimal duration of therapy is not known.

Upon treatment initiation, the recommended Zometa doses for patients with reduced renal function (mild and moderate renal impairment) are listed in Table 1. These doses are calculated to achieve the same AUC as that achieved in patients with creatinine clearance of 75 mL/min. Creatinine clearance (CrCl) is calculated using the Cockcroft-Gault formula [*see Warnings and Precautions (5.2)*].

Table 1: Reduced Doses for Patients with Baseline CrCl less than or equal to 60 mL/min

Baseline Creatinine Clearance (mL/min)	Zometa Recommended Dose*
greater than 60	4 mg
50 – 60	3.5 mg
40 – 49	3.3 mg
30 – 39	3 mg

*Doses calculated assuming target AUC of 0.66(mg•hr/L) (CrCl = 75 mL/min)

During treatment, serum creatinine should be measured before each Zometa dose and treatment should be withheld for renal deterioration. In the clinical studies, renal deterioration was defined as follows:

For patients with normal baseline creatinine, increase of 0.5 mg/dL

For patients with abnormal baseline creatinine, increase of 1.0 mg/dL

In the clinical studies, Zometa treatment was resumed only when the creatinine returned to within 10% of the baseline value. Zometa should be reinitiated at the same dose as that prior to treatment interruption.

Patients should also be administered an oral calcium supplement of 500 mg and a multiple vitamin containing 400 IU of Vitamin D daily.

2.3 Preparation of Solution

Zometa must not be mixed with calcium or other divalent cation-containing infusion solutions, such as Lactated Ringer's solution, and should be administered as a single intravenous solution in a line separate from all other drugs.

4 mg/100 mL Single-Use Ready-to-Use Bottle

Bottles of Zometa ready-to-use solution for infusion contain overfill allowing for the administration of 100 mL of solution (equivalent to 4 mg zoledronic acid). This solution is ready-to-use and may be administered directly to the patient without further preparation. For single use only

To prepare reduced doses for patients with baseline CrCl less than or equal to 60 mL/min, withdraw the specified volume of the Zometa solution from the bottle (see Table 2) and replace with an equal volume of sterile 0.9% Sodium Chloride, USP, or 5% Dextrose Injection, USP. Administer the newly-prepared dose-adjusted solution to the patient by infusion. Follow proper aseptic technique. Properly discard previously withdrawn volume of ready-to-use solution - do not store or reuse.

Table 2: Preparation of Reduced Doses – Zometa ready-to-use bottle

Remove and discard the following Zometa ready-to-use solution (mL)	Replace with the following volume of sterile 0.9% Sodium Chloride, USP or 5% Dextrose Injection, USP (mL)	Dose (mg)
12.0	12.0	3.5
18.0	18.0	3.3
25.0	25.0	3.0

If not used immediately after dilution with infusion media, for microbiological integrity, the solution should be refrigerated at 2°C - 8°C (36°F 46°F). The refrigerated solution should then be equilibrated to room temperature prior to administration. The total time between dilution, storage in the refrigerator, and end of administration must not exceed 24 hours.

4 mg/5 mL Single-Use Vial

Vials of Zometa concentrate for infusion contain overfill allowing for the withdrawal of 5 mL of concentrate (equivalent to 4 mg zoledronic acid). This concentrate should immediately be diluted in 100 mL of sterile 0.9% Sodium Chloride, USP, or 5% Dextrose Injection, USP, following proper aseptic technique, and administered to the patient by infusion. Do not store undiluted concentrate in a syringe, to avoid inadvertent injection.

To prepare reduced doses for patients with baseline CrCl less than or equal to 60 mL/min, withdraw the specified volume of the Zometa concentrate from the vial for the dose required (see Table 3).

Table 3: Preparation of Reduced Doses – Zometa concentrate

Remove and Use Zometa Volume (mL)	Dose (mg)
4.4	3.5
4.1	3.3
3.8	3.0

The withdrawn concentrate must be diluted in 100 mL of sterile 0.9% Sodium Chloride, USP, or 5% Dextrose Injection, USP.

If not used immediately after dilution with infusion media, for microbiological integrity, the solution should be refrigerated at 2°C-8°C (36°F-46°F). The refrigerated solution should then be equilibrated to room temperature prior to administration. The total time between dilution, storage in the refrigerator, and end of administration must not exceed 24 hours.

2.4 Method of Administration

Due to the risk of clinically significant deterioration in renal function, which may progress to renal failure, single doses of Zometa should not exceed 4 mg and the duration of infusion should be no less than 15 minutes [*see Warnings and Precautions (5.3)*]. In the trials and in postmarketing experience, renal deterioration, progression to renal failure and dialysis, have occurred in patients, including those treated with the approved dose of 4 mg infused over 15 minutes. There have been instances of this occurring after the initial Zometa dose.

3 DOSAGE FORMS AND STRENGTHS

4 mg/100 mL single-use ready-to-use bottle
4 mg/5 mL single-use vial of concentrate

4 CONTRAINDICATIONS

4.1 Hypersensitivity to Zoledronic Acid or Any Components of Zometa

Hypersensitivity reactions including rare cases of urticaria and angioedema, and very rare cases of anaphylactic reaction/shock have been reported [*see Adverse Reactions (6.2)*].

5 WARNINGS AND PRECAUTIONS

5.1 Drugs with Same Active Ingredient or in the Same Drug Class

Zometa contains the same active ingredient as found in Reclast® (zoledronic acid). Patients being treated with Zometa should not be treated with Reclast or other bisphosphonates.

5.2 Hydration and Electrolyte Monitoring

Patients with hypercalcemia of malignancy must be adequately rehydrated prior to administration of Zometa. Loop diuretics should not be used until the patient is adequately rehydrated and should be used with caution in combination with Zometa in order to avoid hypocalcemia. Zometa should be used with caution with other nephrotoxic drugs.

Standard hypercalcemia-related metabolic parameters, such as serum levels of calcium, phosphate, and magnesium, as well as serum creatinine, should be carefully monitored following initiation of therapy with Zometa. If hypocalcemia, hypophosphatemia, or hypomagnesemia occur, short-term supplemental therapy may be necessary.

5.3 Renal Impairment

Zometa is excreted intact primarily via the kidney, and the risk of adverse reactions, in particular renal adverse reactions, may be greater in patients with impaired renal function. Safety and pharmacokinetic data are limited in patients with severe renal impairment and the risk of renal deterioration is increased [*see Adverse Reactions (6.1)*]. Preexisting renal insufficiency and multiple cycles of Zometa and other bisphosphonates are risk factors for subsequent renal deterioration with Zometa. Factors predisposing to renal deterioration, such as dehydration or the use of other nephrotoxic drugs, should be identified and managed, if possible.

Zometa treatment in patients with hypercalcemia of malignancy with severe renal impairment should be considered only after evaluating the risks and benefits of treatment. In the clinical studies, patients with serum creatinine greater than 400 µmol/L or greater than 4.5 mg/dL were excluded.

Zometa treatment is not recommended in patients with bone metastases with severe renal impairment. In the clinical studies, patients with serum creatinine greater than 265 µmol/L or greater than 3.0 mg/dL were excluded and there were only 8 of 564 patients treated with Zometa 4 mg by 15-minute infusion with a baseline creatinine greater than 2 mg/dL. Limited pharmacokinetic data exists in patients with creatinine clearance less than 30 mL/min [*see Clinical Pharmacology (12.3)*].

5.4 Osteonecrosis of the Jaw

Osteonecrosis of the jaw (ONJ) has been reported predominantly in cancer patients treated with intravenous bisphosphonates, including Zometa. Many of these patients were also receiving chemotherapy and corticosteroids which may be risk factors for ONJ. Postmarketing experience and the literature suggest a greater frequency of reports of ONJ based on tumor type (advanced breast cancer, multiple myeloma), and dental status (dental extraction, periodontal disease, local trauma including poorly fitting dentures). Many reports of ONJ involved patients with signs of local infection including osteomyelitis.

Cancer patients should maintain good oral hygiene and should have a dental examination with preventive dentistry prior to treatment with bisphosphonates.

While on treatment, these patients should avoid invasive dental procedures if possible. For patients who develop ONJ while on bisphosphonate therapy, dental surgery may exacerbate the condition. For patients requiring dental procedures, there are no data available to suggest whether discontinuation of bisphosphonate treatment reduces the risk of ONJ. Clinical judgment of the treating physician should guide the management plan of each patient based on individual benefit/risk assessment [*see Adverse Reactions (6.2)*].

5.5 Musculoskeletal Pain

In postmarketing experience, severe and occasionally incapacitating bone, joint, and/or muscle pain has been reported in patients taking bisphosphonates, including Zometa. The time to onset of symptoms varied from one day to several months after starting the drug. Discontinue use if severe symptoms develop. Most patients had relief of symptoms after stopping. A subset had recurrence of symptoms when rechallenged with the same drug or another bisphosphonate [*see Adverse Reactions (6.2)*].

5.6 Atypical Subtrochanteric and Diaphyseal Femoral Fractures

Atypical subtrochanteric and diaphyseal femoral fractures have been reported in patients receiving bisphosphonate therapy, including Zometa. These fractures can occur anywhere in the femoral shaft from just below the lesser trochanter to just above the supracondylar flare and are transverse or short oblique in orientation without evidence of comminution. These fractures occur after minimal or no trauma. Patients may experience thigh or groin pain weeks to months before presenting with a completed femoral fracture. Fractures are often bilateral; therefore the contralateral femur should be examined in bisphosphonate-treated patients who have sustained a femoral shaft fracture. Poor healing of these fractures has also been reported. A number of case reports noted that patients were also receiving treatment with glucocorticoids (such as prednisone or dexamethasone) at the time of fracture. Causality with bisphosphonate therapy has not been established.

Any patient with a history of bisphosphonate exposure who presents with thigh or groin pain in the absence of trauma should be suspected of having an atypical fracture and should be evaluated. Discontinuation of Zometa therapy in patients suspected to have an atypical femur fracture should be considered pending evaluation of the patient, based on an individual benefit risk assessment. It is unknown whether the risk of atypical femur fracture continues after stopping therapy.

5.7 Patients with Asthma

While not observed in clinical trials with Zometa, there have been reports of bronchoconstriction in aspirin sensitive patients receiving bisphosphonates.

5.8 Hepatic Impairment

Only limited clinical data are available for use of Zometa to treat hypercalcemia of malignancy in patients with hepatic insufficiency, and these data are not adequate to provide guidance on dosage selection or how to safely use Zometa in these patients.

5.9 Use in Pregnancy

Bisphosphonates, such as Zometa, are incorporated into the bone matrix, from where they are gradually released over periods of weeks to years. There may be a risk of fetal harm (e.g., skeletal and other abnormalities) if a woman becomes pregnant after completing a course of bisphosphonate therapy.

Zometa may cause fetal harm when administered to a pregnant woman. In reproductive studies in pregnant rats, subcutaneous doses equivalent to 2.4 or 4.8 times the human systemic exposure resulted in pre- and post-implantation losses, decreases in viable fetuses and fetal skeletal, visceral, and external malformations. There are no adequate and well controlled studies in pregnant women. If this drug is used during pregnancy, or if the patient becomes pregnant while taking this drug, the patient should be apprised of the potential hazard to a fetus *[see Use in Specific Populations (8.1)]*.

6 ADVERSE REACTIONS

6.1 Clinical Studies Experience

Because clinical trials are conducted under widely varying conditions, adverse reaction rates observed in the clinical trials of a drug cannot be directly compared to rates in the clinical trials of another drug and may not reflect the rates observed in practice.

Hypercalcemia of Malignancy

The safety of Zometa was studied in 185 patients with hypercalcemia of malignancy (HCM) who received either Zometa 4 mg given as a 5-minute intravenous infusion (n=86) or pamidronate 90 mg given as a 2-hour intravenous infusion (n=103). The population was aged 33-84 years, 60% male and 81% Caucasian, with breast, lung, head and neck, and renal cancer as the most common forms of malignancy. NOTE: pamidronate 90 mg was given as a 2-hour intravenous infusion. The relative safety of pamidronate 90 mg given as a 2-hour intravenous infusion compared to the same dose given as a 24-hour intravenous infusion has not been adequately studied in controlled clinical trials.

Renal Toxicity

Administration of Zometa 4 mg given as a 5-minute intravenous infusion has been shown to result in an increased risk of renal toxicity, as measured by increases in serum creatinine, which can progress to renal failure. The incidence of renal toxicity and renal failure has been shown to be reduced when Zometa 4 mg is given as a 15-minute intravenous infusion. Zometa should be administered by intravenous infusion over no less than 15 minutes *[see Warnings and Precautions (5) and Dosage and Administration (2)]*.

The most frequently observed adverse events were fever, nausea, constipation, anemia, and dyspnea (see Table 4).

Table 4 provides adverse events that were reported by 10% or more of the 189 patients treated with Zometa 4 mg or pamidronate 90 mg from the two HCM trials. Adverse events are listed regardless of presumed causality to study drug.

[See table 4 above]

Table 4: Percentage of Patients with Adverse Events ≥10% Reported in Hypercalcemia of Malignancy Clinical Trials by Body System

	Zometa 4 mg n	(%)	Pamidronate 90 mg n	(%)
Patients Studied				
Total No. of Patients Studied	86	(100)	103	(100)
Total No. of Patients with any AE	81	(94)	95	(92)
Body as a Whole				
Fever	38	(44)	34	(33)
Progression of Cancer	14	(16)	21	(20)
Cardiovascular				
Hypotension	9	(11)	2	(2)
Digestive				
Nausea	25	(29)	28	(27)
Constipation	23	(27)	13	(13)
Diarrhea	15	(17)	17	(17)
Abdominal Pain	14	(16)	13	(13)
Vomiting	12	(14)	17	(17)
Anorexia	8	(9)	14	(14)
Hemic and Lymphatic System				
Anemia	19	(22)	18	(18)
Infections				
Moniliasis	10	(12)	4	(4)
Laboratory Abnormalities				
Hypophosphatemia	11	(13)	2	(2)
Hypokalemia	10	(12)	16	(16)
Hypomagnesemia	9	(11)	5	(5)
Musculoskeletal				
Skeletal Pain	10	(12)	10	(10)
Nervous				
Insomnia	13	(15)	10	(10)
Anxiety	12	(14)	8	(8)
Confusion	11	(13)	13	(13)
Agitation	11	(13)	8	(8)
Respiratory				
Dyspnea	19	(22)	20	(19)
Coughing	10	(12)	12	(12)
Urogenital				
Urinary Tract Infection	12	(14)	15	(15)

The following adverse events from the two controlled multicenter HCM trials (n=189) were reported by a greater percentage of patients treated with Zometa 4 mg than with pamidronate 90 mg and occurred with a frequency of greater than or equal to 5% but less than 10%. Adverse events are listed regardless of presumed causality to study drug: asthenia, chest pain, leg edema, mucositis, dysphagia, granulocytopenia, thrombocytopenia, pancytopenia, nonspecific infection, hypocalcemia, dehydration, arthralgias, headache and somnolence.

Rare cases of rash, pruritus, and chest pain have been reported following treatment with Zometa.

Acute Phase Reaction

Within three days after Zometa administration, an acute phase reaction has been reported in patients, with symptoms including pyrexia, fatigue, bone pain and/or arthralgias, myalgias, chills, and influenza-like illness; these symptoms usually resolve within a few days. Pyrexia has been the most commonly associated symptom, occurring in 44% of patients.

Mineral and Electrolyte Abnormalities

Electrolyte abnormalities, most commonly hypocalcemia, hypophosphatemia and hypomagnesemia, can occur with bisphosphonate use.

Grade 3 and Grade 4 laboratory abnormalities for serum creatinine, serum calcium, serum phosphorus, and serum magnesium observed in two clinical trials of Zometa in patients with HCM are shown in Table 5 and 6.

[See table 5 above]

[See table 6 above]

Table 5: Grade 3 Laboratory Abnormalities for Serum Creatinine, Serum Calcium, Serum Phosphorus, and Serum Magnesium in Two Clinical Trials in Patients with HCM

Laboratory Parameter	Grade 3 Zometa 4 mg n/N	(%)	Pamidronate 90 mg n/N	(%)
Serum Creatinine[1]	2/86	(2%)	3/100	(3%)
Hypocalcemia[2]	1/86	(1%)	2/100	(2%)
Hypophosphatemia[3]	36/70	(51%)	27/81	(33%)
Hypomagnesemia[4]	0/71	—	0/84	—

Table 6: Grade 4 Laboratory Abnormalities for Serum Creatinine, Serum Calcium, Serum Phosphorus, and Serum Magnesium in Two Clinical Trials in Patients with HCM

Laboratory Parameter	Grade 4 Zometa 4 mg n/N	(%)	Pamidronate 90 mg n/N	(%)
Serum Creatinine[1]	0/86	—	1/100	(1%)
Hypocalcemia[2]	0/86	—	0/100	—
Hypophosphatemia[3]	1/70	(1%)	4/81	(5%)
Hypomagnesemia[4]	0/71	—	1/84	(1%)

1 Grade 3 (greater than 3× Upper Limit of Normal); Grade 4 (greater than 6× Upper Limit of Normal)
2 Grade 3 (less than 7 mg/dL); Grade 4 (less than 6 mg/dL)
3 Grade 3 (less than 2 mg/dL); Grade 4 (less than 1 mg/dL)
4 Grade 3 (less than 0.8 mEq/L); Grade 4 (less than 0.5 mEq/L)

Injection Site Reactions

Local reactions at the infusion site, such as redness or swelling, were observed infrequently. In most cases, no specific treatment is required and the symptoms subside after 24-48 hours.

Ocular Adverse Events

Ocular inflammation such as uveitis and scleritis can occur with bisphosphonate use, including Zometa. No cases of iritis, scleritis or uveitis were reported during these clinical trials. However, cases have been seen in postmarketing use *[see Adverse Reactions (6.2)]*.

Multiple Myeloma and Bone Metastases of Solid Tumors

The safety analysis includes patients treated in the core and extension phases of the trials. The analysis includes the 2042 patients treated with Zometa 4 mg, pamidronate 90 mg, or placebo in the three controlled multicenter bone metastases trials, including 969 patients completing the efficacy phase of the trial, and 619 patients that continued in the safety extension phase. Only 347 patients completed the extension phases and were followed for 2 years (or 21 months for the other solid tumor patients). The median duration of exposure for safety analysis for Zometa 4 mg (core plus extension phases) was 12.8 months for breast cancer and multiple myeloma, 10.8 months for prostate cancer, and 4.0 months for other solid tumors.

Table 7 describes adverse events that were reported by 10% or more of patients. Adverse events are listed regardless of presumed causality to study drug.

[See table 7 at top of next page]

Grade 3 and Grade 4 laboratory abnormalities for serum creatinine, serum calcium, serum phosphorus, and serum magnesium observed in three clinical trials of Zometa in patients with bone metastases are shown in Tables 8 and 9.

Table 7: Percentage of Patients with Adverse Events ≥10% Reported in Three Bone Metastases Clinical Trials by Body System

	Zometa 4 mg n	(%)	Pamidronate 90 mg n	(%)	Placebo n	(%)
Patients Studied						
Total No. of Patients	1031	(100)	556	(100)	455	(100)
Total No. of Patients with any AE	1015	(98)	548	(99)	445	(98)
Blood and Lymphatic						
Anemia	344	(33)	175	(32)	128	(28)
Neutropenia	124	(12)	83	(15)	35	(8)
Thrombocytopenia	102	(10)	53	(10)	20	(4)
Gastrointestinal						
Nausea	476	(46)	266	(48)	171	(38)
Vomiting	333	(32)	183	(33)	122	(27)
Constipation	320	(31)	162	(29)	174	(38)
Diarrhea	249	(24)	162	(29)	83	(18)
Abdominal Pain	143	(14)	81	(15)	48	(11)
Dyspepsia	105	(10)	74	(13)	31	(7)
Stomatitis	86	(8)	65	(12)	14	(3)
Sore Throat	82	(8)	61	(11)	17	(4)
General Disorders and Administration Site						
Fatigue	398	(39)	240	(43)	130	(29)
Pyrexia	328	(32)	172	(31)	89	(20)
Weakness	252	(24)	108	(19)	114	(25)
Edema Lower Limb	215	(21)	126	(23)	84	(19)
Rigors	112	(11)	62	(11)	28	(6)
Infections						
Urinary Tract Infection	124	(12)	50	(9)	41	(9)
Upper Respiratory Tract Infection	101	(10)	82	(15)	30	(7)
Metabolism						
Anorexia	231	(22)	81	(15)	105	(23)
Weight Decreased	164	(16)	50	(9)	61	(13)
Dehydration	145	(14)	60	(11)	59	(13)
Appetite Decreased	130	(13)	48	(9)	45	(10)
Musculoskeletal						
Bone Pain	569	(55)	316	(57)	284	(62)
Myalgia	239	(23)	143	(26)	74	(16)
Arthralgia	216	(21)	131	(24)	73	(16)
Back Pain	156	(15)	106	(19)	40	(9)
Pain in Limb	143	(14)	84	(15)	52	(11)
Neoplasms						
Malignant Neoplasm Aggravated	205	(20)	97	(17)	89	(20)
Nervous						
Headache	191	(19)	149	(27)	50	(11)
Dizziness (excluding vertigo)	180	(18)	91	(16)	58	(13)
Insomnia	166	(16)	111	(20)	73	(16)
Paresthesia	149	(15)	85	(15)	35	(8)
Hypoesthesia	127	(12)	65	(12)	43	(10)
Psychiatric						
Depression	146	(14)	95	(17)	49	(11)
Anxiety	112	(11)	73	(13)	37	(8)
Confusion	74	(7)	39	(7)	47	(10)
Respiratory						
Dyspnea	282	(27)	155	(28)	107	(24)
Cough	224	(22)	129	(23)	65	(14)
Skin						
Alopecia	125	(12)	80	(14)	36	(8)
Dermatitis	114	(11)	74	(13)	38	(8)

Table 8: Grade 3 Laboratory Abnormalities for Serum Creatinine, Serum Calcium, Serum Phosphorus, and Serum Magnesium in Three Clinical Trials in Patients with Bone Metastases

Laboratory Parameter	Grade 3 Zometa 4 mg n/N	(%)	Pamidronate 90 mg n/N	(%)	Placebo n/N	(%)
Serum Creatinine[1*]	7/529	(1%)	4/268	(2%)	4/241	(2%)
Hypocalcemia[2]	6/973	(<1%)	4/536	(<1%)	0/415	—
Hypophosphatemia[3]	115/973	(12%)	38/537	(7%)	14/415	(3%)
Hypermagnesemia[4]	19/971	(2%)	2/535	(<1%)	8/415	(2%)
Hypomagnesemia[5]	1/971	(<1%)	0/535	—	1/415	(<1%)

1 Grade 3 (greater than 3× Upper Limit of Normal); Grade 4 (greater than 6× Upper Limit of Normal)
* Serum creatinine data for all patients randomized after the 15-minute infusion amendment
2 Grade 3 (less than 7 mg/dL); Grade 4 (less than 6 mg/dL)
3 Grade 3 (less than 2 mg/dL); Grade 4 (less than 1 mg/dL)
4 Grade 3 (greater than 3 mEq/L); Grade 4 (greater than 8 mEq/L)
5 Grade 3 (less than 0.9 mEq/L); Grade 4 (less than 0.7 mEq/L)

[See table 8 above]
[See table 9 at top of next page]
Among the less frequently occurring adverse events (less than 15% of patients), rigors, hypokalemia, influenza-like illness, and hypocalcemia showed a trend for more events with bisphosphonate administration (Zometa 4 mg and pamidronate groups) compared to the placebo group.
Less common adverse events reported more often with Zometa 4 mg than pamidronate included decreased weight, which was reported in 16% of patients in the Zometa 4 mg group compared with 9% in the pamidronate group. Decreased appetite was reported in slightly more patients in the Zometa 4 mg group (13%) compared with the pamidronate (9%) and placebo (10%) groups, but the clinical significance of these small differences is not clear.

Renal Toxicity

In the bone metastases trials, renal deterioration was defined as an increase of 0.5 mg/dL for patients with normal baseline creatinine (less than 1.4 mg/dL) or an increase of 1.0 mg/dL for patients with an abnormal baseline creatinine (greater than or equal to1.4 mg/dL). The following are data on the incidence of renal deterioration in patients receiving Zometa 4 mg over 15 minutes in these trials (see Table 10).
[See table 10 at top of next page]
The risk of deterioration in renal function appeared to be related to time on study, whether patients were receiving Zometa (4 mg over 15 minutes), placebo, or pamidronate.
In the trials and in postmarketing experience, renal deterioration, progression to renal failure and dialysis have occurred in patients with normal and abnormal baseline renal function, including patients treated with 4 mg infused over a 15-minute period. There have been instances of this occurring after the initial Zometa dose.

6.2 Postmarketing Experience

The following adverse reactions have been reported during postapproval use of Zometa. Because these reports are from a population of uncertain size and are subject to confounding factors, it is not possible to reliably estimate their frequency or establish a causal relationship to drug exposure.

Osteonecrosis of the Jaw

Cases of osteonecrosis (primarily involving the jaws) have been reported predominantly in cancer patients treated with intravenous bisphosphonates including Zometa. Many of these patients were also receiving chemotherapy and corticosteroids which may be a risk factor for ONJ. Data suggests a greater frequency of reports of ONJ in certain cancers, such as advanced breast cancer and multiple myeloma. The majority of the reported cases are in cancer patients following invasive dental procedures, such as tooth extraction. It is therefore prudent to avoid invasive dental procedures as recovery may be prolonged [*see Warnings and Precautions (5)*].

Acute Phase Reaction

Within three days after Zometa administration, an acute phase reaction has been reported, with symptoms including pyrexia, fatigue, bone pain and/or arthralgias, myalgias, chills, and influenza-like illness; these symptoms usually resolve within three days of onset, but resolution could take up to 7 to 14 days. However, some of these symptoms have been reported to persist for a longer duration.

Musculoskeletal Pain

Severe and occasionally incapacitating bone, joint, and/or muscle pain has been reported with bisphosphonate use [*see Warnings and Precautions (5)*].

Atypical Subtrochanteric and Diaphyseal Femoral Fractures

Atypical subtrochanteric and diaphyseal femoral fractures have been reported with bisphosphonate therapy, including Zometa [*see Warnings and Precautions (5.6)*].

Ocular Adverse Events

Cases of uveitis, scleritis, episcleritis, conjunctivitis, iritis, and orbital inflammation including orbital edema have been reported during postmarketing use. In some cases, symptoms resolved with topical steroids.

Hypersensitivity Reactions

There have been rare reports of allergic reaction with intravenous zoledronic acid including angioedema and bronchoconstriction. Very rare cases of anaphylactic reaction/shock have also been reported.
Additional adverse reactions reported in postmarketing use include:
CNS: taste disturbance, hyperesthesia, tremor; ***Special Senses:*** blurred vision; ***Gastrointestinal:*** dry mouth; ***Skin:*** Increased sweating; ***Musculoskeletal:*** muscle cramps; ***Cardiovascular:*** hypertension, bradycardia, hypotension (associated with syncope or circulatory collapse primarily in patients with underlying risk factors); ***Respiratory:*** bronchospasms, interstitial lung disease (ILD) with positive re-challenge; ***Renal:*** hematuria, proteinuria; ***General Disorders and Administration Site:*** weight increase, influenza-like illness (pyrexia, asthenia, fatigue or malaise) persisting for greater than 30 days; ***Laboratory Abnormalities:*** hyperkalemia, hypernatremia.

7 DRUG INTERACTIONS

In-vitro studies indicate that the plasma protein binding of zoledronic acid is low, with the unbound fraction ranging from 60-77%. *In-vitro* studies also indicate that zoledronic acid does not inhibit microsomal CYP450 enzymes. *In-vivo* studies showed that zoledronic acid is not metabolized, and is excreted into the urine as the intact drug.

7.1 Aminoglycosides

Caution is advised when bisphosphonates are administered with aminoglycosides, since these agents may have an additive effect to lower serum calcium level for prolonged periods. This effect has not been reported in Zometa clinical trials.

7.2 Loop Diuretics

Caution should also be exercised when Zometa is used in combination with loop diuretics due to an increased risk of hypocalcemia.

7.3 Nephrotoxic Drugs
Caution is indicated when Zometa is used with other potentially nephrotoxic drugs.

7.4 Thalidomide
No dose adjustment for Zometa 4 mg is needed when co-administered with thalidomide. In a pharmacokinetic study of 24 patients with multiple myeloma, Zometa 4 mg given as a 15 minute infusion was administered either alone or with thalidomide (100 mg once daily on days 1-14 and 200 mg once daily on days 15-28). Co-administration of thalidomide with Zometa did not significantly change the pharmacokinetics of zoledronic acid or creatinine clearance.

8 USE IN SPECIFIC POPULATIONS

8.1 Pregnancy

Pregnancy Category D *[see Warnings and Precaution (5.9)]*
There are no adequate and well-controlled studies of Zometa in pregnant women. Zometa may cause fetal harm when administered to a pregnant woman. Bisphosphonates, such as Zometa, are incorporated into the bone matrix and are gradually released over periods of weeks to years. The extent of bisphosphonate incorporation into adult bone, and hence, the amount available for release back into the systemic circulation, is directly related to the total dose and duration of bisphosphonate use. Although there are no data on fetal risk in humans, bisphosphonates do cause fetal harm in animals, and animal data suggest that uptake of bisphosphonates into fetal bone is greater than into maternal bone. Therefore, there is a theoretical risk of fetal harm (e.g., skeletal and other abnormalities) if a woman becomes pregnant after completing a course of bisphosphonate therapy. The impact of variables such as time between cessation of bisphosphonate therapy to conception, the particular bisphosphonate used, and the route of administration (intravenous versus oral) on this risk has not been established. If this drug is used during pregnancy or if the patient becomes pregnant while taking or after taking this drug, the patient should be apprised of the potential hazard to the fetus.

In female rats given subcutaneous doses of zoledronic acid of 0.01, 0.03, or 0.1 mg/kg/day beginning 15 days before mating and continuing through gestation, the number of stillbirths was increased and survival of neonates was decreased in the mid- and high-dose groups (≥0.2 times the human systemic exposure following an intravenous dose of 4 mg, based on an AUC comparison). Adverse maternal effects were observed in all dose groups (with a systemic exposure of ≥0.07 times the human systemic exposure following an intravenous dose of 4 mg, based on an AUC comparison) and included dystocia and periparturient mortality in pregnant rats allowed to deliver. Maternal mortality may have been related to drug-induced inhibition of skeletal calcium mobilization, resulting in periparturient hypocalcemia. This appears to be a bisphosphonate-class effect.

In pregnant rats given a subcutaneous dose of zoledronic acid of 0.1, 0.2, or 0.4 mg/kg/day during gestation, adverse fetal effects were observed in the mid- and high-dose groups (with systemic exposures of 2.4 and 4.8 times, respectively, the human systemic exposure following an intravenous dose of 4 mg, based on an AUC comparison). These adverse effects included increases in pre- and postimplantation losses, decreases in viable fetuses, and fetal skeletal, visceral, and external malformations. Fetal skeletal effects observed in the high-dose group included unossified or incompletely ossified bones, thickened, curved or shortened bones, wavy ribs, and shortened jaw. Other adverse fetal effects observed in the high-dose group included reduced lens, rudimentary cerebellum, reduction or absence of liver lobes, reduction of lung lobes, vessel dilation, cleft palate, and edema. Skeletal variations were also observed in the low-dose group (with systemic exposure of 1.2 times the human systemic exposure following an intravenous dose of 4 mg, based on an AUC comparison). Signs of maternal toxicity were observed in the high-dose group and included reduced body weights and food consumption, indicating that maximal exposure levels were achieved in this study.

In pregnant rabbits given subcutaneous doses of zoledronic acid of 0.01, 0.03, or 0.1 mg/kg/day during gestation (≤0.5 times the human intravenous dose of 4 mg, based on a comparison of relative body surface areas), no adverse fetal effects were observed. Maternal mortality and abortion occurred in all treatment groups (at doses ≥0.05 times the human intravenous dose of 4 mg, based on a comparison of relative body surface areas). Adverse maternal effects were associated with, and may have been caused by, drug-induced hypocalcemia.

8.3 Nursing Mothers

It is not known whether zoledronic acid is excreted in human milk. Because many drugs are excreted in human milk, and because of the potential for serious adverse reactions in nursing infants from Zometa, a decision should be made to discontinue nursing or to discontinue the drug, taking into account the importance of the drug to the mother. Zoledronic acid binds to bone long term and may be released over weeks to years.

Table 9: Grade 4 Laboratory Abnormalities for Serum Creatinine, Serum Calcium, Serum Phosphorus, and Serum Magnesium in Three Clinical Trials in Patients with Bone Metastases

Laboratory Parameter	Zometa 4 mg n/N	(%)	Grade 4 Pamidronate 90 mg n/N	(%)	Placebo n/N	(%)
Serum Creatinine[1*]	2/529	(<1%)	1/268	(<1%)	0/241	—
Hypocalcemia[2]	7/973	(<1%)	3/536	(<1%)	2/415	(<1%)
Hypophosphatemia[3]	5/973	(<1%)	0/537	—	1/415	(<1%)
Hypermagnesemia[4]	0/971	—	0/535	—	2/415	(<1%)
Hypomagnesemia[5]	2/971	(<1%)	1/535	(<1%)	0/415	—

1 Grade 3 (greater than 3× Upper Limit of Normal); Grade 4 (greater than 6× Upper Limit of Normal)
* Serum creatinine data for all patients randomized after the 15-minute infusion amendment
2 Grade 3 (less than 7 mg/dL); Grade 4 (less than 6 mg/dL)
3 Grade 3 (less than 2 mg/dL); Grade 4 (less than 1 mg/dL)
4 Grade 3 (greater than 3 mEq/L); Grade 4 (greater than 8 mEq/L)
5 Grade 3 (less than 0.9 mEq/L); Grade 4 (less than 0.7 mEq/L)

Table 10: Percentage of Patients with Treatment Emergent Renal Function Deterioration by Baseline Serum Creatinine*

Patient Population/Baseline Creatinine				
Multiple Myeloma and Breast Cancer	**Zometa 4 mg n/N**	**(%)**	**Pamidronate 90 mg n/N**	**(%)**
Normal	27/246	(11%)	23/246	(9%)
Abnormal	2/26	(8%)	2/22	(9%)
Total	29/272	(11%)	25/268	(9%)
Solid Tumors	**Zometa 4 mg n/N**	**(%)**	**Placebo n/N**	**(%)**
Normal	17/154	(11%)	10/143	(7%)
Abnormal	1/11	(9%)	1/20	(5%)
Total	18/165	(11%)	11/163	(7%)
Prostate Cancer	**Zometa 4 mg n/N**	**(%)**	**Placebo n/N**	**(%)**
Normal	12/82	(15%)	8/68	(12%)
Abnormal	4/10	(40%)	2/10	(20%)
Total	16/92	(17%)	10/78	(13%)

*Table includes only patients who were randomized to the trial after a protocol amendment that lengthened the infusion duration of Zometa to 15 minutes.

8.4 Pediatric Use

Zometa is not indicated for use in children.

The safety and effectiveness of zoledronic acid was studied in a one-year active-controlled trial of 152 pediatric subjects (74 receiving zoledronic acid). The enrolled population was subjects with severe osteogenesis imperfecta, aged 1-17 years, 55% male, 84% Caucasian, with a mean lumbar spine BMD of 0.431 gm/cm^2, which is 2.7 standard deviations below the mean for age-matched controls (BMD Z-score of -2.7). At one year, increases in BMD were observed in the zoledronic acid treatment group. However, changes in BMD in individual patients with severe osteogenesis imperfecta did not necessarily correlate with the risk for fracture or the incidence or severity of chronic bone pain. The adverse events observed with Zometa use in children did not raise any new safety findings beyond those previously seen in adults treated for hypercalcemia of malignancy or bone metastases. However, adverse reactions seen more commonly in pediatric patients included pyrexia (61%), arthralgia (26%), hypocalcemia (22%) and headache (22%). These reactions, excluding arthralgia, occurred most frequently within 3 days after the first infusion and became less common with repeat dosing. Because of long-term retention in bone, Zometa should only be used in children if the potential benefit outweighs the potential risk.

Plasma zoledronic acid concentration data was obtained from 10 patients with severe osteogenesis imperfecta (4 in the age group of 3-8 years and 6 in the age group of 9-17 years) infused with 0.05 mg/kg dose over 30 min. Mean C_{max} and $AUC_{(0\text{-last})}$ was 167 ng/mL and 220 ng•h/mL, respectively. The plasma concentration time profile of zoledronic acid in pediatric patients represent a multi-exponential decline, as observed in adult cancer patients at an approximately equivalent mg/kg dose.

8.5 Geriatric Use

Clinical studies of Zometa in hypercalcemia of malignancy included 34 patients who were 65 years of age or older. No significant differences in response rate or adverse reactions were seen in geriatric patients receiving Zometa as compared to younger patients. Controlled clinical studies of Zometa in the treatment of multiple myeloma and bone metastases of solid tumors in patients over age 65 revealed similar efficacy and safety in older and younger patients. Because decreased renal function occurs more commonly in the elderly, special care should be taken to monitor renal function.

10 OVERDOSAGE

Clinical experience with acute overdosage of Zometa is limited. Two patients received Zometa 32 mg over 5 minutes in clinical trials. Neither patient experienced any clinical or laboratory toxicity. Overdosage may cause clinically significant hypocalcemia, hypophosphatemia, and hypomagnesemia. Clinically relevant reductions in serum levels of calcium, phosphorus, and magnesium should be corrected by intravenous administration of calcium gluconate, potassium or sodium phosphate, and magnesium sulfate, respectively.

In an open-label study of zoledronic acid 4 mg in breast cancer patients, a female patient received a single 48-mg dose of zoledronic acid in error. Two days after the overdose, the patient experienced a single episode of hyperthermia (38°C), which resolved after treatment. All other evaluations were normal, and the patient was discharged seven days after the overdose.

A patient with non-Hodgkin's lymphoma received zoledronic acid 4 mg daily on four successive days for a total dose of 16 mg. The patient developed paresthesia and abnormal liver function tests with increased GGT (nearly 100U/L, each value unknown). The outcome of this case is not known.

In controlled clinical trials, administration of Zometa 4 mg as an intravenous infusion over 5 minutes has been shown to increase the risk of renal toxicity compared to the same dose administered as a 15-minute intravenous infusion. In controlled clinical trials, Zometa 8 mg has been shown to be associated with an increased risk of renal toxicity compared to Zometa 4 mg, even when given as a 15-minute intravenous infusion, and was not associated with added benefit in patients with hypercalcemia of malignancy [*see Dosage and Administration (2.4)*].

11 DESCRIPTION

Zometa contains zoledronic acid, a bisphosphonic acid which is an inhibitor of osteoclastic bone resorption. Zoledronic acid is designated chemically as (1-Hydroxy-2-imidazol-1-yl-phosphonoethyl) phosphonic acid monohydrate and its structural formula is

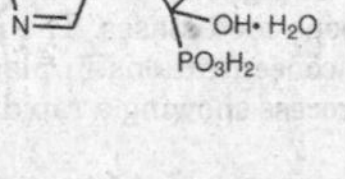

$$CrCl = \frac{[140\text{-age (years)}] \times \text{weight (kg)}}{[72 \times \text{serum creatinine (mg/dL)}]} \quad \{\times 0.85 \text{ for female patients}\}$$

Zoledronic acid is a white crystalline powder. Its molecular formula is $C_5H_{10}N_2O_7P_2 \bullet H_2O$ and its molar mass is 290.1g/Mol. Zoledronic acid is highly soluble in 0.1N sodium hydroxide solution, sparingly soluble in water and 0.1N hydrochloric acid, and practically insoluble in organic solvents. The pH of a 0.7% solution of zoledronic acid in water is approximately 2.0.

Zometa is available in 100-mL bottles as a sterile liquid ready-to-use solution for intravenous infusion and in 5-mL vials as a sterile liquid concentrate solution for intravenous infusion.

- Each 100 mL ready-to-use bottle contains 4.264 mg zoledronic acid monohydrate, corresponding to 4 mg zoledronic acid on an anhydrous basis, 5100 mg of mannitol, USP, water for injection, and 24 mg of sodium citrate, USP.
- Each 5 mL concentrate vial contains 4.264 mg zoledronic acid monohydrate, corresponding to 4 mg zoledronic acid on an anhydrous basis, 220 mg of mannitol, USP, water for injection, and 24 mg of sodium citrate, USP.

Inactive Ingredients: mannitol, USP, as bulking agent, water for injection and sodium citrate, USP, as buffering agent.

12 CLINICAL PHARMACOLOGY

12.1 Mechanism of Action

The principal pharmacologic action of zoledronic acid is inhibition of bone resorption. Although the antiresorptive mechanism is not completely understood, several factors are thought to contribute to this action. *In vitro*, zoledronic acid inhibits osteoclastic activity and induces osteoclast apoptosis. Zoledronic acid also blocks the osteoclastic resorption of mineralized bone and cartilage through its binding to bone. Zoledronic acid inhibits the increased osteoclastic activity and skeletal calcium release induced by various stimulatory factors released by tumors.

12.2 Pharmacodynamics

Clinical studies in patients with hypercalcemia of malignancy (HCM) showed that single-dose infusions of Zometa are associated with decreases in serum calcium and phosphorus and increases in urinary calcium and phosphorus excretion.

Osteoclastic hyperactivity resulting in excessive bone resorption is the underlying pathophysiologic derangement in hypercalcemia of malignancy (HCM, tumor-induced hypercalcemia) and metastatic bone disease. Excessive release of calcium into the blood as bone is resorbed results in polyuria and gastrointestinal disturbances, with progressive dehydration and decreasing glomerular filtration rate. This, in turn, results in increased renal resorption of calcium, setting up a cycle of worsening systemic hypercalcemia. Reducing excessive bone resorption and maintaining adequate fluid administration are, therefore, essential to the management of hypercalcemia of malignancy.

Patients who have hypercalcemia of malignancy can generally be divided into two groups according to the pathophysiologic mechanism involved: humoral hypercalcemia and hypercalcemia due to tumor invasion of bone. In humoral hypercalcemia, osteoclasts are activated and bone resorption is stimulated by factors such as parathyroid hormone-related protein, which are elaborated by the tumor and circulate systemically. Humoral hypercalcemia usually occurs in squamous cell malignancies of the lung or head and neck or in genitourinary tumors such as renal cell carcinoma or ovarian cancer. Skeletal metastases may be absent or minimal in these patients.

Extensive invasion of bone by tumor cells can also result in hypercalcemia due to local tumor products that stimulate bone resorption by osteoclasts. Tumors commonly associated with locally mediated hypercalcemia include breast cancer and multiple myeloma.

Total serum calcium levels in patients who have hypercalcemia of malignancy may not reflect the severity of hypercalcemia, since concomitant hypoalbuminemia is commonly present. Ideally, ionized calcium levels should be used to diagnose and follow hypercalcemic conditions; however, these are not commonly or rapidly available in many clinical situations. Therefore, adjustment of the total serum calcium value for differences in albumin levels (corrected serum calcium, CSC) is often used in place of measurement of ionized calcium; several nomograms are in use for this type of calculation [*see Dosage and Administration (2)*].

12.3 Pharmacokinetics

Pharmacokinetic data in patients with hypercalcemia are not available.

Distribution

Single or multiple (q 28 days) 5-minute or 15-minute infusions of 2, 4, 8 or 16 mg Zometa were given to 64 patients with cancer and bone metastases. The postinfusion decline of zoledronic acid concentrations in plasma was consistent with a triphasic process showing a rapid decrease from peak concentrations at end of infusion to less than 1% of C_{max} 24 hours postinfusion with population half-lives of $t_{1/2\alpha}$ 0.24 hours and $t_{1/2\beta}$ 1.87 hours for the early disposition phases of the drug. The terminal elimination phase of zoledronic acid was prolonged, with very low concentrations in plasma between Days 2 and 28 postinfusion, and a terminal elimination half-life $t_{1/2\gamma}$ of 146 hours. The area under the plasma concentration versus time curve ($AUC_{0\text{-}24h}$) of zoledronic acid was dose proportional from 2-16 mg. The accumulation of zoledronic acid measured over three cycles was low, with mean $AUC_{0\text{-}24h}$ ratios for cycles 2 and 3 versus 1 of 1.13 ± 0.30 and 1.16 ± 0.36, respectively.

In-vitro and *ex-vivo* studies showed low affinity of zoledronic acid for the cellular components of human blood, with a mean blood to plasma concentration ratio of 0.59 in a concentration range of 30 ng/mL to 5000 ng/mL. *In-vitro*, the plasma protein binding is low, with the unbound fraction ranging from 60% at 2 ng/mL to 77% at 2000 ng/mL of zoledronic acid.

Metabolism

Zoledronic acid does not inhibit human P450 enzymes *in vitro*. Zoledronic acid does not undergo biotransformation *in vivo*. In animal studies, less than 3% of the administered intravenous dose was found in the feces, with the balance either recovered in the urine or taken up by bone, indicating that the drug is eliminated intact via the kidney. Following an intravenous dose of 20 nCi ^{14}C-zoledronic acid in a patient with cancer and bone metastases, only a single radioactive species with chromatographic properties identical to those of parent drug was recovered in urine, which suggests that zoledronic acid is not metabolized.

Excretion

In 64 patients with cancer and bone metastases, on average (± s.d.) 39 ± 16% of the administered zoledronic acid dose was recovered in the urine within 24 hours, with only trace amounts of drug found in urine post-Day 2. The cumulative percent of drug excreted in the urine over 0-24 hours was independent of dose. The balance of drug not recovered in urine over 0-24 hours, representing drug presumably bound to bone, is slowly released back into the systemic circulation, giving rise to the observed prolonged low plasma concentrations. The 0-24 hour renal clearance of zoledronic acid was 3.7 ± 2.0 L/h.

Zoledronic acid clearance was independent of dose but dependent upon the patient's creatinine clearance. In a study in patients with cancer and bone metastases, increasing the infusion time of a 4-mg dose of zoledronic acid from 5 minutes (n=5) to 15 minutes (n=7) resulted in a 34% decrease in the zoledronic acid concentration at the end of the infusion ([mean ± SD] 403 ± 118 ng/mL versus 264 ± 86 ng/mL) and a 10% increase in the total AUC (378 ± 116 ng × h/mL versus 420 ± 218 ng × h/mL). The difference between the AUC means was not statistically significant.

Special Populations

Pediatrics

Zometa is not indicated for use in children [*see Pediatric Use (8.4)*].

Geriatrics

The pharmacokinetics of zoledronic acid were not affected by age in patients with cancer and bone metastases who ranged in age from 38 years to 84 years.

Race

Population pharmacokinetic analyses did not indicate any differences in pharmacokinetics among Japanese and North American (Caucasian and African American) patients with cancer and bone metastases.

Hepatic Insufficiency

No clinical studies were conducted to evaluate the effect of hepatic impairment on the pharmacokinetics of zoledronic acid.

Renal Insufficiency

The pharmacokinetic studies conducted in 64 cancer patients represented typical clinical populations with normal to moderately impaired renal function. Compared to patients with normal renal function (N=37), patients with mild renal impairment (N=15) showed an average increase in plasma AUC of 15%, whereas patients with moderate renal impairment (N=11) showed an average increase in plasma AUC of 43%. Limited pharmacokinetic data are available for Zometa in patients with severe renal impairment (creatinine clearance less than 30 mL/min). Based on population PK/PD modeling, the risk of renal deterioration appears to increase with AUC, which is doubled at a creatinine clearance of 10 mL/min. Creatinine clearance is calculated by the Cockcroft-Gault formula:

[See table above]

Zometa systemic clearance in individual patients can be calculated from the population clearance of Zometa, CL $(L/h)=6.5(CL_{cr}/90)^{0.4}$. These formulae can be used to predict the Zometa AUC in patients, where CL = Dose/$AUC_{0\text{-}\infty}$. The average $AUC_{0\text{-}24}$ in patients with normal renal function was 0.42 mg•h/L and the calculated $AUC_{0\text{-}\infty}$ for a patient with creatinine clearance of 75 mL/min was 0.66 mg•h/L following a 4-mg dose of Zometa. However, efficacy and safety of adjusted dosing based on these formulae have not been prospectively assessed [*see Warnings and Precautions (5.2)*].

13 NONCLINICAL TOXICOLOGY

13.1 Carcinogenesis, Mutagenesis, Impairment of Fertility

Standard lifetime carcinogenicity bioassays were conducted in mice and rats. Mice were given oral doses of zoledronic acid of 0.1, 0.5, or 2.0 mg/kg/day. There was an increased incidence of Harderian gland adenomas in males and females in all treatment groups (at doses ≥0.002 times a human intravenous dose of 4 mg, based on a comparison of relative body surface areas). Rats were given oral doses of zoledronic acid of 0.1, 0.5, or 2.0 mg/kg/day. No increased incidence of tumors was observed (at doses ≤0.2 times the human intravenous dose of 4 mg, based on a comparison of relative body surface areas).

Zoledronic acid was not genotoxic in the Ames bacterial mutagenicity assay, in the Chinese hamster ovary cell assay, or in the Chinese hamster gene mutation assay, with or without metabolic activation. Zoledronic acid was not genotoxic in the *in-vivo* rat micronucleus assay.

Female rats were given subcutaneous doses of zoledronic acid of 0.01, 0.03, or 0.1 mg/kg/day beginning 15 days before mating and continuing through gestation. Effects observed in the high-dose group (with systemic exposure of 1.2 times the human systemic exposure following an intravenous dose of 4 mg, based on AUC comparison) included inhibition of ovulation and a decrease in the number of pregnant rats. Effects observed in both the mid-dose group (with systemic exposure of 0.2 times the human systemic exposure following an intravenous dose of 4 mg, based on an AUC comparison) and high-dose group included an increase in preimplantation losses and a decrease in the number of implantations and live fetuses.

14 CLINICAL STUDIES

14.1 Hypercalcemia of Malignancy

Two identical multicenter, randomized, double-blind, double-dummy studies of Zometa 4 mg given as a 5-minute intravenous infusion or pamidronate 90 mg given as a 2-hour intravenous infusion were conducted in 185 patients with hypercalcemia of malignancy (HCM). NOTE: Administration of Zometa 4 mg given as a 5-minute intravenous infusion has been shown to result in an increased risk of renal toxicity, as measured by increases in serum creatinine, which can progress to renal failure. The incidence of renal toxicity and renal failure has been shown to be reduced when Zometa 4 mg is given as a 15-minute intravenous infusion. Zometa should be administered by intravenous infusion over no less than 15 minutes [*see Warnings and Precautions (5.1 and 5.2) and Dosage and Administration (2.4)*]. The treatment groups in the clinical studies were generally well balanced with regards to age, sex, race, and tumor types. The mean age of the study population was 59 years; 81% were Caucasian, 15% were Black, and 4% were of other races. 60% of the patients were male. The most common tumor types were lung, breast, head and neck, and renal.

In these studies, HCM was defined as a corrected serum calcium (CSC) concentration of greater than or equal to 12.0 mg/dL (3.00 mmol/L). The primary efficacy variable was the proportion of patients having a complete response, defined as the lowering of the CSC to less than or equal to 10.8 mg/dL (2.70 mmol/L) within 10 days after drug infusion.

To assess the effects of Zometa versus those of pamidronate, the two multicenter HCM studies were combined in a preplanned analysis. The results of the primary analysis revealed that the proportion of patients that had normalization of corrected serum calcium by Day 10 were 88% and 70% for Zometa 4 mg and pamidronate 90 mg, respectively (P=0.002) (see Figure 1). In these studies, no additional benefit was seen for Zometa 8 mg over Zometa 4 mg; however, the risk of renal toxicity of Zometa 8 mg was significantly greater than that seen with Zometa 4 mg.

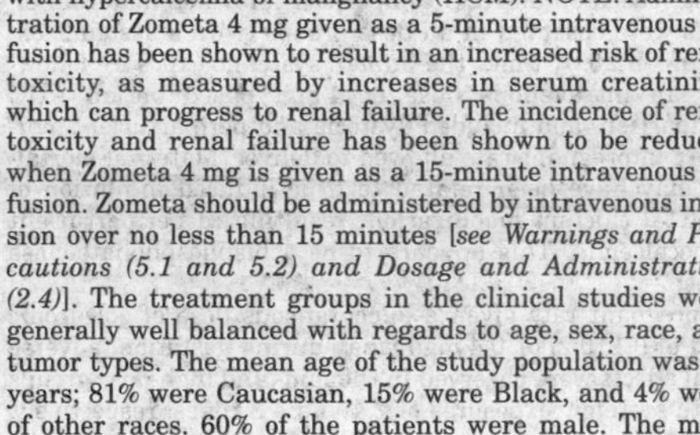

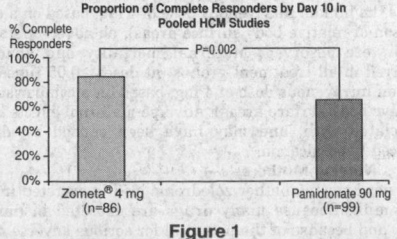

Figure 1

Secondary efficacy variables from the pooled HCM studies included the proportion of patients who had normalization of corrected serum calcium (CSC) by Day 4; the proportion of patients who had normalization of CSC by Day 7; time to relapse of HCM; and duration of complete response. Time to relapse of HCM was defined as the duration (in days) of normalization of serum calcium from study drug infusion until the last CSC value less than 11.6 mg/dL (less than 2.90 mmol/L). Patients who did not have a complete response were assigned a time to relapse of 0 days. Duration of complete response was defined as the duration (in days) from the occurrence of a complete response until the last CSC ≤10.8 mg/dL (2.70 mmol/L). The results of these secondary analyses for Zometa 4 mg and pamidronate 90 mg are shown in Table 11.

[See table 11 above]

14.2 Clinical Trials in Multiple Myeloma and Bone Metastases of Solid Tumors

Table 12 describes an overview of the efficacy population in three randomized Zometa trials in patients with multiple myeloma and bone metastases of solid tumors. These trials included a pamidronate-controlled study in breast cancer and multiple myeloma, a placebo-controlled study in prostate cancer, and a placebo-controlled study in other solid tumors. The prostate cancer study required documentation of previous bone metastases and 3 consecutive rising PSAs while on hormonal therapy. The other placebo-controlled solid tumor study included patients with bone metastases from malignancies other than breast cancer and prostate cancer, including NSCLC, renal cell cancer, small cell lung cancer, colorectal cancer, bladder cancer, GI/genitourinary cancer, head and neck cancer, and others. These trials were comprised of a core phase and an extension phase. In the solid tumor, breast cancer and multiple myeloma trials, only the core phase was evaluated for efficacy as a high percentage of patients did not choose to participate in the extension phase. In the prostate cancer trials, both the core and extension phases were evaluated for efficacy showing the Zometa effect during the first 15 months was maintained without decrement or improvement for another 9 months. The design of these clinical trials does not permit assessment of whether more than one-year administration of Zometa is beneficial. The optimal duration of Zometa administration is not known.

The studies were amended twice because of renal toxicity. The Zometa infusion duration was increased from 5 minutes to 15 minutes. After all patients had been accrued, but while dosing and follow-up continued, patients in the 8 mg Zometa treatment arm were switched to 4 mg due to toxicity. Patients who were randomized to the Zometa 8 mg group are not included in these analyses.

[See table 12 above]

Each study evaluated skeletal-related events (SREs), defined as any of the following: pathologic fracture, radiation therapy to bone, surgery to bone, or spinal cord compression. Change in antineoplastic therapy due to increased pain was a SRE in the prostate cancer study only. Planned analyses included the proportion of patients with a SRE during the study and time to the first SRE. Results for the two Zometa placebo-controlled studies are given in Table 13.

[See table 13 above]

In the breast cancer and myeloma trial, efficacy was determined by a noninferiority analysis comparing Zometa to pamidronate 90 mg for the proportion of patients with a SRE. This analysis required an estimation of pamidronate efficacy. Historical data from 1,128 patients in three pamidronate placebo-controlled trials demonstrated that pamidronate decreased the proportion of patients with a SRE by 13.1% (95% CI = 7.3%, 18.9%). Results of the comparison of treatment with Zometa compared to pamidronate are given in Table 14.

[See table 14 above]

Table 11: Secondary Efficacy Variables in Pooled HCM Studies

	Zometa 4 mg		Pamidronate 90 mg	
Complete Response	**N**	**Response Rate**	**N**	**Response Rate**
By Day 4	86	45.3%	99	33.3%
By Day 7	86	82.6%*	99	63.6%
Duration of Response	**N**	**Median Duration (Days)**	**N**	**Median Duration (Days)**
Time to Relapse	86	30*	99	17
Duration of Complete Response	76	32	69	18

* P less than 0.05 versus pamidronate 90 mg.

Table 12: Overview of Efficacy Population for Phase III Studies

Patient Population	No. of Patients	Zometa Dose	Control	Median Duration (Planned Duration) Zometa 4 mg
Multiple myeloma or metastatic breast cancer	1,648	4 and 8* mg Q3-4 weeks	Pamidronate 90 mg Q3-4 weeks	12.0 months (13 months)
Metastatic prostate cancer	643	4 and 8* mg Q3 weeks	Placebo	10.5 months (15 months)
Metastatic solid tumor other than breast or prostate cancer	773	4 and 8* mg Q3 weeks	Placebo	3.8 months (9 months)

* Patients who were randomized to the 8 mg Zometa group are not included in any of the analyses in this package insert.

Table 13: Zometa Compared to Placebo in Patients with Bone Metastases from Prostate Cancer or Other Solid Tumors

	I. Analysis of Proportion of Patients with a SRE[1]				II. Analysis of Time to the First SRE		
Study	**Study Arm & Patient Number**	**Proportion**	**Difference[2] & 95% CI**	**P-value**	**Median (Days)**	**Hazard Ratio[3] & 95% CI**	**P-value**
Prostate Cancer	Zometa 4 mg (n=214)	33%	-11% (-20%, -1%)	0.02	Not Reached	0.67 (0.49, 0.91)	0.011
	Placebo (n=208)	44%			321		
Solid Tumors	Zometa 4 mg (n=257)	38%	-7% (-15%, 2%)	0.13	230	0.73 (0.55, 0.96)	0.023
	Placebo (n=250)	44%			163		

1SRE=Skeletal-Related Event
2Difference for the proportion of patients with a SRE of Zometa 4 mg versus placebo.
3Hazard ratio for the first occurrence of a SRE of Zometa 4 mg versus placebo.

Table 14: Zometa Compared to Pamidronate in Patients with Multiple Myeloma or Bone Metastases from Breast Cancer

	I. Analysis of Proportion of Patients with a SRE[1]				II. Analysis of Time to the First SRE		
Study	**Study Arm & Patient Number**	**Proportion**	**Difference[2] & 95% CI**	**P-value**	**Median (Days)**	**Hazard Ratio[3] & 95% CI**	**P-value**
Multiple Myeloma & Breast Cancer	Zometa 4 mg (n=561)	44%	-2% (-7.9%, 3.7%)	0.46	373	0.92 (0.77, 1.09)	0.32
	Pamidronate (n=555)	46%			363		

1SRE=Skeletal-Related Event
2Difference for the proportion of patients with a SRE of Zometa 4 mg versus pamidronate 90 mg.
3Hazard ratio for the first occurrence of a SRE of Zometa 4 mg versus pamidronate 90 mg.

16 HOW SUPPLIED/STORAGE AND HANDLING

4 mg/100 mL single-use ready-to-use bottle

Carton of 1 bottle ....NDC 0078-0590-61

Store at 25°C (77°F); excursions permitted to 15-30°C (59-86°F) [see USP Controlled Room Temperature].

4 mg/5 mL single-use vial of concentrate

Carton of 1 vial..NDC 0078-0387-25

Store at 25°C (77°F); excursions permitted to 15-30°C (59-86°F) [see USP Controlled Room Temperature].

17 PATIENT COUNSELING INFORMATION

- Patients should be instructed to tell their doctor if they have kidney problems before being given Zometa.
- Patients should be informed of the importance of getting their blood tests (serum creatinine) during the course of their Zometa therapy.
- Zometa should not be given if the patient is pregnant or plans to become pregnant, or if she is breast-feeding.
- Patients should be advised to have a dental examination prior to treatment with Zometa and should avoid invasive dental procedures during treatment.
- Patients should be informed of the importance of good dental hygiene and routine dental care.
- Patients with multiple myeloma and bone metastasis of solid tumors should be advised to take an oral calcium supplement of 500 mg and a multiple vitamin containing 400 IU of Vitamin D daily.
- Patients should be advised to report any thigh, hip or groin pain. It is unknown whether the risk of atypical femur fracture continues after stopping therapy.
- Patients should be aware of the most common side effects including: anemia, nausea, vomiting, constipation, diarrhea, fatigue, fever, weakness, lower limb edema, anorexia, decreased weight, bone pain, myalgia, arthralgia, back pain, malignant neoplasm aggravated, headache, dizziness, insomnia, paresthesia, dyspnea, cough, and abdominal pain.
- There have been reports of bronchoconstriction in aspirin-sensitive patients receiving bisphosphonates, including zoledronic acid. Before being given zoledronic acid, patients should tell their doctor if they are aspirin-sensitive.

Manufactured by
Novartis Pharma Stein AG
Stein, Switzerland for
Novartis Pharmaceuticals Corporation
East Hanover, New Jersey 07936
© Novartis

T2012-216
November 2012

Shown in Product Identification Guide, page 311

ZORTRESS® ℞
[*ZOR-tres*]
(everolimus)
Tablets for oral use

The following prescribing information is based on official labeling in effect July 2013.

HIGHLIGHTS OF PRESCRIBING INFORMATION

These highlights do not include all the information needed to use ZORTRESS® (everolimus) safely and effectively. See full prescribing information for ZORTRESS.

ZORTRESS (everolimus) tablets for oral use.
Initial U.S. Approval: 2010

WARNING: MALIGNANCIES AND SERIOUS INFECTIONS, KIDNEY GRAFT THROMBOSIS; NEPHROTOXICITY; AND MORTALITY IN HEART TRANSPLANTATION

See Full Prescribing Information for Complete Boxed Warning

- **Only physicians experienced in immunosuppressive therapy and management of transplant patients should use Zortress. (5.1)**
- **Increased susceptibility to infection and the possible development of malignancies may result from immunosuppression. (5.2, 5.3)**
- **Increased incidence of kidney graft thrombosis. (5.4)**
- **Reduced doses of cyclosporine are required for use in combination with Zortress in order to reduce nephrotoxicity. (2.1, 2.3, 5.6, 12.7, 12.8)**
- **Increased mortality in a heart transplant clinical trial. Use in heart transplantation is not recommended. (5.7)**

RECENT MAJOR CHANGES

Boxed Warning: Mortality in Heart Transplantation	04/2012
Indications and Usage: Prophylaxis of Organ Rejection in Liver Transplantation (1.2)	02/2013
Warnings and Precautions (5.5)	02/2013
Warnings and Precautions (5.7, 5.13)	04/2012

INDICATIONS AND USAGE

- Zortress is indicated for the prophylaxis of organ rejection in adult patients:
- Kidney transplant: at low-moderate immunologic risk. (1.1) Use in combination with basiliximab, cyclosporine (reduced doses) and corticosteroids.
- Liver transplant: Administer no earlier than 30 days post-transplant. Use in combination with tacrolimus (reduced doses) and corticosteroids. (1.2, 5.5)

Limitations of Use (1.3)

Safety and efficacy has not been established in the following:

- Kidney transplant patients at high immunologic risk.
- Recipients of transplanted organs other than kidney or liver
- Pediatric patients (<18 years)

DOSAGE AND ADMINISTRATION

- Kidney transplantation: starting oral dose of 0.75 mg twice daily as soon as possible after transplantation. (2.1)
- Liver transplantation: starting oral dose of 1.0 mg twice daily starting 30 days after transplantation. (2.2)
- Monitor everolimus concentrations: Adjust maintenance dose to achieve trough concentrations within the 3-8 ng/mL target range (using LC/MS/MS assay method (2.1, 2.2, 2.3)
- Administer consistently with or without food at the same time as cyclosporine or tacrolimus. (2.6, 12.5)
- Mild hepatic impairment: Reduce initial daily dose by one-third (2.7)
- Moderate or Severe hepatic impairment: Reduce initial daily dose by one-half. (2.7)

DOSAGE FORMS AND STRENGTHS

Zortress is available as 0.25 mg, 0.5 mg, and 0.75 mg tablets. (3)

CONTRAINDICATIONS

- Hypersensitivity to everolimus, sirolimus, or to components of the drug product. (4)

WARNINGS AND PRECAUTIONS

- Angioedema (increased risk with concomitant ACE inhibitors): Monitor for symptoms and treat promptly. (5.8)
- Delayed Wound Healing/Fluid Accumulation: Monitor symptoms; treat promptly to minimize complications. (5.9)
- Interstitial Lung Disease/Non-Infectious Pneumonitis: Monitor for symptoms or radiologic changes; manage by dose reduction or discontinuation until symptoms resolve; consider use of corticosteroids. (5.10)
- Hyperlipidemia (elevations of serum cholesterol and triglycerides): Monitor and consider anti-lipid therapy. (5.11)
- Proteinuria (increased risk with higher trough concentrations): Monitor urine protein. (5.12)
- Polyoma Virus Infections (activation of latent viral infections; BK-virus associated nephropathy): Consider reducing immunosuppression. (5.13)
- TMA/TTP/HUS (concomitant use with cyclosporine may increase risk): Monitor for hematological changes or symptoms. (5.15)
- New Onset Diabetes After Transplantation: Monitor serum glucose. (5.16)
- Male Infertility: Azospermia or oligospermia may occur. (5.17, 13.1)
- Immunizations: Avoid live vaccines. (5.18)

ADVERSE REACTIONS

Most common adverse reactions were as follows:
Kidney transplantation (incidence ≥20%): peripheral edema, constipation, hypertension, nausea, anemia, UTI, and hyperlipidemia. (6.1);
Liver transplantation (incidence>10%): diarrhea, headache, peripheral edema, hypertension, nausea, pyrexia, abdominal pain, and leukopenia (6.1)

To report SUSPECTED ADVERSE REACTIONS, contact Novartis Pharmaceuticals Corporation at 1-888-669-6682 or FDA at 1-800-FDA-1088 or www.fda.gov/medwatch.

DRUG INTERACTIONS

Strong-moderate CYP3A4 inhibitors (e.g., cyclosporine, ketoconazole, erythromycin, verapamil) and CYP3A4 inducers (e.g., rifampin) may affect everolimus concentrations. Consider Zortress dose adjustment (5.14)

USE IN SPECIFIC POPULATIONS

- Pregnancy: Based on animal data may cause fetal harm. (8.1)
- Nursing Mothers: Discontinue drug or nursing. (8.3)

See 17 for PATIENT COUNSELING INFORMATION and Medication Guide

Revised: 02/2013

FULL PRESCRIBING INFORMATION: CONTENTS*

*** Sections or subsections omitted from the full prescribing information are not listed**

FULL PRESCRIBING INFORMATION

WARNING: MALIGNANCIES AND SERIOUS INFECTIONS, KIDNEY GRAFT THROMBOSIS; NEPHROTOXICITY; AND MORTALITY IN HEART TRANSPLANTATION

Malignancies and Serious Infections

- Only physicians experienced in immunosuppressive therapy and management of transplant patients should prescribe Zortress. Patients receiving the drug should be managed in facilities equipped and staffed with adequate laboratory and supportive medical resources. The physician responsible for maintenance therapy should have complete information requisite for the follow-up of the patient. [*See Warnings and Precautions (5.1)*]
- Increased susceptibility to infection and the possible development of malignancies such as lymphoma and skin cancer may result from immunosuppression. [*See Warnings and Precautions (5.2 and 5.3)*]

Kidney Graft Thrombosis

- An increased risk of kidney arterial and venous thrombosis, resulting in graft loss, was reported, mostly within the first 30 days post-transplantation. [*See Warnings and Precautions (5.4)*]

Nephrotoxicity

- Increased nephrotoxicity can occur with use of standard doses of cyclosporine in combination with Zortress. Therefore reduced doses of cyclosporine should be used in combination with Zortress in order to reduce renal dysfunction. It is important to monitor the cyclosporine and everolimus whole blood trough concentrations. [*See Dosage and Administration (2.2 and 2.3) and Warnings and Precautions (5.5) and Clinical Pharmacology (12.7 and 12.8)*]

Mortality in Heart Transplantation

- Increased mortality, often associated with serious infections, within the first three months post-transplantation was observed in a clinical trial of *de novo* heart transplant patients receiving immunosuppressive regimens with or without induction therapy. Use in heart transplantation is not recommended. [*See Warnings and Precautions (5.7)*]

1 INDICATIONS AND USAGE

1.1 Prophylaxis of Organ Rejection in Kidney Transplantation

Zortress is indicated for the prophylaxis of organ rejection in adult patients at low-moderate immunologic risk receiving a kidney transplant. [*See Clinical Studies (14.1)*]
Zortress is to be administered in combination with basiliximab induction and concurrently with reduced doses of cyclosporine and with corticosteroids. Therapeutic drug monitoring of everolimus and cyclosporine is recommended for all patients receiving these products. [*See Dosage and Administration (2.2 and 2.3)*]

1.2 Prophylaxis of Organ Rejection in Liver Transplantation

Zortress is indicated for the prophylaxis of allograft rejection in adult patients receiving a liver transplant. Zortress is to be administered no earlier than 30 days post-transplant concurrently in combination with reduced doses of tacrolimus and with corticosteroids [*See Warnings and Precautions (5.5) and Clinical Studies (14.2)*]. Therapeutic drug monitoring of everolimus and tacrolimus is recommended for all patients receiving these products. [*See Dosage and Administration (2.3 and 2.5)*]

1.3 Limitations of Use

The safety and efficacy of Zortress has not been established in the following populations:

Kidney transplant patients at high immunologic risk
Recipients of transplanted organs other than kidney and liver [*See Warnings and Precautions (5.7)*]
Pediatric patients (<18 years).

2 DOSAGE AND ADMINISTRATION

Patients receiving Zortress may require dose adjustments based on everolimus blood concentrations achieved, tolerability, individual response, change in concomitant medications and the clinical situation. Optimally, dose adjustments of Zortress should be based on trough concentrations obtained 4 or 5 days after a previous dosing change. [*See Therapeutic Drug Monitoring (2.3)*]

2.1 Dosage in Adult Kidney Transplant Patients

An initial Zortress dose of 0.75 mg orally twice daily (1.5 mg per day) is recommended for adult kidney transplant patients in combination with reduced dose cyclosporine, administered as soon as possible after transplantation. [*See Therapeutic Drug Monitoring (2.3 and 2.4), Clinical Studies (14.1)*]
Oral prednisone should be initiated once oral medication is tolerated. Steroid doses may be further tapered on an individualized basis depending on the clinical status of patient and function of graft.

2.2 Dosage in Adult Liver Transplant Patients

Start Zortress at least 30 days post-transplant. An initial dose of 1.0 mg orally twice daily (2.0 mg per day) is recommended for adult liver transplant patients in combination with reduced dose tacrolimus. [*See Therapeutic Drug Monitoring (2.3 and 2.5), Clinical Studies (14.2)*]
Steroid doses may be further tapered on an individualized basis depending on the clinical status of patient and function of graft.

2.3 Therapeutic Drug Monitoring - Everolimus

Routine everolimus whole blood therapeutic drug concentration monitoring is recommended for all patients. The recommended everolimus therapeutic range is 3 to 8 ng/mL. [*See Clinical Pharmacology (12.7)*] Careful attention should be made to clinical signs and symptoms, tissue biopsies, and laboratory parameters. It is important to monitor everolimus blood concentrations, in patients with hepatic impairment, during concomitant administration of CYP3A4 inducers or inhibitors, when switching cyclosporine formulations and/or when cyclosporine dosing is reduced according to recommended target concentrations. [*See Clinical Pharmacology (12.7 and 12.8)*]
There is an interaction of cyclosporine on everolimus, and consequently, everolimus concentrations may decrease if cyclosporine exposure is reduced. There is little to no pharmacokinetic interaction of tacrolimus on everolimus, and thus, everolimus concentrations do not decrease if the tacrolimus exposure is reduced. [*See Drug Interactions (7.2)*]
The everolimus recommended therapeutic range of 3 to 8 ng/mL is based on an LC/MS/MS assay method. Currently in clinical practice, everolimus whole blood trough concentrations may be measured by chromatographic or immunoassay methodologies. Because the measured everolimus whole blood trough concentrations depend on the assay used, individual patient sample concentration values from different assays may not be interchangeable. Consideration of assay results must be made with knowledge of the specific assay used. Therefore, communication should be maintained with the laboratory performing the assay.

2.4 Therapeutic Drug Monitoring- Cyclosporine in Kidney Transplant Patients

Both cyclosporine doses and the target range for whole blood trough concentrations should be reduced, when given in a regimen with Zortress, in order to minimize the risk of nephrotoxicity. [*See Warnings and Precautions (5.6) and Drug Interactions (7.2), Clinical Pharmacology (12.8)*]
The recommended cyclosporine therapeutic ranges when administered with Zortress are 100 to 200 ng/mL through Month 1 post-transplant, 75 to 150 ng/mL at Months 2 and 3 post-transplant, 50 to 100 ng/mL at Month 4 post-transplant, and 25 to 50 ng/mL from Month 6 through Month 12 post-transplant. The median trough concentrations observed in the clinical trial ranged between 161 to 185 ng/mL through Month 1 post-transplant and between 111 to 140 ng/mL at Months 2 and 3 post-transplant. The median trough concentration was 99 ng/mL at Month 4 post-transplant and ranged between 46 to 75 ng/mL from Months 6 through Month 12 post-transplant. [*See Clinical Pharmacology (12.8) and Clinical Studies (14.1)*]
Cyclosporine, USP Modified is to be administered as oral capsules twice daily unless cyclosporine oral solution or intravenous administration of cyclosporine cannot be avoided. Cyclosporine, USP Modified should be initiated as soon as possible - and no later than 48 hours - after reperfusion of the graft and dose adjusted to target concentrations from Day 5 onwards.
If impairment of renal function is progressive the treatment regimen should be adjusted. In renal transplant patients, the cyclosporine dose should be based on cyclosporine whole blood trough concentrations. [*See Clinical Pharmacology (12.8)*]
In renal transplantation, there are limited data regarding dosing Zortress with reduced cyclosporine trough concentrations of 25 to 50 ng/mL after 12 months. Zortress has not been evaluated in clinical trials with other formulations of cyclosporine. Prior to dose reduction of cyclosporine it should be ascertained that steady-state everolimus whole blood trough concentration is at least 3 ng/mL. There is an interaction of cyclosporine on everolimus, and consequently, everolimus concentrations may decrease if cyclosporine exposure is reduced. [See *Drug Interactions (7.2)*]

2.5 Therapeutic Drug Monitoring- Tacrolimus in Liver Transplant Patients

Both tacrolimus doses and the target range for whole blood trough concentrations should be reduced, when given in a regimen with Zortress, in order to minimize the potential risk of nephrotoxicity. [*See Warnings and Precautions (5.6) and Clinical Pharmacology (12.9)*]
The recommended tacrolimus therapeutic range when administered with Zortress are whole blood trough (C-0h) concentrations of 3 to 5 ng/mL by three weeks after the first dose of Zortress (approximately Month 2) and through Month 12 post transplant.
The median tacrolimus trough concentrations observed in the clinical trial ranged between 8.6 to 9.5 ng/mL at Weeks 2 and 4 post-transplant (prior to initiation of everolimus). The median tacrolimus trough concentrations ranged between 7 to 8.1 ng/mL at Weeks 5 and 6 post-transplant, between 5.2 to 5.6 ng/mL at Months 2 and 3 post-transplant, and between 4.3 to 4.9 ng/mL between Months 4 and 12 post-transplant. [*See Clinical Pharmacology (12.9) and Clinical Studies (14.2)*]
Tacrolimus is to be administered as oral capsules twice daily unless intravenous administration of tacrolimus cannot be avoided.
In liver transplant patients, the tacrolimus dose should be based on tacrolimus whole blood trough concentrations. [*See Clinical Pharmacology (12.9)*]
In liver transplantation, there are limited data regarding dosing Zortress with reduced tacrolimus trough concentrations of 3 to 5 ng/mL after 12 months. Prior to dose reduction of tacrolimus it should be ascertained that the steady-state everolimus whole blood trough concentration is at least 3 ng/mL. Unlike the interaction between cyclosporine and everolimus, tacrolimus does not affect everolimus trough concentrations, and consequently, everolimus concentrations do not decrease if the tacrolimus exposure is reduced.

2.6 Administration

Zortress tablets should be swallowed whole with a glass of water and not crushed before use.
Administer Zortress consistently approximately 12 hours apart with or without food to minimize variability in absorption and at the same time as cyclosporine or tacrolimus. [*See Clinical Pharmacology (12.5)*]

2.7 Hepatic Impairment

Whole blood trough concentrations of everolimus should be closely monitored in patients with impaired hepatic function. For patients with mild hepatic impairment (Child-Pugh Class A), the initial daily dose should be reduced by approximately one-third of the normally recommended daily dose. For patients with moderate or severe hepatic impairment (Child-Pugh B or C), the initial daily dose should be reduced to approximately one-half of the normally recommended daily dose. Further dose adjustment and/or dose titration should be made if a patient's whole blood trough concentration of everolimus, as measured by an LC/MS/MS assay, is not within the target trough concentration range of 3 to 8 ng/mL. [*See Clinical Pharmacology (12.5)*]

3 DOSAGE FORMS AND STRENGTHS

Zortress is available as 0.25 mg, 0.5 mg, and 0.75 mg tablets.

Table 1. Description of Zortress (everolimus) Tablets

Dosage Strength	0.25 mg	0.5 mg	0.75 mg
Appearance	White to yellowish, marbled, round, flat tablets with bevelled edge		
Imprint	"C" on one side and "NVR" on the other	"CH" on one side and "NVR" on the other	"CL" on one side and "NVR" on the other

4 CONTRAINDICATIONS

4.1 Hypersensitivity Reactions

Zortress is contraindicated in patients with known hypersensitivity to everolimus, sirolimus, or to components of the drug product.

5 WARNINGS AND PRECAUTIONS

5.1 Management of Immunosuppression

Only physicians experienced in management of systemic immunosuppressant therapy in transplantation should prescribe Zortress. Patients receiving the drug should be managed in facilities equipped and staffed with adequate laboratory and supportive medical resources. The physician responsible for the maintenance therapy should have complete information requisite for the follow-up of the patient.

5.2 Lymphomas and Other Malignancies

Patients receiving immunosuppressants, including Zortress, are at increased risk of developing lymphomas and other malignancies, particularly of the skin. The risk appears to be related to the intensity and duration of immunosuppression rather than to the use of any specific agent.
As usual for patients with increased risk for skin cancer, exposure to sunlight and ultraviolet light should be limited by wearing protective clothing and using a sunscreen with a high protection factor.

5.3 Serious Infections

Patients receiving immunosuppressants, including Zortress, are at increased risk of developing bacterial, viral, fungal, and protozoal infections, including opportunistic infections. [*See Warnings and Precautions (5.13) and Adverse Reactions (6.1, 6.2)*] These infections may lead to serious, including fatal, outcomes. Because of the danger of over immunosuppression, which can cause increased susceptibility to infection, combination immunosuppressant therapy should be used with caution.
Antimicrobial prophylaxis for *Pneumocystis jiroveci (carinii)* pneumonia and prophylaxis for cytomegalovirus (CMV) is recommended in transplant recipients.

5.4 Kidney Graft Thrombosis

An increased risk of kidney arterial and venous thrombosis, resulting in graft loss, has been reported, usually within the first 30 days post-transplantation. [*See Boxed Warning*]

5.5 Hepatic Artery Thrombosis

Mammalian target of rapamycin (mTOR) inhibitors are associated with an increase in hepatic artery thrombosis (HAT). Reported cases mostly have occurred within the first 30 days post-transplant and most also lead to graft loss or death. Therefore, Zortress should not be administered earlier than 30 days after liver transplant.

5.6 Zortress and Calcineurin Inhibitor-Induced Nephrotoxicity

In kidney transplant recipients, Zortress with standard dose cyclosporine increases the risk of nephrotoxicity resulting in a lower glomerular filtration rate. Reduced doses of cyclosporine are required for use in combination with Zortress in order to reduce renal dysfunction. [*See Boxed Warning, Indications and Usage (1.1), Clinical Pharmacology (12.8)*]
In liver transplant recipients, Zortress has not been studied with standard dose tacrolimus. Reduced doses of tacrolimus should be used in combination with Zortress in order to minimize the potential risk of nephrotoxicity. [*See Indications and Usage (1.2), Clinical Pharmacology (12.9)*]
Renal function should be monitored during the administration of Zortress. Consider switching to other immunosuppressive therapies if renal function does not improve after

dose adjustments or if the dysfunction is thought to be drug related. Caution should be exercised when using other drugs which are known to impair renal function.

5.7 Heart Transplantation

In a clinical trial of *de novo* heart transplant patients, Zortress in an immunosuppressive regimen with or without induction therapy, resulted in an increased mortality often associated with serious infections within the first three months post-transplantation compared to the control regimen. Use of Zortress in heart transplantation is not recommended.

5.8 Angioedema

Zortress has been associated with the development of angioedema. The concomitant use of Zortress with other drugs known to cause angioedema, such as angiotensin converting enzyme (ACE) inhibitors may increase the risk of developing angioedema.

5.9 Wound Healing and Fluid Accumulation

Zortress increases the risk of delayed wound healing and increases the occurrence of wound-related complications like wound dehiscence, wound infection, incisional hernia, lymphocele and seroma. These wound-related complications may require more surgical intervention. Generalized fluid accumulation, including peripheral edema (e.g., lymphoedema) and other types of localized fluid collection, such as pericardial and pleural effusions and ascites have also been reported.

5.10 Interstitial Lung Disease/Non-Infectious Pneumonitis

A diagnosis of interstitial lung disease (ILD) should be considered in patients presenting with symptoms consistent with infectious pneumonia but not responding to antibiotic therapy and in whom infectious, neoplastic and other non-drug causes have been ruled-out through appropriate investigations. Cases of ILD have been reported with Zortress, which generally resolve on drug interruption with or without glucocorticoid therapy. However, fatal cases have also occurred.

5.11 Hyperlipidemia

Increased serum cholesterol and triglycerides, requiring the need for anti-lipid therapy, have been reported to occur following initiation of Zortress and the risk of hyperlipidemia is increased with higher everolimus whole blood trough concentrations. [*See Adverse Reactions (6.2)*] Use of anti-lipid therapy may not normalize lipid levels in patients receiving Zortress.

Any patient who is administered Zortress should be monitored for hyperlipidemia. If detected, interventions, such as diet, exercise, and lipid-lowering agents should be initiated as outlined by the National Cholesterol Education Program guidelines. The risk/benefit should be considered in patients with established hyperlipidemia before initiating an immunosuppressive regimen containing Zortress. Similarly, the risk/benefit of continued Zortress therapy should be reevaluated in patients with severe refractory hyperlipidemia. Zortress has not been studied in patients with baseline cholesterol levels >350 mg/dL.

Due to an interaction with cyclosporine, clinical trials of Zortress and cyclosporine in kidney transplant patients strongly discouraged patients from receiving the HMG-CoA reductase inhibitors simvastatin and lovastatin. During Zortress therapy with cyclosporine, patients administered an HMG-CoA reductase inhibitor and/or fibrate should be monitored for the possible development of rhabdomyolysis and other adverse effects, as described in the respective labeling for these agents. [*See Drug Interactions (7.7)*]

5.12 Proteinuria

The use of Zortress in transplant patients has been associated with increased proteinuria. The risk of proteinuria increased with higher everolimus whole blood trough concentrations. Patients receiving Zortress should be monitored for proteinuria. [See *Adverse Reactions (6.2)*]

5.13 Polyoma Virus Infections

Patients receiving immunosuppressants, including Zortress, are at increased risk for opportunistic infections; including polyoma virus infections. Polyoma virus infections in transplant patients may have serious, and sometimes fatal, outcomes. These include polyoma virus-associated nephropathy (PVAN), mostly due to BK virus infection, and JC virus associated progressive multiple leukoencephalopathy (PML). PVAN has been observed in patients receiving immunosuppressants, including Zortress. PVAN is associated with serious outcomes; including deteriorating renal function and kidney graft loss. [*See Adverse Reactions (6.2)*] Patient monitoring may help detect patients at risk for PVAN. Reductions in immunosuppression should be considered for patients who develop evidence of PVAN or PML. Physicians should also consider the risk that reduced immunosuppression represents to the functioning allograft.

5.14 Interaction with Strong Inhibitors and Inducers of CYP3A4

Co-administration of Zortress with strong CYP3A4-inhibitors (e.g., ketoconazole, itraconazole, voriconazole, clarithromycin, telithromycin, ritonavir, boceprevir, telaprevir) and strong CYP3A4 inducers (e.g., rifampin, rifabutin) is not recommended without close monitoring of everolimus whole blood trough concentrations. [*See Drug Interactions (7)*]

5.15 Thrombotic Microangiopathy/Thrombotic Thrombocytopenic Purpura/Hemolytic Uremic Syndrome (TMA/TTP/HUS)

The concomitant use of Zortress with cyclosporine may increase the risk of thrombotic microangiopathy/thrombotic thrombocytopenic purpura/hemolytic uremic syndrome. Monitor hematologic parameters. [*See Adverse Reactions (6.2)*]

5.16 New Onset Diabetes After Transplant

Zortress has been shown to increase the risk of new onset diabetes mellitus after transplant. Blood glucose concentrations should be monitored closely in patients using Zortress.

5.17 Male Infertility

Azospermia or oligospermia may be observed. [*See* Adverse Reactions *(6.2) and Carcinogenesis, Mutagenesis, Impairment of Fertility (13.1)*] Zortress is an anti-proliferative drug and affects rapidly dividing cells like the germ cells.

5.18 Immunizations

The use of live vaccines should be avoided during treatment with Zortress; examples include (not limited to) the following: intranasal influenza, measles, mumps, rubella, oral polio, BCG, yellow fever, varicella, and TY21a typhoid vaccines.

5.19 Interaction with Grapefruit Juice

Grapefruit and grapefruit juice inhibit cytochrome P450 3A4 and P-gp activity and should therefore be avoided with concomitant use of Zortress and cyclosporine or tacrolimus.

5.20 Patients with Hereditary Disorders/Other

Patients with rare hereditary problems of galactose intolerance, the Lapp lactase deficiency or glucose-galactose malabsorption should not take Zortress as this may result in diarrhea and malabsorption.

6 ADVERSE REACTIONS

6.1 Serious and Otherwise Important Adverse Reactions

The following adverse reactions are discussed in greater detail in other sections of the label.

- Hypersensitivity reactions [*See Contraindications (4.1)*]
- Lymphomas and Other Malignancies [*See Boxed Warning, Warnings and Precautions (5.2)*]
- Serious Infections [*See Warnings and Precautions (5.3)*]
- Kidney Graft Thrombosis [*See Warnings and Precautions (5.4)*]
- Hepatic Artery Thrombosis [*See Warnings and Precautions (5.5)*]
- Zortress and Calcineurin Inhibitor-Induced Nephrotoxicity [*See Warnings and Precautions (5.6)*]
- Heart Transplantation [*See Warnings and Precautions (5.7)*]
- Angioedema [*See Warnings and Precautions (5.8)*]
- Wound Healing and Fluid Accumulation [*See Warnings and Precautions (5.9)*]
- Interstitial Lung Disease/Non-Infectious Pneumonitis [*See Warnings and Precautions (5.10)*]
- Hyperlipidemia [*See Warnings and Precautions (5.11)*]
- Proteinuria [*See Warnings and Precautions (5.12)*]
- Polyoma Virus Infections [*See Warnings and Precautions (5.13)*]
- Thrombotic Microangiopathy/Thrombotic Thrombocytopenic Purpura/Hemolytic Uremic Syndrome (TMA/TTP/HUS) [*See Warnings and Precautions (5.15)*]
- New Onset Diabetes After Transplant [*See Warnings and Precautions (5.16)*]
- Male Infertility [*See Warnings and Precautions (5.17)*]

6.2 Clinical Studies Experience

Because clinical trials are conducted under widely varying conditions, the adverse reaction rates observed cannot be directly compared to rates in other trials and may not reflect the rates observed in clinical practice.

Kidney transplantation

The data described below reflect exposure to Zortress in an open-label, randomized trial of *de novo* kidney transplant patients of concentration-controlled everolimus at an initial Zortress starting dose of 1.5 mg per day [target trough concentrations 3 to 8 ng/mL with reduced exposure cyclosporine (N=274) compared to mycophenolic acid (N=273) with standard exposure cyclosporine]. All patients received basiliximab induction therapy and corticosteroids. The population was between 18 and 70 years, more than 43% were 50 years of age or older (mean age was 46 years in the Zortress group, 47 years control group); a majority of recipients were male (64% in the Zortress group, 69% control group); and a majority of patients were Caucasian (70% in the Zortress group, 69% control group). Demographic characteristics were comparable between treatment groups. The most frequent diseases leading to transplantation were balanced between groups and included hypertension/nephrosclerosis, glomerulonephritis/glomerular disease and diabetes mellitus. Significantly more patients discontinued Zortress 1.5 mg per day treatment (83/277, 30%) than discontinued the control regimen (60/277, 22%). Of those patients who prematurely discontinued treatment, most discontinuations were due to adverse reactions: 18% in the Zortress group compared to 9% in the control group (p-value = 0.004). This difference was more prominent between treatment groups among female patients. In those patients discontinuing study medication, adverse reactions were collected up to 7 days after study medication discontinuation and serious adverse reactions up to 30 days after study medication discontinuation.

Discontinuation of Zortress at a higher dose (3 mg per day) was 95/279, 34%, including 20% due to adverse reactions, and this regimen is not recommended (see below).

The overall incidences of serious adverse reactions were 57% (159/278) in the Zortress group and 52% (141/273) in the mycophenolic acid group. Infections and infestations reported as serious adverse reactions had the highest incidence in both groups [20% (54/274) in the Zortress group and 25% (69/273) in the control group]. The difference was mainly due to the higher incidence of viral infections in the mycophenolic acid group, mainly CMV and BK virus infections. Injury, poisoning and procedural complications reported as serious adverse reactions had the second highest incidence in both groups [14% (39/274) in the Zortress group and 12% (32/273) in the control group] followed by renal and urinary disorders [10% (28/274) in the Zortress group and 13% (36/273) in the control group] and vascular disorders [10% (26/274) in the Zortress group and 7% (20/273) in the control group].

A total of 13 patients died during the first 12 months of study; 7 (3%) in the Zortress group and 6 (2%) in the control group. The most common causes of death across the study groups were related to cardiac conditions and infections.

There were 12 (4%) graft losses in the Zortress group and 8 (3%) in the control group over the 12 month study period. Of the graft losses, 4 were due to renal artery and two due to renal vein thrombosis in the Zortress group (2%) compared to two renal artery thromboses in the control group (1%). [*See Boxed Warning and Warnings and Precautions (5.4)*]

The most common (≥20%) adverse reactions observed in the Zortress group were: peripheral edema, constipation, hypertension, nausea, anemia, urinary tract infection, and hyperlipidemia.

<u>Infections</u>

The overall incidence of bacterial, fungal and viral infections reported as adverse reactions was higher in the control group (68%) compared to the Zortress group (64%) and was primarily due to an increased number of viral infections (21% in the control group and 10% in the Zortress group). The incidence of cytomegalovirus (CMV) infections reported as adverse reactions was 8% in the control group compared to 1% in the Zortress group; and 3% of the serious CMV infections in the control group versus 0% in the Zortress group were considered serious. [*See Warnings and Precautions (5.3)*]

<u>BK Virus</u>

BK virus infections were lower in incidence in the Zortress group (2 patients, 1%) compared to the control group (11 patients, 4%). One of the two BK virus infections in the Zortress group and two of the 11 BK virus infections in the control group were also reported as serious adverse reactions. BK virus infections did not result in graft loss in any of the groups in the clinical trial.

<u>Wound Healing and Fluid Collections</u>

Wound healing-related reactions were identified through a retrospective search and request for additional data. The overall incidence of wound-related reactions, including lymphocele, seroma, hematoma, dehiscence, incisional hernia, and infections was 35% in the Zortress group compared to 26% in the control group. More patients required intraoperative repair debridement or drainage of incisional wound complications and more required drainage of lymphoceles and seromas in the Zortress group compared to control.

Adverse reactions due to major fluid collections such as edema and other types of fluid collections was 45% in the Zortress group and 40% in the control group. [*See Warnings and Precautions (5.9)*]

<u>Neoplasms</u>

Adverse reactions due to malignant and benign neoplasms were reported in 3% of patients in the Zortress group and 6% in the control group. The most frequently reported neoplasms in the control group were basal cell carcinoma, squamous cell carcinoma, skin papilloma and seborrheic keratosis. One patient in the Zortress group who underwent a melanoma excision prior to transplantation died due to metastatic melanoma. [*See Boxed Warning and Warnings and Precautions (5.2)*]

<u>New Onset Diabetes Mellitus (NODM)</u>

NODM reported based on adverse reactions and random serum glucose values, was 9% in the Zortress group compared to 7% in the control group.

Endocrine Effects in Males
In the Zortress group, serum testosterone levels significantly decreased while the FSH levels significantly increased without significant changes being observed in the control group. In both the Zortress and the control groups mean testosterone and FSH levels remained within the normal range with the mean FSH level in the Zortress group being at the upper limit of the normal range (11.1 U/L). More patients were reported with erectile dysfunction in the Zortress treatment group compared to the control group (5% compared to 2%, respectively).
Table 2 compares the incidence of treatment-emergent adverse reactions reported with an incidence of ≥10% for patients receiving Zortress with reduced dose cyclosporine or mycophenolic acid with standard dose cyclosporine. Within each MedDRA system organ class, the adverse reactions are presented in order of decreasing frequency.
[See table 2 above and on next page]
Adverse reaction that occurred with at least a 5% higher frequency in the Zortress 1.5 mg group compared to the control group were: peripheral edema (45% compared to 40%), hyperlipidemia (21% compared to 16%), dyslipidemia (15% compared to 9%), and stomatitis/mouth ulceration (8% compared to 3%).
A third treatment group of Zortress 3.0 mg per day (1.5 mg twice daily; target trough concentrations 6 to 12 ng/mL) with reduced exposure cyclosporine was included in the study described above. Although as effective as the lower dose Zortress group, the overall safety was worse and consequently higher doses of Zortress cannot be recommended. Out of 279 patients, 95 (34%) discontinued the study medication with 57 (20%) doing so because of adverse reactions. The most frequent adverse reactions leading to discontinuation of Zortress when used at this higher dose were injury, poisoning and procedural complications (Zortress 1.5 mg: 5%, Zortress 3.0 mg: 7%, and control: 2%), infections (2%, 6%, and 3%, respectively), renal and urinary disorders (4%, 7%, and 4%, respectively) and gastrointestinal disorders (1%, 3%, and 2%).
The combination of fixed dose Zortress and standard doses cyclosporine in previous kidney clinical trials resulted in frequent elevations of serum creatinine with higher mean and median serum creatinine values was observed than in the current study with reduced exposure cyclosporine. These results indicate that Zortress increases the cyclosporine-induced nephrotoxicity; and therefore should only be used in a concentration-controlled regimen with reduced exposure cyclosporine. [*See Boxed Warnings, Indications and Usage (1.1) and Warnings and Precautions (5.6)*]

Liver transplantation
The data described below reflect exposure to Zortress starting 30 days after transplantation in an open-label, randomized trial of liver transplant patients. Seven hundred and nineteen (719) patients who fulfilled the inclusion/exclusion criteria [see Clinical Trials section (14.2)] were randomized into one of the three treatment groups of the study. During the first 30 days prior to randomization patients received tacrolimus and corticosteroids, with or without mycophenolate mofetil (about 70 to 80% received MMF). No induction antibody was administered. At randomization, MMF was discontinued and patients were randomized to Zortress initial dose of 1.0 mg twice per day (2.0 mg daily) and adjusted to protocol specified target trough concentrations of 3 to 8 ng/mL with reduced exposure tacrolimus [protocol specified target troughs 3 to 5 ng/mL] (N=245) or to a control group of standard exposure tacrolimus [protocol specified target troughs 8 to 12 ng/mL up to Month 4 post-transplant, then 6 to 10 ng/mL Month 4 through Month 12 post-transplant] (N=241). A third randomized group was discontinued prematurely [*See Clinical Studies (14.2)*] and is not described in this section.
The population was between 18 and 70 years, more than 50% were 50 years of age (mean age was 54 years in the Zortress group, 55 years in the tacrolimus control group); 74% were male in both Zortress and control groups, respectively, and a majority were Caucasian (86% Zortress group, 80% control group). Demographic characteristics were comparable between treatment groups. The most frequent diseases leading to transplantation were balanced between groups. The most frequent causes of end-stage liver disease (ESLD) were alcoholic cirrhosis, hepatitis C, and hepatocellular carcinoma and were balanced between groups.
Twenty-seven percent discontinued study drug in the Zortress group compared with 22% for the tacrolimus control group. The most common reason for discontinuation of study medication was due to adverse reactions (19% and 11%, respectively), including proteinuria, recurrent hepatitis C, and pancytopenia in the Zortress group.
The overall incidences of serious adverse reactions were 50% (122/245) in the Zortress group and 43% (104/241) in the control group. Infections and infestations were reported as serious adverse reactions with the highest incidence followed by Gastrointestinal disorders and Hepatobiliary disorders.

Table 2. Incidence Rates of Frequent (≥10% in Any Treatment Group) Adverse Reactions by Primary System Organ Class and Preferred Term

Primary System Organ Class Preferred Term	Zortress (everolimus) 1.5 mg With reduced exposure cyclosporine N=274 n (%)	Mycophenolic acid 1.44 g With standard exposure cyclosporine N=273 n (%)
Any Adverse Reactions*	271 (99)	270 (99)
Blood lymphatic system disorders	93 (34)	111 (41)
Anemia	70 (26)	68 (25)
Leukopenia	8 (3)	33 (12)
Gastrointestinal disorders	196 (72)	207 (76)
Constipation	105 (38)	117 (43)
Nausea	79 (29)	85 (31)
Diarrhea	51 (19)	54 (20)
Vomiting	40 (15)	60 (22)
Abdominal pain	36 (13)	42 (15)
Dyspepsia	12 (4)	31 (11)
Abdominal pain upper	9 (3)	30 (11)
General disorders and administrative site conditions	181 (66)	160 (59)
Edema peripheral	123 (45)	108 (40)
Pyrexia	51 (19)	40 (15)
Fatigue	25 (9)	28 (10)
Infections and infestations	169 (62)	185 (68)
Urinary tract infection	60 (22)	63 (23)
Upper respiratory tract infection	44 (16)	49 (18)
Injury, poisoning and procedural complications	163 (60)	163 (60)
Incision site pain	45 (16)	47 (17)
Procedural pain	40 (15)	37 (14)
Investigations	137 (50)	133 (49)
Blood creatinine increased	48 (18)	59 (22)
Metabolism and nutrition disorders	222 (81)	199 (73)
Hyperlipidemia	57 (21)	43 (16)
Hyperkalemia	49 (18)	48 (18)
Hypercholesterolemia	47 (17)	34 (13)
Dyslipidemia	41 (15)	24 (9)
Hypomagnesemia	37 (14)	40 (15)
Hypophosphatemia	35 (13)	35 (13)
Hyperglycemia	34 (12)	38 (14)
Hypokalemia	32 (12)	32 (12)
Musculoskeletal and connective tissue disorders	112 (41)	105 (39)
Pain in extremity	32 (12)	29 (11)
Back pain	30 (11)	28 (10)

(Table continued on next page)

During the first 12 months of study, 13 deaths were reported in the Zortress group (one patient never took Zortress). In the same 12 month period, 7 deaths were reported in the tacrolimus control group. Deaths occurred in both groups for a variety of reasons and were mostly associated with liver-related issues, infections and sepsis.
The most common adverse reactions (reported for ≥10% patients in any group) in the Zortress group were: diarrhea, headache, peripheral edema, hypertension, nausea, pyrexia, abdominal pain, and leukopenia (see Table 3).

Infections
The overall incidence of infections reported as adverse reactions was 50% for Zortress and 44% in the control group. The types of infections were reported as follows: bacterial 16% vs 12%, viral 17% vs 13%; and fungal infections 2% vs 5% for Zortress and control, respectively. [*See Warnings and Precautions (5.3)*]

Wound Healing and Fluid Collections
Wound healing complications were reported as adverse reactions for 11% of patients in the Zortress group compared

Table 2 *(cont.)*. Incidence Rates of Frequent (≥10% in Any Treatment Group) Adverse Reactions by Primary System Organ Class and Preferred Term

Primary System Organ Class Preferred Term	Zortress (everolimus) 1.5 mg With reduced exposure cyclosporine N=274 n (%)	Mycophenolic acid 1.44 g With standard exposure cyclosporine N=273 n (%)
Nervous system disorders	92 (34)	109 (40)
Headache	49 (18)	40 (15)
Tremor	23 (8)	38 (14)
Psychiatric disorders	90 (33)	72 (26)
Insomnia	47 (17)	43 (16)
Renal and urinary disorders	112 (41)	124 (45)
Hematuria	33 (12)	33 (12)
Dysuria	29 (11)	28 (10)
Respiratory, thoracic and mediastinal disorders	86 (31)	93 (34)
Cough	20 (7)	30 (11)
Vascular disorders	122 (45)	124 (45)
Hypertension	81 (30)	82 (30)

* As reported in the safety analysis population defined as all randomized patients who received at least one dose of treatment and had at least one post-baseline safety assessment.

Table 3. Incidence Rates of most Frequent (≥ 10% in Any Treatment Group) Adverse Reactions by Primary System Organ Class and Preferred Term and treatment (Safety population – 12 month analysis)

Primary System Organ Class Preferred Term	Zortress (everolimus) with reduced exposure Tacrolimus N=245 n (%)	Tacrolimus (standard exposure) N=241 n (%)
Any Adverse Reaction/Infection	232 (95)	229 (95)
Blood & lymphatic system disorders	66 (27)	47 (20)
Leukopenia	29 (12)	12 (5)
Gastrointestinal disorders	136 (56)	121 (50)
Diarrhea	47 (19)	50 (21)
Nausea	33 (14)	28 (12)
Abdominal pain	32 (13)	22 (9)
General disorders and administration site conditions	94 (38)	85 (35)
Peripheral edema	43 (18)	26 (11)
Pyrexia	32 (13)	25 (10)
Fatigue	22 (9)	26 (11)
Infections and infestations	123 (50)	105 (44)
Hepatitis C*	28 (11)	19 (8)
Investigations	81 (33)	78 (32)
Liver function test abnormal	16 (7)	24 (10)
Nervous system disorders	89 (36)	85 (35)
Headache	47 (19)	46 (19)
Tremor	23 (9)	29 (12)
Vascular disorders	56 (23)	57 (24)
Hypertension	42 (17)	38 (16)

to 8% of patients in the control group. Pleural effusions were reported in 5% in both groups, and ascites in 4% of patients in the Zortress group and 3% in the control arm.

Neoplasms

Malignant and benign neoplasms were reported as adverse reactions in 4% of patients in the Zortress group and 7% in the control group. In the Zortress group 3 malignant tumors were reported compared to 9 cases in the control group. For the Zortress group this included lymphoma, lymphoproliferative disorder and a hepatocellular carcinoma, and for the control group included Kaposi's sarcoma (2), metastatic colorectal cancer, glioblastoma, malignant hepatic neoplasm, pancreatic neuroendocrine tumor, hemophagocytic histiocytosis, and squamous cell carcinomas. [*See Boxed Warning and Warnings and Precautions (5.2)*]

Lipid abnormalities

Hyperlipidemia adverse reactions (including the preferred terms: hyperlipidemia, hypercholesterolemia, blood cholesterol increased, blood triglycerides increased, hypertriglyceridemia lipids increased, total cholesterol/HDL ratio increased, and dyslipidemia) were reported for 24% Zortress patients, and 10% control patients.

New Onset of Diabetes After Transplant (NODAT)

Of the patients without diabetes mellitus at randomization, NODAT was reported in 32% in the Zortress group compared to 29% in the control group.

Table 3 compares the incidence of treatment-emergent adverse reactions reported with an incidence of ≥10% for patients receiving Zortress with reduced exposure tacrolimus or standard dose tacrolimus. Within each MedDRA system organ class, the adverse reactions are presented in order of decreasing frequency.

[See table 3 below]

Primary system organ classes are presented alphabetically.

* No *de novo* hepatitis C cases were reported

Less common adverse reactions, occurring overall in ≥1% to <10% of kidney and liver transplant patients treated with Zortress include:

Blood and Lymphatic System Disorders: leukocytosis, lymphadenopathy, neutropenia, pancytopenia, thrombocythemia, thrombocytopenia

Cardiac and Vascular Disorders: angina pectoris, atrial fibrillation, cardiac failure congestive, palpitations, tachycardia, hypertension including hypertensive crisis, hypotension, deep vein thrombosis

Endocrine Disorders: Cushingoid, hyperparathyroidism

Eye Disorders: cataract, conjunctivitis, vision blurred

Gastrointestinal Disorders: abdominal distention, dyspepsia, dysphagia, epigastric discomfort, flatulence, gastroesophageal reflux disease, gingival hypertrophy, hematemesis, hemorrhoids, ileus, mouth ulceration, peritonitis, stomatitis

General Disorders and Administrative Site Conditions: chest discomfort, chest pain, chills, fatigue, incisional hernia, malaise, edema including generalized edema, pain

Hepatobiliary Disorders: hepatic enzyme increased, bilirubin increased

Infections and Infestations: BK virus infection [*See Warnings and Precautions (5.13)*], bacteremia, bronchitis, candidiasis, cellulitis, folliculitis, gastroenteritis, herpes infections, influenza, lower respiratory tract, nasopharyngitis, onychomycosis, oral candidiasis, oral herpes, osteomyelitis, pneumonia, pyelonephritis, sepsis, sinusitis, tinea pedis, urethritis, wound infection [*See Boxed Warning and Warnings and Precautions (5.3)*]

Injury Poisoning and Procedural Complications: incision site complications including infections, perinephric collection, seroma, wound dehiscence, incisional hernia, perinephric hematoma, localized intraabdominal fluid collection, impaired healing, lymophocele, lymphorrhea

Investigations: blood alkaline phosphatase increased, white blood cell count decreased, transaminases increased

Metabolism and Nutrition Disorders: blood urea increased, acidosis, anorexia, dehydration, diabetes mellitus [*See Warnings and Precautions (5.16)*], decreased appetite, fluid retention, gout, hypercalcemia, hypertriglyceridemia, hyperuricemia, hypocalcemia, hypoglycemia, hyponatremia, iron deficiency, new onset diabetes mellitus, vitamin B12 deficiency

Musculoskeletal and Connective Tissues Disorders: arthralgia, joint swelling, muscle spasms, muscular weakness, musculoskeletal pain, myalgia, osteonecrosis, osteopenia, osteoporosis, spondylitis

Nervous System Disorders: dizziness, hemiparesis, hypoaesthesia, lethargy, migraine, neuralgia, paresthesia, somnolence, syncope, tremor

Psychiatric Disorders: agitation, anxiety, depression, hallucination

Renal and Urinary Disorders: bladder spasm, hydronephrosis, micturation urgency, nephritis interstitial, pollakiuria, polyuria, proteinuria [*See Warnings and Precautions (5.12)*], pyuria, renal artery thrombosis [*See Boxed Warning and Warnings and Precautions (5.4)*], acute renal failure, renal impairment [*See Warnings and Precautions (5.6)*], urinary retention

Reproductive System and Breast Disorders: erectile dysfunction, ovarian cyst, scrotal edema

Respiratory, Thoracic, Mediastinal Disorders: atelectasis, dyspnea, epistaxis, nasal congestion, oropharyngeal pain, pleural effusions, pulmonary edema, rhinorrhea, sinus congestion, wheezing

Skin and Subcutaneous Tissue Disorders: acne, alopecia, dermatitis acneiform, hirsutism, hyperhydrosis, hypertrichosis, night sweats, pruritus, rash

Vascular Disorders: venous thromboembolism (including deep vein thrombosis), pulmonary embolism

Less common, serious adverse reactions include:

- Interstitial Lung Disease/Non-infectious Pneumonitis [*See Warnings and Precautions (5.10) and Adverse Reactions (6.1)*]
- Thrombotic Microangiopathy (TMA), Thrombotic Thrombocytopenic Purpura (TTP), and Hemolytic Uremic Syndrome (HUS) [*See Warnings and Precautions (5.15)*]

6.3 Post Marketing Experience

Adverse reactions identified from the post-marketing use of the combination regimen of Zortress and cyclosporine that are not specific to any one transplant indication include angioedema [*See Warnings and Precautions (5.8)*], pancreatitis and pulmonary embolism. There have also been reports of male infertility with mTOR inhibitors including Zortress. [*See Warnings and Precautions (5.17)*]

7 DRUG INTERACTIONS

7.1 Interactions with Strong Inhibitors or Inducers of CYP3A4 and P-glycoprotein

Everolimus is mainly metabolized by CYP3A4 in the liver and to some extent in the intestinal wall and is a substrate for the multidrug efflux pump, P-glycoprotein (P-gp). Therefore, absorption and subsequent elimination of systemically absorbed everolimus may be influenced by medicinal products that affect CYP3A4 and/or P-gp. Concurrent treatment with strong inhibitors (e.g., ketoconazole, itraconazole, voriconazole, clarithromycin, telithromycin, ritonavir, boceprevir, telaprevir) and inducers (e.g., rifampin, rifabutin) of CYP3A4 is not recommended. Inhibitors of P-gp (e.g., digoxin, cyclosporine) may decrease the efflux of everolimus from intestinal cells and increase everolimus blood concentrations. *In vitro*, everolimus was a competitive inhibitor of CYP3A4 and of CYP2D6, potentially increasing the concentrations of medicinal products eliminated by these enzymes. Thus, caution should be exercised when co-administering Zortress with CYP3A4 and CYP2D6 substrates with a narrow therapeutic index. [*See Therapeutic Drug Monitoring (2.3)*]

All *in vivo* interaction studies were conducted without concomitant cyclosporine. Pharmacokinetic interactions between Zortress and concomitantly administered drugs are discussed below. Drug interaction studies have not been conducted with drugs other than those described below.

7.2 Cyclosporine (CYP3A4/P-gp inhibitor and CYP3A4 substrate)

The steady-state C_{max} and AUC estimates of everolimus were significantly increased by co-administration of single dose cyclosporine. [*See Clinical Pharmacology (12.5)*] Dose adjustment of Zortress might be needed if the cyclosporine dose is altered. [*See Dosage and Administration (2.3)*] Zortress had a clinically minor influence on cyclosporine pharmacokinetics in transplant patients receiving cyclosporine (Neoral).

7.3 Ketoconazole and Other Strong CYP3A4 Inhibitors

Multiple-dose ketoconazole administration to healthy volunteers significantly increased single dose estimates of everolimus C_{max}, AUC, and half-life. It is recommended that strong inhibitors of CYP3A4 (e.g., ketoconazole, itraconazole, voriconazole, clarithromycin, telithromycin, ritonavir, boceprevir, telaprevir) should not be co-administered with Zortress. [*See Warnings and Precautions (5.14), and Clinical Pharmacology (12.5)*]

7.4 Erythromycin (Moderate CYP3A4 Inhibitor)

Multiple-dose erythromycin administration to healthy volunteers significantly increased single dose estimates of everolimus C_{max}, AUC, and half-life. If erythromycin is co-administered, everolimus blood concentrations should be monitored and a dose adjustment made as necessary. [*See* Clinical *Pharmacology (12.5)*]

7.5 Verapamil (CYP3A4 and P-gp Substrate)

Multiple-dose verapamil administration to healthy volunteers significantly increased single dose estimates of everolimus C_{max} and AUC. Everolimus half-life was not changed. If verapamil is co-administered, everolimus blood concentrations should be monitored and a dose adjustment made as necessary. [*See Clinical Pharmacology (12.5)*]

7.6 Atorvastatin (CYP3A4 substrate) and Pravastatin (P-gp substrate)

Single-dose administration of Zortress with either atorvastatin or pravastatin to healthy subjects did not influence the pharmacokinetics of atorvastatin, pravastatin and everolimus, as well as total HMG-CoA reductase bioreactivity in plasma to a clinically relevant extent. However, these results cannot be extrapolated to other HMG-CoA reductase inhibitors. Patients should be monitored for the development of rhabdomyolysis and other adverse reactions as described in the respective labeling for these products.

7.7 Simvastatin and Lovastatin

Due to an interaction with cyclosporine, clinical studies of Zortress with cyclosporine conducted in kidney transplant patients strongly discouraged patients with receiving HMG-CoA reductase inhibitors such as simvastatin and lovastatin. [*See Warnings and Precautions (5.11)*]

7.8 Rifampin (CYP3A4/P-gp Inducers)

Pretreatment of healthy subjects with multiple-dose rifampin followed by a single dose of Zortress increased everolimus clearance and decreased the everolimus C_{max} and AUC estimates. Combination with rifampin is not recommended. [*See Warnings and Precautions (5.14) and Clinical Pharmacology (12.5)*]

7.9 Midazolam (CYP3A4/5 substrate)

Single-dose administration of midazolam to healthy volunteers following administration of multiple-dose Zortress indicated that everolimus is a weak inhibitor of CYP3A4/5. Dose adjustment of midazolam or other CYP3A4/5 substrates is not necessary when Zortress is coadministered with midazolam or other CYP3A4/5 substrates. [*See Clinical Pharmacology (12.5)*]

7.10 Other Possible Interactions

Moderate inhibitors of CYP3A4 and P-gp may increase everolimus blood concentrations (e.g., fluconazole; macrolide antibiotics; nicardipine, diltiazem; nelfinavir, indinavir, amprenavir). Inducers of CYP3A4 may increase the metabolism of everolimus and decrease everolimus blood concentrations (e.g., St. John's Wort [*Hypericum perforatum*]; anticonvulsants: carbamazepine, phenobarbital, phenytoin; efavirenz, nevirapine).

7.11 Tacrolimus

There is little to no pharmacokinetic interaction of tacrolimus on everolimus, and consequently, dose adjustment of Zortress is not necessary when Zortress is co-administered with tacrolimus.

8 USE IN SPECIFIC POPULATIONS

8.1 Pregnancy

Pregnancy Category C

There are no adequate and well-controlled studies of Zortress in pregnant women. In rats and rabbits, everolimus crossed the placenta and was toxic to the conceptus. The potential risk for humans is unknown. Zortress should be given to pregnant women only if the potential benefit to the mother justifies the potential risk to the fetus. Women of childbearing potential should be advised to use effective contraception methods while they are receiving Zortress and up to 8 weeks after treatment has been stopped.

Everolimus administered daily to pregnant rats by oral gavage at 0.1 mg/kg from before mating through organogenesis resulted in increased preimplantation loss and early resorptions of fetal implants. AUCs in rats at this dose were approximately one-third those in humans administered the starting dose (0.75 mg twice daily). Everolimus administered daily by oral gavage at 0.8 mg/kg to pregnant rabbits during organogenesis resulted in increased late resorptions of fetal implants. At this dose, AUCs in rabbits were slightly less than the AUCs in humans administered the starting clinical dose.

8.3 Nursing Mothers

It is not known whether everolimus is excreted in human milk. Everolimus and/or its metabolites readily transferred into milk of lactating rats at a concentration 3.5 times higher than in maternal serum. Because many drugs are excreted in human milk and because of the potential for serious adverse reactions in nursing infants from everolimus, women should avoid breast-feeding during treatment with Zortress.

8.4 Pediatric Use

The safe and effective use of Zortress in kidney or liver transplant patients younger than 18 years of age has not been established. [*See Clinical Pharmacology (12.5)*]

8.5 Geriatric Use

There is limited clinical experience on the use of Zortress in patients of age 65 or older. There is no evidence to suggest that elderly patients will require a different dosage recommendation from younger adult patients. [*See Clinical Pharmacology (12.5)*]

8.6 Hepatic Impairment

Everolimus whole blood trough concentrations should be closely monitored in patients with impaired hepatic function. For patients with mild hepatic impairment (Child-Pugh Class A), the dose should be reduced by approximately one-third of the normally recommended daily dose. For patients with moderate or severe hepatic impairment (Child-Pugh B or C), the initial daily dose should be reduced to approximately half of the normally recommended daily dose. Further dose adjustment and/or dose titration should be made if a patient's whole blood trough concentration of everolimus, as measured by an LC/MS/MS assay, is not within the target trough concentration range of 3 to 8 ng/mL. [*See Clinical Pharmacology (12.5)*]

8.7 Renal Impairment

No dose adjustment is needed in patients with renal impairment. [*See Clinical Pharmacology (12.5)*]

10 OVERDOSAGE

Reported experience with overdose in humans is very limited. There is a single case of an accidental ingestion of 1.5 mg everolimus in a 2-year-old child where no adverse reactions were observed. Single doses up to 25 mg have been administered to transplant patients with acceptable acute tolerability. Single doses up to 70 mg (without cyclosporine) have been given with acceptable acute tolerability. General supportive measures should be followed in all cases of overdose. Everolimus is not considered dialyzable to any relevant degree (<10% of everolimus removed within 6 hours of hemodialysis). In animal studies, everolimus showed a low acute toxic potential. No lethality or severe toxicity was observed after single oral doses of 2000 mg/kg (limit test) in either mice or rats.

11 DESCRIPTION

Zortress (everolimus) is a macrolide immunosuppressant.

The chemical name of everolimus is

(1R, 9S, 12S, 15R, 16E, 18R, 19R, 21R, 23S, 24E, 26E, 28E, 30S, 32S, 35R)-1, 18-dihydroxy-12 -{(1R)-2-[(1S,3R,4R)-4-(2-hydroxyethoxy)-3-methoxycyclohexyl]-1-methylethyl}-19,30-dimethoxy-15, 17, 21, 23, 29, 35-hexamethyl-11, 36-dioxa-4-aza-tricyclo[30.3.1.$0^{4,9}$] hexatriaconta-16,24,26,28-tetraene-2, 3,10,14,20-pentaone.

The molecular formula is $C_{53}H_{83}NO_{14}$ and the molecular weight is 958.25. The structural formula is:

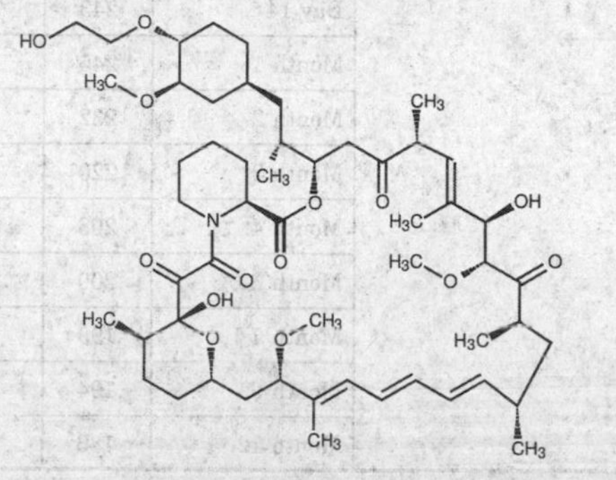

Zortress is supplied as tablets for oral administration containing 0.25 mg, 0.5 mg, and 0.75 mg of everolimus together with butylated hydroxytoluene, magnesium stearate, lactose monohydrate, hypromellose, crospovidone and lactose anhydrous as inactive ingredients.

12 CLINICAL PHARMACOLOGY

12.1 Mechanism of Action

Everolimus inhibits antigenic and interleukin (IL-2 and IL-15) stimulated activation and proliferation of T and B lymphocytes.

In cells, everolimus binds to a cytoplasmic protein, the FK506 Binding Protein-12 (FKBP-12), to form an immunosuppressive complex (everolimus: FKBP-12) that binds to and inhibits the mammalian Target Of Rapamycin (mTOR), a key regulatory kinase. In the presence of everolimus phosphorylation of p70 S6 ribosomal protein kinase (p70S6K), a substrate of mTOR, is inhibited. Consequently, phosphorylation of the ribosomal S6 protein and subsequent protein synthesis and cell proliferation are inhibited. The everolimus: FKBP-12 complex has no effect on calcineurin activity.

In rats and nonhuman primate models, everolimus effectively reduces kidney allograft rejection resulting in prolonged graft survival.

12.3 Pharmacokinetics

Everolimus pharmacokinetics have been characterized after oral administration of single and multiple doses to adult kidney transplant patients, hepatically-impaired patients, and healthy subjects.

Absorption

After oral dosing, peak everolimus concentrations occur 1 to 2 h post dose. Over the dose range of 0.5 mg to 2 mg twice daily, everolimus C_{max} and AUC are dose proportional in transplant patients at steady-state.

Food Effect

In 24 healthy subjects, a high-fat breakfast (44.5 g fat) reduced everolimus C_{max} by 60%, delayed t_{max} by a median 1.3 hours, and reduced AUC by 16% compared with a fasting administration. To minimize variability, everolimus should be taken consistently with or without food. [*See Dosage and Administration (2.6)*]

Distribution

The blood-to-plasma ratio of everolimus is concentration dependent ranging from 17% to 73% over the range of 5 ng/mL to 5000 ng/mL. Plasma protein binding is approximately 74% in healthy subjects and in patients with moderate hepatic impairment. The apparent distribution volume associated with the terminal phase (Vz/F) from a single-dose pharmacokinetic study in maintenance kidney transplant patients is 342 to 107 L (range 128 to 589 L).

Metabolism

Everolimus is a substrate of CYP3A4 and P-gp. The main metabolic pathways identified in man were monohydroxylations and O-dealkylations. Two main metabolites were formed by hydrolysis of the cyclic lactone. Everolimus was

Table 4. Steady-State Pharmacokinetic Parameters (mean +/- SD) Following the Administration of 0.75 mg Twice Daily

C_{max}	T_{max}	AUC	CL/F[1]	Vc/F[1]	Half-life ($T_{1/2}$)
11.1 ± 4.6 ng/mL	1-2 h	75 + 31 ng•h/mL	8.8 L/h	110 L	30 ± 11h

[1] population pharmacokinetic analysis

Table 5. Cyclosporine Trough Concentrations Over 12 Months - Kidney Study Median Values (ng/mL) with 10th and 90th Percentiles

Treatment group	Visit	N	Target (ng/mL)	Median	10th Percentile	90th Percentile
Zortress 0.75 mg twice daily	Day 3	242	100-200	172	46	388
	Day 7	265	100-200	185	75	337
	Day 14	243	100-200	182	97	309
	Month 1	245	100-200	161	85	274
	Month 2	232	75-150	140	84	213
	Month 3	220	75-150	111	68	187
	Month 4	208	50-100	99	56	156
	Month 6	200	25-50	75	43	142
	Month 7	199	25-50	59	36	117
	Month 9	194	25-50	49	28	91
	Month 12	186	25-50	46	25	100

the main circulating component in blood. None of the main metabolites contribute significantly to the immunosuppressive activity of everolimus.

Excretion

After a single dose of radiolabeled everolimus was given to transplant patients receiving cyclosporine, the majority (80%) of radioactivity was recovered from the feces and only a minor amount (5%) was excreted in urine. Parent drug was not detected in urine and feces.

Pharmacokinetics in Kidney Transplant Patients

Steady-state is reached by Day 4 with an accumulation in blood levels of 2- to 3-fold compared with the exposure after the first dose. Table 4 below provides a summary of the steady-state pharmacokinetic parameters.

[See table 4 above]

The half-life estimates from 12 maintenance renal transplant patients who received single doses of everolimus capsules at 0.75 mg or 2.5 mg with their maintenance cyclosporine regimen indicate that the pharmacokinetics of everolimus are linear over the clinically-relevant dose range. Results indicate the half-life of everolimus in maintenance renal transplant patients receiving single doses of 0.75 mg or 2.5 mg Zortress during steady-state cyclosporine treatment was 30 ± 11 hours (range 19 to 53 hours).

12.5 Drug-Drug Interactions

Everolimus is known to be a substrate for both cytochrome CYP3A4 and P-gp. The pharmacokinetic interaction between everolimus and concomitantly administered drugs is discussed below. Drug interaction studies have not been conducted with drugs other than those described below. *[See Warnings and Precautions (5.14), and Drug Interactions (7)]*

Cyclosporine (CYP3A4/P-gp inhibitor and CYP3A4 substrate): Zortress should be taken concomitantly with cyclosporine in kidney transplant patients. Everolimus concentrations may decrease when doses of cyclosporine are reduced, unless the Zortress dose is increased. *[See Dosage and Administration (2.1), Drug Interactions (7.2)]*

In a single-dose study in healthy subjects, cyclosporine (Neoral) administered at a dose of 175 mg increased everolimus AUC by 168% (range, 46% to 365%) and C_{max} by 82% (range, 25% to 158%) when administered with 2 mg Zortress compared with administration of Zortress alone. *[See Drug Interactions (7.2)]*

Ketoconazole and Other Strong CYP3A4 Inhibitors: Multiple-dose administration of 200 mg ketoconazole twice daily for 5 days to 12 healthy volunteers significantly increased everolimus C_{max}, AUC, and half-life by 3.9-fold, 15-fold, and 89%, respectively, when co-administered with 2 mg Zortress. It is recommended that strong inhibitors of CYP3A4 (e.g., ketoconazole, itraconazole, voriconazole, clarithromycin, telithromycin, ritonavir, boceprevir, telaprevir) should not be co-administered with Zortress. *[See Warnings and Precautions (5.14) and Drug Interactions (7.3)]*

Erythromycin *(Moderate CYP3A4 Inhibitor)*: Multiple-dose administration of 500 mg erythromycin three times daily for 5 days to 16 healthy volunteers significantly increased everolimus C_{max}, AUC, and half-life by 2.0-fold, 4.4-fold, and 39%, respectively, when co-administered with 2 mg Zortress. If erythromycin is co-administered, everolimus blood concentrations should be monitored and a dose adjustment made as necessary. *[See Drug Interactions (7.4)]*

Verapamil *(CYP3A4 Inhibitor and P-gp Substrate)*: Multiple-dose administration of 80 mg verapamil three times daily for 5 days to 16 healthy volunteers significantly increased everolimus C_{max} and AUC by 2.3-fold and 3.5-fold, respectively, when co-administered with 2 mg Zortress. Everolimus half-life was not changed. If verapamil is co-administered, everolimus blood concentrations should be monitored and a dose adjustment made as necessary. *[See Drug Interactions (7.5)]*

Atorvastatin *(CYP3A4 Substrate) and* ***Pravastatin*** *(P-gp Substrate)*: Following administration of a single dose of 2 mg Zortress to 12 healthy subjects, the concomitant administration of a single oral dose administration of atorvastatin 20 mg or pravastatin 20 mg only slightly decreased everolimus C_{max} and AUC by 9% and 10%, respectively. There was no apparent change in the mean $T_{1/2}$ or median T_{max}. In the same study, the concomitant Zortress dose slightly increased the mean C_{max} of atorvastatin by 11% and slightly decreased the AUC by 7%. The concomitant Zortress dose decreased the mean C_{max} and AUC of pravastatin by 10% and 5%, respectively. No dosage adjustments are needed for concomitant administration of Zortress and atorvastatin and pravastatin. *[See Drug Interactions (7.6)]*

Midazolam *(CYP3A4/5 Substrate)*: In 25 healthy male subjects, co-administration of a single dose of midazolam 4 mg oral solution with steady-state everolimus (10 mg daily dose for 5 days) resulted in a 25% increase in midazolam C_{max} and a 30% increase in midazolam AUC; whereas, the terminal half-life of midazolam and the metabolic AUC-ratio (1-hydroxymidazolam/midazolam) were not affected. *[See Drug Interactions (7.9)]*

Rifampin *(Strong CYP3A4 and P-gp Inducer)*: Pretreatment of 12 healthy subjects with multiple-dose rifampin (600 mg once-daily for 8 days) followed by a single dose of 4 mg Zortress increased everolimus clearance nearly 3-fold, and decreased C_{max} by 58% and AUC by 63%. Combination with rifampin is not recommended. *[See Drug Interactions (7.8)]*

12.6 Specific Populations

Hepatic Impairment

Relative to the AUC of everolimus in subjects with normal hepatic function, the average AUC in 6 patients with mild hepatic impairment (Child-Pugh Class A) was 1.6-fold higher following administration of a 10 mg single-dose. In two independently studied groups of 8 and 9 patients with moderate hepatic impairment (Child-Pugh Class B) the average AUC was 2.1-fold and 3.3-fold higher following administration of a 2 mg or a 10 mg single-dose, respectively; and in 6 patients with severe hepatic impairment (Child-Pugh Class C) the average AUC was 3.6-fold higher following administration of a 10 mg single-dose. For patients with mild hepatic impairment (Child-Pugh Class A), the dose should be reduced by approximately one-third of the normally recommended daily dose. For patients with moderate or severe hepatic impairment (Child-Pugh B or C), the initial daily dose should be reduced to approximately one-half of the normally recommended daily dose. Further dose adjustment and/or dose titration should be made if a patient's whole blood trough concentration of everolimus, as measured by an LC/MS/MS assay, is not within the target trough concentration range of 3 to 8 ng/mL. *[See Dosage and Administration (2.7)]*

Renal Impairment

No pharmacokinetic studies in patients with renal impairment were conducted. Post-transplant renal function (creatinine clearance range 11 to 107 mL/min) did not affect the pharmacokinetics of everolimus, therefore, no dosage adjustments are needed in patients with renal impairment.

Pediatrics

The safety and efficacy of Zortress has not been established in pediatric patients.

Geriatrics

A limited reduction in everolimus oral CL of 0.33% per year was estimated in adults (age range studied was 16 to 70 years). There is no evidence to suggest that elderly patients will require a different dosage recommendation from younger adult patients.

Race

Based on analysis of population pharmacokinetics, oral clearance (CL/F) is, on average, 20% higher in black transplant patients.

12.7 Everolimus Whole Blood Concentrations Observed in Kidney and in Liver Transplant Patients

Everolimus in Kidney Transplantation

Based on exposure-efficacy and exposure-safety analyses of clinical trials and using an LC/MS/MS assay method, kidney transplant patients achieving everolimus whole blood trough concentrations ≥3.0 ng/mL have been found to have a lower incidence of treated biopsy-proven acute rejection compared with patients whose trough concentrations were below 3.0 ng/mL. Patients who attained everolimus trough concentrations within the range of 6 to 12 ng/mL had similar efficacy and more adverse reactions than patients who attained lower trough concentrations between 3 to 8 ng/mL. *[See Dosage and Administration (2.3)]*

In the kidney clinical trial *[See Clinical Studies (14.1)]*, everolimus whole blood trough concentrations were measured at Days 3, 7, and 14 and Months 1, 2, 3, 4, 6, 7, 9, and 12. The proportion of patients receiving 0.75 mg twice daily Zortress treatment regimen who had everolimus whole blood trough concentrations within the protocol specified target range of 3 to 8 ng/mL at Days 3, 7, and 14 were 55%, 71% and 69%, respectively. Approximately 80% of patients had everolimus whole blood trough concentrations within the 3 to 8 ng/mL target range by Month 1 and remained stable within range through Month 12. The median everolimus trough concentration for the 0.75 mg twice daily treatment group was between 3 and 8 ng/mL throughout the study duration.

Everolimus in Liver Transplantation

In the liver clinical trial *[See Clinical Studies (14.2)]* Zortress dosing was initiated after 30 days following transplantation. Whole blood trough everolimus concentrations were measured within 5 days after first dose, followed by weekly intervals for 3 to 4 weeks, and then monthly thereafter. Approximately 49%, 37%, and 18% of patients, respectively, were below 3 ng/mL at 1, 2, and 4 weeks after initiation of Zortress dosing. The majority of patients (approximately 70 to 80%) had everolimus trough blood concentrations within the target range of 3-8 ng/mL after Month 2 through Month 12.

12.8 Cyclosporine Concentrations Observed in Kidney Transplant Patients

In the kidney transplant clinical trial *[See Clinical Studies (14.1)]*, the target cyclosporine whole blood trough concentration for the Zortress treatment arm of 0.75 mg twice daily were 100 to 200 ng/mL through Month 1 post-transplant, 75 to 150 ng/mL at Months 2 and 3 post-transplant, 50 to 100 ng/mL at Month 4 post-transplant, and 25 to 50 ng/mL from Month 6 through Month 12 post-transplant. Table 5 below provides a summary of the observed cyclosporine whole blood trough concentrations during the study.

[See table 5 above]

12.9 Tacrolimus Concentrations in Liver Transplant

In the liver transplant clinical trial [See Clinical Studies (14.2)], the target tacrolimus whole blood trough concentrations were greater than or equal to 8 ng/mL in the first 30 days post-transplant. The protocol required that patients had a tacrolimus trough concentration of at least 8 ng/mL in the week prior to initiation of Zortress. Zortress was initiated after 30 days post-transplant. At that time, the target tacrolimus trough concentrations were reduced to 3 to 5 ng/mL. Table 6 below provides a summary of the tacrolimus whole blood trough concentrations observed during the study.

[See table 6 above]

13 NONCLINICAL TOXICOLOGY

13.1 Carcinogenesis, Mutagenesis, Impairment of Fertility

Everolimus was not carcinogenic in mice or rats when administered daily by oral gavage for 2 years at doses of 0.9 mg/kg. In these studies, AUCs in mice were much higher (at least 20 times) than those in humans receiving 0.75 mg twice daily, and AUCs in rats were in the same range as those in humans receiving 0.75 mg twice daily.

Everolimus was not mutagenic in the bacterial reverse mutation, the mouse lymphoma thymidine kinase assay, or the chromosome aberration assay using V79 Chinese hamster cells, or *in vivo* following two daily doses of 500 mg/kg in the mouse micronucleus assay.

In a 13-week male fertility oral gavage study in rats, testicular morphology was affected at 0.5 mg/kg and above, and sperm motility, sperm head count and plasma testosterone concentrations were diminished at 5 mg/kg which caused a decrease in male fertility. There was evidence of reversibility of these findings in animals examined after 13 weeks post-dosing. The 0.5 mg/kg dose in male rats resulted in AUCs in the range of clinical exposures, and the 5 mg/kg dose resulted in AUCs approximately 5 times the AUCs in humans receiving 0.75 mg twice daily. Everolimus did not affect female fertility in nonclinical studies, but everolimus crossed the placenta and was toxic to the conceptus. [*See Pregnancy (8.1)*]

14 CLINICAL STUDIES

14.1 Prevention of Organ Rejection after Renal Transplantation

A 24-month, multi-national, open-label, randomized (1:1:1) trial was conducted comparing two concentration-controlled Zortress regimens of 1.5 mg per day starting dose (targeting 3 to 8 ng/mL using an LC/MS/MS assay method and 3.0 mg per day starting dose (targeting 6 to 12 ng/mL using an LC/MS/MS assay method) with reduced exposure cyclosporine and corticosteroids, to 1.44 g per day of mycophenolic acid with standard exposure cyclosporine and corticosteroids. The mean cyclosporine starting dose was 5.2, 5.0 and 5.7 mg/kg body weight/day in the Zortress 1.5 mg, 3.0 mg and in mycophenolic acid groups, respectively. The cyclosporine dose in the Zortress group was then adjusted to the blood trough concentration ranges indicated in Table 5, whereas in the mycophenolic acid group the target ranges were 200-300 ng/mL starting Day 5: 200-300 ng/mL, and 100-250 ng/mL from Month 2 to Month 12.

All patients received basiliximab induction therapy. The study population consisted of 18 to 70 year old male and female low to moderate risk renal transplant recipients undergoing their first transplant. Low to moderate immunologic risk was defined in the study as an ABO blood type compatible first organ or tissue transplant recipient with anti-HLA Class I PRA <20% by a complement dependent cytotoxicity-based assay, or <50% by a flow cytometry or ELISA-based assay, and with a negative T-cell cross match. Eight hundred thirty-three (833) patients were randomized after transplantation; 277 randomized to the Zortress 1.5 mg per day group, 279 to the Zortress 3.0 mg per day group and 277 to the mycophenolic acid 1.44 g per day group. The study was conducted at 79 renal transplant centers across Europe, South Africa, North and South America, and Asia-Pacific. There were no major baseline differences between treatment groups with regard to recipient or donor disease characteristics. The majority of transplant recipients in all groups (70% to 76%) had three or more HLA mismatches; mean percentage of panel reactive antibodies ranged from 1% to 2%. The rate of premature treatment discontinuation at 12 months was 30% and 22% in the Zortress 1.5 mg and control groups, respectively, (p=0.03, Fisher's exact test) and was more prominent between groups among female patients. Results at 12 months indicated that Zortress 1.5 mg per day is comparable to control with respect to efficacy failure, defined as treated biopsy-proven acute rejection*, graft loss, death or loss to follow-up. The percentage of patients experiencing this endpoint and each individual variable in the Zortress and control groups is shown in Table 7.

[See table 7 above]

The estimated mean glomerular filtration rate (using the MDRD equation) for Zortress 1.5 mg (target trough concentrations 3 to 8 ng/mL) and mycophenolic acid groups were comparable at Month 12 in the ITT population (Table 8).

[See table 8 above]

Two earlier studies compared fixed doses of Zortress 1.5 mg per day and 3 mg per day, without therapeutic drug monitoring, combined with standard exposure cyclosporine and corticosteroids to mycophenolate mofetil 2.0 g per day and corticosteroids. Antilymphocyte antibody induction was prohibited in both studies. Both were multicenter, double-blind (for first 12 months), randomized trials (1:1:1) of 588 and 583 *de novo* renal transplant patients, respectively. The 12 month analysis of GFR showed increased rates of renal impairment in both the Zortress groups compared to the mycophenolate mofetil group in both studies. Therefore, reduced exposure cyclosporine should be used in combination with Zortress in order to avoid renal dysfunction and everolimus trough concentrations should be adjusted using therapeutic drug monitoring to maintain trough concentrations between 3 to 8 ng/mL. [*See Boxed Warning, Dosage and Administration (2.4) and Warnings and Precautions (5.6)*]

14.2 Prevention of Organ Rejection after Liver Transplantation

A 24-month, multinational, open-label, randomized (1:1:1) trial was conducted in liver transplant patients starting 30 days post-transplant. During the first 30 days, after transplant and prior to randomization, patients received tacrolimus and corticosteroids, with or without mycophenolate mofetil. No induction antibody was administered. Approximately 70 to 80% of patients received at least one dose of mycophenolate mofetil at a median total daily dose of 1.5 g during the first 30 days. For eligibility, patients had to have a tacrolimus trough concentration of at least 8 ng/mL in the week prior to randomization.

At randomization, mycophenolate mofetil was discontinued and patients were randomized to one of two Zortress treatment groups [initial dose of 1 mg twice per day (2 mg daily)

Table 6. Tacrolimus Trough Concentrations Over 12 Months – Liver Study Median Values (ng/mL) with 10th and 90th Percentiles

Treatment group	Visit	N	Target (ng/mL)	Median	10th Percentile	90th Percentile
Predose group	Week 4	234	3-5	9.5	5.8	14.6
Zortress 1.0 mg twice daily (initiated at month 1)	Week 5	219	3-5	8.1	4.5	13.8
	Week 6	233	3-5	7.0	4.1	12.0
	Month 2	219	3-5	5.6	3.4	10.3
	Month 3	218	3-5	5.2	3.1	9.7
	Month 4	196	3-5	4.9	2.9	7.7
	Month 5	195	3-5	4.8	2.7	7.3
	Month 6	200	3-5	4.6	3.0	7.5
	Month 9	186	3-5	4.4	2.9	8.0
	Month 12	175	3-5	4.3	2.6	7.3

Table 7. Efficacy Failure by Treatment Group (ITT Population) at 12 Months

	Zortress (everolimus) 1.5 mg per day With reduced exposure CsA N=277 n (%)	Mycophenolic Acid 1.44 g per day With standard exposure CsA N=277 n (%)
Efficacy Endpoints[1]		
Efficacy Failure Endpoint[2]	70 (25.3)	67 (24.2)
Treated Biopsy Proven Acute Rejection	45 (16.2)	47 (17.0)
Death	7 (2.5)	6 (2.2)
Graft Loss	12 (4.3)	9 (3.2)
Loss to Follow-up	12 (4.3)	9 (3.2)
Graft Loss or Death or Loss to Follow-up[3]	32 (11.6)	26 (9.4)
Graft Loss or Death	18 (6.5)	15 (5.4)
Loss to Follow-up[3]	14 (5.1)	11 (4.0)

* Treated biopsy-proven acute rejection (tBPAR) was defined as a histologically confirmed acute rejection with a biopsy graded as IA, IB, IIA, IIB, or III according to 1997 Banff criteria that was treated with anti-rejection medication.

[1] The difference in rates (Zortress–mycophenolic acid) with 95% CI for primary efficacy failure endpoint is 1.1% (-6.1%, 8.3%); and for the graft loss, death or loss to follow-up endpoint is 2.2% (-2.9%, 7.3%).

[2] Includes treated BPAR, graft loss, death or loss to follow-up by Month 12 where loss to follow-up represents patient who did not experience treated BPAR, graft loss or death and whose last contact date is prior to 12 month visit

[3] Loss to follow-up (for Graft Loss, Death, or Loss to Follow-up) represents patient who did not experience death or graft loss and whose last contact date is prior to 12 month visit

Table 8. Estimated Glomerular Filtration Rates (mL/min/1.73m²) by MDRD at 12 Months Post-Transplant*

Month 12 GFR (MDRD)	Zortress (everolimus) 1.5 mg per day with reduced exposure CsA N=276	Mycophenolic Acid 1.44 g per day with standard exposure CsA N=277
Mean (SD)**	54.6 (21.7)	52.3 (26.5)
Median (Range)	55.0 (0-140.9)	50.1 (0.0-366.4)

* Analysis based on using a subject's last observation carried forward for missing data at 12 months due to death or lost to follow-up data, a value of zero is used for subjects who experienced a graft loss.

** SD=standard deviation

Table 9. Efficacy Failure by Treatment Group (ITT Population) at 12 Months

	Zortress (everolimus) With reduced Exposure Tacrolimus N=245 n (%)		Tacrolimus (standard exposure) N=243 n (%)	
Efficacy Endpoints[1]				
Efficacy Failure Endpoint[2]	22 (9.0)		33 (13.6)	
Treated Biopsy Proven Acute Rejection*		7 (2.9)		17 (7.0)
Death		13 (5.3)		7 (2.9)
Graft Loss		6 (2.4)		3 (1.2)
Loss to Follow-up		4 (1.6)		9 (3.7)
Graft Loss or Death or Loss to Follow-up[3]	18 (7.3)		18 (7.4)	
Graft Loss or Death		14 (5.7)		8 (3.3)
Loss to Follow-up[3]		4 (1.6)		10 (4.1)

* Treated biopsy-proven acute rejection (tBPAR) was defined as histologically confirmed acute rejection with a rejection activity index (RAI) ≥ RAI score 3 that received anti-rejection treatment.
[1] The difference in rates (Zortress – control) with 97.5% CI for efficacy failure endpoint is -4.6% (-11.4%, 2.2%); and for the graft loss, death or loss to follow-up endpoint is -0.1% (-5.4%, 5.3%).
[2] Includes treated BPAR, graft loss, death or loss to follow-up by Month 12 where loss to follow-up represents patients who did not experience treated BPAR, graft loss or death and whose last contact date is prior to 12 month visit
[3] Loss to follow-up (for Graft Loss, Death, or Loss to Follow-up) represents patients who did not experience death or graft loss and whose last contact date is prior to 12 month visit

and adjusted to target trough concentrations using an LC/MS/MS assay of 3 to 8 ng/mL) either with reduced exposure of tacrolimus (target trough whole blood concentrations of 3 to 5 ng/mL) or tacrolimus elimination. In the tacrolimus elimination group, at Month 4 post-transplant, once the everolimus trough concentrations were within the target range of 6 to 10 ng/mL, reduced exposure tacrolimus was eliminated. The Zortress with tacrolimus elimination group was discontinued early due to higher incidence of acute rejection. In the control group, patients received standard exposure tacrolimus (target trough whole blood concentrations of 8 to 12 ng/mL tapered to 6 to 10 ng/mL by month 4 post-transplant). All patients received corticosteroids during the trial.

The study population consisted of 18 to 70 year old male and female liver transplant recipients undergoing their first transplant, mean age was approximately 54 years, more than 70% of patients were male, and the majority of patients were Caucasian, with approximately 89% of patients per treatment group completing the study. Key stratification parameters of HCV status (31-32% HCV positive across groups) and renal function (mean baseline eGFR range 79-83 mL/min/1.73m²) were also balanced between groups.

A total of 1147 patients were enrolled into the run-in period of this trial. At 30 days post-transplant a total 719 patients, who were eligible according to study inclusion/exclusion criteria, were randomized into one of three treatment groups: Zortress with reduced exposure tacrolimus; N=245, Zortress with tacrolimus elimination (tacrolimus elimination group); N=231, or standard dose/exposure tacrolimus (tacrolimus control); N=243. The study was conducted at 89 liver transplant centers across Europe, including the United Kingdom and Ireland, North and South America, and Australia.

Key inclusion criteria were recipients 18-70 years of age, eGFR ≥30 mL/min/1.73m², tacrolimus trough level of ≥8 ng/mL in the week prior to randomization, and the ability to take oral medication.

Key exclusion criteria were recipients of multiple solid organ transplants, history of malignancy (except hepatocellular carcinoma within Milan criteria), human immunodeficiency virus, and any surgical or medical condition which significantly alter the absorption, distribution, metabolism and excretion of study drug.

There were no major baseline differences between treatment groups with regard to recipient or donor disease characteristics. Mean MELD scores at time of transplantation, cold ischemia times (CIT), and ABO matching were similar across groups. Overall the treatment groups were comparable with respect to the key determinants of liver transplantation.

The tacrolimus elimination group was stopped prematurely due to a higher incidence of acute rejection and adverse reactions leading to treatment discontinuation reported during the elimination phase of tacrolimus. Therefore, a treatment regimen of Zortress with tacrolimus elimination is not recommended.

Results at 12 months indicated that Zortress with reduced exposure tacrolimus is comparable to standard exposure tacrolimus with respect to efficacy failure, defined as treated biopsy-proven acute rejection, graft loss, death or loss to follow-up. The percentage of patients experiencing this endpoint and each individual variable in the Zortress and control group is shown in Table 9.

[See table 9 above]

The estimated mean glomerular filtration rate (using the MDRD equation) for the Zortress group was 80.9 mL/min/1.73m² and the tacrolimus control was 70.3 mL/min/1.73m² at Month 12 for patients with estimated GFR (eGFR) in the ITT population (Table 10).

Table 10. Estimated Glomerular Filtration Rates (mL/min/1.73m²) by MDRD at 12 Months Post-Transplant

Month 12 GFR (MDRD)	Zortress (everolimus) with reduced exposure Tacrolimus N=215	Tacrolimus (standard exposure) N=209
Mean (SD)	80.9 (27.3)	70.3 (23.1)
Median* (Range)	78.3 (28.4-153.1)	66.4 (27.9-155.8)

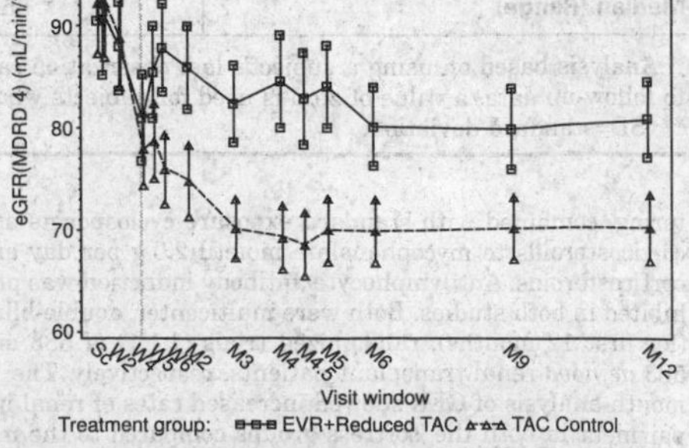

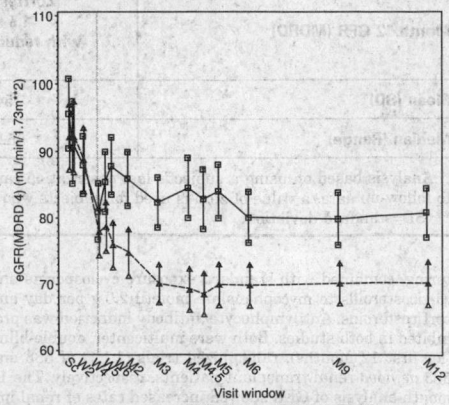

Figure 1. Mean and 95% CI of eGFR (MDRD 4) [mL/min/1.73m²] by Visit Window and Treatment (ITT population – 12 Month Analysis)*

* Zortress dosing was initiated 30 days after transplantation

16 HOW SUPPLIED/STORAGE AND HANDLING

Zortress (everolimus) Tablets are packed in child-resistant blisters.

Table 11. Description of Zortress (everolimus) Tablets

Dosage Strength	0.25 mg	0.5 mg	0.75 mg
Appearance	White to yellowish, marbled, round, flat tablets with beveled edge		
Imprint	"C" on one side and "NVR" on the other	"CH" on one side and "NVR" on the other	"CL" on one side and "NVR" on the other
NDC Number	0078-0417-20	0078-0414-20	0078-0415-20

Each strength is available in boxes of 60 tablets (6 blister strips of 10 tablets each).

Storage

Store at 25°C (77°F); excursions permitted to 15-30°C (59-86°F). [see USP Controlled Room Temperature]
Protect from light and moisture.

17 PATIENT COUNSELING INFORMATION

17.1 Administration

Inform patients that Zortress should be taken orally twice a day approximately 12 hours apart consistently either with or without food.

Inform patients to avoid grapefruit and grapefruit juice which increase blood drug concentrations of Zortress. [*See Warnings and Precautions (5.19)*]

Advise patients that Zortress should be used concurrently with reduced doses of cyclosporine and that any change in doses of these medications should be made under physician supervision. A change in the cyclosporine dose may also require a change in the dosage of Zortress.

Inform patients of the necessity of repeated laboratory tests according to physician recommendations while they are taking Zortress.

17.2 Development of Lymphomas and Other Malignancies

Inform patients they are at risk of developing lymphomas and other malignancies, particularly of the skin, due to immunosuppression. Advise patients to limit exposure to sunlight and ultraviolet (UV) light by wearing protective clothing and using a sunscreen with a high protection factor. [*See Warnings and Precautions (5.2)*]

17.3 Increased Risk of Infection

Inform patients they are at increased risk of developing a variety of infections, including opportunistic infections, due to immunosuppression. Advise patients to contact their physician if they develop any symptoms of infection. [*See Warnings and Precautions (5.3, 5.13)*]

17.4 Kidney Graft Thrombosis

Inform patients that Zortress has been associated with an increased risk of kidney arterial and venous thrombosis, resulting in graft loss, usually within the first 30 days post-transplantation. [*See Warnings and Precautions (5.4)*]

17.5 Zortress and Calcineurin Inhibitor-Induced Nephrotoxicity

Advise patients of the risks of impaired kidney function with the combination of Zortress and cyclosporine as well as the need for routine blood concentration monitoring for both drugs. Advise patients of the importance of serum creatinine monitoring. [*See Warnings and Precautions (5.6)*]

17.6 Angioedema

Inform patients of the risk of angioedema and that concomitant use of angiotensin converting enzyme (ACE) inhibitors may increase this risk. Advise patients to seek prompt medical attention if symptoms occur. [*See Warnings and Precautions (5.8)*]

17.7 Wound Healing Complications and Fluid Accumulation

Inform patients the use of Zortress has been associated with impaired or delayed wound healing, fluid accumulation and the need for careful observation of their incision site. [*See Warnings and Precautions (5.9)*]

17.8 Interstitial lung disease/Non-Infectious Pneumonitis

Inform patients the use of Zortress may increase the risk of non-infectious pneumonitis. Advise patients to seek medical attention if they develop clinical symptoms consistent with pneumonia. [*See Warnings and Precautions (5.10)*]

17.9 Hyperlipidemia

Inform patients the use of Zortress has been associated with increased serum cholesterol and triglycerides that may require treatment and the need for monitoring of blood lipid concentrations. [*See Warnings and Precautions (5.11)*]

17.10 Proteinuria

Inform patients the use of Zortress has been associated with an increased risk of proteinuria. [*See Warnings and Precautions (5.12)*]

17.11 Pregnancy

Advise women of childbearing age to avoid becoming pregnant throughout treatment and for 8 weeks after Zortress therapy has stopped.

17.12 Medications that Interfere with Zortress
Some medications can increase or decrease blood concentrations of Zortress. Advise patients to inform their physician if they are taking any of the following: antifungals, antibiotics, antivirals, anti-epileptic medicines including carbamazepine, phenytoin and barbiturates, herbal/dietary supplements (St. John's Wort), and/or rifampin. [*See Warnings and Precautions (5.14)*]

17.13 New Onset Diabetes
Inform patients the use of Zortress may increase the risk of diabetes mellitus and to contact their physician if they develop symptoms. [*See Warnings and Precautions (5.16)*]

17.14 Immunizations
Inform patients that vaccinations may be less effective while they are being treated with Zortress. Advise patients live vaccines should be avoided. [*See Warnings and Precautions (5.18)*]

17.15 Patient with Hereditary Disorders
Advise patients to inform their physicians that if they have hereditary disorders of galactose intolerance (Lapp-lactase deficiency or glucose-galactose malabsorption) not to take Zortress. [*See Warnings and Precautions (5.20)*]

Manufactured by:
Novartis Pharma Stein AG
Stein, Switzerland
Distributed by:
Novartis Pharmaceuticals Corporation
East Hanover, New Jersey 07936

T2013-09
February 2013

MEDICATION GUIDE
ZORTRESS (ZOR-tres)
(everolimus)
Tablets

Read this Medication Guide before you start using ZORTRESS and each time you get a refill. There may be new information. This information does not take the place of talking with your doctor about your medical condition or treatment.

What is the most important information I should know about ZORTRESS?

ZORTRESS can cause serious side effects, including:
- **Increased risk of getting certain cancers.** People who take ZORTRESS have a higher chance of getting lymphoma and other cancers, especially skin cancer. Talk to your doctor about your risk for cancer.
- **Increased risk of serious infections.** ZORTRESS weakens the body's immune system and affects your ability to fight infections. Serious infections can happen with ZORTRESS that may lead to death. People taking ZORTRESS have a higher chance of getting infections caused by viruses, bacteria, and fungi (yeast).
  - Call your doctor if you have symptoms of infection including fever or chills.
- **Blood clot in the blood vessels of your transplanted kidney.** If this happens, it usually occurs within the first 30 days after your kidney transplant. Tell your doctor right away if you:
  - have pain in your groin, lower back, side or stomach (abdomen)
  - make less urine or you do not pass any urine
  - have blood in your urine or dark colored urine (tea-colored)
  - have fever, nausea, or vomiting
- **Serious problems with your transplanted kidney (nephrotoxicity).** You will need to start with a lower dose of cyclosporine when you take it with ZORTRESS. Your Doctor should do regular blood tests to check your levels of both ZORTRESS and cyclosporine.
- **Increased risk of death that can be related to infection, in people who have had a heart transplant.** You should not take Zortress if you have had a heart transplant without talking to your doctor.

See the section "What are the possible side effects of ZORTRESS?" for information about other serious side effects.

What is ZORTRESS?

ZORTRESS is a prescription medicine used to prevent transplant rejection (antirejection medicine) in people who have received a kidney transplant or liver transplant. Transplant rejection happens when the body's immune system perceives the new transplanted kidney as "foreign" and attacks it.

ZORTRESS is used with other medicines called cyclosporine, corticosteroids and certain other transplant medicines to prevent rejection of your transplanted kidney. Zortress is used with other medicines called tacrolimus and corticosteroids to prevent rejection of your transplanted liver.

It is not known if ZORTRESS is safe and effective in transplanted organs other than the kidney and liver.

It is not known if ZORTRESS is safe and effective in children under 18 years of age.

Who should not take ZORTRESS?

Do not take ZORTRESS if you are allergic to:
- everolimus (ZORTRESS/AFINITOR®) or any of the ingredients in ZORTRESS. See the end of this Medication Guide for a complete list of ingredients in ZORTRESS.
- sirolimus (Rapamune®)

What should I tell my doctor before taking ZORTRESS?

Before taking ZORTRESS, tell your doctor if you:
- have liver problems
- have skin cancer or it runs in your family
- have high cholesterol or triglycerides (fat in your blood)
- have Lapp lactase deficiency or glucose-galactose malabsorption. You should not take ZORTRESS if you have this disorder.
- have any other medical conditions
- are pregnant or plan to become pregnant. It is not known if ZORTRESS will harm your unborn baby. Talk with your doctor if you are pregnant or plan to become pregnant.
  - Women who may become pregnant should use effective birth control (contraception) while taking ZORTRESS and for 8 weeks after stopping ZORTRESS.
- are breastfeeding or plan to breastfeed. It is not known if ZORTRESS passes into your breast milk. You and your doctor should decide if you will take ZORTRESS or breastfeed. You should not do both.

Tell your doctor about all the medicines you take, including prescription and non-prescription medicines, vitamins, and herbal supplements. ZORTRESS may affect the way other medicines work, and other medicines may affect how ZORTRESS works.

Especially tell your doctor if you take:
- antifungal medicine
- antibiotic medicine
- heart medicine
- high blood pressure medicine
- a medicine to lower cholesterol or triglycerides
- cyclosporine (Sandimmune, Gengraf, Neoral)
- tuberculosis (TB) medicine
- HIV medicine
- St. John's Wort
- seizure (anticonvulsant) medicine

Know the medicines you take. Keep a list of them to show your doctor and pharmacist when you get a new medicine. Do not take any new medicine without talking with your doctor first.

How should I take ZORTRESS?
- Take ZORTRESS exactly as your doctor tells you.
- **Do not** stop taking ZORTRESS or change your dose unless your doctor tells you to.
- Take ZORTRESS at the same time as your dose of cyclosporine medicine.
- **Do not** stop taking or change your dose of cyclosporine or tacrolimus medicine unless your doctor tells you to.
- If your doctor changes your dose of cyclosporine your dose of ZORTRESS may change.
- Take ZORTRESS 2 times a day about 12 hours apart.
- Swallow ZORTRESS tablets whole with a glass of water. Do not crush or chew ZORTRESS tablets.
- Take ZORTRESS tablets with or without food. If you take ZORTRESS tablets **with food**, always take ZORTRESS tablets **with food**. If you take ZORTRESS tablets **without food**, always take ZORTRESS tablets **without food.**
- **Your doctor will do regular blood tests to check your kidney function while you take ZORTRESS. It is important that you get these tests done when your doctor tells you to. Blood tests will monitor how your kidneys are working and make sure you are getting the right dose of ZORTRESS and other transplant medications they may be on (cyclosporine and tacrolimus).**
- If you take too much ZORTRESS, call your doctor or go to the nearest hospital emergency room right away.

What should I avoid while taking ZORTRESS?
- Avoid receiving any live vaccines while taking ZORTRESS. Some vaccines may not work as well while you are taking ZORTRESS.
- Do not eat grapefruit or drink grapefruit juice while you are taking ZORTRESS. Grapefruit may increase your blood level of ZORTRESS.
- Limit the amount of time you spend in the sunlight. Avoid using tanning beds or sunlamps. People who take ZORTRESS have a higher risk of getting skin cancer. See the section "What is the most important information I should know about ZORTRESS?" Wear protective clothing when you are in the sun and use a sunscreen with a high protection factor (SPF 30 and above). This is especially important if you have fair skin or if you have a family history of skin cancer.
- Avoid becoming pregnant. See the section "What should I tell my doctor before taking ZORTRESS?"

What are possible side effects of ZORTRESS?

ZORTRESS can cause serious side effects, including:
- See **"What is the most important information I should know about ZORTRESS?"**
- **swelling under your skin especially around your mouth, eyes and in your throat (angioedema).** Your chance of having swelling under your skin is higher if you take ZORTRESS along with certain other medicines. Tell your doctor right away or go to the nearest emergency room if you have any of these symptoms of angioedema:
  - sudden swelling of your face, mouth, throat, tongue or hands
  - hives or welts
  - itchy or painful swollen skin
  - trouble breathing
- **delayed wound healing.** ZORTRESS can cause your incision to heal slowly or not heal well. Call your doctor right away if you have any of the following symptoms:
  - your incision is red, warm or painful
  - blood, fluid, or pus in your incision
  - your incision opens up
  - swelling of your incision
- **lung or breathing problems.** Tell your doctor right away if you have new or worsening cough, shortness of breath, difficulty breathing or wheezing. In some patients lung or breathing problems have been severe, and can even lead to death. Your doctor may need to stop ZORTRESS or lower your dose.
- **increased cholesterol and triglycerides (fat in your blood).** If your cholesterol and triglyceride levels are high your doctor may want to lower them with diet, exercise and certain medicines.
- **protein in your urine (proteinuria).**
- **change in kidney function.** ZORTRESS may cause kidney problems when taken along with a standard dose of cyclosporine medicine instead of a lower dose.

Your doctor should do blood and urine tests to monitor your cholesterol, triglycerides and kidney function.
- **viral infections.** Certain viruses can live in your body and cause active infections when your immune system is weak. Viral infections that can happen with ZORTRESS include BK virus-associated nephropathy. BK virus can affect how your kidney works and cause your transplanted kidney to fail.
- **blood clotting problems.**
- **diabetes.** Tell your doctor if you have frequent urination, increased thirst or hunger.
- **male infertility (low or no sperm count).**

The most common side effects of ZORTRESS in people who have had a kidney or liver transplant include:

These common side effects have been reported in both kidney and liver transplant patients:
- nausea
- swelling of the lower legs, ankles and feet
- high blood pressure

The most common side effects of ZORTRESS in people who have had a kidney transplant include:
- constipation
- low red blood cell count (anemia)
- urinary tract infection
- increased fat in the blood (cholesterol and triglycerides)

The most common side effects of ZORTRESS in people who have had a liver transplant include:
- diarrhea
- headache
- fever
- abdominal pain
- low white blood cells

These are not all of the possible side effects of ZORTRESS. Tell your doctor about any side effect that bothers you or that does not go away.

Call your doctor for medical advice about side effects. You may report side effects to the FDA at 1-800-FDA-1088.

How do I store ZORTRESS?
- Store ZORTRESS tablets between 59°F to 86°F (15°C to 30°C).
- Keep ZORTRESS out of the light.
- Keep ZORTRESS tablets dry.

Keep ZORTRESS and all medicines out of the reach of children.

General information about the safe and effective use of ZORTRESS.

Medicines are sometimes prescribed for purposes other than those listed in a Medication Guide. Do not use ZORTRESS for a condition for which it was not prescribed. Do not give ZORTRESS to other people, even if they have the same symptoms you have. It may harm them.

This Medication Guide summarizes the most important information about ZORTRESS. For more information, talk with your doctor. You can ask your doctor or pharmacist for information about ZORTRESS that is written for healthcare professionals. For more information, call 1-888-669-6682 or visit **www.zortress.com.**

What are the ingredients in ZORTRESS?

Active ingredient: everolimus

Inactive ingredients: butylated hydroxytoluene, magnesium stearate, lactose monohydrate, hypromellose, crospovidone and lactose anhydrous.

This Medication Guide has been approved by the U.S. Food and Drug Administration.

Any other trademarks in this document are the property of their respective owners.
Manufactured by:
Novartis Pharma Stein AG
Stein, Switzerland
Distributed by:
Novartis Pharmaceuticals Corporation
East Hanover, New Jersey 07936

Rapamune® is a registered trademark of Pfizer Inc
Gengraf® is a registered trademark of Abbott Laboratories
T2013-10
February 2013

Shown in Product Identification Guide, page 311

Novo Nordisk Inc.
800 SCUDDERS MILL ROAD
PLAINSBORO, NJ 08536

Direct Inquiries to:
Novo Nordisk Inc.
(800) 727-6500
8:30 AM - 6 PM EST M–F
In Emergencies after hours and weekends:
609-987-5800

LEVEMIR® ℞
[lev'e-mīr]
(insulin detemir [rDNA origin] injection)
solution for subcutaneous injection

HIGHLIGHTS OF PRESCRIBING INFORMATION
These highlights do not include all the information needed to use LEVEMIR® safely and effectively.
See full prescribing information for LEVEMIR.
LEVEMIR® (insulin detemir [rDNA origin] injection) solution for subcutaneous injection
Initial U.S. Approval: 2005

RECENT MAJOR CHANGES

Warnings and Precautions (5.8) 3/2013

INDICATIONS AND USAGE

LEVEMIR is a long-acting human insulin analog indicated to improve glycemic control in adults and children with diabetes mellitus. (1)
Important Limitations of Use:
- Not recommended for treating diabetic ketoacidosis. Use intravenous, rapid-acting or short-acting insulin instead.

DOSAGE AND ADMINISTRATION

- The starting dose should be individualized based on the type of diabetes and whether the patient is insulin-naïve (2.1, 2.2, 2.3)
- Administer subcutaneously once daily or in divided doses twice daily. Once daily administration should be given with the evening meal or at bedtime (2.1)
- Rotate injection sites within an injection area (abdomen, thigh, or deltoid) to reduce the risk of lipodystrophy (2.1)
- Converting from other insulin therapies may require adjustment of timing and dose of LEVEMIR. Closely monitor glucoses especially upon converting to LEVEMIR and during the initial weeks thereafter (2.3)

DOSAGE FORMS AND STRENGTHS

Solution for injection 100 Units/mL (U-100) in
- 3 mL LEVEMIR FlexPen®
- 10 mL vial (3)

CONTRAINDICATIONS

- Do not use in patients with hypersensitivity to LEVEMIR or any of its excipients (4)

WARNINGS AND PRECAUTIONS

- Dose adjustment and monitoring: Monitor blood glucose in all patients treated with insulin. Insulin regimens should be modified cautiously and only under medical supervision (5.1)
- Administration: Do not dilute or mix with any other insulin or solution. Do not administer subcutaneously via an insulin pump, intramuscularly, or intravenously because severe hypoglycemia can occur (5.2)
- Hypoglycemia is the most common adverse reaction of insulin therapy and may be life-threatening (5.3, 6.1)
- Allergic reactions: Severe, life-threatening, generalized allergy, including anaphylaxis, can occur (5.4)
- Renal or hepatic impairment: May require adjustment of the LEVEMIR dose (5.5, 5.6)
- Fluid retention and heart failure can occur with concomitant use of thiazolidinediones (TZDs), which are PPAR-gamma agonists, and insulin, including LEVEMIR (5.8)

ADVERSE REACTIONS

Adverse reactions associated with LEVEMIR include hypoglycemia, allergic reactions, injection site reactions, lipodystrophy, rash and pruritus (6)

To report SUSPECTED ADVERSE REACTIONS, contact Novo Nordisk Inc. at 1-800-727-6500 or FDA at 1-800-FDA-1088 or *www.fda.gov/medwatch*

DRUG INTERACTIONS

- Certain drugs may affect glucose metabolism requiring insulin dose adjustment and close monitoring of blood glucose (7)
- The signs of hypoglycemia may be reduced or absent in patients taking anti-adrenergic drugs (e.g., beta-blockers, clonidine, guanethidine, and reserpine) (7)

USE IN SPECIFIC POPULATIONS

Pediatric: Has not been studied in children with type 2 diabetes. Has not been studied in children with type 1 diabetes < 2 years of age (8.4)

See 17 for PATIENT COUNSELING INFORMATION and FDA-approved patient labeling

Revised: 04/2013

FULL PRESCRIBING INFORMATION: CONTENTS*

* Sections or subsections omitted from the full prescribing information are not listed.

FULL PRESCRIBING INFORMATION

1 INDICATIONS AND USAGE

LEVEMIR is indicated to improve glycemic control in adults and children with diabetes mellitus.
Important Limitations of Use:
- LEVEMIR is not recommended for the treatment of diabetic ketoacidosis. Intravenous rapid-acting or short-acting insulin is the preferred treatment for this condition.

2 DOSAGE AND ADMINISTRATION

2.1 Dosing

LEVEMIR is a recombinant human insulin analog for once- or twice-daily subcutaneous administration.

Patients treated with LEVEMIR once-daily should administer the dose with the evening meal or at bedtime.

Patients who require twice-daily dosing can administer the evening dose with the evening meal, at bedtime, or 12 hours after the morning dose.

The dose of LEVEMIR must be individualized based on clinical response. Blood glucose monitoring is essential in all patients receiving insulin therapy.

Patients adjusting the amount or timing of dosing with LEVEMIR should only do so under medical supervision with appropriate glucose monitoring *[see Warnings and Precautions (5.1)]*.

In patients with type 1 diabetes, LEVEMIR must be used in a regimen with rapid-acting or short-acting insulin.

As with all insulins, injection sites should be rotated within the same region (abdomen, thigh, or deltoid) from one injection to the next to reduce the risk of lipodystrophy *[see Adverse Reactions (6.1)]*.

LEVEMIR can be injected subcutaneously in the thigh, abdominal wall, or upper arm. As with all insulins, the rate of absorption, and consequently the onset and duration of action, may be affected by exercise and other variables, such as stress, intercurrent illness, or changes in co-administered medications or meal patterns.

When using LEVEMIR with a glucagon-like peptide (GLP)-1 receptor agonist, administer as separate injections. Never mix. It is acceptable to inject LEVEMIR and a GLP-1 receptor agonist in the same body region but the injections should not be adjacent to each other.

2.2 Initiation of LEVEMIR Therapy

The recommended starting dose of LEVEMIR in patients with type 1 diabetes should be approximately one-third of the total daily insulin requirements. Rapid-acting or short-acting, pre-meal insulin should be used to satisfy the remainder of the daily insulin requirements.

The recommended starting dose of LEVEMIR in patients with type 2 diabetes inadequately controlled on oral antidiabetic medications is 10 Units (or 0.1-0.2 Units/kg) given once daily in the evening or divided into a twice daily regimen.

The recommended starting dose of LEVEMIR in patients with type 2 diabetes inadequately controlled on a GLP-1 receptor agonist is 10 Units given once daily in the evening.

LEVEMIR doses should subsequently be adjusted based on blood glucose measurements. The dosages of LEVEMIR should be individualized under the supervision of a healthcare provider.

2.3 Converting to LEVEMIR from Other Insulin Therapies

If converting from insulin glargine to LEVEMIR, the change can be done on a unit-to-unit basis.

If converting from NPH insulin, the change can be done on a unit-to-unit basis. However, some patients with type 2 diabetes may require more LEVEMIR than NPH insulin, as observed in one trial *[see Clinical Studies (14)]*.

As with all insulins, close glucose monitoring is recommended during the transition and in the initial weeks thereafter. Doses and timing of concurrent rapid-acting or short-acting insulins or other concomitant antidiabetic treatment may need to be adjusted.

3 DOSAGE FORMS AND STRENGTHS

LEVEMIR solution for injection 100 Unit per mL is available as:
- 3 mL LEVEMIR FlexPen®
- 10 mL vial

4 CONTRAINDICATIONS

LEVEMIR is contraindicated in patients with hypersensitivity to LEVEMIR or any of its excipients. Reactions have included anaphylaxis *[see Warnings and Precautions (5.4) and Adverse Reactions (6.1)]*.

5 WARNINGS AND PRECAUTIONS

5.1 Dosage Adjustment and Monitoring

Glucose monitoring is essential for all patients receiving insulin therapy. Changes to an insulin regimen should be made cautiously and only under medical supervision.

Changes in insulin strength, manufacturer, type, or method of administration may result in the need for a change in the insulin dose or an adjustment of concomitant anti-diabetic treatment.

As with all insulin preparations, the time course of action for LEVEMIR may vary in different individuals or at different times in the same individual and is dependent on many conditions, including the local blood supply, local temperature, and physical activity.

5.2 Administration

LEVEMIR should only be administered subcutaneously.

Do not administer LEVEMIR intravenously or intramuscularly. The intended duration of activity of LEVEMIR is dependent on injection into subcutaneous tissue. Intravenous or intramuscular administration of the usual subcutaneous dose could result in severe hypoglycemia *[see Warnings and Precautions (5.3)]*.

Do not use LEVEMIR in insulin infusion pumps.

Do not dilute or mix LEVEMIR with any other insulin or solution. If LEVEMIR is diluted or mixed, the pharmacokinetic or pharmacodynamic profile (e.g., onset of action, time to peak effect) of LEVEMIR and the mixed insulin may be altered in an unpredictable manner.

5.3 Hypoglycemia

Hypoglycemia is the most common adverse reaction of insulin therapy, including LEVEMIR. The risk of hypoglycemia increases with intensive glycemic control.

When a GLP-1 receptor agonist is used in combination with LEVEMIR, the LEVEMIR dose may need to be lowered or more conservatively titrated to minimize the risk of hypoglycemia *[see Adverse Reactions (6.1)]*.

All patients must be educated to recognize and manage hypoglycemia. Severe hypoglycemia can lead to unconsciousness or convulsions and may result in temporary or permanent impairment of brain function or death. Severe hypoglycemia requiring the assistance of another person or parenteral glucose infusion, or glucagon administration has been observed in clinical trials with insulin, including trials with LEVEMIR.

The timing of hypoglycemia usually reflects the time-action profile of the administered insulin formulations. Other factors such as changes in food intake (e.g., amount of food or timing of meals), exercise, and concomitant medications may also alter the risk of hypoglycemia *[see Drug Interactions (7)]*.

The prolonged effect of subcutaneous LEVEMIR may delay recovery from hypoglycemia.

As with all insulins, use caution in patients with hypoglycemia unawareness and in patients who may be predisposed to hypoglycemia (e.g., the pediatric population and patients who fast or have erratic food intake). The patient's ability to concentrate and react may be impaired as a result of hypoglycemia. This may present a risk in situations where these abilities are especially important, such as driving or operating other machinery.

Early warning symptoms of hypoglycemia may be different or less pronounced under certain conditions, such as long-standing diabetes, diabetic neuropathy, use of medications such as beta-blockers, or intensified glycemic control *[see Drug Interactions (7)]*. These situations may result in severe hypoglycemia (and, possibly, loss of consciousness) prior to the patient's awareness of hypoglycemia.

5.4 Hypersensitivity and Allergic Reactions

Severe, life-threatening, generalized allergy, including anaphylaxis, can occur with insulin products, including LEVEMIR.

5.5 Renal Impairment

No difference was observed in the pharmacokinetics of insulin detemir between non-diabetic individuals with renal impairment and healthy volunteers. However, some studies with human insulin have shown increased circulating insulin concentrations in patients with renal impairment. Careful glucose monitoring and dose adjustments of insulin, including LEVEMIR, may be necessary in patients with renal impairment *[see Clinical Pharmacology (12.3)]*.

5.6 Hepatic Impairment

Non-diabetic individuals with severe hepatic impairment had lower systemic exposures to insulin detemir compared to healthy volunteers. However, some studies with human insulin have shown increased circulating insulin concentrations in patients with liver impairment. Careful glucose monitoring and dose adjustments of insulin, including LEVEMIR, may be necessary in patients with hepatic impairment *[see Clinical Pharmacology (12.3)]*.

5.7 Drug Interactions

Some medications may alter insulin requirements and subsequently increase the risk for hypoglycemia or hyperglycemia *[see Drug Interactions (7)]*.

5.8 Fluid retention and heart failure with concomitant use of PPAR-gamma agonists

Thiazolidinediones (TZDs), which are peroxisome proliferator-activated receptor (PPAR)-gamma agonists, can cause dose-related fluid retention, particularly when used in combination with insulin. Fluid retention may lead to or exacerbate heart failure. Patients treated with insulin, including LEVEMIR, and a PPAR-gamma agonist should be observed for signs and symptoms of heart failure. If heart failure develops, it should be managed according to current standards of care, and discontinuation or dose reduction of the PPAR-gamma agonist must be considered.

6 ADVERSE REACTIONS

The following adverse reactions are discussed elsewhere:

- Hypoglycemia *[see Warnings and Precautions (5.3)]*
- Hypersensitivity and allergic reactions *[see Warnings and Precautions (5.4)]*

6.1 Clinical Trial Experience

Because clinical trials are conducted under widely varying designs, the adverse reaction rates reported in one clinical trial may not be easily compared to those rates reported in another clinical trial, and may not reflect the rates actually observed in clinical practice.

The frequencies of adverse reactions (excluding hypoglycemia) reported during LEVEMIR clinical trials in patients with type 1 diabetes mellitus and type 2 diabetes mellitus are listed in Tables 1-4 below. See Tables 5 and 6 for the hypoglycemia findings.

In the LEVEMIR add-on to liraglutide+metformin trial, all patients received liraglutide 1.8 mg + metformin during a 12-week run-in period. During the run-in period, 167 patients (17% of enrolled total) withdrew from the trial: 76 (46% of withdrawals) of these patients doing so because of gastrointestinal adverse reactions and 15 (9% of withdrawals) doing so due to other adverse events. Only those patients who completed the run-in period with inadequate glycemic control were randomized to 26 weeks of add-on therapy with LEVEMIR or continued, unchanged treatment with liraglutide 1.8 mg + metformin. During this randomized 26-week period, diarrhea was the only adverse reaction reported in ≥5% of patients treated with liraglutide 1.8 mg + metformin (11.7%) and greater than in patients treated with liraglutide 1.8 mg and metformin alone (6.9%).

In two pooled trials, a total of 1155 adults with type 1 diabetes were exposed to individualized doses of LEVEMIR (n=767) or NPH (n=388). The mean duration of exposure to LEVEMIR was 153 days, and the total exposure to LEVEMIR was 321 patient-years. The most common adverse reactions are summarized in Table 1.

Table 1: Adverse reactions (excluding hypoglycemia) in two pooled clinical trials of 16 weeks and 24 weeks duration in adults with type 1 diabetes (adverse reactions with incidence ≥ 5%)

	LEVEMIR, % (n = 767)	NPH, % (n = 388)
Upper respiratory tract infection	26.1	21.4
Headache	22.6	22.7
Pharyngitis	9.5	8.0
Influenza-like illness	7.8	7.0
Abdominal Pain	6.0	2.6

A total of 320 adults with type 1 diabetes were exposed to individualized doses of LEVEMIR (n=161) or insulin glargine (n=159). The mean duration of exposure to LEVEMIR was 176 days, and the total exposure to LEVEMIR was 78 patient-years. The most common adverse reactions are summarized in Table 2.

Table 2: Adverse reactions (excluding hypoglycemia) in a 26-week trial comparing insulin aspart + LEVEMIR to insulin aspart + insulin glargine in adults with type 1 diabetes (adverse reactions with incidence ≥ 5%)

	LEVEMIR, % (n = 161)	Glargine, % (n = 159)
Upper respiratory tract infection	26.7	32.1
Headache	14.3	19.5
Back pain	8.1	6.3
Influenza-like illness	6.2	8.2
Gastroenteritis	5.6	4.4
Bronchitis	5.0	1.9

In two pooled trials, a total of 869 adults with type 2 diabetes were exposed to individualized doses of LEVEMIR (n=432) or NPH (n=437). The mean duration of exposure to LEVEMIR was 157 days, and the total exposure to LEVEMIR was 186 patient-years. The most common adverse reactions are summarized in Table 3.

Table 3: Adverse reactions (excluding hypoglycemia) in two pooled clinical trials of 22 weeks and 24 weeks duration in adults with type 2 diabetes (adverse reactions with incidence ≥ 5%)

	LEVEMIR, % (n = 432)	NPH, % (n = 437)
Upper respiratory tract infection	12.5	11.2
Headache	6.5	5.3

A total of 347 children and adolescents (6-17 years) with type 1 diabetes were exposed to individualized doses of LEVEMIR (n=232) or NPH (n=115). The mean duration of exposure to LEVEMIR was 180 days, and the total exposure to LEVEMIR was 114 patient-years. The most common adverse reactions are summarized in Table 4.

Table 4: Adverse reactions (excluding hypoglycemia) in one 26-week clinical trial of children and adolescents with type 1 diabetes (adverse reactions with incidence ≥ 5%)

	LEVEMIR, % (n = 232)	NPH, % (n = 115)
Upper respiratory tract infection	35.8	42.6
Headache	31.0	32.2
Pharyngitis	17.2	20.9
Gastroenteritis	16.8	11.3
Influenza-like illness	13.8	20.9
Abdominal pain	13.4	13.0
Pyrexia	10.3	6.1
Cough	8.2	4.3
Viral infection	7.3	7.8
Nausea	6.5	7.0
Rhinitis	6.5	3.5
Vomiting	6.5	10.4

Pregnancy

A randomized, open-label, controlled clinical trial has been conducted in pregnant women with type 1 diabetes. *[see Use in Specific Populations (8.1)]*

• *Hypoglycemia*

Hypoglycemia is the most commonly observed adverse reaction in patients using insulin, including LEVEMIR *[see Warnings and Precautions (5.3)]*.

Tables 5 and 6 summarize the incidence of severe and non-severe hypoglycemia in the LEVEMIR clinical trials.

For the adult trials and one of the pediatric trials (Study D), severe hypoglycemia was defined as an event with symptoms consistent with hypoglycemia requiring assistance of another person and associated with either a plasma glucose value below 56 mg/dL (blood glucose below 50 mg/dL) or prompt recovery after oral carbohydrate, intravenous glucose or glucagon administration. For the other pediatric trial (Study I), severe hypoglycemia was defined as an event with semi-consciousness, unconsciousness, coma and/or convulsions in a patient who could not assist in the treatment and who may have required glucagon or intravenous glucose.

For the adult trials and pediatric Study D, non-severe hypoglycemia was defined as an asymptomatic or symptomatic plasma glucose < 56 mg/dL (or equivalently blood glucose <50 mg/dL as used in Study A and C) that was self-treated by the patient. For pediatric Study I, non-severe hypoglycemia included asymptomatic events with plasma glucose <65 mg/dL as well as symptomatic events that the patient could self-treat or treat by taking oral therapy provided by the caregiver.

The rates of hypoglycemia in the LEVEMIR clinical trials (see Section 14 for a description of the study designs) were comparable between LEVEMIR-treated patients and non-LEVEMIR-treated patients (see Tables 5 and 6).

[See table 5 at top of next page]
[See table 6 at top of next page]

• *Insulin Initiation and Intensification of Glucose Control*

Intensification or rapid improvement in glucose control has been associated with a transitory, reversible ophthalmologic refraction disorder, worsening of diabetic retinopathy, and acute painful peripheral neuropathy. However, long-term glycemic control decreases the risk of diabetic retinopathy and neuropathy.

• *Lipodystrophy*

Long-term use of insulin, including LEVEMIR, can cause lipodystrophy at the site of repeated insulin injections. Lipodystrophy includes lipohypertrophy (thickening of adipose tissue) and lipoatrophy (thinning of adipose tissue), and may affect insulin absorption. Rotate insulin injection sites within the same region to reduce the risk of lipodystrophy *[see Dosage and Administration (2.1)]*.

• *Weight Gain*

Weight gain can occur with insulin therapy, including LEVEMIR, and has been attributed to the anabolic effects of insulin and the decrease in glucosuria *[see Clinical Studies (14)]*.

• *Peripheral Edema*

Insulin, including LEVEMIR, may cause sodium retention and edema, particularly if previously poor metabolic control is improved by intensified insulin therapy.

Table 5: Hypoglycemia in Patients with Type 1 Diabetes

		Severe Hypoglycemia		Non-severe Hypoglycemia	
		Percent of patients with at least 1 event (n/total N)	Event/patient/ year	Percent of patients (n/total N)	Event/patient/ year
Study A Type 1 Diabetes Adults 16 weeks In combination with insulin aspart	Twice-daily LEVEMIR	8.7 (24/276)	0.52	88.0 (243/276)	26.4
	Twice-daily NPH	10.6 (14/132)	0.43	89.4 (118/132)	37.5
Study B Type 1 Diabetes Adults 26 weeks In combination with insulin aspart	Twice-daily LEVEMIR	5.0 (8/161)	0.13	82.0 (132/161)	20.2
	Once-daily Glargine	10.1 (16/159)	0.31	77.4 (123/159)	21.8
Study C Type 1 Diabetes Adults 24 weeks In combination with regular insulin	Once-daily LEVEMIR	7.5 (37/491)	0.35	88.4 (434/491)	31.1
	Once-daily NPH	10.2 (26/256)	0.32	87.9 (225/256)	33.4
Study D Type 1 Diabetes Pediatrics 26 weeks In combination with insulin aspart	Once- or Twice-daily LEVEMIR	15.9 (37/232)	0.91	93.1 (216/232)	31.6
	Once- or Twice-daily NPH	20.0 (23/115)	0.99	95.7 (110/115)	37.0
Study I Type 1 Diabetes Pediatrics 52 weeks In combination with insulin aspart	Once- or Twice-daily LEVEMIR	1.7 (3/177)	0.02	94.9 (168/177)	56.1
	Once- or Twice-daily NPH	7.1 (12/170)	0.09	97.6 (166/170)	70.7

Table 6: Hypoglycemia in Patients with Type 2 Diabetes

		Study E Type 2 Diabetes Adults 24 weeks In combination with oral agents		Study F Type 2 Diabetes Adults 22 weeks In combination with insulin aspart		Study H Type 2 Diabetes Adults 26 weeks In combination with Liraglutide and Metformin	
		Twice-daily LEVEMIR	Twice-daily NPH	Once- or Twice-daily LEVEMIR	Once- or Twice-daily NPH	Once- daily LEVEMIR + Liraglutide + Metformin	Liraglutide + Metformin
Severe hypoglycemia	Percent of patients with at least 1 event (n/total N)	0.4 (1/237)	2.5 (6/238)	1.5 (3/195)	4.0 (8/199)	0	0
	Event/patient/year	0.01	0.08	0.04	0.13	0	0
Non-severe hypoglycemia	Percent of patients (n/total N)	40.5 (96/237)	64.3 (153/238)	32.3 (63/195)	32.2 (64/199)	9.2 (15/163)	1.3 (2/158*)
	Event/patient/year	3.5	6.9	1.6	2.0	0.29	0.03

* One subject is an outlier and was excluded due to 25 hypoglycemic episodes that the patient was able to self-treat. This patient had a history of frequent hypoglycemia prior to the study

• *Allergic Reactions*

Local Allergy

As with any insulin therapy, patients taking LEVEMIR may experience injection site reactions, including localized erythema, pain, pruritus, urticaria, edema, and inflammation. In clinical studies in adults, three patients treated with LEVEMIR reported injection site pain (0.25%) compared to one patient treated with NPH insulin (0.12%). The reports of pain at the injection site did not result in discontinuation of therapy.

Rotation of the injection site within a given area from one injection to the next may help to reduce or prevent these reactions. In some instances, these reactions may be related to factors other than insulin, such as irritants in a skin cleansing agent or poor injection technique. Most minor reactions to insulin usually resolve in a few days to a few weeks.

Systemic Allergy

Severe, life-threatening, generalized allergy, including anaphylaxis, generalized skin reactions, angioedema, bronchospasm, hypotension, and shock may occur with any insulin, including LEVEMIR, and may be life-threatening *[see Warnings and Precautions (5.4)]*.

• *Antibody Production*

All insulin products can elicit the formation of insulin antibodies. These insulin antibodies may increase or decrease the efficacy of insulin and may require adjustment of the insulin dose. In phase 3 clinical trials of LEVEMIR, antibody development has been observed with no apparent impact on glycemic control.

6.2 Postmarketing Experience

The following adverse reactions have been identified during post approval use of LEVEMIR. Because these reactions are reported voluntarily from a population of uncertain size, it is not always possible to reliably estimate their frequency or establish a causal relationship to drug exposure.

Medication errors have been reported during post-approval use of LEVEMIR in which other insulins, particularly rapid-acting or short-acting insulins, have been accidentally administered instead of LEVEMIR *[see Patient Counseling Information (17)]*. To avoid medication errors between LEVEMIR and other insulins, patients should be instructed always to verify the insulin label before each injection.

7 DRUG INTERACTIONS

A number of medications affect glucose metabolism and may require insulin dose adjustment and particularly close monitoring.

The following are examples of medications that may increase the blood-glucose-lowering effect of insulins including LEVEMIR and, therefore, increase the susceptibility to hypoglycemia: oral antidiabetic medications, pramlintide acetate, angiotensin converting enzyme (ACE) inhibitors, disopyramide, fibrates, fluoxetine, monoamine oxidase (MAO) inhibitors, propoxyphene, pentoxifylline, salicylates, somatostatin analogs, and sulfonamide antibiotics.

The following are examples of medications that may reduce the blood-glucose-lowering effect of insulins including LEVEMIR: corticosteroids, niacin, danazol, diuretics, sympathomimetic agents (e.g., epinephrine, albuterol, terbutaline), glucagon, isoniazid, phenothiazine derivatives, somatropin, thyroid hormones, estrogens, progestogens (e.g., in oral contraceptives), protease inhibitors and atypical antipsychotic medications (e.g. olanzapine and clozapine).

Beta-blockers, clonidine, lithium salts, and alcohol may either increase or decrease the blood-glucose-lowering effect of insulin. Pentamidine may cause hypoglycemia, which may sometimes be followed by hyperglycemia.

The signs of hypoglycemia may be reduced or absent in patients taking anti-adrenergic drugs such as beta-blockers, clonidine, guanethidine, and reserpine.

8 USE IN SPECIFIC POPULATIONS

8.1 Pregnancy

Pregnancy Category B

Risk Summary

The background risk of birth defects, pregnancy loss, or other adverse events that exists for all pregnancies is increased in pregnancies complicated by hyperglycemia. Female patients should be advised to tell their physician if they intend to become, or if they become pregnant while taking LEVEMIR. A randomized controlled clinical trial of pregnant women with type 1 diabetes using LEVEMIR during pregnancy did not show an increase in the risk of fetal abnormalities. Reproductive toxicology studies in non-diabetic rats and rabbits that included concurrent human insulin control groups indicated that insulin detemir and human insulin had similar effects regarding embryotoxicity and teratogenicity that were attributed to maternal hypoglycemia.

Clinical Considerations

The increased risk of adverse events in pregnancies complicated by hyperglycemia may be decreased with good glucose control before conception and throughout pregnancy. Because insulin requirements vary throughout pregnancy and in the post-partum period, careful monitoring of glucose control is essential in pregnant women.

Human Data

In an open-label clinical study, women with type 1 diabetes who were (between weeks 8 and 12 of gestation) or intended to become pregnant were randomized 1:1 to LEVEMIR (once or twice daily) or NPH insulin (once, twice or thrice daily). Insulin aspart was administered before each meal. A total of 152 women in the LEVEMIR arm and 158 women in the NPH arm were or became pregnant during the study (total pregnant women = 310). Approximately one half of the study participants in each arm were randomized as pregnant and were exposed to NPH or to other insulins prior to conception and in the first 8 weeks of gestation. In the 310 pregnant women, the mean glycosylated hemoglobin (HbA_{1c}) was < 7% at 10, 12, and 24 weeks of gestation in both arms. In the intent-to-treat population, the adjusted mean HbA_{1c} (standard error) at gestational week 36 was 6.27% (0.053) in LEVEMIR-treated patient (n=138) and 6.33% (0.052) in NPH-treated patients (n=145); the difference was not clinically significant.

Adverse reactions in pregnant patients occurring at an incidence of ≥5% are shown in Table 7. The two most common adverse reactions were nasopharyngitis and headache. These are consistent with findings from other type 1 diabetes trials (see Table 1, Section 6.1.), and are not repeated in Table 7.

Table 8: Hypoglycemia in Pregnant Women with Type 1 Diabetes

		Study G Type 1 Diabetes Pregnancy In combination with insulin aspart	
		LEVEMIR	NPH
Severe hypoglycemia*	Percent of patients with at least 1 event (n/total N)	16.4 (25/152)	20.9 (33/158)
	Events/patient/year	1.1	1.2
Non-severe hypoglycemia*	Percent of patients with at least 1 event (n/total N)	94.7 (144/152)	92.4 (146/158)
	Events/patient/year	114.2	108.4

* For definition regarding severe and non-severe hypoglycemia see section 6, Hypoglycemia.

Figure 1: Structural Formula of insulin detemir

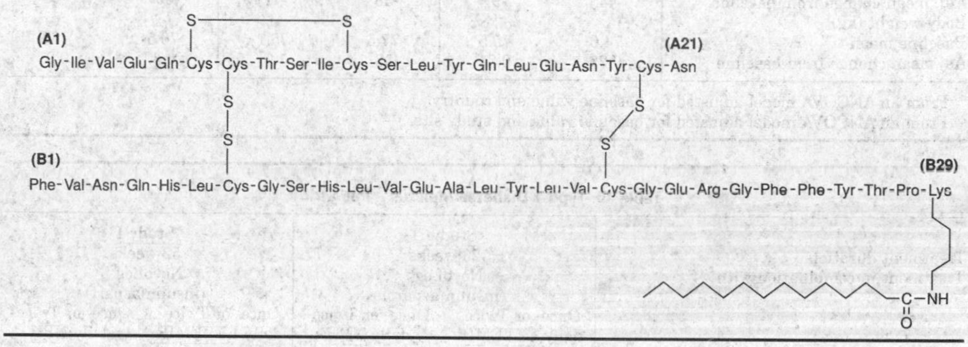

The incidence of adverse reactions of pre-eclampsia was 10.5% (16 cases) and 7.0% (11 cases) in the LEVEMIR and NPH insulin groups respectively. Out of the total number of cases of pre-eclampsia, eight (8) cases in the LEVEMIR group and 1 case in the NPH insulin group required hospitalization. The rates of pre-eclampsia observed in the study are within expected rates for pregnancy complicated by diabetes. Pre-eclampsia is a syndrome defined by symptoms, hypertension and proteinuria; the definition of pre-eclampsia was not standardized in the trial making it difficult to establish a link between a given treatment and an increased risk of pre-eclampsia. All events were considered unlikely related to trial treatment. In all nine (9) cases requiring hospitalization the women had healthy infants. Events of hypertension, proteinuria and edema were reported less frequently in the LEVEMIR group than in the NPH insulin group as a whole. There was no difference between the treatment groups in mean blood pressure during pregnancy and there was no indication of a general increase in blood pressure.

In the NPH insulin group there were 6 serious adverse reactions in four mothers of the following placental disorders, 'Placenta previa', 'Placenta previa hemorrhage', and 'Premature separation of placenta' and 1 serious adverse reaction of 'Antepartum haemorrhage'. There were none reported in the LEVEMIR group.

The incidence of early fetal death (abortions) was similar in LEVEMIR and NPH treated patients; 6.6% and 5.1%, respectively. The abortions were reported under the following terms: 'Abortion spontaneous', 'Abortion missed', 'Blighted ovum', 'Cervical incompetence' and 'Abortion incomplete'.

Table 7: Adverse reactions during pregnancy in a trial comparing insulin aspart + LEVEMIR to insulin aspart + NPH insulin in pregnant women with type 1 diabetes (adverse reactions with incidence ≥ 5%)*

	LEVEMIR, % (n = 152)	NPH, % (n = 158)
Anemia	13.2	10.8
Diarrhea	11.8	5.1
Pre-eclampsia	10.5	7.0
Urinary tract infection	9.9	5.7
Gastroenteritis	8.6	5.1
Abdominal pain upper	5.9	3.8
Vomiting	5.3	4.4
Abortion spontaneous	5.3	2.5
Abdominal pain	5.3	6.3
Oropharyngeal pain	5.3	6.3

* Because clinical trials are conducted under widely varying designs, the adverse reaction rates reported in one clinical trial may not be easily compared to those rates reported in another clinical trial, and may not reflect the rates actually observed in clinical practice.

The proportion of subjects experiencing severe hypoglycemia was 16.4% and 20.9% in LEVEMIR and NPH treated patients respectively. The rate of severe hypoglycemia was 1.1 and 1.2 events per patient-year in LEVEMIR and NPH treated patients respectively. Proportion and incidence rates for non-severe episodes of hypoglycemia were similar in both treatment groups (Table 8).

[See table 8 above]

In about a quarter of infants, LEVEMIR was detected in the infant cord blood at levels above the lower level of quantification (<25 pmol/L).

No differences in pregnancy outcomes or the health of the fetus and newborn were seen with LEVEMIR use.

Animal Data

In a fertility and embryonic development study, insulin detemir was administered to female rats before mating, during mating, and throughout pregnancy at doses up to 300 nmol/kg/day (3 times a human dose of 0.5 Units/kg/day, based on plasma area under the curve (AUC) ratio). Doses of 150 and 300 nmol/kg/day produced numbers of litters with visceral anomalies. Doses up to 900 nmol/kg/day (approximately 135 times a human dose of 0.5 Units/kg/day based on AUC ratio) were given to rabbits during organogenesis. Drug and dose related increases in the incidence of fetuses with gallbladder abnormalities such as small, bilobed, bifurcated, and missing gallbladders were observed at a dose of 900 nmol/kg/day. The rat and rabbit embryofetal development studies that included concurrent human insulin control groups indicated that insulin detemir and human insulin had similar effects regarding embryotoxicity and teratogenicity suggesting that the effects seen were the result of hypoglycemia resulting from insulin exposure in normal animals.

8.3 Nursing Mothers

It is unknown whether LEVEMIR is excreted in human milk. Because many drugs, including human insulin, are excreted in human milk, use caution when administering LEVEMIR to a nursing woman. Women with diabetes who are lactating may require adjustments of their insulin doses.

8.4 Pediatric Use

The pharmacokinetics, safety and effectiveness of subcutaneous injections of LEVEMIR have been established in pediatric patients (age 2 to 17 years) with type 1 diabetes *[see Clinical Pharmacology (12.3) and Clinical Studies (14)]*. LEVEMIR has not been studied in pediatric patients younger than 2 years of age with type 1 diabetes. LEVEMIR has not been studied in pediatric patients with type 2 diabetes.

The dose recommendation when converting to LEVEMIR is the same as that described for adults *[see Dosage and Administration (2) and Clinical Studies (14)]*. As in adults, the dosage of LEVEMIR must be individualized in pediatric patients based on metabolic needs and frequent monitoring of blood glucose.

8.5 Geriatric Use

In controlled clinical trials comparing LEVEMIR to NPH insulin or insulin glargine, 64 of 1624 patients (3.9%) in the type 1 diabetes trials and 309 of 1082 patients (28.6%) in the type 2 diabetes trials were ≥65 years of age. A total of 52 (7 type 1 and 45 type 2) patients (1.9%) were ≥75 years of age. No overall differences in safety or effectiveness were observed between these patients and younger patients, but small sample sizes, particularly for patients ≥65 years of age in the type 1 diabetes trials and for patients ≥75 years of age in all trials limits conclusions. Greater sensitivity of some older individuals cannot be ruled out. In elderly patients with diabetes, the initial dosing, dose increments, and maintenance dosage should be conservative to avoid hypoglycemia. Hypoglycemia may be difficult to recognize in the elderly.

10 OVERDOSAGE

An excess of insulin relative to food intake, energy expenditure, or both may lead to severe and sometimes prolonged and life-threatening hypoglycemia. Mild episodes of hypoglycemia usually can be treated with oral glucose. Adjustments in drug dosage, meal patterns, or exercise may be needed.

More severe episodes with coma, seizure, or neurologic impairment may be treated with intramuscular/subcutaneous glucagon or concentrated intravenous glucose. After apparent clinical recovery from hypoglycemia, continued observation and additional carbohydrate intake may be necessary to avoid recurrence of hypoglycemia *[see Warnings and Precautions (5.3)]*.

11 DESCRIPTION

LEVEMIR (insulin detemir [rDNA origin] injection) is a sterile solution of insulin detemir for use as a subcutaneous injection. Insulin detemir is a long-acting (up to 24-hour duration of action) recombinant human insulin analog. LEVEMIR is produced by a process that includes expression of recombinant DNA in *Saccharomyces cerevisiae* followed by chemical modification.

Insulin detemir differs from human insulin in that the amino acid threonine in position B30 has been omitted, and a C14 fatty acid chain has been attached to the amino acid B29. Insulin detemir has a molecular formula of $C_{267}H_{402}O_{76}N_{64}S_6$ and a molecular weight of 5916.9. It has the following structure:

[See figure 1 above]

LEVEMIR is a clear, colorless, aqueous, neutral sterile solution. Each milliliter of LEVEMIR contains 100 units (14.2 mg/mL) insulin detemir, 65.4 mcg zinc, 2.06 mg m-cresol, 16.0 mg glycerol, 1.80 mg phenol, 0.89 mg disodium phosphate dihydrate, 1.17 mg sodium chloride, and water for injection. Hydrochloric acid and/or sodium hydroxide may be added to adjust pH. LEVEMIR has a pH of approximately 7.4.

12 CLINICAL PHARMACOLOGY

12.1 Mechanism of Action

The primary activity of insulin detemir is the regulation of glucose metabolism. Insulins, including insulin detemir, exert their specific action through binding to insulin receptors. Receptor-bound insulin lowers blood glucose by facilitating cellular uptake of glucose into skeletal muscle and adipose tissue and by inhibiting the output of glucose from the liver. Insulin inhibits lipolysis in the adipocyte, inhibits proteolysis, and enhances protein synthesis.

12.2 Pharmacodynamics

Insulin detemir is a soluble, long-acting basal human insulin analog with up to a 24-hour duration of action. The pharmacodynamic profile of LEVEMIR is relatively constant with no pronounced peak.

The duration of action of LEVEMIR is mediated by slowed systemic absorption of insulin detemir molecules from the injection site due to self-association of the drug molecules. In addition, the distribution of insulin detemir to peripheral target tissues is slowed because of binding to albumin.

Table 9: Type 1 Diabetes Mellitus – Adult

Treatment duration / Treatment in combination with	Study A 16 weeks NovoLog® (insulin aspart)		Study B 26 weeks NovoLog® (insulin aspart)		Study C 24 weeks Human Soluble Insulin (regular insulin)	
	Twice-daily LEVEMIR	Twice-daily NPH	Twice-daily LEVEMIR	Once-daily insulin glargine	Once-daily LEVEMIR	Once-daily NPH
Number of patients treated	276	133	161	159	492	257
HbA_{1c} (%)						
Baseline HbA_{1c}	8.6	8.5	8.9	8.8	8.4	8.3
Adj. mean change from baseline	-0.8*	-0.7*	-0.6†	-0.5†	-0.1*	0.0*
LEVEMIR – NPH	-0.2		-0.0		-0.1	
95% CI for treatment difference	(-0.3, -0.0)		(-0.2, 0.2)		(-0.3, 0.0)	
Basal insulin dose (units/day)						
Baseline mean	21	24	27	23	12	24
Mean change from baseline	16	10	10	4	9	2
Total insulin dose (units/day)						
Baseline mean	48	54	56	51	46	57
Mean change from baseline	17	10	9	6	11	3
Fasting blood glucose (mg/dL)						
Baseline mean	209	220	153	150	213	206
Adj. mean change from baseline	-44*	-9*	-38†	-41†	-30*	-9*
Body weight (kg)						
Baseline mean	74.6	75.5	77.5	75.1	76.5	76.9
Adj.mean change from baseline	0.2*	0.8*	0.5†	1.0†	-0.3*	0.3*

* From an ANCOVA model adjusted for baseline value and country.
† From an ANCOVA model adjusted for baseline value and study site.

Table 10: Type 1 Diabetes Mellitus – Pediatric

Treatment duration / Treatment in combination with	Study D 26 weeks NovoLog® (insulin aspart)		Study I 52 weeks NovoLog® (insulin aspart)	
	Once- or Twice-daily LEVEMIR	Once- or Twice-daily NPH	Once- or Twice-daily LEVEMIR	Once- or Twice-daily NPH
Number of subjects treated	232	115	177	170
HbA_{1c} (%)				
Baseline HbA_{1c}	8.8	8.8	8.4	8.4
Adj. mean change from baseline	-0.7*	-0.8*	0.3†	0.2†
LEVEMIR – NPH	0.1		0.1	
95% CI for treatment difference	(-0.1; 0.3)		(-0.1; 0.4)	
Basal insulin dose (units/day)				
Baseline mean	24	26	17	17
Mean change from baseline	8	6	8	7
Total insulin dose (units/day)				
Baseline mean	48	50	35	34
Mean change from baseline	9	7	10	8
Fasting blood glucose (mg/dL)				
Baseline mean	181	181	135	141
Adj. mean change from baseline	-39	-21	-10†	0†
Body weight (kg)				
Baseline mean	46.3	46.2	37.4	36.5
Adj.mean change from baseline	1.6*	2.7*	2.7†	3.6†

* From an ANCOVA model adjusted for baseline value, geographical region, gender and age (covariate)
† From an ANCOVA model adjusted for baseline value, country, pubertal status at baseline and age (stratification factor).

Figure 2 shows results from a study in patients with type 1 diabetes conducted for a maximum of 24 hours after the subcutaneous injection of LEVEMIR or NPH insulin. The mean time between injection and the end of pharmacological effect for insulin detemir ranged from 7.6 hours to > 24 hours (24 hours was the end of the observation period).

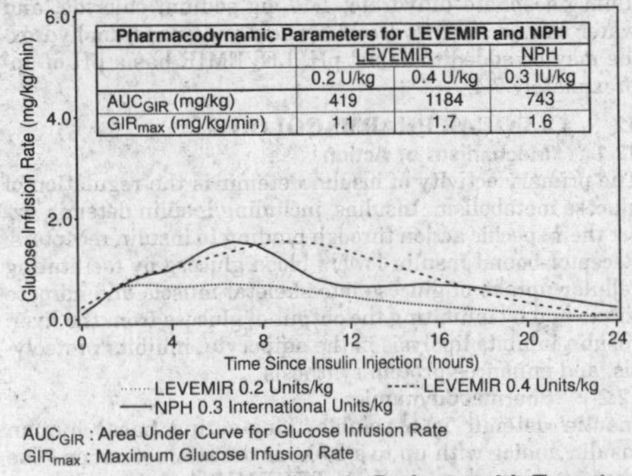

Figure 2: Activity Profiles in Patients with Type 1 Diabetes in a 24-hour Glucose Clamp Study

For doses in the interval of 0.2 to 0.4 Units/kg, insulin detemir exerts more than 50% of its maximum effect from 3 to 4 hours up to approximately 14 hours after dose administration.

Figure 3 shows glucose infusion rate results from a 16-hour glucose clamp study in patients with type 2 diabetes. The clamp study was terminated at 16 hours according to protocol.

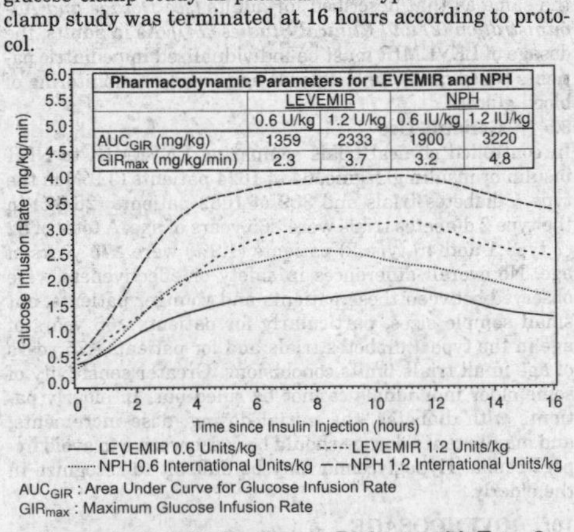

Figure 3: Activity Profiles in Patients with Type 2 Diabetes in a 16-hour Glucose Clamp Study

12.3 Pharmacokinetics

Absorption and Bioavailability

After subcutaneous injection of LEVEMIR in healthy subjects and in patients with diabetes, insulin detemir serum concentrations had a relatively constant concentration/time profile over 24 hours with the maximum serum concentration (C_{max}) reached between 6-8 hours post-dose. Insulin detemir was more slowly absorbed after subcutaneous administration to the thigh where $AUC_{0\text{-}5h}$ was 30-40% lower and $AUC_{0\text{-}inf}$ was 10% lower than the corresponding AUCs with subcutaneous injections to the deltoid and abdominal regions.

The absolute bioavailability of insulin detemir is approximately 60%.

Distribution and Elimination

More than 98% of insulin detemir in the bloodstream is bound to albumin. The results of *in vitro* and *in vivo* protein binding studies demonstrate that there is no clinically relevant interaction between insulin detemir and fatty acids or other protein-bound drugs.

Insulin detemir has an apparent volume of distribution of approximately 0.1 L/kg. After subcutaneous administration in patients with type 1 diabetes, insulin detemir has a terminal half-life of 5 to 7 hours depending on dose.

Specific Populations

Children and Adolescents- The pharmacokinetic properties of LEVEMIR were investigated in children (6-12 years), adolescents (13-17 years), and adults with type 1 diabetes. In children, the insulin detemir plasma area under the curve (AUC) and C_{max} were increased by 10% and 24%, respectively, as compared to adults. There was no difference in pharmacokinetics between adolescents and adults.

Geriatrics- In a clinical trial investigating differences in pharmacokinetics of a single subcutaneous dose of LEVEMIR in young (20 to 35 years) versus elderly (≥68 years) healthy subjects, the insulin detemir AUC was up to 35% higher among the elderly subjects due to reduced clearance. As with other insulin preparations, LEVEMIR should always be titrated according to individual requirements.

Gender- No clinically relevant differences in pharmacokinetic parameters of LEVEMIR are observed between males and females.

Race- In two clinical pharmacology studies conducted in healthy Japanese and Caucasian subjects, there were no clinically relevant differences seen in pharmacokinetic parameters. The pharmacokinetics and pharmacodynamics of LEVEMIR were investigated in a clamp study comparing patients with type 2 diabetes of Caucasian, African-American, and Latino origin. Dose-response relationships for LEVEMIR were comparable in these three populations.

Renal impairment- A single subcutaneous dose of 0.2 Units/kg (1.2 nmol/kg) of LEVEMIR was administered to healthy subjects and those with varying degrees of renal impairment (mild, moderate, severe, and hemodialysis-dependent). In this study, there were no differences in the pharmacokinetics of LEVEMIR between healthy subjects and those with renal impairment. However, some studies with human insulin have shown increased circulating levels of insulin in patients with renal impairment. Careful glucose monitoring and dose adjustments of insulin, including LEVEMIR, may be necessary in patients with renal impairment *[see Warnings and Precautions (5.5)]*.

Hepatic impairment- A single subcutaneous dose of 0.2 Units/kg (1.2 nmol/kg) of LEVEMIR was administered to healthy subjects and those with varying degrees of hepatic impairment (mild, moderate and severe). LEVEMIR exposure as estimated by AUC decreased with increasing degrees of hepatic impairment with a corresponding increase in apparent clearance. However, some studies with human insulin have shown increased circulating levels of insulin in patients with liver impairment. Careful glucose monitoring and dose adjustments of insulin, including LEVEMIR, may be necessary in patients with hepatic impairment *[see Warnings and Precautions (5.6)]*.

Pregnancy- The effect of pregnancy on the pharmacokinetics and pharmacodynamics of LEVEMIR has not been studied *[see Use in Specific Populations (8.1)]*.

Smoking- The effect of smoking on the pharmacokinetics and pharmacodynamics of LEVEMIR has not been studied.

Liraglutide- No pharmacokinetic interaction was observed between liraglutide and LEVEMIR when separate subcutaneous injections of LEVEMIR 0.5 Unit/kg (single-dose) and liraglutide 1.8 mg (steady state) were administered in patients with type 2 diabetes.

13 NONCLINICAL TOXICOLOGY

13.1 Carcinogenesis, Mutagenesis, Impairment of Fertility

Standard 2-year carcinogenicity studies in animals have not been performed. Insulin detemir tested negative for genotoxic potential in the *in vitro* reverse mutation study in bacteria, human peripheral blood lymphocyte chromosome aberration test, and the *in vivo* mouse micronucleus test.

In a fertility and embryonic development study, insulin detemir was administered to female rats before mating, during mating, and throughout pregnancy at doses up to 300 nmol/kg/day (3 times a human dose of 0.5 Units/kg/day, based on plasma AUC ratio). There were no effects on fertility in the rat.

14 CLINICAL STUDIES

The efficacy and safety of LEVEMIR given once-daily at bedtime or twice-daily (before breakfast and at bedtime, before breakfast and with the evening meal, or at 12-hour intervals) was compared to that of once-daily or twice-daily NPH insulin in open-label, randomized, parallel studies of 1155 adults with type 1 diabetes mellitus, 347 pediatric patients with type 1 diabetes mellitus, and 869 adults with type 2 diabetes mellitus. The efficacy and safety of LEVEMIR given twice-daily was compared to once-daily insulin glargine in an open-label, randomized, parallel study of 320 patients with type 1 diabetes. The evening LEVEMIR dose was titrated in all trials according to pre-defined targets for fasting blood glucose. The pre-dinner blood glucose was used to titrate the morning LEVEMIR dose in those trials that also administered LEVEMIR in the morning. In general, the reduction in glycosylated hemoglobin (HbA_{1c}) with LEVEMIR was similar to that with NPH insulin or insulin glargine.

Type 1 Diabetes – Adult

In a 16-week open-label clinical study (Study A, n=409), adults with type 1 diabetes were randomized to treatment with either LEVEMIR at 12-hour intervals, LEVEMIR administered in the morning and bedtime or NPH insulin administered in the morning and bedtime. Insulin aspart was also administered before each meal. At 16 weeks of treatment, the combined LEVEMIR-treated patients had similar HbA_{1c} and fasting plasma glucose (FPG) reductions compared to the NPH-treated patients (Table 9). Differences in timing of LEVEMIR administration had no effect on HbA_{1c}, fasting plasma glucose (FPG), or body weight.

In a 26-week, open-label clinical study (Study B, n=320), adults with type 1 diabetes were randomized to twice-daily LEVEMIR (administered in the morning and bedtime) or once-daily insulin glargine (administered at bedtime). Insulin aspart was administered before each meal. LEVEMIR-treated patients had a decrease in HbA_{1c} similar to that of insulin glargine-treated patients.

In a 24-week, open-label clinical study (Study C, n=749), adults with type 1 diabetes were randomized to once-daily LEVEMIR or once-daily NPH insulin, both administered at bedtime and in combination with regular human insulin before each meal. LEVEMIR and NPH insulin had a similar effect on HbA_{1c}.

[See table 9 at top of previous page]

Type 1 Diabetes – Pediatric

Two open-label, randomized, controlled clinical studies have been conducted in pediatric patients with type 1 diabetes. One study was 26 weeks in duration and enrolled patients 6-17 years of age. The other study was 52 weeks in duration and enrolled patients 2-16 years of age. In both studies, LEVEMIR and NPH insulin were administered once- or twice-daily. Bolus insulin aspart was administered before each meal. In the 26-week study, LEVEMIR-treated patients had a mean decrease in HbA_{1c} similar to that of NPH insulin (Table 10). In the 52-week study, the randomization was stratified by age (2-5 years, n=82, and 6-16 years, n=265) and the mean HbA_{1c} increased in both treatment arms, with similar findings in the 2-5 year-old age group (n=80) and the 6-16 year-old age group (n=258) (Table 10).

[See table 10 at top of previous page]

Type 2 Diabetes – Adult

In a 24-week, open-label, randomized, clinical study (Study E, n=476), LEVEMIR administered twice-daily (before breakfast and evening) was compared to NPH insulin administered twice-daily (before breakfast and evening) as part of a regimen of stable combination therapy with one or two of the following oral antidiabetic medications: metformin, an insulin secretagogue, or an alpha–glucosidase inhibitor. All patients were insulin-naïve at the time of randomization. LEVEMIR and NPH insulin similarly lowered HbA_{1c} from baseline (Table 11).

In a 22-week, open-label, randomized, clinical study (Study F, n=395) in adults with type 2 diabetes, LEVEMIR and NPH insulin were given once- or twice-daily as part of a basal-bolus regimen with insulin aspart. As measured by HbA_{1c} or FPG, LEVEMIR had efficacy similar to that of NPH insulin.

[See table 11 above]

Combination Therapy with Metformin and Liraglutide

This 26-week open-label trial enrolled 988 patients with inadequate glycemic control (HbA_{1c} 7-10%) on metformin (≥1500 mg/day) alone or inadequate glycemic control (HbA_{1c} 7-8.5%) on metformin (≥1500 mg/day) and a sulfonylurea. Patients who were on metformin and a sulfonylurea discontinued the sulfonylurea then all patients entered a 12-week run-in period during which they received add-on therapy with liraglutide titrated to 1.8 mg once-daily. At the end of the run-in period, 498 patients (50%) achieved HbA_{1c} <7% with liraglutide 1.8 mg and metformin and continued treatment in a non-randomized, observational arm. Another 167 patients (17%) withdrew from the trial during the run-in period with approximately one-half of these patients doing so because of gastrointestinal adverse reactions *[see Adverse Reactions (6.1)]*. The remaining 323 patients with HbA_{1c} ≥7% (33% of those who entered the run-in period) were randomized to 26 weeks of once-daily LEVEMIR administered in the evening as add-on therapy (N=162) or to continued, unchanged treatment with liraglutide 1.8 mg and metformin (N=161). The starting dose of LEVEMIR was 10 units/day and the mean dose at the end of the 26-week randomized period was 39 units/day. During the 26-week randomized treatment period, the percentage of patients who discontinued due to ineffective therapy was 11.2% in the group randomized to continued treatment with liraglutide 1.8 mg and metformin and 1.2% in the group randomized to add-on therapy with LEVEMIR.

Treatment with LEVEMIR as add-on to liraglutide 1.8 mg + metformin resulted in statistically significant reductions in HbA_{1c} and FPG compared to continued, unchanged treatment with liraglutide 1.8 mg + metformin alone (Table 12). From a mean baseline body weight of 96 kg after randomization, there was a mean reduction of 0.3 kg in the patients who received LEVEMIR add-on therapy compared to a mean reduction of 1.1 kg in the patients who continued on unchanged treatment with liraglutide 1.8 mg + metformin alone.

[See table 12 above]

Table 11: Type 2 Diabetes Mellitus – Adult

	Study E 24 weeks oral agents		Study F 22 weeks insulin aspart	
Treatment duration / Treatment in combination with	Twice-daily LEVEMIR	Twice-daily NPH	Once- or Twice-daily LEVEMIR	Once- or Twice-daily NPH
Number of subjects treated	237	239	195	200
HbA_{1c} (%)				
Baseline HbA_{1c}	8.6	8.5	8.2	8.1
Adj. mean change from baseline	-2.0*	-2.1*	$-0.6^{\dagger}$	$-0.6^{\dagger}$
LEVEMIR – NPH	0.1		-0.1	
95% CI for treatment difference	(-0.0, 0.3)		(-0.2, 0.1)	
Basal insulin dose (units/day)				
Baseline mean	18	17	22	22
Mean change from baseline	48	28	26	15
Total insulin dose‡ (units/day)				
Baseline mean	-	-	22	22
Mean change from baseline	-	-	57	42
Fasting blood glucose§ (mg/dL)				
Baseline mean	179	173	-	-
Adj. mean change from baseline	-69*	-74*	-	-
Body weight (kg)				
Baseline mean	82.5	82.3	82.0	79.6
Adj. mean change from baseline	1.2*	2.8*	$0.5^{\dagger}$	$1.2^{\dagger}$

* From an ANCOVA model adjusted for baseline value, country and oral antidiabetic treatment category
† From an ANCOVA model adjusted for baseline value and country
‡ Study E – Conducted in insulin-naïve patients
§ Study F - Fasting blood glucose data not collected

Table 12: Results of a 26-week open-label trial of LEVEMIR as add on to liraglutide + metformin compared to continued treatment with liraglutide + metformin alone in patients not achieving HbA_{1c} < 7% after 12 weeks of metformin and liraglutide

	Study H	
	LEVEMIR + Liraglutide +Metformin	Liraglutide+ Metformin
Intent-to-Treat Population (N)*	162	157
HbA_{1c} (%) (Mean)		
Baseline (week 0)	7.6	7.6
Adjusted mean change from baseline	$-0.5^{\dagger}$	$0^{\dagger}$
Difference from liraglutide + metformin arm (LS mean)‡	$-0.5^{\S}$	
95% Confidence interval	(-0.7, -0.4)	
Percentage of patients achieving A_{1c} <7%	43¶	17¶
Fasting Plasma Glucose (mg/dL) (Mean)		
Baseline (week 0)	166	159
Adjusted mean change from baseline	$-38^{\dagger}$	$-7^{\dagger}$
Difference from liraglutide + metformin arm (LS mean)‡	$-31^{\S}$	
95% Confidence interval	(-39 , -23)	

* Intent-to-treat population using last observation on study
† From an ANCOVA model adjusted for baseline value, country and previous oral antidiabetic treatment category
‡ Least squares mean adjusted for baseline value
§ p-value <0.0001
¶ From a logistic regression model adjusted for baseline HbA_{1c}.

Pregnancy

A randomized, open-label, controlled clinical trial has been conducted in pregnant women with type 1 diabetes. *[see Use in Specific Populations (8.1)]*

16 HOW SUPPLIED/STORAGE AND HANDLING

16.1 How Supplied

LEVEMIR is available in the following package sizes: each presentation containing 100 Units of insulin detemir per mL (U-100).

3 mL LEVEMIR FlexPen® NDC 0169-6439-10
10 mL vial NDC 0169-3687-12

FlexPen is for use with NovoFine® disposable needles. Each FlexPen is for use by a single patient. LEVEMIR FlexPen should never be shared between patients, even if the needle is changed.

16.2 Storage

Unused (unopened) LEVEMIR should be stored in the refrigerator between 2° and 8°C (36° to 46°F). Do not store in the freezer or directly adjacent to the refrigerator cooling element. Do not freeze. Do not use LEVEMIR if it has been frozen.

Unused (unopened) LEVEMIR can be kept until the expiration date printed on the label if it is stored in a refrigerator. Keep unused LEVEMIR in the carton so that it stays clean and protected from light.

If refrigeration is not possible, unused (unopened) LEVEMIR can be kept unrefrigerated at room temperature, below 30°C (86°F) as long as it is kept as cool as possible and away from direct heat and light. Unrefrigerated LEVEMIR should be discarded 42 days after it is first kept out of the refrigerator, even if the FlexPen or vial still contains insulin.

Vials:
After initial use, vials should be stored in a refrigerator, never in a freezer. If refrigeration is not possible, the in-use vial can be kept unrefrigerated at room temperature, below 30°C (86°F) as long as it is kept as cool as possible and away from direct heat and light. Refrigerated LEVEMIR vials should be discarded 42 days after initial use. Unrefrigerated LEVEMIR vials should be discarded 42 days after they are first kept out of the refrigerator.

LEVEMIR FlexPen:
After initial use, the LEVEMIR FlexPen must NOT be stored in a refrigerator and must NOT be stored with the needle in place. Keep the opened (in use) LEVEMIR FlexPen away from direct heat and light at room temperature, below 30°C (86°F). Unrefrigerated LEVEMIR FlexPens should be discarded 42 days after they are first kept out of the refrigerator.

The storage conditions are summarized in Table 13:

Table 13: Storage Conditions for LEVEMIR FlexPen and vial

	Not in-use (unopened) Refrigerated	Not in-use (unopened) Room Temperature (below 30°C)	In-use (opened)
3 mL LEVEMIR FlexPen	Until expiration date	42 days*	42 days* Room Temperature (below 30°C) **(Do not refrigerate)**
10 mL vial	Until expiration date	42 days*	42 days * Refrigerated or Room Temperature (below 30°C)

* The total time allowed at room temperature (below 30°C) is 42 days regardless of whether the product is in-use or not in-use.

16.3 Preparation and Handling

Parenteral drug products should be inspected visually for particulate matter and discoloration prior to administration, whenever solution and container permit. LEVEMIR should be inspected visually prior to administration and should only be used if the solution appears clear and colorless.

Mixing and diluting: LEVEMIR must NOT be mixed or diluted with any other insulin or solution *[See Warnings and Precautions (5.2)]*.

17 PATIENT COUNSELING INFORMATION

See FDA-Approved Patient Labeling (Patient Information and Instructions for Use)

17.1 Instructions for Patients

Patients should be informed that changes to insulin regimens must be made cautiously and only under medical supervision. Patients should be informed about the potential side effects of insulin therapy, including hypoglycemia, weight gain, lipodystrophy (and the need to rotate injection sites within the same body region), and allergic reactions. Patients should be informed that the ability to concentrate and react may be impaired as a result of hypoglycemia. This may present a risk in situations where these abilities are especially important, such as driving or operating other machinery. Patients who have frequent hypoglycemia or reduced or absent warning signs of hypoglycemia should be advised to use caution when driving or operating machinery.

Accidental mix-ups between LEVEMIR and other insulins, particularly short-acting insulins, have been reported. To avoid medication errors between LEVEMIR and other insulins, patients should be instructed to always check the insulin label before each injection.

LEVEMIR must only be used if the solution is clear and colorless with no particles visible. Patients must be advised that LEVEMIR must NOT be diluted or mixed with any other insulin or solution.

Patients should be instructed on self-management procedures including glucose monitoring, proper injection technique, and management of hypoglycemia and hyperglycemia. Patients should be instructed on handling of special situations such as intercurrent conditions (illness, stress, or emotional disturbances), an inadequate or skipped insulin dose, inadvertent administration of an increased insulin dose, inadequate food intake, and skipped meals.

Patients with diabetes should be advised to inform their healthcare professional if they are pregnant or are contemplating pregnancy. Refer patients to the LEVEMIR "Patient Information" for additional information.

17.2 Never Share a LEVEMIR FlexPen Between Patients

Counsel patients that they should never share a LEVEMIR FlexPen with another person, even if the needle is changed. Sharing of the FlexPen between patients may pose a risk of transmission of infection.

Novo Nordisk®, Levemir®, NovoLog®, FlexPen®, and NovoFine® are registered trademarks of Novo Nordisk A/S.

LEVEMIR® is covered by US Patent Nos. 5,750,497, 5,866,538, 6,011,007, 6,869,930 and other patents pending.

FlexPen® is covered by US Patent Nos. 6,004,297, RE 43,834, RE 41,956 and other patents pending.

Manufactured by:
Novo Nordisk A/S
DK-2880 Bagsvaerd, Denmark

For information about LEVEMIR contact:
Novo Nordisk Inc.
800 Scudders Mill Road
Plainsboro, New Jersey 08536
1-800-727-6500
www.novonordisk-us.com

Patient Information
LEVEMIR® (LEV–uh-mere)
(insulin detemir [rDNA origin] injection)
solution for subcutaneous injection

Read the Patient Information that comes with LEVEMIR® before you start taking it and each time you get a refill. There may be new information. This leaflet does not take the place of talking with your healthcare provider about your diabetes or your treatment. Make sure that you know how to manage your diabetes. Ask your healthcare provider, if you have any questions about managing your diabetes.

What is LEVEMIR®?

LEVEMIR® is a man-made long-acting insulin used to control high blood sugar in adults and children with diabetes mellitus.

It is not recommended to use LEVEMIR® to treat diabetic ketoacidosis.

Who should not use LEVEMIR®?

Do not use LEVEMIR® if:

- you are allergic to any of the ingredients in LEVEMIR®. See the end of this leaflet for a complete list of ingredients in LEVEMIR®.

What should I tell my healthcare provider before using LEVEMIR®?

Before you use LEVEMIR®, tell your healthcare provider if you:

- have liver or kidney problems
- take any other medicines, especially ones commonly called TZDs (thiazolidinediones).
- have heart failure or other heart problems. If you have heart failure, it may get worse while you take TZDs with LEVEMIR®.
- have any other medical conditions. Some medical conditions can affect your insulin needs and your dose of LEVEMIR®.
- are pregnant or plan to become pregnant. You and your healthcare provider should talk about the best way to manage your diabetes while you are pregnant.
- are breastfeeding or plan to breast-feed. It is not known if LEVEMIR® passes into breast milk. You and your healthcare provider should decide if you will take LEVEMIR® while you breastfeed.

Tell your healthcare provider about all the medicines you take, including prescription and non-prescription medicines, vitamins and herbal supplements. LEVEMIR® may affect the way other medicines work, and other medicines may affect how LEVEMIR® works.

Know the medicines you take. Keep a list of your medicines with you to show your healthcare provider and pharmacist when you get a new medicine.

How should I use LEVEMIR®?

- Use LEVEMIR® exactly as your healthcare provider told you to use it.
- Your healthcare provider will tell you how much LEVEMIR® to use and when to use it.
- Do not make any changes to your dose or type of insulin unless you are told to do so by your healthcare provider.

Know your insulin. **Make sure you know:**

- the type and strength of insulin prescribed for you.
- the amount of insulin you take.
- the best time for you to take your insulin. This may change if you take a different type of insulin.

- Do not dilute or mix LEVEMIR® with any other insulin or injectable diabetes medicine. Your LEVEMIR® will not work the right way and you may lose control of your blood sugar, which can be serious. Give yourself separate injections. You may give the separate injections in the same body area (for example, your stomach area), but you should not give the injections right next to each other.
- Do not use LEVEMIR® in an insulin pump.
- Inject LEVEMIR® under your skin (subcutaneously) in your upper arm, abdomen (stomach area), or thigh. Never inject LEVEMIR® into a vein or muscle.
- Change injection sites within the area you choose with each dose. Do not inject into the exact same spot for each injection.
- **Read the instructions for use that comes with your LEVEMIR®.** Talk to your healthcare provider if you have any questions. Your healthcare provider should show you how to inject LEVEMIR® before you start taking it.
- Your healthcare provider will decide which type of LEVEMIR® to prescribe for you.

LEVEMIR® comes in:

- 10 mL vials (small bottles) for use with a syringe
- 3 mL LEVEMIR® FlexPen®

Ask your healthcare provider how you should use LEVEMIR®.

- **If you use too much LEVEMIR®, your blood sugar may fall low (hypoglycemia).** You can treat mild low blood sugar (hypoglycemia) by drinking or eating something sugary right away (fruit juice, sugar candies, or glucose tablets). It is important to treat low blood sugar (hypoglycemia) right away because it could get worse and you could pass out (lose consciousness).

If you pass out you will need help from another person or emergency medical services right away. See "What are the possible side effects of LEVEMIR®?" for more information on low blood sugar (hypoglycemia).

- **If you forget to take your dose of LEVEMIR®, your blood sugar may go too high (hyperglycemia).** If high blood sugar (hyperglycemia) is not treated it can lead to serious problems, like loss of consciousness (passing out), coma or even death.

Follow your healthcare provider's instructions for treating high blood sugar.

Know your symptoms of high blood sugar, which may include:

- increased thirst
- frequent urination
- drowsiness
- loss of appetite
- a hard time breathing
- fruity smell on the breath
- high amounts of sugar and ketones in your urine
- nausea, vomiting (throwing up) or stomach pain
- Do not share needles, insulin pens or syringes with others.
- **Check your blood sugar levels.** Ask your healthcare provider what your blood sugars should be and when you should check your blood sugar levels.

Your insulin dosage may need to change because of:

- illness
- stress
- other medicines you take
- change in diet
- change in physical activity or exercise

What should I avoid while taking LEVEMIR®?

- **Alcohol.** Drinking alcohol may affect your blood sugar when you use LEVEMIR®.
- **Driving and operating machinery.** You may have trouble paying attention or reacting if you have low blood sugar (hypoglycemia). Be careful when you drive a car or operate machinery. Ask your healthcare provider if it is alright for you to drive if you often have:
  - low blood sugar (hypoglycemia)
  - decreased or no warning signs of low blood sugar

What are the possible side effects of LEVEMIR®?

LEVEMIR® can cause serious side effects, including:

- **Low blood sugar (hypoglycemia).** Signs and symptoms of low blood sugar may include:
  - dizziness or lightheadedness
  - shakiness
  - hunger
  - fast heart beat
  - tingling in your hands, feet, lips or tongue
  - trouble concentrating or confusion
  - blurred vision
  - slurred speech
  - anxiety or mood changes
  - headache
  - sweating

Very low blood sugar (hypoglycemia) can cause loss of consciousness (passing out), seizures, and death. In some people their blood sugar may get so low that they need another person to help them. Talk to your healthcare provider about how to tell if you have low blood sugar and what to do if this happens while taking LEVEMIR®. Know your symptoms of low blood sugar. Follow your healthcare provider's instructions for treating low blood sugar.

If you are using LEVEMIR® with another diabetes medicine, your LEVEMIR® dose may need to be changed to reduce your chance of getting low blood sugar.

Talk to your healthcare provider if low blood sugar is a problem for you. Your dose of LEVEMIR® may need to be changed.

- **Skin thickening or pits at the injection site (lipodystrophy).** Change (rotate) the area where you inject your insulin to help prevent these skin changes from happening. Do not inject insulin into areas of skin that have thickening or pits.
- **Serious allergic reactions. LEVEMIR® can cause life threatening symptoms.** Get medical help right away if you have any of these symptoms of an allergic reaction:
  - a rash all over your body
  - itching
  - shortness of breath
  - trouble breathing (wheezing)
  - fast heartbeat
  - sweating
  - feel faint
- **Swelling of your hands and feet**
- **Heart Failure.** Taking certain diabetes pills called thiazolidinediones or "TZDs" with LEVEMIR® may cause heart failure in some people. This can happen even if you have never had heart failure or heart problems before. If you already have heart failure it may get worse while you take TZDs with LEVEMIR®. Your healthcare provider should monitor you closely while you are taking TZDs with LEVEMIR®. Tell your healthcare provider if you have any new or worse symptoms of heart failure including:
  - shortness of breath
  - swelling of your ankles or feet
  - sudden weight gain

  Treatment with TZDs and LEVEMIR® may need to be adjusted or stopped by your healthcare provider if you have new or worse heart failure.

Common side effects of LEVEMIR® include:

- **Low blood sugar (hypoglycemia). See "What are the possible side effects of LEVEMIR®?" for more information on low blood sugar (hypoglycemia).**
- **Reactions at the injection site (local allergic reaction).** You may get redness, swelling, and itching at the injection site. If you keep having skin reactions or they are serious, talk to your healthcare provider.
- **Weight gain.** This can occur with any insulin therapy. Talk to your healthcare provider about how LEVEMIR® can affect your weight.

Tell your healthcare provider if you have any side effect that bothers you or does not go away.

These are not all of the possible side effects from LEVEMIR®. Ask your healthcare provider or pharmacist for more information.

Call your doctor for medical advice about side effects.

You may report side effects to FDA at 1-800-FDA-1088.

How should I store LEVEMIR®?

Unopened LEVEMIR®:

- **Keep all unopened LEVEMIR® in the refrigerator between 36°F to 46°F (2°C to 8°C).**
- Unopened LEVEMIR® can be kept until the expiration date on the label if the medicine has been stored in a refrigerator.
- If refrigeration is not possible, you can keep the unopened LEVEMIR® at room temperature below 86°F (30°C).
- Throw away LEVEMIR® 42 days after it is first kept out of the refrigerator.
- Do not freeze. Do not use LEVEMIR® if it has been frozen.
- Keep unopened LEVEMIR® in the carton to protect it from light.

LEVEMIR® in use:

- **Vials**
  - Keep opened vials of LEVEMIR® in the refrigerator or at room temperature below 86°F (30°C) away from direct heat or light.
  - Throw away a vial that has always been kept in the refrigerator after 42 days of use, even if there is insulin left in the vial.
  - Throw away a vial that has been kept at room temperature 42 days after it is first kept out of the refrigerator, even if there is insulin left in the vial.
- **LEVEMIR® FlexPen**
  - Keep at room temperature below 86°F (30°C) for up to 42 days.
  - Do not store a LEVEMIR® FlexPen® that you are using in the refrigerator.
  - Do not store LEVEMIR® with the needle attached.
  - Keep LEVEMIR® FlexPen® away from direct heat or light.
  - Throw away used LEVEMIR® FlexPens after 42 days, even if there is insulin left in them.

Keep LEVEMIR® and all medicines out of the reach of children.

General information about LEVEMIR®

Medicines are sometimes prescribed for conditions that are not mentioned in the patient leaflet. Do not use LEVEMIR® for a condition for which it was not prescribed. Do not give LEVEMIR® to other people, even if they have the same symptoms you have. It may harm them.

This leaflet summarizes the most important information about LEVEMIR®. If you would like more information about LEVEMIR® or diabetes, talk with your healthcare provider. You can ask your healthcare provider for information about LEVEMIR® that is written for healthcare professionals.

For more information about LEVEMIR®, call 1-800-727-6500 or go to www.novonordisk-us.com.

What are the ingredients in LEVEMIR®?

Active Ingredient: Insulin detemir

Inactive Ingredients: zinc, m-cresol, glycerol, phenol, disodium phosphate dihydrate, sodium chloride and water for injection. Hydrochloric acid or sodium hydroxide may be added.

This Patient Information has been approved by the U.S. Food and Drug Administration.

Novo Nordisk®, LEVEMIR®, and FlexPen® are registered trademarks of Novo Nordisk A/S.

LEVEMIR® is covered by US Patent Nos. 5,750,497, 5,866,538, 6,011,007, 6,869,930 and other patents pending.

FlexPen® is covered by US Patent Nos. 6,004,297, RE 43,834, RE 41,956 and other patents pending.

Manufactured by:
Novo Nordisk A/S
DK-2880 Bagsvaerd, Denmark

For information about LEVEMIR® contact:
Novo Nordisk Inc.
800 Scudders Mill Road
Plainsboro, New Jersey 08536
www.novonordisk-us.com
1-800-727-6500

Revised: April 16, 2013

Patient Instructions For Use

LEVEMIR® 10 mL vial

Please read the following Instructions for use carefully before using your LEVEMIR® 10 mL vial and each time you get a refill. You should read the instructions in this manual even if you have used an insulin 10 mL vial before.

How should I use the LEVEMIR 10 mL vial?

Using the 10 mL vial:

1. Check to make sure that you have the correct type of insulin. This is especially important if you use different types of insulin.

2. Look at the vial and the insulin. The LEVEMIR insulin should be clear and colorless. The tamper-resistant cap should be in place before the first use. If the cap has been removed before your first use of the vial, or if the insulin is cloudy or colored, **Do not** use the insulin and return it to your pharmacy.

3. Wash your hands with soap and water.

4. If you are using a new vial, pull off the tamper-resistant cap.

Before each use, wipe the rubber stopper with an alcohol wipe.

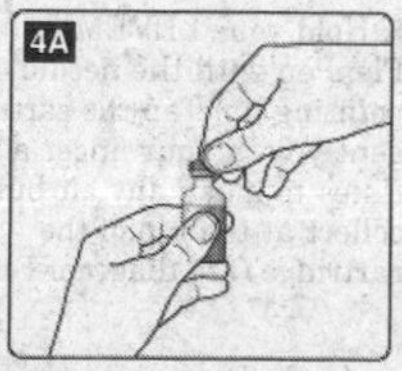

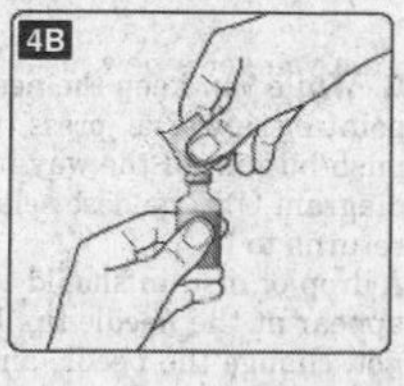

5. Do not roll or shake the vial. Shaking the vial right before the dose is drawn into the syringe may cause bubbles or foam. This can cause you to draw up the wrong dose of insulin. The insulin should be used only if it is clear and colorless.

6. Pull back the plunger on your syringe until the black tip reaches the marking for the number of units you will inject.

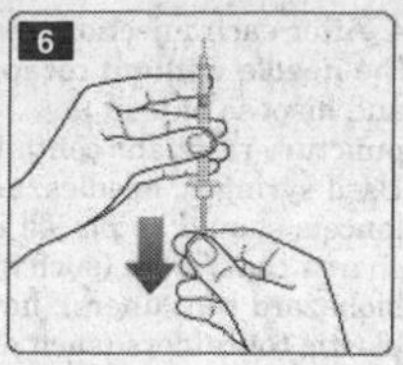

7. Push the needle through the rubber stopper into the vial.

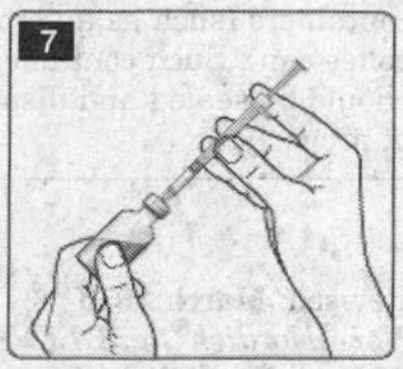

8. Push the plunger all the way in. This inserts air into the vial.

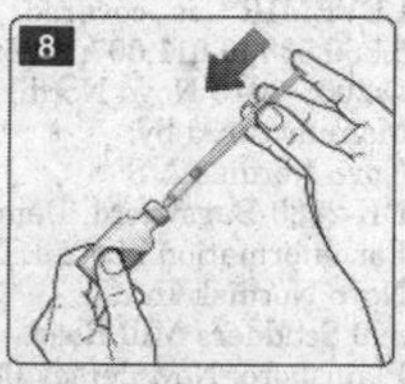

9. Turn the vial and syringe upside down and slowly pull the plunger back to a few units beyond the correct dose that you need.

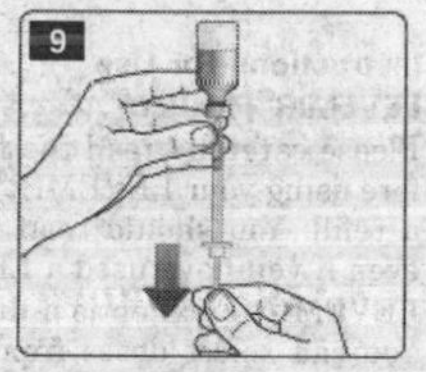

10. If there are air bubbles, tap the syringe gently with your finger to raise the air bubbles to the top of the needle. Then slowly push the plunger to the correct unit marking for your dose.

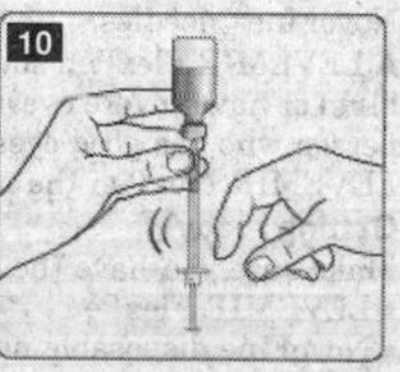

11. Check to make sure you have the right dose of LEVEMIR in the syringe.

12. Pull the syringe out of the vial

13. Inject your LEVEMIR right away as instructed by your healthcare provider.

How should I inject LEVEMIR with a syringe?

If you clean your injection site with an alcohol swab, let the injection site dry before you inject. Talk with your healthcare provider about how to rotate injection sites and how to give an injection.

1. Pinch your skin between two fingers, push the needle into the skinfold, using a dart-like motion and push the plunger to inject the insulin under your skin. The needle will be straight in.

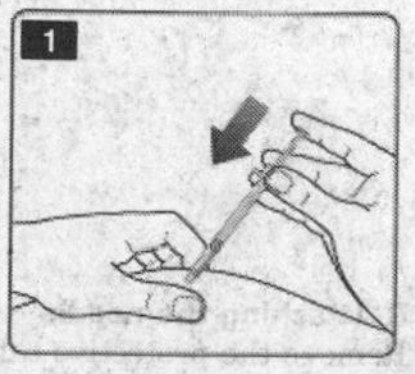

2. Keep the needle under your skin for at least 6 seconds to make sure you have injected all the insulin. After you pull the needle from your skin you may see a drop of Levemir at the needle tip. This is normal and has no effect on the dose you just received.

3. If blood appears after you pull the needle from your skin, press the injection site lightly with an alcohol swab. Do not rub the area.

4. After each injection, **remove the needle without recapping** and dispose of it in a puncture-resistant container. Used syringes, needles, and lancets should be placed in sharps containers (such as red biohazard containers), hard plastic containers (such as detergent bottles), or metal containers (such as an empty coffee can). Such containers should be sealed and disposed of properly.

Revised: March 2013

Novo Nordisk® and LEVEMIR® are registered trademarks of Novo Nordisk A/S.

LEVEMIR® is covered by US Patent Nos. 5,750,497, 5,866,538, 6,011,007, 6,869,930, and other patents pending.

Manufactured by:
Novo Nordisk A/S
DK-2880 Bagsvaerd, Denmark
For information about LEVEMIR® contact:
Novo Nordisk Inc.
800 Scudders Mill Road
Plainsboro, New Jersey 08536

Instructions For Use
LEVEMIR®FlexPen®

Please carefully read the following Instructions for use before using your LEVEMIR® FlexPen® and each time you get a refill. You should read the instructions in this manual even if you have used a LEVEMIR FlexPen before.

LEVEMIR FlexPen is a disposable dial-a-dose insulin pen. You can select doses from 1 to 60 units in increments of 1 unit. LEVEMIR FlexPen is designed to be used with NovoFine® needles.

Δ LEVEMIR FlexPen should not be used by people who are blind or have severe eyesight problems without the help of a person who has good eyesight and who is trained to use the LEVEMIR FlexPen the right way.

Getting ready

Make sure you have the following items:
- LEVEMIR FlexPen
- NovoFine disposable needles
- Alcohol swab

[See figure above]

PREPARING YOUR LEVEMIR FLEXPEN

Wash your hands with soap and water. Before you start to prepare your injection, check the label to make sure that you are taking the right type of insulin. This is especially important if you take more than 1 type of insulin. LEVEMIR should look clear and colorless.

A. Pull off the pen cap (see diagram A).
Wipe the rubber stopper with an alcohol swab.

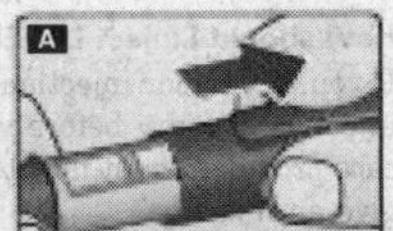

B.Attaching the needle
Remove the protective tab from a new disposable needle.

Attach the needle tightly onto your FlexPen. It is important that the needle is put on straight (see diagram B). Never place a disposable needle on your LEVEMIR FlexPen until you are ready to give your injection.

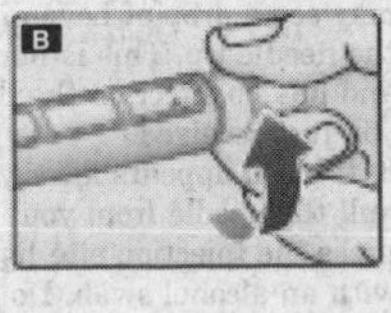

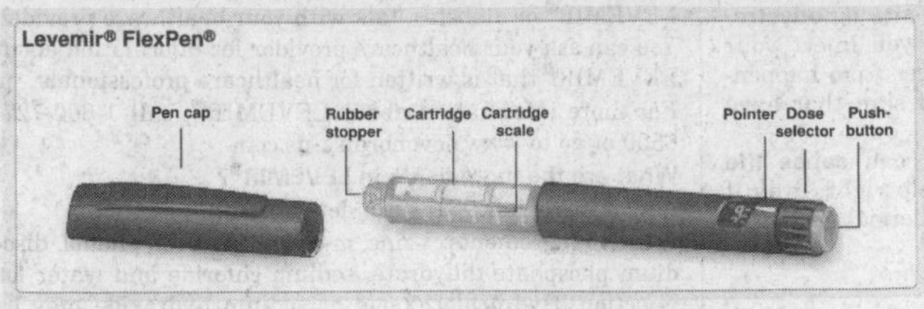

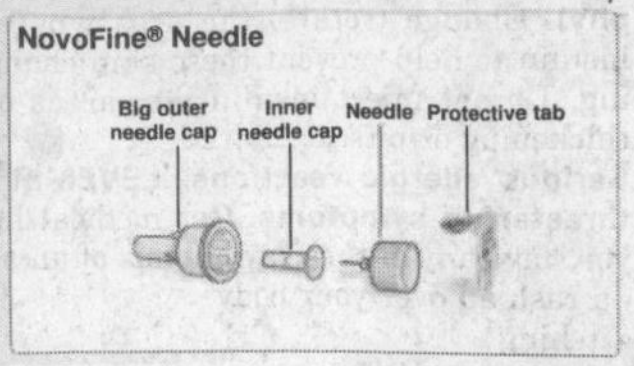

C. Pull off the big outer needle cap (see diagram C).

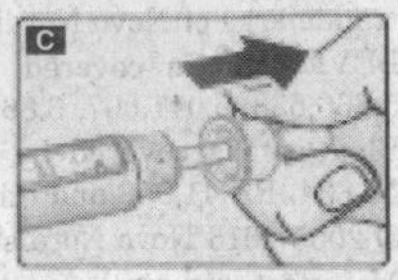

D. Pull off the inner needle cap and throw it away (see diagram D).

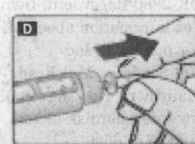

Δ Always use a new needle for each injection to cut down the chance of infection and to prevent blocked needles.

Δ Be careful not to bend or damage the needle before use.

Δ To reduce the risk of needle sticks, never put the inner needle cap back on the needle.

Giving the airshot before each injection

Before each injection, small amounts of air may collect in the cartridge during normal use. To avoid injecting air and to ensure you take the right dose of insulin:

E. Turn the dose selector to select 2 units (see diagram E).

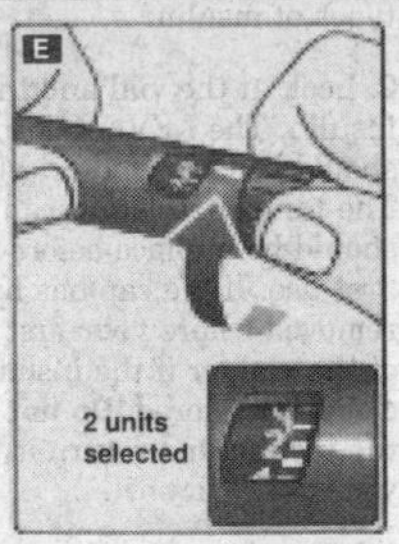

F. Hold your LEVEMIR FlexPen with the needle pointing up. Tap the cartridge gently with your finger a few times to make any air bubbles collect at the top of the cartridge (see diagram F).

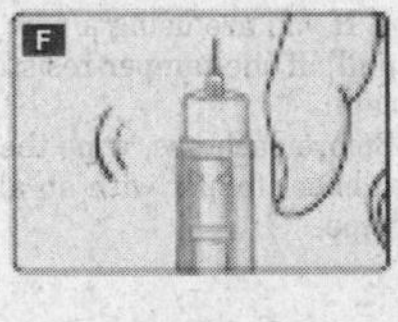

G. While you keep the needle pointing upwards, press the push-button all the way in (see diagram G). The dose selector returns to 0.
A drop of insulin should appear at the needle tip. If not, change the needle and repeat the procedure no more than 6 times.
If you do not see a drop of insulin after 6 times, do not use the LEVEMIR FlexPen and contact Novo Nordisk at 1-800-727-6500.
A small air bubble may remain at the needle tip, but it will not be injected.

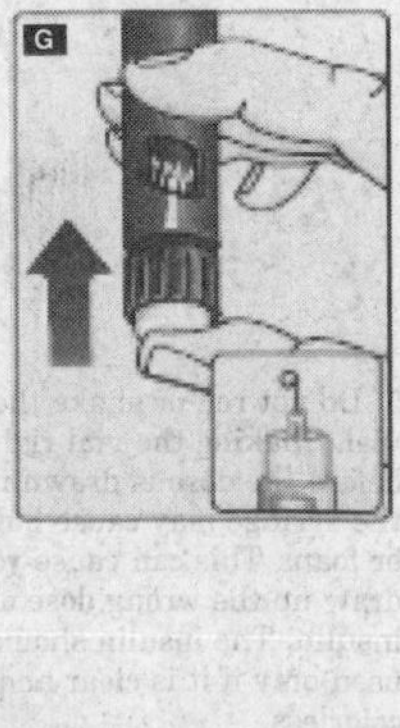

SELECTING YOUR DOSE

Check and make sure that the dose selector is set at 0.

H. Turn the dose selector to the number of units you need to inject. The pointer should line up with your dose.
The dose can be corrected either up or down by turning the dose selector in either direction until the correct dose lines up with the pointer (see diagram H). When turning the dose selector, be careful not to press the push-button as insulin will come out.
You cannot select a dose larger than the number of units left in the cartridge.
You will hear a click for every single unit dialed. Do not set the dose by counting the number of clicks you hear.
Δ Do not use the cartridge scale printed on the cartridge to measure your dose of insulin.

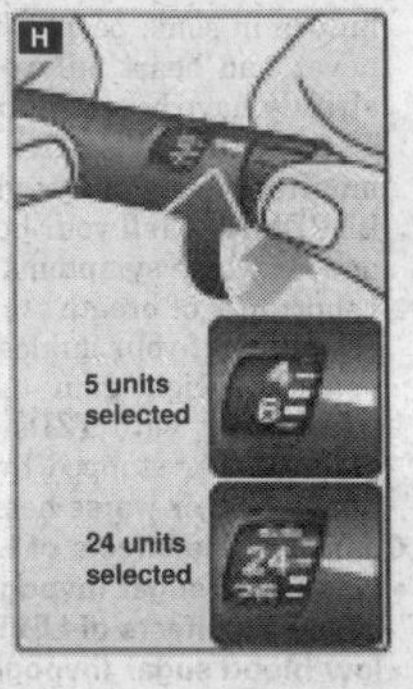

GIVING THE INJECTION

Do the injection exactly as shown to you by your healthcare provider. Your healthcare provider should tell you if you need to pinch the skin before injecting. Wipe the skin with an alcohol swab and let the area dry.

I. Insert the needle into your skin.
Inject the dose by pressing the push-button all the way in until the 0 lines up with the pointer (see diagram I). Be careful only to push the button after the needle is in the skin. Turning the dose selector will not inject insulin.

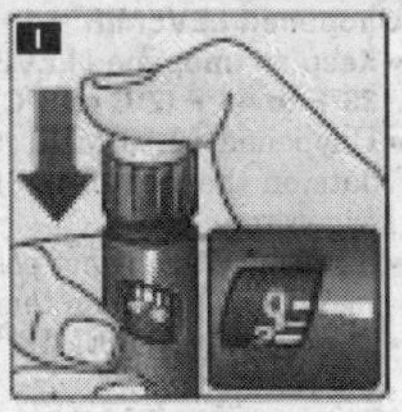

J. Keep the needle in the skin for at least 6 seconds, and keep the push-button pressed all the way in until the needle has been pulled out from the skin (see diagram J). This will make sure that the full dose has been given.
You may see a drop of LEVEMIR at the needle tip. This is normal and has no effect on the dose you just received. If blood appears after you take the needle out of your skin, press the injection site lightly with an alcohol swab. **Do not rub the area.**

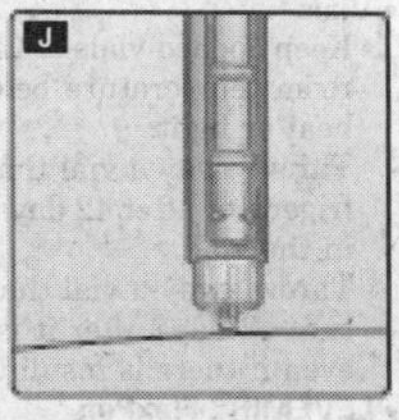

After the injection

Carefully remove the needle from the pen after each injection. This helps to prevent infection and leakage of insulin. You can carefully recap the needle with the bigger outer cap to help make it easier to remove the needle.

Δ **Do not recap the needle with the small inner cap.** Recapping with this small part can increase your chances of having a needle stick injury.

Δ Put the needle in a sharps container or some type of hard plastic or metal container with a screw top such as a detergent bottle or empty coffee can. These containers should be sealed and thrown away the right way. Check with your healthcare provider about the right way to throw away used syringes and needles. There may be local or state laws about how to throw away used needles and syringes. Do not throw away used needles and syringes in household trash or recycling bins.

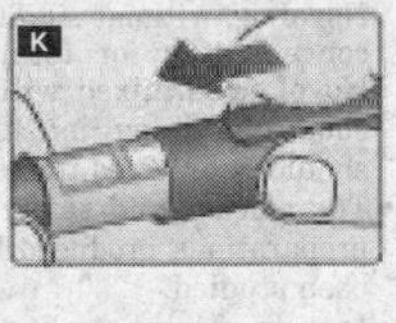

K. Put the pen cap on the LEVEMIR FlexPen and store the LEVEMIR FlexPen without the needle attached (see diagram K).
The LEVEMIR FlexPen prevents the cartridge from being completely emptied. It can deliver 300 units then you should throw it away in a sharps container or some type of hard plastic or metal container with a screw top, such as a detergent bottle or empty coffee can.

FUNCTION CHECK

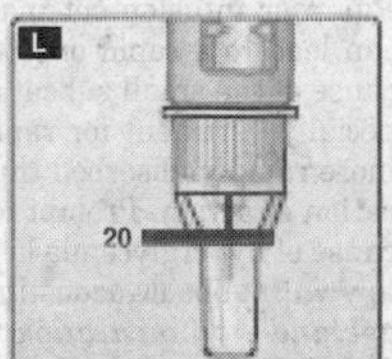

L. If your LEVEMIR FlexPen is not working the right way, follow the steps below:

- Attach a new NovoFine needle.
- Remove the big outer needle cap and the inner needle cap.
- Do an airshot as described in "Giving the airshot before each injection" (see diagram E through G).
- Put the big outer needle cap onto the needle. Do not put on the inner needle cap.
- Turn the dose selector so the dose indicator window shows 20 units.
- Hold the LEVEMIR FlexPen so the needle is pointing down.
- Press the push-button all the way in.

The insulin should fill the lower part of the big outer needle cap to the marker (see diagram L). If LEVEMIR FlexPen has released too much or too little insulin, do the function check again. If the same problem happens again, do not use your LEVEMIR FlexPen and contact Novo Nordisk at 1-800-727-6500.

Maintenance

Your FlexPen is designed to work accurately and safely. It must be handled with care. If you drop your FlexPen it could get damaged. If you are concerned that your FlexPen is damaged, use a new one. You can clean the outside of your FlexPen by wiping it with a damp cloth. Do not soak or wash your FlexPen. Soaking or washing the FlexPen could damage it. Do not refill your FlexPen.

Δ Remove the needle from the LEVEMIR FlexPen after each injection. This helps to cut down your chance of infection, prevent leakage of insulin. Be careful when handling used needles to avoid needle sticks and transfer of infections.

Δ Keep your LEVEMIR FlexPen and needles out of the reach of children.

Δ Use LEVEMIR FlexPen as directed to treat your diabetes. Needles and LEVEMIR FlexPen must not be shared.

Δ Always use a new needle for each injection.

Δ Novo Nordisk is not responsible for harm due to using this insulin pen with products not recommended by Novo Nordisk.

Δ As a safety measure, always carry a spare insulin delivery device in case your LEVEMIR FlexPen is lost or damaged.

Δ Remember to keep the disposable LEVEMIR FlexPen with you. Do not leave it in a car or other location where it can get too hot or too cold.

Revised: May 2013

Novo Nordisk®, LEVEMIR®, FlexPen®, and NovoFine® are registered trademarks of Novo Nordisk A/S.

LEVEMIR® is covered by US Patent Nos. 5,750,497, 5,866,538, 6,011,007, 6,869,930, and other patents pending. FlexPen® is covered by US Patent Nos. 6,004,297, RE 43,834, RE 41,956, and other patents pending.

Manufactured by:
Novo Nordisk A/S
DK-2880 Bagsvaerd, Denmark

For information about LEVEMIR® contact:
Novo Nordisk Inc.
800 Scudders Mill Road
Plainsboro, New Jersey 08536

NOVOLOG® ℞

[NŌ vō log]

(insulin aspart [rDNA origin] injection) solution for subcutaneous use

HIGHLIGHTS OF PRESCRIBING INFORMATION

These highlights do not include all the information needed to use NovoLog safely and effectively.
See full prescribing information for NovoLog.
See full prescribing information for NovoLog.
NovoLog® (insulin aspart [rDNA origin] injection) solution for subcutaneous use
Initial U.S. Approval: 2000

RECENT MAJOR CHANGES

- Warnings and Precautions (5.10) 3/2013

INDICATIONS AND USAGE

- NovoLog is an insulin analog indicated to improve glycemic control in adults and children with diabetes mellitus (1.1).

DOSAGE AND ADMINISTRATION

- The dosage of NovoLog must be individualized.
- *Subcutaneous injection:* NovoLog should generally be given immediately (within 5-10 minutes) prior to the start of a meal (2.2).
- *Use in pumps:* Change the NovoLog in the reservoir at least every 6 days, change the infusion set, and the infusion set insertion site at least every 3 days. NovoLog should not be mixed with other insulins or with a diluent when it is used in the pump (2.3).
- *Intravenous use:* NovoLog should be used at concentrations from 0.05 U/mL to 1.0 U/mL insulin aspart in infusion systems using polypropylene infusion bags. NovoLog has been shown to be stable in infusion fluids such as 0.9% sodium chloride (2.4).

DOSAGE FORMS AND STRENGTHS

Each presentation contains 100 Units of insulin aspart per mL (U-100)

- 10 mL vials (3)
- 3 mL PenFill® cartridges for the 3 mL PenFill cartridge device (3)
- 3 mL NovoLog FlexPen® (3)

CONTRAINDICATIONS

- Do not use during episodes of hypoglycemia (4).
- Do not use in patients with hypersensitivity to NovoLog or one of its excipients.

WARNINGS AND PRECAUTIONS

- Hypoglycemia is the most common adverse effect of insulin therapy. Glucose monitoring is recommended for all patients with diabetes. Any change of insulin dose should be made cautiously and only under medical supervision (5.1, 5.2).
- Insulin, particularly when given intravenously or in settings of poor glycemic control, can cause hypokalemia. Use caution in patients predisposed to hypokalemia (5.3).
- Like all insulins, NovoLog requirements may be reduced in patients with renal impairment or hepatic impairment (5.4, 5.5).
- Severe, life-threatening, generalized allergy, including anaphylaxis, may occur with insulin products, including NovoLog (5.6).
- Fluid retention and heart failure can occur with concomitant use of thiazolidinediones (TZDs), which are PPAR-gamma agonists, and insulin, including NovoLog (5.10).

ADVERSE REACTIONS

Adverse reactions observed with NovoLog include hypoglycemia, allergic reactions, local injection site reactions, lipodystrophy, rash and pruritus (6).

To report SUSPECTED ADVERSE REACTIONS, contact Novo Nordisk Inc. at 1-800-727-6500 or FDA at 1-800-FDA-1088 or www.fda.gov/medwatch.

DRUG INTERACTIONS

- The following may increase the blood-glucose-lowering effect and susceptibility to hypoglycemia: oral antidiabetic products, pramlintide, ACE inhibitors, disopyramide, fibrates, fluoxetine, monoamine oxidase inhibitors, propoxyphene, salicylates, somatostatin analogs, sulfonamide antibiotics (7).
- The following may reduce the blood-glucose-lowering effect: corticosteroids, niacin, danazol, diuretics, sympathomimetic agents (e.g., epinephrine, salbutamol, terbutaline), isoniazid, phenothiazine derivatives, somatropin, thyroid hormones, estrogens, progestogens (e.g., in oral contraceptives), atypical antipsychotics (7).
- Beta-blockers, clonidine, lithium salts, and alcohol may either potentiate or weaken the blood-glucose-lowering effect of insulin (7).
- Pentamidine may cause hypoglycemia, which may sometimes be followed by hyperglycemia (7).
- The signs of hypoglycemia may be reduced or absent in patients taking sympatholytic products such as beta-blockers, clonidine, guanethidine, and reserpine (7).

USE IN SPECIFIC POPULATIONS

- Pediatric: Has not been studied in children with type 2 diabetes. Has not been studied in children with type 1 diabetes <2 years of age (8.4).

See 17 for PATIENT COUNSELING INFORMATION and FDA-approved patient labeling

Revised: 03/2013

FULL PRESCRIBING INFORMATION: CONTENTS*

* Sections or subsections omitted from the full prescribing information are not listed

FULL PRESCRIBING INFORMATION

1 INDICATIONS AND USAGE

1.1 Treatment of Diabetes Mellitus

NovoLog is an insulin analog indicated to improve glycemic control in adults and children with diabetes mellitus.

2 DOSAGE AND ADMINISTRATION

2.1 Dosing

NovoLog is an insulin analog with an earlier onset of action than regular human insulin. The dosage of NovoLog must be individualized. NovoLog given by subcutaneous injection should generally be used in regimens with an intermediate or long-acting insulin [*see Warnings and Precautions (5), How Supplied/Storage and Handling (16.2)*]. The total daily insulin requirement may vary and is usually between 0.5 to 1.0 units/kg/day. When used in a meal-related subcutaneous injection treatment regimen, 50 to 70% of total insulin requirements may be provided by NovoLog and the remainder provided by an intermediate-acting or long-acting insulin. Because of NovoLog's comparatively rapid onset and short duration of glucose lowering activity, some patients may require more basal insulin and more total insulin to prevent pre-meal hyperglycemia when using NovoLog than when using human regular insulin.

Do not use NovoLog that is viscous (thickened) or cloudy; use only if it is clear and colorless. NovoLog should not be used after the printed expiration date.

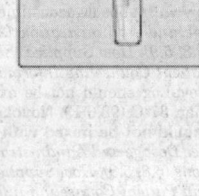

2.2 Subcutaneous Injection
NovoLog should be administered by subcutaneous injection in the abdominal region, buttocks, thigh, or upper arm. Because NovoLog has a more rapid onset and a shorter duration of activity than human regular insulin, it should be injected immediately (within 5-10 minutes) before a meal. Injection sites should be rotated within the same region to reduce the risk of lipodystrophy. As with all insulins, the duration of action of NovoLog will vary according to the dose, injection site, blood flow, temperature, and level of physical activity.
NovoLog may be diluted with Insulin Diluting Medium for NovoLog for subcutaneous injection. Diluting one part NovoLog to nine parts diluent will yield a concentration one-tenth that of NovoLog (equivalent to U-10). Diluting one part NovoLog to one part diluent will yield a concentration one-half that of NovoLog (equivalent to U-50).

2.3 Continuous Subcutaneous Insulin Infusion (CSII) by External Pump
NovoLog can also be infused subcutaneously by an external insulin pump [see *Warnings and Precautions (5.8, 5.9), How Supplied/Storage and Handling (16.2)*]. Diluted insulin should not be used in external insulin pumps. Because NovoLog has a more rapid onset and a shorter duration of activity than human regular insulin, pre-meal boluses of NovoLog should be infused immediately (within 5-10 minutes) before a meal. Infusion sites should be rotated within the same region to reduce the risk of lipodystrophy. The initial programming of the external insulin infusion pump should be based on the total daily insulin dose of the previous regimen. Although there is significant interpatient variability, approximately 50% of the total dose is usually given as meal-related boluses of NovoLog and the remainder is given as a basal infusion. **Change the NovoLog in the reservoir at least every 6 days, change the infusion sets and the infusion set insertion site at least every 3 days.**
The following insulin pumps† have been used in NovoLog clinical or *in vitro* studies conducted by Novo Nordisk, the manufacturer of NovoLog:
- Medtronic Paradigm® 512 and 712
- MiniMed 508
- Disetronic® D-TRON® and H-TRON®

Before using a different insulin pump with NovoLog, read the pump label to make sure the pump has been evaluated with NovoLog.

2.4 Intravenous Use
NovoLog can be administered intravenously under medical supervision for glycemic control with close monitoring of blood glucose and potassium levels to avoid hypoglycemia and hypokalemia [*see Warnings and Precautions (5), How Supplied/Storage and Handling (16.2)*]. For intravenous use, NovoLog should be used at concentrations from 0.05 U/mL to 1.0 U/mL insulin aspart in infusion systems using polypropylene infusion bags. NovoLog has been shown to be stable in infusion fluids such as 0.9% sodium chloride.
Inspect NovoLog for particulate matter and discoloration prior to parenteral administration.

3 DOSAGE FORMS AND STRENGTHS
NovoLog is available in the following package sizes: each presentation contains 100 units of insulin aspart per mL (U-100).
- 10 mL vials
- 3 mL PenFill cartridges for the 3 mL PenFill cartridge delivery device (with or without the addition of a NovoPen® 3 PenMate®) with NovoFine® disposable needles
- 3 mL NovoLog FlexPen

4 CONTRAINDICATIONS
NovoLog is contraindicated
- during episodes of hypoglycemia
- in patients with hypersensitivity to NovoLog or one of its excipients.

5 WARNINGS AND PRECAUTIONS
5.1 Administration
NovoLog has a more rapid onset of action and a shorter duration of activity than regular human insulin. An injection of NovoLog should immediately be followed by a meal within 5-10 minutes. Because of NovoLog's short duration of action, a longer acting insulin should also be used in patients with type 1 diabetes and may also be needed in patients with type 2 diabetes. Glucose monitoring is recommended for all patients with diabetes and is particularly important for patients using external pump infusion therapy.
Any change of insulin dose should be made cautiously and only under medical supervision. Changing from one insulin product to another or changing the insulin strength may result in the need for a change in dosage. As with all insulin preparations, the time course of NovoLog action may vary in different individuals or at different times in the same individual and is dependent on many conditions, including the site of injection, local blood supply, temperature, and physical activity. Patients who change their level of physical activity or meal plan may require adjustment of insulin dosages. Insulin requirements may be altered during illness, emotional disturbances, or other stresses.
Patients using continuous subcutaneous insulin infusion pump therapy must be trained to administer insulin by injection and have alternate insulin therapy available in case of pump failure.
Needles and NovoLog FlexPen must not be shared.

5.2 Hypoglycemia
Hypoglycemia is the most common adverse effect of all insulin therapies, including NovoLog. Severe hypoglycemia may lead to unconsciousness and/or convulsions and may result in temporary or permanent impairment of brain function or death. Severe hypoglycemia requiring the assistance of another person and/or parenteral glucose infusion or glucagon administration has been observed in clinical trials with insulin, including trials with NovoLog.
The timing of hypoglycemia usually reflects the time-action profile of the administered insulin formulations [*see Clinical Pharmacology (12)*]. Other factors such as changes in food intake (e.g., amount of food or timing of meals), injection site, exercise, and concomitant medications may also alter the risk of hypoglycemia [*see Drug Interactions (7)*]. As with all insulins, use caution in patients with hypoglycemia unawareness and in patients who may be predisposed to hypoglycemia (e.g., patients who are fasting or have erratic food intake). The patient's ability to concentrate and react may be impaired as a result of hypoglycemia. This may present a risk in situations where these abilities are especially important, such as driving or operating other machinery.
Rapid changes in serum glucose levels may induce symptoms of hypoglycemia in persons with diabetes, regardless of the glucose value. Early warning symptoms of hypoglycemia may be different or less pronounced under certain conditions, such as longstanding diabetes, diabetic nerve disease, use of medications such as beta-blockers, or intensified diabetes control [*see Drug Interactions (7)*]. These situations may result in severe hypoglycemia (and, possibly, loss of consciousness) prior to the patient's awareness of hypoglycemia. Intravenously administered insulin has a more rapid onset of action than subcutaneously administered insulin, requiring more close monitoring for hypoglycemia.

5.3 Hypokalemia
All insulin products, including NovoLog, cause a shift in potassium from the extracellular to intracellular space, possibly leading to hypokalemia that, if left untreated, may cause respiratory paralysis, ventricular arrhythmia, and death. Use caution in patients who may be at risk for hypokalemia (e.g., patients using potassium-lowering medications, patients taking medications sensitive to serum potassium concentrations, and patients receiving intravenously administered insulin).

5.4 Renal Impairment
As with other insulins, the dose requirements for NovoLog may be reduced in patients with renal impairment [*see Clinical Pharmacology (12.3)*].

5.5 Hepatic Impairment
As with other insulins, the dose requirements for NovoLog may be reduced in patients with hepatic impairment [*see Clinical Pharmacology (12.3)*].

5.6 Hypersensitivity and Allergic Reactions
Local Reactions - As with other insulin therapy, patients may experience redness, swelling, or itching at the site of NovoLog injection. These reactions usually resolve in a few days to a few weeks, but in some occasions, may require discontinuation of NovoLog. In some instances, these reactions may be related to factors other than insulin, such as irritants in a skin cleansing agent or poor injection technique. Localized reactions and generalized myalgias have been reported with injected metacresol, which is an excipient in NovoLog.
Systemic Reactions - Severe, life-threatening, generalized allergy, including anaphylaxis, may occur with any insulin product, including NovoLog. Anaphylactic reactions with NovoLog have been reported post-approval. Generalized allergy to insulin may also cause whole body rash (including pruritus), dyspnea, wheezing, hypotension, tachycardia, or diaphoresis. In controlled clinical trials, allergic reactions were reported in 3 of 735 patients (0.4%) treated with regular human insulin and 10 of 1394 patients (0.7%) treated with NovoLog. In controlled and uncontrolled clinical trials, 3 of 2341 (0.1%) NovoLog-treated patients discontinued due to allergic reactions.

5.7 Antibody Production
Increases in anti-insulin antibody titers that react with both human insulin and insulin aspart have been observed in patients treated with NovoLog. Increases in anti-insulin antibodies are observed more frequently with NovoLog than with regular human insulin. Data from a 12-month controlled trial in patients with type 1 diabetes suggest that the increase in these antibodies is transient, and the differences in antibody levels between the regular human insulin and insulin aspart treatment groups observed at 3 and 6 months were no longer evident at 12 months. The clinical significance of these antibodies is not known. These antibodies do not appear to cause deterioration in glycemic control or necessitate increases in insulin dose.

5.8 Mixing of Insulins
- Mixing NovoLog with NPH human insulin immediately before injection attenuates the peak concentration of NovoLog, without significantly affecting the time to peak concentration or total bioavailability of NovoLog. If NovoLog is mixed with NPH human insulin, NovoLog should be drawn into the syringe first, and the mixture should be injected immediately after mixing.
- The efficacy and safety of mixing NovoLog with insulin preparations produced by other manufacturers have not been studied.
- Insulin mixtures should not be administered intravenously.

5.9 Continuous Subcutaneous Insulin Infusion by External Pump
When used in an external subcutaneous insulin infusion pump, NovoLog should not be mixed with any other insulin or diluent. When using NovoLog in an external insulin pump, the NovoLog-specific information should be followed (e.g., in-use time, frequency of changing infusion sets) because NovoLog-specific information may differ from general pump manual instructions.
Pump or infusion set malfunctions or insulin degradation can lead to a rapid onset of hyperglycemia and ketosis because of the small subcutaneous depot of insulin. This is especially pertinent for rapid-acting insulin analogs that are more rapidly absorbed through skin and have a shorter duration of action. Prompt identification and correction of the cause of hyperglycemia or ketosis is necessary. Interim therapy with subcutaneous injection may be required [*see Dosage and Administration (2.3), Warnings and Precautions (5.8, 5.9), How Supplied/Storage and Handling (16.2), and Patient Counseling Information (17.2)*].
NovoLog should not be exposed to temperatures greater than 37°C (98.6°F). **NovoLog that will be used in a pump should not be mixed with other insulin or with a diluent** [*see Dosage and Administration (2.3), Warnings and Precautions (5.8, 5.9), How Supplied/Storage and Handling (16.2), and Patient Counseling Information (17.2)*].

5.10 Fluid retention and heart failure with concomitant use of PPAR-gamma agonists
Thiazolidinediones (TZDs), which are peroxisome proliferator-activated receptor (PPAR)-gamma agonists, can cause dose-related fluid retention, particularly when used in combination with insulin. Fluid retention may lead to or exacerbate heart failure. Patients treated with insulin, including NovoLog, and a PPAR-gamma agonist should be observed for signs and symptoms of heart failure. If heart failure develops, it should be managed according to current standards of care, and discontinuation or dose reduction of the PPAR-gamma agonist must be considered.

6 ADVERSE REACTIONS
Clinical Trial Experience
Because clinical trials are conducted under widely varying designs, the adverse reaction rates reported in one clinical trial may not be easily compared to those rates reported in another clinical trial, and may not reflect the rates actually observed in clinical practice.
- *Hypoglycemia*

Hypoglycemia is the most commonly observed adverse reaction in patients using insulin, including NovoLog [*see Warnings and Precautions (5)*].
- *Insulin initiation and glucose control intensification*

Intensification or rapid improvement in glucose control has been associated with a transitory, reversible ophthalmologic refraction disorder, worsening of diabetic retinopathy, and acute painful peripheral neuropathy. However, long-term glycemic control decreases the risk of diabetic retinopathy and neuropathy.
- *Lipodystrophy*

Long-term use of insulin, including NovoLog, can cause lipodystrophy at the site of repeated insulin injections or infusion. Lipodystrophy includes lipohypertrophy (thickening of adipose tissue) and lipoatrophy (thinning of adipose tissue), and may affect insulin absorption. Rotate insulin injection or infusion sites within the same region to reduce the risk of lipodystrophy.
- *Weight gain*

Weight gain can occur with some insulin therapies, including NovoLog, and has been attributed to the anabolic effects of insulin and the decrease in glucosuria.
- *Peripheral Edema*

Insulin may cause sodium retention and edema, particularly if previously poor metabolic control is improved by intensified insulin therapy.
- *Frequencies of adverse drug reactions*

The frequencies of adverse drug reactions during NovoLog clinical trials in patients with type 1 diabetes mellitus and type 2 diabetes mellitus are listed in the tables below.

[See table 1 at right]
[See table 2 below]

Postmarketing Data

The following additional adverse reactions have been identified during postapproval use of NovoLog. Because these adverse reactions are reported voluntarily from a population of uncertain size, it is generally not possible to reliably estimate their frequency. Medication errors in which other insulins have been accidentally substituted for NovoLog have been identified during postapproval use [*see Patient Counseling Information (17)*].

7 DRUG INTERACTIONS

A number of substances affect glucose metabolism and may require insulin dose adjustment and particularly close monitoring.

- The following are examples of substances that may increase the blood-glucose-lowering effect and susceptibility to hypoglycemia: oral antidiabetic products, pramlintide, ACE inhibitors, disopyramide, fibrates, fluoxetine, monoamine oxidase (MAO) inhibitors, propoxyphene, salicylates, somatostatin analog (e.g., octreotide), sulfonamide antibiotics.
- The following are examples of substances that may reduce the blood-glucose-lowering effect: corticosteroids, niacin, danazol, diuretics, sympathomimetic agents (e.g., epinephrine, salbutamol, terbutaline), isoniazid, phenothiazine derivatives, somatropin, thyroid hormones, estrogens, progestogens (e.g., in oral contraceptives), atypical antipsychotics.
- Beta-blockers, clonidine, lithium salts, and alcohol may either potentiate or weaken the blood-glucose-lowering effect of insulin.
- Pentamidine may cause hypoglycemia, which may sometimes be followed by hyperglycemia.
- The signs of hypoglycemia may be reduced or absent in patients taking sympatholytic products such as beta-blockers, clonidine, guanethidine, and reserpine.

8 USE IN SPECIFIC POPULATIONS

8.1 Pregnancy

Pregnancy Category B. All pregnancies have a background risk of birth defects, loss, or other adverse outcome regardless of drug exposure. This background risk is increased in pregnancies complicated by hyperglycemia and may be decreased with good metabolic control. It is essential for patients with diabetes or history of gestational diabetes to maintain good metabolic control before conception and throughout pregnancy. Insulin requirements may decrease during the first trimester, generally increase during the second and third trimesters, and rapidly decline after delivery. Careful monitoring of glucose control is essential in these patients. Therefore, female patients should be advised to tell their physician if they intend to become, or if they become pregnant while taking NovoLog.

An open-label, randomized study compared the safety and efficacy of NovoLog (n=157) versus regular human insulin (n=165) in 322 pregnant women with type 1 diabetes. Two-thirds of the enrolled patients were already pregnant when they entered the study. Because only one-third of the patients enrolled before conception, the study was not large enough to evaluate the risk of congenital malformations. Both groups achieved a mean HbA_{1c} of ~ 6% during pregnancy, and there was no significant difference in the incidence of maternal hypoglycemia.

Subcutaneous reproduction and teratology studies have been performed with NovoLog and regular human insulin in rats and rabbits. In these studies, NovoLog was given to female rats before mating, during mating, and throughout pregnancy, and to rabbits during organogenesis. The effects of NovoLog did not differ from those observed with subcutaneous regular human insulin. NovoLog, like human insulin, caused pre- and post-implantation losses and visceral/skeletal abnormalities in rats at a dose of 200 U/kg/day (approximately 32 times the human subcutaneous dose of 1.0 U/kg/day, based on U/body surface area) and in rabbits at a dose of 10 U/kg/day (approximately three times the human subcutaneous dose of 1.0 U/kg/day, based on U/body surface area). The effects are probably secondary to maternal hypoglycemia at high doses. No significant effects were observed in rats at a dose of 50 U/kg/day and in rabbits at a dose of 3 U/kg/day. These doses are approximately 8 times the human subcutaneous dose of 1.0 U/kg/day for rats and equal to the human subcutaneous dose of 1.0 U/kg/day for rabbits, based on U/body surface area.

8.3 Nursing Mothers

It is unknown whether insulin aspart is excreted in human milk. Use of NovoLog is compatible with breastfeeding, but women with diabetes who are lactating may require adjustments of their insulin doses.

8.4 Pediatric Use

NovoLog is approved for use in children for subcutaneous daily injections and for subcutaneous continuous infusion by external insulin pump. NovoLog has not been studied in pediatric patients younger than 2 years of age. NovoLog has not been studied in pediatric patients with type 2 diabetes. Please see *Section 14 **CLINICAL STUDIES*** for summaries of clinical studies.

8.5 Geriatric Use

Of the total number of patients (n= 1,375) treated with NovoLog in 3 controlled clinical studies, 2.6% (n=36) were 65 years of age or over. One-half of these patients had type 1 diabetes (18/1285) and the other half had type 2 diabetes (18/90). The HbA_{1c} response to NovoLog, as compared to human insulin, did not differ by age, particularly in patients with type 2 diabetes. Additional studies in larger populations of patients 65 years of age or over are needed to permit conclusions regarding the safety of NovoLog in elderly compared to younger patients. Pharmacokinetic/pharmacodynamic studies to assess the effect of age on the onset of NovoLog action have not been performed.

10 OVERDOSAGE

Excess insulin administration may cause hypoglycemia and, particularly when given intravenously, hypokalemia. Mild episodes of hypoglycemia usually can be treated with oral glucose. Adjustments in drug dosage, meal patterns, or exercise, may be needed. More severe episodes with coma, seizure, or neurologic impairment may be treated with intramuscular/subcutaneous glucagon or concentrated intravenous glucose. Sustained carbohydrate intake and observation may be necessary because hypoglycemia may recur after apparent clinical recovery. Hypokalemia must be corrected appropriately.

11 DESCRIPTION

NovoLog (insulin aspart [rDNA origin] injection) is a rapid-acting human insulin analog used to lower blood glucose. NovoLog is homologous with regular human insulin with the exception of a single substitution of the amino acid proline by aspartic acid in position B28, and is produced by recombinant DNA technology utilizing *Saccharomyces cerevisiae* (baker's yeast). Insulin aspart has the empirical formula $C_{256}H_{381}N_{65}O_{79}S_6$ and a molecular weight of 5825.8.

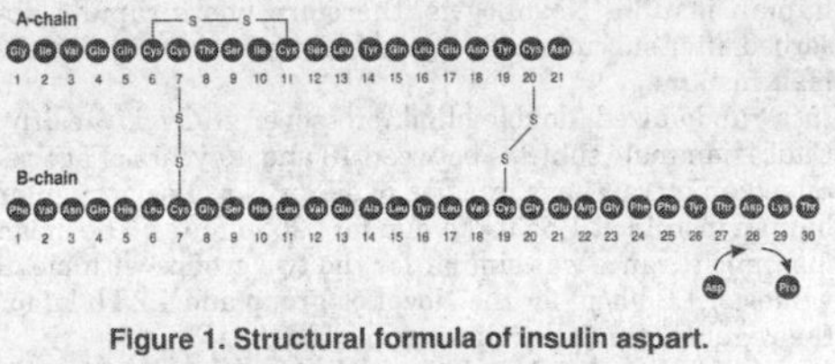

Figure 1. Structural formula of insulin aspart.

NovoLog is a sterile, aqueous, clear, and colorless solution, that contains insulin aspart 100 Units/mL, glycerin 16 mg/mL, phenol 1.50 mg/mL, metacresol 1.72 mg/mL, zinc 19.6 mcg/mL, disodium hydrogen phosphate dihydrate 1.25 mg/mL, sodium chloride 0.58 mg/mL and water for injection. NovoLog has a pH of 7.2-7.6. Hydrochloric acid 10% and/or sodium hydroxide 10% may be added to adjust pH.

12 CLINICAL PHARMACOLOGY

12.1 Mechanism of Action

The primary activity of NovoLog is the regulation of glucose metabolism. Insulins, including NovoLog, bind to the insulin receptors on muscle and fat cells and lower blood glucose by facilitating the cellular uptake of glucose and simultaneously inhibiting the output of glucose from the liver.

12.2 Pharmacodynamics

Studies in normal volunteers and patients with diabetes demonstrated that subcutaneous administration of NovoLog has a more rapid onset of action than regular human insulin.

In a study in patients with type 1 diabetes (n=22), the maximum glucose-lowering effect of NovoLog occurred between 1 and 3 hours after subcutaneous injection (see Figure 2). The duration of action for NovoLog is 3 to 5 hours. The time course of action of insulin and insulin analogs such as NovoLog may vary considerably in different individuals or within the same individual. The parameters of NovoLog activity (time of onset, peak time and duration) as designated in Figure 2 should be considered only as general guidelines.

Table 1: Treatment-Emergent Adverse Events in Patients with Type 1 Diabetes Mellitus (Adverse events with frequency ≥ 5% and occurring more frequently with NovoLog compared to human regular insulin are listed)

	NovoLog + NPH N= 596		Human Regular Insulin + NPH N= 286	
Preferred Term	**N**	**(%)**	**N**	**(%)**
Hypoglycemia*	448	75%	205	72%
Headache	70	12%	28	10%
Injury accidental	65	11%	29	10%
Nausea	43	7%	13	5%
Diarrhea	28	5%	9	3%

* Hypoglycemia is defined as an episode of blood glucose concentration <45 mg/dL, with or without symptoms. See Section 14 for the incidence of serious hypoglycemia in the individual clinical trials.

Table 2: Treatment-Emergent Adverse Events in Patients with Type 2 Diabetes Mellitus (except for hypoglycemia, adverse events with frequency ≥ 5% and occurring more frequently with NovoLog compared to human regular insulin are listed)

	NovoLog + NPH N= 91		Human Regular Insulin + NPH N= 91	
	N	**(%)**	**N**	**(%)**
Hypoglycemia*	25	27%	33	36%
Hyporeflexia	10	11%	6	7%
Onychomycosis	9	10%	5	5%
Sensory disturbance	8	9%	6	7%
Urinary tract infection	7	8%	6	7%
Chest pain	5	5%	3	3%
Headache	5	5%	3	3%
Skin disorder	5	5%	2	2%
Abdominal pain	5	5%	1	1%
Sinusitis	5	5%	1	1%

* Hypoglycemia is defined as an episode of blood glucose concentration <45 mg/dL, with or without symptoms. See Section 14 for the incidence of serious hypoglycemia in the individual clinical trials.

The rate of insulin absorption and onset of activity is affected by the site of injection, exercise, and other variables [*see Warnings and Precautions (5.1)*].

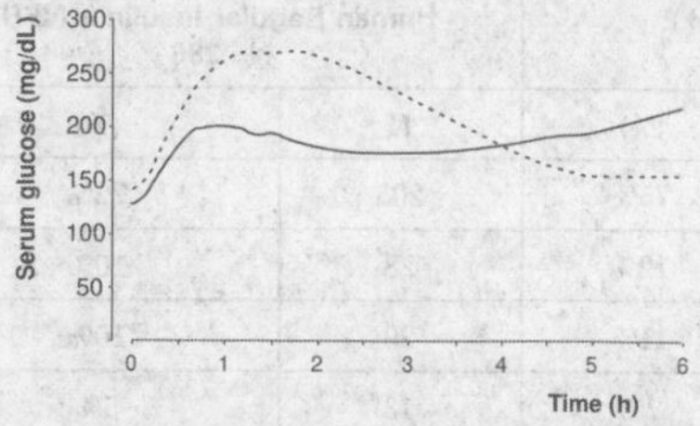

Figure 2. Serial mean serum glucose collected up to 6 hours following a single pre-meal dose of NovoLog (solid curve) or regular human insulin (hatched curve) injected immediately before a meal in 22 patients with type 1 diabetes.

A double-blind, randomized, two-way cross-over study in 16 patients with type 1 diabetes demonstrated that intravenous infusion of NovoLog resulted in a blood glucose profile that was similar to that after intravenous infusion with regular human insulin. NovoLog or human insulin was infused until the patient's blood glucose decreased to 36 mg/dL, or until the patient demonstrated signs of hypoglycemia (rise in heart rate and onset of sweating), defined as the time of autonomic reaction (R) (see Figure 3).

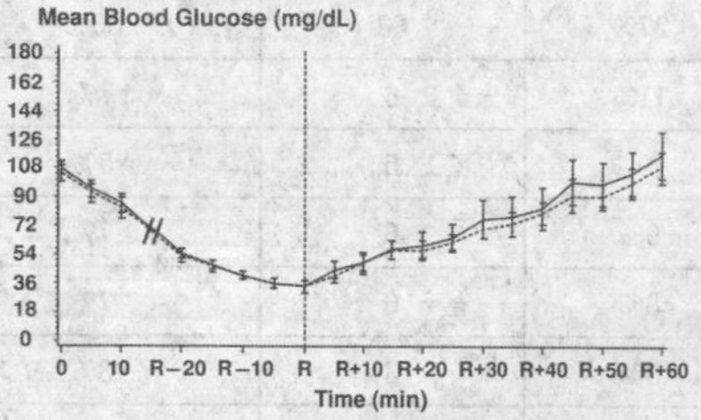

Note: The slashes on the mean profile indicate a jump on the time axis

Figure 3. Mean blood glucose profiles following intravenous infusion of NovoLog (hatched curve) and regular human insulin (solid curve) in 16 patients with type 1 diabetes. R represents the time of autonomic reaction.

12.3 Pharmacokinetics

The single substitution of the amino acid proline with aspartic acid at position B28 in NovoLog reduces the molecule's tendency to form hexamers as observed with regular human insulin. NovoLog is, therefore, more rapidly absorbed after subcutaneous injection compared to regular human insulin.

In a randomized, double-blind, crossover study 17 healthy Caucasian male subjects between 18 and 40 years of age received an intravenous infusion of either NovoLog or regular human insulin at 1.5 mU/kg/min for 120 minutes. The mean insulin clearance was similar for the two groups with mean values of 1.2 l/h/kg for the NovoLog group and 1.2 l/h/kg for the regular human insulin group.

Bioavailability and Absorption - NovoLog has a faster absorption, a faster onset of action, and a shorter duration of action than regular human insulin after subcutaneous injection (see Figure 2 and Figure 4). The relative bioavailability of NovoLog compared to regular human insulin indicates that the two insulins are absorbed to a similar extent.

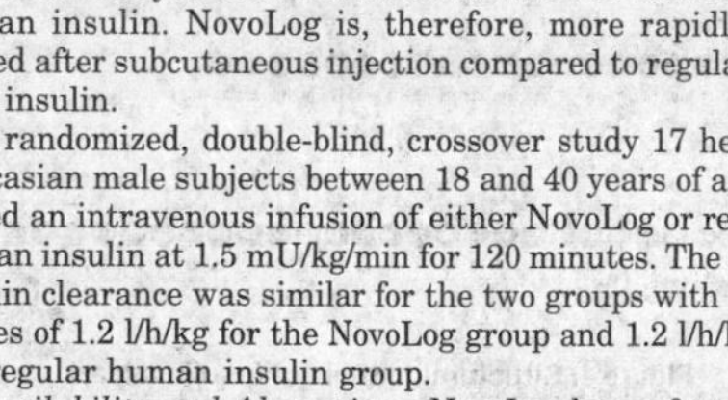

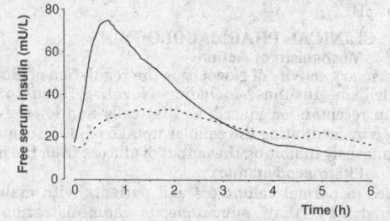

Figure 4. Serial mean serum free insulin concentration collected up to 6 hours following a single pre-meal dose of NovoLog (solid curve) or regular human insulin (hatched curve) injected immediately before a meal in 22 patients with type 1 diabetes.

In studies in healthy volunteers (total n=107) and patients with type 1 diabetes (total n=40), NovoLog consistently reached peak serum concentrations approximately twice as fast as regular human insulin. The median time to maximum concentration in these trials was 40 to 50 minutes for NovoLog versus 80 to 120 minutes for regular human insulin. In a clinical trial in patients with type 1 diabetes, NovoLog and regular human insulin, both administered subcutaneously at a dose of 0.15 U/kg body weight, reached mean maximum concentrations of 82 and 36 mU/L, respectively. Pharmacokinetic/pharmacodynamic characteristics of insulin aspart have not been established in patients with type 2 diabetes.

The intra-individual variability in time to maximum serum insulin concentration for healthy male volunteers was significantly less for NovoLog than for regular human insulin. The clinical significance of this observation has not been established.

In a clinical study in healthy non-obese subjects, the pharmacokinetic differences between NovoLog and regular human insulin described above, were observed independent of the site of injection (abdomen, thigh, or upper arm).

Distribution and Elimination - NovoLog has low binding to plasma proteins (<10%), similar to that seen with regular human insulin. After subcutaneous administration in normal male volunteers (n=24), NovoLog was more rapidly eliminated than regular human insulin with an average apparent half-life of 81 minutes compared to 141 minutes for regular human insulin.

Specific Populations

Children and Adolescents - The pharmacokinetic and pharmacodynamic properties of NovoLog and regular human insulin were evaluated in a single dose study in 18 children (6-12 years, n=9) and adolescents (13-17 years [Tanner grade ≥ 2], n=9) with type 1 diabetes. The relative differences in pharmacokinetics and pharmacodynamics in children and adolescents with type 1 diabetes between NovoLog and regular human insulin were similar to those in healthy adult subjects and adults with type 1 diabetes.

Gender - In healthy volunteers, no difference in insulin aspart levels was seen between men and women when body weight differences were taken into account. There was no significant difference in efficacy noted (as assessed by HbA_{1c}) between genders in a trial in patients with type 1 diabetes.

Obesity - A single subcutaneous dose of 0.1 U/kg NovoLog was administered in a study of 23 patients with type 1 diabetes and a wide range of body mass index (BMI, 22-39 kg/m^2). The pharmacokinetic parameters, AUC and C_{max}, of NovoLog were generally unaffected by BMI in the different groups – BMI 19-23 kg/m^2 (N=4); BMI 23-27 kg/m^2 (N=7); BMI 27-32 kg/m^2 (N=6) and BMI >32 kg/m^2 (N=6). Clearance of NovoLog was reduced by 28% in patients with BMI >32 kg/m^2 compared to patients with BMI <23 kg/m^2.

Renal Impairment - Some studies with human insulin have shown increased circulating levels of insulin in patients with renal failure. A single subcutaneous dose of 0.08 U/kg NovoLog was administered in a study to subjects with either normal (N=6) creatinine clearance (CLcr) (> 80 ml/min) or mild (N=7; CLcr = 50-80 ml/min), moderate (N=3; CLcr = 30-50 ml/min) or severe (but not requiring hemodialysis) (N=2; CLcr = <30 ml/min) renal impairment. In this small study, there was no apparent effect of creatinine clearance values on AUC and C_{max} of NovoLog. Careful glucose monitoring and dose adjustments of insulin, including NovoLog, may be necessary in patients with renal dysfunction [*see Warnings and Precautions (5.4)*].

Hepatic Impairment - Some studies with human insulin have shown increased circulating levels of insulin in patients with liver failure. A single subcutaneous dose of 0.06 U/kg NovoLog was administered in an open-label, single-dose study of 24 subjects (N=6/group) with different degree of hepatic impairment (mild, moderate and severe) having Child-Pugh Scores ranging from 0 (healthy volunteers) to 12 (severe hepatic impairment). In this small study, there was no correlation between the degree of hepatic failure and any NovoLog pharmacokinetic parameter. Careful glucose monitoring and dose adjustments of insulin, including NovoLog, may be necessary in patients with hepatic dysfunction [*see Warnings and Precautions (5.5)*].

The effect of age, ethnic origin, pregnancy and smoking on the pharmacokinetics and pharmacodynamics of NovoLog has not been studied.

13 NONCLINICAL TOXICOLOGY

13.1 Carcinogenesis, Mutagenesis, Impairment of Fertility

Standard 2-year carcinogenicity studies in animals have not been performed to evaluate the carcinogenic potential of NovoLog. In 52-week studies, Sprague-Dawley rats were dosed subcutaneously with NovoLog at 10, 50, and 200 U/kg/day (approximately 2, 8, and 32 times the human subcutaneous dose of 1.0 U/kg/day, based on U/body surface area, respectively). At a dose of 200 U/kg/day, NovoLog increased the incidence of mammary gland tumors in females when compared to untreated controls. The incidence of mammary tumors for NovoLog was not significantly different than for regular human insulin. The relevance of these findings to humans is not known. NovoLog was not genotoxic in the following tests: Ames test, mouse lymphoma cell forward gene mutation test, human peripheral blood lymphocyte chromosome aberration test, *in vivo* micronucleus test in mice, and in *ex vivo* UDS test in rat liver hepatocytes. In fertility studies in male and female rats, at subcutaneous doses up to 200 U/kg/day (approximately 32 times the human subcutaneous dose, based on U/body surface area), no direct adverse effects on male and female fertility, or general reproductive performance of animals was observed.

13.2 Animal Toxicology and/or Pharmacology

In standard biological assays in mice and rabbits, one unit of NovoLog has the same glucose-lowering effect as one unit of regular human insulin. In humans, the effect of NovoLog is more rapid in onset and of shorter duration, compared to regular human insulin, due to its faster absorption after subcutaneous injection (see *Section 12 CLINICAL PHARMACOLOGY* Figure 2 and Figure 4).

14 CLINICAL STUDIES

14.1 Subcutaneous Daily Injections

Two six-month, open-label, active-controlled studies were conducted to compare the safety and efficacy of NovoLog to Novolin R in adult patients with type 1 diabetes. Because the two study designs and results were similar, data are shown for only one study (see Table 3). NovoLog was administered by subcutaneous injection immediately prior to meals and regular human insulin was administered by subcutaneous injection 30 minutes before meals. NPH insulin was administered as the basal insulin in either single or divided daily doses. Changes in HbA_{1c} and the incidence rates of severe hypoglycemia (as determined from the number of events requiring intervention from a third party) were comparable for the two treatment regimens in this study (Table 3) as well as in the other clinical studies that are cited in this section. Diabetic ketoacidosis was not reported in any of the adult studies in either treatment group.

Table 3. Subcutaneous NovoLog Administration in Type 1 Diabetes (24 weeks; n=882)

	NovoLog + NPH	Novolin R + NPH
N	596	286
Baseline HbA_{1c} (%)*	7.9 ±1.1	8.0 ± 1.2
Change from Baseline HbA_{1c} (%)	-0.1 ± 0.8	0.0 ± 0.8
Treatment Difference in HbA_{1c}, Mean (95% confidence interval)	-0.2 (-0.3, -0.1)	
Baseline insulin dose (IU/kg/24 hours)*	0.7 ± 0.2	0.7 ± 0.2
End-of-Study insulin dose (IU/kg/24 hours)*	0.7 ± 0.2	0.7 ± 0.2
Patients with severe hypoglycemia (n, %)†	104 (17%)	54 (19%)
Baseline body weight (kg)*	75.3 ± 14.5	75.9 ± 13.1
Weight Change from baseline (kg)*	0.5 ± 3.3	0.9 ± 2.9

* Values are Mean ± SD

† Severe hypoglycemia refers to hypoglycemia associated with central nervous system symptoms and requiring the intervention of another person or hospitalization.

A 24-week, parallel-group study of children and adolescents with type 1 diabetes (n = 283) aged 6 to 18 years compared two subcutaneous multiple-dose treatment regimens: NovoLog (n = 187) or Novolin R (n = 96). NPH insulin was administered as the basal insulin. NovoLog achieved glycemic control comparable to Novolin R, as measured by change in HbA_{1c} (Table 4) and both treatment groups had a comparable incidence of hypoglycemia. Subcutaneous administration of NovoLog and regular human insulin have also been compared in children with type 1 diabetes (n=26) aged 2 to 6 years with similar effects on HbA_{1c} and hypoglycemia.

Table 4. Pediatric Subcutaneous Administration of NovoLog in Type 1 Diabetes (24 weeks; n=283)

	NovoLog + NPH	Novolin R + NPH
N	187	96
Baseline HbA_{1c} (%)*	8.3 ± 1.2	8.3 ± 1.3

Change from Baseline HbA_{1c} (%)	0.1± 1.0	0.1± 1.1
Treatment Difference in $HbA_{1c,}$ Mean (95% confidence interval)	0.1 (-0.5, 0.1)	
Baseline insulin dose (IU/kg/24 hours)*	0.4 ± 0.2	0.6 ± 0.2
End-of-Study insulin dose (IU/kg/24 hours)*	0.4 ± 0.2	0.7 ± 0.2
Patients with severe hypoglycemia (n, %)†	11 (6%)	9 (9%)
Diabetic ketoacidosis (n, %)	10 (5%)	2 (2%)
Baseline body weight (kg)*	50.6 ± 19.6	48.7 ± 15.8
Weight Change from baseline (kg)*	2.7 ± 3.5	2.4 ± 2.6

* Values are Mean ± SD
† Severe hypoglycemia refers to hypoglycemia associated with central nervous system symptoms and requiring the intervention of another person or hospitalization.

One six-month, open-label, active-controlled study was conducted to compare the safety and efficacy of NovoLog to Novolin R in patients with type 2 diabetes (Table 5). NovoLog was administered by subcutaneous injection immediately prior to meals and regular human insulin was administered by subcutaneous injection 30 minutes before meals. NPH insulin was administered as the basal insulin in either single or divided daily doses. Changes in HbA_{1c} and the rates of severe hypoglycemia (as determined from the number of events requiring intervention from a third party) were comparable for the two treatment regimens.

Table 5. Subcutaneous NovoLog Administration in Type 2 Diabetes (6 months; n=176)

	NovoLog + NPH	Novolin R + NPH
N	90	86
Baseline HbA_{1c} (%)*	8.1 ± 1.2	7.8 ± 1.1
Change from Baseline HbA_{1c} (%)	-0.3 ± 1.0	-0.1 ± 0.8
Treatment Difference in $HbA_{1c,}$ Mean (95% confidence interval)	- 0.1 (-0.4, -0.1)	
Baseline insulin dose (IU/kg/24 hours)*	0.6 ± 0.3	0.6 ± 0.3
End-of-Study insulin dose (IU/kg/24 hours)*	0.7 ± 0.3	0.7 ± 0.3
Patients with severe hypoglycemia (n, %)†	9 (10%)	5 (8%)
Baseline body weight (kg)*	88.4 ± 13.3	85.8 ± 14.8
Weight Change from baseline (kg)*	1.2 ± 3.0	0.4 ± 3.1

* Values are Mean ± SD
† Severe hypoglycemia refers to hypoglycemia associated with central nervous system symptoms and requiring the intervention of another person or hospitalization.

14.2 Continuous Subcutaneous Insulin Infusion (CSII) by External Pump
Two open-label, parallel design studies (6 weeks [n=29] and 16 weeks [n=118]) compared NovoLog to buffered regular human insulin (Velosulin) in adults with type 1 diabetes receiving a subcutaneous infusion with an external insulin pump. The two treatment regimens had comparable changes in HbA_{1c} and rates of severe hypoglycemia.

Table 6. Adult Insulin Pump Study in Type 1 Diabetes (16 weeks; n=118)

	NovoLog	Buffered human insulin
N	59	59
Baseline HbA_{1c} (%)*	7.3 ± 0.7	7.5 ± 0.8
Change from Baseline HbA_{1c} (%)	0.0 ± 0.5	0.2 ± 0.6
Treatment Difference in $HbA_{1c,}$ Mean (95% confidence interval)	0.3 (-0.1, 0.4)	
Baseline insulin dose (IU/kg/24 hours)*	0.7 ± 0.8	0.6 ± 0.2
End-of-Study insulin dose (IU/kg/24 hours)*	0.7 ± 0.7	0.6 ± 0.2
Patients with severe hypoglycemia (n, %)†	1 (2%)	2 (3%)
Baseline body weight (kg)*	77.4 ± 16.1	74.8 ± 13.8
Weight Change from baseline (kg)*	0.1 ± 3.5	-0.0 ± 1.7

* Values are Mean ± SD
† Severe hypoglycemia refers to hypoglycemia associated with central nervous system symptoms and requiring the intervention of another person or hospitalization.

A randomized, 16-week, open-label, parallel design study of children and adolescents with type 1 diabetes (n=298) aged 4-18 years compared two subcutaneous infusion regimens administered via an external insulin pump: NovoLog (n=198) or insulin lispro (n=100). These two treatments resulted in comparable changes from baseline in HbA_{1c} and comparable rates of hypoglycemia after 16 weeks of treatment (see Table 7).

Table 7. Pediatric Insulin Pump Study in Type 1 Diabetes (16 weeks; n=298)

	NovoLog	Lispro
N	198	100
Baseline HbA_{1c} (%)*	8.0 ± 0.9	8.2 ± 0.8
Change from Baseline HbA_{1c} (%)	-0.1 ± 0.8	-0.1 ± 0.7
Treatment Difference in $HbA_{1c,}$ Mean (95% confidence interval)	-0.1 (-0.3, 0.1)	
Baseline insulin dose (IU/kg/24 hours)*	0.9 ± 0.3	0.9 ± 0.3
End-of-Study insulin dose (IU/kg/24 hours)*	0.9 ± 0.2	0.9 ± 0.2
Patients with severe hypoglycemia (n, %)†	19 (10%)	8 (8%)
Diabetic ketoacidosis (n, %)	1 (0.5%)	0 (0)
Baseline body weight (kg)*	54.1 ± 19.7	55.5 ± 19.0
Weight Change from baseline (kg)*	1.8 ± 2.1	1.6 ± 2.1

* Values are Mean ± SD
† Severe hypoglycemia refers to hypoglycemia associated with central nervous system symptoms and requiring the intervention of another person or hospitalization.

An open-label, 16-week parallel design trial compared preprandial NovoLog injection in conjunction with NPH injections to NovoLog administered by continuous subcutaneous infusion in 127 adults with type 2 diabetes. The two treatment groups had similar reductions in HbA_{1c} and rates of severe hypoglycemia (Table 8) [*see Indications and Usage (1), Dosage and Administration (2), Warnings and Precautions (5) and How Supplied/Storage and Handling (16.2)*].

Table 8. Pump Therapy in Type 2 Diabetes (16 weeks; n=127)

	NovoLog pump	NovoLog + NPH
N	66	61
Baseline HbA_{1c} (%)*	8.2 ± 1.4	8.0 ± 1.1
Change from Baseline HbA_{1c} (%)	-0.6 ± 1.1	-0.5 ± 0.9
Treatment Difference in $HbA_{1c,}$ Mean (95% confidence interval)	0.1 (0.4, 0.3)	
Baseline insulin dose (IU/kg/24 hours)*	0.7 ± 0.3	0.8 ± 0.5
End-of-Study insulin dose (IU/kg/24 hours)*	0.9 ± 0.4	0.9 ± 0.5
Baseline body weight (kg)*	96.4 ± 17.0	96.9 ± 17.9
Weight Change from baseline (kg)*	1.7 ± 3.7	0.7 ± 4.1

* Values are Mean ± SD

14.3 Intravenous Administration of NovoLog
See *Section 12.2 CLINICAL PHARMACOLOGY/Pharmacodynamics*.

16 HOW SUPPLIED/STORAGE AND HANDLING
16.1 How Supplied
NovoLog is available in the following package sizes: each presentation containing 100 Units of insulin aspart per mL (U-100).

10 mL vials	NDC 0169-7501-11
3 mL PenFill cartridges*	NDC 0169-3303-12
3 mL NovoLog FlexPen	NDC 0169-6339-10

* NovoLog PenFill cartridges are designed for use with Novo Nordisk 3 mL PenFill cartridge compatible insulin delivery devices (with or without the addition of a NovoPen 3 PenMate) with NovoFine disposable needles.

16.2 Recommended Storage
Unused NovoLog should be stored in a refrigerator between 2° and 8°C (36° to 46°F). Do not store in the freezer or directly adjacent to the refrigerator cooling element. **Do not freeze NovoLog and do not use NovoLog if it has been frozen.** NovoLog should not be drawn into a syringe and stored for later use.
Vials: After initial use a vial may be kept at temperatures below 30°C (86°F) for up to 28 days, but should not be exposed to excessive heat or sunlight. Opened vials may be refrigerated.
Unpunctured vials can be used until the expiration date printed on the label if they are stored in a refrigerator. Keep unused vials in the carton so they will stay clean and protected from light.
PenFill cartridges or NovoLog FlexPen:
Once a cartridge or a NovoLog FlexPen is punctured, it should be kept at temperatures below 30°C (86°F) for up to 28 days, but should not be exposed to excessive heat or sunlight. A NovoLog FlexPen or cartridge in use must NOT be stored in the refrigerator. Keep the NovoLog FlexPen and all PenFill cartridges away from direct heat and sunlight. Unpunctured NovoLog FlexPen and PenFill cartridges can be used until the expiration date printed on the label if they are stored in a refrigerator. Keep unused NovoLog FlexPen and PenFill cartridges in the carton so they will stay clean and protected from light.
Always remove the needle after each injection and store the 3 mL PenFill cartridge delivery device or NovoLog FlexPen without a needle attached. This prevents contamination and/or infection, or leakage of insulin, and will ensure accurate dosing. Always use a new needle for each injection to prevent contamination.
Pump:
NovoLog in the pump reservoir should be discarded after at least every 6 days of use or after exposure to temperatures that exceed 37°C (98.6°F). The infusion set and the infusion set insertion site should be changed at least every 3 days.
Summary of Storage Conditions:
The storage conditions are summarized in the following table:
[See table 9 at top of next page]
Storage of Diluted NovoLog
NovoLog diluted with Insulin Diluting Medium for NovoLog to a concentration equivalent to U-10 or equivalent to U-50 may remain in patient use at temperatures below 30°C (86°F) for 28 days.
Storage of NovoLog in Infusion Fluids
Infusion bags prepared as indicated under *Dosage and Administration (2)* are stable at room temperature for 24 hours. Some insulin will be initially adsorbed to the material of the infusion bag.

17 PATIENT COUNSELING INFORMATION
[See *FDA-Approved Patient Labeling (17.3)*]
17.1 Physician Instructions
Maintenance of normal or near-normal glucose control is a treatment goal in diabetes mellitus and has been associated with a reduction in diabetic complications. Patients should be informed about potential risks and benefits of NovoLog therapy including the possible adverse reactions. Patients should also be offered continued education and advice on

Table 9. Storage conditions for vial, PenFill cartridges and NovoLog FlexPen

NovoLog presentation	**Not in-use (unopened)** Room Temperature (below 30°C)	**Not in-use (unopened)** Refrigerated	**In-use (opened)** Room Temperature (below 30°C)
10 mL vial	28 days	Until expiration date	28 days (refrigerated/room temperature)
3 mL PenFill cartridges	28 days	Until expiration date	28 days (Do not refrigerate)
3 mL NovoLog FlexPen	28 days	Until expiration date	28 days (Do not refrigerate)

insulin therapies, injection technique, life-style management, regular glucose monitoring, periodic glycosylated hemoglobin testing, recognition and management of hypo- and hyperglycemia, adherence to meal planning, complications of insulin therapy, timing of dose, instruction in the use of injection or subcutaneous infusion devices, and proper storage of insulin. Patients should be informed that frequent, patient-performed blood glucose measurements are needed to achieve optimal glycemic control and avoid both hyper- and hypoglycemia.

The patient's ability to concentrate and react may be impaired as a result of hypoglycemia. This may present a risk in situations where these abilities are especially important, such as driving or operating other machinery. Patients who have frequent hypoglycemia or reduced or absent warning signs of hypoglycemia should be advised to use caution when driving or operating machinery.

Accidental substitutions between NovoLog and other insulin products have been reported. Patients should be instructed to always carefully check that they are administering the appropriate insulin to avoid medication errors between NovoLog and any other insulin. **The written prescription for NovoLog should be written clearly, to avoid confusion with other insulin products, for example, NovoLog Mix 70/30.**

17.2 Patients Using Pumps

Patients using external pump infusion therapy should be trained in intensive insulin therapy with multiple injections and in the function of their pump and pump accessories.

The following insulin pumps† have been used in NovoLog clinical or *in vitro* studies conducted by Novo Nordisk, the manufacturer of NovoLog:

- Medtronic Paradigm® 512 and 712
- MiniMed 508
- Disetronic® D-TRON® and H-TRON®

Before using another insulin pump with NovoLog, read the pump label to make sure the pump has been evaluated with NovoLog.

NovoLog is recommended for use in any reservoir and infusion sets that are compatible with insulin and the specific pump. Please see recommended reservoir and infusion sets in the pump manual.

To avoid insulin degradation, infusion set occlusion, and loss of the preservative (metacresol), insulin in the reservoir should be replaced at least every 6 days; infusion sets and infusion set insertion sites should be changed at least every 3 days.

Insulin exposed to temperatures higher than 37°C (98.6°F) should be discarded. The temperature of the insulin may exceed ambient temperature when the pump housing, cover, tubing, or sport case is exposed to sunlight or radiant heat. Infusion sites that are erythematous, pruritic, or thickened should be reported to medical personnel, and a new site selected because continued infusion may increase the skin reaction and/or alter the absorption of NovoLog. Pump or infusion set malfunctions or insulin degradation can lead to hyperglycemia and ketosis in a short time because of the small subcutaneous depot of insulin. This is especially pertinent for rapid-acting insulin analogs that are more rapidly absorbed through skin and have shorter duration of action. These differences are particularly relevant when patients are switched from multiple injection therapy. Prompt identification and correction of the cause of hyperglycemia or ketosis is necessary. Problems include pump malfunction, infusion set occlusion, leakage, disconnection or kinking, and degraded insulin. Less commonly, hypoglycemia from pump malfunction may occur. If these problems cannot be promptly corrected, patients should resume therapy with subcutaneous insulin injection and contact their physician [*see Dosage and Administration (2), Warnings and Precautions (5) and How Supplied/Storage and Handling (16.2)*].

17.3 FDA-Approved Patient Labeling

See separate leaflet.

Rx Only

Date of Issue: March 9, 2013

Version: 20

Novo Nordisk®, NovoLog®, NovoPen® 3, PenFill®, Novolin®, FlexPen®, PenMate® and NovoFine® are registered trademarks of Novo Nordisk A/S.

NovoLog® is covered by US Patent Nos. 5,618,913, 5,866,538, and other patents pending.

FlexPen® is covered by US Patent Nos. 6,582,404, 6,004,297, 6,235,004, and other patents pending.

PenFill® is covered by US Patent No. 5,693,027.

†The brands listed are the registered trademarks of their respective owners and are not trademarks of Novo Nordisk A/S.

Manufactured by:
Novo Nordisk A/S
DK-2880 Bagsvaerd, Denmark

For information about NovoLog contact:
Novo Nordisk Inc.
Plainsboro, New Jersey 08536
1-800-727-6500
www.novonordisk-us.com

PATIENT INFORMATION

NovoLog® (NŌ-vō-log)

(insulin aspart [rDNA origin] Injection)

Important:

Know your insulin. Do not change the type of insulin you use unless told to do so by your healthcare provider. The amount of insulin you take as well as the best time for you to take your insulin may need to change if you take a different type of insulin.

Make sure you know the type and strength of insulin prescribed for you.

Read the Patient Information that comes with NovoLog® before you start taking it and each time you get a refill. There may be new information. This leaflet does not take the place of talking with your healthcare provider about your diabetes or your treatment. Make sure you know how to manage your diabetes. Ask your healthcare provider if you have any questions about managing your diabetes.

What is NovoLog®?

NovoLog® is a man-made insulin that is used to control high blood sugar in adults and children with diabetes mellitus.

Who should not use NovoLog®?

Do not take NovoLog® if:

- Your blood sugar is too low (hypoglycemia).
- You are allergic to anything in NovoLog®. See the end of this leaflet for a complete list of ingredients in NovoLog®. Check with your healthcare provider if you are not sure.

Tell your healthcare provider:

- **about all of your medical conditions.** Medical conditions can affect your insulin needs and your dose of NovoLog®.
- **if you are pregnant or breastfeeding.** You and your healthcare provider should talk about the best way to manage your diabetes while you are pregnant or breastfeeding. NovoLog® has not been studied in nursing women.
- **about all medicines you take,** including prescriptions and non-prescription medicines, vitamins and herbal supplements. Your NovoLog® dose may change if you take other medicines.
- **if you take any other medicines,** especially ones commonly called TZDs (thiazolidinediones).
- **if you have heart failure or other heart problems.** If you have heart failure, it may get worse while you take TZDs with NovoLog®.

Know the medicines you take. Keep a list of your medicines with you to show your healthcare providers when you get a new medicine.

How should I take NovoLog®?

Only use NovoLog® if it appears clear and colorless. There may be air bubbles. This is normal. If it looks cloudy, thickened, or colored, or if it contains solid particles do not use it and call Novo Nordisk at 1-800-727-6500.

NovoLog® comes in:

- 10 mL vials (small bottles) for use with syringe
- 3 mL PenFill® cartridges for use with the Novo Nordisk 3 mL PenFill® cartridge compatible insulin delivery devices and NovoFine® disposable needles. The cartridge delivery device can be used with a NovoPen® 3 PenMate®
- 3 mL NovoLog® FlexPen®

Read the instructions for use that come with your NovoLog® product. Talk to your healthcare provider if you have any questions. Your healthcare provider should show you how to inject NovoLog® before you start taking it.

- **Take NovoLog® exactly as prescribed.** You should eat a meal within 5 to 10 minutes after using NovoLog® to avoid low blood sugar.
- **NovoLog® is a fast-acting insulin.** The effects of NovoLog® start working 10 to 20 minutes after injection or bolus pump infusion.
- **Do not inject NovoLog® if you do not plan to eat right after your injection or bolus pump infusion.**
- The greatest blood sugar lowering effect is between 1 and 3 hours after the injection or infusion. This blood sugar lowering lasts for 3 to 5 hours.
- **While using NovoLog® you may have to change** your total dose of insulin, your dose of longer-acting insulin, or the number of injections of longer-acting insulin you use. Pump users given NovoLog® may need to change the amount of total insulin given as a basal infusion.
- **Do not mix NovoLog®:**
  - with any other insulins when used in a pump
  - with any insulins other than NPH when used with injections by syringe

If your healthcare provider recommends diluting NovoLog®, follow your healthcare provider's instructions exactly so that you know:

- How to make NovoLog® more dilute (that is, a smaller number of units of NovoLog® for a given amount of liquid) and
- How to use this more dilute form of NovoLog®. **Do not use dilute insulin in a pump.**
- **Inject NovoLog® into the skin of your stomach area, upper arms, buttocks or upper legs.** NovoLog® may affect your blood sugar levels sooner if you inject it into the skin of your stomach area. **Never inject NovoLog® into a vein or into a muscle.**
- **Change (rotate) your injection site within the chosen area (for example, stomach or upper arm) with each dose. Do not inject into the exact same spot for each injection.**
- **If you take too much NovoLog®, your blood sugar may fall low (hypoglycemia).** You can treat mild low blood sugar (hypoglycemia) by drinking or eating something sugary right away (fruit juice, sugar candies, or glucose tablets). It is important to treat low blood sugar (hypoglycemia) right away because it could get worse and you could pass out (become unconscious). If you pass out you will need help from another person or emergency medical services right away, and will need treatment with a glucagon injection or treatment at a hospital. See "What are the possible side effects of NovoLog®?" for more information on low blood sugar (hypoglycemia).
- **If you forget to take your dose of NovoLog®, your blood sugar may go too high (hyperglycemia).** If high blood sugar (hyperglycemia) is not treated it can lead to serious problems, like loss of consciousness (passing out), coma or even death. Follow your healthcare provider's instructions for treating high blood sugar. Know your symptoms of high blood sugar which may include:

• increased thirst	• fruity smell on the breath
• frequent urination	• high amounts of sugar and ketones in your urine
• drowsiness	• nausea, vomiting (throwing up) or stomach pain
• loss of appetite	
• a hard time breathing	

Check your blood sugar levels. Ask your healthcare provider what your blood sugars should be and when you should check your blood sugar levels.

Your insulin dosage may need to change because of:

• illness	• change in diet
• stress	• change in physical activity or exercise
• other medicines you take	

What should I avoid while using NovoLog®?

- **Alcohol.** Alcohol, including beer and wine, may affect your blood sugar when you take NovoLog®.
- **Driving and operating machinery.** You may have difficulty concentrating or reacting if you have low blood sugar (hypoglycemia). Be careful when you drive a car or operate machinery. Ask your healthcare provider if it is alright to drive if you often have:
  - low blood sugar
  - decreased or no warning signs of low blood sugar

What are the possible side effects of NovoLog®?

- **Low blood sugar (hypoglycemia).** Symptoms of low blood sugar may include:

• sweating	• trouble concentrating or confusion
• dizziness or lightheadedness	• blurred vision
• shakiness	• slurred speech
• hunger	• anxiety, irritability or mood changes
• fast heart beat	• headache
• tingling of lips and tongue	

Severe low blood sugar can cause unconsciousness (passing out), seizures, and death. Know your symptoms of low blood sugar. Follow your healthcare provider's instructions for treating low blood sugar. Talk to your healthcare provider if low blood sugar is a problem for you.

- **Serious allergic reaction (whole body reaction). Get medical help right away, if you develop** a rash over your whole body, have trouble breathing, a fast heartbeat, or sweating.
- **Reactions at the injection site (local allergic reaction).** You may get redness, swelling, and itching at the injection site. If you keep having skin reactions or they are serious talk to your healthcare provider. You may need to stop using NovoLog® and use a different insulin. Do not inject insulin into skin that is red, swollen, or itchy.
- **Skin thickens or pits at the injection site (lipodystrophy).** Change (rotate) where you inject your insulin to help to prevent these skin changes from happening. Do not inject insulin into this type of skin.
- **Swelling of your hands and feet**
- **Heart Failure.** Taking certain diabetes pills called thiazolidinediones or "TZDs" with NovoLog® may cause heart failure in some people. This can happen even if you have never had heart failure or heart problems before. If you already have heart failure it may get worse while you take TZDs with NovoLog®. Your healthcare provider should monitor you closely while you are taking TZDs with NovoLog®. Tell your healthcare provider if you have any new or worse symptoms of heart failure including:
  - **shortness of breath**
  - **swelling of your ankles or feet**
  - **sudden weight gain**

  Treatment with TZDs and NovoLog® may need to be adjusted or stopped by your healthcare provider if you have new or worse heart failure.
- **Vision changes**
- **Low potassium in your blood (hypokalemia)**
- **Weight gain**

These are not all of the possible side effects from NovoLog®. Ask your healthcare provider or pharmacist for more information.

Call your healthcare provider for medical advice about side effects. You may report side effects to FDA at 1-800-FDA-1088.

How should I store NovoLog®?

All Unopened NovoLog®:

- **Keep all unopened NovoLog® in the refrigerator between 36° to 46°F (2° to 8°C).**
- Do not freeze. Do not use NovoLog® if it has been frozen.
- Keep unopened NovoLog® in the carton to protect from light.

NovoLog® in use:

- **Vials**
  - Keep in the refrigerator or at room temperature below 86°F (30°C) for up to 28 days.
  - Keep vials away from direct heat or light.
  - Throw away an opened vial after 28 days of use, even if there is insulin left in the vial.
  - Do not draw up NovoLog® into a syringe and store for later use.
  - Unopened vials can be used until the expiration date on the NovoLog® label, if the medicine has been stored in a refrigerator.
- **PenFill® Cartridges or NovoLog® FlexPen®**
  - Keep at room temperature below 86°F (30°C) for up to 28 days.
  - Do not store a PenFill® cartridge or NovoLog® FlexPen® that you are using in the refrigerator.
  - Keep PenFill® cartridges and NovoLog® FlexPen® away from direct heat or light.
  - Throw away a used PenFill® cartridge or NovoLog® FlexPen® after 28 days, even if there is insulin left in the cartridge or syringe.
- **NovoLog® in the pump reservoir and the complete external pump infusion set**
  - The infusion set and the infusion site should be changed **at least every 3 days**. The insulin in the reservoir should be changed **at least every 6 days** even if you have not used all of the insulin. Change the infusion set and the infusion site more often than every 3 days if you have high blood sugar (hyperglycemia), the pump alarm sounds, or the insulin flow is blocked (occlusion).

General advice about NovoLog®

Medicines are sometimes prescribed for conditions that are not mentioned in the patient leaflet. Do not use NovoLog® for a condition for which it was not prescribed. Do not give NovoLog® to other people, even if they have the same symptoms you have. It may harm them.

This leaflet summarizes the most important information about NovoLog®. If you would like more information about NovoLog® or diabetes, talk with your healthcare provider. You can ask your healthcare provider or pharmacist for information about NovoLog® that is written for healthcare professionals. Call 1-800-727-6500 or visit www.novonordisk-us.com for more information.

Helpful information for people with diabetes is published by the American Diabetes Association, 1701 N Beauregard Street, Alexandria, VA 22311 and on www.diabetes.org.

NovoLog® ingredients include:

• insulin aspart	• zinc
• glycerin	• disodium hydrogen phosphate dihydrate
• phenol	• sodium chloride
• metacresol	• water for injection

All NovoLog® vials, PenFill® cartridges and NovoLog® FlexPen® are latex free.

Date of Issue: March 9, 2013

Version: 12

Novo Nordisk®, NovoLog®, PenFill®, FlexPen®, NovoPen®, NovoFine®, and PenMate® are registered trademarks of Novo Nordisk A/S.

NovoLog® is covered by US Patent Nos. 5,618,913, 5,866,538, and other patents pending.

FlexPen® is covered by US Patent Nos. 6,582,404, 6,004,297, 6,235,004, and other patents pending.

PenFill® is covered by US Patent No. 5,693,027.

Manufactured by:
Novo Nordisk A/S
DK-2880 Bagsvaerd, Denmark

For information about NovoLog® contact:
Novo Nordisk Inc.
800 Scudders Mill Road
Plainsboro, New Jersey 08536

PATIENT INSTRUCTIONS FOR USE

NovoLog® (NŌ-vō-log)

(insulin aspart [rDNA origin] injection)

10 mL vial (100 Units/mL, U-100)

Read this Instructions for Use before you start taking NovoLog® and each time you get a refill. There may be new information. This information does not take the place of talking to your healthcare provider about your medical condition or your treatment.

Supplies you will need to give your NovoLog® injection:

- 10 mL NovoLog® vial
- insulin syringe and needle
- alcohol swab

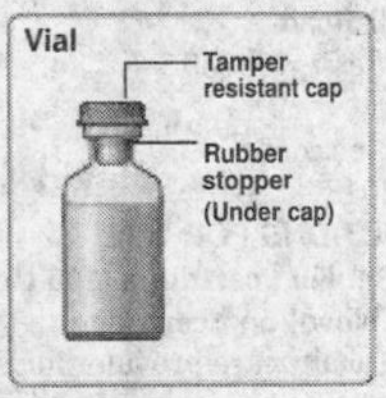

Preparing your NovoLog® dose:

- Wash your hands with soap and water.
- Before you start to prepare your injection, check the NovoLog® label to make sure that you are taking the right type of insulin. This is especially important if you use more than 1 type of insulin.
- NovoLog® should look clear and colorless. **Do not** use NovoLog® if it is thick, cloudy, or is colored.
- **Do not** use NovoLog® past the expiration date printed on the label.

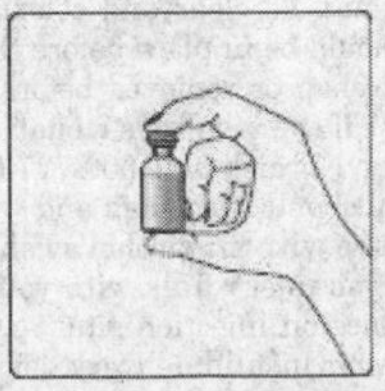

Step 1: Pull off the tamper resistant cap (See Figure A).

Step 2: Wipe the rubber stopper with an alcohol swab (See Figure B).

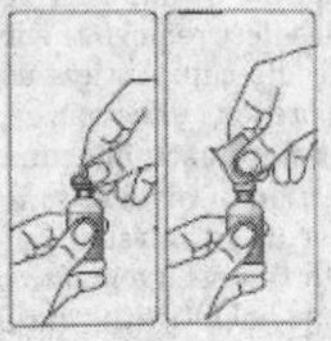

(Figure A Figure B)

Step 3: Hold the syringe with the needle pointing up.Pull down on the plunger until the black tip reaches the line for the number of units for your prescribed dose (See Figure C).

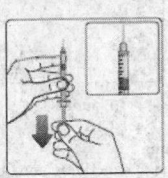

(Figure C)

Step 4: Push the needle through the rubber stopper of the NovoLog® vial (See Figure D).

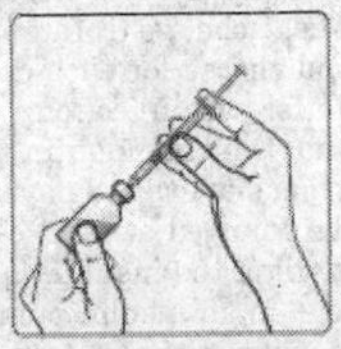

(Figure D)

Step 5: Push the plunger all the way in. This puts air into the NovoLog® vial (See Figure E).

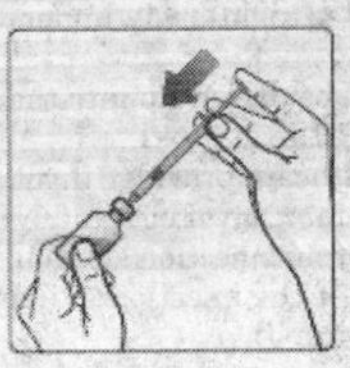

(Figure E)

Step 6: Turn the NovoLog® vial and syringe upside down and slowly pull the plunger down until the black tip is a few units past the line for your dose (See Figure F).

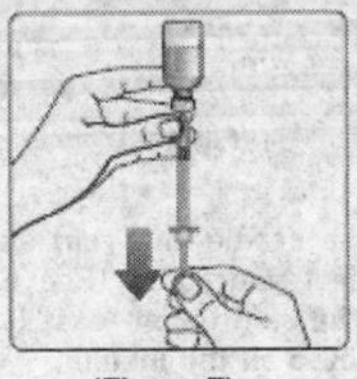

(Figure F)

- If there are air bubbles, tap the syringe gently a few times to let any air bubbles rise to the top (See Figure G).

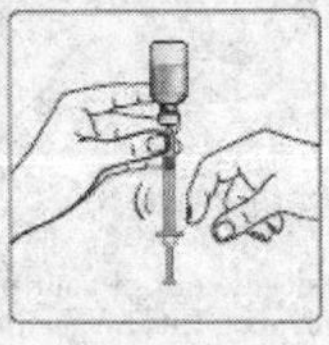

(Figure G)

Step 7: Slowly push the plunger up until the black tip reaches the line for your NovoLog® dose (See Figure H).

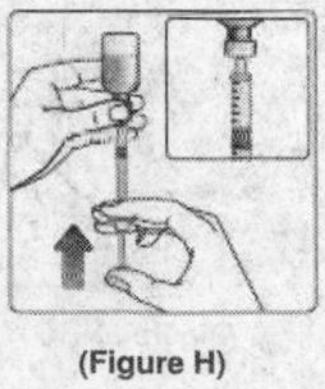

(Figure H)

Step 8: Check the syringe to make sure you have the right dose of NovoLog®.

Step 9: Pull the syringe out of the vial's rubber stopper (See Figure I).

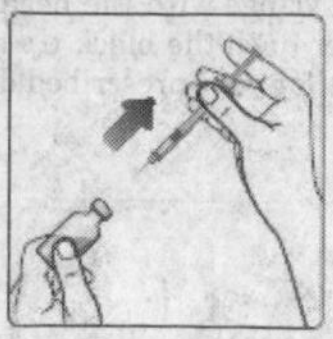

(Figure I)

Giving your Injection:

- Inject your NovoLog® exactly as your healthcare provider has shown you. Your healthcare provider should tell you if you need to pinch the skin before injecting.
- NovoLog® can be injected under the skin (subcutaneously) of your stomach area, buttocks, upper legs or upper arms, infused in an insulin pump, or given through a needle in your arm (intravenously) by your healthcare provider.
- If you inject NovoLog®,change (rotate) your injection sites within the area you choose for each dose. **Do not** use the same injection site for each injection.
- If you use NovoLog® in an insulin pump, you should change your insertion site every 3 days. The insulin in the reservoir should be changed at least every 6 days even if you have not used all of the insulin.
- If you use NovoLog® in an insulin pump, see your insulin pump manual for instructions or talk to your healthcare provider.
- NPH insulin is the only type of insulin that can be mixed with NovoLog®. **Do not** mix NovoLog® with any other type of insulin.
- NovoLog® should **only** be mixed with NPH insulin if it is going to be injected right away under your skin (subcutaneously).
- NovoLog® should be drawn up into the syringe **before** you draw up your NPH insulin.
- Talk to your healthcare provider if you are not sure about the right way to mix NovoLog® and NPH insulin.

Step 10: Choose your injection site and wipe the skin with an alcohol swab. Let the injection site dry before you inject your dose (See Figure J).

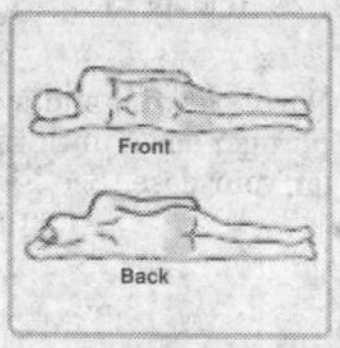

(Figure J)

Step 11: Insert the needle into your skin. Push down on the plunger to inject your dose (See Figure K). **Needle should remain in the skin for at least 6 seconds to make sure you have injected all the insulin.**

(Figure K)

Step 12: Pull the needle out of your skin. After that, you may see a drop of NovoLog® at the needle tip. This is normal and does not affect the dose you just received (See Figure L).

- If you see blood after you take the needle out of your skin, press the injection site lightly with a piece of gauze or an alcohol swab. **Do not** rub the area.

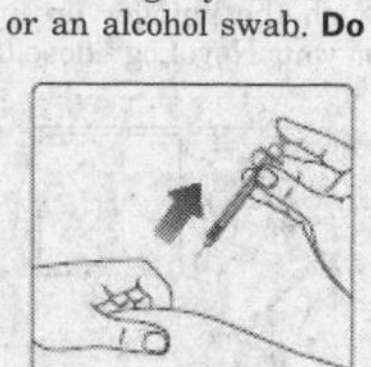

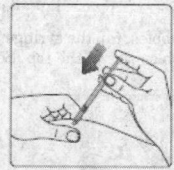

(Figure L)

After your injection:

- **Do not** recap the needle. Recapping the needle can lead to a needle stick injury.
- Throw away empty insulin vials, used syringes, and needles in a sharps container or some type of hard plastic or metal container with a screw on cap such as a detergent bottle or empty coffee can. Check with your healthcare provider about the right way to throw away the container. There may be local or state laws about how to throw away used syringes and needles. Do not throw away used syringes and needles in household trash or recycling bins.

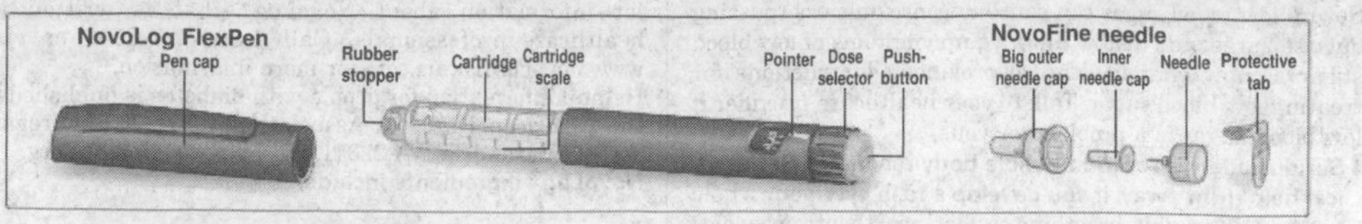

How should I store NovoLog®?

Do not freeze NovoLog®. **Do not** use NovoLog® if it has been frozen.

- Keep NovoLog® away from heat or light.
- Store opened and unopened NovoLog® vials in the refrigerator at 36°F to 46°F (2°C to 8°C). Opened NovoLog® vials can also be stored out of the refrigerator below 86°F (30°C).
- Unopened vials may be used until the expiration date printed on the label, if they are kept in the refrigerator.
- Opened NovoLog® vials should be thrown away after 28 days, even if they still have insulin left in them.

General information about the safe and effective use of NovoLog®

- Always use a new syringe and needle for each injection.
- Do not share syringes or needles.
- Keep NovoLog® vials, syringes, and needles out of the reach of children.

This Instructions for Use has been approved by the U.S. Food and Drug Administration.

Manufactured by:
Novo Nordisk A/S
DK-2880 Bagsvaerd, Denmark

NovoLog® is a registered trademark of Novo Nordisk A/S.

NovoLog® is covered by US Patent Nos. 5,618,913, 5,866,538, and other patents pending.

For information about NovoLog® contact:
Novo Nordisk Inc.
800 Scudders Mill Road
Plainsboro, New Jersey 08536
1-800-727-6500
www.novonordisk-us.com

Revised: March 2013

PATIENT INSTRUCTIONS FOR USE

NovoLog® 3 mL PenFill® cartridge (100 Units/mL, U-100)

Before using the NovoLog® cartridge

1. Talk with your healthcare provider for information about where to inject NovoLog® (injection sites) and how to give an injection with your insulin delivery device.
2. Read the instruction manual that comes with your insulin delivery device for complete instructions on how to use the PenFill® cartridge with the device.

How to use the NovoLog® cartridge

1. **Check your insulin.** Just before using your NovoLog® cartridge, check to make sure that you have the right type of insulin. This is especially important if you use different types of insulin.
2. **Carefully look at the cartridge and the insulin inside it.** The insulin should be clear and colorless. The tamper-resistant foil should be in place before the first use. If the foil has been broken or removed before your first use of the cartridge, or if the insulin is cloudy or colored, do not use it. Call Novo Nordisk at 1-800-727-6500.
3. **Wash your hands** well with soap and water. If you clean your injection site with an alcohol swab, let the injection site dry before you inject. Talk with your healthcare provider for guidance on injection sites and how to give an injection with your insulin delivery device.
4. Gather your supplies for injecting NovoLog®.
5. Insert a 3 mL cartridge into your Novo Nordisk 3 mL PenFill® cartridge compatible insulin delivery device. Wipe the front rubber stopper of the 3 mL PenFill® cartridge with an alcohol swab, then attach a new needle. For NovoFine® needles, remove the big outer needle cap and the inner needle cap. Always use a new needle for each injection to prevent infection.

Giving the airshot before each injection:

To prevent the injection of air and to make sure insulin is delivered, you must do an airshot before each injection. Hold the device with the needle pointing up and gently tap the PenFill® cartridge holder with your finger a few times to raise any air bubbles to the top of the cartridge. Do the airshot as described in the device instruction manual.

Giving the injection

6. Dial the number of units on the insulin delivery device that you need to inject. Inject the right way as shown to you by your healthcare provider.
7. Insert the needle into the skin. Inject the dose by pressing the push button all the way in. Keep the needle in the skin for at least 6 seconds, and keep the push button pressed all the way in until the needle has been pulled out from the skin. This will make sure that the full dose has been given. You may see a drop of NovoLog® at the needle tip. This is normal and has no effect on the dose you just received. If blood appears after you take the needle out of your skin, press the injection site lightly with a finger. **Do not rub the area.**

After the injection

8. **Do not recap the needle.** Recapping can lead to a needle stick injury.
9. Remove the needle from the PenFill® cartridge after each injection. Keep the 3 mL PenFill® cartridge in the insulin delivery device. The needle should not be attached to the 3 mL PenFill® cartridge during storage. This will prevent infection or leakage of insulin and will help ensure that you receive the right dose of NovoLog®.
10. Put the used needle and cartridge in a sharps container, or some type of hard plastic or metal container with a screw on top such as a detergent bottle or coffee can. Check with your healthcare provider about the right way to throw away used needles and cartridges. There may be local or state laws about how to throw away used needles and syringes. Do not throw used needles and cartridges in household trash or recycling bins.
11. Put the pen cap back on the Novo Nordisk 3 mL PenFill® cartridge compatible insulin delivery device.

Date of Issue: March 2013
Version: 9

Novo Nordisk®, NovoLog®, PenFill®, and NovoFine® are registered trademarks of Novo Nordisk A/S.

NovoLog® is covered by US Patent Nos. 5,618,913, 5,866,538, and other patents pending.
PenFill® is covered by US Patent No. 5,693,027.

Manufactured by:
Novo Nordisk A/S
DK-2880 Bagsvaerd, Denmark

For information about NovoLog® contact:
Novo Nordisk Inc.
800 Scudders Mill Road
Plainsboro, New Jersey 08536

PATIENT INSTRUCTIONS FOR USE

NovoLog® FlexPen®

Introduction

Please read the following instructions carefully before using your NovoLog® FlexPen®.

NovoLog FlexPen is a disposable dial-a-dose insulin pen. You can select doses from 1 to 60 units in increments of 1 unit. NovoLog FlexPen is designed to be used with NovoFine® needles.

Δ NovoLog FlexPen should not be used by people who are blind or have severe visual problems without the help of a person who has good eyesight and who is trained to use the NovoLog FlexPen the right way.

Getting ready

Make sure you have the following items:

- NovoLog FlexPen
- New NovoFine needle
- Alcohol swab

[See figure above]

Preparing Your NovoLog FlexPen

Wash your hands with soap and water. Before you start to prepare your injection, check the label to make sure that you are taking the right type of insulin. This is especially important if you take more than 1 type of insulin. NovoLog should look clear.

A. Pull off the pen cap (see diagram A).

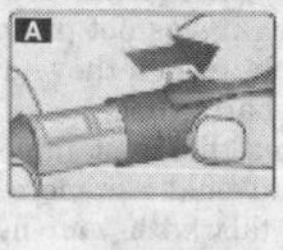

Wipe the rubber stopper with an alcohol swab.

B. Attaching the needle
Remove the protective tab from a disposable needle.
Screw the needle tightly onto your FlexPen. It is important that the needle is put on straight (see diagram B).

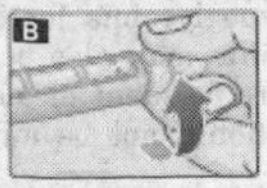

Never place a disposable needle on your NovoLog FlexPen until you are ready to take your injection.
C. Pull off the big outer needle cap (see diagram C).

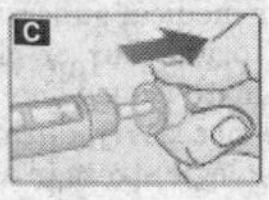

D. Pull off the inner needle cap and dispose of it (see diagram D).

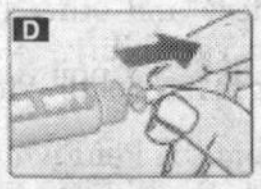

Δ Always use a new needle for each injection to help ensure sterility and prevent blocked needles.
Δ Be careful not to bend or damage the needle before use.
Δ To reduce the risk of unexpected needle sticks, never put the inner needle cap back on the needle.

Giving the airshot before each injection
Before each injection small amounts of air may collect in the cartridge during normal use. To avoid injecting air and to ensure proper dosing:
E. Turn the dose selector to select 2 units (see diagram E).

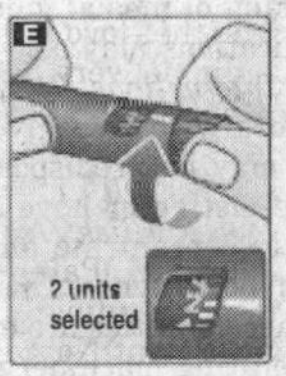

F. Hold your NovoLog FlexPen with the needle pointing up. Tap the cartridge gently with your finger a few times to make any air bubbles collect at the top of the cartridge (see diagram F).

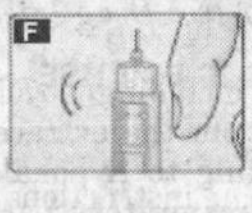

G. Keep the needle pointing upwards, press the push-button all the way in (see diagram G). The dose selector returns to 0.

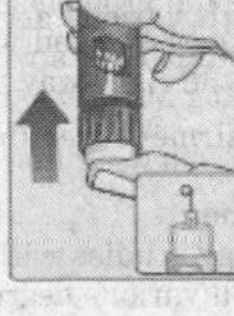

A drop of insulin should appear at the needle tip. If not, change the needle and repeat the procedure no more than 6 times.
If you do not see a drop of insulin after 6 times, do not use the NovoLog FlexPen and contact Novo Nordisk at 1-800-727-6500.
A small air bubble may remain at the needle tip, but it will not be injected.

Selecting your dose
Check and make sure that the dose selector is set at 0.
H. Turn the dose selector to the number of units you need to inject. The pointer should line up with your dose.
The dose can be corrected either up or down by turning the dose selector in either direction until the correct dose lines up with the pointer (see diagram H). When turning the dose selector, be careful not to press the push-button as insulin will come out.

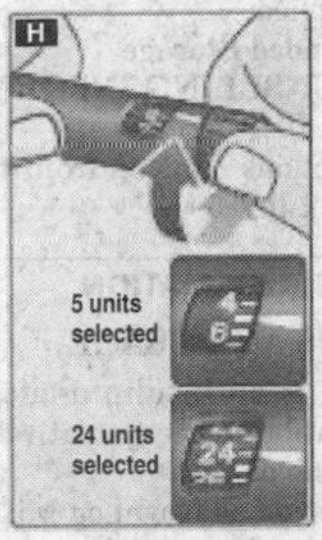

You cannot select a dose larger than the number of units left in the cartridge.
You will hear a click for every single unit dialed. Do not set the dose by counting the number of clicks you hear.
Δ Do not use the cartridge scale printed on the cartridge to measure your dose of insulin.

Giving the injection
Do the injection exactly as shown to you by your healthcare provider. Your healthcare provider should tell you if you need to pinch the skin before injecting.
I. Insert the needle into your skin.
Inject the dose by pressing the push-button all the way in until the 0 lines up with the pointer (see diagram I). Be careful only to push the button when injecting.

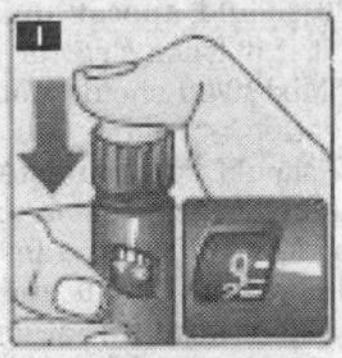

Turning the dose selector will not inject insulin.
J. Keep the needle in the skin for at least 6 seconds, and keep the push-button pressed all the way in until the needle has been pulled out from the skin (see diagram J). This will make sure that the full dose has been given.
You may see a drop of NovoLog at the needle tip. This is normal and has no effect on the dose you just received. If blood appears after you take the needle out of your skin, press the injection site lightly with a finger. **Do not rub the area.**

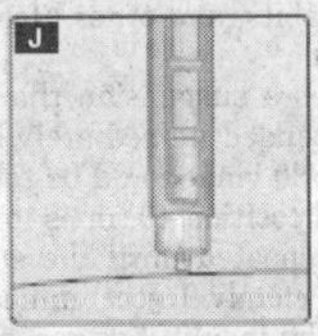

After the injection
Do not recap the needle. Recapping can lead to a needle stick injury. Remove the needle from the NovoLog FlexPen after each injection. This helps to prevent infection, leakage of insulin, and will help to make sure you inject the right dose of insulin.
Δ Put the needle and any empty NovoLog FlexPen or any used NovoLog FlexPen still containing insulin in a sharps container or some type of hard plastic or metal container with a screw top such as a detergent bottle or empty coffee can. These containers should be sealed and thrown away the right way. Check with your healthcare provider about the right way to throw away used syringes and needles. There may be local or state laws about how to throw away used needles and syringes. Do not throw away used needles and syringes in household trash or recycling bins.
The NovoLog FlexPen prevents the cartridge from being completely emptied. It is designed to deliver 300 units.
K. Put the pen cap on the NovoLog FlexPen and store the NovoLog FlexPen without the needle attached (see diagram K).

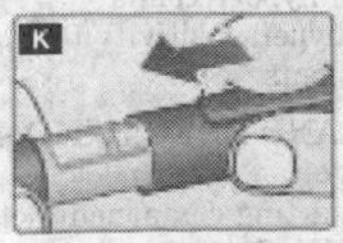

Function Check
L. If your NovoLog FlexPen is not working the right way, follow the steps below:
- Screw on a new NovoFine needle.
- Remove the big outer needle cap and the inner needle cap.
- Do an airshot as described in "Giving the airshot before each injection".
- Put the big outer needle cap onto the needle. Do not put on the inner needle cap.
- Turn the dose selector so the dose indicator window shows 20 units.
- Hold the NovoLog FlexPen so the needle is pointing down.
- Press the push-button all the way in.

The insulin should fill the lower part of the big outer needle cap (see diagram L). If the NovoLog FlexPen has released too much or too little insulin, do the function check again. If the same problem happens again, do not use your NovoLog FlexPen and contact Novo Nordisk at 1-800-727-6500.

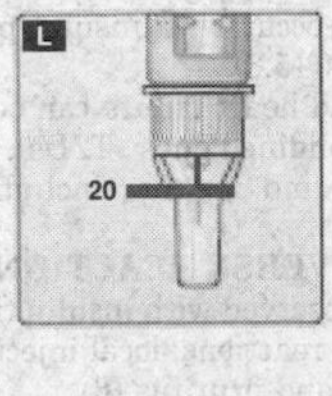

Maintenance
Your FlexPen is designed to work accurately and safely. It must be handled with care. Avoid dropping your FlexPen as it may damage it. If you are concerned that your FlexPen is damaged, use a new one. You can clean the outside of your FlexPen by wiping it with a damp cloth. Do not soak or wash your FlexPen as it may damage it. Do not refill your FlexPen.
Δ Remove the needle from the NovoLog FlexPen after each injection. This helps to ensure sterility, prevent leakage of insulin, and will help to make sure you inject the right dose of insulin for future injections.
Δ Be careful when handling used needles to avoid needle sticks and transfer of infectious diseases.
Δ Keep your NovoLog FlexPen and needles out of the reach of children.
Δ Use NovoLog FlexPen as directed to treat your diabetes.
Δ Needles and NovoLog FlexPen must not be shared. Always use a new needle for each injection.
Δ Novo Nordisk is not responsible for harm due to using this insulin pen with products not recommended by Novo Nordisk.
Δ As a precautionary measure, always carry a spare insulin delivery device in case your NovoLog FlexPen is lost or damaged.
Δ Remember to keep the disposable NovoLog FlexPen with you. Do not leave it in a car or other location where it can get too hot or too cold.

NOVOLOG® MIX 70/30 ℞

[*NŌ-vō-log-MIX-SEV-en-tee-THIR-tee*]
(70% insulin aspart protamine suspension and 30% insulin aspart injection, [rDNA origin])
Suspension for subcutaneous injection

HIGHLIGHTS OF PRESCRIBING INFORMATION
These highlights do not include all the information needed to use NovoLog Mix 70/30 safely and effectively. See full prescribing information for NovoLog Mix 70/30.
NovoLog® Mix 70/30 (70% insulin aspart protamine suspension and 30% insulin aspart injection, [rDNA origin])
Suspension for subcutaneous injection
Initial U.S. Approval: 2001

RECENT MAJOR CHANGES
- Warnings and Precautions (5.8) 3/2013

INDICATIONS AND USAGE
NovoLog Mix 70/30 is an insulin analog indicated to improve glycemic control in patients with diabetes mellitus.
Important Limitations of Use: In premix insulins, such as NovoLog Mix 70/30, the proportions of rapid acting and long acting insulins are fixed and do not allow for basal versus prandial dose adjustments (1).

DOSAGE AND ADMINISTRATION
- Only for subcutaneous injection (2.1).
  Type 1 DM: dose within 15 minutes before meal initiation.
  Type 2 DM: dose within 15 minutes before or after starting a meal.
- Do not administer intravenously (2.1).
- Do not use in insulin infusion pumps (2.1).
- Must be resuspended immediately before use (2.2).

DOSAGE FORMS AND STRENGTHS
Each presentation contains 100 Units of insulin aspart per mL (U-100) (3)
- 10 mL vials
- 3 mL NovoLog Mix 70/30 FlexPen

CONTRAINDICATIONS

- Do not use during episodes of hypoglycemia (4).
- Do not use in patients with hypersensitivity to NovoLog Mix 70/30 or one of its excipients (4).

WARNINGS AND PRECAUTIONS

- NovoLog Mix 70/30 should not be mixed with any other insulin product (5.1).
- Hypoglycemia is the most common adverse effect of insulin therapy. Glucose monitoring is recommended for all patients with diabetes. Any change of insulin dose should be made cautiously and only under medical supervision (5.1, 5.2).
- Insulin, particularly when given in settings of poor glycemic control, can cause hypokalemia. Use caution in patients predisposed to hypokalemia (5.3).
- Like all insulins, NovoLog Mix 70/30 requirements may be reduced in patients with renal impairment or hepatic impairment (5.4, 5.5).
- Severe, life-threatening, generalized allergy, including anaphylaxis, may occur with insulin products, including NovoLog Mix 70/30 (5.6).
- Fluid retention and heart failure can occur with concomitant use of thiazolidinediones (TZDs), which are PPAR-gamma agonists, and insulin, including NovoLog Mix 70/30 (5.8).

ADVERSE REACTIONS

Adverse reactions observed with insulin therapy include hypoglycemia, allergic reactions, local injection site reactions, lipodystrophy, rash and pruritus (6).

To report SUSPECTED ADVERSE REACTIONS, contact Novo Nordisk Inc. at 1-800-727-6500 or FDA at 1-800-FDA-1088 or *www.fda.gov/medwatch*.

DRUG INTERACTIONS

- The following may increase the blood-glucose-lowering effect and susceptibility to hypoglycemia: oral antidiabetic products, pramlintide, ACE inhibitors, disopyramide, fibrates, fluoxetine, monoamine oxidase (MAO) inhibitors, propoxyphene, salicylates, somatostatin analog (e.g. octreotide), sulfonamide antibiotics (7).
- The following may reduce the blood-glucose-lowering effect: corticosteroids, niacin, danazol, diuretics, sympathomimetic agents (e.g., epinephrine, salbutamol, terbutaline), isoniazid, phenothiazine derivatives, somatropin, thyroid hormones, estrogens, progestogens (e.g., in oral contraceptives), atypical antipsychotics (7).
- Beta-blockers, clonidine, lithium salts, and alcohol may either potentiate or weaken the blood-glucose-lowering effect of insulin (7).
- Pentamidine may cause hypoglycemia, which may be followed by hyperglycemia (7).
- The signs of hypoglycemia may be reduced or absent in patients taking sympatholytic products such as beta-blockers, clonidine, guanethidine, and reserpine (7).

See 17 for PATIENT COUNSELING INFORMATION and FDA-approved patient labeling

Revised: 03/2013

FULL PRESCRIBING INFORMATION: CONTENTS*

* Sections or subsections omitted from the full prescribing information are not listed

FULL PRESCRIBING INFORMATION

1 INDICATIONS AND USAGE

NovoLog Mix 70/30 is an insulin analog indicated to improve glycemic control in patients with diabetes mellitus.

Important Limitations of Use:

In premix insulins, such as NovoLog Mix 70/30, the proportions of rapid acting and long acting insulins are fixed and do not allow for basal versus prandial dose adjustments.

2 DOSAGE AND ADMINISTRATION

2.1 Dosing

NovoLog Mix 70/30 is an insulin analog with an earlier onset and intermediate duration of action in comparison to the basal human insulin premix. The addition of protamine to the rapid-acting aspart insulin analog (NovoLog) results in insulin activity that is 30% short-acting and 70% long-acting. NovoLog Mix 70/30 is typically dosed on a twice-daily basis (with each dose intended to cover 2 meals or a meal and a snack). The dosage of NovoLog Mix 70/30 must be individualized. The written prescription for NovoLog Mix 70/30 should include the full name, to avoid confusion with NovoLog (insulin aspart) and Novolin 70/30 (human premix).

NovoLog Mix 70/30 should appear uniformly white and cloudy. Do not use it if it looks clear or if it contains solid particles. NovoLog Mix 70/30 should not be used after the printed expiration date.

NovoLog Mix 70/30 should be administered by subcutaneous injection in the abdominal region, buttocks, thigh, or upper arm. NovoLog Mix 70/30 has a faster onset of action than human insulin premix 70/30 and should be dosed within 15 minutes before meal initiation for patients with type 1 diabetes. For patients with type 2 diabetes, dosing should occur within 15 minutes before or after meal initiation. Injection sites should be rotated within the same region to reduce the risk of lipodystrophy. As with all insulins, the duration of action may vary according to the dose, injection site, blood flow, temperature, and level of physical activity.

NovoLog Mix 70/30 should not be administered intravenously or used in insulin infusion pumps. Dose regimens of NovoLog Mix 70/30 will vary among patients and should be determined by the health care professional familiar with the patient's recommended glucose treatment goals, metabolic needs, eating habits, and other lifestyle variables.

2.2 Resuspension

NovoLog Mix 70/30 is a suspension that must be visually inspected and resuspended immediately before use.

The NovoLog Mix 70/30 vial should be rolled gently in your hands in a horizontal position 10 times to mix it. The rolling procedure must be repeated until the suspension appears uniformly white and cloudy. Inject immediately. Resuspension is easier when the insulin has reached room temperature.

The NovoLog Mix 70/30 FlexPen should be rolled 10 times gently between your hands in a horizontal position. Thereafter, turn the NovoLog Mix 70/30 FlexPen upside down so that the glass ball moves from one end of the reservoir to the other. Do this at least 10 times. The rolling and turning procedure must be repeated until the suspension appears uniformly white and cloudy. Inject immediately. Before each subsequent injection, turn the disposable NovoLog Mix 70/30 FlexPen upside down so that the glass ball moves from one end of the reservoir to the other at least 10 times and until the suspension appears uniformly white and cloudy. Inject immediately.

3 DOSAGE FORMS AND STRENGTHS

NovoLog Mix 70/30 is available in the following package sizes: each presentation contains 100 units of insulin aspart per mL (U-100).

- 10 mL vials
- 3 mL NovoLog Mix 70/30 FlexPen

4 CONTRAINDICATIONS

NovoLog Mix 70/30 is contraindicated

- during episodes of hypoglycemia
- in patients with hypersensitivity to NovoLog Mix 70/30 or one of its excipients.

5 WARNINGS AND PRECAUTIONS

5.1 Administration

The short and long-acting components of insulin mixes, including NovoLog Mix 70/30, cannot be titrated independently. Because NovoLog Mix 70/30 has peak pharmacodynamic activity between 1-4 hours after injection, it should be administered within 15 minutes of meal initiation *[see Clinical Pharmacology (12)]*. The dose of insulin required to provide adequate glycemic control for one of the meals may result in hyper- or hypoglycemia for the other meal. The pharmacodynamic profile may also be inadequate for patients who require more frequent meals.

NovoLog Mix 70/30 should not be mixed with any other insulin product.

NovoLog Mix 70/30 should not be used intravenously.

NovoLog Mix 70/30 should not be used in insulin infusion pumps.

Glucose monitoring is recommended for all patients with diabetes. Any change of insulin dose should be made cautiously and only under medical supervision. Changing from one insulin product to another or changing the insulin strength may result in the need for a change in dosage. Changes may also be necessary during illness, emotional stress, and other physiologic stress in addition to changes in meals and exercise.

The pharmacokinetic and pharmacodynamic profiles of all insulins may be altered by the site used for injection and the degree of vascularization of the site. Smoking, temperature, and exercise contribute to variations in blood flow and insulin absorption. These and other factors contribute to inter- and intra-patient variability.

Needles and NovoLog Mix 70/30 FlexPen must not be shared.

5.2 Hypoglycemia

Hypoglycemia is the most common adverse effect of insulin therapy, including NovoLog Mix 70/30. Severe hypoglycemia may lead to unconsciousness and/or convulsions and may result in temporary or permanent impairment of brain function or even death. Severe hypoglycemia requiring the assistance of another person and/or parenteral glucose infusion or glucagon administration has been observed in clinical trials with insulin, including trials with NovoLog Mix 70/30.

The timing of hypoglycemia may reflect the time-action profile of the insulin formulation *[see Clinical Pharmacology (12)]*. Other factors, such as changes in dietary intake (e.g., amount of food or timing of meals), injection site, exercise, and concomitant medications may also alter the risk of hypoglycemia *[see Drug Interactions (7)]*. As with all insulins, use caution in patients with hypoglycemia unawareness and in patients who may be predisposed to hypoglycemia (e.g. patients who are fasting or have erratic food intake). The patient's ability to concentrate and react may be impaired as a result of hypoglycemia. This may present a risk in situations where these abilities are especially important, such as driving or operating machinery.

Rapid changes in serum glucose levels may induce symptoms of hypoglycemia in persons with diabetes, regardless of the glucose value. Early warning symptoms of hypoglycemia may be different or less pronounced under certain conditions, such as long duration of diabetes, diabetic nerve disease, use of medications such as beta-blockers, or intensified diabetes control *[see Drug Interactions (7)]*.

5.3 Hypokalemia

All insulin products, including NovoLog Mix 70/30, cause a shift in potassium from the extracellular to intracellular space, possibly leading to hypokalemia that, if left untreated, may cause respiratory paralysis, ventricular arrhythmia, and death. Use caution in patients who may be at risk for hypokalemia (e.g. patients using potassium-lowering medications or patients taking medications sensitive to potassium concentrations).

5.4 Renal Impairment

Clinical or pharmacology studies with NovoLog Mix 70/30 in diabetic patients with various degrees of renal impairment have not been conducted. As with other insulins, the requirements for NovoLog Mix 70/30 may be reduced in patients with renal impairment *[see Clinical Pharmacology (12.3)]*.

5.5 Hepatic Impairment

Clinical or pharmacology studies with NovoLog Mix 70/30 in diabetic patients with various degrees of hepatic impairment have not been conducted. As with other insulins, the requirements for NovoLog Mix 70/30 may be reduced in patients with hepatic impairment *[see Clinical Pharmacology (12.3)]*.

5.6 Hypersensitivity and Allergic Reactions

Local Reactions- As with other insulin therapy, patients may experience reactions such as erythema, edema or pruritus at the site of NovoLog Mix 70/30 injection. These reactions usually resolve in a few days to a few weeks, but in some occasions, may require discontinuation of NovoLog Mix 70/30. In some instances, these reactions may be related to the insulin molecule, other components in the insulin preparation including protamine and cresol, components in skin cleansing agents, or injection techniques. Localized reactions and generalized myalgias have been reported with the use of cresol as an injectable excipient.

Systemic Reactions- Less common, but potentially more serious, is generalized allergy to insulin, which may cause rash (including pruritus) over the whole body, shortness of breath, wheezing, reduction in blood pressure, rapid pulse, or sweating. Severe cases of generalized allergy, including anaphylactic reaction, may be life threatening.

5.7 Antibody Production

Specific anti-insulin antibodies as well as cross-reacting anti-insulin antibodies were monitored in a 3-month, open-label comparator trial as well as in a long-term extension trial. Changes in cross-reactive antibodies were more common after NovoLog Mix 70/30 than with Novolin 70/30 but these changes did not correlate with change in HbA_{1c} or increase in insulin dose. The clinical significance of these antibodies has not been established. Antibodies did not increase further after long-term exposure (>6 months) to NovoLog Mix 70/30.

5.8 Fluid retention and heart failure can occur with concomitant use of PPAR-gamma agonists

Thiazolidinediones (TZDs), which are peroxisome proliferator-activated receptor (PPAR)-gamma agonists, can cause dose-related fluid retention, particularly when used in combination with insulin. Fluid retention may lead to or exacerbate heart failure. Patients treated with insulin, including NovoLog Mix 70/30, and a PPAR-gamma agonist should be observed for signs and symptoms of heart failure. If heart failure develops, it should be managed according to current standards of care, and discontinuation or dose reduction of the PPAR-gamma agonist must be considered.

6 ADVERSE REACTIONS

Clinical Trial Experience

Clinical trials are conducted under widely varying designs, therefore, the adverse reaction rates reported in one clinical trial may not be easily compared to those rates reported in another clinical trial, and may not reflect the rates actually observed in clinical practice.

• Hypoglycemia

Hypoglycemia is the most commonly observed adverse reaction in patients using insulin, including NovoLog Mix 70/30 *[see Warnings and Precautions (5.2)]*. NovoLog Mix 70/30 should not be used during episodes of hypoglycemia *[see Contraindications (4)* and *Warnings and Precautions (5)]*.

• Insulin initiation and glucose control intensification

Intensification or rapid improvement in glucose control has been associated with transitory, reversible ophthalmologic refraction disorder, worsening of diabetic retinopathy, and acute painful peripheral neuropathy. However, long-term glycemic control decreases the risk of diabetic retinopathy and neuropathy.

• Lipodystrophy

Long-term use of insulin, including NovoLog Mix 70/30, can cause lipodystrophy at the site of repeated insulin injections. Lipodystrophy includes lipohypertrophy (thickening of adipose tissue) and lipoatrophy (thinning of adipose tissue), and may affect insulin absorption. Rotate insulin injection sites within the same region to reduce the risk of lipodystrophy.

• Weight gain

Weight gain can occur with some insulin therapies, including NovoLog Mix 70/30, and has been attributed to the anabolic effects of insulin and the decrease in glycosuria.

• Peripheral Edema

Insulin may cause sodium retention and edema, particularly if previously poor metabolic control is improved by intensified insulin therapy.

• Frequencies of adverse drug reactions

The frequencies of adverse drug reactions during a clinical trial with NovoLog Mix 70/30 in patients with type 1 diabetes mellitus and type 2 diabetes mellitus are listed in the tables below. The trial was a three-month, open-label trial in patients with Type 1 or Type 2 diabetes who were treated twice daily (before breakfast and before supper) with NovoLog Mix 70/30.

[See table 1 above]

[See table 2 above]

Table 1: Treatment-Emergent Adverse Events in Patients with Type 1 diabetes mellitus (Adverse events with frequency ≥5% are included.)

	NovoLog Mix 70/30 (N=55)		Novolin 70/30 (N=49)	
Preferred Term	**N**	**%**	**N**	**%**
Hypoglycemia	38	69	37	76
Headache	19	35	6	12
Influenza-like symptoms	7	13	1	2
Dyspepsia	5	9	3	6
Back pain	4	7	2	4
Diarrhea	4	7	3	6
Pharyngitis	4	7	1	2
Rhinitis	3	5	6	12
Skeletal pain	3	5	2	4
Upper respiratory tract infection	3	5	1	2

Table 2: Treatment-Emergent Adverse Events in Patients with Type 2 diabetes mellitus (Adverse events with frequency ≥5% are included.)

	NovoLog Mix 70/30 (N=85)		Novolin 70/30 (N=102)	
Preferred Term	**N**	**%**	**N**	**%**
Hypoglycemia	40	47	51	50
Upper respiratory tract infection	10	12	6	6
Headache	8	9	8	8
Diarrhea	7	8	2	2
Neuropathy	7	8	2	2
Pharyngitis	5	6	4	4
Abdominal pain	4	5	0	0
Rhinitis	4	5	2	2

Postmarketing Data

Additional adverse reactions have been identified during post-approval use of NovoLog Mix 70/30. Because these adverse reactions are reported voluntarily from a population of uncertain size, it is generally not possible to reliably estimate their frequency. They include medication errors in which other insulins have been accidentally substituted for NovoLog Mix 70/30 *[see Patient Counseling Information (17)]*.

7 DRUG INTERACTIONS

A number of substances affect glucose metabolism and may require insulin dose adjustment and particularly close monitoring.

• The following are examples of substances that may increase the blood-glucose-lowering effect and susceptibility to hypoglycemia: oral antidiabetic products, pramlintide, ACE inhibitors, disopyramide, fibrates, fluoxetine, monoamine oxidase (MAO) inhibitors, propoxyphene, salicylates, somatostatin analog (e.g. octreotide), sulfonamide antibiotics.

• The following are examples of substances that may reduce the blood-glucose-lowering effect: corticosteroids, niacin, danazol, diuretics, sympathomimetic agents (e.g., epinephrine, salbutamol, terbutaline), isoniazid, phenothiazine derivatives, somatropin, thyroid hormones, estrogens, progestogens (e.g., in oral contraceptives), atypical antipsychotics.

• Beta-blockers, clonidine, lithium salts, and alcohol may either potentiate or weaken the blood-glucose-lowering effect of insulin.

• Pentamidine may cause hypoglycemia, which may sometimes be followed by hyperglycemia.

• The signs of hypoglycemia may be reduced or absent in patients taking sympatholytic products such as beta-blockers, clonidine, guanethidine, and reserpine.

8 USE IN SPECIFIC POPULATIONS

8.1 Pregnancy

Pregnancy Category B.

All pregnancies have a background risk of birth defects, loss, or other adverse outcome regardless of drug exposure. This background risk is increased in pregnancies complicated by hyperglycemia and may be decreased with good metabolic control. It is essential for patients with diabetes or history of gestational diabetes to maintain good metabolic control before conception and throughout pregnancy. Insulin requirements may decrease during the first trimester, generally increase during the second and third trimesters, and rapidly decline after delivery. Careful monitoring of glucose control is essential in such patients.

An open-label, randomized study compared the safety and efficacy of NovoLog (the rapid-acting component of NovoLog Mix 70/30) versus human insulin in the treatment of pregnant women with Type 1 diabetes (322 exposed pregnancies (NovoLog: 157, human insulin: 165)). Two-thirds of the enrolled patients were already pregnant when they entered the study. Since only one-third of the patients enrolled before conception, the study was not large enough to evaluate the risk of congenital malformations. Mean HbA_{1c} of ~ 6% was observed in both groups during pregnancy, and there was no significant difference in the incidence of maternal hypoglycemia.

Animal reproduction studies have not been conducted with NovoLog Mix 70/30. However, subcutaneous reproduction and teratology studies have been performed with NovoLog (the rapid-acting component of NovoLog Mix 70/30) and regular human insulin in rats and rabbits. In these studies, NovoLog was given to female rats before mating, during mating, and throughout pregnancy, and to rabbits during organogenesis. The effects of NovoLog did not differ from those observed with subcutaneous regular human insulin. NovoLog, like human insulin, caused pre- and post-implantation losses and visceral/skeletal abnormalities in rats at a dose of 200 U/kg/day (approximately 32-times the human subcutaneous dose of 1.0 U/kg/day, based on U/body surface area), and in rabbits at a dose of 10 U/kg/day (approximately three times the human subcutaneous dose of 1.0 U/kg/day, based on U/body surface area). The effects are probably secondary to maternal hypoglycemia at high doses. No significant effects were observed in rats at a dose of 50 U/kg/day and rabbits at a dose of 3 U/kg/day. These doses are approximately 8 times the human subcutaneous dose of 1.0 U/kg/day for rats and equal to the human subcutaneous dose of 1.0 U/kg/day for rabbits based on U/body surface area.

Female patients should be advised to discuss with their physician if they intend to, or if they become pregnant. There are no adequate and well-controlled studies of the use of NovoLog Mix 70/30 in pregnant women.

8.3 Nursing Mothers

It is unknown whether insulin aspart is excreted in human milk as occurs with human insulin. There are no adequate and well-controlled studies of the use of NovoLog Mix 70/30 or NovoLog in lactating women. Women with diabetes who are lactating may require adjustments of their insulin doses.

8.4 Pediatric Use

Safety and effectiveness of NovoLog Mix 70/30 have not been established in pediatric patients.

8.5 Geriatric Use

Clinical studies of NovoLog Mix 70/30 did not include sufficient numbers of patients aged 65 and over to determine whether they respond differently than younger patients. In general, dose selection for an elderly patient should be cautious, usually starting at the low end of the dosing range reflecting the greater frequency of decreased hepatic, renal, or cardiac function, and of concomitant disease or other drug therapy in this population.

10 OVERDOSAGE

Hypoglycemia may occur as a result of an excess of insulin relative to food intake, energy expenditure, or both. Mild episodes of hypoglycemia usually can be treated with oral glucose. Adjustments in drug dosage, meal patterns, or exercise, may be needed. More severe episodes with coma, seizure, or neurologic impairment may be treated with intramuscular/subcutaneous glucagon or concentrated intravenous glucose. Sustained carbohydrate intake and observation may be necessary because hypoglycemia may recur after apparent clinical recovery.

11 DESCRIPTION

NovoLog Mix 70/30 (70% insulin aspart protamine suspension and 30% insulin aspart injection, [rDNA origin]) is a human insulin analog suspension containing 70% insulin aspart protamine crystals and 30% soluble insulin aspart. NovoLog Mix 70/30 is a blood-glucose-lowering agent with an earlier onset and an intermediate duration of action. Insulin aspart is homologous with regular human insulin with the exception of a single substitution of the amino acid proline by aspartic acid in position B28, and is produced by recombinant DNA technology utilizing *Saccharomyces cerevisiae* (baker's yeast). Insulin aspart (NovoLog) has the empirical formula $C_{256}H_{381}N_{65}O_{79}S_6$ and a molecular weight of 5825.8 Da.

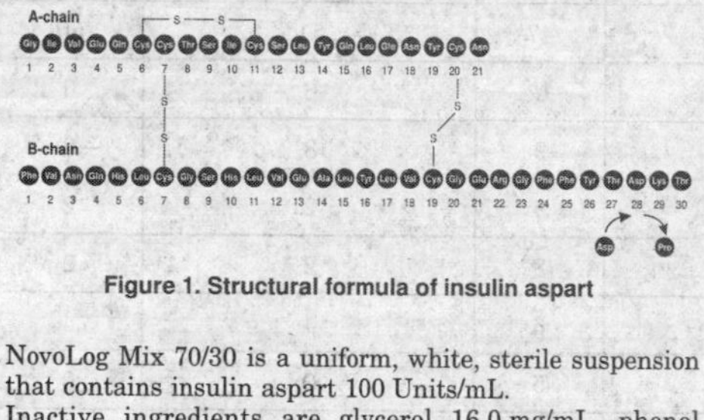

Figure 1. Structural formula of insulin aspart

NovoLog Mix 70/30 is a uniform, white, sterile suspension that contains insulin aspart 100 Units/mL.

Inactive ingredients are glycerol 16.0 mg/mL, phenol 1.50 mg/mL, metacresol 1.72 mg/mL, zinc 19.6 µg/mL, disodium hydrogen phosphate dihydrate 1.25 mg/mL, sodium chloride 0.877 mg/mL, and protamine sulfate 0.32 mg/mL. NovoLog Mix 70/30 has a pH of 7.20 - 7.44. Hydrochloric acid or sodium hydroxide may be added to adjust pH.

12 CLINICAL PHARMACOLOGY

12.1 Mechanism of Action

The primary activity of NovoLog Mix 70/30 is the regulation of glucose metabolism. Insulins, including NovoLog Mix 70/30, bind to the insulin receptors on muscle, liver and fat cells and lower blood glucose by facilitating the cellular uptake of glucose and simultaneously inhibiting the output of glucose from the liver.

12.2 Pharmacodynamics

The two euglycemic clamp studies described below *[see Clinical Pharmacology (12.3)]* assessed glucose utilization after dosing of healthy volunteers. NovoLog Mix 70/30 has an earlier onset of action than human premix 70/30 in studies of normal volunteers and patients with diabetes. The onset of action is between 10-20 minutes for NovoLog Mix 70/30 compared to 30 minutes for Novolin 70/30. The mean ± SD time to peak activity for NovoLog Mix 70/30 is 2.4 hr ± 0.8 hr compared to 4.2 hr ± 0.4 hr for Novolin 70/30. The duration of action may be as long as 24 hours (see Figure 2).

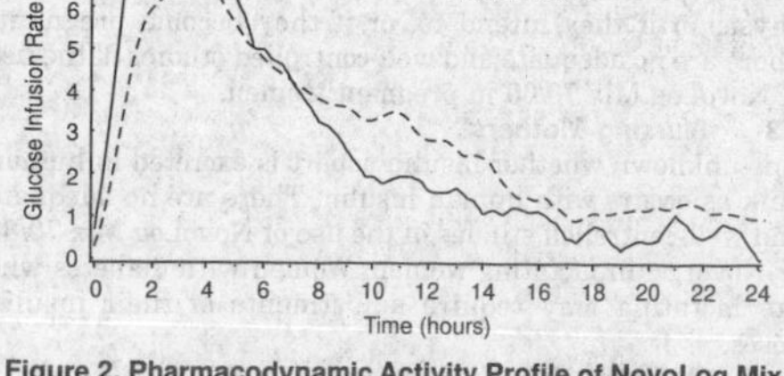

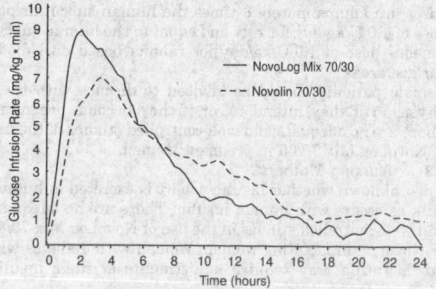

Figure 2. Pharmacodynamic Activity Profile of NovoLog Mix 70/30 and Novolin 70/30 in healthy subjects.

Table 4: Combination Therapy with Oral Agents and Insulin in Patients with Type 2 Diabetes Mellitus [Mean (SD)]

Treatment duration 24-weeks	NovoLog Mix 70/30 + Metformin + Pioglitazone	Metformin + Pioglitazone
HbA_{1c}		
Baseline mean ± SD (n)	8.1 ± 1.0 (102)	8.1 ± 1.0 (98)
End-of-study mean ± SD (n) - LOCF	6.6 ± 1.0 (93)	7.8 ± 1.2 (87)
Adjusted Mean change from baseline ± SE (n)*	-1.6 ± 0.1 (93)	-0.3 ± 0.1 (87)
Treatment difference mean ± SE* 95% CI*	-1.3 ± 0.1 (-1.6, -1.0)	
Percentage of subjects reaching HbA_{1c} <7.0%	76%	24%
Percentage of subjects reaching HbA_{1c} ≤6.5%	59%	12%
Fasting Blood Glucose (mg/dL)		
Baseline Mean ± SD (n)	173 ± 39.8 (93)	163 ± 35.4 (88)
End of Study Mean ± SD (n) - LOCF	130 ± 50.0 (90)	162 ± 40.8 (84)
Adjusted Mean change from baseline ± SE (n)*	-43.0 ± 5.3 (90)	-3.9 ± 5.3 (84)
End-of-Study Blood Glucose (Plasma) (mg/dL)		
2 Hour Post Breakfast	138 ± 42.8 (86)	188 ± 57.7 (74)
2 Hour Post Lunch	150 ± 41.5 (86)	176 ± 56.5 (74)
2 Hour Post Dinner	141 ± 57.8 (86)	195 ± 60.1 (74)
% of patients with severe hypoglycemia**	3	0
% of patients with minor hypoglycemia**	52	3
Weight gain at end of study (kg)**	4.6 ± 4.3 (92)	0.8 ± 3.2 (86)

*Adjusted mean per group, treatment difference, and 95% CI were obtained based on an ANCOVA model with treatment, FPG stratum, and secretagogue stratum as fixed factors and baseline HbA_{1c} as the covariate.

**If metabolic control is improved by intensified insulin therapy, an increased risk of hypoglycemia and weight gain may occur.

12.3 Pharmacokinetics

The single substitution of the amino acid proline with aspartic acid at position B28 in insulin aspart (NovoLog) reduces the molecule's tendency to form hexamers as observed with regular human insulin. The rapid absorption characteristics of NovoLog are maintained by NovoLog Mix 70/30. The insulin aspart in the soluble component of NovoLog Mix 70/30 is absorbed more rapidly from the subcutaneous layer than regular human insulin. The remaining 70% is in crystalline form as insulin aspart protamine which has a prolonged absorption profile after subcutaneous injection.

Bioavailability and Absorption- The relative bioavailability of NovoLog Mix 70/30 compared to NovoLog and Novolin 70/30 indicates that the insulins are absorbed to similar extent. In euglycemic clamp studies in healthy volunteers (n=23) after dosing with NovoLog Mix 70/30 (0.2 U/kg), a mean maximum serum concentration (C_{max}) of 23.4 ± 5.3 mU/L was reached after 60 minutes. The mean half-life ($t_{1/2}$) of NovoLog Mix 70/30 was about 8 to 9 hours. Serum insulin levels returned to baseline 15 to 18 hours after a subcutaneous dose of NovoLog Mix 70/30. Similar data were seen in a separate euglycemic clamp study in healthy volunteers (n=24) after dosing with NovoLog Mix 70/30 (0.3 U/kg). A C_{max} of 61.3 ± 20.1 mU/L was reached after 85 minutes. Serum insulin levels returned to baseline 12 hours after a subcutaneous dose.

The C_{max} and the area under the insulin concentration-time curve (AUC) after administration of NovoLog Mix 70/30 was approximately 20% greater than those after administration of Novolin 70/30, (see Fig. 3 for pharmacokinetic profiles). [See figure 3 at top of next column]

Distribution and Elimination- NovoLog has a low binding to plasma proteins, 0 to 9%, similar to regular human insulin. After subcutaneous administration in normal male volunteers (n=24), NovoLog was more rapidly eliminated than regular human insulin with an average apparent half-life of 81 minutes compared to 141 minutes for regular human insulin.

The effect of sex, age, obesity, ethnic origin, renal and hepatic impairment, pregnancy, or smoking, on the pharmacodynamics and pharmacokinetics of NovoLog Mix 70/30 has not been studied.

13 NONCLINICAL TOXICOLOGY

13.1 Carcinogenesis, Mutagenesis, Impairment of Fertility

Standard 2-year carcinogenicity studies in animals have not been performed to evaluate the carcinogenic potential of

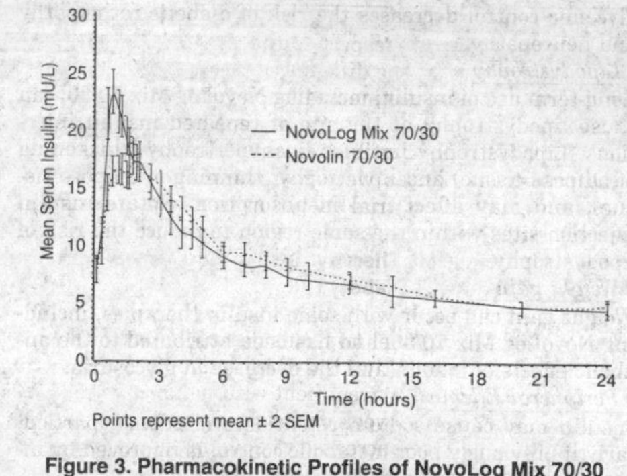

Figure 3. Pharmacokinetic Profiles of NovoLog Mix 70/30 and Novolin 70/30

NovoLog Mix 70/30. In 52-week studies, Sprague-Dawley rats were dosed subcutaneously with NovoLog, the rapid-acting component of NovoLog Mix 70/30, at 10, 50, and 200 U/kg/day (approximately 2, 8, and 32 times the human subcutaneous dose of 1.0 U/kg/day, based on U/body surface area, respectively). At a dose of 200 U/kg/day, NovoLog increased the incidence of mammary gland tumors in females when compared to untreated controls. The incidence of mammary tumors found with NovoLog was not significantly different from that found with regular human insulin. The relevance of these findings to humans is not known.

NovoLog was not genotoxic in the following tests: Ames test, mouse lymphoma cell forward gene mutation test, human peripheral blood lymphocyte chromosome aberration test, *in vivo* micronucleus test in mice, and in *ex vivo* UDS test in rat liver hepatocytes.

In fertility studies in male and female rats, NovoLog at subcutaneous doses up to 200 U/kg/day (approximately 32 times the human subcutaneous dose, based on U/body surface area) had no direct adverse effects on male and female fertility, or on general reproductive performance of animals.

13.2 Animal Toxicology and/or Pharmacology

In standard biological assays in mice and rabbits, one unit of NovoLog has the same glucose-lowering effect as one unit of regular human insulin. However, the effect of NovoLog

Mix 70/30 is more rapid in onset compared to Novolin (human insulin) 70/30 due to its faster absorption after subcutaneous injection.

14 CLINICAL STUDIES

14.1 NovoLog Mix 70/30 versus Novolin 70/30

In a three-month, open-label trial, patients with Type 1 (n=104) or Type 2 (n=187) diabetes were treated twice daily (before breakfast and before supper) with NovoLog Mix 70/30 or Novolin 70/30. Patients had received insulin for at least 24 months before the study. Oral hypoglycemic agents were not allowed within 1 month prior to the study or during the study. The small changes in HbA_{1c} were comparable across the treatment groups (see Table 3).

Table 3: Glycemic Parameters at the End of Treatment [Mean ± SD (N subjects)]

	NovoLog Mix 70/30	Novolin 70/30
Type 1, N=104		
Fasting Blood Glucose (mg/dL)	174 ± 64 (48)	142 ± 59 (44)
1.5 Hour Post Breakfast (mg/dL)	187 ± 82 (48)	200 ± 82 (42)
1.5 Hour Post Dinner (mg/dL)	162 ± 77 (47)	171 ± 66 (41)
HbA_{1c} (%) Baseline	8.4 ± 1.2 (51)	8.5 ± 1.1 (46)
HbA_{1c} (%) Week 12	8.4 ± 1.1 (51)	8.3 ± 1.0 (47)
Type 2, N=187		
Fasting Blood Glucose (mg/dL)	153 ± 40 (76)	152 ± 69 (93)
1.5 Hour Post Breakfast (mg/dL)	182 ± 65 (75)	200 ± 80 (92)
1.5 Hour Post Dinner (mg/dL)	168 ± 51 (75)	191 ± 65 (93)
HbA_{1c} (%) Baseline	8.1 ± 1.2 (82)	8.2 ± 1.3 (98)
HbA_{1c} (%) Week 12	7.9 ± 1.0 (81)	8.1 ± 1.1 (96)

The significance, with respect to the long-term clinical sequelae of diabetes, of the differences in postprandial hyperglycemia between treatment groups has not been established.

Specific anti-insulin antibodies as well as cross-reacting anti-insulin antibodies were monitored in the 3-month, open-label comparator trial as well as in a long-term extension trial.

14.2 Combination Therapy: Insulin and Oral Agents in Patients with Type 2 Diabetes

Trial 1:

In a 34-week, open-label trial, insulin-naïve patients with type 2 diabetes currently treated with 2 oral antidiabetic agents were switched to treatment with metformin and pioglitazone. During an 8-week optimization period metformin and pioglitazone were increased to 2500 mg per day and 30 or 45 mg per day, respectively. After the optimization period, subjects were randomized to receive either NovoLog Mix 70/30 twice daily added on to the metformin and pioglitazone regimen or continue the current optimized metformin and pioglitazone therapy. NovoLog Mix 70/30 was started at a dose of 6 IU twice daily (before breakfast and before supper). Insulin doses were titrated to a pre-meal glucose goal of 80-110 mg/dL. The total daily insulin dose at the end of the study was 56.9 ± 30.5 IU.

[See table 4 at top of previous page]

Trial 2:

In a 28-week, open-label trial, insulin-naïve patients with type 2 diabetes with fasting plasma glucose above 140 mg/dL currently treated with metformin ± thiazolidinedione therapy were randomized to receive either NovoLog Mix 70/30 twice daily [before breakfast and before supper] or insulin glargine once daily[1] (see Table 5). NovoLog Mix 70/30 was started at an average dose of 5-6 IU (0.07 ± 0.03 IU/kg) twice daily (before breakfast and before supper), and bedtime insulin glargine was started at 10-12 IU (0.13 ± 0.03 IU/kg). Insulin doses were titrated weekly by decrements or increments of -2 to +6 units per injection to a pre-meal glucose goal of 80-110 mg/dL. The metformin dose was adjusted to 2550 mg/day. Approximately one-third of the patients in each group were also treated with pioglitazone (30 mg/day). Insulin secretagogues were discontinued in order to reduce the risk of hypoglycemia. Most patients were Caucasian (53%), and the mean initial weight was 90 kg.

	Not in-use (unopened) Room Temperature (below 30°C [86°F])	Not in-use (unopened) Refrigerated (2°C - 8°C [36°F- 46°F])	In-use (opened) Room Temperature (below 30°C [86°F])
10 mL vial	28 days	Until expiration date	28 days (refrigerated/room temperature)
3 mL NovoLog Mix 70/30 FlexPen	14 days	Until expiration date	14 days (Do not refrigerate)

Table 5: Combination Therapy with Oral Agents and Two Types of Insulin in Patients with Type 2 Diabetes Mellitus [Mean (SD)]

Treatment duration 28-weeks	NovoLog Mix 70/30 + Metformin ± Pioglitazone	Insulin Glargine + Metformin ± Pioglitazone
Number of patients	117	116
HbA_{1c}		
Baseline mean (%)	9.7 ± 1.5 (117)	9.8 ± 1.4 (114)
End-of-study mean (± SD)	6.9 ± 1.2 (108)	7.4 ± 1.2 (114)
Mean change from baseline	-2.7 ± 1.6 (108)	-2.4 ± 1.5 (114)
Percentage of subjects reaching HbA_{1c} <7.0%	66%	40%
Total Daily Insulin Dose at end of study (U)	78 ± 40 (117)	51 ± 27 (116)
% of patients with severe hypoglycemia	0	0
% of minor hypoglycemia	43	16
Weight gain at end of study	5.4 ± 4.8 (117)	3.5 ± 4.5 (116)

15 REFERENCES

1. Raskin R, Allen E, Hollander P, et al. Initiating insulin therapy in type 2 diabetes: a comparison of biphasic and basal insulin analogs. *Diabetes Care*. 2005; 28:260-265.

16 HOW SUPPLIED/STORAGE AND HANDLING

16.1 How Supplied

NovoLog Mix 70/30 is available in the following package sizes: each presentation contains 100 Units of insulin aspart per mL (U-100).

10 mL vials	NDC 0169-3685-12
3 mL NovoLog Mix 70/30 FlexPen	NDC 0169-3696-19

NovoLog Mix 70/30 vials and NovoLog Mix 70/30 FlexPen are latex free.

16.2 Recommended Storage

Unused NovoLog Mix 70/30 should be stored in a refrigerator between 2°C and 8°C (36°F to 46°F). Do not store in the freezer or directly adjacent to the refrigerator cooling element. **Do not freeze NovoLog Mix 70/30 or use NovoLog Mix 70/30 if it has been frozen.**

Vials: After initial use, a vial may be kept at temperatures below 30°C (86°F) for up to 28 days, but should not be exposed to excessive heat or sunlight. Open vials may be refrigerated.

Unpunctured vials can be used until the expiration date printed on the label if they are stored in a refrigerator. Keep unused vials in the carton so they will stay clean and protected from light.

NovoLog Mix 70/30 FlexPen: Once a NovoLog Mix 70/30 FlexPen is punctured, it should be kept at temperatures below 30°C (86°F) for up to 14 days, but should not be exposed to excessive heat or sunlight. A NovoLog Mix 70/30 FlexPen in use must NOT be stored in the refrigerator. Keep the disposable NovoLog Mix 70/30 FlexPen away from direct heat and sunlight. An unpunctured NovoLog Mix 70/30 FlexPen can be used until the expiration date printed on the label if they are stored in a refrigerator. Keep any unused NovoLog Mix 70/30 FlexPen in the carton so it will stay clean and protected from light.

These storage conditions are summarized in the following table:

[See table above]

17 PATIENT COUNSELING INFORMATION

[see FDA-Approved Patient Labeling]

17.1 Physician Instructions

Maintenance of normal or near-normal glucose control is a treatment goal in diabetes mellitus and has been associated with a reduction in diabetic complications. Patients should be informed about potential risks and advantages of NovoLog Mix 70/30 therapy including the possible adverse reactions. Patients should also be offered continued education and advice on insulin therapies, injection technique, life-style management, regular glucose monitoring, periodic glycosylated hemoglobin testing, recognition and management of hypo- and hyperglycemia, adherence to meal planning, complications of insulin therapy, timing of dose, instruction for use of injection devices, and proper storage of insulin. See Patient Information supplied with the product.

Patients should be informed that frequent, patient-performed blood glucose measurements are needed to achieve optimal glycemic control and avoid both hyper- and hypoglycemia, and diabetic ketoacidosis.

The patient's ability to concentrate and react may be impaired as a result of hypoglycemia. This may present a risk in situations where these abilities are especially important, such as driving or operating other machinery. Patients who have frequent hypoglycemia or reduced or absent warning signs of hypoglycemia should be advised to use caution when driving or operating machinery.

Accidental substitutions between NovoLog Mix 70/30 and other insulin products have been reported. Patients should be instructed to always carefully check that they are administering the appropriate insulin to avoid medication errors between NovoLog Mix 70/30 and any other insulin. **The prescription for NovoLog Mix 70/30 should be written clearly in order to avoid confusion with other insulin products, for example, NovoLog or Novolin 70/30.** In addition, the written prescription should clearly indicate the presentation, for example FlexPen or vial.

Rx only

Date of Issue: March 9, 2013
Version: 11

Manufactured by:
Novo Nordisk A/S
DK-2880 Bagsvaerd, Denmark

For information about NovoLog Mix 70/30 contact:
Novo Nordisk Inc.
800 Scudders Mill Road
Plainsboro, New Jersey 08536
1-800-727-6500
www.novonordisk-us.com

PATIENT INFORMATION

NovoLog® Mix 70/30

(NŌ-vō-log-MIX-SEV-en-tee-THIR-tee)

(70% insulin aspart protamine suspension and 30% insulin aspart injection, [rDNA origin])

Read the Patient Information leaflet that comes with NovoLog® Mix 70/30 before you start taking it and each time you get a refill. There may be new information. This leaflet does not take the place of talking with your healthcare provider about your diabetes or your treatment. Make sure you know how to manage your diabetes. Ask your healthcare provider if you have any questions about managing your diabetes.

What is NovoLog® Mix 70/30?

NovoLog® Mix 70/30 is a man-made insulin that is used to control high blood sugar in adults with diabetes mellitus.

It is not known if NovoLog® Mix 70/30 is safe or effective in children.

Who should not use NovoLog® Mix 70/30?

Do not take NovoLog® Mix 70/30 if:

- Your blood sugar is too low (hypoglycemia)
- You are allergic to any of the ingredients in NovoLog® Mix 70/30. See the end of this leaflet for a complete list of ingredients in NovoLog® Mix 70/30. Check with your healthcare provider if you are not sure.

What should I tell my healthcare provider before taking NovoLog® Mix 70/30?

Before you use NovoLog® Mix 70/30, tell your healthcare provider if you:

- have kidney or liver problems
- take any other medicines, especially ones commonly called TZDs (thiazolidinediones).
- **have heart failure or other heart problems.** If you have heart failure, it may get worse while you take TZDs with NovoLog® Mix 70/30.
- **have any other medical conditions.** Medical conditions can affect your insulin needs and your dose of NovoLog® Mix 70/30.
- **are pregnant or plan to become pregnant.** It is not known if NovoLog® Mix 70/30 will harm your unborn baby. Talk to your healthcare provider if you are pregnant or plan to become pregnant. You and your healthcare provider should decide about the best way to manage your diabetes while you are pregnant.
- **are breastfeeding or plan to breastfeed.** It is not known if NovoLog® Mix 70/30 passes into your breast milk. You and your healthcare provider should decide if you will take NovoLog® Mix 70/30 while you breastfeed.

Tell your healthcare provider about all medicines you take, including prescriptions and non-prescription medicines, vitamins and herbal supplements.

NovoLog® Mix 70/30 may affect the way other medicines work, and other medicines may affect how NovoLog® Mix 70/30 works. Your NovoLog® Mix 70/30 dose may change if you take other medicines.

Know the medicines you take. Keep a list of your medicines with you to show your healthcare providers and pharmacist when you get a new medicine.

How should I take NovoLog® Mix 70/30?

- Take NovoLog® Mix 70/30 exactly as your healthcare provider tells you to take it.
- Your healthcare provider will tell you how much NovoLog® Mix 70/30 to take and when to take it.
- Do not make any changes to your dose or type of insulin unless your healthcare provider tells you to.
- **NovoLog® Mix 70/30 starts acting fast. If you have Type 1 diabetes, inject it up to 15 minutes before you eat a meal.** Do not inject NovoLog® Mix 70/30 if you are not planning to eat within 15 minutes.
- **If you have Type 2 diabetes, you may inject NovoLog® Mix 70/30 up to 15 minutes before or after starting your meal.**
- **Do Not mix** NovoLog® Mix 70/30 with other insulin products.
- **Do Not** use NovoLog® Mix 70/30 in an insulin pump.
- **Inject NovoLog® Mix 70/30 under the skin (subcutaneously) of your stomach area, upper arms, buttocks or upper legs.** NovoLog® Mix 70/30 may affect your blood sugar levels faster if you inject it under the skin of your stomach area. Never inject NovoLog® Mix 70/30 into a vein or into a muscle.
- **Change (rotate) injection sites** within the area you choose with each dose. **Do not** inject into the exact same spot for each injection.
- **Read the instructions for use that come with your NovoLog® Mix 70/30.** Talk to your healthcare provider if you have any questions. Your healthcare provider should show you how to inject NovoLog® Mix 70/30 before you start using it.
- NovoLog® Mix 70/30 comes in:
  - 10 mL vials for use with a syringe
  - 3 mL NovoLog® Mix 70/30 FlexPen®
- **If you take too much NovoLog® Mix 70/30, your blood sugar may fall too low (hypoglycemia).** You can treat mild low blood sugar (hypoglycemia) by drinking or eating something sugary right away (fruit juice, sugar candies, or glucose tablets). It is important to treat low blood sugar (hypoglycemia) right away because it could get worse and you could pass out (loss of consciousness).
- **If you forget to take your dose of NovoLog® Mix 70/30, your blood sugar may go too high (hyperglycemia).** If high blood sugar (hyperglycemia) is not treated it can lead to serious problems, like passing out (loss of consciousness), coma or even death. Follow your healthcare provider's instructions for treating high blood sugar. Know your symptoms of high blood sugar which may include:

• increased thirst	• a hard time breathing
• frequent urination	• fruity smell on the breath
• drowsiness	• high amounts of sugar and ketones in your urine
• loss of appetite	• nausea, vomiting (throwing up) or stomach pain

- Do not share needles, insulin pens or syringes with others.
- **Check your blood sugar levels.** Ask your healthcare provider what your blood sugars should be and when you should check your blood sugar levels.

Your insulin dosage may need to change because of:

• illness	• change in diet
• stress	• change in physical activity or exercise
• other medicines you take	

See the end of this patient information for instructions about preparing and giving your injection.

What should I consider while using NovoLog® Mix 70/30?

- **Alcohol.** Drinking alcohol may affect your blood sugar when you take NovoLog® Mix 70/30.
- **Driving and operating machinery.** You may have trouble paying attention or reacting if you have low blood sugar (hypoglycemia). Be careful when you drive a car or operate machinery. Ask your healthcare provider if it is alright for you to drive if you often have:
  - low blood sugar
  - decreased or no warning signs of low blood sugar

What are the possible side effects of NovoLog® Mix 70/30?

NovoLog® Mix 70/30 may cause serious side effects, including:

- **low blood sugar (hypoglycemia).** Symptoms of low blood sugar may include:

• sweating	• trouble concentrating or confusion
• dizziness or lightheadedness	• blurred vision
• shakiness	• slurred speech
• hunger	• anxiety, irritability or mood changes
• fast heart beat	
• tingling of lips and tongue	• headache

Very low blood sugar can cause you to pass out (loss of consciousness), seizures, and death. Talk to your healthcare provider about how to tell if you have low blood sugar and what to do if this happens while taking NovoLog® Mix 70/30. Know your symptoms of low blood sugar. Follow your healthcare provider's instructions for treating low blood sugar.

Talk to your healthcare provider if low blood sugar is a problem for you. Your dose of NovoLog® Mix 70/30 may need to be changed.

- **Low potassium in your blood (hypokalemia)**
- **Reactions at the injection site (local allergic reaction).** You may get redness, swelling, and itching at the injection site. If you keep having skin reactions or they are serious talk to your healthcare provider.
- **Serious allergic reaction (whole body reaction). Get medical help right away, if you have any of these symptoms of an allergic reaction:**
  - a rash over your whole body
  - have trouble breathing
  - a fast heartbeat
  - sweating
  - feel faint
- **Swelling of your hands and feet**
- **Heart Failure.** Taking certain diabetes pills called thiazolidinediones or "TZDs" with NovoLog® Mix 70/30 may cause heart failure in some people. This can happen even if you have never had heart failure or heart problems before. If you already have heart failure it may get worse while you take TZDs with NovoLog® Mix 70/30. Your healthcare provider should monitor you closely while you are taking TZDs with NovoLog® Mix 70/30. Tell your healthcare provider if you have any new or worse symptoms of heart failure including:
  - shortness of breath
  - swelling of your ankles or feet
  - sudden weight gain

  Treatment with TZDs and NovoLog® Mix 70/30 may need to be adjusted or stopped by your healthcare provider if you have new or worse heart failure.

The most common side effects of NovoLog® Mix 70/30 include:

- **Skin thickening or pits at the injection site (lipodystrophy).** Change (rotate) where you inject your insulin to help to prevent these skin changes from happening. Do not inject insulin into this type of skin.
- **Weight gain**
- **Swelling of your hands and feet**
- **Vision changes**

These are not all of the possible side effects from NovoLog® Mix 70/30. Ask your healthcare provider or pharmacist for more information.

Call your doctor for medical advice about side effects. You may report side effects to FDA at 1-800-FDA-1088.

How should I store NovoLog® Mix 70/30?

All Unopened NovoLog® Mix 70/30:

- Keep all unopened NovoLog® Mix 70/30 in the refrigerator between 36°F to 46°F (2°C to 8°C).
- **Do not freeze or store next to the refrigerator cooling element.** Do not use NovoLog® Mix 70/30 if it has been frozen.
- Keep unopened NovoLog® Mix 70/30 in the carton to protect from light.
- Unopened vials can be used until the expiration date on the NovoLog® Mix 70/30 label, if the medicine has been stored in a refrigerator.
- Unused NovoLog® Mix 70/30 FlexPen® can be used until the expiration date on the NovoLog® Mix 70/30 FlexPen® label, if the medicine has been stored in a refrigerator.

After NovoLog® Mix 70/30 has been opened:

- **Vials**
  - Keep in the refrigerator or at room temperature below 86°F (30°C) for up to 28 days.
  - Keep vials away from direct heat or light.
  - Throw away an opened vial after 28 days of use, even if there is insulin left in the vial.
- **NovoLog® Mix 70/30 FlexPen®**
  - Keep at room temperature below 86°F (30°C) for up to 14 days.
  - **Do not** store a NovoLog® Mix 70/30 FlexPen® that you are using in the refrigerator.
  - Keep NovoLog® Mix 70/30 FlexPen® away from direct heat or light.
  - Throw away a used NovoLog® Mix 70/30 FlexPen® after 14 days, even if there is insulin left in the syringe.

Never use insulin after the expiration date that is printed on the label and carton.

Keep NovoLog® Mix 70/30 and all medicines out of the reach of children.

General advice about NovoLog® Mix 70/30

Medicines are sometimes prescribed for conditions that are not mentioned in the patient leaflet. Do not use NovoLog® Mix 70/30 for a condition for which it was not prescribed. Do not give NovoLog® Mix 70/30 to other people, even if they have the same symptoms you have. It may harm them.

This leaflet summarizes the most important information about NovoLog® Mix 70/30. If you would like more information about NovoLog® Mix 70/30 or diabetes, talk with your healthcare provider. You can ask your healthcare provider or pharmacist for information about NovoLog® Mix 70/30 that is written for healthcare professionals. For more information call 1-800-727-6500 or go to www.novonordisk-us.com.

What are the ingredients in NovoLog® Mix 70/30?

- **Active Ingredients in NovoLog® Mix 70/30:** 70% insulin aspart protamine suspension and 30% insulin aspart injection (rDNA origin).
- **Inactive Ingredients in NovoLog® Mix 70/30:** glycerol, phenol, metacresol, zinc, disodium hydrogen phosphate dihydrate, sodium chloride, protamine sulfate, water for injection, hydrochloric acid or sodium hydroxide.

All NovoLog® Mix 70/30 vials and NovoLog® Mix 70/30 FlexPen® are latex free.

Helpful information for people with diabetes is published by the American Diabetes Association, 1701 N Beauregard Street, Alexandria, VA 22311 and is available at www.diabetes.org.

Date of Issue: March 9, 2013

Version: 9

Novo Nordisk®, NovoLog®, and FlexPen® are registered trademarks of Novo Nordisk A/S.

NovoLog® Mix 70/30 is covered by US Patent Nos. 5,547,930, 5,618,913, 5,834,422, 5,840,680, 5,866,538 and other patents pending.

FlexPen® is covered by US Patent Nos. 6,582,404, 6,004,297, 6,235,004 and other patents pending.

Manufactured by:
Novo Nordisk A/S
DK-2880 Bagsvaerd, Denmark

For information about NovoLog® Mix 70/30 contact:
Novo Nordisk Inc.
800 Scudders Mill Road
Plainsboro, New Jersey 08536
1-800-727-6500
www.novonordisk-us.com

PATIENT INSTRUCTIONS FOR USE

NovoLog® Mix 70/30 (NŌvōLog-MIX-SEV-en-tee-THIR-tee)
(70% insulin aspart protamine suspension and 30% insulin aspart [rDNA origin] injection)
10 mL vial (100 Units/mL, U-100)

Read this Instructions for Use before you start taking NovoLog® Mix 70/30 and each time you get a refill. There may be new information. This information does not take the place of talking to your healthcare provider about your medical condition or your treatment.

Supplies you will need to give your NovoLog® Mix 70/30 injection:

- 10 mL NovoLog® Mix 70/30 vial
- insulin syringe and needle
- alcohol swab

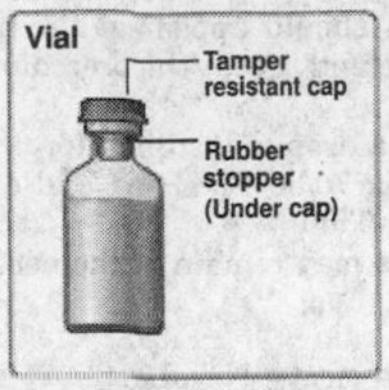

Preparing your NovoLog® Mix 70/30 dose:

- Wash your hands with soap and water.
- Before you start to prepare your injection, check the NovoLog® Mix 70/30 label to make sure that you are taking the right type of insulin. This is especially important if you use more than 1 type of insulin.
- NovoLog® Mix 70/30 should look white and cloudy after mixing. **Do not** use NovoLog Mix 70/30 if it looks clear or contains any lumps or particles.
- NovoLog® Mix 70/30 is easier to mix when it is at room temperature.
- After mixing NovoLog® Mix 70/30, inject your dose right away. If you wait to inject your dose, the insulin will need to be mixed again.
- **Do not** use NovoLog® Mix 70/30 past the expiration date printed on the label.

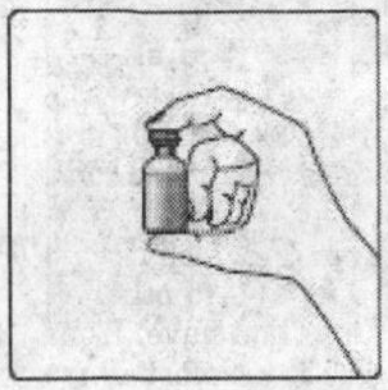

Step 1: If you are using a new vial, pull off the tamper-resistant cap (See Figure A).

Step 2: Wipe the rubber stopper with an alcohol swab (See Figure B).

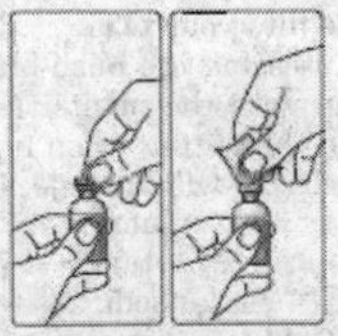

(Figure A Figure B)

Step 3: Roll the NovoLog Mix 70/30 vial between your hands 10 times. Keep the vial in a horizontal (flat) position (See Figure C). Roll the vial between your hands until the NovoLog® Mix 70/30 looks white and cloudy. Do not shake the vial.

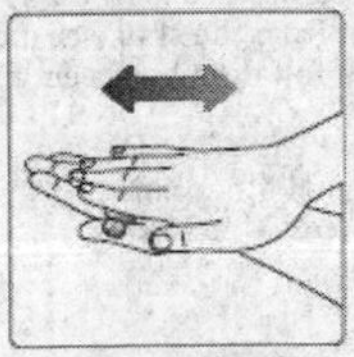

(Figure C)

Step 4: Hold the syringe with the needle pointing up. Pull down on the plunger until the black tip reaches the line for the number of units for your prescribed dose (See Figure D).

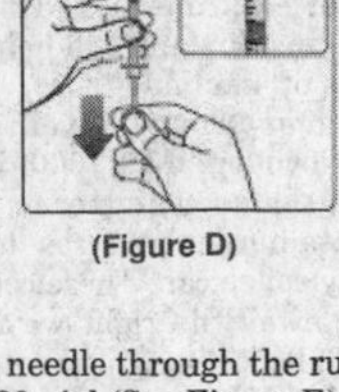

(Figure D)

Step 5: Push the needle through the rubber stopper of the NovoLog® Mix 70/30 vial (See Figure E).

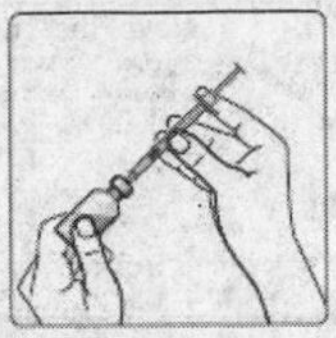

(Figure E)

Step 6: Push the plunger all the way in. This puts air into the NovoLog® Mix 70/30 vial (See Figure F).

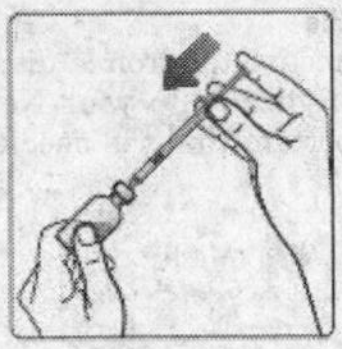

(Figure F)

Step 7: Turn the NovoLog® Mix 70/30 vial and syringe upside down and slowly pull the plunger down until the black tip is a few units past the line for your dose (See Figure G).

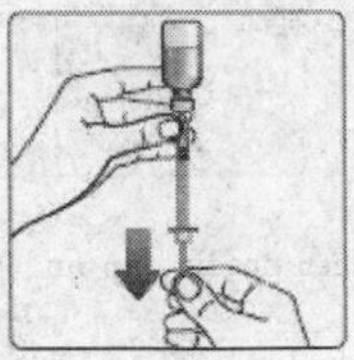

(Figure G)

- If there are air bubbles, tap the syringe gently a few times to let any air bubbles rise to the top (See Figure H).

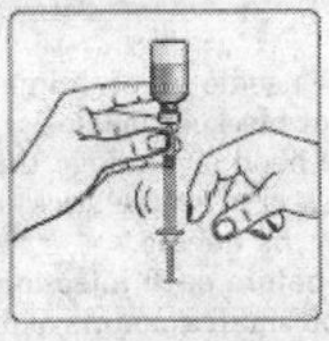

(Figure H)

Step 8: Slowly push the plunger up until the black tip reaches the line for your NovoLog® Mix 70/30 dose (See Figure I).

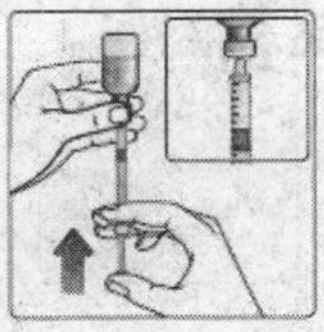

(Figure I)

Step 9: Check the syringe to make sure you have the right dose of NovoLog® Mix 70/30.

Step 10: Pull the syringe out of the vial's rubber stopper (See Figure J).

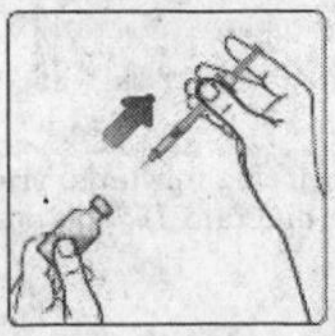

(Figure J)

Giving your injection:

- Inject your NovoLog® Mix 70/30 exactly as your healthcare provider has shown you. Your healthcare provider should tell you if you need to pinch the skin before injecting.
- NovoLog® Mix 70/30 is injected under the skin (subcutaneously) of your stomach area, buttocks, upper legs, or upper arms.
- Change (rotate) your injection sites within the area you choose for each dose. **Do not** use the same injection site for each injection.

Step 11: Choose your injection site and wipe the skin with an alcohol swab. Let the injection site dry before you inject your dose (See Figure K).

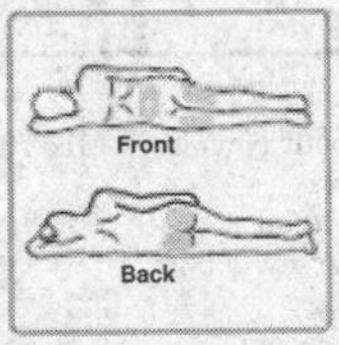

(Figure K)

Step 12: Insert the needle into your skin. Push down on the plunger to inject your dose (See Figure L). Needle should remain in the skin for at least 6 seconds to make sure you have injected all the insulin.

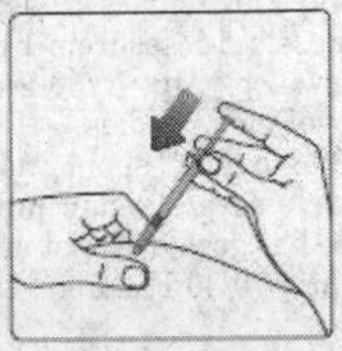

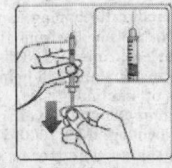

(Figure L)

Step 13: Pull the needle out of your skin. After that, you may see a drop of NovoLog® Mix 70/30 at the needle tip. This is normal and does not affect the dose you just received (See Figure M).

- If you see blood after you take the needle out of your skin, press the injection site lightly with a piece of gauze or an alcohol swab. **Do not** rub the area.

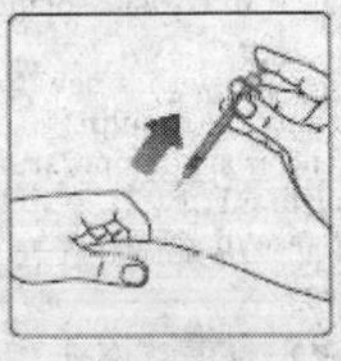

(Figure M)

After your injection:

- **Do not** recap the needle. Recapping the needle can lead to a needle stick injury.
- Throw away empty insulin vials,used syringes and needles in a sharps container or some type of hard plastic or metal container with a screw on cap such as a detergent bottle or coffee can. Check with your healthcare provider about the right way to throw away the container. There may be local or state laws about how to throw away used syringes and needles. **Do not** throw away used syringes and needles in household trash or recycling bins.

How should I store NovoLog®Mix 70/30?

- **Do not** freeze NovoLog® Mix 70/30. **Do not** use NovoLog® Mix 70/30 if it has been frozen.
- Keep NovoLog® Mix 70/30 away from heat or light.
- Store opened and unopened NovoLog® Mix 70/30 vials in the refrigerator at 36°F to 46°F (2°C to 8°C). Opened NovoLog® Mix 70/30 vials can also be stored out of the refrigerator below 86°F (30°C).
- Unopened vials may be used until the expiration date printed on the label, if they are kept in the refrigerator.
- Opened NovoLog® Mix 70/30 vials should be thrown away after 28 days, even if they still have insulin left in them.

General information about the safe and effective use of NovoLog® Mix 70/30

- Always use a new syringe and needle for each injection.
- Do not share syringes or needles.
- Keep NovoLog® Mix 70/30 vials, syringes, and needles out of the reach of children.

This Instructions for Use has been approved by the U.S. Food and Drug Administration.

Manufactured by:
Novo Nordisk A/S
DK-2880 Bagsvaerd, Denmark
Revised: March 2013

NovoLog® is a registered trademark of Novo Nordisk A/S.
NovoLog® Mix 70/30 is covered by US Patent Nos. 5,547,930, 5,618,913, 5,834,422, 5,840,680, 5,866,538 and other patents pending.

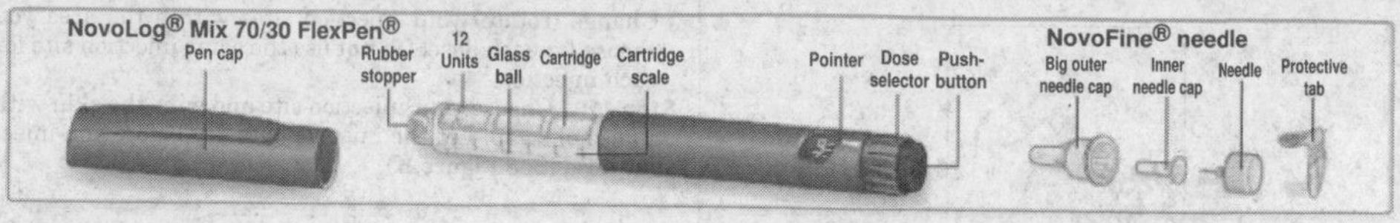

For information about NovoLog® Mix 70/30 contact:
Novo Nordisk Inc.
800 Scudders Mill Road
Plainsboro, New Jersey 08536
1-800-727-6500
www.novonordisk-us.com

PATIENT INSTRUCTIONS FOR USE

NovoLog® Mix 70/30 FlexPen®

Read the following instructions carefully before you start using your NovoLog® Mix 70/30 FlexPen® and each time you get a refill. There may be new information. You should read the instructions even if you have used NovoLog® Mix 70/30 FlexPen® before.

NovoLog® Mix 70/30 FlexPen® is a disposable dial-a-dose insulin pen. You can select doses from 1 to 60 units in increments of 1 unit. NovoLog® Mix 70/30 FlexPen® is designed to be used with NovoFine® needles.

NovoLog Mix® 70/30 FlexPen® should not be used by people who are blind or have severe visual problems without the help of a person who has good eyesight and who is trained to use the NovoLog® Mix 70/30 FlexPen® the right way.

Getting ready

Make sure you have the following items:
- NovoLog® Mix 70/30 FlexPen®
- New NovoFine® needle
- Alcohol swab

[See figure above]

PREPARING YOUR NOVOLOG® MIX 70/30 FLEXPEN®
- Wash your hands with soap and water.
- Before you start to prepare your injection, check the label to make sure that you are taking the right type of insulin. This is especially important if you take more than 1 type of insulin. NovoLog® Mix 70/30 should look cloudy after mixing.

Before your first injection with a new NovoLog® Mix 70/30 FlexPen® you must mix the insulin:

A. Let the insulin reach room temperature before you use it. This makes it easier to mix.

Pull off the pen cap (see diagram A).

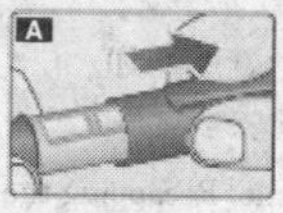

B. Roll the pen between your palms 10 times - it is important that the pen is kept horizontal (see diagram B).

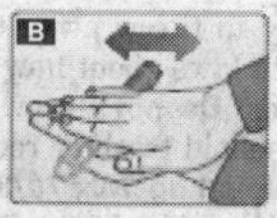

C. Then gently move the pen up and down ten times between position **1** and **2** as shown, so the glass ball moves from one end of the cartridge to the other (see diagram C).

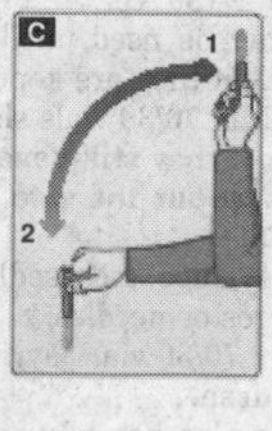

Repeat rolling and moving the pen until the liquid appears white and cloudy.

For every following injection move the pen up and down between positions 1 and 2 at least ten times until the liquid appears white and cloudy.

After mixing, complete all the following steps of the injection right away. If there is a delay, the insulin will need to be mixed again.

Wipe the rubber stopper with an alcohol swab.

Δ Before you inject, there must be at least 12 units of insulin left in the cartridge to make sure the remaining insulin is evenly mixed. If there are less than 12 units left, use a new NovoLog® Mix 70/30 FlexPen®.

Attaching the needle

D. Remove the protective tab from a disposable needle. Screw the needle tightly onto your NovoLog® Mix 70/30 FlexPen®. It is important that the needle is put on straight (see diagram D).

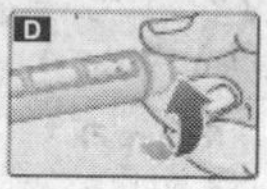

Never place a disposable needle on your NovoLog® Mix 70/30 FlexPen® until you are ready to take your injection.

E. Pull off the big outer needle cap (see diagram E).

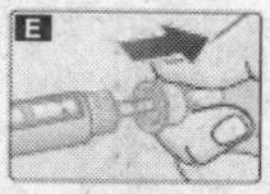

F. Pull off the inner needle cap and dispose of it (see diagram F).

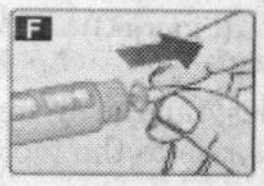

Δ Always use a new needle for each injection to help ensure sterility and prevent blocked needles.

Δ Be careful not to bend or damage the needle before use.

Δ To reduce the risk of a needle stick, **never put the inner needle cap back on the needle.**

Giving the airshot before each injection

Before each injection small amounts of air may collect in the cartridge during normal use. **To avoid injecting air and to make sure you take the right dose of insulin:**

G. Turn the dose selector to select 2 units (see diagram G).

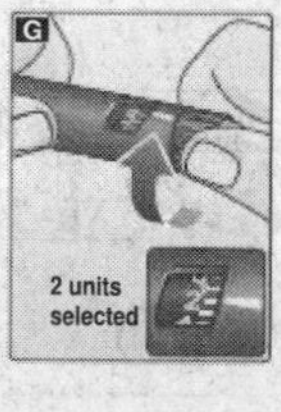

H. Hold your NovoLog® Mix 70/30 FlexPen® with the needle pointing up. Tap the cartridge gently with your finger a few times to make any air bubbles collect at the top of the cartridge (see diagram H).

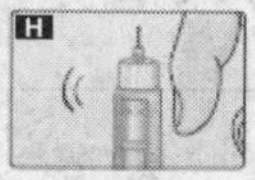

I. Keep the needle pointing upwards, press the push-button all the way in (see diagram I). The dose selector returns to 0.

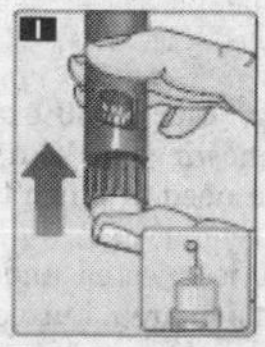

A drop of insulin should appear at the needle tip. If not, change the needle and repeat the procedure no more than 6 times.

If you do not see a drop of insulin after 6 times, do not use the NovoLog® Mix 70/30 FlexPen® and contact Novo Nordisk at 1-800-727-6500.

A small air bubble may remain at the needle tip, but it will not be injected.

SELECTING YOUR DOSE

Check and make sure that the dose selector is set at 0.

J. Turn the dose selector to the number of units you need to inject. The pointer should line up with your dose.

The dose can be corrected either up or down by turning the dose selector in either direction until the correct dose lines up with the pointer (see diagram J). When turning the dose selector, be careful not to press the push-button as insulin will come out.

You cannot select a dose larger than the number of units left in the cartridge.

You will hear a click for every single unit dialed. Do not set the dose by counting the number of clicks you hear.

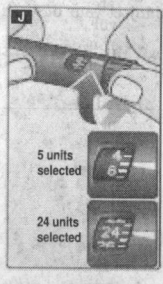

Δ Do not use the cartridge scale printed on the cartridge to measure your dose of insulin.

GIVING THE INJECTION

Do the injection exactly as shown to you by your healthcare provider. Your healthcare provider should tell you if you need to pinch the skin before injecting. Wipe the skin with an alcohol swab and let the area dry.

K. Insert the needle into your skin.

Inject the dose by pressing the push-button all the way in until the 0 lines up with the pointer (see diagram K). Be careful only to push the button when injecting.

Turning the dose selector will not inject insulin.

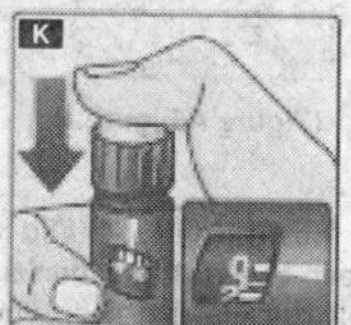

L. Keep the needle in the skin for at least 6 seconds, and keep the push-button pressed all the way in until the needle has been pulled out from the skin (see diagram L). This will make sure that the full dose has been given.

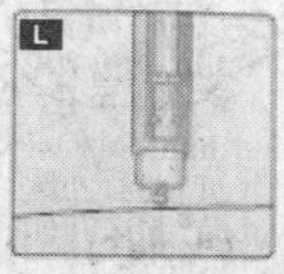

You may see a drop of NovoLog® Mix 70/30 at the needle tip. This is normal and has no effect on the dose you just received. If blood appears after you take the needle out of your skin, press the injection site lightly with an alcohol swab. **Do not rub the area.**

After the injection

Do not recap the needle. Recapping can lead to a needle stick injury. Remove the needle from the NovoLog® Mix 70/30 FlexPen® after each injection. This helps to prevent infection, leakage of insulin, and will help to make sure you inject the right dose of insulin.

Δ Put the needle and any empty NovoLog® Mix 70/30 FlexPen® or any used NovoLog® Mix 70/30 FlexPen® still containing insulin in a sharps container or some type of hard plastic or metal container with a screw top such as a detergent bottle or empty coffee can. These containers should be sealed and thrown away the right way. Check with your healthcare provider about the right way to throw away used syringes and needles. There may be local or state laws about how to throw away used needles and syringes. Do not throw away used needles and syringes in household trash or recycling bins.

The NovoLog® Mix 70/30 FlexPen® prevents the cartridge from being completely emptied. It is designed to deliver 300 units.

M. Put the pen cap on the NovoLog® Mix 70/30 FlexPen® and store the NovoLog® Mix 70/30 FlexPen® without the needle attached (see diagram M).

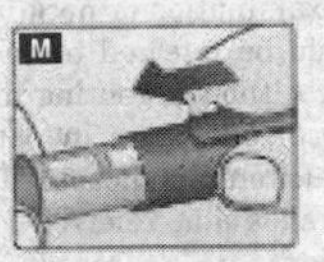

FUNCTION CHECK

N. If your NovoLog® Mix 70/30 FlexPen® is not working the right way, follow the steps below:

- Screw on a new NovoFine® needle.
- Remove the big outer needle cap and the inner needle cap.
- Do an airshot as described in "Giving the airshot before each injection".
- Put the big outer needle cap onto the needle. Do not put on the inner needle cap.
- Turn the dose selector so the dose indicator window shows 20 units.
- Hold the NovoLog® Mix 70/30 FlexPen® so the needle is pointing down.
- Press the push-button all the way in.

The insulin should fill the lower part of the big outer needle cap (see diagram N). If NovoLog® Mix 70/30 FlexPen® has released too much or too little insulin, do the function check again. If the same problem happens again, do not use your NovoLog® Mix 70/30 FlexPen® and contact Novo Nordisk at 1-800-727-6500.

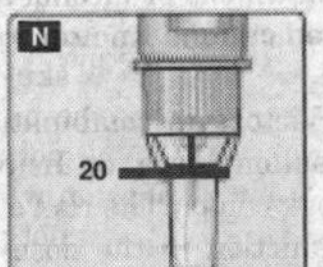

Maintenance

Your NovoLog® Mix 70/30 FlexPen® is designed to work accurately and safely. It must be handled with care. Avoid dropping your NovoLog® Mix 70/30 FlexPen® as it may damage it. If you are concerned that your NovoLog® Mix 70/30 FlexPen® is damaged, use a new one. You can clean the outside of your NovoLog® Mix 70/30 FlexPen® by wiping it with a damp cloth. Do not soak or wash your NovoLog® Mix 70/30 FlexPen® as it may damage it. Do not refill your NovoLog® Mix 70/30 FlexPen®.

Δ Remove the needle from the NovoLog® Mix 70/30 FlexPen® after each injection. This helps to ensure sterility, prevent leakage of insulin, and will help to make sure you inject the right dose of insulin for future injections.

Δ Be careful when handling used needles to avoid needle sticks and transfer of infectious diseases.

Δ Keep your NovoLog® Mix 70/30 FlexPen® and needles out of the reach of children.

Δ Use NovoLog® Mix 70/30 FlexPen® as directed to treat your diabetes. Needles and NovoLog® Mix 70/30 FlexPen® must not be shared.

Δ Always use a new needle for each injection.

Δ Novo Nordisk is not responsible for harm due to using this insulin pen with products not recommended by Novo Nordisk.

Δ As a precautionary measure, always carry a spare insulin delivery device in case your NovoLog® Mix 70/30 FlexPen® is lost or damaged.

Δ Remember to keep the disposable NovoLog® Mix 70/30 FlexPen® with you. Do not leave it in a car or other location where it can get too hot or too cold.

Date of Issue: March 2013

Version: 9

Novo Nordisk®, NovoLog®, FlexPen®, and NovoFine® are registered trademarks of Novo Nordisk A/S.

NovoLog® Mix 70/30 is covered by US Patent Nos. 5,547,930, 5,618,913, 5,834,422, 5,840,680, 5,866,538 and other patents pending.

FlexPen® is covered by US Patent Nos. 6,582,404, 6,004,297, 6,235,004 and other patents pending.

Manufactured by:
Novo Nordisk A/S
DK-2880 Bagsvaerd, Denmark

For information about NovoLog® Mix 70/30 contact:
Novo Nordisk Inc.
800 Scudders Mill Road
Plainsboro, New Jersey 08536
1-800-727-6500
www.novonordisk-us.com

VICTOZA® ℞

[VIC-tow-za]
(liraglutide (rDNA origin) injection)
solution for subcutaneous use

HIGHLIGHTS OF PRESCRIBING INFORMATION

These highlights do not include all the information needed to use Victoza safely and effectively. See full prescribing information for Victoza.

Victoza® (liraglutide [rDNA origin] injection), solution for subcutaneous use

Initial U.S. Approval: 2010

> **WARNING: RISK OF THYROID C-CELL TUMORS**
>
> ***See full prescribing information for complete boxed warning.***
>
> - **Liraglutide causes thyroid C-cell tumors at clinically relevant exposures in rodents. It is unknown whether Victoza causes thyroid C-cell tumors, including medullary thyroid carcinoma (MTC), in humans, as human relevance could not be determined by clinical or nonclinical studies (5.1).**
> - **Victoza is contraindicated in patients with a personal or family history of MTC or in patients with Multiple Endocrine Neoplasia syndrome type 2 (MEN 2) (5.1).**

RECENT MAJOR CHANGES

Indications and Usage: Important Limitations of Use (1.1) 04/2013

Warnings and Precautions: Pancreatitis (5.2) 04/2013

INDICATIONS AND USAGE

Victoza is a glucagon-like peptide-1 (GLP-1) receptor agonist indicated as an adjunct to diet and exercise to improve glycemic control in adults with type 2 diabetes mellitus (1).

Important Limitations of Use (1.1):

- Not recommended as first-line therapy for patients inadequately controlled on diet and exercise (5.1).
- Has not been studied in patients with a history of pancreatitis. Consider other antidiabetic therapies in patients with a history of pancreatitis (5.2).
- Not for treatment of type 1 diabetes mellitus or diabetic ketoacidosis.
- Has not been studied in combination with prandial insulin.

DOSAGE AND ADMINISTRATION

- Administer once daily at any time of day, independently of meals (2).
- Inject subcutaneously in the abdomen, thigh or upper arm (2).
- The injection site and timing can be changed without dose adjustment (2).
- Initiate at 0.6 mg per day for one week. This dose is intended to reduce gastrointestinal symptoms during initial titration, and is not effective for glycemic control. After one week, increase the dose to 1.2 mg. If the 1.2 mg dose does not result in acceptable glycemic control, the dose can be increased to 1.8 mg (2).

DOSAGE FORMS AND STRENGTHS

- Solution for subcutaneous injection, pre-filled, multi-dose pen that delivers doses of 0.6 mg, 1.2 mg, or 1.8 mg (6 mg/mL, 3 mL) (3).

CONTRAINDICATIONS

Do not use in patients with a personal or family history of medullary thyroid carcinoma or in patients with Multiple Endocrine Neoplasia syndrome type 2 (4).

Do not use if history of serious hypersensitivity to Victoza or any product components (4).

WARNINGS AND PRECAUTIONS

- Thyroid C-cell tumors in animals: Counsel patients regarding the risk of medullary thyroid carcinoma and the symptoms of thyroid tumors (5.1).
- Pancreatitis: Postmarketing reports, including fatal and non-fatal hemorrhagic or necrotizing pancreatitis. Discontinue promptly if pancreatitis is suspected. Do not restart if pancreatitis is confirmed. Consider other antidiabetic therapies in patients with a history of pancreatitis (5.2).
- Serious hypoglycemia: Can occur when Victoza is used with an insulin secretagogue (e.g. a sulfonylurea) or insulin. Consider lowering the dose of the insulin secretagogue or insulin to reduce the risk of hypoglycemia (5.3).
- Renal Impairment: Has been reported postmarketing, usually in association with nausea, vomiting, diarrhea, or dehydration which may sometimes require hemodialysis. Use caution when initiating or escalating doses of Victoza in patients with renal impairment (5.4).
- Hypersensitivity: Postmarketing reports of serious hypersensitivity reactions (e.g., anaphylactic reactions and angioedema). The patient should discontinue Victoza and other suspect medications and promptly seek medical advice (5.5).
- Macrovascular outcomes: There have been no studies establishing conclusive evidence of macrovascular risk reduction with Victoza or any other antidiabetic drug (5.6).

ADVERSE REACTIONS

- The most common adverse reactions, reported in ≥5% of patients treated with Victoza and more commonly than in patients treated with placebo, are: headache, nausea, diarrhea and anti-liraglutide antibody formation (6).
- Immunogenicity-related events, including urticaria, were more common among Victoza-treated patients (0.8%) than among comparator-treated patients (0.4%) in clinical trials (6).

To report SUSPECTED ADVERSE REACTIONS, contact Novo Nordisk Inc. at 1-877-484-2869 or FDA at 1-800-FDA-1088 or www.fda.gov/medwatch.

DRUG INTERACTIONS

- Victoza delays gastric emptying. May impact absorption of concomitantly administered oral medications. Use caution (7).

USE IN SPECIFIC POPULATIONS

- Limited data in patients with renal or hepatic impairment. (8.6, 8.7).

See 17 for PATIENT COUNSELING INFORMATION and FDA-Approved Medication Guide

Revised: 4/2013

FULL PRESCRIBING INFORMATION: CONTENTS*

* Sections or subsections omitted from the full prescribing information are not listed

FULL PRESCRIBING INFORMATION

WARNING: RISK OF THYROID C-CELL TUMORS

Liraglutide causes dose-dependent and treatment-duration-dependent thyroid C-cell tumors at clinically relevant exposures in both genders of rats and mice. It is unknown whether Victoza causes thyroid C-cell tumors, including medullary thyroid carcinoma (MTC), in humans, as human relevance could not be ruled out by clinical or nonclinical studies. Victoza is contraindicated in patients with a personal or family history of MTC and in patients with Multiple Endocrine Neoplasia syndrome type 2 (MEN 2). Based on the findings in rodents, monitoring with serum calcitonin or thyroid ultrasound was performed during clinical trials, but this may have increased the number of unnecessary thyroid surgeries. It is unknown whether monitoring with serum calcitonin or thyroid ultrasound will mitigate human risk of thyroid C-cell tumors. Patients should be counseled regarding the risk and symptoms of thyroid tumors *[see Contraindications (4), Warnings and Precautions (5.1) and Nonclinical Toxicology (13.1)]*.

1 INDICATIONS AND USAGE

Victoza is indicated as an adjunct to diet and exercise to improve glycemic control in adults with type 2 diabetes mellitus.

1.1 Important Limitations of Use

Because of the uncertain relevance of the rodent thyroid C-cell tumor findings to humans, prescribe Victoza only to patients for whom the potential benefits are considered to outweigh the potential risk. Victoza is not recommended as first-line therapy for patients who have inadequate glycemic control on diet and exercise.

Based on spontaneous postmarketing reports, acute pancreatitis, including fatal and non-fatal hemorrhagic or necrotizing pancreatitis has been observed in patients treated with Victoza. Victoza has not been studied in patients with a history of pancreatitis. It is unknown whether patients with a history of pancreatitis are at increased risk for pancreatitis while using Victoza. Other antidiabetic therapies should be considered in patients with a history of pancreatitis.

Victoza is not a substitute for insulin. Victoza should not be used in patients with type 1 diabetes mellitus or for the treatment of diabetic ketoacidosis, as it would not be effective in these settings.

The concurrent use of Victoza and prandial insulin has not been studied.

2 DOSAGE AND ADMINISTRATION

Victoza can be administered once daily at any time of day, independently of meals, and can be injected subcutaneously in the abdomen, thigh or upper arm. The injection site and timing can be changed without dose adjustment.

For all patients, Victoza should be initiated with a dose of 0.6 mg per day for one week. The 0.6 mg dose is a starting dose intended to reduce gastrointestinal symptoms during initial titration, and is not effective for glycemic control. After one week at 0.6 mg per day, the dose should be increased to 1.2 mg. If the 1.2 mg dose does not result in acceptable glycemic control, the dose can be increased to 1.8 mg.

When initiating Victoza, consider reducing the dose of concomitantly administered insulin secretagogues (such as sulfonylureas) to reduce the risk of hypoglycemia *[see Warnings and Precautions (5.3) and Adverse Reactions (6)]*.

When using Victoza with insulin, administer as separate injections. Never mix. It is acceptable to inject Victoza and insulin in the same body region but the injections should not be adjacent to each other.

Victoza solution should be inspected prior to each injection, and the solution should be used only if it is clear, colorless, and contains no particles.

If a dose is missed, the once-daily regimen should be resumed as prescribed with the next scheduled dose. An extra dose or increase in dose should not be taken to make-up for the missed dose.

Based on the elimination half-life, patients should be advised to reinitiate Victoza at 0.6 mg if more than 3 days have elapsed since the last Victoza dose. This approach will mitigate any gastrointestinal symptoms associated with reinitiation of treatment. Upon reinitiation, Victoza should be titrated at the discretion of the prescribing healthcare provider.

3 DOSAGE FORMS AND STRENGTHS

Solution for subcutaneous injection, pre-filled, multi-dose pen that delivers doses of 0.6 mg, 1.2 mg, or 1.8 mg (6 mg/mL, 3 mL).

4 CONTRAINDICATIONS

Do not use in patients with a personal or family history of medullary thyroid carcinoma (MTC) or in patients with Multiple Endocrine Neoplasia syndrome type 2 (MEN 2).

Do not use in patients with a prior serious hypersensitivity reaction to Victoza or to any of the product components.

5 WARNINGS AND PRECAUTIONS

5.1 Risk of Thyroid C-cell Tumors

Liraglutide causes dose-dependent and treatment-duration-dependent thyroid C-cell tumors (adenomas and/or carcinomas) at clinically relevant exposures in both genders of rats and mice *[see Nonclinical Toxicology (13.1)]*. Malignant thyroid C-cell carcinomas were detected in rats and mice. A statistically significant increase in cancer was observed in rats receiving liraglutide at 8-times clinical exposure compared to controls. It is unknown whether Victoza will cause thyroid C-cell tumors, including medullary thyroid carcinoma (MTC), in humans, as the human relevance of liraglutide-induced rodent thyroid C-cell tumors could not be determined by clinical or nonclinical studies *[see Boxed Warning, Contraindications (4)]*.

In the clinical trials, there have been 6 reported cases of thyroid C-cell hyperplasia among Victoza-treated patients and 2 cases in comparator-treated patients (1.3 vs. 1.0 cases per 1000 patient-years). One comparator-treated patient with MTC had pre-treatment serum calcitonin concentrations >1000 ng/L suggesting pre-existing disease. All of these cases were diagnosed after thyroidectomy, which was prompted by abnormal results on routine, protocol-specified measurements of serum calcitonin. Five of the six Victoza-treated patients had elevated calcitonin concentrations at baseline and throughout the trial. One Victoza and one non-Victoza-treated patient developed elevated calcitonin concentrations while on treatment.

Calcitonin, a biological marker of MTC, was measured throughout the clinical development program. The serum calcitonin assay used in the Victoza clinical trials had a lower limit of quantification (LLOQ) of 0.7 ng/L and the upper limit of the reference range was 5.0 ng/L for women and 8.4 ng/L for men. At Weeks 26 and 52 in the clinical trials, adjusted mean serum calcitonin concentrations were higher in Victoza-treated patients compared to placebo-treated patients but not compared to patients receiving active comparator. At these timepoints, the adjusted mean serum calcitonin values (~ 1.0 ng/L) were just above the LLOQ with between-group differences in adjusted mean serum calcitonin values of approximately 0.1 ng/L or less. Among patients with pre-treatment serum calcitonin below the upper limit of the reference range, shifts to above the upper limit of the reference range which persisted in subsequent measurements occurred most frequently among patients treated with Victoza 1.8 mg/day. In trials with on-treatment serum calcitonin measurements out to 5-6 months, 1.9% of patients treated with Victoza 1.8 mg/day developed new and persistent calcitonin elevations above the upper limit of the reference range compared to 0.8-1.1% of patients treated with control medication or the 0.6 and 1.2 mg doses of Victoza. In trials with on-treatment serum calcitonin measurements out to 12 months, 1.3% of patients treated with Victoza 1.8 mg/day had new and persistent elevations of calcitonin from below or within the reference range to above the upper limit of the reference range, compared to 0.6%, 0% and 1.0% of patients treated with Victoza 1.2 mg, placebo and active control, respectively. Otherwise, Victoza did not produce consistent dose-dependent or time-dependent increases in serum calcitonin.

Patients with MTC usually have calcitonin values >50 ng/L. In Victoza clinical trials, among patients with pre-treatment serum calcitonin <50 ng/L, one Victoza-treated patient and no comparator-treated patients developed serum calcitonin >50 ng/L. The Victoza-treated patient who developed serum calcitonin >50 ng/L had an elevated pre-treatment serum calcitonin of 10.7 ng/L that increased to 30.7 ng/L at Week 12 and 53.5 ng/L at the end of the 6-month trial. Follow-up serum calcitonin was 22.3 ng/L more than 2.5 years after the last dose of Victoza. The largest increase in serum calcitonin in a comparator-treated patient was seen with glimepiride in a patient whose serum calcitonin increased from 19.3 ng/L at baseline to 44.8 ng/L at Week 65 and 38.1 ng/L at Week 104. Among patients who began with serum calcitonin <20 ng/L, calcitonin elevations to >20 ng/L occurred in 0.7% of Victoza-treated patients, 0.3% of placebo-treated patients, and 0.5% of active-comparator-treated patients, with an incidence of 1.1% among patients treated with 1.8 mg/day of Victoza. The clinical significance of these findings is unknown.

Counsel patients regarding the risk for MTC and the symptoms of thyroid tumors (e.g. a mass in the neck, dysphagia, dyspnea or persistent hoarseness). It is unknown whether monitoring with serum calcitonin or thyroid ultrasound will mitigate the potential risk of MTC, and such monitoring may increase the risk of unnecessary procedures, due to low test specificity for serum calcitonin and a high background incidence of thyroid disease. Patients with thyroid nodules noted on physical examination or neck imaging obtained for other reasons should be referred to an endocrinologist for further evaluation. Although routine monitoring of serum calcitonin is of uncertain value in patients treated with Victoza, if serum calcitonin is measured and found to be elevated, the patient should be referred to an endocrinologist for further evaluation.

5.2 Pancreatitis

Based on spontaneous postmarketing reports, acute pancreatitis, including fatal and non-fatal hemorrhagic or necrotizing pancreatitis, has been observed in patients treated with Victoza. After initiation of Victoza, observe patients carefully for signs and symptoms of pancreatitis (including persistent severe abdominal pain, sometimes radiating to the back and which may or may not be accompanied by vomiting). If pancreatitis is suspected, Victoza should promptly be discontinued and appropriate management should be initiated. If pancreatitis is confirmed, Victoza should not be restarted. Consider antidiabetic therapies other than Victoza in patients with a history of pancreatitis.

In clinical trials of Victoza, there have been 13 cases of pancreatitis among Victoza-treated patients and 1 case in a comparator (glimepiride) treated patient (2.7 vs. 0.5 cases per 1000 patient-years). Nine of the 13 cases with Victoza were reported as acute pancreatitis and four were reported as chronic pancreatitis. In one case in a Victoza-treated patient, pancreatitis, with necrosis, was observed and led to death; however clinical causality could not be established. Some patients had other risk factors for pancreatitis, such as a history of cholelithiasis or alcohol abuse.

5.3 Use with Medications Known to Cause Hypoglycemia

Patients receiving Victoza in combination with an insulin secretagogue (e.g., sulfonylurea) or insulin may have an increased risk of hypoglycemia. The risk of hypoglycemia may be lowered by a reduction in the dose of sulfonylurea (or other concomitantly administered insulin secretagogues) or insulin *[see Adverse Reactions (6.1)]*.

5.4 Renal Impairment

Victoza has not been found to be directly nephrotoxic in animal studies or clinical trials. There have been postmarketing reports of acute renal failure and worsening of chronic renal failure, which may sometimes require hemodialysis in Victoza-treated patients *[see Adverse Reactions (6.2)]*. Some of these events were reported in patients without known underlying renal disease. A majority of the reported events occurred in patients who had experienced nausea, vomiting, diarrhea, or dehydration *[see Adverse Reactions (6.1)]*. Some of the reported events occurred in patients receiving one or more medications known to affect renal function or hydration status. Altered renal function has been reversed in many of the reported cases with supportive treatment and discontinuation of potentially causative agents, including Victoza. Use caution when initiating or escalating doses of Victoza in patients with renal impairment *[see Use in Specific Populations (8.6)]*.

5.5 Hypersensitivity Reactions

There have been postmarketing reports of serious hypersensitivity reactions (e.g., anaphylactic reactions and angioedema) in patients treated with Victoza. If a hypersensitivity reaction occurs, the patient should discontinue Victoza and other suspect medications and promptly seek medical advice.

Angioedema has also been reported with other GLP-1 receptor agonists. Use caution in a patient with a history of angioedema with another GLP-1 receptor agonist because it is unknown whether such patients will be predisposed to angioedema with Victoza.

5.6 Macrovascular Outcomes

There have been no clinical studies establishing conclusive evidence of macrovascular risk reduction with Victoza or any other antidiabetic drug.

6 ADVERSE REACTIONS

6.1 Clinical Trials Experience

Because clinical trials are conducted under widely varying conditions, adverse reaction rates observed in the clinical trials of a drug cannot be directly compared to rates in the clinical trials of another drug and may not reflect the rates observed in practice.

Table 2 Adverse reactions reported in ≥5% of Victoza-treated patients and occurring more frequently with Victoza compared to placebo: 26-week combination therapy trials

Add-on to Metformin Trial

	All Victoza + Metformin N = 724	Placebo + Metformin N = 121	Glimepiride + Metformin N = 242
Adverse Reaction	(%)	(%)	(%)
Nausea	15.2	4.1	3.3
Diarrhea	10.9	4.1	3.7
Headache	9.0	6.6	9.5
Vomiting	6.5	0.8	0.4

Add-on to Glimepiride Trial

	All Victoza + Glimepiride N = 695	Placebo + Glimepiride N = 114	Rosiglitazone + Glimepiride N = 231
Adverse Reaction	(%)	(%)	(%)
Nausea	7.5	1.8	2.6
Diarrhea	7.2	1.8	2.2
Constipation	5.3	0.9	1.7
Dyspepsia	5.2	0.9	2.6

Add-on to Metformin + Glimepiride

	Victoza 1.8 + Metformin + Glimepiride N = 230	Placebo + Metformin + Glimepiride N = 114	Glargine + Metformin + Glimepiride N = 232
Adverse Reaction	(%)	(%)	(%)
Nausea	13.9	3.5	1.3
Diarrhea	10.0	5.3	1.3
Headache	9.6	7.9	5.6
Dyspepsia	6.5	0.9	1.7
Vomiting	6.5	3.5	0.4

Add-on to Metformin + Rosiglitazone

	All Victoza + Metformin + Rosiglitazone N = 355	Placebo + Metformin + Rosiglitazone N = 175
Adverse Reaction	(%)	(%)
Nausea	34.6	8.6
Diarrhea	14.1	6.3
Vomiting	12.4	2.9
Headache	8.2	4.6
Constipation	5.1	1.1

The safety of Victoza has been evaluated in 8 clinical trials *[see Clinical Studies (14)]*:

- A double-blind 52-week monotherapy trial compared Victoza 1.2 mg daily, Victoza 1.8 mg daily, and glimepiride 8 mg daily.
- A double-blind 26 week add-on to metformin trial compared Victoza 0.6 mg once-daily, Victoza 1.2 mg once-daily, Victoza 1.8 mg once-daily, placebo, and glimepiride 4 mg once-daily.
- A double-blind 26 week add-on to glimepiride trial compared Victoza 0.6 mg daily, Victoza 1.2 mg once-daily, Victoza 1.8 mg once-daily, placebo, and rosiglitazone 4 mg once-daily.
- A 26 week add-on to metformin + glimepiride trial, compared double-blind Victoza 1.8 mg once-daily, double-blind placebo, and open-label insulin glargine once-daily.
- A double-blind 26-week add-on to metformin + rosiglitazone trial compared Victoza 1.2 mg once-daily, Victoza 1.8 mg once-daily and placebo.
- An open-label 26-week add-on to metformin and/or sulfonylurea trial compared Victoza 1.8 mg once-daily and exenatide 10 mcg twice-daily.
- An open-label 26-week add-on to metformin trial compared Victoza 1.2 mg once-daily, Victoza 1.8 mg once-daily, and sitagliptin 100 mg once-daily.
- An open-label 26-week trial compared insulin detemir as add-on to Victoza 1.8 mg + metformin to continued treatment with Victoza + metformin alone.

Withdrawals

The incidence of withdrawal due to adverse events was 7.8% for Victoza-treated patients and 3.4% for comparator-treated patients in the five double-blind controlled trials of 26 weeks duration or longer. This difference was driven by withdrawals due to gastrointestinal adverse reactions, which occurred in 5.0% of Victoza-treated patients and 0.5% of comparator-treated patients. In these five trials, the most common adverse reactions leading to withdrawal for Victoza-treated patients were nausea (2.8% versus 0% for comparator) and vomiting (1.5% versus 0.1% for comparator). Withdrawal due to gastrointestinal adverse events mainly occurred during the first 2-3 months of the trials.

Common adverse reactions

Tables 1, 2, 3 and 4 summarize common adverse reactions (hypoglycemia is discussed separately) reported in seven of the eight controlled trials of 26 weeks duration or longer. Most of these adverse reactions were gastrointestinal in nature.

In the five double-blind clinical trials of 26 weeks duration or longer, gastrointestinal adverse reactions were reported in 41% of Victoza-treated patients and were dose-related. Gastrointestinal adverse reactions occurred in 17% of comparator-treated patients. Common adverse reactions that occurred at a higher incidence among Victoza-treated patients included nausea, vomiting, diarrhea, dyspepsia and constipation.

In the five double-blind and three open-label clinical trials of 26 weeks duration or longer, the percentage of patients who reported nausea declined over time. In the five double-blind trials approximately 13% of Victoza-treated patients and 2% of comparator-treated patients reported nausea during the first 2 weeks of treatment.

In the 26-week open-label trial comparing Victoza to exenatide, both in combination with metformin and/or sulfonylurea, gastrointestinal adverse reactions were reported at a similar incidence in the Victoza and exenatide treatment groups (Table 3).

In the 26-week open-label trial comparing Victoza 1.2 mg, Victoza 1.8 mg and sitagliptin 100 mg, all in combination with metformin, gastrointestinal adverse reactions were reported at a higher incidence with Victoza than sitagliptin (Table 4).

In the remaining 26-week trial, all patients received Victoza 1.8 mg + metformin during a 12-week run-in period. During the run-in period, 167 patients (17% of enrolled total) withdrew from the trial: 76 (46% of withdrawals) of these patients doing so because of gastrointestinal adverse reactions and 15 (9% of withdrawals) doing so due to other adverse events. Only those patients who completed the run-in period with inadequate glycemic control were randomized to 26 weeks of add-on therapy with insulin detemir or continued, unchanged treatment with Victoza 1.8 mg + metformin. During this randomized 26-week period, diarrhea was the only adverse reaction reported in ≥5% of patients treated with Victoza 1.8 mg + metformin + insulin detemir (11.7%) and greater than in patients treated with Victoza 1.8 mg and metformin alone (6.9%).

Table 1 Adverse reactions reported in ≥5% of Victoza-treated patients in a 52-week monotherapy trial

	All Victoza N = 497	Glimepiride N = 248
Adverse Reaction	(%)	(%)
Nausea	28.4	8.5
Diarrhea	17.1	8.9
Vomiting	10.9	3.6
Constipation	9.9	4.8
Headache	9.1	9.3

[See table 2 above]

Table 3 Adverse Reactions reported in ≥5% of Victoza-treated patients in a 26-Week Open-Label Trial versus Exenatide

	Victoza 1.8 mg once daily + metformin and/or sulfonylurea N = 235	**Exenatide 10 mcg twice daily + metformin and/or sulfonylurea** N = 232
Adverse Reaction	(%)	(%)
Nausea	25.5	28.0
Diarrhea	12.3	12.1
Headache	8.9	10.3
Dyspepsia	8.9	4.7
Vomiting	6.0	9.9
Constipation	5.1	2.6

Table 4 Adverse Reactions in ≥5% of Victoza-treated patients in a 26-Week Open-Label Trial versus Sitagliptin

	All Victoza + metformin N = 439	**Sitagliptin 100 mg/day + metformin** N = 219
Adverse Reaction	(%)	(%)
Nausea	23.9	4.6
Headache	10.3	10.0
Diarrhea	9.3	4.6
Vomiting	8.7	4.1

Immunogenicity

Consistent with the potentially immunogenic properties of protein and peptide pharmaceuticals, patients treated with Victoza may develop anti-liraglutide antibodies. Approximately 50-70% of Victoza-treated patients in the five double-blind clinical trials of 26 weeks duration or longer were tested for the presence of anti-liraglutide antibodies at the end of treatment. Low titers (concentrations not requiring dilution of serum) of anti-liraglutide antibodies were detected in 8.6% of these Victoza-treated patients. Sampling was not performed uniformly across all patients in the clinical trials, and this may have resulted in an underestimate of the actual percentage of patients who developed antibodies. Cross-reacting anti-liraglutide antibodies to native glucagon-like peptide-1 (GLP-1) occurred in 6.9% of the Victoza-treated patients in the double-blind 52-week monotherapy trial and in 4.8% of the Victoza-treated patients in the double-blind 26-week add-on combination therapy trials. These cross-reacting antibodies were not tested for neutralizing effect against native GLP-1, and thus the potential for clinically significant neutralization of native GLP-1 was not assessed. Antibodies that had a neutralizing effect on liraglutide in an *in vitro* assay occurred in 2.3% of the Victoza-treated patients in the double-blind 52-week monotherapy trial and in 1.0% of the Victoza-treated patients in the double-blind 26-week add-on combination therapy trials.

Among Victoza-treated patients who developed anti-liraglutide antibodies, the most common category of adverse events was that of infections, which occurred among 40% of these patients compared to 36%, 34% and 35% of antibody-negative Victoza-treated, placebo-treated and active-control-treated patients, respectively. The specific infections which occurred with greater frequency among Victoza-treated antibody-positive patients were primarily nonserious upper respiratory tract infections, which occurred among 11% of Victoza-treated antibody-positive patients; and among 7%, 7% and 5% of antibody-negative Victoza-treated, placebo-treated and active-control-treated patients, respectively. Among Victoza-treated antibody-negative patients, the most common category of adverse events was that of gastrointestinal events, which occurred in 43%, 18% and 19% of antibody-negative Victoza-treated, placebo-treated and active-control-treated patients, respectively. Antibody formation was not associated with reduced efficacy of Victoza when comparing mean HbA_{1c} of all antibody-positive and all antibody-negative patients. However, the 3 patients with the highest titers of anti-liraglutide antibodies had no reduction in HbA_{1c} with Victoza treatment.

In the five double-blind clinical trials of Victoza, events from a composite of adverse events potentially related to immunogenicity (e.g. urticaria, angioedema) occurred among 0.8% of Victoza-treated patients and among 0.4% of comparator-treated patients. Urticaria accounted for approximately one-half of the events in this composite for Victoza-treated patients. Patients who developed anti-liraglutide antibodies were not more likely to develop events from the immunogenicity events composite than were patients who did not develop anti-liraglutide antibodies.

Injection site reactions

Injection site reactions (e.g., injection site rash, erythema) were reported in approximately 2% of Victoza-treated patients in the five double-blind clinical trials of at least 26 weeks duration. Less than 0.2% of Victoza-treated patients discontinued due to injection site reactions.

Papillary thyroid carcinoma

In clinical trials of Victoza, there were 7 reported cases of papillary thyroid carcinoma in patients treated with Victoza and 1 case in a comparator-treated patient (1.5 vs. 0.5 cases per 1000 patient-years). Most of these papillary thyroid carcinomas were <1 cm in greatest diameter and were diagnosed in surgical pathology specimens after thyroidectomy prompted by findings on protocol-specified screening with serum calcitonin or thyroid ultrasound.

Hypoglycemia

In the eight clinical trials of at least 26 weeks duration, hypoglycemia requiring the assistance of another person for treatment occurred in 11 Victoza-treated patients (2.3 cases per 1000 patient-years) and in two exenatide-treated patients. Of these 11 Victoza-treated patients, six patients were concomitantly using metformin and a sulfonylurea, one was concomitantly using a sulfonylurea, two were concomitantly using metformin (blood glucose values were 65 and 94 mg/dL) and two were using Victoza as monotherapy (one of these patients was undergoing an intravenous glucose tolerance test and the other was receiving insulin as treatment during a hospital stay). For these two patients on Victoza monotherapy, the insulin treatment was the likely explanation for the hypoglycemia.

In the 26-week open-label trial comparing Victoza to sitagliptin, the incidence of hypoglycemic events defined as symptoms accompanied by a fingerstick glucose <56 mg/dL was comparable among the treatment groups (approximately 5%).

[See table 5 below]

Table 5 Incidence (%) and Rate (episodes/patient year) of Hypoglycemia in the 52-Week Monotherapy Trial and in the 26-Week Combination Therapy Trials

	Victoza Treatment	**Active Comparator**	**Placebo Comparator**
Monotherapy	**Victoza** (N = 497)	**Glimepiride** (N = 248)	**None**
Patient not able to self-treat	0	0	-
Patient able to self-treat	9.7 (0.24)	25.0 (1.66)	-
Not classified	1.2 (0.03)	2.4 (0.04)	-
Add-on to Metformin	**Victoza + Metformin** (N = 724)	**Glimepiride + Metformin** (N = 242)	**Placebo + Metformin** (N = 121)
Patient not able to self-treat	0.1 (0.001)	0	0
Patient able to self-treat	3.6 (0.05)	22.3 (0.87)	2.5 (0.06)
Add-on to Victoza + Metformin	**Insulin detemir + Victoza + Metformin** (N = 163)	**Continued Victoza + Metformin alone** (N = 158*)	**None**
Patient not able to self-treat	0	0	-
Patient able to self-treat	9.2 (0.29)	1.3 (0.03)	-
Add-on to Glimepiride	**Victoza + Glimepiride** (N = 695)	**Rosiglitazone + Glimepiride** (N = 231)	**Placebo + Glimepiride** (N = 114)
Patient not able to self-treat	0.1 (0.003)	0	0
Patient able to self-treat	7.5 (0.38)	4.3 (0.12)	2.6 (0.17)
Not classified	0.9 (0.05)	0.9 (0.02)	0
Add-on to Metformin + Rosiglitazone	**Victoza + Metformin + Rosiglitazone** (N = 355)	**None**	**Placebo + Metformin + Rosiglitazone** (N = 175)
Patient not able to self-treat	0	-	0
Patient able to self-treat	7.9 (0.49)	-	4.6 (0.15)
Not classified	0.6 (0.01)	-	1.1 (0.03)
Add-on to Metformin + Glimepiride	**Victoza + Metformin + Glimepiride** (N = 230)	**Insulin glargine + Metformin + Glimepiride** (N = 232)	**Placebo + Metformin + Glimepiride** (N = 114)
Patient not able to self-treat	2.2 (0.06)	0	0
Patient able to self-treat	27.4 (1.16)	28.9 (1.29)	16.7 (0.95)
Not classified	0	1.7 (0.04)	0

* One patient is an outlier and was excluded due to 25 hypoglycemic episodes that the patient was able to self-treat. This patient had a history of frequent hypoglycemia prior to the study.

In a pooled analysis of clinical trials, the incidence rate (per 1,000 patient-years) for malignant neoplasms (based on investigator-reported events, medical history, pathology reports, and surgical reports from both blinded and open-label study periods) was 10.9 for Victoza, 6.3 for placebo, and 7.2 for active comparator. After excluding papillary thyroid carcinoma events *[see Adverse Reactions (6.1)]*, no particular cancer cell type predominated. Seven malignant neoplasm events were reported beyond 1 year of exposure to study medication, six events among Victoza-treated patients (4 colon, 1 prostate and 1 nasopharyngeal), no events with placebo and one event with active comparator (colon). Causality has not been established.

Laboratory Tests

In the five clinical trials of at least 26 weeks duration, mildly elevated serum bilirubin concentrations (elevations to no more than twice the upper limit of the reference range) occurred in 4.0% of Victoza-treated patients, 2.1% of placebo-treated patients and 3.5% of active-comparator-treated patients. This finding was not accompanied by abnormalities in other liver tests. The significance of this isolated finding is unknown.

Vital signs

Victoza did not have adverse effects on blood pressure. Mean increases from baseline in heart rate of 2 to 3 beats per minute have been observed with Victoza compared to placebo. The long-term clinical effects of the increase in pulse rate have not been established *[see Warnings and Precautions (5.6)]*.

6.2 Post-Marketing Experience

The following additional adverse reactions have been reported during post-approval use of Victoza. Because these events are reported voluntarily from a population of uncertain size, it is generally not possible to reliably estimate their frequency or establish a causal relationship to drug exposure.

- Dehydration resulting from nausea, vomiting and diarrhea. *[see Warnings and Precautions (5.4) and Patient Counseling Information (17.3)]*
- Increased serum creatinine, acute renal failure or worsening of chronic renal failure, sometimes requiring hemodialysis. *[see Warnings and Precautions (5.4) and Patient Counseling Information (17.3)]*
- Angioedema and anaphylactic reactions. *[see Contraindications (4), Warnings and Precautions (5.5), Patient counseling Information (17.5)]*
- Allergic reactions: rash and pruritus
- Acute pancreatitis, hemorrhagic and necrotizing pancreatitis sometimes resulting in death *[see Warnings and Precautions (5.2)]*

7 DRUG INTERACTIONS

7.1 Oral Medications

Victoza causes a delay of gastric emptying, and thereby has the potential to impact the absorption of concomitantly administered oral medications. In clinical pharmacology trials, Victoza did not affect the absorption of the tested orally administered medications to any clinically relevant degree. Nonetheless, caution should be exercised when oral medications are concomitantly administered with Victoza.

8 USE IN SPECIFIC POPULATIONS

8.1 Pregnancy

Pregnancy Category C.

There are no adequate and well-controlled studies of Victoza in pregnant women. Victoza should be used during pregnancy only if the potential benefit justifies the potential risk to the fetus. Liraglutide has been shown to be teratogenic in rats at or above 0.8 times the human systemic exposures resulting from the maximum recommended human dose (MRHD) of 1.8 mg/day based on plasma area under the time-concentration curve (AUC). Liraglutide has been shown to cause reduced growth and increased total major abnormalities in rabbits at systemic exposures below human exposure at the MRHD based on plasma AUC.

Female rats given subcutaneous doses of 0.1, 0.25 and 1.0 mg/kg/day liraglutide beginning 2 weeks before mating through gestation day 17 had estimated systemic exposures 0.8-, 3-, and 11-times the human exposure at the MRHD based on plasma AUC comparison. The number of early embryonic deaths in the 1 mg/kg/day group increased slightly. Fetal abnormalities and variations in kidneys and blood vessels, irregular ossification of the skull, and a more complete state of ossification occurred at all doses. Mottled liver and minimally kinked ribs occurred at the highest dose. The incidence of fetal malformations in liraglutide-treated groups exceeding concurrent and historical controls were misshapen oropharynx and/or narrowed opening into larynx at 0.1 mg/kg/day and umbilical hernia at 0.1 and 0.25 mg/kg/day.

Pregnant rabbits given subcutaneous doses of 0.01, 0.025 and 0.05 mg/kg/day liraglutide from gestation day 6 through day 18 inclusive, had estimated systemic exposures less than the human exposure at the MRHD of 1.8 mg/day at all doses, based on plasma AUC. Liraglutide decreased fetal weight and dose-dependently increased the incidence of total major fetal abnormalities at all doses. The incidence of malformations exceeded concurrent and historical controls at 0.01 mg/kg/day (kidneys, scapula), ≥ 0.01 mg/kg/day (eyes, forelimb), 0.025 mg/kg/day (brain, tail and sacral vertebrae, major blood vessels and heart, umbilicus), ≥ 0.025 mg/kg/day (sternum) and at 0.05 mg/kg/day (parietal bones, major blood vessels). Irregular ossification and/or skeletal abnormalities occurred in the skull and jaw, vertebrae and ribs, sternum, pelvis, tail, and scapula; and dose-dependent minor skeletal variations were observed. Visceral abnormalities occurred in blood vessels, lung, liver, and esophagus. Bilobed or bifurcated gallbladder was seen in all treatment groups, but not in the control group.

In pregnant female rats given subcutaneous doses of 0.1, 0.25 and 1.0 mg/kg/day liraglutide from gestation day 6 through weaning or termination of nursing on lactation day 24, estimated systemic exposures were 0.8-, 3-, and 11-times human exposure at the MRHD of 1.8 mg/day, based on plasma AUC. A slight delay in parturition was observed in the majority of treated rats. Group mean body weight of neonatal rats from liraglutide-treated dams was lower than neonatal rats from control group dams. Bloody scabs and agitated behavior occurred in male rats descended from dams treated with 1 mg/kg/day liraglutide. Group mean body weight from birth to postpartum day 14 trended lower in F_2 generation rats descended from liraglutide-treated rats compared to F_2 generation rats descended from controls, but differences did not reach statistical significance for any group.

8.3 Nursing Mothers

It is not known whether Victoza is excreted in human milk. Because many drugs are excreted in human milk and because of the potential for tumorigenicity shown for liraglutide in animal studies, a decision should be made whether to discontinue nursing or to discontinue Victoza, taking into account the importance of the drug to the mother. In lactating rats, liraglutide was excreted unchanged in milk at concentrations approximately 50% of maternal plasma concentrations.

8.4 Pediatric Use

Safety and effectiveness of Victoza have not been established in pediatric patients. Victoza is not recommended for use in pediatric patients.

8.5 Geriatric Use

In the Victoza clinical trials, a total of 797 (20%) of the patients were 65 years of age and over and 113 (2.8%) were 75 years of age and over. No overall differences in safety or effectiveness were observed between these patients and younger patients, but greater sensitivity of some older individuals cannot be ruled out.

8.6 Renal Impairment

There is limited experience with Victoza in patients with mild, moderate, and severe renal impairment, including end-stage renal disease. However, there have been postmarketing reports of acute renal failure and worsening of chronic renal failure, which may sometimes require hemodialysis *[see Warnings and Precautions (5.4) and Adverse Reactions (6.2)]*. Victoza should be used with caution in this patient population. No dose adjustment of Victoza is recommended for patients with renal impairment *[see Clinical Pharmacology (12.3)]*.

8.7 Hepatic Impairment

There is limited experience in patients with mild, moderate or severe hepatic impairment. Therefore, Victoza should be used with caution in this patient population. No dose adjustment of Victoza is recommended for patients with hepatic impairment *[see Clinical Pharmacology (12.3)]*.

8.8 Gastroparesis

Victoza slows gastric emptying. Victoza has not been studied in patients with pre-existing gastroparesis.

10 OVERDOSAGE

Overdoses have been reported in clinical trials and postmarketing use of Victoza. Effects have included severe nausea and severe vomiting. In the event of overdosage, appropriate supportive treatment should be initiated according to the patient's clinical signs and symptoms.

11 DESCRIPTION

Victoza contains liraglutide, an analog of human GLP-1 and acts as a GLP-1 receptor agonist. The peptide precursor of liraglutide, produced by a process that includes expression of recombinant DNA in *Saccharomyces cerevisiae*, has been engineered to be 97% homologous to native human GLP-1 by substituting arginine for lysine at position 34. Liraglutide is made by attaching a C-16 fatty acid (palmitic acid) with a glutamic acid spacer on the remaining lysine residue at position 26 of the peptide precursor. The molecular formula of liraglutide is $C_{172}H_{265}N_{43}O_{51}$ and the molecular weight is 3751.2 Daltons. The structural formula (Figure 1) is:

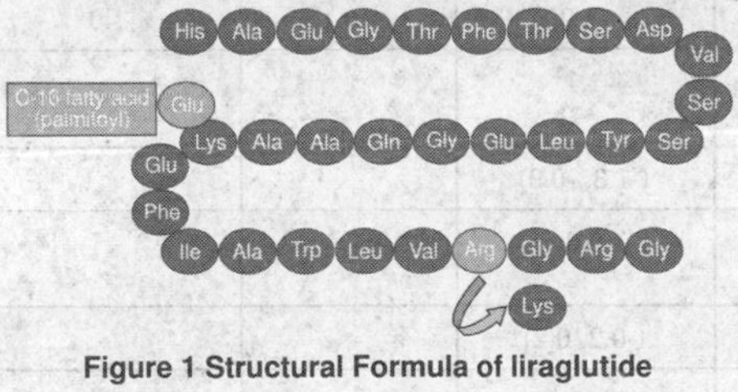

Figure 1 Structural Formula of liraglutide

Victoza is a clear, colorless solution. Each 1 mL of Victoza solution contains 6 mg of liraglutide. Each pre-filled pen contains a 3 mL solution of Victoza equivalent to 18 mg liraglutide (free-base, anhydrous) and the following inactive ingredients: disodium phosphate dihydrate, 1.42 mg; propylene glycol, 14 mg; phenol, 5.5 mg; and water for injection.

12 CLINICAL PHARMACOLOGY

12.1 Mechanism of Action

Liraglutide is an acylated human Glucagon-Like Peptide-1 (GLP-1) receptor agonist with 97% amino acid sequence homology to endogenous human GLP-1(7-37). GLP-1(7-37) represents <20% of total circulating endogenous GLP-1. Like GLP-1(7-37), liraglutide activates the GLP-1 receptor, a membrane-bound cell-surface receptor coupled to adenylyl cyclase by the stimulatory G-protein, Gs, in pancreatic beta cells. Liraglutide increases intracellular cyclic AMP (cAMP) leading to insulin release in the presence of elevated glucose concentrations. This insulin secretion subsides as blood glucose concentrations decrease and approach euglycemia. Liraglutide also decreases glucagon secretion in a glucose-dependent manner. The mechanism of blood glucose lowering also involves a delay in gastric emptying.

GLP-1(7-37) has a half-life of 1.5-2 minutes due to degradation by the ubiquitous endogenous enzymes, dipeptidyl peptidase IV (DPP-IV) and neutral endopeptidases (NEP). Unlike native GLP-1, liraglutide is stable against metabolic degradation by both peptidases and has a plasma half-life of 13 hours after subcutaneous administration. The pharmacokinetic profile of liraglutide, which makes it suitable for once daily administration, is a result of self-association that delays absorption, plasma protein binding and stability against metabolic degradation by DPP-IV and NEP.

12.2 Pharmacodynamics

Victoza's pharmacodynamic profile is consistent with its pharmacokinetic profile observed after single subcutaneous administration as Victoza lowered fasting, premeal and postprandial glucose throughout the day *[see Clinical Pharmacology (12.3)]*.

Fasting and postprandial glucose was measured before and up to 5 hours after a standardized meal after treatment to steady state with 0.6, 1.2 and 1.8 mg Victoza or placebo. Compared to placebo, the postprandial plasma glucose $AUC_{0\text{-}300min}$ was 35% lower after Victoza 1.2 mg and 38% lower after Victoza 1.8 mg.

Glucose-dependent insulin secretion

The effect of a single dose of 7.5 mcg/kg (~ 0.7 mg) Victoza on insulin secretion rates (ISR) was investigated in 10 patients with type 2 diabetes during graded glucose infusion. In these patients, on average, the ISR response was increased in a glucose-dependent manner (Figure 2).

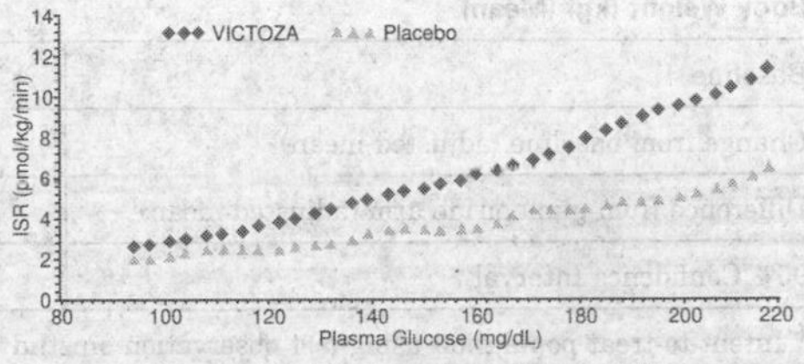

Figure 2 Mean Insulin Secretion Rate (ISR) versus Glucose Concentration Following Single-Dose Victoza 7.5 mcg/kg (~ 0.7 mg) or Placebo in Patients with Type 2 Diabetes (N=10) During Graded Glucose Infusion

Glucagon secretion

Victoza lowered blood glucose by stimulating insulin secretion and lowering glucagon secretion. A single dose of Victoza 7.5 mcg/kg (~ 0.7 mg) did not impair glucagon response to low glucose concentrations.

Gastric emptying

Victoza causes a delay of gastric emptying, thereby reducing the rate at which postprandial glucose appears in the circulation.

Cardiac Electrophysiology (QTc)

The effect of Victoza on cardiac repolarization was tested in a QTc study. Victoza at steady state concentrations with daily doses up to 1.8 mg did not produce QTc prolongation.

12.3 Pharmacokinetics

Absorption - Following subcutaneous administration, maximum concentrations of liraglutide are achieved at 8-12 hours post dosing. The mean peak (C_{max}) and total (AUC) exposures of liraglutide were 35 ng/mL and 960 ng•h/mL, respectively, for a subcutaneous single dose of 0.6 mg. After subcutaneous single dose administrations, C_{max} and AUC of liraglutide increased proportionally over the therapeutic dose range of 0.6 mg to 1.8 mg. At 1.8 mg Victoza, the average steady state concentration of liraglutide over 24 hours was approximately 128 ng/mL. $AUC_{0-\infty}$ was equivalent between upper arm and abdomen, and between upper arm and thigh. $AUC_{0-\infty}$ from thigh was 22% lower than that from abdomen. However, liraglutide exposures were considered comparable among these three subcutaneous injection sites. Absolute bioavailability of liraglutide following subcutaneous administration is approximately 55%.

Distribution - The mean apparent volume of distribution after subcutaneous administration of Victoza 0.6 mg is approximately 13 L. The mean volume of distribution after intravenous administration of Victoza is 0.07 L/kg. Liraglutide is extensively bound to plasma protein (>98%).

Metabolism - During the initial 24 hours following administration of a single [^{3}H]-liraglutide dose to healthy subjects, the major component in plasma was intact liraglutide. Liraglutide is endogenously metabolized in a similar manner to large proteins without a specific organ as a major route of elimination.

Elimination - Following a [^{3}H]-liraglutide dose, intact liraglutide was not detected in urine or feces. Only a minor part of the administered radioactivity was excreted as liraglutide-related metabolites in urine or feces (6% and 5%, respectively). The majority of urine and feces radioactivity was excreted during the first 6-8 days. The mean apparent clearance following subcutaneous administration of a single

Table 6 Results of a 52-week monotherapy trial*

	Victoza 1.8 mg	Victoza 1.2 mg	Glimepiride 8 mg
Intent-to-Treat Population (N)	246	251	248
HbA_{1c} (%) (Mean)			
Baseline	8.2	8.2	8.2
Change from baseline (adjusted mean)†	-1.1	-0.8	-0.5
Difference from glimepiride arm (adjusted mean)†	-0.6‡	-0.3§	
95% Confidence Interval	(-0.8, -0.4)	(-0.5, -0.1)	
Percentage of patients achieving A_{1c} <7%	51	43	28
Fasting Plasma Glucose (mg/dL) (Mean)			
Baseline	172	168	172
Change from baseline (adjusted mean)†	-26	-15	-5
Difference from glimepiride arm (adjusted mean)†	-20‡	-10§	
95% Confidence Interval	(-29, -12)	(-19, -1)	
Body Weight (kg) (Mean)			
Baseline	92.6	92.1	93.3
Change from baseline (adjusted mean)†	-2.5	-2.1	+1.1
Difference from glimepiride arm (adjusted mean)†	-3.6‡	-3.2‡	
95% Confidence Interval	(-4.3, -2.9)	(-3.9, -2.5)	

* Intent-to-treat population using last observation on study
† Least squares mean adjusted for baseline value
‡ p-value <0.0001
§ p-value <0.05

Table 7 Results of a 26-week trial of Victoza as add-on to metformin*

	Victoza 1.8 mg + Metformin	Victoza 1.2 mg + Metformin	Placebo + Metformin	Glimepiride 4 mg† + Metformin
Intent-to-Treat Population (N)	242	240	121	242
HbA_{1c} (%) (Mean)				
Baseline	8.4	8.3	8.4	8.4
Change from baseline (adjusted mean)‡	-1.0	-1.0	+0.1	-1.0
Difference from placebo + metformin arm (adjusted mean)‡	-1.1§	-1.1§		
95% Confidence Interval	(-1.3, -0.9)	(-1.3, -0.9)		
Difference from glimepiride + metformin arm (adjusted mean)‡	0.0	0.0		
95% Confidence Interval	(-0.2, 0.2)	(-0.2, 0.2)		
Percentage of patients achieving A_{1c} <7%	42	35	11	36
Fasting Plasma Glucose (mg/dL) (Mean)				
Baseline	181	179	182	180
Change from baseline (adjusted mean)‡	-30	-30	+7	-24
Difference from placebo + metformin arm (adjusted mean)‡	-38§	-37§		
95% Confidence Interval	(-48, -27)	(-47, -26)		
Difference from glimepiride + metformin arm (adjusted mean)‡	-7	-6		
95% Confidence Interval	(-16, 2)	(-15, 3)		

(Table continued on next page)

dose of liraglutide is approximately 1.2 L/h with an elimination half-life of approximately 13 hours, making Victoza suitable for once daily administration.

Specific Populations

Elderly - Age had no effect on the pharmacokinetics of Victoza based on a pharmacokinetic study in healthy elderly subjects (65 to 83 years) and population pharmacokinetic analyses of patients 18 to 80 years of age *[see Use in Specific Populations (8.5)]*.

Gender - Based on the results of population pharmacokinetic analyses, females have 34% lower weight-adjusted clearance of Victoza compared to males. Based on the exposure response data, no dose adjustment is necessary based on gender.

Race and Ethnicity - Race and ethnicity had no effect on the pharmacokinetics of Victoza based on the results of population pharmacokinetic analyses that included Caucasian, Black, Asian and Hispanic/Non-Hispanic subjects.

Body Weight - Body weight significantly affects the pharmacokinetics of Victoza based on results of population pharmacokinetic analyses. The exposure of liraglutide decreases with an increase in baseline body weight. However, the 1.2 mg and 1.8 mg daily doses of Victoza provided adequate systemic exposures over the body weight range of 40 – 160 kg evaluated in the clinical trials. Liraglutide was not studied in patients with body weight >160 kg.

Pediatric - Victoza has not been studied in pediatric patients *[see Use in Specific Populations (8.4)]*.

Renal Impairment - The single-dose pharmacokinetics of Victoza were evaluated in subjects with varying degrees of renal impairment. Subjects with mild (estimated creatinine clearance 50-80 mL/min) to severe (estimated creatinine clearance <30 mL/min) renal impairment and subjects with end-stage renal disease requiring dialysis were included in the trial. Compared to healthy subjects, liraglutide AUC in mild, moderate, and severe renal impairment and in end-stage renal disease was on average 35%, 19%, 29% and 30% lower, respectively *[see Use in Specific Populations (8.6)]*.

Hepatic Impairment - The single-dose pharmacokinetics of Victoza were evaluated in subjects with varying degrees of hepatic impairment. Subjects with mild (Child Pugh score 5-6) to severe (Child Pugh score > 9) hepatic impairment were included in the trial. Compared to healthy subjects, liraglutide AUC in subjects with mild, moderate and severe hepatic impairment was on average 11%, 14% and 42% lower, respectively *[see Use in Specific Populations (8.7)]*.

Drug Interactions

In vitro assessment of drug-drug interactions

Victoza has low potential for pharmacokinetic drug-drug interactions related to cytochrome P450 (CYP) and plasma protein binding.

In vivo assessment of drug-drug interactions

The drug-drug interaction studies were performed at steady state with Victoza 1.8 mg/day. Before administration of concomitant treatment, subjects underwent a 0.6 mg weekly dose increase to reach the maximum dose of 1.8 mg/day. Administration of the interacting drugs was timed so that C_{max} of Victoza (8-12 h) would coincide with the absorption peak of the co-administered drugs.

Digoxin

A single dose of digoxin 1 mg was administered 7 hours after the dose of Victoza at steady state. The concomitant administration with Victoza resulted in a reduction of digoxin AUC by 16%; C_{max} decreased by 31%. Digoxin median time to maximal concentration (T_{max}) was delayed from 1 h to 1.5 h.

Lisinopril

A single dose of lisinopril 20 mg was administered 5 minutes after the dose of Victoza at steady state. The co-administration with Victoza resulted in a reduction of lisinopril AUC by 15%; C_{max} decreased by 27%. Lisinopril median T_{max} was delayed from 6 h to 8 h with Victoza.

Atorvastatin

Victoza did not change the overall exposure (AUC) of atorvastatin following a single dose of atorvastatin 40 mg, administered 5 hours after the dose of Victoza at steady state. Atorvastatin C_{max} was decreased by 38% and median T_{max} was delayed from 1 h to 3 h with Victoza.

Acetaminophen

Victoza did not change the overall exposure (AUC) of acetaminophen following a single dose of acetaminophen 1000 mg, administered 8 hours after the dose of Victoza at steady state. Acetaminophen C_{max} was decreased by 31% and median T_{max} was delayed up to 15 minutes.

Griseofulvin

Victoza did not change the overall exposure (AUC) of griseofulvin following co-administration of a single dose of griseofulvin 500 mg with Victoza at steady state. Griseofulvin C_{max} increased by 37% while median T_{max} did not change.

Oral Contraceptives

A single dose of an oral contraceptive combination product containing 0.03 mg ethinylestradiol and 0.15 mg levonorgestrel was administered under fed conditions and 7 hours after the dose of Victoza at steady state. Victoza lowered ethinylestradiol and levonorgestrel C_{max} by 12% and 13%, respectively. There was no effect of Victoza on the overall exposure (AUC) of ethinylestradiol. Victoza increased the levonorgestrel $AUC_{0-\infty}$ by 18%. Victoza delayed T_{max} for both ethinylestradiol and levonorgestrel by 1.5 h.

Insulin Detemir

No pharmacokinetic interaction was observed between Victoza and insulin detemir when separate subcutaneous injections of insulin detemir 0.5 Unit/kg (single-dose) and Victoza 1.8 mg (steady state) were administered in patients with type 2 diabetes.

13 NONCLINICAL TOXICOLOGY

13.1 Carcinogenesis, Mutagenesis, Impairment of Fertility

A 104-week carcinogenicity study was conducted in male and female CD-1 mice at doses of 0.03, 0.2, 1.0, and 3.0 mg/kg/day liraglutide administered by bolus subcutaneous injection yielding systemic exposures 0.2-, 2-, 10- and 45-times the human exposure, respectively, at the MRHD of 1.8 mg/day based on plasma AUC comparison. A dose-related increase in benign thyroid C-cell adenomas was seen in the 1.0 and the 3.0 mg/kg/day groups with incidences of 13% and 19% in males and 6% and 20% in females, respectively. C-cell adenomas did not occur in control groups or 0.03 and 0.2 mg/kg/day groups. Treatment-related malignant C-cell carcinomas occurred in 3% of females in the 3.0 mg/kg/day group. Thyroid C-cell tumors are rare findings during carcinogenicity testing in mice. A treatment-related increase in fibrosarcomas was seen on the dorsal skin and subcutis, the body surface used for drug injection, in males in the 3 mg/kg/day group. These fibrosarcomas were attributed to the high local concentration of drug near the injection site. The liraglutide concentration in the clinical formulation (6 mg/mL) is 10-times higher than the concentration in the formulation used to administer 3 mg/kg/day liraglutide to mice in the carcinogenicity study (0.6 mg/mL).

A 104-week carcinogenicity study was conducted in male and female Sprague Dawley rats at doses of 0.075, 0.25 and 0.75 mg/kg/day liraglutide administered by bolus subcutaneous injection with exposures 0.5-, 2- and 8-times the human exposure, respectively, resulting from the MRHD based on plasma AUC comparison. A treatment-related increase in benign thyroid C cell adenomas was seen in males in 0.25 and 0.75 mg/kg/day liraglutide groups with incidences of 12%, 16%, 42%, and 46% and in all female liraglutide-treated groups with incidences of 10%, 27%, 33%, and 56% in 0 (control), 0.075, 0.25, and 0.75 mg/kg/day groups, respectively. A treatment-related increase in malignant thyroid C-cell carcinomas was observed in all male liraglutide-treated groups with incidences of 2%, 8%, 6%, and 14% and in females at 0.25 and 0.75 mg/kg/day with incidences of 0%, 0%, 4%, and 6% in 0 (control), 0.075, 0.25, and 0.75 mg/kg/day groups, respectively. Thyroid C-cell carcinomas are rare findings during carcinogenicity testing in rats.

Human relevance of thyroid C-cell tumors in mice and rats is unknown and could not be determined by clinical studies or nonclinical studies *[see Boxed Warning and Warnings and Precautions (5.1)]*.

Liraglutide was negative with and without metabolic activation in the Ames test for mutagenicity and in a human peripheral blood lymphocyte chromosome aberration test for clastogenicity. Liraglutide was negative in repeat-dose *in vivo* micronucleus tests in rats.

In rat fertility studies using subcutaneous doses of 0.1, 0.25 and 1.0 mg/kg/day liraglutide, males were treated for 4 weeks prior to and throughout mating and females were treated 2 weeks prior to and throughout mating until gestation day 17. No direct adverse effects on male fertility was observed at doses up to 1.0 mg/kg/day, a high dose yielding an estimated systemic exposure 11- times the human exposure at the MRHD, based on plasma AUC. In female rats, an increase in early embryonic deaths occurred at 1.0 mg/kg/day. Reduced body weight gain and food consumption were observed in females at the 1.0 mg/kg/day dose.

14 CLINICAL STUDIES

A total of 6090 patients with type 2 diabetes participated in 8 phase 3 trials. There were 5 double-blind (one of these trials had an open-label active control insulin glargine arm), randomized, controlled clinical trials, one of 52 weeks duration and four of 26 weeks duration. There were also three 26 week open-label trials; one comparing Victoza to twice-daily exenatide, one comparing Victoza to sitagliptin and one comparing Victoza+metformin+insulin detemir to Victoza+metformin alone. These multinational trials were conducted to evaluate the glycemic efficacy and safety of Victoza in type 2 diabetes as monotherapy and in combination with one or two oral anti-diabetic medications or insulin detemir. The 7 add-on combination therapy trials enrolled patients who were previously treated with anti-diabetic therapy, and approximately two-thirds of patients in the monotherapy trial also were previously treated with anti-diabetic therapy. In total, 272 (4%) of the 6090 patients in these 8 trials were new to anti-diabetic therapy. In these 8 clinical trials, patients ranged in age from 18-80 years old and 54% were men. Approximately 82% of patients were Caucasian, and 6% were Black. In the 5 trials where ethnicity was captured, 10% of patients were Hispanic/Latino (n=630).

In each of the placebo controlled trials, treatment with Victoza produced clinically and statistically significant improvements in hemoglobin A_{1c} and fasting plasma glucose (FPG) compared to placebo.

Table 7 *(cont.)* Results of a 26-week trial of Victoza as add-on to metformin*

	Victoza 1.8 mg + Metformin	Victoza 1.2 mg + Metformin	Placebo + Metformin	Glimepiride 4 mg† + Metformin
Intent-to-Treat Population (N)	242	240	121	242
Body Weight (kg) (Mean)				
Baseline	88.0	88.5	91.0	89.0
Change from baseline (adjusted mean)‡	-2.8	-2.6	-1.5	+1.0
Difference from placebo + metformin arm (adjusted mean)‡	-1.3¶	-1.1¶		
95% Confidence Interval	(-2.2, -0.4)	(-2.0, -0.2)		
Difference from glimepiride + metformin arm (adjusted mean)‡	-3.8§	-3.5§		
95% Confidence Interval	(-4.5, -3.0)	(-4.3, -2.8)		

* Intent-to-treat population using last observation on study
† For glimepiride, one-half of the maximal approved United States dose.
‡ Least squares mean adjusted for baseline value
§ p-value <0.0001
¶ p-value <0.05

Table 8 Results of a 26-week open-label trial of Victoza Compared to Sitagliptin (both in combination with metformin)*

	Victoza 1.8 mg + Metformin	Victoza 1.2 mg + Metformin	Sitagliptin 100 mg+ Metformin
Intent-to-Treat Population (N)	218	221	219
HbA_{1c} (%) (Mean)			
Baseline	8.4	8.4	8.5
Change from baseline (adjusted mean)	-1.5	-1.2	-0.9
Difference from sitagliptin arm (adjusted mean)†	-0.6‡	-0.3‡	
95% Confidence Interval	(-0.8, -0.4)	(-0.5, 0.2)	
Percentage of patients achieving A_{1c} <7%	56	44	22
Fasting Plasma Glucose (mg/dL) (Mean)			
Baseline	179	182	180
Change from baseline (adjusted mean)	-39	-34	-15
Difference from sitagliptin arm (adjusted mean)†	-24‡	-19‡	
95% Confidence Interval	(-31, -16)	(-26, -12)	

* Intent-to-treat population using last observation on study
† Least squares mean adjusted for baseline value
‡ p-value <0.0001

All Victoza-treated patients started at 0.6 mg/day. The dose was increased in weekly intervals by 0.6 mg to reach 1.2 mg or 1.8 mg for patients randomized to these higher doses. Victoza 0.6 mg is not effective for glycemic control and is intended only as a starting dose to reduce gastrointestinal intolerance *[see Dosage and Administration (2)]*.

14.1 Monotherapy

In this 52-week trial, 746 patients were randomized to Victoza 1.2 mg, Victoza 1.8 mg, or glimepiride 8 mg. Patients who were randomized to glimepiride were initially treated with 2 mg daily for two weeks, increasing to 4 mg daily for another two weeks, and finally increasing to 8 mg daily. Treatment with Victoza 1.8 mg and 1.2 mg resulted in a statistically significant reduction in HbA_{1c} compared to glimepiride (Table 6). The percentage of patients who discontinued due to ineffective therapy was 3.6% in the Victoza 1.8 mg treatment group, 6.0% in the Victoza 1.2 mg treatment group, and 10.1% in the glimepiride-treatment group.

[See table 6 at top of previous page]
[See figure 3 at top of next column]

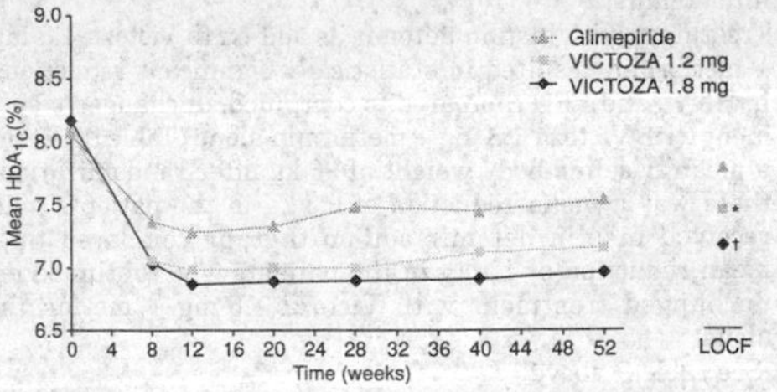

*p-value = 0.0014 for VICTOZA 1.2 mg compared to glimepiride.
†p-value < 0.0001 for VICTOZA 1.8 mg compared to glimepiride.
P values derived from change from baseline ANCOVA model.

Figure 3 Mean HbA_{1c} for patients who completed the 52-week trial and for the Last Observation Carried Forward (LOCF, intent-to-treat) data at Week 52 (Monotherapy)

14.2 Combination Therapy

Add-on to Metformin

In this 26-week trial, 1091 patients were randomized to Victoza 0.6 mg, Victoza 1.2 mg, Victoza 1.8 mg, placebo, or glimepiride 4 mg (one-half of the maximal approved dose in the United States), all as add-on to metformin. Randomization occurred after a 6-week run-in period consisting of a 3-week initial forced metformin titration period followed by a maintenance period of another 3 weeks. During the titration period, doses of metformin were increased up to 2000 mg/day.

Treatment with Victoza 1.2 mg and 1.8 mg as add-on to metformin resulted in a significant mean HbA_{1c} reduction relative to placebo add-on to metformin and resulted in a similar mean HbA_{1c} reduction relative to glimepiride 4 mg add-on to metformin (Table 7). The percentage of patients who discontinued due to ineffective therapy was 5.4% in the Victoza 1.8 mg + metformin treatment group, 3.3% in the Victoza 1.2 mg + metformin treatment group, 23.8% in the placebo + metformin treatment group, and 3.7% in the glimepiride + metformin treated group.

[See table 7 on previous page and above]

Victoza Compared to Sitagliptin, Both as Add-on to Metformin

In this 26–week, open-label trial, 665 patients on a background of metformin ≥1500 mg per day were randomized to Victoza 1.2 mg once-daily, Victoza 1.8 mg once-daily or sitagliptin 100 mg once-daily, all dosed according to approved labeling. Patients were to continue their current treatment on metformin at a stable, pre-trial dose level and dosing frequency.

The primary endpoint was the change in HbA_{1c} from baseline to Week 26. Treatment with Victoza 1.2 mg and Victoza 1.8 mg resulted in statistically significant reductions in HbA_{1c} relative to sitagliptin 100 mg (Table 8). The percentage of patients who discontinued due to ineffective therapy was 3.1% in the Victoza 1.2 mg group, 0.5% in the Victoza 1.8 mg treatment group, and 4.1% in the sitagliptin 100 mg treatment group. From a mean baseline body weight of 94 kg, there was a mean reduction of 2.7 kg for Victoza 1.2 mg, 3.3 kg for Victoza 1.8 mg, and 0.8 kg for sitagliptin 100 mg.

[See table 8 at top of previous page]

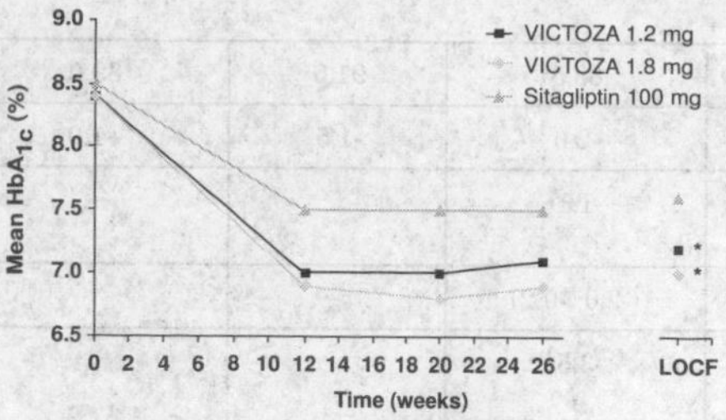

*p-value <0.0001 for Victoza compared with sitagliptin

P values derived from change from baseline ANCOVA model

Figure 4 Mean HbA_{1c} for patients who completed the 26-week trial and for the Last Observation Carried Forward (LOCF, intent-to-treat) data at Week 26

Combination Therapy with Metformin and Insulin

This 26-week open-label trial enrolled 988 patients with inadequate glycemic control (HbA_{1c} 7-10%) on metformin (≥1500 mg/day) alone or inadequate glycemic control (HbA_{1c} 7-8.5%) on metformin (≥1500 mg/day) and a sulfonylurea. Patients who were on metformin and a sulfonylurea discontinued the sulfonylurea then all patients entered a 12-week run-in period during which they received add-on therapy with Victoza titrated to 1.8 mg once-daily. At the end of the run-in period, 498 patients (50%) achieved HbA_{1c} <7% with Victoza 1.8 mg and metformin and continued treatment in a non-randomized, observational arm. Another 167 patients (17%) withdrew from the trial during the run-in period with approximately one-half of these patients doing so because of gastrointestinal adverse reactions *[see Adverse Reactions (6.1)]*. The remaining 323 patients with HbA_{1c} ≥7% (33% of those who entered the run-in period) were randomized to 26 weeks of once-daily insulin detemir administered in the evening as add-on therapy (N=162) or to continued, unchanged treatment with Victoza 1.8 mg and metformin (N=161). The starting dose of insulin detemir was 10 units/day and the mean dose at the end of the 26-week randomized period was 39 units/day. During the 26 week randomized treatment period, the percentage of patients who discontinued due to ineffective therapy was 11.2% in the group randomized to continued treatment with Victoza 1.8 mg and metformin and 1.2% in the group randomized to add-on therapy with insulin detemir.

Treatment with insulin detemir as add-on to Victoza 1.8 mg + metformin resulted in statistically significant reductions in HbA_{1c} and FPG compared to continued, unchanged treatment with Victoza 1.8 mg + metformin alone (Table 9). From a mean baseline body weight of 96 kg after randomization, there was a mean reduction of 0.3 kg in the patients who received insulin detemir add-on therapy compared to a mean reduction of 1.1 kg in the patients who continued on unchanged treatment with Victoza 1.8 mg + metformin alone.

[See table 9 above]

Table 9 Results of a 26-week open label trial of Insulin detemir as add on to Victoza + metformin compared to continued treatment with Victoza + metformin alone in patients not achieving HbA_{1c} < 7% after 12 weeks of Metformin and Victoza*

	Insulin detemir + Victoza + Metformin	Victoza + Metformin
Intent-to-Treat Population (N)	162	157
HbA_{1c} (%) (Mean)		
Baseline (week 0)	7.6	7.6
Change from baseline (adjusted mean)	-0.5	0
Difference from Victoza + metformin arm (LS mean)†	-0.5‡	
95% Confidence Interval	(-0.7, -0.4)	
Percentage of patients achieving A_{1c} <7%	43	17
Fasting Plasma Glucose (mg/dL) (Mean)		
Baseline (week 0)	166	159
Change from baseline (adjusted mean)	-39	-7
Difference from Victoza + metformin arm (LS mean)†	-31‡ (-39 , -23)	
95% Confidence Interval		

* Intent-to-treat population using last observation on study
† Least squares mean adjusted for baseline value
‡ p-value <0.0001

Table 10 Results of a 26-week trial of Victoza as add-on to sulfonylurea*

	Victoza 1.8 mg + Glimepiride	Victoza 1.2 mg + Glimepiride	Placebo + Glimepiride	Rosiglitazone 4 mg† + Glimepiride
Intent-to-Treat Population (N)	234	228	114	231
HbA_{1c} (%) (Mean)				
Baseline	8.5	8.5	8.4	8.4
Change from baseline (adjusted mean)‡	-1.1	-1.1	+0.2	-0.4
Difference from placebo + glimepiride arm (adjusted mean)‡	-1.4§	-1.3§		
95% Confidence Interval	(-1.6, -1.1)	(-1.5, -1.1)		
Percentage of patients achieving A_{1c} <7%	42	35	7	22
Fasting Plasma Glucose (mg/dL) (Mean)				
Baseline	174	177	171	179
Change from baseline (adjusted mean)‡	-29	-28	+18	-16
Difference from placebo + glimepiride arm (adjusted mean)‡	-47§	-46§		
95% Confidence Interval	(-58, -35)	(-58, -35)		
Body Weight (kg) (Mean)				
Baseline	83.0	80.0	81.9	80.6
Change from baseline (adjusted mean)‡	-0.2	+0.3	-0.1	+2.1
Difference from placebo + glimepiride arm (adjusted mean)‡	-0.1	0.4		
95% Confidence Interval	(-0.9, 0.6)	(-0.4, 1.2)		

* Intent-to-treat population using last observation on study
† For rosiglitazone, one-half of the maximal approved United States dose.
‡ Least squares mean adjusted for baseline value
§ p-value <0.0001

Add-on to Sulfonylurea

In this 26-week trial, 1041 patients were randomized to Victoza 0.6 mg, Victoza 1.2 mg, Victoza 1.8 mg, placebo, or rosiglitazone 4 mg (one-half of the maximal approved dose in the United States), all as add-on to glimepiride. Randomization occurred after a 4-week run-in period consisting of an initial, 2-week, forced-glimepiride titration period followed by a maintenance period of another 2 weeks. During the titration period, doses of glimepiride were increased to 4 mg/day. The doses of glimepiride could be reduced (at the discretion of the investigator) from 4 mg/day to 3 mg/day or 2 mg/day (minimum) after randomization, in the event of unacceptable hypoglycemia or other adverse events.

Treatment with Victoza 1.2 mg and 1.8 mg as add-on to glimepiride resulted in a statistically significant reduction in mean HbA_{1c} compared to placebo add-on to glimepiride (Table 10). The percentage of patients who discontinued due to ineffective therapy was 3.0% in the Victoza 1.8 mg + glimepiride treatment group, 3.5% in the Victoza 1.2 mg + glimepiride treatment group, 17.5% in the placebo + glimepiride treatment group, and 6.9% in the rosiglitazone + glimepiride treatment group.

[See table 10 above]

Add-on to Metformin and Sulfonylurea

In this 26-week trial, 581 patients were randomized to Victoza 1.8 mg, placebo, or insulin glargine, all as add-on to metformin and glimepiride. Randomization took place after a 6-week run-in period consisting of a 3-week forced metformin and glimepiride titration period followed by a maintenance period of another 3 weeks. During the titration period, doses of metformin and glimepiride were to be increased up to 2000 mg/day and 4 mg/day, respectively. After randomization, patients randomized to Victoza 1.8 mg underwent a 2 week period of titration with Victoza. During the trial, the Victoza and metformin doses were fixed, although glimepiride and insulin glargine doses could be adjusted. Patients titrated glargine twice-weekly during the first 8 weeks of treatment based on self-measured fasting plasma glucose on the day of titration. After Week 8, the frequency of insulin glargine titration was left to the discretion of the investigator, but, at a minimum, the glargine dose was to be revised, if necessary, at Weeks 12 and 18. Only 20% of glargine-treated patients achieved the pre-specified target fasting plasma glucose of ≤100 mg/dL. Therefore, optimal titration of the insulin glargine dose was not achieved in most patients.

Treatment with Victoza as add-on to glimepiride and metformin resulted in a statistically significant mean reduction in HbA_{1c} compared to placebo add-on to glimepiride and metformin (Table 11). The percentage of patients who discontinued due to ineffective therapy was 0.9% in the Victoza 1.8 mg + metformin + glimepiride treatment group, 0.4% in the insulin glargine + metformin + glimepiride treatment group, and 11.3% in the placebo + metformin + glimepiride treatment group.

[See table 11 at top of next page]

Victoza Compared to Exenatide, Both as Add-on to Metformin and/or Sulfonylurea Therapy

In this 26–week, open-label trial, 464 patients on a background of metformin monotherapy, sulfonylurea monotherapy or a combination of metformin and sulfonylurea were randomized to once daily Victoza 1.8 mg or exenatide 10 mcg twice daily. Maximally tolerated doses of background therapy were to remain unchanged for the duration of the trial. Patients randomized to exenatide started on a dose of 5 mcg twice-daily for 4 weeks and then were escalated to 10 mcg twice daily.

Treatment with Victoza 1.8 mg resulted in statistically significant reductions in HbA_{1c} and FPG relative to exenatide (Table 12). The percentage of patients who discontinued for ineffective therapy was 0.4% in the Victoza treatment group and 0% in the exenatide treatment group. Both treatment groups had a mean decrease from baseline in body weight of approximately 3 kg.

[See table 12 below]

Add-on to Metformin and Thiazolidinedione

In this 26-week trial, 533 patients were randomized to Victoza 1.2 mg, Victoza 1.8 mg or placebo, all as add-on to rosiglitazone (8 mg) plus metformin (2000 mg). Patients underwent a 9 week run-in period (3-week forced dose escalation followed by a 6-week dose maintenance phase) with rosiglitazone (starting at 4 mg and increasing to 8 mg/day within 2 weeks) and metformin (starting at 500 mg with increasing weekly increments of 500 mg to a final dose of 2000 mg/day). Only patients who tolerated the final dose of rosiglitazone (8 mg/day) and metformin (2000 mg/day) and completed the 6-week dose maintenance phase were eligible for randomization into the trial.

Treatment with Victoza as add-on to metformin and rosiglitazone produced a statistically significant reduction in mean HbA_{1c} compared to placebo add-on to metformin and rosiglitazone (Table 13). The percentage of patients who discontinued due to ineffective therapy was 1.7% in the Victoza 1.8 mg + metformin + rosiglitazone treatment group, 1.7% in the Victoza 1.2 mg + metformin + rosiglitazone treatment group, and 16.4% in the placebo + metformin + rosiglitazone treatment group.

[See table 13 at top of next page]

16 HOW SUPPLIED/STORAGE AND HANDLING

16.1 How Supplied

Victoza is available in the following package sizes containing disposable, pre-filled, multi-dose pens. Each individual pen delivers doses of 0.6 mg, 1.2 mg, or 1.8 mg (6 mg/mL, 3 mL).

2 × Victoza pen NDC 0169-4060-12

3 × Victoza pen NDC 0169-4060-13

Each Victoza pen is for use by a single patient. A Victoza pen should never be shared between patients, even if the needle is changed.

16.2 Recommended Storage

Prior to first use, Victoza should be stored in a refrigerator between 36°F to 46°F (2°C to 8°C) (Table 14). Do not store in the freezer or directly adjacent to the refrigerator cooling element. Do not freeze Victoza and do not use Victoza if it has been frozen.

After initial use of the Victoza pen, the pen can be stored for 30 days at controlled room temperature (59°F to 86°F; 15°C to 30°C) or in a refrigerator (36°F to 46°F; 2°C to 8°C). Keep the pen cap on when not in use. Victoza should be protected from excessive heat and sunlight. Always remove and safely discard the needle after each injection and store the Victoza pen without an injection needle attached. This will reduce the potential for contamination, infection, and leakage while also ensuring dosing accuracy.

Table 14 Recommended Storage Conditions for the Victoza Pen

Prior to first use	After first use	
Refrigerated 36°F to 46°F (2°C to 8°C)	Room Temperature 59°F to 86°F (15°C to 30°C)	Refrigerated 36°F to 46°F (2°C to 8°C)
Until expiration date	30 days	

17 PATIENT COUNSELING INFORMATION

17.1 FDA-Approved Medication Guide

See separate leaflet.

17.2 Risk of Thyroid C-cell Tumors

Patients should be informed that liraglutide causes benign and malignant thyroid C-cell tumors in mice and rats and that the human relevance of this finding is unknown. Patients should be counseled to report symptoms of thyroid tumors (e.g., a lump in the neck, hoarseness, dysphagia or dyspnea) to their physician.

17.3 Dehydration and Renal Failure

Patients treated with Victoza should be advised of the potential risk of dehydration due to gastrointestinal adverse reactions and take precautions to avoid fluid depletion. Patients should be informed of the potential risk for worsening renal function, which in some cases may require dialysis.

Table 11 Results of a 26-week trial of Victoza as add-on to metformin and sulfonylurea*

	Victoza 1.8 mg + Metformin + Glimepiride	Placebo + Metformin + Glimepiride	Insulin glargine† + Metformin + Glimepiride
Intent-to-Treat Population (N)	230	114	232
HbA_{1c} (%) (Mean)			
Baseline	8.3	8.3	8.1
Change from baseline (adjusted mean)‡	-1.3	-0.2	-1.1
Difference from placebo + metformin + glimepiride arm (adjusted mean)‡	-1.1§		
95% Confidence Interval	(-1.3, -0.9)		
Percentage of patients achieving A_{1c} <7%	53	15	46
Fasting Plasma Glucose (mg/dL) (Mean)			
Baseline	165	170	164
Change from baseline (adjusted mean)‡	28	+10	-32
Difference from placebo + metformin + glimepiride arm (adjusted mean)‡	-38§		
95% Confidence Interval	(-46, -30)		
Body Weight (kg) (Mean)			
Baseline	85.8	85.4	85.2
Change from baseline (adjusted mean)‡	-1.8	-0.4	1.6
Difference from placebo + metformin + glimepiride arm (adjusted mean)‡	-1.4¶		
95% Confidence Interval	(-2.1, -0.7)		

* Intent-to-treat population using last observation on study
† For insulin glargine, optimal titration regimen was not achieved for 80% of patients.
‡ Least squares mean adjusted for baseline value
§ p-value <0.0001
¶ p-value <0.05

Table 12 Results of a 26-week open-label trial of Victoza versus Exenatide (both in combination with metformin and/or sulfonylurea)*

	Victoza 1.8 mg once daily + metformin and/or sulfonylurea	Exenatide 10 mcg twice daily + metformin and/or sulfonylurea
Intent-to-Treat Population (N)	233	231
HbA_{1c} (%) (Mean)		
Baseline	8.2	8.1
Change from baseline (adjusted mean)†	-1.1	-0.8
Difference from exenatide arm (adjusted mean)†	-0.3‡	
95% Confidence Interval	(-0.5, -0.2)	
Percentage of patients achieving A_{1c} <7%	54	43
Fasting Plasma Glucose (mg/dL) (Mean)		
Baseline	176	171
Change from baseline (adjusted mean)†	-29	-11
Difference from exenatide arm (adjusted mean)†	-18‡	
95% Confidence Interval	(-25, -12)	

* Intent-to-treat population using last observation carried forward
† Least squares mean adjusted for baseline value
‡ p-value <0.0001

17.4 Pancreatitis

Patients should be informed of the potential risk for pancreatitis. Explain that persistent severe abdominal pain that may radiate to the back and which may or may not be accompanied by vomiting, is the hallmark symptom of acute pancreatitis. Instruct patients to discontinue Victoza promptly and contact their physician if persistent severe abdominal pain occurs *[see Warnings and Precautions (5.2)]*.

17.5 Hypersensitivity Reactions

Patients should be informed that serious hypersensitivity reactions have been reported during postmarketing use of Victoza. If symptoms of hypersensitivity reactions occur, patients must stop taking Victoza and seek medical advice promptly *[see Warnings and Precautions (5.5)]*.

17.6 Never Share a Victoza Pen Between Patients

Counsel patients that they should never share a Victoza pen with another person, even if the needle is changed. Sharing of the pen between patients may pose a risk of transmission of infection.

17.7 Instructions

Patients should be informed of the potential risks and benefits of Victoza and of alternative modes of therapy. Patients should also be informed about the importance of adherence to dietary instructions, regular physical activity, periodic blood glucose monitoring and A_{1c} testing, recognition and management of hypoglycemia and hyperglycemia, and assessment for diabetes complications. During periods of stress such as fever, trauma, infection, or surgery, medication requirements may change and patients should be advised to seek medical advice promptly.

Table 13 Results of a 26-week trial of Victoza as add-on to metformin and thiazolidinedione*

	Victoza 1.8 mg + Metformin + Rosiglitazone	Victoza 1.2 mg + Metformin + Rosiglitazone	Placebo + Metformin + Rosiglitazone
Intent-to-Treat Population (N)	178	177	175
HbA_{1c} (%) (Mean)			
Baseline	8.6	8.5	8.4
Change from baseline (adjusted mean)†	-1.5	-1.5	-0.5
Difference from placebo + metformin + rosiglitazone arm (adjusted mean)†	-0.9‡	-0.9‡	
95% Confidence Interval	(-1.1, -0.8)	(-1.1, -0.8)	
Percentage of patients achieving A_{1c} <7%	54	57	28
Fasting Plasma Glucose (mg/dL) (Mean)			
Baseline	185	181	179
Change from baseline (adjusted mean)†	-44	-40	-8
Difference from placebo + metformin + rosiglitazone arm (adjusted mean)†	-36‡	-32‡	
95% Confidence Interval	(-44, -27)	(-41, -23)	
Body Weight (kg) (Mean)			
Baseline	94.9	95.3	98.5
Change from baseline (adjusted mean)†	-2.0	-1.0	+0.6
Difference from placebo + metformin + rosiglitazone arm (adjusted mean)†	-2.6‡	-1.6‡	
95% Confidence Interval	(-3.4, -1.8)	(-2.4, -1.0)	

* Intent-to-treat population using last observation on study
† Least squares mean adjusted for baseline value
‡ p-value <0.0001

Patients should be advised that the most common side effects of Victoza are headache, nausea and diarrhea. Nausea is most common when first starting Victoza, but decreases over time in the majority of patients and does not typically require discontinuation of Victoza.

Physicians should instruct their patients to read the Patient Medication Guide before starting Victoza therapy and to reread each time the prescription is renewed. Patients should be instructed to inform their doctor or pharmacist if they develop any unusual symptom, or if any known symptom persists or worsens.

Inform patients not to take an extra dose of Victoza to make up for a missed dose. If a dose is missed, the once-daily regimen should be resumed as prescribed with the next scheduled dose.

If more than 3 days have elapsed since the last dose, the patient should be advised to reinitiate Victoza at 0.6 mg to mitigate any gastrointestinal symptoms associated with reinitiation of treatment. Victoza should be titrated at the discretion of the prescribing physician *[see Dosage and Administration (2)]*.

17.8 Laboratory Tests

Patients should be informed that response to all diabetic therapies should be monitored by periodic measurements of blood glucose and A_{1c} levels, with a goal of decreasing these levels towards the normal range. A_{1c} is especially useful for evaluating long-term glycemic control.

Date of Issue: April 16, 2013
Version: 6

Victoza® is a registered trademark of Novo Nordisk A/S.

Victoza® is covered by US Patent Nos. 6,268,343, 6,458,924, 7,235,627, 8,114,833 and other patents pending.

Victoza® Pen is covered by US Patent Nos. 6,004,297, RE 43,834, RE 41,956 and other patents pending.

Manufactured by:
Novo Nordisk A/S
DK-2880 Bagsvaerd, Denmark

For information about Victoza contact:
Novo Nordisk Inc.
800 Scudders Mill Road
Plainsboro, NJ 08536
1-877-484-2869

Medication Guide

Victoza® (VIC-tow-za)
(liraglutide [rDNA origin]) Injection

Read this Medication Guide and Patient Instructions for Use that come with Victoza before you start using Victoza and each time you get a refill. There may be new information. This Medication Guide does not take the place of talking with your healthcare provider about your medical condition or your treatment. If you have questions about Victoza after reading this information, ask your healthcare provider or pharmacist.

What is the most important information I should know about Victoza?

Serious side effects may happen in people who take Victoza, including:

1. Possible thyroid tumors, including cancer. During the drug testing process, the medicine in Victoza caused rats and mice to develop tumors of the thyroid gland. Some of these tumors were cancers. It is not known if Victoza will cause thyroid tumors or a type of thyroid cancer called medullary thyroid cancer in people. If medullary thyroid cancer occurs, it may lead to death if not detected and treated early. If you develop tumors or cancer of the thyroid, your thyroid may have to be surgically removed.

- Before you start taking Victoza, tell your healthcare provider if you or any of your family members have had thyroid cancer, especially medullary thyroid cancer, or Multiple Endocrine Neoplasia syndrome type 2. Do not take Victoza if you or any of your family members have medullary thyroid cancer, or if you have Multiple Endocrine Neoplasia syndrome type 2. People with these conditions already have a higher chance of developing medullary thyroid cancer in general and should not take Victoza.
- While taking Victoza, tell your healthcare provider if you get a lump or swelling in your neck, hoarseness, trouble swallowing, or shortness of breath. These may be symptoms of thyroid cancer.

2. Inflammation of the pancreas (pancreatitis), which may be severe and lead to death.

Before taking Victoza, tell your healthcare provider if you have had:

- pancreatitis
- stones in your gallbladder (gallstones)
- a history of alcoholism
- high blood triglyceride levels

These medical conditions can make you more likely to get pancreatitis in general. It is not known if having these conditions will lead to a higher chance of getting pancreatitis while taking Victoza.

While taking Victoza:

Stop taking Victoza and call your healthcare provider right away if you have pain in your stomach area (abdomen) that is severe and will not go away. The pain may happen with or without vomiting. The pain may be felt going from your abdomen through to your back. This type of pain may be a symptom of pancreatitis.

What is Victoza?

- Victoza is an injectable prescription medicine that may improve blood sugar (glucose) in adults with type 2 diabetes mellitus, and should be used along with diet and exercise.
- Victoza is not recommended as the first choice of medication for treating diabetes.
- Victoza is not a substitute for insulin.
- Victoza is not for use in people with type 1 diabetes or people with diabetic ketoacidosis.
- It is not known if Victoza is safe and effective in children. Victoza is not recommended for use in children.

Who should not use Victoza?

Do not use Victoza if:

- you or any of your family members have a history of medullary thyroid cancer.
- you have Multiple Endocrine Neoplasia syndrome type 2 (MEN 2). This is a disease where people have tumors in more than one gland in their body.
- you are allergic to liraglutide or any of the ingredients in Victoza. See the end of this Medication Guide for a complete list of ingredients in Victoza. Symptoms of a serious allergic reaction may include:
  - swelling of your face, lips, tongue, or throat
  - fainting or feeling dizzy
  - very rapid heartbeat
  - problems breathing or swallowing
  - severe rash or itching

Talk with your healthcare provider if you are not sure if you have any of these conditions.

What should I tell my healthcare provider before using Victoza?

Before taking Victoza, tell your healthcare provider if you:

- have any of the conditions listed in the section "What is the most important information I should know about Victoza?"
- are allergic to liraglutide or any of the other ingredients in Victoza. See the end of this Medication Guide for a list of ingredients in Victoza.
- have severe problems with your stomach, such as slowed emptying of your stomach (gastroparesis) or problems with digesting food.
- have or have had kidney or liver problems.
- have any other medical conditions.
- are pregnant or plan to become pregnant. It is not known if Victoza will harm your unborn baby. Tell your healthcare provider if you become pregnant while taking Victoza.
- are breastfeeding or plan to breastfeed. It is not known if Victoza passes into your breast milk. You and your healthcare provider should decide if you will take Victoza or breastfeed. You should not do both without talking with your healthcare provider first.

Tell your healthcare provider about all the medicines you take including prescription and non-prescription medicines, vitamins, and herbal supplements. Victoza slows stomach emptying and can affect medicines that need to pass through the stomach quickly. Victoza may affect the way some medicines work and some other medicines may affect the way Victoza works. Tell your healthcare provider if you take other diabetes medicines, especially sulfonylurea medicines or insulin.

Know the medicines you take. Keep a list of them with you to show your healthcare provider and pharmacist each time you get a new medicine.

How should I use Victoza?

- Use Victoza exactly as prescribed by your healthcare provider. Your dose should be increased after using Victoza for one week. After that, do not change your dose unless your healthcare provider tells you to.
- Victoza is injected 1 time each day, at any time during the day.
- You can take Victoza with or without food.
- Victoza comes in a prefilled pen.
- Your healthcare provider must teach you how to inject Victoza before you use it for the first time. If you have questions or do not understand the instructions, talk to your healthcare provider or pharmacist. See the Patient Instructions for Use that come with this Medication Guide for detailed information about the right way to use your Victoza pen.

- Pen needles are not included. Use the Victoza pen with Novo Nordisk disposable needles. You may need a prescription to get pen needles from your pharmacist. Ask your healthcare provider which needle size is best for you.
- When starting a new prefilled Victoza pen, you must follow the "First Time Use for Each New Pen" (see the detailed Patient Instructions for Use that comes with this Medication Guide). You only need to do this 1 time with each new pen. You should also do this if you drop your pen. If you do the "First Time Use for Each New Pen" before each injection, you will run out of medicine too soon.
- Inject your dose of Victoza under the skin (subcutaneous injection) in your stomach area (abdomen), upper leg (thigh), or upper arm, as instructed by your healthcare provider. **Do not inject into a vein or muscle.**
- If you also give yourself insulin injections in addition to Victoza, **never mix insulin and Victoza together**. Give yourself 2 separate injections. You may give both injections in the same body area (for example, your stomach area), but you should not give the injections right next to each other.
- If you take too much Victoza, call your healthcare provider right away. Too much Victoza may cause severe nausea and vomiting.
- If you miss your daily dose of Victoza, use Victoza as soon as you remember. Then take your next daily dose as usual on the following day. Do not take an extra dose of Victoza or increase your dose on the following day to make up for your missed dose. If you miss your dose of Victoza for **3 days or more**, call your healthcare provider to talk about how to restart your treatment.
- Follow your healthcare provider's instructions for diet, exercise, how often to test your blood sugar, and when to get your HbA_{1c} checked. If you stop using Victoza your blood sugar levels may increase. First talk to your healthcare provider if you want to stop taking Victoza.
- Your dose of diabetes medicines may need to be changed if your body is under certain types of stress. Tell your healthcare provider if you:
  - have fever
  - have trauma
  - have an infection
  - plan to have or have had surgery
- Never share your Victoza pen or needles with another person. You may give an infection to them, or get an infection from them.

What are the possible side effects of Victoza?

Victoza may cause serious side effects, including:

- See "What is the most important information I should know about Victoza?"
- **Low blood sugar (hypoglycemia).** Your risk for getting low blood sugar is higher if you take Victoza with another medicine that can cause low blood sugar, such as a sulfonylurea or insulin. In some people, the blood sugar may get so low that they need another person to help them. The dose of your sulfonylurea medicine or insulin may need to be lowered while you use Victoza. Signs and symptoms of low blood sugar may include:
- shakiness
- sweating
- headache
- drowsiness
- weakness
- dizziness
- confusion
- irritability
- hunger
- fast heartbeat
- feeling jittery

Talk to your healthcare provider about how to recognize and treat low blood sugar. Make sure that your family and other people who are around you a lot know how to recognize and treat low blood sugar.

- **Kidney problems (kidney failure).** Victoza may cause nausea, vomiting or diarrhea leading to loss of fluids (dehydration). Dehydration may cause kidney failure which can lead to the need for dialysis. This can happen in people who have never had kidney problems before. Drinking plenty of fluids may reduce your chance of dehydration.

Call your healthcare provider right away if you have nausea, vomiting, or diarrhea that does not go away, or if you cannot drink liquids by mouth.

- **Serious allergic reactions.** Serious allergic reactions can happen with Victoza. Stop using Victoza, and get medical help right away if you have any symptom of a serious allergic reaction **See "Who should not use Victoza?"**

Common side effects of Victoza include:

- headache
- nausea
- diarrhea

Nausea is most common when first starting Victoza, but decreases over time in most people as their body gets used to the medicine.

Tell your healthcare provider if you have any side effect that bothers you or that does not go away.

These are not all the side effects with Victoza. For more information, ask your healthcare provider or pharmacist.

Call your doctor for medical advice about side effects. You may report side effects to FDA at 1-800-FDA-1088.

How should I store Victoza?

Before use:

- Store your new, unused Victoza pen in the refrigerator at 36°F to 46°F (2°C to 8°C).
- Do not freeze Victoza or use Victoza if it has been frozen. Do not store Victoza near the refrigerator cooling element.

Pen in use:

- Store your Victoza pen for 30 days either at 59°F to 86°F (15°C to 30°C), or in a refrigerator at 36°F to 46°F (2°C to 8°C).
- When carrying the pen away from home, store the pen at a temperature between 59°F to 86°F (15°C to 30°C) and keep it dry.
- If Victoza has been exposed to temperatures above 86°F (30°C), it should be thrown away.
- Protect your Victoza pen from heat and sunlight.
- Keep the pen cap on when your Victoza pen is not in use.
- Use your Victoza pen within 30 days after the first day it is stored outside the refrigerator. After these 30 days, throw away your Victoza pen even if some medicine is left in the pen.
- Do not use Victoza after the expiration date printed on the carton.

Do not store the Victoza pen with the needle attached. Always safely remove and safely throw away the needle after each injection. This may help prevent contamination, infection and leakage. It also helps to make sure that you get the correct dose of Victoza. See the Patient Instructions for Use for information about how to dispose of used pen needles and used Victoza pens.

Keep your Victoza pen, pen needles, and all medicines out of the reach of children.

General information about Victoza

Medicines are sometimes prescribed for purposes other than those listed in a Medication Guide. Do not use Victoza for a condition for which it was not prescribed. Do not give Victoza to other people, even if they have the same symptoms you have. It may harm them.

This Medication Guide summarizes the most important information you should know about using Victoza. If you would like more information, talk with your healthcare provider. You can ask your pharmacist or healthcare provider for information about Victoza that is written for health professionals.

For more information, go to victoza.com or call 1-877-484-2869.

What are the ingredients in Victoza?

Active Ingredient: liraglutide

Inactive Ingredients: disodium phosphate dihydrate, propylene glycol, phenol and water for injection

Manufactured by:
Novo Nordisk A/S
DK-2880 Bagsvaerd, Denmark

For information about Victoza contact:
Novo Nordisk Inc.
800 Scudders Mill Road
Plainsboro, NJ 08536
1-877-484-2869

Issued: April 2013
Version: 4

This Medication Guide has been approved by the U.S. Food and Drug Administration.

Victoza® is a registered trademark of Novo Nordisk A/S.

Victoza® is covered by US Patent Nos. 6,268,343, 6,458,924, 7,235,627, 8,114,833 and other patents pending.

Victoza® pen is covered by US Patent Nos. 6,004,297, RE 43,834, RE 41,956 and other patents pending.

PATIENT INSTRUCTIONS FOR USE

Victoza (liraglutide [rDNA origin]) injection

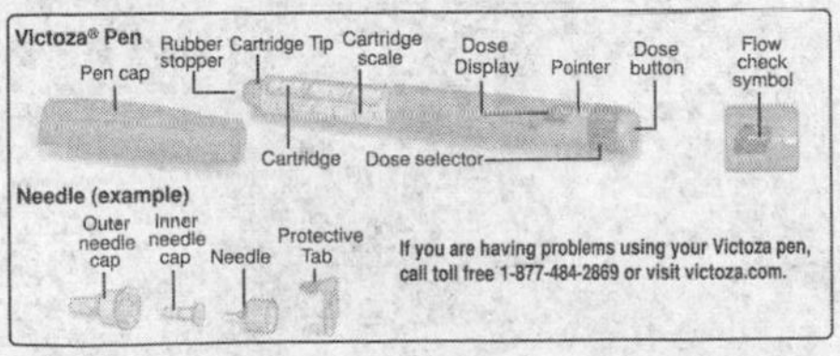

First read the Medication Guide that comes with your Victoza pen and then read these Patient Instructions for Use for information about how to use your Victoza pen the right way.

These instructions do not take the place of talking with your healthcare provider about your medical condition or your treatment.

Your Victoza pen contains 3 mL of Victoza and will deliver doses of 0.6 mg, 1.2 mg or 1.8 mg. The number of doses that you can take with a Victoza pen depends on the dose of medicine that is prescribed for you. Your healthcare provider will tell you how much Victoza to take.

Victoza pen should be used with Novo Nordisk disposable needles. Talk to your healthcare provider or pharmacist for more information about needles for your Victoza pen.

Important Information

- Δ Do not share your Victoza pen or needles with anyone else. You may give an infection to them or get an infection from them.
- Δ Always use a new needle for each injection.
- Δ Keep your Victoza pen and all medicines out of the reach of children.
- Δ If you drop your Victoza pen, repeat "First Time Use For Each New Pen" (steps A through D).
- Δ Be careful not to bend or damage the needle.
- Δ Do not use the cartridge scale to measure how much Victoza to inject.
- Δ Be careful when handling used needles to avoid needle stick injuries.
- Δ You can use your Victoza pen for up to 30 days after you use it the first time.

Caring for your Victoza pen

- After removing the needle, put the pen cap on your Victoza pen and store your Victoza pen without the needle attached.

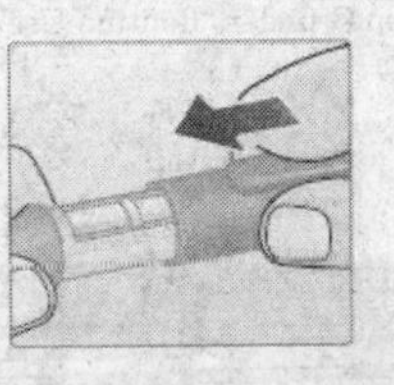

- Do not try to refill your Victoza pen - it is prefilled and is disposable.
- Do not try to repair your pen or pull it apart.
- Keep your Victoza pen away from dust, dirt and liquids.
- If cleaning is needed, wipe the outside of the pen with a clean, damp cloth.

How should I store Victoza?

Before use:

- Store your new, unused Victoza pen in the refrigerator at 36°F to 46°F (2°C to 8°C).
- If Victoza is stored outside of refrigeration (by mistake) prior to first use, it should be used or thrown away within 30 days.
- Do not freeze Victoza or use Victoza if it has been frozen. Do not store Victoza near the refrigerator cooling element.

Pen in use:

- Store your Victoza pen for 30 days at 59°F to 86°F (15°C to 30°C), or in a refrigerator at 36°F to 46°F (2°C to 8°C).
- When carrying the pen away from home, store the pen at a temperature between 59°F to 86°F (15°C to 30°C).
- If Victoza has been exposed to temperatures above 86°F (30°C), it should be thrown away.
- Protect your Victoza pen from heat and sunlight.
- Keep the pen cap on when your Victoza pen is not in use.
- Use a Victoza pen for only 30 days. Throw away a used Victoza pen after 30 days, even if some medicine is left in the pen.

First Time Use for Each New Pen

Step A. Check the Pen

- Take your new Victoza pen out of the refrigerator.
- Wash hands with soap and water before use.
- Check pen label before each use to make sure it is your Victoza pen.
- Pull off pen cap.

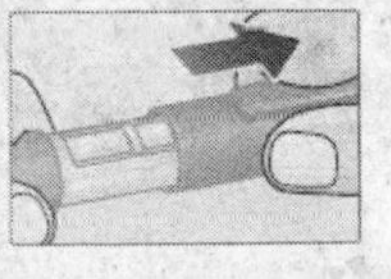

- Check Victoza in the cartridge. The liquid should be clear, colorless and free of particles. If not, do not use.
- Wipe the rubber stopper with an alcohol swab.

Step B. Attach the Needle

- Remove protective tab from outer needle cap.
- Push outer needle cap containing the needle straight onto the pen, then screw needle on until secure.

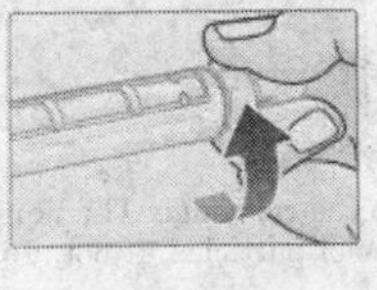

- Pull off outer needle cap. Do not throw away.

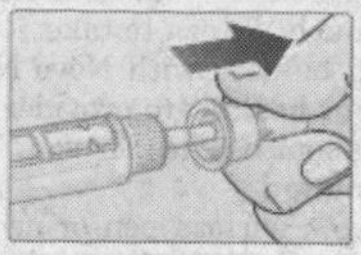

- Pull off inner needle cap and throw away. A small drop of liquid may appear. This is normal.

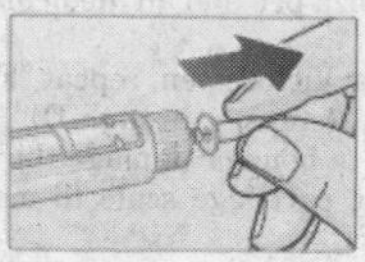

Step C. Dial to the Flow Check Symbol

This step is done only ONCE for each new pen and is ONLY required the first time you use a new pen.

- Turn dose selector until flow check symbol (--) lines up with pointer. The flow check symbol does not administer the dose as prescribed by your healthcare provider.
- To select the dose prescribed by your healthcare provider, continue to Step G under "Routine Use".

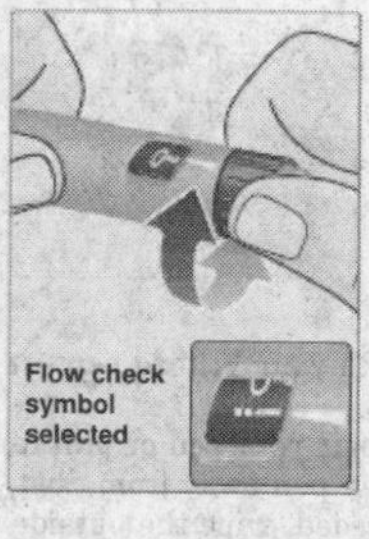

Step D. Prepare the Pen

- Hold pen with needle pointing up.
- Tap cartridge gently with your finger a few times to bring any air bubbles to the top of the cartridge.

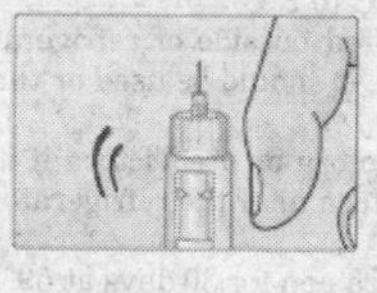

- Keep needle pointing up and press dose button until 0 mg lines up with pointer. Repeat steps C and D, up to 6 times, until a drop of Victoza appears at the needle tip.

If you still see no drop of Victoza, use a new pen and contact Novo Nordisk at 1-877-484-2869.

Continue to Step G under "Routine Use" →

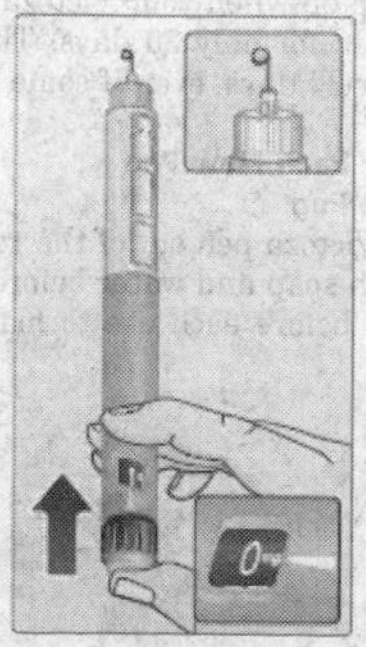

Routine Use

Step E. Check the Pen

- Take your Victoza pen from where it is stored.
- Wash hands with soap and water before use.
- Check pen label before each use to make sure it is your Victoza pen.
- Pull off pen cap.

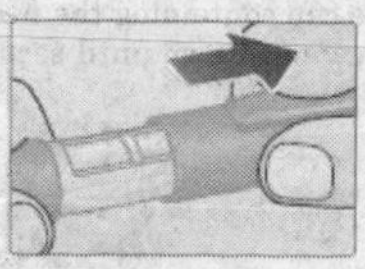

- Check Victoza in the cartridge. The liquid should be clear, colorless and free of particles. If not, do not use.
- Wipe the rubber stopper with an alcohol swab.

Step F. Attach the Needle

- Remove protective tab from outer needle cap.
- Push outer needle cap containing the needle straight onto the pen, then screw needle on until secure.

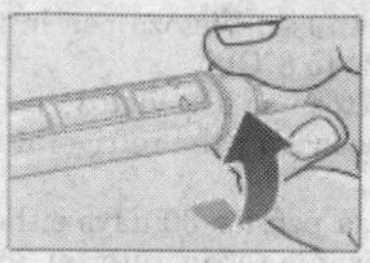

- Pull off outer needle cap. Do not throw away.

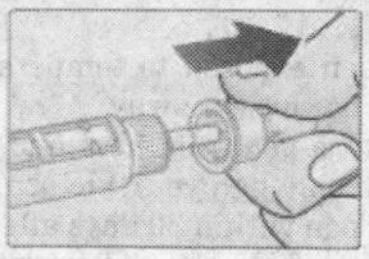

- Pull off inner needle cap and throw away. A small drop of liquid may appear. This is normal.

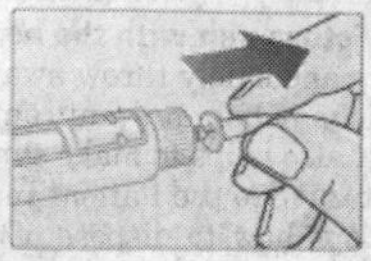

Step G. Dial the Dose

- Victoza pen can give a dose of 0.6 mg (starting dose), 1.2 mg or 1.8 mg. Be sure that you know the dose of Victoza that is prescribed for you.

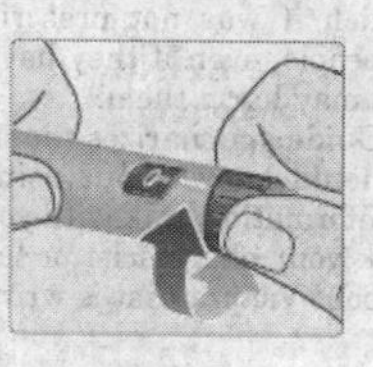

- Turn the dose selector until your needed dose lines up with the pointer (0.6 mg, 1.2 mg or 1.8 mg).

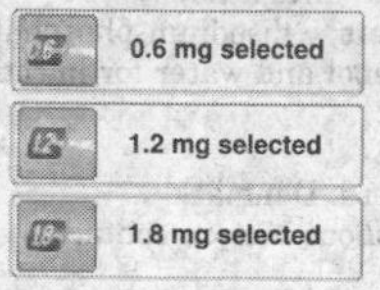

- You will hear a "click" every time you turn the dose selector. **Do not set the dose by counting the number of clicks you hear.**
- If you select a wrong dose, change it by turning the dose selector backwards or forwards until the correct dose lines up with the pointer. Be careful not to press the dose button when turning the dose selector. This may cause Victoza to come out.

Step H. Injecting the Dose

- Insert needle into your skin in the stomach, thigh or upper arm. Use the injection technique shown to you by your healthcare provider. **Do not inject Victoza into a vein or muscle.**

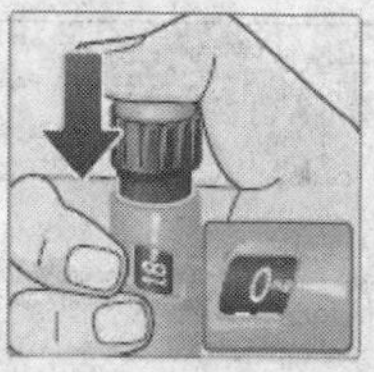

- Press down on the center of the dose button to inject until 0 mg lines up with the pointer.
- Be careful not to touch the dose display with your other fingers. This may block the injection.
- Keep the dose button pressed down and make sure that you keep the needle under the skin for a full count of 6 seconds to make sure the full dose is injected. Keep your thumb on the injection button until you remove the needle from your skin.

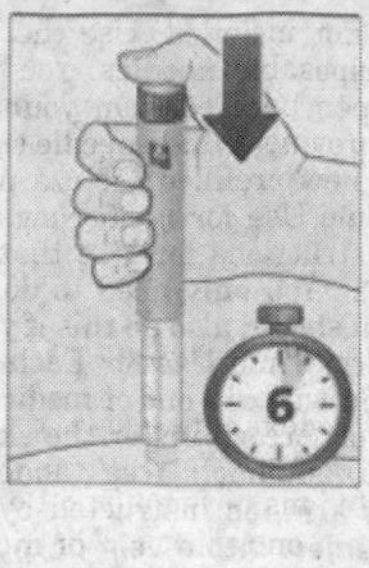

- Change (rotate) your injection sites within the area you choose for each dose. **Do not** use the same injection site for each injection.

Step I. Withdraw Needle

- You may see a drop of Victoza at the needle tip. This is normal and it does not affect the dose you just received. If blood appears after you take the needle out of your skin, apply light pressure, but **do not rub the area.**

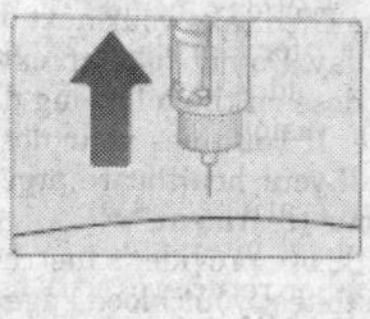

Step J. Remove and Dispose of the Needle

- Carefully put the outer needle cap over the needle. Unscrew the needle.

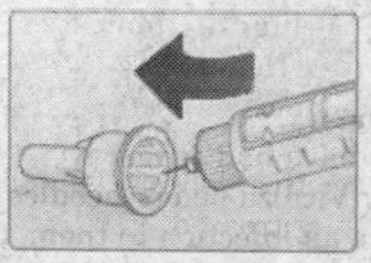

- Safely remove the needle from your Victoza pen after each use.
- Place used needles in a closeable, puncture-resistant container. If your Victoza pen is empty or if you have been using it for 30 days (even if it is not empty), throw away the used pen. You may use a sharps container (such as a red biohazard container), a hard plastic container (such as an empty detergent bottle), or metal container with a screw top (such as an empty coffee can).
- Ask your healthcare provider for instructions on the right way to dispose of your used needles, pens, and the container. Do not throw the disposal container in the household trash. Do not recycle.

Shown in Product Identification Guide, page 311

Onyx Pharmaceuticals, Inc.

249 E. GRAND AVENUE
SOUTH SAN FRANCISCO, CA 94080

Direct Inquires to:
Phone: 877-ONYX-121(669-9121)
Fax: 877-ONX-PHRM(669-7476)
medinfo@onyx.com

KYPROLIS ℞

HIGHLIGHTS OF PRESCRIBING INFORMATION

These highlights do not include all the information needed to use KYPROLIS safely and effectively. See full prescribing information for KYPROLIS.

Initial U.S. Approval: [2012]

INDICATIONS AND USAGE

KYPROLIS is a proteasome inhibitor indicated for the treatment of patients with multiple myeloma who have received at least two prior therapies including bortezomib and an immunomodulatory agent and have demonstrated disease progression on or within 60 days of completion of the last therapy. Approval is based on response rate. Clinical benefit, such as improvement in survival or symptoms, has not been verified. (1, 14)

DOSAGE AND ADMINISTRATION

- Administer intravenously over 2 to 10 minutes, on two consecutive days each week for three weeks (Days 1, 2, 8, 9, 15, and 16), followed by a 12-day rest period (Days 17 to 28). (2.1)
- Recommended Cycle 1 dose is 20 mg/m^2/day and if tolerated increase Cycle 2 dose and subsequent cycles doses to 27 mg/m^2/day. (2.1)
- Hydrate patients prior to and following administration. (2.2)
- Pre-medicate with dexamethasone prior to all Cycle 1 doses, during the first cycle of dose escalation, and if infusion reaction symptoms develop or reappear. (2.3)
- Modify dosing based on toxicity. (2.4)

DOSAGE FORMS AND STRENGTHS

Single-use vial: 60 mg sterile lyophilized powder (3)

CONTRAINDICATIONS

None (4)

WARNINGS AND PRECAUTIONS

- Cardiac Adverse Reactions including heart failure and ischemia: Monitor for cardiac complications. Treat promptly and withhold KYPROLIS. (2.4, 5.1)
- Pulmonary Hypertension: Withhold dosing if suspected. (2.4, 5.2)
- Pulmonary Complications: Monitor for and manage dyspnea immediately; interrupt KYPROLIS until symptoms have resolved or returned to baseline. (2.4, 5.3)
- Infusion Reactions: Pre-medicate with dexamethasone to prevent. (2.3) Advise patients to seek immediate medical attention if symptoms develop. (5.4)
- Tumor Lysis Syndrome (TLS): Hydrate patients to prevent. (2.2) Monitor for TLS and treat promptly. (5.5)
- Thrombocytopenia: Monitor platelet counts; reduce or interrupt dosing as clinically indicated. (2.4, 5.6)
- Hepatic Toxicity and Hepatic Failure: Monitor liver enzymes and withhold dosing if suspected. (2.4, 5.7)
- Embryo-fetal Toxicity: KYPROLIS can cause fetal harm. Females of reproductive potential should avoid becoming pregnant while being treated. (5.8, 8.1)

ADVERSE REACTIONS

Most commonly reported adverse reactions (incidence ≥ 30%) are fatigue, anemia, nausea, thrombocytopenia, dyspnea, diarrhea, and pyrexia. (6)

To report SUSPECTED ADVERSE REACTIONS, contact Onyx Pharmaceuticals, Inc. at 1-877-669-9121or FDA at 1-800-FDA-1088 or *www.fda.gov/medwatch*.

USE IN SPECIFIC POPULATIONS

- Patients on dialysis: Administer KYPROLIS after the dialysis procedure. (8.6)

See 17 for PATIENT COUNSELING INFORMATION

Revised: 07/2012

FULL PRESCRIBING INFORMATION: CONTENTS*

*** Sections or subsections omitted from the full prescribing information are not listed**

FULL PRESCRIBING INFORMATION

1 INDICATIONS AND USAGE

KYPROLIS is indicated for the treatment of patients with multiple myeloma who have received at least two prior therapies including bortezomib and an immunomodulatory agent and have demonstrated disease progression on or within 60 days of completion of the last therapy. Approval is based on response rate [see *Clinical Studies (14.1)*]. Clinical benefit, such as improvement in survival or symptoms, has not been verified.

2 DOSAGE AND ADMINISTRATION

2.1 Dosing Guidelines

KYPROLIS is administered intravenously over 2 to 10 minutes, on two consecutive days, each week for three weeks (Days 1, 2, 8, 9, 15, and 16), followed by a 12-day rest period (Days 17 to 28). Each 28-day period is considered one treatment cycle (Table 1).

In Cycle 1, KYPROLIS is administered at a dose of 20 mg/m^2. If tolerated in Cycle 1, the dose should be escalated to 27 mg/m^2 beginning in Cycle 2 and continued at 27 mg/m^2 in subsequent cycles. Treatment may be continued until disease progression or until unacceptable toxicity occurs [see *Dosage and Administration (2.4)*].

The dose is calculated using the patient's actual body surface area at baseline. Patients with a body surface area greater than 2.2 m^2 should receive a dose based upon a body surface are of 2.2 m^2. Dose adjustments do not need to be made for weight changes of less than or equal to 20%.

[See table 1 above]

Table 1: KYPROLIS Dosage Regimen for Patients with Multiple Myeloma

	Cycle 1									
	Week 1			Week 2			Week 3			Week 4
KYPROLIS (20 mg/m^2):	Day 1	Day 2	Days 3-7	Day 8	Day 9	Days 10-14	Day 15	Day 16	Days 17-21	Days 22-28
	20	20	No Dosing	20	20	No Dosing	20	20	No Dosing	No Dosing
	Cycles 2 and Beyond*									
	Week 1			Week 2			Week 3			Week 4
KYPROLIS (27 mg/m^2):	Day 1	Day 2	Days 3-7	Day 8	Day 9	Days 10-14	Day 15	Day 16	Days 17-21	Days 22-28
	27	27	No Dosing	27	27	No Dosing	27	27	No Dosing	No Dosing

* If previous cycle dosage is tolerated.

2.2 Hydration and Fluid Monitoring

Hydrate patients to reduce the risk of renal toxicity and of tumor lysis syndrome (TLS) with KYPROLIS treatment [see *Warnings and Precautions (5.5)*]. Maintain adequate fluid volume status throughout treatment and monitor blood chemistries closely. Prior to each dose in Cycle 1, give 250 mL to 500 mL of intravenous normal saline or other appropriate intravenous fluid. Give an additional 250 mL to 500 mL of intravenous fluids as needed following KYPROLIS administration. Continue intravenous hydration, as needed, in subsequent cycles. Also monitor patients during this period for fluid overload [see *Warnings and Precautions (5.1)*].

2.3 Dexamethasone Premedication

Pre-medicate with dexamethasone 4 mg orally or intravenously prior to all doses of KYPROLIS during Cycle 1 and prior to all KYPROLIS doses during the first cycle of dose escalation to 27 mg/m^2 to reduce the incidence and severity of infusion reactions [see *Warnings and Precautions (5.4)*]. Reinstate dexamethasone premedication (4 mg orally or intravenously) if these symptoms develop or reappear during subsequent cycles.

2.4 Dose Modifications Based on Toxicities

Recommended actions and dose modifications are presented in Table 2.

Table 2: Dose Modifications for Toxicity* during KYPROLIS Treatment

Hematologic Toxicity	Recommended Action
• Grade 3[a] or 4 Neutropenia • Grade 4 Thrombocytopenia [see *Warnings and Precautions (5.6)*]	• Withhold dose. • If fully recovered before next scheduled dose, continue at same dose level. • If recovered to Grade 2 neutropenia or Grade 3 thrombocytopenia, reduce dose by one dose level (from 27 mg/m^2 to 20 mg/m^2, OR from 20 mg/m^2 to 15 mg/m^2). • If tolerated, the reduced dose may be escalated to the previous dose at the discretion of the physician.
Non-Hematologic Toxicity	**Recommended Action**
Cardiac Toxicity Grade 3 or 4, new onset or worsening of: • congestive heart failure; • decreased left ventricular function; • or myocardial ischemia [see *Warnings and Precautions (5.1)*]	• Withhold until resolved or returned to baseline. • After resolution, consider if restarting KYPROLIS at a reduced dose is appropriate (from 27 mg/m^2 to 20 mg/m^2, OR from 20 mg/m^2 to 15 mg/m^2). • If tolerated, the reduced dose may be escalated to the previous dose at the discretion of the physician.
Pulmonary Hypertension [see *Warnings and Precautions (5.2)*]	• Withhold until resolved or returned to baseline. • Restart at the dose used prior to the event or reduced dose (from 27 mg/m^2 to 20 mg/m^2, OR from 20 mg/m^2 to 15 mg/m^2), at the discretion of the physician. • If tolerated, the reduced dose may be escalated to the previous dose at the discretion of the physician.
Pulmonary Complications • Grade 3 or 4 [see *Warnings and Precautions (5.3)*]	• Withhold until resolved or returned to baseline. • Consider restarting at the next scheduled treatment with one dose level reduction (from 27 mg/m^2 to 20 mg/m^2, OR from 20 mg/m^2 to 15 mg/m^2). • If tolerated, the reduced dose may be escalated to the previous dose at the discretion of the physician.

Hepatic Toxicity • Grade 3 or 4 elevation of transaminases, bilirubin or other liver abnormalities [see *Warnings and Precautions (5.7)*]	• Withhold until resolved or returned to baseline. • After resolution, consider if restarting KYPROLIS is appropriate; may be reinitiated at a reduced dose (from 27 mg/m^2 to 20 mg/m^2, OR from 20 mg/m^2 to 15 mg/m^2) with frequent monitoring of liver function. • If tolerated, the reduced dose may be escalated to the previous dose at the discretion of the physician.
Renal Toxicity • Serum creatinine equal to or greater than 2 × baseline [see *Adverse Reactions (6.1)*]	• Withhold until renal function has recovered to Grade 1 or to baseline and monitor renal function. • If attributable to KYPROLIS, restart at the next scheduled treatment at a reduced dose (from 27 mg/m^2 to 20 mg/m^2, OR from 20 mg/m^2 to 15 mg/m^2). • If not attributable to KYPROLIS, restart at the dose used prior to the event. • If tolerated, the reduced dose may be escalated to the previous dose at the discretion of the physician.
Peripheral Neuropathy • Grade 3 or 4 [see *Adverse Reactions (6.1)*]	• Withhold until resolved or returned to baseline. • Restart at the dose used prior to the event or reduced dose (from 27 mg/m^2 to 20 mg/m^2, OR from 20 mg/m^2 to 15 mg/m^2), at the discretion of the physician. • If tolerated, the reduced dose may be escalated to the previous dose at the discretion of the physician.
Other • Grade 3 or 4 non-hematological toxicities	• Withhold until resolved or returned to baseline. • Consider restarting at the next scheduled treatment with one dose level reduction (from 27 mg/m^2 to 20 mg/m^2, OR from 20 mg/m^2 to 15 mg/m^2). • If tolerated, the reduced dose may be escalated to the previous dose at the discretion of the physician.

* National Cancer Institute Common Terminology Criteria for Adverse Events (NCI CTCAE) Version 3.0

2.5 Administration Precautions

The quantity of KYPROLIS contained in one single-use vial (60 mg carfilzomib) may exceed the required dose. Caution should be used in calculating the quantity delivered to prevent overdosing.

Do not mix KYPROLIS with or administer as an infusion with other medicinal products.

The intravenous administration line should be flushed with normal saline or 5% Dextrose Injection, USP immediately before and after KYPROLIS administration. KYPROLIS should not be administered as a bolus. KYPROLIS should be administered over 2 to 10 minutes.

2.6 Reconstitution and Preparation for Intravenous Administration

KYPROLIS vials contain no antimicrobial preservatives and are intended only for single use. Unopened vials of KYPROLIS are stable until the date indicated on the package when stored in the original package at 2°C to 8°C (36°F to 46°F). The reconstituted solution contains carfilzomib at a concentration of 2 mg/mL. Read the complete preparation instructions prior to reconstitution.

Reconstitution/Preparation Steps:

1. Remove vial from refrigerator just prior to use.
2. Aseptically reconstitute each vial by slowly injecting **29 mL** Sterile Water for Injection, USP, directing the solution onto the INSIDE WALL OF THE VIAL to minimize foaming.

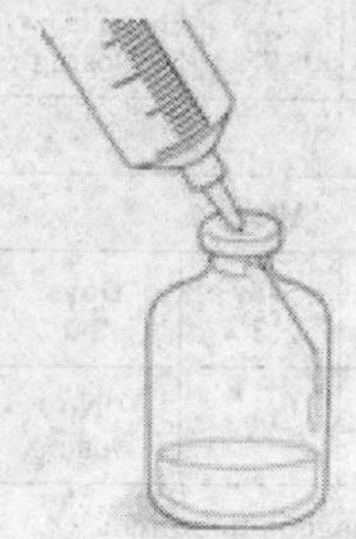

3. Gently swirl and/or invert the vial slowly for about 1 minute, or until complete dissolution of any cake or powder occurs. DO NOT SHAKE to avoid foam generation. If foaming occurs, allow solution to rest in vial for about 2 to 5 minutes, until foaming subsides.
4. After reconstitution, KYPROLIS is ready for intravenous administration. The reconstituted product should be a clear, colorless solution. If any discoloration or particulate matter is observed, do not use the reconstituted product.
5. When administering in an intravenous bag, withdraw the calculated dose [see *Dosage and Administration (2.1)*] from the vial and dilute into **50 mL** 5% Dextrose Injection, USP intravenous bag.
6. Immediately discard the vial containing the unused portion.

The stabilities of reconstituted KYPROLIS under various temperature and container conditions are shown in Table 3. [See table 3 below]

3 DOSAGE FORMS AND STRENGTHS

KYPROLIS single-use vial contains 60 mg of carfilzomib as a sterile, white to off-white lyophilized cake or powder.

4 CONTRAINDICATIONS

None.

5 WARNINGS AND PRECAUTIONS

5.1 Cardiac Arrest, Congestive Heart Failure, Myocardial Ischemia

Death due to cardiac arrest has occurred within a day of KYPROLIS administration. New onset or worsening of preexisting congestive heart failure with decreased left ventricular function or myocardial ischemia have occurred following administration of KYPROLIS. Cardiac failure events (e.g., cardiac failure congestive, pulmonary edema, ejection fraction decreased) were reported in 7% of patients. Monitor for cardiac complications and manage promptly. Withhold KYPROLIS for Grade 3 or 4 cardiac events until recovery and consider whether to restart KYPROLIS based on a benefit/risk assessment [see *Dosage and Administration (2.4)*]. Patients with New York Heart Association Class III and IV heart failure, myocardial infarction in the preceding 6 months, and conduction abnormalities uncontrolled by medications were not eligible for the clinical trials. These patients may be at greater risk for cardiac complications.

5.2 Pulmonary Hypertension

Pulmonary arterial hypertension (PAH) was reported in 2% of patients treated with KYPROLIS and was Grade 3 or greater in less than 1% of patients. Evaluate with cardiac imaging and/or other tests as indicated. Withhold KYPROLIS for pulmonary hypertension until resolved or returned to baseline and consider whether to restart KYPROLIS based on a benefit/risk assessment [see *Dosage and Administration (2.4)*].

5.3 Pulmonary Complications

Dyspnea was reported in 35% of patients enrolled in clinical trials. Grade 3 dyspnea occurred in 5%; no Grade 4 events, and 1 death (Grade 5) was reported. Monitor and manage dyspnea immediately; interrupt KYPROLIS until symptoms have resolved or returned to baseline [see *Dosage and Administration (2.4) and Adverse Reactions (6.1)*].

5.4 Infusion Reactions

Infusion reactions were characterized by a spectrum of systemic symptoms including fever, chills, arthralgia, myalgia, facial flushing, facial edema, vomiting, weakness, shortness of breath, hypotension, syncope, chest tightness, or angina. These reactions can occur immediately following or up to 24 hours after administration of KYPROLIS. Administer dexamethasone prior to KYPROLIS to reduce the incidence and severity of reactions [see *Dosage and Administration (2.3)*]. Inform patients of the risk and symptoms and to contact physician if symptoms of an infusion reaction occur [see *Patient Counseling Information (17)*].

5.5 Tumor Lysis Syndrome

Tumor lysis syndrome (TLS) occurred following KYPROLIS administration in < 1% of patients. Patients with multiple myeloma and a high tumor burden should be considered to be at greater risk for TLS. Prior to receiving KYPROLIS, ensure that patients are well hydrated [see *Dosage and Administration (2.2)*]. Monitor for evidence of TLS during treatment, and manage promptly. Interrupt KYPROLIS until TLS is resolved [see *Dosage and Administration (2.4)*].

5.6 Thrombocytopenia

KYPROLIS causes thrombocytopenia with platelet nadirs occurring around Day 8 of each 28-day cycle and recovery to baseline by the start of the next 28-day cycle. In patients with multiple myeloma, 36% of patients experienced thrombocytopenia, including Grade 4 in 10%. Thrombocytopenia following KYPROLIS administration resulted in a dose reduction in 1% of patients and discontinuation of treatment with KYPROLIS in < 1% of patients. Monitor platelet counts frequently during treatment with KYPROLIS. Reduce or interrupt dose as clinically indicated [see *Dosage and Administration (2.4)*].

5.7 Hepatic Toxicity and Hepatic Failure

Cases of hepatic failure, including fatal cases, have been reported (< 1%). KYPROLIS can cause elevations of serum transaminases and bilirubin. Withhold KYPROLIS in patients experiencing Grade 3 or greater elevations of transaminases, bilirubin, or other liver abnormalities until resolved or returned to baseline. After resolution, consider if restarting KYPROLIS is appropriate. Monitor liver enzymes frequently [see *Dosage and Administration (2.4) and Adverse Reactions (6.1)*].

5.8 Embryo-fetal Toxicity

KYPROLIS can cause fetal harm when administered to a pregnant woman based on its mechanism of action and findings in animals. There are no adequate and well-controlled studies in pregnant women using KYPROLIS. Carfilzomib caused embryo-fetal toxicity in pregnant rabbits at doses that were lower than in patients receiving the recommended dose.

Females of reproductive potential should be advised to avoid becoming pregnant while being treated with KYPROLIS. If this drug is used during pregnancy, or if the patient becomes pregnant while taking this drug, the patient should be apprised of the potential hazard to the fetus [see *Use in Specific Populations (8.1)*].

6 ADVERSE REACTIONS

The following adverse reactions are discussed in greater detail in other sections of the labeling:

- Cardiac Arrest, Congestive Heart Failure, Myocardial Ischemia [see *Warnings and Precautions (5.1)*]
- Pulmonary Hypertension [see *Warnings and Precautions (5.2)*]
- Pulmonary Complications [see *Warnings and Precautions (5.3)*]
- Infusion Reactions [see *Warnings and Precautions (5.4)*]
- Tumor Lysis Syndrome [see *Warnings and Precautions (5.5)*]
- Thrombocytopenia [see *Warnings and Precautions (5.6)*]
- Hepatic Toxicity and Hepatic Failure [see *Warnings and Precautions (5.7)*]

The most common adverse reactions (incidence of 30% or greater) to KYPROLIS observed in clinical trials of patients with multiple myeloma were fatigue, anemia, nausea, thrombocytopenia, dyspnea, diarrhea, and pyrexia.

6.1 Clinical Trials Safety Experience

Because clinical trials are conducted under widely varying conditions, adverse reaction rates observed in the clinical trials of a drug cannot be directly compared with rates in the clinical trials of another drug, and may not reflect the rates observed in medical practice.

A total of 526 patients with relapsed and/or refractory multiple myeloma received KYPROLIS as monotherapy or with pre-dose dexamethasone. Patients received a median of four

Table 3: Stability of Reconstituted KYPROLIS

Storage Conditions of Reconstituted KYPROLIS	Stability* per Container		
	Vial	Syringe	IV Bag (D5W†)
Refrigerated (2°C to 8°C; 36°F to 46°F)	24 hours	24 hours	24 hours
Room Temperature (15°C to 30°C; 59°F to 86°F)	4 hours	4 hours	4 hours

* Total time from reconstitution to administration should not exceed 24 hours.
† 5% Dextrose Injection, USP.

treatment cycles with a median cumulative KYPROLIS dose of 993.4 mg.

Deaths due to all causes within 30 days of the last dose of KYPROLIS occurred in 37/526 (7%) of patients. Deaths not attributed to disease progression were cardiac in 5 patients (acute coronary syndrome, cardiac arrest, cardiac disorder), end-organ failure in 4 patients (multi-organ failure, hepatic failure, renal failure), infection in 4 patients (sepsis, pneumonia, respiratory tract bacterial infection), dyspnea and intracranial hemorrhage in 1 patient each, and 1 patient found dead of unknown causes.

Serious adverse reactions were reported in 45% patients. The most common serious adverse reactions were pneumonia (10%), acute renal failure (4%), pyrexia (3%), and congestive heart failure (3%). Adverse reactions leading to discontinuation of KYPROLIS occurred in 15% of patients and included congestive heart failure (2%), cardiac arrest, dyspnea, increased blood creatinine, and acute renal failure (1% each).

Adverse reactions occurring at a rate of 10% or greater are presented in Table 4.

Table 4: Incidence of Adverse Reactions Occurring in ≥ 10% of Multiple Myeloma Patients Treated with KYPROLIS

Event	Patients (N = 526) [n (%)] All Grades*	Grade 3 Events	Grade 4 Events
Fatigue	292 (55.5)	38 (7.2)	2 (0.4)
Anemia	246 (46.8)	111 (21.1)	7 (1.3)
Nausea	236 (44.9)	7 (1.3)	0
Thrombocytopenia	191 (36.3)	69 (13.1)	54 (10.3)
Dyspnea	182 (34.6)	25 (4.8)	1 (0.2)†
Diarrhea	172 (32.7)	4 (0.8)	1 (0.2)
Pyrexia	160 (30.4)	7 (1.3)	2 (0.4)
Upper respiratory tract infection	149 (28.3)	17 (3.2)	0
Headache	145 (27.6)	7 (1.3)	0
Cough	137 (26.0)	1 (0.2)	0
Blood creatinine increased	127 (24.1)	13 (2.5)	1 (0.2)
Lymphopenia	126 (24.0)	84 (16.0)	11 (2.1)
Edema peripheral	126 (24.0)	3 (0.6)	0
Vomiting	117 (22.2)	5 (1.0)	0
Constipation	110 (20.9)	1 (0.2)	0
Neutropenia	109 (20.7)	50 (9.5)	4 (0.8)
Back pain	106 (20.2)	15 (2.9)	0
Insomnia	94 (17.9)	0	0
Chills	84 (16.0)	1 (0.2)	0
Arthralgia	83 (15.8)	7 (1.3)	0
Muscle spasms	76 (14.4)	2 (0.4)	0
Hypertension	75 (14.3)	15 (2.9)	2 (0.4)
Asthenia	73 (13.9)	12 (2.3)	1 (0.2)
Hypokalemia	72 (13.7)	14 (2.7)	3 (0.6)
Hypomagnesemia	71 (13.5)	2 (0.4)	0
Leukopenia	71 (13.5)	27 (5.1)	1 (0.2)
Pain in extremity	70 (13.3)	7 (1.3)	0
Pneumonia	67 (12.7)	52 (9.9)	3 (0.6)†
Aspartate aminotransferase increased	66 (12.5)	15 (2.9)	1 (0.2)
Dizziness	66 (12.5)	5 (1.0)	1 (0.2)
Hypoesthesia	64 (12.2)	3 (0.6)	0
Anorexia	63 (12.0)	1 (0.2)	0
Pain	63 (12.0)	12 (2.3)	1 (0.2)
Hyperglycemia	62 (11.8)	16 (3.0)	3 (0.6)
Chest wall pain	60 (11.4)	3 (0.6)	0
Hypercalcemia	58 (11.0)	13 (2.5)	8 (1.5)
Hypophosphatemia	55 (10.5)	24 (4.6)	3 (0.6)
Hyponatremia	54 (10.3)	31 (5.9)	3 (0.6)

* National Cancer Institute Common Terminology Criteria for Adverse Events (NCI CTCAE) Version 3.0
† One event was Grade 5 severity.

Description of Selected Adverse Drug Reactions

Renal Events

The most common renal adverse reactions were increase in blood creatinine (24%) and renal failure (9%), which were mostly Grade 1 or Grade 2 in severity. Grade 3 renal adverse reactions occurred in 6% of patients and Grade 4 events occurred in 1%. Discontinuations due to increased blood creatinine and acute renal failure were 1% each. In one patient, death occurred with concurrent sepsis and worsening renal function [see *Dosage and Administration (2.4)*].

Peripheral Neuropathy

Peripheral neuropathy (including all events of peripheral sensory neuropathy and peripheral motor neuropathy) occurred in 14% of patients enrolled in clinical trials. Grade 3 peripheral neuropathy occurred in 1% of patients. Serious peripheral neuropathy events occurred in < 1% of patients, which resulted in dose reduction in < 1% and treatment discontinuation in < 1%. Withhold or discontinue treatment as recommended [see *Dosage and Administration (2.4)*].

Herpes Virus Infection

Herpes zoster reactivation was reported in 2% of patients. Consider antiviral prophylaxis for patients who have a history of herpes zoster infection.

7 DRUG INTERACTIONS

Carfilzomib is primarily metabolized via peptidase and epoxide hydrolase activities, and as a result, the pharmacokinetic profile of carfilzomib is unlikely to be affected by concomitant administration of cytochrome P450 inhibitors and inducers. Carfilzomib is not expected to influence exposure of other drugs [see *Clinical Pharmacology (12.3)*].

8 USE IN SPECIFIC POPULATIONS

8.1 Pregnancy

Pregnancy Category D [*see Warnings and Precautions (5.8)*]. Females of reproductive potential should be advised to avoid becoming pregnant while being treated with KYPROLIS. Based on its mechanism of action and findings in animals, KYPROLIS can cause fetal harm when administered to a pregnant woman. Carfilzomib caused embryo-fetal toxicity in pregnant rabbits at doses that were lower than in patients receiving the recommended dose. If KYPROLIS is used during pregnancy, or if the patient becomes pregnant while taking this drug, the patient should be apprised of the potential hazard to the fetus.

Carfilzomib was administered intravenously to pregnant rats and rabbits during the period of organogenesis at doses of 0.5, 1, and 2 mg/kg/day in rats and 0.2, 0.4, and 0.8 mg/kg/day in rabbits. Carfilzomib was not teratogenic at any dose tested. In rabbits, there was an increase in pre-implantation loss at ≥ 0.4 mg/kg/day and an increase in early resorptions and post-implantation loss and a decrease in fetal weight at the maternally toxic dose of 0.8 mg/kg/day. The doses of 0.4 and 0.8 mg/kg/day in rabbits are approximately 20% and 40%, respectively, of the recommended dose in humans of 27 mg/m^2 based on body surface area.

8.3 Nursing Mothers

It is not known whether KYPROLIS is excreted in human milk. Since many drugs are excreted in human milk and because of the potential for serious adverse reactions in nursing infants from KYPROLIS, a decision should be made whether to discontinue nursing or to discontinue the drug, taking into account the importance of the drug to the mother.

8.4 Pediatric Use

The safety and effectiveness of KYPROLIS in pediatric patients have not been established.

8.5 Geriatric Use

In studies of KYPROLIS there were no clinically significant differences observed in safety and efficacy between patients less than 65 years of age and patients 65 years of age and older.

8.6 Renal Impairment

The pharmacokinetics and safety of KYPROLIS were evaluated in a Phase 2 trial in patients with normal renal function and those with mild, moderate, and severe renal impairment and patients on chronic dialysis. On average, patients were treated for 5.5 cycles using KYPROLIS doses of 15 mg/m^2 on Cycle 1, 20 mg/m^2 on Cycle 2, and 27 mg/m^2 on Cycles 3 and beyond. The pharmacokinetics and safety of KYPROLIS were not influenced by the degree of baseline renal impairment, including the patients on dialysis. Since dialysis clearance of KYPROLIS concentrations has not been studied, the drug should be administered after the dialysis procedure [see *Clinical Pharmacology (12.3)*].

8.7 Hepatic Impairment

The safety, efficacy and pharmacokinetics of KYPROLIS have not been evaluated in patients with baseline hepatic impairment. Patients with the following laboratory values were excluded from the KYPROLIS clinical trials: ALT/AST ≥ 3 × upper limit of normal (ULN) and bilirubin > 2 × ULN [see *Clinical Pharmacology (12.3)*].

8.8 Cardiac Impairment

Patients with New York Heart Association Class III and IV heart failure were not eligible for the clinical trials. Safety in this population has not been evaluated.

10 OVERDOSAGE

There is no known specific antidote for KYPROLIS overdosage. In the event of an overdosage, monitor the patient and provide appropriate supportive care.

11 DESCRIPTION

KYPROLIS (carfilzomib) for Injection is an antineoplastic agent available for intravenous use only. KYPROLIS is a sterile, white to off-white lyophilized powder and is available as a single-use vial. Each vial of KYPROLIS contains 60 mg of carfilzomib, 3000 mg sulfobutylether beta-cyclodextrin, 57.7 mg citric acid, and sodium hydroxide for pH adjustment (target pH 3.5).

Carfilzomib is a modified tetrapeptidyl epoxide, isolated as the crystalline free base. The chemical name for carfilzomib is (2S)-N-((S)-1-((S)-4-methyl-1-((R)-2-methyloxiran-2-yl)-1-oxopentan-2-ylcarbamoyl)-2-phenylethyl)-2-((S)-2-(2-morpholinoacetamido)-4-phenylbutanamido)-4-methylpentanamide. Carfilzomib has the following structure:

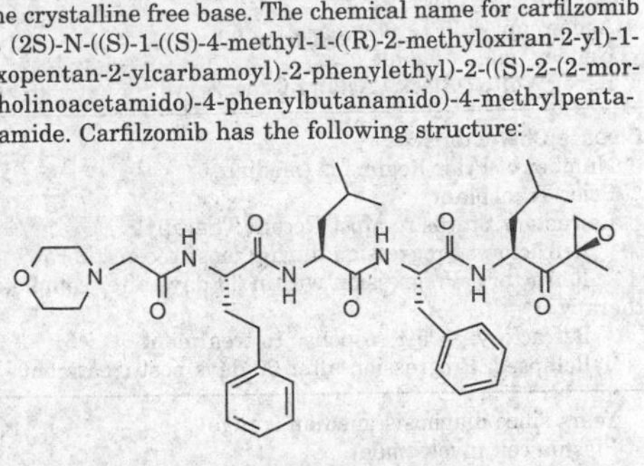

Carfilzomib is a crystalline substance with a molecular weight of 719.9. The molecular formula is $C_{40}H_{57}N_5O_7$. Carfilzomib is practically insoluble in water, and very slightly soluble in acidic conditions.

12 CLINICAL PHARMACOLOGY

12.1 Mechanism of Action

Carfilzomib is a tetrapeptide epoxyketone proteasome inhibitor that irreversibly binds to the N-terminal threonine-containing active sites of the 20S proteasome, the proteolytic core particle within the 26S proteasome. Carfilzomib had antiproliferative and proapoptotic activities *in vitro* in solid and hematologic tumor cells. In animals, carfilzomib inhibited proteasome activity in blood and tissue and delayed tumor growth in models of multiple myeloma, hematologic, and solid tumors.

12.2 Pharmacodynamics

Intravenous carfilzomib administration resulted in suppression of proteasome chymotrypsin-like activity when measured in blood 1 hour after the first dose. On Day 1 of Cycle 1, proteasome inhibition in peripheral blood mononuclear cells (PBMCs) ranged from 79% to 89% at 15 mg/m^2, and from 82% to 83% at 20 mg/m^2. In addition, carfilzomib administration resulted in inhibition of the LMP2 and MECL1 subunits of the immunoproteasome ranging from 26% to 32% and 41% to 49%, respectively, at 20 mg/m^2. Proteasome inhibition was maintained for ≥ 48 hours following the first dose of carfilzomib for each week of dosing.

12.3 Pharmacokinetics

Absorption: The C_{max} and AUC following a single intravenous dose of 27 mg/m^2 was 4232 ng/mL and 379 ng•hr/mL, respectively. Following repeated doses of carfilzomib at 15 and 20 mg/m^2, systemic exposure (AUC) and half-life were similar on Days 1 and 15 or 16 of Cycle 1, suggesting there was no systemic carfilzomib accumulation. At doses between 20 and 36 mg/m^2, there was a dose-dependent increase in exposure.

Distribution: The mean steady-state volume of distribution of a 20 mg/m^2 dose of carfilzomib was 28 L. When tested *in vitro*, the binding of carfilzomib to human plasma proteins averaged 97% over the concentration range of 0.4 to 4 micromolar.

Metabolism: Carfilzomib was rapidly and extensively metabolized. The predominant metabolites measured in human plasma and urine, and generated *in vitro* by human hepatocytes, were peptide fragments and the diol of carfilzomib, suggesting that peptidase cleavage and epoxide hydrolysis were the principal pathways of metabolism. Cytochrome P450-mediated mechanisms played a minor role in overall carfilzomib metabolism. The metabolites have no known biologic activity.

Elimination: Following intravenous administration of doses ≥ 15 mg/m^2, carfilzomib was rapidly cleared from the systemic circulation with a half-life of ≤ 1 hour on Day 1 of Cycle 1. The systemic clearance ranged from 151 to 263 L/hour, and exceeded hepatic blood flow, suggesting that carfilzomib was largely cleared extrahepatically. The pathways of carfilzomib elimination have not been characterized in humans.

Age: Analysis of population pharmacokinetics data after the first dose of Cycle 1 (Day 1) in 154 patients who had received an IV dose of 20 mg/m^2 showed no clinically significant difference in exposure between patients < 65 years and ≥ 65 years of age.

Gender: Mean dose-normalized AUC and C_{max} values were comparable between male and female patients in the population pharmacokinetics study.

Table 5: Demographics and Baseline Disease Characteristics

Characteristic	Number of Patients (%)
Patient Characteristics	
Enrolled patients	266 (100)
Median age, years (range)	63.0 (37, 87)
Age group, < 65 / ≥ 65 (years)	146 (54.9) / 120 (45.1)
Gender (male / female)	155 (58.3) / 111 (41.7)
Race (White / Black / Asian / Other)	190 (71.4) / 53 (19.9) / 6 (2.3) / 17 (6.4)
Disease Characteristics	
Number of Prior Regimens (median)	5*
Prior Transplant	198 (74.4)
Refractory Status to Most Recent Therapy†	
Refractory: Progression during most recent therapy	198 (74.4)
Refractory: Progression within 60 days after completion of most recent therapy	38 (14.3)
Refractory: ≤ 25% response to treatment	16 (6.0)
Relapsed: Progression after 60 days post treatment	14 (5.3)
Years since diagnosis, median (range)	5.35 (0.5, 22.3)
Plasma cell involvement (< 50% / ≥ 50% / unknown or missing)	143 (53.8) / 106 (39.8) / 17 (6.4)
Cytogenetics or FISH analyses	
Normal/Favorable	159 (59.8)
Poor Prognosis	75 (28.2)
Unknown/Not tested	32 (12.0)
Serum Beta-2 Microglobulin median (range)	4.3 (0.4, 20.5)
Creatinine clearance < 30 (mL/min)	6 (2.3)

* Range: 1, 20.
† Categories for refractory status are derived by programmatic assessment using available laboratory data.

Hepatic Impairment: No pharmacokinetic studies were performed with KYPROLIS in patients with hepatic impairment [see *Warnings and Precautions (5.7)*].

Renal Impairment: A pharmacokinetic study was conducted in which 43 multiple myeloma patients who had various degrees of renal impairment and who were classified according to their creatinine clearances (CLcr) into the following groups: normal function (CLcr > 80 mL/min, n = 8), mild impairment (CLcr 50–80 mL/min, n = 12), moderate impairment (CLcr 30–49 mL/min, n = 8), severe impairment (CLcr < 30 mL/min, n = 7), and chronic dialysis (n = 8). KYPROLIS was administered intravenously over 2 to 10 minutes, on two consecutive days, weekly for three weeks (Days 1, 2, 8, 9, 15, and 16), followed by a 12-day rest period every 28 days. Patients received an initial dose of 15 mg/m^2, which could be escalated to 20 mg/m^2 starting in Cycle 2 if 15 mg/m^2 was well tolerated in Cycle 1. In this study, renal function status had no effect on the clearance or exposure of carfilzomib following a single or repeat-dose administration [see *Use in Specific Populations (8.6)*].

Cytochrome P450: In an *in vitro* study using human liver microsomes, carfilzomib showed modest direct and time-dependent inhibitory effect on human cytochrome CYP3A4/5. *In vitro* studies indicated that carfilzomib did not induce human CYP1A2 and CYP3A4 in cultured fresh human hepatocytes. Cytochrome P450-mediated mechanisms play a minor role in the overall metabolism of carfilzomib. A clinical trial of 17 patients using oral midazolam as a CYP3A probe demonstrated that the pharmacokinetics of midazolam were unaffected by concomitant carfilzomib administration. KYPROLIS is not expected to inhibit CYP3A4/5 activities and/or affect the exposure to CYP3A4/5 substrates.

P-gp: Carfilzomib is a P-glycoprotein (P-gp) substrate and showed marginal inhibitory effects on P-gp in a Caco-2 monolayer system. Given that KYPROLIS is administrated intravenously and is extensively metabolized, the pharmacokinetic profile of KYPROLIS is unlikely to be affected by P-gp inhibitors or inducers.

13 NONCLINICAL TOXICOLOGY

13.1 Carcinogenesis, Mutagenesis, Impairment of Fertility

Carcinogenicity studies have not been conducted with carfilzomib.

Carfilzomib was clastogenic in the *in vitro* chromosomal aberration test in peripheral blood lymphocytes. Carfilzomib was not mutagenic in the *in vitro* bacterial reverse mutation (Ames) test and was not clastogenic in the *in vivo* mouse bone marrow micronucleus assay.

Fertility studies with carfilzomib have not been conducted. No effects on reproductive tissues were noted during 28-day repeat-dose rat and monkey toxicity studies or in 6-month rat and 9-month monkey chronic toxicity studies.

13.2 Animal Toxicology and/or Pharmacology

Monkeys administered a single bolus intravenous dose of carfilzomib at 3 mg/kg (approximately 1.3 times recommended dose in humans of 27 mg/m^2 based on body surface area) experienced hypotension, increased heart rate, and increased serum levels of troponin-T. The repeated bolus intravenous administration of carfilzomib at ≥ 2 mg/kg/dose in rats and 2 mg/kg/dose in monkeys using dosing schedules similar to those used clinically resulted in mortalities that were due to toxicities occurring in the cardiovascular (cardiac failure, cardiac fibrosis, pericardial fluid accumulation, cardiac hemorrhage/degeneration), gastrointestinal (necrosis/hemorrhage), renal (glomerulonephropathy, tubular necrosis, dysfunction), and pulmonary (hemorrhage/inflammation) systems. The dose of 2 mg/kg/dose in rats is approximately half the recommended dose in humans of 27 mg/m^2 based on body surface area. The dose of 2 mg/kg/dose in monkeys is approximately equivalent to the recommended dose in humans based on body surface area.

14 CLINICAL STUDIES

14.1 Relapsed Multiple Myeloma

The safety and efficacy of KYPROLIS were evaluated in a single-arm, multicenter clinical trial. Two hundred and sixty-six patients with relapsed multiple myeloma who had received at least two prior therapies (including bortezomib and thalidomide and/or lenalidomide) were enrolled. Patients were enrolled in the trial whose disease had a less than or equal to 25% response to the most recent therapy or had disease progression during or within 60 days of the most recent therapy. Patients were excluded from the trial with total bilirubin levels ≥ 2 × upper limit of normal (ULN); creatinine clearance rates < 30 mL/min; New York Heart Association Class III to IV congestive heart failure; symptomatic cardiac ischemia; myocardial infarction within the last 6 months; peripheral neuropathy Grade 3 or 4, or peripheral neuropathy Grade 2 with pain; active infections requiring treatment; and pleural effusion.

KYPROLIS was administered intravenously over 2 to 10 minutes on two consecutive days each week for three weeks, followed by a 12-day rest period (28-day treatment cycle), until disease progression, unacceptable toxicity, or for a maximum of 12 cycles. Patients received 20 mg/m^2 at each dose in Cycle 1, and 27 mg/m^2 in subsequent cycles. To reduce the incidence and severity of fever, rigors, chills, dyspnea, myalgia, and arthralgia, dexamethasone 4 mg by mouth or by intravenous infusion was administered prior to all KYPROLIS doses during the first cycle and prior to all KYPROLIS doses during the first dose-escalation (27 mg/m^2) cycle. Dexamethasone premedication (4 mg orally or intravenously) was reinstated if these symptoms reappeared during subsequent cycles.

Baseline patient and disease characteristics are summarized in Table 5.

[See table 5 above]

The median number of cycles started was four.

The primary endpoint was the overall response rate (ORR) as determined by Independent Review Committee assessment using International Myeloma Working Group criteria. The ORR (stringent complete response [sCR] + complete response [CR] + very good partial response [VGPR] + partial response [PR]) was 22.9% (95% CI: 18.0, 28.5) (N = 266) (see Table 6). The median duration of response (DOR) was 7.8 months (95% CI: 5.6, 9.2).

Table 6: Response Categories

Characteristic	Study Patients n (%)
Number of patients (%)	266 (100)
Response category*	
Complete response	1 (0.4)
Very good partial response	13 (4.9)
Partial response	47 (17.7)
Overall response	61 (22.9)
95% CI†	(18.0, 28.5)

* As assessed by the Independent Review Committee.
† Exact confidence interval.

16 HOW SUPPLIED/STORAGE AND HANDLING

16.1 How Supplied

KYPROLIS (carfilzomib) for Injection is supplied as an individually cartoned single-use vial containing a dose of 60 mg of carfilzomib as a white to off-white lyophilized cake or powder.

• NDC 76075-101-01, 60 mg carfilzomib per vial

16.2 Storage and Handling

Unopened vials should be stored refrigerated (2°C to 8°C; 36°F to 46°F). Retain in original package to protect from light.

17 PATIENT COUNSELING INFORMATION

Discuss the following with patients prior to treatment with KYPROLIS:

Instruct patients to contact their physician if they develop any of the following symptoms: fever, chills, rigors, chest pain, cough, or swelling of the feet or legs.

Advise patients that KYPROLIS may cause fatigue, dizziness, fainting, and/or drop in blood pressure. Advise patients not to drive or operate machinery if they experience any of these symptoms.

Advise patients that they may experience shortness of breath (dyspnea) during treatment with KYPROLIS. This most commonly occurs within a day of dosing. Advise patients to contact their physicians if they experience shortness of breath.

Counsel patients to avoid dehydration, since patients receiving KYPROLIS therapy may experience vomiting and/or diarrhea. Instruct patients to seek medical advice if they experience symptoms of dizziness, lightheadedness, or fainting spells.

Counsel females of reproductive potential to use effective contraceptive measures to prevent pregnancy during treatment with KYPROLIS. Advise the patient that if she becomes pregnant during treatment, to contact her physician immediately. Advise patients not to take KYPROLIS treatment while pregnant or breastfeeding. If a patient wishes to restart breastfeeding after treatment, advise her to discuss the appropriate timing with her physician.

Advise patients to discuss with their physician any medication they are currently taking prior to starting treatment with KYPROLIS, or prior to starting any new medication(s) during treatment with KYPROLIS.

Manufactured for:
Onyx Pharmaceuticals, Inc.
249 East Grand Avenue
South San Francisco, CA 94080

U.S. Patent Numbers: 7,232,818; 7,417,042; 7,491,704; 7,737,112

05-1088-00

Shown in Product Identification Guide, page 311

Otsuka America Pharmaceutical, Inc.

2440 RESEARCH BOULEVARD
ROCKVILLE, MD 20850

Direct Inquiries to:
Medical Affairs
Otsuka America Pharmaceutical, Inc.
(800) 441-6763
FAX: 301-212-8634
To Request Routine or Emergency Medical Information, or to Report an Adverse Experience:
(800) 438-9927

ABILIFY® ℞
(aripiprazole)
Tablets
ABILIFY DISCMELT®
(aripiprazole)
Orally Disintegrating Tablets
ABILIFY®
(aripiprazole)
Oral Solution
ABILIFY®
(aripiprazole)
Injection FOR INTRAMUSCULAR USE ONLY

HIGHLIGHTS OF PRESCRIBING INFORMATION
These highlights do not include all the information needed to use ABILIFY safely and effectively. See full prescribing information for ABILIFY.
ABILIFY® (aripiprazole) Tablets
ABILIFY DISCMELT® (aripiprazole) Orally Disintegrating Tablets
ABILIFY® (aripiprazole) Oral Solution
ABILIFY® (aripiprazole) Injection FOR INTRAMUSCULAR USE ONLY
Initial U.S. Approval: 2002

WARNINGS: INCREASED MORTALITY IN ELDERLY PATIENTS WITH DEMENTIA-RELATED PSYCHOSIS and SUICIDALITY AND ANTIDEPRESSANT DRUGS
See full prescribing information for complete boxed warning.
- **Elderly patients with dementia-related psychosis treated with antipsychotic drugs are at an increased risk of death. ABILIFY is not approved for the treatment of patients with dementia-related psychosis. (5.1)**
- **Children, adolescents, and young adults taking antidepressants for major depressive disorder (MDD) and other psychiatric disorders are at increased risk of suicidal thinking and behavior. (5.2)**

INDICATIONS AND USAGE

ABILIFY is an atypical antipsychotic indicated as oral formulations for the:
Treatment of schizophrenia (1.1)
- Adults: Efficacy was established in four 4-6 week trials and one maintenance trial in patients with schizophrenia (14.1)
- Adolescents (ages 13-17): Efficacy was established in one 6-week trial in patients with schizophrenia (14.1)

Acute treatment of manic or mixed episodes associated with bipolar I disorder as monotherapy and as an adjunct to lithium or valproate (1.2)
- Adults: Efficacy was established in four 3-week monotherapy trials and one 6-week adjunctive trial in patients with manic or mixed episodes (14.2)
- Pediatric Patients (ages 10-17): Efficacy was established in one 4-week monotherapy trial in patients with manic or mixed episodes (14.2)

Maintenance treatment of bipolar I disorder, both as monotherapy and as an adjunct to lithium or valproate (1.2)
- Adults: Efficacy was established in one maintenance monotherapy trial and in one maintenance adjunctive trial (14.2)

Adjunctive treatment of major depressive disorder (MDD) (1.3)
- Adults: Efficacy was established in two 6-week trials in patients with MDD who had an inadequate response to antidepressant therapy during the current episode (14.3)

Treatment of irritability associated with autistic disorder (1.4)
- Pediatric Patients (ages 6-17 years): Efficacy was established in two 8-week trials in patients with autistic disorder (14.4)

	Initial Dose	Recommended Dose	Maximum Dose
Schizophrenia – adults (2.1)	10-15 mg/day	10-15 mg/day	30 mg/day
Schizophrenia – adolescents (2.1)	2 mg/day	10 mg/day	30 mg/day
Bipolar mania – adults: monotherapy (2.2)	15 mg/day	15 mg/day	30 mg/day
Bipolar mania – adults: adjunct to lithium or valproate (2.2)	10-15 mg/day	15 mg/day	30 mg/day
Bipolar mania – pediatric patients: monotherapy or as an adjunct to lithium or valproate (2.2)	2 mg/day	10 mg/day	30 mg/day
As an adjunct to antidepressants for the treatment of major depressive disorder – adults (2.3)	2-5 mg/day	5-10 mg/day	15 mg/day
Irritability associated with autistic disorder – pediatric patients (2.4)	2 mg/day	5-10 mg/day	15 mg/day
Agitation associated with schizophrenia or bipolar mania – adults (2.5)	9.75 mg/1.3 mL injected IM		30 mg/day injected IM

as an injection for the:
Acute treatment of agitation associated with schizophrenia or bipolar I disorder (1.5)
- Adults: Efficacy was established in three 24-hour trials in agitated patients with schizophrenia or manic/mixed episodes of bipolar I disorder (14.5)

DOSAGE AND ADMINISTRATION

[See table above]
- Oral formulations: Administer once daily without regard to meals (2)
- IM injection: Wait at least 2 hours between doses. Maximum daily dose 30 mg (2.5)

DOSAGE FORMS AND STRENGTHS

- Tablets: 2 mg, 5 mg, 10 mg, 15 mg, 20 mg, and 30 mg (3)
- Orally Disintegrating Tablets: 10 mg and 15 mg (3)
- Oral Solution: 1 mg/mL (3)
- Injection: 9.75 mg/1.3 mL single-dose vial (3)

CONTRAINDICATIONS

Known hypersensitivity to ABILIFY (4)

WARNINGS AND PRECAUTIONS

- *Elderly Patients with Dementia-Related Psychosis:* Increased incidence of cerebrovascular adverse events (eg, stroke, transient ischemic attack, including fatalities) (5.1)
- *Suicidality and Antidepressants:* Increased risk of suicidality in children, adolescents, and young adults with major depressive disorder (5.2)
- *Neuroleptic Malignant Syndrome:* Manage with immediate discontinuation and close monitoring (5.3)
- *Tardive Dyskinesia:* Discontinue if clinically appropriate (5.4)
- *Metabolic Changes:* Atypical antipsychotic drugs have been associated with metabolic changes that include hyperglycemia/diabetes mellitus, dyslipidemia, and body weight gain (5.5)
  - *Hyperglycemia/Diabetes Mellitus:* Monitor glucose regularly in patients with and at risk for diabetes (5.5)
  - *Dyslipidemia:* Undesirable alterations in lipid levels have been observed in patients treated with atypical antipsychotics (5.5)
  - *Weight Gain:* Weight gain has been observed with atypical antipsychotic use. Monitor weight (5.5)
- *Orthostatic Hypotension:* Use with caution in patients with known cardiovascular or cerebrovascular disease (5.6)
- *Leukopenia, Neutropenia, and Agranulocytosis:* have been reported with antipsychotics including ABILIFY. Patients with a history of a clinically significant low white blood cell count (WBC) or a drug-induced leukopenia/neutropenia should have their complete blood count (CBC) monitored frequently during the first few months of therapy and discontinuation of ABILIFY should be considered at the first sign of a clinically significant decline in WBC in the absence of other causative factors (5.7)
- *Seizures/Convulsions:* Use cautiously in patients with a history of seizures or with conditions that lower the seizure threshold (5.8)
- *Potential for Cognitive and Motor Impairment:* Use caution when operating machinery (5.9)
- *Suicide:* The possibility of a suicide attempt is inherent in schizophrenia and bipolar disorder. Closely supervise high-risk patients (5.11)

ADVERSE REACTIONS

Commonly observed adverse reactions (incidence ≥5% and at least twice that for placebo) were (6.2):
- Adult patients with schizophrenia: akathisia
- Pediatric patients (13 to 17 years) with schizophrenia: extrapyramidal disorder, somnolence, and tremor
- Adult patients (monotherapy) with bipolar mania: akathisia, sedation, restlessness, tremor, and extrapyramidal disorder
- Adult patients (adjunctive therapy with lithium or valproate) with bipolar mania: akathisia, insomnia, and extrapyramidal disorder
- Pediatric patients (10 to 17 years) with bipolar mania: somnolence, extrapyramidal disorder, fatigue, nausea, akathisia, blurred vision, salivary hypersecretion, and dizziness
- Adult patients with major depressive disorder (adjunctive treatment to antidepressant therapy): akathisia, restlessness, insomnia, constipation, fatigue, and blurred vision
- Pediatric patients (6 to 17 years) with autistic disorder: sedation, fatigue, vomiting, somnolence, tremor, pyrexia, drooling, decreased appetite, salivary hypersecretion, extrapyramidal disorder, and lethargy
- Adult patients with agitation associated with schizophrenia or bipolar mania: nausea

To report SUSPECTED ADVERSE REACTIONS, contact Bristol-Myers Squibb at 1-800-721-5072 or FDA at 1-800-FDA-1088 or www.fda.gov/medwatch

DRUG INTERACTIONS

- *Strong CYP3A4 (eg, ketoconazole) or CYP2D6 (eg, fluoxetine) inhibitors will increase* ABILIFY drug concentrations; reduce ABILIFY dose to one-half of the usual dose when used concomitantly (2.6, 7.1), except when used as adjunctive treatment with antidepressants (2.6). If a strong CYP3A4 inhibitor and strong CYP2D6 inhibitor are coadministered or a known CYP2D6 poor metabolizer is receiving a concomitant strong CYP3A4 inhibitor, the ABILIFY dose should be reduced to one-quarter (25%) of the usual dose (2.6, 12.3).
- *CYP3A4 inducers (eg, carbamazepine) will decrease* ABILIFY drug concentrations; double ABILIFY dose when used concomitantly (2.6, 7.1)

See 17 for PATIENT COUNSELING INFORMATION and Medication Guide

Revised: 04/2013

FULL PRESCRIBING INFORMATION: CONTENTS*

*** Sections or subsections omitted from the full prescribing information are not listed**

FULL PRESCRIBING INFORMATION

WARNINGS: INCREASED MORTALITY IN ELDERLY PATIENTS WITH DEMENTIA-RELATED PSYCHOSIS and SUICIDALITY AND ANTIDEPRESSANT DRUGS

Elderly patients with dementia-related psychosis treated with antipsychotic drugs are at an increased risk of death. Analyses of seventeen placebo-controlled trials (modal duration of 10 weeks), largely in patients taking atypical antipsychotic drugs, revealed a risk of death in drug-treated patients of between 1.6 to 1.7 times the risk of death in placebo-treated patients. Over the course of a typical 10-week controlled trial, the rate of death in drug-treated patients was about 4.5%, compared to a rate of about 2.6% in the placebo group. Although the causes of death were varied, most of the deaths appeared to be either cardiovascular (eg, heart failure, sudden death) or infectious (eg, pneumonia) in nature. Observational studies suggest that, similar to atypical antipsychotic drugs, treatment with conventional antipsychotic drugs may increase mortality. The extent to which the findings of increased mortality in observational studies may be attributed to the antipsychotic drug as opposed to some characteristic(s) of the patients is not clear. ABILIFY (aripiprazole) is not approved for the treatment of patients with dementia-related psychosis *[see WARNINGS AND PRECAUTIONS (5.1)]*.

Antidepressants increased the risk compared to placebo of suicidal thinking and behavior (suicidality) in children, adolescents, and young adults in short-term studies of major depressive disorder (MDD) and other psychiatric disorders. Anyone considering the use of adjunctive ABILIFY or any other antidepressant in a child, adolescent, or young adult must balance this risk with the clinical need. Short-term studies did not show an increase in the risk of suicidality with antidepressants compared to placebo in adults beyond age 24; there was a reduction in risk with antidepressants compared to placebo in adults aged 65 and older. Depression and certain other psychiatric disorders are themselves associated with increases in the risk of suicide. Patients of all ages who are started on antidepressant therapy should be monitored appropriately and observed closely for clinical worsening, suicidality, or unusual changes in behavior. Families and caregivers should be advised of the need for close observation and communication with the prescriber. ABILIFY is not approved for use in pediatric patients with depression *[see WARNINGS AND PRECAUTIONS (5.2)]*.

1 INDICATIONS AND USAGE

1.1 Schizophrenia

ABILIFY is indicated for the treatment of schizophrenia. The efficacy of ABILIFY was established in four 4-6 week trials in adults and one 6-week trial in adolescents (13 to 17 years). Maintenance efficacy was demonstrated in one trial in adults and can be extrapolated to adolescents *[see CLINICAL STUDIES (14.1)]*.

1.2 Bipolar I Disorder

Acute Treatment of Manic and Mixed Episodes

ABILIFY is indicated for the acute treatment of manic and mixed episodes associated with bipolar I disorder, both as monotherapy and as an adjunct to lithium or valproate. Efficacy as monotherapy was established in four 3-week monotherapy trials in adults and one 4-week monotherapy trial in pediatric patients (10 to 17 years). Efficacy as adjunctive therapy was established in one 6-week adjunctive trial in adults *[see CLINICAL STUDIES (14.2)]*.

Maintenance Treatment of Bipolar I Disorder

ABILIFY is indicated for the maintenance treatment of bipolar I disorder, both as monotherapy and as an adjunct to either lithium or valproate. Maintenance efficacy was demonstrated in one monotherapy maintenance trial and in one adjunctive maintenance trial in adults *[see CLINICAL STUDIES (14.2)]*.

1.3 Adjunctive Treatment of Major Depressive Disorder

ABILIFY is indicated for use as an adjunctive therapy to antidepressants for the treatment of major depressive disorder (MDD). Efficacy was established in two 6-week trials in adults with MDD who had an inadequate response to antidepressant therapy during the current episode *[see CLINICAL STUDIES (14.3)]*.

1.4 Irritability Associated with Autistic Disorder

ABILIFY is indicated for the treatment of irritability associated with autistic disorder. Efficacy was established in two 8-week trials in pediatric patients (aged 6 to 17 years) with irritability associated with autistic disorder (including symptoms of aggression towards others, deliberate self-injuriousness, temper tantrums, and quickly changing moods) *[see CLINICAL STUDIES (14.4)]*.

1.5 Agitation Associated with Schizophrenia or Bipolar Mania

ABILIFY Injection is indicated for the acute treatment of agitation associated with schizophrenia or bipolar disorder, manic or mixed. "Psychomotor agitation" is defined in DSM-IV as "excessive motor activity associated with a feeling of inner tension." Patients experiencing agitation often manifest behaviors that interfere with their diagnosis and care (eg, threatening behaviors, escalating or urgently distressing behavior, or self-exhausting behavior), leading clinicians to the use of intramuscular antipsychotic medications to achieve immediate control of the agitation. Efficacy was established in three short-term (24-hour) trials in adults *[see CLINICAL STUDIES (14.5)]*.

1.6 Special Considerations in Treating Pediatric Schizophrenia, Bipolar I Disorder, and Irritability Associated with Autistic Disorder

Psychiatric disorders in children and adolescents are often serious mental disorders with variable symptom profiles that are not always congruent with adult diagnostic criteria. It is recommended that psychotropic medication therapy for pediatric patients only be initiated after a thorough diagnostic evaluation has been conducted and careful consideration given to the risks associated with medication treatment. Medication treatment for pediatric patients with schizophrenia, bipolar I disorder, and irritability associated with autistic disorder is indicated as part of a total treatment program that often includes psychological, educational, and social interventions.

2 DOSAGE AND ADMINISTRATION

2.1 Schizophrenia

Adults

Dose Selection: The recommended starting and target dose for ABILIFY is 10 mg/day or 15 mg/day administered on a once-a-day schedule without regard to meals. ABILIFY has been systematically evaluated and shown to be effective in a dose range of 10 mg/day to 30 mg/day, when administered as the tablet formulation; however, doses higher than 10 mg/day or 15 mg/day were not more effective than 10 mg/day or 15 mg/day. Dosage increases should generally not be made before 2 weeks, the time needed to achieve steady-state *[see CLINICAL STUDIES (14.1)]*.

Maintenance Treatment: Maintenance of efficacy in schizophrenia was demonstrated in a trial involving patients with schizophrenia who had been symptomatically stable on other antipsychotic medications for periods of 3 months or longer. These patients were discontinued from those medications and randomized to either ABILIFY 15 mg/day or placebo, and observed for relapse *[see CLINICAL STUDIES (14.1)]*. Patients should be periodically reassessed to determine the continued need for maintenance treatment.

Adolescents

Dose Selection: The recommended target dose of ABILIFY is 10 mg/day. Aripiprazole was studied in adolescent patients 13 to 17 years of age with schizophrenia at daily doses of 10 mg and 30 mg. The starting daily dose of the tablet formulation in these patients was 2 mg, which was titrated to 5 mg after 2 days and to the target dose of 10 mg after 2 additional days. Subsequent dose increases should be administered in 5 mg increments. The 30 mg/day dose was not shown to be more efficacious than the 10 mg/day dose. ABILIFY can be administered without regard to meals *[see CLINICAL STUDIES (14.1)]*.

Maintenance Treatment: The efficacy of ABILIFY for the maintenance treatment of schizophrenia in the adolescent population has not been evaluated. While there is no body of evidence available to answer the question of how long the adolescent patient treated with ABILIFY should be maintained on the drug, maintenance efficacy can be extrapolated from adult data along with comparisons of aripiprazole pharmacokinetic parameters in adult and pediatric patients. Thus, it is generally recommended that responding patients be continued beyond the acute response, but at the lowest dose needed to maintain remission. Patients should be periodically reassessed to determine the need for maintenance treatment.

Switching from Other Antipsychotics

There are no systematically collected data to specifically address switching patients with schizophrenia from other antipsychotics to ABILIFY or concerning concomitant administration with other antipsychotics. While immediate discontinuation of the previous antipsychotic treatment may be acceptable for some patients with schizophrenia, more gradual discontinuation may be most appropriate for others. In all cases, the period of overlapping antipsychotic administration should be minimized.

2.2 Bipolar I Disorder

Acute Treatment of Manic and Mixed Episodes

Adults: The recommended starting dose in adults is 15 mg given once daily as monotherapy and 10 mg to 15 mg given once daily as adjunctive therapy with lithium or valproate. ABILIFY can be given without regard to meals. The recommended target dose of ABILIFY is 15 mg/day, as monotherapy or as adjunctive therapy with lithium or valproate. The dose may be increased to 30 mg/day based on clinical response. The safety of doses above 30 mg/day has not been evaluated in clinical trials.

Pediatrics: The recommended starting dose in pediatric patients (10 to 17 years) as monotherapy is 2 mg/day, with titration to 5 mg/day after 2 days, and a target dose of 10 mg/day after 2 additional days. Recommended dosing as adjunctive therapy to lithium or valproate is the same. Subsequent dose increases, if needed, should be administered in 5 mg/day increments. ABILIFY can be given without regard to meals *[see CLINICAL STUDIES (14.2)]*.

Maintenance Treatment
The recommended dose for maintenance treatment, whether as monotherapy or as adjunctive therapy, is the same dose needed to stabilize patients during acute treatment, both for adult and pediatric patients. Patients should be periodically reassessed to determine the continued need for maintenance treatment *[see CLINICAL STUDIES (14.2)]*.

2.3 Adjunctive Treatment of Major Depressive Disorder
Adults
Dose Selection: The recommended starting dose for ABILIFY as adjunctive treatment for patients already taking an antidepressant is 2 mg/day to 5 mg/day. The efficacy of ABILIFY as an adjunctive therapy for major depressive disorder was established within a dose range of 2 mg/day to 15 mg/day. Dose adjustments of up to 5 mg/day should occur gradually, at intervals of no less than 1 week *[see CLINICAL STUDIES (14.3)]*.
Maintenance Treatment: The efficacy of ABILIFY for the adjunctive maintenance treatment of major depressive disorder has not been evaluated. While there is no body of evidence available to answer the question of how long the patient treated with ABILIFY should be maintained, patients should be periodically reassessed to determine the continued need for maintenance treatment.

2.4 Irritability Associated with Autistic Disorder
Pediatric Patients
Dose Selection: The efficacy of aripiprazole has been established in the treatment of pediatric patients 6 to 17 years of age with irritability associated with autistic disorder at doses of 5 mg/day to 15 mg/day. The dosage of ABILIFY should be individualized according to tolerability and response.
Dosing should be initiated at 2 mg/day. The dose should be increased to 5 mg/day, with subsequent increases to 10 mg/day or 15 mg/day if needed. Dose adjustments of up to 5 mg/day should occur gradually, at intervals of no less than 1 week *[see CLINICAL STUDIES (14.4)]*.
Maintenance Treatment: The efficacy of ABILIFY for the maintenance treatment of irritability associated with autistic disorder has not been evaluated. While there is no body of evidence available to answer the question of how long the patient treated with ABILIFY should be maintained, patients should be periodically reassessed to determine the continued need for maintenance treatment.

2.5 Agitation Associated with Schizophrenia or Bipolar Mania (Intramuscular Injection)
Adults
Dose Selection: The recommended dose in these patients is 9.75 mg. The effectiveness of aripiprazole injection in controlling agitation in schizophrenia and bipolar mania was demonstrated over a dose range of 5.25 mg to 15 mg. No additional benefit was demonstrated for 15 mg compared to 9.75 mg. A lower dose of 5.25 mg may be considered when clinical factors warrant. If agitation warranting a second dose persists following the initial dose, cumulative doses up to a total of 30 mg/day may be given. However, the efficacy of repeated doses of aripiprazole injection in agitated patients has not been systematically evaluated in controlled clinical trials. The safety of total daily doses greater than 30 mg or injections given more frequently than every 2 hours have not been adequately evaluated in clinical trials *[see CLINICAL STUDIES (14.5)]*.
If ongoing aripiprazole therapy is clinically indicated, oral aripiprazole in a range of 10 mg/day to 30 mg/day should replace aripiprazole injection as soon as possible *[see DOSAGE AND ADMINISTRATION (2.1 and 2.2)]*.

Administration of ABILIFY Injection
To administer ABILIFY Injection, draw up the required volume of solution into the syringe as shown in Table 1. Discard any unused portion.

Table 1: ABILIFY Injection Dosing Recommendations

Single-Dose	Required Volume of Solution
5.25 mg	0.7 mL
9.75 mg	1.3 mL
15 mg	2 mL

ABILIFY Injection is intended for intramuscular use only. Do not administer intravenously or subcutaneously. Inject slowly, deep into the muscle mass.
Parenteral drug products should be inspected visually for particulate matter and discoloration prior to administration, whenever solution and container permit.

2.6 Dosage Adjustment
Dosage adjustments in adults are not routinely indicated on the basis of age, gender, race, or renal or hepatic impairment status *[see USE IN SPECIFIC POPULATIONS (8.4-8.10)]*.
Dosage adjustment for patients taking aripiprazole concomitantly with strong CYP3A4 inhibitors: When concomitant administration of aripiprazole with strong CYP3A4 inhibitors such as ketoconazole or clarithromycin is indicated, the aripiprazole dose should be reduced to one-half of the usual dose. When the CYP3A4 inhibitor is withdrawn from the combination therapy, the aripiprazole dose should then be increased *[see DRUG INTERACTIONS (7.1)]*.
Dosage adjustment for patients taking aripiprazole concomitantly with potential CYP2D6 inhibitors: When concomitant administration of potential CYP2D6 inhibitors such as quinidine, fluoxetine, or paroxetine with aripiprazole occurs, aripiprazole dose should be reduced at least to one-half of its normal dose. When the CYP2D6 inhibitor is withdrawn from the combination therapy, the aripiprazole dose should then be increased *[see DRUG INTERACTIONS (7.1)]*. When adjunctive ABILIFY is administered to patients with major depressive disorder, ABILIFY should be administered without dosage adjustment as specified in *DOSAGE AND ADMINISTRATION (2.3)*.
Dosing recommendation in patients taking aripiprazole concomitantly with strong CYP3A4 and CYP2D6 inhibitors: When concomitant administration of aripiprazole with strong inhibitors of CYP3A4 (such as ketoconazole or clarithromycin) and CYP2D6 (such as quinidine, fluoxetine, or paroxetine) is indicated, the aripiprazole dose should be reduced to one-quarter (25%) of the usual dose. When the CYP3A4 and/or CYP2D6 inhibitor is withdrawn from the combination therapy, the aripiprazole dose should be increased *[see DRUG INTERACTIONS (7.1)]*.
Dosing recommendation in patients taking aripiprazole concomitantly with strong, moderate, or weak inhibitors of CYP3A4 and CYP2D6: Patients who may be receiving a combination of strong, moderate, and weak inhibitors of CYP3A4 and CYP2D6 (eg, a potent CYP3A4 inhibitor and a moderate CYP2D6 inhibitor or a moderate CYP3A4 inhibitor with a moderate CYP2D6 inhibitor), the dosing may be reduced to one-quarter (25%) of the usual dose initially and then adjusted to achieve a favorable clinical response.
Dosing recommendation in patients who are classified as CYP2D6 poor metabolizers (PM): The aripiprazole dose in PM patients should initially be reduced to one-half (50%) of the usual dose and then adjusted to achieve a favorable clinical response. The dose of aripiprazole for PM patients who are administered a strong CYP3A4 inhibitor should be reduced to one-quarter (25%) of the usual dose *[see CLINICAL PHARMACOLOGY (12.3)]*.
Dosage adjustment for patients taking potential CYP3A4 inducers: When a potential CYP3A4 inducer such as carbamazepine is added to aripiprazole therapy, the aripiprazole dose should be doubled. Additional dose increases should be based on clinical evaluation. When the CYP3A4 inducer is withdrawn from the combination therapy, the aripiprazole dose should be reduced to 10 mg to 15 mg *[see DRUG INTERACTIONS (7.1)]*.

2.7 Dosing of Oral Solution
The oral solution can be substituted for tablets on a mg-per-mg basis up to the 25 mg dose level. Patients receiving 30 mg tablets should receive 25 mg of the solution *[see CLINICAL PHARMACOLOGY (12.3)]*.

2.8 Dosing of Orally Disintegrating Tablets
The dosing for ABILIFY Orally Disintegrating Tablets is the same as for the oral tablets *[see DOSAGE AND ADMINISTRATION (2.1, 2.2, 2.3, and 2.4)]*.

3 DOSAGE FORMS AND STRENGTHS
ABILIFY® (aripiprazole) Tablets are available as described in Table 2.

Table 2: ABILIFY Tablet Presentations

Tablet Strength	Tablet Color/Shape	Tablet Markings
2 mg	green modified rectangle	"A-006" and "2"
5 mg	blue modified rectangle	"A-007" and "5"
10 mg	pink modified rectangle	"A-008" and "10"
15 mg	yellow round	"A-009" and "15"
20 mg	white round	"A-010" and "20"
30 mg	pink round	"A-011" and "30"

ABILIFY DISCMELT® (aripiprazole) Orally Disintegrating Tablets are available as described in Table 3.

Table 3: ABILIFY DISCMELT Orally Disintegrating Tablet Presentations

Tablet Strength	Tablet Color/Shape	Tablet Markings
10 mg	pink (with scattered specks) round	"A" and "640" "10"
15 mg	yellow (with scattered specks) round	"A" and "641" "15"

ABILIFY® (aripiprazole) Oral Solution (1 mg/mL) is a clear, colorless to light-yellow solution, supplied in child-resistant bottles along with a calibrated oral dosing cup.
ABILIFY® (aripiprazole) Injection for Intramuscular Use is a clear, colorless solution available as a ready-to-use, 9.75 mg/1.3 mL (7.5 mg/mL) solution in clear, Type 1 glass vials.

4 CONTRAINDICATIONS
Known hypersensitivity reaction to ABILIFY. Reactions have ranged from pruritus/urticaria to anaphylaxis *[see ADVERSE REACTIONS (6.3)]*.

5 WARNINGS AND PRECAUTIONS
5.1 Use in Elderly Patients with Dementia-Related Psychosis
Increased Mortality
Elderly patients with dementia-related psychosis treated with antipsychotic drugs are at an increased risk of death. ABILIFY (aripiprazole) is not approved for the treatment of patients with dementia-related psychosis *[see BOXED WARNING]*.

Cerebrovascular Adverse Events, Including Stroke
In placebo-controlled clinical studies (two flexible dose and one fixed dose study) of dementia-related psychosis, there was an increased incidence of cerebrovascular adverse events (eg, stroke, transient ischemic attack), including fatalities, in aripiprazole-treated patients (mean age: 84 years; range: 78-88 years). In the fixed-dose study, there was a statistically significant dose response relationship for cerebrovascular adverse events in patients treated with aripiprazole. Aripiprazole is not approved for the treatment of patients with dementia-related psychosis *[see also BOXED WARNING]*.

Safety Experience in Elderly Patients with Psychosis Associated with Alzheimer's Disease
In three, 10-week, placebo-controlled studies of aripiprazole in elderly patients with psychosis associated with Alzheimer's disease (n=938; mean age: 82.4 years; range: 56-99 years), the treatment-emergent adverse events that were reported at an incidence of ≥3% and aripiprazole incidence at least twice that for placebo were lethargy [placebo 2%, aripiprazole 5%], somnolence (including sedation) [placebo 3%, aripiprazole 8%], and incontinence (primarily, urinary incontinence) [placebo 1%, aripiprazole 5%], excessive salivation [placebo 0%, aripiprazole 4%], and lightheadedness [placebo 1%, aripiprazole 4%].
The safety and efficacy of ABILIFY in the treatment of patients with psychosis associated with dementia have not been established. If the prescriber elects to treat such patients with ABILIFY, vigilance should be exercised, particularly for the emergence of difficulty swallowing or excessive somnolence, which could predispose to accidental injury or aspiration *[see also BOXED WARNING]*.

5.2 Clinical Worsening of Depression and Suicide Risk
Patients with major depressive disorder (MDD), both adult and pediatric, may experience worsening of their depression and/or the emergence of suicidal ideation and behavior (suicidality) or unusual changes in behavior, whether or not they are taking antidepressant medications, and this risk may persist until significant remission occurs. Suicide is a known risk of depression and certain other psychiatric disorders, and these disorders themselves are the strongest predictors of suicide. There has been a long-standing concern, however, that antidepressants may have a role in inducing worsening of depression and the emergence of suicidality in certain patients during the early phases of treatment. Pooled analyses of short-term, placebo-controlled trials of antidepressant drugs (SSRIs and others) showed that these drugs increase the risk of suicidal thinking and behavior (suicidality) in children, adolescents, and young adults (ages 18-24) with MDD and other psychiatric disorders. Short-term studies did not show an increase in the risk of suicidality with antidepressants compared to placebo in adults beyond age 24; there was a reduction with antidepressants compared to placebo in adults aged 65 and older.
The pooled analyses of placebo-controlled trials in children and adolescents with MDD, Obsessive Compulsive Disorder (OCD), or other psychiatric disorders included a total of 24

short-term trials of 9 antidepressant drugs in over 4400 patients. The pooled analyses of placebo-controlled trials in adults with MDD or other psychiatric disorders included a total of 295 short-term trials (median duration of 2 months) of 11 antidepressant drugs in over 77,000 patients. There was considerable variation in risk of suicidality among drugs, but a tendency toward an increase in the younger patients for almost all drugs studied. There were differences in absolute risk of suicidality across the different indications, with the highest incidence in MDD. The risk differences (drug vs. placebo), however, were relatively stable within age strata and across indications. These risk differences (drug-placebo difference in the number of cases of suicidality per 1000 patients treated) are provided in Table 4.

Table 4:

Age Range	Drug-Placebo Difference in Number of Cases of Suicidality per 1000 Patients Treated
	Increases Compared to Placebo
<18	14 additional cases
18-24	5 additional cases
	Decreases Compared to Placebo
25-64	1 fewer case
≥65	6 fewer cases

No suicides occurred in any of the pediatric trials. There were suicides in the adult trials, but the number was not sufficient to reach any conclusion about drug effect on suicide.

It is unknown whether the suicidality risk extends to longer-term use, ie, beyond several months. However, there is substantial evidence from placebo-controlled maintenance trials in adults with depression that the use of antidepressants can delay the recurrence of depression.

All patients being treated with antidepressants for any indication should be monitored appropriately and observed closely for clinical worsening, suicidality, and unusual changes in behavior, especially during the initial few months of a course of drug therapy, or at times of dose changes, either increases or decreases.

The following symptoms, anxiety, agitation, panic attacks, insomnia, irritability, hostility, aggressiveness, impulsivity, akathisia (psychomotor restlessness), hypomania, and mania, have been reported in adult and pediatric patients being treated with antidepressants for MDD as well as for other indications, both psychiatric and nonpsychiatric. Although a causal link between the emergence of such symptoms and either the worsening of depression and/or the emergence of suicidal impulses has not been established, there is concern that such symptoms may represent precursors to emerging suicidality.

Consideration should be given to changing the therapeutic regimen, including possibly discontinuing the medication, in patients whose depression is persistently worse, or who are experiencing emergent suicidality or symptoms that might be precursors to worsening depression or suicidality, especially if these symptoms are severe, abrupt in onset, or were not part of the patient's presenting symptoms.

Families and caregivers of patients being treated with antidepressants for major depressive disorder or other indications, both psychiatric and nonpsychiatric, should be alerted about the need to monitor patients for the emergence of agitation, irritability, unusual changes in behavior, and the other symptoms described above, as well as the emergence of suicidality, and to report such symptoms immediately to healthcare providers. Such monitoring should include daily observation by families and caregivers. Prescriptions for ABILIFY should be written for the smallest quantity of tablets consistent with good patient management, in order to reduce the risk of overdose.

Screening Patients for Bipolar Disorder: A major depressive episode may be the initial presentation of bipolar disorder. It is generally believed (though not established in controlled trials) that treating such an episode with an antidepressant alone may increase the likelihood of precipitation of a mixed/manic episode in patients at risk for bipolar disorder. Whether any of the symptoms described above represent such a conversion is unknown. However, prior to initiating treatment with an antidepressant, patients with depressive symptoms should be adequately screened to determine if they are at risk for bipolar disorder; such screening should include a detailed psychiatric history, including a family history of suicide, bipolar disorder, and depression.

It should be noted that ABILIFY is not approved for use in treating depression in the pediatric population.

5.3 Neuroleptic Malignant Syndrome (NMS)

A potentially fatal symptom complex sometimes referred to as Neuroleptic Malignant Syndrome (NMS) may occur with administration of antipsychotic drugs, including aripiprazole. Rare cases of NMS occurred during aripiprazole treatment in the worldwide clinical database. Clinical manifestations of NMS are hyperpyrexia, muscle rigidity, altered mental status, and evidence of autonomic instability (irregular pulse or blood pressure, tachycardia, diaphoresis, and cardiac dysrhythmia). Additional signs may include elevated creatine phosphokinase, myoglobinuria (rhabdomyolysis), and acute renal failure.

The diagnostic evaluation of patients with this syndrome is complicated. In arriving at a diagnosis, it is important to exclude cases where the clinical presentation includes both serious medical illness (eg, pneumonia, systemic infection) and untreated or inadequately treated extrapyramidal signs and symptoms (EPS). Other important considerations in the differential diagnosis include central anticholinergic toxicity, heat stroke, drug fever, and primary central nervous system pathology.

The management of NMS should include: 1) immediate discontinuation of antipsychotic drugs and other drugs not essential to concurrent therapy; 2) intensive symptomatic treatment and medical monitoring; and 3) treatment of any concomitant serious medical problems for which specific treatments are available. There is no general agreement about specific pharmacological treatment regimens for uncomplicated NMS.

If a patient requires antipsychotic drug treatment after recovery from NMS, the potential reintroduction of drug therapy should be carefully considered. The patient should be carefully monitored, since recurrences of NMS have been reported.

5.4 Tardive Dyskinesia

A syndrome of potentially irreversible, involuntary, dyskinetic movements may develop in patients treated with antipsychotic drugs. Although the prevalence of the syndrome appears to be highest among the elderly, especially elderly women, it is impossible to rely upon prevalence estimates to predict, at the inception of antipsychotic treatment, which patients are likely to develop the syndrome. Whether antipsychotic drug products differ in their potential to cause tardive dyskinesia is unknown.

The risk of developing tardive dyskinesia and the likelihood that it will become irreversible are believed to increase as the duration of treatment and the total cumulative dose of antipsychotic drugs administered to the patient increase. However, the syndrome can develop, although much less commonly, after relatively brief treatment periods at low doses.

There is no known treatment for established cases of tardive dyskinesia, although the syndrome may remit, partially or completely, if antipsychotic treatment is withdrawn. Antipsychotic treatment, itself, however, may suppress (or partially suppress) the signs and symptoms of the syndrome and, thereby, may possibly mask the underlying process. The effect that symptomatic suppression has upon the long-term course of the syndrome is unknown.

Given these considerations, ABILIFY should be prescribed in a manner that is most likely to minimize the occurrence of tardive dyskinesia. Chronic antipsychotic treatment should generally be reserved for patients who suffer from a chronic illness that (1) is known to respond to antipsychotic drugs and (2) for whom alternative, equally effective, but potentially less harmful treatments are not available or appropriate. In patients who do require chronic treatment, the smallest dose and the shortest duration of treatment producing a satisfactory clinical response should be sought. The need for continued treatment should be reassessed periodically.

If signs and symptoms of tardive dyskinesia appear in a patient on ABILIFY, drug discontinuation should be considered. However, some patients may require treatment with ABILIFY despite the presence of the syndrome.

Table 5: Changes in Fasting Glucose From Placebo-Controlled Monotherapy Trials in Adult Patients

	Category Change (at least once) from Baseline	Treatment Arm	n/N	%
Fasting Glucose	Normal to High (<100 mg/dL to ≥126 mg/dL)	Aripiprazole	31/822	3.8
		Placebo	22/605	3.6
	Borderline to High (≥100 mg/dL and <126 mg/dL to ≥126 mg/dL)	Aripiprazole	31/176	17.6
		Placebo	13/142	9.2

5.5 Metabolic Changes

Atypical antipsychotic drugs have been associated with metabolic changes that include hyperglycemia/diabetes mellitus, dyslipidemia, and body weight gain. While all drugs in the class have been shown to produce some metabolic changes, each drug has its own specific risk profile.

Hyperglycemia/Diabetes Mellitus

Hyperglycemia, in some cases extreme and associated with ketoacidosis or hyperosmolar coma or death, has been reported in patients treated with atypical antipsychotics. There have been reports of hyperglycemia in patients treated with ABILIFY *[see ADVERSE REACTIONS (6.2, 6.3)]*. Assessment of the relationship between atypical antipsychotic use and glucose abnormalities is complicated by the possibility of an increased background risk of diabetes mellitus in patients with schizophrenia and the increasing incidence of diabetes mellitus in the general population. Given these confounders, the relationship between atypical antipsychotic use and hyperglycemia-related adverse events is not completely understood. However, epidemiological studies suggest an increased risk of treatment-emergent hyperglycemia-related adverse events in patients treated with the atypical antipsychotics. Because ABILIFY was not marketed at the time these studies were performed, it is not known if ABILIFY is associated with this increased risk. Precise risk estimates for hyperglycemia-related adverse events in patients treated with atypical antipsychotics are not available.

Patients with an established diagnosis of diabetes mellitus who are started on atypical antipsychotics should be monitored regularly for worsening of glucose control. Patients with risk factors for diabetes mellitus (eg, obesity, family history of diabetes) who are starting treatment with atypical antipsychotics should undergo fasting blood glucose testing at the beginning of treatment and periodically during treatment. Any patient treated with atypical antipsychotics should be monitored for symptoms of hyperglycemia including polydipsia, polyuria, polyphagia, and weakness. Patients who develop symptoms of hyperglycemia during treatment with atypical antipsychotics should undergo fasting blood glucose testing. In some cases, hyperglycemia has resolved when the atypical antipsychotic was discontinued; however, some patients required continuation of antidiabetic treatment despite discontinuation of the suspect drug.

Adults

In an analysis of 13 placebo-controlled monotherapy trials in adults, primarily with schizophrenia or bipolar disorder, the mean change in fasting glucose in aripiprazole-treated patients (+4.4 mg/dL; median exposure 25 days; N=1057) was not significantly different than in placebo-treated patients (+2.5 mg/dL; median exposure 22 days; N=799). Table 5 shows the proportion of aripiprazole-treated patients with normal and borderline fasting glucose at baseline (median exposure 25 days) that had treatment-emergent high fasting glucose measurements compared to placebo-treated patients (median exposure 22 days).

[See table 5 below]

At 24 weeks, the mean change in fasting glucose in aripiprazole-treated patients was not significantly different than in placebo-treated patients [+2.2 mg/dL (n=42) and +9.6 mg/dL (n=28), respectively].

The mean change in fasting glucose in adjunctive aripiprazole-treated patients with major depressive disorder (+0.7 mg/dL; median exposure 42 days; N=241) was not significantly different than in placebo-treated patients (+0.8 mg/dL; median exposure 42 days; N=246). Table 6 shows the proportion of adult patients with changes in fasting glucose levels from two placebo-controlled, adjunctive trials (median exposure 42 days) in patients with major depressive disorder.

[See table 6 at top of next page]

Pediatric Patients and Adolescents

In an analysis of two placebo-controlled trials in adolescents with schizophrenia (13 to 17 years) and pediatric patients with bipolar disorder (10 to 17 years), the mean change in fasting glucose in aripiprazole-treated patients (+4.8 mg/dL; with a median exposure of 43 days; N=259) was not significantly different than in placebo-treated patients (+1.7 mg/dL; with a median exposure of 42 days; N=123).

In an analysis of two placebo-controlled trials in pediatric and adolescent patients with irritability associated with autistic disorder (6 to 17 years) with median exposure of 56 days, the mean change in fasting glucose in aripiprazole-treated patients (–0.2 mg/dL; N=83) was not significantly different than in placebo-treated patients (–0.6 mg/dL; N=33). Table 7 shows the proportion of patients with changes in fasting glucose levels from the pooled adolescent schizophrenia and pediatric bipolar patients (median exposure of 42-43 days) as well as from two placebo-controlled trials in pediatric patients (6 to 17 years) with irritability associated with autistic disorder (median exposure of 56 days).

[See table 7 at top of next page]

At 12 weeks in the pooled adolescent schizophrenia and pediatric bipolar disorder trials, the mean change in fasting glucose in aripiprazole-treated patients was not significantly different than in placebo-treated patients [+2.4 mg/dL (n=81) and +0.1 mg/dL (n=15), respectively].

Dyslipidemia

Undesirable alterations in lipids have been observed in patients treated with atypical antipsychotics.

There were no significant differences between aripiprazole- and placebo-treated patients in the proportion with changes from normal to clinically significant levels for fasting/nonfasting total cholesterol, fasting triglycerides, fasting LDLs, and fasting/nonfasting HDLs. Analyses of patients with at least 12 or 24 weeks of exposure were limited by small numbers of patients.

Adults

Table 8 shows the proportion of adult patients, primarily from pooled schizophrenia and bipolar disorder monotherapy placebo-controlled trials, with changes in total cholesterol (pooled from 17 trials; median exposure 21 to 25 days), fasting triglycerides (pooled from eight trials; median exposure 42 days), fasting LDL cholesterol (pooled from eight trials; median exposure 39 to 45 days, except for placebo-treated patients with baseline normal fasting LDL measurements, who had median treatment exposure of 24 days) and HDL cholesterol (pooled from nine trials; median exposure 40 to 42 days).

Table 8: Changes in Blood Lipid Parameters From Placebo-Controlled Monotherapy Trials in Adults

	Treatment Arm	n/N	%
Total Cholesterol Normal to High (<200 mg/dL to ≥240 mg/dL)	Aripiprazole	34/1357	2.5
	Placebo	27/973	2.8
Fasting Triglycerides Normal to High (<150 mg/dL to ≥200 mg/dL)	Aripiprazole	40/539	7.4
	Placebo	30/431	7.0
Fasting LDL Cholesterol Normal to High (<100 mg/dL to ≥160 mg/dL)	Aripiprazole	2/332	0.6
	Placebo	2/268	0.7
HDL Cholesterol Normal to Low (≥40 mg/dL to <40 mg/dL)	Aripiprazole	121/1066	11.4
	Placebo	99/794	12.5

In monotherapy trials in adults, the proportion of patients at 12 weeks and 24 weeks with changes from Normal to High in total cholesterol (fasting/nonfasting), fasting triglycerides, and fasting LDL cholesterol were similar between aripiprazole- and placebo-treated patients: at 12 weeks, Total Cholesterol (fasting/nonfasting), 1/71 (1.4%) vs. 3/74 (4.1%); Fasting Triglycerides, 8/62 (12.9%) vs. 5/37 (13.5%); Fasting LDL Cholesterol, 0/34 (0%) vs. 1/25 (4.0%), respectively; and at 24 weeks, Total Cholesterol (fasting/nonfasting), 1/42 (2.4%) vs. 3/37 (8.1%); Fasting Triglycerides, 5/34 (14.7%) vs. 5/20 (25%); Fasting LDL Cholesterol, 0/22 (0%) vs. 1/18 (5.6%), respectively.

Table 9 shows the proportion of patients with changes in total cholesterol (fasting/nonfasting), fasting triglycerides, fasting LDL cholesterol, and HDL cholesterol from two placebo-controlled adjunctive trials in adult patients with major depressive disorder (median exposure 42 days).

Table 9: Changes in Blood Lipid Parameters From Placebo-Controlled Adjunctive Trials in Adult Patients with Major Depressive Disorder

	Treatment Arm	n/N	%
Total Cholesterol Normal to High (<200 mg/dL to ≥240 mg/dL)	Aripiprazole	3/139	2.2
	Placebo	7/135	5.2
Fasting Triglycerides Normal to High (<150 mg/dL to ≥200 mg/dL)	Aripiprazole	14/145	9.7
	Placebo	6/147	4.1
Fasting LDL Cholesterol Normal to High (<100 mg/dL to ≥160 mg/dL)	Aripiprazole	0/54	0
	Placebo	0/73	0
HDL Cholesterol Normal to Low (≥40 mg/dL to <40 mg/dL)	Aripiprazole	17/318	5.3
	Placebo	10/286	3.5

Table 6: Changes in Fasting Glucose From Placebo-Controlled Adjunctive Trials in Adult Patients with Major Depressive Disorder

	Category Change (at least once) from Baseline	Treatment Arm	n/N	%
Fasting Glucose	Normal to High (<100 mg/dL to ≥126 mg/dL)	Aripiprazole	2/201	1.0
		Placebo	2/204	1.0
	Borderline to High (≥100 mg/dL and <126 mg/dL to ≥126 mg/dL)	Aripiprazole	4/34	11.8
		Placebo	3/37	8.1

Table 7: Changes in Fasting Glucose From Placebo-Controlled Trials in Pediatric and Adolescent Patients

Category Change (at least once) from Baseline	Indication	Treatment Arm	n/N	%
Fasting Glucose Normal to High (<100 mg/dL to ≥126 mg/dL)	Pooled Schizophrenia and Bipolar Disorder	Aripiprazole	2/236	0.8
		Placebo	2/110	1.8
	Irritability Associated with Autistic Disorder	Aripiprazole	0/73	0
		Placebo	0/32	0
Fasting Glucose Borderline to High (≥100 mg/dL and <126 mg/dL to ≥126 mg/dL)	Pooled Schizophrenia and Bipolar Disorder	Aripiprazole	1/22	4.5
		Placebo	0/12	0
	Irritability Associated with Autistic Disorder	Aripiprazole	0/9	0
		Placebo	0/1	0

Pediatric Patients and Adolescents

Table 10 shows the proportion of adolescents with schizophrenia (13 to 17 years) and pediatric patients with bipolar disorder (10 to 17 years) with changes in total cholesterol and HDL cholesterol (pooled from two placebo-controlled trials; median exposure 42 to 43 days) and fasting triglycerides (pooled from two placebo-controlled trials; median exposure 42 to 44 days).

Table 10: Changes in Blood Lipid Parameters From Placebo-Controlled Monotherapy Trials in Pediatric and Adolescent Patients

	Treatment Arm	n/N	%
Total Cholesterol Normal to High (<170 mg/dL to ≥200 mg/dL)	Aripiprazole	3/220	1.4
	Placebo	0/116	0
Fasting Triglycerides Normal to High (<150 mg/dL to ≥200 mg/dL)	Aripiprazole	7/187	3.7
	Placebo	4/85	4.7
HDL Cholesterol Normal to Low (≥40 mg/dL to <40 mg/dL)	Aripiprazole	27/236	11.4
	Placebo	22/109	20.2

In monotherapy trials of adolescents with schizophrenia and pediatric patients with bipolar disorder, the proportion of patients at 12 weeks and 24 weeks with changes from Normal to High in total cholesterol (fasting/nonfasting), fasting triglycerides, and fasting LDL cholesterol were similar between aripiprazole- and placebo-treated patients: at 12 weeks, Total Cholesterol (fasting/nonfasting), 0/57 (0%) vs. 0/15 (0%); Fasting Triglycerides, 2/72 (2.8%) vs. 1/14 (7.1%), respectively; and at 24 weeks, Total Cholesterol (fasting/nonfasting), 0/36 (0%) vs. 0/12 (0%); Fasting Triglycerides, 1/47 (2.1%) vs. 1/10 (10.0%), respectively.

Table 11 shows the proportion of patients with changes in total cholesterol (fasting/nonfasting) and fasting triglycerides (median exposure 56 days) and HDL cholesterol (median exposure 55 to 56 days) from two placebo-controlled trials in pediatric patients (6 to 17 years) with irritability associated with autistic disorder.

Table 11: Changes in Blood Lipid Parameters From Placebo-Controlled Trials in Pediatric Patients with Autistic Disorder

	Treatment Arm	n/N	%
Total Cholesterol Normal to High (<170 mg/dL to ≥200 mg/dL)	Aripiprazole	1/95	1.1
	Placebo	0/34	0
Fasting Triglycerides Normal to High (<150 mg/dL to ≥200 mg/dL)	Aripiprazole	0/75	0
	Placebo	0/30	0
HDL Cholesterol Normal to Low (≥40 mg/dL to <40 mg/dL)	Aripiprazole	9/107	8.4
	Placebo	5/49	10.2

Weight Gain

Weight gain has been observed with atypical antipsychotic use. Clinical monitoring of weight is recommended.

Adults

In an analysis of 13 placebo-controlled monotherapy trials, primarily from pooled schizophrenia and bipolar disorder, with a median exposure of 21 to 25 days, the mean change in body weight in aripiprazole-treated patients was +0.3 kg (N=1673) compared to –0.1 kg (N=1100) in placebo-controlled patients. At 24 weeks, the mean change from baseline in body weight in aripiprazole-treated patients was –1.5 kg (n=73) compared to –0.2 kg (n=46) in placebo-treated patients.

In the trials adding aripiprazole to antidepressants, patients first received 8 weeks of antidepressant treatment followed by 6 weeks of adjunctive aripiprazole or placebo in addition to their ongoing antidepressant treatment. The mean change in body weight in patients receiving adjunctive aripiprazole was +1.7 kg (N=347) compared to +0.4 kg (N=330) in patients receiving adjunctive placebo.

Table 12 shows the percentage of adult patients with weight gain ≥7% of body weight by indication.

[See table 12 at top of next page]

Pediatric Patients and Adolescents

In an analysis of two placebo-controlled trials in adolescents with schizophrenia (13 to 17 years) and pediatric patients with bipolar disorder (10 to 17 years) with median exposure of 42 to 43 days, the mean change in body weight in aripiprazole-treated patients was +1.6 kg (N=381) compared to +0.3 kg (N=187) in placebo-treated patients. At 24 weeks, the mean change from baseline in body weight in aripiprazole-treated patients was +5.8 kg (n=62) compared to +1.4 kg (n=13) in placebo-treated patients.

In two short-term, placebo-controlled trials in patients (6 to 17 years) with irritability associated with autistic disorder with median exposure of 56 days, the mean change in body weight in aripiprazole-treated patients was +1.6 kg (n=209) compared to +0.4 kg (n=98) in placebo-treated patients.

Table 13 shows the percentage of pediatric and adolescent patients with weight gain ≥7% of body weight by indication.

[See table 13 at top of next page]

In an open-label trial that enrolled patients from the two placebo-controlled trials of adolescents with schizophrenia (13 to 17 years) and pediatric patients with bipolar disorder (10 to 17 years), 73.2% of patients (238/325) completed 26 weeks of therapy with ABILIFY. After 26 weeks, 32.8% of patients gained ≥7% of their body weight, not adjusted for normal growth. To adjust for normal growth, z-scores were derived (measured in standard deviations [SD]), which normalize for the natural growth of pediatric patients and adolescents by comparisons to age- and gender-matched pop-

Table 12: Percentage of Patients From Placebo-Controlled Trials in Adult Patients with Weight Gain ≥7% of Body Weight

	Indication	Treatment Arm	N	Patients n (%)
Weight gain ≥7% of body weight	Schizophrenia[a]	Aripiprazole	852	69 (8.1)
		Placebo	379	12 (3.2)
	Bipolar Mania[b]	Aripiprazole	719	16 (2.2)
		Placebo	598	16 (2.7)
	Major Depressive Disorder (Adjunctive Therapy)[c]	Aripiprazole	347	18 (5.2)
		Placebo	330	2 (0.6)

[a] 4-6 weeks duration. [b] 3 weeks duration. [c] 6 weeks duration.

Table 13: Percentage of Patients From Placebo-Controlled Monotherapy Trials in Pediatric and Adolescent Patients with Weight Gain ≥7% of Body Weight

	Indication	Treatment Arm	N	Patients n (%)
Weight gain ≥7% of body weight	Pooled Schizophrenia and Bipolar Mania[a]	Aripiprazole	381	20 (5.2)
		Placebo	187	3 (1.6)
	Irritability Associated with Autistic Disorder[b]	Aripiprazole	209	55 (26.3)
		Placebo	98	7 (7.1)

[a] 4-6 weeks duration. [b] 8 weeks duration.

ulation standards. A z-score change <0.5 SD is considered not clinically significant. After 26 weeks, the mean change in z-score was 0.09 SD.

In an open-label trial that enrolled patients from two short-term, placebo-controlled trials, patients (6 to 17 years) with irritability associated with autistic disorder, as well as *de novo* patients, 60.3% (199/330) completed one year of therapy with ABILIFY. The mean change in weight z-score was 0.26 SDs for patients receiving >9 months of treatment.

When treating pediatric patients for any indication, weight gain should be monitored and assessed against that expected for normal growth.

5.6 Orthostatic Hypotension

Aripiprazole may cause orthostatic hypotension, perhaps due to its α_1-adrenergic receptor antagonism. The incidence of orthostatic hypotension-associated events from short-term, placebo-controlled trials of adult patients on oral ABILIFY (n=2467) included (aripiprazole incidence, placebo incidence) orthostatic hypotension (1%, 0.3%), postural dizziness (0.5%, 0.3%), and syncope (0.5%, 0.4%); of pediatric patients 6 to 17 years of age (n=611) on oral ABILIFY included orthostatic hypotension (0.5%, 0%), postural dizziness (0.3%, 0%), and syncope (0.2%, 0%); and of patients on ABILIFY Injection (n=501) included orthostatic hypotension (0.6%, 0%), postural dizziness (0.2%, 0.5%), and syncope (0.4%, 0%).

The incidence of a significant orthostatic change in blood pressure (defined as a decrease in systolic blood pressure ≥20 mmHg accompanied by an increase in heart rate ≥25 when comparing standing to supine values) for aripiprazole was not meaningfully different from placebo (aripiprazole incidence, placebo incidence): in adult oral aripiprazole-treated patients (4%, 2%), in pediatric oral aripiprazole-treated patients aged 6 to 17 years (0.2%, 1%), or in aripiprazole injection-treated patients (3%, 2%).

Aripiprazole should be used with caution in patients with known cardiovascular disease (history of myocardial infarction or ischemic heart disease, heart failure or conduction abnormalities), cerebrovascular disease, or conditions which would predispose patients to hypotension (dehydration, hypovolemia, and treatment with antihypertensive medications).

If parenteral benzodiazepine therapy is deemed necessary in addition to aripiprazole injection treatment, patients should be monitored for excessive sedation and for orthostatic hypotension *[see DRUG INTERACTIONS (7.3)]*.

5.7 Leukopenia, Neutropenia, and Agranulocytosis

Class Effect: In clinical trial and/or postmarketing experience, events of leukopenia/neutropenia have been reported temporally related to antipsychotic agents, including ABILIFY. Agranulocytosis has also been reported.

Possible risk factors for leukopenia/neutropenia include pre-existing low white blood cell count (WBC) and history of drug-induced leukopenia/neutropenia. Patients with a history of a clinically significant low WBC or drug-induced leukopenia/neutropenia should have their complete blood count (CBC) monitored frequently during the first few months of therapy and discontinuation of ABILIFY should be considered at the first sign of a clinically significant decline in WBC in the absence of other causative factors.

Patients with clinically significant neutropenia should be carefully monitored for fever or other symptoms or signs of infection and treated promptly if such symptoms or signs occur. Patients with severe neutropenia (absolute neutrophil count <1000/mm^3) should discontinue ABILIFY and have their WBC followed until recovery.

5.8 Seizures/Convulsions

In short-term, placebo-controlled trials, seizures/convulsions occurred in 0.1% (3/2467) of adult patients treated with oral aripiprazole, in 0.2% (1/611) of pediatric patients (6 to 17 years), and in 0.2% (1/501) of adult aripiprazole injection-treated patients.

As with other antipsychotic drugs, aripiprazole should be used cautiously in patients with a history of seizures or with conditions that lower the seizure threshold, eg, Alzheimer's dementia. Conditions that lower the seizure threshold may be more prevalent in a population of 65 years or older.

5.9 Potential for Cognitive and Motor Impairment

ABILIFY, like other antipsychotics, may have the potential to impair judgment, thinking, or motor skills. For example, in short-term, placebo-controlled trials, somnolence (including sedation) was reported as follows (aripiprazole incidence, placebo incidence): in adult patients (n=2467) treated with oral ABILIFY (11%, 6%), in pediatric patients ages 6 to 17 (n=611) (24%, 6%), and in adult patients (n=501) on ABILIFY Injection (9%, 6%). Somnolence (including sedation) led to discontinuation in 0.3% (8/2467) of adult patients and 3% (15/611) of pediatric patients (6 to 17 years) on oral ABILIFY in short-term, placebo-controlled trials, but did not lead to discontinuation of any adult patients on ABILIFY Injection.

Despite the relatively modest increased incidence of these events compared to placebo, patients should be cautioned about operating hazardous machinery, including automobiles, until they are reasonably certain that therapy with ABILIFY does not affect them adversely.

5.10 Body Temperature Regulation

Disruption of the body's ability to reduce core body temperature has been attributed to antipsychotic agents. Appropriate care is advised when prescribing aripiprazole for patients who will be experiencing conditions which may contribute to an elevation in core body temperature, (eg, exercising strenuously, exposure to extreme heat, receiving concomitant medication with anticholinergic activity, or being subject to dehydration) *[see ADVERSE REACTIONS (6.3)]*.

5.11 Suicide

The possibility of a suicide attempt is inherent in psychotic illnesses, bipolar disorder, and major depressive disorder, and close supervision of high-risk patients should accompany drug therapy. Prescriptions for ABILIFY should be written for the smallest quantity consistent with good patient management in order to reduce the risk of overdose *[see ADVERSE REACTIONS (6.2, 6.3)]*.

In two 6-week, placebo-controlled studies of aripiprazole as adjunctive treatment of major depressive disorder, the incidences of suicidal ideation and suicide attempts were 0% (0/371) for aripiprazole and 0.5% (2/366) for placebo.

5.12 Dysphagia

Esophageal dysmotility and aspiration have been associated with antipsychotic drug use, including ABILIFY. Aspiration pneumonia is a common cause of morbidity and mortality in elderly patients, in particular those with advanced Alzheimer's dementia. Aripiprazole and other antipsychotic drugs should be used cautiously in patients at risk for aspiration pneumonia *[see WARNINGS AND PRECAUTIONS (5.1) and ADVERSE REACTIONS (6.3)]*.

5.13 Use in Patients with Concomitant Illness

Clinical experience with ABILIFY in patients with certain concomitant systemic illnesses is limited *[see USE IN SPECIFIC POPULATIONS (8.6, 8.7)]*.

ABILIFY has not been evaluated or used to any appreciable extent in patients with a recent history of myocardial infarction or unstable heart disease. Patients with these diagnoses were excluded from premarketing clinical studies *[see WARNINGS AND PRECAUTIONS (5.1, 5.6)]*.

6 ADVERSE REACTIONS

6.1 Overall Adverse Reactions Profile

The following are discussed in more detail in other sections of the labeling:

- Use in Elderly Patients with Dementia-Related Psychosis *[see BOXED WARNING and WARNINGS AND PRECAUTIONS (5.1)]*
- Clinical Worsening of Depression and Suicide Risk *[see BOXED WARNING and WARNINGS AND PRECAUTIONS (5.2)]*
- Neuroleptic Malignant Syndrome (NMS) *[see WARNINGS AND PRECAUTIONS (5.3)]*
- Tardive Dyskinesia *[see WARNINGS AND PRECAUTIONS (5.4)]*
- Metabolic Changes *[see WARNINGS AND PRECAUTIONS (5.5)]*
- Orthostatic Hypotension *[see WARNINGS AND PRECAUTIONS (5.6)]*
- Leukopenia, Neutropenia, and Agranulocytosis *[see WARNINGS AND PRECAUTIONS (5.7)]*
- Seizures/Convulsions *[see WARNINGS AND PRECAUTIONS (5.8)]*
- Potential for Cognitive and Motor Impairment *[see WARNINGS AND PRECAUTIONS (5.9)]*
- Body Temperature Regulation *[see WARNINGS AND PRECAUTIONS (5.10)]*
- Suicide *[see WARNINGS AND PRECAUTIONS (5.11)]*
- Dysphagia *[see WARNINGS AND PRECAUTIONS (5.12)]*
- Use in Patients with Concomitant Illness *[see WARNINGS AND PRECAUTIONS (5.13)]*

The most common adverse reactions in adult patients in clinical trials (≥10%) were nausea, vomiting, constipation, headache, dizziness, akathisia, anxiety, insomnia, and restlessness.

The most common adverse reactions in the pediatric clinical trials (≥10%) were somnolence, headache, vomiting, extrapyramidal disorder, fatigue, increased appetite, insomnia, nausea, nasopharyngitis, and weight increased.

Aripiprazole has been evaluated for safety in 13,543 adult patients who participated in multiple-dose, clinical trials in schizophrenia, bipolar disorder, major depressive disorder, Dementia of the Alzheimer's type, Parkinson's disease, and alcoholism, and who had approximately 7619 patient-years of exposure to oral aripiprazole and 749 patients with exposure to aripiprazole injection. A total of 3390 patients were treated with oral aripiprazole for at least 180 days and 1933 patients treated with oral aripiprazole had at least 1 year of exposure.

Aripiprazole has been evaluated for safety in 920 patients (6 to 17 years) who participated in multiple-dose, clinical trials in schizophrenia, bipolar mania, or autistic disorder and who had approximately 517 patient-years of exposure to oral aripiprazole. A total of 465 pediatric patients were treated with oral aripiprazole for at least 180 days and 117 pediatric patients treated with oral aripiprazole had at least 1 year of exposure.

The conditions and duration of treatment with aripiprazole (monotherapy and adjunctive therapy with antidepressants or mood stabilizers) included (in overlapping categories) double-blind, comparative and noncomparative open-label studies, inpatient and outpatient studies, fixed- and flexible-dose studies, and short- and longer-term exposure.

Adverse events during exposure were obtained by collecting volunteered adverse events, as well as results of physical examinations, vital signs, weights, laboratory analyses, and ECG. Adverse experiences were recorded by clinical investigators using terminology of their own choosing. In the tables and tabulations that follow, MedDRA dictionary terminology has been used to classify reported adverse events into a smaller number of standardized event categories, in order to provide a meaningful estimate of the proportion of individuals experiencing adverse events.

The stated frequencies of adverse reactions represent the proportion of individuals who experienced at least once, a treatment-emergent adverse event of the type listed. An event was considered treatment emergent if it occurred for the first time or worsened while receiving therapy following baseline evaluation. There was no attempt to use investigator causality assessments; ie, all events meeting the defined criteria, regardless of investigator causality, are included.

Throughout this section, adverse reactions are reported. These are adverse events that were considered to be reasonably associated with the use of ABILIFY (adverse drug reactions) based on the comprehensive assessment of the available adverse event information. A causal association for ABILIFY often cannot be reliably established in individual cases.

The figures in the tables and tabulations cannot be used to predict the incidence of side effects in the course of usual medical practice where patient characteristics and other factors differ from those that prevailed in the clinical trials. Similarly, the cited frequencies cannot be compared with figures obtained from other clinical investigations involving different treatment, uses, and investigators. The cited figures, however, do provide the prescriber with some basis for estimating the relative contribution of drug and nondrug factors to the adverse reaction incidence in the population studied.

6.2 Clinical Studies Experience

Adult Patients with Schizophrenia

The following findings are based on a pool of five placebo-controlled trials (four 4-week and one 6-week) in which oral aripiprazole was administered in doses ranging from 2 mg/day to 30 mg/day.

Adverse Reactions Associated with Discontinuation of Treatment

Overall, there was little difference in the incidence of discontinuation due to adverse reactions between aripiprazole-treated (7%) and placebo-treated (9%) patients. The types of adverse reactions that led to discontinuation were similar for the aripiprazole-treated and placebo-treated patients.

Commonly Observed Adverse Reactions

The only commonly observed adverse reaction associated with the use of aripiprazole in patients with schizophrenia (incidence of 5% or greater and aripiprazole incidence at least twice that for placebo) was akathisia (aripiprazole 8%; placebo 4%).

Adult Patients with Bipolar Mania

Monotherapy

The following findings are based on a pool of 3-week, placebo-controlled, bipolar mania trials in which oral aripiprazole was administered at doses of 15 mg/day or 30 mg/day.

Adverse Reactions Associated with Discontinuation of Treatment

Overall, in patients with bipolar mania, there was little difference in the incidence of discontinuation due to adverse reactions between aripiprazole-treated (11%) and placebo-treated (10%) patients. The types of adverse reactions that led to discontinuation were similar between the aripiprazole-treated and placebo-treated patients.

Commonly Observed Adverse Reactions

Commonly observed adverse reactions associated with the use of aripiprazole in patients with bipolar mania (incidence of 5% or greater and aripiprazole incidence at least twice that for placebo) are shown in Table 14.

Table 14: Commonly Observed Adverse Reactions in Short-Term, Placebo-Controlled Trials of Adult Patients with Bipolar Mania Treated with Oral ABILIFY Monotherapy

Preferred Term	Percentage of Patients Reporting Reaction Aripiprazole (n=917)	Placebo (n=753)
Akathisia	13	4
Sedation	8	3
Restlessness	6	3
Tremor	6	3
Extrapyramidal Disorder	5	2

Less Common Adverse Reactions in Adults

Table 15 enumerates the pooled incidence, rounded to the nearest percent, of adverse reactions that occurred during acute therapy (up to 6 weeks in schizophrenia and up to 3 weeks in bipolar mania), including only those reactions that occurred in 2% or more of patients treated with aripiprazole (doses ≥2 mg/day) and for which the incidence in patients treated with aripiprazole was greater than the incidence in patients treated with placebo in the combined dataset.

Table 15: Adverse Reactions in Short-Term, Placebo-Controlled Trials in Adult Patients Treated with Oral ABILIFY

System Organ Class Preferred Term	Percentage of Patients Reporting Reaction[a] Aripiprazole (n=1843)	Placebo (n=1166)
Eye Disorders		
Blurred Vision	3	1
Gastrointestinal Disorders		
Nausea	15	11
Constipation	11	7
Vomiting	11	6
Dyspepsia	9	7
Dry Mouth	5	4
Toothache	4	3
Abdominal Discomfort	3	2
Stomach Discomfort	3	2
General Disorders and Administration Site Conditions		
Fatigue	6	4
Pain	3	2
Musculoskeletal and Connective Tissue Disorders		
Musculoskeletal Stiffness	4	3
Pain in Extremity	4	2
Myalgia	2	1
Muscle Spasms	2	1
Nervous System Disorders		
Headache	27	23
Dizziness	10	7
Akathisia	10	4
Sedation	7	4
Extrapyramidal Disorder	5	3
Tremor	5	3
Somnolence	5	3
Psychiatric Disorders		
Agitation	19	17
Insomnia	18	13
Anxiety	17	13
Restlessness	5	3
Respiratory, Thoracic, and Mediastinal Disorders		
Pharyngolaryngeal Pain	3	2
Cough	3	2

[a] Adverse reactions reported by at least 2% of patients treated with oral aripiprazole, except adverse reactions which had an incidence equal to or less than placebo.

An examination of population subgroups did not reveal any clear evidence of differential adverse reaction incidence on the basis of age, gender, or race.

Adult Patients with Adjunctive Therapy with Bipolar Mania

The following findings are based on a placebo-controlled trial of adult patients with bipolar disorder in which aripiprazole was administered at doses of 15 mg/day or 30 mg/day as adjunctive therapy with lithium or valproate.

Adverse Reactions Associated with Discontinuation of Treatment

In a study of patients who were already tolerating either lithium or valproate as monotherapy, discontinuation rates due to adverse reactions were 12% for patients treated with adjunctive aripiprazole compared to 6% for patients treated with adjunctive placebo. The most common adverse drug reactions associated with discontinuation in the adjunctive aripiprazole-treated compared to placebo-treated patients were akathisia (5% and 1%, respectively) and tremor (2% and 1%, respectively).

Commonly Observed Adverse Reactions

The commonly observed adverse reactions associated with adjunctive aripiprazole and lithium or valproate in patients with bipolar mania (incidence of 5% or greater and incidence at least twice that for adjunctive placebo) were: akathisia, insomnia, and extrapyramidal disorder.

Less Common Adverse Reactions in Adult Patients with Adjunctive Therapy in Bipolar Mania

Table 16 enumerates the incidence, rounded to the nearest percent, of adverse reactions that occurred during acute treatment (up to 6 weeks), including only those reactions that occurred in 2% or more of patients treated with adjunctive aripiprazole (doses of 15 mg/day or 30 mg/day) and lithium or valproate and for which the incidence in patients treated with this combination was greater than the incidence in patients treated with placebo plus lithium or valproate.

Table 16: Adverse Reactions in a Short-Term, Placebo-Controlled Trial of Adjunctive Therapy in Patients with Bipolar Disorder

System Organ Class Preferred Term	Percentage of Patients Reporting Reaction[a] Aripiprazole + Li or Val* (n=253)	Placebo + Li or Val* (n=130)
Gastrointestinal Disorders		
Nausea	8	5
Vomiting	4	0
Salivary Hypersecretion	4	2
Dry Mouth	2	1
Infections and Infestations		
Nasopharyngitis	3	2
Investigations		
Weight Increased	2	1
Nervous System Disorders		
Akathisia	19	5
Tremor	9	6
Extrapyramidal Disorder	5	1
Dizziness	4	1
Sedation	4	2
Psychiatric Disorders		
Insomnia	8	4
Anxiety	4	1
Restlessness	2	1

[a] Adverse reactions reported by at least 2% of patients treated with oral aripiprazole, except adverse reactions which had an incidence equal to or less than placebo.

* Lithium or Valproate

Pediatric Patients (13 to 17 years) with Schizophrenia

The following findings are based on one 6-week, placebo-controlled trial in which oral aripiprazole was administered in doses ranging from 2 mg/day to 30 mg/day.

Adverse Reactions Associated with Discontinuation of Treatment

The incidence of discontinuation due to adverse reactions between aripiprazole-treated and placebo-treated pediatric patients (13 to 17 years) was 5% and 2%, respectively.

Commonly Observed Adverse Reactions

Commonly observed adverse reactions associated with the use of aripiprazole in adolescent patients with schizophrenia (incidence of 5% or greater and aripiprazole incidence at least twice that for placebo) were extrapyramidal disorder, somnolence, and tremor.

Pediatric Patients (10 to 17 years) with Bipolar Mania

The following findings are based on one 4-week, placebo-controlled trial in which oral aripiprazole was administered in doses of 10 mg/day or 30 mg/day.

Adverse Reactions Associated with Discontinuation of Treatment

The incidence of discontinuation due to adverse reactions between aripiprazole-treated and placebo-treated pediatric patients (10 to 17 years) was 7% and 2%, respectively.

Commonly Observed Adverse Reactions

Commonly observed adverse reactions associated with the use of aripiprazole in pediatric patients with bipolar mania (incidence of 5% or greater and aripiprazole incidence at least twice that for placebo) are shown in Table 17.

Table 17: Commonly Observed Adverse Reactions in Short-Term, Placebo-Controlled Trials of Pediatric Patients (10 to 17 years) with Bipolar Mania Treated with Oral ABILIFY

Preferred Term	Percentage of Patients Reporting Reaction Aripiprazole (n=197)	Placebo (n=97)
Somnolence	23	3
Extrapyramidal Disorder	20	3
Fatigue	11	4
Nausea	11	4
Akathisia	10	2
Blurred Vision	8	0
Salivary Hypersecretion	6	0
Dizziness	5	1

Pediatric Patients (6 to 17 years) with Autistic Disorder

The following findings are based on two 8-week, placebo-controlled trials in which oral aripiprazole was administered in doses of 2 mg/day to 15 mg/day.

Adverse Reactions Associated with Discontinuation of Treatment

The incidence of discontinuation due to adverse reactions between aripiprazole-treated and placebo-treated pediatric patients (6 to 17 years) was 10% and 8%, respectively.

Commonly Observed Adverse Reactions
Commonly observed adverse reactions associated with the use of aripiprazole in pediatric patients with autistic disorder (incidence of 5% or greater and aripiprazole incidence at least twice that for placebo) are shown in Table 18.

Table 18: Commonly Observed Adverse Reactions in Short-Term, Placebo-Controlled Trials of Pediatric Patients (6 to 17 years) with Autistic Disorder Treated with Oral ABILIFY

Preferred Term	Percentage of Patients Reporting Reaction Aripiprazole (n=212)	Placebo (n=101)
Sedation	21	4
Fatigue	17	2
Vomiting	14	7
Somnolence	10	4
Tremor	10	0
Pyrexia	9	1
Drooling	9	0
Decreased Appetite	7	2
Salivary Hypersecretion	6	1
Extrapyramidal Disorder	6	0
Lethargy	5	0

Less Common Adverse Reactions in Pediatric Patients (6 to 17 years) with Schizophrenia, Bipolar Mania, or Autistic Disorder
Table 19 enumerates the pooled incidence, rounded to the nearest percent, of adverse reactions that occurred during acute therapy (up to 6 weeks in schizophrenia, up to 4 weeks in bipolar mania, and up to 8 weeks in autistic disorder), including only those reactions that occurred in 1% or more of pediatric patients treated with aripiprazole (doses ≥2 mg/day) and for which the incidence in patients treated with aripiprazole was greater than the incidence in patients treated with placebo.

Table 19: Adverse Reactions in Short-Term, Placebo-Controlled Trials of Pediatric Patients (6 to 17 years) Treated with Oral ABILIFY

System Organ Class Preferred Term	Percentage of Patients Reporting Reaction[a] Aripiprazole (n=611)	Placebo (n=298)
Eye Disorders		
Blurred Vision	3	0
Gastrointestinal Disorders		
Vomiting	9	7
Nausea	8	4
Diarrhea	5	3
Salivary Hypersecretion	4	1
Abdominal Pain Upper	3	2
Constipation	3	2
Dry Mouth	1	0
General Disorders and Administration Site Conditions		
Fatigue	10	2
Pyrexia	5	1
Irritability	1	0
Thirst	1	0
Infections and Infestations		
Nasopharyngitis	6	3
Investigations		
Weight Increased	2	1
Metabolism and Nutrition Disorders		
Increased Appetite	7	3
Decreased Appetite	4	2
Musculoskeletal and Connective Tissue Disorders		
Arthralgia	1	0
Musculoskeletal Stiffness	1	0
Nervous System Disorders		
Somnolence	16	4
Extrapyramidal Disorder	14	2
Headache	13	12
Sedation	8	1
Akathisia	6	1
Tremor	6	1
Drooling	4	0
Dizziness	3	1
Lethargy	2	0
Dystonia	1	0
Dyskinesia	1	0
Hypersomnia	1	0
Reproductive System and Breast Disorders		
Dysmenorrhoea*	2	1
Respiratory, Thoracic, and Mediastinal Disorders		
Rhinorrhoea	2	1
Skin and Subcutaneous Tissue Disorders		
Rash	2	1

[a] Adverse reactions reported by at least 1% of pediatric patients treated with oral aripiprazole, except adverse reactions which had an incidence equal to or less than placebo.
* Adjusted for gender.

Adult Patients Receiving ABILIFY as Adjunctive Treatment of Major Depressive Disorder
The following findings are based on a pool of two placebo-controlled trials of patients with major depressive disorder in which aripiprazole was administered at doses of 2 mg to 20 mg as adjunctive treatment to continued antidepressant therapy.
Adverse Reactions Associated with Discontinuation of Treatment
The incidence of discontinuation due to adverse reactions was 6% for adjunctive aripiprazole-treated patients and 2% for adjunctive placebo-treated patients.
Commonly Observed Adverse Reactions
The commonly observed adverse reactions associated with the use of adjunctive aripiprazole in patients with major depressive disorder (incidence of 5% or greater and aripiprazole incidence at least twice that for placebo) were: akathisia, restlessness, insomnia, constipation, fatigue, and blurred vision.
Less Common Adverse Reactions in Adult Patients with Major Depressive Disorder
Table 20 enumerates the pooled incidence, rounded to the nearest percent, of adverse reactions that occurred during acute therapy (up to 6 weeks), including only those adverse reactions that occurred in 2% or more of patients treated with adjunctive aripiprazole (doses ≥2 mg/day) and for which the incidence in patients treated with adjunctive aripiprazole was greater than the incidence in patients treated with adjunctive placebo in the combined dataset.

Table 20: Adverse Reactions in Short-Term, Placebo-Controlled Adjunctive Trials in Patients with Major Depressive Disorder

System Organ Class Preferred Term	Percentage of Patients Reporting Reaction[a] Aripiprazole+ ADT* (n=371)	Placebo+ ADT* (n=366)
Eye Disorders		
Blurred Vision	6	1
Gastrointestinal Disorders		
Constipation	5	2
General Disorders and Administration Site Conditions		
Fatigue	8	4
Feeling Jittery	3	1
Infections and Infestations		
Upper Respiratory Tract Infection	6	4
Investigations		
Weight Increased	3	2
Metabolism and Nutrition Disorders		
Increased Appetite	3	2
Musculoskeletal and Connective Tissue Disorders		
Arthralgia	4	3
Myalgia	3	1
Nervous System Disorders		
Akathisia	25	4
Somnolence	6	4
Tremor	5	4
Sedation	4	2
Dizziness	4	2
Disturbance in Attention	3	1
Extrapyramidal Disorder	2	0
Psychiatric Disorders		
Restlessness	12	2
Insomnia	8	2

[a] Adverse reactions reported by at least 2% of patients treated with adjunctive aripiprazole, except adverse reactions which had an incidence equal to or less than placebo.
* Antidepressant Therapy

Patients with Agitation Associated with Schizophrenia or Bipolar Mania (Intramuscular Injection)
The following findings are based on a pool of three placebo-controlled trials of patients with agitation associated with schizophrenia or bipolar mania in which aripiprazole injection was administered at doses of 5.25 mg to 15 mg.
Adverse Reactions Associated with Discontinuation of Treatment
Overall, in patients with agitation associated with schizophrenia or bipolar mania, there was little difference in the incidence of discontinuation due to adverse reactions between aripiprazole-treated (0.8%) and placebo-treated (0.5%) patients.
Commonly Observed Adverse Reactions
There was one commonly observed adverse reaction (nausea) associated with the use of aripiprazole injection in patients with agitation associated with schizophrenia and bipolar mania (incidence of 5% or greater and aripiprazole incidence at least twice that for placebo).
Less Common Adverse Reactions in Patients with Agitation Associated with Schizophrenia or Bipolar Mania
Table 21 enumerates the pooled incidence, rounded to the nearest percent, of adverse reactions that occurred during acute therapy (24-hour), including only those adverse reactions that occurred in 2% or more of patients treated with aripiprazole injection (doses ≥5.25 mg/day) and for which the incidence in patients treated with aripiprazole injection was greater than the incidence in patients treated with placebo in the combined dataset.

Table 21: Adverse Reactions in Short-Term, Placebo-Controlled Trials in Patients Treated with ABILIFY Injection

System Organ Class Preferred Term	Percentage of Patients Reporting Reaction[a] Aripiprazole (n=501)	Placebo (n=220)
Cardiac Disorders		
Tachycardia	2	<1
Gastrointestinal Disorders		
Nausea	9	3
Vomiting	3	1
General Disorders and Administration Site Conditions		
Fatigue	2	1
Nervous System Disorders		
Headache	12	7
Dizziness	8	5
Somnolence	7	4
Sedation	3	2
Akathisia	2	0

[a] Adverse reactions reported by at least 2% of patients treated with aripiprazole injection, except adverse reactions which had an incidence equal to or less than placebo.

Dose-Related Adverse Reactions
Schizophrenia
Dose response relationships for the incidence of treatment-emergent adverse events were evaluated from four trials in adult patients with schizophrenia comparing various fixed doses (2 mg/day, 5 mg/day, 10 mg/day, 15 mg/day, 20 mg/day, and 30 mg/day) of oral aripiprazole to placebo. This analysis, stratified by study, indicated that the only adverse reaction to have a possible dose response relationship, and then most prominent only with 30 mg, was somnolence [including sedation]; (incidences were placebo, 7.1%; 10 mg, 8.5%; 15 mg, 8.7%; 20 mg, 7.5%; 30 mg, 12.6%).
In the study of pediatric patients (13 to 17 years of age) with schizophrenia, three common adverse reactions appeared to have a possible dose response relationship: extrapyramidal disorder (incidences were placebo, 5.0%; 10 mg, 13.0%; 30 mg, 21.6%); somnolence (incidences were placebo, 6.0%; 10 mg, 11.0%; 30 mg, 21.6%); and tremor (incidences were placebo, 2.0%; 10 mg, 2.0%; 30 mg, 11.8%).
Bipolar Mania
In the study of pediatric patients (10 to 17 years of age) with bipolar mania, four common adverse reactions had a possible dose response relationship at 4 weeks; extrapyramidal disorder (incidences were placebo, 3.1%; 10 mg, 12.2%; 30 mg, 27.3%); somnolence (incidences were placebo, 3.1%; 10 mg, 19.4%; 30 mg, 26.3%); akathisia (incidences were placebo, 2.1%; 10 mg, 8.2%; 30 mg, 11.1%); and salivary hypersecretion (incidences were placebo, 0%; 10 mg, 3.1%; 30 mg, 8.1%).
Autistic Disorder
In a study of pediatric patients (6 to 17 years of age) with autistic disorder, one common adverse reaction had a possible dose response relationship: fatigue (incidences were placebo, 0%; 5 mg, 3.8%; 10 mg, 22.0%; 15 mg, 18.5%).
Extrapyramidal Symptoms
Schizophrenia
In short-term, placebo-controlled trials in schizophrenia in adults, the incidence of reported EPS-related events, excluding events related to akathisia, for aripiprazole-treated patients was 13% vs. 12% for placebo; and the incidence of akathisia-related events for aripiprazole-treated patients was 8% vs. 4% for placebo. In the short-term, placebo-controlled trial of schizophrenia in pediatric patients (13 to 17 years), the incidence of reported EPS-related events, excluding events related to akathisia, for aripiprazole-treated patients was 25% vs. 7% for placebo; and the incidence of akathisia-related events for aripiprazole-treated patients was 9% vs. 6% for placebo.

Objectively collected data from those trials was collected on the Simpson Angus Rating Scale (for EPS), the Barnes Akathisia Scale (for akathisia), and the Assessments of Involuntary Movement Scales (for dyskinesias). In the adult schizophrenia trials, the objectively collected data did not show a difference between aripiprazole and placebo, with the exception of the Barnes Akathisia Scale (aripiprazole, 0.08; placebo, –0.05). In the pediatric (13 to 17 years) schizophrenia trial, the objectively collected data did not show a difference between aripiprazole and placebo, with the exception of the Simpson Angus Rating Scale (aripiprazole, 0.24; placebo, –0.29).

Similarly, in a long-term (26-week), placebo-controlled trial of schizophrenia in adults, objectively collected data on the Simpson Angus Rating Scale (for EPS), the Barnes Akathisia Scale (for akathisia), and the Assessments of Involuntary Movement Scales (for dyskinesias) did not show a difference between aripiprazole and placebo.

Bipolar Mania

In the short-term, placebo-controlled trials in bipolar mania in adults, the incidence of reported EPS-related events, excluding events related to akathisia, for monotherapy aripiprazole-treated patients was 16% vs. 8% for placebo and the incidence of akathisia-related events for monotherapy aripiprazole-treated patients was 13% vs. 4% for placebo. In the 6-week, placebo-controlled trial in bipolar mania for adjunctive therapy with lithium or valproate, the incidence of reported EPS-related events, excluding events related to akathisia for adjunctive aripiprazole-treated patients was 15% vs. 8% for adjunctive placebo and the incidence of akathisia-related events for adjunctive aripiprazole-treated patients was 19% vs. 5% for adjunctive placebo. In the short-term, placebo-controlled trial in bipolar mania in pediatric (10 to 17 years) patients, the incidence of reported EPS-related events, excluding events related to akathisia, for aripiprazole-treated patients was 26% vs. 5% for placebo and the incidence of akathisia-related events for aripiprazole-treated patients was 10% vs. 2% for placebo.

In the adult bipolar mania trials with monotherapy aripiprazole, the Simpson Angus Rating Scale and the Barnes Akathisia Scale showed a significant difference between aripiprazole and placebo (aripiprazole, 0.50; placebo, –0.01 and aripiprazole, 0.21; placebo, –0.05). Changes in the Assessments of Involuntary Movement Scales were similar for the aripiprazole and placebo groups. In the bipolar mania trials with aripiprazole as adjunctive therapy with either lithium or valproate, the Simpson Angus Rating Scale and the Barnes Akathisia Scale showed a significant difference between adjunctive aripiprazole and adjunctive placebo (aripiprazole, 0.73; placebo, 0.07 and aripiprazole, 0.30; placebo, 0.11). Changes in the Assessments of Involuntary Movement Scales were similar for adjunctive aripiprazole and adjunctive placebo. In the pediatric (10 to 17 years), short-term, bipolar mania trial, the Simpson Angus Rating Scale showed a significant difference between aripiprazole and placebo (aripiprazole, 0.90; placebo, –0.05). Changes in the Barnes Akathisia Scale and the Assessments of Involuntary Movement Scales were similar for the aripiprazole and placebo groups.

Major Depressive Disorder

In the short-term, placebo-controlled trials in major depressive disorder, the incidence of reported EPS-related events, excluding events related to akathisia, for adjunctive aripiprazole-treated patients was 8% vs. 5% for adjunctive placebo-treated patients; and the incidence of akathisia-related events for adjunctive aripiprazole-treated patients was 25% vs. 4% for adjunctive placebo-treated patients.

In the major depressive disorder trials, the Simpson Angus Rating Scale and the Barnes Akathisia Scale showed a significant difference between adjunctive aripiprazole and adjunctive placebo (aripiprazole, 0.31; placebo, 0.03 and aripiprazole, 0.22; placebo, 0.02). Changes in the Assessments of Involuntary Movement Scales were similar for the adjunctive aripiprazole and adjunctive placebo groups.

Autistic Disorder

In the short-term, placebo-controlled trials in autistic disorder in pediatric patients (6 to 17 years), the incidence of reported EPS-related events, excluding events related to akathisia, for aripiprazole-treated patients was 18% vs. 2% for placebo and the incidence of akathisia-related events for aripiprazole-treated patients was 3% vs. 9% for placebo.

In the pediatric (6 to 17 years) short-term autistic disorder trials, the Simpson Angus Rating Scale showed a significant difference between aripiprazole and placebo (aripiprazole, 0.1; placebo, –0.4). Changes in the Barnes Akathisia Scale and the Assessments of Involuntary Movement Scales were similar for the aripiprazole and placebo groups.

Agitation Associated with Schizophrenia or Bipolar Mania

In the placebo-controlled trials in patients with agitation associated with schizophrenia or bipolar mania, the incidence of reported EPS-related events excluding events related to akathisia for aripiprazole-treated patients was 2% vs. 2% for placebo and the incidence of akathisia-related events for aripiprazole-treated patients was 2% vs. 0% for placebo. Objectively collected data on the Simpson Angus Rating Scale (for EPS) and the Barnes Akathisia Scale (for akathisia) for all treatment groups did not show a difference between aripiprazole and placebo.

Dystonia

Class Effect: Symptoms of dystonia, prolonged abnormal contractions of muscle groups, may occur in susceptible individuals during the first few days of treatment. Dystonic symptoms include: spasm of the neck muscles, sometimes progressing to tightness of the throat, swallowing difficulty, difficulty breathing, and/or protrusion of the tongue. While these symptoms can occur at low doses, they occur more frequently and with greater severity with high potency and at higher doses of first generation antipsychotic drugs. An elevated risk of acute dystonia is observed in males and younger age groups.

Laboratory Test Abnormalities

A between group comparison for 3-week to 6-week, placebo-controlled trials in adults or 4-week to 8-week, placebo-controlled trials in pediatric patients (6 to 17 years) revealed no medically important differences between the aripiprazole and placebo groups in the proportions of patients experiencing potentially clinically significant changes in routine serum chemistry, hematology, or urinalysis parameters. Similarly, there were no aripiprazole/placebo differences in the incidence of discontinuations for changes in serum chemistry, hematology, or urinalysis in adult or pediatric patients.

ECG Changes

Between group comparisons for a pooled analysis of placebo-controlled trials in patients with schizophrenia, bipolar mania, or major depressive disorder revealed no significant differences between oral aripiprazole and placebo in the proportion of patients experiencing potentially important changes in ECG parameters. Aripiprazole was associated with a median increase in heart rate of 2 beats per minute compared to no increase among placebo patients.

In the pooled, placebo-controlled trials in patients with agitation associated with schizophrenia or bipolar mania, there were no significant differences between aripiprazole injection and placebo in the proportion of patients experiencing potentially important changes in ECG parameters, as measured by standard 12-lead ECGs.

Additional Findings Observed in Clinical Trials

Adverse Reactions in Long-Term, Double-Blind, Placebo-Controlled Trials

The adverse reactions reported in a 26-week, double-blind trial comparing oral ABILIFY and placebo in patients with schizophrenia were generally consistent with those reported in the short-term, placebo-controlled trials, except for a higher incidence of tremor [8% (12/153) for ABILIFY vs. 2% (3/153) for placebo]. In this study, the majority of the cases of tremor were of mild intensity (8/12 mild and 4/12 moderate), occurred early in therapy (9/12 ≤49 days), and were of limited duration (7/12 ≤10 days). Tremor infrequently led to discontinuation (<1%) of ABILIFY. In addition, in a long-term (52-week), active-controlled study, the incidence of tremor was 5% (40/859) for ABILIFY. A similar profile was observed in a long-term monotherapy study and a long-term adjunctive study with lithium and valproate in bipolar disorder.

Other Adverse Reactions Observed During the Premarketing Evaluation of Aripiprazole

Following is a list of MedDRA terms that reflect adverse reactions as defined in *ADVERSE REACTIONS (6.1)* reported by patients treated with oral aripiprazole at multiple doses ≥2 mg/day during any phase of a trial within the database of 13,543 adult patients. All events assessed as possible adverse drug reactions have been included with the exception of more commonly occurring events. In addition, medically/clinically meaningful adverse reactions, particularly those that are likely to be useful to the prescriber or that have pharmacologic plausibility, have been included. Events already listed in other parts of *ADVERSE REACTIONS (6)*, or those considered in *WARNINGS AND PRECAUTIONS (5)* or *OVERDOSAGE (10)* have been excluded. Although the reactions reported occurred during treatment with aripiprazole, they were not necessarily caused by it.

Events are further categorized by MedDRA system organ class and listed in order of decreasing frequency according to the following definitions: those occurring in at least 1/100 patients (only those not already listed in the tabulated results from placebo-controlled trials appear in this listing); those occurring in 1/100 to 1/1000 patients; and those occurring in fewer than 1/1000 patients.

Adults - Oral Administration

Blood and Lymphatic System Disorders:

≥1/1000 patients and <1/100 patients - leukopenia, neutropenia, thrombocytopenia

Cardiac Disorders:

≥1/1000 patients and <1/100 patients - bradycardia, palpitations, cardiopulmonary failure, myocardial infarction, cardio-respiratory arrest, atrioventricular block, extrasystoles, sinus tachycardia, atrial fibrillation, angina pectoris, myocardial ischemia; *<1/1000 patients* - atrial flutter, supraventricular tachycardia, ventricular tachycardia

Eye Disorders:

≥1/1000 patients and <1/100 patients - photophobia, diplopia, eyelid edema, photopsia

Gastrointestinal Disorders:

≥1/1000 patients and <1/100 patients - gastroesophageal reflux disease, swollen tongue, esophagitis; *<1/1000 patients* - pancreatitis

General Disorders and Administration Site Conditions:

≥1/100 patients - asthenia, peripheral edema, chest pain; *≥1/1000 patients and <1/100 patients* - face edema, angioedema; *<1/1000 patients* - hypothermia

Hepatobiliary Disorders:

<1/1000 patients - hepatitis, jaundice

Immune System Disorders:

≥1/1000 patients and <1/100 patients - hypersensitivity

Injury, Poisoning, and Procedural Complications:

≥1/100 patients - fall; *≥1/1000 patients and <1/100 patients* - self mutilation; *<1/1000 patients* - heat stroke

Investigations:

≥1/100 patients - weight decreased, creatine phosphokinase increased; *≥1/1000 patients and <1/100 patients* - hepatic enzyme increased, blood glucose increased, blood prolactin increased, blood urea increased, electrocardiogram QT prolonged, blood creatinine increased, blood bilirubin increased; *<1/1000 patients* - blood lactate dehydrogenase increased, glycosylated hemoglobin increased, gamma-glutamyl transferase increased

Metabolism and Nutrition Disorders:

≥1/1000 patients and <1/100 patients - hyperlipidemia, anorexia, diabetes mellitus (including blood insulin increased, carbohydrate tolerance decreased, diabetes mellitus non-insulin-dependent, glucose tolerance impaired, glycosuria, glucose urine, glucose urine present), hyperglycemia, hypokalemia, hyponatremia, hypoglycemia, polydipsia; *<1/1000 patients* - diabetic ketoacidosis

Musculoskeletal and Connective Tissue Disorders:

≥1/1000 patients and <1/100 patients - muscle rigidity, muscular weakness, muscle tightness, mobility decreased; *<1/1000 patients* - rhabdomyolysis

Nervous System Disorders:

≥1/100 patients - coordination abnormal; *≥1/1000 patients and <1/100 patients* - speech disorder, parkinsonism, memory impairment, cogwheel rigidity, cerebrovascular accident, hypokinesia, tardive dyskinesia, hypotonia, myoclonus, hypertonia, akinesia, bradykinesia; *<1/1000 patients* - Grand Mal convulsion, choreoathetosis

Psychiatric Disorders:

≥1/100 patients - suicidal ideation; *≥1/1000 patients and <1/100 patients* - aggression, loss of libido, suicide attempt, hostility, libido increased, anger, anorgasmia, delirium, intentional self injury, completed suicide, tic, homicidal ideation; *<1/1000 patients* - catatonia, sleep walking

Renal and Urinary Disorders:

≥1/1000 patients and <1/100 patients - urinary retention, polyuria, nocturia

Reproductive System and Breast Disorders:

≥1/1000 patients and <1/100 patients - menstruation irregular, erectile dysfunction, amenorrhea, breast pain; *<1/1000 patients* - gynaecomastia, priapism

Respiratory, Thoracic, and Mediastinal Disorders:

≥1/100 patients - nasal congestion, dyspnea, pneumonia aspiration

Skin and Subcutaneous Tissue Disorders:

≥1/100 patients - rash (including erythematous, exfoliative, generalized, macular, maculopapular, papular rash; acneiform, allergic, contact, exfoliative, seborrheic dermatitis, neurodermatitis, and drug eruption), hyperhydrosis; *≥1/1000 patients and <1/100 patients* - pruritus, photosensitivity reaction, alopecia, urticaria

Vascular Disorders:

≥1/100 patients - hypertension; *≥1/1000 patients and <1/100 patients* - hypotension

Pediatric Patients - Oral Administration

Most adverse events observed in the pooled database of 920 pediatric patients, aged 6 to 17 years, were also observed in the adult population. Additional adverse reactions observed in the pediatric population are listed below.

Gastrointestinal Disorders:

≥1/1000 patients and <1/100 patients - tongue dry, tongue spasm

Investigations:

≥1/100 patients - blood insulin increased

Nervous System Disorders:

≥1/1000 patients and <1/100 patients - sleep talking

Skin and Subcutaneous Tissue Disorders:

≥1/1000 patients and <1/100 patients - hirsutism

Adults - Intramuscular Injection

Most adverse reactions observed in the pooled database of 749 adult patients treated with aripiprazole injection, were also observed in the adult population treated with oral aripiprazole. Additional adverse reactions observed in the aripiprazole injection population are listed below.

General Disorders and Administration Site Conditions:
≥1/100 patients - injection site reaction; *≥1/1000 patients and <1/100 patients* - venipuncture site bruise

6.3 Postmarketing Experience

The following adverse reactions have been identified during postapproval use of ABILIFY. Because these reactions are reported voluntarily from a population of uncertain size, it is not always possible to establish a causal relationship to drug exposure: rare occurrences of allergic reaction (anaphylactic reaction, angioedema, laryngospasm, pruritus/urticaria, or oropharyngeal spasm), and blood glucose fluctuation.

7 DRUG INTERACTIONS

Given the primary CNS effects of aripiprazole, caution should be used when ABILIFY is taken in combination with other centrally-acting drugs or alcohol.

Due to its alpha adrenergic antagonism, aripiprazole has the potential to enhance the effect of certain antihypertensive agents.

7.1 Potential for Other Drugs to Affect ABILIFY

Aripiprazole is not a substrate of CYP1A1, CYP1A2, CYP2A6, CYP2B6, CYP2C8, CYP2C9, CYP2C19, or CYP2E1 enzymes. Aripiprazole also does not undergo direct glucuronidation. This suggests that an interaction of aripiprazole with inhibitors or inducers of these enzymes, or other factors, like smoking, is unlikely.

Both CYP3A4 and CYP2D6 are responsible for aripiprazole metabolism. Agents that induce CYP3A4 (eg, carbamazepine) could cause an increase in aripiprazole clearance and lower blood levels. Inhibitors of CYP3A4 (eg, ketoconazole) or CYP2D6 (eg, quinidine, fluoxetine, or paroxetine) can inhibit aripiprazole elimination and cause increased blood levels.

Ketoconazole and Other CYP3A4 Inhibitors

Coadministration of ketoconazole (200 mg/day for 14 days) with a 15 mg single dose of aripiprazole increased the AUC of aripiprazole and its active metabolite by 63% and 77%, respectively. The effect of a higher ketoconazole dose (400 mg/day) has not been studied. When ketoconazole is given concomitantly with aripiprazole, the aripiprazole dose should be reduced to one-half of its normal dose. Other strong inhibitors of CYP3A4 (itraconazole) would be expected to have similar effects and need similar dose reductions; moderate inhibitors (erythromycin, grapefruit juice) have not been studied. When the CYP3A4 inhibitor is withdrawn from the combination therapy, the aripiprazole dose should be increased.

Quinidine and Other CYP2D6 Inhibitors

Coadministration of a 10 mg single dose of aripiprazole with quinidine (166 mg/day for 13 days), a potent inhibitor of CYP2D6, increased the AUC of aripiprazole by 112% but decreased the AUC of its active metabolite, dehydro-aripiprazole, by 35%. Aripiprazole dose should be reduced to one-half of its normal dose when quinidine is given concomitantly with aripiprazole. Other significant inhibitors of CYP2D6, such as fluoxetine or paroxetine, would be expected to have similar effects and should lead to similar dose reductions. When the CYP2D6 inhibitor is withdrawn from the combination therapy, the aripiprazole dose should be increased. When adjunctive ABILIFY is administered to patients with major depressive disorder, ABILIFY should be administered without dosage adjustment as specified in *DOSAGE AND ADMINISTRATION (2.3)*.

Carbamazepine and Other CYP3A4 Inducers

Coadministration of carbamazepine (200 mg twice daily), a potent CYP3A4 inducer, with aripiprazole (30 mg/day) resulted in an approximate 70% decrease in Cmax and AUC values of both aripiprazole and its active metabolite, dehydro-aripiprazole. When carbamazepine is added to aripiprazole therapy, aripiprazole dose should be doubled. Additional dose increases should be based on clinical evaluation. When carbamazepine is withdrawn from the combination therapy, the aripiprazole dose should be reduced.

7.2 Potential for ABILIFY to Affect Other Drugs

Aripiprazole is unlikely to cause clinically important pharmacokinetic interactions with drugs metabolized by cytochrome P450 enzymes. In *in vivo* studies, 10 mg/day to 30 mg/day doses of aripiprazole had no significant effect on metabolism by CYP2D6 (dextromethorphan), CYP2C9 (warfarin), CYP2C19 (omeprazole, warfarin), and CYP3A4 (dextromethorphan) substrates. Additionally, aripiprazole and dehydro-aripiprazole did not show potential for altering CYP1A2-mediated metabolism *in vitro*.

No effect of aripiprazole was seen on the pharmacokinetics of lithium or valproate.

Alcohol

There was no significant difference between aripiprazole coadministered with ethanol and placebo coadministered with ethanol on performance of gross motor skills or stimulus response in healthy subjects. As with most psychoactive medications, patients should be advised to avoid alcohol while taking ABILIFY.

7.3 Drugs Having No Clinically Important Interactions with ABILIFY

Famotidine

Coadministration of aripiprazole (given in a single dose of 15 mg) with a 40 mg single dose of the H_2 antagonist famotidine, a potent gastric acid blocker, decreased the solubility of aripiprazole and, hence, its rate of absorption, reducing by 37% and 21% the Cmax of aripiprazole and dehydro-aripiprazole, respectively, and by 13% and 15%, respectively, the extent of absorption (AUC). No dosage adjustment of aripiprazole is required when administered concomitantly with famotidine.

Valproate

When valproate (500 mg/day-1500 mg/day) and aripiprazole (30 mg/day) were coadministered, at steady-state the Cmax and AUC of aripiprazole were decreased by 25%. No dosage adjustment of aripiprazole is required when administered concomitantly with valproate.

When aripiprazole (30 mg/day) and valproate (1000 mg/day) were coadministered, at steady-state there were no clinically significant changes in the Cmax or AUC of valproate. No dosage adjustment of valproate is required when administered concomitantly with aripiprazole.

Lithium

A pharmacokinetic interaction of aripiprazole with lithium is unlikely because lithium is not bound to plasma proteins, is not metabolized, and is almost entirely excreted unchanged in urine. Coadministration of therapeutic doses of lithium (1200 mg/day-1800 mg/day) for 21 days with aripiprazole (30 mg/day) did not result in clinically significant changes in the pharmacokinetics of aripiprazole or its active metabolite, dehydro-aripiprazole (Cmax and AUC increased by less than 20%). No dosage adjustment of aripiprazole is required when administered concomitantly with lithium.

Coadministration of aripiprazole (30 mg/day) with lithium (900 mg/day) did not result in clinically significant changes in the pharmacokinetics of lithium. No dosage adjustment of lithium is required when administered concomitantly with aripiprazole.

Lamotrigine

Coadministration of 10 mg/day to 30 mg/day oral doses of aripiprazole for 14 days to patients with bipolar I disorder had no effect on the steady-state pharmacokinetics of 100 mg/day to 400 mg/day lamotrigine, a UDP-glucuronosyltransferase 1A4 substrate. No dosage adjustment of lamotrigine is required when aripiprazole is added to lamotrigine.

Dextromethorphan

Aripiprazole at doses of 10 mg/day to 30 mg/day for 14 days had no effect on dextromethorphan's O-dealkylation to its major metabolite, dextrorphan, a pathway dependent on CYP2D6 activity. Aripiprazole also had no effect on dextromethorphan's N-demethylation to its metabolite 3-methoxymorphinan, a pathway dependent on CYP3A4 activity. No dosage adjustment of dextromethorphan is required when administered concomitantly with aripiprazole.

Warfarin

Aripiprazole 10 mg/day for 14 days had no effect on the pharmacokinetics of R-warfarin and S-warfarin or on the pharmacodynamic end point of International Normalized Ratio, indicating the lack of a clinically relevant effect of aripiprazole on CYP2C9 and CYP2C19 metabolism or the binding of highly protein-bound warfarin. No dosage adjustment of warfarin is required when administered concomitantly with aripiprazole.

Omeprazole

Aripiprazole 10 mg/day for 15 days had no effect on the pharmacokinetics of a single 20 mg dose of omeprazole, a CYP2C19 substrate, in healthy subjects. No dosage adjustment of omeprazole is required when administered concomitantly with aripiprazole.

Lorazepam

Coadministration of lorazepam injection (2 mg) and aripiprazole injection (15 mg) to healthy subjects (n=40: 35 males and 5 females; ages 19-45 years old) did not result in clinically important changes in the pharmacokinetics of either drug. No dosage adjustment of aripiprazole is required when administered concomitantly with lorazepam. However, the intensity of sedation was greater with the combination as compared to that observed with aripiprazole alone and the orthostatic hypotension observed was greater with the combination as compared to that observed with lorazepam alone *[see WARNINGS AND PRECAUTIONS (5.6)]*.

Escitalopram

Coadministration of 10 mg/day oral doses of aripiprazole for 14 days to healthy subjects had no effect on the steady-state pharmacokinetics of 10 mg/day escitalopram, a substrate of CYP2C19 and CYP3A4. No dosage adjustment of escitalopram is required when aripiprazole is added to escitalopram.

Venlafaxine

Coadministration of 10 mg/day to 20 mg/day oral doses of aripiprazole for 14 days to healthy subjects had no effect on the steady-state pharmacokinetics of venlafaxine and O-desmethylvenlafaxine following 75 mg/day venlafaxine XR, a CYP2D6 substrate. No dosage adjustment of venlafaxine is required when aripiprazole is added to venlafaxine.

Fluoxetine, Paroxetine, and Sertraline

A population pharmacokinetic analysis in patients with major depressive disorder showed no substantial change in plasma concentrations of fluoxetine (20 mg/day or 40 mg/day), paroxetine CR (37.5 mg/day or 50 mg/day), or sertraline (100 mg/day or 150 mg/day) dosed to steady-state. The steady-state plasma concentrations of fluoxetine and norfluoxetine increased by about 18% and 36%, respectively, and concentrations of paroxetine decreased by about 27%. The steady-state plasma concentrations of sertraline and desmethylsertraline were not substantially changed when these antidepressant therapies were coadministered with aripiprazole. Aripiprazole dosing was 2 mg/day to 15 mg/day (when given with fluoxetine or paroxetine) or 2 mg/day to 20 mg/day (when given with sertraline).

8 USE IN SPECIFIC POPULATIONS

In general, no dosage adjustment for ABILIFY is required on the basis of a patient's age, gender, race, smoking status, hepatic function, or renal function *[see DOSAGE AND ADMINISTRATION (2.5)]*.

8.1 Pregnancy

Teratogenic Effects

Pregnancy Category C: In animal studies, aripiprazole demonstrated developmental toxicity, including possible teratogenic effects in rats and rabbits.

Pregnant rats were treated with oral doses of 3 mg/kg/day, 10 mg/kg/day, and 30 mg/kg/day (1 times, 3 times, and 10 times the maximum recommended human dose [MRHD] on a mg/m^2 basis) of aripiprazole during the period of organogenesis. Gestation was slightly prolonged at 30 mg/kg. Treatment caused a slight delay in fetal development, as evidenced by decreased fetal weight (30 mg/kg), undescended testes (30 mg/kg), and delayed skeletal ossification (10 mg/kg and 30 mg/kg). There were no adverse effects on embryofetal or pup survival. Delivered offspring had decreased body weights (10 mg/kg and 30 mg/kg), and increased incidences of hepatodiaphragmatic nodules and diaphragmatic hernia at 30 mg/kg (the other dose groups were not examined for these findings). A low incidence of diaphragmatic hernia was also seen in the fetuses exposed to 30 mg/kg. Postnatally, delayed vaginal opening was seen at 10 mg/kg and 30 mg/kg and impaired reproductive performance (decreased fertility rate, corpora lutea, implants, live fetuses, and increased post-implantation loss, likely mediated through effects on female offspring) was seen at 30 mg/kg. Some maternal toxicity was seen at 30 mg/kg; however, there was no evidence to suggest that these developmental effects were secondary to maternal toxicity.

In pregnant rats receiving aripiprazole injection intravenously (3 mg/kg/day, 9 mg/kg/day, and 27 mg/kg/day) during the period of organogenesis, decreased fetal weight and delayed skeletal ossification were seen at the highest dose, which also caused some maternal toxicity.

Pregnant rabbits were treated with oral doses of 10 mg/kg/day, 30 mg/kg/day, and 100 mg/kg/day (2 times, 3 times, and 11 times human exposure at MRHD based on AUC and 6 times, 19 times, and 65 times the MRHD based on mg/m^2) of aripiprazole during the period of organogenesis. Decreased maternal food consumption and increased abortions were seen at 100 mg/kg. Treatment caused increased fetal mortality (100 mg/kg), decreased fetal weight (30 mg/kg and 100 mg/kg), increased incidence of a skeletal abnormality (fused sternebrae at 30 mg/kg and 100 mg/kg), and minor skeletal variations (100 mg/kg).

In pregnant rabbits receiving aripiprazole injection intravenously (3 mg/kg/day, 10 mg/kg/day, and 30 mg/kg/day) during the period of organogenesis, the highest dose, which caused pronounced maternal toxicity, resulted in decreased fetal weight, increased fetal abnormalities (primarily skeletal), and decreased fetal skeletal ossification. The fetal no-effect dose was 10 mg/kg, which produced 5 times the human exposure at the MRHD based on AUC and is 6 times the MRHD based on mg/m^2.

In a study in which rats were treated with oral doses of 3 mg/kg/day, 10 mg/kg/day, and 30 mg/kg/day (1 times, 3 times, and 10 times the MRHD on a mg/m^2 basis) of aripiprazole perinatally and postnatally (from day 17 of gestation through day 21 postpartum), slight maternal toxicity and slightly prolonged gestation were seen at 30 mg/kg. An increase in stillbirths and decreases in pup weight (persisting into adulthood) and survival were seen at this dose.

In rats receiving aripiprazole injection intravenously (3 mg/kg/day, 8 mg/kg/day, and 20 mg/kg/day) from day 6 of gestation through day 20 postpartum, an increase in stillbirths was seen at 8 mg/kg and 20 mg/kg, and decreases in early postnatal pup weights and survival were seen at 20 mg/kg. These doses produced some maternal toxicity. There were no effects on postnatal behavioral and reproductive development.

Non-teratogenic Effects

There are no adequate and well-controlled studies in pregnant women. It is not known whether aripiprazole can cause fetal harm when administered to a pregnant woman or can affect reproductive capacity. Neonates exposed to antipsychotic drugs during the third trimester of pregnancy are at risk for extrapyramidal and/or withdrawal symptoms following delivery. There have been reports of agitation, hypertonia, hypotonia, tremor, somnolence, respiratory distress and feeding disorder in these neonates. These complications have varied in severity; while in some cases symptoms have been self-limited, in other cases neonates have required intensive care unit support and prolonged hospitalization.

Aripiprazole should be used during pregnancy only if the potential benefit justifies the potential risk to the fetus.

8.2 Labor and Delivery

The effect of aripiprazole on labor and delivery in humans is unknown.

8.3 Nursing Mothers

Aripiprazole has been demonstrated to be excreted in milk of rats during lactation. In humans, data on excretion in breast milk is limited. It is recommended that women receiving aripiprazole should not breast-feed.

8.4 Pediatric Use

Safety and effectiveness in pediatric patients with major depressive disorder or agitation associated with schizophrenia or bipolar mania have not been established.

Safety and effectiveness in pediatric patients with schizophrenia were established in a 6-week, placebo-controlled clinical trial in 202 pediatric patients aged 13 to 17 years *[see INDICATIONS AND USAGE (1.1), DOSAGE AND ADMINISTRATION (2.1), ADVERSE REACTIONS (6.2), and CLINICAL STUDIES (14.1)]*. Although maintenance efficacy in pediatric patients has not been systematically evaluated, maintenance efficacy can be extrapolated from adult data along with comparisons of aripiprazole pharmacokinetic parameters in adult and pediatric patients.

Safety and effectiveness in pediatric patients with bipolar mania were established in a 4-week, placebo-controlled clinical trial in 197 pediatric patients aged 10 to 17 years *[see INDICATIONS AND USAGE (1.2), DOSAGE AND ADMINISTRATION (2.2), ADVERSE REACTIONS (6.2), and CLINICAL STUDIES (14.2)]*. Although maintenance efficacy in pediatric patients has not been systematically evaluated, maintenance efficacy can be extrapolated from adult data along with comparisons of aripiprazole pharmacokinetic parameters in adult and pediatric patients.

The efficacy of adjunctive ABILIFY with concomitant lithium or valproate in the treatment of manic or mixed episodes in pediatric patients has not been systematically evaluated. However, such efficacy and lack of pharmacokinetic interaction between aripiprazole and lithium or valproate can be extrapolated from adult data, along with comparisons of aripiprazole pharmacokinetic parameters in adult and pediatric patients.

Safety and effectiveness in pediatric patients demonstrating irritability associated with autistic disorder were established in two 8-week, placebo-controlled clinical trials in 212 pediatric patients aged 6 to 17 years *[see INDICATIONS AND USAGE (1.4), DOSAGE AND ADMINISTRATION (2.4), ADVERSE REACTIONS (6.2), and CLINICAL STUDIES (14.4)]*. Maintenance efficacy in pediatric patients has not been systematically evaluated.

The pharmacokinetics of aripiprazole and dehydro-aripiprazole in pediatric patients, 10 to 17 years of age, were similar to those in adults after correcting for the differences in body weight.

8.5 Geriatric Use

In formal single-dose pharmacokinetic studies (with aripiprazole given in a single dose of 15 mg), aripiprazole clearance was 20% lower in elderly (≥65 years) subjects compared to younger adult subjects (18 to 64 years). There was no detectable age effect, however, in the population pharmacokinetic analysis in schizophrenia patients. Also, the pharmacokinetics of aripiprazole after multiple doses in elderly patients appeared similar to that observed in young, healthy subjects. No dosage adjustment is recommended for elderly patients *[see also BOXED WARNING and WARNINGS AND PRECAUTIONS (5.1)]*.

Of the 13,543 patients treated with oral aripiprazole in clinical trials, 1073 (8%) were ≥65 years old and 799 (6%) were ≥75 years old. The majority (81%) of the 1073 patients were diagnosed with Dementia of the Alzheimer's type.

Placebo-controlled studies of oral aripiprazole in schizophrenia, bipolar mania, or major depressive disorder did not include sufficient numbers of subjects aged 65 and over to determine whether they respond differently from younger subjects.

Of the 749 patients treated with aripiprazole injection in clinical trials, 99 (13%) were ≥65 years old and 78 (10%) were ≥75 years old. Placebo-controlled studies of aripiprazole injection in patients with agitation associated with schizophrenia or bipolar mania did not include sufficient numbers of subjects aged 65 and over to determine whether they respond differently from younger subjects.

Studies of elderly patients with psychosis associated with Alzheimer's disease have suggested that there may be a different tolerability profile in this population compared to younger patients with schizophrenia *[see also BOXED WARNING and WARNINGS AND PRECAUTIONS (5.1)]*. The safety and efficacy of ABILIFY in the treatment of patients with psychosis associated with Alzheimer's disease has not been established. If the prescriber elects to treat such patients with ABILIFY, vigilance should be exercised.

8.6 Renal Impairment

In patients with severe renal impairment (creatinine clearance <30 mL/min), Cmax of aripiprazole (given in a single dose of 15 mg) and dehydro-aripiprazole increased by 36% and 53%, respectively, but AUC was 15% lower for aripiprazole and 7% higher for dehydro-aripiprazole. Renal excretion of both unchanged aripiprazole and dehydro-aripiprazole is less than 1% of the dose. No dosage adjustment is required in subjects with renal impairment.

8.7 Hepatic Impairment

In a single-dose study (15 mg of aripiprazole) in subjects with varying degrees of liver cirrhosis (Child-Pugh Classes A, B, and C), the AUC of aripiprazole, compared to healthy subjects, increased 31% in mild HI, increased 8% in moderate HI, and decreased 20% in severe HI. None of these differences would require dose adjustment.

8.8 Gender

Cmax and AUC of aripiprazole and its active metabolite, dehydro-aripiprazole, are 30% to 40% higher in women than in men, and correspondingly, the apparent oral clearance of aripiprazole is lower in women. These differences, however, are largely explained by differences in body weight (25%) between men and women. No dosage adjustment is recommended based on gender.

8.9 Race

Although no specific pharmacokinetic study was conducted to investigate the effects of race on the disposition of aripiprazole, population pharmacokinetic evaluation revealed no evidence of clinically significant race-related differences in the pharmacokinetics of aripiprazole. No dosage adjustment is recommended based on race.

8.10 Smoking

Based on studies utilizing human liver enzymes *in vitro*, aripiprazole is not a substrate for CYP1A2 and also does not undergo direct glucuronidation. Smoking should, therefore, not have an effect on the pharmacokinetics of aripiprazole. Consistent with these *in vitro* results, population pharmacokinetic evaluation did not reveal any significant pharmacokinetic differences between smokers and nonsmokers. No dosage adjustment is recommended based on smoking status.

9 DRUG ABUSE AND DEPENDENCE

9.1 Controlled Substance

ABILIFY is not a controlled substance.

9.2 Abuse and Dependence

Aripiprazole has not been systematically studied in humans for its potential for abuse, tolerance, or physical dependence. In physical dependence studies in monkeys, withdrawal symptoms were observed upon abrupt cessation of dosing. While the clinical trials did not reveal any tendency for any drug-seeking behavior, these observations were not systematic and it is not possible to predict on the basis of this limited experience the extent to which a CNS-active drug will be misused, diverted, and/or abused once marketed. Consequently, patients should be evaluated carefully for a history of drug abuse, and such patients should be observed closely for signs of ABILIFY misuse or abuse (eg, development of tolerance, increases in dose, drug-seeking behavior).

10 OVERDOSAGE

MedDRA terminology has been used to classify the adverse reactions.

10.1 Human Experience

In clinical trials and in postmarketing experience, adverse reactions of deliberate or accidental overdosage with oral aripiprazole have been reported worldwide. These include overdoses with oral aripiprazole alone and in combination with other substances. No fatality was reported with aripiprazole alone. The largest known dose with a known outcome involved acute ingestion of 1260 mg of oral aripiprazole (42 times the maximum recommended daily dose) by a patient who fully recovered. Deliberate or accidental overdosage was also reported in children (age 12 and younger) involving oral aripiprazole ingestions up to 195 mg with no fatalities.

Common adverse reactions (reported in at least 5% of all overdose cases) reported with oral aripiprazole overdosage (alone or in combination with other substances) include vomiting, somnolence, and tremor. Other clinically important signs and symptoms observed in one or more patients with aripiprazole overdoses (alone or with other substances) include acidosis, aggression, aspartate aminotransferase increased, atrial fibrillation, bradycardia, coma, confusional state, convulsion, blood creatine phosphokinase increased, depressed level of consciousness, hypertension, hypokalemia, hypotension, lethargy, loss of consciousness, QRS complex prolonged, QT prolonged, pneumonia aspiration, respiratory arrest, status epilepticus, and tachycardia.

10.2 Management of Overdosage

No specific information is available on the treatment of overdose with aripiprazole. An electrocardiogram should be obtained in case of overdosage and if QT interval prolongation is present, cardiac monitoring should be instituted. Otherwise, management of overdose should concentrate on supportive therapy, maintaining an adequate airway, oxygenation and ventilation, and management of symptoms. Close medical supervision and monitoring should continue until the patient recovers.

Charcoal: In the event of an overdose of ABILIFY, an early charcoal administration may be useful in partially preventing the absorption of aripiprazole. Administration of 50 g of activated charcoal, one hour after a single 15 mg oral dose of aripiprazole, decreased the mean AUC and Cmax of aripiprazole by 50%.

Hemodialysis: Although there is no information on the effect of hemodialysis in treating an overdose with aripiprazole, hemodialysis is unlikely to be useful in overdose management since aripiprazole is highly bound to plasma proteins.

11 DESCRIPTION

Aripiprazole is a psychotropic drug that is available as ABILIFY® (aripiprazole) Tablets, ABILIFY DISCMELT® (aripiprazole) Orally Disintegrating Tablets, ABILIFY® (aripiprazole) Oral Solution, and ABILIFY® (aripiprazole) Injection, a solution for intramuscular injection. Aripiprazole is 7-[4-[4-(2,3-dichlorophenyl)-1-piperazinyl]butoxy]-3,4-dihydrocarbostyril. The empirical formula is $C_{23}H_{27}Cl_2N_3O_2$ and its molecular weight is 448.38. The chemical structure is:

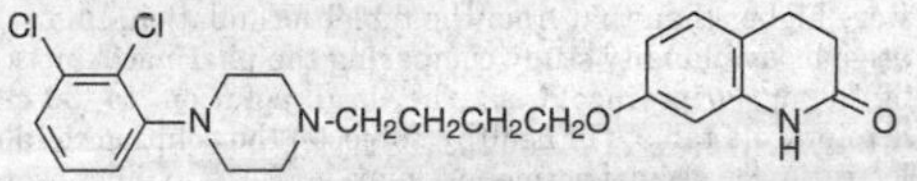

ABILIFY Tablets are available in 2 mg, 5 mg, 10 mg, 15 mg, 20 mg, and 30 mg strengths. Inactive ingredients include cornstarch, hydroxypropyl cellulose, lactose monohydrate, magnesium stearate, and microcrystalline cellulose. Colorants include ferric oxide (yellow or red) and FD&C Blue No. 2 Aluminum Lake.

ABILIFY DISCMELT Orally Disintegrating Tablets are available in 10 mg and 15 mg strengths. Inactive ingredients include acesulfame potassium, aspartame, calcium silicate, croscarmellose sodium, crospovidone, crème de vanilla (natural and artificial flavors), magnesium stearate, microcrystalline cellulose, silicon dioxide, tartaric acid, and xylitol. Colorants include ferric oxide (yellow or red) and FD&C Blue No. 2 Aluminum Lake.

ABILIFY Oral Solution is a clear, colorless to light-yellow solution available in a concentration of 1 mg/mL. The inactive ingredients for this solution include disodium edetate, fructose, glycerin, dl-lactic acid, methylparaben, propylene glycol, propylparaben, sodium hydroxide, sucrose, and purified water. The oral solution is flavored with natural orange cream and other natural flavors.

ABILIFY Injection is available in single-dose vials as a ready-to-use, 9.75 mg/1.3 mL (7.5 mg/mL) clear, colorless, sterile, aqueous solution for intramuscular use only. Inactive ingredients for this solution include 150 mg/mL of sulfobutylether β-cyclodextrin (SBECD), tartaric acid, sodium hydroxide, and water for injection.

12 CLINICAL PHARMACOLOGY

12.1 Mechanism of Action

The mechanism of action of aripiprazole, as with other drugs having efficacy in schizophrenia, bipolar disorder, major depressive disorder, irritability associated with autistic disorder, and agitation associated with schizophrenia or bipolar disorder, is unknown. However, it has been proposed that the efficacy of aripiprazole is mediated through a combination of partial agonist activity at D_2 and 5-HT_{1A} receptors and antagonist activity at 5-HT_{2A} receptors. Actions at receptors other than D_2, 5-HT_{1A}, and 5-HT_{2A} may explain some of the other clinical effects of aripiprazole (eg, the orthostatic hypotension observed with aripiprazole may be explained by its antagonist activity at adrenergic $alpha_1$ receptors).

12.2 Pharmacodynamics

Aripiprazole exhibits high affinity for dopamine D_2 and D_3, serotonin 5-HT_{1A} and 5-HT_{2A} receptors (K_i values of

0.34 nM, 0.8 nM, 1.7 nM, and 3.4 nM, respectively), moderate affinity for dopamine D_4, serotonin 5-HT_{2C} and 5-HT_7, $alpha_1$-adrenergic and histamine H_1 receptors (K_i values of 44 nM, 15 nM, 39 nM, 57 nM, and 61 nM, respectively), and moderate affinity for the serotonin reuptake site (K_i=98 nM). Aripiprazole has no appreciable affinity for cholinergic muscarinic receptors (IC_{50}>1000 nM). Aripiprazole functions as a partial agonist at the dopamine D_2 and the serotonin 5-HT_{1A} receptors, and as an antagonist at serotonin 5-HT_{2A} receptor.

12.3 Pharmacokinetics

ABILIFY activity is presumably primarily due to the parent drug, aripiprazole, and to a lesser extent, to its major metabolite, dehydro-aripiprazole, which has been shown to have affinities for D_2 receptors similar to the parent drug and represents 40% of the parent drug exposure in plasma. The mean elimination half-lives are about 75 hours and 94 hours for aripiprazole and dehydro-aripiprazole, respectively. Steady-state concentrations are attained within 14 days of dosing for both active moieties. Aripiprazole accumulation is predictable from single-dose pharmacokinetics. At steady-state, the pharmacokinetics of aripiprazole are dose-proportional. Elimination of aripiprazole is mainly through hepatic metabolism involving two P450 isozymes, CYP2D6 and CYP3A4.

Pharmacokinetic studies showed that ABILIFY DISCMELT Orally Disintegrating Tablets are bioequivalent to ABILIFY Tablets.

ORAL ADMINISTRATION

Absorption

Tablet: Aripiprazole is well absorbed after administration of the tablet, with peak plasma concentrations occurring within 3 hours to 5 hours; the absolute oral bioavailability of the tablet formulation is 87%. ABILIFY can be administered with or without food. Administration of a 15 mg ABILIFY Tablet with a standard high-fat meal did not significantly affect the Cmax or AUC of aripiprazole or its active metabolite, dehydro-aripiprazole, but delayed Tmax by 3 hours for aripiprazole and 12 hours for dehydro-aripiprazole.

Oral Solution: Aripiprazole is well absorbed when administered orally as the solution. At equivalent doses, the plasma concentrations of aripiprazole from the solution were higher than that from the tablet formulation. In a relative bioavailability study comparing the pharmacokinetics of 30 mg aripiprazole as the oral solution to 30 mg aripiprazole tablets in healthy subjects, the solution to tablet ratios of geometric mean Cmax and AUC values were 122% and 114%, respectively *[see DOSAGE AND ADMINISTRATION (2.6)]*. The single-dose pharmacokinetics of aripiprazole were linear and dose-proportional between the doses of 5 mg to 30 mg.

Distribution

The steady-state volume of distribution of aripiprazole following intravenous administration is high (404 L or 4.9 L/kg), indicating extensive extravascular distribution. At therapeutic concentrations, aripiprazole and its major metabolite are greater than 99% bound to serum proteins, primarily to albumin. In healthy human volunteers administered 0.5 mg/day to 30 mg/day aripiprazole for 14 days, there was dose-dependent D_2 receptor occupancy indicating brain penetration of aripiprazole in humans.

Metabolism and Elimination

Aripiprazole is metabolized primarily by three biotransformation pathways: dehydrogenation, hydroxylation, and N-dealkylation. Based on *in vitro* studies, CYP3A4 and CYP2D6 enzymes are responsible for dehydrogenation and hydroxylation of aripiprazole, and N-dealkylation is catalyzed by CYP3A4. Aripiprazole is the predominant drug moiety in the systemic circulation. At steady-state, dehydro-aripiprazole, the active metabolite, represents about 40% of aripiprazole AUC in plasma.

Approximately 8% of Caucasians and 3–8% of Black/African Americans lack the capacity to metabolize CYP2D6 substrates and are classified as poor metabolizers (PM), whereas the rest are extensive metabolizers (EM). PMs have about an 80% increase in aripiprazole exposure and about a 30% decrease in exposure to the active metabolite compared to EMs, resulting in about a 60% higher exposure to the total active moieties from a given dose of aripiprazole compared to EMs. Coadministration of ABILIFY with known inhibitors of CYP2D6, such as quinidine or fluoxetine in EMs, approximately doubles aripiprazole plasma exposure, and dose adjustment is needed *[see DRUG INTERACTIONS (7.1)]*. Similarly, PMs have higher exposure to aripiprazole compared to EMs; hence, PMs should have their initial dose reduced by one-half. Laboratory tests are available to identify CYP2D6 PMs. The mean elimination half-lives are about 75 hours and 146 hours for aripiprazole in EMs and PMs, respectively. Aripiprazole does not inhibit or induce the CYP2D6 pathway.

Following a single oral dose of [^{14}C]-labeled aripiprazole, approximately 25% and 55% of the administered radioactivity was recovered in the urine and feces, respectively. Less than 1% of unchanged aripiprazole was excreted in the urine and approximately 18% of the oral dose was recovered unchanged in the feces.

INTRAMUSCULAR ADMINISTRATION

In two pharmacokinetic studies of aripiprazole injection administered intramuscularly to healthy subjects, the median times to the peak plasma concentrations were at 1 hour and 3 hours. A 5 mg intramuscular injection of aripiprazole had an absolute bioavailability of 100%. The geometric mean maximum concentration achieved after an intramuscular dose was on average 19% higher than the Cmax of the oral tablet. While the systemic exposure over 24 hours was generally similar between aripiprazole injection given intramuscularly and after oral tablet administration, the aripiprazole AUC in the first 2 hours after an intramuscular injection was 90% greater than the AUC after the same dose as a tablet. In stable patients with schizophrenia or schizoaffective disorder, the pharmacokinetics of aripiprazole after intramuscular administration were linear over a dose range of 1 mg to 45 mg. Although the metabolism of aripiprazole injection was not systematically evaluated, the intramuscular route of administration would not be expected to alter the metabolic pathways.

13 NONCLINICAL TOXICOLOGY

13.1 Carcinogenesis, Mutagenesis, Impairment of Fertility

Carcinogenesis

Lifetime carcinogenicity studies were conducted in ICR mice and in Sprague-Dawley (SD) and F344 rats. Aripiprazole was administered for 2 years in the diet at doses of 1 mg/kg/day, 3 mg/kg/day, 10 mg/kg/day, and 30 mg/kg/day to ICR mice and 1 mg/kg/day, 3 mg/kg/day, and 10 mg/kg/day to F344 rats (0.2 times to 5 times and 0.3 times to 3 times the maximum recommended human dose [MRHD] based on mg/m^2, respectively). In addition, SD rats were dosed orally for 2 years at 10 mg/kg/day, 20 mg/kg/day, 40 mg/kg/day, and 60 mg/kg/day (3 times to 19 times the MRHD based on mg/m^2). Aripiprazole did not induce tumors in male mice or rats. In female mice, the incidences of pituitary gland adenomas and mammary gland adenocarcinomas and adenoacanthomas were increased at dietary doses of 3 mg/kg/day to 30 mg/kg/day (0.1 times to 0.9 times human exposure at MRHD based on AUC and 0.5 times to 5 times the MRHD based on mg/m^2). In female rats, the incidence of mammary gland fibroadenomas was increased at a dietary dose of 10 mg/kg/day (0.1 times human exposure at MRHD based on AUC and 3 times the MRHD based on mg/m^2); and the incidences of adrenocortical carcinomas and combined adrenocortical adenomas/carcinomas were increased at an oral dose of 60 mg/kg/day (14 times human exposure at MRHD based on AUC and 19 times the MRHD based on mg/m^2).

Proliferative changes in the pituitary and mammary gland of rodents have been observed following chronic administration of other antipsychotic agents and are considered prolactin-mediated. Serum prolactin was not measured in the aripiprazole carcinogenicity studies. However, increases in serum prolactin levels were observed in female mice in a 13-week dietary study at the doses associated with mammary gland and pituitary tumors. Serum prolactin was not increased in female rats in 4-week and 13-week dietary studies at the dose associated with mammary gland tumors. The relevance for human risk of the findings of prolactin-mediated endocrine tumors in rodents is unknown.

Mutagenesis

The mutagenic potential of aripiprazole was tested in the *in vitro* bacterial reverse-mutation assay, the *in vitro* bacterial DNA repair assay, the *in vitro* forward gene mutation assay in mouse lymphoma cells, the *in vitro* chromosomal aberration assay in Chinese hamster lung (CHL) cells, the *in vivo* micronucleus assay in mice, and the unscheduled DNA synthesis assay in rats. Aripiprazole and a metabolite (2,3-DCPP) were clastogenic in the *in vitro* chromosomal aberration assay in CHL cells with and without metabolic activation. The metabolite, 2,3-DCPP, produced increases in numerical aberrations in the *in vitro* assay in CHL cells in the absence of metabolic activation. A positive response was obtained in the *in vivo* micronucleus assay in mice; however, the response was due to a mechanism not considered relevant to humans.

Impairment of Fertility

Female rats were treated with oral doses of 2 mg/kg/day, 6 mg/kg/day, and 20 mg/kg/day (0.6 times, 2 times, and 6 times the maximum recommended human dose [MRHD] on a mg/m^2 basis) of aripiprazole from 2 weeks prior to mating through day 7 of gestation. Estrus cycle irregularities and increased corpora lutea were seen at all doses, but no impairment of fertility was seen. Increased pre-implantation loss was seen at 6 mg/kg and 20 mg/kg and decreased fetal weight was seen at 20 mg/kg.

Male rats were treated with oral doses of 20 mg/kg/day, 40 mg/kg/day, and 60 mg/kg/day (6 times, 13 times, and 19 times the MRHD on a mg/m^2 basis) of aripiprazole from 9 weeks prior to mating through mating. Disturbances in spermatogenesis were seen at 60 mg/kg and prostate atrophy was seen at 40 mg/kg and 60 mg/kg, but no impairment of fertility was seen.

13.2 Animal Toxicology and/or Pharmacology

Aripiprazole produced retinal degeneration in albino rats in a 26-week chronic toxicity study at a dose of 60 mg/kg and in a 2-year carcinogenicity study at doses of 40 mg/kg and 60 mg/kg. The 40 mg/kg and 60 mg/kg doses are 13 times and 19 times the maximum recommended human dose (MRHD) based on mg/m^2 and 7 times to 14 times human exposure at MRHD based on AUC. Evaluation of the retinas of albino mice and of monkeys did not reveal evidence of retinal degeneration. Additional studies to further evaluate the mechanism have not been performed. The relevance of this finding to human risk is unknown.

14 CLINICAL STUDIES

14.1 Schizophrenia

Adults

The efficacy of ABILIFY in the treatment of schizophrenia was evaluated in five short-term (4-week and 6-week), placebo-controlled trials of acutely relapsed inpatients who predominantly met DSM-III/IV criteria for schizophrenia. Four of the five trials were able to distinguish aripiprazole from placebo, but one study, the smallest, did not. Three of these studies also included an active control group consisting of either risperidone (one trial) or haloperidol (two trials), but they were not designed to allow for a comparison of ABILIFY and the active comparators.

In the four positive trials for ABILIFY, four primary measures were used for assessing psychiatric signs and symptoms. The Positive and Negative Syndrome Scale (PANSS) is a multi-item inventory of general psychopathology used to evaluate the effects of drug treatment in schizophrenia. The PANSS positive subscale is a subset of items in the PANSS that rates seven positive symptoms of schizophrenia (delusions, conceptual disorganization, hallucinatory behavior, excitement, grandiosity, suspiciousness/persecution, and hostility). The PANSS negative subscale is a subset of items in the PANSS that rates seven negative symptoms of schizophrenia (blunted affect, emotional withdrawal, poor rapport, passive apathetic withdrawal, difficulty in abstract thinking, lack of spontaneity/flow of conversation, stereotyped thinking). The Clinical Global Impression (CGI) assessment reflects the impression of a skilled observer, fully familiar with the manifestations of schizophrenia, about the overall clinical state of the patient.

In a 4-week trial (n=414) comparing two fixed doses of ABILIFY (15 mg/day or 30 mg/day) to placebo, both doses of ABILIFY were superior to placebo in the PANSS total score, PANSS positive subscale, and CGI-severity score. In addition, the 15 mg dose was superior to placebo in the PANSS negative subscale.

In a 4-week trial (n=404) comparing two fixed doses of ABILIFY (20 mg/day or 30 mg/day) to placebo, both doses of ABILIFY were superior to placebo in the PANSS total score, PANSS positive subscale, PANSS negative subscale, and CGI-severity score.

In a 6-week trial (n=420) comparing three fixed doses of ABILIFY (10 mg/day, 15 mg/day, or 20 mg/day) to placebo, all three doses of ABILIFY were superior to placebo in the PANSS total score, PANSS positive subscale, and the PANSS negative subscale.

In a 6-week trial (n=367) comparing three fixed doses of ABILIFY (2 mg/day, 5 mg/day, or 10 mg/day) to placebo, the 10 mg dose of ABILIFY was superior to placebo in the PANSS total score, the primary outcome measure of the study. The 2 mg and 5 mg doses did not demonstrate superiority to placebo on the primary outcome measure.

In a fifth study, a 4-week trial (n=103) comparing ABILIFY in a range of 5 mg/day to 30 mg/day to placebo, ABILIFY was only significantly different compared to placebo in a responder analysis based on the CGI-severity score, a primary outcome for that trial.

Thus, the efficacy of 10 mg, 15 mg, 20 mg, and 30 mg daily doses was established in two studies for each dose. Among these doses, there was no evidence that the higher dose groups offered any advantage over the lowest dose group of these studies.

An examination of population subgroups did not reveal any clear evidence of differential responsiveness on the basis of age, gender, or race.

A longer-term trial enrolled 310 inpatients or outpatients meeting DSM-IV criteria for schizophrenia who were, by history, symptomatically stable on other antipsychotic medications for periods of 3 months or longer. These patients were discontinued from their antipsychotic medications and randomized to ABILIFY 15 mg/day or placebo for up to 26 weeks of observation for relapse. Relapse during the double-blind phase was defined as CGI-Improvement score of ≥5 (minimally worse), scores ≥5 (moderately severe) on the hostility or uncooperativeness items of the PANSS, or ≥20% increase in the PANSS total score. Patients receiving

ABILIFY 15 mg/day experienced a significantly longer time to relapse over the subsequent 26 weeks compared to those receiving placebo.

Pediatric Patients

The efficacy of ABILIFY (aripiprazole) in the treatment of schizophrenia in pediatric patients (13 to 17 years of age) was evaluated in one 6-week, placebo-controlled trial of outpatients who met DSM-IV criteria for schizophrenia and had a PANSS score ≥70 at baseline. In this trial (n=302) comparing two fixed doses of ABILIFY (10 mg/day or 30 mg/day) to placebo, ABILIFY was titrated starting from 2 mg/day to the target dose in 5 days in the 10 mg/day treatment arm and in 11 days in the 30 mg/day treatment arm. Both doses of ABILIFY were superior to placebo in the PANSS total score, the primary outcome measure of the study. The 30 mg/day dosage was not shown to be more efficacious than the 10 mg/day dose. Although maintenance efficacy in pediatric patients has not been systematically evaluated, maintenance efficacy can be extrapolated from adult data along with comparisons of aripiprazole pharmacokinetic parameters in adult and pediatric patients.

14.2 Bipolar Disorder

Acute Treatment of Manic and Mixed Episodes

Adults

Monotherapy

The efficacy of ABILIFY as monotherapy in the acute treatment of manic episodes was established in four 3-week, placebo-controlled trials in hospitalized patients who met the DSM-IV criteria for bipolar I disorder with manic or mixed episodes. These studies included patients with or without psychotic features and two of the studies also included patients with or without a rapid-cycling course.

The primary instrument used for assessing manic symptoms was the Young Mania Rating Scale (Y-MRS), an 11-item clinician-rated scale traditionally used to assess the degree of manic symptomatology (irritability, disruptive/aggressive behavior, sleep, elevated mood, speech, increased activity, sexual interest, language/thought disorder, thought content, appearance, and insight) in a range from 0 (no manic features) to 60 (maximum score). A key secondary instrument included the Clinical Global Impression-Bipolar (CGI-BP) Scale.

In the four positive, 3-week, placebo-controlled trials (n=268; n=248; n=480; n=485) which evaluated ABILIFY in a range of 15 mg to 30 mg, once daily (with a starting dose of 15 mg/day in two studies and 30 mg/day in two studies), ABILIFY was superior to placebo in the reduction of Y-MRS total score and CGI-BP Severity of Illness score (mania). In the two studies with a starting dose of 15 mg/day, 48% and 44% of patients were on 15 mg/day at endpoint. In the two studies with a starting dose of 30 mg/day, 86% and 85% of patients were on 30 mg/day at endpoint.

Adjunctive Therapy

The efficacy of adjunctive ABILIFY with concomitant lithium or valproate in the treatment of manic or mixed episodes was established in a 6-week, placebo-controlled study (n=384) with a 2-week lead-in mood stabilizer monotherapy phase in adult patients who met DSM-IV criteria for bipolar I disorder. This study included patients with manic or mixed episodes and with or without psychotic features.

Patients were initiated on open-label lithium (0.6 mEq/L to 1.0 mEq/L) or valproate (50 µg/mL to 125 µg/mL) at therapeutic serum levels, and remained on stable doses for 2 weeks. At the end of 2 weeks, patients demonstrating inadequate response (Y-MRS total score ≥16 and ≤25% improvement on the Y-MRS total score) to lithium or valproate were randomized to receive either aripiprazole (15 mg/day or an increase to 30 mg/day as early as day 7) or placebo as adjunctive therapy with open-label lithium or valproate. In the 6-week, placebo-controlled phase, adjunctive ABILIFY starting at 15 mg/day with concomitant lithium or valproate (in a therapeutic range of 0.6 mEq/L to 1.0 mEq/L or 50 µg/mL to 125 µg/mL, respectively) was superior to lithium or valproate with adjunctive placebo in the reduction of the Y-MRS total score and CGI-BP Severity of Illness score (mania). Seventy-one percent of the patients coadministered valproate and 62% of the patients coadministered lithium were on 15 mg/day at 6-week endpoint.

Pediatric Patients

The efficacy of ABILIFY in the treatment of bipolar I disorder in pediatric patients (10 to 17 years of age) was evaluated in one 4-week, placebo-controlled trial (n=296) of outpatients who met DSM-IV criteria for bipolar I disorder manic or mixed episodes with or without psychotic features and had a Y-MRS score ≥20 at baseline. This double-blind, placebo-controlled trial compared two fixed doses of ABILIFY (10 mg/day or 30 mg/day) to placebo. The ABILIFY dose was started at 2 mg/day, which was titrated to 5 mg/day after 2 days, and to the target dose in 5 days in the 10 mg/day treatment arm, and in 13 days in the 30 mg/day treatment arm. Both doses of ABILIFY were superior to placebo in change from baseline to week 4 on the Y-MRS total score.

Maintenance Treatment of Bipolar I Disorder

Monotherapy Maintenance Therapy

A maintenance trial was conducted in adult patients meeting DSM-IV criteria for bipolar I disorder with a recent manic or mixed episode who had been stabilized on open-label ABILIFY and who had maintained a clinical response for at least 6 weeks. The first phase of this trial was an open-label stabilization period in which inpatients and outpatients were clinically stabilized and then maintained on open-label ABILIFY (15 mg/day or 30 mg/day, with a starting dose of 30 mg/day) for at least 6 consecutive weeks. One hundred sixty-one outpatients were then randomized in a double-blind fashion, to either the same dose of ABILIFY they were on at the end of the stabilization and maintenance period or placebo and were then monitored for manic or depressive relapse. During the randomization phase, ABILIFY was superior to placebo on time to the number of combined affective relapses (manic plus depressive), the primary outcome measure for this study. A total of 55 mood events were observed during the double-blind treatment phase. Nineteen were from the ABILIFY group and 36 were from the placebo group. The number of observed manic episodes in the ABILIFY group (6) were fewer than that in the placebo group (19), while the number of depressive episodes in the ABILIFY group (9) was similar to that in the placebo group (11).

An examination of population subgroups did not reveal any clear evidence of differential responsiveness on the basis of age and gender; however, there were insufficient numbers of patients in each of the ethnic groups to adequately assess inter-group differences.

Adjunctive Maintenance Therapy

An adjunctive maintenance trial was conducted in adult patients meeting DSM-IV criteria for bipolar I disorder with a recent manic or mixed episode. Patients were initiated on open-label lithium (0.6 mEq/L to 1.0 mEq/L) or valproate (50 µg/mL to 125 µg/mL) at therapeutic serum levels, and remained on stable doses for 2 weeks. At the end of 2 weeks, patients demonstrating inadequate response (Y-MRS total score ≥16 and ≤35% improvement on the Y-MRS total score) to lithium or valproate received aripiprazole with a starting dose of 15 mg/day with the option to increase to 30 mg or reduce to 10 mg as early as day 4, as adjunctive therapy with open-label lithium or valproate. Prior to randomization, patients on the combination of single-blind aripiprazole and lithium or valproate were required to maintain stability (Y-MRS and MADRS total scores ≤12) for 12 consecutive weeks. Three hundred thirty-seven patients were then randomized in a double-blind fashion, to either the same dose of ABILIFY they were on at the end of the stabilization period or placebo plus lithium or valproate and were then monitored for manic, mixed, or depressive relapse for a maximum of 52 weeks. ABILIFY was superior to placebo on the primary endpoint, time from randomization to relapse to any mood event. A mood event was defined as hospitalization for a manic, mixed, or depressive episode, study discontinuation due to lack of efficacy accompanied by Y-MRS score >16 and/or a MADRS >16, or an SAE of worsening disease accompanied by Y-MRS score >16 and/or a MADRS >16. A total of 68 mood events were observed during the double-blind treatment phase. Twenty-five were from the ABILIFY group and 43 were from the placebo group. The number of observed manic episodes in the ABILIFY group (7) were fewer than that in the placebo group (19), while the number of depressive episodes in the ABILIFY group (14) was similar to that in the placebo group (18). The Kaplan-Meier curves of the time from randomization to relapse to any mood event during the 52-week, double-blind treatment phase for ABILIFY and placebo groups are shown in Figure 1.

Figure 1: Kaplan-Meier Estimation of Proportion of Relapses to Any Mood Event for ABILIFY and Placebo Groups

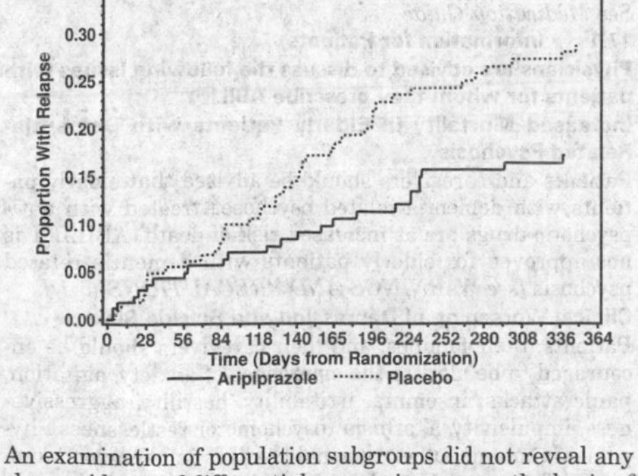

An examination of population subgroups did not reveal any clear evidence of differential responsiveness on the basis of age and gender; however, there were insufficient numbers of patients in each of the ethnic groups to adequately assess inter-group differences.

14.3 Adjunctive Treatment of Major Depressive Disorder

Adults

The efficacy of ABILIFY in the adjunctive treatment of major depressive disorder (MDD) was demonstrated in two short-term (6-week), placebo-controlled trials of adult patients meeting DSM-IV criteria for MDD who had had an inadequate response to prior antidepressant therapy (1 to 3 courses) in the current episode and who had also demonstrated an inadequate response to 8 weeks of prospective antidepressant therapy (paroxetine controlled-release, venlafaxine extended-release, fluoxetine, escitalopram, or sertraline). Inadequate response for prospective treatment was defined as less than 50% improvement on the 17-item version of the Hamilton Depression Rating Scale (HAMD17), minimal HAMD17 score of 14, and a Clinical Global Impressions Improvement rating of no better than minimal improvement. Inadequate response to prior treatment was defined as less than 50% improvement as perceived by the patient after a minimum of 6 weeks of antidepressant therapy at or above the minimal effective dose.

The primary instrument used for assessing depressive symptoms was the Montgomery-Asberg Depression Rating Scale (MADRS), a 10-item clinician-rated scale used to assess the degree of depressive symptomatology (apparent sadness, reported sadness, inner tension, reduced sleep, reduced appetite, concentration difficulties, lassitude, inability to feel, pessimistic thoughts, and suicidal thoughts). The key secondary instrument was the Sheehan Disability Scale (SDS), a 3-item self-rated instrument used to assess the impact of depression on three domains of functioning (work/school, social life, and family life) with each item scored from 0 (not at all) to 10 (extreme).

In the two trials (n=381, n=362), ABILIFY was superior to placebo in reducing mean MADRS total scores. In one study, ABILIFY was also superior to placebo in reducing the mean SDS score.

In both trials, patients received ABILIFY adjunctive to antidepressants at a dose of 5 mg/day. Based on tolerability and efficacy, doses could be adjusted by 5 mg increments, one week apart. Allowable doses were: 2 mg/day, 5 mg/day, 10 mg/day, 15 mg/day, and for patients who were not on potent CYP2D6 inhibitors fluoxetine and paroxetine, 20 mg/day. The mean final dose at the end point for the two trials was 10.7 mg/day and 11.4 mg/day.

An examination of population subgroups did not reveal evidence of differential response based on age, choice of prospective antidepressant, or race. With regard to gender, a smaller mean reduction on the MADRS total score was seen in males than in females.

14.4 Irritability Associated with Autistic Disorder

Pediatric Patients

The efficacy of ABILIFY (aripiprazole) in the treatment of irritability associated with autistic disorder was established in two 8-week, placebo-controlled trials in pediatric patients (6 to 17 years of age) who met the DSM-IV criteria for autistic disorder and demonstrated behaviors such as tantrums, aggression, self-injurious behavior, or a combination of these problems. Over 75% of these subjects were under 13 years of age.

Efficacy was evaluated using two assessment scales: the Aberrant Behavior Checklist (ABC) and the Clinical Global Impression-Improvement (CGI-I) scale. The primary outcome measure in both trials was the change from baseline to endpoint in the Irritability subscale of the ABC (ABC-I). The ABC-I subscale measured the emotional and behavioral symptoms of irritability in autistic disorder, including aggression towards others, deliberate self-injuriousness, temper tantrums, and quickly changing moods.

The results of these trials are as follows:

In one of the 8-week, placebo-controlled trials, children and adolescents with autistic disorder (n=98), aged 6 to 17 years, received daily doses of placebo or ABILIFY 2 mg/day to 15 mg/day. ABILIFY, starting at 2 mg/day with increases allowed up to 15 mg/day based on clinical response, significantly improved scores on the ABC-I subscale and on the CGI-I scale compared with placebo. The mean daily dose of ABILIFY at the end of 8-week treatment was 8.6 mg/day.

In the other 8-week, placebo-controlled trial in children and adolescents with autistic disorder (n=218), aged 6 to 17 years, three fixed doses of ABILIFY (5 mg/day, 10 mg/day, or 15 mg/day) were compared to placebo. ABILIFY dosing started at 2 mg/day and was increased to 5 mg/day after one week. After a second week, it was increased to 10 mg/day for patients in the 10 mg and 15 mg dose arms, and after a third week, it was increased to 15 mg/day in the 15 mg/day treatment arm. All three doses of ABILIFY significantly improved scores on the ABC-I subscale compared with placebo.

Table 22: ABILIFY Tablet Presentations

Tablet Strength	Tablet Color/Shape	Tablet Markings	Pack Size	NDC Code
2 mg	green modified rectangle	"A-006" and "2"	Bottle of 30	59148-006-13
5 mg	blue modified rectangle	"A-007" and "5"	Bottle of 30 Blister of 100	59148-007-13 59148-007-35
10 mg	pink modified rectangle	"A-008" and "10"	Bottle of 30 Blister of 100	59148-008-13 59148-008-35
15 mg	yellow round	"A-009" and "15"	Bottle of 30 Blister of 100	59148-009-13 59148-009-35
20 mg	white round	"A-010" and "20"	Bottle of 30 Blister of 100	59148-010-13 59148-010-35
30 mg	pink round	"A-011" and "30"	Bottle of 30 Blister of 100	59148-011-13 59148-011-35

Table 23: ABILIFY DISCMELT Orally Disintegrating Tablet Presentations

Tablet Strength	Tablet Color	Tablet Markings	Pack Size	NDC Code
10 mg	pink (with scattered specks)	"A" and "640" "10"	Blister of 30	59148-640-23
15 mg	yellow (with scattered specks)	"A" and "641" "15"	Blister of 30	59148-641-23

14.5 Agitation Associated with Schizophrenia or Bipolar Mania

The efficacy of intramuscular aripiprazole for injection for the treatment of agitation was established in three short-term (24-hour), placebo-controlled trials in agitated inpatients from two diagnostic groups: schizophrenia and bipolar I disorder (manic or mixed episodes, with or without psychotic features). Each of the trials included a single active comparator treatment arm of either haloperidol injection (schizophrenia studies) or lorazepam injection (bipolar mania study). Patients could receive up to three injections during the 24-hour treatment periods; however, patients could not receive the second injection until after the initial 2-hour period when the primary efficacy measure was assessed. Patients enrolled in the trials needed to be: (1) judged by the clinical investigators as clinically agitated and clinically appropriate candidates for treatment with intramuscular medication, and (2) exhibiting a level of agitation that met or exceeded a threshold score of ≥15 on the five items comprising the Positive and Negative Syndrome Scale (PANSS) Excited Component (ie, poor impulse control, tension, hostility, uncooperativeness, and excitement items) with at least two individual item scores ≥4 using a 1-7 scoring system (1 = absent, 4 = moderate, 7 = extreme). In the studies, the mean baseline PANSS Excited Component score was 19, with scores ranging from 15 to 34 (out of a maximum score of 35), thus suggesting predominantly moderate levels of agitation with some patients experiencing mild or severe levels of agitation. The primary efficacy measure used for assessing agitation signs and symptoms in these trials was the change from baseline in the PANSS Excited Component at 2 hours post-injection. A key secondary measure was the Clinical Global Impression of Improvement (CGI-I) Scale. The results of the trials follow:

In a placebo-controlled trial in agitated inpatients predominantly meeting DSM-IV criteria for schizophrenia (n=350), four fixed aripiprazole injection doses of 1 mg, 5.25 mg, 9.75 mg, and 15 mg were evaluated. At 2 hours post-injection, the 5.25 mg, 9.75 mg, and 15 mg doses were statistically superior to placebo in the PANSS Excited Component and on the CGI-I Scale.

In a second placebo-controlled trial in agitated inpatients predominantly meeting DSM-IV criteria for schizophrenia (n=445), one fixed aripiprazole injection dose of 9.75 mg was evaluated. At 2 hours post-injection, aripiprazole for injection was statistically superior to placebo in the PANSS Excited Component and on the CGI-I Scale.

In a placebo-controlled trial in agitated inpatients meeting DSM-IV criteria for bipolar I disorder (manic or mixed) (n=291), two fixed aripiprazole injection doses of 9.75 mg and 15 mg were evaluated. At 2 hours post-injection, both doses were statistically superior to placebo in the PANSS Excited Component.

Examination of population subsets (age, race, and gender) did not reveal any differential responsiveness on the basis of these subgroupings.

16 HOW SUPPLIED/STORAGE AND HANDLING

16.1 How Supplied

ABILIFY® (aripiprazole) Tablets have markings on one side and are available in the strengths and packages listed in Table 22.

[See table 22 above]

ABILIFY DISCMELT® (aripiprazole) Orally Disintegrating Tablets are round tablets with markings on either side. ABILIFY DISCMELT is available in the strengths and packages listed in Table 23.

[See table 23 above]

ABILIFY® (aripiprazole) Oral Solution (1 mg/mL) is supplied in child-resistant bottles along with a calibrated oral dosing cup. ABILIFY Oral Solution is available as follows:

150 mL bottle NDC 59148-013-15

ABILIFY® (aripiprazole) Injection for intramuscular use is available as a ready-to-use, 9.75 mg/1.3 mL (7.5 mg/mL) solution in clear, Type 1 glass vials as follows:

9.75 mg/1.3 mL single-dose vial NDC 59148-016-65

16.2 Storage

Tablets

Store at 25°C (77°F); excursions permitted between 15°C to 30°C (59°F to 86°F) [see USP Controlled Room Temperature].

Oral Solution

Store at 25°C (77°F); excursions permitted between 15°C to 30°C (59°F to 86°F) [see USP Controlled Room Temperature]. Opened bottles of ABILIFY Oral Solution can be used for up to 6 months after opening, but not beyond the expiration date on the bottle. The bottle and its contents should be discarded after the expiration date.

Injection

Store at 25°C (77°F); excursions permitted between 15°C to 30°C (59°F to 86°F) [see USP Controlled Room Temperature]. Protect from light by storing in the original container. Retain in carton until time of use.

17 PATIENT COUNSELING INFORMATION

See Medication Guide

17.1 Information for Patients

Physicians are advised to discuss the following issues with patients for whom they prescribe ABILIFY:

Increased Mortality in Elderly Patients with Dementia-Related Psychosis

Patients and caregivers should be advised that elderly patients with dementia-related psychoses treated with antipsychotic drugs are at increased risk of death. ABILIFY is not approved for elderly patients with dementia-related psychosis *[see WARNINGS AND PRECAUTIONS (5.1)]*.

Clinical Worsening of Depression and Suicide Risk

Patients, their families, and their caregivers should be encouraged to be alert to the emergence of anxiety, agitation, panic attacks, insomnia, irritability, hostility, aggressiveness, impulsivity, akathisia (psychomotor restlessness), hypomania, mania, other unusual changes in behavior, worsening of depression, and suicidal ideation, especially early during antidepressant treatment and when the dose is adjusted up or down. Families and caregivers of patients should be advised to look for the emergence of such symptoms on a day-to-day basis, since changes may be abrupt. Such symptoms should be reported to the patient's prescriber or health professional, especially if they are severe, abrupt in onset, or were not part of the patient's presenting symptoms. Symptoms such as these may be associated with an increased risk for suicidal thinking and behavior **and indicate a need for very close monitoring and possibly changes in the medication** *[see WARNINGS AND PRECAUTIONS (5.2)]*.

Prescribers or other health professionals should inform patients, their families, and their caregivers about the benefits and risks associated with treatment with ABILIFY and should counsel them in its appropriate use. A patient Medication Guide including information about "Antidepressant Medicines, Depression and other Serious Mental Illness, and Suicidal Thoughts or Actions" is available for ABILIFY. The prescriber or health professional should instruct patients, their families, and their caregivers to read the Medication Guide and should assist them in understanding its contents. Patients should be given the opportunity to discuss the contents of the Medication Guide and to obtain answers to any questions they may have. It should be noted that ABILIFY is not approved as a single agent for treatment of depression and has not been evaluated in pediatric major depressive disorder.

Use of Orally Disintegrating Tablet

Do not open the blister until ready to administer. For single tablet removal, open the package and peel back the foil on the blister to expose the tablet. Do not push the tablet through the foil because this could damage the tablet. Immediately upon opening the blister, using dry hands, remove the tablet and place the entire ABILIFY DISCMELT Orally Disintegrating Tablet on the tongue. Tablet disintegration occurs rapidly in saliva. It is recommended that ABILIFY DISCMELT be taken without liquid. However, if needed, it can be taken with liquid. Do not attempt to split the tablet.

Interference with Cognitive and Motor Performance

Because aripiprazole may have the potential to impair judgment, thinking, or motor skills, patients should be cautioned about operating hazardous machinery, including automobiles, until they are reasonably certain that aripiprazole therapy does not affect them adversely *[see WARNINGS AND PRECAUTIONS (5.9)]*.

Pregnancy

Patients should be advised to notify their physician if they become pregnant or intend to become pregnant during therapy with ABILIFY *[see USE IN SPECIFIC POPULATIONS (8.1)]*.

Nursing

Patients should be advised not to breast-feed an infant if they are taking ABILIFY *[see USE IN SPECIFIC POPULATIONS (8.3)]*.

Concomitant Medication

Patients should be advised to inform their physicians if they are taking, or plan to take, any prescription or over-the-counter drugs, since there is a potential for interactions *[see DRUG INTERACTIONS (7)]*.

Alcohol

Patients should be advised to avoid alcohol while taking ABILIFY *[see DRUG INTERACTIONS (7.2)]*.

Heat Exposure and Dehydration

Patients should be advised regarding appropriate care in avoiding overheating and dehydration *[see WARNINGS AND PRECAUTIONS (5.10)]*.

Sugar Content

Patients should be advised that each mL of ABILIFY Oral Solution contains 400 mg of sucrose and 200 mg of fructose.

Phenylketonurics

Phenylalanine is a component of aspartame. Each ABILIFY DISCMELT Orally Disintegrating Tablet contains the following amounts: 10 mg - 1.12 mg phenylalanine and 15 mg - 1.68 mg phenylalanine.

Tablets manufactured by Otsuka Pharmaceutical Co, Ltd, Tokyo, 101-8535 Japan or Bristol-Myers Squibb Company, Princeton, NJ 08543 USA

Orally Disintegrating Tablets, Oral Solution, and Injection manufactured by

Bristol-Myers Squibb Company, Princeton, NJ 08543 USA

Distributed and marketed by Otsuka America Pharmaceutical, Inc, Rockville, MD 20850 USA

ABILIFY is a trademark of Otsuka Pharmaceutical Company.

1239550B3 03US13L-1028 Rev April 2013

MEDICATION GUIDE

ABILIFY® (a BIL ĭ fī)

Generic name: aripiprazole

Read this Medication Guide before you start taking ABILIFY and each time you get a refill. There may be new information. This Medication Guide does not take the place of talking to your healthcare provider about your medical condition or treatment.

What is the most important information I should know about ABILIFY?

(For other side effects, also see **"What are the possible side effects of ABILIFY?"**).

Serious side effects may happen when you take ABILIFY, including:

- **Increased risk of death in elderly patients with dementia-related psychosis:** Medicines like ABILIFY can raise the risk of death in elderly people who have lost touch with reality (psychosis) due to confusion and memory loss (dementia). ABILIFY is not approved for the treatment of patients with dementia-related psychosis.
- Risk of suicidal thoughts or actions: Antidepressant medicines, depression and other serious mental illnesses, and suicidal thoughts or actions:

1. **Antidepressant medicines may increase suicidal thoughts or actions in some children, teenagers, and young adults within the first few months of treatment.**
2. **Depression and other serious mental illnesses are the most important causes of suicidal thoughts and actions. Some people may have a particularly high risk of having suicidal thoughts or actions. These include people who have (or have a family history of) bipolar illness (also called manic-depressive illness) or suicidal thoughts or actions.**
3. **How can I watch for and try to prevent suicidal thoughts and actions in myself or a family member?**
   - **Pay close attention to any changes, especially sudden changes, in mood, behaviors, thoughts, or feelings. This is very important when an antidepressant medicine is started or when the dose is changed.**
   - **Call the healthcare provider right away to report new or sudden changes in mood, behavior, thoughts, or feelings.**
   - **Keep all follow-up visits with the healthcare provider as scheduled. Call the healthcare provider between visits as needed, especially if you have concerns about symptoms.**

Call a healthcare provider right away if you or your family member has any of the following symptoms, especially if they are new, worse, or worry you:

- thoughts about suicide or dying
- attempts to commit suicide
- new or worse depression
- new or worse anxiety
- feeling very agitated or restless
- panic attacks
- trouble sleeping (insomnia)
- new or worse irritability
- acting aggressive, being angry, or violent
- acting on dangerous impulses
- an extreme increase in activity and talking (mania)
- other unusual changes in behavior or mood

What else do I need to know about antidepressant medicines?

- **Never stop an antidepressant medicine without first talking to a healthcare provider.** Stopping an antidepressant medicine suddenly can cause other symptoms.
- **Antidepressants are medicines used to treat depression and other illnesses.** It is important to discuss all the risks of treating depression and also the risks of not treating it. Patients and their families or other caregivers should discuss all treatment choices with the healthcare provider, not just the use of antidepressants.
- **Antidepressant medicines have other side effects.** Talk to the healthcare provider about the side effects of the medicine prescribed for you or your family member.
- **Antidepressant medicines can interact with other medicines.** Know all of the medicines that you or your family member takes. Keep a list of all medicines to show the healthcare provider. Do not start new medicines without first checking with your healthcare provider.
- **Not all antidepressant medicines prescribed for children are FDA approved for use in children.** Talk to your child's healthcare provider for more information.

What is ABILIFY?

ABILIFY is a prescription medicine used to treat:

- schizophrenia in people age 13 years and older
- bipolar I disorder in people age 10 years and older, including:
  - manic or mixed episodes that happen with bipolar I disorder
  - manic or mixed episodes that happen with bipolar I disorder, when used with the medicine lithium or valproate
  - long-term treatment of bipolar I disorder
- major depressive disorder in adults, as an add-on treatment to an antidepressant medicine when you do not get better with an antidepressant alone
- irritability associated with autistic disorder in children and adolescents ages 6 to 17 years old
- agitation associated with schizophrenia or bipolar disorder

The symptoms of schizophrenia include:

- losing touch with reality (psychosis)
- seeing things or hearing voices that are not there (hallucinations)
- believing things that are not true (delusions)
- being suspicious (paranoia)
- disorganized speech and thinking
- bizarre behavior

The symptoms of bipolar I disorder include:

- extreme mood swings that include feeling depressed and high or irritable mood
- talking too fast and too much
- impulsive behavior
- having more energy and restlessness than usual
- needing less sleep than usual

The symptoms of major depressive disorder (MDD) include:

- feeling of sadness and emptiness
- loss of interest in activities that you once enjoyed and loss of energy
- problems focusing and making decisions
- feeling of worthlessness or guilt
- changes in sleep or eating patterns
- thoughts of death or suicide

The symptoms of irritability associated with autistic disorder include:

- aggressive behavior towards others
- intentionally trying to harm oneself
- temper tantrums
- quickly changing moods

The symptoms of agitation associated with schizophrenia or bipolar disorder include:

- hostility or aggressive behavior
- agitation and inner tension
- self-exhausting behavior

What should I tell my healthcare provider before taking ABILIFY?

Before taking ABILIFY, tell your healthcare provider if you have or had:

- diabetes or high blood sugar in you or your family; your healthcare provider should check your blood sugar before you start ABILIFY and also during therapy.
- seizures (convulsions).
- low or high blood pressure.
- heart problems or stroke.
- pregnancy or plans to become pregnant. It is not known if ABILIFY will harm your unborn baby.
- breast-feeding or plans to breast-feed. It is not known if ABILIFY will pass into your breast milk. You and your healthcare provider should decide if you will take ABILIFY or breast-feed. You should not do both.
- low white blood cell count.
- phenylketonuria. ABILIFY DISCMELT Orally Disintegrating Tablets contain phenylalanine.
- any other medical conditions.

Tell your healthcare provider about all the medicines that you take or recently have taken, including prescription medicines, non-prescription medicines, herbal supplements, and vitamins.

ABILIFY and other medicines may affect each other causing possible serious side effects. ABILIFY may affect the way other medicines work, and other medicines may affect how ABILIFY works.

Your healthcare provider can tell you if it is safe to take ABILIFY with your other medicines. Do not start or stop any medicines while taking ABILIFY without talking to your healthcare provider first. Know the medicines you take. Keep a list of your medicines to show your healthcare provider and pharmacist when you get a new medicine.

How should I take ABILIFY?

- Take ABILIFY exactly as your healthcare provider tells you to take it. Do not change the dose or stop taking ABILIFY yourself.
- ABILIFY can be taken with or without food.
- ABILIFY tablets should be swallowed whole.
- If you miss a dose of ABILIFY, take the missed dose as soon as you remember. If it is almost time for the next dose, just skip the missed dose and take your next dose at the regular time. Do not take two doses of ABILIFY at the same time.
- If you have been prescribed ABILIFY DISCMELT, take it as follows:
  - Do not open the blister until ready to take the DISCMELT tablet.
  - To remove one DISCMELT tablet, open the package and peel back the foil on the blister to expose the tablet.
  - Do not push the tablet through the foil because this could damage the tablet.
  - Immediately upon opening the blister, using dry hands, remove the tablet and place the entire ABILIFY DISCMELT Orally Disintegrating Tablet on the tongue.
  - Tablet disintegration occurs rapidly in saliva. It is recommended that ABILIFY DISCMELT be taken without liquid. However, if needed, it can be taken with liquid.
  - Do not attempt to split the DISCMELT tablet.

If you take too much ABILIFY, call your healthcare provider or poison control center at 1-800-222-1222 right away, or go to the nearest hospital emergency room.

What should I avoid while taking ABILIFY?

- Do not drive, operate heavy machinery, or do other dangerous activities until you know how ABILIFY affects you. ABILIFY may make you drowsy.
- Do not drink alcohol while taking ABILIFY.
- Avoid getting over-heated or dehydrated.
  - Do not over-exercise.
  - In hot weather, stay inside in a cool place if possible.
  - Stay out of the sun. Do not wear too much or heavy clothing.
  - Drink plenty of water.

What are the possible side effects of ABILIFY?

Serious side effects have been reported with ABILIFY including:

Also see "What is the most important information I should know about ABILIFY?" at the beginning of this Medication Guide.

- **Neuroleptic malignant syndrome (NMS):** Tell your healthcare provider right away if you have some or all of the following symptoms: high fever, stiff muscles, confusion, sweating, changes in pulse, heart rate, and blood pressure. These may be symptoms of a rare and serious condition that can lead to death. Call your healthcare provider right away if you have any of these symptoms.
- **High blood sugar (hyperglycemia):** Increases in blood sugar can happen in some people who take ABILIFY. Extremely high blood sugar can lead to coma or death. If you have diabetes or risk factors for diabetes (such as being overweight or a family history of diabetes), your healthcare provider should check your blood sugar before you start ABILIFY and during therapy.

  Call your healthcare provider if you have any of these symptoms of high blood sugar while taking ABILIFY:
  - feel very thirsty
  - need to urinate more than usual
  - feel very hungry
  - feel weak or tired
  - feel sick to your stomach
  - feel confused, or your breath smells fruity
- **Increase in weight:** Weight gain has been reported in patients taking medicines like ABILIFY, so you and your healthcare provider should check your weight regularly. For children and adolescent patients (6 to 17 years of age) weight gain should be compared against that expected with normal growth.
- **Difficulty swallowing:** may lead to aspiration and choking.
- **Tardive dyskinesia:** Call your healthcare provider about any movements you cannot control in your face, tongue, or other body parts. These may be signs of a serious condition. Tardive dyskinesia may not go away, even if you stop taking ABILIFY. Tardive dyskinesia may also start after you stop taking ABILIFY.
- **Orthostatic hypotension (decreased blood pressure):** lightheadedness or fainting when rising too quickly from a sitting or lying position.
- **Low white blood cell count**
- **Seizures (convulsions)**

Common side effects with ABILIFY in adults include:

• nausea	• inner sense of restlessness/need to move (akathisia)
• vomiting	• anxiety
• constipation	• insomnia
• headache	• restlessness
• dizziness	

Common side effects with ABILIFY in children include:

• feeling sleepy	• insomnia
• headache	• nausea
• vomiting	• stuffy nose
• fatigue	• weight gain
• increased appetite	• uncontrolled movement such as restlessness, tremor, muscle stiffness

These are not all the possible side effects of ABILIFY. For more information, ask your healthcare provider or pharmacist.

Call your doctor for medical advice about side effects. You may report side effects to FDA at 1-800-FDA-1088.

How should I store ABILIFY?

- Store ABILIFY at room temperature, between 59°F to 86°F (15°C to 30°C).
- Opened bottles of ABILIFY Oral Solution can be used for up to 6 months after opening, but not beyond the expiration date on the bottle.

Keep ABILIFY and all medicines out of the reach of children.

General information about ABILIFY

Medicines are sometimes prescribed for purposes other than those listed in a Medication Guide. Do not use ABILIFY for a condition for which it was not prescribed. Do not give ABILIFY to other people, even if they have the same condition. It may harm them.

This Medication Guide summarizes the most important information about ABILIFY. If you would like more information, talk with your healthcare provider. You can ask your healthcare provider or pharmacist for information about ABILIFY that was written for healthcare professionals. For more information about ABILIFY visit www.abilify.com.

What are the ingredients in ABILIFY?

Active ingredient: aripiprazole

Inactive ingredients:

Tablets: cornstarch, hydroxypropyl cellulose, lactose monohydrate, magnesium stearate, and microcrystalline cellulose. Colorants include ferric oxide (yellow or red) and FD&C Blue No. 2 Aluminum Lake.

ABILIFY DISCMELT Orally Disintegrating Tablets: acesulfame potassium, aspartame (which contains phenylalanine), calcium silicate, croscarmellose sodium, crospovidone, crème de vanilla (natural and artificial flavors), magnesium stearate, microcrystalline cellulose, silicon dioxide, tartaric acid, and xylitol. Colorants include ferric oxide (yellow or red) and FD&C Blue No. 2 Aluminum Lake.

ABILIFY Oral Solution: disodium edetate, fructose (200 mg per mL), glycerin, dl-lactic acid, methylparaben, propylene glycol, propylparaben, sodium hydroxide, sucrose (400 mg per mL), and purified water. The oral solution is flavored with natural orange cream and other natural flavors.

This Medication Guide has been approved by the U.S. Food and Drug Administration.

Tablets manufactured by Otsuka Pharmaceutical Co, Ltd, Tokyo, 101-8535 Japan or Bristol-Myers Squibb Company, Princeton, NJ 08543 USA

Orally Disintegrating Tablets, Oral Solution, and Injection manufactured by

Bristol-Myers Squibb Company, Princeton, NJ 08543 USA

Distributed and marketed by Otsuka America Pharmaceutical, Inc, Rockville, MD 20850 USA

ABILIFY is a trademark of Otsuka Pharmaceutical Company.

1239550B3 03US13L-1028C Rev April 2013

ABILIFY MAINTENA™ ℞

(aripiprazole)

for extended-release injectable suspension, for intramuscular use

HIGHLIGHTS OF PRESCRIBING INFORMATION

These highlights do not include all the information needed to use ABILIFY MAINTENA safely and effectively. See full prescribing information for ABILIFY MAINTENA.

ABILIFY MAINTENA™ (aripiprazole) for extended-release injectable suspension, for intramuscular use

Initial U.S. Approval: 2002

WARNING: INCREASED MORTALITY IN ELDERLY PATIENTS WITH DEMENTIA-RELATED PSYCHOSIS

See full prescribing information for complete boxed warning.

- **Elderly patients with dementia-related psychosis treated with antipsychotic drugs are at an increased risk of death (5.1)**
- **ABILIFY MAINTENA is not approved for the treatment of patients with dementia-related psychosis (5.1)**

INDICATIONS AND USAGE

ABILIFY MAINTENA is an atypical antipsychotic indicated for the treatment of schizophrenia (1)

DOSAGE AND ADMINISTRATION

- Only to be administered by intramuscular injection in the gluteal muscle by a healthcare professional (2.1)
- For patients naïve to aripiprazole, establish tolerability with oral aripiprazole prior to initiating ABILIFY MAINTENA (2.1)
- Recommended starting and maintenance dose is 400 mg administered monthly as a single injection (2.1)
- In conjunction with first dose, take 14 consecutive days of concurrent oral aripiprazole (10 mg to 20 mg) or current oral antipsychotic (2.1)
- Some patients may benefit from a reduction to a 300 mg dose (2.1)
- Dosage adjustments are required for missed doses (2.2)
- See instructions for use for reconstitution procedures (2.4, 2.5, 2.6, 2.7, 2.8)
- Dosage adjustments for patients who are CYP2D6 poor metabolizers and for patients taking CYP2D6 inhibitors, CYP3A4 inhibitors, or CYP3A4 inducers for greater than 14 days (2.3):

	Adjusted Dose
CYP2D6 Poor Metabolizers	
CYP2D6 Poor Metabolizers	300 mg
CYP2D6 Poor Metabolizers taking concomitant CYP3A4 inhibitors	200 mg
Patients Taking 400 mg of ABILIFY MAINTENA	
Strong CYP2D6 <u>or</u> CYP3A4 inhibitors	300 mg
CYP2D6 <u>and</u> CYP3A4 inhibitors	200 mg
CYP3A4 inducers	Avoid use
Patients Taking 300 mg of ABILIFY MAINTENA	
Strong CYP2D6 <u>or</u> CYP3A4 inhibitors	200 mg
CYP2D6 <u>and</u> CYP3A4 inhibitors	160 mg
CYP3A4 inducers	Avoid use

DOSAGE FORMS AND STRENGTHS

For extended-release injectable suspension: 400 mg/vial and 300 mg/vial of lyophilized powder for reconstitution (3)

CONTRAINDICATIONS

Known hypersensitivity to aripiprazole (4)

WARNINGS AND PRECAUTIONS

- *Cerebrovascular Adverse Reactions in Elderly Patients with Dementia-Related Psychosis:* Increased incidence of cerebrovascular adverse reactions (e.g., stroke, transient ischemic attack, including fatalities) (5.2)
- *Neuroleptic Malignant Syndrome:* Manage with immediate discontinuation and close monitoring (5.3)
- *Tardive Dyskinesia:* Discontinue if clinically appropriate (5.4)
- *Metabolic Changes:* Atypical antipsychotic drugs have been associated with metabolic changes that may increase cardiovascular/cerebrovascular risk. These metabolic changes include hyperglycemia, dyslipidemia, and weight gain (5.5)
  - *Hyperglycemia and Diabetes Mellitus:* Monitor patients for symptoms of hyperglycemia including polydipsia, polyuria, polyphagia, and weakness. Monitor glucose regularly in patients with and at risk for diabetes (5.5)
  - *Dyslipidemia:* Undesirable alterations have been observed in patients treated with atypical antipsychotics (5.5)
  - *Weight Gain:* Gain in body weight has been observed; clinical monitoring of weight is recommended (5.5)
- *Orthostatic Hypotension:* Use with caution in patients with known cardiovascular or cerebrovascular disease (5.6)
- *Leukopenia, Neutropenia, and Agranulocytosis:* Perform complete blood counts in patients with a history of a clinically significant low white blood cell count (WBC). Consider discontinuation if clinically significant decline in WBC in the absence of other causative factors (5.7)
- *Seizures:* Use cautiously in patients with a history of seizures or with conditions that lower the seizure threshold (5.8)
- *Potential for Cognitive and Motor Impairment:* Use caution when operating machinery (5.9)

ADVERSE REACTIONS

Most commonly observed adverse reaction with oral aripiprazole (incidence ≥5% and at least twice that for placebo) was akathisia (6.1)

To report SUSPECTED ADVERSE REACTIONS, contact Otsuka America Pharmaceutical, Inc. at 1-800-438-9927 or FDA at 1-800-FDA-1088 (*www.fda.gov/medwatch*).

USE IN SPECIFIC POPULATIONS

- *Pregnancy:* Based on animal data, may cause fetal harm (8.1)
- *Nursing Mothers:* Discontinue drug or nursing, taking into consideration importance of drug to the mother (8.3)

See 17 for PATIENT COUNSELING INFORMATION and Medication Guide

Revised: 02/2013

FULL PRESCRIBING INFORMATION: CONTENTS*

*** Sections or subsections omitted from the full prescribing information are not listed**

FULL PRESCRIBING INFORMATION

WARNING: INCREASED MORTALITY IN ELDERLY PATIENTS WITH DEMENTIA-RELATED PSYCHOSIS

Elderly patients with dementia-related psychosis treated with antipsychotic drugs are at an increased

risk of death. ABILIFY MAINTENA is not approved for the treatment of patients with dementia-related psychosis *[see Warnings and Precautions (5.1)]*.

1 INDICATIONS AND USAGE

ABILIFY MAINTENA (aripiprazole) is indicated for the treatment of schizophrenia.

Efficacy was demonstrated in a placebo-controlled, randomized-withdrawal maintenance trial in patients with schizophrenia and additional support for efficacy was derived from oral aripiprazole trials *[see Clinical Studies (14)]*.

2 DOSAGE AND ADMINISTRATION

2.1 Dosing Information

ABILIFY MAINTENA is only to be administered by intramuscular injection by a healthcare professional. For patients who have never taken aripiprazole, establish tolerability with oral aripiprazole prior to initiating treatment with ABILIFY MAINTENA. The recommended starting and maintenance dose of ABILIFY MAINTENA is 400 mg monthly (no sooner than 26 days after the previous injection).

After the first ABILIFY MAINTENA injection, continue treatment with oral aripiprazole (10 mg to 20 mg) or other oral antipsychotic for 14 consecutive days to maintain therapeutic antipsychotic concentrations during initiation of therapy.

If there are adverse reactions with the 400 mg dosage, consider reducing the dosage to 300 mg once monthly.

2.2 Dosage Adjustments for Missed Doses

If the second or third doses are missed:

- **If more than 4 weeks and less than 5 weeks have elapsed since the last injection,** administer the injection as soon as possible.
- **If more than 5 weeks have elapsed since the last injection,** restart concomitant oral aripiprazole for 14 days with the next administered injection.

If the fourth or subsequent doses are missed:

- **If more than 4 weeks and less than 6 weeks have elapsed since the last injection,** administer the injection as soon as possible.
- **If more than 6 weeks have elapsed since the last injection,** restart concomitant oral aripiprazole for 14 days with the next administered injection.

2.3 CYP2D6 Poor Metabolizers and with Concomitant Use of CYP3A4 Inhibitors, CYP2D6 Inhibitors, or CYP3A4 Inducers

Dosage adjustments are recommended in patients who are CYP2D6 poor metabolizers and in patients taking concomitant CYP3A4 inhibitors or CYP2D6 inhibitors for greater than 14 days (see Table 1). If the CYP3A4 inhibitor, or CYP2D6 inhibitor is withdrawn, the ABILIFY MAINTENA dosage may need to be increased *[see Dosage and Administration (2.1)]*.

Avoid the concomitant use of CYP3A4 inducers with ABILIFY MAINTENA for greater than 14 days because the blood levels of aripiprazole are decreased and may be below the effective levels.

Dosage adjustments are not recommended for patients with concomitant use of CYP3A4 inhibitors, CYP2D6 inhibitors or CYP3A4 inducers for less than 14 days.

Table 1: Dose Adjustments of ABILIFY MAINTENA in Patients who are CYP2D6 Poor Metabolizers and Patients Taking Concomitant CYP2D6 Inhibitors, 3A4 Inhibitors, and/or CYP3A4 Inducers for Greater than 14 days

	Adjusted Dose
CYP2D6 Poor Metabolizers	
CYP2D6 Poor Metabolizers	300 mg
CYP2D6 Poor Metabolizers taking concomitant CYP3A4 inhibitors	200 mg
Patients Taking 400 mg of ABILIFY MAINTENA	
Strong CYP2D6 or CYP3A4 inhibitors	300 mg
CYP2D6 and CYP3A4 inhibitors	200 mg
CYP3A4 inducers	Avoid use
Patients Taking 300 mg of ABILIFY MAINTENA	
Strong CYP2D6 or CYP3A4 inhibitors	200 mg
CYP2D6 and CYP3A4 inhibitors	160 mg
CYP3A4 inducers	Avoid use

2.4 Preparation Prior to Reconstitution of the Lyophilized ABILIFY MAINTENA Powder

For deep intramuscular gluteal injection by healthcare professionals only. Do not administer by any other route. Inject immediately after reconstitution. Administer once monthly.

(a) Lay out and confirm that components listed below are provided in the kit:

- Vial of ABILIFY MAINTENA™ (aripiprazole) for extended-release injectable suspension lyophilized powder
- 5 mL vial of Sterile Water for Injection, USP
- One 3 mL Luer Lock syringe with pre-attached 21 gauge, 1.5 inch (38 mm) Hypodermic Needle-Pro® safety needle with needle protection device
- One 3 mL BD Luer-Lok™ disposable syringe with BD Luer-Lok tip
- One vial adapter
- One 21 gauge, 1.5 inch (38 mm) Hypodermic Needle-Pro® safety needle with needle protection device
- One 21 gauge, 2 inch (50 mm) Hypodermic Needle-Pro® safety needle for obese patients with needle protection device

(b) ABILIFY MAINTENA should be suspended using the Sterile Water for Injection as supplied in the kit.

(c) The Sterile Water for Injection and ABILIFY MAINTENA vials are for single-use only.

(d) Use appropriate aseptic techniques throughout reconstitution and reconstitute at room temperature.

(e) Select the amount of Sterile Water for Injection needed for reconstitution (see Table 2).

Table 2: Amount of Sterile Water for Injection Needed for Reconstitution

400 mg Vial		300 mg Vial	
Dose	Sterile Water for Injection	Dose	Sterile Water for Injection
400 mg	1.9 mL	300 mg	1.5 mL

Important: There is more Sterile Water for Injection in the vial than is needed to reconstitute ABILIFY MAINTENA (aripiprazole) for extended-release injectable suspension. The vial will have excess Sterile Water for Injection; discard any unused portion.

2.5 Reconstitution of the Lyophilized Powder

(a) Remove the cap of the vial of Sterile Water for Injection and remove the cap of the vial containing ABILIFY MAINTENA lyophilized powder and wipe the tops with a sterile alcohol swab.

(b) Using the syringe with pre-attached Hypodermic Needle-Pro needle, withdraw the pre-determined Sterile Water for Injection volume from the vial of Sterile Water for Injection into the syringe (see Figure 1). Residual Sterile Water for Injection will remain in the vial following withdrawal; discard any unused portion.

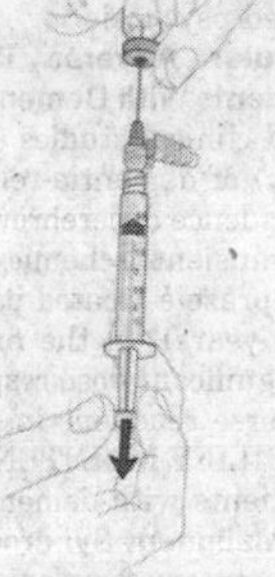

Figure 1

(c) Slowly inject the Sterile Water for Injection into the vial containing the ABILIFY MAINTENA lyophilized powder (see Figure 2).

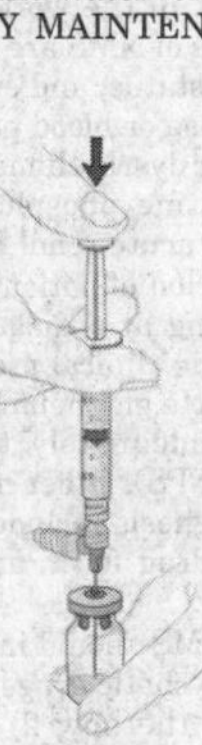

Figure 2

(d) Withdraw air to equalize the pressure in the vial by pulling back slightly on the plunger. Subsequently, remove the needle from the vial. Engage the needle safety device by using the one-handed technique (see Figure 3). Gently press the sheath against a flat surface until the needle is firmly engaged in the needle protection sheath. Visually confirm that the needle is fully engaged into the needle protection sheath, and discard.

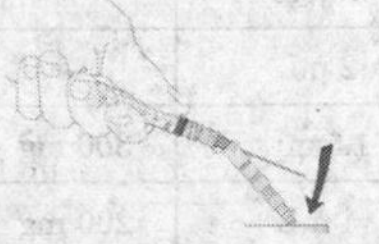

Figure 3

(e) Shake the vial vigorously for 30 seconds until the reconstituted suspension appears uniform (see Figure 4).

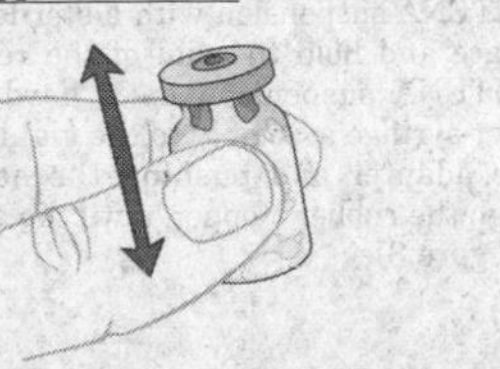

Figure 4

(f) Visually inspect the reconstituted suspension for particulate matter and discoloration prior to administration. The reconstituted ABILIFY MAINTENA is a uniform, homogeneous suspension that is opaque and milky-white in color.

(g) If the injection is not performed immediately after reconstitution keep the vial at room temperature and shake the vial vigorously for at least 60 seconds to re-suspend prior to injection.

(h) Do not store the reconstituted suspension in a syringe.

2.6 Preparation Prior to Injection

(a) Use appropriate aseptic techniques throughout injection of the reconstituted ABILIFY MAINTENA suspension.

(b) Remove the cover from the vial adapter package (see Figure 5). Do not remove the vial adapter from the package.

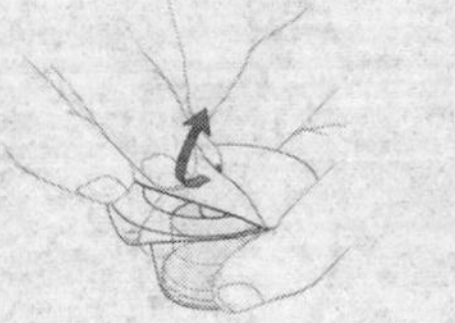

Figure 5

(c) Using the vial adapter package to handle the vial adapter, attach the prepackaged BD Luer-Lok syringe to the vial adapter (see Figure 6).

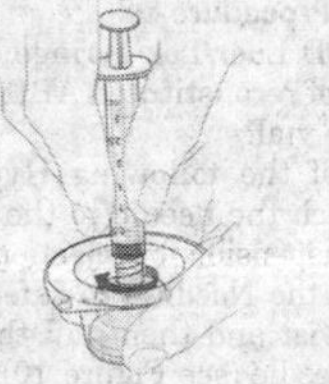

Figure 6

(d) Use the BD Luer-Lok syringe to remove the vial adapter from the package and discard the vial adapter package (see Figure 7). Do not touch the spike tip of the adapter at any time.

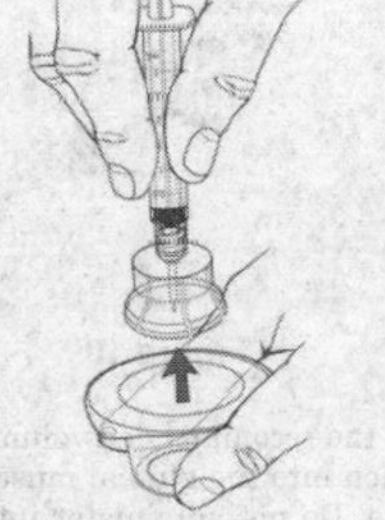

Figure 7

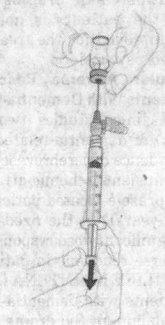

(e) Determine the recommended volume for injection (Table 3).

Table 3: ABILIFY MAINTENA Reconstituted Suspension Volume to Inject

400 mg Vial		300 mg Vial	
Dose	Volume to Inject	Dose	Volume to Inject
400 mg	2 mL	---	---
300 mg	1.5 mL	300 mg	1.5 mL
200 mg	1 mL	200 mg	1 mL
160 mg	0.8 mL	160 mg	0.8 mL

(f) Wipe the top of the vial of the reconstituted ABILIFY MAINTENA suspension with a sterile alcohol swab.
(g) Place and hold the vial of the reconstituted ABILIFY MAINTENA suspension on a hard surface. Attach the adapter-syringe assembly to the vial by holding the outside of the adapter and pushing the adapter's spike firmly through the rubber stopper, until the adapter snaps in place (see Figure 8).

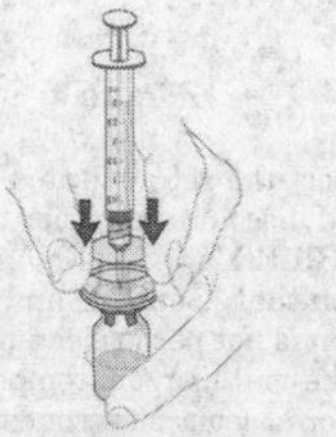

Figure 8

(h) Slowly withdraw the recommended volume from the vial into the BD Luer-Lok syringe to allow for injection (see Figure 9). A small amount of excess product will remain in the vial.

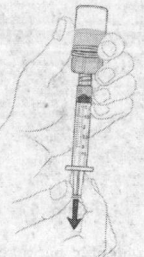

Figure 9

2.7 Injection Procedure
(a) Detach the BD Luer-Lok syringe containing the recommended volume of reconstituted ABILIFY MAINTENA suspension from the vial.
(b) Select one of the following Hypodermic Needle-Pro needles and attach the needle to the BD Luer-Lok syringe containing the suspension for injection. Ensure the needle is firmly seated on the Needle-Pro safety device with a push and clockwise twist and then pull the needle cap straight away from the needle (see Figure 10).
- 21 gauge, 1.5 inch (38 mm) Hypodermic Needle-Pro needle with needle protection device for non-obese patients.
- 21 gauge, 2 inch (50 mm) Hypodermic Needle-Pro safety needle for obese patients.

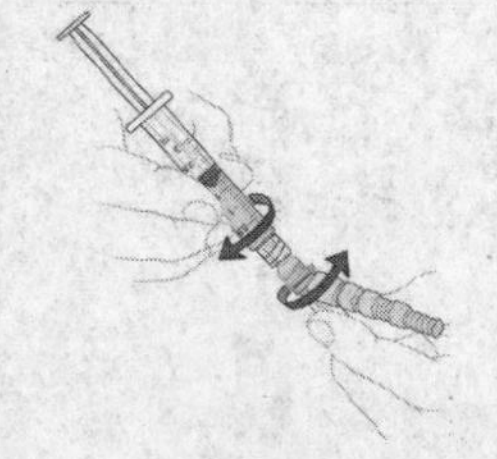

Figure 10

(c) Slowly inject the recommended volume as a single intramuscular injection into the gluteal muscle. Do not massage the injection site. Do not administer intravenously or subcutaneously.

2.8 Procedures After Injection
(a) Engage the needle safety device as described in Section 2.5, Step (d). Dispose of the vials, adapter, needles, and syringe appropriately after injection. **The Sterile Water for Injection and ABILIFY MAINTENA vials are for single-use only.**
(b) Rotate sites of injections between the two gluteal muscles.

2.9 Different Aripiprazole Formulations
There are two aripiprazole formulations for intramuscular use with different dosages, dosing frequencies, and indications. ABILIFY MAINTENA is a long-acting aripiprazole formulation with 4 week dosing intervals indicated for the treatment of schizophrenia. In contrast, aripiprazole injection (9.75 mg per vial) is a short-acting formulation indicated for agitation in patients with schizophrenia or mania. Do not substitute these products. Refer to the prescribing information for aripiprazole injection for more information about aripiprazole injection.

3 DOSAGE FORMS AND STRENGTHS
For extended-release injectable suspension: 300 mg and 400 mg, lyophilized powder in a single-use vial for reconstitution. The reconstituted extended-release injectable suspension is a uniform, homogeneous suspension that is opaque and milky-white in color.

4 CONTRAINDICATIONS
ABILIFY MAINTENA is contraindicated in patients with a known hypersensitivity to aripiprazole. Hypersensitivity reactions ranging from pruritus/urticaria to anaphylaxis have been reported in patients receiving aripiprazole *[see Adverse Reactions (6.2)]*.

5 WARNINGS AND PRECAUTIONS
5.1 Increased Mortality in Elderly Patients with Dementia- Related Psychosis
Elderly patients with dementia-related psychosis treated with antipsychotic drugs are at an increased risk of death. Analyses of 17 placebo-controlled trials (modal duration of 10 weeks), largely in patients taking atypical antipsychotic drugs, revealed a risk of death in drug-treated patients of between 1.6 to 1.7 times the risk of death in placebo-treated patients. Over the course of a typical 10–week controlled trial, the rate of death in drug-treated patients was about 4.5%, compared to a rate of about 2.6% in the placebo group. Although the causes of death were varied, most of the deaths appeared to be either cardiovascular (e.g., heart failure, sudden death) or infectious (e.g., pneumonia) in nature. Observational studies suggest that, similar to atypical antipsychotic drugs, treatment with conventional antipsychotic drugs may increase mortality. The extent to which the findings of increased mortality in observational studies may be attributed to the antipsychotic drug as opposed to some characteristic(s) of the patients is not clear. ABILIFY MAINTENA is not approved for the treatment of patients with dementia-related psychosis.

5.2 Cerebrovascular Adverse Reactions, Including Stroke in Elderly Patients with Dementia-Related Psychosis
In placebo-controlled clinical studies (two flexible dose and one fixed dose study) of dementia-related psychosis, there was an increased incidence of cerebrovascular adverse reactions (e.g., stroke, transient ischemic attack), including fatalities, in oral aripiprazole-treated patients (mean age: 84 years; range: 78–88 years). In the fixed-dose study, there was a statistically significant dose response relationship for cerebrovascular adverse reactions in patients treated with oral aripiprazole. ABILIFY MAINTENA is not approved for the treatment of patients with dementia-related psychosis.

5.3 Neuroleptic Malignant Syndrome
A potentially fatal symptom complex sometimes referred to as Neuroleptic Malignant Syndrome (NMS) may occur with administration of antipsychotic drugs, including ABILIFY MAINTENA. Rare cases of NMS occurred during aripiprazole treatment in the worldwide clinical database. Clinical manifestations of NMS are hyperpyrexia, muscle rigidity, altered mental status, and evidence of autonomic instability (irregular pulse or blood pressure, tachycardia, diaphoresis, and cardiac dysrhythmia). Additional signs may include elevated creatine phosphokinase, myoglobinuria (rhabdomyolysis), and acute renal failure.
The diagnostic evaluation of patients with this syndrome is complicated. In arriving at a diagnosis, it is important to exclude cases where the clinical presentation includes both serious medical illness (e.g., pneumonia, systemic infection) and untreated or inadequately treated extrapyramidal signs and symptoms (EPS). Other important considerations in the differential diagnosis include central anticholinergic toxicity, heat stroke, drug fever, and primary central nervous system pathology.
The management of NMS should include: 1) immediate discontinuation of antipsychotic drugs and other drugs not essential to concurrent therapy; 2) intensive symptomatic treatment and medical monitoring; and 3) treatment of any concomitant serious medical problems for which specific treatments are available. There is no general agreement about specific pharmacological treatment regimens for uncomplicated NMS.
If a patient requires antipsychotic drug treatment after recovery from NMS, the potential reintroduction of drug therapy should be carefully considered. The patient should be carefully monitored, since recurrences of NMS have been reported.

5.4 Tardive Dyskinesia
A syndrome of potentially irreversible, involuntary, dyskinetic movements, may develop in patients treated with antipsychotic drugs. Although the prevalence of the syndrome appears to be highest among the elderly, especially elderly women, it is impossible to rely upon prevalence estimates to predict, at the inception of antipsychotic treatment, which patients are likely to develop the syndrome. Whether antipsychotic drug products differ in their potential to cause tardive dyskinesia is unknown.
The risk of developing tardive dyskinesia and the likelihood that it will become irreversible are believed to increase as the duration of treatment and the total cumulative dose of antipsychotic drugs administered to the patient increase. However, the syndrome can develop, although much less commonly, after relatively brief treatment periods at low doses.
There is no known treatment for established tardive dyskinesia, although the syndrome may remit, partially or completely, if antipsychotic treatment is withdrawn. Antipsychotic treatment, itself, however, may suppress (or partially suppress) the signs and symptoms of the syndrome and, thereby, may possibly mask the underlying process. The effect of symptomatic suppression on the long-term course of the syndrome is unknown.
Given these considerations, ABILIFY MAINTENA should be prescribed in a manner that is most likely to minimize the occurrence of tardive dyskinesia. Chronic antipsychotic treatment should generally be reserved for patients who suffer from a chronic illness that 1) is known to respond to antipsychotic drugs and 2) for whom alternative, equally effective, but potentially less harmful treatments are not available or appropriate. In patients who do require chronic treatment, the smallest dose and the shortest duration of treatment producing a satisfactory clinical response should be sought. The need for continued treatment should be reassessed periodically.
If signs and symptoms of tardive dyskinesia appear in a patient treated with ABILIFY MAINTENA drug discontinuation should be considered. However, some patients may require treatment with ABILIFY MAINTENA despite the presence of the syndrome.

5.5 Metabolic Changes
Atypical antipsychotic drugs have been associated with metabolic changes that include hyperglycemia/diabetes mellitus, dyslipidemia, and weight gain. While all drugs in the class have been shown to produce some metabolic changes, each drug has its own specific risk profile. Although the following metabolic data were collected in patients treated with oral formulations of aripiprazole, the findings pertain to patients receiving ABILIFY MAINTENA as well.

Hyperglycemia/Diabetes Mellitus
Hyperglycemia, in some cases extreme and associated with diabetic ketoacidosis, hyperosmolar coma, or death, has been reported in patients treated with atypical antipsychotics. There have been reports of hyperglycemia in patients treated with aripiprazole *[see Adverse Reactions (6.1)]*. Assessment of the relationship between atypical antipsychotic use and glucose abnormalities is complicated by the possibility of an increased background risk of diabetes mellitus in patients with schizophrenia and the increasing incidence of diabetes mellitus in the general population. Given these confounders, the relationship between atypical antipsychotic use and hyperglycemia-related adverse reactions is not completely understood. However, epidemiological studies suggest an increased risk of hyperglycemia-related adverse reactions in patients treated with the atypical antipsychotics. Because aripiprazole was not marketed at the time these studies were performed, it is not known if aripiprazole is associated with this increased risk. Precise risk estimates for hyperglycemia-related adverse reactions in patients treated with atypical antipsychotics are not available. Patients with an established diagnosis of diabetes mellitus who are started on atypical antipsychotics should be monitored regularly for worsening of glucose control. Patients with risk factors for diabetes mellitus (e.g., obesity, family history of diabetes), who are starting treatment with atypical antipsychotics should undergo fasting blood glucose testing at the beginning of treatment and periodically during treatment. Any patient treated with atypical antipsychotics should be monitored for symptoms of hyperglycemia including polydipsia, polyuria, polyphagia, and weakness. Patients who develop symptoms of hyperglycemia during treatment with atypical antipsychotics should undergo fasting blood glucose testing. In some cases, hyperglycemia has

resolved when the atypical antipsychotic was discontinued; however, some patients required continuation of anti-diabetic treatment despite discontinuation of the atypical antipsychotic drug.

In an analysis of 13 placebo-controlled monotherapy trials in adults, primarily with schizophrenia or bipolar disorder, the mean change in fasting glucose in aripiprazole-treated patients (+4.4 mg/dL; median exposure 25 days; N=1057) was not significantly different than in placebo-treated patients (+2.5 mg/dL; median exposure 22 days; N=799). Table 4 shows the proportion of aripiprazole-treated patients with normal and borderline fasting glucose at baseline (median exposure 25 days) that had high fasting glucose measurements compared to placebo-treated patients (median exposure 22 days).

[See table 4 above]

At 24 weeks, the mean change in fasting glucose in aripiprazole-treated patients was not significantly different than in placebo-treated patients [+2.2 mg/dL (n=42) and +9.6 mg/dL (n=28), respectively].

Dyslipidemia

Undesirable alterations in lipids have been observed in patients treated with atypical antipsychotics.

There were no significant differences between aripiprazole- and placebo-treated patients in the proportion with changes from normal to clinically significant levels for fasting/nonfasting total cholesterol, fasting triglycerides, fasting LDLs, and fasting/nonfasting HDLs. Analyses of patients with at least 12 or 24 weeks of exposure were limited by small numbers of patients.

Table 5 shows the proportion of adult patients, primarily from pooled schizophrenia and bipolar disorder monotherapy placebo-controlled trials, with changes in total cholesterol (pooled from 17 trials; median exposure 21 to 25 days), fasting triglycerides (pooled from eight trials; median exposure 42 days), fasting LDL cholesterol (pooled from eight trials; median exposure 39 to 45 days, except for placebo-treated patients with baseline normal fasting LDL measurements, who had median treatment exposure of 24 days) and HDL cholesterol (pooled from nine trials; median exposure 40 to 42 days).

Table 5: Changes in Blood Lipid Parameters From Placebo-Controlled Monotherapy Trials in Adults

	Treatment Arm	n/N	%
Total Cholesterol Normal to High (<200 mg/dL to ≥240 mg/dL)	Aripiprazole	34/1357	2.5
	Placebo	27/973	2.8
Fasting Triglycerides Normal to High (<150 mg/dL to ≥200 mg/dL)	Aripiprazole	40/539	7.4
	Placebo	30/431	7.0
Fasting LDL Cholesterol Normal to High (<100 mg/dL to ≥160 mg/dL)	Aripiprazole	2/332	0.6
	Placebo	2/268	0.7
HDL Cholesterol Normal to Low (≥40 mg/dL to <40 mg/dL)	Aripiprazole	121/1066	11.4
	Placebo	99/794	12.5

In monotherapy trials in adults, the proportion of patients at 12 weeks and 24 weeks with changes from Normal to High in total cholesterol (fasting/nonfasting), fasting triglycerides, and fasting LDL cholesterol were similar between aripiprazole- and placebo-treated patients: at 12 weeks, Total Cholesterol (fasting/nonfasting), 1/71 (1.4%) vs. 3/74 (4.1%); Fasting Triglycerides, 8/62 (12.9%) vs. 5/37 (13.5%); Fasting LDL Cholesterol, 0/34 (0%) vs. 1/25 (4.0%), respectively; and at 24 weeks, Total Cholesterol (fasting/nonfasting), 1/42 (2.4%) vs. 3/37 (8.1%); Fasting Triglycerides, 5/34 (14.7%) vs. 5/20 (25%); Fasting LDL Cholesterol, 0/22 (0%) vs. 1/18 (5.6%), respectively.

Weight Gain

Weight gain has been observed with atypical antipsychotic use. Clinical monitoring of weight is recommended.

In an analysis of 13 placebo-controlled monotherapy trials, primarily from pooled schizophrenia and bipolar disorder, with a median exposure of 21 to 25 days, the mean change in body weight in aripiprazole-treated patients was +0.3 kg (N=1673) compared to –0.1 kg (N=1100) in placebo-controlled patients. At 24 weeks, the mean change from baseline in body weight in aripiprazole-treated patients was –1.5 kg (n=73) compared to –0.2 kg (n=46) in placebo-treated patients.

Table 6 shows the percentage of adult patients with weight gain ≥7% of body weight in the 13 pooled placebo-controlled monotherapy trials.

Table 4: Changes in Fasting Glucose From Placebo-Controlled Monotherapy Trials in Adult Patients

	Category Change (at least once) from Baseline	Treatment Arm	n/N	%
Fasting Glucose	Normal to High (<100 mg/dL to ≥126 mg/dL)	Aripiprazole	31/822	3.8
		Placebo	22/605	3.6
	Borderline to High (≥100 mg/dL and <126 mg/dL to ≥126 mg/dL)	Aripiprazole	31/176	17.6
		Placebo	13/142	9.2

Table 6: Percentage of Patients From Placebo-Controlled Trials in Adult Patients with Weight Gain ≥7% of Body Weight

	Indication	Treatment Arm	N	Patients n (%)
Weight gain ≥7% of body weight	Schizophrenia*	Aripiprazole	852	69 (8.1)
		Placebo	379	12 (3.2)
	Bipolar Mania†	Aripiprazole	719	16 (2.2)
		Placebo	598	16 (2.7)

* 4–6 weeks duration.
† 3 weeks duration.

[See table 6 above]

5.6 Orthostatic Hypotension

Aripiprazole may cause orthostatic hypotension, perhaps due to its α_1-adrenergic receptor antagonism. Orthostasis occurred in 4/576 (0.7%) patients treated with ABILIFY MAINTENA during the stabilization phase, including abnormal orthostatic blood pressure (1/576, 0.2%), postural dizziness (1/576, 0.2%), presyncope (1/576, 0.2%) and orthostatic hypotension (1/576, 0.2%).

In the stabilization phase, the incidence of significant orthostatic change in blood pressure (defined as a decrease in systolic blood pressure ≥20 mmHg accompanied by an increase in heart rate ≥25 when comparing standing to supine values) was 0.2% (1/575).

5.7 Leukopenia, Neutropenia, and Agranulocytosis

Class Effect: In clinical trials and post-marketing experience, leukopenia and neutropenia have been reported temporally related to antipsychotic agents, including oral aripiprazole. Agranulocytosis has also been reported.

Possible risk factors for leukopenia/neutropenia include pre-existing low white blood cell count (WBC) and history of drug-induced leukopenia/neutropenia. In patients with a history of a clinically significant low WBC or drug-induced leukopenia/neutropenia perform a complete blood count (CBC) frequently during the first few months of therapy. In such patients, consider discontinuation of ABILIFY MAINTENA at the first sign of a clinically significant decline in WBC in the absence of other causative factors.

Monitor patients with clinically significant neutropenia for fever or other symptoms or signs of infection and treat promptly if such symptoms or signs occur. Discontinue ABILIFY MAINTENA in patients with severe neutropenia (absolute neutrophil count <1000/mm^3) and follow their WBC counts until recovery.

5.8 Seizures

As with other antipsychotic drugs, use ABILIFY MAINTENA cautiously in patients with a history of seizures or with conditions that lower the seizure threshold. Conditions that lower the seizure threshold may be more prevalent in a population of 65 years or older.

5.9 Potential for Cognitive and Motor Impairment

ABILIFY MAINTENA, like other antipsychotics, may impair judgment, thinking, or motor skills. Instruct patients to avoid operating hazardous machinery, including automobiles, until they are reasonably certain that therapy with ABILIFY MAINTENA does not affect them adversely.

5.10 Body Temperature Regulation

Disruption of the body's ability to reduce core body temperature has been attributed to antipsychotic agents. Appropriate care is advised when prescribing ABILIFY MAINTENA for patients who will be experiencing conditions which may contribute to an elevation in core body temperature, (e.g., exercising strenuously, exposure to extreme heat, receiving concomitant medication with anticholinergic activity, or being subject to dehydration).

5.11 Dysphagia

Esophageal dysmotility and aspiration have been associated with antipsychotic drug use, including ABILIFY MAINTENA. ABILIFY MAINTENA and other antipsychotic drugs should be used cautiously in patients at risk for aspiration pneumonia *[see Warnings and Precautions (5.1)]*.

6 ADVERSE REACTIONS

The following adverse reactions are discussed in more detail in other sections of the labeling:

- Increased Mortality in Elderly Patients with Dementia-Related Psychosis Use *[see Boxed Warning and Warnings and Precautions (5.1)]*
- Cerebrovascular Adverse Reactions, Including Stroke in Elderly Patients with Dementia-Related Psychosis *[see Boxed Warning and Warnings and Precautions 5.2]*
- Neuroleptic Malignant Syndrome *[see Warnings and Precautions (5.3)]*
- Tardive Dyskinesia *[see Warnings and Precautions (5.4)]*
- Metabolic Changes *[see Warnings and Precautions (5.5)]*
- Orthostatic Hypotension *[see Warnings and Precautions (5.6)]*
- Leukopenia, Neutropenia, and Agranulocytosis *[see Warnings and Precautions (5.7)]*
- Seizures *[see Warnings and Precautions (5.8)]*
- Potential for Cognitive and Motor Impairment *[see Warnings and Precautions (5.9)]*
- Body Temperature Regulation *[see Warnings and Precautions (5.10)]*
- Dysphagia *[see Warnings and Precautions (5.11)]*

6.1 Clinical Trials Experience

Because clinical trials are conducted under widely varying conditions, adverse reaction rates observed in the clinical trials of a drug cannot be directly compared to rates in the clinical trials of another drug and may not reflect the rates observed in practice.

Safety Database of ABILIFY MAINTENA and Oral Aripiprazole

Aripiprazole has been evaluated for safety in 16,114 adult patients who participated in multiple-dose, clinical trials in schizophrenia and other indications, and who had approximately 8,578 patient–years of exposure to oral aripiprazole. A total of 3,901 patients were treated with oral aripiprazole for at least 180 days, 2,259 patients were treated with oral aripiprazole for at least 360 days, and 933 patients continuing aripiprazole treatment for at least 720 days.

ABILIFY MAINTENA 300–400 mg every 4 weeks has been evaluated for safety in 1,287 adult patients in clinical trials in schizophrenia, with approximately 1,281 patient–years of exposure to ABILIFY MAINTENA. A total of 832 patients were treated with ABILIFY MAINTENA for at least 180 days (at least 7 consecutive injections) and 630 patients treated with ABILIFY MAINTENA had at least 1 year of exposure (at least 13 consecutive injections).

The conditions and duration of treatment with ABILIFY MAINTENA included double-blind and open-label studies. The safety profile of ABILIFY MAINTENA is expected to be similar to that of oral aripiprazole. Therefore, most of the safety data presented below are derived from trials with the oral formulation. In patients who tolerated and responded to treatment with oral aripiprazole and single-blind ABILIFY MAINTENA and were then randomized to receive ABILIFY MAINTENA or placebo injections under double-blind conditions, the incidence of adverse reactions was similar between the two treatment groups.

Adverse Reactions of ABILIFY MAINTENA and Oral Aripiprazole

Adverse Reactions Associated with Discontinuation of Oral Aripiprazole

Based on a pool of five placebo-controlled trials (four 4-week and one 6-week) in which oral aripiprazole was administered to adults with schizophrenia in doses ranging from 2 mg/day to 30 mg/day, the incidence of discontinuation due to adverse reactions was 7% in oral aripiprazole-treated and

9% in placebo-treated patients. The types of adverse reactions that led to discontinuation were similar for the aripiprazole-treated and placebo-treated patients.

Commonly Observed Adverse Reactions of Oral Aripiprazole

Based on a pool of five placebo-controlled trials (four 4–week and one 6–week) in which oral aripiprazole was administered to adults with schizophrenia in doses ranging from 2 mg/day to 30 mg/day, the only commonly observed adverse reaction associated with the use of oral aripiprazole in patients with schizophrenia (incidence of 5% or greater and aripiprazole incidence at least twice that for placebo) was akathisia (aripiprazole 8%; placebo 4%).

Less Common Adverse Reactions in Adults Treated with Oral Aripiprazole

Table 7 enumerates the pooled incidence, rounded to the nearest percent, of adverse reactions that occurred during acute therapy (up to 6 weeks in schizophrenia and up to 3 weeks in bipolar mania), including only those reactions that occurred in 2% or more of patients treated with oral aripiprazole (doses ≥2 mg/day) and for which the incidence in patients treated with aripiprazole was greater than the incidence in patients treated with placebo in the combined dataset.

Table 7: Adverse Reactions in Short-Term, Placebo-Controlled Trials in Adult Patients Treated with Oral Aripiprazole

System Organ Class Preferred Term	Percentage of Patients Reporting Reaction* Oral Aripiprazole (n=1843)	Placebo (n=1166)
Eye Disorders		
Blurred Vision	3	1
Gastrointestinal Disorders		
Nausea	15	11
Constipation	11	7
Vomiting	11	6
Dyspepsia	9	7
Dry Mouth	5	4
Toothache	4	3
Abdominal Discomfort	3	2
Stomach Discomfort	3	2
General Disorders and Administration Site Conditions		
Fatigue	6	4
Pain	3	2
Musculoskeletal and Connective Tissue Disorders		
Musculoskeletal Stiffness	4	3
Pain in Extremity	4	2
Myalgia	2	1
Muscle Spasms	2	1
Nervous System Disorders		
Headache	27	23
Dizziness	10	7
Akathisia	10	4
Sedation	7	4
Extrapyramidal Disorder	5	3
Tremor	5	3
Somnolence	5	3
Psychiatric Disorders		
Agitation	19	17
Insomnia	18	13
Anxiety	17	13
Restlessness	5	3
Respiratory, Thoracic, and Mediastinal Disorders		
Pharyngolaryngeal Pain	3	2
Cough	3	2

* Adverse reactions reported by at least 2% of patients treated with oral aripiprazole, except adverse reactions which had an incidence equal to or less than placebo.

An examination of population subgroups did not reveal any clear evidence of differential adverse reaction incidence on the basis of age, gender, or race.

Dose-Related Adverse Reactions of Oral Aripiprazole

Dose response relationships for the incidence of treatment-emergent adverse events were evaluated from four trials in adult patients with schizophrenia comparing various fixed oral doses of aripiprazole (2 mg/day, 5 mg/day, 10 mg/day, 15 mg/day, 20 mg/day, and 30 mg/day) to placebo. This analysis, stratified by study, indicated that the only adverse reaction to have a possible dose response relationship, and then most prominent only with 30 mg, was somnolence [including sedation]; (incidences were placebo, 7.1%; 10 mg, 8.5%; 15 mg, 8.7%; 20 mg, 7.5%; 30 mg, 12.6%).

Injection Site Reactions of ABILIFY MAINTENA

In the open-label, stabilization phase of a study with ABILIFY MAINTENA in patients with schizophrenia, the percent of patients reporting any injection site-related adverse reaction was 6.3% for ABILIFY MAINTENA-treated patients. The mean intensity of injection pain reported by subjects using a visual analog scale (0=no pain to 100=unbearably painful) was minimal and improved in subjects receiving ABILIFY MAINTENA from the first to the last injection in the open-label, stabilization phase (6.1 to 4.9).

Investigator evaluation of the injection site for pain, swelling, redness and induration following injections of ABILIFY MAINTENA in the open-label, stabilization phase were rated as absent for 74%-96% of subjects following the first injection and 77%-96% of subjects following the last injection.

Extrapyramidal Symptoms of Oral Aripiprazole

In short-term, placebo-controlled trials in schizophrenia, the incidence of reported EPS-related events, excluding events related to akathisia, for oral aripiprazole-treated patients was 13% vs. 12% for placebo; and the incidence of akathisia-related events for aripiprazole-treated patients was 8% vs. 4% for placebo.

Objectively collected data from those trials was collected on the Simpson Angus Rating Scale (for EPS), the Barnes Akathisia Scale (for akathisia), and the Abnormal Involuntary Movement Scale (for dyskinesias). In the schizophrenia trials, the objectively collected data did not show a difference between aripiprazole and placebo, with the exception of the Barnes Akathisia Scale (aripiprazole, 0.08; placebo, –0.05). Similarly, in a long-term (26–week), placebo-controlled trial of schizophrenia in adults, objectively collected data on the Simpson Angus Rating Scale (for EPS), the Barnes Akathisia Scale (for akathisia), and the Abnormal Involuntary Movement Scale (for dyskinesias) did not show a difference between aripiprazole and placebo.

Dystonia

Class Effect: Symptoms of dystonia, prolonged abnormal contractions of muscle groups, may occur in susceptible individuals during the first few days of treatment. Dystonic symptoms include: spasm of the neck muscles, sometimes progressing to tightness of the throat, swallowing difficulty, difficulty breathing, and/or protrusion of the tongue. While these symptoms can occur at low doses, they occur more frequently and with greater severity with high potency and at higher doses of first generation antipsychotic drugs. An elevated risk of acute dystonia is observed in males and younger age groups.

Adverse Reactions in Long-Term, Double-Blind, Placebo-Controlled Trials of Oral Aripiprazole

The adverse reactions reported in a 26–week, double-blind trial comparing oral aripiprazole and placebo in patients with schizophrenia were generally consistent with those reported in the short-term, placebo-controlled trials, except for a higher incidence of tremor [8% (12/153) for oral aripiprazole vs. 2% (3/153) for placebo]. In this study, the majority of the cases of tremor were of mild intensity (8/12 mild and 4/12 moderate), occurred early in therapy (9/12 ≤49 days), and were of limited duration (7/12 ≤10 days). Tremor infrequently led to discontinuation (<1%) of oral aripiprazole. In addition, in a long-term, active-controlled study, the incidence of tremor was 5% (40/859) for oral aripiprazole.

Other Adverse Reactions Observed During the Premarketing Evaluation of Oral Aripiprazole

Following is a list of MedDRA terms that reflect adverse reactions reported by patients treated with oral aripiprazole at multiple doses ≥2 mg/day during any phase of a trial within the database of 13,543 adult patients. All events assessed as possible adverse drug reactions have been included with the exception of more commonly occurring events. In addition, medically/clinically meaningful adverse reactions, particularly those that are likely to be useful to the prescriber or that have pharmacologic plausibility, have been included. Events already listed in other parts of *Adverse Reactions (6)*, or those considered in *Warnings and Precautions (5)* or *Overdosage (10)* have been excluded. Although the reactions reported occurred during treatment with aripiprazole, they were not necessarily caused by it. Events are further categorized by MedDRA system organ class and listed in order of decreasing frequency according to the following definitions: those occurring in at least 1/100 patients (only those not already listed in the tabulated results from placebo-controlled trials appear in this listing); those occurring in 1/100 to 1/1000 patients; and those occurring in fewer than 1/1000 patients.

Blood and Lymphatic System Disorders:
≥1/1000 patients and <1/100 patients - thrombocytopenia

Cardiac Disorders:
≥1/1000 patients and <1/100 patients - palpitations, cardiopulmonary failure, myocardial infarction, cardiorespiratory arrest, atrioventricular block, extrasystoles, angina pectoris, myocardial ischemia; *<1/1000 patients* - atrial flutter, supraventricular tachycardia, ventricular tachycardia

Eye Disorders:
≥1/100 patients and <1/100 patients - photophobia, diplopia, eyelid edema, photopsia

Gastrointestinal Disorders:
≥1/1000 patients and <1/100 patients - gastroesophageal reflux disease, swollen tongue, esophagitis; *<1/1000 patients* - pancreatitis

General Disorders and Administration Site Conditions:
≥1/100 patients - asthenia, peripheral edema, chest pain; *≥1/1000 patients and <1/100 patients* - face edema, angioedema; *<1/1000 patients* - hypothermia

Hepatobiliary Disorders:
<1/1000 patients - hepatitis, jaundice

Immune System Disorders:
≥1/1000 patients and <1/100 patients - hypersensitivity

Injury, Poisoning, and Procedural Complications:
≥1/100 patients - fall; *<1/1000 patients* - heat stroke

Investigations:
≥1/1000 patients and <1/100 patients - blood prolactin increased, blood urea increased, blood creatinine increased, blood bilirubin increased; *<1/1000 patients* - blood lactate dehydrogenase increased, glycosylated hemoglobin increased

Metabolism and Nutrition Disorders:
≥1/1000 patients and <1/100 patients - anorexia, hyponatremia, hypoglycemia, polydipsia; *<1/1000 patients* - diabetic ketoacidosis

Musculoskeletal and Connective Tissue Disorders:
≥1/1000 patients and <1/100 patients - muscle rigidity, muscular weakness, muscle tightness, mobility decreased; *<1/1000 patients* - rhabdomyolysis

Nervous System Disorders:
≥1/100 patients - coordination abnormal; *≥1/1000 patients and <1/100 patients* - speech disorder, hypokinesia, hypotonia, myoclonus, akinesia, bradykinesia; *<1/1000 patients* - choreoathetosis

Psychiatric Disorders:
≥1/100 patients - suicidal ideation; *≥1/1000 patients and <1/100 patients* - loss of libido, suicide attempt, hostility, libido increased, anger, anorgasmia, delirium, intentional self injury, completed suicide, tic, homicidal ideation; *<1/1000 patients* - catatonia, sleep walking

Renal and Urinary Disorders:
≥1/1000 patients and <1/100 patients - urinary retention, polyuria, nocturia

Reproductive System and Breast Disorders:
≥1/1000 patients and <1/100 patients - menstruation irregular, erectile dysfunction, amenorrhea, breast pain; *<1/1000 patients* - gynecomastia, priapism

Respiratory, Thoracic, and Mediastinal Disorders:
≥1/100 patients - nasal congestion, dyspnea

Skin and Subcutaneous Tissue Disorders:
≥1/100 patients - rash (including erythematous, exfoliative, generalized, macular, maculopapular, papular rash; acneiform, allergic, contact, exfoliative, seborrheic dermatitis, neurodermatitis, and drug eruption), hyperhydrosis; *≥1/1000 patients and <1/100 patients* - pruritus, photosensitivity reaction, alopecia, urticaria

6.2 Postmarketing Experience

The following adverse reactions have been identified during post-approval use of oral aripiprazole. Because these reactions are reported voluntarily from a population of uncertain size, it is not always possible to reliably estimate their frequency or establish a causal relationship to drug exposure: rare occurrences of allergic reaction (anaphylactic reaction, angioedema, laryngospasm, pruritus/urticaria, or oropharyngeal spasm).

7 DRUG INTERACTIONS

7.1 Carbamazepine or Other CYP3A4 Inducers

Concomitant use of ABILIFY MAINTENA with carbamazepine or other CYP3A4 inducers decreases the concentrations of aripiprazole. Avoid use of ABILIFY MAINTENA in combination with carbamazepine and other inducers of CYP3A4 for greater than 14 days *[see Dosage and Administration (2.3) and Clinical Pharmacology (12.3)]*.

7.2 Ketoconazole or Other Strong CYP3A4 Inhibitors

Concomitant use of ABILIFY MAINTENA with ketoconazole or other CYP3A4 inhibitors for more than 14 days increases the concentrations of aripiprazole and reduction of the ABILIFY MAINTENA dose is recommended *[see Dosage and Administration (2.3) and Clinical Pharmacology (12.3)]*. Due to prolonged-release characteristics of ABILIFY MAINTENA, short-term co-administration of ketoconazole or other inhibitors of CYP3A4 with ABILIFY MAINTENA does not require a dose adjustment.

7.3 Quinidine or Other Strong CYP2D6 Inhibitors

Concomitant use of ABILIFY MAINTENA with quinidine or other CYP2D6 inhibitors increases the concentrations of aripiprazole after longer-term use (i.e., over 14 days) and reduction of the ABILIFY MAINTENA is recommended *[see Dosage and Administration (2.3) and Clinical Pharmacology (12.3)]*. Due to prolonged-release characteristics of ABILIFY MAINTENA, short-term co-administration of quinidine or other CYP2D6 inhibitors with ABILIFY MAINTENA does not require a dose adjustment.

7.4 CNS Depressants
Given the CNS depressant effects of aripiprazole, use caution when ABILIFY MAINTENA is taken in combination with other centrally-acting drugs or alcohol.

7.5 Anti-Hypertensive Agents
Due to its alpha adrenergic antagonism, aripiprazole has the potential to enhance the effect of certain antihypertensive agents.

8 USE IN SPECIFIC POPULATIONS

8.1 Pregnancy
Pregnancy Category C:
Risk Summary
Adequate and well controlled studies with aripiprazole have not been conducted in pregnant women. Neonates exposed to antipsychotic drugs (including ABILIFY MAINTENA) during the third trimester of pregnancy are at risk for extrapyramidal and/or withdrawal symptoms following delivery. In animal studies, aripiprazole demonstrated developmental toxicity, including possible teratogenic effects in rats and rabbits at doses 1 – 10 times the oral maximum recommended human dose [MRHD] of 30 mg/day based on a mg/m^2 body surface area. ABILIFY MAINTENA should be used during pregnancy only if the potential benefit justifies the potential risk to the fetus.
Clinical Considerations
Fetal/Neonatal Adverse Reactions
Monitor neonates exhibiting extrapyramidal or withdrawal symptoms. Some neonates recover within hours or days without specific treatment; others may require prolonged hospitalization.
Animal Data
Pregnant rats were treated with oral doses of 3 mg/kg/day, 10 mg/kg/day, and 30 mg/kg/day (1 times, 3 times, and 10 times the oral maximum recommended human dose [MRHD] of 30 mg/day on a mg/m^2 body surface area) of aripiprazole during the period of organogenesis. Gestation was slightly prolonged at 30 mg/kg. Treatment caused a slight delay in fetal development, as evidenced by decreased fetal weight (30 mg/kg), undescended testes (30 mg/kg), and delayed skeletal ossification (10 mg/kg and 30 mg/kg). There were no adverse effects on embryofetal or pup survival. Delivered offspring had decreased body weights (10 mg/kg and 30 mg/kg), and increased incidences of hepatodiaphragmatic nodules and diaphragmatic hernia at 30 mg/kg (the other dose groups were not examined for these findings). A low incidence of diaphragmatic hernia was also seen in the fetuses exposed to 30 mg/kg. Postnatally, delayed vaginal opening was seen at 10 mg/kg and 30 mg/kg and impaired reproductive performance (decreased fertility rate, corpora lutea, implants, live fetuses, and increased post-implantation loss, likely mediated through effects on female offspring) was seen at 30 mg/kg. Some maternal toxicity was seen at 30 mg/kg; however, there was no evidence to suggest that these developmental effects were secondary to maternal toxicity.
In pregnant rats receiving aripiprazole injection intravenously (3 mg/kg/day, 9 mg/kg/day, and 27 mg/kg/day) during the period of organogenesis, decreased fetal weight and delayed skeletal ossification were seen at the highest dose, which also caused some maternal toxicity.
Pregnant rabbits were treated with oral doses of 10 mg/kg/day, 30 mg/kg/day, and 100 mg/kg/day (2 times, 3 times, and 11 times human exposure at the oral MRHD of 30 mg/day based on AUC and 6 times, 19 times, and 65 times the oral MRHD of 30 mg/day based on mg/m^2 body surface area) of aripiprazole during the period of organogenesis. Decreased maternal food consumption and increased abortions were seen at 100 mg/kg. Treatment caused increased fetal mortality (100 mg/kg), decreased fetal weight (30 mg/kg and 100 mg/kg), increased incidence of a skeletal abnormality (fused sternebrae at 30 mg/kg and 100 mg/kg), and minor skeletal variations (100 mg/kg).
In pregnant rabbits receiving aripiprazole injection intravenously (3 mg/kg/day, 10 mg/kg/day, and 30 mg/kg/day) during the period of organogenesis, the highest dose, which caused pronounced maternal toxicity, resulted in decreased fetal weight, increased fetal abnormalities (primarily skeletal), and decreased fetal skeletal ossification. The fetal no-effect dose was 10 mg/kg, which produced 5 times the human exposure at the oral MRHD based on AUC and is 6 times the oral MRHD of 30 mg/day based on mg/m^2 body surface area.
In a study in which rats were treated with oral doses of 3 mg/kg/day, 10 mg/kg/day, and 30 mg/kg/day (1 times, 3 times, and 10 times the oral MRHD of 30 mg/day on a mg/m^2 body surface area) of aripiprazole perinatally and postnatally (from day 17 of gestation through day 21 postpartum), slight maternal toxicity and slightly prolonged gestation were seen at 30 mg/kg. An increase in stillbirths and decreases in pup weight (persisting into adulthood) and survival were seen at this dose.
In rats receiving aripiprazole injection intravenously (3 mg/kg/day, 8 mg/kg/day, and 20 mg/kg/day) from day 6 of gestation through day 20 postpartum, an increase in stillbirths was seen at 8 mg/kg and 20 mg/kg, and decreases in early postnatal pup weights and survival were seen at 20 mg/kg. These doses produced some maternal toxicity. There were no effects on postnatal behavioral and reproductive development.

8.3 Nursing Mothers
Aripiprazole is excreted in human breast milk. A decision should be made whether to discontinue nursing or to discontinue the drug, taking into account the importance of the drug to the mother.

8.4 Pediatric Use
Safety and effectiveness of ABILIFY MAINTENA in patients <18 years of age have not been evaluated.

8.5 Geriatric Use
Safety and effectiveness of ABILIFY MAINTENA in patients >60 years of age have not been evaluated.
In oral single-dose pharmacokinetic studies (with aripiprazole given in a single oral dose of 15 mg), aripiprazole clearance was 20% lower in elderly (≥65 years) subjects compared to younger adult subjects (18 to 64 years). There was no detectable age effect, however, in the population pharmacokinetic analysis of oral aripiprazole in schizophrenia patients. Also, the pharmacokinetics of oral aripiprazole after multiple doses in elderly patients appeared similar to that observed in young, healthy subjects. No dosage adjustment of ABILIFY MAINTENA is recommended for elderly patients *[see Boxed Warning and Warnings and Precautions (5.1)]*.

8.6 CYP2D6 Poor Metabolizers
Approximately 8% of Caucasians and 3–8% of Black/African Americans cannot metabolize CYP2D6 substrates and are classified as poor metabolizers (PM). Dosage adjustment is recommended in CYP2D6 poor metabolizers due to high aripiprazole concentrations *[see Dosage and Administration (2.3) and Clinical Pharmacology (12.3)]*.

10 OVERDOSAGE

10.1 Human Experience
The largest known case of acute ingestion with a known outcome involved 1260 mg of oral aripiprazole (42 times the maximum recommended daily dose) in a patient who fully recovered.
Common adverse reactions (reported in at least 5% of all overdose cases) reported with oral aripiprazole overdosage (alone or in combination with other substances) include vomiting, somnolence, and tremor. Other clinically important signs and symptoms observed in one or more patients with aripiprazole overdoses (alone or with other substances) include acidosis, aggression, aspartate aminotransferase increased, atrial fibrillation, bradycardia, coma, confusional state, convulsion, blood creatine phosphokinase increased, depressed level of consciousness, hypertension, hypokalemia, hypotension, lethargy, loss of consciousness, QRS complex prolonged, QT prolonged, pneumonia aspiration, respiratory arrest, status epilepticus, and tachycardia.

10.2 Management of Overdosage
In case of overdosage, call the Poison Control Center immediately at 1-800-222-1222.

11 DESCRIPTION

Aripiprazole is an atypical antipsychotic which is present in ABILIFY MAINTENA as its monohydrate polymorphic form. Aripiprazole monohydrate is 7-[4-[4-(2,3-dichlorophenyl)-1-piperazinyl] butoxy]-3,4 dihydrocarbostyril monohydrate. The empirical formula is $C_{23}H_{27}Cl_2N_3O_2.H_2O$ and its molecular weight is 466.40. The chemical structure is:

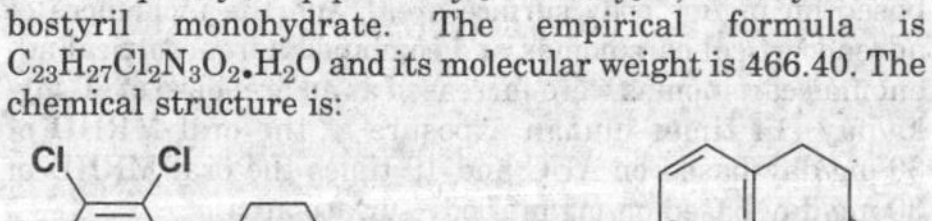

ABILIFY MAINTENA (aripiprazole) is an extended-release injectable suspension available in 400 mg or 300 mg strength vials. The labeled strengths are calculated based on the anhydrous form (aripiprazole). Inactive ingredients include carboxymethyl cellulose sodium, mannitol, sodium phosphate monobasic monohydrate and sodium hydroxide.

12 CLINICAL PHARMACOLOGY

12.1 Mechanism of Action
The mechanism of action of aripiprazole in the treatment of schizophrenia is unknown.
However, the efficacy of aripiprazole may be mediated through a combination of partial agonist activity at D_2 and $5\text{-}HT_{1A}$ receptors and antagonist activity at $5\text{-}HT_{2A}$ receptors. Actions at receptors other than D_2, $5\text{-}HT_{1A}$, and $5\text{-}HT_{2A}$ may explain some of the other adverse reactions of aripiprazole (e.g., the orthostatic hypotension observed with aripiprazole may be explained by its antagonist activity at adrenergic $alpha_1$ receptors).

12.2 Pharmacodynamics
Aripiprazole exhibits high affinity for dopamine D_2 and D_3, serotonin $5\text{-}HT_{1A}$ and $5\text{-}HT_{2A}$ receptors (K_i values of 0.34 nM, 0.8 nM, 1.7 nM, and 3.4 nM, respectively), moderate affinity for dopamine D_4, serotonin $5\text{-}HT_{2C}$ and $5\text{-}HT_7$, $alpha_1$-adrenergic and histamine H_1 receptors (K_i values of 44 nM, 15 nM, 39 nM, 57 nM, and 61 nM, respectively), and moderate affinity for the serotonin reuptake site (K_i=98 nM). Aripiprazole has no appreciable affinity for cholinergic muscarinic receptors (IC_{50}>1000 nM). Aripiprazole functions as a partial agonist at the dopamine D_2 and the serotonin $5\text{-}HT_{1A}$ receptors, and as an antagonist at serotonin $5\text{-}HT_{2A}$ receptor.
Alcohol
There was no significant difference between oral aripiprazole co-administered with ethanol and placebo co-administered with ethanol on performance of gross motor skills or stimulus response in healthy subjects. As with most psychoactive medications, patients should be advised to avoid alcohol while taking ABILIFY MAINTENA.

12.3 Pharmacokinetics
ABILIFY MAINTENA activity is presumably primarily due to the parent drug, aripiprazole, and to a lesser extent, to its major metabolite, dehydro-aripiprazole, which has been shown to have affinities for D_2 receptors similar to the parent drug and represents about 29% of the parent drug exposure in plasma.
Aripiprazole absorption into the systemic circulation is slow and prolonged following intramuscular injection due to low solubility of aripiprazole particles. Following a single intramuscular dose, the plasma concentrations of aripiprazole gradually rise to reach maximum plasma concentrations at a median T_{max} of 5–7 days. The mean aripiprazole terminal elimination half–life was 29.9 days and 46.5 days after every 4–week injection of ABILIFY MAINTENA 300 mg and 400 mg, respectively, and steady state concentrations were attained by the fourth dose. Approximate dose-proportional increases in aripiprazole and dehydro-aripiprazole concentrations and AUC parameters were observed after every four week ABILIFY MAINTENA injections of 300 mg and 400 mg.
Elimination of aripiprazole is mainly through hepatic metabolism involving two P450 isozymes, CYP2D6 and CYP3A4. Aripiprazole is not a substrate of CYP1A1, CYP1A2, CYP2A6, CYP2B6, CYP2C8, CYP2C9, CYP2C19, or CYP2E1 enzymes. Aripiprazole also does not undergo direct glucuronidation.
Drug Interaction Studies
No specific drug interaction studies have been performed with ABILIFY MAINTENA. The information below is obtained from studies with oral aripiprazole.
Potential for Other Drugs to Affect ABILIFY MAINTENA
Ketoconazole and Other Strong CYP3A4 Inhibitors
Co-administration of ketoconazole (200 mg/day for 14 days) with a 15 mg single oral dose of aripiprazole increased the AUC of aripiprazole and its active metabolite by 63% and 77%, respectively. The effect of a higher ketoconazole dose (400 mg/day) has not been studied.
Other strong inhibitors of CYP3A4 (itraconazole) would be expected to have similar effects and need similar dose reductions; moderate inhibitors (erythromycin, grapefruit juice) have not been studied *[see Dosage and Administration (2.3) and Drug Interactions (7.2)]*.
Quinidine and Other Strong CYP2D6 Inhibitors
Co-administration of a 10 mg single oral dose of aripiprazole with quinidine (166 mg/day for 13 days), a potent inhibitor of CYP2D6, increased the AUC of aripiprazole by 112% but decreased the AUC of its active metabolite, dehydro-aripiprazole, by 35%. Other significant inhibitors of CYP2D6, such as fluoxetine or paroxetine, would be expected to have similar effects *[see Dosage and Administration (2.3) and Drug Interactions (7.3)]*.
Carbamazepine and Other CYP3A4 Inducers
Co-administration of carbamazepine (200 mg twice daily), a potent CYP3A4 inducer, with oral aripiprazole (30 mg/day) resulted in an approximate 70% decrease in C_{max} and AUC values of both aripiprazole and its active metabolite, dehydro-aripiprazole *[see Dosage and Administration (2.3) and Drug Interactions (7.1)]*.
Valproate
When valproate (500 mg/day–1500 mg/day) and oral aripiprazole (30 mg/day) were co-administered, at steady-state the C_{max} and AUC of aripiprazole were decreased by 25%. No dosage adjustment of ABILIFY MAINTENA is required when administered concomitantly with valproate.
Lithium
A pharmacokinetic interaction of ABILIFY MAINTENA with lithium is unlikely because lithium is not bound to plasma proteins, is not metabolized, and is almost entirely excreted unchanged in urine. Co-administration of therapeutic doses of lithium (1200 mg/day–1800 mg/day) for 21 days with oral aripiprazole (30 mg/day) did not result in clinically significant changes in the pharmacokinetics of aripiprazole or its active metabolite, dehydro-aripiprazole (C_{max} and AUC increased by less than 20%). No dosage adjustment of ABILIFY MAINTENA is required when administered concomitantly with lithium.

Potential for ABILIFY MAINTENA to Affect Other Drugs
Aripiprazole is unlikely to cause clinically important pharmacokinetic interactions with drugs metabolized by cytochrome P450 enzymes. *In vivo* studies, 10 mg/day to 30 mg/day doses of oral aripiprazole had no significant effect on metabolism by CYP2D6 (dextromethorphan), CYP2C9 (warfarin), CYP2C19 (omeprazole, warfarin), and CYP3A4 (dextromethorphan) substrates. Additionally, aripiprazole and dehydro-aripiprazole did not show potential for altering CYP1A2-mediated metabolism *in vitro*.
No effect of oral aripiprazole was seen on the pharmacokinetics of lithium or valproate.
Valproate
When oral aripiprazole (30 mg/day) and valproate (1000 mg/day) were co-administered, at steady state there were no clinically significant changes in the C_{max} or AUC of valproate. No dosage adjustment of valproate is required when administered concomitantly with ABILIFY MAINTENA.
Lithium
Co-administration of oral aripiprazole (30 mg/day) with lithium (900 mg/day) did not result in clinically significant changes in the pharmacokinetics of lithium. No dosage adjustment of lithium is required when administered concomitantly with ABILIFY MAINTENA.
Dextromethorphan
Oral aripiprazole at doses of 10 mg/day to 30 mg/day for 14 days had no effect on dextromethorphan's O-dealkylation to its major metabolite, dextrorphan, a pathway dependent on CYP2D6 activity. Oral aripiprazole also had no effect on dextromethorphan's N-demethylation to its metabolite 3-methoxymorphinan, a pathway dependent on CYP3A4 activity. No dosage adjustment of dextromethorphan is required when administered concomitantly with ABILIFY MAINTENA.
Warfarin
Oral aripiprazole 10 mg/day for 14 days had no effect on the pharmacokinetics of R-warfarin and S-warfarin or on the pharmacodynamic end-point of International Normalized Ratio, indicating the lack of a clinically relevant effect of aripiprazole on CYP2C9 and CYP2C19 metabolism or the binding of highly protein-bound warfarin. No dosage adjustment of warfarin is required when administered concomitantly with ABILIFY MAINTENA.
Omeprazole
Oral aripiprazole 10 mg/day for 15 days had no effect on the pharmacokinetics of a single 20 mg dose of omeprazole, a CYP2C19 substrate, in healthy subjects. No dosage adjustment of omeprazole is required when administered concomitantly with ABILIFY MAINTENA.
Escitalopram
Co-administration of 10 mg/day doses of oral aripiprazole for 14 days to healthy subjects had no effect on the steady-state pharmacokinetics of 10 mg/day escitalopram, a substrate of CYP2C19 and CYP3A4. No dosage adjustment of escitalopram is required when ABILIFY MAINTENA is added to escitalopram.
Venlafaxine
Co-administration of 10 mg/day to 20 mg/day doses of oral aripiprazole for 14 days to healthy subjects had no effect on the steady-state pharmacokinetics of venlafaxine and O-desmethylvenlafaxine following 75 mg/day venlafaxine XR, a CYP2D6 substrate. No dosage adjustment of venlafaxine is required when ABILIFY MAINTENA is added to venlafaxine.

Specific Population Studies
No specific pharmacokinetic studies have been performed with ABILIFY MAINTENA in specific populations. All the information is obtained from studies with oral aripiprazole.
CYP2D6 Poor Metabolizers
Approximately 8% of Caucasians and 3–8% of Black/African Americans cannot metabolize CYP2D6 substrates and are classified as poor metabolizers (PMs). People who are not PMs are classified as extensive metabolizers (EMs). Laboratory tests are available to identify CYP2D6 PMs. PMs have about an 80% increase in aripiprazole exposure and about a 30% decrease in exposure to the active metabolite compared to EMs, resulting in about a 60% higher exposure to the total active moieties from a given dose of aripiprazole compared to EMs. The mean elimination half-lives for aripiprazole are about 75 and 146 hours in EMs and PMs, respectively. Hence, the recommended dosage of ABILIFY MAINTENA is lower *[see Dosage and Administration (2.3) and Use in Specific Populations (8.6)]*.
Aripiprazole does not inhibit or induce the CYP2D6 pathway.
Gender
C_{max} and AUC of aripiprazole and its active metabolite, dehydro-aripiprazole, are 30% to 40% higher in women than in men, and correspondingly, the apparent oral clearance of aripiprazole is lower in women. These differences, however, are largely explained by differences in body weight (25%) between men and women. No dosage adjustment of ABILIFY MAINTENA is recommended based on gender.
Race
Although no specific pharmacokinetic study was conducted to investigate the effects of race on the disposition of aripiprazole, population pharmacokinetic evaluation revealed no evidence of clinically significant race-related differences in the pharmacokinetics of aripiprazole. No dosage adjustment of ABILIFY MAINTENA is recommended based on race.
Smoking
Based on studies utilizing human liver enzymes *in vitro*, aripiprazole is not a substrate for CYP1A2 and also does not undergo direct glucuronidation. Smoking should, therefore, not have an effect on the pharmacokinetics of aripiprazole. Consistent with these *in vitro* results, population pharmacokinetic evaluation did not reveal any significant pharmacokinetic differences between smokers and nonsmokers. No dosage adjustment of ABILIFY MAINTENA is recommended based on smoking status.
Renal Impairment
In patients with severe renal impairment (creatinine clearance <30 mL/min), C_{max} of aripiprazole (given in a single dose of oral 15 mg) and dehydro-aripiprazole increased by 36% and 53%, respectively, but AUC was 15% lower for aripiprazole and 7% higher for dehydro-aripiprazole. Renal excretion of both unchanged aripiprazole and dehydro-aripiprazole is less than 1% of the dose. No dosage adjustment of ABILIFY MAINTENA is required for doses in subjects with renal impairment.
Hepatic Impairment
In a single-dose trial (15 mg of oral aripiprazole) in subjects with varying degrees of liver cirrhosis (Child-Pugh Classes A, B, and C), the AUC of aripiprazole, compared to healthy subjects, increased 31% in mild hepatic impairment, increased 8% in moderate hepatic impairment, and decreased 20% in severe hepatic impairment. None of these differences would require dose adjustment of ABILIFY MAINTENA.

13 NONCLINICAL TOXICOLOGY

13.1 Carcinogenesis, Mutagenesis, Impairment of Fertility

Carcinogenesis
Lifetime carcinogenicity studies were conducted in ICR mice and in Sprague-Dawley (SD) and F344 rats. Aripiprazole was administered for 2 years in the diet at doses of 1 mg/kg/day, 3 mg/kg/day, 10 mg/kg/day, and 30 mg/kg/day to ICR mice and 1 mg/kg/day, 3 mg/kg/day, and 10 mg/kg/day to F344 rats (0.2 times to 5 times and 0.3 times to 3 times the oral maximum recommended human dose [MRHD] of 30 mg/day based on mg/m^2 body surface area, respectively). In addition, SD rats were dosed orally for 2 years at 10 mg/kg/day, 20 mg/kg/day, 40 mg/kg/day, and 60 mg/kg/day (3 times to 19 times the oral MRHD of 30 mg/day based on mg/m^2 body surface area). Aripiprazole did not induce tumors in male mice or rats. In female mice, the incidences of pituitary gland adenomas and mammary gland adenocarcinomas and adenoacanthomas were increased at dietary doses of 3 mg/kg/day to 30 mg/kg/day (0.1 times to approximately 1 times human exposure at the oral MRHD of 30 mg/day based on AUC and 0.5 times to 5 times the oral MRHD of 30 mg/day based on mg/m^2 body surface area). In female rats, the incidence of mammary gland fibroadenomas was increased at a dietary dose of 10 mg/kg/day (0.1 times human exposure at the oral MRHD of 30 mg/day based on AUC and 3 times the oral MRHD of 30 mg/day based on mg/m^2 body surface area); and the incidences of adrenocortical carcinomas and combined adrenocortical adenomas/carcinomas were increased at an oral dose of 60 mg/kg/day (14 times human exposure at the oral MRHD of 30 mg/day based on AUC and 19 times the oral MRHD of 30 mg/day based on mg/m^2 body surface area).
Proliferative changes in the pituitary and mammary gland of rodents have been observed following chronic administration of other antipsychotic agents and are considered prolactin-mediated. Serum prolactin was not measured in the aripiprazole carcinogenicity studies. However, increases in serum prolactin levels were observed in female mice in a 13–week dietary study at the doses associated with mammary gland and pituitary tumors. Serum prolactin was not increased in female rats in 4–week and 13–week dietary studies at the dose associated with mammary gland tumors. The relevance for human risk of the findings of prolactin-mediated endocrine tumors in rodents is unknown.
Mutagenesis
Aripiprazole was not mutagenic when tested in the *in vitro* bacterial mutation assay, the *in vitro* bacterial DNA repair assay, and the *in vitro* mouse lymphoma gene mutation assay. The clastogenic potential of aripiprazole was tested in the *in vitro* chromosomal aberration assay in Chinese hamster lung (CHL) cells, the *in vivo* micronucleus assay in mice, and the unscheduled DNA synthesis assay in rats. Aripiprazole and its metabolite (2,3-DCPP) were clastogenic in the *in vitro* chromosomal aberration assay in CHL cells both in the presence and absence of metabolic activation. The metabolite, 2,3-DCPP, produced increases in numerical aberrations in the *in vitro* assay in CHL cells in the absence of metabolic activation. A positive response was obtained in the oral *in vivo* micronucleus assay in mice; however, the response was due to a mechanism not considered relevant to humans.
Impairment of Fertility
Female rats were treated with oral doses of 2 mg/kg/day, 6 mg/kg/day, and 20 mg/kg/day (0.6 times, 2 times, and 6 times the oral maximum recommended human dose [MRHD] of 30 mg/day on a mg/m^2 body surface area) of aripiprazole from 2 weeks prior to mating through day 7 of gestation. Estrus cycle irregularities and increased corpora lutea were seen at all doses, but no impairment of fertility was seen. Increased pre-implantation loss was seen at 6 mg/kg and 20 mg/kg and decreased fetal weight was seen at 20 mg/kg.
Male rats were treated with oral doses of 20 mg/kg/day, 40 mg/kg/day, and 60 mg/kg/day (6 times, 13 times, and 19 times the oral MRHD of 30 mg/day on a mg/m^2 body surface area) of aripiprazole from 9 weeks prior to mating through mating. Disturbances in spermatogenesis were seen at 60 mg/kg and prostate atrophy was seen at 40 mg/kg and 60 mg/kg, but no impairment of fertility was seen.

13.2 Animal Toxicity and/or Pharmacology

Oral Aripiprazole
Aripiprazole produced retinal degeneration in albino rats in a 26–week chronic toxicity study at a dose of 60 mg/kg and in a 2–year carcinogenicity study at doses of 40 mg/kg and 60 mg/kg. The 40 mg/kg and 60 mg/kg doses are 13 times and 19 times the oral maximum recommended human dose (MRHD) of 30 mg/day based on mg/m^2 body surface area and 7 times to 14 times human exposure at the oral MRHD based on AUC. Evaluation of the retinas of albino mice and of monkeys did not reveal evidence of retinal degeneration. Additional studies to further evaluate the mechanism have not been performed. The relevance of this finding to human risk is unknown.
Intramuscular Aripiprazole
The toxicological profile for aripiprazole administered to experimental animals by intramuscular injection is generally similar to that seen following oral administration at comparable plasma levels of the drug. With intramuscular injection, however, injection-site tissue reactions are observed that consist of localized inflammation, swelling, scabbing and foreign-body reactions to deposited drug. These effects gradually resolved with discontinuation of dosing.
After 26 weeks of treatment in rats, the no-observed-adverse-effect level (NOAEL) was 50 mg/kg in male rats and 100 mg/kg in female rats, which are approximately 1 and 2 times, respectively, the maximum recommended human 400 mg dose of aripiprazole extended-release injectable suspension on a mg/m^2 body surface area. At the NOAEL in rats, the AUC_{7d} values were 14.4 µg•h/mL in males and 104.1 µg•h/mL in females. In dogs at 52 weeks of treatment at the NOAEL of 40 mg/kg, which is approximately 3 times the MRHD (400 mg) on a mg/m^2 body surface area, the AUC_{7d} values were approximately 59 µg•h/mL in males and 44 µg•h/mL in females. In patients at the MRHD of 400 mg, the AUCτ (0-28 days) was 163 µg•h/mL. For comparison to this human AUC, extrapolating the animal AUC_{7d} values to an AUC_{28d} results in AUC_{28d} values of approximately 58 and 416 µg•h/mL for male and female rats, respectively, and 236 and 175 µg•h/mL for male and female dogs, respectively.

14 CLINICAL STUDIES

The efficacy of ABILIFY MAINTENA in the treatment of patients with schizophrenia was established, in part, on the basis of efficacy data from trials with the oral formulation of aripiprazole. In addition, the efficacy of ABILIFY MAINTENA in maintaining symptomatic control in schizophrenia was established in a randomized-withdrawal, double-blind, placebo-controlled, trial in adult patients who met DSM-IV-TR criteria for schizophrenia and who were being treated with at least one antipsychotic medication. Patients had at least a 3 year history of illness and a history of relapse or symptom exacerbation when not receiving antipsychotic treatment.
Clinical ratings during this trial included:

- The Positive and Negative Syndrome Scale (PANSS). The PANSS is a 30 item scale that measures positive symptoms of schizophrenia (7 items), negative symptoms of schizophrenia (7 items), and general psychopathology (16 items), each rated on a scale of 1 (absent) to 7 (extreme). Total PANSS scores range from 30 to 210.
- The Clinical Global Impression-Severity (CGI-S) scale. The CGI-S rates the severity of mental illness on a scale of 1 (normal) to 7 (among the most extremely ill) based on the total clinical experience of the rater in treating patients with schizophrenia.
- The Clinical Global Impression-Improvement (CGI-I) scale. The CGI-I rates improvement in mental illness on a scale of 1 (very much improved) to 7 (very much worse) based on the change from baseline in clinical condition.

- The Clinical Global Impression- Severity of Suicide (CGI-SS) scale, which is comprised of 2 parts: Part 1 rates the severity of suicidal thoughts and behavior on a scale of 1 (not at all suicidal) to 5 (attempted suicide) based on the most severe level in the last 7 days from all information available to the rater and Part 2 rates the change from baseline in suicidal thoughts and behavior on a scale of 1 (very much improved) to 7 (very much worse).

This trial included:

- A 4–6 week open-label, oral conversion phase for patients on antipsychotic medications other than aripiprazole. A total of 633 patients entered this phase.
- An open-label, oral aripiprazole stabilization phase (target dose of 10 mg to 30 mg once daily). A total of 710 patients entered this phase. Patients were 18 to 60 years old (mean 40 years) and 60% were male. The mean PANSS total score was 66 (range 33 to 124). The mean CGI-S score was 3.5 (mildly to moderately ill). Prior to the next phase, stabilization was required. Stabilization was defined as having all of the following for four consecutive weeks: an outpatient status, PANSS total score ≤80, CGI-S ≤4 (moderately ill), and CGI-SS score ≤2 (mildly suicidal) on Part 1 and ≤5 (minimally worsened) on Part 2; and a score of ≤4 on each of the following PANSS items: conceptual disorganization, suspiciousness, hallucinatory behavior, and unusual thought content.
- A minimum 12–week uncontrolled, single-blind ABILIFY MAINTENA stabilization phase (treatment with 400 mg of ABILIFY MAINTENA given every 4 weeks in conjunction with oral aripiprazole [10 mg to 20 mg/day] for the first 2 weeks). The dose of ABILIFY MAINTENA may have been decreased to 300 mg due to adverse reactions. A total of 576 patients entered this phase. The mean PANSS total score was 59 (range 30 to 80) and the mean CGI-S score was 3.2 (mildly ill). Prior to the next phase, stabilization was required (see above for the definition of stabilization) for 12 consecutive weeks.
- A double-blind, placebo-controlled randomized-withdrawal phase to observe for relapse (defined below). A total of 403 patients were randomized 2:1 to the same dose of ABILIFY MAINTENA they were receiving at the end of the stabilization phase, (400 mg or 300 mg administered once every 4 weeks) or placebo. Patients had a mean PANSS total score of 55 (range 31 to 80) and a CGI-S score of 2.9 (mildly ill) at entry. The dose could be adjusted up and down or down and up within the range of 300 to 400 mg on a one time basis.

The primary efficacy endpoint was time from randomization to relapse. Relapse was defined as the first occurrence of one or more of the following criteria:

1) CGI-I of ≥5 (minimally worse) and
   a) an increase on any of the following individual PANSS items (conceptual disorganization, hallucinatory behavior, suspiciousness, unusual thought content) to a score >4 with an absolute increase of ≥2 on that specific item since randomization or
   b) an increase on any of the following individual PANSS items (conceptual disorganization, hallucinatory behavior, suspiciousness, unusual thought content) to a score >4 and an absolute increase ≥4 on the combined four PANSS items (conceptual disorganization, hallucinatory behavior, suspiciousness, unusual thought content) since randomization
2) Hospitalization due to worsening of psychotic symptoms (including partial hospitalization), but excluding hospitalization for psychosocial reasons
3) CGI-SS of 4 (severely suicidal) or 5 (attempted suicide) on Part 1 and/or 6 (much worse) or 7 (very much worse) on Part 2, or
4) Violent behavior resulting in clinically significant self-injury, injury to another person, or property damage.

A pre-planned interim analysis demonstrated a statistically significantly longer time to relapse in patients randomized to the ABILIFY MAINTENA group compared to placebo-treated patients and the trial was subsequently terminated early because maintenance of efficacy was demonstrated. The final analysis demonstrated a statistically significantly longer time to relapse in patients randomized to the ABILIFY MAINTENA group than compared to placebo-treated patients (log-rank test p<0.0001). The Kaplan-Meier curves of the time from randomization to relapse during the double-blind treatment phase for ABILIFY MAINTENA and placebo groups are shown in Figure 11.

[See figure 11 at top of next column]

The key secondary efficacy endpoint, percentage of subjects meeting the exacerbation of psychotic symptoms/ relapse criteria, was statistically significantly lower in patients randomized to the ABILIFY MAINTENA group (10%) than in the placebo group (40%).

16 HOW SUPPLIED/STORAGE AND HANDLING

16.1 How Supplied

ABILIFY MAINTENA™ (aripiprazole) extended-release injectable suspension is available in 300 mg or 400 mg strength vials.

Figure 11: Time to Relapse *

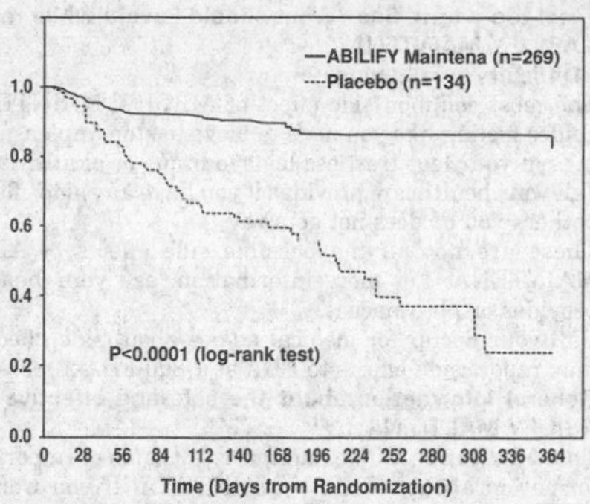

ABILIFY Maintena (n)	269	244	201	186	153	130	104	76	63	54	44	36	30	23
Placebo (n)	134	118	85	68	53	45	37	27	22	14	12	9	5	3

* This figure is based on a total of 80 relapse events

The 300 mg kit includes (NDC 59148-018-71):

- 300 mg vial of ABILIFY MAINTENA (aripiprazole) extended-release injectable suspension lyophilized powder
- 5 mL vial of Sterile Water for Injection, USP
- One 3 mL Luer Lock syringe with pre-attached 21 gauge, 1.5 inch Hypodermic Needle-Pro® safety needle with needle protection device
- One 3 mL BD Luer-Lok™ disposable syringe with BD Luer-Lok tip
- One vial adapter
- One 21 gauge, 1.5 inch (38 mm) Hypodermic Needle-Pro® safety needle with needle protection device
- One 21 gauge, 2 inch (50 mm) Hypodermic Needle-Pro® safety needle with needle protection device

The 400 mg kit includes (NDC 59148-019-71):

- 400 mg vial of ABILIFY MAINTENA (aripiprazole) extended-release injectable suspension lyophilized powder
- 5 mL vial of Sterile Water for Injection, USP
- One 3 mL Luer Lock syringe with pre-attached 21 gauge, 1.5 inch Hypodermic Needle-Pro® safety needle with needle protection device
- One 3 mL BD Luer-Lok™ disposable syringe with BD Luer-Lok tip
- One vial adapter
- One 21 gauge, 1.5 inch (38 mm) Hypodermic Needle-Pro® safety needle with needle protection device
- One 21 gauge, 2 inch (50 mm) Hypodermic Needle-Pro® safety needle with needle protection device

16.2 Storage

Store at 25 °C (77 °F), excursions permitted between 15 °C and 30 °C (59 °F to 86 °F) [see USP Controlled Room Temperature].

Keep out of reach of children.

17 PATIENT COUNSELING INFORMATION

See FDA-approved patient labeling (Medication Guide)

Physicians are advised to discuss the following issues with patients for whom they prescribe ABILIFY MAINTENA.

17.1 Increased Mortality in Elderly Patients with Dementia-Related Psychosis

Patients and caregivers should be advised that elderly patients with dementia-related psychoses treated with antipsychotic drugs are at increased risk of death. Aripiprazole is not approved for elderly patients with dementia-related psychosis *[see Warning and Precautions (5.1)]*.

17.2 Neuroleptic Malignant Syndrome

Counsel patients and caregivers that a potentially fatal symptom complex sometimes referred to as NMS has been reported in association with administration of antipsychotic drugs. Signs and symptoms of NMS include hyperpyrexia, muscle rigidity, altered mental status, and evidence of autonomic instability (irregular pulse or blood pressure, tachycardia, diaphoresis, and cardiac dysrhythmia) *[see Warnings and Precautions (5.3)]*.

17.3 Tardive Dyskinesia

Advise patients that abnormal involuntary movements have been associated with the administration of antipsychotic drugs. Counsel patients to notify their physician if they notice any movements which they cannot control in their face, tongue, or other body part *[see Warnings and Precautions (5.4)]*.

17.4 Hyperglycemia and Diabetes mellitus

Advise patients of the symptoms of hyperglycemia and diabetes mellitus. Patients who are diagnosed with diabetes, those with risk factors for diabetes, or those that develop these symptoms during treatment should have their blood glucose monitored at the beginning of and periodically during treatment *[see Warnings and Precautions (5.5)]*.

17.5 Orthostatic Hypotension

Advise patients of the risk of orthostatic hypotension, particularly at the time of initiating treatment, re-initiating treatment, or increasing the dose *[see Warnings and Precautions (5.6)]*.

17.6 Leukopenia/Neutropenia

Advise patients with a pre-existing low WBC count or a history of drug-induced leukopenia/neutropenia that they should have their CBC monitored while receiving ABILIFY MAINTENA *[see Warnings and Precautions (5.7)]*.

17.7 Interference with Cognitive and Motor Performance

Because ABILIFY MAINTENA may have the potential to impair judgment, thinking, or motor skills, instruct patients to be cautious about operating hazardous machinery, including automobiles, until they are reasonably certain that ABILIFY MAINTENA therapy does not affect them adversely *[see Warnings and Precautions (5.9)]*.

17.8 Heat Exposure and Dehydration

Advise patients regarding appropriate care in avoiding overheating and dehydration *[see Warnings and Precautions (5.10)]*.

17.9 Concomitant Medication

Advise patients to inform their physicians if they are taking, or plan to take, any prescription or over-the-counter drugs, since there is a potential for interactions *[see Drug Interactions (7)]*.

17.10 Pregnancy

Advise patients to notify their physician if they become pregnant or intend to become pregnant during therapy with ABILIFY MAINTENA *[see Use in Specific Populations (8.1)]*.

17.11 Nursing

Aripiprazole is excreted in human breast milk. A decision should be made whether to discontinue nursing or to discontinue ABILIFY MAINTENA, taking into account the importance of the drug to the mother *[see Use in Specific Populations (8.3)]*.

17.12 Alcohol

Advise patients to avoid alcohol while taking ABILIFY MAINTENA *[see Clinical Pharmacology (12.2)]*.

Distributed and marketed by Otsuka America Pharmaceutical, Inc., Rockville, MD 20850 USA
Marketed by Lundbeck, Deerfield, IL 60015 USA

09US12L-1001
February 2013

MEDICATION GUIDE

ABILIFY MAINTENA™ (a-BIL-i-fy main-TEN-a)

(aripiprazole)

extended-release injectable suspension, for intramuscular use

Read this Medication Guide before you receive your first injection of ABILIFY MAINTENA and before each injection. There may be new information. This information does not take the place of talking to your healthcare provider about your medical condition or your treatment.

What is the most important information I should know about ABILIFY MAINTENA?

ABILIFY MAINTENA may cause serious side effects, including:

- **Increased risk of death in elderly people with dementia-related psychosis.** ABILIFY MAINTENA is not for the treatment of people who have lost touch with reality (psychosis) due to confusion and memory loss (dementia).
- **Neuroleptic malignant syndrome (NMS) a serious condition that can lead to death.** Tell your healthcare provider right away if you have some or all of the following symptoms of NMS:
  - high fever
  - stiff muscles
  - confusion
  - sweating
  - changes in pulse, heart rate, and blood pressure

Call your healthcare provider right away if you have any of these symptoms.

What is ABILIFY MAINTENA?

ABILIFY MAINTENA is a prescription medicine used to treat schizophrenia.

It is not known if ABILIFY MAINTENA is safe and effective in children under 18 years of age.

Who should not receive ABILIFY MAINTENA?

Do not receive ABILIFY MAINTENA if you are allergic to aripiprazole or any of the ingredients in ABILIFY MAINTENA. See the end of this leaflet for a complete list of ingredients in ABILIFY MAINTENA.

What should I tell my healthcare provider before receiving ABILIFY MAINTENA?

Before you receive ABILIFY MAINTENA, tell your healthcare provider if you:

- have never taken ABILIFY (aripiprazole) before

- have diabetes or high blood sugar or a family history of diabetes or high blood sugar. Your healthcare provider should check your blood sugar before you start receiving ABILIFY MAINTENA and during your treatment.
- have or had seizures (convulsions)
- have or had low or high blood pressure
- have or had heart problems or a stroke
- have or had a low white blood cell count
- have any other medical problems including problems that may affect you receiving an injection in your buttocks
- are pregnant or plan to become pregnant. It is not known if ABILIFY MAINTENA will harm your unborn baby.
- are breastfeeding or plan to breastfeed. ABILIFY MAINTENA can pass into your milk and may harm your baby. Talk to your healthcare provider about the best way to feed your baby if you receive ABILIFY MAINTENA.

Tell your healthcare provider about all the medicines you take, including prescription medicines, non-prescription medicines, vitamins, and herbal supplements.

ABILIFY MAINTENA and other medicines may affect each other causing possible serious side effects. ABILIFY MAINTENA may affect the way other medicines work, and other medicines may affect how ABILIFY MAINTENA works.

Your healthcare provider can tell you if it is safe to take ABILIFY MAINTENA with your other medicines. Do not start or stop any medicines while taking ABILIFY MAINTENA without talking to your healthcare provider first.

Know the medicines you take. Keep a list of them to show your healthcare provider and pharmacist when you get a new medicine.

How should I receive ABILIFY MAINTENA?

- ABILIFY MAINTENA is an injection given in your buttock by your healthcare provider 1 time a month. You may feel a little pain in your buttock during your injection.
- After your first injection of ABILIFY MAINTENA you should continue your current antipsychotic medicine for 2 weeks.
- You should not miss a dose of ABILIFY MAINTENA. If you miss a dose for some reason, call your healthcare provider right away to discuss what you should do next.

What should I avoid while receiving ABILIFY MAINTENA?

- Do not drive, operate machinery, or do other dangerous activities until you know how ABILIFY MAINTENA affects you. ABILIFY MAINTENA may make you feel drowsy.
- Do not drink alcohol while you receive ABILIFY MAINTENA.
- Do not become too hot or dehydrated while you receive ABILIFY MAINTENA.
  - Do not exercise too much.
  - In hot weather, stay inside in a cool place if possible.
  - Stay out of the sun.
  - Do not wear too much clothing or heavy clothing.
  - Drink plenty of water.

What are the possible side effects of ABILIFY MAINTENA?

ABILIFY MAINTENA may cause serious side effects, including:

- **See "What is the most important information I should know about ABILIFY MAINTENA?"**
- **Uncontrolled body movements (tardive dyskinesia).** ABILIFY MAINTENA may cause movements that you cannot control in your face, tongue, or other body parts. Tardive dyskinesia may not go away, even if you stop receiving ABILIFY MAINTENA. Tardive dyskinesia may also start after you stop receiving ABILIFY MAINTENA.
- **Problems with your metabolism such as:**
  - **High blood sugar (hyperglycemia):** Increases in blood sugar can happen in some people who take ABILIFY MAINTENA. Extremely high blood sugar can lead to coma or death. If you have diabetes or risk factors for diabetes (such as being overweight or a family history of diabetes), your healthcare provider should check your blood sugar before you start receiving ABILIFY MAINTENA and during your treatment.

  Call your healthcare provider if you have any of these symptoms of high blood sugar while receiving ABILIFY MAINTENA:
  - feel very thirsty
  - need to urinate more than usual
  - feel very hungry
  - feel weak or tired
  - feel sick to your stomach
  - feel confused, or your breath smells fruity
  - **Increased fat levels (cholesterol and triglycerides) in your blood.**
  - **Weight gain.** You and your healthcare provider should check your weight regularly.
- **Decreased blood pressure (orthostatic hypotension).** You may feel lightheaded or faint when you rise too quickly from a sitting or lying position.
- **Low white blood cell count**
- **Seizures (convulsions)**
- **Problems controlling your body temperature so that you feel too warm. See "What should I avoid while receiving ABILIFY MAINTENA?"**
- **Difficulty swallowing**

The most common side effect of ABILIFY MAINTENA includes feeling like you need to move to stop unpleasant feelings in your legs (restless leg syndrome or akathisia).

Tell your healthcare provider if you have any side effect that bothers you or does not go away.

These are not all the possible side effects of ABILIFY MAINTENA. For more information, ask your healthcare provider or pharmacist.

Call your doctor for medical advice about side effects. You may report side effects to FDA at 1-800-FDA-1088.

General information about the safe and effective use of ABILIFY MAINTENA

This Medication Guide summarizes the most important information about ABILIFY MAINTENA. If you would like more information, talk with your healthcare provider.

You can ask your healthcare provider or pharmacist for information about ABILIFY MAINTENA. If you would like more information, talk with your healthcare provider. You can ask your pharmacist or healthcare provider for information about ABILIFY MAINTENA that is written for healthcare professionals.

For more information about ABILIFY MAINTENA, go to www.ABILIFYMAINTENA.com or call 1-800-441-6763.

What are the ingredients in ABILIFY MAINTENA?

Active ingredient: aripiprazole monohydrate

Inactive ingredients: carboxymethyl cellulose sodium, mannitol, sodium phosphate monobasic monohydrate and sodium hydroxide

This Medication Guide has been approved by the U.S. Food and Drug Administration.

ABILIFY MAINTENA is a trademark of Otsuka Pharmaceutical Company.

Luer-Lok is a trademark of Becton, Dickinson and Company, NJ

Needle-Pro is a registered trademark of Smiths Medical ASD, Inc., DE

09US12L-1001C

February 2013

SAMSCA® ℞

(tolvaptan)
tablets for oral use

HIGHLIGHTS OF PRESCRIBING INFORMATION

These highlights do not include all the information needed to use SAMSCA safely and effectively. See full prescribing information for SAMSCA.
SAMSCA® (tolvaptan) tablets for oral use
Initial U.S. Approval: 05/2009

WARNING: INITIATE AND RE-INITIATE IN A HOSPITAL AND MONITOR SERUM SODIUM

See full prescribing information for complete boxed warning.

- **SAMSCA should be initiated and re-initiated in patients only in a hospital where serum sodium can be monitored closely.**
- **Too rapid correction of hyponatremia (e.g., >12 mEq/L/24 hours) can cause osmotic demyelination resulting in dysarthria, mutism, dysphagia, lethargy, affective changes, spastic quadriparesis, seizures, coma and death. In susceptible patients, including those with severe malnutrition, alcoholism or advanced liver disease, slower rates of correction may be advisable.**

RECENT MAJOR CHANGES

Warnings and Precautions
Liver Injury (5.2) 04/2013

INDICATIONS AND USAGE

SAMSCA is a selective vasopressin V_2-receptor antagonist indicated for the treatment of clinically significant hypervolemic and euvolemic hyponatremia [serum sodium <125 mEq/L or less marked hyponatremia that is symptomatic and has resisted correction with fluid restriction], including patients with heart failure and Syndrome of Inappropriate Antidiuretic Hormone (SIADH) (1)

Important Limitations:

- Patients requiring intervention to raise serum sodium urgently to prevent or to treat serious neurological symptoms should not be treated with SAMSCA (1)
- It has not been established that SAMSCA provides a symptomatic benefit to patients (1)

DOSAGE AND ADMINISTRATION

- SAMSCA should be initiated and re-initiated in a hospital (2.1)
- The recommended starting dose is 15 mg once daily. Dosage may be increased at intervals ≥24 hr to 30 mg once daily, and to a maximum of 60 mg once daily as needed to raise serum sodium. (2.1)

DOSAGE FORMS AND STRENGTHS

- Tablets: 15 mg and 30 mg (3)

CONTRAINDICATIONS

- Need to raise serum sodium acutely (4.1)
- Patients who are unable to respond appropriately to thirst (4.2)
- Hypovolemic hyponatremia (4.3)
- Concomitant use of strong CYP 3A inhibitors (4.4)
- Anuria (4.5)

WARNINGS AND PRECAUTIONS

- Liver injury: Limit treatment duration to 30 days. If hepatic injury is suspected, discontinue SAMSCA. Avoid use in patients with underlying liver disease (5.2)
- Dehydration and hypovolemia may require intervention (5.3)
- Avoid use with hypertonic saline (5.4)
- Avoid use with CYP 3A inducers and moderate CYP 3A inhibitors (5.5)
- Consider dose reduction if co-administered with P-gp inhibitors (5.5)
- Monitor serum potassium in patients with potassium >5 mEq/L or on drugs known to increase potassium (5.6)

ADVERSE REACTIONS

Most common adverse reactions (≥5% placebo) are thirst, dry mouth, asthenia, constipation, pollakiuria or polyuria, and hyperglycemia (6.1)

To report SUSPECTED ADVERSE REACTIONS, contact Otsuka at 1-877-726-7220 or FDA at 1-800-FDA-1088 (*www.fda.gov/medwatch*).

USE IN SPECIFIC POPULATIONS

- Pregnancy: Based on animal data, may cause fetal harm (8.1)
- Nursing mothers: Discontinue drug or nursing taking into consideration importance of drug to mother (8.3)
- Pediatric Use: There are no studies (8.4)

See 17 for PATIENT COUNSELING INFORMATION and Medication Guide

Revised: 04/2013

FULL PRESCRIBING INFORMATION: CONTENTS*

*** Sections or subsections omitted from the full prescribing information are not listed**

FULL PRESCRIBING INFORMATION

WARNING: INITIATE AND RE-INITIATE IN A HOSPITAL AND MONITOR SERUM SODIUM

SAMSCA should be initiated and re-initiated in patients only in a hospital where serum sodium can be monitored closely.

Too rapid correction of hyponatremia (e.g., >12 mEq/L/24 hours) can cause osmotic demyelination resulting in dysarthria, mutism, dysphagia, lethargy, affective changes, spastic quadriparesis, seizures, coma and death. In susceptible patients, including those with severe malnutrition, alcoholism or advanced liver disease, slower rates of correction may be advisable.

1 INDICATIONS AND USAGE

SAMSCA® is indicated for the treatment of clinically significant hypervolemic and euvolemic hyponatremia (serum sodium <125 mEq/L or less marked hyponatremia that is symptomatic and has resisted correction with fluid restriction), including patients with heart failure and Syndrome of Inappropriate Antidiuretic Hormone (SIADH).

Important Limitations

Patients requiring intervention to raise serum sodium urgently to prevent or to treat serious neurological symptoms should not be treated with SAMSCA.

It has not been established that raising serum sodium with SAMSCA provides a symptomatic benefit to patients.

2 DOSAGE AND ADMINISTRATION

2.1 Usual Dosage in Adults

Patients should be in a hospital for initiation and re-initiation of therapy to evaluate the therapeutic response and because too rapid correction of hyponatremia can cause osmotic demyelination resulting in dysarthria, mutism, dysphagia, lethargy, affective changes, spastic quadriparesis, seizures, coma and death.

The usual starting dose for SAMSCA is 15 mg administered once daily without regard to meals. Increase the dose to 30 mg once daily, after at least 24 hours, to a maximum of 60 mg once daily, as needed to achieve the desired level of serum sodium. Do not administer SAMSCA for more than 30 days to minimize the risk of liver injury *[see Warnings and Precautions (5.2)]*.

During initiation and titration, frequently monitor for changes in serum electrolytes and volume. Avoid fluid restriction during the first 24 hours of therapy. Patients receiving SAMSCA should be advised that they can continue ingestion of fluid in response to thirst *[see Warnings and Precautions (5.1)]*.

2.2 Drug Withdrawal

Following discontinuation from SAMSCA, patients should be advised to resume fluid restriction and should be monitored for changes in serum sodium and volume status.

2.3 Co-Administration with CYP 3A Inhibitors, CYP 3A Inducers and P-gp Inhibitors

CYP 3A Inhibitors

Tolvaptan is metabolized by CYP 3A, and use with strong CYP 3A inhibitors causes a marked (5-fold) increase in exposure *[see Contraindications (4.4)]*. The effect of moderate CYP 3A inhibitors on tolvaptan exposure has not been assessed. Avoid co-administration of SAMSCA and moderate CYP 3A inhibitors *[see Warnings and Precautions (5.5), Drug Interactions (7.1)]*.

CYP 3A Inducers

Co-administration of SAMSCA with potent CYP 3A inducers (e.g., rifampin) reduces tolvaptan plasma concentrations by 85%. Therefore, the expected clinical effects of SAMSCA may not be observed at the recommended dose. Patient response should be monitored and the dose adjusted accordingly *[see Warnings and Precautions (5.5), Drug Interactions (7.1)]*.

P-gp Inhibitors

Tolvaptan is a substrate of P-gp. Co-administration of SAMSCA with inhibitors of P-gp (e.g., cyclosporine) may necessitate a decrease in SAMSCA dose *[see Warnings and Precautions (5.5), Drug Interactions (7.1)]*.

3 DOSAGE FORMS AND STRENGTHS

SAMSCA (tolvaptan) is available in 15 mg and 30 mg tablets *[see How Supplied/Storage and Handling (16)]*.

4 CONTRAINDICATIONS

SAMSCA is contraindicated in the following conditions:

4.1 Urgent need to raise serum sodium acutely

SAMSCA has not been studied in a setting of urgent need to raise serum sodium acutely.

4.2 Inability of the patient to sense or appropriately respond to thirst

Patients who are unable to auto-regulate fluid balance are at substantially increased risk of incurring an overly rapid correction of serum sodium, hypernatremia and hypovolemia.

4.3 Hypovolemic hyponatremia

Risks associated with worsening hypovolemia, including complications such as hypotension and renal failure, outweigh possible benefits.

4.4 Concomitant use of strong CYP 3A inhibitors

Ketoconazole 200 mg administered with tolvaptan increased tolvaptan exposure by 5-fold. Larger doses would be expected to produce larger increases in tolvaptan exposure. There is not adequate experience to define the dose adjustment that would be needed to allow safe use of tolvaptan with strong CYP 3A inhibitors such as clarithromycin, ketoconazole, itraconazole, ritonavir, indinavir, nelfinavir, saquinavir, nefazodone, and telithromycin.

4.5 Anuric patients

In patients unable to make urine, no clinical benefit can be expected.

5 WARNINGS AND PRECAUTIONS

5.1 Too Rapid Correction of Serum Sodium Can Cause Serious Neurologic Sequelae (see BOXED WARNING)

Osmotic demyelination syndrome is a risk associated with too rapid correction of hyponatremia (e.g., >12 mEq/L/24 hours). Osmotic demyelination results in dysarthria, mutism, dysphagia, lethargy, affective changes, spastic quadriparesis, seizures, coma or death. In susceptible patients, including those with severe malnutrition, alcoholism or advanced liver disease, slower rates of correction may be advisable. In controlled clinical trials in which tolvaptan was administered in titrated doses starting at 15 mg once daily, 7% of tolvaptan-treated subjects with a serum sodium <130 mEq/L had an increase in serum sodium greater than 8 mEq/L at approximately 8 hours and 2% had an increase greater than 12 mEq/L at 24 hours. Approximately 1% of placebo-treated subjects with a serum sodium <130 mEq/L had a rise greater than 8 mEq/L at 8 hours and no patient had a rise greater than 12 mEq/L/24 hours. Osmotic demyelination syndrome has been reported in association with SAMSCA therapy *[see Adverse Reactions (6.2)]*. Patients treated with SAMSCA should be monitored to assess serum sodium concentrations and neurologic status, especially during initiation and after titration. Subjects with SIADH or very low baseline serum sodium concentrations may be at greater risk for too-rapid correction of serum sodium. In patients receiving SAMSCA who develop too rapid a rise in serum sodium, discontinue or interrupt treatment with SAMSCA and consider administration of hypotonic fluid. Fluid restriction during the first 24 hours of therapy with SAMSCA may increase the likelihood of overly-rapid correction of serum sodium, and should generally be avoided.

5.2 Liver Injury

SAMSCA can cause serious and potentially fatal liver injury. In a placebo-controlled and open label extension study of chronically administered tolvaptan in patients with autosomal dominant polycystic kidney disease, cases of serious liver injury attributed to tolvaptan were observed. An increased incidence of ALT greater than three times the upper limit of normal was associated with tolvaptan (42/958 or 4.4%) compared to placebo (5/484 or 1.0%). Cases of serious liver injury were generally observed starting 3 months after initiation of tolvaptan although elevations of ALT occurred prior to 3 months.

Patients with symptoms that may indicate liver injury, including fatigue, anorexia, right upper abdominal discomfort, dark urine or jaundice should discontinue treatment with SAMSCA.

Limit duration of therapy with SAMSCA to 30 days. Avoid use in patients with underlying liver disease, including cirrhosis, because the ability to recover from liver injury may be impaired *[see Adverse Reactions (6.1)]*.

5.3 Dehydration and Hypovolemia

SAMSCA therapy induces copious aquaresis, which is normally partially offset by fluid intake. Dehydration and hypovolemia can occur, especially in potentially volume-depleted patients receiving diuretics or those who are fluid restricted. In multiple-dose, placebo-controlled trials in which 607 hyponatremic patients were treated with tolvaptan, the incidence of dehydration was 3.3% for tolvaptan and 1.5% for placebo-treated patients. In patients receiving SAMSCA who develop medically significant signs or symptoms of hypovolemia, interrupt or discontinue SAMSCA therapy and provide supportive care with careful management of vital signs, fluid balance and electrolytes. Fluid restriction during therapy with SAMSCA may increase the risk of dehydration and hypovolemia. Patients receiving SAMSCA should continue ingestion of fluid in response to thirst.

5.4 Co-administration with Hypertonic Saline

Concomitant use with hypertonic saline is not recommended.

5.5 Drug Interactions

Other Drugs Affecting Exposure to Tolvaptan

CYP 3A Inhibitors

Tolvaptan is a substrate of CYP 3A. CYP 3A inhibitors can lead to a marked increase in tolvaptan concentrations *[see Dosage and Administration (2.3), Drug Interactions (7.1)]*. Do not use SAMSCA with strong inhibitors of CYP 3A *[see Contraindications (4.4)]* and avoid concomitant use with moderate CYP 3A inhibitors.

CYP 3A Inducers

Avoid co-administration of CYP 3A inducers (e.g., rifampin, rifabutin, rifapentin, barbiturates, phenytoin, carbamazepine, St. John's Wort) with SAMSCA, as this can lead to a reduction in the plasma concentration of tolvaptan and decreased effectiveness of SAMSCA treatment. If co-administered with CYP 3A inducers, the dose of SAMSCA may need to be increased *[see Dosage and Administration (2.3), Drug Interactions (7.1)]*.

P-gp Inhibitors

The dose of SAMSCA may have to be reduced when SAMSCA is co-administered with P-gp inhibitors, e.g., cyclosporine *[see Dosage and Administration (2.3), Drug Interactions (7.1)]*.

5.6 Hyperkalemia or Drugs that Increase Serum Potassium

Treatment with tolvaptan is associated with an acute reduction of the extracellular fluid volume which could result in increased serum potassium. Serum potassium levels should be monitored after initiation of tolvaptan treatment in patients with a serum potassium >5 mEq/L as well as those who are receiving drugs known to increase serum potassium levels.

6 ADVERSE REACTIONS

6.1 Clinical Trials Experience

Because clinical trials are conducted under widely varying conditions, adverse reactions rates observed in the clinical trials of a drug cannot be directly compared to rates in the clinical trials of another drug and may not reflect the rates observed in practice. The adverse event information from clinical trials does, however, provide a basis for identifying the adverse events that appear to be related to drug use and for approximating rates.

In multiple-dose, placebo-controlled trials, 607 hyponatremic patients (serum sodium <135 mEq/L) were treated with SAMSCA. The mean age of these patients was 62 years; 70% of patients were male and 82% were Caucasian. One hundred eighty nine (189) tolvaptan-treated patients had a serum sodium <130 mEq/L, and 52 patients had a serum sodium <125 mEq/L. Hyponatremia was attributed to cirrhosis in 17% of patients, heart failure in 68% and SIADH/other in 16%. Of these patients, 223 were treated with the recommended dose titration (15 mg titrated to 60 mg as needed to raise serum sodium).

Overall, over 4,000 patients have been treated with oral doses of tolvaptan in open-label or placebo-controlled clinical trials. Approximately 650 of these patients had hyponatremia; approximately 219 of these hyponatremic patients were treated with tolvaptan for 6 months or more.

The most common adverse reactions (incidence ≥5% more than placebo) seen in two 30-day, double-blind, placebo-controlled hyponatremia trials in which tolvaptan was administered in titrated doses (15 mg to 60 mg once daily) were thirst, dry mouth, asthenia, constipation, pollakiuria or polyuria and hyperglycemia. In these trials, 10% (23/223) of tolvaptan-treated patients discontinued treatment because of an adverse event, compared to 12% (26/220) of placebo-treated patients; no adverse reaction resulting in discontinuation of trial medication occurred at an incidence of >1% in tolvaptan-treated patients.

Table 1 lists the adverse reactions reported in tolvaptan-treated patients with hyponatremia (serum sodium <135 mEq/L) and at a rate at least 2% greater than placebo-treated patients in two 30-day, double-blind, placebo-controlled trials. In these studies, 223 patients were exposed to tolvaptan (starting dose 15 mg, titrated to 30 and

60 mg as needed to raise serum sodium). Adverse events resulting in death in these trials were 6% in tolvaptan-treated-patients and 6% in placebo-treated patients.

Table 1. Adverse Reactions (>2% more than placebo) in Tolvaptan-Treated Patients in Double-Blind, Placebo-Controlled Hyponatremia Trials

System Organ Class MedDRA Preferred Term	Tolvaptan 15 mg/ day-60 mg/day (N = 223) n (%)	Placebo (N = 220) n (%)
Gastrointestinal Disorders		
Dry mouth	28 (13)	9 (4)
Constipation	16 (7)	4 (2)
General Disorders and Administration Site Conditions		
Thirst[a]	35 (16)	11 (5)
Asthenia	19 (9)	9 (4)
Pyrexia	9 (4)	2 (1)
Metabolism and Nutrition Disorders		
Hyperglycemia[b]	14 (6)	2 (1)
Anorexia[c]	8 (4)	2 (1)
Renal and Urinary Disorders		
Pollakiuria or polyuria[d]	25 (11)	7 (3)

The following terms are subsumed under the referenced ADR in Table 1:
[a] polydipsia; [b] diabetes mellitus; [c] decreased appetite;
[d] urine output increased, micturition urgency, nocturia

In a subgroup of patients with hyponatremia (N = 475, serum sodium <135 mEq/L) enrolled in a double-blind, placebo-controlled trial (mean duration of treatment was 9 months) of patients with worsening heart failure, the following adverse reactions occurred in tolvaptan-treated patients at a rate at least 2% greater than placebo: mortality (42% tolvaptan, 38% placebo), nausea (21% tolvaptan, 16% placebo), thirst (12% tolvaptan, 2% placebo), dry mouth (7% tolvaptan, 2% placebo) and polyuria or pollakiuria (4% tolvaptan, 1% placebo).

Gastrointestinal bleeding in patients with cirrhosis

In patients with cirrhosis treated with tolvaptan in the hyponatremia trials, gastrointestinal bleeding was reported in 6 out of 63 (10%) tolvaptan-treated patients and 1 out of 57 (2%) placebo treated patients.

The following adverse reactions occurred in <2% of hyponatremic patients treated with SAMSCA and at a rate greater than placebo in double-blind placebo-controlled trials (N = 607 tolvaptan; N = 518 placebo) or in <2% of patients in an uncontrolled trial of patients with hyponatremia (N = 111) and are not mentioned elsewhere in the label.

Blood and Lymphatic System Disorders: Disseminated intravascular coagulation

Cardiac Disorders: Intracardiac thrombus, ventricular fibrillation

Investigations: Prothrombin time prolonged

Gastrointestinal Disorders: Ischemic colitis

Metabolism and Nutrition Disorders: Diabetic ketoacidosis

Musculoskeletal and Connective Tissue Disorders: Rhabdomyolysis

Nervous System: Cerebrovascular accident

Renal and Urinary Disorders: Urethral hemorrhage

Reproductive System and Breast Disorders (female): Vaginal hemorrhage

Respiratory, Thoracic, and Mediastinal Disorders: Pulmonary embolism, respiratory failure

Vascular disorder: Deep vein thrombosis

6.2 Postmarketing Experience

The following adverse reactions have been identified during post-approval use of SAMSCA. Because these reactions are reported voluntarily from a population of an unknown size, it is not always possible to reliably estimate their frequency or establish a causal relationship to drug exposure.

Neurologic: Osmotic demyelination syndrome

Investigations: Hypernatremia

Removal of excess free body water increases serum osmolality and serum sodium concentrations. All patients treated with tolvaptan, especially those whose serum sodium levels become normal, should continue to be monitored to ensure serum sodium remains within normal limits. If hypernatremia is observed, management may include dose decreases or interruption of tolvaptan treatment, combined with modification of free-water intake or infusion. During clinical trials of hyponatremic patients, hypernatremia was reported as an adverse event in 0.7% of patients receiving tolvaptan vs. 0.6% of patients receiving placebo; analysis of laboratory values demonstrated an incidence of hypernatremia of 1.7% in patients receiving tolvaptan vs. 0.8% in patients receiving placebo.

7 DRUG INTERACTIONS

7.1 Effects of Drugs on Tolvaptan

Ketoconazole and Other Strong CYP 3A Inhibitors

SAMSCA is metabolized primarily by CYP 3A. Ketoconazole is a strong inhibitor of CYP 3A and also an inhibitor of P-gp. Co-administration of SAMSCA and ketoconazole 200 mg daily results in a 5-fold increase in exposure to tolvaptan. Co-administration of SAMSCA with 400 mg ketoconazole daily or with other strong CYP 3A inhibitors (e.g., clarithromycin, itraconazole, telithromycin, saquinavir, nelfinavir, ritonavir and nefazodone) at the highest labeled dose would be expected to cause an even greater increase in tolvaptan exposure. Thus, SAMSCA and strong CYP 3A inhibitors should not be co-administered *[see Dosage and Administration (2.3) and Contraindications (4.4)]*.

Moderate CYP 3A Inhibitors

The impact of moderate CYP 3A inhibitors (e.g., erythromycin, fluconazole, aprepitant, diltiazem and verapamil) on the exposure to co-administered tolvaptan has not been assessed. A substantial increase in the exposure to tolvaptan would be expected when SAMSCA is co-administered with moderate CYP 3A inhibitors. Co-administration of SAMSCA with moderate CYP3A inhibitors should therefore generally be avoided *[see Dosage and Administration (2.3) and Warnings and Precautions (5.5)]*.

Grapefruit Juice

Co-administration of grapefruit juice and SAMSCA results in a 1.8-fold increase in exposure to tolvaptan *[see Dose and Administration (2.3) and Warnings and Precautions (5.5)]*.

P-gp Inhibitors

Reduction in the dose of SAMSCA may be required in patients concomitantly treated with P-gp inhibitors, such as e.g., cyclosporine, based on clinical response *[see Dose and Administration (2.3) and Warnings and Precautions (5.5)]*.

Rifampin and Other CYP 3A Inducers

Rifampin is an inducer of CYP 3A and P-gp. Co-administration of rifampin and SAMSCA reduces exposure to tolvaptan by 85%. Therefore, the expected clinical effects of SAMSCA in the presence of rifampin and other inducers (e.g., rifabutin, rifapentin, barbiturates, phenytoin, carbamazepine and St. John's Wort) may not be observed at the usual dose levels of SAMSCA. The dose of SAMSCA may have to be increased *[Dosage and Administration (2.3) and Warnings and Precautions (5.5)]*.

Lovastatin, Digoxin, Furosemide, and Hydrochlorothiazide

Co-administration of lovastatin, digoxin, furosemide, and hydrochlorothiazide with SAMSCA has no clinically relevant impact on the exposure to tolvaptan.

7.2 Effects of Tolvaptan on Other Drugs

Digoxin

Digoxin is a P-gp substrate. Co-administration of SAMSCA with digoxin increased digoxin AUC by 20% and Cmax by 30%.

Warfarin, Amiodarone, Furosemide, and Hydrochlorothiazide

Co-administration of tolvaptan does not appear to alter the pharmacokinetics of warfarin, furosemide, hydrochlorothiazide, or amiodarone (or its active metabolite, desethylamiodarone) to a clinically significant degree.

Lovastatin

SAMSCA is a weak inhibitor of CYP 3A. Co-administration of lovastatin and SAMSCA increases the exposure to lovastatin and its active metabolite lovastatin-β hydroxyacid by factors of 1.4 and 1.3, respectively. This is not a clinically relevant change.

Pharmacodynamic Interactions

Tolvaptan produces a greater 24 hour urine volume/excretion rate than does furosemide or hydrochlorothiazide. Concomitant administration of tolvaptan with furosemide or hydrochlorothiazide results in a 24 hour urine volume/excretion rate that is similar to the rate after tolvaptan administration alone.

Although specific interaction studies were not performed, in clinical studies tolvaptan was used concomitantly with beta-blockers, angiotensin receptor blockers, angiotensin converting enzyme inhibitors and potassium sparing diuretics. Adverse reactions of hyperkalemia were approximately 1-2% higher when tolvaptan was administered with angiotensin receptor blockers, angiotensin converting enzyme inhibitors and potassium sparing diuretics compared to administration of these medications with placebo. Serum potassium levels should be monitored during concomitant drug therapy.

As a V_2 receptor antagonist, tolvaptan may interfere with the V_2 agonist activity of desmopressin (dDAVP). In a male subject with mild Von Willebrand (vW) disease, intravenous infusion of dDAVP 2 hours after administration of oral tolvaptan did not produce the expected increases in vW Factor Antigen or Factor VIII activity. It is not recommended to administer SAMSCA with a V_2 agonist.

8 USE IN SPECIFIC POPULATIONS

There is no need to adjust dose based on age, gender, race, or cardiac function *[see Clinical Pharmacology (12.3)]*.

8.1 Pregnancy

Pregnancy Category C.

There are no adequate and well controlled studies of SAMSCA use in pregnant women. In animal studies, cleft palate, brachymelia, microphthalmia, skeletal malformations, decreased fetal weight, delayed fetal ossification, and embryo-fetal death occurred. SAMSCA should be used during pregnancy only if the potential benefit justifies the potential risk to the fetus.

In embryo-fetal development studies, pregnant rats and rabbits received oral tolvaptan during organogenesis. Rats received 2 to 162 times the maximum recommended human dose (MRHD) of tolvaptan (on a body surface area basis). Reduced fetal weights and delayed fetal ossification occurred at 162 times the MRHD. Signs of maternal toxicity (reduction in body weight gain and food consumption) occurred at 16 and 162 times the MRHD. When pregnant rabbits received oral tolvaptan at 32 to 324 times the MRHD (on a body surface area basis), there were reductions in maternal body weight gain and food consumption at all doses, and increased abortions at the mid and high doses (about 97 and 324 times the MRHD). At 324 times the MRHD, there were increased rates of embryo-fetal death, fetal microphthalmia, open eyelids, cleft palate, brachymelia and skeletal malformations *[see Nonclinical Toxicology (13.3)]*.

8.2 Labor and Delivery

The effect of SAMSCA on labor and delivery in humans is unknown.

8.3 Nursing Mothers

It is not known whether SAMSCA is excreted into human milk. Tolvaptan is excreted into the milk of lactating rats. Because many drugs are excreted into human milk and because of the potential for serious adverse reactions in nursing infants from SAMSCA, a decision should be made to discontinue nursing or SAMSCA, taking into consideration the importance of SAMSCA to the mother.

8.4 Pediatric Use

Safety and effectiveness of SAMSCA in pediatric patients have not been established.

8.5 Geriatric Use

Of the total number of hyponatremic subjects treated with SAMSCA in clinical studies, 42% were 65 and over, while 19% were 75 and over. No overall differences in safety or effectiveness were observed between these subjects and younger subjects, and other reported clinical experience has not identified differences in responses between the elderly and younger patients, but greater sensitivity of some older individuals cannot be ruled out. Increasing age has no effect on tolvaptan plasma concentrations.

8.6 Use in Patients with Hepatic Impairment

Moderate and severe hepatic impairment do not affect exposure to tolvaptan to a clinically relevant extent. Avoid use of tolvaptan in patients with underlying liver disease.

8.7 Use in Patients with Renal Impairment

No dose adjustment is necessary based on renal function. There are no clinical trial data in patients with CrCl <10 mL/min, and, because drug effects on serum sodium levels are likely lost at very low levels of renal function, use in patients with a CrCl <10 mL/min is not recommended. No benefit can be expected in patients who are anuric *[see Contraindications (4.5) and Clinical Pharmacology (12.3)]*.

8.8 Use in Patients with Congestive Heart Failure

The exposure to tolvaptan in patients with congestive heart failure is not clinically relevantly increased. No dose adjustment is necessary.

10 OVERDOSAGE

Single oral doses up to 480 mg and multiple doses up to 300 mg once daily for 5 days have been well tolerated in studies in healthy subjects. There is no specific antidote for tolvaptan intoxication. The signs and symptoms of an acute overdose can be anticipated to be those of excessive pharmacologic effect: a rise in serum sodium concentration, polyuria, thirst, and dehydration/hypovolemia.

The oral LD_{50} of tolvaptan in rats and dogs is >2000 mg/kg. No mortality was observed in rats or dogs following single oral doses of 2000 mg/kg (maximum feasible dose). A single oral dose of 2000 mg/kg was lethal in mice, and symptoms of toxicity in affected mice included decreased locomotor activity, staggering gait, tremor and hypothermia.

If overdose occurs, estimation of the severity of poisoning is an important first step. A thorough history and details of overdose should be obtained, and a physical examination should be performed. The possibility of multiple drug involvement should be considered.

Table 2. Effects of Treatment with Tolvaptan 15 mg/day to 60 mg/day

	Tolvaptan 15 mg/day-60 mg/day	Placebo	Estimated Effect (95% CI)
Subjects with Serum Sodium <135 mEq/L (ITT population)			
Change in average daily serum [Na+] AUC baseline to Day 4 (mEq/L) Mean (SD) N	4.0 (2.8) 213	0.4 (2.4) 203	3.7 (3.3-4.2) *p* <0.0001
Change in average daily serum [Na+] AUC baseline to Day 30 (mEq/L) Mean (SD) N	6.2 (4.0) 213	1.8 (3.7) 203	4.6 (3.9-5.2) *p* <0.0001
Percent of Patients Needing Fluid Restriction*	14% 30/215	25% 51/206	*p* <0.01
Subgroup with Serum Sodium <130 mEq/L			
Change in average daily serum [Na+] AUC baseline to Day 4 (mEq/L) Mean (SD) N	4.8 (3.0) 110	0.7 (2.5) 105	4.2 (3.5-5.0) *p* <0.0001
Change in average daily serum [Na+] AUC baseline to Day 30 (mEq/L) Mean (SD) N	7.9 (4.1) 110	2.6 (4.2) 105	5.5 (4.4-6.5) *p* <0.0001
Percent of Patients Needing Fluid Restriction*	19% 21/110	36% 38/106	*p* <0.01
Subgroup with Serum Sodium <125 mEq/L			
Change in average daily serum [Na+] AUC baseline to Day 4 (mEq/L) Mean (SD) N	5.7 (3.8) 26	1.0 (1.8) 30	5.3 (3.8-6.9) *p* <0.0001
Change in average daily serum [Na+] AUC baseline to Day 30 (mEq/L) Mean (SD) N	10.0 (4.8) 26	4.1 (4.5) 30	5.7 (3.1-8.3) *p* <0.0001
Percent of Patients Needing Fluid Restriction*	35% 9/26	50% 15/30	*p* = 0.14

* Fluid Restriction defined as <1L/day at any time during treatment period.

Treatment should involve symptomatic and supportive care, with respiratory, ECG and blood pressure monitoring and water/electrolyte supplements as needed. A profuse and prolonged aquaresis should be anticipated, which, if not matched by oral fluid ingestion, should be replaced with intravenous hypotonic fluids, while closely monitoring electrolytes and fluid balance.

ECG monitoring should begin immediately and continue until ECG parameters are within normal ranges. Dialysis may not be effective in removing tolvaptan because of its high binding affinity for human plasma protein (>99%). Close medical supervision and monitoring should continue until the patient recovers.

11 DESCRIPTION

Tolvaptan is (±)-4'-[(7-chloro-2,3,4,5-tetrahydro-5-hydroxy-1*H*-1-benzazepin-1-yl) carbonyl]-*o*-tolu-*m*-toluidide. The empirical formula is $C_{26}H_{25}ClN_2O_3$. Molecular weight is 448.94. The chemical structure is:

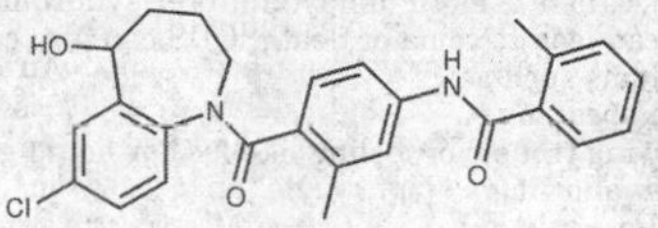

SAMSCA tablets for oral use contain 15 mg or 30 mg of tolvaptan. Inactive ingredients include corn starch, hydroxypropyl cellulose, lactose monohydrate, low-substituted hydroxypropyl cellulose, magnesium stearate and microcrystalline cellulose and FD&C Blue No. 2 Aluminum Lake as colorant.

12 CLINICAL PHARMACOLOGY

12.1 Mechanism of Action

Tolvaptan is a selective vasopressin V_2-receptor antagonist with an affinity for the V_2-receptor that is 1.8 times that of native arginine vasopressin (AVP). Tolvaptan affinity for the V_2-receptor is 29 times greater than for the V_{1a}-receptor. When taken orally, 15 to 60 mg doses of tolvaptan antagonize the effect of vasopressin and cause an increase in urine water excretion that results in an increase in free water clearance (aquaresis), a decrease in urine osmolality, and a resulting increase in serum sodium concentrations. Urinary excretion of sodium and potassium and plasma potassium concentrations are not significantly changed. Tolvaptan metabolites have no or weak antagonist activity for human V_2-receptors compared with tolvaptan.

Plasma concentrations of native AVP may increase (avg. 2-9 pg/mL) with tolvaptan administration.

12.2 Pharmacodynamics

In healthy subjects receiving a single dose of SAMSCA 60 mg, the onset of the aquaretic and sodium increasing effects occurs within 2 to 4 hours post-dose. A peak effect of about a 6 mEq increase in serum sodium and about 9 mL/min increase in urine excretion rate is observed between 4 and 8 hours post-dose; thus, the pharmacological activity lags behind the plasma concentrations of tolvaptan. About 60% of the peak effect on serum sodium is sustained at 24 hours post-dose, but the urinary excretion rate is no longer elevated by this time. Doses above 60 mg tolvaptan do not increase aquaresis or serum sodium further. The effects of tolvaptan in the recommended dose range of 15 to 60 mg once daily appear to be limited to aquaresis and the resulting increase in sodium concentration.

In a parallel-arm, double-blind (for tolvaptan and placebo), placebo- and positive-controlled, multiple dose study of the effect of tolvaptan on the QTc interval, 172 healthy subjects were randomized to tolvaptan 30 mg, tolvaptan 300 mg, placebo, or moxifloxacin 400 mg once daily. At both the 30 mg and 300 mg doses, no significant effect of administering tolvaptan on the QTc interval was detected on Day 1 and Day 5. At the 300 mg dose, peak tolvaptan plasma concentrations were approximately 4-fold higher than the peak concentrations following a 30 mg dose. Moxifloxacin increased the QT interval by 12 ms at 2 hours after dosing on Day 1 and 17 ms at 1 hour after dosing on Day 5, indicating that the study was adequately designed and conducted to detect tolvaptan's effect on the QT interval, had an effect been present.

12.3 Pharmacokinetics

In healthy subjects the pharmacokinetics of tolvaptan after single doses of up to 480 mg and multiple doses up to 300 mg once daily have been examined. Area under the curve (AUC) increases proportionally with dose. After administration of doses ≥60 mg, however, Cmax increases less than proportionally with dose. The pharmacokinetic properties of tolvaptan are stereospecific, with a steady-state ratio of the S-(-) to the R-(+) enantiomer of about 3. The absolute bioavailability of tolvaptan is unknown. At least 40% of the dose is absorbed as tolvaptan or metabolites. Peak concentrations of tolvaptan are observed between 2 and 4 hours post-dose. Food does not impact the bioavailability of tolvaptan. *In vitro* data indicate that tolvaptan is a substrate and inhibitor of P-gp. Tolvaptan is highly plasma protein bound (99%) and distributed into an apparent volume of distribution of about 3 L/kg. Tolvaptan is eliminated entirely by non-renal routes and mainly, if not exclusively, metabolized by CYP 3A. After oral dosing, clearance is about 4 mL/min/kg and the terminal phase half-life is about 12 hours. The accumulation factor of tolvaptan with the once-daily regimen is 1.3 and the trough concentrations amount to ≤16% of the peak concentrations, suggesting a dominant half-life somewhat shorter than 12 hours. There is marked inter-subject variation in peak and average exposure to tolvaptan with a percent coefficient of variation ranging between 30 and 60%.

In patients with hyponatremia of any origin the clearance of tolvaptan is reduced to about 2 mL/min/kg. Moderate or severe hepatic impairment or congestive heart failure decrease the clearance and increase the volume of distribution of tolvaptan, but the respective changes are not clinically relevant. Exposure and response to tolvaptan in subjects with creatinine clearance ranging between 79 and 10 mL/min and patients with normal renal function are not different.

In a study in patients with creatinine clearances ranging from 10-124 mL/min administered a single dose of 60 mg tolvaptan, AUC and Cmax of plasma tolvaptan were less than doubled in patients with severe renal impairment relative to the controls. The peak increase in serum sodium was 5-6 mEq/L, regardless of renal function, but the onset and offset of tolvaptan's effect on serum sodium were slower in patients with severe renal impairment *[see Use in Special Populations (8.7)]*.

13 NONCLINICAL TOXICOLOGY

13.1 Carcinogenesis, Mutagenesis, Impairment of Fertility

Up to two years of oral administration of tolvaptan to male and female rats at doses up to 1000 mg/kg/day (162 times the maximum recommended human dose [MRHD] on a body surface area basis), to male mice at doses up to 60 mg/kg/day (5 times the MRHD) and to female mice at doses up to 100 mg/kg/day (8 times the MRHD) did not increase the incidence of tumors.

Tolvaptan tested negative for genotoxicity in *in vitro* (bacterial reverse mutation assay and chromosomal aberration test in Chinese hamster lung fibroblast cells) and *in vivo* (rat micronucleus assay) test systems.

In a fertility study in which male and female rats were orally administered tolvaptan at 100, 300 or 1000 mg/kg/day, the highest dose level was associated with significantly fewer corpora lutea and implants than control.

13.3 Reproductive and Developmental Toxicology

In pregnant rats, oral administration of tolvaptan at 10, 100 and 1000 mg/kg/day during organogenesis was associated with a reduction in maternal body weight gain and food consumption at 100 and 1000 mg/kg/day, and reduced fetal weight and delayed ossification of fetuses at 1000 mg/kg/day (162 times the MRHD on a body surface area basis). Oral administration of tolvaptan at 100, 300 and 1000 mg/kg/day to pregnant rabbits during organogenesis was associated with reductions in maternal body weight gain and food consumption at all doses, and abortions at mid- and high-doses. At 1000 mg/kg/day (324 times the MRHD), increased incidences of embryo-fetal death, fetal microphthalmia, open eyelids, cleft palate, brachymelia and skeletal malformations were observed. There are no adequate and well-controlled studies of SAMSCA in pregnant women. SAMSCA should be used in pregnancy only if the potential benefit justifies the risk to the fetus.

14 CLINICAL STUDIES

14.1 Hyponatremia

In two double-blind, placebo-controlled, multi-center studies (SALT-1 and SALT-2), a total of 424 patients with euvolemic or hypervolemic hyponatremia (serum sodium <135 mEq/L) resulting from a variety of underlying causes (heart failure, liver cirrhosis, syndrome of inappropriate antidiuretic hormone [SIADH] and others) were treated for 30 days with tolvaptan or placebo, then followed for an additional 7 days after withdrawal. Symptomatic patients, patients likely to require saline therapy during the course of therapy, patients with acute and transient hyponatremia associated with head trauma or postoperative state and patients with hyponatremia due to primary polydipsia, uncontrolled adrenal insufficiency or uncontrolled hypothyroidism were excluded. Patients were randomized to receive either placebo (N = 220) or tolvaptan (N = 223) at an initial oral dose of 15 mg once daily. The mean serum sodium concentration at study entry was 129 mEq/L. Fluid restriction was to be avoided if possible during the first 24 hours of therapy to avoid overly rapid correction of serum sodium, and during the first 24 hours of therapy 87% of patients had no fluid restriction. Thereafter, patients could resume or initiate fluid restriction (defined as daily fluid intake of ≤1.0 liter/day) as clinically indicated.

The dose of tolvaptan could be increased at 24 hour intervals to 30 mg once daily, then to 60 mg once daily, until either the maximum dose of 60 mg or normonatremia (serum sodium >135 mEq/L) was reached. Serum sodium concentrations were determined at 8 hours after study drug initiation and daily up to 72 hours, within which time titration was typically completed. Treatment was maintained for 30 days with additional serum sodium assessments on Days 11, 18, 25 and 30. On the day of study discontinuation, all patients resumed previous therapies for hyponatremia and were reevaluated 7 days later. The primary endpoint for these studies was the average daily AUC for change in serum sodium from baseline to Day 4 and baseline to Day 30 in patients with a serum sodium less than 135 mEq/L. Compared to placebo, tolvaptan caused a statistically greater increase in serum sodium (*p* <0.0001) during both periods in both studies (see Table 2). For patients with a serum sodium of <130 mEq/L or <125 mEq/L, the effects at Day 4 and Day 30 remained significant (see Table 2). This effect was also seen across all disease etiology subsets (e.g., CHF, cirrhosis, SIADH/other).

[See table 2 at top of previous page]

In patients with hyponatremia (defined as <135 mEq/L), serum sodium concentration increased to a significantly greater degree in tolvaptan-treated patients compared to placebo-treated patients as early as 8 hours after the first dose, and the change was maintained for 30 days. The percentage of patients requiring fluid restriction (defined as ≤1 L/day at any time during the treatment period) was also significantly less (p <0.0017) in the tolvaptan-treated group (30/215, 14%) as compared with the placebo-treated group (51/206, 25%).

Figure 1 shows the change from baseline in serum sodium by visit in patients with serum sodium <135 mEq/L. Within 7 days of tolvaptan discontinuation, serum sodium concentrations in tolvaptan-treated patients declined to levels similar to those of placebo-treated patients.

Figure 1: Pooled SALT Studies: Analysis of Mean Serum Sodium (± SD, mEq/L) by Visit - Patients with Baseline Serum Sodium <135 mEq/L

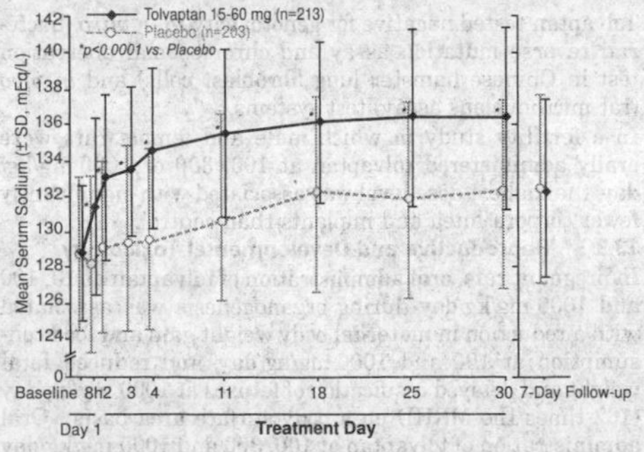

*p-value <0.0001 for all visits during tolvaptan treatment compared to placebo

[See figure 2 at top of next column]

In the open-label study SALTWATER, 111 patients, 94 of them hyponatremic (serum sodium <135 mEq/L), previously on tolvaptan or placebo therapy were given tolvaptan as a titrated regimen (15 to 60 mg once daily) after having returned to standard care for at least 7 days. By this time, their baseline mean serum sodium concentration had fallen to between their original baseline and post-placebo therapy level. Upon initiation of therapy, average serum sodium concentrations increased to approximately the same levels as observed for those previously treated with tolvaptan, and were sustained for at least a year. Figure 3 shows results from 111 patients enrolled in the SALTWATER Study.

[See figure 3 at top of next column]

14.2 Heart Failure

In a phase 3 double-blind, placebo-controlled study (EVEREST), 4133 patients with worsening heart failure were randomized to tolvaptan or placebo as an adjunct to standard of care. Long-term tolvaptan treatment (mean duration of treatment of 0.75 years) had no demonstrated effect, either favorable or unfavorable, on all-cause mortality [HR (95%

Figure 2: Pooled SALT Studies: Analysis of Mean Serum Sodium (± SD, mEq/L) by Visit - Patients with Baseline Serum Sodium <130 mEq/L

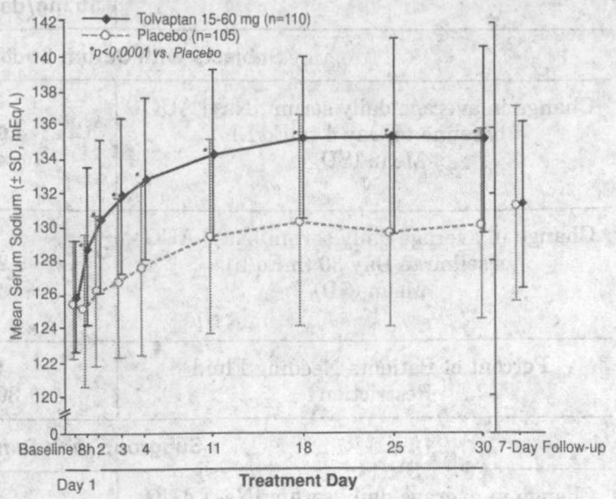

*p-value <0.0001 for all visits during tolvaptan treatment compared to placebo

Figure 3: SALTWATER: Analysis of Mean Serum Sodium (± SD, mEq/L) by Visit

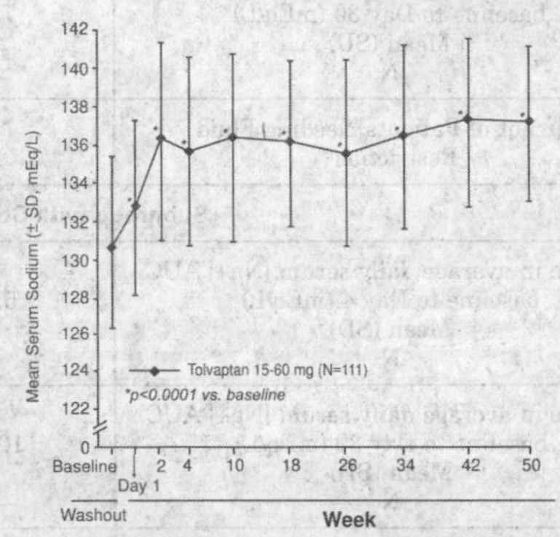

*p-value <0.0001 for all visits during tolvaptan treatment compared to baseline

CI): 0.98 (0.9, 1.1)] or the combined endpoint of CV mortality or subsequent hospitalization for worsening HF [HR (95% CI): 1.0 (0.9, 1.1)].

16 HOW SUPPLIED/STORAGE AND HANDLING

How Supplied

SAMSCA® (tolvaptan) tablets are available in the following strengths and packages.

SAMSCA 15 mg tablets are non-scored, blue, triangular, shallow-convex, debossed with "OTSUKA" and "15" on one side.

Blister of 10 NDC 59148-020-50

SAMSCA 30 mg tablets are non-scored, blue, round, shallow-convex, debossed with "OTSUKA" and "30" on one side.

Blister of 10 NDC 59148-021-50

Storage and Handling

Store at 25°C (77°F), excursions permitted between 15°C and 30°C (59°F to 86°F) [see USP controlled Room Temperature].

Keep out of reach of children.

17 PATIENT COUNSELING INFORMATION

As a part of patient counseling, healthcare providers must review the SAMSCA Medication Guide with every patient *[see FDA-Approved Medication Guide (17.3)]*.

17.1 Concomitant Medication

Advise patients to inform their physician if they are taking or plan to take any prescription or over-the-counter drugs since there is a potential for interactions.

Strong and Moderate CYP 3A inhibitors and P-gp inhibitors

Advise patients to inform their physician if they use strong (e.g., ketoconazole, itraconazole, clarithromycin, telithromycin, nelfinavir, saquinavir, indinavir, ritonavir) or moderate CYP 3A inhibitors (e.g., aprepitant, erythromycin, diltiazem, verapamil, fluconazol) or P-gp inhibitors (e.g., cyclosporine) *[see Dosage and Administration (2.3), Contraindications (4.4), Warnings and Precautions (5.5) and Drug Interactions (7.1)]*.

17.2 Nursing

Advise patients not to breastfeed an infant if they are taking SAMSCA *[see Use In Specific Populations (8.3)]*.

Manufactured by Otsuka Pharmaceutical Co., Ltd., Tokyo, 101-8535 Japan

Distributed and marketed by Otsuka America Pharmaceutical, Inc., Rockville, MD 20850

17.3 FDA-Approved Medication Guide

MEDICATION GUIDE

SAMSCA® (sam-sca)

tolvaptan

Tablets

Read the Medication Guide that comes with SAMSCA before you take it and each time you get a new prescription. There may be new information. This Medication Guide does not take the place of talking to your healthcare provider about your medical condition or your treatment. Share this important information with members of your household.

What is the most important information I should know about SAMSCA?

1) **SAMSCA may make the salt (sodium) level in your blood rise too fast.** This can increase your risk of a serious condition called osmotic demyelination syndrome (ODS). ODS can lead to coma or death. ODS can also cause new symptoms such as:

- trouble speaking
- swallowing trouble or feeling like food or liquid gets stuck while swallowing
- drowsiness
- confusion
- mood changes
- trouble controlling body movement (involuntary movement) and weakness in muscles of the arms and legs
- seizures

You or a family member should tell your healthcare provider right away if you have any of these symptoms even if they begin later in treatment. Also tell you healthcare provider about any other new symptoms while taking SAMSCA.

You may be more at risk for ODS if you have:

- liver disease
- not eaten enough for a long period of time (malnourished)
- very low sodium level in your blood
- been drinking large amounts of alcohol for a long period of time (chronic alcoholism)

To lessen your risk of ODS while taking SAMSCA:

- **Treatment with SAMSCA should be started and re-started only in a hospital, where the sodium levels in your blood can be checked closely.**
- Do not take SAMSCA if you can not tell if you are thirsty.
- To prevent losing too much body water (dehydration), have water available to drink at all times while taking SAMSCA. Unless your healthcare provider tells you otherwise, drink when you are thirsty.
- If your healthcare provider tells you to keep taking SAMSCA after you leave a hospital, it is important that you do not stop and re-start SAMSCA on your own. You may need to go back to a hospital to re-start SAMSCA. Talk to your healthcare provider right away if you stop taking SAMSCA for any reason.
- It is important to stay under the care of your healthcare provider while taking SAMSCA and follow their instructions.

2) **Samsca may cause liver problems, including life-threatening liver failure.** Samsca should not be taken for more than 30 days. Tell your doctor right away if you develop or have worsening of any of these signs and symptoms of liver problems:

- Loss of appetite, nausea, vomiting
- Fever, feeling unwell, unusual tiredness
- Itching
- Yellowing of the skin or the whites of the eyes (jaundice)
- Unusual darkening of the urine
- Right upper stomach area pain or discomfort

What is SAMSCA?

SAMSCA is a prescription medicine used to help increase low sodium levels in the blood, in adults with conditions such as heart failure, and certain hormone imbalances. SAMSCA helps raise salt levels in your blood by removing extra body water as urine.

It is not known if SAMSCA is safe or works in children.

Who should not take SAMSCA?

Do not take SAMSCA if:

- the sodium level in your blood must be increased right away.
- you can not replace fluids by drinking or you can not feel if you are thirsty.
- you are dizzy, faint, or your kidneys are not working normally because you have lost too much body fluid.
- you take certain medicines. These medicines could cause you to have too much SAMSCA in your blood:
  - the antibiotic medicines, clarithromycin (Biaxin, Biaxin XL) or telithromycin (Ketek)
  - the antifungal medicines, ketoconazole (Nizoral) or itraconazole (Sporonox)
  - the anti-HIV medicines, ritonavir (Kaletra, Norvir), indinavir (Crixivan), nelfinavir (Viracept), and saquinavir (Invirase)
  - the antidepressant medicine, nefazodone hydrochloride
- your body is not able to make urine. SAMSCA will not help your condition.

What should I tell my healthcare provider before taking SAMSCA?

Tell your healthcare provider about all your medical conditions, including if you:

- have kidney problems and your body can not make urine.
- have liver problems
- can not feel if you are thirsty. See "What is the most important information I should know about SAMSCA?"
- have any allergies. See the end of this Medication Guide for a list of the ingredients in SAMSCA.
- are pregnant or plan to become pregnant. It is not known if SAMSCA will harm your unborn baby.
- are breast-feeding. It is not known if SAMSCA passes into your breast milk. You and your healthcare provider should decide if you will take SAMSCA or breast-feed. You should not do both.
- are taking desmopressin (dDAVP).

Tell your healthcare provider about all the medicines you take, including prescription and non-prescription medicines, vitamins, and herbal supplements.

Using SAMSCA with certain medicines could cause you to have too much SAMSCA in your blood. See "Who should not take SAMSCA?"

SAMSCA may affect the way other medicines work, and other medicines may affect how SAMSCA works.

Know the medicines you take. Keep a list of them and show it to your healthcare provider and pharmacist when you get a new medicine.

How should I take SAMSCA?

- See "What is the most important information I should know about SAMSCA?"
- Take SAMSCA exactly as prescribed by your healthcare provider.
- Take SAMSCA one time each day.
- You can take SAMSCA with or without food.
- Do not drink grapefruit juice during treatment with SAMSCA. This could cause you to have too much SAMSCA in your blood.
- Certain medicines or illnesses may keep you from drinking fluids or may cause you to lose too much body fluid, such as vomiting or diarrhea. If you have these problems, call your healthcare provider right away.
- Do not miss or skip doses of SAMSCA. If you miss a dose, take it as soon as you remember. If it is near the time of the next dose, skip the missed dose. Just take the next dose at your regular time. Do not take 2 doses at the same time.
- **If you take too much SAMSCA, call your healthcare provider right away.** If you take an overdose of SAMSCA, you may need to go to a hospital.
- If your healthcare provider tells you to stop taking SAMSCA, follow their instructions about limiting the amount of fluid you should drink.

What are the possible side effects of SAMSCA?

SAMSCA can cause serious side effects including:

- **See "What is the most important information I should know about SAMSCA?"**
- **Loss of too much body fluid (dehydration)**. Tell your healthcare provider if you:
  - have vomiting or diarrhea, and cannot drink normally.
  - feel dizzy or faint. These may be symptoms that you have lost too much body fluid.

Call your healthcare provider right away, if you have any of these symptoms.

The most common side effects of SAMSCA are:

- thirst
- dry mouth
- weakness
- constipation
- making large amounts of urine and urinating often
- increased blood sugar levels

These are not all the possible side effects of SAMSCA. Talk to your healthcare provider about any side effect that bothers you or that does not go away while taking SAMSCA.

Call your doctor for medical advice about side effects. You may report side effects to FDA at 1-800-FDA-1088.

How should I store SAMSCA?

Store SAMSCA between 59 °F to 86 °F (15 °C to 30 °C).

Keep SAMSCA and all medicines out of the reach of children.

General Information about SAMSCA

Medicines are sometimes prescribed for purposes other than those listed in a Medication Guide. Do not use SAMSCA for a condition for which it was not prescribed. Do not give SAMSCA to other people, even if they have the same symptoms you have. It may harm them.

This Medication Guide summarizes the most important information about SAMSCA. If you would like more information, talk with your healthcare provider. You can ask your healthcare provider or pharmacist for information about SAMSCA that is written for healthcare professionals. For more information about SAMSCA, call 1-877-726-7220 or go to www.samsca.com.

What are the ingredients in SAMSCA?

Active ingredient: tolvaptan.

Inactive ingredients: corn starch, hydroxypropyl cellulose, lactose monohydrate, low-substituted hydroxypropyl cellulose, magnesium stearate and microcrystalline cellulose, and FD&C Blue No. 2 Aluminum Lake as colorant.

SAMSCA is a registered trademark of Otsuka Pharmaceutical Co., Ltd., Tokyo, 101-8535 Japan

Otsuka

Otsuka America Pharmaceutical, Inc.

07US13L-0916

Rev. 04, 2013

This Medication Guide has been approved by the U.S. Food and Drug Administration.

Shown in Product Identification Guide, page 311

PBM Pharmaceuticals, Inc.

200 GARRETT STREET, SUITE O
CHARLOTTESVILLE, VA 22902

Direct Inquiries to:
Donnatal
PH: 1-800-858-4006
Fax: 1-866-234-6455

DONNATAL® TABLETS ℞

Rx Only
REV 0213

DESCRIPTION: DONNATAL® TABLETS:
Each Donnatal® Tablet contains:

Phenobarbital, USP	16.2 mg
Hyoscyamine Sulfate, USP	0.1037 mg
Atropine Sulfate, USP	0.0194 mg
Scopolamine Hydrobromide, USP	0.0065 mg

INACTIVE INGREDIENTS: Anhydrous Lactose, Calcium Stearate, Colloidal Silicon Dioxide, Corn Starch, and Microcrystalline Cellulose

INDICATIONS AND USAGE: Based on a review of this drug by the National Academy of Sciences-National Research Council and/or other information, FDA has classified the following indications as "possibly" effective: For use as adjunctive therapy in the treatment of irritable bowel syndrome (irritable colon, spastic colon, mucous colitis) and acute enterocolitis. May also be useful as adjunctive therapy in the treatment of duodenal ulcer. IT HAS NOT BEEN SHOWN CONCLUSIVELY WHETHER ANTICHOLINERGIC/ANTISPASMODIC DRUGS AID IN THE HEALING OF A DUODENAL ULCER, DECREASE THE RATE OF RECURRENCES OR PREVENT COMPLICATIONS.

CLINICAL PHARMACOLOGY: This drug combination provides natural belladonna alkaloids in a specific, fixed ratio combined with phenobarbital to provide peripheral anticholinergic/antispasmodic action and mild sedation.

CONTRAINDICATIONS: Glaucoma, obstructive uropathy (for example, bladder neck obstruction due to prostatic hypertrophy); obstructive disease of the gastrointestinal tract (as in achalasia, pyloroduodenal stenosis, etc.); paralytic ileus, intestinal atony of the elderly or debilitated patient; unstable cardiovascular status in acute hemorrhage; severe ulcerative colitis especially if complicated by toxic megacolon; myasthenia gravis; hiatal hernia associated with reflux esophagitis.

Donnatal® is contraindicated in patients with known hypersensitivity to any of the ingredients. Phenobarbital is contraindicated in acute intermittent porphyria and in those patients in whom phenobarbital produces restlessness and/or excitement.

WARNINGS: In the presence of a high environmental temperature, heat prostration can occur with belladonna alkaloids (fever and heatstroke due to decreased sweating). Diarrhea may be an early symptom of incomplete intestinal obstruction, especially in patients with ileostomy or colostomy. In this instance, treatment with this drug would be inappropriate and possibly harmful. Donnatal® may produce drowsiness or blurred vision. The patient should be warned, should these occur, not to engage in activities requiring mental alertness, such as operating a motor vehicle or other machinery, and not to perform hazardous work. Phenobarbital may decrease the effect of anticoagulants, and necessitate larger doses of the anticoagulant for optimal effect. When the phenobarbital is discontinued, the dose of the anticoagulant may have to be decreased. Phenobarbital may be habit forming and should not be administered to individuals known to be addiction prone or to those with a history of physical and/or psychological dependence upon drugs. Since barbiturates are metabolized in the liver, they should be used with caution and initial doses should be small in patients with hepatic dysfunction.

PRECAUTIONS: GENERAL: Use with caution in patients with: autonomic neuropathy, hepatic or renal disease, hyperthyroidism, coronary heart disease, congestive heart failure, cardiac arrhythmias, tachycardia, and hypertension. Belladonna alkaloids may produce a delay in gastric emptying (antral stasis) which would complicate the management of gastric ulcer. Do not rely on the use of the drug in the presence of complication of biliary tract disease. Theoretically, with overdosage, a curare-like action may occur.

CARCINOGENESIS, MUTAGENESIS, IMPAIRMENT OF FERTILITY: Long-term studies in animals have not been performed to evaluate carcinogenic potential.

PREGNANCY: PREGNANCY CATEGORY C: Animal reproduction studies have not been conducted with Donnatal®. It is not known whether Donnatal® can cause fetal harm when administered to a pregnant woman or can affect reproduction capacity. Donnatal® should be given to a pregnant woman only if clearly needed.

NURSING MOTHERS It is not known whether this drug is excreted in human milk. Because many drugs are excreted in human milk, caution should be exercised when Donnatal® is administered to a nursing woman.

ADVERSE REACTIONS: Adverse reactions may include xerostomia; urinary hesitancy and retention; blurred vision; tachycardia; palpitation; mydriasis; cycloplegia; increased ocular tension; loss of taste sense; headache; nervousness; drowsiness; weakness; dizziness; insomnia; nausea; vomiting; impotence; suppression of lactation; constipation; bloated feeling; musculoskeletal pain; severe allergic reaction or drug idiosyncrasies, including anaphylaxis, urticaria and other dermal manifestations; and decreased sweating. Acquired hypersensitivity to barbiturates consists chiefly in allergic reactions that occur especially in persons who tend to have asthma, urticaria, angioedema and similar conditions. Hypersensitivity reactions in this category include localized swelling, particularly of the eyelids, cheeks, or lips, and erythematous dermatitis. Rarely, exfoliative dermatitis (e.g. Stevens-Johnson syndrome and toxic epidermal necrolysis) may be caused by phenobarbital and can prove fatal. The skin eruption may be associated with fever, delirium, and marked degenerative changes in the liver and other parenchymatous organs. In a few cases, megaloblastic anemia has been associated with the chronic use of phenobarbital. Elderly patients may react with symptoms of excitement, agitation, drowsiness, and other untoward manifestations to even small doses of the drug. Phenobarbital may produce excitement in some patients, rather than a sedative effect. In patients habituated to barbiturates, abrupt withdrawal may produce delirium or convulsions.

To report SUSPECTED ADVERSE REACTIONS, contact the IriSys Inc at 1-858-623-1520 or the FDA at 1-800-FDA-1088 or www.fda.gov/medwatch.

OVERDOSAGE: The signs and symptoms of overdose are headache, nausea, vomiting, blurred vision, dilated pupils, hot and dry skin, dizziness, dryness of the mouth, difficulty in swallowing, and CNS stimulation. Treatment should consist of gastric lavage, emetics, and activated charcoal. If indicated, parenteral cholinergic agents such as physostigmine or bethanechol chloride should be used.

DOSAGE AND ADMINISTRATION: The dosage of Donnatal® should be adjusted to the needs of the individual patient to assure symptomatic control with a minimum of adverse effects.

Donnatal® Tablets - Adults: One or two Donnatal® tablets three or four times a day according to condition and severity of symptoms.

HOW SUPPLIED: Donnatal® Tablets are supplied as: White, D-shaped tablets debossed "D" on one side and "Donnatal" on the other side.

- Bottles of 100 tablets- NDC 66213-425-10.
- Bottles of 1000 tablets- NDC 66213-425-11.

AVOID FREEZING

Store at 20-25°C (68-77°F) [See USP Controlled Room Temperature]. Protect from light and moisture. Dispense in a tight, light-resistant container as defined in the USP using a child-resistant closure. Use safety closures when dispensing this product unless otherwise directed by a physician or requested by purchaser.

Also available: Donnatal® Elixir, grape and/or mint flavored liquid, in 4 fl oz (118mL) and 1 pint (473mL) bottles

Manufactured For:
PBM Pharmaceuticals, Inc.
Charlottesville, VA 22902
www.donnatal.com

Manufactured By:
IriSys Inc.
San Diego, CA 92121
8181603
Rev 02/13
R0

Shown in Product Identification Guide, page 311

Pfizer Inc.
235 EAST 42ND STREET
NEW YORK, NY 10017–5755

For updates to the product information listed below, please check the Pfizer Web site, http://www.pfizerpro.com, or call (800) 438-1985. For complete product listing, please see the Manufacturers' Index.

For Medical Information, Contact:
(800) 438-1985
24 hours a day, 7 days a week

Distribution:
1855 Shelby Oaks Drive North
Memphis, TN 38134
(901) 387-5200

Customer Service:
(800) 533-4535

Pfizer Companies Include:
Agouron Pharmaceuticals
King Pharmaceuticals Inc.
Pharmaceuticals Inc.
Parke-Davis
Pharmacia & Upjohn
G.D. Searle & Co.
Wyeth Pharmaceuticals – see Wyeth Pharmaceuticals

VIAGRA® ℞
[vI-AG-ra]
(sildenafil citrate)
Tablets

DESCRIPTION
VIAGRA®, an oral therapy for erectile dysfunction, is the citrate salt of sildenafil, a selective inhibitor of cyclic guanosine monophosphate (cGMP)-specific phosphodiesterase type 5 (PDE5).
Sildenafil citrate is designated chemically as 1-[[3-(6,7-dihydro-1-methyl-7-oxo-3-propyl-1*H*-pyrazolo[4,3-*d*]pyrimidin-5-yl)-4-ethoxyphenyl]sulfonyl]-4-methylpiperazine citrate and has the following structural formula:

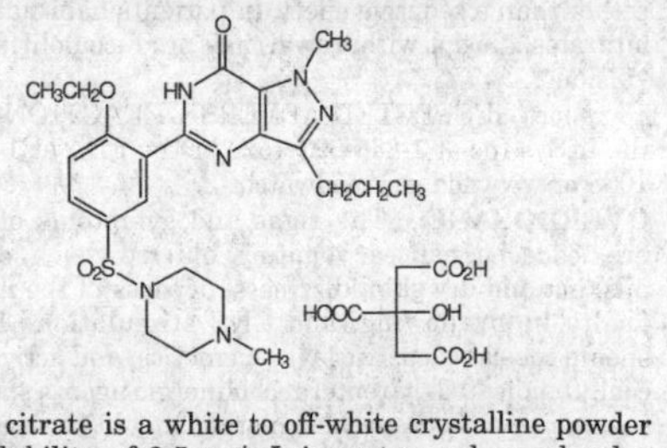

Sildenafil citrate is a white to off-white crystalline powder with a solubility of 3.5 mg/mL in water and a molecular weight of 666.7. VIAGRA (sildenafil citrate) is formulated as blue, film-coated rounded-diamond-shaped tablets equivalent to 25 mg, 50 mg and 100 mg of sildenafil for oral administration. In addition to the active ingredient, sildenafil citrate, each tablet contains the following inactive ingredients: microcrystalline cellulose, anhydrous dibasic calcium phosphate, croscarmellose sodium, magnesium stearate, hypromellose, titanium dioxide, lactose, triacetin, and FD & C Blue #2 aluminum lake.

CLINICAL PHARMACOLOGY
Mechanism of Action
The physiologic mechanism of erection of the penis involves release of nitric oxide (NO) in the corpus cavernosum during sexual stimulation. NO then activates the enzyme guanylate cyclase, which results in increased levels of cyclic guanosine monophosphate (cGMP), producing smooth muscle relaxation in the corpus cavernosum and allowing inflow of blood. Sildenafil has no direct relaxant effect on isolated human corpus cavernosum, but enhances the effect of nitric oxide (NO) by inhibiting phosphodiesterase type 5 (PDE5), which is responsible for degradation of cGMP in the corpus cavernosum. When sexual stimulation causes local release of NO, inhibition of PDE5 by sildenafil causes increased levels of cGMP in the corpus cavernosum, resulting in smooth muscle relaxation and inflow of blood to the corpus cavernosum. Sildenafil at recommended doses has no effect in the absence of sexual stimulation.
Studies *in vitro* have shown that sildenafil is selective for PDE5. Its effect is more potent on PDE5 than on other known phosphodiesterases (10-fold for PDE6, >80-fold for PDE1, >700-fold for PDE2, PDE3, PDE4, PDE7, PDE8, PDE9, PDE10, and PDE11). The approximately 4,000-fold selectivity for PDE5 versus PDE3 is important because PDE3 is involved in control of cardiac contractility. Sildenafil is only about 10-fold as potent for PDE5 compared to PDE6, an enzyme found in the retina which is involved in the phototransduction pathway of the retina. This lower selectivity is thought to be the basis for abnormalities related to color vision observed with higher doses or plasma levels (see **Pharmacodynamics**).
In addition to human corpus cavernosum smooth muscle, PDE5 is also found in lower concentrations in other tissues including platelets, vascular and visceral smooth muscle, and skeletal muscle. The inhibition of PDE5 in these tissues by sildenafil may be the basis for the enhanced platelet antiaggregatory activity of nitric oxide observed *in vitro*, an inhibition of platelet thrombus formation *in vivo* and peripheral arterial-venous dilatation *in vivo*.

Pharmacokinetics and Metabolism
VIAGRA is rapidly absorbed after oral administration, with a mean absolute bioavailability of 41% (range 25–63%). Its pharmacokinetics are dose-proportional over the recommended dose range. It is eliminated predominantly by hepatic metabolism (mainly cytochrome P450 3A4) and is converted to an active metabolite with properties similar to the parent, sildenafil. The concomitant use of potent cytochrome P450 3A4 inhibitors (e.g., erythromycin, ketoconazole, itraconazole) as well as the nonspecific CYP inhibitor, cimetidine, is associated with increased plasma levels of sildenafil (see **DOSAGE AND ADMINISTRATION**). Both sildenafil and the metabolite have terminal half lives of about 4 hours.
Mean sildenafil plasma concentrations measured after the administration of a single oral dose of 100 mg to healthy male volunteers is depicted below:

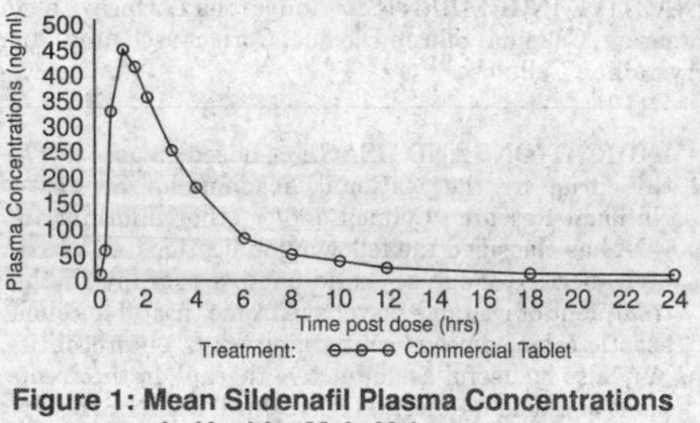

Figure 1: Mean Sildenafil Plasma Concentrations in Healthy Male Volunteers.

Absorption and Distribution
VIAGRA is rapidly absorbed. Maximum observed plasma concentrations are reached within 30 to 120 minutes (median 60 minutes) of oral dosing in the fasted state. When VIAGRA is taken with a high fat meal, the rate of absorption is reduced, with a mean delay in T_{max} of 60 minutes and a mean reduction in C_{max} of 29%. The mean steady state volume of distribution (Vss) for sildenafil is 105 L, indicating distribution into the tissues. Sildenafil and its major circulating N-desmethyl metabolite are both approximately 96% bound to plasma proteins. Protein binding is independent of total drug concentrations.
Based upon measurements of sildenafil in semen of healthy volunteers 90 minutes after dosing, less than 0.001% of the administered dose may appear in the semen of patients.
Metabolism and Excretion
Sildenafil is cleared predominantly by the CYP3A4 (major route) and CYP2C9 (minor route) hepatic microsomal isoenzymes. The major circulating metabolite results from N-desmethylation of sildenafil, and is itself further metabolized. This metabolite has a PDE selectivity profile similar to sildenafil and an *in vitro* potency for PDE5 approximately 50% of the parent drug. Plasma concentrations of this metabolite are approximately 40% of those seen for sildenafil, so that the metabolite accounts for about 20% of sildenafil's pharmacologic effects.
After either oral or intravenous administration, sildenafil is excreted as metabolites predominantly in the feces (approximately 80% of administered oral dose) and to a lesser extent in the urine (approximately 13% of the administered oral dose). Similar values for pharmacokinetic parameters were seen in normal volunteers and in the patient population, using a population pharmacokinetic approach.

Pharmacokinetics in Special Populations
Geriatrics
Healthy elderly volunteers (65 years or over) had a reduced clearance of sildenafil, resulting in approximately 84% and 107% higher plasma AUC values of sildenafil and its active N-desmethyl metabolite, respectively, compared to those seen in healthy younger volunteers (18–45 years). Due to age-differences in plasma protein binding, the corresponding increase in the AUC of free (unbound) sildenafil and its active N-desmethyl metabolite were 45% and 57%, respectively.
Renal Insufficiency
In volunteers with mild (CLcr=50–80 mL/min) and moderate (CLcr=30–49 mL/min) renal impairment, the pharmacokinetics of a single oral dose of VIAGRA (50 mg) were not altered. In volunteers with severe (CLcr=<30 mL/min) renal impairment, sildenafil clearance was reduced, resulting in approximately doubling of AUC and C_{max} compared to age-matched volunteers with no renal impairment.
In addition, N-desmethyl metabolite AUC and Cmax values significantly increased 200% and 79% respectively in subjects with severe renal impairment compared to subjects with normal renal function.
Hepatic Insufficiency
In volunteers with hepatic cirrhosis (Child-Pugh A and B), sildenafil clearance was reduced, resulting in increases in AUC (85%) and C_{max} (47%) compared to age-matched volunteers with no hepatic impairment. The pharmacokinetics of sildenafil in patients with severely impaired hepatic function (Child Pugh class C) have not been studied.
Therefore, age >65, hepatic impairment and severe renal impairment are associated with increased plasma levels of sildenafil. A starting oral dose of 25 mg should be considered in those patients (see **DOSAGE AND ADMINISTRATION**).

Pharmacodynamics
Effects of VIAGRA on Erectile Response
In eight double-blind, placebo-controlled crossover studies of patients with either organic or psychogenic erectile dysfunction, sexual stimulation resulted in improved erections, as assessed by an objective measurement of hardness and duration of erections (RigiScan®), after VIAGRA administration compared with placebo. Most studies assessed the efficacy of VIAGRA approximately 60 minutes post dose. The erectile response, as assessed by RigiScan®, generally increased with increasing sildenafil dose and plasma concentration. The time course of effect was examined in one study, showing an effect for up to 4 hours but the response was diminished compared to 2 hours.
Effects of VIAGRA on Blood Pressure
Single oral doses of sildenafil (100 mg) administered to healthy volunteers produced decreases in sitting blood pressure (mean maximum decrease in systolic/diastolic blood pressure of 8.3/5.3 mmHg). The decrease in sitting blood pressure was most notable approximately 1–2 hours after dosing, and was not different than placebo at 8 hours. Similar effects on blood pressure were noted with 25 mg, 50 mg and 100 mg of VIAGRA, therefore the effects are not related to dose or plasma levels within this dosage range. Larger effects were recorded among patients receiving concomitant nitrates (see **CONTRAINDICATIONS**).

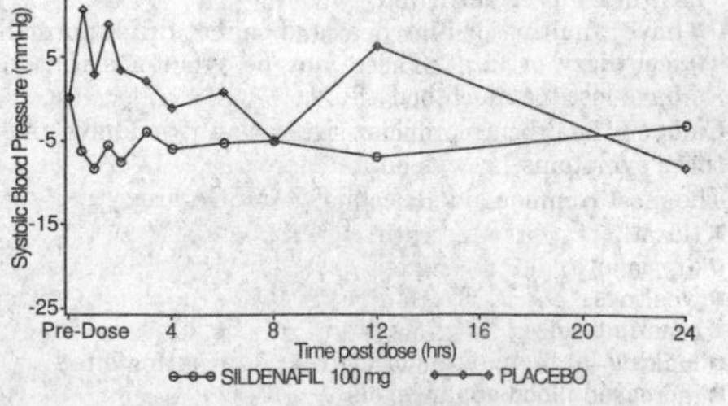

Figure 2: Mean Change from Baseline in Sitting Systolic Blood Pressure, Healthy Volunteers.

Effects of VIAGRA on Cardiac Parameters
Single oral doses of sildenafil up to 100 mg produced no clinically relevant changes in the ECGs of normal male volunteers.
Studies have produced relevant data on the effects of VIAGRA on cardiac output. In one small, open-label, uncontrolled, pilot study, eight patients with stable ischemic heart disease underwent Swan-Ganz catheterization. A total dose of 40 mg sildenafil was administered by four intravenous infusions.
The results from this pilot study are shown in Table 1; the mean resting systolic and diastolic blood pressures decreased by 7% and 10% compared to baseline in these patients. Mean resting values for right atrial pressure, pulmonary artery pressure, pulmonary artery occluded pressure and cardiac output decreased by 28%, 28%, 20% and 7% respectively. Even though this total dosage produced plasma sildenafil concentrations which were approximately 2 to 5 times higher than the mean maximum plasma concentra-

tions following a single oral dose of 100 mg in healthy male volunteers, the hemodynamic response to exercise was preserved in these patients.

[See table 1 above]

TABLE 1. HEMODYNAMIC DATA IN PATIENTS WITH STABLE ISCHEMIC HEART DISEASE AFTER IV ADMINISTRATION OF 40 MG SILDENAFIL

Means ± SD	At rest				After 4 minutes of exercise			
	n	Baseline (B2)	n	Sildenafil (D1)	n	Baseline	n	Sildenafil
PAOP (mmHg)	8	8.1 ± 5.1	8	6.5 ± 4.3	8	36.0 ± 13.7	8	27.8 ± 15.3
Mean PAP (mmHg)	8	16.7 ± 4	8	12.1 ± 3.9	8	39.4 ± 12.9	8	31.7 ± 13.2
Mean RAP (mmHg)	7	5.7 ± 3.7	8	4.1 ± 3.7	-	-	-	-
Systolic SAP (mmHg)	8	150.4 ± 12.4	8	140.6 ± 16.5	8	199.5 ± 37.4	8	187.8 ± 30.0
Diastolic SAP (mmHg)	8	73.6 ± 7.8	8	65.9 ± 10	8	84.6 ± 9.7	8	79.5 ± 9.4
Cardiac output (L/min)	8	5.6 ± 0.9	8	5.2 ± 1.1	8	11.5 ± 2.4	8	10.2 ± 3.5
Heart rate (bpm)	8	67 ± 11.1	8	66.9 ± 12	8	101.9 ± 11.6	8	99.0 ± 20.4

In a double-blind study, 144 patients with erectile dysfunction and chronic stable angina limited by exercise, not receiving chronic oral nitrates, were randomized to a single dose of placebo or VIAGRA 100 mg 1 hour prior to exercise testing. The primary endpoint was time to limiting angina in the evaluable cohort. The mean times (adjusted for baseline) to onset of limiting angina were 423.6 and 403.7 seconds for sildenafil (N=70) and placebo, respectively. These results demonstrated that the effect of VIAGRA on the primary endpoint was statistically non-inferior to placebo.

Effects of VIAGRA on Vision

At single oral doses of 100 mg and 200 mg, transient dose-related impairment of color discrimination (blue/green) was detected using the Farnsworth-Munsell 100-hue test, with peak effects near the time of peak plasma levels. This finding is consistent with the inhibition of PDE6, which is involved in phototransduction in the retina. An evaluation of visual function at doses up to twice the maximum recommended dose revealed no effects of VIAGRA on visual acuity, intraocular pressure, or pupillometry.

Clinical Studies

In clinical studies, VIAGRA was assessed for its effect on the ability of men with erectile dysfunction (ED) to engage in sexual activity and in many cases specifically on the ability to achieve and maintain an erection sufficient for satisfactory sexual activity. VIAGRA was evaluated primarily at doses of 25 mg, 50 mg and 100 mg in 21 randomized, double-blind, placebo-controlled trials of up to 6 months in duration, using a variety of study designs (fixed dose, titration, parallel, crossover). VIAGRA was administered to more than 3,000 patients aged 19 to 87 years, with ED of various etiologies (organic, psychogenic, mixed) with a mean duration of 5 years. VIAGRA demonstrated statistically significant improvement compared to placebo in all 21 studies. The studies that established benefit demonstrated improvements in success rates for sexual intercourse compared with placebo.

The effectiveness of VIAGRA was evaluated in most studies using several assessment instruments. The primary measure in the principal studies was a sexual function questionnaire (the International Index of Erectile Function - IIEF) administered during a 4-week treatment-free run-in period, at baseline, at follow-up visits, and at the end of double-blind, placebo-controlled, at-home treatment. Two of the questions from the IIEF served as primary study endpoints; categorical responses were elicited to questions about (1) the ability to achieve erections sufficient for sexual intercourse and (2) the maintenance of erections after penetration. The patient addressed both questions at the final visit for the last 4 weeks of the study. The possible categorical responses to these questions were (0) no attempted intercourse, (1) never or almost never, (2) a few times, (3) sometimes, (4) most times, and (5) almost always or always. Also collected as part of the IIEF was information about other aspects of sexual function, including information on erectile function, orgasm, desire, satisfaction with intercourse, and overall sexual satisfaction. Sexual function data were also recorded by patients in a daily diary. In addition, patients were asked a global efficacy question and an optional partner questionnaire was administered.

The effect on one of the major end points, maintenance of erections after penetration, is shown in Figure 3, for the pooled results of 5 fixed-dose, dose-response studies of greater than one month duration, showing response according to baseline function. Results with all doses have been pooled, but scores showed greater improvement at the 50 and 100 mg doses than at 25 mg. The pattern of responses was similar for the other principal question, the ability to achieve an erection sufficient for intercourse. The titration studies, in which most patients received 100 mg, showed similar results. Figure 3 shows that regardless of the baseline levels of function, subsequent function in patients treated with VIAGRA was better than that seen in patients treated with placebo. At the same time, on-treatment function was better in treated patients who were less impaired at baseline.

[See figure 3 at top of next column]

The frequency of patients reporting improvement of erections in response to a global question in four of the randomized, double-blind, parallel, placebo-controlled fixed dose studies (1797 patients) of 12 to 24 weeks duration is shown in Figure 4. These patients had erectile dysfunction at baseline that was characterized by median categorical scores of 2 (a few times) on principal IIEF questions. Erectile dysfunction was attributed to organic (58%; generally not characterized, but including diabetes and excluding spinal cord injury), psychogenic (17%), or mixed (24%) etiologies. Sixty-three percent, 74%, and 82% of the patients on 25 mg, 50 mg and 100 mg of VIAGRA, respectively, reported an im-

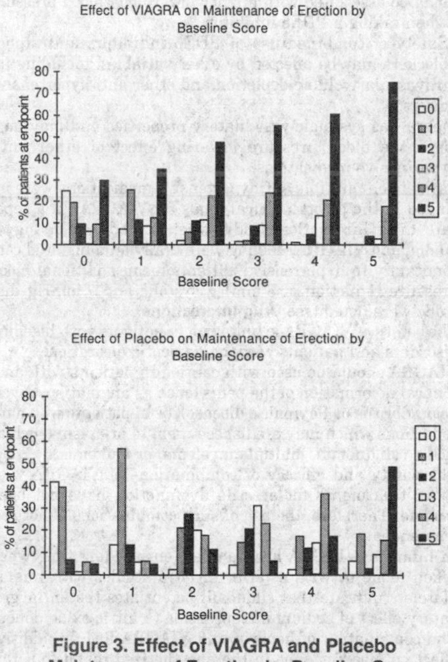

Figure 3. Effect of VIAGRA and Placebo on Maintenance of Erection by Baseline Score.

provement in their erections, compared to 24% on placebo. In the titration studies (n=644) (with most patients eventually receiving 100 mg), results were similar.

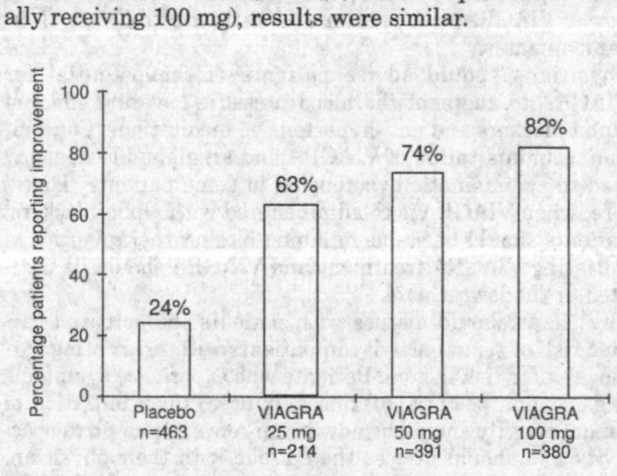

Figure 4. Percentage of Patients Reporting an Improvement in Erections.

The patients in studies had varying degrees of ED. One-third to one-half of the subjects in these studies reported successful intercourse at least once during a 4-week, treatment-free run-in period.

In many of the studies, of both fixed dose and titration designs, daily diaries were kept by patients. In these studies, involving about 1600 patients, analyses of patient diaries showed no effect of VIAGRA on rates of attempted intercourse (about 2 per week), but there was clear treatment-related improvement in sexual function: per patient weekly success rates averaged 1.3 on 50–100 mg of VIAGRA vs 0.4 on placebo; similarly, group mean success rates (total successes divided by total attempts) were about 66% on VIAGRA vs about 20% on placebo.

During 3 to 6 months of double-blind treatment or longer-term (1 year), open-label studies, few patients withdrew from active treatment for any reason, including lack of effectiveness. At the end of the long-term study, 88% of patients reported that VIAGRA improved their erections.

Men with untreated ED had relatively low baseline scores for all aspects of sexual function measured (again using a 5-point scale) in the IIEF. VIAGRA improved these aspects of sexual function: frequency, firmness and maintenance of erections; frequency of orgasm; frequency and level of desire; frequency, satisfaction and enjoyment of intercourse; and overall relationship satisfaction.

One randomized, double-blind, flexible-dose, placebo-controlled study included only patients with erectile dysfunction attributed to complications of diabetes mellitus (n=268). As in the other titration studies, patients were started on 50 mg and allowed to adjust the dose up to 100 mg or down to 25 mg of VIAGRA; all patients, however, were receiving 50 mg or 100 mg at the end of the study. There were highly statistically significant improvements on the two principal IIEF questions (frequency of successful penetration during sexual activity and maintenance of erections after penetration) on VIAGRA compared to placebo. On a global improvement question, 57% of VIAGRA patients reported improved erections versus 10% on placebo. Diary data indicated that on VIAGRA, 48% of intercourse attempts were successful versus 12% on placebo.

One randomized, double-blind, placebo-controlled, crossover, flexible-dose (up to 100 mg) study of patients with erectile dysfunction resulting from spinal cord injury (n=178) was conducted. The changes from baseline in scoring on the two end point questions (frequency of successful penetration during sexual activity and maintenance of erections after penetration) were highly statistically significantly in favor of VIAGRA. On a global improvement question, 83% of patients reported improved erections on VIAGRA versus 12% on placebo. Diary data indicated that on VIAGRA, 59% of attempts at sexual intercourse were successful compared to 13% on placebo.

Across all trials, VIAGRA improved the erections of 43% of radical prostatectomy patients compared to 15% on placebo.

Subgroup analyses of responses to a global improvement question in patients with psychogenic etiology in two fixed-dose studies (total n=179) and two titration studies (total n=149) showed 84% of VIAGRA patients reported improvement in erections compared with 26% of placebo. The changes from baseline in scoring on the two end point questions (frequency of successful penetration during sexual activity and maintenance of erections after penetration) were highly statistically significantly in favor of VIAGRA. Diary data in two of the studies (n=178) showed rates of successful intercourse per attempt of 70% for VIAGRA and 29% for placebo.

A review of population subgroups demonstrated efficacy regardless of baseline severity, etiology, race and age. VIAGRA was effective in a broad range of ED patients, including those with a history of coronary artery disease, hypertension, other cardiac disease, peripheral vascular disease, diabetes mellitus, depression, coronary artery bypass graft (CABG), radical prostatectomy, transurethral resection of the prostate (TURP) and spinal cord injury, and in patients taking antidepressants/antipsychotics and antihypertensives/diuretics.

Analysis of the safety database showed no apparent difference in the side effect profile in patients taking VIAGRA with and without antihypertensive medication. This analysis was performed retrospectively, and was not powered to detect any pre-specified difference in adverse reactions.

INDICATION AND USAGE

VIAGRA is indicated for the treatment of erectile dysfunction.

CONTRAINDICATIONS

Consistent with its known effects on the nitric oxide/cGMP pathway (see **CLINICAL PHARMACOLOGY**), VIAGRA was shown to potentiate the hypotensive effects of nitrates, and its administration to patients who are using organic nitrates, either regularly and/or intermittently, in any form is therefore contraindicated.

After patients have taken VIAGRA, it is unknown when nitrates, if necessary, can be safely administered. Based on the pharmacokinetic profile of a single 100 mg oral dose given to healthy normal volunteers, the plasma levels of sildenafil at 24 hours post dose are approximately 2 ng/mL (compared to peak plasma levels of approximately 440 ng/mL) (see **CLINICAL PHARMACOLOGY: Pharmacokinetics and Metabolism**). In the following patients: age >65, hepatic impairment (e.g., cirrhosis), severe renal impairment (e.g., creatinine clearance <30 mL/min), and concomitant use of potent cytochrome P450 3A4 inhibitors (erythromycin), plasma levels of sildenafil at 24 hours post dose have been found to be 3 to 8 times higher than those seen in healthy volunteers. Although plasma levels of sildenafil at 24 hours post dose are much lower than at peak concentration, it is unknown whether nitrates can be safely coadministered at this time point.

VIAGRA is contraindicated in patients with a known hypersensitivity to any component of the tablet.

WARNINGS

There is a potential for cardiac risk of sexual activity in patients with preexisting cardiovascular disease. Therefore, treatments for erectile dysfunction, including VIAGRA, should not be generally used in men for whom sexual activity is inadvisable because of their underlying cardiovascular status.

VIAGRA has systemic vasodilatory properties that resulted in transient decreases in supine blood pressure in healthy volunteers (mean maximum decrease of 8.4/5.5 mmHg), (see **CLINICAL PHARMACOLOGY: Pharmacodynamics**). While this normally would be expected to be of little consequence in most patients, prior to prescribing VIAGRA, physicians should carefully consider whether their patients with underlying cardiovascular disease could be affected adversely by such vasodilatory effects, especially in combination with sexual activity.

Patients with the following underlying conditions can be particularly sensitive to the actions of vasodilators including VIAGRA – those with left ventricular outflow obstruction (e.g. aortic stenosis, idiopathic hypertrophic subaortic stenosis) and those with severely impaired autonomic control of blood pressure.

There is no controlled clinical data on the safety or efficacy of VIAGRA in the following groups; if prescribed, this should be done with caution.

- Patients who have suffered a myocardial infarction, stroke, or life-threatening arrhythmia within the last 6 months;
- Patients with resting hypotension (BP <90/50) or hypertension (BP >170/110);
- Patients with cardiac failure or coronary artery disease causing unstable angina;
- Patients with retinitis pigmentosa (a minority of these patients have genetic disorders of retinal phosphodiesterases);
- Patients with sickle cell or related anemias.

Prolonged erection greater than 4 hours and priapism (painful erections greater than 6 hours in duration) have been reported infrequently since market approval of VIAGRA. In the event of an erection that persists longer than 4 hours, the patient should seek immediate medical assistance. If priapism is not treated immediately, penile tissue damage and permanent loss of potency could result.

The concomitant administration of the protease inhibitor ritonavir substantially increases serum concentrations of sildenafil (**11-fold increase in AUC**). If VIAGRA is prescribed to patients taking ritonavir, caution should be used. Data from subjects exposed to high systemic levels of sildenafil are limited. Visual disturbances occurred more commonly at higher levels of sildenafil exposure. Decreased blood pressure, syncope, and prolonged erection were reported in some healthy volunteers exposed to high doses of sildenafil (200–800 mg). To decrease the chance of adverse events in patients taking ritonavir, a decrease in sildenafil dosage is recommended (see **Drug Interactions, ADVERSE REACTIONS** and **DOSAGE AND ADMINISTRATION**).

PRECAUTIONS

General

The evaluation of erectile dysfunction should include a determination of potential underlying causes and the identification of appropriate treatment following a complete medical assessment.

Before prescribing VIAGRA, it is important to note the following:

Caution is advised when Phosphodiesterase Type 5 (PDE5) inhibitors are co-administered with alpha-blockers. PDE5 inhibitors, including VIAGRA, and alpha-adrenergic blocking agents are both vasodilators with blood pressure lowering effects. When vasodilators are used in combination, an additive effect on blood pressure may be anticipated. In some patients, concomitant use of these two drug classes can lower blood pressure significantly (see Drug Interactions) leading to symptomatic hypotension (e.g. dizziness, lightheadedness, fainting).

Consideration should be given to the following:

- Patients should be stable on alpha-blocker therapy prior to initiating a PDE5 inhibitor. Patients who demonstrate hemodynamic instability on alpha-blocker therapy alone are at increased risk of symptomatic hypotension with concomitant use of PDE5 inhibitors.
- In those patients who are stable on alpha-blocker therapy, PDE5 inhibitors should be initiated at the lowest dose.
- In those patients already taking an optimized dose of a PDE5 inhibitor, alpha-blocker therapy should be initiated at the lowest dose. Stepwise increase in alpha-blocker dose may be associated with further lowering of blood pressure when taking a PDE5 inhibitor.
- Safety of combined use of PDE5 inhibitors and alpha-blockers may be affected by other variables, including intravascular volume depletion and other anti-hypertensive drugs.

Viagra has systemic vasodilatory properties and may augment the blood pressure lowering effect of other antihypertensive medications.

Patients on multiple antihypertensive medications were included in the pivotal clinical trials for VIAGRA. In a separate drug interaction study, when amlodipine, 5 mg or 10 mg, and VIAGRA, 100 mg were orally administered concomitantly to hypertensive patients mean additional blood pressure reduction of 8 mmHg systolic and 7 mmHg diastolic were noted (see **Drug Interactions**).

The safety of VIAGRA is unknown in patients with bleeding disorders and patients with active peptic ulceration.

VIAGRA should be used with caution in patients with anatomical deformation of the penis (such as angulation, cavernosal fibrosis or Peyronie's disease), or in patients who have conditions which may predispose them to priapism (such as sickle cell anemia, multiple myeloma, or leukemia).

The safety and efficacy of combinations of VIAGRA with other treatments for erectile dysfunction have not been studied. Therefore, the use of such combinations is not recommended.

In humans, VIAGRA has no effect on bleeding time when taken alone or with aspirin. *In vitro* studies with human platelets indicate that sildenafil potentiates the antiaggregatory effect of sodium nitroprusside (a nitric oxide donor). The combination of heparin and VIAGRA had an additive effect on bleeding time in the anesthetized rabbit, but this interaction has not been studied in humans.

Information for Patients

Physicians should discuss with patients the contraindication of VIAGRA with regular and/or intermittent use of organic nitrates.

Physicians should advise patients of the potential for VIAGRA to augment the blood pressure lowering effect of alpha-blockers and anti-hypertensive medications. Concomitant administration of VIAGRA and an alpha-blocker may lead to symptomatic hypotension in some patients. Therefore, when VIAGRA is co-administered with alpha-blockers, patients should be stable on alpha-blocker therapy prior to initiating VIAGRA treatment and VIAGRA should be initiated at the lowest dose.

Physicians should discuss with patients the potential cardiac risk of sexual activity in patients with preexisting cardiovascular risk factors. Patients who experience symptoms (e.g., angina pectoris, dizziness, nausea) upon initiation of sexual activity should be advised to refrain from further activity and should discuss the episode with their physician.

Physicians should advise patients to stop use of all PDE5 inhibitors, including VIAGRA, and seek medical attention in the event of a sudden loss of vision in one or both eyes. Such an event may be a sign of non-arteritic anterior ischemic optic neuropathy (NAION), a cause of decreased vision including permanent loss of vision, that has been reported rarely post-marketing in temporal association with the use of all PDE5 inhibitors. It is not possible to determine whether these events are related directly to the use of PDE5 inhibitors or to other factors. Physicians should also discuss with patients the increased risk of NAION in individuals who have already experienced NAION in one eye, including whether such individuals could be adversely affected by use of vasodilators, such as PDE5 inhibitors (see **POST-MARKETING EXPERIENCE/Special Senses**).

Physicians should advise patients to stop taking PDE5 inhibitors, including VIAGRA, and seek prompt medical attention in the event of sudden decrease or loss of hearing. These events, which may be accompanied by tinnitus and dizziness, have been reported in temporal association to the intake of PDE5 inhibitors, including VIAGRA. It is not possible to determine whether these events are related directly to the use of PDE5 inhibitors or to other factors (see **ADVERSE REACTIONS, CLINICAL TRIALS and POST-MARKETING EXPERIENCE**).

Physicians should warn patients that prolonged erections greater than 4 hours and priapism (painful erections greater than 6 hours in duration) have been reported infrequently since market approval of VIAGRA. In the event of an erection that persists longer than 4 hours, the patient should seek immediate medical assistance. If priapism is not treated immediately, penile tissue damage and permanent loss of potency may result.

Physicians should inform patients not to take VIAGRA with other PDE5 inhibitors including REVATIO. Sildenafil is also marketed as REVATIO for the treatment of pulmonary arterial hypertension. The safety and efficacy of VIAGRA with other PDE5 inhibitors, including REVATIO, have not been studied.

The use of VIAGRA offers no protection against sexually transmitted diseases. Counseling of patients about the protective measures necessary to guard against sexually transmitted diseases, including the Human Immunodeficiency Virus (HIV), may be considered.

Drug Interactions

Effects of Other Drugs on VIAGRA

In vitro studies

Sildenafil metabolism is principally mediated by the cytochrome P450 (CYP) isoforms 3A4 (major route) and 2C9 (minor route). Therefore, inhibitors of these isoenzymes may reduce sildenafil clearance and inducers of these isoenzymes may increase sildenafil clearance.

In vivo studies

Cimetidine (800 mg), a nonspecific CYP inhibitor, caused a 56% increase in plasma sildenafil concentrations when coadministered with VIAGRA (50 mg) to healthy volunteers.

When a single 100 mg dose of VIAGRA was administered with erythromycin, a specific CYP3A4 inhibitor, at steady state (500 mg bid for 5 days), there was a 182% increase in sildenafil systemic exposure (AUC). In addition, in a study performed in healthy male volunteers, coadministration of the HIV protease inhibitor saquinavir, also a CYP3A4 inhibitor, at steady state (1200 mg tid) with VIAGRA (100 mg single dose) resulted in a 140% increase in sildenafil C_{max} and a 210% increase in sildenafil AUC. VIAGRA had no effect on saquinavir pharmacokinetics. Stronger CYP3A4 inhibitors such as ketoconazole or itraconazole would be expected to have still greater effects, and population data from patients in clinical trials did indicate a reduction in sildenafil clearance when it was coadministered with CYP3A4 inhibitors (such as ketoconazole, erythromycin, or cimetidine) (see **DOSAGE AND ADMINISTRATION**).

In another study in healthy male volunteers, coadministration with the HIV protease inhibitor ritonavir, which is a highly potent P450 inhibitor, at steady state (500 mg bid) with VIAGRA (100 mg single dose) resulted in a 300% (4-fold) increase in sildenafil C_{max} and a 1000% (11-fold) increase in sildenafil plasma AUC. At 24 hours the plasma levels of sildenafil were still approximately 200 ng/mL, compared to approximately 5 ng/mL when sildenafil was dosed alone. This is consistent with ritonavir's marked effects on a broad range of P450 substrates. VIAGRA had no effect on ritonavir pharmacokinetics (see **DOSAGE AND ADMINISTRATION**).

Although the interaction between other protease inhibitors and sildenafil has not been studied, their concomitant use is expected to increase sildenafil levels.

In a study of healthy male volunteers, co-administration of sildenafil at steady state (80 mg t.i.d.) with endothelin receptor antagonist bosentan (a moderate inducer of CYP3A4, CYP2C9 and possibly of cytochrome P450 2C19) at steady state (125 mg b.i.d.) resulted in a 63% decrease of sildenafil AUC and a 55% decrease in sildenafil C_{max}. Concomitant administration of strong CYP3A4 inducers, such as rifampin, is expected to cause greater decreases in plasma levels of sildenafil.

Single doses of antacid (magnesium hydroxide/aluminum hydroxide) did not affect the bioavailability of VIAGRA.

Pharmacokinetic data from patients in clinical trials showed no effect on sildenafil pharmacokinetics of CYP2C9 inhibitors (such as tolbutamide, warfarin), CYP2D6 inhibitors (such as selective serotonin reuptake inhibitors, tricyclic antidepressants), thiazide and related diuretics, ACE inhibitors, and calcium channel blockers. The AUC of the active metabolite, N-desmethyl sildenafil, was increased 62% by loop and potassium-sparing diuretics and 102% by nonspecific beta-blockers. These effects on the metabolite are not expected to be of clinical consequence.

Effects of VIAGRA on Other Drugs

In vitro studies

Sildenafil is a weak inhibitor of the cytochrome P450 isoforms 1A2, 2C9, 2C19, 2D6, 2E1 and 3A4 (IC50 >150 μM).

Given sildenafil peak plasma concentrations of approximately 1 μM after recommended doses, it is unlikely that VIAGRA will alter the clearance of substrates of these isoenzymes.

In vivo studies

Three double-blind, placebo-controlled, randomized, two-way crossover studies were conducted to assess the interaction of VIAGRA with doxazosin, an alpha-adrenergic blocking agent.

In the first study, a single oral dose of VIAGRA 100 mg or matching placebo was administered in a 2-period crossover design to 4 generally healthy males with benign prostatic hyperplasia (BPH). Following at least 14 consecutive daily doses of doxazosin, VIAGRA 100 mg or matching placebo was administered simultaneously with doxazosin. Following a review of the data from these first 4 subjects (details provided below), the VIAGRA dose was reduced to 25 mg. Thereafter, 17 subjects were treated with VIAGRA 25 mg or matching placebo in combination with doxazosin 4 mg (15 subjects) or doxazosin 8mg (2 subjects). The mean subject age was 66.5 years.

For the 17 subjects who received VIAGRA 25 mg and matching placebo, the placebo-subtracted mean maximum decreases from baseline (95% CI) in systolic blood pressure were as follows:

Placebo-subtracted mean maximum decrease in systolic blood pressure (mm Hg)	VIAGRA 25 mg
Supine	7.4 (-0.9, 15.7)
Standing	6.0 (-0.8, 12.8)

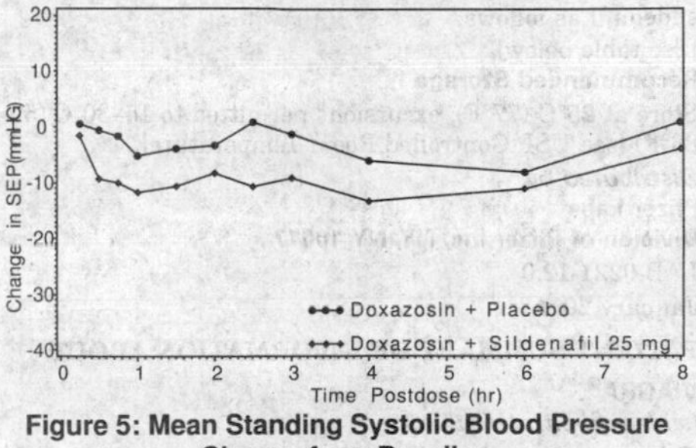

Figure 5: Mean Standing Systolic Blood Pressure Change from Baseline

Blood pressure was measured immediately pre-dose and at 15, 30, 45 minutes, and 1, 1.5, 2, 2.5, 3, 4, 6 and 8 hours after VIAGRA or matching placebo. Outliers were defined as subjects with a standing systolic blood pressure of <85 mmHg or a decrease from baseline in standing systolic blood pressure of >30 mmHg at one or more timepoints. There were no subjects treated with VIAGRA 25 mg who had a standing SBP < 85mmHg. There were three subjects with a decrease from baseline in standing systolic BP >30mmHg following VIAGRA 25 mg, one subject with a decrease from baseline in standing systolic BP > 30 mmHg following placebo and two subjects with a decrease from baseline in standing systolic BP > 30 mmHg following both VIAGRA and placebo. No severe adverse events potentially related to blood pressure effects were reported in this group.

Of the four subjects who received VIAGRA 100 mg in the first part of this study, a severe adverse event related to blood pressure effect was reported in one patient (postural hypotension that began 35 minutes after dosing with VIAGRA with symptoms lasting for 8 hours), and mild adverse events potentially related to blood pressure effects were reported in two others (dizziness, headache and fatigue at 1 hour after dosing; and dizziness, lightheadedness and nausea at 4 hours after dosing). There were no reports of syncope among these patients. For these four subjects, the placebo-subtracted mean maximum decreases from baseline in supine and standing systolic blood pressure were 14.8 mmHg and 21.5 mmHg, respectively. Two of these subjects had a standing SBP < 85mmHg. Both of these subjects were protocol violators, one due to a low baseline standing SBP, and the other due to baseline orthostatic hypotension.

In the second study, a single oral dose of VIAGRA 50 mg or matching placebo was administered in a 2-period crossover design to 20 generally healthy males with BPH. Following at least 14 consecutive days of doxazosin, VIAGRA 50mg or matching placebo was administered simultaneously with doxazosin 4 mg (17 subjects) or with doxazosin 8 mg (3 subjects). The mean subject age in this study was 63.9 years.

Twenty subjects received VIAGRA 50 mg, but only 19 subjects received matching placebo. One patient discontinued the study prematurely due to an adverse event of hypotension following dosing with VIAGRA 50 mg. This patient had been taking minoxidil, a potent vasodilator, during the study.

For the 19 subjects who received both VIAGRA and matching placebo, the placebo-subtracted mean maximum decreases from baseline (95% CI) in systolic blood pressure were as follows:

Placebo-subtracted mean maximum decrease in systolic blood pressure (mm Hg)	VIAGRA 50 mg (95% CI)
Supine	9.08 (5.48, 12.68)
Standing	11.62 (7.34, 15.90)

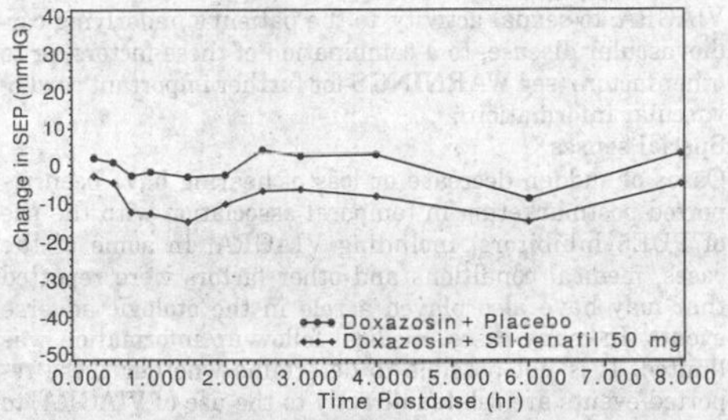

Figure 6: Mean Standing Systolic Blood Pressure Change from Baseline

Blood pressure was measured after administration of VIAGRA at the same times as those specified for the first doxazosin study. There were two subjects who had a standing SBP of < 85 mmHg. In these two subjects, hypotension was reported as a moderately severe adverse event, beginning at approximately 1 hour after administration of VIAGRA 50 mg and resolving after approximately 7.5 hours. There was one subject with a decrease from baseline in standing systolic BP >30mmHg following VIAGRA 50 mg and one subject with a decrease from baseline in standing systolic BP > 30 mmHg following both VIAGRA 50 mg and placebo. There were no severe adverse events potentially related to blood pressure and no episodes of syncope reported in this study.

In the third study, a single oral dose of VIAGRA 100 mg or matching placebo was administered in a 3-period crossover design to 20 generally healthy males with BPH. In dose period 1, subjects were administered open-label doxazosin and a single dose of VIAGRA 50 mg simultaneously, after at least 14 consecutive days of doxazosin. If a subject did not successfully complete this first dosing period, he was discontinued from the study. Subjects who had successfully completed the previous doxazosin interaction study (using VIAGRA 50 mg), including no significant hemodynamic adverse events, were allowed to skip dose period 1. Treatment with doxazosin continued for at least 7 days after dose period 1. Thereafter, VIAGRA 100mg or matching placebo was administered simultaneously with doxazosin 4 mg (14 subjects) or doxazosin 8 mg (6 subjects) in standard crossover fashion. The mean subject age in this study was 66.4 years.

Twenty-five subjects were screened. Two were discontinued after study period 1: one failed to meet pre-dose screening qualifications and the other experienced symptomatic hypotension as a moderately severe adverse event 30 minutes after dosing with open-label VIAGRA 50 mg. Of the twenty subjects who were ultimately assigned to treatment, a total of 13 subjects successfully completed dose period 1, and seven had successfully completed the previous doxazosin study (using VIAGRA 50 mg).

For the 20 subjects who received VIAGRA 100 mg and matching placebo, the placebo-subtracted mean maximum decreases from baseline (95% CI) in systolic blood pressure were as follows:

Placebo-subtracted mean maximum decrease in systolic blood pressure (mm Hg)	VIAGRA 100 mg
Supine	7.9 (4.6, 11.1)
Standing	4.3 (-1.8,10.3)

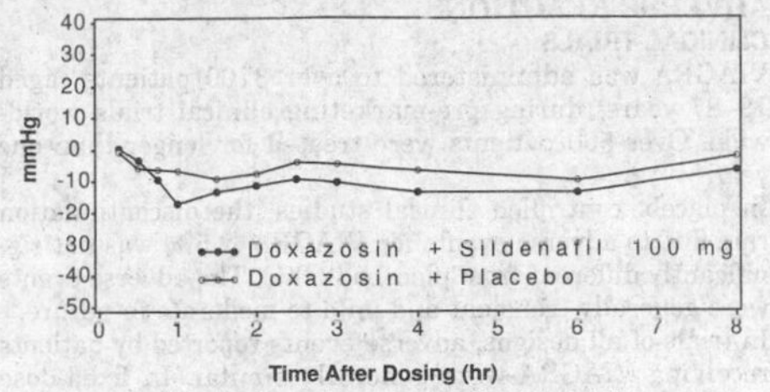

Figure 7: Mean Standing Systolic Blood Pressure Change from Baseline

Blood pressure was measured after administration of VIAGRA at the same times as those specified for the previous doxazosin studies. There were three subjects who had a standing SBP of < 85 mmHg. All three were taking VIAGRA 100 mg, and all three reported mild adverse events at the time of reductions in standing SBP, including vasodilation and lightheadedness. There were four subjects with a decrease from baseline in standing systolic BP >30mmHg following VIAGRA 100 mg, one subject with a decrease from baseline in standing systolic BP > 30 mmHg following placebo and one subject with a decrease from baseline in standing systolic BP > 30 mmHg following both VIAGRA and placebo. While there were no severe adverse events potentially related to blood pressure reported in this study, one subject reported moderate vasodilatation after both VIAGRA 50 mg and 100 mg. There were no episodes of syncope reported in this study.

When VIAGRA 100 mg oral was coadministered with amlodipine, 5 mg or 10 mg oral, to hypertensive patients, the mean additional reduction on supine blood pressure was 8 mmHg systolic and 7 mmHg diastolic.

No significant interactions were shown with tolbutamide (250 mg) or warfarin (40 mg), both of which are metabolized by CYP2C9.

VIAGRA (50 mg) did not potentiate the increase in bleeding time caused by aspirin (150 mg).

VIAGRA (50 mg) did not potentiate the hypotensive effect of alcohol in healthy volunteers with mean maximum blood alcohol levels of 0.08%.

In a study of healthy male volunteers, sildenafil (100 mg) did not affect the steady state pharmacokinetics of the HIV protease inhibitors, saquinavir and ritonavir, both of which are CYP3A4 substrates.

Sildenafil at steady state (80 mg t.i.d.) resulted in a 50% increase in AUC and a 42% increase in C_{max} of bosentan (125 mg b.i.d.).

Carcinogenesis, Mutagenesis, Impairment of Fertility

Sildenafil was not carcinogenic when administered to rats for 24 months at a dose resulting in total systemic drug exposure (AUCs) for unbound sildenafil and its major metabolite of 29- and 42-times, for male and female rats, respectively, the exposures observed in human males given the Maximum Recommended Human Dose (MRHD) of 100 mg. Sildenafil was not carcinogenic when administered to mice for 18–21 months at dosages up to the Maximum Tolerated Dose (MTD) of 10 mg/kg/day, approximately 0.6 times the MRHD on a mg/m^2 basis.

Sildenafil was negative in *in vitro* bacterial and Chinese hamster ovary cell assays to detect mutagenicity, and *in vitro* human lymphocytes and *in vivo* mouse micronucleus assays to detect clastogenicity.

There was no impairment of fertility in rats given sildenafil up to 60 mg/kg/day for 36 days to females and 102 days to males, a dose producing an AUC value of more than 25 times the human male AUC.

There was no effect on sperm motility or morphology after single 100 mg oral doses of VIAGRA in healthy volunteers.

Pregnancy, Nursing Mothers and Pediatric Use

VIAGRA is not indicated for use in newborns, children, or women.

Pregnancy Category B

No evidence of teratogenicity, embryotoxicity or fetotoxicity was observed in rats and rabbits which received up to 200 mg/kg/day during organogenesis. These doses represent, respectively, about 20 and 40 times the MRHD on a mg/m^2 basis in a 50 kg subject. In the rat pre- and postnatal development study, the no observed adverse effect dose was 30 mg/kg/day given for 36 days. In the nonpregnant rat the AUC at this dose was about 20 times human AUC. There are no adequate and well-controlled studies of sildenafil in pregnant women.

Geriatric Use

Healthy elderly volunteers (65 years or over) had a reduced clearance of sildenafil (see **CLINICAL PHARMACOLOGY: Pharmacokinetics in Special Populations**). Since higher plasma levels may increase both the efficacy and incidence of adverse events, a starting dose of 25 mg should be considered (see **DOSAGE AND ADMINISTRATION**).

ADVERSE REACTIONS

CLINICAL TRIALS

VIAGRA was administered to over 3700 patients (aged 19–87 years) during pre-marketing clinical trials worldwide. Over 550 patients were treated for longer than one year.

In placebo-controlled clinical studies, the discontinuation rate due to adverse events for VIAGRA (2.5%) was not significantly different from placebo (2.3%). The adverse events were generally transient and mild to moderate in nature.

In trials of all designs, adverse events reported by patients receiving VIAGRA were generally similar. In fixed-dose studies, the incidence of some adverse events increased with dose. The nature of the adverse events in flexible-dose studies, which more closely reflect the recommended dosage regimen, was similar to that for fixed-dose studies.

When VIAGRA was taken as recommended (on an as-needed basis) in flexible-dose, placebo-controlled clinical trials, the following adverse events were reported:

TABLE 2. ADVERSE EVENTS REPORTED BY ≥2% OF PATIENTS TREATED WITH VIAGRA AND MORE FREQUENT ON DRUG THAN PLACEBO IN PRN FLEXIBLE-DOSE PHASE II/III STUDIES

Adverse Event	Percentage of Patients Reporting Event	
	VIAGRA N=734	PLACEBO N=725
Headache	16%	4%
Flushing	10%	1%
Dyspepsia	7%	2%
Nasal Congestion	4%	2%
Urinary Tract Infection	3%	2%
Abnormal Vision*	3%	0%
Diarrhea	3%	1%
Dizziness	2%	1%
Rash	2%	1%

*Abnormal Vision: Mild and transient, predominantly color tinge to vision, but also increased sensitivity to light or blurred vision. In these studies, only one patient discontinued due to abnormal vision.

Other adverse reactions occurred at a rate of >2%, but equally common on placebo: respiratory tract infection, back pain, flu syndrome, and arthralgia.

In fixed-dose studies, dyspepsia (17%) and abnormal vision (11%) were more common at 100 mg than at lower doses. At doses above the recommended dose range, adverse events were similar to those detailed above but generally were reported more frequently.

The following events occurred in <2% of patients in controlled clinical trials; a causal relationship to VIAGRA is uncertain. Reported events include those with a plausible relation to drug use; omitted are minor events and reports too imprecise to be meaningful:

Body as a whole: face edema, photosensitivity reaction, shock, asthenia, pain, chills, accidental fall, abdominal pain, allergic reaction, chest pain, accidental injury.

Cardiovascular: angina pectoris, AV block, migraine, syncope, tachycardia, palpitation, hypotension, postural hypotension, myocardial ischemia, cerebral thrombosis, cardiac arrest, heart failure, abnormal electrocardiogram, cardiomyopathy.

Digestive: vomiting, glossitis, colitis, dysphagia, gastritis, gastroenteritis, esophagitis, stomatitis, dry mouth, liver function tests abnormal, rectal hemorrhage, gingivitis.

Hemic and Lymphatic: anemia and leukopenia.

Metabolic and Nutritional: thirst, edema, gout, unstable diabetes, hyperglycemia, peripheral edema, hyperuricemia, hypoglycemic reaction, hypernatremia.

Musculoskeletal: arthritis, arthrosis, myalgia, tendon rupture, tenosynovitis, bone pain, myasthenia, synovitis.

Nervous: ataxia, hypertonia, neuralgia, neuropathy, paresthesia, tremor, vertigo, depression, insomnia, somnolence, abnormal dreams, reflexes decreased, hypesthesia.

Respiratory: asthma, dyspnea, laryngitis, pharyngitis, sinusitis, bronchitis, sputum increased, cough increased.

Skin and Appendages: urticaria, herpes simplex, pruritus, sweating, skin ulcer, contact dermatitis, exfoliative dermatitis.

Special Senses: sudden decrease or loss of hearing, mydriasis, conjunctivitis, photophobia, tinnitus, eye pain, ear pain, eye hemorrhage, cataract, dry eyes.

Urogenital: cystitis, nocturia, urinary frequency, breast enlargement, urinary incontinence, abnormal ejaculation, genital edema and anorgasmia.

POST-MARKETING EXPERIENCE

Cardiovascular and cerebrovascular

Serious cardiovascular, cerebrovascular, and vascular events, including myocardial infarction, sudden cardiac death, ventricular arrhythmia, cerebrovascular hemorrhage, transient ischemic attack, hypertension, subarachnoid and intracerebral hemorrhages, and pulmonary hemorrhage have been reported post-marketing in temporal association with the use of VIAGRA. Most, but not all, of these patients had preexisting cardiovascular risk factors. Many of these events were reported to occur during or shortly after sexual activity, and a few were reported to occur shortly after the use of VIAGRA without sexual activity. Others were reported to have occurred hours to days after the use of VIAGRA and sexual activity. It is not possible to determine whether these events are related directly to VIAGRA, to sexual activity, to the patient's underlying cardiovascular disease, to a combination of these factors, or to other factors (see **WARNINGS** for further important cardiovascular information).

Special senses

Cases of sudden decrease or loss of hearing have been reported postmarketing in temporal association with the use of PDE5 inhibitors, including VIAGRA. In some of the cases, medical conditions and other factors were reported that may have also played a role in the otologic adverse events. In many cases, medical follow-up information was limited. It is not possible to determine whether these reported events are related directly to the use of VIAGRA, to the patient's underlying risk factors for hearing loss, a combination of these factors, or to other factors (see **PRECAUTIONS, Information for Patients**).

Other events

Other events reported post-marketing to have been observed in temporal association with VIAGRA and not listed in the clinical trial adverse reactions section above include:

Nervous: seizure, seizure recurrence, anxiety, and transient global amnesia.

Urogenital: prolonged erection, priapism (see **WARNINGS**), and hematuria.

Special Senses: diplopia, temporary vision loss/decreased vision, ocular redness or bloodshot appearance, ocular burning, ocular swelling/pressure, increased intraocular pressure, retinal vascular disease or bleeding, vitreous detachment/traction, paramacular edema and epistaxis.

Non-arteritic anterior ischemic optic neuropathy (NAION), a cause of decreased vision including permanent loss of vision, has been reported rarely post-marketing in temporal association with the use of phosphodiesterase type 5 (PDE5) inhibitors, including VIAGRA. Most, but not all, of these patients had underlying anatomic or vascular risk factors for developing NAION, including but not necessarily limited to: low cup to disc ratio ("crowded disc"), age over 50, diabetes, hypertension, coronary artery disease, hyperlipidemia and smoking. It is not possible to determine whether these events are related directly to the use of PDE5 inhibitors, to the patient's underlying vascular risk factors or anatomical defects, to a combination of these factors, or to other factors (see **PRECAUTIONS/Information for Patients**).

Hemic and Lymphatic: Vaso-occlusive crisis: In a small, prematurely terminated study of REVATIO in patients with pulmonary hypertension (PH) secondary to sickle cell disease, vaso-occlusive crises requiring hospitalization were more commonly reported in patients who received sildenafil than in those randomized to placebo. The clinical relevance of this finding to men treated with VIAGRA for ED is not known.

OVERDOSAGE

In studies with healthy volunteers of single doses up to 800 mg, adverse events were similar to those seen at lower doses but incidence rates and severities were increased.

In cases of overdose, standard supportive measures should be adopted as required. Renal dialysis is not expected to accelerate clearance as sildenafil is highly bound to plasma proteins and it is not eliminated in the urine.

DOSAGE AND ADMINISTRATION

For most patients, the recommended dose is 50 mg taken, as needed, approximately 1 hour before sexual activity. However, VIAGRA may be taken anywhere from 4 hours to 0.5 hour before sexual activity. Based on effectiveness and toleration, the dose may be increased to a maximum recommended dose of 100 mg or decreased to 25 mg. The maximum recommended dosing frequency is once per day.

The following factors are associated with increased plasma levels of sildenafil: age >65 (40% increase in AUC), hepatic impairment (e.g., cirrhosis, 80%), severe renal impairment (creatinine clearance <30 mL/min, 100%), and concomitant use of potent cytochrome P450 3A4 inhibitors [ketoconazole, itraconazole, erythromycin (182%), saquinavir (210%)]. Since higher plasma levels may increase both the efficacy and incidence of adverse events, a starting dose of 25 mg should be considered in these patients.

Ritonavir greatly increased the systemic level of sildenafil in a study of healthy, non-HIV infected volunteers (11-fold increase in AUC, see **Drug Interactions**.) Based on these pharmacokinetic data, it is recommended not to exceed a maximum single dose of 25 mg of VIAGRA in a 48 hour period.

VIAGRA was shown to potentiate the hypotensive effects of nitrates and its administration in patients who use nitric oxide donors or nitrates in any form is therefore contraindicated.

When VIAGRA is co-administered with an alpha-blocker, patients should be stable on alpha-blocker therapy prior to initiating VIAGRA treatment and VIAGRA should be initiated at the lowest dose (see **Drug Interactions**).

HOW SUPPLIED

VIAGRA (sildenafil citrate) is supplied as blue, film-coated, rounded-diamond-shaped tablets containing sildenafil citrate equivalent to the nominally indicated amount of sildenafil as follows:

[See table below]

	25 mg	50 mg	100 mg
Obverse	VGR25	VGR50	VGR100
Reverse	PFIZER	PFIZER	PFIZER
Bottle of 30	NDC-0069-4200-30	NDC-0069-4210-30	NDC-0069-4220-30
Bottle of 100	N/A	NDC-0069-4210-66	NDC-0069-4220-66

Recommended Storage

Store at 25°C (77°F); excursions permitted to 15–30°C (59–86°F) [see USP Controlled Room Temperature].

Distributed by
Pfizer Labs
Division of Pfizer Inc, NY, NY 10017

LAB-0221-12.0
January 2011

PATIENT SUMMARY OF INFORMATION ABOUT

VIAGRA®

(sildenafil citrate) tablets

This summary contains important information about VIAGRA®. It is not meant to take the place of your doctor's instructions. Read this information carefully before you start taking VIAGRA. Ask your doctor or pharmacist if you do not understand any of this information or if you want to know more about VIAGRA.

This medicine can help many men when it is used as prescribed by their doctors. However, VIAGRA is not for everyone. It is intended for use only by men who have a condition called erectile dysfunction. **VIAGRA must never be used by men who are taking medicines that contain nitrates of any kind, at any time. This includes nitroglycerin. If you take VIAGRA with any nitrate medicine your blood pressure could suddenly drop to an unsafe or life threatening level.**

• WHAT IS VIAGRA?

VIAGRA is a pill used to treat erectile dysfunction (impotence) in men. It can help many men who have erectile dysfunction get and keep an erection when they become sexually excited (stimulated).

You will not get an erection just by taking this medicine. VIAGRA helps a man with erectile dysfunction get an erection only when he is sexually excited.

• HOW SEX AFFECTS THE BODY

When a man is sexually excited, the penis rapidly fills with more blood than usual. The penis then expands and hardens. This is called an erection. After the man is done having sex, this extra blood flows out of the penis back into the body. The erection goes away. If an erection lasts for a long time (more than 6 hours), it can permanently damage your penis. You should call a doctor immediately if you ever have a prolonged erection that lasts more than 4 hours.

Some conditions and medicines interfere with this natural erection process. The penis cannot fill with enough blood. The man cannot have an erection. This is called erectile dysfunction if it becomes a frequent problem.

During sex, your heart works harder. Therefore sexual activity may not be advisable for people who have heart problems. Before you start any treatment for erectile dysfunction, ask your doctor if your heart is healthy enough to handle the extra strain of having sex. If you have chest pains, dizziness or nausea during sex, stop having sex and immediately tell your doctor you have had this problem.

• HOW VIAGRA WORKS

VIAGRA enables many men with erectile dysfunction to respond to sexual stimulation. When a man is sexually excited, VIAGRA helps the penis fill with enough blood to cause an erection. After sex is over, the erection goes away.

• VIAGRA IS NOT FOR EVERYONE

As noted above (*How Sex Affects the Body*), ask your doctor if your heart is healthy enough for sexual activity.

If you take any medicines that contain nitrates – either regularly or as needed – you should never take VIAGRA. If you take VIAGRA with any nitrate medicine or recreational drug containing nitrates, your blood pressure could suddenly drop to an unsafe level. You could get dizzy, faint, or even have a heart attack or stroke. Nitrates are found in many prescription medicines that are used to treat angina (chest pain due to heart disease) such as:

- nitroglycerin (sprays, ointments, skin patches or pastes, and tablets that are swallowed or dissolved in the mouth)
- isosorbide mononitrate and isosorbide dinitrate (tablets that are swallowed, chewed, or dissolved in the mouth)

Nitrates are also found in recreational drugs such as amyl nitrate or nitrite ("poppers"). If you are not sure if any of your medicines contain nitrates, or if you do not understand what nitrates are, ask your doctor or pharmacist.

VIAGRA is only for patients with erectile dysfunction. VIAGRA is not for newborns, children, or women. Do not let anyone else take your VIAGRA. VIAGRA must be used only under a doctor's supervision.

• WHAT VIAGRA DOES NOT DO

- VIAGRA does not cure erectile dysfunction. It is a treatment for erectile dysfunction.
- VIAGRA does not protect you or your partner from getting sexually transmitted diseases, including HIV—the virus that causes AIDS.
- VIAGRA is not a hormone or an aphrodisiac.

• WHAT TO TELL YOUR DOCTOR BEFORE YOU BEGIN VIAGRA

Only your doctor can decide if VIAGRA is right for you. VIAGRA can cause mild, temporary lowering of your blood pressure. You will need to have a thorough medical exam to diagnose your erectile dysfunction and to find out if you can safely take VIAGRA alone or with your other medicines. Your doctor should determine if your heart is healthy enough to handle the extra strain of having sex.

Be sure to tell your doctor if you:

- have ever had any heart problems (e.g., angina, chest pain, heart failure, irregular heart beats, heart attack or narrowing of the aortic valve)
- have ever had a stroke
- have low or high blood pressure
- have ever had severe vision loss
- have a rare inherited eye disease called retinitis pigmentosa
- have ever had any kidney problems
- have ever had any liver problems
- have ever had any blood problems, including sickle cell anemia or leukemia
- are allergic to sildenafil or any of the other ingredients of VIAGRA tablets
- have a deformed penis, Peyronie's disease, or ever had an erection that lasted more than 4 hours
- have stomach ulcers or any types of bleeding problems
- are taking any other medicines

• VIAGRA AND OTHER MEDICINES

Some medicines can change the way VIAGRA works. Tell your doctor about **any medicines** you are taking. Do not start or stop taking any medicines before checking with your doctor or pharmacist. This includes prescription and nonprescription medicines or remedies:

- Remember, VIAGRA should never be used with medicines that contain nitrates (see *VIAGRA Is Not for Everyone*).
- If you are taking medicines called alpha-blockers for the treatment of high blood pressure or prostate problems, your blood pressure could suddenly drop. You could get dizzy or faint.
- If you are taking a protease inhibitor, your dose may be adjusted (please see *Finding the Right Dose for You*).
- VIAGRA should not be used with any other medical treatments that cause erections. These treatments include pills, medicines that are injected or inserted into the penis, implants or vacuum pumps.
- VIAGRA contains sildenafil, which is the same medicine found in another drug called REVATIO. REVATIO is used to treat a rare disease called pulmonary arterial hypertension. VIAGRA should not be used with REVATIO.

• FINDING THE RIGHT DOSE FOR YOU

VIAGRA comes in different doses (25 mg, 50 mg and 100 mg). If you do not get the results you expect, talk with your doctor. You and your doctor can determine the dose that works best for you.

- Do not take more VIAGRA than your doctor prescribes.
- If you think you need a larger dose of VIAGRA, check with your doctor.
- VIAGRA should not be taken more than once a day.

Your doctor may prescribe a lower dose of VIAGRA in certain circumstances. For example:

- If you are older than age 65, or have serious liver or kidney problems, your doctor may start you at the lowest dose (25 mg) of VIAGRA.
- If you are taking protease inhibitors, such as for the treatment of HIV, your doctor may recommend a 25 mg dose and may limit you to a maximum single dose of 25 mg of VIAGRA in a 48 hour period.
- If you have prostate problems or high blood pressure for which you take medicines called alpha blockers, your doctor may start you on a lower dose of VIAGRA.

• HOW TO TAKE VIAGRA

Take VIAGRA about one hour before you plan to have sex. Beginning in about 30 minutes and for up to 4 hours, VIAGRA can help you get an erection if you are sexually excited. If you take VIAGRA after a high-fat meal (such as a cheeseburger and french fries), the medicine may take a little longer to start working. VIAGRA can help you get an erection when you are sexually excited. You will not get an erection just by taking the pill.

• POSSIBLE SIDE EFFECTS

Like all medicines, VIAGRA can cause some side effects. These effects are usually mild to moderate and usually don't last longer than a few hours. Some of these side effects are more likely to occur with higher doses. The most common side effects of VIAGRA are headache, flushing of the face, and upset stomach. Less common side effects that may occur are temporary changes in color vision (such as trouble telling the difference between blue and green objects or having a blue color tinge to them), eyes being more sensitive to light, or blurred vision.

In rare instances, men taking PDE5 inhibitors (oral erectile dysfunction medicines, including VIAGRA) reported a sudden decrease or loss of vision in one or both eyes. It is not possible to determine whether these events are related directly to these medicines, to other factors such as high blood pressure or diabetes, or to a combination of these. If you experience sudden decrease or loss of vision, stop taking PDE5 inhibitors, including VIAGRA, and call a doctor right away.

In rare instances, men have reported an erection that lasts many hours. You should call a doctor immediately if you ever have an erection that lasts more than 4 hours. If not treated right away, permanent damage to your penis could occur (see *How Sex Affects the Body*).

Sudden loss or decrease in hearing, sometimes with ringing in the ears and dizziness, has been rarely reported in people taking PDE5 inhibitors, including VIAGRA. It is not possible to determine whether these events are related directly to the PDE5 inhibitors, to other diseases or medications, to other factors, or to a combination of factors. If you experience these symptoms, stop taking VIAGRA and contact a doctor right away.

Heart attack, stroke, irregular heart beats, and death have been reported rarely in men taking VIAGRA. Most, but not all, of these men had heart problems before taking this medicine. It is not possible to determine whether these events were directly related to VIAGRA.

VIAGRA may cause other side effects besides those listed on this sheet. If you want more information or develop any side effects or symptoms you are concerned about, call your doctor.

• ACCIDENTAL OVERDOSE

In case of accidental overdose, call your doctor right away.

• STORING VIAGRA

Keep VIAGRA out of the reach of children. Keep VIAGRA in its original container. Store at 25°C (77°F); excursions permitted to 15–30°C (59–86°F) [see USP Controlled Room Temperature].

• FOR MORE INFORMATION ON VIAGRA

VIAGRA is a prescription medicine used to treat erectile dysfunction. Only your doctor can decide if it is right for you. This sheet is only a summary. If you have any questions or want more information about VIAGRA, talk with your doctor or pharmacist, visit www.viagra.com, or call 1-888-4VIAGRA.

Distributed by
Pfizer Labs
Division of Pfizer Inc, NY, NY 10017
LAB-0220-7.0
January 2010

XELJANZ® ℞

(tofacitinib)
tablets for oral administration

HIGHLIGHTS OF PRESCRIBING INFORMATION
These highlights do not include all the information needed to use XELJANZ safely and effectively. See full prescribing information for XELJANZ.
XELJANZ ® (tofacitinib) tablets for oral administration
Initial U.S. Approval: 2012

WARNING: SERIOUS INFECTIONS AND MALIGNANCY
See* full prescribing information *for complete Boxed Warning.

- **Serious infections leading to hospitalization or death, including tuberculosis and bacterial, invasive fungal, viral, and other opportunistic infections, have occurred in patients receiving XELJANZ. (5.1)**
- **If a serious infection develops, interrupt XELJANZ until the infection is controlled. (5.1)**
- **Prior to starting XELJANZ, perform a test for latent tuberculosis; if it is positive, start treatment for tuberculosis prior to starting XELJANZ. (5.1)**
- **Monitor all patients for active tuberculosis during treatment, even if the initial latent tuberculosis test is negative. (5.1)**
- **Lymphoma and other malignancies have been observed in patients treated with XELJANZ. Epstein Barr Virus- associated post-transplant lymphoproliferative disorder has been observed at an increased rate in renal transplant patients treated with XELJANZ and concomitant immunosuppressive medications. (5.2)**

INDICATIONS AND USAGE

- XELJANZ, an inhibitor of Janus kinases (JAKs), is indicated for the treatment of adult patients with moderately to severely active rheumatoid arthritis who have had an inadequate response or intolerance to methotrexate. It may be used as monotherapy or in combination with methotrexate or other nonbiologic disease-modifying antirheumatic drugs (DMARDs).
- XELJANZ should not be used in combination with biologic DMARDs or potent immunosuppressants such as azathioprine and cyclosporine. (1.1)

DOSAGE AND ADMINISTRATION

Rheumatoid Arthritis (2)
The recommended dose of XELJANZ is 5 mg twice daily. (2)

DOSAGE FORMS AND STRENGTHS

- Tablets: 5 mg (3)

CONTRAINDICATIONS

None (4)

WARNINGS AND PRECAUTIONS

- Serious Infections – Do not administer XELJANZ during an active infection, including localized infections. If a serious infection develops, interrupt XELJANZ until the infection is controlled. (5.1)
- Lymphomas and other malignancies have been reported in patients treated with XELJANZ. (5.2)
- Gastrointestinal Perforations – Use with caution in patients that may be at increased risk. (5.3)
- Laboratory monitoring –Recommended due to potential changes in lymphocytes, neutrophils, hemoglobin, liver enzymes and lipids. (5.4)
- Immunizations –Live vaccines should not be given concurrently with XELJANZ. (5. 5)
- Severe hepatic impairment–Not recommended (5.6)

ADVERSE REACTIONS

The most commonly reported adverse reactions during the first 3 months in controlled clinical trials (occurring in greater than or equal to 2% of patients treated with XELJANZ monotherapy or in combination with DMARDs) were upper respiratory tract infections, headache, diarrhea and nasopharyngitis. (6.1)

To report SUSPECTED ADVERSE REACTIONS, contact Pfizer, Inc at 1-800-438-1985 or FDA at 1-800-FDA-1088 or www.fda.gov/medwatch.

DRUG INTERACTIONS

- Potent inhibitors of Cytochrome P450 3A4 (CYP3A4) (e.g., ketoconazole): Reduce dose to 5 mg once daily. (2.1)
- One or more concomitant medications that result in both moderate inhibition of CYP3A4 and potent inhibition of CYP2C19 (e.g., fluconazole): Reduce dose to 5 mg once daily. (2.1)
- Potent CYP inducers (e.g., rifampin): May result in loss of or reduced clinical response. (2.2)

USE IN SPECIFIC POPULATIONS

Moderate and severe renal impairment and moderate hepatic impairment: Reduce dose to 5 mg once daily. (8.6, 8.7)

See 17 for PATIENT COUNSELING INFORMATION and Medication Guide

Revised: 11/2012

FULL PRESCRIBING INFORMATION: CONTENTS*

*** Sections or subsections omitted from the full prescribing information are not listed**

FULL PRESCRIBING INFORMATION

WARNING: SERIOUS INFECTIONS AND MALIGNANCY

SERIOUS INFECTIONS

Patients treated with XELJANZ are at increased risk for developing serious infections that may lead to hospitalization or death *[see Warnings and Precautions (5.1) and Adverse Reactions (6.1)]*. Most patients who developed these infections were taking concomitant immunosuppressants such as methotrexate or corticosteroids.

If a serious infection develops, interrupt XELJANZ until the infection is controlled.

Reported infections include:

- **Active tuberculosis, which may present with pulmonary or extrapulmonary disease. Patients should be tested for latent tuberculosis before XELJANZ use and during therapy. Treatment for latent infection should be initiated prior to XELJANZ use.**
- **Invasive fungal infections, including cryptococcosis and pneumocystosis. Patients with invasive fungal infections may present with disseminated, rather than localized, disease.**
- **Bacterial, viral, and other infections due to opportunistic pathogens.**

The risks and benefits of treatment with XELJANZ should be carefully considered prior to initiating therapy in patients with chronic or recurrent infection.

Patients should be closely monitored for the development of signs and symptoms of infection during and after treatment with XELJANZ, including the possible development of tuberculosis in patients who tested negative for latent tuberculosis infection prior to initiating therapy *[see Warnings and Precautions (5.1)]*.

MALIGNANCIES

Lymphoma and other malignancies have been observed in patients treated with XELJANZ. Epstein Barr Virus- associated post-transplant lymphoproliferative disorder has been observed at an increased rate in renal transplant patients treated with XELJANZ and concomitant immunosuppressive medications *[see Warnings and Precautions (5.2)]*.

1 INDICATIONS AND USAGE

1.1 Rheumatoid Arthritis

- XELJANZ (tofacitinib) is indicated for the treatment of adult patients with moderately to severely active rheumatoid arthritis who have had an inadequate response or intolerance to methotrexate. It may be used as monotherapy or in combination with methotrexate or other nonbiologic disease-modifying antirheumatic drugs (DMARDs).
- XELJANZ should not be used in combination with biologic DMARDs or with potent immunosuppressants such as azathioprine and cyclosporine.

2 DOSAGE AND ADMINISTRATION

XELJANZ is given orally with or without food.

2.1 Rheumatoid Arthritis

XELJANZ may be used as monotherapy or in combination with methotrexate or other nonbiologic disease modifying antirheumatic drugs (DMARDs). The recommended dose of XELJANZ is 5 mg twice daily.

- Dose interruption is recommended for management of lymphopenia, neutropenia and anemia *[see Dosage and Administration (2.3), Warnings and Precautions (5.4), and Adverse Reactions (6.1)]*.
- XELJANZ dosage should be reduced to 5 mg once daily in patients:
  - with moderate or severe renal insufficiency
  - with moderate hepatic impairment
  - receiving potent inhibitors of Cytochrome P450 3A4 (CYP3A4) (e.g., ketoconazole)
  - receiving one or more concomitant medications that result in both moderate inhibition of CYP3A4 and potent inhibition of CYP2C19 (e.g., fluconazole).

2.2 General Considerations for Administration

- XELJANZ should not be used in patients with severe hepatic impairment.
- It is recommended that XELJANZ not be initiated in patients with a lymphocyte count less than 500 cells/mm^3, an absolute neutrophil count (ANC) less than 1000 cells/mm^3, or who have hemoglobin levels less than 9 g/dL.
- Coadministration of XELJANZ with potent inducers of CYP3A4 (e.g., rifampin) may result in loss of or reduced clinical response to XELJANZ.

2.3 Dosage Modifications

XELJANZ treatment should be interrupted if a patient develops a serious infection until the infection is controlled.

Table 1: Dose Adjustments for Lymphopenia

Low Lymphocyte Count *[see Warnings and Precautions (5.4)]*

Lab Value (cells/mm^3)	Recommendation
Lymphocyte count greater than or equal to 500	Maintain dose
Lymphocyte count less than 500 (Confirmed by repeat testing)	Discontinue XELJANZ

Table 2: Dose Adjustments for Neutropenia

Low ANC *[see Warnings and Precautions (5.4)]*

Lab Value (cells/mm^3)	Recommendation
ANC greater than 1000	Maintain dose
ANC 500–1000	For persistent decreases in this range, interrupt dosing until ANC is greater than 1000 When ANC is greater than 1000, resume XELJANZ 5 mg twice daily
ANC less than 500 (Confirmed by repeat testing)	Discontinue XELJANZ

Table 3: Dose Adjustments for Anemia

Low Hemoglobin Value *[see Warnings and Precautions (5.4)]*

Lab Value (g/dL)	Recommendation
Less than or equal to 2 g/dL decrease and greater than or equal to 9.0 g/dL	Maintain dose
Greater than 2 g/dL decrease or less than 8.0 g/dL (Confirmed by repeat testing)	Interrupt the administration of XELJANZ until hemoglobin values have normalized

3 DOSAGE FORMS AND STRENGTHS

XELJANZ is provided as 5 mg tofacitinib (equivalent to 8 mg tofacitinib citrate) tablets: White, round, immediate-release film-coated tablets, debossed with "Pfizer" on one side, and "JKI 5" on the other side.

4 CONTRAINDICATIONS

None

5 WARNINGS AND PRECAUTIONS

5.1 Serious Infections

Serious and sometimes fatal infections due to bacterial, mycobacterial, invasive fungal, viral, or other opportunistic pathogens have been reported in rheumatoid arthritis patients receiving XELJANZ. The most common serious infections reported with XELJANZ included pneumonia, cellulitis, herpes zoster and urinary tract infection *[see Adverse Reactions (6.1)]*. Among opportunistic infections, tuberculosis and other mycobacterial infections, cryptococcus, esophageal candidiasis, pneumocystosis, multidermatomal herpes zoster, cytomegalovirus, and BK virus were reported with XELJANZ. Some patients have presented with disseminated rather than localized disease, and were often taking concomitant immunomodulating agents such as methotrexate or corticosteroids.

Other serious infections that were not reported in clinical studies may also occur (e.g., histoplasmosis, coccidioidomycosis, and listeriosis).

XELJANZ should not be initiated in patients with an active infection, including localized infections. The risks and benefits of treatment should be considered prior to initiating XELJANZ in patients:

- with chronic or recurrent infection
- who have been exposed to tuberculosis
- with a history of a serious or an opportunistic infection
- who have resided or traveled in areas of endemic tuberculosis or endemic mycoses; or
- with underlying conditions that may predispose them to infection.

Patients should be closely monitored for the development of signs and symptoms of infection during and after treatment with XELJANZ. XELJANZ should be interrupted if a patient develops a serious infection, an opportunistic infection, or sepsis. A patient who develops a new infection during treatment with XELJANZ should undergo prompt and complete diagnostic testing appropriate for an immunocompromised patient; appropriate antimicrobial therapy should be initiated, and the patient should be closely monitored.

Tuberculosis

Patients should be evaluated and tested for latent or active infection prior to administration of XELJANZ.

Anti-tuberculosis therapy should also be considered prior to administration of XELJANZ in patients with a past history of latent or active tuberculosis in whom an adequate course of treatment cannot be confirmed, and for patients with a negative test for latent tuberculosis but who have risk factors for tuberculosis infection. Consultation with a physician with expertise in the treatment of tuberculosis is recommended to aid in the decision about whether initiating anti-tuberculosis therapy is appropriate for an individual patient.

Patients should be closely monitored for the development of signs and symptoms of tuberculosis, including patients who tested negative for latent tuberculosis infection prior to initiating therapy.

Patients with latent tuberculosis should be treated with standard antimycobacterial therapy before administering XELJANZ.

Viral Reactivation

Viral reactivation, including cases of herpes virus reactivation (e.g., herpes zoster), were observed in clinical studies with XELJANZ. The impact of XELJANZ on chronic viral hepatitis reactivation is unknown. Patients who screened positive for hepatitis B or C were excluded from clinical trials.

5.2 Malignancy and Lymphoproliferative Disorder

Consider the risks and benefits of XELJANZ treatment prior to initiating therapy in patients with a known malignancy other than a successfully treated non-melanoma skin cancer (NMSC) or when considering continuing XELJANZ in patients who develop a malignancy. Malignancies were observed in clinical studies of XELJANZ *[see Adverse Reactions (6.1)]*.

In the seven controlled rheumatoid arthritis clinical studies, 11 solid cancers and one lymphoma were diagnosed in 3328 patients receiving XELJANZ with or without DMARD, compared to 0 solid cancers and 0 lymphomas in 809 patients in the placebo with or without DMARD group during the first 12 months of exposure. Lymphomas and solid cancers have also been observed in the long-term extension studies in rheumatoid arthritis patients treated with XELJANZ.

In Phase 2B, controlled dose-ranging trials in *de-novo* renal transplant patients, all of whom received induction therapy with basiliximab, high dose corticosteroids, and mycophenolic acid products, Epstein Barr Virus-associated post-transplant lymphoproliferative disorder was observed in 5 out of 218 patients treated with XELJANZ (2.3%) compared to 0 out of 111 patients treated with cyclosporine.

5.3 Gastrointestinal Perforations

Events of gastrointestinal perforation have been reported in clinical studies with XELJANZ in rheumatoid arthritis patients, although the role of JAK inhibition in these events is not known.

XELJANZ should be used with caution in patients who may be at increased risk for gastrointestinal perforation (e.g., patients with a history of diverticulitis). Patients presenting with new onset abdominal symptoms should be evaluated promptly for early identification of gastrointestinal perforation *[see Adverse Reactions (6.1)]*.

5.4 Laboratory Parameters

Lymphocytes

Treatment with XELJANZ was associated with initial lymphocytosis at one month of exposure followed by a gradual decrease in mean lymphocyte counts below the baseline of approximately 10% during 12 months of therapy. Lymphocyte counts less than 500 cells/mm^3 were associated with an increased incidence of treated and serious infections.

Avoid initiation of XELJANZ treatment in patients with a low lymphocyte count (i.e., less than 500 cells/mm^3). In patients who develop a confirmed absolute lymphocyte count less than 500 cells/mm^3 treatment with XELJANZ is not recommended.

Monitor lymphocyte counts at baseline and every 3 months thereafter. For recommended modifications based on lymphocyte counts *see Dosage and Administration (2.3)*.

Neutrophils

Treatment with XELJANZ was associated with an increased incidence of neutropenia (less than 2000 cells/mm^3) compared to placebo.

Avoid initiation of XELJANZ treatment in patients with a low neutrophil count (i.e., ANC less than 1000 cells/mm^3). For patients who develop a persistent ANC of 500–1000 cells/mm^3, interrupt XELJANZ dosing until ANC is greater than or equal to 1000 cells/mm^3. In patients who develop an ANC less than 500 cells/mm^3, treatment with XELJANZ is not recommended.

Monitor neutrophil counts at baseline and after 4–8 weeks of treatment and every 3 months thereafter. For recommended modifications based on ANC results *see Dosage and Administration (2.3)*.

Hemoglobin

Avoid initiation of XELJANZ treatment in patients with a low hemoglobin level (i.e. less than 9 g/dL). Treatment with XELJANZ should be interrupted in patients who develop hemoglobin levels less than 8 g/dL or whose hemoglobin level drops greater than 2 g/dL on treatment.

Monitor hemoglobin at baseline and after 4–8 weeks of treatment and every 3 months thereafter. For recommended modifications based on hemoglobin results *see Dosage and Administration (2.3)*.

Liver Enzymes

Treatment with XELJANZ was associated with an increased incidence of liver enzyme elevation compared to placebo. Most of these abnormalities occurred in studies with background DMARD (primarily methotrexate) therapy.

Routine monitoring of liver tests and prompt investigation of the causes of liver enzyme elevations is recommended to identify potential cases of drug-induced liver injury. If drug-induced liver injury is suspected, the administration of XELJANZ should be interrupted until this diagnosis has been excluded.

Lipids

Treatment with XELJANZ was associated with increases in lipid parameters including total cholesterol, low-density lipoprotein (LDL) cholesterol, and high-density lipoprotein (HDL) cholesterol. Maximum effects were generally observed within 6 weeks. The effect of these lipid parameter elevations on cardiovascular morbidity and mortality has not been determined.

Assessment of lipid parameters should be performed approximately 4–8 weeks following initiation of XELJANZ therapy.

Manage patients according to clinical guidelines [e.g., National Cholesterol Educational Program (NCEP)] for the management of hyperlipidemia.

5.5 Vaccinations

No data are available on the response to vaccination or on the secondary transmission of infection by live vaccines to patients receiving XELJANZ. Live vaccines should not be given concurrently with XELJANZ.

Update immunizations in agreement with current immunization guidelines prior to initiating XELJANZ therapy.

5.6 Hepatic Impairment

Treatment with XELJANZ is not recommended in patients with severe hepatic impairment *[see Adverse Reactions (6.1) and Use in Specific Populations (8.6)]*.

6 ADVERSE REACTIONS

Because clinical studies are conducted under widely varying conditions, adverse reaction rates observed in the clinical studies of a drug cannot be directly compared to rates in the clinical studies of another drug and may not predict the rates observed in a broader patient population in clinical practice.

The following data includes two Phase 2 and five Phase 3 double-blind, controlled, multicenter trials. In these trials, patients were randomized to doses of XELJANZ 5 mg twice daily (292 patients) and 10 mg twice daily (306 patients) monotherapy, XELJANZ 5 mg twice daily (1044 patients) and 10 mg twice daily (1043 patients) in combination with DMARDs (including methotrexate) and placebo (809 patients). All seven protocols included provisions for patients taking placebo to receive treatment with XELJANZ at Month 3 or Month 6 either by patient response (based on uncontrolled disease activity) or by design, so that adverse events cannot always be unambiguously attributed to a given treatment. Therefore some analyses that follow include patients who changed treatment by design or by patient response from placebo to XELJANZ in both the placebo and XELJANZ group of a given interval. Comparisons between placebo and XELJANZ were based on the first 3 months of exposure, and comparisons between XELJANZ 5 mg twice daily and XELJANZ 10 mg twice daily were based on the first 12 months of exposure.

The long-term safety population includes all patients who participated in a double-blind, controlled trial (including earlier development phase studies) and then participated in one of two long-term safety studies. The design of the long-term safety studies allowed for modification of XELJANZ doses according to clinical judgment. This limits the interpretation of the long-term safety data with respect to dose.

6.1 Clinical Trial Experience

The most common serious adverse reactions were serious infections *[see Warnings and Precautions (5.1)]*.

The proportion of patients who discontinued treatment due to any adverse reaction during the 0 to 3 months exposure in the double-blind, placebo-controlled trials was 4% for patients taking XELJANZ and 3% for placebo-treated patients.

Overall Infections

In the seven controlled trials, during the 0 to 3 months exposure, the overall frequency of infections was 20% and 22% in the 5 mg twice daily and 10 mg twice daily groups, respectively, and 18% in the placebo group.

The most commonly reported infections with XELJANZ were upper respiratory tract infections, nasopharyngitis, and urinary tract infections (4%, 3%, and 2% of patients, respectively).

Serious Infections

In the seven controlled trials, during the 0 to 3 months exposure, serious infections were reported in 1 patient (0.5 events per 100 patient-years) who received placebo and 11 patients (1.7 events per 100 patient-years) who received XELJANZ 5 mg or 10 mg twice daily. The rate difference between treatment groups (and the corresponding 95% confidence interval) was 1.1 (-0.4, 2.5) events per 100 patient-years for the combined 5 mg twice daily and 10 mg twice daily XELJANZ group minus placebo.

In the seven controlled trials, during the 0 to 12 months exposure, serious infections were reported in 34 patients (2.7 events per 100 patient-years) who received 5 mg twice daily of XELJANZ and 33 patients (2.7 events per 100 patient-years) who received 10 mg twice daily of XELJANZ. The rate difference between XELJANZ doses (and the corresponding 95% confidence interval) was -0.1 (-1.3, 1.2) events per 100 patient-years for 10 mg twice daily XELJANZ minus 5 mg twice daily XELJANZ.

The most common serious infections included pneumonia, cellulitis, herpes zoster, and urinary tract infection *[see Warnings and Precautions (5.1)]*.

Tuberculosis

In the seven controlled trials, during the 0 to 3 months exposure, tuberculosis was not reported in patients who received placebo, 5 mg twice daily of XELJANZ, or 10 mg twice daily of XELJANZ.

In the seven controlled trials, during the 0 to 12 months exposure, tuberculosis was reported in 0 patients who received 5 mg twice daily of XELJANZ and 6 patients (0.5 events per 100 patient-years) who received 10 mg twice daily of XELJANZ. The rate difference between XELJANZ doses (and the corresponding 95% confidence interval) was 0.5 (0.1, 0.9) events per 100 patient-years for 10 mg twice daily XELJANZ minus 5 mg twice daily XELJANZ.

Cases of disseminated tuberculosis were also reported. The median XELJANZ exposure prior to diagnosis of tuberculosis was 10 months (range from 152 to 960 days) *[see Warnings and Precautions (5.1)]*.

Opportunistic Infections (excluding tuberculosis)

In the seven controlled trials, during the 0 to 3 months exposure, opportunistic infections were not reported in patients who received placebo, 5 mg twice daily of XELJANZ, or 10 mg twice daily of XELJANZ.

In the seven controlled trials, during the 0 to 12 months exposure, opportunistic infections were reported in 4 patients (0.3 events per 100 patient-years) who received 5 mg twice daily of XELJANZ and 4 patients (0.3 events per 100 patient-years) who received 10 mg twice daily of XELJANZ. The rate difference between XELJANZ doses (and the corresponding 95% confidence interval) was 0 (-0.5, 0.5) events per 100 patient-years for 10 mg twice daily XELJANZ minus 5 mg twice daily XELJANZ.

The median XELJANZ exposure prior to diagnosis of an opportunistic infection was 8 months (range from 41 to 698 days) *[see Warnings and Precautions (5.1)]*.

Malignancy

In the seven controlled trials, during the 0 to 3 months exposure, malignancies excluding NMSC were reported in 0 patients who received placebo and 2 patients (0.3 events per 100 patient-years) who received either XELJANZ 5 mg or 10 mg twice daily. The rate difference between treatment groups (and the corresponding 95% confidence interval) was 0.3 (-0.1, 0.7) events per 100 patient-years for the combined 5 mg and 10 mg twice daily XELJANZ group minus placebo.

In the seven controlled trials, during the 0 to 12 months exposure, malignancies excluding NMSC were reported in 5 patients (0.4 events per 100 patient-years) who received 5 mg twice daily of XELJANZ and 7 patients (0.6 events per 100 patient-years) who received 10 mg twice daily of XELJANZ. The rate difference between XELJANZ doses (and the corresponding 95% confidence interval) was 0.2 (-0.4, 0.7) events per 100 patient-years for 10 mg twice daily XELJANZ minus 5 mg twice daily XELJANZ. One of these malignancies was a case of lymphoma that occurred during the 0 to 12 month period in a patient treated with XELJANZ 10 mg twice daily.

The most common types of malignancy, including malignancies observed during the long-term extension, were lung and breast cancer, followed by gastric, colorectal, renal cell, prostate cancer, lymphoma, and malignant melanoma *[see Warnings and Precautions (5.2)]*.

Laboratory Tests

Lymphocytes

In the controlled clinical trials, confirmed decreases in lymphocyte counts below 500 cells/mm^3 occurred in 0.04% of patients for the 5 mg twice daily and 10 mg twice daily XELJANZ groups combined during the first 3 months of exposure.

Confirmed lymphocyte counts less than 500 cells/mm^3 were associated with an increased incidence of treated and serious infections *[see Warnings and Precautions (5.4)]*.

Neutrophils

In the controlled clinical trials, confirmed decreases in ANC below 1000 cells/mm^3 occurred in 0.07% of patients for the 5 mg twice daily and 10 mg twice daily XELJANZ groups combined during the first 3 months of exposure.

There were no confirmed decreases in ANC below 500 cells/mm^3 observed in any treatment group.

There was no clear relationship between neutropenia and the occurrence of serious infections.

In the long-term safety population, the pattern and incidence of confirmed decreases in ANC remained consistent with what was seen in the controlled clinical trials *[see Warnings and Precautions (5.4)]*.

Liver Enzyme Tests

Confirmed increases in liver enzymes greater than 3 times the upper limit of normal (3× ULN) were observed in patients treated with XELJANZ. In patients experiencing liver enzyme elevation, modification of treatment regimen, such as reduction in the dose of concomitant DMARD, interruption of XELJANZ, or reduction in XELJANZ dose, resulted in decrease or normalization of liver enzymes.

In the controlled monotherapy trials (0–3 months), no differences in the incidence of ALT or AST elevations were observed between the placebo, and XELJANZ 5 mg, and 10 mg twice daily groups.

In the controlled background DMARD trials (0–3 months), ALT elevations greater than 3× ULN were observed in 1.0%, 1.3% and 1.2% of patients receiving placebo, 5 mg, and 10 mg twice daily, respectively. In these trials, AST elevations greater than 3× ULN were observed in 0.6%, 0.5% and 0.4% of patients receiving placebo, 5 mg, and 10 mg twice daily, respectively.

One case of drug-induced liver injury was reported in a patient treated with XELJANZ 10 mg twice daily for approximately 2.5 months. The patient developed symptomatic elevations of AST and ALT greater than 3× ULN and bilirubin elevations greater than 2× ULN, which required hospitalizations and a liver biopsy.

Lipids

In the controlled clinical trials, dose-related elevations in lipid parameters (total cholesterol, LDL cholesterol, HDL cholesterol, triglycerides) were observed at one month of exposure and remained stable thereafter. Changes in lipid parameters during the first 3 months of exposure in the controlled clinical trials are summarized below:

- Mean LDL cholesterol increased by 15% in the XELJANZ 5 mg twice daily arm and 19% in the XELJANZ 10 mg twice daily arm.
- Mean HDL cholesterol increased by 10% in the XELJANZ 5 mg twice daily arm and 12% in the XELJANZ 10 mg twice daily arm.
- Mean LDL/HDL ratios were essentially unchanged in XELJANZ-treated patients.

In a controlled clinical trial, elevations in LDL cholesterol and ApoB decreased to pretreatment levels in response to statin therapy.

In the long-term safety population, elevations in lipid parameters remained consistent with what was seen in the controlled clinical trials.

Serum Creatinine

In the controlled clinical trials, dose-related elevations in serum creatinine were observed with XELJANZ treatment. The mean increase in serum creatinine was <0.1 mg/dL in the 12-month pooled safety analysis; however with increasing duration of exposure in the long-term extensions, up to 2% of patients were discontinued from XELJANZ treatment due to the protocol-specified discontinuation criterion of an increase in creatinine by more than 50% of baseline. The clinical significance of the observed serum creatinine elevations is unknown.

Other Adverse Reactions

Adverse reactions occurring in 2% or more of patients on 5 mg twice daily or 10 mg twice daily XELJANZ and at least 1% greater than that observed in patients on placebo with or without DMARD are summarized in Table 4.

Table 4: Adverse Reactions Occurring in at Least 2% or More of Patients on 5 or 10 mg Twice Daily XELJANZ With or Without DMARD (0–3 months) and at Least 1% Greater Than That Observed in Patients on Placebo

Preferred Term	XELJANZ 5 mg Twice Daily N = 1336 (%)	XELJANZ 10 mg Twice Daily N = 1349 (%)	Placebo N = 809 (%)
Diarrhea	4.0	2.9	2.3
Nasopharyngitis	3.8	2.8	2.8
Upper respiratory tract infection	4.5	3.8	3.3
Headache	4.3	3.4	2.1
Hypertension	1.6	2.3	1.1

N reflects randomized and treated patients from the seven clinical trials

Other adverse reactions occurring in controlled and open-label extension studies included:

Blood and lymphatic system disorders: Anemia
Metabolism and nutrition disorders: Dehydration
Psychiatric disorders: Insomnia
Nervous system disorders: Paresthesia
Respiratory, thoracic and mediastinal disorders: Dyspnea, cough, sinus congestion
Gastrointestinal disorders: Abdominal pain, dyspepsia, vomiting, gastritis, nausea
Hepatobiliary disorders: Hepatic steatosis
Skin and subcutaneous tissue disorders: Rash, erythema, pruritus
Musculoskeletal, connective tissue and bone disorders: Musculoskeletal pain, arthralgia, tendonitis, joint swelling
General disorders and administration site conditions: Pyrexia, fatigue, peripheral edema

7 DRUG INTERACTIONS

7.1 Potent CYP3A4 Inhibitors

Tofacitinib exposure is increased when XELJANZ is coadministered with potent inhibitors of cytochrome P450 (CYP) 3A4 (e.g., ketoconazole) *[see Dosage and Administration (2.1) and Figure 3]*.

7.2 Moderate CYP3A4 and Potent CYP2C19 Inhibitors

Tofacitinib exposure is increased when XELJANZ is coadministered with medications that result in both moderate inhibition of CYP3A4 and potent inhibition of CYP2C19 (e.g., fluconazole) *[see Dosage and Administration (2.1) and Figure 3]*.

7.3 Potent CYP3A4 Inducers

Tofacitinib exposure is decreased when XELJANZ is coadministered with potent CYP3A4 inducers (e.g., rifampin) *[see Dosage and Administration (2.1) and Figure 3]*.

7.4 Immunosuppressive Drugs

There is a risk of added immunosuppression when XELJANZ is coadministered with potent immunosuppressive drugs (e.g., azathioprine, tacrolimus, cyclosporine). Combined use of multiple-dose XELJANZ with potent immunosuppressives has not been studied in rheumatoid arthritis.

8 USE IN SPECIFIC POPULATIONS

8.1 Pregnancy

Teratogenic effects:

Pregnancy Category C. There are no adequate and well-controlled studies in pregnant women. XELJANZ should be used during pregnancy only if the potential benefit justifies the potential risk to the fetus. Tofacitinib has been shown to be fetocidal and teratogenic in rats and rabbits when given at exposures 146 times and 13 times, respectively, the maximum recommended human dose (MRHD).

In a rat embryofetal developmental study, tofacitinib was teratogenic at exposure levels approximately 146 times the MRHD (on an AUC basis at oral doses of 100 mg/kg/day). Teratogenic effects consisted of external and soft tissue malformations of anasarca and membranous ventricular septal defects, respectively, and skeletal malformations or variations (absent cervical arch; bent femur, fibula, humerus, radius, scapula, tibia, and ulna; sternoschisis; absent rib; misshapen femur; branched rib; fused rib; fused sternebra; and hemicentric thoracic centrum). In addition, there was an increase in post-implantation loss, consisting of early and late resorptions, resulting in a reduced number of viable fetuses. Mean fetal body weight was reduced. No developmental toxicity was observed in rats at exposure levels approximately 58 times the MRHD (on an AUC basis at oral doses of 30 mg/kg/day). In the rabbit embryofetal developmental study, tofacitinib was teratogenic at exposure levels approximately 13 times the MRHD (on an AUC basis at oral doses of 30 mg/kg/day) in the absence of signs of maternal toxicity. Teratogenic effects included thoracogastroschisis, omphalocele, membranous ventricular septal defects, and cranial/skeletal malformations (microstomia, microphthalmia), mid-line and tail defects. In addition, there was an increase in post-implantation loss associated with late resorptions. No developmental toxicity was observed in rabbits at exposure levels approximately 3 times the MRHD (on an AUC basis at oral doses of 10 mg/kg/day).

Nonteratogenic effects:

In a peri- and postnatal rat study, there were reductions in live litter size, postnatal survival, and pup body weights at exposure levels approximately 73 times the MRHD (on an AUC basis at oral doses of 50 mg/kg/day). There was no effect on behavioral and learning assessments, sexual maturation or the ability of the F1 generation rats to mate and produce viable F2 generation fetuses in rats at exposure levels approximately 17 times the MRHD (on an AUC basis at oral doses of 10 mg/kg/day).

Pregnancy Registry: To monitor the outcomes of pregnant women exposed to XELJANZ, a pregnancy registry has been established. Physicians are encouraged to register patients and pregnant women are encouraged to register themselves by calling 1-877-311-8972.

8.3 Nursing Mothers

Tofacitinib was secreted in milk of lactating rats. It is not known whether tofacitinib is excreted in human milk. Because many drugs are excreted in human milk and because of the potential for serious adverse reactions in nursing infants from tofacitinib, a decision should be made whether to discontinue nursing or to discontinue the drug, taking into account the importance of the drug for the mother.

8.4 Pediatric Use

The safety and effectiveness of XELJANZ in pediatric patients have not been established.

8.5 Geriatric Use

Of the 3315 patients who enrolled in Studies I to V, a total of 505 rheumatoid arthritis patients were 65 years of age and older, including 71 patients 75 years and older. The frequency of serious infection among XELJANZ-treated subjects 65 years of age and older was higher than among those under the age of 65. As there is a higher incidence of infections in the elderly population in general, caution should be used when treating the elderly.

8.6 Hepatic Impairment

No dose adjustment is required in patients with mild hepatic impairment. XELJANZ dose should be reduced to 5 mg once daily in patients with moderate hepatic impairment. The safety and efficacy of XELJANZ have not been studied in patients with severe hepatic impairment or in patients with positive hepatitis B virus or hepatitis C virus serology *[see Dosage and Administration (2.1) and Warnings and Precautions (5.6)]*.

8.7 Renal Impairment

No dose adjustment is required in patients with mild renal impairment. XELJANZ dose should be reduced to 5 mg once daily in patients with moderate and severe renal impairment *[see Dosage and Administration (2.1)]*. In clinical trials, XELJANZ was not evaluated in rheumatoid arthritis patients with baseline creatinine clearance values (estimated by the Cockroft-Gault equation) less than 40 mL/min.

10 OVERDOSAGE

Signs, Symptoms, and Laboratory Findings of Acute Overdosage in Humans

There is no experience with overdose of XELJANZ.

Treatment or Management of Overdose

Pharmacokinetic data up to and including a single dose of 100 mg in healthy volunteers indicate that more than 95% of the administered dose is expected to be eliminated within 24 hours.

There is no specific antidote for overdose with XELJANZ. In case of an overdose, it is recommended that the patient be monitored for signs and symptoms of adverse reactions. Patients who develop adverse reactions should receive appropriate treatment.

11 DESCRIPTION

XELJANZ is the citrate salt of tofacitinib, a JAK inhibitor. Tofacitinib citrate is a white to off-white powder with the following chemical name: (3R,4R)-4-methyl-3-(methyl-7H-pyrrolo [2,3-d]pyrimidin-4-ylamino)-β-oxo-1-piperidinepropanenitrile, 2-hydroxy-1,2,3-propanetricarboxylate (1:1) . It is freely soluble in water.

Tofacitinib citrate has a molecular weight of 504.5 Daltons (or 312.4 Daltons as the tofacitinib free base) and a molecular formula of $C_{16}H_{20}N_6O \bullet C_6H_8O_7$. The chemical structure of tofacitinib citrate is:

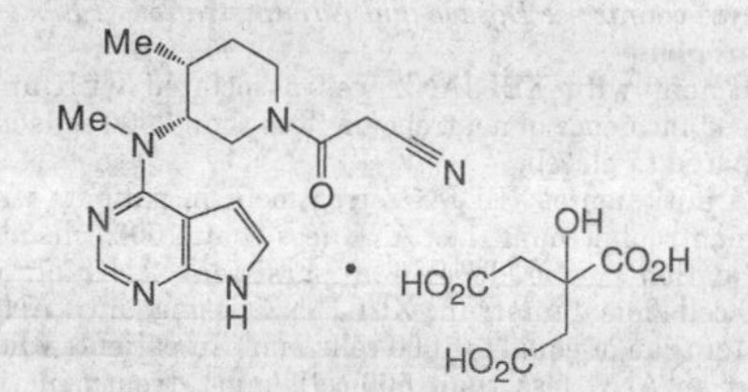

XELJANZ is supplied for oral administration as 5 mg tofacitinib (equivalent to 8 mg tofacitinib citrate) white round, immediate-release film-coated tablet. Each tablet of XELJANZ contains the appropriate amount of XELJANZ as a citrate salt and the following inactive ingredients: microcrystalline cellulose, lactose monohydrate, croscarmellose sodium, magnesium stearate, HPMC 2910/Hypromellose 6cP, titanium dioxide, macrogol/PEG3350, and triacetin.

12 CLINICAL PHARMACOLOGY

12.1 Mechanism of Action

Tofacitinib is a Janus kinase (JAK) inhibitor. JAKs are intracellular enzymes which transmit signals arising from cytokine or growth factor-receptor interactions on the cellular membrane to influence cellular processes of hematopoiesis and immune cell function. Within the signaling pathway, JAKs phosphorylate and activate Signal Transducers and Activators of Transcription (STATs) which modulate intracellular activity including gene expression. Tofacitinib modulates the signaling pathway at the point of JAKs, preventing the phosphorylation and activation of STATs. JAK enzymes transmit cytokine signaling through pairing of JAKs (e.g., JAK1/JAK3, JAK1/JAK2, JAK1/TyK2, JAK2/JAK2). Tofacitinib inhibited the *in vitro* activities of JAK1/JAK2, JAK1/JAK3, and JAK2/JAK2 combinations with IC_{50} of 406, 56, and 1377 nM, respectively. However, the relevance of specific JAK combinations to therapeutic effectiveness is not known.

12.2 Pharmacodynamics

Treatment with XELJANZ was associated with dose-dependent reductions of circulating CD16/56+ natural killer cells, with estimated maximum reductions occurring at approximately 8–10 weeks after initiation of therapy. These changes generally resolved within 2–6 weeks after discontinuation of treatment. Treatment with XELJANZ was associated with dose-dependent increases in B cell counts. Changes in circulating T-lymphocyte counts and T-lymphocyte subsets (CD3+, CD4+ and CD8+) were small and inconsistent. The clinical significance of these changes is unknown.

Total serum IgG, IgM, and IgA levels after 6-month dosing in patients with rheumatoid arthritis were lower than placebo; however, changes were small and not dose-dependent. After treatment with XELJANZ in patients with rheumatoid arthritis, rapid decreases in serum C-reactive protein

Figure 1: Impact of Intrinsic Factors on Tofacitinib Pharmacokinetics

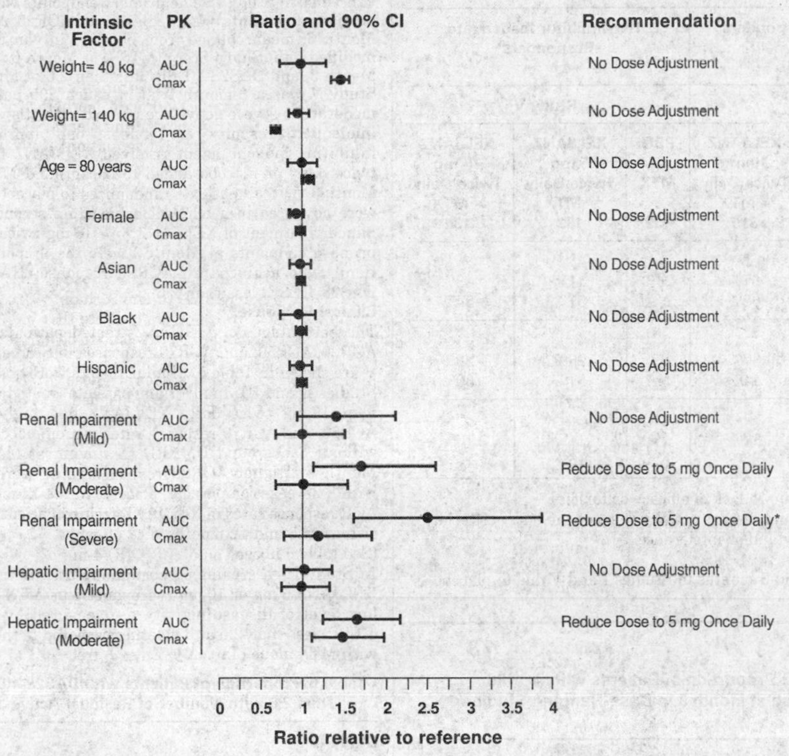

* Supplemental doses are not necessary in patients after dialysis

Figure 3. Impact of Other Drugs on PK of XELJANZ

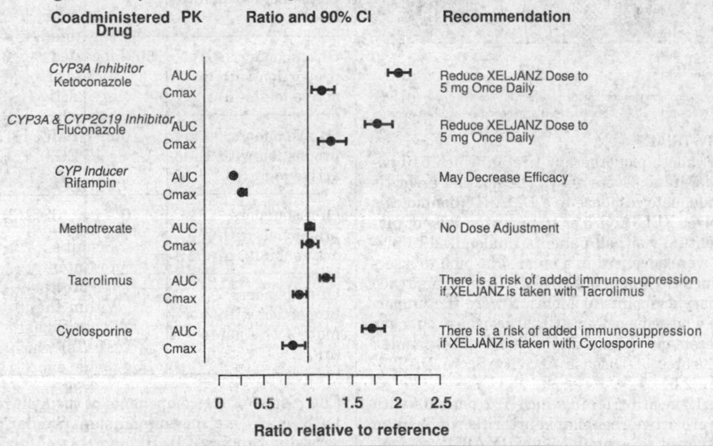

(CRP) were observed and maintained throughout dosing. Changes in CRP observed with XELJANZ treatment do not reverse fully within 2 weeks after discontinuation, indicating a longer duration of pharmacodynamic activity compared to the pharmacokinetic half-life.

12.3 Pharmacokinetics

Following oral administration of XELJANZ, peak plasma concentrations are reached within 0.5–1 hour, elimination half-life is ~3 hours and a dose-proportional increase in systemic exposure was observed in the therapeutic dose range. Steady state concentrations are achieved in 24–48 hours with negligible accumulation after twice daily administration.

Absorption

The absolute oral bioavailability of tofacitinib is 74%. Coadministration of XELJANZ with a high-fat meal resulted in no changes in AUC while C_{max} was reduced by 32%. In clinical trials, XELJANZ was administered without regard to meals.

Distribution

After intravenous administration, the volume of distribution is 87 L. The protein binding of tofacitinib is ~40%. Tofacitinib binds predominantly to albumin and does not appear to bind to α1-acid glycoprotein. Tofacitinib distributes equally between red blood cells and plasma.

Metabolism and Elimination

Clearance mechanisms for tofacitinib are approximately 70% hepatic metabolism and 30% renal excretion of the parent drug. The metabolism of tofacitinib is primarily mediated by CYP3A4 with minor contribution from CYP2C19. In a human radiolabeled study, more than 65% of the total circulating radioactivity was accounted for by unchanged tofacitinib, with the remaining 35% attributed to 8 metabolites, each accounting for less than 8% of total radioactivity. The pharmacologic activity of tofacitinib is attributed to the parent molecule.

Pharmacokinetics in Rheumatoid Arthritis Patients

Population PK analysis in rheumatoid arthritis patients indicated no clinically relevant change in tofacitinib exposure, after accounting for differences in renal function (i.e., creatinine clearance) between patients, based on age, weight, gender and race (Figure 1). An approximately linear relationship between body weight and volume of distribution was observed, resulting in higher peak (C_{max}) and lower trough (C_{min}) concentrations in lighter patients. However, this difference is not considered to be clinically relevant. The between-subject variability (% coefficient of variation) in AUC of tofacitinib is estimated to be approximately 27%.

Specific Populations

The effect of renal and hepatic impairment and other intrinsic factors on the pharmacokinetics of tofacitinib is shown in Figure 1.

[See figure 1 above]

Reference values for weight, age, gender, and race comparisons are 70 kg, 55 years, male, and White, respectively; Reference groups for renal and hepatic impairment data are subjects with normal renal and hepatic function.

Drug Interactions

Potential for XELJANZ to Influence the PK of Other Drugs

In vitro studies indicate that tofacitinib does not significantly inhibit or induce the activity of the major human drug-metabolizing CYPs (CYP1A2, CYP2B6, CYP2C8, CYP2C9, CYP2C19, CYP2D6, and CYP3A4) at concentrations exceeding 185 times the steady state C_{max} of a 5 mg twice daily dose. These *in vitro* results were confirmed by a human drug interaction study showing no changes in the PK of midazolam, a highly sensitive CYP3A4 substrate, when coadministered with XELJANZ.

In rheumatoid arthritis patients, the oral clearance of tofacitinib does not vary with time, indicating that tofacitinib does not normalize CYP enzyme activity in rheumatoid arthritis patients. Therefore, coadministration with XELJANZ is not expected to result in clinically relevant increases in the metabolism of CYP substrates in rheumatoid arthritis patients.

In vitro data indicate that the potential for tofacitinib to inhibit transporters such as P-glycoprotein, organic anionic or cationic transporters at therapeutic concentrations is low.

Dosing recommendations for coadministered drugs following administration with XELJANZ are shown in Figure 2.

Figure 2. Impact of XELJANZ on PK of Other Drugs

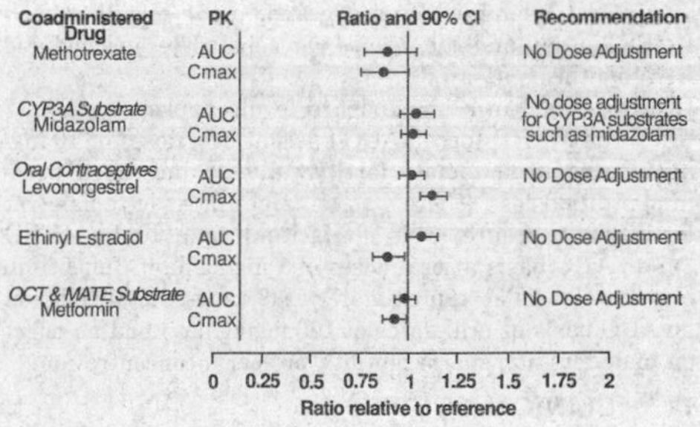

Note: Reference group is administration of concomitant medication alone; OCT = Organic Cationic Transporter; MATE = Multidrug and Toxic Compound Extrusion

Potential for Other Drugs to Influence the PK of Tofacitinib

Since tofacitinib is metabolized by CYP3A4, interaction with drugs that inhibit or induce CYP3A4 is likely. Inhibitors of CYP2C19 alone or P-glycoprotein are unlikely to substantially alter the PK of tofacitinib. Dosing recommendations for XELJANZ for administration with CYP inhibitors or inducers are shown in Figure 3.

[See figure 3 above]

Note: Reference group is administration of tofacitinib alone

13 NONCLINICAL TOXICOLOGY

13.1 Carcinogenesis, Mutagenesis, Impairment of Fertility

In a 39-week toxicology study in monkeys, tofacitinib at exposure levels approximately 6 times the MRHD (on an AUC basis at oral doses of 5 mg/kg twice daily) produced lymphomas. No lymphomas were observed in this study at exposure levels 1 times the MRHD (on an AUC basis at oral doses of 1 mg/kg twice daily).

The carcinogenic potential of tofacitinib was assessed in 6-month rasH2 transgenic mouse carcinogenicity and 2-year rat carcinogenicity studies. Tofacitinib, at exposure levels approximately 34 times the MRHD (on an AUC basis at oral doses of 200 mg/kg/day) was not carcinogenic in mice.

In the 24-month oral carcinogenicity study in Sprague-Dawley rats, tofacitinib caused benign Leydig cell tumors, hibernomas (malignancy of brown adipose tissue), and benign thymomas at doses greater than or equal to 30 mg/kg/

Table 5: Proportion of Patients with an ACR Response

	Percent of Patients								
	Monotherapy in Nonbiologic or Biologic DMARD Inadequate Responders*			MTX Inadequate Responders†			TNF Inhibitor Inadequate Responders‡		
	Study I			Study IV			Study V		
N§	PBO 122	XELJANZ 5 mg Twice Daily 243	XELJANZ 10 mg Twice Daily 245	PBO + MTX 160	XELJANZ 5 mg Twice Daily + MTX 321	XELJANZ 10 mg Twice Daily + MTX 316	PBO + MTX 132	XELJANZ 5 mg Twice Daily + MTX 133	XELJANZ 10 mg Twice Daily + MTX 134
ACR20									
Month 3	26%	59%	65%	27%	55%	67%	24%	41%	48%
Month 6	NA¶	69%	70%	25%	50%	62%	NA	51%	54%
ACR50									
Month 3	12%	31%	36%	8%	29%	37%	8%	26%	28%
Month 6	NA	42%	46%	9%	32%	44%	NA	37%	30%
ACR70									
Month 3	6%	15%	20%	3%	11%	17%	2%	14%	10%
Month 6	NA	22%	29%	1%	14%	23%	NA	16%	16%

* Inadequate response to at least one DMARD (biologic or nonbiologic) due to lack of efficacy or toxicity.
† Inadequate response to MTX defined as the presence of sufficient residual disease activity to meet the entry criteria.
‡ Inadequate response to a least one TNF inhibitor due to lack of efficacy and/or intolerance.
§ N is number of randomized and treated patients.
¶ NA Not applicable, as data for placebo treatment is not available beyond 3 months in Studies I and V due to placebo advancement.

day (approximately 42 times the exposure levels at the MRHD on an AUC basis). The relevance of benign Leydig cell tumors to human risk is not known.

Tofacitinib was not mutagenic in the bacterial reverse mutation assay. It was positive for clastogenicity in the *in vitro* chromosome aberration assay with human lymphocytes in the presence of metabolic enzymes, but negative in the absence of metabolic enzymes. Tofacitinib was negative in the *in vivo* rat micronucleus assay and in the *in vitro* CHO-HGPRT assay and the *in vivo* rat hepatocyte unscheduled DNA synthesis assay.

In rats, tofacitinib at exposure levels approximately 17 times the MRHD (on an AUC basis at oral doses of 10 mg/kg/day) reduced female fertility due to increased post-implantation loss. There was no impairment of female rat fertility at exposure levels of tofacitinib equal to the MRHD (on an AUC basis at oral doses of 1 mg/kg/day). Tofacitinib exposure levels at approximately 133 times the MRHD (on an AUC basis at oral doses of 100 mg/kg/day) had no effect on male fertility, sperm motility, or sperm concentration.

14 CLINICAL STUDIES

The XELJANZ clinical development program included two dose-ranging trials and five confirmatory trials.

DOSE-RANGING TRIALS

Dose selection for XELJANZ was based on two pivotal dose-ranging trials.

Dose-Ranging Study 1 was a 6-month monotherapy trial in 384 patients with active rheumatoid arthritis who had an inadequate response to a DMARD. Patients who previously received adalimumab therapy were excluded. Patients were randomized to 1 of 7 monotherapy treatments: XELJANZ 1, 3, 5, 10 or 15 mg twice daily, adalimumab 40 mg subcutaneously every other week for 10 weeks followed by XELJANZ 5 mg twice daily for 3 months, or placebo.

Dose-Ranging Study 2 was a 6-month trial in which 507 patients with active rheumatoid arthritis who had an inadequate response to MTX alone received one of 6 dose regimens of XELJANZ (20 mg once daily; 1, 3, 5, 10 or 15 mg twice daily), or placebo added to background MTX.

The results of XELJANZ-treated patients achieving ACR20 responses in Studies 1 and 2 are shown in Figure 4. Although a dose-response relationship was observed in Study 1, the proportion of patients with an ACR20 response did not clearly differ between the 10 mg and 15 mg doses. Furthermore, there was a smaller proportion of patients who responded to adalimumab monotherapy compared to those treated with XELJANZ doses 3 mg twice daily and greater. In Study 2, a smaller proportion of patients achieved an ACR20 response in the placebo and XELJANZ 1 mg groups compared to patients treated with the other XELJANZ doses. However, there was no difference in the proportion of responders among patients treated with XELJANZ 3, 5, 10, 15 mg twice daily or 20 mg once daily doses.

Figure 4: Proportion of Patients with ACR20 Response at Month 3 in Dose-Ranging Studies 1 and 2

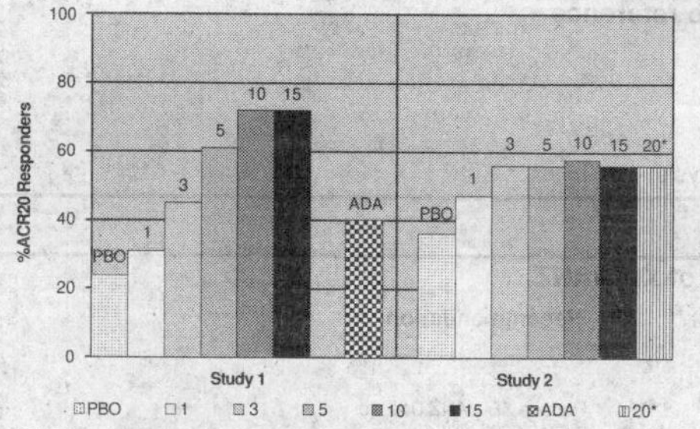

* XELJANZ twice daily dosing in mg, except for 20 mg which is once daily dosing in mg. PBO is placebo; ADA is adalimumab 40 mg subcutaneous injection every other week.

CONFIRMATORY TRIALS

Study I was a 6-month monotherapy trial in which 610 patients with moderate to severe active rheumatoid arthritis who had an inadequate response to a DMARD (nonbiologic or biologic) received XELJANZ 5 or 10 mg twice daily or placebo. At the Month 3 visit, all patients randomized to placebo treatment were advanced in a blinded fashion to a second predetermined treatment of XELJANZ 5 or 10 mg twice daily. The primary endpoints at Month 3 were the proportion of patients who achieved an ACR20 response, changes in Health Assessment Questionnaire – Disability Index (HAQ-DI), and rates of Disease Activity Score DAS28-4(ESR) less than 2.6.

Study II was a 12-month trial in which 792 patients with moderate to severe active rheumatoid arthritis who had an inadequate response to a nonbiologic DMARD received XELJANZ 5 or 10 mg twice daily or placebo added to background DMARD treatment (excluding potent immunosuppressive treatments such as azathioprine or cyclosporine). At the Month 3 visit, nonresponding patients were advanced in a blinded fashion to a second predetermined treatment of XELJANZ 5 or 10 mg twice daily. At the end of Month 6, all placebo patients were advanced to their second predetermined treatment in a blinded fashion. The primary endpoints were the proportion of patients who achieved an ACR20 response at Month 6, changes in HAQ-DI at Month 3, and rates of DAS28-4(ESR) less than 2.6 at Month 6.

Study III was a 12-month trial in 717 patients with moderate to severe active rheumatoid arthritis who had an inadequate response to MTX. Patients received XELJANZ 5 or 10 mg twice daily, adalimumab 40 mg subcutaneously every other week, or placebo added to background MTX. Placebo patients were advanced as in Study II. The primary endpoints were the proportion of patients who achieved an ACR20 response at Month 6, HAQ-DI at Month 3, and DAS28-4(ESR) less than 2.6 at Month 6.

Study IV is an ongoing 2-year trial with a planned analysis at 1 year in which 797 patients with moderate to severe active rheumatoid arthritis who had an inadequate response to MTX received XELJANZ 5 or 10 mg twice daily or placebo added to background MTX. Placebo patients were advanced as in Study II. The primary endpoints were the proportion of patients who achieved an ACR20 response at Month 6, mean change from baseline in van der Heijde-modified total Sharp Score (mTSS) at Month 6, HAQ-DI at Month 3, and DAS28-4(ESR) less than 2.6 at Month 6.

Study V was a 6-month trial in which 399 patients with moderate to severe active rheumatoid arthritis who had an inadequate response to at least one approved TNF-inhibiting biologic agent received XELJANZ 5 or 10 mg twice daily or placebo added to background MTX. At the Month 3 visit, all patients randomized to placebo treatment were advanced in a blinded fashion to a second predetermined treatment of XELJANZ 5 or 10 mg twice daily. The primary endpoints at Month 3 were the proportion of patients who achieved an ACR20 response, HAQ-DI, and DAS28-4(ESR) less than 2.6.

Clinical Response

The percentages of XELJANZ-treated patients achieving ACR20, ACR50, and ACR70 responses in Studies I, IV, and V are shown in Table 5. Similar results were observed with Studies II and III. In all trials, patients treated with either 5 or 10 mg twice daily XELJANZ had higher ACR20, ACR50, and ACR70 response rates versus placebo, with or without background DMARD treatment, at Month 3 and Month 6. Higher ACR20 response rates were observed within 2 weeks compared to placebo. In the 12-month trials, ACR response rates in XELJANZ-treated patients were consistent at 6 and 12 months.

[See table 5 above]

In Study IV, a greater proportion of patients treated with XELJANZ 5 mg or 10 mg twice daily plus MTX achieved a low level of disease activity as measured by a DAS28-4(ESR) less than 2.6 at 6 months compared to those treated with MTX alone (Table 6).

Table 6: Proportion of Patients with DAS28-4(ESR) Less Than 2.6 with Number of Residual Active Joints

Study IV			
DAS28-4(ESR) Less Than 2.6	Placebo + MTX 160	XELJANZ 5 mg Twice Daily + MTX 321	XELJANZ 10 mg Twice Daily + MTX 316
Proportion of responders at Month 6 (n)	1% (2)	6% (19)	13% (42)
Of responders, proportion with 0 active joints (n)	50% (1)	42% (8)	36% (15)
Of responders, proportion with 1 active joint (n)	0	5% (1)	17% (7)
Of responders, proportion with 2 active joints (n)	0	32% (6)	7% (3)
Of responders, proportion with 3 or more active joints (n)	50% (1)	21% (4)	40% (17)

The results of the components of the ACR response criteria for Study IV are shown in Table 7. Similar results were observed in Studies I, II, III, and V.

[See table 7 at top of next page]

The percent of ACR20 responders by visit for Study IV is shown in Figure 5. Similar responses were observed in Studies I, II, III and V.

Figure 5: Percentage of ACR20 Responders by Visit for Study IV

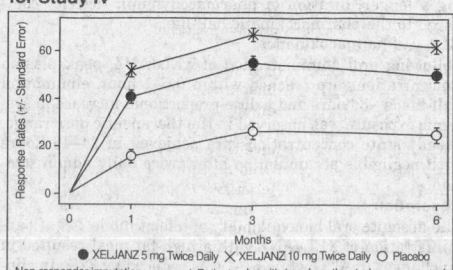

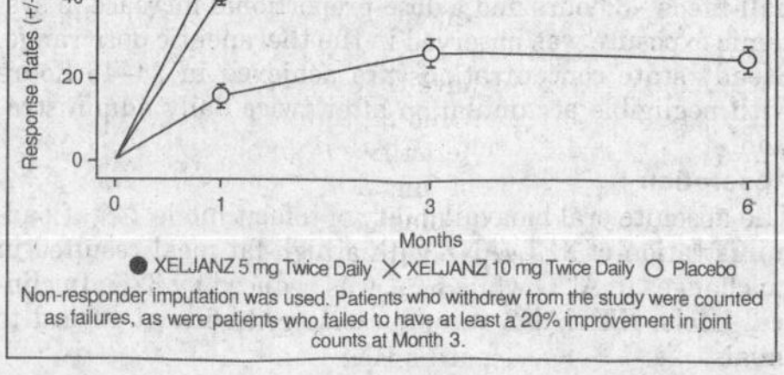

Non-responder imputation was used. Patients who withdrew from the study were counted as failures, as were patients who failed to have at least a 20% improvement in joint counts at Month 3.

Physical Function Response

Improvement in physical functioning was measured by the HAQ-DI. Patients receiving XELJANZ 5 and 10 mg twice daily demonstrated greater improvement from baseline in physical functioning compared to placebo at Month 3.

The mean (95% CI) difference from placebo in HAQ-DI improvement from baseline at Month 3 in Study III was -0.22 (-0.35, -0.10) in patients receiving 5 mg XELJANZ twice daily and -0.32 (-0.44, -0.19) in patients receiving 10 mg XELJANZ twice daily. Similar results were obtained in Studies I, II, IV and V. In the 12-month trials, HAQ-DI results in XELJANZ-treated patients were consistent at 6 and 12 months.

16 HOW SUPPLIED/STORAGE AND HANDLING

XELJANZ is provided as 5 mg tofacitinib (equivalent to 8 mg tofacitinib citrate) tablets: White, round, immediate-release film-coated tablets, debossed with "Pfizer" on one side, and "JKI 5" on the other side, and available in:

Bottles of 28:	NDC 0069-1001-03
Bottles of 60:	NDC 0069-1001-01
Bottles of 180:	NDC 0069-1001-02

Storage and Handling

Store at 20°C to 25°C (68°F to 77°F). [See USP Controlled Room Temperature].

Do not repackage.

17 PATIENT COUNSELING INFORMATION

See FDA-approved patient labeling (Medication Guide).

Inform patients of the availability of a Medication Guide, and instruct them to read the Medication Guide prior to taking XELJANZ. Instruct patients to take XELJANZ only as prescribed.

This product's label may have been updated. For current full prescribing information, please visit www.pfizer.com.

Distributed by
Pfizer Labs
Division of Pfizer Inc, NY, NY 10017
LAB-0445-2.0

Table 7: Components of ACR Response at 3 Months

	Study IV					
	XELJANZ 5 mg Twice Daily + MTX N=321		XELJANZ 10 mg Twice Daily + MTX N=316		Placebo + MTX N=160	
Component (mean) *	**Baseline**	**Month 3***	**Baseline**	**Month 3***	**Baseline**	**Month 3***
Number of tender joints (0–68)	24 (14)	13 (14)	23 (15)	10 (12)	23 (13)	18 (14)
Number of swollen joints (0–66)	14 (8)	6 (8)	14 (8)	6 (7)	14 (9)	10 (9)
Pain†	58 (23)	34 (23)	58 (24)	29 (22)	55 (24)	47 (24)
Patient global assessment†	58 (24)	35 (23)	57 (23)	29 (20)	54 (23)	47 (24)
Disability index (HAQ-DI)‡	1.41 (0.68)	0.99 (0.65)	1.40 (0.66)	0.84 (0.64)	1.32 (0.67)	1.19 (0.68)
Physician global assessment†	59 (16)	30 (19)	58 (17)	24 (17)	56 (18)	43 (22)
CRP (mg/L)	15.3 (19.0)	7.1 (19.1)	17.1 (26.9)	4.4 (8.6)	13.7 (14.9)	14.6 (18.7)

* Data shown is mean (Standard Deviation) at Month 3.
† Visual analog scale: 0 = best, 100 = worst.
‡ Health Assessment Questionnaire Disability Index: 0 = best, 3 = worst; 20 questions; categories: dressing and grooming, arising, eating, walking, hygiene, reach, grip, and activities.

MEDICATION GUIDE
XELJANZ (ZEL' JANS')
(tofacitinib)

Read this Medication Guide before you start taking XELJANZ and each time you get a refill. There may be new information. This Medication Guide does not take the place of talking to your healthcare provider about your medical condition or treatment.

What is the most important information I should know about XELJANZ?

XELJANZ may cause serious side effects including:

1. Serious infections.

XELJANZ is a medicine that affects your immune system. XELJANZ can lower the ability of your immune system to fight infections. Some people have serious infections while taking XELJANZ, including tuberculosis (TB), and infections caused by bacteria, fungi, or viruses that can spread throughout the body. Some people have died from these infections.

- Your healthcare provider should test you for TB before starting XELJANZ.
- Your healthcare provider should monitor you closely for signs and symptoms of TB infection during treatment with XELJANZ.

You should not start taking XELJANZ if you have any kind of infection unless your healthcare provider tells you it is okay.

Before starting XELJANZ, tell your healthcare provider if you:

- think you have an infection or have symptoms of an infection such as:
  - fever, sweating, or chills
  - muscle aches
  - cough
  - shortness of breath
  - blood in phlegm
  - weight loss
  - warm, red, or painful skin or sores on your body
  - diarrhea or stomach pain
  - burning when you urinate or urinating more often than normal
  - feeling very tired
- are being treated for an infection
- get a lot of infections or have infections that keep coming back
- have diabetes, HIV, or a weak immune system. People with these conditions have a higher chance for infections.
- have TB, or have been in close contact with someone with TB
- live or have lived, or have traveled to certain parts of the country (such as the Ohio and Mississippi River valleys and the Southwest) where there is an increased chance for getting certain kinds of fungal infections (histoplasmosis, coccidioidomycosis, or blastomycosis). These infections may happen or become more severe if you use XELJANZ. Ask your healthcare provider if you do not know if you have lived in an area where these infections are common.
- have or have had hepatitis B or C

After starting XELJANZ, call your healthcare provider right away if you have any symptoms of an infection. XELJANZ can make you more likely to get infections or make worse any infection that you have.

2. Cancer and immune system problems.

XELJANZ may increase your risk of certain cancers by changing the way your immune system works.

- Lymphoma and other cancers can happen in patients taking XELJANZ. Tell your healthcare provider if you have ever had any type of cancer.
- Some people who have taken XELJANZ with certain other medicines to prevent kidney transplant rejection have had a problem with certain white blood cells growing out of control (Epstein Barr Virus-associated post transplant lymphoproliferative disorder).

3. Tears (perforation) in the stomach or intestines.

- Tell your healthcare provider if you have had diverticulitis (inflammation in parts of the large intestine) or ulcers in your stomach or intestines. Some people taking XELJANZ get tears in their stomach or intestine. This happens most often in people who also take nonsteroidal anti-inflammatory drugs (NSAIDs), corticosteroids, or methotrexate.
- Tell your healthcare provider right away if you have fever and stomach-area pain that does not go away, and a change in your bowel habits.

4. Changes in certain laboratory test results. Your healthcare provider should do blood tests before you start receiving XELJANZ and while you take XELJANZ to check for the following side effects:

- **changes in lymphocyte counts.** Lymphocytes are white blood cells that help the body fight off infections.
- **low neutrophil counts.** Neutrophils are white blood cells that help the body fight off infections.
- **low red blood cell count.** This may mean that you have anemia, which may make you feel weak and tired.

Your healthcare provider should routinely check certain liver tests.

You should not receive XELJANZ if your lymphocyte count, neutrophil count, or red blood cell count is too low or your liver tests are too high.

Your healthcare provider may stop your XELJANZ treatment for a period of time if needed because of changes in these blood test results.

You may also have changes in other laboratory tests, such as your blood cholesterol levels. Your healthcare provider should do blood tests to check your cholesterol levels 4 to 8 weeks after you start receiving XELJANZ, and as needed after that. Normal cholesterol levels are important to good heart health.

See "What are the possible side effects of XELJANZ?" for more information about side effects.

What is XELJANZ?

XELJANZ is a prescription medicine called a Janus kinase (JAK) inhibitor. XELJANZ is used to treat adults with moderately to severely active rheumatoid arthritis in which methotrexate did not work well.

It is not known if XELJANZ is safe and effective in people with Hepatitis B or C.

XELJANZ is not for people with severe liver problems.

It is not known if XELJANZ is safe and effective in children.

What should I tell my healthcare provider before taking XELJANZ?

XELJANZ may not be right for you. Before taking XELJANZ, tell your healthcare provider if you:

- have an infection. See "What is the most important information I should know about XELJANZ?"
- have liver problems
- have kidney problems
- have any stomach area (abdominal) pain or been diagnosed with diverticulitis or ulcers in your stomach or intestines
- have had a reaction to tofacitinib or any of the ingredients in XELJANZ
- have recently received or are scheduled to receive a vaccine. People who take XELJANZ should not receive live vaccines. People taking XELJANZ can receive non-live vaccines.
- have any other medical conditions
- plan to become pregnant or are pregnant. It is not known if XELJANZ will harm an unborn baby.
  Pregnancy Registry: Pfizer has a registry for pregnant women who take XELJANZ. The purpose of this registry is to check the health of the pregnant mother and her baby. If you are pregnant or become pregnant while taking XELJANZ, talk to your healthcare provider about how you can join this pregnancy registry or you may contact the registry at 1-877-311-8972 to enroll.
- plan to breastfeed or are breastfeeding. You and your healthcare provider should decide if you will take XELJANZ or breastfeed. You should not do both.

Tell your healthcare provider about all the medicines you take, including prescription and non-prescription medicines, vitamins, and herbal supplements. XELJANZ and other medicines may affect each other causing side effects.

Especially tell your healthcare provider if you take:

- any other medicines to treat your rheumatoid arthritis. You should not take tocilizumab (Actemra®), etanercept (Enbrel®), adalimumab (Humira®), infliximab (Remicade®), rituximab (Rituxan®), abatacept (Orencia®), anakinra (Kineret®), certolizumab (Cimzia®), golimumab (Simponi®), azathioprine, cyclosporine, or other immunosuppressive drugs while you are taking XELJANZ. Taking XELJANZ with these medicines may increase your risk of infection.
- medicines that affect the way certain liver enzymes work. Ask your healthcare provider if you are not sure if your medicine is one of these.

Know the medicines you take. Keep a list of them to show your healthcare provider and pharmacist when you get a new medicine.

How should I take XELJANZ?
- Take XELJANZ as your healthcare provider tells you to take it.
- Take XELJANZ 2 times a day with or without food.
- If you take too much XELJANZ, call your healthcare provider or go to the nearest hospital emergency room right away.

What are possible side effects of XELJANZ?
XELJANZ may cause serious side effects, including:
- See "What is the most important information I should know about XELJANZ?"
- **Hepatitis B or C activation infection** in people who carry the virus in their blood. If you are a carrier of the hepatitis B or C virus (viruses that affect the liver), the virus may become active while you use XELJANZ. Your healthcare provider may do blood tests before you start treatment with XELJANZ and while you are using XELJANZ. Tell your healthcare provider if you have any of the following symptoms of a possible hepatitis B or C infection:
  - feel very tired
  - skin or eyes look yellow
  - little or no appetite
  - vomiting
  - clay-colored bowel movements
  - fevers
  - chills
  - stomach discomfort
  - muscle aches
  - dark urine
  - skin rash

Common side effects of XELJANZ include:
- upper respiratory tract infections (common cold, sinus infections)
- headache
- diarrhea
- nasal congestion, sore throat, and runny nose (nasopharyngitis)

Tell your healthcare provider if you have any side effect that bothers you or that does not go away.

These are not all the possible side effects of XELJANZ. For more information, ask your healthcare provider or pharmacist.

Call your doctor for medical advice about side effects. You may report side effects to FDA at 1-800-FDA-1088.

You may also report side effects to Pfizer at 1-800-438-1985.

How should I store XELJANZ?
Store XELJANZ at 68°F to 77°F (room temperature).
Safely throw away medicine that is out of date or no longer needed.

Keep XELJANZ and all medicines out of the reach of children.

General information about the safe and effective use of XELJANZ.
Medicines are sometimes prescribed for purposes other than those listed in a Medication Guide. Do not use XELJANZ for a condition for which it was not prescribed. Do not give XELJANZ to other people, even if they have the same symptoms you have. It may harm them.

This Medication Guide summarizes the most important information about XELJANZ. If you would like more information, talk to your healthcare provider. You can ask your pharmacist or healthcare provider for information about XELJANZ that is written for health professionals.

What are the ingredients in XELJANZ?
Active ingredient: tofacitinib citrate
Inactive ingredients: microcrystalline cellulose, lactose monohydrate, croscarmellose sodium, magnesium stearate, HPMC 2910/Hypromellose 6cP, titanium dioxide, macrogol/PEG3350, and triacetin.

This Medication Guide has been approved by the U.S. Food and Drug Administration.

Distributed by
Pfizer Labs
Division of Pfizer Inc, NY, NY 10017
LAB-0535-1.0
November 2012

Pivotal Therapeutics Inc.

81 ZENWAY BOULEVARD
UNIT #10
WOODBRIDGE, ONTARIO L4H 0S5
CANADA
Telephone: 1-905-856-9797

Pivotal Therapeutics (US), Inc.
3651 FAU Blvd., Suite 400
Boca Raton, FL 33431
United States
Telephone: 1-888-358-2080
Telephone: 1-561-288-5231
Email: info@pivotaltherapeutics.us
Website: www.pivotaltherapeutics.us

VASCAZEN® ℞

RECOMMENDED USE

VASCAZEN® (omega-3-acid ethyl-esters) is a prescription-only medical food intended for the dietary management of Omega-3 deficiency in patients with Cardiovascular Disease (CVD).

VASCAZEN® soft-gelatin capsules, to be administered orally, and is dispensed by prescription only for the dietary management of Omega-3 deficiency in patients with CVD. The adult dose is four (4) capsules daily. **VASCAZEN®** should only be taken under the supervision of a Physician. Do not take **VASCAZEN®** if you have a known allergy to fish or soy.

If you are pregnant or nursing, consult your Physician prior to taking **VASCAZEN®**.

PRODUCT DESCRIPTION

Ingredients
VASCAZEN® consists of a proprietary formulation of eicosapentaenoic acid (EPA) and docosahexaenoic acid (DHA), containing a minimum of 900mg of Omega-3 fatty acid ethyl-esters (680mg EPA and 110mg DHA) per 1.0g capsule.

Other Ingredients
VASCAZEN® contains the following inactive carriers or excipients: Mixed natural tocopherols, gelatin, glycerol, distilled water, and trace amounts of soy.

BACKGROUND
VASCAZEN® is a prescription-only medical food for the dietary management of Omega-3 deficiency in patients with CVD, providing EPA and DHA to levels not attainable through normal dietary modifications alone. This deficiency can be corrected by providing prescription **VASCAZEN®**, reducing key risk factors in patients with CVD.

A review of the scientific and medical literature identifies there are medically determined Omega-3-deficient nutrient requirements in patients with CVD[1,2], supporting the recommendation of consuming 3.0g of EPA and DHA per day. It would be difficult to achieve this high level of EPA and DHA through mere modification of the "normal" diet. Consumption of fatty fish every day may approach the level of 3.0g of EPA and DHA per day. However, the typical American diet consists of approximately 1/15th of these levels[3] and increasing fish consumption 15-fold to reach the clinically beneficial EPA and DHA levels through diet alone, would not be considered "normal", as required under the medical food definition. **VASCAZEN®** delivers 3.0g/day of EPA and DHA, levels not achievable through diet modifications alone and act to elevate and sustain Omega-3 in patients to levels associated with a reduced risk for cardiovascular complications.

Omega-3 Fatty Acids
Omega-3 fatty acids consist of a class of polyunsaturated fatty acids including EPA and DHA.

Structural formulas for EPA and DHA ethyl esters are:

Eicosapentaenoic Acid (EPA)

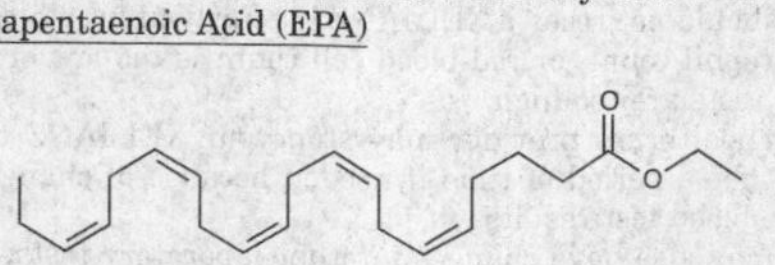

Docosahexaenoic Acid (DHA)

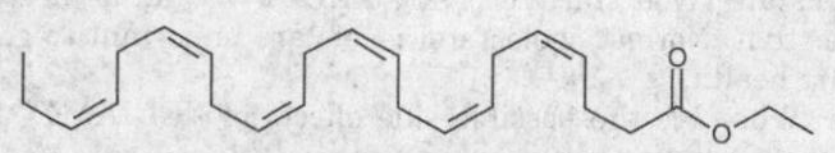

The molecular weight of EPA ethyl ester is 330.5 and has an empirical formula of $C_{22}H_{34}O_2$, and DHA ethyl ester has a molecular weight of 356.6 and an empirical formula of $C_{24}H_{36}O_2$.

Dietary sources of EPA and DHA are largely from cold water, oily fish including anchovies, sardines, mackerel and salmon and have demonstrated therapeutic benefits for overall cardiovascular health. However, to attain the sustained and stable levels of Omega-3 required for cardioprotective effects, a diet consisting predominately of fish can be difficult to maintain. There is also a growing public concern for toxin accumulation in fish (e.g. mercury), contributing to a lower desire to include fish as a regular dietary staple.

Medical Foods
Medical foods are specialized formulations intended for the dietary management of diseases or nutritional deficiencies related to, or caused by a given disease or medical condition and are taken under the supervision of a Physician or other appropriately licensed healthcare professional.

Physical Description
VASCAZEN® is distributed as an ultra-purified, light yellow, fish oil-filled, transparent soft-gelatin capsule in 15-count blister cards. Capsules are intended for oral administration and contain a minimum of 900mg Omega-3 fatty acids by weight comprised of a combination of at least 680mg EPA and 110mg DHA in a weight ratio of 6:1 in each 1.0g capsule. **VASCAZEN®** goes through independent third party testing for safety and purity.

CLINICAL PHARMACOLOGY OF OMEGA-3's

Mechanism of Action:
VASCAZEN® is intended to restore and sustain healthy levels of EPA and DHA in Omega-3 deficient patients with CVD. Increasing dietary levels of EPA and DHA have been shown to have a host of cardio-protective benefits[4,5]. Scientific literature suggests a correlation between high circulating blood levels of EPA and DHA with a reduction in the risk of cardiovascular events[1]. Beneficial effects of EPA and DHA have been documented in a number of clinical studies[4,5]. These include positive effects on lipid metabolism, blood pressure, heart rate, platelet aggregation, inflammation and helping to reduce the risk of cardiovascular disease.

CLINICAL EXPERIENCE
Clinical dietary management of Omega-3 deficiency in patients with CVD can be achieved with **VASCAZEN®** at a dose of four (4) capsules per day.

VASCAZEN® Open Label Safety and Efficacy Study
The safety and efficacy of **VASCAZEN®** was evaluated in an open label clinical study that assessed Omega-3 deficiency and efficacy of **VASCAZEN®** at increasing blood levels of EPA and DHA. The study involved a treatment regime consisting of four (4) capsules of **VASCAZEN®** and monitoring of blood Omega-3 levels over a six-week period. The Open label study consisted of 143 study subjects enrolled for baseline Omega-3 deficiency assessment, of which 63 subjects were scheduled to receive **VASCAZEN®** (3.0g EPA and DHA at a ratio of 6:1 EPA:DHA per day) for two weeks, and 31 patients received **VASCAZEN®** for six weeks. The primary endpoint was the subjects' Omega-Score™[1], measuring EPA, DHA, and docosapentanoic acid (DPA), presented as a percentage of total whole blood fatty acids. Subjects in the study had an average age of 51 years. This study revealed a baseline Omega-3 deficiency[1] in over 84.5% of the study group participants, irrespective of age or sex (Table 1, Figure 1). **VASCAZEN®** treatment resulted in a significant (P<0.0001) improvement in Omega-3 blood levels within two weeks, raising the average Omega-Score™ from 3.4% to 5.7%, and to 7.5% (P<0.0001) within six weeks (Table 2, Figure 2).

[See first table at top of next page]

TABLE 1. Study Participant Baseline Characteristics: The average age of patients was 51 years, with a slightly, but not significant age difference observed between the male (52 years) and female (47 years) groups. Mean Omega-Score™ values were in the "very high risk"[1] quartile and nearly identical between males and females. The vast majority of patients in the study had Omega-Score™ values less than 6.1%, signifying at least a moderate level of risk. 84.5% of patients were at risk, with similar trends in both the male and female groups. Confidence interval (CI), "±" (means ± standard deviation).

[See figure 1 at top of next column]
[See second table at top of next page]

TABLE 2. Timecourse of Study Subject's Omega-Score™ Values. VASCAZEN® rapidly increases patient group Omega-Score™ means with significant improvements (P<0.0001) as early as two weeks after treatment (3.4 at baseline, to 5.7 after two weeks). After four weeks, Omega-Score™ means surpass 6.1% into the "low risk" quartile, and remain in this range through Week 6 (P<0.0001). 84.5% of patients began the study Omega-3 deficient, and by Week Six, only 13.2% of study subjects were deficient, illustrating the efficacy of **VASCAZEN®** for use as an aid in the dietary

	Patient Group		
	Total N=143	Males N=106	Females N=37
Age (years)	46.9±15.0	50.9±14.6	52.1±13.6
Omega-Score™ Mean	3.4±1.3	3.4±1.4	3.5±1.19
95% CI	3.2 to 3.6 (±1.1 to 1.6)	3.2 to 3.7 (±1.1 to 1.6)	3.2 to 3.7 (±1.0 to 1.4)
% of Patients at Risk (<6.1% Omega-Score™)	84.5	82.1	89.2

	Week			
	0	2	4	6
Omega-Score™ Mean	3.4±1.3	5.7±1.9	7.9±2.4	7.5±1.2
95% CI	3.1 to 3.7 (±0.9 to 1.4)	5.4 to 6.3 (±1.4 to 2.3)	6.6 to 9.1 (±1.2 to 3.7)	7.0 to 8.0 (±0.7 to 1.7)
% of Patients at Risk (<6.1% Omega-Score™)	84.5%	43.2%	15.0%	13.2%

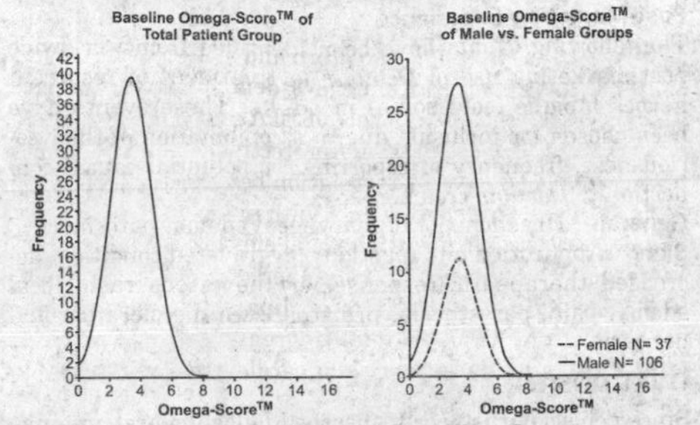

FIGURE 1. Study Participant Baseline Omega-Score™ Values. Out of 143 study participants, the majority of patients had a baseline score less than 6.1%, indicating an Omega-3 deficiency, irrespective of sex.

management of Omega-3 deficiency. Confidence interval (CI), "±" (means ± standard deviation).

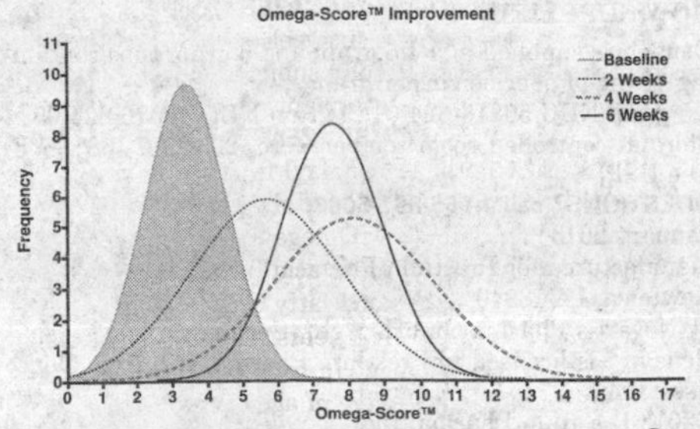

FIGURE 2. Six Week Treatment with VASCAZEN®. Study subjects were administered four capsules per day of **VASCAZEN®**, supplying 3.0g EPA and DHA per day and were monitored for safety and efficacy of increasing Omega-Score™ values from baseline levels. A significant improvement was observed within two weeks, with 86.8% of subjects reaching the low risk Omega-Score™ quartile within six weeks.

FOOD EFFECTS

VASCAZEN® may be taken with or without other foods. Some patients may experience a fish aftertaste/burp, and taking **VASCAZEN®** with food may help reduce this effect.

DRUG INTERACTIONS

Although clinical studies investigating the effect of **VASCAZEN®** plus anticoagulants have not been completed, caution should be taken when taking **VASCAZEN®** with anticoagulant drugs. Omega-3 fatty acids may extend bleeding time and patients receiving treatment with **VASCAZEN®** along with drugs that affect coagulation, should be monitored by a Physician.

ADVERSE REACTIONS

VASCAZEN® contains fish oil and soy products, and there is a risk for allergic reaction in patients with allergies to fish or soy. Patients with known hypersensitivity to fish or soy products should notify their Physician.

In an open label study, for a duration of six weeks, subjects were administered a daily dose of four (4) capsules of **VASCAZEN®**, supplying 3.0g of EPA and DHA Omega-3 fatty acid ethyl esters. Safety was assessed through adverse event reporting during the treatment schedule. **VASCAZEN®** was well tolerated, adverse events were minimal and minor in degree with no severe adverse events reported. Two subjects experienced a mild reflux/aftertaste, while an additional subject showed minor leg bruising that disappeared within three days.

HOW SUPPLIED

VASCAZEN® capsules are supplied as transparent softgelatin capsules, filled with light yellow, ultra-purified fish oil. **VASCAZEN®** is manufactured according to Food and Drug Administration (FDA) current Good Manufacturing Practices (cGMP).

STORAGE

59-77°F (15-25°C). Keep from freezing. Protect from direct sunlight.

Manufactured by: Captek Softgel Inc., Cerritos, CA, 90703
Manufactured for: Pivotal Therapeutics (US), Inc., Boca Raton FL, 33431
P: **561-288-5231**
Website: **www.pivotaltherapeutics.us**

REFERENCES

1. Albert CM, Campos H, Stampfer MJ, et al. (2002). Blood Levels of Long-Chain n-3 Fatty Acids and the Risk of Sudden Death. New England Journal of Medicine. 346: 1113-1118.
2. Danaei G, Ding DL, Mozaffarian D, et al. (2009). The Preventable Causes of Death in the United States: Comparative Risk Assessment of Dietary, Lifestyle, and Metabolic Risk Factors. PLoS Medicine. 6(4): 1-23.
3. Kris-Etherton PM, Taylor DS, et al. (2000). Polyunsaturated Fatty Acids in the Food Chain in the United States. American Journal of Clinical Nutrition. 71(Supp): 179S-188S.
4. GISSI-Prevenzione Investigators (1999). Dietary Supplementation with n-3 Polyunsaturated Fatty Acids and Vitamin E after Myocardial Infarction: Results of the GISSI-Prevenzione Trial. Lancet. 354: 447-455.
5. Yokoyaa M, Origasa H, Matsuzaki M, et al. (2007). Effects of Eicosapentaenoic Acid on Major Coronary Events in Hypercholesterolaemic Patients (JELIS): a randomised open-label, blinded endpoint analysis. Lancet. 369: 1090-1098.

VASCAZEN® is protected by a series of both issued and pending US and foreign patents.

Pivotal THERAPEUTICS

Shown in Product Identification Guide, page 311

Prestium Pharma, Inc.
411 S. STATE ST., SUITE E-100
NEWTOWN, PA 18940

Phone number: (267) 685-0340

DENAVIR® ℞
brand of
penciclovir cream, 1%
For Dermatologic Use Only
Rx only

Prescribing Information

DESCRIPTION

Denavir (penciclovir) cream 1% contains penciclovir, an antiviral agent active against herpes viruses. *Denavir* is available for topical administration as a 1% white cream. Each gram of *Denavir* contains 10 mg of penciclovir and the following inactive ingredients: cetomacrogol 1000 BP, cetostearyl alcohol, mineral oil, propylene glycol, purified water and white petrolatum.

Chemically, penciclovir is known as 9-[4-hydroxy-3-(hydroxymethyl)butyl]guanine. Its molecular formula is $C_{10}H_{15}N_5O_3$; its molecular weight is 253.26. It is a synthetic acyclic guanine derivative and has the following structure:

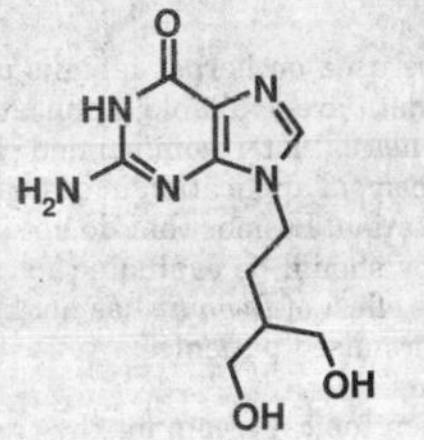

penciclovir

Penciclovir is a white to pale yellow solid. At 20°C it has a solubility of 0.2 mg/mL in methanol, 1.3 mg/mL in propylene glycol, and 1.7 mg/mL in water. In aqueous buffer (pH 2) the solubility is 10.0 mg/mL.

Penciclovir is not hygroscopic. Its partition coefficient in n-octanol/water at pH 7.5 is 0.024 (logP = -1.62).

CLINICAL PHARMACOLOGY

Microbiology

Mechanism of Antiviral Activity: The antiviral compound penciclovir has *in vitro* inhibitory activity against herpes simplex virus types 1 (HSV-1) and 2 (HSV-2). In cells infected with HSV-1 or HSV-2, viral thymidine kinase phosphorylates penciclovir to a monophosphate form which, in turn, is converted to penciclovir triphosphate by cellular kinases. *In vitro* studies demonstrate that penciclovir triphosphate inhibits HSV polymerase competitively with deoxyguanosine triphosphate. Consequently, herpes viral DNA synthesis and, therefore, replication are selectively inhibited.

Antiviral Activity *In Vitro* and *In Vivo*: In cell culture studies, penciclovir has antiviral activity against HSV-1 and HSV-2. Sensitivity test results, expressed as the concentration of the drug required to inhibit growth of the virus by 50% (IC_{50}) or 99% (IC_{99}) in cell culture, vary depending upon a number of factors, including the assay protocols. See Table 1.

[See table 1 at top of next page]

Drug Resistance: Penciclovir-resistant mutants of HSV can result from qualitative changes in viral thymidine kinase or DNA polymerase. The most commonly encountered acyclovir-resistant mutants that are deficient in viral thymidine kinase are also resistant to penciclovir.

Pharmacokinetics

Measurable penciclovir concentrations were not detected in plasma or urine of healthy male volunteers (n=12) following single or repeat application of the 1% cream at a dose of 180 mg penciclovir daily (approximately 67 times the estimated usual clinical dose).

Pediatric Patients: The systemic absorption of penciclovir following topical administration has not been evaluated in patients <18 years of age.

CLINICAL TRIALS

Denavir was studied in two double-blind, placebo (vehicle)-controlled trials for the treatment of recurrent herpes labialis in which otherwise healthy adults were randomized to either *Denavir* or placebo. Therapy was to be initiated by the subjects within 1 hour of noticing signs or symptoms and continued for 4 days, with application of study medication every 2 hours while awake. In both studies, the mean duration of lesions was approximately one-half-day shorter in the subjects treated with *Denavir* (N=1,516) as compared

Table 1

Method of Assay	Virus Type	Cell Type	IC_{50} (mcg/mL)	IC_{99} (mcg/mL)
Plaque Reduction	HSV-1 (c.i.)	MRC-5	0.2-0.6	
	HSV-1 (c.i.)	WISH	0.04-0.5	
	HSV-2 (c.i.)	MRC-5	0.9-2.1	
	HSV-2 (c.i.)	WISH	0.1-0.8	
Virus Yield Reduction	HSV-1 (c.i.)	MRC-5		0.4-0.5
	HSV-2 (c.i.)	MRC-5		0.6-0.7
DNA Synthesis Inhibition	HSV-1 (SC16)	MRC-5	0.04	
	HSV-2 (MS.)	MRC-5	0.05	

(c.i.) = clinical isolates. The latent state of any herpes virus is not known to respond to any viral therapy.

to subjects treated with placebo (N=1,541) (approximately 4.5 days versus 5 days, respectively). The mean duration of lesion pain was also approximately one half-day shorter in the *Denavir* group compared to the placebo group.

INDICATIONS AND USAGE

Denavir (penciclovir cream) is indicated for the treatment of recurrent herpes labialis (cold sores) in adults and children 12 years of age and older.

CONTRAINDICATIONS

Denavir is contraindicated in patients with known hypersensitivity to the product or any of its components.

PRECAUTIONS

General

Denavir should only be used on herpes labialis on the lips and face. Because no data are available, application to human mucous membranes is not recommended. Particular care should be taken to avoid application in or near the eyes since it may cause irritation. Lesions that do not improve or that worsen on therapy should be evaluated for secondary bacterial infection. The effect of *Denavir* has not been established in immunocompromised patients.

Information for Patients

Denavir is a prescription topical cream for the treatment of cold sores (recurrent herpes labialis) that occur on the face and lips. It is not a cure for cold sores and not all patients respond to it. Do not use if you are allergic to *Denavir* (penciclovir) or any of the ingredients in *Denavir* cream. Before you use *Denavir*, tell your doctor if you are pregnant, planning to become pregnant, or are breast-feeding.

Directions: Wash your hands. Your face should be clean and dry. Apply a layer of *Denavir* cream to cover only the cold sore area or the area of tingling (or other symptoms) before the cold sore appears. Rub in the cream until it disappears. Apply the cream every 2 hours during waking hours for 4 days. Even though *Denavir* works at the blister stage, treatment should be started at the earliest sign of a cold sore (i.e., tingling, redness, itching, or bump). Wash your hands with soap and water after using *Denavir* cream. Store *Denavir* cream at room temperature (59°-86°F). Keep out of reach of children.

Possible side effects: *Denavir* cream was well tolerated in clinical studies in patients with cold sores. The most frequently reported side effect was headache. Common skin-related side effects of *Denavir* cream are application site reactions, local anesthesia, taste perversion, and rash.

Carcinogenesis, Mutagenesis, Impairment of Fertility

In clinical trials, systemic drug exposure following the topical administration of penciclovir cream was negligible, as the penciclovir content of all plasma and urine samples was below the limit of assay detection (0.1 mcg/mL and 10 mcg/mL, respectively). However, for the purpose of inter-species dose comparisons presented in the following sections, an assumption of 100% absorption of penciclovir from the topically applied product has been used. Based on use of the maximal recommended topical dose of penciclovir of 0.05 mg/kg/day and an assumption of 100% absorption, the maximum theoretical plasma $AUC_{0\text{-}24\ hrs}$ for penciclovir is approximately 0.129 mcg.hr/mL.

Carcinogenesis: Two-year carcinogenicity studies were conducted with famciclovir (the oral prodrug of penciclovir) in rats and mice. An increase in the incidence of mammary adenocarcinoma (a common tumor in female rats of the strain used) was seen in female rats receiving 600 mg/kg/day (approximately 395× the maximum theoretical human exposure to penciclovir following application of the topical product, based on area under the plasma concentration curve comparisons [24 hr. AUC]). No increases in tumor incidence were seen among male rats treated at doses up to 240 mg/kg/day (approximately 190× the maximum theoretical human AUC for penciclovir), or in male and female mice at doses up to 600 mg/kg/day (approximately 100× the maximum theoretical human AUC for penciclovir).

Mutagenesis: When tested *in vitro*, penciclovir did not cause an increase in gene mutation in the Ames assay using multiple strains of *S. typhimurium* or *E. coli* (at up to 20,000 mcg/plate), nor did it cause an increase in unscheduled DNA repair in mammalian HeLa S3 cells (at up to 5,000 mcg/mL). However, an increase in clastogenic responses was seen with penciclovir in the L5178Y mouse lymphoma cell assay (at doses ≥1000 mcg/mL) and, in human lymphocytes incubated *in vitro* at doses ≥250 mcg/mL. When tested *in vivo*, penciclovir caused an increase in micronuclei in mouse bone marrow following the intravenous administration of doses ≥500 mg/kg (≥810× the maximum human dose, based on body surface area conversion).

Impairment of Fertility: Testicular toxicity was observed in multiple animal species (rats and dogs) following repeated intravenous administration of penciclovir (160 mg/kg/day and 100 mg/kg/day, respectively, approximately 1155 and 3255× the maximum theoretical human AUC). Testicular changes seen in both species included atrophy of the seminiferous tubules and reductions in epididymal sperm counts and/or an increased incidence of sperm with abnormal morphology or reduced motility. Adverse testicular effects were related to an increasing dose or duration of exposure to penciclovir. No adverse testicular or reproductive effects (fertility and reproductive function) were observed in rats after 10 to 13 weeks dosing at 80 mg/kg/day, or testicular effects in dogs after 13 weeks dosing at 30 mg/kg/day (575 and 845× the maximum theoretical human AUC, respectively). Intravenously administered penciclovir had no effect on fertility or reproductive performance in female rats at doses of up to 80 mg/kg/day (260× the maximum human dose [BSA]).

There was no evidence of any clinically significant effects on sperm count, motility or morphology in 2 placebo-controlled clinical trials of Famvir® (famciclovir [the oral prodrug of penciclovir], 250 mg b.i.d.; n=66) in immunocompetent men with recurrent genital herpes, when dosing and follow-up were maintained for 18 and 8 weeks, respectively (approximately 2 and 1 spermatogenic cycles in the human).

Pregnancy

Teratogenic Effects-Pregnancy Category B. No adverse effects on the course and outcome of pregnancy or on fetal development were noted in rats and rabbits following the intravenous administration of penciclovir at doses of 80 and 60 mg/kg/day, respectively (estimated human equivalent doses of 13 and 18 mg/kg/day for the rat and rabbit, respectively, based on body surface area conversion; the body surface area doses being 260 and 355× the maximum recommended dose following topical application of the penciclovir cream). There are, however, no adequate and well-controlled studies in pregnant women. Because animal reproduction studies are not always predictive of human response, penciclovir should be used during pregnancy only if clearly needed.

Nursing Mothers

There is no information on whether penciclovir is excreted in human milk after topical administration. However, following oral administration of famciclovir (the oral prodrug of penciclovir) to lactating rats, penciclovir was excreted in breast milk at concentrations higher than those seen in the plasma. Therefore, a decision should be made whether to discontinue the drug, taking into account the importance of the drug to the mother.

There are no data on the safety of penciclovir in newborns.

Pediatric Use

An open-label, uncontrolled trial with penciclovir cream 1% was conducted in 102 patients, ages 12-17 years, with recurrent herpes labialis. The frequency of adverse events was generally similar to the frequency previously reported for adult patients. Safety and effectiveness in pediatric patients less than 12 years of age have not been established.

Geriatric Use

In 74 patients ≥65 years of age, the adverse events profile was comparable to that observed in younger patients.

ADVERSE REACTIONS

In two double-blind, placebo-controlled trials, 1516 patients were treated with *Denavir* (penciclovir cream) and 1541 with placebo. The most frequently reported adverse event was headache, which occurred in 5.3% of the patients treated with *Denavir* and 5.8% of the placebo-treated patients. The rates of reported local adverse reactions are shown in Table 2 below. One or more local adverse reactions were reported by 2.7% of the patients treated with *Denavir* and 3.9% of placebo-treated patients.

Table 2 - Local Adverse Reactions Reported in Phase III Trials

	Penciclovir n=1516 %	Placebo N=1541 %
Applications site reaction	1.3	1.8
Hypesthesia/Local anesthesia	0.9	1.4
Taste perversion	0.2	0.3
Pruritus	0.0	0.3
Pain	0.0	0.1
Rash (erythematous)	0.1	0.1
Allergic reaction	0.0	0.1

Two studies, enrolling 108 healthy subjects, were conducted to evaluate the dermal tolerance of 5% penciclovir cream (a 5-fold higher concentration than the commercial formulation) compared to vehicle using repeated occluded patch testing methodology. The 5% penciclovir cream induced mild erythema in approximately one-half of the subjects exposed, an irritancy profile similar to the vehicle control in terms of severity and proportion of subjects with a response. No evidence of sensitization was observed.

Post-Marketing Experience

The following events have been identified from worldwide post-marketing use of *Denavir* in treatment of recurrent herpes labialis (cold sores) in adults. These events have been chosen for inclusion due to a combination of their seriousness, frequency of reporting, or potential causal connection to *Denavir* cream.

General: Headache, oral/pharyngeal edema, parosmia.

Skin: Application site reactions, aggravated condition, decreased therapeutic response, erythematous rash, local edema, pain, paresthesia, pruritus, skin discoloration and urticaria.

OVERDOSAGE

Since penciclovir is poorly absorbed following oral administration, adverse reactions related to penciclovir ingestion are unlikely. There is no information on overdose.

DOSAGE AND ADMINISTRATION

Denavir should be applied every 2 hours during waking hours for a period of 4 days. Treatment should be started as early as possible (i.e., during the prodrome or when lesions appear).

HOW SUPPLIED

Denavir is supplied in a 1.5 gram and 5 gram tube containing 10 mg of penciclovir per gram.

1.5 gram NDC 50816-624-01; 5 gram NDC 40076-624-05

Store at controlled room temperature, 20°-25°C (68°-77°F) [see USP]

QUESTIONS? call 1-866-897-5002

January 2013

Manufactured for Prestium Pharma, Inc.
Newtown, PA 18940
by Novartis Pharma GmbH, Wehr, Germany

Denavir® is licensed to Prestium Pharma, Inc. from Denco Asset, LLC.

US 921874-2107436

Shown in Product Identification Guide, page 311

VUSION® ℞

[*Vu-sion*]

(miconazole nitrate, zinc oxide, and white petrolatum) Ointment, for topical use only

HIGHLIGHTS OF PRESCRIBING INFORMATION

These highlights do not include all the information needed to use VUSION Ointment safely and effectively. See full prescribing information for VUSION Ointment.

VUSION® (miconazole nitrate, zinc oxide, and white petrolatum) Ointment, for topical use only

Initial U.S. Approval: 2006

INDICATIONS AND USAGE

- VUSION Ointment is indicated for adjunctive treatment of diaper dermatitis when complicated by documented candidiasis (microscopic evidence of pseudohyphae and /or budding yeast) in immunocompetent pediatric patients 4 weeks and older. (1)
- VUSION Ointment should not be used as a substitute for frequent diaper changes. (1)
- VUSION Ointment should not be used to prevent the occurrence of diaper dermatitis, since preventative use may result in the development of drug resistance. (1)

DOSAGE AND ADMINISTRATION

- VUSION Ointment is for topical use only. VUSION Ointment is not for oral, ophthalmic, or intravaginal use. (2)
- VUSION Ointment should be applied as a thin layer to the affected area at each diaper change for 7 days. (2)
- VUSION Ointment should be used as part of a treatment regimen that includes gentle cleansing of the diaper area and frequent diaper changes. (2)

DOSAGE FORMS AND STRENGTHS

- Ointment with 0.25% miconazole nitrate, 15% zinc oxide, and 81.35% white petrolatum. (3)

CONTRAINDICATIONS

- None

WARNINGS AND PRECAUTIONS

- If irritation occurs or if the disease worsens, discontinue use of the medication, and contact the health care provider. (5)

ADVERSE REACTIONS

To report SUSPECTED ADVERSE REACTIONS, contact Stiefel Laboratories, Inc. at 1-888-784-3335 (1-888-STIEFEL) or FDA at 1-800-FDA-1088 or www.fda.gov/medwatch.

See 17 for PATIENT COUNSELING INFORMATION and FDA-approved patient labeling

Revised: 09/2012

FULL PRESCRIBING INFORMATION: CONTENTS*

*** Sections or subsections omitted from the full prescribing information are not listed**

FULL PRESCRIBING INFORMATION

1 INDICATIONS AND USAGE

1.1 Indication

VUSION Ointment is indicated for the adjunctive treatment of diaper dermatitis only when complicated by documented candidiasis (microscopic evidence of pseudohyphae and/or budding yeast), in immunocompetent pediatric patients 4 weeks and older. A positive fungal culture for *Candida albicans*is not adequate evidence of candidal infection since colonization with *C. albicans* can result in a positive culture. The presence of candidal infection should be established by microscopic evaluation prior to initiating treatment.

VUSION should be used as part of a treatment regimen that includes measures directed at the underlying diaper dermatitis, including gentle cleansing of the diaper area and frequent diaper changes.

VUSION should not be used as a substitute for frequent diaper changes. VUSION should not be used to prevent the occurrence of diaper dermatitis, since preventative use may result in the development of drug resistance.

1.2 Limitations of Use

The safety and efficacy of VUSION have not been demonstrated in immunocompromised patients, or in infants less than 4 weeks of age (premature or term).

The safety and efficacy of VUSION have not been evaluated in incontinent adult patients. **VUSION should not be used to prevent the occurrence of diaper dermatitis, such as in an adult institutional setting, since preventative use may result in the development of drug resistance.**

2 DOSAGE AND ADMINISTRATION

VUSION is not for oral, ophthalmic, or intravaginal use.

Before applying VUSION, gently cleanse the skin with lukewarm water and pat dry with a soft towel. Avoid using any scented soaps, shampoos, or lotions on the diaper area.

Apply VUSION to the affected area at each diaper change for 7 days. Continue treatment for the full 7 days, even if there is improvement. The safety of VUSION when used for longer than 7 days is not known. Do not use VUSION for longer than 7 days. If symptoms have not improved by day 7, see your health care provider.

Gently apply a thin layer of VUSION to the diaper area with the fingertips. Do not rub VUSION into the skin as this may cause additional irritation. Thoroughly wash hands after applying VUSION.

3 DOSAGE FORMS AND STRENGTHS

White ointment containing 0.25% miconazole nitrate, 15% zinc oxide, and 81.35% white petrolatum.

4 CONTRAINDICATIONS

None

5 WARNINGS AND PRECAUTIONS

If irritation occurs or if the disease worsens, discontinue use of the medication, and contact the health care provider.

The safety and efficacy of VUSION have not been evaluated in incontinent adult patients. **VUSION should not be used to prevent the occurrence of diaper dermatitis, such as in an adult institutional setting, since preventative use may result in the development of drug resistance.**

6 ADVERSE REACTIONS

6.1 Clinical Trials Experience

Because clinical trials are conducted under widely varying conditions, adverse reaction rate observed in the clinical trials of a drug cannot be directly compared to rates in the clinical trials of another drug and may not reflect the rates observed in clinical practice.

A total of 835 infants and young children were evaluated in the clinical development program. Of 418 subjects in the VUSION group, 58 (14%) reported one or more adverse events. Of 417 subjects in the zinc oxide/white petrolatum control group, 85 (20%) reported one or more adverse events. Adverse events that occurred at a rate of $\geq 1\%$ for subjects who were treated with VUSION were approximately the same in type and frequency as for subjects who were treated with zinc oxide/white petrolatum ointment.

6.2 Post-marketing Experience

The following adverse reactions have been identified during post approval use of VUSION.

GASTROINTESTINAL DISORDERS: vomiting

GENERAL DISORDERS AND ADMINISTRATION SITE CONDITIONS: burning sensation, condition aggravated, inflammation, pain

INJURY, POISONING AND PROCEDURAL COMPLICATIONS: accidental exposure

SKIN AND SUBCUTANEOUS TISSUE DISORDERS: blister, dermatitis contact, diaper dermatitis, dry skin, erythema, pruritus, rash, skin exfoliation

Because these reactions are reported voluntarily from a population of uncertain size, it is not always possible to reliably estimate their frequency or establish a causal relationship to drug exposure.

7 DRUG INTERACTIONS

Drug-drug interaction studies were not conducted. Women who take a warfarin anticoagulant and use a miconazole intravaginal cream or suppository may be at risk for developing an increased prothrombin time, international normalized ratio (INR), and bleeding. The potential for this interaction between warfarin and VUSION is unknown.

8 USE IN SPECIFIC POPULATIONS

8.1 Pregnancy

Pregnancy Category C

There are no adequate and well-controlled studies of VUSION in pregnant women. Therefore, VUSION should be used during pregnancy only if the potential benefit justifies the potential risk to the fetus.

Miconazole nitrate administration has been shown to result in prolonged gestation and decreased numbers of live young in rats and in increased number of resorptions and decreased number of live young in rabbits at oral doses of 100 mg/kg/day and 80 mg/kg/day, which are 28 and 45 times the maximum possible topical exposure of caregivers, respectively, assuming 100% absorption.

8.3 Nursing Mothers

Safety and efficacy of VUSION have not been established in nursing mothers. It is not known if the active components of VUSION may be present in milk.

8.4 Pediatric Use

Efficacy was not demonstrated in infants less than 4 weeks of age. Safety and efficacy have not been established in very-low-birth-weight infants.

VUSION should not be used to prevent diaper dermatitis.

The safety of VUSION when used for longer than 7 days is not known. Do not use more than 7 days.

8.5 Geriatric Use

Safety and efficacy in a geriatric population have not been evaluated.

11 DESCRIPTION

VUSION contains the synthetic antifungal agent, miconazole nitrate (0.25%) USP, zinc oxide (15%) USP, and white petrolatum (81.35%) USP.

The chemical name of miconazole nitrate is 1-[2, 4-dichloro-ß-[(2,4-dichlorobenzyl)oxy] phenethyl] imidazole mononitrate with empirical formula $C_{18}H_{14}Cl_4N_2O \bullet HNO_3$ and molecular weight of 479.15. The structural formula of miconazole nitrate is as follows:

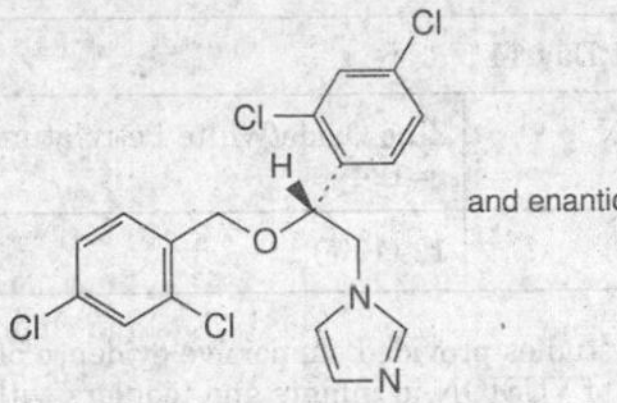

and enantiomer, HNO_3

The zinc oxide has an empirical formula of ZnO and a molecular weight of 81.39.

The white petrolatum, which is obtained from petroleum and is wholly or nearly decolorized, is a purified mixture of semisolid saturated hydrocarbons having the general chemical formula C_nH_{2n+2}. The hydrocarbons consist mainly of branched and unbranched chains. White petrolatum contains butylated hydroxytoluene (BHT) as stabilizer.

Each gram of VUSION contains 2.5 mg of miconazole nitrate USP, 150 mg of zinc oxide USP, and 813.5 mg of white petrolatum USP containing butylated hydroxytoluene, trihydroxystearin, and Chemoderm® 1001/B fragrance.[1]

VUSION is a smooth, uniform, white ointment.

[1]Chemoderm is a registered trademark of Firmenich Inc.

12 CLINICAL PHARMACOLOGY

12.1 Mechanism of Action

The miconazole component of VUSION is an antifungal agent [see Clinical Pharmacology (12.4)]. The mechanism of action of white petrolatum and zinc oxide for the adjunctive treatment of diaper dermatitis is unknown.

12.2 Pharmacodynamics

The human pharmacodynamics of Vusion is unknown [see Clinical Pharmacology (12.4) for fungal pharmacodynamics].

12.3 Pharmacokinetics

The topical absorption of miconazole from VUSION was studied in immunocompetent male and female infants and children (n=17) with diaper dermatitis complicated by documented candidiasis (microscopic evidence of pseudohyphae and/or budding yeast) ranging in age from 1 month to 21 months. After multiple daily applications to the affected area at every diaper change (approximately 5-12 times per day) for 7 days, the plasma concentrations of miconazole were below the lower limit of quantitation (LOQ) of 0.5 ng/mL in 15 out of 17 (88%) subjects. In the other 2 remaining subjects, the plasma concentrations of miconazole were 0.57 and 0.58 ng/mL, respectively at a single timepoint (4 hours after the last application) on Day 7.

12.4 Microbiology

The miconazole nitrate component in this product has been shown to have *in vitro* activity against *Candida albicans*, an organism that is associated with diaper dermatitis. The activity of miconazole nitrate against *C. albicans* is based on the inhibition of the ergosterol biosynthesis in the cell membrane. The accumulation of ergosterol precursors and toxic peroxides results in cytolysis of the cell. *In vitro* minimal inhibitory concentration (MIC) test results for *C. albicans* isolates obtained from treatment failures in Clinical Study 1 (*see Clinical Studies (14)*) does not appear to indicate that resistance to miconazole nitrate was the reason for treatment failure. The clinical significance of the *in vitro* activity of miconazole nitrate against *C. albicans* in the setting of diaper dermatitis is unclear.

13 NONCLINICAL TOXICOLOGY

13.1 Carcinogenesis, Mutagenesis, Impairment of Fertility

The carcinogenic potential of VUSION in animals has not been evaluated.

Miconazole nitrate was negative in a bacterial reverse mutation test, a chromosome aberration test in mice, and micronucleus assays in mice and rats.

Miconazole nitrate had no adverse effect on fertility in a study in rats at oral doses of up to 320 mg/kg/day, which is 89 times the maximum possible topical exposure of caregivers, assuming 100% absorption.

14 CLINICAL STUDIES

Study 1 was a double-blind, multicenter study in which VUSION was compared to the zinc oxide and white petrolatum combination treatment and included 236 infants and toddlers with diaper dermatitis, complicated by candidiasis as documented by KOH tests that demonstrated psuedohyphae and/or budding yeasts. Study medication was applied at every diaper change for 7 days.

The primary endpoint was "Overall Cure" and required that subjects be both clinically cured (total resolution of all signs and symptoms of infection) and microbiologically cured (eradication of candidiasis). Primary efficacy was assessed 1 week following the end of treatment, at Day 14.

Study results are shown in the following table.

Overall Cure at Day 14

	VUSION n=112	Zinc Oxide/White Petrolatum n=124
	26 (23%)	12 (10%)

Two additional studies provided supportive evidence of the clinical efficacy of VUSION in infants and toddlers with diaper dermatitis, some of whom cultured positive for *C. albicans*. However, candidal infection was not documented in the culture-positive subjects, as microscopic testing (e.g. KOH) was not done. Therefore, the positive culture results may have reflected colonization rather than infection.

16 HOW SUPPLIED/STORAGE AND HANDLING

16.1 How Supplied

VUSION is a smooth, uniform, white ointment supplied in an aluminum tube, as follows:

50g (NDC 0145-0002-04)

16.2 Storage Conditions

Store at controlled room temperature between 20°C and 25°C (68°F and 77°F); with excursions permitted between 15°C and 30°C (59°F and 86°F).

Keep out of reach of children.

17 PATIENT COUNSELING INFORMATION

See FDA-Approved Patient Labeling

Patients using VUSION should be informed about the following information:

- VUSION is to be used only for diaper dermatitis that is complicated by documented candidiasis (i.e. documented by microscopic testing).
- VUSION should not be used as a substitute for frequent diaper changes.
- VUSION should not be used to prevent diaper dermatitis.
- VUSION should not be used long term.
- VUSION should be used only as directed by the health care provider.
- VUSION is for external use only. It is not for oral, ophthalmic, or intravaginal use.
- Gently cleanse the diaper area with lukewarm water or a very mild soap and pat the area dry with a soft towel before applying VUSION.
- Gently apply VUSION to the diaper area with the fingertips after each diaper change. Do not rub VUSION into the skin as this may cause additional irritation.
- Thoroughly wash hands after applying VUSION.
- Treatment should be continued for 7 days, even if there is improvement. Do not use VUSION for longer than 7 days. If symptoms have not improved by day 7, see your health care provider.
- VUSION should not be used on children for whom it is not prescribed.

VSN:3PI

FDA-Approved Patient Labeling

VUSION® (Vu-sion) Ointment

(0.25% miconazole nitrate, 15% zinc oxide and 81.35% white petrolatum)

IMPORTANT: For Skin Use Only. Do not use in the mouth, eyes, or vagina.

Read the Patient Information that comes with VUSION before you use it on your child. This leaflet does not take the place of talking to your health care provider about your child's medical condition or treatment. If you have any questions or if you are not sure about any of the information on VUSION, ask your health care provider, or pharmacist.

What is VUSION?

VUSION is a prescription skin medicine used to treat diaper rash that also has a yeast infection in children who are at least 4 weeks old and who have a normal immune system. VUSION contains medicines that will help treat the yeast infection and the diaper rash, *but you must also change your child's diapers very often so that your child is not wearing a wet or soiled diaper.* Even if you use VUSION, *diaper rash will not go away if you do not keep your child's diaper area clean and dry.* You should use water or a very mild cleanser to clean your child's diaper area. VUSION is not to be used to prevent diaper rash or to be used for more than 7 days.

Your health care provider will need to do a special test to tell if your child's diaper rash also has a yeast infection. Do not use VUSION on your child's diaper rash unless your health care provider tells you that there is also a yeast infection.

Who should not use VUSION?

VUSION is not for treatment of all cases of diaper rash. VUSION is only for diaper rash that also has a yeast infection. Most cases of diaper rash do not need the yeast medicine that is in VUSION because most cases of diaper rash do not also have a yeast infection.

Do not use VUSION on any other children or other family member.

Do not use VUSION on your child's diaper rash if they are allergic to anything in it. See the end of this leaflet for a list of ingredients in VUSION.

Do not use on infants less than 4 weeks of age.

Do not use in infants or children who do not have a normal immune system.

How should I use VUSION on my child?

VUSION is applied to the skin on your child's diaper area at each diaper change for 7 days.

Apply VUSION for the full 7 days even if the diaper rash starts to go away. Call your child's health care provider if the diaper rash gets worse or does not go away with 7 days of treatment with VUSION. *VUSION should not be used for more than 7 days.*

To apply VUSION:

- Gently, clean the skin on your child's diaper area with warm (*not hot*) water. You may also use a very mild soap. Pat the area dry with a soft towel.
- Use your fingertips and gently apply a thin layer of VUSION to your child's diaper area at each diaper change. Do not rub VUSION into your child's skin. Rubbing the skin can cause more irritation.
- Wash your hands after applying VUSION on your child.

VUSION is for skin use only.

Call your child's health care provider or poison control center right away if any VUSION is swallowed. Call your child's health care provider if VUSION gets in the eye.

Keep out of reach of children.

What other steps will help diaper rash go away?

- Check your child's diaper often. Change the diaper at the first sign of wetness.
- Clean your child's diaper area after each diaper change. Gently wipe the diaper area from the front to back using warm (*not hot*)water. You may also use a mild soap. Rinse the diaper area well. Pat dry with a soft towel.
- Keep the diaper area open to air when possible.
- Even if you use VUSION, *diaper rash will not go away if you do not keep your child's diaper area clean and dry.*

What are the possible side effects of VUSION?

VUSION may cause irritation. You should call your child's health care provider if irritation appears or if the diaper rash gets worse.

How should I store VUSION?

- *Keep VUSION out of the reach of children to avoid the risk of accidental ingestion.*
- Store VUSION at room temperature between 68°F to 77°F (20°C to 25°C).

General information about VUSION

Medicines are sometimes prescribed for conditions that are not mentioned in patient information leaflets.

Do not use VUSION for a condition for which it was not prescribed. Do not give VUSION to other children or family members, even if they have the same symptoms your child has. It may harm them.

This leaflet summarizes the most important information about VUSION. If you would like more information, talk to your child's health care provider. You can ask your child's health care provider or pharmacist for information about VUSION that is written for healthcare professionals.

Side effects may be reported to Stiefel Laboratories, Inc. at 1-888-784-3335 (1-888-STIEFEL) or the FDA at 1-800-FDA-1088.

What are the ingredients in VUSION?

Active Ingredients: miconazole nitrate, zinc oxide, and white petrolatum

Inactive Ingredients: trihydroxystearin, butylated hydroxyltoluene (BHT), and Chemoderm® 1001/B fragrance

This Patient Information leaflet has been approved by the U.S. Food and Drug Administration.

The Patient Information leaflet was last revised: May 2011

VSN:3PIL

Manufactured for:
Stiefel Laboratories, Inc.
Research Triangle Park, NC 27709

Manufactured by:
DSM Pharmaceuticals, Inc.
Greenville, NC 27834

Revised May 2011

Shown in Product Identification Guide, page 311

Purdue Pharma L.P.

ONE STAMFORD FORUM
STAMFORD, CT 06901-3431

For Medical Inquiries:
888-726-7535
Adverse Drug Experiences:
888-726-7535
Customer Service:
800-877-5666
FAX 800-877-3210

BUTRANS® CIII

[*BYOO-trans*]
(buprenorphine)
Transdermal System for transdermal administration

HIGHLIGHTS OF PRESCRIBING INFORMATION

These highlights do not include all the information needed to use BUTRANS® safely and effectively. See full prescribing information for BUTRANS.

BUTRANS (buprenorphine) Transdermal System for transdermal administration CIII Initial U.S. Approval: 1981

WARNING: ABUSE POTENTIAL, LIFE-THREATENING RESPIRATORY DEPRESSION, and ACCIDENTAL EXPOSURE

See full prescribing information for complete boxed warning.

- **BUTRANS contains buprenorphine, a Schedule III controlled substance. Monitor for signs of misuse, abuse, and addiction during BUTRANS therapy (5.1, 9).**
- **Fatal respiratory depression may occur, with highest risk at initiation and with dose increases. Instruct patients on proper administration of BUTRANS to reduce the risk (5.2).**
- **Accidental exposure to BUTRANS can result in fatal overdose of buprenorphine, especially in children (5.3).**

INDICATIONS AND USAGE

BUTRANS is a partial opioid agonist product indicated for the management of moderate to severe chronic pain in patients requiring a continuous, around-the-clock opioid analgesic for an extended period of time. (1)

Limitations of Use

- BUTRANS is not for use:
  - As an as-needed (prn) analgesic (1)
  - For pain that is mild or not expected to persist for an extended period of time (1)
  - For acute pain (1)
  - For postoperative pain, unless the patient is already receiving chronic opioid therapy prior to surgery, or if the postoperative pain is expected to be moderate to severe and persist for an extended period of time (1)

DOSAGE AND ADMINISTRATION

- Individualize dosing based on patient's prior analgesic treatment experience, and titrate as needed to provide adequate analgesia and minimize adverse reactions. (2.1, 2.2)
- Instruct patients to wear BUTRANS for 7 days and to wait a minimum of 3 weeks before applying to the same site. (2.1)
- Do not abruptly discontinue BUTRANS in a physically dependent patient. (2.3, 5.17)

DOSAGE FORMS AND STRENGTHS

- **Transdermal system**, 5 mcg/hour, 10 mcg/hour, 15 mcg/hour, and 20 mcg/hour. (3)

CONTRAINDICATIONS

- Significant respiratory depression (4)
- Acute or severe bronchial asthma (4)
- Known or suspected paralytic ileus (4)
- Hypersensitivity to buprenorphine (4)

WARNINGS AND PRECAUTIONS

- Elderly, cachectic, and debilitated patients, and patients with chronic pulmonary disease: Monitor closely because of increased risk of respiratory depression. (5.4, 5.5)

- Interaction with CNS depressants, especially benzodiazepines: Consider dose reduction of one or both drugs because of additive effects. (5.6, 7.2, 7.3)
- Avoid in patients with Long QT Syndrome, family history of Long QT Syndrome, or those taking Class IA or Class III antiarrhythmic medications. (5.7, 12.2)
- Hypotensive effects: Monitor during dose initiation and titration. (5.8)
- Patients with head injury or increased intracranial pressure: Monitor for sedation and respiratory depression and avoid use of BUTRANS in patients with impaired consciousness or coma susceptible to intracranial effects of CO_2 retention. (5.9)

ADVERSE REACTIONS

Most common adverse reactions (≥ 5%) include: nausea, headache, application site pruritus, dizziness, constipation, somnolence, vomiting, application site erythema, dry mouth, and application site rash. (6.1)

To report SUSPECTED ADVERSE REACTIONS, contact Purdue Pharma L.P. at 1-888-726-7535 or FDA at 1-800-FDA-1088 or *www.fda.gov/medwatch*.

DRUG INTERACTIONS

- CYP3A4 inducers: May increase clearance of buprenorphine. (7.1)
- Interaction with CNS depressants: Consider dose reduction of one or both drugs because of additive effects. (5.6, 7.3)
- Muscle relaxants may enhance the action of BUTRANS and produce an increased degree of respiratory depression. (7.4)

USE IN SPECIFIC POPULATIONS

- Pregnancy: BUTRANS is not recommended for use during pregnancy. (8.1)
- Nursing Mothers: Buprenorphine has been detected in human milk. Closely monitor infants of nursing women receiving BUTRANS. (8.3)

See 17 for PATIENT COUNSELING INFORMATION and Medication Guide

Revised: 07/2013

FULL PRESCRIBING INFORMATION: CONTENTS*

*** Sections or subsections omitted from the full prescribing information are not listed**

FULL PRESCRIBING INFORMATION

WARNING: ABUSE POTENTIAL, LIFE-THREATENING RESPIRATORY DEPRESSION, and ACCIDENTAL EXPOSURE

Abuse Potential

BUTRANS contains buprenorphine, an opioid agonist and Schedule III controlled substance with an abuse liability similar to other Schedule III opioids, legal or illicit *[see Warnings and Precautions (5.1)]*. Assess each patient's risk for opioid abuse or addiction prior to prescribing BUTRANS. The risk for opioid abuse is increased in patients with a personal or family history of substance abuse (including drug or alcohol abuse or addiction) or mental illness (e.g., major depressive disorder). Routinely monitor all patients receiving BUTRANS for signs of misuse, abuse, and addiction during treatment *[see Drug Abuse and Dependence (9)]*.

Life-Threatening Respiratory Depression

Respiratory depression, including fatal cases, may occur with use of BUTRANS, even when the drug has been used as recommended and not misused or abused *[see Warnings and Precautions (5.2)]*. Proper dosing and titration are essential and BUTRANS should only be prescribed by healthcare professionals who are knowledgeable in the use of potent opioids for the management of chronic pain. Monitor for respiratory depression, especially during initiation of BUTRANS or following a dose increase.

Accidental Exposure

Accidental exposure to BUTRANS, especially in children, can result in a fatal overdose of buprenorphine *[see Warnings and Precautions (5.3)]*.

1 INDICATIONS AND USAGE

BUTRANS is indicated for the management of moderate to severe chronic pain when a continuous, around-the-clock opioid analgesic is needed for an extended period of time.

Limitations of Use

BUTRANS is not for use:

- As an as-needed (prn) analgesic
- For pain that is mild or not expected to persist for an extended period of time
- For acute pain
- For postoperative pain unless the patient is already receiving chronic opioid therapy prior to surgery or if the postoperative pain is expected to be moderate to severe and persist for an extended period of time

2 DOSAGE AND ADMINISTRATION

2.1 Initial Dosing

Initiate the dosing regimen for each patient individually, taking into account the patient's prior analgesic treatment experience. Monitor patients closely for respiratory depression, especially within the first 24-72 hours of initiating therapy with BUTRANS *[see Warnings and Precautions (5.2)]*. Overestimating the BUTRANS dose when converting patients from another opioid medication can result in fatal overdose with the first dose *[see Overdosage (10)]*.

Consider the following factors when selecting an initial dose of BUTRANS:

- Total daily dose, potency, and any prior opioid the patient has been taking previously;
- Reliability of the relative potency estimate used to calculate the equivalent dose of buprenorphine needed (Note: potency estimates may vary with the route of administration);
- Patient's degree of opioid experience and opioid tolerance;
- General condition and medical status of the patient;
- Concurrent medication;
- Type and severity of the patient's pain.

BUTRANS is for transdermal use (on intact skin) only. Each BUTRANS is intended to be worn for 7 days.

Instruct patients not to use BUTRANS if the pouch seal is broken or the patch is cut, damaged, or changed in any way and not to cut BUTRANS.

BUTRANS as the First Opioid Analgesic

Initiate treatment with BUTRANS 5 mcg/hour.

Conversion from Other Opioids to BUTRANS

There is a potential for buprenorphine to precipitate withdrawal in patients who are already on opioids.

Prior Total Daily Dose of Opioid Less than 30 mg of Oral Morphine Equivalents per Day:

Initiate treatment with BUTRANS 5 mcg/hour.

Prior Total Daily Dose of Opioid Between 30 mg to 80 mg of Oral Morphine Equivalents per Day:

Taper the patient's current around-the-clock opioids for up to 7 days to no more than 30 mg of morphine or equivalent per day before beginning treatment with BUTRANS. Then initiate treatment with BUTRANS 10 mcg/hour. Patients may use short-acting analgesics as needed until analgesic efficacy with BUTRANS is attained.

Prior Total Daily Dose of Opioid Greater than 80 mg of Oral Morphine Equivalents per Day:

BUTRANS 20 mcg/hour may not provide adequate analgesia for patients requiring greater than 80 mg/day oral morphine equivalents. Consider the use of an alternate analgesic.

Table 1: Initial BUTRANS Dose

Current Opioid Analgesic	**Current Daily Dose**	
Oral Morphine Equivalent	<30 mg	30-80 mg
Recommended BUTRANS Starting Dose	**5 mcg/hour**	**10 mcg/hour**

2.2 Titration and Maintenance of Therapy

Individually titrate BUTRANS to a dose that provides adequate analgesia and minimizes adverse reactions. The minimum BUTRANS titration interval is 72 hours, based on the pharmacokinetic profile and time to reach steady state levels *[see Clinical Pharmacology (12.3)]*.

The maximum BUTRANS dose is 20 mcg/hour. **Do not exceed a dose of one 20 mcg/hour BUTRANS system due to the risk of QTc interval prolongation.** In a clinical trial, BUTRANS 40 mcg/hour (given as two BUTRANS 20 mcg/hour systems) resulted in prolongation of the QTc interval *[see Warnings and Precautions (5.7), and Clinical Pharmacology (12.2)]*.

If the level of pain increases, attempt to identify the source of increased pain, while adjusting the BUTRANS dose to decrease the level of pain. Because steady-state plasma concentrations are approximated within 72 hours, BUTRANS dosage adjustments may be done every 3 days. Patients who experience breakthrough pain may require dosage adjustment or rescue medication with an appropriate dose of an immediate-release opioid or non-opioid medication.

If signs of excessive opioid-related adverse reactions are observed, the current patch may be removed or next dose may be reduced. Adjust the dose to obtain an appropriate balance between the management of pain and opioid-related adverse reactions.

2.3 Cessation of Therapy

When the patient no longer requires therapy with BUTRANS, use a gradual downward titration of the dose every 7 days to prevent signs and symptoms of withdrawal in the physically dependent patient; consider introduction of an appropriate immediate-release opioid medication. Do not abruptly discontinue BUTRANS.

2.4 Patients with Hepatic Impairment

BUTRANS has not been evaluated in patients with severe hepatic impairment. As BUTRANS is only intended for 7-day application, consider use of an alternate analgesic that may permit more flexibility with the dosing in patients with severe hepatic impairment *[see Warnings and Precautions (5.10), Use in Specific Populations (8.6), and Clinical Pharmacology (12.3)]*.

2.5 Administration of BUTRANS

Instruct patients to apply immediately after removal from the individually sealed pouch. Instruct patients not to use BUTRANS if the pouch seal is broken or the patch is cut, damaged, or changed in any way.

Apply BUTRANS to the upper outer arm, upper chest, upper back or the side of the chest. These 4 sites (each present on both sides of the body) provide 8 possible application sites. Rotate BUTRANS among the 8 described skin sites.

After BUTRANS removal, wait a minimum of 21 days before reapplying to the same skin site *[see Clinical Pharmacology (12.3)]*.
Apply BUTRANS to a hairless or nearly hairless skin site. If none are available, the hair at the site should be clipped, not shaven. Do not apply BUTRANS to irritated skin. If the application site must be cleaned, clean the site with water only. Do not use soaps, alcohol, oils, lotions, or abrasive devices. Allow the skin to dry before applying BUTRANS.
If problems with adhesion of BUTRANS occur, the edges may be taped with first aid tape.
If BUTRANS falls off during the 7 days dosing interval, dispose of the transdermal system properly and place a new BUTRANS on at a different skin site.
When changing the system, instruct patients to remove BUTRANS, fold it over on itself, and flush it down the toilet. Alternatively, BUTRANS can be sealed in the Patch-Disposal Unit provided and then disposed of in the trash. Never throw BUTRANS away in the trash without sealing it in the Patch-Disposal Unit.
See the Instructions for Use for step-by-step instructions for applying BUTRANS.
If the buprenorphine-containing adhesive matrix accidentally contacts the skin, instruct patients or caregivers to wash the area with water and not to use soap, alcohol, or other solvents to remove the adhesive because they may enhance the absorption of the drug.

3 DOSAGE FORMS AND STRENGTHS

BUTRANS is a rectangular or square, beige-colored system consisting of a protective liner and functional layers.
BUTRANS is available in four strengths:

- BUTRANS 5 mcg/hour Transdermal System (dimensions: 45 mm by 45 mm)
- BUTRANS 10 mcg/hour Transdermal System (dimensions: 45 mm by 68 mm)
- BUTRANS 15 mcg/hour Transdermal System (dimensions: 59 mm by 72 mm)
- BUTRANS 20 mcg/hour Transdermal System (dimensions: 72 mm by 72 mm)

4 CONTRAINDICATIONS

BUTRANS is contraindicated in patients with:

- Significant respiratory depression
- Acute or severe bronchial asthma in an unmonitored setting or in the absence of resuscitative equipment
- Known or suspected paralytic ileus
- Hypersensitivity (e.g., anaphylaxis) to buprenorphine *[see Warnings and Precautions (5.12), and Adverse Reactions (6)]*

5 WARNINGS AND PRECAUTIONS

5.1 Abuse Potential

BUTRANS contains buprenorphine, a partial agonist at the mu opioid receptor and a Schedule III controlled substance. Buprenorphine can be abused in a manner similar to other opioid agonists, legal or illicit. Opioid agonists are sought by drug abusers and people with addiction disorders and are subject to criminal diversion. Consider these risks when prescribing or dispensing BUTRANS in situations where there is concern about increased risks of misuse, abuse, or diversion. Concerns about abuse, addiction, and diversion should not, however, prevent the proper management of pain.
Assess each patient's risk for opioid abuse or addiction prior to prescribing BUTRANS. The risk for opioid abuse is increased in patients with a personal or family history of substance abuse (including drug or alcohol abuse or addiction) or mental illness (e.g., major depression). Patients at increased risk may still be appropriately treated with modified-release opioid formulations; however these patients will require intensive monitoring for signs of misuse, abuse, or addiction. Routinely monitor all patients receiving opioids for signs of misuse, abuse, and addiction because these drugs carry a risk for addiction even under appropriate medical use.
Misuse or abuse of BUTRANS by chewing, swallowing, snorting or injecting buprenorphine extracted from the transdermal system will result in the uncontrolled delivery of the opioid and pose a significant risk that could result in overdose and death *[see Overdosage (10)]*.
Contact local state professional licensing board or state controlled substances authority for information on how to prevent and detect abuse or diversion of this product.

5.2 Life-Threatening Respiratory Depression

Respiratory depression is the primary risk of BUTRANS. Respiratory depression, if not immediately recognized and treated, may lead to respiratory arrest and death. Respiratory depression from opioids is manifested by a reduced urge to breathe and a decreased rate of respiration, often associated with a "sighing" pattern of breathing (deep breaths separated by abnormally long pauses). Carbon dioxide (CO_2) retention from opioid-induced respiratory depression can exacerbate the sedating effects of opioids. Management of respiratory depression may include close observation, supportive measures, and use of opioid antagonists, depending on the patient's clinical status *[see Overdosage (10)]*.
While serious, life-threatening, or fatal respiratory depression can occur at any time during the use of BUTRANS, the risk is greatest during the initiation of therapy or following a dose increase. Closely monitor patients for respiratory depression when initiating therapy with BUTRANS and following dose increases. Instruct patients against use by individuals other than the patient for whom BUTRANS was prescribed and to keep BUTRANS out of the reach of children, as such inappropriate use may result in fatal respiratory depression.
To reduce the risk of respiratory depression, proper dosing and titration of BUTRANS are essential *[see Dosage and Administration (2.1, 2.2)]*. Overestimating the BUTRANS dose when converting patients from another opioid product can result in fatal overdose with the first dose. Respiratory depression has also been reported with use of modified-release opioids when used as recommended and not misused or abused.
To further reduce the risk of respiratory depression, consider the following:

- Proper dosing and titration are essential and BUTRANS should only be prescribed by healthcare professionals who are knowledgeable in the use of potent opioids for the management of chronic pain.
- BUTRANS is contraindicated in patients with respiratory depression and in patients with conditions that increase the risk of life-threatening respiratory depression *[see Contraindications (4)]*.

5.3 Accidental Exposure

Accidental exposure to BUTRANS, especially in children, can result in a fatal overdose of buprenorphine.

5.4 Elderly, Cachectic, and Debilitated Patients

Respiratory depression is more likely to occur in elderly, cachectic, or debilitated patients as they may have altered pharmacokinetics due to poor fat stores, muscle wasting, or altered clearance compared to younger, healthier patients. Therefore, monitor such patients closely, particularly when initiating and titrating BUTRANS and when BUTRANS is given concomitantly with other drugs that depress respiration *[see Warnings and Precautions (5.2)]*.

5.5 Use in Patients with Chronic Pulmonary Disease

Monitor patients with significant chronic obstructive pulmonary disease or cor pulmonale, and patients having a substantially decreased respiratory reserve, hypoxia, hypercapnia, or pre-existing respiratory depression for respiratory depression, particularly when initiating therapy and titrating with BUTRANS, as in these patients, even usual therapeutic doses of BUTRANS may decrease respiratory drive to the point of apnea *[see Warnings and Precautions (5.2)]*. Consider the use of alternative non-opioid analgesics in these patients if possible.

5.6 Interactions with Alcohol, CNS Depressants, and Illicit Drugs

Hypotension, profound sedation, coma or respiratory depression may result if BUTRANS is added to a regimen that includes other CNS depressants (e.g., sedatives, anxiolytics, hypnotics, neuroleptics, muscle relaxants, other opioids). When considering the use of BUTRANS in a patient taking a CNS depressant, assess the duration of use of the CNS depressant and the patient's response, including the degree of tolerance that has developed to CNS depression. Additionally, consider the patient's use, if any, of alcohol or illicit drugs that cause CNS depression. If BUTRANS therapy is to be initiated in a patient taking a CNS depressant, start with a lower BUTRANS dose than usual and monitor patients for signs of sedation and respiratory depression and consider using a lower dose of the concomitant CNS depressant *[see Drug Interactions (7.3)]*.

5.7 QTc Prolongation

A positive-controlled study of the effects of BUTRANS on the QTc interval in healthy subjects demonstrated no clinically meaningful effect at a BUTRANS dose of 10 mcg/hour; however, a BUTRANS dose of 40 mcg/hour (given as two BUTRANS 20 mcg/hour Transdermal Systems) was observed to prolong the QTc interval *[see Clinical Pharmacology (12.2)]*.
Consider these observations in clinical decisions when prescribing BUTRANS to patients with hypokalemia or clinically unstable cardiac disease, including: unstable atrial fibrillation, symptomatic bradycardia, unstable congestive heart failure, or active myocardial ischemia. Avoid the use of BUTRANS in patients with a history of Long QT Syndrome or an immediate family member with this condition, or those taking Class IA antiarrhythmic medications (e.g., quinidine, procainamide, disopyramide) or Class III antiarrhythmic medications (e.g., sotalol, amiodarone, dofetilide).

5.8 Hypotensive Effects

BUTRANS may cause severe hypotension including orthostatic hypotension and syncope in ambulatory patients. There is an increased risk in patients whose ability to maintain blood pressure has already been compromised by a reduced blood volume or concurrent administration of certain CNS depressant drugs (e.g., phenothiazines or general anesthetics) *[see Drug Interactions (7.3)]*. Monitor these patients for signs of hypotension after initiating or titrating the dose of BUTRANS.

5.9 Use in Patients with Head Injury or Increased Intracranial Pressure

Monitor patients taking BUTRANS who may be susceptible to the intracranial effects of CO_2 retention (e.g., those with evidence of increased intracranial pressure or brain tumors) for signs of sedation and respiratory depression, particularly when initiating therapy with BUTRANS. BUTRANS may reduce respiratory drive, and the resultant CO_2 retention can further increase intracranial pressure. Opioids may also obscure the clinical course in a patient with a head injury.
Avoid the use of BUTRANS in patients with impaired consciousness or coma.

5.10 Hepatotoxicity

Although not observed in BUTRANS chronic pain clinical trials, cases of cytolytic hepatitis and hepatitis with jaundice have been observed in individuals receiving sublingual buprenorphine for the treatment of opioid dependence, both in clinical trials and in post-marketing adverse event reports. The spectrum of abnormalities ranges from transient asymptomatic elevations in hepatic transaminases to case reports of hepatic failure, hepatic necrosis, hepatorenal syndrome, and hepatic encephalopathy. In many cases, the presence of pre-existing liver enzyme abnormalities, infection with hepatitis B or hepatitis C virus, concomitant usage of other potentially hepatotoxic drugs, and ongoing injection drug abuse may have played a causative or contributory role. For patients at increased risk of hepatotoxicity (e.g., patients with a history of excessive alcohol intake, intravenous drug abuse or liver disease), obtain baseline liver enzyme levels and monitor periodically and during treatment with BUTRANS.

5.11 Application Site Skin Reactions

In rare cases, severe application site skin reactions with signs of marked inflammation including "burn," "discharge," and "vesicles" have occurred. Time of onset varies, ranging from days to months following the initiation of BUTRANS treatment. Instruct patients to promptly report the development of severe application site reactions and discontinue therapy.

5.12 Anaphylactic/Allergic Reactions

Cases of acute and chronic hypersensitivity to buprenorphine have been reported both in clinical trials and in the post-marketing experience. The most common signs and symptoms include rashes, hives, and pruritus. Cases of bronchospasm, angioneurotic edema, and anaphylactic shock have been reported. A history of hypersensitivity to buprenorphine is a contraindication to the use of BUTRANS.

5.13 Application of External Heat

Advise patients and their caregivers to avoid exposing the BUTRANS application site and surrounding area to direct external heat sources, such as heating pads or electric blankets, heat or tanning lamps, saunas, hot tubs, and heated water beds while wearing the system because an increase in absorption of buprenorphine may occur *[see Clinical Pharmacology (12.3)]*. Advise patients against exposure of the BUTRANS application site and surrounding area to hot water or prolonged exposure to direct sunlight. There is a potential for temperature-dependent increases in buprenorphine released from the system resulting in possible overdose and death.

5.14 Patients with Fever

Monitor patients wearing BUTRANS systems who develop fever or increased core body temperature due to strenuous exertion for opioid side effects and adjust the BUTRANS dose if signs of respiratory or central nervous system depression occur.

5.15 Use in Patients with Gastrointestinal Conditions

BUTRANS is contraindicated in patients with paralytic ileus. Avoid the use of BUTRANS in patients with other GI obstruction.

The buprenorphine in BUTRANS may cause spasm of the sphincter of Oddi. Monitor patients with biliary tract disease, including acute pancreatitis, for worsening symptoms. Opioids may cause increases in the serum amylase.

5.16 Use in Patients with Convulsive or Seizure Disorders

The buprenorphine in BUTRANS may aggravate convulsions in patients with convulsive disorders, and may induce or aggravate seizures in some clinical settings. Monitor patients with a history of seizure disorders for worsened seizure control during BUTRANS therapy.

5.17 Avoidance of Withdrawal

Symptoms of withdrawal include restlessness, lacrimation, rhinorrhea, yawning, perspiration, chills, myalgia, and mydriasis. Significant fluid losses from vomiting and diarrhea can require intravenous fluid administration.

When discontinuing BUTRANS, gradually taper the dose *[see Dosage and Administration (2.3)]*. Do not abruptly discontinue BUTRANS.

5.18 Driving and Operating Machinery

BUTRANS may impair the mental and physical abilities needed to perform potentially hazardous activities such as driving a car or operating machinery. Warn patients not to drive or operate dangerous machinery unless they are tolerant to the effects of BUTRANS and know how they will react to the medication.

5.19 Use in Addiction Treatment

BUTRANS has not been studied and is not approved for use in the management of addictive disorders.

6 ADVERSE REACTIONS

The following adverse reactions described elsewhere in the labeling include:

- Respiratory Depression *[see Warnings and Precautions (5.2)]*
- QTc Prolongation *[see Warnings and Precautions (5.7)]*
- Hypotensive Effects *[see Warnings and Precautions (5.8)]*
- Application Site Skin Reactions *[see Warnings and Precautions (5.11)]*
- Anaphylactic/Allergic Reactions *[see Warnings and Precautions (5.12)]*
- Gastrointestinal Effects *[see Warnings and Precautions (5.15)]*
- Seizures *[see Warnings and Precautions (5.16)]*

6.1 Clinical Trial Experience

Because clinical trials are conducted under widely varying conditions, adverse reaction rates observed in the clinical trials of a drug cannot be directly compared to rates in the clinical trials of another drug and may not reflect the rates observed in practice.

A total of 5,415 patients were treated with BUTRANS in controlled and open-label chronic pain clinical trials. Nine hundred twenty-four subjects were treated for approximately six months and 183 subjects were treated for approximately one year. The clinical trial population consisted of patients with persistent moderate to severe pain.

The most common serious adverse drug reactions (all <0.1%) occurring during clinical trials with BUTRANS were: chest pain, abdominal pain, vomiting, dehydration, and hypertension/blood pressure increased.

The most common adverse events (≥ 2%) leading to discontinuation were: nausea, dizziness, vomiting, headache, and somnolence.

The most common adverse reactions (≥ 5%) reported by patients in clinical trials comparing BUTRANS 10 or 20 mcg/hour to placebo are shown in Table 2, and comparing BUTRANS 20 mcg/hour to BUTRANS 5 mcg/hour are shown in Table 3 below:

Table 2: Adverse Reactions Reported in ≥ 5% of Patients during the Open-Label Titration Period and Double-Blind Treatment Period: Opioid-Naïve Patients

	Open-Label Titration Period	Double-Blind	Treatment Period
	BUTRANS	BUTRANS	Placebo
MedDRA Preferred Term	(N = 1024)	(N = 256)	(N = 283)
Nausea	23%	13%	10%
Dizziness	10%	4%	1%
Headache	9%	5%	5%
Application site pruritus	8%	4%	7%
Somnolence	8%	2%	2%
Vomiting	7%	4%	1%
Constipation	6%	4%	1%

Table 3: Adverse Reactions Reported In ≥ 5% of Patients during the Open-Label Titration Period and Double-Blind Treatment Period: Opioid-Experienced Patients

	Open-Label Titration Period	Double-Blind	Treatment Period
	BUTRANS	BUTRANS 20	BUTRANS 5
MedDRA Preferred Term	(N = 1160)	(N = 219)	(N = 221)
Nausea	14%	11%	6%
Application site pruritus	9%	13%	5%
Headache	9%	8%	3%
Somnolence	6%	4%	2%
Dizziness	5%	4%	2%
Constipation	4%	6%	3%
Application site erythema	3%	10%	5%
Application site rash	3%	8%	6%
Application site irritation	2%	6%	2%

The following table lists adverse reactions that were reported in at least 2.0% of patients in four placebo/active-controlled titration-to-effect trials.

Table 4: Adverse Reactions Reported in Titration-to-Effect Placebo/Active-Controlled Clinical Trials with Incidence ≥ 2%

MedDRA Preferred Term	BUTRANS (N = 392)	Placebo (N = 261)
Nausea	21%	6%
Application site pruritus	15%	12%
Dizziness	15%	7%
Headache	14%	9%
Somnolence	13%	4%
Constipation	13%	5%
Vomiting	9%	1%
Application site erythema	7%	2%
Application site rash	6%	6%
Dry mouth	6%	2%
Fatigue	5%	1%
Hyperhidrosis	4%	1%
Peripheral edema	3%	1%
Pruritus	3%	0%
Stomach discomfort	2%	0%

The adverse reactions seen in controlled and open-label studies are presented below in the following manner: most common (≥ 5%), common (≥ 1% to < 5%), and less common (< 1%).

The most common adverse reactions (≥ 5%) reported by patients treated with BUTRANS in the clinical trials were nausea, headache, application site pruritus, dizziness, constipation, somnolence, vomiting, application site erythema, dry mouth, and application site rash.

The common (≥ 1% to < 5%) adverse reactions reported by patients treated with BUTRANS in the clinical trials organized by MedDRA (Medical Dictionary for Regulatory Activities) System Organ Class were:

Gastrointestinal disorders: diarrhea, dyspepsia, and upper abdominal pain

General disorders and administration site conditions: fatigue, peripheral edema, application site irritation, pain, pyrexia, chest pain, and asthenia

Infections and infestations: urinary tract infection, upper respiratory tract infection, nasopharyngitis, influenza, sinusitis, and bronchitis

Injury, poisoning and procedural complications: fall

Metabolism and nutrition disorders: anorexia

Musculoskeletal and connective tissue disorders: back pain, arthralgia, pain in extremity, muscle spasms, musculoskeletal pain, joint swelling, neck pain, and myalgia

Nervous system disorders: hypoesthesia, tremor, migraine, and paresthesia

Psychiatric disorders: insomnia, anxiety, and depression

Respiratory, thoracic and mediastinal disorders: dyspnea, pharyngolaryngeal pain, and cough

Skin and subcutaneous tissue disorders: pruritus, hyperhidrosis, rash, and generalized pruritus

Vascular disorders: hypertension

Other less common adverse reactions, including those known to occur with opioid treatment, that were seen in < 1% of the patients in the BUTRANS trials include the following in alphabetical order:

Abdominal distention, abdominal pain, accidental injury, affect lability, agitation, alanine aminotransferase increased, angina pectoris, angioedema, apathy, application site dermatitis, asthma aggravated, bradycardia, chills, confusional state, contact dermatitis, coordination abnormal, dehydration, depersonalization, depressed level of consciousness, depressed mood, disorientation, disturbance in attention, diverticulitis, drug hypersensitivity, drug withdrawal syndrome, dry eye, dry skin, dysarthria, dysgeusia, dysphagia, euphoric mood, face edema, flatulence, flushing, gait disturbance, hallucination, hiccups, hot flush, hyperventilation, hypotension, hypoventilation, ileus, insomnia, libido decreased, loss of consciousness, malaise, memory impairment, mental impairment, mental status changes, miosis, muscle weakness, nervousness, nightmare, orthostatic hypotension, palpitations, psychotic disorder, respiration abnormal, respiratory depression, respiratory distress, respiratory failure, restlessness, rhinitis, sedation, sexual dysfunction, syncope, tachycardia, tinnitus, urinary hesitation, urinary incontinence, urinary retention, urticaria, vasodilatation, vertigo, vision blurred, visual disturbance, weight decreased, and wheezing.

7 DRUG INTERACTIONS

7.1 Hepatic Enzyme Inhibitors and Inducers

<u>*CYP3A4 Inhibitors*</u>

Co-administration of ketoconazole, a strong CYP3A4 inhibitor, with BUTRANS, did not have any effect on C_{max} (maximum concentration) and AUC (area under the curve) of buprenorphine. Based on this observation, the pharmacokinetics of BUTRANS are not expected to be affected by co-administration of CYP3A4 inhibitors.

However, certain protease inhibitors (PIs) with CYP3A4 inhibitory activity such as atazanavir and atazanavir/ritonavir resulted in elevated levels of buprenorphine and norbuprenorphine following sublingual administration of buprenorphine and naloxone. Patients in this study reported increased sedation, and symptoms of opiate excess have been found in post-marketing reports of patients receiving sublingual buprenorphine and atazanavir with and without ritonavir concomitantly. Atazanavir is both a CYP3A4 and UGT1A1 inhibitor. As such, the drug-drug interaction potential for buprenorphine with CYP3A4 inhibitors is likely to be dependent on the route of administration as well as the specificity of enzyme inhibition *[see Clinical Pharmacology (12.3)]*.

<u>*CYP3A4 Inducers*</u>

The interaction between buprenorphine and CYP3A4 enzyme inducers has not been studied. Monitor patients receiving concurrent therapy with BUTRANS and CYP3A4 inducers (e.g., phenobarbital, carbamazepine, phenytoin, rifampin) closely for reduced efficacy or signs of withdrawal *[see Clinical Pharmacology (12.3)]*.

7.2 Benzodiazepines

There have been a number of reports regarding coma and death associated with the misuse and abuse of the combination of buprenorphine and benzodiazepines. In many, but not all of these cases, buprenorphine was misused by self-injection of crushed buprenorphine tablets. Preclinical studies have shown that the combination of benzodiazepines and buprenorphine altered the usual ceiling effect on buprenorphine-induced respiratory depression, making the respiratory effects of buprenorphine appear similar to those of full opioid agonists. Closely monitor patients with concurrent use of BUTRANS and benzodiazepines. Warn patients that it is extremely dangerous to self-administer benzodiazepines while taking BUTRANS, and warn patients to use benzodiazepines concurrently with BUTRANS only as directed by their physician.

7.3 CNS Depressants

Concurrent use of BUTRANS and other central nervous system (CNS) depressants (e.g., sedatives, hypnotics, general anesthetics, antiemetics, phenothiazines, other tranquilizers, and alcohol) can increase the risk of respiratory depression, hypotension, and profound sedation or coma. Monitor patients receiving CNS depressants and BUTRANS for signs of respiratory depression and hypotension. When such combined therapy is contemplated, reduce the initial dose of one or both agents.

7.4 Skeletal Muscle Relaxants

BUTRANS, like other opioids, may interact with skeletal muscle relaxants to enhance neuromuscular blocking action and increase respiratory depression.

7.5 Anticholinergics

Anticholinergics or other drugs with anticholinergic activity when used concurrently with opioid analgesics may result in increased risk of urinary retention and/or severe constipation, which may lead to paralytic ileus. Monitor patients for signs of urinary retention or reduced gastric motility when BUTRANS is used concurrently with anticholinergic drugs.

8 USE IN SPECIFIC POPULATIONS

8.1 Pregnancy

<u>*Teratogenic Effects (Pregnancy Category C)*</u>

There are no adequate and well-controlled studies with BUTRANS in pregnant women. BUTRANS should be used during pregnancy only if the potential benefit justifies the potential risk to the mother and the fetus. In animal studies, buprenorphine caused an increase in the number of stillborn offspring, reduced litter size, and reduced offspring growth in rats at maternal exposure levels that were approximately 10 times that of human subjects who received one BUTRANS 20 mcg/hour, the maximum recommended human dose (MRHD).

Studies in rats and rabbits demonstrated no evidence of teratogenicity following BUTRANS or subcutaneous (SC) administration of buprenorphine during the period of major organogenesis. Rats were administered up to one BUTRANS 20 mcg/hour every 3 days (gestation days 6, 9, 12, & 15) or received daily SC buprenorphine up to 5 mg/kg (gestation days 6-17). Rabbits were administered four BUTRANS 20 mcg/hour every 3 days (gestation days 6, 9, 12, 15, 18, & 19) or received daily SC buprenorphine up to 5 mg/kg (gestation days 6-19). No teratogenicity was observed at any dose. AUC values for buprenorphine with BUTRANS application and SC injection were approximately 110 and 140 times, respectively, that of human subjects who received the MRHD of one BUTRANS 20 mcg/hour.

Non-Teratogenic Effects

In a peri- and post-natal study conducted in pregnant and lactating rats, administration of buprenorphine either as BUTRANS or SC buprenorphine was associated with toxicity to offspring. Buprenorphine was present in maternal milk. Pregnant rats were administered 1/4 of one BUTRANS 5 mcg/hour every 3 days or received daily SC buprenorphine at doses of 0.05, 0.5, or 5 mg/kg from gestation day 6 to lactation day 21 (weaning). Administration of BUTRANS or SC buprenorphine at 0.5 or 5 mg/kg caused maternal toxicity and an increase in the number of stillborns, reduced litter size, and reduced offspring growth at maternal exposure levels that were approximately 10 times that of human subjects who received the MRHD of one BUTRANS 20 mcg/hour. Maternal toxicity was also observed at the no observed adverse effect level (NOAEL) for offspring.

8.2 Labor and Delivery

BUTRANS is not for use in women immediately prior to and during labor, where use of short-acting analgesics or other analgesic techniques are more appropriate *[see Indications and Usage (1)]*. Occasionally, opioid analgesics may prolong labor through actions which temporarily reduce the strength, duration and frequency of uterine contractions. However this effect is not consistent and may be offset by an increased rate of cervical dilatation, which tends to shorten labor.

Opioids cross the placenta and may produce respiratory depression and psychophysiologic effects in neonates. Closely observe neonates whose mothers received opioid analgesics during labor for signs of respiratory depression. An opioid antagonist, such as naloxone, should be available for reversal of opioid-induced respiratory depression in the neonate in such situations.

8.3 Nursing Mothers

Buprenorphine is excreted in breast milk. The amount of buprenorphine received by the infant varies depending on the maternal plasma concentration, the amount of milk ingested by the infant, and the extent of first pass metabolism.

Withdrawal symptoms can occur in breast-feeding infants when maternal administration of buprenorphine is stopped. Because of the potential for adverse reactions in nursing infants from BUTRANS, a decision should be made whether to discontinue nursing or discontinue the drug, taking into account the importance of the drug to the mother.

8.4 Pediatric Use

The safety and efficacy of BUTRANS in patients under 18 years of age has not been established.

8.5 Geriatric Use

Of the total number of subjects in the clinical trials (5,415), BUTRANS was administered to 1,377 patients aged 65 years and older. Of those, 457 patients were 75 years of age and older. In the clinical program, the incidences of selected BUTRANS-related AEs were higher in older subjects. The incidences of application site AEs were slightly higher among subjects < 65 years of age than those ≥ 65 years of age for both BUTRANS and placebo treatment groups.

In a single-dose study of healthy elderly and healthy young subjects treated with BUTRANS 10 mcg/hour, the pharmacokinetics were similar. In a separate dose-escalation safety study, the pharmacokinetics in the healthy elderly and hypertensive elderly subjects taking thiazide diuretics were similar to those in the healthy young adults. In the elderly groups evaluated, adverse event rates were similar to or lower than rates in healthy young adult subjects, except for constipation and urinary retention, which were more common in the elderly. Although specific dose adjustments on the basis of advanced age are not required for pharmacokinetic reasons, use caution in the elderly population to ensure safe use *[see Clinical Pharmacology (12.3)]*.

8.6 Hepatic Impairment

In a study utilizing intravenous buprenorphine, peak plasma levels (C_{max}) and exposure (AUC) of buprenorphine in patients with mild and moderate hepatic impairment did not increase as compared to those observed in subjects with normal hepatic function. BUTRANS has not been evaluated in patients with severe hepatic impairment. As BUTRANS is intended for 7-day dosing, consider the use of alternate analgesic therapy in patients with severe hepatic impairment *[see Dosage and Administration (2.4), and Clinical Pharmacology (12.3)]*.

8.7 Neonatal Opioid Withdrawal Syndrome

Chronic maternal use of buprenorphine during pregnancy can affect the fetus with subsequent withdrawal signs. Neonatal withdrawal syndrome presents as irritability, hyperactivity and abnormal sleep pattern, high pitched cry, tremor, vomiting, diarrhea and failure to gain weight. The onset, duration and severity of neonatal withdrawal syndrome vary based on the drug used, duration of use, the dose of last maternal use, and rate of elimination drug by the newborn. Neonatal opioid withdrawal syndrome, unlike opioid withdrawal syndrome in adults, may be life-threatening and should be treated according to protocols developed by neonatology experts.

9 DRUG ABUSE AND DEPENDENCE

9.1 Controlled Substance

BUTRANS contains buprenorphine, a mu opioid partial agonist and Schedule III controlled substance with an abuse potential similar to other Schedule III opioids. BUTRANS can be abused and is subject to misuse, abuse, addiction and criminal diversion.

9.2 Abuse

Abuse of BUTRANS poses a hazard of overdose and death. This risk is increased with compromise of the BUTRANS Transdermal System and with concurrent abuse of alcohol or other substances. BUTRANS has been diverted for non-medical use.

All patients treated with opioids, including BUTRANS, require careful monitoring for signs of abuse and addiction, because use of opioid analgesic products carries the risk of addiction even under appropriate medical use.

All patients treated with opioids require careful monitoring for signs of abuse and addiction, since use of opioid analgesic products carries the risk of addiction even under appropriate medical use. Drug abuse is the intentional non-therapeutic use of an over-the-counter or prescription drug, even once, for its rewarding psychological or physiological effects. Drug abuse includes, but is not limited to, the following examples: the use of a prescription or over-the-counter drug to get "high", or the use of steroids for performance enhancement and muscle build up.

Drug addiction is a cluster of behavioral, cognitive, and physiological phenomena that develop after repeated substance use and includes: a strong desire to take the drug, difficulties in controlling its use, persisting in its use despite harmful consequences, a higher priority given to drug use than to other activities and obligations, increased tolerance, and sometimes a physical withdrawal.

"Drug-seeking" behavior is very common in persons with substance use disorders. Drug-seeking tactics include, but are not limited to, emergency calls or visits near the end of office hours, refusal to undergo appropriate examination, testing or referral, repeated "loss" of prescriptions, tampering with prescriptions and reluctance to provide prior medical records or contact information for other treating physician(s). "Doctor shopping" (visiting multiple prescribers) to obtain additional prescriptions is common among drug abusers and people suffering from untreated addiction.

Preoccupation with achieving adequate pain relief can be appropriate behavior in a patient with poor pain control.

Abuse and addiction are separate and distinct from physical dependence and tolerance. Physicians should be aware that addiction may not be accompanied by concurrent tolerance and symptoms of physical dependence in all addicts. In addition, abuse of opioids can occur in the absence of true addiction.

BUTRANS may be diverted for non-medical use into illicit channels of distribution. Careful record-keeping of prescribing information, including quantity, frequency, and renewal requests, as required by state law, is strongly advised.

The risks of misuse and abuse should be considered when prescribing or dispensing BUTRANS. Concerns about abuse and addiction, should not prevent the proper management of pain, however. Treatment of pain should be individualized, balancing the potential benefits and risks for each patient.

Risks Specific to the Abuse of BUTRANS

BUTRANS is intended for transdermal use only. Abuse of BUTRANS poses a risk of overdose and death. This risk is increased with concurrent abuse of BUTRANS with alcohol and other substances including other opioids and benzodiazepines *[see Warnings and Precautions (5.6), and Drug Interactions (7.2)]*. Compromising the transdermal delivery system will result in the uncontrolled delivery of buprenorphine and pose a significant risk to the abuser that could result in overdose and death *[see Warnings and Precautions (5.1)]*. Abuse may occur by applying the transdermal system in the absence of legitimate purpose, or by swallowing, snorting or injecting buprenorphine extracted from the transdermal system.

9.3 Dependence

Both tolerance and physical dependence can develop during chronic opioid therapy. Tolerance is the need for increasing doses of opioids to maintain a defined effect such as analgesia (in the absence of disease progression or other external factors). Tolerance may occur to both the desired and undesired effects of drugs, and may develop at different rates for different effects.

Physical dependence results in withdrawal symptoms after abrupt discontinuation or a significant dose reduction of a drug. Withdrawal also may be precipitated through the administration of drugs with opioid antagonist activity, e.g., naloxone, nalmefene, or mixed agonist/antagonist analgesics (pentazocine, butorphanol, nalbuphine). Physical dependence may not occur to a clinically significant degree until after several days to weeks of continued opioid usage.

BUTRANS should not be abruptly discontinued *[see Dosage and Administration (2.3)]*. If BUTRANS is abruptly discontinued in a physically-dependent patient, an abstinence syndrome may occur. Some or all of the following can characterize this syndrome: restlessness, lacrimation, rhinorrhea, yawning, perspiration, chills, myalgia, and mydriasis. Other signs and symptoms also may develop, including: irritability, anxiety, backache, joint pain, weakness, abdominal cramps, insomnia, nausea, anorexia, vomiting, diarrhea, or increased blood pressure, respiratory rate, or heart rate.

Infants born to mothers physically dependent on opioids will also be physically dependent and may exhibit respiratory difficulties and withdrawal symptoms *[see Use in Specific Populations (8.7)]*.

10 OVERDOSAGE

Clinical Presentation

Acute overdosage with BUTRANS is manifested by respiratory depression, somnolence progressing to stupor or coma, skeletal muscle flaccidity, cold and clammy skin, constricted pupils, bradycardia, hypotension, partial or complete airway obstruction, atypical snoring and death. Marked mydriasis rather than miosis may be seen due to severe hypoxia in overdose situations.

Treatment of Overdose

In case of overdose, priorities are the re-establishment of a patent and protected airway and institution of assisted or controlled ventilation if needed. Employ other supportive measures (including oxygen, vasopressors) in the management of circulatory shock and pulmonary edema as indicated. Cardiac arrest or arrhythmias will require advanced life support techniques.

Naloxone may not be effective in reversing any respiratory depression produced by buprenorphine. High doses of naloxone, 10-35 mg/70 kg, may be of limited value in the management of buprenorphine overdose. The onset of naloxone effect may be delayed by 30 minutes or more. Doxapram hydrochloride (a respiratory stimulant) has also been used.

Remove BUTRANS immediately. Because the duration of reversal would be expected to be less than the duration of action of buprenorphine from BUTRANS, carefully monitor the patient until spontaneous respiration is reliably re-established. Even in the face of improvement, continued medical monitoring is required because of the possibility of extended effects as buprenorphine continues to be absorbed from the skin. After removal of BUTRANS, the mean buprenorphine concentrations decrease approximately 50% in 12 hours (range 10-24 hours) with an apparent terminal half-life of approximately 26 hours. Due to this long apparent terminal half-life, patients may require monitoring and treatment for at least 24 hours.

In an individual physically dependent on opioids, administration of an opioid receptor antagonist may precipitate an acute withdrawal. The severity of the withdrawal produced will depend on the degree of physical dependence and the dose of the antagonist administered. If a decision is made to treat serious respiratory depression in the physically dependent patient with an opioid antagonist, administration of the antagonist should be begun with care and by titration with smaller than usual doses of the antagonist.

11 DESCRIPTION

BUTRANS is a transdermal system providing systemic delivery of buprenorphine, a mu opioid partial agonist analgesic, continuously for 7 days. The chemical name of buprenorphine is 6,14-ethenomorphinan-7-methanol, 17-(cyclopropylmethyl)- α-(1,1-dimethylethyl)-4, 5-epoxy-18, 19-dihydro-3-hydroxy-6-methoxy-α-methyl-, [5α, 7α, (S)]. The structural formula is:

[See chemical structure at top of next column]

The molecular weight of buprenorphine is 467.6; the empirical formula is $C_{29}H_{41}NO_4$. Buprenorphine occurs as a white or almost white powder and is very slightly soluble in water, freely soluble in acetone, soluble in methanol and ether, and slightly soluble in cyclohexane. The pKa is 8.5 and the melting point is about 217°C.

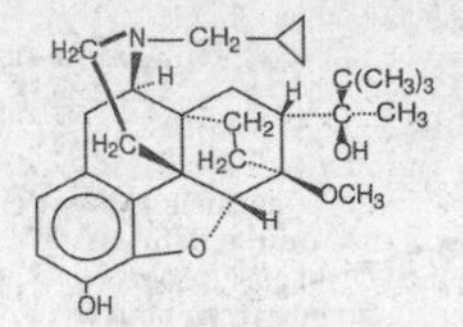

System Components and Structure

Four different strengths of BUTRANS are available: 5, 10, 15, and 20 mcg/hour (Table 5). The proportion of buprenorphine mixed in the adhesive matrix is the same in each of the four strengths. The amount of buprenorphine released from each system per hour is proportional to the active surface area of the system. The skin is the limiting barrier to diffusion from the system into the bloodstream.

Table 5: BUTRANS Product Specifications

Buprenorphine Delivery Rate (mcg/hour)	Active Surface Area (cm^2)	Total Buprenorphine Content (mg)
BUTRANS 5	6.25	5
BUTRANS 10	12.5	10
BUTRANS 15	18.75	15
BUTRANS 20	25	20

BUTRANS is a rectangular or square, beige-colored system consisting of a protective liner and functional layers. Proceeding from the outer surface toward the surface adhering to the skin, the layers are (1) a beige-colored web backing layer; (2) an adhesive rim without buprenorphine; (3) a separating layer over the buprenorphine-containing adhesive matrix; (4) the buprenorphine-containing adhesive matrix; and (5) a peel-off release liner. Before use, the release liner covering the adhesive layer is removed and discarded.

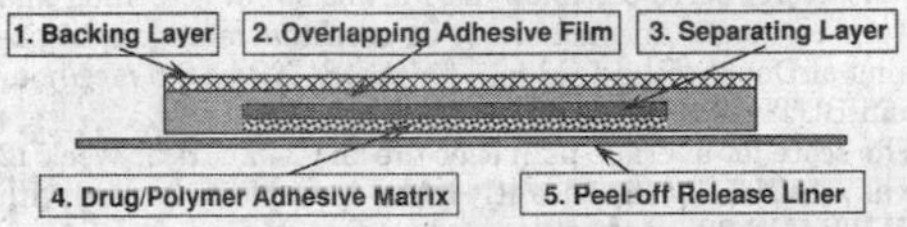

Figure 1: Cross-Section Diagram of BUTRANS (not to scale).

The active ingredient in BUTRANS is buprenorphine. The inactive ingredients in each system are: levulinic acid, oleyl oleate, povidone, and polyacrylate cross-linked with aluminum.

12 CLINICAL PHARMACOLOGY

12.1 Mechanism of Action

Buprenorphine is a partial agonist at mu opioid receptors. Buprenorphine is also an antagonist at kappa opioid receptors, an agonist at delta opioid receptors, and a partial agonist at ORL-1 (nociceptin) receptors. Its clinical actions result from binding to the opioid receptors.

12.2 Pharmacodynamics

Effects on the Central Nervous System

The principal actions of therapeutic value of buprenorphine are analgesia and sedation. Specific CNS opiate receptors and endogenous compounds with morphine-like activity have been identified throughout the brain and spinal cord and are likely to play a role in the expression of analgesic effects.

Buprenorphine produces respiratory depression by direct action on brainstem respiratory centers. The mechanism of respiratory depression involves a reduction in the responsiveness of the brainstem respiratory centers to increases in carbon dioxide tension, and to electrical stimulation.

Buprenorphine causes miosis, even in total darkness, and little tolerance develops to this effect. Pinpoint pupils are a sign of opioid overdose but are not pathognomonic (e.g., pontine lesions of hemorrhagic or ischemic origins may produce similar findings). Marked mydriasis rather than miosis may be seen with worsening hypoxia in the setting of buprenorphine overdose.

Effects on the Gastrointestinal Tract and Other Smooth Muscle

Gastric, biliary, and pancreatic secretions are decreased by buprenorphine. Buprenorphine causes a reduction in motility associated with an increase in tone in the antrum of the stomach and duodenum. Digestion of food in the small intestine is delayed and propulsive contractions are decreased. Propulsive peristaltic waves in the colon are decreased, while tone is increased to the point of spasm. The end result is constipation. Buprenorphine can cause a marked increase in biliary tract pressure as a result of spasm of the sphincter of Oddi.

Effects on the Cardiovascular System

Buprenorphine may cause a reduction in blood pressure.

Effects on Cardiac Electrophysiology

The effect of BUTRANS 10 mcg/hour and 2 × BUTRANS 20 mcg/hour on QTc interval was evaluated in a double-blind (BUTRANS vs. placebo), randomized, placebo and active-controlled (moxifloxacin 400 mg, open label), parallel-group, dose escalating, single dose study in 132 healthy male and female subjects aged 18 to 55 years. The dose escalation sequence for BUTRANS during the titration period was: BUTRANS 5 mcg/hour for 3 days, then BUTRANS 10 mcg/hour for 3 days, then BUTRANS 20 mcg/hour for 3 days, then 2 × BUTRANS 20 mcg/hour for 4 days. The QTc evaluation was performed during the third day of BUTRANS 10 mcg/hour and the fourth day of 2 × BUTRANS 20 mcg/hour when the plasma levels of buprenorphine were at steady state for the corresponding doses *[see Warnings and Precautions (5.7)]*.

There was no clinically meaningful effect on mean QTc with a BUTRANS dose of 10 mcg/hour. A BUTRANS dose of 40 mcg/hour (given as two 20 mcg/hour BUTRANS Transdermal Systems) prolonged mean QTc by a maximum of 9.2 (90% CI: 5.2-13.3) msec across the 13 assessment time points.

Effects on the Endocrine System

Opioids inhibit the secretion of ACTH, cortisol, and luteinizing hormone (LH) in humans. They also stimulate prolactin, growth hormone (GH) secretion, and pancreatic secretion of insulin and glucagon.

Effects on the Immune System

Opioids have been shown to have a variety of effects on components of the immune system in *in vitro* and animal models. The clinical significance of these findings is unknown. Overall, the effects of opioids appear to be modestly immunosuppressive.

12.3 Pharmacokinetics

Absorption

Each BUTRANS system provides delivery of buprenorphine for 7 days. Steady state was achieved during the first application by Day 3 (see Figure 2).

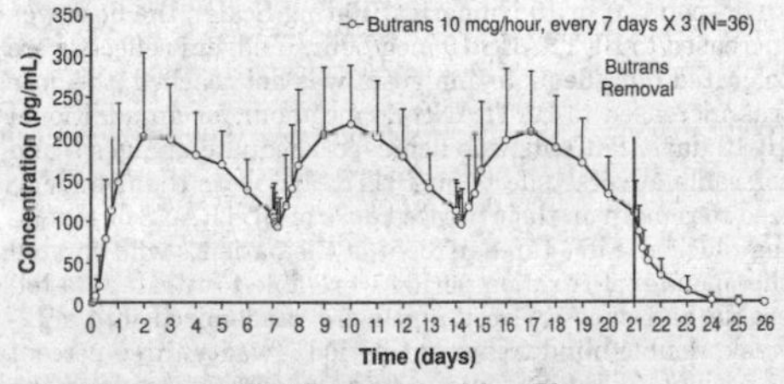

Figure 2 Mean (SD) Buprenorphine Plasma Concentrations Following Three Consecutive Applications of BUTRANS 10 mcg/hour (N = 36 Healthy Subjects)

BUTRANS 5, 10, and 20 mcg/hour provide dose-proportional total buprenorphine exposures (AUC) following 7-day applications. BUTRANS single 7-day application and steady-state pharmacokinetic parameters are summarized in Table 6. Plasma buprenorphine concentrations after titration showed no further change over the 60-day period studied. After removal of BUTRANS, mean buprenorphine concentrations decrease approximately 50% within 10 - 24 hours, followed by decline with an apparent terminal half-life of approximately 26 hours.

Table 6: Pharmacokinetic Parameters of BUTRANS in Healthy Subjects, Mean (%CV)

Single 7-day Application	AUC_{inf} (pg.h/mL)	C_{max} (pg/mL)
BUTRANS 5 mcg/hour	12087 (37)	176 (67)
BUTRANS 10 mcg/hour	27035 (29)	191 (34)
BUTRANS 20 mcg/hour	54294 (36)	471 (49)
Multiple 7-day Applications	**$AUC_{tau,ss}$ (pg.h/mL)**	**$C_{max,ss}$ (pg/mL)**
BUTRANS 10 mcg/hour, steady-state	27543 (33)	224 (35)

Transdermal delivery studies showed that intact human skin is permeable to buprenorphine. In clinical pharmacology studies, the median time for BUTRANS 10 mcg/hour to deliver quantifiable buprenorphine concentrations (≥ 25 pg/mL) was approximately 17 hours. The absolute bioavailability of BUTRANS relative to IV administration, following a 7-day application, is approximately 15% for all doses (BUTRANS 5, 10, and 20 mcg/hour).

Distribution

Buprenorphine is approximately 96% bound to plasma proteins, mainly to alpha- and beta-globulin.

Studies of IV buprenorphine have shown a large volume of distribution (approximately 430 L), implying extensive distribution of buprenorphine.

Following IV administration, buprenorphine and its metabolites are secreted into bile and excreted in urine. CSF buprenorphine concentrations appear to be approximately 15-25% of concurrent plasma concentrations.

Metabolism

Buprenorphine metabolism in the skin following BUTRANS application is negligible. Following transdermal application, buprenorphine is eliminated via hepatic metabolism, with subsequent biliary excretion and renal excretion of soluble metabolites.

Buprenorphine primarily undergoes *N*-dealkylation by CYP3A4 to norbuprenorphine and glucuronidation by UGT-isoenzymes (mainly UGT1A1 and 2B7) to buprenorphine 3β-*O*-glucuronide. Norbuprenorphine, the major metabolite, is also glucuronidated (mainly UGT1A3) prior to excretion. Norbuprenorphine is the only known active metabolite of buprenorphine. It has been shown to be a respiratory depressant in rats, but only at concentrations at least 50-fold greater than those observed following application to humans of BUTRANS 20 mcg/hour.

Since metabolism and excretion of buprenorphine occur mainly via hepatic elimination, reductions in hepatic blood flow induced by some general anesthetics (e.g., halothane) and other drugs may result in a decreased rate of hepatic elimination of the drug, resulting in increased plasma concentrations.

Excretion

Following intramuscular administration of 2 mcg/kg dose of buprenorphine, approximately 70% of the dose was excreted in feces within 7 days. Approximately 27% was excreted in urine. The total clearance of buprenorphine is approximately 55 L/hour in postoperative patients.

Drug Interactions

Effect of CYP3A4 inhibitors

In a drug-drug interaction study, BUTRANS 10 mcg/hour (single dose × 7 days) was co-administered with 200 mg ketoconazole, a strong CYP3A4 inhibitor or ketoconazole placebo twice daily for 11 days and the pharmacokinetics of buprenorphine and its metabolites were evaluated. Plasma buprenorphine concentrations did not accumulate during co-medication with ketoconazole 200 mg twice daily. Based on the results from this study, metabolism during therapy with BUTRANS is not expected to be affected by co-administration of CYP3A4 inhibitors *[see Drug Interactions (7.1)]*.

Antiretroviral agents have been evaluated for CYP3A4 mediated interactions with sublingual buprenorphine. Nucleoside reverse transcriptase inhibitors (NRTIs) and non-nucleoside reverse transcriptase inhibitors (NNRTIs) do not appear to have clinically significant interactions with buprenorphine. However, certain protease inhibitors (PIs) with CYP3A4 inhibitory activity such as atazanavir and atazanavir/ritonavir resulted in elevated levels of buprenorphine and norbuprenorphine when buprenorphine and naloxone were administered sublingually. C_{max} and AUC for buprenorphine increased by up to 1.6 and 1.9 fold, and C_{max} and AUC for norbuprenorphine increased by up to 1.6 and 2.0 fold respectively, when sublingual buprenorphine was administered with these PIs. Patients in this study reported increased sedation, and symptoms of opiate excess have been found in post-marketing reports of patients receiving buprenorphine and atazanavir with and without ritonavir concomitantly. It should be noted that atazanavir is both a CYP3A4 and UGT1A1 inhibitor. As such, the drug-drug interaction potential for buprenorphine with CYP3A4 inhibitors is likely to be dependent on the route of administration as well as the specificity of enzyme inhibition *[see Drug Interactions (7.1)]*.

Effect of CYP3A4 Inducers

The interaction between buprenorphine and CYP3A4 inducers has not been studied.

Effects of Application Site

A study in healthy subjects demonstrated that the pharmacokinetic profile of buprenorphine delivered by BUTRANS 10 mcg/hour is similar when applied to the upper outer arm, upper chest, upper back, or the side of the chest *[see Dosage and Administration (2.5)]*.

The reapplication of BUTRANS 10 mcg/hour after various rest periods to the same application site in healthy subjects showed that the minimum rest period needed to avoid variability in drug absorption is 3 weeks (21 days) *[see Dosage and Administration (2.5)]*.

Effects of Heat

In a study of healthy subjects, application of a heating pad directly on the BUTRANS 10 mcg/hour system caused a 26% - 55% increase in blood concentrations of buprenorphine. Concentrations returned to normal within 5 hours after the heat was removed. For this reason, instruct patients not to apply heating pads directly to the BUTRANS system during system wear *[see Warnings and Precautions (5.13)]*.

Fever may increase the permeability of the skin, leading to increased buprenorphine concentrations during BUTRANS treatment. As a result, febrile patients are at increased risk for the possibility of BUTRANS-related reactions during treatment with BUTRANS. Monitor patients with febrile illness for adverse effects and consider dose adjustment *[see Warnings and Precautions (5.14)]*. In a crossover study of healthy subjects receiving endotoxin or placebo challenge during BUTRANS 10 mcg/hour wear, the AUC and C_{max} were similar despite a physiologic response of mild fever to endotoxin.

Special Populations

Geriatric Patients

Following a single application of BUTRANS 10 mcg/hour to 12 healthy young adults (mean age 32 years) and 12 healthy elderly subjects (mean age 72 years), the pharmacokinetic profile of BUTRANS was similar in healthy elderly and healthy young adult subjects, though the elderly subjects showed a trend toward higher plasma concentrations immediately after BUTRANS removal. Both groups eliminated buprenorphine at similar rates after system removal *[see Use in Specific Populations (8.5)]*.

In a study of healthy young subjects, healthy elderly subjects, and elderly subjects treated with thiazide diuretics, BUTRANS at a fixed dose-escalation schedule (BUTRANS 5 mcg/hour for 3 days, followed by BUTRANS 10 mcg/hour for 3 days and BUTRANS 20 mcg/hour for 7 days) produced similar mean plasma concentration vs. time profiles for each of the three subject groups. There were no significant differences between groups in buprenorphine C_{max} or AUC *[see Use in Specific Populations (8.5)]*.

Pediatric Patients

BUTRANS has not been studied in children and is not recommended for pediatric use.

Gender

In a pooled data analysis utilizing data from several studies that administered BUTRANS 10 mcg/hour to healthy subjects, no differences in buprenorphine C_{max} and AUC or body-weight normalized C_{max} and AUC were observed between males and females treated with BUTRANS.

Renal Impairment

No studies in patients with renal impairment have been performed with BUTRANS.

In an independent study, the effect of impaired renal function on buprenorphine pharmacokinetics after IV bolus and after continuous IV infusion administrations was evaluated. It was found that plasma buprenorphine concentrations were similar in patients with normal renal function and in patients with impaired renal function or renal failure. In a separate investigation of the effect of intermittent hemodialysis on buprenorphine plasma concentrations in chronic pain patients with end-stage renal disease who were treated with a transdermal buprenorphine product (marketed outside the US) up to 70 mcg/hour, no significant differences in buprenorphine plasma concentrations before or after hemodialysis were observed.

No notable relationship was observed between estimated creatinine clearance rates and steady-state buprenorphine concentrations among patients during BUTRANS therapy.

Hepatic Impairment

The pharmacokinetics of buprenorphine following an IV infusion of 0.3 mg of buprenorphine were compared in 8 patients with mild impairment (Child-Pugh A), 4 patients with moderate impairment (Child-Pugh B) and 12 subjects with normal hepatic function. Buprenorphine and norbuprenorphine exposure did not increase in the mild and moderate hepatic impairment patients.

BUTRANS has not been evaluated in patients with severe (Child-Pugh C) hepatic impairment *[see Dosage and Administration (2.4), Warnings and Precautions (5.10), and Use in Specific Populations (8.6)]*.

13 NONCLINICAL TOXICOLOGY

13.1 Carcinogenesis, Mutagenesis, Impairment of Fertility

Carcinogenesis

Buprenorphine administered daily by skin painting to Sprague Dawley rats for 100 weeks at dosages (20, 60, or 200 mg/kg) produced systemic exposures (based on AUC) that ranged from approximately 130 to 350 times that of human subjects administered the maximum recommended human dose (MRHD) of BUTRANS 20 mcg/hour. An increased incidence of benign testicular interstitial cell tumors, considered buprenorphine treatment-related, was observed in male rats compared with concurrent controls. The tumor incidence was also above the highest incidence in the historical control database of the testing facility. These tumors were noted at 60 mg/kg/day and higher at approximately 220 times the proposed MRHD based on AUC. The no observed effect level (NOEL) was 20 mg/kg/day (approximately 140 times the proposed MRHD based on AUC). The mechanism leading to the tumor findings and the relevance to humans is unknown.

Buprenorphine was administered by skin painting to hemizygous Tg.AC mice over a 6-month study period. At the dosages administered daily (18.75, 37.5, 150, or 600 mg/kg/day), buprenorphine was not carcinogenic or tumorigenic at systemic exposure to buprenorphine, based on AUC, of up to approximately 1000 times that of human subjects administered BUTRANS 20 mcg/hour, the MRHD.

Mutagenesis

Buprenorphine was not genotoxic in 3 *in vitro* genetic toxicology studies (bacterial mutagenicity test, mouse lymphoma assay, chromosomal aberration assay in human peripheral blood lymphocytes), and in one *in vivo* mouse micronucleus test.

Impairment of Fertility

BUTRANS (1/4 of a BUTRANS 5 mcg/hour, one BUTRANS 5 mcg/hour, or one BUTRANS 20 mcg/hour every 3 days in males for 4 weeks prior to mating for a total of 10 weeks and in females for 2 weeks prior to mating through gestation day 7) had no effect on fertility or general reproductive performance of rats at AUC-based exposure levels as high as approximately 65 times (females) and 100 times (males) that for human subjects who received BUTRANS 20 mcg/hour, the MRHD.

14 CLINICAL STUDIES

The efficacy of BUTRANS has been evaluated in four 12-week double-blind, controlled clinical trials in opioid-naïve and opioid-experienced patients with moderate to severe chronic low back pain or osteoarthritis using pain scores as the primary efficacy variable. Two of these studies, described below, demonstrated efficacy in patients with low back pain. One study in low back pain failed to show efficacy. One study in osteoarthritis, that included an active comparator, failed to show efficacy for BUTRANS and the active comparator.

12-Week Study in Opioid-Naïve Patients with Chronic Low Back Pain

A total of 1,024 patients with chronic low back pain who were suboptimally responsive to their non-opioid therapy entered an open-label, dose-titration period for up to four weeks. Patients initiated therapy with three days of treatment with BUTRANS 5 mcg/hour. After three days, if adverse events were tolerated but the pain persisted (≥ 5 on an 11-point, 0 to 10 Numerical Rating Scale), the dose was increased to BUTRANS 10 mcg/hour. If adverse effects were tolerated but adequate analgesia was not reached, the dose was increased to BUTRANS 20 mcg/hour for an additional 10-12 days. Patients who achieved adequate analgesia and tolerable adverse effects on BUTRANS were then randomized to remain on their titrated dose of BUTRANS or matching placebo. Fifty-three percent of the patients who entered the open-label titration period were able to titrate to a tolerable and effective dose and were randomized into a 12-week, double-blind treatment period. Twenty-three percent of patients discontinued due to an adverse event from the open-label titration period and 14% discontinued due to lack of a therapeutic effect. The remaining 10% of patients were dropped due to various administrative reasons.

During the first seven days of double-blind treatment patients were allowed up to two tablets per day of immediate-release oxycodone 5 mg as supplemental analgesia to minimize opioid withdrawal symptoms in patients randomized to placebo. Thereafter, the supplemental analgesia was limited to either acetaminophen 500 mg or ibuprofen 200 mg at a maximum of four tablets per day. Sixty-six percent of the patients treated with BUTRANS completed the 12-week treatment compared to 70% of the patients treated with placebo. Of the 256 patients randomized to BUTRANS, 9% discontinued due to lack of efficacy and 16% due to adverse events. Of the 283 patients randomized to placebo, 13% discontinued due to lack of efficacy and 7% due to adverse events.

Of the patients who were randomized, the mean pain (SE) NRS scores were 7.2 (0.08) and 7.2 (0.07) at screening and 2.6 (0.08) and 2.6 (0.07) at pre-randomization (beginning of double-blind phase) for the BUTRANS and placebo groups, respectively.

The score for average pain over the last 24 hours at the end of the study (Week 12/Early Termination) was statistically significantly lower for patients treated with BUTRANS compared with patients treated with placebo. The proportion of patients with various degrees of improvement, from screening to study endpoint, is shown in Figure 3 below.

[See figure 3 at top of next column]

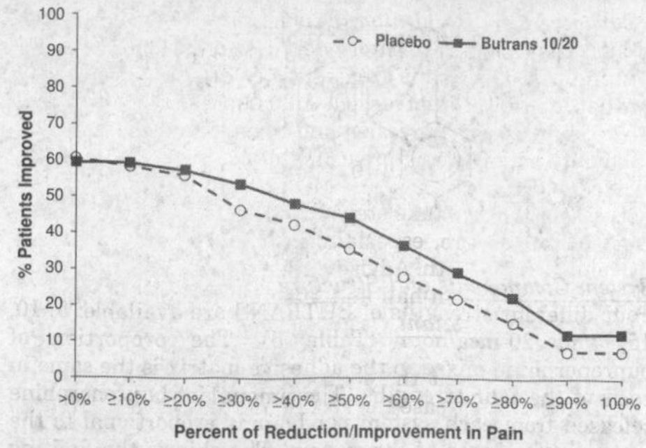

Figure 3: Percent Reduction in Pain Intensity

12-Week Study in Opioid-Experienced Patients with Chronic Low Back Pain

One thousand one hundred and sixty (1,160) patients on chronic opioid therapy (total daily dose 30-80 mg morphine equivalent) entered an open-label, dose-titration period with BUTRANS for up to 3 weeks, following taper of prior opioids. Patients initiated therapy with BUTRANS 10 mcg/hour for three days. After three days, if the patient tolerated the adverse effects, the dose was increased to BUTRANS 20 mcg/hour for up to 18 days. Patients with adequate analgesia and tolerable adverse effects on BUTRANS 20 mcg/hour were randomized to remain on BUTRANS 20 mcg/hour or were switched to a low-dose control (BUTRANS 5 mcg/hour) or an active control. Fifty-seven percent of the patients who entered the open-label titration period were able to titrate to and tolerate the adverse effects of BUTRANS 20 mcg/hour and were randomized into a 12-week double-blind treatment phase. Twelve percent of patients discontinued due to an adverse event and 21% discontinued due to lack of a therapeutic effect during the open-label titration period.

During the double-blind period, patients were permitted to take ibuprofen (200 mg tablets) or acetaminophen (500 mg tablets) every 4 hours as needed for supplemental analgesia (up to 3200 mg of ibuprofen and 4 grams of acetaminophen daily). Sixty-seven percent of patients treated with BUTRANS 20 mcg/hour and 58% of patients treated with BUTRANS 5 mcg/hour completed the 12-week treatment. Of the 219 patients randomized to BUTRANS 20 mcg/hour, 11% discontinued due to lack of efficacy and 13% due to adverse events. Of the 221 patients randomized to BUTRANS 5 mcg/hour, 24% discontinued due to lack of efficacy and 6% due to adverse events. Of the patients who were able to be randomized in the double-blind period, the mean pain (SE) NRS scores were 6.4 (0.08) and 6.5 (0.08) at screening and were 2.8 (0.08) and 2.9 (0.08) at pre-randomization (beginning of Double-Blind Period) for the BUTRANS 5 mcg/hour and BUTRANS 20 mcg/hour, respectively.

The score for average pain over the last 24 hours at Week 12 was statistically significantly lower for subjects treated with BUTRANS 20 mcg/hour compared to subjects treated with BUTRANS 5 mcg/hour. A higher proportion of BUTRANS 20 mcg/hour patients (49%) had at least a 30% reduction in pain score from screening to study endpoint when compared to BUTRANS 5 mcg/hour patients (33%). The proportion of patients with various degrees of improvement from screening to study endpoint is shown in Figure 4 below.

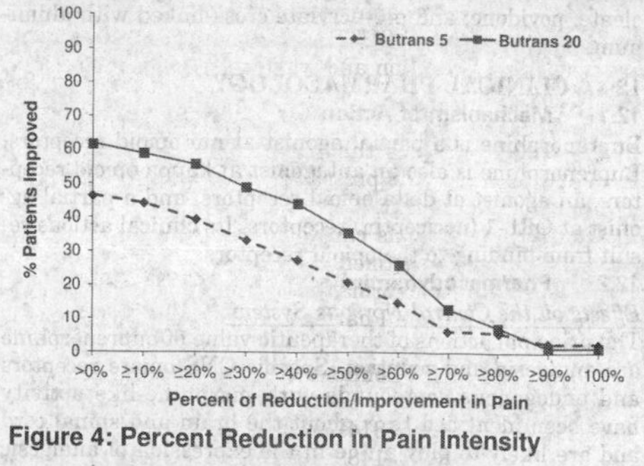

Figure 4: Percent Reduction in Pain Intensity

16 HOW SUPPLIED/STORAGE AND HANDLING

BUTRANS (buprenorphine) Transdermal System is supplied in cartons containing 4 individually-packaged systems and a pouch containing 4 Patch-Disposal Units.

BUTRANS 5 mcg/hour Transdermal System, 4-count carton
NDC 59011-750-04

BUTRANS 10 mcg/hour Transdermal System, 4-count carton
NDC 59011-751-04

BUTRANS 15 mcg/hour Transdermal System, 4-count carton
NDC 59011-758-04

BUTRANS 20 mcg/hour Transdermal System, 4-count carton
NDC 59011-752-04

Store at 25°C (77°F); excursions permitted between 15°C - 30°C (59°F - 86°F).

17 PATIENT COUNSELING INFORMATION

See FDA-approved patient labeling (Medication Guide)

Abuse Potential

Inform patients that BUTRANS contains buprenorphine, a Schedule III controlled substance that is subject to abuse. Instruct patients not to share BUTRANS with others and to take steps to protect BUTRANS from theft or misuse.

Life-Threatening Respiratory Depression

Discuss the risk of respiratory depression with patients, explaining that the risk is greatest when starting BUTRANS or when the dose is increased. Advise patients how to recognize respiratory depression and to seek medical attention if they are experiencing breathing difficulties.

Accidental Exposure

Instruct patients to take steps to store BUTRANS securely. Accidental exposure, especially in children, may result in serious harm or death. Advise patients to dispose of unused BUTRANS folding in half and flushing down the toilet.

Risks from Concomitant Use of Alcohol and other CNS Depressants

Inform patients that the concomitant use of alcohol with BUTRANS can increase the risk of life-threatening respiratory depression.

Inform patients that potentially serious additive effects may occur if BUTRANS is used with other CNS depressants, and not to use such drugs unless supervised by a health care provider.

Important Administration Instructions

Instruct patients how to properly use BUTRANS, including the following:

1. To carefully follow instructions for the application, removal, and disposal of BUTRANS. Each week, apply BUTRANS to a different site based on the 8 described skin sites, with a minimum of 3 weeks between applications to a previously used site.
2. To apply BUTRANS to a hairless or nearly hairless skin site. If none are available, instruct patients to clip the hair at the site and not to shave the area. Instruct patients not to apply to irritated skin. If the application site must be cleaned, use clear water only. Soaps, alcohol, oils, lotions, or abrasive devices should not be used. Allow the skin to dry before applying BUTRANS.

Hypotension

Inform patients that BUTRANS may cause orthostatic hypotension and syncope. Instruct patients how to recognize symptoms of low blood pressure and how to reduce the risk of serious consequences should hypotension occur (e.g., sit or lie down, carefully rise from a sitting or lying position).

Driving or Operating Heavy Machinery

Inform patients that BUTRANS may impair the ability to perform potentially hazardous activities such as driving a car or operating heavy machinery. Advise patients not to perform such tasks until they know how they will react to the medication.

Constipation

Advise patients of the potential for severe constipation, including management instructions and when to seek medical attention.

Anaphylaxis

Inform patients that anaphylaxis has been reported with ingredients contained in BUTRANS. Advise patients how to recognize such a reaction and when to seek medical attention.

Pregnancy

Advise female patients that BUTRANS can cause fetal harm and to inform the prescriber if they are pregnant or plan to become pregnant.

Healthcare professionals can telephone Purdue Pharma's Medical Services Department (1-888-726-7535) for information on this product.

Distributed by: Purdue Pharma L.P., Stamford, CT 06901-3431

Manufactured by: LTS Lohmann Therapie-Systeme AG, Andernach, Germany

U.S. Patent Numbers 5681413; 5804215; 6264980; 6315854; 6344211; RE41408; RE41489; RE41571.

Medication Guide
BUTRANS® (BYOO-trans)
(buprenorphine) Transdermal System, CIII

BUTRANS is:

- A strong prescription pain medicine that contains an opioid (narcotic) that is used to treat moderate to severe around-the-clock pain.

Important information about BUTRANS:

- Get emergency help right away if you take too much BUTRANS (overdose). BUTRANS overdose can cause life-threatening breathing problems that can lead to death.
- Never give anyone else your BUTRANS. They could die from taking it. Store BUTRANS away from children and in a safe place to prevent stealing or abuse. Selling or giving away BUTRANS is against the law.

Do not use BUTRANS if you have:

- severe asthma, trouble breathing, or other lung problems.
- a bowel blockage or have narrowing of the stomach or intestines.

Before applying BUTRANS, tell your healthcare provider if you have a history of:

- head injury, seizures
- liver, kidney, thyroid problems
- problems urinating
- heart rhythm problems (Long QT syndrome)
- pancreas or gallbladder problems
- abuse of street or prescription drugs, alcohol addiction, or mental health problems.

Tell your healthcare provider if you:

- have a fever.
- **are pregnant or planning to become pregnant.** BUTRANS may harm your unborn baby.
- **are breastfeeding.** BUTRANS passes into breast milk and may harm your baby.
- are taking prescription or over-the-counter medicines, vitamins, or herbal supplements.

While using BUTRANS:

- Do not change your dose. Apply BUTRANS exactly as prescribed by your healthcare provider.
- See the detailed Instructions for Use for information about how to apply and dispose of the BUTRANS patch.
- Do not apply a BUTRANS patch if the pouch seal is broken, or the patch is cut, damaged, or changed in any way.
- Do not apply more than 1 patch at the same time unless your healthcare provider tells you to.
- You should wear 1 BUTRANS patch continuously for 7 days.
- **Call your healthcare provider if the dose you are taking does not control your pain.**
- **Do not stop using BUTRANS without talking to your healthcare provider.**

While using BUTRANS Do Not:

- Take hot baths or sunbathe, use hot tubs, saunas, heating pads, electric blankets, heated waterbeds, or tanning lamps. These can cause an overdose that can lead to death.
- Drive or operate heavy machinery, until you know how BUTRANS affects you. BUTRANS can make you sleepy, dizzy, or lightheaded.
- Drink alcohol or use prescription or over-the-counter medicines that contain alcohol.

The possible side effects of BUTRANS are:

- constipation, nausea, sleepiness, vomiting, tiredness, headache, dizziness, itching, redness or rash where the patch is applied. Call your healthcare provider if you have any of these symptoms and they are severe.

Get emergency medical help if you have:

- trouble breathing, shortness of breath, fast heartbeat, chest pain, swelling of your face, tongue or throat, extreme drowsiness, or you are feeling faint.

These are not all the possible side effects of BUTRANS. Call your doctor for medical advice about side effects. You may report side effects to FDA at 1-800-FDA-1088. **For more information go to dailymed.nlm.nih.gov**

Distributed by: Purdue Pharma L.P., Stamford, CT 06901-3431, **www.purduepharma.com or call 1-888-726-7535**

This Medication Guide has been approved by the U.S. Food and Drug Administration. Issue: July 2012

Instructions for Use
Butrans® (BYOO-trans) CIII
(buprenorphine)
Transdermal System

Be sure that you read, understand, and follow these Instructions for Use before you use Butrans. Talk to your doctor or pharmacist if you have any questions.

Before Applying Butrans:

- Do not use soap, alcohol, lotions, oils, or other products to remove any leftover medicine gel from a patch because this may cause more Butrans to pass through the skin.
- Each patch is sealed in its own protective pouch. Do not remove a patch from the pouch until you are ready to use it.
- Do not use a patch if the seal on the protective pouch is broken or if the patch is cut, damaged or changed in any way.
- Butrans patches are available in different strengths and patch sizes. Make sure you have the right strength patch that has been prescribed for you.

Where to apply Butrans:

- Butrans should be applied to the **upper outer arm, upper chest, upper back, or the side of the chest** (See Figure 1). These 4 sites (located on both sides of the body) provide 8 possible Butrans application sites. You should change the skin site where you apply Butrans each week, making sure that at least 3 weeks (21 days) pass before you re-use the same skin site.

Figure 1

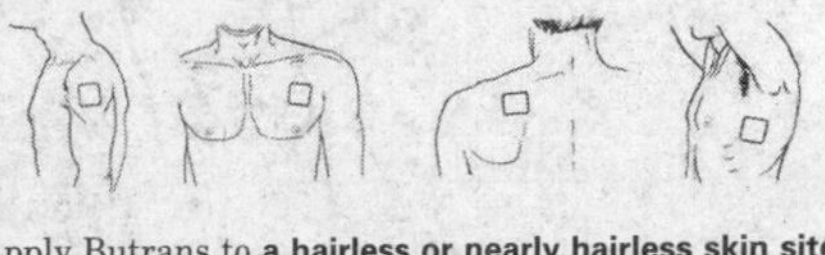

- Apply Butrans to **a hairless or nearly hairless skin site.** If needed, you can clip the hair at the skin site (See Figure 2). Do not shave the area. The skin site should not be irritated. **Use only water to clean** the application site. You should not use soaps, alcohol, oils, lotions, or abrasive devices. Allow the skin to dry before you apply the patch.

Figure 2

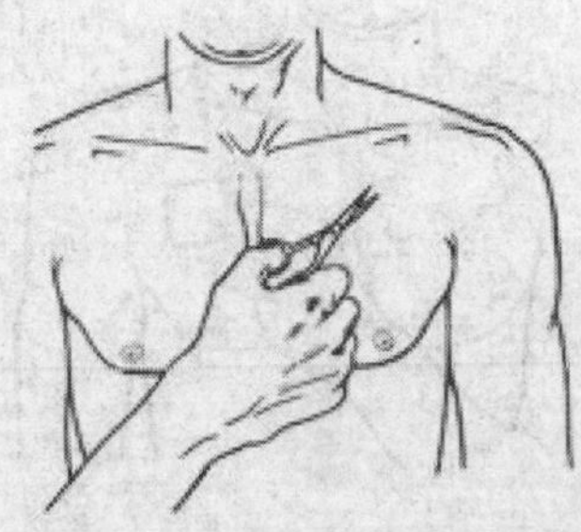

- The skin site should be free of cuts and irritation (rashes, swelling, redness, or other skin problems).

When to apply a new patch:

- When you apply a new patch, write down the date and time that the patch is applied. Use this to remember when the patch should be removed.
- Change the patch at the same time of day, one week (exactly 7 days) after you apply it.
- After removing and disposing of the patch, write down the time it was removed and how it was disposed.

How to apply Butrans:

- If you are wearing a patch, remember to remove it before applying a new one.
- Each patch is sealed in its own protective pouch.
- Use scissors to cut open the pouch along the dotted line (See Figure 3) and remove the patch. Do not remove the patch from the pouch until you are ready to use it. Do not use patches that have been cut or damaged in any way.

Figure 3

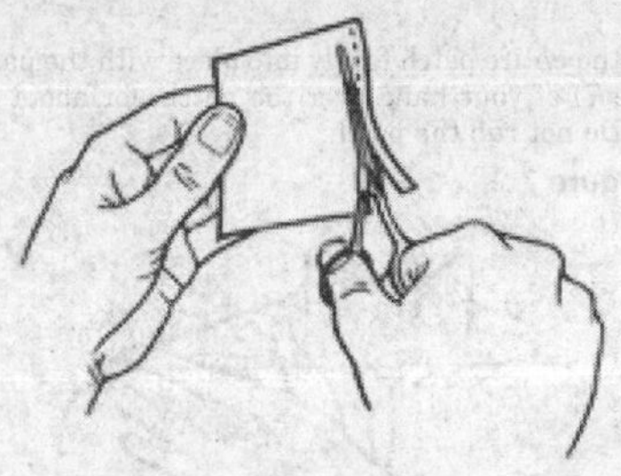

- Hold the patch with the protective liner facing you.
- Gently bend the patch (See Figures 4a and 4b) along the faint line and slowly peel the larger portion of the liner, which covers the sticky surface of the patch.

Figure 4a

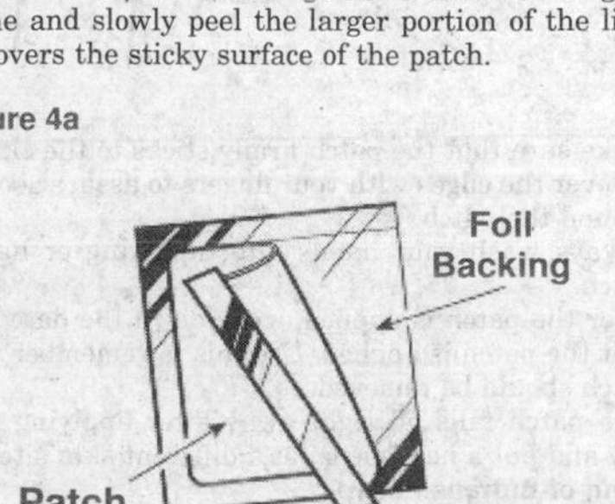

Figure 4b

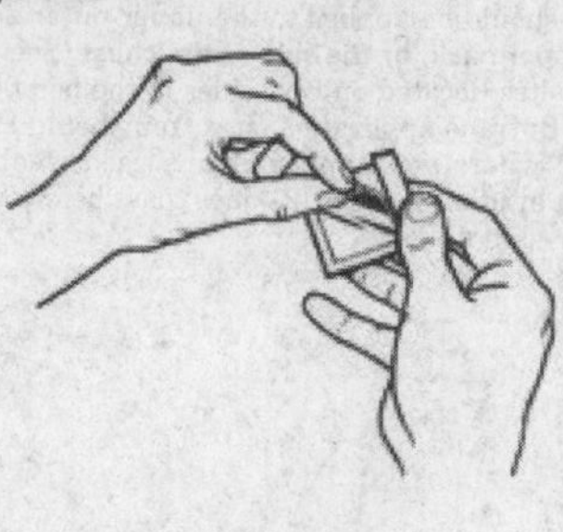

- Do not touch the sticky side of the patch with your fingers.
- Using the smaller portion of the protective liner as a handle (See Figure 5), apply the sticky side of the patch to one of the 8 body locations described above (see **Where to apply Butrans?**).

Figure 5

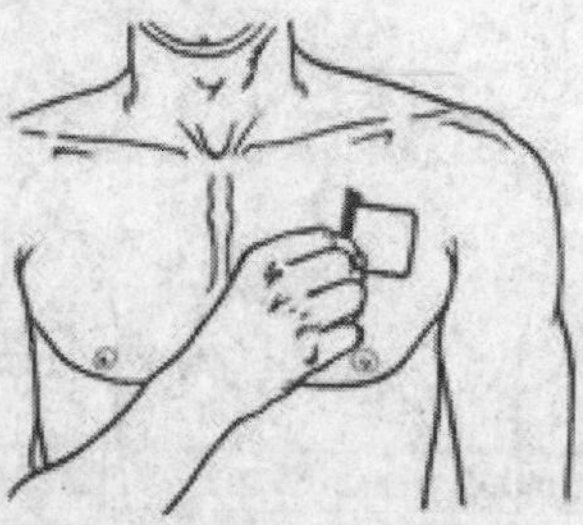

- While still holding the sticky side down, gently fold back the smaller portion of the patch. Grasp an edge of the remaining protective liner and slowly peel it off (See Figure 6).

Figure 6

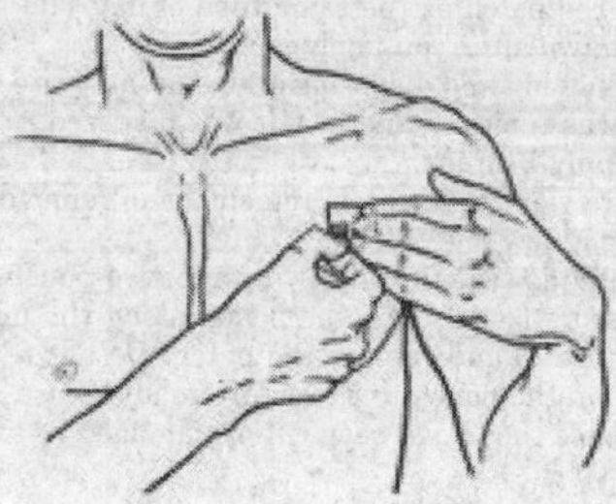

- Press the entire patch firmly into place with the palm (See Figure 7) of your hand over the patch, for about 15 seconds. Do not rub the patch.

Figure 7

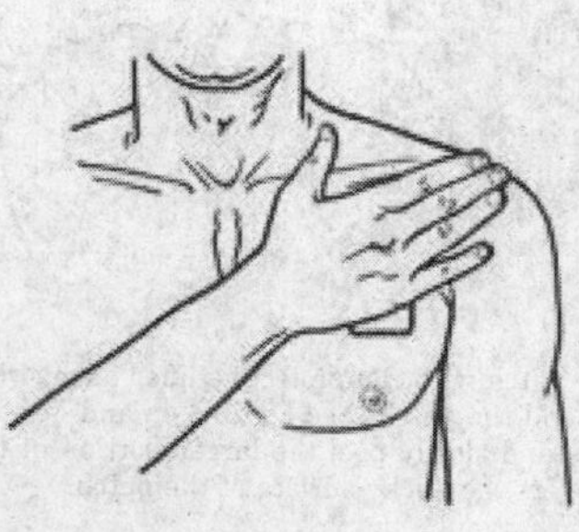

- Make sure that the patch firmly sticks to the skin.
- Go over the edges with your fingers to assure good contact around the patch.
- Always wash your hands after applying or handling a patch.
- After the patch is applied, write down the date and time that the patch is applied. Use this to remember when the patch should be removed.

If the patch falls off right away after applying, throw it away and put a new one on at a different skin site (see **Disposing of Butrans Patch**).

If a patch falls off, do not touch the sticky side of the patch with your fingers. A new patch should be applied to a different site. **Patches that fall off should not be re-applied.** They must be thrown away correctly.

If the edges of the Butrans patch start to loosen:

- Apply first aid tape only to the edges of the patch.
- If problems with the patch not sticking continue, cover the patch with special see-through adhesive dressings (for example Bioclusive or Tegaderm).
  - Remove the backing from the transparent adhesive dressing and place it carefully and completely over the Butrans patch, smoothing it over the patch and your skin.
- **Never cover a Butrans patch with any other bandage or tape. It should only be covered with a special see-through adhesive dressing. Talk to your doctor or pharmacist about the kinds of dressing that should be used.**

If your patch falls off later, but before 1 week (7 days) of use, throw it away properly (see **Disposing of a Butrans Patch**) and apply a new patch at a different skin site. Be sure to let your doctor know that this has happened. Do not replace the new patch until 1 week (7 days) after you put it on (or as directed by your doctor).

Disposing of Butrans Patch:

Butrans patches must be disposed of by flushing them down the toilet or using the Patch-Disposal Unit.

To flush your Butrans patches down the toilet:

Remove your Butrans patch, fold the sticky sides of a used patch together (See Figure 8) and flush it down the toilet right away.

Figure 8

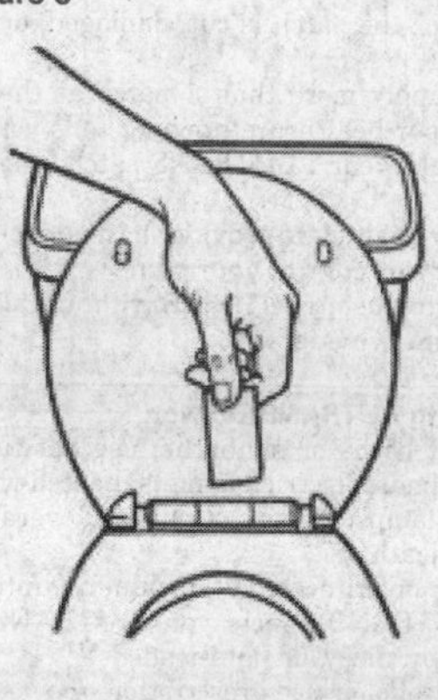

When disposing of unused Butrans patches you no longer need, remove the leftover patches from their protective pouch and remove the protective liner. Fold the patches in half with the sticky sides together, and flush the patches down the toilet.

Do not flush the pouch or the protective liner down the toilet. These items can be thrown away in the trash.

If you prefer not to flush the used patch down the toilet, you must use the Patch-Disposal Unit provided to you to discard the patch.

Never put used Butrans patches in the trash without first sealing them in the Patch-Disposal Unit.

To dispose of Butrans patches in household trash using the Patch-Disposal Unit:

Remove your patch and follow the directions printed on the Patch-Disposal Unit (See Figure 9) or see complete instructions below. **Use one Patch-Disposal Unit for each patch.**

Figure 9

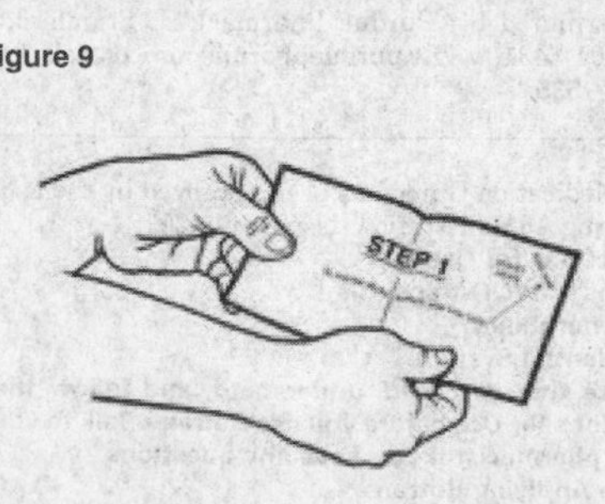

1. Peel back the disposal unit liner to show the sticky surface (See Figure 10).
[See figure 10 at top of next column]
2. Place the sticky side of the used or unused patch to the indicated area on the disposal unit (See Figure 11).
[See figure 11 at top of next column]
3. Close the disposal unit by folding the sticky sides together (See Figure 12). Press firmly and smoothly over the entire disposal unit so that the patch is sealed within.
[See figure 12 at top of next column]

Figure 10

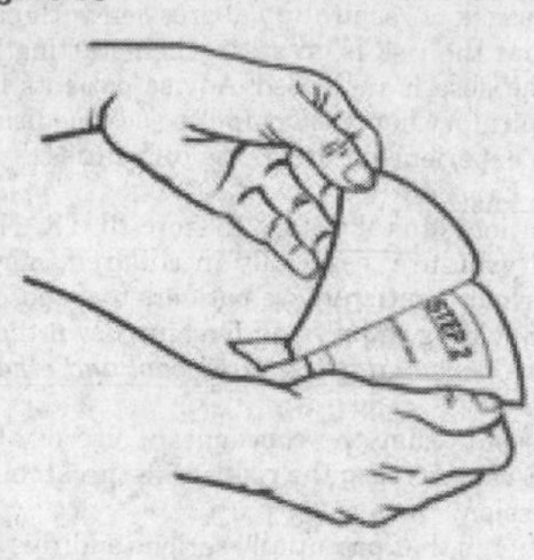

Figure 11

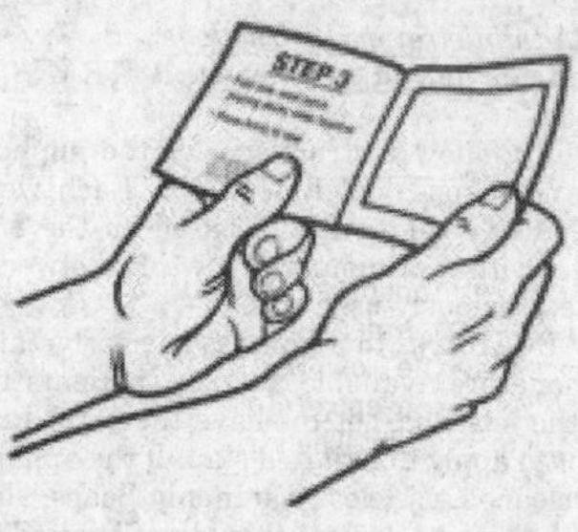

Figure 12

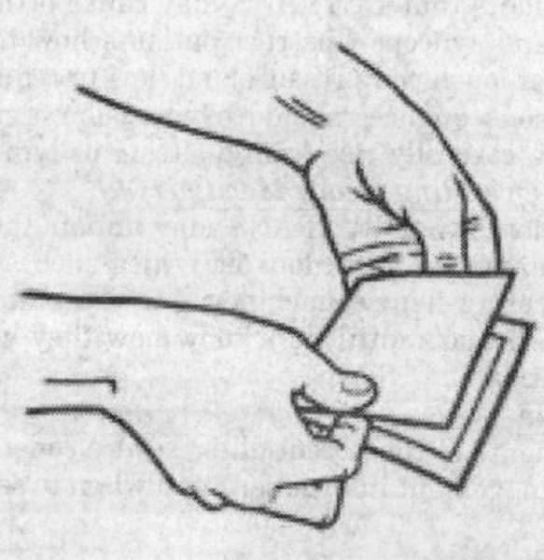

4. The closed disposal unit, with the patch sealed inside may be thrown away in the trash (See Figure 13).

Figure 13

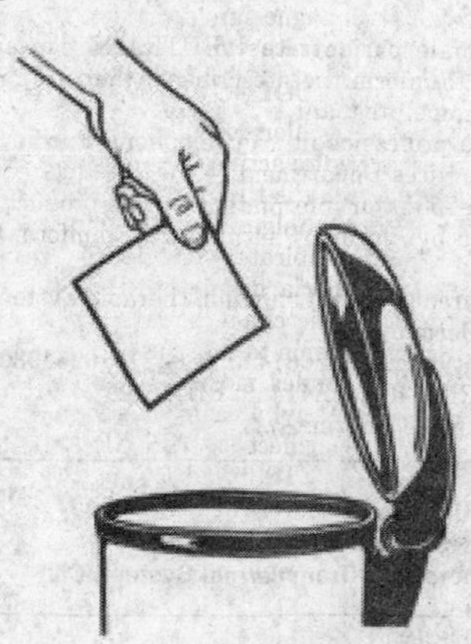

Do not put unused patches in household trash without first sealing them in the Patch-Disposal Unit.

Always remove the leftover patches from their protective pouch and remove the protective liner. The pouch and liner can be disposed of separately in the trash and should not be sealed in the Patch-Disposal Unit.

Distributed by:
Purdue Pharma L.P.
Stamford, CT 06901-3431
Issued: July 2012

Shown in Product Identification Guide, page 311

DILAUDID CII
[di-law-did]
(hydromorphone hydrochloride)
Oral Liquid
DILAUDID
(hydromorphone hydrochloride)
Tablets

WARNING: DILAUDID ORAL LIQUID AND DILAUDID TABLETS CONTAIN HYDROMORPHONE, WHICH IS A POTENT SCHEDULE II CONTROLLED OPIOID AGONIST. SCHEDULE II OPIOID AGONISTS, INCLUDING MORPHINE, OXYMORPHONE, OXYCODONE, FENTANYL, AND METHADONE, HAVE THE HIGHEST POTENTIAL FOR ABUSE AND RISK OF PRODUCING RESPIRATORY DEPRESSION. ALCOHOL, OTHER OPIOIDS AND CENTRAL NERVOUS SYSTEM DEPRESSANTS (SEDATIVE-HYPNOTICS) POTENTIATE THE RESPIRATORY DEPRESSANT EFFECTS OF HYDROMORPHONE, INCREASING THE RISK OF RESPIRATORY DEPRESSION THAT MIGHT RESULT IN DEATH.

DESCRIPTION

DILAUDID (hydromorphone hydrochloride), a hydrogenated ketone of morphine, is an opioid analgesic.

The chemical name of DILAUDID (hydromorphone hydrochloride) is 4,5α-epoxy-3-hydroxy-17-methylmorphinan-6-one hydrochloride. The structural formula is:

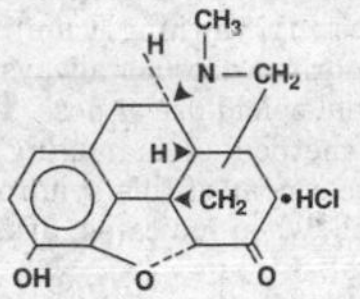

M.W. 321.8

Each 5 mL (1 teaspoon) of DILAUDID ORAL LIQUID contains 5 mg of hydromorphone hydrochloride. In addition, other ingredients include purified water, methylparaben, propylparaben, sucrose, and glycerin. DILAUDID ORAL LIQUID may contain traces of sodium metabisulfite.

Color Coded Tablets (for oral administration) contain:

2 mg hydromorphone hydrochloride (orange tablet) and D&C red #30 Lake dye, D&C yellow #10 Lake dye, lactose, and magnesium stearate. DILAUDID 2 mg TABLET may contain traces of sodium metabisulfite.

4 mg hydromorphone hydrochloride (yellow tablet) and D&C yellow #10 Lake dye, lactose, and magnesium stearate. DILAUDID 4 mg TABLET may contain traces of sodium metabisulfite.

8 mg hydromorphone hydrochloride (white tablet) and lactose anhydrous, and magnesium stearate. DILAUDID 8 mg TABLET may contain traces of sodium metabisulfite.

CLINICAL PHARMACOLOGY

Hydromorphone hydrochloride is a pure opioid agonist with the principal therapeutic activity of analgesia. A significant feature of the analgesia is that it can occur without loss of consciousness. Opioid analgesics also suppress the cough reflex and may cause respiratory depression, mood changes, mental clouding, euphoria, dysphoria, nausea, vomiting and electroencephalographic changes. Many of the effects described below are common to this class of mu-opioid agonist analgesics which includes morphine, oxycodone, hydrocodone, codeine and fentanyl. In some instances, data may not exist to distinguish the effects of DILAUDID ORAL LIQUID and DILAUDID TABLETS from those observed with other opioid analgesics. However, in the absence of data to the contrary, it is assumed that DILAUDID ORAL LIQUID and DILAUDID TABLETS would possess all the actions of mu-agonist opioids.

Central Nervous System

The precise mode of analgesic action of opioid analgesics is unknown. However, specific CNS opiate receptors have been identified. Opioids are believed to express their pharmacological effects by combining with these receptors.

Hydromorphone depresses the cough reflex by direct effect on the cough center in the medulla.

Hydromorphone depresses the respiratory reflex by a direct effect on brain stem respiratory centers. The mechanism of respiratory depression also involves a reduction in the responsiveness of the brain stem respiratory centers to increases in carbon dioxide tension.

Hydromorphone causes miosis. Pinpoint pupils are a common sign of opioid overdose but are not pathognomonic (e.g., pontine lesions of hemorrhagic or ischemic origin may produce similar findings). Marked mydriasis rather than miosis may be seen with hypoxia in the setting of DILAUDID overdose.

Gastrointestinal Tract and Other Smooth Muscle

Gastric, biliary and pancreatic secretions are decreased by opioids such as hydromorphone. Hydromorphone causes a reduction in motility associated with an increase in tone in the gastric antrum and duodenum. Digestion of food in the small intestine is delayed and propulsive contractions are decreased. Propulsive peristaltic waves in the colon are decreased, and tone may be increased to the point of spasm. The end result is constipation. Hydromorphone can cause a marked increase in biliary tract pressure as a result of spasm of the sphincter of Oddi.

Cardiovascular System

Hydromorphone may produce hypotension as a result of either peripheral vasodilation or release of histamine, or both. Other manifestations of histamine release and/or peripheral vasodilation may include pruritus, flushing, and red eyes.

Pharmacokinetics and Metabolism

The analgesic activity of DILAUDID (hydromorphone hydrochloride) is due to the parent drug, hydromorphone. Hydromorphone is rapidly absorbed from the gastrointestinal tract after oral administration and undergoes extensive first-pass metabolism. Exposure of hydromorphone (C_{max} and $AUC_{0\text{-}24}$) is dose-proportional at a dose range of 2 and 8 mg. *In vivo* bioavailability following single-dose administration of the 8 mg tablet is approximately 24% (coefficient of variation 21%). Bioequivalence between the DILAUDID 8 mg TABLET and an equivalent dose of DILAUDID ORAL LIQUID has been demonstrated.

Absorption

After oral administration of DILAUDID 8 mg liquid or tablets, peak plasma hydromorphone concentrations are generally attained within ½ to 1-hour.

Mean (%cv) Dosage Form	C_{max} (ng)	T_{max} (hrs)	AUC (ng*hr/mL)	T ½ (hrs)
8 mg Tablet	5.5 (33%)	0.74 (34%)	23.7 (28%)	2.6 (18%)
8 mg Oral Liquid	5.7 (31%)	0.73 (71%)	24.6 (29%)	2.8 (20%)

Food Effects

In a study conducted with a single 8 mg dose of hydromorphone (2 mg DILAUDID® IR tablets), food lowered C_{max} by 25%, prolonged T_{max} by 0.8 hour, and increased AUC by 35%. The effects may not be clinically relevant.

Distribution

At therapeutic plasma levels, hydromorphone is approximately 8-19% bound to plasma proteins. After an intravenous bolus dose, the steady state of volume distribution [mean (%cv)] is 302.9 (32%) liters.

Metabolism

Hydromorphone is extensively metabolized via glucuronidation in the liver, with greater than 95% of the dose metabolized to hydromorphone-3-glucuronide along with minor amounts of 6-hydroxy reduction metabolites.

Elimination

Only a small amount of the hydromorphone dose is excreted unchanged in the urine. Most of the dose is excreted as hydromorphone-3-glucuronide along with minor amounts of 6-hydroxy reduction metabolites. The systemic clearance is approximately 1.96 (20%) liters/minute. The terminal elimination half-life of hydromorphone after an intravenous dose is about 2.3 hours.

Special Populations

Hepatic Impairment

After oral administration of hydromorphone at a single 4 mg dose (2 mg Dilaudid IR Tablets), mean exposure to hydromorphone (C_{max} and AUC_{∞}) is increased 4-fold in patients with moderate (Child-Pugh Group B) hepatic impairment compared with subjects with normal hepatic function. Due to increased exposure of hydromorphone, patients with moderate hepatic impairment should be started at a lower dose and closely monitored during dose titration. Pharmacokinetics of hydromorphone in severe hepatic impairment patients has not been studied. Further increase in C_{max} and AUC of hydromorphone in this group is expected. As such, starting dose should be even more conservative. Use of oral liquid is recommended to adjust the dose (see **DOSAGE AND ADMINISTRATION**).

Renal Impairment

After oral administration of hydromorphone at a single 4 mg dose (2 mg Dilaudid IR Tablets), exposure to hydromorphone (C_{max} and $AUC_{0\text{-}48}$) is increased in patients with impaired renal function by 2-fold in moderate (CLcr = 40 - 60 mL/min) and 3-fold in severe (CLcr < 30 mL/min) renal impairment compared with normal subjects (CLcr > 80 mL/min). In addition, in patients with severe renal impairment hydromorphone appeared to be more slowly eliminated with longer terminal elimination half-life (40 hr) compared to patients with normal renal function (15 hr). Patients with moderate renal impairment should be started on a lower dose. Starting doses for patients with severe renal impairment should be even lower. Patients with renal impairment should be closely monitored during dose titration. Use of oral liquid is recommended to adjust the dose (see **DOSAGE AND ADMINISTRATION**).

Pediatrics

Pharmacokinetics of hydromorphone have not been evaluated in children.

Geriatric

Age has no effect on the pharmacokinetics of hydromorphone.

Gender

Gender has little effect on the pharmacokinetics of hydromorphone. Females appear to have higher C_{max} (25%) than males with comparable $AUC_{0\text{-}24}$ values. The difference observed in C_{max} may not be clinically relevant.

Pregnancy and Nursing Mothers

Hydromorphone crosses the placenta. Hydromorphone is also found in low levels in breast milk, and may cause respiratory compromise in newborns when administered during labor or delivery.

CLINICAL TRIALS

Analgesic effects of single doses of DILAUDID ORAL LIQUID administered to patients with post-surgical pain have been studied in double-blind controlled trials. In one study, both 5 mg and 10 mg of DILAUDID ORAL LIQUID provided significantly more analgesia than placebo. In another trial, 5 mg and 10 mg of DILAUDID ORAL LIQUID were compared to 30 mg and 60 mg of morphine sulfate oral liquid. The pain relief provided by 5 mg and 10 mg DILAUDID ORAL LIQUID was comparable to 30 mg and 60 mg oral morphine sulfate, respectively.

INDICATIONS AND USAGE

DILAUDID ORAL LIQUID and DILAUDID TABLETS are indicated for the management of pain in patients where an opioid analgesic is appropriate.

CONTRAINDICATIONS

DILAUDID ORAL LIQUID and DILAUDID TABLETS are contraindicated in: patients with known hypersensitivity to hydromorphone, patients with respiratory depression in the absence of resuscitative equipment, and in patients with status asthmaticus. DILAUDID ORAL LIQUID and DILAUDID TABLETS are also contraindicated for use in obstetrical analgesia.

WARNINGS

Respiratory Depression

Respiratory depression is the chief hazard of DILAUDID ORAL LIQUID and DILAUDID TABLETS. Respiratory depression is more likely to occur in the elderly, in the debilitated, and in those suffering from conditions accompanied by hypoxia or hypercapnia when even moderate therapeutic doses may dangerously decrease pulmonary ventilation.

DILAUDID ORAL LIQUID and DILAUDID TABLETS should be used with extreme caution in patients with chronic obstructive pulmonary disease or cor pulmonale, patients having a substantially decreased respiratory reserve, hypoxia, hypercapnia, or in patients with preexisting respiratory depression. In such patients even usual therapeutic doses of opioid analgesics may decrease respiratory drive while simultaneously increasing airway resistance to the point of apnea.

DILAUDID ORAL LIQUID and DILAUDID TABLETS contain hydromorphone, which is a potent Schedule II controlled opioid agonist. Schedule II opioid agonists, including morphine, oxymorphone, oxycodone, fentanyl, and methadone, have the highest potential for abuse and risk of producing respiratory depression. Alcohol, other opioids and central nervous system depressants (sedative-hypnotics) potentiate the respiratory depressant effects of hydromorphone, increasing the risk of respiratory depression that might result in death.

Misuse, Abuse, and Diversion of Opioids

Hydromorphone is an opioid agonist of the morphine-type. Such drugs are sought by drug abusers and people with addiction disorders and are subject to criminal diversion. DILAUDID can be abused in a manner similar to other opioid agonists, legal or illicit. This should be considered when prescribing or dispensing DILAUDID in situations where the physician or pharmacist is concerned about an increased risk of misuse, abuse, or diversion. Prescribers should monitor all patients receiving opioids for signs of abuse, misuse, and addiction. Furthermore, patients should be assessed for their potential for opioid abuse prior to being prescribed opioid therapy. Persons at increased risk for opioid abuse include those with a personal or family history of substance abuse (including drug or alcohol abuse) or mental illness (e.g., depression). Opioids may still be appropriate for use in these patients, however, they will require intensive monitoring for signs of abuse DILAUDID has been reported as being abused by crushing, chewing, snorting, or injecting the dissolved product. These practices pose a significant risk to the abuser that could result in overdose or death (see **WARNINGS** and **DRUG ABUSE AND DEPENDENCE**). Concerns about abuse, addiction, and diversion should not prevent the proper management of pain. Healthcare professionals should contact their State Professional Licensing Board or State Controlled Substances Authority for information on how to prevent and detect abuse or diversion of this product.

Interactions with Alcohol and Drugs of Abuse

Hydromorphone may be expected to have additive effects when used in conjunction with alcohol, other opioids, or illicit drugs that cause central nervous system depression.

Neonatal Withdrawal Syndrome

Infants born to mothers physically dependent on DILAUDID will also be physically dependent and may exhibit respiratory difficulties and withdrawal symptoms (see **DRUG ABUSE AND DEPENDENCE**).

Head Injury and Increased Intracranial Pressure

The respiratory depressant effects of DILAUDID ORAL LIQUID and DILAUDID TABLETS with carbon dioxide retention and secondary elevation of cerebrospinal fluid pressure may be markedly exaggerated in the presence of head injury, other intracranial lesions, or preexisting increase in intracranial pressure. Opioid analgesics including DILAUDID ORAL LIQUID and DILAUDID TABLETS (hydromorphone hydrochloride) may produce effects on pupillary response and consciousness which can obscure the clinical course and neurologic signs of further increase in intracranial pressure in patients with head injuries.

Hypotensive Effect

Opioid analgesics, including DILAUDID ORAL LIQUID and DILAUDID TABLETS, may cause severe hypotension in an individual whose ability to maintain blood pressure has already been compromised by a depleted blood volume, or a concurrent administration of drugs such as phenothiazines or general anesthetics (see **PRECAUTIONS - Drug Interactions**). Therefore, DILAUDID ORAL LIQUID and DILAUDID TABLETS should be administered with caution to patients in circulatory shock, since vasodilation produced by the drug may further reduce cardiac output and blood pressure.

Sulfites

Contains sodium metabisulfite, a sulfite that may cause allergic-type reactions including anaphylactic symptoms and life-threatening or less severe asthmatic episodes in certain susceptible people. The overall prevalence of sulfite sensitivity in the general population is unknown and probably low. Sulfite sensitivity is seen more frequently in asthmatic than in nonasthmatic people.

PRECAUTIONS

Special Risk Patients

DILAUDID ORAL LIQUID and DILAUDID TABLETS should be given with caution and the initial dose should be reduced in the elderly or debilitated and those with severe impairment of hepatic, pulmonary or renal functions; myxedema or hypothyroidism; adrenocortical insufficiency (e.g., Addison's Disease); CNS depression or coma; toxic psychoses; prostatic hypertrophy or urethral stricture; gall bladder disease; acute alcoholism; delirium tremens; kyphoscoliosis or following gastrointestinal surgery.

The administration of opioid analgesics including DILAUDID ORAL LIQUID and DILAUDID TABLETS may obscure the diagnoses or clinical course in patients with acute abdominal conditions and may aggravate preexisting convulsions in patients with convulsive disorders.

Reports of mild to severe seizures and myoclonus have been reported in severely compromised patients, administered high doses of parenteral hydromorphone, for cancer and severe pain. Opioid administration at very high doses is associated with seizures and myoclonus in a variety of diseases where pain control is the primary focus.

Use in Drug and Alcohol Dependent Patients

DILAUDID should be used with caution in patients with alcoholism and other drug dependencies due to the increased frequency of opioid tolerance, dependence, and the risk of addiction observed in these patient populations. Abuse of DILAUDID in combination with other CNS depressant drugs can result in serious risk to the patient.

Hydromorphone is an opioid with no approved use in the management of addictive disorders.

Use in Ambulatory Patients

DILAUDID ORAL LIQUID and DILAUDID TABLETS may impair mental and/or physical ability required for the performance of potentially hazardous tasks (e.g. driving, operating machinery). Patients should be cautioned accordingly. DILAUDID may produce orthostatic hypotension in ambulatory patients.

Use in Biliary Tract Disease

Opioid analgesics, including DILAUDID ORAL LIQUID and DILAUDID TABLETS, should also be used with caution in patients about to undergo surgery of the biliary tract since it may cause spasm of the sphincter of Oddi.

Tolerance and Physical Dependence

Tolerance is the need for increasing doses of opioids to maintain a defined effect such as analgesia (in the absence of disease progression or other external factors). Physical dependence is manifested by withdrawal symptoms after abrupt discontinuation of a drug or upon administration of an antagonist. Physical dependence and tolerance are not unusual during chronic opioid therapy.

The opioid abstinence or withdrawal syndrome is characterized by some or all of the following: restlessness, lacrimation, rhinorrhea, yawning, perspiration, chills, myalgia, mydriasis. Other symptoms also may develop, including: irritability, anxiety, backache, joint pain, weakness, abdominal cramps, insomnia, nausea, anorexia, vomiting, diarrhea, or increased blood pressure, respiratory rate, or heart rate.

In general, opioids used regularly should not be abruptly discontinued.

Information for Patients/Caregivers

Patients receiving DILAUDID (hydromorphone hydrochloride) ORAL LIQUID or DILAUDID TABLETS or their caregivers should be given the following information by the physician, nurse, or pharmacist:

1. Patients should be aware that DILAUDID tablets contain hydromorphone, which is a morphine-like substance and which could cause severe adverse effects including respiratory depression and even death if not taken according to the prescriber's directions.
2. Patients should be advised to report pain and adverse experiences occurring during therapy. Individualization of dosage is essential to make optimal use of this medication.
3. Patients should be advised not to adjust the dose of DILAUDID without consulting the prescribing professional.
4. Patients should be advised that DILAUDID may impair mental and/or physical ability required for the performance of potentially hazardous tasks (e.g., driving, operating heavy machinery).
5. Patients should not combine DILAUDID with alcohol or other central nervous system depressants (sleep aids, tranquilizers) except by the orders of the prescribing physician, because dangerous additive effects may occur, resulting in serious injury or death.
6. Women of childbearing potential who become, or are planning to become pregnant should be advised to consult their physician regarding the effects of analgesics and other drug use during pregnancy on themselves and their unborn child.
7. Patients should be advised that DILAUDID is a potential drug of abuse. They should protect it from theft, and it should never be given to anyone other than the individual for whom it was prescribed.
8. Patients should be advised that if they have been receiving treatment with DILAUDID for more than a few weeks and cessation of therapy is indicated, it may be appropriate to taper the DILAUDID dose, rather than abruptly discontinue it, due to the risk of precipitating withdrawal symptoms. Their physician can provide a dose schedule to accomplish a gradual discontinuation of the medication.
9. Patients should be instructed to keep DILAUDID in a secure place out of the reach of children. When DILAUDID is no longer needed, the unused tablets should be destroyed by flushing down the toilet.

Drug Interactions

Drug Interactions with Other CNS Depressants

The concomitant use of other central nervous system depressants including sedatives or hypnotics, general anesthetics, phenothiazines, tranquilizers and alcohol may produce additive depressant effects. Respiratory depression, hypotension and profound sedation or coma may occur. When such combined therapy is contemplated, the dose of one or both agents should be reduced. DILAUDID should not be taken with alcohol. Opioid analgesics, including DILAUDID ORAL LIQUID and DILAUDID TABLETS, may enhance the action of neuromuscular blocking agents and produce an excessive degree of respiratory depression.

Interactions with Mixed Agonist/Antagonist Opioid Analgesics

Agonist/antagonist analgesics (i.e., pentazocine, nalbuphine, butorphanol, and buprenorphine) should be administered with caution to a patient who has received or is receiving a course of therapy with a pure opioid agonist analgesic such as hydromorphone. In this situation, mixed agonist/antagonist analgesics may reduce the analgesic effect of hydromorphone and/or may precipitate withdrawal symptoms in these patients.

Carcinogenesis, Mutagenesis, Impairment of Fertility

No carcinogenicity studies have been conducted in animals. Hydromorphone was not mutagenic in the *in vitro* Ames reverse mutation assay or the human lymphocyte chromosome aberration assay. Hydromorphone was not clastogenic in the *in vivo* mouse micronucleus assay.

No effects on fertility, reproductive performance, or reproductive organ morphology were observed in male or female rats given oral doses up to 7 mg/kg/day, which is equivalent to the human dose of 2.5-10 mg every 3 to 6 hours for oral liquid, and 3-fold higher than the human dose of 2-4 mg every 4 to 6 hours for the tablet on a body surface area basis.

Pregnancy

Pregnancy Category C

No effects on teratogenicity or embryotoxicity were observed in female rats given oral doses up to 7 mg/kg/day, which is approximately equivalent to the human dose of 2.5-10 mg every 3 to 6 hours for oral liquid, and 3-fold higher than the human dose of 2-4 mg every 4 to 6 hours for the tablet on a body surface area basis. Hydromorphone produced skull malformations (exencephaly and cranioschisis) in Syrian hamsters given oral doses up to 20 mg/kg during the peak of organogenesis (gestation days 8-9). The skull malformations were observed at doses approximately 2-fold higher the human dose of 2.5-10 mg every 3 to 6 hours for oral liquid, and 7-fold higher than the human dose of 2-4 mg every 4 to 6 hours for the tablet on a body surface area basis. There are no adequate and well-controlled studies of DILAUDID in pregnant women.

Hydromorphone crosses the placenta, resulting in fetal exposure. DILAUDID ORAL LIQUID and DILAUDID TABLETS should be used in pregnant women only if the potential benefit justifies the potential risk to the fetus (see **Labor and Delivery** and **DRUG ABUSE AND DEPENDENCE**).

Nonteratogenic Effects

Babies born to mothers who have been taking opioids regularly prior to delivery will be physically dependent. The withdrawal signs include irritability and excessive crying, tremors, hyperactive reflexes, increased respiratory rate, increased stools, sneezing, yawning, vomiting, and fever. The intensity of the syndrome does not always correlate with the duration of maternal opioid use or dose. There is no consensus on the best method of managing withdrawal. Approaches to the treatment of this syndrome have included supportive care and, when indicated, drugs such as paregoric or phenobarbital.

Labor and Delivery

DILAUDID ORAL LIQUID and DILAUDID TABLETS are contraindicated in Labor and Delivery (see **CONTRAINDICATIONS**).

Nursing Mothers

Low levels of opioid analgesics have been detected in human milk. As a general rule, nursing should not be undertaken while a patient is receiving DILAUDID ORAL LIQUID and DILAUDID TABLETS since it, and other drugs in this class, may be excreted in the milk.

Pediatric Use

Safety and effectiveness in children have not been established.

Geriatric Use

Clinical studies of DILAUDID did not include sufficient numbers of subjects aged 65 and over to determine whether they respond differently from younger subjects. In general, dose selection for an elderly patient should be cautious, usually starting at the low end of the dosing range, reflecting the greater frequency of decreased hepatic, renal, or cardiac function, and of concomitant disease or other drug therapy (see **INDIVIDUALIZATION OF DOSAGE** and **PRECAUTIONS**).

ADVERSE REACTIONS

The major hazards of DILAUDID ORAL LIQUID and DILAUDID TABLETS include respiratory depression and apnea. To a lesser degree, circulatory depression, respiratory arrest, shock and cardiac arrest have occurred.

The most frequently observed adverse effects are lightheadedness, dizziness, sedation, nausea, vomiting, sweating, flushing, dysphoria, euphoria, dry mouth, and pruritus. These effects seem to be more prominent in ambulatory patients and in those not experiencing severe pain.

Less Frequently Observed Adverse Reactions

General and CNS

Weakness, headache, agitation, tremor, uncoordinated muscle movements, alterations of mood (nervousness, apprehension, depression, floating feelings, dreams), muscle rigidity, paresthesia, muscle tremor, blurred vision, nystagmus, diplopia and miosis, transient hallucinations and disorientation, visual disturbances, insomnia, increased intracranial pressure

Cardiovascular

Flushing of the face, chills, tachycardia, bradycardia, palpitation, faintness, syncope, hypotension, hypertension

Respiratory

Bronchospasm and laryngospasm

Gastrointestinal

Constipation, biliary tract spasm, ileus, anorexia, diarrhea, cramps, taste alteration

Genitourinary

Urinary retention or hesitancy, antidiuretic effects

Dermatologic

Urticaria, other skin rashes, diaphoresis

OVERDOSAGE

Serious overdosage with DILAUDID ORAL LIQUID and DILAUDID TABLETS is characterized by respiratory depression, somnolence progressing to stupor or coma, skeletal muscle flaccidity, cold and clammy skin, constricted pupils, and sometimes bradycardia and hypotension. In serious overdosage, particularly following intravenous injection, apnea, circulatory collapse, cardiac arrest and death may occur.

In the treatment of overdosage, primary attention should be given to the reestablishment of adequate respiratory exchange through provision of a patent airway and institution of assisted or controlled ventilation. A potentially serious oral ingestion, if recent, should be managed with gut decontamination. In unconscious patients with a secure airway, instill activated charcoal (30-100 g in adults, 1-2 g/kg in infants) via a nasogastric tube. A saline cathartic or sorbitol may be added to the first dose of activated charcoal.

Supportive measures (including oxygen, vasopressors) should be employed in the management of circulatory shock and pulmonary edema accompanying overdose as indicated. Cardiac arrest or arrhythmias may require cardiac massage or defibrillation.

The opioid antagonist, naloxone, is a specific antidote against respiratory depression which may result from overdosage, or unusual sensitivity to DILAUDID ORAL LIQUID and DILAUDID TABLETS. Therefore, an appropriate dose of this antagonist should be administered, preferably by the intravenous route, simultaneously with efforts at respiratory resuscitation. Naloxone should not be administered in the absence of clinically significant respiratory or circulatory depression. Naloxone should be administered cautiously to persons who are known, or suspected to be physically dependent on DILAUDID ORAL LIQUID and DILAUDID TABLETS. In such cases, an abrupt or complete reversal of narcotic effects may precipitate an acute withdrawal syndrome. Since the duration of action of DILAUDID ORAL LIQUID and DILAUDID TABLETS may exceed that of the antagonist, the patient should be kept under continued surveillance; repeated doses of the antagonist may be required to maintain adequate respiration. Apply other supportive measures when indicated.

DOSAGE AND ADMINISTRATION

Dilaudid Oral Liquid

The usual adult oral dosage of DILAUDID ORAL LIQUID is one-half (2.5 mL) to two teaspoonfuls (10 mL) (2.5 mg - 10 mg) every 3 to 6 hours as directed by the clinical situation. Oral dosages higher than the usual dosages may be required in some patients.

Dilaudid Tablets

The usual starting dose for DILAUDID tablets is 2 mg to 4 mg, orally, every 4 to 6 hours. Appropriate use of the DILAUDID TABLETS must be decided by careful evaluation of each clinical situation.

A gradual increase in dose may be required if analgesia is inadequate, as tolerance develops, or if pain severity increases. The first sign of tolerance is usually a reduced duration of effect. Patients with hepatic and renal impairment should be started on a lower starting dose (See **CLINICAL PHARMACOLOGY - Pharmacokinetics and Metabolism**).

INDIVIDUALIZATION OF DOSAGE

The dosage of opioid analgesics like hydromorphone hydrochloride should be individualized for any given patient, since adverse events can occur at doses that may not provide complete freedom from pain.

Safe and effective administration of opioid analgesics to patients with acute or chronic pain depends upon a comprehensive assessment of the patient. The nature of the pain (severity, frequency, etiology, and pathophysiology) as well as the concurrent medical status of the patient will affect selection of the starting dosage.

In non-opioid-tolerant patients, therapy with hydromorphone is typically initiated at an oral dose of 2-4 mg every four hours, but elderly patients may require lower doses (see **PRECAUTIONS - Geriatric Use**).

In patients receiving opioids, both the dose and duration of analgesia will vary substantially depending on the patient's opioid tolerance. The dose should be selected and adjusted so that at least 3-4 hours of pain relief may be achieved. In patients taking opioid analgesics, the starting dose of DILAUDID should be based on prior opioid usage. This should be done by converting the total daily usage of the previous opioid to an equivalent total daily dosage of oral DILAUDID using an equianalgesic table (see below). For opioids not in the table, first estimate the equivalent total daily usage of oral morphine, then use the table to find the equivalent total daily dosage of DILAUDID.

Once the total daily dosage of DILAUDID has been estimated, it should be divided into the desired number of doses. Since there is individual variation in response to different opioid drugs, only 1/2 to 2/3 of the estimated dose of DILAUDID calculated from equivalence tables should be given for the first few doses, then increased as needed according to the patient's response.

Since the pharmacokinetics of hydromorphone are affected in hepatic and renal impairment with a consequent increase in exposure, patients with hepatic and renal impairment should be started on a lower starting dose (See **CLINICAL PHARMACOLOGY - Pharmacokinetics and Metabolism**).

In chronic pain, doses should be administered around-the-clock. A supplemental dose of 5-15% of the total daily usage may be administered every two hours on an "as-needed" basis.

Periodic reassessment after the initial dosing is always required. If pain management is not satisfactory and in the absence of significant opioid-induced adverse events, the hydromorphone dose may be increased gradually. If excessive opioid side effects are observed early in the dosing interval, the hydromorphone dose should be reduced. If this results in breakthrough pain at the end of the dosing interval, the dosing interval may need to be shortened. Dose titration should be guided more by the need for analgesia than the absolute dose of opioid employed.

OPIOID ANALGESIC EQUIVALENTS WITH APPROXIMATELY EQUIANALGESIC POTENCY*

Nonproprietary (Trade) Name	IM or SC Dose	ORAL Dose
Morphine sulfate	10 mg	40-60 mg
Hydromorphone HCl (DILAUDID)	1.3-2 mg	6.5-7.5 mg
Oxymorphone HCl (Numorphan)	1-1.1 mg	6.6 mg
Levorphanol tartrate (Levo-Dromoran)	2-2.3 mg	4 mg
Meperidine, pethidine HCl (Demerol)	75-100 mg	300-400 mg
Methadone HCl (Dolophine)	10 mg	10-20 mg

* Dosages, and ranges of dosages represented, are a compilation of estimated equipotent dosages from published references comparing opioid analgesics in cancer and severe pain.

DRUG ABUSE AND DEPENDENCE

DILAUDID ORAL LIQUID and DILAUDID TABLETS contain hydromorphone, a Schedule II controlled opioid agonist. Schedule II opioid substances which include morphine, oxycodone, oxymorphone, fentanyl, and methadone have the highest potential for abuse and risk of fatal overdose. Hydromorphone can be abused and is subject to criminal diversion.

Opioid analgesics may cause psychological and physical dependence. Physical dependence results in withdrawal symptoms in patients who abruptly discontinue the drug. Physical dependence usually does not occur to a clinically significant degree until after several weeks of continued opioid usage, but it may occur after as little as a week of opioid use. Physical dependence and tolerance are separate and distinct from abuse and addiction.

Addiction is a chronic, neurobiologic disease, with genetic, psychosocial, and environmental factors influencing its development and manifestations. It is characterized by behaviors that include one or more of the following: impaired control over drug use, compulsive use, continued use despite harm, and craving. Drug addiction is a treatable disease, utilizing a multidisciplinary approach, but relapse is common.

"Drug seeking" behavior is very common in addicts and drug abusers. Drug-seeking tactics include emergency calls or visits near the end of office hours, refusal to undergo appropriate examination, testing or referral, repeated "loss" of prescriptions, tampering with, forging or counterfeiting prescriptions and reluctance to provide prior medical records or contact information for other treating physician(s). "Doctor shopping" to obtain additional prescriptions is common among drug abusers, people suffering from untreated addiction and criminals seeking drugs to sell.

Physicians should be aware that addiction may not be accompanied by concurrent tolerance and symptoms of physical dependence in all addicts. In addition, abuse of opioids can occur in the absence of addiction and is characterized by misuse for non-medical purposes, often in combination with other psychoactive substances. Since DILAUDID ORAL LIQUID and DILAUDID TABLETS may be diverted for non-medical use, careful record keeping of prescribing information, including quantity, frequency, and renewal requests is strongly advised.

Proper assessment of the patient, proper prescribing practices, periodic re-evaluation of therapy, and proper dispensing and storage are appropriate measures that help to limit abuse of opioid drugs.

DILAUDID ORAL LIQUID and DILAUDID TABLETS are intended for oral use only. Misuse or abuse of DILAUDID ORAL LIQUID and DILAUDID TABLETS pose a risk of overdose and death. This risk is increased with concurrent abuse of alcohol and other CNS depressants. Parenteral drug abuse can potentially result in local tissue necrosis, infection, pulmonary granulomas, and increased risk of endocarditis and valvular heart injury. In addition, parenteral abuse is commonly associated with transmission of infectious diseases such as hepatitis and HIV.

SAFETY AND HANDLING INSTRUCTIONS

DILAUDID ORAL LIQUID and DILAUDID TABLETS pose little risk of direct exposure to health care personnel and should be handled and disposed of prudently in accordance with hospital or institutional policy. Significant absorption from dermal exposure is unlikely; accidental dermal exposure to DILAUDID ORAL LIQUID should be treated by removal of any contaminated clothing and rinsing the affected area with cool water. Patients and their families should be instructed to flush any DILAUDID ORAL LIQUID and DILAUDID TABLETS that are no longer needed.

Access to abuseable drugs such as DILAUDID ORAL LIQUID and DILAUDID TABLETS presents an occupational hazard for addiction in the health care industry. Routine procedures for handling controlled substances developed to protect the public may not be adequate to protect health care workers. Implementation of more effective accounting procedures and measures to restrict access to drugs of this class (appropriate to the practice setting) may minimize the risk of self-administration by health care providers.

HOW SUPPLIED

DILAUDID ORAL LIQUID is a clear, sweet, slightly viscous liquid. It is available in: Bottles of 1 pint (473 mL) - NDC# 59011-451-01

DILAUDID 2 mg TABLETS are light orange, round, flat-faced tablets, with beveled edges, debossed with a "P" on one side and the number "2" on the opposite side. They are available in:

Bottles of 100 - NDC # 59011-452-10
Unit Dose Packages of 100 (4×25) - NDC # 59011-452-01

DILAUDID 4 mg TABLETS are light yellow, round, flat-faced tablets, with beveled edges, debossed with a "P" on one side and the number "4" on the opposite side. They are available in:

Bottles of 100 - NDC # 59011-454-10
Unit Dose Packages of 100 (4×25) - NDC # 59011-454-01
Bottles of 500 - NDC # 59011-454-05

DILAUDID 8 mg TABLETS are white, triangular shaped tablets debossed with a "P" and an inverted "P" separated with a bisect on one side of the tablet and debossed with the number "8" on the other side of the tablet. They are available in:

Bottles of 100 - NDC# 59011-458-10

Healthcare professionals can telephone Purdue Pharma's Medical Services Department (1-888-726-7535) for information on this product.

Storage

Store at 25°C (77°F); excursions permitted to 15°-30°C (59°-86°F). [See USP Controlled Room Temperature]. Protect from light. A schedule **CS-II** Narcotic. DEA Order Form is Required.

Manufactured for Purdue Pharma L.P. Stamford, CT 06901-3431
By Halo Pharmaceutical, Inc.
Whippany, NJ 07981
Revised: 6/2013

Shown in Product Identification Guide, page 311

DILAUDID® and DILAUDID-HP® INJECTION ℂⅡ

[Di-law-did]

DILAUDID® INJECTION (hydromorphone hydrochloride), CII
DILAUDID-HP® INJECTION (hydromorphone hydrochloride), CII
For intravenous, intramuscular and subcutaneous use

HIGHLIGHTS OF PRESCRIBING INFORMATION
These highlights do not include all the information needed to use DILAUDID® INJECTION and DILAUDID-HP® INJECTION safely and effectively. See full prescribing information for DILAUDID® INJECTION and DILAUDID-HP® INJECTION.
DILAUDID® INJECTION (hydromorphone hydrochloride)
DILAUDID-HP® INJECTION
(hydromorphone hydrochloride)
CII
For intravenous, intramuscular and subcutaneous use
Initial U.S. Approval: January 1984

WARNING: RISK OF RESPIRATORY DEPRESSION, ABUSE, AND MEDICATION ERRORS
DILAUDID-HP® INJECTION IS FOR USE IN OPIOID-TOLERANT PATIENTS ONLY
See full prescribing information for complete boxed warning.
- **Do not confuse DILAUDID-HP INJECTION with standard parenteral formulations of DILAUDID or other opioids, as overdose and death could result.** (5)
- **Hydromorphone is a potent Schedule II opioid agonist. Schedule II opioid agonists have the highest potential for abuse and risk of producing respiratory depression. Ethanol, other opioids, and other central nervous system depressants can potentiate the respiratory-depressant effects of hydromorphone and increase the risk of adverse outcomes, including death.** (5.1, 7.1)

INDICATIONS AND USAGE
- DILAUDID INJECTION is an opioid analgesic indicated for the management of pain where an opioid analgesic is appropriate. (1)
- DILAUDID-HP INJECTION is indicated for the management of moderate-to-severe pain in opioid-tolerant patients who require higher doses of opioids. (1)

DOSAGE AND ADMINISTRATION
- DILAUDID INJECTION: The usual starting dose is 1 mg to 2 mg *subcutaneously* or *intramuscularly* every 2 to 3 hours as necessary. (2.3)
- DILAUDID-HP INJECTION should be used only if the amount of hydromorphone required can be delivered accurately with this formulation. (2.5)
- For patients already receiving opioids, use standard conversion ratio estimates. (2.4)
- The dose should be adjusted according to the severity of pain, as well as the patient's underlying disease state and age. (2.1, 2.2)
- Should intravenous administration be necessary, the injection should be given slowly, over at least 2 to 3 minutes and the usual starting dose is 0.2 to 1 mg. (2.3.2)

DOSAGE FORMS AND STRENGTHS
- DILAUDID INJECTION: 1 mg/mL, 2 mg/mL, or 4 mg/mL. (3)
- DILAUDID-HP INJECTION: 10 mg/mL in 1 mL or 5 mL ampule or 50 mL single-dose vial. (3)
- DILAUDID-HP INJECTION Sterile Lyophilized Powder: 250 mg of sterile, lyophilized hydromorphone hydrochloride to be reconstituted to provide a solution containing 10 mg/mL. (3)

CONTRAINDICATIONS
- Known hypersensitivity to hydromorphone, hydromorphone salts, any components of the product, or in any situation where opioids are contraindicated (4)
- Patients with respiratory depression in the absence of resuscitative equipment or in unmonitored settings; patients with status asthmaticus (4)
- Gastrointestinal obstruction, especially paralytic ileus (4)
- DILAUDID-HP INJECTION: Patients who are not opioid tolerant (4)

WARNINGS AND PRECAUTIONS
- DILAUDID-HP INJECTION is a concentrated formulation of hydromorphone. Do NOT confuse DILAUDID-HP INJECTION with DILAUDID INJECTION. Overdose and death could result. (5.1)
- May cause respiratory depression, use with extreme caution in patients at risk of respiratory depression, elderly, and debilitated patients. (5.2)
- Abuse of DILAUDID INJECTION and DILAUDID-HP INJECTION poses a hazard of overdose and death. (5.3)
- Risk of medication errors: Morphine does not convert to hydromorphone on a milligram per milligram basis. Use Table 1 to convert. (5.1)
- Alcohol, other opioids and central nervous system depressants potentiate the respiratory depressant effects of hydromorphone. (5.4)
- Infants born to mothers physically dependent on DILAUDID INJECTION or DILAUDID-HP INJECTION will also be physically dependent and may exhibit respiratory difficulties and withdrawal symptoms. (5.5)
- Respiratory depression may be markedly increased in patients with head injury, other intracranial lesions, or preexisting increase in intracranial pressure. (5.6)
- May cause hypotension, use with caution in patients at increased risk of hypotension and in patients in circulatory shock. (5.7)
- DILAUDID INJECTION and DILAUDID-HP INJECTION contain sodium metabisulfite. There is a risk of anaphylactic symptoms and life-threatening asthmatic episodes in susceptible people. (5.8)
- Use with caution in patients with biliary tract disease including pancreatitis. (5.9)
- Use with caution and in reduced initial doses in the elderly, debilitated, or other patient populations with increased risk of adverse reactions from opioids. (5.10)
- Use with caution in patients with alcoholism or other drug dependencies. (5.11)
- May impair the mental and physical abilities needed to perform potentially hazardous activities such as driving a car or operating machinery. (5.12)

ADVERSE REACTIONS
Most common adverse reactions are lightheadedness, dizziness, sedation, nausea, vomiting, sweating, flushing, dysphoria, euphoria, dry mouth, and pruritus. (6)
To report Suspected Adverse Reactions, contact Purdue Pharma L.P. at 1-888-726-7535 or FDA at 1-800-FDA-1088 or *www.fda.gov/medwatch*.

DRUG INTERACTIONS
- Concurrent use of other CNS depressants may cause respiratory depression, hypotension, and profound sedation or coma. (7.1)
- Mixed agonist/antagonist analgesics may reduce the analgesic effect of hydromorphone and may precipitate withdrawal symptoms in these patients. (7.2)

USE IN SPECIFIC POPULATIONS
- Pregnancy: Based on animal data, may cause fetal harm. (8.1)
- Labor and Delivery: Use with caution during labor. (8.2)
- Nursing Mothers: Nursing should not be undertaken while a patient is receiving DILAUDID INJECTION or DILAUDID-HP INJECTION. (8.3)
- Pediatrics: Safety and effectiveness in pediatric patients have not been established. (8.4)
- Geriatrics: Use with caution in elderly patients, initiate dose at low end of dosing range. (8.5)
- Hepatic and Renal Impairment: Patients with hepatic and renal impairment should be started on a lower starting dose. (8.6, 8.7, 12.2)

Revised: 07/2011

FULL PRESCRIBING INFORMATION: CONTENTS*

*** Sections or subsections omitted from the full prescribing information are not listed**

FULL PRESCRIBING INFORMATION
DILAUDID® INJECTION (hydromorphone hydrochloride), CII
DILAUDID-HP® INJECTION (hydromorphone hydrochloride), CII
For intravenous, intramuscular, and subcutaneous use

WARNING: RISK OF RESPIRATORY DEPRESSION, ABUSE, AND MEDICATION ERRORS
DILAUDID-HP INJECTION IS FOR USE IN OPIOID-TOLERANT PATIENTS ONLY
Patients considered opioid tolerant are those who are taking at least 60 mg oral morphine/day, 25 mcg transdermal fentanyl/hour, 30 mg oral oxycodone/day, 8 mg oral hydromorphone/day, 25 mg oral oxymorphone/day, or an equianalgesic dose of another opioid for one week or longer.
DILAUDID-HP INJECTION is a more concentrated solution of hydromorphone than DILAUDID INJECTION, and is for use in opioid-tolerant patients only. Do not confuse DILAUDID-HP INJECTION with standard parenteral formulations of DILAUDID INJECTION or other opioids, as overdose and death could result.
DILAUDID INJECTION and DILAUDID-HP INJECTION contain hydromorphone, an opioid agonist and a Schedule II controlled substance with an abuse liability similar to other opioid analgesics. DILAUDID INJECTION and DILAUDID-HP INJECTION can be abused in a manner similar to other opioid agonists, legal or illicit. These risks should be considered when administering, prescribing, or dispensing DILAUDID INJECTION and DILAUDID-HP INJECTION in situations where the healthcare professional is concerned about increased risk of misuse, abuse, or diversion.
Schedule II opioid agonists, including morphine, oxymorphone, hydromorphone, oxycodone, fentanyl and methadone, have the highest potential for abuse and risk of producing fatal overdose due to respiratory depression. Ethanol, other opioids, and other central nervous system depressants (e.g., sedative-hypnotics, skeletal muscle relaxants) can potentiate the respiratory-depressant effects of hydromorphone and increase the risk of adverse outcomes, including death.

1 INDICATIONS AND USAGE

DILAUDID INJECTION is indicated for the management of pain in patients where an opioid analgesic is appropriate. DILAUDID-HP INJECTION is indicated for the management of moderate-to-severe pain in opioid-tolerant patients who require higher doses of opioids.

2 DOSAGE AND ADMINISTRATION

2.1 General Dosing Considerations

Take care when prescribing and administering Dilaudid and Dilaudid-HP Injection to avoid dosing errors due to confusion between the different concentrations and between mg and mL, which could result in accidental overdose and death. Take care to ensure the proper dose is communicated and dispensed. When writing prescriptions, include both the total dose in mg and the total volume of the dose.
Selection of patients and administration of Dilaudid and Dilaudid-HP injection should be governed by the same principles that apply to the use of similar opioid analgesics to treat patients with acute or chronic pain, and depends upon a comprehensive assessment of the patient. Individualize treatment in every case, using non-opioid analgesics, opioids on an as-needed basis and/or combination products, and chronic opioid therapy in a progressive plan of pain management such as outlined by the World Health Organization, the Agency for Healthcare Research and Quality, and the American Pain Society.
The nature of the pain (severity, frequency, etiology, and pathophysiology), as well as the medical status of the patient, will affect selection of the starting dosage. Opioid analgesics, including DILAUDID INJECTION and DILAUDID-HP INJECTION, have a narrow therapeutic index in certain patient populations, especially when combined with CNS depressant drugs, and should be reserved for cases where the benefits of opioid analgesia outweigh the known risks.

2.2 Individualization of Dosing

Initiate the dosing regimen for each patient individually, taking into account the patient's prior analgesic treatment. Give attention to the following:

- the age, general condition and medical status of the patient;
- the patient's degree of opioid tolerance;
- the daily dose, potency, and specific characteristics of the opioid the patient has been taking previously;
- concurrent medications
- the type and severity of the patient's pain
- risk factors for abuse or addiction; including whether the patient has a previous or current substance abuse problem, a family history of substance abuse, or a history of mental illness or depression;
- the balance between pain control and adverse reactions.

Periodic reassessment after the initial dosing of DILAUDID INJECTION and DILAUDID-HP INJECTION is required. If pain management is not satisfactory, and opioid-induced adverse events are tolerable, the hydromorphone dose may be increased gradually. If excessive opioid side effects are observed early in the dosing interval, reduce the hydromorphone hydrochloride dose. If this results in breakthrough pain at the end of the dosing interval, the dosing interval may need to be shortened. Dose titration should be guided more by the need for analgesia and the severity of adverse events than the absolute dose of opioid employed.

2.3 Initiation of Therapy in Opioid-Naïve Patients

Always initiate dosing in opioid-naïve patients using Dilaudid Injection. Never administer Dilaudid-HP injection to opioid-naïve patients.

2.3.1 Subcutaneous or Intramuscular Administration

The usual starting dose of Dilaudid Injection is 1 mg to 2 mg every 2 to 3 hours as necessary. Depending on the clinical situation, the initial starting dose may be lowered in patients who are opioid naïve. Adjust the dose according to the severity of pain, the severity of adverse events, as well as the patient's underlying disease and age.

2.3.2 Intravenous Administration

The initial starting dose is 0.2 to 1 mg every 2 to 3 hours. Intravenous administration should be given **slowly**, over at least 2 to 3 minutes, depending on the dose. Titrate the dose to achieve acceptable analgesia and tolerable adverse events. The initial dose should be reduced in the elderly or debilitated and may be lowered to 0.2 mg.

2.3.3 Hepatic Impairment

Start patients with hepatic impairment on one-fourth to one-half the usual DILAUDID INJECTION starting dose depending on the extent of impairment *[see CLINICAL PHARMACOLOGY, Pharmacokinetics (12.2)]*.

2.3.4 Renal Impairment

Start patients with renal impairment on one-fourth to one-half the usual DILAUDID INJECTION starting dose depending on the degree of impairment *[see CLINICAL PHARMACOLOGY, Pharmacokinetics (12.2)]*.

2.4 Conversion From Prior Opioid

Use the equianalgesic dose table below (Table 1) as a guide to determine the appropriate dose of DILAUDID INJECTION. Convert the current total daily amount(s) of opioid(s) received to an equivalent total daily dose of DILAUDID INJECTION and reduce by one-half due to the possibility of incomplete cross tolerance. Divide the new total amount by the number of doses permitted based on dosing interval (e.g., 8 doses for every-three-hour dosing). Titrate the dose according to the patient's response. For opioids not in Table 1, first estimate the daily amount of morphine that is equivalent to the current total daily amount of other opioid(s) received, then use Table 1 to find the approximate equivalent total daily dose of DILAUDID INJECTION.

Table 1. OPIOID ANALGESIC EQUIVALENTS WITH APPROXIMATELY EQUIANALGESIC POTENCY FOR CONVERSION TO DILAUDID INJECTION*

DRUG SUBSTANCE	PARENTERAL DOSE	ORAL DOSE
Morphine sulfate	10 mg	40 – 60 mg
Hydromorphone HCl	1.3 – 2 mg	6.5 – 7.5 mg
Oxymorphone HCl	1 – 1.1 mg	6.6 mg
Levorphanol tartrate	2 – 2.3 mg	4 mg
Meperidine HCl (Pethidine HCl)	75 – 100 mg	300 – 400 mg
Methadone HCl	10 mg	10 – 20 mg
Nalbuphine HCl	10 – 12 mg	–
Butorphanol tartrate	1.5 – 2.5 mg	–

* Dosages, and ranges of dosages represented, are a compilation of estimated equipotent dosages from published references comparing opioid analgesics in cancer and severe pain.

2.5 DILAUDID-HP Injection (for use in opioid-tolerant patients only)

Do not use DILAUDID-HP for patients who are not tolerant to the respiratory depressant or sedating effects of opioids.

Patients considered opioid tolerant are those who are taking at least 60 mg oral morphine/day, 25 mcg transdermal fentanyl/hour, 30 mg oral oxycodone/day, 8 mg oral hydromorphone/day, 25 mg oral oxymorphone/day, or an equianalgesic dose of another opioid for one week or longer.

Use DILAUDID-HP ONLY for patients who require the higher concentration and lower total volume of DILAUDID-HP.

Because of its high concentration, the delivery of precise doses of DILAUDID-HP INJECTION may be difficult if low doses of hydromorphone are required. Therefore, use DILAUDID-HP INJECTION only if the amount of hydromorphone required can be delivered accurately with this formulation.

Base the starting dose for DILAUDID-HP INJECTION on the prior dose of DILAUDID INJECTION or on the prior dose of an alternate opioid as described above in Section 2.4 Conversion From Prior Opioid and Table 1.

2.6 Administration and Reconstitution

Inspect parenteral drug products visually for particulate matter and discoloration prior to administration, whenever solution and container permit. A slight yellowish discoloration may develop in DILAUDID INJECTION and DILAUDID-HP INJECTION ampules. No loss of potency has been demonstrated. DILAUDID INJECTION and DILAUDID-HP INJECTION are physically compatible and chemically stable for at least 24 hours at 25°C, protected from light in most common large-volume parenteral solutions.

500 mg/50 mL Vial

To use this single dose presentation, do not penetrate the stopper with a syringe. Instead, remove both the aluminum flipseal and rubber stopper in a suitable work area such as under a laminar flow hood (or equivalent clean air compounding area). The contents may then be withdrawn for preparation of a single, large-volume parenteral solution. Discard any unused portion in an appropriate manner.

Reconstitution of Sterile Lyophilized DILAUDID-HP INJECTION 250 mg

Reconstitute immediately prior to use with 25 mL of Sterile Water for Injection USP to provide a sterile solution containing 10 mg/mL of hydromorphone hydrochloride.

3 DOSAGE FORMS AND STRENGTHS

DILAUDID INJECTION:

Each 1 mL colorless ampule contains 1 mg/mL, 2 mg/mL, or 4 mg/mL of hydromorphone hydrochloride in a sterile, aqueous solution.

DILAUDID-HP INJECTION (for use in opioid-tolerant patients only):

Each amber ampule and amber single-dose vial contains 10 mg/mL of hydromorphone hydrochloride in a sterile, aqueous solution and is available in 1 mL or 5 mL ampules or in 50 mL single-dose vials†.

DILAUDID-HP INJECTION Sterile Lyophilized Powder:

Each amber, single-dose vial† contains 250 mg of sterile, lyophilized hydromorphone hydrochloride to be reconstituted with 25 mL of Sterile Water for Injection USP to provide a solution containing 10 mg/mL.

†The Stoppers Of These Products Contain Natural Rubber Latex.

4 CONTRAINDICATIONS

Both DILAUDID INJECTION and DILAUDID-HP INJECTION are contraindicated:

- In patients with known hypersensitivity to hydromorphone, hydromorphone salts, any other components of the product, or sulfite-containing medications *[see WARNINGS AND PRECAUTIONS, Sulfites (5.8)]*.
- In any situation where opioids are contraindicated, e.g., in patients with respiratory depression in the absence of resuscitative equipment or in unmonitored settings; or patients with acute or severe bronchial asthma.
- In patients with, or at risk of developing, gastrointestinal obstruction, especially paralytic ileus because hydromorphone diminishes the propulsive peristaltic wave in the gastrointestinal tract and may prolong the obstruction.

DILAUDID-HP INJECTION is contraindicated in patients who are not opioid tolerant *[see WARNINGS AND PRECAUTIONS (5.1)]*.

5 WARNINGS AND PRECAUTIONS

5.1 Risk of Medication Errors

DILAUDID-HP INJECTION is a 10 mg/mL concentrated solution of hydromorphone, and is intended for use in opioid-tolerant patients only. Patients considered opioid tolerant are those who are taking at least 60 mg oral morphine/day, 25 mcg transdermal fentanyl/hour, 30 mg oral oxycodone/day, 8 mg oral hydromorphone/day, 25 mg oral oxymorphone/day, or an equianalgesic dose of another opioid for one week or longer.

Do not confuse DILAUDID-HP INJECTION with standard parenteral formulations of DILAUDID INJECTION (1 mg/mL, 2 mg/mL, 4 mg/mL) or other opioids, as overdose and death could result.

Morphine does not convert to hydromorphone on a mg per mg basis. Use Table 1 when converting a patient from morphine to hydromorphone to avoid errors that can lead to overdose or death.

5.2 Respiratory Depression

Respiratory depression is the chief hazard of DILAUDID INJECTION and DILAUDID-HP INJECTION. Respiratory depression occurs most frequently in the elderly, in the debilitated, and in those suffering from conditions accompanied by hypoxia or hypercapnia, or upper airway obstruction, in whom even moderate therapeutic doses may dangerously decrease pulmonary ventilation. Respiratory depression is also a particular problem following large initial doses in non opioid-tolerant patients or when opioids are given in conjunction with other agents that depress respiration.

Use DILAUDID INJECTION and DILAUDID-HP INJECTION with extreme caution in patients with chronic obstructive pulmonary disease or cor pulmonale, patients having a substantially decreased respiratory reserve, hypoxia, hypercapnia, or preexisting respiratory depression. In such patients, even usual therapeutic doses of opioid analgesics may decrease respiratory drive while simultaneously increasing airway resistance to the point of apnea. Consider using non-opioid analgesics, and administer DILAUDID only under careful medical supervision at the lowest effective dose in such patients.

5.3 Misuse, Abuse and Diversion of Opioids

DILAUDID INJECTION and DILAUDID-HP INJECTION contain hydromorphone, an opioid agonist with an abuse liability similar to morphine, and a Schedule II, controlled substance. Hydromorphone has the potential for being abused, is sought by drug abusers and people with addiction disorders, and is subject to criminal diversion. Diversion of Schedule II products is an act subject to criminal penalty.

Abuse of DILAUDID INJECTION and DILAUDID-HP INJECTION, poses a hazard of overdose and death. This risk is increased with concurrent abuse of alcohol or other substances. Schedule II opioid agonists have the highest potential for abuse and risk of fatal respiratory depression.

DILAUDID INJECTION and DILAUDID-HP INJECTION can be abused in a manner similar to other opioid agonists, legal or illicit. This should be considered when prescribing or dispensing DILAUDID INJECTION and DILAUDID-HP INJECTION in situations where the physician or pharmacist is concerned about an increased risk of misuse, abuse or diversion.

Concerns about abuse, addiction, and diversion should not prevent the proper management of pain. Healthcare professionals should contact their State Professional Licensing Board or State Controlled Substances Authority for information on how to prevent and detect abuse or diversion of this product.

5.4 Interactions with Alcohol and other CNS Depressants

The concurrent use of DILAUDID INJECTION or DILAUDID-HP INJECTION with other central nervous system (CNS) depressants, including, but not limited to, other opioids, illicit drugs, sedatives, hypnotics, general anesthetics, phenothiazines, muscle relaxants, other tranquilizers, and alcohol, increases the risk of respiratory depression, hypotension, and profound sedation, potentially resulting in coma or death. Use with caution and in reduced dosages in patients taking CNS depressants.

5.5 Neonatal Withdrawal Syndrome

Infants born to mothers physically dependent on DILAUDID INJECTION or DILAUDID-HP INJECTION will also be physically dependent and may exhibit signs of withdrawal. The withdrawal signs include irritability and excessive crying, tremors, hyperactive reflexes, increased respiratory rate, increased stools, sneezing, yawning, vomiting, and fever. The intensity of the syndrome does not always correlate with the duration of maternal opioid use or dose. Neonatal opioid withdrawal syndrome may be life-threatening and should be treated according to protocols developed by neonatology experts *[see DRUG ABUSE AND DEPENDENCE (9.3)]*.

5.6 Use in Increased Intracranial Pressure or Head Injury

The respiratory depressant effects of DILAUDID INJECTION and DILAUDID-HP INJECTION promote carbon dioxide retention which results in elevation of cerebrospinal fluid pressure. This increase in intracranial pressure may be markedly exaggerated in the presence of head injury, intracranial lesions, or other conditions that predispose patients to increased intracranial pressure.

DILAUDID INJECTION and DILAUDID-HP INJECTION may produce effects on pupillary response and consciousness which can obscure the clinical course and neurologic signs of further increase in pressure in patients with head injuries.

5.7 Hypotensive Effect

DILAUDID INJECTION and DILAUDID-HP INJECTION may cause severe hypotension in patients whose ability to maintain blood pressure is compromised by a depleted blood volume, or a concurrent administration of drugs such as phenothiazines, general anesthetics, or other agents which compromise vasomotor tone *[see DRUG INTERACTIONS (7.1)]*.

DILAUDID INJECTION and DILAUDID-HP INJECTION may produce orthostatic hypotension in ambulatory patients.

Administer DILAUDID INJECTION and DILAUDID-HP INJECTION with caution to patients in circulatory shock, since vasodilation produced by the drug may further reduce cardiac output and blood pressure.

5.8 Sulfites

DILAUDID INJECTION and DILAUDID-HP INJECTION contain sodium metabisulfite, a sulfite that may cause allergic-type reactions including anaphylactic symptoms and life-threatening or less severe asthmatic episodes in certain susceptible people. The overall prevalence of sulfite sensitivity in the general population is unknown and probably low. Sulfite sensitivity is seen more frequently in asthmatic than in nonasthmatic people.

5.9 Use in Pancreatic/Biliary Tract Disease and Other Gastrointestinal Conditions

The administration of DILAUDID INJECTION or DILAUDID-HP INJECTION may obscure the diagnosis or clinical course in patients with acute abdominal conditions *[see CONTRAINDICATIONS (4.0)]*.

Use DILAUDID INJECTION and DILAUDID-HP with caution in patients who are at risk of developing ileus.

Use DILAUDID INJECTION and DILAUDID-HP INJECTION with caution in patients with biliary tract disease, including acute pancreatitis, as hydromorphone may cause spasm of the sphincter of Oddi and diminish biliary and pancreatic secretions.

5.10 Special Risk Patients

Give DILAUDID INJECTION and DILAUDID-HP INJECTION with caution and the initial dose should be reduced in the elderly or debilitated and those with severe impairment of hepatic, pulmonary, or renal function; myxedema or hypothyroidism; adrenocortical insufficiency (e.g., Addison's Disease); CNS depression or coma; toxic psychoses; prostatic hypertrophy or urethral stricture; acute alcoholism; delirium tremens; or kyphoscoliosis associated with respiratory depression.

The administration of opioid analgesics including DILAUDID INJECTION and DILAUDID-HP INJECTION may aggravate preexisting convulsions in patients with convulsive disorders.

DILAUDID INJECTION and DILAUDID-HP INJECTION, as with other opioids, may aggravate convulsions in patients with convulsive disorders, and may induce or aggravate seizures in some clinical settings.

Reports of mild to severe seizures and myoclonus have been reported in severely compromised patients administered high doses of parenteral hydromorphone.

5.11 Use in Drug and Alcohol Dependent Patients

Use DILAUDID INJECTION and DILAUDID-HP INJECTION with caution in patients with alcoholism and other drug dependencies due to the increased frequency of opioid tolerance, dependence, and the risk of addiction observed in these patient populations. Abuse of DILAUDID INJECTION or DILAUDID-HP INJECTION in combination with other CNS depressant drugs can result in serious risk to the patient.

DILAUDID INJECTION and DILAUDID-HP INJECTION contain hydromorphone, an opioid with no approved use in the management of addiction disorders. Its proper usage in individuals with drug or alcohol dependence, either active or in remission, is for the management of pain requiring opioid analgesia.

5.12 Use in Ambulatory Patients

DILAUDID INJECTION and DILAUDID-HP INJECTION may impair mental and/or physical ability required for the performance of potentially hazardous tasks (e.g., driving, operating machinery). Patients should be cautioned accordingly. DILAUDID INJECTION and DILAUDID-HP INJECTION may produce orthostatic hypotension in ambulatory patients.

5.13 Parenteral Administration

DILAUDID INJECTION may be given intravenously, but the injection should be given very slowly. Rapid intravenous injection of opioid analgesics increases the possibility of side effects such as hypotension and respiratory depression *[see DOSAGE AND ADMINSTRATION (2.3)]*.

6 ADVERSE REACTIONS

Because clinical trials are conducted under widely varying conditions, adverse reaction rates observed in the clinical trials of a drug cannot be directly compared to rates in the clinical trials of another drug and may not reflect the rates observed in clinical practice.

Serious adverse reactions associated with DILAUDID INJECTION and DILAUDID-HP INJECTION include respiratory depression and apnea and, to a lesser degree, circulatory depression, respiratory arrest, shock, and cardiac arrest.

The following serious adverse reactions described elsewhere in the labeling include:

- Respiratory depression and secondary effects on intracranial pressure *[see WARNINGS AND PRECAUTIONS (5.2, 5.6)]*
- Hypotension *[see WARNINGS AND PRECAUTIONS (5.7)]*
- Gastrointestinal effects and effects in sphincter of Oddi *[see WARNINGS AND PRECAUTIONS (5.9)]*
- Drug abuse, addiction, and dependence *[see DRUG ABUSE AND DEPENDENCE (9.2, 9.3)]*
- Effects on the ability to drive and operate machinery *[see WARNINGS AND PRECAUTIONS (5.12)]*

The most common adverse effects are lightheadedness, dizziness, sedation, nausea, vomiting, sweating, flushing, dysphoria, euphoria, dry mouth, and pruritus. These effects seem to be more prominent in ambulatory patients and in those not experiencing severe pain.

Less Frequently Observed Adverse Reactions

Cardiac disorders: tachycardia, bradycardia, palpitations

Eye disorders: vision blurred, diplopia, miosis, visual impairment

Gastrointestinal disorders: constipation, ileus, diarrhea, abdominal pain

General disorders and administration site conditions: weakness, feeling abnormal, chills, injection site urticaria

Hepatobiliary disorders: biliary colic

Metabolism and nutrition disorders: decreased appetite

Musculoskeletal and connective tissue disorders: muscle rigidity

Nervous system disorders: headache, tremor, paraesthesia, nystagmus, increased intracranial pressure, syncope, taste alteration, involuntary muscle contractions, presyncope

Psychiatric disorders: agitation, mood altered, nervousness, anxiety, depression, hallucination, disorientation, insomnia, abnormal dreams

Renal and urinary disorders: urinary retention, urinary hesitation, antidiuretic effects

Respiratory, thoracic, and mediastinal disorders: bronchospasm, laryngospasm

Skin and subcutaneous tissue disorders: injection site pain, urticaria, rash, hyperhidrosis

Vascular disorders: flushing, hypotension, hypertension

Postmarketing Experience

The following adverse reactions have been identified during post-approval use of hydromorphone. Because these events are reported voluntarily from a population of uncertain size, it is not always possible to reliably estimate their frequency or establish a causal relationship to drug exposure: anaphylactic reactions, confusional state, convulsions, drowsiness, dyskinesia, dyspnea, erectile dysfunction, fatigue, hepatic enzymes increased, hyperalgesia, hypersensitivity reaction, injection site reactions, lethargy, myoclonus, oropharyngeal swelling, peripheral edema, and somnolence.

7 DRUG INTERACTIONS

7.1 Drug Interactions with other CNS Depressants

DILAUDID INJECTION and DILAUDID-HP INJECTION should be used with caution and in reduced dosages when administered to patients concurrently receiving other central nervous system depressants including sedatives or hypnotics, general anesthetics, phenothiazines, centrally acting anti-emetics, tranquilizers, and alcohol because respiratory depression, hypotension, and profound sedation or coma may result.

When such combined therapy is contemplated, the dose of one or both agents should be reduced. Opioid analgesics, including DILAUDID INJECTION and DILAUDID-HP INJECTION, may enhance the action of neuromuscular blocking agents and produce an increased degree of respiratory depression.

7.2 Interactions with Mixed Agonist/Antagonist Opioid Analgesics

Agonist/antagonist analgesics (e.g., pentazocine, nalbuphine, and butorphanol) and partial agonist analgesics (buprenorphine) should be administered with caution to a patient who has received or is receiving a course of therapy with a pure opioid agonist analgesic such as DILAUDID INJECTION and DILAUDID-HP INJECTION. In this situation, mixed agonist/antagonist analgesics may reduce the analgesic effect of DILAUDID INJECTION and DILAUDID-HP INJECTION and/or may precipitate withdrawal symptoms in these patients.

7.3 Monoamine Oxidase Inhibitors (MAOIs)

MAOIs may potentiate the action of DILAUDID INJECTION and DILAUDID-HP INJECTION. Allow at least 14 days after stopping treatment with MAOIs before initiating treatment with DILAUDID INJECTION and DILAUDID-HP INJECTION.

7.4 Anticholinergics

Anticholinergics or other medications with anticholinergic activity when used concurrently with DILAUDID INJECTION and DILAUDID-HP INJECTION may result in increased risk of urinary retention and severe constipation, which may lead to paralytic ileus.

8 USE IN SPECIFIC POPULATIONS

8.1 Pregnancy

Teratogenic Effects

Pregnancy Category C: There are no adequate and well-controlled studies in pregnant women. Hydromorphone crosses the placenta. DILAUDID INJECTION or DILAUDID-HP INJECTION should be used during pregnancy only if the potential benefit justifies the potential risk to the fetus.

No effects on teratogenicity or embryotoxicity were observed in pregnant rats given oral doses up to 7 mg/kg/day which is 3-fold higher than the human dose of 24 mg DILAUDID INJECTION (4 mg every 4 hours), on a body surface area basis. Hydromorphone administration to pregnant Syrian hamsters and CF-1 mice during major organ development revealed teratogenic effects likely the result of maternal toxicity associated with sedation and hypoxia. In Syrian hamsters given single subcutaneous doses from 14 to 258 mg/kg during organogenesis (gestation days 8-10), doses ≥ 19 mg/kg of hydromorphone produced skull malformations (exencephaly and cranioschisis). In CF-1 mice, continuous infusion of hydromorphone (≥ 15 mg/kg over 24 hours) via implanted osmotic pumps during organogenesis (gestation days 7-10) produced soft tissue malformations (cryptorchidism, cleft palate, malformed ventricles and retina), and skeletal variations (split supraoccipital, checkerboard and split sternebrae, delayed ossification of the paws and ectopic ossification sites). The malformations and variations observed in the hamsters and mice were observed at doses approximately 6-fold and 3-fold higher, respectively, than the human dose of 24 mg DILAUDID INJECTION (4 mg every 4 hours) on a body surface area basis.

8.2 Labor and Delivery

DILAUDID should be used with caution during labor. Opioids cross the placenta and may produce respiratory depression and physiologic effects in neonates. Sinusoidal fetal heart rate patterns may occur with the use of opioid analgesics.

Occasionally, opioid analgesics, including DILAUDID INJECTION and DILAUDID-HP INJECTION, may prolong labor through actions which temporarily reduce the strength, duration, and frequency of uterine contractions. However, this effect is not consistent and may be offset by an increased rate of cervical dilatation, which tends to shorten labor.

Opioid analgesics, including DILAUDID INJECTION and DILAUDID-HP INJECTION, may cause respiratory depression in the newborn. Closely observe neonates whose mothers received opioid analgesics during labor for signs of respiratory depression. Have a specific opioid antagonist, such as naloxone or nalmefene, available for reversal of opioid-induced respiratory depression in the neonate.

Neonates whose mothers have been taking opioids chronically may also exhibit withdrawal signs, either at birth or in the nursery, because they have developed physical dependence. This is not, however, synonymous with addiction *[see DRUG ABUSE AND DEPENDENCE (9.3)]*. Neonatal opioid withdrawal syndrome, unlike opioid withdrawal syndrome in adults, may be life-threatening and should be treated according to protocols developed by neonatology experts *[see WARNINGS AND PRECAUTIONS (5.3)]*.

The effect of DILAUDID, if any, on the later growth, development, and functional maturation of the child is unknown.

8.3 Nursing Mothers

Low levels of opioid analgesics have been detected in human milk. As a general rule, nursing should not be undertaken while a patient is receiving DILAUDID INJECTION or DILAUDID-HP INJECTION since it, and other drugs in this class, may be excreted in the milk.

8.4 Pediatric Use

The safety and effectiveness of DILAUDID INJECTION and DILAUDID-HP INJECTION in pediatric patients has not been established.

8.5 Geriatric Use

Clinical studies of DILAUDID INJECTION and DILAUDID-HP INJECTION did not include sufficient numbers of subjects aged 65 and over to determine whether they respond differently from younger subjects. In general, dose selection for an elderly patient should be cautious, usually starting at the low end of the dosing range, reflecting the greater frequency of decreased hepatic, renal, or cardiac function, and of concomitant disease or other drug therapy. Respiratory depression is the chief risk in elderly or debilitated patients, usually the result of large initial doses in non opioid-tolerant patients. Titration in these patients should proceed cautiously *[see DOSAGE AND ADMINISTRATION (2.4) and WARNINGS AND PRECAUTIONS (5.10)]*.

8.6 Renal Impairment

The pharmacokinetics of hydromorphone following an oral administration of hydromorphone at a single 4 mg dose (2 mg hydromorphone immediate-release tablets) are affected by renal impairment. Mean exposure to hydromorphone (C_{max} and $AUC_{0-\infty}$) is increased by 2-fold in patients with moderate (CLcr = 40 - 60 mL/min) renal impairment and increased by 4-fold in patients with severe (CLcr < 30 mL/min) renal impairment compared with normal subjects (CLcr > 80 mL/min). In addition, in patients with severe renal impairment, hydromorphone appeared to be more slowly eliminated with a longer terminal elimination half-life (40 hr) compared to patients with normal renal function (15 hr). Start patients with renal impairment on one-fourth to one-half the usual starting dose depending on the degree of impairment. Patients with renal impairment should be closely monitored during dose titration *[see CLINICAL PHARMACOLOGY (12.2)]*.

8.7 Hepatic Impairment

The pharmacokinetics of hydromorphone following an oral administration of hydromorphone at a single 4 mg dose (2 mg hydromorphone immediate-release tablets) are affected by hepatic impairment. Mean exposure to hydromorphone (C_{max} and AUC_{∞}) is increased 4-fold in patients with moderate (Child-Pugh Group B) hepatic impairment compared with subjects with normal hepatic function. Due to increased exposure of hydromorphone, patients with moderate hepatic impairment should be started at one-fourth to one-half the recommended starting dose depending on the degree of hepatic dysfunction and closely monitored during dose titration. The pharmacokinetics of hydromorphone in patients with severe hepatic impairment has not been studied. A further increase in C_{max} and AUC of hydromorphone in this group is expected and should be taken into consideration when selecting a starting dose *[see CLINICAL PHARMACOLOGY (12.2)]*.

9 DRUG ABUSE AND DEPENDENCE

9.1 Controlled Substance

DILAUDID INJECTION and DILAUDID-HP INJECTION contain hydromorphone, which is a Schedule II controlled substance with an abuse liability similar to morphine. DILAUDID can be abused and is subject to criminal diversion.

9.2 Abuse

DILAUDID INJECTION and DILAUDID-HP INJECTION are intended for parenteral use only under the direct supervision of an appropriately licensed health care professional. Abuse of DILAUDID INJECTION and DILAUDID-HP INJECTION poses a hazard of overdose and death. This risk is increased with concurrent abuse of alcohol or other substances. Parenteral drug abuse is commonly associated with transmission of infectious diseases, such as hepatitis and HIV.

DILAUDID INJECTION and DILAUDID-HP INJECTION can be abused in a manner similar to other opioid agonists, legal or illicit. This should be considered when prescribing, dispensing, ordering, or administering DILAUDID INJECTION or DILAUDID-HP INJECTION in situations where the physician or pharmacist is concerned about an increased risk of misuse, abuse, or diversion. Prescribers should monitor all patients receiving opioids for signs of abuse, misuse, and addiction. Furthermore, patients should be assessed for their potential for opioid abuse prior to being prescribed opioid therapy. Persons at increased risk for opioid abuse include those with a personal or family history of substance abuse (including drug or alcohol abuse) or mental illness (e.g., depression). Opioids may still be appropriate for use in these patients, however, they will require intensive monitoring for indications of abuse.

Opioid drugs are sought by people with substance use disorders (abuse or addiction, the latter of which is also called "substance dependence") and criminals who supply them by diverting medicines out of legitimate distribution channels. DILAUDID INJECTION and DILAUDID-HP INJECTION are targets for diversion.

"Drug-seeking" behavior is very common in persons with substance use disorders. Drug-seeking tactics include, but are not limited to, emergency calls or visits near the end of office hours, refusal to undergo appropriate examination, testing or referral, repeated "loss" of prescriptions, altering or forging of prescriptions and reluctance to provide prior medical records or contact information for other treating physician(s). "Doctor shopping" to obtain additional prescriptions is common among people with untreated substance use disorders and criminals who divert controlled substances.

The risks of misuse and abuse should be considered when prescribing or dispensing DILAUDID INJECTION or DILAUDID-HP INJECTION. Concerns about abuse and addiction, should not prevent the proper management of pain, however. Treatment of pain should be individualized, balancing the potential benefits and risks for each patient.

Addiction is defined as a chronic, neurobiological disorder with genetic, psychosocial, and environmental aspects, characterized by one or more of the following: impaired control over drug use, compulsive use, continued use despite harm, and craving. Drug addiction is a treatable disease, utilizing a multidisciplinary approach, but relapse is common.

Abuse and addiction are separate and distinct from physical dependence and tolerance. Physicians should be aware that addiction may not be accompanied by concurrent tolerance and symptoms of physical dependence in all addicts. In addition, abuse of opioids can occur in the absence of addiction and is characterized by misuse for non-medical purposes, often in combination with other psychoactive substances. Careful record keeping of prescribing information, including quantity, frequency, and renewal requests is strongly advised.

Proper assessment of the patient, proper prescribing practices, periodic re-evaluation of therapy, proper dispensing and correct storage and handling are appropriate measures that help to limit misuse and abuse of opioid drugs. Careful record-keeping of prescribing information, including quantity, frequency, and renewal requests is strongly advised.

Healthcare professionals should contact their State Professional Licensing Board or State Controlled Substances Authority for information on how to prevent and detect abuse or diversion of this product.

9.3 Dependence

Tolerance to opioids is demonstrated by the need for increasing doses to maintain a defined effect such as analgesia (in the absence of disease progression or other external factors). Tolerance to different effects of opioids may develop to varying degrees and at varying rates in a given individual. There is also inter-patient variability in the rate and extent of tolerance that develops to various opioid effects, whether the effect is desirable (e.g., analgesia) or undesirable (e.g., nausea). In general, patients taking opioid analgesics that are appropriately titrated for pain control develop tolerance to the respiratory depressant effects fairly reliably. Conversely, tolerance to the constipating effects of opioids rarely develops, even when they are administered over long periods of time.

Physical dependence is manifested by withdrawal symptoms after abrupt discontinuation of a drug or upon administration of an antagonist. Physical dependence and tolerance are not unusual during chronic opioid therapy.

The opioid abstinence or withdrawal syndrome is characterized by some or all of the following: restlessness, lacrimation, rhinorrhea, yawning, perspiration, chills, myalgia, and mydriasis. Other signs and symptoms also may develop, including: irritability, anxiety, backache, joint pain, weakness, abdominal cramps, insomnia, nausea, anorexia, vomiting, diarrhea, or increased blood pressure, respiratory rate, or heart rate.

In general, opioids used regularly should not be abruptly discontinued.

10 OVERDOSAGE

10.1 Signs and Symptoms

Signs and symptoms of acute overdosage with DILAUDID INJECTION or DILAUDID-HP INJECTION include: respiratory depression, somnolence progressing to stupor or coma, skeletal muscle flaccidity, cold and clammy skin, constricted pupils, bradycardia, hypotension, partial or complete airway obstruction, atypical snoring, apnea, circulatory collapse, cardiac arrest, and death.

Hydromorphone may cause miosis, even in total darkness. Pinpoint pupils are a sign of opioid overdose but are not pathognomonic (pontine lesions of hemorrhagic or ischemic origin may produce similar findings). Marked mydriasis, rather than miosis, may be seen with hypoxia in overdose situations.

10.2 Treatment

In the treatment of overdosage, primary attention should be given to the reestablishment of a patent airway and institution of assisted or controlled ventilation. Supportive measures (including oxygen, vasopressors) should be employed in the management of circulatory shock and pulmonary edema accompanying overdose as indicated. Cardiac arrest or arrhythmias may require cardiac massage or defibrillation.

The opioid antagonist, naloxone, is a specific antidote against respiratory depression which may result from overdosage, or unusual sensitivity to DILAUDID INJECTION or DILAUDID-HP INJECTION. Therefore, an appropriate dose of this antagonist should be administered, preferably by the intravenous route, simultaneously with efforts at respiratory resuscitation. Naloxone should not be administered in the absence of clinically significant respiratory or circulatory depression. Naloxone should be administered cautiously to persons who are known, or suspected, to be physically dependent on DILAUDID INJECTION or DILAUDID-HP INJECTION. In such cases, an abrupt or complete reversal of opioid effects may precipitate an acute withdrawal syndrome.

Since the duration of action of DILAUDID INJECTION and DILAUDID-HP INJECTION may exceed that of the antagonist, the patient should be kept under continued surveillance; repeated doses of the antagonist may be required to maintain adequate respiration. Apply other supportive measures when indicated.

11 DESCRIPTION

DILAUDID (hydromorphone hydrochloride), a hydrogenated ketone of morphine, is an opioid analgesic. The chemical name of DILAUDID is 4,5α-epoxy-3-hydroxy-17-methylmorphinan-6-one hydrochloride. The structural formula is:

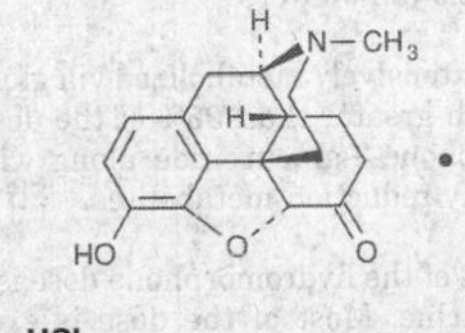

$C_{17}H_{19}NO_3 \cdot HCl$ 321.80

DILAUDID INJECTION is available as a sterile, aqueous solution in COLORLESS ampules for parenteral administration. Each 1 mL ampule contains 1 mg, 2 mg, or 4 mg of hydromorphone hydrochloride with 0.2% sodium citrate and 0.2% citric acid added as a buffer to maintain a pH between 3.5 and 5.5.

DILAUDID-HP INJECTION is available as a sterile, aqueous solution in AMBER ampules and in AMBER, single-dose vials for intravenous, subcutaneous, or intramuscular administration. Each ampule and single-dose vial contains 10 mg/mL of hydromorphone hydrochloride with 0.2% sodium citrate and 0.2% citric acid added as a buffer to maintain a pH of between 3.5 and 5.5. The single dose vials are capped with stoppers containing natural rubber latex.

DILAUDID-HP INJECTION is also available as sterile, lyophilized powder in an AMBER, single-dose vial for reconstitution for intravenous, subcutaneous, or intramuscular administration. Each single dose vial contains 250 mg sterile, lyophilized hydromorphone HCl with either hydrochloric acid or sodium hydroxide added to adjust the pH. Each vial is to be reconstituted with 25 mL of Sterile Water for Injection USP to provide a solution containing 10 mg/mL with a pH between 4.5 and 6.5. The single dose vials are capped with stoppers containing natural rubber latex.

12 CLINICAL PHARMACOLOGY

12.1 Mechanism of Action

The precise mode of analgesic action of opioid analgesics is unknown. However, specific CNS opiate receptors have been identified. Opioids are believed to express their pharmacological effects by combining with these receptors.

Hydromorphone hydrochloride is a mu-opioid receptor agonist whose principal therapeutic action is analgesia. Other members of the class known as opioid agonists include substances such as morphine, oxycodone, fentanyl, codeine, hydrocodone, and oxymorphone.

Central Nervous System

Pharmacological effects of opioid agonists include anxiolysis, euphoria, feelings of relaxation, and cough suppression, as well as analgesia.

Hydromorphone produces respiratory depression by direct effect on brain stem respiratory centers. The mechanism of respiratory depression also involves a reduction in the responsiveness of the brain stem respiratory centers to increases in carbon dioxide tension.

Hydromorphone causes miosis. Pinpoint pupils are a common sign of opioid overdose but are not pathognomonic (pontine lesions of hemorrhagic or ischemic origin may produce similar findings).

Gastrointestinal Tract and Other Smooth Muscle

Gastric, biliary and pancreatic secretions are decreased by opioids such as hydromorphone. Hydromorphone causes a reduction in motility associated with an increase in tone in the gastric antrum and duodenum. Digestion of food in the small intestine is delayed and propulsive contractions are decreased. Propulsive peristaltic waves in the colon are decreased, and tone may be increased to the point of spasm. The end result is constipation. Hydromorphone can cause a marked increase in biliary tract pressure as a result of spasm of the sphincter of Oddi.

Cardiovascular System

Hydromorphone may produce hypotension as a result of either peripheral vasodilation, release of histamine, or both. Other manifestations of histamine release and/or peripheral vasodilation may include pruritus, flushing, and red eyes.

Effects on the myocardium after intravenous administration of opioids are not significant in normal persons, vary with different opioid analgesic agents and vary with the hemodynamic state of the patient, state of hydration and sympathetic drive.

Endocrine System

Opioids may influence the hypothalamic-pituitary-adrenal or -gonadal axes. Some changes that can be seen include an increase in serum prolactin, and decreases in plasma cortisol and testosterone. Clinical signs and symptoms may be manifest from these hormonal changes.

Immune System

In vitro and animal studies indicate that opioids have a variety of effects on immune functions. The clinical significance of these findings is unknown.

12.2 Pharmacokinetics

Distribution

At therapeutic plasma levels, hydromorphone is approximately 8-19% bound to plasma proteins. After an intravenous bolus dose, the steady state of volume of distribution [mean (%CV)] is 302.9 (32%) liters.

Metabolism

Hydromorphone is extensively metabolized via glucuronidation in the liver, with greater than 95% of the dose metabolized to hydromorphone-3-glucuronide along with minor amounts of 6-hydroxy reduction metabolites.

Elimination

Only a small amount of the hydromorphone dose is excreted unchanged in the urine. Most of the dose is excreted as hydromorphone-3-glucuronide along with minor amounts of 6-hydroxy reduction metabolites. The systemic clearance is approximately 1.96 (20%) liters/minute. The terminal elimination half-life of hydromorphone after an intravenous dose is about 2.3 hours.

Special Populations

Hepatic Impairment

After oral administration of hydromorphone at a single 4 mg dose (2 mg hydromorphone immediate-release tablets), mean exposure to hydromorphone (C_{max} and AUC_{∞}) is increased 4-fold in patients with moderate (Child-Pugh Group B) hepatic impairment compared with subjects with normal hepatic function. Patients with moderate hepatic impairment should be started at one-fourth to one-half the recommended starting dose and closely monitored during dose titration. The pharmacokinetics of hydromorphone in patients with severe hepatic impairment has not been studied. A further increase in C_{max} and AUC of hydromorphone in this group is expected and should be taken into consideration when selecting a starting dose *[see USE IN SPECIFIC POPULATIONS (8.7)]*.

Renal Impairment

The pharmacokinetics of hydromorphone following an oral administration of hydromorphone at a single 4 mg dose (2 mg hydromorphone immediate-release tablets) are affected by renal impairment. Mean exposure to hydromorphone (C_{max} and $AUC_{0-\infty}$) is increased by 2-fold in patients with moderate (CLcr = 40 - 60 mL/min) renal impairment and increased by 4-fold in patients with severe (CLcr < 30 mL/min) renal impairment compared with normal subjects (CLcr > 80 mL/min). In addition, in patients with severe renal impairment, hydromorphone appeared to be more slowly eliminated with a longer terminal elimination half-life (40 hr) compared to patients with normal renal function (15 hr). Start patients with renal impairment on one-fourth to one-half the usual starting dose depending on the degree of impairment. Patients with renal impairment should be closely monitored during dose titration *[see USE IN SPECIFIC POPULATIONS (8.6)]*.

Pediatrics

Pharmacokinetics of hydromorphone have not been evaluated in children.

Geriatric

In the geriatric population, age has no effect on the pharmacokinetics of hydromorphone.

Gender

Gender has little effect on the pharmacokinetics of hydromorphone. Females appear to have a higher C_{max} (25%) than males with comparable AUC_{0-24} values. The difference observed in C_{max} may not be clinically relevant.

Race

The effect of race on hydromorphone pharmacokinetics has not been studied.

Pregnancy and Nursing Mothers

Hydromorphone crosses the placenta. Hydromorphone is also found in low levels in breast milk, and may cause respiratory compromise in newborns when administered during labor or delivery.

13 NONCLINICAL TOXICOLOGY

13.1 Carcinogenesis, Mutagenesis, Impairment of Fertility

Carcinogenesis

Long term studies in animals to evaluate the carcinogenic potential of hydromorphone have not been conducted.

Mutagenesis

Hydromorphone was not mutagenic in the *in vitro* bacterial reverse mutation assay (Ames assay). Hydromorphone was not clastogenic in either the *in vitro* human lymphocyte chromosome aberration assay or the *in vivo* mouse micronucleus assay.

Impairment of Fertility

No effects on fertility, reproductive performance, or reproductive organ morphology were observed in male or female rats given oral doses up to 7 mg/kg/day which is 3-fold higher than the human dose of 24 mg DILAUDID INJECTION (4 mg every 4 hours), on a body surface area basis.

14 CLINICAL STUDIES

Analgesic effects of single doses of DILAUDID ORAL LIQUID administered to patients with post-surgical pain have been studied in double-blind controlled trials. In one study, both 5 mg and 10 mg of DILAUDID ORAL LIQUID provided significantly more analgesia than placebo.

16 HOW SUPPLIED/STORAGE AND HANDLING

16.1 Safety and Handling Instructions

DILAUDID INJECTION and DILAUDID-HP INJECTION pose little risk of direct exposure to health care personnel and should be handled and disposed of prudently in accordance with hospital or institutional policy. When DILAUDID INJECTION or DILAUDID-HP INJECTION is no longer needed, any unused liquid should be destroyed by flushing it down the toilet.

Access to drugs with a potential for abuse such as DILAUDID INJECTION and DILAUDID-HP INJECTION presents an occupational hazard for addiction in the health care industry. Routine procedures for handling controlled substances developed to protect the public may not be adequate to protect health care workers. Implementation of more effective accounting procedures and measures to restrict access to drugs of this class (appropriate to the practice setting) may minimize the risk of self-administration by health care providers.

16.2 How Supplied

DILAUDID INJECTION

DILAUDID INJECTION (hydromorphone hydrochloride) is supplied in COLORLESS ampules. Each 1 mL of sterile, aqueous solution contains 1 mg, 2 mg, or 4 mg hydromorphone hydrochloride with 0.2% sodium citrate and 0.2% citric acid solution. DILAUDID INJECTION contains no added preservative and is supplied as follows:

NDC 59011-441-10: Box of ten 1 mL (1 mg/mL) ampules

NDC 59011-442-10: Box of ten 1 mL (2 mg/mL) ampules

NDC 59011-442-25: Box of twenty-five 1 mL (2 mg/mL) ampules

NDC 59011-444-10: Box of ten 1 mL (4 mg/mL) ampules

DILAUDID-HP INJECTION

DILAUDID-HP INJECTION (hydromorphone hydrochloride) is supplied in AMBER ampules, and AMBER single-dose vials. Each ampule and single-dose vial of sterile aqueous solution contains 10 mg of hydromorphone hydrochloride with 0.2% sodium citrate and 0.2% citric acid solution.

DILAUDID-HP INJECTION Sterile Lyophilized Powder is supplied in an AMBER single-dose vial. Each vial contains 250 mg of sterile, lyophilized hydromorphone hydrochloride. DILAUDID-HP INJECTION contains no added preservative and is supplied as follows:

NDC 59011-445-01: Box of ten 1 mL (10 mg/mL) ampules

NDC 59011-445-05: Box of ten 5 mL (10 mg/mL) ampules

†**NDC** 59011-445-50: One 50 mL (10 mg/mL) single-dose vial with black rubber stopper and white flip-top/tear-off seal.

†**NDC** 59011-446-25: One 250 mg single-dose vial with black rubber stopper and black flip-top seal.

†**The Stoppers for These Products Contain Natural Rubber Latex**

16.3 Storage

PROTECT FROM LIGHT.

Keep covered in carton until time of use. Store at 20° to 25°C (68° to 77°F); excursions permitted to 15° to 30°C (59° to 86°F) [See USP Controlled Room Temperature].

Healthcare professionals can telephone Purdue Pharma L.P.'s Medical Services Department (1-888-726-7535) for information on this product.

CAUTION: DEA Order Form Required.

Manufactured by
Hospira, Inc., Lake Forest, IL 60045, U.S.A.
For
Purdue Pharma L.P. Stamford, CT 06901-3431
U.S. Patent Number 6,589,960
302703-0A

Shown in Product Identification Guide, page 312

INTERMEZZO® Ⓒ
[in ter mét zoh]
(zolpidem tartrate)
sublingual tablets

HIGHLIGHTS OF PRESCRIBING INFORMATION
These highlights do not include all the information needed to use INTERMEZZO safely and effectively. See full prescribing information for INTERMEZZO.
INTERMEZZO® (zolpidem tartrate) sublingual tablets, CIV
Initial U.S. Approval: 1992

INDICATIONS AND USAGE

Intermezzo is a $GABA_A$ agonist indicated for use as needed for the treatment of insomnia when a middle-of-the-night awakening is followed by difficulty returning to sleep (1)

Limitation of Use: Not indicated for the treatment of middle-of-the night awakening when the patient has fewer than 4 hours of bedtime remaining before the planned time of waking (1)

DOSAGE AND ADMINISTRATION

- Take only if 4 hours of bedtime remain before the planned time of waking (2.1, 5.1)
- Intermezzo should be placed under the tongue and allowed to disintegrate completely before swallowing. The tablet should not be swallowed whole. (2.1)
- The effect of Intermezzo may be slowed if taken with or immediately after a meal (2.1)
- Recommended dose is 1.75 mg for women and 3.5 mg for men, taken only once per night if needed (2.2)
- Lower doses of CNS depressants may be necessary when taken concomitantly with Intermezzo (2.3)
- Co-administration with CNS depressants: Recommended dose is 1.75 mg for men and women (2.3)
- Geriatric patients and patients with hepatic impairment: Recommended dose is 1.75 mg for men and women (2.4, 2.5)

DOSAGE FORMS AND STRENGTHS

1.75 mg and 3.5 mg sublingual tablets (3)

CONTRAINDICATIONS

Known hypersensitivity to zolpidem (4)

WARNINGS AND PRECAUTIONS

- CNS depressant effects: Impairs alertness and motor coordination. Instruct patients on correct use (5.1)
- Evaluate for co-morbid diagnoses: Re-evaluate if insomnia persists after 7 to 10 days of use (5.2)
- Severe anaphylactic/anaphylactoid reactions: Angioedema and anaphylaxis have been reported. Do not rechallenge if such reactions occur (5.3)
- "Sleep-driving" and other complex behaviors while not fully awake. Risk increases with dose and use with other CNS depressants and alcohol. Immediately evaluate any new onset behavioral changes (5.4)
- Depression: Worsening of depression or suicidal thinking may occur. Prescribe the least number of tablets feasible to avoid intentional overdose (5.5)
- Respiratory Depression: Consider this risk before prescribing in patients with compromised respiratory function (5.6)

ADVERSE REACTIONS

Most commonly observed adverse reactions (> 1% in adult patients) are headache, nausea, and fatigue. (6.1)

To report SUSPECTED ADVERSE REACTIONS, contact Purdue Pharma at 1-888-726-7535 or FDA at 1-800-FDA-1088 or www.fda.gov/medwatch

DRUG INTERACTIONS

- CNS depressants, including alcohol: Possible adverse additive CNS depressant effects (5.1, 7.1)
- Imipramine: Decreased alertness observed (7.1)
- Chlorpromazine: Impaired alertness and psychomotor performance observed (7.1)
- Rifampin: Combination use may decrease effect (7.2)
- Ketoconazole: Combination use may increase effects (7.2)

USE IN SPECIFIC POPULATIONS

- Pregnancy: Based on animal data, zolpidem may cause fetal harm. (8.1)
- Pediatric use: Safety and effectiveness of Intermezzo not established. With bedtime dosing of zolpidem, hallucinations observed (incidence 7%) (8.4)

See 17 for PATIENT COUNSELING INFORMATION and Medication Guide

Revised: 07/2012

FULL PRESCRIBING INFORMATION: CONTENTS*

*** Sections or subsections omitted from the full prescribing information are not listed**

FULL PRESCRIBING INFORMATION

1 INDICATIONS AND USAGE

Intermezzo® (zolpidem tartrate) sublingual tablet is indicated for use as needed for the treatment of insomnia when a middle-of-the-night awakening is followed by difficulty returning to sleep.

Limitations of Use: Intermezzo is not indicated for the treatment of middle-of-the-night insomnia when the patient has fewer than 4 hours of bedtime remaining before the planned time of waking.

2 DOSAGE AND ADMINISTRATION

2.1 Important Administration Instructions

Intermezzo is to be taken in bed when a patient wakes in the middle of the night and has difficulty returning to sleep. Intermezzo should only be taken if the patient has at least 4 hours of bedtime remaining before the planned time of waking *[see Warnings and Precautions (5.1)]*.

Intermezzo should be placed under the tongue and allowed to disintegrate completely before swallowing. The tablet should not be swallowed whole. For optimal effect, Intermezzo should not be administered with or immediately after a meal. The blister should be removed from the pouch just prior to dosing.

2.2 Basic Dosing Information

The recommended and maximum dose of Intermezzo is 1.75 mg for women and 3.5 mg for men, taken only once per night as needed if a middle-of-the-night awakening is followed by difficulty returning to sleep. The recommended doses for women and men are different because women clear zolpidem from the body at a lower rate than men *[see Use in Specific Populations (8.6)]*.

2.3 Use with CNS Depressants

The recommended Intermezzo dose for men and women who are taking concomitant CNS depressants is 1.75 mg. Dose adjustment of concomitant CNS depressants may be necessary when co-administered with Intermezzo because of potentially additive effects. The use of Intermezzo with other sedative-hypnotics (including other zolpidem products) at bedtime or the middle of the night is not recommended *[see Warnings and Precautions (5.1)]*.

2.4 Use in Geriatric Patients

Geriatric patients may be especially sensitive to the effects of zolpidem. The recommended dose of Intermezzo in men and women over 65 years old is 1.75 mg, taken only once per night if needed *[see Use in Specific Populations (8.5)]*.

2.5 Use in Patients with Hepatic Impairment

The recommended dose of Intermezzo in patients with hepatic impairment is 1.75 mg, taken only once per night if needed *[see Clinical Pharmacology (12.3)]*.

3 DOSAGE FORMS AND STRENGTHS

Intermezzo is available as 1.75 mg and 3.5 mg tablets for sublingual administration.

Intermezzo 1.75 mg tablets are yellow, round, uncoated, biconvex, debossed with ZZ on one side.

Intermezzo 3.5 mg tablets are beige, round, uncoated, biconvex, debossed with ZZ on one side.

4 CONTRAINDICATIONS

Intermezzo is contraindicated in patients with known hypersensitivity to zolpidem. Observed reactions with zolpidem include anaphylaxis and angioedema *[see Warnings and Precautions (5.3)]*.

5 WARNINGS AND PRECAUTIONS

5.1 CNS Depressant Effects and Next-Day Impairment

Intermezzo, like other sedative-hypnotic drugs, has central nervous system (CNS) depressant effects. Co-administration with other CNS depressants (e.g., benzodiazepines, opioids, tricyclic antidepressants, alcohol) increases the risk of CNS depression. Dosage adjustments of Intermezzo and of other concomitant CNS depressants may be necessary when Intermezzo is administered with such agents because of the potentially additive effects. The use of Intermezzo with other sedative-hypnotics (including other zolpidem products) at bedtime or the middle of the night is not recommended *[see Dosage and Administration (2.3)]*.

In a driving study, healthy subjects who received Intermezzo with fewer than four hours of bedtime remaining had evidence of impaired driving compared to subjects who received placebo *[see Clinical Studies (14.2)]*. The risk of next-day driving impairment (and psychomotor impairment) is increased if Intermezzo is taken with less than 4 hours of bedtime remaining; if higher than recommended dose is taken; if co-administered with other CNS depressants; or co-administered with other drugs that increase the blood levels of zolpidem.

5.2 Need to Evaluate for Co-morbid Diagnoses

Because sleep disturbances may be the presenting manifestation of a physical and/or psychiatric disorder, symptomatic treatment of insomnia should be initiated only after a careful evaluation of the patient. *The failure of insomnia to remit after 7 to 10 days of treatment may indicate the presence of a primary psychiatric and/or medical illness that should be evaluated.* Worsening of insomnia or the emergence of new thinking or behavior abnormalities may be the consequence of an unrecognized psychiatric or physical disorder. Such findings have emerged during the course of treatment with sedative-hypnotic drugs, including zolpidem.

5.3 Severe Anaphylactic and Anaphylactoid Reactions

Cases of angioedema involving the tongue, glottis, or larynx have been reported in patients after taking the first or subsequent doses of zolpidem. Some patients have had additional symptoms such as dyspnea, throat closing, or nausea and vomiting that suggest anaphylaxis. Some patients have required medical therapy in the emergency department. If angioedema involves the throat, glottis or larynx, airway obstruction may occur and be fatal. Patients who develop angioedema or anaphylaxis after treatment with zolpidem should not be rechallenged with Intermezzo.

5.4 Abnormal Thinking and Behavioral Changes

Abnormal thinking and behavior changes have been reported in patients treated with sedative-hypnotics including zolpidem. Some of these changes included decreased inhibition (e.g., aggressiveness and extroversion that seemed out of character), bizarre behavior, agitation, and depersonalization. Visual and auditory hallucinations have also been reported.

In controlled trials of zolpidem tartrate 10 mg taken at bedtime, < 1% of adults with insomnia who received zolpidem reported hallucinations. In a clinical trial, 7% of pediatric patients treated with zolpidem tartrate 0.25 mg/kg taken at bedtime, reported hallucinations, versus 0% treated with placebo *[see Use in Specific Populations (8.4)]*.

Complex behaviors such as "sleep-driving" (i.e., driving while not fully awake after ingestion of a sedative-hypnotic, with amnesia for the event) have been reported in sedative-hypnotic-naive as well as in sedative-hypnotic-experienced persons. Although behaviors such as "sleep-driving" have occurred with zolpidem alone at therapeutic doses, the co-administration of zolpidem with alcohol and other CNS depressants increases the risk of such behaviors, as does the use of zolpidem at doses exceeding the maximum recommended dose. Due to the risk to the patient and the community, discontinuation of Intermezzo should be strongly considered for patients who report a "sleep-driving" episode.

Other complex behaviors (e.g., preparing and eating food, making phone calls, or having sex) have been reported in patients who are not fully awake after taking a sedative-hypnotic. As with "sleep-driving", patients usually do not remember these events. Amnesia, anxiety and other neuro-psychiatric symptoms may also occur.

The emergence of any new behavioral sign or symptom of concern requires careful and immediate evaluation.

5.5 Use in Patients with Depression

In primarily depressed patients treated with sedative-hypnotics, worsening of depression, and suicidal thoughts and actions (including completed suicides), have been reported. Suicidal tendencies may be present in such patients and protective measures may be required. Intentional overdosage is more common in this group of patients; therefore, the lowest number of tablets that is feasible should be prescribed for the patient at any one time.

5.6 Respiratory Depression

Although studies with 10 mg zolpidem tartrate did not reveal respiratory depressant effects at hypnotic doses in healthy subjects or in patients with mild-to-moderate chronic obstructive pulmonary disease (COPD), a reduction in the Total Arousal Index, together with a reduction in lowest oxygen saturation and increase in the times of oxygen desaturation below 80% and 90%, was observed in patients with mild-to-moderate sleep apnea when treated with zolpidem compared to placebo. Since sedative-hypnotics have the capacity to depress respiratory drive, precautions should be taken if Intermezzo is prescribed to patients with compromised respiratory function. Post-marketing reports of respiratory insufficiency in patients receiving 10 mg of zolpidem tartrate, most of whom had pre-existing respiratory impairment, have been reported. The risks of respiratory depression should be considered prior to prescribing Intermezzo in patients with respiratory impairment including sleep apnea and myasthenia gravis.

5.7 Withdrawal Effects

There have been reports of withdrawal signs and symptoms following the rapid dose decrease or abrupt discontinuation of zolpidem. Monitor patients for tolerance, abuse, and dependence *[see Drug Abuse and Dependence (9.2) and (9.3)]*.

6 ADVERSE REACTIONS

The following serious adverse reactions in zolpidem-treated patients are discussed in greater detail in other sections of the labeling:

- CNS-depressant effects and next-day impairment *[see Warnings and Precautions (5.1)]*
- Serious anaphylactic and anaphylactoid reactions *[see Warnings and Precautions (5.3)]*
- Abnormal thinking and behavioral changes, and complex behaviors *[see Warnings and Precautions (5.4)]*
- Withdrawal effects *[see Warnings and Precautions (5.7)]*

6.1 Clinical Trials Experience

The safety data described below are based on two double-blind placebo-controlled trials of Intermezzo in adult patients with insomnia characterized by difficulty returning to sleep after a middle-of-the-night awakening *[see Clinical Studies (14.1)]*. These two trials included 230 and 82 patients treated with 3.5 mg and 1.75 mg of Intermezzo, respectively. The first study was a 3-way crossover sleep-laboratory study in 82 patients (58 female and 24 male; median age 47 years; 51% Caucasian, 44% African-American) of 1.75 mg and 3.5 mg of Intermezzo compared to placebo (Study 1). The second study was a 4-week, parallel-group at-home study in 295 patients (201 female and 94 male; median age 43 years) of 3.5 mg of Intermezzo compared to placebo, used on an as-needed basis after spontaneous middle-of-the-night awakenings (Study 2). In Study 2, patients took Intermezzo during the night on 62% of study nights.

Because clinical trials are conducted under widely varying conditions, adverse reaction rates observed in the clinical trials of a drug cannot be directly compared to rates in the clinical trials of another drug and may not reflect the rates observed in actual practice.

Table 1 shows the incidence of adverse reactions reported in Study 2 that occurred in 2% or more of Intermezzo-treated (3.5 mg) patients in which the incidence was greater than the incidence in placebo-treated patients. For women and other patients taking the 1.75 mg dose in Study 1, the incidence of adverse reactions was similar to the incidence seen with 3.5 mg of Intermezzo in Table 1.

The most commonly reported adverse reactions in all treatment groups were headache, nausea, and fatigue.

Table 1: Summary of Adverse Reactions (≥ 2%) in Outpatient, Double-Blind, Parallel-Group, Placebo-Controlled Study (Study 2)

MedDRA System Organ Class Preferred Term	3.5 mg Intermezzo (n=150)	Placebo (n=145)
Gastrointestinal Disorders	**4%**	**2%**
Nausea	1%	1%

General Disorders and Administration Site Conditions	**3%**	**0%**
Fatigue	1%	0%
Nervous System Disorders	**5%**	**3%**
Headache	3%	1%

7 DRUG INTERACTIONS

7.1 CNS-active Drugs

Co-administration of zolpidem with other CNS depressants increases the risk of CNS depression *[see Warnings and Precautions (5.1)]*. Zolpidem tartrate was evaluated in healthy volunteers in single-dose interaction studies for several CNS drugs.

Imipramine

Imipramine in combination with zolpidem produced no pharmacokinetic interaction other than a 20% decrease in peak levels of imipramine, but there was an additive effect of decreased alertness. Similarly, chlorpromazine in combination with zolpidem produced no pharmacokinetic interaction, but there was an additive effect of decreased alertness and psychomotor performance.

Haloperidol

A study involving haloperidol and zolpidem revealed no effect of haloperidol on the pharmacokinetics or pharmacodynamics of zolpidem. The lack of a drug interaction following single-dose administration does not predict the absence of an effect following chronic administration.

Alcohol

An additive adverse effect on psychomotor performance between alcohol and oral zolpidem was demonstrated *[see Warnings and Precautions (5.1)]*.

Sertraline

Concomitant administration of zolpidem and sertraline increases exposure to zolpidem and may increase the pharmacodynamic effect of zolpidem.

Fluoxetine

After multiple doses of zolpidem tartrate and fluoxetine an increase in the zolpidem half-life (17%) was observed. There was no evidence of an additive effect in psychomotor performance *[see Clinical Pharmacology (12.3)]*.

7.2 Drugs that Affect Drug Metabolism via Cytochrome P450

Some compounds known to inhibit CYP3A may increase exposure to zolpidem. The effect of other P450 enzymes on the exposure to zolpidem is not known.

Rifampin

Rifampin, a CYP3A4 inducer, significantly reduced the exposure to and the pharmacodynamic effects of zolpidem. Use of Rifampin in combination with zolpidem may decrease the efficacy of zolpidem.

Ketoconazole

Ketoconazole, a potent CYP3A4 inhibitor, increased the pharmacodynamic effects of zolpidem. Consideration should be given to using a lower dose of zolpidem when ketoconazole and zolpidem are given together.

8 USE IN SPECIFIC POPULATIONS

8.1 Pregnancy

Pregnancy Category C

There are no adequate and well-controlled studies of zolpidem in pregnant women. Studies in children to assess the effects of prenatal exposure to zolpidem have not been conducted; however, cases of severe neonatal respiratory depression have been reported when zolpidem was used at the end of pregnancy, especially when taken with other CNS-depressants. Children born to mothers taking sedative-hypnotic drugs may be at risk for withdrawal symptoms during the postnatal period. Neonatal flaccidity has also been reported in infants born to mothers who received sedative-hypnotic drugs during pregnancy. Intermezzo should be used during pregnancy only if the potential benefit outweighs the potential risk to the fetus.

Administration of zolpidem to pregnant rats and rabbits resulted in adverse effects on offspring at doses greater than the recommended human dose (RHD) of 3.5 mg/day (approximately 2.8 mg/day zolpidem base); however, teratogenicity was not observed.

When zolpidem was administered at oral doses of 4, 20, and 100 mg base/kg/day to pregnant rats during the period of organogenesis, dose-related decreases in fetal skull ossification were observed at all but the lowest dose, which is approximately 15 times the RHD on a mg/m^2 basis. In rabbits treated during organogenesis with zolpidem at oral doses of 1, 4, and 16 mg base/kg/day, increased embryo-fetal death and incomplete fetal skull ossification were seen at the highest dose tested. The no-effect dose for embryo-fetal toxicity in rabbits is approximately 30 times the RHD on a mg/m^2 basis. Administration of zolpidem to rats at oral doses of 4, 20, and 100 mg base/kg/day during the latter part of pregnancy and throughout lactation produced decreased offspring growth and survival at all but the lowest dose, which is approximately 15 times the RHD on a mg/m^2 basis.

8.3 Nursing Mothers

Zolpidem is excreted in human milk. The effect of zolpidem on the nursing infant is not known.

8.4 Pediatric Use

Intermezzo is not recommended for use in children. Safety and effectiveness of Intermezzo have not been established in pediatric patients below the age of 18.

In an 8-week study in pediatric patients (aged 6 to 17 years) with insomnia associated with ADHD, an oral solution of zolpidem tartrate dosed at 0.25 mg/kg at bedtime did not decrease sleep latency compared to placebo. Hallucinations were reported in 7% of the pediatric patients who received zolpidem; none of the pediatric patients who received placebo reported hallucinations.

8.5 Geriatric Use

Intermezzo dosage adjustment is necessary in geriatric patients. Sedating drugs may cause confusion and oversedation in the elderly; elderly patients generally should be started on low doses of Intermezzo and observed closely *[see Dosage and Administration (2.4), and Clinical Pharmacology (12.3)]*.

Clinical trial experience with other zolpidem formulations (5 mg to 10 mg oral zolpidem tartrate) given at bedtime:

A total of 154 patients in U.S. controlled clinical trials and 897 patients in non-U.S. clinical trials who received oral zolpidem were ≥ 60 years of age. For a pool of U.S. patients receiving oral zolpidem tartrate at doses of ≤ 10 mg or placebo, there were three adverse reactions occurring at an incidence of at least 3% for zolpidem and for which the zolpidem incidence was at least twice the placebo incidence (see Table 2).

Table 2: Adverse Reactions in Geriatric Patients in Pooled Trials of 5 mg to 10 mg of Oral Zolpidem Tartrate Given at Bedtime

Adverse Reaction	5 to 10 mg Oral Zolpidem tartrate	Placebo
Dizziness	3%	0%
Drowsiness	5%	2%
Diarrhea	3%	1%

Falls in geriatric patients:

A total of 30/1,959 (2%) non-U.S. patients receiving other zolpidem formulations (5 mg to 10 mg oral zolpidem tartrate) reported falls, including 28/30 (93%) who were ≥ 70 years of age. Of these 28 patients, 23 (82%) were receiving zolpidem tartrate doses > 10 mg. A total of 24/1,959 (1%) non-U.S. patients receiving zolpidem reported confusion, including 18/24 (75%) who were ≥70 years of age. Of these 18 patients, 14 (78%) were receiving zolpidem tartrate doses >10 mg.

The dose of Intermezzo in elderly patients is 1.75 mg to minimize adverse effects related to impaired motor and/or cognitive performance and unusual sensitivity to sedative-hypnotic drugs.

8.6 Gender Difference in Pharmacokinetics

Women cleared zolpidem tartrate from the body after sublingual administration of a 3.5 mg dose of Intermezzo at a lower rate than men (2.7 mL/min/kg vs. 4.0 mL/min/kg). C_{max} and AUC parameters of zolpidem were approximately 45% higher at the same dose in female subjects compared with male subjects. Given the higher blood levels of zolpidem tartrate in women compared to men at a given dose, the recommended dose of Intermezzo for women is 1.75 mg, and the recommended dose for adult men is 3.5 mg.

9 DRUG ABUSE AND DEPENDENCE

9.1 Controlled Substance

Zolpidem tartrate is classified as a Schedule IV controlled substance by federal regulation.

9.2 Abuse

Abuse and addiction are separate and distinct from physical dependence and tolerance. Abuse is characterized by misuse of the drug for non-medical purposes, often in combination with other psychoactive substances. Tolerance is a state of adaptation in which exposure to a drug induces changes that result in diminution of one or more of the drug effects over time. Tolerance may occur to both desired and undesired effects of drugs and may develop at different rates for different effects.

Addiction is a primary, chronic, neurobiological disease with genetic, psychosocial, and environmental factors influencing its development and manifestations. It is characterized by behaviors that include one or more of the following: impaired control over drug use, compulsive use, continued use despite harm, and craving. Drug addiction is a treatable disease, using a multidisciplinary approach, but relapse is common.

Studies of abuse potential in former drug abusers found that the effects of single doses of 40 mg of oral zolpidem tartrate were similar, but not identical, to diazepam 20 mg, while 10 mg of oral zolpidem tartrate was difficult to distinguish from placebo.

Because persons with a history of addiction to or abuse of drugs or alcohol are at increased risk for misuse, abuse and addiction of zolpidem, they should be monitored carefully when receiving Intermezzo.

9.3 Dependence

Physical dependence is a state of adaptation that is manifested by a specific withdrawal syndrome that can be produced by abrupt cessation, rapid dose reduction, decreasing blood level of the drug, and/or administration of an antagonist.

Sedative-hypnotics have produced withdrawal signs and symptoms following abrupt discontinuation. These reported symptoms range from mild dysphoria and insomnia to a withdrawal syndrome that may include abdominal and muscle cramps, vomiting, sweating, tremors, and convulsions. The following adverse events which are considered to meet the DSM-III-R criteria for uncomplicated sedative-hypnotic withdrawal were reported during U.S. clinical trials with other oral zolpidem formulations following placebo substitution occurring within 48 hours following the last zolpidem treatment: fatigue, nausea, flushing, lightheadedness, uncontrolled crying, emesis, stomach cramps, panic attack, nervousness, and abdominal discomfort. These reported adverse events occurred at an incidence of 1% or less. However, available data cannot provide a reliable estimate of the incidence, if any, of dependence during treatment at recommended doses. Post-marketing reports of abuse, dependence, and withdrawal resulting from use of oral zolpidem tartrate have been received.

10 OVERDOSAGE

10.1 Signs and Symptoms

In post-marketing experience of overdose with oral zolpidem tartrate alone, or in combination with CNS-depressant agents, impairment of consciousness ranging from somnolence to coma, cardiovascular and/or respiratory compromise, and fatal outcomes have been reported.

10.2 Recommended Treatment

General symptomatic and supportive measures should be used along with immediate gastric lavage where appropriate. Intravenous fluids should be administered as needed. Zolpidem's sedative-hypnotic effect was shown to be reduced by flumazenil and therefore flumazenil may be useful; however, flumazenil administration may contribute to the appearance of neurological symptoms (convulsions). As in all cases of drug overdose, respiration, pulse, blood pressure, and other appropriate signs should be monitored and general supportive measures employed. Hypotension and CNS depression should be treated by appropriate medical intervention. Sedating drugs should be withheld following zolpidem overdosage, even if excitation occurs. The value of dialysis in the treatment of overdosage has not been determined, although hemodialysis studies in patients with renal failure receiving therapeutic doses have demonstrated that zolpidem is not dialyzable.

As with management of all overdosage, the possibility of multiple drug ingestion should be considered. The healthcare provider may wish to consider contacting a poison control center for up-to-date information on the management of hypnotic drug overdosage.

11 DESCRIPTION

Intermezzo contains zolpidem tartrate, a non-benzodiazepine hypnotic of the imidazopyridine class. Intermezzo is available in 1.75 mg and 3.5 mg strength tablets for sublingual administration. Intermezzo sublingual tablets are intended to be placed under the tongue where they will disintegrate.

Intermezzo sublingual tablets contain a bicarbonate-carbonate buffer.

Chemically, zolpidem tartrate is *N,N*-6-trimethyl-2-*p*-tolylimidazo[1,2-α]pyridine-3-acetamide L-(+)-tartrate (2:1).

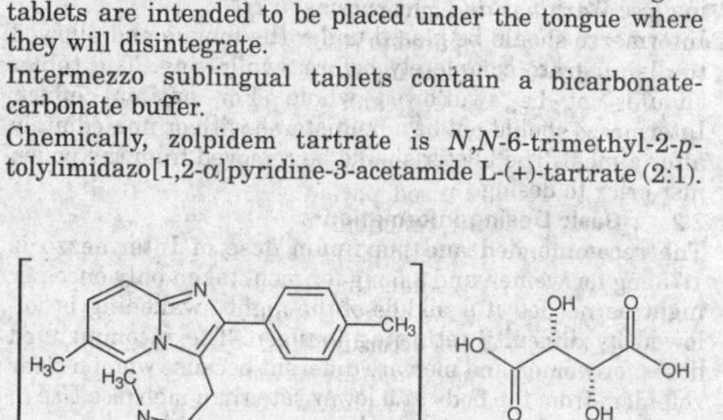

Zolpidem tartrate is a white to off-white crystalline powder that is sparingly soluble in water, alcohol, and propylene glycol. It has a molecular weight of 764.88.

Each Intermezzo tablet includes the following inactive ingredients: mannitol, sorbitol, crospovidone, silicon dioxide, sodium carbonate, sodium bicarbonate, croscarmellose sodium, sodium stearyl fumarate, silicon dioxide, natural and artificial spearmint flavor, silicon dioxide-colloidal, and sucralose. The 1.75 mg tablet also contains yellow iron oxide, and the 3.5 mg tablet contains beige iron oxide.

12 CLINICAL PHARMACOLOGY

12.1 Mechanism of Action

Zolpidem, the active moiety of zolpidem tartrate, is a hypnotic agent with a chemical structure unrelated to benzodiazepines, barbiturates, or other drugs with known hypnotic properties. It interacts with a GABA-BZ complex and shares some of the pharmacological properties of the benzodiazepines. In contrast to the benzodiazepines, which nonselectively bind to and activate all BZ receptor subtypes, zolpidem *in vitro* binds the BZ_1 receptor preferentially with a high affinity ratio of the $alpha_1/alpha_5$ subunits. This selective binding of zolpidem on the BZ_1 receptor is not absolute, but it may explain the relative absence of myorelaxant and anticonvulsant effects in animal studies as well as the preservation of deep sleep (stages 3 and 4) in human studies of zolpidem at hypnotic doses.

12.3 Pharmacokinetics

Absorption

Intermezzo disintegrates in the sublingual cavity after administration. On average, Intermezzo is rapidly absorbed in both genders, with a mean T_{max} across studies of about 35 minutes to about 75 minutes.

In healthy normal volunteers (age 21 to 45 years) dosed with 3.5 mg Intermezzo, the average C_{max} and AUC were 77 ng/mL and 296 ng•h/mL, respectively in women. The average C_{max} and AUC were 53 ng/mL and 198 ng•h/mL, respectively in men. In women, the average C_{max} and AUC of the 1.75 mg Intermezzo dose were 37 ng/mL and 151 ng•h/mL, respectively.

Food decreased the overall C_{max} and AUC of Intermezzo 3.5 mg by 42% and 19%, respectively, and increased the time to peak exposure (T_{max}) to nearly 3 hours. For optimal effect, Intermezzo should not be administered with or immediately after a meal.

Distribution

Based on data obtained with oral zolpidem, the total protein binding was found to be 93% ± 0.1% and remained constant independent of concentration between 40 ng/mL and 790 ng/mL.

Metabolism

Based on data obtained with oral zolpidem, zolpidem tartrate is converted to inactive metabolites that are eliminated primarily by renal excretion.

Elimination

The elimination half-life of a single dose of a 3.5 mg Intermezzo sublingual tablet is approximately 2.5 hours (range 1.4 to 3.6 hours).

Special Populations

Elderly: The recommended dose for Intermezzo is 1.75 mg. A pharmacokinetic study of 1.75 mg and 3.5 mg doses of Intermezzo showed that the plasma C_{max} and $AUC_{0\text{-}4\ hr}$ in elderly subjects following the 3.5 mg dose was higher by 34% and 30%, respectively, than the non-elderly subjects. The C_{max} and AUC of 1.75 mg in elderly subjects were consistently lower than those observed for the 3.5 mg dose in non-elderly subjects but consistently higher than the 1.75 mg dose in non-elderly subjects. The elimination half-life remained unchanged.

Hepatic Impairment: The pharmacokinetics of oral zolpidem tartrate in eight patients with chronic hepatic insufficiency were compared to results in subjects with normal hepatic function. Following a single 20 mg oral zolpidem tartrate dose, mean C_{max} and AUC were found to be two times (250 ng/mL vs. 499 ng/mL) and five times (788 ng•hr/mL vs. 4203 ng•hr/mL) higher, respectively, in hepatically compromised patients compared to subjects with normal hepatic function. T_{max} did not change. The mean half-life in cirrhotic patients of 9.9 hr (range: 4.1 to 25.8 hr) was greater than that observed in subjects with normal hepatic function of 2.2 hr (range: 1.6 to 2.4 hr). Dosing should be modified accordingly in patients with hepatic insufficiency *[see Dosage and Administration (2.5)]*.

Renal Impairment: The pharmacokinetics of zolpidem tartrate were studied in 11 patients with end-stage renal failure (mean Cl_{Cr} = 6.5 ± 1.5 mL/min) undergoing hemodialysis three times a week, who were dosed with zolpidem tartrate 10 mg orally each day for 14 or 21 days. No statistically significant differences were observed for C_{max}, T_{max}, half-life, and AUC between the first and last day of drug administration when baseline concentration adjustments were made. Zolpidem was not hemodialyzable. No accumulation of unchanged drug appeared after 14 or 21 days. Zolpidem pharmacokinetics were not significantly different in renally-impaired patients. No dosage adjustment is necessary in patients with renal impairment.

Drug Interactions

CNS-depressants

Co-administration of zolpidem with other CNS depressants increases the risk of CNS depression *[see Warnings and Precautions (5.1)]*. Zolpidem tartrate was evaluated in healthy volunteers in single-dose interaction studies for several CNS drugs. Imipramine in combination with zolpidem produced no pharmacokinetic interaction other than a 20% decrease in peak levels of imipramine, but there was an additive effect of decreased alertness. Similarly, chlorpromazine in combination with zolpidem produced no pharmacokinetic interaction, but there was an additive effect of decreased alertness and psychomotor performance.

A study involving haloperidol and zolpidem revealed no effect of haloperidol on the pharmacokinetics or pharmacodynamics of zolpidem. The lack of a drug interaction following single-dose administration does not predict the absence of an effect following chronic administration.

An additive adverse effect on psychomotor performance between alcohol and oral zolpidem was demonstrated *[see Warnings and Precautions (5.1)]*.

Following five consecutive nightly doses at bedtime of oral zolpidem tartrate 10 mg in the presence of sertraline 50 mg (17 consecutive daily doses, at 7:00 am, in healthy female volunteers), zolpidem C_{max} was significantly higher (43%) and T_{max} was significantly decreased (-53%). Pharmacokinetics of sertraline and N-desmethylsertraline were unaffected by zolpidem.

A single-dose interaction study with zolpidem tartrate 10 mg and fluoxetine 20 mg at steady-state levels in male volunteers did not demonstrate any clinically significant pharmacokinetic or pharmacodynamic interactions. When multiple doses of zolpidem and fluoxetine were given at steady state and the concentrations evaluated in healthy females, an increase in the zolpidem half-life (17%) was observed. There was no evidence of an additive effect in psychomotor performance.

Drugs that Affect Drug Metabolism via Cytochrome P450

Some compounds known to inhibit CYP3A may increase exposure to zolpidem. The effect of inhibitors of other P450 enzymes on the pharmacokinetics of zolpidem is unknown.

A single-dose interaction study with zolpidem tartrate 10 mg and itraconazole 200 mg at steady-state levels in male volunteers resulted in a 34% increase in $AUC_{0-\infty}$ of zolpidem tartrate. There were no pharmacodynamic effects of zolpidem detected on subjective drowsiness, postural sway, or psychomotor performance.

A single-dose interaction study with zolpidem tartrate 10 mg and rifampin 600 mg at steady-state levels in female subjects showed significant reductions of the AUC (-73%), C_{max} (-58%), and $T_{1/2}$ (-36 %) of zolpidem together with significant reductions in the pharmacodynamic effects of zolpidem tartrate. Rifampin, a CYP3A4 inducer, significantly reduced the exposure to and the pharmacodynamic effects of zolpidem.

A single-dose interaction study with zolpidem tartrate 5 mg and ketoconazole, a potent CYP3A4 inhibitor, given as 200 mg twice daily for 2 days increased C_{max} of zolpidem (30%) and the total AUC of zolpidem (70%) compared to zolpidem alone and prolonged the elimination half-life (30%) along with an increase in the pharmacodynamic effects of zolpidem. Consideration should be given to using a lower dose of zolpidem when ketoconazole and zolpidem are given together.

Other Drugs with No Interactions with Zolpidem

A study involving cimetidine/zolpidem tartrate and ranitidine/zolpidem tartrate combinations revealed no effect of either drug on the pharmacokinetics or pharmacodynamics of zolpidem.

Zolpidem tartrate had no effect on digoxin pharmacokinetics and did not affect prothrombin time when given with warfarin in healthy subjects.

13 NONCLINICAL TOXICOLOGY

13.1 Carcinogenesis, Mutagenesis, Impairment of Fertility

Carcinogenesis: Zolpidem was administered in the diet to rats and mice for 2 years at doses of 4, 18, and 80 mg base/kg/day. In mice, these doses are approximately 7, 30, and 140 times, respectively, the recommended human dose (RHD) of 3.5 mg/day (approximately 2.8 mg zolpidem base) on a mg/m^2 basis. In rats, these doses are approximately 15, 60, and 280 times, respectively, the RHD on a mg/m^2 basis. No evidence of carcinogenic potential was observed in mice. In rats, renal tumors (lipoma, liposarcoma) were seen at the mid- and high doses.

Mutagenesis: Zolpidem was negative in *in vitro* (bacterial reverse mutation, mouse lymphoma, and chromosomal aberration) and *in vivo* (mouse micronucleus) genetic toxicology assays.

Impairment of fertility: Oral administration of zolpidem (doses of 4, 20, and 100 mg base/kg/day) to rats prior to and during mating, and continuing in females through postpartum day 25, resulted in irregular estrus cycles and prolonged precoital intervals at the highest dose tested. The no-effect dose for these findings is approximately 70 times the RHD on a mg/m^2 basis. There was no impairment of fertility at any dose tested.

14 CLINICAL STUDIES

14.1 Middle-of-the-Night Awakening Trials

Intermezzo was evaluated in two randomized, double-blind, placebo-controlled studies (Studies 1 and 2) in patients with insomnia characterized by difficulty returning to sleep after a middle-of-the-night (MOTN) awakening. In these studies, patients met the diagnosis for primary insomnia as defined by the Diagnostic and Statistical Manual of Mental Disorders (DSM-IV-TR) and had at least three prolonged MOTN awakenings per week that were at least 30 minutes in duration.

Sleep Laboratory Study (Scheduled Dosing)

Adult patients aged 19 to 64 years (N=82; 58 female, 24 male) with a history of difficulty returning to sleep after middle-of-the-night awakenings were evaluated in a double-blind, placebo-controlled, 3-period cross-over sleep laboratory study (Study 1). The primary outcome measure was latency to persistent sleep (LPS).

Doses of 3.5 mg and 1.75 mg of Intermezzo significantly decreased both objective (by polysomnography) and subjective (patient-estimated) sleep latency after a scheduled middle-of-the-night awakening as compared to placebo. The effect on sleep latency was similar for females receiving 1.75 mg of Intermezzo and males receiving 3.5 mg of Intermezzo.

Outpatient Study (As-needed Dosing)

Adult patients aged 18 to 64 years (N=295; 201 women, 94 men) with difficulty returning to sleep after middle-of-the-night awakenings were evaluated in a double-blind, placebo-controlled 4-week outpatient study of Intermezzo. Patients took study drug (3.5 mg of Intermezzo or placebo) on an as-needed (prn) basis, when they had difficulty returning to sleep after waking in the middle of the night, provided they had at least 4 hours time remaining in bed. Subjective (patient-estimated) time to fall back to sleep after middle-of-the-night awakening was significantly shorter for Intermezzo 3.5 mg compared to placebo.

14.2 Special Safety Studies

Driving Study

A randomized, double-blind, placebo-controlled, active-control, single-center, four-period, crossover study in 40 healthy subjects was conducted to evaluate the effects of middle-of-the-night administration of Intermezzo on next-morning driving performance. The four randomized treatments included Intermezzo 3.5 mg four hours before driving, Intermezzo 3.5 mg three hours before driving, placebo, and a positive control (an unapproved sedative-hypnotic) given nine hours before driving.

The primary outcome measure was the change in the standard deviation of lateral position (SDLP), a measure of driving impairment. The results were analyzed using a symmetry analysis, which determined the proportion of subjects whose change from their own SDLP in the placebo condition was statistically significantly above a threshold thought to reflect clinically meaningful driving impairment.

When driving began 3 hours after taking Intermezzo, testing had to be terminated for one subject (a 23-year old woman) due to somnolence. Overall, the symmetry analysis showed a statistically significant impairing effect at 3 hours. When driving began 4 hours after taking Intermezzo, statistically significant impairment was not found, but numerically Intermezzo was worse than placebo. Zolpidem blood levels were not measured in the driving study, and the study was not designed to correlate specific blood level with degree of impairment. However, the estimated blood level of zolpidem in patients whose SDLP worsened according to the symmetry analysis is considered to present a risk for driving impairment. In some women, the 3.5 mg dose of Intermezzo results in zolpidem blood levels that remain at or sometimes considerably above this level 4 or more hours after dosing. Therefore, the recommended dose for women is 1.75 mg. A small negative effect on SDLP may remain in some patients 4 hours after the 1.75 mg dose in women, and after the 3.5 mg dose in men, such that a potential negative effect on driving cannot be completely excluded.

Rebound effects

In studies performed with other zolpidem formulations (5 mg to 10 mg oral zolpidem tartrate) given at bedtime, there was no objective (polysomnographic) evidence of rebound insomnia at recommended doses seen in studies evaluating sleep on the nights following discontinuation. There was subjective evidence of impaired sleep in the elderly on the first post-treatment night at doses above the recommended elderly dose of 5 mg oral zolpidem tartrate.

Memory impairment in controlled studies

Controlled studies in adults utilizing objective measures of memory yielded no consistent evidence of next-day memory impairment following the administration at bedtime of 5 mg to 10 mg oral zolpidem tartrate. However, in one study involving zolpidem tartrate doses of 10 mg and 20 mg, there was a significant decrease in next-morning recall of information presented to subjects during peak drug effect (90 minutes post-dose), i.e., these subjects experienced anterograde amnesia. There was also subjective evidence from adverse event data for anterograde amnesia occurring in association with the administration of oral zolpidem tartrate, predominantly at doses above 10 mg.

16 HOW SUPPLIED/STORAGE AND HANDLING

Each sublingual tablet is individually packaged in a foil blister inside a unit-dose pouch.

Intermezzo 1.75 mg tablets are yellow, round, uncoated, biconvex, debossed with ZZ on one side and supplied as:

NDC 59011-256-30: Carton of 30 unit-dose pouches

Intermezzo 3.5 mg tablets are beige, round, uncoated, biconvex, debossed with ZZ on one side and supplied as:

NDC 59011-255-30: Carton of 30 unit-dose pouches

Storage and Handling

Store between 20°C to 25°C (68°F to 77°F). Excursions permitted between 15°C and 30°C (59°F and 86°F). Protect from moisture.

The patient should be instructed not to remove the blister from the unit-dose pouch until the patient is ready to consume the sublingual tablet inside.

17 PATIENT COUNSELING INFORMATION

See FDA-approved patient labeling (Medication Guide).

Inform patients and their families about the benefits and risks of treatment with Intermezzo. Inform patients of the availability of a Medication Guide and instruct them to read the Medication Guide prior to initiating treatment with Intermezzo and with each prescription refill. Review the Intermezzo Medication Guide with every patient prior to initiation of treatment. Instruct patients or caregivers that Intermezzo should be taken only as prescribed.

CNS depressant Effects and Next-Day Impairment

Tell patients that Intermezzo has the potential to cause next-day impairment, and that this risk is increased if dosing instructions are not carefully followed. Tell patients to wait for at least 4 hours after dosing and until they feel fully awake before driving or engaging in other activities requiring full mental alertness.

Severe Anaphylactic and Anaphylactoid Reactions

Inform patients that severe anaphylactic and anaphylactoid reactions have occurred with zolpidem. Describe the signs/symptoms of these reactions and advise patients to seek medical attention immediately if any of them occur.

Sleep-driving and Other Complex Behaviors

Instruct patients to inform their families that zolpidem has been associated with "sleep-driving" and other complex behaviors while not being fully awake (preparing and eating food, making phone calls, or having sex), and tell patients and their families to call their healthcare providers immediately if they develop any of these symptoms.

Suicide

Tell patients to immediately report any suicidal thoughts.

Administration Instructions

For detailed instructions on how to use Intermezzo, tell patients to refer to the Patient Instructions for Use.

Tell patients that Intermezzo is to be taken only once per night if needed if they wake in the middle of the night and have difficulty returning to sleep. Tell patients that Intermezzo should only be taken if they have 4 hours of bedtime remaining before the planned time of waking.

Instruct the patient to place the tablet under the tongue, allowing it to disintegrate completely before swallowing. Tell the patient that Intermezzo should not be swallowed whole.

Tell patients that the effect of Intermezzo may be slowed if taken with or immediately after a meal.

Instruct patients to remove the blister from the unit-dose pouch just prior to dosing.

Advise patients NOT to take Intermezzo if they drank alcohol that day or before bed.

Healthcare professionals can telephone Purdue Pharma's Medical Services Department (1-888-726-7535) for information on this product.

Distributed by:
Purdue Pharma L.P.
Stamford, CT 06901-3431
Manufactured by: Patheon Pharmaceuticals, Inc., Cincinnati, OH 45237
U.S. Patent Numbers 7658945;7682628

MEDICATION GUIDE
Intermezzo® (in ter mét zoh)
(zolpidem tartrate) sublingual tablet CIV

Read the Medication Guide that comes with Intermezzo® before you start taking it and each time you get a refill. There may be new information. This Medication Guide does not take the place of talking to your doctor about your medical condition or treatment.

What is the most important information I should know about Intermezzo?

Follow the Instructions for Use at the end of this Medication Guide when you take Intermezzo. If you do not follow the Instructions for Use, you might be drowsy in the morning without knowing it.

- **Only take one tablet a night, if needed.**
- **Only take Intermezzo if you have at least 4 hours of bedtime left.**

Intermezzo may cause serious side effects, including:

- **After taking Intermezzo, you may get up out of bed while not being fully awake and do an activity that you do not know you are doing. The next morning, you may not remember that you did anything during the night.** You have a higher chance for doing these activities if you drank alcohol that day or take other medicines that make you sleepy with Intermezzo. Reported activities include:
  - driving a car ("sleep-driving")
  - making and eating food
  - talking on the phone
  - having sex
  - sleep-walking

Call your healthcare provider right away if you find out that you have done any of the above activities after taking Intermezzo.

Important:

1. **Take Intermezzo exactly as prescribed**
2. **Do not take Intermezzo if you:**
   - drank alcohol that day or before bed.
   - took another medicine to help you sleep.
   - do not have at least 4 hours of bedtime remaining.

What is Intermezzo?

Intermezzo is a sedative-hypnotic (sleep) medicine. Intermezzo is used in adults for the treatment of a sleep problem called insomnia. Many people have difficulty returning to sleep after awakening in the middle of the night. Intermezzo is designed to specifically treat this problem.

It is not known if Intermezzo is safe and effective in children.

Intermezzo is a federally controlled substance (CIV) because it can be abused or lead to dependence. Keep Intermezzo in a safe place to prevent misuse and abuse. Selling or giving away Intermezzo may harm others, and is against the law. Tell your doctor if you have ever abused or have been dependent on alcohol, prescription medicines, or street drugs.

Who should not take Intermezzo?

- Do not take Intermezzo if you are allergic to zolpidem or any other ingredients in Intermezzo. See the end of this Medication Guide for a complete list of ingredients in Intermezzo.
- Do not take Intermezzo if you have had an allergic reaction to drugs containing zolpidem, such as Ambien, Ambien CR, Edluar, or Zolpimist.

Symptoms of a serious allergic reaction to Intermezzo can include:

- **swelling of your face, lips, and throat that may cause difficulty breathing or swallowing**
- **nausea and vomiting**

Intermezzo may not be right for you. Before starting Intermezzo, tell your doctor about all of your health conditions, including if you:

- have a history of depression, mental illness, or suicidal thoughts
- have a history of drug or alcohol abuse or addiction
- have kidney or liver disease
- have a lung disease or breathing problems
- are pregnant, planning to become pregnant, or breastfeeding

Tell your doctor about all of the medicines you take, including prescription and nonprescription medicines, vitamins, and herbal supplements. Medicines can interact with each other, sometimes causing serious side effects. Your doctor will tell you if you can take Intermezzo with your other medicines.

Know the medicines you take. Keep a list of your medicines with you to show your doctor and pharmacist each time you get a new medicine.

How should I take Intermezzo?

- See **"What is the most important information I should know about Intermezzo"**
- Read the **"Instructions for Use"** at the end of this Medication Guide for detailed instructions on how to take Intermezzo.
- Take Intermezzo exactly as prescribed. Only take one Intermezzo tablet per night if needed.
- Do not take Intermezzo if you drank alcohol that evening or before bed.
- While in bed, place the tablet under your tongue and allow it to break apart completely. Do not swallow it whole.
- You should not take Intermezzo with or right after a meal. Intermezzo may help you fall asleep faster when you take it on an empty stomach.
- Call your health care provider if your insomnia worsens or is not better within 7 to 10 days. This may mean that there is another condition causing your sleep problem.
- If you take too much Intermezzo or overdose get emergency treatment.

What are the possible side effects of Intermezzo?

Intermezzo may cause serious side effects, including:

- **getting out of bed while not being fully awake and doing an activity that you do not know you are doing.** (See **"What is the most important information I should know about Intermezzo?"**)
- **abnormal thoughts and behavior.** Symptoms include more outgoing or aggressive behavior than normal, confusion, agitation, hallucinations, worsening of depression, and suicidal thoughts or actions.
- **memory loss**
- **anxiety**
- **severe allergic reactions.** Symptoms include swelling of the tongue or throat, trouble breathing, and nausea and vomiting. Get emergency medical help if you get these symptoms after taking Intermezzo.

Call your health care provider right away if you have any of the above side effects or any other side effects that worry you while using Intermezzo.

The most common side effects of Intermezzo are:

- Headache
- Nausea
- Fatigue

Even if you follow the Instructions for Use, you may still feel drowsy in the morning after taking Intermezzo. Do not drive or do other dangerous activities after taking Intermezzo until you are fully awake.

These are not all the side effects of Intermezzo. Ask your health care provider or pharmacist for more information.

You may report side effects to FDA at 1-800-FDA-1088.

How should I store Intermezzo?

- Store Intermezzo at room temperature, 68° to 77°F (20° to 25°C). Protect from moisture.
- Only open the pouch when you are ready to use Intermezzo.

Keep Intermezzo and all medicines out of reach of children.

General Information about Intermezzo

Medicines are sometimes prescribed for purposes other than those listed in a Medication Guide. Do not use Intermezzo for a condition for which it was not prescribed. Do not give Intermezzo to other people, even if you think they have the same symptoms that you have. It may harm them and it is against the law.

This Medication Guide summarizes the most important information about Intermezzo. If you would like more information, talk with your doctor. You can ask your doctor or pharmacist for information about Intermezzo that is written for healthcare professionals. For more information about Intermezzo, call Purdue Pharma at 1-888-726-7535 or go to www.purduepharma.com or www.intermezzorx.com.

What are the ingredients in Intermezzo?

Active Ingredient: Zolpidem tartrate

Inactive Ingredients: Each Intermezzo tablet includes the following inactive ingredients: mannitol, sorbitol, crospovidone, silicon dioxide, sodium carbonate, sodium bicarbonate, croscarmellose sodium, sodium stearyl fumarate, silicon dioxide, natural and artificial spearmint flavor, silicon dioxide-colloidal, and sucralose. The 1.75 mg tablet also contains yellow iron oxide, and the 3.5 mg tablet contains beige iron oxide.

Rx only

This Medication Guide has been approved by the U.S. Food and Drug Administration.

Distributed by:
Purdue Pharma L.P.
Stamford, CT 06901-3431
Issued: July 2012

Instructions for Use
Intermezzo® (in ter mét zoh)
(zolpidem tartrate) sublingual tablet CIV

Read these Instructions for Use before you start taking Intermezzo and each time you get a refill. There may be new information. This information does not take the place of talking to your healthcare provider about your medical condition or your treatment.

What is the most important Information I should know about Intermezzo?

Follow these Instructions for Use when you take Intermezzo. If you do not follow these instructions, you might be drowsy in the morning without knowing it.

- Only take 1 tablet a night if needed
- Only take Intermezzo if you have at least 4 hours of bedtime left

Using Intermezzo the wrong way can make you drowsy in the morning.

Before you go to bed:

- Place only 1 Intermezzo pouch by your bed, and have a clock or watch nearby (see Figure A).

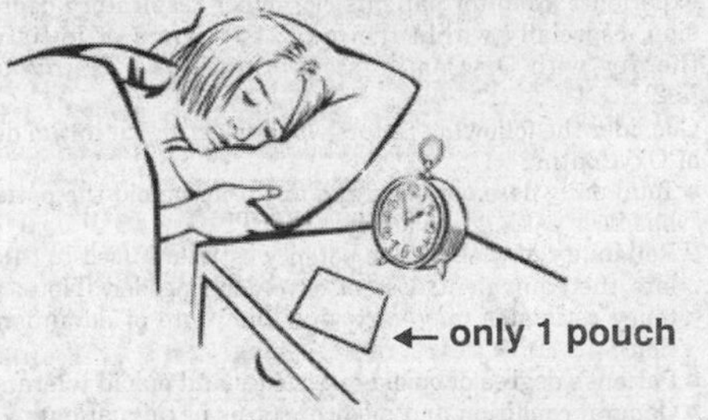

Figure A

- Store all other unopened Intermezzo pouches with your other medicines away from your bedside.
- Only open the Intermezzo pouch when you are ready to use it.
- You can either use the **Intermezzo Dosing Time Chart** (see Figure B) or the **Dosing Time Tool** (see Figure C) that comes with Intermezzo to find the latest time during the night you can take Intermezzo.

Intermezzo Dosing Time Chart (see Figure B):
- You can take Intermezzo if you have at least 4 hours of bedtime left before you must be awake.
- Find the earliest time you have to be up and awake in the column on the left.
- Find the latest time you can take Intermezzo on the same line in the column on the right.

Intermezzo Dosing Time Chart

If you must be awake by:	Take Intermezzo before:
4 am	12 midnight
5 am	1 am
6 am	2 am
7 am	3 am
8 am	4 am
9 am	5 am

Figure B

Intermezzo Dosing Time Tool (see Figure C):
- Turn the Intermezzo Dosing Time Tool wheel to show the earliest time that you must be awake under the green arrow.
- Take Intermezzo before the time under the brown arrow.

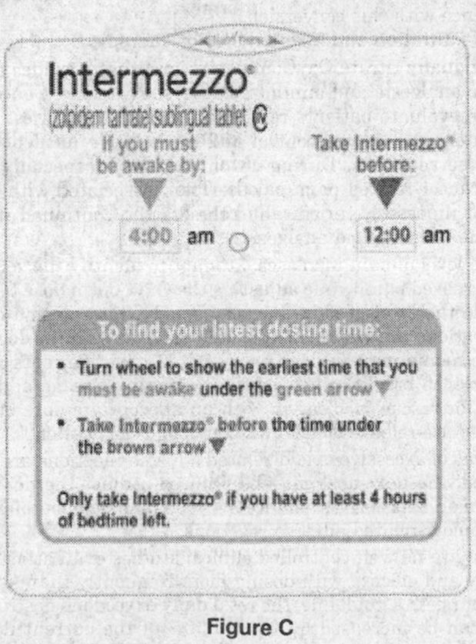

Figure C

During the night when you take Intermezzo:

Step 1. Check the current time and use the Intermezzo Dosing Time Chart or the Intermezzo Dosing Time Tool to decide if you should take Intermezzo.
- Only take Intermezzo if you have at least 4 hours of bedtime left before you have to be awake (see Figure B).

Step 2. Open the Intermezzo pouch you placed by your bed.
- Fold the Intermezzo pouch along the dotted line. While the Intermezzo pouch is folded, tear the pouch open at the notch at the center of the dotted line (see Figure D).

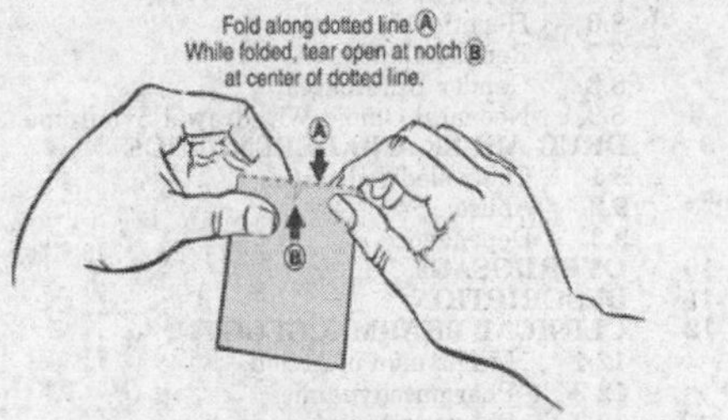

Fold along dotted line. Ⓐ
While folded, tear open at notch Ⓑ
at center of dotted line.
A
B

Figure D

Step 3. Remove the foil blister from the Intermezzo pouch. Push the Intermezzo tablet through the foil (see Figure E).

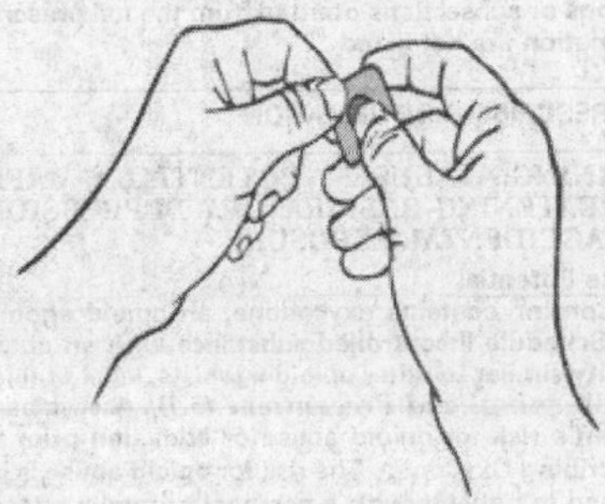

Figure E

Step 4. Leave the empty Intermezzo pouch where you can see it. The empty pouch will help remind you that you already took your Intermezzo dose (see Figure F).

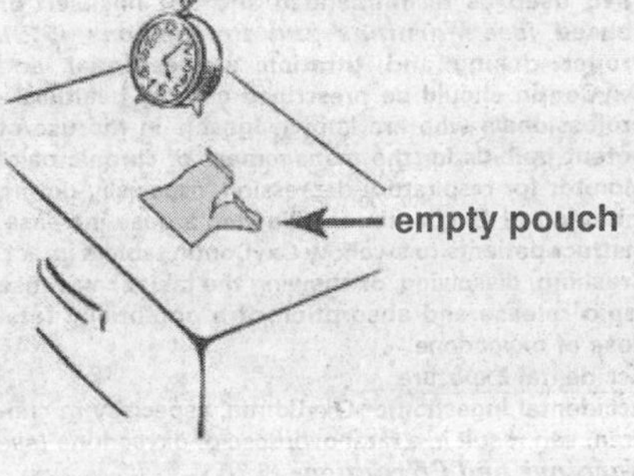

Figure F

Step 5. While in bed, place the Intermezzo tablet under your tongue and allow it to break apart completely, then swallow. Do not swallow it whole (see Figure G).

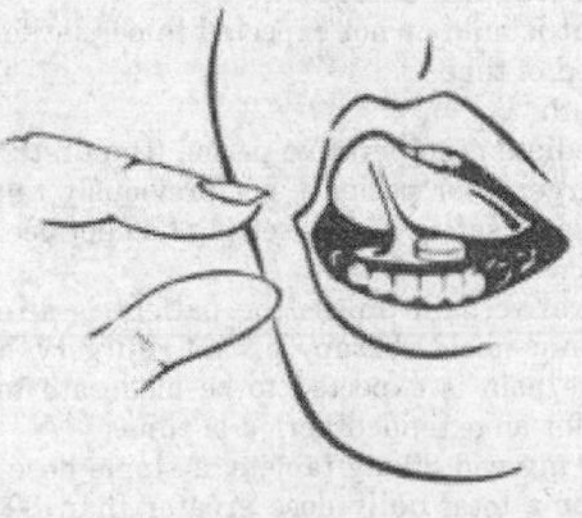

Figure G

Step 6. Throw the empty Intermezzo pouch away in the morning.

When you wake up in the morning, be sure that at least 4 hours have passed since you have taken Intermezzo and you feel fully awake before driving. Do not do dangerous activities until you know how Intermezzo affects you.

This Medication Guide and Instructions for Use have been approved by the U.S. Food and Drug Administration.

Distributed by:
Purdue Pharma L.P.
Stamford, CT 06901-3431
Issued: July 2012

Shown in Product Identification Guide, page 312

OXYCONTIN® CII

[ŏks′ē-kŏn-tĭn]

(oxycodone hydrochloride controlled-release)
Tablets, for oral use

HIGHLIGHTS OF PRESCRIBING INFORMATION

These highlights do not include all the information needed to use OxyContin® safely and effectively. See full prescribing information for OxyContin.

OxyContin® (oxycodone hydrochloride controlled-release) Tablets, for oral use, CII
Initial U.S. Approval: 1950

> **WARNING: ABUSE POTENTIAL, LIFE-THREATENING RESPIRATORY DEPRESSION, and ACCIDENTAL EXPOSURE**
> ***See full prescribing information for complete boxed warning.***
> - **OxyContin contains oxycodone, a Schedule II controlled substance. Monitor for signs of misuse, abuse, and addiction during OxyContin therapy (5.1, 9).**
> - **Fatal respiratory depression may occur, with highest risk at initiation and with dose increases. Instruct patients on proper administration of OxyContin tablets to reduce the risk (5.2).**
> - **Accidental ingestion of OxyContin can result in fatal overdose of oxycodone, especially in children (5.3).**

RECENT MAJOR CHANGES

Dosage and Administration (2) 09/2012

INDICATIONS AND USAGE

OxyContin is an opioid agonist product indicated for the management of moderate to severe pain when a continuous, around-the-clock opioid analgesic is needed for an extended period of time. (1)

Limitations of Use
- OxyContin is not for use:
  - As an as-needed (prn) analgesic (1)
  - For pain that is mild or not expected to persist for an extended period of time (1)
  - For acute pain (1)
  - In the immediate postoperative period (1)
  - For postoperative pain, unless the patient is already receiving chronic opioid therapy prior to surgery, or if the postoperative pain is expected to be moderate to severe and persist for an extended period of time (1)
- OxyContin 60 mg and 80 mg tablets are only for patients in whom tolerance to an opioid of comparable potency is established. (1)

DOSAGE AND ADMINISTRATION

- Individualize dosing based on patient's prior analgesic treatment experience, and titrate as needed to provide adequate analgesia and minimize adverse reactions. (2.1, 2.2)
- Do not abruptly discontinue OxyContin in a physically dependent patient. (2.4)
- Tablets must be swallowed intact and are not to be cut, broken, chewed, crushed, or dissolved (risk of potentially fatal dose). (2.5, 5.1)
- OxyContin tablets should be taken one tablet at a time, with enough water to ensure complete swallowing immediately after placing in the mouth. (2.5, 5.9, 17)

DOSAGE FORMS AND STRENGTHS

- Tablets: 10 mg, 15 mg, 20 mg, 30 mg, 40 mg, 60 mg, and 80 mg (3)

CONTRAINDICATIONS

- Significant respiratory depression (4)
- Acute or severe bronchial asthma (4)
- Known or suspected paralytic ileus and GI obstruction (4)
- Hypersensitivity to oxycodone (4)

WARNINGS AND PRECAUTIONS

- Elderly, cachectic, and debilitated patients, and patients with chronic pulmonary disease: Monitor closely because of increased risk of respiratory depression. (5.4, 5.5)
- Interaction with CNS depressants: Consider dose reduction of one or both drugs because of additive effects. (5.6, 7.1)
- Hypotensive effects: Monitor during dose initiation and titration. (5.7)
- Patients with head injury or increased intracranial pressure: Monitor for sedation and respiratory depression.

Avoid use of OxyContin in patients with impaired consciousness or coma susceptible to intracranial effects of CO_2 retention. (5.8)

- Use with caution in patients who have difficulty swallowing or have underlying GI disorders that may predispose them to obstruction. (5.9)
- Concomitant use of CYP3A4 inhibitors may increase opioid effects. (5.14)

ADVERSE REACTIONS

Most common adverse reactions (>5%) are constipation, nausea, somnolence, dizziness, vomiting, pruritus, headache, dry mouth, asthenia, and sweating. (6.1)

To report SUSPECTED ADVERSE REACTIONS, contact Purdue Pharma L.P. at 1-888-726-7535 or FDA at 1-800-FDA-1088 or *www.fda.gov/medwatch*.

DRUG INTERACTIONS

- Muscle relaxants: Avoid use with OxyContin because of increased risk of respiratory depression. (7.2)
- The CYP3A4 isoenzyme plays a major role in the metabolism of OxyContin. Drugs that inhibit CYP3A4 activity may cause decreased clearance of oxycodone which could lead to an increase in oxycodone plasma concentrations. (7.3)
- Mixed agonist/antagonist opioid analgesics: Avoid use with OxyContin because they may reduce analgesic effect of OxyContin or precipitate withdrawal symptoms. (7.4)

USE IN SPECIFIC POPULATIONS

- Nursing mothers: Oxycodone has been detected in human milk. Closely monitor infants of nursing women receiving OxyContin. (8.3)
- Geriatrics: The initial dose may need to be reduced to 1/3 to 1/2 of the usual doses. (8.5)
- Hepatic impairment: Initiate therapy at 1/3 to 1/2 the usual doses and titrate carefully. (8.6)

See 17 for PATIENT COUNSELING INFORMATION and Medication Guide

Revised: 07/2013

FULL PRESCRIBING INFORMATION: CONTENTS*

*** Sections or subsections omitted from the full prescribing information are not listed**

FULL PRESCRIBING INFORMATION

WARNING: ABUSE POTENTIAL, LIFE-THREATENING RESPIRATORY DEPRESSION, and ACCIDENTAL EXPOSURE

Abuse Potential

OxyContin® contains oxycodone, an opioid agonist and Schedule II controlled substance with an abuse liability similar to other opioid agonists, legal or illicit *[see Warnings and Precautions (5.1)]*. Assess each patient's risk for opioid abuse or addiction prior to prescribing OxyContin. The risk for opioid abuse is increased in patients with a personal or family history of substance abuse (including drug or alcohol abuse or addiction) or mental illness (e.g., major depressive disorder). Routinely monitor all patients receiving OxyContin for signs of misuse, abuse, and addiction during treatment *[see Drug Abuse and Dependence (9)]*.

Life-Threatening Respiratory Depression

Respiratory depression, including fatal cases, may occur with use of OxyContin, even when the drug has been used as recommended and not misused or abused *[see Warnings and Precautions (5.2)]*. Proper dosing and titration are essential and OxyContin should be prescribed only by healthcare professionals who are knowledgeable in the use of potent opioids for the management of chronic pain. Monitor for respiratory depression, especially during initiation of OxyContin or following a dose increase. Instruct patients to swallow OxyContin tablets intact. Crushing, dissolving, or chewing the tablet can cause rapid release and absorption of a potentially fatal dose of oxycodone.

Accidental Exposure

Accidental ingestion of OxyContin, especially in children, can result in a fatal overdose of oxycodone *[see Warnings and Precautions (5.3)]*.

1 INDICATIONS AND USAGE

OxyContin is indicated for the management of moderate to severe pain when a continuous, around-the-clock opioid analgesic is needed for an extended period of time.

Limitations of Use

OxyContin is not for use:

- As an as-needed (prn) analgesic
- For pain that is mild or not expected to persist for an extended period of time
- For acute pain
- In the immediate postoperative period (the first 24 hours following surgery) for patients not previously taking the drug, because its safety in this setting has not been established.
- For postoperative pain unless the patient is already receiving chronic opioid therapy prior to surgery, or if the postoperative pain is expected to be moderate to severe and persist for an extended period of time.

OxyContin 60 mg and 80 mg tablets, a single dose greater than 40 mg, or a total daily dose greater than 80 mg are only for patients in whom tolerance to an opioid of comparable potency is established. Patients considered opioid tolerant are those who are taking at least 60 mg oral morphine/day, 25 mcg transdermal fentanyl/hour, 30 mg oral oxycodone/day, 8 mg oral hydromorphone/day, 25 mg oral oxymorphone/day, or an equianalgesic dose of another opioid for one week or longer.

2 DOSAGE AND ADMINISTRATION

2.1 Initial Dosing

Initiate the dosing regimen for each patient individually, taking into account the patient's prior analgesic treatment experience. Monitor patients closely for respiratory depression, especially within the first 24-72 hours of initiating therapy with OxyContin *[see Warnings and Precautions (5.2)]*.

Consider the following factors when selecting an initial dose of OxyContin:

- Total daily dose, potency, and any prior opioid the patient has been taking previously;
- Reliability of the relative potency estimate used to calculate the equivalent dose of oxycodone needed (Note: potency estimates may vary with the route of administration);
- Patient's degree of opioid experience and opioid tolerance;
- General condition and medical status of the patient;
- Concurrent medication;
- Type and severity of the patient's pain.

Use of OxyContin as the First Opioid Analgesic

Initiate therapy with 10 mg every 12 hours.

Conversion from other Oral Oxycodone Formulations to OxyContin

Patients receiving other oral oxycodone formulations may be converted to OxyContin by administering one-half of the patient's total daily oral oxycodone dose as OxyContin every 12 hours.

Conversion from other Opioids to OxyContin

While there are useful tables of oral and parenteral equivalents, there is substantial inter-patient variation in the relative potency of different opioid drugs and formulations. Specific recommendations are not available because of a lack of systematic evidence for these types of analgesic substitutions. As such, it is safer to underestimate a patient's 24-hour oral oxycodone requirement and provide rescue medication (e.g., immediate-release oxycodone) than to overestimate and precipitate an adverse reaction. In general, begin with half of the estimated daily oxycodone requirement as the initial daily OxyContin estimate, then divide into two doses taken 12 hours apart, and manage inadequate analgesia by supplementation with immediate-release oxycodone.

Published relative potency data are available and may be referred to in clinical practice guidelines such as those published by authorities in the field of pain medicine, but such ratios are approximations. Consider contacting your specific state medical or pharmacy professional societies for further information on how to safely convert patients from one opioid to another.

Conversion from Transdermal Fentanyl to OxyContin

Eighteen hours following the removal of the transdermal fentanyl patch, OxyContin treatment can be initiated. Although there has been no systematic assessment of such conversion, a conservative oxycodone dose, approximately 10 mg every 12 hours of OxyContin, should be initially substituted for each 25 mcg/hr fentanyl transdermal patch. Follow the patient closely during conversion from transdermal fentanyl to OxyContin, as there is limited documented experience with this conversion.

2.2 Titration and Maintenance of Therapy

Individually titrate OxyContin to a dose that provides adequate analgesia and minimizes adverse reactions. Continually reevaluate patients receiving OxyContin to assess the maintenance of pain control and the relative incidence of adverse reactions. During chronic therapy, especially for non-cancer-related pain (or other pain associated with terminal illnesses), periodically reassess the continued need for the use of opioid analgesics.

If the level of pain increases, attempt to identify the source of increased pain, while adjusting the OxyContin dose to decrease the level of pain. Because steady-state plasma concentrations are approximated in 1 day, OxyContin dosage adjustments may be done every 1 to 2 days. Patients who experience breakthrough pain may require dosage adjustment or rescue medication with an appropriate dose of an immediate-release opioid and non-opioid medication.

If signs of excessive opioid-related adverse reactions are observed, the next dose may be reduced. Adjust the dose to obtain an appropriate balance between management of pain and opioid-related adverse reactions.

There are no well-controlled clinical studies evaluating the safety and efficacy with dosing more frequently than every 12 hours. As a guideline, the total daily oxycodone dose usually can be increased by 25% to 50% of the current dose, each time an increase is clinically indicated.

2.3 Patients with Hepatic Impairment

For patients with hepatic impairment, start dosing patients at 1/3 to 1/2 the usual starting dose followed by careful dose titration *[see Clinical Pharmacology (12.3)]*.

2.4 Discontinuation of OxyContin

When the patient no longer requires therapy with OxyContin tablets, use a gradual downward titration of the dose to prevent signs and symptoms of withdrawal in the physically dependent patient. Do not abruptly discontinue OxyContin.

2.5 Administration of OxyContin

Instruct patients to swallow OxyContin tablets intact. The tablets are not to be crushed, dissolved, or chewed due to the risk of rapid release and absorption of a potentially fatal dose of oxycodone *[see Warnings and Precautions (5.1, 5.2)]*. Instruct patients to take OxyContin one tablet at a time and with enough water to ensure complete swallowing immediately after placing in the mouth *[see Warnings and Precautions (5.9), and Patient Counseling Information (17)]*.

3 DOSAGE FORMS AND STRENGTHS

- 10 mg film-coated tablets (round, white-colored, bi-convex tablets debossed with OP on one side and 10 on the other)
- 15 mg film-coated tablets (round, gray-colored, bi-convex tablets debossed with OP on one side and 15 on the other)
- 20 mg film-coated tablets (round, pink-colored, bi-convex tablets debossed with OP on one side and 20 on the other)
- 30 mg film-coated tablets (round, brown-colored, bi-convex tablets debossed with OP on one side and 30 on the other)
- 40 mg film-coated tablets (round, yellow-colored, bi-convex tablets debossed with OP on one side and 40 on the other)
- 60 mg film-coated tablets* (round, red-colored, bi-convex tablets debossed with OP on one side and 60 on the other)
- 80 mg film-coated tablets* (round, green-colored, bi-convex tablets debossed with OP on one side and 80 on the other)

*** 60 mg and 80 mg tablets for use in opioid-tolerant patients only**

4 CONTRAINDICATIONS

OxyContin is contraindicated in patients with:
- Significant respiratory depression
- Acute or severe bronchial asthma in an unmonitored setting or in the absence of resuscitative equipment
- Known or suspected paralytic ileus and gastrointestinal obstruction
- Hypersensitivity (e.g., anaphylaxis) to oxycodone *[see Adverse Reactions (6.2)]*

5 WARNINGS AND PRECAUTIONS

5.1 Abuse Potential

OxyContin contains oxycodone, an opioid agonist and a Schedule II controlled substance. Oxycodone can be abused in a manner similar to other opioid agonists legal or illicit. Opioid agonists are sought by drug abusers and people with addiction disorders and are subject to criminal diversion. Consider these risks when prescribing or dispensing OxyContin in situations where there is concern about increased risks of misuse, abuse, or diversion. Concerns about abuse, addiction, and diversion should not, however, prevent the proper management of pain.

Assess each patient's risk for opioid abuse or addiction prior to prescribing OxyContin. The risk for opioid abuse is increased in patients with a personal or family history of substance abuse (including drug or alcohol abuse or addiction) or mental illness (e.g., major depression). Patients at increased risk may still be appropriately treated with modified-release opioid formulations; however these patients will require intensive monitoring for signs of misuse, abuse, or addiction. Routinely monitor all patients receiving opioids for signs of misuse, abuse, and addiction because these drugs carry a risk for addiction even under appropriate medical use.

Misuse or abuse of OxyContin by crushing, chewing, snorting, or injecting the dissolved product will result in the uncontrolled delivery of the opioid and pose a significant risk that could result in overdose and death *[see Drug Abuse and Dependence (9), and Overdosage (10)]*.

Contact local state professional licensing board or state controlled substances authority for information on how to prevent and detect abuse or diversion of this product.

5.2 Life-Threatening Respiratory Depression

Respiratory depression is the chief hazard of opioid agonists, including OxyContin. Respiratory depression, if not immediately recognized and treated, may lead to respiratory arrest and death. Respiratory depression from opioids is manifested by a reduced urge to breathe and a decreased rate of respiration, often associated with a "sighing" pattern of breathing (deep breaths separated by abnormally long pauses). Carbon dioxide (CO_2) retention from opioid-induced respiratory depression can exacerbate the sedating effects of opioids. Management of respiratory depression may include close observation, supportive measures, and use of opioid antagonists, depending on the patient's clinical status *[see Overdosage (10)]*.

While serious, life-threatening, or fatal respiratory depression can occur at any time during the use of OxyContin, the risk is greatest during the initiation of therapy or following a dose increase. Closely monitor patients for respiratory depression when initiating therapy with OxyContin and following dose increases. Instruct patients against use by individuals other than the patient for whom OxyContin was prescribed and to keep OxyContin out of the reach of children, as such inappropriate use may result in fatal respiratory depression.

To reduce the risk of respiratory depression, proper dosing and titration of OxyContin are essential *[see Dosage and Administration (2)]*. Overestimating the OxyContin dose when converting patients from another opioid product can result in fatal overdose with the first dose. Respiratory depression has also been reported with use of modified-release opioids when used as recommended and not misused or abused.

To further reduce the risk of respiratory depression, consider the following:
- Proper dosing and titration are essential and OxyContin should only be prescribed by healthcare professionals who are knowledgeable in the use of potent opioids for the management of chronic pain.
- OxyContin 60 mg and 80 mg tablets are for use in opioid-tolerant patients only. Ingestion of these strengths of OxyContin tablets may cause fatal respiratory depression when administered to patients not already tolerant to high doses of opioids.
- Instruct patients to swallow OxyContin tablets intact. The tablets are not to be crushed, dissolved, or chewed. The resulting oxycodone dose may be fatal, particularly in opioid-naïve individuals.
- OxyContin is contraindicated in patients with respiratory depression and in patients with conditions that increase the risk of life-threatening respiratory depression *[see Contraindications (4)]*.

5.3 Accidental Exposure

Accidental ingestion of OxyContin, especially in children, can result in a fatal overdose of oxycodone.

5.4 Elderly, Cachectic, and Debilitated Patients

Respiratory depression is more likely to occur in elderly, cachectic, or debilitated patients as they may have altered pharmacokinetics or altered clearance compared to younger, healthier patients. Therefore, monitor such patients closely, particularly when initiating and titrating OxyContin and when OxyContin is given concomitantly with other drugs that depress respiration *[see Warnings and Precautions (5.2)]*.

5.5 Use in Patients with Chronic Pulmonary Disease

Monitor patients with significant chronic obstructive pulmonary disease or cor pulmonale, and patients having a substantially decreased respiratory reserve, hypoxia, hypercapnia, or pre-existing respiratory depression for respiratory depression, particularly when initiating therapy and titrating with OxyContin, as in these patients, even usual therapeutic doses of OxyContin may decrease respiratory drive to the point of apnea *[see Warnings and Precautions (5.2)]*. Consider the use of alternative non-opioid analgesics in these patients if possible.

5.6 Interactions with Alcohol, CNS Depressants, and Illicit Drugs

Hypotension and profound sedation, coma, or respiratory depression may result if OxyContin is used concomitantly with other CNS depressants (e.g., sedatives, anxiolytics, hypnotics, neuroleptics, muscle relaxants, other opioids). When considering the use of OxyContin in a patient taking a CNS depressant, assess the duration of use of the CNS depressant and the patient's response, including the degree of tolerance that has developed to CNS depression. Additionally, consider the patient's use, if any, of alcohol and/or illicit drugs that can cause CNS depression. If OxyContin therapy is to be initiated in a patient taking a CNS depressant, start with a lower OxyContin dose than usual and monitor patients for signs of sedation and respiratory depression and consider using a lower dose of the concomitant CNS depressant *[see Drug Interactions (7.1)]*.

5.7 Hypotensive Effects

OxyContin may cause severe hypotension, including orthostatic hypotension and syncope in ambulatory patients. There is an increased risk in patients whose ability to maintain blood pressure has already been compromised by a reduced blood volume or concurrent administration of certain CNS depressant drugs (e.g., phenothiazines or general anesthetics) *[see Drug Interactions (7.1)]*. Monitor these patients for signs of hypotension after initiating or titrating the dose of OxyContin. In patients with circulatory shock, OxyContin may cause vasodilation that can further reduce cardiac output and blood pressure. Avoid the use of OxyContin in patients with circulatory shock.

5.8 Use in Patients with Head Injury or Increased Intracranial Pressure

Monitor patients taking OxyContin who may be susceptible to the intracranial effects of CO_2 retention (e.g., those with evidence of increased intracranial pressure or brain tumors) for signs of sedation and respiratory depression, particularly when initiating therapy with OxyContin. OxyContin may reduce respiratory drive, and the resultant CO_2 retention can further increase intracranial pressure. Opioids may also obscure the clinical course in a patient with a head injury.

Avoid the use of OxyContin in patients with impaired consciousness or coma.

5.9 Difficulty in Swallowing and Risk for Obstruction in Patients at Risk for a Small Gastrointestinal Lumen

There have been post-marketing reports of difficulty in swallowing OxyContin tablets. These reports included choking, gagging, regurgitation and tablets stuck in the throat. Instruct patients not to pre-soak, lick or otherwise wet OxyContin tablets prior to placing in the mouth, and to take one tablet at a time with enough water to ensure complete swallowing immediately after placing in the mouth.

There have been rare post-marketing reports of cases of intestinal obstruction, and exacerbation of diverticulitis, some of which have required medical intervention to remove the tablet. Patients with underlying GI disorders such as esophageal cancer or colon cancer with a small gastrointestinal lumen are at greater risk of developing these complications. Consider use of an alternative analgesic in patients who have difficulty swallowing and patients at risk for underlying GI disorders resulting in a small gastrointestinal lumen.

5.10 Use in Patients with Gastrointestinal Conditions

OxyContin is contraindicated in patients with GI obstruction, including paralytic ileus. The oxycodone in OxyContin may cause spasm of the sphincter of Oddi. Monitor patients with biliary tract disease, including acute pancreatitis, for worsening symptoms. Opioids may cause increases in the serum amylase.

5.11 Use in Patients with Convulsive or Seizure Disorders

The oxycodone in OxyContin may aggravate convulsions in patients with convulsive disorders, and may induce or aggravate seizures in some clinical settings. Monitor patients with a history of seizure disorders for worsened seizure control during OxyContin therapy.

5.12 Avoidance of Withdrawal

Avoid the use of mixed agonist/antagonist analgesics (i.e., pentazocine, nalbuphine, and butorphanol) in patients who have received or are receiving a course of therapy with a full opioid agonist analgesic, including OxyContin. In these patients, mixed agonist/antagonist analgesics may reduce the analgesic effect and/or may precipitate withdrawal symptoms.

When discontinuing OxyContin, gradually taper the dose *[see Dosage and Administration (2.4)]*. Do not abruptly discontinue OxyContin.

5.13 Driving and Operating Machinery

OxyContin may impair the mental or physical abilities needed to perform potentially hazardous activities such as driving a car or operating machinery. Warn patients not to drive or operate dangerous machinery unless they are tolerant to the effects of OxyContin and know how they will react to the medication.

5.14 Cytochrome P450 3A4 Inhibitors and Inducers

Since the CYP3A4 isoenzyme plays a major role in the metabolism of OxyContin, drugs that alter CYP3A4 activity may cause changes in clearance of oxycodone which could lead to changes in oxycodone plasma concentrations.

Inhibition of CYP3A4 activity by its inhibitors, such as macrolide antibiotics (e.g., erythromycin), azole-antifungal agents (e.g., ketoconazole), and protease inhibitors (e.g., ritonavir), may increase plasma concentrations of oxycodone and prolong opioid effects.

CYP450 inducers, such as rifampin, carbamazepine, and phenytoin, may induce the metabolism of oxycodone and, therefore, may cause increased clearance of the drug which could lead to a decrease in oxycodone plasma concentrations, lack of efficacy or, possibly, development of an abstinence syndrome in a patient who had developed physical dependence to oxycodone.

If co-administration is necessary, caution is advised when initiating OxyContin treatment in patients currently taking, or discontinuing, CYP3A4 inhibitors or inducers. Evaluate these patients at frequent intervals and consider dose adjustments until stable drug effects are achieved *[see Drug Interactions (7.3), and Clinical Pharmacology (12.3)]*.

5.15 Laboratory Monitoring

Not every urine drug test for "opioids" or "opiates" detects oxycodone reliably, especially those designed for in-office use. Further, many laboratories will report urine drug concentrations below a specified "cut off" value as "negative". Therefore, if urine testing for oxycodone is considered in the clinical management of an individual patient, ensure that the sensitivity and specificity of the assay is appropriate, and consider the limitations of the testing used when interpreting results.

6 ADVERSE REACTIONS

The following adverse reactions described elsewhere in the labeling include:
- Respiratory depression *[see Boxed Warning, Warnings and Precautions (5.2, 5.5), and Overdosage (10)]*
- CNS depression *[see Drug Interactions (7.1), and Overdosage (10)]*
- Hypotensive effects *[see Warnings and Precautions (5.7), and Overdosage (10)]*

- Drug abuse, addiction, and dependence *[see Drug Abuse and Dependence (9.2, 9.3)]*
- Gastrointestinal Effects *[see Warnings and Precautions (5.9, 5.10)]*
- Seizures *[see Warnings and Precautions (5.11)]*

6.1 Clinical Trial Experience

Because clinical trials are conducted under widely varying conditions, adverse reaction rates observed in the clinical trials of a drug cannot be directly compared to rates in the clinical trials of another drug and may not reflect the rates observed in practice.

The safety of OxyContin was evaluated in double-blind clinical trials involving 713 patients with moderate to severe pain of various etiologies. In open-label studies of cancer pain, 187 patients received OxyContin in total daily doses ranging from 20 mg to 640 mg per day. The average total daily dose was approximately 105 mg per day.

OxyContin may increase the risk of serious adverse reactions such as those observed with other opioid analgesics, including respiratory depression, apnea, respiratory arrest, circulatory depression, hypotension, or shock *[see Overdosage (10)]*.

The most common adverse reactions (>5%) reported by patients in clinical trials comparing OxyContin with placebo are shown in Table 1 below:

TABLE 1: Common Adverse Reactions (>5%)

Adverse Reaction	OxyContin (n=227) (%)	Placebo (n=45) (%)
Constipation	(23)	(7)
Nausea	(23)	(11)
Somnolence	(23)	(4)
Dizziness	(13)	(9)
Pruritus	(13)	(2)
Vomiting	(12)	(7)
Headache	(7)	(7)
Dry Mouth	(6)	(2)
Asthenia	(6)	-
Sweating	(5)	(2)

In clinical trials, the following adverse reactions were reported in patients treated with OxyContin with an incidence between 1% and 5%:

Gastrointestinal disorders: abdominal pain, diarrhea, dyspepsia, gastritis

General disorders and administration site conditions: chills, fever

Metabolism and nutrition disorders: anorexia

Musculoskeletal and connective tissue disorders: twitching

Psychiatric disorders: abnormal dreams, anxiety, confusion, dysphoria, euphoria, insomnia, nervousness, thought abnormalities

Respiratory, thoracic and mediastinal disorders: dyspnea, hiccups

Skin and subcutaneous tissue disorders: rash

Vascular disorders: postural hypotension

The following adverse reactions occurred **in less than 1% of patients** involved in clinical trials:

Blood and lymphatic system disorders: lymphadenopathy

Ear and labyrinth disorders: tinnitus

Eye disorders: abnormal vision

Gastrointestinal disorders: dysphagia, eructation, flatulence, gastrointestinal disorder, increased appetite, stomatitis

General disorders and administration site conditions: withdrawal syndrome (with and without seizures), edema, peripheral edema, thirst, malaise, chest pain, facial edema

Injury, poisoning and procedural complications: accidental injury

Investigations: ST depression

Metabolism and nutrition disorders: dehydration

Nervous system disorders: syncope, migraine, abnormal gait, amnesia, hyperkinesia, hypesthesia, hypotonia, paresthesia, speech disorder, stupor, tremor, vertigo, taste perversion

Psychiatric disorders: depression, agitation, depersonalization, emotional lability, hallucination

Renal and urinary disorders: dysuria, hematuria, polyuria, urinary retention

Reproductive system and breast disorders: impotence

Respiratory, thoracic and mediastinal disorders: cough increased, voice alteration

Skin and subcutaneous tissue disorders: dry skin, exfoliative dermatitis

6.2 Postmarketing Experience

The following adverse reactions have been identified during post-approval use of controlled-release oxycodone: abuse, addiction, amenorrhea, cholestasis, death, dental caries, increased hepatic enzymes, hyperalgesia, hypogonadism, hyponatremia, ileus, muscular hypertonia, overdose, palpitations (in the context of withdrawal), seizures, syndrome of inappropriate antidiuretic hormone secretion, and urticaria.

Anaphylaxis has been reported with ingredients contained in OxyContin. Advise patients how to recognize such a reaction and when to seek medical attention.

In addition to the events listed above, the following have also been reported, potentially due to the swelling and hydrogelling property of the tablet: choking, gagging, regurgitation, tablets stuck in the throat and difficulty swallowing the tablet.

7 DRUG INTERACTIONS

7.1 CNS Depressants

Concurrent use of OxyContin and other central nervous system (CNS) depressants including sedatives or hypnotics, general anesthetics, phenothiazines, tranquilizers, and alcohol can increase the risk of respiratory depression, hypotension, profound sedation or coma. Monitor patients receiving CNS depressants and OxyContin for signs of respiratory depression and hypotension. When such combined therapy is contemplated, start OxyContin at 1/3 to 1/2 of the usual dosage and consider using a lower dose of the concomitant CNS depressant.

7.2 Muscle Relaxants

Oxycodone may enhance the neuromuscular blocking action of true skeletal muscle relaxants and produce an increased degree of respiratory depression. Monitor patients receiving muscle relaxants and OxyContin for signs of respiratory depression that may be greater than otherwise expected.

7.3 Agents Affecting Cytochrome P450 Isoenzymes

Inhibitors of CYP3A4

Co-administration of a strong CYP3A4 inhibitor ketoconazole, with OxyContin, significantly increased the plasma concentrations of oxycodone. Inhibition of CYP3A4 activity by its inhibitors, such as macrolide antibiotics (e.g., erythromycin), azole-antifungal agents (e.g., ketoconazole), and protease inhibitors (e.g., ritonavir), may prolong opioid effects. If co-administration is necessary, caution is advised when initiating therapy with, currently taking, or discontinuing CYP3A4 inhibitors. Evaluate these patients at frequent intervals and consider dose adjustments until stable drug effects are achieved *[see Clinical Pharmacology (12.3)]*.

Inducers of CYP3A4

A published study showed that the co-administration of rifampin, a drug metabolizing enzyme inducer, significantly decreased plasma oxycodone concentrations. CYP450 inducers, such as rifampin, carbamazepine, and phenytoin, may induce the metabolism of oxycodone and, therefore, may cause increased clearance of the drug which could lead to a decrease in oxycodone plasma concentrations, lack of efficacy or, possibly, development of an abstinence syndrome in a patient who had developed physical dependence to oxycodone. If co-administration with OxyContin is necessary, caution is advised when initiating therapy with, currently taking, or discontinuing CYP3A4 inducers. Evaluate these patients at frequent intervals and consider dose adjustments until stable drug effects are achieved *[see Clinical Pharmacology (12.3)]*.

Inhibitors of CYP2D6

Oxycodone is metabolized in part to oxymorphone via CYP2D6. While this pathway may be blocked by a variety of drugs such as certain cardiovascular drugs (e.g., quinidine) and antidepressants (e.g., fluoxetine), such blockade has not been shown to be of clinical significance during oxycodone treatment. However, clinicians should be aware of this possible interaction.

7.4 Mixed Agonist/Antagonist Opioid Analgesics

Mixed agonist/antagonist analgesics (i.e., pentazocine, nalbuphine, and butorphanol) should generally not be administered to a patient who has received or is receiving a course of therapy with a pure opioid agonist analgesic such as OxyContin. In this situation, mixed agonist/antagonist analgesics may reduce the analgesic effect of oxycodone and may precipitate withdrawal symptoms in these patients.

7.5 Diuretics

Opioids can reduce the efficacy of diuretics by inducing the release of antidiuretic hormone. Opioids may also lead to acute retention of urine by causing spasm of the sphincter of the bladder, particularly in men with enlarged prostates.

7.6 Anticholinergics

Anticholinergics or other medications with anticholinergic activity when used concurrently with opioid analgesics may result in increased risk of urinary retention and/or severe constipation, which may lead to paralytic ileus. Monitor patients for signs of urinary retention or reduced gastric motility when OxyContin is used concurrently with anticholinergic drugs.

8 USE IN SPECIFIC POPULATIONS

8.1 Pregnancy

Pregnancy Category B

There are no adequate and well-controlled studies of oxycodone use during pregnancy. Based on limited human data in the literature, oxycodone does not appear to increase the risk of congenital malformations. In animal reproduction and developmental toxicology studies, no evidence of fetal harm was observed. Because animal reproduction studies are not always predictive of human response, oxycodone should be used during pregnancy only if clearly needed.

Teratogenic Effects

The effect of oxycodone in human reproduction has not been adequately studied. Studies with oral doses of oxycodone hydrochloride in rats up to 8 mg/kg/day and rabbits up to 125 mg/kg/day, equivalent to 0.5 and 2.0 times an adult human dose of 160 mg/day, respectively on a mg/m^2 basis, did not reveal evidence of harm to the fetus due to oxycodone. In a pre- and postnatal toxicity study, female rats received oxycodone during gestation and lactation. There were no long-term developmental or reproductive effects in the pups *[see Nonclinical Toxicology (13.1)]*.

Non-Teratogenic Effects

Oxycodone hydrochloride was administered orally to female rats during gestation and lactation in a pre- and postnatal toxicity study. There were no drug-related effects on reproductive performance in these females or any long-term developmental or reproductive effects in pups born to these rats. Decreased body weight was found during lactation and the early post-weaning phase in pups nursed by mothers given the highest dose used (6 mg/kg/day, equivalent to approximately 0.4-times an adult human dose of 160 mg/day, on a mg/m^2 basis). However, body weight of these pups recovered.

8.2 Labor and Delivery

Opioids cross the placenta and may produce respiratory depression and psycho-physiologic effects in neonates. OxyContin is not recommended for use in women immediately prior to and during labor, when use of shorter-acting analgesics or other analgesic techniques are more appropriate. Occasionally, opioid analgesics may prolong labor through actions which temporarily reduce the strength, duration and frequency of uterine contractions. However this effect is not consistent and may be offset by an increased rate of cervical dilatation, which tends to shorten labor.

Closely observe neonates whose mothers received opioid analgesics during labor for signs of respiratory depression. Have a specific opioid antagonist, such as naloxone or nalmefene, available for reversal of opioid-induced respiratory depression in the neonate.

8.3 Nursing Mothers

Oxycodone has been detected in breast milk. Instruct patients not to undertake nursing while receiving OxyContin. Do not initiate OxyContin therapy while nursing because of the possibility of sedation or respiratory depression in the infant.

Withdrawal signs can occur in breast-fed infants when maternal administration of an opioid analgesic is stopped, or when breast-feeding is stopped.

8.4 Pediatric Use

Safety and effectiveness of OxyContin in pediatric patients below the age of 18 years have not been established.

8.5 Geriatric Use

In controlled pharmacokinetic studies in elderly subjects (greater than 65 years) the clearance of oxycodone was slightly reduced. Compared to young adults, the plasma concentrations of oxycodone were increased approximately 15% *[see Clinical Pharmacology (12.3)]*. Of the total number of subjects (445) in clinical studies of oxycodone hydrochloride controlled-release tablets, 148 (33.3%) were age 65 and older (including those age 75 and older) while 40 (9.0%) were age 75 and older. In clinical trials with appropriate initiation of therapy and dose titration, no untoward or unexpected adverse reactions were seen in the elderly patients who received oxycodone hydrochloride controlled-release tablets. Thus, the usual doses and dosing intervals may be appropriate for elderly patients. However, reduce the starting dose to 1/3 to 1/2 the usual dosage in debilitated, non-opioid-tolerant patients. Respiratory depression is the chief risk in elderly or debilitated patients, usually the result of large initial doses in patients who are not tolerant to opioids, or when opioids are given in conjunction with other agents that depress respiration. Titrate the dose of OxyContin cautiously in these patients.

8.6 Hepatic Impairment

A study of OxyContin in patients with hepatic impairment demonstrated greater plasma concentrations than those seen at equivalent doses in persons with normal hepatic function. Therefore, in the setting of hepatic impairment, start dosing patients at 1/3 to 1/2 the usual starting dose followed by careful dose titration *[see Clinical Pharmacology (12.3)]*.

8.7 Renal Impairment

In patients with renal impairment, as evidenced by decreased creatinine clearance (<60 mL/min), the concentrations of oxycodone in the plasma are approximately 50% higher than in subjects with normal renal function. Follow a conservative approach to dose initiation and adjust according to the clinical situation *[see Clinical Pharmacology (12.3)]*.

8.8 Gender Differences

In pharmacokinetic studies with OxyContin, opioid-naïve females demonstrate up to 25% higher average plasma concentrations and greater frequency of typical opioid adverse events than males, even after adjustment for body weight. The clinical relevance of a difference of this magnitude is low for a drug intended for chronic usage at individualized dosages, and there was no male/female difference detected for efficacy or adverse events in clinical trials.

8.9 Neonatal Opioid Withdrawal Syndrome

Chronic maternal use of oxycodone during pregnancy can affect the fetus with subsequent withdrawal signs. Neonatal withdrawal syndrome presents as irritability, hyperactivity and abnormal sleep pattern, high pitched cry, tremor, vomiting, diarrhea and failure to gain weight. The onset, duration and severity of neonatal withdrawal syndrome vary based on the drug used, duration of use, the dose of last maternal use, and rate of elimination of drug by the newborn. Neonatal opioid withdrawal syndrome, unlike opioid withdrawal syndrome in adults, may be life-threatening and should be treated according to protocols developed by neonatology experts.

9 DRUG ABUSE AND DEPENDENCE

9.1 Controlled Substance

OxyContin contains oxycodone, a Schedule II controlled substance with a high potential for abuse similar to other opioids including fentanyl, hydromorphone, methadone, morphine, and oxymorphone. OxyContin can be abused and is subject to misuse, addiction, and criminal diversion *[see Warnings and Precautions (5.1)]*.

The high drug content in extended-release formulations adds to the risk of adverse outcomes from abuse and misuse.

9.2 Abuse

Abuse of OxyContin poses a hazard of overdose and death. This risk is increased with compromising the tablet and with concurrent abuse of alcohol or other substances.

All patients treated with opioids require careful monitoring for signs of abuse and addiction, since use of opioid analgesic products carries the risk of addiction even under appropriate medical use. Drug addiction is a treatable disease, utilizing a multidisciplinary approach, but relapse is common.

Drug abuse is the intentional non-therapeutic use of an over-the-counter or prescription drug, even once, for its rewarding psychological or physiological effects. Drug abuse includes, but is not limited to, the following examples: the use of a prescription or over-the-counter drug to get "high", or the use of steroids for performance enhancement and muscle build up.

Drug addiction is a cluster of behavioral, cognitive, and physiological phenomena that develop after repeated substance use and include: a strong desire to take the drug, difficulties in controlling its use, persisting in its use despite harmful consequences, a higher priority given to drug use than to other activities and obligations, increased tolerance, and sometimes a physical withdrawal.

"Drug-seeking" behavior is very common to addicts and drug abusers. Drug-seeking tactics include emergency calls or visits near the end of office hours, refusal to undergo appropriate examination, testing or referral, repeated claims of loss of prescriptions, tampering with prescriptions and reluctance to provide prior medical records or contact information for other treating physician(s). "Doctor shopping" (visiting multiple prescribers) to obtain additional prescriptions is common among drug abusers and people suffering from untreated addiction.

Preoccupation with achieving adequate pain relief can be appropriate behavior in a patient with poor pain control.

Abuse and addiction are separate and distinct from physical dependence and tolerance. Physicians should be aware that addiction may not be accompanied by concurrent tolerance and symptoms of physical dependence in all addicts. In addition, abuse of opioids can occur in the absence of true addiction.

OxyContin, like other opioids, can be diverted for non-medical use into illicit channels of distribution. Careful recordkeeping of prescribing information, including quantity, frequency, and renewal requests as required by state law, is strongly advised.

Proper assessment of the patient, proper prescribing practices, periodic reevaluation of therapy, and proper dispensing and storage are appropriate measures that help to reduce abuse of opioid drugs.

Risks Specific to Abuse of OxyContin

OxyContin is for oral use only. Abuse of OxyContin poses a risk of overdose and death. Abuse may occur by taking intact tablets in quantities greater than prescribed or without legitimate purpose, by crushing and chewing or snorting the crushed formulation, or by injecting a solution made from the crushed formulation. The risk of overdose or death is increased with concurrent use of OxyContin with alcohol and other central nervous system depressants. Taking cut, broken, chewed, crushed, or dissolved OxyContin enhances drug release and increases the risk of overdose and death. With parenteral abuse, the inactive ingredients in OxyContin can result in death, local tissue necrosis, infection, pulmonary granulomas, and increased risk of endocarditis and valvular heart injury. Parenteral drug abuse is commonly associated with transmission of infectious diseases, such as hepatitis and HIV.

Abuse Deterrence Studies

OxyContin is formulated with inactive ingredients intended to make the tablet more difficult to manipulate for misuse and abuse. For the purposes of describing the results of studies of the abuse-deterrent characteristics of OxyContin resulting from a change in formulation, in this section, the original formulation of OxyContin, which is no longer marketed, will be referred to as "original OxyContin" and the reformulated, currently marketed product will be referred to as "OxyContin".

In Vitro Testing

In vitro physical and chemical tablet manipulation studies were performed to evaluate the success of different extraction methods in defeating the extended-release formulation. Results support that, relative to original OxyContin, there is an increase in the ability of OxyContin to resist crushing, breaking, and dissolution using a variety of tools and solvents. The results of these studies also support this finding for OxyContin relative to an immediate-release oxycodone. When subjected to an aqueous environment, OxyContin gradually forms a viscous hydrogel (i.e., a gelatinous mass) that resists passage through a needle.

Clinical Studies

In a randomized, double-blind, placebo-controlled 5-period crossover pharmacodynamic study, 30 recreational opioid users with a history of intranasal drug abuse received intranasally administered active and placebo drug treatments. The five treatment arms were finely crushed OxyContin 30 mg tablets, coarsely crushed OxyContin 30 mg tablets, finely crushed original OxyContin 30 mg tablets, powdered oxycodone HCl 30 mg, and placebo. Data for finely crushed OxyContin, finely crushed original OxyContin, and powdered oxycodone HCl are described below.

Drug liking was measured on a bipolar drug liking scale of 0 to 100 where 50 represents a neutral response of neither liking nor disliking, 0 represents maximum disliking and 100 represents maximum liking. Response to whether the subject would take the study drug again was also measured on a bipolar scale of 0 to 100 where 50 represents a neutral response, 0 represents the strongest negative response ("definitely would not take drug again") and 100 represents the strongest positive response ("definitely would take drug again").

Twenty-seven of the subjects completed the study. Incomplete dosing due to granules falling from the subjects' nostrils occurred in 34% (n = 10) of subjects with finely crushed OxyContin, compared with 7% (n = 2) of subjects with finely crushed original OxyContin and no subjects with powdered oxycodone HCl.

The intranasal administration of finely crushed OxyContin was associated with a numerically lower mean and median drug liking score and a lower mean and median score for take drug again, compared to finely crushed original OxyContin or powdered oxycodone HCl as summarized in Table 2.

[See table 2 above]

Table 2: Summary of Maximum Drug Liking (E_{max}) Data Following Intranasal Administration

VAS Scale (100 mm)*		OxyContin (finely crushed)	Original OxyContin (finely crushed)	Oxycodone HCl (powdered)
Drug Liking	Mean (SE)	80.4 (3.9)	94.0 (2.7)	89.3 (3.1)
	Median (Range)	88 (36-100)	100 (51-100)	100 (50-100)
Take Drug Again	Mean (SE)	64.0 (7.1)	89.6 (3.9)	86.6 (4.4)
	Median (Range)	78 (0-100)	100 (20-100)	100 (0-100)

* Bipolar scales (0 = maximum negative response, 50 = neutral response, 100 = maximum positive response)

Figure 1 demonstrates a comparison of drug liking for finely crushed OxyContin compared to powdered oxycodone HCl in subjects who received both treatments. The Y-axis represents the percent of subjects attaining a percent reduction in drug liking for OxyContin vs. oxycodone HCl powder greater than or equal to the value on the X-axis. Approximately 44% (n = 12) had no reduction in liking with OxyContin relative to oxycodone HCl. Approximately 56% (n = 15) of subjects had some reduction in drug liking with OxyContin relative to oxycodone HCl. Thirty-three percent (n = 9) of subjects had a reduction of at least 30% in drug liking with OxyContin compared to oxycodone HCl, and approximately 22% (n = 6) of subjects had a reduction of at least 50% in drug liking with OxyContin compared to oxycodone HCl.

Figure 1: Percent Reduction Profiles for E_{max} of Drug Liking VAS for OxyContin vs. oxycodone HCl, N=27 Following Intranasal Administration

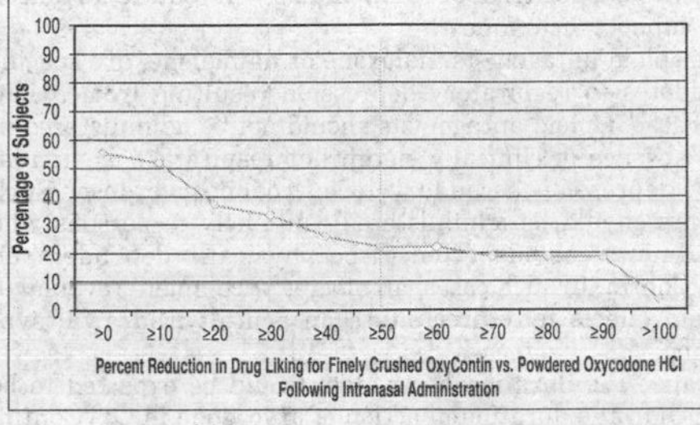

The results of a similar analysis of drug liking for finely crushed OxyContin relative to finely crushed original OxyContin were comparable to the results of finely crushed OxyContin relative to powdered oxycodone HCl. Approximately 43% (n = 12) of subjects had no reduction in liking with OxyContin relative to original OxyContin. Approximately 57% (n = 16) of subjects had some reduction in drug liking, 36% (n = 10) of subjects had a reduction of at least 30% in drug liking, and approximately 29% (n = 8) of subjects had a reduction of at least 50% in drug liking with OxyContin compared to original OxyContin.

Summary

The *in vitro* data demonstrate that OxyContin has physicochemical properties expected to make abuse via injection difficult. The data from the clinical study, along with support from the *in vitro* data, also indicate that OxyContin has physicochemical properties that are expected to reduce abuse via the intranasal route. However, abuse of OxyContin by these routes, as well as by the oral route is still possible.

Additional data, including epidemiological data, when available, may provide further information on the impact of the current formulation of OxyContin on the abuse liability of the drug. Accordingly, this section may be updated in the future as appropriate.

OxyContin contains oxycodone, an opioid agonist and Schedule II controlled substance with an abuse liability similar to other opioid agonists, legal or illicit, including fentanyl, hydromorphone, methadone, morphine, and oxymorphone. OxyContin can be abused and is subject to misuse, addiction, and criminal diversion *[See Warnings and Precautions (5.1), and Drug Abuse and Dependence (9.1)]*.

9.3 Dependence

Both tolerance and physical dependence can develop during chronic opioid therapy. Tolerance is the need for increasing doses of opioids to maintain a defined effect such as analgesia (in the absence of disease progression or other external factors). Tolerance may occur to both the desired and undesired effects of drugs, and may develop at different rates for different effects.

Physical dependence results in withdrawal symptoms after abrupt discontinuation or a significant dose reduction of a drug. Withdrawal also may be precipitated through the administration of drugs with opioid antagonist activity, e.g., naloxone, nalmefene, or mixed agonist/antagonist analgesics (pentazocine, butorphanol, nalbuphine). Physical dependence may not occur to a clinically significant degree until after several days to weeks of continued opioid usage.

OxyContin should not be abruptly discontinued *[see Dosage and Administration (2.4)]*. If OxyContin is abruptly discontinued in a physically-dependent patient, an abstinence syndrome may occur. Some or all of the following can characterize this syndrome: restlessness, lacrimation, rhinorrhea, yawning, perspiration, chills, myalgia, and mydriasis. Other signs and symptoms also may develop, including: irritability, anxiety, backache, joint pain, weakness, abdominal cramps, insomnia, nausea, anorexia, vomiting, diarrhea, or increased blood pressure, respiratory rate, or heart rate.

Infants born to mothers physically dependent on opioids will also be physically dependent and may exhibit respiratory difficulties and withdrawal signs *[see Use in Specific Populations (8.9)]*.

10 OVERDOSAGE

Clinical Presentation

Acute overdosage with OxyContin can be manifested by respiratory depression, somnolence progressing to stupor or coma, skeletal muscle flaccidity, cold and clammy skin, constricted pupils, and in some cases, pulmonary edema, bradycardia, hypotension, partial or complete airway obstruction, atypical snoring and death. Marked mydriasis rather than miosis may be seen due to severe hypoxia in overdose situations.

Treatment of Overdose

In case of overdose, priorities are the reestablishment of a patent and protected airway and institution of assisted or controlled ventilation if needed. Employ other supportive measures (including oxygen, vasopressors) in the management of circulatory shock and pulmonary edema as indicated. Cardiac arrest or arrhythmias will require advanced life support techniques.

The opioid antagonists, naloxone or nalmefene, are specific antidotes to respiratory depression resulting from opioid overdose. Opioid antagonists should not be administered in the absence of clinically significant respiratory or circulatory depression secondary to oxycodone overdose. Such agents should be administered cautiously to persons who are known, or suspected to be physically dependent on OxyContin. In such cases, an abrupt or complete reversal of opioid effects may precipitate an acute withdrawal syndrome.

Because the duration of reversal would be expected to be less than the duration of action of oxycodone in OxyContin, carefully monitor the patient until spontaneous respiration is reliably reestablished. OxyContin will continue to release oxycodone and add to the oxycodone load for 24 to 48 hours or longer following ingestion necessitating prolonged monitoring. If the response to opioid antagonists is suboptimal or not sustained, additional antagonist should be administered as directed in the product's prescribing information.

In an individual physically dependent on opioids, administration of the usual dose of the antagonist will precipitate an acute withdrawal syndrome. The severity of the withdrawal symptoms experienced will depend on the degree of physical dependence and the dose of the antagonist administered. If a decision is made to treat serious respiratory depression in the physically dependent patient, administration of the antagonist should be begun with care and by titration with smaller than usual doses of the antagonist.

11 DESCRIPTION

OxyContin (oxycodone hydrochloride controlled-release) is an opioid analgesic supplied in 10 mg, 15 mg, 20 mg, 30 mg, 40 mg, 60 mg, and 80 mg tablets for oral administration. The tablet strengths describe the amount of oxycodone per tablet as the hydrochloride salt. The structural formula for oxycodone hydrochloride is as follows:

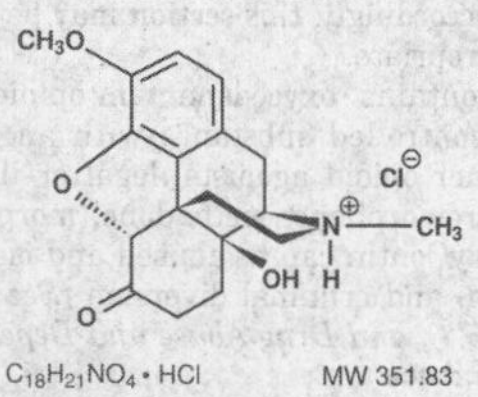

$C_{18}H_{21}NO_4 \cdot HCl$ MW 351.83

The chemical name is 4, 5α-epoxy-14-hydroxy-3-methoxy-17-methylmorphinan-6-one hydrochloride.

Oxycodone is a white, odorless crystalline powder derived from the opium alkaloid, thebaine. Oxycodone hydrochloride dissolves in water (1 g in 6 to 7 mL). It is slightly soluble in alcohol (octanol water partition coefficient 0.7).

The 10 mg, 15 mg, 20 mg, 30 mg, 40 mg, 60 mg and 80 mg tablets contain the following inactive ingredients: butylated hydroxytoluene (BHT), hypromellose, polyethylene glycol 400, polyethylene oxide, magnesium stearate, titanium dioxide.

The 10 mg tablets also contain hydroxypropyl cellulose.

The 15 mg tablets also contain black iron oxide, yellow iron oxide, and red iron oxide.

The 20 mg tablets also contain polysorbate 80 and red iron oxide.

The 30 mg tablets also contain polysorbate 80, red iron oxide, yellow iron oxide, and black iron oxide.

The 40 mg tablets also contain polysorbate 80 and yellow iron oxide.

The 60 mg tablets also contain polysorbate 80, red iron oxide and black iron oxide.

The 80 mg tablets also contain hydroxypropyl cellulose, yellow iron oxide and FD&C Blue #2/Indigo Carmine Aluminum Lake.

12 CLINICAL PHARMACOLOGY

Oxycodone is primarily a mu receptor opioid agonist whose principal therapeutic action is analgesia. Other members of the class known as opioid agonists include substances such as morphine, hydromorphone, fentanyl, codeine, hydrocodone and oxymorphone. Pharmacological effects of opioid agonists include anxiolysis, euphoria, feelings of relaxation, respiratory depression, constipation, miosis, and cough suppression, as well as analgesia. In general, increasing doses of mu receptor agonists are associated with increasing analgesia. There is no defined maximum dose; the ceiling to analgesic effectiveness is imposed only by adverse reactions, the more serious of which may include somnolence and respiratory depression.

12.1 Mechanism of Action

Central Nervous System

The precise mechanism of the analgesic action is unknown. However, specific CNS opioid receptors for endogenous compounds with opioid-like activity have been identified throughout the brain and spinal cord and are thought to play a role in the analgesic effects of this drug.

12.2 Pharmacodynamics

A single-dose, double-blind, placebo- and dose-controlled study was conducted using OxyContin (10, 20, and 30 mg) in an analgesic pain model involving 182 patients with moderate to severe pain. OxyContin doses of 20 mg and 30 mg produced statistically significant pain reduction compared to placebo.

Effects on the Central Nervous System

Oxycodone produces respiratory depression by direct action on brain stem respiratory centers. The respiratory depression involves both a reduction in the responsiveness of the brain stem respiratory centers to increases in CO_2 tension and to electrical stimulation.

Oxycodone depresses the cough reflex by direct effect on the cough center in the medulla. Antitussive effects may occur with doses lower than those usually required for analgesia.

Oxycodone causes miosis, even in total darkness. Pinpoint pupils are a sign of opioid overdose but are not pathognomonic (e.g., pontine lesions of hemorrhagic or ischemic origin may produce similar findings). Marked mydriasis rather than miosis may be seen with hypoxia in the setting of oxycodone overdose *[see Overdosage (10)]*.

Effects on the Gastrointestinal Tract and Other Smooth Muscle

Oxycodone causes a reduction in motility associated with an increase in smooth muscle tone in the antrum of the stomach and duodenum. Digestion of food in the small intestine is delayed and propulsive contractions are decreased. Propulsive peristaltic waves in the colon are decreased, while tone may be increased to the point of spasm resulting in constipation. Other opioid-induced effects may include a reduction in gastric, biliary and pancreatic secretions, spasm of sphincter of Oddi, and transient elevations in serum amylase.

Effects on the Cardiovascular System

Oxycodone may produce release of histamine with or without associated peripheral vasodilation. Manifestations of histamine release and/or peripheral vasodilation may include pruritus, flushing, red eyes, sweating, and/or orthostatic hypotension.

Effects on the Endocrine System

Opioids inhibit the secretion of ACTH, cortisol, testosterone, and luteinizing hormone (LH) in humans. They also stimulate prolactin, growth hormone (GH) secretion, and pancreatic secretion of insulin and glucagon.

Effects on the Immune System

Opioids have been shown to have a variety of effects on components of the immune system in *in vitro* and animal models. The clinical significance of these findings is unknown. Overall, the effects of opioids appear to be modestly immunosuppressive.

Concentration –Efficacy Relationships

Studies in normal volunteers and patients reveal predictable relationships between oxycodone dosage and plasma oxycodone concentrations, as well as between concentration and certain expected opioid effects, such as pupillary constriction, sedation, overall subjective "drug effect", analgesia and feelings of relaxation.

The minimum effective analgesic concentration will vary widely among patients, especially among patients who have been previously treated with potent agonist opioids. As a result, patients must be treated with individualized titration of dosage to the desired effect. The minimum effective analgesic concentration of oxycodone for any individual patient may increase over time due to an increase in pain, the development of a new pain syndrome and/or the development of analgesic tolerance.

Concentration –Adverse Reaction Relationships

There is a relationship between increasing oxycodone plasma concentration and increasing frequency of dose-related opioid adverse reactions such as nausea, vomiting, CNS effects, and respiratory depression. In opioid-tolerant patients, the situation may be altered by the development of tolerance to opioid-related side effects.

The dose of OxyContin must be individualized because the effective analgesic dose for some patients will be too high to be tolerated by other patients *[see Dosage and Administration (2.1)]*.

12.3 Pharmacokinetics

The activity of OxyContin is primarily due to the parent drug oxycodone. OxyContin is designed to provide delivery of oxycodone over 12 hours.

Cutting, breaking, chewing, crushing or dissolving OxyContin impairs the controlled-release delivery mechanism and results in the rapid release and absorption of a potentially fatal dose of oxycodone.

Oxycodone release from OxyContin is pH independent. The oral bioavailability of oxycodone is 60% to 87%. The relative oral bioavailability of oxycodone from OxyContin to that from immediate-release oral dosage forms is 100%. Upon repeated dosing with OxyContin in healthy subjects in pharmacokinetic studies, steady-state levels were achieved within 24-36 hours. Oxycodone is extensively metabolized and eliminated primarily in the urine as both conjugated and unconjugated metabolites. The apparent elimination half-life ($t_{1/2}$) of oxycodone following the administration of OxyContin was 4.5 hours compared to 3.2 hours for immediate-release oxycodone.

Absorption

About 60% to 87% of an oral dose of oxycodone reaches the central compartment in comparison to a parenteral dose. This high oral bioavailability is due to low pre-systemic and/or first-pass metabolism.

Plasma Oxycodone Concentration over Time

Dose proportionality has been established for OxyContin 10 mg, 15 mg, 20 mg, 30 mg, 40 mg, 60 mg, and 80 mg tablet strengths for both peak plasma concentrations (C_{max}) and extent of absorption (AUC) *(see Table 3)*. Given the short elimination $t_{1/2}$ of oxycodone, steady-state plasma concentrations of oxycodone are achieved within 24-36 hours of initiation of dosing with OxyContin. In a study comparing 10 mg of OxyContin every 12 hours to 5 mg of immediate-release oxycodone every 6 hours, the two treatments were found to be equivalent for AUC and C_{max}, and similar for C_{min} (trough) concentrations.

TABLE 3

Mean [% coefficient of variation]

Regimen	Dosage Form	AUC (ng-hr/mL)*	Cmax (ng/mL)	Tmax (hr)
Single Dose†	10 mg	136 [27]	11.5 [27]	5.11 [21]
	15 mg	196 [28]	16.8 [29]	4.59 [19]
	20 mg	248 [25]	22.7 [25]	4.63 [22]
	30 mg	377 [24]	34.6 [21]	4.61 [19]
	40 mg	497 [27]	47.4 [30]	4.40 [22]
	60 mg	705 [22]	64.6 [24]	4.15 [26]
	80 mg	908 [21]	87.1 [29]	4.27 [26]

* for single-dose AUC = AUC_{0-inf}

†data obtained while subjects received naltrexone, which can enhance absorption

Food Effects

Food has no significant effect on the extent of absorption of oxycodone from OxyContin.

Distribution

Following intravenous administration, the steady-state volume of distribution (Vss) for oxycodone was 2.6 L/kg. Oxycodone binding to plasma protein at 37°C and a pH of 7.4 was about 45%. Once absorbed, oxycodone is distributed to skeletal muscle, liver, intestinal tract, lungs, spleen, and brain. Oxycodone has been found in breast milk *[see Use in Specific Populations (8.3)]*.

Metabolism

Oxycodone is extensively metabolized by multiple metabolic pathways to produce noroxycodone, oxymorphone and noroxymorphone, which are subsequently glucuronidated. Noroxycodone and noroxymorphone are the major circulating metabolites. CYP3A mediated *N*-demethylation to noroxycodone is the primary metabolic pathway of oxycodone with a lower contribution from CYP2D6 mediated *O*-demethylation to oxymorphone. Therefore, the formation of these and related metabolites can, in theory, be affected by other drugs *[see Drug Interactions (7.3)]*.

Noroxycodone exhibits very weak anti-nociceptive potency compared to oxycodone, however, it undergoes further oxidation to produce noroxymorphone, which is active at opioid receptors. Although noroxymorphone is an active metabolite and present at relatively high concentrations in circulation, it does not appear to cross the blood-brain barrier to a significant extent. Oxymorphone is present in the plasma only at low concentrations and undergoes further metabolism to form its glucuronide and noroxymorphone. Oxymorphone has been shown to be active and possessing analgesic activity but its contribution to analgesia following oxycodone administration is thought to be clinically insignificant. Other metabolites (α- and β-oxycodol, noroxycodol and oxymorphol) may be present at very low concentrations and demonstrate limited penetration into the brain as compared to oxycodone. The enzymes responsible for keto-reduction and glucuronidation pathways in oxycodone metabolism have not been established.

Excretion

Oxycodone and its metabolites are excreted primarily via the kidney. The amounts measured in the urine have been reported as follows: free and conjugated oxycodone 8.9%, free noroxycodone 23%, free oxymorphone less than 1%, conjugated oxymorphone 10%, free and conjugated noroxymorphone 14%, reduced free and conjugated metabolites up to 18%. The total plasma clearance was approximately 1.4 L/min in adults.

Special Populations

Elderly (≥ 65 years)

The plasma concentrations of oxycodone are only nominally affected by age, being 15% greater in elderly as compared to young subjects (age 21-45).

Gender

Across individual pharmacokinetic studies, average plasma oxycodone concentrations for female subjects were up to 25% higher than for male subjects on a body weight-adjusted basis. The reason for this difference is unknown *[see Use in Specific Populations (8.8)]*.

Renal Impairment

Data from a pharmacokinetic study involving 13 patients with mild to severe renal dysfunction (creatinine clearance <60 mL/min) showed peak plasma oxycodone and noroxycodone concentrations 50% and 20% higher, respectively, and AUC values for oxycodone, noroxycodone, and oxymorphone 60%, 50%, and 40% higher than normal subjects, respectively. This was accompanied by an increase in sedation but not by differences in respiratory rate, pupillary constriction, or several other measures of drug effect. There was an increase in mean elimination $t_{1/2}$ for oxycodone of 1 hour.

Hepatic Impairment

Data from a study involving 24 patients with mild to moderate hepatic dysfunction show peak plasma oxycodone and noroxycodone concentrations 50% and 20% higher, respectively, than healthy subjects. AUC values are 95% and 65% higher, respectively. Oxymorphone peak plasma concentrations and AUC values are lower by 30% and 40%. These differences are accompanied by increases in some, but not other, drug effects. The mean elimination $t_{1/2}$ for oxycodone increased by 2.3 hours.

Drug-Drug Interactions

CYP3A4 Inhibitors

CYP3A4 is the major enzyme involved in noroxycodone formation. Co-administration of OxyContin (10 mg single dose) and the CYP3A4 inhibitor ketoconazole (200 mg BID) increased oxycodone AUC and C_{max} by 170% and 100%, respectively *[see Drug Interactions (7.3)]*.

CYP3A4 Inducers

A published study showed that the co-administration of rifampin, a drug metabolizing enzyme inducer, decreased oxycodone AUC and C_{max} values by 86% and 63%, respectively *[see Drug Interactions (7.3)]*.

CYP2D6 Inhibitors

Oxycodone is metabolized in part to oxymorphone via CYP2D6. While this pathway may be blocked by a variety of drugs such as certain cardiovascular drugs (e.g., quinidine) and antidepressants (e.g., fluoxetine), such blockade has not been shown to be of clinical significance with OxyContin *[see Drug Interactions (7.3)]*.

13 NONCLINICAL TOXICOLOGY

13.1 Carcinogenesis, Mutagenesis, Impairment of Fertility

Carcinogenesis

No animal studies to evaluate the carcinogenic potential of oxycodone have been conducted.

Mutagenesis

Oxycodone was genotoxic in the mouse lymphoma assay at concentrations of 50 mcg/mL or greater with metabolic activation and at 400 mcg/mL or greater without metabolic activation. Clastogenicity was observed with oxycodone in the presence of metabolic activation in one chromosomal aberration assay in human lymphocytes at concentrations greater than or equal to 1250 mcg/mL at 24 but not 48 hours of exposure. In a second chromosomal aberration assay with human lymphocytes, no structural clastogenicity was observed either with or without metabolic activation; however, in the absence of metabolic activation, oxycodone increased numerical chromosomal aberrations (polyploidy). Oxycodone was not genotoxic in the following assays: Ames *S. typhimurium* and *E. coli* test with and without metabolic activation at concentrations up to 5000 μg/plate, chromosomal aberration test in human lymphocytes (in the absence of metabolic activation) at concentrations up to 1500 μg/mL, and with activation after 48 hours of exposure at concentrations up to 5000 μg/mL, and in the *in vivo* bone marrow micronucleus assay in mice (at plasma levels up to 48 μg/mL).

Impairment of Fertility

In a study of reproductive performance, rats were administered a once daily gavage dose of the vehicle or oxycodone hydrochloride (0.5, 2, and 8 mg/kg). Male rats were dosed for 28 days before cohabitation with females, during the cohabitation and until necropsy (2-3 weeks post-cohabitation). Females were dosed for 14 days before cohabitation with males, during cohabitation and up to gestation day 6. Oxycodone hydrochloride did not affect reproductive function in male or female rats at any dose tested (≤ 8 mg/kg/day).

14 CLINICAL STUDIES

A double-blind, placebo-controlled, fixed-dose, parallel group, two-week study was conducted in 133 patients with persistent, moderate to severe pain, who were judged as having inadequate pain control with their current therapy. In this study, OxyContin 20 mg, but not 10 mg, was statistically significant in pain reduction compared with placebo.

16 HOW SUPPLIED/STORAGE AND HANDLING

OxyContin (oxycodone hydrochloride controlled-release) Tablets 10 mg are round, white-colored, bi-convex tablets debossed with OP on one side and 10 on the other and are supplied as child-resistant closure, opaque plastic bottles of 100 (**NDC 59011-410-10**) and unit dose packaging with 10 individually numbered tablets per card; two cards per glue end carton (**NDC 59011-410-20**).

OxyContin (oxycodone hydrochloride controlled-release) Tablets 15 mg are round, gray-colored, bi-convex tablets debossed with OP on one side and 15 on the other and are supplied as child-resistant closure, opaque plastic bottles of 100 (**NDC 59011-415-10**) and unit dose packaging with 10 individually numbered tablets per card; two cards per glue end carton (**NDC 59011-415-20**).

OxyContin (oxycodone hydrochloride controlled-release) Tablets 20 mg are round, pink-colored, bi-convex tablets debossed with OP on one side and 20 on the other and are supplied as child-resistant closure, opaque plastic bottles of 100 (**NDC 59011-420-10**) and unit dose packaging with 10 individually numbered tablets per card; two cards per glue end carton (**NDC 59011-420-20**).

OxyContin (oxycodone hydrochloride controlled-release) Tablets 30 mg are round, brown-colored, bi-convex tablets debossed with OP on one side and 30 on the other and are supplied as child-resistant closure, opaque plastic bottles of 100 (**NDC 59011-430-10**) and unit dose packaging with 10 individually numbered tablets per card; two cards per glue end carton (**NDC 59011-430-20**).

OxyContin (oxycodone hydrochloride controlled-release) Tablets 40 mg are round, yellow-colored, bi-convex tablets debossed with OP on one side and 40 on the other and are supplied as child-resistant closure, opaque plastic bottles of 100 (**NDC 59011-440-10**) and unit dose packaging with 10 individually numbered tablets per card; two cards per glue end carton (**NDC 59011-440-20**).

OxyContin (oxycodone hydrochloride controlled-release) Tablets 60 mg are round, red-colored, bi-convex tablets debossed with OP on one side and 60 on the other and are supplied as child-resistant closure, opaque plastic bottles of 100 (**NDC 59011-460-10**) and unit dose packaging with 10 individually numbered tablets per card; two cards per glue end carton (**NDC 59011-460-20**).

OxyContin (oxycodone hydrochloride controlled-release) Tablets 80 mg are round, green-colored, bi-convex tablets debossed with OP on one side and 80 on the other and are supplied as child-resistant closure, opaque plastic bottles of 100 (**NDC 59011-480-10**) and unit dose packaging with 10 individually numbered tablets per card; two cards per glue end carton (**NDC 59011-480-20**).

Store at 25°C (77°F); excursions permitted between 15°-30°C (59°-86°F).

Dispense in tight, light-resistant container.

CAUTION

DEA FORM REQUIRED

17 PATIENT COUNSELING INFORMATION

See FDA-approved patient labeling (Medication Guide)

Abuse Potential

Inform patients that OxyContin contains oxycodone, a Schedule II controlled substance that is subject to abuse. Instruct patients not to share OxyContin with others and to take steps to protect OxyContin from theft or misuse.

Life-Threatening Respiratory Depression

Discuss the risk of respiratory depression with patients, explaining that the risk is greatest when starting OxyContin or when the dose is increased. Advise patients how to recognize respiratory depression and to seek medical attention if they are experiencing breathing difficulties.

Accidental Exposure

Instruct patients to take steps to store OxyContin securely. Accidental exposure, especially in children, may result in serious harm or death. Advise patients to dispose of unused OxyContin by flushing the tablets down the toilet.

Risks from Concomitant Use of Alcohol and other CNS Depressants

Inform patients that the concomitant use of alcohol with OxyContin can increase the risk of life-threatening respiratory depression. Instruct patients not to consume alcoholic beverages, as well as prescription and over-the-counter drug products that contain alcohol, during treatment with OxyContin.

Inform patients that potentially serious additive effects may occur if OxyContin is used with other CNS depressants, and not to use such drugs unless supervised by a health care provider.

Important Administration Instructions

Instruct patients how to properly take OxyContin, including the following:

- OxyContin is designed to work properly only if swallowed intact. Taking cut, broken, chewed, crushed, or dissolved OxyContin tablets can result in a fatal overdose.
- OxyContin tablets should be taken one tablet at a time.
- Do not pre-soak, lick or otherwise wet the tablet prior to placing in the mouth.
- Take each tablet with enough water to ensure complete swallowing immediately after placing in the mouth.

Hypotension

Inform patients that OxyContin may cause orthostatic hypotension and syncope. Instruct patients how to recognize symptoms of low blood pressure and how to reduce the risk of serious consequences should hypotension occur (e.g., sit or lie down, carefully rise from a sitting or lying position).

Driving or Operating Heavy Machinery

Inform patients that OxyContin may impair the ability to perform potentially hazardous activities such as driving a car or operating heavy machinery. Advise patients not to perform such tasks until they know how they will react to the medication.

Constipation

Advise patients of the potential for severe constipation, including management instructions and when to seek medical attention.

Anaphylaxis

Inform patients that anaphylaxis has been reported with ingredients contained in OxyContin. Advise patients how to recognize such a reaction and when to seek medical attention.

Pregnancy

Advise female patients that OxyContin can cause fetal harm and to inform the prescriber if they are pregnant or plan to become pregnant.

Healthcare professionals can telephone Purdue Pharma's Medical Services Department (1-888-726-7535) for information on this product.

Purdue Pharma L.P.

Stamford, CT 06901-3431

U.S. Patent Numbers 6,488,963; 7,129,248; 7,674,799; 7,674,800; 7,683,072; 7,776,314; 8,114,383; 8,309,060; and 8,337,888.

Medication Guide

OXYCONTIN® (ox-e-KON-tin)

(oxycodone hydrochloride controlled-release) Tablets, CII

OXYCONTIN is:

- A strong prescription pain medicine that contains an opioid (narcotic) that is used to treat moderate to severe around-the-clock pain.

Important information about OXYCONTIN:

- Get emergency help right away if you take too much OXYCONTIN (overdose). OXYCONTIN overdose can cause life-threatening breathing problems that can lead to death.
- Never give anyone else your OXYCONTIN. They could die from taking it. Store OXYCONTIN away from children and in a safe place to prevent stealing or abuse. Selling or giving away OXYCONTIN is against the law.

Do not take OXYCONTIN if you have:

- severe asthma, trouble breathing, or other lung problems.

- a bowel blockage or have narrowing of the stomach or intestines.

Before taking OXYCONTIN, tell your healthcare provider if you have a history of:
- head injury, seizures
- liver, kidney, thyroid problems
- problems urinating
- pancreas or gallbladder problems
- abuse of street or prescription drugs, alcohol addiction, or mental health problems.

Tell your healthcare provider if you are:
- **pregnant or planning to become pregnant.** OXYCONTIN may harm your unborn baby.
- **breastfeeding.** OXYCONTIN passes into breast milk and may harm your baby.
- taking prescription or over-the-counter medicines, vitamins, or herbal supplements.

When taking OXYCONTIN:
- Do not change your dose. Take OXYCONTIN exactly as prescribed by your healthcare provider.
- Take each dose every 12 hours at the same time every day. If you miss a dose, take OXYCONTIN as soon as possible and then take your next dose 12 hours later. If it is almost time for your next dose, skip the missed dose and go back to your regular dosing schedule. Do not take more than 1 dose in 12 hours.
- Swallow OXYCONTIN whole. Do not cut, break, chew, crush, dissolve, or inject OXYCONTIN.
- OXYCONTIN should be taken 1 tablet at a time. Do not pre-soak, lick, or wet the tablet before placing in your mouth.
- **Call your healthcare provider if the dose you are taking does not control your pain.**
- **Do not stop taking OXYCONTIN without talking to your healthcare provider.**
- After you stop taking OXYCONTIN, flush any unused tablets down the toilet.

While taking OXYCONTIN Do Not:
- Drive or operate heavy machinery, until you know how OXYCONTIN affects you. OXYCONTIN can make you sleepy, dizzy, or lightheaded.
- Drink alcohol or use prescription or over-the-counter medicines that contain alcohol.

The possible side effects of OXYCONTIN are:
- constipation, nausea, sleepiness, vomiting, tiredness, headache, dizziness, abdominal pain. Call your healthcare provider if you have any of these symptoms and they are severe.

Get emergency medical help if you have:
- trouble breathing, shortness of breath, fast heartbeat, chest pain, swelling of your face, tongue or throat, extreme drowsiness, or you are feeling faint.

These are not all the possible side effects of OXYCONTIN. Call your doctor for medical advice about side effects. You may report side effects to FDA at 1-800-FDA-1088. **For more information go to dailymed.nlm.nih.gov**

Manufactured by: Purdue Pharma L.P., Stamford, CT 06901-3431, **www.purduepharma.com or call 1-888-726-7535**

This Medication Guide has been approved by the U.S. Food and Drug Administration. Issue: July 2012

Shown in Product Identification Guide, page 312

Ranbaxy Laboratories Inc.

9431 FLORIDA MINING BOULEVARD EAST
JACKSONVILLE, FL 32257

Main Phone: (609) 720-9200

ABSORICA™ ℞
(isotretinoin)
capsules, for oral use

HIGHLIGHTS OF PRESCRIBING INFORMATION
These highlights do not include all the information needed to use ABSORICA™ safely and effectively. See full prescribing information for ABSORICA™.
ABSORICA™ (isotretinoin) capsules, for oral use
Initial U.S. Approval: 1982

WARNING: CAUSES BIRTH DEFECTS
See full prescribing information for complete boxed warning.
Pregnancy Category X.
- **Absorica™ must not be used by female patients who are or may become pregnant (5, 8.1, 8.6).**
- **There is an extremely high risk that severe birth defects will result if pregnancy occurs while taking Absorica™ in any amount, even for short periods of time. Potentially any fetus exposed during pregnancy can be affected (5.1, 8.1).**
- **There are no accurate means of determining whether an exposed fetus has been affected (5.1, 8.1).**
- **Absorica™ is available only through a restricted program called the iPLEDGE program. Prescribers, patients, pharmacies, and distributors must enroll in the program (5.2).**

INDICATIONS AND USAGE
Absorica™ is a retinoid indicated for the treatment of severe recalcitrant nodular acne in patients 12 years of age and older (1).
Limitations of Use
Absorica™ may only be administered to patients enrolled in the iPLEDGE program (1, 5.2).

DOSAGE AND ADMINISTRATION
- Recommended dosage of 0.5 to 1 mg/kg/day given in two divided doses without regards to meals for 15 to 20 weeks (2.1).
- Once daily dosing is **not** recommended (2.1).
- Perform pregnancy tests prior to prescribing, each month during therapy, end of therapy, and one month after discontinuation (2.4, 8.6).
- Prior to prescribing, perform fasting lipid profile and liver function tests (2.4).
- Absorica™ is not substitutable with other forms of isotretinoin (12.3).

DOSAGE FORMS AND STRENGTHS
Capsules: 10 mg, 20 mg, 30 mg and 40 mg (3)

CONTRAINDICATIONS
- Pregnancy (4.1, 8.1)
- Hypersensitivity to this product or any of its components (4.2, 5.14)

WARNINGS AND PRECAUTIONS
- Unacceptable Contraception: Micro-dosed progesterone preparations are not an acceptable method of contraception during Absorica™ therapy (5.3)
- Psychiatric Disorders: Depression, psychosis, suicidal thoughts and behavior, and aggressive and/or violent behaviors (5.4)
- Pseudotumor cerebri, some cases with concomitant tetracyclines (5.5)
- Serious skin reactions: Stevens-Johnson syndrome (SJS), toxic epidermal necrolysis (TEN) (5.6)
- Acute pancreatitis, rarely fatal hemorrhagic pancreatitis, in patients with either elevated or normal serum triglyceride levels (5.7)
- Lipid Abnormalities: Triglyceridemia low HDL and elevation of cholesterol. Monitor lipid levels at regular intervals (5.8, 5.15)
- Hearing Impairment (5.9)
- Hepatotoxicity: Monitor liver function tests at regular intervals (5.10, 5.15)
- Inflammatory Bowel Disease (5.11)
- Skeletal Abnormalities: Arthralgias, back pain, decreases in bone mineral density and premature epiphyseal closure (5.12)
- Ocular Abnormalities: corneal opacities, decreased night vision (5.13)
- Glucose and CPK Abnormalities (5.15)

ADVERSE REACTIONS
Most common adverse reactions (incidence ≥5%) are: lip dry, dry skin, back pain, dry eye, arthralgia, epistaxis, headache, nasopharyngitis, chapped lips, dermatitis, blood creatine kinase increased, cheilitis, musculoskeletal discomfort, upper respiratory tract infection, visual acuity reduced (6.1).

To report SUSPECTED ADVERSE REACTIONS, contact Ranbaxy, Inc. at 1-800-406-7984 or FDA at 1-800-FDA-1088 or *www.fda.gov/medwatch* or iPLEDGE at (1-866-495-0654 and *www.ipledgeprogram.com*).

DRUG INTERACTIONS
- Vitamin A: may cause additive adverse reactions (7.1)
- Tetracyclines: avoid concomitant use (7.2)
- St. John's Wort: may interfere with oral contraceptives (7.4)

See 17 for PATIENT COUNSELING INFORMATION
Revised: 05/2012

FULL PRESCRIBING INFORMATION: CONTENTS*

*** Sections or subsections omitted from the full prescribing information are not listed**

FULL PRESCRIBING INFORMATION

WARNING: CAUSES BIRTH DEFECTS
Pregnancy Category X.
- **Absorica™ must not be used by female patients who are or may become pregnant [(See *Warnings and Precautions* (5) and *Use in Specific Populations* (8.1, 8.6)].**

- **There is an extremely high risk that severe birth defects will result if pregnancy occurs while taking Absorica™ in any amount, even for short periods of time [See *Warnings and Precautions* (5.1) and *Use in Specific Populations* (8.1)].**
- **Potentially any fetus exposed during pregnancy can be affected [See *Use in Specific Populations* (8.1)].**
- **There are no accurate means of determining whether an exposed fetus has been affected [See *Warning and Precautions* (5.1) and *Use in Specific Populations* (8.1)].**
- **Birth defects which have been documented following isotretinoin exposure include abnormalities of the face, eyes, ears, skull, central nervous system, cardiovascular system, and thymus and parathyroid glands. Cases of IQ scores less than 85 with or without other abnormalities have been reported. There is an increased risk of spontaneous abortion and premature births have been reported [See *Use in Specific Populations* (8.1)].**
- **Documented external abnormalities include: skull abnormality; ear abnormalities (including anotia, micropinna, small or absent external auditory canals); eye abnormalities (including microphthalmia); facial dysmorphia; cleft palate. Documented internal abnormalities include: CNS abnormalities (including cerebral abnormalities, cerebellar malformation, hydrocephalus, microcephaly, cranial nerve deficit); cardiovascular abnormalities; thymus gland abnormality; parathyroid hormone deficiency. In some cases death has occurred with certain abnormalities previously noted [See *Use in Specific Populations* (8.1)].**
- **If pregnancy does occur during the treatment of a female patient who is taking Absorica™, Absorica™ must be discontinued immediately and she should be referred to an obstetrician-gynecologist experienced in reproductive toxicity for further evaluation and counseling [See *Use in Specific Populations* (8.1)].**

Special Prescribing Requirements

- **Because of the risk of teratogenicity and to minimize fetal exposure, Absorica™ is available only through a restricted program under a Risk Evaluation and Mitigation Strategy (REMS) called iPLEDGE™. Under the Absorica™ REMS, prescribers, patients, pharmacies, and distributors must enroll and be registered in the program [See *Warnings and Precautions* (5.2)].**

1 INDICATIONS AND USAGE

Absorica™ is a retinoid indicated for the treatment of severe recalcitrant nodular acne in patients 12 years of age and older. Nodules are inflammatory lesions with a diameter of 5 mm or greater. The nodules may become suppurative or hemorrhagic. "Severe," by definition, means "many" as opposed to "few or several" nodules. Because of significant adverse reactions associated with its use, Absorica™ should be reserved for patients with multiple severe nodular acne who are unresponsive to conventional therapy, including systemic antibiotics. In addition, Absorica™ is indicated only for those female patients who are not pregnant, because Absorica™ can cause severe birth defects [see *Contraindications* (4.1)].

Limitations of Use

A single course of therapy for 15 to 20 weeks has been shown to result in complete and prolonged remission of disease in many patients. If a second course of therapy is needed, it should not be initiated until at least 8 weeks after completion of the first course, because experience with isotretinoin has shown that patients may continue to improve following treatment with isotretinoin. The optimal interval before retreatment has not been defined for patients who have not completed skeletal growth [see *Warnings and Precautions* (5.12)].

As a part of the iPLEDGE program, Absorica™ may only be administered to patients enrolled in the program [see *Warnings and Precautions* (5.2)].

2 DOSAGE AND ADMINISTRATION

Healthcare professionals who prescribe Absorica™ must be certified in the iPLEDGE program and must comply with the required monitoring to ensure safe use of Absorica™ [see *Warnings and Precautions* (5.2)].

The required laboratory testing must be completed prior to dosing Absorica™ [see *Dosage and Administration* (2.4)].

Pregnancy Testing, and Contraceptive measures must be followed prior to dosing Absorica™ [see *Use in Specific Populations* (8.6)].

2.1 Recommended Dosage

The recommended dosage range for Absorica™ is 0.5 to 1 mg/kg/day given in two divided doses without regard to meals for 15 to 20 weeks (see Table 1). To decrease the risk of esophageal irritation, patients should swallow the capsules with a full glass of liquid [see *Patient Counseling Information* (17.1)].

The safety of once daily dosing with Absorica™ has not been established. Once daily dosing is **not** recommended.

Table 1: Absorica™ Dosing by Body Weight (Based on Administration With or Without Food)

Body Weight		Total Daily (mg)		
Kilograms	Pounds	0.5 mg/kg	1 mg/kg	2 mg/kg
40	88	20	40	80
50	110	25	50	100
60	132	30	60	120
70	154	35	70	140
80	176	40	80	160
90	198	45	90	180
100	220	50	100	200

2.2 Dosage Range

In trials comparing 0.1, 0.5, and 1 mg/kg/day, it was found that all dosages provided initial clearing of disease, but there was a greater need for retreatment with the lower dosages. During treatment, the dose may be adjusted according to response of the disease and/or the appearance of clinical side effects, some of which may be dose-related. Adult patients whose disease is very severe with scarring or is primarily manifested on the trunk may require dose adjustments up to 2 mg/kg/day, as tolerated.

2.3 Duration of Use

A normal course of treatment is 15 – 20 weeks. If the total nodule count has been reduced by more than 70% prior to completing 15 to 20 weeks of treatment, the drug may be discontinued. After a period of 2 months or more off therapy, and if warranted by persistent or recurring severe nodular acne, a second course of therapy may be initiated. The optimal interval before retreatment has not been defined for patients who have not completed skeletal growth. Long-term use of Absorica™, even in low doses, has not been studied, and is not recommended. It is important that Absorica™ be given at the recommended doses for no longer than the recommended duration. The effect of long-term use of Absorica™ on bone loss is unknown [see *Warnings and Precautions* (5.12)].

2.4 Laboratory Testing

Pregnancy Testing

[see *Use in Specific Populations* (8.6)]

Lipid Profile

Perform a fasting lipid profile including triglycerides prior to use of Absorica™ [see *Warnings and Precautions* (5.8, 5.15)].

Liver Function Test

Perform liver function tests prior to use of Absorica™ [see *Warnings and Precautions* (5.10, 5.15)].

3 DOSAGE FORMS AND STRENGTHS

Absorica™ is available in 10 mg, 20 mg, 30 mg and 40 mg capsules.

- **10 mg capsules:** Dark yellow capsule imprinted with black ink "**G 240**" on cap and "**10**" on the body
- **20 mg capsules:** Red opaque capsule imprinted with black ink "**G 241**" on cap and "**20**" on the body
- **30 mg capsules:** Brown opaque capsule imprinted with white ink "**G 242**" on cap and "**30**" on the body
- **40 mg capsules:** Brown and red capsule imprinted with white ink "**G 325**" on cap and "**40**" on the body

4 CONTRAINDICATIONS

4.1 Pregnancy

Absorica™ can cause fetal harm when administered to a pregnant woman. Major congenital malformations, spontaneous abortions, and premature births have been documented following pregnancy exposure to isotretinoin in any amount and even for short periods of time. Absorica™ is contraindicated in females who are or may become pregnant. If this drug is used during pregnancy, or if the patient becomes pregnant while taking this drug, treatment should be discontinued and the patient should be apprised of the potential hazard to the fetus [see *Use in Specific Populations* (8.1)].

4.2 Hypersensitivity

Hypersensitivity to this product (or Vitamin A, given the chemical similarity to isotretinoin) or to any of its components [see *Warnings and Precautions* (5.14)].

5 WARNINGS AND PRECAUTIONS

Absorica™ must not be used by female patients who are or may become pregnant. There is an extremely high risk that severe birth defects will result if pregnancy occurs while taking Absorica™ in any amount, even for short periods of time.

5.1 Embryofetal Toxicity

Teratogenicity

Major congenital malformations, spontaneous abortions, and premature births have been documented following pregnancy exposure to isotretinoin [see *Use in Specific Populations* (8.1)]. Females of childbearing potential must comply with the pregnancy testing and contraception requirements described in the iPLEDGE program [see *Warnings and Precautions* (5.2) and *Use in Specific Populations* (8.6)]. There are no accurate means of determining whether an exposed fetus has been affected.

No Blood Donation

Patients must be informed not to donate blood during isotretinoin therapy and for 1 month following discontinuation of the drug because the blood might be given to a pregnant female patient whose fetus must not be exposed to isotretinoin.

5.2 iPLEDGE Program

Because of the risk of teratogenicity and to minimize fetal exposure, Absorica™ is available only through a restricted program under a REMS called iPLEDGE. Under the Absorica™ REMS, prescribers, patients, pharmacies, and distributors must enroll and be registered in the program. Absorica™ must not be prescribed, dispensed or otherwise obtained through the internet or any other means outside of the iPLEDGE program. Only FDA-approved isotretinoin products must be distributed, prescribed, dispensed, and used.

Required components of the iPLEDGE Program are:

- Absorica™ must only be prescribed by prescribers who are registered and activated with the iPLEDGE program and agree to comply with the REMS requirements described in the booklets entitled *The Guide to Best Practices for the iPLEDGE Program, The iPLEDGE Program Prescriber Contraception Counseling Guide,* and *Recognizing Psychiatric Disorders in Adolescents and Young Adults: A Guide for Prescribers of Isotretinoin.*
- Male patients and Female patients not of childbearing potential: To obtain Absorica™, these patients must understand the risks and benefits of Absorica™, comply with the REMS requirements described in the booklet entitled *The iPLEDGE Program Guide to Isotretinoin for Male Patients and Female Patients Who Cannot Get Pregnant,* and sign a Patient Information/Informed Consent form.
- Female patients of childbearing potential: Absorica™ is contraindicated in female patients who are or may become pregnant [see *Contraindications* (4.1)].
- Female patients of childbearing potential who are not pregnant must understand the risks and benefits, comply with the REMS requirements described in the booklet entitled *The iPLEDGE Program Guide to Isotretinoin for Female Patients Who Can Get Pregnant* and *The iPLEDGE Program Birth Control Workbook* (including the pregnancy testing and contraception requirements [see *Use in Specific Populations* (8.6) and *Patient Counseling Information* (17.1)]), and sign a Patient Information/Informed Consent form and Patient Information/ Informed Consent About Birth Defects form. Additionally, the patient must answer questions about the iPLEDGE program and pregnancy prevention monthly.
- Pharmacies that dispense Absorica™ must be registered and activated with iPLEDGE, must only dispense to patients who are authorized to receive Absorica™, and agree to comply with the REMS requirements described in the booklet entitled *The Pharmacist Guide for the iPLEDGE Program.*
- Female patients of childbearing potential must fill and pick up the prescription within 7 days of the specimen collection for the pregnancy test; male patients and female patients not of childbearing potential must fill and pick up the prescription within 30 days of the office visit.
- Absorica™ must only be dispensed in no more than a 30-day supply with a Medication Guide. Refills require a new prescription and a new authorization from the iPLEDGE system.
- Wholesalers and distributors that distribute Absorica™ must be registered with iPLEDGE and agree to comply with the REMS requirements.

If a pregnancy does occur during Absorica™ treatment, Absorica™ must be discontinued immediately. The patient should be referred to an obstetrician-gynecologist experienced in reproductive toxicity for further evaluation and counseling. Any suspected fetal exposure during or 1 month after Absorica™ therapy must be reported immediately to the FDA via the MedWatch telephone number 1-800-FDA-1088 and also to the iPLEDGE pregnancy registry at 1-866-495-0654 or via the internet (*www.ipledgeprogram.com*). Further information, including a list of qualified pharmacies, is available at *www.ipledgeprogram.com* or 1-866-495-0654.

5.3 Unacceptable Contraception

Micro-dosed Progesterone Preparations

Micro-dosed progesterone preparations ("minipills" that do not contain an estrogen) are an inadequate method of contraception during Absorica™ therapy.

5.4 Psychiatric Disorders

Isotretinoin may cause depression, psychosis and, rarely, suicidal ideation, suicide attempts, suicide, and aggressive and/or violent behaviors. No mechanism of action has been established for these reactions [see *Adverse Reactions* (6.1)]. Prescribers should read the brochure, *Recognizing Psychiatric Disorders in Adolescents and Young Adults: A Guide for Prescribers of Isotretinoin.* Prescribers should be alert to the warning signs of psychiatric disorders to guide patients to receive the help they need. Therefore, prior to initiation of Absorica™ therapy, patients and family members should be asked about any history of psychiatric disorder, and at each visit during therapy patients should be assessed for symptoms of depression, mood disturbance, psychosis, or aggression to determine if further evaluation may be necessary. Signs and symptoms of depression, as described in the brochure (*Recognizing Psychiatric Disorders in Adolescents and Young Adults*), include sad mood, hopelessness, feelings of guilt, worthlessness or helplessness, loss of pleasure or interest in activities, fatigue, difficulty concentrating, change in sleep pattern, change in weight or appetite, suicidal thoughts or attempts, restlessness, irritability, acting on dangerous impulses, and persistent physical symptoms unresponsive to treatment. Patients should stop Absorica™ and the patient or a family member should promptly contact their prescriber if the patient develops depression, mood disturbance, psychosis, or aggression, without waiting until the next visit. Discontinuation of Absorica™ therapy may be insufficient; further evaluation may be necessary. While such monitoring may be helpful, it may not detect all patients at risk. Patients may report mental health problems or family history of psychiatric disorders. These reports should be discussed with the patient and/or the patient's family. A referral to a mental health professional may be necessary. The physician should consider whether Absorica™ therapy is appropriate in this setting; for some patients the risks may outweigh the benefits of Absorica™ therapy.

5.5 Pseudotumor Cerebri

Isotretinoin use has been associated with cases of pseudotumor cerebri (benign intracranial hypertension), some of which involved concomitant use of tetracyclines. Concomitant treatment with tetracyclines should therefore be avoided. Early signs and symptoms of pseudotumor cerebri include papilledema, headache, nausea and vomiting, and visual disturbances. Patients with these symptoms should be screened for papilledema and, if present, they should be told to discontinue Absorica™ immediately and be referred to a neurologist for further diagnosis and care [see *Adverse Reactions* (6.1)].

5.6 Serious Skin Reactions

There have been post-marketing reports of erythema multiforme and severe skin reactions [e.g., Stevens-Johnson syndrome (SJS), toxic epidermal necrolysis (TEN)] associated with isotretinoin use. These reactions may be serious and result in death, life-threatening events, hospitalization, or disability. Patients should be monitored closely for severe skin reactions, and discontinuation of Absorica™ should be considered if warranted.

5.7 Pancreatitis

Acute pancreatitis has been reported in isotretinoin-treated patients with either elevated or normal serum triglyceride levels. In rare instances, fatal hemorrhagic pancreatitis has been reported. Absorica™ should be stopped if hypertriglyceridemia cannot be controlled at an acceptable level or if symptoms of pancreatitis occur.

5.8 Lipid Abnormalities

Elevations of serum triglycerides in excess of 800 mg/dL have been reported in patients treated with isotretinoin. Marked elevations of serum triglycerides were reported in approximately 25% of patients receiving isotretinoin in clinical trials. In addition, approximately 15% developed a decrease in high-density lipoproteins and about 7% showed an increase in cholesterol levels. In clinical trials, the effects of triglycerides, HDL and cholesterol were reversible upon cessation of isotretinoin therapy. Some patients have been able to reverse triglyceride elevation by reduction in weight, restriction of dietary fat and alcohol, and reduction in the dose while continuing isotretinoin.

Blood lipid determinations should be performed before Absorica™ is given and then at intervals until the lipid response to Absorica™ is established, which usually occurs within 4 weeks. Especially careful consideration must be given to risk/benefit for patients who may be at high risk of triglyceridemia during Absorica™ therapy (patients with diabetes, obesity, increased alcohol intake, lipid metabolism disorder or familial history of lipid metabolism disorder). If Absorica™ therapy is instituted, more frequent checks of serum values for lipids and/or blood sugar are recommended [see *Warnings and Precautions* (5.15)].

The cardiovascular consequences of hypertriglyceridemia associated with isotretinoin are unknown.

5.9 Hearing Impairment

Impaired hearing has been reported in patients taking isotretinoin; in some cases, the hearing impairment has been reported to persist after therapy has been discontinued. Mechanism(s) and causality for this reaction have not been established. Patients who experience tinnitus or hearing impairment should discontinue Absorica™ treatment and be referred for specialized care for further evaluation. [see *Adverse Reactions* (6.1)].

5.10 Hepatotoxicity

Clinical hepatitis considered to be possibly or probably related to isotretinoin therapy has been reported. Additionally, mild to moderate elevations of liver enzymes have been observed in approximately 15% of individuals treated during clinical trials with isotretinoin, some of which normalized with dosage reduction or continued administration of the drug. If normalization does not readily occur or if hepatitis is suspected during treatment with Absorica™, the drug should be discontinued and the etiology further investigated.

5.11 Inflammatory Bowel Disease

Isotretinoin has been associated with inflammatory bowel disease (including regional ileitis) in patients without a prior history of intestinal disorders. In some instances, symptoms have been reported to persist after isotretinoin treatment has been stopped. Patients experiencing abdominal pain, rectal bleeding or severe diarrhea should discontinue Absorica™ immediately [see *Adverse Reactions* (6.1)].

5.12 Skeletal Abnormalities

Bone Mineral Density Changes

Isotretinoin may have a negative effect on bone mineral density (BMD) in some patients. In a clinical trial of Absorica™ and a generic product of Accutane® (isotretinoin), 27/306 (8.8%) of adolescents had BMD declines, defined as ≥ 4% lumbar spine or total hip, or ≥ 5% femoral neck, during the 20 week treatment period. Repeat scans conducted within 2-3 months after the post-treatment scan showed no recovery of BMD. Longer term data at 4–11 months showed that 3 out of 7 patients had total hip and femoral neck BMD below pre-treatment baseline, and 2 others did not show the increase in BMD above baseline expected in this adolescent population. Therefore, physicians should use caution when prescribing Absorica™ to patients with a history of childhood osteoporosis conditions, osteomalacia, or other disorders of bone metabolism. This would include patients diagnosed with anorexia nervosa and those who are on chronic drug therapy that causes drug-induced osteoporosis/osteomalacia and/or affects vitamin D metabolism, such as systemic corticosteroids and any anticonvulsant [see *Use in Specific Populations* (8.4)].

Musculoskeletal Abnormalities

Approximately 16% of patients treated with isotretinoin in a clinical trial developed musculoskeletal symptoms (including arthralgia) during treatment. In general, these symptoms were mild to moderate, but occasionally required discontinuation of the drug.

In a trial of pediatric patients treated with isotretinoin, approximately 29% (104/358) developed back pain. Back pain was severe in 13.5% (14/104) of the cases and occurred at a higher frequency in female patients than male patients. Arthralgias were experienced in 22% (79/358) of pediatric patients. Arthralgias were severe in 7.6% (6/79) of patients. Appropriate evaluation of the musculoskeletal system should be done in patients who present with these symptoms during or after a course of Absorica™. Consideration should be given to discontinuation of Absorica™ if any significant abnormality is found.

There have been spontaneous reports of osteoporosis, osteopenia, bone fractures and/or delayed healing of bone fractures in patients while on therapy with isotretinoin or following cessation of therapy with isotretinoin. While causality to isotretinoin has not been established, an effect cannot be ruled out.

Patients may be at an increased risk when participating in sports with repetitive impact where the risks of spondylolisthesis with and without pars fractures and hip growth plate injures in early and late adolescence are known.

Effects of multiple courses of isotretinoin on the developing musculoskeletal system are unknown. There is some evidence that long-term, high-dose, or multiple courses of therapy with isotretinoin have more of an effect than a single course of therapy on the musculoskeletal system.

Longer term effects have not been studied. It is important that Absorica™ be given at the recommended doses for no longer than the recommended duration.

Hyperostosis

A high prevalence of skeletal hyperostosis was noted in clinical trials for disorders of keratinization with a mean dose of 2.24 mg/kg/day of isotretinoin. Additionally, skeletal hyperostosis was noted in 6 of 8 patients in a prospective trial of disorders of keratinization. Minimal skeletal hyperostosis and calcification of ligaments and tendons have also been observed by x-ray in prospective trials of nodular acne patients treated with a single course of therapy at recommended doses. The skeletal effects of multiple isotretinoin treatment courses for acne are unknown.

In a clinical trial of 217 pediatric patients (12 to 17 years) with severe recalcitrant nodular acne, hyperostosis was not observed after 16 to 20 weeks of treatment with approximately 1 mg/kg/day of isotretinoin given in two divided doses. Hyperostosis may require a longer time frame to appear. The clinical course and significance remain unknown.

Premature Epiphyseal Closure

There are spontaneous literature reports of premature epiphyseal closure in acne patients receiving recommended doses of isotretinoin. The effect of multiple courses of isotretinoin on epiphyseal closure is unknown.

In a 20-week clinical trial that included 289 adolescents on Absorica™ or a generic product of Accutane® (isotretinoin) who had hand radiographs taken to assess bone age, a total of 9 (3.11%) patients had bone age changes that were clinically significant and for which a drug-related effect cannot be excluded.

5.13 Ocular Abnormalities

Visual problems should be carefully monitored. All Absorica™ patients experiencing visual difficulties should discontinue Absorica™ treatment and have an ophthalmological examination [see *Adverse Reactions* (6.1)].

Corneal Opacities

Corneal opacities have occurred in patients receiving isotretinoin for acne and more frequently when higher drug dosages were used in patients with disorders of keratinization. The corneal opacities that have been observed in clinical trial patients treated with isotretinoin have either completely resolved or were resolving at follow-up 6 to 7 weeks after discontinuation of the drug [see *Adverse Reactions* (6.1)].

Decreased Night Vision

Decreased night vision has been reported during isotretinoin therapy and in some instances the event has persisted after therapy was discontinued. Because the onset in some patients was sudden, patients should be advised of this potential problem and warned to be cautious when driving or operating any vehicle at night.

Dry Eye

Dry eye has been reported in subjects during isotretinoin therapy. Patients who wear contact lenses may have trouble wearing them while on Absorica™ treatment and afterwards.

5.14 Hypersensitivity

Anaphylactic reactions and other allergic reactions have been reported in isotretinoin-treated patients. Cutaneous allergic reactions and serious cases of allergic vasculitis, often with purpura (bruises and red patches) of the extremities and extracutaneous involvement (including renal) have been reported. Severe allergic reaction necessitates discontinuation of therapy and appropriate medical management.

5.15 Laboratory Monitoring for Adverse Reactions

Lipids Test

Pretreatment and follow-up blood lipids should be obtained under fasting conditions. After consumption of alcohol, at least 36 hours should elapse before these determinations are made. It is recommended that these tests be performed at weekly or biweekly intervals until the lipid response to Absorica™ is established. The incidence of hypertriglyceridemia is 1 patient in 4 on isotretinoin [see *Warnings and Precautions* (5.8)].

Liver Function Test

Since elevations of liver enzymes have been observed during clinical trials, and hepatitis has been reported in patients on isotretinoin, pretreatment and follow-up liver function tests should be performed at weekly or biweekly intervals until the response to Absorica™ has been established [see *Warnings and Precautions* (5.10)].

Glucose

Some patients receiving isotretinoin have experienced problems in the control of their blood sugar. In addition, new cases of diabetes have been diagnosed during isotretinoin therapy, although no causal relationship has been established.

CPK

Some patients undergoing vigorous physical activity while on isotretinoin therapy have experienced elevated CPK levels; however, the clinical significance is unknown. There have been rare postmarketing reports of rhabdomyolysis, some associated with strenuous physical activity. In an isotretinoin clinical trial of 924 patients, marked elevations in CPK (≥350 U/L) were observed in approximately 24% of patients. In another clinical trial of 217 pediatric patients (12 – 17 years) elevations in CPK were observed in 12% of patients, including those undergoing strenuous physical activity in association with reported musculoskeletal adverse events such as back pain, arthralgia, limb injury, or muscle sprain. In these patients, approximately half of the CPK elevations returned to normal within 2 weeks and half returned to normal within 4 weeks. No cases of rhabdomyolysis were reported in this clinical trial.

6 ADVERSE REACTIONS

The following adverse reactions with Absorica™ or other isotretinoin products are described in more detail in other sections of the labeling:

- Embryofetal Toxicity [see *Warnings and Precautions* (5.1)]
- Psychiatric Disorders [see *Warnings and Precautions* (5.4)]
- Pseudotumor Cerebri [see *Warnings and Precautions* (5.5)]
- Serious Skin Reactions [see *Warnings and Precautions* (5.6)]
- Pancreatitis [see *Warnings and Precautions* (5.7)]
- Lipid Abnormalities [see *Warnings and Precautions* (5.8)]
- Hearing Impairment [see *Warnings and Precautions* (5.9)]
- Hepatotoxicity [see *Warnings and Precautions* (5.10)]
- Inflammatory Bowel Disease [see *Warnings and Precautions* (5.11)]
- Skeletal Abnormalities [see *Warnings and Precautions* (5.12)]
- Ocular Abnormalities [see *Warnings and Precautions* (5.13)]
- Hypersensitivity [see *Warnings and Precautions* (5.14)]

6.1 Clinical Trials Experience

Because clinical trials are conducted under widely varying conditions, adverse reaction rates observed in the clinical trials of Absorica™ cannot be directly compared to rates in clinical trials of other drugs and may not reflect the rates observed in practice.

The adverse reactions listed below reflect both clinical experience with Absorica™, and consider other adverse reactions that are known from clinical trials and the postmarketing surveillance with oral isotretinoin. The relationship of some of these events to isotretinoin therapy is unknown. Many of the side effects and adverse events seen in patients receiving isotretinoin are similar to those described in patients taking very high doses of vitamin A (dryness of the skin and mucous membranes, e.g., of the lips, nasal passage, and eyes).

Dose Relationship

Cheilitis and hypertriglyceridemia are adverse reactions that are usually dose related. Most adverse reactions reported in clinical trials with isotretinoin were reversible when therapy was discontinued; however, some persisted after cessation of therapy.

Body as a Whole

The following adverse reactions have been reported in a clinical trial conducted with Absorica™ and a generic product of Accutane® (isotretinoin): fatigue, irritability, pain. In addition to the above adverse reactions, the following adverse reactions have been reported with isotretinoin: allergic reactions, including vasculitis, systemic hypersensitivity, edema, lymphadenopathy, weight loss.

Cardiovascular

The following adverse reactions have been reported with isotretinoin: vascular thrombotic disease, stroke, palpitation, tachycardia.

Endocrine/Metabolism and Nutritional

The following adverse reactions have been reported in a clinical trial conducted with Absorica™ and a generic product of Accutane® (isotretinoin): decreased appetite, weight fluctuation, hyperlipidaemia. In addition to the above adverse reactions, the following adverse reactions have been reported with isotretinoin: hypertriglyceridemia, alterations in blood sugar.

Gastrointestinal

The following adverse reactions have been reported in a clinical trial conducted with Absorica™ and a generic product of Accutane® (isotretinoin): lip dry, chapped lips, cheilitis, nausea, constipation, diarrhea, abdominal pain, vomiting. In addition to the above adverse reactions, the following adverse reactions have been reported with isotretinoin: inflammatory bowel disease, hepatitis, pancreatitis, bleeding and inflammation of the gums, colitis, esophagitis/esophageal ulceration, ileitis, and other nonspecific gastrointestinal symptoms.

Hematologic

The following adverse reactions have been reported with isotretinoin: allergic reactions, anemia, thrombocytopenia, neutropenia, rare reports of agranulocytosis.

Infections and infestations

The following adverse reactions have been reported in a clinical trial conducted with Absorica™ and a generic product of Accutane® (isotretinoin): nasopharyngitis, hordeolum, upper respiratory tract infection. In addition to the above adverse reactions, the following adverse reaction has been reported with isotretinoin: infections (including disseminated herpes simplex).

Laboratory Abnormalities

The following changes in laboratory tests have been noted in a clinical trial conducted with Absorica™ and a generic product of Accutane® (isotretinoin): blood creatine phosphokinase (CPK) increased, blood triglycerides increased, alanine aminotransferase (SGPT) increased, aspartate aminotransferase (SGOT) increased, gamma-glutamyltransferase (GGTP) increased, blood cholesterol increased, low density lipoprotein (LDL) increased, white blood cell count decreased, blood alkaline phosphatase increased, blood bilirubin increased, blood glucose increased, high density lipoprotein (HDL) decreased, bone mineral density decreased. In addition to the above adverse reactions, the following adverse reactions have been reported with isotretinoin: increased LDH, elevation of fasting blood sugar, hyperuricemia, decreases in red blood cell parameters, decreases in white blood cell counts (including severe neutropenia and rare reports of agranulocytosis), elevated sedimentation rates, elevated platelet counts, thrombocytopenia, white cells in the urine, proteinuria, microscopic or gross hematuria.

Musculoskeletal and Connective Tissue

The following adverse reactions have been reported in a clinical trial conducted with Absorica™ and a generic product of Accutane® (isotretinoin): decreases in bone mineral density, musculoskeletal symptoms (sometimes severe) including back pain, athralgia, musculoskeletal discomfort, musculoskeletal pain, neck pain, pain in extremity, myalgia, musculoskeletal stiffness [see *Warnings and Precautions* (5.12)]. In addition to the above adverse reactions, the following adverse reactions have been reported with isotretinoin: skeletal hyperostosis, calcification of tendons and ligaments, premature epiphyseal closure, tendonitis, arthritis, transient pain in the chest, and rare reports of rhabdomyolysis.

Neurological

The following adverse reactions have been reported in a clinical trial conducted with Absorica™ and a generic product of Accutane® (isotretinoin): headache, syncope. In addition to the above adverse reactions, other adverse reactions reported with isotretinoin include: pseudotumor cerebri, dizziness, drowsiness, lethargy, malaise, nervousness, paresthesias, seizures, stroke, weakness.

Psychiatric

The following adverse reactions have been reported in clinical trials conducted with Absorica™ and a generic product of Accutane® (isotretinoin): suicidal ideation, insomnia, anxiety, depression, irritability, panic attack, anger, euphoria, violent behaviors, emotional instability. In addition to the above adverse reactions, the following adverse reactions have been reported with isotretinoin: suicide attempts, suicide, aggression, psychosis and hallucination auditory. Of the patients reporting depression, some reported that the depression subsided with discontinuation of therapy and recurred with reinstitution of therapy.

Reproductive System

The following adverse reaction has been reported with isotretinoin: abnormal menses.

Respiratory

The following adverse reactions have been reported in a clinical trial conducted with Absorica™ and a generic product of Accutane® (isotretinoin): epistaxis, nasal dryness. In addition to the above adverse reactions, the following adverse reactions have been reported with isotretinoin: bronchospasms (with or without a history of asthma), respiratory infection, voice alteration.

Skin and Subcutaneous Tissue

The following adverse reactions have been reported in a clinical trial conducted with Absorica™ and a generic product of Accutane® (isotretinoin): dry skin, dermatitis, eczema, rash, dermatitis contact, alopecia, pruritus, sunburn, erythema. In addition to the above adverse reactions, the following adverse reactions have been reported with isotretinoin: acne fulminans, alopecia (which in some cases persists), bruising, dry nose, eruptive xanthomas, erythema multiforme, flushing, fragility of skin, hair abnormalities, hirsutism, hyperpigmentation and hypopigmentation, nail dystrophy, paronychia, peeling of palms and soles, photoallergic/photosensitizing reactions, pruritus, pyogenic granuloma, rash (including facial erythema, seborrhea, and eczema), Stevens-Johnson syndrome, sunburn susceptibility increased, sweating, toxic epidermal necrolysis, urticaria, vasculitis (including Wegener's granulomatosis), abnormal wound healing (delayed healing or exuberant granulation tissue with crusting).

Special Senses

Hearing: The following adverse reactions have been reported with isotretinoin: tinnitus and hearing impairment.

Ocular: The following adverse reactions have been reported in clinical trials conducted with Absorica™ and a generic product of Accutane® (isotretinoin): dry eye, visual acuity reduced, vision blurred, eye pruritis, eye irritation, asthenopia, decreased night vision, ocular hyperemia, increased lacrimation, and conjunctivitis. In addition to the above adverse reactions, the following adverse reactions have been reported with isotretinoin: corneal opacities, decreased night vision which may persist, cataracts, color vision disorder, conjunctivitis, eyelid inflammation, keratitis, optic neuritis, photobia, visual disturbances.

Renal and Urinary

The following adverse reactions have been reported in clinical trials conducted with isotretinoin: glomerulonephritis, nonspecific urogenital findings.

7 DRUG INTERACTIONS

7.1 Vitamin A

Absorica™ is closely related to vitamin A. Therefore, the use of both vitamin A and Absorica™ at the same time may lead to vitamin A side effects. Patients should be advised against taking vitamin supplements containing Vitamin A to avoid additive toxic effects.

7.2 Tetracyclines

Concomitant treatment with Absorica™ and tetracyclines should be avoided because isotretinoin use has been associated with a number of cases of pseudotumor cerebri (benign intracranial hypertension), some of which involved concomitant use of tetracyclines.

7.3 Phenytoin

Isotretinoin has not been shown to alter the pharmacokinetics of phenytoin in a trial in seven healthy volunteers. These results are consistent with the in vitro finding that neither isotretinoin nor its metabolites induce or inhibit the activity of the CYP2C9 human hepatic P450 enzyme. Phenytoin is known to cause osteomalacia. No formal clinical trials have been conducted to assess if there is an interactive effect on bone loss between phenytoin and isotretinoin. Therefore, caution should be exercised when using these drugs together.

7.4 St. John's Wort

Isotretinoin use is associated with depression in some patients. Patients should be prospectively cautioned not to self-medicate with the herbal supplement St. John's Wort because a possible interaction has been suggested with hormonal contraceptives based on reports of breakthrough bleeding on oral contraceptives shortly after starting St. John's Wort. Pregnancies have been reported by users of combined hormonal contraceptives who also used some form of St. John's Wort.

7.5 Systemic Corticosteroids

Systemic corticosteroids are known to cause osteoporosis. No formal clinical trials have been conducted to assess if there is an interactive effect on bone loss between systemic corticosteroids and isotretinoin. Therefore, caution should be exercised when using these drugs together.

7.6 Norethindrone/ethinyl estradiol

In a trial of 31 premenopausal female patients with severe recalcitrant nodular acne receiving Norethindrone/ethinyl estradiol as an oral contraceptive agent, isotretinoin at the recommended dose of 1 mg/kg/day, did not induce clinically relevant changes in the pharmacokinetics of ethinyl estradiol and norethindrone and in the serum levels of progesterone, follicle-stimulating hormone (FSH) and luteinizing hormone (LH). Prescribers are advised to consult the package insert of medication administered concomitantly with hormonal contraceptives, since some medications may decrease the effectiveness of these birth control products.

8 USE IN SPECIFIC POPULATIONS

8.1 Pregnancy

Pregnancy Category X.

Risk Summary

Absorica™ is contraindicated during pregnancy because isotretinoin can cause can cause fetal harm when administered to a pregnant woman. There is an increased risk of major congenital malformations, spontaneous abortions, and premature births following isotretinoin exposure during pregnancy in humans. If this drug is used during pregnancy, or if the patient becomes pregnant while taking the drug, the patient should be apprised of the potential hazard to a fetus.

Clinical Considerations

If pregnancy does occur during treatment of a female patient who is taking Absorica™, Absorica™ must be discontinued immediately and she should be referred to an obstetrician-gynecologist experienced in reproductive toxicity for further evaluation and counseling.

Human Data

Major congenital malformations that have been documented following isotretinoin exposure include malformations of the face, eyes, ears, skull, central nervous system, cardiovascular system, and thymus and parathyroid glands. External malformations include: skull; ear (including anotia, micropinna, small or absent external auditory canals); eye (including microphthalmia); facial dysmorphia and cleft palate. Internal abnormalities include: CNS (including cerebral and cerebellar malformations, hydrocephalus, microcephaly, cranial nerve deficit); cardiovascular; thymus gland; parathyroid hormone deficiency. In some cases death has occurred as a result of the malformations.

Isotretinoin is found in the semen of male patients taking isotretinoin, but the amount delivered to a female partner would be about one million times lower than an oral dose of 40 mg. While the no-effect limit for isotretinoin induced embryopathy is unknown and 20 years of post-marketing reports include four reports with isolated defects compatible with features of retinoid exposed fetuses, two of these reports were incomplete and two had other possible explanations for the defects observed.

Cases of IQ scores less than 85 with or without other abnormalities have been reported. An increased risk of spontaneous abortion and premature births have been documented with isotretinoin exposure during pregnancy.

8.3 Nursing Mothers

It is not known whether this drug is present in human milk. Because many drugs are present in human milk and because of the potential for serious adverse reactions in nursing infants from Absorica™, a decision should be made whether to discontinue nursing or to discontinue the drug, taking into account the importance of the drug to the mother.

8.4 Pediatric Use

The use of Absorica™ in pediatric patients less than 12 years of age has not been studied. The use of Absorica™ for the treatment of severe recalcitrant nodular acne in pediatric patients ages 12 to 17 years should be given careful consideration, especially for those patients where a known metabolic or structural bone disease exists [see *Warnings and Precautions* (5.12)]. Use of Absorica™ in this age group for severe recalcitrant nodular acne is supported by evidence from a clinical trial of Absorica™ compared to a generic product of Accutane® (isotretinoin) in 397 pediatric patients (12 to 17 years). Results from this trial demonstrated that both Absorica™ and the other isotretinoin drug product, at a dose of 1 mg/kg/day given in two divided doses, was effective in treating severe recalcitrant nodular acne in pediatric patients.

In trials with isotretinoin, adverse reactions reported in pediatric patients were similar to those described in adults except for the increased incidence of back pain and arthralgia (both of which were sometimes severe) and myalgia in pediatric patients. In a trial of pediatric patients treated with isotretinoin, approximately 29% (104/358) developed back pain. Back pain was severe in 13.5% (14/104) of the cases and occurred at a higher frequency in female patients than male patients. Arthralgias were experienced in 22% (79/358) of pediatric patients. Arthralgias were severe in 7.6% (6/79) of patients. Appropriate evaluation of the musculoskeletal system should be done in patients who present with these symptoms during or after a course of Absorica™. Consideration should be given to discontinuation of Absorica™ if any significant abnormality is found.

The effect on bone mineral density (BMD) of a 20-week course of therapy with Absorica™ or a generic product of Accutane® (isotretinoin) was evaluated in a double-blind, randomized clinical trial involving 396 adolescents with severe recalcitrant nodular acne (mean age 15.4, range 12-17, 80% males). Following 20 weeks of treatment, there were no statistically significant differences between the treatment groups. The mean changes in BMD from baseline for the overall trial population were 1.8% for lumbar spine, -0.1% for total hip and -0.3% for femoral neck. Mean BMD Z-scores declined from baseline at each of these sites (-0.053, -0.109 and -0.104 respectively). Out of 306 adolescents, 27 (8.8%) had clinically significant BMD declines defined as ≥4% lumbar spine or total hip, or ≥5% femoral neck, including 2 subjects for lumbar spine, 17 for total hip and 20 for femoral neck. Repeat DXA scans within 2-3 months after the post treatment scan showed no recovery of BMD. Longer-term follow up at 4-11 months showed that 3 out of 7 patients had total hip and femoral neck BMD below pretreatment baseline, and 2 others did not show the increase in BMD above baseline expected in this adolescent population. The significance of these changes in regard to long-term bone health and future fracture risk is unknown [see *Warnings and Precautions* (5.12)].

In an open-label clinical trial (N=217) of a single course of therapy with isotretinoin for adolescents with severe recalcitrant nodular acne, bone density measurements at several skeletal sites were not significantly decreased (lumbar spine change >-4% and total hip change >-5%) or were increased in the majority of patients. One patient had a decrease in lumbar spine bone mineral density >4% based on unadjusted data. Sixteen (7.9%) patients had decreases in lumbar spine bone mineral density >4%, and all the other patients (92%) did not have significant decreases or had increases (adjusted for body mass index). Nine patients (4.5%) had a decrease in total hip bone mineral density >5% based on unadjusted data. Twenty-one (10.6%) patients had decreases in total hip bone mineral density >5%, and all the other patients (89%) did not have significant decreases or had increases (adjusted for body mass index). Follow-up trials performed in 8 of the patients with decreased bone mineral density for up to 11 months thereafter demonstrated increasing bone density in 5 patients at the lumbar spine, while the other 3 patients had lumbar spine bone density measurements below baseline values. Total hip bone mineral densities remained below baseline (range –1.6% to –7.6%) in 5 of 8 patients (62.5%).

In a separate open-label extension trial of 10 patients, ages 13 to 18 years, who started a second course of isotretinoin 4 months after the first course, two patients showed a decrease in mean lumbar spine bone mineral density up to 3.25%.

There are spontaneous literature reports of premature epiphyseal closure in acne patients receiving recommended doses of isotretinoin. The effect of multiple courses of isotretinoin on epiphyseal closure is unknown. In a 20-week clinical trial that included 289 adolescents who had hand radiographs taken to assess bone age, a total of 9 patients had bone age changes that were clinically significant and for which a drug-related effect cannot be excluded [see *Warnings and Precautions* (5.12)].

8.5 Geriatric Use

Clinical trials of Absorica™ did not include sufficient numbers of subjects aged 65 years and over to determine whether they respond differently from younger subjects. Although reported clinical experience has not identified differences in responses between elderly and younger patients, effects of aging might be expected to increase some risks associated with Absorica™ therapy.

8.6 Females of Childbearing Potential

All females of childbearing potential must comply with the iPLEDGE program requirements [see *Warnings and Precautions* (5.2)].

Pregnancy Testing

Absorica™ must only be prescribed to female patients who are known not to be pregnant as confirmed by a negative CLIA-certified laboratory conducted pregnancy test. Female patients of childbearing potential must have had two negative urine or serum pregnancy tests with a sensitivity of at least 25 mIU/mL before receiving the initial Absorica™ prescription. The first test (a screening test) is obtained by the prescriber when the decision is made to pursue qualification of the patient for Absorica™. The second pregnancy test (a confirmation test) must be done in a CLIA-certified laboratory. The interval between the two tests must be at least 19 days.

- For patients with regular menstrual cycles, perform the second pregnancy test during the first 5 days of the menstrual period immediately preceding the beginning of Absorica™ therapy and after the patient has used 2 forms of contraception for 1 month.
- For patients with amenorrhea, irregular cycles, or using a contraceptive method that precludes withdrawal bleeding, perform the second pregnancy test immediately preceding the beginning of Absorica™ therapy and after the patient has used 2 forms of contraception for 1 month.

Each month of continued Absorica™ therapy, patients must have a negative result from a urine or serum pregnancy test. A pregnancy test must be repeated each month, in a CLIA-certified laboratory, prior to the female patient receiving each prescription. A pregnancy test must also be completed at the end of the entire course of isotretinoin therapy and 1 month after the discontinuation of isotretinoin.

Contraception

Females of childbearing potential must use 2 forms of effective contraception simultaneously, at least 1 of which must be a primary form, unless the patient commits to continuous abstinence from heterosexual contact, or the patient has undergone a hysterectomy or bilateral oophorectomy, or has been medically confirmed to be post-menopausal. Patients must use 2 forms of effective contraception for at least 1 month prior to initiation of Absorica™ therapy, during Absorica™ therapy, and for 1 month after discontinuing Absorica™ therapy. Micro-dosed progesterone preparations ("minipills" that do not contain an estrogen) are an inadequate method of contraception during isotretinoin therapy [see *Warnings and Precautions* (5.3)].

Effective forms of contraception include both primary and secondary forms of contraception:

Primary forms	Secondary forms
• Tubal sterilization • Partner's vasectomy • Intrauterine device • Hormonal (combination oral contraceptives, transdermal patch, injectables, implantables, or vaginal ring)	Barrier: • male latex condom with or without spermicide • diaphragm with spermicide • cervical cap with spermicide Other: • Vaginal sponge (contains spermicide)

Any birth control method can fail. There have been reports of pregnancy from female patients who have used combination oral contraceptives, as well as transdermal patch/ injectable/ implantable/ vaginal ring hormonal birth control products; these pregnancies occurred while taking isotretinoin. These reports are more frequent for female patients who use only a single method of contraception. Therefore, it is critically important for female patients of childbearing potential use 2 effective forms of contraception simultaneously.

Using two forms of contraception simultaneously substantially reduces the chances that a female will become pregnant over the risk of pregnancy with either form alone. A drug interaction that decreases effectiveness of hormonal contraceptives has not been entirely ruled out for isotretinoin. Although hormonal contraceptives are highly effective, prescribers are advised to consult the package insert of any medication administered concomitantly with hormonal contraceptives, since some medications may decrease the effectiveness of these birth control products.

Patients should be prospectively cautioned not to self-medicate with the herbal supplement St. John's Wort because a possible interaction has been suggested with hormonal contraceptives based on reports of breakthrough bleeding on oral contraceptives shortly after starting St. John's Wort. Pregnancies have been reported by users of combined hormonal contraceptives who also used some form of St. John's Wort [see *Drug Interactions* (7.4)].

If the patient has unprotected heterosexual intercourse at any time 1 month before, during, or 1 month after therapy, she must:

a. Stop taking Absorica™ immediately, if on therapy
b. Have a pregnancy test at least 19 days after the last act of unprotected heterosexual intercourse
c. Start using 2 forms of effective contraception simultaneously again for 1 month before resuming Absorica™ therapy
d. Have a second pregnancy test after using 2 forms of effective contraception for 1 month as described above depending on whether she has regular menses or not.

If a pregnancy does occur during Absorica™ treatment, Absorica™ must be discontinued immediately. The patient should be referred to an obstetrician-gynecologist experienced in reproductive toxicity for further evaluation and counseling. Any suspected fetal exposure during or 1 month after Absorica™ therapy must be reported immediately to the FDA via the MedWatch number 1-800-FDA-1088 and also to the iPLEDGE pregnancy registry at 1-866-495-0654 or via the internet (*www.ipledgeprogram.com*) [see *Warnings and Precautions* (5.2)].

10 OVERDOSAGE

In humans, overdosage has been associated with vomiting, facial flushing, cheilosis, abdominal pain, headache, dizziness, and ataxia. These symptoms quickly resolve without apparent residual effects.

Absorica™ causes serious birth defects at any dosage (see Boxed CONTRAINDICATIONS AND WARNINGS). Female patients of childbearing potential who present with Absorica™ overdose must be evaluated for pregnancy. Patients who are pregnant should receive counseling about the risks to the fetus, as described in the Boxed CONTRAINDICATIONS AND WARNINGS. Non-pregnant patients must be warned to avoid pregnancy for at least one month and receive contraceptive counseling as described in *Warnings and Precautions* (5). Educational materials for such patients can be obtained by calling the manufacturer. Because an overdose would be expected to result in higher levels of isotretinoin in semen than found during a normal treatment course, male patients should use a condom, or avoid reproductive sexual activity with a female patient who is or might become pregnant, for 1 month after the overdose. All patients with Absorica™ overdose should not donate blood for at least 1 month.

11 DESCRIPTION

Absorica™ (isotretinoin), a retinoid, is available in 10 mg, 20 mg, 30 mg and 40 mg hard gelatin capsules for oral administration. Each capsule contains isotretinoin USP, stearoyl macrogolglycerides, soybean oil, sorbitan monooleate and propyl gallate. Gelatin capsules contain the following dye systems: 10 mg – iron oxide (yellow) and titanium dioxide; 20 mg – iron oxide (red) and titanium dioxide; 30 mg – iron oxide (yellow, red and black) and titanium dioxide; and 40 mg – iron oxide (yellow, red and black) and titanium dioxide.

Chemically, isotretinoin is 13-*cis*-retinoic acid and is related to both retinoic acid and retinol (vitamin A). It is a yellow to orange crystalline powder with a molecular weight of 300.44. The structural formula is:

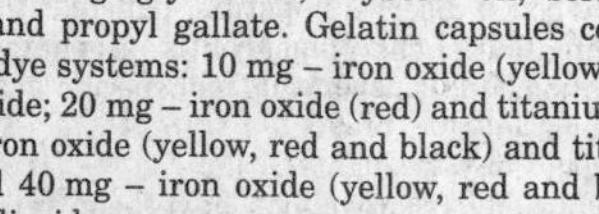

12 CLINICAL PHARMACOLOGY

12.1 Mechanism of Action

Absorica™ is a retinoid, which when administered in pharmacologic dosages of 0.5 to 1 mg/kg/day, inhibits sebaceous gland function and keratinization. Clinical improvement in nodular acne patients occurs in association with a reduction in sebum secretion. The decrease in sebum secretion is temporary and is related to the dose and duration of treatment with isotretinoin and reflects a reduction in sebaceous gland size and an inhibition of sebaceous gland differentiation. The exact mechanism of action of Absorica™ is unknown.

12.2 Pharmacodynamics

The pharmacodynamics of Absorica™ are unknown.

12.3 Pharmacokinetics

Absorption

Due to its high lipophilicity, oral absorption of isotretinoin is enhanced when given with a high-fat meal. Absorica™ is bioequivalent to Accutane® (isotretinoin) capsule when both drugs are taken with a high-fat meal. Absorica™ is more bioavailable than Accutane® (isotretinoin) capsules when both drugs are taken fasted; the $AUC_{0\text{-}t}$ of Absorica™ is approximately 83% greater than that of Accutane®. Absorica™ is therefore not interchangeable with generic products of Accutane®.

A single dose two-way crossover pharmacokinetic trial was conducted in 14 healthy adult male subjects comparing Absorica™ 40 mg (1 × 40 mg capsules), dosed under fasted and fed conditions. Under fed conditions after a high-fat meal, it was observed that the mean $AUC_{0\text{-}t}$ and C_{max} were approximately 50% and 26% higher, than that observed under fasting conditions (Table 2). The observed elimination half-life ($T_{1/2}$) was slightly lower in the fed state versus fasted. The time to peak concentration (T_{max}) increased with food and this may be related to a longer absorption phase.

Table 2: Pharmacokinetic parameters of Absorica™ mean (%CV) following administration of 40 mg strength, N=14

Absorica™ (1 × 40 mg capsules)	$AUC_{0\text{-}t}$ (ng × hr/mL)	C_{max} (ng/mL)	T_{max} (hr)	$T_{1/2}$ (hr)
Fed	6095 (26 %)	395 (39 %)	6.4 (47 %)	22 (25 %)
Fasted	4055 (20 %)	314 (26 %)	2.9 (34 %)	24 (28 %)

Published clinical literature has shown that there is no difference in the pharmacokinetics of isotretinoin between patients with nodular acne and healthy subjects with normal skin.

Distribution

Isotretinoin is more than 99.9% bound to plasma proteins, primarily albumin.

Metabolism

Following oral administration of isotretinoin, at least three metabolites have been identified in human plasma: 4-*oxo*-isotretinoin, retinoic acid (tretinoin), and 4-*oxo*-retinoic acid (4-*oxo*-tretinoin). Retinoic acid and 13-cis-retinoic acid are geometric isomers and show reversible interconversion. The administration of one isomer will give rise to the other. Isotretinoin is also irreversibly oxidized to 4-*oxo*-isotretinoin, which forms its geometric isomer 4-*oxo*-tretinoin.

After a single 40 mg oral dose of Absorica™ to 57 healthy adult subjects, concurrent administration of food increased the extent of formation of all metabolites in plasma when compared to the extent of formation under fasted conditions.

All of these metabolites possess retinoid activity that is in some in vitro models more than that of the parent isotretinoin. However, the clinical significance of these models is unknown.

In vitro studies indicate that the primary P450 isoforms involved in isotretinoin metabolism are 2C8, 2C9, 3A4, and 2B6. Isotretinoin and its metabolites are further metabolized into conjugates, which are then excreted in urine and feces.

Elimination

Following oral administration of an 80 mg dose of 14C-isotretinoin as a liquid suspension, 14C-activity in blood declined with a half-life of 90 hours. The metabolites of isotretinoin and any conjugates are ultimately excreted in the feces and urine in relatively equal amounts (total of 65% to 83%).

After a single 40 mg (2 × 20 mg) oral dose of Absorica™ to 57 healthy adult subjects under fed conditions, the mean ± SD elimination halflives ($T_{1/2}$) of isotretinoin and 4-*oxo*-isotretinoin under fed states were 18 hours and 38 hours, respectively.

Special Patient Populations

The pharmacokinetics of isotretinoin were evaluated after single and multiple doses in 38 pediatric patients (12 to 15 years) and 19 adult patients (≥18 years) who received isotretinoin for the treatment of severe recalcitrant nodular acne. In both age groups, 4-*oxo*-isotretinoin was the major metabolite; tretinoin and 4-*oxo*-tretinoin were also observed. There were no statistically significant differences in the pharmacokinetics of isotretinoin between pediatric and adult patients.

13 NONCLINICAL TOXICOLOGY

13.1 Carcinogenesis, Mutagenesis and Impairment of Fertility

In male and female Fischer 344 rats given oral isotretinoin at dosages of 8 or 32 mg/kg/day (1.3 to 5.3 times the recommended clinical dose of 1 mg/kg/day, respectively, after normalization for total body surface area) for greater than 18 months, there was a dose-related increased incidence of pheochromocytoma relative to controls. The incidence of adrenal medullary hyperplasia was also increased at the higher dosage in both sexes. The relatively high level of spontaneous pheochromocytomas occurring in the male Fischer 344 rat makes it an equivocal model for study of this tumor; therefore, the relevance of this tumor to the human population is uncertain.

The Ames test was conducted with isotretinoin in two laboratories. The results of the tests in one laboratory were negative while in the second laboratory a weakly positive response (less than 1.6 × background) was noted in *S. typhimurium* TA100 when the assay was conducted with metabolic activation. No dose response effect was seen and all other strains were negative. Additionally, other tests designed to assess genotoxicity (Chinese hamster cell assay, mouse micronucleus test, *S. cerevisiae* D7 assay, in vitro clastogenesis assay with human-derived lymphocytes, and unscheduled DNA synthesis assay) were all negative.

In rats, no adverse effects on gonadal function, fertility, conception rate, gestation or parturition were observed at oral dosages of isotretinoin of 2, 8, or 32 mg/kg/day (0.3, 1.3, or 5.3 times the recommended clinical dose of 1 mg/kg/day, respectively, after normalization for total body surface area).

In dogs, testicular atrophy was noted after treatment with oral isotretinoin for approximately 30 weeks at dosages of 20 or 60 mg/kg/day (10 or 30 times the recommended clinical dose of 1 mg/kg/day, respectively, after normalization for total body surface area). In general, there was microscopic evidence for appreciable depression of spermatogenesis but some sperm were observed in all testes examined and in no instance were completely atrophic tubules seen.

In trials of 66 men, 30 of whom were patients with nodular acne under treatment with oral isotretinoin, no significant changes were noted in the count or motility of spermatozoa in the ejaculate. In a study of 50 men (ages 17 to 32 years) receiving isotretinoin therapy for nodular acne, no significant effects were seen on ejaculate volume, sperm count, total sperm motility, morphology or seminal plasma fructose.

13.2 Animal Toxicology

In rats given 8 or 32 mg/kg/day of isotretinoin (1.3 to 5.3 times the recommended clinical dose of 1 mg/kg/day after normalization for total body surface area) for 18 months or longer, the incidences of focal calcification, fibrosis and inflammation of the myocardium, calcification of coronary, pulmonary and mesenteric arteries, and metastatic calcification of the gastric mucosa were greater than in control rats of similar age. Focal endocardial and myocardial calcifications associated with calcification of the coronary arteries were observed in two dogs after approximately 6 to 7 months of treatment with isotretinoin at a dosage of 60 to 120 mg/kg/day (30 to 60 times the recommended clinical dose of 1 mg/kg/day, respectively, after normalization for total body surface area).

14 CLINICAL STUDIES

A double-blind, randomized, parallel group trial (Study 1) was conducted in patients with severe recalcitrant nodular acne to evaluate the efficacy and safety of Absorica™ compared to a generic product of Accutane® under fed conditions. Enrolled patients had a weight of 40 to 110 kg with at least 10 nodular lesions on the face and/or trunk. A total of 925 patients were randomized 1:1 to receive Absorica™ or a generic product of Accutane® (isotretinoin). Study patients ranged from 12 to 54 years of age, were approximately 60% male, 40% female, and were 87% White, 4% Black, 6% Asian, and 3% Other. Patients were treated an initial dose of 0.5 mg/kg/day in two divided doses for the first 4 weeks followed by 1 mg/kg/day in two divided doses for the following 16 weeks.

Change from Baseline to Week 20 in total nodular lesion count and proportion of patients with at least a 90% reduction in total nodular lesion count from Baseline to Week 20 are presented in Table 3. Total nodular lesion counts by visit are presented in Figure 1.

Table 3: Efficacy Results at Week 20 (Study 1)

	Absorica™ N=464	Isotretinoin* N=461
Nodular Lesions		
Mean Baseline Count	18.4	17.7
Mean Reduction	-15.68	-15.62
Patients Achieving 90% Reduction	324 (70%)	344 (75%)

*A generic product of Accutane®

Figure 1: Total Nodular (Facial and Truncal) Lesion Count by Visit in Study 1

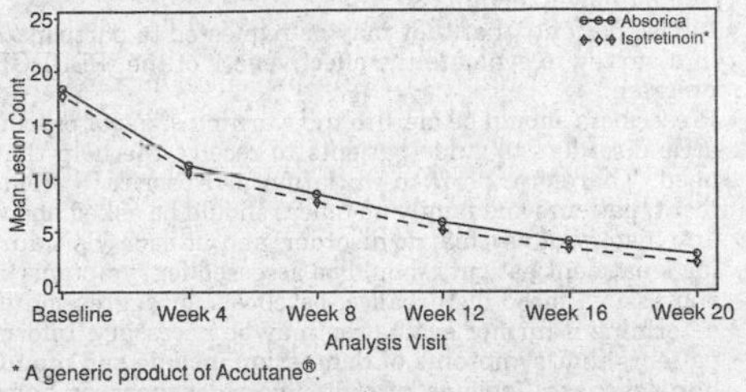

* A generic product of Accutane®.

16 HOW SUPPLIED/STORAGE AND HANDLING

Absorica™ capsules (isotretinoin) are supplied as opaque hard gelatin capsules, imprinted as follows:

- **10 mg capsules**; Dark yellow capsule imprinted with black ink **"G 240"** on cap and **"10"** on the body
  Box of 30 capsules (3 × 10 Prescription Packs): NDC 10631-115-31
- **20 mg capsules**; Red opaque capsule imprinted with black ink **"G 241"** on cap and **"20"** on the body
  Box of 30 capsules (3 × 10 Prescription Packs): NDC 10631-116-31
- **30 mg capsules**; Brown opaque capsule imprinted with white ink **"G 242"** on cap and **"30"** on the body
  Box of 30 capsules (3 × 10 Prescription Packs): NDC 10631-117-31
- **40 mg capsules**; Brown and red capsule imprinted with white ink **"G 325"** on cap and **"40"** on the body
  Box of 30 capsules (3 × 10 Prescription Packs): NDC 10631-118-31

Storage and Handling

Store at 20° C - 25° C (68° F - 77° F), excursion permitted between 15° C - 30° C (59° F - 86° F) [see USP controlled room temperature]. Protect from light.

17 PATIENT COUNSELING INFORMATION

See FDA-Approved Patient Labeling (Medication Guide)

17.1 Information for Patients

Advise the patient that Absorica™ is only available through a restricted program called iPLEDGE.

- As a component of the iPLEDGE program, prescribers must instruct patients to read the Medication Guide, the iPLEDGE program patient educational booklets, and watch the DVD with the following videos "Be Prepared, Be Protected" and "Be Aware: The Risk of Pregnancy While on Isotretinoin". The DVD includes information about contraception, the most common reasons that contraception fails, and the importance of using 2 forms of effective contraception when taking teratogenic drugs and comprehensive information about types of potential birth defects which could occur if a female patient who is pregnant takes Absorica™ at any time during pregnancy.
- Male patients and Female patients not of childbearing potential must understand the risks and benefits of Absorica™, comply with the REMS requirements described in the booklet entitled *The iPLEDGE Program Guide to Isotretinoin for Male Patients and Female Patients Who Cannot Get Pregnant,* and sign a Patient Information/Informed Consent form.
- Female patients of childbearing potential must be instructed that they must not be pregnant when Absorica™ therapy is initiated or plan to become pregnant while receiving Absorica™ therapy. Additionally, they must use 2 forms of effective contraception simultaneously for 1 month before starting Absorica™, while taking Absorica™, and for 1 month after Absorica™ has been stopped, unless they commit to continuous abstinence from heterosexual intercourse. They should also sign a Patient Information/Informed Consent form and Patient Information/ Informed Consent About Birth Defects (for female patients who can get pregnant) form prior to beginning Absorica™ therapy. Female patients should be seen by their prescribers monthly and have a urine or serum pregnancy test, in a CLIA-certified laboratory, performed each month during treatment to confirm negative pregnancy status before another Absorica™ prescription is written. Additionally, a pregnancy test must be completed at the end of the entire course of Absorica™ therapy and 1 month after discontinuation of therapy.
- Advise the patient that isotretinoin is found in the semen of male patients taking isotretinoin, but the amount delivered to a female partner would be about one million times lower than an oral dose of 40 mg. While the no-effect limit for isotretinoin induced embryopathy is unknown, 20 years of post-marketing reports include four with isolated defects compatible with features of retinoid exposed fetuses; however two of these reports were incomplete and two had other possible explanations for the defects observed.
- Advise the patient that Absorica™ is available only from pharmacies that are certified in the iPLEDGE program,

and provide them with the telephone number (1-866-495-0654) and website (*www.ipledgeprogram.com*) for information on how to obtain.

- Advise patients that they may be requested to participate in a survey to evaluate the effectiveness of the iPLEDGE program.
- Prescribers should be alert to the warning signs of psychiatric disorders to guide patients to receive the help they need. Therefore, prior to initiation of Absorica™ treatment, patients and family members should be asked about any history of psychiatric disorder, and at each visit during treatment patients should be assessed for symptoms of depression, mood disturbance, psychosis, or aggression to determine if further evaluation may be necessary. Inform patients that **symptoms of depression include sad mood, hopelessness, feelings of guilt, worthlessness or helplessness, loss of pleasure or interest in activities, fatigue, difficulty concentrating, change in sleep pattern, change in weight or appetite, suicidal thoughts or attempts, restlessness, irritability, acting on dangerous impulses, and persistent physical symptoms unresponsive to treatment.** Patients should stop treatment and the patient or a family member should promptly contact their prescriber if the patient develops depression, mood disturbance, psychosis, or aggression, without waiting until the next visit. Discontinuation of Absorica™ treatment may be insufficient; further evaluation may be necessary. While such monitoring may be helpful, it may not detect all patients at risk. Patients may report mental health problems or family history of psychiatric disorders. These reports should be discussed with the patient and/or the patient's family. A referral to a mental health professional may be necessary. The physician should consider whether Absorica™ therapy is appropriate in this setting; for some patients the risks may outweigh the benefits of Absorica™ therapy.
- Patients must be informed that some patients, while taking isotretinoin or soon after stopping isotretinoin, have become depressed or developed other serious mental problems. Symptoms of depression include sad, "anxious" or empty mood, irritability, acting on dangerous impulses, anger, loss of pleasure or interest in social or sports activities, sleeping too much or too little, changes in weight or appetite, school or work performance going down, or trouble concentrating. Some patients taking isotretinoin have had thoughts about hurting themselves or putting an end to their own lives (suicidal thoughts), some have tried to end their own lives, and some have ended their own lives. There were reports that some of these people did not appear depressed. There have been reports of patients on isotretinoin becoming aggressive or violent. There have also been reports of psychotic symptoms, which indicate a loss of contact with reality. Psychotic symptoms include feelings of suspiciousness toward others, strange beliefs, hearing voices or other noises without an obvious source, and seeing unusual objects or people with no explanation. No one knows if isotretinoin caused these behaviors and symptoms or if they would have happened even if the person did not take isotretinoin. If any of these behaviors or symptoms occur, the patient should stop treatment and the patient or family member should contact the prescriber promptly without waiting until the next visit [see *Warnings and Precautions* (5.4)]. Some people have had other signs of depression while taking isotretinoin.
- Patients must be informed that they must not share Absorica™ with anyone else because of the risk of birth defects and other serious adverse reactions.
- Patients must be informed not to donate blood during therapy and for 1 month following discontinuation of the drug because the blood might be given to a pregnant female patient whose fetus must not be exposed to Absorica™.
- Absorica™ may be taken without regard to meals [see *Dosage and Administration* (2.1)]. To decrease the risk of esophageal irritation, patients should swallow the capsules with a full glass of liquid.
- Patients should be informed that inflammatory bowel disease (including regional ileitis) may occur without a prior history of intestinal disorders. In rare instances, symptoms have been reported to persist after treatment has stopped. Patients should be informed that if they experience abdominal pain, rectal bleeding or severe diarrhea, they should discontinue Absorica™ immediately.
- Patients should be informed that transient exacerbation (flare) of acne has been seen, generally during the initial period of therapy.
- Wax epilation and skin resurfacing procedures (such as dermabrasion, laser) should be avoided during Absorica™ therapy and for at least 6 months thereafter due to the possibility of scarring.
- Patients should be advised to avoid prolonged exposure to UV rays or sunlight.
- Patients should be informed that they may experience dry eye, corneal opacities, and decreased night vision. Contact lens wearers may experience decreased tolerance to contact lenses during and after therapy.
- Patients should be informed that 16% of patients treated with isotretinoin in a clinical trial developed musculoskeletal symptoms (including arthralgia) during treatment. In general, these symptoms were mild to moderate, but occasionally required discontinuation of the drug. Transient pain in the chest has been reported less frequently. In the clinical trial, these symptoms generally cleared rapidly after discontinuation of therapy, but in some cases persisted.
- There have been rare postmarketing reports of rhabdomyolysis, some associated with strenuous physical activity.
- Pediatric patients and their caregivers should be informed that approximately 17% to 29% of pediatric patients treated with isotretinoin developed back pain. In a clinical trial, back pain was severe in 13.5% of the cases and occurred at a higher frequency in female patients than male patients. Arthralgias were experienced in 22% (79/358) of pediatric patients. Arthralgias were severe in 7.6% (6/79) of patients. Appropriate evaluation of the musculoskeletal system should be done in patients who present with these symptoms during or after a course of treatment. Consideration should be given to discontinuation of isotretinoin if any significant abnormality is found.
- Neutropenia and rare cases of agranulocytosis have been reported in patients treated with isotretinoin. Absorica™ should be discontinued if clinically significant decreases in white cell counts occur.
- Patients should be advised that severe skin reactions (Stevens-Johnson syndrome and toxic epidermal necrolysis) have been reported in post marketing data in patients treated with isotretinoin. Treatment with Absorica™ should be discontinued if clinically significant skin reactions occur.
- Adolescent patients who participate in sports with repetitive impact should be informed that isotretinoin use may increase their risk of spondylolisthesis or hip growth plate injuries. There are spontaneous reports of fractures and/or delayed healing in patients while on therapy with isotretinoin or following cessation of therapy with isotretinoin while involved in these activities [see *Warnings and Precautions* (5.12)].

Manufactured for: Ranbaxy Laboratories Inc.
Jacksonville, FL 32257 USA
By: Galephar P R, Inc.
Juncos, Puerto Rico 00777

GK-067

Shown in Product Identification Guide, page 312

HALOG® ℞

(Halcinonide Cream, USP) 0.1%
FOR TOPICAL USE ONLY.
NOT FOR OPHTHALMIC, ORAL, OR INTRAVAGINAL USE.

Rx only

DESCRIPTION

The topical corticosteroids constitute a class of primarily synthetic steroids used as anti-inflammatory and antipruritic agents. The steroids in this class include halcinonide. Halcinonide is designated chemically as 21-Chloro-9-fluoro-11β,16α, 17-trihydroxypregn-4-ene-3,20-dione cyclic 16,17-acetal with acetone. Graphic formula:

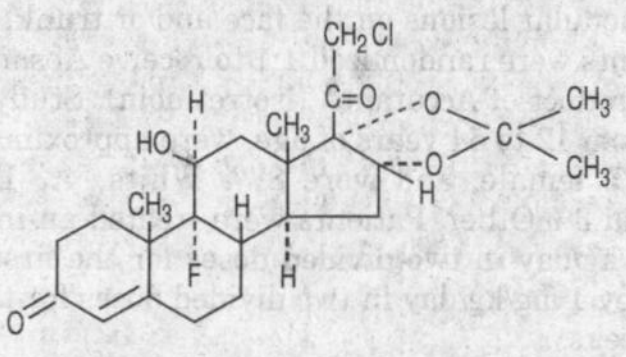

$C_{24}H_{32}ClFO_5$, MW 454.96, CAS-3093-35-4

Each gram of 0.1% HALOG (Halcinonide Cream, USP) contains 1 mg halcinonide in a specially formulated cream base consisting of cetyl alcohol, dimethicone 350, glyceryl monostearate NF XII, isopropyl palmitate, polysorbate 60, propylene glycol, purified water, and titanium dioxide.

CLINICAL PHARMACOLOGY

Topical corticosteroids share anti-inflammatory, antipruritic and vasoconstrictive actions.

The mechanism of anti-inflammatory activity of the topical corticosteroids is unclear. Various laboratory methods, including vasoconstrictor assays, are used to compare and predict potencies and/or clinical efficacies of the topical corticosteroids. There is some evidence to suggest that a recognizable correlation exists between vasoconstrictor potency and therapeutic efficacy in man.

Pharmacokinetics

The extent of percutaneous absorption of topical corticosteroids is determined by many factors including the vehicle, the integrity of the epidermal barrier, and the use of occlusive dressings.

Topical corticosteroids can be absorbed from normal intact skin. Inflammation and/or other disease processes in the skin increase percutaneous absorption. Occlusive dressings substantially increase the percutaneous absorption of topical corticosteroids. Thus, occlusive dressings may be a valuable therapeutic adjunct for treatment of resistant dermatoses (see **DOSAGE AND ADMINISTRATION**).

Once absorbed through the skin, topical corticosteroids are handled through pharmacokinetic pathways similar to systemically administered corticosteroids. Corticosteroids are bound to plasma proteins in varying degrees. Corticosteroids are metabolized primarily in the liver and are then excreted by the kidneys. Some of the topical corticosteroids and their metabolites are also excreted into the bile.

INDICATIONS AND USAGE

HALOG (Halcinonide Cream, USP) 0.1% is indicated for the relief of the inflammatory and pruritic manifestations of corticosteroid-responsive dermatoses.

CONTRAINDICATIONS

Topical corticosteroids are contraindicated in those patients with a history of hypersensitivity to any of the components of the preparations.

PRECAUTIONS

General

Systemic absorption of topical corticosteroids has produced reversible hypothalamic-pituitary-adrenal (HPA) axis suppression, manifestations of Cushing's syndrome, hyperglycemia, and glucosuria in some patients.

Conditions which augment systemic absorption include the application of the more potent steroids, use over large surface areas, prolonged use, and the addition of occlusive dressings.

Therefore, patients receiving a large dose of any potent topical steroid applied to a large surface area or under an occlusive dressing should be evaluated periodically for evidence of HPA axis suppression by using the urinary free cortisol and ACTH stimulation tests, and for impairment of thermal homeostasis. If HPA axis suppression or elevation of the body temperature occurs, an attempt should be made to withdraw the drug, to reduce the frequency of application, substitute a less potent steroid, or use a sequential approach when utilizing the occlusive technique.

Recovery of HPA axis function and thermal homeostasis are generally prompt and complete upon discontinuation of the drug. Infrequently, signs and symptoms of steroid withdrawal may occur, requiring supplemental systemic corticosteroids. Occasionally, a patient may develop a sensitivity reaction to a particular occlusive dressing material or adhesive and a substitute material may be necessary.

Children may absorb proportionally larger amounts of topical corticosteroids and thus be more susceptible to systemic toxicity (see **PRECAUTIONS: Pediatric Use**).

If irritation develops, topical corticosteroids should be discontinued and appropriate therapy instituted.

In the presence of dermatological infections, the use of an appropriate antifungal or antibacterial agent should be instituted. If a favorable response does not occur promptly, the corticosteroid should be discontinued until the infection has been adequately controlled.

This preparation is not for ophthalmic, oral, or intravaginal use.

Information for the Patient

Patients using topical corticosteroids should receive the following information and instructions:

1. This medication is to be used as directed by the physician. It is for dermatologic use only. Avoid contact with the eyes.
2. Patients should be advised not to use this medication for any disorder other than for which it was prescribed.
3. The treated skin area should not be bandaged or otherwise covered or wrapped as to be occlusive unless directed by the physician.
4. Patients should report any signs of local adverse reactions especially under occlusive dressing.
5. Parents of pediatric patients should be advised not to use tight-fitting diapers or plastic pants on a child being treated in the diaper area, as these garments may constitute occlusive dressings.

Laboratory Tests

A urinary free cortisol test and ACTH stimulation test may be helpful in evaluating HPA axis suppression.

Carcinogenesis, Mutagenesis, and Impairment of Fertility

Long-term animal studies have not been performed to evaluate the carcinogenic potential or the effect on fertility of topical corticosteroids.

Studies to determine mutagenicity with prednisolone and hydrocortisone showed negative results.

Pregnancy

Teratogenic Effects: Category C

Corticosteroids are generally teratogenic in laboratory animals when administered systemically at relatively low dosage levels. The more potent corticosteroids have been shown to be teratogenic after dermal application in laboratory animals. There are no adequate and well-controlled studies in pregnant women on teratogenic effects from topically applied corticosteroids. Therefore, topical corticosteroids should be used during pregnancy only if the potential benefit justifies the potential risk to the fetus. Drugs of this class should not be used extensively on pregnant patients, in large amounts, or for prolonged periods of time.

Nursing Mothers

It is not known whether topical administration of corticosteroids could result in sufficient systemic absorption to produce detectable quantities in breast milk. Systemically administered corticosteroids are secreted into breast milk in quantities **not** likely to have a deleterious effect on the infant. Nevertheless, caution should be exercised when topical corticosteroids are administered to a nursing woman.

Pediatric Use

Pediatric patients may demonstrate greater susceptibility to topical corticosteroid-induced HPA axis suppression and Cushing's syndrome than mature patients because of a larger skin surface area to body weight ratio.

HPA axis suppression, Cushing's syndrome, and intracranial hypertension have been reported in children receiving topical corticosteroids. Manifestations of adrenal suppression in children include linear growth retardation, delayed weight gain, low plasma cortisol levels, and absence of response to ACTH stimulation. Manifestations of intracranial hypertension include bulging fontanelles, headaches, and bilateral papilledema.

Administration of topical corticosteroids to children should be limited to the least amount compatible with an effective therapeutic regimen. Chronic corticosteroid therapy may interfere with the growth and development of children.

Geriatric Use

Of approximately 3000 patients included in clinical studies of 0.1% HALOG CREAM, 14% were 60 years or older, while 4% were 70 years or older. No overall differences in safety were observed between these patients and younger patients. Efficacy data have not been evaluated for differences between elderly and younger patients. Other reported clinical experience has not identified differences in responses between the elderly and younger patients, but greater sensitivity of some older individuals cannot be ruled out.

ADVERSE REACTIONS

The following local adverse reactions are reported infrequently with topical corticosteroids, but may occur more frequently with the use of occlusive dressings (reactions are listed in an approximate decreasing order of occurrence): burning, itching, irritation, dryness, folliculitis, hypertrichosis, acneiform eruptions, hypopigmentation, perioral dermatitis, allergic contact dermatitis, maceration of the skin, secondary infection, skin atrophy, striae, and miliaria.

OVERDOSAGE

Topically applied corticosteroids can be absorbed in sufficient amounts to produce systemic effects (see **PRECAUTIONS: General**).

DOSAGE AND ADMINISTRATION

Apply the 0.1% HALOG (Halcinonide Cream, USP) to the affected area two to three times daily. Rub in gently.

Occlusive Dressing Technique

Occlusive dressings may be used for the management of psoriasis or other recalcitrant conditions. Gently rub a small amount of cream into the lesion until it disappears. Reapply the preparation leaving a thin coating on the lesion, cover with a pliable nonporous film, and seal the edges. If needed, additional moisture may be provided by covering the lesion with a dampened clean cotton cloth before the nonporous film is applied or by briefly wetting the affected area with water immediately prior to applying the medication. The frequency of changing dressings is best determined on an individual basis. It may be convenient to apply HALOG under an occlusive dressing in the evening and to remove the dressing in the morning (i.e., 12-hour occlusion). When utilizing the 12-hour occlusion regimen, additional cream should be applied, without occlusion, during the day. Reapplication is essential at each dressing change. If an infection develops, the use of occlusive dressings should be discontinued and appropriate antimicrobial therapy instituted.

HOW SUPPLIED

HALOG® (Halcinonide Cream, USP) 0.1% is smooth, soft homogeneous white to off-white cream, essentially free of foreign matter and is supplied as:

NDC 10631-094-20	Tube containing 30 g
NDC 10631-094-30	Tube containing 60 g
NDC 10631-094-76	Jar containing 216 g

Storage

Store at room temperature; avoid excessive heat (104° F).

To report SUSPECTED ADVERSE REACTIONS, contact the FDA at 1-800-FDA-1088 or www.fda.gov/medwatch.

RANBAXY

Jacksonville, FL 32257 USA

129769

Revised September 2012

HALOG® OINTMENT ℞

(Halcinonide Ointment, USP) 0.1%

FOR TOPICAL USE ONLY.

NOT FOR OPHTHALMIC, ORAL, OR INTRAVAGINAL USE.

Rx only

DESCRIPTION

The topical corticosteroids constitute a class of primarily synthetic steroids used as anti-inflammatory and antipruritic agents. The steroids in this class include halcinonide. Halcinonide is designated chemically as 21-Chloro-9-fluoro-11β,16α, 17-trihydroxypregn-4-ene-3,20-dione cyclic 16,17-acetal with acetone. Graphic formula:

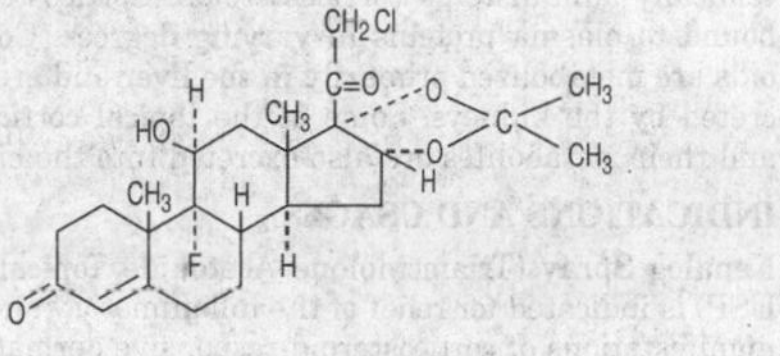

$C_{24}H_{32}ClFO_5$, MW 454.96, CAS-3093-35-4

Each gram of 0.1% HALOG OINTMENT (Halcinonide Ointment, USP) contains 1 mg halcinonide in Plastibase® (Plasticized Hydrocarbon Gel), a mineral oil and polyethylene gel base, polyethylene glycol 300, polyethylene glycol 400, polyethylene glycol 1450, and polyethylene glycol 6000 distearate with butylated hydroxytoluene as an antioxidant.

CLINICAL PHARMACOLOGY

Topical corticosteroids share anti-inflammatory, antipruritic and vasoconstrictive actions.

The mechanism of anti-inflammatory activity of the topical corticosteroids is unclear. Various laboratory methods, including vasoconstrictor assays, are used to compare and predict potencies and/or clinical efficacies of the topical corticosteroids. There is some evidence to suggest that a recognizable correlation exists between vasoconstrictor potency and therapeutic efficacy in man.

Pharmacokinetics

The extent of percutaneous absorption of topical corticosteroids is determined by many factors including the vehicle, the integrity of the epidermal barrier, and the use of occlusive dressings.

Topical corticosteroids can be absorbed from normal intact skin. Inflammation and/or other disease processes in the skin increase percutaneous absorption. Occlusive dressings substantially increase the percutaneous absorption of topical corticosteroids. Thus, occlusive dressings may be a valuable therapeutic adjunct for treatment of resistant dermatoses (see **DOSAGE AND ADMINISTRATION**).

Once absorbed through the skin, topical corticosteroids are handled through pharmacokinetic pathways similar to systemically administered corticosteroids. Corticosteroids are bound to plasma proteins in varying degrees. Corticosteroids are metabolized primarily in the liver and are then excreted by the kidneys. Some of the topical corticosteroids and their metabolites are also excreted into the bile.

INDICATIONS AND USAGE

HALOG OINTMENT (Halcinonide Ointment, USP) 0.1% is indicated for the relief of the inflammatory and pruritic manifestations of corticosteroidresponsive dermatoses.

CONTRAINDICATIONS

Topical corticosteroids are contraindicated in those patients with a history of hypersensitivity to any of the components of the preparations.

PRECAUTIONS

General

Systemic absorption of topical corticosteroids has produced reversible hypothalamic-pituitary-adrenal (HPA) axis suppression, manifestations of Cushing's syndrome, hyperglycemia, and glucosuria in some patients.

Conditions which augment systemic absorption include the application of the more potent steroids, use over large surface areas, prolonged use, and the addition of occlusive dressings.

Therefore, patients receiving a large dose of any potent topical steroid applied to a large surface area or under an occlusive dressing should be evaluated periodically for evidence of HPA axis suppression by using the urinary free cortisol and ACTH stimulation tests, and for impairment of thermal homeostasis. If HPA axis suppression or elevation of the body temperature occurs, an attempt should be made to withdraw the drug, to reduce the frequency of application, substitute a less potent steroid, or use a sequential approach when utilizing the occlusive technique.

Recovery of HPA axis function and thermal homeostasis are generally prompt and complete upon discontinuation of the drug. Infrequently, signs and symptoms of steroid withdrawal may occur, requiring supplemental systemic corticosteroids. Occasionally, a patient may develop a sensitivity reaction to a particular occlusive dressing material or adhesive and a substitute material may be necessary.

Children may absorb proportionally larger amounts of topical corticosteroids and thus be more susceptible to systemic toxicity (see **PRECAUTIONS: Pediatric Use**).

If irritation develops, topical corticosteroids should be discontinued and appropriate therapy instituted.

In the presence of dermatological infections, the use of an appropriate antifungal or antibacterial agent should be instituted. If a favorable response does not occur promptly, the corticosteroid should be discontinued until the infection has been adequately controlled.

This preparation is not for ophthalmic, oral, or intravaginal use.

Information for the Patient

Patients using topical corticosteroids should receive the following information and instructions:

1. This medication is to be used as directed by the physician. It is for dermatologic use only. Avoid contact with the eyes.
2. Patients should be advised not to use this medication for any disorder other than for which it was prescribed.
3. The treated skin area should not be bandaged or otherwise covered or wrapped as to be occlusive unless directed by the physician.
4. Patients should report any signs of local adverse reactions especially under occlusive dressing.
5. Parents of pediatric patients should be advised not to use tight-fitting diapers or plastic pants on a child being treated in the diaper area, as these garments may constitute occlusive dressings.

Laboratory Tests

A urinary free cortisol test and ACTH stimulation test may be helpful in evaluating HPA axis suppression.

Carcinogenesis, Mutagenesis, and Impairment of Fertility

Long-term animal studies have not been performed to evaluate the carcinogenic potential or the effect on fertility of topical corticosteroids.

Studies to determine mutagenicity with prednisolone and hydrocortisone showed negative results.

Pregnancy

Teratogenic Effects: Category C

Corticosteroids are generally teratogenic in laboratory animals when administered systemically at relatively low dosage levels. The more potent corticosteroids have been shown to be teratogenic after dermal application in laboratory animals. There are no adequate and well-controlled studies in pregnant women on teratogenic effects from topically applied corticosteroids. Therefore, topical corticosteroids should be used during pregnancy only if the potential benefit justifies the potential risk to the fetus. Drugs of this class should not be used extensively on pregnant patients, in large amounts, or for prolonged periods of time.

Nursing Mothers

It is not known whether topical administration of corticosteroids could result in sufficient systemic absorption to produce detectable quantities in breast milk. Systemically administered corticosteroids are secreted into breast milk in quantities **not** likely to have a deleterious effect on the infant. Nevertheless, caution should be exercised when topical corticosteroids are administered to a nursing woman.

Pediatric Use

Pediatric patients may demonstrate greater susceptibility to topical corticosteroid-induced HPA axis suppression and Cushing's syndrome than mature patients because of a larger skin surface area to body weight ratio.

HPA axis suppression, Cushing's syndrome, and intracranial hypertension have been reported in children receiving topical corticosteroids. Manifestations of adrenal suppression in children include linear growth retardation, delayed weight gain, low plasma cortisol levels, and absence of response to ACTH stimulation. Manifestations of intracranial hypertension include bulging fontanelles, headaches, and bilateral papilledema.

Administration of topical corticosteroids to children should be limited to the least amount compatible with an effective therapeutic regimen. Chronic corticosteroid therapy may interfere with the growth and development of children.

Geriatric Use

Clinical studies of 0.1% HALOG OINTMENT did not include sufficient numbers of patients aged 65 years and over to determine whether they respond differently from younger patients. Other reported clinical experience has not identified differences in responses between the elderly and younger patients. In general, dose selection for an elderly patient should be cautious, usually starting at the low end of the dosing range.

ADVERSE REACTIONS

The following local adverse reactions are reported infrequently with topical corticosteroids, but may occur more frequently with the use of occlusive dressings (reactions are listed in an approximate decreasing order of occurrence): burning, itching, irritation, dryness, folliculitis, hypertrichosis, acneiform eruptions, hypopigmentation, perioral dermatitis, allergic contact dermatitis, maceration of the skin, secondary infection, skin atrophy, striae, and miliaria.

OVERDOSAGE

Topically applied corticosteroids can be absorbed in sufficient amounts to produce systemic effects (see **PRECAUTIONS: General**).

DOSAGE AND ADMINISTRATION

Apply a thin film of 0.1% HALOG OINTMENT (Halcinonide Ointment, USP) to the affected area two to three times daily.

Occlusive Dressing Technique

Occlusive dressings may be used for the management of psoriasis or other recalcitrant conditions. Apply a thin film of ointment to the lesion, cover with a pliable nonporous film, and seal the edges. If needed, additional moisture may be provided by covering the lesion with a dampened clean cotton cloth before the nonporous film is applied or by briefly wetting the affected area with water immediately prior to applying the medication. The frequency of changing dressings is best determined on an individual basis. It may be convenient to apply HALOG OINTMENT under an occlusive dressing in the evening and to remove the dressing in the morning (i.e., 12-hour occlusion). When utilizing the 12-hour occlusion regimen, additional ointment should be applied, without occlusion, during the day. Reapplication is essential at each dressing change.

If an infection develops, the use of occlusive dressings should be discontinued and appropriate antimicrobial therapy instituted.

HOW SUPPLIED

HALOG® OINTMENT (Halcinonide Ointment, USP) 0.1% is translucent white to off-white, smooth, soft homogeneous ointment type material, essentially free of foreign matter and is supplied as:

NDC 10631-096-20	Tube containing 30 g
NDC 10631-096-30	Tube containing 60 g

Storage

Store at room temperature; avoid excessive heat (104° F).

To report SUSPECTED ADVERSE REACTIONS, contact the FDA at 1-800-FDA-1088 or www.fda.gov/medwatch.

RANBAXY
Jacksonville, FL 32257 USA
129745
Revised September 2012

KENALOG® SPRAY ℞

Triamcinolone Acetonide Topical Aerosol, USP (0.147 mg/g)
Rx only
For dermatologic use only
Not for ophthalmic use

DESCRIPTION

The topical corticosteroids constitute a class of primarily synthetic steroids used as anti-inflammatory and antipruritic agents. The steroids in this class include triamcinolone acetonide. Triamcinolone acetonide is designated chemically as 9-fluoro-11β, 16α, 17, 21-tetrahydroxypregna-1, 4-diene-3, 20-dione cyclic 16, 17-acetal with acetone. The structural formula is:

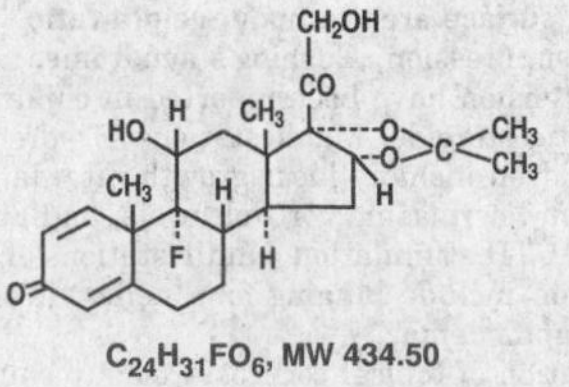

$C_{24}H_{31}FO_6$, MW 434.50

A two-second application, which covers an area approximately the size of the hand, delivers an amount of triamcinolone acetonide not exceeding 0.2 mg. After spraying, the nonvolatile vehicle remaining on the skin contains approximately 0.2% triamcinolone acetonide. Each gram of spray provides 0.147 mg triamcinolone acetonide in a vehicle of isopropyl palmitate, dehydrated alcohol (10.3%), and isobutane propellant.

CLINICAL PHARMACOLOGY

Topical corticosteroids share anti-inflammatory, antipruritic and vasoconstrictive actions.

The mechanism of anti-inflammatory activity of the topical corticosteroids is unclear. Various laboratory methods, including vasoconstrictor assays, are used to compare and predict potencies and/or clinical efficacies of the topical corticosteroids. There is some evidence to suggest that a recognizable correlation exists between vasoconstrictor potency and therapeutic efficacy in man.

Pharmacokinetics

The extent of percutaneous absorption of topical corticosteroids is determined by many factors including the vehicle, the integrity of the epidermal barrier, and the use of occlusive dressings.

Topical corticosteroids can be absorbed from normal intact skin. Inflammation and/or other disease processes in the skin increase percutaneous absorption.

Once absorbed through the skin, topical corticosteroids are handled through pharmacokinetic pathways similar to systemically administered corticosteroids. Corticosteroids are bound to plasma proteins in varying degrees. Corticosteroids are metabolized primarily in the liver and are then excreted by the kidneys. Some of the topical corticosteroids and their metabolites are also excreted into the bile.

INDICATIONS AND USAGE

Kenalog Spray (Triamcinolone Acetonide Topical Aerosol, USP) is indicated for relief of the inflammatory and pruritic manifestations of corticosteroid-responsive dermatoses.

CONTRAINDICATIONS

Topical corticosteroids are contraindicated in those patients with a history of hypersensitivity to any of the components of the preparations.

PRECAUTIONS

General

Systemic absorption of topical corticosteroids has produced reversible hypothalamic-pituitary-adrenal (HPA) axis suppression, manifestations of Cushing's syndrome, hyperglycemia, and glucosuria in some patients.

Conditions which augment systemic absorption include the application of the more potent steroids, use over large surface areas, prolonged use, and the addition of occlusive dressings.

Therefore, patients receiving a large dose of any potent topical steroid applied to a large surface area or under an occlusive dressing should be evaluated periodically for evidence of HPA axis suppression by using the urinary free cortisol and ACTH stimulation tests, and for impairment of thermal homeostasis. If HPA axis suppression or elevation of the body temperature occurs, an attempt should be made to withdraw the drug, to reduce the frequency of application, substitute a less potent steroid, or use a sequential approach.

Recovery of HPA axis function and thermal homeostasis are generally prompt and complete upon discontinuation of the drug. Infrequently, signs and symptoms of steroid withdrawal may occur, requiring supplemental systemic corticosteroids.

Children may absorb proportionally larger amounts of topical corticosteroids and thus be more susceptible to systemic toxicity (see **PRECAUTIONS, Pediatric Use**).

If irritation develops, topical corticosteroids should be discontinued and appropriate therapy instituted.

In the presence of dermatological infections, the use of an appropriate antifungal or antibacterial agent should be instituted. If a favorable response does not occur promptly, the corticosteroid should be discontinued until the infection has been adequately controlled.

Information for the Patient

Patients using Kenalog Spray should receive the following information and instructions:

1. This medication is to be used as directed by the physician. It is for external use only; avoid contact with the eyes and inhalation of the spray.
2. Patients should be advised not to use this medication for any disorder other than for which it was prescribed.
3. The treated skin area should not be bandaged or otherwise covered or wrapped as to be occlusive unless directed by the physician.
4. Patients should report any signs of local adverse reactions.
5. Parents of pediatric patients should be advised not to use tight-fitting diapers or plastic pants on a child being treated in the diaper area, as these garments may constitute occlusive dressings.
6. Do not use Kenalog Spray on the underarms or groin areas unless directed by your physician.
7. If no improvement is seen within 2 weeks, contact your physician.
8. Do not use other corticosteroid-containing products while using Kenalog Spray without first consulting your physician.
9. Kenalog Spray is flammable. Avoid heat, flames or smoking when applying Kenalog Spray.

Laboratory Tests

A urinary free cortisol test and ACTH stimulation test may be helpful in evaluating HPA axis suppression.

Carcinogenesis, Mutagenesis, Impairment of Fertility

Long-term animal studies have not been performed to evaluate the carcinogenic potential or the effect on fertility of topical corticosteroids.

Studies to determine mutagenicity with prednisolone and hydrocortisone showed negative results.

Pregnancy: Teratogenic Effects

Category C. Corticosteroids are generally teratogenic in laboratory animals when administered systemically at relatively low dosage levels. The more potent corticosteroids have been shown to be teratogenic after dermal application in laboratory animals. There are no adequate and well-controlled studies in pregnant women on teratogenic effects from topically applied corticosteroids. Therefore, topical corticosteroids should be used during pregnancy only if the potential benefit justifies the potential risk to the fetus. Drugs of this class should not be used extensively on pregnant patients, in large amounts, or for prolonged periods of time.

Nursing Mothers

It is not known whether topical administration of corticosteroids could result in sufficient systemic absorption to produce detectable quantities in breast milk. Systemically administered corticosteroids are secreted into breast milk in quantities not likely to have a deleterious effect on the infant. Nevertheless, caution should be exercised when topical corticosteroids are administered to a nursing woman.

Pediatric Use

Pediatric patients may demonstrate greater susceptibility to topical corticosteroid-induced HPA axis suppression and Cushing's syndrome than mature patients because of a larger skin surface area to body weight ratio.

HPA axis suppression, Cushing's syndrome, and intracranial hypertension have been reported in children receiving topical corticosteroids. Manifestations of adrenal suppression in children include linear growth retardation, delayed weight gain, low plasma cortisol levels, and absence of response to ACTH stimulation. Manifestations of intracranial hypertension include bulging fontanelles, headaches, and bilateral papilledema.

Administration of topical corticosteroids to children should be limited to the least amount compatible with an effective therapeutic regimen. Chronic corticosteroid therapy may interfere with the growth and development of children.

ADVERSE REACTIONS

The following local adverse reactions are reported infrequently with topical corticosteroids, but may occur more frequently with the use of occlusive dressings (reactions are listed in an approximate decreasing order of occurrence): burning, itching, irritation, dryness, folliculitis, hypertrichosis, acneiform eruptions, hypopigmentation, perioral dermatitis, allergic contact dermatitis, maceration of the skin, secondary infection, skin atrophy, striae, and miliaria.

OVERDOSAGE

Topically applied corticosteroids can be absorbed in sufficient amounts to produce systemic effects (see **PRECAUTIONS, General**).

DOSAGE AND ADMINISTRATION

Directions for use of the spray can are provided on the label. The preparation may be applied to any area of the body, but when it is sprayed about the face, care should be taken to see that the eyes are covered, and that inhalation of the spray is avoided.

Spray is flammable; avoid heat, flame or smoking when using this product.

Three or four applications daily of Kenalog Spray (Triamcinolone Acetonide Topical Aerosol) are generally adequate.

HOW SUPPLIED

Kenalog Spray (Triamcinolone Acetonide Topical Aerosol, USP)

63 g (NDC 10631-093-62) aerosol can.
100 g (NDC 10631-093-07) aerosol can.

Storage and Handling

Store at room temperature; avoid excessive heat. Contents under pressure; do not puncture or incinerate. Keep out of reach of children.

To report SUSPECTED ADVERSE REACTIONS, contact the FDA at 1-800-FDA-1088 or www.fda.gov/medwatch.

RANBAXY
Jacksonville, FL 32257 USA
Revised August 2011

Recordati Rare Diseases, Inc.
100 Corporate Drive
Lebanon, NJ 08833

(908) 437-1210

CHEMET® ℞
(succimer)
Capsule 100 mg

R_x only

DESCRIPTION

CHEMET (succimer) is an orally active, heavy metal chelating agent. The chemical name for succimer is *meso* 2, 3-dimercaptosuccinic acid (DMSA). Its empirical formula is $C_4H_6O_4S_2$ and molecular weight is 182.2. The *meso*-structural formula is:

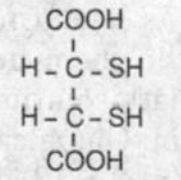

Succimer is a white crystalline powder with an unpleasant, characteristic mercaptan odor and taste.

Each CHEMET opaque white capsule for oral administration, contains beads coated with 100 mg of succimer and is imprinted black with CHEMET 100. Inactive ingredients in medicated beads are: povidone, sodium starch glycolate, starch and sucrose. Inactive ingredients in capsule are: gelatin, iron oxide, titanium dioxide and other ingredients.

CLINICAL PHARMACOLOGY

Succimer is a lead chelator; it forms water soluble chelates and, consequently, increases the urinary excretion of lead.

Preclinical Toxicology

CHEMET has low acute oral toxicity, with oral median lethal doses in rodents in excess of 3.6 g/kg. In a 28-day toxicity study, dogs receiving 30 and 100 mg/kg/day had lower urinary specific gravity and an increase in renal tubular regenerative hyperplasia. No renal toxicity was noted in dogs given 50 mg/kg/day orally for 14 consecutive days. In a chronic 6-month oral toxicity study, one male dog died (out of 7) at a dose of 200 mg/kg/day attributed to associated renal toxicity. Treatment related renal tubule epithelial changes in this study were observed in dogs after chronic (6-month) exposure to 110 and 200 mg/kg/day for 17 days then to 80 and 140 mg/kg/day for the remainder of the study. These changes were dose-dependent and correlated with increased kidney weights in male and female dogs at the 10 mg/kg/day dose. Nephropathy was not observed in dogs treated at 10 mg/kg/day. Reduced platelet counts were noted in 5 of 7 dogs receiving either 80 or 140 mg/kg/day for 3 or 6 months, although group means were not statistically different from concurrent controls. Platelets had not been quantified in earlier studies. Normal megakaryocytes in the bone marrow, plus the absence of fibrin degradation products or histologic evidence for DIC, suggested an autoimmune-mediated thrombocytopenia, a finding common in dogs but not in other species. However, serum antibody tests were inconclusive. Rats dosed chronically to 500 mg/kg/day developed no evidence for nephropathy or thrombocytopenia.

Pharmacokinetics

In a study performed in healthy adult volunteers, after a single dose of ^{14}C-succimer at 16, 32, or 48 mg/kg, absorption was rapid but variable with peak blood radioactivity levels between one and two hours. On average, 49% of the radiolabeled dose was excreted: 39% in the feces, 9% in the urine and 1% as carbon dioxide from the lungs. Since fecal excretion probably represented nonabsorbed drug, most of the absorbed drug was excreted by the kidneys. The apparent elimination half-life of the radiolabeled material in the blood was about two days.

In other studies of healthy adult volunteers receiving a single oral dose of 10 mg/kg, the chemical analysis of succimer and its metabolites in the urine showed that succimer was rapidly and extensively metabolized. Approximately 25% of the administered dose was excreted in the urine with the peak blood level and urinary excretion occurring between two and four hours. Of the total amount of drug eliminated in the urine, approximately 90% was eliminated in altered form as mixed succimer-cysteine disulfides; the remaining 10% was eliminated unchanged. The majority of mixed disulfides consisted of succimer in disulfide linkages with two molecules of L-cysteine, the remaining disulfides contained one L-cysteine per succimer molecule.

Pharmacodynamics

Dose ranging studies were performed in 18 men with blood lead levels of 44-96 mcg/dL. Three groups of 6 patients received either 10.0, 6.7 or 3.3 mg/kg succimer orally every 8 hours for 5 days. After five days the mean blood levels of the three groups decreased 72.5%, 58.3% and 35.5% respectively. The mean urinary lead excretions in the initial 24 hours were 28.6, 18.6 and 12.3 times the pretreatment 24 hour urinary lead excretion. As the chelatable pool was reduced during therapy, urinary lead output decreased. A mean of 19 mg of lead was excreted during a five day course of 30 mg/kg/day succimer. Clinical symptoms, such as headache and colic, and biochemical indices of lead toxicity also improved. Decrease in urinary excretion of d-aminolevulinic acid (ALA) and coproporphyrin paralleled the improvement in erythrocyte d-aminolevulinic acid dehydratase (ALA-D). Three control patients with lead poisoning of similar severity received $CaNa_2EDTA$ intravenously at a dose of 50 mg/kg/day for five days. The mean blood lead level decreased 47.4% and the mean urinary lead excretion was 21 mg in the control patients.

Effect on Essential Minerals

In the above studies succimer had no significant effect on the urinary elimination of iron, calcium or magnesium. Zinc excretion doubled during treatment. The effect of succimer on the excretion of essential minerals was small compared to that of $CaNa_2EDTA$, which can induce more than a tenfold increase in urinary excretion of zinc and doubling of copper and iron excretion.

Efficacy

A dose ranging study was performed in 15 pediatric patients aged 2 to 7 years with blood lead levels of 30-49 mcg/dL and positive $CaNa_2EDTA$ lead mobilization tests. Each group of five patients received 350, 233 or 116 mg/m² succimer every 8 hours for 5 days. These doses corresponded to 10, 6.7 and 3.3 mg/kg. Six control patients received 1000 mg/m²/day $CaNa_2EDTA$ intravenously for 5 days. Following therapy, the mean blood lead levels decreased 78, 63 and 42% respectively in the three groups treated with succimer. The response of the 350 mg/m² every 8 hours (10 mg/kg every 8 hours) group was significantly better than that of the other succimer treated groups as well as that of the control group, whose mean blood lead level fell 48%. No adverse reactions or changes in essential mineral excretion were reported in the succimer treated groups. In the $CaNa_2EDTA$ treated group, the cumulative amount of urinary lead excreted was slightly but significantly greater than in the succimer group. After $CaNa_2EDTA$, the urinary excretion of copper, zinc, iron and calcium were significantly increased.

As with other chelators, both adults and pediatric patients experienced a rebound in blood lead levels after discontinuation of CHEMET. In these studies, after treatment with a dose of 350 mg/m² (10 mg/kg) every 8 hours for five days, the mean lead level rebounded and plateaued at 60-85% of pretreatment levels two weeks after therapy. The rebound plateau was somewhat higher with lower doses of succimer and with intravenous $CaNa_2EDTA$.

In an attempt to control rebound of blood lead levels, 19 pediatric patients, ages 1-7 years, with blood lead levels of 42-67 mcg/dL, were treated with 350 mg/m² succimer every 8 hours for five days and then divided into three groups. One group was followed for two weeks with no further therapy, the second group was treated for two weeks with 350 mg/m² daily, and the third with 350 mg/m² every 12 hours. After the initial 5 days of therapy, the mean blood lead level in all subjects declined 61%. While the untreated group and the group treated with 350 mg/m² daily experienced rebound during the ensuing two weeks, the group who received the 350 mg/m² every 12 hours experienced no such rebound during the treatment period and less rebound following cessation of therapy.

In another study, ten pediatric patients, ages 21 to 72 months, with blood lead levels of 30-57 mcg/dL were treated with succimer 350 mg/m² every eight hours for five days followed by an additional 19-22 days of therapy at a dose of 350 mg/m² every 12 hours. The mean blood lead levels decreased and remained stable at under 15 mcg/dL during the extended dosing period.

In addition to the controlled studies, approximately 250 patients with lead poisoning have been treated with succimer either orally or parenterally in open U.S. and foreign studies with similar results reported. Succimer has been used for the treatment of lead poisoning in one patient with sickle cell anemia and in five patients with glucose-6-phosphodehydrogenase (G6PD) deficiency without adverse reactions.

Lead Encephalopathy

Three adults with lead encephalopathy have been reported in the literature to have improved with succimer therapy. However, data are not available regarding the use of succimer for the treatment of this rare and sometimes fatal complication of lead poisoning in pediatric patients.

Other Heavy Metal Poisoning

No controlled clinical studies have been conducted with succimer in poisoning with other heavy metals. A limited number of patients have received succimer for mercury or arsenic poisoning. These patients showed increased urinary excretion of the heavy metal and varying degrees of symptomatic improvement.

INDICATIONS AND USAGE

CHEMET is indicated for the treatment of lead poisoning in pediatric patients with blood lead levels above 45 mcg/dL. CHEMET is not indicated for prophylaxis of lead poisoning in a lead-containing environment; the use of CHEMET should always be accompanied by identification and removal of the source of the lead exposure.

CONTRAINDICATIONS

CHEMET should not be administered to patients with a history of allergy to the drug.

WARNINGS

Keep out of reach of pediatric patients. CHEMET is not a substitute for effective abatement of lead exposure.

Mild to moderate neutropenia has been observed in some patients receiving succimer. While a causal relationship to succimer has not been definitely established, neutropenia has been reported with other drugs in the same chemical class. A complete blood count with white blood cell differential and direct platelet counts should be obtained prior to and weekly during treatment with succimer. Therapy should either be withheld or discontinued if the absolute neutrophil count (ANC) is below 1200/mcL and the patient followed closely to document recovery of the ANC to above 1500/mcL or to the patient's baseline neutrophil count. There is limited experience with reexposure in patients who have developed neutropenia. Therefore, such patients should be rechallenged only if the benefit of succimer therapy clearly outweighs the potential risk of another episode of neutropenia and then only with careful patient monitoring.

Patients treated with succimer should be instructed to promptly report any signs of infection. If infection is suspected, the above laboratory tests should be conducted immediately.

PRECAUTIONS

The extent of clinical experience with CHEMET is limited. Therefore, patients should be carefully observed during treatment.

General

Elevated blood lead levels and associated symptoms may return rapidly after discontinuation of CHEMET because of redistribution of lead from bone stores to soft tissues and blood. After therapy, patients should be monitored for rebound of blood lead levels, by measuring blood lead levels at least once weekly until stable. However, the severity of lead intoxication (as measured by the initial blood lead level and the rate and degree of rebound of blood lead) should be used as a guide for more frequent blood lead monitoring.

All patients undergoing treatment should be adequately hydrated. Caution should be exercised in using CHEMET therapy in patients with compromised renal function. Limited data suggests that CHEMET is dialyzable, but that the lead chelates are not.

Transient mild elevations of serum transaminases have been observed in 6-10% of patients during the course of succimer therapy. Serum transaminases should be monitored before the start of therapy and at least weekly during therapy. Patients with a history of liver disease should be monitored closely. No data are available regarding the metabolism of succimer in patients with liver disease.

Clinical experience with repeated courses is limited. The safety of uninterrupted dosing longer than three weeks has not been established and it is not recommended.

The possibility of allergic or other mucocutaneous reactions to the drug must be borne in mind on readministration (as well as during initial courses). Patients requiring repeated courses of CHEMET should be monitored during each treatment course. One patient experienced recurrent mucocutaneous vesicular eruptions of increasing severity affecting the oral mucosa, the external urethral meatus and the perianal area on the third, fourth and fifth courses of the drug. The reaction resolved between courses and upon discontinuation of therapy.

Information for Patients

Patients should be instructed to maintain adequate fluid intake. If rash occurs, patients should consult their physician. Patients should be instructed to promptly report any indication of infection, which may be a sign of neutropenia (see WARNINGS and ADVERSE REACTIONS).

In young pediatric patients unable to swallow capsules, the contents of the capsule can be administered in a small amount of food (see DOSAGE AND ADMINISTRATION).

Drug Interaction

CHEMET is not known to interact with other drugs including iron supplements; interactions have not been systematically studied. Concomitant administration of CHEMET with other chelation therapy, such as $CaNa_2EDTA$ is not recommended.

TABLE I INCIDENCE OF ADVERSE EVENTS IN DOMESTIC STUDIES REGARDLESS OF ATTRIBUTION OR SUCCIMER DOSAGE

	Pediatric Patients (191)		Adults (134)	
	%	(n)	%	(n)
Digestive:	12.0	23	20.9	28
Nausea, vomiting, diarrhea, appetite loss, hemorrhoidal symptoms, loose stools, metallic taste in mouth.				
Body as a Whole:	5.2	10	15.7	21
Back pain, abdominal cramps, stomach pains, head pain, rib pain, chills, flank pain, fever, flu-like symptoms, heavy head/tired, head cold, headache, moniliasis.				
Metabolic:	4.2	8	10.4	14
Elevated SGPT, SGOT, alkaline phosphatase, elevated serum cholesterol.				
Nervous:	1.0	2	12.7	17
Drowsiness, dizziness, sensorimotor neuropathy, sleepiness, paresthesia.				
Skin and Appendages:	2.6	5	11.2	15
Papular rash, herpetic rash, rash, mucocutaneous eruptions, pruritus.				
Special Senses:	1.0	2	3.7	5
Cloudy film in eye, ears plugged, otitis media, eyes watery.				
Respiratory	3.7	7	0.7	1
Throat sore, rhinorrhea, nasal congestion, cough.				
Urogenital:	0.0	-	3.7	5
Decreased urination, voiding difficulty, proteinuria increased.				
Cardiovascular:	0.0	-	1.8	2
Arrhythmia				
Heme/Lymphatic:	0.5*	1	1.5*	2
Mild to moderate neutropenia, increased platelet count, intermittent eosinophilia.				
Musculoskeletal:	0.0	-	3.0	4
Kneecap pain, leg pains.				

*Does not include neutropenia - see WARNINGS.

Drug/Laboratory Tests Interaction

Succimer may interfere with serum and urinary laboratory tests. *In vitro* studies have shown succimer to cause false positive results for ketones in urine using nitroprusside reagents such as Ketostix[1] and falsely decreased measurements of serum uric acid and CPK.

[1]Ketostix is a registered trademark of Bayer Diagnostics.

Carcinogenesis, Mutagenesis and Impairment of Fertility

CHEMET has not been tested for carcinogenic potential in long-term animal studies. CHEMET up to a dose of 510 mg/kg/day in males and 100 mg/kg/day in females did not show any adverse effect on fertility and reproductive performance. It was not mutagenic in the Ames bacterial assay and in the mammalian cell forward gene mutation assay.

Pregnancy

Teratogenic Effects

Pregnancy Category C.

CHEMET has been shown to be teratogenic and fetotoxic in pregnant mice when given subcutaneously in a dose range of 410 to 1640 mg/kg/day during the period of organogenesis. In a developmental study in rats, CHEMET produced maternal toxicity and deaths at the dose of 720 mg/kg/day or more during organogenesis.

The dose of 510 mg/kg/day was the highest tolerable dose in pregnant rats. Impaired development of reflexes was noted in pups of 720 mg/kg/day group dam. There are no adequate and well controlled studies in pregnant women. CHEMET should be used during pregnancy only if the potential benefit justifies the potential risk to the fetus.

Nursing Mothers

It is not known whether this drug is excreted in human milk. Because many drugs and heavy metals are excreted in human milk, nursing mothers requiring CHEMET therapy should be discouraged from nursing their infants.

Pediatric Use

Refer to the INDICATIONS and DOSAGE AND ADMINISTRATION sections. Safety and efficacy in pediatric patients less than 12 months of age have not been established.

ADVERSE REACTIONS

Clinical experience with CHEMET has been limited. Consequently, the full spectrum and incidence of adverse reactions including the possibility of hypersensitivity or idiosyncratic reactions have not been determined. The most common events attributable to succimer, i.e., gastrointestinal symptoms or increases in serum transaminases, have been observed in about 10% of patients (see PRECAUTIONS). Rashes, some necessitating discontinuation of therapy, have been reported in about 4% of patients. If rash occurs, other causes (e.g. measles) should be considered before ascribing the reaction to succimer. Rechallenge with succimer may be considered if lead levels are high enough to warrant retreatment. One allergic mucocutaneous reaction has been reported on repeated administration of the drug (see PRECAUTIONS). Mild to moderate neutropenia has been observed in some patients receiving succimer (see WARNINGS). Table I presents adverse events reported with the administration of succimer for the treatment of lead and other heavy metal intoxication.

[See table above]

To report SUSPECTED ADVERSE REACTIONS, contact Recordati Rare Diseases Inc. at 1-888-575-8344 or FDA at 1-800-FDA-1088 or www.fda.gov/medwatch.

OVERDOSAGE

Doses of 2300 mg/kg in the rat and 2400 mg/kg in the mouse produced ataxia, convulsions, labored respiration and frequently death. No case of overdosage has been reported in humans. Limited data indicate that succimer is dialyzable. In case of acute overdosage, induction of vomiting or gastric lavage followed by administration of an activated charcoal slurry and appropriate supportive therapy are recommended.

DOSAGE AND ADMINISTRATION

Start dosage at 10 mg/kg or 350 mg/m^2 every eight hours for five days. Initiation of therapy at higher doses is not recommended. (See Table II for Dosing chart and number of capsules.) Reduce frequency of administration to 10 mg/kg or 350 mg/m^2 every 12 hours (two-thirds of initial daily dosage) for an additional two weeks of therapy. A course of treatment lasts 19 days. Repeated courses may be necessary if indicated by weekly monitoring of blood lead concentration. A minimum of two weeks between courses is recommended unless blood lead levels indicate the need for more prompt treatment.

TABLE II CHEMET (SUCCIMER) PEDIATRIC DOSING CHART

LBS	KG	DOSE (MG)*	Number of CAPSULES*
18-35	8-15	100	1
36-55	16-23	200	2
56-75	24-34	300	3
76-100	35-44	400	4
> 100	> 45	500	5

*To be administered every 8 hours for 5 days, followed by dosing every 12 hours for 14 days.

In young pediatric patients who cannot swallow capsules, CHEMET can be administered by separating the capsule and sprinkling the medicated beads on a small amount of soft food or putting them in a spoon and following with fruit drink.

Identification of the source of lead in the pediatric patient's environment and its abatement are critical to a successful therapy outcome. Chelation therapy is not a substitute for preventing further exposure to lead and should not be used to permit continued exposure to lead.

Patients who have received $CaNa_2EDTA$ with or without BAL may use CHEMET for subsequent treatment after an interval of four weeks. Data on the concomitant use of CHEMET with $CaNa_2EDTA$ with or without BAL are not available, and such use is not recommended.

HOW SUPPLIED

100 mg capsules in bottle of 100 (NDC 55292-201-11).

Store between 15°C and 25°C and avoid excessive heat.

Manufactured by:
Kremers Urban Pharmaceuticals Inc.
Seymour, IN 47274, USA
For: Recordati Rare Diseases Inc., Lebanon, NJ 08833, U.S.A.
® Trademark of Recordati Rare Diseases Inc.
Revised: February 2013
CIA72289C

Shown in Product Identification Guide, page 312

PANHEMATIN® ℞

Hemin For Injection
Rx only
For intravenous infusion only.

> PANHEMATIN (hemin for injection) should only be used by physicians experienced in the management of porphyrias in hospitals where the recommended clinical and laboratory diagnostic and monitoring techniques are available.
> PANHEMATIN therapy should be considered after an appropriate period of alternate therapy (i.e., 400 g glucose/day for 1 to 2 days). (See "WARNINGS", "PRECAUTIONS" and "DOSAGE AND ADMINISTRATION" sections.)

DESCRIPTION

PANHEMATIN (hemin for injection) is an enzyme inhibitor derived from processed red blood cells. Hemin for injection was known previously as hematin. The term hematin has been used to describe the chemical reaction product of hemin and sodium carbonate solution. Hemin is an iron containing metalloporphyrin. Chemically hemin is represented as chloro [7,12-diethenyl-3,8,13,17-tetramethyl-21H,23H-porphine-2,18-dipropanoato(2-)-N^{21},N^{22},N^{23},N^{24}] iron. The structural formula for hemin is:

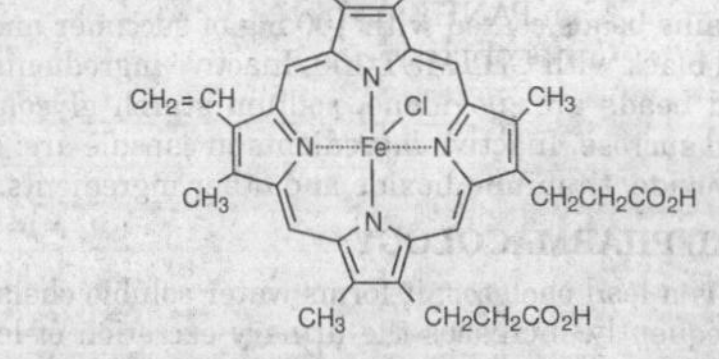

PANHEMATIN is a sterile, lyophilized powder suitable for intravenous administration after reconstitution. Each dispensing vial of PANHEMATIN contains the equivalent of 313 mg hemin, 215 mg sodium carbonate and 300 mg of sorbitol. The pH may have been adjusted with hydrochloric acid; the product contains no preservatives. When mixed as directed with Sterile Water for Injection, USP, each 43 mL provides the equivalent of approximately 301 mg hematin (7 mg/mL).

CLINICAL PHARMACOLOGY

Heme acts to limit the hepatic and/or marrow synthesis of porphyrin. This action is likely due to the inhibition of δ-aminolevulinic acid synthetase, the enzyme which limits the rate of the porphyrin/heme biosynthetic pathway. The exact mechanism by which hematin produces symptomatic improvement in patients with acute episodes of the hepatic porphyrias has not been elucidated.[1,9]

Following intravenous administration of hematin in non-jaundiced human patients, an increase in fecal urobilinogen can be observed which is roughly proportional to the amount of hematin administered. This suggests an enterohepatic pathway as at least one route of elimination. Bilirubin metabolites are also excreted in the urine following hematin injections.[2]

PANHEMATIN (hemin for injection) therapy for the acute porphyrias is not curative. After discontinuation of PANHEMATIN treatment, symptoms generally return although in some cases remission is prolonged. Some neurological symptoms have improved weeks to months after therapy although little or no response was noted at the time of treatment.

Other aspects of human pharmacokinetics have not been defined.

INDICATIONS AND USAGE

PANHEMATIN (hemin for injection) is indicated for the amelioration of recurrent attacks of acute intermittent porphyria temporally related to the menstrual cycle in susceptible women.

Manifestations such as pain, hypertension, tachycardia, abnormal mental status and mild to progressive neurologic signs may be controlled in selected patients with this disorder.

Similar findings have been reported in other patients with acute intermittent porphyria, porphyria variegata and hereditary coproporphyria. PANHEMATIN is not indicated in porphyria cutanea tarda.

CONTRAINDICATIONS

PANHEMATIN is contraindicated in patients with known hypersensitivity to this drug.

WARNINGS

PANHEMATIN is made from human blood. Products made from human blood may contain infectious agents, such as

viruses, that can cause disease. The risk that such products will transmit an infectious agent has been reduced by screening blood donors for prior exposure to certain viruses, by testing for the presence of certain current virus infections, and by inactivating certain viruses. Despite these measures, such products can still potentially transmit disease. There is also the possibility that unknown infectious agents may be present in such products. ALL infections thought by a physician possibly to have been transmitted by this product should be reported by the physician or other healthcare provider to Recordati Rare Diseases, (1-888-575-8344). The physician should discuss the risks and benefits of this product with the patient.

Because this product is made from human blood, it may carry a risk of transmitting infectious agents, e.g., viruses, and theoretically, the Creutzfeldt-Jakob disease (CJD) agent.

PANHEMATIN therapy is intended to limit the rate of porphyria/heme biosynthesis possibly by inhibiting the enzyme δ-aminolevulinic acid synthetase. For this reason, drugs such as estrogens, barbituric acid derivatives and steroid metabolites which increase the activity of δ-aminolevulinic acid synthetase should be avoided.

Also, because hemin for injection has exhibited transient, mild anticoagulant effects during clinical studies, concurrent anticoagulant therapy should be avoided.[9] The extent and duration of the hypocoagulable state induced by PANHEMATIN has not been established.

PRECAUTIONS

General

Clinical benefit from PANHEMATIN depends on prompt administration. Attacks of porphyria may progress to a point where irreversible neuronal damage has occurred. PANHEMATIN therapy is intended to prevent an attack from reaching the critical stage of neuronal degeneration. PANHEMATIN is not effective in repairing neuronal damage.[9]

Recommended dosage guidelines should be strictly followed. Reversible renal shutdown has been observed in a case where an excessive hematin dose (12.2 mg/kg) was administered in a single infusion. Oliguria and increased nitrogen retention occurred although the patient remained asymptomatic.[4] No worsening of renal function has been seen with administration of recommended dosages of hematin.[9]

A large arm vein or a central venous catheter should be utilized for the administration of PANHEMATIN to avoid the possibility of phlebitis.

Since reconstituted PANHEMATIN is not transparent, any undissolved particulate matter is difficult to see when inspected visually. Therefore, terminal filtration through a sterile 0.45 micron or smaller filter is recommended.

Because increased levels of iron and serum ferritin have been reported in post-marketing experience, physicians should monitor iron and serum ferritin in patients receiving multiple administrations of PANHEMATIN (See "ADVERSE REACTIONS" section).

Tests for Diagnosis and Monitoring of Therapy

Before PANHEMATIN therapy is begun, the presence of acute porphyria must be diagnosed using the following criteria:[9]

a. Presence of clinical symptoms.

b. Positive Watson-Schwartz or Hoesch test. (A negative Watson-Schwartz or Hoesch test indicates a porphyric attack is highly unlikely. When in doubt quantitative measures of δ-aminolevulinic acid and porphobilinogen in serum or urine may aid in diagnosis.)

Urinary concentrations of the following compounds may be *monitored* during PANHEMATIN therapy. Drug effect will be demonstrated by a decrease in one or more of the following compounds.[3-6]

ALA - δ-aminolevulinic acid
UPG - uroporphyrinogen
PBG - porphobilinogen
coproporphyrin

Carcinogenesis, Mutagenesis, Impairment of Fertility

PANHEMATIN was not mutagenic in bacteria systems *in vitro* and was not clastogenic in mammalian systems *in vitro* and *in vivo*. No data are available on potential for carcinogenicity or impairment of fertility in animals or humans.

Pregnancy

Teratogenic effects-Pregnancy Category C: Animal reproduction studies have not been conducted with hematin. It is also not known whether hematin can cause fetal harm when administered to a pregnant woman or can affect reproduction capacity. For this reason PANHEMATIN should not be given to a pregnant woman unless the expected benefits are sufficiently important to the health and welfare of the patient to outweigh the unknown hazard to the fetus.

Nursing Mothers

It is not known whether this drug is excreted in human milk. Because many drugs are excreted in human milk, caution should be exercised when PANHEMATIN is administered to a nursing woman.

Pediatric Use

Safety and effectiveness in pediatric patients under 16 years of age have not been established.

Geriatric Use

Clinical studies in PANHEMATIN did not include sufficient numbers of subjects aged 65 and over to determine whether they respond differently from younger subjects. Other reported clinical experience has not identified differences in response between the elderly and younger patients. In general, dose selection for an elderly patient should be cautious, usually starting at the low end of the dosing range, reflecting the greater frequency of decreased hepatic, renal, or cardiac function, and of concomitant disease or other drug therapy.

ADVERSE REACTIONS

Clinical Trials Experience

Phlebitis with or without leucocytosis and with or without mild pyrexia has occurred after administration of hematin through small arm veins.

Post-marketing Experience

Reversible renal shutdown has occurred with administration of excessive doses (See "PRECAUTIONS" section).

There have been post-marketing literature reports of thrombocytopenia and coagulopathy (including prolonged prothrombin time and prolonged partial thromboplastin time) in patients receiving PANHEMATIN.[8] Iron overload and serum ferritin increased have also been reported (See "PRECAUTIONS" section).

To report SUSPECTED ADVERSE REACTIONS, contact Recordati Rare Diseases at 1-888-575-8344 or FDA at 1-800-FDA-1088 or www.fda.gov/medwatch.

OVERDOSAGE

Reversible renal shutdown has been observed in a case where an excessive hematin dose (12.2 mg/kg) was administered in a single infusion. Treatment of this case consisted of ethacrynic acid and mannitol.[7]

DOSAGE AND ADMINISTRATION

Before administering PANHEMATIN, an appropriate period of alternate therapy (i.e., 400 g glucose/day for 1 to 2 days) must be considered. If improvement is unsatisfactory for the treatment of acute attacks of porphyria, an intravenous infusion of PANHEMATIN containing a dose of 1 to 4 mg/kg/day of hematin should be given over a period of 10 to 15 minutes for 3 to 14 days based on the clinical signs. In more severe cases this dose may be repeated no earlier than every 12 hours. No more than 6 mg/kg of hematin should be given in any 24 hour period.

After reconstitution each mL of PANHEMATIN contains the equivalent of approximately 7 mg of hematin. The drug may be administered directly from the vial.

Dosage Calculation Table

1 mg hematin equivalent = 0.14 mL PANHEMATIN
2 mg hematin equivalent = 0.28 mL PANHEMATIN
3 mg hematin equivalent = 0.42 mL PANHEMATIN
4 mg hematin equivalent = 0.56 mL PANHEMATIN

Since reconstituted PANHEMATIN is not transparent, any undissolved particulate matter is difficult to see when inspected visually. Therefore, terminal filtration through a sterile 0.45 micron or smaller filter is recommended.

Preparation of Solution:

Reconstitute PANHEMATIN by aseptically adding 43 mL of Sterile Water for Injection, USP, to the dispensing vial. Immediately after adding diluent, the product should be shaken well for a period of 2 to 3 minutes to aid dissolution.

NOTE: Because PANHEMATIN contains no preservative and because PANHEMATIN undergoes rapid chemical decomposition in solution, it should not be reconstituted until immediately before use. After the first withdrawal from the vial, any solution remaining must be discarded.

No drug or chemical agent should be added to a PANHEMATIN fluid admixture unless its effect on the chemical and physical stability has first been determined.

HOW SUPPLIED

PANHEMATIN is supplied as a sterile, lyophilized black powder in single dose dispensing vials (NDC 55292-701-54) in a carton (NDC 55292-701-55). When mixed as directed with Sterile Water for Injection, USP, each 43 mL provides the equivalent of approximately 301 mg hematin (7 mg/mL). Store lyophilized powder at 20-25°C (68-77°F). See USP controlled room temperature.

Caution: The packaging (vial stopper) of this product contains natural rubber latex which may cause allergic reactions.

REFERENCES

1. Bickers, D., Treatment of the Porphyrias: Mechanisms of Action, J Invest Dermatol 77(1):107-113, 1981.
2. Watson, C. J., Hematin and Porphyria, editorial, N Engl J Med 293(12): 605-607, September 18, 1975.
3. Lamon, J. M., Hematin Therapy for Acute Porphyria, Medicine 58(3): 252-269, 1979.
4. Dhar, G J., et al., Effects of Hematin in Hepatic Porphyria, Ann Intern Med 83: 20-30, 1975.
5. Watson, C. J., et al., Use of Hematin in the Acute Attack of the "Inducible" Hepatic Porphyrias, Adv Intern Med 23: 265-286, 1978.
6. McColl, K. E., et al., Treatment with Haematin in Acute Hepatic Porphyria, Q J Med, New Series L (198): 161-174, Spring, 1981.
7. Dhar, G. J., et al., Transitory Renal Failure Following Rapid Administration of a Relatively Large Amount of Hematin in a Patient with Acute Intermittent Porphyria in Clinical Remission, Acta Med Scand 203: 437-443, 1978.
8. Morris, D.L., et al., Coagulopathy Associated with Hematin Treatment for Acute Intermittent Porphyria, Ann Intern Med 95: 700-701, 1981.
9. Pierach, C. A., Hematin Therapy for the Porphyric Attack, Semin Liver Dis 2(2): 125-131, May, 1982.

Manufactured by: Fresenius Kabi USA, LLC
Raleigh, NC 27616
For: Recordati Rare Diseases Inc.
Lebanon, NJ 08833, U.S.A.
U.S. Lic. No. 1899
RECORDATI RARE DISEASES GROUP
® Trademark of Recordati Rare Diseases Inc.
Revised: February 2013
750-04243-7

Shown in Product Identification Guide, page 312

Regeneron Pharmaceuticals, Inc.

777 OLD SAW MILL RIVER ROAD
TARRYTOWN, NY 10591

For Medical Information Contact:
1-877-REGN-777 (1-877-734-6777)

ARCALYST® ℞

[ARK-a-list]
(rilonacept)
Injection for Subcutaneous Use

HIGHLIGHTS OF PRESCRIBING INFORMATION
These highlights do not include all the information needed to use ARCALYST safely and effectively. See full prescribing information for ARCALYST.
ARCALYST® (rilonacept)
Injection for Subcutaneous Use
Initial U.S. Approval: 2008

INDICATIONS AND USAGE

ARCALYST (rilonacept) is an interleukin-1 blocker indicated for the treatment of Cryopyrin-Associated Periodic Syndromes (CAPS), including Familial Cold Autoinflammatory Syndrome (FCAS) and Muckle-Wells Syndrome (MWS) in adults and children 12 and older. (1)

DOSAGE AND ADMINISTRATION

- Adult patients 18 yrs and older: Initiate treatment with a loading dose of 320 mg delivered as two, 2-mL, subcutaneous injections of 160 mg on the same day at two different sites. Continue dosing with a once-weekly injection of 160 mg administered as a single, 2-mL, subcutaneous injection. Do not administer ARCALYST more often than once weekly. (2)
- Pediatric patients aged 12 to 17 years: Initiate treatment with a loading dose of 4.4 mg/kg, up to a maximum of 320 mg, delivered as one or two subcutaneous injections with a maximum single-injection volume of 2 mL. Continue dosing with a once-weekly injection of 2.2 mg/kg, up to a maximum of 160 mg, administered as a single subcutaneous injection, up to 2 mL. If the initial dose is given as two injections, they should be given on the same day at two different sites. Do not administer ARCALYST more often than once weekly. (2)

DOSAGE FORMS AND STRENGTHS

Sterile, single-use 20-mL, glass vial containing 220 mg of rilonacept as a lyophilized powder for reconstitution. (3)

CONTRAINDICATIONS

None. (4)

WARNINGS AND PRECAUTIONS

- Interleukin-1 blockade may interfere with immune response to infections. Serious, life-threatening infections have been reported in patients taking ARCALYST. Discon-

tinue treatment with ARCALYST if a patient develops a serious infection. Do not initiate treatment with ARCALYST in patients with active or chronic infections. (5.1)
- Hypersensitivity reactions associated with ARCALYST administration have been rare. If a hypersensitivity reaction occurs, discontinue administration of ARCALYST and initiate appropriate therapy. (5.5)
- Live vaccines should not be given concurrently with ARCALYST. Prior to initiation of therapy with ARCALYST, patients should receive all recommended vaccinations. (5.3)

ADVERSE REACTIONS

The most common adverse reactions reported by patients with CAPS treated with ARCALYST are injection-site reactions and upper respiratory tract infections. (6.2, 6.3)

To report SUSPECTED ADVERSE REACTIONS, contact Regeneron at 1-877-REGN-777 (1-877-734-6777) or FDA at 1-800-FDA-1088 or www.fda.gov/medwatch.

DRUG INTERACTIONS

No formal drug interaction studies have been conducted with ARCALYST. (7)

USE IN SPECIFIC POPULATIONS

Pregnancy – No human data. Based on animal data, may cause fetal harm. (8.1)

See 17 for PATIENT COUNSELING INFORMATION and FDA-approved patient labeling

Revised: 04/2010

FULL PRESCRIBING INFORMATION: CONTENTS*

*** Sections or subsections omitted from the full prescribing information are not listed**

FULL PRESCRIBING INFORMATION

1 INDICATIONS AND USAGE

ARCALYST® (rilonacept) is an interleukin-1 blocker indicated for the treatment of Cryopyrin-Associated Periodic Syndromes (CAPS), including Familial Cold Autoinflammatory Syndrome (FCAS) and Muckle-Wells Syndrome (MWS) in adults and children 12 and older.

2 DOSAGE AND ADMINISTRATION

2.1 General Dosing Information

INJECTION FOR SUBCUTANEOUS USE ONLY.

2.2 Dosing

Adult patients 18 years and older: Treatment should be initiated with a loading dose of 320 mg delivered as two, 2 mL, subcutaneous injections of 160 mg each given on the same day at two different sites. Dosing should be continued with a once-weekly injection of 160 mg administered as a single, 2-mL, subcutaneous injection. ARCALYST should not be given more often than once weekly. Dosage modification is not required based on advanced age or gender.

Pediatric patients aged 12 to 17 years: Treatment should be initiated with a loading dose of 4.4 mg/kg, up to a maximum of 320 mg, delivered as one or two subcutaneous injections with a maximum single-injection volume of 2 mL. Dosing should be continued with a once-weekly injection of 2.2 mg/kg, up to a maximum of 160 mg, administered as a single subcutaneous injection, up to 2 mL. If the initial dose is given as two injections, they should be given on the same day at two different sites. ARCALYST should not be given more often than once weekly.

2.3 Preparation for Administration

Each single-use vial of ARCALYST contains a sterile, white to off-white, preservative-free, lyophilized powder. Reconstitution with 2.3 mL of preservative-free Sterile Water for Injection (supplied separately) is required prior to subcutaneous administration of the drug.

2.4 Administration

Using aseptic technique, withdraw 2.3 mL of preservative-free Sterile Water for Injection through a 27-gauge, ½-inch needle attached to a 3-mL syringe and inject the preservative-free Sterile Water for Injection into the drug product vial for reconstitution. The needle and syringe used for reconstitution with preservative-free Sterile Water for Injection should then be discarded and should not be used for subcutaneous injections. After the addition of preservative-free Sterile Water for Injection, the vial contents should be reconstituted by shaking the vial for approximately one minute and then allowing it to sit for one minute. The resulting 80-mg/mL solution is sufficient to allow a withdrawal volume of up to 2 mL for subcutaneous administration. The reconstituted solution is viscous, clear, colorless to pale yellow, and essentially free from particulates. Prior to injection, the reconstituted solution should be carefully inspected for any discoloration or particulate matter. If there is discoloration or particulate matter in the solution, the product in that vial should not be used.

Using aseptic technique, withdraw the recommended dose volume, up to 2 mL (160 mg), of the solution with a new 27-gauge, ½-inch needle attached to a new 3-mL syringe for subcutaneous injection. EACH VIAL SHOULD BE USED FOR A SINGLE DOSE ONLY. Discard the vial after withdrawal of drug.

Sites for subcutaneous injection, such as the abdomen, thigh, or upper arm, should be rotated. Injections should never be made at sites that are bruised, red, tender, or hard.

2.5 Stability and Storage

The lyophilized ARCALYST product is to be stored refrigerated at 2° to 8°C (36° to 46°F) inside the original carton to protect it from light. Do not use beyond the date stamped on the label. After reconstitution, ARCALYST may be kept at room temperature, should be protected from light, and should be used within three hours of reconstitution. ARCALYST does not contain preservatives; therefore, unused portions of ARCALYST should be discarded.

3 DOSAGE FORMS AND STRENGTHS

ARCALYST is supplied in sterile, single-use, 20-mL, glass vials. Each vial contains 220 mg of rilonacept as a white to off-white, preservative-free, lyophilized powder. Reconstitution with 2.3 mL of preservative-free Sterile Water for Injection is required prior to subcutaneous administration of the drug. The reconstituted ARCALYST is a viscous, clear, colorless to pale yellow, essentially free from particulates, 80-mg/mL solution.

4 CONTRAINDICATIONS

None.

5 WARNINGS AND PRECAUTIONS

5.1 Infections

Interleukin -1 (IL-1) blockade may interfere with the immune response to infections. Treatment with another medication that works through inhibition of IL-1 has been associated with an increased risk of serious infections, and serious infections have been reported in patients taking ARCALYST [*see Clinical Studies (14)*]. There was a greater incidence of infections in patients on ARCALYST compared with placebo. In the controlled portion of the study, one infection was reported as severe, which was bronchitis in a patient on ARCALYST.

In an open-label extension study, one patient developed bacterial meningitis and died [*see Adverse Reactions (6.3)*]. ARCALYST should be discontinued if a patient develops a serious infection. Treatment with ARCALYST should not be initiated in patients with an active or chronic infection.

In clinical studies, ARCALYST has not been administered concomitantly with tumor necrosis factor (TNF) inhibitors. An increased incidence of serious infections has been associated with administration of an IL-1 blocker in combination with TNF inhibitors. **Taking ARCALYST with TNF inhibitors is not recommended because this may increase the risk of serious infections.**

Drugs that affect the immune system by blocking TNF have been associated with an increased risk of reactivation of latent tuberculosis (TB). It is possible that taking drugs such as ARCALYST that block IL-1 increases the risk of TB or other atypical or opportunistic infections. Healthcare providers should follow current CDC guidelines both to evaluate for and to treat possible latent tuberculosis infections before initiating therapy with ARCALYST.

5.2 Immunosuppression

The impact of treatment with ARCALYST on active and/or chronic infections and the development of malignancies is not known [*see Adverse Reactions (6.3)*]. However, treatment with immunosuppressants, including ARCALYST, may result in an increase in the risk of malignancies.

5.3 Immunizations

Since no data are available on either the efficacy of live vaccines or on the risks of secondary transmission of infection by live vaccines in patients receiving ARCALYST, live vaccines should not be given concurrently with ARCALYST. In addition, because ARCALYST may interfere with normal immune response to new antigens, vaccinations may not be effective in patients receiving ARCALYST. No data are available on the effectiveness of vaccination with inactivated (killed) antigens in patients receiving ARCALYST.

Because IL-1 blockade may interfere with immune response to infections, it is recommended that prior to initiation of therapy with ARCALYST adult and pediatric patients receive all recommended vaccinations, as appropriate, including pneumococcal vaccine and inactivated influenza vaccine. (See current Recommended Immunizations schedules at the website of the Centers for Disease Control. http://www.cdc.gov/vaccines/recs/schedules/).

5.4 Lipid Profile Changes

Patients should be monitored for changes in their lipid profiles and provided with medical treatment if warranted [*see Adverse Reactions (6.7)*].

5.5 Hypersensitivity

Hypersensitivity reactions associated with ARCALYST administration in the clinical studies were rare. If a hypersensitivity reaction occurs, administration of ARCALYST should be discontinued and appropriate therapy initiated.

6 ADVERSE REACTIONS

Six serious adverse reactions were reported by four patients during the clinical program. These serious adverse reactions were *Mycobacterium intracellulare* infection; gastrointestinal bleeding and colitis; sinusitis and bronchitis; and *Streptococcus pneumoniae* meningitis [*see Adverse Reactions (6.3)*].

The most commonly reported adverse reaction associated with ARCALYST was injection-site reaction (ISR) [*see Adverse Reactions (6.2)*]. The next most commonly reported adverse reaction was upper respiratory infection [*see Adverse Reactions (6.3)*].

Because clinical trials are conducted under widely varying conditions, adverse reaction rates observed in the clinical trials of a drug cannot be directly compared to rates in the clinical trials of another drug and may not reflect the rates observed in practice.

The data described herein reflect exposure to ARCALYST in 600 patients, including 85 exposed for at least 6 months and 65 exposed for at least one year. These included patients with CAPS, patients with other diseases, and healthy volunteers. Approximately 60 patients with CAPS have been treated weekly with 160 mg of ARCALYST. The pivotal trial population included 47 patients with CAPS. These patients were between the ages of 22 and 78 years (average 51 years). Thirty-one patients were female and 16 were male. All of the patients were White/Caucasian. Six pediatric patients (12-17 years) were enrolled directly into the open-label extension phase.

6.1 Clinical Trial Experience

Part A of the clinical trial was conducted in patients with CAPS who were naïve to treatment with ARCALYST. Part A of the study was a randomized, double-blind, placebo-controlled, six-week study comparing ARCALYST to placebo [*see Clinical Studies (14)*]. Table 1 reflects the frequency of adverse events reported by at least two patients during Part A.

Table 1: Most Frequent Adverse Reactions (Part A, Reported by at Least Two Patients)

Adverse Event	ARCALYST 160 mg (n = 23)	Placebo (n= 24)
Any AE	17 (74%)	13 (54%)
Injection-site reactions	11 (48%)	3 (13%)

Upper respiratory tract infection	6 (26%)	1 (4%)
Nausea	1 (4%)	3 (13%)
Diarrhea	1 (4%)	3 (13%)
Sinusitis	2 (9%)	1 (4%)
Abdominal pain upper	0	2 (8%)
Cough	2 (9%)	0
Hypoesthesia	2 (9%)	0
Stomach discomfort	1 (4%)	1 (4%)
Urinary tract infection	1 (4%)	1 (4%)

6.2 Injection-Site Reactions
In patients with CAPS, the most common and consistently reported adverse event associated with ARCALYST was injection-site reaction (ISR). The ISRs included erythema, swelling, pruritis, mass, bruising, inflammation, pain, edema, dermatitis, discomfort, urticaria, vesicles, warmth and hemorrhage. Most injection-site reactions lasted for one to two days. No ISRs were assessed as severe, and no patient discontinued study participation due to an ISR.

6.3 Infections
During Part A, the incidence of patients reporting infections was greater with ARCALYST (48%) than with placebo (17%). In Part B, randomized withdrawal, the incidence of infections were similar in the ARCALYST (18%) and the placebo patients (22%). Part A of the trial was initiated in the winter months, while Part B was predominantly performed in the summer months.
In placebo-controlled studies across a variety of patient populations encompassing 360 patients treated with rilonacept and 179 treated with placebo, the incidence of infections was 34% and 27% (2.15 per patient-exposure year and 1.81 per patient-exposure year), respectively, for rilonacept and placebo.
Serious Infections: One patient receiving ARCALYST for an unapproved indication in another study developed an infection in his olecranon bursa with *Mycobacterium intracellulare*. The patient was on chronic glucocorticoid treatment. The infection occurred after an intraarticular glucocorticoid injection into the bursa with subsequent local exposure to a suspected source of mycobacteria. The patient recovered after the administration of the appropriate antimicrobial therapy. One patient treated for another unapproved indication developed bronchitis/sinusitis, which resulted in hospitalization. One patient died in an open-label study of CAPS from *Streptococcus pneumoniae* meningitis.

6.4 Malignancies
[*see Warnings and Precautions (5.2)*].

6.5 Hematologic Events
One patient in a study in an unapproved indication developed transient neutropenia (ANC < 1×10^9/L) after receiving a large dose (2000 mg intravenously) of ARCALYST. The patient did not experience any infection associated with the neutropenia.

6.6 Immunogenicity
Antibodies directed against the receptor domains of rilonacept were detected by an ELISA assay in patients with CAPS after treatment with ARCALYST. Nineteen of 55 patients (35%) who had received ARCALYST for at least 6 weeks tested positive for treatment-emergent binding antibodies on at least one occasion. Of the 19, seven tested positive at the last assessment (Week 18 or 24 of the open-label extension period), and five patients tested positive for neutralizing antibodies on at least one occasion. There was no correlation of antibody activity and either clinical effectiveness or safety.
The data reflect the percentage of patients whose test results were positive for antibodies to the rilonacept receptor domains in specific assays, and are highly dependent on the sensitivity and specificity of the assays. The observed incidence of antibody (including neutralizing antibody) positivity in an assay is highly dependent on several factors including assay sensitivity and specificity, assay methodology, sample handling, timing of sample collection, concomitant medications, and underlying disease. For these reasons, comparison of the incidence of antibodies to rilonacept with the incidence of antibodies to other products may be misleading.

6.7 Lipid profiles
Cholesterol and lipid levels may be reduced in patients with chronic inflammation. Patients with CAPS treated with ARCALYST experienced increases in their mean total cholesterol, HDL cholesterol, LDL cholesterol, and triglycerides. The mean increases from baseline for total cholesterol, HDL cholesterol, LDL cholesterol, and triglycerides were 19 mg/dL, 2 mg/dL, 10 mg/dL, and 57 mg/dL respectively after 6 weeks of open-label therapy. Physicians should monitor the lipid profiles of their patients (for example after 2-3 months) and consider lipid-lowering therapies as needed based upon cardiovascular risk factors and current guidelines.

7 DRUG INTERACTIONS

7.1 TNF-blocking agent and IL-1 blocking agent
Specific drug interaction studies have not been conducted with ARCALYST. Concomitant administration of another drug that blocks IL-1 with a TNF-blocking agent in another patient population has been associated with an increased risk of serious infections and an increased risk of neutropenia. The concomitant administration of ARCALYST with TNF-blocking agents may also result in similar toxicities and is not recommended [*see Warnings and Precautions (5.1)*]. The concomitant administration of ARCALYST with other drugs that block IL-1 has not been studied. Based upon the potential for pharmacologic interactions between rilonacept and a recombinant IL-1ra, concomitant administration of ARCALYST and other agents that block IL-1 or its receptors is not recommended.

7.2 Cytochrome P450 Substrates
The formation of CYP450 enzymes is suppressed by increased levels of cytokines (e.g., IL-1) during chronic inflammation. Thus it is expected that for a molecule that binds to IL-1, such as rilonacept, the formation of CYP450 enzymes could be normalized. This is clinically relevant for CYP450 substrates with a narrow therapeutic index, where the dose is individually adjusted (e.g., warfarin). Upon initiation of ARCALYST, in patients being treated with these types of medicinal products, therapeutic monitoring of the effect or drug concentration should be performed and the individual dose of the medicinal product may need to be adjusted as needed.

8 USE IN SPECIFIC POPULATIONS

8.1 Pregnancy
Pregnancy Category C. There are no adequate and well-controlled studies of ARCALYST in pregnant women. Based on animal data, ARCALYST may cause fetal harm. An embryo-fetal developmental toxicity study was performed in cynomolgus monkeys treated with 0, 5, 15 or 30 mg/kg given twice a week (highest dose is approximately 3.7-fold higher than the human doses of 160 mg based on body surface area). The fetus of the only monkey with exposure to rilonacept during the later period of gestation showed multiple fusion and absence of the ribs and thoracic vertebral bodies and arches. Exposure to rilonacept during this time period was below that expected clinically. Likewise, in the cynomolgus monkey, all doses of rilonacept reduced serum levels of estradiol up to 64% compared to controls and increased the incidence of lumbar ribs compared to both control animals and historical control incidences. In perinatal and postnatal developmental toxicology studies in the mouse model using a murine analog of rilonacept (0, 20, 100 or 200 mg/kg), there was a 3-fold increase in the number of stillbirths in dams treated with 200 mg/kg three times per week (the highest dose is approximately 6-fold higher than the 160 mg maintenance dose based on body surface area). ARCALYST should be used during pregnancy only if the benefit justifies the potential risk to the fetus.
Nonteratogenic effects. A peri- and post-natal reproductive toxicology study was performed in which mice were subcutaneously administered a murine analogue of rilonacept at doses of 20, 100, 200 mg/kg three times per week (the highest dose is approximately 6-fold higher than the 160 mg maintenance dose based on body surface area). Results indicated an increased incidence in unscheduled deaths of the F_1 offspring during maturation at all doses tested.

8.3 Nursing Mothers
It is not known whether rilonacept is excreted in human milk. Because many drugs are excreted in human milk, caution should be exercised when ARCALYST is administered to a nursing woman.

8.4 Pediatric Use
Six pediatric patients with CAPS between the ages of 12 and 16 were treated with ARCALYST at a weekly, subcutaneous dose of 2.2 mg/kg (up to a maximum of 160 mg) for 24-weeks during the open-label extension phase. These patients showed improvement from baseline in their symptom scores and in objective markers of inflammation (e.g. Serum Amyloid A and C-Reactive Protein). The adverse events included injection site reactions and upper respiratory symptoms as were commonly seen in the adult patients.
The trough drug levels for four pediatric patients measured at the end of the weekly dose interval (mean 20 mcg/mL, range 3.6 to 33 mcg/mL) were similar to those observed in adult patients with CAPS (mean 24 mcg/mL, range 7 to 56 mcg/mL).
Safety and effectiveness in pediatric patients below the age of 12 have not been established.
When administered to pregnant primates, rilonacept treatment may have contributed to alterations in bone ossification in the fetus. It is not known if ARCALYST will alter bone development in pediatric patients. Pediatric patients treated with ARCALYST should undergo appropriate monitoring for growth and development. [*see Use in Specific Populations (8.1)*]

8.5 Geriatric Use
In the placebo-controlled clinical studies in patients with CAPS and other indications, 70 patients randomized to treatment with ARCALYST were ≥ 65 years of age, and 6 were ≥ 75 years of age. In the CAPS clinical trial, efficacy, safety and tolerability were generally similar in elderly patients as compared to younger adults; however, only ten patients ≥ 65 years old participated in the trial. In an open-label extension study of CAPS, a 71 year old woman developed bacterial meningitis and died [*see Adverse Reactions (6.3)*]. Age did not appear to have a significant effect on steady-state trough concentrations in the clinical study.

8.6 Patients with Renal Impairment
No formal studies have been conducted to examine the pharmacokinetics of rilonacept administered subcutaneously in patients with renal impairment.

8.7 Patients with Hepatic Impairment
No formal studies have been conducted to examine the pharmacokinetics of rilonacept administered subcutaneously in patients with hepatic impairment.

10 OVERDOSAGE

There have been no reports of overdose with ARCALYST. Maximum weekly doses of up to 320 mg have been administered subcutaneously for up to approximately 18 months in a small number of patients with CAPS and up to 6 months in patients with an unapproved indication in clinical trials without evidence of dose-limiting toxicities. In addition, ARCALYST given intravenously at doses up to 2000 mg monthly in another patient population for up to six months were tolerated without dose-limiting toxicities. The maximum amount of ARCALYST that can be safely administered has not been determined.
In case of overdose, it is recommended that the patient be monitored for any signs or symptoms of adverse reactions or effects, and appropriate symptomatic treatment instituted immediately.

11 DESCRIPTION

Rilonacept is a dimeric fusion protein consisting of the ligand-binding domains of the extracellular portions of the human interleukin-1 receptor component (IL-1RI) and IL-1 receptor accessory protein (IL-1RAcP) linked in-line to the Fc portion of human IgG1. Rilonacept has a molecular weight of approximately 251 kDa. Rilonacept is expressed in recombinant Chinese hamster ovary (CHO) cells.
ARCALYST is supplied in single-use, 20-mL glass vials containing a sterile, white to off-white, lyophilized powder. Each vial of ARCALYST is to be reconstituted with 2.3 mL of Sterile Water for Injection. A volume of up to 2 mL can be withdrawn, which is designed to deliver 160 mg for subcutaneous administration only. The resulting solution is viscous, clear, colorless to pale yellow, and essentially free from particulates. Each vial contains 220 mg rilonacept. After reconstitution, each vial contains 80 mg/mL rilonacept, 40 mM histidine, 50 mM arginine, 3.0% (w/v) polyethylene glycol 3350, 2.0% (w/v) sucrose, and 1.0% (w/v) glycine at a pH of 6.5 ± 0.3. No preservatives are present.

12 CLINICAL PHARMACOLOGY

12.1 Mechanism of Action
CAPS refer to rare genetic syndromes generally caused by mutations in the NLRP-3 [Nucleotide-binding domain, leucine rich family (NLR), pyrin domain containing 3] gene (also known as Cold-Induced Auto-inflammatory Syndrome-1 [*CIAS1*]). CAPS disorders are inherited in an autosomal dominant pattern with male and female offspring equally affected. Features common to all disorders include fever, urticaria-like rash, arthralgia, myalgia, fatigue, and conjunctivitis.
In most cases, inflammation in CAPS is associated with mutations in the NLRP-3 gene which encodes the protein cryopyrin, an important component of the inflammasome. Cryopyrin regulates the protease caspase-1 and controls the activation of interleukin-1 beta (IL-1β). Mutations in NLRP-3 result in an overactive inflammasome resulting in excessive release of activated IL-1β that drives inflammation.
Rilonacept blocks IL-1β signaling by acting as a soluble decoy receptor that binds IL-1β and prevents its interaction with cell surface receptors. Rilonacept also binds IL-1α and IL-1 receptor antagonist (IL-1ra) with reduced affinity. The equilibrium dissociation constants for rilonacept binding to IL-1β, IL-1α and IL-1ra were 0.5 pM, 1.4 pM and 6.1 pM, respectively.

12.2 Pharmacodynamics
C-Reactive Protein (CRP) and Serum Amyloid A (SAA) are indicators of inflammatory disease activity that are elevated in patients with CAPS. Elevated SAA has been associated with the development of systemic amyloidosis in patients with CAPS. Compared to placebo, treatment with ARCALYST resulted in sustained reductions from baseline in mean serum CRP and SAA to normal levels during the clinical trial. ARCALYST also normalized mean SAA from elevated levels.

12.3 Pharmacokinetics
The average trough levels of rilonacept were approximately 24 mcg/mL at steady-state following weekly subcutaneous doses of 160 mg for up to 48 weeks in patients with CAPS. The steady-state appeared to be reached by 6 weeks.

Table 2: Mean Symptom Scores

Part A	Placebo (n=24)	ARCALYST (n=23)	Part B	Placebo (n=23)	ARCALYST (n=22)
Pre-treatment Baseline Period (Weeks -3 to 0)	2.4	3.1	Active ARCALYST Baseline Period (Weeks 13 to 15)	0.2	0.3
Endpoint Period (Weeks 4 to 6)	2.1	0.5	Endpoint Period (Weeks 22 to 24)	1.2	0.4
LS* Mean Change from Baseline to Endpoint	-0.5	-2.4	LS* Mean Change from Baseline to Endpoint	0.9	0.1
95% confidence interval for difference between treatment groups	(-2.4, -1.3)**		95% confidence interval for difference between treatment groups	(-1.3, -0.4)**	

*Differences are adjusted using an analysis of covariance model with terms for treatment and Part A baseline.
** A confidence interval lying entirely below zero indicates a statistical difference favoring ARCALYST versus placebo.

No pharmacokinetic data are available in patients with hepatic or renal impairment.
No study was conducted to evaluate the effect of age, gender, or body weight on rilonacept exposure. Based on limited data obtained from the clinical study, steady state trough concentrations were similar between male and female patients. Age (26-78 years old) and body weight (50-120 kg) did not appear to have a significant effect on trough rilonacept concentrations. The effect of race could not be assessed because only Caucasian patients participated in the clinical study, reflecting the epidemiology of the disease.

13 NONCLINICAL TOXICOLOGY

13.1 Carcinogenesis, Mutagenesis, Impairment of Fertility

Long-term animal studies have not been performed to evaluate the carcinogenic potential of rilonacept. The mutagenic potential of rilonacept was not evaluated.
Male and female fertility was evaluated in a mouse surrogate model using a murine analog of rilonacept. Male mice were treated beginning 8 weeks prior to mating and continuing through female gestation day 15. Female mice were treated for 2 weeks prior to mating and on gestation days 0, 3, and 6. The murine analog of rilonacept did not alter either male or female fertility parameters at doses up to 200 mg/kg (this dose is approximately 6-fold higher than the 160 mg maintenance dose based on body surface area).

14 CLINICAL STUDIES

The safety and efficacy of ARCALYST for the treatment of CAPS was demonstrated in a randomized, double-blind, placebo-controlled study with two parts (A and B) conducted sequentially in the same patients with FCAS and MWS.
Part A was a 6-week, randomized, double-blind, parallel-group period comparing ARCALYST at a dose of 160 mg weekly after an initial loading dose of 320 mg to placebo. Part B followed immediately after Part A and consisted of a 9-week, patient-blind period during which all patients received ARCALYST 160 mg weekly, followed by a 9-week, double-blind, randomized withdrawal period in which patients were randomly assigned to either remain on ARCALYST 160 mg weekly or to receive placebo. Patients were then given the option to enroll in a 24-week, open-label treatment extension phase in which all patients were treated with ARCALYST 160 mg weekly.
Using a daily diary questionnaire, patients rated the following five signs and symptoms of CAPS: joint pain, rash, feeling of fever/chills, eye redness/pain, and fatigue, each on a scale of 0 (none, no severity) to 10 (very severe). The study evaluated the mean symptom score using the change from baseline to the end of treatment.
The changes in mean symptom scores for the randomized parallel-group period (Part A) and the randomized withdrawal period (Part B) of the study are shown in Table 2. ARCALYST-treated patients had a larger reduction in the mean symptom score in Part A compared to placebo-treated patients. In Part B, mean symptom scores increased more in patients withdrawn to placebo compared to patients who remained on ARCALYST.
[See table 2 above]
Daily mean symptom scores over time for Part A are shown in Figure 1.
[See figure 1 at top of next column]
Improvement in symptom scores was noted within several days of initiation of ARCALYST therapy in most patients.
In Part A, patients treated with ARCALYST experienced more improvement in each of the five components of the composite endpoint (joint pain, rash, feeling of fever/chills, eye redness/pain, and fatigue) than placebo-treated patients.
In Part A, a higher proportion of patients in the ARCALYST group experienced improvement from baseline in the composite score by at least 30% (96% vs. 29% of patients), by at least 50% (87% vs. 8%) and by at least 75% (70% vs. 0%) compared to the placebo group.

Figure 1: Group Mean Daily Symptom Scores by Treatment Group in Part A and Single-blind ARCALYST Treatment Phase from Week -3 to Week 15

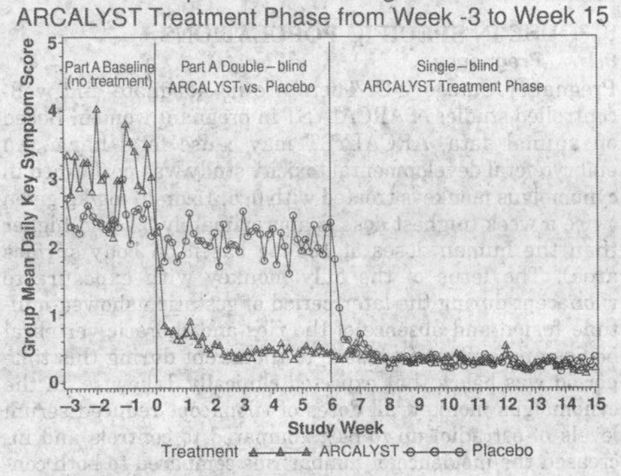

Serum Amyloid A (SAA) and C-Reactive Protein (CRP) levels are acute phase reactants that are typically elevated in patients with CAPS with active disease. During Part A, mean levels of CRP decreased versus baseline for the ARCALYST treated patients, while there was no change for those on placebo (Table 3). ARCALYST also led to a decrease in SAA versus baseline to levels within the normal range.

Table 3. Mean Serum Amyloid A and C-Reactive Protein Levels Over Time in Part A

Part A	ARCALYST	Placebo
SAA (normal range: 0.7 – 6.4 mg/L)	(n=22)	(n=24)
Pre-treatment Baseline	60	110
Week 6	4	110
CRP (normal range: 0.0 – 8.4 mg/L)	(n= 21)	(n=24)
Pre-treatment Baseline	22	30
Week 6	2	28

During the open-label extension, reductions in mean symptom scores, serum CRP, and serum SAA levels were maintained for up to one year.

16 HOW SUPPLIED/ STORAGE AND HANDLING

Each 20-mL glass vial of ARCALYST contains a sterile, white to off-white, preservative-free, lyophilized powder. ARCALYST is supplied in a carton containing four vials (NDC 61755-001-01).
The lyophilized ARCALYST product is to be stored refrigerated at 2° to 8°C (36° to 46°F) inside the original carton to protect from light. Do not use beyond the date stamped on the label. After reconstitution, ARCALYST may be kept at room temperature, should be kept from light, and should be used within three hours of reconstitution. ARCALYST does not contain preservatives; therefore, unused portions of ARCALYST should be discarded. Discard the vial after a single withdrawal of drug.

17 PATIENT COUNSELING INFORMATION

See FDA-approved patient labeling.
The first injection of ARCALYST should be performed under the supervision of a qualified healthcare professional. If a patient or caregiver is to administer ARCALYST, he/she should be instructed on aseptic reconstitution of the lyophilized product and injection technique. The ability to inject subcutaneously should be assessed to ensure proper administration of ARCALYST, including rotation of injection sites. (*See Patient Information Leaflet for ARCALYST®*).
ARCALYST should be reconstituted with preservative-free Sterile Water for Injection to be provided by the pharmacy. A puncture-resistant container for disposal of vials, needles and syringes should be used. Patients or caregivers should be instructed in proper vial, syringe, and needle disposal, and should be cautioned against reuse of these items.
Injection-site Reactions: Physicians should explain to patients that almost half of the patients in the clinical trials experienced a reaction at the injection site. Injection-site reactions may include pain, erythema, swelling, pruritis, bruising, mass, inflammation, dermatitis, edema, urticaria, vesicles, warmth, and hemorrhage. Patients should be cautioned to avoid injecting into an area that is already swollen or red. Any persistent reaction should be brought to the attention of the prescribing physician.
Infections: Patients should be cautioned that ARCALYST has been associated with serious, life-threatening infections, and not to initiate treatment with ARCALYST if they have a chronic or active infection. Patients should be counseled to contact their healthcare professional immediately if they develop an infection after starting ARCALYST. Treatment with ARCALYST should be discontinued if a patient develops a serious infection. Patients should be counseled not to take any IL-1 blocking drug, including ARCALYST, if they are also taking a drug that blocks TNF such as etanercept, infliximab, or adalimumab. Use of ARCALYST with other IL-1 blocking agents, such as anakinra, is not recommended.
Vaccinations: Prior to initiation of therapy with ARCALYST physicians should review with adult and pediatric patients their vaccination history relative to current medical guidelines for vaccine use, including taking into account the potential of increased risk of infection during treatment with ARCALYST.

REGENERON

Manufactured and distributed by:
Regeneron Pharmaceuticals, Inc.
777 Old Saw Mill River Road,
Tarrytown, NY 10591-6707, 1-877-REGN-777 (1-877-734-6777)
U.S. License Number 1760
NDC 61755-001-01

V3.0
Revised: 04/2010
Regeneron U.S. Patent 6,927,044 B2, 6,472,179 B2, 5,844,099 and other pending patents

Patient Information
ARCALYST® (ARK-a-list)
(rilonacept)
Injection for Subcutaneous Use

Read the patient information that comes with ARCALYST before you start taking it and each time you refill your prescription. There may be new information. The information in this leaflet does not take the place of talking with your healthcare provider about your medical condition and your treatment.

What is the most important information I should know about ARCALYST?

ARCALYST can affect your immune system. ARCALYST can lower the ability of your immune system to fight infections. Serious infections, including life-threatening infections and death have happened in patients taking ARCALYST. **Taking ARCALYST can make you more likely to get infections, including life-threatening serious infections, or may make any infection that you have worse.**

You should not begin treatment with ARCALYST if you have an infection or have infections that keep coming back (chronic infection).

After starting ARCALYST, if you get an infection, any sign of an infection including a fever, cough, flu-like symptoms, or have any open sores on your body, call your healthcare provider right away. **Treatment with ARCALYST should be stopped if you develop a serious infection.**

You should not take medicines that block Tumor Necrosis Factor (TNF), such as ENBREL® (etanercept), Humira® (adalimumab), or Remicade® (infliximab), while you are taking ARCALYST. You should also not take other medicines that block Interleukin -1 (IL-1), such as Kineret® (anakinra), while taking ARCALYST. Taking ARCALYST with any of these medicines may increase your risk of getting a serious infection.

Before starting treatment with ARCALYST, tell your healthcare provider if you:
- think you have an infection
- are being treated for an infection
- have signs of an infection, such as fever, cough, or flu-like symptoms
- have any open sores on your body
- have a history of infections that keep coming back
- have asthma. Patients with asthma may have an increased risk of infection.
- have diabetes or an immune system problem. People with these conditions have a higher chance for infections.
- have tuberculosis (TB), or if you have been in close contact with someone who has had tuberculosis.
- have or have had HIV, Hepatitis B, or Hepatitis C
- take other medicines that affect your immune system

Before you begin treatment with ARCALYST, talk with your healthcare provider about your vaccination history. Ask your healthcare provider whether you should receive any vaccinations, including pneumonia vaccine and flu vaccine, before you begin treatment with ARCALYST.

What is ARCALYST?

ARCALYST is a prescription medicine called an interleukin-1 (IL-1) blocker. ARCALYST is used to treat adults and children 12 years and older with Cryopyrin-Associated Periodic Syndromes (CAPS), including Familial Cold Auto-inflammatory Syndrome (FCAS) and Muckle Wells Syndrome (MWS). ARCALYST can help lessen the signs and symptoms of CAPS, such as rash, joint pain, fever, and tiredness, but it can also lead to serious side effects because of the effects on your immune system.

What should I tell my healthcare provider before taking ARCALYST?

ARCALYST may not be right for you. **Before taking ARCALYST, tell your healthcare provider about all of your medical conditions, including if you:**
- are scheduled to receive any vaccines. You should not receive live vaccines if you take ARCALYST.
- are pregnant or planning to become pregnant. It is not known if ARCALYST will harm your unborn child. Tell your healthcare provider right away if you become pregnant while taking ARCALYST.
- are breast-feeding or planning to breast-feed. It is not known if ARCALYST passes into your breast milk.

See "What is the most important information I should know about ARCALYST?"

Tell your healthcare provider about all the medicines you take, including prescription and non-prescription medicines, vitamins, and herbal supplements. Especially tell your healthcare provider if you take other medicines that affect your immune system, such as:
- other medicines that block IL-1, such as Kineret® (anakinra).
- medicines that block Tumor Necrosis Factor (TNF), such as ENBREL® (etanercept), Humira® (adalimumab), or Remicade® (infliximab).
- corticosteroids.

See "What is the most important information I should know about ARCALYST?"

Know the medicines you take. Keep a list of your medicines and show it to your healthcare provider and pharmacist every time you get a new prescription.

If you are not sure or have any questions about any of this information, ask your healthcare provider.

How should I take ARCALYST?

See the "Patient Instructions for Use" at the end of this leaflet.
- Take ARCALYST exactly as prescribed by your healthcare provider.
- ARCALYST is given by injection under the skin (subcutaneous injection) one time each week.
- Your healthcare provider will tell and show you or your caregiver:
  - how much ARCALYST to inject
  - how to prepare your dose
  - how to give the injection
- Do not try to give ARCALYST injections until you are sure that you or your caregiver understands how to prepare and inject your dose. Call your healthcare provider or pharmacist if you have any questions about preparing and injecting your dose, or if you or your caregiver would like more training.
- If you miss a dose of ARCALYST, inject it as soon as you remember, up to the day before your next scheduled dose. The next dose should be taken at the next regularly scheduled time. If you have any questions, contact your healthcare provider.
- If you accidentally take more ARCALYST than prescribed, call your healthcare provider.

What are the possible side effects of ARCALYST?

Serious side effects may occur while you are taking and after you finish taking ARCALYST including:
- **Serious Infections. See "What is the most important information I should know about taking ARCALYST?"** Treatment with ARCALYST should be discontinued if you develop a serious infection.
- **Allergic Reaction.** Call your healthcare provider or seek emergency care right away if you get any of the following symptoms of an allergic reaction while taking ARCALYST:
  - rash
  - swollen face
  - trouble breathing

Common side effects with ARCALYST include:
- **Injection-site reaction.** This includes: pain, redness, swelling, itching, bruising, lumps, inflammation, skin rash, blisters, warmth, and bleeding at the injection site.
- **Upper respiratory infection.**
- **Changes in your blood cholesterol and triglycerides (lipids).** Your healthcare provider will check you for this.

These are not all the possible side effects of ARCALYST. Tell your healthcare provider about any side effects that bother you or that do not go away. For more information ask your healthcare provider or pharmacist. Call your doctor for medical advice about side effects. You may report side effects to FDA at 1-800-FDA-1088.

How should I store ARCALYST?
- Keep ARCALYST in the carton it comes in.
- Store ARCALYST in a refrigerator between 36°F to 46°F (2°C to 8°C). Call your pharmacy if you have any questions.
- Always keep ARCALYST away from light.
- Refrigerated ARCALYST can be used until the expiration date printed on the vial and carton.
- ARCALYST may be kept at room temperature after mixing. ARCALYST should be used within **three hours** of mixing. Keep ARCALYST away from light.
- If you need to take ARCALYST with you when traveling, store the carton in a cool carrier with a cold pack and protect it from light.

Keep ARCALYST, injection supplies, and all other medicines out of reach of children.

What are the ingredients in ARCALYST?

Active ingredient: rilonacept.

Inactive ingredients: histidine, arginine, polyethylene glycol 3350, sucrose, and glycine.

General Information about ARCALYST

Medicines are sometimes prescribed for conditions other than those listed in patient information leaflets. Do not use ARCALYST for a condition for which it was not prescribed. Do not give ARCALYST to other people even if they have the same condition. It may harm them.

This leaflet summarizes the most important information about ARCALYST. If you would like more information, speak with your healthcare provider. You can ask your healthcare provider or pharmacist for information about ARCALYST that was written for healthcare professionals. For more information about ARCALYST, call 1-877-REGN-777 (1-877-734-6777), or visit www.ARCALYST.com.

Patient Instructions for Use

It is important for you to read, understand and follow the instructions below exactly. Following the instructions correctly will help to make sure that you use prepare and inject the medicine the right way to prevent infection.

How do I prepare and give an injection of ARCALYST?

STEP 1: Setting up for an injection
1. Choose a table or other flat surface area to set up the supplies for your injection. Be sure that the area is clean or clean it with an antiseptic or soap and water first.
2. Wash your hands well with soap and water, and dry with a clean towel.
3. Put the following items on a table, or other flat surface, for each injection (see Figure 1):

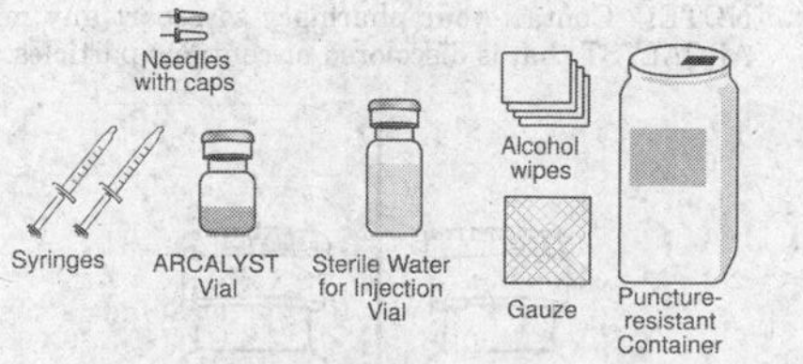

Figure 1

- 2 sterile, 3-milliliter (mL) disposable syringes with markings at each 0.1 mL (see Figure 2):
  - one needed for mixing (reconstitution) ARCALYST
  - one needed for injection

[See figure 2 at top of next column]
- 2 sterile disposable needles (27 gauge ½ inches)
  - one needed for mixing
  - one needed for injection
- 4 alcohol wipes
- 1 2×2 gauze pad
- 1 vial of ARCALYST (powder in vial)
- 1 vial of preservative-free Sterile Water for Injection
- 1 puncture-resistant container for disposal of used needles , syringes, and vials

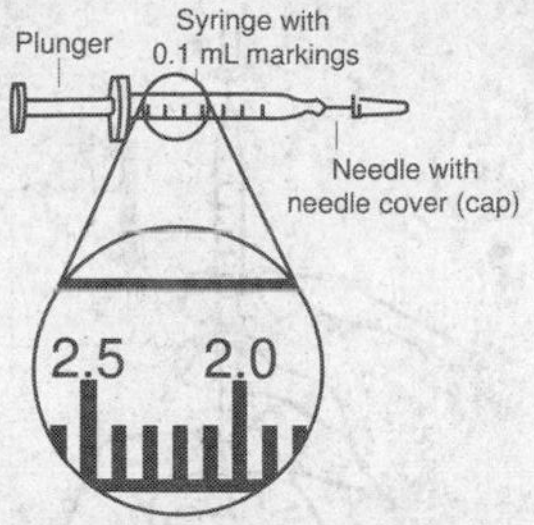

Figure 2

Note:
- Do not use Sterile Water for Injection, syringes or needles other than those provided by your pharmacy. Contact your pharmacy if you need replacement syringes or needles.
- Do not touch the needles or the rubber stoppers on the vials with your hands. If you do touch a stopper, clean it with a fresh alcohol wipe.
- If you touch a needle or the needle touches any surface, throw away the entire syringe into the puncture resistant container and start over with a new syringe.
- **Do not reuse needles or syringes.**
- To protect yourself and others from possible needle sticks, it is very important to throw away every syringe, with the needle attached, in the puncture proof container right after use. ***Do not try to recap the needle.***

STEP 2: Preparing Vials
1. Check the expiration date on the carton of ARCALYST. Do not use the vial if the expiration date has passed. Contact your pharmacy for assistance.
2. Check the expiration date on the vial of Sterile Water for Injection. Do not use the vial if the expiration date has passed. Contact your pharmacy for assistance.
3. Remove the protective plastic cap from both vials.
4. Clean the top of each vial with an alcohol wipe. Use one wipe for each vial and wipe in one direction around the top of the vial (see Figure 3).

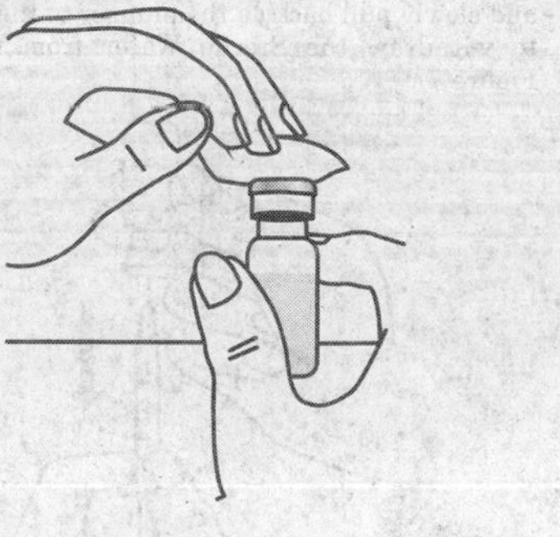

Figure 3

5. Open the wrapper that contains the 27-gauge needle by pulling apart the tabs and set it aside for later use. Do not remove the needle cover. This needle will be used to mix the water with powder. Open the wrapper that contains the syringe by pulling apart the tabs. Hold the barrel of the syringe with one hand and twist the 27-gauge needle onto the tip of the syringe until it fits snugly with the other hand (see Figure 4).

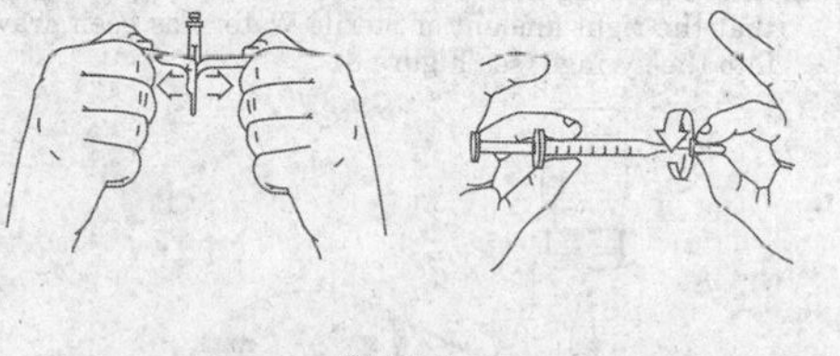

Figure 4

6. Hold the syringe at eye level. With the needle covered pull back the plunger to the 2.3 mL mark, filling the syringe with air (see Figure 5).

[See figure 5 at top of next column]

7. Hold the syringe in one hand, use the other hand to pull the needle cover straight off. Do not twist the needle as you pull off the cover. Place the needle cover aside. Hold the syringe in the hand that you will use to mix (reconstitute) your medicine. Hold the Sterile Water vial on a firm surface with your other hand. Slowly insert the

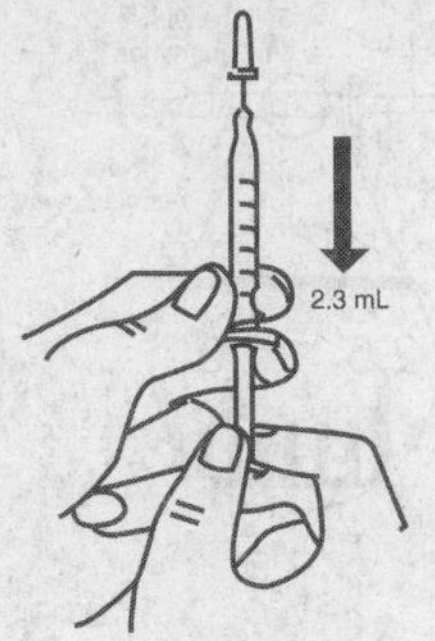

Figure 5

needle straight through the rubber stopper. Do not bend the needle. Push the plunger in all the way to push the air into the vial (see Figure 6).

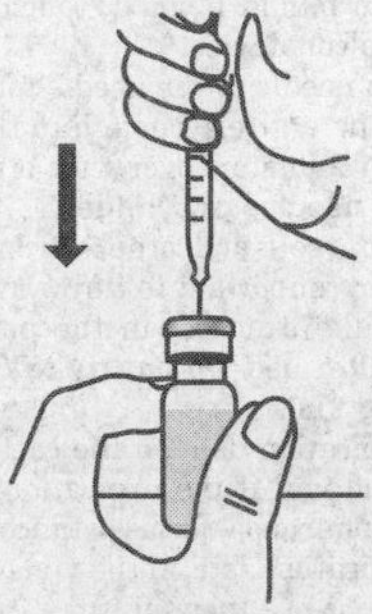

Figure 6

8. Hold the vial in one hand and the syringe in the other hand and carefully turn the vial upside down so that the needle is pointing straight up.
9. Make sure the tip of the needle is covered by the liquid and slowly pull back on the plunger to the 2.3 mL mark to withdraw the Sterile Water from the vial (see Figure 7).

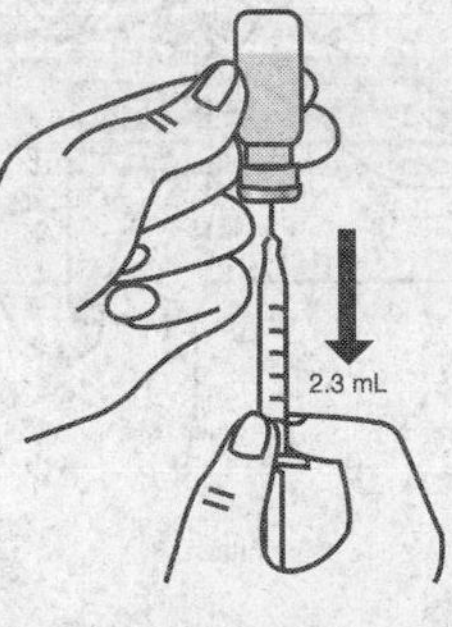

Figure 7

10. Keep the vial upside down and tap or flick the syringe with your fingers until any air bubbles rise to the top of the syringe.
11. To remove the air bubbles, gently push in the plunger so only the air is pushed out of the syringe and back into the bottle.
12. After removing the bubbles, check the syringe to be sure that the right amount of Sterile Water has been drawn into the syringe (see Figure 8).

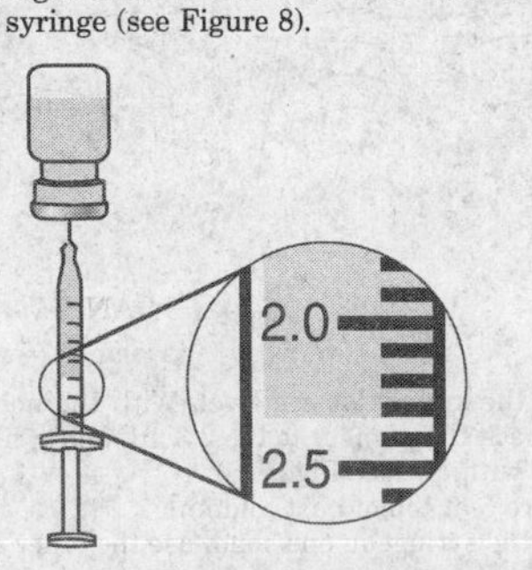

Figure 8

13. Carefully remove the syringe with needle from the Sterile Water vial. Do not touch the needle.

STEP 3: Mixing (Reconstituting) ARCALYST

1. With one hand, hold the ARCALYST vial on a firm surface.
2. With the other hand, take the syringe with the Sterile Water and the same needle, and slowly insert the needle straight down through the rubber stopper of the ARCALYST vial. Push the plunger in all the way to inject the Sterile Water into the vial.
3. Direct the water stream to gently go down the side of the vial into the powder (see Figure 9).

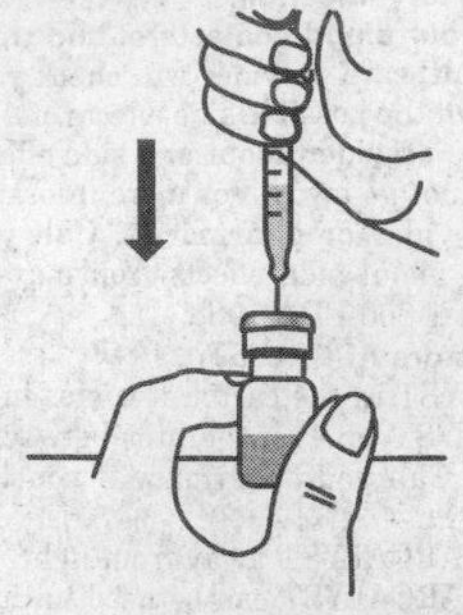

Figure 9

4. Remove the syringe and needle from the stopper and throw away the needle, syringe, and Sterile Water vial in the puncture resistant container. Do not try to put the needle cover back on the needle.
5. Hold the vial containing the ARCALYST and sterile water for injection sideways (not upright) with your thumb and a finger at the top and bottom of the vial, and quickly shake the vial back and forth (side-to-side) for about 1 minute (see Figure 10).

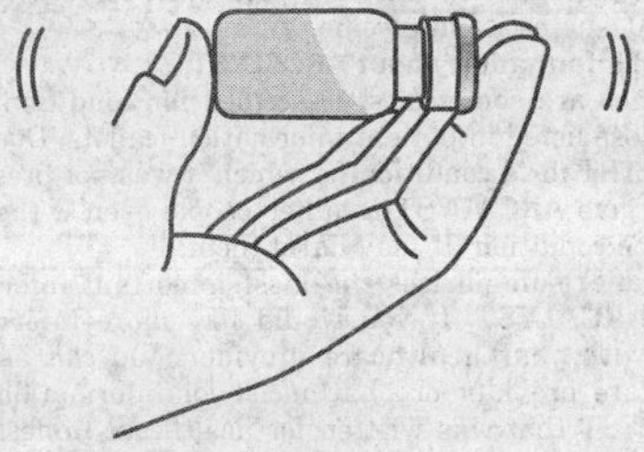

Figure 10

6. Put the vial back on the table and let the vial sit for about 1 minute.
7. Look at the vial for any particles or clumps of powder which have not dissolved.
8. If the powder has not completely dissolved, shake the vial quickly back and forth for 30 seconds more. Let the vial sit for about 1 minute.
9. Repeat Step 8 until the powder is completely dissolved and the solution is clear.
10. The mixed ARCALYST should be thick, clear, and colorless to pale yellow. Do not use the mixed liquid if it is discolored or cloudy, or if small particles are in it (see Figure 11).
NOTE: Contact your pharmacy to report any mixed ARCALYST that is discolored or contains particles.

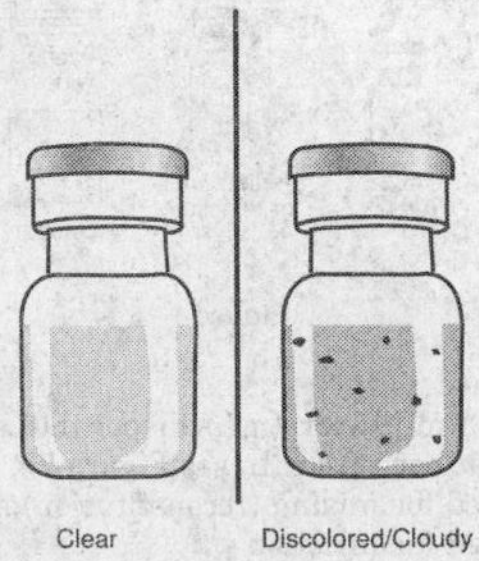

Figure 11

11. ARCALYST may be kept at room temperature after mixing. ARCALYST should be used within **three hours** of mixing. Keep ARCALYST away from light.

STEP 4: Preparing the injection

1. Hold the ARCALYST vial on a firm surface and wipe the top of the ARCALYST vial with a new alcohol wipe (see Figure 12).

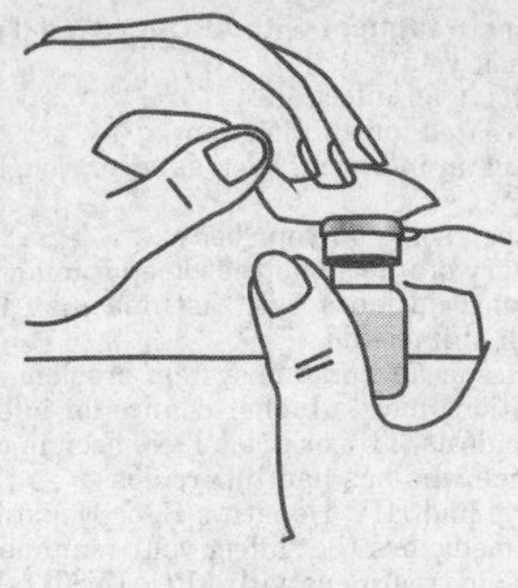

Figure 12

2. Take a new sterile, disposable needle and attach securely to a new syringe without removing the needle cover (see Figure 13).

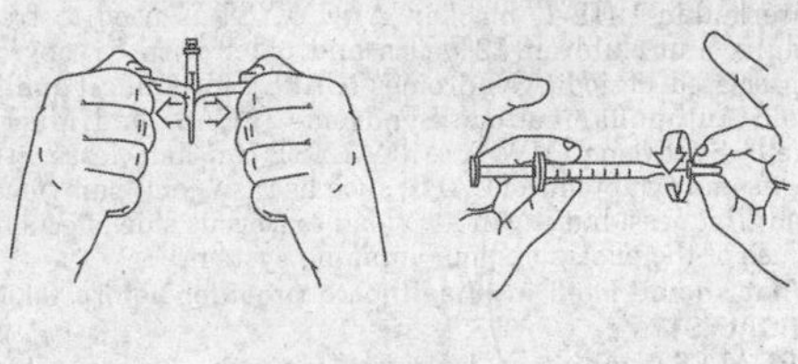

Figure 13

3. The amount of air you draw into the syringe should equal the amount of mixed ARCALYST that your healthcare provider has prescribed for you to inject.
4. To draw air into the syringe, hold the syringe at eye level. Do not remove the needle cover. Pull back the plunger on the syringe to the mark that is equal to the amount of mixed ARCALYST that your healthcare provider has prescribed for you to inject (see Figure 14).

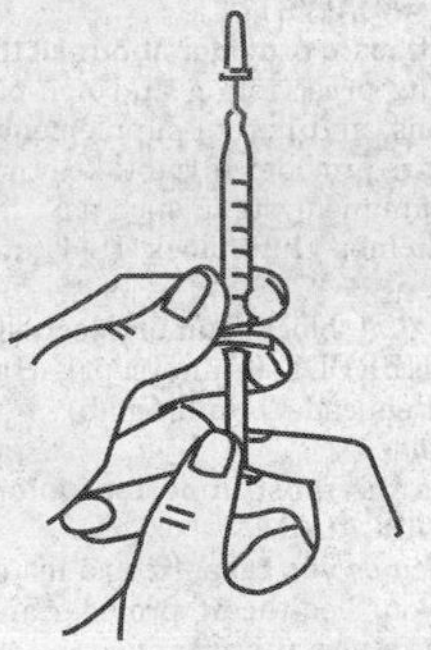

Figure 14

5. Remove the needle cover and be careful not to touch the needle. Keep the ARCALYST vial on a flat surface and slowly insert the needle straight down through the stopper. Push the plunger down and inject all the air into the vial (see Figure 15).

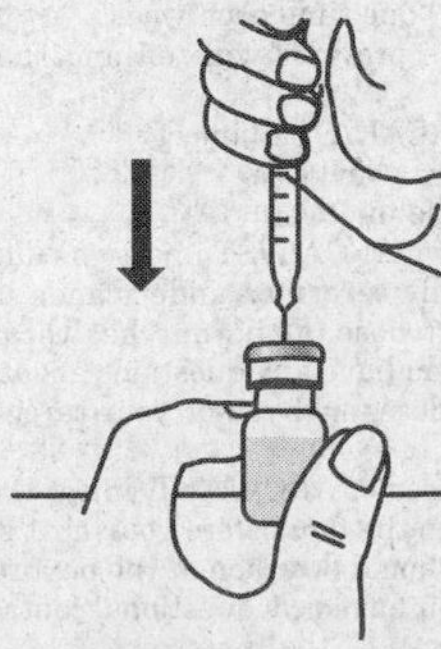

Figure 15

6. Hold the vial in one hand and the syringe in the other hand and carefully turn the vial upside down so that the needle is pointing straight up. Hold the vial at eye level.
7. Keep the tip of the needle in the liquid and slowly pull back on the plunger to the mark on the syringe that matches the amount of medicine prescribed by your healthcare provider (see Figure 16).

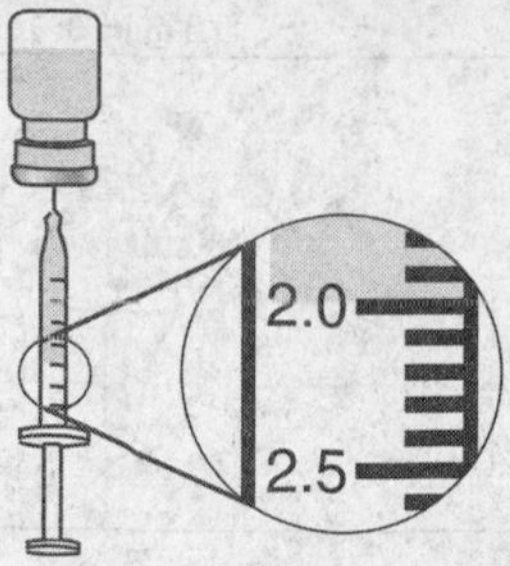

Figure 16

NOTE: The maximum adult dose of ARCALYST is 2 mL.

8. Keep the vial upside down with the needle straight up, and gently tap the syringe until any air bubbles rise to the top of the syringe (see Figure 17).
   It is important to remove air bubbles so that you withdraw up the right amount of medicine from the vial.

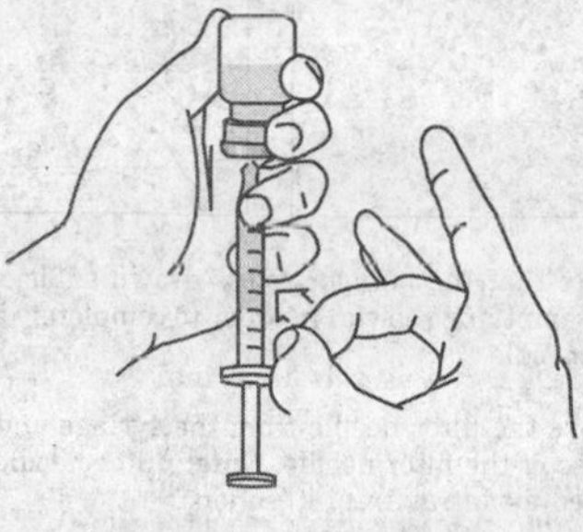

Figure 17

9. To remove the air bubbles, slowly and gently push in the plunger so only the air is pushed through the needle.
10. Check to make sure that you have the amount of medicine prescribed by your healthcare provider in the syringe.
11. Throw away the ARCALYST vial in the puncture resistant container even if there is any medicine left in the vial (see Figure 18). Do not use any vial of ARCALYST more than one time.

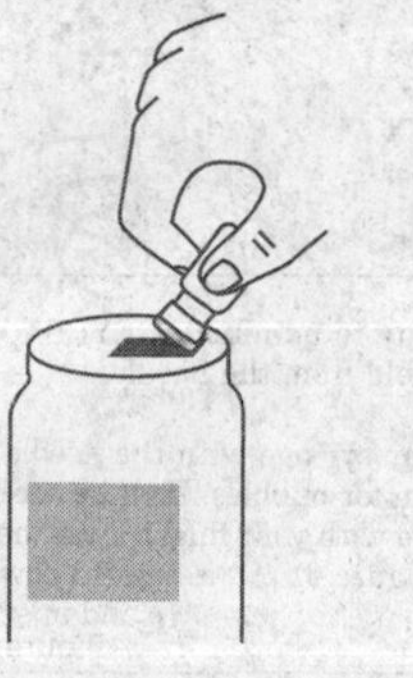

Figure 18

STEP 5: Giving the Injection

1. ARCALYST is given by subcutaneous injection, an injection that is given into the tissue directly below the layers of skin. It is not meant to go into any muscle, vein, or artery.
   You should change (rotate) the sites and inject in a different place each time in order to keep your skin healthy.
   Rotating injection sites helps to prevent irritation and allows the medicine to be completely absorbed. Ask your healthcare provider any questions that you have about rotating injection sites.
   - Do not inject into skin that is tender, red, or hard. If an area is tender or feels hardened, choose another site for injection until the tenderness or "hardening" goes away.
   - Tell your healthcare provider about any skin reactions including redness, swelling, or hardening of the skin.
   - Areas where you may inject ARCALYST include the left and right sides of the abdomen, and left and right thighs. If someone else is giving the injection, the upper left and right arms may also be used for injection (see Figure 19):
   (Do not inject within a 2-inch area around the navel)

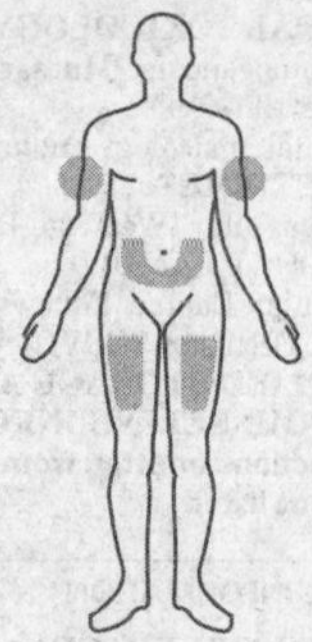

Figure 19

2. Choose the area for the injection. Clean the area in a circular motion with a new alcohol wipe. Begin at the center of the site and move outward. Let the alcohol air dry completely.
3. Take the cover off the needle and be careful not to touch the needle.
4. Hold the syringe in one hand like you would hold a pencil.
5. With the other hand gently pinch a fold of skin at the cleaned site for injection (see Figure 20).

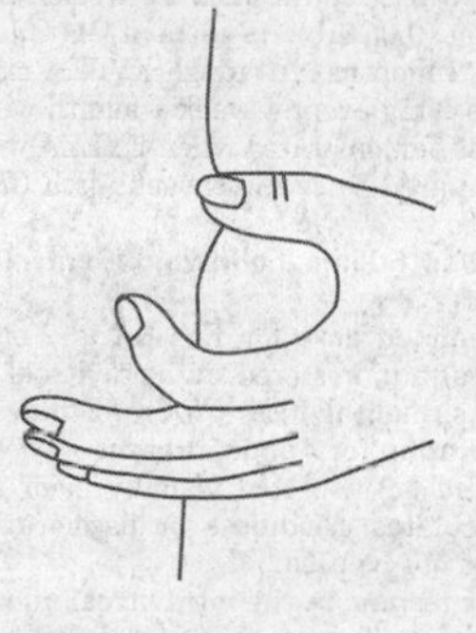

Figure 20

6. Use a quick "dart like" motion to insert the needle straight into the skin (90 degree angle) (see Figure 21). Do not push down on the plunger while inserting the needle into the skin.
   For small children or persons with little fat under the skin, you may need to hold the syringe and needle at a 45 degree angle (see Figure 21).

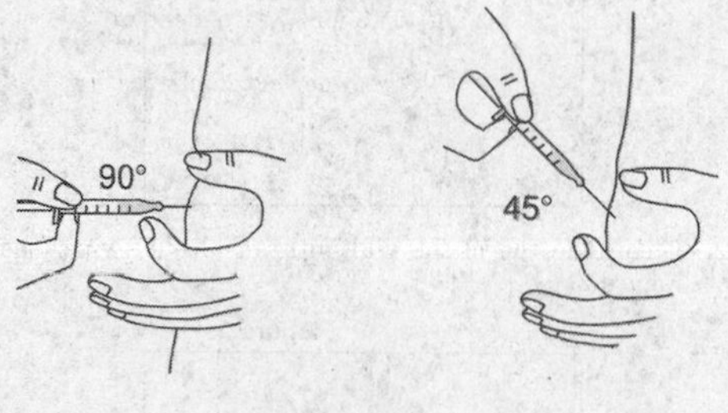

Figure 21

7. After the needle is completely in the skin, let go of the skin that you are pinching.
8. With your free hand hold the syringe near its base. Gently pull back the plunger. If blood comes into the syringe, the needle has entered a blood vessel. Remove the needle, discard the syringe and needle. Start over with "STEP 1: Setting up for an injection" using new supplies (syringes, needles, vials, alcohol swabs and gauze pad).
9. If no blood appears, inject all the medicine n the syringe at a slow, steady rate, pushing the plunger all the way down. It may take up to 30 seconds to inject the entire dose.
10. Pull the needle out of the skin, and hold a piece of sterile gauze over the injection site for several seconds (see Figure 22).

[See figure 22 at top of next column]

11. Do not replace the needle cover. Throw away the vials, used syringes and needles in the puncture-resistant container (see Figure 23). Do not recycle the container. DO

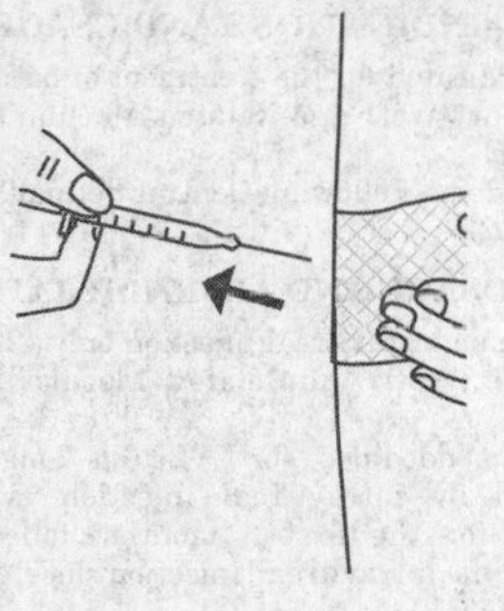

Figure 22

NOT throw away vials, needles, or syringes in the household trash or recycle.

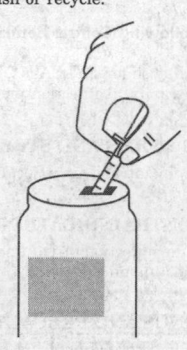

Figure 23

12. Keep the puncture-resistant container out of reach of children. When the container is about two-thirds full, dispose of it as instructed by your healthcare provider. Follow any special state or local laws about the right way to throw away needles and syringes.
13. Used alcohol wipes can be thrown away in the household trash.

Contact your healthcare provider right away with any questions or concerns about ARCALYST.

Issued April, 2009

Notes: 1. ENBREL®, Humira®, Kineret®, and Remicade®, respectively, are trademarks of Immunex Corporation, Abbott Laboratories, Amgen, and Centocor, Inc., respectively.

REGENERON

Manufactured and distributed by:
Regeneron Pharmaceuticals, Inc.
777 Old Saw Mill River Road
Tarrytown, NY 10591-6707
U.S. License Number 1760
NDC 61755-001-01

V2.0
Issue Date: 04/24/2009
Regeneron U.S. Patents 6,927,044 B2, 6,472,179 B2, 5,844,099 and other pending patents

Shown in Product Identification Guide, page 312

EYLEA® ℞

(aflibercept)
Injection
For Intravitreal Injection

HIGHLIGHTS OF PRESCRIBING INFORMATION

These highlights do not include all the information needed to use EYLEA safely and effectively. See full prescribing information for EYLEA.

EYLEA® (aflibercept) Injection
For Intravitreal Injection
Initial U.S. Approval: 2011

RECENT MAJOR CHANGES

- Indications and Usage, Macular Edema Following Central Retinal Vein Occlusion (CRVO) (1.2) 09/2012
- Dosage and Administration, Macular Edema Following Central Retinal Vein Occlusion (CRVO) (2.3) 09/2012
- Dosage and Administration, Preparation for Administration (2.4) 09/2012
- Contraindications, Hypersensitivity (4.3) 09/2012
- Warnings and Precautions, Thromboembolic Events (5.3) 09/2012

INDICATIONS AND USAGE

EYLEA is indicated for the treatment of patients with:
- Neovascular (Wet) Age-Related Macular Degeneration (AMD) (1.1)
- Macular Edema Following Central Retinal Vein Occlusion (CRVO) (1.2)

DOSAGE AND ADMINISTRATION

For ophthalmic intravitreal injection only. (2.1)

Neovascular (Wet) Age-Related Macular Degeneration (AMD)
- The recommended dose for EYLEA is 2 mg (0.05 mL) administered by intravitreal injection every 4 weeks (monthly) for the first 3 months, followed by 2 mg (0.05 mL) via intravitreal injection once every 8 weeks (2 months). (2.2)
- Although EYLEA may be dosed as frequently as 2 mg every 4 weeks (monthly), additional efficacy was not demonstrated when EYLEA was dosed every 4 weeks compared to every 8 weeks. (2.2)

Macular Edema Following Central Retinal Vein Occlusion (CRVO)
- The recommended dose for EYLEA is 2 mg (0.05 mL) administered by intravitreal injection once every 4 weeks (monthly). (2.3)

DOSAGE FORMS AND STRENGTHS

40 mg/mL solution for intravitreal injection in a single-use vial (3)

CONTRAINDICATIONS

- Ocular or periocular infection (4.1)
- Active intraocular inflammation (4.2)
- Hypersensitivity (4.3)

WARNINGS AND PRECAUTIONS

- Endophthalmitis and retinal detachments may occur following intravitreal injections. Patients should be instructed to report any symptoms suggestive of endophthalmitis or retinal detachment without delay and should be managed appropriately. (5.1)
- Increases in intraocular pressure have been seen within 60 minutes of an intravitreal injection. (5.2)
- There is a potential risk of arterial thromboembolic events following intravitreal use of VEGF inhibitors. (5.3)

ADVERSE REACTIONS

The most common adverse reactions (≥5%) reported in patients receiving EYLEA were conjunctival hemorrhage, eye pain, cataract, vitreous detachment, vitreous floaters, and increased intraocular pressure. (6.2)

To report SUSPECTED ADVERSE REACTIONS, contact Regeneron at 1-855-395-3248 or FDA at 1-800-FDA-1088 or *www.fda.gov/medwatch.*

See 17 for PATIENT COUNSELING INFORMATION

Revised: 06/2013

FULL PRESCRIBING INFORMATION: CONTENTS*

*** Sections or subsections omitted from the full prescribing information are not listed**

FULL PRESCRIBING INFORMATION

1 INDICATIONS AND USAGE

EYLEA is indicated for the treatment of patients with:

1.1 Neovascular (Wet) Age-Related Macular Degeneration (AMD)

1.2 Macular Edema Following Central Retinal Vein Occlusion (CRVO)

2 DOSAGE AND ADMINISTRATION

2.1 General Dosing Information

FOR OPHTHALMIC INTRAVITREAL INJECTION ONLY.
EYLEA must only be administered by a qualified physician.

2.2 Neovascular (Wet) Age-Related Macular Degeneration (AMD)

The recommended dose for EYLEA is 2 mg (0.05 mL or 50 microliters) administered by intravitreal injection every 4 weeks (monthly) for the first 12 weeks (3 months), followed by 2 mg (0.05 mL) via intravitreal injection once every 8 weeks (2 months). Although EYLEA may be dosed as frequently as 2 mg every 4 weeks (monthly), additional efficacy was not demonstrated when EYLEA was dosed every 4 weeks compared to every 8 weeks [*see Clinical Studies (14.1)*].

2.3 Macular Edema Following Central Retinal Vein Occlusion (CRVO)

The recommended dose for EYLEA is 2 mg (0.05 mL or 50 microliters) administered by intravitreal injection once every 4 weeks (monthly) [*see Clinical Studies (14.2)*].

2.4 Preparation for Administration

EYLEA should be inspected visually prior to administration. If particulates, cloudiness, or discoloration are visible, the vial must not be used.

Using aseptic technique, the intravitreal injection should be performed with a 30-gauge × ½-inch injection needle.

Vial

The glass vial is for single use only.

1. Remove the protective plastic cap from the vial (see Figure 1).

Figure 1:

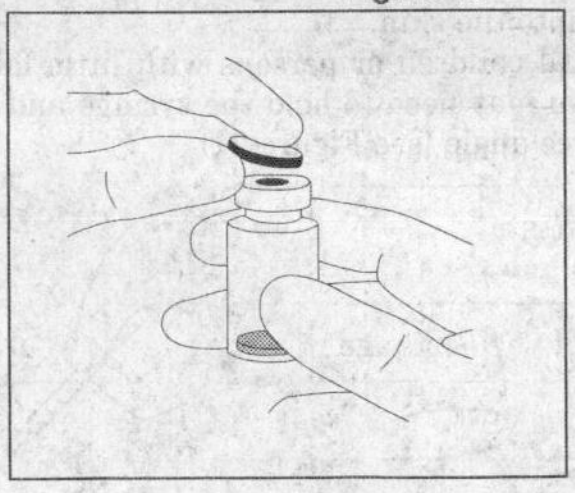

2. Clean the top of the vial with an alcohol wipe (see Figure 2).

Figure 2:

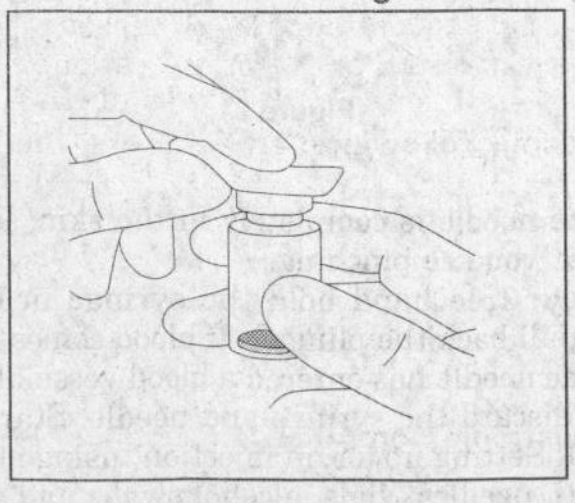

3. Remove the 19-gauge × 1½-inch, 5-micron, filter needle from its pouch and remove the 1-mL syringe supplied in the carton from its pouch. Attach the filter needle to the syringe by twisting it onto the Luer lock syringe tip (see Figure 3).

[See figure 3 at top of next column]

4. Push the filter needle into the center of the vial stopper until the needle is completely inserted into the vial and the tip touches the bottom or bottom edge of the vial.
5. Using aseptic technique withdraw all of the EYLEA vial contents into the syringe, keeping the vial in an upright position, slightly inclined to ease complete withdrawal. To deter the introduction of air, ensure the bevel of the filter needle is submerged into the liquid. Continue to tilt the vial during withdrawal keeping the bevel of the filter needle submerged in the liquid (see Figures 4a and 4b).

Figure 3:

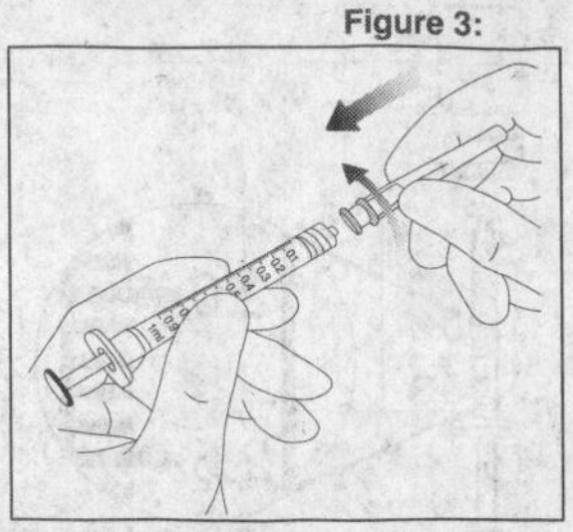

Figure 4a:

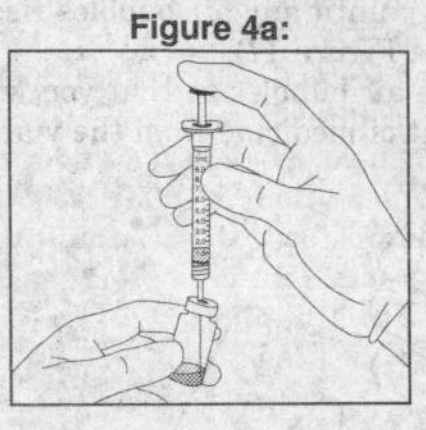

Figure 4b:

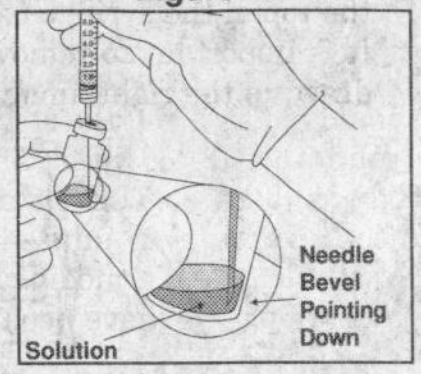

6. Ensure that the plunger rod is drawn sufficiently back when emptying the vial in order to completely empty the filter needle.
7. Remove the filter needle from the syringe and properly dispose of the filter needle. **Note**: Filter needle is **not** to be used for intravitreal injection.
8. Remove the 30-gauge × ½-inch injection needle from the plastic pouch and attach the injection needle to the syringe by firmly twisting the injection needle onto the Luer lock syringe tip (see Figure 5).

Figure 5:

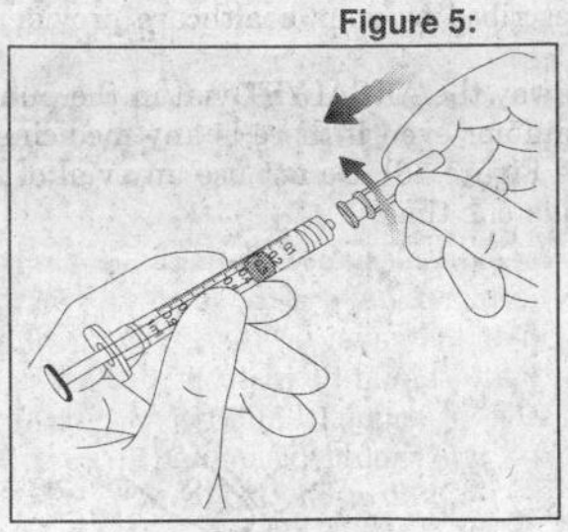

9. When ready to administer EYLEA, remove the plastic needle shield from the needle.
10. Holding the syringe with the needle pointing up, check the syringe for bubbles. If there are bubbles, gently tap the syringe with your finger until the bubbles rise to the top (see Figure 6).

Figure 6:

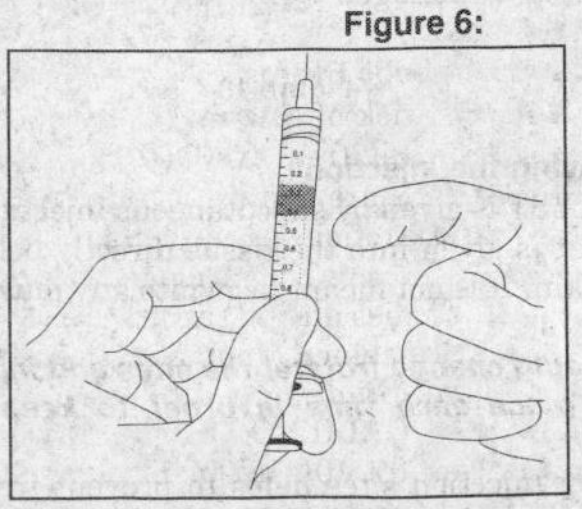

11. To eliminate all of the bubbles and to expel excess drug, SLOWLY depress the plunger so that the plunger tip aligns with the line that marks 0.05 mL on the syringe (see Figures 7a and 7b).

[See figure 7 at top of next column]

2.5 Administration

The intravitreal injection procedure should be carried out under controlled aseptic conditions, which include surgical hand disinfection and the use of sterile gloves, a sterile drape, and a sterile eyelid speculum (or equivalent). Adequate anesthesia and a topical broad–spectrum microbicide should be given prior to the injection.

Immediately following the intravitreal injection, patients should be monitored for elevation in intraocular pressure.

Figure 7a: Figure 7b:

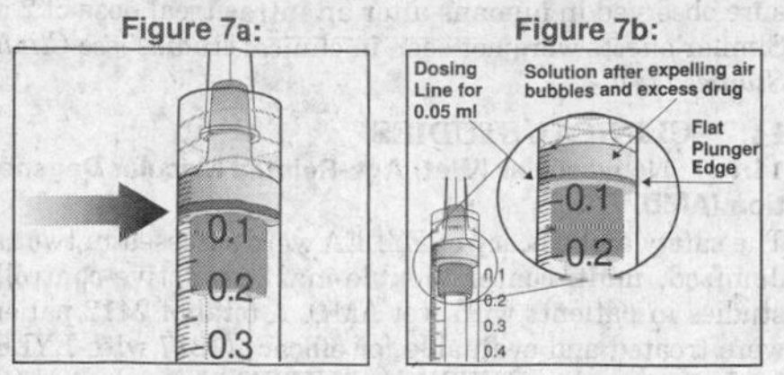

Appropriate monitoring may consist of a check for perfusion of the optic nerve head or tonometry. If required, a sterile paracentesis needle should be available.

Following intravitreal injection, patients should be instructed to report any symptoms suggestive of endophthalmitis or retinal detachment (e.g., eye pain, redness of the eye, photophobia, blurring of vision) without delay [*see Patient Counseling Information (17)*].

Each vial should only be used for the treatment of a single eye. If the contralateral eye requires treatment, a new vial should be used and the sterile field, syringe, gloves, drapes, eyelid speculum, filter, and injection needles should be changed before EYLEA is administered to the other eye.

After injection, any unused product must be discarded.

No special dosage modification is required for any of the populations that have been studied (e.g., gender, elderly).

3 DOSAGE FORMS AND STRENGTHS

Single-use, glass vial designed to provide 0.05 mL of 40 mg/mL solution for intravitreal injection.

4 CONTRAINDICATIONS

4.1 Ocular or Periocular Infections

EYLEA is contraindicated in patients with ocular or periocular infections.

4.2 Active Intraocular Inflammation

EYLEA is contraindicated in patients with active intraocular inflammation.

4.3 Hypersensitivity

EYLEA is contraindicated in patients with known hypersensitivity to aflibercept or any of the excipients in EYLEA. Hypersensitivity reactions may manifest as severe intraocular inflammation.

5 WARNINGS AND PRECAUTIONS

5.1 Endophthalmitis and Retinal Detachments

Intravitreal injections, including those with EYLEA, have been associated with endophthalmitis and retinal detachments [*see Adverse Reactions (6.1)*]. Proper aseptic injection technique must always be used when administering EYLEA. Patients should be instructed to report any symptoms suggestive of endophthalmitis or retinal detachment without delay and should be managed appropriately [*see Dosage and Administration (2.5) and Patient Counseling Information (17)*].

5.2 Increase in Intraocular Pressure

Acute increases in intraocular pressure have been seen within 60 minutes of intravitreal injection, including with EYLEA [*see Adverse Reactions (6.1)*]. Sustained increases in intraocular pressure have also been reported after repeated intravitreal dosing with VEGF inhibitors. Intraocular pressure and the perfusion of the optic nerve head should be monitored and managed appropriately [*see Dosage and Administration (2.5)*].

5.3 Thromboembolic Events

There is a potential risk of arterial thromboembolic events (ATEs) following intravitreal use of VEGF inhibitors, including EYLEA. ATEs are defined as nonfatal stroke, nonfatal myocardial infarction, or vascular death (including deaths of unknown cause). The incidence in the VIEW1 and VIEW2 wet AMD studies during the first year was 1.8% (32 out of 1824) in the combined group of patients treated with EYLEA [*see Clinical Studies (14.1)*]. The incidence in the COPERNICUS and GALILEO CRVO studies during the first 6 months was 0% (0/218) in patients treated with EYLEA 2 mg every 4 weeks compared with 1.4% (2/142) in patients receiving sham treatment [*see Clinical Studies (14.2)*].

6 ADVERSE REACTIONS

The following adverse reactions are discussed in greater detail in the *Warnings and Precautions (5)* section of the labeling:

- Endophthalmitis and retinal detachments
- Increased intraocular pressure
- Thromboembolic events

The most common adverse reactions (≥5%) reported in patients receiving EYLEA were conjunctival hemorrhage, eye pain, cataract, vitreous detachment, vitreous floaters, and increased intraocular pressure.

6.1 Injection Procedure

Serious adverse reactions related to the injection procedure have occurred in <0.1% of intravitreal injections with EYLEA including endophthalmitis, traumatic cataract, increased intraocular pressure, and vitreous detachment.

6.2 Clinical Studies Experience

Because clinical trials are conducted under widely varying conditions, adverse reaction rates observed in the clinical trials of a drug cannot be directly compared to rates in other clinical trials of the same or another drug and may not reflect the rates observed in practice.

A total of 2042 patients treated with EYLEA constituted the safety population in four phase 3 studies. Among those, 1441 patients were treated with the recommended dose of 2 mg.

Neovascular (Wet) Age-Related Macular Degeneration (AMD)

The data described below reflect exposure to EYLEA in 1824 patients with wet AMD, including 1223 patients treated with the 2-mg dose, in 2 double-masked, active-controlled clinical studies (VIEW1 and VIEW2) for 12 months [*see Clinical Studies (14.1)*].

Table 1: Most Common Adverse Reactions (≥1%) in Wet AMD Studies

Adverse Reactions	EYLEA (N=1824)	Active Control (ranibizumab) (N=595)
Conjunctival hemorrhage	25%	28%
Eye pain	9%	9%
Cataract	7%	7%
Vitreous detachment	6%	6%
Vitreous floaters	6%	7%
Intraocular pressure increased	5%	7%
Conjunctival hyperemia	4%	8%
Corneal erosion	4%	5%
Detachment of the retinal pigment epithelium	3%	3%
Injection site pain	3%	3%
Foreign body sensation in eyes	3%	4%
Lacrimation increased	3%	1%
Vision blurred	2%	2%
Intraocular inflammation	2%	3%
Retinal pigment epithelium tear	2%	1%
Injection site hemorrhage	1%	2%
Eyelid edema	1%	2%
Corneal edema	1%	1%

Less common serious adverse reactions reported in <1% of the patients treated with EYLEA were retinal detachment, retinal tear, and endophthalmitis. Hypersensitivity has also been reported in less than 1% of the patients treated with EYLEA.

Macular Edema Following Central Retinal Vein Occlusion (CRVO)

The data described below reflect exposure to EYLEA in 218 patients with macular edema following CRVO treated with 2 mg dose in 2 double-masked, controlled clinical studies (COPERNICUS and GALILEO) for 6 months [*see Clinical Studies (14.2)*].

Table 2: Most Common Adverse Reactions (≥1%) in CRVO Studies

Adverse Reactions	EYLEA (N=218)	Control (N=142)
Eye pain	13%	5%
Conjunctival hemorrhage	12%	11%
Intraocular pressure increased	8%	6%
Corneal erosion	5%	4%
Vitreous floaters	5%	1%
Conjunctival hyperemia	5%	3%
Foreign body sensation in eyes	3%	5%
Vitreous detachment	3%	4%
Lacrimation increased	3%	4%
Injection site pain	3%	1%
Vision blurred	1%	<1%
Intraocular inflammation	1%	1%

Less common adverse reactions reported in <1% of the patients treated with EYLEA were cataract, eyelid edema, corneal edema, retinal tear, hypersensitivity, and endophthalmitis.

6.3 Immunogenicity

As with all therapeutic proteins, there is a potential for an immune response in patients treated with EYLEA. The immunogenicity of EYLEA was evaluated in serum samples. The immunogenicity data reflect the percentage of patients whose test results were considered positive for antibodies to EYLEA in immunoassays. The detection of an immune response is highly dependent on the sensitivity and specificity of the assays used, sample handling, timing of sample collection, concomitant medications, and underlying disease. For these reasons, comparison of the incidence of antibodies to EYLEA with the incidence of antibodies to other products may be misleading.

In the wet AMD and CRVO studies, the pre-treatment incidence of immunoreactivity to EYLEA was 1% to 3% across treatment groups. After dosing with EYLEA for 52 weeks (wet AMD), or 24 weeks (CRVO), antibodies to EYLEA were detected in a similar percentage range of patients. Both in the wet AMD and in the CRVO studies, there were no differences in efficacy or safety between patients with or without immunoreactivity.

8 USE IN SPECIFIC POPULATIONS

8.1 Pregnancy

Pregnancy Category C. Aflibercept produced embryo-fetal toxicity when administered every three days during organogenesis to pregnant rabbits at intravenous doses ≥3 mg per kg, or every six days at subcutaneous doses ≥0.1 mg per kg. Adverse embryo-fetal effects included increased incidences of postimplantation loss and fetal malformations, including anasarca, umbilical hernia, diaphragmatic hernia, gastroschisis, cleft palate, ectrodactyly, intestinal atresia, spina bifida, encephalomeningocele, heart and major vessel defects, and skeletal malformations (fused vertebrae, sternebrae, and ribs; supernumerary vertebral arches and ribs; and incomplete ossification). The maternal No Observed Adverse Effect Level (NOAEL) in these studies was 3 mg per kg. Aflibercept produced fetal malformations at all doses assessed in rabbits and the fetal NOAEL was less than 0.1 mg per kg. Administration of the lowest dose assessed in rabbits (0.1 mg per kg) resulted in systemic exposure (AUC) that was approximately 10 times the systemic exposure observed in humans after an intravitreal dose of 2 mg.

There are no adequate and well-controlled studies in pregnant women. EYLEA should be used during pregnancy only if the potential benefit justifies the potential risk to the fetus.

8.3 Nursing Mothers

It is unknown whether aflibercept is excreted in human milk. Because many drugs are excreted in human milk, a risk to the breastfed child cannot be excluded. EYLEA is not recommended during breastfeeding. A decision must be made whether to discontinue nursing or to discontinue treatment with EYLEA, taking into account the importance of the drug to the mother.

8.4 Pediatric Use

The safety and effectiveness of EYLEA in pediatric patients have not been established.

8.5 Geriatric Use

In the clinical studies, approximately 85% (1728/2034) of patients randomized to treatment with EYLEA were ≥65 years of age and approximately 58% (1177/2034) were ≥75 years of age. No significant differences in efficacy or safety were seen with increasing age in these studies.

11 DESCRIPTION

EYLEA (aflibercept) is a recombinant fusion protein consisting of portions of human VEGF receptors 1 and 2 extracellular domains fused to the Fc portion of human IgG1 formulated as an iso-osmotic solution for intravitreal administration. Aflibercept is a dimeric glycoprotein with a protein molecular weight of 97 kilodaltons (kDa) and contains glycosylation, constituting an additional 15% of the total molecular mass, resulting in a total molecular weight of

Table 3: Efficacy Outcomes at Week 52 (Full Analysis Set with LOCF) in VIEW1 and VIEW2 Studies

	VIEW1			VIEW2		
	EYLEA 2 mg Q8 weeks *	EYLEA 2 mg Q4 weeks	ranibizumab 0.5 mg Q4 weeks	EYLEA 2 mg Q8 weeks *	EYLEA 2 mg Q4 weeks	ranibizumab 0.5 mg Q4 weeks
Full Analysis Set	N=301	N=304	N=304	N=306	N=309	N=291
Efficacy Outcomes						
Proportion of patients who maintained visual acuity (%) (<15 letters of BCVA loss)	94%	95%	94%	95%	95%	95%
Difference† (%) (95.1% CI)	0.6 (-3.2, 4.4)	1.3 (-2.4, 5.0)		0.6 (-2.9, 4.0)	-0.3 (-4.0, 3.3)	
Mean change in BCVA as measured by ETDRS letter score from Baseline	7.9	10.9	8.1	8.9	7.6	9.4
Difference† in LS mean (95.1% CI)	0.3 (-2.0, 2.5)	3.2 (0.9, 5.4)		-0.9 (-3.1, 1.3)	-2.0 (-4.1, 0.2)	
Number of patients who gained at least 15 letters of vision from Baseline (%)	92 (31%)	114 (38%)	94 (31%)	96 (31%)	91 (29%)	99 (34%)
Difference† (%) (95.1% CI)	-0.4 (-7.7, 7.0)	6.6 (-1.0, 14.1)		-2.6 (-10.2, 4.9)	-4.6 (-12.1, 2.9)	

BCVA = Best Corrected Visual Acuity; CI = Confidence Interval; ETDRS = Early Treatment Diabetic Retinopathy Study; LOCF = Last Observation Carried Forward (baseline values are not carried forward); 95.1% confidence intervals were presented to adjust for safety assessment conducted during the study.
* After treatment initiation with 3 monthly doses
† EYLEA group minus the ranibizumab group

115 kDa. Aflibercept is produced in recombinant Chinese hamster ovary (CHO) cells.
EYLEA is a sterile, clear, and colorless to pale yellow solution. EYLEA is supplied as a preservative-free, sterile, aqueous solution in a single-use, glass vial designed to deliver 0.05 mL (50 microliters) of EYLEA (40 mg/mL in 10 mM sodium phosphate, 40 mM sodium chloride, 0.03% polysorbate 20, and 5% sucrose, pH 6.2).

12 CLINICAL PHARMACOLOGY

12.1 Mechanism of Action

Vascular endothelial growth factor-A (VEGF-A) and placental growth factor (PlGF) are members of the VEGF family of angiogenic factors that can act as mitogenic, chemotactic, and vascular permeability factors for endothelial cells. VEGF acts via two receptor tyrosine kinases, VEGFR-1 and VEGFR-2, present on the surface of endothelial cells. PlGF binds only to VEGFR-1, which is also present on the surface of leucocytes. Activation of these receptors by VEGF-A can result in neovascularization and vascular permeability.
Aflibercept acts as a soluble decoy receptor that binds VEGF-A and PlGF, and thereby can inhibit the binding and activation of these cognate VEGF receptors.

12.2 Pharmacodynamics

Neovascular (Wet) Age-Related Macular Degeneration (AMD)

In the clinical studies anatomic measures of disease activity improved similarly in all treatment groups from baseline to week 52. Anatomic data were not used to influence treatment decisions. [*see Clinical Studies (14.1)*].

Macular Edema Following Central Retinal Vein Occlusion (CRVO)

Reductions in mean retinal thickness were observed in COPERNICUS and GALILEO at Week 24 compared to baseline. Anatomic data were not used to influence treatment decisions. [*see Clinical Studies (14.2)*].

12.3 Pharmacokinetics

EYLEA is administered intravitreally to exert local effects in the eye. In patients with wet AMD or CRVO, following intravitreal administration of EYLEA, a fraction of the administered dose is expected to bind with endogenous VEGF in the eye to form an inactive aflibercept: VEGF complex. Once absorbed into the systemic circulation, aflibercept presents in the plasma as free aflibercept (unbound to VEGF) and a more predominant stable inactive form with circulating endogenous VEGF (i.e., aflibercept: VEGF complex).

Absorption/Distribution

Following intravitreal administration of 2 mg per eye of EYLEA to patients with wet AMD and CRVO, the mean C_{max} of free aflibercept in the plasma was 0.02 mcg/mL (range: 0 to 0.054 mcg/mL) and 0.05 mcg/mL (range 0 to 0.081 mcg/mL), respectively and was attained in 1 to 3 days. The free aflibercept plasma concentrations were undetectable two weeks post-dosing in all patients. Aflibercept did not accumulate in plasma when administered as repeated doses intravitreally every 4 weeks. It is estimated that after intravitreal administration of 2 mg to patients, the mean maximum plasma concentration of free aflibercept is more than 100 fold lower than the concentration of aflibercept required to half-maximally bind systemic VEGF.
The volume of distribution of free aflibercept following intravenous (I.V.) administration of aflibercept has been determined to be approximately 6L.

Metabolism/Elimination

Aflibercept is a therapeutic protein and no drug metabolism studies have been conducted. Aflibercept is expected to undergo elimination through both target-mediated disposition via binding to free endogenous VEGF and metabolism via proteolysis. The terminal elimination half-life (t1/2) of free aflibercept in plasma was approximately 5 to 6 days after I.V. administration of doses of 2 to 4 mg/kg aflibercept.

Specific Populations

Renal Impairment

Pharmacokinetic analysis of a subgroup of patients (n=492) in one wet AMD study, of which 43% had renal impairment (mild n=120, moderate n=74, and severe n=16), revealed no differences with respect to plasma concentrations of free aflibercept after intravitreal administration every 4 or 8 weeks. Similar results were seen in patients in a CRVO study. No dose adjustment based on renal impairment status is needed for either wet AMD or CRVO patients.

13 NONCLINICAL TOXICOLOGY

13.1 Carcinogenesis, Mutagenesis, Impairment of Fertility

No studies have been conducted on the mutagenic or carcinogenic potential of aflibercept. Effects on male and female fertility were assessed as part of a 6-month study in monkeys with intravenous administration of aflibercept at weekly doses ranging from 3 to 30 mg per kg. Absent or irregular menses associated with alterations in female reproductive hormone levels and changes in sperm morphology and motility were observed at all dose levels. In addition, females showed decreased ovarian and uterine weight accompanied by compromised luteal development and reduction of maturing follicles. These changes correlated with uterine and vaginal atrophy. A No Observed Adverse Effect Level (NOAEL) was not identified. Intravenous administration of the lowest dose of aflibercept assessed in monkeys (3 mg per kg) resulted in systemic exposure (AUC) that was approximately 1500 times higher than the systemic exposure observed in humans after an intravitreal dose of 2 mg. All changes were reversible within 20 weeks after cessation of treatment.

13.2 Animal Toxicology and/or Pharmacology

Erosions and ulcerations of the respiratory epithelium in nasal turbinates in monkeys treated with aflibercept intravitreally were observed at intravitreal doses of 2 or 4 mg per eye. At the NOAEL of 0.5 mg per eye in monkeys, the systemic exposure (AUC) was 56 times higher than the exposure observed in humans after an intravitreal dose of 2 mg. Similar effects were not seen in clinical studies [*see Clinical Studies (14)*].

14 CLINICAL STUDIES

14.1 Neovascular (Wet) Age-Related Macular Degeneration (AMD)

The safety and efficacy of EYLEA were assessed in two randomized, multi-center, double-masked, active-controlled studies in patients with wet AMD. A total of 2412 patients were treated and evaluable for efficacy (1817 with EYLEA) in the two studies (VIEW1 and VIEW2). In each study, patients were randomly assigned in a 1:1:1:1 ratio to 1 of 4 dosing regimens: 1) EYLEA administered 2 mg every 8 weeks following 3 initial monthly doses (EYLEA 2Q8); 2) EYLEA administered 2 mg every 4 weeks (EYLEA 2Q4); 3) EYLEA 0.5 mg administered every 4 weeks (EYLEA 0.5Q4); and 4) ranibizumab administered 0.5 mg every 4 weeks (ranibizumab 0.5 mg Q4). Patient ages ranged from 49 to 99 years with a mean of 76 years.
In both studies, the primary efficacy endpoint was the proportion of patients who maintained vision, defined as losing fewer than 15 letters of visual acuity at week 52 compared to baseline. Data are available through week 52. Both EYLEA 2Q8 and EYLEA 2Q4 groups were shown to have efficacy that was clinically equivalent to the ranibizumab 0.5 mg Q4 group.
Detailed results from the analysis of the VIEW1 and VIEW2 studies are shown in Table 3 and Figure 8 below.
[See table 3 above]

Figure 8: Mean Change in Visual Acuity from Baseline to Week 52 in VIEW1 and VIEW2 Studies

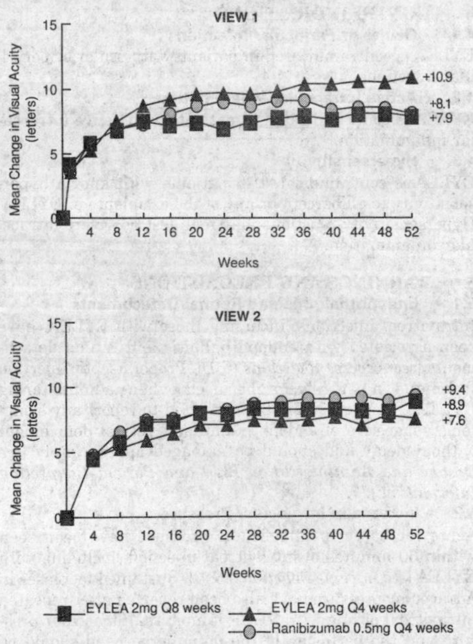

14.2 Macular Edema Following Central Retinal Vein Occlusion (CRVO)

The safety and efficacy of EYLEA were assessed in two randomized, multi-center, double-masked, sham-controlled studies in patients with macular edema following CRVO. A total of 358 patients were treated and evaluable for efficacy (217 with EYLEA) in the two studies (COPERNICUS and GALILEO). In both studies, patients were randomly assigned in a 3:2 ratio to either 2 mg EYLEA administered every 4 weeks (2Q4), or sham injections (control group) administered every 4 weeks for a total of 6 injections. Patient ages ranged from 22 to 89 years with a mean of 64 years.
In both studies, the primary efficacy endpoint was the proportion of patients who gained at least 15 letters in BCVA compared to baseline. At week 24, the EYLEA 2 mg Q4 group was superior to the control group for the primary endpoint.
Results from the analysis of the COPERNICUS and GALILEO studies are shown in Table 4 and Figure 9 below.
[See table 4 at top of next page]
[See figure 9 at top of next column]
Treatment effects in evaluable subgroups (e.g., age, gender, race, baseline visual acuity, retinal perfusion status, and CRVO duration) in each study and in the combined analysis were in general consistent with the results in the overall populations.

Table 4: Efficacy Outcomes at Week 24 (Full Analysis Set with LOCF) in COPERNICUS and GALILEO Studies

	COPERNICUS		GALILEO	
	Control	EYLEA 2 mg Q4 weeks	Control	EYLEA 2 mg Q4 weeks
	N=73	N=114	N=68	N=103
Efficacy Outcomes				
Proportion of patients who gained at least 15 letters in BCVA from Baseline (%)	12%	56%	22%	60%
Weighted Difference *,† (%) (95.1% CI)		44.8%‡ (32.9, 56.6)		38.3%‡ (24.4, 52.1)
Mean change in BCVA as measured by ETDRS letter score from Baseline (SD)	-4.0 (18.0)	17.3 (12.8)	3.3 (14.1)	18.0 (12.2)
Difference in LS mean *,§ (95.1% CI)		21.7‡ (17.3, 26.1)		14.7‡ (10.7, 18.7)

* Difference is EYLEA 2 mg Q4 weeks minus Control
† Difference and CI are calculated using Cochran-Mantel-Haenszel (CMH) test adjusted for baseline factors; 95.1% confidence intervals were presented to adjust for the multiple assessments conducted during the study.
‡ p<0.01 compared with control
§ LS mean and CI based on an ANCOVA model

Figure 9: Mean Change in BCVA as Measured by ETDRS Letter Score from Baseline to Week 24 in COPERNICUS and GALILEO Studies

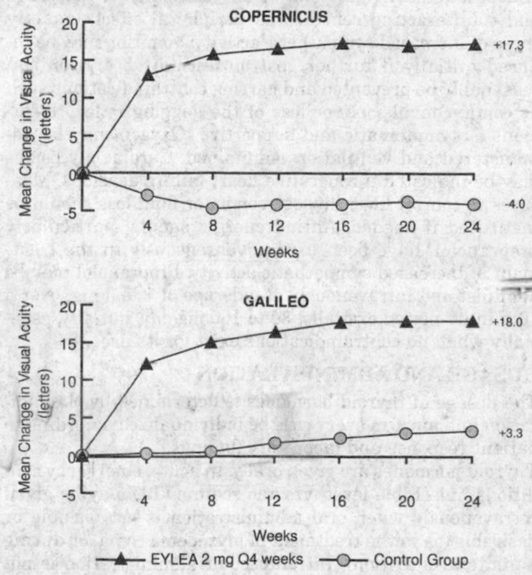

16 HOW SUPPLIED/STORAGE AND HANDLING

Each Vial is for single eye use only. EYLEA is supplied in the following presentation [*see Dosage and Administration (2.4) and (2.5)*].

NDC NUMBER	CARTON TYPE	CARTON CONTENTS
61755-005-02	Vial	one single-use, sterile, 3-mL, glass vial designed to deliver 0.05 mL of 40 mg/mL EYLEA one 19-gauge × 1½-inch, 5-micron, filter needle for withdrawal of the vial contents one 30-gauge × ½-inch injection needle for intravitreal injection one 1-mL syringe for administration one package insert

Storage

EYLEA should be refrigerated at 2°C to 8°C (36°F to 46°F). Do Not Freeze. Do not use beyond the date stamped on the carton and container label. Protect from light. Store in the original carton until time of use.

17 PATIENT COUNSELING INFORMATION

In the days following EYLEA administration, patients are at risk of developing endophthalmitis or retinal detachment. If the eye becomes red, sensitive to light, painful, or develops a change in vision, advise patient to seek immediate care from an ophthalmologist [*see Warnings and Precautions (5.1)*].

Patients may experience temporary visual disturbances after an intravitreal injection with EYLEA and the associated eye examinations [*see Adverse Reactions (6)*]. Advise patients not to drive or use machinery until visual function has recovered sufficiently.

REGENERON

Manufactured by:
Regeneron Pharmaceuticals, Inc.
777 Old Saw Mill River Road
Tarrytown, NY 10591-6707
U.S. License Number 1760

EYLEA is a registered trademark of Regeneron Pharmaceuticals, Inc.

Issue Date: June 2013
Initial U.S. Approval: 2011
Regeneron U.S. Patents 7,306,799; 7,531,173; 7,608,261; 7,070,959; 7,374,757; 7,374,758, and other pending patents

Shown in Product Identification Guide, page 312

RLC Labs, Inc.
CAVE CREEK, AZ 85331

For Product Information:
(877) 797-7997
sales@rlclabs.com
For Customer Service & Ordering Information:
(877) 797-7997
(623) 879-8683 (Fax)
customerservice@rlclabs.com
www.rlclabs.com

NATURE-THROID® ℞
(Thyroid USP) Tablets

DESCRIPTION

Nature-Throid® (Thyroid USP) Tablets, micro-coated, easy to swallow with a reduced odor, for oral use are natural preparations derived from porcine thyroid glands (T3 liothyronine is approximately four times as potent as T4 levothyroxine on a microgram for microgram basis). They provide 38 mcg levothyroxine (T4) and 9 mcg liothyronine (T3) for each 65 mg (1 Grain) of the labeled content of thyroid.

INACTIVE INGREDIENTS

Colloidal Silicon Dioxide, Dicalcium Phosphate, Lactose Monohydrate[1], Magnesium Stearate, Microcrystalline Cellulose, Croscarmellose Sodium, Stearic Acid, Opadry II 85F19316 Clear.

The structural formulas of liothyronine (T3) and levothyroxine (T4) are as follows:

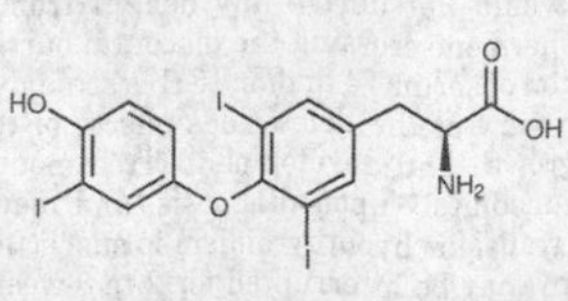

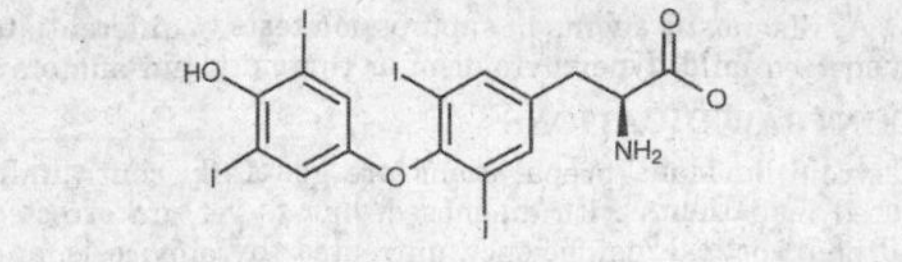

[1]Present in traceable amount as part of Thyroid USP (diluent)

CLINICAL PHARMACOLOGY

The steps in the synthesis of the thyroid hormones are controlled by thyrotropin (Thyroid Stimulating Hormone, TSH) secreted by the anterior pituitary. This hormone's secretion is in turn controlled by a feedback mechanism affected by the thyroid hormones themselves and by thyrotropin releasing hormone (TRH), a tripeptide of hypothalamic origin. Endogenous thyroid hormone secretion is suppressed when exogenous thyroid hormones are administered to euthyroid individuals in excess of the normal gland's secretion.

The mechanisms by which thyroid hormones exert their physiologic action are not well understood. These hormones enhance oxygen consumption by most tissues of the body, increase the basal metabolic rate, and the metabolism of carbohydrates, lipids, and proteins. Thus, they exert a profound influence on every organ system in the body and are of particular importance in the development of the central nervous system.

The normal thyroid gland contains approximately 200 mcg of levothyroxine (T4) per gram of gland, and 15 mcg of liothyronine (T3) per gram. The ratio of these two hormones in the circulation does not represent the ratio in the thyroid gland, since about 80 percent of peripheral liothyronine (T3) comes from monodeiodination of levothyroxine (T4). Peripheral monodeiodination of levothyroxine (T4) at the 5 position (inner ring) also results in the formation of reverse liothyronine (T3), which is calorigenically inactive. Liothyronine (T3) levels are low in the fetus and newborn, in old age, in chronic caloric deprivation, hepatic cirrhosis, renal failure, surgical stress, and chronic illnesses representing what has been called the "T3 thyronine syndrome".

Pharmacokinetics

Animal studies have shown that levothyroxine (T4) is only partially absorbed from the gastrointestinal tract. The degree of absorption is dependent on the vehicle used for its administration and by the character of the intestinal contents, the intestinal flora, including plasma protein, and soluble dietary factors, all of which bind thyroid, thereby making it unavailable for diffusion. Only 41 percent is absorbed when given in a gelatin capsule, as opposed to 74 percent absorption when given with an albumin carrier.

Depending on other factors, absorption has varied from 48 to 79 percent of the administered dose. Fasting increases absorption. Malabsorption syndromes, as well as dietary factors, (children's soybean formula, concomitant use of anionic exchange resins such as cholestyramine) cause excessive fecal loss. Liothyronine (T3) is almost totally absorbed, 95 percent in 4 hours. The hormones contained in the natural preparations are absorbed in a manner similar to the synthetic hormones.

More than 99 percent of circulating hormones are bound to serum proteins, including thyroid-binding globulin (TBg), thyroid-binding pre-albumin (TBPA), and albumin (TBa), whose capacities and affinities vary for the hormones. The higher affinity of levothyroxine (T4) for both TBg and TBPA, as compared to liothyronine (T3), partially explains the higher serum levels and longer half-life of the former hormone. Both protein-bound hormones exist in reverse equilibrium with minute amounts of free hormone, the latter accounting for the metabolic activity. Deiodination of levothyroxine (T4) occurs at a number of sites, including liver, kidney, and other tissues. The conjugated hormone, in the form of glucuronide or sulfate, is found in the bile and gut where it may complete an enterohepatic circulation. Eighty-five percent of levothyroxine (T4) metabolized daily is deiodinated.

INDICATIONS AND USAGE

1. As replacement of supplemental therapy in patients with hypothyroidism of any etiology, except transient hypothyroidism during the recovery phase of subacute thyroiditis. This category includes cretinism, myxedema, and ordinary hypothyroidism in patients of any age (children, adults, the elderly), or state (including pregnancy); primary hypothyroidism resulting from functional deficiency, primary atrophy, partial or total absence of thyroid gland, or the effects of surgery, radiation, or drugs, with or without the presence of goiter; and secondary (pituitary), or tertiary (hypothalamic) hypothyroidism (See WARNINGS).
2. As pituitary TSH suppressants, in the treatment or prevention of various types of euthyroid goiters, including thyroid nodules, subacute, or chronic lymphocytic thyroiditis (Hashimoto's), multinodular goiter, and in the management of thyroid cancer.

3. As diagnostic agents in suppression tests to differentiate suspected mild hyperthyroidism or thyroid gland anatomy.

CONTRAINDICATIONS

Thyroid hormone preparations are generally contraindicated in patients with diagnosed, but as yet, uncorrected adrenal cortical insufficiency, untreated thyrotoxicosis, and apparent hypersensitivity to any of their active or extraneous constituents. There is no well documented evidence in the literature of true allergic or idiosyncratic reactions to thyroid hormone.

WARNINGS

Drugs with thyroid hormone activity, alone or together with other therapeutic agents, have been used for the treatment of obesity. In euthyroid patients, doses within the range of daily hormonal requirements are ineffective for weight reduction. Larger doses may produce serious or even life-threatening manifestations of toxicity, particularly when given in association with sympathomimetic amines such as those used for their anorectic effects.

The use of thyroid hormones in the therapy of obesity, alone or combined with other drugs, is unjustified and has been shown to be ineffective. Neither is their use justified for the treatment of male or female infertility unless this condition is accompanied by hypothyroidism.

PRECAUTIONS

General: Thyroid hormones should be used with great caution in a number of circumstances where the integrity of the cardiovascular system, particularly the coronary arteries, is suspected. These include patients with angina pectoris or the elderly, whom have a greater likelihood of occult cardiac disease. With these patients, therapy should be initiated with low doses, i.e. 16.25 - 32.5 mg. When, in such patients, a euthyroid state can only be reached at the expense of an aggravation of the cardiovascular disease, thyroid hormone dosage should be reduced.

Thyroid hormone therapy in patients with concomitant diabetes mellitus or diabetes insipidus or adrenal cortical insufficiency aggravates the intensity of their symptoms. Appropriate adjustments of the various therapeutic measures directed at these concomitant endocrine diseases are required. The therapy of myxedema coma requires simultaneous administration of glucorticoids (See DOSAGE AND ADMINISTRATION).

Hypothyroidism decreases and hyperthyroidism increases the sensitivity to oral anticoagulants. Prothrombin time should be closely monitored in thyroid treated patients on oral anticoagulants and dosage of the latter agents should be adjusted on the basis of frequent prothrombin time determinations. In infants, excessive doses of thyroid hormone preparations may produce craniosynostosis.

Information for the Patient: Patients on thyroid hormone preparations and parents of children on thyroid therapy should be informed that:

1. Replacement therapy is to be taken essentially for life, with the exception of cases of transient hypothyroidism, usually associated with thyroiditis, and in those patients receiving a therapeutic trial of the drug.
2. They should immediately report, during the course of therapy, any signs or symptoms of thyroid hormone toxicity, e.g., chest pain, increased pulse rate, palpitations, excessive sweating, heat intolerance, nervousness, or any other unusual event.
3. In case of concomitant diabetes mellitus, the daily dosage of antidiabetic medication may need readjustment as thyroid hormone replacement is achieved. If thyroid medication is stopped, a downward readjustment of the dosage of insulin or oral hypoglycemic agent may be necessary to avoid hypoglycemia. At all times, close monitoring of urinary glucose levels is mandatory in such patients.
4. In case of concomitant oral anticoagulant therapy, the prothrombin time should be measured frequently to determine if the dosage of oral anticoagulants is to be readjusted.
5. Partial loss of hair may be experienced by children in the first few months of thyroid therapy, but this is usually a transient phenomenon and later recovery is usually the rule.

Laboratory Tests: Treatment of patients with thyroid hormones requires the periodic assessment of thyroid status by means of appropriate laboratory tests, besides the full clinical evaluation. The TSH suppression test can be used to test the effectiveness of any thyroid preparation, bearing in mind the relative insensitivity of the infant pituitary to the negative feedback effect of thyroid hormones. SerumT4 levels can be used to test the effectiveness of all thyroid medications except T3. When the total serum T4 is low but TSH is normal, a test specific to assess unbound (free) T4 levels is warranted. Specific measurements of T4 and T3 by competitive protein binding or radioimmunoassay are not influenced by blood levels of organic or inorganic iodine.

Drug Interactions: Oral Anticoagulants—Thyroid hormones appear to increase catabolism of vitamin K-dependent clotting factors. If oral anticoagulants are also being given, compensatory increases in clotting factor synthesis are impaired. Patients stabilized on oral anticoagulants that are found to require thyroid replacement therapy should be watched very closely when thyroid is started. If a patient is truly hypothyroid, it is likely that a reduction in anticoagulant dosage will be required. No special precautions appear to be necessary when oral anticoagulant therapy is begun in a patient already stabilized on maintenance thyroid replacement therapy.

Insulin or Oral Hypoglycemic—Initiating thyroid replacement therapy may cause increases in insulin or oral hypoglycemic requirements. The effects seen are poorly understood and depend upon a variety of factors such as dose and type of thyroid preparations and endocrine status of the patient. Patients receiving insulin or oral hypoglycemic should be closely watched during initiation of thyroid replacement therapy.

Cholestyramine or Colestipol—Cholestyramine or Colestipol binds both levothyroxine (T4) and liothyronine (T3) in the intestine, thus impairing absorption of these thyroid hormones. In vitro studies indicate that the binding is not easily removed. Therefore, four to five hours should elapse between administration of Cholestyramine or Colestipol and thyroid hormones.

Estrogen, Oral Contraceptives—Estrogens tend to increase serum thyroxine-binding globulin (TBg). In a patient with a nonfunctioning thyroid gland who is receiving thyroid replacement therapy, free levothyroxine (T4) may be decreased when estrogens are started thus increasing thyroid requirements. However, if the patient's thyroid gland has sufficient function, the decreased free levothyroxine (T4) will result in a compensatory increase in levothyroxine (T4) output by the thyroid. Therefore, patients without a functioning thyroid gland who are on thyroid replacement therapy, may need to increase their thyroid dose if estrogens or estrogen-containing oral contraceptives are given.

Drug/Laboratory Test Interactions: The following drugs or moieties are known to interfere with laboratory tests performed in patients on thyroid hormone therapy: androgens, corticosteroids, estrogens, oral contraceptives containing estrogens, iodine-containing preparations, and the numerous preparations containing salicylates.

1. Changes in TBg concentration should be taken into consideration in the interpretation of levothyroxine (T4) and liothyronine (T3) values. In such cases, the unbound (free) hormone should be measured. Pregnancy, estrogens, and estrogen-containing oral contraceptives increase TBg concentrations. TBg may also be increased during infectious hepatitis. Decreases in TBg concentrations are observed in nephrosis, acromegaly, and after androgen or corticosteroid therapy. Familial hyper or hypothyroxine-binding-globulinemias have been described. The incidence of TBg deficiency approximates 1 in 9,000. The binding of levothyroxine by TBPA is inhibited by salicylates.
2. Medicinal or dietary iodine interferes with all in vivo tests of radio-iodine uptake, producing low uptakes which may not be relative of a true decrease in hormone synthesis.
3. The persistence of clinical and laboratory evidence of hypothyroidism in spite of adequate dosage replacement indicates; either poor patient compliance, poor absorption, excessive fecal loss, or inactivity of the preparation. Intracellular resistance to thyroid hormone is quite rare.

Carcinogenesis, Mutagenesis, and Impairment of Fertility: A reportedly apparent association between prolonged thyroid therapy and breast cancer has not been confirmed and patients on thyroid for established indications should not discontinue therapy. No confirmatory long-term studies in animals have been performed to evaluate carcinogenic potential, mutagenicity, or impairment of fertility in either males or females.

Pregnancy-Category A: Thyroid hormones do not readily cross the placental barrier. The clinical experience to date does not indicate any adverse effect on fetuses when thyroid hormones are administered to pregnant women. On the basis of current knowledge, thyroid replacement therapy to hypothyroid women should not be discontinued during pregnancy.

Nursing Mothers: Minimal amounts of thyroid hormones are excreted in human milk. Thyroid is not associated with serious adverse reactions and does not have a known tumorigenic potential. However, caution should be exercised when thyroid is administered to a nursing woman.

Pediatric Use: Pregnant mothers provide little or no thyroid hormone to the fetus. The incidence of congenital hypothyroidism is relatively high (1:4,000) and the hypothyroid fetus would not derive any benefit from the small amounts of hormone crossing the placental barrier. Routine determination of serumT4 and/or TSH is strongly advised in neonates in view of the deleterious effects of thyroid deficiency on growth and development. Treatment should be initiated immediately upon diagnosis, and maintained for life, unless transient hypothyroidism is suspected; in which case, therapy may be interrupted for 2 to 8 weeks after the age of 3 years to reassess the condition. Cessation of therapy is justified in patients who have maintained a normal TSH during those 2 to 8 weeks.

Geriatric use: Clinical studies of Thyroid Tablets, USP did not include sufficient numbers of subjects aged 65 and over to determine whether they respond differently from younger subjects. Other reported clinical experience has not identified differences in responses between the elderly and younger patients. In general, dose selection for an elderly patient should be cautious, usually starting at the low end of the dosing range, reflecting the greater frequency of decreased hepatic, renal, or cardiac function, and of concomitant disease or other drug therapy.

ADVERSE REACTIONS

Adverse reactions other than those indicative of hyperthyroidism because of therapeutic overdosage, either initially or during the maintenance period, are rare (See OVERDOSAGE).

OVERDOSAGE

Signs and Symptoms: Excessive doses of thyroid result in a hypermetabolic state resembling in every respect the condition of endogenous origin. The condition may be self induced.

Treatment of Overdosage: Dosage should be reduced or therapy temporarily discontinued signs and symptoms of overdosage appear.

Treatment may be reinstituted at a lower dosage. In normal individuals, normal hypothalamic-pituitary-thyroid axis function is restored in 6 to 8 weeks after thyroid suppression.

Treatment of acute massive thyroid hormone overdosage is aimed at reducing gastrointestinal absorption of the drugs and counteracting central and peripheral effects, mainly those of increased sympathetic activity. Vomiting may be induced initially if further gastrointestinal absorption can reasonably be prevented and barring contraindications such as coma, convulsions, or loss of the gagging reflex. Treatment is symptomatic and supportive. Oxygen may be administered and ventilation maintained. Cardiac glycosides may be indicated if congestive heart failure develops. Measures to control fever, hypoglycemia, or fluid loss should be instituted if needed. Antiadrenergic agents, particularly propranolol, have been used advantageously in the treatment of increased sympathetic activity. Propranolol may be administered intravenously at a dosage of 1 to 3 mg, over a 10 minute period or orally, 80 to 160 mg/day, initially, especially when no contraindications exist for its use.

DOSAGE AND ADMINISTRATION

The dosage of thyroid hormones is determined by the indication and must in every case be individualized according to patient response and laboratory findings.

Thyroid hormones are given orally. In acute, emergency conditions, injectable levothyroxine sodium (T4) may be given intravenously when oral administration is not feasible or desirable (as in the treatment of myxedema coma, or during parenteral nutrition). Intramuscular administration is not advisable because of reported poor absorption.

Hypothyroidism: Therapy is usually instituted using low doses, with increments which depend on the cardiovascular status of the patient. The usual starting dose is 32.5 mg, with increment of 16.25 mg every 2 to 3 weeks. A lower starting dosage, 16.25 mg/day, is recommended in patients with longstanding myxedema, particularly if cardiovascular impairment is suspected, in which case extreme caution is recommended. The appearance of angina is an indication for reduction in dosage. Most patients require 65 - 130 mg/day. Failure to respond to doses of 195 mg suggests lack of compliance or malabsorption. Maintenance dosages 65 - 130 mg/day usually result in normal serum T4 and T3 levels. Adequate therapy usually results in normal TSH and T4 levels after 2 or 3 weeks of therapy.

Readjustment of thyroid hormone dosage should be made within the first four weeks of therapy, after proper clinical and laboratory evaluations, including serum levels of T4, bound and free, and TSH.

Liothyronine (T3) may be used in preference to levothyroxine (T4) during radio-isotope scanning procedures, since induction of hypothyroidism in those cases is more abrupt and can be of shorter duration. It may also be preferred when impairment of peripheral conversion of levothyroxine (T4) and liothyronine (T3) is suspected.

Myxedema Coma: Myxedema coma is usually precipitated in the hypothyroid patient of longstanding by intercurrent illness or drugs such as sedatives and anesthetics and should be considered a medical emergency. Therapy should be directed at the correction of electrolyte disturbances and possible infection, besides the administration of thyroid hormones. Corticosteroids should be administered routinely. Levothyroxine (T4) and Liothyronine (T3) may be administered via a nasogastric tube, but the preferred route of administration of both hormones is intravenous. Levothyroxine sodium (T4) is given at a starting dose of

400 mcg (100 mcg/mL) given rapidly, and is usually well tolerated, even in the elderly. This initial dose is followed by daily supplements of 100 to 200 mcg given IV. Normal T4 levels are achieved in 24 hours, followed in 3 days by threefold elevation of T3. Oral therapy with thyroid hormone would be resumed as soon as the clinical situation has been stabilized and the patient is able to take oral medication.

Thyroid Cancer: Exogenous thyroid hormone may produce regression of metastases from follicular and papillary carcinoma of the thyroid and is used as ancillary therapy of these conditions with radioactive iodine. TSH should be suppressed to low or undetectable levels. Therefore, larger amounts of thyroid hormone than those used for replacement therapy are required. Medullary carcinoma of the thyroid is usually unresponsive to this therapy.

Thyroid Suppression Therapy: Administration of thyroid hormone in doses higher than those produced physiologically by the gland results in suppression of the production of endogenous hormone. This is the basis for the thyroid suppression test and is used as an aid in the diagnosis of patients with signs of mild hyperthyroidism, in whom base line laboratory tests appear normal, or to demonstrate thyroid gland autonomy in patients with Grave's ophthalmopathy. 1 uptake is determined before and after the administration of the exogenous hormone. A fifty percent or greater suppression of uptake indicates a normal thyroid pituitary axis, and thus rules out thyroid gland autonomy.

For adults, the usual suppressive dose of levothyroxine (T4) is 1.56 mg/kg of body weight per day given for 7 to 10 days. These doses usually yield normal serum T4 and T3 levels and lack of response to TSH.

Thyroid hormones should be administered cautiously to patients in whom there is strong suspicion of thyroid gland autonomy, in view of the fact that the exogenous hormone effects will be additive to the endogenous source.

Pediatric Dosage: Pediatric dosage should follow the recommendations summarized in Table 1. In infants with congenital hypothyroidism, therapy with full doses should be instituted as soon as the diagnosis has been made.

TABLE 1. Recommended Pediatric Dosage for Congenital Hypothyroidism

Age	Dose per day	Daily dose per kg of body weight
0 - 6 months	16.25 - 32.5 mg	4.8-6.0 mg
6 - 12 months	32.5 - 48.75 mg	3.6-4.8 mg
1 - 5 years	48.75 - 65 mg	3.0-3.6 mg
6 - 12 years	65 - 97.5 mg	2.4-3.0 mg
Over 12 years	Over 97.5 mg	1.2-1.8 mg

HOW SUPPLIED

Nature-Throid® (Thyroid USP) Tablets are supplied as follows:

16.25 mg. (1/4 gr.) in bottles of 30 Count (NDC 64727-3298-4), 60 Count (NDC 64727-3298-5), 90 Count (NDC 64727-3298-6), 100 Count (NDC 64727-3298-1), 1,000 Count (NDC 64727-3298-2), 990 Count (NDC 64727-3298-3) & 1,008 Count (NDC 64727-3298-8)

32.5 mg. (1/2 gr.) in bottles of 30 Count (NDC 64727-3299-4), 60 Count (NDC 64727-3299-5), 90 Count (NDC 64727-3299-6), 100 Count (NDC 64727-3299-1), 1,000 Count (NDC 64727-3299-2), 990 Count (NDC 64727-3299-3) & 1,008 Count (NDC 64727-3299-8)

48.75 mg. (3/4 gr.) in bottles of 30 Count (NDC 64727-3302-4), 60 Count (NDC 64727-3302-5), 90 Count (NDC 64727-3302-6), 100 Count (NDC 64727-3302-1), 1,000 Count (NDC 64727-3302-2), 990 Count (NDC 64727-3302-3) & 1,008 Count (NDC 64727-3302-8)

65 mg. (1 gr.) in bottles of 30 Count (NDC 64727-3300-4), 60 Count (NDC 64727-3300-5), 90 Count (NDC 64727-3300-6), 100 Count (NDC 64727-3300-1), 1,000 Count (NDC 64727-3300-2), 990 Count (NDC 64727-3300-3) & 1,008 Count (NDC 64727-3300-8)

81.25 mg. (1 1/4 gr.) in bottles of 30 Count (NDC 64727-3303-4), 60 Count (NDC 64727-3303-5), 90 Count (NDC 64727-3303-6), 100 Count (NDC 64727-3303-1), 1,000 Count (NDC 64727-3303-2), 990 Count (NDC 64727-3303-3) & 1,008 Count (NDC 64727-3303-8)

97.5 mg. (1 1/2 gr.) in bottles of 30 Count (NDC 64727-3305-4), 60 Count (NDC 64727-3305-5), 90 Count (NDC 64727-3305-6), 100 Count (NDC 64727-3305-1), 1,000 Count (NDC 64727-3305-2), 990 Count (NDC 64727-3305-3) & 1,008 Count (NDC 64727-3305-8)

113.75 mg. (1 3/4 gr.) in bottles of 30 Count (NDC 64727-3307-4), 60 Count (NDC 64727-3307-5), 90 Count (NDC 64727-3307-6), 100 Count (NDC 64727-3307-1), 1,000 Count (NDC 64727-3307-2), 990 Count (NDC 64727-3307-3) & 1,008 Count (NDC 64727-3307-8)

130 mg. (2 gr.) in bottles of 30 Count (NDC 64727-3308-4), 60 Count (NDC 64727-3308-5), 90 Count (NDC 64727-3308-6), 100 Count (NDC 64727-3308-1), 1,000 Count (NDC 64727-3308-2), 990 Count (NDC 64727-3308-3) & 1,008 Count (NDC 64727-3308-8)

146.25 mg. (2 1/4 gr.) in bottles of 30 Count (NDC 64727-3309-4), 60 Count (NDC 64727-3309-5), 90 Count (NDC 64727-3309-6), 100 Count (NDC 64727-3309-1), 1,000 Count (NDC 64727-3309-2), 990 Count (NDC 64727-3309-3) & 1,008 Count (NDC 64727-3309-8)

162.5 mg. (2 1/2 gr.) in bottles of 30 Count (NDC 64727-3310-4), 60 Count (NDC 64727-3310-5), 90 Count (NDC 64727-3310 6), 100 Count (NDC 64727-3310-1), 1,000 Count (NDC 64727-3310-2), 990 Count (NDC 64727 3310-3) & 1,008 Count (NDC 64727-3310-8)

195 mg. (3 gr.) in bottles of 30 Count (NDC 64727-3312-4), 60 Count (NDC 64727-3312-5), 90 Count (NDC 64727-3312-6), 100 Count (NDC 64727-3312-1), 1,000 Count (NDC 64727-3312-2), 990 Count (NDC 64727-3312-3) & 1,008 Count (NDC 64727-3312-8)

260 mg. (4 gr.) in bottles of 30 Count (NDC 64727-3320-4), 60 Count (NDC 64727-3320-5), 90 Count (NDC 64727-3320-6), 100 Count (NDC 64727-3320-1), 1,000 Count (NDC 64727-3320-2), 990 Count (NDC 64727-3320-3) & 1,008 Count (NDC 64727-3320-8)

325 mg. (5 gr.) in bottles of 30 Count (NDC 64727-3340-4), 60 Count (NDC 64727-3340-5), 90 Count (NDC 64727-3340-6), 100 Count (NDC 64727-3340-1), 1,000 Count (NDC 64727-3340-2), 990 Count (NDC 64727-3340-3) & 1,008 Count (NDC 64727-3340-8)

STORAGE: Store at controlled room temperature; 15°-30°C (59°-86°F)

Dispense in tight, light-resistant containers as defined in the USP/NF

Rx Only.

Distributed by:
RLC LABS
Cave Creek, AZ 85331
Rev051309/01 SCD#700809-1

Shown in Product Identification Guide, page 312

WP THYROID® ℞
(Thyroid USP)
Tablets

DESCRIPTION

WP Thyroid® (Thyroid USP) Tablets, for oral use, are natural preparations derived from porcine thyroid glands (T3 liothyronine is approximately four times as potent as T4 levothyroxine on a microgram for microgram basis). They provide 38 mcg levothyroxine (T4) and 9 mcg liothyronine (T3) for each 65 mg (1 Grain) of the labeled content of thyroid.

INACTIVE INGREDIENTS

Inulin, Medium Chain Triglycerides, Lactose Monohydrate[1]

The structural formulas of liothyronine (T3) and levothyroxine (T4) are as follows:

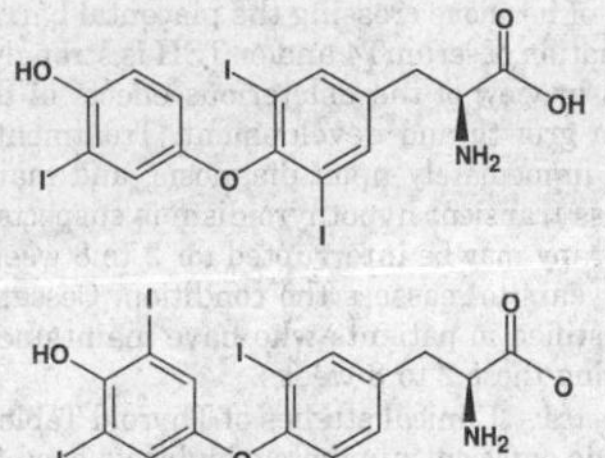

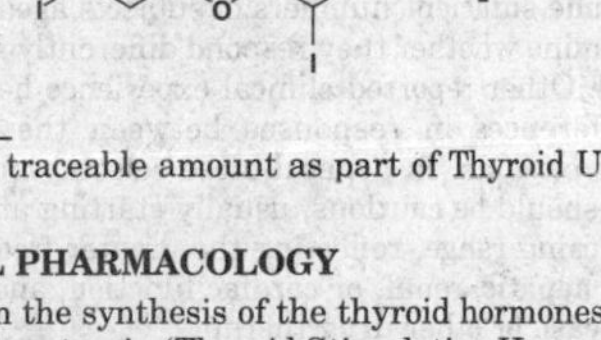

[1]Present in traceable amount as part of Thyroid USP (diluent)

CLINICAL PHARMACOLOGY

The steps in the synthesis of the thyroid hormones are controlled by thyrotropin (Thyroid Stimulating Hormone, TSH) secreted by the anterior pituitary. This hormone's secretion is in turn controlled by a feedback mechanism affected by the thyroid hormones themselves and by thyrotropin releasing hormone (TRH), a tripeptide of hypothalamic origin. Endogenous thyroid hormone secretion is suppressed when exogenous thyroid hormones are administered to euthyroid individuals in excess of the normal gland's secretion.

The mechanisms by which thyroid hormones exert their physiologic action are not well understood. These hormones enhance oxygen consumption by most tissues of the body, increase the basal metabolic rate, and the metabolism of carbohydrates, lipids, and proteins. Thus, they exert a profound influence on every organ system in the body and are of particular importance in the development of the central nervous system.

The normal thyroid gland contains approximately 200 mcg of levothyroxine (T4) per gram of gland, and 15 mcg of liothyronine (T3) per gram. The ratio of these two hormones in the circulation does not represent the ratio in the thyroid gland, since about 80 percent of peripheral liothyronine (T3) comes from monodeiodination of levothyroxine (T4). Peripheral monodeiodination of levothyroxine (T4) at the 5 position (inner ring) also results in the formation of reverse liothyronine (T3), which is calorigenically inactive. Liothyronine (T3) levels are low in the fetus and newborn, in old age, in chronic caloric deprivation, hepatic cirrhosis, renal failure, surgical stress, and chronic illnesses representing what has been called the "T3 thyronine syndrome".

Pharmacokinetics

Animal studies have shown that levothyroxine (T4) is only partially absorbed from the gastrointestinal tract. The degree of absorption is dependent on the vehicle used for its administration and by the character of the intestinal contents, the intestinal flora, including plasma protein, and soluble dietary factors, all of which bind thyroid, thereby making it unavailable for diffusion. Only 41 percent is absorbed when given in a gelatin capsule, as opposed to 74 percent absorption when given with an albumin carrier.

Depending on other factors, absorption has varied from 48 to 79 percent of the administered dose. Fasting increases absorption. Malabsorption syndromes, as well as dietary factors, (children's soybean formula, concomitant use of anionic exchange resins such as cholestyramine) cause excessive fecal loss. Liothyronine (T3) is almost totally absorbed, 95 percent in 4 hours. The hormones contained in the natural preparations are absorbed in a manner similar to the synthetic hormones.

More than 99 percent of circulating hormones are bound to serum proteins, including thyroid-binding globulin (TBg), thyroid-binding pre-albumin (TBPA), and albumin (TBa), whose capacities and affinities vary for the hormones. The higher affinity of levothyroxine (T4) for both TBg and TBPA, as compared to liothyronine (T3), partially explains the higher serum levels and longer half-life of the former hormone. Both protein-bound hormones exist in reverse equilibrium with minute amounts of free hormone, the latter accounting for the metabolic activity. Deiodination of levothyroxine (T4) occurs at a number of sites, including liver, kidney, and other tissues. The conjugated hormone, in the form of glucuronide or sulfate, is found in the bile and gut where it may complete an enterohepatic circulation. Eighty-five percent of levothyroxine (T4) metabolized daily is deiodinated.

INDICATIONS AND USAGE

1. As replacement of supplemental therapy in patients with hypothyroidism of any etiology, except transient hypothyroidism during the recovery phase of subacute thyroiditis. This category includes cretinism, myxedema, and ordinary hypothyroidism in patients of any age (children, adults, the elderly), or state (including pregnancy); primary hypothyroidism resulting from functional deficiency, primary atrophy, partial or total absence of thyroid gland, or the effects of surgery, radiation, or drugs, with or without the presence of goiter; and secondary (pituitary), or tertiary (hypothalamic) hypothyroidism (See WARNINGS).

2. As pituitary TSH suppressants, in the treatment or prevention of various types of euthyroid goiters, including thyroid nodules, subacute, or chronic lymphocytic thyroiditis (Hashimoto's), multinodular goiter, and in the management of thyroid cancer.

3. As diagnostic agents in suppression tests to differentiate suspected mild hyperthyroidism or thyroid gland anatomy.

CONTRAINDICATIONS

Thyroid hormone preparations are generally contraindicated in patients with diagnosed, but as yet, uncorrected adrenal cortical insufficiency, untreated thyrotoxicosis, and apparent hypersensitivity to any of their active or extraneous constituents. There is no well documented evidence in the literature of true allergic or idiosyncratic reactions to thyroid hormone.

WARNINGS

Drugs with thyroid hormone activity, alone or together with other therapeutic agents, have been used for the treatment of obesity. In euthyroid patients, doses within the range of daily hormonal requirements are ineffective for weight reduction. Larger doses may produce serious or even life-threatening manifestations of toxicity, particularly when given in association with sympathomimetic amines such as those used for their anorectic effects.

The use of thyroid hormones in the therapy of obesity, alone or combined with other drugs, is unjustified and has been shown to be ineffective. Neither is their use justified for the treatment of male or female infertility unless this condition is accompanied by hypothyroidism.

PRECAUTIONS

General: Thyroid hormones should be used with great caution in a number of circumstances where the integrity of the cardiovascular system, particularly the coronary arteries, is suspected. These include patients with angina pectoris or the elderly, whom have a greater likelihood of occult cardiac disease. With these patients, therapy should be initiated with low doses, i.e. 16.25 - 32.5 mg. When, in such patients, a euthyroid state can only be reached at the expense of an aggravation of the cardiovascular disease, thyroid hormone dosage should be reduced.

Thyroid hormone therapy in patients with concomitant diabetes mellitus or diabetes insipidus or adrenal cortical insufficiency aggravates the intensity of their symptoms. Appropriate adjustments of the various therapeutic measures directed at these concomitant endocrine diseases are required. The therapy of myxedema coma requires simultaneous administration of glucorticoids (See DOSAGE AND ADMINISTRATION).

Hypothyroidism decreases and hyperthyroidism increases the sensitivity to oral anticoagulants. Prothrombin time should be closely monitored in thyroid treated patients on oral anticoagulants and dosage of the latter agents should be adjusted on the basis of frequent prothrombin time determinations. In infants, excessive doses of thyroid hormone preparations may produce craniosynostosis.

Information for the Patient: Patients on thyroid hormone preparations and parents of children on thyroid therapy should be informed that:

1. Replacement therapy is to be taken essentially for life, with the exception of cases of transient hypothyroidism, usually associated with thyroiditis, and in those patients receiving a therapeutic trial of the drug.
2. They should immediately report, during the course of therapy, any signs or symptoms of thyroid hormone toxicity, e.g., chest pain, increased pulse rate, palpitations, excessive sweating, heat intolerance, nervousness, or any other unusual event.
3. In case of concomitant diabetes mellitus, the daily dosage of antidiabetic medication may need readjustment as thyroid hormone replacement is achieved. If thyroid medication is stopped, a downward readjustment of the dosage of insulin or oral hypoglycemic agent may be necessary to avoid hypoglycemia. At all times, close monitoring of urinary glucose levels is mandatory in such patients.
4. In case of concomitant oral anticoagulant therapy, the prothrombin time should be measured frequently to determine if the dosage of oral anticoagulants is to be readjusted.
5. Partial loss of hair may be experienced by children in the first few months of thyroid therapy, but this is usually a transient phenomenon and later recovery is usually the rule.

Laboratory Tests: Treatment of patients with thyroid hormones requires the periodic assessment of thyroid status by means of appropriate laboratory tests, besides the full clinical evaluation. The TSH suppression test can be used to test the effectiveness of any thyroid preparation, bearing in mind the relative insensitivity of the infant pituitary to the negative feedback effect of thyroid hormones. Serum T4 levels can be used to test the effectiveness of all thyroid medications except T3. When the total serum T4 is low but TSH is normal, a test specific to assess unbound (free) T4 levels is warranted. Specific measurements of T4 and T3 by competitive protein binding or radioimmunoassay are not influenced by blood levels of organic or inorganic iodine.

Drug Interactions: Oral Anticoagulants-Thyroid hormones appear to increase catabolism of vitamin K- dependent clotting factors. If oral anticoagulants are also being given, compensatory increases in clotting factor synthesis are impaired. Patients stabilized on oral anticoagulants that are found to require thyroid replacement therapy should be watched very closely when thyroid is started. If a patient is truly hypothyroid, it is likely that a reduction in anticoagulant dosage will be required. No special precautions appear to be necessary when oral anticoagulant therapy is begun in a patient already stabilized on maintenance thyroid replacement therapy.

Insulin or Oral Hypoglycemic-Initiating thyroid replacement therapy may cause increases in insulin or oral hypoglycemic requirements. The effects seen are poorly understood and depend upon a variety of factors such as dose and type of thyroid preparations and endocrine status of the patient. Patients receiving insulin or oral hypoglycemic should be closely watched during initiation of thyroid replacement therapy.

Cholestyramine or Colestipol- Cholestyramine or Colestipol binds both levothyroxine (T4) and liothyronine (T3) in the intestine, thus impairing absorption of these thyroid hormones. In vitro studies indicate that the binding is not easily removed. Therefore, four to five hours should elapse between administration of Cholestyramine or Colestipol and thyroid hormones.

Estrogen, Oral Contraceptives- Estrogens tend to increase serum thyroxine-binding globulin (TBg). In a patient with a nonfunctioning thyroid gland who is receiving thyroid replacement therapy, free levothyroxine (T4) may be decreased when estrogens are started thus increasing thyroid requirements. However, if the patient's thyroid gland has sufficient function, the decreased free levothyroxine (T4) will result in a compensatory increase in levothyroxine (T4) output by the thyroid. Therefore, patients without a functioning thyroid gland who are on thyroid replacement therapy, may need to increase their thyroid dose if estrogens or estrogen-containing oral contraceptives are given.

Drug/Laboratory Test Interactions: The following drugs or moieties are known to interfere with laboratory tests performed in patients on thyroid hormone therapy: androgens, corticosteroids, estrogens, oral contraceptives containing estrogens, iodine-containing preparations, and the numerous preparations containing salicylates.

1. Changes in TBg concentration should be taken into consideration in the interpretation of levothyroxine (T4) and liothyronine (T3) values. In such cases, the unbound (free) hormone should be measured. Pregnancy, estrogens, and estrogen-containing oral contraceptives increase TBg concentrations. TBg may also be increased during infectious hepatitis. Decreases in TBg concentrations are observed in nephrosis, acromegaly, and after androgen or corticosteroid therapy. Familial hyper or hypothyroxine-binding-globulinemias have been described. The incidence of TBg deficiency approximates 1 in 9,000. The binding of levothyroxine by TBPA is inhibited by salicylates.
2. Medicinal or dietary iodine interferes with all in vivo tests of radio-iodine uptake, producing low uptakes which may not be relative of a true decrease in hormone synthesis.
3. The persistence of clinical and laboratory evidence of hypothyroidism in spite of adequate dosage replacement indicates; either poor patient compliance, poor absorption, excessive fecal loss, or inactivity of the preparation. Intracellular resistance to thyroid hormone is quite rare.

Carcinogenesis, Mutagenesis, and Impairment of Fertility: A reportedly apparent association between prolonged thyroid therapy and breast cancer has not been confirmed and patients on thyroid for established indications should not discontinue therapy. No confirmatory long-term studies in animals have been performed to evaluate carcinogenic potential, mutagenicity, or impairment of fertility in either males or females.

Pregnancy-Category A: Thyroid hormones do not readily cross the placental barrier. The clinical experience to date does not indicate any adverse effect on fetuses when thyroid hormones are administered to pregnant women. On the basis of current knowledge, thyroid replacement therapy to hypothyroid women should not be discontinued during pregnancy.

Nursing Mothers: Minimal amounts of thyroid hormones are excreted in human milk. Thyroid is not associated with serious adverse reactions and does not have a known tumorigenic potential. However, caution should be exercised when thyroid is administered to a nursing woman.

Pediatric Use: Pregnant mothers provide little or no thyroid hormone to the fetus. The incidence of congenital hypothyroidism is relatively high (1:4,000) and the hypothyroid fetus would not derive any benefit from the small amounts of hormone crossing the placental barrier. Routine determination of serumT4 and/or TSH is strongly advised in neonates in view of the deleterious effects of thyroid deficiency on growth and development. Treatment should be initiated immediately upon diagnosis, and maintained for life, unless transient hypothyroidism is suspected; in which case, therapy may be interrupted for 2 to 8 weeks after the age of 3 years to reassess the condition. Cessation of therapy is justified in patients who have maintained a normal TSH during those 2 to 8 weeks.

Geriatric use: Clinical studies of Thyroid Tablets, USP did not include sufficient numbers of subjects aged 65 and over to determine whether they respond differently from younger subjects. Other reported clinical experience has not identified differences in responses between the elderly and younger patients. In general, dose selection for an elderly patient should be cautious, usually starting at the low end of the dosing range, reflecting the greater frequency of decreased hepatic, renal, or cardiac function, and of concomitant disease or other drug therapy.

ADVERSE REACTIONS

Adverse reactions other than those indicative of hyperthyroidism because of therapeutic overdosage, either initially or during the maintenance period, are rare (See OVERDOSAGE).

OVERDOSAGE

Signs and Symptoms: Excessive doses of thyroid result in a hypermetabolic state resembling in every respect the condition of endogenous origin. The condition may be self induced.

Treatment of Overdosage: Dosage should be reduced or therapy temporarily discontinued signs and symptoms of overdosage appear.

Treatment may be reinstituted at a lower dosage. In normal individuals, normal hypothalamic-pituitary-thyroid axis function is restored in 6 to 8 weeks after thyroid suppression.

Treatment of acute massive thyroid hormone overdosage is aimed at reducing gastrointestinal absorption of the drugs and counteracting central and peripheral effects, mainly those of increased sympathetic activity. Vomiting may be induced initially if further gastrointestinal absorption can reasonably be prevented and barring contraindications such as coma, convulsions, or loss of the gagging reflex. Treatment is symptomatic and supportive. Oxygen may be administered and ventilation maintained. Cardiac glycosides may be indicated if congestive heart failure develops. Measures to control fever, hypoglycemia, or fluid loss should be instituted if needed. Antiadrenergic agents, particularly propranolol, have been used advantageously in the treatment of increased sympathetic activity. Propranolol may be administered intravenously at a dosage of 1 to 3 mg, over a 10 minute period or orally, 80 to 160 mg/day, initially, especially when no contraindications exist for its use.

DOSAGE AND ADMINISTRATION

The dosage of thyroid hormones is determined by the indication and must in every case be individualized according to patient response and laboratory findings.

Thyroid hormones are given orally. In acute, emergency conditions, injectable levothyroxine sodium (T4) may be given intravenously when oral administration is not feasible or desirable (as in the treatment of myxedema coma, or during parenteral nutrition). Intramuscular administration is not advisable because of reported poor absorption.

Hypothyroidism: Therapy is usually instituted using low doses, with increments which depend on the cardiovascular status of the patient. The usual starting dose is 32.5 mg, with increment of 16.25 mg every 2 to 3 weeks. A lower starting dosage, 16.25 mg/day, is recommended in patients with longstanding myxedema, particularly if cardiovascular impairment is suspected, in which case extreme caution is recommended. The appearance of angina is an indication for reduction in dosage. Most patients require 65 - 130 mg/day. Failure to respond to doses of 195 mg suggests lack of compliance or malabsorption. Maintenance dosages 65 - 130 mg/day usually result in normal serum T4 and T3 levels. Adequate therapy usually results in normal TSH and T4 levels after 2 or 3 weeks of therapy.

Readjustment of thyroid hormone dosage should be made within the first four weeks of therapy, after proper clinical and laboratory evaluations, including serum levels of T4, bound and free, and TSH.

Liothyronine (T3) may be used in preference to levothyroxine (T4) during radio-isotope scanning procedures, since induction of hypothyroidism in those cases is more abrupt and can be of shorter duration. It may also be preferred when impairment of peripheral conversion of levothyroxine (T4) and liothyronine (T3) is suspected.

Myxedema Coma: Myxedema coma is usually precipitated in the hypothyroid patient of longstanding by intercurrent illness or drugs such as sedatives and anesthetics and should be considered a medical emergency. Therapy should be directed at the correction of electrolyte disturbances and possible infection, besides the administration of thyroid hormones. Corticosteroids should be administered routinely. Levothyroxine (T4) and Liothyronine (T3) may be administered via a nasogastric tube, but the preferred route of administration of both hormones is intravenous. Levothyroxine sodium (T4) is given at a starting dose of 400 mcg (100 mcg/mL) given rapidly, and is usually well tolerated, even in the elderly. This initial dose is followed by daily supplements of 100 to 200 mcg given IV. Normal T4 levels are achieved in 24 hours, followed in 3 days by threefold elevation of T3. Oral therapy with thyroid hormone would be resumed as soon as the clinical situation has been stabilized and the patient is able to take oral medication.

Thyroid Cancer: Exogenous thyroid hormone may produce regression of metastases from follicular and papillary carcinoma of the thyroid and is used as ancillary therapy of these conditions with radioactive iodine. TSH should be suppressed to low or undetectable levels. Therefore, larger amounts of thyroid hormone than those used for replacement therapy are required. Medullary carcinoma of the thyroid is usually unresponsive to this therapy.

Thyroid Suppression Therapy: Administration of thyroid hormone in doses higher than those produced physiologically by the gland results in suppression of the production of endogenous hormone. This is the basis for the thyroid suppression test and is used as an aid in the diagnosis of patients with signs of mild hyperthyroidism, in whom base line laboratory tests appear normal, or to demonstrate thyroid gland autonomy in patients with Grave's ophthalmopathy. 131I uptake is determined before and after the administration of the exogenous hormone. A fifty percent or greater suppression of uptake indicates a normal thyroid pituitary axis, and thus rules out thyroid gland autonomy.

For adults, the usual suppressive dose of levothyroxine (T4) is 1.56 mg/kg of body weight per day given for 7 to 10 days. These doses usually yield normal serum T4 and T3 levels and lack of response to TSH.

Thyroid hormones should be administered cautiously to patients in whom there is strong suspicion of thyroid gland autonomy, in view of the fact that the exogenous hormone effects will be additive to the endogenous source.

Pediatric Dosage: Pediatric dosage should follow the recommendations summarized in Table 1. In infants with congenital hypothyroidism, therapy with full doses should be instituted as soon as the diagnosis has been made.

TABLE 1. Recommended Pediatric Dosage for Congenital Hypothyroidism

Age	Dose per day	Daily dose per kg of body weight
0 - 6 months	16.25 - 32.5 mg	4.8-6.0 mg
6 - 12 months	32.5 - 48.75 mg	3.6-4.8 mg
1 - 5 years	48.75 - 65 mg	3.0-3.6 mg
6 - 12 years	65 - 97.5 mg	2.4-3.0 mg
Over 12 years	Over 97.5 mg	1.2-1.8 mg

HOW SUPPLIED

WP Thyroid® (Thyroid USP) Tablets are supplied as follows:

16.25 mg. (1/4 gr.) in bottles of 30 Count (NDC 64727-5450-4), 60 Count (NDC 64727-5450-5), 90 Count (NDC 64727-5450-6), 100 Count (NDC 64727-5450-1) & 1,000 Count (NDC 64727-5450-2)

32.5 mg. (1/2 gr.) in bottles of 30 Count (NDC 64727-5550-4), 60 Count (NDC 64727-5550-5), 90 Count (NDC 64727-5550-6), 100 Count (NDC 64727-5550-1) & 1,000 Count (NDC 64727-5550-2)

48.75 mg. (3/4 gr.) in bottles of 30 Count (NDC 64727-5650-4), 60 Count (NDC 64727-5650-5), 90 Count (NDC 64727-5650-6), 100 Count (NDC 64727-5650-1) & 1,000 Count (NDC 64727-5650-2)

65 mg. (1 gr.) in bottles of 30 Count (NDC 64727-5750-4), 60 Count (NDC 64727-5750-5), 90 Count (NDC 64727-5750-6), 100 Count (NDC 64727-5750-1) & 1,000 Count (NDC 64727-5750-2)

81.25 mg. (1 1/4 gr.) in bottles of 30 Count (NDC 64727-6050-4), 60 Count (NDC 64727-6050-5), 90 Count (NDC 64727-6050-6), 100 Count (NDC 64727-6050-1) & 1,000 Count (NDC 64727-6050-2)

97.5 mg. (1 1/2 gr.) in bottles of 30 Count (NDC 64727-5850-4), 60 Count (NDC 64727-5850-5), 90 Count (NDC 64727-5850-6), 100 Count (NDC 64727-5850-1) & 1,000 Count (NDC 64727-5850-2)

113.75 mg. (1 3/4 gr.) in bottles of 30 Count (NDC 64727-6150-4), 60 Count (NDC 64727-6150-5), 90 Count (NDC 64727-6150-6), 100 Count (NDC 64727-6150-1) & 1,000 Count (NDC 64727-6150-2)

130 mg. (2 gr.) in bottles of 30 Count (NDC 64727-5950-4), 60 Count (NDC 64727-5950-5), 90 Count (NDC 64727-5950-6), 100 Count (NDC 64727-5950-1) & 1,000 Count (NDC 64727-5950-2)

146.25 mg. (2 1/4 gr.) in bottles of 30 Count (NDC 64727-6250-4), 60 Count (NDC 64727-6250-5), 90 Count (NDC 64727-6250-6), 100 Count (NDC 64727-6250-1) & 1,000 Count (NDC 64727-6250-2)

162.5 mg. (2 1/2 gr.) in bottles of 30 Count (NDC 64727-6350-4), 60 Count (NDC 64727-6350-5), 90 Count (NDC 64727-6350-6), 100 Count (NDC 64727-6350-1) & 1,000 Count (NDC 64727-6350-2)

195 mg. (3 gr.) in bottles of 30 Count (NDC 64727-6450-4), 60 Count (NDC 64727-6450-5), 90 Count (NDC 64727-6450-6), 100 Count (NDC 64727-6450-1) & 1,000 Count (NDC 64727-6450-2)

STORAGE: Store at controlled room temperature; 15°-30°C (59°-86°F)

Dispense in tight, light-resistant containers as defined in the USP/NF

Rx Only.

Distributed by:
RLC® LABS
Cave Creek, AZ 85331
Rev:063191/01
SCD#700809-3

Shown in Product Identification Guide, page 312

Salix Pharmaceuticals, Inc.

8510 COLONNADE CENTER DRIVE
RALEIGH, NC 27615

Direct Inquiries to:
(866) 669-7597 Phone
(919) 862-1817 Fax
www.salix.com

For adverse events, product quality complaints and patient information requests:
Product Information Center
(800) 508-0024 Phone
(510) 595-8183 Fax
E-mail: salix@medcomsol.com

APRISO™ ℞
(mesalamine)
extended-release capsules

HIGHLIGHTS OF PRESCRIBING INFORMATION
These highlights do not include all the information needed to use APRISO safely and effectively. See full prescribing information for APRISO.
APRISO™ (mesalamine) extended-release capsules
Initial U.S. Approval: 1987

INDICATIONS AND USAGE

- APRISO is a locally-acting aminosalicylate indicated for the maintenance of remission of ulcerative colitis in adults (1)

DOSAGE AND ADMINISTRATION

- Four APRISO capsules once daily (1.5 g/day) in the morning with or without food. Do not co-administer with antacids (2)

DOSAGE FORMS AND STRENGTHS

- Extended-release capsules: 0.375 g (3)

CONTRAINDICATIONS

- Hypersensitivity to salicylates, aminosalicylates, or any component of APRISO capsules (4)

WARNINGS AND PRECAUTIONS

- Renal impairment may occur. Assess renal function at the beginning of treatment and periodically during therapy (5.1)
- Acute exacerbation of colitis symptoms can occur (5.2)
- Use caution with pre-existing liver disease (5.4)

ADVERSE REACTIONS

- The most common adverse reactions (incidence ≥3%) are headache, diarrhea, upper abdominal pain, nausea, nasopharyngitis, flu or flu-like illness, sinusitis (6.1)

To report SUSPECTED ADVERSE REACTIONS, contact Salix Pharmaceuticals, Inc. at 1-800-508-0024 or FDA at 1-800-FDA-1088 or www.fda.gov/medwatch.

DRUG INTERACTIONS

- Do not co-administer with antacids (7.1)

USE IN SPECIFIC POPULATIONS

- Use with caution in patients with renal disease (5.1)
- Monitor blood cell counts in geriatric patients (8.5)
- Advise patients with phenylketonuria that APRISO contains aspartame (17.1)

See 17 for PATIENT COUNSELING INFORMATION

Revised: 07/2009

FULL PRESCRIBING INFORMATION: CONTENTS*

*** Sections or subsections omitted from the full prescribing information are not listed**

FULL PRESCRIBING INFORMATION

1 INDICATIONS AND USAGE

APRISO capsules are indicated for the maintenance of remission of ulcerative colitis in patients 18 years of age and older.

2 DOSAGE AND ADMINISTRATION

The recommended dose for maintenance of remission of ulcerative colitis in adult patients is 1.5 g (four APRISO capsules) orally once daily in the morning. APRISO may be taken without regard to meals. APRISO should not be co-administered with antacids. An evaluation of renal function is recommended before initiating therapy with APRISO.

3 DOSAGE FORMS AND STRENGTHS

Extended-release capsules containing 0.375 g mesalamine.

4 CONTRAINDICATIONS

APRISO is contraindicated in patients with hypersensitivity to salicylates or aminosalicylates or to any of the components of APRISO capsules.

5 WARNINGS AND PRECAUTIONS

5.1 Renal Impairment

Renal impairment, including minimal change nephropathy, acute and chronic interstitial nephritis, and, rarely, renal failure, has been reported in patients given products such as APRISO that contain mesalamine or are converted to mesalamine.

It is recommended that patients have an evaluation of renal function prior to initiation of APRISO therapy and periodically while on therapy. Exercise caution when using APRISO in patients with known renal dysfunction or a history of renal disease.

In animal studies, the kidney was the principal organ for toxicity *[See Nonclinical Toxicology (13.2)]*

5.2 Mesalamine-Induced Acute Intolerance Syndrome

Mesalamine has been associated with an acute intolerance syndrome that may be difficult to distinguish from a flare of inflammatory bowel disease. Although the exact frequency of occurrence has not been determined, it has occurred in 3% of patients in controlled clinical trials of mesalamine or sulfasalazine. Symptoms include cramping, acute abdominal pain and bloody diarrhea, sometimes fever, headache, and rash. If acute intolerance syndrome is suspected, promptly discontinue treatment with APRISO.

5.3 Hypersensitivity

Some patients who have experienced a hypersensitivity reaction to sulfasalazine may have a similar reaction to APRISO capsules or to other compounds that contain or are converted to mesalamine.

5.4 Hepatic Impairment

There have been reports of hepatic failure in patients with pre-existing liver disease who have been administered mesalamine. Caution should be exercised when administering APRISO to patients with liver disease.

6 ADVERSE REACTIONS

6.1 Clinical Studies Experience

The data described below reflect exposure to APRISO in 557 patients, including 354 exposed for at least 6 months and 250 exposed for greater than one year. APRISO was studied in two placebo-controlled trials (n = 367 treated with APRISO) and in one open-label, long-term study (n = 190 additional patients). The population consisted of patients with ulcerative colitis; the mean age was 47 years, 54% were female, and 93% were white. Patients received doses of APRISO 1.5 g administered orally once per day for six months in the placebo-controlled trials and for up to 24 months in the open-label study.

Because clinical studies are conducted under widely varying conditions, adverse reaction rates observed in the clinical trials of a drug cannot be directly compared to rates in the clinical trials of another drug and may not reflect the rates observed in practice.

In the two placebo-controlled trials, 59% of APRISO-treated patients experienced an adverse reaction compared with 64% of placebo patients. Most adverse reactions with APRISO were mild or moderate in severity. Severe adverse reactions occurred in 6% of APRISO-treated patients and 5% of placebo-treated patients. Discontinuations due to adverse reactions occurred in 11% of APRISO-treated patients and 17% of placebo-treated patients; the most common adverse reaction resulting in study discontinuation was recurrence of ulcerative colitis (APRISO 6%, placebo 14%). The most common reactions reported with APRISO (≥3%) are shown in Table 1 below.

Table 1: Treatment-Emergent Adverse Reactions during Clinical Trials Occurring in at Least 3% of APRISO-Treated Patients and at a Greater Rate than with Placebo

MedDRA Preferred Term	APRISO 1.5g/day N=367	Placebo N=185
Headache	11%	8%
Diarrhea	8%	7%
Abdominal Pain Upper	5%	3%
Nausea	4%	3%
Nasopharyngitis	4%	3%
Influenza & Influenza-like illness	4%	4%
Sinusitis	3%	3%

The following adverse reactions, presented by body system, were reported at a frequency less than 3% in patients treated with APRISO for up to 24 months in controlled and open-label trials.

Ear and Labyrinth Disorders: tinnitus, vertigo
Dermatological Disorder: alopecia
Gastrointestinal: abdominal pain lower, rectal hemorrhage
Laboratory Abnormalities: increased triglycerides, decreased hematocrit and hemoglobin
General Disorders and Administration Site Disorders: fatigue
Hepatic: hepatitis cholestatic, transaminases increased
Renal Disorders: creatinine clearance decreased, hematuria
Musculoskeletal: pain, arthralgia
Respiratory: dyspnea

6.2 Adverse Reaction Information from Other Sources

The following adverse reactions have been identified during clinical trials of a product similar to APRISO and post approval use of other mesalamine-containing products such as APRISO. Because many of these reactions are reported voluntarily from a population of unknown size, it is not always possible to reliably estimate their frequency or establish a causal relationship to drug exposure.

Body as a Whole: lupus-like syndrome, drug fever
Cardiovascular: pericarditis, pericardial effusion, myocarditis
Gastrointestinal: pancreatitis, cholecystitis, gastritis, gastroenteritis, gastrointestinal bleeding, perforated peptic ulcer
Hepatic: jaundice, cholestatic jaundice, hepatitis, liver necrosis, liver failure, Kawasaki-like syndrome including changes in liver enzymes
Hematologic: agranulocytosis, aplastic anemia
Neurological/Psychiatric: peripheral neuropathy, Guillain-Barré syndrome, transverse myelitis
Respiratory/Pulmonary: eosinophilic pneumonia, interstitial pneumonitis
Skin: psoriasis, pyoderma gangrenosum, erythema nodosum
Renal/Urogenital: reversible oligospermia

7 DRUG INTERACTIONS

Based on in vitro studies, APRISO is not expected to inhibit the metabolism of drugs that are substrates of CYP1A2, CYP2C9, CYP2C19, CYP2D6, or CYP3A4.

7.1 Antacids

Because the dissolution of the coating of the granules in APRISO capsules depends on pH, APRISO capsules should not be co-administered with antacids.

8 USE IN SPECIFIC POPULATIONS

8.1 Pregnancy

Pregnancy Category B. Reproduction studies with mesalamine have been performed in rats at oral doses up to 320 mg/kg/day (about 1.7 times the recommended human dose based on a body surface area comparison) and rabbits at doses up to 495 mg/kg/day (about 5.4 times the recommended human dose based on a body surface area comparison) and have revealed no evidence of impaired fertility or harm to the fetus due to mesalamine. There are, however, no adequate and well-controlled studies in pregnant women. Because animal reproduction studies are not always predictive of human response, this drug should be used during pregnancy only if clearly needed.

Mesalamine is known to cross the placental barrier.

8.3 Nursing Mothers

Low concentrations of mesalamine and higher concentrations of its N-acetyl metabolite have been detected in human breast milk. The clinical significance of this has not been determined and there is limited experience of nursing women using mesalamine. Caution should be exercised when APRISO is administered to a nursing woman.

8.4 Pediatric Use

Safety and effectiveness of APRISO capsules in pediatric patients have not been established.

8.5 Geriatric Use

Clinical studies of APRISO did not include sufficient numbers of subjects aged 65 and over to determine whether they respond differently than younger subjects. Other reported clinical experience has not identified differences in responses between elderly and younger patients. In general, the greater frequency of decreased hepatic, renal, or cardiac function, and of concomitant disease or other drug therapy in elderly patients should be considered when prescribing APRISO.

Reports from uncontrolled clinical studies and post-marketing reporting systems suggested a higher incidence of blood dyscrasias, i.e., neutropenia, pancytopenia, in patients who were 65 years or older who were taking mesalamine-containing products such as APRISO. Caution should be taken to closely monitor blood cell counts during mesalamine therapy.

Mesalamine is known to be substantially excreted by the kidney, and the risk of adverse reactions to this drug may be greater in patients with impaired renal function. Because elderly patients are more likely to have decreased renal function, care should be taken when prescribing this drug therapy. *[see Warning and Precautions (5.1)].*

10 OVERDOSAGE

APRISO is an aminosalicylate, and symptoms of salicylate toxicity include hematemesis, tachypnea, hyperpnea, tinnitus, deafness, lethargy, seizures, confusion, or dyspnea. Severe intoxication may lead to electrolyte and blood pH imbalance and potentially to other organ (e.g., renal and liver) involvement. There is no specific antidote for mesalamine overdose; however, conventional therapy for salicylate toxicity may be beneficial in the event of acute overdosage. This includes prevention of further gastrointestinal tract absorption by emesis and, if necessary, by gastric lavage. Fluid and electrolyte imbalance should be corrected by the administration of appropriate intravenous therapy. Adequate renal function should be maintained. APRISO is a pH-dependent delayed-release product and this factor should be considered when treating a suspected overdose.

11 DESCRIPTION

Each APRISO capsule is a delayed- and extended-release dosage form for oral administration. Each capsule contains 0.375 g of mesalamine USP (5-aminosalicylic acid, 5-ASA), an anti-inflammatory drug. The structural formula of mesalamine is:

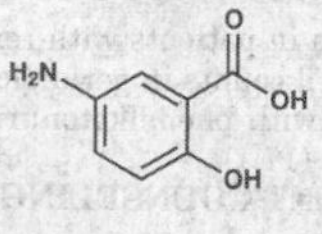

Molecular Weight: 153.14
Molecular Formula: $C_7H_7NO_3$

Each APRISO capsule contains granules composed of mesalamine in a polymer matrix with an enteric coating that dissolves at pH 6 and above.

The inactive ingredients of APRISO capsules are colloidal silicon dioxide, magnesium stearate, microcrystalline cellulose, simethicone emulsion, ethylacrylate/methylmethacrylate copolymer nonoxynol 100 dispersion, hypromellose, methacrylic acid copolymer, talc, titanium dioxide, triethyl citrate, aspartame, anhydrous citric acid, povidone, vanilla flavor, and edible black ink.

12 CLINICAL PHARMACOLOGY

12.1 Mechanism of Action

The mechanism of action of mesalamine (5-ASA) is unknown, but appears to be local to the intestinal mucosa rather than systemic. Mucosal production of arachidonic acid metabolites, both through the cyclooxygenase pathways, i.e., prostanoids, and through the lipoxygenase pathways, i.e., leukotrienes and hydroxyeicosatetraenoic acids, is increased in patients with ulcerative colitis, and it is possible that 5-ASA diminishes inflammation by blocking production of arachidonic acid metabolites.

12.3 Pharmacokinetics

Absorption

The pharmacokinetics of 5-ASA and its metabolite, N-acetyl-5-aminosalicylic acid (N-Ac-5-ASA), were studied after a single and multiple oral doses of 1.5 g APRISO in a crossover study in healthy subjects under fasting conditions. In the multiple-dose period, each subject received APRISO 1.5 g (4 × 0.375 g capsules) every 24 hours (QD) for 7 consecutive days. Steady state was reached on Day 6 of QD dosing based on trough concentrations.

After single and multiple doses of APRISO, peak plasma concentrations were observed at about 4 hours post dose. At steady state, moderate increases (1.5-fold and 1.7-fold) in systemic exposure (AUC_{0-24}) to 5-ASA and N-Ac-5-ASA were observed when compared with a single-dose of APRISO.

Pharmacokinetic parameters after a single dose of 1.5 g APRISO and at steady state in healthy subjects under fasting condition are shown in Table 2.

Table 2: Single Dose and Multiple Dose Mean (±SD) Plasma Pharmacokinetic Parameters of Mesalamine (5-ASA) and N-Ac-5-ASA after 1.5 g APRISO Administration in Healthy Subjects

Mesalamine (5-ASA)	Single Dose (n=24)	Multiple Dose[c] (n=24)
AUC_{0-24} (μg*h/mL)	11 ± 5	17 ± 6
AUC_{0-inf} (μg*h/mL)	14 ± 5	-
C_{max} (μg/mL)	2.1 ± 1.1	2.7 ± 1.1
T_{max} (h) [a]	4 (2, 16)	4 (2, 8)
$t_{1/2}$ (h)[b]	9 ± 7	10 ± 8
N-Ac-5-ASA		
AUC_{0-24} (μg*h/mL)	26 ± 6	37 ± 9
AUC_{0-inf} (μg*h/mL)	51 ± 23	-
C_{max} (μg/mL)	2.8 ± 0.8	3.4 ± 0.9
T_{max} (h)[a]	4 (4, 12)	5 (2, 8)
$t_{1/2}$ (h)[b]	12 ± 11	14 ± 10

[a] Median (range); [b] Harmonic mean (pseudo SD); [c] after 7 days of treatment

In a separate study (n = 30), it was observed that under fasting conditions about 32% ± 11% (mean ± SD) of the administered dose was systemically absorbed based on the combined cumulative urinary excretion of 5-ASA and N-Ac-5-ASA over 96 hours post-dose.

The effect of a high fat meal intake on absorption of mesalamine granules (the same granules contained in APRISO capsules) was evaluated in 30 healthy subjects. Subjects received 1.6 g of mesalamine granules in sachet (2 × 0.8 g) following an overnight fast or a high fat meal in a crossover study. Under fed conditions, t_{max} for both 5-ASA and N-Ac-5-ASA was prolonged by 4 and 2 hours, respectively. A high fat meal did not affect C_{max} for 5-ASA, but a 27% increase in the cumulative urinary excretion of 5-ASA was observed with a high fat meal. The overall extent of absorption of N-Ac-5-ASA was not affected by a high fat meal. As APRISO and mesalamine granules in sachet were bioequivalent, APRISO can be taken without regard to food.

Distribution

In an *in vitro* study, at 2.5 μg/mL, mesalamine and N-Ac-5-ASA are 43 ± 6% and 78 ± 1% bound, respectively, to plasma proteins. Protein binding of N-Ac-5-ASA does not appear to be concentration dependent at concentrations ranging from 1 to 10 μg/mL.

Metabolism

The major metabolite of mesalamine is N-acetyl-5-aminosalicylic acid (N-Ac-5-ASA). It is formed by N-acetyltransferase activity in the liver and intestinal mucosa.

Elimination

Following single and multiple doses of APRISO, the mean half-lives were 9 to 10 hours for 5-ASA, and 12 to 14 hours for N-Ac-5-ASA. Of the approximately 32% of the dose absorbed, about 2% of the dose was excreted unchanged in the urine, compared with about 30% of the dose excreted as N-Ac-5-ASA.

In Vitro Drug-Drug Interaction Study

In an *in vitro* study using human liver microsomes, 5-ASA and its metabolite, N-Ac-5-ASA, were shown not to inhibit the major CYP enzymes evaluated (CYP1A2, CYP2C9, CYP2C19, CYP2D6, and CYP3A4). Therefore, mesalamine and its metabolite are not expected to inhibit the metabolism of other drugs that are substrates of CYP1A2, CYP2C9, CYP2C19, CYP2D6, or CYP3A4.

13 NONCLINICAL TOXICOLOGY

13.1 Carcinogenesis, Mutagenesis, Impairment of Fertility

Dietary mesalamine was not carcinogenic in rats at doses as high as 480 mg/kg/day, or in mice at 2000 mg/kg/day. These doses are about 2.6 and 5.4 times the recommended human dose of granulated mesalamine capsules of 1.5 g/day (30 mg/kg if 50 kg body weight assumed or 1110 mg/m^2), respectively, based on body surface area. Mesalamine was negative in the Ames test, the mouse lymphoma cell (L5178Y/TK+/-) forward mutation test, the sister chromatid exchange assay in the Chinese hamster bone marrow test, and the mouse bone marrow micronucleus test. Mesalamine at oral doses up to 320 mg/kg (about 1.7 times the recommended human dose based on body surface area) was found to have no effect on fertility or reproductive performance in rats.

13.2 Animal Toxicology and/or Pharmacology

Renal Toxicity

Animal studies with mesalamine (13-week and 26-week oral toxicity studies in rats, and 26-week and 52-week oral toxicity studies in dogs) have shown the kidney to be the major target organ of mesalamine toxicity. Oral doses of 40 mg/kg/day (about 0.20 times the human dose, on the basis of body surface area) produced minimal to slight tubular injury, and doses of 160 mg/kg/day (about 0.90 times the human dose, on the basis of body surface area) or higher in rats produced renal lesions including tubular degeneration, tubular mineralization, and papillary necrosis. Oral doses of 60 mg/kg/day (about 1.1 times the human dose, on the basis of body surface area) or higher in dogs also produced renal lesions including tubular atrophy, interstitial cell infiltration, chronic nephritis, and papillary necrosis.

Overdosage

Single oral doses of 800 mg/kg (about 2.2 times the recommended human dose, on the basis of body surface area) and 1800 mg/kg (about 9.7 times the recommended human dose, on the basis of body surface area) of mesalamine were lethal to mice and rats, respectively, and resulted in gastrointestinal and renal toxicity.

14 CLINICAL STUDIES

14.1 Ulcerative Colitis

Two similar, randomized, double-blind, placebo-controlled, multi-center studies were conducted in a total of 562 adult patients in remission from ulcerative colitis. The study populations had a mean age of 46 years (11% age 65 years or older), were 53% female, and were primarily white (92%).

Ulcerative colitis disease activity was assessed using a modified Sutherland Disease Activity Index[1] (DAI), which is a sum of four subscores based on stool frequency, rectal bleeding, mucosal appearance on endoscopy, and physician's rating of disease activity. Each subscore can range from 0 to 3, for a total possible DAI score of 12.

At baseline, approximately 80% of patients had a total DAI score of 0 or 1.0. Patients were randomized 2:1 to receive either APRISO 1.5 g or placebo once daily in the morning for six months. Patients were assessed at baseline, 1 month, 3 months, and 6 months in the clinic, with endoscopy performed at baseline, at end of study, or if clinical symptoms developed. Relapse was defined as a rectal bleeding subscale score of 1 or more and a mucosal appearance subscale score of 2 or more using the DAI. The analysis of the intent-to-treat population was a comparison of the proportions of patients who remained relapse-free at the end of six months of treatment. For the table below (Table 3) all patients who prematurely withdrew from the study for any reason were counted as relapses.

In both studies, the proportion of patients who remained relapse-free at six months was greater for APRISO than for placebo.

Table 3: Percentage of Patients Relapse-Free* through 6 Months in APRISO Maintenance Studies

	APRISO 1.5 g/day % (# no relapse/N)	Placebo % (# no relapse/N)	Difference (95% C.I.)	P-value
Study 1	68% (143/209)	51% (49/96)	17% (5.5, 29.2)	<0.001
Study 2	71% (117/164)	59% (55/93)	12% (0, 24.5)	0.046

* Relapse counted as rectal bleeding score ≥1 and mucosal appearance score ≥2, or premature withdrawal from study.

Examination of gender subgroups did not identify difference in response to APRISO among these subgroups. There were too few elderly and too few African-American patients to adequately assess difference in effects in those populations.

The use of APRISO for treating ulcerative colitis beyond six months has not been evaluated in controlled clinical trials.

15 REFERENCES

1. Sutherland LR, Martin F, Greer S, Robinson M, Greenberger N, Saibil F, *et al.* 5-Aminosalicylic acid enema in the treatment of distal ulcerative colitis, proctosigmoiditis, and proctitis. Gastroenterology 1987;92(6):1894-1898.

16 HOW SUPPLIED/STORAGE AND HANDLING

APRISO is available as light blue opaque hard gelatin capsules containing 0.375 g mesalamine and with the letters "G" and "M" on either side of a black band imprinted on the capsule.

NDC 65649-103-02 Bottles of 120 capsules
NDC 65649-103-01 Bottles of 4 capsules

Storage:
Store at 20° to 25°C (68° to 77°F); excursions permitted between 15° and 30°C (59° and 86°F). See USP Controlled Room Temperature.

17 PATIENT COUNSELING INFORMATION

17.1 Patients with Phenylketonuria

- Inform patients with phenylketonuria (PKU) or their caregivers that each APRISO capsule contains aspartame equivalent to 0.56 mg of phenylalanine, so that the recommended adult dosing provides an equivalent of 2.24 mg of phenylalanine per day.

17.2 General Counseling Information

- Instruct patients not to take APRISO capsules with antacids, because it could affect the way APRISO dissolves.
- Instruct patients to contact a health care provider if they experience a worsening of ulcerative colitis symptoms, because it could be due to a reaction to APRISO.

Manufactured by: Catalent Pharma Solutions
Manufactured for: Salix Pharmaceuticals, Inc., Raleigh, NC 27615
* APRISO™ is a trademark of Salix Pharmaceuticals, Inc.
Product protected by U.S. Patent No. 6,551,620 and U.S. Patent No. 7,547,451
Please see www.salix.com for patent information
VENART-113-2 / FEB 2012

Shown in Product Identification Guide, page 312

FULYZAQ™ ℞

(crofelemer)
delayed-release tablets, for oral use

HIGHLIGHTS OF PRESCRIBING INFORMATION
These highlights do not include all the information needed to use FULYZAQ safely and effectively. See full prescribing information for FULYZAQ.
FULYZAQ™ (crofelemer) delayed-release tablets, for oral use
Initial U.S. Approval: 2012

INDICATIONS AND USAGE

FULYZAQ is an anti-diarrheal indicated for the symptomatic relief of non-infectious diarrhea in adult patients with HIV/AIDS on anti-retroviral therapy. (1)

DOSAGE AND ADMINISTRATION

One 125 mg delayed-release tablet taken orally twice a day, with or without food. (2)

DOSAGE FORMS AND STRENGTHS

Delayed-Release Tablets: 125 mg (3)

CONTRAINDICATIONS

None. (4)

WARNINGS AND PRECAUTIONS

Rule out infectious etiologies of diarrhea before starting crofelemer. If infectious etiologies are not considered, there is a risk that patients with infectious etiologies will not receive the appropriate therapy and their disease may worsen. (5.1)

ADVERSE REACTIONS

Most common adverse reactions (incidence ≥ 3%) are upper respiratory tract infection, bronchitis, cough, flatulence and increased bilirubin. (6)

To report SUSPECTED ADVERSE REACTIONS, contact Salix Pharmaceuticals at 1-800-508-0024 or FDA at 1-800-FDA-1088 or *www.fda.gov/medwatch*

USE IN SPECIFIC POPULATIONS

- *Pregnancy:* Based on animal data, may cause fetal harm. (8.1)
- *Pediatric Use:* Safety and effectiveness of FULYZAQ has not been established in patients less than 18 years of age. (8.4)

See 17 for PATIENT COUNSELING INFORMATION
Revised: 02/2013

FULL PRESCRIBING INFORMATION: CONTENTS*

*** Sections or subsections omitted from the full prescribing information are not listed**

FULL PRESCRIBING INFORMATION

1 INDICATIONS AND USAGE

FULYZAQ is indicated for symptomatic relief of non-infectious diarrhea in patients with HIV/AIDS on anti-retroviral therapy.

2 DOSAGE AND ADMINISTRATION

The recommended dose of FULYZAQ is one 125 mg delayed-release tablet taken orally two times a day, with or without food. FULYZAQ tablets should **not be crushed or chewed.** Tablets should be swallowed whole.

3 DOSAGE FORMS AND STRENGTHS

FULYZAQ is a white, oval, enteric-coated 125 mg delayed-release tablet printed on one side with 125SLXP.

4 CONTRAINDICATIONS

None.

5 WARNINGS AND PRECAUTIONS

5.1 Risks of Treatment in Patients with Infectious Diarrhea

If infectious etiologies are not considered, and FULYZAQ is initiated based on a presumptive diagnosis of non-infectious diarrhea, then there is a risk that patients with infectious etiologies will not receive the appropriate treatments, and their disease may worsen. Before starting FULYZAQ, rule out infectious etiologies of diarrhea. FULYZAQ is not indicated for the treatment of infectious diarrhea.

6 ADVERSE REACTIONS

6.1 Clinical Trials Experience

Because clinical trials are conducted under widely varying conditions, adverse reaction rates observed in the clinical trials of a drug cannot be directly compared to rates in the clinical trials of another drug and may not reflect the rates observed in practice.

A total of 696 HIV-positive patients in three placebo-controlled trials received FULYZAQ for a mean duration of 78 days. Of the total population across the three trials, 229 patients received a dose of 125 mg twice a day for a mean duration of 141 days, 69 patients received a dose of 250 mg twice a day for a mean duration of 139 days, 102 patients received a dose of 250 mg four times a day for a mean duration of 14 days, 54 patients received a dose of 500 mg twice a day for a mean duration of 146 days, and 242 patients received a dose of 500 mg four times a day for a mean duration of 14 days.

Adverse reactions for FULYZAQ that occurred in at least 2% of patients and at a higher incidence than placebo are provided in Table 1.

Table 1: Adverse Reactions Occurring in at Least 2% of Patients in the 125 mg Twice Daily Group

Adverse Reaction	Crofelemer 125 mg BID* N = 229 n (%)	Placebo N = 274 n (%)
Upper respiratory tract infection	13 (5.7)	4 (1.5)
Bronchitis	9 (3.9)	0
Cough	8 (3.5)	3 (1.1)
Flatulence	7 (3.1)	3 (1.1)

Increased bilirubin	7 (3.1)	3 (1.1)
Nausea	6 (2.6)	4 (1.5)
Back pain	6 (2.6)	4 (1.5)
Arthralgia	6 (2.6)	0
Urinary tract infection	5 (2.2)	2 (0.7)
Nasopharyngitis	5 (2.2)	2 (0.7)
Musculoskeletal pain	5 (2.2)	1 (0.4)
Hemorrhoids	5 (2.2)	0
Giardiasis	5 (2.2)	0
Anxiety	5 (2.2)	1 (0.4)
Increased alanine aminotransferase	5 (2.2)	3 (1.1)
Abdominal distension	5 (2.2)	1 (0.4)

* Twice daily

Adverse reactions that occurred in between 1% and 2% of patients taking a 250 mg daily dose of FULYZAQ were abdominal pain, acne, increased aspartate aminotransferase, increased conjugated bilirubin, increased unconjugated blood bilirubin, constipation, depression, dermatitis, dizziness, dry mouth, dyspepsia, gastroenteritis, herpes zoster, nephrolithiasis, pain in extremity, pollakiuria, procedural pain, seasonal allergy, sinusitis and decreased white blood cell count.

Adverse reactions were similar in patients who received doses greater than 250 mg daily.

7 DRUG INTERACTIONS

7.1 Drug Interaction Potential

In vitro studies have shown that crofelemer has the potential to inhibit cytochrome P450 isoenzyme 3A and transporters MRP2 and OATP1A2 at concentrations expected in the gut. Due to the minimal absorption of crofelemer, it is unlikely to inhibit cytochrome P450 isoenzymes 1A2, 2A6, 2B6, 2C9, 2C19, 2D6, 2E1 and CYP3A4 systemically *[see Clinical Pharmacology (12.3)]*.

7.2 Nelfinavir, Zidovudine, and Lamivudine

FULYZAQ administration did not have a clinically relevant interaction with nelfinavir, zidovudine, or lamivudine in a drug-drug interaction trial.

8 USE IN SPECIFIC POPULATIONS

8.1 Pregnancy

Pregnancy Category C

Reproduction studies performed with crofelemer in rats at oral doses up to 177 times the recommended daily human dose of 4.2 mg/kg revealed no evidence of impaired fertility or harm to the fetus. In pregnant rabbits, crofelemer at an oral dose of about 96 times the recommended daily human dose of 4.2 mg/kg, caused abortions and resorptions of fetuses. However, it is not clear whether these effects are related to the maternal toxicity observed. A pre- and postnatal development study performed with crofelemer in rats at oral doses of up to 177 times the recommended daily human dose of 4.2 mg/kg revealed no evidence of adverse pre- and postnatal effects in offspring. There are, however, no adequate, well-controlled studies in pregnant women. Because animal reproduction studies are not always predictive of human response, this drug should be used during pregnancy only if clearly needed.

8.3 Nursing Mothers

It is not known whether crofelemer is excreted in human milk. Because many drugs are excreted in human milk and because of the potential for adverse reactions in nursing infants from FULYZAQ, a decision should be made whether to discontinue nursing or to discontinue the drug, taking into account the importance of the drug to the mother.

8.4 Pediatric Use

The safety and effectiveness of FULYZAQ have not been established in pediatric patients less than 18 years of age.

8.5 Geriatric Use

Clinical studies with crofelemer did not include sufficient numbers of patients aged 65 and over to determine whether they respond differently than younger patients.

8.6 Use in Patients with Low CD4 Counts and High Viral Loads

No dose modifications are recommended with respect to CD4 cell count and HIV viral load, based on the findings in subgroups of patients defined by CD4 cell count and HIV viral load.

The safety profile of crofelemer was similar in patients with baseline CD4 cell count less than 404 cells/µL (lower limit of normal range) (N=388) and patients with baseline CD4 cell counts greater than or equal to 404 cells/µL (N=289).

The safety profile of crofelemer was similar in patients with baseline HIV viral loads less than 400 copies/mL (N = 412) and patients with baseline HIV viral loads greater than or equal to 400 copies/mL (N = 278).

10 OVERDOSAGE

There has been no reported experience with overdosage of crofelemer.

11 DESCRIPTION

FULYZAQ (crofelemer) delayed-release tablets is an anti-diarrheal, enteric-coated drug product for oral administration. It contains 125 mg of crofelemer, a botanical drug substance that is derived from the red latex of *Croton lechleri* Müll. Arg. Crofelemer is an oligomeric proanthocyanidin mixture primarily composed of (+)–catechin, (–)–epicatechin, (+)–gallocatechin, and (–)–epigallocatechin monomer units linked in random sequence, as represented below. The average degree of polymerization for the oligomers ranges between 5 and 7.5, as determined by phloroglucinol degradation.

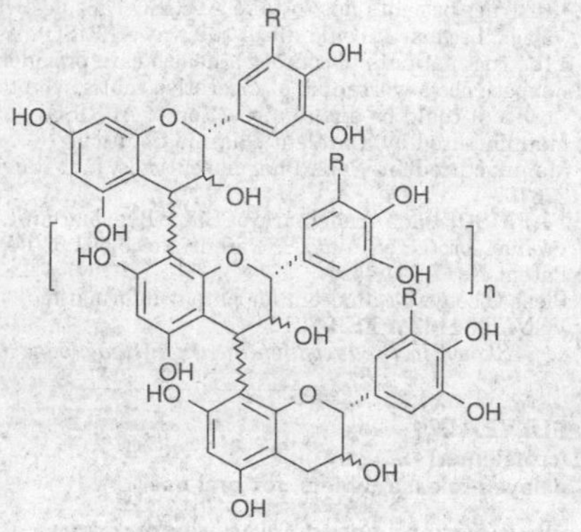

R = H or OH

range n = 3 to 5.5

Inactive ingredients: microcrystalline cellulose, croscarmellose sodium, colloidal silicon dioxide, and magnesium stearate.

Coating ingredients: ethylacrylate and methylacrylate copolymer dispersion, talc, triethyl citrate, and white dispersion which contains xanthan gum, titanium dioxide, propyl paraben, and methyl paraben.

12 CLINICAL PHARMACOLOGY

12.1 Mechanism of Action

Crofelemer is an inhibitor of both the cyclic adenosine monophosphate (cAMP)-stimulated cystic fibrosis transmembrane conductance regulator (CFTR) chloride ion (Cl^-) channel, and the calcium-activated Cl^- channels (CaCC) at the luminal membrane of enterocytes. The CFTR Cl^- channel and CaCC regulate Cl^- and fluid secretion by intestinal epithelial cells. Crofelemer acts by blocking Cl^- secretion and accompanying high volume water loss in diarrhea, normalizing the flow of Cl^- and water in the GI tract.

12.2 Pharmacodynamics

Consistent with the mechanism of action of crofelemer (i.e., inhibition of CFTR and CaCC in the GI lumen), data suggest stool chloride concentrations decreased in patients treated with FULYZAQ (500 mg four times daily) (n=25) for four days relative to placebo (n=24); stool chloride concentrations decreased in both African American patients treated with FULYZAQ (n=3) relative to placebo (n=5) and non-African American patients treated with FULYZAQ (n=22) relative to placebo (n=19).

At a dose 10 times the maximum recommended dose, crofelemer does not prolong the QTc interval to any clinically relevant extent.

12.3 Pharmacokinetics

Absorption

The absorption of crofelemer is minimal following oral dosing in healthy adults and HIV–positive patients and concentrations of crofelemer in plasma are below the level of quantitation (50 ng/mL). Therefore, standard pharmacokinetic parameters such as area under the curve, maximum concentration, and half-life cannot be estimated.

Distribution

The distribution of crofelemer has not been determined.

Metabolism

No metabolites of crofelemer have been identified in healthy subjects or patients in clinical trials.

Elimination

The elimination route has not been identified in humans.

Food Effect

Administration of crofelemer with a high-fat meal was not associated with an increase in systemic exposure of crofelemer in healthy volunteers. In the clinical trial, a single 500 mg dose of crofelemer was administered one-half hour before the morning and evening meals. Therefore, crofelemer may be administered with or without a meal.

Drug–Drug Interactions

Results of a crossover study in healthy volunteers showed crofelemer 500 mg administered four times daily for five days had no effect on the exposure of zidovudine and nelfinavir when administered as a single dose. A 20% decrease in lamivudine exposure was also observed in the same study but was not considered to be clinically important.

13 NONCLINICAL TOXICOLOGY

13.1 Carcinogenesis, Mutagenesis, Impairment of Fertility

Carcinogenesis

Long-term studies in animals have not been performed to evaluate the carcinogenic potential of crofelemer.

Mutagenesis

Crofelemer was negative in the bacterial reverse mutation assay, chromosomal aberration assay, and rat bone marrow micronucleus assay.

Impairment of Fertility

Crofelemer, at oral doses of up to 738 mg/kg/day (177 times the recommended human daily dose of 4.2 mg/kg), had no effects on fertility or reproductive performance of male and female rats.

14 CLINICAL STUDIES

The efficacy of FULYZAQ 125 mg delayed-release tablets twice daily was evaluated in a randomized, double-blind, placebo-controlled (one month) and placebo-free (five month), multi-center study. The study enrolled 374 HIV-positive patients on stable anti-retroviral therapy (ART) with a history of diarrhea for one month or more. Diarrhea was defined as either persistently loose stools despite regular use of anti-diarrheal medication (ADM) (e.g., loperamide, diphenoxylate, and bismuth subsalicylate) or one or more watery bowel movements per day without regular ADM use.

Patients were excluded if they had a positive gastrointestinal (GI) biopsy, GI culture, or stool test for multiple bacteria (*Salmonella*, *Shigella*, *Campylobacter*, *Yersinia*, *Mycobacterium*), bacterial toxin (*Clostridium difficile*), ova and parasites (*Giardia*, *Entamoeba*, *Isospora*, *Cyclospora*, *Cryptosporidium*, *Microsporidium*), or viruses (*Cytomegalovirus*). Patients were also excluded if they had a history of ulcerative colitis, Crohn's disease, celiac sprue (gluten-enteropathy), chronic pancreatitis, malabsorption, or any other GI disease associated with diarrhea.

The study had a two-stage adaptive design. In both stages, patients received placebo for 10 days (screening period) followed by randomization to crofelemer or placebo for 31 days of treatment (double-blind period). Only patients with 1 or more watery bowel movements per day on at least 5 of the last 7 days in the screening period were randomized to the double-blind period. Each stage enrolled patients separately; the dose for the second stage was selected based on an interim analysis of data from the first stage. In the first stage, patients were randomized 1:1:1:1 to one of three crofelemer dose regimens (125, 250, or 500 mg twice daily) or placebo. In the second stage, patients were randomized 1:1 to crofelemer 125 mg twice daily or placebo. The efficacy analysis was based on results from the double-blind portion of both stages.

Each study stage also had a five month period (placebo-free period) that followed the double-blind period. Patients treated with crofelemer continued the same dose in the placebo-free period. In the first stage, patients that received placebo were re-randomized 1:1:1 to one of the three crofelemer dose regimens (125, 250, or 500 mg twice daily) in the placebo-free period. In the second stage, patients that received placebo were treated with crofelemer 125 mg twice daily in the placebo-free period.

The median time since diagnosis of HIV was 12 years. The percentage of patients with a CD4 cell count of less than 404 was 39%. The percentage of patients with a HIV viral load greater than or equal to 1000, 400 to 999, and less than 400 HIV copies/mL was 7%, 3%, and 9%, respectively; the remainder had a viral load that was not detectable. The median time since diarrhea started was 4 years. The median number of daily watery bowel movements was 2.5 per day. Most patients were male (85%). The percentage of patients that were Caucasian was 46%; the percentage of patients that were African-American was 32%. The median age was 45 years with a range of 21 to 68 years.

In the double-blind period of the study, 136 patients received crofelemer 125 mg twice daily, 54 patients received 250 mg twice daily, 47 patients received 500 mg twice daily, and 138 patients received placebo. The percentages of patients that completed the double-blind period were 92%, 100%, 85%, and 94% in the 125 mg, 250 mg, 500 mg, and placebo arms, respectively.

Most patients received concomitant protease inhibitors (PI) during the double-blind period (Table 2). The most frequently used ARTs in each group were tenofovir/emtricitabine, ritonavir, and lopinavir/ritonavir.

Table 2: Concomitant ART Use in the Double-Blind Period

	125 mg BID (N = 136) n (%)	250 mg BID (N = 54) n (%)	500 mg BID (N = 46) n (%)	Placebo BID (N = 138) n (%)
Any ART	135 (99)	53 (98)	45 (98)	134 (97)
Any PI	87 (64)	41 (76)	33 (72)	97 (70)
Tenofovir/Emtricitabine	45 (33)	22 (41)	16 (35)	52 (38)
Ritonavir	46 (34)	18 (33)	15 (33)	49 (36)
Lopinavir/Ritonavir	30 (22)	21 (39)	15 (33)	40 (29)
Efavirenz/Tenofovir/ Emtricitabine	30 (22)	7 (13)	7 (15)	21 (15)
Tenofovir disoproxil fumarate	18 (13)	8 (15)	5 (11)	14 (10)
Atazanavir sulfate	19 (14)	3 (6)	6 (13)	22 (16)
Abacavir w/ lamivudine	17 (13)	5 (9)	5 (11)	18 (13)
Darunavir	19 (14)	4 (7)	4 (9)	14 (10)
Raltegravir	16 (12)	4 (7)	5 (11)	11 (8)
Valaciclovir hydrochloride	12 (9)	8 (15)	5 (11)	16 (12)
Fosamprenavir	12 (9)	6 (11)	4 (9)	13 (9)
Zidovudine w/ lamivudine	12 (9)	3 (6)	3 (7)	15 (11)
Lamivudine	7 (5)	6 (11)	4 (9)	6 (4)
Nevirapine	8 (6)	6 (11)	3 (7)	9 (7)
Atazanavir	5 (4)	6 (11)	2 (4)	2 (1)

Abbreviations: ART = antiretroviral therapy; PI = Protease Inhibitor; BID = twice daily.

[See table 2 above]

The primary efficacy endpoint was the proportion of patients with a clinical response, defined as less than or equal to 2 watery bowel movements per week during at least 2 of the 4 weeks of the placebo-controlled phase. Patients who received concomitant ADMs or opiates were counted as clinical non-responders.

A significantly larger proportion of patients in the crofelemer 125 mg twice daily group experienced clinical response compared with patients in the placebo group (17.6% vs. 8.0%, 1–sided $p < 0.01$).

In the randomized clinical study, examination of duration of diarrhea, baseline number of daily watery bowel movements, use of protease inhibitors, CD4 cell count and age subgroups did not identify differences in the consistency of the crofelemer treatment effect among these subgroups. There were too few female subjects and subjects with an HIV viral load > 400 copies/mL to adequately assess differences in effects in these populations. Among race subgroups, there were no differences in the consistency of the crofelemer treatment effect except for the subgroup of African-Americans; crofelemer was less effective in African-Americans than non-African-Americans.

Although the CD4 cell count and HIV viral load did not appear to change over the one month placebo-controlled period, the clinical significance of this finding is unknown because of the short duration of the placebo-controlled period. Of the 24 clinical responders to crofelemer (125 mg twice daily), 22 entered the placebo-free period; 16 were responding at the end of month 3, and 14 were responding at the end of month 5.

16 HOW SUPPLIED/STORAGE AND HANDLING

Crofelemer delayed release tablets, 125 mg, are white, oval enteric-coated tablets printed on one side with 125SLXP. They are available in the following package size:

Bottles of 60: NDC 65649-802-02

Store at 20°C-25°C (68°F-77°F); excursions permitted between 15°C-30°C (59°F-86°F). See USP Controlled Room Temperature.

17 PATIENT COUNSELING INFORMATION

- Instruct patients that FULYZAQ tablets may be taken with or without food.
- Instruct patients that FULYZAQ tablets should not be crushed or chewed. Tablets should be swallowed whole.

Rx Only

Manufactured by Patheon, Inc. for
Salix Pharmaceuticals, Inc., Raleigh, NC 27615

US Patent Nos. 7,341,744 and 7,323,195.

FULYZAQ is distributed by Salix Pharmaceuticals, Inc. under license from Napo Pharmaceuticals, Inc.

The botanical drug substance of FULYZAQ is extracted from *Croton lechleri* (the botanical raw material) that is harvested from the wild in South America.

Shown in Product Identification Guide, page 312

MOVIPREP® ℞

(PEG-3350, sodium sulfate, sodium chloride, potassium chloride, sodium ascorbate, and ascorbic acid for oral solution)

HIGHLIGHTS OF PRESCRIBING INFORMATION

These highlights do not include all the information needed to use MOVIPREP safely and effectively. See full prescribing information for MOVIPREP.

MOVIPREP® (PEG-3350, sodium sulfate, sodium chloride, potassium chloride, sodium ascorbate, and ascorbic acid for oral solution)

Initial U.S. Approval: 2006

RECENT MAJOR CHANGES

Adverse Reactions (6.2) (08/2013)
Warnings and Precautions (5.9) (07/2012)

INDICATIONS AND USAGE

MoviPrep is an osmotic laxative indicated for cleansing of the colon as a preparation for colonoscopy in adults 18 years or older. (1)

DOSAGE AND ADMINISTRATION

- Split-dose regimen: The evening before the colonoscopy, take the first liter of MoviPrep solution (one 8 ounce glass every 15 minutes) and then drink 16 ounces of clear liquid. On the morning of the colonoscopy, take the second liter of MoviPrep solution over one hour and then drink 16 ounces of clear liquid at least one hour prior to the start of the colonoscopy. (2)
- Evening only (full-dose) regimen: Around 6 PM in the evening before the colonoscopy, take the first liter of MoviPrep solution (one 8 ounce glass every 15 minutes) and then about 1½ hours later take the second liter of MoviPrep solution (one 8 ounce glass every 15 minutes). In addition, drink 32 ounces of clear liquid during the evening before the colonoscopy. (2)

DOSAGE FORMS AND STRENGTHS

- Powdered Form: 2 × Pouch A and 2 × Pouch B to be administered as an oral solution. (3)

CONTRAINDICATIONS

- Gastrointestinal (GI) obstruction (4)
- Bowel perforation (4)
- Gastric retention (4)
- Ileus (4)
- Toxic colitis or toxic megacolon (4)
- Hypersensitivity to any components of MoviPrep (4)

WARNINGS AND PRECAUTIONS

- Risk of fluid and electrolyte abnormalities, arrhythmias, seizures and renal impairment – encourage adequate hydration, assess concurrent medications, and consider laboratory assessments prior to and after use (5.1, 5.2, 5.3)
- Patients with impaired renal function or patients taking concomitant medications that affect renal function – use caution, ensure adequate hydration and consider testing (5.4)
- Suspected GI obstruction or perforation – rule out the diagnosis before administration (5.6)
- Patients at risk for aspiration — observe during administration (5.7)
- Glucose-6-phosphate dehydrogenase deficiency (G-6-PD) – use with caution (5.8)
- Contains phenylalanine (233 mg per treatment) (5.9)

ADVERSE REACTIONS

Most common adverse reactions for split dosing (incidence ≥ 5%) are malaise, nausea, abdominal pain, vomiting, and upper abdominal pain (6). The most common adverse reactions for evening only dosing (incidence ≥ 5%) are abdominal distension, anal discomfort, thirst, nausea, abdominal pain, sleep disorder, rigors, hunger, malaise, vomiting, and dizziness (6).

To report SUSPECTED ADVERSE REACTIONS, contact Salix Pharmaceuticals, Inc. at 1-800-508-0024 or FDA at 1-800-FDA-1088 or *www.fda.gov/medwatch*.

DRUG INTERACTIONS

- Oral medications may not be absorbed when administered while taking MoviPrep. (7)

USE IN SPECIFIC POPULATIONS

- Pregnancy: No human or animal data. Use only if clearly needed. (8.1)

See 17 for PATIENT COUNSELING INFORMATION

Revised: 08/2013

FULL PRESCRIBING INFORMATION: CONTENTS*

*** Sections or subsections omitted from the full prescribing information are not listed**

FULL PRESCRIBING INFORMATION

1 INDICATIONS AND USAGE

MoviPrep is an osmotic laxative indicated for cleansing of the colon as a preparation for colonoscopy in adults 18 years of age or older.

2 DOSAGE AND ADMINISTRATION

The MoviPrep dose for colon cleansing for adult patients is 2 liters (approximately 64 ounces) of MoviPrep solution (with 1 additional liter of clear liquid) taken orally prior to the colonoscopy in one of the following ways:

1) **Split-dose MoviPrep regimen:** The evening before the colonoscopy, take the first liter of MoviPrep solution over one hour (one 8 ounce glass every 15 minutes) and then drink 0.5 liters (approximately 16 ounces) of clear liquid. Then, on the morning of the colonoscopy, take the second liter of MoviPrep solution over one hour and then drink 0.5 liters of clear liquid at least one hour prior to the start of the colonoscopy; or

2) **Evening only (full-dose) MoviPrep regimen:** Around 6 PM in the evening before the colonoscopy, take the first liter of MoviPrep solution over one hour (one 8 ounce glass every 15 minutes) and then about 1.5 hours later take the second liter of MoviPrep solution over one hour. In addition, take 1 liter (approximately 32 ounces) of additional clear liquid during the evening before the colonoscopy.

Preparation of the MoviPrep solution:
MoviPrep solution is prepared by emptying the contents of 1 pouch A and 1 pouch B into a suitable glass container (or the container provided) and adding to the container 1 liter of lukewarm water. Mix the solution to ensure that the ingredients are completely dissolved. If the patient prefers, the MoviPrep solution can be refrigerated prior to drinking. The reconstituted solution should be used within 24 hours.
No additional ingredients (e.g., flavorings) should be added to the MoviPrep solution.
After consumption of the first liter of MoviPrep solution, the above mixing procedure should be repeated with the second pouch A and pouch B to reconstitute the second liter of the MoviPrep solution.

3 DOSAGE FORMS AND STRENGTHS

MoviPrep is available in a carton that contains 4 separate pouches (2 of pouch A and 2 of pouch B). Each pouch A contains 100 grams of polyethylene glycol (PEG) 3350, NF, 7.5 grams of sodium sulfate, USP, 2.691 grams of sodium chloride, USP, and 1.015 grams of potassium chloride, USP, plus the following excipients: aspartame, NF (sweetener), acesulfame potassium, NF (sweetener), and lemon flavoring. Each pouch B contains 4.7 grams of ascorbic acid, USP and 5.9 grams of sodium ascorbate, USP.

4 CONTRAINDICATIONS

MoviPrep is contraindicated in the following conditions:
- Gastrointestinal (GI) obstruction
- Bowel perforation
- Gastric retention
- Ileus
- Toxic colitis or toxic megacolon
- Hypersensitivity to any components of MoviPrep *[see DESCRIPTION (11)]*

5 WARNINGS AND PRECAUTIONS

5.1 Serious Fluid and Electrolyte Abnormalities

Advise patients to hydrate adequately before, during, and after the use of MoviPrep. If a patient develops significant vomiting or signs of dehydration after taking MoviPrep consider performing post-colonoscopy lab tests (electrolytes, creatinine, and BUN). Fluid and electrolyte disturbances can lead to serious adverse events including cardiac arrhythmias, seizures and renal impairment.
Patients with electrolyte abnormalities should have them corrected before treatment with MoviPrep. MoviPrep should be used with caution in patients using concomitant medications that increase the risk of electrolyte abnormalities [such as diuretics, angiotensin converting enzyme (ACE)-inhibitors or angiotensin receptor blockers (ARBs)] or in patients with known or suspected hyponatremia. Consider performing pre-dose and post-colonoscopy laboratory tests (sodium, potassium, calcium, creatinine, and BUN) in these patients. *[See DRUG INTERACTIONS* (7.1)*]*

5.2 Cardiac Arrhythmias

There have been rare reports of serious arrhythmias associated with the use of ionic osmotic laxative products for bowel preparation. Use caution when prescribing MoviPrep for patients at increased risk of arrhythmias (e.g., patients with a history of prolonged QT, uncontrolled arrhythmias, recent myocardial infarction, unstable angina, congestive heart failure, or cardiomyopathy). Pre-dose and post-colonoscopy ECGs should be considered in patients at increased risk of serious cardiac arrhythmias.

5.3 Seizures

There have been rare reports of generalized tonic-clonic seizures and/or loss of consciousness associated with use of bowel preparation products in patients with no prior history of seizures. The seizure cases were associated with electrolyte abnormalities (e.g., hyponatremia, hypokalemia, hypocalcemia, and hypomagnesemia) and low serum osmolality. The neurologic abnormalities resolved with correction of fluid and electrolyte abnormalities.
Use caution when prescribing MoviPrep for patients with a history of seizures and in patients at increased risk of seizure, such as patients taking medications that lower the seizure threshold (e.g., tricyclic antidepressants), patients withdrawing from alcohol or benzodiazepines, or patients with known or suspected hyponatremia.

5.4 Renal Impairment

Use with caution in patients with impaired renal function or patients taking concomitant medications that affect renal function (such as diuretics, angiotensin converting enzyme inhibitors, angiotensin receptor blockers, or non-steroidal anti-inflammatory drugs). Advise these patients of the importance of adequate hydration, and consider performing pre-dose and post-colonoscopy laboratory tests (electrolytes, creatinine, and BUN) in these patients.

5.5 (Colonic) Mucosal Ulceration, Ischemic Colitis and Ulcerative Colitis

Osmotic laxatives may produce colonic mucosal aphthous ulcerations and there have been reports of more serious cases of ischemic colitis requiring hospitalization. Concurrent use of stimulant laxatives and MoviPrep may increase the risk and is not recommended. The potential for mucosal ulcerations resulting from the bowel preparation should be considered when interpreting colonoscopy findings in patients with known or suspected inflammatory bowel disease.

5.6 Use in Patients with Significant Gastrointestinal Disease

If gastrointestinal obstruction or perforation is suspected, perform appropriate diagnostic studies to rule out these conditions before administering MoviPrep. If a patient experiences severe bloating, abdominal distension, or abdominal pain, administration should be slowed or temporarily discontinued until symptoms abate.
Use with caution in patients with severe ulcerative colitis.

5.7 Aspiration

Patients with impaired gag reflex and patients prone to regurgitation or aspiration should be observed during the administration of MoviPrep. Use with caution in these patients.

5.8 Glucose-6-phosphate dehydrogenase (G-6-PD) deficiency

Since MoviPrep contains sodium ascorbate and ascorbic acid, MoviPrep should be used with caution in patients with glucose-6-phosphate dehydrogenase (G-6-PD) deficiency, especially G-6-PD deficiency patients with an active infection, with a history of hemolysis, or taking concomitant medications known to precipitate hemolytic reactions.

5.9 Contains Phenylalanine

Phenylketonurics: Contains aspartame 233 mg per treatment which corresponds to 131 mg of phenylalanine per treatment (after hydrolysis of the aspartame molecule in-vivo to aspartic acid and phenylalanine).

6 ADVERSE REACTIONS

6.1 Clinical Studies Experience

Because clinical trials are conducted under widely varying conditions, adverse reaction rates observed in the clinical trials of a drug cannot be directly compared to rates in the clinical trials of another drug and may not reflect the rates observed in clinical practice.
In the MoviPrep trials, abdominal distension, anal discomfort, thirst, nausea, and abdominal pain were some of the most common adverse reactions to MoviPrep administration. Since diarrhea was considered as a part of the efficacy of MoviPrep, diarrhea was not defined as an adverse reaction in the clinical studies. Tables 1 and 2 display the most common drug-related adverse reactions of MoviPrep and its comparator in the controlled MoviPrep trials.

Table 1: The Most Common Drug-Related Adverse Reactions[1] (≥ 2%) in the Study of MoviPrep vs. 4 Liter Polyethylene Glycol plus Electrolytes Solution

	MoviPrep® (split dose) N=180	4L PEG + E[2] N=179
	n (% = n/N)	n (% = n/N)
Malaise	35 (19.4)	32 (17.9)
Nausea	26 (14.4)	36 (20.1)
Abdominal pain	24 (13.3)	27 (15.1)
Vomiting	14 (7.8)	23 (12.8)
Upper abdominal pain	10 (5.6)	11 (6.1)
Dyspepsia	5 (2.8)	2 (1.1)

[1] Drug-related adverse reactions were adverse events that were possibly, probably, or definitely related to the study drug.
[2] 4L PEG + E is 4 liter Polyethylene Glycol plus Electrolytes Solution

Table 2: The Most Common Drug-Related Adverse Reactions[1] (≥ 5%) in the Study of MoviPrep vs. 90 mL Oral Sodium Phosphate Solution

	MoviPrep® (evening-only) (full dose) N=169	90 mL OSPS[2] N=171
	n (% = n/N)	n (% = n/N)
Abdominal distension	101 (59.8)	70 (40.9)
Anal discomfort	87 (51.5)	89 (52.0)
Thirst	80 (47.3)	112 (65.5)
Nausea	80 (47.3)	80 (46.8)
Abdominal pain	66 (39.1)	55 (32.2)
Sleep disorder	59 (34.9)	49 (28.7)
Rigors	57 (33.7)	51 (29.8)
Hunger	51 (30.2)	121 (70.8)
Malaise	45 (26.6)	90 (52.6)
Vomiting	12 (7.1)	14 (8.2)
Dizziness	11 (6.5)	31 (18.1)
Headache	3 (1.8)	9 (5.3)
Hypokalemia	0 (0)	10 (5.8)
Hyperphosphatemia	0 (0)	10 (5.8)

[1] Drug-related adverse reactions were adverse events that were possibly, probably, or definitely related to the study drug. In addition to the recording of spontaneous adverse events, patients were also specifically asked about the occurrence of the following symptoms: shivering, anal irritations, abdominal bloating or fullness, sleep loss, nausea, vomiting, weakness, hunger sensation, abdominal cramps or pain, thirst sensation, and dizziness.
[2] OSPS is Oral Sodium Phosphate Solution

Isolated cases of urticaria, rhinorrhea, dermatitis, and anaphylactic reaction have been reported with PEG-based products and may represent allergic reactions.
Published literature contains isolated reports of serious adverse events following the administration of PEG-based products in patients over 60 years of age. These adverse events included upper gastrointestinal bleeding from a Mallory-Weiss tear, esophageal perforation, asystole, and acute pulmonary edema after aspirating PEG-based preparation.

6.2 Postmarketing Experience

In addition to adverse reactions reported from clinical trials, the following adverse events have been identified during post-approval use of MoviPrep. Because they are reported voluntarily from a population of uncertain size, it is not always possible to reliably estimate their frequency or establish a causal relationship to drug exposure. These events have been chosen for inclusion due to either their seriousness, frequency of reporting or causal connection to MoviPrep, or a combination of these factors.
Cardiovascular: Tachycardia, palpitations, hypertension, arrhythmia, atrial fibrillation, peripheral edema.
General: Hypersensitivity reactions including anaphylaxis (some of which were severe, including shock), rash, urticaria, pruritus, lip, tongue and facial swelling, dyspnea, chest tightness and throat tightness. Fever, chills and dehydration.
Nervous system: Syncope, tremor, seizure.
Renal: Renal impairment and/or failure.

7 DRUG INTERACTIONS

7.1 Drugs That May Increase Risks Due to Fluid and Electrolyte Abnormalities

Use caution when prescribing MoviPrep for patients with conditions, or who are using medications that increase the risk for fluid and electrolyte disturbances or may increase the risk of adverse events of seizure, arrhythmias, and prolonged QT in the setting of fluid and electrolyte abnormalities. Consider additional patient evaluations as appropriate. *[See WARNINGS (5)]*

7.2 Potential for Altered Drug Absorption

Oral medication administered within 1 hour of the start of administration of MoviPrep may be flushed from the gastrointestinal tract and the medication may not be absorbed.

8 USE IN SPECIFIC POPULATIONS

8.1 Pregnancy

Pregnancy Category C. Animal reproduction studies have not been performed with MoviPrep. It is also not known if

MoviPrep can cause fetal harm when administered to a pregnant woman or can affect reproductive capacity. MoviPrep should be given to a pregnant woman only if clearly needed.

8.3 Nursing Mothers

It is not known whether this drug is excreted in human milk. Because many drugs are excreted in human milk, caution should be exercised when MoviPrep is administered to a nursing woman.

8.4 Pediatric Use

The safety and effectiveness of MoviPrep in pediatric patients has not been established.

8.5 Geriatric Use

Of the 413 patients in clinical studies receiving MoviPrep, 91 (22%) patients were aged 65 or older, while 25 (6%) patients were over 75 years of age. No overall differences in safety or effectiveness were observed between geriatric patients and younger patients, and other reported clinical experience has not identified differences in responses between geriatric patients and younger patients, but greater sensitivity of some older individuals cannot be ruled out.

10 OVERDOSAGE

There have been no reported cases of overdose with MoviPrep. Purposeful or gross accidental ingestion of more than the recommended dose of MoviPrep might be expected to lead to severe electrolyte disturbances, including hyponatremia and/or hypokalemia, as well as dehydration and hypovolemia, with signs and symptoms of these disturbances. The patient who has taken an overdose should be monitored carefully, and treated symptomatically for complications.

11 DESCRIPTION

MoviPrep (PEG-3350, sodium sulfate, sodium chloride, potassium chloride, sodium ascorbate, and ascorbic acid for oral solution) is an osmotic laxative consisting of 4 separate pouches (2 of pouch A and 2 of pouch B) containing white to yellow powder for reconstitution. Each pouch A contains 100 grams of polyethylene glycol (PEG) 3350, NF, 7.5 grams of sodium sulfate, USP, 2.691 grams of sodium chloride, USP, and 1.015 grams of potassium chloride, USP, plus the following excipients: aspartame, NF (sweetener), acesulfame potassium, NF (sweetener), and lemon flavoring. Each pouch B contains 4.7 grams of ascorbic acid, USP and 5.9 grams of sodium ascorbate, USP. When 1 pouch A and 1 pouch B are dissolved together in water to a volume of 1 liter, MoviPrep (PEG-3350, sodium sulfate, sodium chloride, potassium chloride, sodium ascorbate, and ascorbic acid) is an oral solution having a lemon taste.

The entire, reconstituted, 2-liter MoviPrep colon preparation contains 200 grams of PEG-3350, 15 grams of sodium sulfate, 5.38 grams of sodium chloride, 2.03 grams of potassium chloride, 9.4 grams of ascorbic acid, and 11.8 grams of sodium ascorbate plus the following excipients: aspartame (sweetener), acesulfame potassium (sweetener), and lemon flavoring.

A container for reconstitution is enclosed.

12 CLINICAL PHARMACOLOGY

12.1 Mechanism of Action

The primary mode of action is thought to be through the osmotic effect of polyethylene glycol 3350, sodium sulfate, sodium chloride, potassium chloride, sodium ascorbate, and ascorbic acid, which causes water to be retained in the colon and produces a watery stool.

12.3 Pharmacokinetics

The pharmacokinetics of MoviPrep have not been studied in patients with renal or hepatic insufficiency.

13 NONCLINICAL TOXICOLOGY

13.1 Carcinogenesis, Mutagenesis, Impairment of Fertility

Long-term studies in animals to evaluate the carcinogenic potential have not been performed with MoviPrep. Studies to evaluate potential for impairment of fertility or mutagenic potential have not been performed with MoviPrep

14 CLINICAL STUDIES

The colon cleansing efficacy and safety of MoviPrep was evaluated in two randomized, actively-controlled, multicenter, investigator-blinded, phase 3 trials in patients scheduled to have an elective colonoscopy.

In the first study, patients were randomized to one of the following two colon preparation treatments: 1) 2 liters of MoviPrep with 1 additional liter of clear liquid split into two doses (during the evening before and the morning of the colonoscopy) and 2) 4 liters of polyethylene glycol plus electrolytes solution (4L PEG + E) split into two doses (during the evening before and the morning of the colonoscopy). Patients were allowed to have a morning breakfast, a light lunch, clear soup and/or plain yogurt for dinner. Dinner had to be completed at least one hour prior to initiation of the colon preparation administration.

The primary efficacy endpoint was the proportion of patients with effective colon cleansing as judged by blinded gastroenterologists on the basis of videotapes recorded during the colonoscopy.

The blinded gastroenterologists graded the colon cleansing twice (during introduction and withdrawal of the colonoscope) and the poorer of the two assessments was used in the primary efficacy analysis.

The efficacy analysis included 308 adult patients who had an elective colonoscopy. Patients ranged in age from 18 to 88 years old (mean age about 59 years old) with 52% female and 48% male patients. Table 3 displays the results.

Table 3: Effectiveness of Overall Colon Cleansing in the Study of MoviPrep vs 4 Liter Polyethylene Glycol plus Electrolytes Solution

	Responders A[2] or B[3] (%)	C[4] (%)	D[5] (%)
MoviPrep® (N=153)	88.9	9.8	1.3
4L PEG + E[1] (N=155)	94.8	4.5	0.6

[1] 4L PEG + E is 4 Liter Polyethylene Glycol plus Electrolytes Solution

[2] A: colon empty and clean or presence of clear liquid, but easily removed by suction

[3] B: brown liquid or semisolid remaining amounts of stool, fully removable by suction or displaceable, thus allowing a complete visualization of the gut mucosa

[4] C: semisolid amounts of stool, only partially removable with a risk of incomplete visualization of the gut mucosa

[5] D: semisolid or solid amounts of stool; consequently colonoscopy incomplete or needed to be terminated.

4 L PEG+E's responder rate was not significantly higher than MoviPrep's responder rate.

In the second study, patients were randomized to one of the following two colon preparation treatments: 1) 2 liters of MoviPrep with 1 additional liter of clear liquid in the evening prior to the colonoscopy and 2) 90 mL of oral sodium phosphate solution (90 mL OSPS) with at least 2 liters of additional clear liquid during the day and evening prior to the colonoscopy. Patients randomized to MoviPrep therapy were allowed to have a morning breakfast; a light lunch; and clear soup and/or plain yogurt for dinner. Dinner had to be completed at least one hour prior to initiation of the colon preparation administration.

The primary efficacy endpoint was the proportion of patients with effective colon cleansing as judged by the colonoscopist and one blinded gastroenterologist (on the basis of videotapes recorded during the colonoscopy). In case of a discrepancy between the colonoscopist and the blinded gastroenterologist, a second blinded gastroenterologist made the final efficacy determination.

The efficacy analysis included 280 adult patients who had an elective colonoscopy. Patients ranged in age from 21 to 76 years old (mean age about 53 years old) with 47% female and 53% male patients. Table 4 displays the results.

Table 4: Effectiveness of Overall Colon Cleansing in the Study of MoviPrep vs 90mL Oral Sodium Phosphate Solution

	Responders A[2] or B[3] (%)	C[4] (%)	D[5] (%)
MoviPrep® (N=137)	73.0	23.4	3.6
90 mL OSPS[1] (N=143)	64.4	29.4	6.3

[1] OSPS is Oral Sodium Phosphate Solution

[2] A: empty and clean or clear liquid (transparent, yellow, or green)

[3] B: brown liquid or semisolid remaining small amounts of stool, fully removable by suction or displaceable allowing a complete visualization of the underlying mucosa

[4] C: semi solid only partially removable/displaceable stools; risk of incomplete examination of the underlying mucosa

[5] D: heavy and hard stool making the segment examination uninterpretable and, consequently, the colonoscopy needed to be terminated

MoviPrep's responder rate was not significantly higher than OSPS's responder rate.

16 HOW SUPPLIED/STORAGE AND HANDLING

MoviPrep is supplied as a white to yellow powder. MoviPrep is administered as an oral solution after reconstitution.

NDC 65649-201-75, MoviPrep, single use carton.

NDC 65649-201-76, MoviPrep, professional sample carton.

Each carton contains a disposable container for reconstitution of MoviPrep and 4 pouches (2 of pouch A and 2 of pouch B).

STORAGE

Store carton/container at 25°C (77°F); excursions permitted to 15-30°C (59-86°F). When reconstituted, store upright and keep solution refrigerated. Use within 24 hours.

17 PATIENT COUNSELING INFORMATION

- Advise patients who require a diet low in phenylalanine that MoviPrep contains aspartame – a maximum of 233 mg per treatment. This sweetener, after hydrolysis in the body, provides 131 mg of phenylalanine to the patient.
- Ask patients to inform you if they have trouble swallowing or are prone to regurgitation or aspiration.
- Instruct patients that each pouch needs to be diluted in water before ingestion and that they need to drink additional clear liquid (e.g., water, clear soup, fruit juice without pulp, soft drinks, tea and/or coffee without milk) according to instructions.
- Inform patients that oral medications may not be absorbed properly if they are taken within one hour of starting each dose of MoviPrep.
- Tell patients not to take other laxatives while they are taking MoviPrep.
- Tell patients that MoviPrep produces a watery stool (diarrhea) which cleanses the colon before colonoscopy. Advise patients receiving MoviPrep to adequately hydrate before, during, and after the use of MoviPrep. Patients may have clear soup and/or plain yogurt for dinner, finishing the evening meal at least one hour prior to the start of MoviPrep treatment. No solid food should be taken from the start of MoviPrep treatment until after the colonoscopy.
- Tell patients that the first bowel movement may occur approximately 1 hour after the start of MoviPrep administration. Abdominal bloating and distention may occur before the first bowel movement. If severe abdominal discomfort or distention occurs, stop drinking MoviPrep temporarily or drink each portion at longer intervals until these symptoms diminish. If severe symptoms persist, notify your health provider.

Manufactured by:
Novel Laboratories, Inc.
Somerset, NJ 08873

For:
Salix Pharmaceuticals, Inc.
Raleigh, NC 27615

Rev AUG 2013

Product protected by U.S. Patent Nos. 7,169,381 and 7,658,914.

Please see www.salix.com for patent information.

Medication Guide

MoviPrep® (moo-vee-prp)

(polyethylene glycol (PEG) 3350, sodium sulfate, sodium chloride, potassium chloride, sodium ascorbate, and ascorbic acid for oral solution)

Read this Medication Guide before you start taking MoviPrep and each time you get a new prescription. There may be new information. This Medication Guide does not take the place of talking with your healthcare provider about your medical condition or your treatment.

What is the most important information I should know about MoviPrep?

MoviPrep can cause serious side effects, including:

Serious loss of body fluid (dehydration) and changes in blood salts (electrolytes) in your blood.

These changes can cause:

- **abnormal heartbeats that can cause death**
- **seizures.** This can happen even if you have never had a seizure.
- **kidney problems**

Your chance of having fluid loss and changes in body salts with MoviPrep is higher if you:

- have heart problems
- have kidney problems
- take water pills (diuretics), high blood pressure medication, or non-steroidal anti-inflammatory drugs (NSAIDS)

Tell your healthcare provider right away if you have any of these symptoms of a loss of too much body fluid (dehydration) while taking MoviPrep:

- vomiting
- dizziness
- urinating less often than normal
- headache

See "What are the possible side effects of MoviPrep?" for more information about side effects.

What is MoviPrep?

MoviPrep is a prescription medicine used by adults 18 years and older to clean the colon before a colonoscopy. MoviPrep cleans your colon by causing you to have diarrhea. Cleaning your colon helps your healthcare provider see the inside of your colon more clearly during your colonoscopy.

It is not known if MoviPrep is safe and effective in children.

Who should not take MoviPrep?
Do not take MoviPrep if your healthcare provider has told you that you have:
- a blockage in your bowel (obstruction)
- an opening in the wall of your stomach or intestine (bowel perforation)
- problems with food and fluid emptying from your stomach (gastric retention)
- a very dilated intestine (bowel)
- an allergy to any of the ingredients in MoviPrep. See the end of this leaflet for a complete list of ingredients in MoviPrep.

What should I tell my healthcare provider before taking MoviPrep?
Before you take MoviPrep, tell your healthcare provider if you:
- have heart problems
- have a history of seizures
- have kidney problems
- have stomach or bowel problems, including ulcerative colitis
- have problems with swallowing or gastric reflux
- have a condition that destroys red blood cells called Glucose-6-phosphate dehydrogenase (G6PD) deficiency
- are withdrawing from drinking alcohol
- have a low blood salt (sodium) level (hyponatremia)
- are on a diet low in phenylalanine
- have any other medical conditions
- are pregnant. It is not known if MoviPrep will harm your unborn baby. Talk to your healthcare provider if you are pregnant or plan to become pregnant.
- are breastfeeding or plan to breast-feed. It is not known if MoviPrep passes into your breast milk. You and your healthcare provider should decide if you will take MoviPrep while breastfeeding.

Tell your healthcare provider about all the medicines you take, including prescription and non-prescription medicines, vitamins, and herbal supplements.
MoviPrep may affect how other medicines work. Medicines taken by mouth may not be absorbed properly when taken within 1 hour before the start of MoviPrep.
Especially tell your healthcare provider if you take:
- medicines for blood pressure or heart problems
- medicines for kidney problems
- medicines for seizures
- water pills (diuretics)
- non-steroidal anti-inflammatory medicines (NSAID); pain medicines
- laxatives

Ask your healthcare provider or pharmacist for a list of these medicines if you are not sure if you are taking any of the medicines listed above.
Know the medicines you take. Keep a list of them to show your healthcare provider and pharmacist when you get a new medicine.

How should I take MoviPrep?
See the Patient Instructions on the outer product carton for dosing instructions. You must read, understand, and follow these instructions to take MoviPrep the right way.
- Take MoviPrep exactly as your healthcare provider tells you to take it.
- It is important for you to drink the additional prescribed amount of clear liquid (e.g. water, clear soup, fruit juice without pulp, soft drinks, tea and/or coffee without milk) listed in the Patient Instructions to prevent fluid loss (dehydration).
- Do not take MoviPrep that has not been mixed with water (diluted).
- Do not take other laxatives while taking MoviPrep.
- Do not eat solid foods while taking MoviPrep. Only clear liquids are allowed while taking and after taking MoviPrep until your colonoscopy.
- Stop drinking MoviPrep solution temporarily or allow for longer time between each dose if you have stomach discomfort, pain or bloating until your symptoms improve. If symptoms continue, tell your healthcare provider.
- If you take too much MoviPrep, call your healthcare provider or get medical help right away.

What are the possible side effects of MoviPrep?
MoviPrep can cause serious side effects, including:
- **See Section "What is the most important information I should know about MoviPrep?"**
- **Changes in certain blood tests.** Your healthcare provider may do blood tests after you take MoviPrep to check your blood for changes. Tell your healthcare provider if you have any symptoms of too much fluid loss, including:
  - vomiting
  - nausea
- **Heart problems (arrhythmias). MoviPrep may cause irregular heartbeats.**
- **Seizures or fainting (black-outs)**
- **Ulcers of the bowel or bowel problems**

The most common side effects of MoviPrep for split dosing include:
- malaise
- nausea
- stomach (abdominal) pain
- vomiting, bloating

The most common side effects of MoviPrep for evening-only full dosing include:
- stomach swelling (abdominal distention)
- anal discomfort
- thirst
- nausea
- stomach (abdominal) pain
- sleep disorder
- rigors
- hunger
- malaise
- vomiting
- dizziness

Tell your healthcare provider if you have any side effect that bothers you or that does not go away.
These are not all the possible side effects of MoviPrep. For more information, ask your healthcare provider or pharmacist. Call your healthcare provider for medical advice about side effects. You may report side effects to FDA at 1-800-FDA-1088.

How should I store MoviPrep?
- Store MoviPrep between 59°F to 86°F (15°C to 30°C).
- MoviPrep solution that has been mixed with water may be refrigerated. Mixed solution should be taken within 24 hours.

Keep MoviPrep and all medicines out of the reach of children.

General information about the safe and effective use of MoviPrep.
Medicines are sometimes prescribed for purposes other than those listed in a Medication Guide. Do not use MoviPrep for a condition for which it was not prescribed. Do not give MoviPrep to other people, even if they are going to have the same procedure you are. It may harm them.
This Medication Guide summarizes the most important information about MoviPrep. If you would like more information, talk with your healthcare provider or pharmacist. You can ask your pharmacist or healthcare provider for information that is written for healthcare professionals.
For more information, call 1-866-669-7597 or go to www.MoviPrep.com.

What are the ingredients in MoviPrep?
Active ingredients:
Pouch A: polyethylene glycol (PEG) 3350, sodium sulfate, sodium chloride, potassium chloride.
Pouch B: ascorbic acid and sodium ascorbate.
Inactive ingredients:
Pouch A: aspartame, acesulfame potassium, and lemon flavor.
This Medication Guide has been approved by the U.S. Food and Drug Administration.
Revised October 2012
Salix Pharmaceuticals, Inc.
Raleigh, NC 27615
OCT 2012

Shown in Product Identification Guide, page 312

RELISTOR® ℞
(methylnaltrexone bromide)
Subcutaneous Injection

HIGHLIGHTS OF PRESCRIBING INFORMATION
These highlights do not include all the information needed to use RELISTOR safely and effectively. See full prescribing information for RELISTOR.
RELISTOR (methylnaltrexone bromide) Subcutaneous Injection
Initial U.S. Approval: 2008

RECENT MAJOR CHANGES

General Dosing Information *(2.1)*	[08/2013]
Dosing *(2.2)*	[08/2013]
Use in Patients with Severe Renal Impairment *(2.3)*	[08/2013]
Administration and Storage *(2.4)*	[08/2013]
Gastrointestinal Perforation *(5.1)*	[08/2013]
Severe or Persistent Diarrhea *(5.2)*	[08/2013]

INDICATIONS AND USAGE
RELISTOR is indicated for the treatment of opioid-induced constipation in patients with advanced illness who are receiving palliative care, when response to laxative therapy has not been sufficient. Use of RELISTOR beyond four months has not been studied. *(1)*

DOSAGE AND ADMINISTRATION
RELISTOR is administered as a subcutaneous injection. The usual schedule is one dose every other day, as needed, but no more frequently than one dose in a 24-hour period. *(2.2)*
The recommended dose of RELISTOR is 8 mg for patients weighing 38 to less than 62 kg or 12 mg for patients weighing 62 to 114 kg. Patients whose weights fall outside of these ranges should be dosed at 0.15 mg/kg. See the table below to determine the correct injection volume. *(2.2)*

Patient Weight	Injection Volume	Dose
Less than 38 kg	**See below***	0.15 mg/kg
38 kg to less than 62 kg	**0.4 mL**	8 mg
62 kg to 114 kg	**0.6 mL**	12 mg
More than 114 kg	**See below***	0.15 mg/kg

* The injection volume for these patients should be calculated using one of the following *(2.2)*:
- Multiply the patient weight in kilograms by 0.0075 and round up the volume to the nearest 0.1 mL.

Only patients requiring an 8 mg or 12 mg dose should be prescribed pre-filled syringes *(2.2, 3)*.
In patients with severe renal impairment (creatinine clearance less than 30 mL/min), dose reductions of RELISTOR by one half is recommended. *(8.6)*

DOSAGE FORMS AND STRENGTHS
RELISTOR is available in the following dosage forms:
- Single-use vial containing 12 mg/0.6 mL solution for subcutaneous injection, for use with a 27 gauge × ½-inch needle and 1 mL syringe
- Single-use vial containing 12 mg/0.6 mL solution for subcutaneous injection with one 1 mL syringe with retractable 27 gauge × ½-inch needle, two alcohol swabs.
- Single-use pre-filled syringe containing 8 mg/0.4 mL solution for subcutaneous injection.
- Single-use pre-filled syringe containing 12 mg/0.6 mL solution for subcutaneous injection.

CONTRAINDICATIONS
- RELISTOR is contraindicated in patients with known or suspected mechanical gastrointestinal obstruction. *(4)*

WARNINGS AND PRECAUTIONS
- Rare cases of gastrointestinal (GI) perforation have been reported in advanced illness patients. Use RELISTOR with caution in patients with known or suspected lesions of the GI tract. *(5.1)*
- If severe or persistent diarrhea occurs during treatment, advise patients to discontinue therapy with RELISTOR and consult their physician. *(5.2)*

ADVERSE REACTIONS
The most common (≥ 5%) adverse reactions reported with RELISTOR are abdominal pain, flatulence, nausea, dizziness, diarrhea and hyperhidrosis. *(6.1)*
To report SUSPECTED ADVERSE REACTIONS, contact Salix Pharmaceuticals Inc. at 1-800-508-0024 or FDA at 1-800-FDA-1088 or www.fda.gov/medwatch

DRUG INTERACTIONS
In an *in vivo* study Relistor did not significantly affect the metabolism of the CYP2D6 substrate, dextromethorphan. In vitro methylnaltrexone did not significantly inhibit or induce cytochrome P450 (CYP) isozymes including CYP 1A2, 2A6, 2B6, 2C9, 2C19, or 3A4 *(7.1)*

USE IN SPECIFIC POPULATIONS
Pediatric Use: Safety and efficacy of RELISTOR have not been established in pediatric patients. *(8.4)*
See 17 for PATIENT COUNSELING INFORMATION and FDA-approved patient labeling

Revised: 08/2013

FULL PRESCRIBING INFORMATION: CONTENTS*

*** Sections or subsections omitted from the full prescribing information are not listed**

FULL PRESCRIBING INFORMATION

1 INDICATIONS AND USAGE

RELISTOR® is indicated for the treatment of opioid-induced constipation in patients with advanced illness who are receiving palliative care, when response to laxative therapy has not been sufficient.

Limitation of use: Use of RELISTOR beyond four months has not been studied in the advanced illness population.

2 DOSAGE AND ADMINISTRATION

2.1 General Dosing Information

RELISTOR is for subcutaneous use only.

2.2 Dosing

For adult patients with opioid-induced constipation and advanced illness, the usual schedule is one dose every other day, as needed, but no more frequently than one dose in a 24-hour period [*see Clinical Studies (14)*].

The recommended dose of RELISTOR is 8 mg subcutaneously for opioid-induced constipation and advanced illness adult patients weighing 38 kg to less than 62 kg or 12 mg subcutaneously for patients weighing 62 kg to 114 kg. Adult patients whose weight falls outside of these ranges should be dosed at 0.15 mg/kg. See Table 1 to determine the correct injection volume. The prefilled syringe is designed to deliver a fixed dose; therefore, adult patients requiring dosing calculated on a mg/kg basis should not be prescribed pre-filled syringes.

Table 1: Weight of Adult Patient with Opioid-Induced Constipation and Advanced Illness	Injection Volume	Subcutaneous Dose
Less than 38 kg	**See below***	0.15 mg/kg
38 kg to less than 62 kg	**0.4 mL**	8 mg
62 kg to 114 kg	**0.6 mL**	12 mg
More than 114 kg	**See below***	0.15 mg/kg

* The injection volume for these patients should be calculated using the following method:
Multiply the patient weight in kilograms by 0.0075 and round up the volume to the nearest 0.1 mL.

2.3 Use in Patients with Severe Renal Impairment

In adult patients with severe renal impairment (creatinine clearance less than 30 mL/min as estimated by Cockcroft-Gault), dose reduction of RELISTOR by one-half is recommended [*see Use in Specific Populations (8.6)*]. No dosage adjustment is recommended for adult patients with mild to moderate renal impairment.

The pre-filled syringe is designed to deliver a fixed dose; therefore, adult patients with severe renal impairment should only be prescribed single-use vials to ensure correct dosing.

2.4 Administration and Storage

RELISTOR is a sterile, clear, and colorless to pale yellow aqueous solution. Inspect parenteral drug product visually for particulate matter and discoloration prior to administration, whenever solution and container permit. Do not use the vial if any of these are present.

Inject RELISTOR subcutaneously in the upper arm, abdomen or thigh. Do not inject at the same spot each time (rotate injection sites).

Single-use Vials

Once drawn into the 1 mL syringe with a 27-gauge × ½-inch needle, if immediate administration is not possible, store at ambient room temperature and administer within 24 hours. Discard any unused portion that remains in the vial. Advise patients concerning proper training in subcutaneous technique.

Single-use Pre-filled Syringes

Only adult patients requiring an 8 mg or 12 mg dose should be prescribed pre-filled syringes. Do not remove the pre-filled syringe from the tray until ready to administer.

3 DOSAGE FORMS AND STRENGTHS

- Single-use vial containing 12 mg/0.6 mL solution for subcutaneous injection, for use with a 27 gauge × ½-inch needle and 1 mL syringe
- Single-use vial containing 12 mg/0.6 mL solution for subcutaneous injection, with one 1 mL syringe with retractable 27 gauge × ½-inch needle, two alcohol swabs
- Single-use pre-filled syringe containing 8 mg/0.4 mL solution for subcutaneous injection, with a 29-gauge × ½-inch fixed needle and a needle guard
- Single-use pre-filled syringe containing 12 mg/0.6 mL solution for subcutaneous injection, with a 29-gauge × ½-inch fixed needle and a needle guard

4 CONTRAINDICATIONS

RELISTOR is contraindicated in patients with known or suspected mechanical gastrointestinal obstruction.

5 WARNINGS AND PRECAUTIONS

5.1 Gastrointestinal Perforation

Cases of gastrointestinal (GI) perforation have been reported in adult patients with opioid-induced constipation and advanced illness with conditions that may be associated with localized or diffuse reduction of structural integrity in the wall of the GI tract (i.e., cancer, peptic ulcer, Ogilvie's syndrome). Perforations have involved varying regions of the GI tract (e.g., stomach, duodenum, or colon).

Use RELISTOR with caution in patients with known or suspected lesions of the GI tract. Advise patients to discontinue therapy with RELISTOR and promptly notify their physician if they develop severe, persistent, or worsening abdominal symptoms.

5.2 Severe or Persistent Diarrhea

If severe or persistent diarrhea occurs during treatment, advise patients to discontinue therapy with RELISTOR and consult their physician.

6 ADVERSE REACTIONS

6.1 Clinical Trial Experience

Because clinical trials are conducted under widely varying conditions, adverse reaction rates observed in the clinical trials of a drug cannot be directly compared to rates in the clinical trials of another drug and may not reflect the rates observed in clinical practice.

The safety of RELISTOR was evaluated in two, double-blind, placebo-controlled trials in patients with advanced illness receiving palliative care: Study 1 included a single-dose, double-blind, placebo-controlled period, whereas Study 2 included a 14-day multiple dose, double-blind, placebo-controlled period [see *Clinical Studies (14)*]. The majority of patients had a primary diagnosis of incurable cancer; other primary diagnoses included end-stage COPD/emphysema, cardiovascular disease/heart failure, Alzheimer's disease/dementia, HIV/AIDS, or other advanced illnesses. Patients were receiving opioid therapy (median daily baseline oral morphine equivalent dose = 172 mg), and had opioid-induced constipation (either <3 bowel movements in the preceding week or no bowel movement for 2 days). Both the methylnaltrexone bromide and placebo patients were on a stable laxative regimen for at least 3 days prior to study entry and continued on their regimen throughout the study.

The most common (≥5%) adverse reactions in patients receiving RELISTOR are shown in Table 2 below.

Table 2: Adverse Reactions from all Doses in Double-Blind, Placebo-Controlled Clinical Studies of RELISTOR in Adult Patients with Opioid-Induced Constipation and Advanced Illness*

Adverse Reaction	RELISTOR N = 165	Placebo N = 123
Abdominal Pain	47 (28.5%)	12 (9.8%)
Flatulence	22 (13.3%)	7 (5.7%)
Nausea	19 (11.5%)	6 (4.9%)
Dizziness	12 (7.3%)	3 (2.4%)
Diarrhea	9 (5.5%)	3 (2.4%)
Hyperhidrosis	11 (6.7%)	8 (6.5%)

* Doses: 0.075, 0.15, and 0.30 mg/kg/dose

The rates of discontinuation due to adverse events during the double-blind placebo controlled clinical trials (Study 1 and Study 2) were comparable between RELISTOR (1.2%) and placebo (2.4%).

6.2 Postmarketing Experience

The following additional adverse reactions have been identified during post-approval use of RELISTOR. Because they are reported voluntarily from a population of unknown size, estimates of frequency cannot be made. These events have been chosen for inclusion due to either their seriousness, frequency of reporting or causal connection to RELISTOR, or a combination of these factors.

Gastrointestinal

Perforation, cramping, vomiting

General Disorders and Administrative Site Disorders

Diaphoresis, flushing, malaise, pain. Cases of opioid withdrawal have been reported.

7 DRUG INTERACTIONS

7.1 Drugs Metabolized by Cytochrome P450 Isozymes

In healthy subjects, a subcutaneous dose of 0.30 mg/kg of methylnaltrexone did not significantly affect the metabolism of dextromethorphan, a CYP2D6 substrate.

In vitro methylnaltrexone did not significantly inhibit or induce the activity of cytochrome P450 (CYP) isozymes CYP1A2, CYP2A6, CYP2B6, CYP2C9, CYP2C19, or CYP3A4.

In vitro, methylnaltrexone did not induce the enzymatic activity of CYP2E1.

7.2 Drugs Renally Excreted

Methylnaltrexone is actively secreted in the kidney. The potential of drug interactions between methylnaltrexone bromide and other drugs that are inhibitors of transporters in the kidney has not been fully investigated [*see Pharmacokinetics (12.3)*].

7.3 Cimetidine

Cimetidine given 400 mg three times daily did not significantly affect the systemic exposure to methylnaltrexone. The effect of a higher cimetidine dose (e.g., 800 mg) on the systemic exposure of methylnaltrexone has not been evaluated.

8 USE IN SPECIFIC POPULATIONS

8.1 Pregnancy

Pregnancy Category B

Reproduction studies have been performed in pregnant rats at intravenous doses up to about 14 times the recommended maximum human subcutaneous dose of 0.3 mg/kg based on the body surface area and in pregnant rabbits at intravenous doses up to about 17 times the recommended maximum human subcutaneous dose based on the body surface area and have revealed no evidence of impaired fertility or harm to the fetus due to methylnaltrexone bromide. There are no adequate and well-controlled studies in pregnant women. Because animal reproduction studies are not always predictive of human response, methylnaltrexone bromide should be used during pregnancy only if clearly needed.

8.2 Labor and Delivery

Effects of RELISTOR on mother, fetus, duration of labor, and delivery are unknown. There were no effects on the mother, labor, delivery, or on offspring survival and growth in rats following subcutaneous injection of methylnaltrexone bromide at dosages up to 25 mg/kg/day.

8.3 Nursing Mothers

Results from an animal study using [^{3}H]-labeled methylnaltrexone bromide indicate that methylnaltrexone bromide is excreted via the milk of lactating rats. It is not known whether this drug is excreted in human milk. Because many drugs are excreted in human milk, caution should be exercised when RELISTOR is administered to a nursing woman.

8.4 Pediatric Use

Safety and effectiveness of RELISTOR have not been established in pediatric patients.

8.5 Geriatric Use

In the phase 2 and 3 double-blind studies, a total of 77 (24%) patients aged 65-74 years (54 methylnaltrexone bromide, 23 placebo) and a total of 100 (31.2%) patients aged 75 years or older (61 methylnaltrexone bromide, 39 placebo) were enrolled. Pharmacokinetics of methylnaltrexone was similar between the elderly (mean age 72 years old) and young adults (mean age 30 years old). No overall differences in safety or effectiveness were observed between these patients and younger patients, and other reported clinical experience has not identified differences in responses between the elderly and younger patients, but greater sensitivity of some older individuals cannot be ruled out.

Based on pharmacokinetic data, and safety and efficacy data from controlled clinical trials, no dose adjustment based on age is recommended.

8.6 Renal Impairment

No dose adjustment is required in patients with mild or moderate renal impairment. Dose-reduction by one half is recommended in patients with severe renal impairment (creatinine clearance less than 30 mL/min as estimated by Cockcroft-Gault).

In a study of volunteers with varying degrees of renal impairment receiving a single dose of 0.30 mg/kg methylnaltrexone bromide, renal impairment had a marked effect on the renal excretion of methylnaltrexone bromide. Severe renal impairment decreased the renal clearance of methylnaltrexone bromide by 8- to 9-fold and resulted in a 2-fold increase in total methylnaltrexone bromide exposure (AUC). C_{max} was not significantly changed. No studies were performed in patients with end-stage renal impairment requiring dialysis.

8.7 Hepatic Impairment

No dose adjustment is required for patients with mild or moderate hepatic impairment. The effect of severe hepatic impairment on the pharmacokinetics of methylnaltrexone has not been studied.

10 OVERDOSAGE

During clinical trials of RELISTOR administered subcutaneously, no cases of methylnaltrexone bromide overdose were reported. A study of healthy volunteers noted orthostatic hypotension associated with a dose of 0.64 mg/kg administered as an intravenous bolus.

Signs or symptoms of orthostatic hypotension should be monitored, and treatment should be initiated, as appropriate.

11 DESCRIPTION

RELISTOR (methylnaltrexone bromide) injection, a peripherally-acting mu-opioid receptor antagonist, is a sterile, clear and colorless to pale yellow aqueous solution. The chemical name for methylnaltrexone bromide is (*R*)-*N*-(cyclopropylmethyl) noroxymorphone methobromide. The molecular formula is $C_{21}H_{26}NO_4Br$, and the molecular weight is 436.36.

Each 3 mL vial contains 12 mg of methylnaltrexone bromide in 0.6 mL of water. The excipients are 3.9 mg sodium chloride USP, 0.24 mg edetate calcium disodium USP, and 0.18 mg glycine hydrochloride. During manufacture, the pH may have been adjusted with hydrochloric acid and/or sodium hydroxide.

Each 8 mg/0.4 mL pre-filled syringe (1 mL syringe) contains 8 mg of methylnaltrexone bromide in 0.4 mL of water. The excipients are 2.6 mg sodium chloride USP, 0.16 mg edetate calcium disodium USP, and 0.12 mg glycine hydrochloride.

Each 12 mg/0.6 mL pre-filled syringe (1 mL syringe) contains 12 mg of methylnaltrexone bromide in 0.6 mL of water. The excipients are 3.9 mg sodium chloride USP, 0.24 mg edetate calcium disodium USP, and 0.18 mg glycine hydrochloride.

The structural formula is:

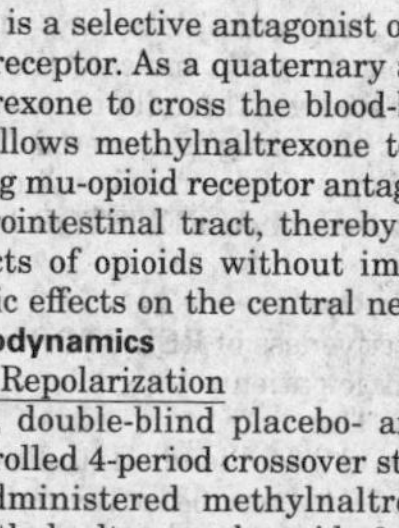

12 CLINICAL PHARMACOLOGY

12.1 Mechanism of Action

Methylnaltrexone is a selective antagonist of opioid binding at the mu-opioid receptor. As a quaternary amine, the ability of methylnaltrexone to cross the blood-brain barrier is restricted. This allows methylnaltrexone to function as a peripherally-acting mu-opioid receptor antagonist in tissues such as the gastrointestinal tract, thereby decreasing the constipating effects of opioids without impacting opioid-mediated analgesic effects on the central nervous system.

12.2 Pharmacodynamics

Effect on Cardiac Repolarization

In a randomized, double-blind placebo- and (open-label) moxifloxacin-controlled 4-period crossover study, 56 healthy subjects were administered methylnaltrexone bromide 0.3 mg/kg and methylnaltrexone bromide 0.64 mg/kg by intravenous infusion over 20 minutes, placebo, and a single oral dose of moxifloxacin. At both the 0.3 mg/kg and 0.64 mg/kg methylnaltrexone bromide doses, no significant effect on the QTc interval was detected.

12.3 Pharmacokinetics

Absorption

Following subcutaneous administration, methylnaltrexone achieved peak concentrations (C_{max}) at approximately 0.5 hours. Across the range of doses from 0.15 mg/kg to 0.50 mg/kg, mean C_{max} and area under the plasma concentration-time curve (AUC) increased in a dose-proportional manner. There was no accumulation of methylnaltrexone following once-daily subcutaneous dosing of methylnaltrexone bromide 12 mg for seven consecutive days in healthy subjects.

Table 3: Pharmacokinetic Parameters of Methylnaltrexone Following Subcutaneous Doses

Parameter	0.15 mg/kg single dose	12 mg single dose	12 mg at steady-state
C_{max} (ng/mL) [i]	117 (32.7)	140 (35.6)	119 (27.2)
t_{max} (hr) [ii]	0.5 (0.25-0.75)	0.25 (0.25-0.5)	0.25 (0.25-0.5)
AUC_{24} (ng•hr/mL) [i]	175 (36.6)	218 (28.3)	223 (28.2)

[i] Expressed as mean (SD).
[ii] Expressed as median (range).

Distribution

The steady-state volume of distribution (Vss) of methylnaltrexone is approximately 1.1 L/kg. The fraction of methylnaltrexone bound to human plasma proteins is 11.0% to 15.3%, as determined by equilibrium dialysis.

Metabolism

In a mass balance study, approximately 44% of the administered radioactivity was recovered in the urine over 24 hours with 5 distinct metabolites and none of the detected metabolites was in amounts over 6% of administered radioactivity. Conversion to methyl-6-naltrexol isomers (5% of total) and methylnaltrexone sulfate (1.3% of total) appear to be the primary pathways of metabolism. N-demethylation of methylnaltrexone to produce naltrexone is not significant.

After 12 mg once daily dosing the mean $AUC_{0\text{-}24}$ ratio of metabolites to methylnaltrexone at steady-state was 30%, 19%, and 9% for methylnaltrexone sulfate, methyl-6α-naltrexol, and methyl-6β-naltrexol, respectively. Methyl-6α-naltrexol, and methyl-6β-naltrexol were active mu-opioid receptor antagonists and methylnaltrexone sulfate is a weak mu-opioid receptor antagonist.

Methylnaltrexone is conjugated by sulfotransferase SULT1E1 and SULT2A1 isoforms to methylnaltrexone sulfate. Conversion to methyl-6-naltrexol isomers is mediated by aldo-keto reductase 1C enzymes.

Excretion

After intravenous administration, approximately half of the dose was excreted in the urine (53.6%) and 17.3% of administered dose was excreted in the feces up to 168 hours post-dose. Methylnaltrexone is excreted primarily as the unchanged drug in the urine and feces. The terminal half-life ($t_{1/2}$) is approximately 8 hours. Active renal secretion of methylnaltrexone is suggested by renal clearance of methylnaltrexone that is approximately 4-5 fold higher than creatinine clearance.

Specific Populations

Geriatric

A study was conducted to characterize the pharmacokinetics of methylnaltrexone after single dose of 24 mg methylnaltrexone via intravenous infusion over 20 min in healthy adults between 18 and 45 years of age and in healthy adults aged 65 years and older. In elderly subjects, mean clearance was about 20% lower (56 L/h versus 70 L/h) and AUC_{∞} was 26% higher than in subjects between 18 and 45 years of age.

Renal impairment

In a study of volunteers with varying degrees of renal impairment receiving a single dose of 0.30 mg/kg methylnaltrexone bromide, renal impairment had a marked effect on the renal excretion of methylnaltrexone. Severe renal impairment decreased the renal clearance of methylnaltrexone by 8- to 9-fold and resulted in a 2-fold increase in total methylnaltrexone exposure (AUC). Mean C_{max} was not significantly changed.

Hepatic impairment

The effect of mild and moderate hepatic impairment on the systemic exposure to methylnaltrexone has been studied in 8 subjects each, with Child-Pugh Class A and B, compared to healthy subjects. Results showed no meaningful effect of hepatic impairment on the AUC or C_{max} of methylnaltrexone.

Drug Interactions

In vitro studies suggested that methylnaltrexone was a substrate of Organic Cation Transporter 1 but not a substrate of Organic Anion Transporter 1 or of P-glycoprotein.

Cimetidine

A clinical drug interaction study in healthy adult subjects evaluated the effects of cimetidine, a drug that inhibits the active renal secretion of organic cations, on the pharmacokinetics of methylnaltrexone (24 mg administered as an IV infusion over 20 minutes). A single dose of methylnaltrexone was administered before cimetidine dosing and with the last dose of cimetidine (400 mg every 8 hours for 6 days). Mean C_{max} and AUC of methylnaltrexone increased by 10% with concomitant cimetidine administration. The renal clearance of methylnaltrexone decreased about 40%.

13 NONCLINICAL TOXICOLOGY

13.1 Carcinogenesis, Mutagenesis, Impairment of Fertility

Carcinogenesis

Two-year oral carcinogenicity studies have been conducted with methylnaltrexone in CD-1 mice at doses up to 200 mg/kg/day (about 108 times the recommended human dose of 0.15 mg/kg based on body surface area) in males and 400 mg/kg/day (about 216 times the recommended human dose of 0.15 mg/kg based on body surface area) in females and in Sprague Dawley rats at oral doses up to 300 mg/kg/day (about 324 times the recommended human dose of 0.15 mg/kg based on body surface area). Oral administration of methylnaltrexone for 104 weeks did not produce tumors in mice and rats.

Mutagenesis

Methylnaltrexone bromide was negative in the Ames test, chromosome aberration tests in Chinese hamster ovary cells and human lymphocytes, in the mouse lymphoma cell forward mutation tests and in the *in vivo* mouse micronucleus test.

Impairment of Fertility

Methylnaltrexone bromide at subcutaneous doses up to 150 mg/kg/day (about 81 times the recommended maximum human subcutaneous dose based on the body surface area) was found to have no adverse effect on fertility and reproductive performance of male and female rats.

13.2 Animal Toxicology and/or Pharmacology

In an *in vitro* human cardiac potassium ion channel (hERG) assay, methylnaltrexone bromide caused concentration-dependent inhibition of hERG current (1%, 12%, 13% and 40% inhibition at 30, 100, 300 and 1000 µM concentrations, respectively). Methylnaltrexone bromide had a hERG IC_{50} of > 1000 µM. In isolated dog Purkinje fibers, methylnaltrexone bromide caused prolongations in action potential duration (APD). The highest tested concentration (10 µM) in the dog Purkinje fiber study was about 18 and 37 times the C_{max} at human subcutaneous (SC) doses of 0.3 and 0.15 mg/kg, respectively. In isolated rabbit Purkinje fibers, methylnaltrexone bromide (up to 100 µM) did not have an effect on APD, compared to vehicle control. The highest methylnaltrexone bromide concentration (100 µM) tested was about 186 and 373 times the human C_{max} at SC doses of 0.3 and 0.15 mg/kg, respectively. In anesthetized dogs, methylnaltrexone bromide caused decreases in blood pressure, heart rate, cardiac output, left ventricular pressure, left ventricular end diastolic pressure, and +dP/dt at ≥ 1 mg/kg. In conscious dogs, methylnaltrexone bromide caused a dose-related increase in QTc interval. After a single intravenous dosage of 20 mg/kg to beagle dogs, predicted C_{max} and AUC values were approximately 482 and 144 times, respectively, the exposure at human SC dose of 0.15 mg/kg and 241 times and 66 times, respectively, the exposure at a human SC dose of 0.3 mg/kg. In conscious guinea pigs, methylnaltrexone caused mild prolongation of QTc (4% over baseline) at 20 mg/kg, intravenous. A thorough QTc assessment was conducted in humans [*see Clinical Pharmacology (12.2)*].

In juvenile rats administered intravenous methylnaltrexone bromide for 13 weeks, adverse clinical signs such as convulsions, tremors and labored breathing occurred at dosages of 3 and 10 mg/kg/day (about 3.2 and 11 times, respectively, the recommended human dose of 0.15 mg/kg based on the body surface area). Similar adverse clinical signs were seen in adult rats at 20 mg/kg/day (about 22 times the recommended human dose of 0.15 mg/kg based on the body surface area). Juvenile rats were found to be more sensitive to the toxicity of methylnaltrexone bromide when compared to adults. The no observed adverse effect levels (NOAELs) in juvenile and adult rats were 1 and 5 mg/kg/day, respectively (about 1.1 and 5.4 times respectively, the recommended human dose of 0.15 mg/kg based on the body surface area).

In juvenile dogs administered intravenous methylnaltrexone bromide for 13 weeks, juvenile dogs had a toxicity profile similar to adult dogs. Following intravenous administration of methylnaltrexone bromide for 13 weeks, decreased heart rate (13.2% reduction compared to pre-dose) in juvenile dogs and prolonged QTc interval in juvenile (9.6% compared to control) and adult (up to 15% compared to control) dogs occurred at 20 mg/kg/day (about 72 times the recommended human subcutaneous doses of 0.15 mg/kg based on the body surface area). Clinical signs consistent with effects on the CNS (including tremors and decreased activity) occurred in both juvenile and adult dogs. The NOAELs in juvenile and adult dogs were 5 mg/kg/day (about 18 times the recommended human subcutaneous doses of 0.15 mg/kg based on the body surface area).

14 CLINICAL STUDIES

The efficacy and safety of RELISTOR in the treatment of opioid-induced constipation in advanced illness patients receiving palliative care was demonstrated in two randomized, double-blind, placebo-controlled studies. In these studies, the median age was 68 years (range 21-100); 51% were females. The majority of patients had a primary diagnosis of incurable cancer; other primary diagnoses included end-stage COPD/emphysema, cardiovascular disease/heart failure, Alzheimer's disease/dementia, HIV/AIDS, or other advanced illnesses. Prior to screening, patients had been receiving palliative opioid therapy (median daily baseline oral morphine equivalent dose = 172 mg), and had opioid-induced constipation (either <3 bowel movements in the preceding week or no bowel movement for >2 days). Patients were on a stable opioid regimen ≥ 3 days prior to randomization (not including PRN or rescue pain medication) and received their opioid medication during the study as clinically needed. Patients maintained their regular laxative regimen for at least 3 days prior to study entry, and throughout the study. Rescue laxatives were prohibited from 4 hours before to 4 hours after taking an injection of study medication.

Study 1 compared a single, double-blind, subcutaneous dose of RELISTOR 0.15 mg/kg, or RELISTOR 0.3 mg/kg versus placebo. The double blind dose was followed by an open-label 4-week dosing period, where RELISTOR could be used as needed, no more frequently than 1 dose in a 24 hour period. Throughout both study periods, patients maintained their regular laxative regimen. A total of 154 patients (47 RELISTOR 0.15 mg/kg, 55 RELISTOR 0.3 mg/kg, 52 placebo) were enrolled and treated in the double-blind period. The primary endpoint was the proportion of patients with a rescue-free laxation within 4 hours of the double-blind dose of study medication. RELISTOR-treated patients had a significantly higher rate of laxation within 4 hours of the double-blind dose (62% for 0.15 mg/kg and 58% for 0.3 mg/kg) than did placebo-treated patients (14%); $p < 0.0001$ for each dose versus placebo (Figure 1).

Study 2 compared double-blind, subcutaneous doses of RELISTOR given every other day for 2 weeks versus placebo. Patients received opioid medication ≥ 2 weeks prior to receiving study medication. During the first week (days 1, 3, 5, 7) patients received either 0.15 mg/kg RELISTOR or placebo. In the second week the patient's assigned dose could be increased to 0.30 mg/kg if the patient had 2 or fewer rescue-free laxations up to day 8. At any time, the patient's assigned dose could be reduced based on tolerability. Data from 133 (62 RELISTOR, 71 placebo) patients were analyzed. There were 2 primary endpoints: proportion of patients with a rescue-free laxation within 4 hours of the first dose of study medication and proportion of patients with a rescue-free laxation within 4 hours after at least 2 of the first 4 doses of study medication. RELISTOR-treated patients had a higher rate of laxation within 4 hours of the first dose (48%) than placebo-treated patients (16%); $p < 0.0001$ (Figure 1). RELISTOR-treated patients also had significantly higher rates of laxation within 4 hours after at least 2 of the first 4 doses (52%) than did placebo-treated patients (9%); $p < 0.0001$. In both studies, in approximately 30% of patients, laxation was reported within 30 minutes of a dose of RELISTOR.

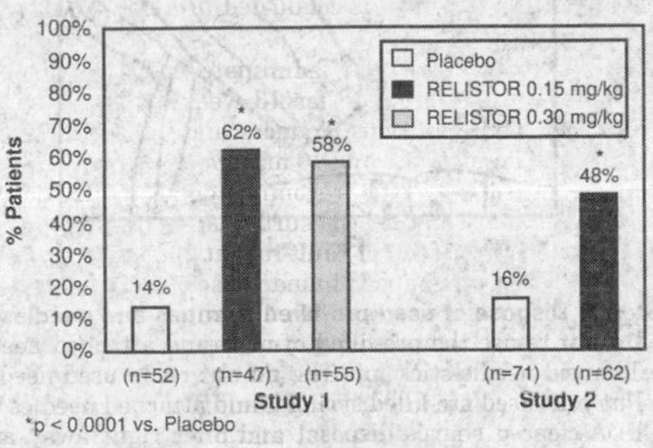

Figure 1. Laxation Response Within 4 Hours of the First Dose

In both studies, there was no evidence of differential effects of age or gender on safety or efficacy. No meaningful subgroup analysis could be conducted on race because the study population was predominantly Caucasian (88%).

Durability of Response

Durability of response was explored in Study 2 and the laxation response rate was consistent from dose 1 through dose 7 over the course of the 2-week, double-blind period.

The efficacy and safety of methylnaltrexone bromide was also demonstrated in open-label treatment administered from Day 2 through Week 4 in Study 1, and in two open-label extension studies (Study 1EXT and Study 2EXT) in which RELISTOR was given as needed for up to 4 months. During open-label treatment, patients maintained their regular laxative regimen. A total of 136, 21, and 82 patients received at least 1 open-label dose in studies 1, 1EXT, and 2EXT, respectively. Laxation response was also explored in this open-label setting and appeared to be maintained over the course of 3 to 4 months of open-label treatment.

Opioid Use and Pain Scores

No relationship between baseline opioid dose and laxation response in methylnaltrexone bromide-treated patients was identified in exploratory analyses of these studies. In addition, median daily opioid dose did not vary meaningfully from baseline in either RELISTOR -treated patients or in placebo-treated patients. There were no clinically relevant changes in pain scores from baseline in either the methylnaltrexone bromide or placebo-treated patients.

16 HOW SUPPLIED/STORAGE AND HANDLING

How Supplied

[See table above]

NDC NUMBER	PACK SIZE	CONTENTS
65649-551-02	1 vial per carton	one 12 mg/0.6 mL single-use vial
65649-553-05	7 trays per kit	Each tray contains: one 12 mg/0.6 mL single-use vial, one 1 cc (mL) syringe with retractable (27-gauge × ½-inch) needle (VanishPoint®), two alcohol swabs
65649-552-04	7 pre-filled syringes per carton	seven 8 mg/0.4 mL single-use pre-filled syringes with needle guard system
65649-551-03	7 pre-filled syringes per carton	seven 12 mg/0.6 mL single-use pre-filled syringes with needle guard system
65649-551-07	1 pre-filled syringe per carton	one 12mg/0.6 mL single-use pre-filled syringe with needle guard system

16.1 Storage

RELISTOR should be stored at 20°C to 25°C (68°F to 77°F); excursions permitted to 15°C to 30°C (59°F to 86°F) [see USP Controlled Room Temperature]. Do not freeze. **Protect from light.**

17 PATIENT COUNSELING INFORMATION

See FDA-approved patient labeling (Patient Information and Instructions for Use)

- Instruct patients not to continue taking RELISTOR and to promptly notify their physician if they experience severe, persistent, or worsening abdominal symptoms because these could be symptoms of gastrointestinal perforation [*see Warnings and Precautions (5.1)*].
- Instruct patients not to continue taking RELISTOR if they experience severe or persistent diarrhea. Inform patients that common side effects of RELISTOR include abdominal pain, flatulence, nausea, dizziness, and diarrhea.
- Advise patients to be within close proximity to toilet facilities once the drug is administered.
- Instruct patients with opioid-induced constipation and advanced illness to administer one dose subcutaneously every other day, as needed, but no more frequently than one dose in a 24-hour period.
- Instruct patients to discontinue RELISTOR if they stop taking their opioid pain medication.
- Instruct patients to use the RELISTOR single-use vial with a 27 gauge × ½-inch needle and 1 mL syringe.

Patient Information

RELISTOR® (rel - *i* – *store*)

(methylnaltrexone bromide)

Subcutaneous Injection

Read this Patient Information that comes with RELISTOR before you start using it and each time you get a refill. There may be new information. This leaflet does not take the place of talking with your healthcare provider about your medical condition or your treatment.

What is RELISTOR?

RELISTOR is a prescription medicine used to treat constipation that is caused by prescription pain medicines, called opioids, in patients receiving supportive care for their advanced illness, when other medicines for constipation, called laxatives, have not worked well enough.

It is not known if RELISTOR is safe and effective if used for longer than 4 months in people with advanced illness.

It is not known if RELISTOR is safe and effective in children.

Who should not use RELISTOR?

Do not use RELISTOR if you have or may have a blockage in your intestines called a mechanical bowel obstruction. Symptoms of this blockage are vomiting, stomach pain, and swelling of your stomach-area (abdomen). Talk to your healthcare provider if you have any of these symptoms before using RELISTOR.

What should I tell my healthcare provider before using RELISTOR?

Before you start using RELISTOR, tell your healthcare provider if you:

- have kidney problems
- have or had cancer of the stomach or intestine
- have or had a stomach ulcer
- have had a blockage in your intestine
- have any other medical condition
- are pregnant or plan to become pregnant. It is not known if RELISTOR can harm your unborn baby.
- are breast-feeding or plan to breast-feed. It is not known if RELISTOR passes into your breast milk.

Tell your healthcare provider about all medicines you take, including prescription and non-prescription medicines, vitamins, and herbal supplements. Continue taking your other medicines for constipation unless your healthcare provider tells you to stop taking them.

How should I use RELISTOR?

- RELISTOR is injected under the skin (subcutaneous injection) of the upper arm, abdomen, or thigh.
- Inject RELISTOR exactly as your healthcare provider tells you.
- RELISTOR is usually used every other day. Do not inject more than one dose of RELISTOR in a 24-hour period.
- Stay close to a toilet after using RELISTOR.
- Stop using RELISTOR if you stop taking your prescription opioid pain medicine.
- If you inject more RELISTOR than prescribed, talk to your healthcare provider right away.

See the detailed Instructions for Use that comes with RELISTOR for information about how to prepare and inject RELISTOR, and properly throw away (dispose of) used needles and syringes the right way.

What are the possible side effects of RELISTOR?

RELISTOR can cause serious side effects, including:

- **Tear in your stomach or intestinal wall (perforation). Stop using RELISTOR and call your healthcare provider right away** if you develop swelling or pain in your stomach-area (abdomen) that is severe, gets worse, or that does not go away, nausea or vomiting that does not go away, or if you vomit blood or have black sticky stools.
- **Diarrhea that is severe or that will not go away.** Stop using RELISTOR and call your healthcare provider if you get diarrhea that is severe or that does not go away during treatment with RELISTOR.

The most common side effects of RELISTOR include:

- stomach-area (abdomen) pain
- gas
- nausea
- dizziness
- diarrhea
- sweating

Tell your healthcare provider if you have any side effect that bothers you or that does not go away.

These are not all of the possible side effects of RELISTOR. Call your doctor for medical advice about side effects. You may report side effects to FDA at 1-800-FDA-1088.

How should I store RELISTOR?

- Store RELISTOR vials and pre-filled syringes at room temperature between 68°F to 77°F (20°C to 25°C).
- Do not freeze RELISTOR.
- Keep RELISTOR away from light until you are ready to use it.
- If RELISTOR has been drawn into a syringe and you are unable to use the medicine right away, keep the syringe at room temperature for up to 24 hours. The syringe does not need to be kept away from light during the 24-hour period.

Keep RELISTOR and all medicines, needles and syringes out of the reach of children.

General information about RELISTOR

Medicines are sometimes prescribed for purposes other than those listed in a Patient Information leaflet. Do not use

RELISTOR for a condition for which it was not prescribed. Do not give RELISTOR to other people, even if they have the same symptoms that you have. It may harm them.

This leaflet summarizes the most important information about RELISTOR. If you would like more information, talk with your healthcare provider. You can ask your pharmacist or healthcare provider for information about RELISTOR that is written for health professionals.

For more information, go to WWW.RELISTOR.COM.

What are the ingredients in RELISTOR?

Active ingredient: methylnaltrexone bromide

Inactive ingredients: sodium chloride, edetate calcium disodium USP, glycine hydrochloride.

During manufacture, the pH may have been adjusted with hydrochloric acid and/or sodium hydroxide.

This Patient Information has been approved by the U.S. Food and Drug Administration.

Manufactured for:
Salix Pharmaceuticals, Inc.
Raleigh, NC 27615
Under license from:
Progenics Pharmaceuticals, Inc.
Tarrytown, NY 10591
Revised: AUG 2013

Product protected by U.S. Patent Nos. 6,559,158, 8,247,425, and 8,420,663.

Please see www.salix.com for patent information

Instructions for Use
RELISTOR® (rel-i-store)
(methylnaltrexone bromide)
Pre-filled Syringe

Read this Instructions for Use before you start using RELISTOR and each time you get a refill. There may be new information. This information does not take the place of talking to your healthcare provider about your medical condition or your treatment.

The following instructions explain how to prepare and give an injection of RELISTOR the right way, when using a pre-filled syringe of RELISTOR.

Important information:

- **Do not** use a RELISTOR pre-filled syringe and attached needle more than one time, even if there is medicine left in the syringe. **See Step 4 "Dispose of used pre-filled syringes and needles."**
- Safely throw away RELISTOR pre-filled syringes and attached needle after use.
- To avoid needle-stick injuries, **do not** recap used needles.
- Avoid touching the trigger fingers of the RELISTOR pre-filled syringe to keep from activating the needle guard (safety device) too soon. The needle guard is activated by pressure from the plunger on the trigger fingers (See Figure A).

Gather the supplies you will need for your injection (See Figure A). These include:

- 1 RELISTOR pre-filled syringe with attached needle
- 1 alcohol swab
- 1 cotton ball or gauze
- 1 adhesive bandage
- a container to dispose of used pre-filled syringes and needles. See Step 4: "Dispose of used pre-filled syringes and needles."

Pre-filled Syringe Parts

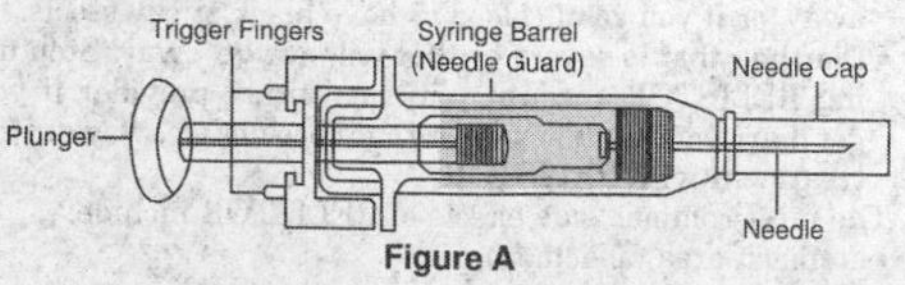

Figure A

Step 1: Choose and prepare the injection site

- Choose an injection site on your abdomen, thighs, or upper arms. See the shaded areas in Figures B and C below. Do not inject at the exact same spot each time (rotate injection sites). Do not inject into areas where the skin is tender, bruised, red or hard. Avoid areas with scars or stretch marks.

  Figure B Abdomen or thigh – use these sites when injecting yourself or another person.

  Figure C Upper arm – use this site only when injecting another person.

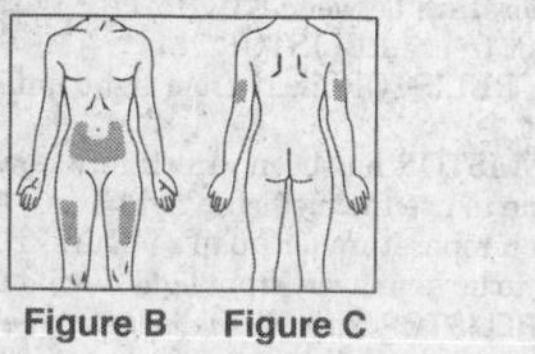
Figure B Figure C

- Clean the injection site with an alcohol swab and let it air dry. Do not touch this area again before giving the injection (See Figure D).

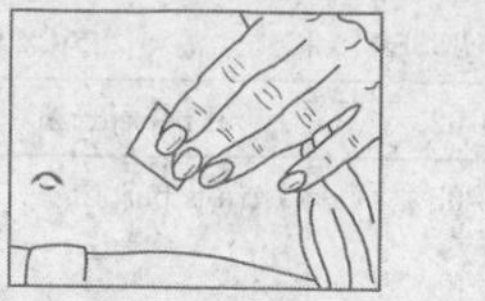
Figure D

Step 2: Prepare the pre-filled syringe

- Choose a flat, clean, well-lit work surface.
- Wash your hands with soap and water before preparing for the injection.
- Look at the pre-filled syringe of RELISTOR (See Figure E). Make sure that the dose prescribed by your healthcare provider matches the dose on the pre-filled syringe label. Look at the plunger rod of the syringe. If the dose prescribed by your healthcare provider is 8 mg, the plunger rod will be yellow; if the prescribed dose is 12 mg, the plunger rod of the syringe will be dark blue (See Figure E).

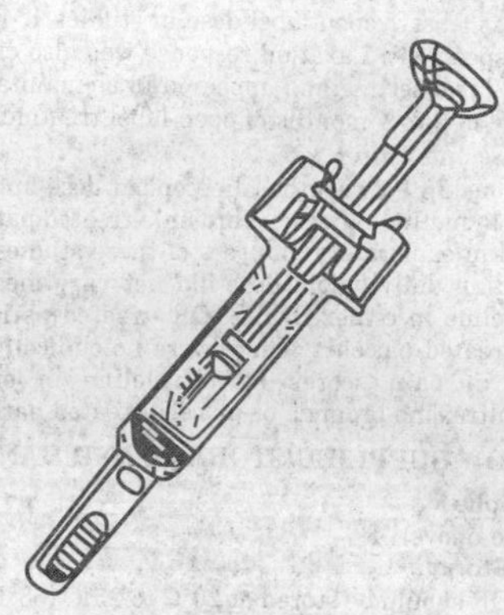
Figure E

- The liquid in the pre-filled syringe should be clear and colorless to pale yellow, and should not have any particles in it. Do not use the pre-filled syringe if it looks discolored, cloudy, or has any particles.
- Use one hand to firmly hold the barrel of the pre-filled syringe. Use your other hand to pull the needle cap straight off (Figure F). Do not touch the needle or allow it to touch anything.

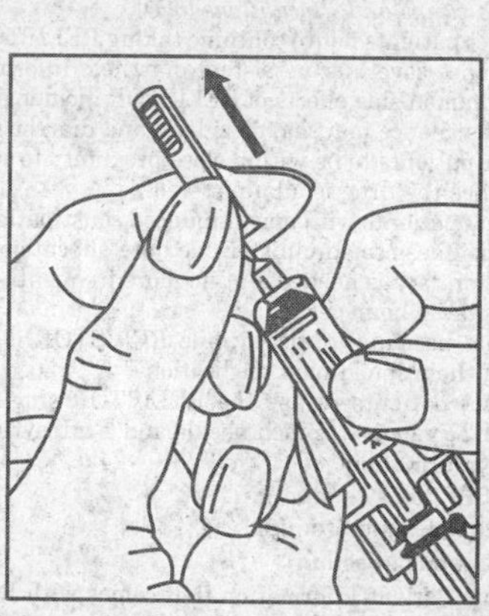
Figure F

Step 3: Inject RELISTOR

- Use one hand to pinch the skin around the injection site (See Figure G).

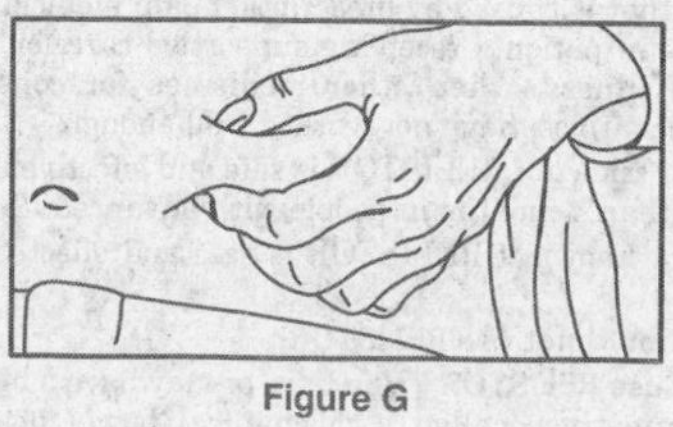
Figure G

- Use your other hand to hold the pre-filled syringe. Insert the full length of the needle into the skin at a 45-degree angle with a quick "dart-like" motion (See Figure H).

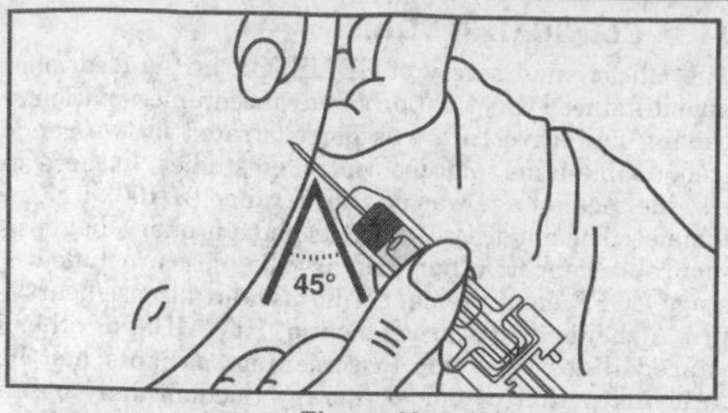

Figure H

- Let go of the skin and slowly push the plunger in with your thumb until the pre-filled syringe is empty (See Figure I). This will release the needle guard (safety device).

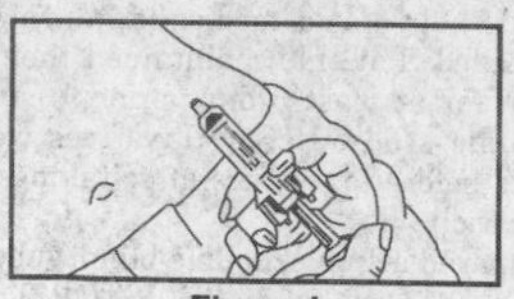
Figure I

- Continue to hold pressure on the plunger with your thumb and quickly pull the needle out of the skin. Be careful to keep the needle at the same angle as it was inserted. Remove your thumb from the plunger to allow the protective sleeve to cover the needle (See Figure J). There may be a little bleeding at the injection site.

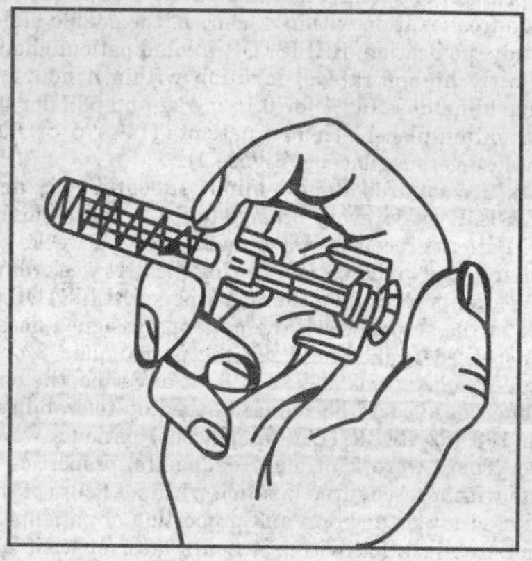
Figure J

- Hold a cotton ball or gauze over the injection site (See Figure K). Do not rub the injection site. Apply an adhesive bandage to the injection site if needed.

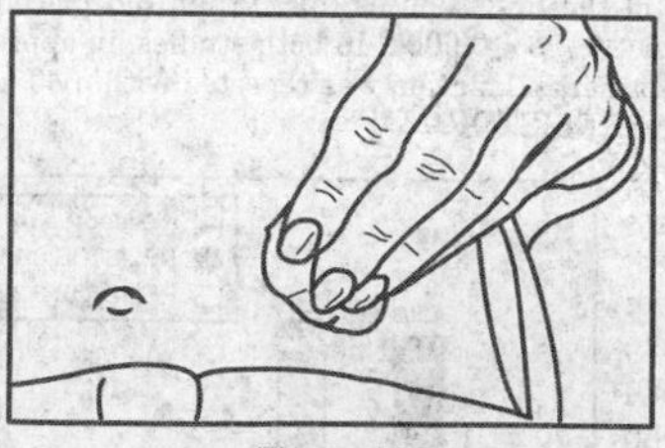
Figure K

Step 4: Dispose of used pre-filled syringes and needles

- **Do not** re-use the pre-filled syringe and attached needle.
- To avoid needle-stick injuries, **do not** recap used needles.
- Put your used pre-filled syringes and attached needles **in a** FDA-cleared sharps disposal container right away after use. **Do not throw away (dispose of) loose needles and syringes in your household trash.**
- If you do not have a FDA-cleared sharps disposal container, you may use a household container that is:
  - made of a heavy-duty plastic,
  - can be closed with a tight-fitting, puncture-resistant lid, without sharps being able to come out,
  - upright and stable during use,
  - leak-resistant, and
  - properly labeled to warn of hazardous waste inside the container.
- When your sharps disposal container is almost full, you will need to follow your community guidelines for the right way to dispose of your sharps disposal container. There may be state or local laws about how you should throw away used needles and syringes. For more information about safe sharps disposal, and for

specific information about sharps disposal in the state that you live in, go to the FDA's website at: http://www.fda.gov/safesharpsdisposal

- Do not dispose of your used sharps disposal container in your household trash unless your community guidelines permit this. Do not recycle your used sharps disposal container.
- If you have any questions, talk to your healthcare provider or pharmacist.

How should I store RELISTOR?

- Store pre-filled syringes at room temperature between 68°F to 77°F (20°C to 25°C).
- Do not freeze RELISTOR.
- Keep RELISTOR away from light until you are ready to use it.

Keep RELISTOR and all medicines, needles and syringes out of the reach of children.

This Instructions for Use has been approved by the U.S. Food and Drug Administration.

Manufactured for:
Salix Pharmaceuticals, Inc.
Raleigh, NC 27615
Under license from:
Progenics Pharmaceuticals, Inc.
Tarrytown, NY 10591
Revised AUG 2013
Product protected by U.S. Patent Nos. 6,559,158, 8,247,425, and 8,420,663.
See www.salix.com for patent information

Instructions for Use
RELISTOR® (rel-i-store)
(methylnaltrexone bromide)
Vial and Syringe with Retractable Needle in Tray

Read this Instructions for Use before you start using RELISTOR and each time you get a refill. There may be new information. This information does not take the place of talking to your healthcare provider about your medical condition or your treatment.

The following instructions explain how to prepare and give an injection of RELISTOR the right way, when using a RELISTOR tray containing a syringe with a retractable needle. A retractable needle is one that is pulled back so that it is covered after use, to prevent needle-stick injury.

Important information:

- **Do not** use a RELISTOR vial more than one time, even if there is medicine left in the vial.
- If RELISTOR has been drawn into a syringe and you are unable to use the medicine right away, carefully recap the needle and keep the syringe at room temperature for up to 24 hours. The syringe does not need to be kept away from light during the 24-hour period. For more information about how to store RELISTOR, see the section called **"How should I store RELISTOR?"** at the end of this Instructions for Use.
- Safely throw away RELISTOR vials after use.
- **Do not** reuse syringes and needles. **See Step 5: "Dispose of used syringes and needles"** for information about how to safely throw away used needles and syringes.
- To avoid needle-stick injuries, **do not** recap used needles.

Your tray should include (See Figure A):

- 1 RELISTOR vial
- 1 1 mL syringe with retractable needle (VanishPoint®)
- 2 alcohol swabs

You will also need:

- 1 cotton ball or gauze
- 1 adhesive bandage
- a container to dispose of your used syringes and needles. See Step 5: "Dispose of used syringes and needles."

Vial and Syringe Parts

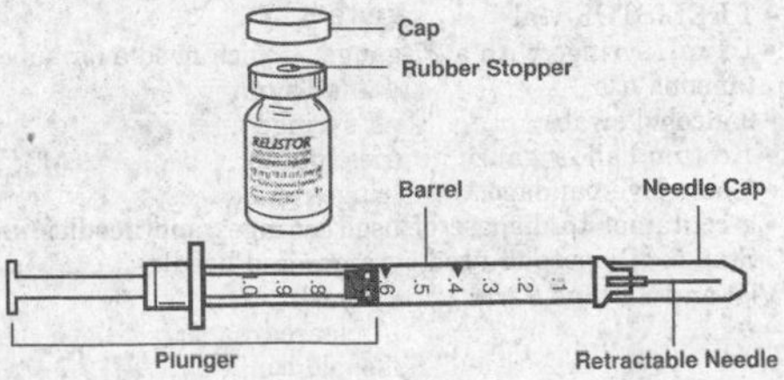

Figure A

Step 1: Choose and prepare the injection site

- Choose an injection site on your abdomen, thighs, or upper arms. See the shaded areas in B and C below. Do not inject at the exact same spot each time (rotate injection sites). Do not inject into areas where the skin is tender, bruised, red, or hard. Avoid areas with scars or stretch marks.

Figure B Abdomen or thigh – use these sites when injecting yourself or another person.

Figure C Upper arm – use this site only when injecting another person.

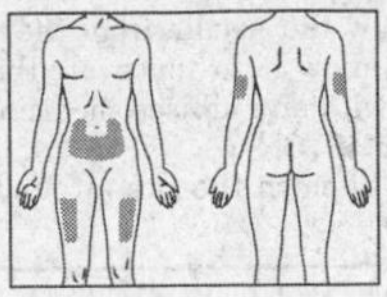

Figure B Figure C

- Clean the injection site with an alcohol swab and let it air dry. Do not touch this area again before giving the injection (See Figure D).

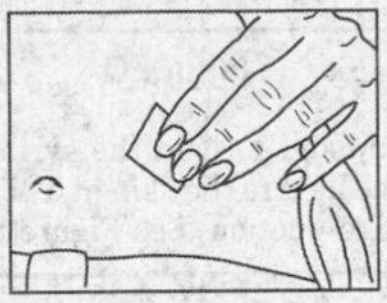

Figure D

Step 2: Prepare the injection

- Choose a flat, clean, well-lit work surface.
- Wash your hands with soap and water before preparing for the injection.
- Look at the vial of RELISTOR (See Figure E). The liquid in the vial should be clear and colorless to pale yellow, and should not have any particles in it. Do not use the vial if it looks discolored, cloudy, or has any particles.

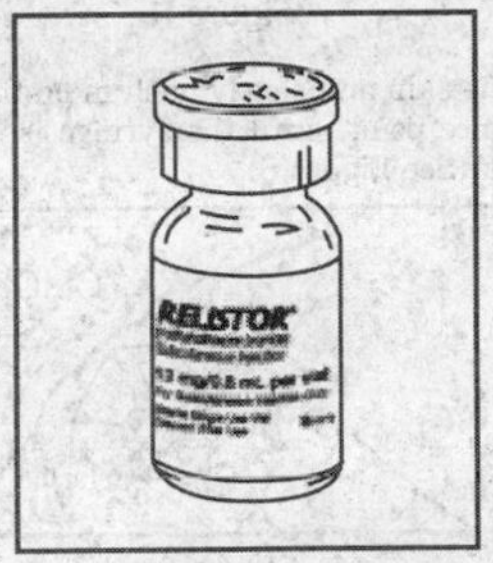

Figure E

Step 3: Prepare the syringe

- Remove the cap from the vial containing RELISTOR (See Figure F).

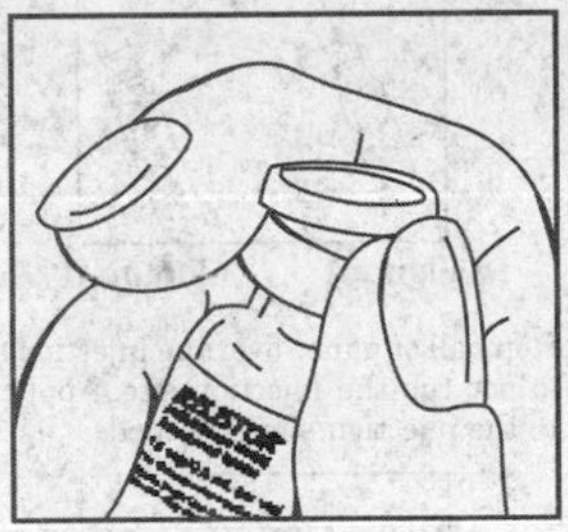

Figure F

- Wipe the rubber stopper with an alcohol swab (See Figure G).

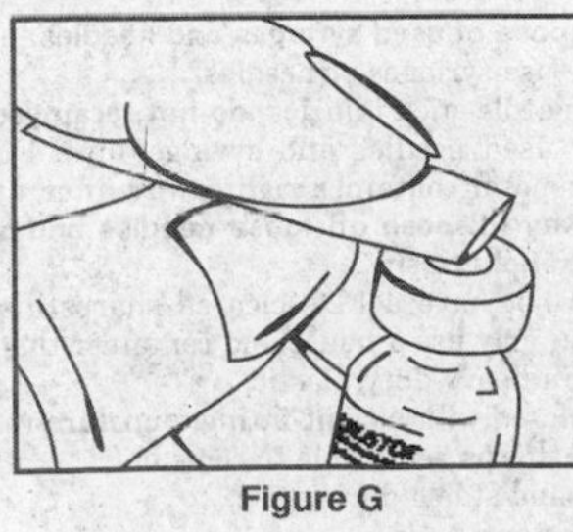

Figure G

- Firmly hold the barrel of the syringe with one hand. With your other hand, pull the needle cap straight off (See Figure H). Do not touch the needle or allow it to touch anything

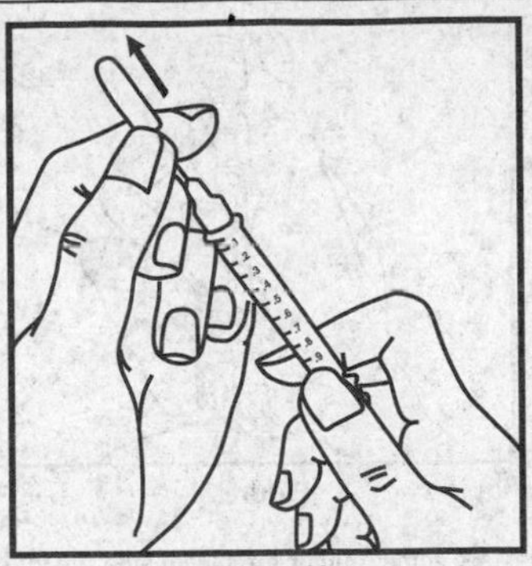

Figure H

- Carefully pull back on the plunger to the line that matches the dose prescribed by your healthcare provider (See Figures I and J). For most people, this will be the 0.4 mL mark which is an 8 mg dose or the 0.6 mL mark which is a 12 mg dose.

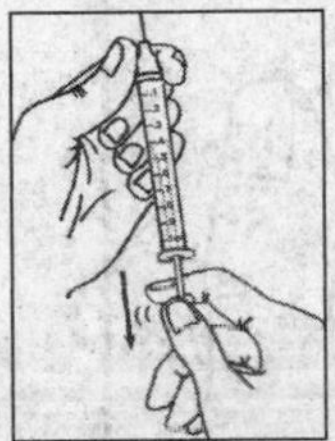

Figure I

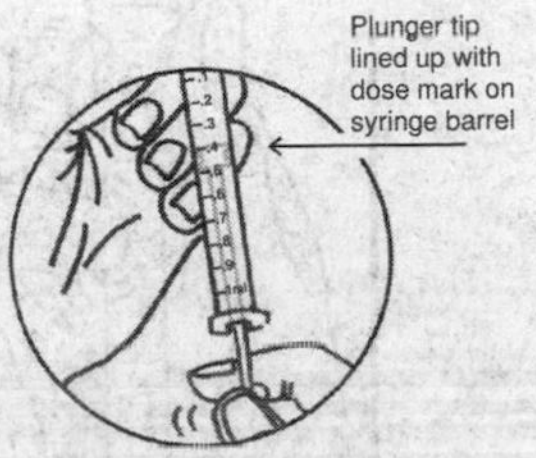

Figure J

- Use one hand to hold the vial steady. Use your other hand to insert the needle straight down into the rubber top of the RELISTOR vial (See Figure K). Do not insert it at an angle. This may cause the needle to bend or break. You will feel some resistance as the needle passes through the rubber top.

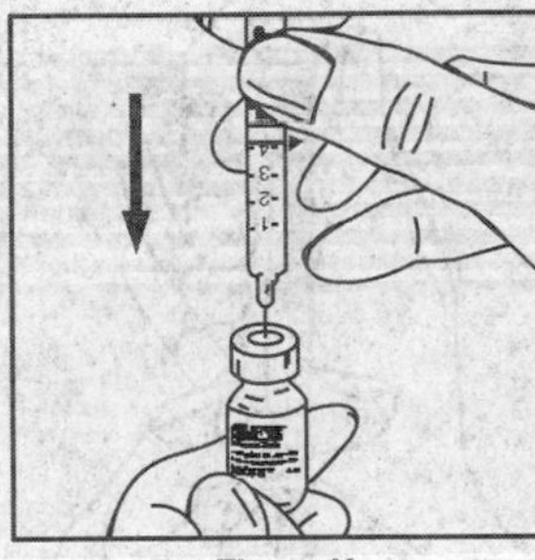

Figure K

- Gently push down on the plunger until you feel resistance, and most of the air has gone from the syringe into the vial (See Figure L). Stop pushing down on the plunger when you feel resistance. If you continue to push down on the plunger when you feel resistance, the needle will pull back (retract) into the syringe barrel.

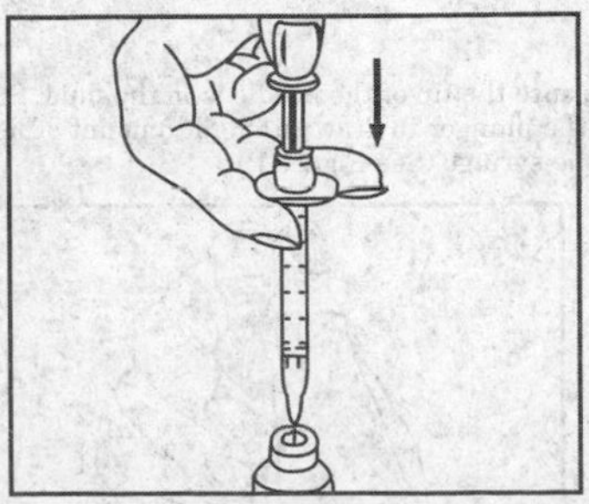

Figure L

- With the needle still in the vial, turn the vial and syringe upside down. Hold the syringe at eye level. Make sure the tip of the needle is in the fluid. Slowly pull back on the plunger (See Figure M) until the tip lines up with the mark that matches your prescribed dose. For most people, this will be the 0.4 mL mark which is an 8 mg dose or the 0.6 mL mark which is a 12 mg dose.

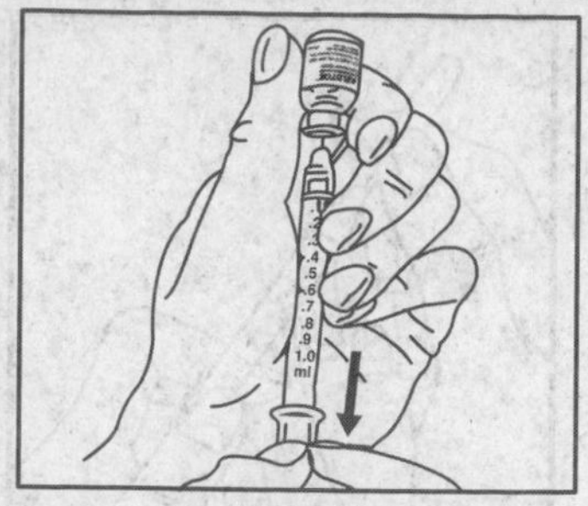

Figure M

- You may see some fluid or bubbles inside the vial when the syringe is filled. This is normal.
- With the needle still in the vial, gently tap the syringe to make any air bubbles rise to the top (See Figure N).

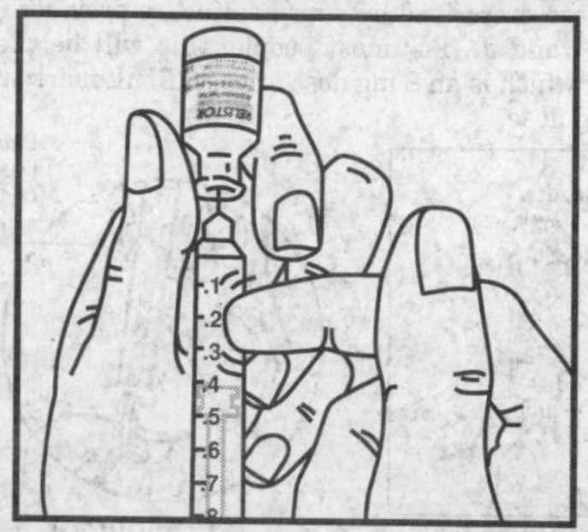

Figure N

- Gently push the plunger up until all air bubbles are out of the syringe (See Figure O). A small air bubble may stay in the syringe. This is okay and it will not affect the dose of medicine in the syringe.

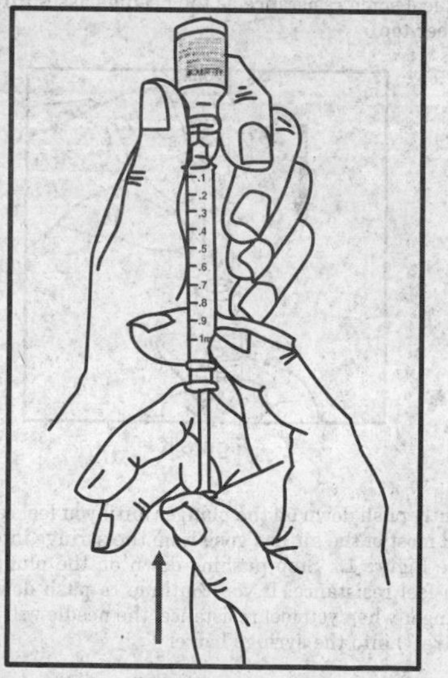

Figure O

- Make sure the tip of the needle is in the fluid. Slowly pull back the plunger to draw the right amount of liquid back into the syringe (See Figure P).

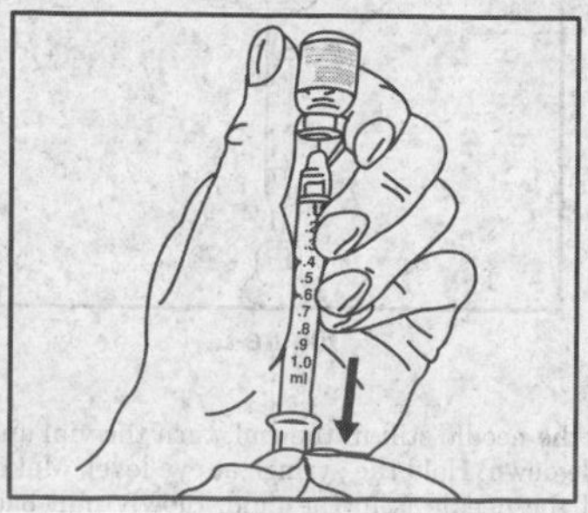

Figure P

Check to be sure that you have the right dose of RELISTOR in the syringe.

- Slowly withdraw the needle from the vial. Do not touch the needle or allow it to touch anything). Safely throw away the vial with any unused medicine.

Step 4: Inject RELISTOR

- Use one hand to pinch the skin around the injection site (See Figure Q).

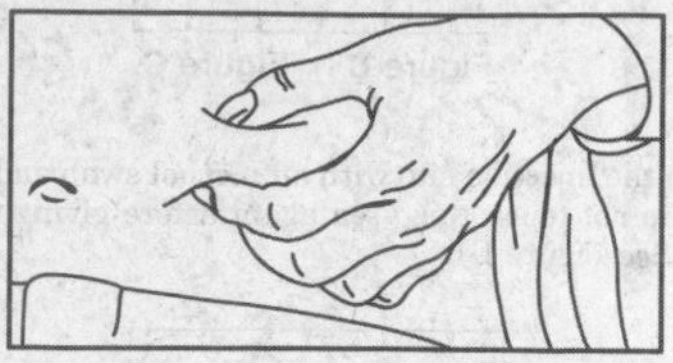

Figure Q

- Use your other hand to hold the syringe. Insert the full length of the needle into the skin at a 45-degree angle with a "quick dart-like" motion (See Figure R).

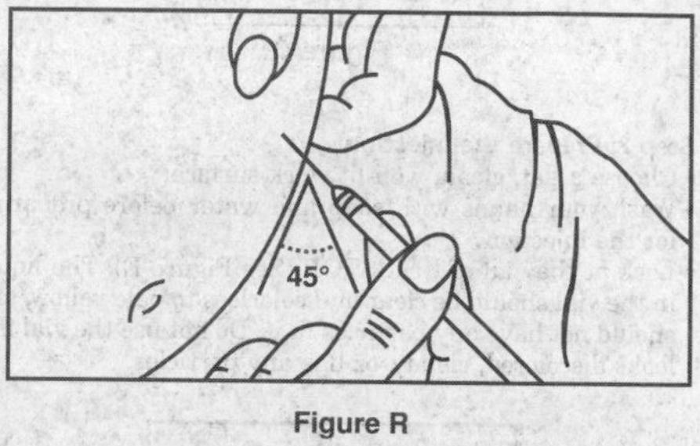

Figure R

- Let go of the skin and slowly push in on the plunger past the resistance point, until the syringe is empty and you hear a click (See Figure S).

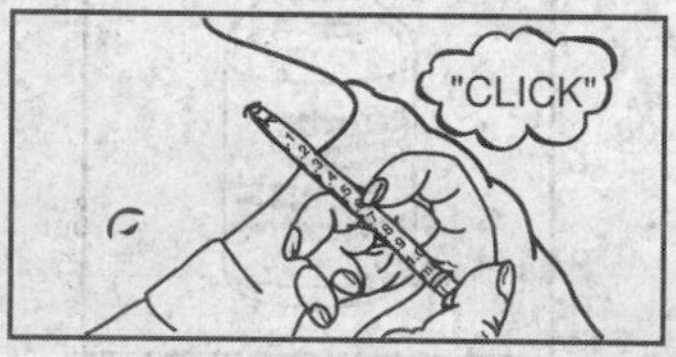

Figure S

- The click sound means that the needle (T) has been pulled back (retracted) into the syringe barrel (See Figure U). You can now remove the syringe from your skin.

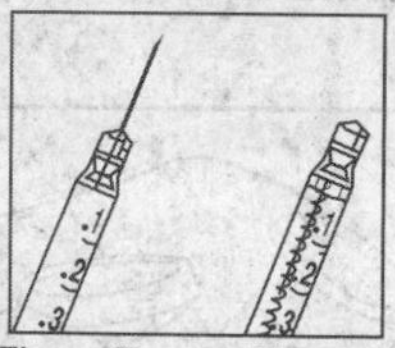

Figure T Figure U

- Hold a cotton ball or gauze over the injection site (See Figure V). Do not rub the injection site. Apply an adhesive bandage to the injection site if needed.

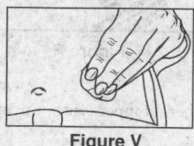

Figure V

Step 5: Dispose of used syringes and needles

- **Do not** re-use syringes or needles.
- To avoid needle-stick injuries, **do not** recap used needles.
- Put your used needles and syringes in a FDA-cleared sharps disposal container right away after use. **Do not throw away (dispose of) loose needles and syringes in your household trash.**
- If you do not have a FDA-cleared sharps disposal container, you may use a household container that is:
  - made of a heavy-duty plastic,
  - can be closed with a tight-fitting, puncture-resistant lid, without sharps being able to come out,
  - upright and stable during use,
  - leak-resistant, and
  - properly labeled to warn of hazardous waste inside the container.
- When your sharps disposal container is almost full, you will need to follow your community guidelines for the right way to dispose of your sharps disposal container. There may be state or local laws about how you should throw away used needles and syringes. For more information about safe sharps disposal, and for specific information about sharps disposal in the state that you live in, go to the FDA's website at: http://www.fda.gov/safesharpsdisposal.
- Do not dispose of your used sharps disposal container in your household trash unless your community guidelines permit this. Do not recycle your used sharps disposal container.
- If you have any questions, talk to your healthcare provider or pharmacist.

How should I store RELISTOR?

- Store RELISTOR vials at room temperature between 68°F to 77°F (20 °C to 25°C).
- Do not freeze RELISTOR.
- Keep RELISTOR away from light until you are ready to use it.
- If RELISTOR has been drawn into a syringe and you are unable to use the medicine right away, keep the syringe at room temperature for up to 24 hours. The syringe does not need to be kept away from light during the 24-hour period.

Keep RELISTOR and all medicines, needles and syringes out of the reach of children.

This Instructions for Use has been approved by the U.S. Food and Drug Administration.

Manufactured for:
Salix Pharmaceuticals, Inc.
Raleigh, NC 27615
Under license from:
Progenics Pharmaceuticals, Inc.
Tarrytown, NY 10591
Revised AUG 2013
Product protected by U.S. Patent Nos. 6,559,158, 8,247,425, and 8,420,663.
See www.salix.com for patent information

Instructions for Use
RELISTOR® (rel-i-store)
(methylnaltrexone bromide)
Subcutaneous Injection
Vial

Read this Instructions for Use before you start using RELISTOR and each time you get a refill. There may be new information. This information does not take the place of talking to your healthcare provider about your medical condition or your treatment.

The following instructions explain how to prepare and give an injection of RELISTOR the right way, when using a vial of RELISTOR.

Important information:

- Use the syringes and needles prescribed by your healthcare provider.
- **Do not** use a RELISTOR vial more than one time, even if there is medicine left in the vial.
- If RELISTOR has been drawn into a syringe and you are unable to use the medicine right away, carefully recap the needle and keep the syringe at room temperature for up to 24 hours. The syringe does not need to be kept away from light during the 24-hour period. For more information about how to store RELISTOR, see the section **"How should I store RELISTOR?"** at the end of this Instructions for Use.
- Safely throw away RELISTOR vials after use.
- **Do not** re-use syringes or needles. **See Step 5 "Dispose of used syringes and needles"** for information about how to safely throw away used needles and syringes.
- To avoid needle-stick injuries, **do not** recap used needles.

Gather the supplies you will need for your injection (See Figure A.). These include:

- 1 RELISTOR vial
- 1 1 mL syringe with a 27-gauge, ½ inch needle for subcutaneous use
- 2 alcohol swabs
- 1 cotton ball or gauze
- 1 adhesive bandage
- a container to dispose of used syringes and needles. See Step 5: "Dispose of used syringes and needles."

Vial and Syringe Parts

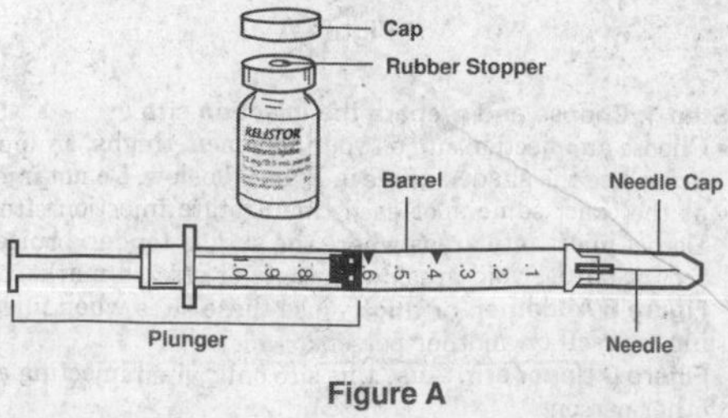

Figure A

Step 1: Choose and prepare the injection site

- Choose an injection site on your abdomen, thighs, or upper arms. See the shaded areas in Figures B and C below. Do not inject at the exact same spot each time (rotate injection sites). Do not inject into areas where the skin is tender, bruised, red or hard. Avoid areas with scars or stretch marks.

Figure B Abdomen or thigh – use these sites when injecting yourself or another person.

Figure C Upper arm – use this site only when injecting another person.

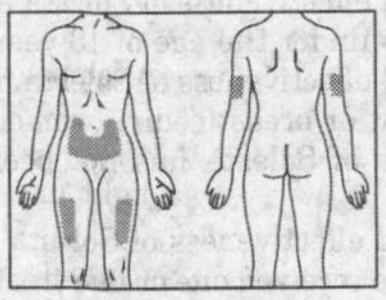

Figure B Figure C

- Clean the injection site with an alcohol swab and let it air dry. Do not touch this area again before giving the injection (See Figure D).

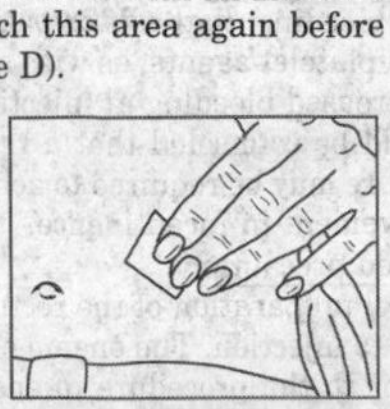

Figure D

Step 2: Prepare the injection

- Choose a flat, clean, well-lit work surface.
- Wash your hands with soap and water before preparing for the injection.
- Look at the vial of RELISTOR (See Figure E). The liquid in the vial should be clear and colorless to pale yellow, and should not have any particles in it. Do not use the vial if it looks discolored, cloudy, or has any particles.

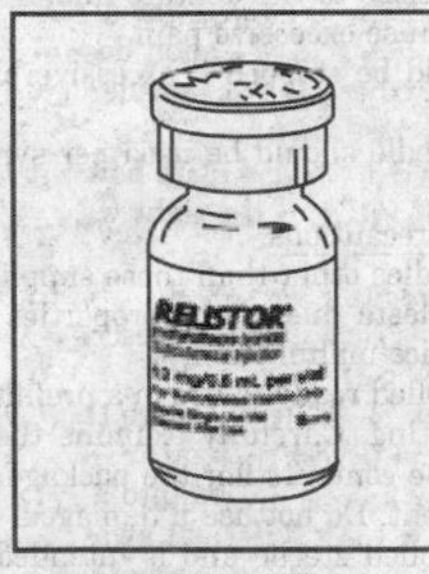

Figure E

Step 3: Prepare the syringe

- Remove the cap from the RELISTOR vial (See Figure F).

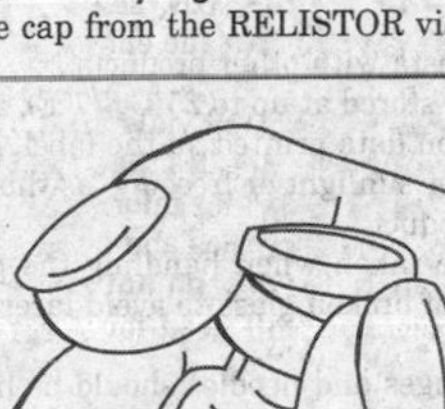

Figure F

- Wipe the rubber stopper with an alcohol swab (See Figure G).

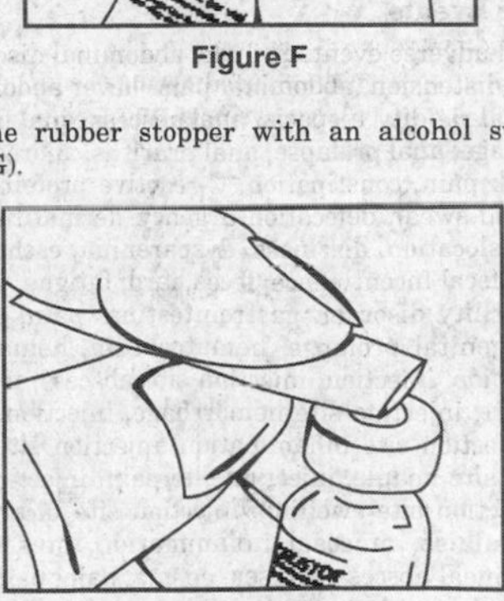

Figure G

- Firmly hold the barrel of the syringe with one hand. With your other hand, pull the needle cap straight off (See Figure H). Do not touch the needle or allow it to touch anything.

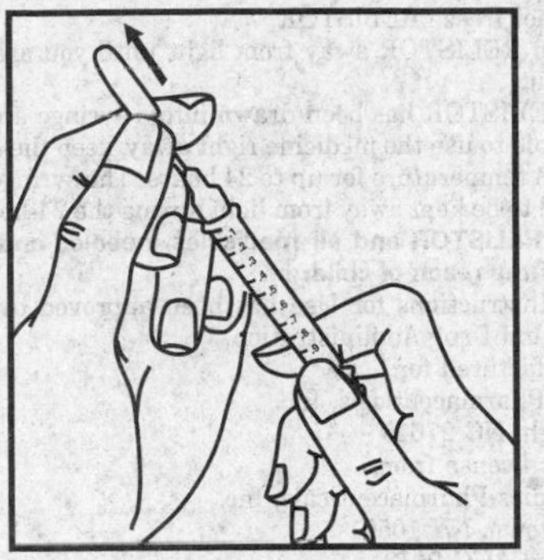

Figure H

- Carefully pull back on the plunger to the line that matches the dose prescribed by your healthcare provider (See Figures I and J). For most people, this will be the 0.4 mL mark which is an 8 mg dose or the 0.6 mL mark which is a 12 mg dose.

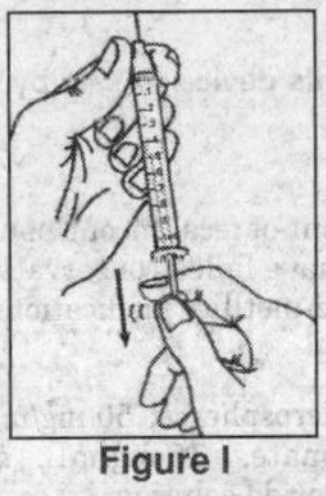

Figure I

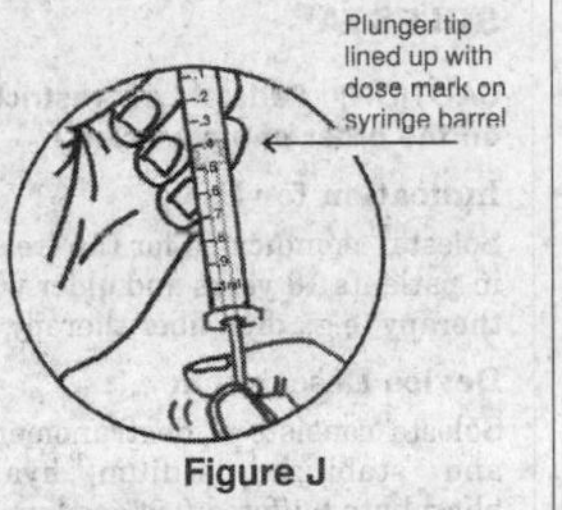

Figure J

- Use one hand to hold the vial steady. Use your other hand to insert the needle straight down into the rubber top of the vial (See Figure K). Do not insert it at an angle. This may cause the needle to bend or break. You will feel some resistance as the needle passes through the rubber top.

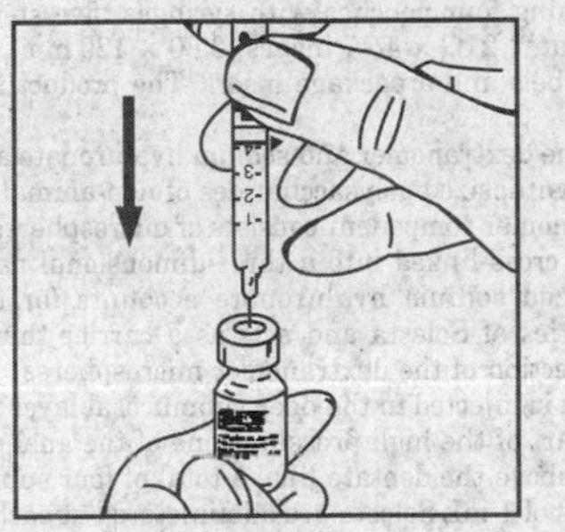

Figure K

- Gently push down the plunger until all of the air has gone from the syringe into the vial (See Figure L).

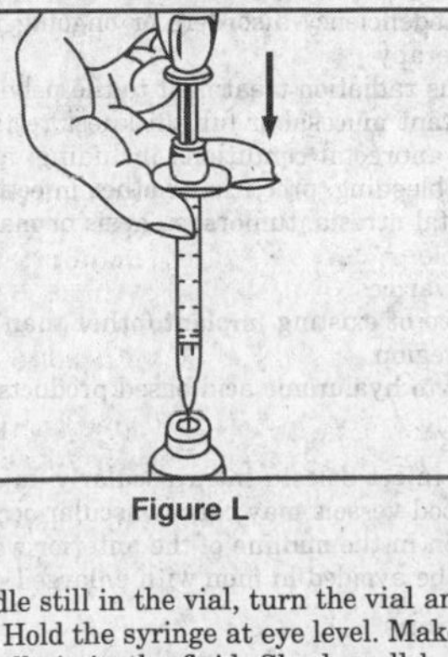

Figure L

- With the needle still in the vial, turn the vial and syringe upside down. Hold the syringe at eye level. Make sure the tip of the needle is in the fluid. Slowly pull back on the plunger (See Figure M) until the tip lines up with the mark that matches your prescribed dose. For most people, this will be the 0.4 mL mark which is an 8 mg dose or the 0.6 mL mark which is a 12 mg dose.

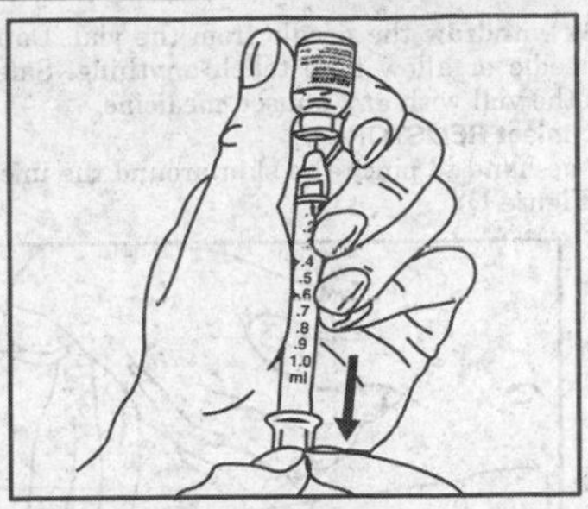

Figure M

- You may see some fluid or bubbles inside the vial when the syringe is filled. This is normal.
- With the needle still in the vial, gently tap the side of the syringe to make any air bubbles rise to the top (See Figure N).

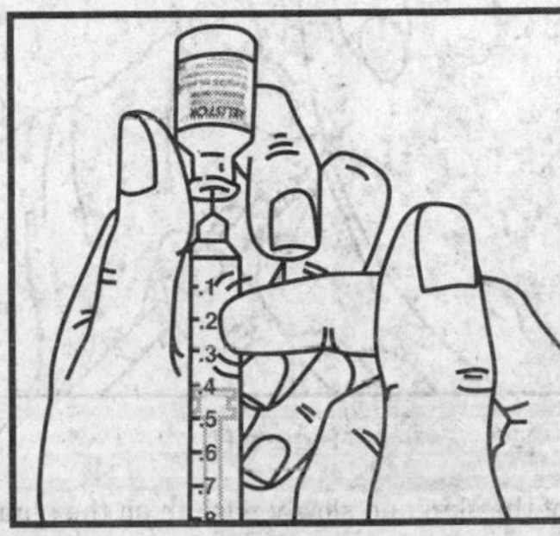

Figure N

- Slowly push the plunger up until all air bubbles are out of the syringe (See Figure O). A small air bubble may stay in the syringe. This is okay and it will not affect the dose of medicine in the syringe.

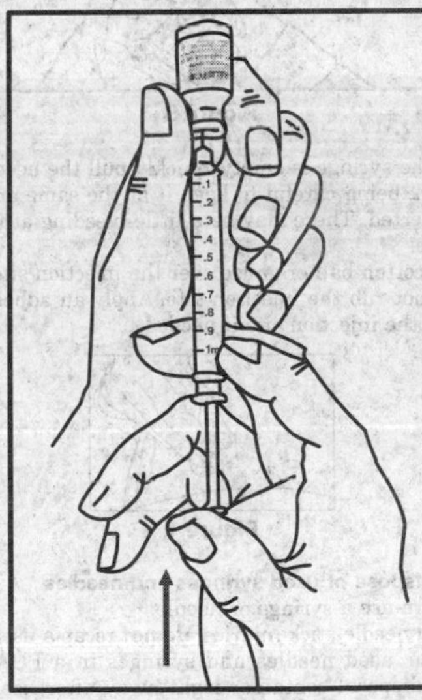

Figure O

- Make sure the tip of the needle is in the fluid. Slowly pull back the plunger to draw the right amount of liquid back into the syringe (See Figure P).

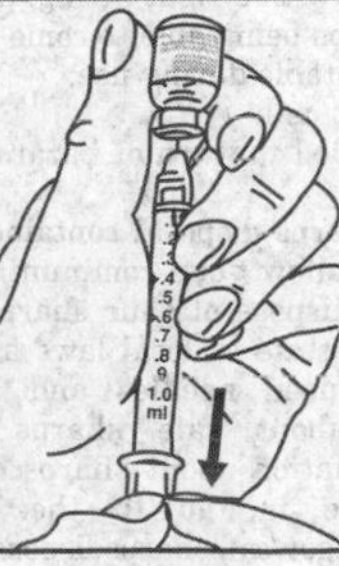

Figure P

Check to be sure that you have the right dose of RELISTOR in the syringe.

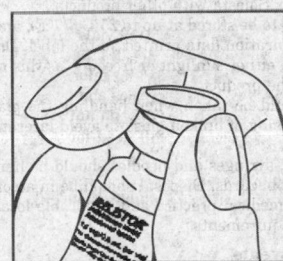

- Slowly withdraw the needle from the vial. Do not touch the needle or allow it to touch anything. Safely throw away the vial with any unused medicine.

Step 4: Inject RELISTOR

- Use one hand to pinch the skin around the injection site (See Figure Q).

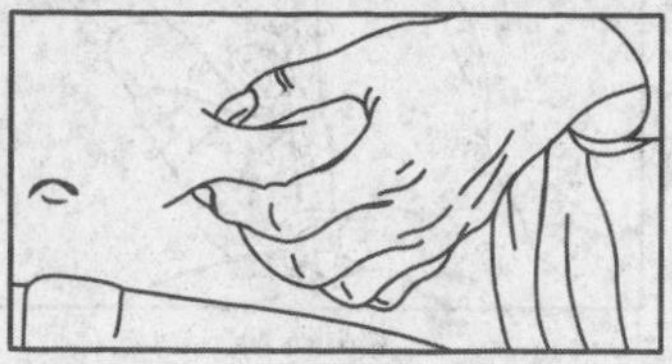

Figure Q

- Use your other hand to hold the syringe. Insert the full length of the needle into the skin at a 45-degree angle with a quick "dart-like" motion (See Figure R).

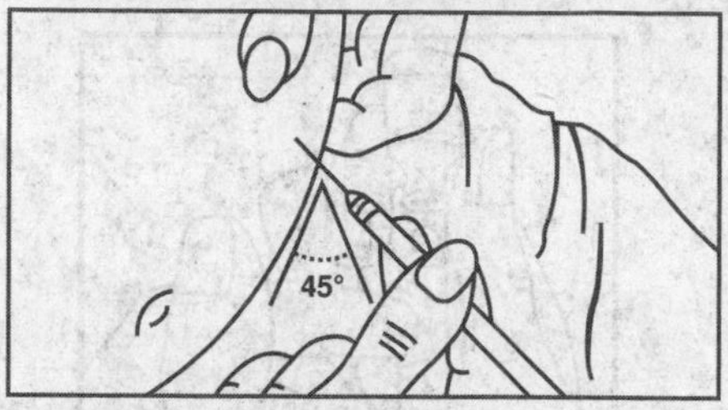

Figure R

- Let go of the skin and slowly push in on the plunger until the syringe is empty (Figure S).

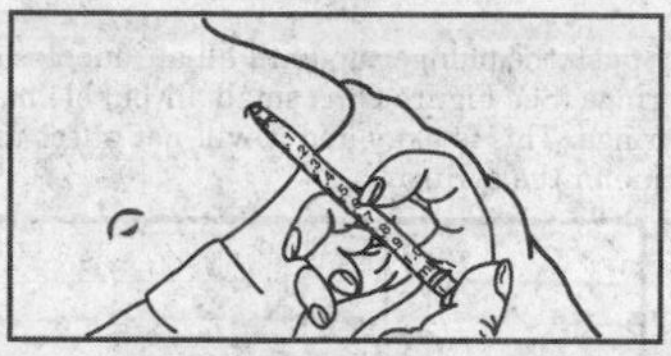

Figure S

- When the syringe is empty, quickly pull the needle out of the skin, being careful to keep it at the same angle as it was inserted. There may be a little bleeding at the injection site.
- Hold a cotton ball or gauze over the injection site (Figure T). Do not rub the injection site. Apply an adhesive bandage to the injection site if needed.

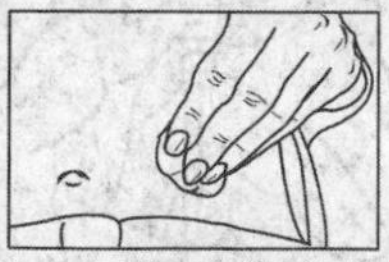

Figure T

Step 5: Dispose of used syringes and needles

- **Do not** re-use a syringe or needle.
- To avoid needle-stick injuries, **do not** recap a used needle.
- Put your used needles and syringes in a FDA-cleared sharps disposal container right away after use. **Do not throw away (dispose of) loose needles and syringes in your household trash.**
- If you do not have a FDA-cleared sharps disposal container, you may use a household container that is:
  - made of a heavy-duty plastic,
  - can be closed with a tight-fitting, puncture-resistant lid, without sharps being able to come out,
  - upright and stable during use,
  - leak-resistant, and
  - properly labeled to warn of hazardous waste inside the container.
- When your sharps disposal container is almost full, you will need to follow your community guidelines for the right way to dispose of your sharps disposal container. There may be state or local laws about how you should throw away used needles and syringes. For more information about safe sharps disposal, and for specific information about sharps disposal in the state that you live in, go to the FDA's website at: http://www.fda.gov/safesharpsdisposal.
- Do not dispose of your used sharps disposal container in your household trash unless your community guidelines permit this. Do not recycle your used sharps disposal container.
- If you have any questions, talk to your healthcare provider or pharmacist.

How should I store RELISTOR?

- Store RELISTOR vials at room temperature between 68°F to 77°F (20°C to 25°C).
- Do not freeze RELISTOR.
- Keep RELISTOR away from light until you are ready to use it.
- If RELISTOR has been drawn into a syringe and you are unable to use the medicine right away, keep the syringe at room temperature for up to 24 hours. The syringe does not need to be kept away from light during the 24-hour period.

Keep RELISTOR and all medicines, needles and syringes out of the reach of children.

This Instructions for Use has been approved by the U.S. Food and Drug Administration.

Manufactured for:
Salix Pharmaceuticals, Inc.
Raleigh, NC 27615
Under license from:
Progenics Pharmaceuticals, Inc.
Tarrytown, NY 10591
Revised AUG 2013
Product protected by U.S. Patent Nos. 6,559,158, 8,247,425, and 8,420,663.
See www.salix.com for patent information

Shown in Product Identification Guide, page 313

SOLESTA® ℞

CAUTION: Federal Law restricts this device to sale by or on the order of a physician.

Indication for Use

Solesta® is indicated for the treatment of fecal incontinence in patients 18 years and older who have failed conservative therapy (e.g., diet, fiber therapy, anti-motility medications).

Device Description

Solesta consists of dextranomer microspheres, 50 mg/mL, and stabilized sodium hyaluronate, 15 mg/mL, in phosphate-buffered 0.9% sodium chloride solution.

Solesta is a sterile, viscous, biocompatible bulking agent contained in a disposable 1 mL assembled glass syringe with a standard Luer-lock fitting. The syringe is equipped with a plunger stopper, a plunger rod and a finger grip. The labeled syringe is packed in a pouch and terminally sterilized by moist heat. The final product consists of a carton containing four pouches with syringes, five sterile needles (Sterican®, 21G × 4 ¾ inches, 0.80 × 120 mm), patient record labels and a package insert. The product is for single use.

Both the dextranomer and sodium hyaluronate are made up of biosynthesized polysaccharides of non-animal origin. The dextranomer component consists of microspheres of dextran chains cross-linked into a three-dimensional network. The stabilized sodium hyaluronate accounts for the viscous properties of Solesta and acts as a carrier that facilitates the injection of the dextranomer microspheres.

Solesta is injected in the deep submucosal layer in the proximal part of the high pressure zone of the anal canal about 5 mm above the dentate line. A total of four submucosal injections of 1 mL Solesta are administered at each treatment session.

Contraindications

Solesta is contraindicated in patients with the following conditions:

- Active inflammatory bowel disease
- Immunodeficiency disorders or ongoing immunosuppressive therapy
- Previous radiation treatment to the pelvic area
- Significant mucosal or full thickness rectal prolapse
- Active anorectal conditions including: abscess, fissures, sepsis, bleeding, proctitis, or other infections
- Anorectal atresia, tumors, stenosis or malformation
- Rectocele
- Rectal varices
- Presence of existing implant (other than Solesta) in anorectal region
- Allergy to hyaluronic acid based products

Warnings

- Do not inject Solesta intravascularly. Injection of Solesta into blood vessels may cause vascular occlusion.
- Injection in the midline of the anterior wall of the rectum should be avoided in men with enlarged prostate.

Precautions

General precautions

- Solesta should only be administered by physicians experienced in performing anorectal procedures and who have successfully completed a comprehensive training and certification program in the Solesta injection procedure.
- The safety and effectiveness of Solesta have not been investigated in patients with complete external sphincter disruption or significant chronic anorectal pain.
- The safety and effectiveness of Solesta have not been investigated in patients with previous procedures involving the anorectal region: rectal anastomosis <12 cm from anal verge, anorectal surgery within previous 12 months, hemorrhoid treatment with rubber band within 3 months, anorectal implants and previous injection therapy, Stapled Transanal Rectal Resection (STARR) or stapled hemorrhoidectomy.
- The safety and effectiveness of Solesta have not been studied in patients under the age of 18 years.
- The safety and effectiveness of Solesta have not been studied in pregnant or breastfeeding women.
- The durability of Solesta has not been studied past 12 months.
- The safety and effectiveness of Solesta have been studied in patients who received one or two treatments. In the Pivotal study, the majority of patients received two treatments, four weeks apart.

Patient related precautions

- Patients with bleeding diathesis or patients using anticoagulant or antiplatelet agents, as with any injections, may experience increased bleeding at injection sites.
- Patients should be counseled that a repeated Solesta injection procedure may be required to achieve a satisfactory level of improvement in incontinence.

Procedure related precautions

- Adequate bowel preparation of the rectum using enema is required prior to injection. The enema should be given immediately prior to the procedure to ensure evacuation of the anorectum. It is recommended that additional cleansing of the injection area with an antiseptic be performed prior to injection. Use of prophylactic antibiotics is recommended.
- Solesta should be injected slowly to avoid undue stress on the Luer-lock connection which could cause leakage of the gel.
- After injection of Solesta, hold the needle at the injection site for an additional 15-30 seconds to minimize leakage of Solesta.
- Injections too close to the dentate line or too deep in the tissue might cause excessive pain.
- Injection should be stopped if excessive bleeding or pain occurs.
- One sterile needle should be used per syringe and injection.

Device related precautions

- The use of needles other than those supplied may impede injection of Solesta due to the properties of the gel and may cause device malfunction.
- Solesta is supplied ready to use in a prefilled syringe with a Luer-lock fitting. Carefully examine the unit to verify that neither the contents nor the package has been damaged in shipment. Do not use if damaged.
- Solesta is supplied sterile and is intended for single use only. Do not re-sterilize, as this may damage or alter the product.
- In the event of accidental contamination of a needle, discard the needle.
- Never mix Solesta with other products.
- Solesta is to be stored at up to 25°C (77°F), and used prior to the expiration date printed on the label. Do not expose Solesta to either sunlight or freezing, as this may damage or alter the product.
- Care should be taken when handling the glass syringes and disposing of broken glass to avoid laceration or other injury.
- After use, syringes and needles should be handled as potential biohazards. Disposal should be in accordance with accepted medical practice and applicable local, state and federal requirements.

Adverse Events

Potential adverse events include: abdominal discomfort, abdominal distension, abdominal pain, lower abdominal pain, abdominal rigidity, alopecia, anal abscess, anal fissure, anal hemorrhage, anal prolapse, anal pruritus, anorectal discomfort, back pain, constipation, C-reactive protein increased, chills, cold sweat, defecation urgency, dermatitis, diarrhea, device dislocation, dizziness, dyspareunia, escherichia bacteremia, fecal incontinence, feces hard, fatigue, gastrointestinal motility disorder, gastrointestinal pain, genital discharge, genital prolapse, hematochezia, hematospermia, hemorrhoids, infection, injection site abscess, injection site discomfort, injection site hemorrhage, injection site hematoma, injection site inflammation, injection site irritation, injection site nodule, injection site pain, injection site pustule, injection site swelling, injection site ulcer, intestinal mass, malaise, mucosal inflammation, musculoskeletal pain, perineal abscess, nausea, edema, pain, painful defecation, pelvic mass, perineal pain, proctalgia, proctitis, pyrexia, rectal abscess, rectal discharge, rectal hemorrhage, rectal lesion, rectal obstruction, rectal prolapse, rectal spasm, rectal tenesmus, rectovaginal septum abscess, urinary retention, vaginal discharge, vulvovaginal pain. The adverse event profile of Solesta beyond 18 months is not known, but is under investigation in post-market studies. The observed adverse events are discussed in the Clinical Studies section below.

Clinical Studies

Introduction

Clinical data supporting the safety and effectiveness of Solesta are available from three clinical studies: 1) a pivotal, prospective, multicenter, randomized, sham-controlled double-blind study of 206 patients conducted under an Investigational Device Exemption (IDE; Pivotal study), 2) a prospective, multicenter, open-label study of 115 patients conducted outside the United States (Open-Label study), and 3) a single center study of 34 patients conducted at one site in Sweden (Proof-of-Concept study). The Pivotal study also included a cross-over option for patients initially randomized to Sham. The majority of patients (over 84%) in all three studies were female.

Table 1 provides an overview of the design of the three studies.

[See table 1 above]

Table 1: Comparison of the three clinical studies supporting safety and effectiveness of Solesta

	Pivotal Study	Open-Label Study	Proof-of-Concept Study
Study Design	Randomized double-blind comparative study of Solesta versus Sham in 2:1 ratio	Open study	Open study
Primary Efficacy Endpoints	Effectiveness: (1) Superiority in proportion $Responder_{50}$ compared with Sham at 6 months (2) Durability of response based on proportion responders at 12 months	Effectiveness: Proportion $Responder_{50}$ at 12 months	Effectiveness: Proportion $Responder_{50}$ at 12 and 24 months
Secondary Efficacy Variables	Fecal Incontinence Quality of Life (FIQL) Scale	FIQL	SF-36 European Organization for Research and Treatment of Cancer (EORTC) QLQ-C30
	Cleveland Clinic Florida Incontinence Score (CCFIS)	CCFIS	Miller Score
	Fecal Incontinence (FI) free days	FI free days	FI free days
	Fecal Incontinence (FI) episodes, controlled bowel emptying medications	FI episodes, controlled bowel emptying medications	FI episodes, global evaluation by patient, patient subjective judgment of treatment effect
Investigational Centers	8 centers in US and 5 centers in Europe	14 centers in Europe and 1 center in Canada	1 center in Sweden
Sample Size	136 patients randomized to Solesta and 70 patients randomized to Sham	115 patients	34 patients
Inclusion Criteria	Age 18-75 years	Age 18-80 years	Age 18-80 years
	≥ 4 FI episodes over 14 days in patient diary	≥ 4 FI episodes over 28 days in patient diary	At least one FI episode weekly
	CCFI ≥ 10	CCFI ≥ 5	Miller score CCFI ≥ 6
	Solid or liquid FI episodes	Solid or liquid FI episodes	Solid or liquid FI episodes
	Failed conservative treatment	Failed conservative treatment	
Exclusion Criteria	Complete external sphincter disruption, significant mucosal prolapse	Complete external sphincter disruption, significant mucosal prolapse	Complete external sphincter disruption, significant mucosal prolapse
Retreatment Criteria	Incontinent at one month after initial treatment and CCFIS ≥ 10	Incontinent at one month after initial treatment	Some subjective improvement but less than 50% reduction in FI episodes

The Pivotal study is the primary data set that demonstrates the safety and effectiveness of Solesta. The Open-Label and Proof-of-Concept studies provide supporting evidence of safety and effectiveness.

Treatment Information

Pre-operative Bowel Preparation

Pre-treatment evacuation of the rectum was done with an enema in the majority of the patients in all 3 studies. A small number of patients received topical antiseptic cleansing at the discretion of the treating physician. Prophylactic antibiotics were administered to individual patients in the Pivotal study at the discretion of the treating investigator and only 15 patients at 3 sites received prophylactic antibiotics in this study. No patients in the Open-Label study received prophylactic antibiotics.

Treatment Procedure

The Solesta injection procedure was the same in all 3 studies. Treatment was administered in an out-patient setting without anesthesia. Four equally spaced injections were administered through an anoscope and placed about 5 mm proximal to the dentate line. Treatment volume was generally 4 × 1 mL per treatment session. A single re-treatment procedure was offered to patients with persistent fecal incontinence after approximately 1 month. The maximum total treatment dose was 8 mL. In the Pivotal study, the sham injection procedure consisted of using 4 separate syringes to pierce the mucosa. The syringes were held in place for the same amount of time as Solesta injection: however, nothing was injected.

Patient Demographics

Both of the multicenter studies enrolled subjects with a broad range of age and body mass index. The majority of patients enrolled in both studies were females. Over 10% of patients enrolled in the Pivotal study were African-Americans, Hispanics or Asians. The causes of FI in both studies were attributed mainly to obstetric cause, neurogenic cause, and iatrogenic cause based on available medical history.

Table 2 provides an overview of the patient demographics in the Pivotal study. The Open-Label study and the Proof-of-Concept study enrolled patients with similar demographics.

Table 2: Demographics in the Pivotal study

		Pivotal Study (n=206)
Female	n (%)	183 (88.8)
Age, years	Mean (range)	60.1 (29.4–76.0)
Body Mass Index (BMI), kg/m^2	Mean (range)	27.1 (17.2–44.8)
Caucasian origin	n (%)	181 (87.9)
Duration of symptoms over 5 years	n (%)	106 (51.7)
Obstetric cause	n (%)	82 (39.8)
Neurogenic cause	n (%)	43 (20.9)
Iatrogenic cause	n (%)	46 (22.3)
Other cause (mostly idiopathic)	n (%)	35 (17.0)

Safety Data

The safety evaluation of Solesta in the treatment of fecal incontinence (FI) is based on the results from the Pivotal clinical study, and is supported by the Open-Label multicenter clinical study and one single site Proof-of-Concept study. The analysis of safety was based on the safety cohort of all 206 patients treated in the Pivotal study with either Solesta or Sham. Safety data for Solesta are available from 359 treatments in 197 total patients followed for up to 18 months post treatment (i.e., 136 subjects from the blinded phase and 61 subjects from the open phase).

The primary safety data set includes data from 206 patients treated with either Solesta or Sham in the Pivotal study. The data show that a total of 232 treatment-related adverse events for either Solesta or Sham were reported up to 18 months after treatment. Three (3) adverse events assessed as related to Solesta, or 1.3% of the treatment-related adverse events, were deemed serious by the investigators. These three (3) serious adverse events occurred in three (3) patients, including one case of an E. coli bacteremia, and two (2) cases of rectal abscesses (one event per patient). All of these serious adverse events resolved following treatment without any sequelae within approximately 30 days of treatment.

Overall, 96% of the 203 Solesta treatment-related adverse events in the Pivotal study were of mild to moderate intensity and 97% of the events required no intervention or required medical or simple non-invasive interventions, including application of local pressure, silicone ointment, water irrigation and warm baths. Seven (7) events required more invasive procedures including: perianal drainage of abscesses (4 events), one (1) case of rubber band ligation of an anal prolapse, one (1) case of lancing of a hemorrhoid, and one (1) case of a Kenalog injection in a pre-existing anal scar. As shown in Table 3, the most frequent adverse events following Solesta treatment pertained to post-treatment proctalgia, minor anal or rectal bleeding, post-treatment fever, abdominal complaints (such as diarrhea and constipation), and events potentially related to peri-operative infection.

Combined with the supportive studies, a total of 346 patients received 566 treatments with Solesta. All three studies utilized similar inclusion/exclusion criteria and all three studies used exactly the same procedure for administering Solesta. The multi-center Open-Label study demonstrated similar safety results as the Pivotal study. A total of 163 AEs were reported by 71 of the 115 patients treated with Solesta in the study. Of these AEs, 79 AEs reported by 44 patients (38%) were assessed by the investigators to be related to the study treatment. Thus, the incidence of treatment-related AEs per total number of performed treatments was 51.3% (79 events/154 treatments). Similar to the Pivotal study, the five (5) most frequently reported types of treatment-related AEs were proctalgia, pyrexia, constipation, diarrhea and injection site pain. Six (6) treatment-related AEs reported in 4 patients were classified as serious in the study. Three (3) of these serious and treatment-related adverse events were cases of abscess reported by three (3) patients and the remaining three (3) were reported by a single patient who had a rectal prolapse with concurrent rectal bleeding and pain. In this latter case, tissues surrounding a Solesta bulge had prolapsed downwards in the anal canal and the Solesta bulge was excised in surgery.

In the Proof-of-Concept study, 34 patients were treated in the study and 33 patients were followed for 24 months. In total, 53 treatments with Solesta were administered in the study. These patients experienced a total of 86 treatment-related adverse events that were reported by 29 patients. No treatment-related adverse event was reported as seri-

Table 3: Related adverse events (including serious AEs) for patients with blinded or open-label treatment with Solesta through month 18 in the Pivotal study. MedDRA Preferred Term. Safety population (n=197)

MedDRA Preferred Term	Number and (%) of patients	Number of events	Maximum intensity			Median (days)		Intervention			% of events resolved
			Mild	Moderate	Severe	Time to onset	Duration	None	Medical treatment	Other*	
Abdominal discomfort	1 (0.5)	1	.	1	.	1.0	6.0	.	.	1	100%
Abdominal distension	1 (0.5)	1	.	1	.	0.0	3.0	1	.	.	100%
Abdominal pain	1 (0.5)	1	.	1	.	68.0	52.0	.	1	.	100%
Abdominal pain lower	2 (1.0)	2	2	.	.	30.5	60.0	2	.	.	100%
Abdominal rigidity	1 (0.5)	1	.	1	.	196.0	.	.	1	.	0% †
Alopecia	1 (0.5)	1	.	.	1	6.0	189.0	1	.	.	100%
Anal abscess	1 (0.5)	1	.	1	.	139.0	44.0	.	.	1	100%
Anal fissure	2 (1.0)	2	1	1	.	90.5	228.0	.	2	.	100%
Anal hemorrhage‡	8 (4.1)	9	7	2	.	1.0	4.0	7	.	2	100%
Anal prolapse	3 (1.5)	3	2	1	.	287.0	2.0	1	.	2	100%
Anal pruritus	3 (1.5)	4	4	.	.	49.0	72.0	3	1	.	100%
Anorectal discomfort	8 (4.1)	8	7	1	.	2.0	21.0	3	5	.	100%
Back pain	1 (0.5)	1	1	.	.	70.0	113.0	.	.	1	100%
C-reactive protein increased	1 (0.5)	1	.	1	.	11.0	18.0	1	.	.	100%
Chills	4 (2.0)	4	1	2	1	0.5	4.5	4	.	.	100%
Cold sweat	1 (0.5)	1	.	1	.	0.0	3.0	1	.	.	100%
Constipation	3 (1.5)	3	3	.	.	3.0	2.0	1	2	.	100%
Defecation urgency	2 (1.0)	2	2	.	.	2.5	4.5	1	1	.	100%
Dermatitis	1 (0.5)	1	1	.	.	90.0	79.0	.	.	1	100%
Device dislocation	1 (0.5)	1	1	.	.	260.0	14.0	.	.	1	100%
Diarrhea	8 (4.1)	10	9	1	.	2.5	5.0	4	6	.	100%
Dyspareunia	2 (1.0)	2	2	.	.	65.0	60.5	2	.	.	100%
Escherichia bacteremia	1 (0.5)	1	.	1	.	0.0	36.0	.	1	.	100%
Fecal incontinence	1 (0.5)	1	.	1	.	0.0	64.0	1	.	.	100%
Feces hard	1 (0.5)	1	1	.	.	15.0	63.0	1	.	.	100%
Fatigue	1 (0.5)	1	.	1	.	0.0	3.0	1	.	.	100%
Gastrointestinal motility disorder	1 (0.5)	1	1	.	.	226.0	117.0	1	.	.	100%
Gastrointestinal pain	1 (0.5)	1	.	1	.	0.0	8.0	1	.	.	100%
Genital prolapse	1 (0.5)	1	.	1	.	1.0	10.0	.	.	1	100%
Hemorrhoids	1 (0.5)	1	.	1	.	0.0	6.0	.	.	1	100%
Injection site hemorrhage‡	16 (8.1)	18	18	.	.	0.0	1.0	17	.	1	100%
Injection site inflammation	1 (0.5)	1	1	.	.	0.0	5.0	.	1	.	100%
Injection site irritation	1 (0.5)	1	1	.	.	28.0	8.0	1	.	.	100%
Injection site nodule	1 (0.5)	1	1	.	.	294.0	99.0	1	.	.	100%
Injection site pain	10 (5.1)	10	7	3	.	0.0	1.5	9	1	.	100%
Injection site pustule	1 (0.5)	1	1	.	.	0.0	22.0	.	1	.	100%
Injection site swelling	1 (0.5)	1	1	.	.	0.0	78.0	1	.	.	100%
Intestinal mass	1 (0.5)	1	1	.	.	196.0	14.0	.	.	1	100%
Mucosal inflammation	1 (0.5)	1	1	.	.	27.0	74.0	1	.	.	100%
Musculoskeletal pain	1 (0.5)	1	1	.	.	358.0	183.0	1	.	.	100%
Nausea	1 (0.5)	1	1	.	.	0.0	3.0	1	.	.	100%
Pain ("body aches")	2 (1.0)	2	.	1	1	1.5	5.0	2	.	.	100%
Painful defecation	2 (1.0)	2	2	.	.	1.5	132.5	1	.	1	100%

(Table continued on next page)

Table 3 *(cont.)*: Related adverse events (including serious AEs) for patients with blinded or open-label treatment with Solesta through month 18 in the Pivotal study. MedDRA Preferred Term. Safety population (n=197)

MedDRA Preferred Term	Number and (%) of patients	Number of events	Maximum intensity			Median (days)		Intervention			% of events resolved
			Mild	Moderate	Severe	Time to onset	Duration	None	Medical treatment	Other*	
Pelvic mass	1 (0.5)	1	.	1	.	2.0	27.0	.	1	.	100%
Perineal pain	1 (0.5)	1	.	1	.	0.0	5.0	1	.	.	100%
Proctalgia	34 (17.3)	41	20	21	.	1.0	8.0	14	19	8	97.6% §
Proctitis	5 (2.5)	5	2	2	1	5.0	16.0	2	3	.	100%
Pyrexia	13 (6.6)	14	12	1	1	1.0	6.0	5	8	1	100%
Rectal abscess	3 (1.5)	3	.	1	2	2.0	6.0	.	1	2	100%
Rectal discharge	7 (3.5)	7	6	1	.	2.0	4.0	4	2	1	100%
Rectal hemorrhage‡	15 (7.6)	15	11	4	.	7.0	3.0	13	1	1	100%
Rectal lesion	1 (0.5)	1	.	1	.	5.0	179.0	.	.	1	100%
Rectal obstruction	2 (1.0)	2	2	.	.	75.5	66.0	2	.	.	100%
Rectal spasm	1 (0.5)	1	.	1	.	133.0	50.0	1	.	.	100%
Urinary retention	1 (0.5)	1	1	.	.	8.0	20.0	1	.	.	100%
Vaginal discharge	1 (0.5)	1	1	.	.	0.0	5.0	1	.	.	100%
Vulvovaginal pain	1 (0.5)	1	.	1	.	0.0	6.0	.	1	.	100%
Totals	**103 (52.3)**	**203**	**136**	**60**	**7**	**1.0**	**6.0**	**115**	**60**	**28**	**99.0%**

* Other intervention included: follow up ultrasound, I & D of rectal abscess, Kenalog injection to anal area scar, rubber band ligation, observation, extra check-up at clinic, Silicone or Xylocaine ointment, examinations, blood tests, feces-Hb screen, outpatient visit to gynecologist, irrigation with water, lanced hemorrhoid, pressure, irrigation-dissection of abscess, flexible sigmoidoscopy, pelvic v/s scan, warm baths, drainage of anal abscess

† Outcome for one event pending at time of this summary report (patient withdrawn and event currently recorded as not recovered)

‡ AEs reported as bleeding were coded as "hemorrhage" at the preferred term level in MedDRA regardless of intensity

§ Outcome for one event pending at time of this summary report

ous. The duration was 1- 4 days for most events and all events were resolved within 1 week. No adverse events occurred after month 12. One (1) patient gave birth to a healthy child approximately 18 months after treatment and the delivery was a normal vaginal delivery. The observed adverse events were similar to those seen in the Pivotal study.

[See table 3 on previous page and above]

Effectiveness

Primary Efficacy Objective - Pivotal Study

The Pivotal study included a primary efficacy objective composed of three parts. All three parts of the primary objective were met. The study was only powered for the primary endpoint and was not designed or powered to demonstrate a statistical difference between Solesta and Sham for the secondary efficacy endpoints.

Superiority was shown for Solesta (53.2%) versus Sham (30.7%) at 6 months (p=0.004; logistic regression), as illustrated in Figure 1, based on analysis of proportion Responder$_{50}$. Responder$_{50}$, defined as proportion of patients with a ≥ 50% reduction in number of incontinence episodes compared to baseline, has been used to objectively evaluate response to treatments for FI in other studies.

The second success criterion required that the results achieve a pre-specified minimum level of responders in the treatment group as defined by a lower confidence limit (LCL) of at least 35%. The LCL of the 95% confidence interval of the proportion Responder$_{50}$ at 6 months was 40.2%, as illustrated in Figure 2.

The third success criterion concerned durability of the treatment effect and required a minimum level of proportion Responder$_{25}$ (≥ 25% improvement from baseline) for Solesta at 12 months, as defined by a lower confidence limit of 50%. The LCL for proportion Responder$_{25}$ at 12 months was 61.4%, as illustrated in Figure 2.

As an additional supporting analysis, the proportion Responder$_{50}$ at 12 months after last treatment was also calculated and it was 57.4%, similar to the results at 6 months. Analyses were performed to determine whether there was any association between baseline or demographic characteristics and treatment response. No such relationship was found.

[See figure 1 at top of next column]

Primary Endpoint Pivotal and Supporting Studies

All three studies show durability of the treatment effect to 12 months as evidenced by the proportion Responder$_{50}$. As shown in Table 4 the proportion Responder$_{50}$ at 6 months and 12 months were similar across all three studies.

Figure 1. Comparison of proportion Responder$_{50}$ at 6 months

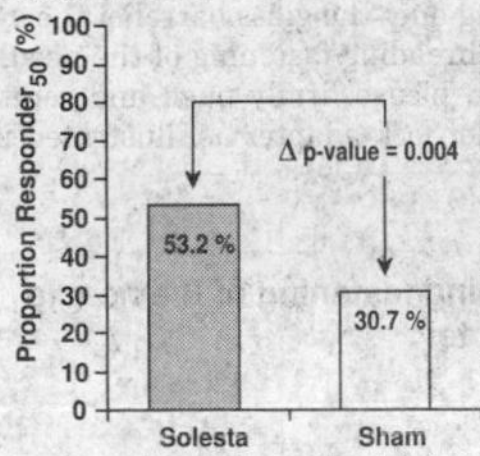

Figure 2. Solesta proportion responders at 6 and 12 months

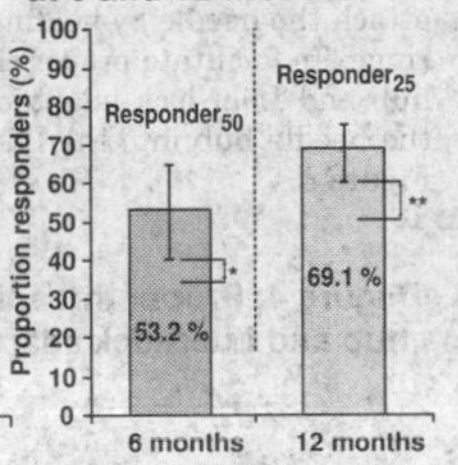

* Responder$_{50}$ LCL = 40.2 % > 35 %
** Responder$_{25}$ LCL = 61.4 % > 50 %

Table 4: Summary of proportion Responder$_{50}$ at 6 and 12 months and at 24 months with Solesta treatment

Proportion Responder$_{50}$ [95% CI]	Pivotal study (ITT, PIM)	Open-Label Study (ITT, OC)	Proof-of-Concept Study (OC)
6 months	53.2% [40.2–65.8] n= 136	57.1% [47.3–66.9] n=98	44.1% [27.4–60.8] n=34
12 months	57.4% [49.0–65.7] n=136	64.0% [53.8–74.1] n=86	55.9% [39.2–72.6] n=34
24 months	N/A	N/A	59.4% [42.4–76.4] n=32

CI = confidence interval; ITT = intent-to-treat; PIM = primary imputation model; OC = observed cases; n = number of subjects

Secondary Endpoints for Pivotal and Supporting Studies

The following secondary endpoints were evaluated in the three clinical studies:

- Fecal incontinence episodes
- Fecal incontinence-free days
- Fecal Incontinence Quality of Life (FIQL) assessment
- Cleveland Clinic Florida Incontinence Score (CCFIS) or Miller Score

Fecal Incontinence Episodes

In the Pivotal study, reductions in number of FI episodes from baseline at both 3 and 6 months were observed in both the Solesta and Sham treatment groups. For the Solesta group the median FI episodes were shown to decrease from 15 episodes at baseline to 7.2 episodes at 6 months and 6.2 episodes at 12 months. For the Sham group the median FI episodes were shown to decrease from 12.5 episodes at baseline to 10.0 episodes at 6 months (see Table 5). Both the Solesta and Sham groups showed a change from baseline at 6 months, and the change from baseline in the Solesta group was larger than that observed for the Sham group. Similar reductions from baseline with Solesta treatment were observed in the Open-Label study and the Proof-of-Concept study.

Figure 3 shows the sustained improvement in Responder$_{50}$ analysis and reduction in fecal incontinence episodes over 12 months in the Pivotal study for the Solesta group only.

Table 5: Median number of fecal incontinence episodes/14 days for each treatment group and change from baseline 6 months. As observed. Last Observation Carried Forward (LOCF). ITT population (n=206 patients: Pivotal study)

Number of episodes	Solesta (n=136) Median	Sham (n=70) Median	Difference in median changes between groups (Solesta-Sham)
Baseline	15.0	12.5	
6 months	7.2	10.0	
Δ from baseline	-6.0	-3.0	-3.0
% Δ from baseline	-50.6	-22.6	-28.0

[See figure 3 at top of next column]

Fecal Incontinence-free Days

In all three studies, an increase in number of fecal incontinence-free days was observed with Solesta treatment. In the Pivotal study at 6 months, both the Solesta and Sham treatment groups experienced an increase in number

Table 6: Secondary efficacy evaluations of difference in change from baseline between Solesta and Sham at 6 months. LOCF. ITT population (n=206 patients: Pivotal study)

Secondary endpoints	Score/Scale range	Estimate of mean change from baseline		Estimate of Difference (95% CI)
		Solesta	Sham	
Fecal Incontinence Quality of Life (FIQL) scale (higher score = increased QoL)				
Lifestyle*	1-4	0.33	0.11	0.22 (0.04:0.40)
Coping/Behavior*	1-4	0.44	0.19	0.25 (0.08:0.43)
Depression/Self perception*	1-6	0.27	0.18	0.09 (-0.08:0.26)
Cleveland Clinic Florida Incontinence Score (CCFIS)				
CCFIS score†	0 = continent; 20 = total incontinence	-3.06	-2.85	-0.21 (-1.15:0.72)

* Positive value indicates improvement; † Negative value indicate improvement

Figure 3. Median number of FI episodes and proportion Responder$_{50}$ at each follow up time point in the Pivotal study. Solesta ITT population (n=136)

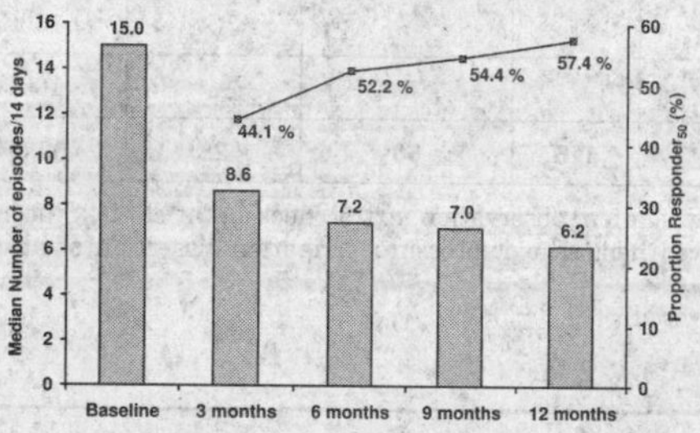

of incontinence free days from their pre-treatment baseline values of 4.4 days and 4.8 days, respectively. However, the Solesta group demonstrated an increase of 3.1 fecal incontinence-free days when compared to the Sham group increase of 2.0 days. At 12 months, the increase in number of fecal incontinence-free days in the Solesta group was maintained at 3.4 days. Similar increases in number of fecal incontinence-free days with Solesta treatment were shown in the Open-Label study and the Proof-of-Concept study.

Fecal Incontinence Quality of Life assessment (FIQL)

The FIQL scale is a validated tool that is specifically designed to assess the impact of FI on a patient's quality of life. In the blinded phase of the Pivotal study, improvement in FIQL scores compared to baseline was observed in both the Solesta and Sham groups at 6 months. The change from baseline score was greater in the Solesta group than the Sham group in all four domains: Lifestyle (Δ=0.22), Coping/Behavior (Δ=0.25), Depression/Self perception (Δ=0.09) and Embarrassment domains (Δ=0.16), (see Table 6). In the Open-Label study, FIQL scores showed a similar improvement. The Proof-of-Concept study did not evaluate FIQL.

Cleveland Clinic Florida Incontinence Score (CCFIS)

The CCFIS is a validated measure of the impact of FI on patients. In the pivotal study, in both the Solesta and Sham groups, the CCFIS was improved as compared to baseline at 6 months. The difference at 6 months in mean change from baseline between the Solesta group and the Sham group was small (see Table 6). Solesta showed improvements from baseline at 12 months in both the Pivotal study and the Open-Label study.

The Proof-of-Concept study did not incorporate CCFIS but instead used the Miller Score, another assessment tool for FI. The Miller Score is based on a subject interview using standardized questions regarding incidence and type of incontinence (solid, liquid or gas). Improvements from baseline and sustained improvements were shown at 6, 12, and 24 months.

[See table 6 above]

Patient Counseling Information

The patient should be advised that Solesta treatment is not effective for all patients with fecal incontinence and that repeat treatment might be required for treatment effect. It should also be made clear to the patient that the available clinical study data are not sufficient to predict in whom Solesta treatment will be effective. The patient should be informed about post-treatment care and potential adverse events. The patient should also be made aware that the implants might be detected during future anorectal examinations and radiographic imaging of the pelvis. Patients should be instructed to inform all future treating physicians about the presence of Solesta gel.

If there should be a need for future surgery (e.g., hemorrhoidectomy) the Solesta implant can be resected.

Directions for Use

Solesta should be administered by qualified physicians with experience in the treatment of anorectal conditions and who have successfully completed a comprehensive training and certification program in the Solesta injection procedure. Solesta should only be used after a thorough physical evaluation of the patient to exclude treatable underlying disorders.

For the safe use of Solesta it is important that a new sterile needle is properly assembled and tightly fastened to each syringe.

Please note that the Luer-lock adapter is snapped onto the syringe and held in place with friction only. It can rotate freely or be pulled off should enough force be applied. Because of this it is recommended that the thumb and forefinger be held firmly around the Luer-lock adapter on the glass syringe while attaching the needle to the syringe. DO NOT attach the needle by holding onto the glass barrel of the syringe. To facilitate proper threading/fastening of the needle hub and Luer-lock adapter, please firmly push and rotate the needle hub into the Luer-lock adapter as illustrated in Figure 4.

Figure 4: Proper threading/fastening of the needle hub and Luer-lock adapter

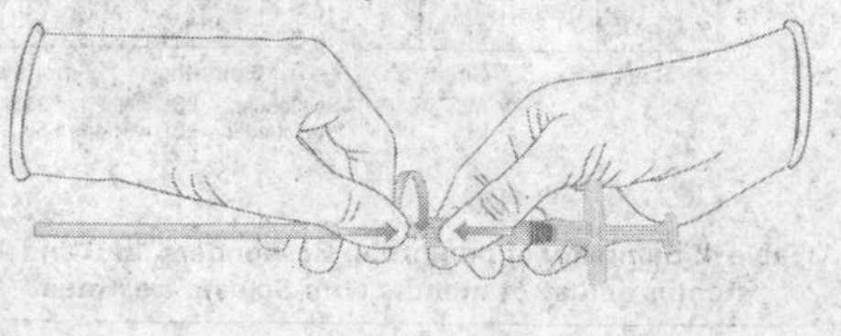

To avoid any interruption in patient treatment or the need to repeat a procedure because of leakage, or accidental contamination or damage of a syringe or needle, it is recommended that extra Solesta cartons be kept in inventory.

Method of Administration

1. The treatment is administered as an outpatient procedure without anesthesia.
2. Prior to treatment, the rectum should be evacuated with an enema. The enema should be given immediately prior to the procedure to ensure evacuation of the anorectum. Additional cleansing of the injection area with an antiseptic may be performed prior to injection.
3. Use of prophylactic antibiotics is recommended.
4. Four Solesta syringes should be made ready with mounted needles under aseptic conditions. Have small swabs and suction prepared and ready for use.
5. The patient is placed in the left lateral position, and a lubricated anoscope is inserted. The obturator is removed and the anoscope withdrawn so that the dentate line is identified.
6. The four injections are to be given in the following order: posterior, left lateral, anterior, and right lateral.
7. The injections should be performed slowly to avoid stress on the Luer-lock connection and allow the tissue to adapt to the injected gel.
8. Under direct vision, the mucosa is penetrated, approximately 5 mm proximal to the dentate line. The needle is advanced a further 5 mm at approximately 30° to the axis of the rectum. If the patient indicates pain at the puncture, the injection site should be adjusted a few mm in the cephalic direction. If the puncture is painless, 1 mL of Solesta is injected in the deep submucosal layer. After injection, the needle should be kept in position for 15-30 seconds to minimize leakage of Solesta.
9. The injection is to be repeated at the remaining three injection sites. A new needle should be used for each syringe and injection site.
10. After completion of the 4 injections, the anoscope is extracted and the patient may rise. The patient should be instructed to rest at the clinic for approximately 60 minutes.
11. If no bleeding or other treatment related symptoms are observed during this time, the patient can be allowed to leave the clinic.
12. Confirming placement of Solesta gel by imaging may be of benefit.

Post-treatment care

1. The patient should be instructed to avoid taking hot baths during the first 24 hours post-treatment.
2. The patient should be informed of the risk of infections and bleeding.
3. The patient should be instructed to contact the clinic or physician's office immediately if symptoms of rectal bleeding, bloody diarrhea, fever, tenesmus or problems with urinating occur.
4. Anti-diarrheal drugs should not be used for one week after treatment.
5. Stool softeners may be used until the first defecation occurs.
6. Analgesics other than Non-steroidal Anti-inflammatory Drugs (NSAIDs) may be prescribed, if needed.
7. The patient should be instructed to:
   - Avoid physical activity for 24 hours
   - Avoid sexual intercourse and strenuous physical activity for one week (e.g., horse back riding, bicycling and jogging, etc.)
   - Avoid anal manipulation for one month (e.g., insertion of suppositories or enemas and rectal temperature recording)

Re-treatment procedure

1. If the patient does not have an adequate response to Solesta after the first injection, a re-injection with a maximum of 4 mL Solesta can be performed, no sooner than 4 weeks after the first injection.
2. The re-treatment procedure and all pretreatment preparations are performed the same way as the initial treatment procedure. All pretreatment preparations and injection procedures should be performed as described in "Methods of Administration" above. However, the point of injection should be made in between the initial injections, shifted one-eighth of a turn (e.g., left posterolateral, left anterolateral, right anterolateral, and right posterolateral).

How Supplied

Solesta is supplied in a glass syringe with a standard Luer-lock fitting containing 1 mL gel. Each syringe is terminally moist heat sterilized in a pouch. Four pouches, each containing one syringe are packed in a carton together with five Sterican needles (21G × 4¾ inches, 0.80 mm × 120 mm), patient record labels and a package insert. The needles are sterilized by ethylene oxide.

Storage

Store at a temperature up to 25°C (77°F) and protect from sunlight and freezing.

For Information

Solesta is marketed by:
Salix Pharmaceuticals, Inc.
Raleigh, NC 27615

For product information, adverse event reports, and product complaint reports, please contact:
Salix Product Information Call Center
Phone: 1-800-508-0024
Fax: 1-510-595-8183
E-mail: Salix@medcomsol.com

Manufacturer

Q-Med AB
Seminariegatan 21
SE-752 28 Uppsala
Sweden

Solesta® is manufactured utilizing the proprietary NASHA® technology.

Solesta and NASHA are registered trademarks of Q-Med AB.

XIFAXAN® ℞
(rifaximin)
Tablets

HIGHLIGHTS OF PRESCRIBING INFORMATION
These highlights do not include all the information needed to use XIFAXAN safely and effectively. See full prescribing information for XIFAXAN.
XIFAXAN® (rifaximin) Tablets
Initial U.S. Approval: 2004

To reduce the development of drug-resistant bacteria and maintain the effectiveness of XIFAXAN and other antibacterial drugs, XIFAXAN should be used only to treat or prevent infections that are proven or strongly suspected to be caused by bacteria.

RECENT MAJOR CHANGES

Indications and Usage, Hepatic Encephalopathy (1.2) 03/2010
Dosage and Administration, Hepatic Encephalopathy (2.2) 03/2010

INDICATIONS AND USAGE

XIFAXAN is a rifamycin antibacterial indicated for:
- The treatment of patients (≥ 12 years of age) with travelers' diarrhea (TD) caused by noninvasive strains of *Escherichia coli* (1.1)
- Reduction in risk of overt hepatic encephalopathy (HE) recurrence in patients ≥ 18 years of age (1.2)

Limitations of Use
- TD: Do not use in patients with diarrhea complicated by fever or blood in the stool or diarrhea due to pathogens other than *Escherichia coli* (1.1)

DOSAGE AND ADMINISTRATION

- Travelers' diarrhea: One 200 mg tablet taken orally three times a day for 3 days, with or without food (2.1)
- Hepatic encephalopathy: One 550 mg tablet taken orally two times a day, with or without food (2.2)

DOSAGE FORMS AND STRENGTHS

- 200 mg and 550 mg tablets (3)

CONTRAINDICATIONS

History of hypersensitivity to rifaximin, rifamycin antimicrobial agents, or any of the components of XIFAXAN (4.1)

WARNINGS AND PRECAUTIONS

- Travelers' Diarrhea Not Caused by *E. coli*: XIFAXAN was not effective in diarrhea complicated by fever and/or blood in the stool or diarrhea due to pathogens other than *E. coli*. If diarrhea symptoms get worse or persist for more than 24-48 hours, discontinue XIFAXAN and consider alternative antibiotics (5.1)
- *Clostridium difficile*-Associated Diarrhea: Evaluate if diarrhea occurs after therapy or does not improve or worsens during therapy (5.2)
- Hepatic Impairment: Use with caution in patients with severe (Child-Pugh C) hepatic impairment (5.4, 8.7)

ADVERSE REACTIONS

- Most common adverse reactions in travelers' diarrhea (≥ 5%): Flatulence, headache, abdominal pain, rectal tenesmus, defecation urgency and nausea (6.1)
- Most common adverse reactions in HE (≥ 10%): Peripheral edema, nausea, dizziness, fatigue, ascites, flatulence, and headache (6.1)

To report suspected adverse reactions, contact Salix Pharmaceuticals at 1-800-508-0024 and www.Salix.com or FDA at 1-800-FDA-1088 or *www.fda.gov/medwatch*

USE IN SPECIFIC POPULATIONS

- Pregnancy: Based on animal data, may cause fetal harm (8.1)
- Nursing Mothers: Discontinue nursing or drug, taking into account the importance of the drug to the mother (8.3)

See 17 for PATIENT COUNSELING INFORMATION

Revised: 11/2010

FULL PRESCRIBING INFORMATION: CONTENTS*

*** Sections or subsections omitted from the full prescribing information are not listed**

FULL PRESCRIBING INFORMATION

1 INDICATIONS AND USAGE

To reduce the development of drug-resistant bacteria and maintain the effectiveness of XIFAXAN and other antibacterial drugs, XIFAXAN when used to treat infection should be used only to treat or prevent infections that are proven or strongly suspected to be caused by susceptible bacteria. When culture and susceptibility information are available, they should be considered in selecting or modifying antibacterial therapy. In the absence of such data, local epidemiology and susceptibility patterns may contribute to the empiric selection of therapy.

1.1 Travelers' Diarrhea

XIFAXAN 200 mg is indicated for the treatment of patients (≥ 12 years of age) with travelers' diarrhea caused by noninvasive strains of *Escherichia coli [see Warnings and Precautions (5), Clinical Pharmacology (12.4) and Clinical Studies (14.1)]*.

Limitations of Use

XIFAXAN should not be used in patients with diarrhea complicated by fever or blood in the stool or diarrhea due to pathogens other than *Escherichia coli*.

1.2 Hepatic Encephalopathy

XIFAXAN 550 mg is indicated for reduction in risk of overt hepatic encephalopathy (HE) recurrence in patients ≥ 18 years of age.

In the trials of XIFAXAN for HE, 91% of the patients were using lactulose concomitantly. Differences in the treatment effect of those patients not using lactulose concomitantly could not be assessed.

XIFAXAN has not been studied in patients with MELD (Model for End-Stage Liver Disease) scores > 25, and only 8.6% of patients in the controlled trial had MELD scores over 19. There is increased systemic exposure in patients with more severe hepatic dysfunction *[see Warnings and Precautions (5.4), Use in Specific Populations (8.7), Clinical Pharmacology (12.3)]*.

2 DOSAGE AND ADMINISTRATION

2.1 Dosage for Travelers' Diarrhea

The recommended dose of XIFAXAN is one 200 mg tablet taken orally three times a day for 3 days. XIFAXAN can be administered orally, with or without food *[see Clinical Pharmacology (12.3)]*.

2.2 Dosage for Hepatic Encephalopathy

The recommended dose of XIFAXAN is one 550 mg tablet taken orally two times a day, with or without food *[see Clinical Pharmacology (12.3)]*.

3 DOSAGE FORMS AND STRENGTHS

XIFAXAN is a pink-colored biconvex tablet and is available in the following strengths:
- 200 mg – a round tablet debossed with "Sx" on one side.
- 550 mg – an oval tablet debossed with "rfx" on one side.

4 CONTRAINDICATIONS

4.1 Hypersensitivity

XIFAXAN is contraindicated in patients with a hypersensitivity to rifaximin, any of the rifamycin antimicrobial agents, or any of the components in XIFAXAN. Hypersensitivity reactions have included exfoliative dermatitis, angioneurotic edema, and anaphylaxis *[see Adverse Reactions (6.2)]*.

5 WARNINGS AND PRECAUTIONS

5.1 Travelers' Diarrhea Not Caused by *Escherichia coli*

XIFAXAN was not found to be effective in patients with diarrhea complicated by fever and/or blood in the stool or diarrhea due to pathogens other than *Escherichia coli*.

Discontinue XIFAXAN if diarrhea symptoms get worse or persist more than 24-48 hours and alternative antibiotic therapy should be considered.

XIFAXAN is not effective in cases of travelers' diarrhea due to *Campylobacter jejuni*. The effectiveness of XIFAXAN in travelers' diarrhea caused by *Shigella* spp. and *Salmonella* spp. has not been proven. XIFAXAN should not be used in patients where *Campylobacter jejuni*, *Shigella* spp., or *Salmonella* spp. may be suspected as causative pathogens.

5.2 *Clostridium difficile*-Associated Diarrhea

Clostridium difficile-associated diarrhea (CDAD) has been reported with use of nearly all antibacterial agents, including XIFAXAN, and may range in severity from mild diarrhea to fatal colitis. Treatment with antibacterial agents alters the normal flora of the colon which may lead to overgrowth of *C. difficile*.

C. difficile produces toxins A and B which contribute to the development of CDAD. Hypertoxin producing strains of *C. difficile* cause increased morbidity and mortality, as these infections can be refractory to antimicrobial therapy and may require colectomy. CDAD must be considered in all patients who present with diarrhea following antibiotic use. Careful medical history is necessary since CDAD has been reported to occur over two months after the administration of antibacterial agents.

If CDAD is suspected or confirmed, ongoing antibiotic use not directed against *C. difficile* may need to be discontinued. Appropriate fluid and electrolyte management, protein supplementation, antibiotic treatment of *C. difficile*, and surgical evaluation should be instituted as clinically indicated.

5.3 Development of Drug Resistant Bacteria

Prescribing XIFAXAN for travelers' diarrhea in the absence of a proven or strongly suspected bacterial infection or a prophylactic indication is unlikely to provide benefit to the patient and increases the risk of the development of drug-resistant bacteria.

5.4 Severe (Child-Pugh C) Hepatic Impairment

There is increased systemic exposure in patients with severe hepatic impairment. Animal toxicity studies did not achieve systemic exposures that were seen in patients with severe hepatic impairment. The clinical trials were limited to patients with MELD scores <25. Therefore, caution should be exercised when administering XIFAXAN to patients with severe hepatic impairment (Child-Pugh C) *[see Use in Specific Populations (8.7), Nonclinical Toxicology (13.2) and Clinical Studies (14.2)]*.

6 ADVERSE REACTIONS

6.1 Clinical Studies Experience

Because clinical trials are conducted under widely varying conditions, adverse reaction rates observed in the clinical trials of a drug cannot be directly compared to rates in the clinical trials of another drug and may not reflect the rates observed in practice.

Travelers' Diarrhea

The safety of XIFAXAN 200 mg taken three times a day was evaluated in patients with travelers' diarrhea consisting of 320 patients in two placebo-controlled clinical trials with 95% of patients receiving three or four days of treatment with XIFAXAN. The population studied had a mean age of 31.3 (18-79) years of which approximately 3% were ≥ 65 years old, 53% were male and 84% were White, 11% were Hispanic.

Discontinuations due to adverse reactions occurred in 0.4% of patients. The adverse reactions leading to discontinuation were taste loss, dysentery, weight decrease, anorexia, nausea and nasal passage irritation.

All adverse reactions for XIFAXAN 200 mg three times daily that occurred at a frequency ≥ 2% in the two placebo-controlled trials combined are provided in Table 1. (These include adverse reactions that may be attributable to the underlying disease.)

Table 1. All Adverse Reactions With an Incidence ≥ 2% Among Patients Receiving XIFAXAN Tablets, 200 mg Three Times Daily, in Placebo-Controlled Studies

	Number (%) of Patients	
MedDRA Preferred Term	XIFAXAN Tablets, 600 mg/day N = 320	Placebo N = 228
Flatulence	36 (11%)	45 (20%)
Headache	31 (10%)	21 (9%)

Abdominal Pain NOS*	23 (7%)	23 (10%)
Rectal Tenesmus	23 (7%)	20 (9%)
Defecation Urgency	19 (6%)	21 (9%)
Nausea	17 (5%)	19 (8%)
Constipation	12 (4%)	8 (4%)
Pyrexia	10 (3%)	10 (4%)
Vomiting NOS	7 (2%)	4 (2%)

*NOS: Not otherwise specified

The following adverse reactions, presented by body system, have also been reported in <2% of patients taking XIFAXAN in the two placebo-controlled clinical trials where the 200 mg tablet was taken three times a day for travelers' diarrhea. The following includes adverse reactions regardless of causal relationship to drug exposure.

Blood and Lymphatic System Disorders: Lymphocytosis, monocytosis, neutropenia

Ear and Labyrinth Disorders: Ear pain, motion sickness, tinnitus

Gastrointestinal Disorders: Abdominal distension, diarrhea NOS, dry throat, fecal abnormality NOS, gingival disorder NOS, inguinal hernia NOS, dry lips, stomach discomfort

General Disorders and Administration Site Conditions: Chest pain, fatigue, malaise, pain NOS, weakness

Infections and Infestations: Dysentery NOS, respiratory tract infection NOS, upper respiratory tract infection NOS

Injury and Poisoning: Sunburn

Investigations: Aspartate aminotransferase increased, blood in stool, blood in urine, weight decreased

Metabolic and Nutritional Disorders: Anorexia, dehydration

Musculoskeletal, Connective Tissue, and Bone Disorders: Arthralgia, muscle spasms, myalgia, neck pain

Nervous System Disorders: Abnormal dreams, dizziness, migraine NOS, syncope, loss of taste

Psychiatric Disorders: Insomnia

Renal and Urinary Disorders: Choluria, dysuria, hematuria, polyuria, proteinuria, urinary frequency

Respiratory, Thoracic, and Mediastinal Disorders: Dyspnea NOS, nasal passage irritation, nasopharyngitis, pharyngitis, pharyngolaryngeal pain, rhinitis NOS, rhinorrhea

Skin and Subcutaneous Tissue Disorders: Clamminess, rash NOS, sweating increased

Vascular Disorders: Hot flashes NOS

Hepatic Encephalopathy

The data described below reflect exposure to XIFAXAN 550 mg in 348 patients, including 265 exposed for 6 months and 202 exposed for more than a year (mean exposure was 364 days). The safety of XIFAXAN 550 mg taken two times a day for reducing the risk of overt hepatic encephalopathy recurrence in adult patients was evaluated in a 6-month placebo-controlled clinical trial (n = 140) and in a long term follow-up study (n = 280). The population studied had a mean age of 56.26 (range: 21-82) years; approximately 20% of the patients were ≥ 65 years old, 61% were male, 86% were White, and 4% were Black. Ninety-one percent of patients in the trial were taking lactulose concomitantly. All adverse reactions that occurred at an incidence ≥ 5% and at a higher incidence in XIFAXAN 550 mg-treated subjects than in the placebo group in the 6-month trial are provided in Table 2. (These include adverse events that may be attributable to the underlying disease).

Table 2: Adverse Reactions Occurring in ≥ 5% of Patients Receiving XIFAXAN and at a Higher Incidence Than Placebo

	Number (%) of Patients	
MedDRA Preferred Term	**XIFAXAN Tablets 550 mg TWICE DAILY N = 140**	**Placebo N = 159**
Edema peripheral	21 (15%)	13 (8%)
Nausea	20 (14%)	21 (13%)
Dizziness	18 (13%)	13 (8%)
Fatigue	17 (12%)	18 (11%)
Ascites	16 (11%)	15 (9%)
Muscle spasms	13 (9%)	11 (7%)
Pruritus	13 (9%)	10 (6%)
Abdominal pain	12 (9%)	13 (8%)
Abdominal distension	11 (8%)	12 (8%)
Anemia	11 (8%)	6 (4%)
Cough	10 (7%)	11 (7%)
Depression	10 (7%)	8 (5%)
Insomnia	10 (7%)	11 (7%)
Nasopharyngitis	10 (7%)	10 (6%)
Abdominal pain upper	9 (6%)	8 (5%)
Arthralgia	9 (6%)	4 (3%)
Back pain	9 (6%)	10 (6%)
Constipation	9 (6%)	10 (6%)
Dyspnea	9 (6%)	7 (4%)
Pyrexia	9 (6%)	5 (3%)
Rash	7 (5%)	6 (4%)

The following adverse reactions, presented by body system, have also been reported in the placebo-controlled clinical trial in greater than 2% but less than 5% of patients taking XIFAXAN 550 mg taken orally two times a day for hepatic encephalopathy. The following includes adverse events occurring at a greater incidence than placebo, regardless of causal relationship to drug exposure.

Ear and Labyrinth Disorders: Vertigo

Gastrointestinal Disorders: Abdominal pain lower, abdominal tenderness, dry mouth, esophageal variceal bleed, stomach discomfort

General Disorders and Administration Site Conditions: Chest pain, generalized edema, influenza like illness, pain NOS

Infections and Infestations: Cellulitis, pneumonia, rhinitis, upper respiratory tract infection NOS

Injury, Poisoning and Procedural Complications: Contusion, fall, procedural pain

Investigations: Weight increased

Metabolic and Nutritional Disorders: Anorexia, dehydration, hyperglycemia, hyperkalemia, hypoglycemia, hyponatremia

Musculoskeletal, Connective Tissue, and Bone Disorders: Myalgia, pain in extremity

Nervous System Disorders: Amnesia, disturbance in attention, hypoesthesia, memory impairment, tremor

Psychiatric Disorders: Confusional state

Respiratory, Thoracic, and Mediastinal Disorders: Epistaxis

Vascular Disorders: Hypotension

6.2 Postmarketing Experience

The following adverse reactions have been identified during post approval use of XIFAXAN. Because these reactions are reported voluntarily from a population of unknown size, estimates of frequency cannot be made. These reactions have been chosen for inclusion due to either their seriousness, frequency of reporting or causal connection to XIFAXAN.

Infections and Infestations

Cases of *C. difficile*-associated colitis have been reported *[see Warnings and Precautions (5.2)]*.

General

Hypersensitivity reactions, including exfoliative dermatitis, rash, angioneurotic edema (swelling of face and tongue and difficulty swallowing), urticaria, flushing, pruritus and anaphylaxis have been reported. These events occurred as early as within 15 minutes of drug administration.

7 DRUG INTERACTIONS

In vitro studies have shown that rifaximin did not inhibit cytochrome P450 isoenzymes 1A2, 2A6, 2B6, 2C9, 2C19, 2D6, 2E1 and CYP3A4 at concentrations ranging from 2 to 200 ng/mL *[see Clinical Pharmacology (12.3)]*. Rifaximin is not expected to inhibit these enzymes in clinical use.

An *in vitro* study has suggested that rifaximin induces CYP3A4 *[see Clinical Pharmacology (12.3)]*. However, in patients with normal liver function, rifaximin at the recommended dosing regimen is not expected to induce CYP3A4. It is unknown whether rifaximin can have a significant effect on the pharmacokinetics of concomitant CYP3A4 substrates in patients with reduced liver function who have elevated rifaximin concentrations.

An *in vitro* study suggested that rifaximin is a substrate of P-glycoprotein. It is unknown whether concomitant drugs that inhibit P-glycoprotein can increase the systemic exposure of rifaximin *[see Clinical Pharmacology (12.3)]*.

8 USE IN SPECIFIC POPULATIONS

8.1 Pregnancy

Pregnancy Category C

There are no adequate and well controlled studies in pregnant women. Rifaximin has been shown to be teratogenic in rats and rabbits at doses that caused maternal toxicity. XIFAXAN tablets should be used during pregnancy only if the potential benefit justifies the potential risk to the fetus.

Administration of rifaximin to pregnant rats and rabbits at dose levels that caused reduced body weight gain resulted in eye malformations in both rat and rabbit fetuses. Additional malformations were observed in fetal rabbits that included cleft palate, lumbar scoliosis, brachygnathia, interventricular septal defect, and large atrium.

The fetal rat malformations were observed in a study of pregnant rats administered a high dose that resulted in 16 times the therapeutic dose to diarrheic patients or 1 times the therapeutic dose to patients with hepatic encephalopathy (based upon plasma AUC comparisons). Fetal rabbit malformations were observed from pregnant rabbits administered mid and high doses that resulted in 1 or 2 times the therapeutic dose to diarrheic patients or less than 0.1 times the dose in patients with hepatic encephalopathy, based upon plasma AUC comparisons.

Post-natal developmental effects were not observed in rat pups from pregnant/lactating female rats dosed during the period from gestation to Day 20 post-partum at the highest dose which resulted in approximately 16 times the human therapeutic dose for travelers' diarrhea (based upon AUCs) or approximately 1 times the AUCs derived from therapeutic doses to patients with hepatic encephalopathy.

8.3 Nursing Mothers

It is not known whether rifaximin is excreted in human milk. Because many drugs are excreted in human milk and because of the potential for adverse reactions in nursing infants from XIFAXAN, a decision should be made whether to discontinue nursing or to discontinue the drug, taking into account the importance of the drug to the mother.

8.4 Pediatric Use

The safety and effectiveness of XIFAXAN 200 mg in pediatric patients with travelers' diarrhea less than 12 years of age have not been established.

The safety and effectiveness of XIFAXAN 550 mg for HE have not been established in patients < 18 years of age.

8.5 Geriatric Use

Clinical studies with rifaximin 200 mg for travelers' diarrhea did not include sufficient numbers of patients aged 65 and over to determine whether they respond differently than younger subjects.

In the controlled trial with XIFAXAN 550 mg for hepatic encephalopathy, 19.4% were 65 and over, while 2.3% were 75 and over. No overall differences in safety or effectiveness were observed between these subjects and younger subjects, and other reported clinical experience has not identified differences in responses between the elderly and younger patients, but greater sensitivity of some older individuals cannot be ruled out.

8.6 Renal Impairment

The pharmacokinetics of rifaximin in patients with impaired renal function has not been studied.

8.7 Hepatic Impairment

Following administration of XIFAXAN 550 mg twice daily to patients with a history of hepatic encephalopathy, the systemic exposure (i.e., AUC_τ) of rifaximin was about 10-, 13-, and 20-fold higher in those patients with mild (Child-Pugh A), moderate (Child-Pugh B) and severe (Child-Pugh C) hepatic impairment, respectively, compared to that in healthy volunteers. No dosage adjustment is recommended because rifaximin is presumably acting locally. Nonetheless, caution should be exercised when XIFAXAN is administered to patients with severe hepatic impairment *[see Warnings and Precautions (5.4), Clinical Pharmacology (12.3), Nonclinical Toxicology (13.2), and Clinical Studies (14.2)]*.

10 OVERDOSAGE

No specific information is available on the treatment of overdosage with XIFAXAN. In clinical studies at doses higher than the recommended dose (> 600 mg/day for travelers' diarrhea or > 1100 mg/day for hepatic encephalopathy), adverse reactions were similar in subjects who received doses higher than the recommended dose and placebo. In the case of overdosage, discontinue XIFAXAN, treat symptomatically, and institute supportive measures as required.

11 DESCRIPTION

XIFAXAN tablets contain rifaximin, a non-aminoglycoside semi-synthetic, nonsystemic antibiotic derived from rifamycin SV. Rifaximin is a structural analog of rifampin. The chemical name for rifaximin is (2*S*,16*Z*,18*E*,20*S*,21*S*,22*R*,23*R*,24*R*,25*S*,26*S*,27*S*,28*E*)-5,6,21,23,25-pentahydroxy-27-methoxy-2,4,11,16,20,22,24,26-octamethyl-2,7-(epoxypentadeca-[1,11,13]trienimino)benzofuro[4,5-e]pyrido[1,2-á]-benzimidazole-1,15(2*H*)-dione,25-acetate. The empirical formula is $C_{43}H_{51}N_3O_{11}$ and its molecular weight is 785.9. The chemical structure is represented below:

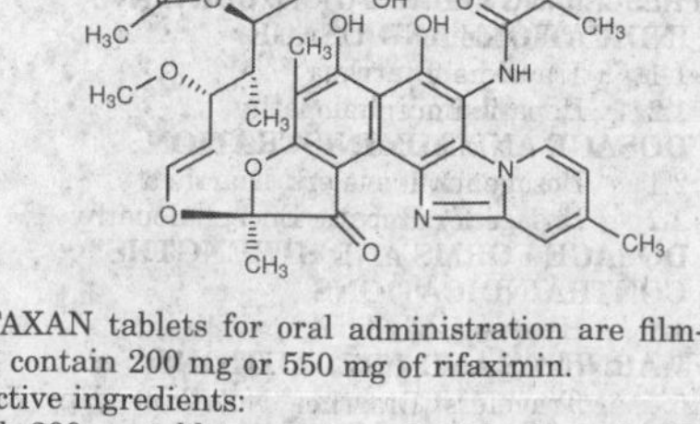

XIFAXAN tablets for oral administration are film-coated and contain 200 mg or 550 mg of rifaximin.

Inactive ingredients:

Each 200 mg tablet contains colloidal silicon dioxide, disodium edetate, glycerol palmitostearate, hypromellose, microcrystalline cellulose, propylene glycol, red iron oxide, sodium starch glycolate, talc, and titanium dioxide.

Each 550 mg tablet contains colloidal silicon dioxide, glycerol palmitostearate, microcrystalline cellulose, polyethylene glycol/macrogol, polyvinyl alcohol, red iron oxide, sodium starch glycolate, talc, and titanium dioxide.

12 CLINICAL PHARMACOLOGY

12.1 Mechanism of Action

Rifaximin is an antibacterial drug *[see Clinical Pharmacology (12.4)]*.

12.3 Pharmacokinetics

Absorption

Travelers' Diarrhea

Systemic absorption of rifaximin (200 mg three times daily) was evaluated in 13 subjects challenged with shigellosis on Days 1 and 3 of a three-day course of treatment. Rifaximin plasma concentrations and exposures were low and variable. There was no evidence of accumulation of rifaximin following repeated administration for 3 days (9 doses). Peak plasma rifaximin concentrations after 3 and 9 consecutive doses ranged from 0.81 to 3.4 ng/mL on Day 1 and 0.68 to 2.26 ng/mL on Day 3. Similarly, $AUC_{0\text{-last}}$ estimates were 6.95 ± 5.15 ng•h/mL on Day 1 and 7.83 ± 4.94 ng•h/mL on Day 3. XIFAXAN is not suitable for treating systemic bacterial infections because of limited systemic exposure after oral administration *[see Warnings and Precautions (5.1)]*.

Hepatic Encephalopathy

After a single dose and multiple doses of rifaximin 550 mg in healthy subjects, the mean time to reach peak plasma concentrations was about an hour. The pharmacokinetic (PK) parameters were highly variable and the accumulation ratio based on AUC was 1.37.

The PK of rifaximin in patients with a history of HE was evaluated after administration of XIFAXAN, 550 mg two times a day. The PK parameters were associated with a high variability and mean rifaximin exposure (AUC_τ) in patients with a history of HE (147 ng•h/mL) was approximately 12-fold higher than that observed in healthy subjects following the same dosing regimen (12.3 ng•h/mL). When PK parameters were analyzed based on Child-Pugh Class A, B, and C, the mean AUC_τ was 10-, 13-, and 20-fold higher, respectively, compared to that in healthy subjects (Table 3).

[See table 3 above]

Table 3. Mean (± SD) Pharmacokinetic Parameters of Rifaximin at Steady-State in Patients with a History of Hepatic Encephalopathy by Child-Pugh Class[1]

	Healthy Subjects (n = 14)	Child-Pugh Class		
		A (n = 18)	B (n = 7)	C (n = 4)
AUC_{tau} (ng•h/mL)	12.3 ± 4.8	118 ± 67.8	161 ± 101	246 ± 120
C_{max} (ng/mL)	3.4 ± 1.6	19.5 ± 11.4	25.1 ± 12.6	35.5 ± 12.5
T_{max}[2] (h)	0.8 (0.5, 4.0)	1 (0.9, 10)	1 (0.97, 1)	1 (0, 2)

[1] Cross-study comparison with PK parameters in healthy subjects
[2] Median (range)

Food Effect in Healthy Subjects

A high-fat meal consumed 30 minutes prior to XIFAXAN dosing in healthy subjects delayed the mean time to peak plasma concentration from 0.75 to 1.5 hours and increased the systemic exposure (AUC) of rifaximin by 2-fold (Table 4).

Table 4. Mean (± SD) Pharmacokinetic Parameters After Single-Dose Administration of XIFAXAN Tablets 550 mg in Healthy Subjects Under Fasting and Fed Conditions (N = 12)

Parameter	Fasting	Fed
C_{max} (ng/mL)	4.1 ± 1.5	4.8 ± 4.3
T_{max}[1] (h)	0.8 (0.5, 2.1)	1.5 (0.5, 4.1)
Half-Life (h)	1.8 ± 1.4	4.8 ± 1.3
AUC (ng•h/mL)	11.1 ± 4.2	22.5 ± 12

[1]Median (range)

XIFAXAN can be administered with or without food *[see Dosage and Administration (2.1 and 2.2)]*.

Distribution

Rifaximin is moderately bound to human plasma proteins. *In vivo*, the mean protein binding ratio was 67.5% in healthy subjects and 62% in patients with hepatic impairment when XIFAXAN 550 mg was administered.

Metabolism and Excretion

In a mass balance study, after administration of 400 mg ^{14}C-rifaximin orally to healthy volunteers, of the 96.94% total recovery, 96.62% of the administered radioactivity was recovered in feces almost exclusively as the unchanged drug and 0.32% was recovered in urine mostly as metabolites with 0.03% as the unchanged drug. Rifaximin accounted for 18% of radioactivity in plasma. This suggests that the absorbed rifaximin undergoes metabolism with minimal renal excretion of the unchanged drug. The enzymes responsible for metabolizing rifaximin are unknown.

In a separate study, rifaximin was detected in the bile after cholecystectomy in patients with intact gastrointestinal mucosa, suggesting biliary excretion of rifaximin.

Specific Populations

Hepatic Impairment

The systemic exposure of rifaximin was markedly elevated in patients with hepatic impairment compared to healthy subjects. The mean AUC in patients with Child-Pugh Class C hepatic impairment was 2-fold higher than in patients with Child-Pugh Class A hepatic impairment (see Table 3), *[see Warnings and Precautions (5.4) and Use in Specific Populations (8.7)]*.

Renal Impairment

The pharmacokinetics of rifaximin in patients with impaired renal function has not been studied.

Drug Interactions

In vitro drug interaction studies have shown that rifaximin, at concentrations ranging from 2 to 200 ng/mL, did not inhibit human hepatic cytochrome P450 isoenzymes 1A2, 2A6, 2B6, 2C9, 2C19, 2D6, 2E1, and 3A4.

In an *in vitro* study, rifaximin was shown to induce CYP3A4 at the concentration of 0.2 μM.

An *in vitro* study suggests that rifaximin is a substrate of P-glycoprotein. In the presence of P-glycoprotein inhibitor verapamil, the efflux ratio of rifaximin was reduced greater than 50% *in vitro*. The effect of P-glycoprotein inhibition on rifaximin was not evaluated *in vivo*.

The inhibitory effect of rifaximin on P-gp transporter was observed in an *in vitro* study. The effect of rifaximin on P-gp transporter was not evaluated *in vivo*.

Midazolam

The effect of rifaximin 200 mg administered orally every 8 hours for 3 days and for 7 days on the pharmacokinetics of a single dose of either midazolam 2 mg intravenous or midazolam 6 mg orally was evaluated in healthy subjects. No significant difference was observed in the metrics of systemic exposure or elimination of intravenous or oral midazolam or its major metabolite, 1′-hydroxymidazolam, between midazolam alone or together with rifaximin. Therefore, rifaximin was not shown to significantly affect intestinal or hepatic CYP3A4 activity for the 200 mg three times a day dosing regimen.

After XIFAXAN 550 mg was administered three times a day for 7 days and 14 days to healthy subjects, the mean AUC of single midazolam 2 mg orally was 3.8% and 8.8% lower, respectively, than when midazolam was administered alone. The mean C_{max} of midazolam was also decreased by 4-5% when XIFAXAN was administered for 7-14 days prior to midazolam administration. This degree of interaction is not considered clinically meaningful.

The effect of rifaximin on CYP3A4 in patients with impaired liver function who have elevated systemic exposure is not known.

Oral Contraceptives Containing 0.07 mg Ethinyl Estradiol and 0.5 mg Norgestimate

The oral contraceptive study utilized an open-label, crossover design in 28 healthy female subjects to determine if rifaximin 200 mg orally administered three times a day for 3 days (the dosing regimen for travelers' diarrhea) altered the pharmacokinetics of a single dose of an oral contraceptive containing 0.07 mg ethinyl estradiol and 0.5 mg norgestimate. Results showed that the pharmacokinetics of single doses of ethinyl estradiol and norgestimate were not altered by rifaximin *[see Drug Interactions (7)]*.

Effect of rifaximin on oral contraceptives was not studied for XIFAXAN 550 mg twice a day, the dosing regimen for hepatic encephalopathy.

12.4 Microbiology

Mechanism of Action

Rifaximin is a non-aminoglycoside semi-synthetic antibacterial derived from rifamycin SV. Rifaximin acts by binding to the beta-subunit of bacterial DNA-dependent RNA polymerase resulting in inhibition of bacterial RNA synthesis.

Escherichia coli has been shown to develop resistance to rifaximin *in vitro*. However, the clinical significance of such an effect has not been studied.

Rifaximin is a structural analog of rifampin. Organisms with high rifaximin minimum inhibitory concentration (MIC) values also have elevated MIC values against rifampin. Cross-resistance between rifaximin and other classes of antimicrobials has not been studied.

Rifaximin has been shown to be active against the following pathogen in clinical studies of infectious diarrhea as described in the *Indications and Usage (1)* section: *Escherichia coli* (enterotoxigenic and enteroaggregative strains).

For HE, rifaximin is thought to have an effect on the gastrointestinal flora.

Susceptibility Tests

In vitro susceptibility testing was performed according to the National Committee for Clinical Laboratory Standards (NCCLS) agar dilution method M7-A6 *[see References (15)]*. However, the correlation between susceptibility testing and clinical outcome has not been determined.

13 NONCLINICAL TOXICOLOGY

13.1 Carcinogenesis, Mutagenesis, Impairment of Fertility

Malignant schwannomas in the heart were significantly increased in male Crl:CD® (SD) rats that received rifaximin by oral gavage for two years at 150 to 250 mg/kg/day (doses equivalent to 2.4 to 4 times the recommended dose of 200 mg three times daily for travelers' diarrhea, and equivalent to 1.3 to 2.2 times the recommended dose of 550 mg twice daily for hepatic encephalopathy, based on relative body surface area comparisons). There was no increase in tumors in Tg.rasH2 mice dosed orally with rifaximin for 26 weeks at 150 to 2000 mg/kg/day (doses equivalent to 1.2 to 16 times the recommended daily dose for travelers' diarrhea and equivalent to 0.7 to 9 times the recommended daily dose for hepatic encephalopathy, based on relative body surface area comparisons).

Rifaximin was not genotoxic in the bacterial reverse mutation assay, chromosomal aberration assay, rat bone marrow micronucleus assay, rat hepatocyte unscheduled DNA synthesis assay, or the CHO/HGPRT mutation assay. There was no effect on fertility in male or female rats following the administration of rifaximin at doses up to 300 mg/kg (approximately 5 times the clinical dose of 600 mg/day, and approximately 2.6 times the clinical dose of 1100 mg/day, adjusted for body surface area).

13.2 Animal Toxicology and/or Pharmacology

Oral administration of rifaximin for 3-6 months produced hepatic proliferation of connective tissue in rats (50 mg/kg/day) and fatty degeneration of liver in dogs (100 mg/kg/day). However, plasma drug levels were not measured in these studies. Subsequently, rifaximin was studied at doses as high as 300 mg/kg/day in rats for 6 months and 1000 mg/kg/day in dogs for 9 months, and no signs of hepatotoxicity were observed. The maximum plasma $AUC_{0\text{-}8\ hr}$ values from the 6 month rat and 9 month dog toxicity studies (range: 42-127 ng•h/mL) was lower than the maximum plasma $AUC_{0\text{-}8\ hr}$ values in cirrhotic patients (range: 19-306 ng•h/mL).

14 CLINICAL STUDIES

14.1 Travelers' Diarrhea

The efficacy of XIFAXAN given as 200 mg orally taken three times a day for 3 days was evaluated in 2 randomized, multi-center, double-blind, placebo-controlled studies in adult subjects with travelers' diarrhea. One study was conducted at clinical sites in Mexico, Guatemala, and Kenya (Study 1). The other study was conducted in Mexico, Guatemala, Peru, and India (Study 2). Stool specimens were collected before treatment and 1 to 3 days following the end of treatment to identify enteric pathogens. The predominant pathogen in both studies was *Escherichia coli*.

The clinical efficacy of XIFAXAN was assessed by the time to return to normal, formed stools and resolution of symptoms. The primary efficacy endpoint was time to last unformed stool (TLUS) which was defined as the time to the last unformed stool passed, after which clinical cure was declared. Table 5 displays the median TLUS and the number of patients who achieved clinical cure for the intent to treat (ITT) population of Study 1. The duration of diarrhea was significantly shorter in patients treated with XIFAXAN than in the placebo group. More patients treated with XIFAXAN were classified as clinical cures than were those in the placebo group.

Table 5. Clinical Response in Study 1 (ITT population)

	XIFAXAN (n=125)	Placebo (n=129)	Estimate (97.5% CI)	P-Value
Median TLUS (hours)	32.5	58.6	1.78[a] (1.26, 2.50)	0.0002
Clinical cure, n (%)	99 (79.2)	78 (60.5)	18.7[b] (5.3, 32.1)	0.001

[a] Hazard Ratio
[b] Difference in rates

Microbiological eradication (defined as the absence of a baseline pathogen in culture of stool after 72 hours of therapy) rates for Study 1 are presented in Table 6 for patients with any pathogen at baseline and for the subset of patients with *Escherichia coli* at baseline. *Escherichia coli* was the only pathogen with sufficient numbers to allow comparisons between treatment groups.

Even though XIFAXAN had microbiologic activity similar to placebo, it demonstrated a clinically significant reduction in duration of diarrhea and a higher clinical cure rate than placebo. Therefore, patients should be managed based on clinical response to therapy rather than microbiologic response.

Table 6. Microbiologic Eradication Rates in Study 1 Subjects with a Baseline Pathogen

	XIFAXAN	Placebo
Overall	48/70 (68.6)	41/61 (67.2)
E. coli	38/53 (71.7)	40/54 (74.1)

The results of Study 2 supported the results presented for Study 1. In addition, this study provided evidence that subjects treated with XIFAXAN with fever and/or blood in the stool at baseline had prolonged TLUS. These subjects had lower clinical cure rates than those without fever or blood in the stool at baseline. Many of the patients with fever and/or blood in the stool (dysentery-like diarrheal syndromes) had invasive pathogens, primarily *Campylobacter jejuni*, isolated in the baseline stool.

Also in this study, the majority of the subjects treated with XIFAXAN who had *Campylobacter jejuni* isolated as a sole pathogen at baseline failed treatment and the resulting clinical cure rate for these patients was 23.5% (4/17). In addition to not being different from placebo, the microbiologic eradication rates for subjects with *Campylobacter jejuni* isolated at baseline were much lower than the eradication rates seen for *Escherichia coli*.

In an unrelated open-label, pharmacokinetic study of oral XIFAXAN 200 mg taken every 8 hours for 3 days, 15 adult subjects were challenged with *Shigella flexneri* 2a, of whom 13 developed diarrhea or dysentery and were treated with XIFAXAN. Although this open-label challenge trial was not adequate to assess the effectiveness of XIFAXAN in the treatment of shigellosis, the following observations were noted: eight subjects received rescue treatment with ciprofloxacin either because of lack of response to XIFAXAN treatment within 24 hours (2), or because they developed severe dysentery (5), or because of recurrence of *Shigella flexneri* in the stool (1); five of the 13 subjects received ciprofloxacin although they did not have evidence of severe disease or relapse.

14.2 Hepatic Encephalopathy

The efficacy of XIFAXAN 550 mg taken orally two times a day was evaluated in a randomized, placebo-controlled, double-blind, multi-center 6-month trial of adult subjects from the U.S., Canada and Russia who were defined as being in remission (Conn score of 0 or 1) from hepatic encephalopathy (HE). Eligible subjects had ≥ 2 episodes of HE associated with chronic liver disease in the previous 6 months.

A total of 299 subjects were randomized to receive either XIFAXAN (n=140) or placebo (n=159) in this study. Patients had a mean age of 56 years (range, 21-82 years), 81% < 65 years of age, 61% were male and 86% White. At baseline, 67% of patients had a Conn score of 0 and 68% had an asterixis grade of 0. Patients had MELD scores of either ≤ 10 (27%) or 11 to 18 (64%) at baseline. No patients were enrolled with a MELD score of > 25. Nine percent of the patients were Child-Pugh Class C. Lactulose was concomitantly used by 91% of the patients in each treatment arm of the study. Per the study protocol, patients were withdrawn from the study after experiencing a breakthrough HE episode. Other reasons for early study discontinuation included: adverse reactions (XIFAXAN 6%; placebo 4%), patient request to withdraw (XIFAXAN 4%; placebo 6%) and other (XIFAXAN 7%; placebo 5%).

The primary endpoint was the time to first breakthrough overt HE episode. A breakthrough overt HE episode was defined as a marked deterioration in neurological function and an increase of Conn score to Grade ≥ 2. In patients with a baseline Conn score of 0, a breakthrough overt HE episode was defined as an increase in Conn score of 1 and asterixis grade of 1.

Breakthrough overt HE episodes were experienced by 31 of 140 subjects (22%) in the XIFAXAN group and by 73 of 159 subjects (46%) in the placebo group during the 6-month treatment period. Comparison of Kaplan-Meier estimates of event-free curves showed XIFAXAN significantly reduced the risk of HE breakthrough by 58% during the 6-month treatment period. Presented below in Figure 1 is the Kaplan-Meier event-free curve for all subjects (n = 299) in the study.

Figure 1: Kaplan-Meier Event-Free Curves[1] in HE Study (Time to First Breakthrough-HE Episode up to 6 Months of Treatment, Day 170) (ITT Population)

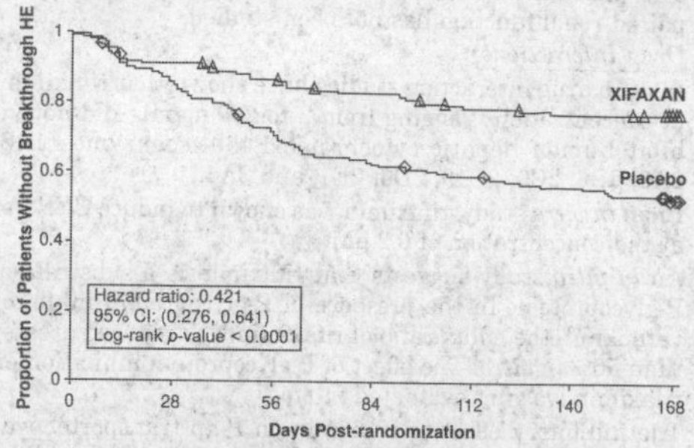

Note: Open diamonds and open triangles represent censored subjects.
[1] Event-free refers to non-occurrence of breakthrough HE.

When the results were evaluated by the following demographic and baseline characteristics, the treatment effect of XIFAXAN 550 mg in reducing the risk of breakthrough overt HE recurrence was consistent for: sex, baseline Conn score, duration of current remission and diabetes. The differences in treatment effect could not be assessed in the following subpopulations due to small sample size: non-White (n=42), baseline MELD > 19 (n=26), Child-Pugh C (n=31), and those without concomitant lactulose use (n=26).

HE-related hospitalizations (hospitalizations directly resulting from HE, or hospitalizations complicated by HE) were reported for 19 of 140 subjects (14%) and 36 of 159 subjects (23%) in the XIFAXAN and placebo groups respectively. Comparison of Kaplan-Meier estimates of event-free curves showed XIFAXAN significantly reduced the risk of HE-related hospitalizations by 50% during the 6-month treatment period. Comparison of Kaplan-Meier estimates of event-free curves is shown in Figure 2.

Figure 2: Kaplan-Meier Event-Free Curves[1] in Pivotal HE Study (Time to First HE-Related Hospitalization in HE Study up to 6 Months of Treatment, Day 170) (ITT Population)

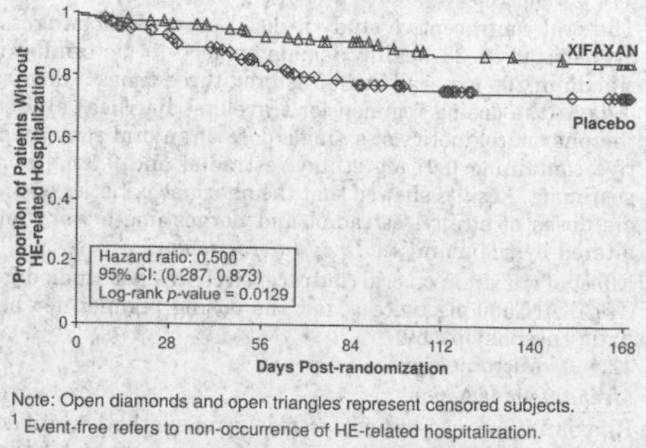

Note: Open diamonds and open triangles represent censored subjects.
[1] Event-free refers to non-occurrence of HE-related hospitalization.

15 REFERENCES

Methods for dilution antimicrobial susceptibility tests for bacteria that grow aerobically. National Committee for Clinical Laboratory Standards, Sixth Edition, Wayne PA. *Approved Standard NCCLS Document M7-A6* January 2003; 23 (2).

16 HOW SUPPLIED/STORAGE AND HANDLING

The 200 mg tablet is a pink-colored, round, biconvex tablet with "Sx" debossed on one side. It is available in the following presentations:

- NDC 65649-301-03, bottles of 30 tablets
- NDC 65649-301-41, bottles of 100 tablets
- NDC 65649-301-05, carton of 100 tablets, Unit Dose

The 550 mg tablet is a pink-colored, oval, biconvex tablet with "rfx" debossed on one side. It is available in the following presentations:

- NDC 65649-303-02, bottles of 60 tablets
- NDC 65649-303-03, carton of 60 tablets, Unit Dose

Storage

Store XIFAXAN Tablets at 20–25°C (68–77°F); excursions permitted to 15–30°C (59-86°F). See USP Controlled Room Temperature.

17 PATIENT COUNSELING INFORMATION

17.1 Persistent Diarrhea

For those patients being treated for travelers' diarrhea, discontinue XIFAXAN if diarrhea persists more than 24-48 hours or worsens. Advise the patient to seek medical care for fever and/or blood in the stool *[see Warnings and Precautions (5.1)]*.

17.2 *Clostridium difficile*-Associated Diarrhea

Clostridium difficile-associated diarrhea (CDAD) has been reported with use of nearly all antibacterial agents, including XIFAXAN, and may range in severity from mild diarrhea to fatal colitis. Treatment with antibiotics alters the normal flora of the colon which may lead to *C. difficile*. Patients can develop watery and bloody stools (with or without stomach cramps and fever) even as late as two or more months after having taken the last dose of the antibiotic. If diarrhea occurs after therapy or does not improve or worsens during therapy, advise patients to contact a physician as soon as possible *[see Warnings and Precautions (5.4)]*.

17.3 Administration with Food

Inform patients that XIFAXAN may be taken with or without food.

17.4 Antibacterial Resistance

Counsel patients that antibacterial drugs including XIFAXAN should only be used to treat bacterial infections. They do not treat viral infections (e.g., the common cold). When XIFAXAN is prescribed to treat a bacterial infection, patients should be told that although it is common to feel better early in the course of therapy, the medication should be taken exactly as directed. Skipping doses or not completing the full course of therapy may (1) decrease the effectiveness of the immediate treatment and (2) increase the likelihood that bacteria will develop resistance and will not be treatable by XIFAXAN or other antibacterial drugs in the future.

17.5 Severe Hepatic Impairment

Patients should be informed that in patients with severe hepatic impairment (Child-Pugh C) there is an increase in systemic exposure to XIFAXAN *[see Warnings and Precautions (5.4)]*.

Manufactured for:
Salix Pharmaceuticals, Inc.
Raleigh, NC 27615

XIFAXAN® is a trademark of Salix Pharmaceuticals, Inc., under license from Alfa Wassermann S.p.A.

Rifaximin for Travelers' Diarrhea and Hepatic encephalopathy is protected by US Patent Nos. 7,045,620; 7,612,199; 7,902,206 and 7,906,542. Rifaximin for Travelers' Diarrhea is also protected by US Patent No. 7,928,115.

Web site: www.Salix.com

VENART-185-1
OCT 2011

Shown in Product Identification Guide, page 313

Schering Corporation

for product information, please see Merck

Smith & Nephew, Inc.
BIOTHERAPEUTICS
3909 HULEN STREET
FORT WORTH, TX 76107

Direct Inquiries to:
800-441-8227

COLLAGENASE SANTYL® OINTMENT ℞
250 units/g

Rx only

DESCRIPTION

Collagenase Santyl® Ointment is a sterile enzymatic debriding ointment which contains 250 collagenase units per gram of white petrolatum USP. The enzyme collagenase is derived from the fermentation by *Clostridium histolyticum*. It possesses the unique ability to digest collagen in necrotic tissue.

CLINICAL PHARMACOLOGY

Since collagen accounts for 75% of the dry weight of skin tissue, the ability of collagenase to digest collagen in the physiological pH and temperature range makes it particularly effective in the removal of detritus.[1] Collagenase thus contributes towards the formation of granulation tissue and subsequent epithelization of dermal ulcers and severely burned areas.[2,3,4,5,6] Collagen in healthy tissue or in newly formed granulation tissue is not attacked.[2,3,4,5,6,7,8] There is no information available on collagenase absorption through skin or its concentration in body fluids associated with therapeutic and/or toxic effects, degree of binding to plasma proteins, degree of uptake by a particular organ or in the fetus, and passage across the blood brain barrier.

INDICATIONS AND USAGE

Collagenase Santyl® Ointment is indicated for debriding chronic dermal ulcers[2,3,4,5,6,8,9,10,11,12,13,14,15,16,17,18] and severely burned areas.[3,4,5,7,16,19,20,21]

CONTRAINDICATIONS

Collagenase Santyl® Ointment is contraindicated in patients who have shown local or systemic hypersensitivity to collagenase.

PRECAUTIONS

The optimal pH range of collagenase is 6 to 8. Higher or lower pH conditions will decrease the enzyme's activity and appropriate precautions should be taken. The enzymatic activity is also adversely affected by certain detergents, and heavy metal ions such as mercury and silver which are used in some antiseptics. When it is suspected such materials have been used, the site should be carefully cleansed by repeated washings with normal saline before Collagenase Santyl® Ointment is applied. Soaks containing metal ions or acidic solutions should be avoided because of the metal ion and low pH. Cleansing materials such as Dakin's solution and normal saline are compatible with Collagenase Santyl® Ointment.

Debilitated patients should be closely monitored for systemic bacterial infections because of the theoretical possibility that debriding enzymes may increase the risk of bacteremia.

A slight transient erythema has been noted occasionally in the surrounding tissue, particularly when Collagenase Santyl® Ointment was not confined to the wound. Therefore, the ointment should be applied carefully within the area of the wound. Safety and effectiveness in pediatric patients have not been established.

ADVERSE REACTIONS

No allergic sensitivity or toxic reactions have been noted in clinical use when used as directed. However, one case of systemic manifestations of hypersensitivity to collagenase in a patient treated for more than one year with a combination of collagenase and cortisone has been reported.

OVERDOSAGE

No systemic or local reaction attributed to overdose has been observed in clinical investigations and clinical use. If deemed necessary the enzyme may be inactivated by washing the area with povidone iodine.

DOSAGE AND ADMINISTRATION

Collagenase Santyl® Ointment should be applied once daily (or more frequently if the dressing becomes soiled, as from incontinence). When clinically indicated, crosshatching thick eschar with a #10 blade allows Collagenase Santyl® Ointment more surface contact with necrotic debris. It is also desirable to remove, with forceps and scissors, as much loosened detritus as can be done readily. Use Collagenase Santyl® Ointment in the following manner:

1. Prior to application the wound should be cleansed of debris and digested material by gently rubbing with a gauze pad saturated with normal saline solution, or with the desired cleansing agent compatible with Collagenase Santyl® Ointment (See **PRECAUTIONS**), followed by a normal saline solution rinse.
2. Whenever infection is present, it is desirable to use an appropriate topical antibiotic powder. The antibiotic should be applied to the wound prior to the application of Collagenase Santyl® Ointment. Should the infection not respond, therapy with Collagenase Santyl® Ointment should be discontinued until remission of the infection.
3. Collagenase Santyl® Ointment may be applied directly to the wound or to a sterile gauze pad which is then applied to the wound and properly secured.
4. Use of Collagenase Santyl® Ointment should be terminated when debridement of necrotic tissue is complete and granulation tissue is well established.

HOW SUPPLIED

Collagenase Santyl® Ointment contains 250 units of collagenase enzyme per gram of white petrolatum USP.

Do not store above 25°C (77°F). Sterility guaranteed until tube is opened.

Collagenase Santyl® Ointment is available in 15 gram and 30 gram tubes.

REFERENCES

1. Mandl, I., Adv Enzymol. 23:163,1961.
2. Boxer, A.M., Gottesman, N., Bernstein, H., & Mandl, I., Geriatrics. 24:75,1969.
3. Mazurek, I., Med. Welt. 22:150, 1971.
4. Zimmerman, WE., in "Collagenase," Mandl, I., ed., Gordon & Breach, Science Publishers, New York, 1971, p. 131, p. 185.
5. Vetra, H., & Whittaker, D., Geriatrics. 30:53, 1975.
6. Rao, D.B., Sane, P.G., & Georgiev, E.L., J. Am. Geriatrics Soc. 23:22, 1975.
7. Vrabec, R., Moserova, J., Konickova, Z., Behounkova, E., & Blaha, J., J. Hyg. Epidemiol. Microbiol. Immunol. 18:496, 1974.
8. Lippmann, H.I., Arch. Phys. Med. Rehabil. 54:588, 1973.
9. German, F.M., in "Collagenase," Mandl, I., ed., Gordon & Breach, Science Publishers, New York, 1971, p. 165.
10. Haimovici, H. & Strauch, B., in "Collagenase," Mandl, I., ed., Gordon & Breach, Science Publishers, New York, 1971, p. 177.
11. Lee, L.K., & Ambrus, J.L., Geriatrics. 30:91, 1975.
12. Locke, R.K., & Heifitz, N.M., J. Am. Pod. Assoc. 65:242, 1975.
13. Varma, A.O., Bugatch, E., & German, F.M., Surg. Gynecol. Obstet. 136:281, 1973.
14. Barrett D., Jr., & Klibanski, A., Am. J. Nurs. 73:849, 1973.
15. Bardfeld, L.A., J. Pod. Ed. 1:41, 1970.
16. Blum, G., Schweiz. Rundschau Med Praxis. 62:820,1973. Abstr. in Dermatology Digest, Feb. 1974, p. 36.
17. Zaruba, F., Lettl, A., Brozkova, L., Skrdlantova, H., & Krs, V., J. Hyg. Epidemiol. Microbiol. Immunol. 18:499, 1974.
18. Altman, M.I., Goldstein, L., & Horwitz, S., J. Am. Pod. Assoc. 68:11, 1978.
19. Rehn, V.J., Med. Klin. 58:799, 1963.
20. Krauss, H., Koslowski, L., & Zimmermann W.E., Langenbecks Arch. Klin. Chir. 303:23, 1963.
21. Gruenagel, H.H., Med. Klin. 58:442, 1963.

MANUFACTURED BY HEALTHPOINT, LTD.
FORT WORTH, TEXAS 76107
US GOV'T LICENSE #1885
Marketed by: HEALTHPOINT® Biotherapeutics
1-800-441-8227
Healthpoint, Biotherapeutics
Fort Worth, Texas 76107
DISTRIBUTED BY:
DPT LABORATORIES, Ltd.
SAN ANTONIO, TEXAS 78215
Reorder Nos.
0064-5010-15 (15g tube)
0064-5010-30 (30g tube)

129915-0812

Shown in Product Identification Guide, page 313

REGRANEX® ℞
(becaplermin)
GEL for TOPICAL use

HIGHLIGHTS OF PRESCRIBING INFORMATION
These highlights do not include all the information needed to use REGRANEX® Gel safely and effectively. See full prescribing information for REGRANEX Gel.
REGRANEX® (becaplermin) GEL for TOPICAL use.
Initial U.S. Approval: 1997

WARNING: INCREASED RATE OF MORTALITY SECONDARY TO MALIGNANCY
An increased rate of mortality secondary to malignancy was observed in patients treated with 3 or more tubes of REGRANEX Gel in a postmarketing retrospective cohort study. REGRANEX Gel should only be used when the benefits can be expected to outweigh the risks. REGRANEX Gel should be used with caution in patients with known malignancy. (5.1)

INDICATIONS AND USAGE

REGRANEX Gel contains becaplermin, a human platelet-derived growth factor that is indicated for the treatment of lower extremity diabetic neuropathic ulcers that extend into the subcutaneous tissue or beyond and have an adequate blood supply. REGRANEX Gel is indicated as an adjunct to, and not a substitute for, good ulcer care practices. (1.1)

Limitations of use:

The efficacy of REGRANEX Gel has not been established for the treatment of pressure ulcers and venous stasis ulcers. (1.2)

The effects of REGRANEX Gel on exposed joints, tendons, ligaments, and bone have not been established in humans. (1.2)

REGRANEX Gel is a non-sterile, low bioburden preserved product. Therefore, it should not be used in wounds that close by primary intention. (1.2)

DOSAGE AND ADMINISTRATION

For topical use; not for oral, ophthalmic or intravaginal use. (2)

To calculate the length of REGRANEX Gel to apply, measure the greatest length of the ulcer by the greatest width of the ulcer in either inches or centimeters. (2)

Formula to Calculate Length of Gel to Be Applied Daily

Tube Size	Inches or Centimeters Formula
15g tube	Inches: ulcer length × ulcer width × 0.6
15g tube	Centimeters: ulcer length × ulcer width ÷ 4

DOSAGE FORMS AND STRENGTHS

Gel: 0.01% (3)

CONTRAINDICATIONS

Known neoplasm(s) at the site(s) of application (4)

WARNINGS AND PRECAUTIONS

Malignancies distant from the site of application have been reported in both a clinical study and in postmarketing use. REGRANEX Gel should be used with caution in patients with a known malignancy. (5.1)

ADVERSE REACTIONS

Erythematous rashes occurred in 2% of patients treated with REGRANEX Gel (6.1)

To report SUSPECTED ADVERSE REACTIONS contact FDA at 1-800-FDA-1088 or www.fda.gov/medwatch, or Healthpoint Biotherapeutics at 1-800-441-8227.

See 17 for PATIENT COUNSELING INFORMATION and Medication Guide

Revised: 09/2012

FULL PRESCRIBING INFORMATION: CONTENTS*

FULL PRESCRIBING INFORMATION

WARNING: INCREASED RATE OF MORTALITY SECONDARY TO MALIGNANCY

An increased rate of mortality secondary to malignancy was observed in patients treated with 3 or more tubes of REGRANEX Gel in a postmarketing retrospective cohort study. REGRANEX Gel should only be used when the benefits can be expected to outweigh the risks. REGRANEX Gel should be used with caution in patients with known malignancy. [*see Warnings and Precautions (5.1)*]

1 INDICATIONS AND USAGE

1.1 Indication

REGRANEX (becaplermin) Gel is indicated for the treatment of lower extremity diabetic neuropathic ulcers that extend into the subcutaneous tissue or beyond and have an adequate blood supply, when used as an adjunct to, and not a substitute for, good ulcer care practices including initial sharp debridement, pressure relief and infection control.

1.2 Limitations of Use

The efficacy of REGRANEX Gel has not been established for the treatment of pressure ulcers and venous stasis ulcers [*see Clinical Studies (14)*] and has not been evaluated for the treatment of diabetic neuropathic ulcers that do not extend through the dermis into subcutaneous tissue (Stage I or II, IAET staging classification) or ischemic diabetic ulcers.

The effects of becaplermin on exposed joints, tendons, ligaments, and bone have not been established in humans. [*see Nonclinical Toxicology (13.2)*]

REGRANEX Gel is a non-sterile, low bioburden preserved product. Therefore, it should not be used in wounds that close by primary intention.

2 DOSAGE AND ADMINISTRATION

For topical use; not for oral, ophthalmic or intravaginal use.

The amount of REGRANEX Gel to be applied will vary depending upon the size of the ulcer area. To calculate the length of gel to apply to the ulcer, measure the greatest length of the ulcer by the greatest width of the ulcer in either inches or centimeters. To calculate the length of gel in inches, use the formula shown below in Table 1, and to calculate the length of gel in centimeters, use the formula shown below in Table 2.

Table 1: Formula to Calculate Length of Gel in Inches to Be Applied Daily

Tube Size	INCHES Formula
15g tube	length × width × 0.6
2g tube (physician sample)	length × width × 1.3

Using the calculation, each square inch of ulcer surface will require approximately 2/3 inch length of gel squeezed from a 15g tube, or approximately 1 1/3 inch length of the gel from a 2g tube (physician sample). For example, if the ulcer measures 1 inch by 2 inches, then a 1 1/4 inch length of gel should be used for 15g tubes (1 × 2 × 0.6 = 1 1/4) and 2 3/4 inch gel length should be used for a 2g tube (1 × 2 × 1.3 = 2 3/4).

Table 2: Formula to Calculate Length of Gel in Centimeters to Be Applied Daily

Tube Size	CENTIMETERS Formula
15g tube	length × width ÷ 4
2g tube (physician sample)	length × width ÷ 2

Using the calculations for ulcer size in centimeters, each square centimeter of ulcer surface will require approximately a 0.25 centimeter length of gel squeezed from a 15g tube, or approximately a 0.5 centimeter length of gel from a 2g tube. For example, if the ulcer measures 4 cm by 2 cm, then a 2 centimeter length of gel should be used for a 15g tube [(4 × 2) ÷ 4 = 2] and a 4 centimeter length of gel should be used for a 2g tube [(4 × 2) ÷ 2 = 4].

The amount of REGRANEX Gel to be applied should be recalculated by the physician or wound caregiver at weekly or biweekly intervals depending on the rate of change in ulcer area. The weight of REGRANEX Gel from 15g tubes is 0.65g per inch length and 0.25g per centimeter length.

To apply REGRANEX Gel, the calculated length of gel should be squeezed on to a clean measuring surface, e.g., wax paper. The measured REGRANEX Gel is transferred from the clean measuring surface using an application aid and then spread over the entire ulcer area to yield a thin continuous layer of approximately 1/16 of an inch thickness. The site(s) of application should then be covered by a saline moistened dressing and left in place for approximately 12 hours. The dressing should then be removed and the ulcer rinsed with saline or water to remove residual gel and covered again with a second moist dressing (without REGRANEX Gel) for the remainder of the day. REGRANEX Gel should be applied once daily to the ulcer until complete healing has occurred. If the ulcer does not decrease in size by approximately 30% after 10 weeks of treatment or complete healing has not occurred in 20 weeks, continued treatment with REGRANEX Gel should be reassessed. The step-by-step instructions for applying REGRANEX Gel for home administration are described under "Patient Counseling Information". [*see Patient Counseling Information (17)*]

3 DOSAGE FORMS AND STRENGTHS

Gel: 0.01%; clear, colorless to straw-colored gel

4 CONTRAINDICATIONS

REGRANEX Gel is contraindicated in patients with known neoplasm(s) at the site(s) of application.

5 WARNINGS AND PRECAUTIONS

5.1 Cancer and Cancer Mortality

REGRANEX Gel contains becaplermin, a recombinant human platelet-derived growth factor, which promotes cellular proliferation and angiogenesis. [*see Clinical Pharmacology (12.1)*] The benefits and risks of becaplermin treatment should be carefully evaluated before prescribing. Becaplermin should be used with caution in patients with a known malignancy.

Malignancies distant from the site of application have occurred in becaplermin users in both a clinical study and postmarketing use, and an increased rate of death from systemic malignancies was seen in patients who have received 3 or more tubes of REGRANEX Gel.

In a follow-up study, 491 (75%) of 651 subjects from two randomized, controlled trials of becaplermin gel 0.01% were followed for a median of approximately 20 months to identify malignancies diagnosed after the end of the trials. Eight of 291 subjects (3%) from the becaplermin group and two of 200 subjects (1%) from the vehicle/standard of care group were diagnosed with cancers during the follow-up period, a relative risk of 2.7 (95% confidence interval 0.6–12.8). The types of cancers varied and all were remote from the treatment site.

In a retrospective study of a medical claims database, cancer rates and overall cancer mortality were compared between 1,622 patients who used REGRANEX Gel and 2,809 matched comparators. Estimates of the incidence rates reported below may be under-reported due to limited follow-up for each individual.

- The incidence rate for all cancers was 10.2 per 1,000 person years for patients treated with REGRANEX Gel and 9.1 per 1,000 person years for the comparators. Adjusted for several possible confounders, the rate ratio was 1.2 (95% confidence interval 0.7–1.9). Types of cancers varied and were remote from the site of treatment.
- The incidence rate for mortality from all cancers was 1.6 per 1,000 person years for those who received REGRANEX Gel and 0.9 per 1,000 person years for the comparators. The adjusted rate ratio was 1.8 (95% confidence interval 0.7–4.9).
- The incidence rate for mortality from all cancers among patients who received 3 or more tubes of REGRANEX Gel was 3.9 per 1,000 person years and 0.9 per 1,000 person years in the comparators. The adjusted rate ratio for cancer mortality among those who received 3 or more tubes relative to those who received none was 5.2 (95% confidence interval 1.6–17.6). [*see Boxed Warning*]

5.2 Application Site Reactions

If application site reactions occur, the possibility of sensitization or irritation caused by parabens or m-cresol should be considered. Consider interruption or discontinuation and further evaluation (e.g. patch testing) as dictated by clinical circumstances.

6 ADVERSE REACTIONS

6.1 Clinical Trials Experience

Because clinical trials are conducted under widely varying conditions, adverse reaction rates observed in the clinical trials of a drug cannot be directly compared to rates in the clinical trials of another drug and may not reflect the rates observed in practice.

In a follow-up study from two randomized, controlled trials, an increased rate of cancer remote from the becaplermin treatment site was observed in subjects treated with REGRANEX Gel. [*see Warnings and Precautions (5.1)*]

In clinical trials, erythematous rashes occurred in 2% of patients treated with REGRANEX Gel (and good ulcer care) or placebo (and good ulcer care), and none in patients receiving good ulcer care alone. Patients treated with REGRANEX Gel did not develop neutralizing antibodies against becaplermin.

6.2 Postmarketing Experience

An increased rate of mortality secondary to malignancy was observed in patients treated with 3 or more tubes of REGRANEX Gel in a postmarketing retrospective cohort study. [*see Boxed Warning and Warnings and Precautions (5.1)*]

Burning sensation at the site of application and erythema have been reported during post-approval use of REGRANEX Gel. Because post approval adverse reactions are reported voluntarily from a population of uncertain size, it is not always possible to reliably estimate their frequency or establish a causal relationship to the drug.

7 DRUG INTERACTIONS

It is not known if REGRANEX Gel interacts with other topical medications applied to the ulcer site. The use of REGRANEX Gel with other topical drugs has not been studied.

8 USE IN SPECIFIC POPULATIONS

8.1 Pregnancy

Pregnancy Category C. There are no adequate and well-controlled studies in pregnant women treated with REGRANEX Gel. REGRANEX Gel should be used during pregnancy only if the potential benefit justifies the potential risk to the fetus. Animal reproduction studies have not been conducted with REGRANEX Gel.

8.3 Nursing Mothers

It is not known whether becaplermin is excreted in human milk. Because many drugs are secreted in human milk, caution should be exercised when REGRANEX Gel is administered to nursing women.

8.4 Pediatric Use

Safety and effectiveness of REGRANEX Gel in pediatric patients below the age of 16 years have not been established.

8.5 Geriatric Use

Among patients receiving any dose of REGRANEX Gel in clinical studies of diabetic lower extremity ulcers, 150 patients were 65 years of age and older. No overall differences in safety or effectiveness were observed between patients < 65 years of age and patients ≥ 65 years of age. The number of patients aged 75 and older were insufficient (n=34) to determine whether they respond differently from younger patients.

10 OVERDOSAGE

There are no data on the effects of becaplermin overdose.

11 DESCRIPTION

REGRANEX Gel contains becaplermin, a recombinant human platelet-derived growth factor for topical administration. Becaplermin is produced by recombinant DNA technology by insertion of the gene for the B chain of platelet-derived growth factor (PDGF) into the yeast, *Saccharomyces cerevisiae*. Becaplermin has a molecular weight of approximately 25 KD and is a homodimer composed of two identical polypeptide chains that are bound together by disulfide bonds. REGRANEX Gel is a non-sterile, low bioburden, preserved, sodium carboxymethylcellulose-based (CMC) topical gel, containing the active ingredient becaplermin and the following inactive ingredients: carboxymethylcellulose sodium, glacial acetic acid, l-lysine hydrochloride, m-cresol, methylparaben, propylparaben, sodium acetate trihydrate, sodium chloride, and water for injection. Each gram of REGRANEX Gel contains 100 mcg of becaplermin.

12 CLINICAL PHARMACOLOGY

12.1 Mechanism of Action

REGRANEX Gel has biological activity similar to that of endogenous platelet-derived growth factor, which includes promoting the chemotactic recruitment and proliferation of cells involved in wound repair and enhancing the formation of granulation tissue.

12.2 Pharmacodynamics

Clinical pharmacodynamic studies have not been conducted.

12.3 Pharmacokinetics

Ten patients with Stage III or IV (as defined in the International Association of Enterostomal Therapy (IAET) guide to chronic wound staging,[1, 2] lower extremity diabetic ulcers received topical applications of becaplermin gel 0.01% at a dose range of 0.32–2.95 μg/kg (7μg/cm^2) daily for 14 days. Six patients had non-quantifiable PDGF levels at baseline and throughout the study, two patients had PDGF levels at baseline which did not increase substantially, and two patients had PDGF levels that increased sporadically above their baseline values during the 14 day study period.

13 NONCLINICAL TOXICOLOGY

13.1 Carcinogenesis, Mutagenesis, Impairment of Fertility

Becaplermin was not genotoxic in a battery of *in vitro* assays (including those for bacterial and mammalian cell point mutation, chromosomal aberration, and DNA damage/repair). Becaplermin was also not mutagenic in an *in vivo* assay for the induction of micronuclei in mouse bone marrow cells.

Carcinogenesis and reproductive toxicity studies have not been conducted with REGRANEX Gel.

13.2 Animal Toxicology and/or Pharmacology

In nonclinical studies, rats injected at the metatarsals with 3 or 10 mcg/site (approximately 60 or 200 mcg/kg) of becaplermin every other day for 13 days displayed histological changes indicative of accelerated bone remodeling consisting of periosteal hyperplasia and subperiosteal bone resorption and exostosis. The soft tissue adjacent to the injection site had fibroplasia with accompanying mononuclear cell infiltration reflective of the ability of PDGF to stimulate connective tissue growth. [*see Indications and Usage (1.2)*]

14 CLINICAL STUDIES

The effects of REGRANEX Gel on the incidence of and time to complete healing in lower extremity diabetic ulcers were assessed in four randomized controlled studies. Of 922 patients studied, 478 received either REGRANEX Gel 0.003% or 0.01%. All study participants had lower extremity diabetic neuropathic ulcers that extended into the subcutaneous tissue or beyond (Stages III and IV of the IAET guide to chronic wound staging). Ninety-three percent of the patients enrolled in these four trials had foot ulcers. The remaining 7% of the patients had ankle or leg ulcers. The diabetic ulcers were of at least 8 weeks duration and had an adequate blood supply (defined as $T_cpO_2 > 30$ mm Hg). In the four trials, ninety-five percent of the ulcers measured in area up to 10 cm^2, and the median ulcer size at baseline ranged from 1.4 cm^2 to 3.5 cm^2. All treatment groups received a program of good ulcer care consisting of initial complete sharp debridement, a non-weight-bearing regimen, systemic treatment for wound-related infection if present, moist saline dressings changed twice a day, and additional debridement as necessary. REGRANEX Gel 0.003% or 0.01% or placebo gel was applied once a day and covered with a saline moistened dressing. After approximately 12 hours, the gel was gently rinsed off and a saline moistened dressing was then applied for the remainder of the day. Patients were treated until complete healing, or for a period of up to 20 weeks. Patients were considered a treatment failure if their ulcer did not show an approximately 30% reduction in initial ulcer area after eight to ten weeks of REGRANEX Gel therapy.

The primary endpoint, incidence of complete ulcer closure within 20 weeks, for all treatment arms is shown in Figure 1. In each study, REGRANEX Gel in conjunction with good ulcer care was compared to placebo gel plus good ulcer care or good ulcer care alone.

In Study 1, a multicenter, double-blind, placebo controlled trial of 118 patients, the incidence of complete ulcer closure for REGRANEX Gel 0.003% (n=61) was 48% versus 25% for placebo gel (n=57; p=0.02, logistic regression analysis).

In Study 2, a multicenter, double-blind, placebo controlled trial of 382 patients, the incidence of complete ulcer closure for REGRANEX Gel 0.01% (n=123) was 50% versus 36% for REGRANEX Gel 0.003% (n=132) and 35% for placebo gel (n=127). Only REGRANEX Gel 0.01% was significantly different from placebo gel (p=0.01, logistic regression analysis).

The primary goal of Study 3, a multicenter controlled trial of 172 patients, was to assess the safety of vehicle gel (placebo; n=70) compared to good ulcer care alone (n=68). The study included a small (n=34) REGRANEX Gel 0.01% arm. Incidences of complete ulcer closure were 44% for REGRANEX Gel, 36% for placebo gel and 22% for good ulcer care alone.

In Study 4, a multicenter, evaluator-blind, controlled trial of 250 patients, the incidences of complete ulcer closure in the REGRANEX Gel 0.01% arm (n=128) (36%) and good ulcer care alone (n=122) (32%) were not statistically different.

[See figure 1 at top of next column]

In general, where REGRANEX Gel was associated with higher incidences of complete ulcer closure, differences in the incidence first became apparent after approximately 10 weeks and increased with continued treatment (Table 3).

Figure 1: Incidence of Complete Healing

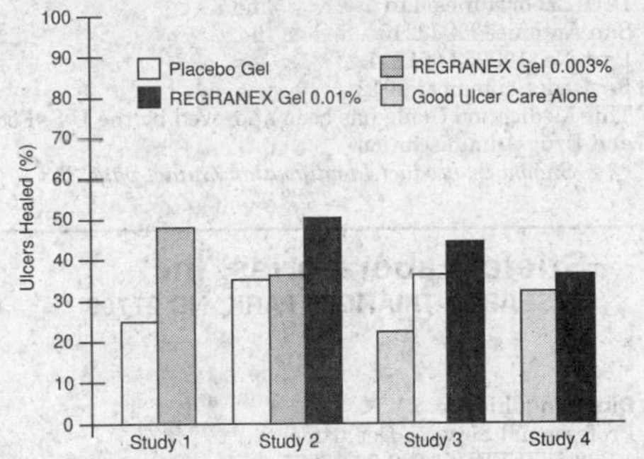

Table 3: Life Table Estimates of the Incidence (%) of Complete Healing over Time for Study 2

	REGRANEX Gel 0.01% (%)	Placebo Gel (%)
Week 2	1	0
Week 4	6	2
Week 6	9	6
Week 8	16	14
Week 10	23	18
Week 12	34	25
Week 14	37	28
Week 16	43	33
Week 18	46	34
Week 20	50	37

In a 3-month follow-up period where no standardized regimen of preventative care was utilized, the incidence of ulcer recurrence was approximately 30% in all treatment groups, demonstrating that the durability of ulcer closure was comparable in all treatment groups.

In a randomized, double-blind study of REGRANEX Gel (100 mcg/g once daily for 16 weeks) in patients with Stage III or IV pressure ulcers, the incidence of complete ulcer closure was 15% (28/189) in the becaplermin group and 12% (22/190) in the vehicle control group. This difference was not statistically significant.

In two small, randomized, double-blinded studies of REGRANEX Gel (100 mcg/g once daily for 16 weeks) in patients with venous stasis ulcers, the combined incidence of complete ulcer closure was 46% (30/65) in the becaplermin group and 39% (26/67) in the vehicle control group. This difference was not statistically significant.

15 REFERENCES

1. *J. Enterostomal Ther* 15:4, 1988
2. *Decubitis* 2:24, 1989

16 HOW SUPPLIED/STORAGE AND HANDLING

REGRANEX Gel is available in a multi use tube in the following size:

15 g tube NDC 0064-0810-15

REGRANEX Gel is for external use only.

Store refrigerated at 2° – 8° C (36° – 46°F). Do not freeze. Do not use the gel after the expiration date shown at the bottom of the tube.

17 PATIENT COUNSELING INFORMATION

[*See FDA-approved patient labeling (Medication Guide)*]

Counsel patients to review and discuss any questions or concerns with their healthcare provider before starting REGRANEX and at regular intervals while receiving REGRANEX.

Patients should be advised that:

- they should read the medication guide;
- hands should be washed thoroughly before applying REGRANEX Gel;
- the tip of the tube should not come into contact with the ulcer or any other surface; the tube should be recapped tightly after each use;
- a cotton swab, tongue depressor, or other application aid should be used to apply REGRANEX Gel;
- REGRANEX Gel should only be applied once a day in a carefully measured quantity [*see Dosage and Administration (2)*]. The measured quantity of gel should be spread evenly over the ulcerated area to yield a thin continuous layer of approximately 1/16 of an inch thickness. The measured length of the gel to be squeezed from the tube should be adjusted according to the size of the ulcer. The amount of REGRANEX Gel to be applied daily should be recalculated at weekly or biweekly intervals by the physician or wound care giver.

Step-by-step instructions for application of REGRANEX Gel are as follows:

- Squeeze the calculated length of gel onto a clean, firm, nonabsorbable surface, e.g., wax paper.
- With a clean cotton swab, tongue depressor, or similar application aid, spread the measured REGRANEX Gel over the ulcer surface to obtain an even layer.
- Cover with a saline moistened gauze dressing.
  - after approximately 12 hours, the ulcer should be gently rinsed with saline or water to remove residual gel and covered with a saline-moistened gauze dressing (without REGRANEX Gel);
  - it is important to use REGRANEX Gel together with a good ulcer care program, including a strict non-weight-bearing program;
  - excess application of REGRANEX Gel has not been shown to be beneficial;
  - REGRANEX Gel should be stored in the refrigerator. Do not freeze REGRANEX Gel;
  - REGRANEX Gel should not be used after the expiration date on the bottom, crimped end of the tube.

Manufactured by:
Healthpoint, Ltd.
Fort Worth, TX 76107
U.S. Gov't License # 1885
Marketed by:
Healthpoint Biotherapeutics
Fort Worth, TX 76107
REGRANEX is a registered trademark of Healthpoint, Ltd.
Distributed by:
DPT Laboratories, Ltd.
San Antonio, TX 78215
Part No. 129953-0912
Revised: September 2012

MEDICATION GUIDE
REGRANEX® (*RE'–GRAN–IX*)
(becaplermin)
Gel

Read this Medication Guide before you start using REGRANEX and each time you get a refill. There may be new information. This information does not take the place of talking to your healthcare provider about your medical condition or your treatment.

What is the most important information I should know about REGRANEX?

People who use 3 or more tubes of REGRANEX may have an increased risk of death from cancer.

- You should talk with your healthcare provider about the possible benefits and risks to you if you use more than 3 tubes of REGRANEX.
- If you already have cancer, you and your healthcare provider should carefully consider whether you will use REGRANEX.

If you decide to use REGRANEX, your healthcare provider will tell you how to use REGRANEX. See the section "How should I use REGRANEX?" below.

What is REGRANEX?

REGRANEX is a man-made protein medicine that is used with other ulcer care practices (such as good wound care) to treat diabetic sores (ulcers) of your legs or feet that are deeper than just your skin, in people who have good blood supply to the legs.

It is not known if REGRANEX is effective for the treatment of pressure ulcers or ulcers that are due to poor blood flow (circulation).

It is not known if REGRANEX is safe and effective in children under 16 years of age.

Who should not use REGRANEX?

Do not use REGRANEX if you have a skin tumor at the area where you apply REGRANEX.

What should I tell my healthcare provider before using REGRANEX?

Before you use REGRANEX tell your healthcare provider if you:

- have cancer
- have poor blood flow to your lower legs and feet
- have allergies to any of the ingredients in REGRANEX. See the end of this Medication Guide for a complete list of ingredients in REGRANEX.
- have any other medical conditions
- are pregnant or plan to become pregnant. It is not known if REGRANEX will harm your unborn baby.
- are breast-feeding or plan to breast-feed. It is not known if REGRANEX passes into your breast milk.

Tell your healthcare provider about all the medicines you take, including prescription and non-prescription medicines, vitamins, and herbal supplements. Especially tell your healthcare provider if you apply other medicines to diabetic ulcers of your legs or feet.

Know the medicines you take. Keep a list of them to show your healthcare provider and pharmacist when you get a new medicine.

How should I use REGRANEX?
Use REGRANEX together with good ulcer care, as prescribed by your healthcare provider. This includes following your healthcare provider's instructions about not putting weight on the affected leg and foot (non-weight bearing).
- Use REGRANEX exactly as your healthcare provider tells you to use it.
- REGRANEX is for use on skin ulcers only. Do not use REGRANEX in your mouth, eyes, or vagina.
- REGRANEX comes as a gel. Your healthcare provider should tell you how often to use REGRANEX and how much REGRANEX to use.
- Your healthcare provider should check the size of your ulcer every 1 to 2 weeks.
- Your healthcare provider may change the amount of REGRANEX to be applied to your ulcer as the size of your ulcer changes. So, the amount of REGRANEX to be squeezed from the tube may change as the size of your ulcer changes.
- Close your REGRANEX tube tightly after each use.
- Put the REGRANEX tube back in the refrigerator after each use.
- Use a cotton swab, tongue depressor, or other application aid when you apply your REGRANEX. Do not let the tip of your REGRANEX tube touch the ulcer or any other surface.
- Apply REGRANEX one time each day.

Apply REGRANEX as follows:
- Wash your hands well before you apply REGRANEX.
- Carefully measure the amount of REGRANEX that your healthcare provider tells you to use.
- Squeeze the amount of REGRANEX needed for your ulcer on to a clean, firm, non-absorbable surface, such as wax paper.
- Use a clean cotton swab, tongue depressor, or similar application aid, to spread the REGRANEX gel in a thin even layer over the surface of the ulcer on your foot or leg.
- Cover the area with a saline-moistened gauze dressing.
- After about 12 hours, gently rinse the ulcer with saline or water to remove the rest of the REGRANEX. Cover the ulcer with a new saline-moistened gauze dressing. Do not apply any more REGRANEX.

What are the possible side effects of REGRANEX?
REGRANEX may cause serious side effects.
- See the section, "What is the most important information I should know about REGRANEX?"
- Common side effects of REGRANEX include:
  - Red skin rash
  - Burning at the application site

Tell your doctor if you have any side effect that bothers you or that does not go away.
These are not all the possible side effects of REGRANEX gel. For more information, ask your doctor or pharmacist.
Call your doctor for medical advice about side effects. You may report side effects to FDA at 1-800-FDA-1088.
You may also report side effects to Healthpoint Biotherapeutics at 1-800-441-8227.

How should I store REGRANEX?
- Store REGRANEX in the refrigerator at 36°F to 46°F (2°C to 8°C).
- Do not freeze REGRANEX.
- Do not use REGRANEX after the expiration date on the bottom (sealed end) of the tube.
- Throw away your REGRANEX that is out of date or no longer needed for your treatment.

Keep REGRANEX and all medicines out of the reach of children.

General information about REGRANEX
Medicines are sometimes prescribed for purposes other than those listed in a Medication Guide. Do not use REGRANEX for a condition for which it was not prescribed. Do not give REGRANEX to other people, even if they have the same symptoms that you have. It may harm them.
This Medication Guide summarizes the most important information about REGRANEX. If you would like more information about REGRANEX, talk to your healthcare provider. You can ask your healthcare provider or pharmacist for information about REGRANEX that is written for health professionals.

What are the ingredients in REGRANEX?
Active ingredient: becaplermin
Inactive ingredients: carboxymethylcellulose sodium, glacial acetic acid, l-lysine hydrochloride, m-cresol, methylparaben, propylparaben, sodium acetate trihydrate, sodium chloride, and water for injection.

Manufactured by:
Healthpoint, Ltd.
Fort Worth, TX 76107
U.S. Gov't License # 1885
Marketed by:
Healthpoint Biotherapeutics
Fort Worth, TX 76107
REGRANEX is a registered trademark of Healthpoint, Ltd.

Distributed by:
DPT Laboratories, Ltd.
San Antonio, TX 78215
Part No. 129953-0912
Revised: September 2012
This Medication Guide has been approved by the U.S. Food and Drug Administration.

Shown in Product Identification Guide, page 313

Stiefel Laboratories, Inc.
RESEARCH TRIANGLE PARK, NC 27709

Direct Inquiries to:
Professional Services Department
1-888-STIEFEL (1-888-784-3335)

ALTABAX ℞
(retapamulin ointment)
1%

HIGHLIGHTS OF PRESCRIBING INFORMATION
These highlights do not include all the information needed to use ALTABAX safely and effectively. See full prescribing information for ALTABAX.
ALTABAX(retapamulin ointment), 1%
For Dermatological use only
Initial U.S. Approval: 2007

———INDICATIONS AND USAGE———
ALTABAX, a pleuromutilin antibacterial, is indicated for the topical treatment of impetigo due to *Staphylococcus aureus* (methicillin-susceptible isolates only) or *Streptococcus pyogenes* in patients aged 9 months or older. Safety in patients younger than 9 months has not been established. (1)

———DOSAGE AND ADMINISTRATION———
- Apply a thin layer of ALTABAX to the affected area (up to 100 cm^2 in total area in adults or 2% total body surface area in pediatric patients aged 9 months or older) twice daily for 5 days. (2)
- The treated area may be covered with a sterile bandage or gauze dressing if desired. (2)

———DOSAGE FORMS AND STRENGTHS———
10 mg retapamulin/1g of ointment in 15-, and 30-gram tubes (3)

———CONTRAINDICATIONS———
None. (4)

———WARNINGS AND PRECAUTIONS———
- Discontinue in the event of sensitization or severe local irritation. (5.1)
- Not intended for ingestion. Not for intraoral, intranasal, ophthalmic, or intravaginal use. (5.2)

———ADVERSE REACTIONS———
The most common drug-related adverse reaction was application site irritation (≤2% of subjects). (6.1)
To report SUSPECTED ADVERSE REACTIONS, contact GlaxoSmithKline at 1-888-825-5249 or FDA at 1-800-FDA-1088 or www.fda.gov/medwatch.
See 17 for PATIENT COUNSELING INFORMATION
Revised: 07/2013

FULL PRESCRIBING INFORMATION: CONTENTS*

*** Sections or subsections omitted from the full prescribing information are not listed**

FULL PRESCRIBING INFORMATION

1 INDICATIONS AND USAGE
ALTABAX® is indicated for use in adults and pediatric patients aged 9 months and older for the topical treatment of impetigo (up to 100 cm^2 in total area in adults or 2% total body surface area in pediatric patients aged 9 months or older) due to *Staphylococcus aureus* (methicillin-susceptible isolates only) or *Streptococcus pyogenes[see Clinical Studies (14)]*. Safety in patients younger than 9 months has not been established.
To reduce the development of drug-resistant bacteria and maintain the effectiveness of ALTABAX and other antibacterial drugs, ALTABAX should be used only to treat or prevent infections that are proven or strongly suspected to be caused by susceptible bacteria.

2 DOSAGE AND ADMINISTRATION
A thin layer of ALTABAX should be applied to the affected area (up to 100 cm^2 in total area in adults or 2% total body surface area in pediatric patients aged 9 months or older) twice daily for 5 days. The treated area may be covered with a sterile bandage or gauze dressing if desired *[see Patient Counseling Information (17)]*.

3 DOSAGE FORMS AND STRENGTHS
10 mg retapamulin/1g of ointment in 15- and 30 gram tubes.

4 CONTRAINDICATIONS
None.

5 WARNINGS AND PRECAUTIONS
5.1 Local Irritation
In the event of sensitization or severe local irritation from ALTABAX, usage should be discontinued, the ointment wiped off, and appropriate alternative therapy for the infection instituted *[see Patient Counseling Information (17)]*.

5.2 Not for Systemic or Mucosal Use
ALTABAX is not intended for ingestion or for oral, intranasal, ophthalmic, or intravaginal use. The efficacy and safety of ALTABAX on mucosal surfaces have not been established. Epistaxis has been reported with the use of ALTABAX on nasal mucosa.

5.3 Potential for Microbial Overgrowth
The use of antibiotics may promote the selection of nonsusceptible organisms. Should superinfection occur during therapy, appropriate measures should be taken.
Prescribing ALTABAX in the absence of a proven or strongly suspected bacterial infection is unlikely to provide benefit to the patient and increases the risk of the development of drug-resistant bacteria.

6 ADVERSE REACTIONS
6.1 Clinical Studies Experience
Because clinical trials are conducted under varying conditions, adverse reaction rates observed in the clinical trials of a drug cannot be directly compared with rates in the clinical trials of another drug and may not reflect the rates observed in practice. The adverse reaction information from the clinical trials does, however, provide a basis for identifying the adverse events that appear to be related to drug use and for approximating rates.
The safety profile of ALTABAX was assessed in 2,115 adult and pediatric subjects ≥9 months who used at least one dose from a 5-day, twice a day regimen of retapamulin ointment. Control groups included 819 adult and pediatric subjects who used at least one dose of the active control (oral cephalexin), 172 subjects who used an active topical comparator (not available in the US), and 71 subjects who used placebo.
Adverse events rated by investigators as drug-related occurred in 5.5% (116/2,115) of subjects treated with retapamulin ointment, 6.6% (54/819) of subjects receiving cephalexin, and 2.8% (2/71) of subjects receiving placebo. The most common drug-related adverse events (≥1% of subjects) were application site irritation (1.4%) in the retapamulin group, diarrhea (1.7%) in the cephalexin group, and application site pruritus (1.4%) and application site paresthesia (1.4%) in the placebo group.
Adults:
The adverse events, regardless of attribution, reported in at least 1% of adults (aged 18 years and older) who received ALTABAX or comparator are presented in Table 1.

Table 1. Adverse Events Reported by ≥1% of Adult Subjects Treated With ALTABAX or Comparator in Phase 3 Clinical Trials

Adverse Event	ALTABAX N = 1,527 %	Cephalexin N = 698 %
Headache	2.0	2.0
Application site irritation	1.6	<1.0
Diarrhea	1.4	2.3
Nausea	1.2	1.9
Nasopharyngitis	1.2	<1.0
Creatinine phosphokinase increased	<1.0	1.0

Pediatrics:
The adverse events, regardless of attribution, reported in at least 1% of pediatric subjects aged 9 months to 17 years who received ALTABAX are presented in Table 2.

Table 2. Adverse Events Reported by ≥1% in Pediatric Subjects Aged 9 Months to 17 Years Treated With ALTABAX in Phase 3 Clinical Trials

Adverse Event	ALTABAX N = 588 %	Cephalexin N = 121 %	Placebo N = 64 %
Application site pruritus	1.9	0	0
Diarrhea	1.7	5.0	0
Nasopharyngitis	1.5	1.7	0
Pruritus	1.5	1.0	1.6
Eczema	1.0	0	0
Headache	1.2	1.7	0
Pyrexia	1.2	<1.0	1.6

Other Adverse Events:
Application site pain, erythema, and contact dermatitis were reported in less than 1% of subjects in clinical trials.

6.2 Postmarketing Experience
In addition to reports in clinical trials, the following events have been identified during postmarketing use of ALTABAX. Because these events are reported voluntarily from a population of uncertain size, it is not possible to reliably estimate their frequency or establish a causal relationship to drug exposure.
General Disorders and Administration Site Conditions: Application site burning.
Immune System Disorders: Hypersensitivity including angioedema.

7 DRUG INTERACTIONS

Coadministration of oral ketoconazole 200 mg twice daily increased retapamulin geometric mean $AUC_{(0-24)}$ and C_{max} by 81% after topical application of retapamulin ointment, 1% on the abraded skin of healthy adult males. Due to low systemic exposure to retapamulin following topical application in adults and pediatric patients aged 2 years and older, dosage adjustments for retapamulin are unnecessary when coadministered with CYP3A4 inhibitors, such as ketoconazole. Based on in vitro P450 inhibition studies and the low systemic exposure observed following topical application of ALTABAX, retapamulin is unlikely to affect the metabolism of other P450 substrates.
Concomitant administration of retapamulin and CYP3A4 inhibitors, such as ketoconazole, has not been studied in pediatric patients. In pediatric subjects aged 2 to 24 months, systemic exposure of retapamulin was higher compared with subjects aged 2 years and older after topical application *[see Pharmacokinetics (12.3)]*. Based on the higher exposure of retapamulin, it is not recommended to coadminister ALTABAX with strong CYP3A4 inhibitors in patients younger than 24 months.
The effect of concurrent application of ALTABAX and other topical products to the same area of skin has not been studied.

8 USE IN SPECIFIC POPULATIONS

8.1 Pregnancy
Pregnancy Category B
Effects on embryo-fetal development were assessed in pregnant rats given 50, 150, or 450 mg/kg/day by oral gavage on days 6 to 17 postcoitus. Maternal toxicity (decreased body weight gain and food consumption) and developmental toxicity (decreased fetal body weight and delayed skeletal ossification) were evident at doses ≥150 mg/kg/day. There were no treatment-related malformations observed in fetal rats. Retapamulin was given as a continuous intravenous infusion to pregnant rabbits at dosages of 2.4, 7.2, or 24 mg/kg/day from day 7 to 19 of gestation. Maternal toxicity (decreased body weight gain, food consumption, and abortions) was demonstrated at dosages ≥7.2 mg/kg/day (8-fold the estimated maximum achievable human exposure, based on AUC, at 7.2 mg/kg/day). There was no treatment-related effect on embryo-fetal development.
There are no adequate and well-controlled trials in pregnant women. Because animal reproduction studies are not always predictive of human response, ALTABAX should be used in pregnancy only when the potential benefits outweigh the potential risk.

8.3 Nursing Mothers
It is not known whether retapamulin is excreted in human milk. Because many drugs are excreted in human milk, caution should be exercised when ALTABAX is administered to a nursing woman. The safe use of retapamulin during breastfeeding has not been established.

8.4 Pediatric Use
The safety and effectiveness of ALTABAX in the treatment of impetigo have been established in pediatric patients aged 9 months to 17 years. Use of ALTABAX in pediatric patients (9 months to 17 years) is supported by evidence from adequate and well-controlled trials of ALTABAX in which 588 pediatric subjects received at least one dose of retapamulin ointment, 1% *[see Adverse Reactions (6.1), Clinical Studies (14)]*. The magnitude of efficacy and the safety profile of ALTABAX in pediatric subjects 9 months and older were similar to those in adults.
The safety and effectiveness of ALTABAX in pediatric patients younger than 9 months of age have not been established. An open-label clinical trial of topical treatment with ALTABAX (twice daily for 5 days) was conducted in patients aged 2 to 24 months. Plasma samples were obtained from 79 subjects. In these pediatric subjects, systemic exposure of retapamulin was higher compared with subjects aged 2 to 17 years. Furthermore, a higher proportion of pediatric subjects aged 2 to 9 months had measurable concentrations (>0.5 ng/mL) of retapamulin compared with subjects aged 9 to 24 months *[see Pharmacokinetics (12.3)]*. The highest levels were seen in subjects aged 2 to 6 months *[see Pharmacokinetics (12.3)]*. The use of retapamulin is not indicated in pediatric patients younger than 9 months.

8.5 Geriatric Use
Of the total number of subjects in the adequate and well-controlled trials of ALTABAX, 234 subjects were 65 years of age and older, of whom 114 subjects were 75 years of age and older. No overall differences in effectiveness or safety were observed between these subjects and younger adult subjects.

10 OVERDOSAGE

Overdosage with ALTABAX has not been reported. Any signs or symptoms of overdose, either topically or by accidental ingestion, should be treated symptomatically consistent with good clinical practice.
There is no known antidote for overdoses of ALTABAX.

11 DESCRIPTION

ALTABAX contains retapamulin, a semisynthetic pleuromutilin antibiotic. The chemical name of retapamulin is acetic acid, [[(3-*exo*)-8-methyl-8-azabicyclo[3.2.1]oct-3-yl]thio]-, (3a*S*,4*R*,5*S*,6*S*,8*R*,9*R*,9a*R*,10*R*)-6-ethenyldecahydro-5-hydroxy-4,6,9,10-tetramethyl-1-oxo-3a,9-propano-3a*H*-cyclopentacycloocten-8-yl ester. Retapamulin, a white to pale-yellow crystalline solid, has a molecular formula of $C_{30}H_{47}NO_4S$, and a molecular weight of 517.78. The chemical structure is:

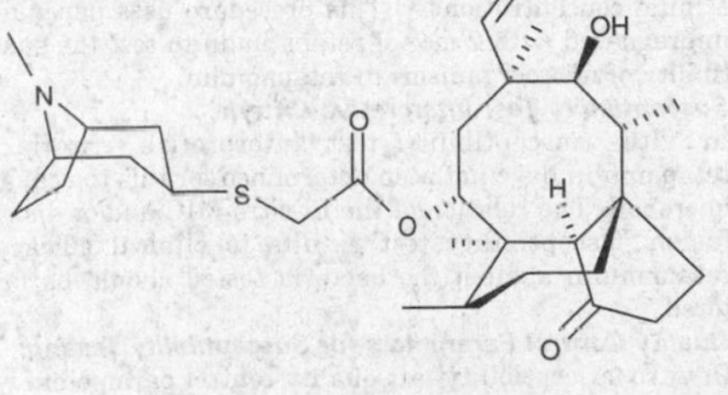

Each gram of ointment for dermatological use contains 10 mg of retapamulin in white petrolatum.

12 CLINICAL PHARMACOLOGY

12.1 Mechanism of Action
ALTABAX is an antibacterial agent *[see Clinical Pharmacology (12.4)]*.

12.2 Pharmacodynamics
In post-hoc analyses of manually over-read 12-lead ECGs from healthy subjects (N = 103), no significant effects on QT/QTc intervals were observed after topical application of retapamulin ointment on intact and abraded skin. Due to the low systemic exposure to retapamulin with topical application, QT prolongation in patients is unlikely *[see Clinical Pharmacology (12.3)]*.

12.3 Pharmacokinetics
Absorption:
In a trial of healthy adult subjects, retapamulin ointment, 1% was applied once daily to intact skin (800 cm^2 surface area) and to abraded skin (200 cm^2 surface area) under occlusion for up to 7 days. Systemic exposure following topical application of retapamulin through intact and abraded skin was low. Three percent of blood samples obtained on Day 1 after topical application to intact skin had measurable retapamulin concentrations (lower limit of quantitation 0.5 ng/mL); thus C_{max} values on Day 1 could not be determined. Eighty-two percent of blood samples obtained on Day 7 after topical application to intact skin and 97% and 100% of blood samples obtained after topical application to abraded skin on Days 1 and 7, respectively, had measurable retapamulin concentrations. The median C_{max} value in plasma after application to 800 cm^2 of intact skin was 3.5 ng/mL on Day 7 (range: 1.2 to 7.8 ng/mL). The median C_{max} value in plasma after application to 200 cm^2 of abraded skin was 11.7 ng/mL on Day 1 (range: 5.6 to 22.1 ng/mL) and 9.0 ng/mL on Day 7 (range: 6.7 to 12.8 ng/mL).
Plasma samples were obtained from 380 adult subjects and 136 pediatric subjects (aged 2 to 17 years) who were receiving topical treatment with ALTABAX topically twice daily. Eleven percent had measurable retapamulin concentrations (lower limit of quantitation 0.5 ng/mL), of which the median concentration was 0.8 ng/mL. The maximum measured retapamulin concentration in adults was 10.7 ng/mL and in pediatric subjects (aged 2 to 17 years) was 18.5 ng/mL.
A single plasma sample was obtained from 79 pediatric subjects (aged 2 to 24 months) who were receiving topical treatment with ALTABAX twice daily. Forty-six percent had measurable retapamulin concentrations (>0.5 ng/mL) compared with 7% in pediatric subjects aged 2 to 17 years. A higher proportion (69%) of pediatric subjects aged 2 to 9 months had measurable concentrations of retapamulin compared with subjects aged 9 to 24 months (32%). Among pediatric subjects aged 2 to 9 months (n = 29), 4 subjects had retapamulin concentrations that were higher (≥26.9 ng/mL) than the maximum concentration observed in pediatric subjects aged 2 to 17 years (18.5 ng/mL). Among pediatric subjects aged 9 to 24 months (n = 50), 1 subject had a retapamulin concentration that was higher (95.1 ng/mL) than the maximum level observed in pediatric subjects aged 2 to 17 years.
Distribution:
Retapamulin is approximately 94% bound to human plasma proteins, and the protein binding is independent of concentration. The apparent volume of distribution of retapamulin has not been determined in humans.
Metabolism:
In vitro studies with human hepatocytes showed that the main routes of metabolism were mono-oxygenation and di-oxygenation. In vitro studies with human liver microsomes demonstrated that retapamulin is extensively metabolized to numerous metabolites, of which the predominant routes of metabolism were mono-oxygenation and N-demethylation. The major enzyme responsible for metabolism of retapamulin in human liver microsomes was cytochrome P450 3A4 (CYP3A4).
Elimination:
Retapamulin elimination in humans has not been investigated due to low systemic exposure after topical application.

12.4 Microbiology
Retapamulin is a semisynthetic derivative of the compound pleuromutilin, which is isolated through fermentation from *Clitopiluspassseckerianus* (formerly *Pleurotuspassseckerianus*). In vitro activity of retapamulin against isolates of *Staphylococcus aureus* as well as *Streptococcus pyogenes* has been demonstrated.
Antimicrobial Mechanism of Action:
Retapamulin selectively inhibits bacterial protein synthesis by interacting at a site on the 50S subunit of the bacterial ribosome through an interaction that is different from that of other antibiotics. This binding site involves ribosomal protein L3 and is in the region of the ribosomal P site and peptidyl transferase center. By virtue of binding to this site, pleuromutilins inhibit peptidyl transfer, block P-site interactions, and prevent the normal formation of active 50S ribosomal subunits. Retapamulin is bacteriostatic against *Staphylococcus aureus* and *Streptococcus pyogenes* at the retapamulin in vitro minimum inhibitory concentration (MIC) for these organisms. At concentrations 1,000× the in vitro MIC, retapamulin is bactericidal against these same organisms. Although cross-resistance between retapamulin

Table 4. Clinical Response at End of Therapy and at Follow-Up by Analysis Population

Analysis Population	ALTABAX		Placebo		Difference in Success Rates (%)	95% CI (%)
	n/N	Success Rate (%)	n/N	Success Rate (%)		
End of Therapy						
PPC	111/124	89.5	33/62	53.2	36.3	(22.8, 49.8)
ITTC	119/139	85.6	37/71	52.1	33.5	(20.5, 46.5)
PPB	96/107	89.7	26/52	50.0	39.7	(25.0, 54.5)
ITTB	101/114	88.6	28/57	49.1	39.5	(25.2, 53.7)
Follow-Up						
PPC	98/119	82.4	25/58	43.1	39.2	(24.8, 53.7)
ITTC	105/139	75.5	28/71	39.4	36.1	(22.7, 49.5)
PPB	86/102	84.3	18/48	37.5	46.8	(31.4, 62.2)
ITTB	91/114	79.8	19/57	33.3	46.5	(32.2, 60.8)

n = number with clinical success outcome, N = number in analysis population, PPC = Clinical Per Protocol Population, ITTC = Clinical Intent to Treat Population, PPB = Bacteriological Per Protocol Population, ITTB = Bacteriological Intent to Treat Population.

Table 5. Clinical Response at End of Therapy and Follow-Up for Subjects With Staphylococcus aureus and Streptococcus pyogenes at Baseline in the Per Protocol Bacteriological Population (PPB)

Pathogen	ALTABAX		Placebo	
	n/N	Success Rate (%)	n/N	Success Rate (%)
End of Therapy				
Staphylococcus aureus (Methicillin-susceptible)	79/88	89.8	25/48	52.1
Streptococcus pyogenes	29/32	90.6	3/7	42.9
Follow-Up				
Staphylococcus aureus (Methicillin-susceptible)	71/84	84.5	19/44	43.2
Streptococcus pyogenes	29/32	90.6	2/6	33.3

n/N = Number of clinical successes/number of pathogens isolated at baseline.

and other antibacterial classes (such as clindamycin and oxazolidones) exist, isolates resistant to these classes may be susceptible to retapamulin.

Mechanisms of Decreased Susceptibility to Retapamulin:

In vitro, 2 mechanisms that cause reduced susceptibility to retapamulin have been identified, specifically, mutations in ribosomal protein L3, the presence of Cfr rRNA methyltransferase or the presence of an efflux mechanism. Decreased susceptibility of *S. aureus* to retapamulin (highest retapamulin MIC was 2 mcg/mL) develops slowly in vitro via multistep mutations in L3 after serial passage in subinhibitory concentrations of retapamulin. There was no apparent treatment-associated reduction in susceptibility to retapamulin in the Phase 3 clinical program. The clinical significance of these findings is not known.

Other:

Based on in vitro broth microdilution susceptibility testing, no differences were observed in susceptibility of *S. aureus* to retapamulin whether the isolates were methicillin-resistant or methicillin-susceptible. Retapamulin susceptibility did not correlate with clinical success rates in patients with methicillin-resistant *S.aureus*. The reason for this is not known but may have been influenced by the presence of particular strains of *S. aureus* possessing certain virulence factors, such as Panton-Valentine Leukocidin (PVL). In the case of treatment failure associated with *S. aureus* (regardless of methicillin susceptibility), the presence of strains possessing additional virulence factors (such as PVL) should be considered.

Retapamulin has been shown to be active against the following microorganisms, both in vitro and in clinical trials *[see Indications and Usage (1)]*.

Aerobic and Facultative Gram-Positive Bacteria:

Staphylococcus aureus (methicillin-susceptible isolates only)

Streptococcus pyogenes

Susceptibility Testing:

The clinical microbiology laboratory should provide cumulative results of the in vitro susceptibility test results for antimicrobial drugs used in local hospitals and practice areas to the physician as periodic reports that describe the susceptibility profile of nosocomial and community-acquired pathogens. These reports should aid the physician in selecting the most effective antimicrobial.

Susceptibility Testing Techniques:

Dilution Techniques:

Quantitative methods can be used to determine the MIC of retapamulin that will inhibit the growth of the bacteria being tested. The MIC provides an estimate of the susceptibility of bacteria to retapamulin. The MIC should be determined using a standardized procedure.[1,2] Standardized procedures are based on a dilution method (broth or agar) or equivalent with standardized inoculum concentrations and standardized concentrations of retapamulin powder.

Diffusion Techniques:

Quantitative methods that require measurement of zone diameters also provide reproducible estimates of the susceptibility of bacteria to antimicrobial compounds. One such standardized procedure requires the use of standardized inoculum concentrations.[2,3] This procedure uses paper disks impregnated with 2 mcg of retapamulin to test the susceptibility of microorganisms to retapamulin.

Susceptibility Test Interpretive Criteria:

In vitro susceptibility test interpretive criteria for retapamulin have not been determined for this topical antimicrobial. The relation of the in vitro MIC and/or disk diffusion susceptibility test results to clinical efficacy of retapamulin against the bacteria tested should be monitored.

Quality Control Parameters for Susceptibility Testing:

In vitro susceptibility test quality control parameters were developed for retapamulin so that laboratories that test the susceptibility of bacterial isolates to retapamulin can determine if the susceptibility test is performing correctly. Standardized dilution techniques and diffusion methods require the use of laboratory control microorganisms to monitor the technical aspects of the laboratory procedures. Standard retapamulin powder should provide the following MIC and a 2 mcg retapamulin disk should produce the following zone diameters with the indicated quality control strains in Table 3.

Table 3. Acceptable Quality Control Ranges for Retapamulin

Microorganism	MIC Range (mcg/mL)	Disk Diffusion Zone Diameter (mm)
Staphylococcus aureus ATCC 29213	0.06-0.25	NA
Staphylococcus aureus ATCC 25923	NA	23-30
Streptococcus pneumoniae ATCC 49619	0.06-0.5[a]	13-19[b]

NA = Not applicable.

[a] This quality control range is applicable using cation-adjusted Mueller-Hinton broth with 2% to 5% lysed horse blood.

[b] This quality control limit is applicable using Mueller-Hinton agar with 5% sheep blood.

13 NONCLINICAL TOXICOLOGY

13.1 Carcinogenesis, Mutagenesis, Impairment of Fertility

Long-term studies in animals to evaluate carcinogenic potential have not been conducted with retapamulin.

Retapamulin showed no genotoxicity when evaluated in vitro for gene mutation and/or chromosomal effects in the mouse lymphoma cell assay, in cultured human peripheral blood lymphocytes, or when evaluated in vivo in a rat micronucleus test.

No evidence of impaired fertility was found in male or female rats given retapamulin 50, 150, or 450 mg/kg/day orally.

14 CLINICAL STUDIES

ALTABAX was evaluated in a placebo-controlled trial that enrolled adult and pediatric subjects aged 9 months and older for treatment of impetigo up to 100 cm^2 in total area (up to 10 lesions) or a total body surface area not exceeding 2%. The majority of subjects enrolled (164/210, 78%) were under the age of 13. The trial was a double-blind, randomized, multi-center, parallel-group comparison of the safety of ALTABAX and placebo ointment, both applied twice daily for 5 days. Patients were randomized to ALTABAX or placebo (2:1). Subjects with underlying skin disease (e.g., preexisting eczematous dermatitis) or skin trauma, with clinical evidence of secondary infection were excluded from these trials. In addition, subjects with any systemic signs and symptoms of infection (such as fever) were excluded from the trial. Clinical success was defined as the absence of treated lesions, or treated lesions had become dry without crusts with or without erythema compared with baseline, or had improved (defined as a decline in the size of the affected area, number of lesions or both) such that no further antimicrobial therapy was required. The intent-to-treat clinical (ITTC) population consisted of all randomized subjects who took at least 1 dose of trial medication. The clinical per protocol (PPC) population included all ITTC subjects who satisfied the inclusion/exclusion criteria and subsequently adhered to the protocol. The intent-to-treat bacteriological (ITTB) population consisted of all randomized subjects who took at least 1 dose of trial medication and had a pathogen identified at trial entry. The bacteriological per protocol (PPB) population included all ITTB subjects who satisfied the inclusion/exclusion criteria and subsequently adhered to the protocol.

Table 4 presents the results for clinical response at end of therapy (2 days after treatment) and follow-up (9 days after treatment), by analysis population:

[See table 4 above]

Table 5 presents the clinical success at end of therapy and follow-up by baseline pathogen:

[See table 5 above]

Examination of age and gender subgroups did not identify differences in response to ALTABAX among these groups. The majority of subjects entered into this trial were classified as White/Caucasian or of Asian heritage; when response rates by racial subgroups were viewed across trials, differences in response to ALTABAX were not identified.

15 REFERENCES

1. Clinical and Laboratory Standards Institute (CLSI) Methods for Dilution Antimicrobial Susceptibility Tests for Bacteria that Grow Aerobically: Approved Standard-Eighth Edition. CLSI Document M07-A9, Vol. 32, No. 2. CLSI, Wayne, PA, Jan. 2012.
2. Clinical and Laboratory Standards Institute (CLSI). Performance Standards for Antimicrobial Susceptibility Test-

ing: Nineteenth Informational Supplement. CLSI Document M100-S22. Vol. 32, No. 3. CLSI, Wayne, PA, Jan. 2012.
3. Clinical and Laboratory Standards Institute (CLSI). Performance Standards for Antimicrobial Disk Susceptibility Tests. Approved Standard-Tenth Edition. CLSI Document M02 A11, Vol. 32, No. 1. CLSI, Wayne, PA, Jan. 2012.

16 HOW SUPPLIED/STORAGE AND HANDLING

ALTABAX is supplied in 15-, and 30-gram tubes.
NDC 0007-5180-22 (15 gram tube)
NDC 0007-5180-25 (30 gram tube)
Store at 25°C (77°F) with excursions permitted to 15°-30°C (59°-86°F).

17 PATIENT COUNSELING INFORMATION

Patients using ALTABAX and/or their guardians should receive the following information and instructions:

- Use ALTABAX as directed by the healthcare practitioner. As with any topical medication, patients and caregivers should wash their hands after application if the hands are not the area for treatment.
- ALTABAX is for external use only. Do not swallow ALTABAX or use it in the eyes, on the mouth or lips, inside the nose, or inside the female genital area.
- The treated area may be covered by a sterile bandage or gauze dressing, if desired. This may also be helpful for infants and young children who accidentally touch or lick the lesion site. A bandage will protect the treated area and avoid accidental transfer of ointment to the eyes or other areas.
- Use the medication for the full time recommended by the healthcare practitioner, even though symptoms may have improved.
- Notify the healthcare practitioner if there is no improvement in symptoms within 3 to 4 days after starting use of ALTABAX.
- ALTABAX may cause reactions at the site of application of the ointment. Inform the healthcare practitioner if the area of application worsens in irritation, redness, itching, burning, swelling, blistering, or oozing.

ALTABAX is a registered trademark of GlaxoSmithKline.
GlaxoSmithKline
Research Triangle Park, NC 27709

ALX:5PI

BACTROBAN CREAM® ℞

(mupirocin calcium cream, 2%)
For Dermatologic Use

DESCRIPTION

BACTROBAN CREAM (mupirocin calcium cream, 2%) contains the dihydrate crystalline calcium hemi-salt of the antibiotic mupirocin. Chemically, it is (*αE*,2*S*,3*R*,4*R*,5*S*)-5-[(2*S*,3*S*,4*S*,5*S*)-2,3-Epoxy-5-hydroxy-4-methylhexyl]tetrahydro-3,4-dihydroxy-β-methyl-2*H*-pyran-2-crotonic acid, ester with 9-hydroxynonanoic acid, calcium salt (2:1), dihydrate.

The molecular formula of mupirocin calcium is $(C_{26}H_{43}O_9)_2Ca \cdot 2H_2O$, and the molecular weight is 1075.3. The molecular weight of mupirocin free acid is 500.6. The structural formula of mupirocin calcium is:

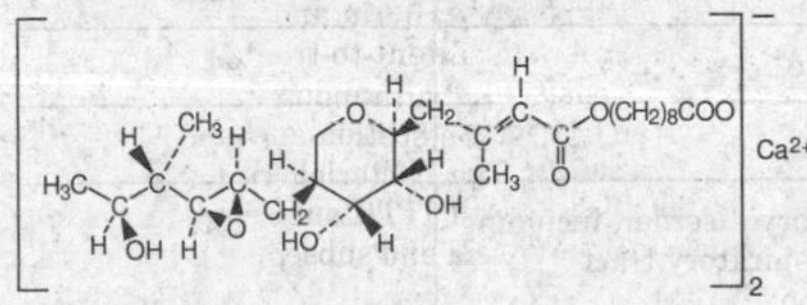

BACTROBAN CREAM is a white cream that contains 2.15% w/w mupirocin calcium (equivalent to 2.0% mupirocin free acid) in an oil and water-based emulsion. The inactive ingredients are benzyl alcohol, cetomacrogol 1000, cetyl alcohol, mineral oil, phenoxyethanol, purified water, stearyl alcohol, and xanthan gum.

CLINICAL PHARMACOLOGY

Pharmacokinetics

Systemic absorption of mupirocin through intact human skin is minimal. The systemic absorption of mupirocin was studied following application of BACTROBAN CREAM 3 times daily for 5 days to various skin lesions (>10 cm in length or 100 cm^2 in area) in 16 adults (aged 29 to 60 years) and 10 children (aged 3 to 12 years). Some systemic absorption was observed as evidenced by the detection of the metabolite, monic acid, in urine. Data from this study indicated more frequent occurrence of percutaneous absorption in children (90% of patients) compared to adults (44% of patients); however, the observed urinary concentrations in children (0.07 - 1.3 mcg/mL [1 pediatric patient had no detectable level]) are within the observed range (0.08 - 10.03 mcg/mL [9 adults had no detectable level]) in the adult population. In general, the degree of percutaneous absorption following multiple dosing appears to be minimal in adults and children. Any mupirocin reaching the systemic circulation is rapidly metabolized, predominantly to inactive monic acid, which is eliminated by renal excretion.

Microbiology

Mupirocin is an antibacterial agent produced by fermentation using the organism *Pseudomonas fluorescens*. It is active against a wide range of gram-positive bacteria including methicillin-resistant *Staphylococcus aureus* (MRSA). It is also active against certain gram-negative bacteria. Mupirocin inhibits bacterial protein synthesis by reversibly and specifically binding to bacterial isoleucyl transfer-RNA synthetase. Due to this unique mode of action, mupirocin demonstrates no in vitro cross-resistance with other classes of antimicrobial agents.

Resistance occurs rarely; however, when mupirocin resistance does occur, it appears to result from the production of a modified isoleucyl-tRNA synthetase. High-level plasmid-mediated resistance (MIC >1024 mcg/mL) has been reported in some strains of *Staphylococcus aureus* and coagulase-negative staphylococci.

Mupirocin is bactericidal at concentrations achieved by topical application. The minimum bactericidal concentration (MBC) against relevant pathogens is generally 8-fold to 30-fold higher than the minimum inhibitory concentration (MIC). In addition, mupirocin is highly protein bound (>97%), and the effect of wound secretions on the MICs of mupirocin has not been determined.

Mupirocin has been shown to be active against most strains of *S. aureus* and *Streptococcus pyogenes*, both in vitro and in clinical studies. (See INDICATIONS AND USAGE.) The following in vitro data are available, BUT THEIR CLINICAL SIGNIFICANCE IS UNKNOWN. Mupirocin is active against most strains of *Staphylococcus epidermidis* and *Staphylococcus saprophyticus*.

INDICATIONS AND USAGE

BACTROBAN CREAM is indicated for the treatment of secondarily infected traumatic skin lesions (up to 10 cm in length or 100 cm^2 in area) due to susceptible strains of *S. aureus* and *S. pyogenes*.

CONTRAINDICATIONS

BACTROBAN CREAM is contraindicated in patients with known hypersensitivity to any of the constituents of the product.

WARNINGS

Avoid contact with the eyes.

In the event of a sensitization or severe local irritation from BACTROBAN CREAM, usage should be discontinued, and appropriate alternative therapy for the infection instituted.

PRECAUTIONS

General

As with other antibacterial products, prolonged use may result in overgrowth of nonsusceptible microorganisms, including fungi. (See DOSAGE AND ADMINISTRATION.)

BACTROBAN CREAM is not formulated for use on mucosal surfaces.

Information for Patients

- Use this medication only as directed by your healthcare provider. It is for external use only. Avoid contact with the eyes.
- The treated area may be covered by gauze dressing if desired.
- Report to your healthcare provider any signs of local adverse reactions. The medication should be stopped and your healthcare provider contacted if irritation, severe itching, or rash occurs.
- If no improvement is seen in 3 to 5 days, contact your healthcare provider.

Drug Interactions

The effect of the concurrent application of topical mupirocin calcium cream and other topical products has not been studied.

Carcinogenesis, Mutagenesis, Impairment of Fertility

Long-term studies in animals to evaluate carcinogenic potential of mupirocin calcium have not been conducted.

Results of the following studies performed with mupirocin calcium or mupirocin sodium in vitro and in vivo did not indicate a potential for mutagenicity: Rat primary hepatocyte unscheduled DNA synthesis, sediment analysis for DNA strand breaks, *Salmonella* reversion test (Ames), *Escherichia coli* mutation assay, metaphase analysis of human lymphocytes, mouse lymphoma assay, and bone marrow micronuclei assay in mice.

Fertility studies were performed in rats with mupirocin administered subcutaneously at doses up to 49 times a human topical dose of 1 gram/day (approximately 20 mg mupirocin per day) on a mg/m^2 basis and revealed no evidence of impaired fertility from mupirocin sodium.

Pregnancy

Teratogenic Effects: Pregnancy Category B. Teratology studies have been performed in rats and rabbits with mupirocin administered subcutaneously at doses up to 78 and 154 times, respectively, a human topical dose of 1 gram/day (approximately 20 mg mupirocin per day) on a mg/m^2 basis and revealed no evidence of harm to the fetus due to mupirocin. There are, however, no adequate and well-controlled studies in pregnant women. Because animal reproduction studies are not always predictive of human response, this drug should be used during pregnancy only if clearly needed.

Nursing Mothers

It is not known whether this drug is excreted in human milk. Because many drugs are excreted in human milk, caution should be exercised when BACTROBAN CREAM is administered to a nursing woman.

Pediatric Use

The safety and effectiveness of BACTROBAN CREAM have been established in the age groups 3 months to 16 years. Use of BACTROBAN CREAM in these age groups is supported by evidence from adequate and well controlled studies of BACTROBAN CREAM in adults with additional data from 93 pediatric patients studied as part of the pivotal trials in adults. (See CLINICAL STUDIES.)

Geriatric Use

In 2 well-controlled studies, 30 patients older than 65 years were treated with BACTROBAN CREAM. No overall difference in the efficacy or safety of BACTROBAN CREAM was observed in this patient population when compared to that observed in younger patients.

ADVERSE REACTIONS

In 2 randomized, double-blind, double-dummy trials, 339 patients were treated with topical BACTROBAN CREAM plus oral placebo. Adverse events thought to be possibly or probably drug-related occurred in 28 (8.3%) patients. The incidence of those events that were reported in at least 1% of patients enrolled in these trials were: Headache (1.7%), rash, and nausea (1.1% each).

Other adverse events thought to be possibly or probably drug-related which occurred in less than 1% of patients were: Abdominal pain, burning at application site, cellulitis, dermatitis, dizziness, pruritus, secondary wound infection, and ulcerative stomatitis.

In a supportive study in the treatment of secondarily infected eczema, 82 patients were treated with BACTROBAN CREAM. The incidence of adverse events thought to be possibly or probably drug-related was as follows: Nausea (4.9%), headache, and burning at application site (3.6% each), pruritus (2.4%) and 1 report each of abdominal pain, bleeding secondary to eczema, pain secondary to eczema, hives, dry skin, and rash.

OVERDOSAGE

Intravenous infusions of 252 mg, as well as single oral doses of 500 mg of mupirocin, have been well tolerated in healthy adult subjects. There is no information regarding overdose of BACTROBAN CREAM.

DOSAGE AND ADMINISTRATION

A small amount of BACTROBAN CREAM should be applied to the affected area 3 times daily for 10 days. The area treated may be covered with gauze dressing if desired. Patients not showing a clinical response within 3 to 5 days should be re-evaluated.

CLINICAL STUDIES

The efficacy of topical BACTROBAN CREAM for the treatment of secondarily infected traumatic skin lesions (e.g., lacerations, sutured wounds, and abrasions not more than 10 cm in length or 100 cm^2 in total area) was compared to that of oral cephalexin in 2 randomized, double-blind, double-dummy clinical trials. Clinical efficacy rates at follow-up in the per protocol populations (adults and pediatric patients included) were 96.1% for BACTROBAN CREAM (n = 231) and 93.1% for oral cephalexin (n = 219). Pathogen eradication rates at follow-up in the per protocol populations were 100% for both BACTROBAN CREAM and oral cephalexin.

Pediatrics: There were 93 pediatric patients aged 2 weeks to 16 years enrolled per protocol in the secondarily infected skin lesion studies, although only 3 were less than 2 years of age in the population treated with BACTROBAN CREAM. Patients were randomized to either 10 days of topical BACTROBAN CREAM 3 times daily or 10 days of oral cephalexin (250 mg 4 times daily for patients >40 kg or 25 mg/kg/day oral suspension in 4 divided doses for patients ≤40 kg). Clinical efficacy at follow-up (7 to 12 days post-therapy) in the per protocol populations was 97.7% (43/44) for BACTROBAN CREAM and 93.9% (46/49) for cephalexin. Only 1 adverse event (headache) was thought to be possibly or probably related to drug therapy with BACTROBAN CREAM in the intent-to-treat pediatric population of 70 children (1.4%).

HOW SUPPLIED

BACTROBAN CREAM is supplied in 15-gram and 30-gram tubes.
NDC 0029-1527-22 (15-gram tube)
NDC 0029-1527-25 (30-gram tube)
Store at or below 25°C (77°F). Do not freeze.
GlaxoSmithKline
Research Triangle Park, NC 27709
BACTROBAN CREAM is a registered trademark of GlaxoSmithKline.

May 2005 BB:L7B

BACTROBAN NASAL® ℞

(mupirocin calcium ointment, 2%)
for intranasal use only

DESCRIPTION

BACTROBAN NASAL (mupirocin calcium ointment, 2%) contains the dihydrate crystalline calcium hemi-salt of the antibiotic mupirocin. Chemically, it is (αE,2S,3R,4R,5S)-5-[(2S,3S,4S,5S)-2,3-Epoxy-5-hydroxy-4-methylhexyl]tetrahydro-3,4-dihydroxy-β-methyl-2H-pyran-2-crotonic acid, ester with 9-hydroxynonanoic acid, calcium salt (2:1), dihydrate.

The molecular formula of mupirocin calcium is $(C_{26}H_{43}O_9)_2Ca{\bullet}2H_2O$, and the molecular weight is 1075.3. The molecular weight of mupirocin free acid is 500.6. The structural formula of mupirocin calcium is:

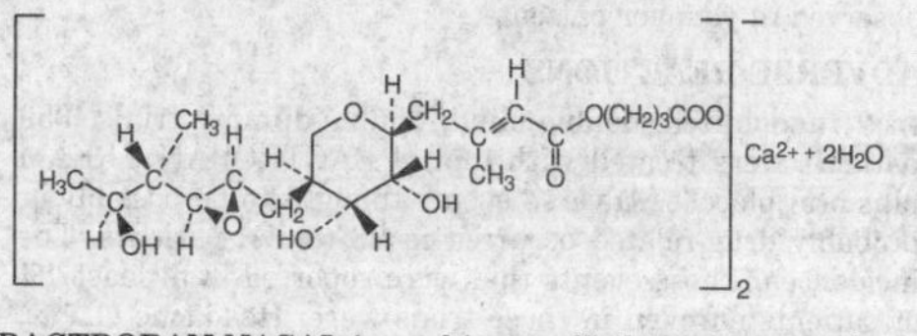

BACTROBAN NASAL is a white to off-white ointment that contains 2.15% w/w mupirocin calcium (equivalent to 2.0% pure mupirocin free acid) in a soft white ointment base. The inactive ingredients are paraffin and a mixture of glycerin esters (SOFTISAN® 649).

CLINICAL PHARMACOLOGY

Pharmacokinetics

Following single or repeated intranasal applications of 0.2 gram of BACTROBAN NASAL 3 times daily for 3 days to 5 healthy adult male subjects, no evidence of systemic absorption of mupirocin was demonstrated. The dosage regimen used in this study was for pharmacokinetic characterization only. (See DOSAGE AND ADMINISTRATION for proper clinical dosing information.)

In this study, the concentrations of mupirocin in urine and of monic acid in urine and serum were below the limit of determination of the assay for up to 72 hours after the applications. The lowest levels of determination of the assay used were 50 ng/mL of mupirocin in urine, 75 ng/mL of monic acid in urine, and 10 ng/mL of monic acid in serum. Based on the detectable limit of the urine assay for monic acid, one can extrapolate that a mean of 3.3% (range: 1.2 to 5.1%) of the applied dose could be systemically absorbed from the nasal mucosa of **adults**.

Data from a report of a pharmacokinetic study in neonates and premature infants indicate that, unlike in adults, significant systemic absorption occurred following intranasal administration of BACTROBAN NASAL in this population. **At this time, the pharmacokinetic properties of mupirocin following intranasal application of BACTROBAN NASAL have not been adequately characterized in neonates or other children less than 12 years of age, and in addition, the safety of the product in children less than 12 years of age has not been established.**

The effect of the concurrent application of intranasal mupirocin calcium ointment, 2% with other intranasal products has not been studied. (See PRECAUTIONS, Drug Interactions.)

Following intravenous or oral administration, mupirocin is rapidly metabolized. The principal metabolite, monic acid, demonstrates no antibacterial activity. In a study conducted in 7 healthy adult male subjects, the elimination half-life after intravenous administration of mupirocin was 20 to 40 minutes for mupirocin and 30 to 80 minutes for monic acid. Monic acid is predominantly eliminated by renal excretion. The pharmacokinetics of mupirocin has not been studied in individuals with renal insufficiency.

Microbiology

Mupirocin is an antibacterial agent produced by fermentation using the organism *Pseudomonas fluorescens*. Mupirocin inhibits bacterial protein synthesis by reversibly and specifically binding to bacterial isoleucyl transfer-RNA synthetase. Due to this mode of action, mupirocin demonstrates no in vitro cross-resistance with other classes of antimicrobial agents.

When mupirocin resistance does occur, it appears to result from the production of a modified isoleucyl-tRNA synthetase. High-level plasmid-mediated resistance (MIC >1,024 mcg/mL) has been reported in some strains of *Staphylococcus aureus* and coagulase-negative staphylococci.

Mupirocin is bactericidal at concentrations achieved topically by intranasal administration. However, the minimum bactericidal concentration (MBC) against relevant intranasal pathogens is generally 8-fold to 30-fold higher than the minimum inhibitory concentration (MIC). In addition, mupirocin is highly protein bound (>97%), and the effect of nasal secretions on the MICs of intranasally applied mupirocin has not been determined.

Mupirocin has been shown to be active against most strains of methicillin-resistant *S. aureus*, both in vitro and in clinical studies of the eradication of nasal colonization. BACTROBAN NASAL only has established clinical utility in nasal eradication as part of a comprehensive program to curtail institutional outbreaks of infections with methicillin-resistant *S. aureus*. (See INDICATIONS AND USAGE.)

The following in vitro data are available, **but their clinical significance is unknown**. Mupirocin exhibits in vitro MICs of 1 mcg/mL or less against most (>90%) strains of methicillin-susceptible *S. aureus*; however, the safety and effectiveness of mupirocin calcium in eradicating nasal colonization of and preventing subsequent infections due to methicillin-susceptible *S. aureus* have not been established.

INDICATIONS AND USAGE

BACTROBAN NASAL is indicated for the eradication of nasal colonization with methicillin-resistant *S. aureus* in adult patients and health care workers as part of a comprehensive infection control program to reduce the risk of infection among patients at high risk of methicillin-resistant *S. aureus* infection during institutional outbreaks of infections with this pathogen.

NOTE:

1. There are insufficient data at this time to establish that this product is safe and effective as part of an intervention program to prevent autoinfection of high-risk patients from their own nasal colonization with *S. aureus*.
2. There are insufficient data at this time to recommend use of BACTROBAN NASAL for general prophylaxis of any infection in any patient population.
3. Greater than 90% of subjects/patients in clinical trials had eradication of nasal colonization 2 to 4 days after therapy was completed. Approximately 30% recolonization was reported in 1 domestic study within 4 weeks after completion of therapy. These eradication rates were clinically and statistically superior to those reported in subjects/patients in the vehicle-treated arms of the adequate and well-controlled studies. Those treated with vehicle had eradication rates of 5% to 30% at 2 to 4 days post-therapy with 85% to 100% recolonization within 4 weeks.

All adequate and well-controlled trials of this product were vehicle-controlled; therefore, no data from direct, head-to-head comparisons with other products are available at this time.

CONTRAINDICATIONS

BACTROBAN NASAL is contraindicated in patients with known hypersensitivity to any of the constituents of the product.

WARNINGS

AVOID CONTACT WITH THE EYES. Application of BACTROBAN NASAL to the eye under testing conditions has caused severe symptoms such as burning and tearing. These symptoms resolved within days to weeks after discontinuation of the ointment.

In the event of a sensitization or severe local irritation from BACTROBAN NASAL, usage should be discontinued.

PRECAUTIONS

General

As with other antibacterial products, prolonged use may result in overgrowth of nonsusceptible microorganisms, including fungi. (See DOSAGE AND ADMINISTRATION.)

Information for Patients

Patients should be given the following instructions:

- Apply approximately one-half of the ointment from the single-use tube directly into 1 nostril and the other half into the other nostril;
- Avoid contact of the medication with the eyes;
- Discard the tube after using, do not re-use;
- Press the sides of the nose together and gently massage after application to spread the ointment throughout the inside of the nostrils; and
- Discontinue usage of the medication and call your healthcare practitioner if sensitization or severe local irritation occurs.

Drug Interactions

The effect of the concurrent application of intranasal mupirocin calcium and other intranasal products has not been studied. Until further information is known, mupirocin calcium ointment, 2% should not be applied concurrently with any other intranasal products.

Carcinogenesis, Mutagenesis, Impairment of Fertility

Long-term studies in animals to evaluate carcinogenic potential of mupirocin calcium have not been conducted.

Results of the following studies performed with mupirocin calcium or mupirocin sodium in vitro and in vivo did not indicate a potential for mutagenicity: Rat primary hepatocyte unscheduled DNA synthesis, sediment analysis for DNA strand breaks, *Salmonella* reversion test (Ames), *Escherichia coli* mutation assay, metaphase analysis of human lymphocytes, mouse lymphoma assay, and bone marrow micronuclei assay in mice.

Reproduction studies were performed in rats with mupirocin administered subcutaneously at doses up to **40** times the human intranasal dose (approximately 20 mg mupirocin per day) on a mg/m[2] basis and revealed no evidence of impaired fertility from mupirocin sodium.

Pregnancy

Teratogenic Effects: Pregnancy Category B

Reproduction studies have been performed in rats and rabbits with mupirocin administered subcutaneously at doses up to 65 and 130 times, respectively, the human intranasal dose (approximately 20 mg mupirocin per day) on a mg/m2 basis and revealed no evidence of harm to the fetus due to mupirocin. There are, however, no adequate and well-controlled studies in pregnant women. Because animal reproduction studies are not always predictive of human response, this drug should be used during pregnancy only if clearly needed.

Nursing Mothers

It is not known whether this drug is excreted in human milk. Because many drugs are excreted in human milk, caution should be exercised when BACTROBAN NASAL is administered to a nursing woman.

Pediatric Use

Safety in children under the age of 12 years has not been established. (See CLINICAL PHARMACOLOGY.)

ADVERSE REACTIONS

Clinical Trials

In clinical trials, 210 domestic and 2,130 foreign adult subjects/patients received BACTROBAN NASAL ointment. Less than 1% of domestic or foreign subjects and patients in clinical trials were withdrawn due to adverse events.

The most frequently reported adverse events in foreign clinical trials were as follows: Rhinitis (1.0%), taste perversion (0.8%), pharyngitis (0.5%).

In domestic clinical trials, 17% (36/210) of adults treated with BACTROBAN NASAL ointment reported adverse events thought to be at least possibly drug-related. The incidence of adverse events that were reported in at least 1% of adults enrolled in domestic clinical trials were as follows:

ADVERSE EVENTS (≥1% INCIDENCE)-ADULTS IN US TRIALS

	% of Subjects/Patients Experiencing Event BACTROBAN NASAL (n=210)
Headache	9%
Rhinitis	6%
Respiratory disorder, including upper respiratory tract congestion	5%
Pharyngitis	4%
Taste perversion	3%
Burning/stinging	2%
Cough	2%
Pruritus	1%

The following events thought possibly drug-related were reported in less than 1% of adults enrolled in domestic clinical trials: Blepharitis, diarrhea, dry mouth, ear pain, epistaxis, nausea, and rash.

All adequate and well-controlled clinical trials have been performed using BACTROBAN NASAL ointment, 2% in 1 arm and the vehicle ointment in the other arm of the study. No adequate and well-controlled safety data are available from direct, head-to-head comparative studies of this product and other products for this indication.

OVERDOSAGE

Following single or repeated intranasal applications of BACTROBAN NASAL to adults, no evidence for systemic absorption of mupirocin was obtained. Intravenous infusions of 252 mg, as well as single oral doses of 500 mg of mupirocin, have been well tolerated in healthy adult subjects. There is no information regarding local overdose of BACTROBAN NASAL or regarding oral ingestion of the nasal ointment formulation.

DOSAGE AND ADMINISTRATION

(See INDICATIONS AND USAGE.)

Adults (12 years of age and older): Approximately one-half of the ointment from the single-use tube should be applied into 1 nostril and the other half into the other nostril twice daily (morning and evening) for 5 days.

After application, the nostrils should be closed by pressing together and releasing the sides of the nose repetitively for approximately 1 minute. This will spread the ointment throughout the nares.

The single-use 1.0 gram tube will deliver a total of approximately 0.5 grams of the ointment (approximately 0.25 grams/nostril).

The tube should be discarded after usage; it should not be re-used.

The safety and effectiveness of applications of this medication for greater than 5 days have not been established. There are no human clinical or pre-clinical animal data to support the use of this product in a chronic manner or in manners other than those described in this package insert. Until further information is known, BACTROBAN NASAL should not be applied concurrently with any other intranasal products.

HOW SUPPLIED

BACTROBAN NASAL is supplied in 1.0-gram tubes.

NDC 0029-1526-11 (package of 10 single-tube cartons).

Store between 20° and 25°C (68° and 77°F); excursions permitted to 15°-30°C (59°-86°F). Do not refrigerate.

REFERENCE

1. Clinical and Laboratory Standards Institute (CLSI). Methods for Dilution Antimicrobial Susceptibility Tests for Bacteria That Grow Aerobically. Approved Standard. CLSI Document M7-A7. CLSI, Wayne, PA, January 2006.

BACTROBAN NASAL is a registered trademark of GlaxoSmithKline.

SOFTISAN is a registered trademark of Sasol Olefins & Surfactants GmbH.

GlaxoSmithKline

Research Triangle Park, NC 27709

April 2009 BBN:2PI

BACTROBAN OINTMENT® ℞

(mupirocin ointment, 2%)

For Dermatologic Use

DESCRIPTION

Each gram of BACTROBAN OINTMENT (mupirocin ointment, 2%) contains 20 mg mupirocin in a bland water miscible ointment base (polyethylene glycol ointment, N.F.) consisting of polyethylene glycol 400 and polyethylene glycol 3350. Mupirocin is a naturally occurring antibiotic. The chemical name is (*E*)-(2*S*,3*R*,4*R*,5*S*)-5-[(2*S*,3*S*,4*S*,5*S*)-2,3-Epoxy-5-hydroxy-4-methylhexyl]tetrahydro-3,4-dihydroxy-β-methyl-2*H*-pyran-2-crotonic acid, ester with 9-hydroxynonanoic acid. The molecular formula of mupirocin is $C_{26}H_{44}O_9$, and the molecular weight is 500.63. The chemical structure is:

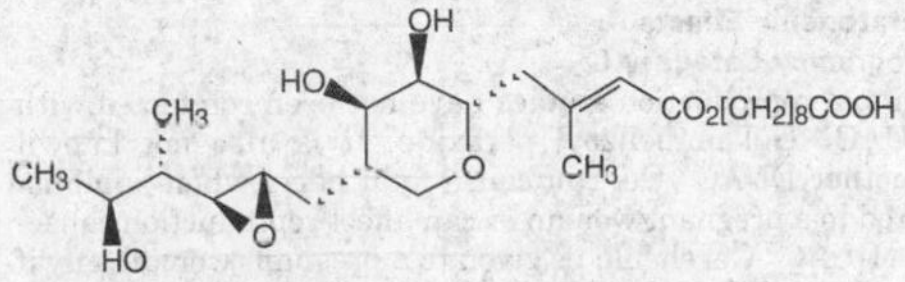

CLINICAL PHARMACOLOGY

Application of ^{14}C-labeled mupirocin ointment to the lower arm of normal male subjects followed by occlusion for 24 hours showed no measurable systemic absorption (<1.1 nanogram mupirocin per milliliter of whole blood). Measurable radioactivity was present in the stratum corneum of these subjects 72 hours after application.

Following intravenous or oral administration, mupirocin is rapidly metabolized. The principal metabolite, monic acid, is eliminated by renal excretion, and demonstrates no antibacterial activity. In a study conducted in 7 healthy adult male subjects, the elimination half-life after intravenous administration of mupirocin was 20 to 40 minutes for mupirocin and 30 to 80 minutes for monic acid. The pharmacokinetics of mupirocin has not been studied in individuals with renal insufficiency.

Microbiology

Mupirocin is an antibacterial agent produced by fermentation using the organism *Pseudomonas fluorescens*. It is active against a wide range of gram-positive bacteria including methicillin-resistant *Staphylococcus aureus* (MRSA). It is also active against certain gram-negative bacteria. Mupirocin inhibits bacterial protein synthesis by reversibly and specifically binding to bacterial isoleucyl transfer-RNA synthetase. Due to this unique mode of action, mupirocin demonstrates no in vitro cross-resistance with other classes of antimicrobial agents.

Resistance occurs rarely. However, when mupirocin resistance does occur, it appears to result from the production of a modified isoleucyl-tRNA synthetase. High-level plasmid-mediated resistance (MIC >1024 mcg/mL) has been reported in some strains of *S. aureus* and coagulase-negative staphylococci.

Mupirocin is bactericidal at concentrations achieved by topical administration. However, the minimum bactericidal concentration (MBC) against relevant pathogens is generally 8-fold to 30-fold higher than the minimum inhibitory concentration (MIC). In addition, mupirocin is highly protein-bound (>97%), and the effect of wound secretions on the MICs of mupirocin has not been determined.

Mupirocin has been shown to be active against most strains of *S. aureus* and *Streptococcus pyogenes*, both in vitro and in clinical studies (see INDICATIONS AND USAGE). The following in vitro data are available, BUT THEIR CLINICAL SIGNIFICANCE IS UNKNOWN. Mupirocin is active against most strains of *Staphylococcus epidermidis* and *Staphylococcus saprophyticus*.

INDICATIONS AND USAGE

BACTROBAN OINTMENT is indicated for the topical treatment of impetigo due to: *S. aureus* and *S. pyogenes*.

CONTRAINDICATIONS

This drug is contraindicated in individuals with a history of sensitivity reactions to any of its components.

WARNINGS

BACTROBAN OINTMENT is not for ophthalmic use.

PRECAUTIONS

If a reaction suggesting sensitivity or chemical irritation should occur with the use of BACTROBAN OINTMENT, treatment should be discontinued and appropriate alternative therapy for the infection instituted.

As with other antibacterial products, prolonged use may result in overgrowth of nonsusceptible organisms, including fungi.

BACTROBAN OINTMENT is not formulated for use on mucosal surfaces. Intranasal use has been associated with isolated reports of stinging and drying. A paraffin-based formulation — BACTROBAN NASAL® (mupirocin calcium ointment) is available for intranasal use.

Polyethylene glycol can be absorbed from open wounds and damaged skin and is excreted by the kidneys. In common with other polyethylene glycol-based ointments, BACTROBAN OINTMENT should not be used in conditions where absorption of large quantities of polyethylene glycol is possible, especially if there is evidence of moderate or severe renal impairment.

Information for Patients

Use this medication only as directed by your healthcare provider. It is for external use only. Avoid contact with the eyes. The medication should be stopped and your healthcare practitioner contacted if irritation, severe itching, or rash occurs.

If impetigo has not improved in 3 to 5 days, contact your healthcare practitioner.

Drug Interactions

The effect of the concurrent application of BACTROBAN OINTMENT and other drug products has not been studied.

Carcinogenesis, Mutagenesis, Impairment of Fertility

Long-term studies in animals to evaluate carcinogenic potential of mupirocin have not been conducted.

Results of the following studies performed with mupirocin calcium or mupirocin sodium in vitro and in vivo did not indicate a potential for genotoxicity: Rat primary hepatocyte unscheduled DNA synthesis, sediment analysis for DNA strand breaks, *Salmonella* reversion test (Ames), *Escherichia coli* mutation assay, metaphase analysis of human lymphocytes, mouse lymphoma assay, and bone marrow micronuclei assay in mice.

Reproduction studies were performed in male and female rats with mupirocin administered subcutaneously at doses up to 14 times a human topical dose (approximately 60 mg mupirocin per day) on a mg/m^2 basis and revealed no evidence of impaired fertility and reproductive performance from mupirocin.

Pregnancy

Teratogenic Effects

Reproduction studies have been performed in rats and rabbits with mupirocin administered subcutaneously at doses up to 22 and 43 times, respectively, the human topical dose (approximately 60 mg mupirocin per day) on a mg/m^2 basis and revealed no evidence of harm to the fetus due to mupirocin. There are, however, no adequate and well-controlled studies in pregnant women. Because animal studies are not always predictive of human response, this drug should be used during pregnancy only if clearly needed.

Nursing Mothers

It is not known whether this drug is excreted in human milk. Because many drugs are excreted in human milk, caution should be exercised when BACTROBAN OINTMENT is administered to a nursing woman.

Pediatric Use

The safety and effectiveness of BACTROBAN OINTMENT have been established in the age range of 2 months to 16 years. Use of BACTROBAN OINTMENT in these age groups is supported by evidence from adequate and well-controlled studies of BACTROBAN OINTMENT in impetigo in pediatric patients studied as a part of the pivotal clinical trials (see CLINICAL STUDIES).

ADVERSE REACTIONS

The following local adverse reactions have been reported in connection with the use of BACTROBAN OINTMENT: Burning, stinging, or pain in 1.5% of patients; itching in 1% of patients; rash, nausea, erythema, dry skin, tenderness, swelling, contact dermatitis, and increased exudate in less than 1% of patients. Systemic reactions to BACTROBAN OINTMENT have occurred rarely.

DOSAGE AND ADMINISTRATION

A small amount of BACTROBAN OINTMENT should be applied to the affected area 3 times daily. The area treated may be covered with a gauze dressing if desired. Patients not showing a clinical response within 3 to 5 days should be re-evaluated.

CLINICAL STUDIES

The efficacy of topical BACTROBAN OINTMENT in impetigo was tested in 2 studies. In the first, patients with impetigo were randomized to receive either BACTROBAN OINTMENT or vehicle placebo 3 times daily for 8 to 12 days. Clinical efficacy rates at end of therapy in the evaluable populations (adults and pediatric patients included) were 71% for BACTROBAN OINTMENT (n = 49) and 35% for vehicle placebo (n = 51). Pathogen eradication rates in the evaluable populations were 94% for BACTROBAN OINTMENT and 62% for vehicle placebo. There were no side effects reported in the group receiving BACTROBAN OINTMENT.

In the second study, patients with impetigo were randomized to receive either BACTROBAN OINTMENT 3 times daily or 30 to 40 mg/kg oral erythromycin ethylsuccinate per day (this was an unblinded study) for 8 days. There was a follow-up visit 1 week after treatment ended. Clinical efficacy rates at the follow-up visit in the evaluable populations (adults and pediatric patients included) were 93% for BACTROBAN OINTMENT (n = 29) and 78.5% for erythromycin (n = 28). Pathogen eradication rates in the evaluable patient populations were 100% for both test groups. There were no side effects reported in the group receiving BACTROBAN OINTMENT.

Pediatrics

There were 91 pediatric patients aged 2 months to 15 years in the first study described above. Clinical efficacy rates at end of therapy in the evaluable populations were 78% for BACTROBAN OINTMENT (n = 42) and 36% for vehicle placebo (n = 49). In the second study described above, all patients were pediatric except 2 adults in the group receiving BACTROBAN OINTMENT. The age range of the pediatric patients was 7 months to 13 years. The clinical efficacy rate for BACTROBAN OINTMENT (n = 27) was 96%, and for erythromycin it was unchanged (78.5%).

HOW SUPPLIED

BACTROBAN OINTMENT is supplied in 22-gram tubes.

NDC 0029-1525-44 (22-gram tube)

Store at controlled room temperature 20° to 25°C (68° to 77°F).

GlaxoSmithKline

Research Triangle Park, NC 27709

BACTROBAN OINTMENT and BACTROBAN NASAL are registered trademarks of GlaxoSmithKline.

MAY 2005 BC:L13C

DUAC® ℞

[dū-ăk]

(clindamycin phosphate and benzoyl peroxide)

Gel, 1.2%/5%

For Dermatological Use Only.
Not for Ophthalmic Use.
Rx Only

DESCRIPTION

DUAC® Gel contains clindamycin phosphate, (7(S)-chloro-7-deoxylincomycin-2-phosphate), equivalent to 1% clindamycin, and 5% benzoyl peroxide.

Clindamycin phosphate is a water soluble ester of the semi-synthetic antibiotic produced by a 7(S)-chloro-substitution of the 7(R)-hydroxyl group of the parent antibiotic lincomycin.

Clindamycin phosphate is $C_{18}H_{34}ClN_2O_8PS$. The structural formula for clindamycin phosphate is represented below:

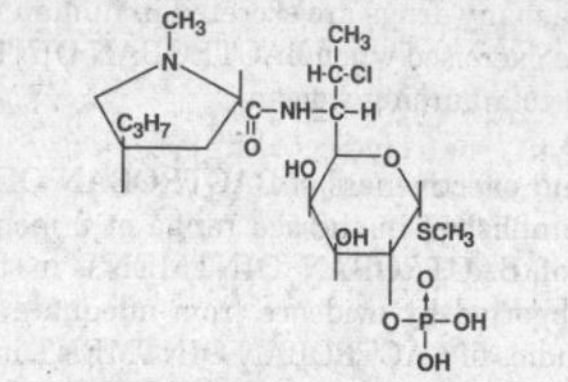

Clindamycin phosphate has a molecular weight of 504.97 and its chemical name is methyl 7-chloro-6,7,8-trideoxy-6-(1-methyl-*trans*-4-propyl-L-2-pyrrolidinecarboxamido)-1-thio-L-*threo*-α-D-*galacto*-octopyranoside 2-(dihydrogen phosphate).

Benzoyl peroxide is $C_{14}H_{10}O_4$. It has the following structural formula:

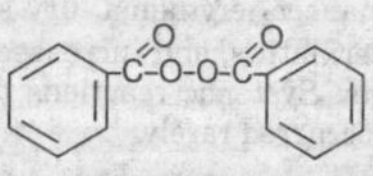

Benzoyl peroxide has a molecular weight of 242.23.

Each gram of DUAC® Gel contains 10 mg (1%) clindamycin, as phosphate, and 50 mg (5%) benzoyl peroxide in a base consisting of carbomer homopolymer (type C), dimethicone, disodium lauryl sulfosuccinate, edetate disodium, glycerin, methylparaben, poloxamer 182, purified water, silicon dioxide, and sodium hydroxide.

CLINICAL PHARMACOLOGY

A comparative study of the pharmacokinetics of DUAC® Gel and 1% clindamycin solution alone in 78 patients indicated that mean plasma clindamycin levels during the four week dosing period were < 0.5 ng/ml for both treatment groups.

Benzoyl peroxide has been shown to be absorbed by the skin where it is converted to benzoic acid. Less than 2% of the dose enters systemic circulation as benzoic acid.

Microbiology

Mechanism of Action

Clindamycin binds to the 50S ribosomal subunits of susceptible bacteria and prevents elongation of peptide chains by interfering with peptidyl transfer, thereby suppressing protein synthesis.

Benzoyl peroxide is a potent oxidizing agent.

***In Vivo* Activity**

No microbiology studies were conducted in the clinical trials with this product.

***In Vitro* Activity**

The clindamycin and benzoyl peroxide components individually have been shown to have *in vitro* activity against *Propionibacterium acnes*, an organism which has been associated with acne vulgaris; however, the clinical significance of this is not known.

Drug Resistance

There are reports of an increase of *P. acnes* resistance to clindamycin in the treatment of acne. In patients with *P. acnes* resistant to clindamycin, the clindamycin component may provide no additional benefit beyond benzoyl peroxide alone.

CLINICAL STUDIES

In five randomized, double-blind clinical studies of 1,319 patients, 397 used DUAC® Gel, 396 used benzoyl peroxide, 349 used clindamycin and 177 used vehicle. DUAC® Gel applied once daily for 11 weeks was significantly more effective than vehicle, benzoyl peroxide, and clindamycin in the treatment of inflammatory lesions of moderate to moderately severe facial acne vulgaris in three of the five studies (Studies 1, 2, and 5).

Patients were evaluated and acne lesions counted at each clinical visit: weeks 2, 5, 8, 11. The primary efficacy measures were the lesion counts and the investigator's global assessment evaluated at week 11. Patients were instructed to wash the face, wait 10 to 20 minutes, and then apply medication to the entire face, once daily, in the evening before retiring. Percent reductions in inflammatory lesion counts after treatment for 11 weeks in these five studies are shown in the following table:

[See table below]

Mean percent reduction in inflammatory lesion counts

	Study 1 (n=120)	Study 2 (n=273)	Study 3 (n=280)	Study 4 (n=288)	Study 5 (n=358)
DUAC® Gel	65%	56%	42%	57%	52%
Benzoyl Peroxide	36%	37%	32%	57%	41%
Clindamycin	34%	30%	38%	49%	33%
Vehicle	19%	-0.4%	29%		29%

The DUAC® Gel group showed greater overall improvement in the investigator's global assessment than the benzoyl peroxide, clindamycin and vehicle groups in three of the five studies (Studies 1, 2, and 5).

Clinical studies have not adequately demonstrated the effectiveness of DUAC® Gel versus benzoyl peroxide alone in the treatment of non-inflammatory lesions of acne.

INDICATIONS AND USAGE

DUAC® Gel is indicated for the topical treatment of inflammatory acne vulgaris.

DUAC® Gel has not been demonstrated to have any additional benefit when compared to benzoyl peroxide alone in the same vehicle when used for the treatment of non-inflammatory acne.

CONTRAINDICATIONS

DUAC® Gel is contraindicated in those individuals who have shown hypersensitivity to any of its components or to lincomycin. It is also contraindicated in those having a history of regional enteritis, ulcerative colitis, pseudomembranous colitis, or antibiotic-associated colitis.

WARNINGS

ORALLY AND PARENTERALLY ADMINISTERED CLINDAMYCIN HAS BEEN ASSOCIATED WITH SEVERE COLITIS WHICH MAY RESULT IN PATIENT DEATH. USE OF THE TOPICAL FORMULATION OF CLINDAMYCIN RESULTS IN ABSORPTION OF THE ANTIBIOTIC FROM THE SKIN SURFACE. DIARRHEA, BLOODY DIARRHEA, AND COLITIS (INCLUDING PSEUDOMEMBRANOUS COLITIS) HAVE BEEN REPORTED WITH THE USE OF TOPICAL AND SYSTEMIC CLINDAMYCIN. STUDIES INDICATE A TOXIN(S) PRODUCED BY CLOSTRIDIA IS ONE PRIMARY CAUSE OF ANTIBIOTIC-ASSOCIATED COLITIS. THE COLITIS IS USUALLY CHARACTERIZED BY SEVERE PERSISTENT DIARRHEA AND SEVERE ABDOMINAL CRAMPS AND MAY BE ASSOCIATED WITH THE PASSAGE OF BLOOD AND MUCUS. ENDOSCOPIC EXAMINATION MAY REVEAL PSEUDOMEMBRANOUS COLITIS. STOOL CULTURE FOR *Clostridium difficile* AND STOOL ASSAY FOR *Clostridium difficile* TOXIN MAY BE HELPFUL DIAGNOSTICALLY. WHEN SIGNIFICANT DIARRHEA OCCURS, THE DRUG SHOULD BE DISCONTINUED. LARGE BOWEL ENDOSCOPY SHOULD BE CONSIDERED TO ESTABLISH A DEFINITIVE DIAGNOSIS IN CASES OF SEVERE DIARRHEA. ANTIPERISTALTIC AGENTS SUCH AS OPIATES AND DIPHENOXYLATE WITH ATROPINE MAY PROLONG AND/OR WORSEN THE CONDITION. DIARRHEA, COLITIS AND PSEUDOMEMBRANOUS COLITIS HAVE BEEN OBSERVED TO BEGIN UP TO SEVERAL WEEKS FOLLOWING CESSATION OF ORAL AND PARENTERAL THERAPY WITH CLINDAMYCIN.

Mild cases of pseudomembranous colitis usually respond to drug discontinuation alone. In moderate to severe cases, consideration should be given to management with fluids and electrolytes, protein supplementation and treatment with an antibacterial drug clinically effective against *Clostridium difficile* colitis.

PRECAUTIONS

General

For dermatological use only; not for ophthalmic use. Concomitant topical acne therapy should be used with caution because a possible cumulative irritancy effect may occur, especially with the use of peeling, desquamating, or abrasive agents.

The use of antibiotic agents may be associated with the overgrowth of nonsusceptible organisms, including fungi. If this occurs, discontinue use of this medication and take appropriate measures.

Avoid contact with eyes and mucous membranes.

Clindamycin and erythromycin containing products should not be used in combination. *In vitro* studies have shown antagonism between these two antimicrobials. The clinical significance of this *in vitro* antagonism is not known.

Information for Patients

Patients using DUAC® Gel should receive the following information and instructions:

1. DUAC® Gel is to be used as directed by the physician. It is for external use only. Avoid contact with eyes, and inside the nose, mouth, and all mucous membranes, as this product may be irritating.
2. This medication should not be used for any disorder other than that for which it was prescribed.
3. Patients should not use any other topical acne preparation unless otherwise directed by their physician.
4. Patients should report any signs of local adverse reactions to their physician. Patients who develop allergic symptoms such as severe swelling or shortness of breath should discontinue use and contact their physician immediately.
5. DUAC® Gel may bleach hair or colored fabric.
6. DUAC® Gel can be stored at room temperature up to 25°C (77°F) for up to 2 months. Do not freeze. Keep tube tightly closed. Keep out of the reach of small children. Discard any unused product after 2 months.
7. Before applying DUAC® Gel to affected areas, wash the skin gently, rinse with warm water, and pat dry.
8. Excessive or prolonged exposure to sunlight should be limited. To minimize exposure to sunlight, a hat or other clothing should be worn.

Carcinogenesis, Mutagenesis, Impairment of Fertility

Benzoyl peroxide has been shown to be a tumor promoter and progression agent in a number of animal studies. Benzoyl peroxide in acetone at doses of 5 and 10 mg administered twice per week induced squamous cell skin tumors in transgenic TgAC mice in a study using 20 weeks of topical treatment. The clinical significance of this is unknown.

In a 2-year dermal carcinogenicity study in mice, treatment with DUAC® Gel at doses up to 8000 mg/kg/day (16 times the highest recommended adult human dose of 2.5 g DUAC® Gel, based on mg/m^2) did not cause an increase in skin tumors. However, topical treatment with another formulation containing 1% clindamycin and 5% benzoyl peroxide at doses of 100, 500, or 2000 mg/kg/day caused a dose-dependent increase in the incidence of keratoacanthoma at the treated skin site of male rats in a 2-year dermal carcinogenicity study in rats.

In a 52-week photocarcinogenicity study in hairless mice (40 weeks of treatment followed by 12 weeks of observation), the median time to onset of skin tumor formation decreased and the number of tumors per mouse increased relative to controls following chronic concurrent topical treatment with DUAC® Gel and exposure to ultraviolet radiation.

Genotoxicity studies were not conducted with DUAC® Gel. Clindamycin phosphate was not genotoxic in *Salmonella typhimurium* or in a rat micronucleus test. Benzoyl peroxide has been found to cause DNA strand breaks in a variety of mammalian cell types, to be mutagenic in *Salmonella typhimurium* tests by some but not all investigators, and to cause sister chromatid exchanges in Chinese hamster ovary cells. Studies have not been performed with DUAC® Gel or benzoyl peroxide to evaluate the effect on fertility. Fertility studies in rats treated orally with up to 300 mg/kg/day of clindamycin (approximately 120 times the amount of clindamycin in the highest recommended adult human dose of 2.5 g DUAC® Gel, based on mg/m^2) revealed no effects on fertility or mating ability.

Pregnancy

Teratogenic Effects

Pregnancy Category C

Animal reproduction studies have not been conducted with DUAC® Gel or benzoyl peroxide. It is also not known whether DUAC® Gel can cause fetal harm when administered to a pregnant woman or can affect reproduction capacity. DUAC® Gel should be given to a pregnant woman only if clearly needed.

Developmental toxicity studies performed in rats and mice using oral doses of clindamycin up to 600 mg/kg/day (240 and 120 times the amount of clindamycin in the highest recommended adult human dose based on mg/m^2, respectively) or subcutaneous doses of clindamycin up to 250 mg/kg/day (100 and 50 times the amount of clindamycin in the highest recommended adult human dose based on mg/m^2, respectively) revealed no evidence of teratogenicity.

Nursing Women

It is not known whether DUAC® Gel is secreted into human milk after topical application. However, orally and parenterally administered clindamycin has been reported to appear

Local reactions with use of DUAC® Gel % of patients using DUAC® Gel with symptom present Combined results from 5 studies (n=397)

	Before Treatment (Baseline)			During Treatment		
	Mild	Moderate	Severe	Mild	Moderate	Severe
Erythema	28%	3%	0	26%	5%	0
Peeling	6%	<1%	0	17%	2%	0
Burning	3%	<1%	0	5%	<1%	0
Dryness	6%	<1%	0	15%	1%	0

in breast milk. Because of the potential for serious adverse reactions in nursing infants, a decision should be made whether to discontinue nursing or to discontinue the drug, taking into account the importance of the drug to the mother.

Pediatric Use

Safety and effectiveness of this product in pediatric patients below the age of 12 have not been established.

ADVERSE REACTIONS

During clinical trials, all patients were graded for facial erythema, peeling, burning, and dryness on the following scale: 0 = absent, 1 = mild, 2 = moderate, and 3 = severe. The percentage of patients that had symptoms present before treatment (at baseline) and during treatment were as follows:

[See table above]

(Percentages derived by # subjects with symptom score/# enrolled DUAC® Gel subjects, n = 397).

Anaphylaxis, as well as allergic reactions leading to hospitalization, has been reported in post-marketing use with DUAC® Gel. Because these reactions are reported voluntarily from a population of uncertain size, it is not always possible to reliably estimate their frequency or establish a causal relationship to a drug exposure.

DOSAGE AND ADMINISTRATION

DUAC® Gel should be applied once daily, in the evening or as directed by the physician, to affected areas after the skin is gently washed, rinsed with warm water and patted dry.

HOW SUPPLIED

DUAC® (clindamycin phosphate and benzoyl peroxide), 1.2%/5% Gel is available in:

- 45 gram tube NDC 0145-2371-05

Prior to Dispensing: Store in a cold place, preferably in a refrigerator, between 2°C and 8°C (36°F and 46°F). Do not freeze.

Dispensing Instructions for the Pharmacist: Dispense DUAC® Gel with a 60 day expiration date and specify "Store at room temperature up to 25°C (77°F). Do not freeze."

Keep tube tightly closed. Keep out of the reach of small children.

Stiefel Laboratories, Inc.
Research Triangle Park, NC 27709
DUA:4PI
Rev. July 2011

DUAC is a registered trademark of Stiefel Laboratories, Inc.

FABIOR™ ℞

(tazarotene)
Foam, 0.1%, for topical use

HIGHLIGHTS OF PRESCRIBING INFORMATION

These highlights do not include all the information needed to use FABIOR Foam safely and effectively. See full prescribing information for FABIOR Foam.

FABIOR™ (tazarotene) Foam, 0.1%, for topical use
Initial U.S. Approval: 1997

INDICATIONS AND USAGE

- FABIOR Foam is a retinoid indicated for the topical treatment of acne vulgaris in patients 12 years of age or older. (1)

DOSAGE AND ADMINISTRATION

- Apply a thin layer to the entire affected areas of the face and/or upper trunk once daily in the evening. Avoid the eyes, lips, and mucous membranes. Wash hands after application. (2)

DOSAGE FORMS AND STRENGTHS

- 0.1%, foam. (3)

CONTRAINDICATIONS

- Pregnancy. (4, 8.1)

WARNINGS AND PRECAUTIONS

- Fetal Risk: FABIOR Foam contains tazarotene, which is a teratogenic substance. FABIOR Foam is contraindicated in pregnancy. Females of childbearing potential should have a negative pregnancy test within 2 weeks prior to initiating treatment and use an effective method of contraception during treatment. (5.1)
- Local Irritation. Use with caution in patients with a history of local tolerability reactions or local hypersensitivity. (5.2)
- Potential Irritant Effect with Concomitant Topical Medications. Use with caution because a cumulative irritant effect may occur. (5.3)
- Photosensitivity and Risk for Sunburn. Avoid exposure to sunlight, sunlamps, and weather extremes. Wear sunscreen daily. (5.4)
- Contents are flammable. Instruct the patient to avoid fire, flame, and smoking during and immediately following application. (5.5)

ADVERSE REACTIONS

- Most common adverse reactions reported at an incidence ≥ 6% are application site irritation, application site dryness, application site erythema, and application site exfoliation. (6.1)

To report SUSPECTED ADVERSE REACTIONS, contact Stiefel Laboratories, Inc at 1-888-784-3335 (1-888-STIEFEL) or FDA at 1-800-FDA-1088 or www.fda.gov/medwatch

DRUG INTERACTIONS

- Avoid concomitant dermatologic medications and cosmetics that have a strong drying effect. (7)

See 17 for PATIENT COUNSELING INFORMATION and FDA-approved patient labeling

Revised: 09/2012

FULL PRESCRIBING INFORMATION: CONTENTS*

*** Sections or subsections omitted from the full prescribing information are not listed**

FULL PRESCRIBING INFORMATION

1 INDICATIONS AND USAGE

FABIOR (tazarotene) Foam, 0.1% is indicated for the topical treatment of acne vulgaris in patients 12 years of age or older.

2 DOSAGE AND ADMINISTRATION

FABIOR Foam is for topical use only. FABIOR Foam is not for oral, ophthalmic, or intravaginal use.

FABIOR Foam should be applied once daily in the evening after washing with a mild cleanser and fully drying the affected area. Dispense a small amount of foam into the palm of the hand. Using fingertips, apply only enough foam to lightly cover the entire affected areas of the face and/or upper trunk with a thin layer; gently massage the foam into the skin until the foam disappears. Avoid the eyes, lips, and mucous membranes. Wash hands after application.

Patients may use moisturizer as needed.

If undue irritation (redness, peeling, or discomfort) occurs, patients should reduce frequency of application or temporarily interrupt treatment. Treatment may be resumed once irritation subsides. Treatment should be discontinued if irritation persists.

3 DOSAGE FORMS AND STRENGTHS

0.1%, white to off-white foam

4 CONTRAINDICATIONS

FABIOR Foam is contraindicated in pregnancy.

FABIOR Foam may cause fetal harm when administered to a pregnant woman. Tazarotene elicits teratogenic and developmental effects associated with retinoids after topical or systemic administration in rats and rabbits *[see Use in Specific Populations (8.1)]*.

If this drug is used during pregnancy, or if the patient becomes pregnant while taking this drug, treatment should be discontinued and the patient apprised of the potential hazard to the fetus *[seeWarnings and Precautions (5.1) and Use in Specific Populations (8.1)]*.

5 WARNINGS AND PRECAUTIONS

5.1 Fetal Risk

Systemic exposure to tazarotenic acid is dependent upon the extent of the body surface area treated. In patients treated topically over sufficient body surface area, exposure could be in the same order of magnitude as in orally treated animals. Tazarotene is a teratogenic substance, and it is not known what level of exposure is required for teratogenicity in humans *[see Clinical Pharmacology (12)]*.

There were five reported pregnancies in patients who participated in clinical trials for topical tazarotene foam. One of the patients was found to have been treated with topical tazarotene for 25 days, two were treated with vehicle foam and the other two did not receive either tazarotene foam or vehicle foam. The patients were discontinued from the trials when their pregnancy was reported. The one pregnant woman who was inadvertently exposed to topical tazarotene during the clinical trial delivered a full-term healthy infant.

Females of Childbearing Potential

Females of child-bearing potential should be warned of the potential risk and use adequate birth-control measures when tazarotene Foam is used. The possibility of pregnancy should be considered in females of child-bearing potential at the time of institution of therapy.

A negative serum or urine result for pregnancy test having a sensitivity down to at least 25 mIU/mL for human chorionic gonadotropin (hCG) should be obtained within 2 weeks prior to FABIOR Foam therapy, which should begin during a normal menstrual period, for females of childbearing potential. Advise patients of the need to use an effective method of contraception to avoid pregnancy *[see Use in Specific Populations (8.1)]*.

5.2 Local Irritation

FABIOR Foam should be used with caution in patients with a history of local tolerability reactions or local hypersensitivity. Retinoids should not be used on abraded or eczematous skin, as they may cause severe irritation. Contact with the mouth, eyes, and mucous membranes should be avoided. In case of accidental contact, rinse well with water. Some individuals may experience skin redness, peeling, burning or excessive pruritus. If these effects occur, the medication should either be discontinued until the integrity of the skin is restored, or the dosing should be reduced to an interval the patient can tolerate. However, efficacy at reduced frequency of application has not been established. Weather extremes, such as wind or cold, may be more irritating to patients using FABIOR Foam.

5.3 Potential Irritant Effect with Concomitant Topical Medications

Concomitant topical acne therapy should be used with caution because a cumulative irritant effect may occur. If irritancy or dermatitis occurs, reduce frequency of application or temporarily interrupt treatment and resume once the irritation subsides. Treatment should be discontinued if the irritation persists.

5.4 Photosensitivity and Risk for Sunburn

Because of heightened burning susceptibility, exposure to sunlight (including sunlamps) should be avoided. Patients must be warned to use sunscreens and protective clothing when using Fabior Foam. Patients with sunburn should be advised not to use FABIOR Foam until fully recovered. Patients who may have considerable sun exposure due to their occupation and those patients with inherent sensitivity to sunlight should exercise particular caution when using FABIOR Foam and ensure that the precautions are observed *[see FDA-approved patient labeling]*. Due to the potential for photosensitivity resulting in greater risk for sunburn, FABIOR Foam should be used with caution in patients with a personal or family history of skin cancer.

FABIOR Foam should be administered with caution if the patient is also taking drugs known to be photosensitizers (e.g., thiazides, tetracyclines, fluoroquinolones, phenothiazines, sulfonamides) because of the increased possibility of augmented photosensitivity.

5.5 Flammability

The propellant in FABIOR Foam is flammable. Instruct the patient to avoid fire, flame, and/or smoking during and immediately following application.

6 ADVERSE REACTIONS

6.1 Clinical Trials Experience

Because clinical trials are conducted under widely varying conditions, adverse reaction rates observed in clinical trials of a drug cannot be directly compared to rates in the clinical trials of another drug and may not reflect the rates observed in clinical practice.

The safety data reflect exposure to FABIOR Foam in 744 patients with acne vulgaris. Patients were 12 years to 45 years of age and were treated once daily in the evening for 12 weeks. Adverse reactions reported in ≥ 1% of patients treated with FABIOR Foam are presented in Table 1. Most adverse reactions were mild to moderate in severity. Severe adverse reactions represented 3.0% of the patients treated. Overall, 2.6% (20/744) of patients discontinued FABIOR Foam because of local skin reactions.

Table 1: Incidence of Adverse Reactions in ≥1 % of Patients Treated with FABIOR Foam

	FABIOR Foam N=744	Vehicle Foam N=741
Patients with any treatment-related adverse reaction, n (%)	163 (22)	19 (3)
Application site irritation	107 (14)	9 (1)
Application site dryness	50 (7)	8 (1)
Application site erythema	48 (6)	3 (<1)
Application site exfoliation	44 (6)	3 (<1)
Application site pain	9 (1)	0
Application site pruritus	7 (1)	3 (<1)
Application site dermatitis	6 (1)	1 (<1)

Additional adverse reactions that were reported in <1% of patients treated with FABIOR Foam included application site reactions (including discoloration, discomfort, edema, rash and swelling), dermatitis, impetigo and pruritus.

Local skin reactions, dryness, erythema, and peeling actively assessed by the investigator and burning/stinging and itching reported by the patient were evaluated at baseline, during treatment, and end of treatment. During the 12 weeks of treatment, each local skin reaction peaked at week 2 and gradually reduced thereafter with the continued use of FABIOR Foam.

7 DRUG INTERACTIONS

No formal drug-drug interaction studies were conducted with FABIOR Foam.

Concomitant dermatologic medications and cosmetics that have a strong drying effect should be avoided. It is recommended to postpone treatment until the effects of these products subside before use of FABIOR Foam is started.

Concomitant use with oxidizing agents, such as benzoyl peroxide, may cause degradation of tazarotene and may reduce the clinical efficacy of tazarotene. If combination therapy is required, they should be applied at different times of the day (e.g. one in the morning and the other in the evening).

The impact of tazarotene on the pharmacokinetics of progestin-only oral contraceptives (i.e., minipills) has not been evaluated.

In a study of 27 healthy female subjects between the ages of 20 to 55 years receiving a combination oral contraceptive tablet containing 1 mg norethindrone and 35 mcg ethinyl estradiol, concomitant use of tazarotene did not affect the pharmacokinetics of norethindrone and ethinyl estradiol over a complete cycle.

8 USE IN SPECIFIC POPULATIONS

8.1 Pregnancy

Pregnancy Category X:

FABIOR Foam is contraindicated in pregnancy *[see Contraindications (4)]*.

There are no adequate and well-controlled studies with FABIOR Foam in pregnant women. FABIOR Foam is contraindicated in females who are or may become pregnant *[see Contraindications (4)]*. Females of child-bearing potential should be warned of the potential risk and use adequate birth-control measures when FABIOR Foam is used. The possibility that a female of child-bearing potential is pregnant at the time of institution of therapy should be considered. A negative serum or urine result for pregnancy test having a sensitivity down to at least 25 mIU/mL for hCG should be obtained within 2 weeks prior to FABIOR Foam therapy, which should begin during a normal menstrual period, for females of childbearing potential.

In rats, tazarotene 0.05% gel administered topically during gestation days 6 through 17 at 0.25 mg/kg/day resulted in reduced fetal body weights and reduced skeletal ossification. Rabbits dosed topically with 0.25 mg/kg/day tazarotene gel during gestation days 6 through 18 were noted with single incidences of known retinoid malformations, including spina bifida, hydrocephaly, and heart anomalies.

Systemic exposure (AUC) to tazarotenic acid at topical doses of 0.25 mg/kg/day tazarotene in a gel formulation in rats and rabbits were 15 and 166 times, respectively, the systemic exposure (AUC) in acne patients treated with 2 mg/cm^2 of FABIOR Foam 0.1% over a 15% body surface area.

As with other retinoids, when tazarotene was administered orally to experimental animals, developmental delays were seen in rats, and teratogenic effects and post-implantation loss were observed in rats and rabbits at doses 13 and 325 times, respectively, the systemic exposure (AUC) to tazarotenic acid in acne patients treated with 2 mg/cm^2 of FABIOR Foam 0.1% over a 15% body surface area.

In female rats orally administered 2 mg/kg/day tazarotene from 15 days before mating through gestation day 7, a number of classic developmental effects of retinoids were observed including decreased number of implantation sites, decreased litter size, decreased numbers of live fetuses, and decreased fetal body weights. A low incidence of retinoid-related malformations was also observed. Systemic exposure (AUC) in rats was 42 times the systemic exposure (AUC) in acne patients treated with 2 mg/cm^2 of FABIOR Foam 0.1% over a 15% body surface area.

8.3 Nursing Mothers

After single topical doses of ^{14}C-tazarotene to the skin of lactating rats, radioactivity was detected in milk, suggesting that there would be transfer of drug-related material to the offspring via milk. It is not known whether this drug is excreted in human milk. The safe use of FABIOR Foam during lactation has not been established. A decision should be made whether to discontinue breast-feeding or to discontinue FABIOR Foam therapy taking into account the benefit of breast-feeding for the child and the benefit of therapy for the woman.

8.4 Pediatric Use

The safety and effectiveness of FABIOR Foam in pediatric patients under 12 years of age have not been established. Clinical studies of FABIOR Foam included 860 patients 12 to 17 years of age with acne vulgaris.

8.5 Geriatric Use

FABIOR Foam for the treatment of acne has not been clinically evaluated in persons over the age of 65.

10 OVERDOSAGE

Excessive topical application of FABIOR Foam may lead to marked redness, peeling, or discomfort. *[See Warnings and Precautions (5.3).]* Management of accidental ingestion or excessive application to the skin should be as clinically indicated.

11 DESCRIPTION

FABIOR (tazarotene) Foam, 0.1% contains the compound tazarotene, a member of the acetylenic class of retinoids. It is for topical use only.

Chemically, tazarotene is ethyl 6-[(4,4-dimethylthiochroman-6-yl)ethynyl]nicotinate. The structural formula is represented below:

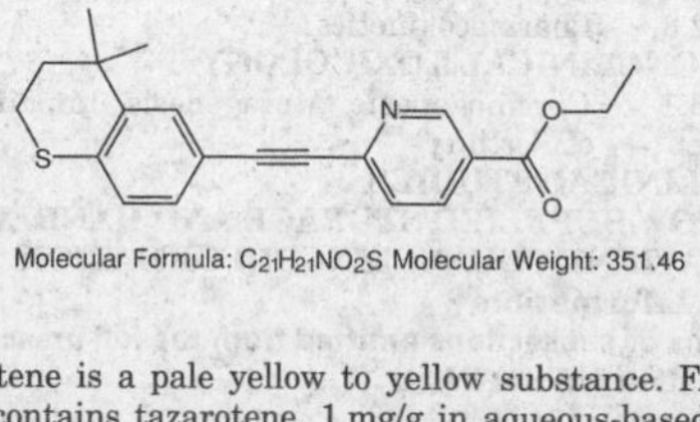

Molecular Formula: $C_{21}H_{21}NO_2S$ Molecular Weight: 351.46

Tazarotene is a pale yellow to yellow substance. FABIOR Foam contains tazarotene, 1 mg/g in aqueous-based white to off-white foam vehicle consisting of butylated hydroxytoluene, ceteareth-12, citric acid anhydrous, diisopropyl adipate, light mineral oil, potassium citrate monohydrate, potassium sorbate, purified water, and sorbic acid. FABIOR Foam is dispensed from an aluminum can pressurized with a hydrocarbon (propane/n-butane/isobutane) propellant.

12 CLINICAL PHARMACOLOGY

12.1 Mechanism of Action

Tazarotene is a retinoid prodrug that is converted to its active form, the cognate carboxylic acid of tazarotene, by rapid deesterification in animals and man. Tazarotenic acid binds to all three members of the retinoic acid receptor (RAR) family: RARα, RARβ, and RARγ but shows relative selectivity for RARβ, and RARγ and may modify gene expression. The clinical significance of these findings is unknown.

The mechanism of tazarotene action in acne vulgaris is not defined. However, the basis of tazarotene's therapeutic effect in acne may be due to its anti-hyperproliferative, normalizing-of-differentiation and anti-inflammatory effects. Tazarotene inhibited corneocyte accumulation in rhino mouse skin and cross-linked envelope formation in cultured human keratinocytes. The clinical significance of these findings is unknown.

12.2 Pharmacodynamics

The pharmacodynamics of FABIOR Foam are unknown.

12.3 Pharmacokinetics

Following topical application, tazarotene undergoes esterase hydrolysis to form its active metabolite, tazarotenic acid. Tazarotenic acid was highly bound to plasma proteins (greater than 99%). Tazarotene and tazarotenic acid were metabolized to sulfoxides, sulfones and other polar metabolites which were eliminated through urinary and fecal pathways.

Systemic exposure following topical application of FABIOR Foam 0.1% was evaluated in one trial. Patients aged 15 years and older with moderate-to-severe acne applied approximately 3.7 grams of FABIOR Foam 0.1% (N=13) to approximately 15% body surface area (face, upper chest, upper back, and shoulders) once daily for 22 days. On day 22, the mean (±SD) tazarotenic acid C_{max} was 0.43 (±0.19) ng/mL, the $AUC_{0\text{-}24h}$ was 6.98 (±3.56) ng•hr/mL and the half-life was 21.7 (±15.7) hours. The median T_{max} was 6 hours (range 4.4 to 12 hours). The $AUC_{0\text{-}24hr}$ for tazarotenic acid was approximately 50 fold higher compared with the parent compound tazarotene. The mean (±SD) half-life of tazarotene was 8.1 (±3.7) hours.

Accumulation was observed upon repeated once-daily dosing as the tazarotenic acid predose concentrations were measurable in the majority of subjects. Steady state was attained within 22 days of daily application. Once-daily dosing resulted in little to no accumulation of tazarotene as predose concentrations were mostly below the quantitation limit throughout the study.

13 NONCLINICAL TOXICOLOGY

13.1 Carcinogenesis, Mutagenesis, Impairment of Fertility

Carcinogenesis

A long-term study of tazarotene following oral administration of 0.025, 0.050, and 0.125 mg/kg/day to rats showed no indications of increased carcinogenic risk. Based on pharmacokinetic data from a shorter-term study in rats, the highest dose of 0.125 mg/kg/day was anticipated to give systemic exposure in rats approximately 2 times the systemic exposure (AUC) in acne patients treated with 2 mg/cm^2 of Fabior Foam 0.1% over a 15% body surface area.

A long-term topical application study of up to 0.1% tazarotene in a gel formulation in mice terminated at 88 weeks showed that dose levels of 0.05, 0.125, 0.25, and 1 mg/kg/day (reduced to 0.5 mg/kg/day for males after 41 weeks due to severe dermal irritation) revealed no apparent carcinogenic effects when compared to vehicle control animals. Systemic exposure (AUC) at the highest dose in mice was 49 times the systemic exposure (AUC) in acne patients treated with 2 mg/cm^2 of FABIOR Foam 0.1% over a 15% body surface area.

In evaluation of photocarcinogenicity, median time to onset of tumors was decreased and the number of tumors increased in hairless mice following chronic topical dosing with exposure to ultraviolet radiation at tazarotene concentrations of 0.001%, 0.005%, and 0.01% in a gel formulation for up to 40 weeks.

Mutagenesis

Tazarotene was non-mutagenic in the Ames assay and did not produce structural chromosomal aberrations in a human lymphocyte assay. Tazarotene was non-mutagenic in the CHO/HGPRT mammalian cell forward gene mutation assay and was non-clastogenic in the in vivo mouse micronucleus test.

Impairment of Fertility

No impairment of fertility was observed in rats when male animals were treated for 70 days prior to mating and female animals were treated for 14 days prior to mating and continuing through gestation and lactation with topical doses of tazarotene gel up to 0.125 mg/kg/day. Based on data from another study, the systemic drug exposure at the 0.125 mg/kg/day dose in rats would be equivalent to 7.6 times the systemic exposure (AUC) in acne patients treated with 2 mg/cm^2 of FABIOR Foam 0.1% over a 15% body surface area.

No impairment of mating performance or fertility was observed in male rats treated for 70 days prior to mating with oral doses of up to 1 mg/kg/day tazarotene. Systemic exposure (AUC) at the highest dose in rats was 23 times the systemic exposure (AUC) in acne patients treated with 2 mg/cm^2 of FABIOR Foam 0.1% over a 15% body surface area.

No effect on parameters of mating performance or fertility was observed in female rats treated for 15 days prior to mating and continuing through gestation day 7 with oral doses of tazarotene up to 2 mg/kg/day. However, there was a significant decrease in the number of estrous stages and an increase in developmental effects at that dose *[see Pregnancy (8.1)]*. Systemic exposure (AUC) at the highest dose in rats was 42 times the systemic exposure (AUC) in acne patients treated with 2 mg/cm^2 of FABIOR Foam 0.1% over a 15% body surface area.

Reproductive capabilities of F1 animals, including F2 survival and development, were not affected by topical administration of tazarotene gel to female F0 parental rats from gestation day 16 through lactation day 20 at the maximum tolerated dose of 0.125 mg/kg/day. Based on data from another study, the systemic drug exposure (AUC) in rats would be equivalent to 7.6 times the systemic exposure (AUC) in acne patients treated with 2 mg/cm^2 of FABIOR Foam 0.1% over a 15% body surface area.

14 CLINICAL STUDIES

In 2 multi-center, randomized, double-blind, vehicle-controlled studies, a total of 1485 patients with moderate-to-severe acne vulgaris were randomized 1:1 to FABIOR Foam or vehicle applied once daily for 12 weeks. Acne severity was evaluated using lesion counts and the 6-point Investigator's Global Assessment (IGA) scale (see Table 2). At baseline, 80% of patients were graded as "moderate" or Grade 3 and 20% were graded as "severe" or Grade 4 on the IGA scale. At baseline, subjects had an average of 79.8 total lesions of which the mean number of inflammatory lesions was 31.9 and the mean number of non inflammatory lesions was 47.8. Patients ranged in age from 12 to 45 years, with 860 (58%) patients 12 to 17 years of age; 428 (29%) patients 18 to 25 years old; 143 (10%) patients 26 to 35 years old and 54 (4%) patients 36 to 45 years old. Patients enrolled in the studies by race were white (77%), Black (15%), Asian (4%) and other (4%). Hispanics comprised 18% of the population. An equal number of males (49%) and females (51%) were enrolled. Treatment success was defined as a score of "clear" (Grade 0) or "almost clear" (Grade 1) and at least 2-grade improvement from the baseline score to week 12.

Table 2: Investigator's Global Assessment Scale

Grade	Description	
0	Clear	Clear skin with no inflammatory or non-inflammatory lesions.
1	Almost clear	Rare non-inflammatory lesions with no more than rare papules.
2	Mild	Greater than Grade 1, some non-inflammatory lesions with no more than a few inflammatory lesions (papules/pustules only, no nodular lesions).
3	Moderate	Greater than Grade 2, up to many non-inflammatory lesions and may have some inflammatory lesions, but no more than one small nodular lesion.
4	Severe	Greater than Grade 3, up to many non-inflammatory and inflammatory lesions, but no more than a few nodular lesions.
5	Very severe	Many non-inflammatory and inflammatory lesions and more than a few nodular lesions. May have cystic lesions.

Absolute and percent reductions in lesion counts and the IGA scale after 12 weeks of treatment in these two studies are shown in Table 3. Each study needed to have a statistically significant reduction in two out of three lesion counts at Week 12.

[See table 3 above]

Table 3: Reductions in Lesion Counts and Improvements in Investigator's Global Assessment at Week 12

	Study 1		Study 2	
	FABIOR Foam N=371	Vehicle Foam N=372	FABIOR Foam N=373	Vehicle Foam N=369
Inflammatory Lesions				
Mean absolute reduction from Baseline	18.0	14.0	18.0	15.0
Mean percent reduction from Baseline	58%	45%	55%	45%
Non-inflammatory Lesions				
Mean absolute reduction from Baseline	28.0	17.0	26.0	18.0
Mean percent reduction from Baseline	55%	33%	57%	41%
Total Lesions				
Mean absolute reduction from Baseline	46.0	31.0	43.0	33.0
Mean percent reduction from Baseline	56%	39%	56%	43%
Investigator's Global Assessment (IGA), n (%)				
Minimum 2-grade improvement *and* IGA of 0 or 1	107 (29%)	60 (16%)	103 (28%)	49 (13%)

16 HOW SUPPLIED/STORAGE AND HANDLING

How Supplied

FABIOR Foam, 0.1% (1 mg/g) is a white to off-white foam, supplied as follows:

50 g aluminum can NDC 0145-0020-03

100 g aluminum can NDC 0145-0020-02

Storage and Handling

- Store at 20°C to 25°C (68°F to 77°F); excursions permitted to 15°C to 30°C (59°F to 86°F). See USP-controlled room temperature.
- Store upright.
- Protect from freezing.
- Flammable. Avoid fire, flame, or smoking during and immediately following application. Contents under pressure. Do not puncture or incinerate. Do not expose to heat or store at temperatures above 120°F (49°C).
- Shake can before use. Hold can at an upright angle and press firmly to dispense.

17 PATIENT COUNSELING INFORMATION

[See FDA-Approved Patient Labeling (Patient Information).]

Inform the patient of the following:

- Fetal risk associated with FABIOR Foam for females of childbearing potential. Advise patients to use an effective method of contraception during treatment to avoid pregnancy. Advise the patient to stop medication if she becomes pregnant and call her doctor.
- If undue irritation (redness, peeling, or discomfort) occurs, reduce frequency of application or temporarily interrupt treatment. Treatment may be resumed once irritation subsides.
- Do not place FABIOR Foam in the freezer.
- Avoid exposure of the treated areas to either natural or artificial sunlight, including tanning beds and sun lamps.
- Avoid contact with the eyes. If FABIOR Foam gets in or near their eyes, to rinse thoroughly with water.
- Wash their hands after applying FABIOR Foam.
- Avoid fire, flame, or smoking during and immediately following application since FABIOR Foam is flammable.
- Keep out of the reach of children.
- Not for ophthalmic, oral, or intravaginal use.

FAB:2PI

Pharmacist-Detach here and Give Instructions to Patient

Patient Information

FABIOR
(fab' ee ore)
(tazarotene)
Foam

IMPORTANT: For skin use only. Do not get FABIOR Foam in your eyes, mouth or vagina.

Read the Patient Information that comes with FABIOR Foam before you start using it and each time you get a refill. There may be new information. This leaflet does not take the place of talking with your doctor about your condition or treatment.

What is FABIOR Foam?

FABIOR Foam is a prescription medicine used on the skin (topical) to treat acne in people 12 years and older.

It is not known if FABIOR Foam is safe and effective in children under 12 years of age.

Who should not use FABIOR Foam?

Do not use FABIOR Foam if you are pregnant or plan to become pregnant. FABIOR Foam may harm your unborn baby, if used during pregnancy.

If you are a female who can become pregnant:

- Use an effective method of birth control during treatment with FABIOR Foam. Talk with your doctor about birth control methods that are right for you during treatment with FABIOR Foam.
- Your doctor should do a blood or urine pregnancy test within 2 weeks before you begin to use FABIOR Foam to be sure you are not pregnant.
- If you have menstrual periods, begin using FABIOR Foam during a normal menstrual period to help assure that you are not pregnant when you begin use.

Stop using FABIOR Foam and call your doctor right away if you become pregnant during treatment with FABIOR Foam.

What should I tell my doctor before using FABIOR Foam?

Before you use FABIOR Foam, tell your doctor if you:

- or a family member have or had skin cancer.
- have eczema.
- have had a reaction to topical products in the past.
- have any condition that makes you sensitive to light.
- have any other medical conditions.
- are pregnant or plan to become pregnant. **See "Who should not use FABIOR Foam?"**
- are breast-feeding or plan to breastfeed. It is not known if tazarotene passes into your breast milk. You and your doctor should decide if you will use FABIOR Foam or breastfeed. You should not do both. Talk to your doctor about the best way to feed your baby if you use FABIOR Foam.

Tell your doctor about all the medicines you take including prescription and nonprescription medicines, vitamins, and herbal supplements.

Especially tell your doctor if you:

- use other medicines or products that make your skin dry
- take other medicines that may increase your sensitivity to sunlight

Ask your doctor or pharmacist if you are not sure if your medicine is one that is listed above.

Know the medicines you take. Keep a list of your medicines and show it to your doctor and pharmacist when you get a new medicine.

How should I use FABIOR Foam?

- Use FABIOR Foam exactly as your doctor tells you to. Do not use more FABIOR Foam than prescribed and do not use it more often than your doctor tells you to.
- If you are a female and have menstrual periods, begin using FABIOR Foam during a normal menstrual period to help assure that you are not pregnant when you begin use. **See "Who should not use FABIOR Foam?"**
- FABIOR Foam is flammable. Avoid fire, flame, and smoking during and right after you apply FABIOR Foam.
- Gently clean the affected area (face and/or upper trunk) with a mild cleanser and dry completely before using FABIOR Foam.
- Apply FABIOR Foam one time each day, before going to bed, to the affected areas (face and/or upper trunk) where you have acne lesions. Use enough foam to cover the entire affected area with a thin film of FABIOR Foam.
- Keep FABIOR Foam away from your eyes, eyelids, mouth, and vagina. If FABIOR Foam comes into contact with your eyes, rinse them well with water.
- Wash your hands after applying FABIOR Foam.
- If you use too much FABIOR Foam, you may get redness, peeling or skin irritation in the treated area. Call your doctor if this happens, or if you accidently swallow FABIOR Foam.
- Follow your doctor's directions for other routine skin care and the use of make-up.
- You may also use a moisturizer as needed.

Instructions for applying FABIOR Foam

1. Shake the FABIOR Foam can before use.
2. Remove cap from can. Nozzle should be lined up with black mark on rim of can. If black mark is not lined up with the nozzle, twist nozzle to line up with black mark. See Figure A.

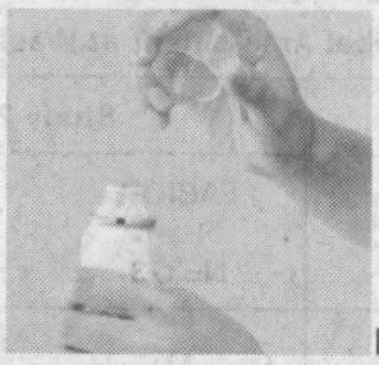

Figure A

3. Hold the FABIOR Foam can upright at a slight angle and press the nozzle. See Figure B.

Figure B

4. Dispense a small amount of FABIOR Foam into the palm of your hand. See Figure C.

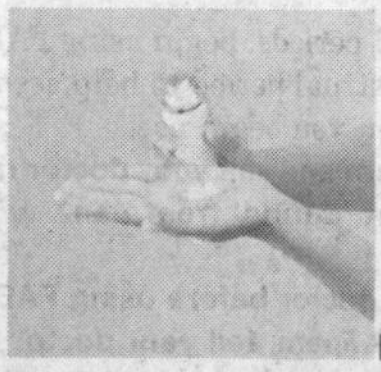

Figure C

5. Use the fingertips of your other hand to apply enough FABIOR Foam to cover the affected area with a thin layer. Gently rub the foam into the affected area until it disappears into the skin. See Figure D.

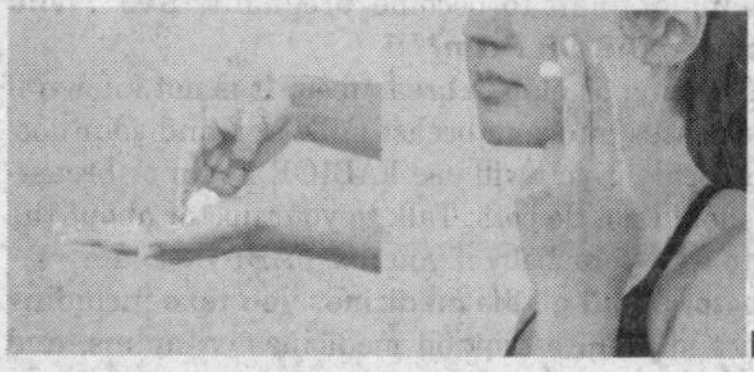

Figure D

6. Wash hands after applying FABIOR Foam. See Figure E.

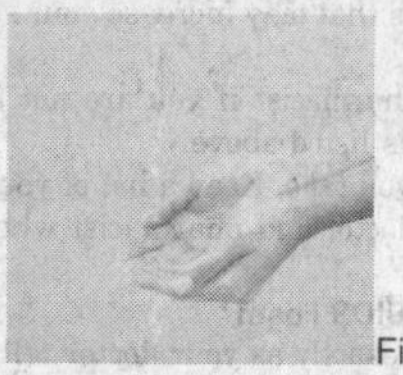

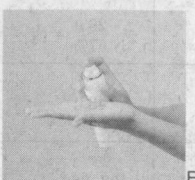

Figure E

Avoid getting FABIOR Foam in your eyes, mouth, or vagina.

What should I avoid while using FABIOR Foam?

- Avoid using abrasive soaps or cleansers that might dry or irritate your skin, unless your doctor tells you it is ok.
- Avoid sunlight. FABIOR Foam can make your skin sensitive to sunlight and the light from sunlamps or tanning beds. You could get a sunburn. Use sunscreen and protective clothing during the day if you must be in sunlight.
- Avoid using FABIOR Foam if you have a sunburn. If you have a sunburn, wait until it is fully healed before using FABIOR Foam.
- Talk to your doctor before using FABIOR Foam if you are sensitive to sunlight, take medications that increase your sensitivity to sunlight, or you must spend a lot of time in the sun for your job.
- Avoid weather extremes, such as wind and cold because they may irritate your skin more while you are using FABIOR Foam.

What are the possible side effects of FABIOR Foam?

FABIOR Foam may harm your unborn baby, if used during pregnancy.

- Do not use FABIOR Foam during pregnancy. See **"Who should not use FABIOR Foam?"**

The most common side effects of FABIOR Foam are:

- burning or stinging
- dry skin
- red skin
- peeling or flaking skin

Sometimes these symptoms can become severe and may be uncomfortable. Tell your doctor if these side effects become uncomfortable for you. Your doctor may tell you to stop using FABIOR Foam until your skin heals and your symptoms improve, or to use FABIOR Foam less often to help you tolerate it better.

These are not all the possible side effects of FABIOR Foam. For more information, ask your doctor or pharmacist.

Call your doctor for medical advice about side effects. You may report side effects to FDA at 1-800-FDA-1088.

You may also report side effects to Stiefel Laboratories, Inc at 1-888-784-3335.

How should I store FABIOR Foam?

- Store FABIOR Foam at room temperature, between 68°F to 77°F (20°C to 25°C).
- Store FABIOR Foam upright.
- Do not freeze FABIOR Foam.
- FABIOR Foam is flammable. Keep the can away from fire and heat. Do not spray FABIOR Foam near fire or direct heat.
- Do not puncture the can or throw it into a fire, even if the can is empty.

Keep FABIOR Foam and all medicines out of the reach of children.

General Information about FABIOR Foam

Medicines are sometimes prescribed for purposes other than those listed in Patient Information leaflets. Do not use FABIOR Foam for a condition for which it was not prescribed. Do not give FABIOR Foam to other people even if they have the same symptoms that you have. It may harm them.

This Patient Information leaflet summarizes the most important information about FABIOR Foam. If you would like more information, talk with your doctor. You can ask your doctor or pharmacist for information about FABIOR Foam that is written for health professionals.

What are the ingredients in FABIOR Foam?

Active ingredient: tazarotene

Inactive ingredients: butylated hydroxytoluene, ceteareth-12, citric acid anhydrous, diisopropyl adipate, light mineral oil, potassium citrate monohydrate, potassium sorbate, purified water, and sorbic acid. The foam is dispensed from an aluminum can pressurized with a hydrocarbon (propane/n-butane/isobutane) propellant.

The Patient Information leaflet has been approved by the U.S. Food and Drug Administration

Manufactured for:
Stiefel Laboratories, Inc.
Research Triangle Park, NC 27709
Manufactured by:
DPT Laboratories, Ltd.
307 E. Josephine Street
San Antonio, TX 78215
Licensed from Allergan, Inc.
FAB:2PIL
Rev: Sept 2012
Issued 05/2012

SORIATANE® ℞

[sōr-ī-ă-tēn]
(acitretin)
CAPSULES

CAUSES BIRTH DEFECTS

DO NOT GET PREGNANT

Rx Only

CONTRAINDICATIONS AND WARNINGS

Soriatane must not be used by females who are pregnant, or who intend to become pregnant during therapy or at any time for at least 3 years following discontinuation of therapy. Soriatane also must not be used by females who may not use reliable contraception while undergoing treatment and for at least 3 years following discontinuation of treatment. Acitretin is a metabolite of etretinate (Tegison®), and major human fetal abnormalities have been reported with the administration of acitretin and etretinate. Potentially, any fetus exposed can be affected.

Clinical evidence has shown that concurrent ingestion of acitretin and ethanol has been associated with the formation of etretinate, which has a significantly longer elimination half-life than acitretin. Because the longer elimination half-life of etretinate would increase the duration of teratogenic potential for female patients, ethanol must not be ingested by female patients either during treatment with Soriatane or for 2 months after cessation of therapy. This allows for elimination of acitretin, thus removing the substrate for transesterification to etretinate. The mechanism of the metabolic process for conversion of acitretin to etretinate has not been fully defined. It is not known whether substances other than ethanol are associated with transesterification.

Acitretin has been shown to be embryotoxic and/or teratogenic in rabbits, mice, and rats at oral doses of 0.6, 3 and 15 mg/kg, respectively. These doses are approximately 0.2, 0.3 and 3 times the maximum recommended therapeutic dose, respectively, based on a mg/m^2 comparison.

Major human fetal abnormalities associated with acitretin and/or etretinate administration have been reported including meningomyelocele, meningoencephalocele, multiple synostoses, facial dysmorphia, syndactyly, absence of terminal phalanges, malformations of hip, ankle and forearm, low-set ears, high palate, decreased cranial volume, cardiovascular malformation and alterations of the skull and cervical vertebrae.

Soriatane should be prescribed only by those who have special competence in the diagnosis and treatment of severe psoriasis, are experienced in the use of systemic retinoids, and understand the risk of teratogenicity.

Because of Soriatane'steratogenicity, a program called the *Do Your P.A.R.T* program, Pregnancy Prevention Actively Required During and After Treatment, has been developed to educate women of childbearing potential and their healthcare providers about the serious risks associated with acitretin and to help prevent pregnancies from occurring with the use of this drug and for 3 years after its discontinuation. The *Do Your P.A.R.T.* program requirements are described below (see also PRECAUTIONS section).

Important Information for Women of Childbearing Potential:

Soriatane should be considered only for women with severe psoriasis unresponsive to other therapies or whose clinical condition contraindicates the use of other treatments.

Females of reproductive potential must not be given a prescription for Soriatane until pregnancy is excluded. Soriatane is contraindicated in females of reproductive potential unless the patient meets ALL of the following conditions:

- **Must have had 2 negative urine or serum pregnancy tests with a sensitivity of at least 25 mIU/mL before receiving the initial Soriatane prescription. The first test (a screening test) is obtained by the prescriber when the decision is made to pursue Soriatane therapy. The second pregnancy test (a confirmation test) should be done during the first 5 days of the menstrual period immediately preceding the beginning of Soriatane therapy. For patients with amenorrhea, the second test should be done at least 11 days after the last act of unprotected sexual intercourse (without using 2 effective forms of contraception [birth control] simultaneously).**
- **Must have a pregnancy test repeated every month during Soriatane treatment. The patient must have a negative result from a urine or serum pregnancy test before receiving a Soriatane prescription. To encourage compliance with this recommendation, a limited supply of the drug should be prescribed. For at least 3 years after discontinuing Soriatane therapy, a pregnancy test must be repeated every 3 months.**
- **Must have selected and have committed to use 2 effective forms of contraception (birth control) simultaneously, at least 1 of which must be a primary form, unless absolute abstinence is the chosen method, or the patient has undergone a hysterectomy or is clearly postmenopausal.**
- **Patients must use 2 effective forms of contraception (birth control) simultaneously for at least 1 month prior to initiation of Soriatane therapy, during Soriatane therapy, and for at least 3 years after discontinuing Soriatane therapy. A Soriatane Patient Referral Form is available so that patients can receive an initial free contraceptive counseling session and pregnancy testing. Counseling about contraception and behaviors associated with an increased risk of pregnancy must be repeated on a monthly basis by the prescriber during Soriatane therapy and every 3 months for at least 3 years following discontinuation of Soriatane therapy.**

Effective forms of contraception include both primary and secondary forms of contraception. Primary forms of contraception include: tubal ligation, partner's vasectomy, intrauterine devices, birth control pills, and injectable/implantable/insertable/topical hormonal birth control products. Secondary forms of contraception include latex condoms (with or without spermicide), diaphragms and cervical caps (which must be used with a spermicide).

Any birth control method can fail. Therefore, it is critically important that women of childbearing potential use 2 effective forms of contraception (birth control) simultaneously. It has not been established if there is a pharmacokinetic interaction between acitretin and combined oral contraceptives. However, it has been established that acitretin interferes with the contraceptive effect of microdosed progestin preparations.[1] Microdosed "minipill" progestin preparations are not recommended for use with Soriatane. *It is not known whether other progestational contraceptives, such as implants and injectables, are adequate methods of contraception during acitretin therapy.*

Prescribers are advised to consult the package insert of any medication administered concomitantly with hormonal contraceptives, since some medications may decrease the effectiveness of these birth control products. Patients should be prospectively cautioned not to self-medicate with the herbal supplement St. John's Wort because a possible interaction has been suggested with hormonal contraceptives based on reports of breakthrough bleeding on oral contraceptives shortly after starting St. John's Wort. Pregnancies have been reported by users of combined hormonal contraceptives who also used some form of St. John's Wort (see PRECAUTIONS).

• Must have signed a Patient Agreement/Informed Consent for Female Patients that contains warnings about the risk of potential birth defects if the fetus is exposed to Soriatane, about contraceptive failure, about the fact that they must not ingest beverages or products containing ethanol while taking Soriatane and for 2 months after Soriatane treatment has been discontinued, and about preventing pregnancy while taking Soriatane and for at least 3 years after discontinuing Soriatane therapy.

If pregnancy does occur during Soriatane therapy or at any time for at least 3 years following discontinuation of Soriatane therapy, the prescriber and patient should discuss the possible effects on the pregnancy. The available information is as follows:

Acitretin, the active metabolite of etretinate, is teratogenic and is contraindicated during pregnancy. The risk of severe fetal malformations is well established when systemic retinoids are taken during pregnancy. Pregnancy must also be prevented after stopping acitretin therapy, while the drug is being eliminated to below a threshold blood concentration that would be associated with an increased incidence of birth defects. Because this threshold has not been established for acitretin in humans and because elimination rates vary among patients, the duration of posttherapy contraception to achieve adequate elimination cannot be calculated precisely. It is strongly recommended that contraception be continued for at least 3 years after stopping treatment with acitretin, based on the following considerations:

• In the absence of transesterification to form etretinate, greater than 98% of the acitretin would be eliminated within 2 months, assuming a mean elimination half-life of 49 hours.

• In cases where etretinate is formed, as has been demonstrated with concomitant administration of acitretin and ethanol,

- **greater than 98% of the etretinate formed would be eliminated in 2 years, assuming a mean elimination half-lie of 120 days.**
- **greater than 98% of the etretinate formed would be eliminated in 3 years, based on the longest demonstrated elimination half-life of 168 days.**

However, etretinate was found in plasma and subcutaneous fat in one patient reported to have had sporadic alcohol intake, 52 months after she stopped acitretin therapy.[2]

• Severe birth defects have been reported where conception occurred during the time interval when the patient was being treated with acitretin and/or etretinate. In addition, severe birth defects have also been reported when conception occurred after the mother completed therapy. These cases have been reported both prospectively (before the outcome was known) and retrospectively (after the outcome was known). The events below are listed without distinction as to whether the reported birth defects are consistent with retinoid-induced embryopathy or not.

Timing of Paternal Acitretin Treatment Relative to Conception	Delivery of Healthy Neonate	Spontaneous Abortion	Induced Abortion	Total
At time of conception	5*	5	1	11
Discontinued ~4 weeks prior	0	0	1**	1
Discontinued ~6 to 8 months prior	0	1	0	1

* Four of 5 cases were prospective.

** With malformation pattern not typical of retinoid embryopathy (bilateral cystic hygromas of neck, hypoplasia of lungs bilateral, pulmonary atresia, VSD with overriding truncus arteriosus).

• There have been 318 prospectively reported cases involving pregnancies and the use of etretinate, acitretin or both. In 238 of these cases, the conception occurred after the last dose of etretinate (103 cases), acitretin (126) or both (9). Fetal outcome remained unknown in approximately one-half of these cases, of which 62 were terminated and 14 were spontaneous abortions. Fetal outcome is known for the other 118 cases and 15 of the outcomes were abnormal (including cases of absent hand/wrist, clubfoot, GI malformation, hypocalcemia, hypotonia, limb malformation, neonatal apnea/anemia, neonatal ichthyosis, placental disorder/death, undescended testicle and 5 cases of premature birth). In the 126 prospectively reported cases where conception occurred after the last dose of acitretin only, 43 cases involved conception at least 1 year but less than 2 years after the last dose. There were 3 reports of abnormal outcomes out of these 43 cases (involving limb malformation, GI tract malformations and premature birth). There were only 4 cases where conception occurred at least 2 years after the last dose but there were no reports of birth defects in these cases.

• There is also a total of 35 retrospectively reported cases where conception occurred at least one year after the last dose of etretinate, acitretin or both. From these cases there are 3 reports of birth defects when the conception occurred at least 1 year but less than 2 years after the last dose of acitretin (including heart malformations, Turner's Syndrome, and unspecified congenital malformations) and 4 reports of birth defects when conception occurred 2 or more years after the last dose of acitretin (including foot malformation, cardiac malformations [2 cases] and unspecified neonatal and infancy disorder). There were 3 additional abnormal outcomes in cases where conception occurred 2 or more years after the last dose of etretinate (including chromosome disorder, forearm aplasia, and stillbirth).

• Females who have taken Tegison (etretinate) must continue to follow the contraceptive recommendations for Tegison. Tegison is no longer marketed in the US; for information, call Stiefel at 1-888-784-3335 (STIEFEL).

• Patients should not donate blood during and for at least 3 years following the completion of Soriatane therapy because women of childbearing potential must not receive blood from patients being treated with Soriatane.

Important Information For Males Taking Soriatane:

• Patients should not donate blood during and for at least 3 years following Soriatane therapy because women of childbearing potential must not receive blood from patients being treated with Soriatane.

• Samples of seminal fluid from 3 male patients treated with acitretin and 6 male patients treated with etretinate have been assayed for the presence of acitretin. The maximum concentration of acitretin observed in the seminal fluid of these men was 12.5 ng/mL. Assuming an ejaculate volume of 10 mL, the amount of drug transferred in semen would be 125 ng, which is 1/200,000 of a single 25 mg capsule. Thus, although it appears that residual acitretin in seminal fluid poses little, if any, risk to a fetus while a male patient is taking the drug or after it is discontinued, the no-effect limit for teratogenicity is unknown and there is no registry for birth defects associated with acitretin. The available data are as follows:

There have been 25 cases of reported conception when the male partner was taking acitretin. The pregnancy outcome is known in 13 of these 25 cases. Of these, 9 reports were retrospective and 4 were prospective (meaning the pregnancy was reported prior to knowledge of the outcome)[3].

[See table above]

***For All Patients:* A SORIATANE MEDICATION GUIDE MUST BE GIVEN TO THE PATIENT EACH TIME SORIATANE IS DISPENSED, AS REQUIRED BY LAW.**

DESCRIPTION

Soriatane (acitretin), a retinoid, is available in 10 mg, 17.5 mg, 22.5 mg, and 25 mg gelatin capsules for oral administration. Chemically, acitretin is all-trans-9-(4-methoxy-2,3,6-trimethylphenyl)-3,7-dimethyl-2,4,6,8-nonatetraenoic acid. It is a metabolite of etretinate and is related to both retinoic acid and retinol (vitamin A). It is a yellow to greenish-yellow powder with a molecular weight of 326.44. The structural formula is:

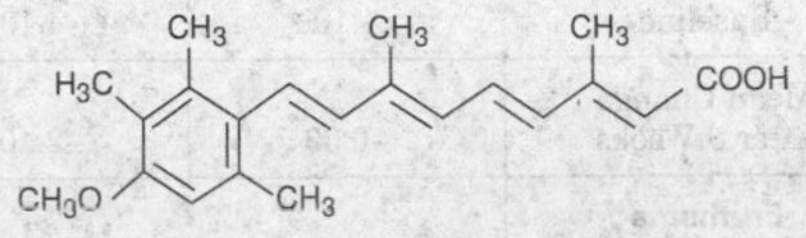

Each capsule contains acitretin, microcrystalline cellulose, sodium ascorbate, gelatin, black monogramming ink and maltodextrin (a mixture of polysaccharides).

Gelatin capsule shells contain gelatin, iron oxide (yellow, black, and red), and titanium dioxide. They may also contain benzyl alcohol, carboxymethylcellulose sodium, edetate calcium disodium.

CLINICAL PHARMACOLOGY

The mechanism of action of Soriatane is unknown.

Pharmacokinetics:

Absorption:

Oral absorption of acitretin is optimal when given with food. For this reason, acitretin was given with food in all of the following studies. After administration of a single 50 mg oral dose of acitretin to 18 healthy subjects, maximum plasma concentrations ranged from 196 to 728 ng/mL (mean 416 ng/mL) and were achieved in 2 to 5 hours (mean 2.7 hours). The oral absorption of acitretin is linear and proportional with increasing doses from 25 to 100 mg. Approximately 72% (range 47% to 109%) of the administered dose was absorbed after a single 50 mg dose of acitretin was given to 12 healthy subjects.

Distribution:

Acitretin is more than 99.9% bound to plasma proteins, primarily albumin.

Metabolism

(see *Pharmacokinetic Drug Interactions: Ethanol*):

Following oral absorption, acitretin undergoes extensive metabolism and interconversion by simple isomerization to its 13-cis form (cis-acitretin). The formation of cis-acitretin relative to parent compound is not altered by dose or fed/fast conditions of oral administration of acitretin. Both parent compound and isomer are further metabolized into chain-shortened breakdown products and conjugates, which are excreted. Following multiple-dose administration of acitretin, steady-state concentrations of acitretin and cis-acitretin in plasma are achieved within approximately 3 weeks.

Elimination:

The chain-shortened metabolites and conjugates of acitretin and cis-acitretin are ultimately excreted in the feces (34% to 54%) and urine (16% to 53%). The terminal elimination half-life of acitretin following multiple-dose administration is 49 hours (range 33 to 96 hours), and that of cis-acitretin under the same conditions is 63 hours (range 28 to 157 hours). The accumulation ratio of the parent compound is 1.2; that of cis-acitretin is 6.6.

Special Populations:

Psoriasis:

In an 8-week study of acitretin pharmacokinetics in patients with psoriasis, mean steady-state trough concentrations of acitretin increased in a dose proportional manner with dosages ranging from 10 to 50 mg daily. Acitretin plasma concentrations were nonmeasurable (<4 ng/mL) in all patients 3 weeks after cessation of therapy.

Elderly:

In a multiple-dose study in healthy young (n=6) and elderly (n=8) subjects, a two-fold increase in acitretin plasma concentrations were seen in elderly subjects, although the elimination half-life did not change.

Table 1. Summary of the Soriatane Efficacy Results of the 8- Week Double- Blind Phase of Studies A and B

Efficacy Variables	Study A		Study B		
	Total daily dose		Total daily dose		
	Placebo (N=29)	50 mg (N=29)	Placebo (N=72)	25 mg (N=74)	50 mg (N=71)
Physician's Global Evaluation					
Baseline	4.62	4.55	4.43	4.37	4.49
Mean Change After 8 Weeks	−0.29	−2.00*	−0.06	−1.06*	−1.57*
Scaling					
Baseline	4.10	3.76	3.97	4.11	4.10
Mean Change After 8 Weeks	−0.22	−1.62*	−0.21	−1.50*	−1.78*
Thickness					
Baseline	4.10	4.10	4.03	4.11	4.20
Mean Change After 8 Weeks	−0.39	−2.10*	−0.18	−1.43*	−2.11*
Erythema					
Baseline	4.21	4.59	4.42	4.24	4.45
Mean Change After 8 Weeks	−0.33	−2.10*	−0.37	−1.12*	−1.65*

* Values were statistically significantly different from placebo and from baseline ($p \leq 0.05$). No adjustment for multiplicity was done for Study B.
The efficacy variables consisted of: the mean severity rating of scale, lesion thickness, erythema, and the physician's global evaluation of the current status of the disease. Ratings of scaling, erythema, and lesion thickness, and the ratings of the global assessments were made using a seven-point scale (0=none, 1=trace, 2=mild, 3=mild-moderate, 4=moderate, 5=moderate-severe, 6=severe).

Renal Failure:
Plasma concentrations of acitretin were significantly (59.3%) lower in end-stage renal failure subjects (n=6) when compared to age-matched controls, following single 50 mg oral doses. Acitretin was not removed by hemodialysis in these subjects.

Pharmacokinetic Drug Interactions
(see also boxed CONTRAINDICATIONS AND WARNINGS and *PRECAUTIONS: Drug Interactions*): In studies of in vivo pharmacokinetic drug interactions, no interaction was seen between acitretin and cimetidine, digoxin, phenprocoumon or glyburide.

Ethanol:
Clinical evidence has shown that etretinate (a retinoid with a much longer half-life, see below) can be formed with concurrent ingestion of acitretin and ethanol. In a two-way crossover study, all 10 subjects formed etretinate with concurrent ingestion of a single 100 mg oral dose of acitretin during a 3-hour period of ethanol ingestion (total ethanol, approximately 1.4 g/kg body weight). A mean peak etretinate concentration of 59 ng/mL (range 22 to 105 ng/mL) was observed, and extrapolation of AUC values indicated that the formation of etretinate in this study was comparable to a single 5 mg oral dose of etretinate. There was no detectable formation of etretinate when a single 100 mg oral dose of acitretin was administered without concurrent ethanol ingestion, although the formation of etretinate without concurrent ethanol ingestion cannot be excluded (see boxed CONTRAINDICATIONS AND WARNINGS). Of 93 evaluable psoriatic patients on acitretin therapy in several foreign studies (10 to 80 mg/day), 16% had measurable etretinate levels (>5 ng/mL).
Etretinate has a much longer elimination half-life compared to that of acitretin. In one study the apparent mean terminal half-life after 6 months of therapy was approximately 120 days (range 84 to 168 days). In another study of 47 patients treated chronically with etretinate, 5 had detectable serum drug levels (in the range of 0.5 to 12 ng/mL) 2.1 to 2.9 years after therapy was discontinued. The long half-life appears to be due to storage of etretinate in adipose tissue.

Progestin-only Contraceptives:
It has not been established if there is a pharmacokinetic interaction between acitretin and combined oral contraceptives. However, it has been established that acitretin interferes with the contraceptive effect of microdosed progestin preparations.[1] Microdosed "minipill" progestin preparations are *not* recommended for use with Soriatane. *It is not known whether other progestational contraceptives, such as implants and injectables, are adequate methods of contraception during acitretin therapy.*

CLINICAL STUDIES

In two double-blind placebo controlled studies, Soriatane was administered once daily to patients with severe psoriasis (ie, covering at least 10% to 20% of the body surface area). At 8 weeks (see Table 1) patients treated in Study A with 50 mg Soriatane per day showed significant improvements ($p \leq 0.05$) relative to baseline and to placebo in the physician's global evaluation and in the mean ratings of severity of psoriasis (scaling, thickness, and erythema). In Study B, differences from baseline and from placebo were statistically significant ($p \leq 0.05$) for all variables at both the 25 mg and 50 mg doses; it should be noted for Study B that no statistical adjustment for multiplicity was carried out.
[See table 1 above]
A subset of 141 patients from both pivotal Studies A and B continued to receive Soriatane in an open fashion for up to 24 weeks. At the end of the treatment period, all efficacy variables, as indicated in Table 2, were significantly improved ($p \leq 0.01$) from baseline, including extent of psoriasis, mean ratings of psoriasis severity and physician's global evaluation.

Table 2. Summary of the First Course of Soriatane Therapy (24 Weeks)

Variables	Study A	Study B
Mean Total Daily Soriatane Dose (mg)	42.8	43.1
Mean Duration of Therapy (Weeks)	21.1	22.6
Physician's Global Evaluation	**N=39**	**N=98**
Baseline	4.51	4.43
Mean Change From Baseline	-2.26*	-2.60*
Scaling	**N=59**	**N=132**
Baseline	3.97	4.07
Mean Change From Baseline	−2.15*	−2.42*
Thickness	**N=59**	**N=132**
Baseline	4.00	4.12
Mean Change From Baseline	−2.44*	−2.66*
Erythema	**N=59**	**N=132**
Baseline	4.35	4.33
Mean Change From Baseline	−2.31*	−2.29*

* Indicates that the difference from baseline was statistically significant ($p \leq 0.01$).
The efficacy variables consisted of: the mean severity rating of scale, lesion thickness, erythema, and the physician's global evaluation of the current status of the disease. Ratings of scaling, erythema, and lesion thickness, and the ratings of the global assessments were made using a seven-point scale (0=none, 1=trace, 2=mild, 3=mild-moderate, 4=moderate, 5=moderate-severe, 6=severe).

All efficacy variables improved significantly in a subset of 55 patients from Study A treated for a second, 6-month maintenance course of therapy (for a total of 12 months of treatment); a small subset of patients (n=4) from Study A continued to improve after a third 6-month course of therapy (for a total of 18 months of treatment).

INDICATIONS AND USAGE

Soriatane is indicated for the treatment of severe psoriasis in adults. Because of significant adverse effects associated with its use, Soriatane should be prescribed only by those knowledgeable in the systemic use of retinoids. In females of reproductive potential, Soriatane should be reserved for non-pregnant patients who are unresponsive to other therapies or whose clinical condition contraindicates the use of other treatments (see boxed CONTRAINDICATIONS AND WARNINGS — Soriatane can cause severe birth defects).
Most patients experience relapse of psoriasis after discontinuing therapy. Subsequent courses, when clinically indicated, have produced efficacy results similar to the initial course of therapy.

CONTRAINDICATIONS

Pregnancy Category X
(see boxed CONTRAINDICATIONS AND WARNINGS).
Soriatane is contraindicated in patients with severely impaired liver or kidney function and in patients with chronic abnormally elevated blood lipid values (see boxed WARNINGS:*Hepatotoxicity*, WARNINGS:*Lipids and Possible Cardiovascular Effects*, and PRECAUTIONS).
An increased risk of hepatitis has been reported to result from combined use of methotrexate and etretinate. Consequently, the combination of methotrexate with Soriatane is also contraindicated (see PRECAUTIONS: *Drug Interactions*).
Since both Soriatane and tetracyclines can cause increased intracranial pressure, their combined use is contraindicated (see WARNINGS: *Pseudotumor Cerebri*).
Soriatane is contraindicated in cases of hypersensitivity to the preparation (acitretin or excipients) or to other retinoids.

WARNINGS

(see also boxed CONTRAINDICATIONS AND WARNINGS)

Hepatotoxicity: **Of the 525 patients treated in US clinical trials, 2 had clinical jaundice with elevated serum bilirubin and transaminases considered related to Soriatane treatment. Liver function test results in these patients returned to normal after Soriatane was discontinued. Two of the 1289 patients treated in European clinical trials developed biopsy-confirmed toxic hepatitis. A second biopsy in one of these patients revealed nodule formation suggestive of cirrhosis. One patient in a Canadian clinical trial of 63 patients developed a three-fold increase of transaminases. A liver biopsy of this patient showed mild lobular disarray, multifocal hepatocyte loss and mild triaditis of the portal tracts compatible with acute reversible hepatic injury. The patient's transaminase levels returned to normal 2 months after Soriatane was discontinued.**
The potential of Soriatane therapy to induce hepatotoxicity was prospectively evaluated using liver biopsies in an open-label study of 128 patients. Pretreatment and posttreatment biopsies were available for 87 patients. A comparison of liver biopsy findings before and after therapy revealed 49 (58%) patients showed no change, 21 (25%) improved and 14 (17%) patients had a worsening of their liver biopsy status. For 6 patients, the classification changed from class 0

(no pathology) to class I (normal fatty infiltration; nuclear variability and portal inflammation; both mild); for 7 patients, the change was from class I to class II (fatty infiltration, nuclear variability, portal inflammation and focal necrosis; all moderate to severe); and for 1 patient, the change was from class II to class IIIb (fibrosis, moderate to severe). No correlation could be found between liver function test result abnormalities and the change in liver biopsy status, and no cumulative dose relationship was found.

Elevations of AST (SGOT), ALT (SGPT), GGT (GGTP) or LDH have occurred in approximately 1 in 3 patients treated with Soriatane. Of the 525 patients treated in clinical trials in the US, treatment was discontinued in 20 (3.8%) due to elevated liver function test results. If hepatotoxicity is suspected during treatment with Soriatane, the drug should be discontinued and the etiology further investigated.

Ten of 652 patients treated in US clinical trials of etretinate, of which acitretin is the active metabolite, had clinical or histologic hepatitis considered to be possibly or probably related to etretinate treatment. There have been reports of hepatitis-related deaths worldwide; a few of these patients had received etretinate for a month or less before presenting with hepatic symptoms or signs.

Hyperostosis:

In adults receiving long-term treatment with Soriatane, appropriate examinations should be periodically performed in view of possible ossification abnormalities (see ADVERSE REACTIONS). Because the frequency and severity of iatrogenic bony abnormality in adults is low, periodic radiography is only warranted in the presence of symptoms or long-term use of Soriatane. If such disorders arise, the continuation of therapy should be discussed with the patient on the basis of a careful risk/benefit analysis. In clinical trials with Soriatane, patients were prospectively evaluated for evidence of development or change in bony abnormalities of the vertebral column, knees and ankles.

Vertebral Results:

Of 380 patients treated with Soriatane, 15% had preexisting abnormalities of the spine which showed new changes or progression of preexisting findings. Changes included degenerative spurs, anterior bridging of spinal vertebrae, diffuse idiopathic skeletal hyperostosis, ligament calcification and narrowing and destruction of a cervical disc space. De novo changes (formation of small spurs) were seen in 3 patients after 1½ to 2½ years.

Skeletal Appendicular Results:

Six of 128 patients treated with Soriatane showed abnormalities in the knees and ankles before treatment that progressed during treatment. In 5, these changes involved the formation of additional spurs or enlargement of existing spurs. The sixth patient had degenerative joint disease which worsened. No patients developed spurs de novo. Clinical complaints did not predict radiographic changes.

Lipids and Possible Cardiovascular Effects:

Blood lipid determinations should be performed before Soriatane is administered and again at intervals of 1 to 2 weeks until the lipid response to the drug is established, usually within 4 to 8 weeks. In patients receiving Soriatane during clinical trials, 66% and 33% experienced elevation in triglycerides and cholesterol, respectively. Decreased high density lipoproteins (HDL) occurred in 40% of patients. These effects of Soriatane were generally reversible upon cessation of therapy.

Patients with an increased tendency to develop hypertriglyceridemia included those with disturbances of lipid metabolism, diabetes mellitus, obesity, increased alcohol intake or a familial history of these conditions. Because of the risk of hypertriglyceridemia, serum lipids must be more closely monitored in high-risk patients and during long term treatment.

Hypertriglyceridemia and lowered HDL may increase a patient's cardiovascular risk status. Although no causal relationship has been established, there have been postmarketing reports of acute myocardial infarction or thromboembolic events in patients on Soriatane therapy. In addition, elevation of serum triglycerides to greater than 800 mg/dL has been associated with fatal fulminant pancreatitis. Therefore, dietary modifications, reduction in Soriatane dose, or drug therapy should be employed to control significant elevations of triglycerides. If, despite these measures, hypertriglyceridemia and low HDL levels persist, the discontinuation of Soriatane should be considered.

Ophthalmologic Effects:

The eyes and vision of 329 patients treated with Soriatane were examined by ophthalmologists. The findings included dry eyes (23%), irritation of eyes (9%) and brow and lash loss (5%). The following were reported in less than 5% of patients: Bell's Palsy, blepharitis and/or crusting of lids, blurred vision, conjunctivitis, corneal epithelial abnormality, cortical cataract, decreased night vision, diplopia, itchy eyes or eyelids, nuclear cataract, pannus, papilledema, photophobia, posterior subcapsular cataract, recurrent sties and subepithelial corneal lesions.

Any patient treated with Soriatane who is experiencing visual difficulties should discontinue the drug and undergo ophthalmologic evaluation.

Pancreatitis:

Lipid elevations occur in 25% to 50% of patients treated with Soriatane. Triglyceride increases sufficient to be associated with pancreatitis are much less common, although fatal fulminant pancreatitis has been reported. There have been rare reports of pancreatitis during Soriatane therapy in the absence of hypertriglyceridemia.

PseudotumorCerebri:

Soriatane and other retinoids administered orally have been associated with cases of pseudotumor cerebri (benign intracranial hypertension). Some of these events involved concomitant use of isotretinoin and tetracyclines. However, the event seen in a single Soriatane patient was not associated with tetracycline use. Early signs and symptoms include papilledema, headache, nausea and vomiting and visual disturbances. Patients with these signs and symptoms should be examined for papilledema and, if present, should discontinue Soriatane immediately and be referred for neurological evaluation and care. Since both Soriatane and tetracyclines can cause increased intracranial pressure, their combined use is contraindicated (see CONTRAINDICATIONS).

PRECAUTIONS

A description of the *Do Your P.A.R.T.* materials is provided below. The main goals of the materials are to explain the program requirements, to reinforce the educational messages, and to assess program effectiveness.

The *Do Your P.A.R.T.* booklet includes:

- The *Do Your P.A.R.T. Patient Brochure:* information on the program requirements, risks of acitretin, and the types of contraceptive methods
- The *Contraceptive Counseling Referral Form* for female patients who want to receive free contraception counseling reimbursed by the manufacturer
- *The Patient Agreement/Informed Consent Form* for female patients
- *Medication Guide*

The *Do Your P.A.R.T.* program also includes a voluntary patient survey for women of childbearing potential to assess the effectiveness of the Soriatane Pregnancy Prevention Program *Do Your P.A.R.T.*

Information for Patients

(see Medication Guide for all patients **and Patient Agreement/Informed Consent for Female Patients at end of professional labeling):**

Patients should be instructed to read the Medication Guide supplied as required by law when Soriatane is dispensed.

Females of reproductive potential:

Soriatane can cause severe birth defects. Female patients must not be pregnant when Soriatane therapy is initiated, they must not become pregnant while taking Soriatane, and for at least 3 years after stopping Soriatane, so that the drug can be eliminated to below a blood concentration that would be associated with an increased incidence of birth defects. Because this threshold has not been established for acitretin in humans and because elimination rates vary among patients, the duration of posttherapy contraception to achieve adequate elimination cannot be calculated precisely (see boxed **CONTRAINDICATIONS AND WARNINGS**).

Females of reproductive potential should also be advised that they must not ingest beverages or products containing ethanol while taking Soriatane and for 2 months after Soriatane treatment has been discontinued. This allows for elimination of the acitretin which can be converted to etretinate in the presence of alcohol.

Female patients should be advised that any method of birth control can fail, including tubal ligation, and that microdosed progestin "minipill" preparations are *not* recommended for use with Soriatane (see *CLINICAL PHARMACOLOGY: Pharmacokinetic Drug Interactions*). Data from one patient who received a very low-dosed progestin contraceptive (levonorgestrel 0.03 mg) had a significant increase of the progesterone level after three menstrual cycles during acitretin treatment.[2]

Female patients should sign a consent form prior to beginning Soriatane therapy (see boxed CONTRAINDICATIONS AND WARNINGS).

Nursing Mothers:

Studies on lactating rats have shown that etretinate is excreted in the milk. There is one prospective case report where acitretin is reported to be excreted in human milk. Therefore, nursing mothers should not receive Soriatane prior to or during nursing because of the potential for serious adverse reactions in nursing infants.

All Patients:

Depression and/or other psychiatric symptoms such as aggressive feelings or thoughts of self-harm have been reported. These events, including self-injurious behavior, have been reported in patients taking other systemically administered retinoids, as well as in patients taking Soriatane. Since other factors may have contributed to these events, it is not known if they are related to Soriatane. Patients should be counseled to stop taking Soriatane and notify their prescriber immediately if they experience psychiatric symptoms.

Patients should be advised that a transient worsening of psoriasis is sometimes seen during the initial treatment period. Patients should be advised that they may have to wait 2 to 3 months before they get the full benefit of Soriatane, although some patients may achieve significant improvements within the first 8 weeks of treatment as demonstrated in clinical trials.

Decreased night vision has been reported with Soriatane therapy. Patients should be advised of this potential problem and warned to be cautious when driving or operating any vehicle at night. Visual problems should be carefully monitored (see WARNINGS and ADVERSE REACTIONS). Patients should be advised that they may experience decreased tolerance to contact lenses during the treatment period and sometimes after treatment has stopped.

Patients should not donate blood during and for at least 3 years following therapy because Soriatane can cause birth defects and women of childbearing potential must not receive blood from patients being treated with Soriatane.

Because of the relationship of Soriatane to vitamin A, patients should be advised against taking vitamin A supplements in excess of minimum recommended daily allowances to avoid possible additive toxic effects.

Patients should avoid the use of sun lamps and excessive exposure to sunlight (non-medical UV exposure) because the effects of UV light are enhanced by retinoids.

Patients should be advised that they must not give their Soriatane to any other person.

For Prescribers:

Soriatane has not been studied in and is not indicated for treatment of acne.

Phototherapy:

Significantly lower doses of phototherapy are required when Soriatane is used because Soriatane-induced effects on the stratum corneum can increase the risk of erythema (burning) (see DOSAGE AND ADMINISTRATION).

Drug Interactions:

Ethanol:

Clinical evidence has shown that etretinate can be formed with concurrent ingestion of acitretin and ethanol (see boxed CONTRAINDICATIONS AND WARNINGS and CLINICAL PHARMACOLOGY: *Pharmacokinetics*).

Glibenclamide:

In a study of 7 healthy male volunteers, acitretin treatment potentiated the blood glucose lowering effect of glibenclamide (a sulfonylurea similar to chlorpropamide) in 3 of the 7 subjects. Repeating the study with 6 healthy male volunteers in the absence of glibenclamide did not detect an effect of acitretin on glucose tolerance. Careful supervision of diabetic patients under treatment with Soriatane is recommended (see CLINICAL PHARMACOLOGY: *Pharmacokinetics* and DOSAGE AND ADMINISTRATION).

Hormonal Contraceptives:

It has not been established if there is a pharmacokinetic interaction between acitretin and combined oral contraceptives. However, it has been established that acitretin interferes with the contraceptive effect of microdosed progestin "minipill" preparations. Microdosed "minipill" progestin preparations are not recommended for use with Soriatane (see CLINICAL PHARMACOLOGY: *Pharmacokinetic Drug Interactions*). *It is not known whether other progestational contraceptives, such as implants and injectables, are adequate methods of contraception during acitretin therapy.*

Methotrexate:

An increased risk of hepatitis has been reported to result from combined use of methotrexate and etretinate. Consequently, the combination of methotrexate with acitretin is also contraindicated (see CONTRAINDICATIONS).

Phenytoin:

If acitretin is given concurrently with phenytoin, the protein binding of phenytoin may be reduced.

Tetracyclines:

Since both acitretin and tetracyclines can cause increased intracranial pressure, their combined use is contraindicated (see *CONTRAINDICATIONS and WARNINGS: Pseudotumor Cerebri*).

Vitamin A and oral retinoids:

Concomitant administration of vitamin A and/or other oral retinoids with acitretin must be avoided because of the risk of hypervitaminosis A.

Table 3. Adverse Events Frequently Reported During Clinical Trials Percent of Patients Reporting (N=525)

BODY SYSTEM	> 75%	50% to 75%	25% to 50%	10% to 25%
CNS				Rigors
Eye Disorders				Xerophthalmia
Mucous Membranes	Cheilitis		Rhinitis	Dry mouth Epistaxis
Musculoskeletal				Arthralgia Spinal hyperostosis (progression of existing lesions)
Skin and Appendages		Alopecia Skin peeling	Dry skin Nail disorder Pruritus	Erythematous rash Hyperesthesia Paresthesia Paronychia Skin atrophy Sticky skin

Other:
There appears to be no pharmacokinetic interaction between acitretin and cimetidine, digoxin, or glyburide. Investigations into the effect of acitretin on the protein binding of anticoagulants of the coumarin type (warfarin) revealed no interaction.

Laboratory Tests:
If significant abnormal laboratory results are obtained, either dosage reduction with careful monitoring or treatment discontinuation is recommended, depending on clinical judgment.

Blood Sugar:
Some patients receiving retinoids have experienced problems with blood sugar control. In addition, new cases of diabetes have been diagnosed during retinoid therapy, including diabetic ketoacidosis. In diabetics, blood-sugar levels should be monitored very carefully.

Lipids:
In clinical studies, the incidence of hypertriglyceridemia was 66%, hypercholesterolemia was 33% and that of decreased HDL was 40%. Pretreatment and follow-up measurements should be obtained under fasting conditions. It is recommended that these tests be performed weekly or every other week until the lipid response to Soriatane has stabilized (see WARNINGS).

Liver Function Tests:
Elevations of AST (SGOT), ALT (SGPT) or LDH were experienced by approximately 1 in 3 patients treated with Soriatane. It is recommended that these tests be performed prior to initiation of Soriatane therapy, at 1- to 2-week intervals until stable and thereafter at intervals as clinically indicated (see CONTRAINDICATIONS and boxed WARNINGS).

Carcinogenesis, Mutagenesis, Impairment of Fertility:
Carcinogenesis:
A carcinogenesis study of acitretin in Wistar rats, at doses up to 2 mg/kg/day administered 7 days/week for 104 weeks, has been completed. There were no neoplastic lesions observed that were considered to have been related to treatment with acitretin. An 80-week carcinogenesis study in mice has been completed with etretinate, the ethyl ester of acitretin. Blood level data obtained during this study demonstrated that etretinate was metabolized to acitretin and that blood levels of acitretin exceeded those of etretinate at all times studied. In the etretinate study, an increased incidence of blood vessel tumors (hemangiomas and hemangiosarcomas at several different sites) was noted in male, but not female, mice at doses approximately one-half the maximum recommended human therapeutic dose based on a mg/m^2 comparison.

Mutagenesis:
Acitretin was evaluated for mutagenic potential in the Ames test, in the Chinese hamster (V79/HGPRT) assay, in unscheduled DNA synthesis assays using rat hepatocytes and human fibroblasts and in an in vivo mouse micronucleus assay. No evidence of mutagenicity of acitretin was demonstrated in any of these assays.

Impairment of Fertility:
In a fertility study in rats, the fertility of treated animals was not impaired at the highest dosage of acitretin tested, 3 mg/kg/day (approximately one-half the maximum recommended therapeutic dose based on a mg/m^2 comparison). Chronic toxicity studies in dogs revealed testicular changes (reversible mild to moderate spermatogenic arrest and appearance of multinucleated giant cells) in the highest dosage group (50 then 30 mg/kg/day).
No decreases in sperm count or concentration and no changes in sperm motility or morphology were noted in 31 men (17 psoriatic patients, 8 patients with disorders of keratinization and 6 healthy volunteers) given 30 to 50 mg/day of acitretin for at least 12 weeks. In these studies, no deleterious effects were seen on either testosterone production, LH or FSH in any of the 31 men.[4-6] No deleterious effects were seen on the hypothalamic-pituitary axis in any of the 18 men where it was measured.[4,5]

Pregnancy:
Teratogenic Effects:
Pregnancy Category X
(see boxed CONTRAINDICATIONS AND WARNINGS).
In a study in which acitretin was administered to male rats only at a dosage of 5 mg/kg/day for 10 weeks (approximate duration of one spermatogenic cycle) prior to and during mating with untreated female rats, no teratogenic effects were observed in the progeny (see boxed CONTRAINDICATIONS AND WARNINGS for information about male use of Soriatane).

Nonteratogenic Effects:
In rats dosed at 3 mg/kg/day (approximately one-half the maximum recommended therapeutic dose based on a mg/m^2 comparison), slightly decreased pup survival and delayed incisor eruption were noted. At the next lowest dose tested, 1 mg/kg/day, no treatment-related adverse effects were observed.

Pediatric Use:
Safety and effectiveness in pediatric patients have not been established. No clinical studies have been conducted in pediatric patients. Ossification of interosseous ligaments and tendons of the extremities, skeletal hyperostoses, decreases in bone mineral density, and premature epiphyseal closure have been reported in children taking other systemic retinoids, including etretinate, a metabolite of Soriatane. A causal relationship between these effects and Soriatane has not been established. While it is not known that these occurrences are more severe or more frequent in children, there is special concern in pediatric patients because of the implications for growth potential (see *WARNINGS: Hyperostosis*).

Geriatric Use:
Clinical studies of Soriatane did not include sufficient numbers of subjects aged 65 and over to determine whether they respond differently than younger subjects. Other reported clinical experience has not identified differences in responses between the elderly and younger patients. In general, dose selection for an elderly patient should be cautious, usually starting at the low end of the dosing range, reflecting the greater frequency of decreased hepatic, renal, or cardiac function, and of concomitant disease or other drug therapy. A twofold increase in acitretin plasma concentrations was seen in healthy elderly subjects compared with young subjects, although the elimination half-life did not change (see *CLINICAL PHARMACOLOGY: Special Populations*).

ADVERSE REACTIONS

Hypervitaminosis A produces a wide spectrum of signs and symptoms primarily of the mucocutaneous, musculoskeletal, hepatic, neuropsychiatric, and central nervous systems. Many of the clinical adverse reactions reported to date with Soriatane administration resemble those of the hypervitaminosis A syndrome.

Adverse Events/Postmarketing Reports:
In addition to the events listed in the tables for the clinical trials, the following adverse events have been identified during postapproval use of Soriatane. Because these events are reported voluntarily from a population of uncertain size, it is not always possible to reliably estimate their frequency or establish a causal relationship to drug exposure.

Cardiovascular:
Acute myocardial infarction, thromboembolism (see WARNINGS), stroke

Nervous System:
Myopathy with peripheral neuropathy has been reported during Soriatane therapy. Both conditions improved with discontinuation of the drug.

Psychiatric:
Aggressive feelings and/or suicidal thoughts have been reported. These events, including self-injurious behavior, have been reported in patients taking other systemically administered retinoids, as well as in patients taking Soriatane. Since other factors may have contributed to these events, it is not known if they are related to Soriatane (see PRECAUTIONS).

Reproductive:
Vulvo-vaginitis due to Candida albicans

Skin and Appendages:
Thinning of the skin, skin fragility and scaling may occur all over the body, particularly on the palms and soles; nail fragility is frequently observed.

Clinical Trials:
During clinical trials with Soriatane, 513/525 (98%) of patients reported a total of 3545 adverse events. One-hundred sixteen patients (22%) left studies prematurely, primarily because of adverse experiences involving the mucous membranes and skin. Three patients died. Two of the deaths were not drug related (pancreatic adenocarcinoma and lung cancer); the other patient died of an acute myocardial infarction, considered remotely related to drug therapy. In clinical trials, Soriatane was associated with elevations in liver function test results or triglyceride levels and hepatitis.
The tables below list by body system and frequency the adverse events reported during clinical trials of 525 patients with psoriasis.
[See table 3 above]
[See table 4 at top of next page]

Laboratory:
Soriatane therapy induces changes in liver function tests in a significant number of patients. Elevations of AST (SGOT), ALT (SGPT) or LDH were experienced by approximately 1 in 3 patients treated with Soriatane. In most patients, elevations were slight to moderate and returned to normal either during continuation of therapy or after cessation of treatment. In patients receiving Soriatane during clinical trials, 66% and 33% experienced elevation in triglycerides and cholesterol, respectively. Decreased high density lipoproteins (HDL) occurred in 40% (see WARNINGS). Transient, usually reversible elevations of alkaline phosphatase have been observed.
Table 5 lists the laboratory abnormalities reported during clinical trials.
[See table 5 at top of page 2302]

OVERDOSAGE

In the event of acute overdosage, Soriatane must be withdrawn at once. Symptoms of overdose are identical to acute hypervitaminosis A, ie, headache and vertigo. The acute oral toxicity (LD_{50}) of acitretin in both mice and rats was greater than 4000 mg/kg.
In one reported case of overdose, a 32-year-old male with Darier's disease took 21 × 25 mg capsules (525 mg single dose). He vomited several hours later but experienced no other ill effects.
All female patients of childbearing potential who have taken an overdose of Soriatane must:
1) Have a pregnancy test at the time of overdose; 2) Be counseled as per the boxed CONTRAINDICATIONS AND WARNINGS and PRECAUTIONS sections regarding birth defects and contraceptive use for at least 3 years' duration after the overdose.

DOSAGE AND ADMINISTRATION

There is intersubject variation in the pharmacokinetics, clinical efficacy and incidence of side effects with Soriatane. A number of the more common side effects are dose related. Individualization of dosage is required to achieve sufficient therapeutic response while minimizing side effects. Soriatane therapy should be initiated at 25 to 50 mg per day, given as a single dose with the main meal. Maintenance doses of 25 to 50 mg per day may be given dependent upon an individual patient's response to initial treatment. Relapses may be treated as outlined for initial therapy.
When Soriatane is used with phototherapy, the prescriber should decrease the phototherapy dose, dependent on the patient's individual response (see *PRECAUTIONS: General*).
Females who have taken Tegison (etretinate) must continue to follow the contraceptive recommendations for Tegison. Tegison is no longer marketed in the US; for information, call Stiefel at 1-888-784-3335 (STIEFEL).

Information for Pharmacists:
A Soriatane Medication Guide must be given to the patient each time Soriatane is dispensed, as required by law.

HOW SUPPLIED

Brown and white capsules, 10 mg, imprinted "A-10 mg"; bottles of 30 (NDC 0145-0090-25).
Rich yellow capsules, 17.5 mg, imprinted "A-17.5 mg"; bottles of 30 (NDC 0145-3817-03).

Brown capsules, 22.5 mg, imprinted "A-22.5 mg"; bottles of 30 (NDC 0145-3821-03).
Brown and yellow capsules, 25 mg, imprinted "A-25 mg"; bottles of 30 (NDC 0145-0091-25).
Store between 15° and 25°C (59° and 77°F). Protect from light. Avoid exposure to high temperatures and humidity after the bottle is opened.

REFERENCES

1. Berbis Ph, et al.: *Arch Dermatol Res* (1988) 280:388-389. **2.** Maier H, Honigsmann H: Concentration of etretinate in plasma and subcutaneous fat after long-term acitretin. *Lancet* 348:1107, 1996. **3.** Geiger JM, Walker M: Is there a reproductive safety risk in male patients treated with acitretin (Neotigason®/Soriatane®)? *Dermatology* 205:105-107, 2002. **4.** Sigg C, et al.: Andrological investigations in patients treated with etretin. *Dermatologica* 175:48-49, 1987. **5.** Parsch EM, et al.: Andrological investigation in men treated with acitretin (Ro 10-1670). *Andrologia* 22:479-482, 1990. **6.** Kadar L, et al.: Spermatological investigations in psoriatic patients treated with acitretin. In: Pharmacology of Retinoids in the Skin; Reichert U. et al., ed, KARGER, Basel, vol. 3, pp 253-254, 1988.

PATIENT AGREEMENT/INFORMED CONSENT FOR FEMALE PATIENTS

To be completed by the patient* and signed by her prescriber

CAUSES BIRTH DEFECTS

DO NOT GET PREGNANT

*Must also be initialed by the parent or guardian of a minor patient (under age 18)
Read each item below and initial in the space provided to show that you understand each item. **Do not sign this consent and do not take SORIATANE® (acitretin) if there is anything that you do not understand.**

____
(Patient's name)

1. I understand that there is a very high risk that my unborn baby could have severe birth defects if I am pregnant or become pregnant while taking SORIATANE in any amount even for short periods of time. Birth defects have also happened in babies of women who became pregnant after stopping SORIATANE treatment.
INITIAL: ________

2. I understand that I must not become pregnant while taking SORIATANE and for at least 3 years after the end of my treatment with SORIATANE.
INITIAL: ________

3. I know that I must avoid all alcohol, including drinks, food, medicines, and over-the-counter products that contain alcohol. I understand that the risk of birth defects may last longer than 3 years if I swallow any form of alcohol during SORIATANE therapy, and for 2 months after I stop taking SORIATANE.
INITIAL: ________

4. I understand that I must not have sexual intercourse, or I must use 2 separate, effective forms of birth control **at the same time.** The only exceptions are if I have had surgery to remove the womb (a hysterectomy) or my prescriber has told me I have gone completely through menopause.
INITIAL: ________

5. I understand that I have to use 2 effective forms of birth control (contraception) at the same time for at least 1 month before starting SORIATANE, for the entire time of SORIATANE therapy, and for at least 3 years after SORIATANE treatment has stopped.
INITIAL: ________

6. I understand that any form of birth control can fail. Therefore, I must use 2 different methods at the same time, every time I have sexual intercourse.
INITIAL: ________

7. I understand that the following are considered effective forms of birth control: Primary: Tubal ligation (having my tubes tied), partner's vasectomy, birth control pills, injectable/implantable/insertable/topical (patch) hormonal birth control products, and IUDs (intrauterine devices). Secondary: Latex condoms (with or without spermicide, which is a special cream or jelly that kills sperm), diaphragms and cervical caps (which must be used with a spermicide). I understand that at least 1 of my 2 methods of birth control must be a primary method.
INITIAL: ________

Table 4. Adverse Events Less Frequently Reported During Clinical Trials (Some of Which May Bear No Relationship to Therapy) Percent of Patients Reporting (N=525)

BODY SYSTEM	1% to 10%		< 1%	
Body as a Whole	Anorexia Edema Fatigue Hot flashes Increased appetite		Alcohol intolerance Dizziness Fever Influenza-like symptoms	Malaise Moniliasis Muscle weakness Weight increase
Cardiovascular	Flushing		Chest pain Cyanosis Increased bleeding time	Intermittent claudication Peripheral ischemia
CNS (also see Psychiatric)	Headache Pain		Abnormal gait Migraine Neuritis	Pseudotumor cerebri (intracranial hypertension)
Eye Disorders	Abnormal/ blurred vision Blepharitis Conjunctivitis/ irritation Corneal epithelial abnormality	Decreased night vision/night blindness Eye abnormality Eye pain Photophobia	Abnormal lacrimation Chalazion Conjunctival hemorrhage Corneal ulceration Diplopia Ectropion	Itchy eyes and lids Papilledema Recurrent sties Subepithelial corneal lesions
Gastrointestinal	Abdominal pain Diarrhea Nausea Tongue disorder		Constipation Dyspepsia Esophagitis Gastritis Gastroenteritis	Glossitis Hemorrhoids Melena Tenesmus Tongue ulceration
Liver and Biliary			Hepatic function abnormal Hepatitis Jaundice	
Mucous Membranes	Gingival bleeding Gingivitis Increased saliva	Stomatitis Thirst Ulcerative stomatitis	Altered saliva Anal disorder Gum hyperplasia	Hemorrhage Pharyngitis
Musculoskeletal	Arthritis Arthrosis Back pain Hypertonia Myalgia	Osteodynia Peripheral joint hyperostosis (progression of existing lesions)	Bone disorder Olecranon bursitis Spinal hyperostosis (new lesions) Tendonitis	
Psychiatric	Depression Insomnia Somnolence		Anxiety Dysphonia Libido decreased Nervousness	
Reproductive			Atrophic vaginitis Leukorrhea	
Respiratory	Sinusitis		Coughing Increased sputum Laryngitis	
Skin and Appendages	Abnormal skin odor Abnormal hair texture Bullous eruption Cold/clammy skin Dermatitis Increased sweating Infection	Psoriasiform rash Purpura Pyogenic granuloma Rash Seborrhea Skin fissures Skin ulceration Sunburn	Acne Breast pain Cyst Eczema Fungal infection Furunculosis Hair discoloration Herpes simplex Hyperkeratosis Hypertrichosis Hypoesthesia Impaired healing Otitis media	Otitis externa Photosensitivity reaction Psoriasis aggravated Scleroderma Skin nodule Skin hypertrophy Skin disorder Skin irritation Sweat gland disorder Urticaria Verrucae
Special Senses/ Other	Earache Taste perversion Tinnitus		Ceruminosis Deafness Taste loss	
Urinary			Abnormal urine Dysuria Penis disorder	

8. I will talk with my prescriber about any medicines or dietary supplements I plan to take during my SORIATANE treatment because certain birth control methods may not work if I am taking certain medicines or herbal products (for example, Saint John's wort).
INITIAL: ________

9. Unless I have had a hysterectomy or my prescriber says I have gone completely through menopause, I understand that I must have 2 negative pregnancy test results before I can get a prescription to start SORIATANE. I will then have pregnancy tests on a monthly basis during my SORIATANE therapy as instructed by my prescriber. In addition, for at

Table 5. Abnormal Laboratory Test Results Reported During Clinical Trials Percent of Patients Reporting

BODY SYSTEM	50% to 75%	25% to 50%	10% to 25%	1% to 10%
Electrolytes			Increased: –Phosphorus –Potassium –Sodium Increased and decreased: –Magnesium	Decreased: –Phosphorus –Potassium –Sodium Increased and decreased: –Calcium –Chloride
Hematologic		Increased: –Reticulocytes	Decreased: –Hematocrit –Hemoglobin –WBC Increased: –Haptoglobin –Neutrophils –WBC	Increased: –Bands –Basophils –Eosinophils –Hematocrit –Hemoglobin –Lymphocytes –Monocytes Decreased: –Haptoglobin –Lymphocytes –Neutrophils –Reticulocytes Increased or decreased: –Platelets –RBC
Hepatic		Increased: –Cholesterol –LDH –SGOT –SGPT Decreased: –HDL cholesterol	Increased: –Alkaline phosphatase –Direct bilirubin –GGTP	Increased: –Globulin –Total bilirubin –Total protein Increased and decreased: –Serum albumin
Miscellaneous	Increased: –Triglycerides	Increased: –CPK –Fasting blood sugar	Decreased: –Fasting blood sugar –High occult blood	Increased and decreased: –Iron
Renal			Increased: –Uric acid	Increased: –BUN –Creatinine
Urinary		WBC in urine	Acetonuria Hematuria RBC in urine	Glycosuria Proteinuria

least 3 years after the end of my treatment with SORIATANE, I will have a pregnancy test every 3 months.
INITIAL: __________

10. I understand that I should not start taking SORIATANE until I am *sure* that I am not pregnant and have negative results from 2 pregnancy tests.
INITIAL: __________

11. I have received information on emergency contraception (birth control).
INITIAL: __________

12. I understand that my prescriber can give me a referral for a free contraceptive (birth control) counseling session and pregnancy testing.
INITIAL: __________

13. I understand that on a monthly basis during SORIATANE therapy and every 3 months for at least 3 years after stopping SORIATANE treatment that I should receive counseling from my prescriber about contraception (birth control) and behaviors associated with an increased risk of pregnancy.
INITIAL: __________

14. I understand that I must stop taking SORIATANE right away and call my prescriber if I get pregnant, miss my menstrual period, stop using birth control, or have sexual intercourse without using my 2 birth control methods during and at least 3 years after stopping SORIATANE treatment.
INITIAL: __________

15. If I do become pregnant while on SORIATANE or at any time within 3 years of stopping SORIATANE, I understand that I should report my pregnancy to Stiefel at 1-888-784-3335 (STIEFEL) or to the Food and Drug Administration (FDA) MedWatch program at 1-800-FDA-1088. The information I share will be kept confidential (private) and will help the company and the FDA evaluate the pregnancy prevention program to prevent birth defects.
INITIAL: __________

I have received a copy of the Do Your P.A.R.T™ brochure. My prescriber has answered all my questions about SORIATANE. I understand that it is my responsibility to follow my doctor's instructions, and not to get pregnant during SORIATANE treatment or for at least 3 years after I stop taking SORIATANE.

I now authorize my prescriber, ______________, to begin my treatment with SORIATANE.
Patient signature: ______________________
Date: __________
Parent/guardian signature (if under age 18): __________
Date: __________
Please print: Patient name and address:
____
____
Telephone: ______________________
I have fully explained to the patient, ____________, the nature and purpose of the treatment described above and the risks to females of childbearing potential. I have asked the patient if she has any questions regarding her treatment with SORIATANE and have answered those questions to the best of my ability.
Prescriber signature: ______________________
Date: __________
March 2011
SRN:1PI

MEDICATION GUIDE FOR PATIENTS

SORIATANE®
[sor-RYE-uh-tane]
(acitretin)
CAPSULES

Read this Medication Guide carefully before you start taking Soriatane and read it each time you get more Soriatane. There may be new information.

The first information in this Guide is about birth defects and how to avoid pregnancy. **After this section there is important safety information about possible effects for any patient taking Soriatane.** ALL patients should read this entire Medication Guide carefully.

This information does not take the place of talking with your prescriber about your medical condition or treatment.

What is the most important information I should know about Soriatane?

Soriatane can cause severe birth defects. If you are a female who can get pregnant, you should use Soriatane only if you are not pregnant now, can avoid becoming pregnant for at least 3 years, and other medicines do not work for your severe psoriasis or you cannot use other psoriasis medicines. Information about effects on unborn babies and about how to avoid pregnancy is found in the next section: "What are the important warnings and instructions for females taking Soriatane?".

CAUSES BIRTH DEFECTS

DO NOT GET PREGNANT

What are the important warnings and instructions for females taking Soriatane?

- **Before you receive your Soriatane prescription, you should have discussed and signed a Patient Information/Consent form with your prescriber. This is to help make sure you understand the risk of birth defects and how to avoid getting pregnant. If you did not talk to your prescriber about this and sign the form, contact your prescriber.**
- **You must not take Soriatane if you are pregnant or might become pregnant during treatment or at any time for at least 3 years after you stop treatment because Soriatane can cause severe birth defects.**
- **During Soriatane treatment and for 2 months after you stop Soriatane treatment, you must avoid drinks, foods, and all medicines that contain alcohol. This includes over-the-counter products that contain alcohol.** Avoiding alcohol is very important, because alcohol changes Soriatane into a drug that may take longer than 3 years to leave your body. The chance of birth defects may last longer than 3 years if you swallow any form of alcohol during Soriatane therapy and for 2 months after you stop taking Soriatane.
- **You and your prescriber must be sure you are not pregnant before you start Soriatane therapy. You must have negative results from 2 pregnancy tests before you start Soriatane treatment.** A negative result shows you are not pregnant. Because it takes a few days after pregnancy begins for a test to show that you are pregnant, the first negative test may not ensure you are not pregnant. Do not start Soriatane until you have negative results from 2 pregnancy tests.
  - The **first pregnancy test** will be done at the time you and your prescriber decide if Soriatane might be right for you.
  - The **second pregnancy test** will usually be done during the first 5 days of your menstrual period, right before you plan to start Soriatane. Your prescriber may suggest another time.
- After you start Soriatane therapy, you must have a pregnancy test repeated each month that you are taking Soriatane. This is to be sure that you are not pregnant during treatment because Soriatane can cause birth defects.
- For at least 3 years after stopping Soriatane treatment, you must have a pregnancy test repeated every three months to make sure that you are not pregnant.
- **Discuss effective birth control (contraception) with your prescriber. You must use 2 effective forms of birth control (contraception) at the same time during all of the following:**
  - for at least 1 month before beginning Soriatane treatment
  - during treatment with Soriatane
  - for at least 3 years after stopping Soriatane treatment
- **If you are sexually active, you must use 2 effective forms of birth control (contraception) at the same time even if you think you cannot become pregnant, unless 1 of the following is true for you:**
  - You had your womb (uterus) removed during an operation (a hysterectomy).
  - Your prescriber said you have gone completely through menopause (the "change of life").
- **You can get a free birth control counseling session and pregnancy testing from a prescriber or family planning expert. Your prescriber can give you a Soriatane Patient Referral Form for this free session.**
- **You must use 2 effective forms of birth control (contraception) at the same time while you are on Soriatane treatment. You must use birth control for at least 1 month before you start Soriatane, during treatment, and at least 3 years after you stop Soriatane treatment.**

The following are considered effective forms of birth control:

Primary Forms:
- having your tubes tied (tubal ligation)
- partner's vasectomy
- IUD (intrauterine device)
- birth control pills that contain both estrogen and progestin (combination oral contraceptives)
- hormonal birth control products that are injected, implanted, or inserted in your body
- birth control patch

Secondary Forms (use with a Primary Form):
- diaphragms with spermicide
- latex condoms (with or without spermicide)
- cervical caps with spermicide

At least 1 of your 2 methods of birth control must be a primary form.

- **If you have sex at any time without using 2 effective forms of birth control (contraception) at the same time, or if you get pregnant or miss your period, stop using Soriatane and call your prescriber right away.**
- **Consider "Emergency Contraception" (EC) if you have sex with a male without correctly using 2 effective forms of birth control (contraception) at the same time.** EC is also called "emergency birth control" or the "morning after" pill. Contact your prescriber **as soon as possible** if you have sex without using 2 effective forms of birth control (contraception) at the same time, because EC works best if it is used within 1 or 2 days after sex. EC is not a replacement for your usual 2 effective forms of birth control (contraception) because it is not as effective as regular birth control methods.
  You can get EC from private doctors or nurse practitioners, women's health centers, or hospital emergency rooms. You can get the name and phone number of EC providers nearest you by calling the free Emergency Contraception Hotline at 1-888-NOT-2-LATE (1-888-668-2528).
- **Stop taking Soriatane right away and contact your prescriber if you get pregnant while taking Soriatane or at any time for at least 3 years after treatment has stopped. You need to discuss the possible effects on the unborn baby with your prescriber.**
- **If you do become pregnant while taking Soriatane or at any time for at least 3 years after stopping Soriatane, you should report your pregnancy to Stiefel Laboratories, Inc. at 1-888-784-3335 (STIEEL) or directly to the Food and Drug Administration (FDA) MedWatch program (1-800-FDA-1088).** Your name will be kept in private (confidential). The information you share will help the FDA and the manufacturer evaluate the Pregnancy Prevention Program for Soriatane.
- **Do not take Soriatane if you are breast feeding.** Soriatane can pass into your milk and may harm your baby. You will need to choose either to breast feed or take Soriatane, but not both.

What should males know before taking Soriatane?

Small amounts of Soriatane are found in the semen of males taking Soriatane. Based upon available information, it appears that these small amounts of Soriatane in semen pose little, if any, risk to an unborn child while a male patient is taking the drug or after it is discontinued. Discuss any concerns you have about this with your prescriber.

All patients should read the rest of this Medication Guide.

What is Soriatane?

Soriatane is a medicine used to treat severe forms of psoriasis in adults. Psoriasis is a skin disease that causes cells in the outer layer of the skin to grow faster than normal and pile up on the skin's surface. In the most common type of psoriasis, the skin becomes inflamed and produces red, thickened areas, often with silvery scales. **Because Soriatane can have serious side effects,** you should talk with your prescriber about whether Soriatane's possible benefits outweigh its possible risks.

Soriatane may not work right away. You may have to wait 2 to 3 months before you get the full benefit of Soriatane. Psoriasis gets worse for some patients when they first start Soriatane treatment.

Soriatane has not been studied in children.

Who should not take Soriatane?

- **Do NOT take Soriatane if you can get pregnant.** Do not take Soriatane if you are pregnant or might get pregnant during Soriatane treatment or at any time for **at least 3 years** after you stop Soriatane treatment (see "What are the important warnings and instructions for females taking Soriatane?").
- **Do NOT take Soriatane if you are breast feeding.** Soriatane can pass into your milk and may harm your baby. You will need to choose either to breast feed or take Soriatane, but not both.
- **Do NOT take Soriatane if you have severe liver or kidney disease.**
- **Do NOT take Soriatane if you have repeated high blood lipids** (fat in the blood).
- **Do NOT take Soriatane if you take these medicines:**
  - methotrexate
  - tetracyclines

  The use of these medicines with Soriatane may cause serious side effects.
- **Do NOT take Soriatane if you are allergic to acitretin,** the active ingredient in Soriatane, to any of the other ingredients in Soriatane (see the end of this Medication Guide for a list of all the ingredients in Soriatane), or to any similar drugs (ask your prescriber or pharmacist whether any drugs you are allergic to are related to Soriatane).

Tell your prescriber if you have or ever had:
- diabetes or high blood sugar
- liver problems
- kidney problems
- high cholesterol or high triglycerides (fat in the blood)
- heart disease
- depression
- alcoholism
- an allergic reaction to a medication

Your prescriber needs this information to decide if Soriatane is right for you and to know what dose is best for you.

Tell your prescriber about all the medicines you take, including prescription and non-prescription medicines, vitamins, and herbal supplements. Some medicines can cause serious side effects if taken while you also take Soriatane. Some medicines may affect how Soriatane works, or Soriatane may affect how your other medicines work. **Be especially sure to tell your prescriber if you are taking the following medicines:**
- methotrexate
- tetracyclines
- phenytoin
- vitamin A supplements
- progestin-only oral contraceptives ("minipills")
- Tegison® or Tigason (etretinate). Tell your prescriber if you have ever taken this medicine in the past.
- St. John's Wort herbal supplement

Tell your prescriber if you are getting phototherapy treatment. Your doses of phototherapy may need to be changed to prevent a burn.

How should I take Soriatane?
- Take Soriatane with food.
- Be sure to take your medicine as prescribed by your prescriber. The dose of Soriatane varies from patient to patient. The number of capsules you must take is chosen specially for you by your prescriber. This dose may change during treatment.
- If you miss a dose, do not double the next dose. Skip the missed dose and resume your normal schedule.
- If you take too much Soriatane (overdose), call your local poison control center or emergency room.

You should have blood tests for liver function, cholesterol and triglycerides before starting treatment and during treatment to check your body's response to Soriatane. Your prescriber may also do other tests.

Once you stop taking Soriatane, your psoriasis may return. Do *not* treat this new psoriasis with leftover Soriatane. It is important to see your prescriber again for treatment recommendations because your situation may have changed.

What should I avoid while taking Soriatane?
- **Avoid pregnancy.** See "What is the most important information I should know about Soriatane?", and "What are the important warnings and instructions for females taking Soriatane?".
- **Avoid breast feeding.** See "What are the important warnings and instructions for females taking Soriatane?".
- **Avoid alcohol.** Females must avoid drinks, foods, medicines, and over-the-counter products that contain alcohol. The risk of birth defects may continue for longer than 3 years if you swallow any form of alcohol during Soriatane treatment and for 2 months after stopping Soriatane (see "What are the important warnings and instructions for females taking Soriatane?").
- **Avoid giving blood. Do not donate blood** while you are taking Soriatane and **for at least 3 years after stopping** Soriatane treatment. Soriatane in your blood can harm an unborn baby if your blood is given to a pregnant woman. Soriatane does not affect your ability to receive a blood transfusion.
- **Avoid progestin-only birth control pills ("minipills").** This type of birth control pill may not work while you take Soriatane. Ask your prescriber if you are not sure what type of pills you are using.
- **Avoid night driving if you develop any sudden vision problems.** Stop taking Soriatane and call your prescriber if this occurs (see "Serious side effects").
- **Avoid non-medical ultraviolet (UV) light.** Soriatane can make your skin more sensitive to UV light. Do not use sunlamps, and avoid sunlight as much as possible. If you are taking light treatment (phototherapy), your prescriber may need to change your light dosages to avoid burns.
- **Avoid dietary supplements containing vitamin A.** Soriatane is related to vitamin A. Therefore, do not take supplements containing vitamin A, because they may add to the unwanted effects of Soriatane. Check with your prescriber or pharmacist if you have any questions about vitamin supplements.
- **DO NOT SHARE Soriatane with anyone else, even if they have the same symptoms.** Your medicine may harm them or their unborn child.

What are the possible side effects of Soriatane?
- **Soriatane can cause birth defects.** See "What is the most important information I should know about Soriatane?" and "What are the important warnings and instructions for females taking Soriatane?"
- Psoriasis gets worse for some patients when they first start Soriatane treatment. Some patients have more redness or itching. If this happens, tell your prescriber. These symptoms usually get better as treatment continues, but your prescriber may need to change the amount of your medicine.

Serious side effects.

These do not happen often, but they can lead to permanent harm, or rarely, to death. Stop taking Soriatane and call your prescriber right away if you get the following signs or symptoms:
- **Bad headaches, nausea, vomiting, blurred vision.** These symptoms can be signs of increased brain pressure that can lead to blindness or even death.
- **Decreased vision in the dark** (night blindness). Since this can start suddenly, you should be very careful when driving at night. This problem usually goes away when Soriatane treatment stops. If you develop any vision problems or eye pain stop taking Soriatane and call your prescriber.
- **Depression.** There have been some reports of patients developing mental problems including a depressed mood, aggressive feelings, or thoughts of ending their own life (suicide). These events, including suicidal behavior, have been reported in patients taking other drugs similar to Soriatane as well as patients taking Soriatane. Since other things may have contributed to these problems, it is not known if they are related to Soriatane. It is very important to stop taking Soriatane and call your prescriber right away if you develop such problems.
- **Yellowing of your skin or the whites of your eyes, nausea and vomiting, loss of appetite, or dark urine.** These can be signs of serious liver damage.
- **Aches or pains in your bones, joints, muscles, or back; trouble moving; loss of feeling in your hands or feet.** These can be signs of abnormal changes to your bones or muscles.
- **Frequent urination, great thirst or hunger.** Soriatane can affect blood sugar control, even if you do not already have diabetes. These are some of the signs of high blood sugar
- **Shortness of breath, dizziness, nausea, chest pain, weakness, trouble speaking, or swelling of a leg. These may be signs of a heart attack, blood clots, or stroke.** Soriatane can cause serious changes in blood fats (lipids). It is possible for these changes to cause blood vessel blockages that lead to heart attacks, strokes, or blood clots.

Common side effects

If you develop any of these side effects or any unusual reaction, check with your prescriber to find out if you need to change the amount of Soriatane you take. These side effects usually get better if the Soriatane dose is reduced or Soriatane is stopped.
- **Chapped lips; peeling fingertips, palms, and soles; itching; scaly skin all over; weak nails; sticky or fragile (weak) skin; runny or dry nose, or nosebleeds.** Your prescriber or pharmacist can recommend a lotion or cream to help treat drying or chapping.
- **Dry mouth**
- **Joint pain**
- **Tight muscles**
- **Hair loss.** Most patients have some hair loss, but this condition varies among patients. No one can tell if you will lose hair, how much hair you may lose or if and when it may grow back.
- **Dry eyes.** Soriatane may dry your eyes. Wearing **contact lenses** may be uncomfortable during and after treatment with Soriatane because of the dry feeling in your eyes. If this happens, remove your contact lenses and call your prescriber. Also read the section about vision under "Serious side effects".
- **Rise in blood fats (lipids).** Soriatane can cause your blood fats (lipids) to rise. Most of the time this is not serious. But sometimes the increase can become a serious problem (see information under "Serious side effects"). You should have blood tests as directed by your prescriber.

These are not all the possible side effects of Soriatane. For more information, ask your prescriber or pharmacist.

How should I store Soriatane?

Keep Soriatane away from sunlight, high temperature, and humidity. **Keep Soriatane away from children.**

What are the ingredients in Soriatane?

Active ingredient: acitretin

Inactive ingredients: microcrystalline cellulose, sodium ascorbate, gelatin, black monogramming ink and maltodextrin (a mixture of polysaccharides). Gelatin capsule shells contain gelatin, iron oxide (yellow, black, and red), and titanium dioxide. They may also contain benzyl alcohol, carboxymethylcellulose sodium, edetate calcium disodium.

General information about the safe and effective use of Soriatane

Medicines are sometimes prescribed for purposes other than those listed in a Medication Guide. Do not use Soriatane for a condition for which it was not prescribed. Do not give Soriatane to other people, even if they have the same symptoms that you have.

This Medication Guide summarizes the most important information about Soriatane. If you would like more information, talk with your prescriber. You can ask your pharmacist or prescriber for information about Soriatane that is written for health professionals.

This Medication Guide has been approved by the U.S. Food and Drug Administration.

Tegison® is a registered trademark of Hoffmann-La Roche Inc.

Do Your P.A.R.T. is a trademark and SORIATANE is a registered trademark of Stiefel Laboratories, Inc.

STIEFEL®
Manufactured for
Stiefel Laboratories, Inc.
Research Triangle Park, NC 27709
March 2011
SRN:1MG

Shown in Product Identification Guide, page 313

SORILUX™ ℞

[SOR-i-lux]
(calcipotriene)
Foam, 0.005%
For topical use

HIGHLIGHTS OF PRESCRIBING INFORMATION

These highlights do not include all the information needed to use SORILUX safely and effectively. See full prescribing information for SORILUX.

SORILUX™ (calcipotriene) foam, 0.005%, for topical use
Initial U.S. Approval: 1993

RECENT MAJOR CHANGES

Indications and Usage, plaque psoriasis of the scalp (1) 9/2012

INDICATIONS AND USAGE

SORILUX Foam is a vitamin D analog indicated for the topical treatment of plaque psoriasis of the scalp and body in patients 18 years and older. (1)

DOSAGE AND ADMINISTRATION

- For topical use only; not for oral, ophthalmic, or intravaginal use. (2)
- Apply twice daily. (2)

DOSAGE FORMS AND STRENGTHS

0.005%, foam. (3)

CONTRAINDICATIONS

Do not use in patients with known hypercalcemia. (4)

WARNINGS AND PRECAUTIONS

- Contents are flammable. Instruct the patient to avoid fire, flame, and smoking during and immediately following application. (5.1)
- If elevation of serum calcium occurs, instruct patients to discontinue treatment until normal calcium levels are restored. (5.2)
- Avoid excessive exposure of the treated areas to natural or artificial sunlight. (5.3)

ADVERSE REACTIONS

Adverse reactions reported in ≥1% of subjects treated with SORILUX Foam and at a higher incidence than subjects treated with vehicle were application site erythema and application site pain. (6.1)

To report SUSPECTED ADVERSE REACTIONS, contact Stiefel Laboratories, Inc. at 1-888-784-3335 (1-888-STIEFEL) or FDA at 1-800-FDA-1088 or www.fda.gov/medwatch.

See 17 for PATIENT COUNSELING INFORMATION and FDA-approved patient labeling

Revised: 09/2012

FULL PRESCRIBING INFORMATION: CONTENTS*

*** Sections or subsections omitted from the full prescribing information are not listed**

FULL PRESCRIBING INFORMATION

1 INDICATIONS AND USAGE

SORILUX Foam is indicated for the topical treatment of plaque psoriasis of the scalp and body in patients 18 years and older.

2 DOSAGE AND ADMINISTRATION

SORILUX Foam is for topical use only. SORILUX Foam is not for oral, ophthalmic, or intravaginal use.

Apply a thin layer of SORILUX Foam twice daily to the affected areas and rub in gently and completely. Avoid contact with the face and eyes.

3 DOSAGE FORMS AND STRENGTHS

0.005%, white foam

4 CONTRAINDICATIONS

SORILUX Foam should not be used by patients with known hypercalcemia.

5 WARNINGS AND PRECAUTIONS

5.1 Flammability

The propellant in SORILUX Foam is flammable. Instruct the patient to avoid fire, flame, and smoking during and immediately following application.

5.2 Effects on Calcium Metabolism

Transient, rapidly reversible elevation of serum calcium has occurred with use of calcipotriene. If elevation in serum calcium outside the normal range should occur, discontinue treatment until normal calcium levels are restored.

5.3 Risk of Ultraviolet Light Exposure

Instruct the patient to avoid excessive exposure of the treated areas to either natural or artificial sunlight, including tanning booths and sun lamps. Physicians may wish to limit or avoid use of phototherapy in patients who use SORILUX Foam. *[See Nonclinical Toxicology (13.1).]*

6 ADVERSE REACTIONS

6.1 Clinical Trials Experience

Because clinical trials are conducted under widely varying conditions, adverse reaction rates observed in clinical trials of a drug cannot be directly compared to rates in the clinical trials of another drug and may not reflect the rates observed in clinical practice.

SORILUX Foam was studied in four vehicle-controlled trials. A total of 1094 subjects with plaque psoriasis, including 654 exposed to SORILUX Foam, were treated twice daily for 8 weeks.

Adverse reactions reported in ≥1% of subjects treated with SORILUX Foam and at a higher incidence than subjects treated with vehicle were application site erythema (2%), application site pain (3%). The incidence of these adverse reactions was similar between the body and scalp.

7 DRUG INTERACTIONS

No drug interaction studies were conducted with SORILUX Foam.

8 USE IN SPECIFIC POPULATIONS

8.1 Pregnancy

Teratogenic Effects, Pregnancy Category C:

There are no adequate and well-controlled trials in pregnant women. Therefore, SORILUX Foam should be used during pregnancy only if the potential benefit justifies the potential risk to the fetus.

Studies of teratogenicity were done by the oral route where bioavailability is expected to be approximately 40-60% of the administered dose. Increased rabbit maternal and fetal toxicity was noted at 12 mcg/kg/day (132 mcg/m²/day). Rabbits administered 36 mcg/kg/day (396 mcg/m²/day) resulted in fetuses with a significant increase in the incidences of incomplete ossification of pubic bones and forelimb phalanges. In a rat study, doses of 54 mcg/kg/day (318 mcg/m²/day) resulted in a significantly higher incidence of skeletal abnormalities consisting primarily of enlarged fontanelles and extra ribs. The enlarged fontanelles are most likely due to calcipotriene's effect upon calcium metabolism. The maternal and fetal no-effect exposures in the rat (43.2 mcg/m²/day) and rabbit (17.6 mcg/m²/day) studies are approximately equal to the expected human systemic exposure level (18.5 mcg/m²/day) from dermal application.

8.3 Nursing Mothers

It is not known whether calcipotriene is excreted in human milk. Because many drugs are excreted in human milk, caution should be exercised when SORILUX Foam is administered to a nursing woman.

8.4 Pediatric Use

Safety and effectiveness of SORILUX Foam in pediatric patients less than 18 years of age have not been established.

8.5 Geriatric Use

Clinical trials of SORILUX Foam did not include sufficient numbers of subjects aged 65 and over to determine whether they respond differently from younger subjects. Other reported clinical experience has not identified differences in responses between the elderly and younger patients.

8.6 Unevaluated Uses

SORILUX Foam has not been evaluated in patients with erythrodermic, exfoliative, or pustular psoriasis.

10 OVERDOSAGE

Topically applied calcipotriene can be absorbed in sufficient amounts to produce systemic effects. Elevated serum calcium has been observed with use of topical calcipotriene. *[See Warnings and Precautions (5.2).]*

11 DESCRIPTION

SORILUX Foam contains the compound calcipotriene, a synthetic vitamin D_3 analog.

Chemically, calcipotriene is (5Z,7E,22E,24S)-24-cyclopropyl-9,10-secochola-5,7,10(19), 22-tetraene-1α,3β,24-triol. The structural formula is represented below:

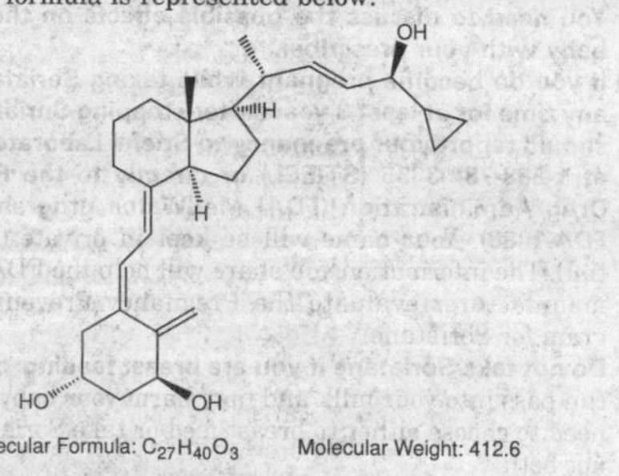

Molecular Formula: $C_{27}H_{40}O_3$ Molecular Weight: 412.6

Calcipotriene is a white or off-white crystalline substance. SORILUX Foam contains calcipotriene 50 mcg/g in an aqueous-based emulsion foam vehicle consisting of cetyl alcohol, dibasic sodium phosphate, edetate disodium, isopropyl myristate, light mineral oil, polyoxyl 20 cetostearyl ether, propylene glycol, purified water, stearyl alcohol, dl-α-tocopherol, and white petrolatum. SORILUX Foam is dispensed from an aluminum can pressurized with a hydrocarbon (propane/n-butane/isobutane) propellant.

12 CLINICAL PHARMACOLOGY

12.1 Mechanism of Action

Calcipotriene is a synthetic vitamin D_3 analog that has a similar receptor binding affinity as natural vitamin D_3. However, the exact mechanism of action contributing to the clinical efficacy in the treatment of psoriasis is unknown.

12.2 Pharmacodynamics

The pharmacodynamics of SORILUX Foam are unknown.

12.3 Pharmacokinetics

The systemic absorption of calcipotriene in subjects with psoriasis of the body was evaluated at steady state following application of either SORILUX Foam or calcipotriene ointment to a body surface area of 5% to 10%. In the SORILUX Foam treatment group, 15 out of 16 subjects had calcipotriene plasma concentrations below the limit of quantitation (10 pg/mL), while in the calcipotriene ointment treated group, 5 out of 16 subjects had measurable calcipotriene plasma concentrations at various time points. All measurable plasma calcipotriene concentrations were below 25 pg/mL.

The systemic disposition of calcipotriene is expected to be similar to that of the naturally occurring vitamin D. Absorbed calcipotriene is known to be converted to inactive metabolites within 24 hours of application and the metabolism occurs via a similar pathway to the natural hormone.

13 NONCLINICAL TOXICOLOGY

13.1 Carcinogenesis, Mutagenesis, Impairment of Fertility

Carcinogenesis

Calcipotriene topically administered to mice for up to 24 months at dose levels of 3, 10, or 30 mcg /kg/day (corresponding to 9, 30, or 90 mcg /m²/day) showed no significant changes in tumor incidence when compared to controls. In a study in which albino hairless mice were exposed to both UVR and topically applied calcipotriene, a reduction in the time required for UVR to induce the formation of skin tumors was observed (statistically significant in males only), suggesting that calcipotriene may enhance the effect of UVR to induce skin tumors. *[See Warnings and Precautions (5.3).]*

Mutagenesis

The genotoxic potential of calcipotriene was evaluated in an Ames assay, a mouse lymphoma TK locus assay, a human lymphocyte chromosome aberration assay, and a mouse micronucleus assay. All assay results were negative.

Impairment of Fertility

Studies in rats at doses up to 54 mcg /kg/day (318 mcg /m²/ day) of calcipotriene indicated no impairment of fertility or general reproductive performance.

14 CLINICAL STUDIES

In two multi-center, randomized, double-blind, vehicle-controlled clinical trials a total of 659 subjects with psoriasis were randomized 2:1 to SORILUX Foam or vehicle; subjects applied the assigned treatment twice daily for 8 weeks. Baseline disease severity was graded using a 5-point Investigator Static Global Assessment scale (ISGA), on which subjects scored either "mild" or "moderate" as shown in Table 1.

Table 1: Investigator Static Global Assessment (ISGA) Scale for Body

Disease Severity	Grade	Definition
Clear	0	No evidence of scaling, erythema, or plaque thickness
almost clear	1	Occasional fine scale, faint erythema, and barely perceptible plaque thickness
Mild	2	Fine scale with light coloration and mild plaque elevation
Moderate	3	Coarse scale with moderate red coloration and moderate plaque thickness
Severe	4	Thick tenacious scale with deep coloration and severe plaque thickness

Efficacy evaluation was carried out at Week 8 with treatment success being defined as a score of "clear" (grade 0) or "almost clear" (grade 1) and at least 2 grade improvement from the baseline score. Approximately 30% of enrolled subjects were graded as "mild" on the ISGA scale. The study population ranged in age from 12 to 89 years with 10 subjects less than 18 years of age at baseline. The subjects were 54% male and 88% Caucasian. Table 2 presents the efficacy results for each trial.

[See table 2 above]

In one trial, subjects graded as "mild" at baseline showed a greater response to vehicle than SORILUX Foam.

Table 3 presents the success rates by disease severity at baseline for each trial.

[See table 3 above]

In another multi-center, randomized, double-blind, vehicle-controlled clinical trial, a total of 363 subjects with moderate plaque psoriasis of the scalp and body were randomized 1:1 to SORILUX Foam or vehicle. Subjects applied the assigned medication to the affected areas twice daily for 8 weeks. Baseline disease severity of the scalp was graded using a 6-point ISGA; a score of "moderate" corresponded to grade 3.

The primary efficacy evaluation for scalp involvement was carried out at Week 8 with treatment success being defined as a score of "clear" (grade 0) or "almost clear" (grade 1). The study population ranged in age from 12 to 97 years with 11 subjects less than 18 years of age at baseline. The subjects were 60% male and 87% Caucasian. Table 4 presents the efficacy results for the trial.

Table 4: Number and Percent of Subjects Achieving Success for Scalp at Week 8

	Trial 3	
	SORILUX Foam N=181	Vehicle Foam N=182
Number (%) of Subjects with Treatment Success	74 (41%)	44 (24%)

Table 2: Number and Percent of Subjects Achieving Success for Body at Week 8 in Each Trial

	Trial 1		Trial 2	
	SORILUX Foam N=223	Vehicle Foam N=113	SORILUX Foam N= 214	Vehicle Foam N=109
Number (%) of Subjects with Treatment Success	31 (14%)	8 (7%)	58 (27%)	17 (16%)

Table 3: Number and Percent of Subjects Achieving Success for Body by Baseline ISGA Score and by Trial

	Trial 1		Trial 2	
ISGA scores at baseline	SORILUX Foam (N=223)	Vehicle Foam (N=113)	SORILUX Foam (N=214)	Vehicle Foam (N=109)
mild	2/73 (2.7%)	3/34 (8.8%)	8/56 (14.3%)	4/31 (12.9%)
moderate	29/150 (19.3%)	5/79 (6.3%)	50/158 (31.6%)	13/78 (16.7%)

The contribution to efficacy of individual components of the vehicle has not been established.

16 HOW SUPPLIED/STORAGE AND HANDLING

16.1 How Supplied

SORILUX (calcipotriene) Foam, 0.005%, is supplied as follows:

60 g aluminum can	NDC 0145-2130-06
120 g aluminum can	NDC 0145-2130-07

16.2 Storage and Handling

- Store at 20°C to 25°C (68°F to 77°F); excursions permitted to 15°C – 30°C (59°F –86°F).
- Flammable. Contents under pressure. Do not puncture or incinerate. Do not expose to heat or store at temperatures above 120°F (49°C).
- Keep out of reach of children.

17 PATIENT COUNSELING INFORMATION

See FDA-Approved Patient Labeling (Patient Information)

Inform the patient to adhere to the following instructions:

- Avoid excessive exposure of the treated areas to either natural or artificial sunlight, including tanning beds and sun lamps.
- Avoid contact with the face and eyes. If SORILUX Foam gets on the face or in or near their eyes, rinse thoroughly with water.
- Apply SORILUX Foam to the scalp when the hair is dry.
- Talk to your doctor if your skin does not improve after treatment with SORILUX Foam for 8 weeks.
- Wash your hands after applying SORILUX Foam unless your hands are the affected site.
- Avoid fire, flame, and smoking during and immediately following application since SORILUX Foam is flammable.
- Do not place SORILUX Foam in the refrigerator or freezer.

SOR:5PI

Patient Information

SORILUX (SOR-i-lux)

(calcipotriene)

Foam

Important: For skin use only. Do not get SORILUX Foam on your face or in your eyes, mouth, or vagina.

Read the Patient Information before you start using SORILUX Foam and each time you get a refill. There may be new information. This information does not take the place of talking with your doctor about your medical condition or treatment.

What is SORILUX Foam?

SORILUX Foam is a prescription medicine used on the skin (topical) to treat plaque psoriasis of the scalp and body in people 18 years and older.

It is not known if SORILUX Foam is safe and effective in people under 18 years old.

Who should not use SORILUX Foam?

Do not use SORILUX Foam if you have been told by your doctor that you have a high level of calcium in your blood (hypercalcemia).

What should I tell my doctor before using SORILUX Foam?

Before you use SORILUX Foam, tell your doctor if you:

- are getting light therapy for your psoriasis
- have any other medical conditions
- are pregnant or planning to become pregnant. It is not known if SORILUX Foam can harm your unborn baby. Talk to your doctor if you are pregnant or plan to become pregnant.
- are breastfeeding. It is not known if SORILUX Foam passes into breast milk. Do not apply SORILUX Foam to the chest area if you are breastfeeding a baby. This will help to prevent the baby from accidentally getting SORILUX Foam into their mouth.

Tell your doctor about all the medicines you take, including prescription and nonprescription medicines, vitamins, and herbal supplements.

Know the medicines you take. Keep a list of your medicines with you to show your doctor and pharmacist when you get a new medicine.

How should I use SORILUX Foam?

- Apply SORILUX Foam exactly as prescribed. SORILUX Foam is usually applied to the affected skin areas two times each day.
- SORILUX Foam is for use on the skin only. Do not get SORILUX Foam in your eyes, mouth or vagina.
- SORILUX Foam is flammable. Avoid fire, flame, or smoking during and right after you apply SORILUX Foam to your skin.
- Avoid excessive natural or artificial sunlight including tanning booths and sunlamps. Wear a hat and clothes that cover the treated areas of your skin if you have to be in sunlight.

Instructions for applying SORILUX Foam

1. Before applying SORILUX Foam for the first time, break the tiny plastic piece at the base of the can's rim by gently pushing back (away from the piece) on the nozzle. See Figure A.

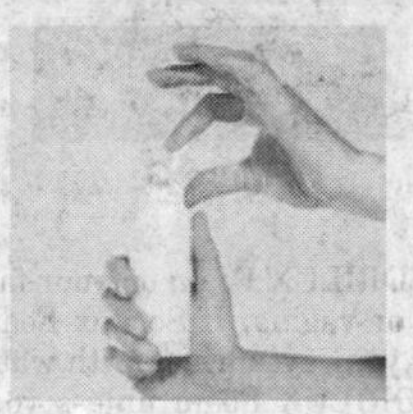

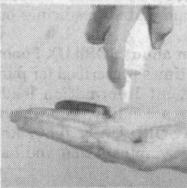

Figure A

2. Shake the SORILUX Foam can before use. See Figure B.

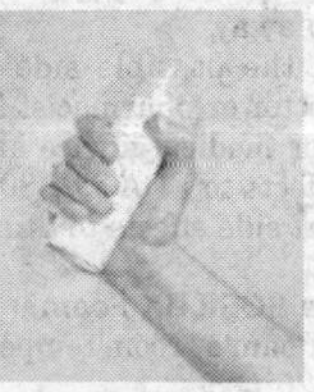

Figure B

3. Turn the SORILUX Foam can upside down and press the nozzle. See Figure C.

Figure C

4. Dispense a small amount of SORILUX Foam into the palm of your hand. See Figure D.

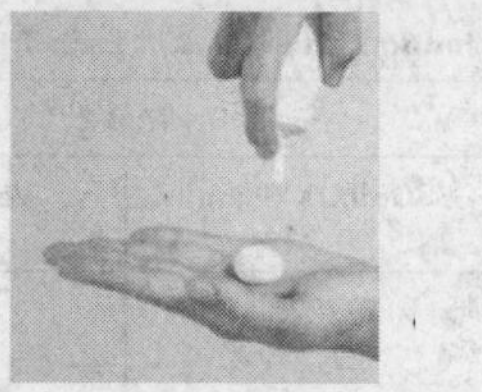

Figure D

5. Use enough SORILUX Foam to cover the affected area with a thin layer. Apply SORILUX Foam to your scalp when your hair is dry. Part your hair and apply directly on the affected area. Gently rub the foam into the affected area until it disappears into the skin. See Figures E, F and G.

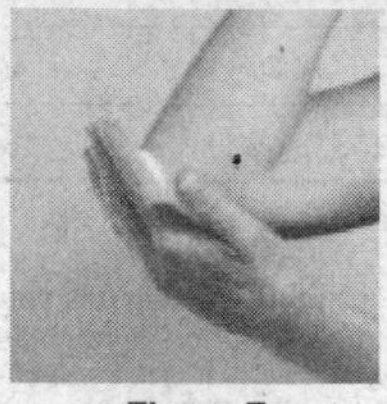

Figure E

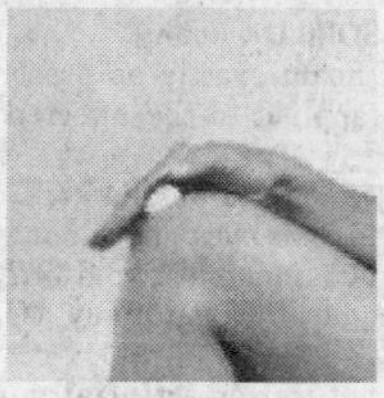

Figure F

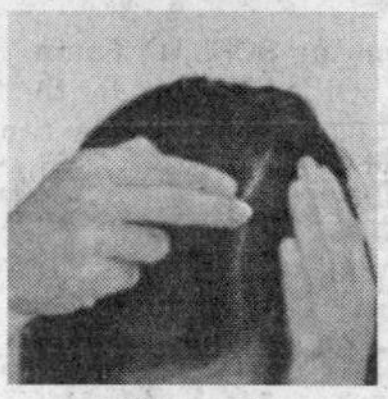

Figure G

6. Avoid getting SORILUX Foam on your face or in or near the eyes, mouth, or vagina. If Sorilux Foam gets on your face or in or near your eyes, rinse with water. Wash hands after applying SORILUX Foam unless your hands are a treated area.

What are the possible side effects of SORILUX Foam?

The most common side effects of SORILUX Foam are redness and pain of the treated skin areas.

Tell your doctor if you have any side effect that bothers you or that does not go away.

These are not all the possible side effects of SORILUX Foam. Ask your doctor or pharmacist for more information. Call your doctor for medical advice about side effects. You may report side effects to FDA at 1-800-FDA-1088.

You may also report side effects to Stiefel Laboratories, Inc. at 1-888-784-3335.

How should I store SORILUX Foam?

- Store SORILUX Foam at room temperature, between 68°F to 77°F (20C° to 25°C).
- SORILUX Foam is flammable. Keep the can away from all sources of fire and heat.
- Do not spray SORILUX Foam near fire or direct heat. Never throw the can into a fire, even if the can is empty.
- Do not puncture the SORILUX Foam can.

Keep SORILUX Foam and all medicines out of the reach of children.

General Information about SORILUX Foam

Medicines are sometimes prescribed for purposes other than those listed in Patient Information leaflets. Do not use SORILUX Foam for a condition for which it was not prescribed. Do not give SORILUX Foam to other people even if they have the same symptoms that you have. It may harm them.

This Patient Information leaflet summarizes the most important information about SORILUX Foam. If you would like more information, talk with your doctor. You can ask your doctor or pharmacist for information about SORILUX Foam that is written for health professionals.

What are the ingredients of SORILUX Foam?

Active ingredient: calcipotriene

Inactive Ingredients: cetyl alcohol, dibasic sodium phosphate, edetate disodium, isopropyl myristate, light mineral oil, polyoxyl 20 cetostearyl ether, propylene glycol, purified water, stearyl alcohol, dl-α-tocopherol, and white petrolatum. The foam is dispensed from an aluminum can pressurized with a hydrocarbon (propane/n-butane/isobutane) propellant.

This Patient Information has been approved by the U.S. Food and Drug Administration.

Manufactured for:
Stiefel Laboratories, Inc.
Research Triangle Park, NC 27709
Manufactured by:
DPT Laboratories, Ltd.
307 E. Josephine Street
San Antonio, TX 78215
Issue: September 2012
SOR:5PIL

VELTIN® ℞

[vel-tin]

(clindamycin phosphate and tretinoin)
Gel 1.2%/0.025%
For topical use only

HIGHLIGHTS OF PRESCRIBING INFORMATION

These highlights do not include all the information needed to use VELTIN Gel safely and effectively. See full prescribing information for VELTIN Gel.

VELTIN® (clindamycin phosphate and tretinoin) Gel 1.2%/0.025%
For topical use only
Initial U.S. Approval: 2006

INDICATIONS AND USAGE

- VELTIN Gel is a lincosamide antibiotic and retinoid combination product indicated for the topical treatment of acne vulgaris in patients 12 years or older. (1)

DOSAGE AND ADMINISTRATION

- Apply a pea size amount once daily in the evening lightly covering the entire affected area. Avoid the eyes, lips, and mucous membranes. (2)
- Not for oral, ophthalmic, or intravaginal use. (2)

DOSAGE FORMS AND STRENGTHS

- Topical gel: clindamycin phosphate 1.2% and tretinoin 0.025% in 30 gram and 60 gram tubes. (3)

CONTRAINDICATIONS

- VELTIN Gel is contraindicated in patients with regional enteritis, ulcerative colitis, or history of antibiotic-associated colitis. (4)

WARNINGS AND PRECAUTIONS

- Colitis: Clindamycin can cause severe colitis, which may result in death. Diarrhea, bloody diarrhea, and colitis (including pseudomembranous colitis) have been reported with the use of clindamycin. VELTIN Gel should be discontinued if significant diarrhea occurs. (5.1)
- Ultraviolet Light and Environmental Exposure: Avoid exposure to sunlight, sunlamps, and weather extremes. Wear sunscreen daily. (5.2)

ADVERSE REACTIONS

- Observed local treatment-related adverse reactions (≥ 1%) in clinical studies with VELTIN Gel were application site reactions, including dryness, irritation, exfoliation, erythema, pruritus, and dermatitis. Sunburn was also reported. (6.1)

To report SUSPECTED ADVERSE REACTIONS, contact Stiefel Laboratories, Inc. at 1-888-784-3335 or FDA at 1-800-FDA-1088 or www.fda.gov/medwatch.

DRUG INTERACTIONS

- VELTIN Gel should not be used in combination with erythromycin-containing products because of its clindamycin component. (7.1)

USE IN SPECIFIC POPULATIONS

- Pediatric Use: The efficacy and safety have not been established in pediatric patients below the age of 12 years. (8.4)

See 17 for PATIENT COUNSELING INFORMATION and FDA-approved patient labeling

Revised: 05/2012

FULL PRESCRIBING INFORMATION: CONTENTS*

*** Sections or subsections omitted from the full prescribing information are not listed**

FULL PRESCRIBING INFORMATION

1 INDICATIONS AND USAGE

VELTIN® (clindamycin phosphate and tretinoin) Gel, 1.2%/0.025% is indicated for the topical treatment of acne vulgaris in patients 12 years or older.

2 DOSAGE AND ADMINISTRATION

VELTIN Gel should be applied once daily in the evening, gently rubbing the medication to lightly cover the entire affected area. Approximately a pea sized amount will be needed for each application. Avoid the eyes, lips, and mucous membranes.

VELTIN Gel is not for oral, ophthalmic, or intravaginal use.

3 DOSAGE FORMS AND STRENGTHS

VELTIN Gel, containing clindamycin phosphate 1.2% and tretinoin 0.025%, is a yellow, opaque topical gel. Each gram of VELTIN Gel contains, as dispensed, 10 mg (1%) clindamycin as clindamycin phosphate, and 0.25 mg (0.025%) tretinoin solubilized in an aqueous based gel.

4 CONTRAINDICATIONS

VELTIN Gel is contraindicated in patients with regional enteritis, ulcerative colitis, or history of antibiotic-associated colitis.

5 WARNINGS AND PRECAUTIONS

5.1 Colitis

Systemic absorption of clindamycin has been demonstrated following topical use. Diarrhea, bloody diarrhea, and colitis (including pseudomembranous colitis) have been reported with the use of topical clindamycin. If significant diarrhea occurs, VELTIN Gel should be discontinued.

Severe colitis has occurred following oral or parenteral administration of clindamycin with an onset of up to several weeks following cessation of therapy. Antiperistaltic agents such as opiates and diphenoxylate with atropine may prolong and/or worsen severe colitis. Severe colitis may result in death.

Studies indicate a toxin(s) produced by clostridia is one primary cause of antibiotic-associated colitis. The colitis is usually characterized by severe persistent diarrhea and severe abdominal cramps and may be associated with the passage of blood and mucus. Stool cultures for *Clostridium difficile* and stool assay for *C. difficile*toxin may be helpful diagnostically.

5.2 Ultraviolet Light and Environmental Exposure

Exposure to sunlight, including sunlamps, should be avoided during the use of VELTIN Gel, and patients with sunburn should be advised not to use the product until fully recovered because of heightened susceptibility to sunlight as a result of the use of tretinoin. Patients who may be required to have considerable sun exposure due to occupation and those with inherent sensitivity to the sun should exercise particular caution. Daily use of sunscreen products and protective apparel (e.g., a hat) are recommended. Weather extremes, such as wind or cold, also may be irritating to patients under treatment with VELTIN Gel.

6 ADVERSE REACTIONS

6.1 Adverse Reactions in Clinical Studies

Because clinical studies are conducted under widely varying conditions, adverse reaction rates observed in clinical studies of a drug cannot be directly compared to rates in the clinical studies of another drug and may not reflect the rates observed in clinical practice.

The safety data reflect exposure to VELTIN Gel in 1,104 patients with acne vulgaris. Patients were 12 years or older and were treated once daily in the evening for 12 weeks. Adverse reactions that were reported in ≥1% of patients treated with VELTIN Gel are presented in Table 1.

[See table 1 above]

Local skin reactions actively assessed at baseline and end of treatment with a score > 0 are presented in Table 2.

[See table 2 above]

During the twelve weeks of treatment, each local skin reaction peaked at week 2 and gradually reduced thereafter.

Table 1: Treatment-Related Adverse Reactions Reported by ≥1% of Subjects

	VELTIN Gel N=1104 n (%)	Clindamycin Gel N=1091 n (%)	Tretinoin Gel N=1084 n (%)	Vehicle Gel N=552 n (%)
Patients with at least one adverse reaction	140 (13)	38 (3)	141 (13)	17 (3)
Application site dryness	64 (6)	12 (1)	62 (6)	3 (1)
Application site irritation	50 (5)	4 (<1)	57 (5)	5 (1)
Application site exfoliation	50 (5)	2 (<1)	56 (5)	2 (<1)
Application site erythema	40 (4)	6 (1)	39 (4)	3 (1)
Application site pruritus	26 (2)	7 (1)	23 (2)	6 (1)
Sunburn	11 (1)	6 (1)	7 (1)	3 (1)
Application site dermatitis	6 (1)	0 (0)	8 (1)	1 (<1)

Table 2: VELTIN GEL-Treated Patients with Local Skin Reactions

	VELTIN GEL		VEHICLE GEL	
Local Reaction	Baseline N= 476 N (%)	End of Treatment N= 409 N (%)	Baseline N= 219 N (%)	End of Treatment N= 209 N (%)
Erythema	24%	21%	31%	35%
Scaling	8%	19%	14%	12%
Dryness	11%	22%	18%	13%
Burning	8%	13%	8%	4%
Itching	17%	15%	22%	14%

7 DRUG INTERACTIONS

7.1 Erythromycin

VELTIN Gel should not be used in combination with erythromycin-containing products due to possible antagonism to the clindamycin component. *In vitro* studies have shown antagonism between these 2 antimicrobials. The clinical significance of this *in vitro* antagonism is not known.

7.2 Neuromuscular Blocking Agents

Clindamycin has been shown to have neuromuscular blocking properties that may enhance the action of other neuromuscular blocking agents. Therefore, VELTIN Gel should be used with caution in patients receiving such agents.

8 USE IN SPECIFIC POPULATIONS

8.1 Pregnancy

Pregnancy Category C. There are no well-controlled studies in pregnant women treated with VELTIN Gel. VELTIN Gel should be used during pregnancy only if the potential benefit justifies the potential risk to the fetus. A limit teratology study performed in Sprague Dawley rats treated topically with VELTIN Gel or 0.025% tretinoin gel at a dose of 2 mL/kg during gestation days 6 to 15 did not result in teratogenic effects. Although no systemic levels of tretinoin were detected, craniofacial and heart abnormalities were described in drug-treated groups. These abnormalities are consistent with retinoid effects and occurred at 16 times the recommended clinical dose assuming 100% absorption and based on body surface area comparison. For purposes of comparison of the animal exposure to human exposure, the recommended clinical dose is defined as 1 g of VELTIN Gel applied daily to a 50 kg person.

Clindamycin

Reproductive developmental toxicity studies performed in rats and mice using oral doses of clindamycin up to 600 mg/kg/day (480 and 240 times the recommended clinical dose based on body surface area comparison, respectively) or subcutaneous doses of clindamycin up to 180 mg/kg/day (140 and 70 times the recommended clinical dose based on body surface area comparison, respectively) revealed no evidence of teratogenicity.

Tretinoin

Oral tretinoin has been shown to be teratogenic in mice, rats, hamsters, rabbits, and primates. It was teratogenic and fetotoxic in Wistar rats when given orally at doses greater than 1 mg/kg/day (32 times the recommended clinical dose based on body surface area comparison). However, variations in teratogenic doses among various strains of rats have been reported. In the cynomologous monkey, a species in which tretinoin metabolism is closer to humans than in other species examined, fetal malformations were reported at oral doses of 10 mg/kg/day or greater, but none were observed at 5 mg/kg/day (324 times the recommended clinical dose based on body surface area comparison), although increased skeletal variations were observed at all doses. Dose-related teratogenic effects and increased abortion rates were reported in pigtail macaques.

With widespread use of any drug, a small number of birth defect reports associated temporally with the administration of the drug would be expected by chance alone. Thirty cases of temporally associated congenital malformations have been reported during two decades of clinical use of an other formulation of topical tretinoin. Although no definite pattern of teratogenicity and no causal association have been established from these cases, 5 of the reports describe the rare birth defect category, holoprosencephaly (defects associated with incomplete midline development of the forebrain). The significance of these spontaneous reports in terms of risk to fetus is not known.

8.3 Nursing Mothers

It is not known whether clindamycin is excreted in human milk following use of VELTIN Gel. However, orally and parenterally administered clindamycin has been reported to appear in breast milk. Because of the potential for serious adverse reactions in nursing infants, a decision should be made whether to discontinue nursing or to discontinue the drug, taking into account the importance of the drug to the mother. It is not known whether tretinoin is excreted in human milk. Because many drugs are excreted in human milk, caution should be exercised when VELTIN Gel is administered to a nursing woman.

8.4 Pediatric Use

Safety and effectiveness of VELTIN Gel in pediatric patients below the age of 12 years have not been established. Clinical trials of VELTIN Gel included 2,086 patients 12-17 years of age with acne vulgaris. *[See Clinical Studies (14).]*

8.5 Geriatric Use

Clinical studies of VELTIN Gel did not include sufficient numbers of subjects aged 65 and over to determine whether they respond differently from younger subjects.

11 DESCRIPTION

VELTIN (clindamycin phosphate and tretinoin) Gel, 1.2%/0.025%, is a fixed combination of two solubilized active ingredients in an aqueous based gel. Clindamycin phosphate is a water soluble ester of the semi-synthetic antibiotic produced by a 7(S)-chloro-substitution of the 7(R)-hydroxyl group of the parent antibiotic lincomycin.

The chemical name for clindamycin phosphate is methyl 7-chloro-6,7,8-trideoxy-6-(1-methyl-*trans*-4-propyl-L-2-pyrrolidinecarboxamido)-1-thio-L-*threo*-α-D-*galacto*-octopyranoside 2-(dihydrogen phosphate). The structural formula for clindamycin phosphate is represented below:

Clindamycin phosphate:

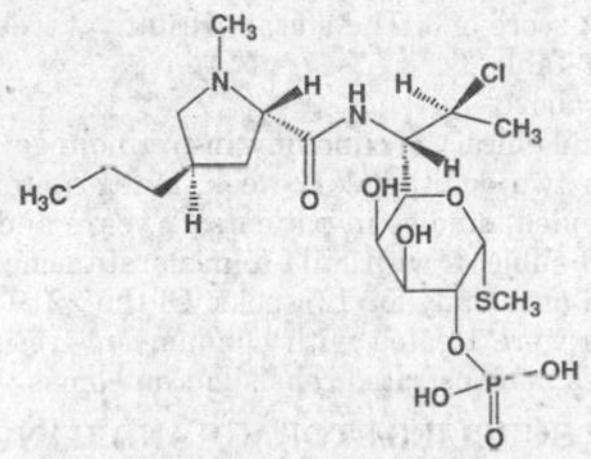

Molecular Formula: $C_{18}H_{34}ClN_2O_8PS$

Molecular Weight: 504.97

The chemical name for tretinoin is all-*trans* 3,7-dimethyl-9-(2,6,6-trimethyl-1-cyclohexen-1-yl)-2,4,6,8-nonatetraenoic acid. It is a member of the retinoid family of compounds. The structural formula for tretinoin is represented below:

Tretinoin:

[See chemical structure at top of next column]

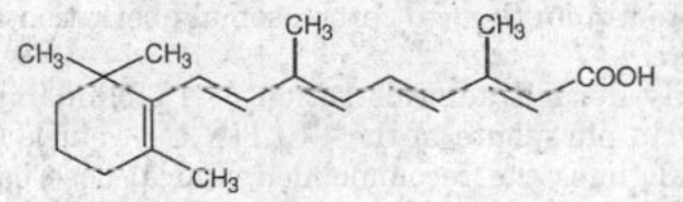

Molecular Formula: $C_{20}H_{28}O_2$

Molecular Weight: 300.44

VELTIN Gel contains the following inactive ingredients: butylated hydroxytoluene, carbomer homopolymer (type C), anhydrous citric acid, edetate disodium, methylparaben, laureth 4, propylene glycol, tromethamine, and purified water.

12 CLINICAL PHARMACOLOGY

12.1 Mechanism of Action

Clindamycin

[See Microbiology (12.4).]

Tretinoin

Although the exact mode of action of tretinoin is unknown, current evidence suggests that topical tretinoin decreases cohesiveness of follicular epithelial cells with decreased microcomedone formation. Additionally, tretinoin stimulates mitotic activity and increased turnover of follicular epithelial cells causing extrusion of the comedones.

12.3 Pharmacokinetics

In an open-label study of 17 patients with moderate-to-severe acne vulgaris, topical administration of approximately 3 grams of VELTIN Gel once daily for 5 days, clindamycin concentrations were quantifiable in all 17 patients starting from 1 hour post dose. All plasma clindamycin concentrations were ≤5.56 ng/mL on day 5, with the exception of one subject who had a maximum clindamycin concentration of 8.73 ng/mL at 4 hours post-dose. There was no appreciable increase in systemic exposure to tretinoin, as compared to the baseline value. The average tretinoin concentration across all sampling times on day 5 ranged from 1.19 to 1.23 ng/mL compared with the corresponding baseline mean tretinoin concentration range of 1.16 to 1.30 ng/mL.

12.4 Microbiology

No microbiology studies were conducted in the clinical trials with this product.

Mechanism of Action

Clindamycin binds to the 50S ribosomal subunit of susceptible bacteria and prevents elongation of peptide chains by interfering with peptidyl transfer, thereby suppressing protein synthesis. Clindamycin has been shown to have *in vitro* activity against *Propionibacterium acnes (P. acnes)*; an organism that has been associated with acne vulgaris; however, the clinical significance of this activity against *P. acnes* was not examined in clinical studies with VELTIN Gel. *P. acnes* resistance to clindamycin has been documented.

Inducible Clindamycin Resistance

The treatment of acne with antimicrobials is associated with the development of antimicrobial resistance in *P. acnes* as well as other bacteria (e.g. *Staphylococcus aureus, Strep-*

Table 3: Efficacy Results at Week 12

Study 1	VELTIN Gel N=476	Clindamycin Gel N=467	Tretinoin Gel N=464	Vehicle Gel N=242
Investigator's Global Assessment				
Percentage of subjects achieving Two Grade Improvement	36.3%	26.6%	26.1%	20.2%
Percentage of subjects achieving an IGA of 0 or 1 with a Two Grade Improvement	33.2%	24.0%	22.6%	17.8%
Inflammatory Lesions:				
Mean absolute reduction	15.5	14.5	13.9	11.1
Mean percentage (%) reduction	60.4%	56.5%	54.5%	43.3%
Non-inflammatory Lesions:				
Mean absolute reduction	23.2	19.5	22.1	17.0
Mean percentage (%) reduction	51.0%	42.9%	47.3%	36.0%
Total Lesions:				
Mean absolute reduction	38.7	34.0	36.0	28.1
Mean percentage (%) reduction	55.0%	49.0%	50.5%	39.1%

tococcus pyogenes). The use of clindamycin may result in developing inducible resistance in these organisms. This resistance is not detected by routine susceptibility testing.

Cross Resistance

Resistance to clindamycin is often associated with resistance to erythromycin.

13 NONCLINICAL TOXICOLOGY

13.1 Carcinogenesis, Mutagenesis, Impairment of Fertility

Long-term animal studies have not been performed to evaluate the carcinogenic potential of VELTIN Gel or the effect of VELTIN Gel on fertility. VELTIN Gel was negative for mutagenic potential when evaluated in an *in vitro* Ames *Salmonella* reversion assay. VELTIN Gel was equivocal for clastogenic potential in the absence of metabolic activation when tested in an *in vitro* chromosomal aberration assay.

Clindamycin

Once daily dermal administration of 1% clindamycin as clindamycin phosphate in the VELTIN Gel vehicle (32 mg/kg/day, 13 times the recommended clinical dose based on body surface area comparison) to mice for up to 2 years did not produce evidence of tumorigenicity.

Fertility studies in rats treated orally with up to 300 mg/kg/day of clindamycin (240 times the recommended clinical dose based on body surface area comparison) revealed no effects on fertility or mating ability.

Tretinoin

In two independent mouse studies where tretinoin was administered topically (0.025% or 0.1%) three times per week for up to two years no carcinogenicity was observed, with maximum effects of dermal amyloidosis. However, in a dermal carcinogenicity study in mice, tretinoin applied at a dose of 5.1 µg (1.4 times the recommended clinical dose based on body surface area comparison) three times per week for 20 weeks acted as a weak promoter of skin tumor formation following a single application of dimethylbenz[α]anthracene (DMBA).

In a study in female SENCAR mice, papillomas were induced by topical exposure to DMBA followed by promotion with 12-O-tetradecanoyl-phorbol 13-acetate or mezerein for up to 20 weeks. Topical application of tretinoin prior to each application of promoting agent resulted in a reduction in the number of papillomas per mouse. However, papillomas resistant to topical tretinoin suppression were at higher risk for pre-malignant progression.

Tretinoin has been shown to enhance photoco-carcinogenicity in properly performed specific studies, employing concurrent or intercurrent exposure to tretinoin and UV radiation. The photoco-carcinogenic potential of the clindamycin tretinoin combination is unknown. Although the significance of these studies to humans is not clear, patients should avoid exposure to sun.

The genotoxic potential of tretinoin was evaluated in an *in vitro* Ames *Salmonella* reversion test and an *in vitro* chromosomal aberration assay in Chinese hamster ovary cells. Both tests were negative.

In oral fertility studies in rats treated with tretinoin, the no-observed-effect-level was 2 mg/kg/day (64 times the recommended clinical dose based on body surface area comparison).

14 CLINICAL STUDIES

The safety and efficacy of VELTIN Gel, applied once daily for the treatment of acne vulgaris, was evaluated in 12-week multicenter, randomized, blinded studies in subjects 12 years and older.

Treatment response was defined as the percent of subjects who had a two grade improvement from baseline to Week 12 based on the Investigator's Global Assessment (IGA) and a mean absolute change from baseline to Week 12 in two out of three (total, inflammatory and non-inflammatory) lesion counts. The IGA scoring scale used in all the clinical trials for VELTIN Gel is as follows:

0	Clear	Normal, clear skin with no evidence of acne vulgaris.
1	Almost Clear	Skin almost clear; rare non-inflammatory lesions present, with rare non-inflamed papules (papules must be resolving and may be hyperpigmented, though not pink-red) requiring no further treatment in the Investigator's opinion.
2	Mild	Some non-inflammatory lesions are present, with few inflammatory lesions (papules/pustules only, no nodulo-cystic lesions).
3	Moderate	Non-inflammatory lesions predominate, with multiple inflammatory lesions evident; several to many comedones and papules/pustules, and there may or may not be 1 small nodulo-cystic lesion.
4	Severe	Inflammatory lesions are more apparent; many comedones and papules/pustules, there may or may not be a few nodulo-cystic lesions.
5	Very Severe	Highly inflammatory lesions predominate; variable numbers of comedones, many papules/pustules and nodulo-cystic lesions.

In Study 1, 1649 subjects were randomized to VELTIN Gel, Clindamycin gel, Tretinoin gel, and vehicle gel. The median age of subjects was 17 years old and 58% were females. At baseline, subjects had an average of 71 total lesions of which the mean number of inflammatory lesions was 25.5 lesions and the mean number of non-inflammatory lesions was 45.1 lesions. The majority of subjects enrolled with a baseline IGA score of 3. The efficacy results at week 12 are presented in Table 3.

[See table 3 above]

The safety and efficacy of clindamycin-tretinoin gel was also evaluated in two additional 12-week, multi-centered, randomized, blinded, studies in patients 12 years and older. A total of 2219 subjects with mild-to-moderate acne vulgaris were treated once daily for 12 weeks. Of the 2219 subjects, 634 subjects were treated with clindamycin-tretinoin gel. These studies demonstrated consistent outcomes.

16 HOW SUPPLIED/STORAGE AND HANDLING

How Supplied

VELTIN Gel is supplied as follows:
30 g aluminum tubes NDC 0145-0071-30
60 g aluminum tubes NDC 0145-0071-60

Storage and Handling

- Store at 25°C (77°F); excursions permitted to 15–30°C (59–86°F).
- Protect from heat.
- Protect from light.
- Protect from freezing.
- Keep out of reach of children.
- Keep tube tightly closed.

17 PATIENT COUNSELING INFORMATION

[See FDA-approved Patient Labeling].

17.1 Instructions for Use

- At bedtime, the face should be gently washed with a mild soap and water. After patting the skin dry, apply VELTIN Gel as a thin layer over the entire affected area (excluding the eyes and lips).
- Patients should be advised not to use more than a pea sized amount to cover the face and not to apply more often than once daily (at bedtime) as this will not make for faster results and may increase irritation.
- A sunscreen should be applied every morning and reapplied over the course of the day as needed. Patients should be advised to avoid exposure to sunlight, sunlamp, ultraviolet light, and other medicines that may increase sensitivity to sunlight.
- Other topical products with a strong drying effect, such as abrasive soaps or cleansers, may cause an increase in skin irritation with VELTIN Gel.

17.2 Skin Irritation

VELTIN Gel may cause irritation such as erythema, scaling, itching, burning, or stinging.

17.3 Colitis

In the event a patient treated with VELTIN Gel experiences severe diarrhea or gastrointestinal discomfort, VELTIN Gel should be discontinued and a physician should be contacted.

VEL:3PI

PATIENT INFORMATION

VELTIN (vel-tin)
(clindamycin phosphate and tretinoin) Gel

IMPORTANT: For use on skin only (topical use). Do not get VELTIN Gel in your mouth, eyes, or vagina.

Read the Patient Information that comes with VELTIN Gel before you start using it and each time you get a refill. There may be new information. This leaflet does not take the place of talking with your doctor about your medical condition or your treatment.

What is VELTIN Gel?

VELTIN Gel is prescription medicine used on the skin to treat acne in people 12 years and older.

It is not known if VELTIN Gel is safe and effective in children under 12 years of age.

Who should not use VELTIN Gel?

Do not use VELTIN Gel if you have:

- Crohn's disease
- ulcerative colitis
- had inflammation of the colon (colitis) with past antibiotic use

Talk to your doctor if you are not sure if you have one of these conditions.

What should I tell my doctor before using VELTIN Gel?

Before using VELTIN Gel, tell your doctor if you:

- **have any allergies**
- **Plan to have surgery with general anesthesia.** One of the medicines in VELTIN Gel can affect how certain anesthesia medicines work.
- **have any other medical conditions**
- **are pregnant or plan to become pregnant.** It is not known if VELTIN Gel may harm your unborn baby.
- **are breast-feeding or plan to breast-feed.** It is not known if VELTIN Gel passes into your breast milk. One of the medicines in VELTIN Gel contains clindamycin. When clindamycin is taken by mouth or injection, it may pass into breast milk. You and your doctor should decide if you will take VELTIN Gel or breast feed. You should not do both.

Tell your doctor about all the medicines and skin products you use. Especially tell your doctor if you take medicine that contains erythromycin. VELTIN Gel should not be used with products that contain erythromycin.

Know the medicines you take. Keep a list of your medicines and show it to your doctor and pharmacist when you get a new medicine.

How should I use VELTIN Gel?

- Use VELTIN Gel exactly as prescribed.
- Your doctor will tell you how long to use VELTIN Gel.
- **Do not** apply VELTIN Gel more than one time each day.
- **Do not** use too much VELTIN Gel, because it may irritate your skin.

Instructions for applying VELTIN Gel:

1. At bedtime, wash your face gently with a mild soap, rinse with water.
2. Pat the skin dry.
3. Squeeze a pea sized amount of medication onto one fingertip. Then, gently rub over the entire affected area. **Do not get VELTIN Gel in your eyes, mouth, or on your lips.**

What should I avoid while using VELTIN Gel?

- Limit your time in sunlight. Avoid using tanning beds or sun lamps. If you have to be in sunlight, wear a wide-brimmed hat or other protective clothing. Apply a sunscreen every morning and re-apply during the day as needed.

- Avoid wind and cold weather during treatment with VELTIN Gel. These may be irritating to your skin.
- Avoid using abrasive soaps and cleansers. These may cause increased skin irritation with VELTIN Gel.

What are the possible side effects of VELTIN Gel?

VELTIN Gel may cause serious side effects, including:

- **Inflammation of the colon (colitis).** Clindamycin, one of the ingredients in VELTIN Gel, can cause severe colitis that may lead to death. Stop taking VELTIN Gel and call your doctor if you develop severe watery diarrhea, or bloody diarrhea.
- **Sunburn.** VELTIN Gel may cause your skin to become sunburned more easily. If your face is sunburned, do not use VELTIN Gel until your sunburn is completely healed. Tretinoin, one of the medicines in VELTIN Gel, makes your skin more sensitive to sunlight. See "What should I avoid while using VELTIN Gel?"

Common side effects of VELTIN Gel include:

- **Skin irritation.** VELTIN Gel may cause skin irritation such as dryness, peeling, burning, or itching.

Talk to your doctor about any side effect that bothers you or that does not go away.

These are not all the side effects with VELTIN Gel. Ask your doctor or pharmacist for more information.

Call your doctor for medical advice about side effects. You may report side effects to FDA at 1-800-FDA-1088.

How should I store VELTIN Gel?

- **Store VELTIN Gel** at room temperature, between 59°F to 86°F (15°C to 30°C).
- Protect from freezing.
- Keep VELTIN Gel away from heat and light.
- **Keep VELTIN Gel and all medicines out of the reach of children.**

General information about VELTIN Gel

Medicines are sometimes prescribed for purposes other than those listed in the patient information leaflet. Do not use VELTIN Gel for a condition for which it was not prescribed. **Do not give VELTIN Gel to other people, even if they have the same symptoms you have. It may harm them.**

This patient information leaflet summarizes the most important information about VELTIN Gel. If you would like more information, talk with your doctor. You can also ask your pharmacist or doctor for information about VELTIN Gel that is written for healthcare professionals. For more information call 1-888-784-3335.

What are the ingredients in VELTIN Gel?

Active Ingredients: clindamycin phosphate and tretinoin

Inactive Ingredients: butylated hydroxytoluene, carbomer homopolymer (type C), anhydrous citric acid, edetate disodium, methylparaben, laureth 4, propylene glycol, tromethamine, and purified water.

Manufactured for:
Stiefel Laboratories, Inc.
Research Triangle Park, NC 27709
Manufactured by:
DPT Laboratories, Ltd.
307 E. Josephine Street
San Antonio, TX 78215
Issued May 2012
VEL:2PIL

Sunovion Pharmaceuticals Inc.

84 WATERFORD DRIVE
MARLBOROUGH, MA 01752
(508) 481-6700

For Medical Information Inquiries:
Medical Information
(800) 739-0565
minfo@sunovion.com
www.SunovionMedical.com
For Adverse Event Reporting
(877) 737-7226
For Customer Service
(888) 394-7377
CAC@sunovion.com

BROVANA®
(arformoterol tartrate)
Inhalation Solution

℞

HIGHLIGHTS OF PRESCRIBING INFORMATION

These highlights do not include all the information needed to use BROVANA® (arformoterol tartrate) Inhalation Solution safely and effectively. See full prescribing information for BROVANA Inhalation Solution.

BROVANA® (arformoterol tartrate) Inhalation Solution
Initial U.S. Approval: 2006

WARNING: ASTHMA-RELATED DEATH

See full prescribing information for complete boxed warning

- **Long-acting $beta_2$-adrenergic agonists (LABA) increase the risk of asthma-related death. (5.1)**
- **A placebo-controlled study with another long-acting $beta_2$-adrenergic agonist (salmeterol) showed an increase in asthma related deaths in patients receiving salmeterol. (5.1)**
- **The finding of an increase in the risk of asthma-related deaths with salmeterol is considered a class effect of LABA, including arformoterol, the active ingredient in BROVANA Inhalation Solution. The safety and efficacy of BROVANA Inhalation Solution in patients with asthma have not been established. All LABA, including BROVANA Inhalation Solution, are contraindicated in patients with asthma without use of a long-term asthma control medication. (4, 5.1)**

INDICATIONS AND USAGE

BROVANA Inhalation Solution is a long-acting $beta_2$-adrenergic agonist ($beta_2$-agonist) indicated for:

- Long-term, twice daily (morning and evening) administration in the maintenance treatment of bronchoconstriction in patients with chronic obstructive pulmonary disease (COPD), including chronic bronchitis and emphysema. (1.1)

Important limitations of use:

- BROVANA Inhalation Solution is not indicated to treat acute deteriorations of chronic obstructive pulmonary disease. (1.2, 5.2)
- BROVANA Inhalation Solution is not indicated to treat asthma. (1.2)

DOSAGE AND ADMINISTRATION

For oral inhalation only.

- A total daily dose of greater than 30 mcg is not recommended. (2)
- One 15 mcg/2 mL vial every 12 hours. (2)
- For use with a standard jet nebulizer (with a face mask or mouthpiece) connected to an air compressor. (2)

DOSAGE FORMS AND STRENGTHS

Inhalation Solution (unit-dose vial for nebulization): 15 mcg/2 mL solution (3)

CONTRAINDICATIONS

BROVANA Inhalation Solution is contraindicated in patients with a history of hypersensitivity to arformoterol, racemic formoterol or to any other components of this product. (4)

All LABA, including BROVANA Inhalation Solution, are contraindicated in patients with asthma without use of a long-term asthma control medication. (4)

WARNINGS AND PRECAUTIONS

- Do not initiate BROVANA Inhalation Solution in acutely deteriorating patients. (5.2)
- Do not use for relief of acute symptoms. Concomitant short-acting $beta_2$-agonists can be used as needed for acute relief. (5.2)
- Do not exceed the recommended dose. Excessive use of BROVANA Inhalation Solution, or use in conjunction with other medications containing long-acting $beta_2$-agonists, can result in clinically significant cardiovascular effects, and may be fatal. (5.3, 5.5)
- Life-threatening paradoxical bronchospasm can occur. Discontinue BROVANA Inhalation Solution immediately. (5.4)
- Use with caution in patients with cardiovascular or convulsive disorders, thyrotoxicosis, or with sensitivity to sympathomimetic drugs. (5.6, 5.7)

ADVERSE REACTIONS

Most common adverse reactions (≥2% incidence and more common than placebo) are pain, chest pain, back pain, diarrhea, sinusitis, leg cramps, dyspnea, rash, flu syndrome, peripheral edema and lung disorder. (6.2)

To report SUSPECTED ADVERSE REACTIONS, contact Sunovion Pharmaceuticals Inc. at 1-877-737-7226 or FDA at 1-800-FDA-1088 or *www.fda.gov/medwatch.*

DRUG INTERACTIONS

- Other adrenergic drugs may potentiate effect. Use with caution. (5.3, 7.1)
- Xanthine derivatives, steroids, diuretics, or non-potassium sparing diuretics may potentiate hypokalemia or ECG changes. Use with caution. (5.7, 7.2, 7.3)
- MAO inhibitors, tricyclic antidepressants and drugs that prolong the QTc interval may potentiate effect on the cardiovascular system. Use with extreme caution. (7.4)
- Beta-blockers may decrease effectiveness. May block bronchodilatory effects of beta-agonists. Use with caution and only when medically necessary. (7.5)

USE IN SPECIFIC POPULATIONS

- Hepatic Impairment
  Use with caution in patients with hepatic impairment. (8.6)

See 17 for PATIENT COUNSELING INFORMATION and Medication Guide

Revised: 02/2012

FULL PRESCRIBING INFORMATION: CONTENTS*

*** Sections or subsections omitted from the full prescribing information are not listed**

FULL PRESCRIBING INFORMATION

WARNING: ASTHMA RELATED DEATH

Long-acting $beta_2$-adrenergic agonists (LABA) increase the risk of asthma-related death. Data from a large placebo-controlled US study that compared the safety of another long-acting $beta_2$-adrenergic agonist (salmeterol) or placebo added to usual asthma therapy showed an increase in asthma-related deaths in patients receiving salmeterol. This finding with salmeterol is considered a class effect of LABA, including arformoterol, the active ingredient in BROVANA Inhalation Solution [see *WARNINGS AND PRECAUTIONS (5.1)*]. The safety and efficacy of BROVANA Inhalation Solution in patients with asthma have not been established. All LABA, including BROVANA Inhalation Solution, are contraindicated in patients with asthma without use of a long-term asthma control medication [see *CONTRAINDICATIONS (4), WARNINGS AND PRECAUTIONS (5.1)*].

1 INDICATIONS AND USAGE

1.1 Maintenance Treatment of COPD

BROVANA (arformoterol tartrate) Inhalation Solution is indicated for the long-term, twice daily (morning and evening) maintenance treatment of bronchoconstriction in patients with chronic obstructive pulmonary disease (COPD), including chronic bronchitis and emphysema. BROVANA Inhalation Solution is for use by nebulization only.

1.2 Important Limitations of Use

BROVANA Inhalation Solution is not indicated to treat acute deteriorations of chronic obstructive pulmonary disease [*see WARNINGS AND PRECAUTIONS (5.2)*].

BROVANA Inhalation Solution is not indicated to treat asthma. The safety and effectiveness of BROVANA Inhalation Solution in asthma have not been established.

2 DOSAGE AND ADMINISTRATION

The recommended dose of BROVANA (arformoterol tartrate) Inhalation Solution is one 15 mcg unit-dose vial administered twice daily (morning and evening) by nebulization. A total daily dose of greater than 30 mcg (15 mcg twice daily) is not recommended.

BROVANA Inhalation Solution should be administered by the orally inhaled route via a standard jet nebulizer connected to an air compressor (see the accompanying **Medication Guide**). BROVANA Inhalation Solution should not be swallowed. BROVANA Inhalation Solution should be stored refrigerated in foil pouches. After opening the pouch, unused unit-dose vials should be returned to, and stored in, the pouch. An opened unit-dose vial should be used right away.

If the recommended maintenance treatment regimen fails to provide the usual response, medical advice should be sought immediately, as this is often a sign of destabilization of COPD. Under these circumstances, the therapeutic regimen should be reevaluated and additional therapeutic options should be considered.

No dose adjustment is required for patients with renal or hepatic impairment. However, since the clearance of BROVANA Inhalation Solution is prolonged in patients with hepatic impairment, they should be monitored closely.

The drug compatibility (physical and chemical), efficacy, and safety of BROVANA Inhalation Solution when mixed with other drugs in a nebulizer have not been established.

The safety and efficacy of BROVANA Inhalation Solution have been established in clinical trials when administered using the PARI LC® Plus nebulizer (with a face mask or mouthpiece) and the PARI DURA NEB™ 3000 compressor. The safety and efficacy of BROVANA Inhalation Solution delivered from non-compressor based nebulizer systems have not been established.

3 DOSAGE FORMS AND STRENGTHS

BROVANA (arformoterol tartrate) Inhalation Solution is supplied as a sterile solution for nebulization in low-density polyethylene unit-dose vials. Each 2 mL vial contains 15 mcg of arformoterol equivalent to 22 mcg of arformoterol tartrate.

4 CONTRAINDICATIONS

BROVANA Inhalation Solution is contraindicated in patients with a history of hypersensitivity to arformoterol, racemic formoterol or to any other components of this product.

All LABA, including BROVANA Inhalation Solution, are contraindicated in patients with asthma without use of a long-term asthma control medication [*see WARNINGS AND PRECAUTIONS (5)*].

5 WARNINGS AND PRECAUTIONS

5.1 Asthma-Related Deaths

[see BOXED WARNING]

Data from a large placebo-controlled study in asthma patients showed that long-acting $beta_2$-adrenergic agonists (LABA) increase the risk of asthma-related death. This finding is considered a class effect of LABA, including arformoterol, the active ingredient in BROVANA Inhalation Solution. The safety and efficacy of BROVANA Inhalation Solution in patients with asthma have not been established. All LABA, including BROVANA Inhalation Solution, are contraindicated in patients with asthma without use of a long-term asthma control medication [*see CONTRAINDICATIONS (4)*]. Data are not available to determine whether the rate of deaths in patients with COPD is increased by long-acting $beta_2$-adrenergic agonists.

A 28-week, placebo-controlled US study comparing the safety of salmeterol with placebo, each added to usual asthma therapy, showed an increase in asthma-related deaths in patients receiving salmeterol (13/13,176 in patients treated with salmeterol vs. 3/13,179 in patients treated with placebo; RR 4.37, 95% CI 1.25, 15.34). The increased risk of asthma-related death is considered a class effect of the long-acting $beta_2$-adrenergic agonists, including BROVANA Inhalation Solution. No study adequate to determine whether the rate of asthma-related death is increased in patients treated with BROVANA Inhalation Solution has been conducted.

Clinical studies with racemic formoterol suggested a higher incidence of serious asthma exacerbations in patients who received racemic formoterol than in those who received placebo. The sizes of these studies were not adequate to precisely quantify the differences in serious asthma exacerbation rates between treatment groups.

5.2 Deterioration of Disease and Acute Episodes

BROVANA Inhalation Solution should not be initiated in patients with acutely deteriorating COPD, which may be a life-threatening condition. The use of BROVANA Inhalation Solution in this setting is inappropriate.

BROVANA Inhalation Solution is not indicated for the treatment of acute episodes of bronchospasm, i.e., as rescue therapy and extra doses should not be used for that purpose. Acute symptoms should be treated with an inhaled short-acting $beta_2$-agonist.

When beginning BROVANA Inhalation Solution, patients who have been taking inhaled short-acting $beta_2$-agonists on a regular basis (e.g., four times a day) should be instructed to discontinue the regular use of these drugs and use them only for symptomatic relief of acute respiratory symptoms. When prescribing BROVANA Inhalation Solution, the healthcare provider should also prescribe an inhaled, short-acting $beta_2$-agonist and instruct the patient how it should be used. Increasing inhaled $beta_2$-agonist use is a signal of deteriorating disease for which prompt medical attention is indicated. COPD may deteriorate acutely over a period of hours or chronically over several days or longer. If BROVANA Inhalation Solution no longer controls the symptoms of bronchoconstriction, or the patient's inhaled, short-acting $beta_2$-agonist becomes less effective or the patient needs more inhalation of short-acting $beta_2$-agonist than usual, these may be markers of deterioration of disease. In this setting, a reevaluation of the patient and the COPD treatment regimen should be undertaken at once. Increasing the daily dosage of BROVANA Inhalation Solution beyond the recommended 15 mcg twice daily dose is not appropriate in this situation.

5.3 Excessive Use of BROVANA Inhalation Solution and Use with Other Long-Acting $Beta_2$-Agonists

Fatalities have been reported in association with excessive use of inhaled sympathomimetic drugs. As with other inhaled $beta_2$-adrenergic drugs, BROVANA Inhalation Solution should not be used more often, at higher doses than recommended, or in conjunction with other medications containing long-acting $beta_2$-agonists.

5.4 Paradoxical Bronchospasm

As with other inhaled $beta_2$-agonists, BROVANA Inhalation Solution can produce paradoxical bronchospasm that may be life-threatening. If paradoxical bronchospasm occurs, BROVANA Inhalation Solution should be discontinued immediately and alternative therapy instituted.

5.5 Cardiovascular Effects

BROVANA Inhalation Solution, like other $beta_2$-agonists, can produce a clinically significant cardiovascular effect in some patients as measured by increases in pulse rate, systolic and/or diastolic blood pressure, and/or symptoms. If such effects occur, the drug may need to be discontinued. In addition, beta-agonists have been reported to produce ECG changes, such as flattening of the T-wave, prolongation of the QTc interval, and ST segment depression. The clinical significance of these findings is unknown. BROVANA Inhalation Solution, as with other sympathomimetic amines, should be used with caution in patients with cardiovascular disorders, especially coronary insufficiency, cardiac arrhythmias, and hypertension.

5.6 Coexisting Conditions

BROVANA Inhalation Solution, like other sympathomimetic amines, should be used with caution in patients with cardiovascular disorders, especially coronary insufficiency, cardiac arrhythmias, and hypertension; in patients with convulsive disorders or thyrotoxicosis, and in patients who are unusually responsive to sympathomimetic amines. In two pooled, 12-week, placebo-controlled trials investigating BROVANA Inhalation Solution doses of 15 µg BID, 25 µg BID, and 50 µg QD, changes in mean predose and 2-hour post dose systolic and/or diastolic blood pressure were seen as a general fall of 2-4 mm/Hg; for pulse rate the mean of maximal increases were 8.8-12.0 beats/min. Over the course of a one-year study measuring serial electrocardiograms while receiving a dose of 50 mcg daily of BROVANA Inhalation Solution resulted in an approximately 3.0 ms increase in QT_{C-F} compared to the active comparator, salmeterol. Doses of the related $beta_2$-agonist albuterol, when administered intravenously, have been reported to aggravate preexisting diabetes mellitus and ketoacidosis.

5.7 Hypokalemia and Hyperglycemia

Beta-agonist medications may produce significant hypokalemia in some patients, possibly through intracellular shunting, which has the potential to produce adverse cardiovascular effects [*see CLINICAL PHARMACOLOGY (12.2)*]. The decrease in serum potassium is usually transient, not requiring supplementation. Beta-agonist medications may produce transient hyperglycemia in some patients.

Clinically significant and dose-related changes in serum potassium and blood glucose were infrequent during clinical trials with long-term administration of BROVANA Inhalation Solution at the recommended dose.

5.8 Immediate Hypersensitivity Reactions

Immediate hypersensitivity reactions may occur after administration of BROVANA Inhalation Solution as demonstrated by cases of anaphylactic reaction, urticaria, angioedema, rash and bronchospasm.

6 ADVERSE REACTIONS

Long-acting $beta_2$-adrenergic agonists increase the risk of asthma-related death *[see BOXED WARNING and WARNINGS AND PRECAUTIONS (5.1)]*.

6.1 $Beta_2$-Agonist Adverse Reaction Profile

Adverse reactions to BROVANA Inhalation Solution are expected to be similar in nature to other $beta_2$-adrenergic receptor agonists including: angina, hypertension or hypotension, tachycardia, arrhythmias, nervousness, headache, tremor, dry mouth, palpitation, muscle cramps, nausea, dizziness, fatigue, malaise, hypokalemia, hyperglycemia, metabolic acidosis and insomnia.

6.2 Clinical Trials Experience

Because clinical trials are conducted under widely varying conditions, adverse reaction rates observed in clinical trials of a drug cannot be directly compared to rates in the clinical trials of another drug and may not reflect the rates observed in clinical practice.

The safety data described below for adults ≥35 years of age are based on 2 clinical trials of 12 weeks. In the 2 trials of 12 weeks duration, 1456 patients (860 males and 596 females, ages 34 to 89 years old) with COPD were treated with BROVANA Inhalation Solution 15 mcg twice daily, 25 mcg twice daily, 50 mcg once daily, salmeterol 42 mcg twice daily, or placebo. The racial/ethnic distribution in these two trials included 1383 Caucasians, 49 Blacks, 10 Asians, and 10 Hispanics, and 4 patients classified as Other.

Adults with COPD

Among 1,456 COPD patients in two 12-week, placebo-controlled trials, 288 were treated with BROVANA Inhalation Solution 15 mcg twice daily and 293 were treated with placebo. Doses of 25 mcg twice daily and 50 mcg once daily were also evaluated.

Table 1 shows adverse reaction rates among patients from these two trials where the frequency was greater than or equal to 2% in the BROVANA Inhalation Solution 15 mcg twice daily group and where the rate in the BROVANA Inhalation Solution 15 mcg twice daily group exceeded the rate in the placebo group. The total number and percent of patients who reported adverse events were 202 (70%) in the 15 mcg twice daily and 219 (75%) in the placebo groups. Ten adverse events demonstrated a dose relationship: asthenia, fever, bronchitis, COPD, headache, vomiting, hyperkalemia, leukocytosis, nervousness, and tremor.

Table 1: Number of Patients Experiencing Adverse Events from Two 12-Week, Double-Blind, Placebo-Controlled Clinical Trials

	BROVANA Inhalation Solution 15 mcg twice daily		Placebo	
	n	(%)	n	(%)
Total Patients	288	(100)	293	(100)
Pain	23	(8)	16	(5)
Chest Pain	19	(7)	19	(6)
Back Pain	16	(6)	6	(2)
Diarrhea	16	(6)	13	(4)
Sinusitis	13	(5)	11	(4)
Leg Cramps	12	(4)	6	(2)
Dyspnea	11	(4)	7	(2)
Rash	11	(4)	5	(2)
Flu Syndrome	10	(3)	4	(1)
Peripheral Edema	8	(3)	7	(2)
Lung Disorder*	7	(2)	2	(1)

* Reported terms coded to "Lung Disorder" were predominantly pulmonary or chest congestion.

Adverse events occurring in patients treated with BROVANA Inhalation Solution 15 mcg twice daily with a frequency of <2%, but greater than placebo, were as follows:

Body as a Whole: abscess, allergic reaction, digitalis intoxication, fever, hernia, injection site pain, neck rigidity, neoplasm, pelvic pain, retroperitoneal hemorrhage

Cardiovascular: arteriosclerosis, atrial flutter, AV block, congestive heart failure, heart block, myocardial infarct, QT interval prolonged, supraventricular tachycardia, inverted T-wave
Digestive: constipation, gastritis, melena, oral moniliasis, periodontal abscess, rectal hemorrhage
Metabolic and Nutritional Disorders: dehydration, edema, glucose tolerance decreased, gout, hyperglycemia, hyperlipemia, hypoglycemia, hypokalemia
Musculoskeletal: arthralgia, arthritis, bone disorder, rheumatoid arthritis, tendinous contracture
Nervous: agitation, cerebral infarct, circumoral paresthesia, hypokinesia, paralysis, somnolence, tremor
Respiratory: carcinoma of the lung, respiratory disorder, voice alteration
Skin and Appendages: dry skin, herpes simplex, herpes zoster, skin discoloration, skin hypertrophy
Special Senses: abnormal vision, glaucoma
Urogenital: breast neoplasm, calcium crystalluria, cystitis, glycosuria, hematuria, kidney calculus, nocturia, PSA increase, pyuria, urinary tract disorder, urine abnormality.

In these trials, the overall frequency of all cardiovascular adverse events was 6.9% in BROVANA Inhalation Solution 15 mcg twice daily and 13.3% in the placebo group. There were no frequently occurring specific cardiovascular adverse events for BROVANA Inhalation Solution (frequency ≥1% and greater than placebo). The rate of COPD exacerbations was also comparable between the BROVANA Inhalation Solution 15 mcg twice daily and placebo groups, 12.2% and 15.1%, respectively.

7 DRUG INTERACTIONS

7.1 Adrenergic Drugs

If additional adrenergic drugs are to be administered by any route, they should be used with caution because the sympathetic effects of arformoterol may be potentiated [*see WARNINGS AND PRECAUTIONS (5.3, 5.5, 5.6, 5.7)*].

7.2 Xanthine Derivatives, Steroids, or Diuretics

Concomitant treatment with methylxanthine (aminophylline, theophylline), steroids, or diuretics may potentiate any hypokalemic effect of adrenergic agonists including BROVANA Inhalation Solution [*see WARNINGS AND PRECAUTIONS (5.7)*].

The concurrent use of intravenously or orally administered methylxanthines (e.g., aminophylline, theophylline) by patients receiving BROVANA Inhalation Solution has not been completely evaluated. In two combined 12-week, placebo-controlled trials that included BROVANA Inhalation Solution doses of 15 mcg twice daily, 25 mcg twice daily, and 50 mcg once daily, 54 of 873 BROVANA Inhalation Solution-treated subjects received concomitant theophylline at study entry. In a 12-month controlled trial that included a 50 mcg once daily BROVANA Inhalation Solution dose, 30 of the 528 BROVANA Inhalation Solution-treated subjects received concomitant theophylline at study entry. In these trials, heart rate and systolic blood pressure were approximately 2-3 bpm and 6-8 mm Hg higher, respectively, in subjects on concomitant theophylline compared with the overall population.

7.3 Non-potassium Sparing Diuretics

The ECG changes and/or hypokalemia that may result from the administration of non-potassium sparing diuretics (such as loop or thiazide diuretics) can be acutely worsened by beta-agonists, especially when the recommended dose of the beta-agonist is exceeded. Although the clinical significance of these effects is not known, caution is advised in the co-administration of beta-agonists, including BROVANA Inhalation Solution, with non-potassium sparing diuretics.

7.4 MAO Inhibitors, Tricyclic Antidepressants, QTc Prolonging Drugs

BROVANA Inhalation Solution, as with other beta-agonists, should be administered with extreme caution to patients being treated with monoamine oxidase inhibitors, tricyclic antidepressants, or drugs known to prolong the QTc interval because of the effect of adrenergic agonists on the cardiovascular system may be potentiated by these agents. Drugs that are known to prolong the QTc interval have an increased risk of ventricular arrhythmias.

7.5 Beta-Blockers

Beta-adrenergic receptor antagonists (beta-blockers) and BROVANA Inhalation Solution may inhibit the effect of each other when administered concurrently. Beta-blockers not only block the therapeutic effects of beta-agonists, but may produce severe bronchospasm in COPD patients. Therefore, patients with COPD should not normally be treated with beta-blockers. However, under certain circumstances, e.g., as prophylaxis after myocardial infarction, there may be no acceptable alternatives to the use of beta-blockers in patients with COPD. In this setting, cardioselective beta-blockers could be considered, although they should be administered with caution.

8 USE IN SPECIFIC POPULATIONS

8.1 Pregnancy

Teratogenic Effects: ***Pregnancy Category C***

There are no adequate and well-controlled studies of BROVANA Inhalation Solution in pregnant women. Arformoterol has been shown to be teratogenic in rats and rabbits. Arformoterol also caused neonatal mortality and developmental delays in rats. Because animal reproduction studies are not always predictive of human response, BROVANA Inhalation Solution should be used during pregnancy, only if the potential benefit justifies the potential risk to the fetus.

Arformoterol has been shown to be teratogenic in rats based upon findings of omphalocele (umbilical hernia), a malformation, at oral doses equal to and greater than approximately 370 times adult exposure at the maximum recommended daily inhalation dose. Increased pup loss at birth and during lactation and decreased pup weights were observed in rats at oral doses equal to and greater than approximately 1100 times adult exposure at the maximum recommended daily inhalation dose. Delays in development were evident with an oral dose approximately 2400 times adult exposure at the maximum recommended daily inhalation dose.

Arformoterol has been shown to be teratogenic in rabbits based upon findings of malpositioned right kidney, a malformation, at oral doses equal to and greater than approximately 8400 times adult exposure at the maximum recommended daily inhalation dose. Malformations including brachydactyly, bulbous aorta, and liver cysts were observed at oral doses equal to and greater than approximately 22,000 times the maximum recommended daily inhalation dose in adults on a mg/m^2 basis. Malformations including adactyly, lobular dysgenesis of the lung, and interventricular septal defect were observed at an oral dose approximately 43,000 times the maximum recommended daily inhalation dose in adults on a mg/m^2 basis. Embryolethality was observed at an oral dose approximately 43,000 times the maximum recommended daily inhalation dose in adults on a mg/m^2 basis. Decreased pup body weights were observed at oral doses equal to and greater than approximately 22,000 times the maximum recommended daily inhalation dose in adults on a mg/m^2 basis. There were no teratogenic findings in rabbits with oral doses equal to or less than approximately 4900 times adult exposure at the maximum recommended daily inhalation dose.

8.2 Labor and Delivery

There are no human studies that have investigated the effects of BROVANA Inhalation Solution on preterm labor or labor at term.

Because beta-agonists may potentially interfere with uterine contractility, BROVANA Inhalation Solution should be used during labor and delivery only if the potential benefit justifies the potential risk.

8.3 Nursing Mothers

In reproductive studies in rats, arformoterol was excreted in the milk. It is not known whether arformoterol is excreted in human milk. Because many drugs are excreted in human milk, caution should be exercised when BROVANA Inhalation Solution is administered to a nursing woman.

8.4 Pediatric Use

BROVANA Inhalation Solution is approved for use in the long-term maintenance treatment of bronchoconstriction associated with chronic obstructive pulmonary disease, including chronic bronchitis and emphysema. This disease does not occur in children. The safety and efficacy of BROVANA Inhalation Solution in pediatric patients have not been established.

8.5 Geriatric Use

Of the 873 patients who received BROVANA Inhalation Solution in two placebo-controlled clinical studies in adults with COPD, 391 (45%) were 65 years of age or older while 96 (11%) were 75 years of age or older. No overall differences in safety or effectiveness were observed between these subjects and younger subjects. Among subjects age 65 years and older, 129 (33%) received BROVANA Inhalation Solution at the recommended dose of 15 mcg twice daily, while the remainder received higher doses. ECG alerts for ventricular ectopy in patients 65 to ≤75 years of age were comparable among patients receiving 15 mcg twice daily, 25 mcg twice daily, and placebo (3.9%, 5.2%, and 7.1%, respectively). A higher frequency (12.4%) was observed when BROVANA Inhalation Solution was dosed at 50 mcg once daily. The clinical significance of this finding is not known. Other reported clinical experience has not identified differences in responses between the elderly and younger patients, but greater sensitivity of some older individuals cannot be ruled out.

8.6 Hepatic Impairment

BROVANA Inhalation Solution should be used cautiously in patients with hepatic impairment due to increased systemic exposure in these patients [*see Pharmacokinetics (12.3)*].

8.7 Renal Impairment

The systemic exposure to arformoterol was similar to renally impaired patients compared with demographically matched healthy control subjects [*see Pharmacokinetics (12.3)*].

9 DRUG ABUSE AND DEPENDENCE

There were no reported cases of abuse or evidence of drug dependence with the use of BROVANA Inhalation Solution in the clinical trials.

10 OVERDOSAGE

The expected signs and symptoms associated with overdosage of BROVANA (arformoterol tartrate) Inhalation Solution are those of excessive beta-adrenergic stimulation and/or occurrence or exaggeration of any of the signs and symptoms listed under **ADVERSE REACTIONS**. Signs and symptoms may include angina, hypertension or hypotension, tachycardia, with rates up to 200 beats/min, arrhythmias, nervousness, headache, tremor, dry mouth, palpitation, muscle cramps, nausea, dizziness, fatigue, malaise, hypokalemia, hyperglycemia, metabolic acidosis and insomnia. As with all inhaled sympathomimetic medications, cardiac arrest and even death may be associated with an overdose of BROVANA Inhalation Solution.

Treatment of overdosage consists of discontinuation of BROVANA Inhalation Solution together with institution of appropriate symptomatic and/or supportive therapy. The judicious use of a cardioselective beta-receptor blocker may be considered, bearing in mind that such medication can produce bronchospasm. There is insufficient evidence to determine if dialysis is beneficial for overdosage of BROVANA Inhalation Solution. Cardiac monitoring is recommended in cases of overdosage.

Clinical signs in dogs included flushing of the body surface and facial area, reddening of the ears and gums, tremor, and increased heart rate. A death was reported in dogs after a single oral dose of 5 mg/kg (approximately 4500 times the maximum recommended daily inhalation dose in adults on a mg/m^2 basis). Death occurred for a rat that received arformoterol at a single inhalation dose of 1600 mcg/kg (approximately 430 times the maximum recommended daily inhalation dose in adults on a mg/m^2 basis).

11 DESCRIPTION

BROVANA (arformoterol tartrate) Inhalation Solution is a sterile, clear, colorless, aqueous solution of the tartrate salt of arformoterol, the (R,R)-enantiomer of formoterol.

Arformoterol is a selective beta$_2$-adrenergic bronchodilator. The chemical name for arformoterol tartrate is formamide, N-[2-hydroxy-5-[(1R)-1-hydroxy-2-[[(1R)-2-(4-methoxyphenyl)-1-methylethyl]amino]ethyl]phenyl]-, (2R,3R)-2,3-dihydroxybutanedioate (1:1 salt), and its established structural formula is as follows:

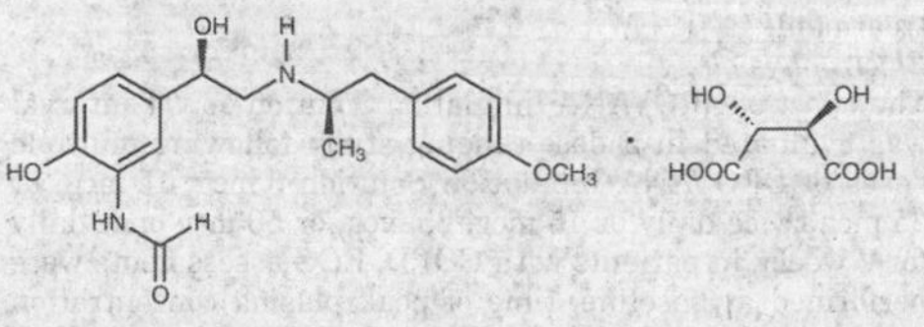

The molecular weight of *arformoterol tartrate* is 494.5 g/mol, and its empirical formula is $C_{19}H_{24}N_2O_4 \bullet C_4H_6O_6$ (1:1 salt). It is a white to off-white solid that is slightly soluble in water.

Arformoterol tartrate is the United States Adopted Name (USAN) for (R,R)-formoterol L-tartrate.

BROVANA (arformoterol tartrate) Inhalation Solution is supplied as 2 mL of arformoterol tartrate solution packaged in 2.1 mL unit-dose, low-density polyethylene (LDPE) unit-dose vials. Each unit-dose vial contains 15 mcg of arformoterol (equivalent to 22 mcg of arformoterol tartrate) in a sterile, isotonic saline solution, pH-adjusted to 5.0 with citric acid and sodium citrate.

BROVANA Inhalation Solution requires no dilution before administration by nebulization. Like all other nebulized treatments, the amount delivered to the lungs will depend upon patient factors, the nebulizer used, and compressor performance. Using the PARI LC® Plus nebulizer (with mouthpiece) connected to a PARI DURA NEB™ 3000 compressor under *in vitro* conditions, the mean delivered dose from the mouthpiece (% nominal) was approximately 4.1 mcg (27.6%) at a mean flow rate of 3.3 L/min. The mean nebulization time was 6 minutes or less. BROVANA Inhalation Solution should be administered from a standard jet nebulizer at adequate flow rates via face mask or mouthpiece.

Patients should be carefully instructed on the correct use of this drug product (please refer to the accompanying **Medication Guide**).

12 CLINICAL PHARMACOLOGY

12.1 Mechanism of Action

Arformoterol, the (R,R)-enantiomer of formoterol, is a selective long-acting beta$_2$-adrenergic receptor agonist (beta$_2$-agonist) that has two-fold greater potency than racemic formoterol (which contains both the (S,S) and (R,R)-enantiomers). The (S,S)-enantiomer is about 1,000-fold less potent as a beta$_2$-agonist than the (R,R)-enantiomer. While it is recognized that $beta_2$-receptors are the predominant adrenergic receptors in bronchial smooth muscle and $beta_1$-receptors are the predominant receptors in the heart, data indicate that there are also $beta_2$-receptors in the human heart comprising 10% to 50% of the total beta-adrenergic receptors. The precise function of these receptors has not been established, but they raise the possibility that even highly selective $beta_2$-agonists may have cardiac effects.

The pharmacologic effects of $beta_2$-adrenoceptor agonist drugs, including arformoterol, are at least in part attributable to stimulation of intracellular adenyl cyclase, the enzyme that catalyzes the conversion of adenosine triphosphate (ATP) to cyclic-3′,5′-adenosine monophosphate (cyclic AMP). Increased intracellular cyclic AMP levels cause relaxation of bronchial smooth muscle and inhibition of release of mediators of immediate hypersensitivity from cells, especially from mast cells.

In vitro tests show that arformoterol is an inhibitor of the release of mast cell mediators, such as histamine and leukotrienes, from the human lung. Arformoterol also inhibits histamine-induced plasma albumin extravasation in anesthetized guinea pigs and inhibits allergen-induced eosinophil influx in dogs with airway hyper-responsiveness. The relevance of these *in vitro* and animal findings to humans is unknown.

12.2 Pharmacodynamics

Systemic Safety and Pharmacokinetic/Pharmacodynamic Relationships

The predominant adverse effects of inhaled $beta_2$-agonists occur as a result of excessive activation of systemic beta-adrenergic receptors. The most common adverse effects may include skeletal muscle tremor and cramps, insomnia, tachycardia, decreases in plasma potassium, and increases in plasma glucose.

Effects on Serum Potassium and Serum Glucose Levels

Changes in serum potassium and serum glucose were evaluated in a dose-ranging study of twice daily (5 mcg, 15 mcg, or 25 mcg; 215 patients with COPD) and once daily (15 mcg, 25 mcg, or 50 mcg; 191 patients with COPD) BROVANA Inhalation Solution in COPD patients. At 2 and 6 hours post dose at week 0 (after the first dose), mean changes in serum potassium ranging from 0 to -0.3 mEq/L were observed in the BROVANA Inhalation Solution groups with similar changes observed after 2 weeks of treatment. Changes in mean serum glucose levels, ranging from a decrease of 1.2 mg/dL to an increase of 32.8 mg/dL were observed for BROVANA Inhalation Solution dose groups at both 2 and 6 hours post dose, both after the first dose and 14 days of daily treatment.

Electrophysiology

The effect of BROVANA Inhalation Solution on QT interval was evaluated in a dose-ranging study following multiple doses of BROVANA Inhalation Solution 5 mcg, 15 mcg, or 25 mcg twice daily or 15 mcg, 25 mcg, or 50 mcg once daily for 2 weeks in patients with COPD. ECG assessments were performed at baseline, time of peak plasma concentration and throughout the dosing interval. Different methods of correcting for heart rate were employed, including a subject-specific method and the Fridericia method.

Relative to placebo, the mean change in subject-specific QTc averaged over the dosing interval ranged from -1.8 to 2.7 msec, indicating little effect of BROVANA Inhalation Solution on cardiac repolarization after 2 weeks of treatment. The maximum mean change in subject-specific QTc for the BROVANA Inhalation Solution 15 mcg twice daily dose was 17.3 msec, compared with 15.4 msec in the placebo group. No apparent correlation of QTc with arformoterol plasma concentration was observed.

Electrocardiographic Monitoring in Patients with COPD

The effect of different doses of BROVANA Inhalation Solution on cardiac rhythm was assessed using 24-hour Holter monitoring in two 12-week, double-blind, placebo-controlled studies of 1,456 patients with COPD (873 received BROVANA Inhalation Solution at 15 or 25 mcg twice daily or 50 mcg once daily doses; 293 received placebo; 290 received salmeterol). The 24-hour Holter monitoring occurred once at baseline, and up to 3 times during the 12-week treatment period. The rates of new-onset cardiac arrhythmias not present at baseline over the double-blind 12-week treatment period were similar (approximately 33-34%) for patients who received BROVANA Inhalation Solution 15 mcg twice daily to those who received placebo. There was a dose-related increase in new, treatment-emergent arrhythmias seen in patients who received BROVANA Inhalation Solution 25 mcg twice daily and 50 mcg once daily, 37.6% and 40.1%, respectively. The frequencies of new treatment-emergent events of non-sustained (3-10 beat run) and sustained (>10 beat run) ventricular tachycardia were 7.4% and 1.1% in BROVANA Inhalation Solution 15 mcg twice daily and 6.9% and 1.0% in placebo. In patients who received BROVANA Inhalation Solution 25 mcg twice daily and 50 mcg once daily, the frequencies of non-sustained (6.2% and 8.2%, respectively) and sustained ventricular tachycardia (1.0% and 1.0%, respectively) were similar. Five cases of ventricular tachycardia were reported as adverse events (1 in BROVANA Inhalation Solution 15 mcg twice daily and 4 in placebo), with two of these events leading to discontinuation of treatment (2 in placebo).

There were no baseline occurrences of atrial fibrillation/flutter observed on 24-hour Holter monitoring in patients treated with BROVANA Inhalation Solution 15 mcg twice daily or placebo. New, treatment-emergent atrial fibrillation/flutter occurred in 0.4% of patients who received BROVANA Inhalation Solution 15 mcg twice daily and 0.3% of patients who received placebo. There was a dose-related increase in the frequency of atrial fibrillation/flutter reported in the BROVANA Inhalation Solution 25 mcg twice daily and 50 mcg once daily dose groups of 0.7% and 1.4%, respectively. Two cases of atrial fibrillation/flutter were reported as adverse events (1 in BROVANA Inhalation Solution 15 mcg twice daily and 1 in placebo).

Dose-related increases in mean maximum change in heart rate in the 12 hours after dosing were also observed following 12 weeks of dosing with BROVANA Inhalation Solution 15 mcg twice daily (8.8 bpm), 25 mcg twice daily (9.9 bpm) and 50 mcg once daily (12 bpm) versus placebo (8.5 bpm).

Tachyphylaxis/Tolerance

Tolerance to the effects of inhaled beta-agonists can occur with regularly-scheduled, chronic use.

In two placebo-controlled clinical trials in patients with COPD involving approximately 725 patients in each, the overall efficacy of BROVANA Inhalation Solution was maintained throughout the 12-week trial duration. However, tolerance to the bronchodilator effect of BROVANA Inhalation Solution was observed after 6 weeks of dosing, as measured by a decrease in trough FEV_1. FEV_1 improvement at the end of the 12-hour dosing interval decreased by approximately one-third (22.1% mean improvement after the first dose compared to 14.6% at week 12). Tolerance to the trough FEV_1 bronchodilator effect of BROVANA Inhalation Solution was not accompanied by other clinical manifestations of tolerance in these trials.

12.3 Pharmacokinetics

The pharmacokinetics (PK) of arformoterol have been investigated in healthy subjects, elderly subjects, renally and hepatically impaired subjects, and COPD patients following the nebulization of the recommended therapeutic dose and doses up to 96 mcg.

Absorption

In COPD patients administered 15 mcg arformoterol every 12 hours for 14 days, the mean steady-state peak (R,R)-formoterol plasma concentration (C_{max}) and systemic exposure ($AUC_{0\text{-}12h}$) were 4.3 pg/mL and 34.5 pg.hr/mL, respectively. The median steady-state peak (R,R)-formoterol plasma concentration time (t_{max}) was observed approximately one-half hour after drug administration.

Systemic exposure to (R,R)-formoterol increased linearly with dose in COPD patients following arformoterol doses of 5 mcg, 15 mcg, or 25 mcg twice daily for 2 weeks or 15 mcg, 25 mcg, or 50 mcg once daily for 2 weeks.

In a crossover study in patients with COPD, when arformoterol 15 mcg inhalation solution and 12 and 24 mcg formoterol fumarate inhalation powder (Foradil® Aerolizer®) was administered twice daily for 2 weeks, the accumulation index was approximately 2.5 based on the plasma (R,R)-formoterol concentrations in all three treatments. At steady- state, geometric means of systemic exposure ($AUC_{0\text{-}12h}$) to (R,R)-formoterol following 15 mcg of arformoterol inhalation solution and 12 mcg of formoterol fumarate inhalation powder were 39.33 pg.hr/mL and 33.93 pg.hr/mL, respectively (ratio 1.16; 90% CI 1.00, 1.35), while the geometric means of the C_{max} were 4.30 pg/mL and 4.75 pg/mL, respectively (ratio 0.91; 90% CI 0.76, 1.09).

In a study in patients with asthma, treatment with arformoterol 50 mcg with pre- and post-treatment with activated charcoal resulted in a geometric mean decrease in (R,R)-formoterol $AUC_{0\text{-}6h}$ by 27% and C_{max} by 23% as compared to treatment with arformoterol 50 mcg alone. This suggests that a substantial portion of systemic drug exposure is due to pulmonary absorption.

Distribution

The binding of arformoterol to human plasma proteins *in vitro* was 52-65% at concentrations of 0.25, 0.5 and 1.0 ng/mL of radiolabeled arformoterol. The concentrations of arformoterol used to assess the plasma protein binding were higher than those achieved in plasma following inhalation of multiple doses of 50 mcg arformoterol.

Metabolism

In vitro profiling studies in hepatocytes and liver microsomes have shown that arformoterol is primarily metabolized by direct conjugation (glucuronidation) and secondarily by O-demethylation. At least five human uridine diphosphoglucuronosyltransferase (UGT) isozymes catalyze arformoterol glucuronidation *in vitro*. Two cytochrome P450 isozymes (CYP2D6 and secondarily CYP2C19) catalyze the O-demethylation of arformoterol.

Arformoterol was almost entirely metabolized following oral administration of 35 mcg of radiolabeled arformoterol in eight healthy subjects. Direct conjugation of arformoterol with glucuronic acid was the major metabolic pathway. Most of the drug-related material in plasma and urine was in the form of glucuronide or sulfate conjugates of arformoterol. O-Desmethylation and conjugates of the O-desmethyl metabolite were relatively minor metabolites accounting for less than 17% of the dose recovered in urine and feces.

Elimination

After administration of a single oral dose of radiolabeled arformoterol to eight healthy male subjects, 63% of the total radioactive dose was recovered in urine and 11% in feces within 48 hours. A total of 89% of the total radioactive dose was recovered within 14 days, with 67% in urine and 22% in feces. Approximately 1% of the dose was recovered as unchanged arformoterol in urine over 14 days. Renal clearance was 8.9 L/hr for unchanged arformoterol in these subjects. In COPD patients given 15 mcg inhaled arformoterol twice a day for 14 days, the mean terminal half-life of arformoterol was 26 hours.

Special Populations:

Gender

A population PK analysis indicated that there was no effect of gender upon the pharmacokinetics of arformoterol.

Race

The influence of race on arformoterol pharmacokinetics was assessed using a population PK analysis and data from healthy subjects. There was no clinically significant impact of race upon the pharmacokinetic profile of arformoterol.

Geriatric

The pharmacokinetic profile of arformoterol in 24 elderly subjects (aged 65 years or older) was compared to a younger cohort of 24 subjects (18-45 years) that were matched for body weight and gender. No significant differences in systemic exposure (AUC and C_{max}) were observed when the two groups were compared.

Pediatric

The pharmacokinetics of arformoterol have not been studied in pediatric subjects.

Hepatic Impairment

The pharmacokinetic profile of arformoterol was assessed in 24 subjects with mild, moderate, and severe hepatic impairment. The systemic exposure (C_{max} and AUC) to arformoterol increased 1.3 to 2.4-fold in subjects with hepatic impairment compared to 16 demographically matched healthy control subjects. No clear relationship between drug exposure and the severity of hepatic impairment was observed. BROVANA Inhalation Solution should be used cautiously in patients with hepatic impairment.

Renal Impairment

The impact of renal disease upon the pharmacokinetics of arformoterol was studied in 24 subjects with mild, moderate, or severe renal impairment. Systemic exposure (AUC and C_{max}) to arformoterol was similar in renally impaired patients compared with demographically matched healthy control subjects.

Drug-Drug Interaction

When paroxetine, a potent inhibitor of CYP2D6, was co-administered with BROVANA Inhalation Solution at steady-state, exposure to either drug was not altered. Dosage adjustments of BROVANA Inhalation Solution are not necessary when the drug is given concomitantly with potent CYP2D6 inhibitors.

Arformoterol did not inhibit CYP1A2, CYP2A6, CYP2C9/10, CYP2C19, CYP2D6, CYP2E1, CYP3A4/5, or CYP4A9/11 enzymes at >1,000-fold higher concentrations than the expected peak plasma concentrations following a therapeutic dose.

12.4 Pharmacogenetics

Arformoterol is eliminated through the action of multiple drug metabolizing enzymes. Direct glucuronidation of arformoterol is mediated by several UGT enzymes and is the primary elimination route. O-Desmethylation is a secondary route catalyzed by the CYP enzymes CYP2D6 and CYP2C19. In otherwise healthy subjects with reduced CYP2D6 and/or UGT1A1 enzyme activity, there was no impact on systemic exposure to arformoterol compared to subjects with normal CYP2D6 and/or UGT1A1 enzyme activities.

13 NONCLINICAL TOXICOLOGY

13.1 Carcinogenesis, Mutagenesis, Impairment of Fertility

Long-term studies were conducted in mice using oral administration and rats using inhalation administration to evaluate the carcinogenic potential of arformoterol.

In a 24-month carcinogenicity study in CD-1 mice, arformoterol caused a dose-related increase in the incidence of uterine and cervical endometrial stromal polyps and stromal cell sarcoma in female mice at oral doses of 1 mg/kg and above (AUC exposure approximately 70 times adult exposure at the maximum recommended daily inhalation dose).

In a 24-month carcinogenicity study in Sprague-Dawley rats, arformoterol caused a statistically significant increase in the incidence of thyroid gland c-cell adenoma and carcinoma in female rats at an inhalation dose of 200 mcg/kg (AUC exposure approximately 130 times adult exposure at the maximum recommended daily inhalation dose). There were no tumor findings with an inhalation dose of 40 mcg/kg (AUC exposure approximately 55 times adult exposure at the maximum recommended daily inhalation dose).

Arformoterol was not mutagenic or clastogenic in the following tests: mutagenicity tests in bacteria, chromosome aberration analyses in mammalian cells, and micronucleus test in mice.

Arformoterol had no effects on fertility and reproductive performance in rats at oral doses up to 10 mg/kg (approximately 2700 times the maximum recommended daily inhalation dose in adults on a mg/m^2 basis).

13.2 Animal Toxicology and/or Pharmacology

Animal Pharmacology

In animal studies investigating its cardiovascular effects, arformoterol induced dose-dependent increases in heart rate and decreases in blood pressure consistent with its pharmacology as a beta-adrenergic agonist. In dogs, at systemic exposures higher than anticipated clinically, arformoterol also induced exaggerated pharmacologic effects of a beta-adrenergic agonist on cardiac function as measured by electrocardiogram (sinus tachycardia, atrial premature beats, ventricular escape beats, PVCs).

Studies in laboratory animals (minipigs, rodents, and dogs) have demonstrated the occurrence of arrhythmias and sudden death (with histologic evidence of myocardial necrosis) when beta-agonists and methylxanthines are administered concurrently. The clinical significance of these findings is unknown.

Reproductive Toxicology Studies

Arformoterol has been shown to be teratogenic in rats based upon findings of omphalocele (umbilical hernia), a malformation, at oral doses of 1 mg/kg and above (AUC exposure approximately 370 times adult exposure at the maximum recommended daily inhalation dose). Increased pup loss at birth and during lactation and decreased pup weights were observed in rats at oral doses of 5 mg/kg and above (AUC exposure approximately 1100 times adult exposure at the maximum recommended daily inhalation dose). Delays in development were evident with an oral dose of 10 mg/kg (AUC exposure approximately 2400 times adult exposure at the maximum recommended daily inhalation dose).

Arformoterol has been shown to be teratogenic in rabbits based upon findings of malpositioned right kidney, a malformation, at oral doses of 20 mg/kg and above (AUC exposure approximately 8400 times adult exposure at the maximum recommended daily inhalation dose). Malformations including brachydactyly, bulbous aorta, and liver cysts were observed at doses of 40 mg/kg and above (approximately 22,000 times the maximum recommended daily inhalation dose in adults on a mg/m^2 basis). Malformations including adactyly, lobular dysgenesis of the lung, and interventricular septal defect were observed at 80 mg/kg (approximately 43,000 times the maximum recommended daily inhalation dose in adults on a mg/m^2 basis). Embryolethality was observed at 80 mg/kg/day (approximately 43,000 times the maximum recommended daily inhalation dose in adults on a mg/m^2 basis). Decreased pup body weights were observed at doses of 40 mg/kg/day and above (approximately 22,000 times the maximum recommended daily inhalation dose in adults on a mg/m^2 basis). There were no teratogenic findings in rabbits with oral dose of 10 mg/kg and lower (AUC exposure approximately 4900 times adult exposure at the maximum recommended daily inhalation dose).

14 CLINICAL STUDIES

14.1 Adult COPD Trials

BROVANA (arformoterol tartrate) Inhalation Solution was studied in two identical, 12-week, double-blind, placebo- and active-controlled, randomized, multi-center, parallel group trials conducted in the United States (Clinical Trial A and Clinical Trial B). A total of 1,456 adult patients (age range: 34 to 89 years; mean age: 63 years; gender: 860 males and 596 females) with COPD who had a mean FEV_1 of 1.3 L (42% of predicted) were enrolled in the two clinical trials. The racial/ethnic distribution in these two trials included 1383 Caucasians, 49 Blacks, 10 Asians, and 10 Hispanics, and 4 patients classified as Other. The diagnosis of COPD was based on a prior clinical diagnosis of COPD, a smoking history (greater than 15 pack-years), age (at least 35 years), spirometry results (baseline $FEV_1 \leq 65\%$ of predicted value and >0.70 L, and a FEV_1/forced vital capacity (FVC) ratio ≤70%). About 80% of patients in these studies had bronchodilator reversibility, defined as a 10% or greater increase in FEV_1 after inhalation of 2 actuations (180 mcg racemic albuterol from a metered dose inhaler). Both trials compared BROVANA Inhalation Solution 15 mcg twice daily (288 patients), 25 mcg twice daily (292 patients), 50 mcg once daily (293 patients) with placebo (293 subjects). Both trials included salmeterol inhalation aerosol, 42 mcg twice daily as an active comparator (290 patients).

In both 12-week trials, BROVANA Inhalation Solution 15 mcg twice daily resulted in a statistically significant change of approximately 11% in mean FEV_1 (as measured by percent change from study baseline FEV_1 at the end of the dosing interval over the 12 weeks of treatment, the primary efficacy endpoint) compared to placebo. Compared to BROVANA Inhalation Solution 15 mcg twice daily, BROVANA Inhalation Solution 25 mcg twice daily and 50 mcg once daily did not provide sufficient additional benefit on a variety of endpoints, including FEV_1, to support the use of higher doses. Plots of the mean change in FEV_1 values obtained over the 12 hours after dosing for the BROVANA Inhalation Solution 15 mcg twice daily dose group and for the placebo group are provided in Figures 1 and 2 for Clinical Trial A, below. The plots include mean FEV_1 change observed after the first dose and after 12 weeks of treatment. The results from Clinical Trial B were similar.

Figure 1 Mean Change in FEV_1 Over Time for Clinical Trial A at Week 0 (Day 1)

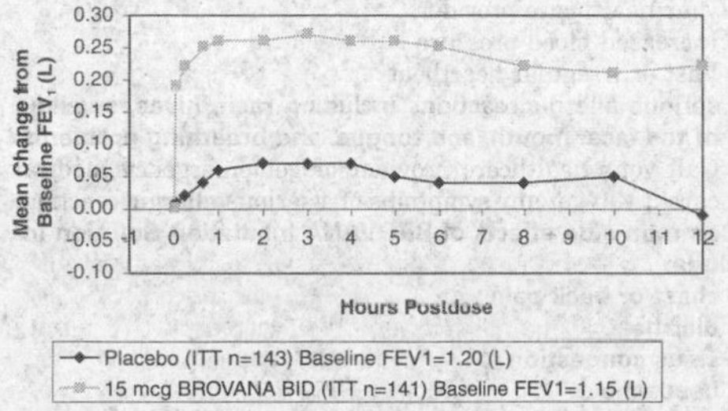

Figure 2 Mean Change in FEV_1 Over Time for Clinical Trial A at Week 12

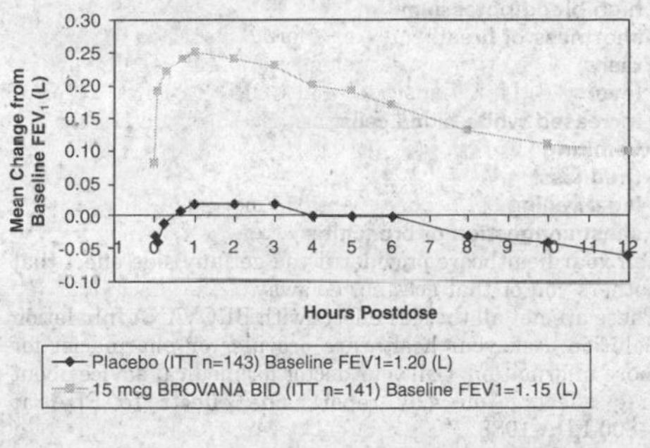

BROVANA Inhalation Solution 15 mcg twice daily significantly improved bronchodilation compared to placebo over the 12 hours after dosing (FEV_1 $AUC_{0\text{-}12h}$). This improvement was maintained over the 12-week study period.

Following the first dose of BROVANA Inhalation Solution 15 mcg, the median time to onset of bronchodilation, defined by an FEV_1 increase of 15%, occurred at 6.7 min. When defined as an increase in FEV_1 of 12% and 200 mL, the time to onset of bronchodilation was 20 min after dosing. Peak bronchodilator effect was generally seen within 1-3 hours of dosing.

In both clinical trials, compared to placebo, patients treated with BROVANA Inhalation Solution demonstrated improvements in peak expiratory flow rates, supplemental ipratropium and rescue albuterol use.

16 HOW SUPPLIED/STORAGE AND HANDLING

BROVANA (arformoterol tartrate) Inhalation Solution is supplied in a single strength (15 mcg of arformoterol, equivalent to 22 mcg of arformoterol tartrate) as 2 mL of a sterile solution in low-density polyethylene (LDPE) unit-dose vials overwrapped in foil. BROVANA Inhalation Solution is available in a shelf-carton containing 30 or 60 unit-dose vials.

NDC 63402-911-30: carton of 30 individually pouched unit-dose vials.

NDC 63402-911-64: carton of 60 unit-dose vials (15×4 unit-dose vial pouches).

Storage and Handling

Store BROVANA Inhalation Solution in the protective foil pouch under refrigeration at 36°-46°F (2°-8°C). Protect from light and excessive heat. After opening the pouch, unused unit-dose vials should be returned to, and stored in, the pouch. An opened unit-dose vial should be used right away. Discard any unit-dose vial if the solution is not colorless. Unopened foil pouches of BROVANA Inhalation Solution can also be stored at room temperature 68°-77°F (20°-25°C) for up to 6 weeks. If stored at room temperature, discard if not used after 6 weeks or if past the expiration date, whichever is sooner.

17 PATIENT COUNSELING INFORMATION

Patients should be instructed to read the accompanying Medication Guide with each new prescription and refill. The complete text of the Medication Guide is reprinted at the end of this document. Patients should be given the following information:

Asthma-Related Deaths, Acute Exacerbations or Deteriorations

Patients should be informed that long-acting $beta_2$-adrenergic agonists, such as BROVANA Inhalation Solution, increase risk of asthma-related death in patients with asthma.

BROVANA Inhalation Solution is not indicated to relieve acute respiratory symptoms and extra doses should not be used for that purpose. Acute symptoms should be treated with an inhaled, short-acting $beta_2$-agonist (the healthcare provider should prescribe the patient with such medication and instruct the patient in how it should be used). Patients should be instructed to seek medical attention if their symptoms worsen despite recommended doses of BROVANA Inhalation Solution, if BROVANA Inhalation Solution treatment becomes less effective, or if they need more inhalations of a short-acting $beta_2$-agonist than usual.

Appropriate Dosing

Patients should not stop using BROVANA Inhalation Solution unless told to do so by a healthcare provider because symptoms may get worse. Patients should not inhale more than one dose at any one time. The daily dosage of BROVANA Inhalation Solution should not exceed one unit-dose vial (15 mcg) by inhalation twice daily (30 mcg total daily dose). Excessive use of sympathomimetics may cause significant cardiovascular effects, and may be fatal.

Concomitant Therapy

Patients who have been taking inhaled, short-acting $beta_2$-agonists (e.g., levalbuterol) on a regular basis should be instructed to discontinue the regular use of these products and use them only for the symptomatic relief of acute symptoms.

BROVANA Inhalation Solution should not be used in conjunction with other inhaled medications containing long-acting $beta_2$-agonists. Patients should be warned not to stop or change the dose of other concomitant COPD therapy without medical advice, even if symptoms improve after initiating treatment with BROVANA Inhalation Solution.

Common Adverse Reactions with $Beta_2$-agonists

Patients should be informed that treatment with $beta_2$-agonists may lead to adverse reactions that include palpitations, chest pain, rapid heart rate, increased or decreased blood pressure, headache, tremor, nervousness, dry mouth, muscle cramps, nausea, dizziness, fatigue, malaise, low blood potassium, high blood sugar, high blood acid, or trouble sleeping [*see ADVERSE REACTIONS (6.1)*].

Instructions for Administration

It is important that patients understand how to use BROVANA Inhalation Solution with a nebulizer appropriately and how it should be used in relation to other medications to treat COPD they are taking *[see the accompanying* ***Medication Guide****]*. Patients should be instructed not to mix other medications with BROVANA Inhalation Solution and not to inject or swallow BROVANA Inhalation Solution. Patients should throw the plastic dispensing vials away immediately after use. Due to their small size, the vials pose a danger of choking to young children.

Women should be advised to contact their physician if they become pregnant or if they are nursing.

FDA-Approved Medication Guide

See the accompanying **Medication Guide**.

SUNOVION

Manufactured for:

Sunovion Pharmaceuticals Inc.

Marlborough, MA 01752 USA

For customer service, call 1-888-394-7377.

To report adverse events, call 1-877-737-7226.

For medical information, call 1-800-739-0565.

February 2012

901552R01

MEDICATION GUIDE

BROVANA® *[Brō vă '-nah]*

(arformoterol tartrate) Inhalation Solution

BROVANA Inhalation Solution is only for use with a nebulizer.

Read the Medication Guide that comes with BROVANA Inhalation Solution before you start using it and each time you get a refill. There may be new information. This Medication Guide does not take the place of talking to your healthcare provider about your medical condition or treatment.

What is the most important information I should know about BROVANA Inhalation Solution?

BROVANA Inhalation Solution can cause serious side effects, including:

- **People with asthma, who take long-acting $beta_2$-adrenergic agonist (LABA) medicines, such as BROVANA Inhalation Solution, have an increased risk of death from asthma problems.**

- It is not known if LABA medicines, such as BROVANA Inhalation Solution, increase the risk of death in people with chronic obstructive pulmonary disease (COPD).
- **Get emergency medical care if:**
  - **breathing problems worsen quickly**
  - **you use your rescue inhaler medicine, but it does not relieve your breathing problems**

What is BROVANA Inhalation Solution?

BROVANA Inhalation Solution is used long term, 2 times each day (morning and evening), in controlling symptoms of chronic obstructive pulmonary disease (COPD) in adults with COPD.

BROVANA Inhalation Solution is only for use with a nebulizer.

LABA medicines such as BROVANA Inhalation Solution help the muscles around the airways in your lungs stay relaxed to prevent symptoms, such as wheezing, cough, chest tightness, and shortness of breath.

BROVANA Inhalation Solution should not be used in children. **It is not known if BROVANA Inhalation Solution is safe and effective in children.**

It is not known if BROVANA Inhalation Solution is safe and effective in people with asthma.

Who should not use BROVANA Inhalation Solution?

Do not use BROVANA Inhalation Solution if you:

- have had a serious allergic reaction to arformoterol, formoterol, or any of the ingredients in BROVANA Inhalation Solution. Ask your healthcare provider if you are not sure. See the end of this Medication Guide for a complete list of ingredients in BROVANA Inhalation Solution.
- have asthma without using a long-term asthma control medicine.

What should I tell my healthcare provider before using BROVANA Inhalation Solution?

Tell your healthcare provider about all of your health conditions, including if you:

- have heart problems
- have high blood pressure
- have seizures
- have thyroid problems
- have diabetes
- have liver problems
- are pregnant or planning to become pregnant. It is not known if BROVANA Inhalation Solution can harm your unborn baby.
- are breastfeeding. It is not known if BROVANA Inhalation Solution passes into your milk and if it can harm your baby.

Tell your healthcare provider about all the medicines you take including prescription and non-prescription medicines, vitamins and herbal supplements. BROVANA Inhalation Solution and certain other medicines may interact with each other. This may cause serious side effects.

Know the medicines you take. Keep a list of them to show your healthcare provider and pharmacist each time you get a new medicine.

How should I use BROVANA Inhalation Solution?

Read the step-by-step instructions for using BROVANA Inhalation Solution at the end of this Medication Guide.

- Use BROVANA Inhalation Solution exactly as prescribed. One ready-to-use vial of BROVANA Inhalation Solution is one dose. The usual dose of BROVANA Inhalation Solution is 1 ready-to-use vial, twice a day (morning and evening) breathed in through your nebulizer machine. The 2 doses should be about 12 hours apart. **Do not use more than 2 ready-to-use vials of BROVANA Inhalation Solution a day.**
- Do not swallow or inject BROVANA Inhalation Solution.
- BROVANA Inhalation Solution is for use with a standard jet nebulizer machine connected to an air compressor. Read the complete instructions for use at the end of this Medication Guide before starting BROVANA Inhalation Solution.
- Do not mix other medicines with BROVANA Inhalation Solution in your nebulizer machine.
- If you miss a dose of BROVANA Inhalation Solution, just skip that dose. Take your next dose at your usual time. Do not take 2 doses at one time.
- While you are using BROVANA Inhalation Solution 2 times each day:
  - **do not use** other medicines that contain a long-acting beta$_2$-agonist (LABA) for any reason.
  - **do not use** your short-acting beta$_2$-agonist medicine on a regular basis (four times a day).
- **BROVANA Inhalation Solution does not relieve sudden symptoms of COPD.** Always have a rescue inhaler medicine with you to treat sudden symptoms. If you do not have a rescue inhaler medicine, call your healthcare provider to have one prescribed for you.
- Do not stop using BROVANA Inhalation Solution or other medicines to control or treat your COPD unless told to do so by your healthcare provider because your symptoms might get worse. Your healthcare provider will change your medicines as needed.
- **Do not use BROVANA Inhalation Solution:**
  - **more often than prescribed**
  - **more medicine than prescribed to you**
  - **with other LABA medicines**

Call your healthcare provider or get emergency medical care right away if:

- your breathing problems worsen with BROVANA Inhalation Solution
- you need to use your rescue inhaler medicine more often than usual
- your rescue inhaler medicine does not work as well for you at relieving symptoms

What are the possible side effects with BROVANA Inhalation Solution?

BROVANA Inhalation Solution can cause serious side effects, including:

- **See "What is the most important information I should know about BROVANA Inhalation Solution?"**
- Sudden shortness of breath immediately after use of BROVANA Inhalation Solution
- If your COPD symptoms worsen over time, do not increase your dose of BROVANA Inhalation Solution; instead, call your healthcare provider.
- Increased blood pressure
- Fast or irregular heartbeat
- **serious allergic reactions including rash, hives, swelling of the face, mouth, and tongue, and breathing problems.** Call your healthcare provider or get emergency medical care if you get any symptoms of a serious allergic reaction.

Common side effects of BROVANA Inhalation Solution include:

- **chest or back pain**
- **diarrhea**
- **sinus congestion**
- **headache**
- **tremor**
- **nervousness**
- **leg cramps**
- **high blood potassium**
- **shortness of breath**
- **rash**
- **fever**
- **increased white blood cells**
- **vomiting**
- **tiredness**
- **leg swelling**
- **chest congestion or bronchitis**

Tell your healthcare provider if you get any side effect that bothers you or that does not go away.

These are not all the side effects with BROVANA Inhalation Solution. Ask your healthcare provider or pharmacist for more information. Call your doctor for medical advice about side effects. You may report side effects to FDA at 1-800-FDA-1088.

How should I store BROVANA Inhalation Solution?

- Store BROVANA Inhalation Solution in a refrigerator between 36° to 46°F (2° to 8°C) in the protective foil pouch. Protect from light and excessive heat. **Do not open a sealed pouch until you are ready to use a dose of BROVANA Inhalation Solution. After opening the pouch, unused ready-to-use vials should be returned to, and stored in, the pouch. An opened ready-to-use vial should be used right away.** BROVANA Inhalation Solution may be used directly from the refrigerator.
- BROVANA Inhalation Solution may also be stored at room temperature between 68° to 77°F (20° to 25°C) for up to 6 weeks (42 days). If stored at room temperature, discard BROVANA Inhalation Solution if it is not used after 6 weeks or if past the expiration date, whichever is sooner. Space is provided on the packaging to record room temperature storage times.
- Do not use BROVANA Inhalation Solution after the expiration date provided on the foil pouch and ready-to-use vial.
- BROVANA Inhalation Solution should be colorless. Discard BROVANA Inhalation Solution if it is not colorless.
- **Keep BROVANA Inhalation Solution and all medicines out of the reach of children.**

General Information about BROVANA Inhalation Solution

Medicines are sometimes prescribed for purposes not mentioned in a Medication Guide. Do not use BROVANA Inhalation Solution for a condition for which it was not prescribed. Do not give BROVANA Inhalation Solution to other people, even if they have the same condition. It may harm them.

This Medication Guide summarizes the most important information about BROVANA Inhalation Solution. If you would like more information, talk with your healthcare provider. You can ask your healthcare provider or pharmacist for information about BROVANA Inhalation Solution that was written for healthcare professionals.

- For customer service, call 1-888-394-7377.
- To report side effects, call 1-877-737-7226.
- For medical information, call 1-800-739-0565.

Instructions for Using BROVANA (arformoterol tartrate) Inhalation Solution

BROVANA Inhalation Solution is used only in a standard jet nebulizer machine connected to an air compressor. Make sure you know how to use your nebulizer machine before you use it to breathe in BROVANA Inhalation Solution or other medicines.

Do not mix BROVANA Inhalation Solution with other medicines in your nebulizer machine.

BROVANA Inhalation Solution comes sealed in a foil pouch. Do not open a sealed pouch until you are ready to use a dose of BROVANA Inhalation Solution. After opening the pouch, unused ready-to-use vials should be returned to, and stored in, the pouch. An opened ready-to-use vial should be used right away.

1. Open the foil pouch by tearing on the rough edge along the seam of the pouch. Remove a ready-to-use vial of BROVANA Inhalation Solution.
2. Carefully twist open the top of the ready-to-use vial and use it right away (**Figure 1**).

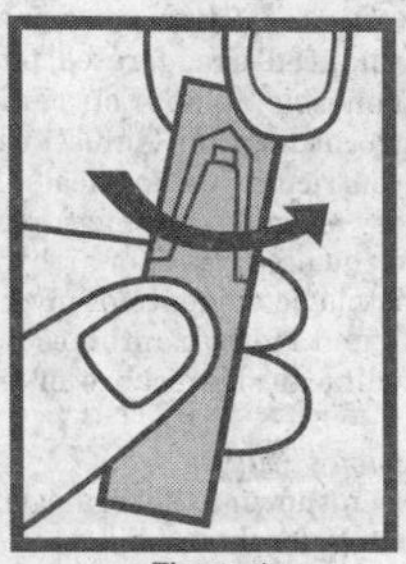

Figure 1

3. Squeeze all of the medicine from the ready-to-use vial into the nebulizer medicine cup (reservoir) (**Figure 2**).

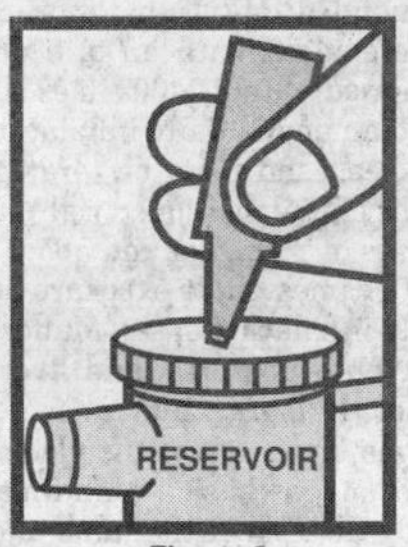

Figure 2

4. Connect the nebulizer reservoir to the mouthpiece (**Figure 3**) or face mask (**Figure 4**).

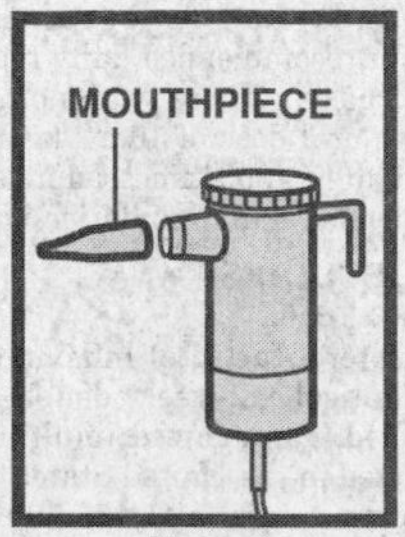

Figure 3

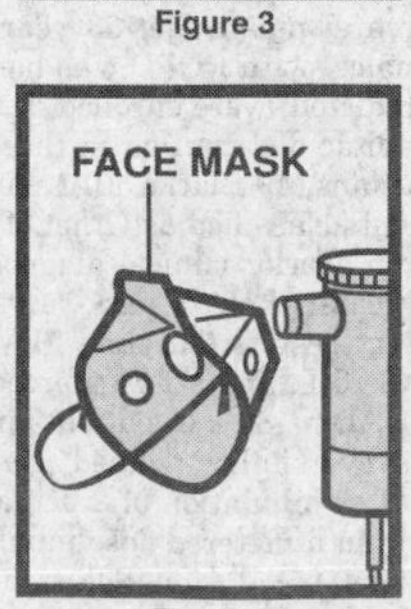

Figure 4

5. Connect the nebulizer to the compressor (**Figure 5**).

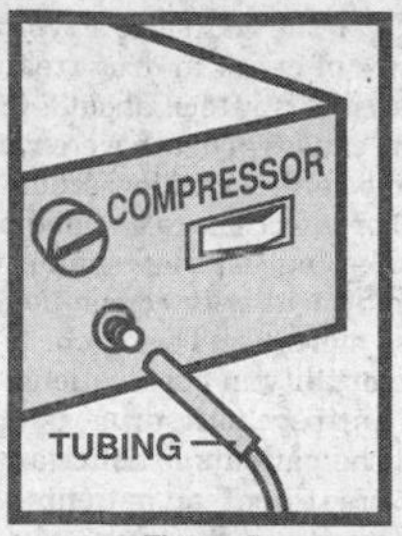

Figure 5

6. Sit in a comfortable, upright position. Place the mouthpiece in your mouth (**Figure 6**) (or put on the face mask) and turn on the compressor.

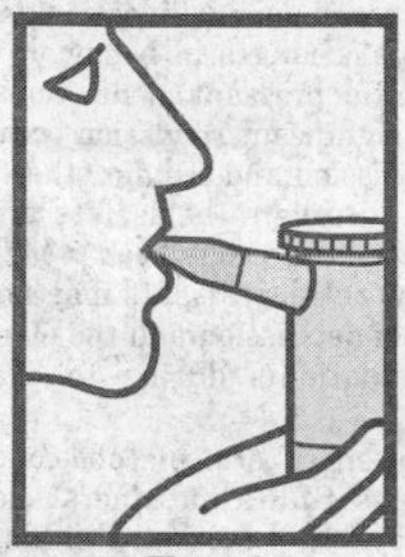
Figure 6

7. Breathe as calmly, deeply, and evenly as possible until no more mist is formed in the nebulizer reservoir. It takes about 5 to 10 minutes for each treatment.
8. Clean the nebulizer (see manufacturer's instructions).

Rx Only
This Medication Guide has been approved by the Food and Drug Administration.
SUNOVION
Manufactured for:
Sunovion Pharmaceuticals Inc.
Marlborough, MA 01752 USA

February 2012
901552R01
Shown in Product Identification Guide, page 313

LATUDA ℞
(lurasidone hydrochloride)
tablets, for oral use

HIGHLIGHTS OF PRESCRIBING INFORMATION
These highlights do not include all the information needed to use LATUDA safely and effectively. See full prescribing information for LATUDA.
LATUDA (lurasidone hydrochloride) tablets, for oral use
Initial U.S. Approval: 2010

WARNINGS: INCREASED MORTALITY IN ELDERLY PATIENTS WITH DEMENTIA-RELATED PSYCHOSIS; AND SUICIDAL THOUGHTS AND BEHAVIORS
See full prescribing information for complete boxed warning.
- **Elderly patients with dementia-related psychosis treated with antipsychotic drugs are at an increased risk of death.**
- **LATUDA is not approved for the treatment of patients with dementia-related psychosis (5.1).**
- **Increased risk of suicidal thinking and behavior in children, adolescents, and young adults taking antidepressants (5.2)**
- **Monitor for worsening and emergence of suicidal thoughts and behaviors (5.2)**

RECENT MAJOR CHANGES

Boxed Warnings, Suicidal Thoughts and Behaviors (5.2) 6/2013
Indications and Usage, Bipolar Depression (1.2) 6/2013
Dosage and Administration, Bipolar Depression (2.1) 6/2013
Dosage Forms and Strengths (3) 7/2013
Warnings and Precautions (5.2, 5.6, 5.7, 5.9, 5.10, 5.11, 5.13, 5.14) 6/2013

INDICATIONS AND USAGE

LATUDA is an atypical antipsychotic for the treatment of:
- Schizophrenia (1.1, 14.1)
- Depressive episodes associated with Bipolar I Disorder (bipolar depression), as monotherapy and as adjunctive therapy with lithium or valproate (1.2, 14.2).

DOSAGE AND ADMINISTRATION

LATUDA should be taken with food (at least 350 calories). Administration with food substantially increases the absorption of LATUDA (2.3, 12.3).

Indication	Starting Dose	Recommended Dose
Schizophrenia (2.1)	40 mg per day	40 mg to 160 mg per day
Bipolar Depression (2.2)	20 mg per day	20 mg to 120 mg per day

- Moderate and Severe Renal Impairment: Recommended starting dose is 20 mg per day, and the maximum recommended dose is 80 mg per day (2.4, 8.6).
- Moderate and Severe Hepatic Impairment: Recommended starting dose is 20 mg per day. The maximum recommended dose is 80 mg per day in moderate hepatic impairment and 40 mg per day in severe hepatic impairment (2.4, 8.6).
- Concomitant Use of a Moderate CYP3A4 inhibitor (e.g., diltiazem): LATUDA dose should be reduced to half of the original dose level. Recommended starting dose is 20 mg per day. Maximum recommended dose is 80 mg per day (2.5, 7.1)
- Concomitant Use of a Moderate CYP3A4 Inducer: It may be necessary to increase the dose of LATUDA (2.5, 7.1)

DOSAGE FORMS AND STRENGTHS

Tablets: 20 mg, 40 mg, 60 mg, 80 mg and 120 mg (3)

CONTRAINDICATIONS

- Known hypersensitivity to LATUDA or any components in the formulation (4).
- Concomitant use with a strong CYP3A4 inhibitor (e.g., ketoconazole) (2.5, 4, 7.1).
- Concomitant use with a strong CYP3A4 inducer (e.g., rifampin) (2.5, 4, 7.1).

WARNINGS AND PRECAUTIONS

- Cerebrovascular Adverse Reactions in Elderly Patients with Dementia-Related Psychosis: Increased incidence of cerebrovascular adverse events (e.g., stroke, transient ischemic attack) (5.2).
- Neuroleptic Malignant Syndrome: Manage with immediate discontinuation and close monitoring (5.4).
- Tardive Dyskinesia: Discontinue if clinically appropriate (5.5).
- Metabolic Changes: Atypical antipsychotic drugs have been associated with metabolic changes that may increase cardiovascular/cerebrovascular risk. These metabolic changes include hyperglycemia, dyslipidemia, and weight gain (5.6).
  - *Hyperglycemia and Diabetes Mellitus:* Monitor patients for symptoms of hyperglycemia including polydipsia, polyuria, polyphagia, and weakness. Monitor glucose regularly in patients with diabetes or at risk for diabetes.
  - *Dyslipidemia:* Undesirable alterations have been observed in patients treated with atypical antipsychotics.
  - *Weight Gain:* Gain in body weight has been observed. Monitor weight.
- Hyperprolactinemia: Prolactin elevations may occur (5.7).
- Leukopenia, Neutropenia, and Agranulocytosis: Perform complete blood counts (CBC) in patients with a pre-existing low white blood cell count (WBC) or a history of leukopenia or neutropenia. Consider discontinuing LATUDA if a clinically significant decline in WBC occurs in the absence of other causative factors (5.8).
- Orthostatic Hypotension and Syncope: Dizziness, tachycardia or bradycardia, and syncope may occur, especially early in treatment. In patients with known cardiovascular or cerebrovascular disease, and in antipsychotic-naïve patients, consider a lower starting dose and slower titration (5.9).

ADVERSE REACTIONS

Commonly observed adverse reactions (incidence ≥ 5% and at least twice the rate for placebo) were (6.1):
- Schizophrenia: somnolence, akathisia, extrapyramidal symptoms, and nausea
- Bipolar depression: akathisia, extrapyramidal symptoms, and somnolence

To report SUSPECTED ADVERSE REACTIONS, contact Sunovion Pharmaceuticals Inc. at 1-877-737-7226 or FDA at 1-800-FDA-1088 or www.fda.gov/medwatch.

USE IN SPECIFIC POPULATIONS

- Pregnancy: Use LATUDA during pregnancy only if the potential benefit justifies the potential risk (8.1).
- Nursing Mothers: Discontinue drug or nursing, considering risk of drug discontinuation to the mother (8.3).

See 17 for PATIENT COUNSELING INFORMATION and Medication Guide

Revised: 07/2013

FULL PRESCRIBING INFORMATION: CONTENTS*

*** Sections or subsections omitted from the full prescribing information are not listed**

FULL PRESCRIBING INFORMATION

WARNINGS: INCREASED MORTALITY IN ELDERLY PATIENTS WITH DEMENTIA-RELATED PSYCHOSIS; AND SUICIDAL THOUGHTS AND BEHAVIORS

- **Elderly patients with dementia-related psychosis treated with antipsychotic drugs are at an increased risk of death *[see Warnings and Precautions (5.1)]*.**
- **LATUDA is not approved for use in patients with dementia-related psychosis *[see Warnings and Precautions (5.1)]*.**
- **Antidepressants increased the risk of suicidal thoughts and behavior in children, adolescents, and young adults in short-term studies. These studies did not show an increase in the risk of suicidal thoughts and behavior with antidepressant use in patients over age 24; there was a reduction in risk with antidepressant use in patients aged 65 and older *[see Warnings and Precautions (5.2)]*.**
- **In patients of all ages who are started on antidepressant therapy, monitor closely for worsening, and for emergence of suicidal thoughts and behaviors. Advise families and caregivers of the need for close observation and communication with the prescriber *[see Warnings and Precautions (5.2)]*.**

1 INDICATIONS AND USAGE

1.1 Schizophrenia

LATUDA is indicated for the treatment of patients with schizophrenia.

The efficacy of LATUDA in schizophrenia was established in five 6-week controlled studies of adult patients with schizophrenia *[see Clinical Studies (14.1)]*.

The effectiveness of LATUDA for longer-term use, that is, for more than 6 weeks, has not been established in controlled studies. Therefore, the physician who elects to use LATUDA for extended periods should periodically re-evaluate the long-term usefulness of the drug for the individual patient *[see Dosage and Administration (2)]*.

1.2 Depressive Episodes Associated with Bipolar I Disorder

Monotherapy: LATUDA is indicated as monotherapy for the treatment of patients with major depressive episodes associated with bipolar I disorder (bipolar depression). The efficacy of LATUDA was established in a 6-week monotherapy study in adult patients with bipolar depression *[see Clinical Studies (14.2)]*.

Adjunctive Therapy with Lithium or Valproate: LATUDA is indicated as adjunctive therapy with either lithium or valproate for the treatment of patients with major depressive episodes associated with bipolar I disorder (bipolar depression). The efficacy of LATUDA as adjunctive therapy was established in a 6-week study in adult patients with bipolar depression who were treated with lithium or valproate *[see Clinical Studies (14.2)]*.

The effectiveness of LATUDA for longer-term use, that is, for more than 6 weeks, has not been established in controlled studies. Therefore, the physician who elects to use LATUDA for extended periods should periodically re-evaluate the long-term usefulness of the drug for the individual patient *[see Dosage and Administration (2.2)]*.

The efficacy of LATUDA in the treatment of mania associated with bipolar disorder has not been established.

2 DOSAGE AND ADMINISTRATION

2.1 Schizophrenia

The recommended starting dose of LATUDA is 40 mg once daily. Initial dose titration is not required. LATUDA has been shown to be effective in a dose range of 40 mg per day to 160 mg per day *[see Clinical Studies (14.1)]*. The maximum recommended dose is 160 mg per day.

2.2 Depressive Episodes Associated with Bipolar I Disorder

The recommended starting dose of LATUDA is 20 mg given once daily as monotherapy or as adjunctive therapy with lithium or valproate. Initial dose titration is not required. LATUDA has been shown to be effective in a dose range of 20 mg per day to 120 mg per day as monotherapy or as adjunctive therapy with lithium or valproate *[see Clinical Studies (14.2)]*. The maximum recommended dose, as monotherapy or as adjunctive therapy with lithium or valproate, is 120 mg per day. In the monotherapy study, the higher dose range (80 mg to 120 mg per day) did not provide additional efficacy, on average, compared to the lower dose range (20 to 60 mg per day) *[see Clinical Studies (14.2)*.

2.3 Administration Instructions

LATUDA should be taken with food (at least 350 calories). Administration with food substantially increases the absorption of LATUDA. Administration with food increases the AUC approximately 2-fold and increases the Cmax approximately 3-fold. In the clinical studies, LATUDA was administered with food *[see Clinical Pharmacology (12.3)]*.

2.4 Dose Modifications in Special Populations

Renal Impairment

Dose adjustment is recommended in moderate (creatinine clearance: 30 to <50 mL/min) and severe renal impairment (creatinine clearance <30 mL/min) patients. The recommended starting dose is 20 mg per day. The dose in these patients should not exceed 80 mg per day *[see Use in Specific Populations (8.6)]*.

Hepatic Impairment

Dose adjustment is recommended in moderate (Child-Pugh Score = 7 to 9) and severe hepatic impairment (Child-Pugh Score = 10 to 15) patients. The recommended starting dose is 20 mg per day. The dose in moderate hepatic impairment patients should not exceed 80 mg per day and the dose in severe hepatic impairment patients should not exceed 40 mg/day *[see Use in Specific Populations (8.6)]*.

2.5 Dose Modifications Due to Drug Interactions

Concomitant Use with CYP3A4 Inhibitors

LATUDA should not be used concomitantly with a strong CYP3A4 inhibitor (e.g., ketoconazole, clarithromycin, ritonavir, voriconazole, mibefradil, etc.) *[see Contraindications (4)]*.

If LATUDA is being prescribed and a moderate CYP3A4 inhibitor (e.g. diltiazem, atazanavir, erythromycin, fluconazole, verapamil etc.) is added to the therapy, the LATUDA dose should be reduced to half of the original dose level. Similarly, if a moderate CYP3A4 inhibitor is being prescribed and LATUDA is added to the therapy, the recommended starting dose of LATUDA is 20 mg per day, and the maximum recommended dose of LATUDA is 80 mg per day *[see Contraindications (4); Drug Interactions (7.1)]*.

Grapefruit and grapefruit juice should be avoided in patients taking LATUDA, since these may inhibit CYP3A4 and alter LATUDA concentrations *[see Drug Interactions (7.1)]*.

Concomitant Use with CYP3A4 Inducers

LATUDA should not be used concomitantly with a strong CYP3A4 inducer (e.g., rifampin, avasimibe, St. John's wort, phenytoin, carbamazepine, etc.) *[see Contraindications (4); Drug Interactions (7.1)]*. If LATUDA is used concomitantly with a moderate CYP3A4 inducer, it may be necessary to increase the LATUDA dose after chronic treatment (7 days or more) with the CYP3A4 inducer.

3 DOSAGE FORMS AND STRENGTHS

LATUDA tablets are available in the following shape and color (Table 1) with respective one-sided debossing:

Table 1: LATUDA Tablet Presentations

Tablet Strength	Tablet Color/ Shape	Tablet Markings
20 mg	white to off-white round	L20
40 mg	white to off-white round	L40
60 mg	white to off white oblong	L60
80 mg	pale green oval	L80
120 mg	white to off-white oval	L120

4 CONTRAINDICATIONS

- Known hypersensitivity to lurasidone HCl or any components in the formulation. Angioedema has been observed with lurasidone *[see Adverse Reactions (6.1)]*.
- Strong CYP3A4 inhibitors (e.g., ketoconazole, clarithromycin, ritonavir, voriconazole, mibefradil, etc.) *[see Drug Interactions (7.1)]*.
- Strong CYP3A4 inducers (e.g., rifampin, avasimibe, St. John's wort, phenytoin, carbamazepine, etc.) *[see Drug Interactions (7.1)]*.

5 WARNINGS AND PRECAUTIONS

5.1 Increased Mortality in Elderly Patients with Dementia-Related Psychosis

Elderly patients with dementia-related psychosis treated with antipsychotic drugs are at an increased risk of death. Analyses of 17 placebo-controlled trials (modal duration of 10 weeks), largely in patients taking atypical antipsychotic drugs, revealed a risk of death in drug-treated patients of between 1.6- to 1.7-times the risk of death in placebo-treated patients. Over the course of a typical 10-week controlled trial, the rate of death in drug-treated patients was about 4.5%, compared to a rate of about 2.6% in the placebo group. Although the causes of death were varied, most of the deaths appeared to be either cardiovascular (e.g., heart failure, sudden death) or infectious (e.g., pneumonia) in nature. Observational studies suggest that, similar to atypical antipsychotic drugs, treatment with conventional antipsychotic drugs may increase mortality. The extent to which the findings of increased mortality in observational studies may be attributed to the antipsychotic drug as opposed to some characteristic(s) of the patients is not clear. LATUDA is not approved for the treatment of patients with dementia-related psychosis *[see Boxed Warning]*.

5.2 Suicidal Thoughts and Behaviors in Adolescents and Young Adults

Patients with major depressive disorder (MDD), both adult and pediatric, may experience worsening of their depression and/or the emergence of suicidal ideation and behavior (suicidality) or unusual changes in behavior, whether or not they are taking antidepressant medications, and this risk may persist until significant remission occurs. Suicide is a known risk of depression and certain other psychiatric disorders, and these disorders themselves are the strongest predictors of suicide. There has been a long-standing concern, however, that antidepressants may have a role in inducing worsening of depression and the emergence of suicidality in certain patients during the early phases of treatment.

Pooled analyses of short-term placebo-controlled trials of antidepressant drugs (SSRIs and others) showed that these drugs increase the risk of suicidal thinking and behavior (suicidality) in children, adolescents, and young adults (ages 18-24) with major depressive disorder (MDD) and other psychiatric disorders. Short-term studies did not show an increase in the risk of suicidality with antidepressants compared to placebo in adults beyond age 24; there was a reduction with antidepressants compared to placebo in adults aged 65 and older.

The pooled analyses of placebo-controlled trials in children and adolescents with MDD, obsessive compulsive disorder (OCD), or other psychiatric disorders included a total of 24 short-term trials of 9 antidepressant drugs in over 4400 patients. The pooled analyses of placebo-controlled trials in adults with MDD or other psychiatric disorders included a total of 295 short-term trials (median duration of 2 months) of 11 antidepressant drugs in over 77,000 patients. There was considerable variation in risk of suicidality among drugs, but a tendency toward an increase in the younger patients for almost all drugs studied. There were differences in absolute risk of suicidality across the different indications, with the highest incidence in MDD. The risk of differences (drug vs. placebo), however, were relatively stable within age strata and across indications. These risk differences (drug-placebo difference in the number of cases of suicidality per 1000 patients treated) are provided in Table 2.

Table 2

Age Range	Drug-Placebo Difference in Number of Cases of Suicidality per 1000 Patients Treated
	Increases Compared to Placebo
<18	14 additional cases
18-24	5 additional cases
	Decreases Compared to Placebo
25-64	1 fewer case
≥65	6 fewer cases

No suicides occurred in any of the pediatric trials. There were suicides in the adult trials, but the number was not sufficient to reach any conclusion about drug effect on suicide.

It is unknown whether the suicidality risk extends to longer-term use, i.e., beyond several months. However, there is substantial evidence from placebo-controlled maintenance trials in adults with depression that the use of antidepressants can delay the recurrence of depression.

All patients being treated with antidepressants for any indication should be monitored appropriately and observed closely for clinical worsening, suicidality, and unusual changes in behavior, especially during the initial few months of a course of drug therapy, or at times of dose changes, either increases or decreases.

The following symptoms, anxiety, agitation, panic attacks, insomnia, irritability, hostility, aggressiveness, impulsivity, akathisia (psychomotor restlessness), hypomania, and mania, have been reported in adult and pediatric patients being treated with antidepressants for major depressive disorder as well as for other indications, both psychiatric and nonpsychiatric. Although a causal link between the emergence of such symptoms and either the worsening of depression and/or the emergence of suicidal impulses has not been established, there is concern that such symptoms may represent precursors to emerging suicidality.

Consideration should be given to changing the therapeutic regimen, including possibly discontinuing the medication, in patients whose depression is persistently worse, or who are experiencing emergent suicidality or symptoms that might be precursors to worsening depression or suicidality, especially if these symptoms are severe, abrupt in onset, or were not part of the patient's presenting symptoms.

Families and caregivers of patients being treated with antidepressants for major depressive disorder or other indications, both psychiatric and nonpsychiatric, should be alerted about the need to monitor patients for the emergence of agitation, irritability, unusual changes in behavior, and the other symptoms described above, as well as the emergence of suicidal thoughts and behaviors, and to report such symptoms immediately to health care providers. Such monitoring should include daily observation by families and caregivers. Prescriptions for LATUDA should be written for the smallest quantity of capsules consistent with good patient management, in order to reduce the risk of overdose.

5.3 Cerebrovascular Adverse Reactions, Including Stroke in Elderly Patients with Dementia-Related Psychosis

In placebo-controlled trials with risperidone, aripiprazole, and olanzapine in elderly subjects with dementia, there was a higher incidence of cerebrovascular adverse reactions (cerebrovascular accidents and transient ischemic attacks), including fatalities, compared to placebo-treated subjects. LATUDA is not approved for the treatment of patients with dementia-related psychosis *[see also Boxed Warning and Warnings and Precautions (5.1)]*.

5.4 Neuroleptic Malignant Syndrome

A potentially fatal symptom complex sometimes referred to as Neuroleptic Malignant Syndrome (NMS) has been reported in association with administration of antipsychotic drugs, including LATUDA.

Clinical manifestations of NMS are hyperpyrexia, muscle rigidity, altered mental status, and evidence of autonomic instability (irregular pulse or blood pressure, tachycardia, diaphoresis, and cardiac dysrhythmia). Additional signs may include elevated creatine phosphokinase, myoglobinuria (rhabdomyolysis), and acute renal failure.

The diagnostic evaluation of patients with this syndrome is complicated. It is important to exclude cases where the clinical presentation includes both serious medical illness (e.g., pneumonia, systemic infection) and untreated or inadequately treated extrapyramidal signs and symptoms (EPS). Other important considerations in the differential diagnosis include central anticholinergic toxicity, heat stroke, drug fever, and primary central nervous system pathology.

The management of NMS should include: 1) immediate discontinuation of antipsychotic drugs and other drugs not essential to concurrent therapy; 2) intensive symptomatic treatment and medical monitoring; and 3) treatment of any concomitant serious medical problems for which specific treatments are available. There is no general agreement about specific pharmacological treatment regimens for NMS.

If a patient requires antipsychotic drug treatment after recovery from NMS, the potential reintroduction of drug therapy should be carefully considered. If reintroduced, the patient should be carefully monitored, since recurrences of NMS have been reported.

5.5 Tardive Dyskinesia

Tardive dyskinesia is a syndrome consisting of potentially irreversible, involuntary, dyskinetic movements that can develop in patients treated with antipsychotic drugs. Although the prevalence of the syndrome appears to be highest among the elderly, especially elderly women, it is impossible to rely upon prevalence estimates to predict, at the inception of antipsychotic treatment, which patients are likely to develop the syndrome. Whether antipsychotic drug products differ in their potential to cause tardive dyskinesia is unknown.

The risk of developing tardive dyskinesia and the likelihood that it will become irreversible are believed to increase as the duration of treatment and the total cumulative dose of antipsychotic drugs administered to the patient increase. However, the syndrome can develop, although much less commonly, after relatively brief treatment periods at low doses.

There is no known treatment for established cases of tardive dyskinesia, although the syndrome may remit, partially or completely, if antipsychotic treatment is withdrawn. Antipsychotic treatment, itself, however, may suppress (or partially suppress) the signs and symptoms of the syndrome and thereby may possibly mask the underlying process. The effect that symptomatic suppression has upon the long-term course of the syndrome is unknown.

Table 3: Change in Fasting Glucose in Schizophrenia Studies

	Placebo	LATUDA 20 mg/day	LATUDA 40 mg/day	LATUDA 80 mg/day	LATUDA 120 mg/day	LATUDA 160 mg/day
Mean Change from Baseline (mg/dL)						
	n=680	n=71	n=478	n=508	n=283	n=113
Serum Glucose	-0.0	-0.6	+2.6	-0.4	+2.5	+ 2.5
Proportion of Patients with Shifts to ≥ 126 mg/dL						
Serum Glucose (≥ 126 mg/dL)	8.3% (52/628)	11.7% (7/60)	12.7% (57/449)	6.8% (32/472)	10.0% (26/260)	5.6% (6/108)

Table 4: Change in Fasting Glucose in the Monotherapy Bipolar Depression Study

	Placebo	LATUDA 20 to 60 mg/day	LATUDA 80 to 120 mg/day
Mean Change from Baseline (mg/dL)			
	n=148	n=140	n=143
Serum Glucose	+1.8	-0.8	+1.8
Proportion of Patients with Shifts to ≥ 126 mg/dL			
Serum Glucose (≥ 126 mg/dL)	4.3% (6/141)	2.2% (3/138)	6.4% (9/141)

Patients were randomized to flexibly dosed LATUDA 20 to 60 mg/day, LATUDA 80 to 120 mg/day, or placebo

Given these considerations, LATUDA should be prescribed in a manner that is most likely to minimize the occurrence of tardive dyskinesia. Chronic antipsychotic treatment should generally be reserved for patients who suffer from a chronic illness that (1) is known to respond to antipsychotic drugs, and (2) for whom alternative, equally effective, but potentially less harmful treatments are not available or appropriate. In patients who do require chronic treatment, the smallest dose and the shortest duration of treatment producing a satisfactory clinical response should be sought. The need for continued treatment should be reassessed periodically.

If signs and symptoms of tardive dyskinesia appear in a patient on LATUDA, drug discontinuation should be considered. However, some patients may require treatment with LATUDA despite the presence of the syndrome.

5.6 Metabolic Changes

Atypical antipsychotic drugs have been associated with metabolic changes that may increase cardiovascular/cerebrovascular risk. These metabolic changes include hyperglycemia, dyslipidemia, and body weight gain. While all of the drugs in the class have been shown to produce some metabolic changes, each drug has its own specific risk profile.

Hyperglycemia and Diabetes Mellitus

Hyperglycemia, in some cases extreme and associated with ketoacidosis or hyperosmolar coma or death, has been reported in patients treated with atypical antipsychotics. Assessment of the relationship between atypical antipsychotic use and glucose abnormalities is complicated by the possibility of an increased background risk of diabetes mellitus in patients with schizophrenia and the increasing incidence of diabetes mellitus in the general population. Given these confounders, the relationship between atypical antipsychotic use and hyperglycemia-related adverse events is not completely understood. However, epidemiological studies suggest an increased risk of treatment-emergent hyperglycemia-related adverse events in patients treated with the atypical antipsychotics. Because LATUDA was not marketed at the time these studies were performed, it is not known if LATUDA is associated with this increased risk.

Patients with an established diagnosis of diabetes mellitus who are started on atypical antipsychotics should be monitored regularly for worsening of glucose control. Patients with risk factors for diabetes mellitus (e.g., obesity, family history of diabetes) who are starting treatment with atypical antipsychotics should undergo fasting blood glucose testing at the beginning of treatment and periodically during treatment. Any patient treated with atypical antipsychotics should be monitored for symptoms of hyperglycemia including polydipsia, polyuria, polyphagia, and weakness. Patients who develop symptoms of hyperglycemia during treatment with atypical antipsychotics should undergo fasting blood glucose testing. In some cases, hyperglycemia has resolved when the atypical antipsychotic was discontinued; however, some patients required continuation of anti-diabetic treatment despite discontinuation of the suspect drug.

Schizophrenia

Pooled data from short-term, placebo-controlled schizophrenia studies are presented in Table 3.

[See table 3 above]

In the uncontrolled, longer-term schizophrenia studies (primarily open-label extension studies), LATUDA was associated with a mean change in glucose of +1.8 mg/dL at week 24 (n=355), +0.8 mg/dL at week 36 (n=299) and +2.3 mg/dL at week 52 (n=307).

Bipolar Depression

Monotherapy

Data from the short-term, flexible-dose, placebo-controlled monotherapy bipolar depression study are presented in Table 4.

[See table 4 above]

In the uncontrolled, open-label, longer-term bipolar depression study, patients who received LATUDA as monotherapy in the short-term study and continued in the longer-term study, had a mean change in glucose of +1.2 mg/dL at week 24 (n=129).

Adjunctive Therapy with Lithium or Valproate

Data from the short-term, flexible-dosed, placebo-controlled adjunctive therapy bipolar depression studies are presented in Table 5.

Table 5: Change in Fasting Glucose in the Adjunctive Therapy Bipolar Depression Studies

	Placebo	LATUDA 20 to 120 mg/day
Mean Change from Baseline (mg/dL)		
	n=302	n=319
Serum Glucose	-0.9	+1.2
Proportion of Patients with Shifts to ≥ 126 mg/dL		
Serum Glucose (≥ 126 mg/dL)	1.0% (3/290)	1.3% (4/316)

Patients were randomized to flexibly dosed LATUDA 20 to 120 mg/day or placebo as adjunctive therapy with lithium or valproate.

In the uncontrolled, open-label, longer-term bipolar depression study, patients who received LATUDA as adjunctive therapy with either lithium or valproate in the short-term study and continued in the longer-term study, had a mean change in glucose of +1.7 mg/dL at week 24 (n=88).

Dyslipidemia

Undesirable alterations in lipids have been observed in patients treated with atypical antipsychotics.

Schizophrenia

Pooled data from short-term, placebo-controlled schizophrenia studies are presented in Table 6.

Table 6: Change in Fasting Lipids in Schizophrenia Studies

	Placebo	LATUDA 20 mg/day	40 mg/day	80 mg/day	120 mg/day	160 mg/day
Mean Change from Baseline (mg/dL)						
	n=660	n=71	n=466	n=499	n=268	n=115
Total Cholesterol	-5.8	-12.3	-5.7	-6.2	-3.8	-6.9
Triglycerides	-13.4	-29.1	-5.1	-13.0	-3.1	-10.6
Proportion of Patients with Shifts						
Total Cholesterol (≥ 240 mg/dL)	5.3% (30/571)	13.8% (8/58)	6.2% (25/402)	5.3% (23/434)	3.8% (9/238)	4.0% (4/101)
Triglycerides (≥ 200 mg/dL)	10.1% (53/526)	14.3% (7/49)	10.8% (41/379)	6.3% (25/400)	10.5% (22/209)	7.0% (7/100)

Table 7: Change in Fasting Lipids in the Monotherapy Bipolar Depression Study

	Placebo	LATUDA 20 to 60 mg/day	80 to 120 mg/day
Mean Change from Baseline (mg/dL)			
	n=147	n=140	n=144
Total cholesterol	-3.2	+1.2	-4.6
Triglycerides	+6.0	+5.6	+0.4
Proportion of Patients with Shifts			
Total cholesterol (≥ 240 mg/dL)	4.2% (5/118)	4.4% (5/113)	4.4% (5/114)
Triglycerides (≥ 200 mg/dL)	4.8% (6/126)	10.1% (12/119)	9.8% (12/122)

Patients were randomized to flexibly dosed LATUDA 20 to 60 mg/day, LATUDA 80 to 120 mg/day, or placebo

Table 9: Mean Change in Weight (kg) from Baseline in Schizophrenia Studies

	Placebo (n=696)	LATUDA 20 mg/day (n=71)	40 mg/day (n=484)	80 mg/day (n=526)	120 mg/day (n=291)	160 mg/day (n=114)
All Patients	-0.02	-0.15	+0.22	+0.54	+0.68	+0.60

[See table 6 above]

In the uncontrolled, longer-term schizophrenia studies (primarily open-label extension studies), LATUDA was associated with a mean change in total cholesterol and triglycerides of -3.8 (n=356) and -15.1 (n=357) mg/dL at week 24, -3.1 (n=303) and -4.8 (n=303) mg/dL at week 36 and -2.5 (n=307) and -6.9 (n=307) mg/dL at week 52, respectively.

Bipolar Depression

Monotherapy

Data from the short-term, flexible-dosed, placebo-controlled, monotherapy bipolar depression study are presented in Table 7.

[See table 7 above]

In the uncontrolled, open-label, longer-term bipolar depression study, patients who received LATUDA as monotherapy in the short-term and continued in the longer-term study had a mean change in total cholesterol and triglycerides of -0.5 (n=130) and -1.0 (n=130) mg/dL at week 24, respectively.

Adjunctive Therapy with Lithium or Valproate

Data from the short-term, flexible-dosed, placebo-controlled, adjunctive therapy bipolar depression studies are presented in Table 8.

Table 8: Change in Fasting Lipids in the Adjunctive Therapy Bipolar Depression Studies

	Placebo	LATUDA 20 to 120 mg/day
Mean Change from Baseline (mg/dL)		
	n=303	n=321
Total cholesterol	-2.9	-3.1
Triglycerides	-4.6	+4.6
Proportion of Patients with Shifts		
Total cholesterol (≥ 240 mg/dL)	5.7% (15/263)	5.4% (15/276)
Triglycerides (≥ 200 mg/dL)	8.6% (21/243)	10.8% (28/260)

Patients were randomized to flexibly dosed LATUDA 20 to 120 mg/day or placebo as adjunctive therapy with lithium or valproate.

In the uncontrolled, open-label, longer-term bipolar depression study, patients who received LATUDA, as adjunctive therapy with either lithium or valproate in the short-term study and continued in the longer-term study, had a mean change in total cholesterol and triglycerides of -0.9 (n=88) and +5.3 (n=88) mg/dL at week 24, respectively.

Weight Gain

Weight gain has been observed with atypical antipsychotic use. Clinical monitoring of weight is recommended.

Schizophrenia

Pooled data from short-term, placebo-controlled schizophrenia studies are presented in Table 9. The mean weight gain was +0.43 kg for LATUDA-treated patients compared to -0.02 kg for placebo-treated patients. Change in weight from baseline for olanzapine was +4.15 kg and for quetiapine extended-release was +2.09 kg in Studies 3 and 5 *[see Clinical Studies (14.1)]*, respectively. The proportion of patients with a ≥ 7% increase in body weight (at Endpoint) was 4.8% for LATUDA-treated patients versus 3.3% for placebo-treated patients.

[See table 9 above]

In the uncontrolled, longer-term schizophrenia studies (primarily open-label extension studies), LATUDA was associated with a mean change in weight of -0.69 kg at week 24 (n=755), -0.59 kg at week 36 (n=443) and -0.73 kg at week 52 (n=377).

Bipolar Depression

Monotherapy

Data from the short-term, flexible-dosed, placebo-controlled monotherapy bipolar depression study are presented in Table 10. The mean weight gain was +0.29 kg for LATUDA-treated patients compared to -0.04 kg for placebo-treated patients. The proportion of patients with a ≥ 7% increase in body weight (at Endpoint) was 2.4% for LATUDA-treated patients versus 0.7% for placebo-treated patients.

Table 10: Mean Change in Weight (kg) from Baseline in the Monotherapy Bipolar Depression Study

	Placebo (n=151)	LATUDA 20 to 60 mg/day (n=143)	80 to 120 mg/day (n=147)
All Patients	-0.04	+0.56	+0.02

Patients were randomized to flexibly dosed LATUDA 20 to 60 mg/day, LATUDA 80 to 120 mg/day, or placebo

In the uncontrolled, open-label, longer-term bipolar depression study, patients who received LATUDA as monotherapy in the short-term and continued in the longer-term study had a mean change in weight of -0.02 kg at week 24 (n=130).

Adjunctive Therapy with Lithium or Valproate

Data from the short-term, flexible-dosed, placebo-controlled adjunctive therapy bipolar depression studies are presented in Table 11. The mean weight gain was +0.11 kg for LATUDA-treated patients compared to +0.16 kg for placebo-treated patients. The proportion of patients with a ≥ 7% increase in body weight (at Endpoint) was 3.1% for LATUDA-treated patients versus 0.3% for placebo-treated patients.

Table 11: Mean Change in Weight (kg) from Baseline in the Adjunctive Therapy Bipolar Depression Studies

	Placebo (n=307)	LATUDA 20 to 120 mg/day (n=327)
All Patients	+0.16	+0.11

Patients were randomized to flexibly dosed LATUDA 20 to 120 mg/day or placebo as adjunctive therapy with lithium or valproate.

In the uncontrolled, open-label, longer-term bipolar depression study, patients who were treated with LATUDA, as adjunctive therapy with either lithium or valproate in the short-term and continued in the longer-term study, had a mean change in weight of +1.28 kg at week 24 (n=86).

5.7 Hyperprolactinemia

As with other drugs that antagonize dopamine D_2 receptors, LATUDA elevates prolactin levels.

Hyperprolactinemia may suppress hypothalamic GnRH, resulting in reduced pituitary gonadotrophin secretion. This, in turn, may inhibit reproductive function by impairing gonadal steroidogenesis in both female and male patients. Galactorrhea, amenorrhea, gynecomastia, and impotence have been reported with prolactin-elevating compounds. Long-standing hyperprolactinemia, when associated with hypogonadism, may lead to decreased bone density in both female and male patients *[see Adverse Reactions (6)]*.

Tissue culture experiments indicate that approximately one-third of human breast cancers are prolactin-dependent *in vitro*, a factor of potential importance if the prescription of these drugs is considered in a patient with previously detected breast cancer. As is common with compounds which increase prolactin release, an increase in mammary gland neoplasia was observed in a LATUDA carcinogenicity study conducted in rats and mice *[see Nonclinical Toxicology (13)]*. Neither clinical studies nor epidemiologic studies conducted to date have shown an association between chronic administration of this class of drugs and tumorigenesis in humans, but the available evidence is too limited to be conclusive.

Schizophrenia

In short-term, placebo-controlled schizophrenia studies, the median change from baseline to endpoint in prolactin levels for LATUDA-treated patients was +0.4 ng/mL and was -1.9 ng/mL in the placebo-treated patients. The median change from baseline to endpoint for males was +0.5 ng/mL and for females was -0.2 ng/mL. Median changes for prolactin by dose are shown in Table 12.

[See table 12 at top of next page]

The proportion of patients with prolactin elevations ≥ 5× upper limit of normal (ULN) was 2.8% for LATUDA-treated patients versus 1.0% for placebo-treated patients. The proportion of female patients with prolactin elevations

≥ 5× ULN was 5.7% for LATUDA-treated patients versus 2.0% for placebo-treated female patients. The proportion of male patients with prolactin elevations ≥ 5× ULN was 1.6% versus 0.6% for placebo-treated male patients.

In the uncontrolled longer-term schizophrenia studies (primarily open-label extension studies), LATUDA was associated with a median change in prolactin of -0.9 ng/mL at week 24 (n=357), -5.3ng/mL at week 36 (n=190) and -2.2 ng/mL at week 52 (n=307).

Bipolar Depression

Monotherapy

The median change from baseline to endpoint in prolactin levels, in the short-term, flexible-dosed, placebo-controlled monotherapy bipolar depression study, was +1.7 ng/mL and +3.5 ng/mL with LATUDA 20 to 60 mg/day and 80 to 120 mg/day, respectively compared to +0.3 ng/mL with placebo-treated patients. The median change from baseline to endpoint for males was +1.5 ng/mL and for females was +3.1 ng/mL. Median changes for prolactin by dose range are shown in Table 13.

[See table 13 above]

The proportion of patients with prolactin elevations ≥ 5× upper limit of normal (ULN) was 0.4% for LATUDA-treated patients versus 0.0% for placebo-treated patients. The proportion of female patients with prolactin elevations ≥ 5× ULN was 0.6% for LATUDA-treated patients versus 0% for placebo-treated female patients. The proportion of male patients with prolactin elevations ≥ 5× ULN was 0% versus 0% for placebo-treated male patients.

In the uncontrolled, open-label, longer-term bipolar depression study, patients who were treated with LATUDA as monotherapy in the short-term and continued in the longer-term study, had a median change in prolactin of -1.15 ng/mL at week 24 (n=130).

Adjunctive Therapy with Lithium or Valproate

The median change from baseline to endpoint in prolactin levels, in the short-term, flexible-dosed, placebo-controlled adjunctive therapy bipolar depression studies was +2.8 ng/mL with LATUDA 20 to 120 mg/day compared to 0.0 ng/mL with placebo-treated patients. The median change from baseline to endpoint for males was +2.4 ng/mL and for females was +3.2 ng/mL. Median changes for prolactin across the dose range are shown in Table 14.

Table 14: Median Change in Prolactin (ng/mL) from Baseline in the Adjunctive Therapy Bipolar Depression Studies

	Placebo	LATUDA 20 to 120 mg/day
All Patients	0.0 (n=301)	+2.8 (n=321)
Females	+0.4 (n=156)	+3.2 (n=162)
Males	-0.1 (n=145)	+2.4 (n=159)

Patients were randomized to flexibly dosed LATUDA 20 to 120 mg/day or placebo as adjunctive therapy with lithium or valproate.

The proportion of patients with prolactin elevations ≥ 5× upper limit of normal (ULN) was 0.0% for LATUDA-treated patients versus 0.0% for placebo-treated patients. The proportion of female patients with prolactin elevations ≥ 5× ULN was 0% for LATUDA-treated patients versus 0% for placebo-treated female patients. The proportion of male patients with prolactin elevations ≥ 5× ULN was 0% versus 0% for placebo-treated male patients.

In the uncontrolled, open-label, longer-term bipolar depression study, patients who were treated with LATUDA, as adjunctive therapy with either lithium or valproate, in the short-term and continued in the longer-term study, had a median change in prolactin of -2.9 ng/mL at week 24 (n=88).

5.8 Leukopenia, Neutropenia and Agranulocytosis

Leukopenia/neutropenia has been reported during treatment with antipsychotic agents. Agranulocytosis (including fatal cases) has been reported with other agents in the class. Possible risk factors for leukopenia/neutropenia include pre-existing low white blood cell count (WBC) and history of drug-induced leukopenia/neutropenia. Patients with a pre-existing low WBC or a history of drug-induced leukopenia/neutropenia should have their complete blood count (CBC) monitored frequently during the first few months of therapy and LATUDA should be discontinued at the first sign of decline in WBC, in the absence of other causative factors.

Patients with neutropenia should be carefully monitored for fever or other symptoms or signs of infection and treated promptly if such symptoms or signs occur. Patients with severe neutropenia (absolute neutrophil count < 1000/mm^3) should discontinue LATUDA and have their WBC followed until recovery.

Table 12: Median Change in Prolactin (ng/mL) from Baseline in Schizophrenia Studies

	Placebo	LATUDA 20 mg/day	40 mg/day	80 mg/day	120 mg/day	160 mg/day
All Patients	-1.9 (n=672)	-1.1 (n=70)	-1.4 (n=476)	-0.2 (n=495)	+3.3 (n=284)	+3.3 (n=115)
Females	-5.1 (n=200)	-0.7 (n=19)	-4.0 (n=149)	-0.2 (n=150)	+6.7 (n=70)	+7.1 (n=36)
Males	-1.3 (n=472)	-1.2 (n=51)	-0.7 (n=327)	-0.2 (n=345)	+3.1 (n=214)	+2.4 (n=79)

Table 13: Median Change in Prolactin (ng/mL) from Baseline in the Monotherapy Bipolar Depression Study

	Placebo	LATUDA 20 to 60 mg/day	LATUDA 80 to 120 mg/day
All Patients	+0.3 (n=147)	+1.7 (n=140)	+3.5 (n=144)
Females	0.0 (n=82)	+1.8 (n=78)	+5.3 (n=88)
Males	+0.4 (n=65)	+1.2 (n=62)	+1.9 (n=56)

Patients were randomized to flexibly dosed LATUDA 20 to 60 mg/day, LATUDA 80 to 120 mg/day, or placebo

5.9 Orthostatic Hypotension and Syncope

LATUDA may cause orthostatic hypotension and syncope, perhaps due to its α1-adrenergic receptor antagonism. Associated adverse reactions can include dizziness, lightheadedness, tachycardia, and bradycardia. Generally, these risks are greatest at the beginning of treatment and during dose escalation. Patients at increased risk of these adverse reactions or at increased risk of developing complications from hypotension include those with dehydration, hypovolemia, treatment with antihypertensive medication, history of cardiovascular disease (e.g., heart failure, myocardial infarction, ischemia, or conduction abnormalities), history of cerebrovascular disease, as well as patients who are antipsychotic-naïve. In such patients, consider using a lower starting dose and slower titration, and monitor orthostatic vital signs.

Orthostatic hypotension, as assessed by vital sign measurement, was defined by the following vital sign changes: ≥ 20 mm Hg decrease in systolic blood pressure and ≥ 10 bpm increase in pulse from sitting to standing or supine to standing position.

Schizophrenia

The incidence of orthostatic hypotension and syncope reported as adverse events from short-term, placebo-controlled schizophrenia studies was (LATUDA incidence, placebo incidence): orthostatic hypotension [0.3% (5/1508), 0.1% (1/708)] and syncope [0.1% (2/1508), 0% (0/708)].

In short-term schizophrenia clinical studies, orthostatic hypotension, as assessed by vital signs, occurred with a frequency of 0.8% with LATUDA 40 mg, 2.1% with LATUDA 80 mg, 1.7% with LATUDA 120 mg and 0.8% with LATUDA 160 mg compared to 0.7% with placebo.

Bipolar Depression

Monotherapy

In the short-term, flexible-dose, placebo-controlled monotherapy bipolar depression study, there were no reported adverse events of orthostatic hypotension and syncope.

Orthostatic hypotension, as assessed by vital signs, occurred with a frequency of 0.6% with LATUDA 20 to 60 mg and 0.6% with LATUDA 80 to 120 mg compared to 0% with placebo.

Adjunctive Therapy with Lithium or Valproate

In the short-term, flexible-dose, placebo-controlled adjunctive therapy bipolar depression therapy studies, there were no reported adverse events of orthostatic hypotension and syncope. Orthostatic hypotension, as assessed by vital signs, occurred with a frequency of 1.1% with LATUDA 20 to 120 mg compared to 0.9% with placebo.

5.10 Seizures

As with other antipsychotic drugs, LATUDA should be used cautiously in patients with a history of seizures or with conditions that lower the seizure threshold, e.g., Alzheimer's dementia. Conditions that lower the seizure threshold may be more prevalent in patients 65 years or older.

Schizophrenia

In short-term, placebo-controlled schizophrenia studies, seizures/convulsions occurred in 0.1% (2/1508) of patients treated with LATUDA compared to 0.1% (1/708) placebo-treated patients.

Bipolar Depression

Monotherapy

In the short-term, flexible-dose, placebo-controlled monotherapy bipolar depression study, no patient experienced seizures/convulsions.

Adjunctive Therapy with Lithium or Valproate

In the short-term, flexible-dose, placebo-controlled adjunctive therapy bipolar depression studies, no patient experienced seizures/convulsions.

5.11 Potential for Cognitive and Motor Impairment

LATUDA, like other antipsychotics, has the potential to impair judgment, thinking or motor skills. Caution patients about operating hazardous machinery, including motor vehicles, until they are reasonably certain that therapy with LATUDA does not affect them adversely.

In clinical studies with LATUDA, somnolence included: hypersomnia, hypersomnolence, sedation and somnolence.

Schizophrenia

In short-term, placebo-controlled schizophrenia studies, somnolence was reported by 17.0% (256/1508) of patients treated with LATUDA (15.5% LATUDA 20 mg, 15.6% LATUDA 40 mg, 15.2% LATUDA 80 mg, 26.5% LATUDA 120 mg and 8.3% LATUDA 160 mg/day) compared to 7.1% (50/708) of placebo patients.

Bipolar Depression

Monotherapy

In the short-term, flexible-dosed, placebo-controlled monotherapy bipolar depression study, somnolence was reported by 7.3% (12/164) and 13.8% (23/167) with LATUDA 20 to 60 mg and 80 to120 mg, respectively compared to 6.5% (11/168) of placebo patients.

Adjunctive Therapy with Lithium or Valproate

In the short-term, flexible-dosed, placebo-controlled adjunctive therapy bipolar depression studies, somnolence was reported by 11.4% (41/360) of patients treated with LATUDA 20-120 mg compared to 5.1% (17/334) of placebo patients.

5.12 Body Temperature Dysregulation

Disruption of the body's ability to reduce core body temperature has been attributed to antipsychotic agents. Appropriate care is advised when prescribing LATUDA for patients who will be experiencing conditions that may contribute to an elevation in core body temperature, e.g., exercising strenuously, exposure to extreme heat, receiving concomitant medication with anticholinergic activity, or being subject to dehydration *[see Patient Counseling Information (17.9)]*.

5.13 Suicide

The possibility of a suicide attempt is inherent in psychotic illness and close supervision of high-risk patients should accompany drug therapy. Prescriptions for LATUDA should be written for the smallest quantity of tablets consistent with good patient management in order to reduce the risk of overdose.

Schizophrenia

In short-term, placebo-controlled schizophrenia studies, the incidence of treatment-emergent suicidal ideation was 0.4% (6/1508) for LATUDA-treated patients compared to 0.8% (6/708) on placebo. No suicide attempts or completed suicides were reported in these studies.

Table 15: Adverse Reactions in 2% or More of LATUDA-Treated Patients and That Occurred at Greater Incidence than in the Placebo-Treated Patients in Short-term Schizophrenia Studies

	Percentage of Patients Reporting Reaction						
		LATUDA					
Body System or Organ Class	Placebo (N=708) (%)	20 mg/day (N=71) (%)	40 mg/day (N=487) (%)	80 mg/day (N=538) (%)	120 mg/day (N=291) (%)	160 mg/day (N=121) (%)	All LATUDA (N=1508) (%)
Gastrointestinal Disorders							
Nausea	5	11	10	9	13	7	10
Vomiting	6	7	6	9	9	7	8
Dyspepsia	5	11	6	5	8	6	6
Salivary Hypersecretion	<1	1	1	2	4	2	2
Musculoskeletal and Connective Tissue Disorders							
Back Pain	2	0	4	3	4	0	3
Nervous System Disorders							
Somnolence*	7	15	16	15	26	8	17
Akathisia	3	6	11	12	22	7	13
Extrapyramidal Disorder**	6	6	11	12	22	13	14
Dizziness	2	6	4	4	5	6	4
Psychiatric Disorders							
Insomnia	8	8	10	11	9	7	10
Agitation	4	10	7	3	6	5	5
Anxiety	4	3	6	4	7	3	5
Restlessness	1	1	3	1	3	2	2

Note: Figures rounded to the nearest integer
* Somnolence includes adverse event terms: hypersomnia, hypersomnolence, sedation, and somnolence
** Extrapyramidal symptoms includes adverse event terms: bradykinesia, cogwheel rigidity, drooling, dystonia, extrapyramidal disorder, hypokinesia, muscle rigidity, oculogyric crisis, oromandibular dystonia, parkinsonism, psychomotor retardation, tongue spasm, torticollis, tremor, and trismus

Table 16: Adverse Reactions in 2% or More of LATUDA-Treated Patients and That Occurred at Greater Incidence than in the Placebo-Treated Patients in a Short-term Monotherapy Bipolar Depression Study

	Percentage of Patients Reporting Reaction			
Body System or Organ Class Dictionary-derived Term	Placebo (N=168) (%)	LATUDA 20-60 mg/day (N=164) (%)	LATUDA 80-120 mg/day (N=167) (%)	All LATUDA (N=331) (%)
Gastrointestinal Disorders				
Nausea	8	10	17	14
Dry Mouth	4	6	4	5
Vomiting	2	2	6	4
Diarrhea	2	5	3	4
Infections and Infestations				
Nasopharyngitis	1	4	4	4
Influenza	1	<1	2	2
Urinary Tract Infection	<1	2	1	2
Musculoskeletal and Connective Tissue Disorders				
Back Pain	<1	3	<1	2
Nervous System Disorders				
Extrapyramidal Symptoms*	2	5	9	7
Akathisia	2	8	11	9
Somnolence**	7	7	14	11
Psychiatric Disorders				
Anxiety	1	4	5	4

Note: Figures rounded to the nearest integer
*Extrapyramidal symptoms includes adverse event terms: bradykinesia, cogwheel rigidity, drooling, dystonia, extrapyramidal disorder, glabellar reflex abnormal, hypokinesia, muscle rigidity, oculogyric crisis, oromandibular dystonia, parkinsonism, psychomotor retardation, tongue spasm, torticollis, tremor, and trismus
** Somnolence includes adverse event terms: hypersomnia, hypersomnolence, sedation, and somnolence

Bipolar Depression

Monotherapy

In the short-term, flexible-dose, placebo-controlled monotherapy bipolar depression study, the incidence of treatment-emergent suicidal ideation was 0.0% (0/331) with LATUDA-treated patients compared to 0.0% (0/168) with placebo-treated patients. No suicide attempts or completed suicides were reported in this study.

Adjunctive Therapy with Lithium or Valproate

In the short-term, flexible-dose, placebo-controlled adjunctive therapy bipolar depression studies, the incidence of treatment-emergent suicidal ideation was 1.1% (4/360) for LATUDA-treated patients compared to 0.3% (1/334) on placebo. No suicide attempts or completed suicides were reported in these studies.

5.14 Activation of Mania/Hypomania

Antidepressant treatment can increase the risk of developing a manic or hypomanic episode, particularly in patients with bipolar disorder. Monitor patients for the emergence of such episodes.

In the bipolar depression monotherapy and adjunctive therapy (with lithium or valproate) studies, less than 1% of subjects in the LATUDA and placebo groups developed manic or hypomanic episodes.

5.15 Dysphagia

Esophageal dysmotility and aspiration have been associated with antipsychotic drug use. Aspiration pneumonia is a common cause of morbidity and mortality in elderly patients, in particular those with advanced Alzheimer's dementia. LATUDA and other antipsychotic drugs should be used cautiously in patients at risk for aspiration pneumonia.

5.16 Neurological Adverse Reactions in Patients with Parkinson's Disease or Dementia with Lewy Bodies

Patients with Parkinson's Disease or Dementia with Lewy Bodies are reported to have an increased sensitivity to antipsychotic medication. Manifestations of this increased sensitivity include confusion, obtundation, postural instability with frequent falls, extrapyramidal symptoms, and clinical features consistent with the neuroleptic malignant syndrome.

6 ADVERSE REACTIONS

The following adverse reactions are discussed in more detail in other sections of the labeling:

- Increased Mortality in Elderly Patients with Dementia-Related Psychosis *[see Boxed Warning and Warnings and Precautions (5.1)]*
- Suicidal Thoughts and Behaviors *[see Boxed Warning and Warnings and Precautions (5.2)]*
- Cerebrovascular Adverse Reactions, Including Stroke, in Elderly Patients with Dementia-related Psychosis *[see Warnings and Precautions (5.23)]*
- Neuroleptic Malignant Syndrome *[see Warnings and Precautions (5.4)]*
- Tardive Dyskinesia *[see Warnings and Precautions (5.5)]*
- Metabolic Changes (Hyperglycemia and Diabetes Mellitus, Dyslipidemia, and Weight Gain) *[see Warnings and Precautions (5.6)]*
- Hyperprolactinemia *[see Warnings and Precautions (5.7)]*
- Leukopenia, Neutropenia, and Agranulocytosis *[see Warnings and Precautions (5.8)]*
- Orthostatic Hypotension and Syncope *[see Warnings and Precautions (5.9)]*
- Seizures *[see Warnings and Precautions (5.10)]*
- Potential for Cognitive and Motor Impairment *[see Warnings and Precautions (5.11)]*
- Body Temperature Dysregulation *[see Warnings and Precautions (5.12)]*
- Suicide *[see Warnings and Precautions (5.13)]*
- Activation of Mania/Hypomania *[see Warnings and Precautions (5.14)]*
- Dysphagia *[see Warnings and Precautions (5.15)]*
- Neurological Adverse Reactions in Patients with Parkinson's Disease or Dementia with Lewy Bodies *[see Warnings and Precautions (5.16)]*

6.1 Clinical Trials Experience

Because clinical trials are conducted under widely varying conditions, adverse reaction rates observed in clinical trials of a drug cannot be directly compared to rates in the clinical trials of another drug and may not reflect the rates observed in clinical practice.

The information below is derived from an integrated clinical study database for LATUDA consisting of 3799 patients exposed to one or more doses of LATUDA for the treatment of schizophrenia and bipolar depression in placebo-controlled studies. This experience corresponds with a total experience of 1250.9 patient-years. A total of 1106 LATUDA-treated patients had at least 24 weeks and 371 LATUDA-treated patients had at least 52 weeks of exposure.

Adverse events during exposure to study treatment were obtained by general inquiry and voluntarily reported adverse experiences, as well as results from physical examinations, vital signs, ECGs, weights and laboratory investigations. Adverse experiences were recorded by clinical investigators using their own terminology. In order to provide a meaningful estimate of the proportion of individuals experiencing adverse events, events were grouped in standardized categories using MedDRA terminology.

Schizophrenia

The following findings are based on the short-term, placebo-controlled premarketing studies for schizophrenia in which LATUDA was administered at daily doses ranging from 20 to 160 mg (n=1508).

Commonly Observed Adverse Reactions: The most common adverse reactions (incidence ≥ 5% and at least twice the rate of placebo) in patients treated with LATUDA were somnolence, akathisia, extrapyramidal symptoms, and nausea.

Adverse Reactions Associated with Discontinuation of Treatment: A total of 9.5% (143/1508) LATUDA-treated patients and 9.3% (66/708) of placebo-treated patients discontinued due to adverse reactions. There were no adverse reactions associated with discontinuation in subjects treated with LATUDA that were at least 2% and at least twice the placebo rate.

Adverse Reactions Occurring at an Incidence of 2% or More in LATUDA-Treated Patients: Adverse reactions associated with the use of LATUDA (incidence of 2% or greater, rounded to the nearest percent and LATUDA incidence greater than placebo) that occurred during acute therapy (up to 6 weeks in patients with schizophrenia) are shown in Table 15.

[See table 15 above]

Table 17: Adverse Reactions in 2% or More of LATUDA-Treated Patients and That Occurred at Greater Incidence than in the Placebo-Treated Patients in the Short-term Adjunctive Therapy Bipolar Depression Studies

Body System or Organ Class Dictionary-derived Term	Percentage of Patients Reporting Reaction Placebo (N=334) (%)	LATUDA 20 to 120 mg/day (N=360) (%)
Gastrointestinal Disorders		
Nausea	10	14
Vomiting	1	4
General Disorders		
Fatigue	1	3
Infections and Infestations		
Nasopharyngitis	2	4
Investigations		
Weight Increased	<1	3
Metabolism and Nutrition Disorders		
Increased Appetite	1	3
Nervous System Disorders		
Extrapyramidal Symptoms*	9	14
Somnolence**	5	11
Akathisia	5	11
Psychiatric Disorders		
Restlessness	<1	4

Note: Figures rounded to the nearest integer
*Extrapyramidal symptoms includes adverse event terms: bradykinesia, cogwheel rigidity, drooling, dystonia, extrapyramidal disorder, glabellar reflex abnormal, hypokinesia, muscle rigidity, oculogyric crisis, oromandibular dystonia, parkinsonism, psychomotor retardation, tongue spasm, torticollis, tremor, and trismus
** Somnolence includes adverse event terms: hypersomnia, hypersomnolence, sedation, and somnolence

Table 18: Incidence of EPS Compared to Placebo in Schizophrenia Studies

Adverse Event Term	Placebo (N=708) (%)	LATUDA 20 mg/day (N=71) (%)	40 mg/day (N=487) (%)	80 mg/day (N=538) (%)	120 mg/day (N=291) (%)	160 mg/day (N=121) (%)
All EPS events	9	10	21	23	39	20
All EPS events, excluding Akathisia/Restlessness	6	6	11	12	22	13
Akathisia	3	6	11	12	22	7
Dystonia*	<1	0	4	5	7	2
Parkinsonism**	5	6	9	8	17	11
Restlessness	1	1	3	1	3	2

Note: Figures rounded to the nearest integer
* Dystonia includes adverse event terms: dystonia, oculogyric crisis, oromandibular dystonia, tongue spasm, torticollis, and trismus
** Parkinsonism includes adverse event terms: bradykinesia, cogwheel rigidity, drooling, extrapyramidal disorder, hypokinesia, muscle rigidity, parkinsonism, psychomotor retardation, and tremor

Table 19: Incidence of EPS Compared to Placebo in the Monotherapy Bipolar Depression Study

Adverse Event Term	Placebo (N=168) (%)	LATUDA 20 to 60 mg/day (N=164) (%)	80 to 120 mg/day (N=167) (%)
All EPS events	5	12	20
All EPS events, excluding Akathisia/Restlessness	2	5	9
Akathisia	2	8	11
Dystonia*	0	0	2
Parkinsonism**	2	5	8
Restlessness	<1	0	3

Note: Figures rounded to the nearest integer
* Dystonia includes adverse event terms: dystonia, oculogyric crisis, oromandibular dystonia, tongue spasm, torticollis, and trismus
** Parkinsonism includes adverse event terms: bradykinesia, cogwheel rigidity, drooling, extrapyramidal disorder, glabellar reflex abnormal, hypokinesia, muscle rigidity, parkinsonism, psychomotor retardation, and tremor

Dose-Related Adverse Reactions in the Schizophrenia Studies

Akathisia and extrapyramidal symptoms were dose-related. The frequency of akathisia increased with dose up to 120 mg/day (5.6% for LATUDA 20 mg, 10.7% for LATUDA 40 mg, 12.3% for LATUDA 80 mg, and 22.0% for LATUDA 120 mg). Akathisia was reported by 7.4% (9/121) of patients receiving 160 mg/day. Akathisia occurred in 3.0% of subjects receiving placebo. The frequency of extrapyramidal symptoms increased with dose up to 120 mg/day (5.6% for LATUDA 20 mg, 11.5% for LATUDA 40 mg, 11.9% for LATUDA 80 mg, and 22.0% for LATUDA 120 mg).

Bipolar Depression (Monotherapy)

The following findings are based on the short-term, placebo-controlled premarketing study for bipolar depression in which LATUDA was administered at daily doses ranging from 20 to 120 mg (n=331).

Commonly Observed Adverse Reactions: The most common adverse reactions (incidence ≥ 5%, in either dose group, and at least twice the rate of placebo) in patients treated with LATUDA were akathisia, extrapyramidal symptoms, somnolence, nausea, vomiting, diarrhea, and anxiety.

Adverse Reactions Associated with Discontinuation of Treatment: A total of 6.0% (20/331) LATUDA-treated patients and 5.4% (9/168) of placebo-treated patients discontinued due to adverse reactions. There were no adverse reactions associated with discontinuation in subjects treated with LATUDA that were at least 2% and at least twice the placebo rate.

Adverse Reactions Occurring at an Incidence of 2% or More in LATUDA-Treated Patients: Adverse reactions associated with the use of LATUDA (incidence of 2% or greater, rounded to the nearest percent and LATUDA incidence greater than placebo) that occurred during acute therapy (up to 6 weeks in patients with bipolar depression) are shown in Table 16.

[See table 16 at top of previous page]

Dose-Related Adverse Reactions in the Monotherapy Study: In the short-term, placebo-controlled study (involving lower and higher LATUDA dose ranges) [see Clinical Studies (14.2)] the adverse reactions that occurred with a greater than 5% incidence in the patients treated with LATUDA in any dose group and greater than placebo in both groups were nausea (10.4%, 17.4%), somnolence (7.3%, 13.8%), akathisia (7.9%, 10.8%), and extrapyramidal symptoms (4.9%, 9.0%) for LATUDA 20 to 60 mg/day and LATUDA 80 to 120 mg/day, respectively.

Bipolar Depression

Adjunctive Therapy with Lithium or Valproate

The following findings are based on two short-term, placebo-controlled premarketing studies for bipolar depression in which LATUDA was administered at daily doses ranging from 20 to 120 mg as adjunctive therapy with lithium or valproate (n=360).

Commonly Observed Adverse Reactions: The most common adverse reactions (incidence ≥ 5% and at least twice the rate of placebo) in subjects treated with LATUDA were akathisia and somnolence.

Adverse Reactions Associated with Discontinuation of Treatment: A total of 5.8% (21/360) LATUDA-treated patients and 4.8% (16/334) of placebo-treated patients discontinued due to adverse reactions. There were no adverse reactions associated with discontinuation in subjects treated with LATUDA that were at least 2% and at least twice the placebo rate.

Adverse Reactions Occurring at an Incidence of 2% or More in LATUDA-Treated Patients: Adverse reactions associated with the use of LATUDA (incidence of 2% or greater, rounded to the nearest percent and LATUDA incidence greater than placebo) that occurred during acute therapy (up to 6 weeks in patients with bipolar depression) are shown in Table 17.

[See table 17 above]

Extrapyramidal Symptoms

Schizophrenia

In the short-term, placebo-controlled schizophrenia studies, for LATUDA-treated patients, the incidence of reported events related to extrapyramidal symptoms (EPS), excluding akathisia and restlessness, was 13.5% versus 5.8% for placebo-treated patients. The incidence of akathisia for LATUDA-treated patients was 12.9% versus 3.0% for placebo-treated patients. Incidence of EPS by dose is provided in Table 18.

[See table 18 above]

Bipolar Depression

Monotherapy

In the short-term, placebo-controlled monotherapy bipolar depression study, for LATUDA-treated patients, the incidence of reported events related to EPS, excluding akathisia and restlessness was 6.9% versus 2.4% for placebo-treated patients. The incidence of akathisia for LATUDA-treated patients was 9.4% versus 2.4% for placebo-treated patients. Incidence of EPS by dose groups is provided in Table 19.

[See table 19 above]

Adjunctive Therapy with Lithium or Valproate

In the short-term, placebo-controlled adjunctive therapy bipolar depression studies, for LATUDA-treated patients, the incidence of EPS, excluding akathisia and restlessness, was

Table 21: Serum Creatinine Shifts from Normal at Baseline to High at Study End-Point in Schizophrenia Studies

Laboratory Parameter	Placebo (N=708)	LATUDA 20 mg/day (N=71)	LATUDA 40 mg/day (N=487)	LATUDA 80 mg/day (N=538)	LATUDA 120 mg/day (N=291)	LATUDA 160 mg/day (N=121)
Serum Creatinine Elevated	2%	1%	2%	2%	5%	7%

13.9% versus 8.7% for placebo. The incidence of akathisia for LATUDA-treated patients was 10.8% versus 4.8% for placebo-treated patients. Incidence of EPS is provided in Table 20.

Table 20: Incidence of EPS Compared to Placebo in the Adjunctive Therapy Bipolar Depression Studies

Adverse Event Term	Placebo (N=334) (%)	LATUDA 20 to 120 mg/day (N=360) (%)
All EPS events	**13**	**24**
All EPS events, excluding Akathisia/ Restlessness	**9**	**14**
Akathisia	5	11
Dystonia*	<1	1
Parkinsonism**	8	13
Restlessness	<1	4

Note: Figures rounded to the nearest integer
* Dystonia includes adverse event terms: dystonia, oculogyric crisis, oromandibular dystonia, tongue spasm, torticollis, and trismus
** Parkinsonism includes adverse event terms: bradykinesia, cogwheel rigidity, drooling, extrapyramidal disorder, glabellar reflex abnormal, hypokinesia, muscle rigidity, parkinsonism, psychomotor retardation, and tremor

In the short-term, placebo-controlled schizophrenia and bipolar depression studies, data was objectively collected on the Simpson Angus Rating Scale (SAS) for extrapyramidal symptoms (EPS), the Barnes Akathisia Scale (BAS) for akathisia and the Abnormal Involuntary Movement Scale (AIMS) for dyskinesias.

Schizophrenia

The mean change from baseline for LATUDA-treated patients for the SAS, BAS and AIMS was comparable to placebo-treated patients, with the exception of the Barnes Akathisia Scale global score (LATUDA, 0.1; placebo, 0.0). The percentage of patients who shifted from normal to abnormal was greater in LATUDA-treated patients versus placebo for the BAS (LATUDA, 14.4%; placebo, 7.1%), the SAS (LATUDA, 5.0%; placebo, 2.3%) and the AIMS (LATUDA, 7.4%; placebo, 5.8%).

Bipolar Depression

Monotherapy

The mean change from baseline for LATUDA-treated patients for the SAS, BAS and AIMS was comparable to placebo-treated patients. The percentage of patients who shifted from normal to abnormal was greater in LATUDA-treated patients versus placebo for the BAS (LATUDA, 8.4%; placebo, 5.6%), the SAS (LATUDA, 3.7%; placebo, 1.9%) and the AIMS (LATUDA, 3.4%; placebo, 1.2%).

Adjunctive Therapy with Lithium or Valproate

The mean change from baseline for LATUDA-treated patients for the SAS, BAS and AIMS was comparable to placebo-treated patients. The percentage of patients who shifted from normal to abnormal was greater in LATUDA-treated patients versus placebo for the BAS (LATUDA, 8.7%; placebo, 2.1%), the SAS (LATUDA, 2.8%; placebo, 2.1%) and the AIMS (LATUDA, 2.8%; placebo, 0.6%).

Dystonia

Class Effect: Symptoms of dystonia, prolonged abnormal contractions of muscle groups, may occur in susceptible individuals during the first few days of treatment. Dystonic symptoms include: spasm of the neck muscles, sometimes progressing to tightness of the throat, swallowing difficulty, difficulty breathing, and/or protrusion of the tongue. While these symptoms can occur at low doses, they occur more frequently and with greater severity with high potency and at higher doses of first-generation antipsychotic drugs. An elevated risk of acute dystonia is observed in males and younger age groups.

Schizophrenia

In the short-term, placebo-controlled schizophrenia clinical studies, dystonia occurred in 4.2% of LATUDA-treated subjects (0.0% LATUDA 20 mg, 3.5% LATUDA 40 mg, 4.5% LATUDA 80 mg, 6.5% LATUDA 120 mg and 2.5% LATUDA 160 mg) compared to 0.8% of subjects receiving placebo. Seven subjects (0.5%, 7/1508) discontinued clinical trials due to dystonic events – four were receiving LATUDA 80 mg/day and three were receiving LATUDA 120 mg/day.

Bipolar Depression

Monotherapy

In the short-term, flexible-dose, placebo-controlled monotherapy bipolar depression study, dystonia occurred in 0.9% of LATUDA-treated subjects (0.0% and 1.8% for LATUDA 20 to 60 mg/day and LATUDA 80 to 120 mg/day, respectively) compared to 0.0% of subjects receiving placebo. No subject discontinued the clinical study due to dystonic events.

Adjunctive Therapy with Lithium or Valproate

In the short-term, flexible-dose, placebo-controlled adjunctive therapy bipolar depression studies, dystonia occurred in 1.1% of LATUDA-treated subjects (20 to 120 mg) compared to 0.6% of subjects receiving placebo. No subject discontinued the clinical study due to dystonic events.

Other Adverse Reactions Observed During the Premarketing Evaluation of LATUDA

Following is a list of adverse reactions reported by patients treated with LATUDA at multiple doses of ≥ 20 mg once daily within the premarketing database of 2905 patients with schizophrenia. The reactions listed are those that could be of clinical importance, as well as reactions that are plausibly drug-related on pharmacologic or other grounds. Reactions listed in Table 15 or those that appear elsewhere in the LATUDA label are not included. Although the reactions reported occurred during treatment with LATUDA, they were not necessarily caused by it.

Reactions are further categorized by organ class and listed in order of decreasing frequency according to the following definitions: those occurring in at least 1/100 patients (frequent) (only those not already listed in the tabulated results from placebo-controlled studies appear in this listing); those occurring in 1/100 to 1/1000 patients (infrequent); and those occurring in fewer than 1/1000 patients (rare).

Blood and Lymphatic System Disorders: **Infrequent:** *anemia*

Cardiac Disorders: **Frequent:** *tachycardia;* **Infrequent:** *AV block 1st degree, angina pectoris, bradycardia*

Ear and Labyrinth Disorders: **Infrequent:** *vertigo*

Eye Disorders: **Frequent:** *blurred vision*

Gastrointestinal Disorders: **Frequent:** *abdominal pain, diarrhea;* **Infrequent:** *gastritis*

General Disorders and Administrative Site Conditions: **Rare:** *sudden death*

Investigations: **Frequent:** *CPK increased*

Metabolism and Nutritional System Disorders: **Frequent:** *decreased appetite*

Musculoskeletal and Connective Tissue Disorders: **Rare:** *rhabdomyolysis*

Nervous System Disorders: **Infrequent:** *cerebrovascular accident, dysarthria*

Psychiatric Disorders: **Infrequent:** *abnormal dreams, panic attack, sleep disorder*

Renal and Urinary Disorders: **Infrequent:** *dysuria;* **Rare:** *renal failure*

Reproductive System and Breast Disorders: **Infrequent:** *amenorrhea, dysmenorrhea;* **Rare:** *breast enlargement, breast pain, galactorrhea, erectile dysfunction*

Skin and Subcutaneous Tissue Disorders: **Frequent:** *rash, pruritus;* **Rare:** *angioedema*

Vascular Disorders: **Frequent:** *hypertension*

Clinical Laboratory Changes

Schizophrenia

Serum Creatinine: In short-term, placebo-controlled trials, the mean change from Baseline in serum creatinine was +0.05 mg/dL for LATUDA-treated patients compared to +0.02 mg/dL for placebo-treated patients. A creatinine shift from normal to high occurred in 3.0% (43/1453) of LATUDA-treated patients and 1.6% (11/681) on placebo. The threshold for high creatinine value varied from > 0.79 to > 1.3 mg/dL based on the centralized laboratory definition for each study (Table 21).

[See table 21 above]

Bipolar Depression

Monotherapy

Serum Creatinine: In the short-term, flexible-dose, placebo-controlled monotherapy bipolar depression study, the mean change from Baseline in serum creatinine was +0.01 mg/dL for LATUDA-treated patients compared to -0.02 mg/dL for placebo-treated patients. A creatinine shift from normal to high occurred in 2.8% (9/322) of LATUDA-treated patients and 0.6% (1/162) on placebo (Table 22).

Table 22: Serum Creatinine Shifts from Normal at Baseline to High at Study End-Point in a Monotherapy Bipolar Depression Study

Laboratory Parameter	Placebo (N=168)	LATUDA 20 to 60 mg/day (N=164)	LATUDA 80 to 120 mg/day (N=167)
Serum Creatinine Elevated	<1%	2%	4%

Adjunctive Therapy with Lithium or Valproate

Serum Creatinine: In short-term, placebo-controlled premarketing adjunctive studies for bipolar depression, the mean change from Baseline in serum creatinine was +0.04 mg/dL for LATUDA-treated patients compared to -0.01 mg/dL for placebo-treated patients. A creatinine shift from normal to high occurred in 4.3% (15/360) of LATUDA-treated patients and 1.6% (5/334) on placebo (Table 23).

Table 23: Serum Creatinine Shifts from Normal at Baseline to High at Study End-Point in the Adjunctive Therapy Bipolar Depression Studies

Laboratory Parameter	Placebo (N=334)	LATUDA 20 to 120 mg/day (N=360)
Serum Creatinine Elevated	2%	4%

7 DRUG INTERACTIONS

7.1 Potential for Other Drugs to Affect LATUDA

LATUDA is predominantly metabolized by CYP3A4. LATUDA should not be used concomitantly with strong CYP3A4 inhibitors (e.g., ketoconazole, clarithromycin, ritonavir, voriconazole, mibefradil, etc.) or strong CYP3A4 inducers (e.g., rifampin, avasimibe, St. John's wort, phenytoin, carbamazepine, etc.) *[see Contraindications (4)]*. The LATUDA dose should be reduced to half of the original level when used concomitantly with moderate inhibitors of CYP3A4 (e.g., diltiazem, atazanavir, erythromycin, fluconazole, verapamil, etc.). If LATUDA is used concomitantly with a moderate CYP3A4 inducer, it may be necessary to increase the LATUDA dose *[see Dosage and Administration (2.5)]*.

Lithium: It is not necessary to adjust the LATUDA dose when used concomitantly with lithium (Figure 1).

Valproate: It is not necessary to adjust the LATUDA dose when used concomitantly with valproate. A dedicated drug-drug interaction study has not been conducted with valproate and LATUDA. Based on pharmacokinetic data from the bipolar depression studies valproate levels were not affected by lurasidone, and lurasidone concentrations were not affected by valproate.

Grapefruit: Grapefruit and grapefruit juice should be avoided in patients taking LATUDA, since these may inhibit CYP3A4 and alter LATUDA concentrations *[see Dosage and Administration (2.5)]*.

[See figure 1 at top of next page]

7.2 Potential for LATUDA to Affect Other Drugs

No dose adjustment is needed for lithium, substrates of P-gp, CYP3A4 (Figure 2) or valproate when coadministered with LATUDA.).

[See figure 2 at top of next page]

8 USE IN SPECIFIC POPULATIONS

8.1 Pregnancy

Pregnancy Category B

Risk Summary

There are no adequate and well controlled studies of LATUDA use in pregnant women. Neonates exposed to antipsychotic drugs during the third trimester of pregnancy are at risk for extrapyramidal and/or withdrawal symptoms following delivery. There have been reports of agitation, hypertonia, hypotonia, tremor, somnolence, respiratory distress and feeding disorder in these neonates. These complications have varied in severity; while in some cases symptoms have been self-limited, in other cases neonates have required intensive care unit support and prolonged hospitalization.

LATUDA should be used during pregnancy only if the potential benefit justifies the potential risk to the fetus.

Human Data

Safe use of LATUDA during pregnancy or lactation has not been established; therefore, use of LATUDA in pregnancy,

Figure 1: Impact of Other Drugs on LATUDA Pharmacokinetics

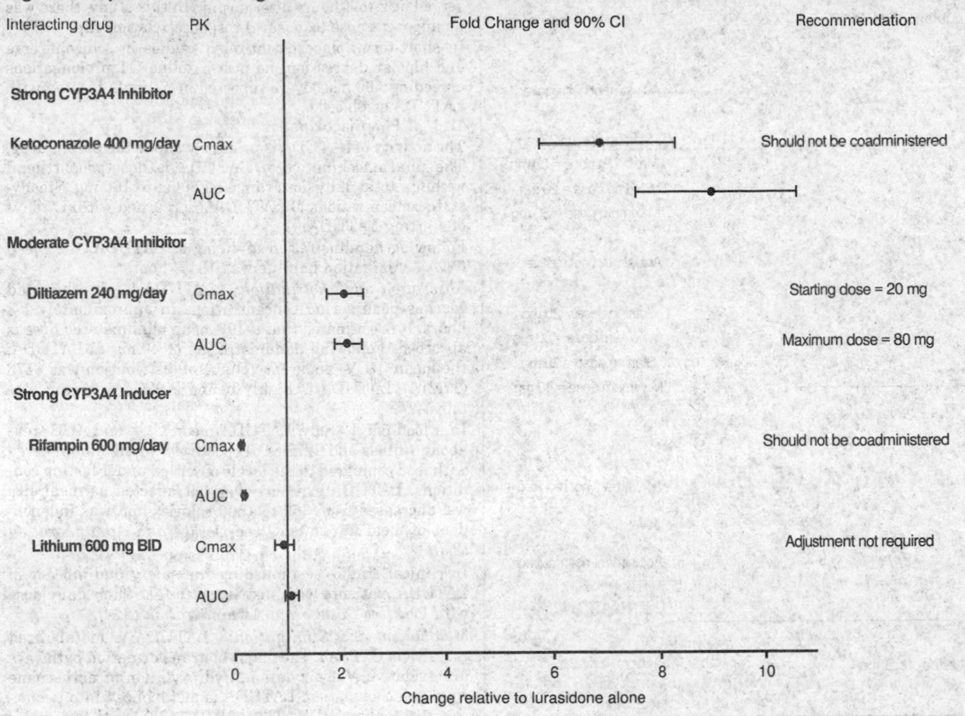

Figure 2: Impact of LATUDA on Other Drugs

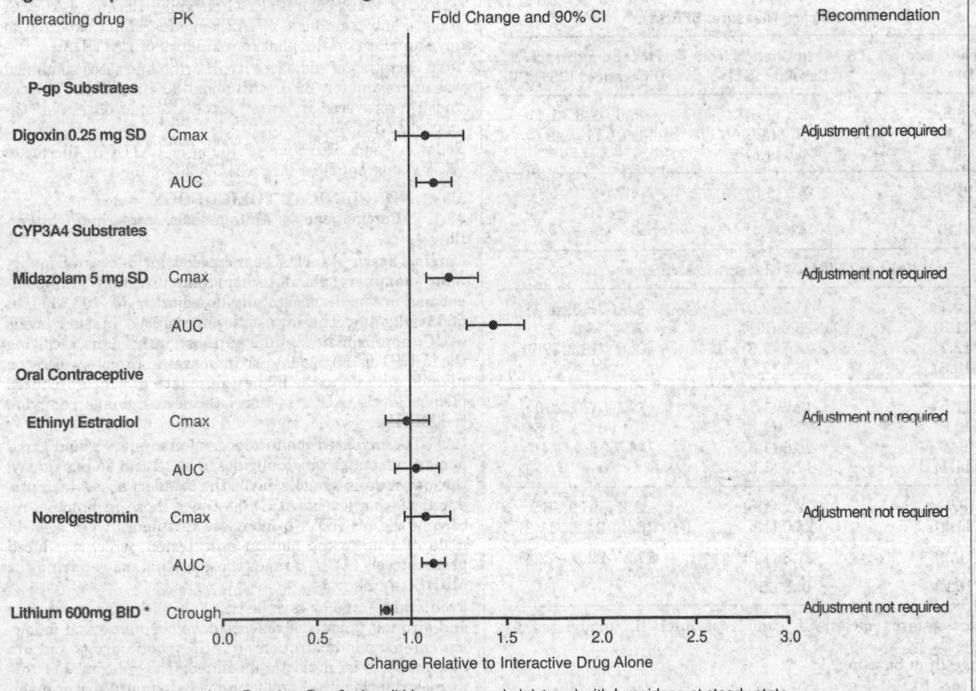

* Steady state lithium Ctrough on Day 4 vs Day 8 when lithium was coadministered with lurasidone at steady state

in nursing mothers, or in women of childbearing potential requires that the benefits of treatment be weighed against the possible risks to mother and child.

Animal Data

No adverse developmental effects were observed in a study in which pregnant rats were given lurasidone during the period of organogenesis and continuing through weaning at doses up to 10 mg/kg/day, which is approximately half of the maximum recommended human dose (MRHD) of 160 mg/day, based on mg/m^2 body surface area.

No teratogenic effects were seen in studies in which pregnant rats and rabbits were given lurasidone during the period of organogenesis at doses up to 25 and 50 mg/kg/day, respectively. These doses are 1.5- and 6-times, in rats and rabbits, respectively, the MRHD of 160 mg/day based on mg/m^2 body surface area.

8.3 Nursing Mothers

LATUDA was excreted in milk of rats during lactation. It is not known whether LATUDA or its metabolites are excreted in human milk. Because of the potential for serious adverse reactions in nursing infants, a decision should be made whether to discontinue nursing or to discontinue the drug, considering the risk of drug discontinuation to the mother.

8.4 Pediatric Use

Safety and effectiveness in pediatric patients have not been established.

8.5 Geriatric Use

Clinical studies with LATUDA did not include sufficient numbers of patients aged 65 and older to determine whether or not they respond differently from younger patients. In elderly patients with psychosis (65 to 85), LATUDA concentrations (20 mg/day) were similar to those in young subjects. It is unknown whether dose adjustment is necessary on the basis of age alone.

Elderly patients with dementia-related psychosis treated with LATUDA are at an increased risk of death compared to placebo. LATUDA is not approved for the treatment of patients with dementia-related psychosis *[see Boxed Warning]*.

8.6 Other Patient Factors

The effect of intrinsic patient factors on the pharmacokinetics of LATUDA is presented in Figure 3.

[See figure 3 at top of next page]

9 DRUG ABUSE AND DEPENDENCE

9.1 Controlled Substance

LATUDA is not a controlled substance.

9.2 Abuse

LATUDA has not been systematically studied in humans for its potential for abuse or physical dependence or its ability to induce tolerance. While clinical studies with LATUDA did not reveal any tendency for drug-seeking behavior, these observations were not systematic and it is not possible to predict the extent to which a CNS-active drug will be misused, diverted and/or abused once it is marketed. Patients should be evaluated carefully for a history of drug abuse, and such patients should be observed carefully for signs of LATUDA misuse or abuse (e.g., development of tolerance, drug-seeking behavior, increases in dose).

10 OVERDOSAGE

10.1 Human Experience

In premarketing clinical studies, accidental or intentional overdosage of LATUDA was identified in one patient who ingested an estimated 560 mg of LATUDA. This patient recovered without sequelae. This patient resumed LATUDA treatment for an additional two months.

10.2 Management of Overdosage

Consult a Certified Poison Control Center for up-to-date guidance and advice. There is no specific antidote to LATUDA, therefore, appropriate supportive measures should be instituted and close medical supervision and monitoring should continue until the patient recovers. Consider the possibility of multiple-drug overdose.

Cardiovascular monitoring should commence immediately, including continuous electrocardiographic monitoring for possible arrhythmias. If antiarrhythmic therapy is administered, disopyramide, procainamide, and quinidine carry a theoretical hazard of additive QT-prolonging effects when administered in patients with an acute overdose of LATUDA. Similarly, the alpha-blocking properties of bretylium might be additive to those of LATUDA, resulting in problematic hypotension.

Hypotension and circulatory collapse should be treated with appropriate measures. Epinephrine and dopamine should not be used, or other sympathomimetics with beta-agonist activity, since beta stimulation may worsen hypotension in the setting of LATUDA-induced alpha blockade. In case of severe extrapyramidal symptoms, anticholinergic medication should be administered.

Gastric lavage (after intubation if patient is unconscious) and administration of activated charcoal together with a laxative should be considered.

The possibility of obtundation, seizures, or dystonic reaction of the head and neck following overdose may create a risk of aspiration with induced emesis.

11 DESCRIPTION

LATUDA is an atypical antipsychotic belonging to the chemical class of benzisothiazol derivatives.

Its chemical name is (3a*R*,4*S*,7*R*,7a*S*)-2-{(1*R*,2*R*)-2-[4-(1,2-benzisothiazol-3-yl)piperazin-1-ylmethyl] cyclohexylmethyl}hexahydro-4,7-methano-2*H*-isoindole-1,3-dione hydrochloride. Its molecular formula is $C_{28}H_{36}N_4O_2S{\cdot}HCl$ and its molecular weight is 529.14.

The chemical structure is:

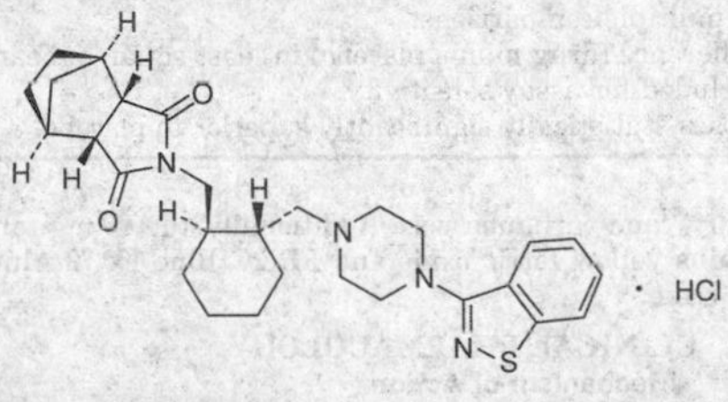

Lurasidone hydrochloride is a white to off-white powder. It is very slightly soluble in water, practically insoluble or insoluble in 0.1 N HCl, slightly soluble in ethanol, sparingly soluble in methanol, practically insoluble or insoluble in toluene and very slightly soluble in acetone.

LATUDA tablets are intended for oral administration only. Each tablet contains 20 mg, 40 mg, 60 mg, 80 mg, or 120 mg of lurasidone hydrochloride.

Inactive ingredients are mannitol, pregelatinized starch, croscarmellose sodium, hypromellose, magnesium stearate,

Figure 3: Impact of Other Patient Factors on LATUDA Pharmacokinetics

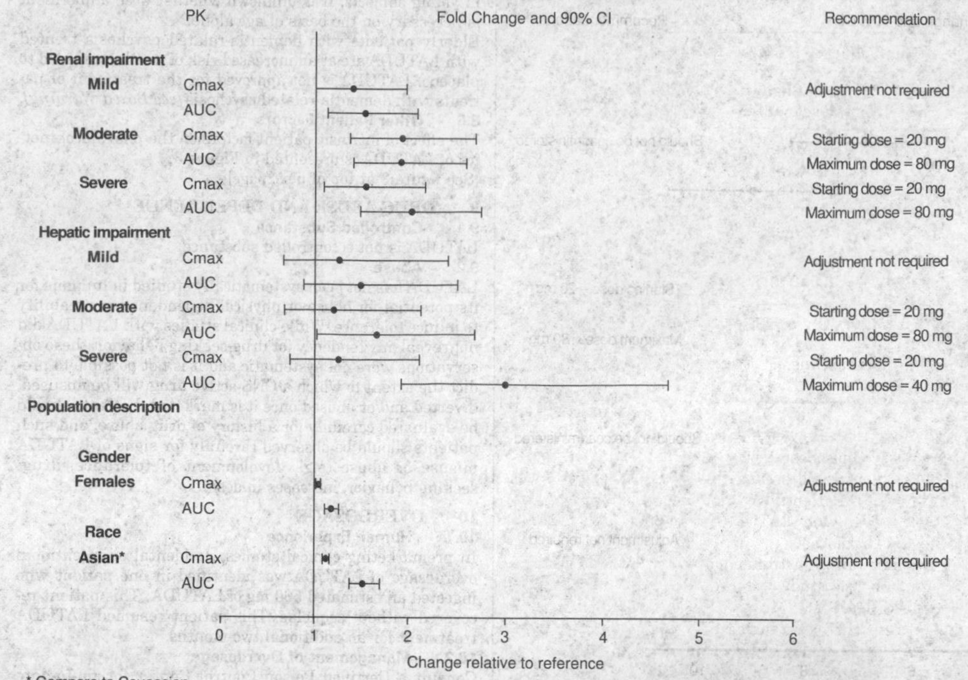

* Compare to Caucasian

Table 24: Primary Efficacy Results for Studies in Schizophrenia (BPRSd or PANSS Scores)

Study	Treatment Group	Mean Baseline Score (SD)	LS Mean Change from Baseline (SE)	Placebo-subtracted Difference[a] (95% CI)
		Primary Efficacy Measure: BPRSd		
1	LATUDA (40 mg/day)*	54.2 (8.8)	-9.4 (1.6)	-5.6 (-9.8, -1.4)
	LATUDA (120 mg/day)*	52.7 (7.6)	-11.0 (1.6)	-6.7 (-11.0, -2.5)
	Placebo	54.7 (8.1)	-3.8 (1.6)	--
2	LATUDA (80 mg/day)*	55.1 (6.0)	-8.9 (1.3)	-4.7 (-8.3, -1.1)
	Placebo	56.1 (6.8)	-4.2 (1.4)	--
		Primary Efficacy Measure: PANSS		
3	LATUDA (40 mg/day)*	96.6 (10.7)	-25.7 (2.0)	-9.7 (-15.3, -4.1)
	LATUDA (120 mg/day)*	97.9 (11.3)	-23.6 (2.1)	-7.5 (-13.4, -1.7)
	Olanzapine (15 mg/day)*[b]	96.3 (12.2)	-28.7 (1.9)	-12.6 (-18.2, -7.9)
	Placebo	95.8 (10.8)	-16.0 (2.1)	--
4	LATUDA (40 mg/day)	96.5 (11.5)	-19.2 (1.7)	-2.1 (-7.0, 2.8)
	LATUDA (80 mg/day)*	96.0 (10.8)	-23.4 (1.8)	-6.4 (-11.3, -1.5)
	LATUDA (120 mg/day)	96.0 (9.7)	-20.5 (1.8)	-3.5 (-8.4, 1.4)
	Placebo	96.8 (11.1)	-17.0 (1.8)	--
5	LATUDA (80 mg/day)*	97.7 (9.7)	-22.2 (1.8)	-11.9 (-16.9, -6.9)
	LATUDA (160 mg/day)*	97.5 (11.8)	-26.5 (1.8)	-16.2 (-21.2, -11.2)
	Quetiapine Extended-release (600 mg/day)*[b]	97.7 (10.2)	-27.8 (1.8)	-17.5 (-22.5, -12.4)
	Placebo	96.6 (10.2)	-10.3 (1.8)	--

SD: standard deviation; SE: standard error; LS Mean: least-squares mean; CI: confidence interval, unadjusted for multiple comparisons.

[a] Difference (drug minus placebo) in least-squares mean change from baseline.

[b] Included for assay sensitivity.

* Doses statistically significantly superior to placebo.

Opadry® and carnauba wax. Additionally, the 80 mg tablet contains yellow ferric oxide and FD&C Blue No. 2 Aluminum Lake.

12 CLINICAL PHARMACOLOGY

12.1 Mechanism of Action

The mechanism of action of LATUDA in the treatment of schizophrenia and bipolar depression is unknown. However, its efficacy in schizophrenia and bipolar depression could be mediated through a combination of central dopamine Type 2 (D_2) and serotonin Type 2 ($5HT_{2A}$) receptor antagonism.

12.2 Pharmacodynamics

LATUDA is an antagonist with high affinity binding at the dopamine D_2 receptors (Ki=1 nM) and the 5-hydroxytryptamine (5-HT, serotonin) receptors 5-HT_{2A} (Ki=0.5 nM) and 5-HT_7 (Ki=0.5 nM) receptors. It also binds with moderate affinity to the human α_{2C} adrenergic receptors (Ki=11 nM), is a partial agonist at serotonin 5-HT_{1A} (Ki=6.4 nM) receptors, and is an antagonist at the α_{2A} adrenergic receptors (Ki=41 nM). LATUDA exhibits little or no affinity for histamine H_1 and muscarinic M_1 receptors (IC_{50} > 1,000 nM).

<u>ECG Changes</u>

The effects of LATUDA on the QTc interval were evaluated in a randomized, double-blind, multiple-dose, parallel-dedicated thorough QT study in 43 patients with schizophrenia or schizoaffective disorder, who were treated with LATUDA doses of 120 mg daily, 600 mg daily and completed the study. The maximum mean (upper 1-sided, 95% CI) increase in baseline-adjusted QTc intervals based on individual correction method (QTcI) was 7.5 (11.7) ms and 4.6 (9.5) ms, for the 120 mg and 600 mg dose groups respectively, observed at 2 to 4 hours after dosing. In this study, there was no apparent dose (exposure)-response relationship.

In short-term, placebo-controlled studies in schizophrenia and bipolar depression, no post-baseline QT prolongations exceeding 500 msec were reported in patients treated with LATUDA or placebo.

12.3 Pharmacokinetics

The activity of LATUDA is primarily due to the parent drug. The pharmacokinetics of LATUDA is dose-proportional within a total daily dose range of 20 mg to 160 mg. Steady-state concentrations of LATUDA are reached within 7 days of starting LATUDA.

Following administration of 40 mg of LATUDA, the mean (%CV) elimination half-life was 18 (7) hours.

Absorption and Distribution: LATUDA is absorbed and reaches peak serum concentrations in approximately 1-3 hours. It is estimated that 9-19% of an administered dose is absorbed. Following administration of 40 mg of LATUDA, the mean (%CV) apparent volume of distribution was 6173 (17.2) L. LATUDA is highly bound (~99%) to serum proteins.

In a food effect study, LATUDA mean C_{max} and AUC were about 3-times and 2-times, respectively, when administered with food compared to the levels observed under fasting conditions. LATUDA exposure was not affected as meal size was increased from 350 to 1000 calories and was independent of meal fat content *[see Dosage and Administration (2.3)]*.

In clinical studies, establishing the safety and efficacy of LATUDA, patients were instructed to take their daily dose with food *[see Dosage and Administration (2.3)]*.

Metabolism and Elimination: LATUDA is metabolized mainly via CYP3A4. The major biotransformation pathways are oxidative *N*-dealkylation, hydroxylation of norbornane ring, and *S*-oxidation. LATUDA is metabolized into two active metabolites (ID-14283 and ID-14326) and two major non-active metabolites (ID-20219 and ID-20220). Based on *in vitro* studies, LATUDA is not a substrate of CYP1A1, CYP1A2, CYP2A6, CYP4A11, CYP2B6, CYP2C8, CYP2C9, CYP2C19, CYP2D6 or CYP2E1 enzymes. Because LATUDA is not a substrate for CYP1A2, smoking is not expected to have an effect on the pharmacokinetics of LATUDA.

Total excretion of radioactivity in urine and feces combined was approximately 89%, with about 80% recovered in feces and 9% recovered in urine, after a single dose of [^{14}C]-labeled LATUDA.

Following administration of 40 mg of LATUDA, the mean (%CV) apparent clearance was 3902 (18.0) mL/min.

13 NONCLINICAL TOXICOLOGY

13.1 Carcinogenesis, Mutagenesis, Impairment of Fertility

Carcinogenesis: LATUDA increased incidences of malignant mammary gland tumors and pituitary gland adenomas in female mice orally dosed with 30, 100, 300, or 650 mg/kg/day. The lowest dose produced plasma levels (AUC) approximately equal to those in humans receiving the MRHD of 160 mg/day. No increases in tumors were seen in male mice up to the highest dose tested, which produced plasma levels (AUC) 14-times those in humans receiving the MRHD.

LATUDA increased the incidence of mammary gland carcinomas in females rats orally dosed at 12 and 36 mg/kg/day: the lowest dose; 3 mg/kg/day is the no-effect dose which produced plasma levels (AUC) 0.4-times those in humans receiving the MRHD. No increases in tumors were seen in male rats up to the highest dose tested, which produced plasma levels (AUC) 6-times those in humans receiving the MRHD.

Proliferative and/or neoplastic changes in the mammary and pituitary glands of rodents have been observed following chronic administration of antipsychotic drugs and are considered to be prolactin-mediated. The relevance of this increased incidence of prolactin-mediated pituitary or mammary gland tumors in rodents to humans is unknown *[see Warnings and Precautions (5.7)]*.

Mutagenesis: LATUDA did not cause mutation or chromosomal aberration when tested *in vitro* and *in vivo*. LATUDA was negative in the Ames gene mutation test, the Chinese Hamster Lung (CHL) cells, and in the *in vivo* mouse bone marrow micronucleus test up to 2000 mg/kg (61 times the MRHD of 160 mg/day based on mg/m^2 body surface area).

Impairment of Fertility: Estrus cycle irregularities were seen in rats orally administered LATUDA at 1.5, 15 and 150 mg/kg/day for 15 consecutive days prior to mating, during the mating period, and through day 7 of gestation. The no-effect dose is 0.1 mg/kg which is approximately 0.006-times the MRHD of 160 mg/day based on body surface area. Fertility was reduced only at the highest dose, which was reversible after a 14-day drug-free period. The no-effect dose for reduced fertility was 15 mg/kg, which is approximately equal to the MRHD based on body surface area.

Table 25: Primary Efficacy Results for Studies in Depressive Episodes Associated with Bipolar I Disorder (MADRS Scores)

Study	Treatment Group	Primary Efficacy Measure: MADRS		
		Mean Baseline Score (SD)	LS Mean Change from Baseline (SE)	Placebo-subtracted Difference[a] (95% CI)
Monotherapy study	LATUDA (20-60 mg/day)*	30.3 (5.0)	-15.4 (0.8)	-4.6 (-6.9, -2.3)
	LATUDA (80-120 mg/day)*	30.6 (4.9)	-15.4 (0.8)	-4.6 (-6.9, -2.3)
	Placebo	30.5 (5.0)	-10.7 (0.8)	--
Adjunctive Therapy study	LATUDA (20-120 mg/day)* + lithium or valproate	30.6 (5.3)	-17.1 (0.9)	-3.6 (-6.0, -1.1)
	Placebo + lithium or valproate	30.8 (4.8)	-13.5 (0.9)	--

SD: standard deviation; SE: standard error; LS Mean: least-squares mean; CI: confidence interval, unadjusted for multiple comparisons.

[a] Difference (drug minus placebo) in least-squares mean change from baseline. * Treatment group statistically significantly superior to placebo.

LATUDA had no effect on fertility in male rats treated orally with LATUDA for 64 consecutive days prior to mating and during the mating period at doses up to 150 mg/kg/day (9-times the MRHD based on mg/m^2 body surface area).

14 CLINICAL STUDIES

14.1 Schizophrenia

The efficacy of LATUDA for the treatment of schizophrenia was established in five short-term (6-week), placebo-controlled studies in adult patients (mean age of 38.4 years, range 18-72) who met DSM-IV criteria for schizophrenia. An active-control arm (olanzapine or quetiapine extended-release) was included in two studies to assess assay sensitivity.

Several instruments were used for assessing psychiatric signs and symptoms in these studies:

1. Positive and Negative Syndrome Scale (PANSS), is a multi-item inventory of general psychopathology used to evaluate the effects of drug treatment in schizophrenia. PANSS total scores may range from 30 to 210.
2. Brief Psychiatric Rating Scale derived (BPRSd), derived from the PANSS, is a multi-item inventory primarily focusing on positive symptoms of schizophrenia, whereas the PANSS includes a wider range of positive, negative and other symptoms of schizophrenia. The BPRSd consists of 18 items rated on a scale of 1 (not present) to 7 (severe). BPRSd scores may range from 18 to 126.
3. The Clinical Global Impression severity scale (CGI-S) is a clinician-rated scale that measures the subject's current illness state on a 1- to 7-point scale.

The endpoint associated with each instrument is change from baseline in the total score to the end of week 6. These changes are then compared to placebo changes for the drug and control groups.

The results of the studies follow:

1. Study 1: In a 6-week, placebo-controlled trial (N=145) involving two fixed doses of LATUDA (40 or 120 mg/day), both doses of LATUDA at Endpoint were superior to placebo on the BPRSd total score, and the CGI-S.
2. Study 2: In a 6-week, placebo-controlled trial (N=180) involving a fixed dose of LATUDA (80 mg/day), LATUDA at Endpoint was superior to placebo on the BPRSd total score, and the CGI-S.
3. Study 3: In a 6-week, placebo- and active-controlled trial (N=473) involving two fixed doses of LATUDA (40 or 120 mg/day) and an active control (olanzapine), both LATUDA doses and the active control at Endpoint were superior to placebo on the PANSS total score, and the CGI-S.
4. Study 4: In a 6-week, placebo-controlled trial (N=489) involving three fixed doses of LATUDA (40, 80 or 120 mg/day), only the 80 mg/day dose of LATUDA at Endpoint was superior to placebo on the PANSS total score, and the CGI-S.
5. Study 5: In a 6-week, placebo- and active-controlled trial (N=482) involving two fixed doses of LATUDA (80 or 160 mg/day) and an active control (quetiapine extended-release), both LATUDA doses and the active control at Endpoint were superior to placebo on the PANSS total score, and the CGI-S.

Thus, the efficacy of LATUDA at doses of 40, 80, 120 and 160 mg/day has been established (Table 24).

[See table 24 at top of previous page]

Examination of population subgroups based on age (there were few patients over 65), gender and race did not reveal any clear evidence of differential responsiveness.

14.2 Depressive Episodes Associated with Bipolar I Disorder

Monotherapy

The efficacy of LATUDA, as monotherapy, was established in a 6-week, multicenter, randomized, double-blind, placebo-controlled study of adult patients (mean age of 41.5 years, range 18 to 74) who met DSM-IV-TR criteria for major depressive episodes associated with bipolar I disorder, with or without rapid cycling, and without psychotic features (N=485). Patients were randomized to one of two flexible-dose ranges of LATUDA (20 to 60 mg/day, or 80 to 120 mg/day) or placebo.

The primary rating instrument used to assess depressive symptoms in this study was the Montgomery-Asberg Depression Rating Scale (MADRS), a 10-item clinician-rated scale with total scores ranging from 0 (no depressive features) to 60 (maximum score). The primary endpoint was the change from baseline in MADRS score at Week 6. The key secondary instrument was the Clinical Global Impression-Bipolar-Severity of Illness scale (CGI-BP-S), a clinician-rated scale that measures the subject's current illness state on a 7-point scale, where a higher score is associated with greater illness severity.

For both dose groups, LATUDA was superior to placebo in reduction of MADRS and CGI-BP-S scores at Week 6. The primary efficacy results are provided in Table 25. The high dose range (80 to 120 mg per day) did not provide additional efficacy on average, compared to the low dose range (20 to 60 mg per day).

Adjunctive Therapy with Lithium or Valproate

The efficacy of LATUDA, as an adjunctive therapy with lithium or valproate, was established in a 6-week, multicenter, randomized, double-blind, placebo-controlled study of adult patients (mean age of 41.7 years, range 18 to 72) who met DSM-IV-TR criteria for major depressive episodes associated with bipolar I disorder, with or without rapid cycling, and without psychotic features (N=340). Patients who remained symptomatic after treatment with lithium or valproate were randomized to flexibly dosed LATUDA 20 to 120 mg/day or placebo.

The primary rating instrument used to assess depressive symptoms in this study was the MADRS. The primary endpoint was the change from baseline in MADRS score at Week 6. The key secondary instrument was the CGI-BP-S scale.

LATUDA was superior to placebo in reduction of MADRS and CGI-BP-S scores at Week 6, as an adjunctive therapy with lithium or valproate (Table 25).

[See table 25 above]

16 HOW SUPPLIED/STORAGE AND HANDLING

LATUDA tablets are white to off-white, round (20 mg or 40 mg), white to off-white, oblong (60 mg), pale green, oval (80 mg) or white to off-white, oval (120 mg) and identified with strength-specific one-sided debossing, "L20" (20 mg), "L40" (40 mg), "L80" (80 mg) or "L120" (120 mg). Tablets are supplied in the following strengths and package configurations (Table 26):

Table 26: Package Configuration for LATUDA Tablets

Tablet Strength	Package Configuration	NDC Code
20 mg	Bottles of 30	63402-302-30
	Bottles of 90	63402-302-90
	Bottles of 500	63402-302-50
	Box of 100 (Hospital Unit Dose) 10 blister cards, 10 tablets each	63402-302-10 Carton 63402-302-01 Blister
40 mg	Bottles of 30	63402-304-30
	Bottles of 90	63402-304-90
	Bottles of 500	63402-304-50
	Box of 100 (Hospital Unit Dose) 10 blister cards, 10 tablets each	63402-304-10 Carton 63402-304-01 Blister
60 mg	Bottles of 30	63402-306-30
	Bottles of 90	63402-306-90
	Bottles of 500	63402-306-50
	Box of 100 (Hospital Unit Dose) 10 blister cards, 10 tablets each	63402-306-10 Carton 63402-306-01 Blister
80 mg	Bottles of 30	63402-308-30
	Bottles of 90	63402-308-90
	Bottles of 500	63402-308-50
	Box of 100 (Hospital Unit Dose) 10 blister cards, 10 tablets each	63402-308-10 Carton 63402-308-01 Blister
120 mg	Bottles of 30	63402-312-30
	Bottles of 90	63402-312-90
	Bottles of 500	63402-312-50
	Box of 100 (Hospital Unit Dose) 10 blister cards, 10 tablets each	63402-312-10 Carton 63402-312-01 Blister

Storage

Store LATUDA tablets at 25°C (77°F); excursions permitted to 15° - 30°C (59° - 86°F) *[See USP Controlled Room Temperature]*.

17 PATIENT COUNSELING INFORMATION

Physicians are advised to discuss with patients for whom they prescribe LATUDA all relevant safety information including, but not limited to, the following:

17.1 Increased Mortality in Elderly Patients with Dementia-Related Psychosis

Advise patients and caregivers that elderly patients with dementia-related psychoses treated with atypical antipsychotic drugs are at increased risk of death compared with placebo. LATUDA is not approved for elderly patients with dementia-related psychosis *[see Boxed Warning; Warnings and Precautions (5.1)]*.

17.2 Suicidal Thoughts and Behaviors; and Activation of Mania or Hypomania

Educate patients, families, and caregivers about the risk of suicidal thoughts and behaviors with antidepressant treatment, as well as the risk of mania and hypomania. Advise them about monitoring for the emergence of suicidal thoughts and behavior, manic/hypomanic symptoms, irritability, agitation, or unusual changes in behavior. Instruct patients, families, and caregivers to report such symptoms to the healthcare provider *[see Warnings and Precautions (5.2 and 5.14)]*.

17.3 Neuroleptic Malignant Syndrome

Advise patients and caregivers that a potentially fatal symptom complex sometimes referred to as NMS has been reported in association with administration of antipsychotic drugs. Signs and symptoms of NMS include hyperpyrexia, muscle rigidity, altered mental status, and evidence of autonomic instability (irregular pulse or blood pressure, tachycardia, diaphoresis, and cardiac dysrhythmia) *[see Warnings and Precautions (5.4)]*.

17.4 Metabolic Changes (Hyperglycemia and Diabetes Mellitus, Dyslipidemia, and Weight Gain)

Educate patients and caregivers about the risk of metabolic changes and the need for specific monitoring. The risks include hyperglycemia and diabetes mellitus, dyslipidemia, weight gain, and cardiovascular reactions. Educate patients and caregivers about the symptoms of hyperglycemia (high blood sugar) and diabetes mellitus (e.g., polydipsia, polyuria, polyphagia, and weakness). Monitor all patients for these symptoms. Patients who are diagnosed with diabetes or have risk factors for diabetes (obesity, family history of diabetes) should have their fasting blood glucose monitored before beginning treatment and periodically during treatment. Patients who develop symptoms of hyperglycemia should have assessments of fasting glucose. Clinical monitoring of weight is recommended *[see Warnings and Precautions (5.6)]*.

17.5 Orthostatic Hypotension

Educate patients about the risk of orthostatic hypotension, particularly at the time of initiating treatment, re-initiating treatment, or increasing the dose *[see Warnings and Precautions (5.9)]*.

17.6 Leukopenia/Neutropenia

Advise patients with a pre-existing low WBC or a history of drug-induced leukopenia/neutropenia that they should have their CBC monitored while taking LATUDA *[see Warnings and Precautions (5.8)]*.

17.7 Interference with Cognitive and Motor Performance

Caution patients about performing activities requiring mental alertness, such as operating hazardous machinery or operating a motor vehicle, until they are reasonably certain that LATUDA therapy does not affect them adversely *[see Warnings and Precautions (5.11)]*.

17.8 Pregnancy and Nursing

Instruct patients to notify their physician if they become pregnant or intend to become pregnant during therapy with LATUDA *[see Use in Specific Populations (8.1)]*.

17.9 Concomitant Medication and Alcohol

Instruct patients to inform their physicians if they are taking, or plan to take, any prescription or over-the-counter drugs, because there is a potential for drug interactions. Advise patients to avoid alcohol while taking LATUDA *[see Drug Interactions (7)]*.

17.10 Heat Exposure and Dehydration

Educate patients regarding appropriate care in avoiding overheating and dehydration *[see Warnings and Precautions (5.12)]*.

SUNOVION

Manufactured for:
Sunovion Pharmaceuticals Inc.
Marlborough, MA 01752 USA
For Customer Service, call 1-888-394-7377.
For Medical Information, call 1-800-739-0565.
To report suspected adverse reactions, call 1-877-737-7226.
Revised: Month Year
901456RXX

Medication Guide
LATUDA (luh-TOO-duh)
(lurasidone hydrochloride)
Tablets

What is the most important information I should know about LATUDA?

LATUDA may cause serious side effects, including:

1. **Increased risk of death in elderly people who are confused, have memory loss and have lost touch with reality (dementia-related psychosis).** Medicines like LATUDA can increase the risk of death in elderly people who are confused, have memory loss and have lost touch with reality (dementia-related psychosis). LATUDA should not be used to treat people with dementia-related psychosis.
2. **Increased risk of suicidal thoughts or actions (antidepressant medicines, depression and other serious mental illnesses, and suicidal thoughts or actions).**
   - **Talk to your, or your family member's, healthcare provider about:**
     - all risks and benefits of treatment with antidepressant medicines.
     - all treatment choices for depression or other serious mental illness.
   - **Antidepressant medicines may increase suicidal thoughts or actions in some children, teenagers, and young adults within the first few months of treatment.**
   - **Depression and other serious mental illnesses are the most important causes of suicidal thoughts and actions. Some people may have a particularly high risk of having suicidal thoughts or actions.** These include people who have (or have a family history of) depression, bipolar illness (also called manic-depressive illness), or a history of suicidal thoughts or actions.
   - **How can I watch for and try to prevent suicidal thoughts and actions in myself or a family member?**
     - Pay close attention to any changes, especially sudden changes, in mood, behaviors, thoughts, or feelings. This is very important when an antidepressant medicine is started or when the dose is changed.
     - Call the healthcare provider right away to report new or sudden changes in mood, behavior, thoughts, or feelings.
     - Keep all follow-up visits with the healthcare provider as scheduled. Call the healthcare provider between visits as needed, especially if you have concerns about symptoms.

Call a healthcare provider right away if you or your family member has any of the following symptoms, especially if they are new, worse, or worry you:

- thoughts about suicide or dying
- attempts to commit suicide
- new or worse depression
- new or worse anxiety
- feeling very agitated or restless
- panic attacks
- trouble sleeping (insomnia)
- new or worse irritability
- acting aggressive, being angry, or violent
- acting on dangerous impulses
- an extreme increase in activity and talking (mania)
- other unusual changes in behavior or mood

What else do I need to know about antidepressant medicines?

- **Never stop an antidepressant medicine without first talking to your healthcare provider.** Stopping an antidepressant medicine suddenly can cause other symptoms.
- **Antidepressants are medicines used to treat depression and other illnesses.** It is important to discuss all the risks of treating depression and also the risks of not treating it. Patients and their families or other caregivers should discuss all treatment choices with the healthcare provider, not just the use of antidepressants.
- **Antidepressant medicines have other side effects.** Talk to the healthcare provider about the side effects of the medicine prescribed for you or your family member.
- **Antidepressant medicines can interact with other medicines.** Know all of the medicines that you or your family member takes. Keep a list of all medicines to show the healthcare provider. Do not start new medicines without first checking with your healthcare provider.
- **Not all antidepressant medicines prescribed for children are FDA approved for use in children.** Talk to your child's healthcare provider for more information.

What is LATUDA?

LATUDA is a prescription medicine used to treat adults with:

- schizophrenia
- depressive episodes associated with bipolar I disorder, alone or with lithium or valproate

It is not known if LATUDA is safe and effective in children.

Who should not take LATUDA?

Do not take LATUDA if you:

- are allergic to lurasidone hydrochloride or any of the ingredients in LATUDA. See the end of this Medication Guide for a complete list of ingredients in LATUDA.
- are taking certain other medicines called CYP3A4 inhibitors or inducers including ketoconazole, clarithromycin, ritonavir, voriconazole, mibefradil, rifampin, avasimibe, St. John's wort, phenytoin, or carbamazepine. Ask your healthcare provider if you are not sure if you are taking any of these medicines.

What should I tell my healthcare provider before taking LATUDA?

Before you take LATUDA, tell your healthcare provider if you:

- have or have had diabetes or high blood sugar in you or your family. Your healthcare provider should check your blood sugar before you start LATUDA and also during therapy.
- have or have had high levels of total cholesterol, triglycerides or LDL-cholesterol or low levels of HDL-cholesterol
- have or have had low or high blood pressure
- have or have had low white blood cell count
- have or have had seizures
- have or have had abnormal thyroid tests
- have or have had high prolactin levels
- have or have had heart problems
- have or have had liver problems
- have or have had any other medical conditions
- are pregnant or plan to become pregnant. It is not known if LATUDA will harm your unborn baby.
- are breastfeeding or plan to breastfeed. It is not known if LATUDA passes into your breast milk. You and your healthcare provider should decide if you will take LATUDA or breastfeed. You should not do both.

Tell the healthcare provider about all the medicines that you take or recently have taken including prescription medicines, over-the-counter medicines, herbal supplements and vitamins.

LATUDA and other medicines may affect each other causing serious side effects. LATUDA may affect the way other medicines work, and other medicines may affect how LATUDA works.

Especially tell your healthcare provider if you take or plan to take medicines for:

- depression
- high blood pressure
- Parkinson's disease
- trouble sleeping
- abnormal heart beats or rhythm
- epilepsy
- inflammation
- psychosis

Know the medicines you take. Keep a list of your medicines to show your healthcare provider and pharmacist when you get a new medicine.

How should I take LATUDA?

- Take LATUDA exactly as your healthcare provider tells you to take it. Do not change the dose yourself.
- Take LATUDA by mouth, with food (at least 350 calories).
- If you take too much LATUDA, call your healthcare provider or poison control center at 1-800-222-1222 right away, or go to the nearest hospital emergency room.

What should I avoid while taking LATUDA?

- Avoid eating grapefruit or drinking grapefruit juice while you take LATUDAsince these can affect the amount of LATUDA in the blood. Do not drive, operate machinery, or do other dangerous activities until you know how LATUDA affects you. LATUDA may make you drowsy.
- Avoid getting overheated or dehydrated.
- Do not over-exercise.
- In hot weather, stay inside in a cool place if possible.
- Stay out of the sun. Do not wear too much or heavy clothing.
- Drink plenty of water.
- Do not drink alcohol while taking LATUDA. It may make some side effects of LATUDA worse.

What are possible side effects of LATUDA?

LATUDA can cause serious side effects, including:

- **See "What is the most important information I should know about LATUDA?"**
- **stroke that can lead to death can happen in elderly people with dementia who take medicines like LATUDA**
- **neuroleptic malignant syndrome (NMS).** NMS is a rare but very serious condition that can happen in people who take antipsychotic medicines, including LATUDA. NMS can cause death and must be treated in a hospital. Call your healthcare provider right away if you become severely ill and have some or all of these symptoms:
  - high fever
  - excessive sweating
  - rigid muscles
  - confusion
  - changes in your breathing, heartbeat, and blood pressure
- **movements you cannot control in your face, tongue, or other body parts (tardive dyskinesia).** These may be signs of a serious condition. Tardive dyskinesia may not go away, even if you stop taking LATUDA. Tardive dyskinesia may also start after you stop taking LATUDA.
- **high blood sugar (hyperglycemia).** High blood sugar can happen if you have diabetes already or if you have never had diabetes. High blood sugar could lead to:
  - build-up of acid in your blood due to ketones (ketoacidosis)
  - coma
  - death

  Increases in blood sugar can happen in some people who take LATUDA. Extremely high blood sugar can lead to coma or death. If you have diabetes or risk factors for diabetes (such as being overweight or a family history of diabetes) your healthcare provider should check your blood sugar before you start LATUDA and during therapy.

  Call your healthcare provider if you have any of these symptoms of high blood sugar (hyperglycemia) while taking LATUDA:
  - feel very thirsty
  - need to urinate more than usual
  - feel very hungry
  - feel weak or tired
  - feel sick to your stomach
  - feel confused, or your breath smells fruity

- **high fat levels in your blood (increased cholesterol and triglycerides).** High fat levels may happen in people treated with LATUDA. You may not have any symptoms,so your healthcare provider may decide to check your cholesterol and triglycerides during your treatment with LATUDA.
- **increase in weight (weight gain).** Weight gain has been reported in patients taking medicines like LATUDA. You and your healthcare provider should check your weight regularly. Talk to your healthcare provider about ways to control weight gain, such as eating a healthy, balanced diet, and exercising.
- **increases in prolactin levels.** Your healthcare provider may do blood tests to check your prolactin levels.
- **low white blood cell count**
- **decreased blood pressure (orthostatic hypotension),** including lightheadedness or fainting caused by a sudden change in heart rate and blood pressure when rising too quickly from a sitting or lying position.
- **seizures**
- **difficulty swallowing**

The most common side effects of LATUDA include:

- sleepiness or drowsiness
- restlessness and feeling like you need to move around (akathisia)
- difficulty moving, slow movements, muscle stiffness, or tremor
- nausea

These are not all the possible side effects of LATUDA. For more information, ask your healthcare provider or pharmacist.

Call your doctor for medical advice about side effects. You may report side effects to FDA at 1-800-FDA-1088.

How should I store LATUDA?

- Store LATUDA tablets at room temperature between 68°F to 77°F (20°C to 25°C).
- Keep LATUDA and all medicines out of the reach of children.

General information about the safe and effective use of LATUDA.

Medicines are sometimes prescribed for purposes other than those listed in a Medication Guide. Do not use LATUDA for a condition for which it was not prescribed. Do not give LATUDA to other people, even if they have the same symptoms you have. It may harm them.

This Medication Guide summarizes the most important information about LATUDA. If you would like more information, talk with your healthcare provider. You can ask your pharmacist or healthcare provider for information about LATUDA that is written for health professionals.

For more information, go to www.LATUDA.com or call 1-888-394-7377.

What are the ingredients in LATUDA?

Active ingredient: lurasidone hydrochloride

Inactive ingredients: mannitol, pregelatinized starch, croscarmellose sodium, hypromellose, magnesium stearate, Opadry® and carnauba wax. Additionally, the 80 mg tablet contains yellow ferric oxide and FD&C Blue No. 2 Aluminum Lake

This Medication Guide has been approved by the U.S. Food and Drug Administration.

Manufactured for:
Sunovion Pharmaceuticals Inc.
Marlborough, MA 01752 USA

LATUDA is a registered trademark of Dainippon Sumitomo Pharma Co. Ltd.,
Sunovion Pharmaceuticals Inc. is a U.S. subsidiary of Dainippon Sumitomo Pharma Co. Ltd.,

Issued: July/2013

Shown in Product Identification Guide, page 313

Supernus Pharmaceuticals, Inc.

**1550 E GUDE DRIVE
ROCKVILLE, MD 20850**

Direct Inquiries: 1-866-398-0833

OXTELLAR XR ℞

**(oxcarbazepine)
extended-release tablets, for oral use**

**HIGHLIGHTS OF PRESCRIBING INFORMATION
These highlights do not include all the information needed to use OXTELLAR XR safely and effectively. See full prescribing information for OXTELLAR XR.
OXTELLAR XR (oxcarbazepine) extended-release tablets, for oral use
Initial U.S. Approval: 2000**

INDICATIONS AND USAGE

Oxtellar XR™ is an antiepileptic drug (AED) indicated for:
- Adults: Adjunctive therapy in the treatment of partial seizures
- Children: Adjunctive therapy in the treatment of partial seizures in children 6 to 17 years *(1)*

DOSAGE AND ADMINISTRATION

- Recommended daily dose is 1,200 mg to 2,400 mg once per day *(2.2)*
- Adults: Initiate with a dose of 600 mg once per day. Dose increases can be made at weekly intervals in 600 mg per day increments to achieve the recommended daily dose *(2.2)*
- Children: Target dose is based upon weight. Titrate to target dose over two to three weeks. Initiate with 8 mg/kg to 10 mg/kg once per day. Increase in weekly increments of 8 mg/kg to 10 mg/kg once daily, not to exceed 600 mg, to achieve target daily dose *(2.3)*
- Patients with creatinine clearance less than 30mL/minute: Start at 300 mg per day and increase slowly *(2.4)*
- Geriatric Patients: Start at lower dose (300 mg or 450 mg per day) and increase slowly *(2.5)*
- In conversion of oxcarbazepine immediate-release to Oxtellar XR™, higher doses of Oxtellar XR™ may be necessary *(2.8, 12.3)*

DOSAGE FORMS AND STRENGTHS

Extended-release tablets: 150 mg, 300 mg and 600 mg *(3)*

CONTRAINDICATIONS

- Known hypersensitivity to oxcarbazepine or to any of its components *(4)*

WARNINGS AND PRECAUTIONS

- *Hyponatremia:* Monitor sodium as recommended. *(5.1)*
- *Anaphylactic Reactions and Angioedema.* Discontinue if occurs *(5.2)*
- *Patients with a Past History of Hypersensitivity Reaction to Carbamazepine:* Only use based upon risk benefit *(5.3)*
- *Serious Dermatological Reactions:* Discontinue if observed *(5.4)*
- *Suicidal Behavior and Ideation:* Monitor for symptoms *(5.5)*
- *Withdrawal of* Oxtellar XR™: Withdrawal gradually *(5.6)*
- *Multi-Organ Hypersensitivity:* Discontinue if suspected *(5.7)*
- *Hematologic Reactions:* Discontinue if suspected *(5.8)*

ADVERSE REACTIONS

Most commonly observed (≥5%) and more frequent than placebo adverse reactions were: dizziness, somnolence, headache, balance disorder, tremor, vomiting, diplopia, asthenia, and fatigue *(6.1)*.

To report SUSPECTED ADVERSE REACTIONS, contact Supernus, Inc. at (1-866-398-0833) or contact FDA at 1-800-FDA-1088 or www.fda.gov/medwatch

DRUG INTERACTIONS

- *Phenytoin, Carbamazepine, and Phenobarbital:* Coadministration decreased blood levels of an active metabolite of Oxtellar XR™: Greater dose of Oxtellar XR™ may be required *(2.6, 7.1)*.
- *Oral Contraceptives:* Advise patients that Oxtellar XR™ may decrease the effectiveness of hormonal contraceptives. Additional non-hormonal forms of contraception are recommended. *(7.2)*

USE IN SPECIFIC POPULATIONS

- *Pregnancy:* Plasma levels of active metabolite may be decreased. Monitor patients. Based on animal data, may cause fetal harm. *(5.9, 8.1)*.
- *Severe Hepatic Impairment:* Not recommended *(8.6)*.

See 17 for PATIENT COUNSELING INFORMATION and Medication Guide

Revised: 10/2012

FULL PRESCRIBING INFORMATION: CONTENTS*

*** Sections or subsections omitted from the full prescribing information are not listed**

FULL PRESCRIBING INFORMATION

1 INDICATIONS AND USAGE

Oxtellar XR™ is indicated as adjunctive therapy of partial seizures in adults and in children 6 years to 17 years of age.

2 DOSAGE AND ADMINISTRATION

2.1 Important Administration Instructions

Administer Oxtellar XR™ as a single daily dose taken on an empty stomach (at least 1 hour before or at least 2 hours after meals) [see *Clinical Pharmacology (12.3)*]. If Oxtellar XR™ is taken with food, adverse reactions are more likely to occur because of increased peak levels [see *Clinical Pharmacology (12.3)*].

Swallow Oxtellar XR™ tablets whole. Do not cut, crush, or chew the tablets. For ease of swallowing in pediatric patients or patients with difficulty swallowing, achieve daily dosages with multiples of appropriate lower strength tablets (e.g., 150 mg tablets).

2.2 Dosing for Adults in Adjunctive Therapy

The recommended daily dose of Oxtellar XR™ is 1,200 mg to 2,400 mg per day, given once daily. The dose of 2,400 mg per day showed slightly greater efficacy than 1,200 mg per day, but was associated with an increase in adverse reactions.

Table 2: Risk by Indication for Antiepileptic Drugs in the Pooled Analysis

Indication	Placebo Patients with Events per 1,000 Patients	Drug Patients with Events per 1,000 Patients	Relative Risk: Incidence of Events in Drug Patients/Incidence in Placebo Patients	Risk Difference: Additional Drug Patients with Events per 1,000 Patients
Epilepsy	1.0	3.4	3.5	2.4
Psychiatric	5.7	8.5	1.5	2.9
Other	1.0	1.8	1.9	0.9
Total	2.4	4.3	1.8	1.9

Initiate treatment at a dose of 600 mg per day given once daily for one week. Subsequent dose increases can be made at weekly intervals in 600 mg per day increments to achieve the recommended daily dose.

2.3 Dosing for Children (6 to 17 years of age) in Adjunctive Therapy

In pediatric patients 6 years to 17 years of age, initiate treatment at a daily dose of 8 mg/kg to 10 mg/kg once daily, not to exceed 600 mg per day in the first week.

Subsequent dose increases can be made at weekly intervals in 8 mg/kg to 10 mg/kg increments once daily, not to exceed 600 mg, to achieve the target daily dose. The target maintenance dose, achieved over two to three weeks, is displayed in Table 1.

Table 1: Target Daily Dose in Pediatric Patients Aged 6 to 17 Years Old

Weight	Target Daily Dose
20 kg to 29 kg	900 mg per day
29.1 kg to 39 kg	1200 mg per day
Greater than 39 kg	1800 mg per day

2.4 Dosage Modifications in Patients with Renal Impairment

In patients with severe renal impairment (creatinine clearance less than 30 mL/minute), initiate Oxtellar XR™ at one-half the usual starting dose (300 mg per day). Subsequent dose increases can be made at weekly intervals in increments of 300 mg to 450 mg per day to achieve the desired clinical response. [see *Use in Specific Populations (8.5)*].

2.5 Dosage Modifications in Geriatric Patients

In geriatric patients, consider starting at a lower dose (300 mg or 450 mg per day). Subsequent dose increases can be made at weekly intervals in increments of 300 mg to 450 mg per day to achieve the desired clinical effect [see *Use in Specific Populations (8.4)*].

2.6 Dosage Modification for use with Concomitant Antiepileptic Drugs

Enzyme inducing antiepileptic drugs such as carbamazepine, phenobarbital, and phenytoin decrease exposure to 10-monohydroxy derivative (MHD), the active metabolite. Dosage increases may be necessary. Consider initiating dose at 900 mg once per day [see *Drug Interactions (7.1)*].

2.7 Withdrawal of AEDs

As with all antiepileptic drugs, Oxtellar XR™ should be withdrawn gradually to minimize the potential of increased seizure frequency [see *Warnings and Precautions (5.6)*].

2.8 Conversion from Immediate-Release Oxcarbazepine to Oxtellar XR™

In conversion of oxcarbazepine immediate-release to Oxtellar XR™, higher doses of Oxtellar XR™ may be necessary [see *Clinical Pharmacology (12.3)*].

3 DOSAGE FORMS AND STRENGTHS

Extended-release tablets:

150 mg: yellow modified-oval shaped with "150" printed on one side

300 mg: brown modified-oval shaped with "300" printed on one side

600 mg: brownish red modified-oval shaped with "600" printed on one side

4 CONTRAINDICATIONS

Oxtellar XR™ is contraindicated in patients with a known hypersensitivity to oxcarbazepine or to any of its components [see *Warnings and Precautions (5.2, 5.3)*].

5 WARNINGS AND PRECAUTIONS

5.1 Hyponatremia

Clinically significant hyponatremia (sodium <125 mmol/L) may develop during Oxtellar XR™ use. Serum sodium levels less than 125 mmol/L have occurred in immediate-release oxcarbazepine-treated patients generally in the first three months of treatment. However, clinically significant hyponatremia may develop more than a year after initiating therapy.

Most immediate-release oxcarbazepine-treated patients who developed hyponatremia were asymptomatic in clinical trials. However, some of these patients had their dose reduced, discontinued, or had their fluid intake restricted for hyponatremia. Serum sodium levels returned toward normal when the dosage was reduced or discontinued, or when the patient was treated conservatively (e.g., fluid restriction). Post-marketing cases of symptomatic hyponatremia have been reported during post-marketing use of immediate-release oxcarbazepine.

Among treated patients in a controlled trial of adjunctive therapy with Oxtellar XR™ in 366 adults with complex partial seizures, 1 patient receiving 2400 mg experienced a severe reduction in serum sodium (117 mEq/L) requiring discontinuation from treatment, while 2 other patients receiving 1200 mg experienced serum sodium concentrations low enough (125 and 126 mEq/L) to require discontinuation from treatment. The overall incidence of clinically significant hyponatremia in patients treated with Oxtellar XR™ was 1.2%, although slight shifts in serum sodium concentrations from Normal to Low (<135 mEq/L) were observed for the 2400 mg (6.5%) and 1200 mg (9.8%) groups compared to placebo (1.7%). Measure serum sodium concentrations if patients develop symptoms of hyponatremia (e.g., nausea, malaise, headache, lethargy, confusion, obtunded consciousness, or increase in seizure frequency or severity). Consider measurement of serum sodium concentrations during treatment with Oxtellar XR™, particularly if the patient receives concomitant medications known to decrease serum sodium levels (for example, drugs associated with inappropriate ADH secretion).

5.2 Anaphylactic Reactions and Angioedema

Rare cases of anaphylaxis and angioedema involving the larynx, glottis, lips and eyelids have been reported in patients after taking the first or subsequent doses of immediate-release oxcarbazepine. Angioedema associated with laryngeal edema can be fatal. If a patient develops any of these reactions after treatment with Oxtellar XR™, discontinue the drug and initiate an alternative treatment. Do not rechallenge these patients with Oxtellar XR™.

5.3 Hypersensitivity Reactions in Patients with Hypersensitivity to Carbamazepine

Inform patients who have had hypersensitivity reactions to carbamazepine that approximately 25%-30% of them will experience hypersensitivity reactions with Oxtellar XR™. Question patients about any prior adverse reactions with carbamazepine. Patients with a history of hypersensitivity reactions to carbamazepine should ordinarily be treated with Oxtellar XR™ only if the potential benefit justifies the potential risk. Discontinue Oxtellar XR™ immediately if signs or symptoms of hypersensitivity develop [see *Warnings and Precautions (5.8)*].

5.4 Serious Dermatological Reactions

Serious dermatological reactions, including Stevens-Johnson syndrome (SJS) and toxic epidermal necrolysis (TEN), have occurred in both children and adults in treated with immediate-release oxcarbazepine use. The median time of onset for reported cases was 19 days. Such serious skin reactions may be life threatening, and some patients have required hospitalization with very rare reports of fatal outcome. Recurrence of the serious skin reactions following rechallenge with immediate-release oxcarbazepine has also been reported.

The reporting rate of TEN and SJS associated with immediate-release oxcarbazepine use, which is generally accepted to be an underestimate due to underreporting, exceeds the background incidence rate estimates by a factor of 3- to 10-fold. Estimates of the background incidence rate for these serious skin reactions in the general population range between 0.5 to 6 cases per million-person years. Therefore, if a patient develops a skin reaction while taking Oxtellar XR™, consider discontinuing Oxtellar XR™ use and prescribing another AED.

5.5 Suicidal Behavior and Ideation

Antiepileptic drugs (AEDs), including Oxtellar XR™, increase the risk of suicidal thoughts or behavior in patients taking these drugs for any indication. Monitor patients treated with any AED for any indication for the emergence or worsening of depression, suicidal thoughts or behavior, and/or any unusual changes in mood or behavior.

Pooled analyses of 199 placebo-controlled clinical trials (mono- and adjunctive therapy) of 11 different AEDs showed that patients randomized to one of the AEDs had approximately twice the risk (adjusted Relative Risk 1.8, 95% CI:1.2, 2.7) of suicidal thinking or behavior compared to patients randomized to placebo. In these trials, which had a median treatment duration of 12 weeks, the estimated incidence rate of suicidal behavior or ideation among 27,863 AED-treated patients was 0.43%, compared to 0.24% among 16,029 placebo-treated patients, representing an increase of approximately one case of suicidal thinking or behavior for every 530 patients treated. There were four suicides in drug-treated patients in the trials and none in placebo-treated patients, but the number is too small to allow any conclusion about drug effect on suicide.

The increased risk of suicidal thoughts or behavior with AEDs was observed as early as one week after starting drug treatment with AEDs and persisted for the duration of treatment assessed. Because most trials included in the analysis did not extend beyond 24 weeks, the risk of suicidal thoughts or behavior beyond 24 weeks could not be assessed.

The risk of suicidal thoughts or behavior was generally consistent among drugs in the data analyzed. The finding of increased risk with AEDs of varying mechanisms of action and across a range of indications suggests that the risk applies to all AEDs used for any indication. The risk did not vary substantially by age (5-100 years) in the clinical trials analyzed. Table 2 shows absolute and relative risk by indication for all evaluated AEDs.

[See table 2 above]

The relative risk for suicidal thoughts or behavior was higher in clinical trials for epilepsy than in clinical trials for psychiatric or other conditions, but the absolute risk differences were similar for the epilepsy and psychiatric indications.

Anyone considering prescribing Oxtellar XR™ or any other AED must balance the risk of suicidal thoughts or behavior with the risk of untreated illness. Epilepsy and many other illnesses for which AEDs are prescribed are themselves associated with morbidity and mortality and an increased risk of suicidal thoughts and behavior. Should suicidal thoughts and behavior emerge during Oxtellar XR™ treatment, the prescriber needs to consider whether the emergence of these symptoms in any given patient may be related to the illness being treated.

Patients, their caregivers, and families should be informed that AEDs increase the risk of suicidal thoughts and behavior and should be advised of the need to be alert for the emergence or worsening of the signs and symptoms of depression, any unusual changes in mood or behavior, or the emergence of suicidal thoughts, behavior, or thoughts about self-harm. Behaviors of concern should be reported immediately to healthcare providers.

5.6 Withdrawal of AEDs

As with all AEDs, Oxtellar XR™ should be withdrawn gradually to minimize the potential of increased seizure frequency.

5.7 Multi-Organ Hypersensitivity

Multi-organ hypersensitivity reactions have occurred in close temporal association (median time to detection 13 days: range 4-60) to the initiation of immediate-release oxcarbazepine therapy in adult and pediatric patients. Although there have been a limited number of reports, many of these cases resulted in hospitalization and some were life-threatening. Signs and symptoms of this disorder were diverse; however, patients typically, although not exclusively, presented with fever and rash associated with other organ system involvement. These included the following: hematologic and lymphatic (e.g., eosinophilia, thrombocytopenia, lymphadenopathy, leukopenia, neutropenia, splenomegaly), hepatobiliary (e.g., hepatitis, liver function test abnormalities), renal (e.g., proteinuria, nephritis, oliguria, renal failure), muscles and joints (e.g., joint swelling, myalgia, arthralgia, asthenia), nervous system (e.g., hepatic encephalopathy), respiratory (e.g., dyspnea, pulmonary edema, asthma, bronchospasm, interstitial lung disease), hepatorenal syndrome, pruritus, and angioedema. Because the disorder is variable in its expression, other organ system symptoms and signs, not noted here, may occur. If this reaction is suspected, discontinue Oxtellar XR™ and initiate an alternative treatment.

5.8 Hematologic Reactions

Rare reports of pancytopenia, agranulocytosis, and leukopenia have been seen in patients treated with immediate-release oxcarbazepine during post-marketing experience. Discontinuation of Oxtellar XR™ should be considered if any evidence of these hematologic reactions develops.

5.9 Risk of Seizures in the Pregnant Patient
Due to physiological changes during pregnancy, plasma concentrations of the active metabolite of oxcarbazepine, the 10-monohydroxy derivative (MHD), may gradually decrease throughout pregnancy. Monitor patients carefully during pregnancy and through the postpartum period because MHD concentrations may increase after delivery.

5.10 Laboratory Tests
Laboratory data from clinical trials suggest that immediate-release oxcarbazepine may be associated with decreases in T4, without changes in T3 or TSH.

6 ADVERSE REACTIONS

The following adverse reactions are described in other sections of the labeling:

- Hyponatremia [see *Warnings and Precautions (5.1)*]
- Anaphylactic Reactions and Angioedema [see *Warnings and Precautions (5.2)*]
- Hypersensitivity Reactions in Patients with Hypersensitivity to Carbamazepine [see *Warnings and Precautions (5.3)*]
- Serious Dermatological Reactions [see *Warnings and Precautions (5.4)*]
- Suicidal Behavior and Ideation [see *Warnings and Precautions (5.5)*]
- Withdrawal of AEDs [see *Warnings and Precautions (5.6)*]
- Multi-Organ Hypersensitivity [see *Warnings and Precautions (5.7)*]
- Hematologic Reactions [see *Warnings and Precautions (5.8)*]
- Risk of Seizures in the Pregnant Patient [see *Warnings and Precautions (5.9)*]
- Laboratory Tests [see *Warnings and Precautions (5.10)*]

6.1 Clinical Trials Experience
Because clinical trials are conducted under widely varying conditions, adverse reaction rates observed in the clinical trials of a drug cannot be directly compared to rates in the clinical trials of another drug and may not reflect the rates observed in clinical practice.

The safety data presented below are from 384 patients with partial epilepsy who received Oxtellar XR™ (366 adults and 18 children) with concomitant AEDs.

In addition, safety data presented below are from a total of 2,288 patients with seizure disorders treated with immediate-release oxcarbazepine; 1,832 were adults and 456 were children.

Most Common Adverse Reactions Reported by Adult Patients Receiving Concomitant AEDs in Oxtellar XR™ Clinical Studies

Table 3 lists adverse reactions that occurred in at least 2% of adult patients with epilepsy treated with Oxtellar XR™ or placebo and concomitant AEDs and that were numerically more common in the patients treated with any dose of Oxtellar XR™ than in patients receiving placebo.

The overall incidence of adverse reactions appeared to be dose related, particularly during the Titration Period. The most commonly observed (≥ 5%) adverse reactions seen in association with Oxtellar XR™ and more frequent than in placebo-treated patients were: dizziness, somnolence, headache, balance disorder, tremor, vomiting, diplopia, and asthenia.

[See table 3 above]

Table 3: Adverse Reaction Incidence in a Controlled Clinical Study of Oxtellar XR™ with Concomitant AEDs in Adults*

	Oxtellar XR 2400 mg/day N=123 %	Oxtellar XR 1200 mg/day N=122 %	Placebo N=121 %
Any System / Any Term	69	57	55
Nervous System Disorders			
Dizziness	41	20	15
Somnolence	14	12	9
Headache	15	8	7
Balance Disorder	7	5	5
Tremor	1	5	2
Nystagmus	3	3	1
Ataxia	1	3	1
Gastrointestinal Disorders			
Vomiting	15	6	9
Abdominal Pain Upper	0	3	1
Dyspepsia	0	3	1
Gastritis	0	3	2
Eye Disorders			
Diplopia	13	10	4
Vision Blurred	1	4	3
Visual Impairment	1	3	0
General Disorders And Administration Site Conditions			
Asthenia	7	3	1
Fatigue	3	6	1
Gait Disturbance	0	3	1
Drug Intolerance	2	0	0
Infections And Infestations			
Nasopharyngitis	0	3	0
Sinusitis	0	3	2

* Reported by ≥ 2% of Patients Treated with Oxtellar XR™ and Numerically More Frequent than in the Placebo Group

Adverse Reactions Associated with Discontinuation of Oxtellar XR™ Treatment: Approximately 23.3% of the 366 adult patients receiving Oxtellar XR™ in clinical studies discontinued treatment because of an adverse reaction. The adverse reactions most commonly associated with discontinuation of Oxtellar XR™ (reported by ≥2%) were: dizziness (9.8%), vomiting (5.3%), nausea (3.7%), diplopia (3.2%), and somnolence (2.4%).

Adjunctive Therapy with Oxtellar XR™ in Pediatric Patients 4 to 16 Years Old Previously Treated with other AEDs

In a pharmacokinetic study in 18 children (age 4-16 years) with partial seizures treated with different doses of Oxtellar XR™, the observed adverse reactions seen in association with Oxtellar XR™ were similar to those seen in adults.

Most Common Adverse Reactions in Immediate-Release Oxcarbazepine Controlled Clinical Studies

Controlled Clinical Studies of Adjunctive Therapy with Immediate-Release Oxcarbazepine in Adults Previously Treated with other AEDs: Table 4 lists adverse reactions that occurred in at least 2% of adult patients with epilepsy treated with immediate-release oxcarbazepine or placebo with concomitant AEDs and that were numerically more common in the patients treated with any dose of immediate-release oxcarbazepine than in placebo. As immediate-release oxcarbazepine and Oxtellar XR™ were not examined in the same trial, adverse event frequencies cannot be directly compared between the two formulations.

[See table 4 on pages 2330 and 2331]

Other Reactions Observed in Association with the Administration of Immediate-Release Oxcarbazepine

In the paragraphs that follow, the adverse reactions, other than those in the preceding tables or text, that occurred in a total of 565 children and 1,574 adults exposed to immediate-release oxcarbazepine and that are reasonably likely to be related to drug use are presented. Events common in the population, events reflecting chronic illness and events likely to reflect concomitant illness are omitted particularly if minor. They are listed in order of decreasing frequency. Because the reports cite reactions observed in open label and uncontrolled trials, the role of immediate-release oxcarbazepine in their causation cannot be reliably determined.

Body as a Whole: fever, malaise, pain chest precordial, rigors, weight decrease.

Cardiovascular System: bradycardia, cardiac failure, cerebral hemorrhage, hypertension, hypotension postural, palpitation, syncope, tachycardia.

Digestive System: appetite increased, blood in stool, cholelithiasis, colitis, duodenal ulcer, dysphagia, enteritis, eructation, esophagitis, flatulence, gastric ulcer, gingival bleeding, gum hyperplasia, hematemesis, hemorrhage rectum, hemorrhoids, hiccup, mouth dry, pain biliary, pain right hypochondrium, retching, sialoadenitis, stomatitis, stomatitis ulcerative.

Hematologic and Lymphatic System: thrombocytopenia.

Laboratory Abnormality: gamma-GT increased, hyperglycemia, hypocalcemia, hypoglycemia, hypokalemia, liver enzymes elevated, serum transaminase increased.

Musculoskeletal System: hypertonia muscle.

Nervous System: aggressive reaction, amnesia, anguish, anxiety, apathy, aphasia, aura, convulsions aggravated, delirium, delusion, depressed level of consciousness, dysphonia, dystonia, emotional lability, euphoria, extrapyramidal disorder, feeling drunk, hemiplegia, hyperkinesia, hyperreflexia, hypoesthesia, hypokinesia, hyporeflexia, hypotonia, hysteria, libido decreased, libido increased, manic reaction, migraine, muscle contractions involuntary, nervousness, neuralgia, oculogyric crisis, panic disorder, paralysis, paroniria, personality disorder, psychosis, ptosis, stupor, tetany.

Respiratory System: asthma, bronchitis, coughing, dyspnea, epistaxis, laryngismus, pleurisy.

Skin and Appendages: acne, alopecia, angioedema, bruising, dermatitis contact, eczema, facial rash, flushing, folliculitis, heat rash, hot flushes, photosensitivity reaction, pruritus genital, psoriasis, purpura, rash erythematous, rash maculopapular, vitiligo, urticaria.

Special Senses: accommodation abnormal, cataract, conjunctival hemorrhage, edema eye, hemianopia, mydriasis, otitis externa, photophobia, scotoma, taste perversion, tinnitus, xerophthalmia.

Urogenital and Reproductive System: dysuria, hematuria, intermenstrual bleeding, leukorrhea, menorrhagia, micturition frequency, pain renal, pain urinary tract, polyuria, priapism, renal calculus, urinary tract infection.

Other: Systemic lupus erythematosus.

6.2 Postmarketing and Other Experience
The following adverse reactions have been identified during post-approval use of immediate-release oxcarbazepine. Because these reactions are reported voluntarily from a population of uncertain size, it is not always possible to reliably estimate their frequency or establish a causal relationship to drug exposure.

Body as a Whole: multi-organ hypersensitivity disorders characterized by features such as rash, fever, lymphadenop-

Table 4: Adverse Reaction Incidence in a Controlled Clinical Study of Immediate Release Oxcarbazepine with Concomitant AEDs in Adults*

	Immediate-Release Oxcarbazepine Dosage (mg/day)			Placebo N = 166%
	OXC 600 N = 163%	OXC 1200 N = 171%	OXC 2400 N = 126%	
Body as a Whole				
Fatigue	15	12	15	7
Asthenia	6	3	6	5
Edema Legs	2	1	2	1
Weight Increase	1	2	2	1
Feeling Abnormal	0	1	2	0
Cardiovascular System				
Hypotension	0	1	2	0
Digestive System				
Nausea	15	25	29	10
Vomiting	13	25	36	5
Pain Abdominal	10	13	11	5
Diarrhea	5	6	7	6
Dyspepsia	5	5	6	2
Constipation	2	2	6	4
Gastritis	2	1	2	1
Metabolic and Nutritional Disorders				
Hyponatremia	3	1	2	1
Musculoskeletal System				
Muscle Weakness	1	2	2	0
Sprains and Strains	0	2	2	1
Nervous System				
Headache	32	28	26	23
Dizziness	36	32	49	13
Somnolence	20	28	36	12
Ataxia	9	17	31	5
Nystagmus	7	20	26	5
Gait Abnormal	5	10	17	1
Insomnia	4	2	3	1
Tremor	3	8	16	5
Nervousness	2	4	2	1
Agitation	1	1	2	1
Coordination Abnormal	1	3	2	1
EEG Abnormal	0	0	2	0
Speech Disorder	1	1	3	0
Confusion	1	1	2	1
Cranial Injury NOS	1	0	2	1
Dysmetria	1	2	3	0
Thinking Abnormal	0	2	4	0

(Table continued on next page)

athy, abnormal liver function tests, eosinophilia and arthralgia [see *Warnings and Precautions (5.7)*]
Anaphylaxis: [see *Warnings and Precautions (5.2)*]
Digestive System: pancreatitis and/or lipase and/or amylase increase
Hematologic and Lymphatic Systems: aplastic anemia [see *Warnings and Precautions (5.8)*]
Skin and Appendages: erythema multiforme, Stevens-Johnson syndrome, toxic epidermal necrolysis [see *Warnings and Precautions (5.4)*]

7 DRUG INTERACTIONS

Oxcarbazepine and MHD induce a subgroup of the cytochrome P450 3A family (CYP3A4 and CYP3A5).
In addition, several AEDs that are cytochrome P450 inducers can decrease plasma concentrations of oxcarbazepine and MHD.
These interactions have implications when Oxtellar XR™ is used with other AEDs or hormonal contraceptives.

7.1 Other Antiepileptic Drugs

Potential interactions between immediate-release oxcarbazepine and other AEDs were assessed in clinical studies. Oxtellar XR™ would be expected to have the same effects on coadministered AEDs as immediate-release oxcarbazepine.
[See table 5 at top of next page]

7.2 Hormonal Contraceptives

Coadministration of immediate-release oxcarbazepine with an oral contraceptive decreased the plasma concentrations of two components of hormonal contraceptives, ethinylestradiol and levonorgestrel. Therefore, concurrent use of Oxtellar XR™ with these hormonal contraceptives and other oral or implant contraceptives may render these contraceptives less effective [see *Clinical Pharmacology (12.3)*]. Additional non-hormonal forms of contraception are recommended.

8 USE IN SPECIFIC POPULATIONS

8.1 Pregnancy

Oxtellar XR™ plasma concentrations may decrease during pregnancy [see *Warnings and Precautions (5.9)*]

Pregnancy Category C

There are no adequate and well-controlled clinical studies of Oxtellar XR™ in pregnant women; however, Oxtellar XR™ is closely related structurally to carbamazepine, which is considered to be teratogenic in humans. Given this fact, and the results of the animal studies described, it is likely that Oxtellar XR™ is a human teratogen. Oxtellar XR™ should be used during pregnancy only if the potential benefit justifies the potential risk to the fetus.
Increased incidences of fetal structural abnormalities and other manifestations of developmental toxicity (embryolethality, growth retardation) were observed in the offspring of animals treated with either oxcarbazepine or its active 10-hydroxy metabolite (MHD) during pregnancy at doses similar to the maximum recommended human dose.
When pregnant rats were given oxcarbazepine (30, 300, or 1000 mg/kg) orally throughout the period of organogenesis, increased incidences of fetal malformations (craniofacial, cardiovascular, and skeletal) and variations were observed at the intermediate and high doses (approximately 1.2 and 4 times, respectively, the maximum recommended human dose [MRHD] on a mg/m^2 basis). Increased embryofetal death and decreased fetal body weights were seen at the high dose. Doses ≥ 300 mg/kg were also maternally toxic (decreased body weight gain, clinical signs), but there is no evidence to suggest that teratogenicity was secondary to the maternal effects.
In a study in which pregnant rabbits were orally administered MHD (20, 100, or 200 mg/kg) during organogenesis, embryofetal mortality was increased at the highest dose (1.5 times the MRHD on a mg/m^2 basis). This dose produced only minimal maternal toxicity.
In a study in which female rats were dosed orally with oxcarbazepine (25, 50, or 150 mg/kg) during the latter part of gestation and throughout the lactation period, a persistent reduction in body weights and altered behavior (decreased activity) were observed in offspring exposed to the highest dose (0.6 times the MRHD on a mg/m^2 basis). Oral administration of MHD (25, 75, or 250 mg/kg) to rats during gestation and lactation resulted in a persistent reduction in offspring weights at the highest dose (equivalent to the MRHD on a mg/m^2 basis).
To provide information regarding the effects of in utero exposure to Oxtellar XR™, physicians are advised to recommend that pregnant patients taking Oxtellar XR™ enroll in the NAAED Pregnancy Registry. This can be done by calling the toll free number 1-888-233-2334, and must be done by patients themselves. Information on the registry can also be found at the website http://www.aedpregnancyregistry.org/.

8.2 Nursing Mothers

Oxcarbazepine and its active metabolite (MHD) are excreted in human milk. A milk-to-plasma concentration ratio of 0.5 was found for both. Because of the potential for serious adverse reactions to Oxtellar XR™ in nursing infants, a decision should be made about whether to discontinue nursing or to discontinue the drug in nursing women, taking into account the importance of the drug to the mother.

8.3 Pediatric Use

The short term safety and effectiveness of Oxtellar XR™ in pediatric patients ages 6 to 16 years with partial onset seizures is supported by:
1) An adequate and well-controlled short term safety and efficacy study of Oxtellar XR™ in adults that included pharmacokinetic sampling [see *Clinical Studies (14.1)*],

2) A pharmacokinetic study of Oxtellar XR™ in pediatric patients ages 4 to 16 years [see *Clinical Pharmacology (12.3)*], and
3) Safety and efficacy studies with the immediate-release formulation in adults and pediatric patients [see *Clinical Studies (14.2)* and *Adverse Reactions (6.1)*].

Oxtellar XR™ is not approved for pediatric patients less than 6 years of age because the size of the tablets are inappropriate for younger children, and has not been studied in patients younger than 4 years of age.

8.4 Geriatric Use

Following administration of single (300 mg) and multiple (600 mg/day) doses of immediate-release oxcarbazepine to elderly volunteers (60-82 years of age), the maximum plasma concentrations and AUC values of MHD were 30%-60% higher than in younger volunteers (18-32 years of age). Comparisons of creatinine clearance in young and elderly volunteers indicate that the difference was due to age-related reductions in creatinine clearance. Consider starting at a lower dose and lower titration [see *Dosage and Administration (2.5)*].

8.5 Renal Impairment

There is a linear correlation between creatinine clearance and the renal clearance of MHD. [see *Clinical Pharmacology (12.3)* and *Dosage and Administration (2.4)*].

The pharmacokinetics of Oxtellar XR™ has not been evaluated in patients with renal impairment. In patients with severe renal impairment (creatinine clearance <30 mL/min) given immediate release oxcarbazepine, the elimination half-life of MHD was prolonged with a corresponding two-fold increase in AUC [see *Clinical Pharmacology (12.3)*]. In these patients initiate Oxtellar XR™ at a lower starting dose and increase, if necessary, at a slower than usual rate until the desired clinical response is achieved [see *Dosage and Administration (2.4)*].

In patients with end-stage renal disease on dialysis, it is recommended that immediate release oxcarbazepine be used instead of Oxtellar XR™.

8.6 Hepatic Impairment

The pharmacokinetics of oxcarbazepine and MHD has not been evaluated in severe hepatic impairment, and therefore is not recommended in these patients. [see *Clinical Pharmacology (12.3)*].

9 DRUG ABUSE AND DEPENDENCE

9.2 Abuse

The abuse potential of Oxtellar XR™ has not been evaluated in human studies. Oxtellar XR™ is not habit forming, and is not expected to encourage abuse.

9.3 Dependence

Intragastric injections of oxcarbazepine to four cynomolgus monkeys demonstrated no signs of physical dependence as measured by the desire to self-administer oxcarbazepine by lever pressing activity.

10 OVERDOSAGE

Human Overdose Experience

Isolated cases of overdose with immediate-release oxcarbazepine have been reported. The maximum dose taken was approximately 24,000 mg. All patients recovered with symptomatic treatment.

Treatment and Management

There is no specific antidote for Oxtellar XR™ overdose. Administer symptomatic and supportive treatment as appropriate. Options include removal of the drug by gastric lavage and/or inactivation by administering activated charcoal.

11 DESCRIPTION

Oxtellar XR™ is an antiepileptic drug (AED). Oxtellar XR™ extended-release tablets contain oxcarbazepine for once-a-day oral administration.

Oxcarbazepine is 10,11-Dihydro-10-oxo-5H-dibenz[b,f]-azepine-5-carboxamide, and its structural formula is

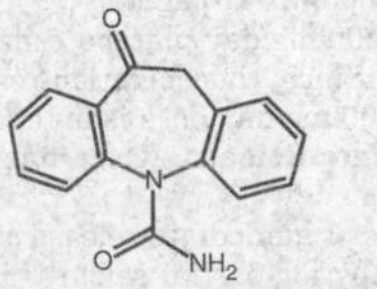

Oxcarbazepine is off-white to yellow crystalline powder. Oxcarbazepine is sparingly soluble in chloroform (30-100 g/L). In aqueous media over pH range 1 to 8, oxcarbazepine is practically insoluble and its solubility is 40 mg/L (0.04 g/L) at pH 7.0, 25°C. The molecular formula is $C_{15}H_{12}N_2O_2$ and its molecular weight is 252.27.

Oxtellar XR™ tablets contain the following inactive ingredients: colloidal silicon dioxide, hypromellose, yellow iron oxide (150 mg, 300 mg tablets only), red iron oxide (300 mg, 600 mg tablets only), black iron oxide (300 mg tablet only), magnesium stearate, methacrylic acid copolymer, microcrystalline cellulose, polyethylene glycol, polyvinyl alcohol, povidone, sodium lauryl sulfate, talc, and titanium dioxide. Each tablet is printed on one side with edible black ink.

Table 4 *(cont.)*: Adverse Reaction Incidence in a Controlled Clinical Study of Immediate Release Oxcarbazepine with Concomitant AEDs in Adults*

	Immediate-Release Oxcarbazepine Dosage (mg/day)			Placebo N = 166%
	OXC 600 N = 163%	OXC 1200 N = 171%	OXC 2400 N = 126%	
Respiratory System				
Rhinitis	2	4	5	4
Skin and Appendages				
Acne	1	2	2	0
Special Senses				
Diplopia	14	30	40	5
Vertigo	6	12	15	2
Vision Abnormal	6	14	13	4
Accommodation Abnormal	0	0	2	0

* Events in at Least 2% of Patients Treated with 2400mg/day of Immediate-Release Oxcarbazepine and Numerically More Frequent than in the Placebo Group

Table 5: AED Drug Interactions with Oxcarbazepine

AED Coadministered (daily dose)	IR-Oxcarbazepine (daily dose)	Influence of IR-Oxcarbazepine on AED Concentration Mean Change [90% Confidence Interval]	Influence of AED on MHD Concentration (Mean Change, 90% Confidence Interval)	Recommendation
Carbamazepine (400 – 2000 mg)	900 mg	nc[1]	40% decrease [CI: 17% decrease, 57% decrease]	Consider initiating Oxtellar XR™ at a higher dose. Monitor and titrate dose to desired clinical effect (see 2.6)
Phenobarbital (100 – 150 mg)	600 – 1800 mg	14% increase [CI: 2% increase, 24% increase]	25% decrease [CI: 12% decrease, 51% decrease]	
Phenytoin (250 – 500 mg)	600 – 1800 >1200-2400	nc[1,2] up to 40% increase[3] [CI: 12% increase, 60% increase]	30% decrease [CI: 3% decrease, 48% decrease]	
Valproic Acid (400 – 2800 mg)	600-1800	nc[1]	18% decrease [CI: 13% decrease, 40% decrease]	Monitor. Dose adjustment of Oxtellar XR™ may not be needed.

[1]nc denotes a mean change of less than 10%
[2]Pediatrics
[3]Mean increase in adults at high doses of immediate-release oxcarbazepine

12 CLINICAL PHARMACOLOGY

12.1 Mechanism of Action

The pharmacological activity of Oxtellar XR™ is primarily exerted through the 10-monohydroxy metabolite (MHD) of oxcarbazepine [see *Clinical Pharmacology (12.3)*]. The precise mechanism by which oxcarbazepine and MHD exert their antiseizure effect is unknown; however, in vitro electrophysiological studies indicate that they produce blockade of voltage-sensitive sodium channels, resulting in stabilization of hyperexcited neural membranes, inhibition of repetitive neuronal firing, and diminution of propagation of synaptic impulses. These actions are thought to be important in the prevention of seizure spread in the intact brain. In addition, increased potassium conductance and modulation of high-voltage activated calcium channels may contribute to the anticonvulsant effects of the drug. No significant interactions of oxcarbazepine or MHD with brain neurotransmitter or modulator receptor sites have been demonstrated.

12.2 Pharmacodynamics

Oxcarbazepine and its active metabolite (MHD) exhibit anticonvulsant properties in animal seizure models. They protected rodents against electrically induced tonic extension seizures and, to a lesser degree, chemically induced clonic seizures, and abolished or reduced the frequency of chronically recurring focal seizures in Rhesus monkeys with aluminum implants. No development of tolerance (i.e., attenuation of anticonvulsive activity) was observed in the maximal electroshock test when mice and rats were treated daily for five days and four weeks, respectively, with oxcarbazepine or MHD.

12.3 Pharmacokinetics

Following oral administration, oxcarbazepine is absorbed and extensively metabolized to its pharmacologically active 10-monohydroxy metabolite (MHD), which is responsible for most antiepileptic activity.

In clinical studies of Oxtellar XR™, the elimination half-life of oxcarbazepine was between 7 and 11 hours; the elimination half-life of MHD is between 9 and 11 hours.

In a mass balance study in human, only 2% of total radioactivity in plasma after administration of immediate-release oxcarbazepine was due to unchanged oxcarbazepine, with approximately 70% present as MHD, and the remainder attributable to minor metabolites.

Absorption

Oxtellar XR™ administered as a once daily dose is not bioequivalent to the same total dose of the immediate release formulation given twice daily at steady state. Steady state plasma concentrations of MHD are reached within 5 days when Oxtellar XR™ is given once daily. At steady state, when 1200 mg Oxtellar XR™ was given once daily, MHD C_{max} occurred 7 hours post-dose. At steady state, Oxtellar XR™ given once daily produced MHD exposures (AUC and C_{max}) about 19% lower and MHD minimum concentrations (C_{min}) about 16% lower than the immediate-release oxcarbazepine given twice daily when administered at the same 1200 mg total daily dose. When Oxtellar XR™ was administered at an equivalent 600 mg single dose (4 × 150 mg tablets, 2 × 300 mg tablets, or 1 × 600 mg tablet), equivalent MHD exposures (AUC) were observed.

Following a single dose of Oxtellar XR™ (1 × 150 mg tablets, 1 × 300 mg tablets, or 1 × 600 mg tablet), the pharmacokinetics of MHD are not linear and show greater than dose proportional increase in AUC and less than proportional increase in C_{max}: AUC increases 2.4-fold and C_{max} increases 1.9-fold with a 2-fold increase in dose.

Effect of Food: Single dose administration of 600 mg Oxtellar XR™ following a high fat meal (800 – 1000 calories) produced MHD exposure (AUC) equivalent to that produced under fasting conditions. Peak MHD concentration (C_{max}) was about 60% higher and occurred 2 hours earlier under fed conditions than under fasting conditions.

The increase in C_{max}, even without a significant change in the overall exposure, should be considered by the prescriber especially during the titration phase, when some adverse reactions are most likely to occur coincidentally with peak levels.

Distribution

The apparent volume of distribution of MHD is 49 L. Approximately 40% of MHD is bound to serum proteins, predominantly to albumin. Binding is independent of the serum concentration within the therapeutically relevant range. Oxcarbazepine and MHD do not bind to alpha-1-acid glycoprotein.

Metabolism

Oxcarbazepine is rapidly reduced by cytosolic enzymes in the liver to MHD, which is primarily responsible for the pharmacological effect of Oxtellar XR™. MHD is metabolized further by conjugation with glucuronic acid. Minor amounts (4% of the dose) are oxidized to the pharmacologically inactive 10,11-dihydroxy metabolite (DHD).

Elimination

Oxcarbazepine is cleared from the body mostly in the form of metabolites which are predominantly excreted by the kidneys. More than 95% of a dose of immediate-release oxcarbazepine appears in the urine, with less than 1% as unchanged oxcarbazepine. Fecal excretion accounts for less than 4% of an administered dose. Approximately 80% of the dose is excreted in the urine either as glucuronides of MHD (49%) or as unchanged MHD (27%); the inactive DHD accounts for approximately 3% and conjugates of MHD and oxcarbazepine account for 13% of the dose.

The half-life of the parent was about two hours, while the half-life of MHD was about nine hours after the immediate release formulation. A population pharmacokinetic model for Oxtellar XR™ was developed in healthy normal adults and applied to pharmacokinetic data in patients with epilepsy. For oxcarbazepine, systemic parameters were scaled allometrically, suggesting that steady state oxcarbazepine exposure will vary inversely with weight.

Special Populations

Elderly

No studies with Oxtellar XR™ in elderly patients have been completed [see *Use in Specific Populations (8.4)*].

Following administration of single (300 mg) and multiple (600 mg/day) doses of immediate-release oxcarbazepine to elderly volunteers (60-82 years of age), the maximum plasma concentrations and AUC values of MHD were 30%-60% higher than in younger volunteers (18-32 years of age). Comparisons of creatinine clearance in young and elderly volunteers indicate that the difference was due to age-related reductions in creatinine clearance.

Pediatric

Oxtellar XR™ is not approved for pediatric patients less than 6 years of age because the size of the tablets are inappropriate for younger children, and has not been studied in patients younger than 4 years of age. A pharmacokinetic study of Oxtellar XR™ was performed in 18 pediatric patients with epilepsy, 4 to 16 years of age, after multiple doses. The population pharmacokinetic model suggested that dosing of pediatric patients with Oxtellar XR™ can be determined based on body weight. Weight-normalized doses in pediatric patients should produce MHD exposures (AUC) comparable to that in typical adults, with oxcarbazepine exposures ~40% higher in children than in adults [see *Use in Specific Populations (8.3)*].

Gender

The effects of gender have not been studied for Oxtellar XR™.

No gender-related pharmacokinetic differences have been observed in children, adults, or the elderly with immediate-release oxcarbazepine.

Race

The effects of race have not been studied for Oxtellar XR™.

Renal or Hepatic Impairment

The effects of renal or hepatic impairment have not been studied for Oxtellar XR™ [see *Use in Specific Populations (8.5, 8.6)*].

Based on investigations with immediate-release oxcarbazepine, there is a linear correlation between creatinine clearance and the renal clearance of MHD. When immediate-release oxcarbazepine is administered as a single 300 mg dose in renally-impaired patients (creatinine clearance <30 mL/min), the elimination half-life of MHD is prolonged to 19 hours, with a two-fold increase in AUC. Dose adjustment is recommended in these patients [see *Dosage and Administration (2.4)* and *Use in Special Populations (8.5)*].

The pharmacokinetics and metabolism of immediate-release oxcarbazepine and MHD were evaluated in healthy volunteers and hepatically impaired subjects after a single 900 mg oral dose. Mild-to-moderate hepatic impairment did not affect the pharmacokinetics of immediate-release oxcarbazepine and MHD. The pharmacokinetics of oxcarbazepine and MHD have not been evaluated in severe hepatic impairment, and therefore it is not recommended in these patients [see *Use in Specific Populations (8.6)*].

Pregnancy

Due to physiological changes during pregnancy, MHD plasma levels may gradually decrease throughout pregnancy [see *Use in Specific Populations (8.1)*]

Drug Interaction Studies

In Vitro: Oxcarbazepine can inhibit CYP2C19 and induce CYP3A4/5 with potentially important effects on plasma concentrations of other drugs. In addition, several AEDs that are cytochrome P450 inducers can decrease plasma concentrations of oxcarbazepine and MHD.

Oxcarbazepine was evaluated in human liver microsomes to determine its capacity to inhibit the major cytochrome P450 enzymes responsible for the metabolism of other drugs. Results demonstrate that oxcarbazepine and its pharmacologically active 10-monohydroxy metabolite (MHD) have little or no capacity to function as inhibitors for most of the human cytochrome P450 enzymes evaluated (CYP1A2, CYP2A6, CYP2C9, CYP2D6, CYP2E1, CYP4A9 and CYP4A11) with the exception of CYP2C19 and CYP3A4/5. Although inhibition of CYP3A4/5 by oxcarbazepine and MHD did occur at high concentrations, it is not likely to be of clinical significance. The inhibition of CYP2C19 by oxcarbazepine and MHD, is clinically relevant.

In vitro, the UDP-glucuronyl transferase level was increased, indicating induction of this enzyme. Increases of 22% with MHD and 47% with oxcarbazepine were observed. As MHD, the predominant plasma substrate, is only a weak inducer of UDP-glucuronyl transferase, it is unlikely to have an effect on drugs that are mainly eliminated by conjugation through UDPglucuronyl transferase (e.g., valproic acid, lamotrigine).

In addition, oxcarbazepine and MHD induce a subgroup of the cytochrome P450 3A family (CYP3A4 and CYP3A5) responsible for the metabolism of dihydropyridine calcium antagonists, oral contraceptives and cyclosporine resulting in a lower plasma concentration of these drugs.

Several AEDs that are cytochrome P450 inducers can decrease plasma concentrations of oxcarbazepine and MHD. No autoinduction has been observed with immediate-release oxcarbazepine.

As binding of MHD to plasma proteins is low (40%), clinically significant interactions with other drugs through competition for protein binding sites are unlikely.

In Vivo:

Hormonal Contraceptives

Coadministration of immediate-release oxcarbazepine with an oral contraceptive has been shown to influence the plasma concentrations of two components of hormonal contraceptives, ethinylestradiol (EE) and levonorgestrel (LNG). The mean AUC values of EE were decreased by 48% [90% CI: 22-65] in one study and 52% [90% CI: 38-52] in another study. The mean AUC values of LNG were decreased by 32% [90% CI: 20-45] in one study and 52% [90% CI: 42-52] in another study. Therefore, concurrent use of oxcarbazepine with hormonal contraceptives may render these contraceptives less effective.

Calcium Channel Antagonists

After repeated coadministration of immediate-release oxcarbazepine, the AUC of felodipine was lowered by 28% [90% CI: 20-33]. Verapamil produced a decrease of 20% [90% CI: 18-27] of the plasma levels of MHD after coadministration with immediate-release oxcarbazepine.

Other Interactions

Cimetidine, erythromycin and dextropropoxyphene had no effect on the pharmacokinetics of MHD after coadministration with immediate-release oxcarbazepine. Results with warfarin show no evidence of interaction with either single or repeated doses of immediate-release oxcarbazepine.

13 NONCLINICAL TOXICOLOGY

13.1 Carcinogenesis, Mutagenesis, Impairment of Fertility

Carcinogenesis

In two-year carcinogenicity studies, oxcarbazepine was administered in the diet at doses of up to 100 mg/kg/day to mice and by gavage at doses of up to 250 mg/kg/day to rats, and the pharmacologically active 10-hydroxy metabolite (MHD) was administered orally at doses of up to 600 mg/kg/day to rats.

In mice, a dose-related increase in the incidence of hepatocellular adenomas was observed at oxcarbazepine doses ≥ 70 mg/kg/day or approximately 0.1 times the maximum recommended human dose (MRHD) on a mg/m^2 basis.

In rats, the incidence of hepatocellular carcinomas was increased in females treated with oxcarbazepine at doses ≥25 mg/kg/day (0.1 times the MRHD on a mg/m^2 basis), and incidences of hepatocellular adenomas and/or carcinomas were increased in males and females treated with MHD at doses of 600 mg/kg/day (2.4 times the MRHD on a mg/m^2 basis) and ≥ 250 mg/kg/day (equivalent to the MRHD on a mg/m^2 basis), respectively.

There was an increase in the incidence of benign testicular interstitial cell tumors in rats at 250 mg oxcarbazepine/kg/day and at ≥ 250 mg MHD/kg/day, and an increase in the incidence of granular cell tumors in the cervix and vagina in rats at 600 mg MHD/kg/day.

Mutagenesis

Oxcarbazepine increased mutation frequencies in the Ames test in vitro in the absence of metabolic activation in one of five bacterial strains. Both oxcarbazepine and MHD produced increases in chromosomal aberrations and polyploidy in the Chinese hamster ovary assay in vitro in the absence of metabolic activation. MHD was negative in the Ames test, and no mutagenic or clastogenic activity was found with either oxcarbazepine or MHD in V79 Chinese hamster cells in vitro. Oxcarbazepine and MHD were both negative for clastogenic or aneugenic effects (micronucleus formation) in an in vivo rat bone marrow assay.

Impairment of Fertility

In a fertility study in which rats were administered MHD (50, 150, or 450 mg/kg) orally prior to and during mating and early gestation, estrous cyclicity was disrupted and numbers of corpora lutea, implantations, and live embryos were reduced in females receiving the highest dose (approximately two times the MRHD on a mg/m^2 basis).

14 CLINICAL STUDIES

Oxtellar XR™ has been evaluated as adjunctive therapy for partial seizures in adults. The use of Oxtellar XR™ for the treatment of partial seizures in children is based on adequate and well-controlled studies of Oxtellar XR™ in adults, along with clinical trials of immediate-release oxcarbazepine in children, and on pharmacokinetic evaluations of the use of Oxtellar XR™ in children.

14.1 Oxtellar XR™ Primary Trial

A multicenter, randomized, double-blind, placebo-controlled, three-arm, parallel-group study (Study 1) in male and female adults with refractory partial epilepsy (18 to 65 years of age, inclusive) was performed to examine the safety and efficacy of Oxtellar XR™.

Patients had at least three partial seizures per 28 days during an 8 week Baseline Period. Subjects were receiving treatment with at least one to three antiepileptic drugs and were on stable treatment for a minimum of 4 weeks. Subjects with a diagnosis other than partial epilepsy were excluded.

The study included an 8 week Baseline Period, followed by a Treatment Period, which included a 4 week Titration Phase followed by a 12 week Maintenance Phase. The primary endpoint of the study was median percentage change from baseline in seizure frequency per 28 days during the treatment period relative to the baseline period. The criterion for statistical significance was $p < 0.05$. A total of 366 patients were enrolled at 88 sites in North America and Eastern Europe. Subjects were randomized to one of three treatment groups and took Oxtellar XR™ (1200 or 2400 mg/day) or placebo.

Table 6 presents the primary efficacy results by treatment group.

[See table 6 at top of next page]

Although the 1200 mg/day-placebo contrast did not reach statistical significance, concentration-response analyses reveal that the 1200 mg/day dose is an effective dose.

14.2 Immediate-Release Oxcarbazepine Adjunctive Therapy Trials

The effectiveness of immediate-release oxcarbazepine as an adjunctive therapy for partial seizures in adults was demonstrated at doses of 600mg per day, 1200mg per day and 2400mg per day (divided twice daily) in a randomized, double-blind, placebo-controlled trial. All doses resulted in a statistically significant reduction in seizure frequency when compared to placebo ($p<0.05$).

The effectiveness of immediate-release oxcarbazepine in doses of 30-46 mg/kg/day, depending on baseline weight, as an adjunctive therapy for partial seizures in children 3 years to 17 years of age was studied in a randomized, double-blind, placebo-controlled trial. Oxcarbazepine in the single weight based dose group resulted in a statistically significant reduction in seizure frequency when compared to placebo ($p<0.05$).

16 HOW SUPPLIED/STORAGE AND HANDLING

16.1 Dosage Form Supplied

150 mg (yellow modified-oval shaped tablet printed "150" on one side with edible black ink).
Bottles of 100 tablets NDC 17772-121-01
300 mg (brown modified-oval shaped tablet printed "300" on one side with edible black ink).
Bottles of 100 tablets NDC 17772-122-01
600 mg (brownish red modified-oval shaped tablet printed "600" on one side with edible black ink).
Bottles of 100 tablets NDC 17772-123-01

16.2 Storage and Handling

Store at 25°C (77°F); excursions permitted between 15°C and 30°C (59°F to 86°F) [See USP controlled room temperature]. Protect from light and moisture. Dispense in a tight, light-resistant container.

17 PATIENT COUNSELING INFORMATION

See FDA-Approved patient labeling (Medication Guide).
Inform patients and caregivers of the availability of a Medication Guide. Instruct patients and caregivers to read the Medication Guide prior to taking Oxtellar XR™.

- Advise patients to take the tablet whole with water or other liquid, and not to cut, chew or crush the tablet. Cutting, chewing or crushing Oxtellar XR™ tablet could affect its performance.
- Advise patients to take Oxtellar XR™ on an empty stomach. This means they should take Oxtellar XR™ at least one hour before food or at least two hours after food [see *Clinical Pharmacology (12.3)*].
- Advise patients that Oxtellar XR™ may reduce serum sodium concentrations especially if they are taking other medications that can lower sodium. Advise patients to report symptoms of low sodium like nausea, tiredness, lack of energy, confusion, and more frequent or more severe seizures [see *Warnings and Precautions (5.1)*].
- Anaphylactic reactions and angioedema may occur during treatment with Oxtellar XR™. Advise patients to immediately report signs and symptoms suggesting angioedema (swelling of the face, eyes, lips, tongue or difficulty in swallowing or breathing) and to stop taking the drug until they have consulted with their physician [see *Warnings and Precautions (5.2)*].
- Inform patients who have exhibited hypersensitivity reactions to carbamazepine that approximately 25%-30% of these patients may also experience hypersensitivity reactions with Oxtellar XR™. If patients experience a hypersensitivity reaction while taking Oxtellar XR™, advise them to consult with their physician immediately [see *Warnings and Precautions (5.3)*].
- Advise patients that serious skin reactions have been reported in association with immediate-release oxcarbazepine. If patients experience a skin reaction while taking Oxtellar XR™, advise patients to consult with their physician immediately [see *Warnings and Precautions (5.4)*].
- Instruct patients that a fever associated with other organ system involvement (rash, lymphadenopathy, etc.) occurring during treatment with Oxtellar XR™ may be drug-related and advise them to consult their physician immediately [see *Warnings and Precautions (5.7)*].
- Advise patients that there have been rare reports of blood disorders reported in patients treated with immediate-release oxcarbazepine. Instruct patients to immediately consult with their physician if they experience symptoms suggestive of blood disorders during treatment with Oxtellar XR™ [see *Warnings and Precautions (5.8)*].
- Warn female patients of childbearing age that the concurrent use of Oxtellar XR™ with hormonal contraceptives may render this method of contraception less effective [see *Drug Interactions (7.2)*]. Additional non-hormonal forms of contraception are recommended when using Oxtellar XR™.
- Counsel patients, their caregivers, and families that AEDs, including Oxtellar XR™, may increase the risk of suicidal thoughts and behavior and that they need to be alert for the emergence or worsening of symptoms of depression, any unusual changes in mood or behavior, or the emergence of suicidal thoughts, behavior, or thoughts about self-harm. Advise them to immediately report behaviors of concern to healthcare providers.
- Advise patients to exercise caution if alcohol is taken in combination with Oxtellar XR™ therapy, due to a possible additive sedative effect.
- Advise patients that Oxtellar XR™ may cause dizziness and somnolence. Accordingly, advise patients not to drive or operate machinery until they have gained sufficient experience on Oxtellar XR™ to gauge whether it adversely affects their ability to drive or operate machinery.
- Encourage patients to enroll in the North American Antiepileptic Drug (NAAED) Pregnancy Registry if they become pregnant. This registry is collecting information about the safety of antiepileptic drugs during pregnancy. To enroll, patients can call the toll free number 1-888-233-2334 [see *Use in Specific Populations (8.1)*].

Table 6: Primary Efficacy Results in Study 1: Percent Change from Baseline in Partial Seizure Frequency in the 16-week Treatment Period

	Median seizure frequency during 8-week baseline period (per 28 days)	Median seizure frequency during 16-week treatment period (per 28 days)	Median percent change in seizure frequency	Seizure frequency percent change effect size	P value vs placebo*
Placebo (N=121)	7.0	5.0	-28.7 %		
Oxtellar XR™ 1200mg/day (N=122)	6.0	4.3	-38.2 %	9.5%	0.078
Oxtellar XR™ 2400mg/day (N=123)	6.0	3.7	-42.9 %	14.2%	0.003

*Wilcoxon rank-sum test of the median percentage change in partial seizure frequency per 28 days during the 16-week Treatment Phase (Titration + Maintenance Periods) relative to the 8-week Baseline Phase.

- Advise patients that they should call their healthcare provider or poison control center (phone number 1-800-222-1222) if they take too much Oxtellar XR™.
- Discuss with your patient what they should do if they miss a dose.

Oxtellar XR™ is manufactured by:
Patheon Inc.
Whitby, Ontario L1N 5Z5 CANADA
Distributed by:
Supernus Pharmaceuticals, Inc.
Rockville, MD 20850 USA
Oxtellar XR™ is a trademark of Supernus Pharmaceuticals, Inc.
Revised: October 2012

MEDICATION GUIDE
Oxtellar XR™((ahks-TEH-lahr eks ahr))
(oxcarbazepine)
Extended-Release Tablets

Read this Medication Guide before you start taking Oxtellar XR™ and each time you get a refill. There may be new information. This information does not take the place of talking to your healthcare provider about your medical condition or treatment.

What is the most important information I should know about Oxtellar XR™?

Do not stop taking Oxtellar XR™ without first talking to your healthcare provider.

Stopping Oxtellar XR™ suddenly can cause serious problems.

Oxtellar XR™ can cause serious side effects, including:

1. Oxtellar XR™ may cause the level of sodium in your blood to be low. Symptoms of low blood sodium include:

- nausea
- tiredness, lack of energy
- headache
- confusion
- more frequent or more severe seizures.

Similar symptoms that are not related to low sodium may occur from taking Oxtellar XR™. You should tell your healthcare provider if you have any of these side effects and if they bother you or they do not go away.

Some other medicines can also cause low sodium in your blood. Be sure to tell your healthcare provider about all the other medicines that you are taking.

2. Oxtellar XR™ may also cause allergic reactions or serious problems which may affect organs and other parts of your body like the liver or blood cells. You may or may not have a rash with these types of reactions.

Call your healthcare provider right away if you have any of the following:

- swelling of your face, eyes, lips, or tongue
- trouble swallowing or breathing
- a skin rash
- hives
- fever, swollen glands, or sore throat that do not go away or come and go
- painful sores in the mouth or around your eyes
- yellowing of your skin or eyes
- unusual bruising or bleeding
- severe fatigue or weakness
- severe muscle pain
- frequent infections or infections that do not go away

Many people who are allergic to carbamazepine are also allergic to Oxtellar XR™. Tell your healthcare provider if you are allergic to carbamazepine.

3. Like other antiepileptic drugs, Oxtellar XR™ may cause suicidal thoughts or actions in a very small number of people, about 1 in 500.

Call your healthcare provider right away if you have any of these symptoms, especially if they are new, worse, or worry you:

- thoughts about suicide or dying
- attempts to commit suicide
- new or worse depression
- new or worse anxiety
- feeling agitated or restless
- panic attacks
- trouble sleeping (insomnia)
- new or worse irritability
- acting aggressive, being angry, or violent
- acting on dangerous impulses
- an extreme increase in activity and talking (mania)
- other unusual changes in behavior or mood

How can I watch for early symptoms of suicidal thoughts and actions?

- Pay attention to any changes, especially sudden changes, in mood, behaviors, thoughts, or feelings.
- Keep all follow-up visits with your healthcare provider as scheduled.

Call your healthcare provider between visits as needed, especially if you are worried about symptoms.

Do not stop taking Oxtellar XR™ without first talking to a healthcare provider.

Stopping Oxtellar XR™ suddenly can cause serious problems. Stopping a seizure medicine suddenly in a patient who has epilepsy may cause seizures that will not stop (status epilepticus).

Suicidal thoughts or actions may be caused by things other than medicines. If you have suicidal thoughts or actions, your healthcare provider may check for other causes.

What is Oxtellar XR™?

Oxtellar XR™ is a prescription medicine used:

- with other medicines to treat partial seizures in adults
- with other medicines to treat partial seizures in children 6 to 17 years of age.

It is not known if Oxtellar XR™ is safe and effective in children under 6 years of age.

Who should not take Oxtellar XR™?

- Do not take Oxtellar XR™ if you are allergic to oxcarbazepine or any of the other ingredients in Oxtellar XR™. See the end of this leaflet for a complete list of ingredients in Oxtellar XR™.

What should I tell my healthcare provider before taking Oxtellar XR™?

Before taking Oxtellar XR™, tell your healthcare provider about all your medical conditions, including if you:

- have or have had suicidal thoughts or actions, depression or mood problems
- have liver problems
- have kidney problems
- use birth control medicine. Oxtellar XR™ may cause your birth control medicine to be less effective. Talk to your healthcare provider about the best birth control method to use.
- are pregnant or plan to become pregnant. Oxtellar XR™ may harm your unborn baby. Tell your healthcare provider right away if you become pregnant while taking Oxtellar XR™. You and your healthcare provider will decide if you should take Oxtellar XR™ while you are pregnant.
  - If you become pregnant while taking Oxtellar XR™, talk to your healthcare provider about registering with the

North American Antiepileptic Drug (NAAED) Pregnancy Registry. The purpose of this registry is to collect information about the safety of antiepileptic medicine during pregnancy. You can enroll in this registry by calling 1-888-233-2334.
- are breastfeeding or plan to breastfeed. Oxtellar XR™ passes into breast milk. You and your healthcare provider should discuss whether you should take Oxtellar XR™ or breastfeed. You should not do both.

Tell your healthcare provider about all the medicines you take, including prescription and non-prescription medicines, vitamins, and herbal supplements.

Taking Oxtellar XR™ with certain other medicines may cause side effects or affect how well they work. Do not start or stop other medicines without talking to your healthcare provider.

Especially tell your healthcare provider if you take: carbamazepine, phenobarbital, phenytoin, or birth control medicine.

Ask your healthcare provider or pharmacist for a list of these medicines, if you are not sure.

Know the medicines you take. Keep a list of them and show it to your healthcare provider and pharmacist when you get a new medicine.

How should I take Oxtellar XR™?

Do not stop taking Oxtellar XR™ without talking to your healthcare provider. Stopping Oxtellar XR™ suddenly can cause serious problems, including seizures that will not stop (status epilepticus).Take Oxtellar XR™ exactly as prescribed. Your healthcare provider may change your dose. Your healthcare provider will tell you how much Oxtellar XR™ to take.

Take Oxtellar XR™ 1 time each day.

Take Oxtellar XR™ on an empty stomach. This means you should take Oxtellar XR™ at least 1 hour before or at least 2 hours after a meal. Take Oxtellar XR™ tablets whole with water or other liquid.

Do not cut, crush, or chew the tablets before swallowing.

If you take too much Oxtellar XR™ call your healthcare provider or call the poison control center at 1-800-222-1222.

Take Oxtellar XR™ at the same time each day.

Talk with your healthcare provider about what you should do if you miss a dose.

What should I avoid while taking Oxtellar XR™?
- Do not drive, operate heavy machinery, or do other dangerous activities until you know how Oxtellar XR™ affects you. Oxtellar XR™ may slow your thinking and motor skills.
- Do not drink alcohol or take other drugs that make you sleepy or dizzy while taking Oxtellar XR™ until you talk to your healthcare provider. Oxtellar XR™ taken with alcohol or drugs that cause sleepiness or dizziness may make your sleepiness or dizziness worse.

What are the possible side effects of Oxtellar XR™?

See **"What is the most important information I should know about Oxtellar XR™?"**

Oxtellar XR™ may cause other serious side effects including:
- your seizures can happen more often or become worse
- trouble concentrating
- problems with your speech and language
- feeling confused
- feeling sleepy and tired
- trouble walking and with coordination

Get medical help right away if you have any of the symptoms listed above or listed in "What is the most important information I should know about Oxtellar XR™?"

The most common side effects of Oxtellar XR™ include:
- dizziness
- sleepiness
- headache
- problems with walking and coordination (unsteadiness)
- shakiness
- nausea
- vomiting
- double vision
- weakness
- tiredness

These are not all the possible side effects of Oxtellar XR™. For more information, ask your healthcare provider or pharmacist.

Tell your healthcare provider if you have any side effect that bothers you or does not go away.

Call your doctor for medical advice about side effects. You may report side effects to FDA at 1-800-FDA-1088.

How should I store Oxtellar XR™?
- Store Oxtellar XR™ at room temperature 68°F to 77°F (20°C and 25°C)
- Keep Oxtellar XR™ in a tightly closed container, and keep Oxtellar XR™ out of the light.
- Keep Oxtellar XR™ tablets dry.

Keep Oxtellar XR™ and all medicines out of the reach of children.

General Information about the safe and effective use of Oxtellar XR™

Medicines are sometimes prescribed for purposes other than those listed in a Medication Guide. Do not use Oxtellar XR™ for a condition for which it was not prescribed. Do not give Oxtellar XR™ to other people, even if they have the same symptoms that you have. It may harm them.

This Medication Guide summarizes the most important information about Oxtellar XR™. If you would like more information, talk with your healthcare provider. You can ask your pharmacist or healthcare provider for the full prescribing information about Oxtellar XR™ that is written for health professionals.

For more information, go to www.supernus.com or call 1-866-398-0833.

What are the ingredients in Oxtellar XR™?

Active ingredient: oxcarbazepine

Inactive ingredients:

150 mg tablets: colloidal silicon dioxide, hypromellose, yellow iron oxide, magnesium stearate, methacrylic acid copolymer, microcrystalline cellulose, polyethylene glycol, polyvinyl alcohol, povidone, sodium lauryl sulfate, talc, and titanium dioxide.

300 mg tablets: colloidal silicon dioxide, hypromellose, yellow iron oxide, red iron oxide, black iron oxide, magnesium stearate, methacrylic acid copolymer, microcrystalline cellulose, polyethylene glycol, polyvinyl alcohol, povidone, sodium lauryl sulfate, talc, and titanium dioxide.

600 mg tablets: red iron oxide, magnesium stearate, methacrylic acid copolymer, microcrystalline cellulose, polyethylene glycol, polyvinyl alcohol, povidone, sodium lauryl sulfate, talc, and titanium dioxide.

This Medication Guide has been approved by the U.S. Food and Drug Administration.

Distributed by:
Supernus Pharmaceuticals, Inc.

Issued October 2012.

Shown in Product Identification Guide, page 313

TROKENDI XR ℞
(topiramate)
extended-release capsules for oral use

HIGHLIGHTS OF PRESCRIBING INFORMATION

These highlights do not include all the information needed to use TROKENDI XR safely and effectively. See full prescribing information for TROKENDI XR.

Trokendi XR (topiramate) extended-release capsules for oral use

Initial U.S. Approval: 1996

INDICATIONS AND USAGE

Trokendi XR™ is an antiepileptic drug indicated for:
- Partial Onset Seizure and Primary Generalized Tonic-Clonic Seizures - initial monotherapy in patients 10 years of age and older with partial onset or primary generalized tonic-clonic seizures and adjunctive therapy in patients 6 years of age and older with partial onset or primary generalized tonic-clonic seizures (1.1)
- Lennox-Gastaut Syndrome (LGS) - adjunctive therapy in patients 6 years of age and older with seizures associated with Lennox-Gastaut syndrome (1.2)

DOSAGE AND ADMINISTRATION

[See table below]

Swallow capsule whole and intact. Do not sprinkle on food, chew or crush (2.9)

DOSAGE FORMS AND STRENGTHS

- Extended-release capsules: 25 mg, 50 mg, 100 mg, and 200 mg (3)

CONTRAINDICATIONS

- With recent alcohol use (i.e., within 6 hours prior to and 6 hours after Trokendi XR use [(4), (5.4)]
- In patients with metabolic acidosis taking concomitant metformin [(4), (5.3)]

WARNINGS AND PRECAUTIONS

- *Acute myopia and secondary angle closure glaucoma:* Untreated elevated intraocular pressure can lead to permanent visual loss. Discontinue Trokendi XR™ if it occurs (5.1)
- *Oligohydrosis and hyperthermia:* Monitor decreased sweating and increased body temperature, especially in pediatric patients (5.2)
- *Metabolic acidosis:* Measure baseline and periodic measurement of serum bicarbonate. Consider dose reduction or discontinuation of Trokendi XR™ if clinically appropriate (5.3)
- *Suicidal behavior and ideation:* Antiepileptic drugs increase the risk of suicidal behavior or ideation (5.5)
- *Cognitive/neuropsychiatric:* Trokendi XR™ may cause cognitive dysfunction. Use caution when operating machinery including automobiles. Depression and mood problems may occur (5.6)
- *Fetal toxicity:* Topiramate use during pregnancy can cause cleft lip and/or palate (5.7)
- *Withdrawal of AEDs:* Withdrawal of Trokendi XR™ should be done gradually (5.8)
- *Hyperammonemia and encephalopathy:* Patients with inborn errors of metabolism or reduced mitochondrial activity may have an increased risk of hyper-ammonemia. Measure ammonia if encephalopathic symptoms occur (5.9)
- *Kidney stones:* Avoid use with other carbonic anhydrase inhibitors, other drugs causing metabolic acidosis, or in patients on a ketogenic diet (5.10)
- *Hypothermia:* Reported with concomitant valproic acid use (5.11)

ADVERSE REACTIONS

The most common (greater than 5% more frequent than placebo or low-dose topiramate in monotherapy) adverse reactions were paresthesia, anorexia, weight decrease, fatigue, dizziness, somnolence, nervousness, psychomotor slowing, difficulty with memory, difficulty with concentration/attention, cognitive problem, confusion, mood problems, fever, infection, and flushing (6.1)

To report SUSPECTED ADVERSE REACTIONS, contact Supernus Pharmaceuticals at 1-866-398-0833- or FDA at 1-800-FDA-1088 or www.fda.gov/medwatch.

DRUG INTERACTIONS

- *Oral contraceptives:* Decreased contraceptive efficacy and increased breakthrough bleeding, especially at doses greater than 200 mg per day (7.2)
- *Phenytoin or carbamazepine:* Concomitant administration with topiramate decreased plasma concentrations of topiramate (7.3)
- *Other carbonic anhydrase inhibitors:* Monitor for the appearance or worsening of metabolic acidosis (7.5)

	Initial Dose	Titration	Recommended Dose
Monotherapy Therapy: Partial Onset or Primary Generalized Tonic-Clonic Seizures			
Adults and pediatric patients 10 years and older (2.1)	50 mg orally once daily	Increase dose weekly by increments of 50 mg for first 4 weeks then 100 mg for weeks 5 to 6	400 mg once daily
Adjunctive Therapy			
Adults with partial onset seizures or LGS (2.2)	25 mg to 50 mg orally once daily	Increase dose weekly by increments of 25 mg to 50 mg to achieve an effective dose	200 mg to 400 mg once daily
Adults with primary generalized tonic-clonic seizures (2.2)	25 mg to 50 mg orally once daily	Increase dose weekly to an effective dose by increments of 25 mg to 50 mg	400 mg once daily
Pediatric patients 6 years and older with partial onset seizures, primary generalized tonic-clonic seizures or LGS (2.2)	25 mg once at night-time (based on a range of 1 mg/kg to 3 mg/kg once daily) for first week	Increase dosage at 1- or 2-week intervals by increments of 1 mg/kg to 3 mg/kg Dose titration should be guided by clinical outcome	5 mg/kg to 9 mg/kg once daily

- *Lithium:* Monitor lithium levels when co-administered with high-dose topiramate (7.7)

USE IN SPECIFIC POPULATIONS

- *Renal Impairment:* (creatinine clearance less than 70 mL/min/1.73m2), one-half of the adult dose is recommended (8.7)
- *Patients undergoing hemodialysis:* Topiramate is cleared by hemodialysis. Dosage adjustment is necessary to avoid rapid drops in topiramate plasma concentration during hemodialysis (8.8)
- *Pregnancy:* Increased risk of cleft lip and/or palate. Pregnancy registry available (8.1)
- *Nursing mothers:* Caution should be exercised when administered to a nursing mother (8.3)
- *Pediatric Use:* Because the capsule must be swallowed whole, and may not be sprinkled on food, crushed or chewed, Trokendi XR™ is recommended only for children ages 6 years and older (8.4)

See 17 for PATIENT COUNSELING INFORMATION and Medication Guide

Revised: 08/2013

FULL PRESCRIBING INFORMATION: CONTENTS*

*** Sections or subsections omitted from the full prescribing information are not listed**

FULL PRESCRIBING INFORMATION

1 INDICATIONS AND USAGE

1.1 Partial Onset Seizure and Primary Generalized Tonic-Clonic Seizures

Trokendi XR™ (topiramate) extended-release capsules are indicated as initial monotherapy in patients 10 years of age and older with partial onset or primary generalized tonic-clonic seizures and adjunctive therapy in patients 6 years of age and older with partial onset or primary generalized tonic-clonic seizures [*see Clinical Studies (14.2, 14.3, 14.4)*]. Safety and effectiveness in patients who were converted to monotherapy from a previous regimen of other anticonvulsant drugs have not been established in controlled trials [*see Clinical Studies (14.2)*].

1.2 Lennox-Gastaut Syndrome

Trokendi XR™ (topiramate) extended-release capsules are indicated as adjunctive therapy in patients 6 years of age and older with seizures associated with Lennox-Gastaut syndrome [*see Clinical Studies (14.5)*].

2 DOSAGE AND ADMINISTRATION

2.1 Monotherapy Use

Adults and Pediatric Patients 10 Years and Older with Partial Onset or Primary Generalized Tonic-Clonic Seizures

The recommended dose for topiramate monotherapy in adults and pediatric patients 10 years of age and older is 400 mg orally once daily. Titrate Trokendi XR™ according to the following schedule:

Week 1	50 mg once daily
Week 2	100 mg once daily
Week 3	150 mg once daily
Week 4	200 mg once daily
Week 5	300 mg once daily
Week 6	400 mg once daily

2.2 Adjunctive Therapy Use

Adults (17 Years of Age and Older) - Partial Onset Seizures, Primary Generalized Tonic-Clonic Seizures, or Lennox-Gastaut Syndrome

The recommended total daily dose of Trokendi XR™ as adjunctive therapy in adults with partial onset seizures or Lennox-Gaustaut Syndrome is 200 mg to 400 mg orally once daily with primary generalized tonic-clonic seizures is 400 mg orally once daily.

Initiate therapy at 25 mg to 50 mg once daily followed by titration to an effective dose in increments of 25 mg to 50mg every week. Daily topiramate doses above 1,600 mg have not been studied.

In the study of primary generalized tonic-clonic seizures using topiramate, the assigned dose was reached at the end of 8 weeks [*see Clinical Studies (14.4)*].

Pediatric Patients (Ages 6 years to 16 Years) - Partial Onset Seizures, Primary Generalized Tonic-Clonic Seizures, or Lennox Gastaut Syndrome

The recommended total daily dose of Trokendi XR™ as adjunctive therapy for pediatric patients with partial onset seizures, primary generalized tonic-clonic seizures, or seizures associated with Lennox-Gastaut syndrome is approximately 5 mg/kg to 9 mg/kg orally once daily. Begin titration at 25 mg once daily (based on a range of 1 mg/kg/day to 3 mg/kg/day) given nightly for the first week. Subsequently, increase the dosage at 1- or 2-week intervals by increments of 1 mg/kg to 3 mg/kg to achieve optimal clinical response. Dose titration should be guided by clinical outcome. If required, longer intervals between dose adjustments can be used.

In the study of primary generalized tonic-clonic seizures, the assigned dose of 6 mg/kg once daily was reached at the end of 8 weeks [*see Clinical Studies (14.4)*].

2.3 Administration with Alcohol

Alcohol use should be completely avoided within 6 hours prior to and 6 hours after Trokendi XR™ administration [see *Warnings and Precautions (5.4)*].

2.4 Dose Modifications in Patients with Renal Impairment

In patients with renal impairment (creatinine clearance less than 70 mL/min/1.73 m^2), one-half of the usual adult dose is recommended. Such patients will require a longer time to reach steady-state at each dose.

Prior to dosing, obtain an estimated GFR measurement in patients at high risk for renal insufficiency (e.g., older patients, or those with diabetes mellitus, hypertension, or autoimmune disease).

2.5 Dosage Modifications in Patients Undergoing Hemodialysis

Topiramate is cleared by hemodialysis at a rate that is 4 to 6 times greater than in patients with normal renal function. Accordingly, a prolonged period of dialysis may cause topiramate concentration to fall below that required to maintain an anti-seizure effect. To avoid rapid drops in topiramate plasma concentration during hemodialysis, a supplemental dose of topiramate may be required. The actual adjustment should take into account the:

- duration of dialysis period
- clearance rate of the dialysis system being used
- effective renal clearance of topiramate in the patient being dialyzed.

2.6 Laboratory Testing Prior to Treatment Initiation

Measurement of baseline and periodic serum bicarbonate during Trokendi XR™ treatment is recommended [*see Warnings and Precautions (5.3)*].

2.7 Dosing Modifications in Patients Taking Phenytoin and/or Carbamazepine

The co-administration of Trokendi XR™ with phenytoin may require an adjustment of the dose of phenytoin to achieve optimal clinical outcome. Addition or withdrawal of phenytoin and/or carbamazepine during adjunctive therapy with Trokendi XR™ may require adjustment of the dose of Trokendi XR™.

2.8 Monitoring for Therapeutic Blood Levels

It is not necessary to monitor topiramate plasma concentrations to optimize Trokendi XR™ therapy.

2.9 Administration Instructions

Trokendi XR™ can be taken without regard to meals. Swallow capsule whole and intact. Do not sprinkle on food, chew or crush.

3 DOSAGE FORMS AND STRENGTHS

Trokendi XR™ (topiramate) extended-release capsules are available in the following strengths and colors:

25 mg: Size 2 capsules, light green opaque body/yellow opaque cap (printed "SPN" on the cap, "25" on the body)

50 mg: Size 0 capsules, light green opaque body/orange opaque cap (printed "SPN" on the cap, "50" on the body)

100 mg: Size 00 capsules, green opaque body/blue opaque cap (printed "SPN" on the cap, "100" on the body)

200 mg: Size 00 capsules, pink opaque body/blue opaque cap (printed "SPN" on the cap, "200" on the body)

4 CONTRAINDICATIONS

Trokendi XR™ is contraindicated in patients:

- With recent alcohol use (i.e., within 6 hours prior to and 6 hours after Trokendi XR™ use) [*see Warnings and Precautions (5. 4)*]
- With metabolic acidosis who are taking concomitant metformin [*see Warnings and Precautions (5.3) and Drug Interactions (7.6)*]

5 WARNINGS AND PRECAUTIONS

5.1 Acute Myopia and Secondary Angle Closure Glaucoma

A syndrome consisting of acute myopia associated with secondary angle closure glaucoma has been reported in patients receiving topiramate. Symptoms include acute onset of decreased visual acuity and/or ocular pain. Ophthalmologic findings can include myopia, anterior chamber shallowing, ocular hyperemia (redness) and increased intraocular pressure. Mydriasis may or may not be present. This syndrome may be associated with supraciliary effusion resulting in anterior displacement of the lens and iris, with secondary angle closure glaucoma. Symptoms typically occur within 1 month of initiating topiramate therapy. In contrast to primary narrow angle glaucoma, which is rare under 40 years of age, secondary angle closure glaucoma associated with topiramate has been reported in pediatric patients as well as adults. The primary treatment to reverse symptoms is discontinuation of Trokendi XR™ as rapidly as possible, according to the judgment of the treating physician. Other measures, in conjunction with discontinuation of Trokendi XR™, may be helpful.

Elevated intraocular pressure of any etiology, if left untreated, can lead to serious sequelae including permanent vision loss.

5.2 Oligohydrosis and Hyperthermia

Oligohydrosis (decreased sweating), resulting in hospitalization in some cases, has been reported in association with topiramate use. Decreased sweating and an elevation in

Table 1: Risk by Indication for Antiepileptic Drugs in the Pooled Analysis

Indication	*Placebo Patients with Events per 1,000 Patients*	*Drug Patients with Events per 1,000 Patients*	*Relative Risk: Incidence of Events in Drug Patients/ Incidence in Placebo Patients*	*Risk Difference: Additional Drug Patients with Events per 1,000 patients*
Epilepsy	1.0	3.4	3.5	2.4
Psychiatric	5.7	8.5	1.5	2.9
Other	1.0	1.8	1.9	0.9
Total	2.4	4.3	1.8	1.9

body temperature above normal characterized these cases. Some of the cases were reported after exposure to elevated environmental temperatures.
The majority of the reports have been in pediatric patients. Patients, especially pediatric patients, treated with Trokendi XR™ should be monitored closely for evidence of decreased sweating and increased body temperature, especially in hot weather. Caution should be used when Trokendi XR™ is prescribed with other drugs that predispose patients to heat-related disorders; these drugs include, but are not limited to, other carbonic anhydrase inhibitors and drugs with anticholinergic activity.

5.3 Metabolic Acidosis

Hyperchloremic, non-anion gap, metabolic acidosis (i.e., decreased serum bicarbonate below the normal reference range in the absence of chronic respiratory alkalosis) is associated with topiramate, and can be expected with treatment with Trokendi XR™. This metabolic acidosis is caused by renal bicarbonate loss due to the inhibitory effect of topiramate on carbonic anhydrase. Such electrolyte imbalance has been observed with the use of topiramate in placebo-controlled clinical trials and in the post-marketing period. Generally, topiramate-induced metabolic acidosis occurs early in treatment although cases can occur at any time during treatment. Bicarbonate decrements are usually mild-moderate (average decrease of 4 mEq/L at daily doses of 400 mg in adults and at approximately 6 mg/kg/day in pediatric patients); rarely, patients can experience severe decrements to values below 10 mEq/L. Conditions or therapies that predispose patients to acidosis (such as renal disease, severe respiratory disorders, status epilepticus, diarrhea, ketogenic diet or specific drugs) may be additive to the bicarbonate lowering effects of topiramate.

Adults

In adults, the incidence of persistent treatment-emergent decreases in serum bicarbonate (levels of less than 20 mEq/L at two consecutive visits or at the final visit) in controlled clinical trials for adjunctive treatment of epilepsy was 32% for 400 mg per day, and 1% for placebo. Metabolic acidosis has been observed at doses as low as 50 mg per day. The incidence of persistent treatment-emergent decreases in serum bicarbonate in adults in the epilepsy controlled clinical trial for monotherapy was 15% for 50 mg per day and 25% for 400 mg per day. The incidence of a markedly abnormally low serum bicarbonate (i.e., absolute value less than 17 mEq/L and greater than 5 mEq/L decrease from pretreatment) in the adjunctive therapy trials was 3% for 400 mg per day, and 0% for placebo and in the monotherapy trial was 1% for 50 mg per day and 7% for 400 mg per day. Serum bicarbonate levels have not been systematically evaluated at daily doses greater than 400 mg per day.

Pediatric Patients (2 years to 16 years of age)

Although Trokendi XR™ is not approved for use in patients below the age of 6, the incidence of persistent treatment-emergent decreases in serum bicarbonate in placebo-controlled trials for adjunctive treatment of Lennox-Gastaut syndrome or refractory partial onset seizures in patients age 2 years to 16 years was 67% for topiramate (at approximately 6 mg/kg/day), and 10% for placebo. The incidence of a markedly abnormally low serum bicarbonate (i.e., absolute value less than17 mEq/L and greater than 5 mEq/L decrease from pretreatment) in these trials was 11% for topiramate and 0% for placebo. Cases of moderately severe metabolic acidosis have been reported in patients as young as 5 months old, especially at daily doses above 5 mg/kg/day.
In pediatric patients (6 years to 15 years of age), the incidence of persistent treatment-emergent decreases in serum bicarbonate in the epilepsy controlled clinical trial for monotherapy performed with topiramate was 9% for 50 mg per day and 25% for 400 mg per day. The incidence of a markedly abnormally low serum bicarbonate (i.e., absolute value less than 17 mEq/L and greater than 5 mEq/L decrease from pretreatment) in this trial was 1% for 50 mg per day and 6% for 400 mg per day.

Pediatric Patients (under 2 years of age)

Although Trokendi XR™ is not approved for use in patients less than 6 years of age with partial onset seizures, a study of topiramate as adjunctive use in patients under 2 years of age revealed that topiramate produced a metabolic acidosis that is notably greater in magnitude than that observed in controlled trials in older children and adults. The mean treatment difference (25 mg/kg/day topiramate-placebo) was -5.9 mEq/L for bicarbonate. The incidence of metabolic acidosis (defined by a serum bicarbonate less than 20 mEq/L) was 0% for placebo, 30% for 5 mg/kg/day, 50% for 15 mg/kg/day, and 45% for 25 mg/kg/day [*see Use in Specific Populations(8.4)*].

Manifestations of Metabolic Acidosis

Some manifestations of acute or chronic metabolic acidosis may include hyperventilation, nonspecific symptoms such as fatigue and anorexia, or more severe sequelae including cardiac arrhythmias or stupor. Chronic, untreated metabolic acidosis may increase the risk for nephrolithiasis or nephrocalcinosis, and may also result in osteomalacia (referred to as rickets in pediatric patients) and/or osteoporosis with an increased risk for fractures. Chronic metabolic acidosis in pediatric patients may also reduce growth rates. A reduction in growth rate may eventually decrease the maximal height achieved. The effect of topiramate on growth and bone-related sequelae has not been systematically investigated in long-term, placebo-controlled trials. Long-term, open-label treatment of infants/toddlers, with intractable partial epilepsy, for up to 1 year, showed reductions from baseline in Z SCORES for length, weight, and head circumference compared to age and sex-matched normative data, although these patients with epilepsy are likely to have different growth rates than normal infants. Reductions in Z SCORES for length and weight were correlated to the degree of acidosis [*see Pediatric Use (8.4)*]. Topiramate treatment that causes metabolic acidosis during pregnancy can possibly produce adverse effects on the fetus and might also cause metabolic acidosis in the neonate from possible transfer of topiramate to the fetus [*see Warnings and Precautions (5.7) and Use in Specific Populations (8.1)*].

Risk Mitigation Strategies

Measurement of baseline and periodic serum bicarbonate during topiramate treatment is recommended. If metabolic acidosis develops and persists, consideration should be given to reducing the dose or discontinuing topiramate (using dose tapering). If the decision is made to continue patients on topiramate in the face of persistent acidosis, alkali treatment should be considered.

5.4 Interaction with Alcohol

In vitro data show that, in the presence of alcohol, the pattern of topiramate release from Trokendi XR™ capsules is significantly altered. As a result, plasma levels of topiramate with Trokendi XR™ may be markedly higher soon after dosing and subtherapeutic later in the day. Therefore, alcohol use should be completely avoided within 6 hours prior to and 6 hours after Trokendi XR™ administration.

5.5 Suicidal Behavior and Ideation

Antiepileptic drugs (AEDs) increase the risk of suicidal thoughts or behavior in patients taking these drugs for any indication. Patients treated with any AED, including Trokendi XR™ for any indication should be monitored for the emergence or worsening of depression, suicidal thoughts or behavior, and/or any unusual changes in mood or behavior.
Pooled analyses of 199 placebo-controlled clinical trials (mono- and adjunctive therapy) of 11 different AEDs showed that patients randomized to one of the AEDs had approximately twice the risk (adjusted Relative Risk 1.8, 95% CI:1.2, 2.7) of suicidal thinking or behavior compared to patients randomized to placebo. In these trials, which had a median treatment duration of 12 weeks, the estimated incidence rate of suicidal behavior or ideation among 27,863 AED-treated patients was 0.43%, compared to 0.24% among 16,029 placebo-treated patients, representing an increase of approximately one case of suicidal thinking or behavior for every 530 patients treated. There were four suicides in drug-treated patients in the trials and none in placebo-treated patients, but the number is too small to allow any conclusion about drug effect on suicide.
The increased risk of suicidal thoughts or behavior with AEDs was observed as early as one week after starting drug treatment with AEDs and persisted for the duration of treatment assessed. Because most trials included in the analysis did not extend beyond 24 weeks, the risk of suicidal thoughts or behavior beyond 24 weeks could not be assessed.
The risk of suicidal thoughts or behavior was generally consistent among drugs in the data analyzed. The finding of increased risk with AEDs of varying mechanisms of action and across a range of indications suggests that the risk applies to all AEDs used for any indication. The risk did not vary substantially by age (5 to 100 years) in the clinical trials analyzed.
Table 1 shows absolute and relative risk by indication for all evaluated AEDs.
[See table 1 above]
The relative risk for suicidal thoughts or behavior was higher in clinical trials for epilepsy than in clinical trials for psychiatric or other conditions, but the absolute risk differences were similar for the epilepsy and psychiatric indications.
Anyone considering prescribing Trokendi XR™ or any other AED must balance the risk of suicidal thoughts or behavior with the risk of untreated illness. Epilepsy and many other illnesses for which AEDs are prescribed are themselves associated with morbidity and mortality and an increased risk of suicidal thoughts and behavior. Should suicidal thoughts and behavior emerge during treatment, the prescriber needs to consider whether the emergence of these symptoms in any given patient may be related to the illness being treated.
Patients, their caregivers, and families should be informed that AEDs increase the risk of suicidal thoughts and behavior and should be advised of the need to be alert for the emergence or worsening of the signs and symptoms of depression, any unusual changes in mood or behavior or the emergence of suicidal thoughts, behavior or thoughts about self-harm. Behaviors of concern should be reported immediately to healthcare providers.

5.6 Cognitive/Neuropsychiatric Adverse Reactions

Adverse reactions most often associated with the use of topiramate, and therefore expected to be associated with the use of Trokendi XR™ were related to the central nervous system and were observed in the epilepsy population. In adults, the most frequent of these can be classified into three general categories: 1) Cognitive-related dysfunction (e.g. confusion, psychomotor slowing, difficulty with concentration/attention, difficulty with memory, speech or language problems, particularly word-finding difficulties), 2) Psychiatric/behavioral disturbances (e.g. depression or mood problems), and 3) Somnolence or fatigue.

Adult Patients

Cognitive Related Dysfunction

The majority of cognitive-related adverse reactions were mild to moderate in severity, and they frequently occurred in isolation. Rapid titration rate and higher initial dose were associated with higher incidences of these reactions. Many of these reactions contributed to withdrawal from treatment [*see Adverse Reactions (6.1)*].
In the adjunctive epilepsy controlled trials conducted with topiramate (using rapid titration such as 100 mg per day to 200mg per day weekly increments), the proportion of patients who experienced one or more cognitive-related adverse reactions was 42% for 200mg per day, 41% for 400mg per day, 52% for 600mg per day, 56% for 800 and 1,000 mg per day, and 14% for placebo. These dose-related adverse reactions began with a similar frequency in the titration or in the maintenance phase, although in some patients the events began during titration and persisted into the maintenance phase. Some patients who experienced one or more cognitive-related adverse reactions in the titration phase had a dose-related recurrence of these reactions in the maintenance phase.
In the monotherapy epilepsy controlled trial conducted with topiramate, the proportion of patients who experienced one or more cognitive-related adverse reactions was 19% for topiramate 50mg per day and 26% for 400mg per day.

Psychiatric/Behavioral Disturbances

Psychiatric/behavioral disturbances (depression or mood) were dose-related for the epilepsy population treated with topiramate [*see Warnings and Precautions (5.6)*].

Somnolence/Fatigue

Somnolence and fatigue were the adverse reactions most frequently reported during clinical trials of topiramate for adjunctive epilepsy. For the adjunctive epilepsy population, the incidence of somnolence did not differ substantially between 200 mg per day and 1,000 mg per day, but the incidence of fatigue was dose-related and increased at dosages above 400 mg per day. For the monotherapy epilepsy population in the 50 mg per day and 400 mg per day groups, the incidence of somnolence was dose-related (9% for the 50 mg per day group and 15% for the 400 mg per day group) and the incidence of fatigue was comparable in both treatment groups (14% each). For other uses not approved for Trokendi XR™, somnolence and fatigue were more common in the titration phase.

Additional nonspecific CNS events commonly observed with topiramate in the adjunctive epilepsy population include dizziness or ataxia.

Pediatric Patients

In double-blind adjunctive therapy and monotherapy epilepsy clinical studies conducted with topiramate, the incidences of cognitive/neuropsychiatric adverse reactions in pediatric patients were generally lower than observed in adults. These reactions included psychomotor slowing, difficulty with concentration/attention, speech disorders/related speech problems and language problems. The most frequently reported neuropsychiatric reactions in pediatric patients during adjunctive therapy double-blind studies were somnolence and fatigue. The most frequently reported neuropsychiatric reactions in pediatric patients in the 50 mg per day and 400 mg per day groups during the monotherapy double-blind study were headache, dizziness, anorexia, and somnolence.

No patients discontinued treatment due to any adverse events in the adjunctive epilepsy double-blind trials. In the monotherapy epilepsy double-blind trial conducted with immediate-release topiramate product, 1 pediatric patient (2%) in the 50 mg per day group and 7 pediatric patients (12%) in the 400 mg per day group discontinued treatment due to any adverse events. The most common adverse reaction associated with discontinuation of therapy was difficulty with concentration/attention; all occurred in the 400 mg per day group.

5.7 Fetal Toxicity

Topiramate can cause fetal harm when administered to a pregnant woman. Data from pregnancy registries indicate that infants exposed to topiramate *in utero* have an increased risk for cleft lip and/or cleft palate (oral clefts). When multiple species of pregnant animals received topiramate at clinically relevant doses, structural malformations, including craniofacial defects, and reduced fetal weights occurred in offspring [*see Use in Specific Populations (8.1)*].

Consider the benefits and risks of topiramate when administering the drug in women of childbearing potential, particularly when topiramate is considered for a condition not usually associated with permanent injury or death [*see Use in Specific Populations (8.9)*]. Topiramate should be used during pregnancy only if the potential benefit outweighs the potential risk. If this drug is used during pregnancy, or if the patient becomes pregnant while taking this drug, the patient should be informed of the potential hazard to a fetus [*see Use in Specific Populations (8.1) and (8.9)*].

5.8 Withdrawal of Antiepileptic Drugs

In patients with or without a history of seizures or epilepsy, antiepileptic drugs including Trokendi XR™ should be gradually withdrawn to minimize the potential for seizures or increased seizure frequency [*see Clinical Studies (14)*]. In situations where rapid withdrawal of Trokendi XR™ is medically required, appropriate monitoring is recommended.

5.9 Hyperammonemia and Encephalopathy

Hyperammonemia/Encephalopathy Without Concomitant Valproic Acid (VPA)

Topiramate treatment has produced hyperammonemia (in some instances dose-related) in clinical investigational programs in very young pediatric patients (1 month to 24 months) who were treated with adjunctive topiramate for partial onset epilepsy (8% for placebo, 10% for 5 mg/kg/day, 0% for 15 mg/kg/day, 9 % for 25 mg/kg/day). Trokendi XR™ is not approved as adjunctive treatment of partial onset seizures in pediatric patients less than 6 years old. In some patients, ammonia was markedly increased (greater than 50 % above upper limit of normal). The hyperammonemia associated with topiramate treatment occurred with and without encephalopathy in placebo-controlled trials, and in an open-label, extension trial. Dose-related hyperammonemia was also observed in the extension trial in pediatric patients up to 2 years old. Clinical symptoms of hyperammonemic encephalopathy often include acute alterations in level of consciousness and/or cognitive function with lethargy or vomiting.

Hyperammonemia with and without encephalopathy has also been observed in post-marketing reports in patients who were taking topiramate without concomitant valproic acid (VPA).

Hyperammonemia/Encephalopathy With Concomitant Valproic Acid (VPA)

Concomitant administration of topiramate and valproic acid (VPA) has been associated with hyperammonemia with or without encephalopathy in patients who have tolerated either drug alone based upon post-marketing reports. Although hyperammonemia may be asymptomatic, clinical symptoms of hyperammonemic encephalopathy often include acute alterations in level of consciousness and/or cognitive function with lethargy or vomiting. In most cases, symptoms and signs abated with discontinuation of either drug. This adverse reaction is not due to a pharmacokinetic interaction.

Although Trokendi XR™ is not indicated for use in infants/toddlers (1month to 24 months), topiramate with concomitant VPA clearly produced a dose-related increase in the incidence of treatment-emergent hyperammonemia (above the upper limit of normal, 0% for placebo, 12% for 5 mg/kg/day, 7% for 15 mg/kg/day, 17% for 25 mg/kg/day) in an investigational program using topiramate. Markedly increased, dose-related hyperammonemia (0% for placebo and 5 mg/kg/day, 7% for 15 mg/kg/day, and 8% for 25 mg/kg/day) also occurred in these infants/toddlers. Dose-related hyperammonemia was similarly observed in a long-term, extension trial utilizing topiramate in these very young, pediatric patients [*see Use in Specific Populations (8.4)*].

Hyperammonemia with and without encephalopathy has also been observed in post-marketing reports in patients taking topiramate with valproic acid (VPA).

The hyperammonemia associated with topiramate treatment appears to be more common when used concomitantly with VPA.

Monitoring for Hyperammonemia

Patients with inborn errors of metabolism or reduced hepatic mitochondrial activity may be at an increased risk for hyperammonemia with or without encephalopathy. Although not studied, topiramate or Trokendi XR™ treatment or an interaction of concomitant topiramate-based product and valproic acid treatment may exacerbate existing defects or unmask deficiencies in susceptible persons.

In patients who develop unexplained lethargy, vomiting, or changes in mental status associated with any topiramate treatment, hyperammonemic encephalopathy should be considered and an ammonia level should be measured.

5.10 Kidney Stones

A total of 32/2086 (1.5%) of adults exposed to topiramate during its adjunctive epilepsy therapy development reported the occurrence of kidney stones, an incidence about 2 to 4 times greater than expected in a similar, untreated population. In the double-blind monotherapy epilepsy study, a total of 4/319 (1.3%) of adults exposed to topiramate reported the occurrence of kidney stones. As in the general population, the incidence of stone formation among topiramate treated patients was higher in men. Kidney stones have also been reported in pediatric patients. During long-term (up to 1 year) topiramate treatment in an open-label extension study of 284 pediatric patients 1 month to 24 months old with epilepsy, 7% developed kidney or bladder stones that were diagnosed clinically or by sonogram. Trokendi XR™ is not approved for pediatric patients less than 6 years old [*see Use in Specific Populations (8.4)*].

Trokendi XR™ would be expected to have the same effect as topiramate on the formation of kidney stones. An explanation for the association of topiramate and kidney stones may lay in the fact that topiramate is a carbonic anhydrase inhibitor. Carbonic anhydrase inhibitors (e.g., zonisamide, acetazolamide or dichlorphenamide) can promote stone formation by reducing urinary citrate excretion and by increasing urinary pH [*see Warnings and Precautions (5.9)*]. The concomitant use of Trokendi XR™ with any other drug producing metabolic acidosis, or potentially in patients on a ketogenic diet may create a physiological environment that increases the risk of kidney stone formation, and should therefore be avoided.

Increased fluid intake increases the urinary output, lowering the concentration of substances involved in stone formation. Hydration is recommended to reduce new stone formation.

5.11 Hypothermia with Concomitant Valproic Acid Use

Hypothermia, defined as an unintentional drop in body core temperature to less than 35°C (95°F) has been reported in association with topiramate use with concomitant valproic acid (VPA) both in the presence and in the absence of hyperammonemia. This adverse reaction in patients using concomitant topiramate and valproate can occur after starting topiramate treatment or after increasing the daily dose of topiramate [*see Drug Interactions (7.5)*]. Consideration should be given to stopping topiramate or valproate in patients who develop hypothermia, which may be manifested by a variety of clinical abnormalities including lethargy, confusion, coma, and significant alterations in other major organ systems such as the cardiovascular and respiratory systems. Clinical management and assessment should include examination of blood ammonia levels.

5.12 Paresthesia

Paresthesia (usually tingling of the extremities), an effect associated with the use of other carbonic anhydrase inhibitors, appears to be a common effect of topiramate. Paresthesia was more frequently reported in the monotherapy epilepsy trials conducted with topiramate than in the adjunctive therapy epilepsy trials conducted with the same product. In the majority of instances, paresthesia did not lead to treatment discontinuation.

5.13 Interaction with Other CNS Depressants

Topiramate is a CNS depressant. Concomitant administration of topiramate with other CNS depressant drugs can result in significant CNS depression. Patients should be watched carefully when Trokendi XR™ is co-administered with other CNS depressant drugs.

6 ADVERSE REACTIONS

The following adverse reactions are discussed in more detail in other sections of the labeling:

- Acute Myopia and Secondary Angle Closure [*see Warnings and Precautions (5.1)*]
- Oligohydrosis and Hyperthermia [*see Warnings and Precautions (5.2)*]
- Metabolic Acidosis [*see Warnings and Precautions (5.3)*]
- Suicidal Behavior and Ideation [*see Warnings and Precautions (5.5)*]
- Cognitive/Neuropsychiatric Adverse Reactions [*see Warnings and Precautions (5.6)*]
- Fetal Toxicity [*see Warnings and Precautions (5.7)*]
- Withdrawal of Antiepileptic Drugs [*see Warnings and Precautions (5.8)*]
- Hyperammonemia and Encephalopathy (Without and With Concomitant Valproic Acid Use [*see Warnings and Precautions (5.9)*]
- Kidney Stones [*see Warnings and Precautions (5.10)*]
- Hypothermia with Concomitant Valproic Acid Use [*see Warnings and Precautions (5.11)*]
- Paresthesia [*see Warnings and Precautions (5.12)*]

The data described in the following sections were obtained using immediate-release topiramate tablets in studies of patients with epilepsy. Trokendi XR™ has not been studied in a randomized, placebo-controlled Phase III clinical study in the epilepsy patient population. However, it is expected that Trokendi XR™ would produce a similar adverse reaction profile as immediate-release topiramate.

6.1 Clinical Trials Experience

Because clinical trials are conducted under widely varying conditions, adverse reaction rates observed in the clinical trials of a drug cannot be directly compared to rates in the clinical trials of another drug and may not reflect the rates observed in clinical practice.

Adverse Reactions Observed in Monotherapy Trial

Adults 17 Years and Older

The adverse reactions in the controlled trial (Study 1) that occurred most commonly in adults in the 400 mg per day group (incidence greater than or equal to 5%) and at a rate higher than the 50 mg per day group were paresthesia, weight decrease, somnolence, anorexia, dizziness, and difficulty with memory (see Table 2) [*see Clinical Studies (14.2)*].

Approximately 21% of the 159 adult patients in the 400 mg per day group who received topiramate as monotherapy in Study 1 discontinued therapy due to adverse reactions. The most common (greater than or equal to 2% more frequent than low-dose 50 mg per day topiramate) adverse reactions causing discontinuation in this trial were difficulty with memory, fatigue, asthenia, insomnia, somnolence and paresthesia.

Pediatric Patients 10 Years to 16 Years of Age

The adverse reactions in the controlled trial (Study 1) that occurred most commonly in children (10 years up to 16 years of age) in the 400 mg per day topiramate group (incidence greater than or equal to 5%) and at a rate higher than in the 50 mg per day group were weight decrease, upper respiratory tract infection, paresthesia, anorexia, diarrhea, and mood problems (see Table 3) [*see Clinical Studies (14.2)*].

Approximately 12% of the 57 pediatric patients in the 400 mg per day group who received topiramate as monotherapy in the controlled clinical trial discontinued therapy due to adverse reactions. The most common (greater than 5%) adverse reactions resulting in discontinuation in this trial were difficulty with concentration/attention.

Table 2: Incidence of Treatment-Emergent Adverse Reaction in the Monotherapy Epilepsy Trial in Adults* Where Incidence Was at Least 2% in the 400 mg/day Immediate-Release Topiramate Group and Greater Than the Rate in the 50 mg/day Immediate-Release Topiramate Group

	Immediate-release topiramate Dosage (mg/day)	
Body System/	**50**	**400**
Adverse Reaction	**(N=160)**	**(N=159)**
Body as a Whole-General Disorders		
Asthenia	4	6
Leg Pain	2	3

Chest Pain	1	2
Central & Peripheral Nervous System Disorders		
Paresthesia	21	40
Dizziness	13	14
Hypoasthesia	4	5
Ataxia	3	4
Hypertonia	0	3
Gastro-intestinal System Disorders		
Diarrhea	5	6
Constipation	1	4
Gastritis	0	3
Dry Mouth	1	3
Gastroesophogeal Reflux	1	2
Liver and Biliary System Disorders		
Gamma-GT Increased	1	3
Metabolic and Nutritional Disorders		
Weight Decrease	6	16
Psychiatric Disorders		
Somnolence	9	15
Anorexia	4	14
Difficulty with Memory NOS	5	10
Insomnia	8	9
Depression	7	9
Difficulty with Concentration/ Attention	7	8
Anxiety	4	6
Pychomotor Slowing	3	5
Mood Problems	2	5
Confusion	3	4
Cognitive Problem NOS	1	4
Libido Decreased	0	3
Reproductive Disorders, Female		
Vaginal Hemorrhage	0	3
Red Blood Cell Disorders		
Anemia	1	2
Resistance Mechanism Disorders		
Infection Viral	6	8
Infection	2	3
Respiratory System Disorders		
Bronchitis	3	4
Rhinitis	2	4
Dyspnea	1	2
Skin and Appendages Disorders		
Rash	1	4
Pruritus	1	4
Acne	2	3
Special Senses Other, Disorders		
Taste Perversion	3	5
Urinary System Disorders		
Cystitis	1	3
Renal Calculus	0	3
Urinary Tract Infection	1	2
Dysuria	0	2
Micturition Frequency	0	2

* Values represent the percentage of patients reporting a given adverse reaction. Patients may have reported more than one adverse reaction during the study and can be included in more than one adverse reaction category

Table 3: Incidence of Treatment-Emergent Adverse Reactions in the Monotherapy Epilepsy Trial in Pediatric Patients (Ages 10 up to 16 Years)* Where Incidence Was at Least 5% in the 400 mg/day Immediate-Release Topiramate Group and Greater than the Rate in the 50mg/day Immediate-Release Topiramate Group

	Immediate-release topiramate Dosage (mg/day)	
Body System/	**50**	**400**
Adverse Reaction	**(N=57)**	**(N=57)**
Body as a Whole-General Disorders		
Fever	0	9
Central & Peripheral Nervous System Disorders		
Paresthesia	2	16
Gastro-Intestinal System Disorders		
Diarrhea	5	11
Metabolic and Nutritional Disorders		
Weight Decrease	7	21
Psychiatric Disorders		
Anorexia	11	14
Mood Problems	2	11
Difficulty with Concentration/ Attention	4	9
Cognitive Problem NOS	0	7
Nervousness	4	5
Resistance Mechanism Disorders		
Infection Viral	4	9
Infection	2	7
Respiratory System Disorders		
Upper Respiratory Tract Infection	16	18
Rhinitis	2	7
Bronchitis	2	7
Sinusitis	2	5
Skin and Appendages Disorders		
Alopecia	2	5

* Values represent the percentage of patients reporting a given adverse event. Patients may have reported more than one adverse event during the study and can be included in more than one adverse event category

Adverse Reactions Observed in Adjunctive Therapy Epilepsy Trials

The most commonly observed adverse reactions associated with the use of topiramate at dosages of 200 to 400 mg per day in controlled trials in adults with partial onset seizures, primary generalized tonic-clonic seizures, or Lennox-Gastaut syndrome that were seen at greater frequency in topiramate-treated patients and did not appear to be dose-related were: somnolence, ataxia, speech disorders and related speech problems, psychomotor slowing, abnormal vision, difficulty with memory, paresthesia and diplopia [see Table 4] [see Clinical Studies (14.3, 14.4, and 14.5)]. The most common dose-related adverse reactions at dosages of 200 mg to 1,000 mg per day were: fatigue, nervousness, difficulty with concentration or attention, confusion, depression, anorexia, language problems, anxiety, mood problems, and weight decrease [*see Table 6*].

Adverse reactions associated with the use of topiramate at dosages of 5 mg/kg/day to 9 mg/kg/day in controlled trials in pediatric patients with partial onset seizures, primary generalized tonic-clonic seizures, or Lennox-Gastaut syndrome that were seen at greater frequency in topiramate-treated patients were: fatigue, somnolence, anorexia, nervousness, difficulty with concentration/attention, difficulty with memory, aggressive reaction, and weight decrease [*see Table 7*].

In controlled clinical trials in adults, 11% of patients receiving topiramate 200 to 400mg per day as adjunctive therapy discontinued due to adverse reactions. This rate appeared to increase at dosages above 400mg per day. Adverse events associated with discontinuing therapy included somnolence, dizziness, anxiety, difficulty with concentration or attention, fatigue, and paresthesia and increased at dosages above 400 mg per day. None of the pediatric patients who received topiramate adjunctive therapy at 5 mg/kg/day to 9 mg/kg/day in controlled clinical trials discontinued due to adverse reactions.

Approximately 28% of the 1757 adults with epilepsy who received topiramate at dosages of 200 mg to 1,600 mg per day in clinical studies discontinued treatment because of adverse reactions; an individual patient could have reported more than one adverse reaction. These adverse reactions were: psychomotor slowing (4.0%), difficulty with memory (3.2%), fatigue (3.2%), confusion (3.1%), somnolence (3.2%), difficulty with concentration/attention (2.9%), anorexia (2.7%), depression (2.6%), dizziness (2.5%), weight decrease (2.5%), nervousness (2.3%), ataxia (2.1%), and paresthesia (2.0%). Approximately 11% of the 310 pediatric patients who received topiramate at dosages up to 30 mg/kg/day discontinued due to adverse reactions. Adverse reactions associated with discontinuing therapy included aggravated convulsions (2.3%), difficulty with concentration/attention (1.6%), language problems (1.3%), personality disorder (1.3%), and somnolence (1.3%).

Incidence in Epilepsy Controlled Clinical Trials – Adjunctive Therapy – Partial Onset Seizures, Primary Generalized Tonic-Clonic Seizures, and Lennox-Gastaut Syndrome

Table 4 lists adverse reactions that occurred in at least 1% of adults treated with 200 to 400 mg per day topiramate in controlled trials that were numerically more common at this dose than in the patients treated with placebo. In general, most patients who experienced adverse reactions during the first eight weeks of these trials no longer experienced them by their last visit. Table 7 lists adverse reactions that occurred in at least 1% of pediatric patients treated with 5 mg/kg to 9 mg/kg topiramate in controlled trials that were numerically more common than in patients treated with placebo.

Other Adverse Reactions Observed During Double-Blind Epilepsy Adjunctive Therapy Trials

Other adverse reactions that occurred in more than 1% of adults treated with 200 mg to 400 mg of topiramate in placebo-controlled epilepsy trials but with equal or greater frequency in the placebo group were headache, injury, anxiety, rash, pain, convulsions aggravated, coughing, fever, diarrhea, vomiting, muscle weakness, insomnia, personality disorder, dysmenorrhea, upper respiratory tract infection, and eye pain.

Table 4: Incidence of Adverse Reactions in Placebo-Controlled, Adjunctive Epilepsy Trials in Adults *,†,‡

	Topiramate Dosage (mg per day)		
Body System/	**Placebo**	**200-400**	**600-1,000**
Adverse Reaction‡	**(N=291)**	**(N=183)**	**(N=414)**
Body as a Whole-General Disorders			
Fatigue	13	15	30
Asthenia	1	6	3
Back pain	4	5	3
Chest pain	3	4	2
Influenza-like symptoms	2	3	4

Leg pain	2	2	4
Hot flushes	1	2	1
Allergy	1	2	3
Edema	1	2	1
Body odor	0	1	0
Rigors	0	1	<1
Central & Peripheral Nervous System Disorders			
Dizziness	15	25	32
Ataxia	7	16	14
Speech disorders/Related speech problems	2	13	11
Paresthesia	4	11	19
Nystagmus	7	10	11
Tremor	6	9	9
Language problems	1	6	10
Coordination abnormal	2	4	4
Hypoaesthesia	1	2	1
Gait abnormal	1	3	2
Muscle contractions involuntary	1	2	2
Stupor	0	2	1
Vertigo	1	1	2
Gastro-intestinal System Disorders			
Nausea	8	10	12
Dyspepsia	6	7	6
Abdominal pain	4	6	7
Constipation	2	4	3
Gastroenteritis	1	2	1
Dry mouth	1	2	4
Gingivitis	<1	1	1
GI disorder	<1	1	0
Hearing and Vestibular Disorders			
Hearing decreased	1	2	1
Metabolic and Nutritional Disorders			
Weight decrease	3	9	13
Musculo-Skeletal System Disorders			
Myalgia	1	2	2
Skeletal pain	0	1	0
Platelet, Bleeding & Clotting Disorders			
Epistaxis	1	2	1
Psychiatric Disorders			
Somnolence	12	29	28
Nervousness	6	16	19
Psychomotor slowing	2	13	21
Difficulty with memory	3	12	14
Anorexia	4	10	12
Confusion	5	11	14
Depression	5	5	13
Difficulty with concentration/attention	2	6	14
Mood problems	2	4	9
Agitation	2	3	3
Aggressive reaction	2	3	3
Emotional liability	1	3	3
Cognitive problems	1	3	3
Libido decreased	1	2	<1
Apathy	1	1	3
Depersonalization	1	1	2
Reproductive Disorders, Female			
Breast pain	2	4	0
Amenorrhea	1	2	2
Menorrhagia	0	2	1
Menstrual disorder	1	2	1
Reproductive Disorders, Male			
Prostatic disorder	<1	2	0
Resistance Mechanism Disorders			
Infection	1	2	1
Infection viral	1	2	<1
Moniliasis	<1	1	0
Respiratory System Disorders			
Pharyngitis	2	6	3
Rhinitis	6	7	6
Sinusitis	4	5	6
Dyspnea	1	1	2
Skin and Appendages Disorders			
Skin disorder	<1	2	1
Sweating increased	<1	1	<1
Rash, erythematous	<1	1	<1
Special Senses Other, Disorders			
Taste perversion	0	2	4
Urinary System Disorders			
Hematuria	1	2	<1
Urinary tract infection	1	2	3
Micturition frequency	1	1	2
Urinary incontinence	<1	2	1
Urine abnormal	0	1	<1
Vision Disorders			
Vision abnormal	2	13	10
Diplopia	5	10	10
White Cell and RES Disorders			
Leukopenia	1	2	1

* Patients in these adjunctive trials were receiving 1 to 2 concomitant antiepileptic drugs in addition to topiramate or placebo

† Values represent the percentage of patients reporting a given reaction. Patient may have reported more than one adverse reaction during the study and can be included in more than one adverse reaction category.

‡ Adverse reactions reported by at least 1% of patients in the topiramate 200 mg to 400 mg per day group and more common than in the placebo group

Adverse Reactions Observed in Adjunctive Therapy Trial in Adults with Partial Onset Seizures (Study 7)

Study 7 was a randomized, double-blind, adjunctive, placebo-controlled, parallel group study with 3 treatment arms: 1) placebo; 2) topiramate 200 mg per day with a 25 mg per day starting dose, increased by 25 mg per day each week for 8 weeks until the 200 mg per day maintenance dose was reached; and 3) topiramate 200 mg per day with a 50 mg per day starting dose, increased by 50 mg per day each week for 4 weeks until the 200 mg per day maintenance dose was reached. All patients were maintained on concomitant carbamazepine with or without another concomitant antiepileptic drug.

The incidence of adverse reactions (Table 5) did not differ significantly between the 2 topiramate regimens. Because the frequencies of adverse reactions reported in this study were markedly lower than those reported in the previous epilepsy studies, they cannot be directly compared with data obtained in other studies.

Table 5: Incidence of Adverse Reactions in Study 7*,†,‡

		Topiramate Dosage (mg per day)
Body System/	**Placebo**	**200**
Adverse Reaction‡	**(N=92)**	**(N=171)**
Body as a Whole-General Disorders		
Fatigue	4	9
Chest pain	1	2
Cardiovasular Disorders, General		
Hypertension	0	2
Central & Peripheral Nervous System Disorders		
Paresthesia	2	9
Dizziness	4	7
Tremor	2	3
Hypoesthesia	0	2
Leg cramps	0	2
Language problems	0	2
Gastro-intestinal System Disorders		
Abdominal pain	3	5
Constipation	0	4
Diarrhea	1	2
Dyspepsia	0	2
Dry mouth	0	2
Hearing and Vestibular Disorders		
Tinnitus	0	2
Metabolic and Nutritional Disorders		
Weight decrease	4	8
Psychiatric Disorders		
Somnolence	9	15
Anorexia	7	9
Nervousness	2	9
Difficulty with concentration/ attention	0	5
Insomnia	3	4
Difficulty with memory	1	2
Aggressive reaction	0	2
Respiratory System Disorders		
Rhinitis	0	4

Urinary System Disorders		
Cystitis	0	2
Vision Disorder		
Diplopia	0	2
Vision abnormal	0	2

* Patients in these adjunctive trials were receiving 1 to 2 concomitant antiepileptic drugs in addition to topiramate or placebo
† Values represent the percentage of patients reporting a given adverse reaction. Patients may have reported more than one adverse reaction during the study and can be included in more than one adverse reaction category
‡ Adverse reactions reported by at least 2% of patients in the topiramate 200 mg per day group and more common than in the placebo group

[See table 6 above]

Table 7: Incidence (%) of Adverse Reaction in Placebo-Controlled, Adjunctive Epilepsy Trial in Pediatric Patients (Ages 2 Years to 16 Years)*,†,‡ (Study 8)

Body System/ Adverse Reaction	Placebo (N=101)	Topiramate (N=98)
Body as a Whole-General Disorders		
Fatigue	5	16
Injury	13	14
Allergic reaction	1	2
Back pain	0	1
Pallor	0	1
Cardiovascular Disorders, General		
Hypertension	0	1
Central & Peripheral Nervous System Disorders		
Gait abnormal	5	8
Ataxia	2	6
Hyperkinesia	4	5
Dizziness	2	4
Speech disorders/Related speech problems	2	4
Hyporeflexia	0	2
Convulsions grand mal	0	1
Fecal incontinence	0	1
Paresthesia	0	1
Gastro-Intestinal System Disorders		
Nausea	5	6
Saliva increased	4	6
Constipation	4	5
Gastroenteritis	2	3
Dysphagia	0	1
Flatulence	0	1
Gastroesophageal reflux	0	1
Glossitis	0	1
Gum hyperplasia	0	1
Heart Rate and Rhythm Disorders		
Bradycardia	0	1
Metabolic and Nutritional Disorders		
Weight decrease	1	9
Thirst	1	2
Hypoglycemia	0	1
Weight increase	0	1
Platelet, Bleeding & Clotting Disorders		
Purpura	4	8
Epistaxis	1	4
Hematoma	0	1
Prothrombin increased	0	1
Thrombocytopenia	0	1
Psychiatric Disorders		
Somnolence	16	26
Anorexia	15	24
Nervousness	7	14
Personality disorder (Behavior Problems)	9	11
Difficulty with concentration/ attention	2	10
Aggressive reaction	4	9
Insomnia	7	8
Difficulty with memory	0	5
Confusion	3	4
Psychomotor slowing	2	3
Appetite increased	0	1
Neurosis	0	1
Reproductive Disorders, Female		
Leukorrhea	0	2
Resistance Mechanism Disorders		
Infection viral	3	7
Respiratory System Disorders		
Pneumonia	1	5
Respiratory disorder	0	1
Skin and Appendages Disorders		
Skin Disorder	2	3
Alopecia	1	2
Dermatitis	0	2
Hypertrichosis	1	2
Rash erythematous	0	2
Eczema	0	1
Seborrhea	0	1
Skin discoloration	0	1
Urinary System Disorders		
Urinary incontinence	2	4
Nocturia	0	1
Vision Disorders		
Eye abnormality	1	2
Vision abnormal	1	2
Diplopia	0	1
Lacrimation abnormal	0	1
Myopia	0	1
White Cell and RES Disorders		
Leukopenia	0	2

* Patients in these adjunctive trials were receiving 1 to 2 concomitant antiepileptic drugs in addition to topiramate or placebo
† Values represent the percentage of patients reporting a given adverse reaction. Patients may have reported more than one adverse reaction during the study and can be included in more than one adverse reaction category
‡ Reactions that Occurred in at Least 1% of Topiramate-Treated Patients and Occurred More Frequently in Topiramate-Treated Than Placebo-Treated Patients

Table 6: Incidence (%) of Dose-Related Adverse Reactions From Placebo-Controlled, Adjunctive Trials in Adults With Partial Onset Seizures (Studies 2 through 7)*

Adverse Reaction	Placebo (N=216)	(Topiramate) Dosage (mg per day) 200 (N=45)	400 (N=68)	600-1,000 (N=414)
Fatigue	13	11	12	30
Nervousness	7	13	18	19
Difficulty with concentration/attention	1	7	9	14
Confusion	4	9	10	14
Depression	6	9	7	13
Anorexia	4	4	6	12
Language Problems	<1	2	9	10
Anxiety	6	2	3	10
Mood Problems	2	0	6	9
Weight Decrease	3	4	9	13

* Dose-response studies were not conducted for other adult indications or for pediatric indications

Laboratory Abnormalities

Topiramate decreases serum bicarbonate *[see Warnings and Precautions (5.3)]*

Immediate-release topiramate treatment was associated with changes in several clinical laboratory analytes in randomized, double-blind, placebo-controlled studies. Similar effects should be anticipated with use of Trokendi XR™. Controlled trials of adjunctive topiramate treatment of adults for partial onset seizures showed an increased incidence of markedly decreased serum phosphorus (6% topiramate, 2% placebo), markedly increased serum alkaline phosphatase (3% topiramate, 1% placebo), and decreased serum potassium (0.4 % topiramate, 0.1 % placebo). The clinical significance of these abnormalities has not been clearly established.

Changes in several clinical laboratory results (increased creatinine, BUN, alkaline phosphatase, total protein, total eosinophil count and decreased potassium) have been observed in a clinical investigational program in very young (2 years and younger) pediatric patients who were treated with adjunctive topiramate for partial onset seizures [*see Use in Specific Populations (8.4)*].

Topiramate treatment produced a dose-related increased shift in serum creatinine from normal at baseline to an increased value at the end of 4 months treatment in adolescent patients (ages 12 years to 16 years) in a double-blind, placebo-controlled study. The incidence of these abnormal shifts was 4% for placebo, 4% for 50 mg, and 18% for 100 mg.

Topiramate treatment with or without concomitant valproic acid (VPA) can cause hyperammonemia with or without encephalopathy [*see Warnings and Precautions (5.9)*].

6.2 Postmarketing Experience

The following adverse reactions have been identified during post-approval use of topiramate. Because these reactions are reported voluntarily from a population of uncertain size, it is not always possible to reliably estimate their frequency or establish a causal relationship to drug exposure. The listing is alphabetized: bullous skin reactions (including erythema multiforme, Stevens-Johnson syndrome, toxic epidermal necrolysis), hepatic failure (including fatalities), hepatitis, maculopathy, pancreatitis, and pemphigus.

7 DRUG INTERACTIONS

7.1 Alcohol

Alcohol use is contraindicated within 6 hours prior to and 6 hours after Trokendi XR™ administration *[see Contraindications (4) and Warnings and Precautions (5.4)]*.

7.2 Oral Contraceptives

Exposure to ethinyl estradiol was statistically significantly decreased when topiramate (at doses above 200 mg) was given as adjunctive therapy in patients taking valproic acid. However, norethindrone exposure was not significantly affected.

In another pharmacokinetic interaction study in healthy volunteers with a concomitantly administered combination oral contraceptive product containing 1 mg norethindrone (NET) plus 35 mcg ethinyl estradiol (EE), topiramate, given in the absence of other medications at doses of 50 to 200 mg per day, was not associated with statistically significant changes in mean exposure to either component of the oral contraceptive.

The possibility of decreased contraceptive efficacy and increased breakthrough bleeding should be considered in patients taking combination oral contraceptive products with Trokendi XR™. Patients taking estrogen-containing contraceptives should be asked to report any change in their bleeding patterns. Contraceptive efficacy can be decreased even in the absence of breakthrough bleeding [*see Clinical Pharmacology (12.3)*].

7.3 Antiepileptic Drugs

Concomitant administration of phenytoin or carbamazepine with topiramate decreased plasma concentrations of topiramate [*see Clinical Pharmacology (12.3)*].

Concomitant administration of valproic acid and topiramate has been associated with hyperammonemia with and without encephalopathy. Concomitant administration of topiramate with valproic acid has also been associated with hypothermia (with and without hyperammonemia) in patients who have tolerated either drug alone. It may be prudent to examine blood ammonia levels in patients in whom the onset of hypothermia has been reported [*see Warnings and Precautions (5.8), (5.10)and Clinical Pharmacology (12.3)*].

Numerous AEDs are substrates of the CYP enzyme system. *In vitro* studies indicate that topiramate does not inhibit enzyme activity for CYP1A2, CYP2A6, CYP2B6, CYP2C9, CYP2D6, CYP2E1, and CYP3A4/5 isozymes. *In vitro* studies indicate that immediate-release topiramate is a mild inhibitor of CYP2C19 and a mild inducer of CYP3A4. The same drug interactions can be expected with the use of Trokendi XR™.

7.4 CNS Depressants

Topiramate is a CNS depressant. Concomitant administration of topiramate with other CNS depressant drugs or alcohol can result in significant CNS depression [*see Warnings and Precautions (5.13)*].

7.5 Other Carbonic Anhydrase Inhibitors

Concomitant use of topiramate, a carbonic anhydrase inhibitor, with any other carbonic anhydrase inhibitor (e.g., zonisamide, acetazolamide or dichlorphenamide), may increase the severity of metabolic acidosis and may also increase the risk of kidney stone formation. Patient should be monitored for the appearance or worsening of metabolic acidosis when Trokendi XR™ is given concomitantly with another carbonic anhydrase inhibitor [*see Clinical Pharmacology (12.3)*].

7.6 Metformin

Topiramate treatment can frequently cause metabolic acidosis, a condition for which the use of metformin is contraindicated. The concomitant use of Trokendi XR™ and metformin is contraindicated in patients with metabolic acidosis. [*see Clinical Pharmacology (12.3)*].

7.7 Lithium

In patients, there was an observed increase in systemic exposure of lithium following topiramate doses of up to 600 mg per day. Lithium levels should be monitored when co-administered with high-dose Trokendi XR™ [*see Clinical Pharmacology (12.3)*].

8 USE IN SPECIFIC POPULATIONS

8.1 Pregnancy

Pregnancy Category D [*see Warnings and Precautions (5.7)*]

Topiramate can cause fetal harm when administered to a pregnant woman. Data from pregnancy registries indicate that infants exposed to topiramate *in utero* have increased risk for cleft lip and/or cleft palate (oral clefts). When multiple species of pregnant animals received topiramate at clinically relevant doses, structural malformations, including craniofacial defects, and reduced fetal weights occurred in offspring. Topiramate should be used during pregnancy only if the potential benefit outweighs the potential risk. If this drug is used during pregnancy, or if the patient becomes pregnant while taking this drug, the patient should be informed of the potential hazard to the fetus [*see Use in Specific Populations (8.9)*].

<u>Pregnancy Registry</u>

Patients should be encouraged to enroll in the North American Antiepileptic Drug (NAAED) Pregnancy Registry if they become pregnant. This registry is collecting information about the safety of antiepileptic drugs during pregnancy. To enroll, patients can call the toll-free number 1-888-233-2334. Information about the North American Drug Pregnancy Registry can be found at *http://www.massgeneral.org/aed/*.

<u>Human Data</u>

Data from the NAAED Pregnancy Registry indicate an increased risk of oral clefts in infants exposed to topiramate monotherapy during the first trimester of pregnancy. The prevalence of oral clefts was 1.2% compared to a prevalence of 0.39% - 0.46% in infants exposed to other AEDs, and a prevalence of 0.12% in infants of mothers without epilepsy or treatment with other AEDs. For comparison, the Centers for Disease Control and Prevention (CDC) reviewed available data on oral clefts in the United States and found a similar background rate of 0.17%. The relative risk of oral clefts in topiramate-exposed pregnancies in the NAAED Pregnancy Registry was 9.6 (95% Confidence Interval=CI 3.6-25.7) as compared to the risk in a background population of untreated women. The UK Epilepsy and Pregnancy Register reported a similarly increased prevalence of oral clefts of 3.2% among infants exposed to topiramate monotherapy. The observed rate of oral clefts was 16 times higher than the background rate in the UK, which is approximately 0.2%.

Topiramate treatment can cause metabolic acidosis (*see Warnings and Precautions (5.3)*]. The effect of topiramate-induced metabolic acidosis has not been studied in pregnancy; however, metabolic acidosis in pregnancy (due to other causes) can cause decreased fetal growth, decreased fetal oxygenation, and fetal death, and may affect the fetus' ability to tolerate labor. Pregnant patients should be monitored for metabolic acidosis and treated as in the nonpregnant state [*see Warnings and Precautions (5.3)*]. Newborns of mothers treated with topiramate should be monitored for metabolic acidosis because of transfer of topiramate to the fetus and possible occurrence of transient metabolic acidosis following birth.

<u>Animal Data</u>

Topiramate has demonstrated selective developmental toxicity, including teratogenicity, in multiple animal species at clinically relevant doses. When oral doses of 20 mg/kg, 100 mg/kg, or 500 mg/kg were administered to pregnant mice during the period of organogenesis, the incidence of fetal malformations (primarily craniofacial defects) was increased at all doses. The low dose is approximately 0.2 times the recommended human dose (RHD) 400mg per day on a mg/m^2 basis. Fetal body weights and skeletal ossification were reduced at 500 mg/kg in conjunction with decreased maternal body weight gain.

In rat studies (oral doses of 20 mg/kg, 100 mg/kg, and 500 mg/kg or 0.2 mg/kg, 2.5 mg/kg, 30 mg/kg, and 400 mg/kg), the frequency of limb malformations (ectrodactyly, micromelia, and amelia) was increased among the offspring of dams treated with 400 mg/kg (10 times the RHD on a mg/m^2 basis) or greater during the organogenesis period of pregnancy. Embryotoxicity (reduced fetal body weights, increased incidence of structural variations) was observed at doses as low as 20 mg/kg (0.5 times the RHD on a mg/m^2 basis). Clinical signs of maternal toxicity were seen at 400 mg/kg and above, and maternal body weight gain was reduced during treatment with 100 mg/kg or greater.

In rabbit studies (20 mg/kg, 60 mg/kg, and 180 mg/kg or 10 mg/kg, 35 mg/kg, and 120 mg/kg orally during organogenesis), embryo/fetal mortality was increased at 35 mg/kg (2 times the RHD on a mg/m^2 basis) or greater, and teratogenic effects (primarily rib and vertebral malformations) were observed at 120 mg/kg (6 times the RHD on a mg/m^2 basis). Evidence of maternal toxicity (decreased body weight gain, clinical signs, and/or mortality) was seen at 35 mg/kg and above.

When female rats were treated during the latter part of gestation and throughout lactation (0.2 mg/kg, 4 mg/kg, 20 mg/kg, and 100 mg/kg or 2, 20, and 200 mg/kg), offspring exhibited decreased viability and delayed physical development at 200 mg/kg (5 times the RHD on a mg/m^2 basis) and reductions in pre-and/or postweaning body weight gain at 2mg/kg (0.05 times the RHD on a mg/m^2 basis) and above. Maternal toxicity (decreased body weight gain, clinical signs) was evident at 100 mg/kg or greater.

In a rat embryo/fetal development study with a postnatal component (0.2 mg/kg, 2.5 mg/kg, 30 mg/kg, or 400mg/kg during organogenesis; noted above), pups exhibited delayed physical development at 400 mg/kg (10 times the RHD on a mg/m^2 basis) and persistent reductions in body weight gain at 30 mg/kg (1 times the RHD on a mg/m^2 basis) and higher.

8.2 Labor and Delivery

Although the effect of topiramate on labor and delivery in humans has not been established, the development of topiramate-induced metabolic acidosis in the mother and/or in the fetus might affect the fetus' ability to tolerate labor [*see Use in Specific Populations (8.1)*].

8.3 Nursing Mothers

Limited data on 5 breastfeeding infants exposed to topiramate showed infant plasma topiramate levels equal to 10-20% of the maternal plasma level. The effects of this exposure on infants are unknown. Caution should be exercised when Trokendi XR™ is administered to a nursing woman.

8.4 Pediatric Use

<u>*Seizures in Pediatric Patients 6 Years of Age and Older*</u>

Because the capsule must be swallowed whole, and may not be sprinkled on food, crushed or chewed, Trokendi XR™ is recommended only for children age 6 or older.

The safety and effectiveness of Trokendi XR™ in pediatric patients is based on controlled trials with immediate-release topiramate *[see Clinical Studies (14)]*.

The adverse reactions (both common and serious) in pediatric patients are similar to those seen in adults *[see Warnings and Precautions (5) and Adverse Reactions (6)]*.

These include, but are not limited to:

- oligohydrosis and hyperthermia *[see Warnings and Precautions (5.2)]*.
- dose-related increased incidence of metabolic acidosis *[see Warnings and Precautions (5.3)]*.
- dose-related increased incidence of hyperammonemia *[see Warnings and Precautions (5.9)]*.

<u>*Adjunctive Treatment for Partial Onset Epilepsy in Infants and Toddlers (1 to 24 months)*</u>

The following pediatric use information is based on studies conducted with immediate-release topiramate.

Safety and effectiveness in patients below the age of 2 years have not been established for the adjunctive therapy treatment of partial onset seizures, primary generalized tonic-clonic seizures, or seizures associated with Lennox-Gastaut syndrome. In a single randomized, double-blind, placebo-controlled investigational trial, the efficacy, safety, and tolerability of immediate-release topiramate oral liquid and sprinkle formulations as an adjunct to concurrent antiepileptic drug therapy in infants 1 to 24 months of age with refractory partial onset seizures, was assessed. After 20 days of double-blind treatment, immediate-release topiramate (at fixed doses of 5 mg/kg, 15 mg/kg, and 25 mg/kg per day) did not demonstrate efficacy compared with placebo in controlling seizures.

In general, the adverse reaction profile in this population was similar to that of older pediatric patients, although results from the above controlled study, and an open-label, long-term extension study in these infants/toddlers (1 to 24 months old) suggested some adverse reactions not previously observed in older pediatric patients and adults; i.e., growth/length retardation, certain clinical laboratory abnormalities, and other adverse reactions that occurred with a greater frequency and/or greater severity than had been recognized previously from studies in older pediatric patients or adults for various indications.

These very young pediatric patients appeared to experience an increased risk for infections (any topiramate dose 12%, placebo 0%) and of respiratory disorders (any topiramate dose 40%, placebo 16%). The following adverse reactions were observed in at least 3% of patients on immediate-release topiramate and were 3% to 7% more frequent than in patients on placebo: viral infection, bronchitis, pharyngitis, rhinitis, otitis media, upper respiratory infection, cough, and bronchospasm. A generally similar profile was observed in older children [*see Adverse Reactions (6)*].

Immediate-release topiramate resulted in an increased incidence of patients with increased creatinine (any topiramate dose 5%, placebo 0%), BUN (any topiramate dose 3%, placebo 0%), and protein (any topiramate dose 34%, placebo 6%), and an increased incidence of decreased potassium (any topiramate dose 7%, placebo 0%). This increased frequency of abnormal values was not dose related. Creatinine was the only analyte showing a noteworthy increased incidence (topiramate 25 mg/kg/day 5%, placebo 0%) of a markedly abnormal increase [*see Adverse Reactions (6.1)*]. The significance of these findings is uncertain.

Immediate-release topiramate treatment also produced a dose-related increase in the percentage of patients who had a shift from normal at baseline to high/increased (above the normal reference range) in total eosinophil count at the end of treatment. The incidence of these abnormal shifts was 6 % for placebo, 10% for 5 mg/kg/day, 9% for 15 mg/kg/day, 14% for 25 mg/kg/day, and 11% for any topiramate dose [*see Adverse Reactions (6.1)*]. There was a mean dose-related increase in alkaline phosphatase. The significance of these findings is uncertain.

Treatment with immediate-release topiramate for up to 1 year was associated with reductions in Z SCORES for length, weight, and head circumference [*see Warnings and Precautions (5.3) and Adverse Reactions (6)*].

In open-label, uncontrolled experience, increasing impairment of adaptive behavior was documented in behavioral testing over time in this population. There was a suggestion that this effect was dose-related. However, because of the absence of an appropriate control group, it is not known if this decrement in function was treatment related or reflects the patient's underlying disease (e.g., patients who received higher doses may have more severe underlying disease) [*see Warnings and Precautions (5.6)*].

In this open-label, uncontrolled study, the mortality was 37 deaths/1000 patient years. It is not possible to know whether this mortality rate is related to immediate-release topiramate treatment, because the background mortality rate for a similar, significantly refractory, young pediatric population (1month to 24 months) with partial epilepsy is not known.

Other Pediatric Studies

Topiramate treatment produced a dose-related increased shift in serum creatinine from normal at baseline to an increased value at the end of 4 months treatment in adolescent patients (ages 12 years to 16 years) in a double-blind, placebo-controlled study [*see Adverse Reactions (6.1)*].

Juvenile Animal Studies

When topiramate (30 mg/kg/day, 90 mg/kg/day or 300 mg/kg/day) was administered orally to rats during the juvenile period of development (postnatal days 12 to 50), bone growth plate thickness was reduced in males at the highest dose, which is approximately 5 to 8 times the maximum recommended pediatric dose (9 mg/kg/day) on a body surface area (mg/m^2) basis.

8.5 Geriatric Use

Clinical studies of immediate-release topiramate did not include sufficient numbers of subjects aged 65 and over to determine whether they respond differently than younger subjects. Dosage adjustment is necessary for elderly with creatinine clearance less than 70 mL/min/1.73 m^2. Estimate GFR should be measured prior to dosing [*see Dosage and Administration (2) and Clinical Pharmacology (12.3)*].

8.6 Race and Gender Effects

Evaluation of effectiveness and safety of topiramate in clinical trials has shown no race- or gender-related effects.

8.7 Renal Impairment

The clearance of topiramate was reduced by 42% in moderately renally impaired (creatinine clearance 30 to 69 mL/min/1.73m^2) and by 54% in severely renally impaired subjects (creatinine clearance less than 30 mL/min/1.73m^2) compared to normal renal function subjects (creatinine clearance greater than70 mL/min/1.73m^2). One-half the usual starting and maintenance dose is recommended in patients with moderate or severe renal impairment [*see Dosage and Administration (2.4) and Clinical Pharmacology (12.3)*].

8.8 Patients Undergoing Hemodialysis

Topiramate is cleared by hemodialysis at a rate that is 4 to 6 times greater than a normal individual. Accordingly, a prolonged period of dialysis may cause topiramate concentration to fall below that required to maintain an anti-seizure effect. To avoid rapid drops in topiramate plasma concentration during hemodialysis, a supplemental dose of topiramate may be required. The actual adjustment should take into account the duration of dialysis period, the clearance rate of the dialysis system being used, and the effective renal clearance of topiramate in the patient being dialyzed [*see Dosage and Administration (2.5) and Clinical Pharmacology (12.3)*].

8.9 Women of Childbearing Potential

Data from pregnancy registries indicate that infants exposed to topiramate *in utero* have an increased risk for cleft lip and/or cleft palate (oral clefts) [*see Warnings and Precautions (5.7) and Use in Specific Populations (8.1)*]. Consider the benefits and risks of topiramate when prescribing this drug to women of childbearing potential, particularly when topiramate is considered for a condition not usually associated with permanent injury or death. Because of the risk of oral clefts to the fetus, which occur in the first trimester of pregnancy before many women know they are pregnant, all women of childbearing potential should be apprised of the potential hazard to the fetus from exposure to topiramate. If the decision is made to use topiramate, women who are not planning a pregnancy would use effective contraception [*see Drug Interactions (7.2)*] Women who are planning a pregnancy would be counseled regarding the relative risks and benefits of topiramate use during pregnancy, and alternative therapeutic options should be considered for these patients.

9 DRUG ABUSE AND DEPENDENCE

9.1 Controlled Substance

Trokendi XR™ (topiramate) extended-release capsule is not a controlled substance.

9.2 Abuse

The abuse and dependence potential of Trokendi XR™ has not been evaluated in human studies.

9.3 Dependence

Trokendi XR™ has not been systematically studied in animals or humans for its potential for tolerance or physical dependence.

10 OVERDOSAGE

Overdoses of topiramate resulted in signs and symptoms which included convulsions, drowsiness, speech disturbance, blurred vision, diplopia, mentation impaired, lethargy, abnormal coordination, stupor, hypotension, abdominal pain, agitation, dizziness and depression. The clinical consequences were not severe in most cases, but deaths have been reported after polydrug overdoses involving topiramate.

Topiramate overdose has resulted in severe metabolic acidosis [*see Warnings and Precautions (5.3)*].

A patient who ingested a dose between 96 g and 110 g of topiramate was admitted to hospital with coma lasting 20 to 24 hours followed by full recovery after 3 to 4 days.

Similar signs, symptoms, and clinical consequences are expected to occur with overdosage of Trokendi XR™. Therefore, in acute Trokendi XR™ overdose, if the ingestion is recent, the stomach should be emptied immediately by lavage or by induction of emesis. Activated charcoal has been shown to adsorb topiramate *in vitro*. Treatment should be appropriately supportive. Hemodialysis is an effective means of removing topiramate from the body.

11 DESCRIPTION

Topiramate, USP, is a sulfamate-substituted monosaccharide. Trokendi XR™ (topiramate) extended-release capsules are available as 25 mg, 50 mg, 100 mg and 200 mg capsules for oral administration.

Topiramate is a white to off-white powder. Topiramate is freely soluble in polar organic solvents such as acetonitrile and acetone; and very slightly soluble to practically insoluble in non-polar organic solvents such as hexanes. Topiramate has the molecular formula $C_{12}H_{21}NO_8S$ and a molecular weight of 339.4. Topiramate is designated chemically as 2,3:4,5-Di-*O*-isopropylidene-β-D-fructopyranose sulfamate and has the following structural formula:

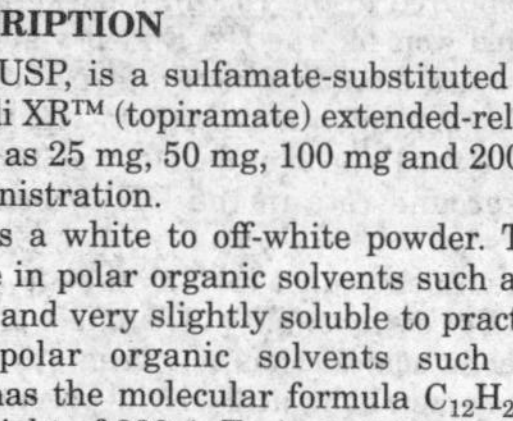

Trokendi XR™ (topiramate) is an extended-release capsule. Trokendi XR™ capsules contain the following inactive ingredients:

Sugar Spheres, NF
Hypromellose (Type 2910), USP
Mannitol, USP
Docusate Sodium, USP
Sodium Benzoate, NF
Ethylcellulose, NF
Oleic Acid, NF
Medium Chain Triglycerides, NF
Polyethylene Glycol, NF
Polyvinyl Alcohol, USP
Titanium Dioxide, USP
Talc, USP
Lecithin, NF
Xanthan Gum, NF

The capsule shells contain gelatin, USP; Titanium Dioxide, USP; and Colorants.

The colorants are:
FD&C Blue #1 (all strength capsules)
Yellow Iron Oxide, USP (25 mg and 50 mg capsules)
FD&C Red #3 (50 mg, 100 mg and 200 mg capsules)
FD&C Yellow #6 (50 mg, 100 mg and 200 mg capsules)
Riboflavin, USP (25 mg capsules)

All capsule shells are imprinted with black print that contains shellac, NF, and black iron oxide, NF.

12 CLINICAL PHARMACOLOGY

12.1 Mechanism of Action

The precise mechanisms by which topiramate exerts its anticonvulsant effects are unknown; however, preclinical studies have revealed four properties that may contribute to topiramate's efficacy for epilepsy. Electrophysiological and biochemical evidence suggests that topiramate, at pharmacologically relevant concentrations, blocks voltage-dependent sodium channels, augments the activity of the neurotransmitter gamma-aminobutyrate at some subtypes of the GABA-A receptor, antagonizes the AMPA/kainate subtype of the glutamate receptor, and inhibits the carbonic anhydrase enzyme, particularly isozymes II and IV.

12.2 Pharmacodynamics

Topiramate has anticonvulsant activity in rat and mouse maximal electroshock seizure (MES) tests. Topiramate is only weakly effective in blocking clonic seizures induced by the GABAA receptor antagonist, pentylenetetrazole. Topiramate is also effective in rodent models of epilepsy, which include tonic and absence-like seizures in the spontaneous epileptic rat (SER) and tonic and clonic seizures induced in rats by kindling of the amygdala or by global ischemia.

12.3 Pharmacokinetics

Absorption and Distribution

Linear pharmacokinetics of topiramate from Trokendi XR™ were observed following a single oral dose over the range of 50 mg to 200 mg. At 25 mg, the pharmacokinetics of Trokendi XR™ is nonlinear possibly due to the binding of topiramate to carbonic anhydrase in red blood cells.

The peak plasma concentrations (Cmax) of topiramate occurred at approximately 24 hours following a single 200 mg oral dose of Trokendi XR™. At steady-state, the ($AUC_{0\text{-}24hr}$, C_{max}, and C_{min}) of topiramate from Trokendi XR™ administered once-daily and the immediate-release tablet administered twice-daily were shown to be bioequivalent. Fluctuation of topiramate plasma concentrations at steady-state for Trokendi XR™ administered once-daily was approximately 26% and 42% in healthy subjects and in epileptic patients, respectively, compared to approximately 40% and 51%, respectively, for immediate-release topiramate [see *Clinical Pharmacology (12.6)*].

Compared to the fasted state, high-fat meal increased the C_{max} of topiramate by 37% and shortened the T_{max} to approximately 8 hour following a single dose of Trokendi XR™, while having no effect on the AUC. Modeling of the observed single dose fed data with simulation to steady state showed that the effect on C_{max} is significantly reduced following repeat administrations. Trokendi XR™ can be taken without regard to meals.

Topiramate is 15% to 41% bound to human plasma proteins over the blood concentration range of 0.5 mcg/mL to 250 mcg/mL. The fraction bound decreased as blood concentration increased.

Carbamazepine and phenytoin do not alter the binding of immediate-release topiramate. Sodium valproate, at 500 mcg/mL (a concentration 5 to 10 times higher than considered therapeutic for valproate) decreased the protein binding of immediate-release topiramate from 23% to 13%. Immediate-release topiramate does not influence the binding of sodium valproate.

Metabolism and Excretion

Topiramate is not extensively metabolized and is primarily eliminated unchanged in the urine (approximately 70% of an administered dose). Six metabolites have been identified in humans, none of which constitutes more than 5% of an administered dose. The metabolites are formed via hydroxylation, hydrolysis, and glucuronidation. There is evidence of renal tubular reabsorption of topiramate. In rats, given probenecid to inhibit tubular reabsorption, along with topiramate, a significant increase in renal clearance of topiramate was observed. This interaction has not been evaluated in humans. Overall, oral plasma clearance (CL/F) is approximately 20 mL/min to 30 mL/min in adults following oral administration. The mean elimination half-life of topiramate was approximately 31 hours following repeat administration of Trokendi XR™.

Specific Populations

Renal Impairment

The clearance of topiramate was reduced by 42% in moderately renally impaired (creatinine clearance 30 to 69 mL/min/1.73m^2) and by 54% in severely renally impaired subjects (creatinine clearance less than 30 mL/min/1.73m^2) compared to normal renal function subjects (creatinine clearance greater than70 mL/min/1.73m^2). Since topiramate is presumed to undergo significant tubular reabsorption, it is uncertain whether this experience can be generalized to all situations of renal impairment. It is conceivable that some forms of renal disease could differentially affect glomerular filtration rate and tubular reabsorption resulting in a clearance of topiramate not predicted by creatinine clearance. In general, however, use of one-half the usual starting and maintenance dose is recommended in patients with creatinine clearance less than 70 mL/min/1.73 m^2 [*see Dosage and Administration (2.3), (2.4)*].

Hemodialysis

Topiramate is cleared by hemodialysis. Using a high-efficiency, counterflow, single pass-dialysate hemodialysis procedure, topiramate dialysis clearance was 120 mL/min with blood flow through the dialyzer at 400 mL/min. This high clearance (compared to 20 mL/min to 30 mL/min total oral clearance in healthy adults) will remove a clinically significant amount of topiramate from the patient over the hemodialysis treatment period. Therefore, a supplemental dose may be required [*see Dosage and Administration (2.5)*].

Hepatic Impairment

In hepatically impaired subjects, the clearance of topiramate may be decreased; the mechanism underlying the decrease is not well understood.

Age, Gender and Race

The pharmacokinetics of topiramate in elderly subjects (65 to 85 years of age, N=16) were evaluated in a controlled clinical study. The elderly subject population had reduced renal function (creatinine clearance [-20%]) compared to young adults. Following a single oral 100 mg dose, maximum plasma concentration for elderly and young adults was achieved at approximately 1 to 2 hours. Reflecting the primary renal elimination of topiramate, topiramate plasma and renal clearance were reduced 21% and 19%, respectively, in elderly subjects, compared to young adults. Similarly, topiramate half-life was longer (13%) in the elderly. Reduced topiramate clearance resulted in slightly higher maximum plasma concentration (23%) and AUC (25%) in elderly subjects than observed in young adults. Topiramate clearance is decreased in the elderly only to the extent that renal function is reduced.

In a study of 13 healthy elderly subjects and 18 healthy young adults who received Trokendi XR™, 30% higher mean C_{max} and 44% higher AUC values were observed in elderly compared to young subjects. Elderly subjects exhibited shorter median T_{max} at 16 hours versus 24 hours in young subjects. The apparent elimination half-life was similar across age groups. As recommended for all patients, dosage adjustment is indicated in elderly patients with a creatinine clearance rate less than 70 mL/min/1.73 m^2) [*see Dosage and Administration (2.4)*].

Clearance of topiramate in adults was not affected by gender or race.

Pediatric Pharmacokinetics

Pharmacokinetics of immediate-release topiramate were evaluated in patients ages 2 years to less than 16 years. Patients received either no or a combination of other antiepileptic drugs. A population pharmacokinetic model was developed on the basis of pharmacokinetic data from relevant topiramate clinical studies. This dataset contained data from 1217 subjects including 258 pediatric patients aged 2 years to less than 16 years (95 pediatric patients less than 10 years of age). Pediatric patients on adjunctive treatment exhibited a higher oral clearance (L/h) of topiramate compared to patients on monotherapy, presumably because of increased clearance from concomitant enzyme-inducing antiepileptic drugs. In comparison, topiramate clearance per kg is greater in pediatric patients than in adults and in young pediatric patients (down to 2 years) than in older pediatric patients. Consequently, the plasma drug concentration for the same mg/kg/day dose would be lower in pediatric patients compared to adults and also in younger pediatric patients compared to older pediatric patients. Clearance was independent of dose.

As in adults, hepatic enzyme-inducing antiepileptic drugs decrease the steady state plasma concentrations of topiramate.

Drug-Drug Interaction Studies

Antiepileptic Drugs

Potential interactions between immediate-release topiramate and standard AEDs were assessed in controlled clinical pharmacokinetic studies in patients with epilepsy. The effects of these interactions on mean plasma AUCs are summarized in Table 8. Interaction of Trokendi XR™ and standard AEDs is not expected to differ from the experience with immediate-release topiramate products.

In Table 8, the second column (AED concentration) describes what happened to the concentration of the AED listed in the first column when topiramate was added. The third column (topiramate concentration) describes how the co-administration of a drug listed in the first column modified the concentration of topiramate in experimental settings when topiramate was given alone.

Table 8: Summary of AED Interactions with topiramate

AED Coadministered	AED Concentration	Topiramate Concentration
Phenytoin	NC or 25% increase*	48% decrease
Carbamazapine (CBZ)	NC	40% decrease
CBZ epoxide†	NC	NE
Valproic acid	11% decrease	14% decrease
Phenobarbital	NC	NE
Primidone	NC	NE
Lamotrigine	NC at TPM doses up to 400mg per day	13% decrease

NC=Less than 10% change in plasma concentration
AED=Antiepileptic drug
NE=Not evaluated
TPM=topiramate
* =Plasma concentration increased 25% in some patients, generally those on a twice a day dosing regimen of phenytoin
† =Is not administered but is an active metabolite of carbamazepine

In addition to the pharmacokinetic interaction described in the above table, concomitant administration of valproic acid and topiramate has been associated with hyperammonemia with and without encephalopathy and hypothermia [*see Warnings and Precautions (5.9), (5.11) and Drug Interactions (7.5)*].

CNS Depressants or Alcohol

Concomitant administration of Trokendi XR™ and other CNS depressant drugs or alcohol has not been evaluated in clinical studies. [*see Contraindications (4), Warnings and Precautions (5.4), (5.13), and Drug Interactions (7.1),(7.4)*].

Oral Contraceptives

In a pharmacokinetic interaction study in healthy volunteers with a concomitantly administered combination oral contraceptive product containing 1 mg norethindrone (NET) plus 35 mcg ethinyl estradiol (EE), topiramate, given in the absence of other medications at doses of 50 to 200 mg per day, was not associated with statistically significant changes in mean exposure (AUC) to either component of the oral contraceptive. In another study, exposure to EE was statistically significantly decreased at doses of 200, 400, and 800 mg per day (18%, 21%, and 30%, respectively) when given as adjunctive therapy in patients taking valproic acid. In both studies, topiramate (50 mg per day to 800 mg per day) did not significantly affect exposure to NET. Although there was a dose-dependent decrease in EE exposure for doses between 200 to 800 mg per day, there was no significant dose-dependent change in EE exposure for doses of 50 to 200 mg per day. The clinical significance of the changes observed is not known. The possibility of decreased contraceptive efficacy and increased breakthrough bleeding should be considered in patients taking combination oral contraceptive products with Trokendi XR™. Patients taking estrogen-containing contraceptives should be asked to report any change in their bleeding patterns. Contraceptive efficacy can be decreased even in the absence of breakthrough bleeding [*see Drug Interactions (7.2)*].

Digoxin

In a single-dose study, serum digoxin AUC was decreased by 12% with concomitant topiramate administration. The clinical relevance of this observation has not been established.

Hydrochlorothiazide

A drug-drug interaction study conducted in healthy volunteers evaluated the steady-state pharmacokinetics of hydrochlorothiazide (HCTZ) (25 mg every 24 hours) and topiramate (96 mg every 12 hours) when administered alone and concomitantly. The results of this study indicate that topiramate C_{max} increased by 27% and AUC increased by 29% when HCTZ was added to topiramate. The clinical significance of this change is unknown. The addition of HCTZ to Trokendi XR™ therapy may require an adjustment of the Trokendi XR™ dose. The steady-state pharmacokinetics of HCTZ were not significantly influenced by the concomitant administration of topiramate. Clinical laboratory results indicated decreases in serum potassium after topiramate or HCTZ administration, which were greater when HCTZ and topiramate were administered in combination.

Metformin

Topiramate treatment can frequently cause metabolic acidosis, a condition for which the use of metformin is contraindicated. Trokendi XR™ is expected to exhibit the same degree of metabolic acidosis as topiramate.

A drug-drug interaction study conducted in healthy volunteers evaluated the steady-state pharmacokinetics of metformin (500 mg every 12 hr) and topiramate in plasma when metformin was given alone and when metformin and topiramate (100 mg every 12 hr) were given simultaneously. The results of this study indicated that the mean metformin C_{max} and AUC_{0-12h} increased by 17% and 25%, respectively, when topiramate was added. Topiramate did not affect metformin tmax. The clinical significance of the effect of topiramate on metformin pharmacokinctics is not known. Oral plasma clearance of topiramate appears to be reduced when administered with metformin. The clinical significance of the effect of metformin on topiramate or Trokendi XR™ pharmacokinetics is unclear. [*see Drug Interactions (7.6)*].

Pioglitazone

A drug-drug interaction study conducted in healthy volunteers evaluated the steady-state pharmacokinetics of topiramate and pioglitazone when administered alone and concomitantly. A 15% decrease in the $AUC_{\tau,ss}$ of pioglitazone with no alteration in $C_{max,ss}$ was observed. This finding was not statistically significant. In addition, a 13% and 16% decrease in $C_{max,ss}$ and $AUC_{\tau,ss}$ respectively, of the active hydroxy-metabolite was noted as well as a 60% decrease in $C_{max,ss}$ and $AUC_{\tau,ss}$ of the active keto-metabolite. The clinical significance of these findings is not known.

When Trokendi XR™ is added to pioglitazone therapy or pioglitazone is added to Trokendi XR™ therapy, careful attention should be given to the routine monitoring of patients for adequate control of their diabetic disease state.

Glyburide

A drug-drug interaction study conducted in patients with type 2 diabetes evaluated the steady-state pharmacokinetics of glyburide (5mg per day) alone and concomitantly with topiramate (150 mg per day). There was a 22% decrease in C_{max} and 25% reduction in AUC_{24} for glyburide during topiramate administration. Systemic exposure (AUC) of the active metabolites, 4-*trans*-hydroxy glyburide (M1) and 3-*cis*-hydroxyglyburide (M2), was also reduced by 13% and 15%, reduced C_{max} by 18% and 25%, respectively. The steady-state pharmacokinetics of topiramate were unaffected by concomitant administration of glyburide.

Lithium

In patients, the pharmacokinetics of lithium were unaffected during treatment with topiramate at doses of 200 mg per day; however, there was an observed increase in systemic exposure of lithium (27% for C_{max} and 26% for AUC) following topiramate doses up to 600 mg per day. Lithium levels should be monitored when co-administered with high-dose Trokendi XR™ [*see Drug Interactions (7.7)*].

Haloperidol

The pharmacokinetics of a single dose of haloperidol (5 mg) were not affected following multiple dosing of topiramate (100 mg every 12 hr) in 13 healthy adults (6 males, 7 females).

Amitriptyline

There was a 12% increase in AUC and C_{max} for amitriptyline (25 mg per day) in 18 normal subjects (9 males, 9 females) receiving 200 mg per day of topiramate. Some subjects may experience a large increase in amitriptyline concentration in the presence of Trokendi XR™ and any adjustments in amitriptyline dose should be made according to the patient's clinical response and not on the basis of plasma levels.

Sumatriptan

Multiple dosing of topiramate (100 mg every 12 hrs) in 24 healthy volunteers (14 males, 10 females) did not affect the pharmacokinetics of single-dose sumatriptan either orally (100 mg) or subcutaneously (6 mg).

Risperidone

When administered concomitantly with topiramate at escalating doses of 100, 250, and 400 mg per day, there was a reduction in risperidone systemic exposure (16% and 33% for steady-state AUC at the 250 and 400 mg per day doses of topiramate). No alterations of 9-hydroxyrisperidone levels were observed. Coadministration of topiramate 400 mg per day with risperidone resulted in a 14% increase in C_{max} and a 12% increase in AUC_{12} of topiramate. There were no clinically significant changes in the systemic exposure of risperidone plus 9-hydroxyrisperidone or of topiramate; therefore, this interaction is not likely to be of clinical significance.

Propranolol

Multiple dosing of topiramate (200 mg per day) in 34 healthy volunteers (17 males, 17 females) did not affect the pharmacokinetics of propranolol following daily 160 mg doses. Propranolol doses of 160 mg per day in 39 volunteers (27 males, 12 females) had no effect on the exposure to topiramate at a dose of 200 mg per day of topiramate.

Dihydroergotamine

Multiple dosing of topiramate (200 mg per day) in 24 healthy volunteers (12 males, 12 females) did not affect the pharmacokinetics of a 1 mg subcutaneous dose of dihydro-

Table 9: Immediate Release Topiramate Dose Summary During the Stabilization Periods of Each of Six Double-Blind, Placebo-Controlled, Adjunctive Trials in Adults with Partial Onset Seizures*

		Target Topiramate Dosage (mg per day)					
Study	**Stabilization Dose**	**Placebo†**	**200**	**400**	**600**	**800**	**1,000**
2	N	42	42	40	41	--	--
	Mean Dose	5.9	200	390	556	--	--
	Median Dose	6.0	200	400	600	--	--
3	N	44	--	--	40	45	40
	Mean Dose	9.7	--	--	544	739	796
	Median Dose	10.0	--	--	600	800	1,000
4	N	23	--	19	--	--	--
	Mean Dose	3.8	--	395	--	--	--
	Median Dose	4.0	--	400	--	--	--
5	N	30	--	--	28	--	--
	Mean Dose	5.7	--	--	522	--	--
	Median Dose	6.0	--	--	600	--	--
6	N	28	--	--	--	25	--
	Mean Dose	8.0	--	--	--	568	--
	Median Dose	8.0	--	--	--	600	--
7	N	90	157	--	--	--	--
	Mean Dose	8	200	--	--	--	--
	Median Dose	8	200	--	--	--	--

* Dose-response studies were not conducted for other indications or pediatric partial-onset seizures
† Placebo dosages are given as the number of tablets. Placebo target dosages were as follows: Study 4 (4 tablets/day); Studies 2 and 5 (6 tablets/day); Studies 6 and 7 (8 tablets/day); Study 3 (10 tablets/day)

ergotamine. Similarly, a 1 mg subcutaneous dose of dihydroergotamine did not affect the pharmacokinetics of a 200 mg per day dose of topiramate in the same study.

Diltiazem

Co-administration of diltiazem (240 mg Cardizem CD®) with topiramate (150 mg per day) resulted in a 10% decrease in C_{max} and 25% decrease in diltiazem AUC, 27% decrease in C_{max} and 18% decrease in des-acetyl diltiazem AUC, and no effect on N-desmethyl diltiazem. Co-administration of topiramate with diltiazem resulted in a 16% increase in C_{max} and a 19% increase in AUC_{12} of topiramate.

Venlafaxine

Multiple dosing of topiramate (150 mg per day) in healthy volunteers did not affect the pharmacokinetics of venlafaxine or O-desmethyl venlafaxine. Multiple dosing of venlafaxine (150 mg) did not affect the pharmacokinetics of topiramate.

Other Carbonic Anhydrase Inhibitors

Concomitant use of Trokendi XR™, a carbonic anhydrase inhibitor, with any other carbonic anhydrase inhibitor (e.g., zonisamide, acetazolamide, or dichlorphenamide), may increase the severity of metabolic acidosis and may also increase the risk of kidney stone formation. Therefore, if Trokendi XR™ is given concomitantly with another carbonic anhydrase inhibitor, the patient should be monitored for the appearance or worsening of metabolic acidosis [*see Drug Interactions (7.5)*].

Drug/Laboratory Tests Interactions

There are no known interactions of Trokendi XR™ with commonly used laboratory tests.

12.6 Relative Bioavailability of Trokendi XR™ Compared to Immediate-Release Topiramate

Study in Healthy Normal Volunteers

Trokendi XR™ taken once a day provides steady state plasma levels comparable to immediate-release topiramate taken every 12 hours, when administered at the same total 200 mg daily dose. In a crossover study, 33 healthy subjects were titrated to a 200mg dose of either Trokendi XR™ or immediate-release topiramate and were maintained at 200mg per day for 10 days.

The 90% CI for the ratios of AUC_{0-24}, C_{max} and C_{min}, as well as partial AUC (the area under the concentration-time curve from time 0 to time p (post dose) for multiple time points were within the 80 to 125% bioequivalence limits, indicating no clinically significant difference between the two formulations. In addition, the 90% CI for the ratios of topiramate plasma concentration at each of multiple time points over 24 hours for the two formulations were within the 80 to 125% bioequivalence limits, except for the initial time points before 1.5 hour post-dose.

Study in Patients with Epilepsy

In a study in epilepsy patients treated with immediate-release topiramate alone or in combination with either enzyme-inducing or neutral AEDs who were switched to an equivalent daily dose of Trokendi XR™, there was a 10% decrease in AUC_{0-24}, C_{max}, and C_{min} on the first day after the switch in all patients. At steady state, AUC_{0-24} and C_{max} were comparable to immediate-release topiramate in all patients. While patients treated with Trokendi XR™ alone or in combination with neutral AEDs showed comparable C_{min} at steady state, patients treated with enzyme-inducers showed a 10% decrease in C_{min}. This difference is likely not clinically significant and probably due to the small number of patients on enzyme-inducers.

13 NON-CLINICAL TOXICOLOGY

13.1 Carcinogenesis, Mutagenesis, and Impairment of Fertility

Carcinogenesis

An increase in urinary bladder tumors was observed in mice given topiramate (20 mg/kg, 75 mg/kg, and 300 mg/kg) in the diet for 21 months. The elevated bladder tumor incidence, which was statistically significant in males and females receiving 300 mg/kg, was primarily due to the increased occurrence of a smooth muscle tumor considered histomorphologically unique to mice. Plasma exposures in mice receiving 300 mg/kg were approximately 0.5 to 1 times steady-state exposures measured in patients receiving topiramate monotherapy at the recommended human dose (RHD) of 400 mg, and 1.5 to 2 times steady-state topiramate exposures in patients receiving 400 mg of topiramate plus phenytoin. The relevance of this finding to human carcinogenic risk is uncertain.

No evidence of carcinogenicity was seen in rats following oral administration of topiramate for 2 years at doses up to 120 mg/kg (approximately 3 times the RHD on a mg/m² basis).

Mutagenesis

Topiramate did not demonstrate genotoxic potential when tested in a battery of *in vitro* and *in vivo* assays. Topiramate was not mutagenic in the Ames test or the *in vitro* mouse lymphoma assay; it did not increase unscheduled DNA synthesis in rat hepatocytes *in vitro;* and it did not increase chromosomal aberrations in human lymphocytes *in vitro* or in rat bone marrow *in vivo.*

Impairment of Fertility

No adverse effects on male or female fertility were observed in rats at doses up to 100 mg/kg (2.5 times the RHD on a mg/m² basis).

14 CLINICAL STUDIES

14.1 Bridging Study to Demonstrate Pharmacokinetic Equivalence between Extended-Release and Immediate-Release Topiramate Formulations

The basis for approval of the extended-release formulation (Trokendi XR™) included the studies described below using an immediate-release formulation and the demonstration of the pharmacokinetic equivalence of Trokendi XR™ to immediate-release topiramate through the analysis of concentrations and cumulative AUCs at multiple time points [*see Clinical Pharmacology (12.6)*].

The clinical studies described in the following sections were conducted using immediate-release topiramate.

14.2 Monotherapy Treatment in Patients with Partial Onset or Primary Generalized Tonic-Clonic Seizures

Adults and Pediatric Patients 10 Years of Age and Older

The effectiveness of topiramate as initial monotherapy in adults and children 10 years of age and older with partial onset or primary generalized tonic-clonic seizures was established in a multicenter, randomized, double-blind, dose-controlled, parallel-group trial (Study 1).

Study 1 was conducted in 487 patients diagnosed with epilepsy (6 to 83 years of age) who had 1 or 2 well-documented seizures during the 3-month retrospective baseline phase who then entered the study and received topiramate 25 mg per day for 7 days in an open-label fashion. Forty-nine percent of subjects had no prior AED treatment and 17% had a diagnosis of epilepsy for greater than 24 months. Any AED therapy used for temporary or emergency purposes was discontinued prior to randomization. In the double-blind phase, 470 patients were randomized to titrate up to 50 mg per day or 400 mg per day of topiramate. If the target dose could not be achieved, patients were maintained on the maximum tolerated dose. Fifty eight percent of patients achieved the maximal dose of 400 mg per day for greater than 2 weeks, and patients who did not tolerate 150 mg per day were discontinued.

The primary efficacy assessment was a between-group comparison of time to first seizure during the double-blind phase. Comparison of the Kaplan-Meier survival curves of time to first seizure favored the topiramate 400 mg per day group over the topiramate 50 mg per day group (p=0.0002, log rank test; Figure 1). The treatment effects with respect to time to first seizure were consistent across various patient subgroups defined by age, sex, geographic region, baseline body weight, baseline seizure type, time since diagnosis, and baseline AED use.

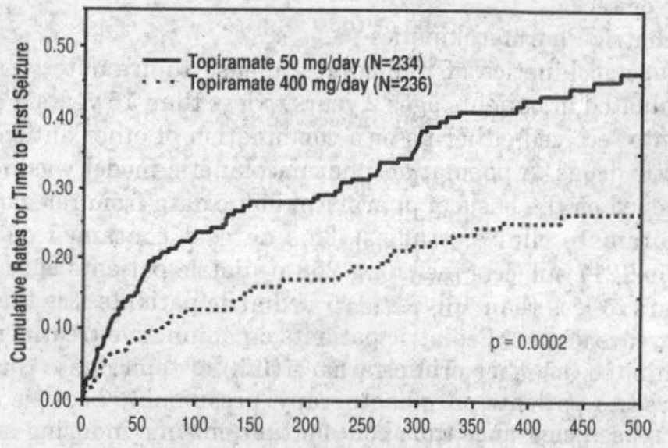

Figure 1: Kaplan-Meier Estimates of Cumulative Rates for Time to First Seizure in Study 1

14.3 Adjunctive Therapy in Patients with Partial Onset Seizures

Adult Patients with Partial Onset Seizures

The effectiveness of topiramate as an adjunctive treatment for adults with partial onset seizures was established in six multicenter, randomized, double-blind, placebo-controlled trials (Studies 2, 3, 4, 5, 6, and 7), two comparing several dosages of topiramate and placebo and four comparing a single dosage with placebo, in patients with a history of partial onset seizures, with or without secondarily generalized seizures.

Patients in these studies were permitted a maximum of two antiepileptic drugs (AEDs) in addition to topiramate tablets or placebo. In each study, patients were stabilized on optimum dosages of their concomitant AEDs during baseline phase lasting between 4 and 12 weeks. Patients who experienced a prespecified minimum number of partial onset seizures, with or without secondary generalization, during the baseline phase (12 seizures for 12-week baseline, 8 for 8-week baseline or 3 for 4-week baseline) were randomly assigned to placebo or a specified dose of topiramate tablets in addition to their other AEDs.

Following randomization, patients began the double-blind phase of treatment. In five of the six studies, patients received active drug beginning at 100 mg per day; the dose was then increased by 100 mg or 200 mg per day increments weekly or every other week until the assigned dose was reached, unless intolerance prevented increases. In Study 7, the 25 or 50 mg per day initial doses of topiramate were followed by respective weekly increments of 25 or 50 mg per day until the target dose of 200 mg per day was reached. After titration, patients entered a 4, 8 or 12-week stabilization period. The numbers of patients randomized to each dose, and the actual mean and median doses in the stabilization period are shown in Table 9.

[See table 9 at top of previous page]

Pediatric Patients Ages 2 to 16 Years with Partial Onset Seizures

The effectiveness of topiramate as an adjunctive treatment for pediatric patients ages 2 to 16 years with partial onset seizures was established in a multicenter, randomized, double-blind, placebo-controlled trial (Study 8), comparing topiramate and placebo in patients with a history of partial onset seizures, with or without secondarily generalized seizures.

Patients in Study 8 were permitted a maximum of two antiepileptic drugs (AEDs) in addition to topiramate tablets or placebo. In Study 8, patients were stabilized on optimum dosages of their concomitant AEDs during an 8-week baseline phase. Patients who experienced at least six partial onset seizures, with or without secondarily generalized seizures, during the baseline phase were randomly assigned to placebo or topiramate in addition to their other AEDs.

Following randomization, patients began the double-blind phase of treatment. Patients received active drug beginning at 25 or 50 mg per day; the dose was then increased by 25 mg to 150 mg per day increments every other week until the assigned dosage of 125, 175, 225 or 400 mg per day based on patients' weight to approximate a dosage of 6 mg/kg/day per day was reached, unless intolerance prevented increases. After titration, patients entered an 8-week stabilization period.

14.4 Adjunctive Therapy in Patients With Primary Generalized Tonic-Clonic Seizures

The effectiveness of topiramate as an adjunctive treatment for primary generalized tonic-clonic seizures in patients 2 years old and older was established in a multicenter, randomized, double-blind, placebo-controlled trial (Study 9), comparing a single dosage of topiramate and placebo.

Patients in Study 9 were permitted a maximum of two antiepileptic drugs (AEDs) in addition to topiramate or placebo. Patients were stabilized on optimum dosages of their concomitant AEDs during an 8-week baseline phase. Patients who experienced at least three primary generalized tonic-clonic seizures during the baseline phase were randomly assigned to placebo or topiramate in addition to their other AEDs.

Following randomization, patients began the double-blind phase of treatment. Patients received active drug beginning at 50 mg per day for four weeks; the dose was then increased by 50 mg to 150 mg per day increments every other week until the assigned dose of 175, 225 or 400 mg per day based on patients' body weight to approximate a dosage of 6 mg/kg/day was reached, unless intolerance prevented increases. After titration, patients entered a 12-week stabilization period.

14.5 Adjunctive Therapy in Patients With Lennox-Gastaut Syndrome

The effectiveness of topiramate as an adjunctive treatment for seizures associated with Lennox-Gastaut syndrome was established in a multicenter, randomized, double-blind, placebo-controlled trial comparing a single dosage of topiramate with placebo in patients 2 years of age and older (Study 10).

Patients in Study 10 were permitted a maximum of two antiepileptic drugs (AEDs) in addition to topiramate or placebo. Patients who were experiencing at least 60 seizures per month before study entry were stabilized on optimum dosages of their concomitant AEDs during a 4 week baseline phase. Following baseline, patients were randomly assigned to placebo or topiramate in addition to their other AEDs. Active drug was titrated beginning at 1 mg/kg/day for a week; the dose was then increased to 3 mg/kg/day for one week then to 6 mg/kg/day. After titration, patients entered an 8-week stabilization period. The primary measures of effectiveness were the percent reduction in drop attacks and a parental global rating of seizure severity.

In all adjunctive topiramate trials, the reduction in seizure rate from baseline during the entire double-blind phase was measured. The median percent reductions in seizure rates and the responder rates (fraction of patients with at least a 50% reduction) by treatment group for each study are shown below in Table 10. As described above, a global improvement in seizure severity was also assessed in the Lennox-Gastaut trial.

[See table 10 above]

Table 10: Efficacy Results in Double-Blind, Placebo-Controlled, Adjunctive Epilepsy Trials

		Target Topiramate Dosage (mg per day)						
Study #	**#**	**Placebo**	**200**	**400**	**600**	**800**	**1,000**	**≈6mg/kg/day***
Partial Onset Seizures Studies in Adults								
2	N	45	45	45	46	--	--	--
	Median % Reduction	11.6	27.2[†]	47.5[‡]	44.7[§]	--	--	--
	% Responders	18	24	44[¶]	46[¶]	--	--	--
3	N	47	--	--	48	48	47	--
	Median % Reduction	1.7	--	--	40.8[§]	41.0[§]	36.0[§]	
	% Responders	9	--	--	40[§]	41[§]	36[¶]	
4	N	24	--	23	--	--	--	--
	Median % Reduction	1.1	--	40.7[#]	--	--	--	--
	% Responders	8	--	35[¶]	--	--	--	--
5	N	30	--	--	30	--	--	--
	Median % Reduction	-12.2	--	--	46.4[Þ]	--	--	--
	% Responders	10	--	--	47[§]	--	--	--
6	N	28	--	--	--	28	--	--
	Median % Reduction	-20.6	--	--	--	24.3[§]	--	--
	% Responders	0	--	--	--	43[§]	--	--
7	N	91	168	--	--	--	--	--
	Median % Reduction	20.0	44.2[§]	--	--	--	--	--
	% Responders	24	45[§]	--	--	--	--	--
Studies in Pediatric Patients								
8	N	45	--	--	--	--	--	41
	Median % Reduction	10.5	--	--	--	--	--	33.1[¶]
	% Responders	20	--	--	--	--	--	39
Primary Generalized Tonic-Clonic[ß]								
9	N	40	--	--	--	--	--	39
	Median % Reduction	9.0	--	--	--	--	--	56.7[¶]
	% Responders	20	--	--	--	--	--	56[§]
Lennox-Gastaut Syndrome[à]								
10	N	49	--	--	--	--	--	46
	Median % Reduction	-5.1	--	--	--	--	--	14.8[¶]
	% Responders	14	--	--	--	--	--	28[è]
	Improvement in Seizure Severity[ð]	28						52[¶]

* For Studies 8 and 9, specified target dosages (less than 9.3 mg/kg/day) were assigned based on subject's weight to approximate a dosage of 6mg/kg per day; these dosages corresponded to mg per day dosages of 125 mg per day, 175 mg per day, 225 mg per day, and 400 mg per day

† Comparisons with placebo: p=0.080;

‡ p ≤ 0.010;

§ p ≤ 0.001;

¶ p ≤ 0.050;

\# p=0.065;

Þ p ≤0.005;

ß Median % reduction and % responders are reported for PGTC seizures;

à Median % reduction and % responders for drop attacks, i.e., tonic or atonic seizures

è p=0.071;

ð Percent of subjects who were minimally, much, or very much improved from baseline.

Subset analyses of the antiepileptic efficacy of topiramate tablets in these studies showed no differences as a function of gender, race, age, baseline seizure rate, or concomitant AED.

In clinical trials for epilepsy, daily dosages were decreased in weekly intervals by 50 mg per day to 100 mg per day in adults and over a 2- to 8-week period in children; transition was permitted to a new antiepileptic regimen when clinically indicated.

16 HOW SUPPLIED/STORAGE AND HANDLING

16.1 Trokendi XR™ Capsules

Trokendi XR™ (topiramate) extended-release capsules are available as extended-release capsules in the following strengths and colors:

Bottles

25 mg (light green opaque body/yellow opaque cap) topiramate extended-release capsules (black print "SPN" and "25") - bottles of 100 count (NDC-17772-101-01)

50 mg (light green opaque body/orange opaque cap) topiramate extended-release capsules (black print "SPN" and "50") - bottles of 100 count (NDC-17772-102-01)
100 mg (green opaque body/blue opaque cap) topiramate extended-release capsules (black print "SPN" and "100") - bottles of 100 count (NDC-17772-103-01)
200 mg (pink opaque body/blue opaque cap) topiramate extended-release capsules (black print "SPN" and "200") - bottles of 100 count (NDC-17772-104-01)

Blister package

25 mg (light green opaque body/yellow opaque cap) topiramate extended-release capsules (black print "SPN" and "25") – blister packages of 30-count (NDC-17772-101-15)
50 mg (light green opaque body/orange opaque cap) topiramate extended-release capsules (black print "SPN" and "50") – blister packages of 30-count (NDC-17772-102-15)
100 mg (green opaque body/blue opaque cap) topiramate extended-release capsules (black print "SPN" and "100") – blister packages of 30-count (NDC-17772-103-15)
200 mg (pink opaque body/blue opaque cap) topiramate extended-release capsules (black print "SPN" and "200") – blister packages of 30-count (NDC-17772-104-15)

16.2 Storage and Handling

Trokendi XR™ (topiramate) extended-release capsules should be stored in well closed containers at controlled room temperature [25°C (77°F); excursions 15°C-30°C (59°F-86°F)]. Protect from moisture and light.

17 PATIENT COUNSELING INFORMATION

See FDA-approved patient labeling (Medication Guide)

Administration Instructions

Counsel patients to swallow Trokendi XR™ capsules whole and intact. Trokendi XR™ should not be sprinkled on food, chewed or crushed. *[See Dosage and Administration (2.9)]*.

Consumption of Alcohol

Advise patients to completely avoid consumption of alcohol at least 6 hours prior to and 6 hours after taking Trokendi XR™*[see Warnings and Precautions (5.4)]*.

Acute Myopia and Secondary Angle Closure Glaucoma

Advise patients taking Trokendi XR™ to seek immediate medical attention if they experience blurred vision, visual disturbances or periorbital pain *[see Warnings and Precautions (5.1)]*.

Oligohydrosis and Hyperthermia

Counsel patients that Trokendi XR™, especially pediatric patients, can cause decreased sweating and increased body temperature, especially in hot weather, and they should seek medical attention if this is noticed *[see Warnings and Precautions (5.2)]*.

Metabolic Acidosis

Inform patients about the potentially significant risk for metabolic acidosis that may be asymptomatic and may be associated with adverse effects on kidneys (e.g., kidney stones, nephrocalcinosis), bones (e.g., osteoporosis, osteomalacia, and/or rickets in children), and growth (e.g., growth delay/retardation) in pediatric patients, and on the fetus *[see Warnings and Precautions (5.3)*

Suicidal Behavior and Ideation

Counsel patients, their caregivers, and families that AEDs, including Trokendi XR™, may increase the risk of suicidal thoughts and behavior and they should be advised of the need to be alert for the emergence or worsening of the signs and symptoms of depression, any unusual changes in mood or behavior or the emergence of suicidal thoughts, behavior or thoughts about self-harm. Behaviors of concern should be reported immediately to healthcare providers. *[see Warnings and Precautions (5.5)]*.

Interference with Cognitive and Motor Performance

Warn patients about the potential for somnolence, dizziness, confusion, difficulty concentrating, visual effects and advise them not to drive or operate machinery until they have gained sufficient experience on Trokendi XR™ to gauge whether it adversely affects their mental performance, motor performance, and/or vision. *[see Warnings and Precautions (5.6)]*.

Advise patients that even when taking Trokendi XR™ or other anticonvulsants, some patients with epilepsy will continue to have unpredictable seizures. Therefore, counsel all patients taking Trokendi XR™ for epilepsy to exercise appropriate caution when engaging in any activities where loss of consciousness could result in serious danger to themselves or those around them (including swimming, driving a car, climbing in high places, etc.). Some patients with refractory epilepsy will need to avoid such activities altogether. Physicians should discuss the appropriate level of caution with their patients, before patients with epilepsy engage in such activities.

Fetal Toxicity

Counsel pregnant women and women of childbearing potential that use of topiramate during pregnancy can cause fetal harm, including an increased risk for cleft lip and/or cleft palate (oral clefts), which occur early in pregnancy before many women know they are pregnant. When appropriate, prescribers should counsel pregnant women and women of childbearing potential about alternative therapeutic options.

Advise women of childbearing potential who are not planning a pregnancy to use effective contraception while using topiramate, keeping in mind that there is a potential for decreased contraceptive efficacy when using estrogen-containing birth control with topiramate *[see Warnings and Precautions (5.7) and Drug Interactions (7.2)]*.

Encourage pregnant women using topiramate to enroll in the North American Antiepileptic Drug (NAAED) Pregnancy Registry. The registry is collecting information about the safety of antiepileptic drugs during pregnancy. To enroll, patients can call the toll free number, 1-888-233-2334. Information about the North American Drug Pregnancy Registry can be found at http://www.massgeneral.org/aed/ *[see Use in Specific Populations (8.1)]*.

Hyperammonemia and Encephalopathy

Warn patients about the possible development of hyperammonemia with or without encephalopathy. Although hyperammonemia may be asymptomatic, clinical symptoms of hyperammonemic encephalopathy often include acute alterations in level of consciousness and/or cognitive function with lethargy or vomiting. This hyperammonemia and encephalopathy can develop with topiramate treatment alone or with topiramate treatment with concomitant valproic acid (VPA). Patients should be instructed to contact their physician if they develop unexplained lethargy, vomiting, or changes in mental status *[see Warnings and Precautions (5.9)]*.

Kidney Stones

Instruct patients, particularly those with predisposing factors, to maintain an adequate fluid intake in order to minimize the risk of kidney stone formation *[see Warnings and Precautions (5.10)]*.

Hypothermia

Counsel patients that Trokendi XR™ can cause a reduction in body temperature, which can lead to alterations in mental status. If they note such changes, they should call their health care professional and measure their body temperature. Patients taking concomitant valproic acid should be specifically counseled on this potential adverse reaction *[see Warnings and Precautions (5.11)]*.

Paresthesia

Counsel patients that they may experience tingling in the arms and legs. If this symptom occurs, they should consult with their physician *[see Warnings and Precautions (5.12)]*.

Manufactured by: Catalent Pharma Solutions, Winchester, Kentucky 40391
Manufactured for: Supernus Pharmaceuticals, Inc., Rockville, Maryland 20850
RA-TRO-V1
Revised: August 2013

MEDICATION GUIDE

Trokendi XR™ (tro-KEN-dee eks ahr)
(topiramate)
Extended-release Capsules

Read this Medication Guide before you start taking Trokendi XR™ and each time you get a refill. There may be new information. This information does not take the place of talking to your healthcare provider about your medical condition or treatment. If you have any questions about Trokendi XR™, talk to your healthcare provider or pharmacist.

What is the most important information I should know about Trokendi XR™?

Take Trokendi XR™ capsules whole. Do not sprinkle Trokendi XR™ on food, or break, crush, dissolve, or chew Trokendi XR™ capsules before swallowing. If you cannot swallow Trokendi XR™ capsules whole, tell your healthcare provider. You may need a different medicine.

Do not drink alcohol within 6 hours prior to and 6 hours after Trokendi XR™ administration.

Trokendi XR™ may cause eye problems. Serious eye problems include:

- any sudden decrease in vision with or without eye pain and redness,
- a blockage of fluid in the eye causing increased pressure in the eye (secondary angle closure glaucoma).
- These eye problems can lead to permanent loss of vision if not treated. You should call your healthcare provider right away if you have any new eye symptoms.

Trokendi XR™ may cause decreased sweating and increased body temperature (fever). People, especially children, should be watched for signs of decreased sweating and fever, especially in hot temperatures. Some people may need to be hospitalized for this condition.

Trokendi XR™ can increase the level of acid in your blood (metabolic acidosis). If left untreated, metabolic acidosis can cause brittle or soft bones (osteoporosis, osteomalacia, osteopenia), kidney stones, can slow the rate of growth in children, and may possibly harm your baby if you are pregnant. Metabolic acidosis can happen with or without symptoms. Sometimes people with metabolic acidosis will:

- feel tired
- not feel hungry (loss of appetite)
- feel changes in heartbeat
- have trouble thinking clearly

Your healthcare provider should do a blood test to measure the level of acid in your blood before and during your treatment with Trokendi XR™. If you are pregnant, you should talk to your healthcare provider about whether you have metabolic acidosis.

Like other antiepileptic drugs, Trokendi XR™ may cause suicidal thoughts or actions in a very small number of people, about 1 in 500.

Call a healthcare provider right away if you have any of these symptoms, especially if they are new, worse, or worry you:

- thoughts about suicide or dying
- attempts to commit suicide
- new or worse depression
- new or worse anxiety
- feeling agitated or restless
- panic attacks
- trouble sleeping (insomnia)
- new or worse irritability
- acting aggressive, being angry, or violent
- acting on dangerous impulses
- an extreme increase in activity and talking (mania)
- other unusual changes in behavior or mood

Do not stop Trokendi XR™ without first talking to a healthcare provider.

- Stopping Trokendi XR™ suddenly can cause serious problems.
- Suicidal thoughts or actions can be caused by things other than medicines. If you have suicidal thoughts or actions, your healthcare provider may check for other causes.

How can I watch for early symptoms of suicidal thoughts and actions?

- Pay attention to any changes, especially sudden changes, in mood, behaviors, thoughts, or feelings.
- Keep all follow-up visits with your healthcare provider as scheduled.
- Call your healthcare provider between visits as needed, especially if you are worried about symptoms.

Trokendi XR™ can harm your unborn baby.

- If you take Trokendi XR™ during pregnancy, your baby has a higher risk for birth defects called cleft lip and cleft palate. These defects can begin early in pregnancy, even before you know you are pregnant.
- Cleft lip and cleft palate may happen even in children born to women who are not taking any medicines and do not have other risk factors.
- There may be other medicines to treat your condition that have a lower chance of birth defects.
- All women of childbearing age should talk to their healthcare providers about using other possible treatments instead of Trokendi XR™. If the decision is made to use Trokendi XR™, you should use effective birth control (contraception) unless you are planning to become pregnant. You should talk to your doctor about the best kind of birth control to use while you are taking Trokendi XR™.
- Tell your healthcare provider right away if you become pregnant while taking Trokendi XR™. You and your healthcare provider should decide if you will continue to take Trokendi XR™ while you are pregnant.
- Metabolic acidosis may have harmful affects on your baby. Talk to your healthcare provider if Trokendi XR™ has caused metabolic acidosis during your pregnancy.
- Pregnancy Registry: If you become pregnant while taking Trokendi XR™, talk to your healthcare provider about registering with the North American Antiepileptic Drug Pregnancy Registry. You can enroll in this registry by calling 1-888-233-2334. The purpose of this registry is to collect information about the safety of Trokendi XR™ and other antiepileptic drugs during pregnancy.

What is Trokendi XR™?

Trokendi XR™ is a prescription medicine used:

- to treat certain types of seizures (partial onset seizures and primary generalized tonic-clonic seizures) in people 10 years and older,
- with other medicines to treat certain types of seizures (partial onset seizures, primary generalized tonic-clonic seizures, and seizures associated with Lennox-Gastaut syndrome) in adults and children 6 years and older.

What should I tell my healthcare provider before taking Trokendi XR™?

Before taking Trokendi XR™, tell your healthcare provider about all your medical conditions, including if you:

- have or have had depression, mood problems or suicidal thoughts or behavior
- have kidney problems, kidney stones or are getting kidney dialysis

- have a history of metabolic acidosis (too much acid in the blood)
- have liver problems
- have weak, brittle or soft bones (osteomalacia, osteoporosis, osteopenia, or decreased bone density)
- have lung or breathing problems
- have eye problems, especially glaucoma
- have diarrhea
- have a growth problem
- are on a diet high in fat and low in carbohydrates, which is called a ketogenic diet
- are having surgery
- are pregnant or plan to become pregnant
- are breastfeeding. Trokendi XR™ passes into your breast milk. It is not known if the Trokendi XR™ that passes into breast milk can harm your baby. Talk to your healthcare provider about the best way to feed your baby if you take Trokendi XR™.

Tell your healthcare provider about all the medicines you take, including prescription and non-prescription medicines, vitamins, and herbal supplements. Trokendi XR™ and other medicines may affect each other causing side effects.

Especially, tell your healthcare provider if you take:

- Metformin (such as Glucophage)
- Valproic acid (such as DEPAKENE® or DEPAKOTE®)
- any medicines that impair or decrease your thinking, concentration, or muscle coordination
- birth control pills. Trokendi XR™ may make your birth control pills less effective. Tell your healthcare provider if your menstrual bleeding changes while you are taking birth control pills and Trokendi XR™.

Ask your healthcare provider if you are not sure if your medicine is listed above.

Know the medicines you take. Keep a list of them to show your healthcare provider and pharmacist each time you get a new medicine. Do not start a new medicine without talking with your healthcare provider.

How should I take Trokendi XR™?

- Take Trokendi XR™ exactly as prescribed.
- Your healthcare provider may change your dose. **Do not** change your dose without talking to your healthcare provider.
- Take Trokendi XR™ capsules whole. **Do not** sprinkle Trokendi XR™ on food, or break, crush, dissolve, or chew Trokendi XR™ capsules before swallowing.
- Trokendi XR™ can be taken before, during, or after a meal. Drink plenty of fluids during the day. This may help prevent kidney stones while taking Trokendi XR™.
- If you take too much Trokendi XR™, call your healthcare provider or poison control center right away or go to the nearest emergency room.
- If you miss a single dose of Trokendi XR™, take it as soon as you can. Do not double your dose. If you have missed more than one dose, you should call your healthcare professional for advice.
- Do not stop taking Trokendi XR™ without talking to your healthcare provider. Stopping Trokendi XR™ suddenly may cause serious problems. If you have epilepsy and you stop taking Trokendi XR™ suddenly, you may have seizures that do not stop. Your healthcare provider will tell you how to stop taking Trokendi XR™ slowly.
- Your healthcare provider may do blood tests while you take Trokendi XR™.

What should I avoid while taking Trokendi XR™?

- Do not drink alcohol within 6 hours before or 6 hours after taking Trokendi XR™ capsules. Trokendi XR and alcohol can cause serious side effects such as severe sleepiness and dizziness and an increase in seizures.
- Do not drive a car or operate heavy machinery until you know how Trokendi XR™ affects you. Trokendi XR™ can slow your thinking and motor skills, and may affect vision.

What are the possible side effects of Trokendi XR™?

Trokendi XR™ may cause serious side effects including:

See "What is the most important information I should know about Trokendi XR™?"

- **High blood ammonia levels.** High ammonia in the blood can affect your mental activities, slow your alertness, make you feel tired, or cause vomiting. This has happened when Trokendi XR™ is taken with a medicine called valproic acid (DEPAKENE ® and DEPAKOTE®).
- **Kidney stones.** Drink plenty of fluids when taking Trokendi XR™ to decrease your chances of getting kidney stones.
- **Low body temperature.** Taking Trokendi XR™ when you are also taking valproic acid cause a drop in body temperature to less than 95°F, feeling tired, confusion, or coma.
- **Effects on thinking and alertness.** Trokendi XR™ may affect how you think, and cause confusion, problems with concentration, attention, memory, or speech. Trokendi XR™ may cause depression or mood problems, tiredness, and sleepiness.
- **Dizziness or loss of muscle coordination.**

Call your healthcare provider right away if you have any of the symptoms above.

The most common side effects of Trokendi XR™ include:

- tingling of the arms and legs (paresthesia)
- not feeling hungry
- nausea
- a change in the way foods taste
- diarrhea
- weight loss
- nervousness
- upper respiratory tract infection

Tell your healthcare provider about any side effect that bothers you or that does not go away.

These are not all the possible side effects of Trokendi XR™. For more information, ask your healthcare provider or pharmacist.

Call your doctor for medical advice about side effects. You may report side effects to FDA at 1 800-FDA-1088.

You may also report side effects to Supernus Pharmaceuticals, Inc. at 1-866-398-0833.

How should I store Trokendi XR™?

- Store Trokendi XR™ tablets at room temperature between 59°F to 86°F (15°C to 30°C).
- Keep Trokendi XR™ in a tightly closed container.
- Keep Trokendi XR™ dry and away from moisture and light.
- **Keep Trokendi XR™ and all medicines out of the reach of children.**

General information about Trokendi XR™

Medicines are sometimes prescribed for purposes other than those listed in a Medication Guide. Do not use Trokendi XR™ for a condition for which it was not prescribed. Do not give Trokendi XR™ to other people, even if they have the same symptoms that you have. It may harm them.

This Medication Guide summarizes the most important information about Trokendi XR™. If you would like more information, talk with your healthcare provider. You can ask your pharmacist or healthcare provider for information about Trokendi XR™ that is written for health professionals.

For more information, go to www.trokendixrcom or call 1-866-398-0833.

What are the ingredients in Trokendi XR™?

Active ingredient: topiramate

Inactive ingredients:

Sugar Spheres, NF, Hypromellose (Type 2910), USP, mannitol, USP, docusate sodium, USP, sodium benzoate, NF,, ethylcellulose, NF, oleic acid, NF, medium chain triglycerides, NF, polyethylene glycol, NF, polyvinyl alcohol, USP titanium dioxide, USP, talc, USP, lecithin, NF, xanthan gum, NF

Capsule shells: Gelatin, USP; titanium Dioxide, USP, and Colorants.

Colorants:

FD&C Blue #1 (all strength capsules)
Yellow iron oxide, USP (25 mg and 50 mg capsules)
FD&C red #3 (50 mg, 100 mg and 200 mg capsules)
FD&C yellow #6 (50 mg, 100 mg and 200 mg capsules)
Riboflavin, USP (25 mg capsules)

All capsule shells are imprinted with black print that contains shellac, NF, and black iron oxide, NF.

This Medication Guide has been approved by the U.S. Food and Drug Administration.

Manufactured by: Catalent Pharma Solutions, Winchester, KY USA 40391
Manufactured for: Supernus Pharmaceuticals, Inc. Rockville, MD USA 20850

RA-TRO-MGV1
Issued: August 2013

Shown in Product Identification Guide, page 313

Takeda Pharmaceuticals U.S.A., Inc.

ONE TAKEDA PARKWAY
DEERFIELD, IL 60015

Direct Inquiries to:
Sales and Ordering:
Customer Service
(877) TAKEDA7
(877) 825-3327
For Medical Information:
(877) TAKEDA7
(877) 825-3327
To Report Adverse Drug Experiences:
(877) TAKEDA7
(877) 825-3327

AMITIZA ℞

[ahm-i-TEE-za]
(lubiprostone)
capsules, for oral use

HIGHLIGHTS OF PRESCRIBING INFORMATION
These highlights do not include all the information needed to use AMITIZA safely and effectively. See full prescribing information for AMITIZA.
AMITIZA (lubiprostone) capsules, for oral use
Initial U.S. Approval: 2006

RECENT MAJOR CHANGES

Indications and Usage (1.2)	04/2013
Dosage and Administration (2.1)	04/2013
Warnings and Precautions, Pregnancy (5.1)	removed 11/2012

INDICATIONS AND USAGE

Amitiza is a chloride channel activator indicated for:

- Treatment of chronic idiopathic constipation in adults (1.1)
- Treatment of opioid-induced constipation in adults with chronic, non-cancer pain (1.2)
- Treatment of irritable bowel syndrome with constipation in women ≥ 18 years old (1.3)

Limitations of Use:

Effectiveness of Amitiza in the treatment of opioid-induced constipation in patients taking diphenylheptane opioids (e.g., methadone) has not been established (1) (14.2)

DOSAGE AND ADMINISTRATION

Capsules should be swallowed whole and should not be broken apart or chewed (2)

Chronic Idiopathic Constipation and Opioid-induced Constipation

- 24 mcg taken twice daily orally with food and water (2.1)

Reduce the dosage in patients with moderate and severe hepatic impairment (2.1)

Irritable Bowel Syndrome with Constipation

- 8 mcg taken twice daily orally with food and water (2.2)

Reduce the dosage in patients with severe hepatic impairment (2.2)

DOSAGE FORMS AND STRENGTHS

- Capsules: 8 mcg and 24 mcg (3)

CONTRAINDICATIONS

- Amitiza is contraindicated in patients with known or suspected mechanical gastrointestinal obstruction. (4)

WARNINGS AND PRECAUTIONS

- Patients may experience nausea; concomitant administration of food may reduce this symptom (5.1)
- Do not prescribe for patients that have severe diarrhea (5.2)
- Patients taking Amitiza may experience dyspnea within an hour of first dose. This symptom generally resolves within 3 hours, but may recur with repeat dosing (5.3)
- Evaluate patients with symptoms suggestive of mechanical gastrointestinal obstruction prior to initiating treatment with Amitiza (5.4)

ADVERSE REACTIONS

- Most common adverse reactions (incidence > 4%) in chronic idiopathic constipation are nausea, diarrhea, headache, abdominal pain, abdominal distension, and flatulence (6.1)
- Most common adverse reactions (incidence > 4%) in opioid-induced constipation are nausea and diarrhea (6.1)

- Most common adverse reactions (incidence > 4%) in irritable bowel syndrome with constipation are nausea, diarrhea, and abdominal pain (6.1)

To report SUSPECTED ADVERSE REACTIONS, contact Takeda Pharmaceuticals at 1-877-825-3327 or FDA at 1-800-FDA-1088 or www.fda.gov/medwatch.

DRUG INTERACTIONS

- Concomitant use of diphenylheptane opioids (e.g., methadone) may interfere with the efficacy of Amitiza (7)

USE IN SPECIFIC POPULATIONS

- Pregnancy: Based on animal data, may cause fetal harm (8.1)
- Nursing Mothers: Caution should be exercised when administering to a nursing woman (8.3)

See 17 for PATIENT COUNSELING INFORMATION

Revised: 04/2013

FULL PRESCRIBING INFORMATION: CONTENTS*

*** Sections or subsections omitted from the full prescribing information are not listed**

FULL PRESCRIBING INFORMATION

1 INDICATIONS AND USAGE

1.1 Chronic Idiopathic Constipation

Amitiza® is indicated for the treatment of chronic idiopathic constipation in adults.

1.2 Opioid-induced Constipation

Amitiza is indicated for the treatment of opioid-induced constipation (OIC) in adults with chronic non-cancer pain.

Limitations of Use:

- Effectiveness of Amitiza in the treatment of opioid-induced constipation in patients taking diphenylheptane-opioids (e.g., methadone) has not been established. *[see Clinical Studies (14.2)]*

1.3 Irritable Bowel Syndrome with Constipation

Amitiza is indicated for the treatment of irritable bowel syndrome with constipation (IBS-C) in women ≥ 18 years old.

2 DOSAGE AND ADMINISTRATION

Take Amitiza orally with food and water. Swallow capsules whole and do not break apart or chew. Physicians and patients should periodically assess the need for continued therapy.

2.1 Chronic Idiopathic Constipation and Opioid-induced Constipation

The recommended dose is 24 mcg twice daily orally with food and water.

Dosage in patients with hepatic impairment

For patients with moderately impaired hepatic function (Child-Pugh Class B), the recommended starting dose is 16 mcg twice daily. For patients with severely impaired hepatic function (Child-Pugh Class C), the recommended starting dose is 8 mcg twice daily. If this dose is tolerated and an adequate response has not been obtained after an appropriate interval, doses can then be escalated to full dosing with appropriate monitoring of patient response *[see Use in Specific Populations (8.7) and Clinical Pharmacology (12.3)]*.

2.2 Irritable Bowel Syndrome with Constipation

The recommended dose is 8 mcg twice daily orally with food and water.

Dosage in patients with hepatic impairment

For patients with severely impaired hepatic function (Child-Pugh Class C), the recommended starting dose is 8 mcg once daily. If this dose is tolerated and an adequate response has not been obtained after an appropriate interval, doses can then be escalated to full dosing with appropriate monitoring of patient response. Dosage adjustment is not required for patients with moderately impaired hepatic function (Child-Pugh Class B) *[see Use in Specific Populations (8.7) and Clinical Pharmacology (12.3)]*.

3 DOSAGE FORMS AND STRENGTHS

Amitiza is available as an oval, gelatin capsule containing 8 mcg or 24 mcg of lubiprostone.

- 8 mcg capsules are pink and are printed with "SPI" on one side
- 24 mcg capsules are orange and are printed with "SPI" on one side

4 CONTRAINDICATIONS

Amitiza is contraindicated in patients with known or suspected mechanical gastrointestinal obstruction.

5 WARNINGS AND PRECAUTIONS

5.1 Nausea

Patients taking Amitiza may experience nausea. Concomitant administration of food with Amitiza may reduce symptoms of nausea [see *Adverse Reactions (6.1)*].

5.2 Diarrhea

Amitiza should not be prescribed to patients that have severe diarrhea. Patients should be aware of the possible occurrence of diarrhea during treatment. Patients should be instructed to discontinue Amitiza and inform their physician if severe diarrhea occurs [see *Adverse Reactions (6.1)*].

5.3 Dyspnea

In clinical trials, dyspnea was reported by 3%, 1%, and < 1% of the treated CIC, OIC, and IBS-C populations receiving Amitiza, respectively, compared to 0%, 1%, and < 1% of placebo-treated patients. There have been postmarketing reports of dyspnea when using Amitiza 24 mcg twice daily. Some patients have discontinued treatment because of dyspnea. These events have usually been described as a sensation of chest tightness and difficulty taking in a breath, and generally have an acute onset within 30–60 minutes after taking the first dose. They generally resolve within a few hours after taking the dose, but recurrence has been frequently reported with subsequent doses.

5.4 Bowel Obstruction

In patients with symptoms suggestive of mechanical gastrointestinal obstruction, perform a thorough evaluation to confirm the absence of an obstruction prior to initiating therapy with Amitiza.

6 ADVERSE REACTIONS

The following adverse reactions are described below and elsewhere in labeling:

- Nausea *[see Warnings and Precautions (5.1)]*
- Diarrhea *[see Warnings and Precautions (5.2)]*
- Dyspnea *[see Warnings and Precautions (5.3)]*

6.1 Clinical Studies Experience

Because clinical studies are conducted under widely varying conditions, adverse reaction rates observed in the clinical studies of a drug cannot be directly compared to rates in the clinical studies of another drug and may not reflect the rates observed in practice.

During clinical development of Amitiza for CIC, OIC, and IBS-C, 1234 patients were treated with Amitiza for 6 months and 524 patients were treated for 1 year (not mutually exclusive).

Chronic Idiopathic Constipation

Adverse reactions in dose-finding, efficacy, and long-term clinical studies: The data described below reflect exposure to Amitiza 24 mcg twice daily in 1113 patients with chronic idiopathic constipation over 3- or 4-week, 6-month, and 12-month treatment periods; and from 316 patients receiving placebo over short-term exposure (≤ 4 weeks). The placebo population (N = 316) had a mean age of 47.8 (range 21–81) years; was 87.3% female; 80.7% Caucasian, 10.1% African American, 7.3% Hispanic, 0.9% Asian; and 11.7% elderly (≥ 65 years of age). Of those patients treated with Amitiza 24 mcg twice daily (N=1113), the mean age was 50.3 (range 19-86) years; 86.9% were female; 86.1% Caucasian, 7.6% African American, 4.7% Hispanic, 1.0% Asian; and 16.7% elderly (≥ 65 years of age). Table 1 presents data for the adverse reactions that occurred in at least 1% of patients who received Amitiza 24 mcg twice daily and that occurred more frequently with study drug than placebo.

Table 1: Percent of Patients with Adverse Reactions (Chronic Idiopathic Constipation)

System/Adverse Reaction*	Placebo N = 316 %	Amitiza 24 mcg Twice Daily N = 1113 %
Gastrointestinal disorders		
Nausea	3	29
Diarrhea	1	12
Abdominal pain	3	8
Abdominal distension	2	6
Flatulence	2	6
Vomiting	0	3
Loose stools	0	3
Abdominal discomfort†	1	3
Dyspepsia	< 1	2
Dry mouth	< 1	1
Nervous system disorders		
Headache	5	11
Dizziness	1	3
General disorders and site administration conditions		
Edema	< 1	3
Fatigue	1	2
Chest discomfort/pain	0	2
Respiratory, thoracic, and mediastinal disorders		
Dyspnea	0	2

* Includes only those events associated with treatment (possibly, probably, or definitely related, as assessed by the investigator).

† This term combines "abdominal tenderness," "abdominal rigidity," "gastrointestinal discomfort," "stomach discomfort", and "abdominal discomfort."

The most common adverse reactions (incidence > 4%) in CIC were nausea, diarrhea, headache, abdominal pain, abdominal distension, and flatulence.

Nausea: Approximately 29% of patients who received Amitiza 24 mcg twice daily experienced nausea; 4% of patients had severe nausea and 9% of patients discontinued treatment due to nausea. The rate of nausea associated with Amitiza 24 mcg twice daily was lower among male (8%) and elderly (19%) patients. No patients in the clinical studies were hospitalized due to nausea.

Diarrhea: Approximately 12% of patients who received Amitiza 24 mcg twice daily experienced diarrhea; 2% of patients had severe diarrhea and 2% of patients discontinued treatment due to diarrhea.

Electrolytes: No serious adverse reactions of electrolyte imbalance were reported in clinical studies, and no clinically significant changes were seen in serum electrolyte levels in patients receiving Amitiza.

Less common adverse reactions: The following adverse reactions (assessed by investigator as probably or definitely related to treatment) occurred in less than 1% of patients receiving Amitiza 24 mcg twice daily in clinical studies, occurred in at least two patients, and occurred more frequently in patients receiving study drug than those receiving placebo: fecal incontinence, muscle cramp, defecation urgency, frequent bowel movements, hyperhidrosis, pharyngolaryngeal pain, intestinal functional disorder, anxiety, cold sweat, constipation, cough, dysgeusia, eructation, influenza, joint swelling, myalgia, pain, syncope, tremor, decreased appetite.

Opioid-induced Constipation

Adverse reactions in efficacy and long-term clinical studies: The data described below reflect exposure to Amitiza 24 mcg twice daily in 860 patients with OIC for up to 12 months and from 632 patients receiving placebo twice daily for up to 12 weeks. The total population (N = 1492) had a mean age of 50.4 (range 20–89) years; was 62.7% female; 82.7% Caucasian, 14.2% African American, 0.8% American Indian/Alaska Native, 0.8% Asian; 5.2% were of Hispanic ethnicity; and 8.8% were elderly (≥ 65 years of age). Table 2 presents data for the adverse reactions that occurred in at least 1% of patients who received Amitiza 24 mcg twice daily and that occurred more frequently with study drug than placebo.

Table 2: Percent of Patients with Adverse Reactions (OIC Studies)

System/Adverse Reaction*	Placebo N = 632 %	Amitiza 24 mcg Twice Daily N = 860 %
Gastrointestinal disorders		
Nausea	5	11
Diarrhea	2	8
Abdominal pain	1	4
Flatulence	3	4
Abdominal distension	2	3
Vomiting	2	3
Abdominal discomfort†	1	1
Nervous system disorders		
Headache	1	2
General disorders and site administration conditions		
Peripheral edema	< 1	1

* Includes only those events associated with treatment (possibly, probably, or definitely related, as assessed by the investigator).

† This term combines "abdominal tenderness," "abdominal rigidity," "gastrointestinal discomfort," "stomach discomfort", and "abdominal discomfort."

The most common adverse reactions (incidence > 4%) in OIC were nausea and diarrhea.

Nausea: Approximately 11% of patients who received Amitiza 24 mcg twice daily experienced nausea; 1% of patients had severe nausea and 2% of patients discontinued treatment due to nausea.

Diarrhea: Approximately 8% of patients who received Amitiza 24 mcg twice daily experienced diarrhea; 2% of patients had severe diarrhea and 1% of patients discontinued treatment due to diarrhea.

Less common adverse reactions: The following adverse reactions (assessed by investigator as probably or definitely related to treatment) occurred in less than 1% of patients receiving Amitiza 24 mcg twice daily in clinical studies, occurred in at least two patients, and occurred more frequently in patients receiving study drug than those receiving placebo: fecal incontinence, blood potassium decreased.

Irritable Bowel Syndrome with Constipation

Adverse reactions in dose-finding, efficacy, and long-term clinical studies: The data described below reflect exposure to Amitiza 8 mcg twice daily in 1011 patients with IBS-C for up to 12 months and from 435 patients receiving placebo twice daily for up to 16 weeks. The total population (N = 1267) had a mean age of 46.5 (range 18–85) years; was 91.6% female; 77.5% Caucasian, 12.9% African American, 8.6% Hispanic, 0.4% Asian; and 8.0% elderly (≥ 65 years of age). Table 3 presents data for the adverse reactions that occurred in at least 1% of patients who received Amitiza 8 mcg twice daily and that occurred more frequently with study drug than placebo.

Table 3: Percent of Patients with Adverse Reactions (IBS-C Studies)

System/Adverse Reaction*	Placebo N = 435 %	Amitiza 8 mcg Twice Daily N = 1011 %
Gastrointestinal disorders		
Nausea	4	8
Diarrhea	4	7
Abdominal pain	5	5
Abdominal distension	2	3

* Includes only those events associated with treatment (possibly or probably related, as assessed by the investigator).

The most common adverse reactions (incidence > 4%) in IBS-C were nausea, diarrhea, and abdominal pain.

Nausea: Approximately 8% of patients who received Amitiza 8 mcg twice daily experienced nausea; 1% of patients had severe nausea and 1% of patients discontinued treatment due to nausea.

Diarrhea: Approximately 7% of patients who received Amitiza 8 mcg twice daily experienced diarrhea; <1% of patients had severe diarrhea and <1% of patients discontinued treatment due to diarrhea.

Less common adverse reactions: The following adverse reactions (assessed by investigator as probably related to treatment) occurred in less than 1% of patients receiving Amitiza 8 mcg twice daily in clinical studies, occurred in at least two patients, and occurred more frequently in patients receiving study drug than those receiving placebo: dyspepsia, loose stools, vomiting, fatigue, dry mouth, edema, increased alanine aminotransferase, increased aspartate aminotransferase, constipation, eructation, gastroesophageal reflux disease, dyspnea, erythema, gastritis, increased weight, palpitations, urinary tract infection, anorexia, anxiety, depression, fecal incontinence, fibromyalgia, hard feces, lethargy, rectal hemorrhage, pollakiuria.

6.2 Postmarketing Experience

The following additional adverse reactions have been identified during post-approval use of Amitiza. Because these reactions are reported voluntarily from a population of uncertain size, it is not always possible to reliably estimate their frequency or establish a causal relationship to drug exposure.

Voluntary reports of adverse reactions occurring with the use of Amitiza include the following: syncope, ischemic colitis, hypersensitivity/allergic-type reactions (including rash, swelling, and throat tightness), malaise, tachycardia, muscle cramps or muscle spasms, and asthenia.

7 DRUG INTERACTIONS

No *in vivo* drug-drug interaction studies have been performed with Amitiza.

Based upon the results of *in vitro* human microsome studies, there is low likelihood of pharmacokinetic drug-drug interactions. *In vitro* studies using human liver microsomes indicate that cytochrome P450 isoenzymes are not involved in the metabolism of lubiprostone. Further *in vitro* studies indicate microsomal carbonyl reductase may be involved in the extensive biotransformation of lubiprostone to the metabolite M3 [see *Clinical Pharmacology (12.3)*]. Additionally, *in vitro* studies in human liver microsomes demonstrate that lubiprostone does not inhibit cytochrome P450 isoforms 3A4, 2D6, 1A2, 2A6, 2B6, 2C9, 2C19, or 2E1, and *in vitro* studies of primary cultures of human hepatocytes show no induction of cytochrome P450 isoforms 1A2, 2B6, 2C9, and 3A4 by lubiprostone. Based on the available information, no protein binding–mediated drug interactions of clinical significance are anticipated.

Interaction potential with diphenylheptane opioids (e.g. methadone): Non-clinical studies have shown opioids of the diphenylheptane chemical class (e.g., methadone) to dose-dependently reduce the activation of ClC-2 by lubiprostone in the gastrointestinal tract. There is a possibility of a dose-dependent decrease in the efficacy of Amitiza in patients using diphenylheptane opioids.

8 USE IN SPECIFIC POPULATIONS

8.1 Pregnancy

Pregnancy Category C.

Risk Summary

There are no adequate and well-controlled studies with Amitiza in pregnant women. A dose dependent increase in fetal loss was observed in pregnant guinea pigs that received lubiprostone doses equivalent to 0.2 to 6 times the maximum recommended human dose (MRHD) based on body surface area (mg/m^2). Animal studies did not show an increase in structural malformations. Amitiza should be used during pregnancy only if the potential benefit justifies the potential risk to the fetus.

Clinical Considerations

Current available data suggest that miscarriage occurs in 15-18% of clinically recognized pregnancies, regardless of any drug exposure. Consider the risks and benefits of available therapies when treating a pregnant woman for chronic idiopathic constipation, opioid-induced constipation or irritable bowel syndrome with constipation.

Animal Data

In developmental toxicity studies, pregnant rats and rabbits received oral lubiprostone during organogenesis at doses up to approximately 338 times (rats) and approximately 34 times (rabbits) the maximum recommended human dose (MHRD) based on body surface area (mg/m^2). Maximal animal doses were 2000 mcg/kg/day (rats) and 100 mcg/kg/day (rabbits). In rats, there were increased incidences of early resorptions and soft tissue malformations (*situs inversus*, cleft palate) at the 2000 mcg/kg/day dose; however, these effects were probably secondary to maternal toxicity. A dose-dependent increase in fetal loss occurred when guinea pigs received lubiprostone after the period of organogenesis, on days 40 to 53 of gestation, at daily oral doses of 1, 10, and 25 mcg/kg/day (approximately 0.2, 2 and 6 times the MRHD based on body surface area (mg/m^2)). The potential of lubiprostone to cause fetal loss was also examined in pregnant Rhesus monkeys. Monkeys received lubiprostone post-organogenesis on gestation days 110 through 130 at daily oral doses of 10 and 30 mcg/kg/day (approximately 3 and 10 times the MHRD based on body surface area (mg/m^2)). Fetal loss was noted in one monkey from the 10-mcg/kg dose group, which is within normal historical rates for this species. There was no drug-related adverse effect seen in monkeys.

8.3 Nursing Mothers

It is not known whether lubiprostone is excreted in human milk. In rats, neither lubiprostone nor its active metabolites were detectable in breast milk following oral administration of lubiprostone. Because lubiprostone increases fluid secretion in the intestine and intestinal motility, human milk-fed infants should be monitored for diarrhea. Caution should be exercised when Amitiza is administered to a nursing woman.

8.4 Pediatric Use

Safety and effectiveness in pediatric patients have not been established.

8.5 Geriatric Use

Chronic Idiopathic Constipation

The efficacy of Amitiza in the elderly (≥ 65 years of age) subpopulation was consistent with the efficacy in the overall study population. Of the total number of constipated patients treated in the dose-finding, efficacy, and long-term studies of Amitiza, 15.5% were ≥ 65 years of age, and 4.2% were ≥ 75 years of age. Elderly patients taking Amitiza 24 mcg twice daily experienced a lower rate of associated nausea compared to the overall study population taking Amitiza (19% vs. 29%, respectively).

Opioid-induced Constipation

The safety profile of Amitiza in the elderly (≥ 65 years of age) subpopulation (8.8% were ≥ 65 years of age and 1.6% were ≥ 75 years of age) was consistent with the safety profile in the overall study population. Clinical studies of Amitiza did not include sufficient numbers of patients aged 65 years and over to determine whether they respond differently from younger patients.

Irritable Bowel Syndrome with Constipation

The safety profile of Amitiza in the elderly (≥ 65 years of age) subpopulation (8.0% were ≥ 65 years of age and 1.8% were ≥ 75 years of age) was consistent with the safety profile in the overall study population. Clinical studies of Amitiza did not include sufficient numbers of patients aged 65 years and over to determine whether they respond differently from younger patients.

8.6 Renal Impairment

No dosage adjustment is required in patients with renal impairment [see *Clinical Pharmacology (12.3)*].

8.7 Hepatic Impairment

Patients with moderate hepatic impairment (Child-Pugh Class B) and severe hepatic impairment (Child-Pugh Class C) experienced markedly higher systemic exposure of lubiprostone active metabolite M3, when compared to normal subjects [see *Clinical Pharmacology (12.3)*]. Clinical safety results demonstrated an increased incidence and severity of adverse events in subjects with greater severity of hepatic impairment.

In case of chronic idiopathic constipation or opioid-induced constipation indications, the starting dosage of Amitiza should be reduced in patients with moderate hepatic impairment. The starting dose of Amitiza should be reduced in all patients with severe hepatic impairment, regardless of the indication [see *Dosage and Administration (2.1, 2.2)*]. No dosing adjustment is required in patients with mild hepatic impairment (Child-Pugh Class A).

10 OVERDOSAGE

There have been two confirmed reports of overdosage with Amitiza. The first report involved a 3-year-old child who accidentally ingested 7 or 8 capsules of 24 mcg of Amitiza and fully recovered. The second report was a study patient who self-administered a total of 96 mcg of Amitiza per day for 8 days. The patient experienced no adverse reactions during this time. Additionally, in a Phase 1 cardiac repolarization study, 38 of 51 healthy volunteers given a single oral dose of 144 mcg of Amitiza (6 times the highest recommended dose) experienced an adverse event that was at least possibly related to the study drug. Adverse reactions that occurred in at least 1% of these volunteers included the following: nausea (45%), diarrhea (35%), vomiting (27%), dizziness (14%), headache (12%), abdominal pain (8%), flushing/hot flash (8%), retching (8%), dyspnea (4%), pallor (4%), stomach discomfort (4%), anorexia (2%), asthenia (2%), chest discomfort (2%), dry mouth (2%), hyperhidrosis (2%), and syncope (2%).

11 DESCRIPTION

Amitiza (lubiprostone) is a chloride channel activator for oral use.

The chemical name for lubiprostone is (–)-7-[(2*R*,4a*R*,5*R*,7a*R*)-2-(1,1-difluoropentyl)-2-hydroxy-6-oxo-octahydrocyclopenta[*b*]pyran-5-yl]heptanoic acid. The molecular formula of lubiprostone is $C_{20}H_{32}F_2O_5$ with a molecular weight of 390.46 and a chemical structure as follows:

Table 4: Pharmacokinetic Parameters of the Metabolite M3 for Subjects with Normal or Impaired Liver Function following Dosing with Amitiza

Liver Function Status	Mean (SD) AUC_{0-t} (pg·hr/mL)	% Change vs. Normal	Mean (SD) C_{max} (pg/mL)	% Change vs. Normal
Normal (n=8)	39.6 (18.7)	n.a.	37.5 (15.9)	n.a.
Child-Pugh Class B (n=8)	119 (104)	+119	70.9 (43.5)	+66
Child-Pugh Class C (n=8)	234 (61.6)	+521	114 (59.4)	+183

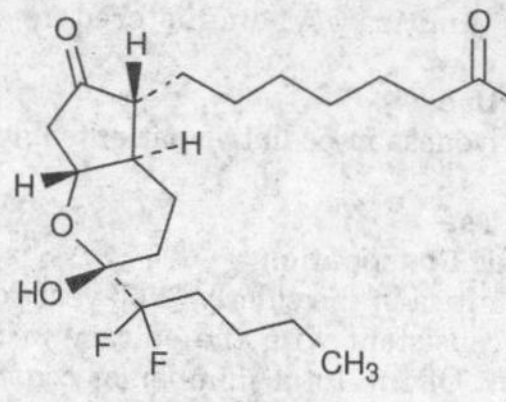

Lubiprostone drug substance occurs as white, odorless crystals or crystalline powder, is very soluble in ether and ethanol, and is practically insoluble in hexane and water. Amitiza is available as an imprinted, oval, soft gelatin capsule in two strengths. Pink capsules contain 8 mcg of lubiprostone and the following inactive ingredients: medium-chain triglycerides, gelatin, sorbitol, ferric oxide, titanium dioxide, and purified water. Orange capsules contain 24 mcg of lubiprostone and the following inactive ingredients: medium-chain triglycerides, gelatin, sorbitol, FD&C Red #40, D&C Yellow #10, and purified water.

12 CLINICAL PHARMACOLOGY

12.1 Mechanism of Action

Lubiprostone is a locally acting chloride channel activator that enhances a chloride-rich intestinal fluid secretion without altering sodium and potassium concentrations in the serum. Lubiprostone acts by specifically activating ClC-2, which is a normal constituent of the apical membrane of the human intestine, in a protein kinase A–independent fashion.

By increasing intestinal fluid secretion, lubiprostone increases motility in the intestine, thereby facilitating the passage of stool and alleviating symptoms associated with chronic idiopathic constipation. Patch clamp cell studies in human cell lines have indicated that the majority of the beneficial biological activity of lubiprostone and its metabolites is observed only on the apical (luminal) portion of the gastrointestinal epithelium.

Lubiprostone, via activation of apical ClC-2 channels in intestinal epithelial cells, bypasses the antisecretory action of opiates that results from suppression of secretomotor neuron excitability.

Activation of ClC-2 by lubiprostone has also been shown to stimulate recovery of mucosal barrier function and reduce intestinal permeability via the restoration of tight junction protein complexes in *ex vivo* studies of ischemic porcine intestine.

12.2 Pharmacodynamics

Although the pharmacologic effects of lubiprostone in humans have not been fully evaluated, animal studies have shown that oral administration of lubiprostone increases chloride ion transport into the intestinal lumen, enhances fluid secretion into the bowels, and improves fecal transit.

12.3 Pharmacokinetics

Lubiprostone has low systemic availability following oral administration and concentrations of lubiprostone in plasma are below the level of quantitation (10 pg/mL). Therefore, standard pharmacokinetic parameters such as area under the curve (AUC), maximum concentration (C_{max}), and half-life ($t_{1/2}$) cannot be reliably calculated. However, the pharmacokinetic parameters of M3 (only measurable active metabolite of lubiprostone) have been characterized. Gender has no effect on the pharmacokinetics of M3 following the oral administration of lubiprostone.

Absorption

Concentrations of lubiprostone in plasma are below the level of quantitation (10 pg/mL) because lubiprostone has a low systemic availability following oral administration. Peak plasma levels of M3, after a single oral dose with 24 mcg of lubiprostone, occurred at approximately 1.10 hours. The C_{max} was 41.5 pg/mL and the mean AUC_{0-t} was 57.1 pg·hr/mL. The AUC_{0-t} of M3 increases dose proportionally after single 24-mcg and 144-mcg doses of lubiprostone.

Distribution

In vitro protein binding studies indicate lubiprostone is approximately 94% bound to human plasma proteins. Studies in rats given radiolabeled lubiprostone indicate minimal distribution beyond the gastrointestinal tissues. Concentrations of radiolabeled lubiprostone at 48 hours post-administration were minimal in all tissues of the rats.

Metabolism

The results of both human and animal studies indicate that lubiprostone is rapidly and extensively metabolized by 15-position reduction, α-chain β-oxidation, and ω-chain ω-oxidation. These biotransformations are not mediated by the hepatic cytochrome P450 system but rather appear to be mediated by the ubiquitously expressed carbonyl reductase. M3, a metabolite of lubiprostone found in both humans and animals, is formed by the reduction of the carbonyl group at the 15-hydroxy moiety that consists of both α-hydroxy and β-hydroxy epimers. M3 makes up less than 10% of the dose of radiolabeled lubiprostone. Animal studies have shown that metabolism of lubiprostone rapidly occurs within the stomach and jejunum, most likely in the absence of any systemic absorption.

Elimination

Lubiprostone could not be detected in plasma; however, M3 has a $t_{1/2}$ ranging from 0.9 to 1.4 hours. After a single oral dose of 72 mcg of ^{3}H-labeled lubiprostone, 60% of total administered radioactivity was recovered in the urine within 24 hours and 30% of total administered radioactivity was recovered in the feces by 168 hours. Lubiprostone and M3 are only detected in trace amounts in human feces.

Food Effect

A study was conducted with a single 72-mcg dose of ^{3}H-labeled lubiprostone to evaluate the potential of a food effect on lubiprostone absorption, metabolism, and excretion. Pharmacokinetic parameters of total radioactivity demonstrated that C_{max} decreased by 55% while $AUC_{0-\infty}$ was unchanged when lubiprostone was administered with a high-fat meal. The clinical relevance of the effect of food on the pharmacokinetics of lubiprostone is not clear. However, lubiprostone was administered with food and water in a majority of clinical trials.

Special Populations

Renal Impairment

Sixteen subjects, 34–47 years old (8 severe renally impaired subjects [creatinine clearance (CrCl) < 20 mL/min] who required hemodialysis and 8 control subjects with normal renal function [CrCl > 80 mL/min]), received a single oral 24-mcg dose of Amitiza. Following administration, lubiprostone plasma concentrations were below the limit of quantitation (10 pg/mL). Plasma concentrations of M3 were within the range of exposure from previous clinical experience with Amitiza.

Hepatic Impairment

Twenty-five subjects, 38–78 years old (9 with severe hepatic impairment [Child-Pugh Class C], 8 with moderate impairment [Child-Pugh Class B], and 8 with normal liver function), received either 12 mcg or 24 mcg of Amitiza under fasting conditions. Following administration, lubiprostone plasma concentrations were below the limit of quantitation (10 pg/mL) except for two subjects. In moderately and severely impaired subjects, the C_{max} and AUC_{0-t} of the active lubiprostone metabolite M3 were increased, as shown in Table 4.

[See table 4 above]

These results demonstrate that there is a correlation between increased exposure of M3 and severity of hepatic impairment. *[see Use in Specific Populations (8.7)]*

13 NONCLINICAL TOXICOLOGY

13.1 Carcinogenesis, Mutagenesis, Impairment of Fertility

Carcinogenesis

Two 2-year oral (gavage) carcinogenicity studies (one in Crl:B6C3F1 mice and one in Sprague-Dawley rats) were conducted with lubiprostone. In the 2-year carcinogenicity study in mice, lubiprostone doses of 25, 75, 200, and 500 mcg/kg/day (approximately 2, 6, 17, and 42 times the highest recommended human dose, respectively, based on body surface area) were used. In the 2-year rat carcinogenicity study, lubiprostone doses of 20, 100, and 400 mcg/kg/day (approximately 3, 17, and 68 times the highest recommended human dose, respectively, based on body surface area) were used. In the mouse carcinogenicity study, there was no significant increase in any tumor incidences. There was a significant increase in the incidence of interstitial cell adenoma of the testes in male rats at the 400 mcg/kg/day dose. In female rats, treatment with lubiprostone produced hepatocellular adenoma at the 400 mcg/kg/day dose.

Mutagenesis

Lubiprostone was not genotoxic in the *in vitro* Ames reverse mutation assay, the *in vitro* mouse lymphoma (L5178Y TK $^{+/-}$) forward mutation assay, the *in vitro* Chinese hamster lung (CHL/IU) chromosomal aberration assay, and the *in vivo* mouse bone marrow micronucleus assay.

Impairment of Fertility

Lubiprostone, at oral doses of up to 1000 mcg/kg/day, had no effect on the fertility and reproductive function of male and female rats. However, the number of implantation sites and live embryos were significantly reduced in rats at the 1000 mcg/kg/day dose as compared to control. The number of dead or resorbed embryos in the 1000 mcg/kg/day group was higher compared to the control group, but was not statistically significant. The 1000 mcg/kg/day dose in rats is approximately 169 times the highest recommended human dose of 48 mcg/day, based on body surface area.

14 CLINICAL STUDIES

14.1 Chronic Idiopathic Constipation

Two double-blinded, placebo-controlled studies of identical design were conducted in patients with chronic idiopathic constipation. Chronic idiopathic constipation was defined as, on average, less than 3 spontaneous bowel movements (SBMs) per week (a SBM is a bowel movement occurring in the absence of laxative use) along with one or more of the following symptoms of constipation for at least 6 months prior to randomization: 1) very hard stools for at least a quarter of all bowel movements; 2) sensation of incomplete evacuation following at least a quarter of all bowel movements; and 3) straining with defecation at least a quarter of the time.

Following a 2-week baseline/washout period, a total of 479 patients (mean age 47.2 [range 20–81] years; 88.9% female; 80.8% Caucasian, 9.6% African American, 7.3% Hispanic, 1.5% Asian; 10.9% ≥ 65 years of age) were randomized and received Amitiza 24 mcg twice daily or placebo twice daily for 4 weeks. The primary endpoint of the studies was SBM frequency. The studies demonstrated that patients treated with Amitiza had a higher frequency of SBMs during Week 1 than the placebo patients. In both studies, results similar to those in Week 1 were also observed in Weeks 2, 3, and 4 of therapy (Table 5).

[See table 5 at top of next page]

In both studies, Amitiza demonstrated increases in the percentage of patients who experienced SBMs within the first 24 hours after administration when compared to placebo (56.7% vs. 36.9% in Study 1 and 62.9% vs. 31.9% in Study 2, respectively). Similarly, the time to first SBM was shorter for patients receiving Amitiza than for those receiving placebo.

Signs and symptoms related to constipation, including abdominal bloating, abdominal discomfort, stool consistency, and straining, as well as constipation severity ratings, were also improved with Amitiza versus placebo. The results were consistent in subpopulation analyses for gender, race, and elderly patients (≥ 65 years of age).

During a 7-week randomized withdrawal study, patients who received Amitiza during a 4-week treatment period were then randomized to receive either placebo or to continue treatment with Amitiza. In Amitiza-treated patients randomized to placebo, SBM frequency rates returned toward baseline within 1 week and did not result in worsening compared to baseline. Patients who continued on Amitiza maintained their response to therapy over the additional 3 weeks of treatment.

14.2 Opioid-induced Constipation

The efficacy of Amitiza in the treatment of opioid-induced constipation in patients receiving opioid therapy for chronic, non-cancer-related pain was assessed in three randomized, double-blinded, placebo-controlled studies. In Study 1, the median age was 52 years (range 20–82) and 63.1% were female. In Study 2, the median age was 50 years (range 21–77) and 64.4% were female. In Study 3, the median age was 50 years (range 21–89) and 60.1% were female. Patients had been receiving stable opioid therapy for at least 30 days prior to screening, which was to continue throughout the 12-week treatment period. At baseline, mean oral morphine equivalent daily doses (MEDDs) were 99 mg and 130 mg for placebo-treated and Amitiza-treated patients, respectively, in Study 1. Baseline mean MEDDs were 237 mg and 265 mg for placebo-treated and Amitiza-treated patients, respectively, in Study 2. In Study 3, baseline mean MEDDs were 330 mg and 373 mg for placebo-treated and Amitiza-treated patients, respectively. The Brief Pain Inventory-Short Form (BPI-SF) questionnaire was administered to patients at baseline and monthly during the treatment period to assess pain control. Patients had documented opioid-induced constipation at baseline, defined as having less than 3 spontaneous bowel movements (SBMs) per week, with at least 25% of SBMs associated with one or more of the following conditions: (1) hard to very hard stool consistency; (2) moderate to very severe straining; and/or (3) having a sensation of incomplete evacuation. Laxative use was discontinued at the

Table 5: Spontaneous Bowel Movement Frequency Rates* (Efficacy Studies)

Trial	Study Arm	Baseline *Mean ± SD Median*	Week 1 *Mean ± SD Median*	Week 2 *Mean ± SD Median*	Week 3 *Mean ± SD Median*	Week 4 *Mean ± SD Median*	Week 1 Change from Baseline *Mean ± SD Median*	Week 4 Change from Baseline *Mean ± SD Median*
Study 1	Placebo	1.6 ± 1.3 1.5	3.5 ± 2.3 3.0	3.2 ± 2.5 3.0	2.8 ± 2.2 2.0	2.9 ± 2.4 2.3	1.9 ± 2.2 1.5	1.3 ± 2.5 1.0
	Amitiza 24 mcg Twice Daily	1.4 ± 0.8 1.5	5.7 ± 4.4 5.0	5.1 ± 4.1 4.0	5.3 ± 4.9 5.0	5.3 ± 4.7 4.0	4.3 ± 4.3 3.5	3.9 ± 4.6 3.0
Study 2	Placebo	1.5 ± 0.8 1.5	4.0 ± 2.7 3.5	3.6 ± 2.7 3.0	3.4 ± 2.8 3.0	3.5 ± 2.9 3.0	2.5 ± 2.6 1.5	1.9 ± 2.7 1.5
	Amitiza 24 mcg Twice Daily	1.3 ± 0.9 1.5	5.9 ± 4.0 5.0	5.0 ± 4.2 4.0	5.6 ± 4.6 5.0	5.4 ± 4.8 4.3	4.6 ± 4.1 3.8	4.1 ± 4.8 3.0

* Frequency rates are calculated as 7 times (number of SBMs) / (number of days observed for that week).

beginning of the screening period and throughout the study. With the exception of the 48-hour period prior to first dose and for at least 72 hours (Study 1) or 1 week (Study 2 and Study 3) following first dose, use of rescue medication was allowed in cases where no bowel movement had occurred in a 3-day period. Median weekly SBM frequencies at baseline were 1.5 for placebo patients and 1.0 for Amitiza patients in Study 1 and, for both Study 2 and Study 3, median weekly SBM frequencies at baseline were 1.5 for both treatment groups.

In Study 1, patients receiving non-diphenylheptane (e.g., non-methadone) opioids (n = 431) were randomized to receive placebo (n = 217) or Amitiza 24 mcg twice daily (n = 214) for 12 weeks. The primary efficacy analysis was a comparison of the proportion of "overall responders" in each treatment arm. A patient was considered an "overall responder" if ≥1 SBM improvement over baseline were reported for all treatment weeks for which data were available *and* ≥3 SBMs/week were reported for at least 9 of 12 treatment weeks. The proportion of patients in Study 1 qualifying as an "overall responder" was 27.1% in the group receiving Amitiza 24 mcg twice daily compared to 18.9% of patients receiving placebo twice daily (treatment difference = 8.2%; p-value = 0.03). Examination of gender and race subgroups did not identify differences in response to Amitiza among these subgroups. There were too few elderly patients (≥ 65 years of age) to adequately assess differences in effects in that population.

In Study 2, patients receiving opioids (N = 418) were randomized to receive placebo (n = 208) or Amitiza 24 mcg twice daily (n = 210) for 12 weeks. Study 2 did not exclude patients receiving diphenylheptane opioids (e.g., methadone). The primary efficacy endpoint was the mean change from baseline in SBM frequency at Week 8; 3.3 vs. 2.4 for Amitiza and placebo-treated patients, respectively; treatment difference = 0.9; p-value = 0.004. The proportion of patients in Study 2 qualifying as an "overall responder," as prespecified in Study 1, was 24.3% in the group receiving Amitiza compared to 15.4% of patients receiving placebo. In the subgroup of patients in Study 2 taking diphenylheptane opioids (baseline mean [median] MEDDs of 691 [403] mg and 672 [450] mg for placebo and Amitiza patients, respectively), the proportion of patients qualifying as an "overall responder" was 20.5% (8/39) in the group receiving Amitiza compared to 6.3% (2/32) of patients receiving placebo. Examination of gender and race subgroups did not identify differences in response to Amitiza among these subgroups. There were too few elderly patients (≥ 65 years of age) to adequately assess differences in effects in that population.

In Study 3, patients receiving opioids (N = 451) were randomized to placebo (n = 216) or Amitiza 24 mcg twice daily (n = 235) for 12 weeks. Study 3 did not exclude patients receiving diphenylheptane opioids (e.g., methadone). The primary efficacy endpoint was the change from baseline in SBM frequency at Week 8. The study did not demonstrate a statistically significant improvement in SBM frequency rates at Week 8 (mean change from baseline of 2.7 vs. 2.5 for Amitiza and placebo-treated patients, respectively; treatment difference = 0.2; p-value = 0.76). The proportion of patients in Study 3 qualifying as an "overall responder," as prespecified in Study 1, was 15.3% in the patients receiving Amitiza compared to 13.0% of patients receiving placebo. In the subgroup of patients in Study 3 taking diphenylheptane opioids (baseline mean [median] MEDDs of 730 [518] mg and 992 [480] mg for placebo and Amitiza patients, respectively), the proportion of patients qualifying as an "overall responder" was 2.1% (1/47) in the group receiving Amitiza compared to 12.2% (5/41) of patients receiving placebo.

14.3 Irritable Bowel Syndrome with Constipation

Two double-blinded, placebo-controlled studies of similar design were conducted in patients with IBS-C. IBS was defined as abdominal pain or discomfort occurring over at least 6 months with two or more of the following: 1) relieved with defecation; 2) onset associated with a change in stool frequency; and 3) onset associated with a change in stool form. Patients were sub-typed as having IBS-C if they also experienced two of three of the following: 1) < 3 spontaneous bowel movements (SBMs) per week, 2) > 25% hard stools, and 3) > 25% SBMs associated with straining.

Following a 4-week baseline/washout period, a total of 1154 patients (mean age 46.6 [range 18–85] years; 91.6% female; 77.4% Caucasian, 13.2% African American, 8.5% Hispanic, 0.4% Asian; 8.3% ≥ 65 years of age) were randomized and received Amitiza 8 mcg twice daily (16 mcg/day) or placebo twice daily for 12 weeks. The primary efficacy endpoint was assessed weekly utilizing the patient's response to a global symptom relief question based on a 7-point, balanced scale ("significantly worse" to "significantly relieved"): "How would you rate your relief of IBS symptoms (abdominal discomfort/pain, bowel habits, and other IBS symptoms) over the past week compared to how you felt before you entered the study?"

The primary efficacy analysis was a comparison of the proportion of "overall responders" in each arm. A patient was considered an "overall responder" if the criteria for being designated a "monthly responder" were met in at least 2 of the 3 months on study. A "monthly responder" was defined as a patient who had reported "significantly relieved" for at least 2 weeks of the month or at least "moderately relieved" in all 4 weeks of that month. During each monthly evaluation period, patients reporting "moderately worse" or "significantly worse" relief, an increase in rescue medication use, or those who discontinued due to lack of efficacy, were deemed non-responders.

The percentage of patients in Study 1 qualifying as an "overall responder" was 13.8% in the group receiving Amitiza 8 mcg twice daily compared to 7.8% of patients receiving placebo twice daily. In Study 2, 12.1% of patients in the Amitiza 8 mcg group were "overall responders" versus 5.7% of patients in the placebo group. In both studies, the treatment differences between the placebo and Amitiza groups were statistically significant.

Results in men: The two randomized, placebo-controlled, double-blinded studies comprised 97 (8.4%) male patients, which is insufficient to determine whether men with IBS-C respond differently to Amitiza from women.

During a 4-week randomized withdrawal period following Study 1, patients who received Amitiza during the 12-week treatment period were re-randomized to receive either placebo or to continue treatment with Amitiza. In Amitiza-treated patients who were "overall responders" during Study 1 and who were re-randomized to placebo, SBM frequency rates did not result in worsening compared to baseline.

16 HOW SUPPLIED/STORAGE AND HANDLING

Amitiza is available as an oval, soft gelatin capsule containing 8 mcg or 24 mcg of lubiprostone with "SPI" printed on one side. Amitiza is available as follows:

8 mcg pink capsule
- Bottles of 60 (NDC 64764-080-60)

24 mcg orange capsule
- Bottles of 60 (NDC 64764-240-60)
- Bottles of 100 (NDC 64764-240-10)

Store at 25°C (77°F); excursions permitted to 15° to 30°C (59° to 86°F).

Protect from light and extreme temperatures.

17 PATIENT COUNSELING INFORMATION

Physicians and patients should periodically assess the need for continued therapy.

17.1 Nausea, Dyspnea or Diarrhea

Instruct patients to take Amitiza twice daily with food and water to reduce the occurrence of nausea. Patients taking Amitiza may experience dyspnea within an hour of the first dose. Dyspnea generally resolves within 3 hours, but may recur with repeat dosing. Patients on treatment who experience severe nausea, dyspnea, or diarrhea should notify their physician.

17.2 Nursing Mothers

Advise lactating women to monitor their human milk-fed infants for diarrhea while taking Amitiza [see *Use in Specific Populations (8.3)*].

Marketed by:
Sucampo Pharma Americas, LLC
Bethesda, MD 20814
and
Takeda Pharmaceuticals America, Inc.
Deerfield, IL 60015
Amitiza® is a registered trademark of Sucampo AG.

Shown in Product Identification Guide, page 313

BRINTELLIX ℞
(vortioxetine)
tablets, for oral use

HIGHLIGHTS OF PRESCRIBING INFORMATION
These highlights do not include all the information needed to use BRINTELLIX safely and effectively. See full prescribing information for BRINTELLIX.
BRINTELLIX (vortioxetine) tablets, for oral use
Initial U.S. Approval: 2013

WARNING: SUICIDAL THOUGHTS AND BEHAVIORS
See full prescribing information for complete boxed warning.
- **Increased risk of suicidal thinking and behavior in children, adolescents, and young adults taking antidepressants (5.1).**
- **Monitor for worsening and emergence of suicidal thoughts and behaviors (5.1).**
- **BRINTELLIX has not been evaluated for use in pediatric patients (8.4).**

INDICATIONS AND USAGE

BRINTELLIX is indicated for the treatment of major depressive disorder (MDD) (1,14).

DOSAGE AND ADMINISTRATION
- The recommended starting dose is 10 mg administered orally once daily without regard to meals (2.1).
- The dose should then be increased to 20 mg/day, as tolerated (2.1).
- Consider 5 mg/day for patients who do not tolerate higher doses (2.1).
- BRINTELLIX can be discontinued abruptly. However, it is recommended that doses of 15 mg/day or 20 mg/day be reduced to 10 mg/day for one week prior to full discontinuation if possible (2.3).
- The maximum recommended dose is 10 mg/day in known CYP2D6 poor metabolizers (2.6).

DOSAGE FORMS AND STRENGTHS

BRINTELLIX is available as 5 mg, 10 mg, 15 mg, and 20 mg immediate release tablets (3).

CONTRAINDICATIONS
- Hypersensitivity to vortioxetine or any components of the BRINTELLIX formulation (4).
- Monoamine Oxidase Inhibitors (MAOIs): Do not use MAOIs intended to treat psychiatric disorders with BRINTELLIX or within 21 days of stopping treatment with BRINTELLIX. Do not use BRINTELLIX within 14 days of stopping an MAOI intended to treat psychiatric disorders. In addition, do not start BRINTELLIX in a patient who is being treated with linezolid or intravenous methylene blue (4).

WARNINGS AND PRECAUTIONS
- Serotonin Syndrome has been reported with serotonergic antidepressants (SSRIs, SNRIs, and others), including

with BRINTELLIX, both when taken alone, but especially when co-administered with other serotonergic agents (including triptans, tricyclic antidepressants, fentanyl, lithium, tramadol, tryptophan, buspirone, and St. John's Wort). If such symptoms occur, discontinue BRINTELLIX and initiate supportive treatment. If concomitant use of BRINTELLIX with other serotonergic drugs is clinically warranted, patients should be made aware of a potential increased risk for serotonin syndrome, particularly during treatment initiation and dose increases (5.2).
- Treatment with serotonergic antidepressants (SSRIs, SNRIs, and others) may increase the risk of abnormal bleeding. Patients should be cautioned about the increased risk of bleeding when BRINTELLIX is coadministered with nonsteroidal anti-inflammatory drugs (NSAIDs), aspirin, or other drugs that affect coagulation (5.3).
- Activation of Mania/Hypomania can occur with antidepressant treatment. Screen patients for bipolar disorder (5.4).
- Hyponatremia can occur in association with the syndrome of inappropriate antidiuretic hormone secretion (SIADH) (5.5).

ADVERSE REACTIONS

Most common adverse reactions (incidence ≥5% and at least twice the rate of placebo) were: nausea, constipation and vomiting (6).

To report SUSPECTED ADVERSE REACTIONS, contact Takeda Pharmaceuticals at 1-877-TAKEDA-7 (1-877-825-3327) or FDA at 1-800-FDA-1088 or www.fda.gov/medwatch.

DRUG INTERACTIONS

- Strong inhibitors of CYP2D6: Reduce BRINTELLIX dose by half when a strong CYP2D6 inhibitor (e.g., bupropion, fluoxetine, paroxetine, or quinidine) is coadministered (2.6 and 7.3).
- Strong CYP Inducers: Consider increasing BRINTELLIX dose when a strong CYP inducer (e.g., rifampin, carbamazepine, or phenytoin) is coadministered for more than 14 days. The maximum recommended dose should not exceed 3 times the original dose (2.7 and 7.3).

USE IN SPECIFIC POPULATIONS

- Pregnancy: Based on animal data, BRINTELLIX may cause fetal harm (8.1).
- Nursing Mothers: Discontinue BRINTELLIX or nursing (8.3).

See 17 for PATIENT COUNSELING INFORMATION and Medication Guide

Revised: 09/2013

FULL PRESCRIBING INFORMATION: CONTENTS*

*** Sections or subsections omitted from the full prescribing information are not listed**

FULL PRESCRIBING INFORMATION

WARNING: SUICIDAL THOUGHTS AND BEHAVIORS

Antidepressants increased the risk of suicidal thoughts and behavior in children, adolescents, and young adults in short-term studies. These studies did not show an increase in the risk of suicidal thoughts and behavior with antidepressant use in patients over age 24; there was a trend toward reduced risk with antidepressant use in patients aged 65 and older *[see Warnings and Precautions (5.1)]*.

In patients of all ages who are started on antidepressant therapy, monitor closely for worsening, and for emergence of suicidal thoughts and behaviors. Advise families and caregivers of the need for close observation and communication with the prescriber *[see Warnings and Precautions (5.1)]*.

BRINTELLIX has not been evaluated for use in pediatric patients *[see Use in Specific Populations (8.4)]*.

1 INDICATIONS AND USAGE

1.1 Major Depressive Disorder

BRINTELLIX is indicated for the treatment of major depressive disorder (MDD). The efficacy of BRINTELLIX was established in six 6 to 8 week studies (including one study in the elderly) and one maintenance study in adults *[see Clinical Studies (14)]*.

2 DOSAGE AND ADMINISTRATION

2.1 General Instruction for Use

The recommended starting dose is 10 mg administered orally once daily without regard to meals. Dosage should then be increased to 20 mg/day, as tolerated, because higher doses demonstrated better treatment effects in trials conducted in the United States. The efficacy and safety of doses above 20 mg/day have not been evaluated in controlled clinical trials. A dose decrease down to 5 mg/day may be considered for patients who do not tolerate higher doses *[see Clinical Studies (14)]*.

2.2 Maintenance/Continuation/Extended Treatment

It is generally agreed that acute episodes of major depression should be followed by several months or longer of sustained pharmacologic therapy. A maintenance study of BRINTELLIX demonstrated that BRINTELLIX decreased the risk of recurrence of depressive episodes compared to placebo.

2.3 Discontinuing Treatment

Although BRINTELLIX can be abruptly discontinued, in placebo-controlled trials patients experienced transient adverse reactions such as headache and muscle tension following abrupt discontinuation of BRINTELLIX 15 mg/day or 20 mg/day. To avoid these adverse reactions, it is recommended that the dose be decreased to 10 mg/day for one week before full discontinuation of BRINTELLIX 15 mg/day or 20 mg/day *[see Adverse Reactions (6)]*.

2.4 Switching a Patient To or From a Monoamine Oxidase Inhibitor (MAOI) Intended to Treat Psychiatric Disorders

At least 14 days should elapse between discontinuation of a MAOI intended to treat psychiatric disorders and initiation of therapy with BRINTELLIX to avoid the risk of Serotonin Syndrome *[see Warnings and Precautions (5.2)]*. Conversely, at least 21 days should be allowed after stopping BRINTELLIX before starting an MAOI intended to treat psychiatric disorders *[see Contraindications (4)]*.

2.5 Use of BRINTELLIX with Other MAOIs such as Linezolid or Methylene Blue

Do not start BRINTELLIX in a patient who is being treated with linezolid or intravenous methylene blue because there is an increased risk of serotonin syndrome. In a patient who requires more urgent treatment of a psychiatric condition, other interventions, including hospitalization, should be considered *[see Contraindications (4)]*.

In some cases, a patient already receiving BRINTELLIX therapy may require urgent treatment with linezolid or intravenous methylene blue. If acceptable alternatives to linezolid or intravenous methylene blue treatment are not available and the potential benefits of linezolid or intravenous methylene blue treatment are judged to outweigh the risks of serotonin syndrome in a particular patient, BRINTELLIX should be stopped promptly, and linezolid or intravenous methylene blue can be administered. The patient should be monitored for symptoms of serotonin syndrome for 21 days or until 24 hours after the last dose of linezolid or intravenous methylene blue, whichever comes first. Therapy with BRINTELLIX may be resumed 24 hours after the last dose of linezolid or intravenous methylene blue *[see Warnings and Precautions (5.2)]*.

The risk of administering methylene blue by non-intravenous routes (such as oral tablets or by local injection) or in intravenous doses much lower than 1 mg/kg with BRINTELLIX is unclear. The clinician should, nevertheless, be aware of the possibility of emergent symptoms of serotonin syndrome with such use *[see Warnings and Precautions (5.2)]*.

2.6 Use of BRINTELLIX in Known CYP2D6 Poor Metabolizers or in Patients Taking Strong CYP2D6 Inhibitors

The maximum recommended dose of BRINTELLIX is 10 mg/day in known CYP2D6 poor metabolizers. Reduce the dose of BRINTELLIX by one half when patients are receiving a CYP2D6 strong inhibitor (e.g., bupropion, fluoxetine, paroxetine, or quinidine) concomitantly. The dose should be increased to the original level when the CYP2D6 inhibitor is discontinued *[see Drug Interactions (7.3)]*.

2.7 Use of BRINTELLIX in Patients Taking Strong CYP Inducers

Consider increasing the dose of BRINTELLIX when a strong CYP inducer (e.g., rifampin, carbamazepine, or phenytoin) is coadministered for greater than 14 days. The maximum recommended dose should not exceed three times the original dose. The dose of BRINTELLIX should be reduced to the original level within 14 days, when the inducer is discontinued *[see Drug Interactions (7.3)]*.

3 DOSAGE FORMS AND STRENGTHS

BRINTELLIX is available as immediate-release, film-coated tablets in the following strengths:
- 5 mg: pink, almond shaped biconvex film coated tablet, debossed with "5" on one side and "TL" on the other side
- 10 mg: yellow, almond shaped biconvex film coated tablet, debossed with "10" on one side and "TL" on the other side
- 15 mg: orange, almond shaped biconvex film coated tablet, debossed with "15" on one side and "TL" on the other side
- 20 mg: red, almond shaped biconvex film coated tablet, debossed with "20" on one side and "TL" on the other side

4 CONTRAINDICATIONS

- Hypersensitivity to vortioxetine or any components of the formulation. Angioedema has been reported in patients treated with BRINTELLIX.
- The use of MAOIs intended to treat psychiatric disorders with BRINTELLIX or within 21 days of stopping treatment with BRINTELLIX is contraindicated because of an increased risk of serotonin syndrome. The use of BRINTELLIX within 14 days of stopping an MAOI intended to treat psychiatric disorders is also contraindicated *[see Dosage and Administration (2.4) and Warnings and Precautions (5.2)]*.

Starting BRINTELLIX in a patient who is being treated with MAOIs such as linezolid or intravenous methylene blue is also contraindicated because of an increased risk of serotonin syndrome *[see Dosage and Administration (2.5) and Warnings and Precautions (5.2)]*.

5 WARNINGS AND PRECAUTIONS

5.1 Clinical Worsening and Suicide Risk

Patients with major depressive disorder (MDD), both adult and pediatric, may experience worsening of their depression and/or the emergence of suicidal ideation and behavior (suicidality) or unusual changes in behavior, whether or not they are taking antidepressant medications, and this risk may persist until significant remission occurs. Suicide is a known risk of depression and certain other psychiatric disorders, and these disorders themselves are the strongest predictors of suicide. There has been a long-standing concern, however, that antidepressants may have a role in inducing worsening of depression and the emergence of suicidality in certain patients during the early phases of treatment. Pooled analyses of short-term placebo-controlled studies of antidepressant drugs (selective serotonin reuptake inhibitors [SSRIs] and others) showed that these drugs increase the risk of suicidal thinking and behavior (suicidality) in children, adolescents, and young adults (ages 18 to 24) with MDD and other psychiatric disorders. Short-term studies did not show an increase in the risk of suicidality with antidepressants compared to placebo in adults beyond age 24; there was a trend toward reduction with antidepressants compared to placebo in adults aged 65 and older.

The pooled analyses of placebo-controlled studies in children and adolescents with MDD, obsessive compulsive disorder (OCD), or other psychiatric disorders included a total of 24 short-term studies of nine antidepressant drugs in over 4,400 patients. The pooled analyses of placebo-controlled studies in adults with MDD or other psychiatric disorders included a total of 295 short-term studies (median duration of two months) of 11 antidepressant drugs in over 77,000 patients. There was considerable variation in risk of suicidality among drugs, but a tendency toward an increase in the younger patients for almost all drugs studied. There were differences in absolute risk of suicidality across the different indications, with the highest incidence in MDD. The risk differences (drug vs. placebo), however, were relatively stable within age strata and across indications. These risk differences (drug-placebo difference in the number of cases of suicidality per 1000 patients treated) are provided in *Table 1.*

Table 1. Drug-Placebo Difference in Number of Cases of Suicidality per 1000 Patients Treated

Age Range	
Increases Compared to Placebo	
<18	14 additional cases
18-24	5 additional cases
Decreases Compared to Placebo	
25-64	1 fewer case
≥65	6 fewer cases

No suicides occurred in any of the pediatric studies. There were suicides in the adult studies, but the number was not sufficient to reach any conclusion about drug effect on suicide. It is unknown whether the suicidality risk extends to longer-term use, i.e., beyond several months. However, there is substantial evidence from placebo-controlled maintenance studies in adults with depression that the use of antidepressants can delay the recurrence of depression.

All patients being treated with antidepressants for any indication should be monitored appropriately and observed closely for clinical worsening, suicidality, and unusual changes in behavior, especially during the initial few months of a course of drug therapy, or at times of dose changes, either increases or decreases.

The following symptoms anxiety, agitation, panic attacks, insomnia, irritability, hostility, aggressiveness, impulsivity, akathisia (psychomotor restlessness), hypomania, and mania have been reported in adult and pediatric patients being treated with antidepressants for MDD as well as for other indications, both psychiatric and nonpsychiatric. Although a causal link between the emergence of such symptoms and either the worsening of depression and/or the emergence of suicidal impulses has not been established, there is concern that such symptoms may represent precursors to emerging suicidality.

Consideration should be given to changing the therapeutic regimen, including possibly discontinuing the medication, in patients whose depression is persistently worse, or who are experiencing emergent suicidality or symptoms that might be precursors to worsening depression or suicidality, especially if these symptoms are severe, abrupt in onset, or were not part of the patient's presenting symptoms.

Families and caregivers of patients being treated with antidepressants for MDD or other indications, both psychiatric and nonpsychiatric, should be alerted about the need to monitor patients for the emergence of agitation, irritability, unusual changes in behavior, and the other symptoms described above, as well as the emergence of suicidality, and to report such symptoms immediately to healthcare providers. Such monitoring should include daily observation by families and caregivers.

Screening Patients for Bipolar Disorder

A major depressive episode may be the initial presentation of bipolar disorder. It is generally believed (though not established in controlled studies) that treating such an episode with an antidepressant alone may increase the likelihood of precipitation of a mixed/manic episode in patients at risk for bipolar disorder. Whether any of the symptoms described above represent such a conversion is unknown. However, prior to initiating treatment with an antidepressant, patients with depressive symptoms should be adequately screened to determine if they are at risk for bipolar disorder; such screening should include a detailed psychiatric history, including a family history of suicide, bipolar disorder, and depression. It should be noted that BRINTELLIX is not approved for use in treating bipolar depression.

5.2 Serotonin Syndrome

The development of a potentially life-threatening serotonin syndrome has been reported with serotonergic antidepressants including BRINTELLIX, when used alone but more often when used concomitantly with other serotonergic drugs (including triptans, tricyclic antidepressants, fentanyl, lithium, tramadol, tryptophan, buspirone, and St. John's Wort), and with drugs that impair metabolism of serotonin (in particular, MAOIs, both those intended to treat psychiatric disorders and also others, such as linezolid and intravenous methylene blue).

Serotonin syndrome symptoms may include mental status changes (e.g., agitation, hallucinations, delirium, and coma), autonomic instability (e.g., tachycardia, labile blood pressure, dizziness, diaphoresis, flushing, hyperthermia), neuromuscular symptoms (e.g., tremor, rigidity, myoclonus, hyperreflexia, incoordination), seizures, and/or gastrointestinal symptoms (e.g., nausea, vomiting, diarrhea). Patients should be monitored for the emergence of serotonin syndrome.

The concomitant use of BRINTELLIX with MAOIs intended to treat psychiatric disorders is contraindicated. BRINTELLIX should also not be started in a patient who is being treated with MAOIs such as linezolid or intravenous methylene blue. All reports with methylene blue that provided information on the route of administration involved intravenous administration in the dose range of 1 mg/kg to 8 mg/kg. No reports involved the administration of methylene blue by other routes (such as oral tablets or local tissue injection) or at lower doses. There may be circumstances when it is necessary to initiate treatment with a MAOI such as linezolid or intravenous methylene blue in a patient taking BRINTELLIX. BRINTELLIX should be discontinued before initiating treatment with the MAOI *[see Contraindications (4) and Dosage and Administration (2.4)]*.

If concomitant use of BRINTELLIX with other serotonergic drugs, including triptans, tricyclic antidepressants, fentanyl, lithium, tramadol, buspirone, tryptophan, and St. John's Wort is clinically warranted, patients should be made aware of a potential increased risk for serotonin syndrome, particularly during treatment initiation and dose increases. Treatment with BRINTELLIX and any concomitant serotonergic agents should be discontinued immediately if the above events occur and supportive symptomatic treatment should be initiated.

5.3 Abnormal Bleeding

The use of drugs that interfere with serotonin reuptake inhibition, including BRINTELLIX, may increase the risk of bleeding events. Concomitant use of aspirin, nonsteroidal anti-inflammatory drugs (NSAIDs), warfarin, and other anticoagulants may add to this risk. Case reports and epidemiological studies (case-control and cohort design) have demonstrated an association between use of drugs that interfere with serotonin reuptake and the occurrence of gastrointestinal bleeding. Bleeding events related to drugs that inhibit serotonin reuptake have ranged from ecchymosis, hematoma, epistaxis, and petechiae to life-threatening hemorrhages.

Patients should be cautioned about the increased risk of bleeding when BRINTELLIX is coadministered with NSAIDs, aspirin, or other drugs that affect coagulation or bleeding *[see Drug Interactions (7.2)]*.

5.4 Activation of Mania/Hypomania

Symptoms of mania/hypomania were reported in <0.1% of patients treated with BRINTELLIX in pre-marketing clinical studies. Activation of mania/hypomania has been reported in a small proportion of patients with major affective disorder who were treated with other antidepressants. As with all antidepressants, use BRINTELLIX cautiously in patients with a history or family history of bipolar disorder, mania, or hypomania.

5.5 Hyponatremia

Hyponatremia has occurred as a result of treatment with serotonergic drugs. In many cases, hyponatremia appears to be the result of the syndrome of inappropriate antidiuretic hormone secretion (SIADH). One case with serum sodium lower than 110 mmol/L was reported in a subject treated with BRINTELLIX in a pre-marketing clinical study. Elderly patients may be at greater risk of developing hyponatremia with a serotonergic antidepressant. Also, patients taking diuretics or who are otherwise volume depleted can be at greater risk. Discontinuation of BRINTELLIX in patients with symptomatic hyponatremia and appropriate medical intervention should be instituted. Signs and symptoms of hyponatremia include headache, difficulty concentrating, memory impairment, confusion, weakness, and unsteadiness, which can lead to falls. More severe and/or acute cases have included hallucination, syncope, seizure, coma, respiratory arrest, and death.

6 ADVERSE REACTIONS

The following adverse reactions are discussed in greater detail in other sections of the label.

- Hypersensitivity *[see Contraindications (4)]*
- Clinical Worsening and Suicide Risk *[see Warnings and Precautions (5.1)]*
- Serotonin Syndrome *[see Warnings and Precautions (5.2)]*
- Abnormal Bleeding *[see Warnings and Precautions (5.3)]*
- Activation of Mania/Hypomania *[see Warnings and Precautions (5.4)]*
- Hyponatremia *[see Warnings and Precautions (5.5)]*

6.1 Clinical Studies Experience

Because clinical trials are conducted under widely varying conditions, adverse reaction rates observed in the clinical trials of a drug cannot be directly compared to rates in the clinical studies of another drug and may not reflect the rates observed in clinical practice.

Patient Exposure

BRINTELLIX was evaluated for safety in 4746 patients (18 years to 88 years of age) diagnosed with MDD who participated in pre-marketing clinical studies; 2616 of those patients were exposed to BRINTELLIX in 6 to 8 week, placebo-controlled studies at doses ranging from 5 mg to

Table 2. Common Adverse Reactions Occurring in ≥2% of Patients Treated with any BRINTELLIX Dose and at Least 2% Greater than the Incidence in Placebo-treated Patients

System Organ Class Preferred Term	BRINTELLIX 5 mg/day	BRINTELLIX 10 mg/day	BRINTELLIX 15 mg/day	BRINTELLIX 20 mg/day	Placebo
	N=1013 %	N=699 %	N=449 %	N=455 %	N=1621 %
Gastrointestinal disorders					
Nausea	21	26	32	32	9
Diarrhea	7	7	10	7	6
Dry mouth	7	7	6	8	6
Constipation	3	5	6	6	3
Vomiting	3	5	6	6	1
Flatulence	1	3	2	1	1
Nervous system disorders					
Dizziness	6	6	8	9	6
Psychiatric disorders					
Abnormal dreams	<1	<1	2	3	1
Skin and subcutaneous tissue disorders					
Pruritus*	1	2	3	3	1

*includes pruritus generalized

Table 3. ASEX Incidence of Treatment Emergent Sexual Dysfunction*

	BRINTELLIX 5 mg/day N=65:67†	BRINTELLIX 10 mg/day N=94:86†	BRINTELLIX 15 mg/day N=57:67†	BRINTELLIX 20 mg/day N=67:59†	Placebo N=135:162†
Females	22%	23%	33%	34%	20%
Males	16%	20%	19%	29%	14%

*Incidence based on number of subjects with sexual dysfunction during the study / number of subjects without sexual dysfunction at baseline. Sexual dysfunction was defined as a subject scoring any of the following on the ASEX scale at two consecutive visits during the study: 1) total score ≥19; 2) any single item ≥5; 3) three or more items each with a score ≥4

†Sample size for each dose group is the number of patients (females:males) without sexual dysfunction at baseline

Figure 1. Impact of Other Drugs on Vortioxetine PK

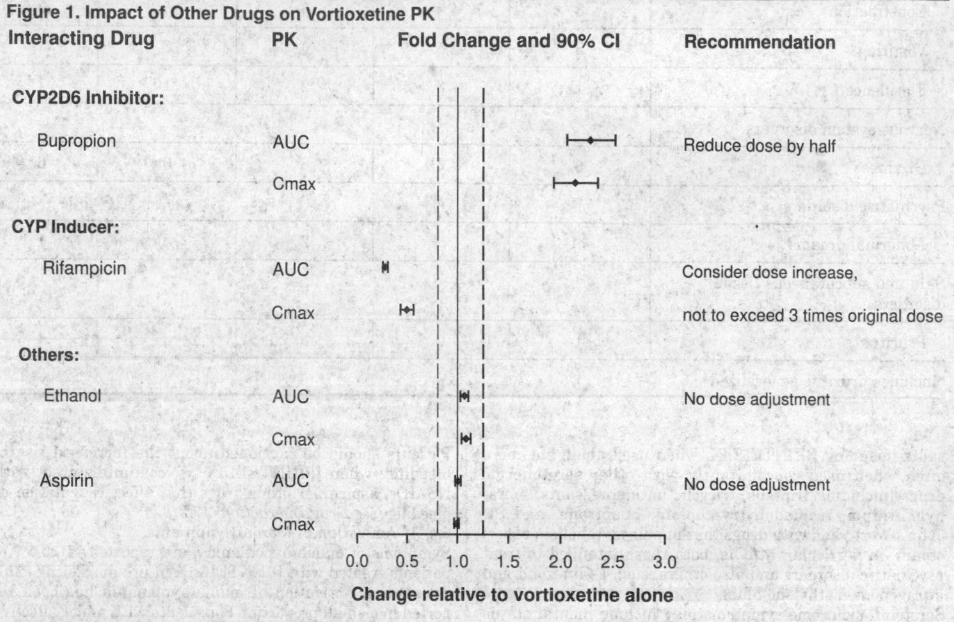

20 mg once daily and 204 patients were exposed to BRINTELLIX in a 24 week to 64 week placebo-controlled maintenance study at doses of 5 mg to 10 mg once daily. Patients from the 6 to 8 week studies continued into 12-month open-label studies. A total of 2586 patients were exposed to at least one dose of BRINTELLIX in open-label studies, 1727 were exposed to BRINTELLIX for six months and 885 were exposed for at least one year.

Adverse Reactions Reported as Reasons for Discontinuation of Treatment

In pooled 6 to 8 week placebo-controlled studies the incidence of patients who received BRINTELLIX 5 mg/day, 10 mg/day, 15 mg/day and 20 mg/day and discontinued treatment because of an adverse reaction was 5%, 6%, 8% and 8%, respectively, compared to 4% of placebo-treated patients. Nausea was the most common adverse reaction reported as a reason for discontinuation.

Common Adverse Reactions in Placebo-Controlled MDD Studies

The most commonly observed adverse reactions in MDD patients treated with BRINTELLIX in 6 to 8 week placebo-controlled studies (incidence ≥5% and at least twice the rate of placebo) were nausea, constipation and vomiting.

Table 2 shows the incidence of common adverse reactions that occurred in ≥2% of MDD patients treated with any BRINTELLIX dose and at least 2% more frequently than in placebo-treated patients in the 6 to 8 week placebo-controlled studies.

[See table 2 at top of previous page]

Nausea

Nausea was the most common adverse reaction and its frequency was dose-related *(Table 2)*. It was usually considered mild or moderate in intensity and the median duration was 2 weeks. Nausea was more common in females than males. Nausea most commonly occurred in the first week of BRINTELLIX treatment with 15 to 20% of patients experiencing nausea after 1 to 2 days of treatment. Approximately 10% of patients taking BRINTELLIX 10 mg/day to 20 mg/day had nausea at the end of the 6 to 8 week placebo-controlled studies.

Sexual Dysfunction

Difficulties in sexual desire, sexual performance and sexual satisfaction often occur as manifestations of psychiatric disorders, but they may also be consequences of pharmacologic treatment.

In the MDD 6 to 8 week controlled trials of BRINTELLIX, voluntarily reported adverse reactions related to sexual dysfunction were captured as individual event terms. These event terms have been aggregated and the overall incidence was as follows. In male patients the overall incidence was 3%, 4%, 4%, 5% in BRINTELLIX 5 mg/day, 10 mg/day, 15 mg/day, 20 mg/day, respectively, compared to 2% in placebo. In female patients, the overall incidence was <1%, 1%, <1%, 2% in BRINTELLIX 5 mg/day, 10 mg/day, 15 mg/day, 20 mg/day, respectively, compared to <1% in placebo.

Because voluntarily reported adverse sexual reactions are known to be underreported, in part because patients and physicians may be reluctant to discuss them, the Arizona Sexual Experiences Scale (ASEX), a validated measure designed to identify sexual side effects, was used prospectively in seven placebo-controlled trials. The ASEX scale includes five questions that pertain to the following aspects of sexual function: 1) sex drive, 2) ease of arousal, 3) ability to achieve erection (men) or lubrication (women), 4) ease of reaching orgasm, and 5) orgasm satisfaction.

The presence or absence of sexual dysfunction among patients entering clinical studies was based on their ASEX scores. For patients without sexual dysfunction at baseline (approximately 1/3 of the population across all treatment groups in each study), *Table 3* shows the incidence of patients that developed treatment-emergent sexual dysfunction when treated with BRINTELLIX or placebo in any fixed dose group. Physicians should routinely inquire about possible sexual side effects.

[See table 3 above]

Adverse Reactions Following Abrupt Discontinuation of BRINTELLIX Treatment

Discontinuation symptoms have been prospectively evaluated in patients taking BRINTELLIX 10 mg/day, 15 mg/day, and 20 mg/day using the Discontinuation-Emergent Signs and Symptoms (DESS) scale in clinical trials. Some patients experienced discontinuation symptoms such as headache, muscle tension, mood swings, sudden outbursts of anger, dizziness, and runny nose in the first week of abrupt discontinuation of BRINTELLIX 15 mg/day and 20 mg/day.

Laboratory Tests

BRINTELLIX has not been associated with any clinically important changes in laboratory test parameters in serum chemistry (except sodium), hematology and urinalysis as measured in the 6 to 8 week placebo-controlled studies. Hyponatremia has been reported with the treatment of BRINTELLIX *[see Warnings and Precautions (5.5)]*. In the 6-month, double-blind, placebo-controlled phase of a long-term study in patients who had responded to BRINTELLIX during the initial 12-week, open-label phase, there were no clinically important changes in lab test parameters between BRINTELLIX and placebo-treated patients.

Weight

BRINTELLIX had no significant effect on body weight as measured by the mean change from baseline in the 6 to 8 week placebo-controlled studies. In the 6-month, double-blind, placebo-controlled phase of a long-term study in patients who had responded to BRINTELLIX during the initial 12-week, open-label phase, there was no significant effect on body weight between BRINTELLIX and placebo-treated patients.

Vital Signs

BRINTELLIX has not been associated with any clinically significant effects on vital signs, including systolic and diastolic blood pressure and heart rate, as measured in placebo-controlled studies.

Other Adverse Reactions Observed in Clinical Studies

The following listing does not include reactions: 1) already listed in previous tables or elsewhere in labeling, 2) for which a drug cause was remote, 3) which were so general as to be uninformative, 4) which were not considered to have significant clinical implications, or 5) which occurred at a rate equal to or less than placebo.

Ear and labyrinth disorders — vertigo
Gastrointestinal disorders — dyspepsia
Nervous system disorders — dysgeusia
Vascular disorders — flushing

7 DRUG INTERACTIONS

7.1 CNS Active Agents

Monoamine Oxidase Inhibitors

Adverse reactions, some of which are serious or fatal, can develop in patients who use MAOIs or who have recently been discontinued from an MAOI and started on a serotonergic antidepressant(s) or who have recently had SSRI or SNRI therapy discontinued prior to initiation of an MAOI *[see Dosage and Administration (2.4), Contraindications (4) and Warnings and Precautions (5.2)]*.

Serotonergic Drugs

Based on the mechanism of action of BRINTELLIX and the potential for serotonin toxicity, serotonin syndrome may occur when BRINTELLIX is coadministered with other drugs that may affect the serotonergic neurotransmitter systems (e.g., SSRIs, SNRIs, triptans, buspirone, tramadol, and tryptophan products etc.). Closely monitor symptoms of serotonin syndrome if BRINTELLIX is co-administered with other serotonergic drugs. Treatment with BRINTELLIX and any concomitant serotonergic agents should be discontinued immediately if serotonin syndrome occurs *[see Warnings and Precautions (5.2)]*.

Other CNS Active Agents

No clinically relevant effect was observed on steady state lithium exposure following coadministration with multiple daily doses of BRINTELLIX. Multiple doses of BRINTELLIX did not affect the pharmacokinetics or pharmacodynamics (composite cognitive score) of diazepam. A clinical study has shown that BRINTELLIX (single dose of 20 or 40 mg) did not increase the impairment of mental and motor skills caused by alcohol (single dose of 0.6 g/kg). Details on the potential pharmacokinetic interactions between BRINTELLIX and bupropion can be found in Section 7.3.

7.2 Drugs that Interfere with Hemostasis (e.g., NSAIDs, Aspirin, and Warfarin)

Serotonin release by platelets plays an important role in hemostasis. Epidemiological studies of case-control and cohort design have demonstrated an association between use of psychotropic drugs that interfere with serotonin reuptake and the occurrence of upper gastrointestinal bleeding. These studies have also shown that concurrent use of an NSAID or aspirin may potentiate this risk of bleeding. Altered anticoagulant effects, including increased bleeding, have been reported when SSRIs and SNRIs are coadministered with warfarin.

Following coadministration of stable doses of warfarin (1 to 10 mg/day) with multiple daily doses of BRINTELLIX, no significant effects were observed in INR, prothrombin values or total warfarin (protein bound plus free drug) pharmacokinetics for both R- and S-warfarin *[see Drug Interactions (7.4)]*. Coadministration of aspirin 150 mg/day with multiple daily doses of BRINTELLIX had no significant inhibitory effect on platelet aggregation or pharmacokinetics of aspirin and salicylic acid *[(see Drug Interactions (7.4)]*. Patients receiving other drugs that interfere with hemostasis should be carefully monitored when BRINTELLIX is initiated or discontinued *[see Warnings and Precautions (5.3)]*.

7.3 Potential for Other Drugs to Affect BRINTELLIX

Reduce BRINTELLIX dose by half when a strong CYP2D6 inhibitor (e.g., bupropion, fluoxetine, paroxetine, quinidine)

is coadministered. Consider increasing the BRINTELLIX dose when a strong CYP inducer (e.g., rifampicin, carbamazepine, phenytoin) is coadministered. The maximum dose is not recommended to exceed three times the original dose *[see Dosage and Administration (2.5 and 2.6)]* (*Figure 1*).

[See figure 1 at top of previous page]

7.4 Potential for BRINTELLIX to Affect Other Drugs

No dose adjustment for the comedications is needed when BRINTELLIX is coadministered with a substrate of CYP1A2 (e.g., duloxetine), CYP2A6, CYP2B6 (e.g., bupropion), CYP2C8 (e.g., repaglinid), CYP2C9 (e.g., S-warfarin), CYP2C19 (e.g., diazepam), CYP2D6 (e.g., venlafaxine), CYP3A4/5 (e.g., budesonide), and P-gp (e.g., digoxin). In addition, no dose adjustment for lithium, aspirin, and warfarin is necessary.

Vortioxetine and its metabolites are unlikely to inhibit the following CYP enzymes and transporter based on *in vitro* data: CYP1A2, CYP2A6, CYP2B6, CYP2C8, CYP2C9, CYP2C19, CYP2D6, CYP2E1, CYP3A4/5, and P-gp. As such, no clinically relevant interactions with drugs metabolized by these CYP enzymes would be expected.

In addition, vortioxetine did not induce CYP1A2, CYP2A6, CYP2B6, CYP2C8, CYP2C9, CYP2C19, and CYP3A4/5 in an *in vitro* study in cultured human hepatocytes. Chronic administration of BRINTELLIX is unlikely to induce the metabolism of drugs metabolized by these CYP isoforms. Furthermore, in a series of clinical drug interaction studies, coadministration of BRINTELLIX with substrates for CYP2B6 (e.g., bupropion), CYP2C9 (e.g., warfarin), and CYP2C19 (e.g., diazepam), had no clinical meaningful effect on the pharmacokinetics of these substrates *(Figure 2)*.

Because vortioxetine is highly bound to plasma protein, coadministration of BRINTELLIX with another drug that is highly protein bound may increase free concentrations of the other drug. However, in a clinical study with coadministration of BRINTELLIX (10 mg/day) and warfarin (1 mg/day to 10 mg/day), a highly protein-bound drug, no significant change in INR was observed *[see Drug Interactions (7.2)]*.

[See figure 2 above]

Figure 2. Impact of Vortioxetine on PK of Other Drugs

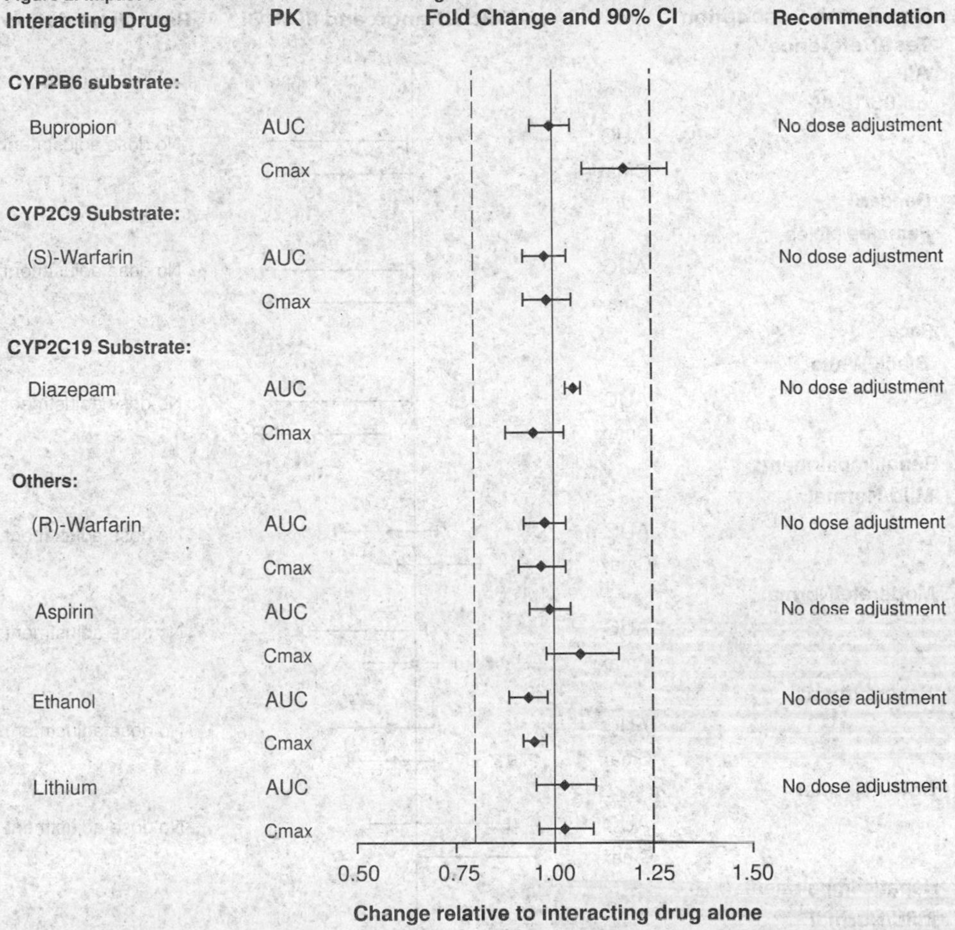

8 USE IN SPECIFIC POPULATIONS

8.1 Pregnancy

Pregnancy Category C

Risk Summary

There are no adequate and well-controlled studies of BRINTELLIX in pregnant women. Vortioxetine caused developmental delays when administered during pregnancy to rats and rabbits at doses 15 and 10 times the maximum recommended human dose (MRHD) of 20 mg, respectively. Developmental delays were also seen after birth in rats at doses 20 times the MRHD of vortioxetine given during pregnancy and through lactation. There were no teratogenic effects in rats or rabbits at doses up to 77 and 58 times, the MRHD of vortioxetine, respectively, given during organogenesis. The incidence of malformations in human pregnancies has not been established for BRINTELLIX. All human pregnancies, regardless of drug exposure, have a background rate of 2 to 4% for major malformations, and 15 to 20% for pregnancy loss. BRINTELLIX should be used during pregnancy only if the potential benefit justifies the potential risk to the fetus.

Clinical Considerations

Neonates exposed to SSRIs or SNRIs, late in the third trimester have developed complications requiring prolonged hospitalization, respiratory support and tube feeding. Such complications can arise immediately upon delivery. Reported clinical findings have included respiratory distress, cyanosis, apnea, seizures, temperature instability, feeding difficulty, vomiting, hypoglycemia, hypotonia, hypertonia, hyperreflexia, tremor, jitteriness, irritability and constant crying. These features are consistent with either a direct toxic effect of these classes of drugs or possibly, a drug discontinuation syndrome. It should be noted that in some cases, the clinical picture is consistent with serotonin syndrome *[see Warnings and Precautions 5.2]*. When treating a pregnant woman with BRINTELLIX during the third trimester, the physician should carefully consider the potential risks and benefits of treatment.

Neonates exposed to SSRIs in pregnancy may have an increased risk for persistent pulmonary hypertension of the newborn (PPHN). PPHN occurs in one to two per 1,000 live births in the general population and is associated with substantial neonatal morbidity and mortality. Several recent epidemiologic studies suggest a positive statistical association between SSRI use in pregnancy and PPHN. Other studies do not show a significant statistical association.

A prospective longitudinal study was conducted of 201 pregnant women with a history of major depression, who were either on antidepressants or had received antidepressants less than 12 weeks prior to their last menstrual period, and were in remission. Women who discontinued antidepressant medication during pregnancy showed a significant increase in relapse of their major depression compared to those women who remained on antidepressant medication throughout pregnancy. When treating a pregnant woman with BRINTELLIX, the physician should carefully consider both the potential risks of taking a serotonergic antidepressant, along with the established benefits of treating depression with an antidepressant.

Animal Data

In pregnant rats and rabbits, no teratogenic effects were seen when vortioxetine was given during the period of organogenesis at oral doses up to 160 and 60 mg/kg/day, respectively. These doses are 77 and 58 times, in rats and rabbits, respectively, the maximum recommended human dose (MRHD) of 20 mg on a mg/m^2 basis. Developmental delay, seen as decreased fetal body weight and delayed ossification, occurred in rats and rabbits at doses equal to and greater than 30 and 10 mg/kg (15 and 10 times the MRHD, respectively) in the presence of maternal toxicity (decreased food consumption and decreased body weight gain). When vortioxetine was administered to pregnant rats at oral doses up to 120 mg/kg (58 times the MRHD) throughout pregnancy and lactation, the number of live-born pups was decreased and early postnatal pup mortality was increased at 40 and 120 mg/kg. Additionally, pup weights were decreased at birth to weaning at 120 mg/kg and development (specifically eye opening) was slightly delayed at 40 and 120 mg/kg. These effects were not seen at 10 mg/kg (5 times the MRHD).

8.3 Nursing Mothers

It is not known whether vortioxetine is present in human milk. Vortioxetine is present in the milk of lactating rats. Because many drugs are present in human milk and because of the potential for serious adverse reactions in nursing infants from BRINTELLIX, a decision should be made whether to discontinue nursing or to discontinue the drug, taking into account the importance of the drug to the mother.

8.4 Pediatric Use

Clinical studies on the use of BRINTELLIX in pediatric patients have not been conducted; therefore, the safety and effectiveness of BRINTELLIX in the pediatric population have not been established.

8.5 Geriatric Use

No dose adjustment is recommended on the basis of age *(Figure 3)*. Results from a single-dose pharmacokinetic study in elderly (>65 years old) vs. young (24 to 45 years old) subjects demonstrated that the pharmacokinetics were generally similar between the two age groups.

Of the 2616 subjects in clinical studies of BRINTELLIX, 11% (286) were 65 and over, which included subjects from a placebo-controlled study specifically in elderly patients *[see Clinical Studies (14)]*. No overall differences in safety or effectiveness were observed between these subjects and younger subjects, and other reported clinical experience has not identified differences in responses between the elderly and younger patients.

Serotonergic antidepressants have been associated with cases of clinically significant hyponatremia in elderly patients, who may be at greater risk for this adverse event *[see Warnings and Precautions (5.5)]*.

8.6 Use in Other Patient Populations

No dose adjustment of BRINTELLIX on the basis of race, gender, ethnicity, or renal function (from mild renal impairment to end-stage renal disease) is necessary. In addition, the same dose can be administered in patients with mild to moderate hepatic impairment *(Figure 3)*. BRINTELLIX has not been studied in patients with severe hepatic impairment. Therefore, BRINTELLIX is not recommended in patients with severe hepatic impairment.

[See figure 3 at top of next page]

9 DRUG ABUSE AND DEPENDENCE

BRINTELLIX is not a controlled substance.

10 OVERDOSAGE

10.1 Human Experience

There is limited clinical trial experience regarding human overdosage with BRINTELLIX. In premarketing clinical studies, cases of overdose were limited to patients who accidentally or intentionally consumed up to a maximum dose of 40 mg of BRINTELLIX. The maximum single dose tested was 75 mg in men. Ingestion of BRINTELLIX in the dose range of 40 to 75 mg was associated with increased rates of nausea, dizziness, diarrhea, abdominal discomfort, generalized pruritus, somnolence, and flushing.

Figure 3. Impact of Intrinsic Factors on Vortioxetine PK

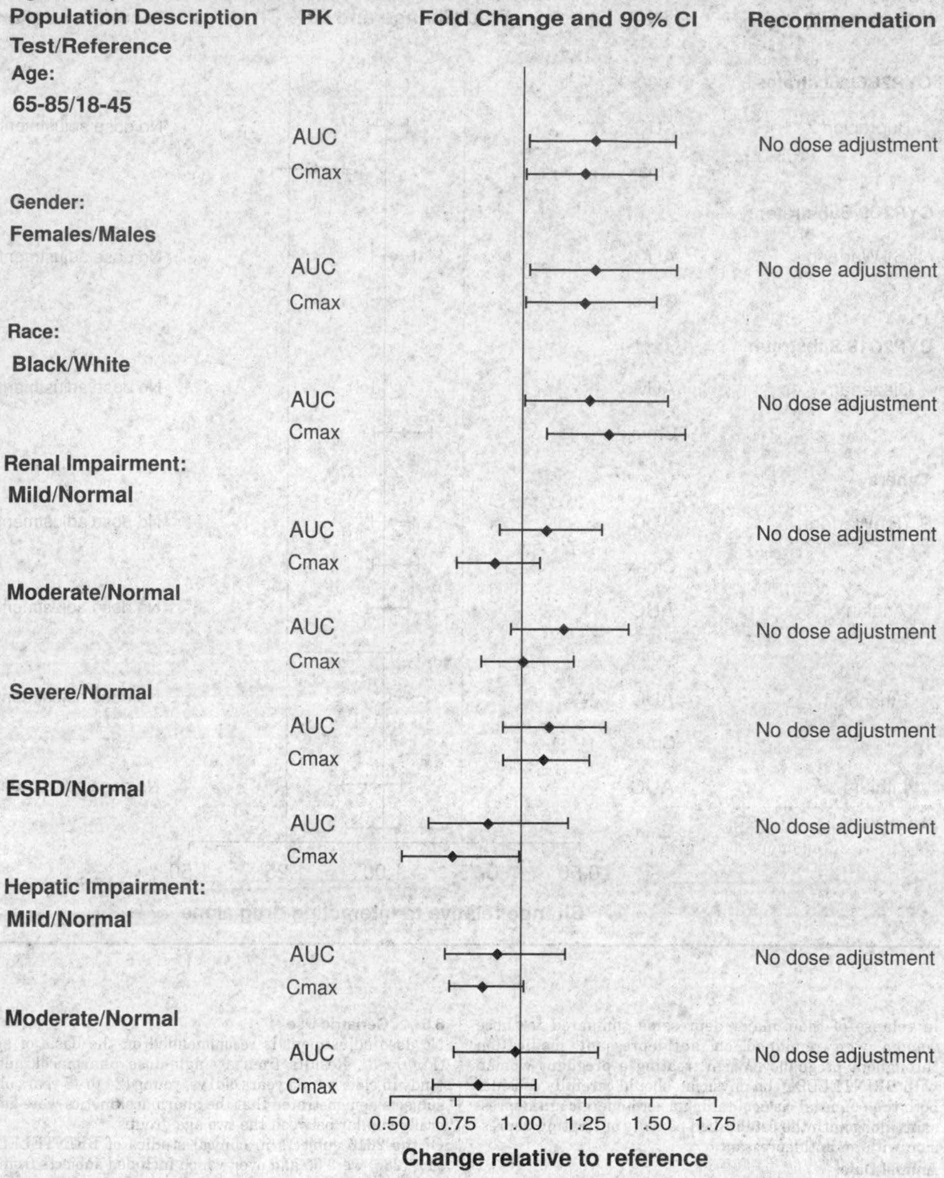

10.2 Management of Overdose

No specific antidotes for BRINTELLIX are known. In managing over dosage, consider the possibility of multiple drug involvement. In case of overdose, call Poison Control Center at 1-800-222-1222 for latest recommendations.

11 DESCRIPTION

BRINTELLIX is an immediate-release tablet for oral administration that contains the beta (β) polymorph of vortioxetine hydrobromide (HBr), an antidepressant. Vortioxetine HBr is known chemically as 1-[2-(2,4-Dimethyl-phenylsulfanyl)-phenyl]-piperazine, hydrobromide. The empirical formula is $C_{18}H_{22}N_2S$, HBr with a molecular weight of 379.36 g/mol. The structural formula is:

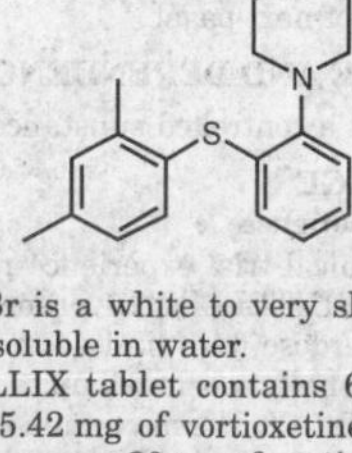

Vortioxetine HBr is a white to very slightly beige powder that is slightly soluble in water.

Each BRINTELLIX tablet contains 6.355 mg, 12.71 mg, 19.065 mg, or 25.42 mg of vortioxetine HBr equivalent to 5 mg, 10 mg, 15 mg, or 20 mg of vortioxetine, respectively. The inactive ingredients in BRINTELLIX tablets include mannitol, microcrystalline cellulose, hydroxypropyl cellulose, sodium starch glycolate, magnesium stearate and film coating which consists of hypromellose, titanium dioxide, polyethylene glycol 400, iron oxide red (5 mg, 15 mg, and 20 mg) and iron oxide yellow (10 mg and 15 mg).

12 CLINICAL PHARMACOLOGY

12.1 Mechanism of Action

The mechanism of the antidepressant effect of vortioxetine is not fully understood, but is thought to be related to its enhancement of serotonergic activity in the CNS through inhibition of the reuptake of serotonin (5-HT). It also has several other activities including 5-HT3 receptor antagonism and 5-HT1A receptor agonism. The contribution of these activities to vortioxetine's antidepressant effect has not been established.

12.2 Pharmacodynamics

Vortioxetine binds with high affinity to the human serotonin transporter (Ki=1.6 nM), but not to the norepinephrine (Ki=113 nM) or dopamine (Ki>1000 nM) transporters. Vortioxetine potently and selectively inhibits reuptake of serotonin (IC50=5.4 nM). Vortioxetine binds to 5-HT3 (Ki=3.7 nM), 5-HT1A (Ki=15 nM), 5-HT7 (Ki=19 nM), 5-HT1D (Ki=54 nM), and 5-HT1B (Ki=33 nM), receptors and is a 5-HT3, 5-HT1D, and 5-HT7 receptor antagonist, 5-HT1B receptor partial agonist, and 5-HT1A receptor agonist.

In humans, the mean 5-HT transporter occupancy, based on the results from 2 clinical PET studies using 5-HTT ligands ([^{11}C]-MADAM or [^{11}C]-DASB), was approximately 50% at 5 mg/day, 65% at 10 mg/day and approximately 80% at 20 mg/day in the regions of interest.

Effect on Cardiac Repolarization

The effect of vortioxetine 10 mg and 40 mg administered once daily on QTc interval was evaluated in a randomized, double-blind, placebo-, and active-controlled (moxifloxacin 400 mg), four-treatment-arm parallel study in 340 male subjects. In the study the upper bound of the one-sided 95% confidence interval for the QTc was below 10 ms, the threshold for regulatory concern. The oral dose of 40 mg is sufficient to assess the effect of metabolic inhibition.

Effect on Driving Performance

In a clinical study in healthy subjects, BRINTELLIX did not impair driving performance, or have adverse psychomotor or cognitive effects following single and multiple doses of 10 mg/day. Because any psychoactive drug may impair judgment, thinking, or motor skills, however, patients should be cautioned about operating hazardous machinery, including automobiles, until they are reasonably certain that BRINTELLIX therapy does not affect their ability to engage in such activities.

12.3 Pharmacokinetics

Vortioxetine pharmacological activity is due to the parent drug. The pharmacokinetics of vortioxetine (2.5 mg to 60 mg) are linear and dose-proportional when vortioxetine is administered once daily. The mean terminal half-life is approximately 66 hours, and steady-state plasma concentrations are typically achieved within two weeks of dosing.

Absorption

The maximal plasma vortioxetine concentration (Cmax) after dosing is reached within 7 to 11 hours postdose (Tmax). Steady state mean Cmax values were 9, 18, and 33 ng/mL following doses of 5, 10, and 20 mg/day. Absolute bioavailability is 75%. No effect of food on the pharmacokinetics was observed.

Distribution

The apparent volume of distribution of vortioxetine is approximately 2600 L, indicating extensive extravascular distribution. The plasma protein binding of vortioxetine in humans is 98%, independent of plasma concentrations. No apparent difference in the plasma protein binding between healthy subjects and subjects with hepatic (mild, moderate) or renal (mild, moderate, severe, ESRD) impairment is observed.

Metabolism and Elimination

Vortioxetine is extensively metabolized primarily through oxidation via cytochrome P450 isozymes CYP2D6, CYP3A4/5, CYP2C19, CYP2C9, CYP2A6, CYP2C8 and CYP2B6 and subsequent glucuronic acid conjugation. CYP2D6 is the primary enzyme catalyzing the metabolism of vortioxetine to its major, pharmacologically inactive, carboxylic acid metabolite, and poor metabolizers of CYP2D6 have approximately twice the vortioxetine plasma concentration of extensive metabolizers.

Following a single oral dose of [14C]-labeled vortioxetine, approximately 59% and 26% of the administered radioactivity was recovered in the urine and feces, respectively as metabolites. Negligible amounts of unchanged vortioxetine were excreted in the urine up to 48 hours. The presence of hepatic (mild or moderate) or renal impairment (mild, moderate, severe and ESRD) did not affect the apparent clearance of vortioxetine.

13 NONCLINICAL TOXICOLOGY

13.1 Carcinogenesis, Mutagenesis, Impairment of Fertility

Carcinogenesis

Carcinogenicity studies were conducted in which CD-1 mice and Wistar rats were given oral doses of vortioxetine up to 50 and 100 mg/kg/day for male and female mice, respectively, and 40 and 80 mg/kg/day for male and female rats, respectively, for 2 years. The doses in the two species were approximately 12, 24, 20, and 39 times, respectively, the maximum recommended human dose (MRHD) of 20 mg on a mg/m^2 basis.

In rats, the incidence of benign polypoid adenomas of the rectum was statistically significantly increased in females at doses 39 times the MRHD, but not at 15 times the MRHD. These were considered related to inflammation and hyperplasia and possibly caused by an interaction with a vehicle component of the formulation used for the study. The finding did not occur in male rats at 20 times the MRHD.

In mice, vortioxetine was not carcinogenic in males or females at doses up to 12 and 24 times, respectively, the MRHD.

Mutagenicity

Vortioxetine was not genotoxic in the *in vitro* bacterial reverse mutation assay (Ames test), an *in vitro* chromosome aberration assay in cultured human lymphocytes, and an *in vivo* rat bone marrow micronucleus assay.

Impairment of Fertility

Treatment of rats with vortioxetine at doses up to 120 mg/kg/day had no effect on male or female fertility, which is 58 times the maximum recommended human dose (MRHD) of 20 mg on a mg/m^2 basis.

14 CLINICAL STUDIES

The efficacy of BRINTELLIX in treatment for MDD was established in six 6 to 8 week randomized, double-blind, placebo-controlled, fixed-dose studies (including one study in the elderly) and one maintenance study in adult inpatients and outpatients who met the Diagnostic and Statistical Manual of Mental Disorders (DSM-IV-TR) criteria for MDD.

Adults (aged 18 years to 75 years)

The efficacy of BRINTELLIX in patients aged 18 years to 75 years was demonstrated in five 6 to 8 week, placebo-controlled studies (Studies 1 to 5 in *Table 4*). In these studies, patients were randomized to BRINTELLIX 5 mg, 10 mg, 15 mg or 20 mg or placebo once daily. For patients who were randomized to BRINTELLIX 15 mg/day or 20 mg/day, the final doses were titrated up from 10 mg/day after the first week.

The primary efficacy measures were the Hamilton Depression Scale (HAMD-24) total score in Study 2 and the Montgomery-Asberg Depression Rating Scale (MADRS) total score in all other studies. In each of these studies, at least one dose group of BRINTELLIX was superior to placebo in improvement of depressive symptoms as measured by mean change from baseline to endpoint visit on the primary efficacy measurement *(see Table 4)*. Subgroup analysis by age, gender or race did not suggest any clear evidence of differential responsiveness. Two studies of the 5 mg dose in the U.S. (not represented in *Table 4*) failed to show effectiveness.

Elderly Study (aged 64 years to 88 years)

The efficacy of BRINTELLIX for the treatment of MDD was also demonstrated in a randomized, double-blind, placebo-controlled, fixed-dose study of BRINTELLIX in elderly patients (aged 64 years to 88 years) with MDD (Study 6 in *Table 4*). Patients meeting the diagnostic criteria for recurrent MDD with at least one previous major depressive episode before the age of 60 years and without comorbid cognitive impairment (Mini Mental State Examination score <24) received BRINTELLIX 5 mg or placebo.

[See table 4 above]

Time Course of Treatment Response

In the 6 to 8 week placebo-controlled studies, an effect of BRINTELLIX based on the primary efficacy measure was generally observed starting at week 2 and increased in subsequent weeks with the full antidepressant effect of BRINTELLIX generally not seen until Study week 4 or later. *Figure 4* depicts time course of response in U.S. based on the primary efficacy measure (MADRS) in Study 5.

Figure 4. Change from Baseline in MADRS Total Score by Study Visit (Week) in Study 5

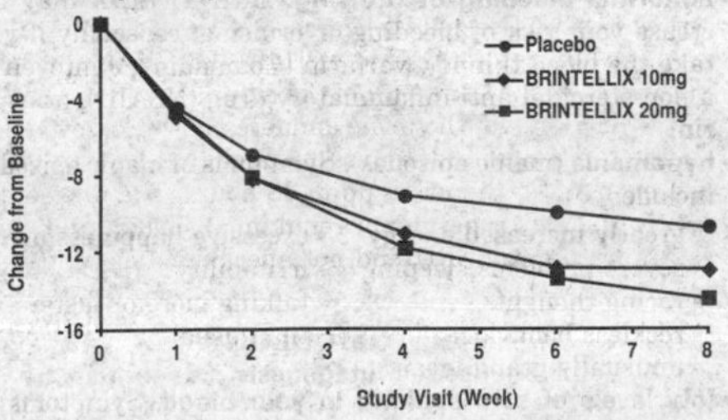

Figure 5. Difference from Placebo in Mean Change from Baseline in MADRS Total Score at Week 6 or Week 8

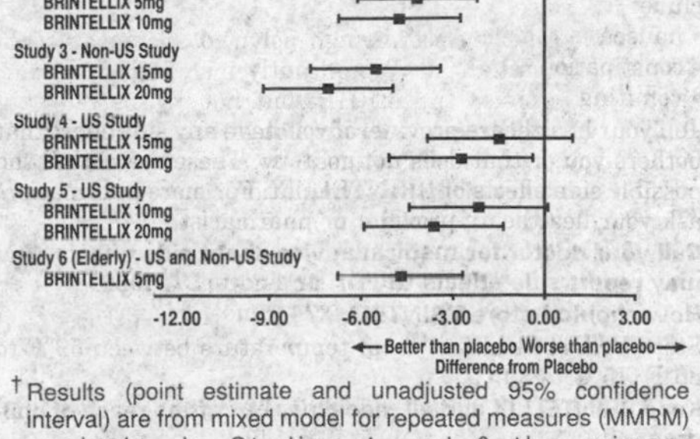

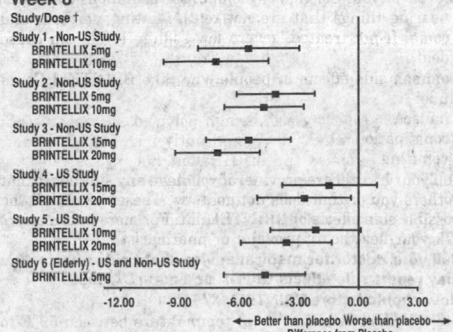

† Results (point estimate and unadjusted 95% confidence interval) are from mixed model for repeated measures (MMRM) analysis. In Studies 1 and 6 the primary analysis was not based on MMRM and in Studies 2 and 6 the primary efficacy measure was not based on MADRS.

Maintenance Study

In a non-US maintenance study (Study 7 in *Figure 6*), 639 patients meeting DSM-IV-TR criteria for MDD received flexible doses of BRINTELLIX (5 mg or 10 mg) once daily during an initial 12 week open-label treatment phase; the dose of BRINTELLIX was fixed during Weeks 8 to 12. Three hundred ninety six (396) patients who were in remission (MADRS total score ≤10 at both Weeks 10 and 12) after open-label treatment were randomly assigned to continuation of a fixed dose of BRINTELLIX at the final dose they responded to (about 75% of patients were on 10 mg/day) during the open-label phase or to placebo for 24 to 64 weeks. Approximately 61% of randomized patients satisfied remission criterion (MADRS total score ≤10) for at least 4 weeks (since Week 8), and 15% for at least 8 weeks (since Week 4). Patients on BRINTELLIX experienced a statistically significantly longer time to recurrence of depressive episodes than did patients on placebo. Recurrence of depressive episode was defined as a MADRS total score ≥22 or lack of efficacy as judged by the investigator.

[See figure 6 at top of next column]

Table 4. Primary Efficacy Results of 6 Week to 8 Week Clinical Trials

Study No. [Primary Measure]	Treatment Group	Number of Patients	Mean Baseline Score (SD)	LS Mean Change from Baseline (SE)	Placebo-subtracted Difference† (95% CI)
Study 1 [MADRS] Non-US Study	BRINTELLIX (5 mg/day)‡	108	34.1 (2.6)	-20.4 (1.0)	-5.9 (-8.6, -3.2)
	BRINTELLIX (10 mg/day)‡	100	34.0 (2.8)	-20.2 (1.0)	-5.7 (-8.5, -2.9)
	Placebo	105	33.9 (2.7)	-14.5 (1.0)	--
Study 2 [HAMD-24] Non-US Study	BRINTELLIX (5 mg/day)	139	32.2 (5.0)	-15.4 (0.7)	-4.1 (-6.2, -2.1)
	BRINTELLIX (10 mg/day)‡	139	33.1 (4.8)	-16.2 (0.8)	-4.9 (-7.0, -2.9)
	Placebo	139	32.7 (4.4)	-11.3 (0.7)	--
Study 3 [MADRS] Non-US Study	BRINTELLIX (15 mg/day) ‡	149	31.8 (3.4)	-17.2 (0.8)	-5.5 (-7.7, -3.4)
	BRINTELLIX (20 mg/day) ‡	151	31.2 (3.4)	18.8 (0.8)	-7.1 (-9.2, -5.0)
	Placebo	158	31.5 (3.6)	-11.7 (0.8)	--
Study 4 [MADRS] US Study	BRINTELLIX (15 mg/day)	145	31.9 (4.1)	-14.3 (0.9)	-1.5 (-3.9, 0.9)
	BRINTELLIX (20 mg/day) ‡	147	32.0 (4.4)	-15.6 (0.9)	-2.8 (-5.1, -0.4)
	Placebo	153	31.5 (4.2)	-12.8 (0.8)	--
Study 5 [MADRS] US Study	BRINTELLIX (10 mg/day)	154	32.2 (4.5)	-13.0 (0.8)	-2.2 (-4.5, 0.1)
	BRINTELLIX (20 mg/day) ‡	148	32.5 (4.3)	-14.4 (0.9)	-3.6 (-5.9, -1.4)
	Placebo	155	32.0 (4.0)	-10.8 (0.8)	--
Study 6 (elderly) [HAMD-24] US and Non-US	BRINTELLIX (5 mg/day) ‡	155	29.2 (5.0)	-13.7 (0.7)	-3.3 (-5.3, -1.3)
	Placebo	145	29.4 (5.1)	-10.3 (0.8)	--

SD; standard deviation; SE: standard error; LS Mean: least-squares mean; CI: unadjusted confidence interval.

†Difference (drug minus placebo) in least-squares mean change from baseline.

‡Doses that are statistically significantly superior to placebo after adjusting for multiplicity.

Features	Strengths			
	5 mg	10 mg	15 mg	20 mg
Color	pink	yellow	orange	red
Debossment	"5" on one side of tablet "TL" on other side of tablet	"10" on one side of tablet "TL" on other side of tablet	"15" on one side of tablet "TL" on other side of tablet	"20" on one side of tablet "TL" on other side of tablet
Presentations and NDC Codes				
Bottles of 30*	64764-550-30	64764-560-30	64764-570-30	64764-580-30
Bottles of 90*	64764-550-90	64764-560-90	64764-570-90	64764-580-90
Bottles of 500	64764-550-77	64764-560-77	64764-570-77	64764-580-77

***The unit-of-use package is intended to be dispensed as a unit.**

16 HOW SUPPLIED/STORAGE AND HANDLING

BRINTELLIX tablets are available as follows:

[See second table above]

Storage: Store at 77°F (25°C); excursions permitted to 59°F to 86°F (15°C to 30°C) [see USP Controlled Room Temperature].

17 PATIENT COUNSELING INFORMATION

See FDA-approved patient labeling (Medication Guide)

Advise patients and their caregivers about the benefits and risks associated with treatment with BRINTELLIX and counsel them in its appropriate use. Advise patients and

Figure 6. Kaplan-Meier Estimates of Proportion of Patients with Recurrence (Study 7)

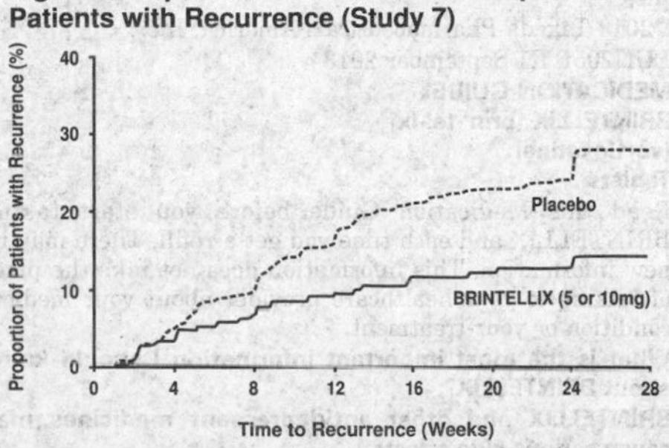

their caregivers to read the Medication Guide and assist them in understanding its contents. The complete text of the Medication Guide is reprinted at the end of this document.

Suicide Risk

Advise patients and caregivers to look for the emergence of suicidal ideation and behavior, especially early during treatment and when the dose is adjusted up or down *[see Boxed Warning and Warnings and Precautions (5.1)]*.

Discontinuation of Treatment

Patients who are on BRINTELLIX 15 mg/day or 20 mg/day may experience headache, muscle tension, mood swings, sudden outburst of anger, dizziness and runny nose if they abruptly stop their medicine. Advise patients not stopping BRINTELLIX without talking to their healthcare provider *[see Adverse Reactions (6)]*.

Concomitant Medication

Advise patients to inform their physicians if they are taking, or plan to take, any prescription or over-the-counter medications because of a potential for interactions. Instruct patients not to take BRINTELLIX with an MAOI or within 14 days of stopping an MAOI and to allow 21 days after stopping BRINTELLIX before starting an MAOI *[see Dosage and Administration (2.4), Contraindications (4), Warnings and Precautions (5.2), and Drug Interactions (7.1)]*.

Serotonin Syndrome

Caution patients about the risk of serotonin syndrome, particularly with the concomitant use of BRINTELLIX and triptans, tricyclic antidepressants, fentanyl, Lithium, tramadol, tryptophan supplements, and St. John's Wort supplements *[see Warnings and Precautions (5.2) and Drug Interactions (7.1, 7.2)]*.

Abnormal Bleeding

Caution patients about the increased risk of abnormal bleeding when BRINTELLIX is given with NSAIDs, aspirin, warfarin, or other drugs that affect coagulation *[see Warnings and Precautions (5.3)]*.

Activation of Mania/Hypomania

Advise patients and their caregivers to look for signs of activation of mania/hypomania *[see Warnings and Precautions (5.4)]*.

Hyponatremia

Advise patients that if they are treated with diuretics, or are otherwise volume depleted, or are elderly, they may be at greater risk of developing hyponatremia while taking BRINTELLIX *[see Warnings and Precautions (5.5)]*.

Nausea

Advise patients that nausea is the most common adverse reaction, and is dose related. Nausea commonly occurs within the first week of treatment, then decreases in frequency but can persist in some patients.

Alcohol

A clinical study has shown that BRINTELLIX (single dose of 20 or 40 mg/day) did not increase the impairment of mental and motor skills caused by alcohol.

Allergic Reactions

Advise patients to notify their healthcare provider if they develop an allergic reaction such as rash, hives, swelling, or difficulty breathing.

Pregnancy

Advise patients to notify their healthcare provider if they become pregnant or intend to become pregnant during therapy with BRINTELLIX *[see Use in Specific Populations (8.1)]*.

Nursing Mothers

Advise patients to notify their healthcare provider if they are breast-feeding an infant and would like to continue or start BRINTELLIX *[see Use in Specific Populations (8.3)]*.

Distributed and marketed by:
Takeda Pharmaceuticals America, Inc.
Deerfield, IL 60015
Marketed by:
Lundbeck
Deerfield, IL 60015

LUN205P R1 September 2013

MEDICATION GUIDE
BRINTELLIX [brin'-tel-ix]
(vortioxetine)
Tablets

Read this Medication Guide before you start taking BRINTELLIX and each time you get a refill. There may be new information. This information does not take the place of talking to your healthcare provider about your medical condition or your treatment.

What is the most important information I should know about BRINTELLIX?

BRINTELLIX and other antidepressant medicines may cause serious side effects.

1. **Antidepressant medicines may increase suicidal thoughts or actions in some children, teenagers, or young adults within the first few months of treatment.**
2. **Depression or other serious mental illnesses are the most important causes of suicidal thoughts or actions. Some people may have a particularly high risk of having suicidal thoughts or actions.** These include people who have (or have a family history of) bipolar illness (also called manic-depressive illness) or suicidal thoughts or actions.
3. **How can I watch for and try to prevent suicidal thoughts and actions?**
   - Pay close attention to any changes, especially sudden changes in mood, behavior, thoughts, or feelings. This is very important when an antidepressant medicine is started or when the dose is changed.
   - Call your healthcare provider right away to report new or sudden changes in mood, behavior, thoughts, or feelings.
   - Keep all follow-up visits with your healthcare provider as scheduled. Call your healthcare provider between visits as needed, especially if you have concerns about symptoms.

Call your healthcare provider right away if you have any of the following symptoms, especially if they are new, worse, or worry you:

- attempts to commit suicide
- acting on dangerous impulses
- acting aggressive, being angry or violent
- thoughts about suicide or dying
- new or worse depression
- new or worse anxiety
- feeling agitated, restless, angry or irritable
- trouble sleeping
- an extreme increase in activity or talking (mania)
- other unusual changes in behavior or mood
- panic attacks
- new or worse irritability

What is BRINTELLIX?

BRINTELLIX is a prescription medicine used to treat a certain type of depression called Major Depressive Disorder (MDD).

It is important to talk with your healthcare provider about the risks of treating depression and also the risk of not treating it. You should discuss all treatment choices with your healthcare provider.

- Talk to your healthcare provider if you do not think that your condition is getting better with BRINTELLIX treatment.

Who should not take BRINTELLIX?

Do not take BRINTELLIX if you:

- are allergic to vortioxetine, or any of the ingredients in BRINTELLIX. See the end of this Medication Guide for a complete list of ingredients in BRINTELLIX.
- take a Monoamine Oxidase Inhibitor (MAOI). Ask your healthcare provider or pharmacist if you are not sure if you take an MAOI, including the antibiotic linezolid.
- Do not take an MAOI within 21 days of stopping BRINTELLIX.
- Do not start BRINTELLIX if you stopped taking an MAOI in the last 14 days.

What should I tell my healthcare provider before taking BRINTELLIX?

Tell your healthcare provider if you:

- have liver problems
- have or had seizures or convulsions
- have mania or bipolar disorder (manic depression)
- have low salt (sodium) levels in your blood
- have or had bleeding problems
- drink alcohol
- have any other medical conditions
- are pregnant or plan to become pregnant. It is not known if BRINTELLIX will harm your unborn baby.
- are breastfeeding or plan to breastfeed. It is not known if BRINTELLIX passes into breast milk. Talk to your healthcare provider about the best way to feed your baby if you take BRINTELLIX.

Tell your healthcare provider about all the medicines that you take, including prescription and over-the-counter medicines, vitamins, and herbal supplements. BRINTELLIX and some medicines may interact with each other, may not work as well, or may cause serious side effects when taken together.

Especially tell your healthcare provider if you take:

- medicines used to treat migraine headache (e.g. triptans)
- medicines used to treat mood, anxiety, psychotic or thought disorders, including tricyclics, lithium, selective serotonin reuptake inhibitors (SSRIs), serotonin norepinephrine reuptake inhibitors (SNRIs), buspirone, or antipsychotics
- MAOIs (including linezolid, an antibiotic)
- Tramadol or fentanyl
- over-the-counter supplements such as tryptophan or St. John's Wort
- nonsteroidal anti-inflammatory drugs (NSAIDs)
- aspirin
- warfarin (Coumadin, Jantoven)
- diuretics
- rifampicin
- carbamazepine
- phenytoin
- quinidine

Ask your healthcare provider if you are not sure if you are taking any of these medicines.

Before you take BRINTELLIX with any of these medicines, talk to your healthcare provider about serotonin syndrome. See "What are the possible side effects of BRINTELLIX?"

Know the medicines you take. Keep a list of them to show your healthcare provider or pharmacist when you get new medicine.

How should I take BRINTELLIX?

- Take BRINTELLIX exactly as your healthcare providers tells you to take it.
- Take BRINTELLIX at about the same time each day.
- Your healthcare provider may need to change the dose of BRINTELLIX until it is the right dose for you.
- Do not start or stop taking BRINTELLIX without talking to your healthcare provider first. Suddenly stopping BRINTELLIX when you take higher doses may cause you to have side effects, including:
  - headache
  - stiff muscles
  - mood swings
  - sudden outburst of anger
  - dizziness or feeling lightheaded
  - runny nose
- BRINTELLIX may be taken with or without food.
- If you take too much BRINTELLIX, call the Poison Control Center at 1-800-222-1222 or go to the nearest hospital emergency room right away.

What should I avoid while taking BRINTELLIX?

- Do not drive, operate heavy machinery, or do other dangerous activities until you know how BRINTELLIX affects you.
- Avoid drinking alcohol while taking BRINTELLIX.

What are the possible side effects of BRINTELLIX?

BRINTELLIX may cause serious side effects, including:

- **See "What is the most important information I should know about BRINTELLIX?"**
- **serotonin syndrome.** A potentially life-threatening problem called serotonin syndrome can happen when medicines such as BRINTELLIX are taken with certain other medicines. Symptoms of serotonin syndrome may include:
  - agitation, hallucinations, coma or other changes in mental status
  - problems controlling your movements or muscle twitching
  - fast heartbeat
  - high or low blood pressure
  - sweating or fever
  - nausea or vomiting
  - diarrhea
  - muscle stiffness or tightness
- **abnormal bleeding or bruising.** BRINTELLIX may increase your risk of bleeding or bruising, especially if you take the blood thinner warfarin (Coumadin®, Jantoven®), a non-steroidal anti-inflammatory drug (NSAID), or aspirin.
- **hypomania** (manic episodes). Symptoms of manic episodes include:
  - greatly increased energy
  - severe problems sleeping
  - racing thoughts
  - reckless behavior
  - unusually grand ideas
  - excessive happiness or irritability
  - talking more or faster than usual
- **low levels of salt (sodium) in your blood.** Symptoms of this may include: headache, difficulty concentrating, memory changes, confusion, weakness and unsteadiness on your feet. Symptoms of severe or sudden cases of low salt levels in your blood may include: hallucinations (seeing or hearing things that are not real), fainting, seizures and coma. If not treated, severe low sodium levels can cause death.

Common side effects in people who take BRINTELLIX include:

- nausea
- constipation
- vomiting

Tell your healthcare provider if you have any side effect that bothers you or that does not go away. These are not all the possible side effects of BRINTELLIX. For more information, ask your healthcare provider or pharmacist.

Call your doctor for medical advice about side effects. You may report side effects to FDA at 1-800-FDA-1088.

How should I store BRINTELLIX?

Store BRINTELLIX at room temperature between 59°F to 86°F (15°C to 30°C).

Keep BRINTELLIX and all medicines out of the reach of children.

General information about the safe and effective use of BRINTELLIX.

Medicines are sometimes prescribed for purposes other than those listed in a Medication Guide. Do not use BRINTELLIX for a condition for which it was not prescribed. Do not give BRINTELLIX to other people, even if they have the same condition. It may harm them.

This Medication Guide summarizes the most important information about BRINTELLIX. If you would like more information, talk with your healthcare provider. You may ask your healthcare provider or pharmacist for information about BRINTELLIX that is written for healthcare professionals.

For more information, go to www.BRINTELLIX.com or call 1-877-TAKEDA-7 (1-877-825-3327).

What are the ingredients in BRINTELLIX?

Active ingredient: vortioxetine hydrobromide

Inactive ingredients: mannitol, microcrystalline cellulose, hydroxypropyl cellulose, sodium starch glycolate, magnesium stearate and film coating consisting of hypromellose, titanium dioxide, polyethylene glycol 400, iron oxide red (5 mg, 15 mg, and 20 mg) and iron oxide yellow (10 mg and 15 mg)

This Medication Guide has been approved by the U.S. Food and Drug Administration.

Distributed and Marketed by:
Takeda Pharmaceuticals America, Inc.
Deerfield, IL 60015
Marketed by:
Lundbeck
Deerfield, IL 60015

BRINTELLIX is a trademark of H. Lundbeck A/S and is used under license by Takeda Pharmaceuticals America, Inc.

All other trademarks are the property of their respective owners.

LUN205M R1 September 2013

COLCRYS® ℞

(colchicine, USP)
tablets for Oral use

HIGHLIGHTS OF PRESCRIBING INFORMATION

These highlights do not include all the information needed to use colchicine safely and effectively. See full prescribing information for COLCRYS®.

COLCRYS® (colchicine, USP) tablets for Oral use
Initial U.S. Approval: 1961

INDICATIONS AND USAGE

COLCRYS (colchicine, USP) tablets are an alkaloid indicated for:

- Prophylaxis and Treatment of Gout Flares in adults (1.1).
- Familial Mediterranean fever (FMF) in adults and children 4 years or older (1.2).

COLCRYS is not an analgesic medication and should not be used to treat pain from other causes.

DOSAGE AND ADMINISTRATION

- **Gout Flares:**
  Prophylaxis of Gout Flares: 0.6 mg once or twice daily in adults and adolescents older than 16 years of age (2.1). Maximum dose 1.2 mg/day.
  Treatment of Gout Flares: 1.2 mg (2 tablets) at the first sign of a gout flare followed by 0.6 mg (1 tablet) one hour later (2.1).
- **FMF:** Adults and Children older than 12 years 1.2 – 2.4 mg; Children 6 to 12 years 0.9 – 1.8 mg; Children 4 to 6 years 0.3 – 1.8 mg (2.2, 2.3).
  - Give total daily dose in one or two divided doses (2.2).
  - Increase or decrease the dose as indicated and as tolerated in increments of 0.3 mg/day, not to exceed the maximum recommended daily dose (2.2).

Colchicine tablets are administered orally, without regard to meals.

See full prescribing information for dose adjustment regarding patients with impaired renal function (2.5), impaired hepatic function (2.6), the patient's age (2.3, 8.5), or use of co-administered drugs (2.4).

DOSAGE FORMS AND STRENGTHS

- 0.6 mg tablets (3).

CONTRAINDICATIONS

Patients with renal or hepatic impairment should not be given COLCRYS in conjunction with P-gp or strong CYP3A4 inhibitors (5.3). In these patients, life-threatening and fatal colchicine toxicity has been reported with colchicine taken in therapeutic doses (7).

WARNINGS AND PRECAUTIONS

- *Fatal overdoses* have been reported with colchicine in adults and children. Keep COLCRYS out of the reach of children (5.1, 10).
- *Blood dyscrasias:* myelosuppression, leukopenia, granulocytopenia, thrombocytopenia, and aplastic anemia have been reported (5.2).
- Monitor for toxicity and if present consider temporary interruption or discontinuation of colchicine (5.2, 5.3, 5.4, 6, 10).
- *Drug interaction P-gp and/or CYP3A4 inhibitors:* Co-administration of colchicine with P-gp and/or strong CYP3A4 inhibitors has resulted in life-threatening interactions and death (5.3, 7).
- *Neuromuscular toxicity:* Myotoxicity including rhabdomyolysis may occur, especially in combination with other drugs known to cause this effect. Consider temporary interruption or discontinuation of COLCRYS (5.4, 7).

ADVERSE REACTIONS

Prophylaxis of Gout Flares: The most commonly reported adverse reaction in clinical trials for the prophylaxis of gout was diarrhea.

Treatment of Gout Flares: The most common adverse reactions reported in the clinical trial for gout were diarrhea (23%) and pharyngolaryngeal pain (3%).

FMF: Most common adverse reactions (up to 20%) are abdominal pain, diarrhea, nausea, and vomiting. These effects are usually mild, transient, and reversible upon lowering the dose (6).

To report SUSPECTED ADVERSE REACTIONS, contact Takeda Pharmaceuticals America, Inc. at 1-877-825-3327 or FDA at 1-800-FDA-1088 or www.fda.gov/medwatch.

DRUG INTERACTIONS

Co-administration of P-gp and/or CYP3A4 inhibitors (*e.g.,* clarithromycin or cyclosporine) have been demonstrated to alter the concentration of colchicine. The potential for drug-drug interactions must be considered prior to and during therapy. See full prescribing information for a complete list of reported and potential interactions (2.4, 5.3, 7).

USE IN SPECIFIC POPULATIONS

- In the presence of mild to moderate renal or hepatic impairment, adjustment of dosing is not required for treatment of gout flare, prophylaxis of gout flare, and FMF but patients should be monitored closely (2.5, 8.6).
- In patients with severe renal impairment for prophylaxis of gout flares the starting dose should be 0.3 mg/day, for gout flares no dose adjustment is required but a treatment course should be repeated no more than once every 2 weeks. In FMF patients, start with 0.3 mg/day and any increase in dose should be done with close monitoring (2.5, 8.6).
- In patients with severe hepatic impairment, a dose reduction may be needed in prophylaxis of gout flares and FMF patients; while a dose reduction may not be needed in gout flares, a treatment course should be repeated no more than once every 2 weeks (2.5, 2.6, 8.6, 8.7).
- For patients undergoing dialysis, the total recommended dose for prophylaxis of gout flares should be 0.3 mg given twice a week with close monitoring. For treatment of gout flares, the total recommended dose should be reduced to 0.6 mg (1 tablet) × 1 dose and the treatment course should not be repeated more than once every two weeks. For FMF patients the starting dose should be 0.3 mg per day and dosing can be increased with close monitoring (2.5, 8.6).
- Pregnancy: Use only if the potential benefit justifies the potential risk to the fetus (8.1).
- Nursing Mothers: Caution should be exercised when administered to a nursing woman (8.3).
- Geriatric Use: The recommended dose of colchicine should be based on renal function (2.5, 8.5).

See 17 for PATIENT COUNSELING INFORMATION and Medication Guide.

Revised: 04/2013

FULL PRESCRIBING INFORMATION: CONTENTS*

* Sections or subsections omitted from the full prescribing information are not listed

FULL PRESCRIBING INFORMATION

1 INDICATIONS AND USAGE

1.1 Gout Flares

COLCRYS® (colchicine, USP) tablets are indicated for prophylaxis and the treatment of acute gout flares.

Prophylaxis of Gout Flares:
COLCRYS is indicated for prophylaxis of gout flares.

Treatment of Gout Flares:
COLCRYS tablets are indicated for treatment of acute gout flares when taken at the first sign of a flare.

1.2 Familial Mediterranean fever (FMF)

COLCRYS® (colchicine, USP) tablets are indicated in adults and children 4 years or older for treatment of familial Mediterranean fever (FMF).

2 DOSAGE AND ADMINISTRATION

The long term use of colchicine is established for FMF and the prophylaxis of gout flares but the safety and efficacy of repeat treatment for gout flares has not been evaluated. The dosing regimens for COLCRYS are different for each indication and must be individualized.

The recommended dosage of COLCRYS depends on the patient's age, renal function, hepatic function, and use of co-administered drugs [*see Dose Modification for Co-administration of Interacting Drugs (2.4)*].

COLCRYS tablets are administered orally, without regard to meals.

COLCRYS is not an analgesic medication and should not be used to treat pain from other causes.

2.1 Gout Flares

Prophylaxis of Gout Flares:

The recommended dosage of COLCRYS for prophylaxis of gout flares for adults and adolescents older than 16 years of age is 0.6 mg once or twice daily. The maximum recommended dose for prophylaxis of gout flares is 1.2 mg/day.

Treatment of Gout Flares:

The recommended dose of COLCRYS for treatment of a gout flare is 1.2 mg (2 tablets) at the first sign of the flare followed by 0.6 mg (1 tablet) one hour later. Higher doses have not been found to be more effective. The maximum recommended dose for treatment of gout flares is 1.8 mg over a 1 hour period. COLCRYS may be administered for treatment of a gout flare during prophylaxis at doses not to exceed 1.2 mg (2 tablets) at the first sign of the flare followed by 0.6 mg (1 tablet) one hour later. Wait 12 hours and then resume the prophylactic dose.

2.2 FMF

The recommended dosage of COLCRYS for FMF in adults is 1.2 mg to 2.4 mg daily.

COLCRYS should be increased as needed to control disease and as tolerated in increments of 0.3 mg/day to a maximum recommended daily dose. If intolerable side effects develop, the dose should be decreased in increments of 0.3 mg/day. The total daily COLCRYS dose may be administered in one to two divided doses.

2.3 Recommended Pediatric Dosage

Prophylaxis and Treatment of Gout Flares:

COLCRYS is not recommended for pediatric use in prophylaxis or treatment of gout flares.

FMF:

The recommended dosage of COLCRYS for FMF in pediatric patients 4 years of age and older is based on age. The following daily doses may be given as a single or divided dose twice daily:

- Children 4 – 6 years: 0.3 mg to 1.8 mg daily
- Children 6 – 12 years: 0.9 mg to 1.8 mg daily
- Adolescents older than 12 years: 1.2 mg to 2.4 mg daily

2.4 Dose Modification for Co-administration of Interacting Drugs

Concomitant Therapy:

Co-administration of COLCRYS with drugs known to inhibit CYP3A4 and/or P-glycoprotein (P-gp) increases the risk of colchicine-induced toxic effects (Table 1). If patients are taking or have recently completed treatment with drugs listed in Table 1 within the prior 14 days, the dose adjustments are as shown on the table below [*see DRUG INTERACTIONS (7)*].

Table 1 COLCRYS Dose Adjustment for Co-administration with Interacting Drugs if no Alternative Available*

Strong CYP3A4 Inhibitors†

Drug	Noted or Anticipated Outcome	Gout Flares				FMF	
		Prophylaxis of Gout Flares		Treatment of Gout Flares			
		Original Intended Dosage	Adjusted Dose	Original Intended Dosage	Adjusted Dose	Original Intended Dosage	Adjusted Dose
Atazanavir Clarithromycin Darunavir/ Ritonavir‡ Indinavir Itraconazole Ketoconazole Lopinavir/ Ritonavir‡ Nefazodone Nelfinavir Ritonavir Saquinavir Telithromycin Tipranavir/ Ritonavir‡	Significant increase in colchicine plasma levels*; fatal colchicine toxicity has been reported with clarithromycin, a strong CYP3A4 inhibitor. Similarly, significant increase in colchicine plasma levels is anticipated with other strong CYP3A4 inhibitors.	0.6 mg twice a day 0.6 mg once a day	0.3 mg once a day 0.3 mg once every other day	1.2 mg (2 tablets) followed by 0.6 mg (1 tablet) 1 hour later. Dose to be repeated no earlier than 3 days.	0.6 mg (1 tablet) × 1 dose, followed by 0.3 mg (1/2 tablet) 1 hour later. Dose to be repeated no earlier than 3 days.	Maximum daily dose of 1.2 – 2.4 mg	Maximum daily dose of 0.6 mg (may be given as 0.3 mg twice a day)

Moderate CYP3A4 Inhibitors

Drug	Noted or Anticipated Outcome	Gout Flares				FMF	
		Prophylaxis of Gout Flares		Treatment of Gout Flares			
		Original Intended Dosage	Adjusted Dose	Original Intended Dosage	Adjusted Dose	Original Intended Dosage	Adjusted Dose
Amprenavir‡ Aprepitant Diltiazem Erythromycin Fluconazole Fosamprenavir‡ (pro-drug of Amprenavir) Grapefruit Juice Verapamil	Significant increase in colchicine plasma concentration is anticipated. Neuromuscular toxicity has been reported with diltiazem and verapamil interactions.	0.6 mg twice a day 0.6 mg once a day	0.3 mg twice a day or 0.6 mg once a day 0.3 mg once a day	1.2 mg (2 tablets) followed by 0.6 mg (1 tablet) 1 hour later. Dose to be repeated no earlier than 3 days.	1.2 mg (2 tablets) × 1 dose. Dose to be repeated no earlier than 3 days.	Maximum daily dose of 1.2 – 2.4 mg.	Maximum daily dose of 1.2 mg (may be given as 0.6 mg twice a day)

P-gp Inhibitors†

Drug	Noted or Anticipated Outcome	Gout Flares				FMF	
		Prophylaxis of Gout Flares		Treatment of Gout Flares			
		Original Intended Dosage	Adjusted Dose	Original Intended Dosage	Adjusted Dose	Original Intended Dosage	Adjusted Dose
Cyclosporine Ranolazine	Significant increase in colchicine plasma levels*; fatal colchicine toxicity has been reported with cyclosporine, a P-gp inhibitor. Similarly, significant increase in colchicine plasma levels is anticipated with other P-gp inhibitors.	0.6 mg twice a day 0.6 mg once a day	0.3 mg once a day 0.3 mg once every other day	1.2 mg (2 tablets) followed by 0.6 mg (1 tablet) 1 hour later. Dose to be repeated no earlier than 3 days.	0.6 mg (1 tablet) × 1 dose. Dose to be repeated no earlier than 3 days.	Maximum daily dose of 1.2 – 2.4 mg	Maximum daily dose of 0.6 mg (may be given as 0.3 mg twice a day)

* For magnitude of effect on colchicine plasma concentrations [*see Pharmacokinetics (12.3)*]
† Patients with renal or hepatic impairment should not be given COLCRYS in conjunction with strong CYP3A4 or P-gp inhibitors [*see CONTRAINDICATIONS (4)*].
‡ When used in combination with Ritonavir, see dosing recommendations for strong CYP3A4 inhibitors [*see CONTRAINDICATIONS (4)*].

[See table 1 above]
[See table 2 on pages 2361 and 2362]
Treatment of gout flares with COLCRYS is not recommended in patients receiving prophylactic dose of COLCRYS and CYP3A4 inhibitors.

2.5 Dose Modification in Renal Impairment

Colchicine dosing must be individualized according to the patient's renal function [*see Renal Impairment (8.6)*].

Clcr in mL/minute may be estimated from serum creatinine (mg/dL) determination using the following formula:
[See second table at top of page 2362]

Gout Flares:

Prophylaxis of Gout Flares:

For prophylaxis of gout flares in patients with mild (estimated creatinine clearance Clcr 50 – 80 mL/min) to moderate (Clcr 30 – 50 mL/min) renal function impairment, adjustment of the recommended dose is not required, but patients should be monitored closely for adverse effects of colchicine. However, in patients with severe impairment, the starting dose should be 0.3 mg per day and any increase in dose should be done with close monitoring. For the prophylaxis of gout flares in patients undergoing dialysis, the starting doses should be 0.3 mg given twice a week with close monitoring [*see Clinical Pharmacology (12.3) and Renal Impairment (8.6)*].

Treatment of Gout Flares:

For treatment of gout flares in patients with mild (Clcr 50 – 80 mL/min) to moderate (Clcr 30 – 50 mL/min) renal function impairment, adjustment of the recommended dose is not required, but patients should be monitored closely for adverse effects of colchicine. However, in patients with severe impairment, while the dose does not need to be adjusted for the treatment of gout flares, a treatment course should be repeated no more than once every 2 weeks. For patients with gout flares requiring repeated courses consideration should be given to alternate therapy. For patients undergoing dialysis, the total recommended dose for the treatment of gout flares should be reduced to a single dose of 0.6 mg (1 tablet). For these patients, the treatment course should not be repeated more than once every 2 weeks [*see Clinical Pharmacology (12.3) and Renal Impairment (8.6)*]. Treatment of gout flares with COLCRYS is not recommended in patients with renal impairment who are receiving COLCRYS for prophylaxis.

FMF:

Caution should be taken in dosing patients with moderate and severe renal impairment and in patients undergoing dialysis. For these patients, the dosage should be reduced [*see Clinical Pharmacology (12.3)*]. Patients with mild (Clcr 50 – 80 mL/min) and moderate (Clcr 30 – 50 mL/min) renal impairment should be monitored closely for adverse effects of COLCRYS. Dose reduction may be necessary. For patients with severe renal failure (Clcr less than 30 mL/minute), start with 0.3 mg/day; any increase in dose should be done with adequate monitoring of the patient for adverse effects of colchicine [*see Renal Impairment (8.6)*]. For patients undergoing dialysis, the total recommended starting dose should be 0.3 mg (half tablet) per day. Dosing can be increased with close monitoring. Any increase in dose should be done with adequate monitoring of the patient for adverse effects of colchicine [*see Clinical Pharmacology (12.3) and Renal Impairment (8.6)*].

2.6 Dose Modification in Hepatic Impairment

Gout Flares

Prophylaxis of Gout Flares:

For prophylaxis of gout flares in patients with mild to moderate hepatic function impairment, adjustment of the recommended dose is not required, but patients should be monitored closely for adverse effects of colchicine. Dose reduction should be considered for the prophylaxis of gout flares in patients with severe hepatic impairment [*see Hepatic Impairment (8.7)*].

Treatment of Gout Flares:

For treatment of gout flares in patients with mild to moderate hepatic function impairment, adjustment of the recommended dose is not required, but patients should be monitored closely for adverse effects of colchicine. However, for the treatment of gout flares in patients with severe impairment while the dose does not need to be adjusted, but a treatment course should be repeated no more than once every 2 weeks. For these patients, requiring repeated courses for the treatment of gout flares, consideration should be given to alternate therapy [*see Hepatic Impairment (8.7)*]. Treatment of gout flares with COLCRYS is not recommended in patients with hepatic impairment who are receiving COLCRYS for prophylaxis.

FMF:

Patients with mild to moderate hepatic impairment should be monitored closely for adverse effects of colchicine. Dose reduction should be considered in patients with severe hepatic impairment [*see Hepatic Impairment (8.7)*].

3 DOSAGE FORMS AND STRENGTHS

0.6 mg tablets — purple capsule-shaped, film-coated with AR 374 debossed on one side and scored on the other side.

4 CONTRAINDICATIONS

Patients with renal or hepatic impairment should not be given COLCRYS in conjunction with P-gp or strong CYP3A4 inhibitors (this includes all protease inhibitors, except fosamprenavir). In these patients, life-threatening and fatal colchicine toxicity has been reported with colchicine taken in therapeutic doses.

5 WARNINGS AND PRECAUTIONS

5.1 Fatal Overdose

Fatal overdoses, both accidental and intentional, have been reported in adults and children who have ingested colchicine [*see OVERDOSAGE (10)*]. COLCRYS should be kept out of the reach of children.

5.2 Blood Dyscrasias
Myelosuppression, leukopenia, granulocytopenia, thrombocytopenia, pancytopenia, and aplastic anemia have been reported with colchicine used in therapeutic doses.

5.3 Drug Interactions
Colchicine is a P-gp and CYP3A4 substrate. Life-threatening and fatal drug interactions have been reported in patients treated with colchicine given with P-gp and strong CYP3A4 inhibitors. If treatment with a P-gp or strong CYP3A4 inhibitor is required in patients with normal renal and hepatic function, the patient's dose of colchicine may need to be reduced or interrupted [*see DRUG INTERACTIONS (7)*]. Use of COLCRYS in conjunction with P-gp or strong CYP3A4 inhibitors (this includes all protease inhibitors, except fosamprenavir) is contraindicated in patients with renal or hepatic impairment [*see CONTRAINDICATIONS (4)*].

5.4 Neuromuscular Toxicity
Colchicine-induced neuromuscular toxicity and rhabdomyolysis have been reported with chronic treatment in therapeutic doses. Patients with renal dysfunction and elderly patients, even those with normal renal and hepatic function, are at increased risk. Concomitant use of atorvastatin, simvastatin, pravastatin, fluvastatin, lovastatin, gemfibrozil, fenofibrate, fenofibric acid, or benzafibrate (themselves associated with myotoxicity) or cyclosporine with COLCRYS may potentiate the development of myopathy [*see DRUG INTERACTIONS (7)*]. Once colchicine is stopped, the symptoms generally resolve within 1 week to several months.

6 ADVERSE REACTIONS

Prophylaxis of Gout Flares:
The most commonly reported adverse reaction in clinical trials of colchicine for the prophylaxis of gout was diarrhea.

Treatment of Gout Flares:
The most common adverse reactions reported in the clinical trial with COLCRYS for treatment of gout flares were diarrhea (23%) and pharyngolaryngeal pain (3%).

FMF:
Gastrointestinal tract adverse effects are the most frequent side effects in patients initiating COLCRYS, usually presenting within 24 hours, and occurring in up to 20% of patients given therapeutic doses. Typical symptoms include cramping, nausea, diarrhea, abdominal pain, and vomiting. These events should be viewed as dose-limiting if severe as they can herald the onset of more significant toxicity.

6.1 Clinical Trials Experience in Gout
Because clinical studies are conducted under widely varying and controlled conditions, adverse reaction rates observed in clinical studies of a drug cannot be directly compared to rates in the clinical studies of another drug, and may not predict the rates observed in a broader patient population in clinical practice.

In a randomized, double-blind, placebo-controlled trial in patients with a gout flare, gastrointestinal adverse reactions occurred in 26% of patients using the recommended dose (1.8 mg over 1 hour) of COLCRYS compared to 77% of patients taking a non-recommended high-dose (4.8 mg over 6 hours) of colchicine and 20% of patients taking placebo. Diarrhea was the most commonly reported drug-related gastrointestinal adverse event. As shown in Table 3, diarrhea is associated with COLCRYS treatment. Diarrhea was more likely to occur in patients taking the high-dose regimen than the low-dose regimen. Severe diarrhea occurred in 19% and vomiting occurred in 17% of patients taking the non-recommended high-dose colchicine regimen but did not occur in the recommended low-dose COLCRYS regimen.

[See table 3 at top of next page]

6.2 Postmarketing Experience
Serious toxic manifestations associated with colchicine include myelosuppression, disseminated intravascular coagulation, and injury to cells in the renal, hepatic, circulatory, and central nervous systems.

These most often occur with excessive accumulation or overdosage [*see OVERDOSAGE (10)*].

The following adverse reactions have been reported with colchicine. These have been generally reversible upon temporarily interrupting treatment or lowering the dose of colchicine.

Neurological: sensory motor neuropathy
Dermatological: alopecia, maculopapular rash, purpura, rash
Digestive: abdominal cramping, abdominal pain, diarrhea, lactose intolerance, nausea, vomiting
Hematological: leukopenia, granulocytopenia, thrombocytopenia, pancytopenia, aplastic anemia
Hepatobiliary: elevated AST, elevated ALT
Musculoskeletal: myopathy, elevated CPK, myotonia, muscle weakness, muscle pain, rhabdomyolysis
Reproductive: azoospermia, oligospermia

7 DRUG INTERACTIONS

COLCRYS (colchicine) is a substrate of the efflux transporter P-glycoprotein (P-gp). Of the cytochrome P450 enzymes tested, CYP3A4 was mainly involved in the metabolism of colchicine. If COLCRYS is administered with drugs that inhibit P-gp, most of which also inhibit CYP3A4, increased concentrations of colchicine are likely. Fatal drug interactions have been reported.

Physicians should ensure that patients are suitable candidates for treatment with COLCRYS and remain alert for signs and symptoms of toxicities related to increased colchicine exposure as a result of a drug interaction. Signs and symptoms of COLCRYS toxicity should be evaluated promptly and, if toxicity is suspected, COLCRYS should be discontinued immediately.

Table 2 COLCRYS Dose Adjustment for Co-administration with Protease Inhibitors

Protease Inhibitor	Clinical Comment	w/Colchicine – Prophylaxis of Gout Flares		w/Colchicine – Treatment of Gout Flares	w/Colchicine – Treatment of FMF
		Original dose	Adjusted dose		
Atazanavir sulfate (Reyataz)	Patients with renal or hepatic impairment should not be given colchicine with Reyataz.	0.6 mg twice a day 0.6 mg once a day	0.3 mg once a day 0.3 mg once every other day	0.6 mg (1 tablet) × 1 dose, followed by 0.3 mg (1/2 tablet) 1 hour later. Dose to be repeated no earlier than 3 days.	Maximum daily dose of 0.6 mg (may be given as 0.3 mg twice a day)
Darunavir (Prezista)	Patients with renal or hepatic impairment should not be given colchicine with Prezista/ritonavir.	0.6 mg twice a day 0.6 mg once a day	0.3 mg once a day 0.3 mg once every other day	0.6 mg (1 tablet) × 1 dose, followed by 0.3 mg (1/2 tablet) 1 hour later. Dose to be repeated no earlier than 3 days.	Maximum daily dose of 0.6 mg (may be given as 0.3 mg twice a day)
Fosamprenavir (Lexiva) with Ritonavir	Patients with renal or hepatic impairment should not be given colchicine with Lexiva/ritonavir.	0.6 mg twice a day 0.6 mg once a day	0.3 mg once a day 0.3 mg once every other day	0.6 mg (1 tablet) × 1 dose, followed by 0.3 mg (1/2 tablet) 1 hour later. Dose to be repeated no earlier than 3 days.	Maximum daily dose of 0.6 mg (may be given as 0.3 mg twice a day)
Fosamprenavir (Lexiva)	Patients with renal or hepatic impairment should not be given colchicine with Lexiva/ritonavir.	0.6 mg twice a day 0.6 mg once a day	0.3 mg twice a day or 0.6 mg once a day 0.3 mg once a day	1.2 mg (2 tablets) × 1 dose. Dose to be repeated no earlier than 3 days.	Maximum daily dose of 1.2 mg (may be given as 0.6 mg twice a day)
Indinavir (Crixivan)	Patients with renal or hepatic impairment should not be given colchicine with Crixivan.	0.6 mg twice a day 0.6 mg once a day	0.3 mg once a day 0.3 mg once every other day	0.6 mg (1 tablet) × 1 dose, followed by 0.3 mg (1/2 tablet) 1 hour later. Dose to be repeated no earlier than 3 days.	Maximum daily dose of 0.6 mg (may be given as 0.3 mg twice a day)
Lopinavir/Ritonavir (Kaletra)	Patients with renal or hepatic impairment should not be given colchicine with Kaletra.	0.6 mg twice a day 0.6 mg once a day	0.3 mg once a day 0.3 mg once every other day	0.6 mg (1 tablet) × 1 dose, followed by 0.3 mg (1/2 tablet) 1 hour later. Dose to be repeated no earlier than 3 days.	Maximum daily dose of 0.6 mg (may be given as 0.3 mg twice a day)
Nelfinavir mesylate (Viracept)	Patients with renal or hepatic impairment should not be given colchicine with Viracept.	0.6 mg twice a day 0.6 mg once a day	0.3 mg once a day 0.3 mg once every other day	0.6 mg (1 tablet) × 1 dose, followed by 0.3 mg (1/2 tablet) 1 hour later. Dose to be repeated no earlier than 3 days.	Maximum daily dose of 0.6 mg (may be given as 0.3 mg twice a day)
Ritonavir (Norvir)	Patients with renal or hepatic impairment should not be given colchicine with Norvir.	0.6 mg twice a day 0.6 mg once a day	0.3 mg once a day 0.3 mg once every other day	0.6 mg (1 tablet) × 1 dose, followed by 0.3 mg (1/2 tablet) 1 hour later. Dose to be repeated no earlier than 3 days.	Maximum daily dose of 0.6 mg (may be given as 0.3 mg twice a day)

(Table continued on next page)

Table 4 provides recommendations as a result of other potentially significant drug interactions. Table 1 provides recommendations for strong and moderate CYP3A4 inhibitors and P-gp inhibitors.

[See table 4 at top of next page]

8 USE IN SPECIFIC POPULATIONS

8.1 Pregnancy
Pregnancy Category C
There are no adequate and well-controlled studies with colchicine in pregnant women. Colchicine crosses the human placenta. While not studied in the treatment of gout flares, data from a limited number of published studies

Table 2 *(cont.)* COLCRYS Dose Adjustment for Co-administration with Protease Inhibitors

Protease Inhibitor	Clinical Comment	w/Colchicine – Prophylaxis of Gout Flares		w/Colchicine – Treatment of Gout Flares	w/Colchicine – Treatment of FMF
		Original dose	Adjusted dose		
Saquinavir mesylate (Invirase)	Patients with renal or hepatic impairment should not be given colchicine with Invirase/ritonavir.	0.6 mg twice a day 0.6 mg once a day	0.3 mg once a day 0.3 mg once every other day	0.6 mg (1 tablet) × 1 dose, followed by 0.3 mg (1/2 tablet) 1 hour later. Dose to be repeated no earlier than 3 days.	Maximum daily dose of 0.6 mg (may be given as 0.3 mg twice a day)
		Original dose	Adjusted dose		
Tipranavir (Aptivus)	Patients with renal or hepatic impairment should not be given colchicine with Aptivus/ritonavir.	0.6 mg twice a day 0.6 mg once a day	0.3 mg once a day 0.3 mg once every other day	0.6 mg (1 tablet) × 1 dose, followed by 0.3 mg (1/2 tablet) 1 hour later. Dose to be repeated no earlier than 3 days.	Maximum daily dose of 0.6 mg (may be given as 0.3 mg twice a day)

$$\text{Clcr} = \frac{[140\text{-age (years)} \times \text{weight (kg)}]}{72 \times \text{serum creatinine (mg/dL)}} \quad \times 0.85 \text{ for female patients}$$

Table 3 Number (%) of Patients with at Least One Drug-Related Treatment Emergent Adverse Events with an Incidence of ≥ 2% of Patients in Any Treatment Group

MedDRA System Organ Class MedDRA Preferred Term	COLCRYS Dose		Placebo (N=59) n (%)
	High (N=52) n (%)	Low (N=74) n (%)	
Number of Patients with at Least One Drug-Related TEAE	40 (77)	27 (37)	16 (27)
Gastrointestinal Disorders	40 (77)	19 (26)	12 (20)
Diarrhea	40 (77)	17 (23)	8 (14)
Nausea	9 (17)	3 (4)	3 (5)
Vomiting	9 (17)	0	0
Abdominal Discomfort	0	0	2 (3)
General Disorders and Administration Site Conditions	4 (8)	1 (1)	1 (2)
Fatigue	2 (4)	1 (1)	1 (2)
Metabolic and Nutrition Disorders	0	3 (4)	2 (3)
Gout	0	3 (4)	1 (2)
Nervous System Disorders	1 (2)	1 (1.4)	2 (3)
Headache	1 (2)	1 (1)	2 (3)
Respiratory Thoracic Mediastinal Disorders	1 (2)	2 (3)	0
Pharyngolaryngeal Pain	1 (2)	2 (3)	0

Table 4 Other Potentially Significant Drug Interactions

Concomitant Drug Class or Food	Noted or anticipated Outcome	Clinical Comment
HMG-Co A Reductase Inhibitors: atorvastatin, fluvastatin, lovastatin, pravastatin, simvastatin	Pharmacokinetic and/or pharmacodynamic interaction: the addition of one drug to a stable long-term regimen of the other has resulted in myopathy and rhabdomyolysis (including a fatality)	Weigh the potential benefits and risks and carefully monitor patients for any signs or symptoms of muscle pain, tenderness, or weakness, particularly during initial therapy; monitoring CPK (creatine phosphokinase) will not necessarily prevent the occurrence of severe myopathy.
Other Lipid Lowering Drugs: fibrates, gemfibrozil		
Digitalis Glycosides: digoxin	P-gp substrate; rhabdomyolysis has been reported	

found no evidence of an increased risk of miscarriage, stillbirth, or teratogenic effects among pregnant women using colchicine to treat familial Mediterranean fever (FMF). Although animal reproductive and developmental studies were not conducted with COLCRYS, published animal reproduction and development studies indicate that colchicine causes embryofetal toxicity, teratogenicity, and altered postnatal development at exposures within or above the clinical therapeutic range. COLCRYS should be used during pregnancy only if the potential benefit justifies the potential risk to the fetus.

8.2 Labor and Delivery

The effect of colchicine on labor and delivery is unknown.

8.3 Nursing Mothers

Colchicine is excreted into human milk. Limited information suggests that exclusively breast-fed infants receive less than 10 percent of the maternal weight-adjusted dose. While there are no published reports of adverse effects in breast-feeding infants of mothers taking colchicine, colchicine can affect gastrointestinal cell renewal and permeability. Caution should be exercised and breast-feeding infants should be observed for adverse effects when COLCRYS is administered to a nursing woman.

8.4 Pediatric Use

The safety and efficacy of colchicine in children of all ages with FMF has been evaluated in uncontrolled studies. There does not appear to be an adverse effect on growth in children with FMF treated long-term with colchicine. Gout is rare in pediatric patients, safety and effectiveness of colchicine in pediatric patients has not been established.

8.5 Geriatric Use

Clinical studies with colchicine for prophylaxis and treatment of gout flares and for treatment of FMF did not include sufficient numbers of patients aged 65 years and older to determine whether they respond differently from younger patients. In general, dose selection for an elderly patient with gout should be cautious, reflecting the greater frequency of decreased renal function, concomitant disease, or other drug therapy [*see Dose Modification for Co-administration of Interacting Drugs (2.4)*].

8.6 Renal Impairment

Colchicine is significantly excreted in urine in healthy subjects. Clearance of colchicine is decreased in patients with impaired renal function. Total body clearance of colchicine was reduced by 75% in patients with end-stage renal disease undergoing dialysis.

Prophylaxis of Gout Flares:

For prophylaxis of gout flares in patients with mild (estimated creatinine clearance Clcr 50 – 80 mL/min) to moderate (Clcr 30 – 50 mL/min) renal function impairment, adjustment of the recommended dose is not required, but patients should be monitored closely for adverse effects of colchicine. However, in patients with severe impairment, the starting dose should be 0.3 mg per day and any increase in dose should be done with close monitoring. For the prophylaxis of gout flares in patients undergoing dialysis, the starting doses should be 0.3 mg given twice a week with close monitoring [*see Dose Modification in Renal Impairment (2.5)*].

Treatment of Gout Flares:

For treatment of gout flares in patients with mild (Clcr 50 – 80 mL/min) to moderate (Clcr 30 – 50 mL/min) renal function impairment, adjustment of the recommended dose is not required, but patients should be monitored closely for adverse effects of COLCRYS. However, in patients with severe impairment, while the dose does not need to be adjusted for the treatment of gout flares, a treatment course should be repeated no more than once every 2 weeks. For patients with gout flares requiring repeated courses consideration should be given to alternate therapy. For patients undergoing dialysis, the total recommended dose for the treatment of gout flares should be reduced to a single dose of 0.6 mg (1 tablet). For these patients, the treatment course should not be repeated more than once every 2 weeks [*see Dose Modification in Renal Impairment (2.5)*].

FMF

Although, pharmacokinetics of colchicine in patients with mild (Clcr 50 – 80 mL/min) and moderate (Clcr 30 – 50 mL/min) renal impairment is not known, these patients should be monitored closely for adverse effects of colchicine. Dose reduction may be necessary. In patients with severe renal failure (Clcr less than 30 mL/minute) and end-stage renal disease requiring dialysis, COLCRYS may be started at the dose of 0.3 mg/day. Any increase in dose should be done with adequate monitoring of the patient for adverse effects of COLCRYS [*see Pharmacokinetics (12.3) and Dose Modification in Renal Impairment (2.5)*].

8.7 Hepatic Impairment

The clearance of colchicine may be significantly reduced and plasma half-life prolonged in patients with chronic hepatic impairment, compared to healthy subjects [*see Pharmacokinetics (12.3)*].

Prophylaxis of Gout Flares:

For prophylaxis of gout flares in patients with mild to moderate hepatic function impairment, adjustment of the recommended dose is not required, but patients should be monitored closely for adverse effects of colchicine. Dose reduction should be considered for the prophylaxis of gout flares in patients with severe hepatic impairment [*see Dose Modification in Hepatic Impairment (2.6)*].

Treatment of Gout Flares:

For treatment of gout flares in patients with mild to moderate hepatic function impairment, adjustment of the recommended COLCRYS dose is not required, but patients should be monitored closely for adverse effects of COLCRYS. However, for the treatment of gout flares in patients with severe impairment while the dose does not need to be adjusted, the treatment course should be repeated no more than once every 2 weeks. For these patients, requiring repeated courses for the treatment of gout flares, consideration should be given to alternate therapy [*see Dose Modification in Hepatic Impairment (2.6)*].

FMF

In patients with severe hepatic disease, dose reduction should be considered with careful monitoring [*see Pharmacokinetics (12.3) and Dose Modification in Hepatic Impairment (2.6)*].

9 DRUG ABUSE AND DEPENDENCE

Tolerance, abuse, or dependence with colchicine has not been reported.

10 OVERDOSAGE

The exact dose of colchicine that produces significant toxicity is unknown. Fatalities have occurred after ingestion of a dose as low as 7 mg over a 4-day period, while other patients have survived after ingesting more than 60 mg. A review of 150 patients who overdosed on colchicine found that those who ingested less than 0.5 mg/kg survived and tended to have milder toxicities, such as gastrointestinal symptoms, whereas those who took 0.5 to 0.8 mg/kg had more severe reactions, such as myelosuppression. There was 100% mortality in those who ingested more than 0.8 mg/kg.

The first stage of acute colchicine toxicity typically begins within 24 hours of ingestion and includes gastrointestinal symptoms, such as abdominal pain, nausea, vomiting, diarrhea, and significant fluid loss, leading to volume depletion. Peripheral leukocytosis may also be seen. Life-threatening complications occur during the second stage, which occurs 24 to 72 hours after drug administration, attributed to multi-organ failure and its consequences. Death is usually a result of respiratory depression and cardiovascular collapse. If the patient survives, recovery of multi-organ injury may be accompanied by rebound leukocytosis and alopecia starting about 1 week after the initial ingestion.

Treatment of colchicine poisoning should begin with gastric lavage and measures to prevent shock. Otherwise, treatment is symptomatic and supportive. No specific antidote is known. Colchicine is not effectively removed by dialysis [*see Pharmacokinetics (12.3)*].

11 DESCRIPTION

Colchicine is an alkaloid chemically described as (S)N-(5,6,7,9-tetrahydro- 1,2,3, 10-tetramethoxy-9-oxobenzo [alpha] heptalen-7-yl) acetamide with a molecular formula of $C_{22}H_{25}NO_6$ and a molecular weight of 399.4. The structural formula of colchicine is given below.

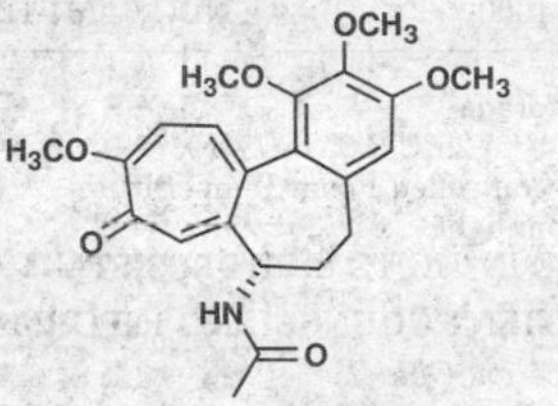

Colchicine occurs as a pale yellow powder that is soluble in water.

COLCRYS® (colchicine, USP) tablets are supplied for oral administration as purple, film-coated, capsule-shaped tablets (0.1575″ × 0.3030″), debossed with 'AR 374' on one side and scored on the other, containing 0.6 mg of the active ingredient colchicine USP. Inactive ingredients: carnauba wax, FD&C blue #2, FD&C red #40, hypromellose, lactose monohydrate, magnesium stearate, microcrystalline cellulose, polydextrose, polyethylene glycol, pregelatinized starch, sodium starch glycolate, titanium dioxide, and triacetin.

12 CLINICAL PHARMACOLOGY

12.1 Mechanism of Action

The mechanism by which COLCRYS exerts its beneficial effect in patients with FMF has not been fully elucidated; however, evidence suggests that colchicine may interfere with the intracellular assembly of the inflammasome complex present in neutrophils and monocytes that mediates activation of interleukin-1β. Additionally, colchicine disrupts cytoskeletal functions through inhibition of β-tubulin polymerization into microtubules, and consequently prevents the activation, degranulation, and migration of neutrophils thought to mediate some gout symptoms.

12.3 Pharmacokinetics

Absorption

In healthy adults, COLCRYS is absorbed when given orally, reaching a mean C_{max} of 2.5 ng/mL (range 1.1 to 4.4 ng/mL) in 1 to 2 hours (range 0.5 to 3 hours) after a single dose administered under fasting conditions.

Following oral administration of COLCRYS given as 1.8 mg colchicine over 1 hour to healthy, young adults under fasting conditions, colchicine appears to be readily absorbed, reaching mean maximum plasma concentrations of 6.2 ng/mL at a median 1.81 hours (range: 1.0 to 2.5 hours). Following administration of the non-recommended high-dose regimen (4.8 mg over 6 hours), mean maximal plasma concentrations were 6.8 ng/mL, at a median 4.47 hours (range: 3.1 to 7.5 hours).

After 10 days on a regimen of 0.6 mg twice daily, peak concentrations are 3.1 to 3.6 ng/mL (range 1.6 to 6.0 ng/mL), occurring 1.3 to 1.4 hours post-dose (range 0.5 to 3.0 hours). Mean pharmacokinetic parameter values in healthy adults are shown in Table 5 below.

[See table 5 above]

Table 5 Mean (%CV) Pharmacokinetic Parameters in Healthy Adults Given COLCRYS

C_{max} (colchicine ng/mL)	T_{max}* (h)	Vd/F (L)	CL/F (L/hr)	$t_{1/2}$ (h)
COLCRYS 0.6 mg Single Dose (N=13)				
2.5 (28.7)	1.5 (1.0 – 3.0)	341.5 (54.4)	54.1 (31.0)	--
COLCRYS 0.6 mg b.i.d. × 10 days (N=13)				
3.6 (23.7)	1.3 (0.5 – 3.0)	1150 (18.7)	30.3 (19.0)	26.6 (16.3)

CL= Dose/AUC_{0-t} (Calculated from mean values)
Vd = CL/Ke (Calculated from mean values)

* T_{max} mean (range)

In some subjects, secondary colchicine peaks are seen, occurring between 3 and 36 hours post-dose and ranging from 39% to 155% of the height of the initial peak. These observations are attributed to intestinal secretion and reabsorption and/or biliary recirculation.

Absolute bioavailability is reported to be approximately 45%.

Administration of COLCRYS with food has no effect on the rate of colchicine absorption, but did decrease the extent of colchicine by approximately 15%. This is without clinical significance.

Distribution

The mean apparent volume of distribution in healthy young volunteers was approximately 5 to 8 L/kg.

Colchicine binding to serum protein is low, 39 ± 5%, primarily to albumin regardless of concentration.

Colchicine crosses the placenta (plasma levels in the fetus are reported to be approximately 15% of the maternal concentration). Colchicine also distributes into breast milk at concentrations similar to those found in the maternal serum [*see Pregnancy (8.1) and Nursing Mothers (8.3)*].

Metabolism

Colchicine is demethylated to two primary metabolites, 2-O-demethylcolchicine and 3-O-demethylcolchicine (2- and 3-DMC, respectively), and one minor metabolite, 10-O-demethylcolchicine (also known as colchiceine). *In vitro* studies using human liver microsomes have shown that CYP3A4 is involved in the metabolism of colchicine to 2- and 3-DMC. Plasma levels of these metabolites are minimal (less than 5% of parent drug).

Elimination/Excretion

In healthy volunteers (n=12) 40 – 65% of 1 mg orally administered colchicine was recovered unchanged in urine. Enterohepatic recirculation and biliary excretion are also postulated to play a role in colchicine elimination. Following multiple oral doses (0.6 mg twice daily), the mean elimination half-lives in young healthy volunteers (mean age 25 to 28 years of age) is 26.6 to 31.2 hours. Colchicine is a substrate of P-gp.

Extracorporeal Elimination: Colchicine is not removed by hemodialysis.

Special Populations

There is no difference between men and women in the pharmacokinetic disposition of colchicine.

Pediatric Patients: Pharmacokinetics of colchicine was not evaluated in pediatric patients.

Elderly: Pharmacokinetics of colchicine has not been determined in elderly patients. A published report described the pharmacokinetics of 1 mg oral colchicine tablet in four elderly women compared to six young healthy males. The mean age of the four elderly women was 83 years (range 75 – 93), mean weight was 47 kg (38 – 61 kg) and mean creatinine clearance was 46 mL/min (range 25 – 75 mL/min). Mean peak plasma levels and AUC of colchicine were two times higher in elderly subjects compared to young healthy males. However, it is possible that the higher exposure in the elderly subjects was due to decreased renal function.

Renal impairment: Pharmacokinetics of colchicine in patients with mild and moderate renal impairment is not known. A published report described the disposition of colchicine (1 mg) in young adult men and women with FMF who had normal renal function or end-stage renal disease requiring dialysis. Patients with end-stage renal disease had 75% lower colchicine clearance (0.17 *vs* 0.73 L/hr/kg) and prolonged plasma elimination half-life (18.8 hrs *vs* 4.4 hrs) as compared to subjects with FMF and normal renal function [*see Dose Modification in Renal Impairment (2.5) and Renal Impairment (8.6)*].

Hepatic impairment: Published reports on the pharmacokinetics of IV colchicine in patients with severe chronic liver disease, as well as those with alcoholic or primary biliary cirrhosis, and normal renal function suggest wide interpatient variability. In some subjects with mild to moderate cirrhosis, the clearance of colchicine is significantly reduced and plasma half-life prolonged compared to healthy subjects. In subjects with primary biliary cirrhosis, no consistent trends were noted [*see Dose Modification in Hepatic Impairment (2.6) and Hepatic Impairment (8.7)*]. No pharmacokinetic data are available for patients with severe hepatic impairment (Child-Pugh C).

Drug interactions:

In vitro drug interactions:

In vitro studies in human liver microsomes have shown that colchicine is not an inhibitor or inducer of CYP1A2, CYP2A6, CYP2B6, CYP2C8, CYP2C9, CYP2C19, CYP2D6, CYP2E1, or CYP3A4 activity.

Table 6 Drug Interactions: Pharmacokinetic Parameters for COLCRYS (colchicine, USP) tablets in the Presence of the Co-Administered Drug

Co-administered Drug	Dose of Co-administered Drug (mg)	Dose of COLCRYS (mg)	N	% Change in Colchicine Concentrations from Baseline (Range: Min - Max)	
				C_{max}	AUC_{0-t}
Cyclosporine	100 mg single-dose	0.6 mg single-dose	23	270.0 (62.0 to 606.9)	259.0 (75.8 to 511.9)
Clarithromycin	250 mg BID, 7 days	0.6 mg single-dose	23	227.2 (65.7 to 591.1)	281.5 (88.7 to 851.6)
Ketoconazole	200 mg BID, 5 days	0.6 mg single-dose	24	101.7 (19.6 to 219.0)	212.2 (76.7 to 419.6)
Ritonavir	100 mg BID, 5 days	0.6 mg single-dose	18	184.4 (79.2 to 447.4)	296.0 (53.8 to 924.4)
Verapamil	240 mg daily, 5 days	0.6 mg single-dose	24	40.1 (-47.1 to 149.5)	103.3 (-9.8 to 217.2)
Diltiazem	240 mg daily, 7 days	0.6 mg single-dose	20	44.2 (-46.0 to 318.3)	93.4 (-30.2 to 338.6)
Azithromycin	500 mg × 1 day, then 250 mg × 4 days	0.6 mg single-dose	21	21.6 (-41.7 to 222.0)	57.1 (-24.3 to 241.1)
Grapefruit Juice	240 mL BID, 4 days	0.6 mg single-dose	21	-2.55 (-53.4 to 55.0)	-2.36 (-46.4 to 62.2)

Table 7 Drug Interactions: Pharmacokinetic Parameters for Co-Administration of Drug in the Presence of COLCRYS (colchicine, USP) tablets

Co-administered Drug	Dose of Co-administered Drug (mg)	Dose of COLCRYS (mg)	N	% Change in Co-Administered Drug Concentrations from Baseline (Range: Min - Max)	
				C_{max}	AUC_{0-t}
Theophylline	300 mg (elixir) single-dose	0.6 mg BID × 14 days	27	1.6 (-30.4 to 23.1)	1.6 (-28.5 to 27.1)
Ethinyl Estradiol (Ortho-Novum® 1/35)	21-Day Cycle (Active Treatment) + 7-Day Placebo	0.6 mg BID × 14 days	27*	-6.7 (-40.3 to 44.7)	-3.0† (-25.3 to 24.9)
Norethindrone (Ortho-Novum® 1/35)				0.94 (-37.3 to 59.4)	-1.6† (-32.0 to 33.7)

* Conducted in healthy adult females
† AUCτ

Table 8 Number (%) of Responders Based on Target Joint Pain Score at 24 Hours Post First Dose

COLCRYS Dose Responders n (%)		Placebo n (%) (n=58)	% Differences in Proportion	
Low-dose (n=74)	High-dose (n=52)		Low-dose vs Placebo (95% CI)	High-dose vs Placebo (95% CI)
28 (38%)	17 (33%)	9 (16%)	22 (8, 37)	17 (1, 33)

In vivo drug interactions:
The effects of co-administration of other drugs with COLCRYS on C_{max}, AUC, and C_{min} are summarized in Table 6 (effect of other drugs on colchicine) and Table 7 (effect of colchicine on other drugs). For information regarding clinical recommendations, see Table 1 in Dose Modification for Co-administration of Interacting Drugs [*see Dose Modification for Co-administration of Interacting Drugs (2.4)*].
[See table 6 at top of previous page]
Estrogen-containing oral contraceptives: In healthy female volunteers given ethinyl estradiol and norethindrone (Ortho-Novum® 1/35) co-administered with COLCRYS (0.6 mg b.i.d. × 14 days), hormone concentrations are not affected.
In healthy volunteers given theophylline co-administered with COLCRYS (0.6 mg b.i.d. × 14 days), theophylline concentrations were not affected.
[See table 7 above]

13 NONCLINICAL TOXICOLOGY

13.1 Carcinogenesis, Mutagenesis, Impairment of Fertility

Carcinogenesis
Carcinogenicity studies of colchicine have not been conducted. Due to the potential for colchicine to produce aneuploid cells (cells with an unequal number of chromosomes), there is theoretically an increased risk of malignancy.
Mutagenesis
Colchicine was negative for mutagenicity in the bacterial reverse mutation assay. In a chromosomal aberration assay in cultured human white blood cells, colchicine treatment resulted in the formation of micronuclei. Since published studies demonstrated that colchicine induces aneuploidy from the process of mitotic nondisjunction without structural DNA changes, colchicine is not considered clastogenic, although micronuclei are formed.
Impairment of Fertility
No studies of colchicine effects on fertility were conducted with COLCRYS. However, published nonclinical studies demonstrated that colchicine-induced disruption of microtubule formation affects meiosis and mitosis. Reproductive studies also reported abnormal sperm morphology and reduced sperm counts in males, and interference with sperm penetration, second meiotic division, and normal cleavage in females when exposed to colchicine. Colchicine administered to pregnant animals resulted in fetal death and teratogenicity. These effects were dose dependent, with the timing of exposure critical for the effects on embryofetal development. The nonclinical doses evaluated were generally higher than an equivalent human therapeutic dose, but safety margins for reproductive and developmental toxicity could not be determined.
Case reports and epidemiology studies in human male subjects on colchicine therapy indicated that infertility from colchicine is rare. A case report indicated that azoospermia was reversed when therapy was stopped. Case reports and epidemiology studies in female subjects on colchicine therapy have not established a clear relationship between colchicine use and female infertility. However, since the progression of FMF without treatment may result in infertility, the use of colchicine needs to be weighed against the potential risks.

14 CLINICAL STUDIES

The evidence for the efficacy of colchicine in patients with chronic gout is derived from the published literature. Two randomized clinical trials assessed the efficacy of colchicine 0.6 mg twice a day for the prophylaxis of gout flares in patients with gout initiating treatment with urate lowering therapy. In both trials, treatment with colchicine decreased the frequency of gout flares.
The efficacy of a low dosage regimen of oral colchicine (COLCRYS total dose 1.8 mg over 1 hour) for treatment of gout flares was assessed in a multicenter, randomized, double-blind, placebo-controlled, parallel group, 1 week, dose comparison study. Patients meeting American College of Rheumatology criteria for gout were randomly assigned to three groups: high-dose colchicine (1.2 mg, then 0.6 mg hourly × 6 hours [4.8 mg total]); low-dose colchicine (1.2 mg, then 0.6 mg in 1 hour [1.8 mg total] followed by 5 placebo doses hourly); or placebo (2 capsules, then 1 capsule hourly × 6 hours). Patients took the first dose within 12 hours of the onset of the flare and recorded pain intensity (11-point Likert scale) and adverse events over 72 hours. The efficacy of colchicine was measured based on response to treatment in the target joint, using patient self assessment of pain at 24 hours following the time of first dose as recorded in the diary. A responder was one who achieved at least a 50% reduction in pain score at the 24-hour post-dose assessment relative to the pre-treatment score and did not use rescue medication prior to the actual time of 24-hour post-dose assessment.
Rates of response were similar for the recommended low-dose treatment group (38%) and the non-recommended high-dose group (33%) but were higher as compared to the placebo group (16%) as shown in Table 8.
[See table 8 above]
Figure 1 below shows the percentage of patients achieving varying degrees of improvement in pain from baseline at 24 hours.

Figure 1
Pain Relief on Low and High Doses of COLCRYS and Placebo (Cumulative)

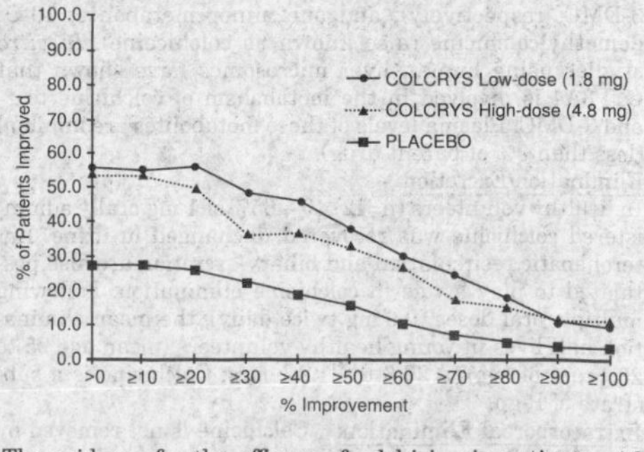

The evidence for the efficacy of colchicine in patients with FMF is derived from the published literature. Three randomized, placebo-controlled studies were identified. The three placebo-controlled studies randomized a total of 48 adult patients diagnosed with FMF and reported similar efficacy endpoints as well as inclusion and exclusion criteria. One of the studies randomized 15 patients with FMF to a 6-month crossover study during which 5 patients discontinued due to study non-compliance. The 10 patients completing the study experienced 5 attacks over the course of 90 days while treated with colchicine compared to 59 attacks over the course of 90 days while treated with placebo. Similarly, the second study randomized 22 patients with FMF to a 4-month crossover study during which 9 patients discontinued due to lack of efficacy while receiving placebo or study non-compliance. The 13 patients completing the study experienced 18 attacks over the course of 60 days while treated with colchicine compared to 68 attacks over the course of 60 days while treated with placebo. The third study was discontinued after an interim analysis of 6 of the 11 patients enrolled had completed the study; results could not be confirmed.
Open-label experience with colchicine in adults and children with FMF is consistent with the randomized, controlled trial experience, and was utilized to support information on the safety profile of colchicine and for dosing recommendations.

16 HOW SUPPLIED/STORAGE AND HANDLING

16.1 How Supplied

COLCRYS® (colchicine, USP) tablets 0.6 mg, are purple, film-coated, capsule-shaped tablets, debossed with 'AR 374' on one side and scored on the other side.

Bottles of 30	NDC 64764-119-07
Bottles of 60	NDC 64764-119-06
Bottles of 100	NDC 64764-119-01
Bottles of 250	NDC 64764-119-03
Bottles of 500	NDC 64764-119-05
Bottles of 1000	NDC 64764-119-10

16.2 Storage

Store at 20° to 25°C (68° to 77°F).
[See USP Controlled Room Temperature]
Protect from light.
DISPENSE IN TIGHT, LIGHT-RESISTANT CONTAINER.

17 PATIENT COUNSELING INFORMATION

[See Medication Guide]

17.1 Dosing Instructions

Patients should be advised to take COLCRYS as prescribed, even if they are feeling better. Patients should not alter the dose or discontinue treatment without consulting with their doctor. If a dose of COLCRYS is missed:

- For treatment of a gout flare when the patient is not being dosed for prophylaxis, take the missed dose as soon as possible.
- For treatment of a gout flare during prophylaxis, take the missed dose immediately, wait twelve hours, then resume the previous dosing schedule.
- For prophylaxis without treatment for a gout flare, or FMF, take the dose as soon as possible and then return to the normal dosing schedule. However, if a dose is skipped the patient should not double the next dose.

17.2 Fatal Overdose

Instruct patient that fatal overdoses, both accidental and intentional, have been reported in adults and children who have ingested colchicine. COLCRYS should be kept out of the reach of children.

17.3 Blood Dyscrasias

Patients should be informed that bone marrow depression with agranulocytosis, aplastic anemia, and thrombocytopenia may occur with COLCRYS.

17.4 Drug and Food Interactions

Patients should be advised that many drugs or other substances may interact with COLCRYS and some interactions could be fatal. Therefore, patients should report to their healthcare provider all of the current medications they are taking, and check with their healthcare provider before starting any new medications, particularly antibiotics. Patients should also be advised to report the use of nonprescription medication or herbal products. Grapefruit and grapefruit juice may also interact and should not be consumed during COLCRYS treatment.

17.5 Neuromuscular Toxicity

Patients should be informed that muscle pain or weakness, tingling or numbness in fingers or toes may occur with COLCRYS alone or when it is used with certain other drugs. Patients developing any of these signs or symptoms must discontinue COLCRYS and seek medical evaluation immediately.

17.6 Medication Guide

Distributed by:
Takeda Pharmaceuticals America, Inc.
Deerfield, IL 60015
Rev 01, June 2012

MEDICATION GUIDE
COLCRYS
(KOL-kris)
(colchicine) tablets

Read the Medication Guide that comes with COLCRYS before you start taking it and each time you get a refill. There may be new information. This Medication Guide does not take the place of talking to your healthcare provider about your medical condition or treatment. You and your healthcare provider should talk about COLCRYS when you start taking it and at regular checkups.

What is the most important information I should know about COLCRYS?

COLCRYS can cause serious side effects or death if levels of COLCRYS are too high in your body.

- Taking certain medicines with COLCRYS can cause your level of COLCRYS to be too high, especially if you have kidney or liver problems.
- Tell your healthcare provider about all your medical conditions, including if you have kidney or liver problems. Your dose of COLCRYS may need to be changed.
- Tell your healthcare provider about all the medicines you take, including prescription and non-prescription medicines, vitamins and herbal supplements.
- Even medicines that you take for a short period of time, such as antibiotics, can interact with COLCRYS and cause serious side effects or death.
- Talk to your healthcare provider or pharmacist before taking any new medicine.
- Especially tell your healthcare provider if you take:

• atazanavir sulfate (Reyataz®)	• clarithromycin (Biaxin®)
• cyclosporine (Neoral®, Gengraf®, Sandimmune®)	• darunavir (Prezista®)
• fosamprenavir (Lexiva®) with ritonavir	• fosamprenavir (Lexiva®)
• indinavir (Crixivan®)	• itraconazole (Sporanox®)
• ketoconazole (Nizoral®)	• lopinavir/ritonavir (Kaletra®)
• nefazodone (Serzone®)	• nelfinavir mesylate (Viracept®)
• ritonavir (Norvir®)	• saquinavir mesylate (Invirase®)
• telithromycin (Ketek®)	• tipranavir (Aptivus®)

Ask your healthcare provider or pharmacist if you are not sure if you take any of the medicines listed above. This is not a complete list of all the medicines that can interact with COLCRYS.

- Know the medicines you take. Keep a list of them and show it to your healthcare provider and pharmacist when you get a new medicine.
- Keep COLCRYS out of the reach of children.

What is COLCRYS?

COLCRYS is a prescription medicine used to:

- prevent and treat gout flares in adults
- treat familial Mediterranean fever (FMF) in adults and children age four or older

COLCRYS is not a pain medicine and it should not be taken to treat pain related to other conditions unless specifically prescribed for those conditions.

Who should not take COLCRYS?

Do not take COLCRYS if you have liver or kidney problems and you take certain other medicines. Serious side effects, including death, have been reported in these patients even when taken as directed. See "What is the most important information I should know about COLCRYS?"

What should I tell my healthcare provider before starting COLCRYS?

See "What is the most important information I should know about COLCRYS?"

Before you take COLCRYS tell your healthcare provider about all your medical conditions including if you:

- have liver or kidney problems
- are pregnant or plan to become pregnant. It is not known if COLCRYS will harm your unborn baby. Talk to your healthcare provider if you are pregnant or plan to become pregnant.
- are breast-feeding or plan to breast-feed. COLCRYS passes into your breast milk. You and your healthcare provider should decide if you will take COLCRYS or breast-feed. If you take COLCRYS and breast-feed, you should talk to your child's healthcare provider about how to watch for side effects in your child.

Tell your healthcare provider about all the medicines you take, including ones that you may only be taking for a short time, such as antibiotics. See "What is the most important information I should know about COLCRYS?" Do not start a new medicine without talking to your healthcare provider.

Using COLCRYS with certain other medicines, such as cholesterol-lowering medications and digoxin, can affect each other causing serious side effects. Your healthcare provider may need to change your dose of COLCRYS. Talk to your healthcare provider about whether the medications you are taking might interact with COLCRYS, and what side effects to look for.

How should I take COLCRYS?

- Take COLCRYS exactly as your healthcare provider tells you to take it. **If you are not sure about your dosing**, call your healthcare provider.
- COLCRYS can be taken with or without food.
- If you take too much COLCRYS go to the nearest hospital emergency room right away.
- Do not stop taking COLCRYS even if you start to feel better, unless your healthcare provider tells you.
- Your healthcare provider may do blood tests while you take COLCRYS.
- If you take COLCRYS daily and you miss a dose, then take it as soon as you remember. If it is almost time for your next dose, just skip the missed dose. Take the next dose at your regular time. Do not take 2 doses at the same time.
- If you have a gout flare while taking COLCRYS daily, report this to your healthcare provider.

What should I avoid while taking COLCRYS?

- Avoid eating grapefruit or drinking grapefruit juice while taking COLCRYS. It can increase your chances of getting serious side effects.

What are the possible side effects of COLCRYS?

COLCRYS can cause serious side effects or even cause death. See "What is the most important information I should know about COLCRYS?"

Get medical help right away, if you have:

- Muscle weakness or pain
- Numbness or tingling in your fingers or toes
- Unusual bleeding or bruising
- Increased infections
- Feel weak or tired
- Pale or gray color to your lips, tongue, or palms of your hands
- Severe diarrhea or vomiting

Gout Flares: The most common side effect of COLCRYS in people who have gout flares is diarrhea.

FMF: The most common side effects of COLCRYS in people who have FMF are abdominal pain, diarrhea, nausea and vomiting.

Tell your healthcare provider if you have any side effect that bothers you or that does not go away.

These are not all of the possible side effects of COLCRYS. For more information, ask your healthcare provider or pharmacist.

Call your doctor for medical advice about side effects. You may report side effects to FDA at 1-800-FDA-1088.

How should I store COLCRYS?

- Store COLCRYS at room temperature between 68° and 77°F (20° to 25°C).
- Keep COLCRYS in a tightly closed container.
- Keep COLCRYS out of the light.

Keep COLCRYS and all medicines out of the reach of children.

General Information about COLCRYS

Medicines are sometimes prescribed for purposes other than those listed in a Medication Guide. Do not use COLCRYS for a condition for which it was not prescribed. Do not give COLCRYS to other people, even if they have the same symptoms that you have. It may harm them. This Medication Guide summarizes the most important information about COLCRYS. If you would like more information, talk with your healthcare provider. You can ask your healthcare provider or pharmacist for information about COLCRYS that is written for healthcare professionals.

For more information, go to www.COLCRYS.com or call 1-877-825-3327.

What are the ingredients in COLCRYS?

Active Ingredient: Colchicine

Inactive Ingredients: carnauba wax, FD&C blue #2, FD&C red #40, hypromellose, lactose monohydrate, magnesium stearate, microcrystalline cellulose, polydextrose, polyethylene glycol, pregelatinized starch, sodium starch glycolate, titanium dioxide, and triacetin.

This Medication Guide has been approved by the U.S. Food and Drug Administration.

All trademarks are the property of their respective owners.

Distributed by:
Takeda Pharmaceuticals America, Inc.
Deerfield, IL 60015
Rev 01, June 2012

Shown in Product Identification Guide, page 313

DEXILANT ℞

[decks-ĭ-launt]
(dexlansoprazole)
delayed-release capsules for oral use

HIGHLIGHTS OF PRESCRIBING INFORMATION

These highlights do not include all the information needed to use DEXILANT safely and effectively. See full prescribing information for DEXILANT.

DEXILANT (dexlansoprazole) delayed-release capsules for oral use.
Initial U.S. Approval: 1995 (lansoprazole)

RECENT MAJOR CHANGES

Dosage and Administration:
• Important Administration Information (2.3) 8/2013
Warnings and Precautions
• *Clostridium difficile* associated diarrhea (5.2) 9/2012

INDICATIONS AND USAGE

DEXILANT is a proton pump inhibitor (PPI) indicated for:

- Healing of all grades of erosive esophagitis (EE). (1.1)
- Maintaining healing of EE and relief of heartburn. (1.2)
- Treating heartburn associated with symptomatic non-erosive gastroesophageal reflux disease (GERD). (1.3)

DOSAGE AND ADMINISTRATION

- Healing of EE: 60 mg once daily for up to 8 weeks. (2.1)
- Maintenance of healed EE: 30 mg once daily for up to 6 months. (2.1)
- Symptomatic non-erosive GERD: 30 mg once daily for 4 weeks. (2.1)
- Hepatic impairment: Consider 30 mg maximum daily dose for patients with moderate hepatic impairment (Child-Pugh Class B). No studies were conducted in patients with severe hepatic impairment (Child-Pugh Class C). (2.2, 8.7)
- DEXILANT can be taken without regard to food. (2.3)
- DEXILANT should be swallowed whole. See full prescribing information for administration options. (2.3)

DOSAGE FORMS AND STRENGTHS

- Delayed-Release Capsules: 30 mg and 60 mg. (3)

CONTRAINDICATIONS

- Patients with known hypersensitivity to any component of the formulation. (4)

WARNINGS AND PRECAUTIONS

- Gastric Malignancy: Symptomatic response with DEXILANT does not preclude the presence of gastric malignancy. (5.1)
- *Clostridium difficile* associated diarrhea: PPI therapy may be associated with increased risk of *Clostridium difficile* associated diarrhea. (5.2)
- Bone Fracture: Long-term and multiple daily dose PPI therapy may be associated with an increased risk for osteoporosis-related fractures of the hip, wrist or spine. (5.3)
- Hypomagnesemia: Hypomagnesemia has been reported rarely with prolonged treatment with PPIs. (5.4)

ADVERSE REACTIONS

Most commonly reported adverse reactions (≥2%): diarrhea, abdominal pain, nausea, upper respiratory tract infection, vomiting, and flatulence. (6.1)

To report SUSPECTED ADVERSE REACTIONS, contact Takeda Pharmaceuticals America, Inc. at 1-877-TAKEDA-7 (1-877-825-3327) or FDA at 1-800-FDA-1088 or www.fda.gov/medwatch.

DRUG INTERACTIONS

- Atazanavir: Do not co-administer with DEXILANT because atazanavir systemic concentrations may be substantially decreased. (7.1)
- Drugs with pH-dependent absorption (e.g., Ampicillin esters, Digoxin, iron salts, ketoconazole, erlotinib): DEXILANT may interfere with absorption of drugs for which gastric pH is important for bioavailability. (7.1)
- Warfarin: Patients taking concomitant warfarin may require monitoring for increases in international normalized ratio (INR) and prothrombin time. (7.2)
- Tacrolimus: Concomitant tacrolimus use may increase tacrolimus whole blood concentrations. (7.3)
- Methotrexate: DEXILANT may increase serum levels of methotrexate. (7.5)

See 17 for PATIENT COUNSELING INFORMATION and Medication Guide

Revised: 08/2013

FULL PRESCRIBING INFORMATION: CONTENTS*

*** Sections or subsections omitted from the full prescribing information are not listed**

FULL PRESCRIBING INFORMATION

1 INDICATIONS AND USAGE

1.1 Healing of Erosive Esophagitis

DEXILANT is indicated for healing of all grades of erosive esophagitis (EE) for up to eight weeks.

1.2 Maintenance of Healed Erosive Esophagitis

DEXILANT is indicated to maintain healing of EE and relief of heartburn for up to six months.

1.3 Symptomatic Non-Erosive Gastroesophageal Reflux Disease

DEXILANT is indicated for the treatment of heartburn associated with symptomatic non-erosive gastroesophageal reflux disease (GERD) for four weeks.

2 DOSAGE AND ADMINISTRATION

2.1 Recommended Dose

DEXILANT is available as capsules in 30 mg and 60 mg strengths for adult use. Directions for use in each indication are summarized in Table 1.

Table 1. DEXILANT Dosing Recommendations

Indication	Recommended Dose	Frequency
Healing of EE	60 mg	Once daily for up to 8 weeks
Maintenance of Healed EE and relief of heartburn	30 mg	Once daily*
Symptomatic Non-Erosive GERD	30 mg	Once daily for 4 weeks

*Controlled studies did not extend beyond 6 months.

2.2 Hepatic Impairment

No adjustment for DEXILANT is necessary for patients with mild hepatic impairment (Child-Pugh Class A). Consider a maximum daily dose of 30 mg for patients with moderate hepatic impairment (Child-Pugh Class B). No studies have been conducted in patients with severe hepatic impairment (Child-Pugh Class C) *[see Use in Specific Populations (8.7) and Clinical Pharmacology (12.3)]*.

2.3 Important Administration Information

- DEXILANT can be taken without regard to food.
- DEXILANT should be swallowed whole.
- DEXILANT should not be chewed.

Table 2. Incidence of Adverse Reactions in Controlled Studies

Adverse Reaction	Placebo (N=896) %	DEXILANT 30 mg (N=455) %	DEXILANT 60 mg (N=2218) %	DEXILANT Total (N=2621) %	Lansoprazole 30 mg (N=1363) %
Diarrhea	2.9	5.1	4.7	4.8	3.2
Abdominal Pain	3.5	3.5	4.0	4.0	2.6
Nausea	2.6	3.3	2.8	2.9	1.8
Upper Respiratory Tract Infection	0.8	2.9	1.7	1.9	0.8
Vomiting	0.8	2.2	1.4	1.6	1.1
Flatulence	0.6	2.6	1.4	1.6	1.2

For patients who have difficulty swallowing capsules, follow the instructions below for administration:

Administration with Applesauce

1. Place one tablespoon of applesauce into a clean container.
2. Open capsule.
3. Sprinkle intact granules on applesauce.
4. Swallow applesauce and granules immediately. Do not chew granules. Do not save the applesauce and granules for later use.

Administration with Water in an Oral Syringe

1. Open the capsule and empty the granules into a clean container with 20 mL of water.
2. Withdraw the entire mixture into a syringe.
3. Gently swirl the syringe in order to keep granules from settling.
4. Administer the mixture immediately into the mouth. Do not save the water and granule mixture for later use.
5. Refill the syringe with 10 mL of water, swirl gently, and administer.
6. Refill the syringe again with 10 mL of water, swirl gently, and administer.

Administration with Water via a Nasogastric Tube (≥16 French)

1. Open the capsule and empty the granules into a clean container with 20 mL of water.
2. Withdraw the entire mixture into a catheter-tip syringe.
3. Swirl the syringe gently in order to keep the granules from settling, and immediately inject the mixture through the nasogastric tube into the stomach. Do not save the water and granule mixture for later use.
4. Refill the syringe with 10 mL of water, swirl gently, and flush the tube.
5. Refill the syringe again with 10 mL of water, swirl gently, and administer.

3 DOSAGE FORMS AND STRENGTHS

- 30 mg delayed-release capsules are opaque, blue and gray with TAP and "30" imprinted on the capsule.
- 60 mg delayed-release capsules are opaque, blue with TAP and "60" imprinted on the capsule.

4 CONTRAINDICATIONS

DEXILANT is contraindicated in patients with known hypersensitivity to any component of the formulation *[see Description (11)]*. Hypersensitivity and anaphylaxis have been reported with DEXILANT use *[see Adverse Reactions (6.1)]*.

5 WARNINGS AND PRECAUTIONS

5.1 Gastric Malignancy

Symptomatic response with DEXILANT does not preclude the presence of gastric malignancy.

5.2 *Clostridium difficile* Associated Diarrhea

Published observational studies suggest that PPI therapy like DEXILANT may be associated with an increased risk of *Clostridium difficile* associated diarrhea, especially in hospitalized patients. This diagnosis should be considered for diarrhea that does not improve *[see Adverse Reactions (6.2)]*.

Patients should use the lowest dose and shortest duration of PPI therapy appropriate to the condition being treated.

5.3 Bone Fracture

Several published observational studies suggest that PPI therapy may be associated with an increased risk for osteoporosis-related fractures of the hip, wrist or spine. The risk of fracture was increased in patients who received high-dose, defined as multiple daily doses, and long-term PPI therapy (a year or longer). Patients should use the lowest dose and shortest duration of PPI therapy appropriate to the conditions being treated. Patients at risk for osteoporosis-related fractures should be managed according to established treatment guidelines *[see Dosage and Administration (2) and Adverse Reactions (6)]*.

5.4 Hypomagnesemia

Hypomagnesemia, symptomatic and asymptomatic, has been reported rarely in patients treated with PPIs for at least three months, in most cases after a year of therapy. Serious adverse events include tetany, arrhythmias, and seizures. In most patients, treatment of hypomagnesemia required magnesium replacement and discontinuation of the PPI.

For patients expected to be on prolonged treatment or who take PPIs with medications such as digoxin or drugs that may cause hypomagnesemia (e.g., diuretics), health care professionals may consider monitoring magnesium levels prior to initiation of PPI treatment and periodically *[see Adverse Reactions (6.2)]*.

5.5 Concomitant Use of DEXILANT with Methotrexate

Literature suggests that concomitant use of PPIs with methotrexate (primarily at high dose; see methotrexate prescribing information) may elevate and prolong serum levels of methotrexate and/or its metabolite, possibly leading to methotrexate toxicities. In high-dose methotrexate administration, a temporary withdrawal of the PPI may be considered in some patients *[see Drug Interactions (7.5)]*.

6 ADVERSE REACTIONS

6.1 Clinical Trials Experience

Because clinical trials are conducted under widely varying conditions, adverse reaction rates observed in the clinical trials of a drug cannot be directly compared to rates in the clinical trials of another drug and may not reflect the rates observed in practice.

The safety of DEXILANT was evaluated in 4548 patients in controlled and uncontrolled clinical studies, including 863 patients treated for at least six months and 203 patients treated for one year. Patients ranged in age from 18 to 90 years (median age 48 years), with 54% female, 85% Caucasian, 8% Black, 4% Asian, and 3% other races. Six randomized controlled clinical trials were conducted for the treatment of EE, maintenance of healed EE, and symptomatic GERD, which included 896 patients on placebo, 455 patients on DEXILANT 30 mg, 2218 patients on DEXILANT 60 mg, and 1363 patients on lansoprazole 30 mg once daily.

Most Commonly Reported Adverse Reactions

The most common adverse reactions (≥2%) that occurred at a higher incidence for DEXILANT than placebo in the controlled studies are presented in Table 2.

[See table 2 above]

Adverse Reactions Resulting in Discontinuation

In controlled clinical studies, the most common adverse reaction leading to discontinuation from DEXILANT therapy was diarrhea (0.7%).

Other Adverse Reactions

Other adverse reactions that were reported in controlled studies at an incidence of less than 2% are listed below by body system:

Blood and Lymphatic System Disorders: anemia, lymphadenopathy

Cardiac Disorders: angina, arrhythmia, bradycardia, chest pain, edema, myocardial infarction, palpitation, tachycardia

Ear and Labyrinth Disorders: ear pain, tinnitus, vertigo

Endocrine Disorders: goiter

Eye Disorders: eye irritation, eye swelling

Gastrointestinal Disorders: abdominal discomfort, abdominal tenderness, abnormal feces, anal discomfort, Barrett's esophagus, bezoar, bowel sounds abnormal, breath odor, colitis microscopic, colonic polyp, constipation, dry mouth, duodenitis, dyspepsia, dysphagia, enteritis, eructation, esophagitis, gastric polyp, gastritis, gastroenteritis, gastrointestinal disorders, gastrointestinal hypermotility disorders, GERD, GI ulcers and perforation, hematemesis, hematochezia, hemorrhoids, impaired gastric emptying, irritable bowel syndrome, mucus stools, oral mucosal blistering, painful defecation, proctitis, paresthesia oral, rectal hemorrhage, retching

General Disorders and Administration Site Conditions: adverse drug reaction, asthenia, chest pain, chills, feeling abnormal, inflammation, mucosal inflammation, nodule, pain, pyrexia

Hepatobiliary Disorders: biliary colic, cholelithiasis, hepatomegaly

Immune System Disorders: hypersensitivity
Infections and Infestations: candida infections, influenza, nasopharyngitis, oral herpes, pharyngitis, sinusitis, viral infection, vulvo-vaginal infection
Injury, Poisoning and Procedural Complications: falls, fractures, joint sprains, overdose, procedural pain, sunburn
Laboratory Investigations: ALP increased, ALT increased, AST increased, bilirubin decreased/increased, blood creatinine increased, blood gastrin increased, blood glucose increased, blood potassium increased, liver function test abnormal, platelet count decreased, total protein increased, weight increase
Metabolism and Nutrition Disorders: appetite changes, hypercalcemia, hypokalemia
Musculoskeletal and Connective Tissue Disorders: arthralgia, arthritis, muscle cramps, musculoskeletal pain, myalgia
Nervous System Disorders: altered taste, convulsion, dizziness, headaches, migraine, memory impairment, paresthesia, psychomotor hyperactivity, tremor, trigeminal neuralgia
Psychiatric Disorders: abnormal dreams, anxiety, depression, insomnia, libido changes
Renal and Urinary Disorders: dysuria, micturition urgency
Reproductive System and Breast Disorders: dysmenorrhea, dyspareunia, menorrhagia, menstrual disorder
Respiratory, Thoracic and Mediastinal Disorders: aspiration, asthma, bronchitis, cough, dyspnoea, hiccups, hyperventilation, respiratory tract congestion, sore throat
Skin and Subcutaneous Tissue Disorders: acne, dermatitis, erythema, pruritis, rash, skin lesion, urticaria
Vascular Disorders: deep vein thrombosis, hot flush, hypertension

Additional adverse reactions that were reported in a long-term uncontrolled study and were considered related to DEXILANT by the treating physician included: anaphylaxis, auditory hallucination, B-cell lymphoma, bursitis, central obesity, cholecystitis acute, dehydration, diabetes mellitus, dysphonia, epistaxis, folliculitis, gout, herpes zoster, hyperlipidemia, hypothyroidism, increased neutrophils, MCHC decrease, neutropenia, rectal tenesmus, restless legs syndrome, somnolence, tonsillitis.

Other adverse reactions not observed with DEXILANT, but occurring with the racemate lansoprazole can be found in the lansoprazole prescribing information, ADVERSE REACTIONS section.

6.2 Postmarketing Experience

The following adverse reactions have been identified during post-approval of DEXILANT. As these reactions are reported voluntarily from a population of uncertain size, it is not always possible to reliably estimate their frequency or establish a causal relationship to drug exposure.

Blood and Lymphatic System Disorders: autoimmune hemolytic anemia, idiopathic thrombocytopenic purpura
Ear and Labyrinth Disorders: deafness
Eye Disorders: blurred vision
Gastrointestinal Disorders: oral edema, pancreatitis
General Disorders and Administration Site Conditions: facial edema
Hepatobiliary Disorders: drug-induced hepatitis
Immune System Disorders: anaphylactic shock (requiring emergency intervention), exfoliative dermatitis, Stevens-Johnson syndrome, toxic epidermal necrolysis (some fatal)
Infections and Infestations: Clostridium difficile associated diarrhea
Metabolism and Nutrition Disorders: hypomagnesemia, hyponatremia
Musculoskeletal System Disorders: bone fracture
Nervous System Disorders: cerebrovascular accident, transient ischemic attack
Renal and Urinary Disorders: acute renal failure
Respiratory, Thoracic and Mediastinal Disorders: pharyngeal edema, throat tightness
Skin and Subcutaneous Tissue Disorders: generalized rash, leukocytoclastic vasculitis

7 DRUG INTERACTIONS

7.1 Drugs with pH-Dependent Absorption Pharmacokinetics

DEXILANT causes inhibition of gastric acid secretion. DEXILANT is likely to substantially decrease the systemic concentrations of the HIV protease inhibitor atazanavir, which is dependent upon the presence of gastric acid for absorption, and may result in a loss of therapeutic effect of atazanavir and the development of HIV resistance. Therefore, DEXILANT should not be co-administered with atazanavir.

DEXILANT may interfere with the absorption of other drugs where gastric pH is an important determinant of oral bioavailability (e.g., ampicillin esters, digoxin, iron salts, ketoconazole, erlotinib).

7.2 Warfarin

Co-administration of DEXILANT 90 mg and warfarin 25 mg did not affect the pharmacokinetics of warfarin or INR *[see Clinical Pharmacology (12.3)]*. However, there have been reports of increased INR and prothrombin time in patients receiving PPIs and warfarin concomitantly. Increases in INR and prothrombin time may lead to abnormal bleeding and even death. Patients treated with DEXILANT and warfarin concomitantly may need to be monitored for increases in INR and prothrombin time.

7.3 Tacrolimus

Concomitant administration of dexlansoprazole and tacrolimus may increase whole blood levels of tacrolimus, especially in transplant patients who are intermediate or poor metabolizers of CYP2C19.

7.4 Clopidogrel

Concomitant administration of dexlansoprazole and clopidogrel in healthy subjects had no clinically important effect on exposure to the active metabolite of clopidogrel or clopidogrel-induced platelet inhibition *[see Clinical Pharmacology (12.3)]*. No dose adjustment of clopidogrel is necessary when administered with an approved dose of DEXILANT.

7.5 Methotrexate

Case reports, published population pharmacokinetic studies, and retrospective analyses suggest that concomitant administration of PPIs and methotrexate (primarily at high dose; see methotrexate prescribing information) may elevate and prolong serum levels of methotrexate and/or its metabolite hydroxymethotrexate. However, no formal drug interaction studies of high-dose methotrexate with PPIs have been conducted *[see Warnings and Precautions (5.5)]*.

8 USE IN SPECIFIC POPULATIONS

8.1 Pregnancy

Teratogenic Effects

Pregnancy Category B. There are no adequate and well-controlled studies with dexlansoprazole in pregnant women. There were no adverse fetal effects in animal reproduction studies of dexlansoprazole in rabbits. Because animal reproduction studies are not always predictive of human response, DEXILANT should be used during pregnancy only if clearly needed.

A reproduction study conducted in rabbits at oral dexlansoprazole doses up to approximately nine times the maximum recommended human dexlansoprazole dose (60 mg/day) revealed no evidence of impaired fertility or harm to the fetus due to dexlansoprazole. In addition, reproduction studies performed in pregnant rats with oral lansoprazole at doses up to 40 times the recommended human lansoprazole dose and in pregnant rabbits at oral lansoprazole doses up to 16 times the recommended human lansoprazole dose revealed no evidence of impaired fertility or harm to the fetus due to lansoprazole *[see Nonclinical Toxicology (13.2)]*.

8.3 Nursing Mothers

It is not known whether dexlansoprazole is excreted in human milk. However, lansoprazole and its metabolites are present in rat milk following the administration of lansoprazole. As many drugs are excreted in human milk, and because of the potential for tumorigenicity shown for lansoprazole in rat carcinogenicity studies *[see Nonclinical Toxicology (13.1)]*, a decision should be made whether to discontinue nursing or to discontinue the drug, taking into account the importance of the drug to the mother.

8.4 Pediatric Use

Safety and effectiveness of DEXILANT in pediatric patients (less than 18 years of age) have not been established.

8.5 Geriatric Use

In clinical studies of DEXILANT, 11% of patients were aged 65 years and over. No overall differences in safety or effectiveness were observed between these patients and younger patients, and other reported clinical experience has not identified significant differences in responses between geriatric and younger patients, but greater sensitivity of some older individuals cannot be ruled out *[see Clinical Pharmacology (12.3)]*.

8.6 Renal Impairment

No dosage adjustment of DEXILANT is necessary in patients with renal impairment. The pharmacokinetics of dexlansoprazole in patients with renal impairment are not expected to be altered since dexlansoprazole is extensively metabolized in the liver to inactive metabolites, and no parent drug is recovered in the urine following an oral dose of dexlansoprazole *[see Clinical Pharmacology (12.3)]*.

8.7 Hepatic Impairment

No dosage adjustment for DEXILANT is necessary for patients with mild hepatic impairment (Child-Pugh Class A). DEXILANT 30 mg should be considered for patients with moderate hepatic impairment (Child-Pugh Class B). No studies have been conducted in patients with severe hepatic impairment (Child-Pugh Class C) *[see Clinical Pharmacology (12.3)]*.

10 OVERDOSAGE

There have been no reports of significant overdose of DEXILANT. Multiple doses of DEXILANT 120 mg and a single dose of DEXILANT 300 mg did not result in death or other severe adverse events. However, serious adverse events of hypertension have been reported in association with twice daily doses of DEXILANT 60 mg. Non-serious adverse reactions observed with twice daily doses of DEXILANT 60 mg include hot flashes, contusion, oropharyngeal pain, and weight loss. Dexlansoprazole is not expected to be removed from the circulation by hemodialysis. If an overdose occurs, treatment should be symptomatic and supportive.

11 DESCRIPTION

The active ingredient in DEXILANT (dexlansoprazole) delayed-release capsules, a proton pump inhibitor, is (+)-2-[(*R*)-{[3-methyl-4-(2,2,2-trifluoroethoxy)pyridin-2-yl] methyl} sulfinyl]-*1H*-benzimidazole, a compound that inhibits gastric acid secretion. Dexlansoprazole is the *R*-enantiomer of lansoprazole (a racemic mixture of the *R*- and *S*-enantiomers). Its empirical formula is: $C_{16}H_{14}F_3N_3O_2S$, with a molecular weight of 369.36. The structural formula is:

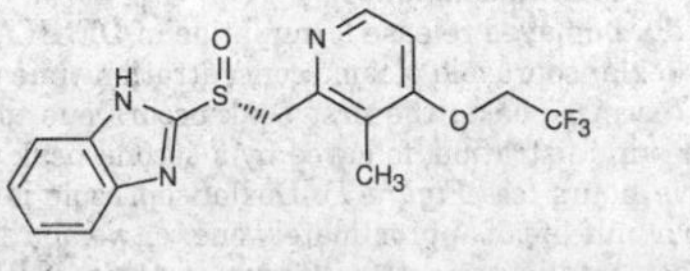

Dexlansoprazole is a white to nearly white crystalline powder which melts with decomposition at 140°C. Dexlansoprazole is freely soluble in dimethylformamide, methanol, dichloromethane, ethanol, and ethyl acetate; and soluble in acetonitrile; slightly soluble in ether; and very slightly soluble in water; and practically insoluble in hexane.

Dexlansoprazole is stable when exposed to light. Dexlansoprazole is more stable in neutral and alkaline conditions than acidic conditions.

DEXILANT is supplied as a dual delayed-release formulation in capsules for oral administration. The capsules contain dexlansoprazole in a mixture of two types of enteric-coated granules with different pH-dependent dissolution profiles *[see Clinical Pharmacology (12.3)]*.

DEXILANT is available in two dosage strengths: 30 mg and 60 mg, per capsule. Each capsule contains enteric-coated granules consisting of dexlansoprazole (active ingredient) and the following inactive ingredients: sugar spheres, magnesium carbonate, sucrose, low-substituted hydroxypropyl cellulose, titanium dioxide, hydroxypropyl cellulose, hypromellose 2910, talc, methacrylic acid copolymers, polyethylene glycol 8000, triethyl citrate, polysorbate 80, and colloidal silicon dioxide. The components of the capsule shell include the following inactive ingredients: hypromellose, carrageenan and potassium chloride. Based on the capsule shell color, blue contains FD&C Blue No. 2 aluminum lake; gray contains black ferric oxide; and both contain titanium dioxide.

12 CLINICAL PHARMACOLOGY

12.1 Mechanism of Action

Dexlansoprazole is a PPI that suppresses gastric acid secretion by specific inhibition of the (H^+, K^+)-ATPase in the gastric parietal cell. By acting specifically on the proton pump, dexlansoprazole blocks the final step of acid production.

12.2 Pharmacodynamics

Antisecretory Activity

The effects of DEXILANT 60 mg (n=20) or lansoprazole 30 mg (n=23) once daily for five days on 24 hour intragastric pH were assessed in healthy subjects in a multiple-dose crossover study. The results are summarized in Table 3.

Table 3. Effect on 24 Hour Intragastric pH on Day 5 After Administration of DEXILANT or Lansoprazole

DEXILANT 60 mg	Lansoprazole 30 mg
Mean Intragastric pH	
4.55	4.13
% Time Intragastric pH >4 (hours)	
71 (17 hours)	60 (14 hours)

Serum Gastrin Effects

The effect of DEXILANT on serum gastrin concentrations was evaluated in approximately 3460 patients in clinical trials up to eight weeks and in 1023 patients for up to six to 12 months. The mean fasting gastrin concentrations increased from baseline during treatment with DEXILANT 30 mg and 60 mg doses. In patients treated for more than six months, mean serum gastrin levels increased during approximately the first three months of treatment and were stable for the remainder of treatment. Mean serum gastrin levels returned to pre-treatment levels within one month of discontinuation of treatment.

Enterochromaffin-Like Cell (ECL) Effects

There were no reports of ECL cell hyperplasia in gastric biopsy specimens obtained from 653 patients treated with DEXILANT 30 mg, 60 mg or 90 mg for up to 12 months.

During lifetime exposure of rats dosed daily with up to 150 mg/kg/day of lansoprazole, marked hypergastrinemia was observed followed by ECL cell proliferation and formation of carcinoid tumors, especially in female rats *[see Nonclinical Toxicology (13.1)]*.

Effect on Cardiac Repolarization

A study was conducted to assess the potential of DEXILANT to prolong the QT/QT_c interval in healthy adult subjects. DEXILANT doses of 90 mg or 300 mg did not delay cardiac repolarization compared to placebo. The positive control (moxifloxacin) produced statistically significantly greater mean maximum and time-averaged QT/QT_c intervals compared to placebo.

12.3 Pharmacokinetics

The dual delayed release formulation of DEXILANT results in a dexlansoprazole plasma concentration-time profile with two distinct peaks; the first peak occurs one to two hours after administration, followed by a second peak within four to five hours *(see Figure 1)*. Dexlansoprazole is eliminated with a half-life of approximately one to two hours in healthy subjects and in patients with symptomatic GERD. No accumulation of dexlansoprazole occurs after multiple, once daily doses of DEXILANT 30 mg or 60 mg, although mean AUC_t and C_{max} values of dexlansoprazole were slightly higher (less than 10%) on Day 5 than on Day 1.

Figure 1: Mean Plasma Dexlansoprazole Concentration — Time Profile Following Oral Administration of 30 or 60 mg DEXILANT Once Daily for 5 Days in Healthy Subjects

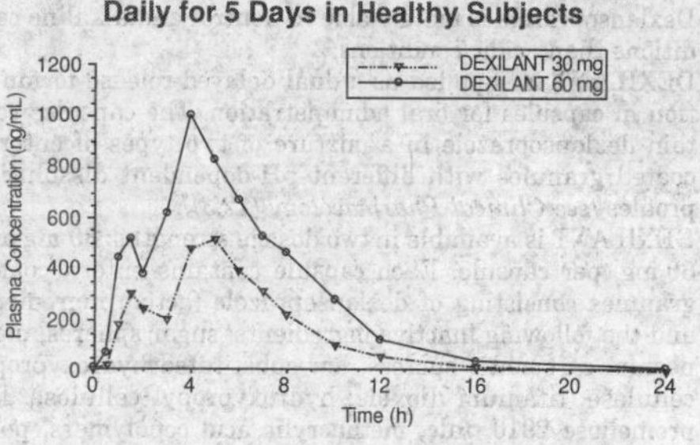

The pharmacokinetics of dexlansoprazole are highly variable, with percent coefficient of variation (CV%) values for C_{max}, AUC, and CL/F of greater than 30% *(see Table 4)*.

Table 4. Mean (CV%) Pharmacokinetic Parameters for Subjects on Day 5 After Administration of DEXILANT

Dose (mg)	C_{max} (ng/mL)	AUC_{24} (ng·h/mL)	CL/F (L/h)
30	658 (40%) (N=44)	3275 (47%) (N=43)	11.4 (48%) (N=43)
60	1397 (51%) (N=79)	6529 (60%) (N=73)	11.6 (46%) (N=41)

Absorption

After oral administration of DEXILANT 30 mg or 60 mg to healthy subjects and symptomatic GERD patients, mean C_{max} and AUC values of dexlansoprazole increased approximately dose proportionally *(see Figure 1)*.

When granules of DEXILANT 60 mg are mixed with water and dosed via NG tube or orally via syringe, the bioavailability (C_{max} and AUC) of dexlansoprazole was similar to that when DEXILANT 60 mg was administered as an intact capsule.

Distribution

Plasma protein binding of dexlansoprazole ranged from 96.1% to 98.8% in healthy subjects and was independent of concentration from 0.01 to 20 mcg/mL. The apparent volume of distribution (V_z/F) after multiple doses in symptomatic GERD patients was 40.3 L.

Metabolism

Dexlansoprazole is extensively metabolized in the liver by oxidation, reduction, and subsequent formation of sulfate, glucuronide and glutathione conjugates to inactive metabolites. Oxidative metabolites are formed by the cytochrome P450 (CYP) enzyme system including hydroxylation mainly by CYP2C19, and oxidation to the sulfone by CYP3A4.

CYP2C19 is a polymorphic liver enzyme which exhibits three phenotypes in the metabolism of CYP2C19 substrates; extensive metabolizers (*1/*1), intermediate metabolizers (*1/mutant) and poor metabolizers (mutant/mutant). Dexlansoprazole is the major circulating component in plasma regardless of CYP2C19 metabolizer status. In CYP2C19 intermediate and extensive metabolizers, the major plasma metabolites are 5-hydroxy dexlansoprazole and its glucuronide conjugate, while in CYP2C19 poor metabolizers dexlansoprazole sulfone is the major plasma metabolite.

Elimination

Following the administration of DEXILANT, no unchanged dexlansoprazole is excreted in urine. Following the administration of [^{14}C] dexlansoprazole to six healthy male subjects, approximately 50.7% (standard deviation (SD): 9.0%) of the administered radioactivity was excreted in urine and 47.6% (SD: 7.3%) in the feces. Apparent clearance (CL/F) in healthy subjects was 11.4 to 11.6 L/h, respectively, after five days of 30 or 60 mg once daily administration.

Effect of Food on Pharmacokinetics and Pharmacodynamics

In food-effect studies in healthy subjects receiving DEXILANT under various fed conditions compared to fasting, increases in C_{max} ranged from 12% to 55%, increases in AUC ranged from 9% to 37%, and t_{max} varied (ranging from a decrease of 0.7 hours to an increase of three hours). No significant differences in mean intragastric pH were observed between fasted and various fed conditions. However, the percentage of time intragastric pH exceeded four over the 24 hour dosing interval decreased slightly when DEXILANT was administered after a meal (57%) relative to fasting (64%), primarily due to a decreased response in intragastric pH during the first four hours after dosing. Because of this, while DEXILANT can be taken without regard to food, some patients may benefit from administering the dose prior to a meal if post-meal symptoms do not resolve under post-fed conditions.

Special Populations

Pediatric Use

The pharmacokinetics of dexlansoprazole in patients under the age of 18 years have not been studied.

Geriatric Use

The terminal elimination half-life of dexlansoprazole is significantly increased in geriatric subjects compared to younger subjects (2.23 and 1.5 hours, respectively); this difference is not clinically relevant. Dexlansoprazole exhibited higher systemic exposure (AUC) in geriatric subjects (34.5% higher) than younger subjects. No dosage adjustment is needed in geriatric patients *[see Use in Specific Populations (8.5)]*.

Renal Impairment

Dexlansoprazole is extensively metabolized in the liver to inactive metabolites, and no parent drug is recovered in the urine following an oral dose of dexlansoprazole. Therefore, the pharmacokinetics of dexlansoprazole are not expected to be altered in patients with renal impairment, and no studies were conducted in subjects with renal impairment *[see Use in Specific Populations (8.6)]*. In addition, the pharmacokinetics of lansoprazole were studied in patients with mild, moderate or severe renal impairment; results demonstrated no need for a dose adjustment for this patient population.

Hepatic Impairment

In a study of 12 patients with moderately impaired hepatic function who received a single oral dose of DEXILANT 60 mg, plasma exposure (AUC) of bound and unbound dexlansoprazole in the hepatic impairment group was approximately two times greater compared to subjects with normal hepatic function. This difference in exposure was not due to a difference in protein binding between the two liver function groups. No adjustment for DEXILANT is necessary for patients with mild hepatic impairment (Child-Pugh Class A). DEXILANT 30 mg should be considered for patients with moderate hepatic impairment (Child-Pugh Class B). No studies have been conducted in patients with severe hepatic impairment (Child-Pugh Class C) *[see Use in Specific Populations (8.7)]*.

Gender

In a study of 12 male and 12 female healthy subjects who received a single oral dose of DEXILANT 60 mg, females had higher systemic exposure (AUC) (42.8% higher) than males. No dosage adjustment is necessary in patients based on gender.

Drug-Drug Interactions

Warfarin

In a study of 20 healthy subjects, co-administration of DEXILANT 90 mg once daily for 11 days with a single 25 mg oral dose of warfarin on Day 6 did not result in any significant differences in the pharmacokinetics of warfarin or INR compared to administration of warfarin with placebo. However, there have been reports of increased INR and prothrombin time in patients receiving PPIs and warfarin concomitantly *[see Drug Interactions (7.2)]*.

Cytochrome P 450 Interactions

Dexlansoprazole is metabolized, in part, by CYP2C19 and CYP3A4 *[see Clinical Pharmacology (12.3)]*.

In vitro studies have shown that dexlansoprazole is not likely to inhibit CYP isoforms 1A1, 1A2, 2A6, 2B6, 2C8, 2C9, 2D6, 2E1 or 3A4. As such, no clinically relevant interactions with drugs metabolized by these CYP enzymes would be expected. Furthermore, *in vivo* studies showed that DEXILANT did not have an impact on the pharmacokinetics of coadministered phenytoin (CYP2C9 substrate) or theophylline (CYP1A2 substrate). The subjects' CYP1A2 genotypes in the drug-drug interaction study with theophylline were not determined. Although *in vitro* studies indicated that DEXILANT has the potential to inhibit CYP2C19 *in vivo*, an *in vivo* drug-drug interaction study in mainly CYP2C19 extensive and intermediate metabolizers has shown that DEXILANT does not affect the pharmacokinetics of diazepam (CYP2C19 substrate).

Clopidogrel

Clopidogrel is metabolized to its active metabolite in part by CYP2C19. A study of healthy subjects who were CYP2C19 extensive metabolizers, receiving once daily administration of clopidogrel 75 mg alone or concomitantly with DEXILANT 60 mg (n=40), for nine days was conducted. The mean AUC of the active metabolite of clopidogrel was reduced by approximately 9% (mean AUC ratio was 91%, with 90% CI of 86-97%) when DEXILANT was coadministered compared to administration of clopidogrel alone. Pharmacodynamic parameters were also measured and demonstrated that the change in inhibition of platelet aggregation (induced by 5 mcM ADP) was related to the change in the exposure to clopidogrel active metabolite. The clinical significance of this finding is not clear.

12.5 Pharmacogenomics

Effect of CYP2C19 Polymorphism on Systemic Exposure of Dexlansoprazole

Systemic exposure of dexlansoprazole is generally higher in intermediate and poor metabolizers. In male Japanese subjects who received a single dose of DEXILANT 30 mg or 60 mg (N=2 to 6 subjects/group), mean dexlansoprazole C_{max} and AUC values were up to two times higher in intermediate compared to extensive metabolizers; in poor metabolizers, mean C_{max} was up to four times higher and mean AUC was up to 12 times higher compared to extensive metabolizers. Though such study was not conducted in Caucasians and African Americans, it is expected dexlansoprazole exposure in these races will be affected by CYP2C19 phenotypes as well.

13 NONCLINICAL TOXICOLOGY

13.1 Carcinogenesis, Mutagenesis, Impairment of Fertility

The carcinogenic potential of dexlansoprazole was assessed using lansoprazole studies. In two 24-month carcinogenicity studies, Sprague-Dawley rats were treated orally with lansoprazole at doses of 5 to 150 mg/kg/day, about one to 40 times the exposure on a body surface (mg/m^2) basis of a 50 kg person of average height [1.46 m^2 body surface area (BSA)] given the recommended human dose of lansoprazole 30 mg/day.

Lansoprazole produced dose-related gastric ECL cell hyperplasia and ECL cell carcinoids in both male and female rats *[see Clinical Pharmacology (12.2)]*.

In rats, lansoprazole also increased the incidence of intestinal metaplasia of the gastric epithelium in both sexes. In male rats, lansoprazole produced a dose-related increase of testicular interstitial cell adenomas. The incidence of these adenomas in rats receiving doses of 15 to 150 mg/kg/day (4 to 40 times the recommended human lansoprazole dose based on BSA) exceeded the low background incidence (range = 1.4 to 10%) for this strain of rat.

In a 24 month carcinogenicity study, CD-1 mice were treated orally with lansoprazole doses of 15 to 600 mg/kg/day, two to 80 times the recommended human lansoprazole dose based on BSA. Lansoprazole produced a dose-related increased incidence of gastric ECL cell hyperplasia. It also produced an increased incidence of liver tumors (hepatocellular adenoma plus carcinoma). The tumor incidences in male mice treated with 300 and 600 mg lansoprazole/kg/day (40 to 80 times the recommended human lansoprazole dose based on BSA) and female mice treated with 150 to 600 mg lansoprazole/kg/day (20 to 80 times the recommended human lansoprazole dose based on BSA) exceeded the ranges of background incidences in historical controls for this strain of mice. Lansoprazole treatment produced adenoma of rete testis in male mice receiving 75 to 600 mg/kg/day (10 to 80 times the recommended human lansoprazole dose based on BSA).

A 26 week p53 (+/-) transgenic mouse carcinogenicity study of lansoprazole was not positive.

Lansoprazole was positive in the Ames test and the *in vitro* human lymphocyte chromosomal aberration assay. Lansoprazole was not genotoxic in the *ex vivo* rat hepatocyte unscheduled DNA synthesis (UDS) test, the *in vivo* mouse micronucleus test or the rat bone marrow cell chromosomal aberration test.

Dexlansoprazole was positive in the Ames test and in the *in vitro* chromosome aberration test using Chinese hamster lung cells. Dexlansoprazole was negative in the *in vivo* mouse micronucleus test.

The potential effects of dexlansoprazole on fertility and reproductive performance were assessed using lansoprazole studies. Lansoprazole at oral doses up to 150 mg/kg/day (40 times the recommended human lansoprazole dose based on BSA) was found to have no effect on fertility and reproductive performance of male and female rats.

13.2 Animal Toxicology and/or Pharmacology

Reproductive Toxicology Studies

A reproduction study conducted in rabbits at oral dexlansoprazole doses up to 30 mg/kg/day (approximately nine times the maximum recommended human dexlansoprazole dose [60 mg/day] based on BSA) revealed no evidence of impaired fertility or harm to the fetus due to dexlansoprazole. In addition, reproduction studies performed in pregnant rats with oral lansoprazole at doses up to 150 mg/kg/day (40 times the recommended human lansoprazole dose based on BSA) and in pregnant rabbits at oral lansoprazole doses up to 30 mg/kg/day (16 times the recommended human lansoprazole dose based on BSA) revealed no evidence of impaired fertility or harm to the fetus due to lansoprazole.

14 CLINICAL STUDIES

14.1 Healing of Erosive Esophagitis

Two multi-center, double-blind, active-controlled, randomized, eight week studies were conducted in patients with endoscopically confirmed EE. Severity of the disease was classified based on the Los Angeles Classification Grading System (Grades A-D). Patients were randomized to one of the following three treatment groups: DEXILANT 60 mg daily, DEXILANT 90 mg daily or lansoprazole 30 mg daily. Patients who were *H. pylori* positive or who had Barrett's Esophagus and/or definite dysplastic changes at baseline were excluded from these studies. A total of 4092 patients were enrolled and ranged in age from 18 to 90 years (median age 48 years) with 54% male. Race was distributed as follows: 87% Caucasian, 5% Black and 8% other. Based on the Los Angeles Classification, 71% of patients had mild EE (Grades A and B) and 29% of patients had moderate to severe EE (Grades C and D) before treatment.

The studies were designed to test non-inferiority. If non-inferiority was demonstrated then superiority would be tested. Although non-inferiority was demonstrated in both studies, the finding of superiority in one study was not replicated in the other.

The proportion of patients with healed EE at Week 4 or 8 is presented below in Table 5.

[See table 5 above]

Table 5. EE Healing Rates*: All Grades

Study	Number of Patients (N)†	Treatment Group (daily)	Week 4 % Healed	Week 8‡ % Healed	(95% CI) for the Treatment Difference (DEXILANT–Lansoprazole) by Week 8
1	657	DEXILANT 60 mg	70	87	(-1.5, 6.1)§
	648	Lansoprazole 30 mg	65	85	
2	639	DEXILANT 60 mg	66	85	(2.2, 10.5)§
	656	Lansoprazole 30 mg	65	79	

CI = Confidence interval

*Based on crude rate estimates, patients who did not have endoscopically documented healed EE and prematurely discontinued were considered not healed.

†Patients with at least one post baseline endoscopy

‡Primary efficacy endpoint

§Demonstrated non-inferiority to lansoprazole

DEXILANT 90 mg was studied and did not provide additional clinical benefit over DEXILANT 60 mg.

14.2 Maintenance of Healed Erosive Esophagitis

A multi-center, double-blind, placebo-controlled, randomized study was conducted in patients who successfully completed an EE study and showed endoscopically confirmed healed EE. Maintenance of healing and symptom resolution over a six month period were evaluated with DEXILANT 30 mg or 60 mg once daily compared to placebo. A total of 445 patients were enrolled and ranged in age from 18 to 85 years (median age 49 years), with 52% female. Race was distributed as follows: 90% Caucasian, 5% Black and 5% other.

Sixty-six percent of patients treated with 30 mg of DEXILANT remained healed over the six-month time period as confirmed by endoscopy (*see Table 6*).

Table 6. Maintenance Rates* of Healed EE at Month 6

Number of Patients (N)†	Treatment Group (daily)	Maintenance Rate (%)
125	DEXILANT 30 mg	66.4‡
119	Placebo	14.3

*Based on crude rate estimates, patients who did not have endoscopically documented relapse and prematurely discontinued were considered to have relapsed.

†Patients with at least one post baseline endoscopy

‡Statistically significant vs placebo

DEXILANT 60 mg was studied and did not provide additional clinical benefit over DEXILANT 30 mg.

The effect of DEXILANT 30 mg on maintenance of relief of heartburn was also evaluated. Upon entry into the maintenance study, a majority of patients' baseline heartburn severity was rated as none. DEXILANT 30 mg demonstrated a statistically significantly higher percent of 24 hour heartburn-free periods compared to placebo over the six month treatment period (*see Table 7*). The majority of patients treated with placebo discontinued due to relapse of EE between month two and month six.

[See table 7 above]

Table 7. Median Percentage of 24 Hour Heartburn-Free Periods of the Maintenance of Healed EE Study

Treatment Group (daily)	Overall Treatment* N	Overall Treatment* Heartburn-Free 24-hour Periods (%)	Month 1 N	Month 1 Heartburn-Free 24-hour Periods (%)	Month 6 N	Month 6 Heartburn-Free 24-hour Periods (%)
DEXILANT 30 mg	132	96.1†	126	96.7	80	98.3
Placebo	141	28.6	117	28.6	23	73.3

*Secondary efficacy endpoint

†Statistically significant vs placebo

14.3 Symptomatic Non-Erosive GERD

A multi-center, double-blind, placebo-controlled, randomized, four week study was conducted in patients with a diagnosis of symptomatic non-erosive GERD made primarily by presentation of symptoms. These patients who identified heartburn as their primary symptom, had a history of heartburn for 6 months or longer, had heartburn on at least four of seven days immediately prior to randomization and had no esophageal erosions as confirmed by endoscopy. However, patients with symptoms which were not acid-related may not have been excluded using these inclusion criteria. Patients were randomized to one of the following treatment groups: DEXILANT 30 mg daily, 60 mg daily, or placebo. A total of 947 patients were enrolled and ranged in age from 18 to 86 years (median age 48 years) with 71% female. Race was distributed as follows: 82% Caucasian, 14% Black and 4% other.

DEXILANT 30 mg provided statistically significantly greater percent of days with heartburn-free 24 hour periods over placebo as assessed by daily diary over four weeks (*see Table 8*). DEXILANT 60 mg was studied and provided no additional clinical benefit over DEXILANT 30 mg.

Table 8. Median Percentages of 24 Hour Heartburn-Free Periods During the 4 Week Treatment Period of the Symptomatic Non-Erosive GERD Study

N	Treatment Group (daily)	Heartburn-Free 24-hour Periods (%)
312	DEXILANT 30 mg	54.9*
310	Placebo	18.5

*Statistically significant vs placebo

A higher percentage of patients on DEXILANT 30 mg had heartburn-free 24 hour periods compared to placebo as early as the first three days of treatment and this was sustained throughout the treatment period (percentage of patients on Day 3: DEXILANT 38% versus placebo 15%; on Day 28: DEXILANT 63% versus placebo 40%).

16 HOW SUPPLIED/STORAGE AND HANDLING

DEXILANT delayed-release capsules, 30 mg, are opaque, blue and gray with TAP and "30" imprinted on the capsule and supplied as:

NDC Number	Size
64764-171-11	Unit dose package of 100
64764-171-30	Bottle of 30
64764-171-90	Bottle of 90
64764-171-19	Bottle of 1000

DEXILANT delayed-release capsules, 60 mg, are opaque, blue with TAP and "60" imprinted on the capsule and supplied as:

NDC Number	Size
64764-175-11	Unit dose package of 100
64764-175-30	Bottle of 30
64764-175-90	Bottle of 90
64764-175-19	Bottle of 1000

Store at 25°C (77°F); excursions permitted to 15 to 30°C (59 to 86°F) [see USP Controlled Room Temperature].

17 PATIENT COUNSELING INFORMATION

See FDA-approved patient labeling (Medication Guide and Instructions for Use)

To ensure the safe and effective use of DEXILANT, this information and instructions provided in the FDA-Approved Medication Guide should be discussed with the patient.

Inform the patient to watch for signs of an allergic reaction as these could be serious and may require that DEXILANT be discontinued.

Advise patients to immediately report and seek care for diarrhea that does not improve. This may be a sign of *Clostridium difficile* associated diarrhea *[see Warnings and Precautions (5.2)]*.

Advise the patient to immediately report and seek care for any cardiovascular or neurological symptoms including palpitations, dizziness, seizures, and tetany as these may be signs of hypomagnesemia *[see Warnings and Precautions (5.4)]*.

Advise the patient to tell their health care provider if they take atazanavir, tacrolimus, warfarin, methotrexate and drugs that are affected by gastric pH changes *[see Drug Interactions (7)]*.

Advise the patient to follow the dosing instructions in the Medication Guide and inform the patient of the following administration options:

- DEXILANT is available as a delayed-release capsule.
- DEXILANT can be taken without regard to food.
- DEXILANT should be swallowed whole.
- DEXILANT should not be chewed.

Counsel patients who have difficulty swallowing capsules according to instructions provided in Dosage and Administration (2.3). Advise patients to follow the Instructions for Use that comes with the product.

MEDICATION GUIDE

DEXILANT (decks-i-launt)
(dexlansoprazole)
delayed-release capsules

Read this Medication Guide before you start taking DEXILANT and each time you get a refill. There may be new information. This information does not take the place of talking to your doctor about your medical condition or your treatment.

What is the most important information that I should know about DEXILANT?

DEXILANT may help your acid-related symptoms, but you could still have serious stomach problems. Talk with your doctor.

DEXILANT can cause serious side effects, including:

- **Diarrhea.** DEXILANT may increase your risk of getting severe diarrhea. This diarrhea may be caused by an infection (*Clostridium difficile*) in your intestines.
  Call your doctor right away if you have watery stool, stomach pain, and fever that does not go away.
- **Bone fractures.** People who take multiple daily doses of proton pump inhibitor medicines for a long period of time (a year or longer) may have an increased risk of fractures of the hip, wrist or spine. You should take DEXILANT exactly as prescribed, at the lowest dose possible for your treatment and for the shortest time needed. Talk to your doctor about your risk of bone fracture if you take DEXILANT.

DEXILANT can have other serious side effects. See **"What are the possible side effects of DEXILANT?"**

What is DEXILANT?

DEXILANT is a prescription medicine called a proton pump inhibitor (PPI). DEXILANT reduces the amount of acid in your stomach.

DEXILANT is used in adults:

- for up to 8 weeks to heal acid-related damage to the lining of the esophagus (called erosive esophagitis or EE).
- for up to 6 months to continue healing of erosive esophagitis and relief of heartburn.
- for 4 weeks to treat heartburn related to gastroesophageal reflux disease (GERD).

GERD happens when acid from your stomach enters the tube (esophagus) that connects your mouth to your stomach. This may cause a burning feeling in your chest or throat, sour taste or burping.

It is not known if DEXILANT is safe and effective in children under 18 years of age.

Who should not take DEXILANT?

Do not take DEXILANT if you are allergic to dexlansoprazole or any of the other ingredients in DEXILANT. See the end of this Medication Guide for a complete list of ingredients in DEXILANT.

What should I tell my doctor before taking DEXILANT?

Before you take DEXILANT, tell your doctor if you:

- have been told that you have low magnesium levels in your blood
- have liver problems
- have any other medical conditions
- are pregnant or plan to become pregnant. It is not known if DEXILANT will harm your unborn baby.
- are breastfeeding or planning to breastfeed. It is not known if DEXILANT passes into your breast milk. You and your doctor should decide if you will take DEXILANT or breastfeed. You should not do both. Talk to your doctor about the best way to feed your baby if you take DEXILANT.

Tell your doctor about all the medicines you take, including prescription and non-prescription medicines, vitamins, and herbal supplements. DEXILANT may affect how other medicines work, and other medicines may affect how DEXILANT works.

Especially tell your doctor if you take:

- an antibiotic that contains ampicillin
- atazanavir (Reyataz)
- erlotinib (Tarceva)
- digoxin (Lanoxin)
- a product that contains iron
- ketoconazole (Nizoral)
- warfarin (Coumadin, Jantoven)
- tacrolimus (Prograf)
- methotrexate

Ask your doctor or pharmacist for a list of these medicines, if you are not sure.

Know the medicines that you take. Keep a list of them to show your doctor and pharmacist when you get a new medicine.

How should I take DEXILANT?

- Take DEXILANT exactly as prescribed by your doctor.
- Do not change your dose or stop taking DEXILANT without talking to your doctor first.
- You can take DEXILANT with or without food.
- Swallow DEXILANT capsules whole. Do not chew DEXILANT capsules or the granules that are in the capsules.
- If you have trouble swallowing DEXILANT capsules whole, you can open the capsules and sprinkle the contents on a tablespoon of applesauce.

See the "Instructions for Use" at the end of this Medication Guide for instructions about how to take DEXILANT capsules with applesauce, and how to give DEXILANT capsules using an oral syringe or through a nasogastric tube.

- If you forget to take a dose of DEXILANT, take it as soon as you remember. If it is almost time for your next dose, do not take the missed dose. Take the next dose on time. Do not take 2 doses at the same time to make up for the missed dose.
- If you take too much DEXILANT, call your doctor right away or go to the nearest hospital emergency room.

What are the possible side effects of DEXILANT?

DEXILANT may cause serious side effects, including:

- **See "What is the most important information I should know about DEXILANT?"**
- **Low magnesium levels in your body.** This problem can be serious. Low magnesium can happen in some people who take a proton pump inhibitor medicine for at least 3 months. If low magnesium levels happen, it is usually after a year of treatment. You may or may not have symptoms of low magnesium.
  Tell your doctor right away if you develop any of these symptoms
  - seizures
  - dizziness
  - abnormal or fast heartbeat
  - jitteriness
  - jerking movements or shaking (tremors)
  - muscle weakness
  - spasms of the hands and feet
  - cramps or muscle aches
  - spasm of the voice box

  Your doctor may check the level of magnesium in your body before you start taking DEXILANT, or during treatment, if you will be taking DEXILANT for a long period of time.

The most common side effects of DEXILANT include:

- diarrhea
- stomach pain
- nausea
- common cold
- vomiting
- gas

Other side effects:

- **Serious allergic reactions.** Tell your doctor if you get any of the following symptoms with DEXILANT:
  - rash
  - face swelling
  - throat tightness
  - difficulty breathing

Your doctor may stop DEXILANT if these symptoms happen.

Tell your doctor if you have any side effect that bothers you or that does not go away.

These are not all the possible side effects of DEXILANT. For more information, ask your doctor or pharmacist.

Call your doctor for medical advice about side effects. You may report side effects to FDA at 1-800-FDA-1088.

How should I store DEXILANT?

- Store DEXILANT at room temperature between 68°F to 77°F (20°C to 25°C).

Keep DEXILANT and all medicines out of the reach of children.

General information about DEXILANT

Medicines are sometimes prescribed for purposes other than those listed in a Medication Guide. Do not use DEXILANT for a condition for which it was not prescribed. Do not give DEXILANT to other people, even if they have the same symptoms you have. It may harm them.

This Medication Guide summarizes the most important information about DEXILANT. If you would like more information, talk with your doctor. You can ask your doctor or pharmacist for information about DEXILANT that is written for healthcare professionals.

For more information, go to www.DEXILANT.com or call 1-877-825-3327.

What are the ingredients in DEXILANT?

Active ingredient: dexlansoprazole.

Inactive ingredients: sugar spheres, magnesium carbonate, sucrose, low-substituted hydroxypropyl cellulose, titanium dioxide, hydroxypropyl cellulose, hypromellose 2910, talc, methacrylic acid copolymers, polyethylene glycol 8000, triethyl citrate, polysorbate 80, and colloidal silicon dioxide. The capsule shell is made of hypromellose, carrageenan and potassium chloride. Based on the capsule shell color, blue contains FD&C Blue No. 2 aluminum lake; gray contains black ferric oxide; and both contain titanium dioxide.

Instructions for Use

- DEXILANT may be taken with or without food.
- Swallow DEXILANT capsules whole.
- Do not chew DEXILANT capsules or the granules that are in the capsules.

If you have trouble swallowing DEXILANT capsules whole, you may take or give them as follows:

Taking DEXILANT with applesauce:

1. Place 1 tablespoon of applesauce into a clean container.
2. Carefully open the capsule and sprinkle the granules onto the applesauce.
3. Swallow the applesauce and granules right away. Do not chew the granules. Do not save the applesauce and granules for later use.

Giving DEXILANT with water using an oral syringe:

1. Place 20 mL of water into a clean container.
2. Carefully open the capsule and empty the granules into the container of water.
3. Use an oral syringe to draw up the water and granule mixture.
4. Gently swirl the syringe to keep the granules from settling.
5. Give the mixture into the mouth right away. Do not save the water and granule mixture for later use.
6. Refill the syringe with 10 mL of water and swirl gently. Give the water into the mouth.
7. Repeat step 6 above.

Giving DEXILANT with water through a nasogastric tube (NG tube):

For people who have a nasogastric (NG) tube that is **size 16 French or larger,** DEXILANT may be given as follows:

1. Place 20 mL of water into a clean container.
2. Carefully open the capsule and empty the granules into the container of water.
3. Use a 60 mL catheter-tip syringe to draw up the water and granule mixture.
4. Gently swirl the syringe to keep the granules from settling.
5. Connect the catheter-tip syringe to the nasogastric tube.
6. Give the mixture right away through the nasogastric tube into the stomach. Do not save the water and granule mixture for later use.
7. Refill the syringe with 10 mL of water and swirl gently. Flush the nasogastric tube with the water.
8. Repeat step 7 above.

This Medication Guide and Instructions for Use have been approved by the U.S. Food and Drug Administration.

Distributed by:

Takeda Pharmaceuticals America, Inc.

Deerfield, IL 60015

Revised: August 2013

DEX006 R20

Shown in Product Identification Guide, page 313

EDARBI ℞

[*eh-DAR-bee*]

(azilsartan medoxomil)

tablets

HIGHLIGHTS OF PRESCRIBING INFORMATION

These HIGHLIGHTS do not include all the information needed to use EDARBI safely and effectively. See full prescribing information for EDARBI.

Edarbi (azilsartan medoxomil) tablets

Initial U.S. Approval: 2011

WARNING: FETAL TOXICITY

See full prescribing information for complete boxed warning.

- **When pregnancy is detected, discontinue Edarbi as soon as possible. (5.1)**
- **Drugs that act directly on the renin-angiotensin system can cause injury and death to the developing fetus. (5.1)**

RECENT MAJOR CHANGES

Boxed Warning	11/2011
Contraindications (4)	10/2012
Warnings and Precautions	
Fetal Toxicity (5.1)	11/2011

INDICATIONS AND USAGE

Edarbi is an angiotensin II receptor blocker indicated for the treatment of hypertension to lower blood pressure. Lowering blood pressure reduces the risk of fatal and nonfatal cardiovascular events, primarily strokes and myocardial infarctions. Edarbi may be used either alone or in combination with other antihypertensive agents. (1)

—DOSAGE AND ADMINISTRATION—

The recommended dose in adults is 80 mg taken once daily. Consider a starting dose of 40 mg for patients who are treated with high doses of diuretics. (2.1)

Edarbi may be administered with or without food. (2.1)

Edarbi may be administered with other antihypertensive agents. (2.1)

—DOSAGE FORMS AND STRENGTHS—

Tablets: 40 mg and 80 mg. (3)

—CONTRAINDICATIONS—

- Do not coadminister aliskiren with Edarbi in patients with diabetes. (4)

—WARNINGS AND PRECAUTIONS—

- Correct volume or salt depletion prior to administration of Edarbi. (5.2)
- Monitor for worsening renal function in patients with renal impairment. (5.3)

—ADVERSE REACTIONS—

The most common adverse reaction in adults was diarrhea (2%). (6.1)

To report SUSPECTED ADVERSE REACTIONS, contact Takeda Pharmaceuticals at 1-877-825-3327 or FDA at 1-800-FDA-1088 or www.fda.gov/medwatch.

—DRUG INTERACTIONS—

Dual inhibition of the renin angiotensin system: Increased risk of renal impairment, hypotension, and hyperkalemia. (7)

—USE IN SPECIFIC POPULATIONS—

- **Nursing Mothers:** Discontinue nursing or drug. (8.3)
- **Geriatric Patients:** Abnormally high serum creatinine values were more likely to be reported for patients age 75 or older. No overall difference in efficacy versus younger patients, but greater sensitivity of some older individuals cannot be ruled out. (8.5)
- In patients with an activated renin-angiotensin system, as by volume- or salt-depletion, renin-angiotensin-aldosterone system (RAAS) blockers such as azilsartan medoxomil can cause excessive hypotension. In susceptible patients, e.g., with renal artery stenosis, RAAS blockers can cause renal failure (5.2, 5.3).
- **Pediatrics:** Safety and efficacy in children have not been established.

See 17 for PATIENT COUNSELING INFORMATION

Revised: 10/2012

FULL PRESCRIBING INFORMATION: CONTENTS*

*** Sections or subsections omitted from the full prescribing information are not listed**

FULL PRESCRIBING INFORMATION

WARNING: FETAL TOXICITY

- **When pregnancy is detected, discontinue Edarbi as soon as possible *[see Warnings and Precautions (5.1)]*.**
- **Drugs that act directly on the renin-angiotensin system can cause injury and death to the developing fetus *[see Warnings and Precautions (5.1)]*.**

1 INDICATIONS AND USAGE

Edarbi is an angiotensin II receptor blocker (ARB) indicated for the treatment of hypertension to lower blood pressure. Lowering blood pressure reduces the risk of fatal and nonfatal cardiovascular events, primarily strokes and myocardial infarctions. These benefits have been seen in controlled trials of antihypertensive drugs from a wide variety of pharmacologic classes, including the class to which this drug principally belongs. There are no controlled trials demonstrating risk reduction with Edarbi.

Control of high blood pressure should be part of comprehensive cardiovascular risk management, including, as appropriate, lipid control, diabetes management, antithrombotic therapy, smoking cessation, exercise, and limited sodium intake. Many patients will require more than one drug to achieve blood pressure goals. For specific advice on goals and management, see published guidelines, such as those of the National High Blood Pressure Education Program's Joint National Committee on Prevention, Detection, Evaluation, and Treatment of High Blood Pressure (JNC).

Numerous antihypertensive drugs, from a variety of pharmacologic classes and with different mechanisms of action, have been shown in randomized controlled trials to reduce cardiovascular morbidity and mortality, and it can be concluded that it is blood pressure reduction, and not some other pharmacologic property of the drugs, that is largely responsible for those benefits. The largest and most consistent cardiovascular outcome benefit has been a reduction in the risk of stroke, but reductions in myocardial infarction and cardiovascular mortality also have been seen regularly.

Elevated systolic or diastolic pressure causes increased cardiovascular risk, and the absolute risk increase per mmHg is greater at higher blood pressures, so that even modest reductions of severe hypertension can provide substantial benefit. Relative risk reduction from blood pressure reduction is similar across populations with varying absolute risk, so the absolute benefit is greater in patients who are at higher risk independent of their hypertension (for example, patients with diabetes or hyperlipidemia), and such patients would be expected to benefit from more aggressive treatment to a lower blood pressure goal.

Some antihypertensive drugs have smaller blood pressure effects (as monotherapy) in black patients, and many antihypertensive drugs have additional approved indications and effects (e.g., on angina, heart failure, or diabetic kidney disease). These considerations may guide selection of therapy.

Edarbi may be used alone or in combination with other antihypertensive agents.

2 DOSAGE AND ADMINISTRATION

2.1 Recommended Dose

The recommended dose in adults is 80 mg taken orally once daily. Consider a starting dose of 40 mg for patients who are treated with high doses of diuretics.

If blood pressure is not controlled with Edarbi alone, additional blood pressure reduction can be achieved by taking Edarbi with other antihypertensive agents.

Edarbi may be taken with or without food *[see Clinical Pharmacology (12.3)]*.

2.2 Handling Instructions

Do not repackage Edarbi. Dispense and store Edarbi in its original container to protect Edarbi from light and moisture.

2.3 Special Populations

No initial dose adjustment is recommended for elderly patients, patients with mild-to-severe renal impairment, end-stage renal disease, or mild-to-moderate hepatic dysfunction. Edarbi has not been studied in patients with severe hepatic impairment *[see Clinical Pharmacology (12.3)]*.

3 DOSAGE FORMS AND STRENGTHS

Edarbi is supplied as white to nearly white round tablets in the following dosage strengths:

- 40-mg tablets - debossed "ASL" on one side and "40" on the other
- 80-mg tablets - debossed "ASL" on one side and "80" on the other

4 CONTRAINDICATIONS

Do not coadminister aliskiren with Edarbi in patients with diabetes *[see Drug Interactions (7)]*.

5 WARNINGS AND PRECAUTIONS

5.1 Fetal Toxicity

Use of drugs that act on the renin-angiotensin system during the second and third trimesters of pregnancy reduces fetal renal function and increases fetal and neonatal morbidity and death. Resulting oligohydramnios can be associated with fetal lung hypoplasia and skeletal deformations. Potential neonatal adverse effects include skull hypoplasia, anuria, hypotension, renal failure, and death. When pregnancy is detected, discontinue Edarbi as soon as possible *[see Use in Specific Populations (8.1)]*.

5.2 Hypotension in Volume- or Salt-Depleted Patients

In patients with an activated renin-angiotensin system, such as volume- and/or salt-depleted patients (e.g., those being treated with high doses of diuretics), symptomatic hypotension may occur after initiation of treatment with Edarbi. Correct volume or salt depletion prior to administration of Edarbi, or start treatment at 40 mg. If hypotension does occur, the patient should be placed in the supine position and, if necessary, given an intravenous infusion of normal saline. A transient hypotensive response is not a contraindication to further treatment, which usually can be continued without difficulty once the blood pressure has stabilized.

5.3 Impaired Renal Function

As a consequence of inhibiting the renin-angiotensin system, changes in renal function may be anticipated in susceptible individuals treated with Edarbi. In patients whose renal function may depend on the activity of the renin-angiotensin system (e.g., patients with severe congestive heart failure, renal artery stenosis, or volume depletion), treatment with angiotensin-converting enzyme inhibitors and angiotensin receptor blockers has been associated with oliguria or progressive azotemia and rarely with acute renal failure and death. Similar results may be anticipated in patients treated with Edarbi *[see Drug Interactions (7), Use in Specific Populations (8.6), and Clinical Pharmacology (12.3)]*.

In studies of ACE inhibitors in patients with unilateral or bilateral renal artery stenosis, increases in serum creatinine or blood urea nitrogen have been reported. There has been no long-term use of Edarbi in patients with unilateral or bilateral renal artery stenosis, but similar results may be expected.

6 ADVERSE REACTIONS

6.1 Clinical Trials Experience

Because clinical trials are conducted under widely varying conditions, adverse reaction rates observed in the clinical trials of a drug cannot be directly compared to rates in the clinical trials of another drug and may not reflect the rates observed in practice.

A total of 4814 patients were evaluated for safety when treated with Edarbi at doses of 20, 40, or 80 mg in clinical trials. This includes 1704 patients treated for at least six months; of these, 588 were treated for at least one year.

Treatment with Edarbi was well-tolerated with an overall incidence of adverse reactions similar to placebo. The rate of withdrawals due to adverse events in placebo-controlled monotherapy and combination therapy trials was 2.4% (19/801) for placebo, 2.2% (24/1072) for Edarbi 40 mg, and 2.7% (29/1074) for Edarbi 80 mg. The most common adverse event leading to discontinuation, hypotension/orthostatic hypotension, was reported by 0.4% (8/2146) patients randomized to Edarbi 40 mg or 80 mg compared to 0% (0/801) patients randomized to placebo. Generally, adverse reactions were mild, not dose related, and similar regardless of age, gender, and race.

In placebo-controlled monotherapy trials, diarrhea was reported up to 2% in patients treated with Edarbi 80 mg daily compared with 0.5% of patients on placebo.

Other adverse reactions with a plausible relationship to treatment that have been reported with an incidence of ≥0.3% and greater than placebo in more than 3300 patients treated with Edarbi in controlled trials are listed below:

Gastrointestinal Disorders: nausea

General Disorders and Administration Site Conditions: asthenia, fatigue

Musculoskeletal and Connective Tissue Disorders: muscle spasm

Nervous System Disorders: dizziness, dizziness postural

Respiratory, Thoracic, and Mediastinal Disorders: cough

6.2 Clinical Laboratory Findings

In controlled clinical trials, clinically relevant changes in standard laboratory parameters were uncommon with administration of Edarbi.

Serum creatinine

Small reversible increases in serum creatinine are seen in patients receiving 80 mg of Edarbi. The increase may be larger when coadministered with chlorthalidone or hydrochlorothiazide.

In addition, patients taking Edarbi who had moderate to severe renal impairment at baseline or who were >75 years of age were more likely to report serum creatinine increases.

Hemoglobin/Hematocrit

Low hemoglobin, hematocrit, and RBC counts were observed in 0.2%, 0.4%, and 0.3% of Edarbi-treated subjects, respectively. None of these abnormalities were reported in the placebo group. Low and high markedly abnormal platelet and WBC counts were observed in <0.1% of subjects.

7 DRUG INTERACTIONS

No clinically significant drug interactions have been observed in studies of azilsartan medoxomil or azilsartan given with amlodipine, antacids, chlorthalidone, digoxin, fluconazole, glyburide, ketoconazole, metformin, pioglitazone, and warfarin. Therefore, Edarbi may be used concomitantly with these medications.

Non-steroidal Anti-Inflammatory Agents, including Selective Cyclooxygenase-2 Inhibitors (COX-2 Inhibitors)

In patients who are elderly, volume-depleted (including those on diuretic therapy), or who have compromised renal function, coadministration of NSAIDs, including selective COX-2 inhibitors, with angiotensin II receptor antagonists, including azilsartan, may result in deterioration of renal function, including possible acute renal failure. These effects are usually reversible. Monitor renal function periodically in patients receiving azilsartan and NSAID therapy.

The antihypertensive effect of angiotensin II receptor antagonists, including azilsartan, may be attenuated by NSAIDs, including selective COX-2 inhibitors.

Dual Blockade of the Renin-Angiotensin System (RAS)

Dual blockade of the RAS with angiotensin receptor blockers, ACE inhibitors, or aliskiren is associated with increased risks of hypotension, hyperkalemia, and changes in renal function (including acute renal failure) compared to monotherapy. Closely monitor blood pressure, renal function and electrolytes in patients on Edarbi and other agents that affect the RAS.

Do not coadminister aliskiren with Edarbi in patients with diabetes. Avoid use of aliskiren with Edarbi in patients with renal impairment (GFR <60 mL/min).

8 USE IN SPECIFIC POPULATIONS

8.1 Pregnancy

Pregnancy Category D

Use of drugs that affect the renin-angiotensin system during the second and third trimesters of pregnancy reduces fetal renal function and increases fetal and neonatal morbidity and death. Resulting oligohydramnios can be associated with fetal lung hypoplasia and skeletal deformations. Potential neonatal adverse effects include skull hypoplasia, anuria, hypotension, renal failure, and death. When pregnancy is detected, discontinue Edarbi as soon as possible. These adverse outcomes are usually associated with use of these drugs in the second and third trimester of pregnancy. Most epidemiologic studies examining fetal abnormalities after exposure to antihypertensive use in the first trimester have not distinguished drugs affecting the renin-angiotensin system from other antihypertensive agents. Appropriate management of maternal hypertension during pregnancy is important to optimize outcomes for both mother and fetus.

In the unusual case that there is no appropriate alternative to therapy with drugs affecting the renin-angiotensin system for a particular patient, apprise the mother of the potential risk to the fetus. Perform serial ultrasound examinations to assess the intra-amniotic environment. If oligohydramnios is observed, discontinue Edarbi, unless it is considered lifesaving for the mother. Fetal testing may be appropriate, based on the week of pregnancy. Patients and physicians should be aware, however, that oligohydramnios may not appear until after the fetus has sustained irreversible injury. Closely observe infants with histories of *in utero* exposure to Edarbi for hypotension, oliguria, and hyperkalemia *[see Use in Specific Populations (8.4)]*.

8.3 Nursing Mothers

It is not known if azilsartan is excreted in human milk, but azilsartan is excreted at low concentrations in the milk of lactating rats. Because of the potential for adverse effects on the nursing infant, a decision should be made whether to discontinue nursing or discontinue the drug, taking into account the importance of the drug to the mother.

8.4 Pediatric Use

Neonates with a history of *in utero* exposure to Edarbi

If oliguria or hypotension occurs, support blood pressure and renal function. Exchange transfusions or dialysis may be required.

Safety and effectiveness in pediatric patients under 18 years of age have not been established.

8.5 Geriatric Use

No dose adjustment with Edarbi is necessary in elderly patients. Of the total patients in clinical studies with Edarbi, 26% were elderly (65 years of age and older); 5% were 75 years of age and older. Abnormally high serum creatinine values were more likely to be reported for patients age 75 or older. No other differences in safety or effectiveness were observed between elderly patients and younger patients, but greater sensitivity of some older individuals cannot be ruled out *[see Clinical Pharmacology (12.3)]*.

8.6 Renal Impairment

Dose adjustment is not required in patients with mild-to-severe renal impairment or end-stage renal disease. Patients with moderate to severe renal impairment are more likely to report abnormally high serum creatinine values.

8.7 Hepatic Impairment

No dose adjustment is necessary for subjects with mild or moderate hepatic impairment. Edarbi has not been studied in patients with severe hepatic impairment *[see Clinical Pharmacology (12.3)]*.

10 OVERDOSAGE

Limited data are available related to overdosage in humans. During controlled clinical trials in healthy subjects, once-daily doses up to 320 mg of Edarbi were administered for seven days and were well tolerated. In the event of an overdose, supportive therapy should be instituted as dictated by the patient's clinical status. Azilsartan is not dialyzable *[see Clinical Pharmacology (12.3)]*.

11 DESCRIPTION

Edarbi (azilsartan medoxomil), a prodrug, is hydrolyzed to azilsartan in the gastrointestinal tract during absorption. Azilsartan is a selective AT_1 subtype angiotensin II receptor antagonist.

The drug substance used in the drug product formulation is the potassium salt of azilsartan medoxomil, also known by the US accepted name of azilsartan kamedoxomil and is chemically described as (5-Methyl-2-oxo-1,3-dioxol-4-yl) methyl 2-ethoxy-1-{[2′-(5-oxo-4,5-dihydro-1,2,4-oxadiazol-3-yl)biphenyl-4-yl]methyl}-1*H*-benzimidazole-7-carboxylate monopotassium salt.

Its empirical formula is $C_{30}H_{23}KN_4O_8$ and its structural formula is:

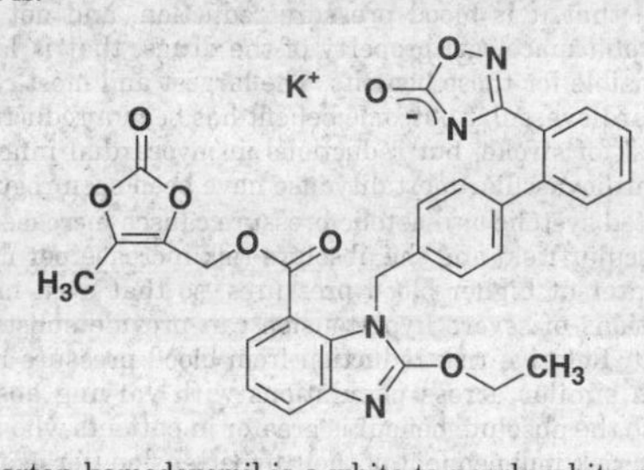

Azilsartan kamedoxomil is a white to nearly white powder with a molecular weight of 606.62. It is practically insoluble in water and freely soluble in methanol.

Edarbi is available for oral use as tablets. The tablets have a characteristic odor. Each Edarbi tablet contains 42.68 or 85.36 mg of azilsartan kamedoxomil, which is equivalent to containing 40 mg or 80 mg respectively, of azilsartan medoxomil and the following inactive ingredients: mannitol, fumaric acid, sodium hydroxide, hydroxypropyl cellulose, croscarmellose sodium, microcrystalline cellulose, and magnesium stearate.

12 CLINICAL PHARMACOLOGY

12.1 Mechanism of Action

Angiotensin II is formed from angiotensin I in a reaction catalyzed by angiotensin-converting enzymes (ACE, kinase II). Angiotensin II is the principal pressor agent of the renin-angiotensin system, with effects that include vasoconstriction, stimulation of synthesis and release of aldosterone, cardiac stimulation, and renal reabsorption of sodium. Azilsartan blocks the vasoconstrictor and aldosterone-secreting effects of angiotensin II by selectively blocking the binding of angiotensin II to the AT_1 receptor in many tissues, such as vascular smooth muscle and the adrenal gland. Its action is, therefore, independent of the pathway for angiotensin II synthesis.

An AT_2 receptor is also found in many tissues, but this receptor is not known to be associated with cardiovascular homeostasis. Azilsartan has more than a 10,000-fold greater affinity for the AT_1 receptor than for the AT_2 receptor.

Blockade of the renin-angiotensin system with ACE inhibitors, which inhibit the biosynthesis of angiotensin II from angiotensin I, is widely used in the treatment of hypertension. ACE inhibitors also inhibit the degradation of bradykinin, a reaction catalyzed by ACE. Because azilsartan does not inhibit ACE (kinase II), it should not affect bradykinin levels. Whether this difference has clinical relevance is not yet known. Azilsartan does not bind to or block other receptors or ion channels known to be important in cardiovascular regulation.

Blockade of the angiotensin II receptor inhibits the negative regulatory feedback of angiotensin II on renin secretion, but the resulting increased plasma renin activity and angiotensin II circulating levels do not overcome the effect of azilsartan on blood pressure.

12.2 Pharmacodynamics

Azilsartan inhibits the pressor effects of an angiotensin II infusion in a dose-related manner. An azilsartan single dose equivalent to 32 mg azilsartan medoxomil inhibited the maximal pressor effect by approximately 90% at peak, and approximately 60% at 24 hours. Plasma angiotensin I and II concentrations and plasma renin activity increased while plasma aldosterone concentrations decreased after single and repeated administration of Edarbi to healthy subjects; no clinically significant effects on serum potassium or sodium were observed.

Effect on Cardiac Repolarization

A thorough QT/QTc study was conducted to assess the potential of azilsartan to prolong the QT/QTc interval in healthy subjects. There was no evidence of QT/QTc prolongation at a dose of 320 mg of Edarbi.

12.3 Pharmacokinetics

Absorption

Azilsartan medoxomil is hydrolyzed to azilsartan, the active metabolite, in the gastrointestinal tract during absorption. Azilsartan medoxomil is not detected in plasma after oral administration. Dose proportionality in exposure was established for azilsartan in the azilsartan medoxomil dose range of 20 mg to 320 mg after single or multiple dosing.

The estimated absolute bioavailability of azilsartan following administration of azilsartan medoxomil is approximately 60%. After oral administration of azilsartan medoxomil, peak plasma concentrations (C_{max}) of azilsartan are reached within 1.5 to 3 hours. Food does not affect the bioavailability of azilsartan.

Distribution

The volume of distribution of azilsartan is approximately 16 L. Azilsartan is highly bound to human plasma proteins (>99%), mainly serum albumin. Protein binding is constant at azilsartan plasma concentrations well above the range achieved with recommended doses.

In rats, minimal azilsartan-associated radioactivity crossed the blood-brain barrier. Azilsartan passed across the placental barrier in pregnant rats and was distributed to the fetus.

Metabolism and Elimination

Azilsartan is metabolized to two primary metabolites. The major metabolite in plasma is formed by *O*-dealkylation, referred to as metabolite M-II, and the minor metabolite is formed by decarboxylation, referred to as metabolite M-I. Systemic exposures to the major and minor metabolites in humans were approximately 50% and less than 1% of azilsartan, respectively. M-I and M-II do not contribute to the pharmacologic activity of Edarbi. The major enzyme responsible for azilsartan metabolism is CYP2C9.

Following an oral dose of ^{14}C-labeled azilsartan medoxomil, approximately 55% of radioactivity was recovered in feces and approximately 42% in urine, with 15% of the dose excreted in urine as azilsartan. The elimination half-life of azilsartan is approximately 11 hours and renal clearance is approximately 2.3 mL/min. Steady-state levels of azilsartan are achieved within five days, and no accumulation in plasma occurs with repeated once-daily dosing.

Special Populations

The effect of demographic and functional factors on the pharmacokinetics of azilsartan was studied in single and multiple dose studies. Pharmacokinetic measures indicating the magnitude of the effect on azilsartan are presented in Figure 1 as change relative to reference (test/reference). Effects are modest and do not call for dosage adjustment.

Figure 1. Impact of intrinsic factors on the pharmacokinetics of azilsartan

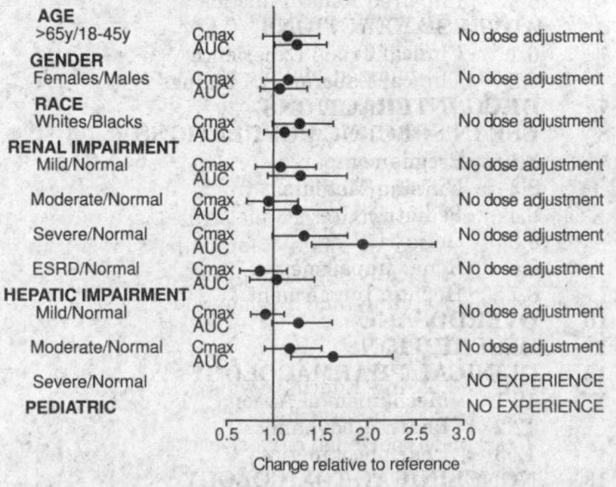

13 NONCLINICAL TOXICOLOGY

13.1 Carcinogenesis, Mutagenesis, Impairment of Fertility

Carcinogenesis

Azilsartan medoxomil was not carcinogenic when assessed in 26-week transgenic (Tg.rasH2) mouse and two-year rat studies. The highest doses tested (450 mg azilsartan medoxomil/kg/day in the mouse and 600 mg azilsartan medoxomil/kg/day in the rat) produced exposures to azilsartan that are 12 (mice) and 27 (rats) times the average exposure to azilsartan in humans given the maximum recommended human dose (MRHD, 80 mg azilsartan medoxomil/day). M-II was not carcinogenic when assessed in 26-week Tg.rasH2 mouse and two-year rat studies. The highest doses tested (approximately 8000 mg M-II/kg/day [males] and 11,000 mg M-II/kg/day [females] in the mouse and 1000 mg M-II/kg/day [males] and up to 3000 mg M-II/kg/day [females] in the rat) produced exposures that are, on average, about 30 (mice) and seven (rats) times the average exposure to M-II in humans at the MRHD.

Mutagenesis

Azilsartan medoxomil, azilsartan, and M-II were positive for structural aberrations in the Chinese Hamster Lung Cytogenetic Assay. In this assay, structural chromosomal aberrations were observed with the prodrug, azilsartan medoxomil, without metabolic activation. The active moiety, azilsartan was also positive in this assay both with and without metabolic activation. The major human metabolite, M-II was also positive in this assay during a 24-hour assay without metabolic activation.

Azilsartan medoxomil, azilsartan, and M-II were devoid of genotoxic potential in the Ames reverse mutation assay with *Salmonella typhimurium* and *Escherichia coli*, the *in vitro* Chinese Hamster Ovary Cell forward mutation assay, the *in vitro* mouse lymphoma (tk) gene mutation test, the *ex vivo* unscheduled DNA synthesis test, and the *in vivo* mouse and/or rat bone marrow micronucleus assay.

Impairment of Fertility

There was no effect of azilsartan medoxomil on the fertility of male or female rats at oral doses of up to 1000 mg azilsartan medoxomil/kg/day (6000 mg/m^2 [approximately 122 times the MRHD of 80 mg azilsartan medoxomil/60 kg on a mg/m^2 basis]). Fertility of rats also was unaffected at doses of up to 3000 mg M-II/kg/day.

13.2 Animal Toxicology and/or Pharmacology

Reproductive Toxicology

In peri- and postnatal rat development studies, adverse effects on pup viability, delayed incisor eruption and dilatation of the renal pelvis along with hydronephrosis were seen when azilsartan medoxomil was administered to pregnant and nursing rats at 1.2 times the MRHD on a mg/m^2 basis. Reproductive toxicity studies indicated that azilsartan medoxomil was not teratogenic when administered at oral doses up to 1000 mg azilsartan medoxomil/kg/day to pregnant rats (122 times the MRHD on a mg/m^2 basis) or up to 50 mg azilsartan medoxomil/kg/day to pregnant rabbits (12 times the MRHD on a mg/m^2 basis). M-II also was not teratogenic in rats or rabbits at doses up to 3000 mg M-II/kg/day. Azilsartan crossed the placenta and was found in the fetuses of pregnant rats and was excreted into the milk of lactating rats.

14 CLINICAL STUDIES

The antihypertensive effects of Edarbi have been demonstrated in a total of seven double-blind, randomized studies, which included five placebo-controlled and four active comparator-controlled studies (not mutually exclusive). The studies ranged from six weeks to six months in duration, at doses ranging from 20 mg to 80 mg once daily. A total of 5941 patients (3672 given Edarbi, 801 given placebo, and 1468 given active comparator) with mild, moderate or severe hypertension were studied. Overall, 51% of patients were male and 26% were 65 years or older; 67% were white and 19% were black.

Two 6-week, randomized, double-blind studies compared the effect on blood pressure of Edarbi at doses of 40 mg and 80 mg, with placebo and with active comparators. Blood pressure reductions compared to placebo based on clinic blood pressure measurements at trough and 24-hour mean blood pressure by ambulatory blood pressure monitoring (ABPM) are shown in Table 1 for both studies. Edarbi, 80 mg, was statistically superior to placebo and active comparators for both clinic and 24-hour mean blood pressure measurements.

[See table 1 above]

Table 1. Placebo Corrected Mean Change from Baseline in Systolic/Diastolic Blood Pressure at 6 Weeks (mm Hg)

	Study 1 N=1285		Study 2 N=989	
	Clinic Blood Pressure (Mean Baseline 157.4/92.5)	**24 Hour Mean by ABPM** (Mean Baseline 144.9/88.7)	**Clinic Blood Pressure** (Mean Baseline 159.0/91.8)	**24 Hour Mean by ABPM** (Mean Baseline 146.2/87.6)
Edarbi 40 mg	-14.6/-6.2	-13.2/-8.6	-12.4/-7.1	-12.1/-7.7
Edarbi 80 mg	-14.9/-7.5	-14.3/-9.4	-15.5/-8.6	-13.2/-7.9
Olmesartan 40 mg	-11.4/-5.3	-11.7/-7.7	-12.8/-7.1	-11.2/-7.0
Valsartan 320 mg	-9.5/-4.4	-10.0/-7.0		

In a study comparing Edarbi to valsartan over 24 weeks, similar results were observed.

Most of the antihypertensive effect occurs within the first two weeks of dosing.

Figure 2 shows the 24-hour ambulatory systolic and diastolic blood pressure profiles at endpoint.

[See figure 2 at top of next column]

Other studies showed similar 24-hour ambulatory blood pressure profiles.

Edarbi has a sustained and consistent antihypertensive effect during long-term treatment, as shown in a study that randomized patients to placebo or continued Edarbi after 26 weeks. No rebound effect was observed following the abrupt cessation of Edarbi therapy.

Figure 2. Mean Ambulatory Blood Pressure at 6 Weeks by Dose and Hour

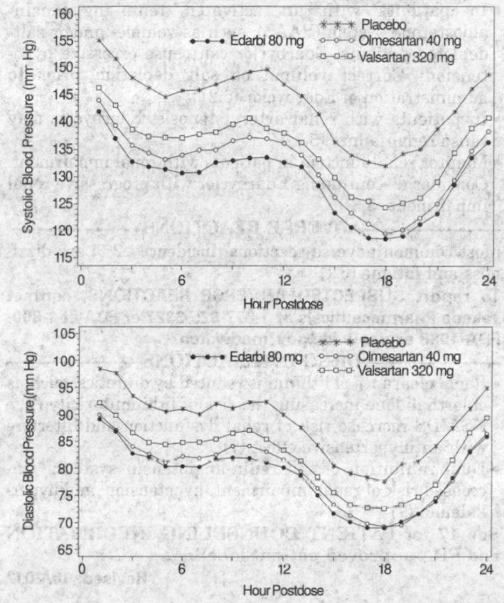

Edarbi was effective in reducing blood pressure regardless of the age, gender, or race of patients, but the effect, as monotherapy, was smaller, approximately half, in black patients, who tend to have low renin levels. This has been generally true for other angiotensin II antagonists and ACE inhibitors.

Edarbi has about its usual blood pressure lowering effect size when added to a calcium channel blocker (amlodipine) or a thiazide-type diuretic (chlorthalidone).

There are no trials of Edarbi demonstrating reductions in cardiovascular risk in patients with hypertension, but at least one pharmacologically similar drug has demonstrated such benefits.

16 HOW SUPPLIED/STORAGE AND HANDLING

Edarbi tablets are unscored and white to nearly white, debossed with "ASL" on one side and "40" or "80" on the other.

Tablet	NDC 64764-xxx-xx	
	Bottle/30	Bottle/90
40 mg	844-30	844-90
80 mg	884-30	884-90

Storage

Store at 25°C (77°F); excursions permitted to 15°-30°C (59°-86°F) *[see USP Controlled Room Temperature]*. Keep container tightly closed. Protect from moisture and light. Do not repackage; dispense and store in original container.

17 PATIENT COUNSELING INFORMATION

See FDA-approved patient labeling (17.2).

17.1 General Information

Pregnancy

Tell female patients of childbearing potential about the consequences of exposure to Edarbi during pregnancy. Discuss treatment options with women planning to become pregnant. Tell patients to report pregnancies to their physicians as soon as possible.

17.2 FDA-Approved Patient Labeling

Patient Information

Edarbi (eh-DAR-bee)

(azilsartan medoxomil)

Tablets

Read this Patient Information leaflet before you start taking Edarbi and each time you get a refill. There may be new information. This information does not take the place of talking to your doctor about your medical condition or your treatment.

What is the most important information I should know about Edarbi?

- Edarbi can cause harm or death to your unborn baby.
- Talk to your doctor about other ways to lower your blood pressure if you plan to become pregnant.
- If you become pregnant while taking Edarbi, tell your doctor right away. Your doctor may switch you to a different medicine to treat your high blood pressure.

What is Edarbi?

Edarbi is a prescription medicine called an angiotensin II receptor blocker (ARB) used to treat high blood pressure (hypertension) in adults.

Your doctor may prescribe other medicines for you to take along with Edarbi to treat your high blood pressure.

It is not known if Edarbi is safe and effective in children under 18 years of age.

What should I tell my doctor before taking Edarbi?

Before you take Edarbi, tell your doctor if you:

- have been told that you have abnormal body salt (electrolytes) levels in your blood
- are pregnant or plan to become pregnant. See **"What is the most important information I should know about Edarbi?"**
- are breastfeeding or plan to breastfeed. It is not known if Edarbi passes into your breast milk. You and your doctor should decide if you will take Edarbi or breastfeed. You should not do both. Talk with your doctor about the best way to feed your baby if you take Edarbi.

Tell your doctor about all the medicines you take, including prescription and nonprescription medicines, vitamins, and herbal supplements.

Especially tell your doctor if you take:

- other medicines used to treat your high blood pressure or heart problem
- water pills (diuretic)

Ask your doctor if you are not sure if you are taking a medicine listed above.

Know the medicines you take. Keep a list of them and show it to your doctor or pharmacist when you get a new medicine.

How should I take Edarbi?

- Your doctor will tell you how much Edarbi to take and when to take it. Follow his/her instructions.
- Edarbi can be taken with or without food.
- If you take too much Edarbi, call your doctor or go to the nearest hospital emergency room right away.

What are the possible side effects of Edarbi?

Edarbi may cause side effects, including:

- **Harm or death to your unborn fetus if taken in the second or third trimester.** See **"What is the most important information I should know about Edarbi?"**
- **Low blood pressure (hypotension) and dizziness** is most likely to happen if you also:
  - take water pills (diuretics)
  - are on a low-salt diet
  - take other medicines that affect your blood pressure
  - get sick with vomiting or diarrhea
  - do not drink enough fluids

If you feel faint or dizzy, lie down and call your doctor right away.

These are not all the possible side effects with Edarbi. Tell your doctor if you have any side effect that bothers you or that does not go away.

Call your doctor for medical advice about side effects. You may report side effects to FDA at 1-800-FDA-1088.

How do I store Edarbi?

- Store Edarbi at 59°F to 86°F (15°C to 30°C).
- Store Edarbi in the original container that you received from your pharmacist or doctor. Do not put Edarbi into a different container.
- Keep Edarbi in a tightly closed container, and keep Edarbi out of the light.

Keep Edarbi and all medicines out of the reach of children.

General information about Edarbi.

Medicines are sometimes prescribed for purposes other than those listed in a Patient Information leaflet. Do not give Edarbi to other people, even if they have the same symptoms you have. It may harm them.

This Patient Information leaflet summarizes the most important information about Edarbi. If you would like more information, talk with your doctor. You can ask your pharmacist or doctor for information about Edarbi that is written for health professionals.

For more information, go to www.edarbi.com or call 1-877-825-3327.

What is high blood pressure (hypertension)?

Blood pressure is the force in your blood vessels when your heart beats and when your heart rests. You have high blood pressure when the force is too great.

High blood pressure makes the heart work harder to pump blood through the body and causes damage to the blood vessels. Edarbi tablets can help your blood vessels relax so your blood pressure is lower. Medicines that lower your blood pressure may lower your chance of having a stroke or heart attack.

What are the ingredients in Edarbi?

Active ingredient: azilsartan medoxomil

Inactive ingredients: mannitol, fumaric acid, sodium hydroxide, hydroxypropyl cellulose, croscarmellose sodium, microcrystalline cellulose, and magnesium stearate.

Distributed by

Takeda Pharmaceuticals America, Inc.
Deerfield, IL 60015
Revised: October 2012

AZL069 R4

Shown in Product Identification Guide, page 313

EDARBYCLOR ℞

(azilsartan medoxomil and chlorthalidone) tablets, for oral use

HIGHLIGHTS OF PRESCRIBING INFORMATION

These highlights do not include all the information needed to use EDARBYCLOR safely and effectively. See full prescribing information for EDARBYCLOR.

EDARBYCLOR (azilsartan medoxomil and chlorthalidone) tablets, for oral use

Initial U.S. Approval: 2011

> **WARNING: FETAL TOXICITY**
> ***See full prescribing information for complete boxed warning.***
> - **When pregnancy is detected, discontinue EDARBYCLOR as soon as possible (5.1)**
> - **Drugs that act directly on the renin-angiotensin system can cause injury and death to the developing fetus (5.1)**

RECENT MAJOR CHANGES

Contraindications (4) 10/2012

INDICATIONS AND USAGE

Edarbyclor is an angiotensin II receptor blocker (ARB) and a thiazide-like diuretic combination product indicated for the treatment of hypertension, to lower blood pressure:

- In patients not adequately controlled with monotherapy (1)
- As initial therapy in patients likely to need multiple drugs to help achieve blood pressure goals (1)

Lowering blood pressure reduces the risk of fatal and nonfatal cardiovascular events, primarily strokes and myocardial infarctions (1)

DOSAGE AND ADMINISTRATION

- Starting dose is 40/12.5 mg once daily (2.1)
- Edarbyclor may be used to provide additional blood pressure lowering for patients not adequately controlled on azilsartan medoxomil 80 mg or chlorthalidone 25 mg (2.1)
- Dose may be increased to 40/25 mg after 2 to 4 weeks as needed to achieve blood pressure goals (2.1)
- Maximal dose is 40/25 mg (2.1)
- May be administered with other antihypertensive agents (2.1)
- Edarbyclor may be administered with or without food (2.1)
- Replace volume in volume-depleted patients prior to use (2.2)

DOSAGE FORMS AND STRENGTHS

Tablets (azilsartan/chlorthalidone): 40/12.5 mg and 40/25 mg (3)

CONTRAINDICATIONS

- Anuria (4)
- Do not coadminister aliskiren with Edarbyclor in patients with diabetes (4)

WARNINGS AND PRECAUTIONS

- In patients with an activated renin-angiotensin-aldosterone system (RAAS), such as volume- and/or salt-depleted patients, Edarbyclor can cause excessive hypotension. Correct volume or salt depletion prior to administration of Edarbyclor (5.2)
- In patients with renal artery stenosis, Edarbyclor may cause renal failure (5.3)
- Monitor renal function in patients with renal impairment. Consider discontinuing Edarbyclor with progressive renal impairment (5.3)

ADVERSE REACTIONS

Most common adverse reactions (incidence ≥2%) are dizziness and fatigue (6.1)

To report SUSPECTED ADVERSE REACTIONS, contact Takeda Pharmaceuticals at 1-877-825-3327 or FDA at 1-800-FDA-1088 or www.fda.gov/medwatch.

DRUG INTERACTIONS

- Renal clearance of lithium is reduced by diuretics, such as chlorthalidone increasing the risk of lithium toxicity (7)
- NSAIDS increase risk of renal dysfunction and interfere with antihypertensive effect (7)
- Dual inhibition of the renin-angiotensin system: Increased risk of renal impairment, hypotension, and hyperkalemia (7)

See 17 for PATIENT COUNSELING INFORMATION and FDA-approved patient labeling.

Revised: 10/2012

FULL PRESCRIBING INFORMATION: CONTENTS*

*** Sections or subsections omitted from the full prescribing information are not listed.**

FULL PRESCRIBING INFORMATION

> **WARNING: FETAL TOXICITY**
> - **When pregnancy is detected, discontinue Edarbyclor as soon as possible *[see Warnings and Precautions (5.1)]*.**
> - **Drugs that act directly on the renin-angiotensin system can cause injury and death to the developing fetus *[see Warnings and Precautions (5.1)]*.**

1 INDICATIONS AND USAGE

Edarbyclor contains an angiotensin II receptor blocker (ARB) and a thiazide-like diuretic and is indicated for the treatment of hypertension, to lower blood pressure.

Edarbyclor may be used in patients whose blood pressure is not adequately controlled on monotherapy.

Edarbyclor may be used as initial therapy if a patient is likely to need multiple drugs to achieve blood pressure goals.

Lowering blood pressure reduces the risk of fatal and nonfatal cardiovascular events, primarily strokes and myocardial infarctions. These benefits have been seen in controlled trials of antihypertensive drugs from a wide variety of pharmacologic classes including thiazide-like diuretics such as chlorthalidone and ARBs such as azilsartan medoxomil. There are no controlled trials demonstrating risk reduction with Edarbyclor.

Control of high blood pressure should be part of comprehensive cardiovascular risk management, including, as appropriate, lipid control, diabetes management, antithrombotic therapy, smoking cessation, exercise, and limited sodium intake. Many patients will require more than one drug to achieve blood pressure goals. For specific advice on goals and management of high blood pressure, see published guidelines, such as those of the National High Blood Pressure Education Program's Joint National Committee on Prevention, Detection, Evaluation, and Treatment of High Blood Pressure (JNC).

Numerous antihypertensive drugs, from a variety of pharmacologic classes and with different mechanisms of action, have been shown in randomized controlled trials to reduce cardiovascular morbidity and mortality, and it can be concluded that it is blood pressure reduction, and not some other pharmacologic property of the drugs, that is largely responsible for those benefits. The largest and most consistent cardiovascular outcome benefit has been a reduction in the risk of stroke, but reductions in myocardial infarction and cardiovascular mortality also have been seen regularly.

Elevated systolic or diastolic pressure causes increased cardiovascular risk, and the absolute risk increase per mmHg is greater at higher blood pressures, so that even modest reductions of severe hypertension can provide substantial benefit. Relative risk reduction from blood pressure reduction is similar across populations with varying absolute risk, so the absolute benefit is greater in patients who are at higher risk independent of their hypertension (for example, patients with diabetes or hyperlipidemia), and such patients would be expected to benefit from more aggressive treatment to a lower blood pressure goal.

Some antihypertensive drugs have smaller blood pressure effects (as monotherapy) in black patients; however, the blood pressure effect of Edarbyclor in blacks is similar to that in non-blacks. Many antihypertensive drugs have additional approved indications and effects (e.g., on angina, heart failure, or diabetic kidney disease). These considerations may guide selection of therapy.

The choice of Edarbyclor as initial therapy for hypertension should be based on an assessment of potential benefits and risks including whether the patient is likely to tolerate the starting dose of Edarbyclor.

Patients with moderate-to-severe hypertension are at a relatively high risk of cardiovascular events (e.g., stroke, heart attack, and heart failure), kidney failure, and vision problems, so prompt treatment is clinically relevant. Consider the patient's baseline blood pressure, target goal and the incremental likelihood of achieving the goal with a combination product, such as Edarbyclor, versus a monotherapy product when deciding upon initial therapy. Individual blood pressure goals may vary based on the patient's risk.

Data from an 8-week, active-controlled, factorial trial provide estimates of the probability of reaching a target blood pressure with Edarbyclor compared with azilsartan medoxomil or chlorthalidone monotherapy [see *Clinical Studies (14)*].

Figures 1.a-1.d provide estimates of the likelihood of achieving target clinic systolic and diastolic blood pressure control with Edarbyclor 40/25 mg tablets after 8 weeks, based on baseline systolic or diastolic blood pressure. The curve for each treatment group was estimated by logistic regression modeling and is more variable at the tails.

Table 1. Adverse Reactions Occurring at an Incidence of ≥2% of Edarbyclor-treated Patients and > Azilsartan medoxomil or Chlorthalidone

Preferred Term	Azilsartan medoxomil 20, 40, 80 mg (N=470)	Chlorthalidone 12.5, 25 mg (N=316)	Edarbyclor 40 / 12.5, 40 / 25 mg (N=302)
Dizziness	1.7%	1.9%	8.9%
Fatigue	0.6%	1.3%	2.0%

Figure 1.a Probability of Achieving Systolic Blood Pressure <140 mmHg at Week 8

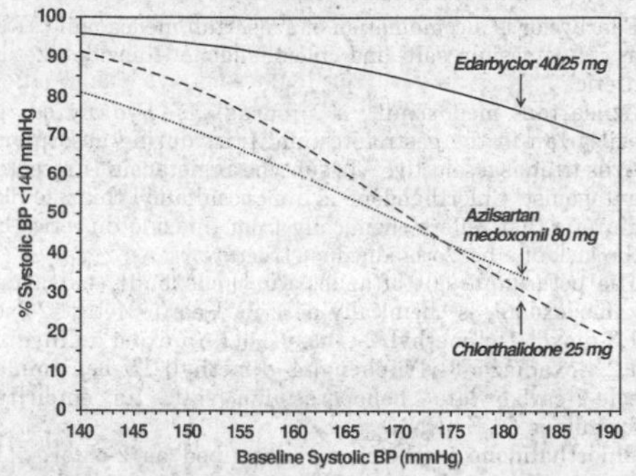

Figure 1.b Probability of Achieving Systolic Blood Pressure <130 mmHg at Week 8

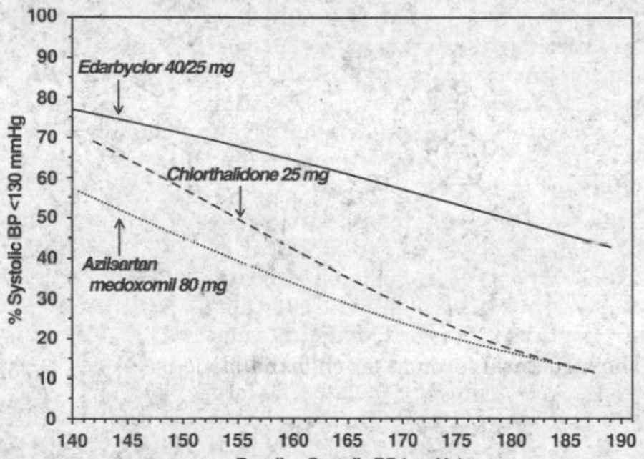

Figure 1.c Probability of Achieving Diastolic Blood Pressure <90 mmHg at Week 8

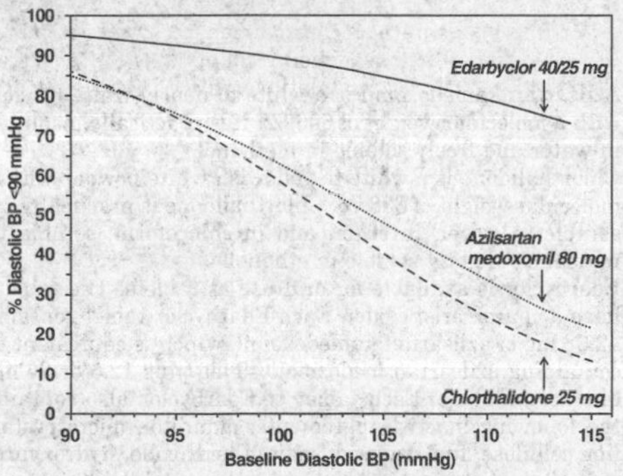

Figure 1.d Probability of Achieving Diastolic Blood Pressure <80 mmHg at Week 8

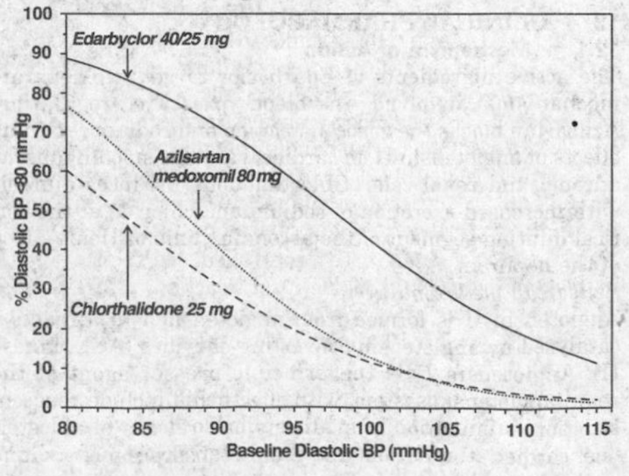

For example, a patient with a baseline blood pressure of 170/105 mm Hg has approximately a 48% likelihood of achieving a goal of <140 mm Hg (systolic) and 48% likelihood of achieving <90 mm Hg (diastolic) on azilsartan medoxomil 80 mg. The likelihood of achieving these same goals on chlorthalidone 25 mg is approximately 51% (systolic) and 40% (diastolic). These likelihoods rise to 85% (systolic) and 85% (diastolic) with Edarbyclor 40/25 mg.

2 DOSAGE AND ADMINISTRATION

2.1 Dosing Information

The recommended starting dose of Edarbyclor is 40/12.5 mg taken orally once daily. Most of the antihypertensive effect is apparent within 1 to 2 weeks. The dosage may be increased to 40/25 mg after 2 to 4 weeks as needed to achieve blood pressure goals. Edarbyclor doses above 40/25 mg are probably not useful.

Edarbyclor may be used to provide additional blood pressure lowering for patients not adequately controlled on ARB or diuretic monotherapy treatment. Patients not controlled with azilsartan medoxomil 80 mg may have an additional systolic / diastolic clinic blood pressure reduction of 13/6 mm Hg when switched to Edarbyclor 40/12.5 mg. Patients not controlled with chlorthalidone 25 mg may have an additional clinic blood pressure reduction of 10/7 mm Hg when switched to Edarbyclor 40/12.5 mg.

Edarbyclor may be used as initial therapy if a patient is likely to need multiple drugs to achieve blood pressure goals.

Patients titrated to the individual components (azilsartan medoxomil and chlorthalidone) may instead receive the corresponding dose of Edarbyclor.

Edarbyclor may be taken with or without food *[see Clinical Pharmacology (12.3)]*.

Edarbyclor may be administered with other antihypertensive agents as needed.

2.2 Prior to Dosing

Correct any volume depletion prior to administration of Edarbyclor, particularly in patients with impaired renal function or those treated with high doses of diuretics *[see Warnings and Precautions (5.2)]*.

Patients who experience dose-limiting adverse reactions on chlorthalidone may be switched to Edarbyclor, initially with a lower dose of chlorthalidone *[see Warnings and Precautions (5.4)]*.

2.3 Handling Instructions

As Edarbyclor is moisture sensitive, dispense and store Edarbyclor in its original container to protect Edarbyclor from light and moisture.

3 DOSAGE FORMS AND STRENGTHS

Edarbyclor is supplied in the following dosage strengths:

- 40/12.5 mg: pale red, round, biconvex, film-coated tablets, approximately 9.7 mm in diameter, with "A/C" and "40/12.5" imprinted on one side. Each tablet contains 40 mg of azilsartan medoxomil and 12.5 mg of chlorthalidone.
- 40/25 mg: light red, round, biconvex, film-coated tablets, approximately 9.7 mm in diameter, with "A/C" and "40/25" imprinted on one side. Each tablet contains 40 mg of azilsartan medoxomil and 25 mg of chlorthalidone.

4 CONTRAINDICATIONS

- Edarbyclor is contraindicated in patients with anuria *[see Warnings and Precautions (5.3)]*.
- Do not coadminister aliskiren with Edarbyclor in patients with diabetes *[see Drug Interactions (7)]*.

5 WARNINGS AND PRECAUTIONS

5.1 Fetal Toxicity

Azilsartan medoxomil

Use of drugs that act on the renin-angiotensin system during the second and third trimesters of pregnancy reduces fetal renal function and increases fetal and neonatal morbidity and death. Resulting oligohydramnios can be associated with fetal lung hypoplasia and skeletal deformations. Potential neonatal adverse effects include skull hypoplasia, anuria, hypotension, renal failure, and death. When pregnancy is detected, discontinue Edarbyclor as soon as possible *[see Use in Specific Populations (8.1)]*.

Chlorthalidone

Thiazides cross the placental barrier and appear in cord blood. Adverse reactions include fetal or neonatal jaundice and thrombocytopenia.

5.2 Hypotension in Volume- or Salt-Depleted Patients

In patients with an activated renin-angiotensin system, such as volume- or salt-depleted patients (e.g., those being treated with high doses of diuretics), symptomatic hypotension may occur after initiation of treatment with Edarbyclor. Such patients are probably not good candidates to start therapy with more than one drug; therefore, correct volume prior to administration of Edarbyclor. If hypotension does occur, the patient should be placed in the supine position and, if necessary, given an intravenous infusion of normal saline. A transient hypotensive response is not a contraindication to further treatment, which usually can be continued without difficulty once the blood pressure has stabilized.

5.3 Impaired Renal Function

Edarbyclor

Monitor for worsening renal function in patients with renal impairment. Consider withholding or discontinuing Edarbyclor if progressive renal impairment becomes evident.

Azilsartan medoxomil

As a consequence of inhibiting the renin-angiotensin system, changes in renal function may be anticipated in susceptible individuals treated with Edarbyclor. In patients whose renal function may depend on the activity of the renin-angiotensin system (e.g., patients with severe congestive heart failure, renal artery stenosis, or volume depletion), treatment with angiotensin-converting enzyme inhibitors and angiotensin receptor blockers has been associated with oliguria or progressive azotemia and rarely with acute renal failure and death. Similar results may be anticipated in patients treated with Edarbyclor *[see Drug Interactions (7), Use in Specific Populations (8.6) and Clinical Pharmacology (12.3)]*.

In studies of ACE inhibitors in patients with unilateral or bilateral renal artery stenosis, increases in serum creatinine or blood urea nitrogen have been reported. There has been no long-term use of azilsartan medoxomil in patients with unilateral or bilateral renal artery stenosis, but similar results are expected.

Chlorthalidone

In patients with renal disease, chlorthalidone may precipitate azotemia. If progressive renal impairment becomes evident, as indicated by increased blood urea nitrogen, consider withholding or discontinuing diuretic therapy.

5.4 Hypokalemia

Chlorthalidone

Hypokalemia is a dose-dependent adverse reaction that may develop with chlorthalidone. Co-administration of digitalis may exacerbate the adverse effects of hypokalemia.

Edarbyclor attenuates chlorthalidone-associated hypokalemia. In patients with normal potassium levels at baseline, 1.7% of Edarbyclor-treated patients, 0.9% of azilsartan medoxomil-treated patients, and 13.4% of chlorthalidone-treated patients shifted to low potassium values (less than 3.4 mmol/L).

5.5 Hyperuricemia

Chlorthalidone

Hyperuricemia may occur or frank gout may be precipitated in certain patients receiving chlorthalidone or other thiazide diuretics.

6 ADVERSE REACTIONS

The following potential adverse reactions with Edarbyclor, azilsartan medoxomil, or chlorthalidone and similar agents are included in more detail in the Warnings and Precautions section of the label:

- Fetal toxicity *[see Warnings and Precautions (5.1)]*
- Hypotension in Volume- or Salt-Depleted Patients *[see Warnings and Precautions (5.2)]*
- Impaired Renal Function *[see Warnings and Precautions (5.3)]*
- Hypokalemia *[see Warnings and Precautions (5.4)]*
- Hyperuricemia *[see Warnings and Precautions (5.5)]*

6.1 Clinical Trials Experience

Because clinical trials are conducted under widely varying conditions, adverse reaction rates observed in the clinical trials of a drug cannot be directly compared to rates in the clinical trials of another drug and may not reflect the rates observed in practice.

Edarbyclor has been evaluated for safety in more than 3900 patients with hypertension; more than 700 patients were treated for at least 6 months and more than 280 for at least 1 year. Adverse reactions have generally been mild and transient in nature.

Common adverse reactions that occurred in the 8-week factorial design trial in at least 2% of Edarbyclor-treated patients and greater than azilsartan medoxomil or chlorthalidone are presented in Table 1.

[See table 1 above]

Hypotension and syncope were reported in 1.7% and 0.3%, respectively, of patients treated with Edarbyclor.

Study discontinuation because of adverse reactions occurred in 8.3% of patients treated with the recommended doses of Edarbyclor compared with 3.2% of patients treated with azilsartan medoxomil and 3.2% of patients treated with chlorthalidone. The most common reasons for discontinuation of therapy with Edarbyclor were serum creatinine increased (3.6%) and dizziness (2.3%).
The adverse reaction profile obtained from 52 weeks of open-label combination therapy with azilsartan medoxomil plus chlorthalidone or Edarbyclor was similar to that observed during the double-blind, active controlled trials.
In 3 double-blind, active controlled, titration studies, in which Edarbyclor was titrated to higher doses in a step-wise manner, adverse reactions and discontinuations for adverse events were less frequent than in the fixed-dose factorial trial.
Azilsartan medoxomil
A total of 4814 patients were evaluated for safety when treated with azilsartan medoxomil at doses of 20, 40 or 80 mg in clinical trials. This includes 1704 patients treated for at least 6 months, of these, 588 were treated for at least 1 year. Generally, adverse reactions were mild, not dose related and similar regardless of age, gender and race.
Adverse reactions with a plausible relationship to treatment that have been reported with an incidence of ≥0.3% and greater than placebo in more than 3300 patients treated with azilsartan medoxomil in controlled trials are listed below:
Gastrointestinal Disorders: diarrhea, nausea
General Disorders and Administration Site Conditions: asthenia, fatigue
Musculoskeletal and Connective Tissue Disorders: muscle spasm
Nervous System Disorders: dizziness, dizziness postural
Respiratory, Thoracic and Mediastinal Disorders: cough
Chlorthalidone
The following adverse reactions have been observed in clinical trials of chlorthalidone: rash, headache, dizziness, GI upset, and elevations of uric acid and cholesterol.
Clinical Laboratory Findings with Edarbyclor
In the factorial design trial, clinically relevant changes in standard laboratory parameters were uncommon with administration of the recommended doses of Edarbyclor.
Renal parameters:
Increased blood creatinine is a known pharmacologic effect of renin-angiotensin aldosterone system (RAAS) blockers, such as ARBs and ACE inhibitors, and is related to the magnitude of blood pressure reduction. The incidence of consecutive increases of creatinine ≥50% from baseline and >ULN was 2.0% in patients treated with the recommended doses of Edarbyclor compared with 0.4% and 0.3% with azilsartan medoxomil and chlorthalidone, respectively. Elevations of creatinine were typically transient, or non-progressive and reversible, and associated with large blood pressure reductions.
Mean increases in blood urea nitrogen (BUN) were observed with Edarbyclor (5.3 mg/dL) compared with azilsartan medoxomil (1.5 mg/dL) and with chlorthalidone (2.5 mg/dL).

7 DRUG INTERACTIONS

Edarbyclor
The pharmacokinetics of azilsartan medoxomil and chlorthalidone are not altered when the drugs are co-administered.
No drug interaction studies have been conducted with other drugs and Edarbyclor, although studies have been conducted with azilsartan medoxomil and chlorthalidone.
Azilsartan medoxomil
No clinically significant drug interactions have been observed in studies of azilsartan medoxomil or azilsartan given with amlodipine, antacids, chlorthalidone, digoxin, fluconazole, glyburide, ketoconazole, metformin, pioglitazone, and warfarin. Therefore, azilsartan medoxomil may be used concomitantly with these medications.
Non-Steroidal Anti-Inflammatory Agents including Selective Cyclooxygenase-2 Inhibitors (COX-2 Inhibitors)
In patients who are elderly, volume-depleted (including those on diuretic therapy), or who have compromised renal function, co-administration of NSAIDs, including selective COX-2 inhibitors, with angiotensin II receptor antagonists, including azilsartan, may result in deterioration of renal function, including possible acute renal failure. These effects are usually reversible. Monitor renal function periodically in patients receiving Edarbyclor and NSAID therapy.
The antihypertensive effect of Edarbyclor may be attenuated by NSAIDs, including selective COX-2 inhibitors.
Dual Blockade of the Renin-Angiotensin System (RAS)
Dual blockade of the RAS with angiotensin receptor blockers, ACE inhibitors, or aliskiren is associated with increased risks of hypotension, hyperkalemia, and changes in renal function (including acute renal failure) compared to monotherapy. Closely monitor blood pressure, renal function and electrolytes in patients on Edarbyclor and other agents that affect the RAS.
Do not coadminister aliskiren with Edarbyclor in patients with diabetes. Avoid use of aliskiren with Edarbyclor in patients with renal impairment (GFR <60 mL/min).
Chlorthalidone
Lithium renal clearance is reduced by diuretics, such as chlorthalidone, increasing the risk of lithium toxicity. Consider monitoring lithium levels when using Edarbyclor.

8 USE IN SPECIFIC POPULATIONS

8.1 Pregnancy

Pregnancy Category D
Use of drugs that affect the renin-angiotensin system during the second and third trimesters of pregnancy reduces fetal renal function and increases fetal and neonatal morbidity and death. Resulting oligohydramnios can be associated with fetal lung hypoplasia and skeletal deformations. Potential neonatal adverse effects include skull hypoplasia, anuria, hypotension, renal failure, and death. When pregnancy is detected, discontinue Edarbyclor as soon as possible. These adverse outcomes are usually associated with use of these drugs in the second and third trimester of pregnancy. Most epidemiologic studies examining fetal abnormalities after exposure to antihypertensive use in the first trimester have not distinguished drugs affecting the renin-angiotensin system from other antihypertensive agents. Appropriate management of maternal hypertension during pregnancy is important to optimize outcomes for both mother and fetus.
In the unusual case that there is no appropriate alternative to therapy with drugs affecting the renin-angiotensin system for a particular patient, apprise the mother of the potential risk to the fetus. Perform serial ultrasound examinations to assess the intra-amniotic environment. If oligohydramnios is observed, discontinue Edarbyclor, unless it is considered lifesaving for the mother. Fetal testing may be appropriate, based on the week of pregnancy. Patients and physicians should be aware, however, that oligohydramnios may not appear until after the fetus has sustained irreversible injury. Closely observe infants with histories of *in utero* exposure to Edarbyclor for hypotension, oliguria, and hyperkalemia *[see Use in Specific Populations (8.4)]*.

8.3 Nursing Mothers

It is not known if azilsartan is excreted in human milk, but azilsartan is excreted at low concentrations in the milk of lactating rats and thiazide-like diuretics like chlorthalidone are excreted in human milk. Because of the potential for adverse effects on the nursing infant, a decision should be made whether to discontinue nursing or discontinue the drug, taking into account the importance of the drug to the mother.

8.4 Pediatric Use

Safety and effectiveness of Edarbyclor in pediatric patients under 18 years of age have not been established.
Neonates with a history of *in utero* exposure to Edarbyclor: If oliguria or hypotension occurs, support blood pressure and renal function. Exchange transfusions or dialysis may be required.

8.5 Geriatric Use

Edarbyclor
No dose adjustment with Edarbyclor is necessary in elderly patients. Of the total patients in clinical studies with Edarbyclor, 24% were elderly (65 years of age or older); 5.7% were 75 years and older. No overall differences in safety or effectiveness were observed between elderly patients and younger patients, but greater sensitivity of some older individuals cannot be ruled out *[see Clinical Pharmacology (12.3)]*.

8.6 Renal Impairment

Edarbyclor
Safety and effectiveness of Edarbyclor in patients with severe renal impairment (eGFR <30 mL/min/1.73 m^2) have not been established. No dose adjustment is required in patients with mild (eGFR 60-90 mL/min/1.73 m^2) or moderate (eGFR 30-60 mL/min/1.73 m^2) renal impairment.
Chlorthalidone
Chlorthalidone may precipitate azotemia.

8.7 Hepatic Impairment

Azilsartan medoxomil
No dose adjustment is necessary for subjects with mild or moderate hepatic impairment. Azilsartan medoxomil has not been studied in patients with severe hepatic impairment *[see Clinical Pharmacology (12.3)]*.
Chlorthalidone
Minor alterations of fluid and electrolyte balance may precipitate hepatic coma in patients with impaired hepatic function or progressive liver disease.

10 OVERDOSAGE

Limited data are available related to overdosage in humans.
Azilsartan medoxomil
Limited data are available related to overdosage in humans. During controlled clinical trials in healthy subjects, once daily doses up to 320 mg of azilsartan medoxomil were administered for 7 days and were well tolerated. In the event of an overdose, supportive therapy should be instituted as dictated by the patient's clinical status. Azilsartan is not dialyzable.
Chlorthalidone
Symptoms of acute overdosage include nausea, weakness, dizziness, and disturbances of electrolyte balance. The oral LD50 of the drug in the mouse and the rat is more than 25,000 mg/kg body weight. The minimum lethal dose (MLD) in humans has not been established. There is no specific antidote, but gastric lavage is recommended, followed by supportive treatment. Where necessary, this may include intravenous dextrose-saline with potassium, administered with caution.

11 DESCRIPTION

Edarbyclor is a combination of azilsartan medoxomil (ARB; as its potassium salt) and chlorthalidone (thiazide-like diuretic).
Azilsartan medoxomil, a prodrug, is hydrolyzed to azilsartan in the gastrointestinal tract during absorption. Azilsartan is a selective AT_1 subtype angiotensin II receptor antagonist. Chlorthalidone is a monosulfamyl thiazide-like diuretic that differs chemically from thiazide diuretics by the lack of a benzothiadiazine structure.
The potassium salt of azilsartan medoxomil, azilsartan kamedoxomil, is chemically described as (5-Methyl-2-oxo-1,3-dioxol-4-yl)methyl 2-ethoxy-1-{[2′-(5-oxo-4,5-dihydro-1,2,4-oxadiazol-3-yl)biphenyl-4-yl]methyl}-1*H*-benzimidazole-7-carboxylate monopotassium salt. Its empirical formula is $C_{30}H_{23}KN_4O_8$.
Chlorthalidone is chemically described as 2-chloro-5(1-hydroxy-3-oxo-1- isoindolinyl) benzenesulfonamide. Its empirical formula is $C_{14}H_{11}ClN_2O_4S$.
The structural formula for azilsartan medoxomil is

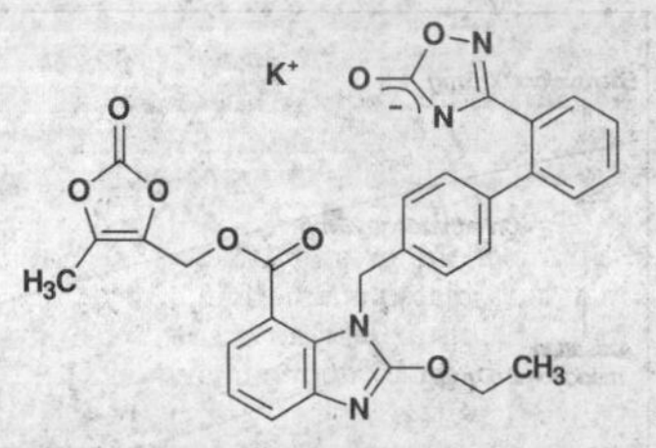

The structural formula for chlorthalidone is

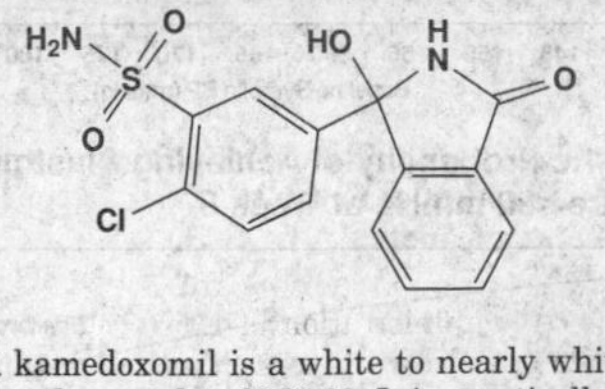

Azilsartan kamedoxomil is a white to nearly white powder with a molecular weight of 606.62. It is practically insoluble in water and freely soluble in methanol.
Chlorthalidone is a white to yellowish white powder with a molecular weight of 338.76. Chlorthalidone is practically insoluble in water, in ether, and in chloroform; soluble in methanol; slightly soluble in ethanol.
Edarbyclor is available for oral use as tablets. The tablets have a characteristic odor. Each Edarbyclor tablet contains 42.68 mg of azilsartan kamedoxomil, which is equivalent to containing azilsartan medoxomil 40 mg plus 12.5 or 25 mg of chlorthalidone. Each tablet of Edarbyclor also contains the following inactive ingredients: mannitol, microcrystalline cellulose, fumaric acid, sodium hydroxide, hydroxypropyl cellulose, crospovidone, magnesium stearate, hypromellose 2910, talc, titanium dioxide, ferric oxide red, polyethylene glycol 8000, and printing ink gray F1.

12 CLINICAL PHARMACOLOGY

12.1 Mechanism of Action

The active ingredients of Edarbyclor target two separate mechanisms involved in blood pressure regulation. Azilsartan blocks the vasoconstriction and sodium retaining effects of angiotensin II on cardiac, vascular smooth muscle, adrenal and renal cells. Chlorthalidone produces diuresis with increased excretion of sodium and chloride at the cortical diluting segment of the ascending limb of Henle's loop of the nephron.
Azilsartan medoxomil
Angiotensin II is formed from angiotensin I in a reaction catalyzed by angiotensin-converting enzymes (ACE, kinase II). Angiotensin II is the principle pressor agent of the renin-angiotensin system, with effects that include vasoconstriction, stimulation of synthesis and release of aldosterone, cardiac stimulation, and renal reabsorption of sodium. Azilsartan blocks the vasoconstrictor and aldosterone-secreting effects of angiotensin II by selectively blocking the binding of angiotensin II to the AT_1 receptor in many tis-

sues, such as vascular smooth muscle and the adrenal gland. Its action is, therefore, independent of the pathway for angiotensin II synthesis.

An AT_2 receptor is also found in many tissues, but this receptor is not known to be associated with cardiovascular homeostasis. Azilsartan has more than a 10,000-fold greater affinity for the AT_1 receptor than for the AT_2 receptor.

Blockade of the renin-angiotensin system with ACE inhibitors, which inhibit the biosynthesis of angiotensin II from angiotensin I, is widely used in the treatment of hypertension. ACE inhibitors also inhibit the degradation of bradykinin, a reaction catalyzed by ACE. Because azilsartan does not inhibit ACE (kinase II), it should not affect bradykinin levels. Whether this difference has clinical relevance is not yet known. Azilsartan does not bind to or block other receptors or ion channels known to be important in cardiovascular regulation.

Blockade of the angiotensin II receptor inhibits the negative regulatory feedback of angiotensin II on renin secretion, but the resulting increased plasma renin activity and angiotensin II circulating levels do not overcome the effect of azilsartan on blood pressure.

Chlorthalidone

Chlorthalidone produces diuresis with increased excretion of sodium and chloride. The site of action appears to be the cortical diluting segment of the ascending limb of Henle's loop of the nephron. The diuretic effects of chlorthalildone lead to decreased extracellular fluid volume, plasma volume, cardiac output, total exchangeable sodium, glomerular filtration rate, and renal plasma flow. Although the mechanism of action of chlorthalidone and related drugs is not wholly clear, sodium and water depletion appear to provide a basis for its antihypertensive effect.

12.2 Pharmacodynamics

Edarbyclor

Edarbyclor tablets have been shown to be effective in lowering blood pressure. Both azilsartan medoxomil and chlorthalidone lower blood pressure by reducing peripheral resistance but through complementary mechanisms.

Azilsartan medoxomil

Azilsartan inhibits the pressor effects of an angiotensin II infusion in a dose-related manner. An azilsartan single dose equivalent to 32 mg azilsartan medoxomil inhibited the maximal pressor effect by approximately 90% at peak, and approximately 60% at 24 hours. Plasma angiotensin I and II concentrations and plasma renin activity increased while plasma aldosterone concentrations decreased after single and repeated administration of azilsartan medoxomil to healthy subjects; no clinically significant effects on serum potassium or sodium were observed.

Chlorthalidone

The diuretic effect of chlorthalidone occurs in approximately 2.6 hours and continues for up to 72 hours.

12.3 Pharmacokinetics

Edarbyclor

Following oral administration of Edarbyclor, peak plasma concentrations of azilsartan and chlorthalidone are reached at 3 and 1 hours, respectively. The rate (C_{max} and T_{max}) and extent (AUC) of absorption of azilsartan are similar when it is administered alone or with chlorthalidone. The extent (AUC) of absorption of chlorthalidone is similar when it is administered alone or with azilsartan medoxomil; however, the C_{max} of chlorthalidone from Edarbyclor was 47% higher. The elimination half-lives of azilsartan and chlorthalidone are approximately 12 hours and 45 hours, respectively.

There is no clinically significant effect of food on the bioavailability of Edarbyclor.

Azilsartan medoxomil

Absorption: Azilsartan medoxomil is rapidly hydrolyzed to azilsartan, the active metabolite, in the gastrointestinal tract during absorption. Azilsartan medoxomil is not detected in plasma after oral administration. Dose proportionality in exposure was established for azilsartan in the azilsartan medoxomil dose range of 20 mg to 320 mg after single or multiple dosing.

The estimated absolute bioavailability of azilsartan following administration of azilsartan medoxomil is approximately 60%. After oral administration of azilsartan medoxomil, peak plasma concentrations (C_{max}) of azilsartan are reached within 1.5 to 3 hours. Food does not affect the bioavailability of azilsartan.

Distribution

Azilsartan medoxomil: The volume of distribution of azilsartan is approximately 16L. Azilsartan is highly bound to human plasma proteins (>99%), mainly serum albumin. Protein binding is constant at azilsartan plasma concentrations well above the range achieved with recommended doses.

In rats, minimal azilsartan-associated radioactivity crossed the blood-brain barrier. Azilsartan passed across the placental barrier in pregnant rats and was distributed to the fetus.

Chlorthalidone: In whole blood, chlorthalidone is predominantly bound to erythrocyte carbonic anhydrase. In the plasma, approximately 75% of chlorthalidone is bound to plasma proteins, 58% of the drug being bound to albumin.

Metabolism and Elimination

Azilsartan medoxomil: Azilsartan is metabolized to two primary metabolites. The major metabolite in plasma is formed by *O*-dealkylation, referred to as metabolite M-II, and the minor metabolite is formed by decarboxylation, referred to as metabolite M-I. Systemic exposures to the major and minor metabolites in humans were approximately 50% and less than 1% of azilsartan, respectively. M-I and M-II do not contribute to the pharmacologic activity of azilsartan medoxomil. The major enzyme responsible for azilsartan metabolism is CYP2C9.

Following an oral dose of ^{14}C-labeled azilsartan medoxomil, approximately 55% of radioactivity was recovered in feces and approximately 42% in urine, with 15% of the dose excreted in urine as azilsartan. The elimination half-life of azilsartan is approximately 11 hours and renal clearance is approximately 2.3 mL/min. Steady-state levels of azilsartan are achieved within 5 days and no accumulation in plasma occurs with repeated once-daily dosing.

Chlorthalidone: The major portion of the drug is excreted unchanged by the kidneys. Nonrenal routes of elimination have yet to be clarified. Data are not available regarding percentage of dose as unchanged drug and metabolites, concentration of the drug in body fluids, degree of uptake by a particular organ or in the fetus, or passage across the blood-brain barrier.

Special Populations

Azilsartan medoxomil: The effect of demographic and functional factors on the pharmacokinetics of azilsartan was studied in single and multiple dose studies. Pharmacokinetic measures indicating the magnitude of the effect on azilsartan are presented in Figure 2 as change relative to reference (test/reference).

Figure 2. Impact of intrinsic factors on the pharmacokinetics of azilsartan

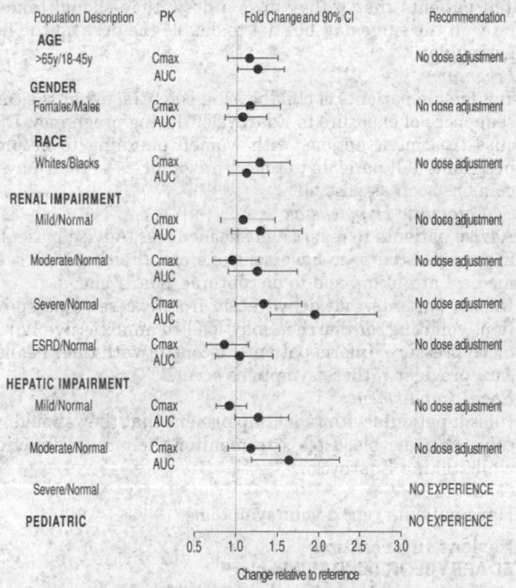

13 NONCLINICAL TOXICOLOGY

13.1 Carcinogenesis, Mutagenesis, Impairment of Fertility

No carcinogenicity, mutagenicity, or fertility studies have been conducted with the combination of azilsartan medoxomil and chlorthalidone. However, these studies have been conducted for azilsartan medoxomil alone.

Azilsartan medoxomil

Carcinogenesis: Azilsartan medoxomil was not carcinogenic when assessed in 26-week transgenic (Tg.rasH2) mouse and 2-year rat studies. The highest doses tested (450 mg azilsartan medoxomil/kg/day in the mouse and 600 mg azilsartan medoxomil/kg/day in the rat) produced exposures to azilsartan that are 12 (mice) and 27 (rats) times the average exposure to azilsartan in humans given the maximum recommended human dose (MRHD, 80 mg azilsartan medoxomil/day). M-II was not carcinogenic when assessed in 26-week Tg.rasH2 mouse and 2-year rat studies. The highest doses tested (approximately 8000 mg M-II/kg/day (males) and 11,000 mg M-II/kg/day (females) in the mouse and 1000 mg M-II/kg/day (males) and up to 3000 mg M-II/kg/day (females) in the rat) produced exposures that are, on average, about 30 (mice) and 7 (rats) times the average exposure to M-II in humans at the MRHD.

Mutagenesis: Azilsartan medoxomil, azilsartan, and M-II were positive for structural aberrations in the Chinese Hamster Lung Cytogenic Assay. In this assay, structural chromosomal aberrations were observed with the prodrug, azilsartan medoxomil, without metabolic activation. The active moiety, azilsartan, was also positive in this assay both with and without metabolic activation. The major human metabolite, M-II was also positive in this assay during a 24-hr assay without metabolic activation.

Azilsartan medoxomil, azilsartan, and M-II were devoid of genotoxic potential in the Ames reverse mutation assay with *Salmonella typhimurium* and *Escherichia coli*, the *in vitro* Chinese Hamster Ovary Cell forward mutation assay, the *in vitro* mouse lymphoma (tk) gene mutation test, the *ex vivo* unscheduled DNA synthesis test, and the *in vivo* mouse and/or rat bone marrow micronucleus assay.

Impairment of Fertility: There was no effect of azilsartan medoxomil on the fertility of male or female rats at oral doses of up to 1000 mg azilsartan medoxomil/kg/day [6000 mg/m^2 (approximately 122 times the MRHD of 80 mg azilsartan medoxomil/60 kg on a mg/m^2 basis)]. Fertility of rats also was unaffected at doses of up to 3000 mg M-II/kg/day.

13.2 Animal Toxicology and/or Pharmacology

Edarbyclor

The safety profiles of azilsartan medoxomil and chlorthalidone monotherapy have been individually established. To characterize the toxicological profile for Edarbyclor, a 13-week repeat-dose toxicity study was conducted in rats. The results of this study indicated that the combined administration of azilsartan medoxomil, M-II, and chlorthalidone resulted in increased exposures to chlorthalidone. Pharmacologically-mediated toxicity, including suppression of body weight gain and decreased food consumption in male rats, and increases in blood urea nitrogen in both sexes, was enhanced by coadministration of azilsartan medoxomil, M-II, and chlorthalidone. With the exception of these findings, there were no toxicologically synergistic effects in this study.

In an embryo-fetal developmental study in rats, there was no teratogenicity or increase in fetal mortality in the litters of dams receiving azilsartan medoxomil, M-II and chlorthalidone concomitantly at maternally toxic doses.

Azilsartan medoxomil

Reproductive Toxicology: In peri- and postnatal rat development studies, adverse effects on pup viability, delayed incisor eruption and dilatation of the renal pelvis along with hydronephrosis were seen when azilsartan medoxomil was administered to pregnant and nursing rats at 1.2 times the MRHD on a mg/m^2 basis. Reproductive toxicity studies indicated that azilsartan medoxomil was not teratogenic when administered at oral doses up to 1000 mg azilsartan medoxomil/kg/day to pregnant rats (122 times the MRHD on a mg/m^2 basis) or up to 50 mg azilsartan medoxomil/kg/day to pregnant rabbits (12 times the MRHD on a mg/m^2 basis). M-II also was not teratogenic in rats or rabbits at doses up to 3000 mg M-II/kg/day. Azilsartan crossed the placenta and was found in the fetuses of pregnant rats and was excreted into the milk of lactating rats.

Chlorthalidone

Reproductive toxicology: Reproduction studies have been performed in the rat and the rabbit at doses up to 420 times the human dose and have revealed no evidence of harm to the fetus. Thiazides cross the placental barrier and appear in cord blood.

Pharmacology: Biochemical studies in animals have suggested reasons for the prolonged effect of chlorthalidone. Absorption from the gastrointestinal tract is slow because of its low solubility. After passage to the liver, some of the drug enters the general circulation, while some is excreted in the bile, to be reabsorbed later. In the general circulation, it is distributed widely to the tissue, but is taken up in highest concentrations by the kidneys, where amounts have been found 72 hours after ingestion, long after it has disappeared from other tissues. The drug is excreted unchanged in the urine.

14 CLINICAL STUDIES

The antihypertensive effects of Edarbyclor have been demonstrated in a total of 5 randomized controlled studies, which included 4 double-blind, active-controlled studies and 1 open-label, long-term active-controlled study. The studies ranged from 8 weeks to 12 months in duration, at doses ranging from 20/12.5 mg to 80/25 mg once daily. A total of 5310 patients (3082 given Edarbyclor and 2228 given active comparator) with moderate or severe hypertension were studied. Overall, randomized patients had a mean age of 57 years, and included 52% males, 72% whites, 21% blacks, 15% with diabetes, 70% with mild or moderate renal impairment, and a mean BMI of 31.6 kg/m^2.

An 8-week, multicenter, randomized, double-blind, active-controlled, parallel group factorial trial in patients with moderate to severe hypertension compared the effect on blood pressure of Edarbyclor with the respective monotherapies. The trial randomized 1714 patients with baseline systolic blood pressure between 160 and 190 mm Hg (mean 165 mm Hg) and a baseline diastolic blood pressure <119 mm Hg (mean 95 mm Hg) to one of the 11 active treatment arms.

Strength	Color	Imprinting	NDC Number 64764-xxx-xx	
			Bottle of 30	Bottle of 90
40 / 12.5 mg	Pale red	A/C 40 / 12.5	944-30	944-90
40 / 25 mg	Light red	A/C 40 / 25	994-30	994-90

The 6 treatment combinations of azilsartan medoxomil 20, 40, or 80 mg and chlorthalidone 12.5 or 25 mg resulted in statistically significant reduction in systolic and diastolic blood pressure as determined by ambulatory blood pressure monitoring (ABPM) (Table 2) and clinic measurement (Table 3) at trough compared with the respective individual monotherapies. The clinic blood pressure reductions appear larger than those observed with ABPM, because the former include a placebo effect, which was not directly measured. Most of the antihypertensive effect of Edarbyclor occurs within 1-2 weeks of dosing. The blood pressure lowering effect was maintained throughout the 24-hour period (Figure 3).

Table 2. Mean Change from Baseline in Systolic/Diastolic Blood Pressure (mm Hg) as Measured by ABPM at Trough (22-24 Hours Post-Dose) at Week 8: Combination Therapy vs Monotherapy

Chlorthalidone, mg	Azilsartan Medoxomil, mg			
	0	20	40	80
0	N/A	-12 / -8	-13 / -7	-15 / -9
12.5	-13 / -7	-23 / -13	-24 / -14	-26 / -17
25	-16 / -8	-26 / -15	-30 / -17	-28 / -16

Table 3. Mean Change from Baseline in Clinic Systolic/ Diastolic Blood Pressure (mm Hg) at Week 8: Combination Therapy vs Monotherapy

Chlorthalidone, mg	Azilsartan Medoxomil, mg			
	0	20	40	80
0	N/A	-20 / -7	-23 / -9	-24 / -10
12.5	-21 / -7	-34 / -14	-37 / -16	-37 / -17
25	-27 / -9	-37 / -16	-40 / -17	-40 / -19

Figure 3. Mean Change from Baseline at Week 8 in Ambulatory Systolic Blood Pressure (mm Hg) by Treatment and Hour

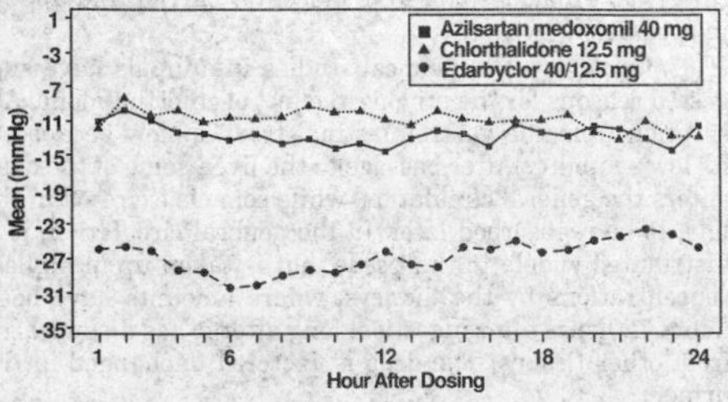

Edarbyclor was effective in reducing blood pressure regardless of age, gender, or race.

Edarbyclor was effective in treating black patients (usually a low-renin population).

In a 12-week, double-blind forced-titration trial, Edarbyclor 40/25 mg was statistically superior (P<0.001) to olmesartan medoxomil – hydrochlorothiazide (OLM/HCTZ) 40/25 mg in reducing systolic blood pressure in patients with moderate to severe hypertension (Table 4). Similar results were observed in all subgroups, including age, gender, or race of patients.

Table 4. Mean Change in Systolic/Diastolic Blood Pressure (mm Hg) at Week 12

	Edarbyclor 40/25 mg N=355	OLM/HCTZ 40/25 mg N=364
Clinic (Mean Baseline 165/96 mm Hg)	-43 / -19	-37 / -16
Trough by ABPM (22-24 hours) (Mean Baseline 153/92 mm Hg)	-33 / -20	-26 / -16

Edarbyclor lowered blood pressure more effectively than OLM/HCTZ at each hour of the 24-hour interdosing period as measured by ABPM.

Cardiovascular Outcomes

There are no trials of Edarbyclor demonstrating reductions in cardiovascular risk in patients with hypertension; however, trials with chlorthalidone and at least one drug pharmacologically similar to azilsartan medoxomil have demonstrated such benefits.

16 HOW SUPPLIED/STORAGE AND HANDLING

Edarbyclor is supplied as fixed dose combination tablets that are round, biconvex, film-coated, and 9.7 mm in diameter.

[See table above]

Store at 25°C (77°F), excursions permitted to 15°-30°C (59°-86°F) *[see USP Controlled Room Temperature]*. Keep container tightly closed. Protect from moisture and light. Do not repackage; dispense and store in original container.

17 PATIENT COUNSELING INFORMATION

See FDA-approved patient labeling (Patient Information).

Tell patients that if they miss a dose, they should take it later in the same day, but not to double the dose on the following day.

Pregnancy

Tell female patients of childbearing potential about the consequences of exposure to Edarbyclor during pregnancy. Discuss treatment options with women planning to become pregnant. Tell patients to report pregnancies to their physicians as soon as possible.

Symptomatic Hypotension

Advise patients to report light-headedness. Advise patients, if syncope occurs, to have someone call the doctor or seek medical attention, and to discontinue Edarbyclor.

Inform patients that dehydration from excessive perspiration, vomiting, or diarrhea may lead to an excessive fall in blood pressure. Inform patients to consult with their healthcare provider if these symptoms occur.

Renal Impairment

Inform patients with renal impairment that they should receive periodic blood tests to monitor their renal function while taking Edarbyclor.

Gout

Have patients report gout symptoms.

Patient Information
EDARBYCLOR (eh-DAR-bih-clor)
(Azilsartan medoxomil and chlorthalidone)
tablets

Read this Patient Information leaflet before you start taking Edarbyclor and each time you get a refill. There may be new information. This information does not take the place of talking to your doctor about your medical condition or your treatment.

What is the most important information I should know about Edarbyclor?

- Edarbyclor can cause harm or death to your unborn baby.
- Talk to your doctor about other ways to lower your blood pressure if you plan to become pregnant.
- If you become pregnant while taking Edarbyclor, tell your doctor right away. Your doctor may switch you to a different medicine to treat your high blood pressure.

What Is Edarbyclor?

Edarbyclor is a prescription medicine that contains azilsartan medoxomil, an angiotensin receptor blocker (ARB) and chlorthalidone, a water pill (diuretic).

Edarbyclor is used to treat high blood pressure (hypertension):

- when one medicine to lower your high blood pressure is not enough
- as the first medicine to lower your high blood pressure if your doctor decides you are likely to need more than one medicine.

It is not known if Edarbyclor is safe and effective in children under 18 years of age.

Who should not take Edarbyclor?

Do not take Edarbyclor if you:

- make less urine because of kidney problems

What should I tell my doctor before taking Edarbyclor?

Before you take Edarbyclor, tell your doctor if you:

- have been told that you have abnormal body salt (electrolytes) levels in your blood
- have liver or kidney problems
- have heart problems or stroke
- are vomiting or have diarrhea
- have gout
- are pregnant or plan to become pregnant. See **"What is the most important information I should know about Edarbyclor?"**
- are breastfeeding or plan to breastfeed. It is not known if Edarbyclor passes into your breast milk. You and your doctor should decide if you will take Edarbyclor or breastfeed. You should not do both. Talk with your doctor about the best way to feed your baby if you take Edarbyclor.

Tell your doctor about all the medicines you take, including prescription and nonprescription medicines, vitamins, and herbal supplements.

Especially tell your doctor if you take:

- other medicines used to treat your high blood pressure or heart problem
- water pills (diuretics)
- lithium carbonate (Lithobid), lithium citrate
- digoxin (Lanoxin)

Ask your doctor if you are not sure if you are taking a medicine listed above.

Know the medicines you take. Keep a list of them and show it to your doctor or pharmacist when you get a new medicine.

How should I take Edarbyclor?

- Take Edarbyclor exactly as your doctor tells you to.
- Your doctor will tell you how much Edarbyclor to take and when to take it.
- Your doctor may prescribe other medicines for you to take along with Edarbyclor to treat your high blood pressure.
- Edarbyclor can be taken with or without food.
- If you miss a dose, take it later in the same day. Do not take more than 1 dose of Edarbyclor in a day.
- If you take too much Edarbyclor and have symptoms of low blood pressure (hypotension) and dizziness, call your doctor for advice. See "What are the possible side effects of Edarbyclor?"

What are the possible side effects of Edarbyclor?

Edarbyclor may cause serious side effects, including:

- **See "What is the most important information I should know about Edarbyclor?"**
- **Low blood pressure (hypotension) and dizziness** is most likely to happen if you also:
    - take water pills (diuretics)
    - are on a low-salt diet
    - take other medicines that affect your blood pressure
    - sweat a lot
    - get sick with vomiting or diarrhea
    - do not drink enough fluids

If you feel faint or dizzy, lie down and call your doctor right away. If you pass out (faint) have someone call your doctor or get medical help. Stop taking Edarbyclor.

- **Kidney problems.** Kidney problems may become worse in people that already have kidney disease. Some people have changes in blood tests for kidney function and may need a lower dose of Edarbyclor or may need to stop treatment with Edarbyclor. During treatment with Edarbyclor, certain people who have severe heart failure, narrowing of the artery to the kidney, or who lose too much body fluid such as with nausea, vomiting, bleeding, or trauma, may develop sudden kidney failure and in rare instances, death.
- **Fluid and body salt (electrolyte) problems.** Tell your doctor if you get any of the following symptoms:

• dry mouth • thirst • lack of energy (lethargic) • weakness • drowsiness	• confusion • seizures • muscle pain or cramps • restlessness • muscle tiredness (fatigue)	• passing very little urine or passing large amounts of urine • fast or abnormal heartbeat • nausea and vomiting • constipation

- **Increased uric acid levels in the blood.** People who have increased levels of uric acid in the blood may develop gout. If you already have gout, tell your doctor about worsening of your gout symptoms.

The most common side effects of Edarbyclor are:

- dizziness, and
- tiredness

These are not all the possible side effects with Edarbyclor. Tell your doctor if you have any side effect that bothers you or that does not go away.

Call your doctor for medical advice about side effects. You may report side effects to FDA at 1-800-FDA-1088.

How should I store Edarbyclor?

- Store Edarbyclor at room temperature between 68°F to 77°F (20°C to 25°C).
- Store Edarbyclor in the original container that you received from your pharmacist or doctor. Do not put Edarbyclor into a different container.
- Keep the container closed tightly, and keep Edarbyclor out of the light.

Keep Edarbyclor and all medicines out of the reach of children.

General information about Edarbyclor

Medicines are sometimes prescribed for purposes other than those listed in the Patient Information leaflet. Do not use Edarbyclor for a condition for which it was not prescribed. Do not give Edarbyclor to other people, even if they have the same symptoms you have. It may harm them.

This Patient Information leaflet summarizes the most important information about Edarbyclor. If you would like more information, talk with your doctor. You can ask your pharmacist or doctor for information about Edarbyclor that is written for health professionals.

For more information, go to www.edarbyclor.com or call 1-877-825-3327.

What is high blood pressure (hypertension)?

Blood pressure is the force in your blood vessels when your heart beats and when your heart rests. You have high blood pressure when the force is too great.

High blood pressure makes the heart work harder to pump blood through the body and causes damage to the blood vessels. Edarbyclor tablets can help your blood vessels relax so your blood pressure is lower. Medicines that lower your blood pressure may lower your chance of having a stroke or heart attack.

What are the ingredients in Edarbyclor?

Active ingredients: azilsartan medoxomil and chlorthalidone

Inactive ingredients: mannitol, microcrystalline cellulose, fumaric acid, sodium hydroxide, hydroxypropyl cellulose, crospovidone, magnesium stearate, hypromellose 2910, talc, titanium dioxide, ferric oxide red, polyethylene glycol 8000, and printing ink gray F1.

This Patient Information has been approved by the U.S. Food and Drug Administration.

Distributed by
Takeda Pharmaceuticals America, Inc.
Deerfield, IL 60015
Revised: October 2012

Edarbyclor is a trademark of Takeda Pharmaceutical Company Limited registered with the U.S. Patent and Trademark Office and used under license by Takeda Pharmaceuticals America, Inc.

AZC066 R2

Shown in Product Identification Guide, page 313

KAZANO ℞

(alogliptin and metformin HCl)
tablets for oral administration

HIGHLIGHTS OF PRESCRIBING INFORMATION

These highlights do not include all the information needed to use KAZANO safely and effectively. See full prescribing information for KAZANO.

KAZANO (alogliptin and metformin HCl) tablets for oral administration

Initial U.S. Approval: 2013

> **WARNING: LACTIC ACIDOSIS**
> *See full prescribing information for complete boxed warning*
> - **Lactic acidosis can occur due to metformin accumulation. The risk increases with conditions such as sepsis, dehydration, excess alcohol intake, hepatic impairment, renal impairment and acute congestive heart failure. (5.1)**
> - **Symptoms include malaise, myalgias, respiratory distress, increasing somnolence and nonspecific abdominal distress. Laboratory abnormalities include low pH, increased anion gap and elevated blood lactate. (5.1)**
> - **If acidosis is suspected, discontinue KAZANO and hospitalize the patient immediately. (5.1)**

INDICATIONS AND USAGE

KAZANO is a dipeptidyl-peptidase-4 (DPP-4) inhibitor and a biguanide combination product indicated as an adjunct to diet and exercise to improve glycemic control in adults with type 2 diabetes mellitus. (1.1)

Important Limitation of Use: Not for treatment of type 1 diabetes or diabetic ketoacidosis. (1.2)

DOSAGE AND ADMINISTRATION

- Individualize the starting dose of KAZANO based on the patient's current regimen. (2.1)
- KAZANO should be taken twice daily with food. (2.1)
- May adjust the dosing based on effectiveness and tolerability while not exceeding the maximum recommended daily dose of 25 mg alogliptin and 2000 mg metformin HCl. (2.1)

DOSAGE FORMS AND STRENGTHS

Tablets: 12.5 mg alogliptin and 500 mg metformin HCl, 12.5 mg alogliptin and 1000 mg metformin HCl. (3)

CONTRAINDICATIONS

- Renal impairment. (4, 5.5)
- Metabolic acidosis, including diabetic ketoacidosis. (4, 5.1)
- History of a serious hypersensitivity reaction to alogliptin or metformin, components of KAZANO, such as anaphylaxis, angioedema or severe cutaneous adverse reactions. (4)

WARNINGS AND PRECAUTIONS

- Lactic acidosis: Warn against excessive alcohol intake. KAZANO is not recommended in hepatic impairment and is contraindicated in renal impairment. Ensure normal renal function before initiating and at least annually thereafter. (5.1)
- Acute pancreatitis: There have been postmarketing reports of acute pancreatitis. If pancreatitis is suspected, promptly discontinue KAZANO. (5.2)
- Hypersensitivity: There have been postmarketing reports of serious hypersensitivity reactions in patients treated with alogliptin such as anaphylaxis, angioedema and severe cutaneous adverse reactions. In such cases, promptly discontinue KAZANO, assess for other potential causes, institute appropriate monitoring and treatment and initiate alternative treatment for diabetes. (5.3)
- Hepatic effects: Postmarketing reports of hepatic failure, sometimes fatal. Causality cannot be excluded. If liver injury is detected, promptly interrupt KAZANO and assess patient for probable cause, then treat cause if possible, to resolution or stabilization. Do not restart KAZANO if liver injury is confirmed and no alternative etiology can be found. (5.4)
- Temporarily discontinue in patients undergoing radiologic studies with intravascular administration of iodinated contrast materials or any surgical procedures necessitating restricted intake of food and fluids. (5.5)
- Vitamin B_{12} deficiency: Metformin may lower vitamin B_{12} levels. Monitor hematologic parameters annually. (5.8)
- Hypoglycemia: When used with an insulin secretagogue (e.g., sulfonylurea) or with insulin, a lower dose of the insulin secretagogue or insulin may be required to reduce the risk of hypoglycemia. (5.9)
- Macrovascular outcomes: There have been no clinical studies establishing conclusive evidence of macrovascular risk reduction with KAZANO or any other antidiabetic drug. (5.10)

ADVERSE REACTIONS

Common adverse reactions reported in ≥4% of patients treated with coadministration of alogliptin with metformin were: upper respiratory tract infection, nasopharyngitis, diarrhea, hypertension, headache, back pain and urinary tract infection. (6.1)

To report SUSPECTED ADVERSE REACTIONS, contact Takeda Pharmaceuticals at 1-877-TAKEDA-7 or FDA at 1-800-FDA-1088 or www.fda.gov/medwatch.

DRUG INTERACTIONS

Cationic drugs eliminated by renal tubular secretion: Use with caution. (7.2)

USE IN SPECIFIC POPULATIONS

- Pregnancy Category B: There are no adequate and well-controlled studies in pregnant women. (8.1)
- Pediatrics: Safety and effectiveness of KAZANO in patients below the age of 18 have not been established. (8.4)
- Geriatric Use: Caution should be used when prescribing KAZANO to elderly patients because reduced renal functions are associated with increasing age. (8.5)

See 17 for PATIENT COUNSELING INFORMATION and FDA-approved patient labeling

Revised: 08/2013

FULL PRESCRIBING INFORMATION: CONTENTS*

*** Sections or subsections omitted from the full prescribing information are not listed**

FULL PRESCRIBING INFORMATION

> **WARNING: LACTIC ACIDOSIS**
> - **Lactic acidosis is a rare but serious complication that can occur due to metformin accumulation. The risk increases with conditions such as sepsis, dehydration, excess alcohol intake, hepatic impairment, renal impairment and acute congestive heart failure *[see Warnings and Precautions (5.1)]*.**
> - **The onset is often subtle, accompanied only by nonspecific symptoms such as malaise, myalgias, respiratory distress, increasing somnolence and nonspecific abdominal distress. Laboratory abnormalities include low pH, increased anion gap and elevated blood lactate *[see Warnings and Precautions (5.1)]*.**
> - **If acidosis is suspected, KAZANO (alogliptin and metformin HCl) should be discontinued and the patient hospitalized immediately *[see Warnings and Precautions (5.1)]*.**

1 INDICATIONS AND USAGE

1.1 Monotherapy and Combination Therapy

KAZANO is indicated as an adjunct to diet and exercise to improve glycemic control in adults with type 2 diabetes mellitus in multiple clinical settings when treatment with both alogliptin and metformin is appropriate *[see Clinical Studies (14)]*.

1.2 Limitation of Use

KAZANO should not be used in patients with type 1 diabetes mellitus or for the treatment of diabetic ketoacidosis, as it would not be effective in these settings.

2 DOSAGE AND ADMINISTRATION

2.1 Recommendations for All Patients

- Healthcare providers should individualize the starting dose of KAZANO based on the patient's current regimen.
- KAZANO should be taken twice daily with food with gradual dose escalation to reduce the gastrointestinal (GI) side effects due to metformin. KAZANO tablets must not be split before swallowing.
- Dosing may be adjusted based on effectiveness and tolerability while not exceeding the maximum recommended daily dose of 25 mg alogliptin and 2000 mg metformin HCl.
- The following doses are available:
  12.5 mg alogliptin and 500 mg metformin HCl
  12.5 mg alogliptin and 1000 mg metformin HCl

3 DOSAGE FORMS AND STRENGTHS

- 12.5 mg/500 mg tablets are pale yellow, oblong, film-coated tablets with "12.5/500" debossed on one side and "322M" debossed on the other side
- 12.5 mg/1000 mg tablets are pale yellow, oblong, film-coated tablets with "12.5/1000" debossed on one side and "322M" debossed on the other side

4 CONTRAINDICATIONS

KAZANO is contraindicated in patients with:

- Renal impairment (e.g., serum creatinine levels ≥1.5 mg/dL for men, ≥1.4 mg/dL for women or abnormal creatinine clearance), which may also result from conditions such as cardiovascular collapse (shock), acute myocardial infarction and septicemia *[see Warnings and Precautions (5.5)]*.
- Acute or chronic metabolic acidosis, including diabetic ketoacidosis. Diabetic ketoacidosis should be treated with insulin.
- History of a serious hypersensitivity reaction to alogliptin or metformin, components of KAZANO, such as anaphylaxis, angioedema or severe cutaneous adverse reactions.

5 WARNINGS AND PRECAUTIONS

5.1 Lactic Acidosis

Lactic acidosis is a rare but serious metabolic complication that can occur due to metformin accumulation during treatment with KAZANO and is fatal in approximately 50% of cases. Lactic acidosis may also occur in association with a number of pathophysiologic conditions, including diabetes mellitus, and whenever there is significant tissue hypoperfusion and hypoxemia. Lactic acidosis is characterized by elevated blood lactate levels (more than 5 mmol/L), decreased blood pH, electrolyte disturbances with an increased anion gap, and an increased lactate/pyruvate ratio. When metformin is implicated as the cause of lactic acidosis, metformin plasma levels of more than 5 mcg/mL are generally found.

The reported incidence of lactic acidosis in patients receiving metformin HCl is very low (approximately 0.03 cases per 1000 patient-years, with approximately 0.015 fatal cases per 1000 patient-years). In more than 20,000 patient-years' exposure to metformin in clinical trials, there were no reports of lactic acidosis. Reported cases have occurred primarily in diabetic patients with significant renal impairment, including both intrinsic renal disease and renal hypoperfusion, often in the setting of multiple concomitant medical/surgical problems and multiple concomitant medications. Patients with congestive heart failure requiring pharmacologic management, particularly when accompanied by hypoperfusion and hypoxemia due to unstable or acute failure, are at increased risk of lactic acidosis. The risk of lactic acidosis increases with the degree of renal dysfunction and the patient's age. The risk of lactic acidosis may, therefore, be significantly decreased by regular monitoring of renal function in patients taking metformin. In particular, treatment of the elderly should be accompanied by careful monitoring of renal function. Metformin treatment should not be initiated in any patients unless measurement of creatinine clearance demonstrates that renal function is not reduced, as these patients are more susceptible to developing lactic acidosis. In addition, metformin should be promptly withheld in the presence of any condition associated with hypoxemia, dehydration or sepsis. Because impaired hepatic function may significantly limit the ability to clear lactate, metformin should generally be avoided in patients with clinical or laboratory evidence of hepatic impairment. Patients should be cautioned against excessive alcohol intake when taking metformin, because alcohol potentiates the effects of metformin on lactate metabolism. In addition, metformin should be temporarily discontinued prior to any intravascular radiocontrast study and for any surgical procedure necessitating restricted intake of food or fluids. Use of topiramate, a carbonic anhydrase inhibitor, in epilepsy and migraine prophylaxis may frequently cause dose-dependent metabolic acidosis (in controlled trials, 32% and 67% for adjunctive treatment in adult and pediatric patients, respectively, and 15% to 25% for monotherapy of epilepsy, with decrease in serum bicarbonate to less than 20 mEq/L; 3% and 11% for adjunctive treatment in adult and pediatric patients, respectively, and 1% to 7% for monotherapy of epilepsy, with decrease in serum bicarbonate to less than 17 mEq/L) and may exacerbate the risk of metformin-induced lactic acidosis *[see Drug Interactions (7.1) and Clinical Pharmacology (12.3)]*.

The onset of lactic acidosis often is subtle and accompanied only by nonspecific symptoms such as malaise, myalgias, respiratory distress, increasing somnolence and nonspecific abdominal distress. There may be associated hypothermia, hypotension and resistant bradyarrhythmias with more marked acidosis.

Patients should be educated to promptly report these symptoms should they occur. If present, KAZANO should be withdrawn until lactic acidosis is ruled out. Serum electrolytes, ketones, blood glucose, blood pH, lactate levels and blood metformin levels may be useful. Once a patient is stabilized on any dose level of metformin, GI symptoms, which are common during initiation of therapy, are unlikely to recur. Later occurrence of GI symptoms could be due to lactic acidosis or other serious disease.

Levels of fasting venous plasma lactate above the upper limit of normal but less than 5 mmol/L in patients taking metformin do not necessarily indicate impending lactic acidosis and may be explainable by other mechanisms such as poorly controlled diabetes or obesity, vigorous physical activity or technical problems in sample handling.

Lactic acidosis should be suspected in any diabetic patient with metabolic acidosis lacking evidence of ketoacidosis (ketonuria and ketonemia).

Lactic acidosis is a medical emergency that must be treated in a hospital setting. In a patient with lactic acidosis who is taking metformin, the drug should be discontinued immediately and general supportive measures promptly instituted. Because metformin is dialyzable (with a clearance of up to 170 mL/min under good hemodynamic conditions), prompt hemodialysis is recommended to correct the acidosis and remove the accumulated metformin. Such management often results in prompt reversal of symptoms and recovery *[see Contraindications (4)]*.

5.2 Pancreatitis

There have been postmarketing reports of acute pancreatitis in patients taking alogliptin. After initiation of KAZANO, patients should be observed carefully for signs and symptoms of pancreatitis. If pancreatitis is suspected, alogliptin should promptly be discontinued and appropriate management should be initiated. It is unknown whether patients with a history of pancreatitis are at increased risk for the development of pancreatitis while using KAZANO.

5.3 Hypersensitivity Reactions

There have been postmarketing reports of serious hypersensitivity reactions in patients treated with alogliptin. These reactions include anaphylaxis, angioedema and severe cutaneous adverse reactions, including Stevens-Johnson syndrome. If a serious hypersensitivity reaction is suspected, discontinue KAZANO, assess for other potential causes for the event and institute alternative treatment for diabetes *[see Adverse Reactions (6.3)]*. Use caution in patients with a history of angioedema to another DPP-4 inhibitor because it is unknown whether such patients will be predisposed to angioedema with KAZANO.

5.4 Hepatic Effects

There have been postmarketing reports of fatal and nonfatal hepatic failure in patients taking alogliptin, although the reports contain insufficient information necessary to establish the probable cause *[see Adverse Reactions (6.3)]*. In randomized controlled studies, serum alanine aminotransferase (ALT) elevations greater than three times the upper limit of normal (ULN) were observed: 1.3% in alogliptin-treated patients and 1.5% in all comparator-treated patients.

Patients with type 2 diabetes may have fatty liver disease, which may cause liver test abnormalities, and they may also have other forms of liver disease, many of which can be treated or managed. Therefore, obtaining a liver test panel and assessing the patient before initiating KAZANO therapy is recommended. Because impaired hepatic function has been associated with some cases of lactic acidosis with use of metformin, KAZANO should generally be avoided in patients with clinical or laboratory evidence of hepatic disease.

Measure liver tests promptly in patients who report symptoms that may indicate liver injury, including fatigue, anorexia, right upper abdominal discomfort, dark urine or jaundice. In this clinical context, if the patient is found to have clinically significant liver enzyme elevations and if abnormal liver tests persist or worsen, KAZANO should be interrupted and investigation done to establish the probable cause. KAZANO should not be restarted in these patients without another explanation for the liver test abnormalities.

5.5 Monitoring of Renal Function

Metformin is substantially excreted by the kidney, and the risk of metformin accumulation and lactic acidosis increases with the degree of impairment. Therefore, KAZANO is contraindicated in patients with renal impairment.

Before initiation of KAZANO therapy and at least annually thereafter, renal function should be assessed and verified as normal. In patients in whom development of renal dysfunction is anticipated, renal function should be assessed more frequently and KAZANO discontinued if evidence of renal impairment is present. Metformin treatment should not be initiated in patients ≥80 years of age unless measurement of creatinine clearance demonstrates that renal function is not reduced, as these patients are more susceptible to developing lactic acidosis.

Use of Concomitant Medications that May Affect Renal Function or Metformin Disposition

Concomitant medication(s) that may affect renal function or result in significant hemodynamic change or may interfere with the disposition of metformin, such as cationic drugs that are eliminated by renal tubular secretion *[see Drug Interactions (7.2)]*, should be used with caution.

Radiological Studies and Surgical Procedures

Radiological studies involving the use of intravascular iodinated contrast materials (for example, intravenous urogram, intravenous cholangiography, angiography and computed tomography) can lead to acute alteration of renal function and have been associated with lactic acidosis in patients receiving metformin. Therefore, in patients in whom any such study is planned, KAZANO should be temporarily discontinued at the time of or prior to the procedure and withheld for 48 hours subsequent to the procedure and reinstituted only after renal function has been re-evaluated and found to be normal.

KAZANO therapy should be temporarily suspended for any surgical procedure (except minor procedures not associated with restricted intake of food and fluids) and should not be restarted until the patient's oral intake has resumed and renal function has been evaluated as normal.

5.6 Hypoxic States

Cardiovascular collapse (shock) from whatever cause, acute congestive heart failure, acute myocardial infarction and other conditions characterized by hypoxemia have been associated with lactic acidosis and may also cause prerenal azotemia. When such events occur in patients on KAZANO therapy, the drug should be promptly discontinued.

5.7 Alcohol Intake

Alcohol is known to potentiate the effect of metformin on lactate metabolism. Patients, therefore, should be warned against excessive alcohol intake while receiving KAZANO.

5.8 Vitamin B_{12} Levels

In controlled, 29-week clinical trials of immediate-release metformin, a decrease to subnormal levels of previously normal serum vitamin B_{12} levels, without clinical manifestations, was observed in approximately 7% of patients. Such decrease, possibly due to interference with B_{12} absorption from the B_{12}-intrinsic factor complex is, however, very rarely associated with anemia and appears to be rapidly reversible with discontinuation of metformin or vitamin B_{12} supplementation. Measurement of hematologic parameters on an annual basis is advised in patients on KAZANO, and any apparent abnormalities should be appropriately investigated and managed. Certain individuals (those with inadequate vitamin B_{12} or calcium intake or absorption) appear to be predisposed to developing subnormal vitamin B_{12} levels. In these patients, routine serum vitamin B_{12} measurements at two- to three-year intervals may be useful.

5.9 Use with Medications Known to Cause Hypoglycemia

Alogliptin

Insulin and insulin secretagogues, such as sulfonylureas, are known to cause hypoglycemia. Therefore, a lower dose of insulin or insulin secretagogue may be required to reduce the risk of hypoglycemia when used in combination with KAZANO.

Metformin Hydrochloride

Hypoglycemia does not occur in patients receiving metformin alone under usual circumstances of use but could occur when caloric intake is deficient, when strenuous exercise is not compensated by caloric supplementation or during concomitant use with other glucose-lowering agents (such as sulfonylureas and insulin) or ethanol. Elderly, debilitated or malnourished patients and those with adrenal or pituitary insufficiency or alcohol intoxication are particularly susceptible to hypoglycemic effects. Hypoglycemia may be difficult to recognize in the elderly and in people who are taking β-adrenergic blocking drugs.

5.10 Macrovascular Outcomes

There have been no clinical studies establishing conclusive evidence of macrovascular risk reduction with KAZANO or any other antidiabetic drug.

6 ADVERSE REACTIONS

6.1 Clinical Studies Experience

Because clinical trials are conducted under widely varying conditions, adverse reaction rates observed in the clinical trials of a drug cannot be directly compared to rates in the clinical trials of another drug and may not reflect the rates observed in practice.

Alogliptin and Metformin Hydrochloride

Over 2700 patients with type 2 diabetes have received alogliptin coadministered with metformin in four large, randomized, double-blind controlled clinical trials. The mean exposure to KAZANO was 58 weeks, with more than 1400 subjects treated for more than one year. These included two 26-week placebo-controlled studies, one 52-week active control study and an interim analysis of a 104-week active-controlled study. In the KAZANO arm, the mean duration of diabetes was approximately six years, the mean body mass index (BMI) was 31 kg/m^2 (56% of patients had a BMI ≥30 kg/m^2) and the mean age was 55 years (18% of patients ≥65 years of age).

In a pooled analysis of these four controlled clinical studies, the overall incidence of adverse reactions was 74% in patients treated with KAZANO compared to 75% treated with placebo. Overall discontinuation of therapy due to adverse events was 6.2% with KAZANO compared to 1.9% in placebo, 6.4% in metformin and 5.0% in alogliptin.

Adverse reactions reported in ≥4% of patients treated with KAZANO and more frequently than in patients who received alogliptin, metformin or placebo are summarized in *Table 1*.

[See table 1 above]

Hypoglycemia

In a 26-week, double-blind, placebo-controlled study of alogliptin in combination with metformin, the number of patients reporting hypoglycemia was 1.9% in the alogliptin 12.5 mg with metformin HCl 500 mg, 5.3% in the alogliptin 12.5 mg with metformin HCl 1000 mg, 1.8% in the metformin HCl 500 mg and 6.3% in the metformin HCl 1000 mg treatment groups.

In a 26-week placebo-controlled study of alogliptin 25 mg administered once daily as add-on to metformin regimen, the number of patients reporting hypoglycemic events was 0% in the alogliptin with metformin and 2.9% in the placebo treatment groups.

In a 52-week, active-controlled, double-blind study of alogliptin once daily as add-on therapy to the combination of pioglitazone 30 mg and metformin compared to the titration of pioglitazone 30 mg to 45 mg and metformin, the number of patients reporting hypoglycemia was 4.5% in the alogliptin 25 mg with pioglitazone 30 mg and metformin group versus 1.5% in the pioglitazone 45 mg with metformin group.

In an interim analysis conducted in a 104-week, double-blind, active-controlled study of alogliptin 25 mg in combination with metformin, the number of patients reporting hypoglycemia was 1.4% in the alogliptin 25 mg with metformin group versus 23.8% in the glipizide with metformin group.

Alogliptin

Approximately 8500 patients with type 2 diabetes have been treated with alogliptin in 14 randomized, double-blind, controlled clinical trials with approximately 2900 subjects randomized to placebo and approximately 2200 to an active comparator. The mean exposure to alogliptin was 40 weeks, with more than 2400 subjects treated for more than one year. Among these patients, 63% had a history of hypertension, 51% had a history of dyslipidemia, 25% had a history of myocardial infarction, 8% had a history of unstable angina and 7% had a history of congestive heart failure. The mean duration of diabetes was seven years, the mean BMI was 31 kg/m^2 (51% of patients had a BMI ≥30 kg/m^2) and the mean age was 57 years (24% of patients ≥65 years of age).

Two placebo-controlled monotherapy trials of 12 and 26 weeks of duration were conducted in patients treated with alogliptin 12.5 mg daily, alogliptin 25 mg daily and placebo. Four placebo-controlled add-on combination therapy trials of 26 weeks' duration were also conducted: with metformin, with a sulfonylurea, with a thiazolidinedione and with insulin.

Four placebo-controlled and one active-controlled trials of 16 weeks up through two years in duration were conducted in combination with metformin, in combination with pioglitazone and with pioglitazone added to a background of metformin therapy.

Three active-controlled trials of 52 weeks in duration were conducted in patients treated with pioglitazone and metformin, in combination with metformin and as monotherapy compared to glipizide.

In a pooled analysis of these 14 controlled clinical trials, the overall incidence of adverse events was 66% in patients treated with alogliptin 25 mg compared to 62% with placebo and 70% with active comparator. Overall discontinuation of therapy due to adverse events was 4.7% with alogliptin 25 mg compared to 4.5% with placebo or 6.2% with active comparator.

Adverse reactions reported in ≥4% of patients treated with alogliptin 25 mg and more frequently than in patients who received placebo are summarized in *Table 2*.

Table 2. Adverse Reactions Reported in ≥4% Patients Treated with Alogliptin 25 mg and More Frequently than in Patients Given Placebo in Pooled Studies

	Number of Patients (%)		
	Alogliptin 25 mg	Placebo	Active Comparator
	N=5902	N=2926	N=2257
Nasopharyngitis	257 (4.4)	89 (3.0)	113 (5.0)
Headache	247 (4.2)	72 (2.5)	121 (5.4)
Upper respiratory tract infection	247 (4.2)	61 (2.1)	113 (5.0)

Pancreatitis

In the clinical trial program, pancreatitis was reported in 11 of 5902 (0.2%) patients receiving alogliptin 25 mg daily compared to five of 5183 (<0.1%) patients receiving all comparators.

Table 1. Adverse Reactions Reported in ≥4% of Patients Treated with KAZANO and More Frequently than in Patients Receiving Either Alogliptin, Metformin or Placebo

	Number of Patients (%)			
	KAZANO*	Alogliptin†	Metformin‡	Placebo
	N=2794	N=222	N=1592	N=106
Upper respiratory tract infection	224 (8.0)	6 (2.7)	105 (6.6)	3 (2.8)
Nasopharyngitis	191 (6.8)	7 (3.2)	93 (5.8)	2 (1.9)
Diarrhea	155 (5.5)	4 (1.8)	105 (6.6)	3 (2.8)
Hypertension	154 (5.5)	5 (2.3)	96 (6.0)	6 (5.7)
Headache	149 (5.3)	11 (5.0)	74 (4.6)	3 (2.8)
Back pain	119 (4.3)	1 (0.5)	72 (4.5)	1 (0.9)
Urinary tract infection	116 (4.2)	4 (1.8)	59 (3.7)	2 (1.9)

* KAZANO – includes data pooled for patients receiving alogliptin 25 and 12.5 mg combined with various dose of metformin

† Alogliptin – includes data pooled for patients receiving alogliptin 25 and 12.5 mg

‡ Metformin – includes data pooled for patients receiving various doses of metformin

Hypersensitivity Reactions

In a pooled analysis, the overall incidence of hypersensitivity reactions was 0.6% with alogliptin 25 mg compared to 0.8% with all comparators. A single event of serum sickness was reported in a patient treated with alogliptin 25 mg.

Hypoglycemia

Hypoglycemic events were documented based upon a blood glucose value and/or clinical signs and symptoms of hypoglycemia.

In the monotherapy study, the incidence of hypoglycemia was 1.5% in patients treated with alogliptin compared to 1.6% with placebo. The use of alogliptin as add-on therapy to glyburide or insulin did not increase the incidence of hypoglycemia compared to placebo. In a monotherapy study comparing alogliptin to a sulfonylurea in elderly patients, the incidence of hypoglycemia was 5.4% with alogliptin compared to 26% with glipizide.

Metformin Hydrochloride

Table 3. Most Common Adverse Reactions (≥5%) in a Placebo-Controlled Clinical Study of Metformin Monotherapy*

	Metformin Monotherapy (n=141)	Placebo (n=145)
Adverse Reaction	% of Patients	
Diarrhea	53.2	11.7
Nausea/vomiting	25.5	8.3
Flatulence	12.1	5.5
Asthenia	9.2	5.5
Indigestion	7.1	4.1
Abdominal discomfort	6.4	4.8
Headache	5.7	4.8

* Reactions that were more common in metformin than placebo-treated patients

6.2 Laboratory Abnormalities

Alogliptin and Metformin Hydrochloride

No clinically meaningful differences were observed among treatment groups regarding hematology, serum chemistry or urinalysis results.

Alogliptin

No clinically meaningful changes in hematology, serum chemistry or urinalysis were observed in patients treated with alogliptin.

Metformin Hydrochloride

Metformin may lower serum vitamin B12 concentrations. Measurement of hematologic parameters on an annual basis is advised in patients on KAZANO, and any apparent abnormalities should be appropriately investigated and managed *[see Warnings and Precautions (5.8)]*.

6.3 Postmarketing Experience

Alogliptin

The following adverse reactions have been identified during the postmarketing use of alogliptin outside the United States. Because these reactions are reported voluntarily from a population of uncertain size, it is not always possible to reliably estimate their frequency or establish a causal relationship to drug exposure.

Hypersensitivity reactions include anaphylaxis, angioedema, rash, urticaria, and severe cutaneous adverse reactions, including Stevens-Johnson syndrome, hepatic enzyme elevations, fulminant hepatic failure and acute pancreatitis.

7 DRUG INTERACTIONS

Alogliptin

Alogliptin is primarily renally excreted and CYP-related metabolism is negligible. No drug-drug interactions were observed with the CYP-substrates or inhibitors tested or with renally excreted drugs *[see Clinical Pharmacology (12.3)]*.

Metformin Hydrochloride

7.1 Carbonic Anhydrase Inhibitors

Topiramate or other carbonic anhydrase inhibitors (e.g., zonisamide, acetazolamide or dichlorphenamide) frequently decrease serum bicarbonate and induce nonanion gap, hyperchloremic metabolic acidosis. Concomitant use of these drugs may induce metabolic acidosis. Use these drugs with caution in patients treated with metformin, as the risk of lactic acidosis may increase.

7.2 Cationic Drugs

Cationic drugs (e.g., amiloride, digoxin, morphine, procainamide, quinidine, quinine, ranitidine, triamterene, trimethoprim or vancomycin) that are eliminated by renal tubular secretion theoretically have the potential for interaction with metformin by competing for common renal tubular transport systems. Although such interactions remain theoretical (except for cimetidine), careful patient monitoring and dose adjustment of KAZANO and/or the interfering drug is recommended in patients who are taking cationic medications that are excreted via the proximal renal tubular secretory system.

7.3 The Use of Metformin with Other Drugs

Certain drugs tend to produce hyperglycemia and may lead to loss of glycemic control. These drugs include the thiazides and other diuretics, corticosteroids, phenothiazines, thyroid products, estrogens, oral contraceptives, phenytoin, nicotinic acid, sympathomimetics, calcium channel blocking drugs and isoniazid. When such drugs are administered to a patient receiving KAZANO, the patient should be closely observed for loss of blood glucose control. When such drugs are withdrawn from a patient receiving KAZANO, the patient should be observed closely for hypoglycemia.

8 USE IN SPECIFIC POPULATIONS

8.1 Pregnancy

Pregnancy Category B

Alogliptin and Metformin Hydrochloride

There are no adequate and well-controlled studies in pregnant women with KAZANO or its individual components. Based on animal data, KAZANO is not predicted to increase the risk of developmental abnormalities. Because animal reproduction studies are not always predictive of human risk and exposure, KAZANO, like other antidiabetic medications, should be used during pregnancy only if clearly needed.

No treatment-related fetal abnormalities occurred following concomitant administration of 100 mg/kg alogliptin with 150 mg/kg metformin to pregnant rats, or approximately 28 and two times the clinical dose of alogliptin (25 mg) and metformin (2000 mg), respectively (based on AUC).

Alogliptin

Alogliptin administered to pregnant rabbits and rats during the period of organogenesis was not teratogenic at doses of up to 200 and 500 mg/kg, or 149 times and 180 times, respectively, the clinical dose based on plasma drug exposure (AUC).

Doses of alogliptin up to 250 mg/kg (approximately 95 times clinical exposure based on AUC) given to pregnant rats from gestation Day 6 to lactation Day 20 did not harm the developing embryo or adversely affect growth and development of offspring.

Placental transfer of alogliptin into the fetus was observed following oral dosing to pregnant rats.

Metformin Hydrochloride

Metformin was not teratogenic in rats and rabbits at doses up to 600 mg/kg, which represents an exposure of about two and six times the MRHD dose of 2000 mg based on body surface area comparisons for rats and rabbits, respectively. Metformin HCl should not be used during pregnancy unless clearly needed.

8.3 Nursing Mothers

No studies have been conducted with the combined components of KAZANO. In studies performed with the individual components, both alogliptin and metformin are secreted in the milk of lactating rats. It is not known whether alogliptin and/or metformin are secreted in human milk. Because many drugs are excreted in human milk, caution should be exercised when KAZANO is administered to a nursing woman.

8.4 Pediatric Use

Safety and effectiveness of KAZANO in pediatric patients have not been established.

8.5 Geriatric Use

Alogliptin and Metformin Hydrochloride

Elderly patients are more likely to have decreased renal function. Because metformin is contraindicated in patients with renal impairment, carefully monitor renal function in the elderly and use KAZANO with caution as age increases *[see Warnings and Precautions (5.5) and Clinical Pharmacology (12.3)]*.

Of the total number of patients (N = 2095) in clinical safety and efficacy studies, 343 (16.4%) patients were 65 years and older and 37 (1.8%) patients were 75 years and older. No overall differences in safety or effectiveness were observed between these patients and younger patients. While this and other reported clinical experiences have not identified differences in responses between the elderly and younger patients, greater sensitivity of some older individuals cannot be excluded.

Alogliptin

Of the total number of patients (N=8507) in clinical safety and efficacy studies treated with alogliptin, 2064 (24.3%) patients were 65 years and older and 341 (4%) patients were 75 years and older. No overall differences in safety or effectiveness were observed between patients 65 years and over and younger patients.

Metformin Hydrochloride

Controlled studies of metformin did not include sufficient numbers of subjects age 65 and over to determine whether they respond differently from younger patients. Other reported clinical experience has not identified differences in responses between the elderly and younger patients.

Metformin should only be used in patients with normal renal function. The initial and maintenance dosing of metformin should be conservative in patients with advanced age due to the potential for decreased renal function in this population *[see Contraindications (4), Warnings and Precautions (5.5) and Clinical Pharmacology (12.3)]*.

10 OVERDOSAGE

Alogliptin

The highest doses of alogliptin administered in clinical trials were single doses of 800 mg to healthy subjects and doses of 400 mg once daily for 14 days to patients with type 2 diabetes (equivalent to 32 times and 16 times the recommended clinical dose, respectively). No dose-limiting adverse events were observed at these doses.

In the event of an overdose, it is reasonable to institute the necessary clinical monitoring and supportive therapy as dictated by the patient's clinical status. Per clinical judgment, it may be reasonable to initiate removal of unabsorbed material from the gastrointestinal tract.

Alogliptin is minimally dialyzable; over a three-hour hemodialysis session, approximately 7% of the drug was removed. Therefore, hemodialysis is unlikely to be beneficial in an overdose situation. It is not known if alogliptin is dialyzable by peritoneal dialysis.

Metformin Hydrochloride

Overdose of metformin has occurred, including ingestion of amounts greater than 50 grams. Hypoglycemia was reported in approximately 10% of cases, but no causal association with metformin has been established. Lactic acidosis has been reported in approximately 32% of metformin overdose cases *[see Warnings and Precautions (5.1)]*. Metformin is dialyzable with a clearance of up to 170 mL/min under good hemodynamic conditions. Therefore, hemodialysis may be useful for removal of accumulated drug from patients in whom metformin overdosage is suspected.

11 DESCRIPTION

KAZANO tablets contain two oral antihyperglycemic drugs used in the management of type 2 diabetes: alogliptin and metformin hydrochloride.

Alogliptin

Alogliptin is a selective, orally bioavailable inhibitor of the enzymatic activity of dipeptidyl peptidase-4 (DPP-4). Chemically, alogliptin is prepared as a benzoate salt, which is identified as 2-({6-[(3*R*)-3-aminopiperidin-1-yl]-3-methyl-2,4-dioxo-3,4-dihydropyrimidin-1(2*H*)-yl}methyl) benzonitrile monobenzoate. It has a molecular formula of $C_{18}H_{21}N_5O_2 \bullet C_7H_6O_2$ and a molecular weight of 461.51 daltons; the structural formula is:

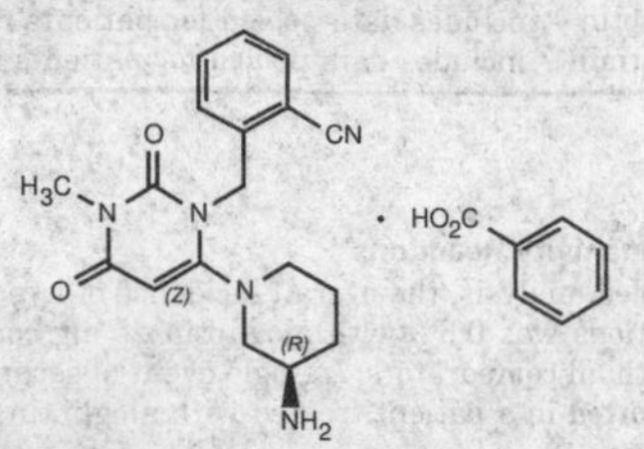

Alogliptin benzoate is a white to off-white crystalline powder, containing one asymmetric carbon in the aminopiperidine moiety. It is soluble in dimethylsulfoxide, sparingly soluble in water and methanol, slightly soluble in ethanol and very slightly soluble in octanol and isopropyl acetate.

Metformin Hydrochloride

Metformin hydrochloride (*N,N*-dimethylimidodicarbonimidic diamide hydrochloride) is not chemically or pharmacologically related to any other classes of oral antihyperglycemic agents. Metformin hydrochloride is a white to off-white crystalline compound with a molecular formula of $C_4H_{11}N_5 \bullet HCl$ and a molecular weight of 165.63. Metformin hydrochloride is freely soluble in water and is practically insoluble in acetone, ether and chloroform. The pKa of metformin is 12.4. The pH of a 1% aqueous solution of metformin hydrochloride is 6.68. The structural formula is as shown:

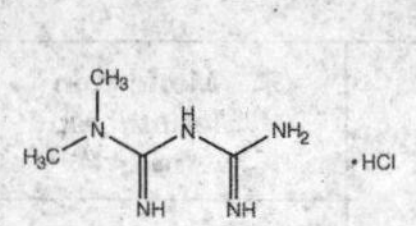

KAZANO is available as a tablet for oral administration containing 17 mg alogliptin benzoate equivalent to 12.5 mg alogliptin and:

- 500 mg metformin hydrochloride (12.5 mg/500 mg) or
- 1000 mg metformin hydrochloride (12.5 mg/1000 mg).

KAZANO tablets contain the following inactive ingredients: mannitol, microcrystalline cellulose, povidone, crospovidone, and magnesium stearate; the tablets are film-coated with hypromellose 2910, talc, titanium dioxide and ferric oxide yellow.

12 CLINICAL PHARMACOLOGY

12.1 Mechanism of Action

Alogliptin and Metformin Hydrochloride

KAZANO combines two antihyperglycemic agents with complementary and distinct mechanisms of action to improve glycemic control in patients with type 2 diabetes: alogliptin, a selective inhibitor of DPP-4, and metformin HCl, a member of the biguanide class.

Alogliptin

Increased concentrations of the incretin hormones such as glucagon-like peptide-1 (GLP-1) and glucose-dependent insulinotropic polypeptide (GIP) are released into the bloodstream from the small intestine in response to meals. These hormones cause insulin release from the pancreatic beta cells in a glucose-dependent manner but are inactivated by the DPP-4 enzyme within minutes. GLP-1 also lowers glucagon secretion from pancreatic alpha cells, reducing hepatic glucose production. In patients with type 2 diabetes, concentrations of GLP-1 are reduced but the insulin response to GLP-1 is preserved. Alogliptin is a DPP-4 inhibitor that slows the inactivation of the incretin hormones, thereby increasing their bloodstream concentrations and reducing fasting and postprandial glucose concentrations in a glucose-dependent manner in patients with type 2 diabetes mellitus. Alogliptin selectively binds to and inhibits DPP-4 but not DPP-8 or DPP-9 activity *in vitro* at concentrations approximating therapeutic exposures.

Metformin Hydrochloride

Metformin is a biguanide that improves glucose tolerance in patients with type 2 diabetes, lowering both basal and postprandial plasma glucose. Metformin decreases hepatic glucose production, decreases intestinal absorption of glucose and improves insulin sensitivity by increasing peripheral glucose uptake and utilization. Metformin does not produce hypoglycemia in patients with type 2 diabetes or in healthy subjects except in special circumstances *[see Warnings and Precautions (5.9)]* and does not cause hyperinsulinemia. With metformin therapy, insulin secretion remains unchanged while fasting insulin levels and daylong plasma insulin response may actually decrease.

12.2 Pharmacodynamics

Alogliptin

Single-dose administration of alogliptin to healthy subjects resulted in a peak inhibition of DPP-4 within two to three hours after dosing. The peak inhibition of DPP-4 exceeded 93% across doses of 12.5 mg to 800 mg. Inhibition of DPP-4 remained above 80% at 24 hours for doses greater than or equal to 25 mg. Peak and total exposure over 24 hours to active GLP-1 were three- to four-fold greater with alogliptin (at doses of 25 to 200 mg) than placebo. In a 16-week, double-blind, placebo-controlled study, alogliptin 25 mg demonstrated decreases in postprandial glucagon while increasing postprandial active GLP-1 levels compared to placebo over an eight-hour period following a standardized meal. It is unclear how these findings relate to changes in overall glycemic control in patients with type 2 diabetes mellitus. In this study, alogliptin 25 mg demonstrated decreases in two-hour postprandial glucose compared to placebo (-30 mg/dL versus 17 mg/dL, respectively).

Multiple-dose administration of alogliptin to patients with type 2 diabetes also resulted in a peak inhibition of DPP-4 within one to two hours and exceeded 93% across all doses (25 mg, 100 mg and 400 mg) after a single dose and after 14 days of once-daily dosing. At these doses of alogliptin, inhibition of DPP-4 remained above 81% at 24 hours after 14 days of dosing.

12.3 Pharmacokinetics

Absorption and Bioavailability

Alogliptin and Metformin Hydrochloride

In bioequivalence studies of KAZANO, the area under the curve (AUC) and maximum concentration (C_{max}) of both the alogliptin and the metformin component following a single dose of the combination tablet were bioequivalent to the alogliptin 12.5 mg concomitantly administered with metformin HCl 500 or 1000 mg tablets under fasted conditions in healthy subjects. Administration of KAZANO with food resulted in no change in total exposure (AUC) of alogliptin and metformin. Mean peak plasma concentrations of alogliptin and metformin were decreased by 13% and 28%, respectively, when administered with food. There was no change in time to peak plasma concentrations (T_{max}) for alogliptin under fed conditions, however, there was a delayed T_{max} for metformin of 1.5 hours. These changes are not likely to be clinically significant.

Alogliptin

The absolute bioavailability of alogliptin is approximately 100%. Administration of alogliptin with a high-fat meal resulted in no change in total and peak exposure to alogliptin. Alogliptin may therefore be administered with or without food.

Metformin Hydrochloride

The absolute bioavailability of metformin following administration of a 500 mg metformin HCl tablet given under fasting conditions is approximately 50% to 60%. Studies using single oral doses of metformin HCl tablets 500 mg to 1500 mg and 850 mg to 2550 mg indicate that there is a lack of dose proportionality with increasing doses, which is due to decreased absorption rather than an alteration in elimination. Food decreases the extent of and slightly delays the absorption of metformin, as shown by approximately a 40% lower mean peak plasma concentration (C_{max}), a 25% lower area under the plasma concentration versus time curve (AUC), and a 35-minute prolongation of time to peak plasma concentration (T_{max}) following administration of a single 850 mg tablet of metformin HCl with food compared to the same tablet strength administered fasting. The clinical relevance of these decreases is unknown.

Distribution

Alogliptin

Following a single, 12.5 mg intravenous dose of alogliptin to healthy subjects, the volume of distribution during the terminal phase was 417 L, indicating that the drug is well distributed into tissues.

Alogliptin is 20% bound to plasma proteins.

Metformin Hydrochloride

The apparent volume of distribution (V/F) of metformin following single oral doses of immediate release metformin HCl tablets 850 mg averaged 654 ± 358 L. Metformin is negligibly bound to plasma proteins. Metformin partitions into erythrocytes, most likely as a function of time. At usual clinical doses and dosing schedules of metformin, steady-state plasma concentrations of metformin are reached within 24 to 48 hours and are generally less than 1 mcg/mL. During controlled clinical trials, which served as the basis for approval for metformin, maximum metformin plasma levels did not exceed 5 mcg/mL, even at maximum doses.

Metabolism

Alogliptin

Alogliptin does not undergo extensive metabolism and 60% to 71% of the dose is excreted as unchanged drug in the urine.

Two minor metabolites were detected following administration of an oral dose of [^{14}C] alogliptin, *N*-demethylated, M-I (less than 1% of the parent compound), and *N*-acetylated alogliptin, M-II (less than 6% of the parent compound). M-I is an active metabolite and is an inhibitor of DPP-4 similar to the parent molecule; M-II does not display any inhibitory activity toward DPP-4 or other DPP-related enzymes. *In vitro* data indicate that CYP2D6 and CYP3A4 contribute to the limited metabolism of alogliptin.

Alogliptin exists predominantly as the (*R*)-enantiomer (more than 99%) and undergoes little or no chiral conversion *in vivo* to the (*S*)-enantiomer. The (*S*)-enantiomer is not detectable at the 25 mg dose.

Metformin Hydrochloride

Intravenous single-dose studies in healthy subjects demonstrate that metformin is excreted unchanged in the urine and does not undergo hepatic metabolism (no metabolites have been identified in humans) or biliary excretion.

Excretion and Elimination

Alogliptin

The primary route of elimination of [^{14}C] alogliptin-derived radioactivity occurred via renal excretion (76%) with 13% recovered in the feces, achieving a total recovery of 89% of the administered radioactive dose. The renal clearance of alogliptin (9.6 L/hr) indicates some active renal tubular secretion and systemic clearance was 14.0 L/hr.

Metformin Hydrochloride

Renal clearance is approximately 3.5 times greater than creatinine clearance, which indicates that tubular secretion is the major route of metformin elimination. Following oral administration, approximately 90% of the absorbed drug is eliminated via the renal route within the first 24 hours, with a plasma elimination half-life of approximately 6.2 hours. In blood, the elimination half-life is approximately 17.6 hours, suggesting that the erythrocyte mass may be a compartment of distribution.

Special Populations

Renal Impairment

Alogliptin and Metformin Hydrochloride

Use of KAZANO in patients with renal impairment increases the risk for lactic acidosis. Because KAZANO contains metformin, KAZANO is contraindicated in patients with renal impairment *[see Contraindications (4) and Warnings and Precautions (5.5)]*.

Hepatic Impairment

KAZANO is not recommended in patients with hepatic impairment. KAZANO contains metformin and use of metformin in patients with hepatic impairment has been associated with some cases of lactic acidosis *[see Warnings and Precautions (5.4)]*.

Alogliptin

Total exposure to alogliptin was approximately 10% lower and peak exposure was approximately 8% lower in patients with moderate hepatic impairment (Child-Pugh Grade B) compared to healthy subjects. The magnitude of these reductions is not considered to be clinically meaningful. Patients with severe hepatic impairment (Child-Pugh Grade C) have not been studied.

Metformin Hydrochloride

No pharmacokinetic studies of metformin have been conducted in subjects with hepatic impairment.

Gender

Alogliptin

No dose adjustment is necessary based on gender. Gender did not have any clinically meaningful effect on the pharmacokinetics of alogliptin.

Metformin Hydrochloride

Metformin pharmacokinetic parameters did not differ significantly between normal subjects and patients with type 2 diabetes when analyzed according to gender. Similarly, in controlled clinical studies in patients with type 2 diabetes, the antihyperglycemic effect of metformin hydrochloride tablets was comparable in males and females.

Geriatric

KAZANO contains metformin, which is contraindicated in patients with renal impairment *[see Warnings and Precautions (5.5)]*. Due to declining renal function in the elderly, measurement of creatinine clearance should be obtained prior to initiation of therapy. Do not use KAZANO if renal function is not within normal range.

Alogliptin

No dose adjustment is necessary based on age. Age did not have any clinically meaningful effect on the pharmacokinetics of alogliptin.

Figure 1. Effect of Alogliptin on the Pharmacokinetic Exposure to Other Drugs

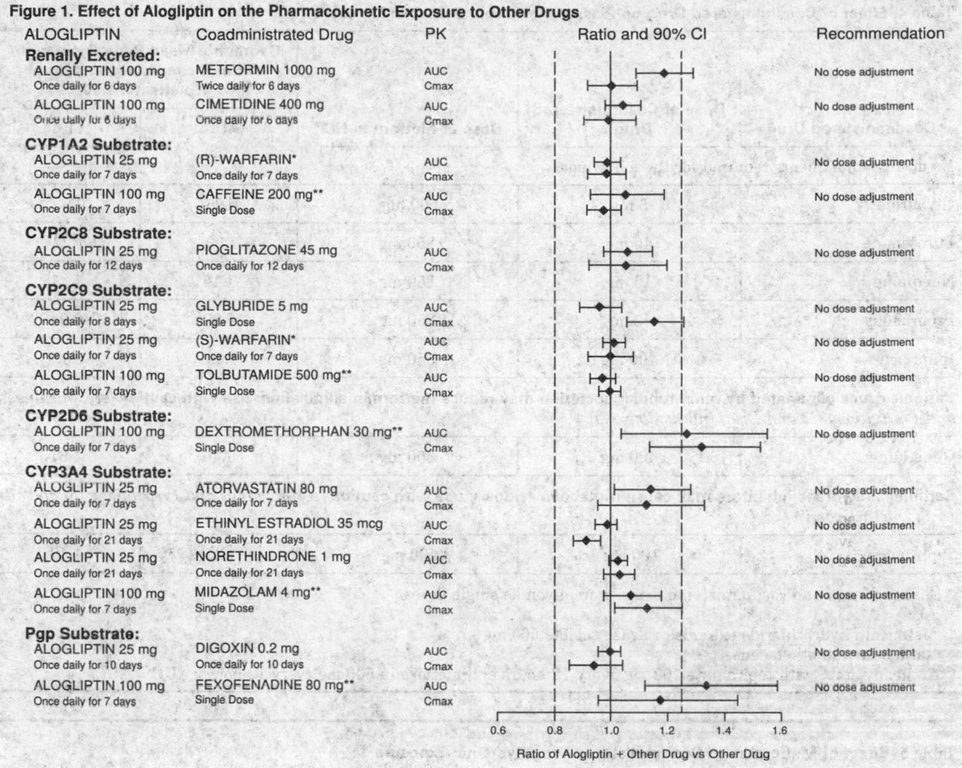

*Warfarin was given once daily at a stable dose in the range of 1 mg to 10 mg. Alogliptin had no significant effect on the prothrombin time (PT) or International Normalized Ratio (INR).

**Caffeine (1A2 substrate), tolbutamide (2C9 substrate), dextromethorphan (2D6 substrate), midazolam (3A4 substrate) and fexofenadine (P-gp substrate) were administered as a cocktail.

Figure 2. Effect of Other Drugs on the Pharmacokinetic Exposure of Alogliptin

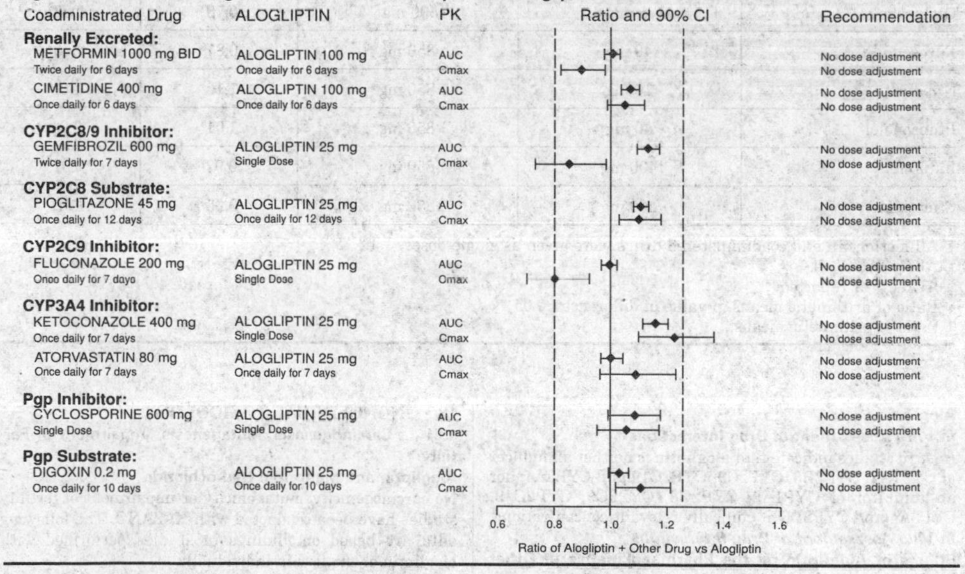

Metformin Hydrochloride

Limited data from controlled pharmacokinetic studies of metformin in healthy elderly subjects suggest that total plasma clearance of metformin is decreased, the half-life is prolonged, and C_{max} is increased, compared to healthy young subjects. From these data it appears that the change in metformin pharmacokinetics with aging is primarily accounted for by a change in renal function.

Pediatrics

Studies characterizing the pharmacokinetics of alogliptin in pediatric patients have not been performed.

Race

Alogliptin

No dose adjustment of alogliptin is necessary based on race. Race (white, black and Asian) did not have any clinically meaningful effect on the pharmacokinetics of alogliptin.

Metformin Hydrochloride

No studies of metformin pharmacokinetic parameters according to race have been performed. In controlled clinical studies of metformin in patients with type 2 diabetes, the antihyperglycemic effect was comparable in whites (n=249), blacks (n=51) and Hispanics (n=24).

Drug Interactions

Alogliptin and Metformin Hydrochloride

Administration of alogliptin 100 mg once daily with metformin HCl 1000 mg twice daily for six days had no meaningful effect on the pharmacokinetics of alogliptin or metformin.

Specific pharmacokinetic drug interaction studies with KAZANO have not been performed, although such studies have been conducted with the individual components of KAZANO (alogliptin and metformin).

Table 4. Effect of Coadministered Drug on Plasma Metformin Systemic Exposure

Coadministered Drug	Dose of Coadministered Drug*	Dose of Metformin HCl*	Geometric Mean Ratio (ratio with/without coadministered drug) No effect = 1.00	
			AUC†	C_{max}
No dosing adjustments required for the following:				
Glyburide	5 mg	500 mg‡	0.98§	0.99§
Furosemide	40 mg	850 mg	1.09§	1.22§
Nifedipine	10 mg	850 mg	1.16	1.21
Propranolol	40 mg	850 mg	0.90	0.94
Ibuprofen	400 mg	850 mg	1.05§	1.07§
Cationic drugs eliminated by renal tubular secretion may reduce metformin elimination: use with caution *[see Warnings and Precautions (5) and Drug Interactions (7)]*				
Cimetidine	400 mg	850 mg	1.40	1.61
Carbonic anhydrase inhibitors may cause metabolic acidosis: use with caution *[see Warnings and Precautions (5) and Drug Interactions (7)]*				
Topiramate	100 mg¶	500 mg¶	1.25¶	1.17

* All metformin and coadministered drugs were given as single doses
† AUC = $AUC_{(0-\infty)}$
‡ Metformin hydrochloride extended-release tablets 500 mg
§ Ratio of arithmetic means
¶ At steady-state with topiramate 100 mg every 12 hours and metformin 500 mg every 12 hours; AUC = AUC_{0-12h}

Table 5. Effect of Metformin on Coadministered Drug Systemic Exposure

Coadministered Drug	Dose of Coadministered Drug*	Dose of Metformin HCl*	Geometric Mean Ratio (ratio with/without coadministered drug) No effect = 1.00	
			AUC†	C_{max}
No dosing adjustments required for the following:				
Glyburide	5 mg	500 mg‡	0.78§	0.63§
Furosemide	40 mg	850 mg	0.87§	0.69§
Nifedipine	10 mg	850 mg	1.10‡	1.08
Propranolol	40 mg	850 mg	1.01‡	0.94
Ibuprofen	400 mg	850 mg	0.97¶	1.01¶
Cimetidine	400 mg	850 mg	0.95‡	1.01

* All metformin and coadministered drugs were given as single doses
† AUC = $AUC_{(0-\infty)}$
‡ AUC_{0-24} hr reported
§ Ratio of arithmetic means, p-value of difference <0.05
¶ Ratio of arithmetic means

Alogliptin

***In Vitro* Assessment of Drug Interactions**

In vitro studies indicate that alogliptin is neither an inducer of CYP1A2, CYP2B6, CYP2C9, CYP2C19 and CYP3A4, nor an inhibitor of CYP1A2, CYP2C8, CYP2C9, CYP2C19, CYP3A4 and CYP2D6 at clinically relevant concentrations.

***In Vivo* Assessment of Drug Interactions**

Effects of Alogliptin on the Pharmacokinetics of Other Drugs

In clinical studies, alogliptin did not meaningfully increase the systemic exposure to the following drugs that are metabolized by CYP isozymes or excreted unchanged in urine *(Figure 1)*. No dose adjustment of alogliptin is recommended based on results of the described pharmacokinetic studies.

[See figure 1 at top of previous page]

Effects of Other Drugs on the Pharmacokinetics of Alogliptin

There are no clinically meaningful changes in the pharmacokinetics of alogliptin when alogliptin is administered concomitantly with the drugs described below *(Figure 2)*.

[See figure 2 at top of previous page]

Metformin Hydrochloride

Pharmacokinetic drug interaction studies have been performed on metformin *(Tables 4 and 5)*.

[See table 4 above]
[See table 5 above]

13 NONCLINICAL TOXICOLOGY

13.1 Carcinogenesis, Mutagenesis, Impairment of Fertility

Alogliptin and Metformin Hydrochloride

No carcinogenicity, mutagenicity or impairment of fertility studies have been conducted with KAZANO. The following data are based on findings in studies performed with alogliptin or metformin individually.

Alogliptin

Rats were administered oral doses of 75, 400 and 800 mg/kg alogliptin for two years. No drug-related tumors were observed up to 75 mg/kg or approximately 32 times the maximum recommended clinical dose of 25 mg, based on AUC exposure. At higher doses (approximately 308 times the maximum recommended clinical dose of 25 mg), a combination of thyroid C-cell adenomas and carcinomas increased in male but not female rats. No drug-related tumors were observed in mice after administration of 50, 150 or 300 mg/kg alogliptin for two years, or up to approximately 51 times the maximum recommended clinical dose of 25 mg, based on AUC exposure.

Alogliptin was not mutagenic or clastogenic, with and without metabolic activation, in the Ames test with *S. typhimurium* and *E. coli* or the cytogenetic assay in mouse lymphoma cells. Alogliptin was negative in the *in vivo* mouse micronucleus study.

In a fertility study in rats, alogliptin had no adverse effects on early embryonic development, mating or fertility, at doses up to 500 mg/kg, or approximately 172 times the clinical dose based on plasma drug exposure (AUC).

Metformin Hydrochloride

Long-term carcinogenicity studies have been performed in rats (dosing duration of 104 weeks) and mice (dosing duration of 91 weeks) at doses up to and including 900 mg/kg and 1500 mg/kg, respectively. These doses are both approximately four times the maximum recommended human daily dose of 2000 mg based on body surface area comparisons. No evidence of carcinogenicity with metformin was found in either male or female mice. Similarly, there was no tumorigenic potential observed with metformin in male rats. There was an increased incidence of benign stromal uterine polyps in female rats treated with 900 mg/kg.

There was no evidence of a mutagenic potential of metformin in the following *in vitro* tests: Ames test (*S. typhimurium*), gene mutation test (mouse lymphoma cells) or chromosomal aberrations test (human lymphocytes). Results in the *in vivo* mouse micronucleus test were also negative.

Fertility of male or female rats was unaffected by metformin when administered at doses as high as 600 mg/kg, which is approximately three times the maximum recommended human daily dose based on body surface area comparisons.

14 CLINICAL STUDIES

The coadministration of alogliptin and metformin has been studied in patients with type 2 diabetes inadequately controlled on either diet and exercise alone, on metformin alone or metformin in combination with a thiazolidinedione.

There have been no clinical efficacy studies conducted with KAZANO; however, bioequivalence of KAZANO with coadministered alogliptin and metformin tablets was demonstrated, and efficacy of the combination of alogliptin and metformin has been demonstrated in three Phase 3 efficacy studies.

A total of 2095 patients with type 2 diabetes were randomized in three double-blind, placebo- or active-controlled clinical safety and efficacy studies conducted to evaluate the effects of KAZANO on glycemic control. The racial distribution of patients exposed to study medication was 69.2% white, 16.3% Asian, 6.5% black and 8.0% other racial groups. The ethnic distribution was 24.3% Hispanic. Patients had an overall mean age of approximately 54.4 years (range 22 to 80 years). In patients with type 2 diabetes, treatment with KAZANO produced clinically meaningful and statistically significant improvements in A1C versus comparator. As is typical for trials of agents to treat type 2 diabetes, the mean reduction in A1C with KAZANO appears to be related to the degree of A1C elevation at baseline.

Alogliptin and Metformin Coadministration in Patients with Type 2 Diabetes Inadequately Controlled on Diet and Exercise

In a 26-week, double-blind, placebo-controlled study, a total of 784 patients inadequately controlled on diet and exercise alone (mean baseline A1C = 8.4%) were randomized to one of seven treatment groups: placebo; metformin HCl 500 mg or metformin HCl 1000 mg twice daily, alogliptin 12.5 mg twice daily, or alogliptin 25 mg daily; alogliptin 12.5 mg in combination with metformin HCl 500 mg or metformin HCl 1000 mg twice daily. Both coadministration treatment arms (alogliptin 12.5 mg + metformin HCl 500 mg and alogliptin 12.5 mg + metformin HCl 1000 mg) resulted in significant improvements in A1C *(Figure 3)* and FPG when compared with their respective individual alogliptin and metformin component regimens *(Table 6)*. Coadministration treatment arms demonstrated improvements in two-hour postprandial glucose (PPG) compared to alogliptin alone or metformin alone *(Table 6)*. A total of 12% of patients receiving alogliptin 12.5 mg + metformin HCl 500 mg, 3% of patients receiving alogliptin 12.5 mg + metformin HCl 1000 mg, 17% of patients receiving alogliptin 12.5 mg, 23% of patients receiving metformin HCl 500 mg, 11% of patients receiving metformin HCl 1000 mg and 39% of patients receiving placebo required glycemic rescue.

Improvements in A1C were not affected by gender, age, race or baseline BMI. The mean decrease in body weight was similar between metformin alone and alogliptin when coadministered with metformin. Lipid effects were neutral.

[See table 6 at top of next page]
[See figure 3 at top of next column]

Alogliptin and Metformin Coadministration in Patients with Type 2 Diabetes Inadequately Controlled on Metformin Alone

In a 26-week, double-blind, placebo-controlled study, a total of 527 patients already on metformin (mean baseline A1C = 8%) were randomized to receive alogliptin 12.5 mg, alogliptin 25 mg, or placebo once daily. Patients were maintained on a stable dose of metformin HCl (median daily dose = 1700 mg) during the treatment period. Alogliptin 25 mg in combination with metformin resulted in statistically significant improvements from baseline in A1C and FPG at Week 26, when compared to placebo *(Table 7)*. A to-

Figure 3. Change from Baseline A1C at Week 26 with Alogliptin and Metformin Alone and Alogliptin in Combination with Metformin

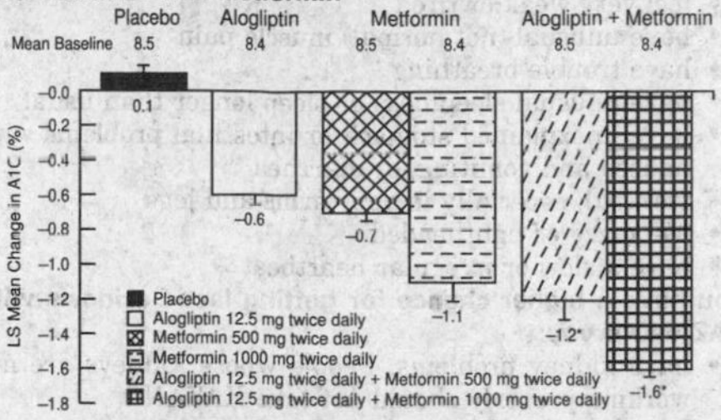

Intent-to-treat population using last observation on study prior to discontinuation of double-blind study medication or sulfonylurea rescue therapy for patients needing rescue.
*P<0.001 when compared to metformin and alogliptin alone.

tal of 8% of patients receiving alogliptin 25 mg and 24% of patients receiving placebo required glycemic rescue. Improvements in A1C were not affected by gender, age, race, baseline BMI or baseline metformin dose.

The mean decrease in body weight was similar between alogliptin 25 mg and placebo when given in combination with metformin. Lipid effects were also neutral.

[See table 7 at top of next page]

Alogliptin Add-On Therapy in Patients with Type 2 Diabetes Inadequately Controlled on the Combination of Metformin and Pioglitazone

In a 52-week, active-comparator study, a total of 803 patients inadequately controlled (mean baseline A1C = 8.2%) on a current regimen of pioglitazone 30 mg and metformin were randomized to either receive the addition of once-daily alogliptin 25 mg or the titration of pioglitazone 30 mg to 45 mg following a four-week single-blind, placebo run-in period. Patients were maintained on a stable dose of metformin HCl (median daily dose = 1700 mg). Patients who failed to meet prespecified hyperglycemic goals during the 52-week treatment period received glycemic rescue therapy.

In combination with pioglitazone and metformin, alogliptin 25 mg was shown to be statistically superior in lowering A1C and FPG compared with the titration of pioglitazone from 30 to 45 mg at Week 26 and at Week 52 *(Table 8)*. A total of 11% of patients in the alogliptin 25 mg in combination with pioglitazone 30 mg and metformin treatment group and 22% of patients in the up titration of pioglitazone in combination with metformin treatment group required glycemic rescue. Improvements in A1C were not affected by gender, age, race or baseline BMI.

The mean increase in body weight was similar in both treatment arms. Lipid effects were neutral.

[See table 8 at top of next page]

16 HOW SUPPLIED/STORAGE AND HANDLING

KAZANO tablets are available in the following strengths and packages:

12.5 mg/500 mg tablet: pale yellow, oblong, film-coated tablets with "12.5/500" debossed on one side and "322M" debossed on the other side, available in:

NDC 64764-335-60	Bottles of 60 tablets
NDC 64764-335-80	Bottles of 180 tablets
NDC 64764-335-77	Bottles of 500 tablets

12.5 mg/1000 mg tablet: pale yellow, oblong, film-coated tablets with "12.5/1000" debossed on one side and "322M" debossed on the other side, available in:

NDC 64764-337-60	Bottles of 60 tablets
NDC 64764-337-80	Bottles of 180 tablets
NDC 64764-337-77	Bottles of 500 tablets

Storage

Store at 25°C (77°F); excursions permitted to 15° to 30°C (59° to 86°F) [see USP Controlled Room Temperature]. Keep container tightly closed.

17 PATIENT COUNSELING INFORMATION

See FDA-Approved Patient Labeling (Medication Guide).

17.1 Instructions

- Inform patients of the potential risks and benefits of KAZANO.
- The risks of lactic acidosis, its symptoms, and conditions that predispose to its development, as noted in *Warnings and Precautions (5.1)*, should be explained to patients. Patients should be advised to discontinue KAZANO immediately and to promptly notify their health practitioner if unexplained hyperventilation, myalgias, malaise, unusual somnolence or other nonspecific symptoms occur. Once a patient is stabilized on

Table 6. Glycemic Parameters at Week 26 for Alogliptin and Metformin Alone and in Combination in Patients with Type 2 Diabetes

	Placebo	Alogliptin 12.5 mg twice daily	Metformin HCl 500 mg twice daily	Metformin HCl 1000 mg twice daily	Alogliptin 12.5 mg + Metformin HCl 500 mg twice daily	Alogliptin 12.5 mg + Metformin HCl 1000 mg twice daily
A1C (%)*	**N=102**	**N=104**	**N=103**	**N=108**	**N=102**	**N=111**
Baseline (mean)	8.5	8.4	8.5	8.4	8.5	8.4
Change from baseline (adjusted mean†)	0.1	-0.6	-0.7	-1.1	-1.2	-1.6
Difference from metformin (adjusted mean† with 95% confidence interval)	-	-	-	-	-0.6‡ (-0.9, -0.3)	-0.4‡ (-0.7, -0.2)
Difference from alogliptin (adjusted mean† with 95% confidence interval)	-	-	-	-	-0.7‡ (-1.0, -0.4)	-1.0‡ (-1.3, -0.7)
% of Patients (n/N) achieving A1C <7%§	4% (4/102)	20% (21/104)	27% (28/103)	34% (37/108)	47%‡ (48/102)	59%‡ (66/111)
FPG (mg/dL)*	**N=105**	**N=106**	**N=106**	**N=110**	**N=106**	**N=112**
Baseline (mean)	187	177	180	181	176	185
Change from baseline (adjusted mean†)	12	-10	-12	-32	-32	-46
Difference from metformin (adjusted mean† with 95% confidence interval)	-	-	-	-	-20‡ (-33, -8)	-14‡ (-26, -2)
Difference from alogliptin (adjusted mean† with 95% confidence interval)	-	-	-	-	-22‡ (-35, -10)	-36‡ (-49, -24)
2-Hour PPG (mg/dL)¶	**N=26**	**N=34**	**N=28**	**N=37**	**N=31**	**N=37**
Baseline (mean)	263	272	247	266	261	268
Change from baseline (adjusted mean†)	-21	-43	-49	-54	-68	-86‡
Difference from metformin (adjusted mean† with 95% confidence interval)	-	-	-	-	-19 (-49, 11)	-32‡ (-58, -5)
Difference from alogliptin (adjusted mean† with 95% confidence interval)	-	-	-	-	-25 (-53, 3)	-43‡ (-70, -16)

* Intent-to-treat population using last observation on study prior to discontinuation of double-blind study medication or sulfonylurea rescue therapy for patients needing rescue
† Least squares means adjusted for treatment, geographic region and baseline value
‡ p<0.05 when compared to metformin and alogliptin alone
§ Compared using logistic regression
¶ Intent-to-treat population using data available at Week 26

Table 7. Glycemic Parameters at Week 26 in a Placebo-Controlled Study of Alogliptin as Add-on Therapy to Metformin*

	Alogliptin 25 mg + Metformin	Placebo + Metformin
A1C (%)	**N=203**	**N=103**
Baseline (mean)	7.9	8.0
Change from baseline (adjusted mean†)	-0.6	-0.1
Difference from placebo (adjusted mean† with 95% confidence interval)	-0.5‡ (-0.7, -0.3)	-
% of patients (n/N) achieving A1C ≤7%†	44% (92/207)‡	18% (19/104)
FPG (mg/dL)	**N=204**	**N=104**
Baseline (mean)	172	180
Change from baseline (adjusted mean†)	-17	0
Difference from placebo (adjusted mean† with 95% confidence interval)	-17‡ (-26, -9)	-

* Intent-to-treat population using last observation on study.
† Least squares means adjusted for treatment, baseline value, geographic region and baseline metformin dose.
‡ p<0.001 compared to placebo.

Table 8. Glycemic Parameters at Week 52 in an Active-Controlled Study of Alogliptin as Add-On Combination Therapy to Metformin and Pioglitazone*

	Alogliptin 25 mg + Pioglitazone 30 mg + Metformin	Pioglitazone 45 mg + Metformin
A1C (%)	**N=397**	**N=394**
Baseline (mean)	8.2	8.1
Change from baseline (adjusted mean†)	-0.7	-0.3
Difference from pioglitazone 45 mg + metformin* (adjusted mean† with 95% confidence interval)	-0.4‡ (-0.5, -0.3)	-
% of Patients (n/N) achieving A1C ≤7%	33% (134/404)§	21% (85/399)
FPG (mg/dL)‡	**N=399**	**N=396**
Baseline (mean)	162	162
Change from baseline (adjusted mean†)	-15	-4
Difference from pioglitazone 45 mg + metformin (adjusted mean† with 95% confidence interval)	-11§ (-16, -6)	-

* Intent-to-treat population using last observation on study
† Least squares means adjusted for treatment, baseline value, geographic region, and baseline metformin dose
‡ Non-inferior and statistically superior to metformin plus pioglitazone at the 0.025 one-sided significance level
§ p<0.001 compared to pioglitazone 45 mg + metformin

any dose level of KAZANO, gastrointestinal symptoms, which are common during initiation of metformin therapy, are unlikely to recur. Later occurrence of gastrointestinal symptoms could be due to lactic acidosis or other serious disease.

- Patients should be informed that acute pancreatitis has been reported during use of alogliptin. Patients should be informed that persistent, severe abdominal pain, sometimes radiating to the back, which may or may not be accompanied by vomiting, is the hallmark symptom of acute pancreatitis. Patients should be instructed to promptly discontinue KAZANO and contact their physician if persistent severe abdominal pain occurs.
- Patients should be informed that allergic reactions have been reported during use of alogliptin and metformin. If symptoms of allergic reactions (including skin rash, hives and swelling of the face, lips, tongue and throat that may cause difficulty in breathing or swallowing) occur, patients should be instructed to discontinue KAZANO and seek medical advice promptly.
- Patients should be informed that postmarketing reports of liver injury, sometimes fatal, have been reported during use of alogliptin. If signs or symptoms of liver injury occur, patients should be instructed to discontinue KAZANO and seek medical advice promptly.
- Patients should be informed about the importance of regular testing of renal function and hematological parameters when receiving treatment with KAZANO.
- Patients should be counseled against excessive alcohol intake, either acute or chronic, while receiving KAZANO.
- Inform patients that hypoglycemia can occur, particularly when an insulin secretagogue or insulin is used in combination with KAZANO. Explain the risks, symptoms and appropriate management of hypoglycemia.
- Instruct patients to take KAZANO only as prescribed twice daily. KAZANO should be taken with food. If a dose is missed, advise patients not to double their next dose.
- Patients should be informed that the tablets must never be split.

Instruct patients to read the Medication Guide before starting KAZANO therapy and to reread each time the prescription is refilled. Instruct patients to inform their healthcare provider if an unusual symptom develops or if a symptom persists or worsens.

Revised: June 2013
ALM143P R3

MEDICATION GUIDE
KAZANO (Kah-ZAHN-oh)
(alogliptin and metformin HCl)
tablets

Read this Medication Guide carefully before you start taking KAZANO and each time you get a refill. There may be new information. This information does not take the place of talking with your doctor about your medical condition or treatment. If you have any questions about KAZANO, ask your doctor or pharmacist.

What is the most important information I should know about KAZANO?

KAZANO can cause serious side effects, including:

1. Lactic Acidosis. Metformin, one of the medicines in KAZANO, can cause a rare but serious condition called lactic acidosis (a buildup of an acid in the blood) that can cause death. Lactic acidosis is a medical emergency and must be treated in the hospital.

Stop taking KAZANO and call your doctor right away if you get any of the following symptoms of lactic acidosis:

- feel very weak or tired
- have unusual (not normal) muscle pain
- have trouble breathing
- have unusual sleepiness or sleep longer than usual
- have unexplained stomach or intestinal problems with nausea and vomiting, or diarrhea
- feel cold, especially in your arms and legs
- feel dizzy or lightheaded
- have a slow or irregular heartbeat

You have a higher chance for getting lactic acidosis with KAZANO if you:

- have kidney problems. People whose kidneys are not working properly should not take KAZANO
- have liver problems
- have congestive heart failure that requires treatment with medicines
- drink a lot of alcohol (very often or short-term "binge" drinking)
- get dehydrated (lose a large amount of body fluids). This can happen if you are sick with a fever, vomiting or diarrhea. Dehydration can also happen when you sweat a lot with activity or exercise and do not drink enough fluids
- have certain x-ray tests with injectable dyes or contrast agents
- have surgery
- have a heart attack, severe infection or stroke

2. Inflammation of the pancreas (pancreatitis). Alogliptin, one of the medicines in KAZANO, may cause pancreatitis, which may be severe.

Certain medical conditions make you more likely to get pancreatitis.

Before you start taking KAZANO:

Tell your doctor if you have ever had:

- pancreatitis
- stones in your gallbladder (gallstones)
- a history of alcoholism
- kidney problems
- liver problems

Stop taking KAZANO and call your doctor right away if you have pain in your stomach area (abdomen) that is severe and will not go away. The pain may be felt going from your abdomen through to your back. The pain may happen with or without vomiting. These may be symptoms of pancreatitis.

What is KAZANO?

- KAZANO contains 2 prescription diabetes medicines, alogliptin (NESINA) and metformin hydrochloride.
- KAZANO is a prescription medicine used with diet and exercise to improve blood sugar (glucose) control in adults with type 2 diabetes.
- KAZANO is not for people with type 1 diabetes.
- KAZANO is not for people with diabetic ketoacidosis (increased ketones in blood or urine).

It is not known if KAZANO is safe and effective in children under the age of 18.

Who should not take KAZANO?

Do not take KAZANO if you:

- have kidney problems
- have a condition called metabolic acidosis or have had diabetic ketoacidosis (increased ketones in your blood or urine)
- are going to get an injection of dye or contrast agents for an x-ray procedure, KAZANO will need to be stopped for a short time. Talk to your doctor about when you should stop KAZANO and when you should start KAZANO again
- are allergic to alogliptin (NESINA) or metformin or any of the ingredients in KAZANO or have had a serious allergic (hypersensitivity) reaction to alogliptin or metformin. See the end of this Medication Guide for a complete list of the ingredients in KAZANO

  Symptoms of a serious allergic reaction to KAZANO may include:
  - swelling of your face, lips, throat and other areas on your skin
  - difficulty with swallowing or breathing
  - raised, red areas on your skin (hives)
  - skin rash, itching, flaking or peeling

  If you have any of these symptoms, stop taking KAZANO and contact your doctor right away or go to the nearest hospital emergency room.

What should I tell my doctor before and during treatment with KAZANO?

Before you take KAZANO, tell your doctor if you:

- have or have had inflammation of your pancreas (pancreatitis)
- have kidney or liver problems
- have heart problems, including congestive heart failure
- are older than 80 years, you should not take KAZANO unless your kidneys have been checked and they are normal

- drink alcohol very often or drink a lot of alcohol in short-term "binge" drinking
- have other medical conditions
- are pregnant or plan to become pregnant. It is not known if KAZANO will harm your unborn baby. Talk with your doctor about the best way to control your blood sugar while you are pregnant or if you plan to become pregnant
- are breastfeeding or plan to breastfeed. It is not known whether KAZANO passes into your breast milk. Talk with your doctor about the best way to feed your baby if you are taking KAZANO

Tell your doctor about all the medicines you take, including prescription and nonprescription medicines, vitamins and herbal supplements. Know the medicines you take. Keep a list of them and show it to your doctor and pharmacist before you start any new medicine.

KAZANO may affect the way other medicines work, and other medicines may affect how KAZANO works. Contact your doctor before you start or stop other types of medicines.

How should I take KAZANO?

- Take KAZANO exactly as your doctor tells you to take it.
- Take KAZANO 2 times each day.
- Take KAZANO with food to lower your chances of having an upset stomach.
- Do not break or cut KAZANO tablets before swallowing.
- Your doctor may need to change your dose of KAZANO to control your blood glucose. Do not change your dose unless told to do so by your doctor.
- If you miss a dose, take it as soon as you remember. If you do not remember until it is time for your next dose, skip the missed dose, and take the next dose at your regular schedule. Do not take 2 doses of KAZANO at the same time.
- If you take too much KAZANO, call your doctor or go to the nearest hospital emergency room right away.
- If your body is under stress, such as from fever, infection, accident or surgery, the dose of your diabetes medicines may need to be changed. Call your doctor right away.
- Stay on your diet and exercise programs and check your blood sugar as your doctor tells you to.
- Your doctor may do certain blood tests before you start KAZANO and during treatment as needed. Your doctor may ask you to stop taking KAZANO based on the results of your blood tests due to how well your kidneys are working.
- Your doctor will check your diabetes with regular blood tests, including your blood sugar levels and your hemoglobin A1C.

What are the possible side effects of KAZANO?

KAZANO can cause serious side effects, including:

- See **"What is the most important information I should know about KAZANO?"**
- **Allergic (hypersensitivity) reactions,** such as:
  - ○ swelling of your face, lips, throat and other areas on your skin
  - ○ difficulty swallowing or breathing
  - ○ raised, red areas on your skin (hives)
  - ○ skin rash, itching, flaking or peeling

  If you have these symptoms, stop taking KAZANO and contact your doctor right away.
- **Liver problems.** Call your doctor right away if you have symptoms, such as:
  - ○ nausea or vomiting
  - ○ stomach pain
  - ○ unusual or unexplained tiredness
  - ○ loss of appetite
  - ○ dark urine
  - ○ yellowing of your skin or the whites of your eyes
- **Low blood sugar (hypoglycemia).** If you take KAZANO with another medicine that can cause low blood sugar, such as a sulfonylurea or insulin, your risk of getting low blood sugar is higher. The dose of your sulfonylurea medicine or insulin may need to be lowered while you take KAZANO. If you have symptoms of low blood sugar, you should check your blood sugar and treat if low, and then call your doctor. Signs and symptoms of low blood sugar may include:

• shaking or feeling jittery	• headache
• sweating	• change in mood
• fast heartbeat	• confusion
• change in vision	• dizziness
• hunger	

The most common side effects of KAZANO include:

- cold-like symptoms (upper respiratory tract infection)
- stuffy or runny nose and sore throat
- diarrhea
- increase in blood pressure
- headache
- back pain
- urinary tract infection

Taking KAZANO with food can help lessen the common stomach side effects of metformin that usually happen at the beginning of treatment. If you have unexplained stomach problems, tell your doctor. Stomach problems that start later, during treatment, may be a sign of something more serious.

Tell your doctor if you have any side effect that bothers you or that does not go away.

These are not all the possible side effects of KAZANO. For more information, ask your doctor or pharmacist.

Call your doctor for medical advice about side effects. You may report side effects to FDA at 1-800-FDA-1088.

How should I store KAZANO?

- Store KAZANO at room temperature between 68°F to 77°F (20°C to 25°C).
- Keep the container of KAZANO tightly closed.

Keep KAZANO and all medicines out of the reach of children.

General information about the safe and effective use of KAZANO

Medicines are sometimes prescribed for purposes other than those listed in the Medication Guide. Do not take KAZANO for a condition for which it was not prescribed. Do not give KAZANO to other people, even if they have the same symptoms you have. It may harm them.

This Medication Guide summarizes the most important information about KAZANO. If you would like more information, talk with your doctor. You can ask your doctor or pharmacist for information about KAZANO that is written for health professionals.

For more information go to www.kazano.com or call 1-877-TAKEDA-7 (1-877-825-3327).

What are the ingredients in KAZANO?

Active ingredients: alogliptin and metformin hydrochloride

Inactive ingredients: mannitol, microcrystalline cellulose, povidone, crospovidone and magnesium stearate; the tablets are film-coated with hypromellose 2910, talc, titanium dioxide and ferric oxide yellow.

This Medication Guide has been approved by the U.S. Food and Drug Administration.

Distributed by:
Takeda Pharmaceuticals America, Inc.
Deerfield, IL 60015
Revised: June 2013

KAZANO and NESINA are trademarks of Takeda Pharmaceutical Company Limited registered with the U.S. Patent and Trademark Office and are used under license by Takeda Pharmaceuticals America, Inc.

ALM143P R3

Shown in Product Identification Guide, page 313

NESINA ℞
(alogliptin)
tablets

HIGHLIGHTS OF PRESCRIBING INFORMATION
These highlights do not include all the information needed to use NESINA safely and effectively. See full prescribing information for NESINA.
NESINA (alogliptin) tablets
Initial U.S. Approval: 2013

INDICATIONS AND USAGE

NESINA is a dipeptidyl peptidase-4 (DPP-4) inhibitor indicated as an adjunct to diet and exercise to improve glycemic control in adults with type 2 diabetes mellitus. (1.1, 14)

Limitation of Use: Not for treatment of type 1 diabetes or diabetic ketoacidosis. (1.2)

DOSAGE AND ADMINISTRATION

- The recommended dose in patients with normal renal function or mild renal impairment is 25 mg once daily. (2.1)
- Can be taken with or without food. (2.1)
- Adjust dose if moderate or severe renal impairment or end-stage renal disease (ESRD). (2.2)

Degree of Renal Impairment	Creatinine Clearance (mL/min)	Recommended Dosing
Moderate	≥30 to <60	12.5 mg once daily
Severe/ESRD	<30	6.25 mg once daily

DOSAGE FORMS AND STRENGTHS

Tablets: 25 mg, 12.5 mg and 6.25 mg (3)

CONTRAINDICATIONS

History of a serious hypersensitivity reaction to alogliptin-containing products, such as anaphylaxis, angioedema or severe cutaneous adverse reactions. (4)

WARNINGS AND PRECAUTIONS

- Acute pancreatitis: There have been postmarketing reports of acute pancreatitis. If pancreatitis is suspected, promptly discontinue NESINA. (5.1)
- Hypersensitivity: There have been postmarketing reports of serious hypersensitivity reactions in patients treated with NESINA such as anaphylaxis, angioedema and severe cutaneous adverse reactions. In such cases, promptly discontinue NESINA, assess for other potential causes, institute appropriate monitoring and treatment and initiate alternative treatment for diabetes. (5.2)
- Hepatic effects: Postmarketing reports of hepatic failure, sometimes fatal. Causality cannot be excluded. If liver injury is detected, promptly interrupt NESINA and assess patient for probable cause, then treat cause if possible, to resolution or stabilization. Do not restart NESINA if liver injury is confirmed and no alternative etiology can be found. (5.3)
- Hypoglycemia: When an insulin secretagogue (e.g., sulfonylurea) or insulin is used in combination with NESINA, a lower dose of the insulin secretagogue or insulin may be required to minimize the risk of hypoglycemia. (5.4)
- Macrovascular outcomes: There have been no clinical studies establishing conclusive evidence of macrovascular risk reduction with NESINA or any other antidiabetic drug. (5.5)

ADVERSE REACTIONS

Common adverse reactions (reported in ≥4% of patients treated with NESINA 25 mg and more frequently than in patients who received placebo) are: nasopharyngitis, headache and upper respiratory tract infection. (6.1)

To report SUSPECTED ADVERSE REACTIONS, contact Takeda Pharmaceuticals at 1-877-TAKEDA-7 (1-877-825-3327) or FDA at 1-800-FDA-1088 or www.fda.gov/medwatch.

See 17 for PATIENT COUNSELING INFORMATION and Medication Guide

Revised: 06/2013

FULL PRESCRIBING INFORMATION: CONTENTS*

*** Sections or subsections omitted from the full prescribing information are not listed**

FULL PRESCRIBING INFORMATION

1 INDICATIONS AND USAGE

1.1 Monotherapy and Combination Therapy

NESINA is indicated as an adjunct to diet and exercise to improve glycemic control in adults with type 2 diabetes mellitus in multiple clinical settings *[see Clinical Studies (14)]*.

Table 1. Adverse Reactions Reported in ≥4% Patients Treated with NESINA 25 mg and More Frequently Than in Patients Given Placebo in Pooled Studies

	Number of Patients (%)		
	NESINA 25 mg	Placebo	Active Comparator
	N=5902	N=2926	N=2257
Nasopharyngitis	257 (4.4)	89 (3.0)	113 (5.0)
Headache	247 (4.2)	72 (2.5)	121 (5.4)
Upper Respiratory Tract Infection	247 (4.2)	61 (2.1)	113 (5.0)

1.2 Limitation of Use

NESINA should not be used in patients with type 1 diabetes mellitus or for the treatment of diabetic ketoacidosis, as it would not be effective in these settings.

2 DOSAGE AND ADMINISTRATION

2.1 Recommended Dosing

The recommended dose of NESINA is 25 mg once daily. NESINA may be taken with or without food.

2.2 Patients with Renal Impairment

No dose adjustment of NESINA is necessary for patients with mild renal impairment (creatinine clearance [CrCl] ≥60 mL/min).

The dose of NESINA is 12.5 mg once daily for patients with moderate renal impairment (CrCl ≥30 to <60 mL/min).

The dose of NESINA is 6.25 mg once daily for patients with severe renal impairment (CrCl ≥15 to <30 mL/min) or with end-stage renal disease (ESRD) (CrCl <15 mL/min or requiring hemodialysis). NESINA may be administered without regard to the timing of dialysis. NESINA has not been studied in patients undergoing peritoneal dialysis *[see Clinical Pharmacology (12.3)]*.

Because there is a need for dose adjustment based upon renal function, assessment of renal function is recommended prior to initiation of NESINA therapy and periodically thereafter.

3 DOSAGE FORMS AND STRENGTHS

- 25 mg tablets are light red, oval, biconvex, film-coated, with "TAK ALG-25" printed on one side.
- 12.5 mg tablets are yellow, oval, biconvex, film-coated, with "TAK ALG-12.5" printed on one side.
- 6.25 mg tablets are light pink, oval, biconvex, film-coated, with "TAK ALG-6.25" printed on one side.

4 CONTRAINDICATIONS

History of a serious hypersensitivity reaction to alogliptin-containing products, such as anaphylaxis, angioedema or severe cutaneous adverse reactions.

5 WARNINGS AND PRECAUTIONS

5.1 Pancreatitis

There have been postmarketing reports of acute pancreatitis in patients taking NESINA. After initiation of NESINA, patients should be observed carefully for signs and symptoms of pancreatitis. If pancreatitis is suspected, NESINA should promptly be discontinued and appropriate management should be initiated. It is unknown whether patients with a history of pancreatitis are at increased risk for the development of pancreatitis while using NESINA.

5.2 Hypersensitivity Reactions

There have been postmarketing reports of serious hypersensitivity reactions in patients treated with NESINA. These reactions include anaphylaxis, angioedema and severe cutaneous adverse reactions, including Stevens-Johnson syndrome. If a serious hypersensitivity reaction is suspected, discontinue NESINA, assess for other potential causes for the event and institute alternative treatment for diabetes *[see Adverse Reactions (6.2)]*. Use caution in a patient with a history of angioedema with another DPP-4 inhibitor because it is unknown whether such patients will be predisposed to angioedema with NESINA.

5.3 Hepatic Effects

There have been postmarketing reports of fatal and nonfatal hepatic failure in patients taking NESINA, although some of the reports contain insufficient information necessary to establish the probable cause *[see Adverse Reactions (6.2)]*. In randomized controlled studies, serum alanine aminotransferase (ALT) elevations greater than three times the upper limit of normal (ULN) were observed: 1.3% in alogliptin-treated patients and 1.5% in all comparator-treated patients.

Patients with type 2 diabetes may have fatty liver disease, which may cause liver test abnormalities, and they may also have other forms of liver disease, many of which can be treated or managed. Therefore, obtaining a liver test panel and assessing the patient before initiating NESINA therapy is recommended. In patients with abnormal liver tests, NESINA should be initiated with caution.

Measure liver tests promptly in patients who report symptoms that may indicate liver injury, including fatigue, anorexia, right upper abdominal discomfort, dark urine or jaundice. In this clinical context, if the patient is found to have clinically significant liver enzyme elevations and if abnormal liver tests persist or worsen, NESINA should be interrupted and investigation done to establish the probable cause. NESINA should not be restarted in these patients without another explanation for the liver test abnormalities.

5.4 Use with Medications Known to Cause Hypoglycemia

Insulin and insulin secretagogues, such as sulfonylureas, are known to cause hypoglycemia. Therefore, a lower dose of insulin or insulin secretagogue may be required to minimize the risk of hypoglycemia when used in combination with NESINA.

5.5 Macrovascular Outcomes

There have been no clinical studies establishing conclusive evidence of macrovascular risk reduction with NESINA or any other antidiabetic drug.

6 ADVERSE REACTIONS

6.1 Clinical Studies Experience

Because clinical trials are conducted under widely varying conditions, adverse reaction rates observed in the clinical trials of a drug cannot be directly compared to rates in the clinical trials of another drug and may not reflect the rates observed in clinical practice.

Approximately 8500 patients with type 2 diabetes have been treated with NESINA in 14 randomized, double-blind, controlled clinical trials with approximately 2900 subjects randomized to placebo and approximately 2200 to an active comparator. The mean exposure to NESINA was 40 weeks with more than 2400 subjects treated for more than one year. Among these patients, 63% had a history of hypertension, 51% had a history of dyslipidemia, 25% had a history of myocardial infarction, 8% had a history of unstable angina and 7% had a history of congestive heart failure. The mean duration of diabetes was seven years, the mean body mass index (BMI) was 31 kg/m^2 (51% of patients had a BMI ≥30 kg/m^2), and the mean age was 57 years (24% of patients ≥65 years of age).

Two placebo-controlled monotherapy trials of 12 and 26 weeks of duration were conducted in patients treated with NESINA 12.5 mg daily, NESINA 25 mg daily and placebo. Four placebo-controlled add-on combination therapy trials of 26 weeks duration were also conducted: with metformin, with a sulfonylurea, with a thiazolidinedione and with insulin.

Four placebo-controlled and one active-controlled trials of 16 weeks up through two years in duration were conducted in combination with metformin, in combination with pioglitazone and with pioglitazone added to a background of metformin therapy.

Three active-controlled trials of 52 weeks in duration were conducted in patients treated with pioglitazone and metformin, in combination with metformin and as monotherapy compared to glipizide.

In a pooled analysis of these 14 controlled clinical trials, the overall incidence of adverse events was 66% in patients treated with NESINA 25 mg compared to 62% with placebo and 70% with active comparator. Overall discontinuation of therapy due to adverse events was 4.7% with NESINA 25 mg compared to 4.5% with placebo or 6.2% with active comparator.

Adverse reactions reported in ≥4% of patients treated with NESINA 25 mg and more frequently than in patients who received placebo are summarized in *Table 1*.

[See table 1 above]

Pancreatitis

In the clinical trial program, pancreatitis was reported in 11 of 5902 (0.2%) patients receiving NESINA 25 mg daily compared to five of 5183 (<0.1%) patients receiving all comparators.

Hypersensitivity Reactions

In a pooled analysis, the overall incidence of hypersensitivity reactions was 0.6% with NESINA 25 mg compared to 0.8% with all comparators. A single event of serum sickness was reported in a patient treated with NESINA 25 mg.

Hypoglycemia

Hypoglycemic events were documented based upon a blood glucose value and/or clinical signs and symptoms of hypoglycemia.

In the monotherapy study, the incidence of hypoglycemia was 1.5% in patients treated with NESINA compared to 1.6% with placebo. The use of NESINA as add-on therapy to glyburide or insulin did not increase the incidence of hypoglycemia compared to placebo. In a monotherapy study comparing NESINA to a sulfonylurea in elderly patients, the incidence of hypoglycemia was 5.4% with NESINA compared to 26% with glipizide *(Table 2)*.

[See table 2 at top of next page]

Vital Signs

No clinically meaningful changes in vital signs or in electrocardiograms were observed in patients treated with NESINA.

Laboratory Tests

No clinically meaningful changes in hematology, serum chemistry or urinalysis were observed in patients treated with NESINA.

6.2 Postmarketing Experience

The following adverse reactions have been identified during the postmarketing use of NESINA outside the United States. Because these reactions are reported voluntarily from a population of uncertain size, it is not always possible to reliably estimate their frequency or establish a causal relationship to drug exposure.

Hypersensitivity reactions including anaphylaxis, angioedema, rash, urticaria and severe cutaneous adverse reactions, including Stevens-Johnson syndrome, hepatic enzyme elevations, fulminant hepatic failure and acute pancreatitis.

7 DRUG INTERACTIONS

NESINA is primarily renally excreted. Cytochrome (CYP) P450-related metabolism is negligible. No significant drug-drug interactions were observed with the CYP-substrates or inhibitors tested or with renally excreted drugs *[see Clinical Pharmacology (12.3)]*.

8 USE IN SPECIFIC POPULATIONS

8.1 Pregnancy

Pregnancy Category B

No adequate or well-controlled studies in pregnant women have been conducted with NESINA. Based on animal data, NESINA is not predicted to increase the risk of developmental abnormalities. Because animal reproduction studies are not always predictive of human risk and exposure, NESINA, like other antidiabetic medications, should be used during pregnancy only if clearly needed.

Alogliptin administered to pregnant rabbits and rats during the period of organogenesis was not teratogenic at doses of up to 200 mg/kg and 500 mg/kg, or 149 times and 180 times, respectively, the clinical dose based on plasma drug exposure (AUC).

Doses of alogliptin up to 250 mg/kg (approximately 95 times clinical exposure based on AUC) given to pregnant rats from gestation Day 6 to lactation Day 20 did not harm the developing embryo or adversely affect growth and development of offspring.

Placental transfer of alogliptin into the fetus was observed following oral dosing to pregnant rats.

8.3 Nursing Mothers

Alogliptin is secreted in the milk of lactating rats in a 2:1 ratio to plasma. It is not known whether alogliptin is excreted in human milk. Because many drugs are excreted in human milk, caution should be exercised when NESINA is administered to a nursing woman.

8.4 Pediatric Use

Safety and effectiveness of NESINA in pediatric patients have not been established.

8.5 Geriatric Use

Of the total number of patients (N=8507) in clinical safety and efficacy studies treated with NESINA, 2064 (24.3%) patients were 65 years and older and 341 (4%) patients were 75 years and older. No overall differences in safety or effectiveness were observed between patients 65 years and over and younger patients. While this clinical experience has not identified differences in responses between the elderly and younger patients, greater sensitivity of some older individuals cannot be ruled out.

8.6 Hepatic Impairment

No dose adjustments are required in patients with mild to moderate hepatic impairment (Child-Pugh Grade A and B) based on insignificant change in systemic exposures (e.g., AUC) compared to subjects with normal hepatic function in a pharmacokinetic study. NESINA has not been studied in patients with severe hepatic impairment (Child-Pugh Grade C). Use caution when administering NESINA to patients with liver disease *[see Warnings and Precautions (5.3)]*.

10 OVERDOSAGE

The highest doses of NESINA administered in clinical trials were single doses of 800 mg to healthy subjects and doses of 400 mg once daily for 14 days to patients with type 2 diabetes (equivalent to 32 times and 16 times the maximum recommended clinical dose of 25 mg, respectively). No serious adverse events were observed at these doses.

In the event of an overdose, it is reasonable to institute the necessary clinical monitoring and supportive therapy as dictated by the patient's clinical status. Per clinical judgment, it may be reasonable to initiate removal of unabsorbed material from the gastrointestinal tract.

Alogliptin is minimally dialyzable; over a three-hour hemodialysis session, approximately 7% of the drug was removed. Therefore, hemodialysis is unlikely to be beneficial in an overdose situation. It is not known if NESINA is dialyzable by peritoneal dialysis.

11 DESCRIPTION

NESINA tablets contain the active ingredient alogliptin, which is a selective, orally bioavailable inhibitor of the enzymatic activity of dipeptidyl peptidase-4 (DPP-4).

Chemically, alogliptin is prepared as a benzoate salt, which is identified as 2-({6-[(3*R*)-3-aminopiperidin-1-yl]-3-methyl-2,4-dioxo-3,4-dihydropyrimidin-1(2*H*)-yl}methyl)benzonitrile monobenzoate. It has a molecular formula of $C_{18}H_{21}N_5O_2 \bullet C_7H_6O_2$ and a molecular weight of 461.51 daltons. The structural formula is:

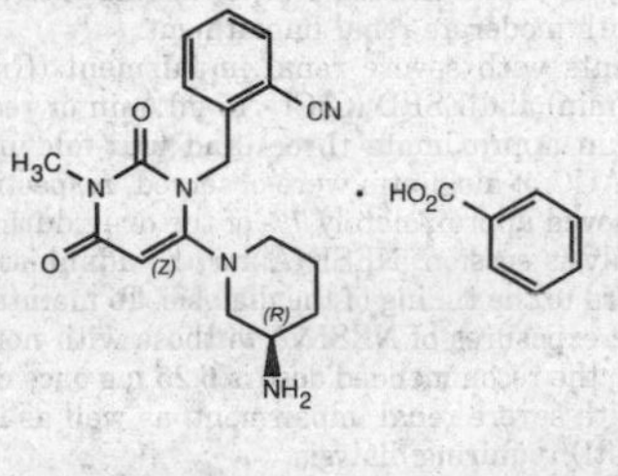

Alogliptin benzoate is a white to off-white crystalline powder containing one asymmetric carbon in the aminopiperidine moiety. It is soluble in dimethylsulfoxide, sparingly soluble in water and methanol, slightly soluble in ethanol and very slightly soluble in octanol and isopropyl acetate.

Each NESINA tablet contains 34 mg, 17 mg or 8.5 mg alogliptin benzoate, which is equivalent to 25 mg, 12.5 mg or 6.25 mg, respectively, of alogliptin and the following inactive ingredients: mannitol, microcrystalline cellulose, hydroxypropyl cellulose, croscarmellose sodium and magnesium stearate. In addition, the film coating contains the following inactive ingredients: hypromellose, titanium dioxide, ferric oxide (red or yellow) and polyethylene glycol, and is marked with printing ink (Gray F1).

12 CLINICAL PHARMACOLOGY

12.1 Mechanism of Action

Increased concentrations of the incretin hormones such as glucagon-like peptide-1 (GLP-1) and glucose-dependent insulinotropic polypeptide (GIP) are released into the bloodstream from the small intestine in response to meals. These hormones cause insulin release from the pancreatic beta cells in a glucose-dependent manner but are inactivated by the DPP-4 enzyme within minutes. GLP-1 also lowers glucagon secretion from pancreatic alpha cells, reducing hepatic glucose production. In patients with type 2 diabetes, concentrations of GLP-1 are reduced but the insulin response to GLP-1 is preserved. Alogliptin is a DPP-4 inhibitor that slows the inactivation of the incretin hormones, thereby increasing their bloodstream concentrations and reducing fasting and postprandial glucose concentrations in a glucose-dependent manner in patients with type 2 diabetes mellitus. Alogliptin selectively binds to and inhibits DPP-4 but not DPP-8 or DPP-9 activity *in vitro* at concentrations approximating therapeutic exposures.

12.2 Pharmacodynamics

Single-dose administration of NESINA to healthy subjects resulted in a peak inhibition of DPP-4 within two to three hours after dosing. The peak inhibition of DPP-4 exceeded 93% across doses of 12.5 mg to 800 mg. Inhibition of DPP-4

Table 2. Incidence and Rate of Hypoglycemia* in Placebo and Active-Controlled Studies when NESINA Was Used as Add-On Therapy to Glyburide, Insulin, Metformin, Pioglitazone or Compared to Glipizide

Add-On to Glyburide (26 Weeks)	**NESINA 25 mg + Glyburide**	**Placebo + Glyburide**
	N=198	N=99
Overall (%)	19 (9.6)	11 (11.1)
Severe (%)†	0	1 (1)
Add-On to Insulin (± Metformin) (26 Weeks)	**NESINA 25 mg + Insulin (± Metformin)**	**Placebo + Insulin (± Metformin)**
	N=129	N=129
Overall (%)	35 (27)	31 (24)
Severe (%)†	1 (0.8)	2 (1.6)
Add-On to Metformin (26 Weeks)	**NESINA 25 mg + Metformin**	**Placebo + Metformin**
	N=207	N=104
Overall (%)	0	3 (2.9)
Severe (%)†	0	0
Add-On to Pioglitazone (± Metformin or Sulfonylurea) (26 Weeks)	**NESINA 25 mg + Pioglitazone**	**Placebo + Pioglitazone**
	N=199	N=97
Overall (%)	14 (7.0)	5 (5.2)
Severe (%)†	0	1 (1)
Compared to Glipizide (52 Weeks)	**NESINA 25 mg**	**Glipizide**
	N=222	N=219
Overall (%)	12 (5.4)	57 (26)
Severe (%)†	0	3 (1.4)
Add-On to Metformin (26 Weeks)	**NESINA 25 mg**	**Metformin 500 mg twice daily**
	N=112	N=109
Overall (%)	2 (1.8)	2 (1.8)
Severe (%)†	0	0
Add-On to Metformin Compared to Glipizide (52 Weeks)	**NESINA 25 mg + Metformin**	**Glipizide + Metformin**
	N=877	N=869
Overall (%)	12 (1.4)	207 (23.8)
Severe (%)†	0	4 (0.5)

* Adverse reactions of hypoglycemia were based on all reports of symptomatic and asymptomatic hypoglycemia; a concurrent glucose measurement was not required; intent-to-treat population.

† Severe events of hypoglycemia were defined as those events requiring medical assistance or exhibiting depressed level or loss of consciousness or seizure.

remained above 80% at 24 hours for doses greater than or equal to 25 mg. Peak and total exposure over 24 hours to active GLP-1 were three- to four-fold greater with NESINA (at doses of 25 to 200 mg) than placebo. In a 16-week, double-blind, placebo-controlled study, NESINA 25 mg demonstrated decreases in postprandial glucagon while increasing postprandial active GLP-1 levels compared to placebo over an eight-hour period following a standardized meal. It is unclear how these findings relate to changes in overall glycemic control in patients with type 2 diabetes mellitus. In this study, NESINA 25 mg demonstrated decreases in two-hour postprandial glucose compared to placebo (-30 mg/dL versus 17 mg/dL, respectively).

Multiple-dose administration of alogliptin to patients with type 2 diabetes also resulted in a peak inhibition of DPP-4 within one to two hours and exceeded 93% across all doses (25 mg, 100 mg and 400 mg) after a single dose and after 14 days of once-daily dosing. At these doses of NESINA, inhibition of DPP-4 remained above 81% at 24 hours after 14 days of dosing.

Cardiac Electrophysiology

In a randomized, placebo-controlled, four-arm, parallel-group study, 257 subjects were administered either alogliptin 50 mg, alogliptin 400 mg, moxifloxacin 400 mg or placebo once daily for a total of seven days. No increase in QTc was observed with either dose of alogliptin. At the 400 mg dose, peak alogliptin plasma concentrations were 19-fold higher than the peak concentrations following the maximum recommended clinical dose of 25 mg.

12.3 Pharmacokinetics

The pharmacokinetics of NESINA has been studied in healthy subjects and in patients with type 2 diabetes. After administration of single, oral doses up to 800 mg in healthy

Figure 1. Effect of Alogliptin on the Pharmacokinetic Exposure to Other Drugs

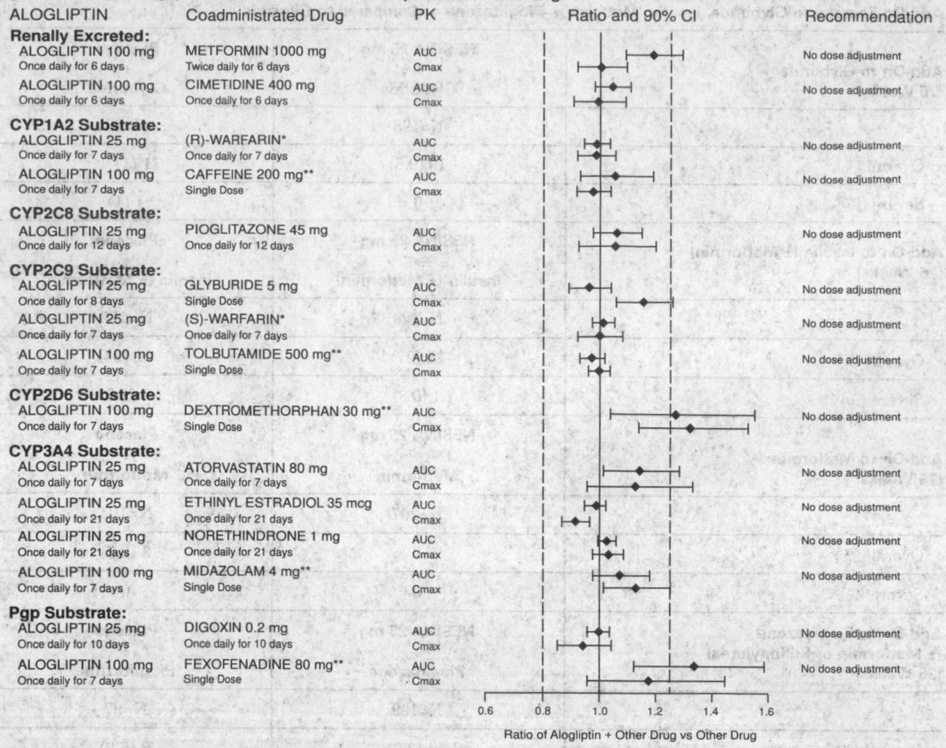

ALOGLIPTIN
Coadministrated Drug
PK
Ratio and 90% CI
Recommendation
Renally Excreted:
ALOGLIPTIN 100 mg Once daily for 6 days | METFORMIN 1000 mg Twice daily for 6 days | AUC Cmax | No dose adjustment
ALOGLIPTIN 100 mg Once daily for 6 days | CIMETIDINE 400 mg Once daily for 6 days | AUC Cmax | No dose adjustment
CYP1A2 Substrate:
ALOGLIPTIN 25 mg Once daily for 7 days | (R)-WARFARIN* Once daily for 7 days | AUC Cmax | No dose adjustment
ALOGLIPTIN 100 mg Once daily for 7 days | CAFFEINE 200 mg** Single Dose | AUC Cmax | No dose adjustment
CYP2C8 Substrate:
ALOGLIPTIN 25 mg Once daily for 12 days | PIOGLITAZONE 45 mg Once daily for 12 days | AUC Cmax | No dose adjustment
CYP2C9 Substrate:
ALOGLIPTIN 25 mg Once daily for 8 days | GLYBURIDE 5 mg Single Dose | AUC Cmax | No dose adjustment
ALOGLIPTIN 25 mg Once daily for 7 days | (S)-WARFARIN* Once daily for 7 days | AUC Cmax | No dose adjustment
ALOGLIPTIN 100 mg Once daily for 7 days | TOLBUTAMIDE 500 mg** Single Dose | AUC Cmax | No dose adjustment
CYP2D6 Substrate:
ALOGLIPTIN 100 mg Once daily for 7 days | DEXTROMETHORPHAN 30 mg** Single Dose | AUC Cmax | No dose adjustment
CYP3A4 Substrate:
ALOGLIPTIN 25 mg Once daily for 7 days | ATORVASTATIN 80 mg Once daily for 7 days | AUC Cmax | No dose adjustment
ALOGLIPTIN 25 mg Once daily for 21 days | ETHINYL ESTRADIOL 35 mcg Once daily for 21 days | AUC Cmax | No dose adjustment
ALOGLIPTIN 25 mg Once daily for 21 days | NORETHINDRONE 1 mg Once daily for 21 days | AUC Cmax | No dose adjustment
ALOGLIPTIN 100 mg Once daily for 7 days | MIDAZOLAM 4 mg** Single Dose | AUC Cmax | No dose adjustment
Pgp Substrate:
ALOGLIPTIN 25 mg Once daily for 10 days | DIGOXIN 0.2 mg Once daily for 10 days | AUC Cmax | No dose adjustment
ALOGLIPTIN 100 mg Once daily for 7 days | FEXOFENADINE 80 mg** Single Dose | AUC Cmax | No dose adjustment
0.6 0.8 1.0 1.2 1.4 1.6
Ratio of Alogliptin + Other Drug vs Other Drug

*Warfarin was given once daily at a stable dose in the range of 1 mg to 10 mg. Alogliptin had no significant effect on the prothrombin time (PT) or International Normalized Ratio (INR).

**Caffeine (1A2 substrate), tolbutamide (2C9 substrate), dextromethorphan (2D6 substrate), midazolam (3A4 substrate) and fexofenadine (P-gp substrate) were administered as a cocktail.

Figure 2. Effect of Other Drugs on the Pharmacokinetic Exposure of Alogliptin

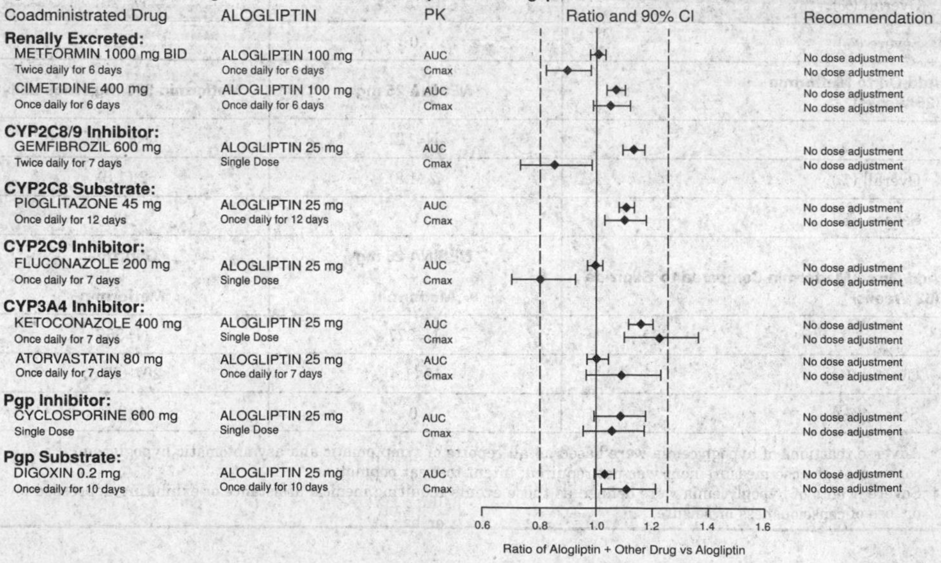

subjects, the peak plasma alogliptin concentration (median T_{max}) occurred one to two hours after dosing. At the maximum recommended clinical dose of 25 mg, NESINA was eliminated with a mean terminal half-life ($T_{1/2}$) of approximately 21 hours.

After multiple-dose administration up to 400 mg for 14 days in patients with type 2 diabetes, accumulation of alogliptin was minimal with an increase in total (i.e., AUC) and peak (i.e., C_{max}) alogliptin exposures of 34% and 9%, respectively. Total and peak exposure to alogliptin increased proportionally across single doses and multiple doses of alogliptin ranging from 25 mg to 400 mg. The intersubject coefficient of variation for alogliptin AUC was 17%. The pharmacokinetics of NESINA was also shown to be similar in healthy subjects and in patients with type 2 diabetes.

Absorption

The absolute bioavailability of NESINA is approximately 100%. Administration of NESINA with a high-fat meal results in no significant change in total and peak exposure to alogliptin. NESINA may therefore be administered with or without food.

Distribution

Following a single, 12.5 mg intravenous infusion of alogliptin to healthy subjects, the volume of distribution during the terminal phase was 417 L, indicating that the drug is well distributed into tissues.

Alogliptin is 20% bound to plasma proteins.

Metabolism

Alogliptin does not undergo extensive metabolism and 60% to 71% of the dose is excreted as unchanged drug in the urine.

Two minor metabolites were detected following administration of an oral dose of [^{14}C] alogliptin, *N*-demethylated, M-I (<1% of the parent compound), and *N*-acetylated alogliptin, M-II (<6% of the parent compound). M-I is an active metabolite and is an inhibitor of DPP-4 similar to the parent molecule; M-II does not display any inhibitory activity toward DPP-4 or other DPP-related enzymes. *In vitro* data indicate that CYP2D6 and CYP3A4 contribute to the limited metabolism of alogliptin.

Alogliptin exists predominantly as the (*R*)-enantiomer (>99%) and undergoes little or no chiral conversion *in vivo* to the (*S*)-enantiomer. The (*S*)-enantiomer is not detectable at the 25 mg dose.

Excretion

The primary route of elimination of [^{14}C] alogliptin-derived radioactivity occurs via renal excretion (76%) with 13% recovered in the feces, achieving a total recovery of 89% of the administered radioactive dose. The renal clearance of alogliptin (9.6 L/hr) indicates some active renal tubular secretion and systemic clearance was 14.0 L/hr.

Specific Populations

Renal Impairment

A single-dose, open-label study was conducted to evaluate the pharmacokinetics of alogliptin 50 mg in patients with chronic renal impairment compared with healthy subjects.

In patients with mild renal impairment (creatinine clearance [CrCl] ≥60 to <90 mL/min), an approximate 1.2-fold increase in plasma AUC of alogliptin was observed. Because increases of this magnitude are not considered clinically relevant, dose adjustment for patients with mild renal impairment is not recommended.

In patients with moderate renal impairment (CrCl ≥30 to <60 mL/min), an approximate two-fold increase in plasma AUC of alogliptin was observed. To maintain similar systemic exposures of NESINA to those with normal renal function, the recommended dose is 12.5 mg once daily in patients with moderate renal impairment.

In patients with severe renal impairment (CrCl ≥15 to <30 mL/min) and ESRD (CrCl <15 mL/min or requiring dialysis), an approximate three- and four-fold increase in plasma AUC of alogliptin were observed, respectively. Dialysis removed approximately 7% of the drug during a three-hour dialysis session. NESINA may be administered without regard to the timing of the dialysis. To maintain similar systemic exposures of NESINA to those with normal renal function, the recommended dose is 6.25 mg once daily in patients with severe renal impairment, as well as in patients with ESRD requiring dialysis.

Hepatic Impairment

Total exposure to alogliptin was approximately 10% lower and peak exposure was approximately 8% lower in patients with moderate hepatic impairment (Child-Pugh Grade B) compared to healthy subjects. The magnitude of these reductions is not considered to be clinically meaningful. Patients with severe hepatic impairment (Child-Pugh Grade C) have not been studied. Use caution when administering NESINA to patients with liver disease *[see Use in Specific Populations (8.6) and Warnings and Precautions (5.3)]*.

Gender

No dose adjustment of NESINA is necessary based on gender. Gender did not have any clinically meaningful effect on the pharmacokinetics of alogliptin.

Geriatric

No dose adjustment of NESINA is necessary based on age. Age did not have any clinically meaningful effect on the pharmacokinetics of alogliptin.

Pediatric

Studies characterizing the pharmacokinetics of alogliptin in pediatric patients have not been performed.

Race

No dose adjustment of NESINA is necessary based on race. Race (White, Black, and Asian) did not have any clinically meaningful effect on the pharmacokinetics of alogliptin.

Drug Interactions

In Vitro Assessment of Drug Interactions

In vitro studies indicate that alogliptin is neither an inducer of CYP1A2, CYP2B6, CYP2C9, CYP2C19 and CYP3A4, nor an inhibitor of CYP1A2, CYP2C8, CYP2C9, CYP2C19, CYP3A4 and CYP2D6 at clinically relevant concentrations.

In Vivo Assessment of Drug Interactions

Effects of Alogliptin on the Pharmacokinetics of Other Drugs

In clinical studies, alogliptin did not meaningfully increase the systemic exposure to the following drugs that are metabolized by CYP isozymes or excreted unchanged in urine (*Figure 1*). No dose adjustment of NESINA is recommended based on results of the described pharmacokinetic studies.
[See figure 1 above]

Effects of Other Drugs on the Pharmacokinetics of Alogliptin

There are no clinically meaningful changes in the pharmacokinetics of alogliptin when NESINA is administered concomitantly with the drugs described below *(Figure 2)*.

[See figure 2 at top of previous page]

13 NONCLINICAL TOXICOLOGY

13.1 Carcinogenesis, Mutagenesis, Impairment of Fertility

Rats were administered oral doses of 75, 400 and 800 mg/kg alogliptin for two years. No drug-related tumors were observed up to 75 mg/kg or approximately 32 times the maximum recommended clinical dose of 25 mg, based on AUC exposure. At higher doses (approximately 308 times the maximum recommended clinical dose of 25 mg), a combination of thyroid C-cell adenomas and carcinomas increased in male but not female rats. No drug-related tumors were observed in mice after administration of 50, 150 or 300 mg/kg alogliptin for two years, or up to approximately 51 times the maximum recommended clinical dose of 25 mg, based on AUC exposure.

Alogliptin was not mutagenic or clastogenic, with and without metabolic activation, in the Ames test with *S. typhimurium* and *E. coli* or the cytogenetic assay in mouse lymphoma cells. Alogliptin was negative in the *in vivo* mouse micronucleus study.

In a fertility study in rats, alogliptin had no adverse effects on early embryonic development, mating or fertility at doses up to 500 mg/kg, or approximately 172 times the clinical dose based on plasma drug exposure (AUC).

14 CLINICAL STUDIES

NESINA has been studied as monotherapy and in combination with metformin, a sulfonylurea, a thiazolidinedione (either alone or in combination with metformin or a sulfonylurea) and insulin (either alone or in combination with metformin).

A total of 8673 patients with type 2 diabetes were randomized in 10 double-blind, placebo- or active-controlled clinical safety and efficacy studies conducted to evaluate the effects of NESINA on glycemic control. The racial distribution of patients exposed to study medication was 68% Caucasian, 15% Asian, 7% Black and 9% other racial groups. The ethnic distribution was 30% Hispanic. Patients had an overall mean age of 55 years (range 21 to 80 years).

In patients with type 2 diabetes, treatment with NESINA produced clinically meaningful and statistically significant improvements in A1C compared to placebo. As is typical for trials of agents to treat type 2 diabetes, the mean reduction in A1C with NESINA appears to be related to the degree of A1C elevation at baseline.

NESINA had similar changes from baseline in serum lipids compared to placebo.

14.1 Patients with Inadequate Glycemic Control on Diet and Exercise

A total of 1768 patients with type 2 diabetes participated in three double-blind studies to evaluate the efficacy and safety of NESINA in patients with inadequate glycemic control on diet and exercise. All three studies had a four-week, single-blind, placebo run-in period followed by a 26-week randomized treatment period. Patients who failed to meet prespecified hyperglycemic goals during the 26-week treatment periods received glycemic rescue therapy.

In a 26-week, double-blind, placebo-controlled study, a total of 329 patients (mean baseline A1C = 8%) were randomized to receive NESINA 12.5 mg, NESINA 25 mg or placebo once daily. Treatment with NESINA 25 mg resulted in statistically significant improvements from baseline in A1C and fasting plasma glucose (FPG) compared to placebo at Week 26 *(Table 3)*. A total of 8% of patients receiving NESINA 25 mg and 30% of those receiving placebo required glycemic rescue therapy.

Improvements in A1C were not affected by gender, age or baseline BMI.

The mean change in body weight with NESINA was similar to placebo.

[See table 3 above]

In a 26-week, double-blind, active-controlled study, a total of 655 patients (mean baseline A1C = 8.8%) were randomized to receive NESINA 25 mg alone, pioglitazone 30 mg alone, NESINA 12.5 mg with pioglitazone 30 mg or NESINA 25 mg with pioglitazone 30 mg once daily. Coadministration of NESINA 25 mg with pioglitazone 30 mg resulted in statistically significant improvements from baseline in A1C and FPG compared to NESINA 25 mg alone and to pioglitazone 30 mg alone (*Table 4*). A total of 3% of patients receiving NESINA 25 mg coadministered with pioglitazone 30 mg, 11% of those receiving NESINA 25 mg alone and 6% of those receiving pioglitazone 30 mg alone required glycemic rescue.

Table 3. Glycemic Parameters at Week 26 in a Placebo-Controlled Monotherapy Study of NESINA*

	NESINA 25 mg	Placebo
A1C (%)	N=128	N=63
Baseline (mean)	7.9	8.0
Change from baseline (adjusted mean†)	-0.6	0
Difference from placebo (adjusted mean† with 95% confidence interval)	-0.6‡ (-0.8, -0.3)	-
% of patients (n/N) achieving A1C ≤7%	44% (58/131)‡	23% (15/64)
FPG (mg/dL)	N=129	N=64
Baseline (mean)	172	173
Change from baseline (adjusted mean†)	-16	11
Difference from placebo (adjusted mean† with 95% confidence interval)	-28‡ (-40, -15)	-

* Intent-to-treat population using last observation on study
† Least squares means adjusted for treatment, baseline value, geographic region and duration of diabetes
‡ p<0.01 compared to placebo

Table 4. Glycemic Parameters at Week 26 in an Active-Controlled Study of NESINA, Pioglitazone, and NESINA in Combination with Pioglitazone*

	NESINA 25 mg	Pioglitazone 30 mg	NESINA 25 mg + Pioglitazone 30 mg
A1C (%)	N=160	N=153	N=158
Baseline (mean)	8.8	8.8	8.8
Change from baseline (adjusted mean†)	-1.0	-1.2	-1.7
Difference from NESINA 25 mg (adjusted mean† with 95% confidence interval)	-	-	-0.8‡ (-1.0, -0.5)
Difference from pioglitazone 30 mg (adjusted mean† with 95% confidence interval)	-	-	-0.6‡ (-0.8, -0.3)
% of patients (n/N) achieving A1C ≤7%	24% (40/164)	34% (55/163)	63% (103/164)‡
FPG (mg/dL)	N=162	N=157	N=162
Baseline (mean)	189	189	185
Change from baseline (adjusted mean†)	-26	-37	-50
Difference from NESINA 25 mg (adjusted mean† with 95% confidence interval)	-	-	-24‡ (-34, -15)
Difference from pioglitazone 30 mg (adjusted mean† with 95% confidence interval)	-	-	-13‡ (-22, -4)

* Intent-to-treat population using last observation carried forward
† Least squares means adjusted for treatment, geographic region and baseline value
‡ p<0.01 compared to NESINA 25 mg or pioglitazone 30 mg

Improvements in A1C were not affected by gender, age or baseline BMI.

The mean increase in body weight was similar between pioglitazone alone and NESINA when coadministered with pioglitazone.

[See table 4 above]

In a 26-week, double-blind, placebo-controlled study, a total of 784 patients inadequately controlled on diet and exercise alone (mean baseline A1C = 8.4%) were randomized to one of seven treatment groups: placebo; metformin HCl 500 mg or metformin HCl 1000 mg twice daily; NESINA 12.5 mg twice daily; NESINA 25 mg daily; or NESINA 12.5 mg in combination with metformin HCl 500 mg or metformin HCl 1000 mg twice daily. Both coadministration treatment arms (NESINA 12.5 mg + metformin HCl 500 mg and NESINA 12.5 mg + metformin HCl 1000 mg) resulted in statistically significant improvements in A1C and FPG when compared with their respective individual alogliptin and metformin component regimens *(Table 5)*. Coadministration treatment arms demonstrated improvements in two-hour postprandial glucose (PPG) compared to NESINA alone or metformin alone *(Table 5)*. A total of 12.3% of patients receiving NESINA 12.5 mg + metformin HCl 500 mg, 2.6% of patients receiving NESINA 12.5 mg + metformin HCl 1000 mg, 17.3% of patients receiving NESINA 12.5 mg, 22.9% of patients receiving metformin HCl 500 mg, 10.8% of patients receiving metformin HCl 1000 mg and 38.7% of patients receiving placebo required glycemic rescue.

Improvements in A1C were not affected by gender, age, race or baseline BMI. The mean decrease in body weight was similar between metformin alone and NESINA when coadministered with metformin.

[See table 5 at top of next page]

14.2 Combination Therapy

Add-On Therapy to Metformin

A total of 2081 patients with type 2 diabetes participated in two 26-week, double-blind, placebo-controlled studies to evaluate the efficacy and safety of NESINA as add-on therapy to metformin. In both studies, patients were inadequately controlled on metformin at a dose of at least 1500 mg per day or at the maximum tolerated dose. All patients entered a four-week, single-blind placebo run-in period prior to randomization. Patients who failed to meet prespecified hyperglycemic goals during the 26-week treatment periods received glycemic rescue therapy.

In the first 26-week, placebo-controlled study, a total of 527 patients already on metformin (mean baseline A1C = 8%) were randomized to receive NESINA 12.5 mg, NESINA 25 mg or placebo. Patients were maintained on a stable dose of metformin (median dose = 1700 mg) during the treatment

Table 5. Glycemic Parameters at Week 26 for NESINA and Metformin Alone and in Combination in Patients with Type 2 Diabetes

	Placebo	NESINA 12.5 mg Twice Daily	Metformin HCl 500 mg Twice Daily	Metformin HCl 1000 mg Twice Daily	NESINA 12.5 mg + Metformin HCl 500 mg Twice Daily	NESINA 12.5 mg + Metformin HCl 1000 mg Twice Daily
A1C (%)*	N=102	N=104	N=103	N=108	N=102	N=111
Baseline (mean)	8.5	8.4	8.5	8.4	8.5	8.4
Change from baseline (adjusted mean†)	0.1	-0.6	-0.7	-1.1	-1.2	-1.6
Difference from metformin (adjusted mean† with 95% confidence interval)	-	-	-	-	-0.6‡ (-0.9, -0.3)	-0.4‡ (-0.7, -0.2)
Difference from NESINA (adjusted mean† with 95% confidence interval)	-	-	-	-	-0.7‡ (-1.0, -0.4)	-1.0‡ (-1.3, -0.7)
% of patients (n/N) achieving A1C <7%§	4% (4/102)	20% (21/104)	27% (28/103)	34% (37/108)	47%‡ (48/102)	59%‡ (66/111)
FPG (mg/dL)*	N=105	N=106	N=106	N=110	N=106	N=112
Baseline (mean)	187	177	180	181	176	185
Change from baseline (adjusted mean†)	12	-10	-12	-32	-32	-46
Difference from metformin (adjusted mean† with 95% confidence interval)	-	-	-	-	-20‡ (-33, -8)	-14‡ (-26, -2)
Difference from NESINA (adjusted mean† with 95% confidence interval)	-	-	-	-	-22‡ (-35, -10)	-36‡ (-49, -24)
2-Hour PPG (mg/dL)¶	N=26	N=34	N=28	N=37	N=31	N=37
Baseline (mean)	263	272	247	266	261	268
Change from baseline (adjusted mean†)	-21	-43	-49	-54	-68	-86‡
Difference from metformin (adjusted mean† with 95% confidence interval)	-	-	-	-	-19 (-49, 11)	-32‡ (-58, -5)
Difference from NESINA (adjusted mean† with 95% confidence interval)	-	-	-	-	-25 (-53, -3)	-43‡ (-70, -16)

* Intent-to-treat population using last observation on study prior to discontinuation of double-blind study medication or sulfonylurea rescue therapy for patients needing rescue
† Least squares means adjusted for treatment, geographic region and baseline value
‡ p<0.05 when compared to metformin and NESINA alone
§ Compared using logistic regression
¶ Intent-to-treat population using data available at Week 26

period. NESINA 25 mg in combination with metformin resulted in statistically significant improvements from baseline in A1C and FPG at Week 26, when compared to placebo *(Table 6)*. A total of 8% of patients receiving NESINA 25 mg and 24% of patients receiving placebo required glycemic rescue.

Improvements in A1C were not affected by gender, age, baseline BMI or baseline metformin dose.

The mean decrease in body weight was similar between NESINA and placebo when given in combination with metformin.

[See table 6 at top of next page]

In the second 26-week, double-blind, placebo-controlled study, a total of 1554 patients already on metformin (mean baseline A1C = 8.5%) were randomized to one of 12 double-blind treatment groups: placebo; 12.5 mg or 25 mg of NESINA alone; 15 mg, 30 mg or 45 mg of pioglitazone alone; or 12.5 mg or 25 mg of NESINA in combination with 15 mg, 30 mg or 45 mg of pioglitazone. Patients were maintained on a stable dose of metformin (median dose = 1700 mg) during the treatment period. Coadministration of NESINA and pioglitazone provided statistically significant improvements in A1C and FPG compared to placebo, to NESINA alone or to pioglitazone alone when added to background metformin therapy (*Table 7, Figure 3*). In addition, improvements from baseline A1C were comparable between NESINA alone and pioglitazone alone (15 mg, 30 mg and 45 mg) at Week 26. A total of 4%, 5% or 2% of patients receiving NESINA 25 mg with 15 mg, 30 mg or 45 mg pioglitazone, 33% of patients receiving placebo, 13% of patients receiving NESINA 25 mg and 10%, 15% or 9% of patients receiving pioglitazone 15 mg, 30 mg or 45 mg alone required glycemic rescue.

Improvements in A1C were not affected by gender, age or baseline BMI.

The mean increase in body weight was similar between pioglitazone alone and NESINA when coadministered with pioglitazone.

[See table 7 on pages 2393 and 2394]
[See figure 3 at top of next column]

Add-On Therapy to a Thiazolidinedione

In a 26-week, placebo-controlled study, a total of 493 patients inadequately controlled on a thiazolidinedione alone or in combination with metformin or a sulfonylurea (10 mg) (mean baseline A1C = 8%) were randomized to receive

Figure 3. Change from Baseline in A1C at Week 26 with NESINA and Pioglitazone Alone and NESINA in Combination with Pioglitazone When Added to Metformin

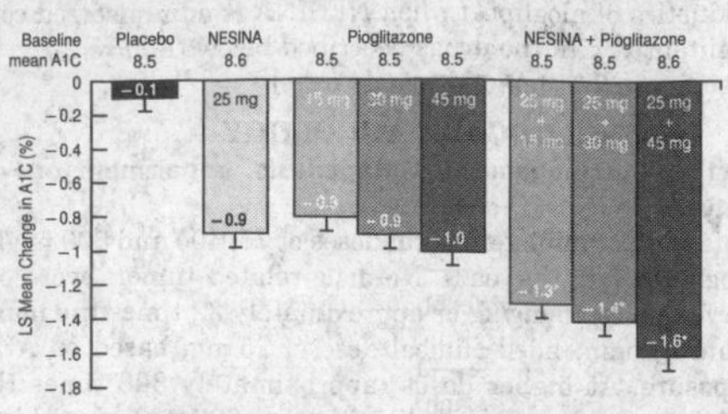

Intent-to-treat population using last observation on study.
*P≤0.001 compared to corresponding doses of NESINA alone or Pioglitazone alone.

NESINA 12.5 mg, NESINA 25 mg or placebo. Patients were maintained on a stable dose of pioglitazone (median dose = 30 mg) during the treatment period; those who were also previously treated on metformin (median dose = 2000 mg) or sulfonylurea (median dose = 10 mg) prior to randomization were maintained on the combination therapy during the treatment period. All patients entered into a four-week, single-blind placebo run-in period prior to randomization. Patients who failed to meet prespecified hyperglycemic goals during the 26-week treatment period received glycemic rescue therapy.

The addition of NESINA 25 mg once daily to pioglitazone therapy resulted in statistically significant improvements from baseline in A1C and FPG at Week 26, compared to placebo (*Table 8*). A total of 9% of patients who were receiving NESINA 25 mg and 12% of patients receiving placebo required glycemic rescue.

Improvements in A1C were not affected by gender, age, baseline BMI or baseline pioglitazone dose.

Clinically meaningful reductions in A1C were observed with NESINA compared to placebo regardless of whether subjects were receiving concomitant metformin or sulfonylurea (-0.2% placebo versus -0.9% NESINA) therapy or pioglitazone alone (0% placebo versus -0.52% NESINA).

The mean increase in body weight was similar between NESINA and placebo when given in combination with pioglitazone.

[See table 8 at top of page 2394]

Add-on Combination Therapy with Pioglitazone and Metformin

In a 52-week, active-comparator study, a total of 803 patients inadequately controlled (mean baseline A1C = 8.2%) on a current regimen of pioglitazone 30 mg and metformin at least 1500 mg per day or at the maximum tolerated dose were randomized to either receive the addition of NESINA 25 mg or the titration of pioglitazone 30 mg to 45 mg following a four-week, single-blind placebo run-in period. Patients were maintained on a stable dose of metformin (median dose = 1700 mg). Patients who failed to meet prespecified hyperglycemic goals during the 52-week treatment period received glycemic rescue therapy.

In combination with pioglitazone and metformin, NESINA 25 mg was shown to be statistically superior in lowering A1C and FPG compared with the titration of pioglitazone from 30 mg to 45 mg at Week 26 and at Week 52 (*Table 9; results shown only for Week 52*). A total of 11% of patients in the NESINA 25 mg treatment group and 22% of patients in the pioglitazone up-titration group required glycemic rescue.

Improvements in A1C were not affected by gender, age, race or baseline BMI.

The mean increase in body weight was similar in both treatment arms.

[See table 9 on pages 2394 and 2395]

Add-On Therapy to a Sulfonylurea

In a 26-week, placebo-controlled study, a total of 500 patients inadequately controlled on a sulfonylurea (mean baseline A1C = 8.1%) were randomized to receive NESINA 12.5 mg, NESINA 25 mg or placebo. Patients were maintained on a stable dose of glyburide (median dose = 10 mg) during the treatment period. All patients entered into a four-week, single-blind, placebo run-in period prior to randomization. Patients who failed to meet prespecified hyperglycemic goals during the 26-week treatment period received glycemic rescue therapy.

The addition of NESINA 25 mg to glyburide therapy resulted in statistically significant improvements from baseline in A1C at Week 26 when compared to placebo *(Table 10)*. Improvements in FPG observed with NESINA 25 mg were not statistically significant compared with placebo. A total of 16% of patients receiving NESINA 25 mg and 28% of those receiving placebo required glycemic rescue.

Improvements in A1C were not affected by gender, age, baseline BMI or baseline glyburide dose.

Table 6. Glycemic Parameters at Week 26 in a Placebo-Controlled Study of NESINA as Add-On Therapy to Metformin*

	NESINA 25 mg + Metformin	Placebo + Metformin
A1C (%)	N=203	N=103
Baseline (mean)	7.9	8.0
Change from baseline (adjusted mean†)	-0.6	-0.1
Difference from placebo (adjusted mean† with 95% confidence interval)	-0.5‡ (-0.7, -0.3)	-
% of patients (n/N) achieving A1C ≤7%	44% (92/207)‡	18% (19/104)
FPG (mg/dL)	N=204	N=104
Baseline (mean)	172	180
Change from baseline (adjusted mean†)	-17	0
Difference from placebo (adjusted mean† with 95% confidence interval)	-17‡ (-26, -9)	-

* Intent-to-treat population using last observation on study
† Least squares means adjusted for treatment, baseline value, geographic region and baseline metformin dose
‡ p<0.001 compared to placebo

Table 7. Glycemic Parameters in a 26-Week Study of NESINA, Pioglitazone and NESINA in Combination with Pioglitazone when Added to Metformin*

	Placebo	NESINA 25 mg	Pioglitazone 15 mg	Pioglitazone 30 mg	Pioglitazone 45 mg	NESINA 25 mg + Pioglitazone 15 mg	NESINA 25 mg + Pioglitazone 30 mg	NESINA 25 mg + Pioglitazone 45 mg
A1C (%)	N=126	N=123	N=127	N=123	N=126	N=127	N=124	N=126
Baseline (mean)	8.5	8.6	8.5	8.5	8.5	8.5	8.5	8.6
Change from baseline (adjusted mean†)	-0.1	-0.9	-0.8	-0.9	-1.0	-1.3‡	-1.4‡	-1.6‡
Difference from pioglitazone (adjusted mean† with 95% confidence interval)	-	-	-	-		-0.5‡ (-0.7, -0.3)	-0.5‡ (-0.7, -0.3)	-0.6‡ (-0.8, -0.4)
Difference from NESINA (adjusted mean† with 95% confidence interval)						-0.4‡ (-0.6, -0.1)	-0.5‡ (-0.7, -0.3)	-0.7‡ (-0.9, -0.5)
Patients (%) achieving A1C ≤7%	6% (8/129)	27% (35/129)	26% (33/129)	30% (38/129)	36% (47/129)	55% (71/130)‡	53% (69/130)‡	60% (78/130)‡
FPG (mg/dL)	N=129	N=126	N=127	N=125	N=129	N=130	N=126	N=127
Baseline (mean)	177	184	177	175	181	179	179	178
Change from baseline (adjusted mean†)	7	-19	-24	-29	-32	-38‡	-42‡	-53‡

(Table continued on next page)

The mean change in body weight was similar between NESINA and placebo when given in combination with glyburide.

[See table 10 at top of page 2395]

Add-On Therapy to Insulin

In a 26-week, placebo-controlled study, a total of 390 patients inadequately controlled on insulin alone (42%) or in combination with metformin (58%) (mean baseline A1C = 9.3%) were randomized to receive NESINA 12.5 mg, NESINA 25 mg or placebo. Patients were maintained on their insulin regimen (median dose = 55 IU) upon randomization and those previously treated with insulin in combination with metformin (median dose = 1700 mg) prior to randomization continued on the combination regimen during the treatment period. Patients entered the trial on short-, intermediate- or long-acting (basal) insulin or premixed insulin. Patients who failed to meet prespecified hyperglycemic goals during the 26-week treatment period received glycemic rescue therapy.

The addition of NESINA 25 mg once daily to insulin therapy resulted in statistically significant improvements from baseline in A1C and FPG at Week 26, when compared to placebo *(Table 11)*. A total of 20% of patients receiving NESINA 25 mg and 40% of those receiving placebo required glycemic rescue.

Improvements in A1C were not affected by gender, age, baseline BMI or baseline insulin dose. Clinically meaningful reductions in A1C were observed with NESINA compared to placebo regardless of whether subjects were receiving concomitant metformin and insulin (-0.2% placebo versus -0.8% NESINA) therapy or insulin alone (0.1% placebo versus -0.7% NESINA).

The mean increase in body weight was similar between NESINA and placebo when given in combination with insulin.

[See table 11 at top of page 2395]

16 HOW SUPPLIED/STORAGE AND HANDLING

NESINA tablets are available as film-coated tablets containing 25 mg, 12.5 mg or 6.25 mg of alogliptin as follows:

25 mg tablet: light red, oval, biconvex, film-coated, with "TAK ALG-25" printed on one side, available in:

NDC 64764-250-30	Bottles of 30 tablets
NDC 64764-250-90	Bottles of 90 tablets
NDC 64764-250-50	Bottles of 500 tablets

12.5 mg tablet: yellow, oval, biconvex, film-coated, with "TAK ALG-12.5" printed on one side, available in:

NDC 64764-125-30	Bottles of 30 tablets
NDC 64764-125-90	Bottles of 90 tablets
NDC 64764-125-50	Bottles of 500 tablets

6.25 mg tablet: light pink, oval, biconvex, film-coated, with "TAK ALG-6.25" printed on one side, available in:

NDC 64764-625-30	Bottles of 30 tablets
NDC 64764-625-90	Bottles of 90 tablets

Storage

Store at 25°C (77°F); excursions permitted to 15° to 30°C (59° to 86°F) [see USP Controlled Room Temperature].

17 PATIENT COUNSELING INFORMATION

See FDA-Approved Patient Labeling (Medication Guide)

17.1 Instructions

Inform patients of the potential risks and benefits of NESINA.

Patients should be informed that acute pancreatitis has been reported during use of NESINA. Patients should be informed that persistent, severe abdominal pain, sometimes radiating to the back, which may or may not be accompanied by vomiting, is the hallmark symptom of acute pancreatitis. Patients should be instructed to promptly discontinue NESINA and contact their physician if persistent severe abdominal pain occurs.

Patients should be informed that allergic reactions have been reported during use of NESINA. If symptoms of allergic reactions (including skin rash, hives and swelling of the face, lips, tongue and throat that may cause difficulty in breathing or swallowing) occur, patients should be instructed to discontinue NESINA and seek medical advice promptly.

Patients should be informed that postmarketing reports of liver injury, sometimes fatal, have been reported during use of NESINA. If signs or symptoms of liver injury occur, patients should be instructed to discontinue NESINA and seek medical advice promptly.

Inform patients that hypoglycemia can occur, particularly when an insulin secretagogue or insulin is used in combination with NESINA. Explain the risks, symptoms and appropriate management of hypoglycemia.

Instruct patients to take NESINA only as prescribed. If a dose is missed, advise patients not to double their next dose. Instruct patients to read the Medication Guide before starting NESINA therapy and to reread each time the prescription is refilled. Instruct patients to inform their healthcare provider if an unusual symptom develops or if a symptom persists or worsens.

Revised: June 2013
NES011 R3

MEDICATION GUIDE
NESINA (nes-see'-na)
(alogliptin)
tablets

Read this Medication Guide carefully before you start taking NESINA and each time you get a refill. There may be new information. This information does not take the place of talking with your doctor about your medical condition or treatment. If you have any questions about NESINA, ask your doctor or pharmacist.

What is the most important information I should know about NESINA?

Serious side effects can happen to people taking NESINA, including inflammation of the pancreas (pancreatitis), which may be severe.

Certain medical conditions make you more likely to get pancreatitis.

Before you start taking NESINA:

Tell your doctor if you have ever had:
- pancreatitis
- stones in your gallbladder (gallstones)
- a history of alcoholism
- kidney problems
- liver problems

Stop taking NESINA and call your doctor right away if you have pain in your stomach area (abdomen) that is severe and will not go away. The pain may be felt going from your abdomen through to your back. The pain may happen with or without vomiting. These may be symptoms of pancreatitis.

What is NESINA?
- NESINA is a prescription medicine used along with diet and exercise to improve blood sugar (glucose) control in adults with type 2 diabetes.
- NESINA is unlikely by itself to cause your blood sugar to be lowered to a dangerous level (hypoglycemia). However, hypoglycemia may still occur with NESINA.
- NESINA is not for people with type 1 diabetes.
- NESINA is not for people with diabetic ketoacidosis (increased ketones in blood or urine).

  It is not known if NESINA is safe and effective in children under the age of 18.

Who should not take NESINA?

Do not take NESINA if you:
- Are allergic to any ingredients in NESINA or have had a serious allergic (hypersensitivity) reaction to NESINA. See the end of this Medication Guide for a complete list of the ingredients in NESINA.
- Symptoms of a serious allergic reaction to NESINA may include:
  - swelling of your face, lips, throat and other areas on your skin
  - difficulty with swallowing or breathing
  - raised, red areas on your skin (hives)
  - skin rash, itching, flaking or peeling

If you have any of these symptoms, stop taking NESINA and contact your doctor or go to the nearest hospital emergency room right away.

What should I tell my doctor before and during treatment with NESINA?

Before you take NESINA, tell your doctor if you:
- have or have had inflammation of your pancreas (pancreatitis)
- have kidney or liver problems
- have other medical conditions
- are pregnant or plan to become pregnant. It is not known if NESINA can harm your unborn baby. Talk with your doctor about the best way to control your blood sugar while you are pregnant or if you plan to become pregnant
- are breastfeeding or plan to breastfeed. It is not known whether NESINA passes into your breast milk. Talk with your doctor about the best way to feed your baby if you are taking NESINA

Tell your doctor about all the medicines you take, including prescription and nonprescription medicines, vitamins and herbal supplements.

Know the medicines you take. Keep a list of them and show it to your doctor and pharmacist before you start any new medicine.

NESINA may affect the way other medicines work, and other medicines may affect how NESINA works. Contact your doctor before you start or stop other types of medicines.

How should I take NESINA?
- Take NESINA exactly as your doctor tells you to take it.
- Take NESINA 1 time each day with or without food.
- If you miss a dose, take it as soon as you remember. If you do not remember until it is time for your next dose, skip the missed dose, and take the next dose at your regular time. **Do not** take 2 doses of NESINA at the same time
- If you take too much NESINA, call your doctor or go to the nearest hospital emergency room right away
- If your body is under stress, such as from fever, infection, accident or surgery, the dose of your diabetes medicines may need to be changed. Call your doctor right away
- Stay on your diet and exercise programs and check your blood sugar as your doctor tells you to
- Your doctor may do certain blood tests before you start NESINA and during treatment as needed. Your doctor

Table 7 *(cont.)*. Glycemic Parameters in a 26-Week Study of NESINA, Pioglitazone and NESINA in Combination with Pioglitazone when Added to Metformin*

	Placebo	NESINA 25 mg	Pioglitazone 15 mg	Pioglitazone 30 mg	Pioglitazone 45 mg	NESINA 25 mg + Pioglitazone 15 mg	NESINA 25 mg + Pioglitazone 30 mg	NESINA 25 mg + Pioglitazone 45 mg
A1C (%)	N=126	N=123	N=127	N=123	N=126	N=127	N=124	N=126
Difference from pioglitazone (adjusted mean† with 95% confidence interval)	-	-	-	-	-	-14‡ (-24, -5)	-13‡ (-23, -3)	-20‡ (-30, -11)
Difference from NESINA (adjusted mean† with 95% confidence interval)	-	-	-	-	-	-19‡ (-29, -10)	-23‡ (-33, -13)	-34‡ (-44, -24)

* Intent-to-treat population using last observation on study
† Least squares means adjusted for treatment, geographic region, metformin dose and baseline value
‡ p≤0.01 when compared to corresponding doses of pioglitazone and NESINA alone

Table 8. Glycemic Parameters in a 26-Week, Placebo-Controlled Study of NESINA as Add-On Therapy to Pioglitazone*

	NESINA 25 mg + Pioglitazone ± Metformin ± Sulfonylurea	Placebo + Pioglitazone ± Metformin ± Sulfonylurea
A1C (%)	N=195	N=95
Baseline (mean)	8	8
Change from baseline (adjusted mean†)	-0.8	-0.2
Difference from placebo (adjusted mean† with 95% confidence interval)	-0.6‡ (-0.8, -0.4)	-
% of patients (n/N) achieving A1C ≤7%	49% (98/199)‡	34% (33/97)
FPG (mg/dL)	N=197	N=97
Baseline (mean)	170	172
Change from baseline (adjusted mean†)	-20	-6
Difference from placebo (adjusted mean† with 95% confidence interval)	-14‡ (-23, -5)	-

* Intent-to-treat population using last observation on study
† Least squares means adjusted for treatment, baseline value, geographic region, baseline treatment regimen (pioglitazone, pioglitazone + metformin or pioglitazone + sulfonylurea) and baseline pioglitazone dose
‡ p<0.01 compared to placebo

Table 9. Glycemic Parameters in a 52-Week, Controlled Study of NESINA as Add-On Combination Therapy with Pioglitazone and Metformin*

	NESINA 25 mg + Pioglitazone 30 mg + Metformin	Pioglitazone 45 mg + Metformin
A1C (%)	N=397	N=394
Baseline (mean)	8.2	8.1
Change from baseline (adjusted mean†)	-0.7	-0.3
Difference from pioglitazone 45 mg + metformin (adjusted mean† with 95% confidence interval)	-0.4‡ (-0.5, -0.3)	-
% of patients (n/N) achieving A1C≤7%	33% (134/404)§	21% (85/399)

(Table continued on next page)

Table 9 *(cont.)*. Glycemic Parameters in a 52-Week, Controlled Study of NESINA as Add-On Combination Therapy with Pioglitazone and Metformin*

	NESINA 25 mg + Pioglitazone 30 mg + Metformin	Pioglitazone 45 mg + Metformin
Fasting Plasma Glucose (mg/dL)	N=399	N=396
Baseline (mean)	162	162
Change from baseline (adjusted mean†)	-15	-4
Difference from pioglitazone 45 mg + metformin (adjusted mean† with 95% confidence interval)	-11§ (-16, -6)	

* Intent-to-treat population using last observation on study
† Least squares means adjusted for treatment, baseline value, geographic region and baseline metformin dose.
‡ Noninferior and statistically superior to metformin + pioglitazone at the 0.025 one-sided significance level
§ p<0.001 compared to pioglitazone 45 mg + metformin

Table 10. Glycemic Parameters in a 26-Week, Placebo-Controlled Study of NESINA as Add-On Therapy to Glyburide*

	NESINA 25 mg + Glyburide	Placebo + Glyburide
A1C (%)	N=197	N=97
Baseline (mean)	8.1	8.2
Change from baseline (adjusted mean†)	-0.5	0
Difference from placebo (adjusted mean† with 95% confidence interval)	-0.5‡ (-0.7, -0.3)	-
% of patients (n/N) achieving A1C ≤7%	35% (69/198)‡	18% (18/99)
FPG (mg/dL)	N=198	N=99
Baseline (mean)	174	177
Change from baseline (adjusted mean†)	-8	2
Difference from placebo (adjusted mean† with 95% confidence interval)	-11 (-22, 1)	-

* Intent-to-treat population using last observation on study
† Least squares means adjusted for treatment, baseline value, geographic region and baseline glyburide dose
‡ p<0.01 compared to placebo

Table 11. Glycemic Parameters in a 26-Week, Placebo-Controlled Study of NESINA as Add-On Therapy to Insulin*

	NESINA 25 mg + Insulin ± Metformin	Placebo + Insulin ± Metformin
A1C (%)	N=126	N=126
Baseline (mean)	9.3	9.3
Change from baseline (adjusted mean†)	-0.7	-0.1
Difference from placebo (adjusted mean† with 95% confidence interval)	-0.6‡ (-0.8, -0.4)	-
% of patients (n/N) achieving A1C ≤7%	8% (10/129)	1% (1/129)
FPG (mg/dL)	N=128	N=127
Baseline (mean)	186	196
Change from baseline (adjusted mean†)	-12	6
Difference from placebo (adjusted mean† with 95% confidence interval)	-18‡ (-33, -2)	-

* Intent-to-treat population using last observation on study
† Least squares means adjusted for treatment, baseline value, geographic region, baseline treatment regimen (insulin or insulin + metformin) and baseline daily insulin dose
‡ p<0.05 compared to placebo

may change your dose of NESINA based on the results of your blood tests due to how well your kidneys are working
- Your doctor will check your diabetes with regular blood tests, including your blood sugar levels and your hemoglobin A1C

What are the possible side effects of NESINA?
NESINA can cause serious side effects, including:
See **"What is the most important information I should know about NESINA?"**

- **Allergic (hypersensitivity) reactions** such as:
  - swelling of your face, lips, throat and other areas on your skin
  - difficulty with swallowing or breathing
  - raised, red areas on your skin (hives)
  - skin rash, itching, flaking or peeling

If you have these symptoms, stop taking NESINA and contact your doctor right away.

- **Liver problems.** Call your doctor right away if you have unexplained symptoms, such as:
  - nausea or vomiting
  - stomach pain
  - unusual or unexplained tiredness
  - loss of appetite
  - dark urine
  - yellowing of your skin or the whites of your eyes
- **Low blood sugar (hypoglycemia).** If you take NESINA with another medicine that can cause low blood sugar, such as a sulfonylurea or insulin, your risk of getting low blood sugar is higher. The dose of your sulfonylurea medicine or insulin may need to be lowered while you take NESINA. If you have symptoms of low blood sugar, you should check your blood sugar and treat if low, then call your doctor. Signs and symptoms of low blood sugar include:

• shaking or feeling jittery	• fast heartbeat
• sweating	• change in vision
• hunger	• confusion
• headache	• dizziness
• change in mood	

The most common side effects of NESINA include:
- stuffy or runny nose and sore throat
- headache
- cold-like symptoms (upper respiratory tract infection)

Tell your doctor if you have any side effect that bothers you or that does not go away.
These are not all the possible side effects of NESINA. For more information, ask your doctor or pharmacist.
Call your doctor for medical advice about side effects. You may report side effects to FDA at 1-800-FDA-1088.

How should I store NESINA?
Store NESINA at room temperature between 68°F to 77°F (20°C to 25°C).
Keep NESINA and all medicines out of the reach of children.

General information about the safe and effective use of NESINA
Medicines are sometimes prescribed for purposes other than those listed in the Medication Guide. Do not take NESINA for a condition for which it was not prescribed. Do not give NESINA to other people, even if they have the same symptoms you have. It may harm them.
This Medication Guide summarizes the most important information about NESINA. If you would like to know more information, talk with your doctor. You can ask your doctor or pharmacist for information about NESINA that is written for health professionals.
For more information go to www.NESINA.com or call 1-877-TAKEDA-7 (1-877-825-3327).

What are the ingredients in NESINA?
Active ingredient: alogliptin
Inactive ingredients: mannitol, microcrystalline cellulose, hydroxypropyl cellulose, croscarmellose sodium and magnesium stearate. In addition, the film-coating contains the following inactive ingredients: hypromellose, titanium dioxide, ferric oxide (red or yellow) and polyethylene glycol and is marked with gray F1 printing ink
This Medication Guide has been approved by the U.S. Food and Drug Administration.
Distributed by:
Takeda Pharmaceuticals America, Inc.
Deerfield, IL 60015
Revised: June 2013
NESINA is a trademark of Takeda Pharmaceutical Company Limited registered with the U.S. Patent and Trademark Office and is used under license by Takeda Pharmaceuticals America, Inc.

NES011 R3
Shown in Product Identification Guide, page 313

OSENI ℞
(alogliptin and pioglitazone)
tablets

HIGHLIGHTS OF PRESCRIBING INFORMATION
These highlights do not include all the information needed to use OSENI safely and effectively. See full prescribing information for OSENI.
OSENI (alogliptin and pioglitazone) tablets
Initial U.S. Approval: 2013

WARNING: CONGESTIVE HEART FAILURE
See full prescribing information for complete boxed warning
- **Thiazolidinediones, including pioglitazone, cause or exacerbate congestive heart failure in some patients. (5.1)**

- **After initiation of OSENI and after dose increases, monitor patients carefully for signs and symptoms of heart failure (e.g., excessive, rapid weight gain, dyspnea and/or edema). If heart failure develops, it should be managed according to current standards of care and discontinuation or dose reduction of pioglitazone in OSENI must be considered.**
- **OSENI is not recommended in patients with symptomatic heart failure.**
- **Initiation of OSENI in patients with established New York Heart Association (NYHA) Class III or IV heart failure is contraindicated. (4, 5.1)**

INDICATIONS AND USAGE

OSENI is a dipeptidyl peptidase-4 inhibitor and thiazolidinedione combination product indicated as an adjunct to diet and exercise to improve glycemic control in adults with type 2 diabetes mellitus. (1.1)
Limitation of Use: Not for treatment of type 1 diabetes or diabetic ketoacidosis. (1.2)

DOSAGE AND ADMINISTRATION

- Individualize the starting dose of OSENI based on the patient's current regimen and concurrent medical condition but do not exceed a daily dose of alogliptin 25 mg and pioglitazone 45 mg.
- Can be taken with or without food. (2.1)
- Limit initial dose of pioglitazone to 15 mg once daily in patients with NYHA Class I or II heart failure. (2.1)
- Adjust dose if moderate renal impairment. (2.2)

Degree of Renal Impairment	Creatinine Clearance (mL/min)	Recommended Dosing
Moderate	≥30 to <60	12.5 mg/15 mg, 12.5 mg/30 mg or 12.5 mg/45 mg once daily

- OSENI is not recommended for patients with severe renal impairment or end-stage renal disease (ESRD) requiring dialysis. (2.2)
- The maximum recommended dose of pioglitazone is 15 mg once daily in patients taking strong CYP2C8 inhibitors (e.g., gemfibrozil). (2.3, 7.1)

DOSAGE FORMS AND STRENGTHS

Tablets:
25 mg alogliptin and 15 mg pioglitazone, 25 mg alogliptin and 30 mg pioglitazone, 25 mg alogliptin and 45 mg pioglitazone. (3)
12.5 mg alogliptin and 15 mg pioglitazone, 12.5 mg alogliptin and 30 mg pioglitazone, 12.5 mg alogliptin and 45 mg pioglitazone. (3)

CONTRAINDICATIONS

- History of a serious hypersensitivity reaction to alogliptin or pioglitazone, components of OSENI, such as anaphylaxis, angioedema or severe cutaneous adverse reactions. (4)
- Do not initiate OSENI in patients with established NYHA Class III or IV heart failure. (4)

WARNINGS AND PRECAUTIONS

- Congestive heart failure: Fluid retention may occur and can exacerbate or lead to congestive heart failure. Combination use with insulin and use in congestive heart failure NYHA Class I and II may increase risk. Monitor patients for signs and symptoms. (5.1)
- Acute pancreatitis: There have been postmarketing reports of acute pancreatitis. If pancreatitis is suspected, promptly discontinue OSENI. (5.2)
- Hypersensitivity: There have been postmarketing reports of serious hypersensitivity reactions in patients treated with alogliptin such as anaphylaxis, angioedema and severe cutaneous adverse reactions. In such cases, promptly discontinue OSENI, assess for other potential causes, institute appropriate monitoring and treatment and initiate alternative treatment for diabetes. (5.3)
- Hepatic effects: Postmarketing reports of hepatic failure, sometimes fatal. Causality cannot be excluded. If liver injury is detected, promptly interrupt OSENI and assess patient for probable cause, then treat cause if possible, to resolution or stabilization. Do not restart OSENI if liver injury is confirmed and no alternative etiology can be found. Use with caution in patients with liver disease. (5.4)
- Edema: Dose-related edema may occur. (5.5)
- Fractures: Increased incidence in female patients. Apply current standards of care for assessing and maintaining bone health. (5.6)
- Bladder cancer: Preclinical and clinical trial data, and results from an observational study suggest an increased risk of bladder cancer in pioglitazone users. The observational data further suggest that the risk increases with duration of use. Do not use in patients with active bladder cancer. Use caution when using in patients with a prior history of bladder cancer. (5.7)
- Hypoglycemia: When an insulin secretagogue (e.g., sulfonylurea) or insulin is used in combination with OSENI, a lower dose of insulin secretagogue or insulin may be required to minimize the risk of hypoglycemia. (5.8)
- Macular edema: Postmarketing reports. Recommend regular eye exams in all patients with diabetes according to current standards of care with prompt evaluation for acute visual changes. (5.9)
- Macrovascular outcomes: There have been no clinical studies establishing conclusive evidence of macrovascular risk reduction with OSENI or any other antidiabetic drug. (5.11)

ADVERSE REACTIONS

Common adverse reactions reported in ≥4% of patients treated with coadministration of alogliptin 25 mg and pioglitazone 15 mg, 30 mg or 45 mg were nasopharyngitis, back pain and upper respiratory tract infection. (6.1)
To report SUSPECTED ADVERSE REACTIONS, contact Takeda Pharmaceuticals at 1-877-TAKEDA-7 (1-877-825-3327) or FDA at 1-800-FDA-1088 or www.fda.gov/medwatch.

DRUG INTERACTIONS

- Strong CYP2C8 inhibitors (e.g., gemfibrozil) increase pioglitazone concentrations. Limit the pioglitazone dose to 15 mg daily. (2.3, 7.1)
- CYP2C8 inducers (e.g., rifampin) may decrease pioglitazone concentrations. (7.2)

USE IN SPECIFIC POPULATIONS

- Nursing mothers: Discontinue drug or nursing, taking into consideration the importance of the drug to the mother. (8.3)

See 17 for PATIENT COUNSELING INFORMATION and Medication Guide

Revised: 07/2013

FULL PRESCRIBING INFORMATION: CONTENTS*

*** Sections or subsections omitted from the full prescribing information are not listed**

FULL PRESCRIBING INFORMATION

WARNING: CONGESTIVE HEART FAILURE

- **Thiazolidinediones, including pioglitazone, which is a component of OSENI, cause or exacerbate congestive heart failure in some patients *[see Warnings and Precautions (5.1)]*.**
- **After initiation of OSENI and after dose increases, monitor patients carefully for signs and symptoms of heart failure (e.g., excessive, rapid weight gain, dyspnea and/or edema). If heart failure develops, it should be managed according to current standards of care and discontinuation or dose reduction of pioglitazone in OSENI must be considered.**
- **OSENI is not recommended in patients with symptomatic heart failure.**
- **Initiation of OSENI in patients with established New York Heart Association (NYHA) Class III or IV heart failure is contraindicated *[see Contraindications (4)* and *Warnings and Precautions (5.1)]*.**

1 INDICATIONS AND USAGE

1.1 Monotherapy and Combination Therapy

OSENI is indicated as an adjunct to diet and exercise to improve glycemic control in adults with type 2 diabetes mellitus in multiple clinical settings when treatment with both alogliptin and pioglitazone is appropriate *[see Clinical Studies (14)]*.

1.2 Limitation of Use

OSENI should not be used in patients with type 1 diabetes mellitus or for the treatment of diabetic ketoacidosis, as it would not be effective in these settings.
Use with caution in patients with liver disease *[see Warnings and Precautions (5.4)]*.

2 DOSAGE AND ADMINISTRATION

2.1 Recommendations for All Patients

OSENI should be taken once daily and can be taken with or without food. The tablets must not be split before swallowing.
The recommended starting dose for OSENI (alogliptin and pioglitazone):
- for patients inadequately controlled on diet and exercise is 25 mg/15 mg or 25 mg/30 mg,
- for patients inadequately controlled on metformin monotherapy is 25 mg/15 mg or 25 mg/30 mg,
- for patients on alogliptin who require additional glycemic control is 25 mg/15 mg or 25 mg/30 mg,
- for patients on pioglitazone who require additional glycemic control is 25 mg/15 mg, 25 mg/30 mg or 25 mg/45 mg as appropriate based upon current therapy,
- for patients switching from alogliptin coadministered with pioglitazone, OSENI may be initiated at the dose of alogliptin and pioglitazone based upon current therapy,
- for patients with congestive heart failure (NYHA Class I or II) is 25 mg/15 mg.

The OSENI dose can be titrated up to a maximum of 25 mg/45 mg once daily based on glycemic response as determined by hemoglobin A1c (A1C).
After initiation of OSENI or with dose increase, monitor patients carefully for adverse reactions related to fluid retention as has been seen with pioglitazone (e.g., weight gain, edema and signs and symptoms of congestive heart failure) *[see Boxed Warning and Warnings and Precautions (5.1)]*.

2.2 Patients with Renal Impairment

No dose adjustment of OSENI is necessary for patients with mild renal impairment (creatinine clearance [CrCl] ≥60 mL/min).
The dose of OSENI is 12.5 mg/15 mg, 12.5 mg/30 mg or 12.5 mg/45 mg once daily for patients with moderate renal impairment (CrCl ≥30 to <60 mL/min).
OSENI is not recommended for patients with severe renal impairment or ESRD *[see Clinical Pharmacology (12.3)]*. Coadministration of pioglitazone and alogliptin 6.25 mg once daily based on individual requirements may be considered in these patients.
Because there is a need for dose adjustment based upon renal function, assessment of renal function is recommended prior to initiation of OSENI therapy and periodically thereafter.

2.3 Coadministration with Strong CYP2C8 Inhibitors

Coadministration of pioglitazone and gemfibrozil, a strong CYP2C8 inhibitor, increases pioglitazone exposure approximately three-fold. Therefore, the maximum recommended dose of OSENI is 25 mg/15 mg daily when used in combination with gemfibrozil or other strong CYP2C8 inhibitors *[see Drug Interactions (7.1) and Clinical Pharmacology (12.3)]*.

3 DOSAGE FORMS AND STRENGTHS

- 25 mg/15 mg tablets are yellow, round, biconvex, and film-coated, with both "A/P" and "25/15" printed on one side.

- 25 mg/30 mg tablets are peach, round, biconvex, and film-coated, with both "A/P" and "25/30" printed on one side.
- 25 mg/45 mg tablets are red, round, biconvex, and film-coated, with both "A/P" and "25/45" printed on one side.
- 12.5 mg/15 mg tablets are pale yellow, round, biconvex, and film-coated, with both "A/P" and "12.5/15" printed on one side.
- 12.5 mg/30 mg tablets are pale peach, round, biconvex, and film-coated, with both "A/P" and "12.5/30" printed on one side.
- 12.5 mg/45 mg tablets are pale red, round, biconvex, and film-coated, with both "A/P" and "12.5/45" printed on one side.

4 CONTRAINDICATIONS

History of a serious hypersensitivity reaction to alogliptin or pioglitazone, components of OSENI, such as anaphylaxis, angioedema or severe cutaneous adverse reactions.
Do not initiate in patients with NYHA Class III or IV heart failure *[see Boxed Warning]*.

5 WARNINGS AND PRECAUTIONS

5.1 Congestive Heart Failure

Pioglitazone

Pioglitazone, like other thiazolidinediones, can cause dose-related fluid retention when used alone or in combination with other antidiabetic medications and is most common when pioglitazone is used in combination with insulin. Fluid retention may lead to or exacerbate congestive heart failure. Patients should be observed for signs and symptoms of congestive heart failure. If congestive heart failure develops, it should be managed according to current standards of care and discontinuation or dose reduction of pioglitazone must be considered *[see Boxed Warning, Contraindications (4) and Adverse Reactions (6.1)]*.

5.2 Pancreatitis

There have been postmarketing reports of acute pancreatitis in patients taking alogliptin. After initiation of OSENI, patients should be observed carefully for signs and symptoms of pancreatitis. If pancreatitis is suspected, OSENI should promptly be discontinued and appropriate management should be initiated. It is unknown whether patients with a history of pancreatitis are at increased risk for the development of pancreatitis while using OSENI.

5.3 Hypersensitivity Reactions

There have been postmarketing reports of serious hypersensitivity reactions in patients treated with alogliptin. These reactions include anaphylaxis, angioedema and severe cutaneous adverse reactions, including Stevens-Johnson syndrome. If a serious hypersensitivity reaction is suspected, discontinue OSENI, assess for other potential causes for the event and institute alternative treatment for diabetes *[see Adverse Reactions (6.3)]*. Use caution in patients with a history of angioedema to another DPP-4 inhibitor because it is unknown whether such patients will be predisposed to angioedema with OSENI.

5.4 Hepatic Effects

There have been postmarketing reports of fatal and nonfatal hepatic events in patients taking pioglitazone or alogliptin, although the reports contain insufficient information necessary to establish the probable cause *[see Adverse Reactions (6.3)]*. There has been no evidence of drug-induced hepatotoxicity in the pioglitazone controlled clinical trial database to date *[see Adverse Reactions (6.1)]*. In randomized controlled studies of alogliptin, serum alanine aminotransferase (ALT) elevations greater than three times the upper limit of normal (ULN) were observed: 1.3% in alogliptin-treated patients and 1.5% in all comparator-treated patients.

Patients with type 2 diabetes may have fatty liver disease or cardiac disease with episodic congestive heart failure, both of which may cause liver test abnormalities, and they may also have other forms of liver disease, many of which can be treated or managed. Therefore, obtaining a liver test panel (ALT, aspartate aminotransferase [AST], alkaline phosphatase and total bilirubin) and assessing the patient is recommended before initiating OSENI therapy. In patients with abnormal liver tests, OSENI should be initiated with caution.

Measure liver tests promptly in patients who report symptoms that may indicate liver injury, including fatigue, anorexia, right upper abdominal discomfort, dark urine or jaundice. In this clinical context, if the patient is found to have abnormal liver tests (ALT greater than three times the upper limit of the reference range), OSENI treatment should be interrupted and an investigation done to establish the probable cause. OSENI should not be restarted in these patients without another explanation for the liver test abnormalities.

5.5 Edema

Pioglitazone

In controlled clinical trials, edema was reported more frequently in patients treated with pioglitazone than in placebo-treated patients and is dose-related *[see Adverse Reactions (6.1)]*. In postmarketing experience, reports of new onset or worsening of edema have been received.

Table 1. Adverse Reactions Reported in ≥4% of Patients Treated with OSENI and More Frequently than in Patients Receiving Either Alogliptin, Pioglitazone or Placebo

	Number of Patients (%)			
	OSENI*	Alogliptin†	Pioglitazone‡	Placebo
	N=1533	N=446	N=949	N=153
Nasopharyngitis	75 (4.9)	21 (4.7)	37 (3.9)	6 (3.9)
Back Pain	64 (4.2)	9 (2.0)	32 (3.4)	5 (3.3)
Upper Respiratory Tract Infection	63 (4.1)	19 (4.3)	26 (2.7)	5 (3.3)

* OSENI – includes data pooled for patients receiving alogliptin 25 mg and 12.5 mg combined with pioglitazone 15 mg, 30 mg and 45 mg
† Alogliptin – includes data pooled for patients receiving alogliptin 25 mg and 12.5 mg
‡ Pioglitazone – includes data pooled for patients receiving pioglitazone 15 mg, 30 mg and 45 mg

OSENI should be used with caution in patients with edema. Because thiazolidinediones, including pioglitazone, can cause fluid retention, which can exacerbate or lead to congestive heart failure, OSENI should be used with caution in patients at risk for congestive heart failure. Patients treated with OSENI should be monitored for signs and symptoms of congestive heart failure *[see Boxed Warning, Warnings and Precautions (5.1) and Patient Counseling Information (17.1)]*.

5.6 Fractures

Pioglitazone

In PROactive (the Prospective Pioglitazone Clinical Trial in Macrovascular Events), 5238 patients with type 2 diabetes and a history of macrovascular disease were randomized to pioglitazone (N=2605), force-titrated up to 45 mg daily or placebo (N=2633) in addition to standard of care. During a mean follow-up of 34.5 months, the incidence of bone fracture in females was 5.1% (44/870) for pioglitazone versus 2.5% (23/905) for placebo. This difference was noted after the first year of treatment and persisted during the course of the study. The majority of fractures observed in female patients were nonvertebral fractures including lower limb and distal upper limb. No increase in the incidence of fracture was observed in men treated with pioglitazone (1.7%) versus placebo (2.1%). The risk of fracture should be considered in the care of patients, especially female patients, treated with pioglitazone and attention should be given to assessing and maintaining bone health according to current standards of care.

5.7 Urinary Bladder Tumors

Pioglitazone

Tumors were observed in the urinary bladder of male rats in the two-year carcinogenicity study *[see Nonclinical Toxicology (13.1)]*. In two 3-year trials in which pioglitazone was compared to placebo or glyburide, there were 16/3656 (0.44%) reports of bladder cancer in patients taking pioglitazone compared to 5/3679 (0.14%) in patients not taking pioglitazone. After excluding patients in whom exposure to study drug was less than one year at the time of diagnosis of bladder cancer, there were six (0.16%) cases on pioglitazone and two (0.05%) cases on placebo.

A five-year interim report of an ongoing 10-year observational cohort study found a nonsignificant increase in the risk for bladder cancer in subjects ever exposed to pioglitazone, compared to subjects never exposed to pioglitazone (HR 1.2 [95% CI 0.9–1.5]). Compared to never exposure, a duration of pioglitazone therapy longer than 12 months was associated with an increase in risk (HR 1.4 [95% CI 0.9–2.1]), which reached statistical significance after more than 24 months of pioglitazone use (HR 1.4 [95% CI 1.03–2.0]). Interim results from this study suggested that taking pioglitazone longer than 12 months increased the relative risk of developing bladder cancer in any given year by 40%, which equates to an absolute increase of three cases in 10,000 (from approximately seven in 10,000 [without pioglitazone] to approximately 10 in 10,000 [with pioglitazone]).

There are insufficient data to determine whether pioglitazone is a tumor promoter for urinary bladder tumors. Consequently, pioglitazone should not be used in patients with active bladder cancer and the benefits of glycemic control versus unknown risks for cancer recurrence with pioglitazone should be considered in patients with a prior history of bladder cancer.

5.8 Use with Medications Known to Cause Hypoglycemia

Insulin and insulin secretagogues, such as sulfonylureas, are known to cause hypoglycemia. Therefore, a lower dose of insulin or insulin secretagogue may be required to minimize the risk of hypoglycemia when used in combination with OSENI.

5.9 Macular Edema

Pioglitazone

Macular edema has been reported in postmarketing experience in diabetic patients who were taking pioglitazone or another thiazolidinedione. Some patients presented with blurred vision or decreased visual acuity, but others were diagnosed on routine ophthalmologic examination.

Most patients had peripheral edema at the time macular edema was diagnosed. Some patients had improvement in their macular edema after discontinuation of their thiazolidinedione.

Patients with diabetes should have regular eye exams by an ophthalmologist according to current standards of care. Patients with diabetes who report any visual symptoms should be promptly referred to an ophthalmologist, regardless of the patient's underlying medications or other physical findings *[see Adverse Reactions (6.1)]*.

5.10 Ovulation

Pioglitazone

Therapy with pioglitazone, like other thiazolidinediones, may result in ovulation in some premenopausal anovulatory women. As a result, these patients may be at an increased risk for pregnancy while taking OSENI *[see Use in Specific Populations (8.1)]*. This effect has not been investigated in clinical trials, so the frequency of this occurrence is not known. Adequate contraception in all premenopausal women treated with OSENI is recommended.

5.11 Macrovascular Outcomes

There have been no clinical studies establishing conclusive evidence of macrovascular risk reduction with OSENI or any other antidiabetic drug.

6 ADVERSE REACTIONS

6.1 Clinical Studies Experience

Because clinical trials are conducted under widely varying conditions, adverse reaction rates observed in the clinical trials of a drug cannot be directly compared to rates in the clinical trials of another drug and may not reflect the rates observed in clinical practice.

Alogliptin and Pioglitazone

Over 1500 patients with type 2 diabetes have received alogliptin coadministered with pioglitazone in four large, randomized, double-blind, controlled clinical trials. The mean exposure to OSENI was 29 weeks with more than 100 subjects treated for more than one year. The studies consisted of two placebo-controlled studies of 16 to 26 weeks in duration and two active-controlled studies of 26 weeks and 52 weeks in duration. In the OSENI arm, the mean duration of diabetes was approximately six years, the mean body mass index (BMI) was 31 kg/m^2 (54% of patients had a BMI ≥30 kg/m^2), and the mean age was 54 years (16% of patients ≥65 years of age).

In a pooled analysis of these four controlled clinical studies, the overall incidence of adverse events was 65% in patients treated with OSENI compared to 57% treated with placebo. Overall discontinuation of therapy due to adverse events was 2.5% with OSENI compared to 2.0% with placebo, 3.7% with pioglitazone or 1.3% with alogliptin.

Adverse reactions reported in ≥4% of patients treated with OSENI and more frequently than in patients who received alogliptin, pioglitazone or placebo are summarized in *Table 1*.

[See table 1 above]

Alogliptin Add-On Therapy to a Thiazolidinedione

In addition, in a 26-week, placebo-controlled, double-blind study, patients inadequately controlled on a thiazolidinedione alone or in combination with metformin or a sulfonylurea were treated with add-on alogliptin therapy or placebo; the adverse reactions reported in ≥5% of patients and more frequently than in patients who received placebo was influenza (alogliptin, 5.5%; placebo, 4.1%).

Hypoglycemia

In a 26-week, placebo-controlled factorial study with alogliptin in combination with pioglitazone on background therapy with metformin, the incidence of subjects reporting

Table 2. Adverse Reactions Reported in ≥4% Patients Treated with Alogliptin 25 mg and More Frequently than in Patients Given Placebo in Pooled Studies

	Number of Patients (%)		
	Alogliptin 25 mg	Placebo	Active Comparator
	N=5902	N=2926	N=2257
Nasopharyngitis	257 (4.4)	89 (3.0)	113 (5.0)
Headache	247 (4.2)	72 (2.5)	121 (5.4)
Upper Respiratory Tract Infection	247 (4.2)	61 (2.1)	113 (5.0)

hypoglycemia was 0.8%, 0% and 3.8% for alogliptin 25 mg with pioglitazone 15 mg, 30 mg or 45 mg, respectively; 2.3% for alogliptin 25 mg; 4.7%, 0.8% and 0.8% for pioglitazone 15 mg, 30 mg or 45 mg, respectively; and 0.8% for placebo. In a 26-week, active-controlled, double-blind study with alogliptin alone, pioglitazone alone or alogliptin coadministered with pioglitazone in patients inadequately controlled on diet and exercise, the incidence of hypoglycemia was 3% on alogliptin 25 mg with pioglitazone 30 mg, 0.6% on alogliptin 25 mg and 1.8% on pioglitazone 30 mg.

In a 52-week, active-controlled, double-blind study of alogliptin as add-on therapy to the combination of pioglitazone 30 mg and metformin compared to the titration of pioglitazone 30 mg to 45 mg and metformin, the incidence of subjects reporting hypoglycemia was 4.5% in the alogliptin 25 mg with pioglitazone 30 mg and metformin group versus 1.5% in the pioglitazone 45 mg and metformin group.

Alogliptin

Approximately 8500 patients with type 2 diabetes have been treated with alogliptin in 14 randomized, double-blind, controlled clinical trials with approximately 2900 subjects randomized to placebo and approximately 2200 to an active comparator. The mean exposure to alogliptin was 40 weeks with more than 2400 subjects treated for more than one year. Among these patients, 63% had a history of hypertension, 51% had a history of dyslipidemia, 25% had a history of myocardial infarction, 8% had a history of unstable angina and 7% had a history of congestive heart failure. The mean duration of diabetes was seven years, the mean BMI was 31 kg/m^2 (51% of patients had a BMI ≥30 kg/m^2) and the mean age was 57 years (24% of patients ≥65 years of age).

Two placebo-controlled monotherapy trials of 12 and 26 weeks in duration were conducted in patients treated with alogliptin 12.5 mg daily, alogliptin 25 mg daily and placebo. Four placebo-controlled add-on combination therapy trials of 26 weeks in duration were also conducted: with metformin, with a sulfonylurea, with a thiazolidinedione and with insulin.

Four placebo-controlled and one active-controlled trials of 16 weeks up through two years in duration were conducted in combination with metformin, in combination with pioglitazone and with pioglitazone added to a background of metformin therapy.

Three active-controlled trials of 52 weeks in duration were conducted in patients treated with pioglitazone and metformin, in combination with metformin and as monotherapy compared to glipizide.

In a pooled analysis of these 14 controlled clinical trials, the overall incidence of adverse events was 66% in patients treated with alogliptin 25 mg compared to 62% with placebo and 70% with active comparator. Overall discontinuation of therapy due to adverse events was 4.7% with alogliptin 25 mg compared to 4.5% with placebo or 6.2% with active comparator.

Adverse reactions reported in ≥4% of patients treated with alogliptin 25 mg and more frequently than in patients who received placebo are summarized in *Table 2*.

[See table 2 above]

Pancreatitis

In the clinical trial program, pancreatitis was reported in 11 of 5902 (0.2%) patients receiving alogliptin 25 mg daily compared to five of 5183 (<0.1%) patients receiving all comparators.

Hypersensitivity Reactions

In a pooled analysis, the overall incidence of hypersensitivity reactions was 0.6% with alogliptin 25 mg compared to 0.8% with all comparators. A single event of serum sickness was reported in a patient treated with alogliptin 25 mg.

Hypoglycemia

Hypoglycemic events were documented based upon a blood glucose value and/or clinical signs and symptoms of hypoglycemia.

In the monotherapy study, the incidence of hypoglycemia was 1.5% in patients treated with alogliptin compared to 1.6% with placebo. The use of alogliptin as add-on therapy to glyburide or insulin did not increase the incidence of hypoglycemia compared to placebo. In a monotherapy study comparing alogliptin to a sulfonylurea in elderly patients, the incidence of hypoglycemia was 5.4% with alogliptin compared to 26% with glipizide.

Pioglitazone

Over 8500 patients with type 2 diabetes have been treated with pioglitazone in randomized, double-blind, controlled clinical trials, including 2605 patients with type 2 diabetes and macrovascular disease treated with pioglitazone in the PROactive clinical trial. In these trials, over 6000 patients have been treated with pioglitazone for six months or longer, over 4500 patients have been treated with pioglitazone for one year or longer, and over 3000 patients have been treated with pioglitazone for at least two years.

Common Adverse Events: 16- to 26-Week Monotherapy Trials

A summary of the incidence and type of common adverse events reported in three pooled 16- to 26-week placebo-controlled monotherapy trials of pioglitazone is provided in *Table 3*. Terms that are reported represent those that occurred at an incidence of >5% and more commonly in patients treated with pioglitazone than in patients who received placebo. None of these adverse events were related to pioglitazone dose.

Table 3. Three Pooled 16- to 26-Week Placebo-Controlled Clinical Trials of Pioglitazone Monotherapy: Adverse Events Reported at an Incidence >5% and More Commonly in Patients Treated with Pioglitazone than in Patients Treated with Placebo

	% of Patients	
	Placebo N=259	Pioglitazone N=606
Upper Respiratory Tract Infection	8.5	13.2
Headache	6.9	9.1
Sinusitis	4.6	6.3
Myalgia	2.7	5.4
Pharyngitis	0.8	5.1

Congestive Heart Failure

A summary of the incidence of adverse events related to congestive heart failure for the 16- to 24-week add-on to sulfonylurea trials, for the 16- to 24-week add-on to insulin trials, and for the 16- to 24-week add-on to metformin trials were (at least one congestive heart failure, 0.2% to 1.7%; hospitalized due to congestive heart failure, 0.2% to 0.9%). None of the events were fatal.

Patients with type 2 diabetes and NYHA class II or early class III congestive heart failure were randomized to receive 24 weeks of double-blind treatment with either pioglitazone at daily doses of 30 mg to 45 mg (N=262) or glyburide at daily doses of 10 mg to 15 mg (N=256). A summary of the incidence of adverse events related to congestive heart failure reported in this study is provided in *Table 4*.

Table 4. Treatment-Emergent Adverse Events of Congestive Heart Failure (CHF) in Patients with NYHA Class II or III Congestive Heart Failure Treated with Pioglitazone or Glyburide

	Number (%) of Subjects	
	Pioglitazone N=262	Glyburide N=256
Death due to cardiovascular causes (adjudicated)	5 (1.9%)	6 (2.3%)
Overnight hospitalization for worsening CHF (adjudicated)	26 (9.9%)	12 (4.7%)
Emergency room visit for CHF (adjudicated)	4 (1.5%)	3 (1.2%)
Patients experiencing CHF progression during study	35 (13.4%)	21 (8.2%)

Congestive heart failure events leading to hospitalization that occurred during the PROactive trial are summarized in *Table 5*.

Table 5. Treatment-Emergent Adverse Events of Congestive Heart Failure (CHF) in PROactive Trial

	Number (%) of Patients	
	Placebo N=2633	Pioglitazone N=2605
At least one hospitalized congestive heart failure event	108 (4.1%)	149 (5.7%)
Fatal	22 (0.8%)	25 (1%)
Hospitalized, nonfatal	86 (3.3%)	124 (4.7%)

Cardiovascular Safety

In the PROactive trial, 5238 patients with type 2 diabetes and a history of macrovascular disease were randomized to pioglitazone (N=2605), force-titrated up to 45 mg daily or placebo (N=2633) in addition to standard of care. Almost all patients (95%) were receiving cardiovascular medications (beta blockers, ACE inhibitors, angiotensin II receptor blockers, calcium channel blockers, nitrates, diuretics, aspirin, statins and fibrates). At baseline, patients had a mean age of 62 years, mean duration of diabetes of 9.5 years and mean A1C of 8.1%. Mean duration of follow-up was 34.5 months.

The primary objective of this trial was to examine the effect of pioglitazone on mortality and macrovascular morbidity in patients with type 2 diabetes mellitus who were at high risk for macrovascular events. The primary efficacy variable was the time to the first occurrence of any event in a cardiovascular composite endpoint that included all-cause mortality, nonfatal myocardial infarction (MI) including silent MI, stroke, acute coronary syndrome, cardiac intervention including coronary artery bypass grafting or percutaneous intervention, major leg amputation above the ankle and bypass surgery or revascularization in the leg. A total of 514 (19.7%) patients treated with pioglitazone and 572 (21.7%) placebo-treated patients experienced at least one event from the primary composite endpoint (hazard ratio 0.90; 95% Confidence Interval: 0.80, 1.02; p=0.10).

Although there was no statistically significant difference between pioglitazone and placebo for the three-year incidence of a first event within this composite, there was no increase in mortality or in total macrovascular events with pioglitazone. The number of first occurrences and total individual events contributing to the primary composite endpoint is shown in *Table 6*.

[See table 6 at top of next page]

Weight Gain

Dose-related weight gain occurs when pioglitazone is used alone or in combination with other antidiabetic medications. The mechanism of weight gain is unclear but probably involves a combination of fluid retention and fat accumulation.

Edema

Edema induced from taking pioglitazone is reversible when pioglitazone is discontinued. The edema usually does not require hospitalization unless there is coexisting congestive heart failure.

Hepatic Effects

There has been no evidence of pioglitazone-induced hepatotoxicity in the pioglitazone controlled clinical trial database to date. One randomized, double-blind, three-year trial comparing pioglitazone to glyburide as add-on to metformin and insulin therapy was specifically designed to evaluate the incidence of serum ALT elevation to greater than three times the upper limit of the reference range, measured every eight weeks for the first 48 weeks of the trial then every 12 weeks thereafter. A total of 3/1051 (0.3%) patients treated with pioglitazone and 9/1046 (0.9%) patients treated with glyburide developed ALT values greater than three times the upper limit of the reference range. None of the patients treated with pioglitazone in the pioglitazone controlled clinical trial database to date have had a serum ALT greater than three times the upper limit of the reference range and a corresponding total bilirubin greater than two times the upper limit of the reference range, a combination predictive of the potential for severe drug-induced liver injury.

Hypoglycemia

In the pioglitazone clinical trials, adverse events of hypoglycemia were reported based on clinical judgment of the investigators and did not require confirmation with fingerstick glucose testing. In the 16-week add-on to sulfonylurea trial, the incidence of reported hypoglycemia was 3.7% with pioglitazone 30 mg and 0.5% with placebo. In the 16-week add-on to insulin trial, the incidence of reported hypoglycemia was 7.9% with pioglitazone 15 mg, 15.4% with pioglitazone 30 mg and 4.8% with placebo. The incidence of reported hypoglycemia was higher with pioglitazone 45 mg compared to pioglitazone 30 mg in both the 24 week add on to sulfonylurea trial (15.7% versus 13.4%) and in the 24-week add-on to insulin trial (47.8% versus 43.5%). Three patients in these four trials were hospitalized due to hypoglycemia. All three patients were receiving pioglitazone 30 mg (0.9%) in the 24-week add-on to insulin trial. An additional 14 patients reported severe hypoglycemia (defined as causing considerable interference with patient's usual activities) that did not require hospitalization. These patients were receiving pioglitazone 45 mg in combination with sulfonylurea (N=2) or pioglitazone 30 mg or 45 mg in combination with insulin (N=12).

Urinary Bladder Tumors

Tumors were observed in the urinary bladder of male rats in the two-year carcinogenicity study *[see Nonclinical Toxicology (13.1)]*. In two 3-year trials in which pioglitazone was compared to placebo or glyburide, there were 16/3656 (0.44%) reports of bladder cancer in patients taking pioglitazone compared to 5/3679 (0.14%) in patients not taking pioglitazone. After excluding patients in whom exposure to study drug was less than one year at the time of diagnosis of bladder cancer, there were six (0.16%) cases on pioglitazone and two (0.05%) cases on placebo. There are too few events of bladder cancer to establish causality.

6.2 Laboratory Abnormalities

Alogliptin

No clinically meaningful changes in hematology, serum chemistry or urinalysis were observed in patients treated with alogliptin.

Pioglitazone

Hematologic Effects

Pioglitazone may cause decreases in hemoglobin and hematocrit. In placebo-controlled monotherapy trials, mean hemoglobin values declined by 2% to 4% in patients treated with pioglitazone compared with a mean change in hemoglobin of -1% to +1% in placebo-treated patients. These changes primarily occurred within the first four to 12 weeks of therapy and remained relatively constant thereafter. These changes may be related to increased plasma volume associated with pioglitazone therapy and are not likely to be associated with any clinically significant hematologic effects.

Creatine Phosphokinase

During protocol-specified measurement of serum creatine phosphokinase (CPK) in pioglitazone clinical trials, an isolated elevation in CPK to greater than 10 times the upper limit of the reference range was noted in nine (0.2%) patients treated with pioglitazone (values of 2150 to 11400 IU/L) and in no comparator-treated patients. Six of these nine patients continued to receive pioglitazone, two patients were noted to have the CPK elevation on the last day of dosing and one patient discontinued pioglitazone due to the elevation. These elevations resolved without any apparent clinical sequelae. The relationship of these events to pioglitazone therapy is unknown.

6.3 Postmarketing Experience

Alogliptin

The following adverse reactions have been identified during the postmarketing use of alogliptin outside the United States. Because these reactions are reported voluntarily from a population of uncertain size, it is not always possible to reliably estimate their frequency or establish a causal relationship to drug exposure.

Hypersensitivity reactions including anaphylaxis, angioedema, rash, urticaria and severe cutaneous adverse reactions, including Stevens-Johnson syndrome, hepatic enzyme elevations, fulminant hepatic failure and acute pancreatitis.

Pioglitazone

The following adverse reactions have been identified during the postmarketing use of pioglitazone. Because these reactions are reported voluntarily from a population of uncertain size, it is generally not possible to reliably estimate their frequency or establish a causal relationship to drug exposure.

New onset or worsening diabetic macular edema with decreased visual acuity *[see Warnings and Precautions (5.9)]*.

Fatal and nonfatal hepatic failure *[see Warnings and Precautions (5.4)]*.

Postmarketing reports of congestive heart failure have been reported in patients treated with pioglitazone, both with and without previously known heart disease and both with and without concomitant insulin administration.

In postmarketing experience, there have been reports of unusually rapid increases in weight and increases in excess of that generally observed in clinical trials. Patients who experience such increases should be assessed for fluid accumulation and volume-related events such as excessive edema and congestive heart failure *[see Boxed Warning and Warnings and Precautions (5.1)]*.

Table 6. PROactive: Number of First and Total Events for Each Component Within the Cardiovascular Composite Endpoint

	Placebo N=2633		Pioglitazone N=2605	
Cardiovascular Events	First Events n (%)	Total Events n	First Events n (%)	Total Events n
Any Event	572 (21.7)	900	514 (19.7)	803
All-Cause Mortality	122 (4.6)	186	110 (4.2)	177
Nonfatal Myocardial Infarction (MI)	118 (4.5)	157	105 (4)	131
Stroke	96 (3.6)	119	76 (2.9)	92
Acute Coronary Syndrome	63 (2.4)	78	42 (1.6)	65
Cardiac Intervention (CABG/PCI)	101 (3.8)	240	101 (3.9)	195
Major Leg Amputation	15 (0.6)	28	9 (0.3)	28
Leg Revascularization	57 (2.2)	92	71 (2.7)	115

CABG=coronary artery bypass grafting; PCI=percutaneous intervention

7 DRUG INTERACTIONS

Alogliptin

Alogliptin is primarily renally excreted. Cytochrome (CYP) P450-related metabolism is negligible. No significant drug-drug interactions were observed with the CYP-substrates or inhibitors tested or with renally excreted drugs *[see Clinical Pharmacology (12.3)]*.

7.1 Strong CYP2C8 Inhibitors

Pioglitazone

An inhibitor of CYP2C8 (e.g., gemfibrozil) significantly increases the exposure (area under the concentration-time curve [AUC]) and half-life of pioglitazone. Therefore, the maximum recommended dose of pioglitazone is 15 mg daily if used in combination with gemfibrozil or other strong CYP2C8 inhibitors *[see Dosage and Administration (2.3) and Clinical Pharmacology (12.3)]*.

7.2 CYP2C8 Inducers

Pioglitazone

An inducer of CYP2C8 (e.g., rifampin) may significantly decrease the exposure (AUC) of pioglitazone. Therefore, if an inducer of CYP2C8 is started or stopped during treatment with OSENI, changes in diabetes treatment may be needed based on clinical response without exceeding the maximum recommended daily dose of 45 mg for pioglitazone *[see Clinical Pharmacology (12.3)]*.

8 USE IN SPECIFIC POPULATIONS

8.1 Pregnancy

Pregnancy Category C

Alogliptin and Pioglitazone

There are no adequate and well-controlled studies in pregnant women with OSENI or its individual components. Based on animal data, the likelihood that OSENI increases the risk of developmental abnormalities is predicted to be low. OSENI should be used during pregnancy only if the potential benefit justifies the potential risk to the fetus.

When administered to rats during organogenesis, the combination treatment with alogliptin and pioglitazone (100 mg/kg alogliptin plus 40 mg/kg pioglitazone) slightly augmented pioglitazone-related fetal effects of delayed development and reduced fetal weights but did not result in embryofetal mortality or teratogenicity.

Alogliptin

Alogliptin administered to pregnant rabbits and rats during the period of organogenesis was not teratogenic at doses of up to 200 and 500 mg/kg, or 149 times and 180 times, respectively, the clinical dose based on plasma drug exposure (AUC).

Doses of alogliptin up to 250 mg/kg (approximately 95 times clinical exposure based on AUC) given to pregnant rats from gestation Day 6 to lactation Day 20 did not harm the developing embryo or adversely affect growth and development of offspring.

Placental transfer of alogliptin into the fetus was observed following oral dosing to pregnant rats.

Pioglitazone

In animal reproductive studies, pregnant rats and rabbits received pioglitazone at doses up to approximately 17 (rat) and 40 (rabbit) times the MRHD based on body surface area (mg/m^2); no teratogenicity was observed. Increases in embryotoxicity (increased postimplantation losses, delayed development, reduced fetal weights and delayed parturition) occurred in rats that received oral doses approximately 10 or more times the MRHD (mg/m^2 basis). No functional or behavioral toxicity was observed in rat offspring. When pregnant rats received pioglitazone during late gestation and lactation, delayed postnatal development, attributed to decreased body weight, occurred in rat offspring at oral maternal doses approximately two or more times the MRHD (mg/m^2 basis). In rabbits, embryotoxicity occurred at oral doses approximately 40 times the MRHD (mg/m^2 basis).

8.3 Nursing Mothers

No studies have been conducted with the combined components of OSENI. In studies performed with the individual components, both alogliptin and pioglitazone are secreted in the milk of lactating rats. It is not known whether alogliptin and/or pioglitazone are secreted in human milk. Because many drugs are excreted in human milk, and because of the potential for OSENI to cause serious adverse reactions in nursing infants, a decision should be made to discontinue nursing or discontinue OSENI, taking into account the importance of OSENI to the mother.

8.4 Pediatric Use

Safety and effectiveness of OSENI in pediatric patients have not been established.

OSENI is not recommended for use in pediatric patients based on adverse effects observed in adults, including fluid retention and congestive heart failure, fractures and urinary bladder tumors *[see Warnings and Precautions (5.1, 5.5, 5.6, 5.7)]*.

8.5 Geriatric Use

Alogliptin and Pioglitazone

Of the total number of patients (N=1533) in clinical safety and efficacy studies treated with alogliptin and pioglitazone, 248 (16.2%) patients were 65 years and older and 15 (1%) patients were 75 years and older. No overall differences in safety or effectiveness were observed between these patients and younger patients. While this and other reported clinical experiences have not identified differences in responses between the elderly and younger patients, greater sensitivity of some older individuals cannot be excluded.

Alogliptin

Of the total number of patients (N=8507) in clinical safety and efficacy studies treated with alogliptin, 2064 (24.3%) patients were ≥65 years old and 341 (4%) patients were ≥75 years old. No overall differences in safety or effectiveness were observed between patients ≥65 years old and younger patients.

Pioglitazone

A total of 92 patients (15.2%) treated with pioglitazone in the three pooled, 16- to 26-week, double-blind, placebo-controlled, monotherapy trials were ≥65 years old and two patients (0.3%) were ≥75 years old. In the two pooled 16- to 24-week add-on to sulfonylurea trials, 201 patients (18.7%) treated with pioglitazone were ≥65 years old and 19 (1.8%) were ≥75 years old. In the two pooled 16- to 24-week add-on to metformin trials, 155 patients (15.5%) treated with pioglitazone were ≥65 years old and 19 (1.9%) were ≥75 years old. In the two pooled 16- to 24-week add-on to insulin trials, 272 patients (25.4%) treated with pioglitazone were ≥65 years old and 22 (2.1%) were ≥75 years old.

In PROactive, 1068 patients (41%) treated with pioglitazone were ≥65 years old and 42 (1.6%) were ≥75 years old.

In pharmacokinetic studies with pioglitazone, no significant differences were observed in pharmacokinetic parameters between elderly and younger patients. These clinical experiences have not identified differences in effectiveness and safety between the elderly (≥65 years) and younger patients although small sample sizes for patients ≥75 years old limit conclusions *[see Clinical Pharmacology (12.3)]*.

8.6 Hepatic Impairment

Alogliptin

No dose adjustments are required in patients with mild to moderate hepatic impairment (Child-Pugh Grade A and B) based on insignificant change in systemic exposures (e.g., AUC) compared to subjects with normal hepatic function in a pharmacokinetic study. Alogliptin has not been studied in patients with severe hepatic impairment (Child-Pugh Grade C). Use caution when administering alogliptin to patients with liver disease *[see Warnings and Precautions (5.4)]*.

Pioglitazone

No dose adjustments are required in patients with hepatic impairment (Child-Pugh Grade B and C) based on insignificant change in systemic exposures (e.g., AUC) compared to subjects with normal hepatic function in a pharmacokinetic study. However, use with caution in patients with liver disease *[see Warnings and Precautions (5.4)]*.

10 OVERDOSAGE

Alogliptin

The highest doses of alogliptin administered in clinical trials were single doses of 800 mg to healthy subjects and doses of 400 mg once daily for 14 days to patients with type 2 diabetes (equivalent to 32 times and 16 times the maximum recommended clinical dose of 25 mg, respectively). No serious adverse events were observed at these doses.

In the event of an overdose, it is reasonable to institute the necessary clinical monitoring and supportive therapy as dictated by the patient's clinical status. Per clinical judgment, it may be reasonable to initiate removal of unabsorbed material from the gastrointestinal tract.

Alogliptin is minimally dialyzable; over a three-hour hemodialysis session, approximately 7% of the drug was removed. Therefore, hemodialysis is unlikely to be beneficial in an overdose situation. It is not known if alogliptin is dialyzable by peritoneal dialysis.

Pioglitazone

During controlled clinical trials, one case of overdose with pioglitazone was reported. A male patient took 120 mg per day for four days, then 180 mg per day for seven days. The patient denied any clinical symptoms during this period.

In the event of overdosage, appropriate supportive treatment should be initiated according to patient's clinical signs and symptoms.

11 DESCRIPTION

OSENI tablets contain two oral antihyperglycemic drugs used in the management of type 2 diabetes: alogliptin and pioglitazone.

Alogliptin

Alogliptin is a selective, orally bioavailable inhibitor of the enzymatic activity of dipeptidyl peptidase-4 (DPP-4). Chemically, alogliptin is prepared as a benzoate salt, which is identified as 2-({6-[(3*R*)-3-aminopiperidin-1-yl]-3-methyl-2,4-dioxo-3,4-dihydropyrimidin-1(2*H*)-yl}methyl)-benzonitrile monobenzoate. It has a molecular formula of $C_{18}H_{21}N_5O_2 \bullet C_7H_6O_2$ and a molecular weight of 461.51 daltons. The structural formula is:

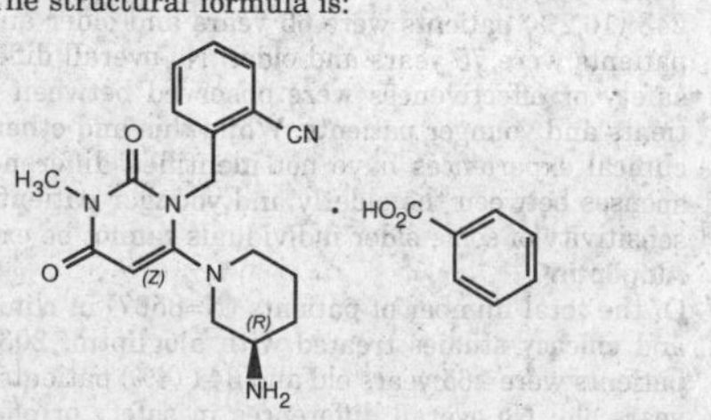

Alogliptin benzoate is a white to off-white crystalline powder that contains one asymmetric carbon in the aminopiperidine moiety. It is soluble in dimethylsulfoxide, sparingly soluble in water and methanol, slightly soluble in ethanol and very slightly soluble in octanol and isopropyl acetate.

Pioglitazone

Pioglitazone is an oral antihyperglycemic agent that acts primarily by decreasing insulin resistance. Chemically, pioglitazone is prepared as hydrochloride salt, which is identified as (±)-5-[[4-[2-(5-ethyl-2-pyridinyl)ethoxy] phenyl]methyl]-2,4-thiazolidinedione monohydrochloride. It has a molecular formula of $C_{19}H_{20}N_2O_3S \bullet HCl$ and a molecular weight of 392.90 daltons. The structural formula is:

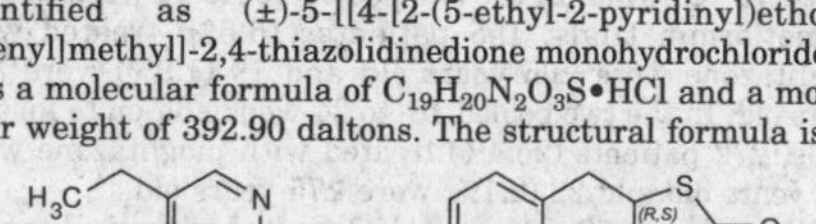

Pioglitazone hydrochloride is an odorless white crystalline powder that contains one asymmetric carbon in the thiazolidinedione moiety. The synthetic compound is a racemate and the two enantiomers of pioglitazone interconvert *in vivo*. It is soluble in *N,N* dimethylformamide, slightly soluble in anhydrous ethanol, very slightly soluble in acetone and acetonitrile, practically insoluble in water and insoluble in ether.

OSENI is available as a fixed-dose combination tablet for oral administration containing 34 mg alogliptin benzoate equivalent to 25 mg alogliptin and any of the following strengths of pioglitazone hydrochloride:

- 16.53 mg pioglitazone hydrochloride equivalent to 15 mg pioglitazone (25 mg/15 mg)
- 33.06 mg pioglitazone hydrochloride equivalent to 30 mg pioglitazone (25 mg/30 mg)
- 49.59 mg pioglitazone hydrochloride equivalent to 45 mg pioglitazone (25 mg/45 mg)

OSENI is also available as a fixed-dose combination tablet for oral administration containing 17 mg alogliptin benzoate equivalent to 12.5 mg alogliptin and any of the following strengths of pioglitazone hydrochloride:

- 16.53 mg pioglitazone hydrochloride equivalent to 15 mg pioglitazone (12.5 mg/15 mg)
- 33.06 mg pioglitazone hydrochloride equivalent to 30 mg pioglitazone (12.5 mg/30 mg)
- 49.59 mg pioglitazone hydrochloride equivalent to 45 mg pioglitazone (12.5 mg/45 mg)

OSENI tablets contain the following inactive ingredients: mannitol, microcrystalline cellulose, hydroxypropyl cellulose, croscarmellose sodium, magnesium stearate and lactose monohydrate; the tablets are film-coated with hypromellose, polyethylene glycol, titanium dioxide, talc and ferric oxide (yellow and/or red) and are marked with printing ink (Red A1 or Gray F1).

12 CLINICAL PHARMACOLOGY

12.1 Mechanism of Action

OSENI combines two antihyperglycemic agents with complementary and distinct mechanisms of action to improve glycemic control in patients with type 2 diabetes: alogliptin, a selective inhibitor of DPP-4, and pioglitazone, a member of the TZD class.

Alogliptin

Increased concentrations of the incretin hormones such as glucagon-like peptide-1 (GLP-1) and glucose-dependent insulinotropic polypeptide (GIP) are released into the bloodstream from the small intestine in response to meals. These hormones cause insulin release from the pancreatic beta cells in a glucose-dependent manner but are inactivated by the DPP-4 enzyme within minutes. GLP-1 also lowers glucagon secretion from pancreatic alpha cells, reducing hepatic glucose production. In patients with type 2 diabetes, concentrations of GLP-1 are reduced but the insulin response to GLP-1 is preserved. Alogliptin is a DPP-4 inhibitor that slows the inactivation of the incretin hormones, thereby increasing their bloodstream concentrations and reducing fasting and postprandial glucose concentrations in a glucose-dependent manner in patients with type 2 diabetes mellitus. Alogliptin selectively binds to and inhibits DPP-4 but not DPP-8 or DPP-9 activity *in vitro* at concentrations approximating therapeutic exposures.

Pioglitazone

Pharmacologic studies indicate that pioglitazone improves insulin sensitivity in muscle and adipose tissue while inhibiting hepatic gluconeogenesis. Unlike sulfonylureas, pioglitazone is not an insulin secretagogue. Pioglitazone is an agonist for peroxisome proliferator-activated receptor-gamma (PPARγ). PPAR receptors are found in tissues important for insulin action such as adipose tissue, skeletal muscle and liver. Activation of PPARγ nuclear receptors modulates the transcription of a number of insulin-responsive genes involved in the control of glucose and lipid metabolism.

In animal models of diabetes, pioglitazone reduces the hyperglycemia, hyperinsulinemia and hypertriglyceridemia characteristic of insulin-resistant states such as type 2 diabetes. The metabolic changes produced by pioglitazone result in increased responsiveness of insulin-dependent tissues and are observed in numerous animal models of insulin resistance.

Because pioglitazone enhances the effects of circulating insulin (by decreasing insulin resistance), it does not lower blood glucose in animal models that lack endogenous insulin.

12.2 Pharmacodynamics

Alogliptin and Pioglitazone

In a 26-week, randomized, active-controlled study, patients with type 2 diabetes received alogliptin 25 mg coadministered with pioglitazone 30 mg, alogliptin 12.5 mg coadministered with pioglitazone 30 mg, alogliptin 25 mg alone or pioglitazone 30 mg alone. Patients who were randomized to alogliptin 25 mg with pioglitazone 30 mg achieved a 26.2% decrease in triglyceride levels from a mean baseline of 214.2 mg/dL compared to an 11.5% decrease for alogliptin alone and a 21.8% decrease for pioglitazone alone. In addition, a 14.4% increase in HDL cholesterol levels from a mean baseline of 43.2 mg/dL was also observed for alogliptin 25 mg with pioglitazone 30 mg compared to a 1.9% increase for alogliptin alone and a 13.2% increase for pioglitazone alone. The changes in measures of LDL cholesterol and total cholesterol were similar between alogliptin 25 mg with pioglitazone 30 mg versus alogliptin alone and pioglitazone alone. A similar pattern of lipid effects was observed in a 26-week, placebo-controlled factorial study.

Alogliptin

Single-dose administration of alogliptin to healthy subjects resulted in a peak inhibition of DPP-4 within two to three hours after dosing. The peak inhibition of DPP-4 exceeded 93% across doses of 12.5 mg to 800 mg. Inhibition of DPP-4 remained above 80% at 24 hours for doses greater than or equal to 25 mg. Peak and total exposure over 24 hours to active GLP-1 were three- to four-fold greater with alogliptin (at doses of 25 to 200 mg) than placebo. In a 16-week, double-blind, placebo-controlled study alogliptin 25 mg demonstrated decreases in postprandial glucagon while increasing postprandial active GLP-1 levels compared to placebo over an eight-hour period following a standardized meal. It is unclear how these findings relate to changes in overall glycemic control in patients with type 2 diabetes mellitus. In this study, alogliptin 25 mg alone demonstrated decreases in two-hour postprandial glucose compared to placebo (-30 mg/dL versus 17.3 mg/dL respectively).

Multiple-dose administration of alogliptin to patients with type 2 diabetes also resulted in a peak inhibition of DPP-4 within one to two hours and exceeded 93% across all doses (25 mg, 100 mg and 400 mg) after a single dose and after 14 days of once-daily dosing). At these doses of alogliptin, inhibition of DPP-4 remained above 81% at 24 hours after 14 days of dosing.

Pioglitazone

Clinical studies demonstrate that pioglitazone improves insulin sensitivity in insulin-resistant patients. Pioglitazone enhances cellular responsiveness to insulin, increases insulin-dependent glucose disposal, and improves hepatic sensitivity to insulin. In patients with type 2 diabetes, the decreased insulin resistance produced by pioglitazone results in lower plasma glucose concentrations, lower plasma insulin concentrations and lower A1C values. In controlled clinical trials, pioglitazone had an additive effect on glycemic control when used in combination with a sulfonylurea, metformin or insulin *[see Clinical Studies (14)]*. Patients with lipid abnormalities were included in clinical trials with pioglitazone. Overall, patients treated with pioglitazone had mean decreases in serum triglycerides, mean increases in HDL cholesterol and no consistent mean changes in LDL and total cholesterol. There is no conclusive evidence of macrovascular benefit with pioglitazone or any other antidiabetic medication *[see Warnings and Precautions (5.11) and Adverse Reactions (6.1)]*.

In a 26-week, placebo-controlled, dose-ranging monotherapy study, mean serum triglycerides decreased in the pioglitazone 15 mg, 30 mg and 45 mg dose groups compared to a mean increase in the placebo group. Mean HDL cholesterol increased to a greater extent in patients treated with pioglitazone than in the placebo-treated patients. There were no consistent differences for LDL and total cholesterol in patients treated with pioglitazone compared to placebo *(Table 7)*.

[See table 7 at top of next page]

In the two other monotherapy studies (16 weeks and 24 weeks) and in combination therapy studies with sulfonylurea (16 weeks and 24 weeks), metformin (16 weeks and 24 weeks) or insulin (16 weeks and 24 weeks), the lipid results were generally consistent with the data above.

12.3 Pharmacokinetics

Absorption and Bioavailability

Alogliptin and Pioglitazone

In bioequivalence studies of OSENI, the AUC and maximum concentration (C_{max}) of both the alogliptin and the pioglitazone component following a single dose of the combination tablet (12.5 mg/15 mg or 25 mg/45 mg) were bioequivalent to alogliptin (12.5 mg or 25 mg) concomitantly administered with pioglitazone (15 mg or 45 mg respectively) tablets under fasted conditions in healthy subjects. Administration of OSENI 25 mg/45 mg with food resulted in no significant change in overall exposure of alogliptin or pioglitazone. OSENI may therefore be administered with or without food.

Alogliptin

The absolute bioavailability of alogliptin is approximately 100%. Administration of alogliptin with a high-fat meal results in no significant change in total and peak exposure to alogliptin. Alogliptin may therefore be administered with or without food.

Pioglitazone

Following oral administration of pioglitazone hydrochloride, peak concentrations of pioglitazone were observed within two hours. Food slightly delays the time to peak serum concentration (T_{max}) to three to four hours but does not alter the extent of absorption (AUC).

Distribution

Alogliptin

Following a single, 12.5 mg intravenous infusion of alogliptin to healthy subjects, the volume of distribution during the terminal phase was 417 L, indicating that the drug is well distributed into tissues.

Alogliptin is 20% bound to plasma proteins.

Pioglitazone

The mean apparent V_d/F of pioglitazone following single-dose administration is 0.63 ± 0.41 (mean ± SD) L/kg of body weight. Pioglitazone is extensively protein bound (>99%) in human serum, principally to serum albumin. Pioglitazone also binds to other serum proteins, but with lower affinity. Metabolites M-III and M-IV also are extensively bound (>98%) to serum albumin.

Metabolism

Alogliptin

Alogliptin does not undergo extensive metabolism, and 60% to 71% of the dose is excreted as unchanged drug in the urine.

Two minor metabolites were detected following administration of an oral dose of [^{14}C] alogliptin, *N*-demethylated, M-I (<1% of the parent compound), and *N*-acetylated alogliptin, M-II (<6% of the parent compound). M-I is an active metabolite and is an inhibitor of DPP-4 similar to the parent molecule; M-II does not display any inhibitory activity toward DPP-4 or other DPP-related enzymes. *In vitro* data indicate that, CYP2D6 and CYP3A4 contribute to the limited metabolism of alogliptin.

Alogliptin exists predominantly as the (*R*)-enantiomer (>99%) and undergoes little or no chiral conversion *in vivo* to the (*S*)-enantiomer. The (*S*)-enantiomer is not detectable at the 25 mg dose.

Pioglitazone

Pioglitazone is extensively metabolized by hydroxylation and oxidation; the metabolites also partly convert to glucuronide or sulfate conjugates. Metabolites M-III and M-IV are the major circulating active metabolites in humans. Following once-daily administration of pioglitazone, steady-state serum concentrations of both pioglitazone and its major active metabolites, M-III (keto derivative of pioglitazone) and M-IV (hydroxyl derivative of pioglitazone), are achieved within seven days. At steady-state, M-III and M-IV reach serum concentrations equal to or greater than that of pioglitazone. At steady-state, in both healthy volunteers and patients with type 2 diabetes, pioglitazone comprises approximately 30% to 50% of the peak total pioglitazone serum concentrations (pioglitazone plus active metabolites) and 20% to 25% of the total AUC.

Maximum serum concentration (C_{max}), AUC and trough serum concentrations (C_{min}) for pioglitazone and M-III and M-IV, increased proportionally with administered doses of 15 mg and 30 mg per day.

In vitro data demonstrate that multiple CYP isoforms are involved in the metabolism of pioglitazone. The cytochrome P450 isoforms involved are CYP2C8 and, to a lesser degree, CYP3A4 with additional contributions from a variety of other isoforms, including the mainly extrahepatic CYP1A1. *In vivo* studies of pioglitazone in combination with gemfibrozil, a strong CYP2C8 inhibitor, showed that pioglitazone is a CYP2C8 substrate *[see Dosage and Administration (2.3) and Drug Interactions (7)]*. Urinary 6β-hydroxycortisol/cortisol ratios measured in patients treated with pioglitazone showed that pioglitazone is not a strong CYP3A4 enzyme inducer.

Excretion and Elimination

Alogliptin

The primary route of elimination of [^{14}C] alogliptin derived radioactivity occurred via renal excretion (76%), with 13% recovered in the feces, achieving a total recovery of 89% of the administered radioactive dose. The renal clearance of alogliptin (9.6 L/hr) indicates some active renal tubular secretion and systematic clearance was 14.0 L/hr.

Pioglitazone

Following oral administration, approximately 15% to 30% of the pioglitazone dose is recovered in the urine. Renal elimination of pioglitazone is negligible, and the drug is excreted primarily as metabolites and their conjugates. It is presumed that most of the oral dose is excreted into the bile either unchanged or as metabolites and eliminated in the feces.

The mean serum half-life of pioglitazone and its metabolites (M-III and M-IV) range from three to seven hours and 16 to 24 hours, respectively. Pioglitazone has an apparent clearance, CL/F, calculated to be 5 to 7 L/hr.

Special Populations

Renal Impairment

Alogliptin

A single-dose, open-label study was conducted to evaluate the pharmacokinetics of alogliptin 50 mg in patients with chronic renal impairment compared with healthy subjects.

In patients with mild renal impairment (creatinine clearance [CrCl] ≥60 to <90 mL/min), an approximate 1.2-fold increase in plasma AUC of alogliptin was observed. Because increases of this magnitude are not considered clinically relevant, dose adjustment for patients with mild renal impairment is not recommended.

In patients with moderate renal impairment (CrCl ≥30 to <60 mL/min), an approximate two-fold increase in plasma AUC of alogliptin was observed. To maintain similar systemic exposures of OSENI to those with normal renal function, the recommended dose of OSENI is 12.5 mg/15 mg, 12.5 mg/30 mg or 12.5 mg/45 mg once daily in patients with moderate renal impairment.

In patients with severe renal impairment (CrCl ≥15 to <30 mL/min) and ESRD (CrCl <15 mL/min or requiring dialysis), approximate three- and four-fold increases in plasma AUC of alogliptin were observed, respectively. Dialysis removed approximately 7% of the drug during a three-hour dialysis session. OSENI is not recommended for patients with severe renal impairment or ESRD. Coadministration of pioglitazone and alogliptin 6.25 mg once daily based on individual requirements may be considered in these patients.

Pioglitazone

The serum elimination half-life of pioglitazone, M-III and M-IV remains unchanged in patients with moderate (creatinine clearance 30 to 50 mL/min) to severe (creatinine clearance <30 mL/min) renal impairment when compared to subjects with normal renal function. Therefore no dose adjustment in patients with renal impairment is required.

Hepatic Impairment

Alogliptin

Total exposure to alogliptin was approximately 10% lower and peak exposure was approximately 8% lower in patients with moderate hepatic impairment (Child-Pugh Grade B) compared to healthy subjects. The magnitude of these reductions is not considered to be clinically meaningful. Patients with severe hepatic impairment (Child-Pugh Grade C) have not been studied. Use caution when administering OSENI to patients with liver disease *[see Use in Specific Populations (8.6) and Warnings and Precautions (5.4)]*.

Pioglitazone

Compared with healthy controls, subjects with impaired hepatic function (Child-Pugh Grade B and C) have an approximate 45% reduction in pioglitazone and total pioglitazone (pioglitazone, M-III and M-IV) mean peak concentrations but no change in the mean AUC values. Therefore, no dose adjustment in patients with hepatic impairment is required.

There are postmarketing reports of liver failure with pioglitazone and clinical trials have generally excluded patients with serum ALT >2.5 times the upper limit of the reference range. Use caution in patients with liver disease *[see Warnings and Precautions (5.4)]*.

Gender

Alogliptin

No dose adjustment is necessary based on gender. Gender did not have any clinically meaningful effect on the pharmacokinetics of alogliptin.

Pioglitazone

The mean C_{max} and AUC values of pioglitazone were increased 20% to 60% in women compared to men. In controlled clinical trials, A1C decreases from baseline were generally greater for females than for males (average mean difference in A1C 0.5%). Because therapy should be individualized for each patient to achieve glycemic control, no dose adjustment is recommended based on gender alone.

Geriatric

Alogliptin

No dose adjustment is necessary based on age. Age did not have any clinically meaningful effect on the pharmacokinetics of alogliptin.

Pioglitazone

In healthy elderly subjects, peak serum concentrations of pioglitazone and total pioglitazone are not significantly different, but AUC values are approximately 21% higher than those achieved in younger subjects. The mean terminal half-life values of pioglitazone were also longer in elderly subjects (about 10 hours) as compared to younger subjects (about seven hours). These changes were not of a magnitude that would be considered clinically relevant.

Pediatrics

Alogliptin

Studies characterizing the pharmacokinetics of alogliptin in pediatric patients have not been performed.

Pioglitazone

Safety and efficacy of pioglitazone in pediatric patients have not been established. Pioglitazone is not recommended for use in pediatric patients *[see Use in Specific Populations (8.4)]*.

Race and Ethnicity

Alogliptin

No dose adjustment is necessary based on race. Race (White, Black and Asian) did not have any clinically meaningful effect on the pharmacokinetics of alogliptin.

Pioglitazone

Pharmacokinetic data among various ethnic groups are not available.

Drug Interactions

Coadministration of alogliptin 25 mg once daily with a CYP2C8 substrate, pioglitazone 45 mg once daily for 12 days had no clinically meaningful effects on the pharmacokinetics of pioglitazone and its active metabolites.

Specific pharmacokinetic drug interaction studies with OSENI have not been performed, although such studies have been conducted with the individual components of OSENI (alogliptin and pioglitazone).

Alogliptin

In Vitro Assessment of Drug Interactions

In vitro studies indicate that alogliptin is neither an inducer of CYP1A2, CYP2B6, CYP2C9, CYP2C19 and CYP3A4, nor an inhibitor of CYP1A2, CYP2C8, CYP2C9, CYP2C19, CYP3A4 and CYP2D6 at clinically relevant concentrations.

In Vivo Assessment of Drug Interactions

Effects of Alogliptin on the Pharmacokinetics of Other Drugs

In clinical studies, alogliptin did not meaningfully increase the systemic exposure to the following drugs that are metabolized by CYP isozymes or excreted unchanged in urine (*Figure 1*). No dose adjustment of alogliptin is recommended based on results of the described pharmacokinetic studies.

Table 7. Lipids in a 26-Week, Placebo-Controlled, Monotherapy, Dose-Ranging Study

	Placebo	Pioglitazone 15 mg Once Daily	Pioglitazone 30 mg Once Daily	Pioglitazone 45 mg Once Daily
Triglycerides (mg/dL)	N=79	N=79	N=84	N=77
Baseline (mean)	263	284	261	260
Percent change from baseline (adjusted mean*)	4.8%	-9%†	-9.6%†	-9.3%†
HDL Cholesterol (mg/dL)	N=79	N=79	N=83	N=77
Baseline (mean)	42	40	41	41
Percent change from baseline (adjusted mean*)	8.1%	14.1%†	12.2%	19.1%†
LDL Cholesterol (mg/dL)	N=65	N=63	N=74	N=62
Baseline (mean)	139	132	136	127
Percent change from baseline (adjusted mean*)	4.8%	7.2%	5.2%	6%
Total Cholesterol (mg/dL)	N=79	N=79	N=84	N=77
Baseline (mean)	225	220	223	214
Percent change from baseline (adjusted mean*)	4.4%	4.6%	3.3%	6.4%

* Adjusted for baseline, pooled center and pooled center by treatment interaction
† p<0.05 versus placebo

[See figure 1 above]

Effects of Other Drugs on the Pharmacokinetics of Alogliptin

There are no clinically meaningful changes in the pharmacokinetics of alogliptin when alogliptin is administered concomitantly with the drugs described below *(Figure 2)*.

[See figure 2 above]

Pioglitazone

[See table 8 at top of next page]

[See table 9 at top of page 2404]

13 NONCLINICAL TOXICOLOGY

13.1 Carcinogenesis, Mutagenesis, Impairment of Fertility

Alogliptin and Pioglitazone

No carcinogenicity, mutagenicity or impairment of fertility studies have been conducted with OSENI. The following data are based on findings in studies performed with alogliptin or pioglitazone individually.

Alogliptin

Rats were administered oral doses of 75, 400 and 800 mg/kg alogliptin for two years. No drug-related tumors were observed up to 75 mg/kg, or approximately 32 times the maximum recommended clinical dose of 25 mg, based on AUC exposure. At higher doses (approximately 308 times the maximum recommended clinical dose of 25 mg), a combination of thyroid C-cell adenomas and carcinomas increased in male but not female rats. No drug-related tumors were observed in mice after administration of 50, 150 or 300 mg/kg alogliptin for two years, or up to approximately 51 times the maximum recommended clinical dose of 25 mg, based on AUC exposure.

Alogliptin was not mutagenic or clastogenic, with and without metabolic activation, in the Ames test with *S. typhimurium* and *E. coli* or the cytogenetic assay in mouse lymphoma cells. Alogliptin was negative in the *in vivo* mouse micronucleus study.

In a fertility study in rats, alogliptin had no adverse effects on early embryonic development, mating or fertility at doses up to 500 mg/kg, or approximately 172 times the clinical dose based on plasma drug exposure (AUC).

Pioglitazone

A two-year carcinogenicity study was conducted in male and female rats at oral doses up to 63 mg/kg (approximately 14 times the MRHD of 45 mg based on mg/m^2). Drug-induced tumors were not observed in any organ except for the urinary bladder. Benign and/or malignant transitional cell neoplasms were observed in male rats at 4 mg/kg and above (approximately equal to the MRHD based on mg/m^2). A two-year carcinogenicity study was conducted in male and female mice at oral doses up to 100 mg/kg (approximately 11 times the MRHD based on mg/m^2). No drug-induced tumors were observed in any organ.

Pioglitazone was not mutagenic in a battery of genetic toxicology studies, including the Ames bacterial assay, a mammalian cell forward gene mutation assay (CHO/HPRT and AS52/XPRT), an *in vitro* cytogenetics assay using CHL cells, an unscheduled DNA synthesis assay and an *in vivo* micronucleus assay.

No adverse effects upon fertility were observed in male and female rats at oral doses up to 40 mg/kg pioglitazone daily prior to and throughout mating and gestation (approximately nine times the MRHD based on mg/m^2).

13.2 Animal Toxicology and/or Pharmacology

Pioglitazone

Heart enlargement has been observed in mice (100 mg/kg), rats (4 mg/kg and above) and dogs (3 mg/kg) treated orally with pioglitazone (approximately 11, one, and two times the MRHD for mice, rats and dogs, respectively, based on mg/m^2). In a one-year rat study, drug-related early death due to apparent heart dysfunction occurred at an oral dose of 160 mg/kg (approximately 35 times the MRHD based on mg/m^2). Heart enlargement was seen in a 13-week study in monkeys at oral doses of 8.9 mg/kg and above (approximately four times the MRHD based on mg/m^2), but not in a 52-week study at oral doses up to 32 mg/kg (approximately 13 times the MRHD based on mg/m^2).

14 CLINICAL STUDIES

The coadministration of alogliptin and pioglitazone has been studied in patients with type 2 diabetes inadequately controlled on either diet and exercise alone or on metformin alone.

There have been no clinical efficacy studies conducted with OSENI; however, bioequivalence of OSENI with coadministered alogliptin and pioglitazone tablets was demonstrated, and efficacy of the combination of alogliptin and pioglitazone has been demonstrated in four Phase 3 efficacy studies.

In patients with type 2 diabetes, treatment with OSENI produced clinically meaningful and statistically significant improvements in A1C compared to either alogliptin or pioglitazone alone. As is typical for trials of agents to treat

Figure 1. Effect of Alogliptin on the Pharmacokinetic Exposure to Other Drugs

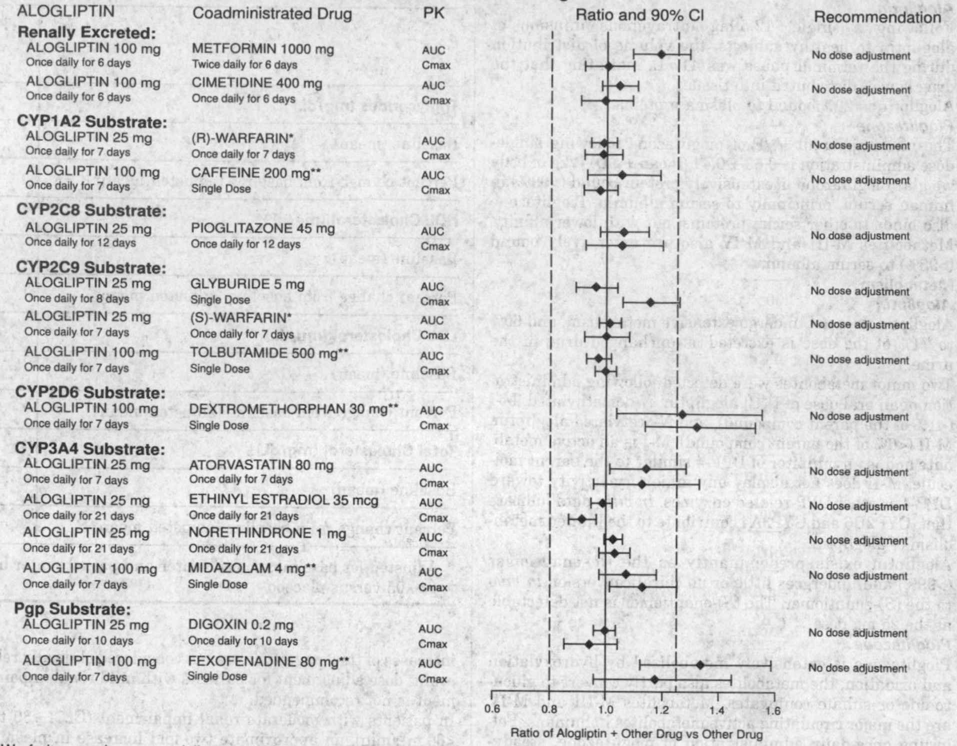

*Warfarin was given once daily at a stable dose in the range of 1 mg to 10 mg. Alogliptin had no significant effect on the prothrombin time (PT) or International Normalized Ratio (INR).

**Caffeine (1A2 substrate), tolbutamide (2C9 substrate), dextromethorphan (2D6 substrate), midazolam (3A4 substrate) and fexofenadine (P-gp substrate) were administered as a cocktail.

Figure 2. Effect of Other Drugs on the Pharmacokinetic Exposure of Alogliptin

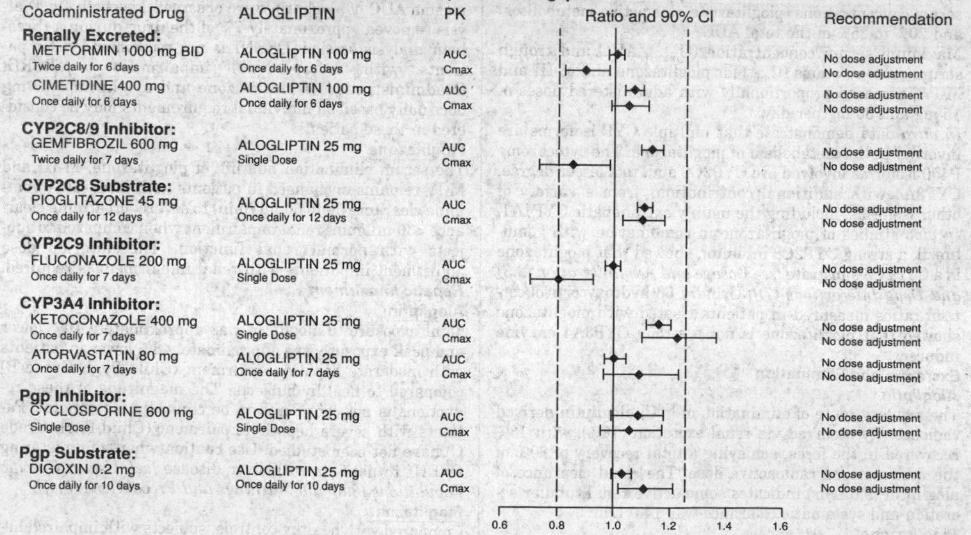

type 2 diabetes, the mean reduction in A1C with OSENI appears to be related to the degree of A1C elevation at baseline.

Alogliptin and Pioglitazone Coadministration in Patients with Type 2 Diabetes Inadequately Controlled on Diet and Exercise

In a 26-week, double-blind, active-controlled study, a total of 655 patients inadequately controlled on diet and exercise alone (mean baseline A1C = 8.8%) were randomized to receive alogliptin 25 mg alone, pioglitazone 30 mg alone, alogliptin 12.5 mg with pioglitazone 30 mg or alogliptin 25 mg with pioglitazone 30 mg once daily. Coadministration of alogliptin 25 mg with pioglitazone 30 mg resulted in statistically significant improvements from baseline in A1C and FPG compared to either alogliptin 25 mg alone or to pioglitazone 30 mg alone *(Table 10)*. Coadministration of alogliptin 25 mg with pioglitazone 30 mg once daily resulted in statistically significant reductions in fasting plasma glucose (FPG) starting from Week 2 through Week 26 compared to either alogliptin 25 mg or pioglitazone 30 mg alone. A total of 3% of patients receiving alogliptin 25 mg coadministered with pioglitazone 30 mg, 11% of those receiving alogliptin 25 mg alone, and 6% of those receiving pioglitazone 30 mg alone required glycemic rescue.

Improvements in A1C were not affected by gender, age or baseline BMI.

The mean increase in body weight was similar between pioglitazone alone and alogliptin when coadministered with pioglitazone.

[See table 10 at top of page 2404]

Alogliptin and Pioglitazone Coadministration in Patients with Type 2 Diabetes Inadequately Controlled on Metformin Alone

In the second 26-week, double-blind, placebo-controlled study, a total of 1554 patients already on metformin (mean

Table 8. Effect of Pioglitazone Coadministration on Systemic Exposure of Other Drugs

Pioglitazone Dosage Regimen (mg)*	Coadministered Drug: Name and Dose Regimens	Change in AUC†		Change in C_{max}†	
45 mg (N=12)	**Warfarin**‡				
	Daily loading then maintenance doses based PT and INR values Quick's Value=35 ± 5%	R-Warfarin	↓3%	R-Warfarin	↓2%
		S-Warfarin	↓1%	S-Warfarin	↑1%
45 mg (N=12)	**Digoxin**				
	0.200 mg twice daily (loading dose) then 0.250 mg daily (maintenance dose, 7 days)	↑15%		↑17%	
45 mg daily for 21 days (N=35)	**Oral Contraceptive**				
	[Ethinyl Estradiol (EE) 0.035 mg plus Norethindrone (NE) 1 mg] for 21 days	EE	↓11%	EE	↓13%
		NE	↑3%	NE	↓7%
45 mg (N=23)	**Fexofenadine**				
	60 mg twice daily for 7 days	↑30%		↑37%	
45 mg (N=14)	**Glipizide**				
	5 mg daily for 7 days	↓3%		↓8%	
45 mg daily for 8 days (N=16)	**Metformin**				
	1000 mg single dose on 8 days	↓3%		↓5%	
45 mg (N=21)	**Midazolam**				
	7.5 mg single dose on day 15	↓26%		↓26%	
45 mg (N=24)	**Ranitidine**				
	150 mg twice daily for 7 days	↑1%		↓1%	
45 mg daily for 4 days (N=24)	**Nifedipine ER**				
	30 mg daily for 4 days	↓13%		↓17%	
45 mg (N=25)	**Atorvastatin Ca**				
	80 mg daily for 7 days	↓14%		↓23%	
45 mg (N=22)	**Theophylline**				
	400 mg twice daily for 7 days	↑2%		↑5%	

* Daily for seven days unless otherwise noted
† % change (with/without coadministered drug and no change=0%); symbols of ↑ and ↓ indicate the exposure increase and decrease, respectively
‡ Pioglitazone had no clinically significant effect on prothrombin time

baseline A1C=8.5%) were randomized to one of 12 double-blind treatment groups: placebo; 12.5 mg or 25 mg of alogliptin alone; 15 mg, 30 mg or 45 mg of pioglitazone alone; or 12.5 mg or 25 mg of alogliptin in combination with 15 mg, 30 mg or 45 mg of pioglitazone. Patients were maintained on a stable dose of metformin (median dose=1700 mg) during the treatment period. Coadministration of alogliptin and pioglitazone provided statistically significant improvements in A1C and FPG compared to placebo, to alogliptin alone, or to pioglitazone alone when added to background metformin therapy *(Table 11, Figure 3)*. A total of 4%, 5% or 2% of patients receiving alogliptin 25 mg with 15 mg, 30 mg or 45 mg pioglitazone, 33% of patients receiving placebo, 13% of patients receiving alogliptin 25 mg, and 10%, 15% or 9% of patients receiving pioglitazone 15 mg, 30 mg or 45 mg alone required glycemic rescue.

Improvements in A1C were not affected by gender, age or baseline BMI.

The mean increase in body weight was similar between pioglitazone alone and alogliptin when coadministered with pioglitazone.

[See table 11 at top of page 2405]
[See figure 3 at top of next column]

Alogliptin Add-On Therapy in Patients with Type 2 Diabetes Inadequately Controlled on Metformin in Combination with Pioglitazone

In a 52-week, active-comparator study, a total of 803 patients inadequately controlled (mean baseline A1C = 8.2%) on a current regimen of pioglitazone 30 mg and metformin at least 1500 mg per day or at the maximum tolerated dose were randomized to either receive the addition of alogliptin

Figure 3. Change from Baseline in A1C at Week 26 with Alogliptin and Pioglitazone Alone and Alogliptin in Combination with Pioglitazone when Added to Metformin

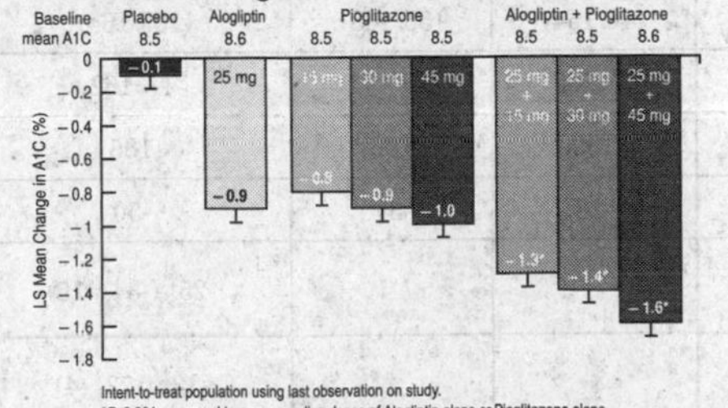

Intent-to-treat population using last observation on study.
*P≤0.001 compared to corresponding doses of Alogliptin alone or Pioglitazone alone.

25 mg or the titration of pioglitazone 30 mg to 45 mg following a four-week, single-blind, placebo run-in period. Patients were maintained on a stable dose of metformin (median dose = 1700 mg). Patients who failed to meet prespecified hyperglycemic goals during the 52-week treatment period received glycemic rescue therapy.

In combination with pioglitazone and metformin, alogliptin 25 mg was shown to be statistically superior in lowering A1C and FPG compared with the titration of pioglitazone from 30 mg to 45 mg at Week 26 and Week 52 (*Table 12, results shown only for Week 52)*. A total of 11% of patients who were receiving alogliptin 25 mg in combination with pioglitazone 30 mg and metformin and 22% of patients receiving a dose titration of pioglitazone from 30 mg to 45 mg in combination with metformin required glycemic rescue.

Improvements in A1C were not affected by gender, age, race or baseline BMI. The mean increase in body weight was similar in both treatment arms. Lipid effects were neutral.

[See table 12 at top of page 2406]

Alogliptin Add-On Therapy to a Thiazolidinedione

A 26-week, placebo-controlled study, was conducted to evaluate the efficacy and safety of alogliptin as add-on therapy to pioglitazone in patients with type 2 diabetes. A total of 493 patients inadequately controlled on a thiazolidinedione alone or in combination with metformin or a sulfonylurea (mean baseline A1C = 8%) were randomized to receive alogliptin 12.5 mg, alogliptin 25 mg or placebo. Patients were maintained on a stable dose of pioglitazone (median dose = 30 mg) during the treatment period and those who were also previously treated on metformin (median dose = 2000 mg) or sulfonylurea (median dose = 10 mg) prior to randomization were maintained on the combination therapy during the treatment period. All patients entered into a four-week, single-blind, placebo run-in period prior to randomization. Following randomization, all patients continued to receive instruction on diet and exercise. Patients who failed to meet prespecified hyperglycemic goals during the 26-week treatment period received glycemic rescue.

The addition of alogliptin 25 mg once daily to pioglitazone therapy resulted in significant improvements from baseline in A1C and FPG at Week 26 when compared to the addition of placebo *(Table 13)*. A total of 9% of patients who were receiving alogliptin 25 mg and 12% of patients receiving placebo required glycemic rescue.

The improvement in A1C was not affected by gender, age, baseline BMI or baseline pioglitazone dose. The mean increase in body weight was similar between alogliptin and placebo when given in combination with pioglitazone. Lipid effects were neutral.

[See table 13 at top of page 2406]

16 HOW SUPPLIED/STORAGE AND HANDLING

OSENI tablets are available in the following strengths and packages:

25 mg/15 mg tablet: yellow, round, biconvex and film-coated with both "A/P" and "25/15" printed on one side, available in:

NDC 64764-251-03	Bottles of 30 tablets
NDC 64764-251-04	Bottles of 90 tablets
NDC 64764-251-05	Bottles of 500 tablets

25 mg/30 mg tablet: peach, round, biconvex and film-coated with both "A/P" and "25/30" printed on one side, available in:

NDC 64764-253-03	Bottles of 30 tablets
NDC 64764-253-04	Bottles of 90 tablets
NDC 64764-253-05	Bottles of 500 tablets

25 mg/45 mg tablet: red, round, biconvex, film-coated and with both "A/P" and "25/45" printed on one side, available in:

NDC 64764-254-03	Bottles of 30 tablets
NDC 64764-254-04	Bottles of 90 tablets
NDC 64764-254-05	Bottles of 500 tablets

12.5 mg/15 mg tablet: pale yellow, round, biconvex and film-coated with both "A/P" and "12.5/15" printed on one side, available in:

NDC 64764-121-03	Bottles of 30 tablets
NDC 64764-121-04	Bottles of 90 tablets
NDC 64764-121-05	Bottles of 500 tablets

12.5 mg/30 mg tablet: pale peach, round, biconvex and film-coated with both "A/P" and "12.5/30" printed on one side, available in:

NDC 64764-123-03	Bottles of 30 tablets
NDC 64764-123-04	Bottles of 90 tablets
NDC 64764-123-05	Bottles of 500 tablets

12.5 mg/45 mg tablet: pale red, round, biconvex and film-coated with both "A/P" and "12.5/45" printed on one side, available in:

NDC 64764-124-03	Bottles of 30 tablets
NDC 64764-124-04	Bottles of 90 tablets
NDC 64764-124-05	Bottles of 500 tablets

Table 9. Effect of Coadministered Drugs on Pioglitazone Systemic Exposure

Coadministered Drug and Dosage Regimen	Pioglitazone		
	Dose Regimen (mg)*	Change in AUC†	Change in C_{max}†
Gemfibrozil 600 mg twice daily for 2 days (N=12)	30 mg single dose	↑3.4-fold‡	↑6%
Ketoconazole 200 mg twice daily for 7 days (N=28)	45 mg	↑34%	↑14%
Rifampin 600 mg daily for 5 days (N=10)	30 mg single dose	↓54%	↓5%
Fexofenadine 60 mg twice daily for 7 days (N=23)	45 mg	↑1%	0%
Ranitidine 150 mg twice daily for 4 days (N=23)	45 mg	↓13%	↓16%
Nifedipine ER 30 mg daily for 7 days (N = 23)	45 mg	↑5%	↑4%
Atorvastatin Ca 80 mg daily for 7 days (N=24)	45 mg	↓24%	↓31%
Theophylline 400 mg twice daily for 7 days (N=22)	45 mg	↓4%	↓2%

* Daily for seven days unless otherwise noted
† Mean ratio (with/without coadministered drug and no change=one-fold) % change (with/without coadministered drug and no change=0%); symbols of ↑ and ↓ indicate the exposure increase and decrease, respectively
‡ The half-life of pioglitazone increased from 6.5 hours to 15.1 hours in the presence of gemfibrozil [see Dosage and Administration (2.3) and Drug Interactions (7)]

Table 10. Glycemic Parameters at Week 26 in a Coadministration Study of Alogliptin and Pioglitazone in Patients Inadequately Controlled on Diet and Exercise*

	Alogliptin 25 mg	Pioglitazone 30 mg	Alogliptin 25 mg + Pioglitazone 30 mg
A1C (%)	N=160	N=153	N=158
Baseline (mean)	8.8	8.8	8.8
Change from Baseline (adjusted mean†)	-1	-1.2	-1.7
Difference from alogliptin 25 mg (adjusted mean† with 95% confidence interval)			-0.8‡ (-1, -0.5)
Difference from pioglitazone 30 mg (adjusted mean† with 95% confidence interval)			-0.6‡ (-0.8, -0.3)
% of Patients (n/N) achieving A1C ≤7%	24% (40/164)	34% (55/163)	63% (103/164)‡
FPG (mg/dL)	N=162	N=157	N=162
Baseline (mean)	189	189	185
Change from Baseline (adjusted mean†)	-26	-37	-50
Difference from alogliptin 25 mg (adjusted mean† with 95% confidence interval)			-25‡ (-34, -15)
Difference from pioglitazone 30 mg (adjusted mean† with 95% confidence interval)			-13‡ (-22, -4)

* Intent-to-treat population using last observation carried forward
† Least squares means adjusted for treatment, geographic region and baseline value
‡ p<0.01 compared to alogliptin 25 mg or pioglitazone 30 mg

Storage

Store at 25°C (77°F); excursions permitted to 15° to 30°C (59°to 86°F) [see USP Controlled Room Temperature]. Keep container tightly closed and protect from moisture and humidity.

17 PATIENT COUNSELING INFORMATION

See FDA-Approved Patient Labeling (Medication Guide).

17.1 Instructions

Inform patients of the potential risks and benefits of OSENI.

Patients who experience an unusually rapid increase in weight or edema or who develop shortness of breath or other symptoms of heart failure while on OSENI should immediately report these symptoms to their physician.

Patients should be informed that acute pancreatitis has been reported during use of alogliptin. Patients should be informed that persistent, severe abdominal pain, sometimes radiating to the back, which may or may not be accompanied by vomiting, is the hallmark symptom of acute pancreatitis. Patients should be instructed to promptly discontinue OSENI and contact their physician if persistent severe abdominal pain occurs.

Patients should be informed that allergic reactions have been reported during use of alogliptin and pioglitazone. If symptoms of allergic reactions (including skin rash, hives and swelling of the face, lips, tongue and throat that may cause difficulty in breathing or swallowing) occur, patients should be instructed to discontinue OSENI and seek medical advice promptly.

Patients should be informed that postmarketing reports of liver injury, sometimes fatal, have been reported during use of alogliptin and pioglitazone. If signs or symptoms of liver injury occur (e.g., unexplained nausea, vomiting, abdominal pain, fatigue, anorexia or dark urine), patients should be instructed to discontinue OSENI and seek medical advice promptly.

Tell patients to promptly report any sign of macroscopic hematuria or other symptoms such as dysuria or urinary urgency that develop or increase during treatment, as these may be due to bladder cancer.

Inform patients that hypoglycemia can occur, particularly when an insulin secretagogue or insulin is used in combination with OSENI. Explain the risks, symptoms and appropriate management of hypoglycemia.

Therapy with thiazolidinediones, including pioglitazone, which is one of the active components of OSENI, may result in ovulation in some premenopausal anovulatory women. As a result, these patients may be at an increased risk for pregnancy while taking OSENI. Therefore, adequate contraception should be recommended for all premenopausal women who are prescribed OSENI.

Instruct patients to take OSENI only as prescribed daily. OSENI can be taken with or without meals. If a dose is missed, advise patients not to double their next dose.

Patients should be informed that the tablets must never be split.

Instruct patients to read the Medication Guide before starting OSENI therapy and to reread each time the prescription is refilled. Instruct patients to inform their healthcare provider if an unusual symptom develops or if a symptom persists or worsens.

Revised: June 2013
ALP008 R3

MEDICATION GUIDE

OSENI (OH-senn-ee)
(alogliptin and pioglitazone)
tablets

Read this Medication Guide carefully before you start taking OSENI and each time you get a refill. There may be new information. This information does not take the place of talking with your doctor about your medical condition or your treatment. If you have any questions about OSENI, ask your doctor or pharmacist.

What is the most important information I should know about OSENI?

OSENI can cause serious side effects, including:

1. **New or worse heart failure:** Pioglitazone, one of the medicines in OSENI, can cause your body to keep extra fluid (fluid retention), which leads to swelling (edema) and weight gain. Extra body fluid can make some heart problems worse or lead to heart failure. Heart failure means your heart does not pump blood well enough.
   - Do not take OSENI if you have severe heart failure.
   - If you have heart failure with symptoms (such as shortness of breath or swelling), even if these symptoms are not severe, OSENI may not be right for you.

   Call your doctor right away if you have any of the following:
   - swelling or fluid retention, especially in the ankles or legs
   - shortness of breath or trouble breathing, especially when you lie down
   - an unusually fast increase in weight
   - unusual tiredness
2. **Inflammation of the pancreas (pancreatitis):** Alogliptin, one of the medicines in OSENI, may cause pancreatitis, which may be severe.

   Certain medical conditions make you more likely to get pancreatitis.

   Before you start taking OSENI:

   Tell your doctor if you have ever had:
   - pancreatitis
   - stones in your gallbladder (gallstones)
   - a history of alcoholism
   - kidney problems
   - liver problems

Stop taking OSENI and call your doctor right away if you have pain in your stomach area (abdomen) that is severe and will not go away. The pain may be felt going from your abdomen through to your back. The pain may happen with or without vomiting. These may be symptoms of pancreatitis.

What is OSENI?

- OSENI contains 2 prescription diabetes medicines, alogliptin (NESINA) and pioglitazone (ACTOS).
- OSENI is a prescription medicine used with diet and exercise to improve blood sugar (glucose) control in adults with type 2 diabetes.
- OSENI is not for people with type 1 diabetes.
- OSENI is not for people with diabetic ketoacidosis (increased ketones in blood or urine).

It is not known if OSENI is safe and effective in children under the age of 18. OSENI is not recommended for use in children.

Who should not take OSENI?

Do not take OSENI if you:

- have severe heart failure
- are allergic to alogliptin (NESINA), pioglitazone (ACTOS) or any ingredient in OSENI or have had a serious allergic (hypersensitivity) reaction to alogliptin or pioglitazone. See the end of this Medication Guide for a complete list of the ingredients in OSENI.

Symptoms of a serious allergic reaction to OSENI may include:

- swelling of your face, lips, throat and other areas on your skin
- difficulty with swallowing or breathing
- raised, red areas on your skin (hives)
- skin rash, itching, flaking or peeling

If you have these symptoms, stop taking OSENI and contact your doctor or go to the nearest hospital emergency room right away.

What should I tell my doctor before and during treatment with OSENI?

Before you start taking OSENI, tell your doctor if you:

- have heart failure
- have a type of diabetic eye disease that causes swelling of the back of the eye (macular edema)
- have kidney or liver problems
- have or have had inflammation of the pancreas (pancreatitis)
- have or have had cancer of the bladder
- have other medical conditions
- **are pregnant or plan to become pregnant.** It is not known if OSENI can harm your unborn baby. Talk to your doctor about the best way to control your blood sugar while you are pregnant or if you plan to become pregnant.
- **are a premenopausal woman who does not have periods regularly or at all.** OSENI may increase your chance of becoming pregnant. Talk to your doctor about birth control choices while taking OSENI. Tell your doctor right away if you become pregnant while taking OSENI.
- **are breastfeeding or plan to breastfeed.** It is not known whether OSENI passes into your breast milk and if it can harm your baby. You should not take OSENI if you breastfeed your baby. Talk with your doctor about the best way to feed your baby if you are taking OSENI.

Tell your doctor about all the medicines you take, including prescription and nonprescription medicines, vitamins and herbal supplements.

Know the medicines you take. Keep a list of them and show it to your doctor and pharmacist before you start a new medicine.

OSENI may affect the way other medicines work, and other medicines may affect how OSENI works. Contact your doctor before you start or stop other types of medicines.

How should I take OSENI?

- Take OSENI exactly as your doctor tells you to take it.
- Take OSENI 1 time each day with or without food.
- Do not break or cut OSENI tablets before swallowing.
- Your doctor may need to change your dose of OSENI to control your blood glucose. Do not change your dose unless told to do so by your doctor.
- If you miss a dose, take it as soon as you remember. If you do not remember until it is time for your next dose, skip the missed dose and take the next dose at your regular time. **Do not** take 2 doses of OSENI at the same time.
- If you take too much OSENI, call your doctor or go to the nearest hospital emergency room right away.
- If your body is under stress, such as from fever, infection, accident or surgery, the dose of your diabetes medicines may need to be changed. Call your doctor right away.
- Stay on your diet and exercise programs and check your blood sugar as your doctor tells you to.
- Your doctor may do certain blood tests before you start OSENI and during treatment as needed. Your doctor may change your dose of OSENI based on the results of your blood tests due to how well your kidneys are working.
- Your doctor will check your diabetes with regular blood tests, including your blood sugar levels and your hemoglobin A1C.
- Your doctor should check your eyes regularly while you take OSENI.

Table 11. Glycemic Parameters at Week 26 for Alogliptin and Pioglitazone Alone and in Combination in Patients with Type 2 Diabetes*

	Placebo	Alogliptin 25 mg	Pioglitazone 15 mg	Pioglitazone 30 mg	Pioglitazone 45 mg	Alogliptin 25 mg + Pioglitazone 15 mg	Alogliptin 25 mg + Pioglitazone 30 mg	Alogliptin 25 mg + Pioglitazone 45 mg
A1C (%)	N=126	N=123	N=127	N=123	N=126	N=127	N=124	N=126
Baseline (mean)	8.5	8.6	8.5	8.5	8.5	8.5	8.5	8.6
Change from baseline (adjusted mean† with 95% confidence interval)	-0.1	-0.9	-0.8	-0.9	-1	-1.3‡	-1.4‡	-1.6‡
Difference from pioglitazone (adjusted mean† with 95% confidence interval)	-	-	-	-	-	-0.5‡ (-0.7, -0.3)	-0.5‡ (-0.7, -0.3)	-0.6‡ (-0.8, -0.4)
Difference from alogliptin (adjusted mean† with 95% confidence interval)	-	-	-	-	-	-0.4‡ (-0.6, -0.1)	-0.5‡ (-0.7, -0.3)	-0.7‡ (-0.9, -0.5)
Patients (%) achieving A1C ≤7%	6% (8/129)	27% (35/129)	26% (33/129)	30% (38/129)	36% (47/129)	55% (71/130)‡	53% (69/130)‡	60% (78/130)‡
FPG (mg/dL)	N=129	N=126	N=127	N=125	N=129	N=130	N=126	N=127
Baseline (mean)	177	184	177	175	181	179	179	178
Change from baseline (adjusted mean† with 95% confidence interval)	7	-19	-24	-29	-32	-38‡	-42‡	-53‡
Difference from pioglitazone (adjusted mean† with 95% confidence interval)	-	-	-	-	-	-14‡ (-24, -5)	-13‡ (-23, -3)	-20‡ (-30, -11)
Difference from alogliptin (adjusted mean† with 95% confidence interval)	-	-	-	-	-	-19‡ (-29, -10)	-23‡ (-33, -13)	-34‡ (-44, -24)

* Intent-to-treat population using last observation carried forward
† Least squares means adjusted for treatment, geographic region, metformin dose and baseline value
‡ p≤0.01 when compared to pioglitazone and alogliptin alone

What are the possible side effects of OSENI?

OSENI can cause serious side effects, including:

- See **"What is the most important information I should know about OSENI?"**
- **Allergic (hypersensitivity) reactions,** such as:
  - swelling of your face, lips, throat and other areas on your skin
  - difficulty with swallowing or breathing
  - raised, red areas on your skin (hives)
  - skin rash, itching, flaking or peeling

If you have these symptoms, stop taking OSENI and contact your doctor right away.

- **Liver problems.** Call your doctor right away if you have unexplained symptoms such as:
  - nausea or vomiting
  - stomach pain
  - unusual or unexplained tiredness
  - loss of appetite
  - dark urine
  - yellowing of your skin or the whites of your eyes
- **Broken bones (fractures).** Usually in the hand, upper arm or foot in women. Talk to your doctor for advice on how to keep your bones healthy.

Table 12. Glycemic Parameters at Week 52 in an Active-Controlled Study of Alogliptin as Add-On Combination Therapy to Metformin and Pioglitazone*

	Alogliptin 25 mg + Pioglitazone 30 mg + Metformin	Pioglitazone 45 mg + Metformin
A1C (%)	N=397	N=394
Baseline (mean)	8.2	8.1
Change from Baseline (adjusted mean†)	-0.7	-0.3
Difference from Pioglitazone 45 mg + Metformin (adjusted mean† with 95% confidence interval)	-0.4‡ (-0.5, -0.3)	—
% of Patients (n/N) achieving A1C ≤7%	33% (134/404)§	21% (85/399)
FPG (mg/dL)	N=399	N=396
Baseline (mean)	162	162
Change from Baseline (adjusted mean†)	-15	-4
Difference from Pioglitazone 45 mg + Metformin (adjusted mean† with 95% confidence interval)	-11§ (-16, -6)	-

* Intent-to-treat population using last observation on study
† Least squares means adjusted for treatment, baseline value, geographic region and baseline metformin dose
‡ Noninferior and statistically superior to metformin plus pioglitazone at the 0.025 one-sided significance level
§ p<0.001 compared to pioglitazone 45 mg + metformin

Table 13. Glycemic Parameters at Week 26 in a Placebo-Controlled Study of Alogliptin as Add-On Therapy to Pioglitazone*

	Alogliptin 25 mg + Pioglitazone	Placebo + Pioglitazone
A1C (%)	N=195	N=95
Baseline (mean)	8	8
Change from baseline (adjusted mean†)	-0.8	-0.2
Difference from placebo (adjusted mean† with 95% confidence interval)	-0.6‡ (-0.8, -0.4)	-
% of patients (n/N) achieving A1C ≤7%	49% (98/199)‡	34% (33/97)
FPG (mg/dL)	N=197	N=97
Baseline (mean)	170	172
Change from baseline (adjusted mean†)	-20	-6
Difference from placebo (adjusted mean† with 95% confidence interval)	-14‡ (-23, -5)	-

* Intent-to-treat population using last observation on study
† Least squares means adjusted for treatment, baseline value, geographic region, baseline treatment regimen (pioglitazone, pioglitazone plus metformin or pioglitazone plus sulfonylurea) and baseline pioglitazone dose
‡ p<0.01 compared to placebo

- **Bladder cancer.** There may be an increased chance of having bladder cancer when you take OSENI. You should not take OSENI if you are receiving treatment for bladder cancer. Tell your doctor right away if you have any of the following symptoms of bladder cancer:
  - blood or a red color in your urine
  - an increased need to urinate
  - pain while you urinate
- **Low blood sugar (hypoglycemia).** If you take OSENI with another medicine that can cause low blood sugar, such as a sulfonylurea or insulin, your risk of getting low blood sugar is higher. The dose of your sulfonylurea medicine or insulin may need to be lowered while you take OSENI. If you have symptoms of low blood sugar, you should check your blood sugar and treat if low, then call your doctor. Signs and symptoms of low blood sugar may include:

shaking or feeling jittery	headache
sweating	change in mood
fast heartbeat	confusion
change in vision	dizziness
hunger	

- **Diabetic eye disease with swelling in the back of the eye (macular edema).** Tell your doctor right away if you have any changes in your vision. Your doctor should check your eyes regularly.
- **Release of an egg from an ovary in a woman (ovulation) leading to pregnancy.** Ovulation may happen when premenopausal women who do not have regular monthly periods take OSENI. This can increase your chance of getting pregnant.

The most common side effects of OSENI include:
- stuffy or runny nose and sore throat
- back pain
- cold-like symptoms (upper respiratory tract infection)

Tell your doctor if you have any side effect that bothers you or that does not go away.
These are not all the possible side effects of OSENI. For more information, ask your doctor or pharmacist.
Call your doctor for medical advice about side effects. You may report side effects to FDA at 1-800-FDA-1088.
How should I store OSENI?
- Store OSENI at room temperature between 68°F to 77°F (20°C to 25°C).
- Keep container tightly closed and protect from moisture and humidity.

Keep OSENI and all medicines out of the reach of children.
General information about the safe and effective use of OSENI
Medicines are sometimes prescribed for purposes other than those listed in the Medication Guide. Do not take OSENI for a condition for which it was not prescribed. Do not give OSENI to other people, even if they have the same symptoms you have. It may harm them.
This Medication Guide summarizes the most important information about OSENI. If you would like more information, talk with your doctor. You can ask your doctor or pharmacist for information about OSENI that is written for health professionals.
For more information, go to www.oseni.com or call 1-877-TAKEDA-7 (1-877-825-3327).
What are the ingredients in OSENI?
Active ingredients: alogliptin and pioglitazone.
Inactive ingredients: mannitol, microcrystalline cellulose, hydroxypropyl cellulose, croscarmellose sodium, magnesium stearate, and lactose monohydrate; the tablets are film-coated with hypromellose, polyethylene glycol, titanium dioxide, talc and ferric oxide (yellow and/or red) and are marked with red A1 or gray F1 printing ink.
This Medication Guide has been approved by the U.S. Food and Drug Administration.
Distributed by:
Takeda Pharmaceuticals America, Inc.
Deerfield, IL 60015
Revised: June 2013

ALP008 R3
Shown in Product Identification Guide, page 313

ULORIC ℞
(febuxostat)
tablet for oral use

HIGHLIGHTS OF PRESCRIBING INFORMATION
These HIGHLIGHTS do not include all the information needed to use ULORIC safely and effectively. See full prescribing information for ULORIC.
ULORIC (febuxostat) tablet for oral use
Initial U.S. Approval: 2009

RECENT MAJOR CHANGES
Warnings and Precautions
Hepatic Effects (5.3) 11/2012

INDICATIONS AND USAGE
ULORIC is a xanthine oxidase (XO) inhibitor indicated for the chronic management of hyperuricemia in patients with gout. (1)
ULORIC is not recommended for the treatment of asymptomatic hyperuricemia. (1)

DOSAGE AND ADMINISTRATION
- ULORIC is recommended at 40 mg or 80 mg once daily. The recommended starting dose of ULORIC is 40 mg once daily. For patients who do not achieve a serum uric acid (sUA) less than 6 mg/dL after 2 weeks with 40 mg, ULORIC 80 mg is recommended. (2.1)
- ULORIC can be administered without regard to food or antacid use. (2.1)
- No dose adjustment is necessary when administering ULORIC to patients with mild to moderate renal or hepatic impairment. (2.2)

DOSAGE FORMS AND STRENGTHS
Tablet: 40 mg, 80 mg. (3)

CONTRAINDICATIONS
ULORIC is contraindicated in patients being treated with azathioprine or mercaptopurine. (4)

WARNINGS AND PRECAUTIONS
- Gout Flare: An increase in gout flares is frequently observed during initiation of anti-hyperuricemic agents, including ULORIC. If a gout flare occurs during treatment, ULORIC need not be discontinued. Prophylactic therapy (i.e., non-steroidal anti-inflammatory drug [NSAID] or colchicine upon initiation of treatment) may be beneficial for up to six months. (2.4, 5.1)
- Cardiovascular Events: A higher rate of cardiovascular thromboembolic events was observed in patients treated with ULORIC than allopurinol in clinical trials. Monitor for signs and symptoms of MI and stroke. (5.2)
- Hepatic Effects: Postmarketing reports of hepatic failure, sometimes fatal. Causality cannot be excluded. If liver injury is detected, promptly interrupt ULORIC and assess patient for probable cause, then treat cause if possible, to resolution or stabilization. Do not restart ULORIC if liver injury is confirmed and no alternate etiology can be found. (5.3)

ADVERSE REACTIONS
Adverse reactions occurring in at least 1% of ULORIC-treated patients, and at least 0.5% greater than placebo, are liver function abnormalities, nausea, arthralgia, and rash. (6.1)
To report SUSPECTED ADVERSE REACTIONS, contact Takeda Pharmaceuticals at 1-877-TAKEDA-7 (1-877-825-3327) or FDA at 1-800-FDA-1088 or www.fda.gov/medwatch.

DRUG INTERACTIONS

Concomitant administration of ULORIC with XO substrate drugs, azathioprine or mercaptopurine could increase plasma concentrations of these drugs resulting in severe toxicity. (7)

USE IN SPECIFIC POPULATIONS

- There is insufficient data in patients with severe renal impairment. No studies have been conducted in patients with severe hepatic impairment. Caution should be exercised in these patients. (8.6, 8.7)
- No studies have been conducted in patients with secondary hyperuricemia (including patients being treated for Lesch-Nyhan syndrome or malignant disease, or in organ transplant recipients); therefore, ULORIC is not recommended for use in these patients. (8.8)

See 17 for PATIENT COUNSELING INFORMATION and FDA-approved patient labeling

Revised: 11/2012

FULL PRESCRIBING INFORMATION: CONTENTS*

*** Sections or subsections omitted from the full prescribing information are not listed**

FULL PRESCRIBING INFORMATION

1 INDICATIONS AND USAGE

ULORIC is a xanthine oxidase (XO) inhibitor indicated for the chronic management of hyperuricemia in patients with gout.

ULORIC is not recommended for the treatment of asymptomatic hyperuricemia.

2 DOSAGE AND ADMINISTRATION

2.1 Recommended Dose

For treatment of hyperuricemia in patients with gout, ULORIC is recommended at 40 mg or 80 mg once daily.

The recommended starting dose of ULORIC is 40 mg once daily. For patients who do not achieve a serum uric acid (sUA) less than 6 mg/dL after two weeks with 40 mg, ULORIC 80 mg is recommended.

ULORIC can be taken without regard to food or antacid use *[see Clinical Pharmacology (12.3)]*.

2.2 Special Populations

No dose adjustment is necessary when administering ULORIC in patients with mild to moderate renal impairment *[see Use in Specific Populations (8.6) and Clinical Pharmacology (12.3)]*. The recommended starting dose of ULORIC is 40 mg once daily. For patients who do not achieve a sUA less than 6 mg/dL after two weeks with 40 mg, ULORIC 80 mg is recommended.

No dose adjustment is necessary in patients with mild to moderate hepatic impairment *[see Use in Specific Populations (8.7) and Clinical Pharmacology (12.3)]*.

Table 1: Adverse Reactions Occurring in ≥1% of ULORIC-Treated Patients and at Least 0.5% Greater than Seen in Patients Receiving Placebo in Controlled Studies

Adverse Reactions	Placebo	ULORIC		allopurinol*
	(N=134)	40 mg daily (N=757)	80 mg daily (N=1279)	(N=1277)
Liver Function Abnormalities	0.7%	6.6%	4.6%	4.2%
Nausea	0.7%	1.1%	1.3%	0.8%
Arthralgia	0%	1.1%	0.7%	0.7%
Rash	0.7%	0.5%	1.6%	1.6%

* Of the subjects who received allopurinol, 10 received 100 mg, 145 received 200 mg, and 1122 received 300 mg, based on level of renal impairment.

2.3 Uric Acid Level

Testing for the target serum uric acid level of less than 6 mg/dL may be performed as early as two weeks after initiating ULORIC therapy.

2.4 Gout Flares

Gout flares may occur after initiation of ULORIC due to changing serum uric acid levels resulting in mobilization of urate from tissue deposits. Flare prophylaxis with a non-steroidal anti-inflammatory drug (NSAID) or colchicine is recommended upon initiation of ULORIC. Prophylactic therapy may be beneficial for up to six months *[see Clinical Studies (14.1)]*.

If a gout flare occurs during ULORIC treatment, ULORIC need not be discontinued. The gout flare should be managed concurrently, as appropriate for the individual patient *[see Warnings and Precautions (5.1)]*.

3 DOSAGE FORMS AND STRENGTHS

- 40 mg tablets, light green to green, round, debossed with "TAP" and "40"
- 80 mg tablets, light green to green, teardrop shaped, debossed with "TAP" and "80"

4 CONTRAINDICATIONS

ULORIC is contraindicated in patients being treated with azathioprine or mercaptopurine *[see Drug Interactions (7)]*.

5 WARNINGS AND PRECAUTIONS

5.1 Gout Flare

After initiation of ULORIC, an increase in gout flares is frequently observed. This increase is due to reduction in serum uric acid levels, resulting in mobilization of urate from tissue deposits.

In order to prevent gout flares when ULORIC is initiated, concurrent prophylactic treatment with an NSAID or colchicine is recommended *[see Dosage and Administration (2.4)]*.

5.2 Cardiovascular Events

In the randomized controlled studies, there was a higher rate of cardiovascular thromboembolic events (cardiovascular deaths, non-fatal myocardial infarctions, and non-fatal strokes) in patients treated with ULORIC (0.74 per 100 P-Y [95% Confidence Interval (CI) 0.36-1.37]) than allopurinol (0.60 per 100 P-Y [95% CI 0.16-1.53]) *[see Adverse Reactions (6.1)]*. A causal relationship with ULORIC has not been established. Monitor for signs and symptoms of myocardial infarction (MI) and stroke.

5.3 Hepatic Effects

There have been postmarketing reports of fatal and non-fatal hepatic failure in patients taking ULORIC, although the reports contain insufficient information necessary to establish the probable cause. During randomized controlled studies, transaminase elevations greater than three times the upper limit of normal (ULN) were observed (AST: 2%, 2%, and ALT: 3%, 2% in ULORIC and allopurinol -treated patients, respectively). No dose-effect relationship for these transaminase elevations was noted *[see Clinical Pharmacology (12.3)]*.

Obtain a liver test panel (serum alanine aminotransferase [ALT], aspartate aminotransferase [AST], alkaline phosphatase , and total bilirubin) as a baseline before initiating ULORIC.

Measure liver tests promptly in patients who report symptoms that may indicate liver injury, including fatigue, anorexia, right upper abdominal discomfort, dark urine or jaundice. In this clinical context, if the patient is found to have abnormal liver tests (ALT greater than three times the upper limit of the reference range), ULORIC treatment should be interrupted and investigation done to establish the probable cause. ULORIC should not be restarted in these patients without another explanation for the liver test abnormalities.

Patients who have serum ALT greater than three times the reference range with serum total bilirubin greater than two times the reference range without alternative etiologies are at risk for severe drug-induced liver injury and should not be restarted on ULORIC. For patients with lesser elevations of serum ALT or bilirubin and with an alternate probable cause, treatment with ULORIC can be used with caution.

6 ADVERSE REACTIONS

6.1 Clinical Trials Experience

Because clinical trials are conducted under widely varying conditions, adverse reaction rates observed in the clinical trials of a drug cannot be directly compared to rates in the clinical trials of another drug and may not reflect the rates observed in practice.

A total of 2757 subjects with hyperuricemia and gout were treated with ULORIC 40 mg or 80 mg daily in clinical studies. For ULORIC 40 mg, 559 patients were treated for ≥6 months. For ULORIC 80 mg, 1377 subjects were treated for ≥6 months, 674 patients were treated for ≥1 year and 515 patients were treated for ≥2 years.

Most Common Adverse Reactions

In three randomized, controlled clinical studies (Studies 1, 2 and 3), which were six to 12 months in duration, the following adverse reactions were reported by the treating physician as related to study drug. Table 1 summarizes adverse reactions reported at a rate of at least 1% in ULORIC treatment groups and at least 0.5% greater than placebo.

[See table 1 above]

The most common adverse reaction leading to discontinuation from therapy was liver function abnormalities in 1.8% of ULORIC 40 mg, 1.2% of ULORIC 80 mg, and in 0.9% of allopurinol-treated subjects.

In addition to the adverse reactions presented in Table 1, dizziness was reported in more than 1% of ULORIC-treated subjects although not at a rate more than 0.5% greater than placebo.

Less Common Adverse Reactions

In Phase 2 and 3 clinical studies the following adverse reactions occurred in less than 1% of subjects and in more than one subject treated with doses ranging from 40 mg to 240 mg of ULORIC. This list also includes adverse reactions (less than 1% of subjects) associated with organ systems from Warnings and Precautions.

Blood and Lymphatic System Disorders: anemia, idiopathic thrombocytopenic purpura, leukocytosis/leukopenia, neutropenia, pancytopenia, splenomegaly, thrombocytopenia.

Cardiac Disorders: angina pectoris, atrial fibrillation/flutter, cardiac murmur, ECG abnormal, palpitations, sinus bradycardia, tachycardia.

Ear and Labyrinth Disorders: deafness, tinnitus, vertigo.

Eye Disorders: vision blurred.

Gastrointestinal Disorders: abdominal distention, abdominal pain, constipation, dry mouth, dyspepsia, flatulence, frequent stools, gastritis, gastroesophageal reflux disease, gastrointestinal discomfort, gingival pain, haematemesis, hyperchlorhydria, hematochezia, mouth ulceration, pancreatitis, peptic ulcer, vomiting.

General Disorders and Administration Site Conditions: asthenia, chest pain/discomfort, edema, fatigue, feeling abnormal, gait disturbance, influenza-like symptoms, mass, pain, thirst.

Hepatobiliary Disorders: cholelithiasis/cholecystitis, hepatic steatosis, hepatitis, hepatomegaly.

Immune System Disorder: hypersensitivity.

Infections and Infestations: herpes zoster.

Procedural Complications: contusion.

Metabolism and Nutrition Disorders: anorexia, appetite decreased/increased, dehydration, diabetes mellitus, hypercholesterolemia, hyperglycemia, hyperlipidemia, hypertriglyceridemia, hypokalemia, weight decreased/increased.

Musculoskeletal and Connective Tissue Disorders: arthritis, joint stiffness, joint swelling, muscle spasms/twitching/tightness/weakness, musculoskeletal pain/stiffness, myalgia.

Nervous System Disorders: altered taste, balance disorder, cerebrovascular accident, Guillain-Barré syndrome, headache, hemiparesis, hypoesthesia, hyposmia, lacunar infarction, lethargy, mental impairment, migraine, paresthesia, somnolence, transient ischemic attack, tremor.

Psychiatric Disorders: agitation, anxiety, depression, insomnia, irritability, libido decreased, nervousness, panic attack, personality change.

Renal and Urinary Disorders: hematuria, nephrolithiasis, pollakiuria, proteinuria, renal failure, renal insufficiency, urgency, incontinence.

Reproductive System and Breast Changes: breast pain, erectile dysfunction, gynecomastia.

Respiratory, Thoracic and Mediastinal Disorders: bronchitis, cough, dyspnea, epistaxis, nasal dryness, paranasal sinus hypersecretion, pharyngeal edema, respiratory tract congestion, sneezing, throat irritation, upper respiratory tract infection.

Skin and Subcutaneous Tissue Disorders: alopecia, angioedema, dermatitis, dermographism, ecchymosis, eczema, hair color changes, hair growth abnormal, hyperhidrosis, peeling skin, petechiae, photosensitivity, pruritus, purpura, skin discoloration/altered pigmentation, skin lesion, skin odor abnormal, urticaria.

Vascular Disorders: flushing, hot flush, hypertension, hypotension.

Laboratory Parameters: activated partial thromboplastin time prolonged, creatine increased, bicarbonate decreased, sodium increased, EEG abnormal, glucose increased, cholesterol increased, triglycerides increased, amylase increased, potassium increased, TSH increased, platelet count decreased, hematocrit decreased, hemoglobin decreased, MCV increased, RBC decreased, creatinine increased, blood urea increased, BUN/creatinine ratio increased, creatine phosphokinase (CPK) increased, alkaline phosphatase increased, LDH increased, PSA increased, urine output increased/decreased, lymphocyte count decreased, neutrophil count decreased, WBC increased/decreased, coagulation test abnormal, low density lipoprotein (LDL) increased, prothrombin time prolonged, urinary casts, urine positive for white blood cells and protein.

Cardiovascular Safety

Cardiovascular events and deaths were adjudicated to one of the pre-defined endpoints from the Anti-Platelet Trialists' Collaborations (APTC) (cardiovascular death, non-fatal myocardial infarction, and non-fatal stroke) in the randomized controlled and long-term extension studies. In the Phase 3 randomized controlled studies, the incidences of adjudicated APTC events per 100 patient-years of exposure were: Placebo 0 (95% CI 0.00-6.16), ULORIC 40 mg 0 (95% CI 0.00-1.08), ULORIC 80 mg 1.09 (95% CI 0.44-2.24), and allopurinol 0.60 (95% CI 0.16-1.53).

In the long-term extension studies, the incidences of adjudicated APTC events were: ULORIC 80 mg 0.97 (95% CI 0.57-1.56), and allopurinol 0.58 (95% CI 0.02-3.24).

Overall, a higher rate of APTC events was observed in ULORIC than in allopurinol-treated patients. A causal relationship with ULORIC has not been established. Monitor for signs and symptoms of MI and stroke.

6.2 Postmarketing Experience

Adverse reactions have been identified during postapproval use of ULORIC. Because these reactions are reported voluntarily from a population of uncertain size, it is not always possible to reliably estimate their frequency or establish a causal relationship.

Hepatobiliary Disorders: hepatic failure (some fatal), jaundice, serious cases of abnormal liver function test results, liver disorder.

Immune System Disorders: anaphylaxis, anaphylactic reaction.

Musculoskeletal and Connective Tissue Disorders: rhabdomyolysis.

Psychiatric Disorders: psychotic behavior including aggressive thoughts.

Renal and Urinary Disorders: tubulointerstitial nephritis.

Skin and Subcutaneous Tissue Disorders: generalized rash, Stevens Johnson Syndrome, hypersensitivity skin reactions.

7 DRUG INTERACTIONS

7.1 Xanthine Oxidase Substrate Drugs

ULORIC is an XO inhibitor. Based on a drug interaction study in healthy subjects, febuxostat altered the metabolism of theophylline (a substrate of XO) in humans *[see Clinical Pharmacology (12.3)]*. Therefore, use with caution when coadministering ULORIC with theophylline.

Drug interaction studies of ULORIC with other drugs that are metabolized by XO (e.g., mercaptopurine and azathioprine) have not been conducted. Inhibition of XO by ULORIC may cause increased plasma concentrations of these drugs leading to toxicity *[see Clinical Pharmacology (12.3)]*. ULORIC is contraindicated in patients being treated with azathioprine or mercaptopurine *[see Contraindications (4)]*.

7.2 Cytotoxic Chemotherapy Drugs

Drug interaction studies of ULORIC with cytotoxic chemotherapy have not been conducted. No data are available regarding the safety of ULORIC during cytotoxic chemotherapy.

7.3 *In Vivo* Drug Interaction Studies

Based on drug interaction studies in healthy subjects, ULORIC does not have clinically significant interactions with colchicine, naproxen, indomethacin, hydrochlorothiazide, warfarin or desipramine *[see Clinical Pharmacology (12.3)]*. Therefore, ULORIC may be used concomitantly with these medications.

8 USE IN SPECIFIC POPULATIONS

8.1 Pregnancy

Pregnancy Category C: There are no adequate and well-controlled studies in pregnant women. ULORIC should be used during pregnancy only if the potential benefit justifies the potential risk to the fetus.

Febuxostat was not teratogenic in rats and rabbits at oral doses up to 48 mg/kg (40 and 51 times the human plasma exposure at 80 mg/day for equal body surface area, respectively) during organogenesis. However, increased neonatal mortality and a reduction in the neonatal body weight gain were observed when pregnant rats were treated with oral doses up to 48 mg/kg (40 times the human plasma exposure at 80 mg/day) during organogenesis and through lactation period.

8.3 Nursing Mothers

Febuxostat is excreted in the milk of rats. It is not known whether this drug is excreted in human milk. Because many drugs are excreted in human milk, caution should be exercised when ULORIC is administered to a nursing woman.

8.4 Pediatric Use

Safety and effectiveness in pediatric patients under 18 years of age have not been established.

8.5 Geriatric Use

No dose adjustment is necessary in elderly patients. Of the total number of subjects in clinical studies of ULORIC, 16% were 65 and over, while 4% were 75 and over. Comparing subjects in different age groups, no clinically significant differences in safety or effectiveness were observed but greater sensitivity of some older individuals cannot be ruled out. The C_{max} and AUC_{24} of febuxostat following multiple oral doses of ULORIC in geriatric subjects (≥65 years) were similar to those in younger subjects (18 to 40 years) *[see Clinical Pharmacology (12.3)]*.

8.6 Renal Impairment

No dose adjustment is necessary in patients with mild or moderate renal impairment (Cl_{cr} 30 to 89 mL/min). The recommended starting dose of ULORIC is 40 mg once daily. For patients who do not achieve a sUA less than 6 mg/dL after two weeks with 40 mg, ULORIC 80 mg is recommended.

There are insufficient data in patients with severe renal impairment (Cl_{cr} less than 30 mL/min); therefore, caution should be exercised in these patients *[see Clinical Pharmacology (12.3)]*.

8.7 Hepatic Impairment

No dose adjustment is necessary in patients with mild or moderate hepatic impairment (Child-Pugh Class A or B). No studies have been conducted in patients with severe hepatic impairment (Child-Pugh Class C); therefore, caution should be exercised in these patients *[see Clinical Pharmacology (12.3)]*.

8.8 Secondary Hyperuricemia

No studies have been conducted in patients with secondary hyperuricemia (including organ transplant recipients); ULORIC is not recommended for use in patients whom the rate of urate formation is greatly increased (e.g., malignant disease and its treatment, Lesch-Nyhan syndrome). The concentration of xanthine in urine could, in rare cases, rise sufficiently to allow deposition in the urinary tract.

10 OVERDOSAGE

ULORIC was studied in healthy subjects in doses up to 300 mg daily for seven days without evidence of dose-limiting toxicities. No overdose of ULORIC was reported in clinical studies. Patients should be managed by symptomatic and supportive care should there be an overdose.

11 DESCRIPTION

ULORIC (febuxostat) is a xanthine oxidase inhibitor. The active ingredient in ULORIC is 2-[3-cyano-4-(2-methylpropoxy) phenyl]-4-methylthiazole-5-carboxylic acid, with a molecular weight of 316.38. The empirical formula is $C_{16}H_{16}N_2O_3S$.

The chemical structure is:

[See chemical structure at top of next column]

Febuxostat is a non-hygroscopic, white crystalline powder that is freely soluble in dimethylformamide; soluble in dimethylsulfoxide; sparingly soluble in ethanol; slightly soluble in methanol and acetonitrile; and practically insoluble in water. The melting range is 205°C to 208°C.

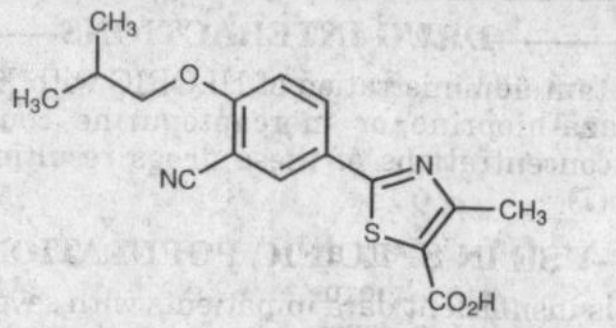

ULORIC tablets for oral use contain the active ingredient, febuxostat, and are available in two dosage strengths, 40 mg and 80 mg. Inactive ingredients include lactose monohydrate, microcrystalline cellulose, hydroxypropyl cellulose, sodium croscarmellose, silicon dioxide and magnesium stearate. ULORIC tablets are coated with Opadry II, green.

12 CLINICAL PHARMACOLOGY

12.1 Mechanism of Action

ULORIC, a xanthine oxidase inhibitor, achieves its therapeutic effect by decreasing serum uric acid. ULORIC is not expected to inhibit other enzymes involved in purine and pyrimidine synthesis and metabolism at therapeutic concentrations.

12.2 Pharmacodynamics

Effect on Uric Acid and Xanthine Concentrations: In healthy subjects, ULORIC resulted in a dose dependent decrease in 24-hour mean serum uric acid concentrations and an increase in 24-hour mean serum xanthine concentrations. In addition, there was a decrease in the total daily urinary uric acid excretion. Also, there was an increase in total daily urinary xanthine excretion. Percent reduction in 24-hour mean serum uric acid concentrations was between 40% and 55% at the exposure levels of 40 mg and 80 mg daily doses.

Effect on Cardiac Repolarization: The effect of ULORIC on cardiac repolarization as assessed by the QTc interval was evaluated in normal healthy subjects and in patients with gout. ULORIC in doses up to 300 mg daily, at steady-state, did not demonstrate an effect on the QTc interval.

12.3 Pharmacokinetics

In healthy subjects, maximum plasma concentrations (C_{max}) and AUC of febuxostat increased in a dose proportional manner following single and multiple doses of 10 mg to 120 mg. There is no accumulation when therapeutic doses are administered every 24 hours. Febuxostat has an apparent mean terminal elimination half-life ($t_{1/2}$) of approximately 5 to 8 hours. Febuxostat pharmacokinetic parameters for patients with hyperuricemia and gout estimated by population pharmacokinetic analyses were similar to those estimated in healthy subjects.

Absorption: The absorption of radiolabeled febuxostat following oral dose administration was estimated to be at least 49% (based on total radioactivity recovered in urine). Maximum plasma concentrations of febuxostat occurred between 1 and 1.5 hours post-dose. After multiple oral 40 mg and 80 mg once daily doses, C_{max} is approximately 1.6 ± 0.6 mcg/mL (N=30), and 2.6 ± 1.7 mcg/mL (N=227), respectively. Absolute bioavailability of the febuxostat tablet has not been studied.

Following multiple 80 mg once daily doses with a high fat meal, there was a 49% decrease in C_{max} and an 18% decrease in AUC, respectively. However, no clinically significant change in the percent decrease in serum uric acid concentration was observed (58% fed vs. 51% fasting). Thus, ULORIC may be taken without regard to food.

Concomitant ingestion of an antacid containing magnesium hydroxide and aluminum hydroxide with an 80 mg single dose of ULORIC has been shown to delay absorption of febuxostat (approximately one hour) and to cause a 31% decrease in C_{max} and a 15% decrease in AUC_{∞}. As AUC rather than C_{max} was related to drug effect, change observed in AUC was not considered clinically significant. Therefore, ULORIC may be taken without regard to antacid use.

Distribution: The mean apparent steady state volume of distribution (V_{ss}/F) of febuxostat was approximately 50 L (CV ~40%). The plasma protein binding of febuxostat is approximately 99.2%, (primarily to albumin), and is constant over the concentration range achieved with 40 mg and 80 mg doses.

Metabolism: Febuxostat is extensively metabolized by both conjugation via uridine diphosphate glucuronosyltransferase (UGT) enzymes including UGT1A1, UGT1A3, UGT1A9, and UGT2B7 and oxidation via cytochrome P450 (CYP) enzymes including CYP1A2, 2C8 and 2C9 and non-P450 enzymes. The relative contribution of each enzyme isoform in the metabolism of febuxostat is not clear. The oxidation of the isobutyl side chain leads to the formation of four pharmacologically active hydroxy metabolites, all of which occur in plasma of humans at a much lower extent than febuxostat.

In urine and feces, acyl glucuronide metabolites of febuxostat (~35% of the dose), and oxidative metabolites, 67M-1 (~10% of the dose), 67M-2 (~11% of the dose), and 67M-4, a secondary metabolite from 67M-1 (~14% of the dose), appeared to be the major metabolites of febuxostat *in vivo*.

Elimination: Febuxostat is eliminated by both hepatic and renal pathways. Following an 80 mg oral dose of ^{14}C-labeled febuxostat, approximately 49% of the dose was recovered in the urine as unchanged febuxostat (3%), the acyl glucuronide of the drug (30%), its known oxidative metabolites and their conjugates (13%), and other unknown metabolites (3%). In addition to the urinary excretion, approximately 45% of the dose was recovered in the feces as the unchanged febuxostat (12%), the acyl glucuronide of the drug (1%), its known oxidative metabolites and their conjugates (25%), and other unknown metabolites (7%).

The apparent mean terminal elimination half-life ($t_{1/2}$) of febuxostat was approximately 5 to 8 hours.

Special Populations

Pediatric Use: The pharmacokinetics of ULORIC in patients under the age of 18 years have not been studied.

Geriatric Use: The C_{max} and AUC of febuxostat and its metabolites following multiple oral doses of ULORIC in geriatric subjects (≥65 years) were similar to those in younger subjects (18 to 40 years). In addition, the percent decrease in serum uric acid concentration was similar between elderly and younger subjects. No dose adjustment is necessary in geriatric patients *[see Use in Specific Populations (8.5)]*.

Renal Impairment: Following multiple 80 mg doses of ULORIC in healthy subjects with mild (Cl_{cr} 50 to 80 mL/min), moderate (Cl_{cr} 30 to 49 mL/min) or severe renal impairment (Cl_{cr} 10 to 29 mL/min), the C_{max} of febuxostat did not change relative to subjects with normal renal function (Cl_{cr} greater than 80 mL/min). AUC and half-life of febuxostat increased in subjects with renal impairment in comparison to subjects with normal renal function, but values were similar among three renal impairment groups. Mean febuxostat AUC values were up to 1.8 times higher in subjects with renal impairment compared to those with normal renal function. Mean C_{max} and AUC values for three active metabolites increased up to 2- and 4-fold, respectively. However, the percent decrease in serum uric acid concentration for subjects with renal impairment was comparable to those with normal renal function (58% in normal renal function group and 55% in the severe renal function group).

No dose adjustment is necessary in patients with mild to moderate renal impairment *[see Dosage and Administration (2) and Use in Specific Populations (8.6)]*. The recommended starting dose of ULORIC is 40 mg once daily. For patients who do not achieve a sUA less than 6 mg/dL after two weeks with 40 mg, ULORIC 80 mg is recommended. There is insufficient data in patients with severe renal impairment; caution should be exercised in those patients *[see Use in Specific Populations (8.6)]*.

ULORIC has not been studied in end stage renal impairment patients who are on dialysis.

Hepatic Impairment: Following multiple 80 mg doses of ULORIC in patients with mild (Child-Pugh Class A) or moderate (Child-Pugh Class B) hepatic impairment, an average of 20% to 30% increase was observed for both C_{max} and AUC_{24} (total and unbound) in hepatic impairment groups compared to subjects with normal hepatic function. In addition, the percent decrease in serum uric acid concentration was comparable between different hepatic groups (62% in healthy group, 49% in mild hepatic impairment group, and 48% in moderate hepatic impairment group). No dose adjustment is necessary in patients with mild or moderate hepatic impairment. No studies have been conducted in subjects with severe hepatic impairment (Child-Pugh Class C); caution should be exercised in those patients *[see Use in Specific Populations (8.7)]*.

Gender: Following multiple oral doses of ULORIC, the C_{max} and AUC_{24} of febuxostat were 30% and 14% higher in females than in males, respectively. However, weight-corrected C_{max} and AUC were similar between the genders. In addition, the percent decrease in serum uric acid concentrations was similar between genders. No dose adjustment is necessary based on gender.

Race: No specific pharmacokinetic study was conducted to investigate the effects of race.

Drug-Drug Interactions

Effect of ULORIC on Other Drugs

Xanthine Oxidase Substrate Drugs-Azathioprine, Mercaptopurine, and Theophylline: Febuxostat is an XO inhibitor. A drug-drug interaction study evaluating the effect of ULORIC upon the pharmacokinetics of theophylline (an XO substrate) in healthy subjects showed that coadministration of febuxostat with theophylline resulted in an approximately 400-fold increase in the amount of 1-methylxanthine, one of the major metabolites of theophylline, excreted in the urine. Since the long-term safety of exposure to 1-methylxanthine in humans is unknown, use with caution when coadministering febuxostat with theophylline.

Drug interaction studies of ULORIC with other drugs that are metabolized by XO (e.g., mercaptopurine and azathioprine) have not been conducted. Inhibition of XO by ULORIC may cause increased plasma concentrations of these drugs leading to toxicity. ULORIC is contraindicated in patients being treated with azathioprine or mercaptopurine *[see Contraindications (4) and Drug Interactions (7)]*.

Azathioprine and mercaptopurine undergo metabolism via three major metabolic pathways, one of which is mediated by XO. Although ULORIC drug interaction studies with azathioprine and mercaptopurine have not been conducted, concomitant administration of allopurinol [a xanthine oxidase inhibitor] with azathioprine or mercaptopurine has been reported to substantially increase plasma concentrations of these drugs. Because ULORIC is a xanthine oxidase inhibitor, it could inhibit the XO-mediated metabolism of azathioprine and mercaptopurine leading to increased plasma concentrations of azathioprine or mercaptopurine that could result in severe toxicity.

P450 Substrate Drugs: In vitro studies have shown that febuxostat does not inhibit P450 enzymes CYP1A2, 2C9, 2C19, 2D6, or 3A4 and it also does not induce CYP1A2, 2B6, 2C9, 2C19, or 3A4 at clinically relevant concentrations. As such, pharmacokinetic interactions between ULORIC and drugs metabolized by these CYP enzymes are unlikely.

Effect of Other Drugs on ULORIC

Febuxostat is metabolized by conjugation and oxidation via multiple metabolizing enzymes. The relative contribution of each enzyme isoform is not clear. Drug interactions between ULORIC and a drug that inhibits or induces one particular enzyme isoform is in general not expected.

In Vivo Drug Interaction Studies

Theophylline: No dose adjustment is necessary for theophylline when coadministered with ULORIC. Administration of ULORIC (80 mg once daily) with theophylline resulted in an increase of 6% in C_{max} and 6.5% in AUC of theophylline. These changes were not considered statistically significant. However, the study also showed an approximately 400-fold increase in the amount of 1-methylxanthine (one of the major theophylline metabolites) excreted in urine as a result of XO inhibition by ULORIC. The safety of long-term exposure to 1-methylxanthine has not been evaluated. This should be taken into consideration when deciding to coadminister ULORIC and theophylline.

Colchicine: No dose adjustment is necessary for either ULORIC or colchicine when the two drugs are coadministered. Administration of ULORIC (40 mg once daily) with colchicine (0.6 mg twice daily) resulted in an increase of 12% in C_{max} and 7% in AUC_{24} of febuxostat. In addition, administration of colchicine (0.6 mg twice daily) with ULORIC (120 mg daily) resulted in a less than 11% change in C_{max} or AUC of colchicine for both AM and PM doses. These changes were not considered clinically significant.

Naproxen: No dose adjustment is necessary for ULORIC or naproxen when the two drugs are coadministered. Administration of ULORIC (80 mg once daily) with naproxen (500 mg twice daily) resulted in a 28% increase in C_{max} and a 40% increase in AUC of febuxostat. The increases were not considered clinically significant. In addition, there were no significant changes in the C_{max} or AUC of naproxen (less than 2%).

Indomethacin: No dose adjustment is necessary for either ULORIC or indomethacin when these two drugs are coadministered. Administration of ULORIC (80 mg once daily) with indomethacin (50 mg twice daily) did not result in any significant changes in C_{max} or AUC of febuxostat or indomethacin (less than 7%).

Hydrochlorothiazide: No dose adjustment is necessary for ULORIC when coadministered with hydrochlorothiazide. Administration of ULORIC (80 mg) with hydrochlorothiazide (50 mg) did not result in any clinically significant changes in C_{max} or AUC of febuxostat (less than 4%), and serum uric acid concentrations were not substantially affected.

Warfarin: No dose adjustment is necessary for warfarin when coadministered with ULORIC. Administration of ULORIC (80 mg once daily) with warfarin had no effect on the pharmacokinetics of warfarin in healthy subjects. INR and Factor VII activity were also not affected by the coadministration of ULORIC.

Desipramine: Coadministration of drugs that are CYP2D6 substrates (such as desipramine) with ULORIC are not expected to require dose adjustment. Febuxostat was shown to be a weak inhibitor of CYP2D6 *in vitro* and *in vivo*. Administration of ULORIC (120 mg once daily) with desipramine (25 mg) resulted in an increase in C_{max} (16%) and AUC (22%) of desipramine, which was associated with a 17% decrease in the 2-hydroxydesipramine to desipramine metabolic ratio (based on AUC).

13 NONCLINICAL TOXICOLOGY

13.1 Carcinogenesis, Mutagenesis, Impairment of Fertility

Carcinogenesis: Two-year carcinogenicity studies were conducted in F344 rats and B6C3F1 mice. Increased transitional cell papilloma and carcinoma of urinary bladder was observed at 24 mg/kg (25 times the human plasma exposure at maximum recommended human dose of 80 mg/day) and 18.75 mg/kg (12.5 times the human plasma exposure at 80 mg/day) in male rats and female mice, respectively. The urinary bladder neoplasms were secondary to calculus formation in the kidney and urinary bladder.

Mutagenesis: Febuxostat showed a positive mutagenic response in a chromosomal aberration assay in a Chinese hamster lung fibroblast cell line with and without metabolic activation *in vitro*. Febuxostat was negative in the *in vitro* Ames assay and chromosomal aberration test in human peripheral lymphocytes, and L5178Y mouse lymphoma cell line, and *in vivo* tests in mouse micronucleus, rat unscheduled DNA synthesis and rat bone marrow cells.

Impairment of Fertility: Febuxostat at oral doses up to 48 mg/kg/day (approximately 35 times the human plasma exposure at 80 mg/day) had no effect on fertility and reproductive performance of male and female rats.

13.2 Animal Toxicology

A 12-month toxicity study in beagle dogs showed deposition of xanthine crystals and calculi in kidneys at 15 mg/kg (approximately four times the human plasma exposure at 80 mg/day). A similar effect of calculus formation was noted in rats in a six-month study due to deposition of xanthine crystals at 48 mg/kg (approximately 35 times the human plasma exposure at 80 mg/day).

14 CLINICAL STUDIES

A serum uric acid level of less than 6 mg/dL is the goal of anti-hyperuricemic therapy and has been established as appropriate for the treatment of gout.

14.1 Management of Hyperuricemia in Gout

The efficacy of ULORIC was demonstrated in three randomized, double-blind, controlled trials in patients with hyperuricemia and gout. Hyperuricemia was defined as a baseline serum uric acid level ≥8 mg/dL.

Study 1 randomized patients to: ULORIC 40 mg daily, ULORIC 80 mg daily, or allopurinol (300 mg daily for patients with estimated creatinine clearance (Cl_{cr}) ≥60 mL/min or 200 mg daily for patients with estimated Cl_{cr} ≥30 mL/min and ≤59 mL/min). The duration of Study 1 was six months.

Study 2 randomized patients to: placebo, ULORIC 80 mg daily, ULORIC 120 mg daily, ULORIC 240 mg daily or allopurinol (300 mg daily for patients with a baseline serum creatinine ≤1.5 mg/dL or 100 mg daily for patients with a baseline serum creatinine greater than 1.5 mg/dL and ≤2 mg/dL). The duration of Study 2 was six months.

Study 3, a 1-year study, randomized patients to: ULORIC 80 mg daily, ULORIC 120 mg daily, or allopurinol 300 mg daily. Subjects who completed Study 2 and Study 3 were eligible to enroll in a phase 3 long-term extension study in which subjects received treatment with ULORIC for over three years.

In all three studies, subjects received naproxen 250 mg twice daily or colchicine 0.6 mg once or twice daily for gout flare prophylaxis. In Study 1 the duration of prophylaxis was six months; in Study 2 and Study 3 the duration of prophylaxis was eight weeks.

The efficacy of ULORIC was also evaluated in a 4 week dose ranging study which randomized patients to: placebo, ULORIC 40 mg daily, ULORIC 80 mg daily, or ULORIC 120 mg daily. Subjects who completed this study were eligible to enroll in a long-term extension study in which subjects received treatment with ULORIC for up to five years.

Patients in these studies were representative of the patient population for which ULORIC use is intended. Table 2 summarizes the demographics and baseline characteristics for the subjects enrolled in the studies.

Table 2: Patient Demographics and Baseline Characteristics in Study 1, Study 2 and Study 3

Male		95%
Race:	Caucasian African American	80% 10%
Ethnicity:	Hispanic or Latino	7%
Alcohol User		67%
Mild to Moderate Renal Insufficiency (percent with estimated Cl_{cr} less than 90 mL/min)		59%
History of Hypertension		49%
History of Hyperlipidemia		38%
BMI ≥30 kg/m^2		63%
Mean BMI		33 kg/m^2

Table 3: Proportion of Patients with Serum Uric Acid Levels less than 6 mg/dL at Final Visit

Study*	ULORIC 40 mg daily	ULORIC 80 mg daily	allopurinol	Placebo	Difference in Proportion (95% CI) ULORIC 40 mg vs allopurinol	Difference in Proportion (95% CI) ULORIC 80 mg vs allopurinol
Study 1 (6 months) (N=2268)	45%	67%	42%		3% (-2%, 8%)	25% (20%, 30%)
Study 2 (6 months) (N=643)		72%	39%	1%		33% (26%, 42%)
Study 3 (12 months) (N=491)		74%	36%			38% (30%, 46%)

* Randomization was balanced between treatment groups, except in Study 2 in which twice as many patients were randomized to each of the active treatment groups compared to placebo.

Table 4: Proportion of Patients with Serum Uric Acid Levels less than 6 mg/dL in Patients with Mild or Moderate Renal Impairment at Final Visit

ULORIC 40 mg daily (N=479)	ULORIC 80 mg daily (N=503)	allopurinol* 300 mg daily (N=501)	Difference in Proportion (95% CI) ULORIC 40 mg vs allopurinol	Difference in Proportion (95% CI) ULORIC 80 mg vs allopurinol
50%	72%	42%	7% (1%, 14%)	29% (23%, 35%)

* Allopurinol patients (n=145) with estimated Cl_{cr} ≥30 mL/min and Cl_{cr} ≤59 mL/min were dosed at 200 mg daily.

Baseline sUA ≥10 mg/dL	36%
Mean baseline sUA	9.7 mg/dL
Experienced a gout flare in previous year	85%

Serum Uric Acid Level less than 6 mg/dL at Final Visit: ULORIC 80 mg was superior to allopurinol in lowering serum uric acid to less than 6 mg/dL at the final visit. ULORIC 40 mg daily, although not superior to allopurinol, was effective in lowering serum uric acid to less than 6 mg/dL at the final visit *(Table 3)*.

[See table 3 above]

In 76% of ULORIC 80 mg patients, reduction in serum uric acid levels to less than 6 mg/dL was noted by the Week 2 visit. Average serum uric acid levels were maintained at 6 mg/dL or below throughout treatment in 83% of these patients.

In all treatment groups, fewer subjects with higher baseline serum urate levels (≥10 mg/dL) and/or tophi achieved the goal of lowering serum uric acid to less than 6 mg/dL at the final visit; however, a higher proportion achieved a serum uric acid less than 6 mg/dL with ULORIC 80 mg than with ULORIC 40 mg or allopurinol.

Study 1 evaluated efficacy in patients with mild to moderate renal impairment (i.e., baseline estimated Cl_{cr} less than 90 mL/min). The results in this sub-group of patients are shown in Table 4.

[See table 4 above]

16 HOW SUPPLIED/STORAGE AND HANDLING

ULORIC 40 mg tablets are light green to green in color, round, debossed with "TAP" on one side and "40" on the other side and supplied as:

NDC Number	Size
64764-918-11	Hospital Unit Dose Pack of 100 Tablets
64764-918-30	Bottle of 30 Tablets
64764-918-90	Bottle of 90 Tablets
64764-918-18	Bottle of 500 Tablets

ULORIC 80 mg tablets are light green to green in color, teardrop shaped, debossed with "TAP" on one side and "80" on the other side and supplied as:

NDC Number	Size
64764-677-11	Hospital Unit Dose Pack of 100 Tablets
64764-677-30	Bottle of 30 Tablets
64764-677-13	Bottle of 100 Tablets
64764-677-19	Bottle of 1000 Tablets

Protect from light. Store at 25°C (77°F); excursions permitted to 15° to 30°C (59° to 86°F) [See USP Controlled Room Temperature].

17 PATIENT COUNSELING INFORMATION

See FDA-Approved Patient Labeling (Patient Information)

17.1 General Information

Patients should be advised of the potential benefits and risks of ULORIC. Patients should be informed about the potential for gout flares, elevated liver enzymes and adverse cardiovascular events after initiation of ULORIC therapy.

Concomitant prophylaxis with an NSAID or colchicine for gout flares should be considered.

Patients should be instructed to inform their healthcare professional if they develop a rash, chest pain, shortness of breath or neurologic symptoms suggesting a stroke. Patients should be instructed to inform their healthcare professional of any other medications they are currently taking with ULORIC, including over-the-counter medications.

Patient Information

ULORIC (Ū–'lor–ik)

(febuxostat) tablets

Read the Patient Information that comes with ULORIC before you start taking it and each time you get a refill. There may be new information. This information does not take the place of talking with your healthcare provider about your medical condition or your treatment.

What is ULORIC?

ULORIC is a prescription medicine called a xanthine oxidase (XO) inhibitor, used to lower blood uric acid levels in adults with gout.

It is not known if ULORIC is safe and effective in children under 18 years of age.

Who should not take ULORIC?

Do not take ULORIC if you:

- take azathioprine (Azasan, Imuran)
- take mercaptopurine (Purinethol)

It is not known if ULORIC is safe and effective in children under 18 years of age.

What should I tell my healthcare provider before taking ULORIC?

Before taking ULORIC tell your healthcare provider about all of your medical conditions, including if you:

- have liver or kidney problems
- have a history of heart disease or stroke
- are pregnant or plan to become pregnant. It is not known if ULORIC will harm your unborn baby. Talk with your healthcare provider if you are pregnant or plan to become pregnant.
- are breastfeeding or plan to breastfeed. It is not known if ULORIC passes into your breast milk. You and your healthcare provider should decide if you should take ULORIC while breastfeeding.

Tell your healthcare provider about all the medicines you take, including prescription and non-prescription medicines, vitamins, and herbal supplements. ULORIC may affect the way other medicines work, and other medicines may affect how ULORIC works.

Know the medicines you take. Keep a list of them and show it to your healthcare provider and pharmacist when you get a new medicine.

How should I take ULORIC?

- Take ULORIC exactly as your healthcare provider tells you to take it.
- ULORIC can be taken with or without food.
- ULORIC can be taken with antacids.
- Your gout may flare up when you start taking ULORIC, do not stop taking your ULORIC even if you have a flare. Your healthcare provider may give you other medicines to help prevent your gout flares.
- Your healthcare provider may do certain tests while you take ULORIC.

What are the possible side effects of ULORIC?

Heart problems. A small number of heart attacks, strokes and heart-related deaths were seen in clinical studies. It is not certain that ULORIC caused these events.

The most common side effects of ULORIC include:

- liver problems
- nausea
- gout flares
- joint pain
- rash

Tell your healthcare provider if you develop a rash, have any side effect that bothers you, or that does not go away. These are not all of the possible side effects of ULORIC. For more information, ask your healthcare provider or pharmacist.

Call your doctor for medical advice about side effects. You may report side effects to the FDA at 1-800-FDA-1088.

How should I store ULORIC?

Store ULORIC between 59°F and 86°F (15°C to 30°C).

Keep ULORIC out of the light.

Keep ULORIC and all medicines out of the reach of children.

General information about the safe and effective use of ULORIC.

Medicines are sometimes prescribed for purposes other than those listed in a patient information leaflet. Do not use ULORIC for a condition for which it was not prescribed. Do not give ULORIC to other people, even if they have the same symptoms that you have. It may harm them.

This patient information leaflet summarizes the most important information about ULORIC. If you would like more information about ULORIC talk with your healthcare provider. You can ask your healthcare provider or pharmacist for information about ULORIC that is written for health professionals. For more information go to www.uloric.com, or call 1-877-825-3327.

What are the ingredients in ULORIC?

Active Ingredient: febuxostat

Inactive ingredients include: lactose monohydrate, microcrystalline cellulose, hydroxypropyl cellulose, sodium croscarmellose, silicon dioxide, magnesium stearate, and Opadry II, green

Distributed by:

Takeda Pharmaceuticals America, Inc.

Deerfield, IL 60015

Revised: November 2012

ULORIC is a registered trademark of Teijin Pharma Limited registered in the U.S. Patent and Trademark Office and used under license by Takeda Pharmaceuticals America, Inc.

All other trademarks are the property of their respective owners.

ULR015 R3

Shown in Product Identification Guide, page 313

Teva
11100 NALL AVENUE
OVERLAND PARK, KS 66221

For Company Inquiries Contact:
1-800-221-4026
For Medical Information Contact:
1-888-4-TEVA-RX
(1-888-483-8279)

AZILECT® ℞
[az-ĭl-ect]
(rasagiline mesylate)
Tablets for Oral Use

HIGHLIGHTS OF PRESCRIBING INFORMATION
These highlights do not include all the information needed to use AZILECT® safely and effectively. See full prescribing information for AZILECT®.
AZILECT® (rasagiline mesylate) Tablets for Oral Use
Initial U.S. Approval: 2006

INDICATIONS AND USAGE

AZILECT is indicated for the treatment of the signs and symptoms of idiopathic Parkinson's disease as initial monotherapy and as adjunct therapy to levodopa. (1)

DOSAGE AND ADMINISTRATION

- Monotherapy: AZILECT 1 mg once daily (2.1)
- As adjunct to levodopa: AZILECT 0.5 mg once daily. Dose increase to 1 mg daily as required for sufficient clinical response. (2.2)
- Patients with mild hepatic impairment: AZILECT 0.5 mg once daily should not be exceeded. AZILECT should not be used in patients with moderate or severe hepatic impairment (2.3)
- AZILECT has not been studied in patients with severe renal impairment (2.4)
- Patients taking ciprofloxacin or other CYP1A2 inhibitors: AZILECT 0.5 mg once daily should not be exceeded. (2.5)

DOSAGE FORMS AND STRENGTHS

- AZILECT 0.5 mg tablets (containing, as the active ingredient, rasagiline mesylate equivalent to 0.5 mg of rasagiline base) (3)
- AZILECT 1 mg tablets (containing, as the active ingredient, rasagiline mesylate equivalent to 1 mg of rasagiline base) (3)

CONTRAINDICATIONS

Concomitant use of :
- meperidine, tramadol, methadone or propoxyphene (4.1)
- dextromethorphan, St. John's wort or cyclobenzaprine (4.2)
- other MAO inhibitors (selective or non-selective) (4.3)

WARNINGS AND PRECAUTIONS

- Risk of severe CNS toxicity (serotonin syndrome) when AZILECT is combined with antidepressants. (5.1)
- Concomitant use of ciprofloxacin or other CYP1A2 inhibitors: Increase in rasagiline plasma concentrations. 0.5 mg rasagiline once daily should not be exceeded (5.2)
- Patients with hepatic impairment: Increase in rasagiline plasma concentrations. Limit dose to 0.5 mg rasagiline in mild hepatic impairment. AZILECT should not be used in patients with moderate or severe hepatic impairment (5.3)
- Risk for Hypertensive Crisis and nonselective MAO inhibition above the recommended Doses (5.4)
- Melanoma (5.4)
- AZILECT may cause lower blood pressure, especially postural hypotension (5.7) or increase blood pressure in different patients (5.8)
- AZILECT may cause or exacerbate hallucinations or potentially other manifestations of psychotic-like behavior (5.9)

ADVERSE REACTIONS

- Most common adverse reactions (treatment difference ≥ 3% greater than placebo); with monotherapy: flu syndrome, arthralgia, depression, dyspepsia. (6.1)
- Most common adverse reactions (treatment difference ≥ 3% greater than placebo); when used as adjunct to levodopa: dyskinesia, accidental injury, weight loss, postural hypotension, vomiting, anorexia, arthralgia, abdominal pain, nausea, constipation, dry mouth, rash, abnormal dreams, fall. (6.1)

To report SUSPECTED ADVERSE REACTIONS, contact TEVA at 1-800-221-4026 or FDA at 1-800-FDA-1088 or *www.fda.gov/medwatch.*

DRUG INTERACTIONS

- Meperidine: Risk of serious, sometimes fatal reactions from serotonin syndrome. See also Contraindications. (7.1)
- Dextromethorphan: Risk of psychosis episodes or bizarre behavior. See also Contraindications. (7.2)
- MAO inhibitors: Risk of non-selective MAO inhibition and hypertensive crisis. See also Contraindications. (7.4)
- Antidepressants (SSRIs, SNRIs, tricyclic, tetracyclic, or triazolopyridine): Concomitant use not recommended. (7.5)
- Levodopa: See also Warnings and Precautions. (7.6)
- Ciprofloxacin and Other CYP1A2 Inhibitors: Increased rasagiline plasma levels possible. Increased risk of adverse events. See also Dosage and Administration and Warnings and Precautions.(7.7)

USE IN SPECIFIC POPULATIONS

- Pregnancy: AZILECT should be used only if the potential benefit justifies the potential risk to the fetus. (8.1)
- Nursing mothers: Rasagiline inhibits prolactin secretion and may inhibit milk secretion. It is not known whether rasagiline is excreted in human milk. Use with caution. (8.3)
- Hepatic impairment: Rasagiline plasma concentrations may be increased. See also Dosage and Administration and Warnings and Precautions. (8.6)

See 17 for PATIENT COUNSELING INFORMATION

Revised: 08/2012

FULL PRESCRIBING INFORMATION: CONTENTS*

*** Sections or subsections omitted from the full prescribing information are not listed**

FULL PRESCRIBING INFORMATION

1 INDICATIONS AND USAGE

AZILECT (rasagiline tablets) is indicated for the treatment of the signs and symptoms of idiopathic Parkinson's disease as initial monotherapy and as adjunct therapy to levodopa. The effectiveness of AZILECT was demonstrated in patients with early Parkinson's disease who were receiving AZILECT as monotherapy and who were not receiving any concomitant dopaminergic therapy. The effectiveness of AZILECT as adjunct therapy was demonstrated in patients with Parkinson's disease who were treated with levodopa.

2 DOSAGE AND ADMINISTRATION

AZILECT is a selective inhibitor of monoamine oxidase (MAO)-B at recommended doses of 0.5 or 1 mg daily. Dietary tyramine restriction is not ordinarily required with recommended doses of AZILECT. However, certain foods (e.g., aged cheeses, such as Stilton cheese) may contain very high amounts (i.e., > 150 mg) of tyramine and could potentially cause a hypertensive "cheese" reaction in patients taking AZILECT even at the recommended dose due to mild increased sensitivity to tyramine. The selectivity for inhibiting MAO-B diminishes in a dose-related manner as the dose is progressively increased above the recommended daily dose *[see Warnings and Precautions (5.4), Clinical Pharmacology (12.3, and Information for Patients (17.3)]*.

2.1 Monotherapy

The recommended AZILECT dose for the treatment of Parkinson's disease patients is 1 mg administered orally once daily.

2.2 Adjunctive Therapy

The recommended initial dose is 0.5 mg administered orally once daily. If a sufficient clinical response is not achieved, the dose may be increased to 1 mg administered once daily.

Change of Levodopa Dose in Adjunct Therapy

When AZILECT is used in combination with levodopa, a reduction of the levodopa dosage may be considered based upon individual response. During the controlled trials of AZILECT as adjunct therapy to levodopa, levodopa dosage was reduced in some patients. In clinical studies, dosage reduction of levodopa was allowed within the first 6 weeks if dopaminergic side effects, including dyskinesia and hallucinations, emerged. In Study 1, levodopa dosage reduction occurred in 8% of patients in the placebo group and in 16% and 17% of patients in the 0.5 mg/day and 1 mg/day rasagiline groups, respectively. In those patients who had levodopa dosage reduced, the dose was reduced on average by about 7%, 9%, and 13% in the placebo, 0.5 mg/day, and 1 mg/day groups, respectively. In Study 2, levodopa dosage reduction occurred in 6% of patients in the placebo group and in 9% in the rasagiline 1 mg/day group. In patients who had their levodopa dosage reduced, the dose was reduced on average by about 13% and 11% in the placebo and the rasagiline groups, respectively.

2.3 Patients with Hepatic Impairment

AZILECT plasma concentrations will increase in patients with hepatic impairment. Patients with mild hepatic impairment should use 0.5 mg daily of AZILECT. AZILECT should not be used in patients with moderate or severe hepatic impairment *[see Warnings and Precautions (5.3), Use in Specific Populations (8.6), and Clinical Pharmacology (12.3)]*.

2.4 Patients with Renal Impairment

Dose adjustment of AZILECT is not required for patients with mild or moderate renal impairment because AZILECT plasma concentrations are not increased in patients with moderate renal impairment. Rasagiline has not been studied in patients with severe renal impairment.

2.5 Patients Taking Ciprofloxacin or Other CYP1A2 Inhibitors

Rasagiline plasma concentrations are expected to double in patients taking concomitant ciprofloxacin and other

CYP1A2 inhibitors. Therefore, patients taking concomitant ciprofloxacin or other CYP1A2 inhibitors should use 0.5 mg daily of AZILECT *[see Warnings and Precautions (5.2), Drug Interactions (7.7), and Clinical Pharmacology (12.3)]*.

3 DOSAGE FORMS AND STRENGTHS

AZILECT 0.5 mg Tablets: White to off-white, round, flat, beveled tablets, debossed with "GIL 0.5" on one side and plain on the other side containing, as the active ingredient, rasagiline mesylate equivalent to 0.5 mg of rasagiline base.
AZILECT 1 mg Tablets: White to off-white, round, flat, beveled tablets, debossed with "GIL 1" on one side and plain on the other side containing, as the active ingredient, rasagiline mesylate equivalent to 1 mg of rasagiline base.

4 CONTRAINDICATIONS

4.1 Meperidine and Certain Other Analgesics

AZILECT is contraindicated for use with meperidine. Serious adverse reactions have been precipitated with concomitant use of meperidine (e.g., Demerol and other tradenames) and MAO inhibitors (MAOIs) including selective MAO-B inhibitors. These adverse reactions are often described as "serotonin syndrome", a potentially serious condition, which can result in death. Typical clinical signs and symptoms include behavioral and cognitive/mental status changes (e.g., confusion, hypomania, hallucinations, agitation, delirium, headache, and coma), autonomic effects (e.g., syncope, shivering, sweating, high fever/hyperthermia, hypertension, hypotension, tachycardia, nausea, diarrhea), and somatic effects (e.g., muscular rigidity, myoclonus, muscle twitching, hyperreflexia manifested by clonus, and tremor). At least 14 days should elapse between discontinuation of AZILECT and initiation of treatment with meperidine.
For similar reasons, AZILECT should not be administered with the analgesic agents tramadol, methadone, and propoxyphene.
In the post-marketing period, serotonin syndrome has been reported in a patient erroneously treated with a higher than recommended dose of AZILECT (4 mg daily) and tramadol.

4.2 Other Drugs

AZILECT should not be used with the antitussive agent dextromethorphan. The combination of MAO inhibitors and dextromethorphan has been reported to cause brief episodes of psychosis or bizarre behavior. AZILECT is also contraindicated for use with St. John's wort, and cyclobenzaprine (a tricyclic muscle relaxant).

4.3 MAO Inhibitors

AZILECT should not be administered along with any other MAO inhibitor (selective or non-selective) because of the increased risk of non-selective MAO inhibition that may lead to a hypertensive crisis. At least 14 days should elapse between discontinuation of AZILECT and initiation of treatment with any MAO inhibitor.

5 WARNINGS AND PRECAUTIONS

5.1 Coadministration with Antidepressants

Severe CNS toxicity associated with hyperpyrexia has been reported with the combined treatment of an antidepressant (e.g., selective serotonin reuptake inhibitors-SSRIs, serotonin-norepinephrine reuptake inhibitors-SNRIs, tricyclic antidepressants, tetracyclic antidepressants, triazolopyridine antidepressants) and a non-selective MAOI (e.g., phenelzine, tranylcypromine) or selective MAO-B inhibitors, such as selegiline (Eldepryl) and rasagiline (AZILECT). These adverse reactions are often described as "serotonin syndrome" which can result in death. In the post-marketing period, non-fatal cases of serotonin syndrome have been reported in patients treated with antidepressants concomitantly with AZILECT.
The symptoms of serotonin syndrome have included behavioral and cognitive/mental status changes (e.g., confusion, hypomania, hallucinations, agitation, delirium, headache, and coma), autonomic effects (e.g., syncope, shivering, sweating, high fever/hyperthermia, hypertension, tachycardia, nausea, diarrhea), and somatic effects (e.g., muscular rigidity, myoclonus, muscle twitching, hyperreflexia manifested by clonus, and tremor).
AZILECT clinical trials did not allow concomitant use of fluoxetine or fluvoxamine with AZILECT, but the following antidepressants and doses were allowed in the AZILECT trials: amitriptyline ≤ 50 mg/daily, trazodone ≤ 100 mg/daily, citalopram ≤ 20 mg/daily, sertraline ≤ 100 mg/daily and paroxetine ≤ 30 mg/daily.
Although a small number of rasagiline-treated patients were concomitantly exposed to antidepressants (tricyclics n=115; SSRIs n=141), the exposure, both in dose and number of subjects, was not adequate to rule out the possibility of an untoward reaction from combining these agents. Furthermore, because the mechanisms of these reactions are not fully understood, it seems prudent, in general, to avoid the combination of AZILECT with any antidepressant. At least 14 days should elapse between discontinuation of AZILECT and initiation of treatment with a SSRI, SNRI, tricyclic, tetracyclic, or triazolopyridine antidepressant. Because of the long half lives of certain antidepressants (e.g., fluoxetine and its active metabolite), at least five weeks (perhaps longer, especially if fluoxetine has been prescribed chronically and/or at higher doses) should elapse between discontinuation of fluoxetine and initiation of AZILECT *[see Drug Interactions (7.5)]*.

5.2 Ciprofloxacin and Other CYP1A2 Inhibitors

Rasagiline plasma concentrations may increase up to 2 fold in patients using concomitant ciprofloxacin and other CYP1A2 inhibitors *[see Dosage and Administration (2.5), Drug Interactions (7.7), and Clinical Pharmacology (12.3)]*.

5.3 Hepatic Impairment

Rasagiline plasma concentration may increase in patients with mild (up to 2 fold, Child-Pugh score 5-6), moderate (up to 7 fold, Child-Pugh score 7-9), and severe (Child-Pugh score 10-15) hepatic impairment. Patients with mild hepatic impairment should be given the dose of 0.5 mg/day. AZILECT should not be used in patients with moderate or severe hepatic impairment *[see Dosage and Administration (2.3) and Clinical Pharmacology (12.3)]*.

5.4 Risk for Hypertensive Crisis and Nonselective Monoamine Oxidase Inhibition Above The Recommended Doses

AZILECT is a selective inhibitor of monoamine oxidase (MAO)-B at the recommended doses of 0.5 or 1 mg daily. AZILECT should not be used at daily doses exceeding 1 mg/day (or 0.5 mg/day for patients with mild hepatic impairment or in patients using concomitant ciprofloxacin or another CYP1A2 inhibitor) because of the risks of hypertensive crisis and other adverse reactions associated with nonselective inhibition of MAO *[see Dosage and Administration (2), Drug Interactions (7.9), and Clinical Pharmacology (12.3)]*.
Dietary tyramine restriction is not ordinarily required with ingestion of most foods and beverages that may contain tyramine, during treatment with recommended doses of AZILECT. However, certain foods (e.g., aged cheeses, such as Stilton cheese) may contain very high amounts (i.e., > 150 mg) of tyramine and could potentially cause a hypertensive "cheese" reaction in patients taking AZILECT even at the recommended doses due to mild increased sensitivity to tyramine. Patients should be advised to avoid foods (e.g., aged cheese) containing a very large amount of tyramine while taking recommended doses of AZILECT because of the potential for large increases in blood pressure. Selectivity for inhibiting MAO-B diminishes in a dose-related manner as the dose is progressively increased above the recommended daily doses.
There were no cases of hypertensive crisis in the clinical development program associated with 1 mg daily rasagiline treatment, in which most patients did not follow dietary tyramine restriction.
Rare cases of hypertensive crisis have been reported in the post-marketing period in patients after ingesting unknown amounts of tyramine-rich foods while taking recommended doses of AZILECT.

5.5 Melanoma

Epidemiological studies have shown that patients with Parkinson's disease have a higher risk (2- to approximately 6-fold higher) of developing melanoma than the general population. Whether the increased risk observed was due to Parkinson's disease or other factors, such as drugs used to treat Parkinson's disease, is unclear.
For the reasons stated above, patients and providers are advised to monitor for melanomas frequently and on a regular basis. Ideally, periodic skin examinations should be performed by appropriately qualified individuals (e.g., dermatologists).

5.6 Dyskinesia

When used as an adjunct to levodopa, AZILECT may cause dyskinesia or potentiate dopaminergic side effects and exacerbate pre-existing dyskinesia (treatment-emergent dyskinesia occurred in about 18% of patients treated with 0.5 mg or 1 mg rasagiline as an adjunct to levodopa, and 10% of patients who received placebo as an adjunct to levodopa). Decreasing the dose of levodopa may ameliorate this side effect.

5.7 Lowering of Blood Pressure and Postural/Orthostatic Hypotension

In placebo controlled studies of AZILECT given in combination with levodopa, the incidence of postural hypotension consisting of a systolic blood pressure decrease (≥ 30 mm Hg) or a diastolic blood pressure decrease (≥ 20 mm Hg) after standing was 13.4 % with AZILECT (1 mg/day) compared to 8.5 % with placebo.
At the 1 mg dose, the frequency of orthostatic hypotension at any time during the study was approximately 44 % for AZILECT vs 33% for placebo for mild to moderate systolic blood pressure decrements (≥ 20 mm Hg), 40 % for AZILECT vs 33 % for placebo for mild to moderate diastolic blood pressure decrements (≥ 10 mm Hg), 7 % for AZILECT vs 3 % for placebo for severe systolic blood pressure decrements (≥ 40 mm Hg), and 9 % for AZILECT vs 6 % for placebo for severe diastolic blood pressure decrements (≥ 20 mm Hg). There was also an increased risk for some of these abnormalities at the lower 0.5 mg daily dose and for an individual patient having mild to moderate or severe postural hypotension for both systolic and diastolic blood pressure.
Clinical trial data further suggest that postural hypotension occurs most frequently in the first two months of AZILECT treatment and tends to decrease over time.
Some patients treated with AZILECT experienced a mildly increased risk for significant decreases in blood pressure unrelated to standing but while supine.
The risk for post-treatment hypotension (e.g., systolic < 90 or diastolic < 50 mm Hg) combined with a significant decrease from baseline (e.g., systolic > 30 or diastolic > 20 mm Hg) was higher for AZILECT 1 mg (3.2 %) compared to placebo (1.3 %).
There was no clear increased risk for lowering of blood pressure or postural hypotension associated with AZILECT 1 mg/day as monotherapy.
When used as an adjunct to levodopa, postural hypotension was also reported as an adverse reaction in approximately 6% of patients treated with 0.5 mg rasagiline, 9% of patients treated with 1 mg rasagiline and 3% of patients treated with placebo. Postural hypotension led to drug discontinuation and premature withdrawal from clinical trials in one (0.7%) patient treated with rasagiline 1 mg/day, no patients treated with rasagiline 0.5 mg/day and no placebo-treated patients.

5.8 Elevation of Blood Pressure

In studies in which AZILECT (1 mg/day) was given in conjunction with levodopa, AZILECT produced an increased incidence of a significant, high blood pressure (e.g., systolic > 180 or diastolic > 100 mm Hg) of 4% compared to 3% for placebo.
The risk for developing post-treatment high blood pressure (e.g., systolic > 180 or diastolic >100 mm Hg) combined with a significant increase from baseline (e.g., systolic > 30 or diastolic > 20 mm Hg) was higher for AZILECT (2 %) compared to placebo (1 %).
There was no increased frequency of the incidence of hypertension as an adverse reaction in the adjunctive treatment pivotal trials for AZILECT treatment vs placebo.
There was no observed increased risk for increasing blood pressure or high blood pressure (based upon various measurements and analyses) or for the development of hypertension as an adverse reaction in the monotherapy study for 1 mg daily AZILECT treatment (vs placebo).

5.9 Hallucinations / Psychotic-Like Behavior

In the monotherapy study, hallucinations were reported as an adverse event in 1.3% of patients treated with 1 mg rasagiline and in 0.7% of patients treated with placebo. In the monotherapy trial, hallucinations led to drug discontinuation and premature withdrawal from clinical trials in 1.3% of the 1 mg rasagiline-treated patients and in none of the placebo-treated patients.
When used as an adjunct to levodopa, hallucinations were reported as an adverse reaction in approximately 5% of patients treated with 0.5 mg/day AZILECT, 4% of patients treated with 1 mg/day AZILECT and 3% of patients treated with placebo. Hallucinations led to drug discontinuation and premature withdrawal from clinical trials in about 1% of patients treated with 0.5 mg/day or 1 mg/day rasagiline and none of the placebo-treated patients.
Patients should be informed of the possibility of developing hallucinations and instructed to report them to their health care provider promptly should they develop.
Patients with a major psychotic disorder should ordinarily not be treated with AZILECT because of the risk of exacerbating the psychosis with an increase in central dopaminergic tone. In addition, many treatments for psychosis that decrease in central dopaminergic tone may decrease the effectiveness of AZILECT.
AZILECT administration may cause or exacerbate psychotic-like behavior based upon post-marketing reports. This adverse reaction has been reported with many anti-Parkinsonian drugs that increase central dopaminergic tone. This abnormal behavior has been exhibited by one or more of a variety of manifestations including paranoia, confusional state/confusion, psychotic disorder, agitation, delusion, and hallucinations.

5.10 Withdrawal-Emergent Hyperpyrexia and Confusion

A symptom complex resembling neuroleptic malignant syndrome (characterized by elevated temperature, muscular rigidity, altered consciousness, and autonomic instability), with no other obvious etiology, has been reported in association with rapid dose reduction, withdrawal of, or changes in drugs that increase central dopaminergic tone. *[see Dosage and Administration (2.2)]*.
Withdrawal emergent hyperpyrexia was not reported in the AZILECT clinical development program.

5.11 Laboratory Tests

No specific laboratory tests are required for the treatment of patients on AZILECT.

6 ADVERSE REACTIONS

6.1 Clinical Studies Experience

During the clinical development of AZILECT, 1361 Parkinson's disease patients received rasagiline as initial monotherapy or as adjunct therapy to levodopa. As these two populations differ, not only in the adjunct use of levodopa during rasagiline treatment, but also in the severity and duration of their disease, they may have differential risks for various adverse reactions. Therefore, most of the adverse reactions data in this section are presented separately for each population.

Because clinical trials are conducted under widely varying conditions, adverse reaction rates observed in the clinical trials of a drug cannot be directly compared to rates in the clinical trials of another drug and may not reflect the rates of adverse reactions observed in practice.

Patients Receiving AZILECT as Initial Monotherapy Treatment

Adverse Reactions Leading to Discontinuation in Controlled Clinical Studies

In the double-blind, placebo-controlled trials conducted in patients receiving AZILECT as monotherapy, approximately 5% of the 149 patients treated with rasagiline discontinued treatment due to adverse reactions compared to 2% of the 151 patients who received placebo.

The only adverse reaction that led to the discontinuation of more than one patient was hallucinations.

Adverse Reaction Incidence in Controlled Clinical Studies

The most commonly observed adverse reactions were those in which the treatment difference for the incidence in AZILECT-treated patients was ≥ 3 % greater than the incidence in the placebo-treated patients and included flu syndrome, arthralgia, depression, and dyspepsia. Table 1 lists treatment-emergent adverse reactions that occurred in ≥ 2% of patients receiving AZILECT as monotherapy participating in the double-blind, placebo-controlled trial and were numerically more frequent than in the placebo group.

Table 1. Treatment-Emergent* Adverse Reactions in AZILECT 1 mg-Treated Monotherapy Patients

Placebo-Controlled Studies Without Levodopa Treatment	AZILECT 1 mg (N=149)	Placebo (N=151)
	% of Patients	% of Patients
Headache	14	12
Arthralgia	7	4
Dyspepsia	7	4
Depression	5	2
Fall	5	3
Flu syndrome	5	1
Conjunctivitis	3	1
Fever	3	1
Gastroenteritis	3	1
Rhinitis	3	1
Arthritis	2	1
Ecchymosis	2	0
Malaise	2	0
Neck Pain	2	0
Paresthesia	2	1
Vertigo	2	1

* Incidence ≥ 2% in AZILECT 1 mg group and numerically more frequent than in placebo group

Other events of potential clinical importance reported by 1% or more of patients receiving AZILECT as monotherapy, and at least as frequent as in the placebo group, in descending order of frequency include: dizziness, diarrhea, chest pain, albuminuria, allergic reaction, alopecia, angina pectoris, anorexia, asthma, hallucinations, impotence, leukopenia, libido decreased, liver function tests abnormal, skin carcinoma, syncope, vesiculobullous rash, vomiting.

There were no significant differences in the safety profile based on age or gender.

Patients Receiving AZILECT as Adjunct to Levodopa Therapy

Adverse Reactions Leading to Discontinuation in Controlled Clinical Studies

In a double-blind, placebo-controlled trial (Study 1) conducted in patients treated with AZILECT as adjunct to levodopa therapy, approximately 9% of the 164 patients treated with AZILECT 0.5 mg/day and 7% of the 149 patients treated with AZILECT 1 mg/day discontinued treatment due to adverse reactions compared to 6% of the 159 patients who received placebo. The adverse reactions that led to discontinuation of more than one rasagiline-treated patient were: diarrhea, weight loss, hallucination, and rash. Adverse event reporting was considered more reliable for Study 1 than for the second controlled trial (Study 2); therefore only the adverse event data from Study 1 are presented in this section of labeling.

Adverse Reactions: Incidence in Controlled Clinical Studies

The most commonly observed adverse reactions were those in which the treatment difference for the incidence in AZILECT-treated patients (n=149) was ≥ 3 % greater than the incidence in the placebo-treated patients (n=159) and included dyskinesia, accidental injury, weight loss, postural hypotension, vomiting, anorexia, arthralgia, abdominal pain, nausea, constipation, dry mouth, rash, abnormal dreams, and fall.

Table 2 lists treatment-emergent adverse reactions that occurred in ≥ 2% of patients treated with AZILECT 1 mg/day as adjunct to levodopa therapy participating in the double-blind, placebo-controlled trial (Study 1) and that were numerically more frequent than the placebo group. The table also shows the rates for the 0.5 mg group in Study 1.

Table 2. Incidence of Treatment-Emergent* Adverse Reactions in Patients Receiving AZILECT as Adjunct to Levodopa Therapy in Study 1

	AZILECT 1 mg + Levodopa (N=149)	AZILECT 0.5 mg + Levodopa (N=164)	Placebo + Levodopa (N=159)
	% of patients	% of patients	% of patients
Dyskinesia	18	18	10
Accidental injury	12	8	5
Nausea	12	10	8
Headache	11	8	10
Fall	11	12	8
Weight loss	9	2	3
Constipation	9	4	5
Postural hypotension	9	6	3
Arthralgia	8	6	4
Vomiting	7	4	1
Dry mouth	6	2	3
Rash	6	3	3
Somnolence	6	4	4
Abdominal pain	5	2	1
Anorexia	5	2	1
Diarrhea	5	7	4
Ecchymosis	5	2	3
Dyspepsia	5	4	4
Paresthesia	5	2	3
Abnormal dreams	4	1	1
Hallucinations	4	5	3
Ataxia	3	6	1
Dyspnea	3	5	2
Infection	3	2	2
Neck pain	3	1	1
Sweating	3	2	1
Tenosynovitis	3	1	0
Dystonia	3	2	1
Gingivitis	2	1	1
Hemorrhage	2	1	1
Hernia	2	1	1
Myasthenia	2	2	1

* Incidence ≥ 2% in AZILECT 1 mg group and numerically more frequent than in placebo group

Several of the more common adverse reactions seemed dose-related, including weight loss, postural hypotension, and dry mouth.

Other adverse reactions of potential clinical importance reported in Study 1 by 1% or more of patients treated with rasagiline 1 mg/day as adjunct to levodopa therapy, and at least as frequent as in the placebo group, in descending order of frequency include : skin carcinoma, anemia, albuminuria, amnesia, arthritis, bursitis, cerebrovascular accident, confusion, dysphagia, epistaxis, leg cramps, pruritus, skin ulcer.

There were no significant differences in the safety profile based on age or gender.

Other Adverse Reactions Observed During All Phase 2/3 Clinical Trials

Rasagiline was administered to approximately 1361 patients during all PD phase 2/3 clinical trials. About 283 patients received rasagiline for at least one year, approximately 410 patients received rasagiline for at least two years, 116 patients received rasagiline for at least 3 years, and 245 patients received rasagiline for more than 3 years, with some patients treated for more than 5 years. The long-term safety profile was similar to that observed with shorter duration exposure.

The frequencies listed below represent the proportion of the 1361 individuals exposed to rasagiline who experienced events of the type cited.

All events that occurred at least twice (or once for serious or potentially serious events), except those already listed above, trivial events, terms too vague to be meaningful, adverse events with no plausible relation to treatment, and events that would be expected in patients of the age studied, were reported without regard to determination of a causal relationship to rasagiline.

Events are further classified within body system categories and enumerated in order of decreasing frequency using the following definitions: frequent adverse events are defined as those occurring in at least 1/100 patients, infrequent adverse events are defined as those occurring in at least 1/100 to 1/1000 patients and rare adverse events are defined as those occurring in fewer than 1/1000 patients.

Body as a whole:

Frequent: asthenia

Infrequent: chills, face edema, flank pain, photosensitivity reaction

Cardiovascular system:

Frequent: bundle branch block

Infrequent: deep thrombophlebitis, heart failure, migraine, myocardial infarct, phlebitis, ventricular tachycardia

Rare: arterial thrombosis, atrial arrhythmia, AV block complete, AV block second degree, bigeminy, cerebral hemorrhage, cerebral ischemia, ventricular fibrillation

Digestive system:

Frequent: gastrointestinal hemorrhage

Infrequent: colitis, esophageal ulcer, esophagitis, fecal incontinence, intestinal obstruction, mouth ulceration, stomach ulcer, stomatitis, tongue edema

Rare: hematemesis, hemorrhagic gastritis, intestinal perforation, intestinal stenosis, jaundice, large intestine perforation, megacolon, melena

Hemic and Lymphatic system:

Infrequent: macrocytic anemia

Rare: purpura, thrombocythemia

Metabolic and Nutritional disorders:

Infrequent: hypocalcemia

Musculoskeletal system:

Infrequent: bone necrosis, muscle atrophy

Rare: arthrosis

Nervous system:

Frequent: abnormal gait, anxiety, hyperkinesia, hypertonia, neuropathy, tremor

Infrequent: agitation, aphasia, circumoral paresthesia, convulsion, delusions, dementia, dysarthria, dysautonomia, dysesthesia, emotional lability, facial paralysis, foot drop, hemiplegia, hypesthesia, incoordination, manic reaction, myoclonus, neuritis, neurosis, paranoid reaction, personality disorder, psychosis, wrist drop

Rare: apathy, delirium, hostility, manic depressive reaction, myelitis, neuralgia, psychotic depression, stupor

Respiratory system:

Frequent: cough increased

Infrequent: apnea, emphysema, laryngismus, pleural effusion, pneumothorax

Rare: interstitial pneumonia, larynx edema, lung fibrosis

Skin and Appendages:

Infrequent: eczema, urticaria

Rare: exfoliative dermatitis, leukoderma

Special senses:

Infrequent: blepharitis, deafness, diplopia, eye hemorrhage, eye pain, glaucoma, keratitis, ptosis, retinal degeneration, taste perversion, visual field defect

Rare: blindness, parosmia, photophobia, retinal detachment, retinal hemorrhage, strabismus, taste loss, vestibular disorder

Urogenital system:

Frequent: hematuria, urinary incontinence

Infrequent: acute kidney failure, dysmenorrhea, dysuria, kidney calculus, nocturia, polyuria, scrotal edema, sexual function abnormal, urinary retention, urination impaired, vaginal hemorrhage, vaginal moniliasis, vaginitis

Rare: abnormal ejaculation, amenorrhea, anuria, epididymitis, gynecomastia, hydroureter, leukorrhea, priapism

6.2 Post-marketing Experience

The following adverse events not described in sections 4 and 5 have been identified during the post-marketing/post-approval use of AZILECT. Because these adverse events are reported voluntarily from a population of uncertain size, it is not possible to reliably estimate their frequency nor to establish unequivocally a causal relationship to drug exposure: Increased libido including hypersexuality, impulse control symptoms, pathological gambling *[see Patient Counseling Information (17.11)]*

7 DRUG INTERACTIONS

7.1 Meperidine

Serious, sometimes fatal reactions have been precipitated with concomitant use of meperidine (e.g., Demerol and other tradenames) and MAO inhibitors including selective MAO-B inhibitors *[see Contraindications (4.1)]*.

7.2 Dextromethorphan

The concomitant use of AZILECT and dextromethorphan was not allowed in clinical studies. The combination of MAO inhibitors and dextromethorphan has been reported to cause brief episodes of psychosis or bizarre behavior. Therefore, in view of AZILECT's MAO inhibitory activity, dextromethorphan should not be used concomitantly with AZILECT *[see Contraindications (4.2)]*.

7.3 Sympathomimetic Medications

The concomitant use of AZILECT and sympathomimetic medications was not allowed in clinical studies. Severe hypertensive reactions have followed the administration of sympathomimetics and non-selective MAO inhibitors. One case of hypertensive crisis has been reported in a patient taking the recommended dose of a selective MAO-B inhibitor and a sympathomimetic medication (ephedrine). Elevated blood pressure was reported in another patient taking the recommended dose of AZILECT and ophthalmic drops with a sympathomimetic medication (tetrahydrozoline).

Because AZILECT is a selective MAOI, hypertensive reactions are not ordinarily expected with the concomitant use of sympathomimetic medications. Nevertheless, caution should be exercised when concomitantly using recommended doses of AZILECT with any sympathomimetic medications including nasal, oral, and ophthalmic decongestants and cold remedies.

7.4 MAO Inhibitors

AZILECT should not be administered along with other MAO inhibitors because of the increased risk of non-selective MAO inhibition that may lead to a hypertensive crisis *[see Contraindications (4.3)]*.

7.5 Antidepressants

Concomitant use of AZILECT with one of many classes of antidepressants (e.g., SSRIs, SNRIs, triazolopyridine, tricyclic or tetracyclic antidepressants) is not recommended *[see Warnings and Precautions (5.1)]*.

7.6 Levodopa/Carbidopa

[see Warnings and Precautions (5.6) and Clinical Pharmacology (12.3)].

7.7 Ciprofloxacin and Other CYP1A2 Inhibitors

Rasagiline plasma concentrations may increase up to 2 fold in patients using concomitant ciprofloxacin and other CYP1A2 inhibitors. This could result in increased adverse events *[see Warnings and Precautions (5.2) and Clinical Pharmacology (12.3)]*.

7.8 Theophylline

[see Clinical Pharmacology (12.3)].

7.9 Tyramine/Rasagiline Interaction

MAO in the gastrointestinal tract and liver (primarily type A) is thought to provide vital protection from exogenous amines (e.g., tyramine) that have the capacity, if absorbed intact, to cause a "hypertensive crisis," the so-called "cheese reaction". If large amounts of certain exogenous amines (e.g., from fermented cheese, herring, over-the-counter cough/cold medications) gain access to the systemic circulation because MAO-A has been inhibited, they cause release of norepinephrine which may result in a rise in systemic blood pressure. MAOIs that selectively inhibit MAO-B are largely devoid of the potential to cause tyramine-induced hypertensive crisis.

Results of a special tyramine challenge study indicate that rasagiline is selective for MAO-B at recommended doses and can ordinarily be used without dietary tyramine restriction. However, certain foods (e.g., aged cheeses, such as Stilton cheese) may contain very high amounts (i.e., > 150 mg) of tyramine and could potentially cause a hypertensive cheese reaction in patients taking AZILECT due to mild increased sensitivity to tyramine. Patients should be advised to avoid foods (e.g., aged cheese) containing a very large amount of tyramine while taking recommended doses of AZILECT because of the potential for large increases in blood pressure. Selectivity for inhibiting MAO-B diminishes in a dose-related manner as the dose is progressively increased above the recommended daily doses.

There were no cases of hypertensive crisis in the clinical development program associated with 1 mg daily rasagiline treatment, in which most patients did not follow dietary tyramine restriction.

Despite the selective inhibition of MAO-B at recommended doses of AZILECT, there have been post-marketing reports of patients who experienced significantly elevated blood pressure (including rare cases of hypertensive crisis) after ingestion of unknown amounts of tyramine-rich foods while taking recommended doses of AZILECT *[see Dosing and Administration (2), and Warnings and Precautions (5.4)]*.

8 USE IN SPECIFIC POPULATIONS

8.1 Pregnancy

Category C

No effect on embryo-fetal development was observed in a combined mating/fertility and embryo-fetal development study in female rats at doses up to 3 mg/kg/day (approximately 30 times the expected plasma rasagiline exposure (AUC) at the maximum recommended human dose [MRHD, 1 mg/day]). Effects on embryo-fetal development in rabbit have not been adequately assessed.

In a study in which pregnant rats were dosed with rasagiline (0.1, 0.3, 1 mg/kg/day) orally, from the beginning of organogenesis to day 20 post-partum, offspring survival was decreased and offspring body weight was reduced at doses of 0.3 mg/kg/day and 1 mg/kg/day (10 and 16 times the expected plasma rasagiline exposure [AUC] at the MRHD). No plasma data were available at the no-effect dose (0.1 mg/kg); however, that dose is 1 times the MRHD on a mg/m^2 basis. Rasagiline's effect on physical and behavioral development was not adequately assessed in this study.

Rasagiline may be given as an adjunct therapy to levodopa/carbidopa treatment. In a study in which pregnant rats were dosed with rasagiline (0.1, 0.3, 1 mg/kg/day) and levodopa/carbidopa (80/20 mg/kg/day) (alone and in combination) throughout the period of organogenesis, there was an increased incidence of wavy ribs in fetuses from rats treated with rasagiline in combination with levodopa/carbidopa at 1/80/20 mg/kg/day (approximately 8 times the plasma AUC expected in humans at the MRHD and 1/1 times the MRHD of levodopa/carbidopa [800/200 mg/day] on a mg/m^2 basis). In a study in which pregnant rabbits were dosed throughout the period of organogenesis with rasagiline alone (3 mg/kg) or in combination with levodopa/carbidopa (rasagiline: 0.1, 0.6, 1.2 mg/kg, levodopa/carbidopa: 80/20 mg/kg/day), an increase in embryo-fetal death was noted at rasagiline doses of 0.6 and 1.2 mg/kg/day when administered in combination with levodopa/carbidopa (approximately 7 and 13 times, respectively, the plasma rasagiline AUC at the MRHD). There was an increase in cardiovascular abnormalities with levodopa/carbidopa alone (1/1 times the MRHD on a mg/m^2 basis) and to a greater extent when rasagiline (at all doses; 1-13 times the plasma rasagiline AUC at the MRHD) was administered in combination with levodopa/carbidopa.

There are no adequate and well-controlled studies of rasagiline in pregnant women. Therefore, AZILECT should be used during pregnancy only if the potential benefit justifies the potential risk to the fetus.

8.3 Nursing Mothers

In rats rasagiline was shown to inhibit prolactin secretion and it may inhibit milk secretion in females.

It is not known whether rasagiline is excreted in human milk. Because many drugs are excreted in human milk, caution should be exercised when AZILECT is administered to a nursing woman.

8.4 Pediatric Use

The safety and effectiveness of AZILECT in the pediatric population have not been studied.

8.5 Geriatric Use

Approximately half of patients in clinical trials were 65 years and over. There were no significant differences in the safety profile of the geriatric and non-geriatric patients.

8.6 Hepatic Impairment

Rasagiline plasma concentration may be increased in patients with mild (up to 2 fold, Child-Pugh score 5-6), moderate (up to 7 fold, Child-Pugh score 7-9), and severe (Child-Pugh score 10-15) hepatic impairment. Patients with mild hepatic impairment should be given the dose of 0.5 mg/day. AZILECT should not be used in patients with moderate or severe hepatic impairment *[see Dosage and Administration (2.3), Warnings and Precautions (5.3) and Clinical Pharmacology (12.3)]*.

8.7 Renal Impairment

Dose adjustment of AZILECT is not required for patients with mild or moderate renal impairment because AZILECT plasma concentrations are not increased in patients with moderate renal impairment. Rasagiline has not been studied in patients with severe renal impairment.

9 DRUG ABUSE AND DEPENDENCE

9.1 Controlled Substance

AZILECT is not a controlled substance.

9.2 Abuse

Studies conducted in mice and rats did not reveal any potential for drug abuse and dependence. Clinical trials have not revealed any evidence of the potential for abuse, tolerance or physical dependence; however, systematic studies in humans designed to evaluate these effects have not been performed.

9.3 Dependence

Studies conducted in mice and rats did not reveal any potential for drug abuse and dependence. Clinical trials have not revealed any evidence of the potential for abuse, tolerance or physical dependence; however, systematic studies in humans designed to evaluate these effects have not been performed.

10 OVERDOSE

No cases of AZILECT overdose were reported in clinical trials.

Rasagiline was well tolerated in a single-dose study in healthy volunteers receiving 20 mg/day and in a ten-day study in healthy volunteers receiving 10 mg/day. Adverse events were mild or moderate. In a dose escalation study in patients on chronic levodopa therapy treated with 10 mg of rasagiline there were three reports of cardiovascular side effects (including hypertension and postural hypotension) which resolved following treatment discontinuation.

Symptoms of overdosage, although not observed with rasagiline during clinical development, may resemble those observed with non-selective MAO inhibitors (MAOIs).

Although no cases of overdose have been observed with rasagiline during the clinical development program, the following description of presenting symptoms and clinical course is based upon overdose descriptions of non-selective MAO inhibitors.

Characteristically, signs and symptoms of non-selective MAOI overdose may not appear immediately. Delays of up to 12 hours between ingestion of drug and the appearance of signs may occur. Importantly, the peak intensity of the syndrome may not be reached for upwards of a day following the overdose. Death has been reported following overdosage. Therefore, immediate hospitalization, with continuous patient observation and monitoring for a period of at least two days following the ingestion of such drugs in overdose, is strongly recommended.

The clinical picture of MAOI overdose varies considerably; its severity may be a function of the amount of drug consumed. The central nervous and cardiovascular systems are prominently involved.

Signs and symptoms of overdosage may include, alone or in combination, any of the following: drowsiness, dizziness, faintness, irritability, hyperactivity, agitation, severe headache, hallucinations, trismus, opisthotonos, convulsions, and coma; rapid and irregular pulse, hypertension, hypotension and vascular collapse; precordial pain, respiratory depression and failure, hyperpyrexia, diaphoresis, and cool, clammy skin.

There is no specific antidote for rasagiline overdose. The following suggestions are offered based upon the assumption that rasagiline overdose may be modeled after non-selective MAO inhibitor poisoning. Treatment of overdose with non-selective MAO inhibitors is symptomatic and supportive. Respiration should be supported by appropriate measures, including management of the airway, use of supplemental oxygen, and mechanical ventilatory assistance, as required. Body temperature should be monitored closely. Intensive management of hyperpyrexia may be required. Maintenance of fluid and electrolyte balance is essential. For this reason, in cases of overdose with AZILECT, dietary tyramine restriction should be observed for several weeks to avoid the risk of a hypertensive/cheese reaction.

A poison control center should be called for the most current treatment guidelines.

A post-marketing report described a single patient who developed a non-fatal serotonin syndrome after ingesting 100 mg of AZILECT in a suicide attempt. Another patient who was treated in error with 4 mg AZILECT daily and tramadol also developed a serotonin syndrome. One patient who was treated in error with 3 mg AZILECT daily experienced alternating episodes of vascular fluctuations consisting of hypertension and orthostatic hypotension.

11 DESCRIPTION

AZILECT® tablets contain rasagiline (as the mesylate), a propargylamine-based drug indicated for the treatment of idiopathic Parkinson's disease. It is designated chemically as: 1H-Inden-1-amine, 2, 3-dihydro-N-2-propynyl-, (1R)-, methanesulfonate. The empirical formula of rasagiline mesylate is $(C_{12}H_{13}N)CH_4SO_3$ and its molecular weight is 267.34.

Its structural formula is:

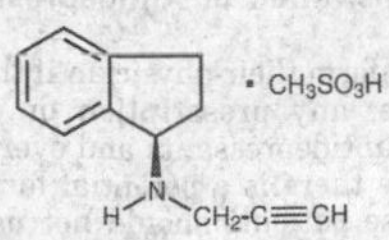

Rasagiline mesylate is a white to off-white powder, freely soluble in water or ethanol and sparingly soluble in isopropanol. Each AZILECT tablet for oral administration contains rasagiline mesylate equivalent to 0.5 mg or 1 mg of rasagiline base.

Each AZILECT tablet also contains the following inactive ingredients: mannitol, starch, pregelatinized starch, colloidal silicon dioxide, stearic acid and talc.

12 CLINICAL PHARMACOLOGY

12.1 Mechanism of Action

AZILECT functions as a selective, irreversible MAO-B inhibitor indicated for the treatment of idiopathic Parkinson's disease. The results of a clinical trial designed to examine the effects of Azilect on blood pressure when it is administered with increasing doses of tyramine indicates the functional selectivity can be incomplete when healthy subjects ingest large amounts of tyramine while receiving recommended doses of AZILECT. The selectivity for inhibiting MAO-B diminishes in a dose-related manner.

MAO, a flavin-containing enzyme, is classified into two major molecular species, A and B, and is localized in mitochondrial membranes throughout the body in nerve terminals, brain, liver and intestinal mucosa. MAO regulates the metabolic degradation of catecholamines and serotonin in the CNS and peripheral tissues. MAO-B is the major form in the human brain. In *ex vivo* animal studies in brain, liver and intestinal tissues, rasagiline was shown to be a potent, irreversible monoamine oxidase type B (MAO-B) selective inhibitor. Rasagiline at the recommended therapeutic dose was also shown to be a potent and irreversible inhibitor of MAO-B in platelets. The precise mechanisms of action of rasagiline are unknown. One mechanism is believed to be related to its MAO-B inhibitory activity, which causes an increase in extracellular levels of dopamine in the striatum. The elevated dopamine level and subsequent increased dopaminergic activity are likely to mediate rasagiline's beneficial effects seen in models of dopaminergic motor dysfunction.

12.2 Pharmacodynamics

Platelet MAO Activity in Clinical Studies

Studies in healthy subjects and in Parkinson's disease patients have shown that rasagiline inhibits platelet MAO-B irreversibly. The inhibition lasts at least 1 week after last dose. Almost 25-35% MAO-B inhibition was achieved after a single rasagiline dose of 1 mg/day and more than 55% of MAO-B inhibition was achieved after a single rasagiline dose of 2 mg/day. Over 90% inhibition was achieved 3 days after rasagiline daily dosing at 2 mg/day and this inhibition level was maintained 3 days post-dose. Multiple doses of rasagiline of 0.5, 1 and 2 mg per day resulted in complete MAO-B inhibition.

12.3 Pharmacokinetics

Rasagiline in the range of 1-6 mg demonstrated a more than proportional increase in AUC, while Cmax was dose proportional. Rasagiline mean steady-state half life is 3 hours but there is no correlation of pharmacokinetics with its pharmacological effect because of its irreversible inhibition of MAO-B.

Absorption

Rasagiline is rapidly absorbed, reaching peak plasma concentration (Cmax) in approximately 1 hour. The absolute bioavailability of rasagiline is about 36%.

Food does not affect the Tmax of rasagiline, although Cmax and exposure (AUC) are decreased by approximately 60% and 20%, respectively, when the drug is taken with a high fat meal. Because AUC is not significantly affected, AZILECT can be administered with or without food *[see Dosage and Administration (2)]*.

Distribution

The mean volume of distribution at steady-state is 87 L, indicating that the tissue binding of rasagiline is in excess of plasma protein binding. Plasma protein binding ranges from 88-94% with mean extent of binding of 61-63% to human albumin over the concentration range of 1-100 ng/mL.

Metabolism and Elimination

Rasagiline undergoes almost complete biotransformation in the liver prior to excretion. The metabolism of rasagiline proceeds through two main pathways: N-dealkylation and/or hydroxylation to yield 1-aminoindan (AI), 3-hydroxy-N-propargyl-1 aminoindan (3-OH-PAI) and 3-hydroxy-1-aminoindan (3-OH-AI). *In vitro* experiments indicate that both routes of rasagiline metabolism are dependent on the cytochrome P450 (CYP) system, with CYP1A2 being the major isoenzyme involved in rasagiline metabolism. Glucuronide conjugation of rasagiline and its metabolites, with subsequent urinary excretion, is the major elimination pathway.

After oral administration of ^{14}C-labeled rasagiline, elimination occurred primarily via urine and secondarily via feces (62% of total dose in urine and 7% of total dose in feces over 7 days), with a total calculated recovery of 84% of the dose over a period of 38 days. Less than 1% of rasagiline was excreted as unchanged drug in urine.

Special Populations

Hepatic Impairment

Following repeat dose administration (7 days) of rasagiline (1 mg/day) in subjects with mild hepatic impairment (Child-Pugh score 5-6), AUC and Cmax were increased by 2 fold and 1.4 fold, respectively, compared to healthy subjects. In subjects with moderate hepatic impairment (Child-Pugh score 7-9), AUC and Cmax were increased by 7 fold and 2 fold, respectively, compared to healthy subjects *[see Dosage and Administration (2.3) and Warnings and Precautions (5.3)]*.

Renal Impairment

Following repeat dose administration (8 days) of rasagiline (1 mg/day) in subjects with moderate renal impairment, rasagiline exposure (AUC) was similar to rasagiline exposure in healthy subjects, while the major metabolite 1-AI exposure (AUC) was increased 1.5- fold in subjects with moderate renal impairment, compared to healthy subjects. Because 1-AI is not an MAO inhibitor, no dose adjustment is needed for patients with mild and moderate renal impairment. Data are not available for patients with severe renal impairment.

Elderly

Since age has little influence on rasagiline pharmacokinetics, it can be administered at the recommended dose in the elderly (≥ 65 years).

Pediatric

AZILECT has not been investigated in patients below 18 years of age.

Gender

The pharmacokinetic profile of rasagiline is similar in men and women.

Drug Drug Interactions

Tyramine Effect

[see Dosage and Administration (2), Warnings and Precautions (5.4), and Drug Interactions (7.9)].

Levodopa

Data from population pharmacokinetic studies comparing rasagiline clearance in the presence and absence of levodopa have given conflicting results. Although there may be some increase in rasagiline blood levels in the presence of levodopa, the effect is modest and rasagiline dosing need not be modified in the presence of levodopa.

Effect of Other Drugs on the Metabolism of AZILECT

In vitro metabolism studies showed that CYP1A2 was the major enzyme responsible for the metabolism of rasagiline. There is the potential for inhibitors of this enzyme to alter AZILECT clearance when coadministered *[see Dosage and Administration (2.5) and Warnings and Precautions (5.2)]*.

Ciprofloxacin: When ciprofloxacin, an inhibitor of CYP1A2, was administered to healthy volunteers (n=12) at 500 mg (BID) with rasagiline at 2 mg/day, the AUC of rasagiline increased by 83% and there was no change in the elimination half life *[see Dosage and Administration (2.5) and Warnings and Precautions (5.2)]*.

Theophylline: Coadministration of rasagiline 1 mg/day and theophylline, a substrate of CYP1A2, up to 500 mg twice daily to healthy subjects (n=24) did not affect the pharmacokinetics of either drug.

Antidepressants: Severe CNS toxicity (occasionally fatal) associated with hyperpyrexia as part of a serotonin syndrome, has been reported with combined treatment of an antidepressant (e.g., from one of many classes including tricyclic or tetracyclic antidepressants, SSRIs, SNRIs, triazolopyridine antidepressants) and non-selective MAOI or a selective MAO-B inhibitor *[see Warnings and Precautions (5.1)]*.

Effect of AZILECT on Other Drugs

No additional *in vivo* trials have investigated the effect of AZILECT on other drugs metabolized by the cytochrome P450 enzyme system. *In vitro* studies showed that rasagiline at a concentration of 1mcg/ml (equivalent to a level that is 160 times the average Cmax ~ 5.9-8.5 ng/mL in Parkinson's disease patients after 1 mg rasagiline multiple dosing) did not inhibit cytochrome P450 isoenzymes, CYP1A2, CYP2A6, CYP2C9, CYP2C19, CYP2D6, CYP2E1, CYP3A4 and CYP4A. These results indicate that rasagiline is unlikely to cause any clinically significant interference with substrates of these enzymes.

13 NONCLINICAL TOXICOLOGY

13.1 Carcinogenesis, Mutagenesis, Impairment of Fertility

Carcinogenesis

Two year carcinogenicity studies were conducted in CD-1 mice at oral (gavage) doses of 1, 15, and 45 mg/kg and in Sprague-Dawley rats at oral (gavage) doses of 0.3, 1, and 3 mg/kg (males) or 0.5, 2, 5, and 17 mg/kg (females). In rats, there was no increase in tumors at any dose tested. Plasma exposures at the highest dose tested were approximately 33 and 260 times, in male and female rats, respectively, the expected plasma exposures in humans at the maximum recommended dose (MRD) of 1 mg/day.

In mice, there was an increase in lung tumors (combined adenomas/carcinomas) at 15 and 45 mg/kg males and females. Plasma exposures associated with the no-effect dose (1 mg/kg) were approximately 5 times those expected in humans at the MRD.

The carcinogenic potential of rasagiline administered in combination with levodopa/carbidopa has not been examined.

Mutagenesis

Rasagiline was reproducibly clastogenic in *in vitro* chromosomal aberration assays in human lymphocytes in the presence of metabolic activation and was mutagenic and clastogenic in the *in vitro* mouse lymphoma tk assay in the absence and presence of metabolic activation. Rasagiline was negative in the *in vitro* bacterial reverse mutation (Ames) assay, the *in vivo* unscheduled DNA synthesis assay, and the *in vivo* micronucleus assay in CD-1 mice. Rasagiline was also negative in the *in vivo* micronucleus assay in CD-1 mice when administered in combination with levodopa/carbidopa.

Impairment of Fertility

Rasagiline had no effect on mating performance or fertility in male rats treated prior to and throughout the mating period, or in female rats treated from prior to mating through day 17 of gestation at oral doses up to 3 mg/kg/day (approximately 30 times the expected plasma rasagiline exposure (AUC) at the maximum recommended human dose [1 mg/day]). The effect of rasagiline administered in combination with levodopa/carbidopa on mating and fertility has not been examined.

14 CLINICAL TRIALS

The effectiveness of AZILECT for the treatment of Parkinson's disease was established in three 18- to 26-week, randomized, placebo-controlled trials. In one of these trials AZILECT was given as initial monotherapy and in the other two as adjunctive therapy to levodopa.

14.1 Monotherapy Use of AZILECT

The monotherapy trial was a double-blind, randomized, fixed-dose parallel group, 26-week study in early Parkinson's disease patients not receiving any concomitant dopaminergic therapy at the start of the study. The majority of the patients were not treated with any anti-Parkinson's disease medication before receiving rasagiline treatment.

In this trial, 404 patients were randomly assigned to receive placebo (138 patients), rasagiline 1 mg/day (134 patients) or rasagiline 2 mg/day (132 patients). Patients were not allowed to take levodopa, dopamine agonists, selegiline or amantadine, but if necessary, could take stable doses of anticholinergic medication. The average Parkinson's disease duration was approximately 1 year (range 0 to 11 years).

The primary measure of effectiveness was the change from baseline in the total score of the Unified Parkinson's Disease Rating Scale (UPDRS), [mentation (Part I) + activities of daily living (ADL) (Part II) + motor function (Part III)]. The UPDRS is a multi-item rating scale that measures the ability of a patient to perform mental and motor tasks as well as activities of daily living. A reduction in the score represents improvement and a beneficial change from baseline appears as a negative number.

Rasagiline (1 or 2 mg once daily) had a significant beneficial effect relative to placebo on the primary measure of effectiveness in patients receiving six months of treatment and not on dopaminergic therapy. Patients who received rasagiline had significantly less worsening in the UPDRS score, compared to those who received placebo. The effectiveness of rasagiline 1 mg and 2 mg was comparable. Table 3 displays the results of the monotherapy trial.

Table 3. Parkinson's Disease Patients not on Dopaminergic Therapy (Monotherapy)

Primary Measure of Effectiveness: Change in total UPDRS score			
	Baseline score	Change from baseline to termination score	p-value vs. placebo
Placebo	24.5	3.9	---
1.0 mg/day	24.7	0.1	0.0001
2.0 mg/day	25.9	0.7	0.0001

For the comparison between rasagiline 1 mg/day and placebo, no differences in effectiveness based on age or gender were detected.

14.2 Adjunctive Use of AZILECT

Two multicenter, randomized, multinational trials were conducted in more advanced Parkinson's disease patients treated chronically with levodopa and experiencing motor fluctuations (including but not limited to, end of dose "wearing off," sudden or random "off," etc.). The first (Study 1) was conducted in North America (U.S. and Canada) and compared two doses (0.5 mg and 1 mg daily) of rasagiline and placebo while the second (Study 2) was conducted outside of North America (several European countries, Argentina, Israel) and studied only a single dose (1 mg daily) of rasagiline and placebo. Patients had had Parkinson's disease for an average of 9 years (range 5 months to 33 years), had been taking levodopa for an average of 8 years (range 5 months to 32 years), and had been experiencing motor fluctuations for approximately 3 to 4 years (range 1 month to 23 years). Patients kept home diaries just prior to baseline and at specified intervals during the trial. Diaries recorded one of the following four conditions for each half-hour interval over a 24-hour period: "ON" (period of relatively good function and mobility) as either "ON" with no dyskinesia or without troublesome dyskinesia, or "ON" with troublesome dyskinesia, "OFF" (period of relatively poor function and mobility) or asleep. "Troublesome" dyskinesia is defined as that which interferes with the patient's daily activity. All patients had been inadequately controlled and were experiencing motor fluctuations typical of advanced stage disease despite receiving levodopa/decarboxylase inhibitor. The average dose of levodopa/decarboxylase inhibitor was approximately 700 to 800 mg (range 150 to 3000 mg/day). Patients were also allowed to take stable doses of additional anti-PD medications at entry into the trials. In both trials, approximately 65% of patients were on dopamine agonists and in the North American study (Study 1) approximately 35% were on entacapone. The majority of patients taking entacapone were taking a dopamine agonist as well.

In both trials the primary measure of effectiveness was the change in the mean number of hours that were spent in the "OFF" state at baseline compared to the mean number of hours that were spent in the "OFF" state during the treatment period.

The first adjunct study (Study 1) was a double-blind, randomized, fixed-dose, parallel group trial conducted in 472 levodopa-treated Parkinson's disease patients who were experiencing motor fluctuations. Patients were randomly assigned to receive placebo (159 patients), rasagiline 0.5 mg/day (164 patients), or rasagiline 1 mg/day (149 patients), and were treated for 26 weeks. Patients averaged approximately 6 hours daily in the "OFF" state at baseline, as confirmed by home diaries.

The second adjunct study (Study 2) was a double-blind, randomized, parallel group trial conducted in 687 levodopa-treated Parkinson's disease patients who were experiencing motor fluctuations. Patients were randomly assigned to receive placebo (229 patients), rasagiline 1 mg/day (231 patients) or an active comparator, a COMT inhibitor taken along with scheduled doses of levodopa/decarboxylase inhibitor (227 patients). Patients were treated for 18 weeks. Patients averaged approximately 5.6 hours daily in the "OFF" state at baseline as confirmed by home diaries.

In both studies, rasagiline 1 mg once daily reduced "OFF" time compared to placebo when added to levodopa in patients experiencing motor fluctuations (Tables 4 and 5). The lower dose (0.5 mg) of rasagiline also significantly reduced "OFF" time (Table 4), but had a numerically smaller effect than the 1 mg dose of rasagiline. In Study 2, the active comparator also reduced "OFF" time when compared to placebo.

Table 4. Parkinson's Disease Patients Receiving AZILECT as Adjunct Therapy (Study 1)

Primary Measure of Effectiveness: Change in mean total daily "OFF" time			
	Baseline (hours)	Change from baseline to treatment period (hours)	p-value vs. placebo
Placebo	6.0	-0.9	---
0.5 mg/day	6.0	-1.4	0.0199
1.0 mg/day	6.3	-1.9	< 0.0001

Table 5. Parkinson's Disease Patients Receiving AZILECT as Adjunct Therapy (Study 2)

Primary Measure of Effectiveness: Change in mean total daily "OFF" time			
	Baseline (hours)	Change from baseline to treatment period (hours)	p-value vs. placebo
Placebo	5.5	- 0.40	---
1.0 mg/day	5.6	-1.2	0.0001

In both studies, dosage reduction of levodopa was allowed within the first 6 weeks if dopaminergic side effects, including dyskinesia and hallucinations, emerged. In Study 1, levodopa dosage reduction occurred in 8% of patients in the placebo group and in 16% and 17% of patients in the 0.5 mg/day and 1 mg/day rasagiline groups, respectively. In those patients who had levodopa dosage reduced, the dose was reduced on average by about 7%, 9%, and 13% in the placebo, 0.5 mg/day, and 1 mg/day groups, respectively. In Study 2, levodopa dosage reduction occurred in 6% of patients in the placebo group and in 9% in the rasagiline 1 mg/day group. In patients who had their levodopa dosage reduced, the dose was reduced on average by about 13% and 11% in the placebo and the rasagiline groups, respectively.

For the comparison between rasagiline 1 mg/day and placebo in both studies, no differences in effectiveness based on age or gender were detected.

Several secondary outcome assessments in the two studies showed statistically significant improvements with rasagiline. These included effects on the activities of daily living (ADL) subscale of the UPDRS performed during an "OFF" period and the motor subscale of the UPDRS performed during an "ON" period. In both scales, a negative response represents improvement. Tables 6 and 7 show these results for Studies 1 and 2.

Table 6. Secondary Measures of Effectiveness (Study 1)

	Baseline (score)	Change from baseline to last value
UPDRS ADL (Activities of Daily Living) subscale score while "OFF"		
Placebo	15.5	0.68
0.5 mg/day	15.8	-0.60
1.0 mg/day	15.5	-0.68
UPDRS Motor subscale score while "ON"		
Placebo	20.8	1.21
0.5 mg/day	21.5	-1.43
1.0 mg/day	20.9	-1.30

Table 7. Secondary Measures of Effectiveness (Study 2)

	Baseline (score)	Change from baseline to last value
UPDRS ADL (Activities of Daily Living) subscale score while "OFF"		
Placebo	18.7	-0.89
1.0 mg/day	19.0	-2.61
UPDRS Motor subscale score while "ON"		
Placebo	23.5	-0.82
1.0 mg/day	23.8	-3.87

16 HOW SUPPLIED

AZILECT 0.5 mg Tablets:
White to off-white, round, flat, beveled tablets, debossed with "GIL 0.5" on one side and plain on the other side. Supplied as bottles of 30 tablets (NDC 68546-142-56).
AZILECT 1 mg Tablets:
White to off-white, round, flat, beveled tablets, debossed with "GIL 1" on one side and plain on the other side. Supplied as bottles of 30 tablets (NDC 68546-229-56).
Storage:
Store at 25°C (77°F) with excursions permitted to 15°-30°C (59°-86°F).

17 INFORMATION FOR PATIENTS

17.1 Coadministration of Antidepressants and Other Drugs

Patients should inform their physician if they are taking, or planning to take, any prescription or over-the-counter drugs, especially antidepressants and over-the-counter cold medications, since there is a potential for interaction with AZILECT. Because patients should not use meperidine or certain other analgesics with AZILECT, they should contact their healthcare provider before taking analgesics *[see Warnings and Precautions (5.1)]*.

17.2 Ciprofloxacin or Other CYP1A2 Inhibitors

Patients should be informed that they should contact their healthcare provider of AZILECT if they take ciprofloxacin or a similar drug that could increase blood levels of rasagiline because of the need to adjust the dose of AZILECT *[see Warnings and Precautions (5.2)]*.

17.3 Risk of Hypertensive Crisis and Nonselective Monoamine Oxidase Inhibition Above the Recommended Doses

Patients should be advised not to exceed the maximum recommended daily dose of 1 mg/day (0.5 mg/day for subjects with mild hepatic impairment and subjects using concomitant ciprofloxacin and other CYP1A2 inhibitors).

The risk of using higher than recommended daily doses of AZILECT should be explained, and a brief description of the hypertensive/cheese reaction provided.

The possibility exists that very tyramine-rich foods (e.g., aged cheese such as Stilton) could possibly cause an increase in blood pressure. Patients should be advised to avoid certain foods (e.g., aged cheese) containing a very large amount of tyramine while taking recommended doses of AZILECT because of the potential for large increases in blood pressure. If patients eat foods very rich in tyramine and do not feel well soon after eating, they should contact their healthcare provider *[see Warnings and Precautions (5.4)]*.

17.4 Melanoma

It is not known if melanoma is associated with Parkinson's disease or the medicines used to treat Parkinson's disease. Patients being treated with AZILECT should be advised to have periodic skin examinations. *[see Warnings and Precautions (5.5)]*.

17.5 Dyskinesia

Patients taking AZILECT as adjunct to levodopa should be advised that there is a possibility of dyskinesia or increased dyskinesia *[see Warnings and Precautions (5.6)]*.

17.6 Lowering of Blood Pressure and Postural/Orthostatic Hypotension

Patients should be advised that they may develop postural (orthostatic) hypotension with or without symptoms such as dizziness, nausea, syncope, and sometimes sweating. Hypotension and/or orthostatic symptoms may occur more frequently during initial therapy or with an increase in dose at any time (cases have been seen after weeks of treatment). Accordingly, patients should be cautioned against standing up rapidly after sitting or lying down, especially if they have been doing so for prolonged periods, and especially, at the initiation of treatment with AZILECT *[see Warnings and Precautions (5.7)]*.

17.7 Elevation of Blood Pressure

Patients should be alerted to the possibility of increases in blood pressure during treatment with AZILECT. Exacerbation of hypertension may occur. Medication dose adjustment may be necessary if elevation of blood pressure is sustained over multiple evaluations *[see Warnings and Precautions (5.8)]*.

17.8 Hallucinations / Psychotic-Like Behavior

Patients should be informed that hallucinations or other manifestations of psychotic-like behavior can occur when taking AZILECT. Patients should also be advised that, if they have a major psychotic disorder, that AZILECT should not ordinarily be used because of the risk of exacerbating the psychosis. Patients with a major psychotic disorder should also be aware that many treatments for psychosis may decrease the effectiveness of AZILECT *[see Warnings and Precautions (5.9)]*.

17.9 Withdrawal-Emergent Hyperpyrexia and Confusion
Patients should be told to contact their healthcare provider if they wish to discontinue Azilect.

17.10 Missing Dose
Patients should be instructed to take AZILECT as prescribed. If a dose is missed, the patient should not double-up the dose of AZILECT. The next dose should be taken at the usual time on the following day.

17.11 Impulse Control/Compulsive Behaviors
There have been reports of patients experiencing intense urges to gamble, increased sexual urges, other intense urges, and the inability to control these urges while taking one or more of the medications that increase central dopaminergic tone and that are generally used for the treatment of Parkinson's disease (including AZILECT). Although it is not proven that the medications caused these events, these urges were reported to have stopped in some cases when the dose was reduced or the medication was stopped. Prescribers should ask patients about the development of new or increased gambling urges, sexual urges, or other urges while being treated with rasagiline. Patients should inform their physician if they experience new or increased gambling urges, increased sexual urges, or other intense urges while taking rasagiline. Physicians should consider dose reduction or stopping the medication if a patient develops such urges while taking rasagiline.

Marketed by: TEVA Neuroscience, Inc., Kansas City, MO 64131
Distributed by: TEVA Pharmaceuticals USA, Inc., North Wales, PA 19454
Product of Israel
AZT0812G

Shown in Product Identification Guide, page 314

COPAXONE ℞
[*co-PAX-own*]
(glatiramer acetate)
injection, solution for subcutaneous use

HIGHLIGHTS OF PRESCRIBING INFORMATION
These highlights do not include all the information needed to use COPAXONE safely and effectively. See full prescribing information for COPAXONE.
COPAXONE (glatiramer acetate injection), solution for subcutaneous use
Initial U.S. Approval: 1996

INDICATIONS AND USAGE
COPAXONE is indicated for reduction of the frequency of relapses in patients with Relapsing-Remitting Multiple Sclerosis, including patients who have experienced a first clinical episode and have MRI features consistent with multiple sclerosis. (1)

DOSAGE AND ADMINISTRATION
- For subcutaneous injection only (2.1)
- Recommended dose: 20 mg/day (2.1)
- Before use, allow the solution to warm to room temperature (2.2)

DOSAGE FORMS AND STRENGTHS
- Prefilled syringe containing 1 mL solution with 20 mg of glatiramer acetate (3)

CONTRAINDICATIONS
Known hypersensitivity to glatiramer acetate or mannitol (4)

WARNINGS AND PRECAUTIONS
- Immediate Post-Injection Reaction (flushing, chest pain, palpitations, anxiety, dyspnea, throat constriction, and/or urticaria), generally transient and self-limiting (5.1)
- Chest pain, usually transient (5.2)
- Lipoatrophy and skin necrosis may occur. Instruct patient in proper injection technique and to rotate injection sites daily (5.3)
- COPAXONE can modify immune response (5.4)

ADVERSE REACTIONS
- In controlled studies, most common adverse reactions (≥10% and ≥1.5 times higher than placebo) were: injection site reactions, vasodilatation, rash, dyspnea, and chest pain (6.1)

To report SUSPECTED ADVERSE REACTIONS, contact TEVA at 1-800-221-4026 or FDA at 1-800-FDA-1088 or www.fda.gov/medwatch

USE IN SPECIFIC POPULATIONS
- Nursing Mothers: It is not known if COPAXONE is excreted in human milk (8.3)
- Pediatric Use: The safety and effectiveness of COPAXONE have not been established in patients under 18 years of age (8.4)

See 17 for PATIENT COUNSELING INFORMATION and FDA-approved patient labeling

Revised: 08/2012

FULL PRESCRIBING INFORMATION: CONTENTS*

*** Sections or subsections omitted from the full prescribing information are not listed**

FULL PRESCRIBING INFORMATION

1 INDICATIONS AND USAGE
COPAXONE is indicated for reduction of the frequency of relapses in patients with Relapsing-Remitting Multiple Sclerosis (RRMS), including patients who have experienced a first clinical episode and have MRI features consistent with multiple sclerosis.

2 DOSAGE AND ADMINISTRATION
2.1 Recommended Dose
COPAXONE is for subcutaneous use only. Do not administer intravenously. The recommended dose of COPAXONE is 20 mg/day.

2.2 Instructions for Use
Remove one blister that contains the syringe from the COPAXONE prefilled syringes package. Since this product should be refrigerated, let the prefilled syringe stand at room temperature for 20 minutes to allow the solution to warm to room temperature. Inspect the COPAXONE syringe visually for particulate matter and discoloration prior to administration, whenever solution and container permit. The solution in the syringe should appear clear, colorless to slightly yellow. If particulate matter or discoloration is observed, discard the COPAXONE syringe.
Areas for self-injection include arms, abdomen, hips, and thighs. The prefilled syringe is for single use only. Discard unused portions.

3 DOSAGE FORMS AND STRENGTHS
Single-use prefilled syringe containing 1 mL solution with 20 mg of glatiramer acetate and 40 mg of mannitol.

4 CONTRAINDICATIONS
COPAXONE is contraindicated in patients with known hypersensitivity to glatiramer acetate or mannitol.

5 WARNINGS AND PRECAUTIONS
5.1 Immediate Post-Injection Reaction
Approximately 16% of patients exposed to COPAXONE in the 5 placebo-controlled trials compared to 4% of those on placebo experienced a constellation of symptoms immediately after injection that included at least two of the following: flushing, chest pain, palpitations, anxiety, dyspnea, constriction of the throat, and urticaria. The symptoms were generally transient and self-limited and did not require treatment. In general, these symptoms have their onset several months after the initiation of treatment, although they may occur earlier, and a given patient may experience one or several episodes of these symptoms. Whether or not any of these symptoms actually represent a specific syndrome is uncertain. During the postmarketing period, there have been reports of patients with similar symptoms who received emergency medical care.
Whether an immunologic or nonimmunologic mechanism mediates these episodes, or whether several similar episodes seen in a given patient have identical mechanisms, is unknown.

5.2 Chest Pain
Approximately 13% of COPAXONE patients in the 5 placebo-controlled studies compared to 6% of placebo patients experienced at least one episode of what was described as transient chest pain. While some of these episodes occurred in the context of the Immediate Post-Injection Reaction described above, many did not. The temporal relationship of this chest pain to an injection of COPAXONE was not always known. The pain was transient (usually lasting only a few minutes), often unassociated with other symptoms, and appeared to have no clinical sequelae. Some patients experienced more than one such episode, and episodes usually began at least 1 month after the initiation of treatment. The pathogenesis of this symptom is unknown.

5.3 Lipoatrophy and Skin Necrosis
At injection sites, localized lipoatrophy and, rarely, injection site skin necrosis have been reported during the postmarketing experience. Lipoatrophy may occur at various times after treatment onset (sometimes after several months) and is thought to be permanent. There is no known therapy for lipoatrophy. To assist in possibly minimizing these events, the patient should be advised to follow proper injection technique and to rotate injection sites daily.

5.4 Potential Effects on Immune Response
Because COPAXONE can modify immune response, it may interfere with immune functions. For example, treatment with COPAXONE may interfere with the recognition of foreign antigens in a way that would undermine the body's tumor surveillance and its defenses against infection. There is no evidence that COPAXONE does this, but there has not been a systematic evaluation of this risk. Because COPAXONE is an antigenic material, it is possible that its use may lead to the induction of host responses that are untoward, but systematic surveillance for these effects has not been undertaken.
Although COPAXONE is intended to minimize the autoimmune response to myelin, there is the possibility that continued alteration of cellular immunity due to chronic treatment with COPAXONE may result in untoward effects.
Glatiramer acetate-reactive antibodies are formed in most patients exposed to daily treatment with the recommended dose. Studies in both the rat and monkey have suggested that immune complexes are deposited in the renal glomeruli. Furthermore, in a controlled trial of 125 RRMS patients given COPAXONE, 20 mg, subcutaneously every day for 2 years, serum IgG levels reached at least 3 times baseline values in 80% of patients by 3 months of initiation of treatment. By 12 months of treatment, however, 30% of patients still had IgG levels at least 3 times baseline values, and 90% had levels above baseline by 12 months. The antibodies are exclusively of the IgG subtype and predominantly of the IgG-1 subtype. No IgE type antibodies could be detected in any of the 94 sera tested; nevertheless, anaphylaxis can be associated with the administration of most any foreign substance, and therefore, this risk cannot be excluded.

6 ADVERSE REACTIONS
6.1 Clinical Trials Experience
Because clinical trials are conducted under widely varying conditions, adverse reaction rates observed in the clinical trials of a drug cannot be directly compared to rates in the clinical trials of another drug and may not reflect the rates observed in clinical practice.

Incidence in Controlled Clinical Trials
Among 563 patients treated with COPAXONE in blinded placebo controlled trials, approximately 5% of the subjects discontinued treatment because of an adverse reaction. The adverse reactions most commonly associated with discontinuation were: injection site reactions, dyspnea, urticaria, vasodilatation, and hypersensitivity. The most common adverse reactions were: injection site reactions, vasodilatation, rash, dyspnea, and chest pain.
Table 1 lists treatment-emergent signs and symptoms that occurred in at least 2% of patients treated with COPAXONE in the placebo-controlled trials. These signs and symptoms were numerically more common in patients treated with COPAXONE than in patients treated with placebo. Adverse reactions were usually mild in intensity.

Table 1: Adverse reactions in controlled clinical trials with an incidence ≥2% of patients and more frequent with COPAXONE than with placebo

		GA 20 mg (N=563)	Placebo (N=564)
Blood And Lymphatic System Disorders	Lymphadenopathy	7%	3%
Cardiac Disorders	Palpitations	9%	4%
	Tachycardia	5%	2%
Eye Disorders	Eye Disorder	3%	1%
	Diplopia	3%	2%
Gastrointestinal Disorders	Nausea	15%	11%
	Vomiting	7%	4%
	Dysphagia	2%	1%
General Disorders And Administration Site Conditions	Injection Site Erythema	43%	10%
	Injection Site Pain	40%	20%
	Injection Site Pruritus	27%	4%
	Injection Site Mass	26%	6%
	Asthenia	22%	21%
	Pain	20%	17%
	Injection Site Edema	19%	4%
	Chest Pain	13%	6%
	Injection Site Inflammation	9%	1%
	Edema	8%	2%
	Injection Site Reaction	8%	1%
	Pyrexia	6%	5%
	Injection Site Hypersensitivity	4%	0%
	Local Reaction	3%	1%
	Chills	3%	1%
	Face Edema	3%	1%
	Edema Peripheral	3%	2%
	Injection Site Fibrosis	2%	1%
	Injection Site Atrophy*	2%	0%
Immune System Disorders	Hypersensitivity	3%	2%
Infections And Infestations	Infection	30%	28%
	Influenza	14%	13%
	Rhinitis	7%	5%
	Bronchitis	6%	5%
	Gastroenteritis	6%	4%
	Vaginal Candidiasis	4%	2%
Metabolism And Nutrition Disorders	Weight Increased	3%	1%
Musculoskeletal And Connective Tissue Disorders	Back Pain	12%	10%
Neoplasms Benign, Malignant And Unspecified (Incl Cysts And Polyps)	Benign Neoplasm of Skin	2%	1%
Nervous System Disorders	Tremor	4%	2%
	Migraine	4%	2%
	Syncope	3%	2%
	Speech Disorder	2%	1%
Psychiatric Disorders	Anxiety	13%	10%
	Nervousness	2%	1%
Renal And Urinary Disorders	Micturition Urgency	5%	4%
Respiratory, Thoracic And Mediastinal Disorders	Dyspnea	14%	4%
	Cough	6%	5%
	Laryngospasm	2%	1%
Skin And Subcutaneous Tissue Disorders	Rash	19%	11%
	Hyperhidrosis	7%	5%
	Pruritus	5%	4%
	Urticaria	3%	1%
	Skin Disorder	3%	1%
Vascular Disorders	Vasodilatation	20%	5%

* Injection site atrophy comprises terms relating to localized lipoatrophy at injection site

[See table 1 above]
Adverse reactions which occurred only in 4-5 more subjects in the COPAXONE group than in the placebo group (less than 1% difference), but for which a relationship to COPAXONE could not be excluded, were arthralgia and herpes simplex.
Laboratory analyses were performed on all patients participating in the clinical program for COPAXONE. Clinically significant laboratory values for hematology, chemistry, and urinalysis were similar for both COPAXONE and placebo groups in blinded clinical trials. In controlled trials one patient discontinued treatment due to thrombocytopenia (16 $\times 10^9$/L), which resolved after discontinuation of treatment.
Data on adverse reactions occurring in the controlled clinical trials were analyzed to evaluate differences based on sex. No clinically significant differences were identified. Ninety-six percent of patients in these clinical trials were Caucasian. The majority of patients treated with COPAXONE were between the ages of 18 and 45. Consequently, data are inadequate to perform an analysis of the adverse reaction incidence related to clinically relevant age subgroups.

Other Adverse Reactions

In the paragraphs that follow, the frequencies of less commonly reported adverse clinical reactions are presented. Because the reports include reactions observed in open and uncontrolled premarketing studies (n= 979), the role of COPAXONE in their causation cannot be reliably determined. Furthermore, variability associated with adverse reaction reporting, the terminology used to describe adverse reactions, etc., limit the value of the quantitative frequency estimates provided. Reaction frequencies are calculated as the number of patients who used COPAXONE and reported a reaction divided by the total number of patients exposed to COPAXONE. All reported reactions are included except those already listed in the previous table, those too general to be informative, and those not reasonably associated with the use of the drug. Reactions are further classified within body system categories and enumerated in order of decreasing frequency using the following definitions: *Frequent* adverse reactions are defined as those occurring in at least 1/100 patients and *infrequent* adverse reactions are those occurring in 1/100 to 1/1,000 patients.

Body as a Whole:

Frequent: Abscess

Infrequent: Injection site hematoma, injection site fibrosis, moon face, cellulitis, generalized edema, hernia, injection site abscess, serum sickness, suicide attempt, injection site hypertrophy, injection site melanosis, lipoma, and photosensitivity reaction.

Cardiovascular:

Frequent: Hypertension.

Infrequent: Hypotension, midsystolic click, systolic murmur, atrial fibrillation, bradycardia, fourth heart sound, postural hypotension, and varicose veins.

Digestive:

Infrequent: Dry mouth, stomatitis, burning sensation on tongue, cholecystitis, colitis, esophageal ulcer, esophagitis, gastrointestinal carcinoma, gum hemorrhage, hepatomegaly, increased appetite, melena, mouth ulceration, pancreas disorder, pancreatitis, rectal hemorrhage, tenesmus, tongue discoloration, and duodenal ulcer.

Endocrine:

Infrequent: Goiter, hyperthyroidism, and hypothyroidism.

Gastrointestinal:

Frequent: Bowel urgency, oral moniliasis, salivary gland enlargement, tooth caries, and ulcerative stomatitis.

Hemic and Lymphatic:

Infrequent: Leukopenia, anemia, cyanosis, eosinophilia, hematemesis, lymphedema, pancytopenia, and splenomegaly.

Metabolic and Nutritional:

Infrequent: Weight loss, alcohol intolerance, Cushing's syndrome, gout, abnormal healing, and xanthoma.

Musculoskeletal:

Infrequent: Arthritis, muscle atrophy, bone pain, bursitis, kidney pain, muscle disorder, myopathy, osteomyelitis, tendon pain, and tenosynovitis.

Nervous:

Frequent: Abnormal dreams, emotional lability, and stupor.

Infrequent: Aphasia, ataxia, convulsion, circumoral paresthesia, depersonalization, hallucinations, hostility, hypokinesia, coma, concentration disorder, facial paralysis, decreased libido, manic reaction, memory impairment, myoclonus, neuralgia, paranoid reaction, paraplegia, psychotic depression, and transient stupor.

Respiratory:

Frequent: Hyperventilation and hay fever.

Infrequent: Asthma, pneumonia, epistaxis, hypoventilation, and voice alteration.

Skin and Appendages:

Frequent: Eczema, herpes zoster, pustular rash, skin atrophy, and warts.

Infrequent: Dry skin, skin hypertrophy, dermatitis, furunculosis, psoriasis, angioedema, contact dermatitis, erythema nodosum, fungal dermatitis, maculopapular rash, pigmentation, benign skin neoplasm, skin carcinoma, skin striae, and vesiculobullous rash.

Special Senses:

Frequent: Visual field defect.

Infrequent: Dry eyes, otitis externa, ptosis, cataract, corneal ulcer, mydriasis, optic neuritis, photophobia, and taste loss.

Urogenital:

Frequent: Amenorrhea, hematuria, impotence, menorrhagia, suspicious papanicolaou smear, urinary frequency, and vaginal hemorrhage.

Infrequent: Vaginitis, flank pain (kidney), abortion, breast engorgement, breast enlargement, carcinoma *in situ* cervix, fibrocystic breast, kidney calculus, nocturia, ovarian cyst, priapism, pyelonephritis, abnormal sexual function, and urethritis.

6.2 Postmarketing Experience

Reports of adverse events occurring under treatment with COPAXONE not mentioned above that have been received since market introduction and may or may not have causal relationship to COPAXONE are listed below. Because these events are reported voluntarily from a population of uncertain size, it is not always possible to reliably estimate their frequency or establish a causal relationship to drug exposure.

Body as a Whole: sepsis; SLE syndrome; hydrocephalus; enlarged abdomen; injection site hypersensitivity; allergic reaction; anaphylactoid reaction
Cardiovascular System: thrombosis; peripheral vascular disease; pericardial effusion; myocardial infarct; deep thrombophlebitis; coronary occlusion; congestive heart failure; cardiomyopathy; cardiomegaly; arrhythmia; angina pectoris
Digestive System: tongue edema; stomach ulcer; hemorrhage; liver function abnormality; liver damage; hepatitis; eructation; cirrhosis of the liver; cholelithiasis
Hemic and Lymphatic System: thrombocytopenia; lymphoma-like reaction; acute leukemia
Metabolic and Nutritional Disorders: hypercholesterolemia
Musculoskeletal System: rheumatoid arthritis; generalized spasm
Nervous System: myelitis; meningitis; CNS neoplasm; cerebrovascular accident; brain edema; abnormal dreams; aphasia; convulsion; neuralgia
Respiratory System: pulmonary embolus; pleural effusion; carcinoma of lung; hay fever
Special Senses: glaucoma; blindness; visual field defect
Urogenital System: urogenital neoplasm; urine abnormality; ovarian carcinoma; nephrosis; kidney failure; breast carcinoma; bladder carcinoma; urinary frequency

7 DRUG INTERACTIONS

Interactions between COPAXONE and other drugs have not been fully evaluated. Results from existing clinical trials do not suggest any significant interactions of COPAXONE with therapies commonly used in MS patients, including the concurrent use of corticosteroids for up to 28 days. COPAXONE has not been formally evaluated in combination with interferon beta.

8 USE IN SPECIFIC POPULATIONS

8.1 Pregnancy

Pregnancy Category B.

Administration of glatiramer acetate by subcutaneous injection to pregnant rats and rabbits resulted in no adverse effects on offspring development. There are no adequate and well-controlled studies in pregnant women. Because animal reproduction studies are not always predictive of human response, COPAXONE should be used during pregnancy only if clearly needed.

In rats or rabbits receiving glatiramer acetate by subcutaneous injection during the period of organogenesis, no adverse effects on embryo-fetal development were observed at doses up to 37.5 mg/kg/day (18 and 36 times, respectively, the therapeutic human dose of 20 mg/day on a mg/m^2 basis).

In rats receiving subcutaneous glatiramer acetate at doses of up to 36 mg/kg from day 15 of pregnancy throughout lactation, no significant effects on delivery or on offspring growth and development were observed.

8.2 Labor and Delivery

The effects of COPAXONE on labor and delivery in pregnant women are unknown.

8.3 Nursing Mothers

It is not known if glatiramer acetate is excreted in human milk. Because many drugs are excreted in human milk, caution should be exercised when COPAXONE is administered to a nursing woman.

8.4 Pediatric Use

The safety and effectiveness of COPAXONE have not been established in patients under 18 years of age.

8.5 Geriatric Use

COPAXONE has not been studied in elderly patients.

8.6 Use in Patients with Impaired Renal Function

The pharmacokinetics of glatiramer acetate in patients with impaired renal function have not been determined.

11 DESCRIPTION

COPAXONE is the brand name for glatiramer acetate (formerly known as copolymer-1). Glatiramer acetate, the active ingredient of COPAXONE, consists of the acetate salts of synthetic polypeptides, containing four naturally occurring amino acids: L-glutamic acid, L-alanine, L-tyrosine, and L-lysine with an average molar fraction of 0.141, 0.427, 0.095, and 0.338, respectively. The average molecular weight of glatiramer acetate is 5,000 – 9,000 daltons. Glatiramer acetate is identified by specific antibodies.

Chemically, glatiramer acetate is designated L-glutamic acid polymer with L-alanine, L-lysine and L-tyrosine, acetate (salt). Its structural formula is:

(Glu, Ala, Lys, Tyr)$_x$•xCH$_3$COOH
$(C_5H_9NO_4 \bullet C_3H_7NO_2 \bullet C_6H_{14}N_2O_2 \bullet C_9H_{11}NO_3)_x \bullet xC_2H_4O_2$
CAS - 147245-92-9

COPAXONE is a clear, colorless to slightly yellow, sterile, nonpyrogenic solution for subcutaneous injection. Each 1 mL of solution contains 20 mg of glatiramer acetate and 40 mg of mannitol. The pH range of the solution is approximately 5.5 to 7.0. The biological activity of COPAXONE is determined by its ability to block the induction of experimental autoimmune encephalomyelitis (EAE) in mice.

12 CLINICAL PHARMACOLOGY

12.1 Mechanism of Action

The mechanism(s) by which glatiramer acetate exerts its effects in patients with MS are not fully understood. However, glatiramer acetate is thought to act by modifying immune processes that are believed to be responsible for the pathogenesis of MS. This hypothesis is supported by findings of studies that have been carried out to explore the pathogenesis of experimental autoimmune encephalomyelitis, a condition induced in animals through immunization against central nervous system derived material containing myelin and often used as an experimental animal model of MS. Studies in animals and *in vitro* systems suggest that upon its administration, glatiramer acetate-specific suppressor T-cells are induced and activated in the periphery.

Because glatiramer acetate can modify immune functions, concerns exist about its potential to alter naturally occurring immune responses. There is no evidence that glatiramer acetate does this, but this has not been systematically evaluated *[see Warnings and Precautions (5.4)]*.

12.3 Pharmacokinetics

Results obtained in pharmacokinetic studies performed in humans (healthy volunteers) and animals support that a substantial fraction of the therapeutic dose delivered to patients subcutaneously is hydrolyzed locally. Larger fragments of glatiramer acetate can be recognized by glatiramer acetate-reactive antibodies. Some fraction of the injected material, either intact or partially hydrolyzed, is presumed to enter the lymphatic circulation, enabling it to reach regional lymph nodes, and some may enter the systemic circulation intact.

13 NONCLINICAL TOXICOLOGY

13.1 Carcinogenesis, Mutagenesis, Impairment of Fertility

In a 2-year carcinogenicity study, mice were administered up to 60 mg/kg/day glatiramer acetate by subcutaneous injection (up to 15 times the human therapeutic dose of 20 mg/day on a mg/m^2 basis). No increase in systemic neoplasms was observed. In males receiving the 60-mg/kg/day dose, there was an increased incidence of fibrosarcomas at the injection sites. These sarcomas were associated with skin damage precipitated by repetitive injections of an irritant over a limited skin area.

In a 2-year carcinogenicity study, rats were administered up to 30 mg/kg/day glatiramer acetate by subcutaneous injection (up to 15 times the human therapeutic dose on a mg/m^2 basis). No increase in neoplasms was observed.

Glatiramer acetate was not mutagenic in *in vitro* (Ames test, mouse lymphoma tk) assays. Glatiramer acetate was clastogenic in two separate *in vitro* chromosomal aberration assays in cultured human lymphocytes but not clastogenic in an *in vivo* mouse bone marrow micronucleus assay.

When glatiramer acetate was administered by subcutaneous injection prior to and during mating (males and females) and throughout gestation and lactation (females) at doses up to 36 mg/kg/day (18 times the human therapeutic dose on a mg/m^2 basis) no adverse effects were observed on reproductive or developmental parameters.

14 CLINICAL STUDIES

14.1 Relapsing-Remitting Multiple Sclerosis (RRMS)

Evidence supporting the effectiveness of COPAXONE in decreasing the frequency of relapses derives from 3 placebo-controlled trials, all of which used a COPAXONE dose of 20 mg/day.

Study 1 was performed at a single center. Fifty patients were enrolled and randomized to receive daily doses of either COPAXONE, 20 mg subcutaneously, or placebo (COPAXONE: n=25; placebo: n=25). Patients were diagnosed with RRMS by standard criteria, and had had at least 2 exacerbations during the 2 years immediately preceding enrollment. Patients were ambulatory, as evidenced by a score of no more than 6 on the Kurtzke Disability Scale Score (DSS), a standard scale ranging from 0–Normal to 10–Death due to MS. A score of 6 is defined as one at which a patient is still ambulatory with assistance; a score of 7 means the patient must use a wheelchair.

Patients were examined every 3 months for 2 years, as well as within several days of a presumed exacerbation. To confirm an exacerbation, a blinded neurologist had to document objective neurologic signs, as well as document the existence of other criteria (e.g., the persistence of the neurological signs for at least 48 hours).

The protocol-specified primary outcome measure was the proportion of patients in each treatment group who remained exacerbation free for the 2 years of the trial, but two other important outcomes were also specified as endpoints: the frequency of attacks during the trial, and the change in the number of attacks compared with the number which occurred during the previous 2 years.

Table 2 presents the values of the three outcomes described above, as well as several protocol specified secondary measures. These values are based on the intent-to-treat population (i.e., all patients who received at least 1 dose of treatment and who had at least 1 on-treatment assessment):

[See table 2 above]

Table 2: Study 1 Efficacy Results

	COPAXONE (N=25)	Placebo (N=25)	P-Value
% Relapse-Free Patients	14/25 (56%)	7/25 (28%)	0.085
Mean Relapse Frequency	0.6/2 years	2.4/2 years	0.005
Reduction in Relapse Rate Compared to Prestudy	3.2	1.6	0.025
Median Time to First Relapse (days)	>700	150	0.03
% of Progression-Free* Patients	20/25 (80%)	13/25 (52%)	0.07

* Progression was defined as an increase of at least 1 point on the DSS, persisting for at least 3 consecutive months.

Study 2 was a multicenter trial of similar design which was performed in 11 US centers. A total of 251 patients (COPAXONE: n=125; placebo: n=126) were enrolled. The primary outcome measure was the Mean 2-Year Relapse Rate. Table 3 presents the values of this outcome for the intent-to-treat population, as well as several secondary measures:

[See table 3 above]

Table 3: Study 2 Efficacy Results

	COPAXONE (N=125)	Placebo (N=126)	P-Value
Mean No. of Relapses	1.19/2 years	1.68 /2 years	0.055
% Relapse-Free Patients	42/125 (34%)	34/126 (27%)	0.25
Median Time to First Relapse (days)	287	198	0.23
% of Progression-Free Patients	98/125 (78%)	95/126 (75%)	0.48
Mean Change in DSS	-0.05	+0.21	0.023

In both studies, COPAXONE exhibited a clear beneficial effect on relapse rate, and it is based on this evidence that COPAXONE is considered effective.

In Study 3, 481 patients who had recently (within 90 days) experienced an isolated demyelinating event and who had lesions typical of multiple sclerosis on brain MRI were randomized to receive either COPAXONE 20 mg/day (n=243) or placebo (n=238). The primary outcome measure was time to development of a second exacerbation. Patients were followed for up to three years or until they reached the primary endpoint. Secondary outcomes were brain MRI measures, including number of new T2 lesions and T2 lesion volume.

Time to development of a second exacerbation was significantly delayed in patients treated with COPAXONE compared to placebo (Hazard Ratio = 0.55; 95% confidence interval 0.40 to 0.77; Figure 1). The Kaplan-Meier estimates of the percentage of patients developing a relapse within 36 months were 42.9% in the placebo group and 24.7% in the COPAXONE group.

Figure 1: Time to Second Exacerbation

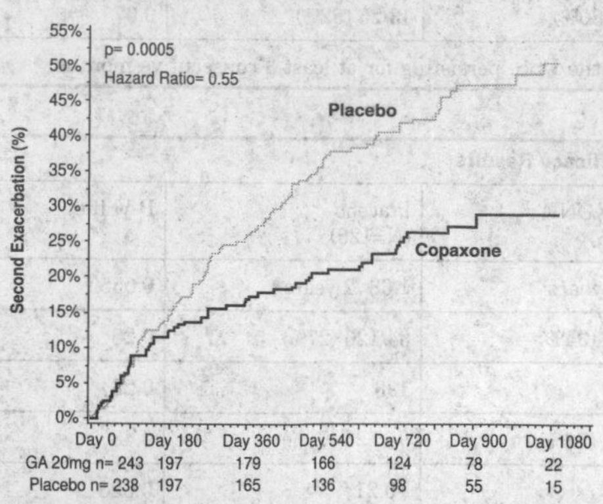

Patients treated with COPAXONE demonstrated fewer new T2 lesions at the last observation (rate ratio 0.41; confidence interval 0.28 to 0.59; $p < 0.0001$). Additionally, baseline-adjusted T2 lesion volume at the last observation was lower for patients treated with COPAXONE (ratio of 0.89; confidence interval 0.84 to 0.94; $p = 0.0001$).

Study 4 was a multinational study in which MRI parameters were used both as primary and secondary endpoints. A total of 239 patients with RRMS (COPAXONE: n=119; and placebo: n=120) were randomized. Inclusion criteria were similar to those in the second study with the additional criterion that patients had to have at least one Gd-enhancing lesion on the screening MRI. The patients were treated in a double-blind manner for nine months, during which they underwent monthly MRI scanning. The primary endpoint for the double-blind phase was the total cumulative number of T1 Gd-enhancing lesions over the nine months. Table 4 summarizes the results for the primary outcome measure monitored during the trial for the intent-to-treat cohort.

Table 4: Study 4 MRI Results

	COPAXONE (N=119)	Placebo (N=120)	P-Value
Medians of the Cumulative Number of T1 Gd-Enhancing Lesions	11	17	0.0030

Figure 2 displays the results of the primary outcome on a monthly basis.

Figure 2: Median Cumulative Number of Gd-Enhancing Lesions

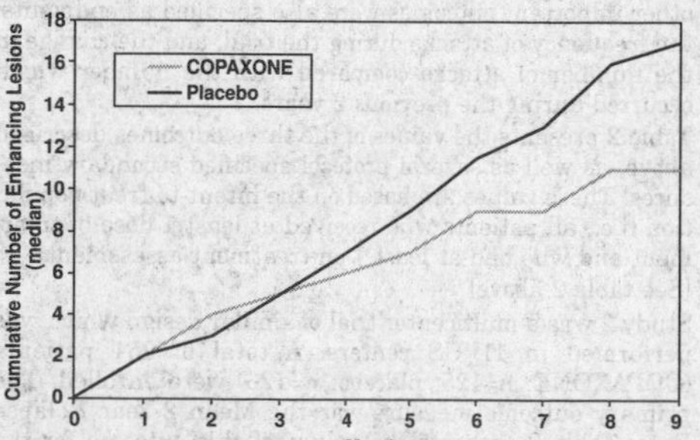

16 HOW SUPPLIED/STORAGE AND HANDLING

COPAXONE is supplied as a single-use prefilled syringe containing 1 mL of a clear, colorless to slightly yellow, sterile, nonpyrogenic solution containing 20 mg of glatiramer acetate and 40 mg of mannitol in cartons of 30 single-use prefilled syringes with 33 alcohol preps (NDC 68546-317-30).

The recommended storage condition for the COPAXONE is refrigeration (2°C to 8°C / 36°F to 46°F). However, excursions from recommended storage conditions (15°C to 30°C / 59°F to 86°F) for up to one month have been shown to have no adverse impact on the product. Exposure to higher temperatures or intense light should be avoided. COPAXONE should not be frozen. If a COPAXONE syringe freezes, it should be discarded.

COPAXONE contains no preservative. Do not use if the solution contains any particulate matter.

17 PATIENT COUNSELING INFORMATION

[See FDA-Approved Patient Labeling (17.7)]

17.1 Pregnancy

Instruct patients that if they are pregnant or plan to become pregnant while taking COPAXONE they should inform their physician.

17.2 Immediate Post-Injection Reaction

Advise patients that COPAXONE may cause various symptoms after injection, include flushing, chest pain, palpitations, anxiety, dyspnea, constriction of the throat, and urticaria. These symptoms are generally transient and self-limited and do not require specific treatment. Inform patients that these symptoms may occur early or may have their onset several months after the initiation of treatment. A patient may experience one or several episodes of these symptoms.

17.3 Chest Pain

Advise patients that they may experience transient chest pain either as part of the Immediate Post-Injection Reaction or in isolation. Inform patients that the pain should be transient (usually only lasting a few minutes). Some patients may experience more than one such episode, usually beginning at least one month after the initiation of treatment. Patient should be advised to seek medical attention if they experience chest pain of unusual duration or intensity.

17.4 Lipoatrophy and Skin Necrosis at Injection Site

Advise patients that localized lipoatrophy, and rarely, injection site necrosis may occur at injections sites. Instruct patients to follow proper injection technique and to rotate injection areas and sites on a daily basis.

17.5 Instructions for Use

Instruct patients to read the COPAXONE Patient Information leaflet carefully. Caution patients to use aseptic technique. The first injection should be performed under the supervision of a health care professional. Instruct patients to rotate injection areas and sites on a daily basis. Caution patients against the reuse of needles or syringes. Instruct patients in safe disposal procedures.

17.6 Storage Conditions

Advise patients that the recommended storage condition for COPAXONE is refrigeration (36-46°F /2-8°C), although COPAXONE can be stored at room temperature (59-86°F /15-30°C) for up to one month. COPAXONE should not be exposed to higher temperatures or intense light.

17.7 FDA-Approved Patient Labeling

Read this information carefully before you use COPAXONE. Read the information you get when you refill your COPAXONE prescriptions because there may be new information. This information does not take the place of your doctor's advice. Ask your doctor or pharmacist if you do not understand some of this information or if you want to know more about this medicine.

What is COPAXONE?

COPAXONE (co-PAX-own) is a medicine you inject to treat Relapsing-Remitting Multiple Sclerosis. Although COPAXONE is not a cure; patients treated with COPAXONE have fewer relapses.

Who should not use COPAXONE?

- Do not use COPAXONE if you are allergic to glatiramer acetate or mannitol.

What are the possible side effects of COPAXONE?

- **Call your doctor right away if you develop any of the following symptoms: hives, skin rash with irritation, dizziness, sweating, chest pain, trouble breathing, or severe pain at the injection site.** Do not give yourself any more injections until your doctor tells you to begin again.
- The most common side effects of COPAXONE are redness, pain, swelling, itching, or a lump at the injection site. These reactions are usually mild and seldom require medical care.
- Some patients report a short-term reaction right after injecting COPAXONE. This reaction can involve flushing (feeling of warmth and/or redness), chest tightness or pain with heart palpitations, anxiety, and trouble breathing. These symptoms generally appear within minutes after an injection, last a few minutes, and then go away by themselves without further problems.
- A permanent depression under the skin at the injection site may occur, due to a local destruction of fat tissue.
- **If symptoms become severe, call the emergency phone number in your area.** Do not give yourself any more injections until your doctor tells you to begin again.

These are not all the possible side effects of COPAXONE. For a complete list, ask your doctor or pharmacist. Tell your doctor about any side effects you have while taking COPAXONE.

Information for pregnant and nursing women

- COPAXONE has not been studied in pregnant women. Talk to your doctor about the risks and benefits of COPAXONE if you are pregnant or planning a pregnancy.
- It is not known if COPAXONE passes into breastmilk. Talk to your baby's doctor about the risks and benefits of breastfeeding while using COPAXONE.

How should I use COPAXONE?

- The recommended dose of COPAXONE for the treatment of Relapsing-Remitting Multiple Sclerosis is 20 mg once a day injected subcutaneously (in the fatty layer under the skin).
- Look at the medicine in the prefilled syringe. If the medicine is cloudy or has particles in it, do not use it. Instead, call Shared Solutions® at 1-800-887-8100 for assistance.
- Have a friend or relative with you if you need help, especially when you first start giving yourself injections.
- Each prefilled syringe should be used for only one injection. Do not reuse the prefilled syringe. After use, throw it away properly.
- Do not change the dose or dosing schedule or stop taking the medicine without talking with your doctor.

How do I inject COPAXONE?

There are 3 basic steps for injecting COPAXONE prefilled syringes:
1. Gather the materials.
2. Choose the injection site.
3. Give yourself the injection.

Step 1: Gather the materials

1. First, place each of the items you will need on a clean, flat surface in a well-lit area:
   - 1 blister pack with COPAXONE Prefilled Syringe
     Remove only 1 blister pack from the COPAXONE Prefilled Syringe carton. Keep all unused syringes in the Prefilled Syringe carton and store them in the refrigerator.
   - Alcohol prep (wipe not supplied)
   - Dry cotton ball (not supplied)
2. Let the blister pack with the syringe inside warm up to room temperature for 20 minutes.
3. To prevent infection, wash and dry your hands. Do not touch your hair or skin after washing.
4. There may be small air bubbles in the syringe. To avoid loss of medicine when using COPAXONE prefilled syringes, do not expel (or do not attempt to expel) the air bubble from the syringe before injecting the medicine.

Step 2: Choose the injection site

- There are 7 possible injection areas on your body: arms, thighs, hips and lower stomach area (abdomen) (See Figure 1).

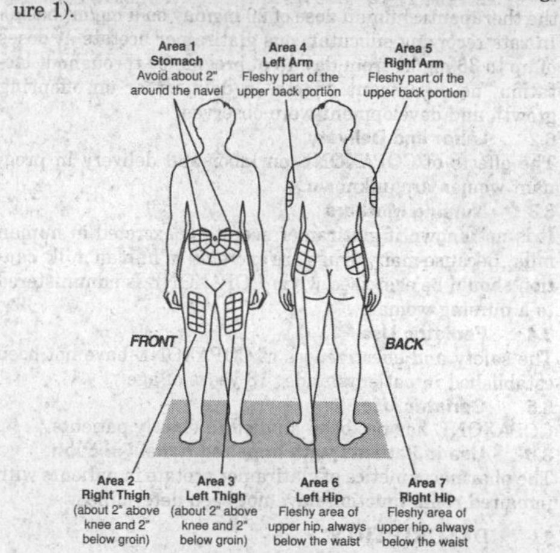

Figure 1

- Each day, pick a different injection area from one of the 7 areas. **Do not inject in the same area more than once a week.**
- Within each injection area there are multiple injection sites. Have a plan for rotating your injection sites. Keep a record of your injection sites, so you know where you have injected.
- There are some sites in your body that may be hard to reach for self-injection (like the back of your arm), and you may need help.
- Do not inject in sites where skin depression has occurred, because further injections in these sites may make the depression deeper.

Step 3: Give yourself the injection

1. Remove the syringe from its protective blister pack by peeling back the paper label. Before use, look at the liquid in the syringe. If it is cloudy or contains any particles, do not use it and call Shared Solutions® at 1-800-887-8100 for assistance. If the liquid is clear, place the syringe on the clean, flat surface.

2. Choose an injection site on your body. Clean the injection site with a new alcohol prep and let the site air dry to reduce stinging.
3. Pick up the syringe as you would a pencil. Remove the needle shield from the needle.
4. With your other hand, pinch about a 2-inch fold of skin between your thumb and index finger (See Figure 2).
5. Insert the needle at a 90-degree angle (straight in), resting the heel of your hand against your body. When the needle is all the way in release the fold of skin (See Figure 3).

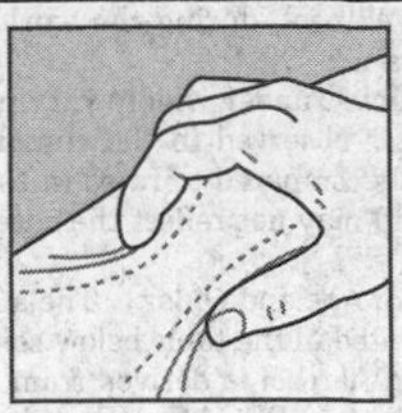
Figure 2

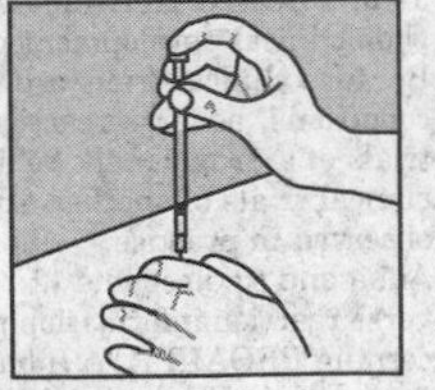
Figure 3

6. To inject the medicine, hold the syringe steady and push down the plunger.
7. When you have injected all of the medicine, pull the needle straight out.
8. Press a dry cotton ball on the injection site for a few seconds. **Do not rub the injection site.**
9. Throw away the syringe in a safe hard-walled plastic container.

What is the proper use and disposal of prefilled syringes?
Each prefilled syringe should be used for only 1 injection. Throw away all used prefilled syringes in a hard-walled plastic container, such as an empty liquid laundry detergent bottle. Keep the container closed tightly and out of the reach of children. When the container is full, check with your doctor, pharmacist, or nurse about proper disposal, as laws vary from state to state.

How should I store COPAXONE prefilled syringes?
Keep the COPAXONE prefilled syringe carton in the refrigerator, out of the reach of children.
The COPAXONE package should be refrigerated at 36-46°F (2-8°C). You can store it at room temperature, 59-86°F (15-30°C), for up to one month. Do not store COPAXONE at room temperature for longer than one month. **Do not freeze COPAXONE.** If a COPAXONE prefilled syringe freezes, throw it away in a proper container.
COPAXONE is light sensitive. Protect it from light when not injecting. Do not use the prefilled syringe if the solution contains particles or is cloudy.

General advice about prescription medicines
Medicines are sometimes prescribed for conditions that are not mentioned in patient information leaflets. Do not use COPAXONE for a condition for which it was not prescribed. Do not give COPAXONE to other people, even if they have the same condition you have. It may harm them.
This leaflet summarizes the most important information about COPAXONE. If you would like more information, talk with your doctor. You can ask your pharmacist or doctor for information about COPAXONE that is written for health professionals. Also, you can call Shared Solutions® for any questions about COPAXONE and its use. The phone number for Shared Solutions® is 1-800-887-8100.
Marketed by: TEVA Neuroscience, Inc., Kansas City, MO 64131
Distributed by: TEVA Pharmaceuticals USA, Inc., North Wales, PA 19454
Product of Israel
COP-40670

Shown in Product Identification Guide, page 314

Teva Respiratory, LLC.
425 PRIVET ROAD
HORSHAM, PA 19044

For All Inquiries Call:
1-888-482-9522

PROAIR HFA ℞
(albuterol sulfate)
Inhalation Aerosol

HIGHLIGHTS OF PRESCRIBING INFORMATION
These highlights do not include all the information needed to use PROAIR HFA safely and effectively. See full prescribing information for PROAIR HFA Inhalation Aerosol
PROAIR HFA (albuterol sulfate) INHALATION AEROSOL
Initial U.S. Approval: 1981

RECENT MAJOR CHANGES
Dosage and Administration (2.3) 03/12

INDICATIONS AND USAGE
PROAIR HFA Inhalation Aerosol is a beta$_2$-adrenergic agonist indicated for:
- Treatment or prevention of bronchospasm in patients 4 years of age and older with reversible obstructive airway disease. (1.1)
- Prevention of exercise-induced bronchospasm in patients 4 years of age and older. (1.2)

DOSAGE AND ADMINISTRATION
For oral inhalation only
- Treatment or prevention of bronchospasm in adults and children 4 years of age and older: 2 inhalations every 4 to 6 hours. In some patients, one inhalation every 4 hours may be sufficient. (2.1)
- Prevention of exercise-induced bronchospasm in adults and children 4 years of age and older: 2 inhalations 15 to 30 minutes before exercise. (2.2)
- Priming information: Prime PROAIR HFA before using for the first time, or when the inhaler has not been used for more than 2 weeks. To prime PROAIR HFA, release 3 sprays into the air away from the face. Shake well before each spray. (2.3)
- Cleaning information: At least once a week, wash the actuator with warm water, shake off excess, and air dry thoroughly. (2.3)
- PROAIR HFA inhaler should be discarded when the dose counter displays 0 or after the expiration date on the product, whichever comes first. (2.3)

DOSAGE FORMS AND STRENGTHS
Inhalation Aerosol: Each actuation delivers 108 mcg of albuterol sulfate from the actuator mouthpiece (equivalent to 90 mcg of albuterol base). Supplied in 8.5-g canister containing 200 actuations. (3)

CONTRAINDICATIONS
Hypersensitivity to albuterol and any other PROAIR HFA Inhalation Aerosol Components. (4)

WARNINGS AND PRECAUTIONS
- Life-threatening paradoxical bronchospasm may occur. Discontinue PROAIR HFA immediately and treat with alternative therapy. (5.1)
- Need for more doses of PROAIR HFA than usual may be a sign of deterioration of asthma and requires reevaluation of treatment. (5.2)
- PROAIR HFA is not a substitute for corticosteroids. (5.3)
- Cardiovascular effects may occur. Use with caution in patients sensitive to sympathomimetic drugs and patients with cardiovascular or convulsive disorders. (5.4, 5.7)
- Excessive use may be fatal. Do not exceed recommended dose. (5.5)
- Immediate hypersensitivity reactions may occur. Discontinue PROAIR HFA immediately. (5.6)
- Hypokalemia and changes in blood glucose may occur. (5.7, 5.8)

ADVERSE REACTIONS
Most common adverse reactions (≥3.0% and >placebo) are headache, tachycardia, pain, dizziness, pharyngitis, and rhinitis. (6.1)
To report SUSPECTED ADVERSE REACTIONS, contact Teva Respiratory, LLC at 1-888-482-9522 or FDA at 1-800-FDA-1088 or *www.fda.gov/medwatch*.

DRUG INTERACTIONS
- Other short-acting sympathomimetic aerosol bronchodilators and adrenergic drugs: May potentiate effect. (7)
- Beta-blockers: May decrease effectiveness of PROAIR HFA and produce severe bronchospasm. Patients with asthma should not normally be treated with beta-blockers. (7.1)
- Diuretics, or non-potassium sparing diuretics: May potentiate hypokalemia or ECG changes. Consider monitoring potassium levels. (7.2)
- Digoxin: May decrease serum digoxin levels. Consider monitoring digoxin levels. (7.3)
- Monoamine oxidase (MAO) inhibitors and tricyclic antidepressants: May potentiate effect of albuterol on the cardiovascular system. Consider alternative therapy in patients taking MAOs or tricyclic antidepressants. (7.4)

See 17 for PATIENT COUNSELING INFORMATION and FDA-approved patient labeling

Revised: 05/2012

FULL PRESCRIBING INFORMATION: CONTENTS*

*** Sections or subsections omitted from the full prescribing information are not listed**

FULL PRESCRIBING INFORMATION

1 INDICATIONS AND USAGE
1.1 Bronchospasm
PROAIR HFA Inhalation Aerosol is indicated for the treatment or prevention of bronchospasm in patients 4 years of age and older with reversible obstructive airway disease.
1.2 Exercise-Induced Bronchospasm
PROAIR HFA Inhalation Aerosol is indicated for the prevention of exercise-induced bronchospasm in patients 4 years of age and older.

2 DOSAGE AND ADMINISTRATION
2.1 Bronchospasm
For treatment of acute episodes of bronchospasm or prevention of symptoms associated with bronchospasm, the usual dosage for adults and children 4 years and older is two inhalations repeated every 4 to 6 hours. More frequent administration or a larger number of inhalations is not recommended. In some patients, one inhalation every 4 hours may be sufficient.

Adverse Experience Incidences (% of Patients) in a Six Week Clinical Trial*

Body System/ Adverse Event (as Preferred Term)		PROAIR HFA Inhalation Aerosol (N = 58)	Marketed active comparator HFA-134a albuterol inhaler (N = 56)	Matched Placebo HFA-134a Inhalation Aerosol (N = 58)
Body as a Whole	Headache	7	5	2
Cardiovascular	Tachycardia	3	2	0
Musculoskeletal	Pain	3	0	0
Nervous System	Dizziness	3	0	0
Respiratory System	Pharyngitis	14	7	9
	Rhinitis	5	4	2

* This table includes all adverse events (whether considered by the investigator drug related or unrelated to drug) which occurred at an incidence rate of at least 3.0% in the PROAIR HFA Inhalation Aerosol group and more frequently in the PROAIR HFA Inhalation Aerosol group than in the placebo HFA Inhalation Aerosol group.

2.2 Exercise-Induced Bronchospasm

The usual dosage for adults and children 4 years of age or older is two inhalations 15 to 30 minutes before exercise.

2.3 Administration Information

Administer PROAIR HFA by oral inhalation only. Shake well before each spray. To maintain proper use of this product and to prevent medication build-up and blockage, it is important to follow the cleaning directions carefully.

Priming: Prime the inhaler before using for the first time and in cases where the inhaler has not been used for more than 2 weeks by releasing three sprays into the air, away from the face.

Cleaning: As with all HFA-containing albuterol inhalers, to maintain proper use of this product and to prevent medication build-up and blockage, it is important to clean the plastic mouthpiece regularly. The inhaler may cease to deliver medication if the plastic actuator mouthpiece is not properly cleaned and dried. To clean: Wash the plastic mouthpiece with warm running water for 30 seconds, shake off excess water, and air dry thoroughly at least once a week. **If the patient has more than one PROAIR HFA inhaler, the patient should wash each one separately to prevent attaching the wrong canister to the wrong plastic actuator. In this way, the patient can be sure to always know the correct number of remaining doses. Never attach a canister of medication from any other inhaler to the PROAIR HFA actuator and never attach the PROAIR HFA canister to an actuator from any other inhaler.** If the mouthpiece becomes blocked, washing the mouthpiece will remove the blockage. If it is necessary to use the inhaler before it is completely dry, shake off excess water, replace canister, spray twice into the air away from face, and take the prescribed dose. After such use, the mouthpiece should be rewashed and allowed to air dry thoroughly. *[see **FDA-Approved Patient Labeling (17.9)**]*.

Dose Counter: PROAIR HFA has a dose counter attached to the actuator. When the patient receives the inhaler, a black dot will appear in the viewing window until it has been primed 3 times, at which point the number 200 will be displayed. The dose counter will count down each time a spray is released. When the dose counter reaches 20, the color of the numbers will change to red to remind the patient to contact their pharmacist for a refill of medication or consult their physician for a prescription refill. When the dose counter reaches 0, the background will change to solid red. PROAIR HFA inhaler should be discarded when the dose counter displays 0 or after the expiration date on the product, whichever comes first.

3 DOSAGE FORMS AND STRENGTHS

PROAIR HFA is an inhalation aerosol. PROAIR HFA is supplied as an 8.5 g/200 actuations pressurized aluminum canister with a red plastic actuator with a dose counter and white dust cap each in boxes of one. Each actuation delivers 120 mcg of albuterol sulfate from the canister valve and 108 mcg of albuterol sulfate from the actuator mouthpiece (equivalent to 90 mcg of albuterol base).

4 CONTRAINDICATIONS

PROAIR HFA Inhalation Aerosol is contraindicated in patients with a history of hypersensitivity to albuterol and any other PROAIR HFA Inhalation Aerosol components. Rare cases of hypersensitivity reactions, including urticaria, angioedema, and rash have been reported after the use of albuterol sulfate *[see **Warnings and Precautions (5.6)**]*.

5 WARNINGS AND PRECAUTIONS

5.1 Paradoxical Bronchospasm

PROAIR HFA Inhalation Aerosol can produce paradoxical bronchospasm that may be life threatening. If paradoxical bronchospasm occurs, PROAIR HFA Inhalation Aerosol should be discontinued immediately and alternative therapy instituted. It should be recognized that paradoxical bronchospasm, when associated with inhaled formulations, frequently occurs with the first use of a new canister.

5.2 Deterioration of Asthma

Asthma may deteriorate acutely over a period of hours or chronically over several days or longer. If the patient needs more doses of PROAIR HFA Inhalation Aerosol than usual, this may be a marker of destabilization of asthma and requires re-evaluation of the patient and treatment regimen, giving special consideration to the possible need for anti-inflammatory treatment, e.g., corticosteroids.

5.3 Use of Anti-inflammatory Agents

The use of beta-adrenergic-agonist bronchodilators alone may not be adequate to control asthma in many patients. Early consideration should be given to adding anti-inflammatory agents, e.g., corticosteroids, to the therapeutic regimen.

5.4 Cardiovascular Effects

PROAIR HFA Inhalation Aerosol, like other beta-adrenergic agonists, can produce clinically significant cardiovascular effects in some patients as measured by pulse rate, blood pressure, and/or symptoms. Although such effects are uncommon after administration of PROAIR HFA Inhalation Aerosol at recommended doses, if they occur, the drug may need to be discontinued. In addition, beta-agonists have been reported to produce ECG changes, such as flattening of the T wave, prolongation of the QTc interval, and ST segment depression. The clinical significance of these findings is unknown. Therefore, PROAIR HFA Inhalation Aerosol, like all sympathomimetic amines, should be used with caution in patients with cardiovascular disorders, especially coronary insufficiency, cardiac arrhythmias, and hypertension.

5.5 Do Not Exceed Recommended Dose

Fatalities have been reported in association with excessive use of inhaled sympathomimetic drugs in patients with asthma. The exact cause of death is unknown, but cardiac arrest following an unexpected development of a severe acute asthmatic crisis and subsequent hypoxia is suspected.

5.6 Immediate Hypersensitivity Reactions

Immediate hypersensitivity reactions may occur after administration of albuterol sulfate, as demonstrated by rare cases of urticaria, angioedema, rash, bronchospasm, anaphylaxis, and oropharyngeal edema. The potential for hypersensitivity must be considered in the clinical evaluation of patients who experience immediate hypersensitivity reactions while receiving PROAIR HFA Inhalation Aerosol.

5.7 Coexisting Conditions

PROAIR HFA Inhalation Aerosol, like all sympathomimetic amines, should be used with caution in patients with cardiovascular disorders, especially coronary insufficiency, cardiac arrhythmias, and hypertension; in patients with convulsive disorders, hyperthyroidism, or diabetes mellitus; and in patients who are unusually responsive to sympathomimetic amines. Clinically significant changes in systolic and diastolic blood pressure have been seen in individual patients and could be expected to occur in some patients after use of any beta-adrenergic bronchodilator. Large doses of intravenous albuterol have been reported to aggravate preexisting diabetes mellitus and ketoacidosis.

5.8 Hypokalemia

As with other beta-agonists, PROAIR HFA Inhalation Aerosol may produce significant hypokalemia in some patients, possibly through intracellular shunting, which has the potential to produce adverse cardiovascular effects. The decrease is usually transient, not requiring supplementation.

6 ADVERSE REACTIONS

Use of PROAIR HFA may be associated with the following:

- Paradoxical bronchospasm *[see **Warnings and Precautions (5.1)**]*
- Cardiovascular Effects *[see **Warnings and Precautions (5.4)**]*
- Immediate hypersensitivity reactions *[see **Warnings and Precautions (5.6)**]*
- Hypokalemia *[see **Warnings and Precautions (5.8)**]*

6.1 Clinical Trials Experience

A total of 1090 subjects were treated with PROAIR HFA Inhalation Aerosol, or with the same formulation of albuterol as in PROAIR HFA Inhalation Aerosol, during the worldwide clinical development program.

Because clinical trials are conducted under widely varying conditions, adverse reaction rates observed in the clinical trials of a drug cannot be directly compared to rates in the clinical trials of another drug and may not reflect the rates observed in practice.

Adult and Adolescents 12 Years of Age and Older: The adverse reaction information presented in the table below concerning PROAIR HFA Inhalation Aerosol is derived from a 6-week, blinded study which compared PROAIR HFA Inhalation Aerosol (180 mcg four times daily) with a double-blinded matched placebo HFA-Inhalation Aerosol and an evaluator-blinded marketed active comparator HFA-134a albuterol inhaler in 172 asthmatic patients 12 to 76 years of age. The table lists the incidence of all adverse events (whether considered by the investigator drug related or unrelated to drug) from this study which occurred at a rate of 3% or greater in the PROAIR HFA Inhalation Aerosol treatment group and more frequently in the PROAIR HFA Inhalation Aerosol treatment group than in the matched placebo group. Overall, the incidence and nature of the adverse events reported for PROAIR HFA Inhalation Aerosol and the marketed active comparator HFA-134a albuterol inhaler were comparable.

[See table above]

Adverse events reported by less than 3% of the patients receiving PROAIR HFA Inhalation Aerosol but by a greater proportion of PROAIR HFA Inhalation Aerosol patients than the matched placebo patients, which have the potential to be related to PROAIR HFA Inhalation Aerosol, included chest pain, infection, diarrhea, glossitis, accidental injury (nervous system), anxiety, dyspnea, ear disorder, ear pain, and urinary tract infection.

In small cumulative dose studies, tremor, nervousness, and headache were the most frequently occurring adverse events.

Pediatric Patients 4 to 11 Years of Age: Adverse events reported in a 3-week pediatric clinical trial comparing the same formulation of albuterol as in PROAIR HFA Inhalation Aerosol (180 mcg albuterol four times daily) to a matching placebo HFA inhalation aerosol occurred at a low incidence rate (no greater than 2% in the active treatment group) and were similar to those seen in adult and adolescent trials.

6.2 Postmarketing Experience

The following adverse reactions have been identified during postapproval use of PROAIR HFA. Because these reactions are reported voluntarily from a population of uncertain size, it is not always possible to reliably estimate their frequency or establish a causal relationship to drug exposure. Reports have included rare cases of aggravated bronchospasm, lack of efficacy, asthma exacerbation (reported fatal in one case), muscle cramps, and various oropharyngeal side-effects such as throat irritation, altered taste, glossitis, tongue ulceration, and gagging.

The following adverse events have been observed in postapproval use of inhaled albuterol: urticaria, angioedema, rash, bronchospasm, hoarseness, oropharyngeal edema, and arrhythmias (including atrial fibrillation, supraventricular tachycardia, extrasystoles). In addition, albuterol, like other sympathomimetic agents, can cause adverse reactions such as: angina, hypertension or hypotension, palpitations, central nervous system stimulation, insomnia, headache, nervousness, tremor, muscle cramps, drying or irritation of the oropharynx, hypokalemia, hyperglycemia, and metabolic acidosis.

7 DRUG INTERACTIONS

Other short-acting sympathomimetic aerosol bronchodilators should not be used concomitantly with PROAIR HFA Inhalation Aerosol. If additional adrenergic drugs are to be administered by any route, they should be used with caution to avoid deleterious cardiovascular effects.

7.1 Beta-Blockers

Beta-adrenergic-receptor blocking agents not only block the pulmonary effect of beta-agonists, such as PROAIR HFA Inhalation Aerosol, but may produce severe bronchospasm in asthmatic patients. Therefore, patients with asthma should not normally be treated with beta-blockers. However, under certain circumstances, e.g., as prophylaxis after myocardial infarction, there may be no acceptable alternatives to the use of beta-adrenergic-blocking agents in patients with asthma. In this setting, consider cardioselective beta-blockers, although they should be administered with caution.

7.2 Diuretics

The ECG changes and/or hypokalemia which may result from the administration of non-potassium sparing diuretics (such as loop or thiazide diuretics) can be acutely worsened by beta-agonists, especially when the recommended dose of the beta-agonist is exceeded. Although the clinical significance of these effects is not known, caution is advised in the coadministration of beta-agonists with non-potassium sparing diuretics. Consider monitoring potassium levels.

7.3 Digoxin

Mean decreases of 16% and 22% in serum digoxin levels were demonstrated after single dose intravenous and oral administration of albuterol, respectively, to normal volunteers who had received digoxin for 10 days. The clinical significance of these findings for patients with obstructive airway disease who are receiving albuterol and digoxin on a chronic basis is unclear. Nevertheless, it would be prudent to carefully evaluate the serum digoxin levels in patients who are currently receiving digoxin and PROAIR HFA Inhalation Aerosol.

7.4 Monoamine Oxidase Inhibitors or Tricyclic Antidepressants

PROAIR HFA Inhalation Aerosol should be administered with extreme caution to patients being treated with monoamine oxidase inhibitors or tricyclic antidepressants, or within 2 weeks of discontinuation of such agents, because the action of albuterol on the cardiovascular system may be potentiated. Consider alternative therapy in patients taking MAO inhibitors or tricyclic antidepressants.

8 USE IN SPECIFIC POPULATIONS

8.1 Pregnancy

Teratogenic Effects: Pregnancy Category C:

There are no adequate and well-controlled studies of PROAIR HFA Inhalation Aerosol or albuterol sulfate in pregnant women. During worldwide marketing experience, various congenital anomalies, including cleft palate and limb defects, have been reported in the offspring of patients treated with albuterol. Some of the mothers were taking multiple medications during their pregnancies. No consistent pattern of defects can be discerned, and a relationship between albuterol use and congenital anomalies has not been established. Animal reproduction studies in mice and rabbits revealed evidence of teratogenicity. PROAIR HFA Inhalation Aerosol should be used during pregnancy only if the potential benefit justifies the potential risk to the fetus.

In a mouse reproduction study, subcutaneously administered albuterol sulfate produced cleft palate formation in 5 of 111 (4.5%) fetuses at an exposure approximately eight-tenths of the maximum recommended human dose (MRHD) for adults on a mg/m^2 basis and in 10 of 108 (9.3%) fetuses at approximately 8 times the MRHD. Similar effects were not observed at approximately one-thirteenth of the MRHD. Cleft palate also occurred in 22 of 72 (30.5%) fetuses from females treated subcutaneously with isoproterenol (positive control).

In a rabbit reproduction study, orally administered albuterol sulfate induced cranioschisis in 7 of 19 fetuses (37%) at approximately 630 times the MRHD.

In a rat reproduction study, an albuterol sulfate/HFA-134a formulation administered by inhalation did not produce any teratogenic effects at exposures approximately 65 times the MRHD *[see* ***Nonclinical Toxicology (13.2)****]*.

8.2 Labor and Delivery

Because of the potential for beta-agonist interference with uterine contractility, use of PROAIR HFA Inhalation Aerosol for relief of bronchospasm during labor should be restricted to those patients in whom the benefits clearly outweigh the risk. PROAIR HFA Inhalation Aerosol has not been approved for the management of pre-term labor. The benefit:risk ratio when albuterol is administered for tocolysis has not been established. Serious adverse reactions, including pulmonary edema, have been reported during or following treatment of premature labor with beta$_2$-agonists, including albuterol.

8.3 Nursing Mothers

Plasma levels of albuterol sulfate and HFA-134a after inhaled therapeutic doses are very low in humans, but it is not known whether the components of PROAIR HFA Inhalation Aerosol are excreted in human milk.

Caution should be exercised when PROAIR HFA Inhalation Aerosol is administered to a nursing woman. Because of the potential for tumorigenicity shown for albuterol in animal studies and lack of experience with the use of PROAIR HFA Inhalation Aerosol by nursing mothers, a decision should be made whether to discontinue nursing or to discontinue the drug, taking into account the importance of the drug to the mother.

8.4 Pediatric Use

The safety and effectiveness of PROAIR HFA Inhalation Aerosol for the treatment or prevention of bronchospasm in children 12 years of age and older with reversible obstructive airway disease is based on one 6-week clinical trial in 116 patients 12 years of age and older with asthma comparing doses of 180 mcg four times daily with placebo, and one single-dose crossover study comparing doses of 90, 180, and 270 mcg with placebo in 58 patients *[see* ***Clinical Studies (14.1)****]*. The safety and effectiveness of PROAIR HFA Inhalation Aerosol for treatment of exercise-induced bronchospasm in children 12 years of age and older is based on one single-dose crossover study in 24 adults and adolescents with exercise-induced bronchospasm comparing doses of 180 mcg with placebo *[see* ***Clinical Studies (14.2)****]*.

The safety of PROAIR HFA Inhalation Aerosol in children 4 to 11 years of age is based on one 3-week clinical trial in 50 patients 4 to 11 years of age with asthma using the same formulation of albuterol as in PROAIR HFA Inhalation Aerosol comparing doses of 180 mcg four times daily with placebo. The effectiveness of PROAIR HFA Inhalation Aerosol in children 4 to 11 years of age is extrapolated from clinical trials in patients 12 years of age and older with asthma and exercise-induced bronchospasm, based on data from a single-dose study comparing the bronchodilatory effect of PROAIR HFA 90 mcg and 180 mcg with placebo in 55 patients with asthma and a 3-week clinical trial using the same formulation of albuterol as in PROAIR HFA Inhalation Aerosol in 95 asthmatic children 4 to 11 years of age comparing a dose of 180 mcg albuterol four times daily with placebo *[see* ***Clinical Studies (14.1)****]*.

The safety and effectiveness of PROAIR HFA Inhalation Aerosol in pediatric patients below the age of 4 years have not been established.

8.5 Geriatric Use

Clinical studies of PROAIR HFA Inhalation Aerosol did not include sufficient numbers of patients aged 65 and over to determine whether they respond differently from younger patients. Other reported clinical experience has not identified differences in responses between elderly and younger patients. In general, dose selection for an elderly patient should be cautious, usually starting at the low end of the dosing range, reflecting the greater frequency of decreased hepatic, renal, or cardiac function, and of concomitant disease or other drug therapy *[see* ***Warnings and Precautions (5.4, 5.7)****]*.

All beta$_2$-adrenergic agonists, including albuterol, are known to be substantially excreted by the kidney, and the risk of toxic reactions may be greater in patients with impaired renal function. Because elderly patients are more likely to have decreased renal function, care should be taken in dose selection, and it may be useful to monitor renal function.

10 OVERDOSAGE

The expected symptoms with overdosage are those of excessive beta-adrenergic stimulation and/or occurrence or exaggeration of any of the symptoms listed under ADVERSE REACTIONS, e.g., seizures, angina, hypertension or hypotension, tachycardia with rates up to 200 beats per minute, arrhythmias, nervousness, headache, tremor, dry mouth, palpitation, nausea, dizziness, fatigue, malaise, and insomnia.

Hypokalemia may also occur. As with all sympathomimetic medications, cardiac arrest and even death may be associated with abuse of PROAIR HFA Inhalation Aerosol.

Treatment consists of discontinuation of PROAIR HFA Inhalation Aerosol together with appropriate symptomatic therapy. The judicious use of a cardioselective beta-receptor blocker may be considered, bearing in mind that such medication can produce bronchospasm. There is insufficient evidence to determine if dialysis is beneficial for overdosage of PROAIR HFA Inhalation Aerosol.

The oral median lethal dose of albuterol sulfate in mice is greater than 2,000 mg/kg (approximately 6,800 times the maximum recommended daily inhalation dose for adults on a mg/m^2 basis and approximately 3,200 times the maximum recommended daily inhalation dose for children on a mg/m^2 basis). In mature rats, the subcutaneous median lethal dose of albuterol sulfate is approximately 450 mg/kg (approximately 3,000 times the maximum recommended daily inhalation dose for adults on a mg/m^2 basis and approximately 1,400 times the maximum recommended daily inhalation dose for children on a mg/m^2 basis). In young rats, the subcutaneous median lethal dose is approximately 2,000 mg/kg (approximately 14,000 times the maximum recommended daily inhalation dose for adults on a mg/m^2 basis and approximately 6,400 times the maximum recommended daily inhalation dose for children on a mg/m^2 basis). The inhalation median lethal dose has not been determined in animals.

11 DESCRIPTION

The active ingredient of PROAIR HFA (albuterol sulfate) Inhalation Aerosol is albuterol sulfate, a racemic salt, of albuterol. Albuterol sulfate has the chemical name α^1-[(*tert*-butylamino) methyl]-4-hydroxy-*m*-xylene-α,α'-diol sulfate (2:1) (salt), and has the following chemical structure:

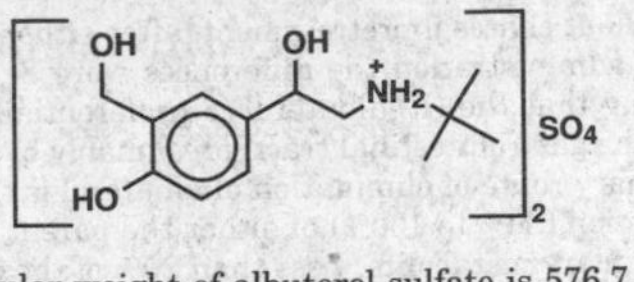

The molecular weight of albuterol sulfate is 576.7, and the empirical formula is $(C_{13}H_{21}NO_3)_2 \bullet H_2SO_4$. Albuterol sulfate is a white to off-white crystalline powder. It is soluble in water and slightly soluble in ethanol. Albuterol sulfate is the official generic name in the United States, and salbutamol sulfate is the World Health Organization recommended generic name. PROAIR HFA Inhalation Aerosol is a pressurized metered-dose aerosol unit with a dose counter. PROAIR HFA is for oral inhalation only. It contains a microcrystalline suspension of albuterol sulfate in propellant HFA-134a (1, 1, 1, 2-tetrafluoroethane) and ethanol.

Prime the inhaler before using for the first time and in cases where the inhaler has not been used for more than 2 weeks by releasing three sprays into the air, away from the face. After priming, each actuation delivers 108 mcg albuterol sulfate, from the actuator mouthpiece (equivalent to 90 mcg of albuterol base). Each canister provides 200 actuations (inhalations).

This product does not contain chlorofluorocarbons (CFCs) as the propellant.

12 CLINICAL PHARMACOLOGY

12.1 Mechanism of Action

Albuterol sulfate is a beta$_2$-adrenergic agonist. The pharmacologic effects of albuterol sulfate are attributable to activation of beta$_2$-adrenergic receptors on airway smooth muscle. Activation of beta$_2$-adrenergic receptors leads to the activation of adenylcyclase and to an increase in the intracellular concentration of cyclic-3', 5'-adenosine monophosphate (cyclic AMP). This increase of cyclic AMP is associated with the activation of protein kinase A, which in turn inhibits the phosphorylation of myosin and lowers intracellular ionic calcium concentrations, resulting in muscle relaxation. Albuterol relaxes the smooth muscle of all airways, from the trachea to the terminal bronchioles. Albuterol acts as a functional antagonist to relax the airway irrespective of the spasmogen involved, thus protecting against all bronchoconstrictor challenges. Increased cyclic AMP concentrations are also associated with the inhibition of release of mediators from mast cells in the airway. While it is recognized that beta$_2$-adrenergic receptors are the predominant receptors on bronchial smooth muscle, data indicate that there are beta-receptors in the human heart, 10% to 50% of which are cardiac beta$_2$-adrenergic receptors. The precise function of these receptors has not been established *[see* ***Warnings and Precautions (5.4)****]*.

Albuterol has been shown in most controlled clinical trials to have more effect on the respiratory tract, in the form of bronchial smooth muscle relaxation, than isoproterenol at comparable doses while producing fewer cardiovascular effects. However, inhaled albuterol, like other beta-adrenergic agonist drugs, can produce a significant cardiovascular effect in some patients, as measured by pulse rate, blood pressure, symptoms, and/or electrocardiographic changes *[see* ***Warnings and Precautions (5.4)****]*.

12.2 Pharmacokinetics

The systemic levels of albuterol are low after inhalation of recommended doses. In a crossover study conducted in healthy male and female volunteers, high cumulative doses of PROAIR HFA Inhalation Aerosol (1,080 mcg of albuterol base administered over one hour) yielded mean peak plasma concentrations (C_{max}) and systemic exposure (AUC_{inf}) of approximately 4,100 pg/mL and 28,426 pg/mL*hr, respectively compared to approximately 3,900 pg/mL and 28,395 pg/mL*hr, respectively following the same dose of an active HFA-134a albuterol inhaler comparator. The terminal plasma half-life of albuterol delivered by PROAIR HFA Inhalation Aerosol was approximately 6 hours. Comparison of the pharmacokinetic parameters demonstrated no differences between the products.

The pharmacokinetic profile of PROAIR HFA Inhalation Aerosol was evaluated in a two-way cross-over study in 11 healthy pediatric volunteers, 4 to 11 years of age. A single dose administration of PROAIR HFA Inhalation Aerosol (180 mcg albuterol base) yielded a least square mean (SE) C_{max} and $AUC_{0-\infty}$ of 1,100 (1.18) pg/mL and 5,120 (1.15) pg/mL*hr, respectively. The least square mean (SE) terminal plasma half-life of albuterol delivered by PROAIR HFA Inhalation Aerosol was 166 (7.8) minutes.

Metabolism and Elimination: Information available in the published literature suggests that the primary enzyme responsible for the metabolism of albuterol in humans is SULTIA3 (sulfotransferase). When racemic albuterol was administered either intravenously or via inhalation after oral charcoal administration, there was a 3- to 4-fold difference in the area under the concentration-time curves between the (R)- and (S)-albuterol enantiomers, with (S)-albuterol concentrations being consistently higher. However, without charcoal pretreatment, after either oral or inhalation administration the differences were 8- to 24-fold, suggesting that the (R)-albuterol is preferentially metabolized in the gastrointestinal tract, presumably by SULTIA3. The primary route of elimination of albuterol is through renal excretion (80% to 100%) of either the parent compound or the primary metabolite. Less than 20% of the drug is detected in the feces. Following intravenous administration of racemic albuterol, between 25% and 46% of the (R)-albuterol fraction of the dose was excreted as unchanged (R)-albuterol in the urine.

Geriatric, Pediatric, Hepatic/Renal Impairment: No pharmacokinetic studies for PROAIR HFA Inhalation Aerosol have been conducted in neonates or elderly subjects.

The effect of hepatic impairment on the pharmacokinetics of PROAIR HFA Inhalation Aerosol has not been evaluated.

The effect of renal impairment on the pharmacokinetics of albuterol was evaluated in 5 subjects with creatinine clearance of 7 to 53 mL/min, and the results were compared with those from healthy volunteers. Renal disease had no effect on the half-life, but there was a 67% decline in albuterol clearance. Caution should be used when administering high doses of PROAIR HFA Inhalation Aerosol to patients with renal impairment *[see **Use in Specific Populations (8.5)**]*.

13 NONCLINICAL TOXICOLOGY

13.1 Carcinogenesis, Mutagenesis, Impairment of Fertility

In a 2-year study in Sprague-Dawley rats, albuterol sulfate caused a dose-related increase in the incidence of benign leiomyomas of the mesovarium at and above dietary doses of 2 mg/kg (approximately 15 times the maximum recommended daily inhalation dose for adults on a mg/m^2 basis and approximately 6 times the maximum recommended daily inhalation dose for children on a mg/m^2 basis). In another study this effect was blocked by the coadministration of propranolol, a non-selective beta-adrenergic antagonist.

In an 18-month study in CD-1 mice, albuterol sulfate showed no evidence of tumorigenicity at dietary doses of up to 500 mg/kg (approximately 1,600 times the maximum recommended daily inhalation dose for adults on a mg/m^2 basis and approximately 740 times the maximum recommended daily inhalation dose for children on a mg/m^2 basis). In a 22-month study in Golden Hamsters, albuterol sulfate showed no evidence of tumorigenicity at dietary doses of up to 50 mg/kg (approximately 210 times the maximum recommended daily inhalation dose for adults on a mg/m^2 basis and approximately 100 times the maximum recommended daily inhalation dose for children on a mg/m^2 basis).

Albuterol sulfate was not mutagenic in the Ames test or a mutation test in yeast. Albuterol sulfate was not clastogenic in a human peripheral lymphocyte assay or in an AH1 strain mouse micronucleus assay.

Reproduction studies in rats demonstrated no evidence of impaired fertility at oral doses up to 50 mg/kg (approximately 310 times the maximum recommended daily inhalation dose for adults on a mg/m^2 basis).

13.2 Animal Toxicology and/or Pharmacology

Preclinical: Intravenous studies in rats with albuterol sulfate have demonstrated that albuterol crosses the blood-brain barrier and reaches brain concentrations amounting to approximately 5% of the plasma concentrations. In structures outside the blood-brain barrier (pineal and pituitary glands), albuterol concentrations were found to be 100 times those in the whole brain.

Studies in laboratory animals (minipigs, rodents, and dogs) have demonstrated the occurrence of cardiac arrhythmias and sudden death (with histologic evidence of myocardial necrosis) when β-agonists and methylxanthines were administered concurrently. The clinical significance of these findings is unknown.

Propellant HFA-134a is devoid of pharmacological activity except at very high doses in animals (380 - 1300 times the maximum human exposure based on comparisons of AUC values), primarily producing ataxia, tremors, dyspnea, or salivation. These are similar to effects produced by the structurally related chlorofluorocarbons (CFCs), which have been used extensively in metered-dose inhalers.

In animals and humans, propellant HFA-134a was found to be rapidly absorbed and rapidly eliminated, with an elimination half-life of 3 - 27 minutes in animals and 5 - 7 minutes in humans. Time to maximum plasma concentration (T_{max}) and mean residence time are both extremely short leading to a transient appearance of HFA-134a in the blood with no evidence of accumulation.

Reproductive Toxicology Studies: A study in CD-1 mice given albuterol sulfate subcutaneously showed cleft palate formation in 5 of 111 (4.5%) fetuses at 0.25 mg/kg (less than the maximum recommended daily inhalation dose for adults on a mg/m^2 basis) and in 10 of 108 (9.3%) fetuses at 2.5 mg/kg (approximately 8 times the maximum recommended daily inhalation dose for adults on a mg/m^2 basis). The drug did not induce cleft palate formation at a dose of 0.025 mg/kg (less than the maximum recommended daily inhalation dose for adults on a mg/m^2 basis). Cleft palate also occurred in 22 of 72 (30.5%) fetuses from females treated subcutaneously with 2.5 mg/kg of isoproterenol (positive control).

A reproduction study in Stride Dutch rabbits revealed cranioschisis in 7 of 19 fetuses (37%) when albuterol sulfate was administered orally at 50 mg/kg (approximately 630 times the maximum recommended daily inhalation dose for adults on a mg/m^2 basis).

In an inhalation reproduction study in Sprague-Dawley rats, the albuterol sulfate/HFA-134a did not exhibit any teratogenic effects at 10.5 mg/kg (approximately 65 times the maximum recommended daily inhalation dose for adults on a mg/m^2 basis).

A study in which pregnant rats were dosed with radiolabeled albuterol sulfate demonstrated that drug-related material is transferred from the maternal circulation to the fetus.

14 CLINICAL STUDIES

14.1 Bronchospasm Associated with Asthma

Adult and Adolescent Patients 12 Years of Age and Older: In a 6-week, randomized, double-blind, placebo-controlled trial, PROAIR HFA Inhalation Aerosol (58 patients) was compared to a matched placebo HFA inhalation aerosol (58 patients) in asthmatic patients 12 to 76 years of age at a dose of 180 mcg albuterol four times daily. An evaluator-blind marketed active comparator HFA-134a albuterol inhaler arm (56 patients) was included.

Serial FEV_1 measurements, shown below as percent change from test-day baseline at Day 1 and at Day 43, demonstrated that two inhalations of PROAIR HFA Inhalation Aerosol produced significantly greater improvement in FEV_1 over the pre-treatment value than the matched placebo, as well as a comparable bronchodilator effect to the marketed active comparator HFA-134a albuterol inhaler.

FEV_1 as Mean Percent Change from Test-Day Pre-Dose in a 6-Week Clinical Trial

Day 1

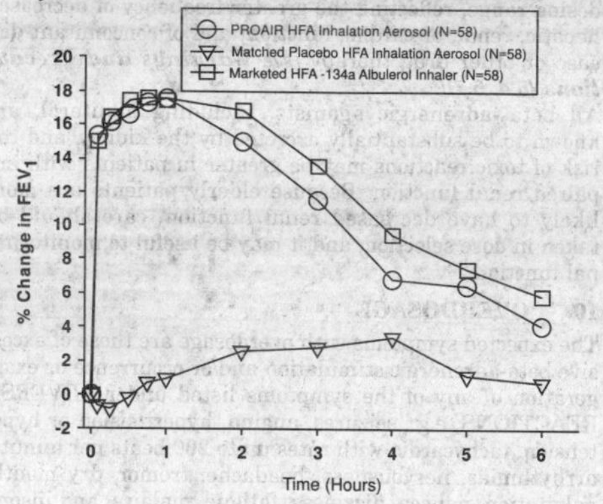

Day 43

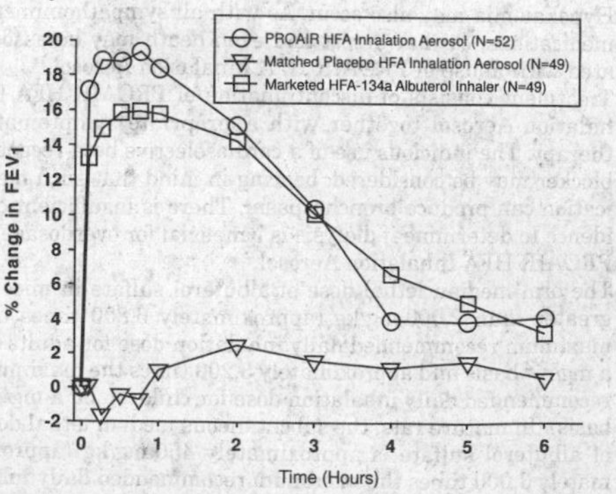

In this study, 31 of 58 patients treated with PROAIR HFA Inhalation Aerosol achieved a 15% increase in FEV_1 within 30 minutes post-dose on Day 1. In these patients, the median time to onset, median time to peak effect, and median duration of effect were 8.2 minutes, 47 minutes, and approximately 3 hours, respectively. In some patients, the duration of effect was as long as 6 hours.

In a placebo-controlled, single-dose, crossover study, PROAIR HFA Inhalation Aerosol, administered at albuterol doses of 90, 180 and 270 mcg, produced bronchodilator responses significantly greater than those observed with a matched placebo HFA inhalation aerosol and comparable to a marketed active comparator HFA-134a albuterol inhaler.

Pediatric Patients 4 to 11 Years of Age: In a 3-week, randomized, double-blind, placebo-controlled trial, the same formulation of albuterol as in PROAIR HFA Inhalation Aerosol (50 patients) was compared to a matched placebo HFA inhalation aerosol (45 patients) in asthmatic children 4 to 11 years of age at a dose of 180 mcg albuterol four times daily. Serial FEV_1 measurements, expressed as the maximum percent change from test-day baseline in percent predicted FEV_1 at Day 1 and at Day 22 observed within two hours post-dose, demonstrated that two inhalations of HFA albuterol sulfate produced significantly greater improvement in FEV_1 over the pre-treatment value than the matched placebo.

In this study, 21 of 50 pediatric patients treated with the same formulation of albuterol as in PROAIR HFA Inhalation Aerosol achieved a 15% increase in FEV_1 within 30 minutes post-dose on Day 1. In these patients, the median time to onset, median time to peak effect and median duration of effect were 10 minutes, 31 minutes, and approximately 4 hours, respectively. In some pediatric patients, the duration of effect was as long as 6 hours.

In a placebo-controlled, single-dose, crossover study in 55 pediatric patients 4 to 11 years of age, PROAIR HFA Inhalation Aerosol, administered at albuterol doses of 90 and 180 mcg, was compared with a matched placebo HFA inhalation aerosol. Serial FEV_1 measurements, expressed as the baseline-adjusted percent predicted FEV_1 observed over 6 hours post-dose, demonstrated that one and two inhalations of PROAIR HFA Inhalation Aerosol produced significantly greater bronchodilator responses than the matched placebo.

14.2 Exercise-Induced Bronchospasm

In a randomized, single-dose, crossover study in 24 adults and adolescents with exercise-induced bronchospasm (EIB), two inhalations of PROAIR HFA taken 30 minutes before exercise prevented EIB for the hour following exercise (defined as maintenance of FEV_1 within 80% of post-dose, pre-exercise baseline values) in 83% (20 of 24) of patients as compared to 25% (6 of 24) of patients when they received placebo.

Some patients who participated in these clinical trials were using concomitant steroid therapy.

16 HOW SUPPLIED/STORAGE AND HANDLING

PROAIR HFA (albuterol sulfate) Inhalation Aerosol is supplied as a pressurized aluminum canister with a red plastic actuator with a dose counter and white dust cap each in boxes of one. Each canister contains 8.5 g of the formulation and provides 200 actuations (NDC 59310-579-22). Each actuation delivers 120 mcg of albuterol sulfate from the canister valve and 108 mcg of albuterol sulfate from the actuator mouthpiece (equivalent to 90 mcg of albuterol base).

SHAKE WELL BEFORE USE. Store between 15° and 25°C (59° and 77°F). Contents under pressure. Do not puncture or incinerate. Protect from freezing temperatures and prolonged exposure to direct sunlight. Exposure to temperatures above 120°F may cause bursting. For best results, canister should be at room temperature before use. Avoid spraying in eyes. Keep out of reach of children.

See **FDA-Approved Patient Labeling (17.9)** for priming and cleaning instructions.

The red actuator supplied with PROAIR HFA Inhalation Aerosol should not be used with the canister from any other inhalation aerosol products. The PROAIR HFA Inhalation Aerosol canister should not be used with the actuator from any other inhalation aerosol products.

PROAIR HFA inhaler has a dose counter attached to the actuator. Patients should never try to alter the numbers for the dose counter or tamper with the pin mechanism inside the actuator. Discard the PROAIR HFA inhaler when the counter displays 0 or after the expiration date on the product, whichever comes first.The labeled amount of medication in each actuation cannot be assured after the counter displays 0, even though the canister is not completely empty and will continue to operate. Never immerse the canister into water to determine how full the canister is ("float test").

PROAIR HFA Inhalation Aerosol does not contain chlorofluorocarbons (CFCs) as the propellant.

17 PATIENT COUNSELING INFORMATION

See **FDA-Approved Patient Labeling (17.9)**

Patients should be given the following information:

17.1 Frequency of Use

The action of PROAIR HFA Inhalation Aerosol should last for 4 to 6 hours. Do not use PROAIR HFA Inhalation Aerosol more frequently than recommended. Instruct patients to not increase the dose or frequency of doses of PROAIR HFA Inhalation Aerosol without consulting the physician. If patients find that treatment with PROAIR HFA Inhalation Aerosol becomes less effective for symptomatic relief, symptoms become worse, and/or they need to use the product more frequently than usual, they should seek medical attention immediately.

17.2 Priming and Cleaning

Priming: Priming is essential to ensure appropriate albuterol content in each actuation. Instruct patients to prime the inhaler before using for the first time and in cases where the inhaler has not been used for more than 2 weeks by releasing three sprays into the air, away from the face.

Cleaning: To ensure proper dosing and prevent actuator orifice blockage, instruct patients to wash the red plastic actuator mouthpiece and dry thoroughly at least once a week. Instruct patients that if they have more than one PROAIR HFA inhaler, they should wash each one at separate times to prevent attaching the wrong canister to the wrong plastic actuator. In this way, they can be sure they will always know the correct number of remaining doses. Patients should be instructed to never attach a canister of medicine from any other inhaler to the PROAIR HFA actuator and never attach the PROAIR HFA canister to an actuator from any other inhaler. Patients should not remove the canister from the actuator except during cleaning because reattachment may release a dose into the air and the dose counter will count down each time a spray is released. Detailed cleaning instructions are included in the illustrated Information for the Patient leaflet.

17.3 Dose Counter

Patients should be informed that PROAIR HFA has a dose counter attached to the actuator. When the patient receives the inhaler, a black dot will appear in the viewing window until it has been primed 3 times, at which point the number 200 will be displayed. The dose counter will count down each time a spray is released. The dose-counter window displays the number of sprays left in the inhaler in units of two (e.g., 200, 198, 196, etc). When the counter displays 20, the color of the numbers will change to red to remind the patient to contact their pharmacist for a refill of medication or consult their physician for a prescription refill. When the dose counter reaches 0, the background will change to solid red. Patients should be informed to discard PROAIR HFA inhaler when the dose counter displays 0 or after the expiration date on the product, whichever comes first.

17.4 Paradoxical Bronchospasm

Inform patients that PROAIR HFA Inhalation Aerosol can produce paradoxical bronchospasm. Instruct patients to discontinue PROAIR HFA Inhalation Aerosol if paradoxical bronchospasm occurs.

17.5 Concomitant Drug Use

While patients are taking PROAIR HFA Inhalation Aerosol, other inhaled drugs and asthma medications should be taken only as directed by a physician.

17.6 Common Adverse Events

Common adverse effects of treatment with inhaled albuterol include palpitations, chest pain, rapid heart rate, tremor, or nervousness.

17.7 Pregnancy

Patients who are pregnant or nursing should contact their physician about the use of PROAIR HFA Inhalation Aerosol.

17.8 General Information on Use

Effective and safe use of PROAIR HFA Inhalation Aerosol includes an understanding of the way that it should be administered.

Shake well before each spray.

Use PROAIR HFA Inhalation Aerosol only with the actuator supplied with the product. Discard the HFA inhaler when the dose counter displays 0 or after the expiration date on the product, whichever comes first. Never immerse the canister in water to determine how full the canister is ("float test").

In general, the technique for administering PROAIR HFA Inhalation Aerosol to children is similar to that for adults. Children should use PROAIR HFA Inhalation Aerosol under adult supervision, as instructed by the patient's physician.

17.9 FDA-Approved Patient Labeling

See tear-off illustrated Information for the Patient leaflet.

Mktd by: Teva Respiratory, LLC
Horsham, PA 19044
Mfd by: IVAX Pharmaceuticals Ireland
Waterford, Ireland

Manufactured In Ireland
PE 2557 05/12

Attention Pharmacist:
Detach Patient's Instructions for use from package insert and dispense with the product.

Patient Information
PROAIR® HFA (*prō´ ār*)
(albuterol sulfate)
Inhalation Aerosol

Read this Patient Information before you start using PROAIR HFA and each time you get a refill. There may be new information. This information does not take the place of talking to your doctor about your medical condition or your treatment.

What is PROAIR HFA?

PROAIR HFA is a prescription medicine used in people 4 years of age and older to:

- treat or prevent bronchospasm in people who have reversible obstructive airway disease
- prevent exercise induced bronchospasm

It is not known if PROAIR HFA is safe and effective in children under 4 years of age.

Who should not use PROAIR HFA?

Do not use PROAIR HFA if you are allergic to albuterol sulfate or any of the ingredients in PROAIR HFA. See the end of this leaflet for a complete list of ingredients in PROAIR HFA.

What should I tell my doctor before I use PROAIR HFA?

Before you use PROAIR HFA, tell your doctor if you:

- have heart problems
- have high blood pressure (hypertension)
- have convulsions (seizures)
- have thyroid problems
- have diabetes
- have low potassium levels in your blood
- are pregnant or plan to become pregnant. It is not known if PROAIR HFA will harm your unborn baby. Talk to your doctor if you are pregnant or plan to become pregnant.
- are breastfeeding or plan to breastfeed. It is not known if PROAIR HFA passes into your breast milk. Talk to your doctor about the best way to feed your baby if you are using PROAIR HFA.

Tell your doctor about all the medicines you take, including prescription and non-prescription medicines, vitamins, and herbal supplements.

PROAIR HFA and other medicines may affect each other and cause side effects. PROAIR HFA may affect the way other medicines work, and other medicines may affect the way PROAIR HFA works.

Especially tell your doctor if you take:

- other inhaled medicines or asthma medicines
- beta blocker medicines
- diuretics
- digoxin
- monoamine oxidase inhibitors
- tricyclic antidepressants

Ask your doctor or pharmacist for a list of these medicines if you are not sure.

Know the medicines you take. Keep a list of them to show your doctor and pharmacist when you get a new medicine.

How should I use PROAIR HFA?

- For detailed instructions, see **"Instructions for Use"** at the end of this Patient Information.
- Use PROAIR HFA exactly as your doctor tells you to use it.
- If your child needs to use PROAIR HFA, watch your child closely to make sure your child uses the inhaler correctly. Your doctor will show you how your child should use PROAIR HFA.
- Each dose of PROAIR HFA should last up to 4 hours to 6 hours.
- **Do not** increase your dose or take extra doses of PROAIR HFA without first talking to your doctor.
- Get medical help right away if PROAIR HFA no longer helps your symptoms.
- Get medical help right away if your symptoms get worse or if you need to use your inhaler more often.
- While you are using PROAIR HFA, **do not** use other inhaled rescue medicines and asthma medicines unless your doctor tells you to do so.
- Call your doctor if your asthma symptoms like wheezing and trouble breathing become worse over a few hours or days. Your doctor may need to give you another medicine (for example, corticosteroids) to treat your symptoms.

What are the possible side effects of PROAIR HFA?

PROAIR HFA may cause serious side effects, including:

- **worsening trouble breathing, coughing and wheezing (paradoxical bronchospasm).** If this happens stop using PROAIR HFA and call your doctor or get emergency help right away. Paradoxical bronchospasm is more likely to happen with your first use of a new canister of medicine.
- **heart problems including faster heart rate and higher blood pressure**
- **possible death in people with asthma who use too much PROAIR HFA**
- **allergic reactions.** Call your doctor right away if you have the following symptoms of an allergic reaction:
  - itchy skin
  - swelling beneath your skin or in your throat
  - rash
  - worsening trouble breathing
- **low potassium levels in your blood**
- **worsening of other medical problems in people who also use PROAIR HFA including increases in blood sugar**

The most common side effects of PROAIR HFA include:

- your heart feels like it is pounding or racing (palpitations)
- chest pain
- fast heart rate
- shakiness
- nervousness
- headache
- dizziness
- sore throat
- runny nose

Tell your doctor if you have any side effect that bothers you or that does not go away.

These are not all of the possible side effects of PROAIR HFA. For more information, ask your doctor or pharmacist.

Call your doctor for medical advice about side effects. You may report side effects to FDA at 1-800-FDA-1088.

How should I store PROAIR HFA?

- Store PROAIR HFA at room temperature between 59° F and 77° F (15° C and 25° C).
- Avoid exposure to extreme heat and cold.
- Shake the PROAIR HFA canister well before use.
- **Do not** puncture the PROAIR HFA canister.
- **Do not** store the PROAIR HFA canister near heat or a flame. Temperatures above 120° F may cause the canister to burst.
- **Do not** throw the PROAIR HFA canister into a fire or an incinerator.
- Avoid spraying PROAIR HFA in your eyes.

Keep PROAIR HFA and all medicines out of the reach of children.

General Information about the safe and effective use of PROAIR HFA

Medicines are sometimes prescribed for purposes other than those listed in a Medication Guide. Do not use PROAIR HFA for a condition for which it was not prescribed. Do not give PROAIR HFA to other people, even if they have the same symptoms that you have. It may harm them.

This Patient Information summarizes the most important information about PROAIR HFA. If you would like more information, talk with your doctor. You can ask your pharmacist or doctor for information about PROAIR HFA that is written for health professionals.

For more information, go to www.ProAirHFA.com or call 1-888-482-9522.

What are the ingredients in PROAIR HFA?

Active ingredient: albuterol sulfate

Inactive ingredients: propellant HFA-134a and ethanol.

Instructions for Use
PROAIR® HFA (*prō´ ār*)
(albuterol sulfate)
Inhalation Aerosol

Read this Instructions for Use before you start using PROAIR HFA and each time you get a refill. There may be new information. This information does not take the place of talking to your doctor about your medical condition or your treatment.

The Parts of Your PROAIR HFA Inhaler Device:

There are 2 main parts of your PROAIR HFA inhaler device including a:

- red plastic actuator that sprays the medicine from the canister. See Figure A.
- protective dust cap that covers the mouthpiece of the actuator. See Figure A.

There is also a metal canister that holds the medicine. See Figure A.

There is also a dose counter attached to the back of the actuator with a viewing window that shows you how many sprays of medicine you have left. See Figure B.

You will see a black dot in the viewing window on the actuator until the device has been primed 3 times. See Figure B and **"Priming Your PROAIR HFA Device"** below.

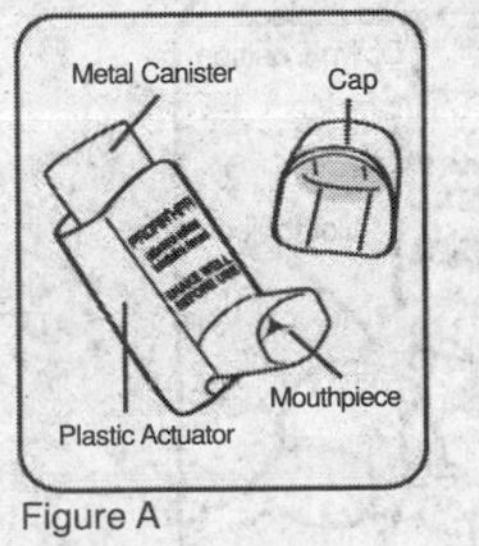

Figure A

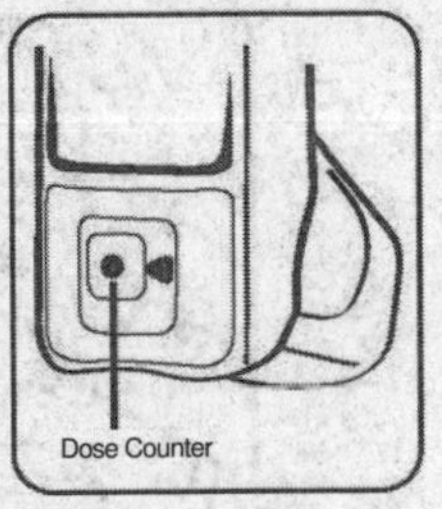

Figure B

- **Do not** use the PROAIR HFA actuator with a canister of medicine from any other inhaler.
- **Do not** use a PROAIR HFA canister with an actuator from any other inhaler, including another PROAIR HFA inhaler.

Priming Your PROAIR HFA Device:

Your PROAIR device must be primed before you use it for the first time or if your device has not been used for more than 14 days in a row. **Do not** prime your PROAIR HFA device every day.

- Remove your PROAIR HFA device from its package.
- Remove the protective dust cap from the mouthpiece.

- Shake the inhaler well, and spray it into the air away from your face. See Figure C.

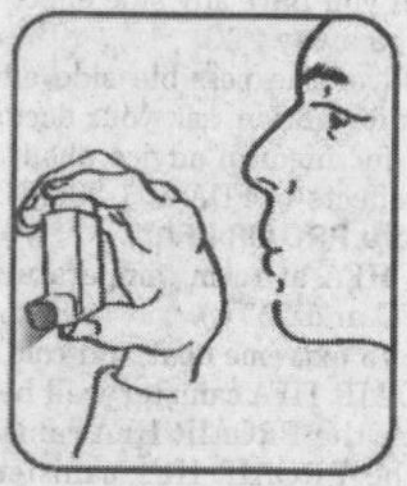

Figure C

- Shake and spray the inhaler like this 2 more times to finish priming it.
  The dose counter on the actuator should display the number 200 after you prime the actuator for the first time. See Figure D.

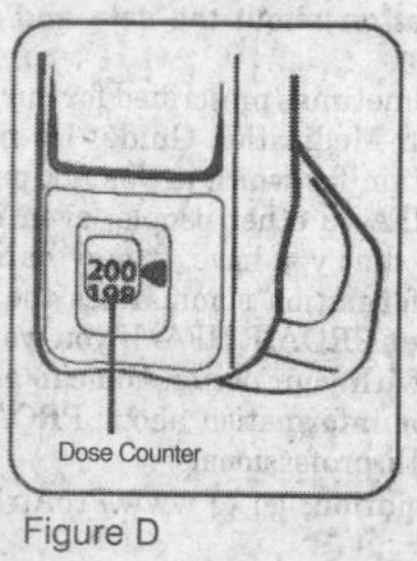

Figure D

Each Time You Use Your PROAIR HFA Device:
- Make sure the canister fits firmly in the plastic actuator.
- Look into the mouthpiece to make sure there are no foreign objects there, especially if the cap has not been used to cover the mouthpiece.

Reading the Dose Counter on Your PROAIR HFA Actuator
- The dose counter will count down each time a spray is released. The dose counter window shows the number of sprays left in your inhaler in units of 2 sprays. For example, there are 190 sprays left if the arrow is exactly opposite the number 190, or 189 sprays left if the arrow points between 190 and 188. See Figure D.
- When the dose counter reaches **0**, it will continue to show **0** and you should replace your PROAIR HFA device.
- The dose counter cannot be reset and is permanently attached to the actuator. **Never** change the numbers for the dose counter or touch the pin inside the actuator.
- **Do not** remove the canister from the plastic actuator except during cleaning. Reattaching the canister to the actuator may accidently release a dose of PROAIR HFA into the air. The dose counter will count down each time a spray is released.

Using Your PROAIR HFA Device:

Step 1. **Shake the inhaler well** before each spray. Take the cap off the mouthpiece of the actuator.

Step 2. Hold the inhaler with the mouthpiece down. See Figure E.

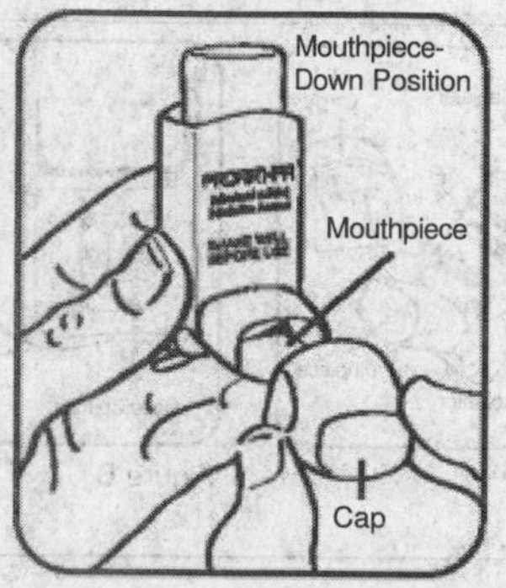

Figure E

Step 3. **Breathe out through your mouth** and push as much air from your lungs as you can. Put the mouthpiece in your mouth and close your lips around it. See Figure F.

Step 4. **Push the top of the canister all the way down while you breathe in deeply and slowly through your mouth.** See Figure F.

[See figure F at top of next column]

Step 5. Right after the spray comes out, take your finger off the canister. After you have breathed in all the way, take the inhaler out of your mouth and close your mouth.

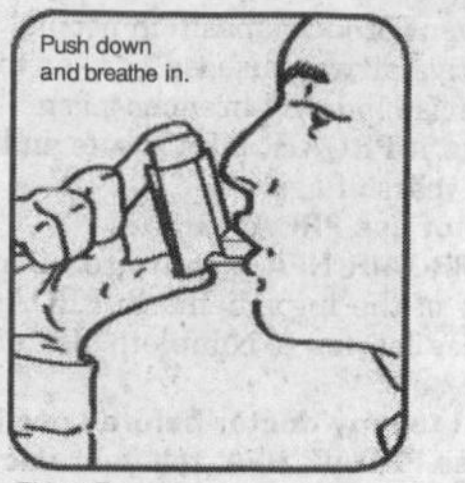

Push down and breathe in.

Figure F

Step 6. **Hold your breath as long as you can**, up to 10 seconds, then breathe normally.

If your doctor has told you to use more sprays, wait 1 minute and shake the inhaler again. Repeat Steps 2 through Step 6.

Step 7. Put the cap back on the mouthpiece after every time you use the inhaler. Make sure the cap snaps firmly into place.

Cleaning Your PROAIR HFA Device:

It is very important to keep the plastic actuator clean so the medicine will not build-up and block the spray. See Figure G and Figure H.

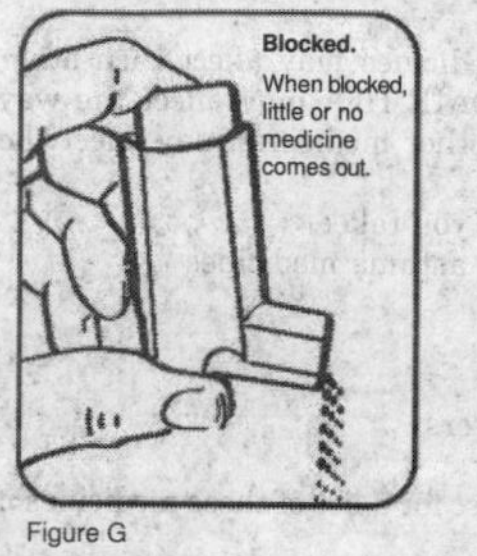

Figure G

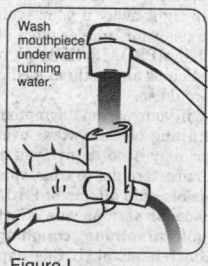

Not Blocked.

Figure H

- **Do not try to clean the metal canister or let it get wet.** The inhaler may stop spraying if it is not cleaned correctly.
- If you have more than 1 PROAIR HFA inhaler, wash each device at separate times to prevent putting the wrong canister together with the wrong plastic actuator. This way you can be sure you will always know the correct number of remaining doses of PROAIR HFA.
- **Wash the actuator** at least 1 time each week as follows:
  - Take the canister out of the actuator, and take the cap off the mouthpiece.
  - Hold the actuator under the faucet and run warm water through it for about 30 seconds. See Figure I.

Figure I

  - Turn the actuator upside down and run warm water through the mouthpiece for about 30 seconds. See Figure J.

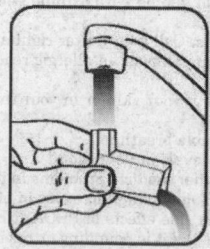

Figure J

  - Shake off as much water from the actuator as you can. Look into the mouthpiece to make sure any medicine build-up has been completely washed away. If there is any build-up, repeat the washing instructions.
  - Let the actuator air-dry completely, such as overnight. See Figure K.

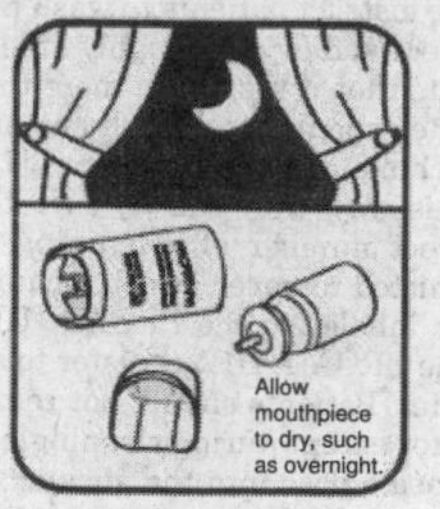

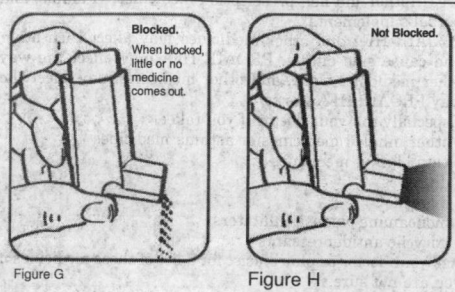

Figure K

  - When the actuator is dry, put the canister in the actuator and make sure it fits firmly. Shake the inhaler well and spray it twice into the air away from your face. Put the cap back on the mouthpiece.

If you need to use your inhaler before the actuator is completely dry:
- Shake as much water off the actuator as you can.
- Put the canister in the actuator and make sure it fits firmly.
- Shake the inhaler well and spray it twice into the air away from your face.
- Take your PROAIR HFA dose as prescribed.
- Follow the Cleaning Instructions above.

Replacing Your PROAIR HFA Device
- **When the dose counter on the actuator says the number 20,** the color of the numbers will change to red. The red numbers are to remind you to refill your prescription or ask your doctor for another prescription for PROAIR HFA. When the dose counter reaches **0**, the background color will change to solid red.
- **Throw the PROAIR HFA inhaler away** as soon as the dose counter says **0** or after the expiration date on the PROAIR HFA packaging, whichever comes first. You should not keep using the inhaler after 200 sprays even though the canister may not be completely empty. You cannot be sure you will receive any medicine after using 200 sprays.
- **Do not use the inhaler** after the expiration date on the PROAIR HFA packaging.

This Patient Information and Instructions for Use has been approved by the U.S. Food and Drug Administration.

Marketed by Teva Respiratory, LLC
Horsham, PA 19044
Manufactured by IVAX Pharmaceuticals Ireland
Waterford, Ireland
Revised 05/12
PE2557

Shown in Product Identification Guide, page 314

QVAR® 40 mcg ℞
(beclomethasone dipropionate HFA, 40 mcg)
INHALATION AEROSOL
For Oral Inhalation Only

QVAR® 80 mcg
(beclomethasone dipropionate HFA, 80 mcg)
INHALATION AEROSOL
For Oral Inhalation Only

DESCRIPTION

The active component of QVAR 40 mcg Inhalation Aerosol and QVAR 80 mcg Inhalation Aerosol is beclomethasone dipropionate, USP, an anti-inflammatory corticosteroid having the chemical name 9-chloro-11β,17,21-trihydroxy-16β-methylpregna-1,4-diene-3,20-dione 17,21-dipropionate. Beclomethasone dipropionate (BDP) is a diester of beclomethasone, a synthetic corticosteroid chemically related to dexamethasone. Beclomethasone differs from dexamethasone in having a chlorine at the 9-alpha carbon in place of a fluorine, and in having a 16 beta-methyl group instead of a 16 alpha-methyl group. Beclomethasone dipropionate is a white to creamy white, odorless powder with a molecular formula of $C_{28}H_{37}ClO_7$ and a molecular weight of 521.1. Its chemical structure is:

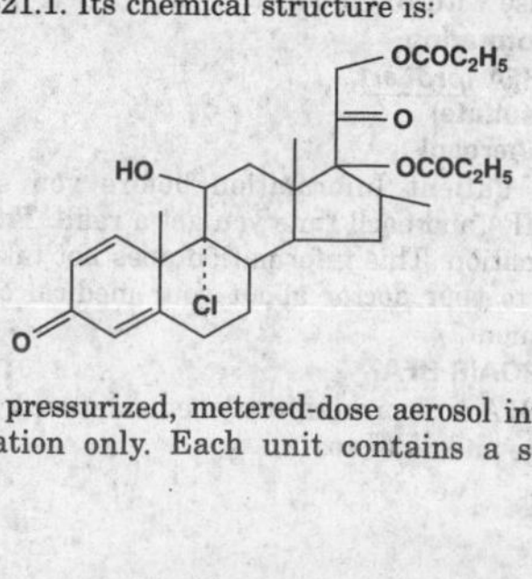

QVAR is a pressurized, metered-dose aerosol intended for oral inhalation only. Each unit contains a solution of beclomethasone dipropionate in propellant HFA-134a (1,1,1,2 tetrafluoroethane) and ethanol. QVAR 40 mcg delivers 40 mcg of beclomethasone dipropionate from the actuator and 50 mcg from the valve. QVAR 80 mcg delivers 80 mcg of beclomethasone dipropionate from the actuator and 100 mcg from the valve. Both products deliver 50 microliters (59 milligrams) of solution formulation from the valve with each actuation. Depending on the product size prescribed, the 40 mcg canisters provide either 100 inhalations or 120 inhalations and the 80 mcg canisters provide either 50 inhalations, 100 inhalations or 120 inhalations. QVAR should be "primed" or actuated twice prior to taking the first dose from a new canister, or when the inhaler has not been used for more than ten days. Avoid spraying in the eyes or face while priming QVAR. This product does not contain chlorofluorocarbons (CFCs).

CLINICAL PHARMACOLOGY

Airway inflammation is known to be an important component in the pathogenesis of asthma. Inflammation occurs in both large and small airways. Corticosteroids have multiple anti-inflammatory effects, inhibiting both inflammatory cells (e.g., mast cells, eosinophils, basophils, lymphocytes, macrophages, and neutrophils) and release of inflammatory mediators (e.g., histamine, eicosanoids, leukotrienes, and cytokines). These anti-inflammatory actions of corticosteroids such as beclomethasone dipropionate contribute to their efficacy in asthma.

Beclomethasone dipropionate is a prodrug that is rapidly activated by hydrolysis to the active monoester, 17 monopropionate (17-BMP). Beclomethasone 17 monopropionate has been shown *in vitro* to exhibit a binding affinity for the human glucocorticoid receptor which is approximately 13 times that of dexamethasone, 6 times that of triamcinolone acetonide, 1.5 times that of budesonide and 25 times that of beclomethasone dipropionate. The clinical significance of these findings is unknown.

Studies in patients with asthma have shown a favorable ratio between topical anti-inflammatory activity and systemic corticosteroid effects with recommended doses of QVAR.

Pharmacokinetics

Beclomethasone dipropionate (BDP) undergoes rapid and extensive conversion to beclomethasone-17-monopropionate (17-BMP) during absorption. The pharmacokinetics of 17-BMP has been studied in asthmatics given single doses.

Absorption

The mean peak plasma concentration (C_{max}) of BDP was 88 pg/ml at 0.5 hour after inhalation of 320 mcg using QVAR (4 actuations of the 80 mcg/actuation strength). The mean peak plasma concentration of the major and most active metabolite, 17-BMP, was 1419 pg/ml at 0.7 hour after inhalation of 320 mcg of QVAR. When the same nominal dose is provided by the two QVAR strengths (40 and 80 mcg/actuation), equivalent systemic pharmacokinetics can be expected. The C_{max} of 17-BMP increased dose proportionally in the dose range of 80 and 320 mcg.

Metabolism

Three major metabolites are formed via cytochrome P450-3A catalyzed biotransformation - beclomethasone-17-monopropionate (17-BMP), beclomethasone-21-monopropionate (21-BMP) and beclomethasone (BOH). Lung slices metabolize BDP rapidly to 17-BMP and more slowly to BOH. 17-BMP is the most active metabolite.

Distribution

The *in vitro* protein binding for 17-BMP was reported to be 94-96% over the concentration range of 1000 to 5000 pg/mL. Protein binding was constant over the concentration range evaluated. There is no evidence of tissue storage of BDP or its metabolites.

Elimination

The major route of elimination of inhaled BDP appears to be via hydrolysis. More than 90% of inhaled BDP is found as 17-BMP in the systemic circulation. The mean elimination half-life of 17-BMP is 2.8 hours. Irrespective of the route of administration (injection, oral or inhalation), BDP and its metabolites are mainly excreted in the feces. Less than 10% of the drug and its metabolites are excreted in the urine.

Special Populations

Formal pharmacokinetic studies using QVAR were not conducted in any special populations.

Pediatrics

The pharmacokinetics of 17-BMP, including dose and strength proportionalities, is similar in children and adults, although the exposure is highly variable. In 17 children (mean age 10 years), the C_{max} of 17-BMP was 787 pg/ml at 0.6 hour after inhalation of 160 mcg (four actuations of the 40 mcg/actuation strength of HFA beclomethasone dipropionate). The systemic exposure to 17-BMP from 160 mcg of HFA-BDP administered without a spacer was comparable to the systemic exposure to 17-BMP from 336 mcg CFC-BDP administered with a large volume spacer in 14 children (mean age 12 years). This implies that approximately twice the systemic exposure to 17-BMP would be expected for comparable mg doses of HFA-BDP without a spacer and CFC-BDP with a large volume spacer.

Pharmacodynamics

Improvement in asthma control following inhalation can occur within 24 hours of beginning treatment in some patients, although maximum benefit may not be achieved for 1 to 2 weeks, or longer. The effects of QVAR on the hypothalamic-pituitary-adrenal (HPA) axis were studied in 40 corticosteroid-naive patients. QVAR, at doses of 80, 160 or 320 mcg twice daily was compared with placebo and 336 mcg twice daily of beclomethasone dipropionate in a CFC propellant based formulation (CFC-BDP). Active treatment groups showed an expected dose-related reduction in 24-hour urinary-free cortisol (a sensitive marker of adrenal production of cortisol). Patients treated with the highest recommended dose of QVAR (320 mcg twice daily) had a 37.3% reduction in 24-hour urinary-free cortisol compared to a reduction of 47.3% produced by treatment with 336 mcg twice daily of CFC-BDP. There was a 12.2% reduction in 24-hour urinary-free cortisol seen in the group of patients that received 80 mcg twice daily of QVAR and a 24.6% reduction in the group of patients that received 160 mcg twice daily. An open label study of 354 asthma patients given QVAR at recommended doses for one year assessed the effect of QVAR treatment on the HPA axis (as measured by both morning and stimulated plasma cortisol). Less than 1% of patients treated for one year with QVAR had an abnormal response (peak less than 18 mcg/dL) to short-cosyntropin test.

CLINICAL TRIALS

Blinded, randomized, parallel, placebo-controlled and active-controlled clinical studies were conducted in 940 adult asthma patients to assess the efficacy and safety of QVAR in the treatment of asthma. Fixed doses ranging from 40 mcg to 160 mcg twice daily were compared to placebo, and doses ranging from 40 mcg to 320 mcg twice daily were compared with doses of 42 mcg to 336 mcg twice daily of an active CFC-BDP comparator. These studies provided information about appropriate dosing through a range of asthma severity. A blinded, randomized, parallel, placebo-controlled study was conducted in 353 pediatric patients (age 5 to 12 years) to assess the efficacy and safety of HFA beclomethasone dipropionate in the treatment of asthma. Fixed doses of 40 mcg and 80 mcg twice daily were compared with placebo in this study. In these adult and pediatric efficacy trials, at the doses studied, measures of pulmonary function [forced expiratory volume in 1 second (FEV_1) and morning peak expiratory flow (AM PEF)] and asthma symptoms were significantly improved with QVAR treatment when compared to placebo.

In controlled clinical trials with adult patients not adequately controlled with beta-agonist alone, QVAR was effective at improving asthma control at doses as low as 40 mcg twice daily (80 mcg/day). Comparable asthma control was achieved at lower daily doses of QVAR than with CFC-BDP. Treatment with increasing doses of both QVAR and CFC-BDP generally resulted in increased improvement in FEV_1. In this trial the improvement in FEV_1 across doses was greater for QVAR than for CFC-BDP, indicating a shift in the dose response curve for QVAR.

Patients Not Previously Receiving Corticosteroid Therapy

In a 6-week clinical trial, 270 steroid-naive patients with symptomatic asthma being treated with as-needed beta-agonist bronchodilators, were randomized to receive either 40 mcg twice daily of QVAR, 80 mcg twice daily of QVAR, or placebo. Both doses of QVAR were effective in improving asthma control with significantly greater improvements in FEV_1, AM PEF, and asthma symptoms than with placebo. Shown below is the change from baseline in AM PEF during this trial.

A 6-Week Clinical Trial in Patients with Mild to Moderate Asthma Not on Corticosteroid Therapy Prior to Study Entry: Mean Change in AM PEF

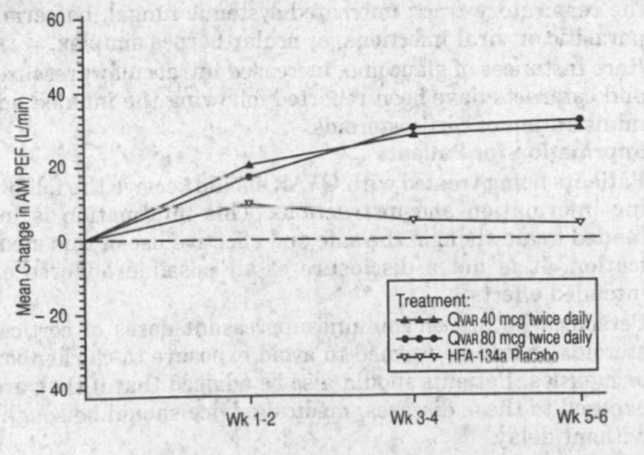

In a 6-week clinical trial, 256 patients with symptomatic asthma being treated with as-needed beta-agonist bronchodilators, were randomized to receive either 160 mcg twice-daily of QVAR (delivered as either 40 mcg/actuation or 80 mcg/actuation) or placebo. Treatment with QVAR significantly improved asthma control, as assessed by FEV_1, AM PEF, and asthma symptoms, when compared to treatment with placebo. Comparable improvement in AM PEF was seen for patients receiving 160 mcg twice-daily QVAR from the 40 mcg and 80 mcg strength products.

Patients Responsive to a Short Course of Oral Corticosteroids

In another clinical trial, 347 patients with symptomatic asthma, being treated with as-needed inhaled beta-agonist bronchodilators and, in some cases, inhaled corticosteroids, were given a 7 to 12 day course of oral corticosteroids and then randomized to receive either 320 mcg daily of QVAR, 672 mcg of CFC-BDP, or placebo. Patients treated with either QVAR or CFC-BDP had significantly better asthma control, as assessed by AM PEF, FEV_1 and asthma symptoms, and fewer study withdrawals due to asthma symptoms, than those treated with placebo over 12 weeks of treatment. A daily dose of 320 mcg QVAR administered in divided doses provided comparable control of AM PEF and FEV_1 as 672 mcg of CFC-BDP. Shown below are the mean AM PEF results from this trial.

A 12-Week Trial in Moderate Symptomatic Patients with Asthma Responding to Oral Corticosteroid Therapy: Mean AM PEF by Study Week

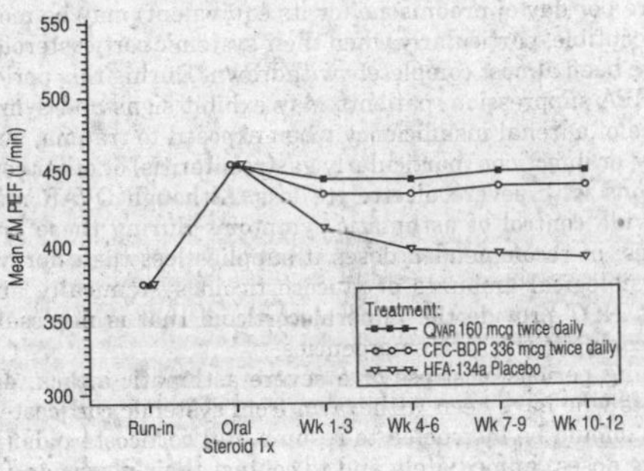

Patients Previously on Inhaled Corticosteroids

In a 6-week clinical trial, 323 patients, who exhibited a deterioration in asthma control during an inhaled corticosteroid washout period were randomized to daily treatment with either 40, 160, or 320 mcg twice-daily QVAR or 42, 168, or 336 mcg twice-daily CFC-BDP. Treatment with increasing doses of both QVAR and CFC-BDP resulted in increased improvement in FEV_1, $FEF_{25\text{-}75\%}$ (forced expiratory flow over 25-75% of the vital capacity), and asthma symptoms. Shown below is the change from baseline in FEV_1 as percent predicted after 6 weeks of treatment.

A 6-Week Dose Response Clinical Trial in Patients with Inhaled Corticosteroid Dependent Asthma: Mean Change in FEV_1 as Percent of Predicted

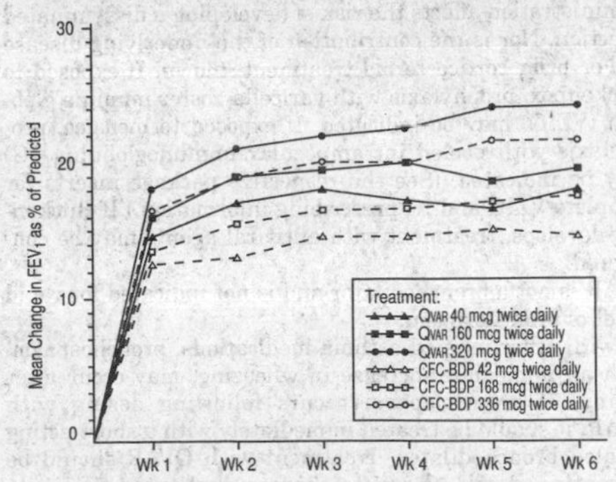

Patients Previously Maintained on Oral Corticosteroids

Clinical experience has shown that some patients with asthma who require oral corticosteroid therapy for control of symptoms can be partially or completely withdrawn from oral corticosteroids if therapy with beclomethasone dipropionate aerosol is substituted. Inhaled corticosteroids may not be effective for all patients with asthma or at all stages of the disease in a given patient.

Pediatric Experience

In one 12-week clinical trial, pediatric patients (age 5 to 12 years) with symptomatic asthma (N=353) being treated with as-needed beta-agonist bronchodilators were randomized to receive either 40 mcg or 80 mcg twice daily of HFA beclomethasone dipropionate or placebo. Both doses were effective in improving asthma control with significantly greater improvements in FEV_1 (9% and 10% predicted change from baseline at week 12 in FEV_1 percent predicted, respectively) than with placebo (4% predicted change).

INDICATIONS AND USAGE

QVAR is indicated in the maintenance treatment of asthma as prophylactic therapy in patients 5 years of age and older. QVAR is also indicated for asthma patients who require systemic corticosteroid administration, where adding QVAR may reduce or eliminate the need for the systemic corticosteroids.

Beclomethasone dipropionate is NOT indicated for the relief of acute bronchospasm.

CONTRAINDICATIONS

QVAR is contraindicated in the primary treatment of status asthmaticus or other acute episodes of asthma where intensive measures are required. Hypersensitivity to any of the ingredients of this preparation contraindicates its use.

WARNINGS

Particular care is needed in patients who are transferred from systemically active corticosteroids to QVAR because deaths due to adrenal insufficiency have occurred in asthmatic patients during and after transfer from systemic corticosteroids to less systemically available inhaled corticosteroids. After withdrawal from systemic corticosteroids, a number of months are required for recovery of hypothalamic-pituitary-adrenal (HPA) function.

Patients who have been previously maintained on 20 mg or more per day of prednisone (or its equivalent) may be most susceptible, particularly when their systemic corticosteroids have been almost completely withdrawn. During this period of HPA suppression, patients may exhibit signs and symptoms of adrenal insufficiency when exposed to trauma, surgery, or infections (particularly gastroenteritis) or other conditions with severe electrolyte loss. Although QVAR may provide control of asthmatic symptoms during these episodes, in recommended doses it supplies less than normal physiological amounts of glucocorticoid systemically and does NOT provide the mineralocorticoid that is necessary for coping with these emergencies.

During periods of stress or a severe asthmatic attack, patients who have been withdrawn from systemic corticosteroids should be instructed to resume oral corticosteroids (in large doses) immediately and to contact their physician for further instruction. These patients should also be instructed to carry a warning card indicating that they may need supplementary systemic steroids during periods of stress or a severe asthma attack.

Transfer of patients from systemic steroid therapy to QVAR may unmask allergic conditions previously suppressed by the systemic steroid therapy, e.g., rhinitis, conjunctivitis, and eczema.

Persons who are on drugs which suppress the immune system are more susceptible to infections than healthy individuals. Chickenpox and measles, for example, can have a more serious or even fatal course in non-immune children or adults on corticosteroids. In such children or adults who have not had these diseases or been properly immunized, particular care should be taken to avoid exposure. It is not known how the dose, route and duration of corticosteroid administration affects the risk of developing a disseminated infection. Nor is the contribution of the underlying disease and/or prior corticosteroid treatment known. If exposed to chickenpox, prophylaxis with varicella-zoster immune globulin (VZIG) may be indicated. If exposed to measles, prophylaxis with pooled intramuscular immunoglobulin (IG) may be indicated. (See the respective package inserts for complete VZIG and IG prescribing information.) If chickenpox develops, treatment with antiviral agents may be considered.

QVAR is not a bronchodilator and is not indicated for rapid relief of bronchospasm.

As with other inhaled asthma medications, bronchospasm, with an immediate increase in wheezing, may occur after dosing. If bronchospasm occurs following dosing with QVAR, it should be treated immediately with a short-acting inhaled bronchodilator. Treatment with QVAR should be discontinued and alternate therapy instituted. Patients should be instructed to contact their physician immediately when episodes of asthma, which are not responsive to bronchodilators, occur during the course of treatment with QVAR. During such episodes, patients may require therapy with oral corticosteroids.

PRECAUTIONS

General

During withdrawal from oral corticosteroids, some patients may experience symptoms of systemically active corticosteroid withdrawal, e.g., joint and/or muscular pain, lassitude and depression, despite maintenance or even improvement of respiratory function. Although suppression of HPA function below the clinical normal range did not occur with doses of QVAR up to and including 640 mcg/day, a dose-dependent reduction of adrenal cortisol production was observed. Since inhaled beclomethasone dipropionate is absorbed into the circulation and can be systemically active, HPA-axis suppression by QVAR could occur when recommended doses are exceeded or in particularly sensitive individuals. Since individual sensitivity to effects on cortisol production exist, physicians should consider this information when prescribing QVAR. Because of the possibility of systemic absorption of inhaled corticosteroids, patients treated with these drugs should be observed carefully for any evidence of systemic corticosteroid effect. Particular care should be taken in observing patients postoperatively or during periods of stress for evidence of inadequate adrenal response.

TABLE 1

	Wait time, seconds	Mean medication delivery through AeroChamber, mcg/actuation *	Body Weight 50th percentile, kg †	Medication delivered per dose, mcg/kg ‡,§
Age 6 months, Flow rate 4.8 L/min	0	11.5	7.6	1.2
Age 2 years, Flow rate 8.2 L/min	0	14.1	13.5	0.83
Age 2 years, Flow rate 8.2 L/min	5	5.4	13.5	0.32
Age 2 years, Flow rate 8.2 L/min	10	3.9	13.5	0.23
Age 5 years, Flow rate 11.0 L/min	0	17.5	18	0.78

* Summary Report; Pediatric Dose Characterization of QVAR with Spacer; 3M Pharmaceutical Development, July 21, 2004.

† CDC Growth charts, developed by the National Center for Health Statistics in collaboration with the National Center for Chronic Disease Prevention and Health Promotion (2000).

‡ Includes an estimated 20% loss in the masks

§ QVAR 40mcg in an average adult without using a spacer delivers approximately 0.4 mcg/kg, or bid, 0.8 mcg/kg/day.

It is possible that systemic corticosteroid effects, such as hypercorticism and adrenal suppression, may appear in a small number of patients, particularly at higher doses. If such changes occur, QVAR should be reduced slowly, consistent with accepted procedures for management of asthma symptoms and for tapering of systemic steroids.

A 12-month, randomized, controlled clinical trial evaluated the effects of HFA beclomethasone dipropionate without spacer versus CFC beclomethasone dipropionate with large volume spacer on growth in children age 5 to 11. A total of 520 patients were enrolled, of whom 394 received HFA-BDP (100 to 400 mcg/day ex-valve) and 126 received CFC-BDP (200 to 800 mcg/day ex-valve). Similar control of asthma was noted in each treatment arm. When comparing results at month 12 to baseline, the mean growth velocity in children treated with HFA-BDP was approximately 0.5 cm/year less than that noted with children treated with CFC-BDP via large volume spacer.

A reduction in growth velocity in growing children may occur as a result of inadequate control of chronic diseases such as asthma or from use of corticosteroids for treatment. Physicians should closely follow the growth of all pediatric patients taking corticosteroids by any route and weigh the benefits of corticosteroid therapy and asthma control against the possibility of growth suppression.

The long-term and systemic effects of QVAR in humans are still not fully known. In particular, the effects resulting from chronic use of the agent on developmental or immunologic processes in the mouth, pharynx, trachea, and lung are unknown.

Inhaled corticosteroids should be used with caution, if at all, in patients with active or quiescent tuberculosis infection of the respiratory tract; untreated systemic fungal, bacterial, parasitic or viral infections; or ocular herpes simplex.

Rare instances of glaucoma, increased intraocular pressure, and cataracts have been reported following the inhaled administration of corticosteroids.

Information for Patients

Patients being treated with QVAR should receive the following information and instructions. This information is intended to aid them in the safe and effective use of this medication. It is not a disclosure of all possible adverse or intended effects.

Persons who are on immunosuppressant doses of corticosteroids should be warned to avoid exposure to chickenpox or measles. Patients should also be advised that if they are exposed to these diseases, medical advice should be sought without delay.

Patients should use QVAR at regular intervals as directed. Results of clinical trials indicated significant improvements may occur within the first 24 hours of treatment in some patients; however, the full benefit may not be achieved until treatment has been administered for 1 to 2 weeks, or longer. The patient should not increase the prescribed dosage but should contact their physician if symptoms do not improve or if the condition worsens.

Patients should be advised that QVAR is not intended for use in the treatment of acute asthma. The patient should be instructed to contact their physician immediately if there is any deterioration of their asthma.

Patients should be instructed on the proper use of their inhaler. Patients may wish to rinse their mouth after QVAR use. The patient should also be advised that QVAR may have a different taste and inhalation sensation than that of an inhaler containing CFC propellant.

QVAR use should not be stopped abruptly. The patient should contact their physician immediately if use of QVAR is discontinued.

For the proper use of QVAR, the patient should read and carefully follow the accompanying Patient's Instructions.

Carcinogenesis, Mutagenesis, Impairment of Fertility

The carcinogenicity of beclomethasone dipropionate was evaluated in rats which were exposed for a total of 95 weeks, 13 weeks at inhalation doses up to 0.4 mg/kg/day and the remaining 82 weeks at combined oral and inhalation doses up to 2.4 mg/kg/day. There was no evidence of carcinogenicity in this study at the highest dose, which is approximately 30 and 55 times the maximum recommended daily inhalation dose in adults and children, respectively, on a mg/m^2 basis.

Beclomethasone dipropionate did not induce gene mutation in the bacterial cells or mammalian Chinese Hamster ovary (CHO) cells *in vitro*. No significant clastogenic effect was seen in cultured CHO cells *in vitro* or in the mouse micronucleus test *in vivo*.

In rats, beclomethasone dipropionate caused decreased conception rates at an oral dose of 16 mg/kg/day (approximately 200 times the maximum recommended daily inhalation dose in adults on a mg/m^2 basis). Impairment of fertility, as evidence by inhibition of the estrous cycle in dogs, was observed following treatment by the oral route at a dose of 0.5 mg/kg/day (approximately 20 times the maximum recommended daily inhalation dose in adults on a mg/m^2 basis). No inhibition of the estrous cycle in dogs was seen following 12 months of exposure to beclomethasone dipropionate by the Inhalation route at an estimated daily dose of 0.33 mg/kg (approximately 15 times the maximum recommended daily inhalation dose in adults on a mg/m^2 basis).

Pregnancy

Teratogenic Effects

Pregnancy Category C

Like other corticosteroids, parenteral (subcutaneous) beclomethasone dipropionate was teratogenic and embryocidal in the mouse and rabbit when given at a dose of 0.1 mg/kg/day in mice or at a dose of 0.025 mg/kg/day in rabbits. These doses in mice and rabbits were approximately one-half the maximum recommended daily inhalation dose in adults on a mg/m^2 basis. No teratogenicity or embryocidal effects were seen in rats when exposed to an inhalation dose of 15 mg/kg/day (approximately 190 times the maximum recommended daily inhalation dose in adults on a mg/m^2 basis). There are no adequate and well-controlled studies in pregnant women. Beclomethasone dipropionate should be used during pregnancy only if the potential benefit justifies the potential risk to the fetus.

Non-teratogenic Effects

Findings of drug-related adrenal toxicity in fetuses following administration of beclomethasone dipropionate to rats suggest that infants born of mothers receiving substantial doses of QVAR during pregnancy should be observed for adrenal suppression.

Nursing Mothers

Corticosteroids are secreted in human milk. Because of the potential for serious adverse reactions in nursing infants from QVAR, a decision should be made whether to discontinue nursing or to discontinue the drug, taking into account the importance of the drug to the mother.

Pediatric Use

Eight-hundred and thirty-four children between the ages of 5 and 12 were treated with HFA beclomethasone dipropionate (HFA BDP) in clinical trials. The safety and effectiveness of QVAR in children below 5 years of age have not been established.

Use of QVAR with a spacer device in children less than 5 years of age is not recommended. *In vitro* dose characterization studies were performed with QVAR 40 mcg/actuation with the Optichamber and AeroChamber Plus® spacer utilizing inspiratory flows representative of children under 5 years old. These studies indicated that the amount of medication delivered through the spacing device decreased rapidly with increasing wait times of 5 to 10 seconds as shown in Table 1. If QVAR is used with a spacer device, it is important to inhale immediately.

Based on the average inspiratory flow rates generated by children 6 months to 5 years old, the projected daily dose derived from QVAR 40 mcg at one puff per day at various wait times is depicted in the table below:

[See table 1 at top of previous page]

Oral inhaled corticosteroids have been shown to cause a reduction in growth velocity in children and teenagers with extended use. If a child or teenager on any corticosteroid appears to have growth suppression, the possibility that they are particularly sensitive to this effect of corticosteroids should be considered (see PRECAUTIONS, General).

Geriatric Use

Clinical studies of QVAR did not include sufficient numbers of subjects aged 65 and over to determine whether they respond differently from younger subjects. Other reported clinical experience has not identified differences in responses between the elderly and younger patients. In general, dose selection for an elderly patient should be cautious, usually starting at the low end of the dosing range, reflecting the greater frequency of decreased hepatic, renal, or cardiac function, and of concomitant disease or other drug therapy.

ADVERSE REACTIONS

The following reporting rates of common adverse experiences are based upon 4 clinical trials in which 1196 Patients (671 female and 525 male adults previously treated with as-needed bronchodilators and/or inhaled corticosteroids) were treated with QVAR (doses of 40, 80, 160, or 320 mcg twice daily) or CFC-BDP (doses of 42, 168, or 336 mcg twice daily) or placebo. The table below includes all events reported by patients taking QVAR (whether considered drug related or not) that occurred at a rate over 3% for either QVAR or CFC-BDP. In considering these data, difference in average duration of exposure and clinical trial design should be taken into account.

[See table above]

Adverse Events Reported by at Least 3% of the Patients for Either QVAR or CFC-BDP by Treatment and Daily Dose

Adverse Events		QVAR				CFC-BDP			
	Placebo (N=289) %	Total (N=624) %	80-160 mcg (N=233) %	320 mcg (N=335) %	640 mcg (N=56) %	Total (N=283) %	84 mcg (N=59) %	336 mcg (N=55) %	672 mcg (N=169) %
HEADACHE	9	12	15	8	25	15	14	11	17
PHARYNGITIS	4	8	6	5	27	10	12	9	10
UPPER RESP TRACT INFECTION	11	9	7	11	5	12	3	9	17
RHINITIS	9	6	8	3	7	11	15	9	10
INCREASED ASTHMA SYMPTOMS	18	3	2	4	0	8	14	5	7
ORAL SYMPTOMS INHALATION ROUTE	2	3	3	3	2	6	7	5	5
SINUSITIS	2	3	3	3	0	4	7	2	4
PAIN	<1	2	1	2	5	3	3	5	2
BACK PAIN	1	1	2	<1	4	4	2	4	4
NAUSEA	0	1	<1	1	2	3	5	5	1
DYSPHONIA	2	<1	1	0	4	4	0	0	6

Other adverse events that occurred in these clinical trials using QVAR with an incidence of 1% to 3% and which occurred at a greater incidence than placebo were: dysphonia, dysmenorrhea and coughing.

No patients treated with QVAR in the clinical development program developed symptomatic oropharyngeal candidiasis. If such an infection develops, treatment with appropriate antifungal therapy or discontinuance of treatment with QVAR may be required.

Pediatric Studies

In two 12-week placebo-controlled studies in steroid naive pediatric patients 5 to 12 years of age, no clinically relevant differences were found in the pattern, severity, or frequency of adverse events compared with those reported in adults, with the exception of conditions which are more prevalent in a pediatric population generally.

Adverse Event Reports from Other Sources

Rare cases of immediate and delayed hypersensitivity reactions, including urticaria, angioedema, rash, and bronchospasm, have been reported following the oral and intranasal inhalation of beclomethasone dipropionate.

During postmarketing experience, psychiatric events and behavioral changes such as aggression, depression, sleep disorders, psychomotor hyperactivity, and suicidal ideation have been reported (primarily in children). Because these events are reported voluntarily from a population of uncertain size, it is not always possible to reliably estimate their frequency or establish a causal relationship to drug exposure.

OVERDOSAGE

There were no deaths over 15 days following the oral administration of a single dose of 3000 mg/kg in mice, 2000 mg/kg in rats, and 1000 mg/kg in rabbits. The doses in mice, rats, and rabbits were 19,000, 25,000, and 25,000 times, respectively, the maximum recommended daily inhalation in adults or 36,000, 48,000, and 48,000 times, respectively the maximum recommended daily inhalation dose in children on a mg/m^2 basis.

DOSAGE AND ADMINISTRATION

Patients should prime QVAR by actuating into the air twice before using for the first time or if QVAR has not been used for over ten days. Avoid spraying in the eyes or face when priming QVAR. QVAR is a solution aerosol, which does not require shaking. Consistent dose delivery is achieved, whether using the 40 or 80 mcg strengths, due to proportionality of the 2 products (i.e., 2 actuations of 40 mcg strength should provide a dose comparable to 1 actuation of the 80 mcg strength).

QVAR should be administered by the oral inhaled route in patients 5 years of age and older. Use of QVAR with a spacer device in children less than 5 years of age is not recommended (see PRECAUTIONS, Pediatric Use). The onset and degree of symptom relief will vary in individual patients. Improvement in asthma symptoms should be expected within the first or second week of starting treatment, but maximum benefit should not be expected until 3 to 4 weeks of therapy. For patients who do not respond adequately to the starting dose after 3 to 4 weeks of therapy, higher doses may provide additional asthma control. The safety and efficacy of QVAR when administered in excess of recommended doses has not been established.

Table 2: Recommended Dosing for Adults and Adolescents

Patient's Previous Therapy	Recommended Starting Dose	Highest Recommended Dose
Bronchodilators Alone	40 to 80 mcg twice daily	320 mcg twice daily
Inhaled Corticosteroids	40 to 160 mcg twice daily	320 mcg twice daily

Table 3: Recommended Dosing for Children 5 to 11 Years

Patient's Previous Therapy	Recommended Starting Dose	Highest Recommended Dose
Bronchodilators Alone	40 mcg twice daily	80 mcg twice daily
Inhaled Corticosteroids	40 mcg twice daily	80 mcg twice daily

As with any inhaled corticosteroid, physicians are advised to titrate the dose of QVAR downward over time to the lowest level that maintains proper asthma control. This is particularly important in children since a controlled study has shown that QVAR has the potential to affect growth in children. Patients should be instructed on the proper use of their inhaler.

Patients Not Receiving Systemic Corticosteroids

Patients who require maintenance therapy of their asthma may benefit from treatment with QVAR at the doses recommended above. In patients who respond to QVAR, improvement in pulmonary function is usually apparent within 1 to 4 weeks after the start of therapy. Once the desired effect is achieved, consideration should be given to tapering to the lowest effective dose.

Patients Maintained on Systemic Corticosteroids

QVAR may be effective in the management of asthmatics maintained on systemic corticosteroids and may permit replacement or significant reduction in the dosage of systemic corticosteroids.

The patient's asthma should be reasonably stable before treatment with QVAR is started. Initially, QVAR should be used concurrently with the patient's usual maintenance dose of systemic corticosteroids. After approximately one week, gradual withdrawal of the systemic corticosteroids is started by reducing the daily or alternate daily dose. Reductions may be made after an interval of one or two weeks, depending on the response of the patient. A slow rate of withdrawal is strongly recommended. Generally these decrements should not exceed 2.5 mg of prednisone or its equivalent. During withdrawal, some patients may experience symptoms of systemic corticosteroid withdrawal, e.g. joint and/or muscular pain, lassitude and depression, despite maintenance or even improvement in pulmonary function. Such patients should be encouraged to continue with the inhaler but should be monitored for objective signs of adrenal insufficiency. If evidence of adrenal insufficiency occurs, the systemic corticosteroid doses should be increased temporarily and thereafter withdrawal should continue more slowly. During periods of stress or a severe asthma attack, transfer patients may require supplementary treatment with systemic corticosteroids.

DIRECTIONS FOR USE

Illustrated Patient's Instructions for proper use accompany each package of QVAR.

HOW SUPPLIED

QVAR is supplied in 2 strengths:

QVAR 40 mcg is supplied either in a 7.3 g canister containing 100 actuations with a beige plastic actuator and gray dust cap, and Patient's Instructions; box of one; 100 Actuations – NDC 59310-175-40 or in an 8.7 g canister containing 120 actuations with a beige plastic actuator and gray dust cap, and Patient's Instructions; box of one; 120 Actuations – NDC 59310-202-40

QVAR 80 mcg is supplied either in a 4.2 g canister, for Institutional Use, containing 50 actuations with a dark mauve plastic actuator and a gray dust cap, and Patient's Instructions; box of one; 50 Actuations – NDC 59310-204-50, a 7.3 g canister containing 100 actuations with a dark mauve plastic actuator and gray dust cap, and Patient's Instructions; box of one; 100 Actuations – NDC 59310-177-80 or in an 8.7 g canister containing 120 actuations with a dark mauve plastic actuator and gray dust cap, and Patient's Instructions; box of one; 120 Actuations – NDC 59310-204-80

The correct amount of medication in each inhalation cannot be assured after 50 actuations from the 4.2 g canister, 100 actuations from the 7.3 g canister or 120 actuations from the 8.7 g canister even though the canister is not completely empty. The canister should be discarded when the labeled number of actuations have been used.

Store QVAR Inhalation Aerosol when not being used, so that the product rests on the concave end of the canister with the plastic actuator on top.

Store at 25°C (77°F).

Excursions between 15° and 30°C (59° and 86°F) are permitted (see USP). For optimal results, the canister should be at room temperature when used. QVAR Inhalation Aerosol canister should only be used with the QVAR Inhalation Aerosol actuator and the actuator should not be used with any other inhalation drug product.

CONTENTS UNDER PRESSURE

Do not puncture. Do not use or store near heat or open flame. Exposure to temperatures above 49°C (120°F) may cause bursting. Never throw container into fire or incinerator.

Keep out of reach of children.

Rx only

Mktd by:
Teva Respiratory, LLC– Horsham, PA 19044
Developed and Manufactured by:
3M Drug Delivery Systems
Northridge, CA 91324
OR
3M Health Care, Ltd.
Loughborough, UK
July 2012

657100
QVAR is a registered trademark of IVAX LLC, a member of the TEVA Group.
Rev. 07/12
OptiChamber is a registered trademark of Respironics Healthscan, Inc. and AeroChamber Plus is a registered trademark of Trudell Medical International Trudell Partnership Holdings Limited and Packard Medical Supply Centre Ltd.

PATIENT'S INSTRUCTIONS

QVAR®
(beclomethasone dipropionate HFA)
INHALATION AEROSOL

Attention Pharmacist: Detach "PATIENT'S INSTRUCTIONS for Use" from package insert and dispense with the product.

PATIENT'S INSTRUCTIONS

It is important that you read these instructions before using QVAR.

Correct and regular use of the inhaler will prevent or lessen the severity of asthma attacks.

1. Remove the plastic cap (see Figure 1) and be sure there are no foreign objects in the mouthpiece.

Figure 1

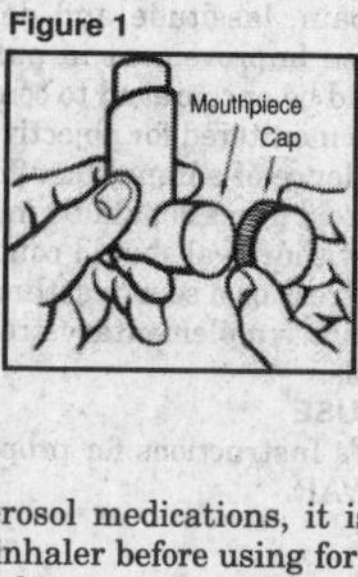

2. As with all aerosol medications, it is recommended to prime the QVAR inhaler before using for the very first time after purchase, and in cases where the inhaler has not been used for more than 10 days. Prime by releasing 2 actuations into the air, away from your eyes and face. Be sure the canister is firmly seated in the plastic mouthpiece adapter before each use.

3. BREATHE OUT AS FULLY AS YOU COMFORTABLY CAN. Hold the inhaler as shown in Figure 2. Close your lips around the mouthpiece, keeping your tongue below it.

Figure 2

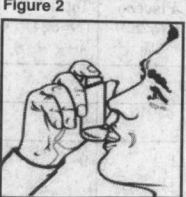

4. WHILE BREATHING IN DEEPLY AND SLOWLY, PRESS DOWN ON THE CAN WITH YOUR FINGER. When you have finished breathing in, hold your breath as long as you comfortably can (i.e., 5 to 10 seconds).

5. TAKE YOUR FINGER OFF THE CAN and remove the inhaler from your mouth. Breathe out gently.

6. If your physician has told you to take more than one inhalation per treatment repeat steps 3 through 5.

7. You should rinse your mouth with water after treatment.

8. For normal hygiene, the mouthpiece of your inhaler should be cleaned weekly with a clean, dry tissue or cloth. DO NOT WASH OR PUT ANY PART OF YOUR INHALER IN WATER.

9. DISCARD THE CANISTER AFTER the date calculated by your physician or pharmacist. The correct amount of medication in each inhalation cannot be assured after 50 actuations from the 4.2 g canister, 100 actuations from the 7.3 g canister or 120 actuations from the 8.7 g canister even though the canister is not completely empty. The canister should be discarded when the labeled number of actuations have been used. Before the discard date you should consult your physician to determine whether a refill is needed. It is advisable to keep track of the number of doses taken from the canister to better predict when a refill is necessary. Just as you should not take extra doses without consulting your physician, you also should not stop taking QVAR without consulting your physician.

IMPORTANT: QVAR is preventive therapy for asthma and must be used regularly and at the times your physician has prescribed.

DO NOT CONFUSE QVAR WITH OTHER ASTHMA MEDICATION. QVAR WILL NOT PROVIDE IMMEDIATE RELIEF IF YOU ARE HAVING AN ASTHMA ATTACK.

Your physician will decide whether other medication is needed should you require immediate relief. If you also use another medicine by inhalation, you should consult your physician for instructions on when to use it in relation to using QVAR. If this is the first time you will be using QVAR, it may take from 1 to 4 weeks before you feel the full benefits.

QVAR Inhalation Aerosol canister should only be used with the QVAR Inhalation Aerosol mouthpiece and the mouthpiece should not be used with any other inhalation drug product.

DOSAGE

Use only as directed by your physician.

CONTENTS UNDER PRESSURE

Do not puncture. Do not use or store near heat or open flame. Exposure to temperatures above 49°C (120°F) may cause bursting. Never throw container into fire or incinerator.

Keep out of reach of children.

Avoid spraying in eyes.

Store at 25°C (77°F). For optimal results, the canister should be at room temperature when used. Store QVAR Inhalation Aerosol when not being used, so that the product rests on the concave end of the canister with the plastic actuator on top.

Mktd by:
Teva Respiratory, LLC
Horsham, PA 19044
Developed and Manufactured by:
3M Drug Delivery Systems
Northridge, CA 91324
OR
3M Health Care, Ltd.
Loughborough, UK

QVAR is a registered trademark of IVAX LLC, a member of the TEVA Group.
657100
Rev. 07/12
QVA-40318

Teva Select Brands
Division of Teva Pharmaceuticals USA
41 MOORES ROAD
FRAZER, PA 19355

For all Inquiries Call:
800-292-4283

ADIPEX-P®

(phentermine hydrochloride USP)
for oral use CIV Ⓒ

HIGHLIGHTS OF PRESCRIBING INFORMATION
These highlights do not include all the information needed to use ADIPEX-P® safely and effectively. See full prescribing information for ADIPEX-P®.
ADIPEX-P® (phentermine hydrochloride USP) for oral use CIV
Initial U.S. Approval: 1959

INDICATIONS AND USAGE

ADIPEX-P® is a sympathomimetic amine anorectic indicated as a short-term adjunct (a few weeks) in a regimen of weight reduction based on exercise, behavioral modification and caloric restriction in the management of exogenous obesity for patients with an initial body mass index ≥ 30 kg/m^2, or ≥ 27 kg/m^2 in the presence of other risk factors (e.g., controlled hypertension, diabetes, hyperlipidemia). (1)

The limited usefulness of agents of this class, including ADIPEX-P®, should be measured against possible risk factors inherent in their use. (1)

DOSAGE AND ADMINISTRATION

- Dosage should be individualized to obtain an adequate response with the lowest effective dose. (2)
- Late evening administration should be avoided (risk of insomnia). (2)
- ADIPEX-P® can be taken with or without food. (12.3)

DOSAGE FORMS AND STRENGTHS

- Capsules containing 37.5 mg phentermine hydrochloride. (3)
- Tablets containing 37.5 mg phentermine hydrochloride. (3)

CONTRAINDICATIONS

- History of cardiovascular disease (e.g., coronary artery disease, stroke, arrhythmias, congestive heart failure, uncontrolled hypertension) (4)
- During or within 14 days following the administration of monoamine oxidase inhibitors (4)
- Hyperthyroidism (4)
- Glaucoma (4)
- Agitated states (4)
- History of drug abuse (4)
- Pregnancy (4, 8.1)
- Nursing (4, 8.3)
- Known hypersensitivity, or idiosyncrasy to the sympathomimetic amines (4)

WARNINGS AND PRECAUTIONS

- Coadministration with other drugs for weight loss is not recommended (safety and efficacy of combination not established). (5.1)
- Rare cases of primary pulmonary hypertension have been reported. ADIPEX-P® should be discontinued in case of new, unexplained symptoms of dyspnea, angina pectoris, syncope or lower extremity edema. (5.2)
- Rare cases of serious regurgitant cardiac valvular disease have been reported. (5.3)
- Tolerance to the anorectic effect usually develops within a few weeks. If this occurs, ADIPEX-P® should be discontinued. The recommended dose should not be exceeded. (5.4)
- ADIPEX-P® may impair the ability of the patient to engage in potentially hazardous activities such as operating machinery or driving a motor vehicle. (5.5)
- Risk of abuse and dependence. The least amount feasible should be prescribed or dispensed at one time in order to minimize the possibility of overdosage. (5.6)
- Concomitant alcohol use may result in an adverse drug reaction. (5.7)
- Use caution in patients with even mild hypertension (risk of increase in blood pressure). (5.8)
- A reduction in dose of insulin or oral hypoglycemic medication may be required in some patients. (5.9)

ADVERSE REACTIONS

Adverse events have been reported in the cardiovascular, central nervous, gastrointestinal, allergic, and endocrine systems. (6)

To report SUSPECTED ADVERSE REACTIONS, contact TEVA USA, PHARMACOVIGILANCE at 1-866-832-8537 or drug.safety@tevapharm.com; or FDA at 1-800-FDA-1088 or www.fda.gov/medwatch.

DRUG INTERACTIONS

- Monoamine oxidase inhibitors: Risk of hypertensive crisis. (4, 7.1)
- Alcohol: Consider potential interaction (7.2)
- Insulin and oral hypoglycemics: Requirements may be altered. (7.3)
- Adrenergic neuron blocking drugs: Hypotensive effect may be decreased by ADIPEX-P®. (7.4)

USE IN SPECIFIC POPULATIONS

- Nursing mothers: Discontinue drug or nursing taking into consideration importance of drug to mother. (4, 8.3)
- Pediatric use: Safety and effectiveness not established. (8.4)
- Geriatric use: Due to substantial renal excretion, use with caution. (8.5)
- Use caution when administering ADIPEX-P® to patients with renal impairment (8.6)

See 17 for PATIENT COUNSELING INFORMATION

Revised: 01/2013

FULL PRESCRIBING INFORMATION: CONTENTS*

*** Sections or subsections omitted from the full prescribing information are not listed**

FULL PRESCRIBING INFORMATION

1 INDICATIONS AND USAGE

ADIPEX-P® is indicated as a short-term (a few weeks) adjunct in a regimen of weight reduction based on exercise, behavioral modification and caloric restriction in the management of exogenous obesity for patients with an initial body mass index ≥ 30 kg/m^2, or ≥ 27 kg/m^2 in the presence of other risk factors (e.g., controlled hypertension, diabetes, hyperlipidemia).

Below is a chart of body mass index (BMI) based on various heights and weights.

BMI is calculated by taking the patient's weight, in kilograms (kg), divided by the patient's height, in meters (m), squared. Metric conversions are as follows: pounds ÷ 2.2 = kg; inches × 0.0254 = meters.

BODY MASS INDEX (BMI), kg/m^2

Height (feet, inches)

Weight (pounds)	5'0"	5'3"	5'6"	5'9"	6'0"	6'3"
140	27	25	23	21	19	18
150	29	27	24	22	20	19
160	31	28	26	24	22	20
170	33	30	28	25	23	21
180	35	32	29	27	25	23
190	37	34	31	28	26	24
200	39	36	32	30	27	25
210	41	37	34	31	29	26
220	43	39	36	33	30	28
230	45	41	37	34	31	29
240	47	43	39	36	33	30
250	49	44	40	37	34	31

The limited usefulness of agents of this class, including ADIPEX-P®, [*see Clinical Pharmacology (12.1, 12.2)*] should be measured against possible risk factors inherent in their use such as those described below.

2 DOSAGE AND ADMINISTRATION

Exogenous Obesity

Dosage should be individualized to obtain an adequate response with the lowest effective dose.

The usual adult dose is one capsule (37.5 mg) daily as prescribed by the physician, administered before breakfast or 1 to 2 hours after breakfast for appetite control.

The usual adult dose is one tablet (37.5 mg) daily, as prescribed by the physician, administered before breakfast or 1 to 2 hours after breakfast. The dosage may be adjusted to the patient's need. For some patients, half tablet (18.75 mg) daily may be adequate, while in some cases it may be desirable to give half tablets (18.75 mg) two times a day.

ADIPEX-P® is not recommended for use in pediatric patients < 16 years of age.

Late evening medication should be avoided because of the possibility of resulting insomnia.

3 DOSAGE FORMS AND STRENGTHS

Capsules containing 37.5 mg phentermine hydrochloride (equivalent to 30 mg phentermine base).

Tablets containing 37.5 mg phentermine hydrochloride (equivalent to 30 mg phentermine base).

4 CONTRAINDICATIONS

- History of cardiovascular disease (e.g., coronary artery disease, stroke, arrhythmias, congestive heart failure, uncontrolled hypertension)
- During or within 14 days following the administration of monoamine oxidase inhibitors
- Hyperthyroidism
- Glaucoma
- Agitated states
- History of drug abuse
- Pregnancy [*see Use in Specific Populations (8.1)*]
- Nursing [*see Use in Specific Populations (8.3)*]
- Known hypersensitivity, or idiosyncrasy to the sympathomimetic amines

5 WARNINGS AND PRECAUTIONS

5.1 Coadministration With Other Drug Products for Weight Loss

ADIPEX-P® is indicated only as short-term (a few weeks) monotherapy for the management of exogenous obesity. The safety and efficacy of combination therapy with ADIPEX-P® and any other drug products for weight loss including prescribed drugs, over-the-counter preparations, and herbal products, or serotonergic agents such as selective serotonin reuptake inhibitors (e.g., fluoxetine, sertraline, fluvoxamine, paroxetine), have not been established. Therefore, coadministration of ADIPEX-P® and these drug products is not recommended.

5.2 Primary Pulmonary Hypertension

Primary Pulmonary Hypertension (PPH) – a rare, frequently fatal disease of the lungs – has been reported to occur in patients receiving a combination of phentermine with fenfluramine or dexfenfluramine. The possibility of an association between PPH and the use of ADIPEX-P® alone cannot be ruled out; there have been rare cases of PPH in patients who reportedly have taken phentermine alone. The initial symptom of PPH is usually dyspnea. Other initial symptoms may include angina pectoris, syncope or lower extremity edema. Patients should be advised to report immediately any deterioration in exercise tolerance. Treatment should be discontinued in patients who develop new, unexplained symptoms of dyspnea, angina pectoris, syncope or lower extremity edema, and patients should be evaluated for the possible presence of pulmonary hypertension.

5.3 Valvular Heart Disease

Serious regurgitant cardiac valvular disease, primarily affecting the mitral, aortic and/or tricuspid valves, has been reported in otherwise healthy persons who had taken a combination of phentermine with fenfluramine or dexfenfluramine for weight loss. The possible role of phentermine in the etiology of these valvulopathies has not been established and their course in individuals after the drugs are stopped is not known. The possibility of an association between valvular heart disease and the use of ADIPEX-P® alone cannot be ruled out; there have been rare cases of valvular heart disease in patients who reportedly have taken phentermine alone.

5.4 Development of Tolerance, Discontinuation in Case of Tolerance

When tolerance to the anorectant effect develops, the recommended dose should not be exceeded in an attempt to increase the effect; rather, the drug should be discontinued.

5.5 Effect on the Ability to Engage in Potentially Hazardous Tasks

ADIPEX-P® may impair the ability of the patient to engage in potentially hazardous activities such as operating machinery or driving a motor vehicle; the patient should therefore be cautioned accordingly.

5.6 Risk of Abuse and Dependence

ADIPEX-P® is related chemically and pharmacologically to amphetamine (d- and d*l*-amphetamine) and other related stimulant drugs that have been extensively abused. The possibility of abuse of ADIPEX-P® should be kept in mind when evaluating the desirability of including a drug as part of a weight reduction program. See *Drug Abuse and Dependence (9)* and *Overdosage (10)*.

The least amount feasible should be prescribed or dispensed at one time in order to minimize the possibility of overdosage.

5.7 Usage With Alcohol

Concomitant use of alcohol with ADIPEX-P® may result in an adverse drug reaction.

5.8 Use in Patients With Hypertension

Use caution in prescribing ADIPEX-P® for patients with even mild hypertension (risk of increase in blood pressure).

5.9 Use in Patients on Insulin or Oral Hypoglycemic Medications for Diabetes Mellitus

A reduction in insulin or oral hypoglycemic medications in patients with diabetes mellitus may be required.

6 ADVERSE REACTIONS

The following adverse reactions are described, or described in greater detail, in other sections:

- Primary pulmonary hypertension [*see Warnings and Precautions (5.2)*]
- Valvular heart disease [*see Warnings and Precautions (5.3)*]
- Effect on the ability to engage in potentially hazardous tasks [*see Warnings and Precautions (5.5)*]
- Withdrawal effects following prolonged high dosage administration [*see Drug Abuse and Dependence (9.3)*]

The following adverse reactions to phentermine have been identified:

Cardiovascular

Primary pulmonary hypertension and/or regurgitant cardiac valvular disease, palpitation, tachycardia, elevation of blood pressure, ischemic events.

Central Nervous System

Overstimulation, restlessness, dizziness, insomnia, euphoria, dysphoria, tremor, headache, psychosis.

Gastrointestinal

Dryness of the mouth, unpleasant taste, diarrhea, constipation, other gastrointestinal disturbances.

Allergic

Urticaria.

Endocrine

Impotence, changes in libido.

7 DRUG INTERACTIONS

7.1 Monoamine Oxidase Inhibitors

Use of ADIPEX-P® is contraindicated during or within 14 days following the administration of monoamine oxidase inhibitors because of the risk of hypertensive crisis.

7.2 Alcohol

Concomitant use of alcohol with ADIPEX-P® may result in an adverse drug reaction.

7.3 Insulin and Oral Hypoglycemic Medications

Requirements may be altered [*see Warnings and Precautions (5.9)*].

7.4 Adrenergic Neuron Blocking Drugs

ADIPEX-P® may decrease the hypotensive effect of adrenergic neuron blocking drugs.

8 USE IN SPECIFIC POPULATIONS

8.1 Pregnancy

Teratogenic Effects

Pregnancy category X

ADIPEX-P® is contraindicated during pregnancy because weight loss offers no potential benefit to a pregnant woman and may result in fetal harm. A minimum weight gain, and no weight loss, is currently recommended for all pregnant women, including those who are already overweight or obese, due to obligatory weight gain that occurs in maternal tissues during pregnancy. Phentermine has pharmacologic activity similar to amphetamine (d- and d/l-amphetamine) [*see Clinical Pharmacology (12.1)*]. Animal reproduction studies have not been conducted with phentermine. If this drug is used during pregnancy, or if the patient becomes pregnant while taking this drug, the patient should be apprised of the potential hazard to a fetus.

8.3 Nursing Mothers

It is not known if ADIPEX-P® is excreted in human milk; however, other amphetamines are present in human milk. Because of the potential for serious adverse reactions in nursing infants, a decision should be made whether to discontinue nursing or to discontinue the drug, taking into account the importance of the drug to the mother.

8.4 Pediatric Use

Safety and effectiveness in pediatric patients have not been established. Because pediatric obesity is a chronic condition requiring long-term treatment, the use of this product, approved for short-term therapy, is not recommended.

8.5 Geriatric Use

In general, dose selection for an elderly patient should be cautious, usually starting at the low end of the dosing range, reflecting the greater frequency of decreased hepatic, renal, or cardiac function, and of concomitant disease or other drug therapy.

This drug is known to be substantially excreted by the kidney, and the risk of toxic reactions to this drug may be greater in patients with impaired renal function. Because elderly patients are more likely to have decreased renal function, care should be taken in dose selection, and it may be useful to monitor renal function.

8.6 Renal Impairment

ADIPEX-P® was not studied in patients with renal impairment. Based on the reported excretion of phentermine in urine, exposure increases can be expected in patients with renal impairment. Use caution when administering ADIPEX-P® to patients with renal impairment [*see Clinical Pharmacology (12.3)*].

9 DRUG ABUSE AND DEPENDENCE

9.1 Controlled Substance

Phentermine is a Schedule IV controlled substance.

9.2 Abuse

Phentermine is related chemically and pharmacologically to the amphetamines. Amphetamines and other stimulant drugs have been extensively abused and the possibility of abuse of phentermine should be kept in mind when evaluating the desirability of including a drug as part of a weight reduction program.

9.3 Dependence

Abuse of amphetamines and related drugs may be associated with intense psychological dependence and severe social dysfunction. There are reports of patients who have increased the dosage of these drugs to many times than recommended. Abrupt cessation following prolonged high dosage administration results in extreme fatigue and mental depression; changes are also noted on the sleep EEG. Manifestations of chronic intoxication with anorectic drugs include severe dermatoses, marked insomnia, irritability, hyperactivity and personality changes. A severe manifestation of chronic intoxication is psychosis, often clinically indistinguishable from schizophrenia.

10 OVERDOSAGE

The least amount feasible should be prescribed or dispensed at one time in order to minimize the possibility of overdosage.

10.1 Acute Overdosage

Manifestations of acute overdosage include restlessness, tremor, hyperreflexia, rapid respiration, confusion, assaultiveness, hallucinations, and panic states. Fatigue and depression usually follow the central stimulation. Cardiovascular effects include tachycardia, arrhythmia, hypertension or hypotension, and circulatory collapse. Gastrointestinal symptoms include nausea, vomiting, diarrhea and abdominal cramps. Overdosage of pharmacologically similar compounds has resulted in fatal poisoning and usually terminates in convulsions and coma.

Management of acute phentermine hydrochloride intoxication is largely symptomatic and includes lavage and sedation with a barbiturate. Experience with hemodialysis or peritoneal dialysis is inadequate to permit recommendations in this regard. Acidification of the urine increases phentermine excretion. Intravenous phentolamine (Regitine®, CIBA) has been suggested on pharmacologic grounds for possible acute, severe hypertension, if this complicates overdosage.

10.2 Chronic Intoxication

Manifestations of chronic intoxication with anorectic drugs include severe dermatoses, marked insomnia, irritability, hyperactivity and personality changes. The most severe manifestation of chronic intoxications is psychosis, often clinically indistinguishable from schizophrenia. See *Drug Abuse and Dependence (9.3)*.

11 DESCRIPTION

Phentermine hydrochloride USP is a sympathomimetic amine anorectic. It has the chemical name of α,α,-Dimethylphenethylamine hydrochloride. The structural formula is as follows:

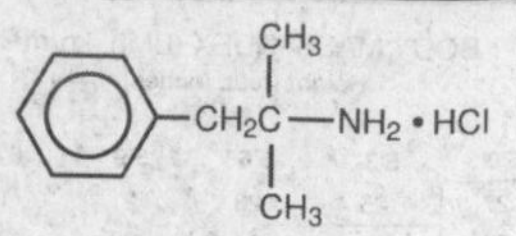

$C_{10}H_{15}N \cdot HCl$ M.W. 185.7

Phentermine hydrochloride is a white, odorless, hygroscopic, crystalline powder which is soluble in water and lower alcohols, slightly soluble in chloroform and insoluble in ether.

ADIPEX-P®, an anorectic agent for oral administration, is available as a capsule or tablet containing 37.5 mg of phentermine hydrochloride (equivalent to 30 mg of phentermine base).

ADIPEX-P® Capsules contain the inactive ingredients Black Iron Oxide, Corn Starch, D&C Red #33, FD&C Blue #1, Gelatin, Lactose Monohydrate, Magnesium Stearate, Propylene Glycol, Shellac, and Titanium Dioxide.

ADIPEX-P® Tablets contain the inactive ingredients Corn Starch, Lactose (Anhydrous), Magnesium Stearate, Microcrystalline Cellulose, Pregelatinized Starch, Sucrose, and FD&C Blue #1.

12 CLINICAL PHARMACOLOGY

12.1 Mechanism of Action

ADIPEX-P® is a sympathomimetic amine with pharmacologic activity similar to the prototype drugs of this class used in obesity, amphetamine (d- and d/l-amphetamine). Drugs of this class used in obesity are commonly known as "anorectics" or "anorexigenics." It has not been established that the primary action of such drugs in treating obesity is one of appetite suppression since other central nervous system actions, or metabolic effects, may also be involved.

12.2 Pharmacodynamics

Typical actions of amphetamines include central nervous system stimulation and elevation of blood pressure. Tachyphylaxis and tolerance have been demonstrated with all drugs of this class in which these phenomena have been looked for.

12.3 Pharmacokinetics

Following the administration of phentermine, phentermine reaches peak concentrations (C_{max}) after 3 to 4.4 hours.

Specific Populations

Renal Impairment

ADIPEX-P® was not studied in patients with renal impairment. The literature reported cumulative urinary excretion of phentermine under uncontrolled urinary pH conditions is 62% to 85%. Exposure increases can be expected in patients with renal impairment. Use caution when administering ADIPEX-P® to patients with renal impairment.

Drug Interactions

In a single-dose study comparing the exposures after oral administration of a combination capsule of 15 mg phentermine and 92 mg topiramate to the exposures after oral administration of a 15 mg phentermine capsule or a 92 mg topiramate capsule, there is no significant topiramate exposure change in the presence of phentermine. However in the presence of topiramate, phentermine C_{max} and AUC increase 13% and 42%, respectively.

13 NONCLINICAL TOXICOLOGY

13.1 Carcinogenesis, Mutagenesis, Impairment of Fertility

Studies have not been performed with phentermine to determine the potential for carcinogenesis, mutagenesis or impairment of fertility.

14 CLINICAL STUDIES

In relatively short-term clinical trials, adult obese subjects instructed in dietary management and treated with "anorectic" drugs lost more weight on the average than those treated with placebo and diet.

The magnitude of increased weight loss of drug-treated patients over placebo-treated patients is only a fraction of a pound a week. The rate of weight loss is greatest in the first weeks of therapy for both drug and placebo subjects and tends to decrease in succeeding weeks. The possible origins of the increased weight loss due to the various drug effects are not established. The amount of weight loss associated with the use of an "anorectic" drug varies from trial to trial, and the increased weight loss appears to be related in part to variables other than the drugs prescribed, such as the physician-investigator, the population treated and the diet prescribed. Studies do not permit conclusions as to the relative importance of the drug and non-drug factors on weight loss.

The natural history of obesity is measured over several years, whereas the studies cited are restricted to a few weeks' duration; thus, the total impact of drug-induced weight loss over that of diet alone must be considered clinically limited.

16 HOW SUPPLIED/STORAGE AND HANDLING

Available in tablets and capsules containing 37.5 mg phentermine hydrochloride (equivalent to 30 mg phentermine base). Each blue and white, oblong, speckled, scored tablet is debossed with "ADIPEX-P" and "9"-"9". The #3 capsule has an opaque white body and an opaque bright blue cap. Each capsule is imprinted with "ADIPEX-P" - "37.5" on the cap and two stripes on the body using dark blue ink.

Tablets are packaged in bottles of 30 (NDC 57844-009-56); 100 (NDC 57844-009-01); and 1000 (NDC 57844-009-10).

Capsules are packaged in bottles of 100 (NDC 57844-019-01).

Store at 20° to 25°C (68° to 77°F) [See USP Controlled Room Temperature].

Dispense in a tight container as defined in the USP, with a child-resistant closure (as required).

KEEP THIS AND ALL MEDICATIONS OUT OF THE REACH OF CHILDREN.

17 PATIENT COUNSELING INFORMATION

Patients must be informed that ADIPEX-P® is a *short-term* (a few weeks) adjunct in a regimen of weight reduction based on exercise, behavioral modification and caloric restriction in the management of exogenous obesity, and that coadministration of phentermine with other drugs for weight loss is not recommended [*see Indications and Usage (1) and Warnings and Precautions (5)*].

Patients must be instructed on how much ADIPEX-P® to take, and when and how to take it [*see Dosage and Administration (2)*].

Advise pregnant women and nursing mothers not to use ADIPEX-P® [*see Use in Specific Populations (8.1, 8.3)*].

Patients must be informed about the risks of use of phentermine (including the risks discussed in Warnings and Precautions), about the symptoms of potential adverse reactions and when to contact a physician and/or take other action. The risks include, but are not limited to:

- Development of primary pulmonary hypertension [*see Warnings and Precautions (5.2)*]
- Development of serious valvular heart disease [*see Warnings and Precautions (5.3)*]
- Effects on the ability to engage in potentially hazardous tasks [*see Warnings and Precautions (5.5)*]
- The risk of an increase in blood pressure [*see Warnings and Precautions (5.8) and Adverse Reactions (6)*]
- The risk of interactions [*see Contraindications (4), Warnings and Precautions (5) and Drug Interactions (7)*]

See also, for example, *Adverse Reactions (6)* and *Use in Specific Populations (8)*.

The patients must also be informed about

- the potential for developing tolerance and actions if they suspect development of tolerance [*see Warnings and Precautions (5.4)*] and
- the risk of dependence and the potential consequences of abuse [*see Warnings and Precautions (5.6), Drug Abuse and Dependence (9), and Overdosage (10)*].

Tell patients to keep ADIPEX-P® in a safe place to prevent theft, accidental overdose, misuse or abuse. Selling or giving away ADIPEX-P® may harm others and is against the law.

All trademarks are the property of their respective owners.

Manufactured by:
TEVA PHARMACEUTICALS USA
Sellersville, PA 18960
Manufactured for:
Teva Select Brands, Horsham, PA 19044
Division of Teva Pharmaceuticals USA
Rev. X 1/2013
ADI-40004

Shown in Product Identification Guide, page 314

PROGLYCEM® ℞

[pro-glī-cem]
brand of diazoxide
Capsules
Suspension, USP
FOR ORAL ADMINISTRATION
Rx only

DESCRIPTION

PROGLYCEM® (diazoxide) is a nondiuretic benzothiadiazine derivative taken orally for the management of symptomatic hypoglycemia. PROGLYCEM® **Capsules** contain 50 mg diazoxide, USP. The **Suspension** contains 50 mg of diazoxide, USP in each milliliter and has a chocolate-mint flavor; alcohol content is approximately 7.25%. Other ingredients: Sorbitol solution, chocolate cream flavor, propylene glycol, magnesium aluminum silicate, carboxymethycellulose sodium, mint flavor, sodium benzoate, methylparaben, poloxamer 188, propylparaben, and purified water. Hydrochloric acid or sodium hydroxide may be added to adjust pH. Diazoxide has the following structural formula:

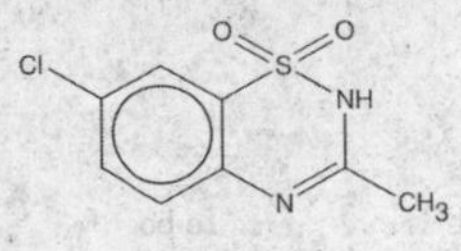

Diazoxide is 7-chloro-3-methyl-2*H*-1,2,4-benzothiadiazine 1,1-dioxide with the empirical formula $C_8H_7ClN_2O_2S$ and the molecular weight 230.7. It is a white powder practically insoluble to sparingly soluble in water.

CLINICAL PHARMACOLOGY

Diazoxide administered orally produces a prompt dose-related increase in blood glucose level, due primarily to an inhibition of insulin release from the pancreas, and also to an extrapancreatic effect.

The hyperglycemic effect begins within an hour and generally lasts no more than eight hours in the presence of normal renal function.

PROGLYCEM® decreases the excretion of sodium and water, resulting in fluid retention which may be clinically significant.

The hypotensive effect of diazoxide on blood pressure is usually not marked with the oral preparation. This contrasts with the intravenous preparation of diazoxide (see ADVERSE REACTIONS).

Other pharmacologic actions of PROGLYCEM® include increased pulse rate; increased serum uric acid levels due to decreased excretion; increased serum levels of free fatty acids' decreased chloride excretion; decreased para-aminohippuric acid; (PAH) clearance with no appreciable effect on glomerular filtration rate.

The concomitant administration of a benzothiazide diuretic may intensify the hyperglycemic and hyperuricemic effects of PROGLYCEM®. In the presence of hypokalemia, hyperglycemic effects are also potentiated.

PROGLYCEM®-induced hyperglycemia is reversed by the administration of insulin or tolbutamide. The inhibition of insulin release by PROGLYCEM® is antagonized by alpha-adrenergic blocking agents.

PROGLYCEM® is extensively bound (more than 90%) to serum proteins, and is excreted in the kidneys. The plasma half-life following I.V. administration is 28 ± 8.3 hours. Limited data on oral administration revealed a half-life of 24 and 36 hours in two adults. In four children aged four months to six years, the plasma half-life varied from 9.5 to 24 hours on long-term oral administration. The half-life may be prolonged following overdosage, and in patients with impaired renal function.

INDICATIONS AND USAGE

PROGLYCEM® (ORAL DIAZOXIDE) is useful in the management of hypoglycemia due to hyperinsulinism associated with the following conditions:

Adults: Inoperable islet cell adenoma or carcinoma, or extrapancreatic malignancy.

Infants and Children: Leucine sensitivity, islet cell hyperplasia, nesidioblastosis, extrapancreatic malignancy, islet cell adenoma, or adenomatosis. PROGLYCEM® may be used preoperatively as a temporary measure, and postoperatively, if hypoglycemia persists.

PROGLYCEM® should be used only after a diagnosis of hypoglycemia due to one of the above conditions has been definitely established. When other specific medical therapy or surgical management either has been unsuccessful or is not feasible, treatment with PROGLYCEM® should be considered.

CONTRAINDICATIONS

The use of PROGLYCEM® for functional hypoglycemia is contraindicated. The drug should not be used in patients hypersensitive to diazoxide or to other thiazides unless the potential benefits outweigh the possible risks.

WARNINGS

The antidiuretic property of diazoxide may lead to significant fluid retention, which in patients with compromised cardiac reserve, may precipitate congestive heart failure. The fluid retention will respond to conventional therapy with diuretics.

It should be noted that concomitantly administered thiazides may potentiate the hyperglycemic and hyperuricemic actions of diazoxide (See DRUG INTERACTIONS and ANIMAL PHARMACOLOGY AND/OR TOXICOLOGY).

Ketoacidosis and nonketotic hyperosmolar coma have been reported in patients treated with recommended doses of PROGLYCEM® usually during intercurrent illness. Prompt recognition and treatment are essential (See OVERDOSAGE), and prolonged surveillance following the acute episode is necessary because of the long drug half-life of approximately 30 hours. The occurrence of these serious events may be reduced by careful education of patients regarding the need for monitoring the urine for sugar and ketones and for prompt reporting of abnormal findings and unusual symptoms to the physician. Transient cataracts occurred in association with hyperosmolar coma in an infant, and subsided on correction of the hyper-osmolarity. Cataracts have been observed in several animals receiving daily doses of intravenous or oral diazoxide.

The development of abnormal facial features in four children treated chronically (>4 years) with PROGLYCEM® for hypoglycemia hyperinsulinism in the same clinic has been reported.

PRECAUTIONS

General: treatment with PROGLYCEM® should be initiated under close clinical supervision, with careful monitoring of blood glucose and clinical response until the patient's condition has stabilized. This usually requires several days. If not effective in two to three weeks, the drug should be discontinued.

Prolonged treatment requires regular monitoring of the urine for sugar and ketones, especially under stress conditions, with prompt reporting of any abnormalities to the physician. Additionally, blood sugar levels should be monitored periodically by the physician to determine the need for dose adjustment.

The effects of diazoxide on the hematopoietic system and the level of serum uric acid should be kept in mind; the latter should be considered particularly in patients with hyperuricemia or a history of gout.

In some patients, higher blood levels have been observed with the oral suspension than with the capsule formulation of PROGLYCEM®. Dosage should be adjusted as necessary in individual patients if changed from one formulation to the other.

Since the plasma half-life of diazoxide is prolonged in patients with impaired renal function, a reduced dosage should be considered. Serum electrolyte levels should also be evaluated for such patients.

The antihypertensive effect of other drugs may be enhanced by PROGLYCEM®, and this should be kept in mind when administering it concomitantly with antihypertensive agents.

Because of the protein binding, administration of PROGLYCEM® with coumarin or its derivatives may require reduction in the dosage of the anticoagulant, although there has been no reported evidence of excessive anticoagulant effect. In addition, PROGLYCEM® may possibly displace bilirubin from albumin; this should be kept in mind particularly when treating newborns with increased bilirubinemia.

Information for Patients: During treatment with PROGLYCEM® the patient should be advised to consult regularly with the physician and to cooperate in the periodic monitoring of his condition by laboratory tests. In addition, the patient should be advised:

- to take the drug on a regular schedule as prescribed, not to skip doses, not to take extra doses;
- not to use this drug with other medications unless this is done with the physician's advice;
- not to allow anyone else to take this medication;
- to follow dietary instructions;
- to report promptly any adverse effects (i.e., increased urinary frequency, increased thirst, fruity breath odor);
- to report pregnancy or to discuss plans for pregnancy.

Laboratory tests: The following procedures may be especially important in patient monitoring (not necessarily inclusive); blood glucose determinations (recommended at periodic intervals in patients taking diazoxide orally for treatment of hypoglycemia, until stabilized); blood urea nitrogen (BUN) determinations and creatinine clearance determinations; hematocrit determinations; platelet count determinations; total and differential leukocyte counts; serum aspartate aminotransferase (AST) level determinations; serum uric acid level determinations; and urine testing for glucose and ketones (in patients being treated with diazoxide for hypoglycemia, semi-quantitative estimation of sugar and ketones in serum performed by the patient and reported to the physician provides frequent and relatively inexpensive monitoring of the condition).

Drug Interactions: Since diazoxide is highly bound to serum proteins, it may displace other substances which are also bound to protein, such as bilirubin or coumarin and its derivatives, resulting in higher blood levels of these substances. Concomitant administration of oral diazoxide and diphenylhydantoin may result in a loss of seizure control. These potential interactions must be considered when administering PROGLYCEM® **Capsules** or **Suspension.**

The concomitant administration of thiazides or other commonly used diuretics may potentiate the hyperglycemic and hyperuricemic effects of diazoxide.

Drug/Laboratory Test Interactions: The hyperglycemic and hyperuricemic effects of diazoxide preclude proper assessment of these metabolic states. Increased renin secretion, IgG concentrations and decreased cortisol secretions have also been noted. Diazoxide inhibits glucagon-stimulated insulin release and causes a false-negative insulin response to glucagon.

Carcinogenesis, mutagenesis, impairment of fertility: No long-term animal dosing study has been done to evaluate the carcinogenic potential of diazoxide. No laboratory study of mutagenic potential or animal study of effects on fertility has been done.

Pregnancy Category C: Reproduction studies using the oral preparation in rats have revealed increased fetal resorptions and delayed parturition, as well as fetal skeletal anomalies; evidence of skeletal and cardiac teratogenic effects in rabbits has been noted with intravenous administration. The drug has also been demonstrated to cross the placental barrier in animals and to cause degeneration of the fetal pancreatic beta cells (See ANIMAL PHARMACOLOGY AND/OR TOXICOLOGY). Since there are no adequate data on fetal effects of this drug when given to pregnant women, safety in pregnancy has not been established. When the use of PROGLYCEM® is considered, the indications should be limited to those specified above for adults (See INDICATIONS AND USAGE), and the potential benefits to the mother must be weighed against possible harmful effects to the fetus.

Non-teratogenic effects: Diazoxide crosses the placental barrier and appears in cord blood. When given to the mother prior to delivery of the infant, the drug may produce fetal or neonatal hyperbilirubinemia, thrombocytopenia, altered carbohydrate metabolism, and possibly other side effects that have occurred in adults.

Alopecia and hypertrichosis lanuginosa have occurred in infants whose mothers received oral diazoxide during the last 19 to 60 days of pregnancy.

Labor and delivery: Since intravenous administration of the drug during labor may cause cessation of uterine contractions, and administration of oxytocic agents may be required to reinstate labor, caution is advised in administering PROGLYCEM® at that time.

Nursing mothers: Information is not available concerning the passage of diazoxide in breast milk. Because many drugs are excreted in human milk and because of the potential for adverse reactions from diazoxide in nursing infants, a decision should be made whether to discontinue nursing or to discontinue the drug, taking into account the importance of the drug to the mother.

Pediatric use: (See INDICATIONS AND USAGE).

ADVERSE REACTIONS

Frequent and Serious: Sodium and fluid retention is most common in young infants and in adults and may precipitate congestive heart failure in patients with compromised cardiac reserve. It usually responds to diuretic therapy (See DRUG INTERACTIONS).

Infrequent but Serious: Diabetic ketoacidosis and hyperosmolar nonketotic coma may develop very rapidly. Conventional therapy with insulin and restoration of fluid and electrolyte balance is usually effective if instituted promptly. Prolonged surveillance is essential in view of the long half-life of PROGLYCEM® (See OVERDOSAGE).

Other frequent adverse reactions: Hirsutism of the lanugo type, mainly on the forehead, back and limbs, occurs most commonly in children and women and may be cosmetically unacceptable. It subsides on discontinuation of the drug.

Hyperglycemia or glycosuria may require reduction in dosage in order to avoid progression to ketoacidosis or hyperosmolar coma.

Gastrointestinal intolerance may include anorexia, nausea, vomiting, abdominal pain, ileus, diarrhea, transient loss of taste.

Tachycardia, palpitations, increased levels of serum uric acid are common.

Thrombocytopenia with or without purpura may require discontinuation of the drug. Neutropenia is transient, is not associated with increased susceptibility to infection, and ordinarily does not require discontinuation of the drug. Skin rash, headache, weakness, and malaise may also occur.

Other adverse reactions which have been observed are:

Cardiovascular: hypotension occurs occasionally, which may be augmented by thiazide diuretics given concurrently. A few cases of transient hypertension, for which no explanation is apparent, have been noted. Chest pain has been reported rarely.

Hematologic: eosinophilia; decreased hemoglobin / hematocrit; excessive bleeding, decreased IgG.

Hepato-renal: increased AST, alkaline phosphatase; azotemia, decreased creatinine clearance, reversible nephrotic syndrome, decreased urinary output, hematuria, albuminuria. Neurologic: anxiety, dizziness, insomnia, polyneuritis, paresthesia, pruritus, extrapyramidal signs. *Ophthalmologic:* transient cataracts, subconjunctival hemorrhage, ring scotoma, blurred vision, diplopia, lacrimation. *Skeletal, integumentary;* monilial dermatitis, herpes, advance in bone age; loss of scalp hair. *Systemic:* fever, lymphadenopathy. *Other;* gout acute pancreatitis/pancreatic necrosis, galactorrhea, enlargement of lump in breast.

OVERDOSAGE

An overdosage of PROGLYCEM® causes marked hyperglycemia which may be associated with ketoacidosis. It will respond to prompt insulin administration and restoration of fluid and electrolyte balance. Because of the drug's long half-life (approximately 30 hours), the symptoms of overdosage require prolonged surveillance for periods up to seven days until the blood sugar level stabilizes within the normal range. One investigator reported successful lowering of diazoxide blood levels by peritoneal dialysis in one patient and by hemodialysis in another.

DOSAGE AND ADMINISTRATION

Patients should be under close clinical observation when treatment with PROGLYCEM® is initiated. The clinical response and blood glucose level should be carefully monitored until the patient's condition has stabilized satisfactory; in most instances, this may be accomplished in several days. If administration of PROGLYCEM® is not effective after two or three weeks, the drug should be discontinued.

The dosage of PROGLYCEM® must be individualized based on the severity of the hypoglycemic condition and the blood glucose level and clinical response of the patient. The dosage should be adjusted until the desired clinical and laboratory effects are produced with the least amount of the drug. Special care should be taken to assure accuracy of dosage in infants and young children.

Adults and children: The usual daily dosage is 3 to 8 mg/kg, divided into two or three equal doses every 8 or 12 hours. In certain instances, patients with refractory hypoglycemia may require higher dosages. Ordinarily, an appropriate starting dosage is 3 mg/kg/day, divided into three equal doses every 8 hours. Thus an average adult would receive a starting dosage of approximately 200 mg daily.

Infants and newborns: The usual daily dosage is 8 to 15 mg/kg divided into two or three equal doses every 8 to 12 hours. An appropriate starting dosage is 10 mg/kg/day, divided into three equal doses every 8 hours.

ANIMAL PHARMACOLOGY AND/OR TOXICOLOGY

Oral diazoxide in the mouse, rat, rabbit, dog, pig, and monkey produces a rapid and transient rise in blood glucose levels. In dogs, increased blood glucose is accompanied by increased free fatty acids, lactate, and pyruvate in the serum. In mice, a marked decrease in liver glycogen and an increase in the blood urea nitrogen level occur.

In acute toxicity studies the LD50 for oral diazoxide suspension is >5000 mg/kg in the rat, >522 mg/kg in the neonatal rat, between 1900 and 2572 mg/kg in the mouse, and 219 mg/kg in the guinea pig. Although the oral LD_{50} was not determined in the dog, a dosage of up to 500 mg/kg was well tolerated.

In subacute oral toxicity studies, diazoxide at 400 mg/kg in the rat produced growth retardation, edema, increases in liver and kidney weights, and adrenal hypertrophy. Daily dosages up to 1080 mg/kg for three months produced hyperglycemia, an increase in liver weight and an increase in mortality. In dogs given oral diazoxide at approximately 40 mg/kg/day for one month, no biologically significant gross or microscopic abnormalities were observed. Cataracts, attributed to markedly disturbed carbohydrate metabolism, have been observed in a few dogs given repeated daily doses of oral or intravenous diazoxide. The lenticular changes resembled those which occur experimentally in animals with increased blood glucose levels. In chronic toxicity studies, rats given a daily dose of 200 mg/kg diazoxide for 52 weeks had a decrease in weight gain and an increase in heart, liver, adrenal and thyroid weights. Mortality in drug-treated and control groups was not different. Dogs treated with diazoxide at dosages of 50, l00, and 200 mg/kg/day for 82 weeks had higher blood glucose levels than controls. Mild bone marrow stimulation and increased pancreas weights were evident in the drug-treated dogs; several developed inguinal hernias, one had a testicular seminoma, and another had a mass near the penis. Two females had inguinal mammary swellings. The etiology of these changes was not established. There was no difference in mortality between drug-treated and control groups. In a second chronic oral toxicity study, dogs given milled diazoxide at 50, l00, and 200 mg/kg/day had anorexia and severe weight loss, causing death in a few. Hematologic, biochemical, and histologic examination did not indicate any cause of death other than inanition. After one year of treatment, there is no evidence of herniation or tissue swelling in any of the dogs.

When diazoxide was administered at high dosages concomitantly with either chlorothiazide to rats or trichlormethiazide to dogs, increased toxicity was observed. In rats, the combination was nephrotoxic; epithelial hyperplasia was observed in the collecting tubules. In dogs, a diabetic syndrome was produced which resulted in ketosis and death. Neither of the drugs given alone produced these effects.

Although the data are inconclusive, reproduction and teratology studies in several species of animals indicate that diazoxide, when administered during the critical period of embryo formation, may interfere with normal fetal development, possibly through altered glucose metabolism. Parturition was occasionally prolonged in animals treated at term. Intravenous administration of diazoxide to pregnant sheep, goats, and swine produced in the fetus an appreciable increase in blood glucose level and degeneration of the beta cells of the Islets of Langerhans. The reversibility of these effects was not studied.

HOW SUPPLIED

PROGLYCEM® (diazoxide capsules, USP), 50 mg, half opaque orange and half clear capsules, branded in black with BNP 6000: bottle of 100 (NDC 0575-6000-01).

PROGLYCEM® suspension, 50 mg/mL, a chocolate-mint flavored suspension; bottle of 30 ml (NDC 0575-6200-30), with dropper calibrated to deliver 10, 20, 30, 40 and 50 mg diazoxide. **Shake well before each use. Protect from light. Store in carton until contents are used. Store in light resistant container as defined in the USP. Store PROGLYCEM® Capsules and Suspension at 25°C (77°F) excursions permitted 15°-30°C (59-86°F). [See USP Controlled Room Temperature].**

Manufactured by:
TEVA PHARMACEUTICALS USA
Sellersville, PA 18960
Manufactured for:
Teva Select Brands
Horsham, PA 19044
Division of Teva Pharmaceuticals USA
Rev. 2/2012
PRG-40004

Shown in Product Identification Guide, page 314

Label intentionally removed due to change in Important Safety Information

Label intentionally removed due to change in Important Safety Information

Label intentionally removed due to change in Important Safety Information

Label intentionally removed due to change in Important Safety Information

Label intentionally removed due to change in Important Safety Information

Label intentionally removed due to change in Important Safety Information

Label intentionally removed due to change in Important Safety Information

Label intentionally removed due to change in Important Safety Information

Label intentionally removed due to change in Important Safety Information

Topical BioMedics, Inc.

6565 SPRING BROOK AVENUE SUITE 11
RHINEBECK, NY 12572-0494

Direct Inquiries to:
Professional Services at Topricin
Phone: (845) 871-4900 ext. 1115
Fax: (845) 876-0818
E-mail: info@topicalbiomedics.com for Free samples and prescription pads

TOPRICIN® **OTC**
[toe-pri-sin]

KEY FACTS
Topricin is patented for the Topical Treatment of Neuropathy and Safe for Diabetics.
Topricin® is an odorless, non-irritating, Pain Relief and Healing cream that provides superior relief of all trauma injuries and excellent adjunctive support in medical treatment protocols such as: post surgical trauma, physical and occupational therapy, physiatry, physical and sports medicine. Greaseless and contains no chemical preservatives, or menthol, camphor, capsaicin, methyl salicylates or fragrances. Topricin is the ideal topical treatment that is safe for the entire family, and the best alternative option for patients who cannot tolerate oral pain medications.

ACTIVE INGREDIENTS (HPUS)
Arnica Montana 6X, Echinacea 6X, Aesculus 6X, Ruta Graveolens 6X, Lachesis 8X, Rhus Tox 6X Belladonna 6X, Crotalus 8X, Heloderma 8X, Naja 8X, Graphites 6X.

MAJOR USES
Superior topical relief of pain edema and a healing treatment for all soft tissue neuropathic pain, repetitive motion and cumulative trauma work/sports injuries.

BENEFITS
Rapidly relieves: stiffness, soreness, numbness, tingling pain/burning pain associated with these soft tissue ailments: carpal tunnel syndrome, other peripheral neuropathic pain, arthritis, lower back pain, muscle spasm of the back, neck, legs, and feet, muscle soreness, strains, sprains. First aid: bruises, minor burns. Use before and after exercise.
*Improves recovery after surgery up to 40%
*Reduces dependency on all classes of oral pain medicine
*Prevents bedsores
*Sufficient success in scar tissue management
*Effective for chemo-induced neuropathy

DIRECTIONS
Apply generously 3–4 times a day or more often if needed. Be sure the application covers the entire joint or area of pain. Massage in until absorbed. Reapply before bed and at the start of the day for best results. Can be used with hot and cold therapy or Phonophoresis. For further information go to www.topicalbiomedics.com

SAFETY INFORMATION
For external use only, use only as directed, if pain persists for more than 7 days or worsens, consult a doctor. This homeopathic medicine has no known side effects or contraindications. This medicine complies with all FDA regulations as an OTC medicine, safe to use for children over 2 years, adults, pregnant women and the elderly. Paraben and Petroleum free

INACTIVE INGREDIENTS
Purified water, purified coconut oil, glycerin, medium chain triglyceride.

HOW SUPPLIED
Consumer size: 2oz tube, 4oz jar, and 8oz flip top bottle.
For Professionals only: 16oz and 32oz pump bottle.
Other products: Topricin Junior 1.5oz tube, Topricin Foot Therapy Cream 2oz, 4oz and 8oz flip top bottle.
Countertop Display available for medical office or pharmacy shelf.

Shown in Product Identification Guide, page 314

Vertex Pharmaceuticals Incorporated

130 WAVERLY STREET
CAMBRIDGE, MA 02139

Direct Health Care Provider Inquiries to:
Vertex Medical Information
1-877-634-VRTX (8789)
Direct Consumer/Patient Inquiries to:
INCIVEK Patient Services: 1-855-837-8394
KALYDECO Patient Services: 1-877-752-5933
For Reporting Adverse Events:
Health Care Providers and Consumer/Patients:
1-877-634-VRTX (8789)

INCIVEK™ ℞
[in-SEE-veck]
(telaprevir)
Film Coated Tablets, for oral use

HIGHLIGHTS OF PRESCRIBING INFORMATION
These highlights do not include all the information needed to use INCIVEK safely and effectively. See full prescribing information for INCIVEK.
INCIVEK™ (telaprevir) Film Coated Tablets, for oral use
Initial U.S. Approval: 2011

WARNING: SERIOUS SKIN REACTIONS
See full prescribing information for complete boxed warning.
Fatal and non-fatal serious skin reactions, including Stevens Johnson Syndrome (SJS), Drug Reaction with Eosinophilia and Systemic Symptoms (DRESS), and Toxic Epidermal Necrolysis (TEN), have been reported in patients treated with INCIVEK combination treatment [*see Warnings and Precautions (5.1)*]. Fatal cases have been reported in patients with progressive rash and systemic symptoms who continued to receive INCIVEK combination treatment after a serious skin reaction was identified. For serious skin reactions, including rash with systemic symptoms or a progressive severe rash, INCIVEK, peginterferon alfa, and ribavirin must be discontinued immediately. Discontinuing other medications known to be associated with serious skin reactions should be considered. Patients should be promptly referred for urgent medical care.

RECENT MAJOR CHANGES

• Boxed Warning	12/2012
• Contraindications (4)	12/2012
• Warnings and Precautions (5.1, 5.2)	12/2012
• Warnings and Precautions (5.5)	04/2013

INDICATIONS AND USAGE
INCIVEK is a hepatitis C virus (HCV) NS3/4A protease inhibitor indicated, in combination with peginterferon alfa and ribavirin, for the treatment of genotype 1 chronic hepatitis C (CHC) in adult patients with compensated liver disease, including cirrhosis, who are treatment-naïve or who have been previously treated with interferon-based treatment, including prior null responders, partial responders, and relapsers. (1)
- INCIVEK must not be used as monotherapy and must only be used in combination with peginterferon alfa and ribavirin. (5.6)
- A high proportion of previous null responders (particularly those with cirrhosis) did not achieve Sustained Virologic Response (SVR) and had telaprevir resistance-associated substitutions emerge on treatment with INCIVEK. (12.4, 14.3)
- INCIVEK efficacy has not been established for patients who have previously failed therapy with a treatment regimen that includes INCIVEK or other HCV NS3/4A protease inhibitors. (12.4)

DOSAGE AND ADMINISTRATION
- 750 mg taken 3 times a day (7-9 hours apart) with food (not low fat). (2, 12.3, 17.4)
- INCIVEK must be administered with both peginterferon alfa and ribavirin for all patients for 12 weeks, followed by a response-guided regimen of either 12 or 36 additional weeks of peginterferon alfa and ribavirin depending on viral response and prior response status. (2)
- For specific dosage instructions for peginterferon alfa and ribavirin, refer to their respective prescribing information. (2)

Table 1: Recommended Treatment Duration (See also Table 2 for Treatment Futility Rules)

HCV RNA*	Triple Therapy INCIVEK, peginterferon alfa and ribavirin	Dual Therapy peginterferon alfa and ribavirin	Total Treatment Duration
Treatment-Naïve and Prior Relapse Patients			
Undetectable (Target Not Detected) at Weeks 4 and 12	First 12 weeks	Additional 12 weeks	24 weeks
Detectable (1000 IU/mL or less) at Weeks 4 and/or 12	First 12 weeks	Additional 36 weeks	48 weeks
Prior Partial and Null Responder Patients			
	Triple Therapy INCIVEK, peginterferon alfa and ribavirin	**Dual Therapy** peginterferon alfa and ribavirin	**Total Treatment Duration**
All Patients	First 12 weeks	Additional 36 weeks	48 weeks

* In clinical trials, HCV RNA in plasma was measured using a COBAS® TaqMan® assay with a lower limit of quantification of 25 IU/mL and a limit of detection of 10 IU/mL. See *Laboratory Tests (5.5)* for a description of HCV RNA assay recommendations.

DOSAGE FORMS AND STRENGTHS

- 375 mg tablets (3)

CONTRAINDICATIONS

- All contraindications to peginterferon alfa and ribavirin also apply since INCIVEK must be administered with peginterferon alfa and ribavirin. (4)
- Pregnant women and men whose female partners are pregnant: Because ribavirin may cause birth defects and fetal death, telaprevir in combination with peginterferon alfa and ribavirin is contraindicated in pregnant women and in men whose female partners are pregnant. (4, 5.3, 8.1, 17.2)
- Co-administration with drugs that:
  - are highly dependent on CYP3A for clearance and for which elevated plasma concentrations are associated with serious and/or life-threatening events. (4)
  - strongly induce CYP3A which may lead to lower exposure and loss of efficacy of INCIVEK. (4)

WARNINGS AND PRECAUTIONS

- Serious Skin Reactions/Rash: Fatal and non-fatal serious skin reactions (including SJS, DRESS, and TEN) have been reported. Patients with mild to moderate rash should be monitored for progression. If rash progresses and becomes severe, INCIVEK should be discontinued. For serious skin reactions, including rash with systemic symptoms or a progressive severe rash, INCIVEK, peginterferon alfa, and ribavirin must be discontinued immediately. Consider discontinuing other medications known to be associated with serious skin reactions. (5.1)
- Anemia: Monitor hemoglobin prior to and at regular intervals during INCIVEK combination treatment. Follow dose modifications for ribavirin; discontinue INCIVEK if required. (5.2)
- **Pregnancy: Use with Ribavirin and Peginterferon alfa: Ribavirin may cause birth defects and fetal death; avoid pregnancy in female patients and female partners of male patients.** Patients must have a negative pregnancy test prior to initiating therapy, use at least 2 effective methods of contraception, and undergo monthly pregnancy tests. (5.3, 8.1, 17.2)

ADVERSE REACTIONS

The most common adverse drug reactions to INCIVEK (incidence at least 5% higher with INCIVEK than in controls) were rash, pruritus, anemia, nausea, hemorrhoids, diarrhea, anorectal discomfort, dysgeusia, fatigue, vomiting, and anal pruritus. (6)

To report SUSPECTED ADVERSE REACTIONS, contact Vertex Pharmaceuticals Incorporated at 877-824-4281 or FDA at 1-800-FDA-1088 or www.fda.gov/medwatch.

DRUG INTERACTIONS

- Co-administration of INCIVEK combination treatment with other drugs can alter the concentration of other drugs and other drugs may alter the concentrations of telaprevir. Consult the full prescribing information prior to and during treatment for potential drug-drug interactions. (4, 7, 12.3)

USE IN SPECIFIC POPULATIONS

- Hepatic Impairment: Safety and efficacy have not been established in patients with Child-Pugh score greater than or equal to 7 (class B and C). (5.7, 8.6)
- Co-infection: Safety and efficacy have not been established in HCV/HIV and HCV/HBV co-infected patients. (8.8)
- Pediatrics: Safety and efficacy have not been established in pediatric patients. (8.4)
- Solid Organ Transplant: Safety and efficacy have not been established in patients undergoing solid organ transplants. (8.9)

See 17 for PATIENT COUNSELING INFORMATION and Medication Guide

Revised: 05/2013

FULL PRESCRIBING INFORMATION: CONTENTS*

*** Sections or subsections omitted from the full prescribing information are not listed**

FULL PRESCRIBING INFORMATION

WARNING: SERIOUS SKIN REACTIONS

Fatal and non-fatal serious skin reactions, including Stevens Johnson Syndrome (SJS), Drug Reaction with Eosinophilia and Systemic Symptoms (DRESS), and Toxic Epidermal Necrolysis (TEN), have been reported in patients treated with INCIVEK combination treatment [*see Warnings and Precautions (5.1)*]. Fatal cases have been reported in patients with progressive rash and systemic symptoms who continued to receive INCIVEK combination treatment after a serious skin reaction was identified. For serious skin reactions, including rash with systemic symptoms or a progressive severe rash, INCIVEK, peginterferon alfa, and ribavirin must be discontinued immediately. Discontinuing other medications known to be associated with serious skin reactions should be considered. Patients should be promptly referred for urgent medical care.

1 INDICATIONS AND USAGE

1.1 Chronic Hepatitis C

INCIVEK™ (telaprevir), in combination with peginterferon alfa and ribavirin, is indicated for the treatment of genotype 1 chronic hepatitis C in adult patients with compensated liver disease, including cirrhosis, who are treatment-naïve or who have previously been treated with interferon-based treatment, including prior null responders, partial responders, and relapsers [*see Clinical Studies (14.2 and 14.3), including definitions of these terms*].

The following points should be considered when initiating treatment with INCIVEK:

- INCIVEK must not be administered as monotherapy and must only be prescribed with both peginterferon alfa and ribavirin [*see Warnings and Precautions (5.6)*].
- A high proportion of previous null responders (particularly those with cirrhosis) did not achieve a Sustained Virologic Response (SVR) and had telaprevir resistance-associated substitutions emerge on treatment with INCIVEK combination treatment [*see Microbiology (12.4) and Clinical Studies (14.3)*].
- INCIVEK efficacy has not been established for patients who have previously failed therapy with a treatment regimen that includes INCIVEK or other HCV NS3/4A protease inhibitors [*see Microbiology (12.4)*].

2 DOSAGE AND ADMINISTRATION

2.1 INCIVEK/Peginterferon Alfa/Ribavirin Combination Treatment

The recommended dose of INCIVEK tablets is 750 mg (two 375-mg tablets) taken orally 3 times a day (7-9 hours apart) with food (not low fat) [*see Clinical Pharmacology (12.3) and Patient Counseling Information (17.4)*].

For specific dosage instructions for peginterferon alfa and ribavirin, refer to their respective prescribing information.

Duration of Treatment

The recommended duration of treatment with INCIVEK is 12 weeks in combination with peginterferon alfa and ribavirin. HCV RNA levels should be monitored at weeks 4 and 12 to determine combination treatment duration and assess for treatment futility (Tables 1 and 2).

[See table 1 above]

For the purpose of assessing response-guided therapy eligibility at weeks 4 and 12 (see Table 1), an "undetectable" HCV RNA (Target Not Detected) result is required; a confirmed "detectable but below limit of quantification" HCV RNA result should not be considered equivalent to an "undetectable" HCV RNA (Target Not Detected) result [*see Laboratory Tests (5.5)*].

Treatment-naïve patients with cirrhosis who have undetectable HCV RNA (Target Not Detected) at weeks 4 and 12 of INCIVEK combination treatment may benefit from an additional 36 weeks of peginterferon alfa and ribavirin (48 weeks total) [*see Clinical Studies (14.2)*].

2.2 Dose Reduction

To prevent treatment failure, the dose of INCIVEK must not be reduced or interrupted. Refer to the respective prescribing information for dose modification of peginterferon alfa and ribavirin [*see Warnings and Precautions (5.6)*].

2.3 Discontinuation of Dosing

Patients with inadequate viral response are unlikely to achieve SVR, and may develop treatment-emergent resistance substitutions [*see Microbiology (12.4)*]. Discontinuation of therapy is recommended in all patients with (1) HCV RNA levels of greater than 1000 IU/mL at Treatment Week 4 or 12; or (2) confirmed detectable HCV RNA levels at Treatment Week 24 (see Table 2).

Table 2: Treatment Futility Rules: All Patients

HCV RNA	Action
Week 4 or Week 12: Greater than 1000 IU/mL	Discontinue INCIVEK and peginterferon alfa and ribavirin (INCIVEK treatment complete at 12 weeks)
Week 24: Detectable	Discontinue peginterferon alfa and ribavirin

If peginterferon alfa or ribavirin is discontinued for any reason, INCIVEK must also be discontinued.

3 DOSAGE FORMS AND STRENGTHS

Each tablet contains 375 mg of telaprevir. Tablets are available as purple, film-coated, capsule-shaped tablets debossed with the characters "V 375" on one side.

4 CONTRAINDICATIONS

Contraindications to peginterferon alfa and ribavirin also apply to INCIVEK combination treatment.

INCIVEK combination treatment is contraindicated in:

- women who are or may become pregnant. Ribavirin may cause fetal harm when administered to a pregnant woman. If this drug is used during pregnancy, or if the patient becomes pregnant while taking this drug treatment, the patient should be apprised of the potential hazard to a fetus [*see Warnings and Precautions (5.3), Use in Specific Populations (8.1), and Patient Counseling Information (17.2)*].
- men whose female partners are pregnant.

INCIVEK is a strong inhibitor of CYP3A. INCIVEK is contraindicated when combined with drugs that are highly dependent on CYP3A for clearance and for which elevated plasma concentrations are associated with serious and/or life-threatening events (narrow therapeutic index). INCIVEK is contraindicated when combined with drugs that strongly induce CYP3A and thus may lead to lower exposure and loss of efficacy of INCIVEK. Contraindicated drugs are listed below in Table 3 [*also see Drug Interactions (7), Table 5 and Clinical Pharmacology (12.3), Tables 6 and 7*].

[See table 3 above]

Table 3: Drugs that are Contraindicated with INCIVEK

Drug Class	Drugs within Class that are Contraindicated with INCIVEK	Clinical Comments
Alpha 1-adrenoreceptor antagonist	Alfuzosin	Potential for hypotension or cardiac arrhythmia
Antimycobacterials	Rifampin	Rifampin significantly reduces telaprevir plasma concentrations.
Ergot derivatives	Dihydroergotamine, ergonovine, ergotamine, methylergonovine	Potential for acute ergot toxicity characterized by peripheral vasospasm or ischemia
GI motility agent	Cisapride	Potential for cardiac arrhythmias
Herbal products	St. John's wort (*Hypericum perforatum*)	Plasma concentrations of telaprevir can be reduced by concomitant use of the herbal preparation St. John's wort.
HMG-CoA reductase inhibitors	Lovastatin, simvastatin	Potential for myopathy including rhabdomyolysis
Neuroleptic	Pimozide	Potential for serious and/or life-threatening adverse reactions such as cardiac arrhythmias
PDE5 inhibitor	Sildenafil (Revatio®) or tadalafil (Adcirca®) [for treatment of pulmonary arterial hypertension]*	Potential for PDE5 inhibitor-associated adverse events, including visual abnormalities, hypotension, prolonged erection, and syncope
Sedatives/hypnotics	Orally administered midazolam†, triazolam	Prolonged or increased sedation or respiratory depression

* See *Drug Interactions, Table 5* for co-administration of sildenafil and tadalafil when dosed for erectile dysfunction.
† See *Drug Interactions, Table 5* for parenterally administered midazolam.

5 WARNINGS AND PRECAUTIONS

5.1 Serious Skin Reactions/Rash

Fatal and non-fatal serious skin reactions, including Stevens Johnson Syndrome (SJS), Drug Reaction with Eosinophilia and Systemic Symptoms (DRESS), and Toxic Epidermal Necrolysis (TEN), have been reported in patients treated with INCIVEK combination treatment. Fatal cases have been reported in patients with progressive rash and systemic symptoms who continued to receive INCIVEK combination treatment after a serious skin reaction was identified.

For serious skin reactions, including rash with systemic symptoms or a progressive severe rash, INCIVEK, peginterferon alfa, and ribavirin must be discontinued immediately. Discontinuing other medications known to be associated with serious skin reactions should be considered. Patients should be promptly referred for urgent medical care.

In clinical trials, serious skin reactions, including DRESS and SJS were reported in less than 1% of subjects who received INCIVEK combination treatment compared to none who received peginterferon alfa and ribavirin alone. These serious skin reactions required hospitalization, and all subjects recovered. The presenting signs of DRESS may include rash, fever, facial edema, and evidence of internal organ involvement (e.g., hepatitis, nephritis). Eosinophilia may or may not be present. The presenting signs of SJS may include fever, target lesions, and mucosal erosions or ulcerations (e.g., conjunctivae, lips).

TEN and Erythema Multiforme (EM) have been observed in post-marketing experience [*see also Boxed Warning and Adverse Reactions (6.2)*].

Rash events (all grades) developed in 56% of subjects who received INCIVEK combination treatment [see *Adverse Reactions (6.1)*] and in 34% of subjects who received peginterferon alfa and ribavirin. Rash most frequently began during the first 4 weeks, but could occur at any time during INCIVEK combination treatment. Rash events led to discontinuation of INCIVEK alone in 6% of subjects and discontinuation of INCIVEK combination treatment in 1% of subjects. Severe rash (e.g., a generalized rash or rash with vesicles or bullae or ulcerations other than SJS) was reported in 4% of subjects who received INCIVEK combination treatment compared to less than 1% who received peginterferon alfa and ribavirin alone. The severe rash may have a prominent eczematous component.

Patients with mild to moderate rashes should be followed for progression of rash or development of systemic symptoms. If rash progresses and becomes severe, INCIVEK should be discontinued. Peginterferon alfa and ribavirin may be continued. If improvement is not observed within 7 days of INCIVEK discontinuation, sequential or simultaneous interruption or discontinuation of ribavirin and/or peginterferon alfa should be considered. If medically indicated, earlier interruption or discontinuation of ribavirin and peginterferon alfa should be considered [*see also Boxed Warning*]. Patients should be monitored until the rash has resolved. INCIVEK must not be reduced or restarted if discontinued due to rash. Treatment of rash with oral antihistamines and/or topical corticosteroids may provide symptomatic relief but effectiveness of these measures has not been established. Treatment of rash with systemic corticosteroids is not recommended [*see Drug Interactions (7)*].

5.2 Anemia

Anemia has been reported with peginterferon alfa and ribavirin therapy. The addition of INCIVEK to peginterferon alfa and ribavirin is associated with an additional decrease in hemoglobin concentrations. A decrease in hemoglobin levels occurred during the first 4 weeks of treatment, with lowest values reached at the end of INCIVEK dosing. Hemoglobin values gradually returned to levels observed with peginterferon alfa and ribavirin after INCIVEK dosing was completed. Hemoglobin values less than or equal to 10 g per dL were observed in 36% of subjects who received INCIVEK combination treatment compared to 17% of subjects who received peginterferon alfa and ribavirin. In clinical trials, the median time to onset of hemoglobin less than or equal to 10 g per dL was faster among subjects treated with INCIVEK combination treatment compared to those who received peginterferon alfa and ribavirin: 56 days (range 8-365 days) versus 63 days (range 13-341 days), respectively. Hemoglobin values less than 8.5 g per dL were observed in 14% of subjects who received INCIVEK combination treatment compared to 5% of subjects receiving peginterferon alfa and ribavirin.

In subjects receiving INCIVEK combination treatment, 32% underwent a ribavirin dose modification (reduction, interruption or discontinuation) due to anemia, 6% received a blood transfusion, 4% discontinued INCIVEK, and 1% discontinued INCIVEK combination treatment. In subjects treated with peginterferon alfa and ribavirin alone, 12% underwent ribavirin dose modification due to anemia, 1% received a blood transfusion, and fewer than 1% discontinued treatment. Anemia requiring ribavirin dose reduction, blood transfusion, and/or erythropoiesis stimulating agent (ESA) has been reported to occur as soon as 10 days following initiation of INCIVEK combination treatment.

Hemoglobin should be monitored prior to and at least at weeks 2, 4, 8 and 12 during INCIVEK combination treatment and as clinically appropriate. Earlier and more frequent monitoring for some patients should be considered. For the management of anemia, ribavirin dose reductions should be used (refer to the prescribing information for ribavirin for its dose reduction guidelines). If ribavirin dose reductions are inadequate, discontinuation of INCIVEK should be considered. If ribavirin is permanently discontinued for the management of anemia, INCIVEK must also be permanently discontinued. Ribavirin may be restarted per the dosing modification guidelines for ribavirin. The dose of INCIVEK must not be reduced and INCIVEK must not be restarted if discontinued.

5.3 Pregnancy: Use with Ribavirin and Peginterferon Alfa

Ribavirin may cause birth defects and/or death of the exposed fetus. Extreme care must be taken to avoid pregnancy in female patients and in female partners of male patients. Ribavirin therapy should not be started unless a report of a negative pregnancy test has been obtained immediately prior to initiation of therapy.

Because INCIVEK must be used in combination with peginterferon alfa and ribavirin, the contraindications and warnings applicable to those drugs are applicable to combination therapy. Female patients of childbearing potential and their male partners as well as male patients and their female partners must use 2 effective contraceptive methods during treatment and for 6 months after all treatment has ended. Female patients should have monthly pregnancy tests during treatment and during the 6-month period after stopping treatment. Extreme care must be taken to avoid pregnancy in female patients and in female partners of male patients as significant teratogenic and/or embryocidal effects have been demonstrated in all animal species exposed to ribavirin [*see Contraindications (4), Use in Specific Populations (8.1), and Patient Counseling Information (17.2)*]. Refer also to the prescribing information for ribavirin.

Female Patients

Hormonal contraceptives may be continued but may not be reliable during INCIVEK dosing and for up to 2 weeks following cessation of INCIVEK [see *Drug Interactions (7)*]. During this time, female patients of childbearing potential should use 2 effective non-hormonal methods of contraception. Examples may include barrier methods or intrauterine devices (IUDs) [*see also Use in Specific Populations: Pregnancy (8.1) and Patient Counseling Information (17.2)*]. Two weeks after completion of INCIVEK treatment, hormonal contraceptives are again appropriate as one of the 2 required effective methods of birth control; however, specific prescribing information recommendations should be followed for the contraceptives.

5.4 Drug Interactions

See Table 3 for a listing of drugs that are contraindicated for use with INCIVEK due to potentially life-threatening adverse events or potential loss of therapeutic effect to INCIVEK [*see Contraindications (4)*]. Refer to Table 5 for established and other potentially significant drug-drug interactions [*see Drug Interactions (7)*].

5.5 Laboratory Tests

HCV RNA levels should be monitored at weeks 4 and 12 and as clinically indicated. Use of a sensitive real-time RT-PCR assay for monitoring HCV RNA levels during treatment is recommended. The assay should have a lower limit of HCV RNA quantification equal to or less than 25 IU per mL and a limit of HCV RNA detection of approximately 10-15 IU per mL. For the purpose of assessing response-guided therapy eligibility, an "undetectable" HCV RNA (Target Not Detected) result is required; a confirmed "detectable but below limit of quantification" HCV RNA result should not be considered equivalent to an "undetectable" HCV RNA result (reported as "Target Not Detected" or "HCV RNA Not Detected").

Hematology evaluations (including hemoglobin, white cell differential, and platelet count) are recommended prior to and at weeks 2, 4, 8 and 12 and as clinically appropriate. Chemistry evaluations (including electrolytes, serum creatinine, uric acid, hepatic enzymes, bilirubin, and TSH) are recommended as frequently as hematology evaluations or as clinically appropriate [*see Adverse Reactions (6)*].

Refer to the prescribing information for peginterferon alfa and ribavirin, including pregnancy testing requirements.

5.6 General

INCIVEK must not be administered as monotherapy and must only be prescribed with both peginterferon alfa and ribavirin. Therefore, the prescribing information for peginterferon alfa and ribavirin must be consulted before starting treatment with INCIVEK.

There are no clinical data on re-treating patients who have failed an HCV NS3/4A protease inhibitor-based treatment, nor are there data on repeated courses of INCIVEK [*see Microbiology (12.4)*].

5.7 Hepatic Impairment

INCIVEK is not recommended for patients with moderate or severe hepatic impairment (Child-Pugh B or C, score greater than or equal to 7) or patients with decompensated liver disease. Refer to prescribing information for peginterferon alfa and ribavirin which must be co-administered with INCIVEK [*see Use in Specific Populations: Hepatic Impairment (8.6)*].

6 ADVERSE REACTIONS

The following adverse reactions are discussed in greater detail in other sections of the label:

- Serious Skin Reactions/Rash [*see Boxed Warning and Warnings and Precautions (5.1)*]
- Anemia [*see Warnings and Precautions (5.2)*]
- Pregnancy: Use with Ribavirin and Peginterferon alfa [*see Contraindications (4), Warnings and Precautions (5.3), Use in Specific Populations (8.1), and Patient Counseling Information (17.2)*]

INCIVEK must be administered with peginterferon alfa and ribavirin. Refer to their respective prescribing information for their associated adverse reactions.

6.1 Clinical Trials Experience

Because clinical trials are conducted under widely varying conditions, adverse reaction rates observed in the clinical trials of a drug cannot be directly compared to rates in the clinical trials of another drug and may not reflect the rates observed in clinical practice.

The safety assessment is based on data from pooled adequate and well-controlled clinical trials including 1797 subjects who received INCIVEK combination treatment and 493 who received peginterferon alfa and ribavirin.

Serious adverse drug reactions occurred in 3% of subjects who received INCIVEK combination treatment compared to none of the subjects treated with peginterferon alfa and ribavirin. The most frequent serious adverse events in subjects treated with INCIVEK combination treatment were skin disorders (rash and/or pruritus) and anemia [*see Warnings and Precautions (5.1 and 5.2)*]. Fourteen percent of subjects discontinued INCIVEK due to adverse drug reactions. Rash, anemia, fatigue, pruritus, nausea, and vomiting were the most frequent adverse drug reactions leading to discontinuation of INCIVEK.

INCIVEK was administered in combination with peginterferon alfa and ribavirin. The following table lists adverse drug reactions that occurred in subjects treated with INCIVEK with an incidence at least 5% greater than in subjects receiving peginterferon alfa and ribavirin alone (Table 4).

Table 4: Clinical Adverse Drug Reactions Reported with at Least 5% Higher Frequency Among Subjects Receiving INCIVEK

	INCIVEK, peginterferon alfa, and ribavirin Combination Treatment N=1797	Peginterferon alfa and ribavirin N=493
Rash*	56%	34%
Fatigue	56%	50%
Pruritus	47%	28%
Nausea	39%	28%
Anemia*	36%	17%
Diarrhea	26%	17%
Vomiting	13%	8%
Hemorrhoids	12%	3%
Anorectal discomfort	11%	3%
Dysgeusia	10%	3%
Anal pruritus	6%	1%

* Rash and anemia based on SSC (Special Search Category) grouped terms.

Description of Selected Adverse Drug Reactions

Anorectal Signs and Symptoms

In the controlled clinical trials, 29% of subjects treated with INCIVEK combination treatment experienced anorectal adverse events, compared to 7% of those treated with peginterferon alfa and ribavirin alone. The majority of these events (e.g., hemorrhoids, anorectal discomfort, anal pruritus, and rectal burning) were mild to moderate in severity; less than 1% led to treatment discontinuation and all resolved during or after completion of INCIVEK dosing.

Laboratory abnormalities

White Blood Cells: Treatment with peginterferon alfa is associated with decreases in mean values for total white blood cell, absolute neutrophil, and absolute lymphocyte count. More subjects treated with INCIVEK had decreases in lymphocyte counts to 499/mm^3 or less (15% compared to 5%). Decreases in total white cell counts to 1,499/mm^3 or less were comparable (8% compared to 5%). The incidence of decreases in absolute neutrophil counts to 749/mm^3 or less was 15% in subjects treated with peginterferon alfa and ribavirin alone compared to 12% among those treated with INCIVEK combination treatment.

Platelets: Treatment with peginterferon alfa is associated with decreases in mean platelet counts. More patients treated with INCIVEK combination treatment had decreases in mean platelet values of all grades: 47% compared to 36% treated with peginterferon alfa and ribavirin alone. Three percent of INCIVEK combination treatment subjects had decreases to 49,999/mm^3 or less compared to 1% of those treated with peginterferon alfa and ribavirin-treated alone.

Bilirubin: Forty one percent of subjects treated with INCIVEK compared to 28% of peginterferon alfa and ribavirin-treated subjects had all grade elevations in bilirubin levels; 4% and 2% of subjects, respectively, had greater than or equal to 2.6 × ULN elevations. Bilirubin levels increased most steeply during the first 1 to 2 weeks of INCIVEK dosing, stabilized and between Weeks 12 and 16 were at baseline levels.

Uric Acid: During the INCIVEK combination treatment period, 73% of subjects had elevated uric acid levels compared to 29% for those treated with peginterferon alfa and ribavirin alone. Shifts to greater than or equal to 12.1 mg per dL from baseline in uric acid levels were also more frequent among subjects treated with INCIVEK (7%) compared to peginterferon alfa and ribavirin (1%). Less than 1% of subjects had clinical events of gout/gouty arthritis; none were serious and none resulted in treatment discontinuation.

6.2 Post-marketing Experience

The following adverse reactions have been identified during post-approval use of INCIVEK. Because these reactions are reported voluntarily from a population of uncertain size, it is not always possible to reliably estimate their frequency or establish a causal relationship to drug exposure.

Skin and Subcutaneous Tissue Disorders: Toxic Epidermal Necrolysis (TEN) and Erythema Multiforme (EM) [*see also Boxed Warning and Warnings and Precautions (5.1)*]

Renal and Urinary Disorders: Pre-renal azotemia with or without acute renal insufficiency/failure, uric acid nephropathy

7 DRUG INTERACTIONS

7.1 Potential for INCIVEK to Affect Other Drugs

INCIVEK is a strong inhibitor of CYP3A. Co-administration of INCIVEK with drugs that are primarily metabolized by CYP3A may result in increased plasma concentrations of such drugs, which could increase adverse reactions (see Table 5). INCIVEK is also an inhibitor of P-gp, OATP1B1, and OATP2B1. Co-administration of INCIVEK with drugs that are substrates for P-gp, OATP1B1, and OATP2B1 transport may result in increased plasma concentrations of such drugs, which could increase adverse reactions (see Table 5). **If dose adjustments of concomitant medications are made during INCIVEK treatment, they should be re-adjusted after administration of INCIVEK is completed.**

7.2 Potential for Other Drugs to Affect INCIVEK

INCIVEK is a substrate of CYP3A and P-gp; therefore, drugs that induce CYP3A and/or P-gp may decrease INCIVEK plasma concentrations and reduce the therapeutic effect of INCIVEK. Co-administration of INCIVEK with drugs that inhibit CYP3A and/or P-gp may increase INCIVEK plasma concentrations.

7.3 Established and Other Potentially Significant Drug Interactions

Table 5 provides effect of concentration of INCIVEK or concomitant drug with INCIVEK. These recommendations are based on either drug interaction trials (indicated with *) or predicted interactions due to the expected magnitude of interaction and potential for serious adverse events or loss of efficacy.

[See table 5 on pages 2441 through 2444]

In addition to the drugs included in Table 5, the interaction between INCIVEK and the following drugs was evaluated in clinical trials and no dose adjustment is needed for any drug [*see Clinical Pharmacology (12.3)*]: esomeprazole, raltegravir, or buprenorphine.

8 USE IN SPECIFIC POPULATIONS

8.1 Pregnancy

Because INCIVEK must be used in combination with ribavirin and peginterferon alfa, the contraindications and warnings applicable to those drugs are applicable to combination treatment. Extreme care must be taken to avoid pregnancy in female patients and in female partners of male patients.

INCIVEK/Peginterferon Alfa/Ribavirin Combination Treatment

Pregnancy Category X: Animal studies have shown that ribavirin causes birth defects and/or fetal deaths while peginterferon alfa is abortifacient [*see Contraindications (4) and Warnings and Precautions (5.3)*]. See the prescribing information for ribavirin.

Significant teratogenic and/or embryocidal effects have been demonstrated in all animal species exposed to ribavirin; and therefore ribavirin is contraindicated in women who are pregnant and in the male partners of women who are pregnant [*see Contraindications (4), Warnings and Precautions (5.3) and ribavirin prescribing information*]. Interferons have abortifacient effects in animals and should be assumed to have abortifacient potential in humans (see peginterferon alfa prescribing information).

Extreme caution must be taken to avoid pregnancy in female patients and female partners of male patients while taking this combination. Women of childbearing potential and their male partners should not receive ribavirin unless they are using effective contraception (2 reliable forms) during treatment with ribavirin and for 6 months after treatment. Systemic hormonal contraceptives may not be as effective in women while taking INCIVEK. Therefore, 2 alternative effective methods of contraception, including intrauterine devices and barrier methods, should be used in women during treatment with INCIVEK and concomitant ribavirin [*see Warnings and Precautions (5.3)*].

A Ribavirin Pregnancy Registry has been established to monitor maternal-fetal outcomes of pregnancies in female patients and female partners of male patients exposed to ribavirin during treatment and for 6 months following cessation of treatment. Health care providers and patients are encouraged to report such cases by calling 1-800-593-2214.

INCIVEK (telaprevir) Tablets

Pregnancy Category B: Telaprevir treatment alone in mice and rats did not result in harm to the fetus. The highest doses tested produced exposures equal to 1.84- and 0.60-fold the exposures in humans at the recommended clinical dose, respectively. Telaprevir treatment alone had effects on fertility parameters in rats. The no observed adverse effect level (NOAEL) for testicular toxicity was established at exposures 0.17-fold the human exposures at the recommended clinical dose. Potential effects on sperm (e.g., decreased %

motile sperm and increased non-motile sperm count) were observed in a rat fertility study at exposures 0.30-fold the human exposures at the recommended clinical dose. Additional effects on fertility include minor increases in percent preimplantation loss, in percent of dams with nonviable embryos and percent of nonviable conceptuses per litter. These effects are likely associated with testicular toxicity in male but contributions of the female cannot be ruled out. There are, however, no adequate and well-controlled trials in pregnant women.

Significant teratogenic and/or embryocidal effects have been demonstrated in all animal species exposed to ribavirin. Extreme care must be taken to avoid pregnancy in female patients and in female partners of male patients—both during treatment and for 6 months after the completion of all treatment. INCIVEK combination treatment should not be started unless a female patient has a negative pregnancy test immediately prior to initiation of treatment. Pregnancy testing should occur monthly during INCIVEK combination treatment and for 6 months after all treatment has ended [*see Contraindications (4) and Patient Counseling Information (17.2)*]. Pregnancy testing in non-pregnant female partners is recommended before INCIVEK combination therapy, every month during INCIVEK combination therapy, and for 6 months after ribavirin therapy has ended.

Hormonal contraceptives may be continued but may not be reliable during INCIVEK dosing and for up to 2 weeks following cessation of INCIVEK [*see Drug Interactions (7)*]. During this time, female patients of childbearing potential should use 2 effective non-hormonal methods of contraception. Examples may include barrier methods or IUDs [*see also Warnings and Precautions (5.3) and Patient Counseling Information (17.2)*]. Refer also to the prescribing information for ribavirin.

Two weeks after completion of INCIVEK treatment, hormonal contraceptives are again appropriate as one of the 2 required effective methods of birth control; however, specific prescribing information recommendations should be followed for the contraceptives. Refer also to the prescribing information for ribavirin.

8.3 Nursing Mothers

It is not known whether telaprevir is excreted in human breast milk. When administered to lactating rats, levels of telaprevir were higher in milk compared to those observed in plasma. Rat offspring exposed to telaprevir in utero showed no effects on body weight at birth. However, when fed via milk from telaprevir-treated dams, body weight gain of pups was lower than pups fed milk from control dams. After weaning, rat pup body weight gain was similar in offspring from telaprevir-treated and control dams. Because of the potential for adverse reactions in nursing infants, nursing must be discontinued prior to initiation of treatment. See also the prescribing information for ribavirin.

8.4 Pediatric Use

The safety, efficacy and pharmacokinetic profile of INCIVEK in pediatric patients have not been established.

8.5 Geriatric Use

Clinical trials of INCIVEK did not include sufficient numbers of subjects aged 65 and over to determine whether they respond differently from younger subjects. In general, caution should be exercised in the administration and monitoring of INCIVEK in geriatric patients reflecting the greater frequency of decreased hepatic function, and of concomitant disease or other drug therapy [*see Clinical Pharmacology (12.3)*].

8.6 Hepatic Impairment

INCIVEK is not recommended for use in patients with moderate or severe hepatic impairment (Child-Pugh B or C, score greater than or equal to 7) because no pharmacokinetic or safety data are available regarding the use of INCIVEK in HCV-infected patients with moderate or severe hepatic impairment, and appropriate doses have not been established [*see Warnings and Precautions (5.7) and Clinical Pharmacology (12.3)*]. No dose adjustment of INCIVEK is necessary for patients with mild hepatic impairment (Child-Pugh A, score 5-6). Refer also to the prescribing information for peginterferon alfa and ribavirin which must be co-administered with INCIVEK.

8.7 Renal Impairment

No dose adjustment is necessary for INCIVEK in HCV-infected patients with mild, moderate or severe renal impairment. INCIVEK has not been studied in HCV-infected patients with CrCl less than or equal to 50 mL per min.

The pharmacokinetics of telaprevir were assessed after administration of a single dose of 750 mg to HCV-negative subjects with severe renal impairment (CrCl less than 30 mL per min). INCIVEK has not been studied in subjects with end-stage renal disease (ESRD) or on hemodialysis [*see Clinical Pharmacology (12.3)*]. Refer also to the prescribing information for peginterferon alfa and ribavirin which must be co-administered with INCIVEK.

8.8 Co-infection

The safety and efficacy of INCIVEK have not been established in patients co-infected with HCV/HIV or HCV/HBV [*see Drug Interactions (7)*].

Table 5: Established and Other Potentially Significant Drug Interactions: Alterations in Dose or Regimen May Be Recommended Based on Drug Interaction Trials or Predicted Interaction [See Clinical Pharmacology (12.3) (Tables 6 and 7) for Magnitude of Interaction.]

Concomitant Drug Class: Drug Name	Effect on concentration of INCIVEK or Concomitant Drug	Clinical Comment
ANTIARRHYTHMICS		
lidocaine (systemic), amiodarone, bepridil, flecainide, propafenone, quinidine	↑ antiarrhythmics	Co-administration with telaprevir has the potential to produce serious and/or life-threatening adverse events and has not been studied. Caution is warranted and clinical monitoring is recommended when co-administered with telaprevir.
digoxin*	↑ digoxin	Concentrations of digoxin were increased when co-administered with telaprevir. The lowest dose of digoxin should be initially prescribed. The serum digoxin concentrations should be monitored and used for titration of digoxin dose to obtain the desired clinical effect.
ANTIBACTERIALS		
clarithromycin erythromycin telithromycin	↑ telaprevir ↑ antibacterials	Concentrations of both telaprevir and the antibacterial may be increased during co-administration. Caution is warranted and clinical monitoring is recommended when co-administered with telaprevir. QT interval prolongation and Torsade de Pointes have been reported with clarithromycin and erythromycin. QT interval prolongation has been reported with telithromycin.
ANTICOAGULANT		
warfarin	↑ or ↓ warfarin	Concentrations of warfarin may be altered when co-administered with telaprevir. The international normalized ratio (INR) should be monitored when warfarin is co-administered with telaprevir.
ANTICONVULSANTS		
carbamazepine phenobarbital phenytoin	↓ telaprevir ↑ carbamazepine ↑ or ↓ phenytoin ↑ or ↓ phenobarbital	Concentrations of the anticonvulsant may be altered and concentrations of telaprevir may be decreased. Caution should be used when prescribing carbamazepine, phenobarbital, and phenytoin. Telaprevir may be less effective in patients taking these agents concomitantly. Clinical or laboratory monitoring of carbamazepine, phenobarbital, and phenytoin concentrations and dose titration are recommended to achieve the desired clinical response.
ANTIDEPRESSANTS		
escitalopram*	↔ telaprevir ↓ escitalopram	Concentrations of escitalopram were decreased when co-administered with telaprevir. Selective serotonin reuptake inhibitors such as escitalopram have a wide therapeutic index, but doses may need to be adjusted when combined with telaprevir.
trazodone	↑ trazodone	Concomitant use of trazodone and telaprevir may increase plasma concentrations of trazodone which may lead to adverse events such as nausea, dizziness, hypotension and syncope. If trazodone is used with telaprevir, the combination should be used with caution and a lower dose of trazodone should be considered.
ANTIFUNGALS		
ketoconazole* itraconazole posaconazole voriconazole	↑ ketoconazole ↑ telaprevir ↑ itraconazole ↑ posaconazole ↑ or ↓ voriconazole	Ketoconazole increases the plasma concentrations of telaprevir. Concomitant systemic use of itraconazole or posaconazole with telaprevir may increase plasma concentration of telaprevir. Plasma concentrations of itraconazole, ketoconazole, or posaconazole may be increased in the presence of telaprevir. When co-administration is required, high doses of itraconazole or ketoconazole (greater than 200 mg/day) are not recommended. Caution is warranted and clinical monitoring is recommended for itraconazole, posaconazole and voriconazole. QT interval prolongation and Torsade de Pointes have been reported with voriconazole and posaconazole. QT interval prolongation has been reported with ketoconazole. Due to multiple enzymes involved with voriconazole metabolism, it is difficult to predict the interaction with telaprevir. Voriconazole should not be administered to patients receiving telaprevir unless an assessment of the benefit/risk ratio justifies its use.

(Table continued on next page)

8.9 Solid Organ Transplantation

The safety and efficacy of INCIVEK have not been established in solid organ transplant patients [*see Drug Interactions (7)*].

10 OVERDOSAGE

The highest documented dose administered is 1875 mg every 8 hours for 4 days in healthy subjects with INCIVEK alone. In that trial, the following common adverse events were reported more frequently with the 1875 mg q8h regimen compared to the 750 mg q8h regimen: nausea, headache, diarrhea, decreased appetite, dysgeusia, and vomiting.

No specific antidote is available for overdose with INCIVEK. Treatment of overdose with INCIVEK consists of general supportive measures including monitoring of vital signs and observation of the clinical status of the patient. In the event of an overdose, it is reasonable to employ the standard supportive measures, such as, removing unabsorbed material from the gastrointestinal tract, employing clinical monitoring (including obtaining an electrocardiogram), and instituting supportive therapy if required.

It is not known whether telaprevir is dialyzable by peritoneal or hemodialysis.

11 DESCRIPTION

INCIVEK (telaprevir) is an inhibitor of the HCV NS3/4A protease.

The IUPAC name for telaprevir is (1*S*,3a*R*,6a*S*)-2-[(2*S*)-2-({(2*S*)-2-cyclohexyl-2-[(pyrazin-2-ylcarbonyl)amino]acetyl} amino)-3,3-dimethylbutanoyl]-*N*-[(3*S*)-1-(cyclopropylamino)-1,2-dioxohexan-3-yl]-3,3a,4,5,6,6a-hexahydro-1H-cyclopenta[c]pyrrole-1-carboxamide. Its molecular formula is $C_{36}H_{53}N_7O_6$ and its molecular weight is 679.85. Telaprevir has the following structural formula:

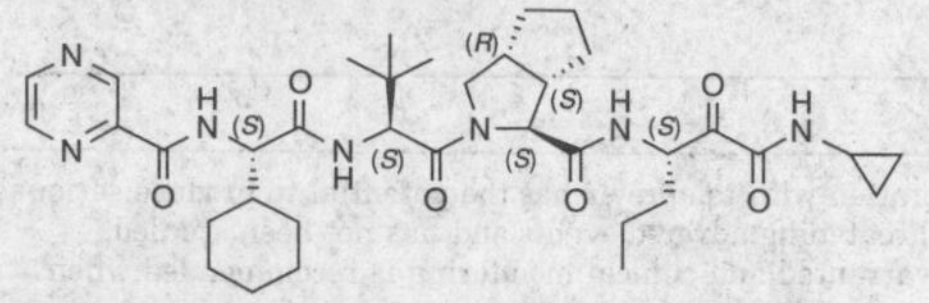

Telaprevir drug substance is a white to off-white powder with a solubility in water of 0.0047 mg/mL.

Telaprevir interconverts to an *R*-diastereomer, VRT-127394, which is the major metabolite in plasma and is approximately 30-fold less potent than telaprevir.

INCIVEK is available as a purple, capsule-shaped, film-coated tablet for oral administration containing 375 mg of telaprevir. Each tablet contains the inactive ingredients colloidal silicon dioxide, croscarmellose sodium, D&C Red No. 40, dibasic calcium phosphate (anhydrous), FD&C Blue No. 2, hypromellose acetate succinate, microcrystalline cellulose, polyethylene glycol, polyvinyl alcohol, sodium lauryl sulfate, sodium stearyl fumarate, talc, and titanium dioxide.

12 CLINICAL PHARMACOLOGY

12.1 Mechanism of Action

Telaprevir is a direct-acting antiviral (DAA) agent against the hepatitis C virus [*see Microbiology (12.4)*].

12.2 Pharmacodynamics

ECG Evaluation

The effect of telaprevir 750 and 1875 mg on QTc interval was evaluated in a double-blind, double-dummy, randomized, placebo-, and active-controlled (moxifloxacin 400 mg) four period crossover thorough QT trial in 44 subjects. In the trial with demonstrated ability to detect small effects, the upper bound of the one-sided 95% confidence interval for the largest placebo adjusted, baseline-corrected QTc based on Fridericia correction method (QTcF) was below 10 ms, the threshold for regulatory concern. The dose of 1875 mg is adequate to represent the high exposure clinical scenario.

12.3 Pharmacokinetics

The pharmacokinetic properties of telaprevir have been evaluated in healthy adult subjects and in subjects with chronic hepatitis C. Following multiple doses of telaprevir (750 mg q8h) in combination with peginterferon alfa and ribavirin in treatment-naïve subjects with genotype 1 chronic hepatitis C, mean (SD) C_{max} was 3510 (1280) ng/mL, C_{min} was 2030 (930) ng/mL, and AUC_{8h} was 22,300 (8650) ng•hr/mL.

Absorption and Bioavailability

Telaprevir is orally available, most likely absorbed in the small intestine, with no evidence for absorption in the colon. Maximum plasma concentrations after a single dose of telaprevir are generally achieved after 4 to 5 hours. *In vitro* studies performed with human Caco-2 cells indicated that telaprevir is a substrate of P-glycoprotein (P-gp). Exposure to telaprevir is higher during co-administration of peginterferon alfa and ribavirin than after administration of telaprevir alone.

Effects of Food on Oral Absorption

The systemic exposure (AUC) to telaprevir was increased by 237% when telaprevir was administered with a standard fat meal (containing 533 kcal and 21 g fat) compared to when telaprevir was administered under fasting conditions. In addition, the type of meal significantly affects exposure to telaprevir. Relative to fasting, when telaprevir was administered with a low-fat meal (249 kcal, 3.6 g fat) and a high-fat meal (928 kcal, 56 g fat), the systemic exposure (AUC) to telaprevir was increased by approximately 117% and 330%, respectively. Doses of INCIVEK were administered within 30 minutes of completing a meal or snack containing approximately 20 grams of fat in the Phase 3 trials. Therefore, INCIVEK should always be taken with food (not low fat).

Distribution

In vitro, within a concentration range of 0.1 µM (68 ng per mL) to 20 µM (13600 ng per mL), telaprevir is approximately 59% to 76% bound to plasma proteins. Telaprevir binds primarily to alpha 1-acid glycoprotein and albumin and the binding is concentration dependent, decreasing with increasing concentrations of telaprevir. After oral administration, the typical apparent volume of distribution (Vd/F) was estimated to be 252 L, with an inter-individual variability of 72%.

Metabolism

Telaprevir is extensively metabolized in the liver, involving hydrolysis, oxidation, and reduction. Multiple metabolites were detected in feces, plasma, and urine. After repeated-oral administration, the R-diastereomer of telaprevir (30-

Table 5 *(cont.)*: Established and Other Potentially Significant Drug Interactions: Alterations in Dose or Regimen May Be Recommended Based on Drug Interaction Trials or Predicted Interaction [See Clinical Pharmacology (12.3) (Tables 6 and 7) for Magnitude of Interaction.]

Concomitant Drug Class: Drug Name	Effect on concentration of INCIVEK or Concomitant Drug	Clinical Comment
ANTI GOUT		
colchicine	↑ colchicine	Patients with renal or hepatic impairment should not be given colchicine with telaprevir, due to the risk of colchicine toxicity. A reduction in colchicine dosage or an interruption of colchicine treatment is recommended in patients with normal renal or hepatic function. Treatment of gout flares: co-administration of colchicine in patients on telaprevir: 0.6 mg (1 tablet) for 1 dose, followed by 0.3 mg (half tablet) 1 hour later. Not to be repeated before 3 days. If used for prophylaxis of gout flares: co-administration of colchicine in patients on telaprevir: If the original regimen was 0.6 mg twice a day, the regimen should be adjusted to 0.3 mg once a day. If the original regimen was 0.6 mg once a day, the regimen should be adjusted to 0.3 mg once every other day. Treatment of familial Mediterranean fever (FMF): co-administration of colchicine in patients on telaprevir: Maximum daily dose of 0.6 mg (may be given as 0.3 mg twice a day).
ANTIMYCOBACTERIAL		
rifabutin	↓ telaprevir ↑ rifabutin	Concentrations of telaprevir may be decreased, while rifabutin concentrations may be increased during co-administration. Telaprevir may be less effective due to decreased concentrations. The concomitant use of rifabutin and telaprevir is not recommended.
BENZODIAZEPINES		
alprazolam*	↑ alprazolam	Concomitant use of alprazolam and telaprevir increases exposure to alprazolam. Clinical monitoring is warranted.
parenterally administered midazolam*	↑ midazolam	Concomitant use of parenterally administered midazolam with telaprevir increased exposure to midazolam. Co-administration should be done in a setting which ensures clinical monitoring and appropriate medical management in case of respiratory depression and/or prolonged sedation. Dose reduction for midazolam should be considered, especially if more than a single dose of midazolam is administered. Co-administration of oral midazolam with telaprevir is contraindicated.
zolpidem (non-benzodiazepine sedative)*	↓ zolpidem	Exposure to zolpidem was decreased when co-administered with telaprevir. Clinical monitoring and dose titration of zolpidem is recommended to achieve the desired clinical response.
CALCIUM CHANNEL BLOCKERS		
amlodipine*	↑ amlodipine	Exposure to amlodipine was increased when co-administered with telaprevir. Caution should be used and dose reduction for amlodipine should be considered. Clinical monitoring is recommended.
diltiazem felodipine nicardipine nifedipine nisoldipine verapamil	↑calcium channel blockers	Concentrations of other calcium channel blockers may be increased when telaprevir is co-administered. Caution is warranted and clinical monitoring of patients is recommended.
CORTICOSTEROIDS		
Systemic prednisone methylprednisolone	↑ prednisone ↑ methylprednisolone	Systemic corticosteroids such as prednisone and methylprednisolone are CYP3A substrates. Since telaprevir is a strong CYP3A inhibitor, plasma concentrations of these corticosteroids can be increased significantly. Co-administration of systemic corticosteroids and telaprevir is not recommended [*see Warnings and Precautions (5.1)*].
Systemic dexamethasone	↓ telaprevir	Systemic dexamethasone induces CYP3A and can thereby decrease telaprevir plasma concentrations. This may result in loss of therapeutic effect of telaprevir. Therefore this combination should be used with caution or alternatives should be considered.
Inhaled/Nasal fluticasone budesonide	↑fluticasone ↑ budesonide	Concomitant use of inhaled fluticasone or budesonide and telaprevir may increase plasma concentrations of fluticasone or budesonide resulting in significantly reduced serum cortisol concentrations. Co-administration of fluticasone or budesonide and telaprevir is not recommended unless the potential benefit to the patient outweighs the risk of systemic corticosteroid side effects.

(Table continued on next page)

fold less active), pyrazinoic acid, and a metabolite that underwent reduction at the α-ketoamide bond of telaprevir (not active) were found to be the predominant metabolites of telaprevir. *In vitro* studies using recombinant human cytochrome P450 (CYP) isoforms indicated that CYP3A4 was the major isoform responsible for CYP-mediated telaprevir metabolism. *In vitro* studies using recombinant aldo-ketoreductases indicated that these and potentially other reductases are also responsible for the reduction of telaprevir. Other proteolytic enzymes are also involved in the hydrolysis of telaprevir. These non-CYP mediated pathways of metabolism likely play a major role after multiple dosing of telaprevir.

Elimination

Following administration of a single oral dose of 750 mg ^{14}C-telaprevir in healthy subjects, 90% of total radioactivity was recovered in feces, urine and expired air within 96 hours post-dose. The median recovery of the administered radioactive dose was approximately 82% in the feces, 9% in exhaled air and 1% in urine. The contribution of unchanged ^{14}C-telaprevir and the R-diastereomer of telaprevir towards total radioactivity recovered in feces was 31.9% and 18.8%, respectively. After oral administration, the apparent total clearance (Cl/F) was estimated to be 32.4 L per hour with an inter-individual variability of 27.2%. The mean elimination half-life after single-dose oral administration of telaprevir 750 mg typically ranged from about 4.0 to 4.7 hours. At steady state, the effective half-life is about 9 to 11 hours.

Specific Populations

Hepatic Impairment

Steady-state exposure to telaprevir was reduced by 46% in HCV-negative subjects with moderate hepatic impairment (Child-Pugh Class B) compared to healthy subjects. The appropriate dose of INCIVEK in HCV-infected subjects with moderate or severe hepatic impairment has not been determined and therefore INCIVEK is not recommended in these populations.

Steady-state exposure to telaprevir was reduced by 15% in HCV-negative subjects with mild hepatic impairment (Child-Pugh Class A) compared to healthy subjects. Dose modification of INCIVEK is not required when administered to subjects with mild hepatic impairment. In previously treated subjects who had compensated liver disease and were treated with INCIVEK in combination with peginterferon alfa and ribavirin, subjects with cirrhosis had similar PK parameters compared to those without cirrhosis.

Renal Impairment

After administration of a single dose of 750 mg to HCV-negative subjects with severe renal impairment (CrCl less than 30 mL per min), the LS means of telaprevir C_{max} and AUC_{inf} were increased by 3% and 21%, respectively, compared to healthy subjects.

Gender

The effect of subject gender on telaprevir pharmacokinetics was evaluated using population pharmacokinetics of data from clinical trials of telaprevir. No dose adjustments are deemed necessary based on gender.

Race

Population pharmacokinetic analysis of telaprevir in HCV-infected subjects indicated that race had no apparent effect on the exposure to telaprevir.

Geriatric Use

Population pharmacokinetic analysis in HCV-infected subjects showed that within the age range (19-70 years) investigated (35 subjects 65 years of age and older), subject age did not have a clinically relevant effect on the exposure to telaprevir.

Pediatric Use

The pharmacokinetics of INCIVEK in pediatric patients have not been evaluated.

Drug Interactions

In vitro studies indicated that telaprevir is a substrate and a strong inhibitor of CYP3A and P-gp. *In vitro* studies indicated that telaprevir is also an inhibitor of OATP1B1 and OATP2B1. No inhibition by telaprevir of CYP1A2, CYP2A6, CYP2B6, CYP2C8, CYP2C9, CYP2C19, CYP2D6, or CYP2E1 isozymes was observed *in vitro*. *In vitro* studies also suggest that telaprevir does not induce CYP1A, CYP3A, CYP2B6, or CYP2C. Furthermore, *in vitro* studies suggest that telaprevir is neither a substrate for BCRP, OATP1B1, OATP2B1, or MRP2, nor an inhibitor of BCRP, MRP2, OCT2, and OAT1 transporters. Clinical trials were conducted to evaluate the effect of drugs that can affect or be affected by telaprevir during co-administration (Tables 6 and 7).

[See table 6 on pages 2444 and 2445]
[See table 7 on pages 2446 and 2447]

12.4 Microbiology

Mechanism of Action

Telaprevir is an inhibitor of the HCV NS3/4A serine protease, necessary for the proteolytic cleavage of the HCV encoded polyprotein into mature forms of the NS4A, NS4B, NS5A and NS5B proteins and essential for viral replication. In a biochemical assay, telaprevir inhibited the proteolytic activity of the recombinant HCV NS3 protease domain with an IC_{50} value of 10 nM.

Antiviral Activity in Cell Culture

In an HCV subtype 1b replicon assay, the telaprevir EC_{50} value against wild-type HCV was 354 nM in a 2-day cell culture assay, and in a subtype 1a infectious virus assay, the EC_{50} value was 280 nM in a 5-day cell culture assay. In biochemical enzymatic assays, the median IC_{50} values of telaprevir against genotype 2, 3a, and 4a were 16 nM (range 6-32 nM; n=5), 40 nM (range 39-88 nM; n=5), and 130 nM (n=1), respectively, compared to a median IC_{50} value of 20 nM (range 16-23; n=2) for genotype 1a and 20 nM for genotype 1b (range 13-33; n=4). The presence of 40% human serum reduced the anti-HCV activity of telaprevir by approximately 10-fold. Evaluation of telaprevir in combination with interferon alfa or ribavirin showed no evidence of antagonism in reducing HCV RNA levels in HCV replicon cells.

Resistance

In Cell Culture

HCV genotype 1b replicons with reduced susceptibility to telaprevir have been selected in cell culture and characterized for telaprevir genotypic and phenotypic resistance. Additionally, resistance to telaprevir was evaluated in both biochemical and HCV genotype 1b replicon assays using site-directed mutants and recombinant NS3/4A from telaprevir Phase 2 clinical trials isolates. Variants V36A/M, T54A/S, R155K/T, A156S, R155T+D168N, and V36A+T54A conferred 3- to 25-fold reduced susceptibility to telaprevir; and A156V/T variants and the V36M/A+R155K/T and T54S/A+A156S/T double variants conferred greater than 62-fold reduced susceptibility to telaprevir. No amino acid substitutions were observed at the proteolytic cleavage sites.

Table 5 *(cont.)*: Established and Other Potentially Significant Drug Interactions: Alterations in Dose or Regimen May Be Recommended Based on Drug Interaction Trials or Predicted Interaction [See Clinical Pharmacology (12.3) (Tables 6 and 7) for Magnitude of Interaction.]

Concomitant Drug Class: Drug Name	Effect on concentration of INCIVEK or Concomitant Drug	Clinical Comment
ENDOTHELIN RECEPTOR ANTAGONIST		
bosentan	↑ bosentan	Concentrations of bosentan may be increased when co-administered with telaprevir. Caution is warranted and clinical monitoring is recommended.
HIV-ANTIVIRAL AGENTS: HIV-PROTEASE INHIBITORS (PIs)		
atazanavir/ritonavir*	↓ telaprevir ↑ atazanavir	Concomitant administration of telaprevir and atazanavir/ritonavir resulted in reduced steady-state telaprevir exposure, while steady-state atazanavir exposure was increased.
darunavir/ritonavir*	↓ telaprevir ↓ darunavir	Concomitant administration of telaprevir and darunavir/ritonavir resulted in reduced steady-state exposures to telaprevir and darunavir. It is not recommended to co-administer darunavir/ritonavir and telaprevir.
fosamprenavir/ritonavir*	↓ telaprevir ↓ fosamprenavir	Concomitant administration of telaprevir and fosamprenavir/ritonavir resulted in reduced steady-state exposures to telaprevir and amprenavir. It is not recommended to co-administer fosamprenavir/ritonavir and telaprevir.
lopinavir/ritonavir*	↓ telaprevir ↔ lopinavir	Concomitant administration of telaprevir and lopinavir/ritonavir resulted in reduced steady-state telaprevir exposure, while the steady-state exposure to lopinavir was not affected. It is not recommended to co-administer lopinavir/ritonavir and telaprevir.
HIV-ANTIVIRAL AGENTS: REVERSE TRANSCRIPTASE INHIBITORS		
efavirenz*	↓ telaprevir ↓ efavirenz	Concomitant administration of telaprevir and efavirenz resulted in reduced steady-state exposures to telaprevir and efavirenz.
tenofovir disoproxil fumarate*	↔ telaprevir ↑ tenofovir	Concomitant administration of telaprevir and tenofovir disoproxil fumarate resulted in increased tenofovir exposure. Increased clinical and laboratory monitoring are warranted. Tenofovir disoproxil fumarate should be discontinued in patients who develop tenofovir-associated toxicities.
HMG-CoA REDUCTASE INHIBITORS		
atorvastatin* fluvastatin pitavastatin pravastatin rosuvastatin	↑ statin	Plasma concentrations of atorvastatin are markedly increased when co-administered with telaprevir. Avoid concomitant administration of telaprevir and atorvastatin. For fluvastatin, pitavastatin, pravastatin, and rosuvastatin, caution is warranted and clinical monitoring is recommended. Refer to *Contraindications (4)* for HMG-CoA reductase inhibitors (lovastatin, simvastatin) that are contraindicated with INCIVEK.
HORMONAL CONTRACEPTIVES/ESTROGEN		
ethinyl estradiol* norethindrone	↓ ethinyl estradiol ↔ norethindrone	Exposure to ethinyl estradiol was decreased when co-administered with telaprevir. Two effective non-hormonal methods of contraception should be used during treatment with telaprevir. Patients using estrogens as hormone replacement therapy should be clinically monitored for signs of estrogen deficiency. Refer also to *Contraindications (4), Warnings and Precautions (5.3), Use in Specific Populations (8.1),* and *Patient Counseling Information (17.2).*
IMMUNOSUPPRESSANTS		
cyclosporine* sirolimus tacrolimus*	↑ cyclosporine ↑ sirolimus ↑ tacrolimus	Plasma concentrations of cyclosporine and tacrolimus are markedly increased when co-administered with telaprevir. Plasma concentration of sirolimus may be increased when co-administered with telaprevir, though this has not been studied. Significant dose reductions and prolongation of the dosing interval of the immunosuppressant to achieve the desired blood levels should be anticipated. Close monitoring of the immunosuppressant blood levels, and frequent assessments of renal function and immunosuppressant-related side effects are recommended when co-administered with telaprevir. Tacrolimus may prolong the QT interval. The use of telaprevir in organ transplant patients has not been studied.

(Table continued on next page)

Table 5 *(cont.)*: Established and Other Potentially Significant Drug Interactions: Alterations in Dose or Regimen May Be Recommended Based on Drug Interaction Trials or Predicted Interaction [See Clinical Pharmacology (12.3) (Tables 6 and 7) for Magnitude of Interaction.]

Concomitant Drug Class: Drug Name	Effect on concentration of INCIVEK or Concomitant Drug	Clinical Comment
INHALED BETA AGONIST		
salmeterol	↑ salmeterol	Concentrations of salmeterol may be increased when co-administered with telaprevir. Concurrent administration of salmeterol and telaprevir is not recommended. The combination may result in increased risk of cardiovascular adverse events associated with salmeterol, including QT prolongation, palpitations and sinus tachycardia.
INSULIN SECRETAGOGUES		
repaglinide	↑ repaglinide	Caution is warranted and clinical monitoring is recommended.
NARCOTIC ANALGESIC		
methadone*	↓ R-methadone	Concentrations of methadone were reduced when co-administered with telaprevir. No adjustment of methadone dose is required when initiating co-administration of telaprevir. However, clinical monitoring is recommended as the dose of methadone during maintenance therapy may need to be adjusted in some patients.
PDE5 INHIBITORS		
sildenafil tadalafil vardenafil	↑ PDE5 inhibitors	Concentrations of PDE5 inhibitors may be increased when co-administered with telaprevir. For the treatment of erectile dysfunction, sildenafil at a single dose not exceeding 25 mg in 48 hours, vardenafil at a single dose not exceeding 2.5 mg dose in 72 hours, or tadalafil at a single dose not exceeding 10 mg dose in 72 hours can be used with increased monitoring for PDE5 inhibitor-associated adverse events. QT interval prolongation has been reported with vardenafil. Caution is warranted and clinical monitoring is recommended. Co-administration of sildenafil or tadalafil and telaprevir in the treatment of pulmonary arterial hypertension is contraindicated [*see Contraindications (4)*].

The direction of the arrow (↑ = *increase*, ↓ = *decrease*, ↔ = *no change*) indicates the direction of the change in PK.
* These interactions have been studied. See *Clinical Pharmacology (12.3),* Tables 6 and 7.

Table 6 Drug Interactions: Summary of Pharmacokinetic Parameters for Telaprevir in the Presence of Co-administered Drugs*

Drug	Dose and Schedule		N	Effect on Telaprevir PK†	LS Mean Ratio (90% CI) of Telaprevir PK With/Without Co-administered Drug		
	Drug	Telaprevir			C_{max}	AUC or $C_{avg,ss}$‡	C_{min}
Escitalopram	10 mg qd for 7 days	750 mg q8h for 14 days	13	↔	1.00 (0.95; 1.05)	0.93 (0.89; 0.97)	0.91 (0.86; 0.97)
Esomeprazole	40 mg qd for 6 days	750 mg single dose	24	↔	0.95 (0.86; 1.06)	0.98 (0.91; 1.05)	NA
Ketoconazole	Ketoconazole 400 mg single dose	750 mg single dose	17	↑	1.24 (1.10; 1.41)	1.62 (1.45; 1.81)	NA
Oral Contraceptive	Norethindrone/ ethinyl estradiol 0.5 mg/ 0.035 mg qd for 21 days	750 mg q8h for 21 days	23	↔	1.00 (0.93; 1.07)	0.99 (0.93; 1.05)	1.00 (0.93; 1.08)
Rifampin	600 mg qd for 8 days	750 mg single dose	16	↓	0.14 (0.11; 0.18)	0.08 (0.07; 0.11)	NA
Anti-HIV Drugs							
Atazanavir (ATV)/ritonavir (rtv)	300 mg ATV/ 100 mg rtv qd for 20 days	750 mg q8h for 10 days	14	↓	0.79 (0.74; 0.84)	0.80 (0.76; 0.85)	0.85 (0.75; 0.98)
Darunavir (DRV)/ritonavir (rtv)	600 mg DRV/ 100 mg rtv bid for 20 days	750 mg q8h for 10 days	11 (N=14 for C_{max})	↓	0.64 (0.61; 0.67)	0.65 (0.61; 0.69)	0.68 (0.63; 0.74)

(Table continued on next page)

In Clinical Trials

In a pooled analysis of subjects who did not achieve SVR (on-treatment virologic failure or relapse) from the controlled Phase 3 clinical trials, NS3 amino acid substitutions V36M/A/L, T54A/S, R155K/T, and A156S/T were determined to emerge frequently on INCIVEK treatment (Table 8). Nearly all of these substitutions have been shown to reduce telaprevir anti-HCV activity in cell culture or biochemical assays. No clear evidence of treatment-emergent substitutions in the NS3 helicase domain or NS4A coding regions of the HCV genome was observed among subjects treated with INCIVEK who did not achieve SVR.

Telaprevir treatment-emergent resistance substitutions emerged in the majority of isolates from subjects who did not achieve SVR (Table 8): in almost 100% of subjects who failed during 12 weeks of T/PR and in the majority of subjects who failed on PR after Week 12 or who relapsed.

HCV genotype 1 subtype-associated patterns of INCIVEK treatment-emergent amino acid substitutions were observed. Subjects with HCV genotype 1a predominately had V36M and R155K or the combination of these variants, while subjects with HCV genotype 1b predominately had V36A, T54A/S, and A156S/T variants (Table 8). Among subjects treated with telaprevir, on-treatment virologic failure was more frequent in subjects with genotype 1a than with genotype 1b and more frequent in prior null responders [*see Clinical Studies (14)*].

Table 8: Treatment-Emergent Substitutions in Pooled Phase 3 Trials: Subjects who did not achieve SVR24 in INCIVEK Combination Treatment Arms

Emerging Substitutions* in NS3	Percent of No SVR Subjects (n) N=525	Percent Subtype 1a No SVR Subjects (n) N=356	Percent Subtype 1b No SVR Subjects (n) N=169
Any substitution at V36, T54, R155, A156 or D168	62% (323)	69% (247)	45% (76)
R155K/T	38% (201)	56% (200)	0.6% (1)
V36M	33% (178)	49% (173)	3% (5)
V36M + R155K†	27% (142)	40% (142)	0% (0)
T54A/S	13% (68)	9% (31)	22% (37)
V36A/L	12% (65)	10% (37)	17% (28)
A156S/T	9% (48)	8% (28)	12% (20)
V36G/I, I132V, R155G/M, A156V/F/N or D168N	Less than 2%	Less than 2%	Less than 2%

* Alone or in combination with other substitutions (includes mixtures)
† Subjects with this combination are also encompassed in two V36M and R155K rows above.

Persistence of Resistance-Associated Substitutions

Persistence of telaprevir-resistant NS3 amino acid substitutions has been observed following treatment failure. Of a combined 255 treatment-naïve and previously treated subjects from Trials 108, 111, and C216 in whom telaprevir-resistant variants had emerged during treatment, 103 (40%) had detectable resistant variants by population sequencing at end of trial (follow-up range 2-70 weeks, median 45 weeks) and results for loss of variants were similar across the 3 trials. In the combined trials, 46% of the telaprevir-resistant substitutions in subtype 1a and 16% of the substitutions in subtype 1b were still detected by the end of trial: 29% of V36, 16% of T54, 38% of R155, 14% of A156, and 44% of V36M+R155K variants were detected at the end of trial.

In a 3-year follow-up trial of 56 treatment-naïve and prior treatment-failure subjects who did not achieve SVR with a telaprevir regimen in a Phase 2 trial and had telaprevir-resistant variants after treatment failure, variants were detected by population sequencing in 11% (6/56) of subjects (median follow-up of 25 months). Telaprevir-resistant variants V36L/M, T54S, and R155K were detectable (present at greater than 25% of the viral population) in some subjects at 24 months. By 36 months, V36M, T54A/S, and A156N/S/T variants had fallen below the level of detection by population sequencing in all subjects. At 36 months, 3% of the subject isolates that had the R155K variant still had detectable R155K variants by population sequencing.

The lack of detection of a substitution based on a population-based assay does not necessarily indicate the substitution has declined to the pre-treatment level. The long-term clinical impact of the emergence or persistence of detectable INCIVEK resistance-associated substitutions is unknown. No data are available regarding INCIVEK efficacy among patients who were previously exposed to INCIVEK, or who previously failed treatment with a regimen containing INCIVEK.

Effect of Baseline HCV Substitutions/Polymorphisms on Treatment Response

A pooled analysis was conducted to explore the association between the detection (population-based assay) of baseline NS3/4A amino acid substitutions/polymorphisms and treatment outcome in Trials 108, 111, and C216. Baseline polymorphisms at NS3 position Q80 (Q80K, Q80L, Q80R), which are frequently observed in HCV genotype 1a-infected subjects and have been reported to reduce the activity of some HCV NS3/4A protease inhibitors, were not associated with reduced INCIVEK efficacy.

Telaprevir-associated resistance substitutions (substitutions at positions V36, T54, R155 or D168) were present at baseline in 5% (117/2217) of the available subject samples in the combined clinical trials. Given the small number of subjects with baseline telaprevir resistance substitutions, conclusions about their effect on response outcomes when these substitutions are present at baseline cannot be determined.

Cross-Resistance

Treatment-emergent NS3 amino acid substitutions detected in subjects treated with INCIVEK who did not achieve SVR in the clinical trials (substitutions at positions V36, T54, R155, A156 or D168) have been demonstrated to reduce the anti-HCV activity of boceprevir and other HCV NS3/4A protease inhibitors. The impact of prior INCIVEK exposure or treatment failure on the efficacy of boceprevir or other HCV NS3/4A protease inhibitors has not been studied. INCIVEK efficacy has not been established for patients with a history of exposure to NS3/4A protease inhibitors.

Cross-resistance is not expected between INCIVEK and interferons, or INCIVEK and ribavirin. HCV replicons expressing telaprevir-associated resistance substitutions remained fully sensitive to interferon-alfa and ribavirin, as well as other direct-acting antivirals with different mechanisms of action, such as NS5B polymerase inhibitors.

12.5 Pharmacogenomics

A genetic variant near the gene encoding interferon-lambda-3 (*IL28B* rs12979860, a C to T change) is a strong predictor of response to peginterferon alfa and ribavirin (PR). rs12979860 was genotyped in 454 of 1088 subjects in Trial 108 (treatment-naïve) and 527 of 662 subjects in Trial C216 (previously treated) [*see Clinical Studies (14.2 and 14.3) for trial descriptions*]. SVR rates tended to be lower in subjects with the CT and TT genotypes compared to those with the CC genotype, particularly among treatment-naïve subjects receiving PR48 (Table 9). Among both treatment-naïve and previous treatment failures, subjects of all IL28B genotypes appeared to have higher SVR rates with regimens containing INCIVEK. The results of this retrospective subgroup analysis should be viewed with caution because of the small sample size and potential differences in demographic or clinical characteristics of the subtrial population relative to the overall trial population.

Table 9: SVR Rates by rs12979860 Genotype

Trial	rs12979860 Genotype	SVR, n/N (%)	
		T12/PR	**Pbo/PR48**
108 (treatment-naïve)	C/C	45/50 (90%)	35/55 (64%)
	C/T	48/68 (71%)	20/80 (25%)
	T/T	16/22 (73%)	6/26 (23%)
		T12 /PR48*	**Pbo/PR48**
C216 (previously treated)	C/C	60/76 (79%)	5/17 (29%)
	C/T	160/266 (60%)	9/58 (16%)
	T/T	49/80 (61%)	4/30 (13%)

* Lead-in and immediate start T12/PR regimens pooled.

Table 6 *(cont.)* Drug Interactions: Summary of Pharmacokinetic Parameters for Telaprevir in the Presence of Co-administered Drugs*

Drug	Dose and Schedule: Drug	Dose and Schedule: Telaprevir	N	Effect on Telaprevir PK†	LS Mean Ratio (90% CI) of Telaprevir PK With/Without Co-administered Drug: C_{max}	AUC or $C_{avg,ss}$‡	C_{min}
Efavirenz	600 mg qd for 20 days	750 mg q8h for 10 days	21	↓	0.91 (0.82; 1.02)	0.74· (0.65; 0.84)	0.53 (0.44; 0.65)
Fosamprenavir (fAPV)/ ritonavir (rtv)	700 mg fAPV/ 100 mg rtv bid for 20 days	750 mg q8h for 10 days	18	↓	0.67 (0.63; 0.71)	0.68 (0.63; 0.72)	0.70 (0.64; 0.77)
Lopinavir (LPV)/ritonavir (rtv)	400 mg LPV/ 100 mg rtv bid for 20 days	750 mg q8h for 10 days	12	↓	0.47 (0.41; 0.52)	0.46 (0.41; 0.52)	0.48 (0.40; 0.56)
Raltegravir	400 mg bid for 11 days	750 mg q8h for 7 days	20	↔	1.07 (0.98; 1.16)	1.07 (1.00; 1.15)	1.14 (1.04; 1.26)
Ritonavir	100 mg single dose	750 mg single dose	14	↑	1.30 (1.15; 1.47)	2.00 (1.72; 2.33)	NA
Ritonavir	100 mg q12h for 14 days	750 mg q12h for 14 days	5	↓	0.85 (0.63; 1.13)	0.76[b,c] (0.60; 0.97)	0.68 (0.57; 0.82)
Tenofovir disoproxil fumarate (TDF)	300 mg qd TDF for 7 days	750 mg q8h for 7 days	16	↔	1.01 (0.96; 1.05)	1.00 (0.94; 1.07)	1.03 (0.93; 1.14)
Tenofovir disoproxil fumarate (TDF) and efavirenz (EFV)	600 mg EFV /300 mg TDF qd for 7 days	1125 mg q8h for 7 days	15	↓	0.86§ (0.76; 0.97)	0.82§ (0.73; 0.92)	0.75§ (0.66; 0.86)
	600 mg EFV /300 mg TDF qd for 7 days	1500 mg q12h for 7 days	16	↓	0.97§ (0.88; 1.06)	0.80‡,§ (0.73; 0.88)	0.52§ (0.42; 0.64)

NA: not available/ not applicable; N = Number of subjects with data; qd = once daily; bid = twice daily; q8h = every 8 hours; q12h = every 12 hours

* Data provided are under fed conditions unless otherwise noted.

† The direction of the arrow (↑ = *increase*, ↓ = *decrease*, ↔ = *no change*) indicates the direction of the change in PK

‡ $C_{avg,ss}$ = Average concentrations at steady state (AUC_τ/τ).

§ Value with co-administered drug and telaprevir / value with telaprevir 750 mg q8h alone

13 NONCLINICAL TOXICOLOGY

13.1 Carcinogenesis, Mutagenesis, Impairment of Fertility

Carcinogenesis and Mutagenesis

INCIVEK /Peginterferon Alfa/Ribavirin Combination Treatment

Ribavirin was shown to be genotoxic in several *in vitro* and *in vivo* assays. Ribavirin was not oncogenic in a 6-month p53+/- transgenic mouse study or a 2-year carcinogenicity study in rat. See the prescribing information for ribavirin.

INCIVEK (telaprevir) Tablets

Evidence of genotoxicity was not observed in a bacterial mutagenicity assay, *in vitro* mammalian chromosomal aberration assay, or *in vivo* micronucleus study in mouse. Telaprevir has not been tested for its carcinogenic potential.

Impairment of Fertility

INCIVEK /Peginterferon Alfa/Ribavirin Combination Treatment

Animal studies have shown that ribavirin induced reversible toxicity in males while peginterferon alfa may impair female fertility. See the prescribing information for ribavirin and peginterferon alfa.

INCIVEK (telaprevir) Tablets

Telaprevir treatment alone had effects on fertility parameters in rats. The no observed adverse effect level (NOAEL) for degenerative testicular toxicity was established at exposures 0.17-fold the human exposures at the recommended clinical dose. Potential effects on sperm (e.g., decreased % motile sperm and increased non-motile sperm count) were observed in a rat fertility study at exposures 0.30-fold the human exposures at the recommended clinical dose. Additional effects on fertility include minor increases in percent preimplantation loss, the percent of dams with nonviable embryos and percent of nonviable conceptuses per litter. These effects are likely associated with testicular toxicity in male rats but contributions of the female cannot be ruled out. Degenerative testicular toxicity was not observed in chronic toxicity studies in the dog. Furthermore, mean changes in proposed hormonal biomarkers of testicular toxicity among subjects who received telaprevir were comparable to placebo.

14 CLINICAL STUDIES

14.1 Description of Adult Clinical Trials

The efficacy and safety of INCIVEK in subjects with genotype 1 chronic hepatitis C were evaluated in 3 adequate and well-controlled clinical trials: 2 in treatment-naïve subjects and one in previously treated subjects (relapsers, partial responders, and null responders). Subjects in these trials had compensated liver disease, detectable HCV RNA, and liver histopathology consistent with chronic hepatitis C. In all 3 trials, INCIVEK was administered at a dosage of 750 mg every 8 hours; the peginterferon alfa-2a (Peg-IFN-alfa-2a) dose was 180 micrograms per week, and the ribavirin (RBV) dose was 1000 mg per day (subjects weighing less than 75 kg) or 1200 mg per day (subjects weighing greater than or equal to 75 kg). Plasma HCV RNA values were measured during the clinical trials using the COBAS® TaqMan® HCV test (version 2.0), for use with the High Pure System. The assay had a lower limit of quantitation of 25 IU per mL. SVR was defined as HCV RNA less than 25 IU per mL at last observation within the SVR visit window (i.e., weeks 32-78 for patients assigned to 24 weeks of treatment and weeks 56-78 for patients assigned to 48 weeks of treatment).

14.2 Treatment-Naïve Adults

Trial 108 (ADVANCE)

Trial 108 was a randomized, double-blind, parallel-group, placebo-controlled trial conducted in treatment-naïve subjects (had received no prior therapy for HCV, including interferon or pegylated interferon monotherapy). INCIVEK was given for the first 8 weeks of treatment (T8/PR regimen) or the first 12 weeks of treatment (T12/PR regimen) in combination with Peg-IFN-alfa-2a/RBV for either 24 or 48 weeks. Subjects who had undetectable HCV RNA (Target Not Detected) at weeks 4 and 12 (extended Rapid Virologic Response [eRVR]) received 24 weeks of Peg-IFN-alfa-2a/RBV treatment, and subjects who did not have undetectable HCV RNA at weeks 4 and 12 (no eRVR) received 48 weeks of Peg-IFN-alfa-2a/RBV treatment. The control regimen (Pbo/PR48) had a fixed treatment duration, with telaprevir-matching placebo for the first 12 weeks and Peg-IFN-alfa-2a/RBV for 48 weeks.

The 1088 enrolled subjects had a median age of 49 years (range: 18 to 69); 59% of the subjects were male; 23% had a body mass index greater than or equal to 30 kg/m²; 9% were Black; 11% were Hispanic or Latino; 77% had baseline HCV RNA levels greater than 800,000 IU per mL; 15% had bridging fibrosis; 6% had cirrhosis; 59% had HCV genotype 1a; and 40% had HCV genotype 1b.

Table 10 shows the response rates for the T12/PR and Pbo/PR48 groups.

Table 10: Response Rates: Trial 108

Treatment Outcome	T12/PR N = 363 n/N (%)	Pbo/PR48 N = 361 n/N (%)
Overall SVR	79% (285/363)	46% (166/361)
eRVR	58% (212/363)	8% (29/361)
SVR in eRVR subjects	92% (195/212)	93% (27/29)
No eRVR	42% (151/363)	92% (332/361)
SVR in no eRVR subjects	60% (90/151)	42% (139/332)
Outcome for Subjects without SVR		
On-treatment virologic failure*	7% (26/363)	29% (105/361)
Relapse†	4% (11/298)	24% (53/220)
Other‡	11% (41/363)	10% (37/361)

* On-treatment virologic failure was defined as meeting a protocol-defined stopping rule and/or having detectable HCV RNA at end of treatment with viral breakthrough.

† Relapse was defined as having less than 25 IU/mL at last observation within the planned end of treatment visit window followed by detectable HCV RNA during follow-up.

‡ Other includes subjects with detectable HCV RNA at the time of their last trial drug but who did not have viral breakthrough, and subjects with a missing SVR assessment.

In the T8/PR group, the overall SVR rate was 72%. The eRVR rate was 57% and the SVR rate for eRVR subjects was 86%. The SVR rate for no eRVR subjects was 52%. More subjects in the T8/PR group experienced virologic failure after Week 12 while receiving peginterferon alfa and ribavirin alone, 7% compared to 4% in T12/PR group.

SVR rates were higher (absolute difference of at least 22%) for the T12/PR group than for the Pbo/PR48 group across subgroups by sex, age, race, ethnicity, body mass index, HCV genotype subtype, baseline HCV RNA (less than 800,000, greater than or equal to 800,000 IU per mL), and extent of liver fibrosis. However, there were small numbers of subjects enrolled in some key subgroups. In the T12/PR group:

- Twenty-one subjects had cirrhosis at baseline and the overall SVR in these subjects was 71% (15/21). Among subjects with cirrhosis, 43% (9/21) were assigned to 24 weeks of treatment and of those 78% (7/9) achieved SVR.
- Twenty-six subjects were Black/African Americans. The overall SVR among Black/African American subjects was 62% (16/26). Among these subjects, 35% (9/26) were assigned to 24 weeks of treatment and of those 89% (8/9) achieved SVR.

Trial 111 (ILLUMINATE)

Trial 111 was a randomized, open-label trial conducted in treatment-naïve subjects. The trial was designed to compare SVR rates in subjects achieving eRVR who were treated with INCIVEK for 12 weeks in combination with Peg-IFN-alfa-2a/RBV for either 24 weeks (T12/PR24 regimen) or 48 weeks (T12/PR48 regimen).

The 540 enrolled subjects had a median age of 51 years (range: 19 to 70); 60% were male; 32% had a body mass index greater than or equal to 30 kg/m^2; 14% were Black; 10% were Hispanic or Latino; 82% had baseline HCV RNA levels greater than 800,000 IU per mL; 16% had bridging fibrosis; 11% had cirrhosis; 72% had HCV genotype 1a; and 27% had HCV genotype 1b.

The SVR rate for all subjects enrolled in the trial was 74%. A total of 352 (65%) subjects achieved eRVR and of those 322 (60%) were randomized to 24 weeks (T12/PR24, n=162) or 48 weeks (T12/PR48, n=160) of treatment. The SVR rates were similar at 92% (T12/PR24) and 90% (T12/PR48), respectively. Again, small numbers of subjects were enrolled in some key subgroups:

- Sixty-one (11%) of subjects had cirrhosis at baseline. Among subjects with cirrhosis, 30 (49%) achieved an eRVR: 18 were randomized to T12/PR24 and 12 to T12/PR48. The SVR rates were 61% (11/18) for the T12/PR24 group and 92% (11/12) for the T12/PR48 group.
- Blacks/African Americans comprised 14% (73/540) of trial subjects. Thirty-four (47%) Black/African American subjects achieved an eRVR and were randomized to T12/PR24 or T12/PR48. The respective SVR rates were 88% (15/17) and 88% (15/17), compared to 92% (244/266) for Caucasians among randomized subjects.

Table 7 Drug Interactions: Summary of Pharmacokinetic Parameters for Co-administered Drugs in the Presence of Telaprevir

Drug	Dose and Schedule: Drug	Dose and Schedule: Telaprevir	N	Effect on Drug PK*	LS Mean Ratio (90% CI) of Drug PK With/Without Telaprevir: C_{max}	AUC	C_{min}
Alprazolam	0.5 mg single dose	750 mg q8h for 10 days	17	↑	0.97 (0.92; 1.03)	1.35 (1.23; 1.49)	NA
Amlodipine	5 mg single dose	750 mg q8h for 7 days	19	↑	1.27 (1.21; 1.33)	2.79 (2.58; 3.01)	NA
Atorvastatin	20 mg single dose	750 mg q8h for 7 days	19	↑	10.60 (8.74; 12.85)	7.88 (6.84; 9.07)	NA
Buprenorphine	Buprenorphine maintenance therapy (4 to 24 mg/daily in combination with naloxone)	750 mg q8h for 7 days	14	↔	0.80 (0.69; 0.93)	0.96 (0.84; 1.10)	1.06 (0.87; 1.30)
Cyclosporine A (CsA)	100 mg single dose when administered alone; 10 mg single dose when co-administered with telaprevir (D8)	750 mg q8h for 11 days	9	↑	0.13 (0.11; 0.16) **Dose norm.:** 1.32 (1.08; 1.60)	0.46 (0.39; 0.55) **Dose norm.:** 4.64 (3.90; 5.51)	NA
Digoxin	0.5 mg single dose	750 mg q8h for 11 days	20	↑	1.50 (1.36; 1.65)	1.85 (1.70; 2.00)	NA
Escitalopram	10 mg qd, for 7 days	750 mg q8h for 14 days	13	↓	0.70 (0.65; 0.76)	0.65 (0.60; 0.70)	0.58 (0.52; 0.64)
Ethinyl estradiol (EE), co-administered with norethindrone (NE)	0.035 mg qd EE/ 0.5 mg qd NE for 21 days	750 mg q8h for 21 days	24	↓	0.74 (0.68; 0.80)	0.72 (0.69; 0.75)	0.67 (0.63; 0.71)
Ketoconazole	400 mg single dose	1250 mg q8h for 4 doses	81	↑	1.23 (1.14; 1.33)	1.46 (1.35; 1.58)	NA
	200 mg single dose	1250 mg q8h for 4 doses	28	↑	1.75 (1.51; 2.03)	2.25 (1.93; 2.61)	NA
R-Methadone	Methadone maintenance therapy (40 to 120 mg/daily)	750 mg q8h for 7 days	15	↓	0.71 (0.66; 0.76)	0.71 (0.66; 0.76)	0.69 (0.64; 0.75)
S-Methadone	Methadone maintenance therapy (40 to 120 mg/daily)	750 mg q8h for 7 days	15	↓	0.65 (0.60; 0.71)	0.64 (0.58; 0.70)	0.60 (0.54; 0.67)
Midazolam (iv)	0.5 mg iv single dose	750 mg q8h for 9 days	22	↑	1.02 (0.8; 1.31)	3.40 (3.04; 3.79)	NA
Midazolam (oral)	2 mg oral single dose	750 mg q8h for 11 days	21	↑	2.86 (2.52; 3.25)	8.96 (7.75; 10.35)	NA
Norethindrone (NE), co-administered with EE	0.035 mg qd EE/ 0.5 mg qd NE for 21 days	750 mg q8h for 21 days	24	↔	0.85 (0.81; 0.89)	0.89 (0.86; 0.93)	0.94 (0.87; 1.0)
Tacrolimus	2 mg single dose when administered alone; 0.5 mg single dose when co-administered with telaprevir (D8)	750 mg q8h for 13 days	9	↑	2.34 (1.68; 3.25) **Dose norm.:** 9.35 (6.73; 13.0)	17.6 (13.2; 23.3) **Dose norm.:** 70.3 (52.9; 93.4)	NA
Zolpidem	5 mg single dose	750 mg q8h for 10 days	19	↓	0.58 (0.52; 0.66)	0.53 (0.45; 0.64)	NA

(Table continued on next page)

14.3 Previously Treated Adults

Trial C216 (REALIZE)

Trial C216 was a randomized, double-blind, placebo-controlled trial conducted in subjects who did not achieve SVR with prior treatment with Peg-IFN-alfa-2a/RBV or Peg-IFN-alfa-2b/RBV. The trial enrolled prior relapsers (subjects with HCV RNA undetectable at end of treatment with a pegylated interferon-based regimen, but HCV RNA detectable within 24 weeks of treatment follow-up) and prior non-responders (subjects who did not have undetectable HCV RNA levels during or at the end of a prior course of at least 12 weeks of treatment). The nonresponder population included 2 subgroups: prior partial responders (greater than or equal to 2-$\log_{10}$ reduction in HCV RNA at week 12, but not achieving HCV RNA undetectable at end of treatment with peginterferon alfa and ribavirin) and prior null responders (less than 2-$\log_{10}$ reduction in HCV RNA at week 12 of prior treatment with peginterferon alfa and ribavirin).

Subjects were randomized in a 2:2:1 ratio to one of 2 INCIVEK combination treatment groups (with and without a Peg-IFN-alfa-2a/RBV lead-in) or a control group. The T12/PR48 group received INCIVEK and Peg-IFN-alfa-2a/RBV for 12 weeks (without a lead-in), followed by placebo and Peg-IFN-alfa-2a/RBV for 4 weeks, followed by Peg-IFN-alfa-2a/RBV for 32 weeks. The T12(DS)/PR48 group had a lead-in (delayed start of INCIVEK) with placebo and Peg-IFN-alfa-2a/RBV for 4 weeks, followed by INCIVEK and Peg-IFN-alfa-2a/RBV for 12 weeks, followed by Peg-IFN-alfa-2a/RBV for 32 weeks. The Pbo/PR48 group received placebo and Peg-IFN-alfa-2a/RBV for 16 weeks, followed by Peg-IFN-alfa-2a/RBV for 32 weeks.

The 662 enrolled subjects had a median age of 51 years (range: 21 to 70); 70% of the subjects were male; 26% had a body mass index greater than or equal to 30 kg/m^2; 5% were Black; 11% were Hispanic or Latino; 89% had baseline HCV RNA levels greater than 800,000 IU per mL; 22% had bridging fibrosis; 26% had cirrhosis; 54% had HCV genotype 1a, and 46% had HCV genotype 1b. Null and partial responders had higher baseline HCV RNA levels and more advanced liver disease (cirrhosis) than relapsers; other characteristics were similar across these populations.

The lead-in and immediate start regimens produced comparable SVR and no SVR rates, so data from these 2 groups were pooled (Table 11).

Table 11: Response Rates: Trial C216

Treatment Outcome	All T12/PR48* % (n/N)	Pbo/PR48 % (n/N)
SVR rate		
Prior relapsers	86% (246/286)	22% (15/68)
Prior partial responders	59% (57/97)	15% (4/27)
Prior null responders	32% (47/147)	5% (2/37)
Treatment Outcomes for Subjects Without SVR		
On-treatment virologic failure†		
Prior relapsers	1% (3/286)	26% (18/68)
Prior partial responders	18% (17/97)	70% (19/27)
Prior null responders	52% (76/147)	84% (31/37)
Relapse‡		
Prior relapsers	3% (8/254)	63% (27/43)
Prior partial responders	20% (14/71)	0% (0/4)
Prior null responders	24% (15/62)	50% (2/4)

* Lead-in and immediate start T12/PR regimens pooled

† On-treatment virologic failure includes subjects who met a protocol-defined virologic stopping rule or who had detectable HCV RNA at the time of their last dose of INCIVEK and subjects who had viral breakthrough on peginterferon alfa/ribavirin.

‡ Relapse rates are calculated with a denominator of subjects with undetectable HCV RNA (Target Not Detected) at the end of treatment.

Among prior relapsers, 76% (218/286) achieved an eRVR and of those 95% (208/218) achieved an SVR. In an earlier, dose-finding clinical trial, 78% (52/67) of prior relapsers achieved an eRVR and were treated with 24 weeks of peginterferon alfa and ribavirin (T12/PR24); of those 94% (49/52) achieved an SVR.

Table 7 *(cont.)* Drug Interactions: Summary of Pharmacokinetic Parameters for Co-administered Drugs in the Presence of Telaprevir

Drug	Dose and Schedule		N	Effect on Drug PK*	LS Mean Ratio (90% CI) of Drug PK With/Without Telaprevir		
	Drug	Telaprevir			C_{max}	AUC	C_{min}
Anti-HIV Drugs							
Atazanavir (ATV), boosted with ritonavir (rtv)	300 mg ATV/ 100 mg rtv qd for 20 days	750 mg q8h for 10 days	7	↑	0.85 (0.73; 0.98)	1.17 (0.97; 1.43)	1.85 (1.40; 2.44)
Darunavir (DRV), boosted with ritonavir (rtv)	600 mg DRV/ 100 mg rtv bid for 20 days	750 mg q8h for 10 days	11 (N=14 for C_{max})	↓	0.60 (0.56; 0.64)	0.60 (0.57; 0.63)	0.58 (0.52; 0.64)
	600 mg DRV/ 100 mg rtv bid for 24 days	1125 mg q12h for 4 days	15	↓	0.53 (0.47; 0.59)	0.49 (0.43; 0.55)	0.42 (0.35; 0.51)
Efavirenz	600 mg qd for 20 days	750 mg q8h for 10 days	21	↔	0.84 (0.76; 0.93)	0.93 (0.87; 0.98)	0.98 (0.94; 1.02)
Efavirenz (EFV), co-administered with tenofovir disoproxil fumarate (TDF)	600 mg EFV /300 mg TDF qd for 7 days	1125 mg q8h for 7 days	15	↓	0.76 (0.68; 0.85)	0.82 (0.74; 0.90)	0.90 (0.81; 1.01)
	600 mg EFV /300 mg TDF qd for 7 days	1500 mg q12h for 7 days	16	↓	0.80 (0.74; 0.86)	0.85 (0.79; 0.91)	0.89 (0.82; 0.96)
Fosamprenavir (fAPV), boosted with ritonavir (rtv)	700 mg fAPV/ 100 mg bid rtv for 20 days	750 mg q8h for 10 days	18	↓	0.65 (0.59; 0.70)	0.53 (0.49; 0.58)	0.44 (0.40; 0.50)
	700 mg fAPV/ 100 mg bid rtv for 24 days	1125 mg q12h for 4 days	17 (N=18 for C_{min})	↓	0.60 (0.55; 0.67)	0.51 (0.47; 0.55)	0.42 (0.37; 0.47)
Lopinavir (LPV), boosted with ritonavir (rtv)	400 mg LPV/ 100 mg rtv bid for 20 days	750 mg q8h for 10 days	12	↔	0.96 (0.87; 1.05)	1.06 (0.96; 1.17)	1.14 (0.96; 1.36)
Raltegravir	400 mg bid for 11 days	750 mg q8h for 7 days	20	↑	1.26 (0.97; 1.62)	1.31 (1.03; 1.67)	1.78 (1.26; 2.53)
Tenofovir disoproxil fumarate	300 mg qd for 7 days	750 mg q8h for 7 days	16	↑	1.30 (1.16; 1.45)	1.30 (1.22; 1.39)	1.41 (1.29; 1.54)
Tenofovir, on co-administration of tenofovir disoproxil fumarate (TDF) and efavirenz (EFV)	600 mg EFV /300 mg TDF qd for 7 days	1125 mg q8h for 7 days	15	↑	1.22 (1.12; 1.33)	1.10 (1.03; 1.18)	1.17 (1.06; 1.28)
	600 mg EFV /300 mg TDF qd for 7 days	1500 mg q12h for 7 days	16	↑	1.24 (1.13; 1.37)	1.10 (1.03; 1.17)	1.06 (0.98; 1.15)

* The direction of the arrow (↑ = *increase*, ↓ = *decrease*, ↔ = *no change*) indicates the direction of the change in PK.

For all populations in the trial (prior relapsers, prior partial responders, and prior null responders), SVR rates were higher for the T12/PR group than for the Pbo/PR48 group across subgroups by sex, age, ethnicity, body mass index, HCV genotype subtype, baseline HCV RNA level, and extent of liver fibrosis.

Twenty-six percent (139/530) of subjects treated with INCIVEK had cirrhosis at baseline. SVR rates among cirrhotic subjects who received INCIVEK combination treatment compared to Pbo/PR48 were: 84% (48/57) compared to 7% (1/15) for prior relapsers, 34% (11/32) compared to 20% (1/5) for prior partial responders, and 14% (7/50) compared to 10% (1/10) for prior null responders.

Four percent (19/530) of treatment experienced subjects who received INCIVEK combination treatment were Black/African Americans; the SVR rate for these subjects was 63% (12/19) compared to 66% (328/498) for Caucasians.

16 HOW SUPPLIED/STORAGE AND HANDLING

INCIVEK™ (telaprevir) is supplied as purple film-coated capsule-shaped tablets containing 375 mg of telaprevir. Each tablet is debossed with the characters "V 375" on one side and is packaged as follows:

28-day packer contains 4 weekly cartons of 7 blister strips each (6 tablets per blister strip) — **NDC 51167-100-01**

Store at 25°C (77°F); excursions permitted to 15-30°C (59-86°F) [see USP Controlled Room Temperature].

17 PATIENT COUNSELING INFORMATION

See FDA-Approved Patient Labeling (Medication Guide)

17.1 Serious Skin Reactions/Rash

Patients should be informed that INCIVEK combination treatment may cause rash. The rash can be serious, may be accompanied by fever and skin breakdown, may require urgent treatment in a hospital, and may result in death [*see also Boxed Warning and Warnings and Precautions (5.1)*]. Patients should promptly report any skin changes or itching to their healthcare provider. Patients should not stop INCIVEK due to rash unless instructed by their healthcare provider.

17.2 Pregnancy

Ribavirin must not be used by women who are pregnant or by men whose female partners are pregnant. Ribavirin therapy should not be initiated until a report of a negative pregnancy test has been obtained immediately before starting therapy. Because INCIVEK must be used in combination with ribavirin and peginterferon alfa, the contraindications and warnings applicable to those drugs are applicable to combination treatment. INCIVEK combination treatment is contraindicated in women who are pregnant and in men whose female partners are pregnant (see also the prescribing information for ribavirin).

Patients must be advised of the teratogenic/embryocidal risks of ribavirin and should be advised that extreme care must be taken to avoid pregnancy in female patients and in female partners of male patients—both during treatment and for 6 months after the completion of all treatment. Women of childbearing potential must be counseled about use of effective contraception (2 methods) prior to initiating treatment. Patients (both male and female) should be advised to notify their health care provider immediately in the event of a pregnancy [*see Contraindications (4), Warnings and Precautions (5.3), and Use in Specific Populations (8.1)*]. Patients should also be advised that hormonal contraceptives may not be reliable during INCIVEK dosing and for up to 2 weeks following cessation of INCIVEK [*see Drug Interactions (7)*]. During this time, female patients of childbearing potential should use 2 non-hormonal methods of effective birth control. Examples of non-hormonal methods of contraception include a male condom with spermicidal jelly OR female condom with spermicidal jelly (a combination of a male condom and a female condom is not suitable), a diaphragm with spermicidal jelly, a cervical cap with spermicidal jelly, or an intrauterine device (IUD).

17.3 Hepatitis C Virus Transmission

Patients should be informed that the effect of treatment of hepatitis C infection on transmission is not known, and that appropriate precautions to prevent transmission of the hepatitis C virus during treatment or in the event of treatment failure should be taken.

17.4 Importance of Hydration

Patients should be informed about the importance of hydration and fluid intake during INCIVEK combination treatment. Patients should be instructed to recognize the signs and symptoms of dehydration such as increased thirst, dry mouth, decreased urine output, and more concentrated urine. Patients should be advised to contact their health care provider if oral fluid intake is poor or if the patient experiences severe vomiting and/or diarrhea.

17.5 Administration

Patients should be advised INCIVEK must be administered in combination with both peginterferon alfa and ribavirin. If peginterferon alfa and/or ribavirin is discontinued for any reason, INCIVEK must also be discontinued.

Patients should be advised that the dose of INCIVEK must not be reduced or interrupted, as it may increase the possibility of treatment failure.

The recommended dose of INCIVEK tablets is 750 mg (two 375-mg tablets) taken orally 3 times a day (7-9 hours apart) with food containing approximately 20 grams of fat. Patients should be advised that the fat content of the meal or snack is critical for the absorption of telaprevir. Food that is taken with INCIVEK should be ingested within 30 minutes prior to each INCIVEK dose. Examples of some foods that could be taken with INCIVEK include: a bagel with cream cheese, ½ cup nuts, 3 tablespoons peanut butter, 1 cup ice cream, 2 ounces American or cheddar cheese, 2 ounces potato chips, or ½ cup trail mix.

Patients should be informed about what to do in the event they miss a dose of INCIVEK:

- In case a dose of INCIVEK is missed within 4 hours of the time it is usually taken, patients should be instructed to take the prescribed dose of INCIVEK with food as soon as possible.
- If more than 4 hours has passed since INCIVEK is usually taken, the missed dose should NOT be taken and the patient should resume the usual dosing schedule.
- Patients should be advised to contact their health care provider if they have questions.

Patients should be advised that they can contact the local Poison Control Center in the event of an overdose.

Manufactured for
Vertex Pharmaceuticals Incorporated
Cambridge, MA 02139
U.S. Patent No. 7,820,671

60884-05

MEDICATION GUIDE
INCIVEK (in-SEE-veck)
(telaprevir)
Film-Coated Tablets

Read this Medication Guide before you start taking INCIVEK™ and each time you get a refill. There may be new information. This information does not take the place of talking with your healthcare provider about your medical condition or your treatment.

INCIVEK is taken along with peginterferon alfa and ribavirin. You should also read those Medication Guides.

What is the most important information I should know about INCIVEK?

INCIVEK combination treatment may cause serious side effects including:

1. **Skin rash and serious skin reactions. Skin rashes are common with INCIVEK combination treatment. Sometimes these skin rashes and other skin reactions can become serious, require treatment in a hospital, and may lead to death.**
   - **Call your healthcare provider right away if you develop any skin changes during treatment with INCIVEK.**
   - Your healthcare provider will decide if your skin changes or any of the following symptoms may be a sign of a serious skin reaction:
     - skin rash, with or without itching
     - fever
     - swelling of your face
     - blisters or skin lesions
     - mouth sores or ulcers
     - red or inflamed eyes, like "pink eye" (conjunctivitis)
   - Your healthcare provider will decide if you need treatment for your skin rash or if you need to stop taking INCIVEK, or any of your other medicines.
   - Never stop taking INCIVEK combination treatment without talking with your healthcare provider first.

   See **"What are the possible side effects of INCIVEK?"** for more information about side effects.
2. **Low red blood cell count (anemia),** which can be severe. Tell your healthcare provider if you have any of these symptoms of anemia:
   - dizziness
   - shortness of breath
   - tiredness
   - weakness

   Your healthcare provider will do blood tests regularly to check your red blood cell count during treatment. If your anemia is severe, your healthcare provider may tell you to stop taking INCIVEK. If INCIVEK is stopped for this reason, **do not** start taking it again.
3. **Birth defects or death of your unborn baby.** INCIVEK in combination with peginterferon alfa and ribavirin may cause birth defects or death of your unborn baby. If you are pregnant or your sexual partner is pregnant or plans to become pregnant, do not take these medicines. You or your sexual partner should not become pregnant while taking INCIVEK with peginterferon alfa and ribavirin and for 6 months after treatment is over.

If you are a female who can become pregnant, or you are a female whose male partner takes these medicines:

- You must have a negative pregnancy test before starting treatment, each month during treatment, and for 6 months after your treatment ends.
- **You must use 2 forms of effective birth control during treatment and for the 6 months after treatment with these medicines.** Hormonal forms of birth control including birth control pills, vaginal rings, implants, or injections may not work during treatment with INCIVEK. You could become pregnant. Talk to your healthcare provider about other forms of birth control that may be used during this time. If your healthcare provider tells you to stop taking INCIVEK, peginterferon alfa and ribavirin, **you must still use 2 forms of birth control for the 6 months after treatment with these medicines. You may use a hormonal form of birth control as one of your 2 forms of birth control after 2 weeks of stopping INCIVEK.**
- If you or your female sexual partner becomes pregnant while taking INCIVEK, peginterferon alfa, and ribavirin or within 6 months after you stop taking these medicines, tell your healthcare provider right away. You or your healthcare provider should contact the Ribavirin Pregnancy Registry by calling 1-800-593-2214. The Ribavirin Pregnancy Registry collects information about what happens to mothers and their babies if the mother takes ribavirin while she is pregnant.

4. **Do not take INCIVEK alone to treat chronic hepatitis C infection. INCIVEK must be used with peginterferon alfa and ribavirin to treat chronic hepatitis C infection.**

What is INCIVEK?

INCIVEK is a prescription medicine used with the medicines peginterferon alfa and ribavirin to treat chronic (lasting a long time) hepatitis C genotype 1 infection in adults with stable liver problems, who have not been treated before or who have failed previous treatment.

It is not known if INCIVEK is safe and effective in children under 18 years of age.

Who should not take INCIVEK?

Do not take INCIVEK if you:

- are pregnant or may become pregnant. See **"What is the most important information I should know about INCIVEK?"**
- are a man with a sexual partner who is pregnant.
- take certain medicines. **INCIVEK may cause serious side effects when taken with certain medicines. Read the section "What should I tell my healthcare provider before taking INCIVEK?"**

Talk to your health care provider before taking INCIVEK if any of the above applies to you.

What should I tell my healthcare provider before taking INCIVEK?

Before you take INCIVEK, tell your healthcare provider if you:

- have certain blood problems, such as low red blood cell count (anemia)
- have liver problems other than hepatitis C infection
- have hepatitis B infection
- have Human Immunodeficiency Virus (HIV) infection or any other problems with your immune system
- history of gout or high uric acid levels in your blood
- have had an organ transplant
- plan to have surgery
- have any other medical condition
- are breastfeeding. It is not known if INCIVEK passes into your breast milk. You and your healthcare provider should decide if you will take INCIVEK or breastfeed. You should not do both.

Tell your healthcare provider about all the medicines you take, including prescription and non-prescription medicines, vitamins, and herbal supplements.

INCIVEK and other medicines can affect each other. This can cause you to have too much or not enough INCIVEK or your other medicines in your body, and cause side effects that can be serious or life-threatening. Your healthcare provider may need to change the amount of medicine you take.

Do not take INCIVEK if you take a medicine that contains:

- alfuzosin hydrochloride (Uroxatral®)
- cisapride (Propulsid®)
- ergot, including:
  - dihydroergotamine mesylate (D.H.E. 45®, Migranal®)
  - ergotamine tartrate (Cafergot®, Migergot®, Ergomar®, Ergostat®, Medihaler Ergotamine, Wigraine®, Wigrettes)
  - methylergonovine maleate (Ergotrate®, Methergine®)
- lovastatin (Advicor®, Altoprev®, Mevacor®)
- pimozide (Orap®)
- rifampin (Rifadin®, Rifamate®, Rifater®)
- sildenafil citrate (Revatio®) or tadalafil (Adcirca®) for the lung problem, pulmonary artery hypertension (PAH)
- simvastatin (Zocor®, Vytorin®, Simcor®)
- St. John's wort (Hypericum perforatum) or products containing St. John's wort
- triazolam (Halcion®)

Tell your healthcare provider if you are taking or starting to take medicines that contain:

- atorvastatin (Lipitor®, Caduet®)
- budesonide (Pulmicort®, Rhinocort®, Symbicort®)
- colchicine (Colcrys®)
- darunavir (Prezista®) and ritonavir (Norvir®)
- fluticasone (Advair®, Flonase®, Flovent®, Veramyst®)
- fosamprenavir (Lexiva®) and ritonavir (Norvir®)
- lopinavir and ritonavir (Kaletra®)
- methylprednisolone (Medrol®)
- prednisone
- rifabutin (Mycobutin®)
- salmeterol (Advair®, Serevent®)

Your healthcare provider may need to monitor your therapy more closely if you take INCIVEK with the following medicines. Talk to your healthcare provider if you are taking or starting to take medicines that contain:

- alprazolam (Xanax®)
- amiodarone (Cordarone®, Pacerone®)
- amlodipine (Norvasc®)
- atazanavir and ritonavir (Reyataz®, Norvir®)
- bepridil hydrochloride (Vascor®, Bepadin)
- bosentan (Tracleer®)
- carbamazepine (Carbatrol®, Equetro®, Tegretol®)
- clarithromycin (Biaxin®, Prevpac®)
- colchicine (Colcrys®)
- cyclosporine (Gengraf®, Neoral®, Sandimmune®)
- dexamethasone
- digoxin (Lanoxin®)
- diltiazem (Cardizem®, Dilacor XR®, Tiazac®)
- efavirenz (Sustiva®, Atripla®)
- erythromycin (E.E.S.®, Eryc®, Ery-Tab®, Erythrocin®, Erythrocin Stearate®)
- escitalopram (Lexapro®)
- ethinyl estradiol containing birth control methods (Lo Loestrin™ FE, Norinyl®, Ortho Tri-Cyclen Lo®)
- felodipine (Plendil®)
- flecainide (Tambocor™)
- fluvastatin (Lescol®, Lescol® XL)
- itraconazole (Sporanox®)
- ketoconazole (Nizoral®)
- methadone (Dolophine®, Methadose™)
- nicardipine (Cardene®)
- nifedipine (Adalat®, Procardia®)
- nisoldipine (Sular®)
- phenobarbital
- phenytoin (Dilantin®, Phenytek®)
- pitavastatin (Livalo®)
- posaconazole (Noxafil®)
- pravastatin (Pravachol®)
- propafenone (Rythmol®)
- quinidine (Nuedexta®)
- repaglinide (Prandin®)
- rosuvastatin (Crestor®)
- sildenafil for the treatment of erectile dysfunction (Viagra®)
- sirolimus (Rapamune®)

- tacrolimus (Prograf®)
- tadalafil for the treatment of erectile dysfunction (Cialis®)
- telithromycin (Ketek®)
- tenofovir disoproxil fumarate (Atripla®, Complera®, Truvada®, Viread®)
- trazodone (Desyrel®, Trialodine, Oleptro™)
- vardenafil for the treatment of erectile dysfunction (Levitra®, Staxyn®)
- verapamil (Calan®, Covera-HS®, Isoptin®, Tarka®)
- voriconazole (Vfend®)
- warfarin (Coumadin®)
- zolpidem (Ambien®, Edluar®)

Know the medicines you take. Keep a list of them with you and show it to your healthcare provider and pharmacist each time you get a new medicine.

How should I take INCIVEK?

- Take INCIVEK exactly as your healthcare provider tells you. Your healthcare provider will tell you how much INCIVEK to take and when to take it.
- Take INCIVEK 3 times a day. Each dose should be taken 7 to 9 hours apart. Eat a meal or snack that contains about 20 grams of fat, within 30 minutes before you take each dose of INCIVEK. Talk to your healthcare provider about examples of foods that you can eat that contain about 20 grams of fat. **Always take INCIVEK with food.**
- If you miss a dose **within 4 hours** of when you usually take it, take your dose with food as soon as possible.
- If you miss a dose and it is **more than 4 hours** after the time you usually take it, **skip that dose only** and take the next dose at your normal dosing schedule.
- Do not stop taking INCIVEK unless your healthcare provider tells you to. If you think there is a reason to stop taking INCIVEK, talk to your healthcare provider before doing so.
- If your healthcare provider tells you to stop taking INCIVEK, you should not start taking it again even if the reason for stopping goes away.
- If you take too much INCIVEK or overdose, call your healthcare provider or local Poison Control Center, or go to the nearest hospital emergency room right away.

What are the possible side effects of INCIVEK?

INCIVEK may cause serious side effects including:

See **"What is the most important information I should know about INCIVEK?"**

Common side effects of INCIVEK in combination with peginterferon alfa and ribavirin include:

- itching
- nausea
- diarrhea
- vomiting
- anal or rectal problems, including:
  - hemorrhoids
  - discomfort or burning around or near the anus
  - itching around or near the anus
- taste changes
- tiredness

It is important to stay hydrated with fluids during INCIVEK combination treatment. Signs and symptoms of dehydration include increased thirst, dry mouth, decreased urine frequency or volume, and dark colored urine.

Tell your healthcare provider about any side effect that bothers you or does not go away.

These are not all the possible side effects of INCIVEK. For more information, ask your healthcare provider or pharmacist.

Call your doctor for medical advice about side effects. You may report side effects to FDA at 1-800-FDA-1088.

You may also report side effects to Vertex Pharmaceuticals Incorporated at 1-877-824-4281.

How should I store INCIVEK?

- Store INCIVEK tablets at room temperature between 68°F to 77°F (20°C to 25°C).

Keep INCIVEK and all medicines out of the reach of children.

General information about INCIVEK

It is not known if treatment with INCIVEK will prevent you from infecting another person with the hepatitis C virus during treatment or if you do not respond to treatment.

Medicines are sometimes prescribed for purposes other than those listed in a Medication Guide. Do not use INCIVEK for a condition for which it was not prescribed. Do not give INCIVEK to other people, even if they have the same symptoms or condition you have. It may harm them.

This Medication Guide summarizes the most important information about INCIVEK. If you would like more information, talk with your healthcare provider. You can ask your healthcare provider or pharmacist for information about INCIVEK that is written for healthcare professionals.

For more information, go to www.incivek.com or call 1-877-824-4281.

What are the ingredients in INCIVEK?

Active ingredient: telaprevir

Inactive ingredients: colloidal silicon dioxide, croscarmellose sodium, D&C Red No. 40, dibasic calcium phosphate (anhydrous), FD&C Blue No. 2, hypromellose acetate succinate, microcrystalline cellulose, polyethylene glycol, polyvinyl alcohol, sodium lauryl sulfate, sodium stearyl fumarate, talc, and titanium dioxide.

This Medication Guide has been approved by the U.S. Food and Drug Administration.

Manufactured for
Vertex Pharmaceuticals Incorporated
Cambridge, MA 02139
Revised April 2013

KALYDECO™ ℞

(ivacaftor)
Tablets

HIGHLIGHTS OF PRESCRIBING INFORMATION

These highlights do not include all the information needed to use KALYDECO safely and effectively. See full prescribing information for KALYDECO.
KALYDECO™ (ivacaftor) Tablets
Initial U.S. Approval: 2012

INDICATIONS AND USAGE

KALYDECO is classified as a cystic fibrosis transmembrane conductance regulator (CFTR) potentiator. KALYDECO is indicated for the treatment of cystic fibrosis (CF) in patients age 6 years and older who have a *G551D* mutation in the *CFTR* gene. If the patient's genotype is unknown, an FDA-cleared CF mutation test should be used to detect the presence of the *G551D* mutation. (1)

Limitations of Use:

- Not effective in patients with CF who are homozygous for the *F508del* mutation in the *CFTR* gene. (1, 14)
- KALYDECO has not been studied in other populations of patients with CF. (1, 14)

DOSAGE AND ADMINISTRATION

- Adults and pediatric patients age 6 years and older: one 150 mg tablet taken orally every 12 hours with fat-containing food. (2, 12.3)
- Reduce dose in patients with moderate and severe hepatic impairment. (8.6, 12.3)
- Reduce dose when co-administered with drugs that are moderate or strong CYP3A inhibitors. (7.1, 12.3)

DOSAGE FORMS AND STRENGTHS

- Tablets: 150 mg (3)

CONTRAINDICATIONS

- None known

WARNINGS AND PRECAUTIONS

- Elevated transaminases (ALT or AST): Transaminases (ALT and AST) should be assessed prior to initiating KALYDECO, every 3 months during the first year of treatment, and annually thereafter. Patients who develop increased transaminase levels should be closely monitored until the abnormalities resolve. Dosing should be interrupted in patients with ALT or AST of greater than 5 times the upper limit of normal (ULN). Following resolution of transaminase elevations, consider the benefits and risks of resuming KALYDECO dosing. (5.1, 6)
- Use with CYP3A inducers: Concomitant use with strong CYP3A inducers (e.g., rifampin, St. John's Wort) substantially decreases exposure of ivacaftor which may diminish effectiveness. Therefore, co-administration is not recommended. (5.2, 7.2, 12.3)

ADVERSE REACTIONS

The most common adverse drug reactions to KALYDECO (occurring ≥8% of patients with CF who have a *G551D* mutation in the *CFTR* gene) were headache, oropharyngeal pain, upper respiratory tract infection, nasal congestion, abdominal pain, nasopharyngitis, diarrhea, rash, nausea, and dizziness. (6.1)

To report SUSPECTED ADVERSE REACTIONS, contact Vertex Pharmaceuticals Incorporated at 1-877-752-5933 or FDA at 1-800-FDA-1088 or *www.fda.gov/medwatch.*

DRUG INTERACTIONS

CYP3A inhibitors: Reduce KALYDECO dose to 150 mg twice-a-week when co-administered with strong CYP3A inhibitors (e.g., ketoconazole). Reduce KALYDECO dose to 150 mg once daily when co-administered with moderate CYP3A inhibitors (e.g., fluconazole). Avoid food containing grapefruit or Seville oranges. (7.1, 12.3)

See 17 for PATIENT COUNSELING INFORMATION and FDA-approved patient labeling

Revised: 09/2012

FULL PRESCRIBING INFORMATION: CONTENTS*

*** Sections or subsections omitted from the full prescribing information are not listed**

FULL PRESCRIBING INFORMATION

1 INDICATIONS AND USAGE

KALYDECO is classified as a cystic fibrosis transmembrane conductance regulator (CFTR) potentiator. KALYDECO is indicated for the treatment of cystic fibrosis (CF) in patients age 6 years and older who have a *G551D* mutation in the *CFTR* gene. If the patient's genotype is unknown, an FDA-cleared CF mutation test should be used to detect the presence of the *G551D* mutation.

Limitations of Use

KALYDECO is not effective in patients with CF who are homozygous for the *F508del* mutation in the *CFTR* gene and has not been studied in other populations of patients with CF.

2 DOSAGE AND ADMINISTRATION

2.1 Dosing Information in Adults and Children Ages 6 Years and Older

The recommended dose of KALYDECO for both adults and pediatric patients age 6 years and older is one 150 mg tablet taken orally every 12 hours (300 mg total daily dose) with fat-containing food. Examples of appropriate fat-containing food include eggs, butter, peanut butter, cheese pizza, etc. [*see Clinical Pharmacology (12.3)* and *Patient Counseling Information (17.4)*].

2.2 Dosage Adjustment for Patients with Hepatic Impairment

The dose of KALYDECO should be reduced to 150 mg once daily for patients with moderate hepatic impairment (Child-

Pugh Class B). KALYDECO should be used with caution in patients with severe hepatic impairment (Child-Pugh Class C) at a dose of 150 mg once daily or less frequently [see *Use in Specific Populations (8.6), Clinical Pharmacology (12.3),* and *Patient Counseling Information (17.3)*].

2.3 Dosage Adjustment for Patients Taking Drugs that are CYP3A Inhibitors

When KALYDECO is being co-administered with strong CYP3A inhibitors (e.g., ketoconazole), the dose should be reduced to 150 mg twice-a-week. The dose of KALYDECO should be reduced to 150 mg once daily when co-administered with moderate CYP3A inhibitors (e.g., fluconazole). Food containing grapefruit or Seville oranges should be avoided [see *Drug Interactions (7.1), Clinical Pharmacology (12.3),* and *Patient Counseling Information (17.2)*].

3 DOSAGE FORMS AND STRENGTHS

150 mg tablets.

4 CONTRAINDICATIONS

None known.

5 WARNINGS AND PRECAUTIONS

5.1 Transaminase (ALT or AST) Elevations

Elevated transaminases have been reported in patients with CF receiving KALYDECO. It is recommended that ALT and AST be assessed prior to initiating KALYDECO, every 3 months during the first year of treatment, and annually thereafter. Patients who develop increased transaminase levels should be closely monitored until the abnormalities resolve. Dosing should be interrupted in patients with ALT or AST of greater than 5 times the upper limit of normal (ULN). Following resolution of transaminase elevations, consider the benefits and risks of resuming KALYDECO dosing [see *Adverse Reactions (6)*].

5.2 Concomitant Use with CYP3A Inducers

Use of KALYDECO with strong CYP3A inducers, such as rifampin, substantially decreases the exposure of ivacaftor, which may reduce the therapeutic effectiveness of KALYDECO. Therefore, co-administration of KALYDECO with strong CYP3A inducers (e.g., rifampin, St. John's Wort) is not recommended [see *Drug Interactions (7.2)* and *Clinical Pharmacology (12.3)*].

6 ADVERSE REACTIONS

The following adverse reaction is discussed in greater detail in other sections of the label:

- Transaminase Elevations [see *Warnings and Precautions (5.1)*]

6.1 Clinical Trials Experience

Because clinical trials are conducted under widely varying conditions, adverse reaction rates observed in the clinical trials of a drug cannot be directly compared to rates in the clinical trials of another drug and may not reflect the rates observed in clinical practice.

The overall safety profile of KALYDECO is based on pooled data from placebo-controlled clinical trials conducted in 353 patients with CF who had a *G551D* mutation in the *CFTR* gene or were homozygous for the *F508del* mutation. Of the 353 patients, 50% of patients were female and 97% were Caucasian; 221 received KALYDECO and 132 received placebo from 16 to 48 weeks. Patients treated with KALYDECO were between the ages of 6 and 53 years.

In these trials, the proportion of patients who prematurely discontinued study drug due to adverse reactions was 2% for KALYDECO-treated patients and 5% for placebo-treated patients. Serious adverse reactions, whether considered drug-related or not by the investigators, which occurred more frequently in KALYDECO-treated patients included abdominal pain, increased hepatic enzymes, and hypoglycemia.

Overall, the most common adverse reactions in 221 patients with CF who had either a *G551D* mutation or were homozygous for the *F508del* mutation in the *CFTR* gene and treated with KALYDECO were headache (17%), upper respiratory tract infection (16%), nasal congestion (16%), nausea (10%), rash (10%), rhinitis (6%), dizziness (5%), arthralgia (5%), and bacteria in sputum (5%).

The incidence of adverse reactions below is based upon two double-blind, placebo-controlled 48-week clinical trials in a total of 213 patients with CF ages 6 to 53 who have a *G551D* mutation in the *CFTR* gene and who were treated with KALYDECO 150 mg orally or placebo twice daily. Table 1 shows adverse reactions occurring in ≥8% of KALYDECO-treated patients with CF who have a *G551D* mutation in the *CFTR* gene that also occurred at a higher rate than in the placebo-treated patients in the two double-blind, placebo-controlled trials.

Table 1: Incidence of Adverse Drug Reactions in ≥8% of KALYDECO-Treated Patients with a G551D Mutation in the CFTR Gene and Greater than Placebo in 2 Placebo-Controlled Phase 3 Clinical Trials of 48 Weeks Duration

	Incidence: Pooled 48-week Trials	
Adverse Reaction (Preferred Term)	KALYDECO N=109 n (%)	Placebo N=104 n (%)
Headache	26 (24)	17 (16)
Oropharyngeal pain	24 (22)	19 (18)
Upper respiratory tract infection	24 (22)	14 (14)
Nasal congestion	22 (20)	16 (15)
Abdominal pain	17 (16)	13 (13)
Nasopharyngitis	16 (15)	12 (12)
Diarrhea	14 (13)	10 (10)
Rash	14 (13)	7 (7)
Nausea	13 (12)	11 (11)
Dizziness	10 (9)	1 (1)

Adverse reactions that occurred in the KALYDECO group at a frequency of 4 to 7% where rates exceeded that in the placebo group include:

Infections and infestations: rhinitis

Investigations: aspartate aminotransferase increased, bacteria in sputum, blood glucose increased, hepatic enzyme increased

Musculoskeletal and connective tissue disorders: arthralgia, musculoskeletal chest pain, myalgia

Nervous system disorders: sinus headache

Respiratory, thoracic and mediastinal disorders: pharyngeal erythema, pleuritic pain, sinus congestion, wheezing

Skin and subcutaneous tissue disorders: acne

Laboratory Abnormalities

Transaminase Elevations: During 48-week, placebo-controlled clinical studies, the incidence of maximum transaminase (ALT or AST) >8, >5 or >3 × ULN was 2%, 3% and 6% in KALYDECO-treated patients and 2%, 2% and 8% in placebo-treated patients, respectively. Two patients (2%) on placebo and 1 patient (0.5 %) on KALYDECO permanently discontinued treatment for elevated transaminases, all >8× ULN. Two patients treated with KALYDECO were reported to have serious adverse reactions of elevated liver transaminases compared to none on placebo [see *Warnings and Precautions (5.1)*].

7 DRUG INTERACTIONS

Potential for other drugs to affect ivacaftor

7.1 Inhibitors of CYP3A

Ivacaftor is a sensitive CYP3A substrate. Co-administration with ketoconazole, a strong CYP3A inhibitor, significantly increased ivacaftor exposure [measured as area under the curve (AUC)] by 8.5-fold. Therefore, a reduction of the KALYDECO dose to 150 mg twice-a-week is recommended for co-administration with strong CYP3A inhibitors, such as ketoconazole, itraconazole, posaconazole, voriconazole, telithromycin, and clarithromycin.

Co-administration with fluconazole, a moderate inhibitor of CYP3A, increased ivacaftor exposure by 3-fold. Therefore, a reduction of the KALYDECO dose to 150 mg once daily is recommended for patients taking concomitant moderate CYP3A inhibitors, such as fluconazole and erythromycin.

Co-administration of KALYDECO with grapefruit juice, which contains one or more components that moderately inhibit CYP3A, may increase exposure of ivacaftor. Therefore, food containing grapefruit or Seville oranges should be avoided during treatment with KALYDECO [see *Clinical Pharmacology (12.3)*].

7.2 Inducers of CYP3A

Co-administration with rifampin, a strong CYP3A inducer, significantly decreased ivacaftor exposure (AUC) by approximately 9-fold. Therefore, co-administration with strong CYP3A inducers, such as rifampin, rifabutin, phenobarbital, carbamazepine, phenytoin, and St. John's Wort is not recommended [see *Warnings and Precautions (5.2)* and *Clinical Pharmacology (12.3)*].

Potential for ivacaftor to affect other drugs

7.3 CYP3A and/or P-gp Substrates

Ivacaftor and its M1 metabolite have the potential to inhibit CYP3A and P-gp. Co-administration with midazolam, a sensitive CYP3A substrate, increased midazolam exposure 1.5-fold, consistent with weak inhibition of CYP3A by ivacaftor. Administration of KALYDECO may increase systemic exposure of drugs which are substrates of CYP3A and/or P-gp, which may increase or prolong their therapeutic effect and adverse events. Therefore, caution is recommended when co-administering KALYDECO with CYP3A and/or P-gp substrates, such as digoxin, cyclosporine, and tacrolimus [see *Clinical Pharmacology (12.3)*].

8 USE IN SPECIFIC POPULATIONS

8.1 Pregnancy

Teratogenic effects: Pregnancy Category B. There are no adequate and well-controlled studies of KALYDECO in pregnant women. Ivacaftor was not teratogenic in rats at approximately 6 times the maximum recommended human dose (MRHD) (based on summed AUCs for ivacaftor and its metabolites at a maternal dose of 200 mg/kg/day). Ivacaftor was not teratogenic in rabbits at approximately 12 times the MRHD (on an ivacaftor AUC basis at a maternal dose of 100 mg/kg/day, respectively). Placental transfer of ivacaftor was observed in pregnant rats and rabbits. Because animal reproduction studies are not always predictive of human response, KALYDECO should be used during pregnancy only if clearly needed.

8.3 Nursing Mothers

Ivacaftor is excreted into the milk of lactating female rats. Excretion of ivacaftor into human milk is probable. There are no human studies that have investigated the effects of ivacaftor on breast-fed infants. Caution should be exercised when KALYDECO is administered to a nursing woman.

8.4 Pediatric Use

The safety and efficacy of KALYDECO in patients 6 to 17 years of age with CF who have a *G551D* mutation in the *CFTR* gene has been demonstrated in 2 placebo-controlled clinical trials. Trial 1 evaluated 161 patients with CF who were 12 years of age or older and Trial 2 evaluated 52 patients with CF who were 6 to 11 years of age [see *Clinical Studies (14.1)*].

The safety and efficacy of KALYDECO in patients with CF younger than age 6 years have not been established.

8.5 Geriatric Use

CF is largely a disease of children and young adults. Clinical trials of KALYDECO did not include sufficient numbers of patients 65 years of age and over to determine whether they respond differently from younger patients.

8.6 Hepatic Impairment

No dose adjustment is necessary for patients with mild hepatic impairment (Child-Pugh Class A). A reduced dose of 150 mg once daily is recommended in patients with moderate hepatic impairment (Child-Pugh Class B). Studies have not been conducted in patients with severe hepatic impairment (Child-Pugh Class C) but exposure is expected to be higher than in patients with moderate hepatic impairment. Therefore, use with caution at a dose of 150 mg once daily or less frequently in patients with severe hepatic impairment after weighing the risks and benefit of treatment [see *Pharmacokinetics (12.3)*].

8.7 Renal Impairment

KALYDECO has not been studied in patients with mild, moderate, or severe renal impairment or in patients with end stage renal disease. No dose adjustment is necessary for patients with mild to moderate renal impairment; however, caution is recommended while using KALYDECO in patients with severe renal impairment (creatinine clearance less than or equal to 30 mL/min) or end stage renal disease.

8.8 Patients with CF who are Homozygous for the *F508del* Mutation in the *CFTR* Gene

Efficacy results from a double-blind, placebo-controlled trial in patients with CF who are homozygous for the *F508del* mutation in the *CFTR* gene showed no statistically significant difference in forced expiratory volume exhaled in one second (FEV_1) over 16 weeks of KALYDECO treatment compared to placebo [see *Clinical Studies (14.2)*]. Therefore, KALYDECO should not be used in patients homozygous for the *F508del* mutation in the *CFTR* gene.

10 OVERDOSAGE

There have been no reports of overdose with KALYDECO. The highest single dose used in a clinical study was 800 mg in a solution formulation without any treatment-related adverse events.

The highest repeated dose was 450 mg (in a tablet formulation) every 12 hours for 4.5 days (9 doses) in a trial evaluating the effect of KALYDECO on ECGs in healthy subjects. Adverse events reported at a higher incidence compared to placebo included dizziness and diarrhea.

No specific antidote is available for overdose with KALYDECO. Treatment of overdose with KALYDECO consists of general supportive measures including monitoring of vital signs and observation of the clinical status of the patient.

11 DESCRIPTION

The active ingredient in KALYDECO tablets is ivacaftor which has the following chemical name: *N*-(2,4-di-tert-butyl-5-hydroxyphenyl)-1,4-dihydro-4-oxoquinoline-3-carboxamide. Its molecular formula is $C_{24}H_{28}N_2O_3$ and its molecular weight is 392.49. Ivacaftor has the following structural formula:

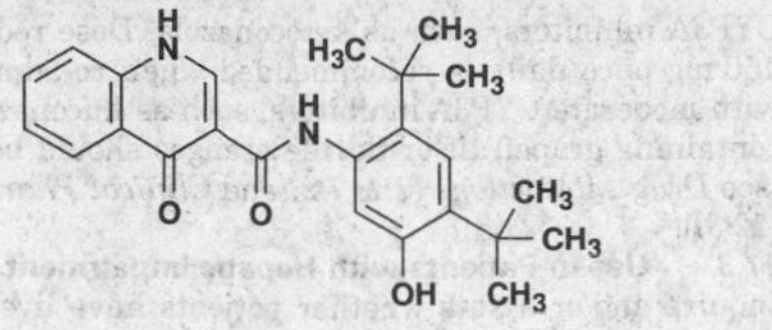

Ivacaftor is a white to off-white powder that is practically insoluble in water (<0.05 microgram/mL).

KALYDECO is available as a light blue capsule-shaped, film-coated tablet for oral administration containing 150 mg of ivacaftor. Each tablet contains the inactive ingredients colloidal silicon dioxide, croscarmellose sodium, hypromellose acetate succinate, lactose monohydrate, magnesium stearate, microcrystalline cellulose, and sodium lauryl sulfate. The tablet film coat contains carnauba wax, FD&C Blue #2, PEG 3350, polyvinyl alcohol, talc, and titanium dioxide. The printing ink contains ammonium hydroxide, iron oxide black, propylene glycol, and shellac.

12 CLINICAL PHARMACOLOGY

12.1 Mechanism of Action

Ivacaftor is a potentiator of the CFTR protein. The CFTR protein is a chloride channel present at the surface of epithelial cells in multiple organs. Ivacaftor facilitates increased chloride transport by potentiating the channel-open probability (or gating) of the G551D-CFTR protein.

In vitro, ivacaftor increased CFTR-mediated transepithelial current (I_T) in rodent cells expressing G551D-CFTR protein following addition of a cyclic adenosine monophosphate (cAMP) agonist with an EC_{50} of 100 ± 47 nM; however, ivacaftor did not increase I_T in the absence of cAMP agonist. Ivacaftor also increased I_T in human bronchial epithelial cells expressing G551D-CFTR protein following addition of a cAMP agonist by 10-fold with an EC_{50} of 236 ±200 nM. Ivacaftor increased the open probability of G551D-CFTR protein in single channel patch clamp experiments using membrane patches from rodent cells expressing G551D-CFTR protein by 6-fold versus untreated cells after addition of PKA and ATP.

12.2 Pharmacodynamics

Sweat Chloride Evaluation

In clinical trials in patients with the *G551D* mutation in the *CFTR* gene, KALYDECO led to statistically significant reductions in sweat chloride concentration. In two randomized, double-blind, placebo-controlled clinical trials (one in patients 12 and older and the other in patients 6-11 years of age), the mean change in sweat chloride from baseline through week 24 was -48 mmol/L (95% CI -51, -45) and -54 mmol/L (95% CI -62, -47) respectively. These changes persisted through 48 weeks. There was no direct correlation between decrease in sweat chloride levels and improvement in lung function (FEV_1).

ECG Evaluation

The effect of multiple doses of ivacaftor 150 mg and 450 mg twice daily on QTc interval was evaluated in a randomized, placebo- and active-controlled (moxifloxacin 400 mg) four-period crossover thorough QT study in 72 healthy subjects. In a study with demonstrated ability to detect small effects, the upper bound of the one-sided 95% confidence interval for the largest placebo adjusted, baseline-corrected QTc based on Fridericia's correction method (QTcF) was below 10 ms, the threshold for regulatory concern.

12.3 Pharmacokinetics

The pharmacokinetics of ivacaftor is similar between healthy adult volunteers and patients with CF.

After oral administration of a single 150 mg dose to healthy volunteers in a fed state, peak plasma concentrations (T_{max}) occurred at approximately 4 hours, and the mean (±SD) for AUC and C_{max} were 10600 (5260) ng*hr/mL and 768 (233) ng/mL, respectively.

After every 12 hour dosing, steady-state plasma concentrations of ivacaftor were reached by days 3 to 5, with an accumulation ratio ranging from 2.2 to 2.9.

Absorption

The exposure of ivacaftor increased approximately 2- to 4-fold when given with food containing fat. Therefore, KALYDECO should be administered with fat-containing food. Examples of fat-containing foods include eggs, butter, peanut butter, and cheese pizza. The median (range) t_{max} is approximately 4.0 (3.0; 6.0) hours in the fed state.

Distribution

Ivacaftor is approximately 99% bound to plasma proteins, primarily to alpha 1-acid glycoprotein and albumin. Ivacaftor does not bind to human red blood cells.

The mean apparent volume of distribution (Vz/F) of ivacaftor after a single dose of 275 mg of KALYDECO in the fed state was similar for healthy subjects and patients with CF. After oral administration of 150 mg every 12 hours for 7 days to healthy volunteers in a fed state, the mean (±SD) for apparent volume of distribution was 353 (122) L.

Metabolism

Ivacaftor is extensively metabolized in humans. In vitro and clinical studies indicate that ivacaftor is primarily metabolized by CYP3A. M1 and M6 are the two major metabolites of ivacaftor in humans. M1 has approximately one-sixth the potency of ivacaftor and is considered pharmacologically active. M6 has less than one-fiftieth the potency of ivacaftor and is not considered pharmacologically active.

Elimination

Following oral administration, the majority of ivacaftor (87.8%) is eliminated in the feces after metabolic conversion. The major metabolites M1 and M6 accounted for approximately 65% of the total dose eliminated with 22% as M1 and 43% as M6. There was negligible urinary excretion of ivacaftor as unchanged parent. The apparent terminal half-life was approximately 12 hours following a single dose. The mean apparent clearance (CL/F) of ivacaftor was similar for healthy subjects and patients with CF. The CL/F (SD) for the 150 mg dose was 17.3 (8.4) L/hr in healthy subjects.

Special populations

Hepatic impairment

Patients with moderately impaired hepatic function (Child-Pugh Class B, score 7 to 9) had similar ivacaftor C_{max}, but an approximately two-fold increase in ivacaftor $AUC_{0-\infty}$ compared with healthy subjects matched for demographics. Therefore, a reduced KALYDECO dose of 150 mg once daily is recommended for patients with moderate hepatic impairment. The impact of mild hepatic impairment (Child-Pugh Class A) on pharmacokinetics of ivacaftor has not been studied, but the increase in ivacaftor $AUC_{0-\infty}$ is expected to be less than two-fold. Therefore, no dose adjustment is necessary for patients with mild hepatic impairment. The impact of severe hepatic impairment (Child-Pugh Class C, score 10-15) on pharmacokinetics of ivacaftor has not been studied. The magnitude of increase in exposure in these patients is unknown but is expected to be substantially higher than that observed in patients with moderate hepatic impairment. When benefits are expected to outweigh the risks, KALYDECO should be used with caution in patients with severe hepatic impairment at a dose of 150 mg given once daily or less frequently.

Renal impairment

KALYDECO has not been studied in patients with mild, moderate or severe renal impairment (creatinine clearance less than or equal to 30 mL/min) or in patients with end stage renal disease. No dose adjustments are recommended for mild and moderate renal impairment patients because of minimal elimination of ivacaftor and its metabolites in urine (only 6.6% of total radioactivity was recovered in the urine in a human PK study); however, caution is recommended when administering KALYDECO to patients with severe renal impairment or end stage renal disease.

Gender

The effect of gender on KALYDECO pharmacokinetics was evaluated using population pharmacokinetics of data from clinical studies of KALYDECO. No dose adjustments are necessary based on gender.

Drug Interactions

Drug interaction studies were performed with KALYDECO and other drugs likely to be co-administered or drugs commonly used as probes for pharmacokinetic interaction studies [see *Drug Interactions (7)*].

Dosing recommendations based on clinical studies or potential drug interactions with KALYDECO are presented below.

Potential for Ivacaftor to Affect Other Drugs

In vitro studies showed that ivacaftor is a weak inhibitor of CYP3A and has potential to inhibit P-gp at therapeutic concentrations, and may also inhibit the CYP2C8 and CYP2C9 isozymes. Metabolite M1, but not M6, also has potential to inhibit CYP3A and P-gp. Ivacaftor, M1, and M6 were not inducers of CYP isozymes. Dosing recommendations for co-administered drugs following administration with KALYDECO are shown in Figure 1.

[See figure 1 at top of next column]

Potential for Other Drugs to Affect Ivacaftor

In vitro studies showed that ivacaftor and metabolite M1 were substrates of CYP3A enzymes (i.e., CYP3A4 and CYP3A5). KALYDECO dosing recommendations for co-administration with CYP3A inhibitors or inducers are shown in Figure 2.

[See figure 2 at top of next column]

13 NONCLINICAL TOXICOLOGY

13.1 Carcinogenesis, Mutagenesis, and Impairment of Fertility

Two-year studies were conducted in mice and rats to assess carcinogenic potential of KALYDECO. No evidence of tumorigenicity was observed in mice or rats at ivacaftor oral doses up to 200 mg/kg/day and 50 mg/kg/day, respectively (approximately equivalent to and 3 to 5 times the MRHD, respectively, based on summed AUCs of ivacaftor and its metabolites).

Figure 1: Impact of KALYDECO on Other Drugs

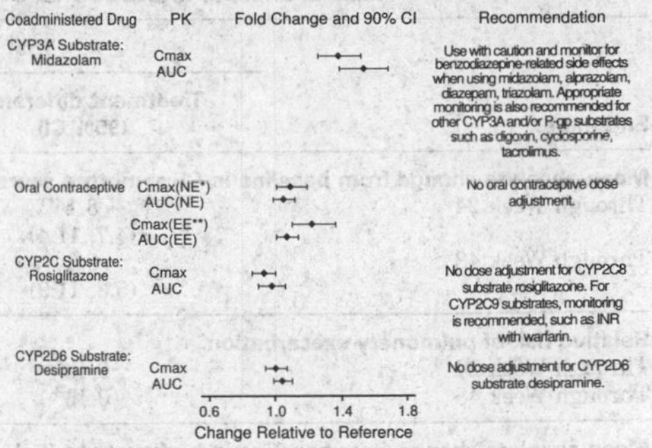

Note: The data obtained with substrates but without co-administration of KALYDECO are used as reference.

*NE: Norethindrone; **EE: Ethinyl Estradiol

The vertical lines are at 0.8, 1.0 and 1.25, respectively.

Figure 2: Impact of Other Drugs on KALYDECO

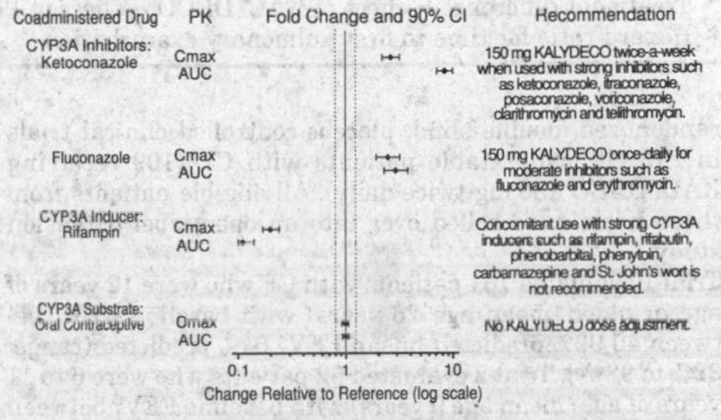

Note: The data obtained for KALYDECO without co-administration of inducers or inhibitors are used as reference.

The vertical lines are at 0.8, 1.0 and 1.25, respectively.

Ivacaftor was negative for genotoxicity in the following assays: Ames test for bacterial gene mutation, in vitro chromosomal aberration assay in Chinese hamster ovary cells, and in vivo mouse micronucleus test.

Ivacaftor impaired fertility and reproductive performance indices in male and female rats at 200 mg/kg/day (approximately 5 and 6 times, respectively, the MRHD based on summed AUCs of ivacaftor and its metabolites). Increases in prolonged diestrus were observed in females at 200 mg/kg/day. Ivacaftor also increased the number of females with all nonviable embryos and decreased corpora lutea, implantations, and viable embryos in rats at 200 mg/kg/day (approximately 6 times the MRHD based on summed AUCs of ivacaftor and its metabolites) when dams were dosed prior to and during early pregnancy. These impairments of fertility and reproductive performance in male and female rats at 200 mg/kg/day were attributed to severe toxicity. No effects on male or female fertility and reproductive performance indices were observed at ≤100 mg/kg/day (approximately 3 times the MRHD based on summed AUCs of ivacaftor and its metabolites).

13.2 Animal Toxicology and/or Pharmacology

Cataracts were seen in juvenile rats dosed with ivacaftor from postnatal day 7-35 at dose levels of 10 mg/kg/day and higher (approximately 0.12 times the MRHD based on summed AUCs of ivacaftor and its metabolites). This finding has not been observed in older animals.

14 CLINICAL STUDIES

14.1 Trials in Patients with CF who have a *G551D* Mutation in the *CFTR* Gene

Dose Ranging:

Dose ranging for the clinical program consisted primarily of one double-blind, placebo-controlled, cross-over trial in 39 adult (mean age 31 years) Caucasian patients with CF who had FEV_1 ≥ 40% predicted. Twenty patients with median predicted FEV_1 at baseline of 56% (range: 42% to 109%) received KALYDECO 25, 75, 150 mg or placebo every 12 hours for 14 days and 19 patients with median predicted FEV_1 at baseline of 69% (range: 40% to 122%) received KALYDECO 150, 250 mg or placebo every 12 hours for 28 days. The selection of the 150 mg every 12 hours dose was primarily based on nominal improvements in lung function (pre-dose FEV_1) and changes in pharmacodynamic parameters (sweat chloride and nasal potential difference). The twice-daily dosing regimen was primarily based on an apparent terminal plasma half-life of approximately 12 hours. Selection of the 150 mg dose of KALYDECO for children 6 to 11 years of age was based on achievement of comparable pharmacokinetics as those observed for adult patients.

Efficacy:

The efficacy of KALYDECO in patients with CF who have a *G551D* mutation in the *CFTR* gene was evaluated in two

Table 2: Effect of KALYDECO on Other Efficacy Endpoints in Trials 1 and 2

Endpoint	Trial 1 Treatment difference* (95% CI)	Trial 1 *P* value	Trial 2 Treatment difference* (95% CI)	Trial 2 *P* value
Mean absolute change from baseline in CF symptom score (points)				
Through Week 24	8.1 (4.7, 11.4)	<0.0001	6.1 (-1.4, 13.5)	0.1092
Through Week 48	8.6 (5.3, 11.9)	<0.0001	5.1 (-1.6, 11.8)	0.1354
Relative risk of pulmonary exacerbation				
Through Week 24	0.40†	0.0016	NA	NA
Through Week 48	0.46†	0.0012	NA	NA
Mean absolute change from baseline in body weight (kg)				
At Week 24	2.8 (1.8, 3.7)	<0.0001	1.9 (0.9, 2.9)	0.0004
At Week 48	2.7 (1.3, 4.1)	0.0001	2.8 (1.3, 4.2)	0.0002

CI: confidence interval; NA: not analyzed due to low incidence of events
* Treatment difference = effect of KALYDECO – effect of Placebo
† Hazard ratio for time to first pulmonary exacerbation

randomized, double-blind, placebo-controlled clinical trials in 213 clinically stable patients with CF (109 receiving KALYDECO 150 mg twice daily). All eligible patients from these trials were rolled over into an open-label extension study.

Trial 1 evaluated 161 patients with CF who were 12 years of age or older (mean age 26 years) with baseline FEV_1 between 40-90% predicted [mean FEV_1 64% predicted (range: 32% to 98%)]. Trial 2 evaluated 52 patients who were 6 to 11 years of age (mean age 9 years) with baseline FEV_1 between 40-105% predicted [mean FEV_1 84% predicted (range: 44% to 134%)]. Patients who had persistent *Burkholderia cenocepacia, dolosa*, or *Mycobacterium abcessus* isolated from sputum at screening and those with abnormal liver function defined as 3 or more liver function tests (ALT, AST, AP, GGT, total bilirubin) ≥3 times the upper limit of normal were excluded.

Patients in both trials were randomized 1:1 to receive either 150 mg of KALYDECO or placebo every 12 hours with food containing fat for 48 weeks in addition to their prescribed CF therapies (e.g., tobramycin, dornase alfa). The use of inhaled hypertonic saline was not permitted.

The primary efficacy endpoint in both studies was improvement in lung function as determined by the mean absolute change from baseline in percent predicted pre-dose FEV_1 through 24 weeks of treatment.

In both studies, treatment with KALYDECO resulted in a significant improvement in FEV_1. The treatment difference between KALYDECO and placebo for the mean absolute change in percent predicted FEV_1 from baseline through Week 24 was 10.6 percentage points ($P < 0.0001$) in Trial 1 and 12.5 percentage points ($P < 0.0001$) in Trial 2 (Figure 3). These changes persisted through 48 weeks. Improvements in percent predicted FEV_1 were observed regardless of age, disease severity, sex, and geographic region.

Figure 3: Mean Absolute Change from Baseline in Percent Predicted FEV_1 *

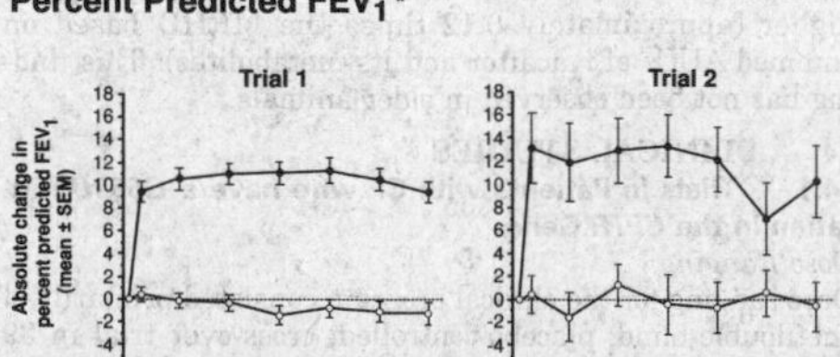

*primary endpoint was assessed at the 24-week time point.

Other efficacy variables included absolute change in sweat chloride from baseline to week 24 [discussed in *Clinical Pharmacology (12.2)*], time to first pulmonary exacerbation through week 48 (Trial 1 only), absolute change in weight from baseline to week 48, and improvement in cystic fibrosis symptoms including relevant respiratory symptoms such as cough, sputum production, and difficulty breathing. For the purpose of the study, a pulmonary exacerbation was defined as a change in antibiotic therapy (IV, inhaled, or oral) as a result of 4 or more of 12 pre-specified sino-pulmonary signs/symptoms. Patients treated with KALYDECO demonstrated statistically significant improvements in risk of pulmonary exacerbations, CF symptoms (in Trial 1 only), and gain in body weight (Table 2). Weight data, when expressed as body mass index normalized for age and sex in patients <20 years of age, was consistent with absolute change from baseline in weight.

[See table 2 above]

14.2 Trial in Patients Homozygous for the *F508del* Mutation in the *CFTR* Gene

Trial 3 was a 16-week randomized, double-blind, placebo-controlled, parallel-group trial in 140 patients with CF age 12 years and older who were homozygous for the *F508del* mutation in the *CFTR* gene and who had FEV_1 ≥40% predicted. Patients were randomized 4:1 to receive KALYDECO 150 mg (n=112) every twelve hours or placebo (n=28) in addition to their prescribed CF therapies. The mean age of patients enrolled was 23 years and the mean baseline FEV_1 was 79% predicted (range 40% to 129%). As in Trials 1 and 2, patients who had persistent *Burkholderia cenocepacia, dolosa*, or *Mycobacterium abcessus* isolated from sputum at screening and those with abnormal liver function defined as 3 or more liver function tests (ALT, AST, AP, GGT, total bilirubin) ≥3 times the upper limit of normal were excluded. The use of inhaled hypertonic saline was not permitted.

The primary endpoint was improvement in lung function as determined by the mean absolute change from baseline through Week 16 in percent predicted FEV_1. Treatment with KALYDECO resulted in no improvement in FEV_1 relative to placebo in patients with CF homozygous for the *F508del* mutation in the *CFTR* gene [mean absolute change from baseline through Week 16 in percent predicted FEV_1 was 1.5% and -0.2% for patients in the KALYDECO and placebo-treated groups, respectively (p = 0.15)]. There were no meaningful differences between patients treated with KALYDECO compared to placebo for secondary endpoints (change in CF symptoms, change in weight, or change in sweat chloride concentration).

16 HOW SUPPLIED/STORAGE AND HANDLING

KALYDECO™ (ivacaftor) is supplied as light blue, film-coated, capsule-shaped tablets containing 150 mg of ivacaftor. Each tablet is printed with the characters "V 150" on one side and plain on the other, and is packaged as follows:

56-count carton (contains 4 individual blister cards of 14 tablets per card)	**NDC** 51167-200-01
60-count bottle	**NDC** 51167-200-02

Store at 20-25ºC (68-77ºF); excursions permitted to 15-30ºC (59-86ºF) [see USP Controlled Room Temperature].

17 PATIENT COUNSELING INFORMATION

17.1 Transaminase (ALT or AST) Elevations and Monitoring

Inform patients that elevation in liver tests have occurred in patients treated with KALYDECO. Liver function tests will be performed prior to initiating KALYDECO, every 3 months during the first year of treatment and annually thereafter [see *Warnings and Precautions (5.1)*].

17.2 Drug Interactions with CYP3A Inducers and Inhibitors

Ask patients to tell you all the medications they are taking including any herbal supplements or vitamins. Co-administration of KALYDECO with strong CYP3A inducers (e.g., rifampin, St. John's Wort) is not recommended as they may reduce the therapeutic effectiveness of KALYDECO. Reduction of the dose of KALYDECO to 150 mg twice-a-week is recommended when co-administered with strong CYP3A inhibitors, such as ketoconazole. Dose reduction to 150 mg once daily is recommended when co-administered with moderate CYP3A inhibitors, such as fluconazole. Food containing grapefruit or Seville oranges should be avoided [see *Drug Interactions (7.1, 7.2)* and *Clinical Pharmacology (12.3)*].

17.3 Use in Patients with Hepatic Impairment

Inquire and/or assess whether patients have liver impairment. Reduce the dose of KALYDECO in patients with moderately impaired hepatic function (Child-Pugh Class B, score 7 to 9) to 150 mg once daily. KALYDECO has not been studied in patients with severe hepatic impairment (Child-Pugh Class C, score 10-15); however, exposure is expected to be substantially higher than that observed in patients with moderate hepatic impairment. When benefits are expected to outweigh the risks, KALYDECO should be used with caution in patients with severe hepatic impairment at a dose of 150 mg given once daily or less frequently. No dose adjustment is recommended for patients with mild hepatic impairment (Child-Pugh Class A, score 5-6) [see *Clinical Pharmacology (12.3)*].

17.4 Take with Fat-containing Food

Inform your patients that KALYDECO is best absorbed by the body when taken with fatty food. A typical CF diet will satisfy this requirement. Examples include eggs, butter, peanut butter, cheese pizza, etc.

Manufactured for
Vertex Pharmaceuticals Incorporated
Cambridge, MA 02139

KALYDECO is a trademark of Vertex Pharmaceuticals Incorporated.

VERTEX and the VERTEX triangle logo are registered trademarks of Vertex Pharmaceuticals Incorporated.

All other trademarks referenced herein are the property of their respective owners.

69264-01
Revised August 2012

Patient Information is perforated for dispensing to the patient.

PATIENT INFORMATION
KALYDECO (kuh-LYE-deh-koh)
(ivacaftor)
Film-Coated Tablets

Read this Patient Information before you start taking KALYDECO and each time you get a refill. There may be new information. This information does not take the place of talking to your doctor about your medical condition or your treatment.

What is KALYDECO?

KALYDECO is a prescription medicine used for the treatment of cystic fibrosis (CF) in patients age 6 years and older who have a certain mutation in their CF gene called the *G551D* mutation.

KALYDECO is not for use in people with CF due to other mutations in the CF gene. It is not effective in CF patients with two copies of the *F508del* mutation (*F508del/F508del*) in the CF gene.

It is not known if KALYDECO is safe and effective in children under 6 years of age.

What should not take KALYDECO?

Do not take KALYDECO if you take certain medicines or herbal supplements such as:

- the antibiotics rifampin (Rifamate®, Rifater®) or rifabutin (Mycobutin®)
- seizure medications such as phenobarbital, carbamazepine (Tegretol®, Carbatrol®, Equetro®) or phenytoin (Dilantin®, Phenytek®)
- St. John's Wort

Talk to your doctor before taking KALYDECO if you take any of the medicines or supplements listed above.

What should I tell my doctor before taking KALYDECO?

Before you take KALYDECO, tell your doctor if you:

- have liver or kidney problems
- drink grapefruit juice, or eat grapefruit or Seville oranges
- are pregnant or plan to become pregnant. It is not known if KALYDECO will harm your unborn baby. You and your doctor should decide if you will take KALYDECO while you are pregnant.
- are breastfeeding or planning to breastfeed. It is not known if KALYDECO passes into your breast milk. You and your doctor should decide if you will take KALYDECO while you are breastfeeding.

KALYDECO may affect the way other medicines work, and other medicines may affect how KALYDECO works.

Tell your doctor about all the medicines you take, including prescription and non-prescription medicines, vitamins, and herbal supplements as the dose of KALYDECO may need to be adjusted when taken with certain medications.

Ask your doctor or pharmacist for a list of these medicines if you are not sure.

Especially tell your doctor if you take:
- antifungal medications such as ketoconazole (e.g., Nizoral®), itraconazole (e.g., Sporanox®), posaconazole (e.g., Noxafil®), voriconazole (e.g., Vfend®), or fluconazole (e.g., Diflucan®)
- antibiotics such as telithromycin (e.g., Ketek®), clarithromycin (e.g., Biaxin®), or erythromycin (e.g., Ery-Tab®)

Know the medicines you take. Keep a list of them to show your doctor and pharmacist when you get a new medicine.

How should I take KALYDECO?
- Take KALYDECO exactly as your doctor tells you to take it.
- Always take KALYDECO with fatty food. Examples of fat-containing food include eggs, butter, peanut butter, cheese pizza, etc.

Your doses of KALYDECO should be taken 12 hours apart.

What should I avoid while taking KALYDECO?
- KALYDECO can cause dizziness in some people who take it. Do not drive a car, use machinery or do anything that needs you to be alert until you know how KALYDECO affects you.
- You should avoid food containing grapefruit or Seville oranges while you are taking KALYDECO.

What are the possible side effects of KALYDECO?

KALYDECO can cause serious side effects.

High liver enzymes in the blood have been reported in patients receiving KALYDECO. Your doctor will do blood tests to check your liver:
- before you start KALYDECO
- every 3 months during your first year of taking KALYDECO
- every year while you are taking KALYDECO

Call your doctor right away if you have any of the following symptoms of liver problems:
- pain or discomfort in the upper right stomach (abdominal) area
- yellowing of your skin or the white part of your eyes
- loss of appetite
- nausea or vomiting
- dark, amber-colored urine

The most common side effects of KALYDECO include:
- headache
- upper respiratory tract infection (common cold), including:
  - sore throat
  - nasal or sinus congestion
  - runny nose
- stomach (abdominal) pain
- diarrhea
- rash
- nausea
- dizziness

Tell your doctor if you have any side effect that bothers you or that does not go away.

These are not all the possible side effects of KALYDECO. For more information, ask your doctor or pharmacist.

Call your doctor for medical advice about side effects. You may report side effects to FDA at 1-800-FDA-1088.

How should I store KALYDECO?
- Store KALYDECO at room temperature between 68°F to 77°F (20°C to 25°C).
- Do not use KALYDECO after the expiration date on the package.

Keep KALYDECO and all medicines out of the reach of children.

General information about KALYDECO

Medicines are sometimes prescribed for purposes other than those listed in a Patient Information leaflet. Do not use KALYDECO for a condition for which it was not prescribed. Do not give KALYDECO to other people, even if they have the same symptoms you have. It may harm them.

This Patient Information summarizes the most important information about KALYDECO. If you would like more information, talk with your doctor. You can ask your pharmacist or doctor for information about KALYDECO that is written for health professionals.

For more information, go to www.kalydeco.com or call 1-877-752-5933.

What are the ingredients in KALYDECO?

Active ingredient: ivacaftor

Inactive ingredients: colloidal silicon dioxide, croscarmellose sodium, hypromellose acetate succinate, lactose monohydrate, magnesium stearate, microcrystalline cellulose, and sodium lauryl sulfate.

The tablet film coat contains: carnauba wax, FD&C Blue #2, PEG 3350, polyvinyl alcohol, talc, and titanium dioxide.

The printing ink contains: ammonium hydroxide, iron oxide black, propylene glycol, and shellac.

This Patient Information has been approved by the U.S. Food and Drug Administration.

Manufactured for:
Vertex Pharmaceuticals Incorporated
130 Waverly Street
Cambridge, MA 02139
Approved August 2012

69264-01

ViiV Healthcare Company
FIVE MOORE DRIVE
RESEARCH TRIANGLE PARK, NC 27709

Direct Inquiries
1-877-ViiVUSA (1-877-844-8872)

COMBIVIR ℞
[kom' bə-vir]
(lamivudine and zidovudine)
Tablets 150 mg/300 mg

HIGHLIGHTS OF PRESCRIBING INFORMATION
These highlights do not include all the information needed to use COMBIVIR safely and effectively. See full prescribing information for COMBIVIR.
COMBIVIR (lamivudine and zidovudine) Tablets 150 mg/300 mg
Initial U.S. Approval: 1997

WARNING: RISK OF HEMATOLOGIC TOXICITY, MYOPATHY, LACTIC ACIDOSIS, EXACERBATIONS OF HEPATITIS B

See full prescribing information for complete boxed warning
- **Hematologic toxicity including neutropenia and anemia have been associated with the use of zidovudine, one of the components of COMBIVIR (5.1)**
- **Symptomatic myopathy associated with prolonged use of zidovudine. (5.2)**
- **Lactic acidosis and hepatomegaly with steatosis, including fatal cases, have been reported with the use of nucleoside analogues including zidovudine. Suspend treatment if clinical or laboratory findings suggestive of lactic acidosis or pronounced hepatotoxicity occur. (5.3)**
- **Severe, acute exacerbations of hepatitis B have been reported in patients who are co-infected with hepatitis B virus (HBV) and human immunodeficiency virus (HIV-1) and have discontinued lamivudine, a component of COMBIVIR. Monitor hepatic function closely in these patients and, if appropriate, initiate anti-hepatitis B treatment. (5.4)**

INDICATIONS AND USAGE

COMBIVIR, a combination of 2 nucleoside analogue reverse transcriptase inhibitors, is indicated in combination with other antiretroviral agents for the treatment of HIV-1 infection. (1)

DOSAGE AND ADMINISTRATION

- Adults and Adolescents weighing ≥30 kg: 1 tablet twice daily. (2.1)
- Pediatrics: Dosage should be based on body weight not to exceed adult doses. (2.2)
- COMBIVIR, a fixed-dose product, should not be prescribed for pediatric patients weighing less than 30 kg or patients requiring dosage adjustment, such as those with renal or hepatic impairment, or patients experiencing dose-limiting adverse reactions. (2.3)

DOSAGE FORMS AND STRENGTHS

Tablets: Scored 150 mg lamivudine and 300 mg zidovudine (3)

CONTRAINDICATIONS

COMBIVIR Tablets are contraindicated in patients with previously demonstrated clinically significant hypersensitivity (e.g., anaphylaxis, Stevens-Johnson syndrome). (4)

WARNINGS AND PRECAUTIONS

- See boxed warning for information about the following: hematologic toxicity, symptomatic myopathy, lactic acidosis and severe hepatomegaly, and severe acute exacerbations of hepatitis B. (5.1, 5.2, 5.3. 5.4)
- COMBIVIR should not be administered with other lamivudine- or zidovudine-containing products or emtricitabine-containing products. (5.5)
- Hepatic decompensation, some fatal, has occurred in HIV-1/HCV co-infected patients receiving combination antiretroviral therapy and interferon alfa with/without ribavirin. Discontinue COMBIVIR as medically appropriate and consider dose reduction or discontinuation of interferon alfa, ribavirin, or both. (5.6)
- Exacerbation of anemia has been reported in HIV-1/HCV co-infected patients receiving ribavirin and zidovudine. Co-administration of ribavirin and zidovudine is not advised. (5.6)
- Pancreatitis: Use with caution in pediatric patients with a history of pancreatitis or other significant risk factors for pancreatitis. Discontinue treatment as clinically appropriate. (5.7)
- Immune reconstitution syndrome (5.8) and redistribution/accumulation of body fat (5.9) have been reported in patients treated with combination antiretroviral therapy.

ADVERSE REACTIONS

- Most commonly reported adverse reactions (incidence greater than or equal to 15%) in adult and pediatric HIV-1 clinical trials of combination lamivudine and zidovudine were headache, nausea, malaise and fatigue, nasal signs and symptoms, diarrhea, and cough. (6.1)

To report SUSPECTED ADVERSE REACTIONS, contact ViiV Healthcare at 1-877-844-8872 or FDA at 1-800-FDA-1088 or www.fda.gov/medwatch.

DRUG INTERACTIONS

- Concomitant use with the following drugs should be avoided: stavudine (7.1), zalcitabine (7.1), doxorubicin (7.2).
- Bone marrow suppressive/cytotoxic agents: May increase the hematologic toxicity of zidovudine. (7.3)

USE IN SPECIFIC POPULATIONS

- Pregnancy: Physicians are encouraged to register patients in the Antiretroviral Pregnancy Registry by calling 1-800-258-4263. (8.1)
- Nursing Mothers: HIV-1 infected mothers in the United States should not breastfeed to avoid potential postnatal transmission of HIV-1. (8.3)

See 17 for PATIENT COUNSELING INFORMATION

Revised: 01/2013

FULL PRESCRIBING INFORMATION: CONTENTS*

FULL PRESCRIBING INFORMATION

WARNING: HEMATOLOGIC TOXICITY, MYOPATHY, LACTIC ACIDOSIS, EXACERBATIONS OF HEPATITIS B

Hematologic Toxicity: Zidovudine, one of the 2 active ingredients in COMBIVIR® (lamivudine and zidovudine) Tablets, has been associated with hematologic toxicity including neutropenia and anemia, particularly in patients with advanced HIV-1 disease *[see Warnings and Precautions (5.1)]*.

Myopathy: Prolonged use of zidovudine has been associated with symptomatic myopathy *[see Warnings and Precautions (5.2)]*.

Lactic Acidosis and Severe Hepatomegaly: Lactic acidosis and hepatomegaly with steatosis, including fatal cases, have been reported with the use of nucleoside analogues alone or in combination, including lamivudine, zidovudine, and other antiretrovirals. Suspend treatment if clinical or laboratory findings suggestive of lactic acidosis or pronounced hepatotoxicity occur *[see Warnings and Precautions (5.3)]*.

Exacerbations of Hepatitis B: Severe, acute exacerbations of hepatitis B have been reported in patients who are co-infected with hepatitis B virus (HBV) and HIV-1 and have discontinued lamivudine, which is one component of COMBIVIR. Hepatic function should be monitored closely with both clinical and laboratory follow-up for at least several months in patients who discontinue COMBIVIR and are co-infected with HIV-1 and HBV. If appropriate, initiation of anti-hepatitis B therapy may be warranted *[see Warnings and Precautions (5.4)]*.

1 INDICATIONS AND USAGE

COMBIVIR, a combination of 2 nucleoside analogues, is indicated in combination with other antiretrovirals for the treatment of HIV-1 infection.

2 DOSAGE AND ADMINISTRATION

2.1 Adults and Adolescents Weighing ≥30 kg

The recommended oral dose of COMBIVIR in HIV-1-infected adults and adolescents weighing greater than or equal to 30 kg is 1 tablet (containing 150 mg of lamivudine and 300 mg of zidovudine) twice daily.

2.2 Pediatric Patients

The recommended oral dosage of scored COMBIVIR Tablets for pediatric patients who weigh greater than or equal to 30 kg and for whom a solid oral dosage form is appropriate is 1 tablet administered twice daily.

Before prescribing COMBIVIR Tablets, children should be assessed for the ability to swallow tablets. If a child is unable to reliably swallow a COMBIVIR Tablet, the liquid oral formulations should be prescribed: EPIVIR® (lamivudine) Oral Solution and RETROVIR® (zidovudine) Syrup.

2.3 Patients Requiring Dosage Adjustment

Because COMBIVIR is a fixed-dose combination tablet, it should not be prescribed for pediatric patients weighing less than 30 kg or patients requiring dosage adjustment, such as those with reduced renal function (creatinine clearance less than 50 mL/min), patients with hepatic impairment, or patients experiencing dose-limiting adverse reactions. Liquid and solid oral formulations of the individual components of COMBIVIR are available for these populations.

3 DOSAGE FORMS AND STRENGTHS

COMBIVIR Tablets contain 150 mg of lamivudine and 300 mg of zidovudine. The tablets are white, scored, film-coated, modified capsule-shaped tablets, debossed on both tablet faces, such that when broken in half, the full "GX FC3" code is present on both halves of the tablet ("GX" on one face and "FC3" on the opposite face of the tablet).

4 CONTRAINDICATIONS

COMBIVIR Tablets are contraindicated in patients with previously demonstrated clinically significant hypersensitivity (e.g., anaphylaxis, Stevens-Johnson syndrome) to any of the components of the product.

5 WARNINGS AND PRECAUTIONS

5.1 Hemotologic Toxicity/Bone Marrow Suppression

Zidovudine, a component of COMBIVIR, has been associated with hematologic toxicity including neutropenia and anemia, particularly in patients with advanced HIV-1 disease. COMBIVIR should be used with caution in patients who have bone marrow compromise evidenced by granulocyte count less than 1,000 cells/mm^3 or hemoglobin less than 9.5 g/dL *[see Adverse Reactions (6.1)]*.

Frequent blood counts are strongly recommended in patients with advanced HIV-1 disease who are treated with COMBIVIR. Periodic blood counts are recommended for other HIV-1-infected patients. If anemia or neutropenia develops, dosage interruption may be needed.

5.2 Myopathy

Myopathy and myositis, with pathological changes similar to that produced by HIV-1 disease, have been associated with prolonged use of zidovudine, and therefore may occur with therapy with COMBIVIR.

5.3 Lactic Acidosis/Hepatomegaly With Steatosis

Lactic acidosis and hepatomegaly with steatosis, including fatal cases, have been reported with the use of nucleoside analogues alone or in combination, including lamivudine, zidovudine, and other antiretrovirals. A majority of these cases have been in women. Obesity and prolonged nucleoside exposure may be risk factors. Particular caution should be exercised when administering COMBIVIR to any patient with known risk factors for liver disease; however, cases have also been reported in patients with no known risk factors. Treatment with COMBIVIR should be suspended in any patient who develops clinical or laboratory findings suggestive of lactic acidosis or pronounced hepatotoxicity (which may include hepatomegaly and steatosis even in the absence of marked transaminase elevations).

5.4 Patients With HIV-1 and Hepatitis B Virus Co-infection

Posttreatment Exacerbations of Hepatitis: In clinical trials in non-HIV-1-infected patients treated with lamivudine for chronic HBV, clinical and laboratory evidence of exacerbations of hepatitis have occurred after discontinuation of lamivudine. These exacerbations have been detected primarily by serum ALT elevations in addition to re-emergence of hepatitis B viral DNA (HBV DNA). Although most events appear to have been self-limited, fatalities have been reported in some cases. Similar events have been reported from post-marketing experience after changes from lamivudine-containing HIV-1 treatment regimens to non-lamivudine-containing regimens in patients infected with both HIV-1 and HBV. The causal relationship to discontinuation of lamivudine treatment is unknown. Patients should be closely monitored with both clinical and laboratory follow-up for at least several months after stopping treatment. There is insufficient evidence to determine whether re-initiation of lamivudine alters the course of posttreatment exacerbations of hepatitis.

Important Differences Among Lamivudine-Containing Products: COMBIVIR Tablets contain a higher dose of the same active ingredient (lamivudine) than EPIVIR-HBV® (lamivudine) Tablets and Oral Solution. EPIVIR-HBV was developed for treating chronic hepatitis B. Safety and efficacy of lamivudine have not been established for treatment of chronic hepatitis B in patients co-infected with HIV-1 and HBV.

Emergence of Lamivudine-Resistant HBV: In non-HIV-infected patients treated with lamivudine for chronic hepatitis B, emergence of lamivudine-resistant HBV has been detected and has been associated with diminished treatment response (see full prescribing information for EPIVIR-HBV for additional information). Emergence of hepatitis B virus variants associated with resistance to lamivudine has also been reported in HIV-1-infected patients who have received lamivudine-containing antiretroviral regimens in the presence of concurrent infection with hepatitis B virus.

5.5 Use With Other, Lamivudine-, Zidovudine-, and/or Emtricitabine-Containing Products

COMBIVIR is a fixed-dose combination of lamivudine and zidovudine. COMBIVIR should not be administered concomitantly with other lamivudine- or zidovudine-containing products including EPIVIR® (lamivudine) Tablets and Oral Solution; EPIVIR-HBV Tablets and Oral Solution; RETROVIR® (zidovudine) Tablets, Capsules, Syrup, and IV Infusion; EPZICOM® (abacavir sulfate and lamivudine) Tablets; or TRIZIVIR® (abacavir sulfate, lamivudine, and zidovudine) Tablets; or emtricitabine-containing products, including ATRIPLA® (efavirenz, emtricitabine, and tenofovir), EMTRIVA® (emtricitabine), TRUVADA® (emtricitabine and tenofovir), or COMPLERA® (rilpivirine/emtricitabine/tenofovir).

5.6 Use With Interferon- and Ribavirin-Based Regimens

In vitro studies have shown ribavirin can reduce the phosphorylation of pyrimidine nucleoside analogues such as lamivudine and zidovudine. Although no evidence of a pharmacokinetic or pharmacodynamic interaction (e.g., loss of HIV-1/HCV virologic suppression) was seen when ribavirin was coadministered with lamivudine or zidovudine in HIV-1/HCV co-infected patients *[see Clinical Pharmacology (12.3)]*, hepatic decompensation (some fatal) has occurred in HIV-1/HCV co-infected patients receiving combination antiretroviral therapy for HIV-1 and interferon alfa with or without ribavirin. Patients receiving interferon alfa with or without ribavirin and COMBIVIR should be closely monitored for treatment-associated toxicities, especially hepatic decompensation, neutropenia, and anemia. Discontinuation of COMBIVIR should be considered as medically appropriate. Dose reduction or discontinuation of interferon alfa, ribavirin, or both should also be considered if worsening clinical toxicities are observed, including hepatic decompensation (e.g., Child-Pugh greater than 6) (see the complete prescribing information for interferon and ribavirin).

Exacerbation of anemia has been reported in HIV-1/HCV co-infected patients receiving ribavirin and zidovudine. Coadministration of ribavirin and zidovudine is not advised.

5.7 Pancreatitis

COMBIVIR should be used with caution in patients with a history of pancreatitis or other significant risk factors for the development of pancreatitis. Treatment with COMBIVIR should be stopped immediately if clinical signs, symptoms, or laboratory abnormalities suggestive of pancreatitis occur *[see Adverse Reactions (6.1)]*.

5.8 Immune Reconstitution Syndrome

Immune reconstitution syndrome has been reported in patients treated with combination antiretroviral therapy, including COMBIVIR. During the initial phase of combination antiretroviral treatment, patients whose immune systems respond may develop an inflammatory response to indolent or residual opportunistic infections (such as *Mycobacterium avium* infection, cytomegalovirus, *Pneumocystis jirovecii* pneumonia [PCP], or tuberculosis), which may necessitate further evaluation and treatment.

Autoimmune disorders (such as Graves' disease, polymyositis, and Guillain-Barré syndrome) have also been reported to occur in the setting of immune reconstitution; however, the time to onset is more variable, and can occur many months after initiation of treatment.

5.9 Fat Redistribution

Redistribution/accumulation of body fat including central obesity, dorsocervical fat enlargement (buffalo hump), peripheral wasting, facial wasting, breast enlargement, and "cushingoid appearance" have been observed in patients receiving antiretroviral therapy. The mechanism and long-term consequences of these events are currently unknown. A causal relationship has not been established.

6 ADVERSE REACTIONS

The following adverse reactions are discussed in greater detail in other sections of the labeling:

- Hematologic toxicity, including neutropenia and anemia *[see Boxed Warning, Warnings and Precautions (5.1)]*.
- Symptomatic myopathy *[see Boxed Warning, Warnings and Precautions (5.2)]*.
- Lactic acidosis and hepatomegaly with steatosis *[see Boxed Warning, Warnings and Precautions (5.3)]*.
- Acute exacerbations of hepatitis B *[see Boxed Warning, Warnings and Precautions (5.4)]*.
- Hepatic decompensation in patients co-infected with HIV-1 and hepatitis C *[see Warnings and Precautions (5.6)]*.
- Exacerbation of anemia in HIV-1/HCV co-infected patients receiving ribavirin and zidovudine *[see Warnings and Precautions (5.6)]*.
- Pancreatitis *[see Warnings and Precautions (5.7)]*.

6.1 Clinical Trials Experience

Because clinical trials are conducted under widely varying conditions, adverse reaction rates observed in the clinical trials of a drug cannot be directly compared with rates in the clinical trials of another drug and may not reflect the rates observed in practice.

Lamivudine Plus Zidovudine Administered As Separate Formulations: In 4 randomized, controlled trials of EPIVIR 300 mg per day plus RETROVIR 600 mg per day, the following selected adverse reactions and laboratory abnormalities were observed (see Tables 1 and 2).

Table 1. Selected Clinical Adverse Reactions (≥5% Frequency) in 4 Controlled Clinical Trials With EPIVIR 300 mg/day and RETROVIR 600 mg/day

Adverse Reaction	EPIVIR plus RETROVIR (n = 251)
Body as a whole	
Headache	35%
Malaise & fatigue	27%
Fever or chills	10%
Digestive	
Nausea	33%

Diarrhea	18%
Nausea & vomiting	13%
Anorexia and/or decreased appetite	10%
Abdominal pain	9%
Abdominal cramps	6%
Dyspepsia	5%
Nervous system	
Neuropathy	12%
Insomnia & other sleep disorders	11%
Dizziness	10%
Depressive disorders	9%
Respiratory	
Nasal signs & symptoms	20%
Cough	18%
Skin	
Skin rashes	9%
Musculoskeletal	
Musculoskeletal pain	12%
Myalgia	8%
Arthralgia	5%

Pancreatitis was observed in 9 of the 2,613 adult subjects (0.3%) who received EPIVIR in controlled clinical trials *[see Warnings and Precautions (5.7)]*.

Selected laboratory abnormalities observed during therapy are listed in Table 2.

Table 2. Frequencies of Selected Laboratory Abnormalities Among Adults in 4 Controlled Clinical Trials of EPIVIR 300 mg/day plus RETROVIR 600 mg/day[a]

Test (Abnormal Level)	EPIVIR plus RETROVIR % (n)
Neutropenia (ANC<750/mm^3)	7.2% (237)
Anemia (Hgb<8.0 g/dL)	2.9% (241)
Thrombocytopenia (platelets<50,000/mm^3)	0.4% (240)
ALT (>5.0 × ULN)	3.7% (241)
AST (>5.0 × ULN)	1.7% (241)
Bilirubin (>2.5 × ULN)	0.8% (241)
Amylase (>2.0 × ULN)	4.2% (72)

ULN = Upper limit of normal.
ANC = Absolute neutrophil count.
n = Number of subjects assessed.
[a] Frequencies of these laboratory abnormalities were higher in subjects with mild laboratory abnormalities at baseline.

6.2 Postmarketing Experience

In addition to adverse reactions reported from clinical trials, the following reactions have been identified during post-approval use of EPIVIR, RETROVIR, and/or COMBIVIR. Because they are reported voluntarily from a population of unknown size, estimates of frequency cannot be made. These events have been chosen for inclusion due to a combination of their seriousness, frequency of reporting, or potential causal connection to EPIVIR, RETROVIR, and/or COMBIVIR.

Body as a Whole: Redistribution/accumulation of body fat *[see Warnings and Precautions (5.9)]*.

Cardiovascular: Cardiomyopathy.

Endocrine and Metabolic: Gynecomastia, hyperglycemia.

Gastrointestinal: Oral mucosal pigmentation, stomatitis.

General: Vasculitis, weakness.

Hemic and Lymphatic: Anemia, (including pure red cell aplasia and anemias progressing on therapy), lymphadenopathy, splenomegaly.

Hepatic and Pancreatic: Lactic acidosis and hepatic steatosis, pancreatitis, posttreatment exacerbation of hepatitis B *[see Boxed Warning, Warnings and Precautions (5.3), (5.4), (5.7)]*.

Hypersensitivity: Sensitization reactions (including anaphylaxis), urticaria.

Musculoskeletal: Muscle weakness, CPK elevation, rhabdomyolysis.

Nervous: Paresthesia, peripheral neuropathy, seizures.

Respiratory: Abnormal breath sounds/wheezing.

Skin: Alopecia, erythema multiforme, Stevens-Johnson syndrome.

7 DRUG INTERACTIONS

No drug interaction trials have been conducted using COMBIVIR Tablets *[see Clinical Pharmacology (12.3)]*.

7.1 Antiretroviral Agents

Lamivudine: *Zalcitabine:* Lamivudine and zalcitabine may inhibit the intracellular phosphorylation of one another. Therefore, use of COMBIVIR in combination with zalcitabine is not recommended.

Zidovudine: *Stavudine:* Concomitant use of COMBIVIR with stavudine should be avoided since an antagonistic relationship with zidovudine has been demonstrated in vitro.

Nucleoside Analogues Affecting DNA Replication: Some nucleoside analogues affecting DNA replication, such as ribavirin, antagonize the in vitro antiviral activity of zidovudine against HIV-1; concomitant use of such drugs should be avoided.

7.2 Doxorubicin

Zidovudine: Concomitant use of COMBIVIR with doxorubicin should be avoided since an antagonistic relationship with zidovudine has been demonstrated in vitro.

7.3 Hematologic/Bone Marrow Suppressive/Cytotoxic Agents

Zidovudine: Coadministration of ganciclovir, interferon alfa, ribavirin, and other bone marrow suppressive or cytotoxic agents may increase the hematologic toxicity of zidovudine.

7.4 Interferon- and Ribavirin-Based Regimens

Lamivudine: Although no evidence of a pharmacokinetic or pharmacodynamic interaction (e.g., loss of HIV-1/HCV virologic suppression) was seen when ribavirin was coadministered with lamivudine in HIV-1/HCV co-infected patients, hepatic decompensation (some fatal) has occurred in HIV-1/HCV co-infected patients receiving combination antiretroviral therapy for HIV-1 and interferon alfa with or without ribavirin *[see Warnings and Precautions (5.5), Clinical Pharmacology (12.3)]*.

7.5 Trimethoprim/Sulfamethoxazole (TMP/SMX)

Lamivudine: No change in dose of either drug is recommended. There is no information regarding the effect on lamivudine pharmacokinetics of higher doses of TMP/SMX such as those used to treat PCP.

8 USE IN SPECIFIC POPULATIONS

8.1 Pregnancy

Pregnancy Category C.

Fetal Risk Summary: There are no adequate and well-controlled trials of COMBIVIR (lamivudine and zidovudine) in pregnant women. Clinical trial data demonstrate that maternal zidovudine treatment during pregnancy reduces vertical transmission of HIV-1 infection to the fetus. Animal reproduction studies performed with lamivudine and zidovudine showed increased embryotoxicity and fetal malformations (zidovudine), and increased embryolethality (lamivudine). COMBIVIR should be used during pregnancy only if the potential benefit justifies the potential risk to the fetus.

Antiretroviral Pregnancy Registry: To monitor maternal-fetal outcomes of pregnant women exposed to COMBIVIR and other antiretroviral agents, an Antiretroviral Pregnancy Registry has been established. Physicians are encouraged to register patients by calling 1-800-258-4263.

Clinical Considerations: Treatment of HIV during pregnancy optimizes the health of both mother and fetus. Clinical trial data reviewed by FDA demonstrate that maternal zidovudine treatment significantly reduces vertical transmission of HIV-1 infection to the fetus *[see Clinical Studies (14.2)]*. Published data suggest that combination antiretroviral regimens may reduce the rate of vertical transmission even further.

Pharmacokinetics of lamivudine and zidovudine in pregnant women are similar to the pharmacokinetics in nonpregnant women. No dose adjustments are needed during pregnancy.

In a clinical trial, adverse events among HIV-1-infected women were not different among untreated women and women treated with zidovudine. It is not known whether risks of adverse events associated with lamivudine are altered in pregnant women compared with other HIV-1-infected patients (see Human data below).

Data: *Human Data: Lamivudine:* Lamivudine pharmacokinetics were studied in pregnant women during 2 clinical trials conducted in South Africa. The trial assessed pharmacokinetics in: 16 women at 36 weeks gestation using 150 mg lamivudine twice daily with zidovudine, 10 women at 38 weeks gestation using 150 mg lamivudine twice daily with zidovudine, and 10 women at 38 weeks gestation using lamivudine 300 mg twice daily without other antiretrovirals. Lamivudine pharmacokinetics in pregnant women were similar to those seen in nonpregnant adults and in postpartum women. Lamivudine concentrations were generally similar in maternal, neonatal, and umbilical cord serum samples.

Zidovudine: A randomized, double-blind, placebo-controlled trial was conducted in HIV-1-infected pregnant women to determine the utility of zidovudine for the prevention of maternal-fetal HIV-1 transmission. Zidovudine treatment during pregnancy reduced the rate of maternal-fetal HIV-1 transmission from 24.9% for infants born to placebo-treated mothers to 7.8% for infants born to mothers treated with zidovudine. There were no differences in pregnancy-related adverse events between the treatment groups. Congenital abnormalities occurred with similar frequency between neonates born to mothers who received zidovudine and neonates born to mothers who received placebo. The observed abnormalities included problems in embryogenesis (prior to 14 weeks) or were recognized on ultrasound before or immediately after initiation of trial drug *[see Clinical Studies (14.2)]*.

Zidovudine pharmacokinetics were studied in a Phase 1 trial of 8 women during the last trimester of pregnancy. As pregnancy progressed, there was no evidence of drug accumulation. The pharmacokinetics of zidovudine were similar to that of nonpregnant adults. Consistent with passive transmission of the drug across the placenta, zidovudine concentrations in neonatal plasma at birth were essentially equal to those in maternal plasma at delivery.

Animal Data: Lamivudine: Animal reproduction studies performed at oral doses up to 130 and 60 times the adult dose in rats and rabbits, respectively, revealed no evidence of teratogenicity due to lamivudine. Increased early embryolethality occurred in rabbits at exposure levels similar to those in humans. However, there was no indication of this effect in rats at exposure levels up to 35 times those in humans. Based on animal studies, lamivudine crosses the placenta and is transferred to the fetus *[see Nonclinical Toxicology (13.2)]*.

Zidovudine: Increased fetal resorptions occurred in pregnant rats and rabbits treated with doses of zidovudine that produced drug plasma concentrations 66 to 226 times (rats) and 12 to 87 times (rabbits) the mean steady-state peak human plasma concentration following a single 100-mg dose of zidovudine. There were no other reported developmental anomalies. In another developmental toxicity study, pregnant rats received zidovudine up to near-lethal doses that produced peak plasma concentrations 350 times peak human plasma concentrations (300 times the daily exposure [AUC] in humans given 600 mg/day zidovudine). This dose was associated with marked maternal toxicity and an increased incidence of fetal malformations. However, there were no signs of teratogenicity at doses up to one-fifth the lethal dose *[see Nonclinical Toxicology(13.2)]*.

8.3 Nursing Mothers

The Centers for Disease Control and Prevention recommend that HIV-1-infected mothers in the United States not breastfeed their infants to avoid risking postnatal transmission of HIV-1 infection. Because of both the potential for HIV-1 transmission and serious adverse reactions in nursing infants, mothers should be instructed not to breastfeed if they are receiving COMBIVIR.

Although no trials of COMBIVIR excretion in breast milk have been performed, lactation trials performed with lamivudine and zidovudine show that both drugs are excreted in human breast milk. Samples of breast milk obtained from 20 mothers receiving lamivudine monotherapy (300 mg twice daily) or combination therapy (150 mg lamivudine twice daily and 300 mg zidovudine twice daily) had measurable concentrations of lamivudine. In another trial, after administration of a single dose of 200 mg zidovudine to 13 HIV–1–infected women, the mean concentration of zidovudine was similar in human milk and serum.

8.4 Pediatric Use

COMBIVIR should not be administered to pediatric patients weighing less than 30 kg, because it is a fixed-dose combination that cannot be adjusted for this patient population.

8.5 Geriatric Use

Clinical trials of COMBIVIR did not include sufficient numbers of subjects aged 65 and over to determine whether they respond differently from younger subjects. In general, dose selection for an elderly patient should be cautious, reflecting the greater frequency of decreased hepatic, renal, or cardiac function, and of concomitant disease or other drug therapy. COMBIVIR is not recommended for patients with impaired renal function (i.e., creatinine clearance less than 50 mL/min) because it is a fixed-dose combination that cannot be adjusted.

8.6 Renal Impairment

Reduction of the dosages of lamivudine and zidovudine is recommended for patients with impaired renal function. Patients with creatinine clearance less than 50 mL/min should not receive COMBIVIR because it is a fixed-dose combination that cannot be adjusted.

8.7 Hepatic Impairment

A reduction in the daily dose of zidovudine may be necessary in patients with mild to moderate impaired hepatic function or liver cirrhosis. COMBIVIR is not recommended for patients with impaired hepatic function because it is a fixed-dose combination that cannot be adjusted.

10 OVERDOSAGE

COMBIVIR: There is no known antidote for COMBIVIR.

Lamivudine: One case of an adult ingesting 6 grams of lamivudine was reported; there were no clinical signs or symptoms noted and hematologic tests remained normal. Because a negligible amount of lamivudine was removed via (4-hour) hemodialysis, continuous ambulatory peritoneal di-

Table 3. Pharmacokinetic Parameters[a] for Lamivudine and Zidovudine in Adults

Parameter	Lamivudine		Zidovudine	
Oral bioavailability (%)	86 ± 16	N = 12	64 ± 10	n = 5
Apparent volume of distribution (L/kg)	1.3 ± 0.4	N = 20	1.6 ± 0.6	n = 8
Plasma protein binding (%)	<36		<38	
CSF:plasma ratio[b]	0.12 [0.04 to 0.47]	n = 38[c]	0.60 [0.04 to 2.62]	N = 39[d]
Systemic clearance (L/hr/kg)	0.33 ± 0.06	N = 20	1.6 ± 0.6	n = 6
Renal clearance (L/hr/kg)	0.22 ± 0.06	N = 20	0.34 ± 0.05	n = 9
Elimination half-life (hr)[e]	5 to 7		0.5 to 3	

[a] Data presented as mean ± standard deviation except where noted.
[b] Median [range].
[c] Children.
[d] Adults.
[e] Approximate range.

alysis, and automated peritoneal dialysis, it is not known if continuous hemodialysis would provide clinical benefit in a lamivudine overdose event.

Zidovudine: Acute overdoses of zidovudine have been reported in pediatric patients and adults. These involved exposures up to 50 grams. The only consistent findings were nausea and vomiting. Other reported occurrences included headache, dizziness, drowsiness, lethargy, confusion, and 1 report of a grand mal seizure. Hematologic changes were transient. All patients recovered. Hemodialysis and peritoneal dialysis appear to have a negligible effect on the removal of zidovudine, while elimination of its primary metabolite, 3′-azido-3′-deoxy-5′-*O*-β-*D*-glucopyranuronosylthymidine (GZDV), is enhanced.

11 DESCRIPTION

COMBIVIR: COMBIVIR Tablets are combination tablets containing lamivudine and zidovudine. Lamivudine (EPIVIR) and zidovudine (RETROVIR, azidothymidine, AZT, or ZDV) are synthetic nucleoside analogues with activity against HIV-1.

COMBIVIR Tablets are for oral administration. Each film-coated tablet contains 150 mg of lamivudine, 300 mg of zidovudine, and the inactive ingredients colloidal silicon dioxide, hypromellose, magnesium stearate, microcrystalline cellulose, polyethylene glycol, polysorbate 80, sodium starch glycolate, and titanium dioxide.

Lamivudine: The chemical name of lamivudine is (2R,cis)-4-amino-1-(2-hydroxymethyl-1,3-oxathiolan-5-yl)-(1H)-pyrimidin-2-one. Lamivudine is the (-)enantiomer of a dideoxy analogue of cytidine. Lamivudine has also been referred to as (-)2′,3′-dideoxy, 3′-thiacytidine. It has a molecular formula of $C_8H_{11}N_3O_3S$ and a molecular weight of 229.3. It has the following structural formula:

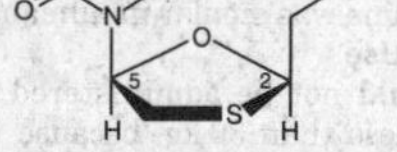

Lamivudine is a white to off-white crystalline solid with a solubility of approximately 70 mg/mL in water at 20°C.

Zidovudine: The chemical name of zidovudine is 3′-azido-3′-deoxythymidine. It has a molecular formula of $C_{10}H_{13}N_5O_4$ and a molecular weight of 267.24. It has the following structural formula:

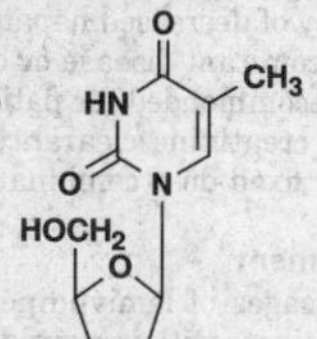

Zidovudine is a white to beige, odorless, crystalline solid with a solubility of 20.1 mg/mL in water at 25°C.

12 CLINICAL PHARMACOLOGY

12.1 Mechanism of Action

COMBIVIR is an antiviral agent *[see Clinical Pharmacology (12.4)]*.

12.3 Pharmacokinetics

Pharmacokinetics in Adults: *COMBIVIR:* One COMBIVIR Tablet was bioequivalent to 1 EPIVIR Tablet (150 mg) plus 1 RETROVIR Tablet (300 mg) following single-dose administration to fasting healthy subjects (n = 24).

Lamivudine: The pharmacokinetic properties of lamivudine in fasting subjects are summarized in Table 3. Following oral administration, lamivudine is rapidly absorbed and extensively distributed. Binding to plasma protein is low. Approximately 70% of an intravenous dose of lamivudine is recovered as unchanged drug in the urine. Metabolism of lamivudine is a minor route of elimination. In humans, the only known metabolite is the trans-sulfoxide metabolite (approximately 5% of an oral dose after 12 hours).

Zidovudine: The pharmacokinetic properties of zidovudine in fasting subjects are summarized in Table 3. Following oral administration, zidovudine is rapidly absorbed and extensively distributed. Binding to plasma protein is low. Zidovudine is eliminated primarily by hepatic metabolism. The major metabolite of zidovudine is GZDV. GZDV area under the curve (AUC) is about 3-fold greater than the zidovudine AUC. Urinary recovery of zidovudine and GZDV accounts for 14% and 74% of the dose following oral administration, respectively. A second metabolite, 3′-amino-3′-deoxythymidine (AMT), has been identified in plasma. The AMT AUC was one fifth of the zidovudine AUC. [See table 3 above]

Effect of Food on Absorption of COMBIVIR: COMBIVIR may be administered with or without food. The lamivudine and zidovudine AUC following administration of COMBIVIR with food was similar when compared with fasting healthy subjects (n = 24).

Special Populations:

Pregnancy: See Use in Specific Populations (8.1).

COMBIVIR: No data are available.

Zidovudine: Zidovudine pharmacokinetics has been studied in a Phase 1 trial of 8 women during the last trimester of pregnancy. As pregnancy progressed, there was no evidence of drug accumulation. The pharmacokinetics of zidovudine was similar to that of nonpregnant adults. Consistent with passive transmission of the drug across the placenta, zidovudine concentrations in neonatal plasma at birth were essentially equal to those in maternal plasma at delivery. Although data are limited, methadone maintenance therapy in 5 pregnant women did not appear to alter zidovudine pharmacokinetics. In a nonpregnant adult population, a potential for interaction has been identified.

Nursing Mothers: See Use in Specific Populations (8.3).

Pediatric Patients: COMBIVIR should not be administered to pediatric patients weighing less than 30 kg.

Geriatric Patients: The pharmacokinetics of lamivudine and zidovudine have not been studied in patients over 65 years of age.

Gender: A pharmacokinetic trial in healthy male (n = 12) and female (n = 12) subjects showed no gender differences in zidovudine AUC_∞ or lamivudine AUC_∞ normalized for body weight.

Race: *Lamivudine:* There are no significant racial differences in lamivudine pharmacokinetics.

Zidovudine: The pharmacokinetics of zidovudine with respect to race have not been determined.

Drug Interactions: *See Drug Interactions (7).*

No drug interaction trials have been conducted using COMBIVIR Tablets. However, Table 4 presents drug interaction information for the individual components of COMBIVIR.

Lamivudine Plus Zidovudine: No clinically significant alterations in lamivudine or zidovudine pharmacokinetics were observed in 12 asymptomatic HIV-1-infected adult subjects given a single dose of zidovudine (200 mg) in combination with multiple doses of lamivudine (300 mg q 12 hr).

[See table 4 at top of next page]

Ribavirin: In vitro data indicate ribavirin reduces phosphorylation of lamivudine, stavudine, and zidovudine. However, no pharmacokinetic (e.g., plasma concentrations or intracellular triphosphorylated active metabolite concentrations) or pharmacodynamic (e.g., loss of HIV-1/HCV virologic suppression) interaction was observed when ribavirin and lamivudine (n = 18), stavudine (n = 10), or zidovudine (n = 6) were coadministered as part of a multi-drug regimen to HIV-1/HCV co-infected subjects *[see Warnings and Precautions (5.5)]*.

12.4 Microbiology

Mechanism of Action: *Lamivudine:* Intracellularly, lamivudine is phosphorylated to its active 5′-triphosphate metabolite, lamivudine triphosphate (3TC-TP). The principal mode of action of 3TC-TP is inhibition of reverse transcriptase (RT) via DNA chain termination after incorporation of the nucleotide analogue. 3TC-TP is a weak inhibitor of cellular DNA polymerases α, β, and γ.

Zidovudine: Intracellularly, zidovudine is phosphorylated to its active 5′-triphosphate metabolite, zidovudine triphosphate (ZDV-TP). The principal mode of action of ZDV-TP is inhibition of RT via DNA chain termination after incorporation of the nucleotide analogue. ZDV-TP is a weak inhibitor of the cellular DNA polymerases α and γ and has been reported to be incorporated into the DNA of cells in culture.

Antiviral Activity: *Lamivudine Plus Zidovudine:* In HIV-1–infected MT-4 cells, lamivudine in combination with zidovudine at various ratios exhibited synergistic antiretroviral activity.

Lamivudine: The antiviral activity of lamivudine against HIV-1 was assessed in a number of cell lines (including monocytes and fresh human peripheral blood lymphocytes) using standard susceptibility assays. EC_{50} values (50% effective concentrations) were in the range of 0.003 to 15 µM (1 µM = 0.23 mcg/mL). HIV-1 from therapy-naive subjects with no amino acid substitutions associated with resistance gave median EC_{50} values of 0.429 µM (range: 0.200 to 2.007 µM) from Virco (n = 92 baseline samples from COL40263) and 2.35 µM (1.37 to 3.68 µM) from Monogram Biosciences (n = 135 baseline samples from ESS30009). The EC_{50} values of lamivudine against different HIV-1 clades (A-G) ranged from 0.001 to 0.120 µM, and against HIV-2 isolates from 0.003 to 0.120 µM in peripheral blood mononuclear cells. Ribavirin (50 µM) decreased the anti-HIV-1 activity of lamivudine by 3.5 fold in MT-4 cells.

Zidovudine: The antiviral activity of zidovudine against HIV-1 was assessed in a number of cell lines (including monocytes and fresh human peripheral blood lymphocytes). The EC_{50} and EC_{90} values for zidovudine were 0.01 to 0.49 µM (1 µM = 0.27 mcg/mL) and 0.1 to 9 µM, respectively. HIV-1 from therapy-naive subjects with no amino acid substitutions associated with resistance gave median EC_{50} values of 0.011 µM (range: 0.005 to 0.110 µM) from Virco (n = 92 baseline samples from COL40263) and 0.0017 µM (0.006 to 0.0340 µM) from Monogram Biosciences (n = 135 baseline samples from ESS30009). The EC_{50} values of zidovudine against different HIV-1 clades (A-G) ranged from 0.00018 to 0.02 µM, and against HIV-2 isolates from 0.00049 to 0.004 µM. In cell culture drug combination studies, zidovudine demonstrates synergistic activity with the nucleoside reverse transcriptase inhibitors (NRTIs) abacavir, didanosine, lamivudine, and zalcitabine; the non-nucleoside reverse transcriptase inhibitors (NNRTIs) delavirdine and nevirapine; and the protease inhibitors (PIs) indinavir, nelfinavir, ritonavir, and saquinavir; and additive activity with interferon alfa. Ribavirin has been found to inhibit the phosphorylation of zidovudine in cell culture.

Resistance: *Lamivudine Plus Zidovudine Administered As Separate Formulations:* In subjects receiving lamivudine monotherapy or combination therapy with lamivudine plus zidovudine, HIV–1 isolates from most subjects became phenotypically and genotypically resistant to lamivudine within 12 weeks. In some subjects harboring zidovudine–resistant virus at baseline, phenotypic sensitivity to zidovudine was restored by 12 weeks of treatment with lamivudine and zidovudine. Combination therapy with lamivudine plus zidovudine delayed the emergence of amino acid substitutions conferring resistance to zidovudine.

HIV-1 strains resistant to both lamivudine and zidovudine have been isolated from subjects after prolonged lamivudine/zidovudine therapy. Dual resistance required the presence of multiple amino acid substitutions, the most essential of which may be G333E. The incidence of dual resistance and the duration of combination therapy required before dual resistance occurs are unknown.

Lamivudine: Lamivudine–resistant isolates of HIV–1 have been selected in cell culture and have also been recovered from subjects treated with lamivudine or lamivudine plus zidovudine. Genotypic analysis of isolates selected in cell culture and recovered from lamivudine–treated subjects showed that the resistance was due to a specific amino acid substitution in the HIV–1 reverse transcriptase at codon 184 changing the methionine to either isoleucine or valine (M184V/I).

Zidovudine: HIV–1 isolates with reduced susceptibility to zidovudine have been selected in cell culture and were also recovered from subjects treated with zidovudine. Genotypic analyses of the isolates selected in cell culture and recovered from zidovudine–treated subjects showed substitutions in the HIV-1 RT gene resulting in 6 amino acid substitutions (M41L, D67N, K70R, L210W, T215Y or F, and K219Q) that confer zidovudine resistance. In general, higher levels of resistance were associated with greater number of amino acid substitutions.

Cross-Resistance: Cross-resistance has been observed among NRTIs.

Lamivudine Plus Zidovudine: Cross–resistance between lamivudine and zidovudine has not been reported. In some subjects treated with lamivudine alone or in combination with zidovudine, isolates have emerged with a substitution at codon 184, which confers resistance to lamivudine. Cross-resistance to abacavir, didanosine, tenofovir, and zalcitabine has been observed in some subjects harboring lamivudine–resistant HIV–1 isolates. In some subjects treated with zidovudine plus didanosine or zalcitabine, isolates resistant to multiple drugs, including lamivudine, have emerged (see under Zidovudine below).

Lamivudine: See Lamivudine Plus Zidovudine (above).

Zidovudine: In a trial of 167 HIV–1–infected subjects, isolates (n = 2) with multi–drug resistance to didanosine, lamivudine, stavudine, zalcitabine, and zidovudine were recovered from subjects treated for ≥1 year with zidovudine plus didanosine or zidovudine plus zalcitabine. The pattern of resistance–associated amino acid substitutions with such combination therapies was different (A62V, V75I, F77L, F116Y, Q151M) from the pattern with zidovudine monotherapy, with the Q151M substitution being most commonly associated with multi–drug resistance. The substitution at codon 151 in combination with substitutions at 62, 75, 77, and 116 results in a virus with reduced susceptibility to didanosine, lamivudine, stavudine, zalcitabine, and zidovudine. Thymidine analogue mutations (TAMs) are selected by zidovudine and confer cross–resistance to abacavir, didanosine, stavudine, tenofovir, and zalcitabine.

13 NONCLINICAL TOXICOLOGY

13.1 Carcinogenesis, Mutagenesis, Impairment of Fertility

Carcinogenicity: *Lamivudine:* Long-term carcinogenicity studies with lamivudine in mice and rats showed no evidence of carcinogenic potential at exposures up to 10 times (mice) and 58 times (rats) those observed in humans at the recommended therapeutic dose for HIV-1 infection.

Zidovudine: Zidovudine was administered orally at 3 dosage levels to separate groups of mice and rats (60 females and 60 males in each group). Initial single daily doses were 30, 60, and 120 mg/kg/day in mice and 80, 220, and 600 mg/kg/day in rats. The doses in mice were reduced to 20, 30, and 40 mg/kg/day after day 90 because of treatment-related anemia, whereas in rats only the high dose was reduced to 450 mg/kg/day on day 91 and then to 300 mg/kg/day on day 279.

In mice, 7 late-appearing (after 19 months) vaginal neoplasms (5 nonmetastasizing squamous cell carcinomas, 1 squamous cell papilloma, and 1 squamous polyp) occurred in animals given the highest dose. One late-appearing squamous cell papilloma occurred in the vagina of a middle-dose animal. No vaginal tumors were found at the lowest dose.

In rats, 2 late-appearing (after 20 months), nonmetastasizing vaginal squamous cell carcinomas occurred in animals given the highest dose. No vaginal tumors occurred at the low or middle dose in rats. No other drug-related tumors were observed in either sex of either species.

At doses that produced tumors in mice and rats, the estimated drug exposure (as measured by AUC) was approximately 3 times (mouse) and 24 times (rat) the estimated human exposure at the recommended therapeutic dose of 100 mg every 4 hours.

It is not known how predictive the results of rodent carcinogenicity studies may be for humans.

Mutagenicity: *Lamivudine:* Lamivudine was mutagenic in an L5178Y/TK$^{+/-}$ mouse lymphoma assay and clastogenic in a cytogenetic assay using cultured human lymphocytes. Lamivudine was negative in a microbial mutagenicity assay, in an in vitro cell transformation assay, in a rat micro nucleus test, in a rat bone marrow cytogenetic assay, and in an assay for unscheduled DNA synthesis in rat liver.

Zidovudine: Zidovudine was mutagenic in an L5178Y/TK$^{+/-}$ mouse lymphoma assay, positive in an in vitro cell transformation assay, clastogenic in a cytogenetic assay using cultured human lymphocytes, and positive in mouse and rat micronucleus tests after repeated doses. It was negative in a cytogenetic study in rats given a single dose.

Impairment of Fertility: *Lamivudine:* In a study of reproductive performance, lamivudine, administered to male and female rats at doses up to 130 times the usual adult dose based on body surface area considerations, revealed no evidence of impaired fertility (judged by conception rates) and no effect on the survival, growth, and development to weaning of the offspring.

Zidovudine: Zidovudine, administered to male and female rats at doses up to 7 times the usual adult dose based on body surface area considerations, had no effect on fertility judged by conception rates.

Table 4. Effect of Coadministered Drugs on Lamivudine and Zidovudine AUC[a]

Note: ROUTINE DOSE MODIFICATION OF LAMIVUDINE AND ZIDOVUDINE IS NOT WARRANTED WITH COADMINISTRATION OF THE FOLLOWING DRUGS.

Drugs That May Alter Lamivudine Blood Concentrations

Coadministered Drug and Dose	Lamivudine Dose	n	Lamivudine Concentrations		Concentration of Coadministered Drug
			AUC	Variability	
Nelfinavir 750 mg q 8 hr × 7 to 10 days	single 150 mg	11	↑AUC 10%	95% CI: 1% to 20%	↔
Trimethoprim 160 mg/Sulfamethoxazole 800 mg daily × 5 days	single 300 mg	14	↑AUC 43%	90% CI: 32% to 55%	

Drugs That May Alter Zidovudine Blood Concentrations

Coadministered Drug and Dose	Zidovudine Dose	n	Zidovudine Concentrations		Concentration of Coadministered Drug
			AUC	Variability	
Atovaquone 750 mg q 12 hr with food	200 mg q 8 hr	14	↑AUC 31%	Range 23% to 78%[b]	↔
Clarithromycin 500 mg twice daily	100 mg q 4 hr × 7 days	4	↓AUC 12%	Range ↓34% to ↑14%	Not Reported
Fluconazole 400 mg daily	200 mg q 8 hr	12	↑AUC 74%	95% CI: 54% to 98%	Not Reported
Methadone 30 to 90 mg daily	200 mg q 4 hr	9	↑AUC 43%	Range 16% to 64%[b]	↔
Nelfinavir 750 mg q 8 hr × 7 to 10 days	single 200 mg	11	↓AUC 35%	Range 28% to 41%	↔
Probenecid 500 mg q 6 hr × 2 days	2 mg/kg q 8 hr × 3 days	3	↑AUC 106%	Range 100% to 170%[b]	Not Assessed
Rifampin 600 mg daily × 14 days	200 mg q 8 hr × 14 days	8	↓AUC 47%	90% CI: 41% to 53%	Not Assessed
Ritonavir 300 mg q 6 hr × 4 days	200 mg q 8 hr × 4 days	9	↓AUC 25%	95% CI: 15% to 34%	↔
Valproic acid 250 mg or 500 mg q 8 hr × 4 days	100 mg q 8 hr × 4 days	6	↑AUC 80%	Range 64% to 130%[b]	Not Assessed

↑ = Increase; ↓= Decrease; ↔ = no significant change; AUC = area under the concentration versus time curve; CI = confidence interval.

[a] This table is not all inclusive.

[b] Estimated range of percent difference.

13.2 Reproductive and Developmental Toxicology Studies

Lamivudine: Reproduction studies have been performed in rats and rabbits at orally administered doses up to 4,000 mg/kg/day and 1,000 mg/kg/day, respectively, producing plasma levels up to approximately 35 times that for the adult HIV dose. No evidence of teratogenicity due to lamivudine was observed. Evidence of early embryolethality was seen in the rabbit at exposure levels similar to those observed in humans, but there was no indication of this effect in the rat at exposure levels up to 35 times those in humans. Studies in pregnant rats and rabbits showed that lamivudine is transferred to the fetus through the placenta.

Zidovudine: Oral teratology studies in the rat and in the rabbit at doses up to 500 mg/kg/day revealed no evidence of teratogenicity with zidovudine. Zidovudine treatment resulted in embryo/fetal toxicity as evidenced by an increase in the incidence of fetal resorptions in rats given 150 or 450 mg/kg/day and rabbits given 500 mg/kg/day. The doses used in the teratology studies resulted in peak zidovudine plasma concentrations (after one half of the daily dose) in rats 66 to 226 times, and in rabbits 12 to 87 times, mean steady-state peak human plasma concentrations (after one sixth of the daily dose) achieved with the recommended daily dose (100 mg every 4 hours). In an in vitro experiment with fertilized mouse oocytes, zidovudine exposure resulted in a dose-dependent reduction in blastocyst formation. In an additional teratology study in rats, a dose of 3,000 mg/kg/day (very near the oral median lethal dose in rats of 3,683 mg/kg) caused marked maternal toxicity and an increase in the incidence of fetal malformations. This dose resulted in peak zidovudine plasma concentrations 350 times peak human plasma concentrations. (Estimated AUC in rats at this dose level was 300 times the daily AUC in humans given 600 mg/day.) No evidence of teratogenicity was seen in this experiment at doses of 600 mg/kg/day or less.

14 CLINICAL STUDIES

There have been no clinical trials conducted with COMBIVIR. See *Clinical Pharmacology (12.3)* for information about bioequivalence. One COMBIVIR Tablet given twice daily is an alternative regimen to EPIVIR Tablets 150 mg twice daily plus RETROVIR 600 mg per day in divided doses.

14.1 Adults

Lamivudine Plus Zidovudine: The NUCB3007 (CAESAR) trial was conducted using EPIVIR 150–mg Tablets (150 mg twice daily) and RETROVIR 100–mg Capsules (2 × 100 mg 3 times daily). CAESAR was a multi-center, double-blind, placebo-controlled trial comparing continued current therapy (zidovudine alone [62% of subjects] or zidovudine with didanosine or zalcitabine [38% of subjects]) to the addition of EPIVIR or EPIVIR plus an investigational non-nucleoside reverse transcriptase inhibitor, randomized 1:2:1. A total of 1,816 HIV–1–infected adults with 25 to 250 (median 122) CD4 cells/mm^3 at baseline were enrolled: median age was 36 years, 87% were male, 84% were nucleoside-experienced, and 16% were therapy–naive. The median duration on trial was 12 months. Results are summarized in Table 5.

[See table 5 at top of next page]

14.2 Prevention of Maternal-Fetal HIV-1 Transmission

The utility of zidovudine alone for the prevention of maternal-fetal HIV-1 transmission was demonstrated in a randomized, double-blind, placebo-controlled trial conducted in HIV-1-infected pregnant women with CD4+ cell

Table 5. Number of Subjects (%) With At Least 1 HIV-1 Disease-Progression Event or Death

Endpoint	Current Therapy (n = 460)	EPIVIR plus Current Therapy (n = 896)	EPIVIR plus a NNRTI[a] plus Current Therapy (n = 460)
HIV-1 progression or death	90 (19.6%)	86 (9.6%)	41 (8.9%)
Death	27 (5.9%)	23 (2.6%)	14 (3.0%)

[a] An investigational non-nucleoside reverse transcriptase inhibitor not approved in the United States.

counts of 200 to 1,818 cells/mm^3 (median in the treated group: 560 cells/mm^3) who had little or no previous exposure to zidovudine. Oral zidovudine was initiated between 14 and 34 weeks of gestation (median 11 weeks of therapy) followed by IV administration of zidovudine during labor and delivery. Following birth, neonates received oral zidovudine syrup for 6 weeks. The trial showed a statistically significant difference in the incidence of HIV–1 infection in the neonates (based on viral culture from peripheral blood) between the group receiving zidovudine and the group receiving placebo. Of 363 neonates evaluated in the trial, the estimated risk of HIV–1 infection was 7.8% in the group receiving zidovudine and 24.9% in the placebo group, a relative reduction in transmission risk of 68.7%. Zidovudine was well tolerated by mothers and infants. There was no difference in pregnancy-related adverse events between the treatment groups.

16 HOW SUPPLIED/STORAGE AND HANDLING

COMBIVIR Tablets, containing 150 mg lamivudine and 300 mg zidovudine, are white, scored, film-coated, modified-capsule-shaped tablets, debossed on both tablet faces, such that when broken in half, the full "GXFC3" code is present on both halves of the tablet ("GX" on one face and "FC3" on the opposite face of the tablet). They are available as follows:

60 Tablets/Bottle (NDC 49702-202-18).

Unit Dose Pack of 120 (NDC 49702-202-29).

Store between 2° and 30°C (36° and 86°F).

17 PATIENT COUNSELING INFORMATION

17.1 Advice for the Patient

Neutropenia and Anemia: Patients should be informed that the important toxicities associated with zidovudine are neutropenia and/or anemia. They should be told of the extreme importance of having their blood counts followed closely while on therapy, especially for patients with advanced HIV-1 disease *[see Boxed Warning, Warnings and Precautions (5.1)]*.

Myopathy: Patients should be informed that myopathy and myositis with pathological changes, similar to that produced by HIV-1 disease, have been associated with prolonged use of zidovudine *[see Warnings and Precautions (5.2)]*.

Lactic Acidosis/Hepatomegaly: Patients should be informed that some HIV medicines, including COMBIVIR, can cause a rare, but serious condition called lactic acidosis with liver enlargement (hepatomegaly) *[see Warnings and Precautions (5.3)]*.

HIV-1/HBV Co-infection: Patients co-infected with HIV-1 and HBV should be informed that deterioration of liver disease has occurred in some cases when treatment with lamivudine was discontinued. Patients should be advised to discuss any changes in regimen with their physician *[see Warnings and Precautions (5.4)]*.

Use With Other Lamivudine-, Zidovudine-, and/or Emtricitabine-Containing Products: COMBIVIR should not be coadministered with drugs containing lamivudine, zidovudine, or emtricitabine, including EPIVIR (lamivudine), EPIVIR-HBV (lamivudine), RETROVIR (zidovudine), EPZICOM (abacavir sulfate and lamivudine), TRIZIVIR (abacavir sulfate, lamivudine, and zidovudine), ATRIPLA (efavirenz, emtricitabine, and tenofovir), EMTRIVA (emtricitabine), TRUVADA (emtricitabine and tenofovir), or COMPLERA™ (rilpivirine/emtricitabine/tenofovir) *[see Warnings and Precautions (5.5)]*.

HIV-1/HCV Co-Infection: Patients with HIV-1/HCV co-infection should be informed that hepatic decompensation (some fatal) has occurred in HIV-1/HCV co-infected patients receiving combination antiretroviral therapy for HIV-1 and interferon alfa with or without ribavirin *[see Warnings and Precautions (5.6)]*.

Drug Interactions: Patients should be cautioned about the use of other medications, including ganciclovir, interferon alfa, and ribavirin, which may exacerbate the toxicity of zidovudine *[see Drug Interactions (7.3)]*.

Redistribution/Accumulation of Body Fat: Patients should be informed that redistribution or accumulation of body fat may occur in patients receiving antiretroviral therapy and that the cause and long-term health effects of these conditions are not known at this time *[see Warnings and Precautions (5.9)]*.

Information About HIV-1 Infection: COMBIVIR is not a cure for HIV-1 infection and patients may continue to experience illnesses associated with HIV-1 infection, including opportunistic infections. Patients should remain under the care of a physician when using COMBIVIR.

Patients should be advised to avoid doing things that can spread HIV-1 infection to others.

- **Do not share needles or other injection equipment.**
- **Do not share personal items that can have blood or body fluids on them, like toothbrushes and razor blades.**
- **Do not have any kind of sex without protection.** Always practice safe sex by using a latex or polyurethane condom or other barrier method to lower the chance of sexual contact with semen, vaginal secretions, or blood.
- **Do not breastfeed.** Lamivudine and zidovudine are excreted in human breast milk. Mothers with HIV-1 should not breastfeed because HIV-1 can be passed to the baby in the breast milk.

Patients should be informed to take all HIV medications exactly as prescribed.

EPIVIR, RETROVIR, EPZICOM, and TRIZIVIR are registered trademarks of ViiV Healthcare.

The other brands listed are trademarks of their respective owners and are not trademarks of ViiV Healthcare. The makers of these brands are not affiliated with and do not endorse ViiV Healthcare or its products.

Manufactured for:
ViiV Healthcare
Research Triangle Park, NC 27709
by GlaxoSmithKline
Research Triangle Park, NC 27709
Lamivudine is manufactured under agreement from
Shire Pharmaceuticals Group plc
Basingstoke, UK

CMB: 5PI

EPIVIR ℞

[ĕp'ə-vir]
(lamivudine)
Tablets and Oral Solution

HIGHLIGHTS OF PRESCRIBING INFORMATION
These highlights do not include all the information needed to use EPIVIR safely and effectively. See full prescribing information for EPIVIR.
EPIVIR (lamivudine) Tablets and Oral Solution
Initial U.S. Approval: 1995

WARNING: LACTIC ACIDOSIS, POSTTREATMENT EXACERBATIONS OF HEPATITIS B IN CO-INFECTED PATIENTS, DIFFERENT FORMULATIONS OF EPIVIR
See full prescribing information for complete boxed warning

- **Lactic acidosis and severe hepatomegaly with steatosis, including fatal cases, have been reported with the use of nucleoside analogues. Suspend treatment if clinical or laboratory findings suggestive of lactic acidosis or pronounced hepatotoxicity occur. (5.1)**
- **Severe acute exacerbations of hepatitis B have been reported in patients who are co-infected with hepatitis B virus (HBV) and human immunodeficiency virus (HIV-1) and have discontinued EPIVIR. Monitor hepatic function closely in these patients and, if appropriate, initiate anti-hepatitis B treatment. (5.2)**
- **Patients with HIV-1 infection should receive only dosage forms of EPIVIR appropriate for treatment of HIV-1. (5.2)**

INDICATIONS AND USAGE

EPIVIR is a nucleoside analogue reverse transcriptase inhibitor indicated in combination with other antiretroviral agents for the treatment of HIV-1 infection. Limitation of Use: The dosage of this product is for HIV-1 and not for HBV. (1)

DOSAGE AND ADMINISTRATION

- Adults and adolescents aged >16 years: 300 mg daily, administered as either 150 mg twice daily or 300 mg once daily. (2.1)
- Pediatric patients aged 3 months 16 years: Dosage should be based on body weight. (2.2)
- Patients With Renal Impairment: Doses of EPIVIR must be adjusted in accordance with renal function. (2.3)

DOSAGE FORMS AND STRENGTHS

- Tablets: 300 mg (3)
- Tablets: Scored 150 mg (3)
- Oral Solution: 10 mg/mL (3)

CONTRAINDICATIONS

EPIVIR Tablets and Oral Solution are contraindicated in patients with previously demonstrated clinically significant hypersensitivity (e.g., anaphylaxis) to any of the components of the products. (4)

WARNINGS AND PRECAUTIONS

- Lactic acidosis and severe hepatomegaly with steatosis: Reported with the use of nucleoside analogues. Suspend treatment if clinical or laboratory findings suggestive of lactic acidosis or pronounced hepatoxicity occur. (5.1)
- Severe acute exacerbations of hepatitis: Reported in patients who are co-infected with hepatitis B virus and HIV-1 and discontinued EPIVIR. Monitor hepatic function closely in these patients and, if appropriate, initiate anti-hepatitis B treatment. (5.2)
- Patients with HIV-1 infection should receive only dosage forms of EPIVIR appropriate for treatment of HIV-1. (5.2)
- Co-infected HIV-1/HBV Patients: Emergence of lamivudine-resistant HBV variants associated with lamivudine-containing antiretroviral regimens has been reported. (5.2)
- Emtricitabine should not be administered concomitantly with lamivudine-containing products. (5.3)
- Hepatic decompensation (some fatal) has occurred in HIV-1/HCV co-infected patients receiving interferon and ribavirin-based regimens. Monitor for treatment-associated toxicities. Discontinue EPIVIR as medically appropriate and consider dose reduction or discontinuation of interferon alfa, ribavirin, or both. (5.4)
- Pancreatitis: Use with caution in pediatric patients with a history of pancreatitis or other significant risk factors for pancreatitis. Discontinue treatment as clinically appropriate. (5.5)
- Immune reconstitution syndrome (5.6) and redistribution/accumulation of body fat (5.7) have been reported in patients treated with combination antiretroviral therapy.

ADVERSE REACTIONS

- **The most common reported adverse reactions (incidence ≥15%) in adults were headache, nausea, malaise and fatigue, nasal signs and symptoms, diarrhea, and cough. (6.1)**
- **The most common reported adverse reactions (incidence ≥15%) in pediatric subjects were fever and cough. (6.1)**

To report SUSPECTED ADVERSE REACTIONS, contact ViiV Healthcare at 1-877-844-8872 or FDA at 1-800-FDA-1088 or www.fda.gov/medwatch.

DRUG INTERACTIONS

Zalcitabine is not recommended for use in combination with EPIVIR. (7.2)

USE IN SPECIFIC POPULATIONS

- Pregnancy: Physicians are encouraged to register patients in the Antiretroviral Pregnancy Registry by calling 1-800-258-4263. (8.1)

Revised: September 2010

See 17 for PATIENT COUNSELING INFORMATION

Revised: 01/2013

FULL PRESCRIBING INFORMATION: CONTENTS*

*** Sections or subsections omitted from the full prescribing information are not listed**

FULL PRESCRIBING INFORMATION

WARNING: RISK OF LACTIC ACIDOSIS, EXACERBATIONS OF HEPATITIS B IN CO-INFECTED PATIENTS UPON DISCONTINUATION OF EPIVIR , DIFFERENT FORMULATIONS OF EPIVIR.

Lactic Acidosis and Severe Hepatomegaly: Lactic acidosis and severe hepatomegaly with steatosis, including fatal cases, have been reported with the use of nucleoside analogues alone or in combination, including lamivudine and other antiretrovirals. Suspend treatment if clinical or laboratory findings suggestive of lactic acidosis or pronounced hepatotoxicity occur *[see Warnings and Precautions (5.1)]*.

Exacerbations of Hepatitis B: Severe acute exacerbations of hepatitis B have been reported in patients who are co-infected with hepatitis B virus (HBV) and human immunodeficiency virus (HIV-1) and have discontinued EPIVIR. Hepatic function should be monitored closely with both clinical and laboratory follow-up for at least several months in patients who discontinue EPIVIR and are co-infected with HIV-1 and HBV. If appropriate, initiation of anti-hepatitis B therapy may be warranted *[see Warnings and Precautions (5.2)]*.

Important Differences Among Lamivudine-Containing Products: EPIVIR Tablets and Oral Solution (used to treat HIV-1 infection) contain a higher dose of the active ingredient (lamivudine) than EPIVIR-HBV® Tablets and Oral Solution (used to treat chronic HBV infection). Patients with HIV-1 infection should receive only dosage forms appropriate for treatment of HIV-1 *[see Warnings and Precautions (5.2)*

1 INDICATIONS AND USAGE

EPIVIR is a nucleoside analogue indicated in combination with other antiretroviral agents for the treatment of human immunodeficiency virus (HIV-1) infection. Limitation of use: The dosage of this product is for HIV-1 and not for HBV.

2 DOSAGE AND ADMINISTRATION

2.1 Adults and Adolescents >16 years of age

The recommended oral dose of EPIVIR in HIV-1-infected adults and adolescents aged >16 years is 300 mg daily, administered as either 150 mg twice daily or 300 mg once daily, in combination with other antiretroviral agents. If lamivudine is administered to a patient infected with HIV-1 and HBV, the dosage indicated for HIV-1 therapy should be used as part of an appropriate combination regimen *[see Warnings and Precautions (5.2)]*.

2.2 Pediatric Patients

The recommended oral dose of EPIVIR Oral Solution in HIV-1-infected pediatric patients aged 3 months to 16 years is 4 mg/kg twice daily (up to a maximum of 150 mg twice a day), administered in combination with other antiretroviral agents.

EPIVIR is also available as a scored tablet for HIV-1-infected pediatric patients who weigh ≥14 kg and for whom a solid dosage form is appropriate. Before prescribing EPIVIR Tablets, children should be assessed for the ability to swallow tablets. If a child is unable to reliably swallow EPIVIR Tablets, the oral solution formulation should be prescribed. The recommended oral dosage of EPIVIR Tablets for HIV-1-infected pediatric patients is presented in Table 1.

Table 1. Dosing Recommendations for EPIVIR Tablets in Pediatric Patients

Weight (kg)	Dosage Regimen Using Scored 150-mg Tablet		Total Daily Dose
	AM Dose	PM Dose	
14 to 21	½ tablet (75 mg)	½ tablet (75 mg)	150 mg
>21 to <30	½ tablet (75 mg)	1 tablet (150 mg)	225 mg
≥30	1 tablet (150 mg)	1 tablet (150 mg)	300 mg

2.3 Patients With Renal Impairment

Dosing of EPIVIR is adjusted in accordance with renal function. Dosage adjustments are listed in Table 2 *[see Clinical Pharmacology (12.3)]*.

Table 2. Adjustment of Dosage of EPIVIR in Adults and Adolescents (≥30 kg) in Accordance With Creatinine Clearance

Creatinine Clearance (mL/min)	Recommended Dosage of EPIVIR
≥50	150 mg twice daily or 300 mg once daily
30-49	150 mg once daily
15-29	150 mg first dose, then 100 mg once daily
5-14	150 mg first dose, then 50 mg once daily
<5	50 mg first dose, then 25 mg once daily

No additional dosing of EPIVIR is required after routine (4-hour) hemodialysis or peritoneal dialysis.

Although there are insufficient data to recommend a specific dose adjustment of EPIVIR in pediatric patients with renal impairment, a reduction in the dose and/or an increase in the dosing interval should be considered.

3 DOSAGE FORMS AND STRENGTHS

• EPIVIR Scored Tablets

150 mg, are white, diamond-shaped, scored, film-coated tablets debossed with "GX CJ7" on both sides.

• EPIVIR Tablets

300 mg, are gray, modified diamond-shaped, film-coated tablets engraved with "GX EJ7" on one side and plain on the reverse side.

• EPIVIR Oral Solution

A clear, colorless to pale yellow, strawberry-banana flavored liquid, containing 10 mg of lamivudine per 1 mL.

4 CONTRAINDICATIONS

EPIVIR Tablets and Oral Solution are contraindicated in patients with previously demonstrated clinically significant hypersensitivity (e.g., anaphylaxis) to any of the components of the products.

5 WARNINGS AND PRECAUTIONS

5.1 Lactic Acidosis/Severe Hepatomegaly With Steatosis

Lactic acidosis and severe hepatomegaly with steatosis, including fatal cases, have been reported with the use of nucleoside analogues alone or in combination, including lamivudine and other antiretrovirals. A majority of these cases have been in women. Obesity and prolonged nucleoside exposure may be risk factors. Particular caution should be exercised when administering EPIVIR to any patient with known risk factors for liver disease; however, cases also have been reported in patients with no known risk factors. Treatment with EPIVIR should be suspended in any patient who develops clinical or laboratory findings suggestive of lactic acidosis or pronounced hepatotoxicity (which may include hepatomegaly and steatosis even in the absence of marked transaminase elevations).

5.2 Patients With HIV-1 and Hepatitis B Virus Co-infection

Posttreatment Exacerbations of Hepatitis: In clinical trials in non-HIV-1-infected patients treated with lamivudine for chronic hepatitis B, clinical and laboratory evidence of exacerbations of hepatitis have occurred after discontinuation of lamivudine. These exacerbations have been detected primarily by serum ALT elevations in addition to re-emergence of HBV DNA. Although most events appear to have been self-limited, fatalities have been reported in some cases. Similar events have been reported from post-marketing experience after changes from lamivudine-containing HIV-1 treatment regimens to non-lamivudine-containing regimens in patients infected with both HIV-1 and HBV. The causal relationship to discontinuation of lamivudine treatment is unknown. Patients should be closely monitored with both clinical and laboratory follow-up for at least several months after stopping treatment. There is insufficient evidence to determine whether re-initiation of lamivudine alters the course of posttreatment exacerbations of hepatitis.

Important Differences Among Lamivudine-Containing Products: EPIVIR Tablets and Oral Solution contain a higher dose of the same active ingredient (lamivudine) than EPIVIR-HBV Tablets and EPIVIR-HBV Oral Solution. EPIVIR-HBV was developed for patients with chronic hepatitis B. The formulation and dosage of lamivudine in EPIVIR-HBV are not appropriate for patients co-infected with HIV-1 and HBV. Safety and efficacy of lamivudine have not been established for treatment of chronic hepatitis B in patients co-infected with HIV-1 and HBV. If treatment with EPIVIR-HBV is prescribed for chronic hepatitis B for a patient with unrecognized or untreated HIV-1 infection, rapid emergence of HIV-1 resistance is likely to result because of the subtherapeutic dose and the inappropriateness of monotherapy HIV-1 treatment. If a decision is made to administer lamivudine to patients co-infected with HIV-1 and HBV, EPIVIR Tablets, EPIVIR Oral Solution, COMBIVIR® (lamivudine/zidovudine) Tablets, EPZICOM® (abacavir sulfate and lamivudine) Tablets, or TRIZIVIR® (abacavir sulfate, lamivudine, and zidovudine) Tablets should be used as part of an appropriate combination regimen.

Emergence of Lamivudine-Resistant HBV: In non–HIV-1-infected patients treated with lamivudine for chronic hepatitis B, emergence of lamivudine-resistant HBV has been detected and has been associated with diminished treatment response (see full prescribing information for EPIVIR-HBV for additional information). Emergence of hepatitis B virus variants associated with resistance to lamivudine has also been reported in HIV-1-infected patients who have received lamivudine-containing antiretroviral regimens in the presence of concurrent infection with hepatitis B virus.

5.3 Use With Other Lamivudine- and Emtricitabine-Containing Products

EPIVIR should not be administered concomitantly with other lamivudine-containing products including EPIVIR-HBV Tablets, EPIVIR Oral Solution, COMBIVIR (lamivudine/zidovudine) Tablets, EPZICOM (abacavir sulfate and lamivudine) Tablets, or TRIZIVIR (abacavir sulfate, lamivudine, and zidovudine) or emtricitabine-containing products, including ATRIPLA® (efavirenz, emtricitabine, and tenofovir), EMTRIVA® (emtricitabine), TRUVADA® (emtricitabine and tenofovir), or COMPLERA® (rilpivirine/emtricitabine/tenofovir).

5.4 Use With Interferon- and Ribavirin-Based Regimens

In vitro studies have shown ribavirin can reduce the phosphorylation of pyrimidine nucleoside analogues such as lamivudine. Although no evidence of a pharmacokinetic or pharmacodynamic interaction (e.g., loss of HIV-1/HCV virologic suppression) was seen when ribavirin was coadministered with lamivudine in HIV-1/HCV co-infected patients *[see Clinical Pharmacology (12.3)]*, hepatic decompensation (some fatal) has occurred in HIV-1/HCV co-infected patients receiving combination antiretroviral therapy for HIV-1 and interferon alfa with or without ribavirin. Patients receiving interferon alfa with or without ribavirin and EPIVIR should be closely monitored for treatment-associated toxicities, especially hepatic decompensation. Discontinuation of EPIVIR should be considered as medically appropriate. Dose reduction or discontinuation of interferon alfa, ribavirin, or both should also be considered if worsening clinical toxicities are observed, including hepatic decompensation (e.g., Child-Pugh >6). See the complete prescribing information for interferon and ribavirin.

5.5 Pancreatitis

In pediatric patients with a history of prior antiretroviral nucleoside exposure, a history of pancreatitis, or other significant risk factors for the development of pancreatitis, EPIVIR should be used with caution. Treatment with EPIVIR should be stopped immediately if clinical signs, symptoms, or laboratory abnormalities suggestive of pancreatitis occur *[see Adverse Reactions (6.1)]*.

5.6 Immune Reconstitution Syndrome

Immune reconstitution syndrome has been reported in patients treated with combination antiretroviral therapy, including EPIVIR. During the initial phase of combination antiretroviral treatment, patients whose immune system responds may develop an inflammatory response to indolent or residual opportunistic infections (such as *Mycobacterium*

Table 4. Frequencies of Selected Grade 3-4 Laboratory Abnormalities in Adults in Four 24-Week Surrogate Endpoint Trials(NUCA3001, NUCA3002, NUCB3001, NUCB3002) and a Clinical Endpoint Trial (NUCB3007)

	24-Week Surrogate Endpoint Trials[a]		Clinical Endpoint Trial[a]	
Test (Threshold Level)	EPIVIR plus RETROVIR	RETROVIR[b]	EPIVIR plus Current Therapy	Placebo plus Current Therapy[c]
Absolute neutrophil count (<750/mm^3)	7.2%	5.4%	15%	13%
Hemoglobin (<8.0 g/dL)	2.9%	1.8%	2.2%	3.4%
Platelets (<50,000/mm^3)	0.4%	1.3%	2.8%	3.8%
ALT (>5.0 × ULN)	3.7%	3.6%	3.8%	1.9%
AST (>5.0 × ULN)	1.7%	1.8%	4.0%	2.1%
Bilirubin (>2.5 × ULN)	0.8%	0.4%	ND	ND
Amylase (>2.0 × ULN)	4.2%	1.5%	2.2%	1.1%

[a] The median duration on study was 12 months.
[b] Either zidovudine monotherapy or zidovudine in combination with zalcitabine.
[c] Current therapy was either zidovudine, zidovudine plus didanosine, or zidovudine plus zalcitabine.
ULN = Upper limit of normal.
ND = Not done.

avium infection, cytomegalovirus, *Pneumocystis jirovecii* pneumonia [PCP], or tuberculosis), which may necessitate further evaluation and treatment.
Autoimmune disorders (such as Graves' disease, polymyositis, and Guillain-Barré syndrome) have also been reported to occur in the setting of immune reconstitution, however, the time to onset is more variable, and can occur many months after initiation of treatment.

5.7 Fat Redistribution

Redistribution/accumulation of body fat including central obesity, dorsocervical fat enlargement (buffalo hump), peripheral wasting, facial wasting, breast enlargement, and "cushingoid appearance" have been observed in patients receiving antiretroviral therapy. The mechanism and long-term consequences of these events are currently unknown. A causal relationship has not been established.

6 ADVERSE REACTIONS

The following adverse reactions are discussed in greater detail in other sections of the labeling:

- Lactic acidosis and severe hepatomegaly with steatosis *[see Boxed Warning, Warnings and Precautions (5.1)]*.
- Severe acute exacerbations of hepatitis B *[see Boxed Warning, Warnings and Precautions (5.2)]*.
- Hepatic decompensation in patients co-infected with HIV-1 and hepatitis C *[see Warnings and Precautions (5.4)]*.
- Pancreatitis *[see Warnings and Precautions (5.5)]*.

6.1 Clinical Trials Experience

Because clinical trials are conducted under widely varying conditions, adverse reaction rates observed in the clinical trials of a drug cannot be directly compared with rates in the clinical trials of another drug and may not reflect the rates observed in practice.
Adults - Clinical Trials in HIV-1: The safety profile of EPIVIR in adults is primarily based on 3,568 HIV-1-infected subjects in 7 clinical trials.
The most common adverse reactions are headache, nausea, malaise, fatigue, nasal signs and symptoms, diarrhea and cough.
Selected clinical adverse reactions in ≥5% of subjects during therapy with EPIVIR 150 mg twice daily plus RETROVIR® 200 mg 3 times daily for up to 24 weeks are listed in Table 3.

Table 3. Selected Clinical Adverse Reactions (≥5% Frequency) in Four Controlled Clinical Trials (NUCA3001, NUCA3002, NUCB3001, NUCB3002)

Adverse Reaction	EPIVIR 150 mg Twice Daily plus RETROVIR (n = 251)	RETROVIR[a] (n = 230)
Body as a Whole		
Headache	35%	27%
Malaise & fatigue	27%	23%
Fever or chills	10%	12%
Digestive		
Nausea	33%	29%
Diarrhea	18%	22%
Nausea & vomiting	13%	12%
Anorexia and/or decreased appetite	10%	7%
Abdominal pain	9%	11%
Abdominal cramps	6%	3%
Dyspepsia	5%	5%
Nervous System		
Neuropathy	12%	10%
Insomnia & other sleep disorders	11%	7%
Dizziness	10%	4%
Depressive disorders	9%	4%
Respiratory		
Nasal signs & symptoms	20%	11%
Cough	18%	13%
Skin		
Skin rashes	9%	6%
Musculoskeletal		
Musculoskeletal pain	12%	10%
Myalgia	8%	6%
Arthralgia	5%	5%

[a] Either zidovudine monotherapy or zidovudine in combination with zalcitabine.

Pancreatitis: Pancreatitis was observed in 9 out of 2,613 adult subjects (0.3%) who received EPIVIR in controlled clinical trials EPV20001, NUCA3001, NUCB3001, NUCA3002, NUCB3002, and NUCB3007 *[see Warnings and Precautions (5.5)]*.
EPIVIR 300 mg Once Daily: The types and frequencies of clinical adverse reactions reported in subjects receiving EPIVIR 300 mg once daily or EPIVIR 150 mg twice daily (in 3-drug combination regimens in EPV20001 and EPV40001) for 48 weeks were similar.
Selected laboratory abnormalities observed during therapy are summarized in Table 4.
[See table 4 above]
The frequencies of selected laboratory abnormalities reported subjects receiving EPIVIR 300 mg once daily or EPIVIR 150 mg twice daily (in 3-drug combination regimens in EPV20001 and EPV40001) were similar.
Pediatric Subjects – Clinical Trials in HIV-1: EPIVIR Oral Solution has been studied in 638 pediatric subjects aged 3 months to 18 years in 3 clinical trials.
Selected clinical adverse reactions and physical findings with a ≥5% frequency during therapy with EPIVIR 4 mg/kg twice daily plus RETROVIR 160 mg/m^2 3 times daily in therapy-naive (≤56 days of antiretroviral therapy) pediatric subjects are listed in Table 5.

Table 5. Selected Clinical Adverse Reactions and Physical Findings (≥5% Frequency) in Pediatric Subjects in Trial ACTG300

Adverse Reaction	EPIVIR plus RETROVIR (n = 236)	Didanosine (n = 235)
Body as a Whole		
Fever	25%	32%
Digestive		
Hepatomegaly	11%	11%
Nausea & vomiting	8%	7%
Diarrhea	8%	6%
Stomatitis	6%	12%
Splenomegaly	5%	8%
Respiratory		
Cough	15%	18%
Abnormal breath sounds/wheezing	7%	9%
Ear, Nose, and Throat		
Signs or symptoms of ears[a]	7%	6%
Nasal discharge or congestion	8%	11%
Other		
Skin rashes	12%	14%
Lymphadenopathy	9%	11%

[a] Includes pain, discharge, erythema, or swelling of an ear.

Pancreatitis: Pancreatitis, which has been fatal in some cases, has been observed in antiretroviral nucleoside–experienced pediatric subjects receiving EPIVIR alone or in combination with other antiretroviral agents. In an open–label dose–escalation trial (NUCA2002), 14 subjects (14%) developed pancreatitis while receiving monotherapy with EPIVIR. Three of these subjects died of complications of pancreatitis. In a second open–label trial (NUCA2005), 12 subjects (18%) developed pancreatitis. In Trial ACTG300, pancreatitis was not observed in 236 subjects randomized to EPIVIR plus RETROVIR. Pancreatitis was observed in 1 subject in this trial who received open–label EPIVIR in combination with RETROVIR and ritonavir following discontinuation of didanosine monotherapy *[see Warnings and Precautions (5.5)]*.
Paresthesias and Peripheral Neuropathies: Paresthesias and peripheral neuropathies were reported in 15 subjects (15%) in Trial NUCA2002, 6 subjects (9%) in Trial NUCA2005, and 2 subjects (<1%) in Trial ACTG300.
Selected laboratory abnormalities experienced by therapy–naive (56 days of antiretroviral therapy) pediatric subjects are listed in Table 6.

Table 6. Frequencies of Selected Grade 3-4 Laboratory Abnormalities in Pediatric Subjects in Trial ACTG300

Test (Threshold Level)	EPIVIR plus RETROVIR	Didanosine
Absolute neutrophil count (<400/mm^3)	8%	3%
Hemoglobin (<7.0 g/dL)	4%	2%
Platelets (<50,000/mm^3)	1%	3%
ALT (>10 × ULN)	1%	3%
AST (>10 × ULN)	2%	4%
Lipase (>2.5 × ULN)	3%	3%
Total Amylase (>2.5 × ULN)	3%	3%

ULN = Upper limit of normal.

Neonates - Clinical Trials in HIV-1: Limited short-term safety information is available from 2 small, uncontrolled trials in South Africa in neonates receiving lamivudine with or without zidovudine for the first week of life following maternal treatment starting at Week 38 or 36 of gestation *[see Clinical Pharmacology (12.3)]*. Selected adverse reactions reported in these neonates included increased liver function tests, anemia, diarrhea, electrolyte disturbances, hypoglycemia, jaundice and hepatomegaly, rash, respiratory infections, and sepsis; 3 neonates died (1 from gastroenteritis with acidosis and convulsions, 1 from traumatic injury, and 1 from unknown causes). Two other nonfatal gastroenteritis or diarrhea cases were reported, including 1 with convulsions; 1 infant had transient renal insufficiency associated with dehydration. The absence of control groups limits assessments of causality, but it should be assumed that perinatally exposed infants may be at risk for adverse reactions comparable to those reported in pediatric and adult HIV-1-infected patients treated with lamivudine-containing combination regimens. Long-term effects of in utero and infant lamivudine exposure are not known.

6.2 Postmarketing Experience

In addition to adverse reactions reported from clinical trials, the following adverse reactions have been reported during postmarketing use of EPIVIR. Because these reactions are reported voluntarily from a population of unknown size, estimates of frequency cannot be made. These reactions have been chosen for inclusion due to a combination of their seriousness, frequency of reporting, or potential causal connection to lamivudine.
Body as a Whole: Redistribution/accumulation of body fat *[see Warnings and Precautions (5.7)]*.
Endocrine and Metabolic: Hyperglycemia.
General: Weakness.
Hemic and Lymphatic: Anemia (including pure red cell aplasia and severe anemias progressing on therapy).
Hepatic and Pancreatic: Lactic acidosis and hepatic steatosis, posttreatment exacerbation of hepatitis B *[see Boxed Warning, Warnings and Precautions (5.1, 5.2)]*.
Hypersensitivity: Anaphylaxis, urticaria.
Musculoskeletal: Muscle weakness, CPK elevation, rhabdomyolysis.
Skin: Alopecia, pruritus.

7 DRUG INTERACTIONS

Lamivudine is predominantly eliminated in the urine by active organic cationic secretion. The possibility of interactions with other drugs administered concurrently should be considered, particularly when their main route of elimination is active renal secretion via the organic cationic transport system (e.g., trimethoprim). No data are available regarding interactions with other drugs that have renal clearance mechanisms similar to that of lamivudine.

7.1 Interferon- and Ribavirin-Based Regimens

Although no evidence of a pharmacokinetic or pharmacodynamic interaction (e.g., loss of HIV-1/HCV virologic suppression) was seen when ribavirin was coadministered with lamivudine in HIV-1/HCV co-infected patients, hepatic decompensation (some fatal) has occurred in HIV-1/HCV co-infected patients receiving combination antiretroviral therapy for HIV-1 and interferon alfa with or without ribavirin *[see Warnings and Precautions (5.4), Clinical Pharmacology (12.3)]*.

7.2 Zalcitabine

Lamivudine and zalcitabine may inhibit the intracellular phosphorylation of one another. Therefore, use of lamivudine in combination with zalcitabine is not recommended.

7.3 Trimethoprim/Sulfamethoxazole (TMP/SMX)

No change in dose of either drug is recommended. There is no information regarding the effect on lamivudine pharmacokinetics of higher doses of TMP/SMX such as those used to treat PCP.

7.4 Drugs with No Observed Interactions With EPIVIR

A drug interaction trial showed no clinically significant interaction between EPIVIR and zidovudine.

8 USE IN SPECIFIC POPULATIONS

8.1 Pregnancy

Pregnancy Category C. There are no adequate and well-controlled trials of EPIVIR in pregnant women. Animal reproduction studies in rats and rabbits revealed no evidence of teratogenicity. Increased early embryolethality occurred in rabbits at exposure levels similar to those in humans. EPIVIR should be used during pregnancy only if the potential benefit justifies the potential risk to the fetus.

Lamivudine pharmacokinetics were studied in pregnant women during 2 clinical trials conducted in South Africa. The trial assessed pharmacokinetics in: 16 women at 36 weeks gestation using 150 mg lamivudine twice daily with zidovudine, 10 women at 38 weeks gestation using 150 mg lamivudine twice daily with zidovudine, and 10 women at 38 weeks gestation using lamivudine 300 mg twice daily without other antiretrovirals. These trials were not designed or powered to provide efficacy information. Lamivudine pharmacokinetics in pregnant women were similar to those seen in non-pregnant adults and in postpartum women. Lamivudine concentrations were generally similar in maternal, neonatal, and umbilical cord serum samples. In a subset of subjects, lamivudine amniotic fluid specimens were collected following natural rupture of membranes. Amniotic fluid concentrations of lamivudine were typically 2 times greater than maternal serum levels and ranged from 1.2 to 2.5 mcg/mL (150 mg twice daily) and 2.1 to 5.2 mcg/mL (300 mg twice daily). It is not known whether risks of adverse events associated with lamivudine are altered in pregnant women compared with other HIV-1-infected patients.

Animal reproduction studies performed at oral doses up to 130 and 60 times the adult dose in rats and rabbits, respectively, revealed no evidence of teratogenicity due to lamivudine. Increased early embryolethality occurred in rabbits at exposure levels similar to those in humans. However, there was no indication of this effect in rats at exposure levels up to 35 times those in humans. Based on animal studies, lamivudine crosses the placenta and is transferred to the fetus *[see Nonclinical Toxicology (13.2)]*.

Antiretroviral Pregnancy Registry: To monitor maternal-fetal outcomes of pregnant women exposed to lamivudine, a Pregnancy Registry has been established. Physicians are encouraged to register patients by calling 1-800-258-4263.

8.3 Nursing Mothers

The Centers for Disease Control and Prevention recommend that HIV-1-infected mothers in the United States not breastfeed their infants to avoid risking postnatal transmission of HIV-1 infection. Because of the potential for serious adverse reactions in nursing infants and HIV-1 transmission, mothers should be instructed not to breastfeed if they are receiving lamivudine.

Lamivudine is excreted into human milk. Samples of breast milk obtained from 20 mothers receiving lamivudine monotherapy (300 mg twice daily) or combination therapy (150 mg lamivudine twice daily and 300 mg zidovudine twice daily) had measurable concentrations of lamivudine.

8.4 Pediatric Use

The safety and effectiveness of twice-daily EPIVIR in combination with other antiretroviral agents have been established in pediatric patients 3 months and older *[see Adverse Reactions (6.1), Clinical Pharmacology (12.3), Clinical Studies (14.2)]*.

8.5 Geriatric Use

Clinical trials of EPIVIR did not include sufficient numbers of subjects aged 65 and over to determine whether they respond differently from younger subjects. In general, dose selection for an elderly patient should be cautious, reflecting the greater frequency of decreased hepatic, renal, or cardiac function, and of concomitant disease or other drug therapy. In particular, because lamivudine is substantially excreted by the kidney and elderly patients are more likely to have decreased renal function, renal function should be monitored and dosage adjustments should be made accordingly *[see Dosage and Administration (2.3), Clinical Pharmacology (12.3)]*.

8.6 Patients With Impaired Renal Function

Reduction of the dosage of EPIVIR is recommended for patients with impaired renal function *[see Dosage and Administration (2.3), Clinical Pharmacology (12.3)]*.

10 OVERDOSAGE

There is no known antidote for EPIVIR. One case of an adult ingesting 6 g of EPIVIR was reported; there were no clinical signs or symptoms noted and hematologic tests remained normal. Two cases of pediatric overdose were reported in Trial ACTG300. One case involved a single dose of 7 mg/kg of EPIVIR; the second case involved use of 5 mg/kg of EPIVIR twice daily for 30 days. There were no clinical signs or symptoms noted in either case. Because a negligible amount of lamivudine was removed via (4-hour) hemodialysis, continuous ambulatory peritoneal dialysis, and automated peritoneal dialysis, it is not known if continuous hemodialysis would provide clinical benefit in a lamivudine overdose event. If overdose occurs, the patient should be monitored, and standard supportive treatment applied as required.

11 DESCRIPTION

EPIVIR (also known as 3TC) is a brand name for lamivudine, a synthetic nucleoside analogue with activity against HIV-1 and HBV. The chemical name of lamivudine is (2R,cis)-4-amino-1-(2-hydroxymethyl-1,3-oxathiolan-5-yl)-(1H)-pyrimidin-2-one. Lamivudine is the (-)enantiomer of a dideoxy analogue of cytidine. Lamivudine has also been referred to as (-)2′,3′-dideoxy, 3′-thiacytidine. It has a molecular formula of $C_8H_{11}N_3O_3S$ and a molecular weight of 229.3. It has the following structural formula:

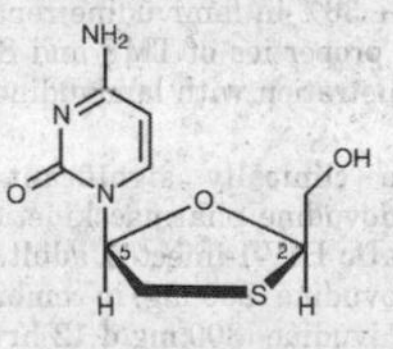

Lamivudine is a white to off-white crystalline solid with a solubility of approximately 70 mg/mL in water at 20°C.

EPIVIR Tablets are for oral administration. Each scored 150-mg film-coated tablet contains 150 mg of lamivudine and the inactive ingredients hypromellose, magnesium stearate, microcrystalline cellulose, polyethylene glycol, polysorbate 80, sodium starch glycolate, and titanium dioxide.

Each 300-mg film-coated tablet contains 300 mg of lamivudine and the inactive ingredients black iron oxide, hypromellose, magnesium stearate, microcrystalline cellulose, polyethylene glycol, polysorbate 80, sodium starch glycolate, and titanium dioxide.

EPIVIR Oral Solution is for oral administration. One milliliter (1 mL) of EPIVIR Oral Solution contains 10 mg of lamivudine (10 mg/mL) in an aqueous solution and the inactive ingredients artificial strawberry and banana flavors, citric acid (anhydrous), methylparaben, propylene glycol, propylparaben, sodium citrate (dihydrate), and sucrose (200 mg).

12 CLINICAL PHARMACOLOGY

12.1 Mechanism of Action

Lamivudine is an antiviral agent *[see Clinical Pharmacology (12.4)]*.

12.3 Pharmacokinetics

Pharmacokinetics in Adults: The pharmacokinetic properties of lamivudine have been studied in asymptomatic, HIV-1-infected adult subjects after administration of single intravenous (IV) doses ranging from 0.25 to 8 mg/kg, as well as single and multiple (twice-daily regimen) oral doses ranging from 0.25 to 10 mg/kg.

The pharmacokinetic properties of lamivudine have also been studied as single and multiple oral doses ranging from 5 mg to 600 mg/day administered to HBV-infected subjects.

The steady-state pharmacokinetic properties of the EPIVIR 300-mg tablet once daily for 7 days compared with the EPIVIR 150-mg tablet twice daily for 7 days were assessed in a crossover trial in 60 healthy subjects. EPIVIR 300 mg once daily resulted in lamivudine exposures that were similar to EPIVIR 150 mg twice daily with respect to plasma $AUC_{24,ss}$; however, $C_{max,ss}$ was 66% higher and the trough value was 53% lower compared with the 150-mg twice-daily regimen. Intracellular lamivudine triphosphate exposures in peripheral blood mononuclear cells were also similar with respect to $AUC_{24,ss}$ and $C_{max24,ss}$; however, trough values were lower compared with the 150-mg twice-daily regimen. Inter-subject variability was greater for intracellular lamivudine triphosphate concentrations versus lamivudine plasma trough concentrations. The clinical significance of observed differences for both plasma lamivudine concentrations and intracellular lamivudine triphosphate concentrations is not known.

Absorption and Bioavailability: Lamivudine was rapidly absorbed after oral administration in HIV-1-infected subjects. Absolute bioavailability in 12 adult subjects was 86% ± 16% (mean ± SD) for the 150-mg tablet and 87% ± 13% for the oral solution. After oral administration of 2 mg/kg twice a day to 9 adults with HIV-1, the peak serum lamivudine concentration (C_{max}) was 1.5 ± 0.5 mcg/mL (mean ± SD). The area under the plasma concentration versus time curve (AUC) and C_{max} increased in proportion to oral dose over the range from 0.25 to 10 mg/kg.

The accumulation ratio of lamivudine in HIV-1-positive asymptomatic adults with normal renal function was 1.50 following 15 days of oral administration of 2 mg/kg twice daily.

Effects of Food on Oral Absorption: An investigational 25-mg dosage form of lamivudine was administered orally to 12 asymptomatic, HIV-1-infected subjects on 2 occasions, once in the fasted state and once with food (1,099 kcal; 75 grams fat, 34 grams protein, 72 grams carbohydrate). Absorption of lamivudine was slower in the fed state (T_{max}: 3.2 ± 1.3 hours) compared with the fasted state (T_{max}: 0.9 ± 0.3 hours); C_{max} in the fed state was 40% ± 23% (mean ± SD) lower than in the fasted state. There was no significant difference in systemic exposure (AUC∞) in the fed and fasted states; therefore, EPIVIR Tablets and Oral Solution may be administered with or without food.

Distribution: The apparent volume of distribution after IV administration of lamivudine to 20 subjects was 1.3 ± 0.4 L/kg, suggesting that lamivudine distributes into extravascular spaces. Volume of distribution was independent of dose and did not correlate with body weight.

Binding of lamivudine to human plasma proteins is low (<36%). In vitro studies showed that over the concentration range of 0.1 to 100 mcg/mL, the amount of lamivudine associated with erythrocytes ranged from 53% to 57% and was independent of concentration.

Metabolism: Metabolism of lamivudine is a minor route of elimination. In man, the only known metabolite of lamivudine is the trans-sulfoxide metabolite. Within 12 hours after a single oral dose of lamivudine in 6 HIV-1-infected adults, 5.2% ± 1.4% (mean ± SD) of the dose was excreted as the trans-sulfoxide metabolite in the urine. Serum concentrations of this metabolite have not been determined.

Elimination: The majority of lamivudine is eliminated unchanged in urine by active organic cationic secretion. In 9 healthy subjects given a single 300-mg oral dose of lamivudine, renal clearance was 199.7 ± 56.9 mL/min (mean ± SD). In 20 HIV-1-infected subjects given a single IV dose, renal clearance was 280.4 ± 75.2 mL/min (mean ± SD), representing 71% ± 16% (mean ± SD) of total clearance of lamivudine.

In most single-dose trials in HIV-1-infected subjects, HBV-infected subjects, or healthy subjects with serum sampling for 24 hours after dosing, the observed mean elimination half-life ($t^{1/2}$) ranged from 5 to 7 hours. In HIV-1-infected subjects, total clearance was 398.5 ± 69.1 mL/min (mean ± SD). Oral clearance and elimination half-life were independent of dose and body weight over an oral dosing range of 0.25 to 10 mg/kg.

Special Populations: *Renal Impairment:* The pharmacokinetic properties of lamivudine have been determined in a small group of HIV-1-infected adults with impaired renal function (Table 7).

[See table 7 at top of next page]

Exposure (AUC∞), C_{max}, and half-life increased with diminishing renal function (as expressed by creatinine clearance). Apparent total oral clearance (Cl/F) of lamivudine decreased as creatinine clearance decreased. T_{max} was not significantly affected by renal function. Based on these observations, it is recommended that the dosage of lamivudine be modified in patients with renal impairment *[see Dosage and Administration (2.3)]*.

Based on a trial in otherwise healthy subjects with impaired renal function, hemodialysis increased lamivudine clearance from a mean of 64 to 88 mL/min; however, the length of time of hemodialysis (4 hours) was insufficient to significantly alter mean lamivudine exposure after a single-dose administration. Continuous ambulatory peritoneal dialysis and automated peritoneal dialysis have negligible effects on lamivudine clearance. Therefore, it is recommended, following correction of dose for creatinine clearance, that no additional dose modification be made after routine hemodialysis or peritoneal dialysis.

Table 7. Pharmacokinetic Parameters (Mean ± SD) After a Single 300-mg Oral Dose of Lamivudine in 3 Groups of Adults With Varying Degrees of Renal Function

Parameter	Creatinine Clearance Criterion (Number of Subjects)		
	>60 mL/min (n = 6)	10-30 mL/min (n = 4)	<10 mL/min (n = 6)
Creatinine clearance (mL/min)	111 ± 14	28 ± 8	6 ± 2
C_{max} (mcg/mL)	2.6 ± 0.5	3.6 ± 0.8	5.8 ± 1.2
AUC∞ (mcg•hr/mL)	11.0 ± 1.7	48.0 ± 19	157 ± 74
Cl/F (mL/min)	464 ± 76	114 ± 34	36 ± 11

It is not known whether lamivudine can be removed by continuous (24-hour) hemodialysis.

The effects of renal impairment on lamivudine pharmacokinetics in pediatric patients are not known.

Hepatic Impairment: The pharmacokinetic properties of lamivudine have been determined in adults with impaired hepatic function. Pharmacokinetic parameters were not altered by diminishing hepatic function; therefore, no dose adjustment for lamivudine is required for patients with impaired hepatic function. Safety and efficacy of lamivudine have not been established in the presence of decompensated liver disease.

Pediatric Patients: In Trial NUCA2002, pharmacokinetic properties of lamivudine were assessed in a subset of 57 HIV-1-infected pediatric subjects (age range: 4.8 months to 16 years, weight range: 5 to 66 kg) after oral and IV administration of 1, 2, 4, 8, 12, and 20 mg/kg/day. In the 9 infants and children (age range: 5 months to 12 years) receiving oral solution 4 mg/kg twice daily (the usual recommended pediatric dose), absolute bioavailability was 66% ± 26% (mean ± SD), which was less than the 86% ± 16% (mean ± SD) observed in adults. The mechanism for the diminished absolute bioavailability of lamivudine in infants and children is unknown.

Systemic clearance decreased with increasing age in pediatric subjects, as shown in Figure 1.

Figure 1. Systemic Clearance (L/hr•kg) of Lamivudine in Relation to Age

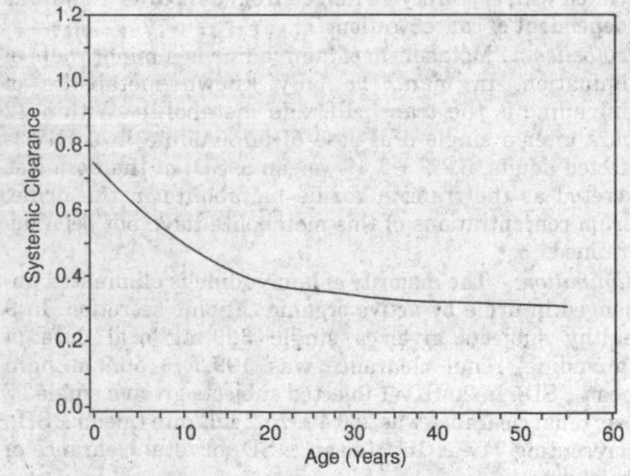

After oral administration of lamivudine 4 mg/kg twice daily to 11 pediatric subjects ranging in age from 4 months to 14 years, C_{max} was 1.1 ± 0.6 mcg/mL and half-life was 2.0 ± 0.6 hours. (In adults with similar blood sampling, the half-life was 3.7 ± 1 hours.) Total exposure to lamivudine, as reflected by mean AUC values, was comparable between pediatric subjects receiving an 8-mg/kg/day dose and adults receiving a 4-mg/kg/day dose.

Distribution of lamivudine into cerebrospinal fluid (CSF) was assessed in 38 pediatric subjects after multiple oral dosing with lamivudine. CSF samples were collected between 2 and 4 hours postdose. At the dose of 8 mg/kg/day, CSF lamivudine concentrations in 8 subjects ranged from 5.6% to 30.9% (mean ± SD of 14.2% ± 7.9%) of the concentration in a simultaneous serum sample, with CSF lamivudine concentrations ranging from 0.04 to 0.3 mcg/mL.

Limited, uncontrolled pharmacokinetic and safety data are available from administration of lamivudine (and zidovudine) to 36 infants aged up to 1 week in 2 trials in South Africa. In these trials, lamivudine clearance was substantially reduced in 1-week-old neonates relative to pediatric subjects (aged >3 months) studied previously. There is insufficient information to establish the time course of changes in clearance between the immediate neonatal period and the age-ranges >3 months old *[see Adverse Reactions (6.1)]*.

Geriatric Patients: The pharmacokinetics of lamivudine after administration of EPIVIR to patients over 65 years have not been studied *[see Use in Specific Populations (8.5)]*.

Gender: There are no significant gender differences in lamivudine pharmacokinetics.

Race: There are no significant racial differences in lamivudine pharmacokinetics.

Drug Interactions: *Interferon Alfa:* There was no significant pharmacokinetic interaction between lamivudine and interferon alfa in a trial of 19 healthy male subjects *[see Warnings and Precautions (5.4)]*.

Ribavirin: In vitro data indicate ribavirin reduces phosphorylation of lamivudine, stavudine, and zidovudine. However, no pharmacokinetic (e.g., plasma concentrations or intracellular triphosphorylated active metabolite concentrations) or pharmacodynamic (e.g., loss of HIV-1/HCV virologic suppression) interaction was observed when ribavirin and lamivudine (n = 18), stavudine (n = 10), or zidovudine (n = 6) were coadministered as part of a multi-drug regimen to HIV-1/HCV co-infected subjects *[see Warnings and Precautions (5.4)]*.

Trimethoprim/Sulfamethoxazole: Lamivudine and TMP/SMX were coadministered to 14 HIV-1-positive subjects in a single-center, open-label, randomized, crossover trial. Each subject received treatment with a single 300-mg dose of lamivudine and TMP 160 mg/SMX 800 mg once a day for 5 days with concomitant administration of lamivudine 300 mg with the fifth dose in a crossover design. Coadministration of TMP/SMX with lamivudine resulted in an increase of 43% ± 23% (mean ± SD) in lamivudine AUC∞, a decrease of 29% ± 13% in lamivudine oral clearance, and a decrease of 30% ± 36% in lamivudine renal clearance. The pharmacokinetic properties of TMP and SMX were not altered by coadministration with lamivudine *[see Drug Interactions (7.3)]*.

Zidovudine: No clinically significant alterations in lamivudine or zidovudine pharmacokinetics were observed in 12 asymptomatic HIV-1-infected adult subjects given a single dose of zidovudine (200 mg) in combination with multiple doses of lamivudine (300 mg q 12 hr) *[see Drug Interactions (7.4)]*.

12.4 Microbiology

Mechanism of Action: Intracellularly, lamivudine is phosphorylated to its active 5′-triphosphate metabolite, lamivudine triphosphate (3TC-TP). The principal mode of action of 3TC-TP is the inhibition of HIV-1 reverse transcriptase (RT) via DNA chain termination after incorporation of the nucleotide analogue into viral DNA. 3TC-TP is a weak inhibitor of mammalian DNA polymerases α, β, and γ.

Antiviral Activity: The antiviral activity of lamivudine against HIV-1 was assessed in a number of cell lines (including monocytes and fresh human peripheral blood lymphocytes) using standard susceptibility assays. EC_{50} values (50% effective concentrations) were in the range of 0.003 to 15 μM (1 μM = 0.23 mcg/mL). HIV-1 from therapy-naive subjects with no amino acid substitutions associated with resistance gave median EC_{50} values of 0.429 μM (range: 0.200 to 2.007 μM) from Virco (n = 92 baseline samples from COLA40263) and 2.35 μM (1.37 to 3.68 μM) from Monogram Biosciences (n = 135 baseline samples from ESS30009). The EC_{50} values of lamivudine against different HIV-1 clades (A-G) ranged from 0.001 to 0.120 μM, and against HIV-2 isolates from 0.003 to 0.120 μM in peripheral blood mononuclear cells. Ribavirin (50 μM) decreased the anti-HIV-1 activity of lamivudine by 3.5 fold in MT-4 cells. In HIV-1-infected MT-4 cells, lamivudine in combination with zidovudine at various ratios exhibited synergistic antiretroviral activity. Please see the full prescribing information for EPIVIR-HBV for information regarding the inhibitory activity of lamivudine against HBV.

Resistance: Lamivudine-resistant variants of HIV-1 have been selected in cell culture. Genotypic analysis showed that the resistance was due to a specific amino acid substitution in the HIV-1 reverse transcriptase at codon 184 changing the methionine to either isoleucine or valine (M184V/I).

HIV-1 strains resistant to both lamivudine and zidovudine have been isolated from subjects. Susceptibility of clinical isolates to lamivudine and zidovudine was monitored in controlled clinical trials. In subjects receiving lamivudine monotherapy or combination therapy with lamivudine plus zidovudine, HIV-1 isolates from most subjects became phenotypically and genotypically resistant to lamivudine within 12 weeks. In some subjects harboring zidovudine-resistant virus at baseline, phenotypic sensitivity to zidovudine was restored by 12 weeks of treatment with lamivudine and zidovudine. Combination therapy with lamivudine plus zidovudine delayed the emergence of mutations conferring resistance to zidovudine.

Lamivudine-resistant HBV isolates develop substitutions (rtM204V/I) in the YMDD motif of the catalytic domain of the viral reverse transcriptase. rtM204V/I substitutions are frequently accompanied by other substitutions (rtV173L, rtL180M) which enhance the level of lamivudine resistance or act as compensatory mutations improving replication efficiency. Other substitutions detected in lamivudine-resistant HBV isolates include: rtL80I and rtA181T. Similar HBV mutants have been reported in HIV-1-infected subjects who received lamivudine-containing antiretroviral regimens in the presence of concurrent infection with hepatitis B virus *[see Warnings and Precautions (5.2)]*.

Cross-Resistance: Lamivudine-resistant HIV-1 mutants were cross-resistant to didanosine (ddI) and zalcitabine (ddC). In some subjects treated with zidovudine plus didanosine or zalcitabine, isolates resistant to multiple reverse transcriptase inhibitors, including lamivudine, have emerged.

Genotypic and Phenotypic Analysis of On-Therapy HIV-1 Isolates From Subjects With Virologic Failure: *Trial EPV20001:* Fifty-three of 554 (10%) subjects enrolled in EPV20001 were identified as virological failures (plasma HIV-1 RNA level 400 copies/mL) by Week 48. Twenty-eight subjects were randomized to the lamivudine once-daily treatment group and 25 to the lamivudine twice-daily treatment group. The median baseline plasma HIV-1 RNA levels of subjects in the lamivudine once-daily group and lamivudine twice-daily group were 4.9 log_{10} copies/mL and 4.6 log_{10} copies/mL, respectively.

Genotypic analysis of on–therapy isolates from 22 subjects identified as virologic failures in the lamivudine once-daily group showed that isolates from 0/22 subjects contained treatment-emergent amino acid substitutions associated with zidovudine resistance (M41L, D67N, K70R, L210W, T215Y/F, or K219Q/E), isolates from 10/22 subjects contained treatment-emergent amino acid substitutions associated with efavirenz resistance (L100I, K101E, K103N, V108I, or Y181C), and isolates from 8/22 subjects contained a treatment-emergent lamivudine resistance-associated substitution (M184I or M184V).

Genotypic analysis of on-therapy isolates from subjects (n = 22) in the lamivudine twice-daily treatment group showed that isolates from 1/22 subjects contained treatment-emergent zidovudine resistance substitutions, isolates from 7/22 contained treatment-emergent efavirenz resistance substitutions, and isolates from 5/22 contained treatment-emergent lamivudine resistance substitutions.

Phenotypic analysis of baseline-matched on-therapy HIV-1 isolates from subjects (n = 13) receiving lamivudine once daily showed that isolates from 12/13 subjects were susceptible to zidovudine; isolates from 8/13 subjects exhibited a 25- to 295-fold decrease in susceptibility to efavirenz, and isolates from 7/13 subjects showed an 85- to 299-fold decrease in susceptibility to lamivudine.

Phenotypic analysis of baseline-matched on-therapy HIV-1 isolates from subjects (n = 13) receiving lamivudine twice daily showed that isolates from all 13 subjects were susceptible to zidovudine; isolates from 3/13 subjects exhibited a 21- to 342-fold decrease in susceptibility to efavirenz, and isolates from 4/13 subjects exhibited a 29- to 159-fold decrease in susceptibility to lamivudine.

Trial EPV40001: Fifty subjects received zidovudine 300 mg twice daily plus abacavir 300 mg twice daily plus lamivudine 300 mg once daily and 50 subjects received zidovudine 300 mg plus abacavir 300 mg plus lamivudine 150 mg all twice-daily. The median baseline plasma HIV-1 RNA levels for subjectsin the 2 groups were 4.79 log_{10} copies/mL and 4.83 log_{10} copies/mL, respectively. Fourteen of 50 subjects in the lamivudine once-daily treatment group and 9 of 50 subjects in the lamivudine twice-daily group were identified as virologic failures.

Genotypic analysis of on-therapy HIV-1 isolates from subjects (n = 9) in the lamivudine once-daily treatment group showed that isolates from 6 subjects had an abacavir and/or lamivudine resistance-associated substitution M184V alone. On-therapy isolates from subjects (n = 6) receiving lamivudine twice daily showed that isolates from 2 subjects had M184V alone, and isolates from 2 subjects harbored the M184V substitution in combination with zidovudine resistance-associated amino acid substitutions.

Phenotypic analysis of on-therapy isolates from subjects (n = 6) receiving lamivudine once daily showed that HIV-1 isolates from 4 subjects exhibited a 32- to 53-fold decrease in susceptibility to lamivudine. HIV-1 isolates from these 6 subjects were susceptible to zidovudine.

Phenotypic analysis of on-therapy isolates from subjects (n = 4) receiving lamivudine twice daily showed that HIV-1 isolates from 1 subject exhibited a 45-fold decrease in susceptibility to lamivudine and a 4.5-fold decrease in susceptibility to zidovudine.

13 NONCLINICAL TOXICOLOGY

13.1 Carcinogenesis, Mutagenesis, Impairment of Fertility

Long-term carcinogenicity studies with lamivudine in mice and rats showed no evidence of carcinogenic potential at exposures up to 10 times (mice) and 58 times (rats) those observed in humans at the recommended therapeutic dose for HIV-1 infection. Lamivudine was not active in a microbial mutagenicity screen or an in vitro cell transformation assay, but showed weak in vitro mutagenic activity in a cytogenetic assay using cultured human lymphocytes and in the mouse lymphoma assay. However, lamivudine showed no evidence of in vivo genotoxic activity in the rat at oral doses of up to 2,000 mg/kg, producing plasma levels of 35 to 45 times those in humans at the recommended dose for HIV-1 infection. In a study of reproductive performance, lamivudine administered to rats at doses up to 4,000 mg/kg/day, producing plasma levels 47 to 70 times those in humans, revealed no evidence of impaired fertility and no effect on the survival, growth, and development to weaning of the offspring.

13.2 Reproductive Toxicology Studies

Reproduction studies have been performed in rats and rabbits at orally administered doses up to 4,000 mg/kg/day and 1,000 mg/kg/day, respectively, producing plasma levels up to approximately 35 times that for the adult HIV dose. No evidence of teratogenicity due to lamivudine was observed. Evidence of early embryolethality was seen in the rabbit at exposure levels similar to those observed in humans, but there was no indication of this effect in the rat at exposure levels up to 35 times those in humans. Studies in pregnant rats and rabbits showed that lamivudine is transferred to the fetus through the placenta.

14 CLINICAL STUDIES

The use of EPIVIR is based on the results of clinical trials in HIV–1-infected subjects in combination regimens with other antiretroviral agents. Information from trials with clinical endpoints or a combination of CD4+ cell counts and HIV-1 RNA measurements is included below as documentation of the contribution of lamivudine to a combination regimen in controlled trials.

14.1 Adults

Clinical Endpoint Trial: NUCB3007 (CAESAR) was a multi-center, double-blind, placebo-controlled trial comparing continued current therapy (zidovudine alone [62% of subjects] or zidovudine with didanosine or zalcitabine [38% of subjects]) to the addition of EPIVIR or EPIVIR plus an investigational non-nucleoside reverse transcriptase inhibitor (NNRTI), randomized 1:2:1. A total of 1,816 HIV-1-infected adults with 25 to 250 CD4+ cells/mm^3 (median = 122 cells/mm^3) at baseline were enrolled: median age was 36 years, 87% were male, 84% were nucleoside-experienced, and 16% were therapy-naive. The median duration on trial was 12 months. Results are summarized in Table 8.

[See table 8 above]

Table 8. Number of Subjects (%) With at Least One HIV-1 Disease Progression Event or Death

Endpoint	Current Therapy (n = 460)	EPIVIR plus Current Therapy (n = 896)	EPIVIR plus an NNRTI[a] plus Current Therapy (n = 460)
HIV-1 progression or death	90 (19.6%)	86 (9.6%)	41 (8.9%)
Death	27 (5.9%)	23 (2.6%)	14 (3.0%)

[a] An investigational non-nucleoside reverse transcriptase inhibitor not approved in the United States.

Surrogate Endpoint Trials: *Dual Nucleoside Analogue Trials:* Principal clinical trials in the initial development of lamivudine compared lamivudine/zidovudine combinations with zidovudine monotherapy or with zidovudine plus zalcitabine. These trials demonstrated the antiviral effect of lamivudine in a 2-drug combination. More recent uses of lamivudine in treatment of HIV-1 infection incorporate it into multiple-drug regimens containing at least 3 antiretroviral drugs for enhanced viral suppression.

Dose Regimen Comparison Surrogate Endpoint Trials in Therapy-Naive Adults: EPV20001 was a multi-center, double-blind, controlled trial in which subjects were randomized 1:1 to receive EPIVIR 300 mg once daily or EPIVIR 150 mg twice daily, in combination with zidovudine 300 mg twice daily and efavirenz 600 mg once daily. A total of 554 antiretroviral treatment-naive HIV-1-infected adults enrolled: male (79%), Caucasian (50%), median age of 35 years, baseline CD4+ cell counts of 69 to 1,089 cells/mm^3 (median = 362 cells/mm^3), and median baseline plasma HIV-1 RNA of 4.66 $\log_{10}$ copies/mL. Outcomes of treatment through 48 weeks are summarized in Figure 2 and Table 9.

[See figure 2 at top of next column]

[See table 9 above]

Table 9. Outcomes of Randomized Treatment Through 48 Weeks (Intent-to-Treat)

Outcome	EPIVIR 300 mg Once Daily plus RETROVIR plus Efavirenz (n = 278)	EPIVIR 150 mg Twice Daily plus RETROVIR plus Efavirenz (n = 276)
Responder[a]	67%	65%
Virologic failure[b]	8%	8%
Discontinued due to clinical progression	<1%	0%
Discontinued due to adverse events	6%	12%
Discontinued due to other reasons[c]	18%	14%

[a] Achieved confirmed plasma HIV-1 RNA <400 copies/mL and maintained through 48 weeks.

[b] Achieved suppression but rebounded by Week 48, discontinued due to virologic failure, insufficient viral response according to the investigator, or never suppressed through Week 48.

[c] Includes consent withdrawn, lost to followup, protocol violation, data outside the trial-defined schedule, and randomized but never initiated treatment.

The proportions of subjects with HIV-1 RNA <50 copies/mL (via Roche Ultrasensitive assay) through Week 48 were 61% for subjects receiving EPIVIR 300 mg once daily and 63% for subjects receiving EPIVIR 150 mg twice daily. Median increases in CD4+ cell counts were 144 cells/mm^3 at Week 48 in subjects receiving EPIVIR 300 mg once daily and 146 cells/mm^3 for subjects receiving EPIVIR 150 mg twice daily.

A small, randomized, open-label pilot trial, EPV40001, was conducted in Thailand. A total of 159 treatment-naive adult subjects (male 32%, Asian 100%, median age 30 years, baseline median CD4+ cell count 380 cells/mm^3, median plasma HIV-1 RNA 4.8 $\log_{10}$ copies/mL) were enrolled. Two of the treatment arms in this trial provided a comparison between lamivudine 300 mg once daily (n = 54) and lamivudine 150 mg twicedaily (n = 52), each in combination with zidovudine 300 mg twice daily and abacavir 300 mg twice daily. In intent-to-treat analyses of 48-week data, the proportions of subjects with HIV-1 RNA below 400 copies/mL were 61% (33/54) in the group randomized to once-daily lamivudine and 75% (39/52) in the group randomized to receive all 3 drugs twice daily; the proportions with HIV-1 RNA below 50 copies/mL were 54% (29/54) in the once-daily lamivudine group and 67% (35/52) in the all-twice-daily group; and the median increases in CD4+ cell counts were 166 cells/mm^3 in the once-daily lamivudine group and 216 cells/mm^3 in the all-twice-daily group.

Figure 2. Virologic Response Through Week 48, EPV20001[ab] (Intent-to-Treat)

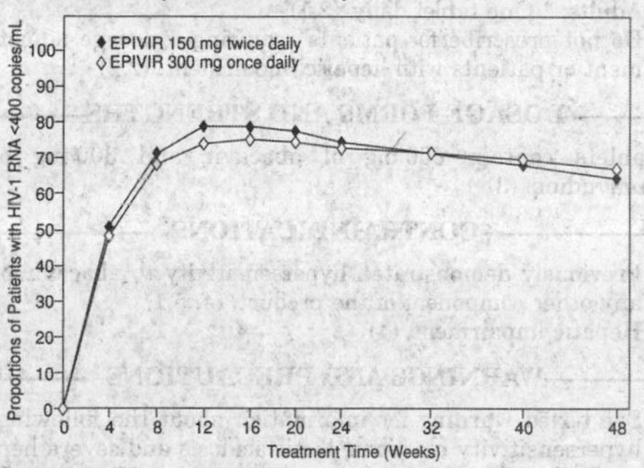

[a] Roche AMPLICOR HIV-1 MONITOR.

[b] Responders at each visit are subjects who had achieved and maintained HIV-1 RNA <400 copies/mL without discontinuation by that visit.

14.2 Pediatric Subjects

Clinical Endpoint Trial: ACTG300 was a multi-center, randomized, double-blind trial that provided for comparison of EPIVIR plus RETROVIR (zidovudine) with didanosine monotherapy. A total of 471 symptomatic, HIV-1-infected therapy-naive (56 days of antiretroviral therapy) pediatric subjects were enrolled in these 2 treatment arms. The median age was 2.7 years (range: 6 weeks to 14 years), 58% were female, and 86% were non-Caucasian. The mean baseline CD4+ cell count was 868 cells/mm^3 (mean: 1,060 cells/mm^3 and range:0 to 4,650 cells/mm^3 for subjects aged 5 years; mean: 419 cells/mm^3 and range: 0 to 1,555 cells/mm^3 for subjects aged >5 years) and the mean baseline plasma HIV-1 RNA was 5.0 $\log_{10}$ copies/mL. The median duration on trial was 10.1 months for the subjects receiving EPIVIR plus RETROVIR and 9.2 months for subjects receiving didanosine monotherapy. Results are summarized in Table 10.

Table 10. Number of Subjects (%) Reaching a Primary Clinical Endpoint (Disease Progression or Death)

Endpoint	EPIVIR plus RETROVIR (n = 236)	Didanosine (n = 235)
HIV-1 disease progression or death (total)	15 (6.4%)	37 (15.7%)
Physical growth failure	7 (3.0%)	6 (2.6%)
Central nervous system deterioration	4 (1.7%)	12 (5.1%)
CDC Clinical Category C	2 (0.8%)	8 (3.4%)
Death	2 (0.8%)	11 (4.7%)

16 HOW SUPPLIED/STORAGE AND HANDLING

EPIVIR Scored Tablets, 150 mg

White, diamond-shaped, scored, film-coated tablets debossed with "GX CJ7" on both sides.

Bottle of 60 tablets (NDC 49702-203-18) with child-resistant closure.

EPIVIR Tablets, 300 mg

Gray, modified diamond-shaped, film-coated tablets engraved with "GX EJ7" on one side and plain on the reverse side.

Bottle of 30 tablets (NDC 49702-204-13) with child-resistant closure.

Recommended Storage:

Store EPIVIR Tablets at 25°C (77°F); excursions permitted to 15° to 30°C (59° to 86°F) [see USP Controlled Room Temperature].

EPIVIR Oral Solution, 10 mg/mL

A clear, colorless to pale yellow, strawberry-banana-flavored liquid, contains 10 mg of lamivudine in each 1 mL.

Plastic bottle of 240 mL (NDC 49702-205-48) with child-resistant closure. This product does not require reconstitution.

Recommended Storage:

Store in tightly closed bottles at 25°C (77°F) [see USP Controlled Room Temperature].

17 PATIENT COUNSELING INFORMATION

17.1 Advice for the Patient

Lactic Acidosis/Hepatomegaly: Patients should be informed that some HIV medicines, including EPIVIR, can cause a rare, but serious condition called lactic acidosis with liver enlargement (hepatomegaly) *[see Warnings and Precautions (5.1)]*.

HIV-1/HBV Co-infection: Patients co-infected with HIV-1 and HBV should be informed that deterioration of liver disease has occurred in some cases when treatment with lamivudine was discontinued. Patients should be advised to discuss any changes in regimen with their physician *[see Warnings and Precautions (5.2)]*.

Differences in Formulations of EPIVIR: Patients should be advised that EPIVIR Tablets and Oral Solution contain a higher dose of the same active ingredient (lamivudine) as EPIVIR-HBV Tablets and Oral Solution. If a decision is made to include lamivudine in the HIV-1 treatment regimen of a patient co-infected with HIV-1 and HBV, the formulation and dosage of lamivudine in EPIVIR (not EPIVIR-HBV) should be used *[see Warnings and Precautions (5.2)]*.

Use With Other Lamivudine- and Emtricitabine-Containing Products: EPIVIR should not be coadministered with drugs containing lamivudine or emtricitabine, including COMBIVIR (lamivudine/zidovudine) Tablets, EPZICOM (abacavir sulfate and lamivudine) Tablets, TRIZIVIR (abacavir sulfate, lamivudine, and zidovudine), ATRIPLA (efavirenz, emtricitabine, and tenofovir), EMTRIVA (emtricitabine), TRUVADA (emtricitabine and tenofovir), or COMPLERA (rilpivirine/emtricitabine/tenofovir) *[see Warnings and Precautions (5.3)]*.

HIV-1/HCV Co-Infection: Patients with HIV-1/HCV co-infection should be informed that hepatic decompensation (some fatal) has occurred in HIV-1/HCV co-infected patients receiving combination antiretroviral therapy for HIV-1 and interferon alfa with or without ribavirin *[see Warnings and Precautions (5.4)]*.

Risk of Pancreatitis: Parents or guardians should be advised to monitor pediatric patients for signs and symptoms of pancreatitis *[see Warnings and Precautions (5.5)]*.

Redistribution/Accumulation of Body Fat: Patients should be informed that redistribution or accumulation of body fat may occur in patients receiving antiretroviral therapy, including EPIVIR, and that the cause and long-term health effects of these conditions are not known at this time *[see Warnings and Precautions (5.7)]*.

Sucrose Content of EPIVIR Oral Solution: Diabetic patients should be advised that each 15-mL dose of EPIVIR Oral Solution contains 3 grams of sucrose *[see Description (11)]*.

Information About HIV-1 Infection: EPIVIR is not a cure for HIV-1 infection and patients may continue to experience illnesses associated with HIV-1 infection, including opportunistic infections. Patients should remain under the care of a physician when using EPIVIR.

Patients should be advised to avoid doing things that can spread HIV-1 infection to others.

- **Do not share needles or other injection equipment.**
- **Do not share personal items that can have blood or body fluids on them, like toothbrushes and razor blades.**
- **Do not have any kind of sex without protection.** Always practice safe sex by using a latex or polyurethane condom or other barrier method to lower the chance of sexual contact with semen, vaginal secretions, or blood.
- **Do not breastfeed.** Lamivudine is excreted in human breast milk. Mothers with HIV-1 should not breastfeed because HIV-1 can be passed to the baby in the breast milk.

Patients should be informed to take all HIV medications exactly as prescribed.

COMBIVIR, EPIVIR, EPZICOM, RETROVIR, and TRIZIVIR are registered trademarks of ViiV Healthcare.

The other brands listed are trademarks of their respective owners and are not trademarks of ViiV Healthcare. The makers of these brands are not affiliated with and do not endorse ViiV Healthcare or its products.

Manufactured for:
ViiV Healthcare
Research Triangle Park, NC 27709
by:
GlaxoSmithKline
Research Triangle Park, NC 27709
Manufactured under agreement from
Shire Pharmaceuticals Group plc
Basingstoke, UK

EPV:5PI

EPZICOM ℞

[ep' zih com]
(abacavir sulfate and lamivudine)
Tablets, for oral use

HIGHLIGHTS OF PRESCRIBING INFORMATION
These highlights do not include all the information needed to use EPZICOM safely and effectively. See full prescribing information for EPZICOM.
EPZICOM (abacavir sulfate and lamivudine) Tablets, for oral use
Initial U.S. Approval: 2004

WARNING: RISK OF HYPERSENSITIVITY REACTIONS, LACTIC ACIDOSIS AND SEVERE HEPATOMEGALY, AND EXACERBATIONS OF HEPATITIS
See full prescribing information for complete boxed warning

- **Serious and sometimes fatal hypersensitivity reactions have been associated with abacavir-containing products (5.1)**
- **Hypersensitivity to abacavir is a multi-organ clinical syndrome. (5.1)**
- **Patients who carry the HLA-B*5701 allele are at high risk for experiencing a hypersensitivity reaction to abacavir. (5.1)**
- **Discontinue EPZICOM as soon as a hypersensitivity reaction is suspected. Regardless of HLA-B*5701 status, permanently discontinue EPZICOM if hypersensitivity cannot be ruled out, even when other diagnoses are possible. (5.1)**
- **Following a hypersensitivity reaction to abacavir, NEVER restart EPZICOM or any other abacavir-containing product. (5.1)**
- **Lactic acidosis and severe hepatomegaly with steatosis, including fatal cases, have been reported with the use of nucleoside analogues. (5.2)**
- **Severe acute exacerbations of hepatitis B have been reported in patients who are co-infected with hepatitis B virus (HBV) and human immunodeficiency virus (HIV-1) and have discontinued lamivudine, a component of EPZICOM. Monitor hepatic function closely in these patients and, if appropriate, initiate anti-hepatitis B treatment. (5.3)**

RECENT MAJOR CHANGES

Dosage and Administration (2) 05/2012
Warnings and Precautions, Hypersensitivity Reaction (5.1) 05/2012
Warnings and Precautions, Immune Reconstitution Syndrome (5.5) 11/2011

INDICATIONS AND USAGE

EPZICOM, a combination of abacavir and lamivudine, both nucleoside analogue HIV-1 reverse transcriptase inhibitors, is indicated in combination with other antiretroviral agents for the treatment of HIV-1 infection. (1)

DOSAGE AND ADMINISTRATION

- A medication guide and warning card should be dispensed with each new prescription and refill. (2)
- Adults: One tablet daily. (2.1)
- Do not prescribe for patients requiring a dosage adjustment or patients with hepatic impairment. (2.2)

DOSAGE FORMS AND STRENGTHS

Tablets contain 600 mg of abacavir and 300 mg of lamivudine. (3)

CONTRAINDICATIONS

- Previously demonstrated hypersensitivity to abacavir or any other component of the product. (4, 5.1)
- Hepatic impairment. (4)

WARNINGS AND PRECAUTIONS

- See boxed warning for information about the following: hypersensitivity reactions, lactic acidosis and severe hepatomegaly, and severe acute exacerbations of hepatitis B. (5.1, 5.2, 5.3)
- Hepatic decompensation, some fatal, has occurred in HIV-1/HCV co-infected patients receiving combination antiretroviral therapy and interferon alfa with or without ribavirin. Discontinue EPZICOM as medically appropriate and consider dose reduction or discontinuation of interferon alfa, ribavirin, or both. (5.4)
- Immune reconstitution syndrome (5.5) and redistribution/accumulation of body fat have been reported in patients treated with combination antiretroviral therapy. (5.6)
- EPZICOM should not be administered with other lamivudine- or zidovudine-containing products or emtricitabine-containing products. (5.8)

ADVERSE REACTIONS

The most commonly reported adverse reactions of at least moderate intensity (incidence >5%) in an adult HIV-1 clinical trial were drug hypersensitivity, insomnia, depression/depressed mood, headache/migraine, fatigue/malaise, dizziness/vertigo, nausea, and diarrhea. (6.1)

To report SUSPECTED ADVERSE REACTIONS, contact ViiV Healthcare at 1-877-844-8872 or FDA at 1-800-FDA-1088 or www.fda.gov/medwatch.

DRUG INTERACTIONS

- Ethanol: Decreases elimination of abacavir. (7.2)
- Methadone: An increased methadone dose may be required in a small number of patients. (7.4)

See 17 for PATIENT COUNSELING INFORMATION and Medication Guide

Revised: 05/2012

FULL PRESCRIBING INFORMATION: CONTENTS*

*** Sections or subsections omitted from the full prescribing information are not listed**

FULL PRESCRIBING INFORMATION

WARNING: RISK OF HYPERSENSITIVITY REACTIONS, LACTIC ACIDOSIS AND SEVERE HEPATOMEGALY, AND EXACERBATIONS OF HEPATITIS B

Hypersensitivity Reactions: Serious and sometimes fatal hypersensitivity reactions have been associated with abacavir sulfate, a component of EPZICOM® (abacavir sulfate and lamivudine) Tablets.

Hypersensitivity to abacavir is a multi-organ clinical syndrome usually characterized by a sign or symptom in 2 or more of the following groups: (1) fever, (2) rash, (3) gastrointestinal (including nausea, vomiting, diarrhea, or abdominal pain), (4) constitutional (including generalized malaise, fatigue, or achiness), and (5) respiratory (including dyspnea, cough, or pharyngitis). Discontinue EPZICOM as soon as a hypersensitivity reaction is suspected.

Patients who carry the HLA-B*5701 allele are at high risk for experiencing a hypersensitivity reaction to abacavir. Prior to initiating therapy with abacavir, screening for the HLA-B*5701 allele is recommended; this approach has been found to decrease the risk of hypersensitivity reaction. Screening is also recommended prior to reinitiation of abacavir in patients of unknown HLA-B*5701 status who have previously tolerated abacavir. HLA-B*5701-negative patients may develop a suspected hypersensitivity reaction to abacavir; however, this occurs significantly less frequently than in HLA-B*5701-positive patients.

Regardless of HLA-B*5701 status, permanently discontinue EPZICOM if hypersensitivity cannot be ruled out, even when other diagnoses are possible.

Following a hypersensitivity reaction to abacavir, NEVER restart EPZICOM or any other abacavir-containing product because more severe symptoms can occur within hours and may include life-threatening hypotension and death.

Reintroduction of EPZICOM or any other abacavir-containing product, even in patients who have no identified history or unrecognized symptoms of hypersensitivity to abacavir therapy, can result in serious or fatal hypersensitivity reactions. Such reactions can occur within hours *[see Warnings and Precautions (5.1)]*.

Lactic Acidosis and Severe Hepatomegaly:Lactic acidosis and severe hepatomegaly with steatosis, including fatal cases, have been reported with the use of nucleoside analogues alone or in combination, including abacavir, lamivudine, and other antiretrovirals*[see Warnings and Precautions (5.2)]*.

Exacerbations of Hepatitis B: Severe acute exacerbations of hepatitis B have been reported in patients who are co-infected with hepatitis B virus (HBV) and human immunodeficiency virus (HIV-1) and have discontinued lamivudine, which is one component of EPZICOM. Hepatic function should be monitored closely with both clinical and laboratory follow-up for at least several months in patients who discontinue EPZICOM and are co-infected with HIV-1 and HBV. If appropriate, initiation of anti-hepatitis B therapy may be warranted *[see Warnings and Precautions (5.3)]*.

1 INDICATIONS AND USAGE

EPZICOM Tablets, in combination with other antiretroviral agents, are indicated for the treatment of HIV-1 infection.

Additional important information on the use of EPZICOM for treatment of HIV-1 infection:

- EPZICOM is one of multiple products containing abacavir. Before starting EPZICOM, review medical history for prior exposure to any abacavir-containing product in order to avoid reintroduction in a patient with a history of hypersensitivity to abacavir *[see Warnings and Precautions (5.1), Adverse Reactions (6)]*.
- As part of a triple-drug regimen, EPZICOM Tablets are recommended for use with antiretroviral agents from different pharmacological classes and not with other nucleoside/nucleotide reverse transcriptase inhibitors.

2 DOSAGE AND ADMINISTRATION

- A Medication Guide and Warning Card that provide information about recognition of hypersensitivity reactions should be dispensed with each new prescription and refill.
- EPZICOM can be taken with or without food.

2.1 Adult Patients

The recommended oral dose of EPZICOM for adults is one tablet daily, in combination with other antiretroviral agents.

2.2 Dosage Adjustment

Because it is a fixed-dose combination, EPZICOM should not be prescribed for:

- patients requiring dosage adjustment such as those with creatinine clearance <50 mL/min,
- patients with hepatic impairment.

Use of EPIVIR® (lamivudine) Oral Solution or Tablets and ZIAGEN® (abacavir sulfate) Oral Solution may be considered.

3 DOSAGE FORMS AND STRENGTHS

EPZICOM Tablets contain 600 mg of abacavir as abacavir sulfate and 300 mg of lamivudine. The tablets are modified capsule-shaped, orange, film-coated, and debossed with "GS FC2" on one side with no markings on the reverse side.

4 CONTRAINDICATIONS

EPZICOM Tablets are contraindicated in patients with:

- previously demonstrated hypersensitivity to abacavir or to any other component of the product. NEVER restart EPZICOM or any other abacavir-containing product following a hypersensitivity reaction to abacavir, regardless of HLA-B*5701 status *[see Warnings and Precautions (5.1), Adverse Reactions (6)]*.
- hepatic impairment *[see Use in Specific Populations (8.7)]*.

5 WARNINGS AND PRECAUTIONS

5.1 Hypersensitivity Reaction

Serious and sometimes fatal hypersensitivity reactions have been associated with EPZICOM and other abacavir-containing products. Patients who carry the HLA-B*5701 allele are at high risk for experiencing a hypersensitivity reaction to abacavir. Prior to initiating therapy with abacavir, screening for the HLA-B*5701 allele is recommended; this approach has been found to decrease the risk of a hypersensitivity reaction. Screening is also recommended prior to reinitiation of abacavir in patients of unknown HLA-B*5701 status who have previously tolerated abacavir. For HLA-B*5701-positive patients, treatment with an abacavir-containing regimen is not recommended and should be considered only with close medical supervision and under exceptional circumstances when the potential benefit outweighs the risk.

HLA-B*5701-negative patients may develop a hypersensitivity reaction to abacavir; however, this occurs significantly less frequently than in HLA-B*5701-positive patients. Regardless of HLA-B*5701 status, permanently discontinue EPZICOM if hypersensitivity cannot be ruled out, even when other diagnoses are possible.

Important information on signs and symptoms of hypersensitivity, as well as clinical management, is presented below.

Signs and Symptoms of Hypersensitivity: Hypersensitivity to abacavir is a multi-organ clinical syndrome usually characterized by a sign or symptom in 2 or more of the following groups.

Group 1: Fever
Group 2: Rash
Group 3: Gastrointestinal (including nausea, vomiting, diarrhea, or abdominal pain)
Group 4: Constitutional (including generalized malaise, fatigue, or achiness)
Group 5: Respiratory (including dyspnea, cough, or pharyngitis)

Hypersensitivity to abacavir following the presentation of a single sign or symptom has been reported infrequently.

Hypersensitivity to abacavir was reported in approximately 8% of 2,670 subjects (n = 206) in 9 clinical trials (range: 2% to 9%) with enrollment from November 1999 to February 2002. Data on time to onset and symptoms of suspected hypersensitivity were collected on a detailed data collection module. The frequencies of symptoms are shown in Figure 1. Symptoms usually appeared within the first 6 weeks of treatment with abacavir, although the reaction may occur at any time during therapy. Median time to onset was 9 days; 89% appeared within the first 6 weeks; 95% of subjects reported symptoms from 2 or more of the 5 groups listed above.

Figure 1: Hypersensitivity-Related Symptoms Reported With ≥10% Frequency in Clinical Trials (n = 206 Subjects)

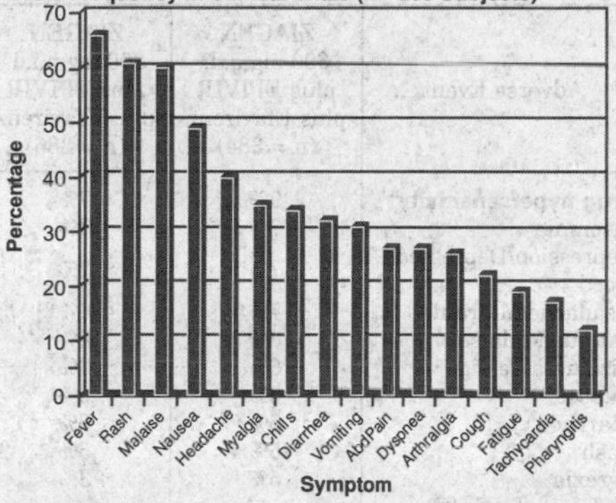

Other less common signs and symptoms of hypersensitivity include lethargy, myolysis, edema, abnormal chest x-ray findings (predominantly infiltrates, which can be localized), and paresthesia. Anaphylaxis, liver failure, renal failure, hypotension, adult respiratory distress syndrome, respiratory failure, and death have occurred in association with hypersensitivity reactions. In one trial, 4 subjects (11%) receiving ZIAGEN 600 mg once daily experienced hypotension with a hypersensitivity reaction compared with 0 subjects receiving ZIAGEN 300 mg twice daily.

Physical findings associated with hypersensitivity to abacavir in some subjects include lymphadenopathy, mucous membrane lesions (conjunctivitis and mouth ulcerations), and rash. The rash usually appears maculopapular or urticarial, but may be variable in appearance. There have been reports of erythema multiforme. Hypersensitivity reactions have occurred without rash.

Laboratory abnormalities associated with hypersensitivity to abacavir in some subjects include elevated liver function tests, elevated creatine phosphokinase, elevated creatinine, and lymphopenia.

Clinical Management of Hypersensitivity: Discontinue EPZICOM as soon as a hypersensitivity reaction is suspected. To minimize the risk of a life-threatening hypersensitivity reaction, permanently discontinue EPZICOM if hypersensitivity cannot be ruled out, even when other diagnoses are possible (e.g., acute onset respiratory diseases such as pneumonia, bronchitis, pharyngitis, or influenza; gastroenteritis; or reactions to other medications).

Following a hypersensitivity reaction to abacavir, NEVER restart EPZICOM or any other abacavir-containing product because more severe symptoms can occur within hours and may include life-threatening hypotension and death.

When therapy with EPZICOM has been discontinued for reasons other than symptoms of a hypersensitivity reaction, and if reinitiation of EPZICOM or any other abacavir-containing product is under consideration, carefully evaluate the reason for discontinuation of EPZICOM to ensure that the patient did not have symptoms of a hypersensitivity reaction. If the patient is of unknown HLA-B*5701 status, screening for the allele is recommended prior to reinitiation of EPZICOM.

If hypersensitivity cannot be ruled out, DO NOT reintroduce EPZICOM or any other abacavir-containing product. Even in the absence of the HLA-B*5701 allele, it is important to permanently discontinue abacavir and not rechallenge with abacavir if a hypersensitivity reaction cannot be ruled out on clinical grounds, due to the potential for a severe or even fatal reaction.

If symptoms consistent with hypersensitivity are not identified, reintroduction can be undertaken with continued monitoring for symptoms of a hypersensitivity reaction. Make patients aware that a hypersensitivity reaction can occur with reintroduction of EPZICOM or any other abacavir-containing product and that reintroduction of EPZICOM or introduction of any other abacavir-containing product needs to be undertaken only if medical care can be readily accessed by the patient or others.

Risk Factor: *HLA-B*5701 Allele:* Trials have shown that carriage of the HLA-B*5701 allele is associated with a significantly increased risk of a hypersensitivity reaction to abacavir.

CNA106030 (PREDICT-1), a randomized, double-blind trial, evaluated the clinical utility of prospective HLA-B*5701 screening on the incidence of abacavir hypersensitivity reaction in abacavir-naive HIV-1-infected adults (n = 1,650). In this trial, use of pre-therapy screening for the HLA-B*5701 allele and exclusion of subjects with this allele reduced the incidence of clinically suspected abacavir hypersensitivity reactions from 7.8% (66/847) to 3.4% (27/803). Based on this trial, it is estimated that 61% of patients with the HLA-B*5701 allele will develop a clinically suspected hypersensitivity reaction during the course of abacavir treatment compared with 4% of patients who do not have the HLA-B*5701 allele.

Screening for carriage of the HLA-B*5701 allele is recommended prior to initiating treatment with abacavir. Screening is also recommended prior to reinitiation of abacavir in patients of unknown HLA-B*5701 status who have previously tolerated abacavir. For HLA-B*5701-positive patients, initiating or reinitiating treatment with an abacavir-containing regimen is not recommended and should be considered only with close medical supervision and under exceptional circumstances where potential benefit outweighs the risk.

Skin patch testing is used as a research tool and should not be used to aid in the clinical diagnosis of abacavir hypersensitivity.

In any patient treated with abacavir, the clinical diagnosis of hypersensitivity reaction must remain the basis of clinical decision-making. Even in the absence of the HLA-B*5701 allele, it is important to permanently discontinue abacavir and not rechallenge with abacavir if a hypersensitivity reaction cannot be ruled out on clinical grounds, due to the potential for a severe or even fatal reaction.

5.2 Lactic Acidosis and Severe Hepatomegaly With Steatosis

Lactic acidosis and severe hepatomegaly with steatosis, including fatal cases, have been reported with the use of nucleoside analogues alone or in combination, including abacavir and lamivudine and other antiretrovirals. A majority of these cases have been in women. Obesity and prolonged nucleoside exposure may be risk factors. Particular caution should be exercised when administering EPZICOM to any patient with known risk factors for liver disease; however, cases have also been reported in patients with no known risk factors. Treatment with EPZICOM should be suspended in any patient who develops clinical or laboratory findings suggestive of lactic acidosis or pronounced hepatotoxicity (which may include hepatomegaly and steatosis even in the absence of marked transaminase elevations).

5.3 Patients With HIV-1 and Hepatitis B Virus Co-Infection

Posttreatment Exacerbations of Hepatitis: In clinical trials in non-HIV-1-infected subjects treated with lamivudine for chronic HBV, clinical and laboratory evidence of exacerbations of hepatitis have occurred after discontinuation of lamivudine. These exacerbations have been detected primarily by serum ALT elevations in addition to re-emergence of HBV DNA. Although most events appear to have been self-limited, fatalities have been reported in some cases. Similar events have been reported from post-marketing experience after changes from lamivudine-containing HIV-1 treatment regimens to non-lamivudine-containing regimens in patients infected with both HIV-1 and HBV. The causal relationship to discontinuation of lamivudine treatment is unknown. Patients should be closely monitored with both clinical and laboratory follow-up for at least several months after stopping treatment. There is insufficient evidence to determine whether re-initiation of lamivudine alters the course of posttreatment exacerbations of hepatitis.

Emergence of Lamivudine-Resistant HBV: Safety and efficacy of lamivudine have not been established for treatment of chronic hepatitis B in subjects dually infected with HIV-1 and HBV. In non–HIV-1-infected subjects treated with lamivudine for chronic hepatitis B, emergence of lamivudine-resistant HBV has been detected and has been associated with diminished treatment response (see full prescribing information for EPIVIR-HBV® [lamivudine]

Tablets and Oral Solution for additional information). Emergence of hepatitis B virus variants associated with resistance to lamivudine has also been reported in HIV-1-infected subjects who have received lamivudine-containing antiretroviral regimens in the presence of concurrent infection with hepatitis B virus.

5.4 Use With Interferon- and Ribavirin-Based Regimens

In vitro studies have shown ribavirin can reduce the phosphorylation of pyrimidine nucleoside analogues such as lamivudine, a component of EPZICOM. Although no evidence of a pharmacokinetic or pharmacodynamic interaction (e.g., loss of HIV-1/HCV virologic suppression) was seen when ribavirin was coadministered with lamivudine in HIV-1/HCV co-infected subjects *[see Clinical Pharmacology (12.3)]*, hepatic decompensation (some fatal) has occurred in HIV-1/HCV co-infected subjects receiving combination antiretroviral therapy for HIV-1 and interferon alfa with or without ribavirin. Patients receiving interferon alfa with or without ribavirin and EPZICOM should be closely monitored for treatment-associated toxicities, especially hepatic decompensation. Discontinuation of EPZICOM should be considered as medically appropriate. Dose reduction or discontinuation of interferon alfa, ribavirin, or both should also be considered if worsening clinical toxicities are observed, including hepatic decompensation (e.g., Child-Pugh >6) (see the complete prescribing information for interferon and ribavirin).

5.5 Immune Reconstitution Syndrome

Immune reconstitution syndrome has been reported in patients treated with combination antiretroviral therapy, including EPZICOM. During the initial phase of combination antiretroviral treatment, patients whose immune systems respond may develop an inflammatory response to indolent or residual opportunistic infections (such as *Mycobacterium avium* infection, cytomegalovirus, *Pneumocystisjirovecii* pneumonia [PCP], or tuberculosis), which may necessitate further evaluation and treatment.

Autoimmune disorders (such as Graves' disease, polymyositis, and Guillain-Barré syndrome) have also been reported to occur in the setting of immune reconstitution; however, the time to onset is more variable, and can occur many months after initiation of treatment.

5.6 Fat Redistribution

Redistribution/accumulation of body fat including central obesity, dorsocervical fat enlargement (buffalo hump), peripheral wasting, facial wasting, breast enlargement, and "cushingoid appearance" have been observed in patients receiving antiretroviral therapy. The mechanism and long-term consequences of these events are currently unknown. A causal relationship has not been established.

5.7 Myocardial Infarction

In a published prospective, observational, epidemiological trial designed to investigate the rate of myocardial infarction in patients on combination antiretroviral therapy, the use of abacavir within the previous 6 months was correlated with an increased risk of myocardial infarction (MI).[1] In a sponsor-conducted pooled analysis of clinical trials, no excess risk of MI was observed in abacavir-treated subjects as compared with control subjects. In totality, the available data from the observational cohort and from clinical trials are inconclusive.

As a precaution, the underlying risk of coronary heart disease should be considered when prescribing antiretroviral therapies, including abacavir, and action taken to minimize all modifiable risk factors (e.g., hypertension, hyperlipidemia, diabetes mellitus, smoking).

5.8 Use With Other Abacavir-, Lamivudine-, and/or Emtricitabine-Containing Products

EPZICOM contains fixed doses of 2 nucleoside analogues, abacavir and lamivudine, and should not be administered concomitantly with other abacavir-containing and/or lamivudine-containing products, including ZIAGEN (abacavir sulfate) Tablets and Oral Solution, EPIVIR (lamivudine) Tablets and Oral Solution, EPIVIR-HBV® (lamivudine) Tablets and Oral Solution COMBIVIR® (lamivudine and zidovudine) Tablets, or TRIZIVIR® (abacavir sulfate, lamivudine, and zidovudine) Tablets; or emtricitabine-containing products, including ATRIPLA® (efavirenz/emtricitabine/tenofovir disoproxil fumarate) Tablets, EMTRIVA® (emtricitabine) Capsules and Oral Solution, TRUVADA® (emtricitabine/tenofovir disoproxil fumarate) Tablets, or COMPLERA™ (emtricitabine/rilpivirine/tenofovir disoproxil fumarate) Tablets.

The complete prescribing information for all agents being considered for use with EPZICOM should be consulted before combination therapy with EPZICOM is initiated.

6 ADVERSE REACTIONS

The following adverse reactions are discussed in greater detail in other sections of the labeling:

- Serious and sometimes fatal hypersensitivity reaction. In one trial, once-daily dosing of abacavir was associated with more severe hypersensitivity reactions *[see Boxed Warning, Warnings and Precautions (5.1)]*.
- Lactic acidosis and severe hepatomegaly *[see Boxed Warning, Warnings and Precautions (5.2)]*.
- Acute exacerbations of hepatitis B *[see Boxed Warning, Warnings and Precautions (5.3)]*.
- Hepatic decompensation in patients co-infected with HIV-1 and Hepatitis C *[see Warnings and Precautions (5.4)]*.
- Immune reconstitution syndrome *[see Warnings and Precautions (5.5)]*.
- Fat redistribution *[see Warnings and Precautions (5.6)]*.
- Myocardial infarction *[see Warnings and Precautions (5.7)]*.

6.1 Clinical Trials Experience

Because clinical trials are conducted under widely varying conditions, adverse reaction rates observed in the clinical trials of a drug cannot be directly compared to rates in the clinical trials of another drug and may not reflect the rates observed in clinical practice.

Therapy-Naive Adults: Treatment-emergent clinical adverse reactions (rated by the investigator as moderate or severe) with a ≥5% frequency during therapy with ZIAGEN 600 mg once daily or ZIAGEN 300 mg twice daily, both in combination with lamivudine 300 mg once daily and efavirenz 600 mg once daily, are listed in Table 1.

Table 1. Treatment-Emergent (All Causality) Adverse Reactions of at Least Moderate Intensity (Grades 2-4, ≥5% Frequency) in Therapy-Naive Adults (CNA30021) Through 48 Weeks of Treatment

Adverse Event	ZIAGEN 600 mg q.d. plus EPIVIR plus Efavirenz (n = 384)	ZIAGEN 300 mg b.i.d. plus EPIVIR plus Efavirenz (n = 386)
Drug hypersensitivity[a,b]	9%	7%
Insomnia	7%	9%
Depression/Depressed mood	7%	7%
Headache/Migraine	7%	6%
Fatigue/Malaise	6%	8%
Dizziness/Vertigo	6%	6%
Nausea	5%	6%
Diarrhea[a]	5%	6%
Rash	5%	5%
Pyrexia	5%	3%
Abdominal pain/gastritis	4%	5%
Abnormal dreams	4%	5%
Anxiety	3%	5%

[a]Subjects receiving ZIAGEN 600 mg once daily, experienced a significantly higher incidence of severe drug hypersensitivity reactions and severe diarrhea compared with subjects who received ZIAGEN 300 mg twice daily. Five percent (5%) of subjects receiving ZIAGEN 600 mg once daily had severe drug hypersensitivity reactions compared with 2% of subjects receiving ZIAGEN 300 mg twice daily. Two percent (2%) of subjects receiving ZIAGEN 600 mg once daily had severe diarrhea while none of the subjects receiving ZIAGEN 300 mg twice daily had this event.

[b]CNA30024 was a multi-center, double-blind, controlled trial in which 649 HIV-1-infected, therapy-naive adults were randomized and received either ZIAGEN (300 mg twice daily), EPIVIR (150 mg twice daily), and efavirenz (600 mg once daily); or zidovudine (300 mg twice daily), EPIVIR (150 mg twice daily), and efavirenz (600 mg once daily). CNA30024 used double-blind ascertainment of suspected hypersensitivity reactions. During the blinded portion of the trial, suspected hypersensitivity to abacavir was reported by investigators in 9% of 324 patients in the abacavir group and 3% of 325 patients in the zidovudine group.

Laboratory Abnormalities: Laboratory abnormalities observed in clinical trials of ZIAGEN were anemia, neutropenia, liver function test abnormalities, and elevations of CPK, blood glucose, and triglycerides. Additional laboratory abnormalities observed in clinical trials of EPIVIR were thrombocytopenia and elevated levels of bilirubin, amylase, and lipase.

The frequencies of treatment-emergent laboratory abnormalities were comparable between treatment groups in CNA30021.

Other Adverse Events: In addition to adverse reactions listed above, other adverse events observed in the expanded access program for abacavir were pancreatitis and increased GGT.

6.2 Postmarketing Experience

In addition to adverse reactions reported from clinical trials, the following reactions have been identified during postmarketing use of abacavir, lamivudine, and/or EPZICOM. Because they are reported voluntarily from a population of unknown size, estimates of frequency cannot be made. These reactions have been chosen for inclusion due to a combination of their seriousness, frequency of reporting, or potential causal connection to abacavir, lamivudine, and/or EPZICOM.

Abacavir: *Cardiovascular:* Myocardial infarction.

Skin: Suspected Stevens-Johnson syndrome (SJS) and toxic epidermal necrolysis (TEN) have been reported in patients receiving abacavir primarily in combination with medications known to be associated with SJS and TEN, respectively. Because of the overlap of clinical signs and symptoms between hypersensitivity to abacavir and SJS and TEN, and the possibility of multiple drug sensitivities in some patients, abacavir should be discontinued and not restarted in such cases.

There have also been reports of erythema multiforme with abacavir use.

Abacavir and Lamivudine: *Body as a Whole:* Redistribution/accumulation of body fat *[see Warnings and Precautions (5.6)]*.

Digestive: Stomatitis.

Endocrine and Metabolic: Hyperglycemia.

General: Weakness.

Hemic and Lymphatic: Aplastic anemia, anemia (including pure red cell aplasia and severe anemias progressing on therapy), lymphadenopathy, splenomegaly.

Hepatic: Lactic acidosis and hepatic steatosis *[see Warnings and Precautions (5.2)]*, posttreatment exacerbation of hepatitis B *[see Warnings and Precautions (5.3)]*.

Hypersensitivity: Sensitization reactions (including anaphylaxis), urticaria.

Musculoskeletal: Muscle weakness, CPK elevation, rhabdomyolysis.

Nervous: Paresthesia, peripheral neuropathy, seizures.

Respiratory: Abnormal breath sounds/wheezing.

Skin: Alopecia, erythema multiforme, Stevens-Johnson syndrome.

7 DRUG INTERACTIONS

- No drug interaction trials have been conducted using EPZICOM Tablets *[see Clinical Pharmacology (12.3)]*.

7.1 Ethanol

Abacavir: Abacavir has no effect on the pharmacokinetic properties of ethanol. Ethanol decreases the elimination of abacavir causing an increase in overall exposure *[see Clinical Pharmacology (12.3)]*.

7.2 Interferon- and Ribavirin-Based Regimens

Lamivudine: Although no evidence of a pharmacokinetic or pharmacodynamic interaction (e.g., loss of HIV-1/HCV virologic suppression) was seen when ribavirin was coadministered with lamivudine in HIV-1/HCV co-infected subjects, hepatic decompensation (some fatal) has occurred in HIV-1/HCV co-infected subjects receiving combination antiretroviral therapy for HIV-1 and interferon alfa with or without ribavirin *[see Warnings and Precautions (5.4), Clinical Pharmacology (12.3)]*.

7.3 Methadone

Abacavir: The addition of methadone has no clinically significant effect on the pharmacokinetic properties of abacavir. In a trial of 11 HIV-1-infected subjects receiving methadone-maintenance therapy with 600 mg of ZIAGEN twice daily (twice the currently recommended dose), oral methadone clearance increased *[see Clinical Pharmacology (12.3)]*. This alteration will not result in a methadone dose modification in the majority of patients; however, an increased methadone dose may be required in a small number of patients.

7.4 Trimethoprim/Sulfamethoxazole (TMP/SMX)

Lamivudine: No change in dose of either drug is recommended *[see Clinical Pharmacology (12.3)]*. There is no information regarding the effect on lamivudine pharmacokinetics of higher doses of TMP/SMX such as those used to treat PCP.

8 USE IN SPECIFIC POPULATIONS

8.1 Pregnancy

EPZICOM: Pregnancy Category C. There are no adequate and well-controlled studies of EPZICOM in pregnant women. Reproduction studies with abacavir and lamivudine have been performed in animals (see Abacavir and Lamivudine sections below). EPZICOM should be used during pregnancy only if the potential benefits outweigh the risks.

Abacavir: Studies in pregnant rats showed that abacavir is transferred to the fetus through the placenta. Fetal malformations (increased incidences of fetal anasarca and skeletal malformations) and developmental toxicity (depressed fetal body weight and reduced crown-rump length) were observed in rats at a dose which produced 35 times the human exposure, based on AUC. Embryonic and fetal toxicities (increased resorptions, decreased fetal body weights) and toxicities to the offspring (increased incidence of stillbirth and lower body weights) occurred at half of the above-mentioned dose in separate fertility studies conducted in rats. In the rabbit, no developmental toxicity and no increases in fetal malformations occurred at doses that produced 8.5 times the human exposure at the recommended dose based on AUC.

Lamivudine: Studies in pregnant rats showed that lamivudine is transferred to the fetus through the placenta. Reproduction studies with orally administered lamivudine have been performed in rats and rabbits at doses producing plasma levels up to approximately 35 times that for the recommended adult HIV dose. No evidence of teratogenicity due to lamivudine was observed. Evidence of early embryolethality was seen in the rabbit at exposure levels similar to those observed in humans, but there was no indication of this effect in the rat at exposure levels up to 35 times those in humans.

Antiretroviral Pregnancy Registry: To monitor maternal-fetal outcomes of pregnant women exposed to EPZICOM or other antiretroviral agents, an Antiretroviral Pregnancy Registry has been established. Physicians are encouraged to register patients by calling 1-800-258-4263.

8.3 Nursing Mothers

The Centers for Disease Control and Prevention recommend that HIV-1-infected mothers not breastfeed their infants to avoid risking postnatal transmission of HIV-1 infection.

Abacavir: Abacavir is secreted into the milk of lactating rats.

Lamivudine: Lamivudine is excreted in human breast milk and into the milk of lactating rats.

Because of both the potential for HIV-1 transmission and the potential for serious adverse reactions in nursing infants, mothers should be instructed not to breastfeed if they are receiving EPZICOM.

8.4 Pediatric Use

Safety and effectiveness of EPZICOM in pediatric patients have not been established. EPZICOM is not recommended for use in patients younger than 18 years because it cannot be dose adjusted.

8.5 Geriatric Use

Clinical studies of abacavir and lamivudine did not include sufficient numbers of subjects aged 65 and over to determine whether they respond differently from younger subjects. In general, dose selection for an elderly patient should be cautious, reflecting the greater frequency of decreased hepatic, renal, or cardiac function, and of concomitant disease or other drug therapy *[see Dosage and Administration (2.2), Use in Specific Populations (8.6, 8.7)]*.

8.6 Patients With Impaired Renal Function

EPZICOM is not recommended for patients with impaired renal function (creatinine clearance <50 mL/min) because EPZICOM is a fixed-dose combination and the dosage of the individual components cannot be adjusted.

8.7 Patients With Impaired Hepatic Function

EPZICOM is contraindicated for patients with hepatic impairment because EPZICOM is a fixed-dose combination and the dosage of the individual components cannot be adjusted.

10 OVERDOSAGE

Abacavir: There is no known antidote for abacavir. It is not known whether abacavir can be removed by peritoneal dialysis or hemodialysis.

Lamivudine: One case of an adult ingesting 6 grams of lamivudine was reported; there were no clinical signs or symptoms noted and hematologic tests remained normal. It is not known whether lamivudine can be removed by peritoneal dialysis or hemodialysis.

11 DESCRIPTION

EPZICOM: EPZICOM Tablets contain the following 2 synthetic nucleoside analogues: abacavir sulfate (ZIAGEN, also a component of TRIZIVIR) and lamivudine (also known as EPIVIR or 3TC) with inhibitory activity against HIV-1. EPZICOM Tablets are for oral administration. Each orange, film-coated tablet contains the active ingredients 600 mg of abacavir as abacavir sulfate and 300 mg of lamivudine, and the inactive ingredients magnesium stearate, microcrystalline cellulose, and sodium starch glycolate. The tablets are coated with a film (OPADRY® orange YS-1-13065-A) that is made of FD&C Yellow No. 6, hypromellose, polyethylene glycol 400, polysorbate 80, and titanium dioxide.

Abacavir Sulfate: The chemical name of abacavir sulfate is *(1S,cis)*-4-[2-amino-6-(cyclopropylamino)-9*H*-purin-9-yl]-2-cyclopentene-1-methanol sulfate (salt) (2:1). Abacavir sulfate is the enantiomer with *1S, 4R* absolute configuration on the cyclopentene ring. It has a molecular formula of $(C_{14}H_{18}N_6O)_2.H_2SO_4$ and a molecular weight of 670.76 daltons. It has the following structural formula:

Table 2. Pharmacokinetic Parameters[a] for Abacavir and Lamivudine in Adults

Parameter	Abacavir		Lamivudine	
Oral bioavailability (%)	86 ± 25	n = 6	86 ± 16	n = 12
Apparent volume of distribution (L/kg)	0.86 ± 0.15	n = 6	1.3 ± 0.4	n = 20
Systemic clearance (L/hr/kg)	0.80 ± 0.24	n = 6	0.33 ± 0.06	n = 20
Renal clearance (L/hr/kg)	.007 ± .008	n = 6	0.22 ± 0.06	n = 20
Elimination half-life (hr)	1.45 ± 0.32	n = 20	5 to 7[b]	

[a]Data presented as mean ± standard deviation except where noted.

[b]Approximate range.

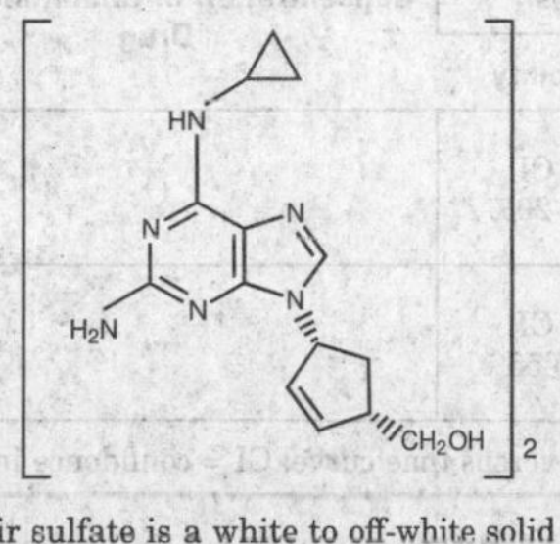

Abacavir sulfate is a white to off-white solid with a solubility of approximately 77 mg/mL in distilled water at 25°C. In vivo, abacavir sulfate dissociates to its free base, abacavir. All dosages for abacavir sulfate are expressed in terms of abacavir.

Lamivudine: The chemical name of lamivudine is (2R,cis)-4-amino-1-(2-hydroxymethyl-1,3-oxathiolan-5-yl)-(1H)-pyrimidin-2-one. Lamivudine is the (-)enantiomer of a dideoxy analogue of cytidine. Lamivudine has also been referred to as (-)2′,3′-dideoxy, 3′-thiacytidine. It has a molecular formula of $C_8H_{11}N_3O_3S$ and a molecular weight of 229.3 daltons. It has the following structural formula:

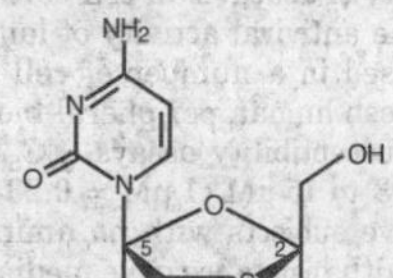

Lamivudine is a white to off-white crystalline solid with a solubility of approximately 70 mg/mL in water at 20°C.

12 CLINICAL PHARMACOLOGY

12.1 Mechanism of Action

EPZICOM is an antiviral agent *[see Clinical Pharmacology (12.4)]*.

12.3 Pharmacokinetics

Pharmacokinetics in Adults:*EPZICOM:* In a single-dose, 3-way crossover bioavailability trial of 1 EPZICOM Tablet versus 2 ZIAGEN Tablets (2 × 300 mg) and 2 EPIVIR Tablets (2 × 150 mg) administered simultaneously in healthy subjects (n = 25), there was no difference in the extent of absorption, as measured by the area under the plasma concentration-time curve (AUC) and maximal peak concentration (C_{max}), of each component.

Abacavir: Following oral administration, abacavir is rapidly absorbed and extensively distributed. After oral administration of a single dose of 600 mg of abacavir in 20 subjects, C_{max} was 4.26 ± 1.19 mcg/mL (mean ± SD) and AUC_∞ was 11.95 ± 2.51 mcg•hr/mL. Binding of abacavir to human plasma proteins is approximately 50% and was independent of concentration. Total blood and plasma drug-related radioactivity concentrations are identical, demonstrating that abacavir readily distributes into erythrocytes. The primary routes of elimination of abacavir are metabolism by alcohol dehydrogenase to form the 5′-carboxylic acid and glucuronyl transferase to form the 5′-glucuronide.

Lamivudine: Following oral administration, lamivudine is rapidly absorbed and extensively distributed. After multiple-dose oral administration of lamivudine 300 mg once daily for 7 days to 60 healthy subjects, steady-state C_{max} ($C_{max,ss}$) was 2.04 ± 0.54 mcg/mL (mean ± SD) and the 24-hour steady-state AUC ($AUC_{24,ss}$) was 8.87 ± 1.83 mcg•hr/mL. Binding to plasma protein is low. Approximately 70% of an intravenous dose of lamivudine is recovered as unchanged drug in the urine. Metabolism of lamivudine is a minor route of elimination. In humans, the only known metabolite is the trans-sulfoxide metabolite (approximately 5% of an oral dose after 12 hours).

The steady-state pharmacokinetic properties of the EPIVIR 300-mg tablet once daily for 7 days compared with the EPIVIR 150-mg tablet twice daily for 7 days were assessed in a crossover trial in 60 healthy subjects. EPIVIR 300 mg once daily resulted in lamivudine exposures that were similar to EPIVIR 150 mg twice daily with respect to plasma $AUC_{24,ss}$; however, $C_{max,ss}$ was 66% higher and the trough value was 53% lower compared with the 150-mg twice-daily regimen. Intracellular lamivudine triphosphate exposures in peripheral blood mononuclear cells were also similar with respect to $AUC_{24,ss}$ and $C_{max24,ss}$; however, trough values were lower compared with the 150-mg twice-daily regimen. Inter-subject variability was greater for intracellular lamivudine triphosphate concentrations versus lamivudine plasma trough concentrations. The clinical significance of observed differences for both plasma lamivudine concentrations and intracellular lamivudine triphosphate concentrations is not known.

In humans, abacavir and lamivudine are not significantly metabolized by cytochrome P450 enzymes.

The pharmacokinetic properties of abacavir and lamivudine in fasting subjects are summarized in Table 2.

[See table 2 above]

Effect of Food on Absorption of EPZICOM: EPZICOM may be administered with or without food. Administration with a high-fat meal in a single-dose bioavailability trial resulted in no change in AUC_{last}, AUC_∞, and C_{max} for lamivudine. Food did not alter the extent of systemic exposure to abacavir (AUC_∞), but the rate of absorption (C_{max}) was decreased approximately 24% compared with fasted conditions (n = 25). These results are similar to those from previous trials of the effect of food on abacavir and lamivudine tablets administered separately.

Special Populations:*Renal Impairment: EPZICOM:* Because lamivudine requires dose adjustment in the presence of renal insufficiency, EPZICOM is not recommended for use in patients with creatinine clearance <50 mL/min *[see Dosage and Administration (2.2)]*.

Hepatic Impairment: EPZICOM: EPZICOM is contraindicated for patients with hepatic impairment because EPZICOM is a fixed-dose combination and the dosage of the individual components cannot be adjusted. Abacavir is contraindicated in patients with moderate to severe hepatic impairment, and dose reduction is required in patients with mild hepatic impairment.

Pregnancy: See Use in Specific Populations (8.1).

Abacavir and Lamivudine: No data are available on the pharmacokinetics of abacavir or lamivudine during pregnancy.

Nursing Mothers: See Use in Specific Populations (8.3).

Abacavir: No data are available on the pharmacokinetics of abacavir in nursing mothers.

Lamivudine: Samples of breast milk obtained from 20 mothers receiving lamivudine monotherapy (300 mg twice daily) or combination therapy (150 mg lamivudine twice daily and 300 mg zidovudine twice daily) had measurable concentrations of lamivudine.

Pediatric Patients: EPZICOM: The pharmacokinetics of EPZICOM in pediatric subjects are under investigation. There are insufficient data at this time to recommend a dose.

Geriatric Patients: The pharmacokinetics of abacavir and lamivudine have not been studied in subjects over 65 years of age.

Gender: Abacavir: A population pharmacokinetic analysis in HIV-1-infected male (n = 304) and female (n = 67) subjects showed no gender differences in abacavir AUC normalized for lean body weight.

Lamivudine: A pharmacokinetic trial in healthy male (n = 12) and female (n = 12) subjects showed no gender differences in lamivudine AUC_∞ normalized for body weight.

Race: Abacavir: There are no significant differences between blacks and Caucasians in abacavir pharmacokinetics.

Lamivudine: There are no significant racial differences in lamivudine pharmacokinetics.

Drug Interactions: The drug interactions described are based on trials conducted with the individual nucleoside

Table 3. Effect of Coadministered Drugs on Abacavir and Lamivudine AUC

Note: ROUTINE DOSE MODIFICATION OF ABACAVIR AND LAMIVUDINE IS NOT WARRANTED WITH COADMINISTRATION OF THE FOLLOWING DRUGS.

Drugs That May Alter Abacavir Blood Concentrations

Coadministered Drug and Dose	Abacavir Dose	n	Abacavir Concentrations		Concentration of Coadministered Drug
			AUC	Variability	
Ethanol 0.7 g/kg	Single 600 mg	24	↑41%	90% CI: 35% to 48%	↔

Drugs That May Alter Lamivudine Blood Concentrations

Coadministered Drug and Dose	Lamivudine Dose	n	Lamivudine Concentrations		Concentration of Coadministered Drug
			AUC	Variability	
Nelfinavir 750 mg q 8 hr × 7 to 10 days	Single 150 mg	11	↑10%	95% CI: 1% to 20%	↔
Trimethoprim 160 mg/ Sulfamethoxazole 800 mg daily × 5 days	Single 300 mg	14	↑43%	90% CI: 32% to 55%	↔

↑ = Increase; ↔ = no significant change; AUC = area under the concentration versus time curve; CI = confidence interval.

analogues. In humans, abacavir and lamivudine are not significantly metabolized by cytochrome P450 enzymes nor do they inhibit or induce this enzyme system; therefore, it is unlikely that clinically significant drug interactions will occur with drugs metabolized through these pathways.

Abacavir: Lamivudine and Zidovudine: Fifteen HIV-1-infected subjects were enrolled in a crossover-designed drug interaction trial evaluating single doses of abacavir (600 mg), lamivudine (150 mg), and zidovudine (300 mg) alone or in combination. Analysis showed no clinically relevant changes in the pharmacokinetics of abacavir with the addition of lamivudine or zidovudine or the combination of lamivudine and zidovudine. Lamivudine exposure (AUC decreased 15%) and zidovudine exposure (AUC increased 10%) did not show clinically relevant changes with concurrent abacavir.

Methadone: In a trial of 11 HIV-1-infected subjects receiving methadone-maintenance therapy (40 mg and 90 mg daily), with 600 mg of ZIAGEN twice daily (twice the currently recommended dose), oral methadone clearance increased 22% (90% CI: 6% to 42%) *[see Drug Interactions (7.4)].*

Lamivudine:Zidovudine: No clinically significant alterations in lamivudine or zidovudine pharmacokinetics were observed in 12 asymptomatic HIV-1-infected adult subjects given a single dose of zidovudine (200 mg) in combination with multiple doses of lamivudine (300 mg q 12 hr).

Ribavirin: In vitro data indicate ribavirin reduces phosphorylation of lamivudine, stavudine, and zidovudine. However, no pharmacokinetic (e.g., plasma concentrations or intracellular triphosphorylated active metabolite concentrations) or pharmacodynamic (e.g., loss of HIV-1/HCV virologic suppression) interaction was observed when ribavirin and lamivudine (n = 18), stavudine (n = 10), or zidovudine (n = 6) were coadministered as part of a multi-drug regimen to HIV-1/HCV co-infected subjects *[see Warnings and Precautions (5.4)].*

The effects of other coadministered drugs on abacavir or lamivudine are provided in Table 3.

[See table 3 above]

12.4 Microbiology

Mechanism of Action:*Abacavir:* Abacavir is a carbocyclic synthetic nucleoside analogue. Abacavir is converted by cellular enzymes to the active metabolite, carbovir triphosphate (CBV-TP), an analogue of deoxyguanosine-5′-triphosphate (dGTP). CBV-TP inhibits the activity of HIV-1 reverse transcriptase (RT) both by competing with the natural substrate dGTP and by its incorporation into viral DNA. The lack of a 3′-OH group in the incorporated nucleotide analogue prevents the formation of the 5′ to 3′ phosphodiester linkage essential for DNA chain elongation, and therefore, the viral DNA growth is terminated. CBV-TP is a weak inhibitor of cellular DNA polymerases α, β, and γ.

Lamivudine: Lamivudine is a synthetic nucleoside analogue. Intracellularly lamivudine is phosphorylated to its active 5′-triphosphate metabolite, lamivudine triphosphate (3TC-TP). The principal mode of action of 3TC-TP is inhibition of RT via DNA chain termination after incorporation of the nucleotide analogue. CBV-TP and 3TC-TP are weak inhibitors of cellular DNA polymerases α, β, and γ.

Antiviral Activity:*Abacavir:* The antiviral activity of abacavir against HIV-1 was evaluated against a T-cell tropic laboratory strain HIV-1_{IIIB} in lymphoblastic cell lines, a monocyte/macrophage tropic laboratory strain HIV-1_{BaL} in primary monocytes/macrophages, and clinical isolates in peripheral blood mononuclear cells. The concentration of drug necessary to effect viral replication by 50 percent (EC_{50}) ranged from 3.7 to 5.8 µM (1 µM = 0.28 mcg/mL) and 0.07 to 1.0 µM against HIV-1_{IIIB} and HIV-1_{BaL}, respectively, and was 0.26 ± 0.18 µM against 8 clinical isolates. The EC_{50} values of abacavir against different HIV-1 clades (A-G) ranged from 0.0015 to 1.05 µM, and against HIV-2 isolates, from 0.024 to 0.49 µM. Ribavirin (50 µM) had no effect on the anti–HIV-1 activity of abacavir in cell culture.

Lamivudine: The antiviral activity of lamivudine against HIV-1 was assessed in a number of cell lines (including monocytes and fresh human peripheral blood lymphocytes) using standard susceptibility assays. EC_{50} values were in the range of 0.003 to 15 µM (1 µM = 0.23 mcg/mL). HIV-1 from therapy-naive subjects with no amino acid substitutions associated with resistance gave median EC_{50} values of 0.429 µM (range: 0.200 to 2.007 µM) from Virco (n = 92 baseline samples from COLA40263) and 2.35 µM (1.37 to 3.68 µM) from Monogram Biosciences (n = 135 baseline samples from ESS30009). The EC_{50} values of lamivudine against different HIV-1 clades (A-G) ranged from 0.001 to 0.120 µM, and against HIV-2 isolates from 0.003 to 0.120 µM in peripheral blood mononuclear cells. Ribavirin (50 µM) decreased the anti–HIV-1 activity of lamivudine by 3.5 fold in MT-4 cells.

The combination of abacavir and lamivudine has demonstrated antiviral activity in cell culture against non-subtype B isolates and HIV-2 isolates with equivalent antiviral activity as for subtype B isolates. Abacavir/lamivudine had additive to synergistic activity in cell culture in combination with the nucleoside reverse transcriptase inhibitors (NRTIs) emtricitabine, stavudine, tenofovir, zalcitabine, zidovudine; the non-nucleoside reverse transcriptase inhibitors (NNRTIs) delavirdine, efavirenz, nevirapine; the protease inhibitors (PIs) amprenavir, indinavir, lopinavir, nelfinavir, ritonavir, saquinavir; or the fusion inhibitor, enfuvirtide. Ribavirin, used in combination with interferon for the treatment of HCV infection, decreased the anti-HIV-1 potency of abacavir/lamivudine reproducibly by 2- to 6-fold in cell culture.

Resistance: HIV-1 isolates with reduced susceptibility to the combination of abacavir and lamivudine have been selected in cell culture and have also been obtained from subjects failing abacavir/lamivudine-containing regimens. Genotypic characterization of abacavir/lamivudine-resistant viruses selected in cell culture identified amino acid substitutions M184V/I, K65R, L74V, and Y115F in HIV-1 RT. Genotypic analysis of isolates selected in cell culture and recovered from abacavir-treated subjects demonstrated that amino acid substitutions K65R, L74V, Y115F, and M184V/I in HIV-1 RT contributed to abacavir resistance. Genotypic analysis of isolates selected in cell culture and recovered from lamivudine-treated subjects showed that the resistance was due to a specific amino acid substitution in HIV-1 RT at codon 184 changing the methionine to either isoleucine or valine (M184V/I). In a trial of therapy-naive adults receiving ZIAGEN 600 mg once daily (n = 384) or 300 mg twice daily (n = 386) in a background regimen of lamivudine 300 mg and efavirenz 600 mg once daily (CNA30021), the incidence of virologic failure at 48 weeks was similar between the 2 groups (11% in both arms). Genotypic (n = 38) and phenotypic analyses (n = 35) of virologic failure isolates from this trial showed that the RT substitutions that emerged during abacavir/lamivudine once-daily and twice-daily therapy were K65R, L74V, Y115F, and M184V/I. The abacavir- and lamivudine-associated resistance substitution M184V/I was the most commonly observed substitution in virologic failure isolates from subjects receiving abacavir/lamivudine once daily (56%, 10/18) and twice daily (40%, 8/20).

Thirty-nine percent (7/18) of the isolates from subjects who experienced virologic failure in the abacavir once-daily arm had a >2.5-fold decrease in abacavir susceptibility with a median-fold decrease of 1.3 (range: 0.5 to 11) compared with 29% (5/17) of the failure isolates in the twice-daily arm with a median-fold decrease of 0.92 (range: 0.7 to 13). Fifty-six percent (10/18) of the virologic failure isolates in the once-daily abacavir group compared with 41% (7/17) of the failure isolates in the twice-daily abacavir group had a >2.5-fold decrease in lamivudine susceptibility with median-fold changes of 81 (range 0.79 to >116) and 1.1 (range 0.68 to >116) in the once-daily and twice-daily abacavir arms, respectively.

Cross-Resistance: Cross-resistance has been observed among NRTIs. Viruses containing abacavir and lamivudine resistance-associated amino acid substitutions, namely, K65R, L74V, M184V, and Y115F, exhibit cross-resistance to didanosine, emtricitabine, lamivudine, tenofovir, and zalcitabine in cell culture and in subjects. The K65R substitution can confer resistance to abacavir, didanosine, emtricitabine, lamivudine, stavudine, tenofovir, and zalcitabine; the L74V substitution can confer resistance to abacavir, didanosine, and zalcitabine; and the M184V substitution can confer resistance to abacavir, didanosine, emtricitabine, lamivudine, and zalcitabine.

The combination of abacavir/lamivudine has demonstrated decreased susceptibility to viruses with the substitutions K65R with or without the M184V/I substitution, viruses with L74V plus the M184V/I substitution, and viruses with thymidine analog mutations (TAMs: M41L, D67N, K70R, L210W, T215Y/F, K219 E/R/H/Q/N) plus M184V. An increasing number of TAMs is associated with a progressive reduction in abacavir susceptibility.

13 NONCLINICAL TOXICOLOGY

13.1 Carcinogenesis, Mutagenesis, Impairment of Fertility

Carcinogenicity:*Abacavir:* Abacavir was administered orally at 3 dosage levels to separate groups of mice and rats in 2-year carcinogenicity studies. Results showed an increase in the incidence of malignant and non-malignant tumors. Malignant tumors occurred in the preputial gland of males and the clitoral gland of females of both species, and in the liver of female rats. In addition, non-malignant tumors also occurred in the liver and thyroid gland of female rats. These observations were made at systemic exposures in the range of 6 to 32 times the human exposure at the recommended dose.

Lamivudine: Long-term carcinogenicity studies with lamivudine in mice and rats showed no evidence of carcinogenic potential at exposures up to 10 times (mice) and 58 times (rats) those observed in humans at the recommended therapeutic dose for HIV-1 infection.

It is not known how predictive the results of rodent carcinogenicity studies may be for humans.

Mutagenicity:*Abacavir:* Abacavir induced chromosomal aberrations both in the presence and absence of metabolic activation in an in vitro cytogenetic study in human lymphocytes. Abacavir was mutagenic in the absence of metabolic activation, although it was not mutagenic in the presence of metabolic activation in an L5178Y mouse lymphoma assay. Abacavir was clastogenic in males and not clastogenic in females in an in vivo mouse bone marrow micronucleus assay. Abacavir was not mutagenic in bacterial mutagenicity assays in the presence and absence of metabolic activation.

Lamivudine: Lamivudine was mutagenic in an L5178Y mouse lymphoma assay and clastogenic in a cytogenetic assay using cultured human lymphocytes. Lamivudine was not mutagenic in a microbial mutagenicity assay, in an in vitro cell transformation assay, in a rat micronucleus test, in a rat bone marrow cytogenetic assay, and in an assay for unscheduled DNA synthesis in rat liver.

Impairment of Fertility: Abacavir or lamivudine induced no adverse effects on the mating performance or fertility of male and female rats at doses producing systemic exposure levels approximately 8 or 130 times, respectively, higher than those in humans at the recommended dose based on body surface area comparisons.

13.2 Animal Toxicology and/or Pharmacology

Myocardial degeneration was found in mice and rats following administration of abacavir for 2 years.The systemic exposures were equivalent to 7 to 24 times the expected systemic exposure in humans. The clinical relevance of this finding has not been determined.

14 CLINICAL STUDIES

EPZICOM: There have been no clinical trials conducted with EPZICOM. One EPZICOM Tablet given once daily is an alternative regimen to EPIVIR Tablets 300 mg once daily plus ZIAGEN Tablets 2 × 300 mg once daily as a component of antiretroviral therapy.

The following trial was conducted with the individual components of EPZICOM.

Therapy-Naive Adults: **CNA30021** was an international, multi-center, double-blind, controlled trial in which 770 HIV-1-infected, therapy-naive adults were randomized and received either ZIAGEN 600 mg once daily or ZIAGEN 300 mg twice daily, both in combination with EPIVIR 300 mg once daily and efavirenz 600 mg once daily. The double-blind treatment duration was at least 48 weeks. Trial participants had a mean age of 37 years; were male (81%), Caucasian (54%), black (27%), and American Hispanic (15%). The median baseline CD4+ cell count was 262 cells/mm^3 (range: 21 to 918 cells/mm^3) and the median baseline plasma HIV-1 RNA was 4.89 $\log_{10}$ copies/mL (range: 2.60 to 6.99 $\log_{10}$ copies/mL).

The outcomes of randomized treatment are provided in Table 4.

Table 4. Outcomes of Randomized Treatment Through Week 48 (CNA30021)

Outcome	ZIAGEN 600 mg q.d. plus EPIVIR plus Efavirenz (n = 384)	ZIAGEN 300 mg b.i.d. plus EPIVIR plus Efavirenz (n = 386)
Responder[a]	64% (71%)	65% (72%)
Virologic failure[b]	11% (5%)	11% (5%)
Discontinued due to adverse reactions	13%	11%
Discontinued due to other reasons[c]	11%	13%

[a]Subjects achieved and maintained confirmed HIV-1 RNA <50 copies/mL (<400 copies/mL) through Week 48 (Roche AMPLICOR Ultrasensitive HIV-1 MONITOR® standard test version 1.0).

[b]Includes viral rebound, failure to achieve confirmed <50 copies/mL (<400 copies/mL) by Week 48, and insufficient viral load response.

[c]Includes consent withdrawn, lost to follow-up, protocol violations, clinical progression, and other.

After 48 weeks of therapy, the median CD4+ cell count increases from baseline were 188 cells/mm^3 in the group receiving ZIAGEN 600 mg once daily and 200 cells/mm^3 in the group receiving ZIAGEN 300 mg twice daily. Through Week 48, 6 subjects (2%) in the group receiving ZIAGEN 600 mg once daily (4 CDC classification C events and 2 deaths) and 10 subjects (3%) in the group receiving ZIAGEN 300 mg twice daily (7 CDC classification C events and 3 deaths) experienced clinical disease progression. None of the deaths were attributed to trial medications.

15 REFERENCES

1. Data Collection on Adverse Events of Anti-HIV Drugs (D:A:D) Study Group. *Lancet*. 2008;371 (9622):1417-1426.

16 HOW SUPPLIED/STORAGE AND HANDLING

EPZICOM is available as tablets. Each tablet contains 600 mg of abacavir as abacavir sulfate and 300 mg of lamivudine. The tablets are orange, film-coated, modified capsule-shaped, and debossed with GS FC2 on one side with no markings on the reverse side. They are packaged as follows:

Bottles of 30 Tablets (NDC 49702-206-13).

Store at 25°C (77°F); excursions permitted to 15° to 30°C (59° to 86°F) (see USP Controlled Room Temperature).

17 PATIENT COUNSELING INFORMATION

See FDA-approved patient labeling (Medication Guide)

Hypersensitivity Reaction: Inform patients:

- that a Medication Guide and Warning Card summarizing the symptoms of the abacavir hypersensitivity reaction and other product information will be dispensed by the pharmacist with each new prescription and refill of EPZICOM, and encourage the patient to read the Medication Guide and Warning Card every time to obtain any new information that may be present about EPZICOM. (The complete text of the Medication Guide is reprinted at the end of this document.)
- to carry the Warning Card with them.
- how to identify a hypersensitivity reaction *[see Warnings and Precautions (5.1), Medication Guide]*.
- that if they develop symptoms consistent with a hypersensitivity reaction they should call their doctor right away to determine if they should stop taking EPZICOM.
- that a hypersensitivity reaction can worsen and lead to hospitalization or death if EPZICOM is not immediately discontinued.
- that in one study, more severe hypersensitivity reactions were seen when ZIAGEN was dosed 600 mg once daily.
- to not restart EPZICOM or any other abacavir-containing product following a hypersensitivity reaction because more severe symptoms can occur within hours and may include life-threatening hypotension and death.
- that a hypersensitivity reaction is usually reversible if it is detected promptly and EPZICOM is stopped right away.
- that if they have interrupted EPZICOM for reasons other than symptoms of hypersensitivity (for example, those who have an interruption in drug supply), a serious or fatal hypersensitivity reaction may occur with reintroduction of abacavir.
- to not restart EPZICOM or any other abacavir-containing product without medical consultation and that restarting abacavir needs to be undertaken only if medical care can be readily accessed by the patient or others.
- EPZICOM should not be administered concomitantly with ATRIPLA, COMBIVIR, COMPLERA, EMTRIVA, EPIVIR, EPIVIR-HBV, TRIZIVIR, TRUVADA, or ZIAGEN.

Lactic Acidosis/Hepatomegaly: Inform patients that some HIV medicines, including EPZICOM, can cause a rare, but serious condition called lactic acidosis with liver enlargement (hepatomegaly) *[see Warnings and Precautions (5.2)]*.

HIV-1/ HBV Co-infection: Patients co-infected with HIV-1 and HBV should be informed that deterioration of liver disease has occurred in some cases when treatment with lamivudine was discontinued. Patients should be advised to discuss any changes in regimen with their physician *[see Warnings and Precautions (5.3)]*.

HIV-1/HCV Co-Infection: Patients with HIV-1/HCV co-infection should be informed that hepatic decompensation (some fatal) has occurred in HIV-1/HCV co-infected patients receiving combination antiretroviral therapy for HIV-1 and interferon alfa with or without ribavirin *[see Warnings and Precautions (5.4)]*.

Redistribution/Accumulation of Body Fat: Inform patients that redistribution or accumulation of body fat may occur in patients receiving antiretroviral therapy and that the cause and long-term health effects of these conditions are not known at this time *[see Warnings and Precautions (5.6)]*.

Information About HIV-1 Infection: EPZICOM is not a cure for HIV-1 infection and patients may continue to experience illnesses associated with HIV-1 infection, including opportunistic infections. Patients should remain under the care of a physician when using EPZICOM.

Patients should be advised to avoid doing things that can spread HIV-1 infection to others.

- **Do not share needles or other injection equipment.**
- **Do not share personal items that can have blood or body fluids on them, like toothbrushes and razor blades.**
- **Do not have any kind of sex without protection.** Always practice safe sex by using a latex or polyurethane condom to lower the chance of sexual contact with semen, vaginal secretions, or blood.
- **Do not breastfeed.** Lamivudine is excreted in human breast milk. It is not known if abacavir can be passed to your baby in your breast milk and whether it could harm your baby. Also, mothers with HIV-1 should not breastfeed because HIV-1 can be passed to the baby in the breast milk.

Patients should be informed to take all HIV medications exactly as prescribed.

COMBIVIR, EPIVIR, EPZICOM, TRIZIVIR, and ZIAGEN are registered trademarks of ViiV Healthcare.

The other brands listed are trademarks of their respective owners and are not trademarks of ViiV Healthcare. The makers of these brands are not affiliated with and do not endorse ViiV Healthcare or its products.

Manufactured for:
ViiV Healthcare
Research Triangle Park, NC 27709
by:
GlaxoSmithKline
Research Triangle Park, NC 27709
Lamivudine is manufactured under agreement from
Shire Pharmaceuticals Group plc
Basingstoke, UK

EPZ:7PI

MEDICATION GUIDE
EPZICOM® (ep' zih com)
(abacavir sulfate and lamivudine)
Tablets

Read this Medication Guide before you start taking EPZICOM and each time you get a refill. There may be new information. This information does not take the place of talking to your healthcare provider about your medical condition or your treatment. Be sure to carry your EPZICOM Warning Card with you at all times.

What is the most important information I should know about EPZICOM?

1. Serious allergic reaction (hypersensitivity reaction). EPZICOM contains abacavir (also contained in ZIAGEN® and TRIZIVIR®). Patients taking EPZICOM may have a serious allergic reaction (hypersensitivity reaction) that can cause death. Your risk of this allergic reaction is much higher if you have a gene variation called HLA-B*5701. Your healthcare provider can determine with a blood test if you have this gene variation.

If you get a symptom from 2 or more of the following groups while taking EPZICOM, call your healthcare provider right away to find out if you should stop taking EPZICOM.

	Symptom(s)
Group 1	**Fever**
Group 2	**Rash**
Group 3	**Nausea, vomiting, diarrhea, abdominal (stomach area) pain**
Group 4	**Generally ill feeling, extreme tiredness, or achiness**
Group 5	**Shortness of breath, cough, sore throat**

A list of these symptoms is on the Warning Card your pharmacist gives you. **Carry this Warning Card with you at all times.**

If you stop EPZICOM because of an allergic reaction, never take EPZICOM (abacavir sulfate and lamivudine) or any other abacavir-containing medicine (ZIAGEN and TRIZIVIR) again. If you take EPZICOM or any other abacavir-containing medicine again after you have had an allergic reaction, **within hours** you may get **life-threatening symptoms** that may include **very low blood pressure or death.** If you stop EPZICOM for any other reason, even for a few days, and you are not allergic to EPZICOM, talk with your healthcare provider before taking it again. Taking EPZICOM again can cause a serious allergic or life-threatening reaction, even if you never had an allergic reaction to it before.

If your healthcare provider tells you that you can take EPZICOM again, start taking it when you are around medical help or people who can call a healthcare provider if you need one.

2. Lactic Acidosis (buildup of acid in the blood). Some human immunodeficiency virus (HIV) medicines, including EPZICOM, can cause a rare but serious condition called lactic acidosis. Lactic acidosis is a serious medical emergency that can cause death and must be treated in the hospital.

Call your healthcare provider right away if you get any of the following signs or symptoms of lactic acidosis:

- you feel very weak or tired
- you have unusual (not normal) muscle pain
- you have trouble breathing
- you have stomach pain with nausea and vomiting
- you feel cold, especially in your arms and legs
- you feel dizzy or light-headed
- you have a fast or irregular heartbeat

3. Serious liver problems. Some people who have taken medicines like EPZICOM have developed serious liver problems called hepatotoxicity, with liver enlargement (hepatomegaly) and fat in the liver (steatosis). Hepatomegaly with steatosis is a serious medical emergency that can cause death.

Call your healthcare provider right away if you get any of the following signs or symptoms of liver problems:

- your skin or the white part of your eyes turns yellow (jaundice)
- your urine turns dark
- your bowel movements (stools) turn light in color
- you don't feel like eating food for several days or longer
- you feel sick to your stomach (nausea)
- you have lower stomach area (abdominal) pain

You may be more likely to get lactic acidosis or serious liver problems if you are female, very overweight, or have been taking nucleoside analogue medicines for a long time.

4. Use with interferon and ribavirin-based regimens. Worsening of liver disease (sometimes resulting in death) has occurred in patients infected with both HIV and hepatitis C virus who are taking anti-HIV medicines and are also being treated for hepatitis C with interferon with or without ribavirin. If you are taking EPZICOM as well as interferon with or without ribavirin and you experience side effects, be sure to tell your healthcare provider.

5. If you have HIV and hepatitis B virus infection, your hepatitis B virus infection may get worse if you stop taking EPZICOM.

- Take EPZICOM exactly as prescribed.
- Do not run out of EPZICOM.
- Do not stop EPZICOM without talking to your healthcare provider.

Your healthcare provider should monitor your health and do regular blood tests to check your liver if you stop taking EPZICOM.

What is EPZICOM?

EPZICOM is a prescription medicine used to treat HIV infection. EPZICOM contains 2 medicines: abacavir (ZIAGEN) and lamivudine or 3TC (EPIVIR®). Both of these medicines are called nucleoside analogue reverse transcriptase inhibitors (NRTIs). When used together, they help lower the amount of HIV in your blood.

- **EPZICOM does not cure HIV infection or AIDS.**
- It is not known if EPZICOM will help you live longer or have fewer of the medical problems that people get with HIV or AIDS.
- It is very important that you see your healthcare provider regularly while you are taking EPZICOM.
- It is not known if EPZICOM is safe or effective in children under the age of 18.

Who should not take EPZICOM?

Do not take EPZICOM if you:

- **are allergic to abacavir or any of the ingredients in EPZICOM. See the end of this Medication Guide for a complete list of ingredients in EPZICOM.**
- **have certain liver problems.**

What should I tell my healthcare provider before taking EPZICOM?

Before you take EPZICOM tell your healthcare provider if you:

- **have been tested and know whether or not you have a particular gene variation called HLA-B*5701.**
- **have hepatitis B virus infection or have other liver problems.**
- **have kidney problems.**
- **have heart problems, smoke, or have diseases that increase your risk of heart disease such as high blood pressure, high cholesterol, or diabetes.**
- **are pregnant or plan to become pregnant.** It is not known if EPZICOM will harm your unborn baby. Talk to your healthcare provider if you are pregnant or plan to become pregnant.

Pregnancy Registry. If you take EPZICOM while you are pregnant, talk to your healthcare provider about how you can take part in the Pregnancy Registry for EPZICOM. The purpose of the pregnancy registry is to collect information about the health of you and your baby.

- **are breastfeeding or plan to breastfeed.Do not breastfeed.** Lamivudine is excreted in human breast milk. We do not know if abacavir can be passed to your baby in your breast milk and whether it could harm your baby. Also, mothers with HIV-1 should not breastfeed because HIV-1 can be passed to the baby in the breast milk.

Tell your healthcare provider about all the medicines you take, including prescription and nonprescription medicines, vitamins, and herbal supplements.

Especially tell your healthcare provider if you take:

- alcohol
- medicines used to treat hepatitis viruses such as interferon or ribavirin.
- methadone
- ATRIPLA® (efavirenz/emtricitabine/tenofovir disoproxil fumarate)
- COMBIVIR® (lamivudine and zidovudine)
- COMPLERA™ (emtricitabine/rilpivirine/tenofovir disoproxil fumarate)
- EMTRIVA® (emtricitabine)
- EPIVIR or EPIVIR-HBV® (lamivudine)
- TRIZIVIR (abacavir sulfate, lamivudine, and zidovudine)
- TRUVADA® (emtricitabine/tenofovir disoproxil fumarate)
- ZIAGEN (abacavir sulfate)

Ask your healthcare provider if you are not sure if you take one of the medicines listed above.

EPZICOM may affect the way other medicines work, and other medicines may affect how EPZICOM works.

Know the medicines you take. Keep a list of your medicines with you to show to your healthcare provider and pharmacist when you get a new medicine.

How should I take EPZICOM?

- **Take EPZICOM exactly as your healthcare provider tells you to take it.**
- EPZICOM may be taken with or without food.
- Do not skip doses.
- **Do not let your EPZICOM run out.**

If you stop your anti-HIV medicines, even for a short time, the amount of virus in your blood may increase and the virus may become harder to treat. If you take too much EPZICOM, call your healthcare provider or poison control center or go to the nearest hospital emergency room right away

What are the possible side effects of EPZICOM?

- **EPZICOM can cause serious side effects including allergic reactions, lactic acidosis, and liver problems. See "What is the most important information I should know about EPZICOM?"**
- **Changes in immune system (Immune Reconstitution Syndrome).** Your immune system may get stronger and begin to fight infections that have been hidden in your body for a long time. Tell your healthcare provider if you start having new or worse symptoms of infection after you start taking EPZICOM.
- **Changes in body fat (fat redistribution).** Changes in body fat (lipoatrophy or lipodystrophy) can happen in some people taking antiretroviral medicines including EPZICOM. These changes may include:
- more fat in or around your trunk, upper back and neck (buffalo hump), breast, or chest
- loss of fat in your legs, arms, or face
- **Heart attack (myocardial infarction).** Some HIV medicines including EPZICOM may increase your risk of heart attack.

The most common side effects of EPZICOM include:

- trouble sleeping
- depression
- headache
- tiredness
- dizziness
- nausea
- diarrhea
- rash
- fever

Tell your healthcare provider if you have any side effect that bothers you or that does not go away.

These are not all the possible side effects of EPZICOM. For more information, ask your healthcare provider or pharmacist.

Call your doctor for medical advice about side effects. You may report side effects to FDA at 1-800-FDA-1088.

How should I store EPZICOM?

Store EPZICOM at 59°F to 86°F (15°C to 30°C).

Keep EPZICOM and all medicines out of the reach of children.

General information for safe and effective use of EPZICOM.

Avoid doing things that can spread HIV infection to others.

- **Do not share needles or other injection equipment.**
- **Do not share personal items that can have blood or body fluids on them, like toothbrushes and razor blades.**
- **Do not have any kind of sex without protection.** Always practice safe sex by using a latex or polyurethane condom to lower the chance of sexual contact with semen, vaginal secretions, or blood.

Medicines are sometimes prescribed for purposes other than those listed in a Medication Guide. Do not use EPZICOM for a condition for which it was not prescribed. Do not give EPZICOM to other people, even if they have the same symptoms that you have. It may harm them.

This Medication Guide summarizes the most important information about EPZICOM. If you would like more information, talk with your healthcare provider. You can ask your healthcare provider or pharmacist for the information about EPZICOM that is written for healthcare professionals.

For more information go to www.EPZICOM.com or call 1-877-844-8872.

What are the ingredients in EPZICOM?

Active ingredients: abacavir sulfate and lamivudine

Inactive ingredients: magnesium stearate, microcrystalline cellulose, sodium starch glycolate, and OPADRY® orange YS-1-13065-A, a film coating made of FD&C Yellow No. 6, hypromellose, polyethylene glycol 400, polysorbate 80, and titanium dioxide.

This Medication Guide has been approved by the US Food and Drug Administration.

COMBIVIR, EPIVIR, EPZICOM, TRIZIVIR, and ZIAGEN are registered trademarks of ViiV Healthcare.

The brands listed are trademarks of their respective owners and are not trademarks of ViiV Healthcare. The makers of these brands are not affiliated with and do not endorse ViiV Healthcare or its products.

Manufactured for:
ViiV Healthcare
Research Triangle Park, NC 27709
by:
GlaxoSmithKline
Research Triangle Park, NC 27709
Lamivudine is manufactured under agreement from
Shire Pharmaceuticals Group plc
Basingstoke, UK

May 2012
EPZ:8MG

LEXIVA ℞

[lex-EE-vah]
(fosamprenavir calcium)
Tablets, for oral use

LEXIVA

(fosamprenavir calcium)
Oral Suspension

HIGHLIGHTS OF PRESCRIBING INFORMATION

These highlights do not include all the information needed to use LEXIVA safely and effectively. See full prescribing information for LEXIVA.

LEXIVA (fosamprenavir calcium) Tablets, for oral use
LEXIVA (fosamprenavir calcium) Oral Suspension
Initial U.S. Approval: 2003

INDICATIONS AND USAGE

LEXIVA is an HIV protease inhibitor indicated in combination with other antiretroviral agents for the treatment of HIV-1 infection. (1)

DOSAGE AND ADMINISTRATION

- Therapy-Naive Adults: LEXIVA 1,400 mg twice daily; LEXIVA 1,400 mg once daily plus ritonavir 200 mg once daily; LEXIVA 1,400 mg once daily plus ritonavir 100 mg once daily; LEXIVA 700 mg twice daily plus ritonavir 100 mg twice daily. (2.1)
- Protease Inhibitor-Experienced Adults: LEXIVA 700 mg twice daily plus ritonavir 100 mg twice daily. (2.1)
- Pediatric Patients (aged at least 4 weeks to 18 years): Dosage should be calculated based on body weight (kg) and should not exceed adult dose. (2.2)
- Hepatic Impairment: Recommended adjustments for patients with mild, moderate, or severe hepatic impairment. (2.3)

Dosing Considerations

- LEXIVA Tablets may be taken with or without food. (2)
- LEXIVA Suspension: Adults should take without food; pediatric patients should take with food. (2)

DOSAGE FORMS AND STRENGTHS

700 mg tablets and 50 mg per mL oral suspension (3)

CONTRAINDICATIONS

- Hypersensitivity to LEXIVA or amprenavir (e.g., Stevens-Johnson syndrome). (4)
- Drugs highly dependent on CYP3A4 for clearance and for which elevated plasma levels may result in serious and/or life-threatening events. (4)
- Review ritonavir contraindications when used in combination. (4)

WARNINGS AND PRECAUTIONS

- Certain drugs should not be coadministered with LEXIVA due to risk of serious or life-threatening adverse reactions. (5.1)
- LEXIVA should be discontinued for severe skin reactions including Stevens-Johnson syndrome. (5.2)
- LEXIVA should be used with caution in patients with a known sulfonamide allergy. (5.3)
- Use of higher than approved doses may lead to transaminase elevations. Patients with hepatitis B or C are at increased risk of transaminase elevations. (5.4)
- Patients receiving LEXIVA may develop new onset or exacerbations of diabetes mellitus, hyperglycemia (5.5), immune reconstitution syndrome (5.6), redistribution/accumulation of body fat (5.7), and elevated triglyceride and cholesterol concentrations (5.8). Monitor cholesterol and triglycerides prior to therapy and periodically thereafter.
- Acute hemolytic anemia has been reported with amprenavir. (5.9)
- Hemophilia: Spontaneous bleeding may occur, and additional factor VIII may be required. (5.10)
- Nephrolithiasis: Cases of nephrolithiasis have been reported with fosamprenavir. (5.11)

ADVERSE REACTIONS

- In adults the most common adverse reactions (incidence greater than or equal to 4%) are diarrhea, rash, nausea, vomiting, headache. (6.1)
- Vomiting and neutropenia were more frequent in pediatrics than in adults. (6.1)

To report SUSPECTED ADVERSE REACTIONS, contact ViiV Healthcare at 1-877-844-8872 or FDA at 1-800-FDA-1088 or www.fda.gov/medwatch.

DRUG INTERACTIONS

- Coadministration of LEXIVA with drugs that induce CYP3A4 may decrease amprenavir (active metabolite) concentrations leading to potential loss of virologic activity. (7, 12.3)
- Coadministration with drugs that inhibit CYP3A4 may increase amprenavir concentrations. (7, 12.3)

• Coadministration of LEXIVA and ritonavir may result in clinically significant interactions with drugs metabolized by CYP2D6. (7)

See 17 for PATIENT COUNSELING INFORMATION and FDA-approved patient labeling

Revised: 04/2013

FULL PRESCRIBING INFORMATION: CONTENTS*

*** Sections or subsections omitted from the full prescribing information are not listed**

FULL PRESCRIBING INFORMATION

1 INDICATIONS AND USAGE

LEXIVA® is indicated in combination with other antiretroviral agents for the treatment of human immunodeficiency virus (HIV-1) infection.

The following points should be considered when initiating therapy with LEXIVA plus ritonavir in protease inhibitor-experienced patients:

- The protease inhibitor-experienced patient trial was not large enough to reach a definitive conclusion that LEXIVA plus ritonavir and lopinavir plus ritonavir are clinically equivalent *[see Clinical Studies (14.2)]*.
- Once-daily administration of LEXIVA plus ritonavir is not recommended for adult protease inhibitor-experienced patients or any pediatric patients *[see Dosage and Administration (2.1, 2.2), Clinical Studies (14.2, 14.3)]*.
- Dosing of LEXIVA plus ritonavir is not recommended for protease inhibitor-experienced pediatric patients younger than 6 months *[see Clinical Pharmacology (12.3)]*.

2 DOSAGE AND ADMINISTRATION

LEXIVA Tablets may be taken with or without food.

Adults should take LEXIVA Oral Suspension without food. Pediatric patients should take LEXIVA Oral Suspension with food *[see Clinical Pharmacology (12.3)]*. If emesis occurs within 30 minutes after dosing, re-dosing of LEXIVA Oral Suspension should occur.

Table 2. Drugs Contraindicated With LEXIVA. (Information in the table applies to LEXIVA with or without ritonavir, unless otherwise indicated.)

Drug Class/Drug Name	Clinical Comment
Alpha 1-adrenoreceptor antagonist: Alfuzosin	Potentially increased alfuzosin concentrations can result in hypotension.
Antiarrhythmics: Flecainide, propafenone	**POTENTIAL** for serious and/or life-threatening reactions such as cardiac arrhythmias secondary to increases in plasma concentrations of antiarrhythmics if LEXIVA is co-prescribed with **ritonavir**.
Antimycobacterials: Rifampin[a]	May lead to loss of virologic response and possible resistance to LEXIVA or to the class of protease inhibitors.
Ergot derivatives: Dihydroergotamine, ergonovine, ergotamine, methylergonovine	**POTENTIAL** for serious and/or life-threatening reactions such as acute ergot toxicity characterized by peripheral vasospasm and ischemia of the extremities and other tissues.
GI motility agents: Cisapride	**POTENTIAL** for serious and/or life-threatening reactions such as cardiac arrhythmias.
Herbal products: St. John's wort (*Hypericum perforatum*)	May lead to loss of virologic response and possible resistance to LEXIVA or to the class of protease inhibitors.
HMG co-reductase inhibitors: Lovastatin, simvastatin	**POTENTIAL** for serious reactions such as risk of myopathy including rhabdomyolysis.
Neuroleptic: Pimozide	**POTENTIAL** for serious and/or life-threatening reactions such as cardiac arrhythmias.
Non-nucleoside reverse transcriptase inhibitor: Delavirdine[a]	May lead to loss of virologic response and possible resistance to delavirdine.
PDE5 inhibitor: Sildenafil (REVATIO®) (for treatment of pulmonary arterial hypertension)	A safe and effective dose has not been established when used with LEXIVA. There is increased potential for sildenafil-associated adverse events (which include visual disturbances, hypotension, prolonged erection, and syncope).
Sedative/hypnotics: Midazolam, triazolam	**POTENTIAL** for serious and/or life-threatening reactions such as prolonged or increased sedation or respiratory depression.

[a] *See Clinical Pharmacology (12.3) Tables 10, 11, 12, or 13 for magnitude of interaction.*

Higher-than-approved dose combinations of LEXIVA plus ritonavir are not recommended due to an increased risk of transaminase elevations *[see Overdosage (10)]*.

When LEXIVA is used in combination with ritonavir, prescribers should consult the full prescribing information for ritonavir.

2.1 Adults

Therapy-Naive Adults:

- LEXIVA 1,400 mg twice daily (without ritonavir).
- LEXIVA 1,400 mg once daily plus ritonavir 200 mg once daily.
- LEXIVA 1,400 mg once daily plus ritonavir 100 mg once daily.
  - Dosing of LEXIVA 1,400 mg once daily plus ritonavir 100 mg once daily is supported by pharmacokinetic data *[see Clinical Pharmacology (12.3)]*.
- LEXIVA 700 mg twice daily plus ritonavir 100 mg twice daily.
  - Dosing of LEXIVA 700 mg twice daily plus 100 mg ritonavir twice daily is supported by pharmacokinetic and safety data *[see Clinical Pharmacology (12.3)]*.

Protease Inhibitor-Experienced Adults:

- LEXIVA 700 mg twice daily plus ritonavir 100 mg twice daily.

2.2 Pediatric Patients (Aged at Least 4 Weeks to 18 Years)

The recommended dosage of LEXIVA in patients aged at least 4 weeks to 18 years should be calculated based on body weight (kg) and should not exceed the recommended adult dose (Table 1).

Table 1. Twice-Daily Dosage Regimens by Weight for Protease Inhibitor-Naive Pediatric Patients (Greater Than or Equal to 4 Weeks of Age) and for Protease Inhibitor-Experienced Pediatric Patients (Greater Than or Equal to 6 Months of Age) Using LEXIVA Oral Suspension With Concurrent Ritonavir

Weight	Twice-Daily Dosage Regimen
<11 kg	LEXIVA 45 mg/kg plus ritonavir 7 mg/kg[a]
11 kg - <15 kg	LEXIVA 30 mg/kg plus ritonavir 3 mg/kg[a]
15 kg - <20 kg	LEXIVA 23 mg/kg plus ritonavir 3 mg/kg[a]
≥20 kg	LEXIVA 18 mg/kg plus ritonavir 3 mg/kg[a]

[a]When dosing with ritonavir, do not exceed the adult dose of LEXIVA 700 mg/ritonavir 100 mg twice-daily dose.

Alternatively, protease inhibitor-naive children aged 2 years and older can be administered LEXIVA (without ritonavir) 30 mg per kg twice daily.

LEXIVA should only be administered to infants born at 38 weeks gestation or greater and who have attained a postnatal age of 28 days.

For pediatric patients, pharmacokinetic and clinical data:

- do not support once-daily dosing of LEXIVA alone or in combination with ritonavir *[see Clinical Studies (14.3)]*.
- do not support administration of LEXIVA alone or in combination with ritonavir for protease inhibitor–experienced children younger than 6 months *[see Clinical Pharmacology (12.3)]*.
- do not support twice-daily dosing of LEXIVA without ritonavir in pediatric patients younger than 2 years *[see Clinical Pharmacology (12.3)]*.

Other Dosing Considerations:

- When administered without ritonavir, the adult regimen of LEXIVA Tablets 1,400 mg twice daily may be used for pediatric patients weighing at least 47 kg.
- When administered in combination with ritonavir, LEXIVA Tablets may be used for pediatric patients weighing at least 39 kg; ritonavir capsules may be used for pediatric patients weighing at least 33 kg.

2.3 Patients With Hepatic Impairment

See Clinical Pharmacology (12.3).

Mild Hepatic Impairment (Child-Pugh Score Ranging From 5 to 6): LEXIVA should be used with caution at a reduced dosage of 700 mg twice daily without ritonavir (therapy-naive) or 700 mg twice daily plus ritonavir 100 mg once daily (therapy-naive or protease inhibitor-experienced).

Moderate Hepatic Impairment (Child-Pugh Score Ranging From 7 to 9): LEXIVA should be used with caution at a reduced dosage of 700 mg twice daily without ritonavir (therapy-naive), or 450 mg twice daily plus ritonavir 100 mg once daily (therapy-naive or protease inhibitor-experienced).

Severe Hepatic Impairment (Child-Pugh Score Ranging From 10 to 15): LEXIVA should be used with caution at a reduced dosage of 350 mg twice daily without ritonavir (therapy-naive) or 300 mg twice daily plus ritonavir 100 mg once daily (therapy-naive or protease inhibitor-experienced).

Table 3. Selected Moderate/Severe Clinical Adverse Reactions Reported in Greater Than or Equal to 2% of Antiretroviral-Naive Adult Subjects

Adverse Reaction	APV30001[a]		APV30002[a]	
	LEXIVA 1,400 mg b.i.d. (n = 166)	Nelfinavir 1,250 mg b.i.d. (n = 83)	LEXIVA 1,400 mg q.d./ Ritonavir 200 mg q.d. (n = 322)	Nelfinavir 1,250 mg b.i.d. (n = 327)
Gastrointestinal				
Diarrhea	5%	18%	10%	18%
Nausea	7%	4%	7%	5%
Vomiting	2%	4%	6%	4%
Abdominal pain	1%	0%	2%	2%
Skin				
Rash	8%	2%	3%	2%
General disorders				
Fatigue	2%	1%	4%	2%
Nervous system				
Headache	2%	4%	3%	3%

[a]All subjects also received abacavir and lamivudine twice daily.

Table 5. Grade 3/4 Laboratory Abnormalities Reported in Greater Than or Equal to 2% of Antiretroviral-Naive Adult Subjects in Trials APV30001 and APV30002

Laboratory Abnormality	APV30001[a]		APV30002[a]	
	LEXIVA 1,400 mg b.i.d. (n = 166)	Nelfinavir 1,250 mg b.i.d. (n = 83)	LEXIVA 1,400 mg q.d./ Ritonavir 200 mg q.d. (n = 322)	Nelfinavir 1,250 mg b.i.d. (n = 327)
ALT (>5 × ULN)	6%	5%	8%	8%
AST (>5 × ULN)	6%	6%	6%	7%
Serum lipase (>2 × ULN)	8%	4%	6%	4%
Triglycerides[b] (>750 mg/dL)	0%	1%	6%	2%
Neutrophil count, absolute (<750 cells/mm^3)	3%	6%	3%	4%

[a]All subjects also received abacavir and lamivudine twice daily.
[b]Fasting specimens.
ULN = Upper limit of normal.

There are no data to support dosing recommendations for pediatric patients with hepatic impairment.

3 DOSAGE FORMS AND STRENGTHS

LEXIVA Tablets, 700 mg, are pink, film-coated, capsule-shaped, biconvex tablets with "GX LL7" debossed on one face.

LEXIVA Oral Suspension, 50 mg per mL, is a white to off-white suspension that has a characteristic grape-bubblegum-peppermint flavor.

4 CONTRAINDICATIONS

LEXIVA is contraindicated:

- in patients with previously demonstrated clinically significant hypersensitivity (e.g., Stevens-Johnson syndrome) to any of the components of this product or to amprenavir.
- when coadministered with drugs that are highly dependent on cytochrome P450 3A4 (CYP3A4) for clearance and for which elevated plasma concentrations are associated with serious and/or life-threatening events (Table 2).

[See table 2 at top of previous page]

- when coadministered with ritonavir in patients receiving the antiarrhythmic agents, flecainide and propafenone. If LEXIVA is coadministered with ritonavir, reference should be made to the full prescribing information for ritonavir for additional contraindications.

5 WARNINGS AND PRECAUTIONS

5.1 Drug Interactions

See Table 2 for listings of drugs that are contraindicated due to potentially life-threatening adverse events, significant drug interactions, or loss of virologic activity *[see Contraindications (4), Drug Interactions (7.2)]*. See Table 7 for a listing of established and other potentially significant drug interactions *[see Drug Interactions (7.3)]*.

5.2 Skin Reactions

Severe and life-threatening skin reactions, including 1 case of Stevens-Johnson syndrome among 700 subjects treated with LEXIVA in clinical trials. Treatment with LEXIVA should be discontinued for severe or life-threatening rashes and for moderate rashes accompanied by systemic symptoms *[see Adverse Reactions (6)]*.

5.3 Sulfa Allergy

LEXIVA should be used with caution in patients with a known sulfonamide allergy. Fosamprenavir contains a sulfonamide moiety. The potential for cross-sensitivity between drugs in the sulfonamide class and fosamprenavir is unknown. In a clinical trial of LEXIVA used as the sole protease inhibitor, rash occurred in 2 of 10 subjects (20%) with a history of sulfonamide allergy compared with 42 of 126 subjects (33%) with no history of sulfonamide allergy. In 2 clinical trials of LEXIVA plus low-dose ritonavir, rash occurred in 8 of 50 subjects (16%) with a history of sulfonamide allergy compared with 50 of 412 subjects (12%) with no history of sulfonamide allergy.

5.4 Hepatic Toxicity

Use of LEXIVA with ritonavir at higher-than-recommended dosages may result in transaminase elevations and should not be used *[see Dosage and Administration (2), Overdosage (10)]*. Patients with underlying hepatitis B or C or marked elevations in transaminases prior to treatment may be at increased risk for developing or worsening of transaminase elevations. Appropriate laboratory testing should be conducted prior to initiating therapy with LEXIVA and patients should be monitored closely during treatment.

5.5 Diabetes/Hyperglycemia

New onset diabetes mellitus, exacerbation of pre-existing diabetes mellitus, and hyperglycemia have been reported during postmarketing surveillance in HIV-1-infected patients receiving protease inhibitor therapy. Some patients required either initiation or dose adjustments of insulin or oral hypoglycemic agents for treatment of these events. In some cases, diabetic ketoacidosis has occurred. In those patients who discontinued protease inhibitor therapy, hyperglycemia persisted in some cases. Because these events have been reported voluntarily during clinical practice, estimates of frequency cannot be made and causal relationships between protease inhibitor therapy and these events have not been established.

5.6 Immune Reconstitution Syndrome

Immune reconstitution syndrome has been reported in patients treated with combination antiretroviral therapy, including LEXIVA. During the initial phase of combination antiretroviral treatment, patients whose immune systems respond may develop an inflammatory response to indolent or residual opportunistic infections (such as *Mycobacterium avium* infection, cytomegalovirus, *Pneumocystis jirovecii* pneumonia [PCP], or tuberculosis), which may necessitate further evaluation and treatment.

Autoimmune disorders (such as Graves' disease, polymyositis, and Guillain-Barré syndrome) have also been reported to occur in the setting of immune reconstitution; however, the time to onset is more variable, and can occur many months after initiation of treatment.

5.7 Fat Redistribution

Redistribution/accumulation of body fat, including central obesity, dorsocervical fat enlargement (buffalo hump), peripheral wasting, facial wasting, breast enlargement, and "cushingoid appearance," have been observed in patients receiving antiretroviral therapy, including LEXIVA. The mechanism and long-term consequences of these events are currently unknown. A causal relationship has not been established.

5.8 Lipid Elevations

Treatment with LEXIVA plus ritonavir has resulted in increases in the concentration of triglycerides and cholesterol *[see Adverse Reactions (6)]*. Triglyceride and cholesterol testing should be performed prior to initiating therapy with LEXIVA and at periodic intervals during therapy. Lipid disorders should be managed as clinically appropriate *[see Drug Interactions (7)]*.

5.9 Hemolytic Anemia

Acute hemolytic anemia has been reported in a patient treated with amprenavir.

5.10 Patients With Hemophilia

There have been reports of spontaneous bleeding in patients with hemophilia A and B treated with protease inhibitors. In some patients, additional factor VIII was required. In many of the reported cases, treatment with protease inhibitors was continued or restarted. A causal relationship between protease inhibitor therapy and these episodes has not been established.

5.11 Nephrolithiasis

Cases of nephrolithiasis were reported during postmarketing surveillance in HIV-1-infected patients receiving LEXIVA.Because these events were reported voluntarily during clinical practice, estimates of frequency cannot be made. If signs or symptoms of nephrolithiasis occur, temporary interruption or discontinuation of therapy may be considered.

5.12 Resistance/Cross-Resistance

Because the potential for HIV cross-resistance among protease inhibitors has not been fully explored, it is unknown what effect therapy with LEXIVA will have on the activity of subsequently administered protease inhibitors. LEXIVA has been studied in patients who have experienced treatment failure with protease inhibitors *[see Clinical Studies (14.2)]*.

6 ADVERSE REACTIONS

- Severe or life-threatening skin reactions have been reported with the use of LEXIVA *[see Warnings and Precautions (5.2)]*.
- The most common moderate to severe adverse reactions in clinical trials of LEXIVA were diarrhea, rash, nausea, vomiting, and headache.
- Treatment discontinuation due to adverse events occurred in 6.4% of subjects receiving LEXIVA and in 5.9% of subjects receiving comparator treatments. The most common adverse reactions leading to discontinuation of LEXIVA (incidence less than or equal to 1% of subjects) included diarrhea, nausea, vomiting, AST increased, ALT increased, and rash.

6.1 Clinical Trials

Because clinical trials are conducted under widely varying conditions, adverse reaction rates observed in the clinical trials of a drug cannot be directly compared to rates in the clinical trials of another drug and may not reflect the rates observed in clinical practice.

Adult Trials: The data for the 3 active-controlled clinical trials described below reflect exposure of 700 HIV-1–infected subjects to LEXIVA Tablets, including 599 subjects exposed to LEXIVA for greater than 24 weeks, and 409 subjects exposed for greater than 48 weeks. The population age ranged from 17 to 72 years. Of these subjects, 26% were female, 51% Caucasian, 31% black, 16% American Hispanic, and 70% were antiretroviral-naive. Sixty-one percent received LEXIVA 1,400 mg once daily plus ritonavir 200 mg once daily; 24% received LEXIVA 1,400 mg twice daily; and 15% received LEXIVA 700 mg twice daily plus ritonavir 100 mg twice daily.

Selected adverse reactions reported during the clinical efficacy trials of LEXIVA are shown in Tables 3 and 4. Each table presents adverse reactions of moderate or severe intensity in subjects treated with combination therapy for up to 48 weeks.

[See table 3 above]

Table 4. Selected Moderate/Severe Clinical Adverse Reactions Reported in Greater Than or Equal to 2% of Protease Inhibitor-Experienced Adult Subjects (Trial APV30003)

Adverse Reaction	LEXIVA 700 mg b.i.d./ Ritonavir 100 mg b.i.d.[a] (n = 106)	Lopinavir 400 mg b.i.d./ Ritonavir 100 mg b.i.d.[a] (n = 103)
Gastrointestinal		
Diarrhea	13%	11%
Nausea	3%	9%
Vomiting	3%	5%
Abdominal pain	<1%	2%
Skin		
Rash	3%	0%
Nervous system		
Headache	4%	2%

[a]All subjects also received 2 reverse transcriptase inhibitors.

Skin rash (without regard to causality) occurred in approximately 19% of subjects treated with LEXIVA in the pivotal efficacy trials. Rashes were usually maculopapular and of mild or moderate intensity, some with pruritus. Rash had a median onset of 11 days after initiation of LEXIVA and had a median duration of 13 days. Skin rash led to discontinuation of LEXIVA in less than 1% of subjects. In some subjects with mild or moderate rash, dosing with LEXIVA was often continued without interruption; if interrupted, reintroduction of LEXIVA generally did not result in rash recurrence.

The percentages of subjects with Grade 3 or 4 laboratory abnormalities in the clinical efficacy trials of LEXIVA are presented in Tables 5 and 6.

[See table 5 at top of previous page]

The incidence of Grade 3 or 4 hyperglycemia in antiretroviral-naive subjects who received LEXIVA in the pivotal trials was less than 1%.

Table 6. Grade 3/4 Laboratory Abnormalities Reported in Greater Than or Equal to 2% of Protease Inhibitor-Experienced Adult Subjects in Trial APV30003

Laboratory Abnormality	LEXIVA 700 mg b.i.d./ Ritonavir 100 mg b.i.d.[a] (n = 104)	Lopinavir 400 mg b.i.d./ Ritonavir 100 mg b.i.d.[a] (n = 103)
Triglycerides[b] (>750 mg/dL)	11%[c]	6%[c]
Serum lipase (>2 × ULN)	5%	12%
ALT (>5 × ULN)	4%	4%
AST (>5 × ULN)	4%	2%
Glucose (>251 mg/dL)	2%[c]	2%[c]

[a]All subjects also received 2 reverse transcriptase inhibitors.
[b]Fasting specimens.
[c]n = 100 for LEXIVA plus ritonavir, n = 98 for lopinavir plus ritonavir.
ULN = Upper limit of normal.

Pediatric Trials: LEXIVA with and without ritonavir was studied in 237 HIV-1–infected pediatric subjects aged at least 4 weeks to 18 years in 3 open–label trials, APV20002, APV20003, and APV29005 *[see Clinical Studies (14.3)]*. Vomiting and neutropenia occurred more frequently in pediatric subjects compared to adults. Other adverse events occurred with similar frequency in pediatric subjects compared with adults.

The frequency of vomiting among pediatric subjects receiving LEXIVA twice daily with ritonavir was 20% in subjects aged at least 4 weeks to less than 2 years and 36% in subjects aged 2 to 18 years compared with 10% in adults. The frequency of vomiting among pediatric subjects receiving LEXIVA twice daily without ritonavir was 60% in subjects aged 2 to 5 years compared with 16% in adults.

The median duration of drug–related vomiting episodes in APV29005 was 1 day (range: 1 to 3 days), in APV20003 was 16 days (range: 1 to 38 days), and in APV20002 was 9 days (range: 4 to 13 days). Vomiting was treatment limiting in 4 pediatric subjects across all 3 trials.

The incidence of Grade 3 or 4 neutropenia (neutrophils less than 750 cells per mm^3) seen in pediatric subjects treated with LEXIVA with and without ritonavir was higher (15%) than the incidence seen in adult subjects (3%). Grade 3/4 neutropenia occurred in 10% (5/51) of subjects aged at least 4 weeks to less than 2 years and 16% (28/170) of subjects aged 2 to 18 years.

6.2 Postmarketing Experience

In addition to adverse reactions reported from clinical trials, the following reactions have been identified during post-approval use of LEXIVA. Because they are reported voluntarily from a population of unknown size, estimates of frequency cannot be made. These reactions have been chosen for inclusion due to a combination of their seriousness, frequency of reporting, or potential causal connection to LEXIVA.

Table 7. Established and Other Potentially Significant Drug Interactions

Concomitant Drug Class: Drug Name	Effect on Concentration of Amprenavir or Concomitant Drug	Clinical Comment
HCV/HIV-Antiviral Agents		
HCV protease inhibitor: Telaprevir[a]	**LEXIVA/ritonavir:** ↓Amprenavir ↓Telaprevir	Coadministration of LEXIVA/ritonavir and telaprevir is not recommended.
HCV protease inhibitor: Boceprevir	**LEXIVA/ritonavir:** ↓Amprenavir (predicted) ↓Boceprevir (predicted)	Coadministration of LEXIVA/ritonavir and boceprevir is not recommended. A pharmacokinetic interaction has been reported between boceprevir and some HIV protease inhibitors in combination with ritonavir, leading to decreased HIV protease inhibitor concentrations and, in some cases, decreased boceprevir concentrations.
Non-nucleoside reverse transcriptase inhibitor: Efavirenz[a]	**LEXIVA:** ↓Amprenavir **LEXIVA/ritonavir:** ↓Amprenavir	Appropriate doses of the combinations with respect to safety and efficacy have not been established. An additional 100 mg/day (300 mg total) of ritonavir is recommended when efavirenz is administered with LEXIVA/ritonavir once daily. No change in the ritonavir dose is required when efavirenz is administered with LEXIVA plus ritonavir twice daily.
Non-nucleoside reverse transcriptase inhibitor: Nevirapine[a]	**LEXIVA:** ↓Amprenavir ↑Nevirapine **LEXIVA/ritonavir:** ↓Amprenavir ↑Nevirapine	Coadministration of nevirapine and LEXIVA without ritonavir is not recommended. No dosage adjustment required when nevirapine is administered with LEXIVA/ritonavir twice daily. The combination of nevirapine administered with LEXIVA/ritonavir once-daily regimen has not been studied.
HIV protease inhibitor: Atazanavir[a]	**LEXIVA:** Interaction has not been evaluated. **LEXIVA/ritonavir:** ↓Atazanavir ↔Amprenavir	Appropriate doses of the combinations with respect to safety and efficacy have not been established.
HIV protease inhibitors: Indinavir[a], nelfinavir[a]	**LEXIVA:** ↑Amprenavir Effect on indinavir and nelfinavir is not well established. **LEXIVA/ritonavir:** Interaction has not been evaluated.	Appropriate doses of the combinations with respect to safety and efficacy have not been established.
HIV protease inhibitors: Lopinavir/ritonavir[a]	↓Amprenavir ↓Lopinavir	An increased rate of adverse events has been observed. Appropriate doses of the combinations with respect to safety and efficacy have not been established.
HIV protease inhibitor: Saquinavir[a]	**LEXIVA:** ↓Amprenavir Effect on saquinavir is not well established. **LEXIVA/ritonavir:** Interaction has not been evaluated.	Appropriate doses of the combination with respect to safety and efficacy have not been established.
HIV integrase inhibitor: Raltegravir[a]	**LEXIVA:** ↓Amprenavir ↓Raltegravir **LEXIVA/ritonavir:** ↓Amprenavir ↓Raltegravir	Appropriate doses of the combination with respect to safety and efficacy have not been established.
HIV CCR5 co-receptor antagonist: Maraviroc[a]	**LEXIVA/ritonavir:** ↓Amprenavir ↑Maraviroc	No dosage adjustment required for LEXIVA/ritonavir. The recommended dose of maraviroc is 150 mg twice daily when coadministered with LEXIVA/ritonavir. LEXIVA should be given with ritonavir when coadministered with maraviroc.
Other Agents		
Antiarrhythmics: Amiodarone, bepridil, lidocaine (systemic), and quinidine	↑Antiarrhythmics	Use with caution. Increased exposure may be associated with life-threatening reactions such as cardiac arrhythmias. Therapeutic concentration monitoring, if available, is recommended for antiarrhythmics.
Anticoagulant: Warfarin		Concentrations of warfarin may be affected. It is recommended that INR (international normalized ratio) be monitored.

(Table continued on next page)

Table 7 *(cont.)*. Established and Other Potentially Significant Drug Interactions

Concomitant Drug Class: Drug Name	Effect on Concentration of Amprenavir or Concomitant Drug	Clinical Comment
Anticonvulsants: Carbamazepine, phenobarbital, phenytoin Phenytoin[a]	**LEXIVA:** ↓Amprenavir **LEXIVA/ritonavir:** ↑Amprenavir ↓Phenytoin	Use with caution. LEXIVA may be less effective due to decreased amprenavir plasma concentrations in patients taking these agents concomitantly. Plasma phenytoin concentrations should be monitored and phenytoin dose should be increased as appropriate. No change in LEXIVA/ritonavir dose is recommended.
Antidepressant: Paroxetine, trazodone	↓Paroxetine ↑Trazodone	Coadministration of paroxetine with LEXIVA/ritonavir significantly decreased plasma levels of paroxetine. Any paroxetine dose adjustment should be guided by clinical effect (tolerability and efficacy). Concomitant use of trazodone and LEXIVA with or without ritonavir may increase plasma concentrations of trazodone. Adverse events of nausea, dizziness, hypotension, and syncope have been observed following coadministration of trazodone and ritonavir. If trazodone is used with a CYP3A4 inhibitor such as LEXIVA, the combination should be used with caution and a lower dose of trazodone should be considered.
Antifungals: Ketoconazole[a], itraconazole	↑Ketoconazole ↑Itraconazole	Increase monitoring for adverse events. **LEXIVA:** Dose reduction of ketoconazole or itraconazole may be needed for patients receiving more than 400 mg ketoconazole or itraconazole per day. **LEXIVA/ritonavir:** High doses of ketoconazole or itraconazole (greater than 200 mg/day) are not recommended.
Anti-gout: Colchicine	↑Colchicine	Patients with renal or hepatic impairment should not be given colchicine with LEXIVA/ritonavir. **LEXIVA/ritonavir and coadministration of colchicine:** **Treatment of gout flares:** 0.6 mg (1 tablet) × 1 dose, followed by 0.3 mg (half tablet) 1 hour later. Dose to be repeated no earlier than 3 days. **Prophylaxis of gout flares:** If the original regimen was 0.6 mg twice a day, the regimen should be adjusted to 0.3 mg once a day. If the original regimen was 0.6 mg once a day, the regimen should be adjusted to 0.3 mg once every other day. **Treatment of familial Mediterranean fever (FMF):** Maximum daily dose of 0.6 mg (may be given as 0.3 mg twice a day). **LEXIVA and coadministration of colchicine:** **Treatment of gout flares:** 1.2 mg (2 tablets) × 1 dose. Dose to be repeated no earlier than 3 days. **Prophylaxis of gout flares:** If the original regimen was 0.6 mg twice a day, the regimen should be adjusted to 0.3 mg twice a day or 0.6 mg once a day. If the original regimen was 0.6 mg once a day, the regimen should be adjusted to 0.3 mg once a day. **Treatment of FMF:** Maximum daily dose of 1.2 mg (may be given as 0.6 mg twice a day).
Antimycobacterial: Rifabutin[a]	↑Rifabutin and rifabutin metabolite	A complete blood count should be performed weekly and as clinically indicated to monitor for neutropenia. **LEXIVA:** A dosage reduction of rifabutin by at least half the recommended dose is required. **LEXIVA/ritonavir:** Dosage reduction of rifabutin by at least 75% of the usual dose of 300 mg/day is recommended (a maximum dose of 150 mg every other day or 3 times per week).
Benzodiazepines: Alprazolam, clorazepate, diazepam, flurazepam	↑Benzodiazepines	Clinical significance is unknown. A decrease in benzodiazepine dose may be needed.
Calcium channel blockers: Diltiazem, felodipine, nifedipine, nicardipine, nimodipine, verapamil, amlodipine, nisoldipine, isradipine	↑Calcium channel blockers	Use with caution. Clinical monitoring of patients is recommended.
Corticosteroid: Dexamethasone	↓Amprenavir	Use with caution. LEXIVA may be less effective due to decreased amprenavir plasma concentrations.

(Table continued on next page)

Cardiac Disorders: Myocardial infarction.
Metabolism and Nutrition Disorders: Hypercholesterolemia.

Nervous System Disorders: Oral paresthesia.
Skin and Subcutaneous Tissue Disorders: Angioedema.
Urogenital: Nephrolithiasis.

7 DRUG INTERACTIONS

See also Contraindications (4), Clinical Pharmacology (12.3).

If LEXIVA is used in combination with ritonavir, see full prescribing information for ritonavir for additional information on drug interactions.

7.1 Cytochrome P450 Inhibitors and Inducers

Amprenavir, the active metabolite of fosamprenavir, is an inhibitor of CYP3A4 metabolism and therefore should not be administered concurrently with medications with narrow therapeutic windows that are substrates of CYP3A4. Data also suggest that amprenavir induces CYP3A4.

Amprenavir is metabolized by CYP3A4. Coadministration of LEXIVA and drugs that induce CYP3A4, such as rifampin, may decrease amprenavir concentrations and reduce its therapeutic effect. Coadministration of LEXIVA and drugs that inhibit CYP3A4 may increase amprenavir concentrations and increase the incidence of adverse effects.

The potential for drug interactions with LEXIVA changes when LEXIVA is coadministered with the potent CYP3A4 inhibitor ritonavir. The magnitude of CYP3A4-mediated drug interactions (effect on amprenavir or effect on coadministered drug) may change when LEXIVA is coadministered with ritonavir. Because ritonavir is a CYP2D6 inhibitor, clinically significant interactions with drugs metabolized by CYP2D6 are possible when coadministered with LEXIVA plus ritonavir.

There are other agents that may result in serious and/or life-threatening drug interactions *[see Contraindications (4)]*.

7.2 Drugs That Should Not Be Coadministered With LEXIVA

See Contraindications (4).

7.3 Established and Other Potentially Significant Drug Interactions

Table 7 provides a listing of established or potentially clinically significant drug interactions. Information in the table applies to LEXIVA with or without ritonavir, unless otherwise indicated.

[See table 7 on pages 2473 through 2476]

8 USE IN SPECIFIC POPULATIONS

8.1 Pregnancy

Pregnancy Category C. Embryo/fetal development studies were conducted in rats (dosed from day 6 to day 17 of gestation) and rabbits (dosed from day 7 to day 20 of gestation). Administration of fosamprenavir to pregnant rats and rabbits produced no major effects on embryo-fetal development; however, the incidence of abortion was increased in rabbits that were administered fosamprenavir. Systemic exposures ($AUC_{0\text{-}24\ hr}$) to amprenavir at these dosages were 0.8 (rabbits) to 2 (rats) times the exposures in humans following administration of the maximum recommended human dose (MRHD) of fosamprenavir alone or 0.3 (rabbits) to 0.7 (rats) times the exposures in humans following administration of the MRHD of fosamprenavir in combination with ritonavir. In contrast, administration of amprenavir was associated with abortions and an increased incidence of minor skeletal variations resulting from deficient ossification of the femur, humerus, and trochlea, in pregnant rabbits at the tested dose approximately one-twentieth the exposure seen at the recommended human dose.

The mating and fertility of the F_1 generation born to female rats given fosamprenavir was not different from control animals; however, fosamprenavir did cause a reduction in both pup survival and body weights. Surviving F_1 female rats showed an increased time to successful mating, an increased length of gestation, a reduced number of uterine implantation sites per litter, and reduced gestational body weights compared with control animals. Systemic exposure ($AUC_{0\text{-}24\ hr}$) to amprenavir in the F_0 pregnant rats was approximately 2 times higher than exposures in humans following administration of the MRHD of fosamprenavir alone or approximately the same as those seen in humans following administration of the MRHD of fosamprenavir in combination with ritonavir.

There are no adequate and well-controlled studies in pregnant women. LEXIVA should be used during pregnancy only if the potential benefit justifies the potential risk to the fetus.

Antiretroviral Pregnancy Registry: To monitor maternal-fetal outcomes of pregnant women exposed to LEXIVA, an Antiretroviral Pregnancy Registry has been established. Physicians are encouraged to register patients by calling 1-800-258-4263.

8.3 Nursing Mothers

The Centers for Disease Control and Prevention recommend that HIV-infected mothers not breastfeed their infants to avoid risking postnatal transmission of HIV. Although it is not known if amprenavir is excreted in human milk, amprenavir is secreted into the milk of lactating rats. Because of both the potential for HIV transmission and the potential for serious adverse reactions in nursing infants, mothers should be instructed not to breastfeed if they are receiving LEXIVA.

8.4 Pediatric Use

The safety, pharmacokinetic profile, virologic, and immunologic responses of LEXIVA with and without ritonavir were evaluated in protease inhibitor-naive and –experienced HIV-1–infected pediatric subjects aged at least 4 weeks to less than 18 years and weighing at least 3 kg in 3 open-label trials *[see Adverse Reactions (6.1), Clinical Pharmacology (12.3), Clinical Studies (14.3)]*. Vomiting and neutropenia, were more frequent in pediatrics than in adults *[see Adverse Reactions (6.1)]*. Other adverse events occurred with similar frequency in pediatric subjects compared with adults.

Treatment with LEXIVA is not recommended in protease inhibitor-experienced pediatric patients younger than 6 months. The pharmacokinetics, safety, tolerability, and efficacy of LEXIVA in pediatric patients younger than 4 weeks have not been established *[see Clinical Pharmacology (12.3)]*. Available pharmacokinetic and clinical data do not support once-daily dosing of LEXIVA alone or in combination with ritonavir for any pediatrics or twice-daily dosing without ritonavir in pediatric patients younger than 2 years*[see Clinical Pharmacology (12.3), Clinical Studies (14.3)]*. See *Dosage and Administration (2.2)* for dosing recommendations for pediatric patients.

8.5 Geriatric Use

Clinical studies of LEXIVA did not include sufficient numbers of patients aged 65 and over to determine whether they respond differently from younger adults. In general, dose selection for an elderly patient should be cautious, reflecting the greater frequency of decreased hepatic, renal, or cardiac function and of concomitant disease or other drug therapy.

8.6 Hepatic Impairment

Amprenavir is principally metabolized by the liver; therefore, caution should be exercised when administering LEXIVA to patients with hepatic impairment because amprenavir concentrations may be increased *[see Clinical Pharmacology (12.3)]*. Patients with impaired hepatic function receiving LEXIVA with or without concurrent ritonavir require dose reduction *[see Dosage and Administration (2.3)]*.

There are no data to support dosing recommendations for pediatric subjects with hepatic impairment.

10 OVERDOSAGE

In a healthy volunteer repeat-dose pharmacokinetic trial evaluating high-dose combinations of LEXIVA plus ritonavir, an increased frequency of Grade 2/3 ALT elevations (greater than 2.5 × ULN) was observed with LEXIVA 1,400 mg twice daily plus ritonavir 200 mg twice daily (4 of 25 subjects). Concurrent Grade 1/2 elevations in AST (greater than 1.25 × ULN) were noted in 3 of these 4 subjects. These transaminase elevations resolved following discontinuation of dosing.

There is no known antidote for LEXIVA. It is not known whether amprenavir can be removed by peritoneal dialysis or hemodialysis. If overdosage occurs, the patient should be monitored for evidence of toxicity and standard supportive treatment applied as necessary.

11 DESCRIPTION

LEXIVA (fosamprenavir calcium) is a prodrug of amprenavir, an inhibitor of HIV protease. The chemical name of fosamprenavir calcium is (3*S*)-tetrahydrofuran-3-yl (1*S*,2*R*)-3-[[(4-aminophenyl) sulfonyl](isobutyl)amino]-1-benzyl-2-(phosphonooxy) propylcarbamate monocalcium salt. Fosamprenavir calcium is a single stereoisomer with the (3*S*)(1*S*,2*R*) configuration. It has a molecular formula of $C_{25}H_{34}CaN_3O_9PS$ and a molecular weight of 623.7. It has the following structural formula:

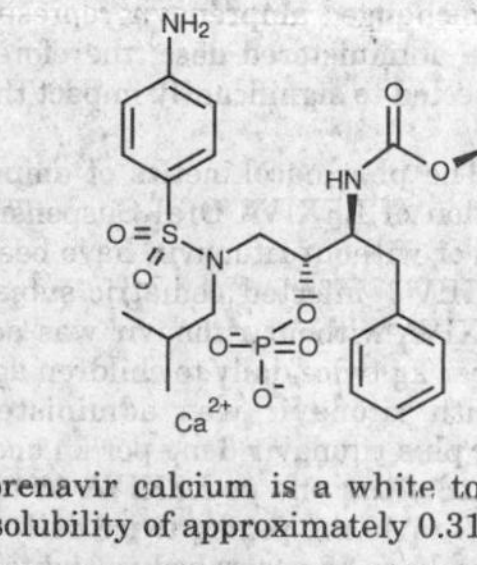

Fosamprenavir calcium is a white to cream-colored solid with a solubility of approximately 0.31 mg per mL in water at 25°C.

LEXIVA Tablets are available for oral administration in a strength of 700 mg of fosamprenavir as fosamprenavir calcium (equivalent to approximately 600 mg of amprenavir). Each 700 mg tablet contains the inactive ingredients colloidal silicon dioxide, croscarmellose sodium, magnesium stearate, microcrystalline cellulose, and povidone K30. The tablet film-coating contains the inactive ingredients hypromellose, iron oxide red, titanium dioxide, and triacetin.

LEXIVA Oral Suspension is available in a strength of 50 mg per mL of fosamprenavir as fosamprenavir calcium equivalent to approximately 43 mg of amprenavir. LEXIVA Oral Suspension is a white to off-white suspension with a grape-bubblegum-peppermint flavor. Each one milliliter (1 mL) contains the inactive ingredients artificial grape-bubblegum flavor, calcium chloride dihydrate, hypromellose, methylparaben, natural peppermint flavor, polysorbate 80, propylene glycol, propylparaben, purified water, and sucralose.

Table 7 *(cont.)*. Established and Other Potentially Significant Drug Interactions

Concomitant Drug Class: Drug Name	Effect on Concentration of Amprenavir or Concomitant Drug	Clinical Comment
Endothelin-receptor antagonists: Bosentan	↑Bosentan	Coadministration of bosentan in patients on LEXIVA: In patients who have been receiving LEXIVA for at least 10 days, start bosentan at 62.5 mg once daily or every other day based upon individual tolerability. Coadministration of LEXIVA in patients on bosentan: Discontinue use of bosentan at least 36 hours prior to initiation of LEXIVA. After at least 10 days following the initiation of LEXIVA, resume bosentan at 62.5 mg once daily or every other day based upon individual tolerability.
Histamine H_2-receptor antagonists: Cimetidine, famotidine, nizatidine, ranitidine[a]	**LEXIVA:** ↓Amprenavir **LEXIVA/ritonavir:** Interaction not evaluated	Use with caution. LEXIVA may be less effective due to decreased amprenavir plasma concentrations.
HMG-CoA reductase inhibitors: Atorvastatin[a]	↑Atorvastatin	Titrate atorvastatin dose carefully and use the lowest necessary dose; do not exceed atorvastatin 20 mg/day.
Immunosuppressants: Cyclosporine, tacrolimus, rapamycin	↑Immunosuppressants	Therapeutic concentration monitoring is recommended for immunosuppressant agents.
Inhaled beta-agonist: Salmeterol	↑Salmeterol	Concurrent administration of salmeterol with LEXIVA is not recommended. The combination may result in increased risk of cardiovascular adverse events associated with salmeterol, including QT prolongation, palpitations, and sinus tachycardia.
Inhaled/nasal steroid: Fluticasone	**LEXIVA:** ↑Fluticasone **LEXIVA/ritonavir:** ↑Fluticasone	Use with caution. Consider alternatives to fluticasone, particularly for long-term use. May result in significantly reduced serum cortisol concentrations. Systemic corticosteroid effects including Cushing's syndrome and adrenal suppression have been reported during postmarketing use in patients receiving ritonavir and inhaled or intranasally administered fluticasone. Coadministration of fluticasone and LEXIVA/ritonavir is not recommended unless the potential benefit to the patient outweighs the risk of systemic corticosteroid side effects.
Narcotic analgesic: Methadone	↓Methadone	Data suggest that the interaction is not clinically relevant; however, patients should be monitored for opiate withdrawal symptoms.
Oral contraceptives: Ethinyl estradiol/ norethindrone[a]	**LEXIVA:** ↓Amprenavir ↓Ethinyl estradiol **LEXIVA/ritonavir:** ↓Ethinyl estradiol	Alternative methods of non-hormonal contraception are recommended. May lead to loss of virologic response. [a] Increased risk of transaminase elevations. No data are available on the use of LEXIVA/ritonavir with other hormonal therapies, such as hormone replacement therapy (HRT) for postmenopausal women.

(Table continued on next page)

12 CLINICAL PHARMACOLOGY

12.1 Mechanism of Action

Fosamprenavir is an antiviral agent *[see Microbiology (12.4)]*.

12.3 Pharmacokinetics

The pharmacokinetic properties of amprenavir after administration of LEXIVA, with or without ritonavir, have been evaluated in both healthy adult volunteers and in HIV-1-infected subjects; no substantial differences in steady-state amprenavir concentrations were observed between the 2 populations.

The pharmacokinetic parameters of amprenavir after administration of LEXIVA (with and without concomitant ritonavir) are shown in Table 8.

[See table 8 at top of next page]

The mean plasma amprenavir concentrations of the dosing regimens over the dosing intervals are displayed in Figure 1.

[See figure 1 at top of next column]

Figure 1. Mean (SD) Steady-State Plasma Amprenavir Concentrations and Mean EC50 Values Against HIV from Protease Inhibitor-Naive Subjects (in the Absence of Human Serum)

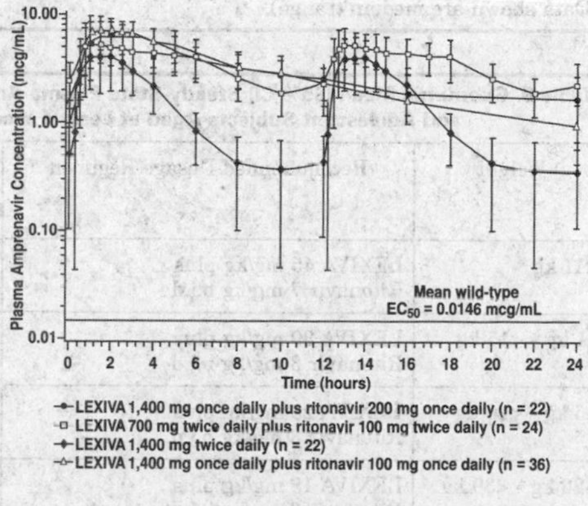

Absorption and Bioavailability: After administration of a single dose of LEXIVA to HIV-1–infected subjects, the time to peak amprenavir concentration (T_{max}) occurred between 1.5 and 4 hours (median 2.5 hours). The absolute oral bioavailability of amprenavir after administration of LEXIVA in humans has not been established.

After administration of a single 1,400-mg dose in the fasted state, LEXIVA Oral Suspension (50 mg per mL) and LEXIVA Tablets (700 mg) provided similar amprenavir exposures (AUC); however, the C_{max} of amprenavir after administration of the suspension formulation was 14.5% higher compared with the tablet.

Effects of Food on Oral Absorption: Administration of a single 1,400-mg dose of LEXIVA Tablets in the fed state (standardized high-fat meal: 967 kcal, 67 grams fat,

Table 7 *(cont.)*. Established and Other Potentially Significant Drug Interactions

Concomitant Drug Class: Drug Name	Effect on Concentration of Amprenavir or Concomitant Drug	Clinical Comment
PDE5 inhibitors: Sildenafil, tadalafil, vardenafil	↑Sildenafil ↑Tadalafil ↑Vardenafil	May result in an increase in PDE5 inhibitor-associated adverse events, including hypotension, syncope, visual disturbances, and priapism. Use of PDE5 inhibitors for pulmonary arterial hypertension (PAH): • Use of sildenafil (REVATIO) is contraindicated when used for the treatment of PAH *[see Contraindications (4)]*. • The following dose adjustments are recommended for use of tadalafil (ADCIRCA®) with LEXIVA: Coadministration of ADCIRCA in patients on LEXIVA: In patients receiving LEXIVA for at least one week, start ADCIRCA at 20 mg once daily. Increase to 40 mg once daily based upon individual tolerability. Coadministration of LEXIVA in patients on ADCIRCA: Avoid use of ADCIRCA during the initiation of LEXIVA. Stop ADCIRCA at least 24 hours prior to starting LEXIVA. After at least one week following the initiation of LEXIVA, resume ADCIRCA at 20 mg once daily. Increase to 40 mg once daily based upon individual tolerability. Use of PDE5 inhibitors for erectile dysfunction: **LEXIVA:** Sildenafil: 25 mg every 48 hours. Tadalafil: no more than 10 mg every 72 hours. Vardenafil: no more than 2.5 mg every 24 hours. **LEXIVA/ritonavir:** Sildenafil: 25 mg every 48 hours. Tadalafil: no more than 10 mg every 72 hours. Vardenafil: no more than 2.5 mg every 72 hours. Use with increased monitoring for adverse events.
Proton pump inhibitors: Esomeprazole[a], lansoprazole, omeprazole, pantoprazole, rabeprazole	**LEXIVA:** ↔Amprenavir ↑Esomeprazole **LEXIVA/ritonavir:** ↔Amprenavir ↔Esomeprazole	Proton pump inhibitors can be administered at the same time as a dose of LEXIVA with no change in plasma amprenavir concentrations.
Tricyclic antidepressants: Amitriptyline, imipramine	↑Tricyclics	Therapeutic concentration monitoring is recommended for tricyclic antidepressants.

[a] *See Clinical Pharmacology (12.3) Tables 10, 11, 12, or 13 for magnitude of interaction.*

Table 8. Geometric Mean (95% CI) Steady-State Plasma Amprenavir Pharmacokinetic Parameters in Adults

Regimen	C_{max} (mcg/mL)	T_{max} (hours)[a]	AUC_{24} (mcg•hr/mL)	C_{min} (mcg/mL)
LEXIVA 1,400 mg b.i.d.	4.82 (4.06-5.72)	1.3 (0.8-4.0)	33.0 (27.6-39.2)	0.35 (0.27-0.46)
LEXIVA 1,400 mg q.d. plus Ritonavir 200 mg q.d.	7.24 (6.32-8.28)	2.1 (0.8-5.0)	69.4 (59.7-80.8)	1.45 (1.16-1.81)
LEXIVA 1,400 mg q.d. plus Ritonavir 100 mg q.d.	7.93 (7.25-8.68)	1.5 (0.75-5.0)	66.4 (61.1-72.1)	0.86 (0.74-1.01)
LEXIVA 700 mg b.i.d. plus Ritonavir 100 mg b.i.d.	6.08 (5.38-6.86)	1.5 (0.75-5.0)	79.2 (69.0-90.6)	2.12 (1.77-2.54)

[a]Data shown are median (range).

Table 9. Geometric Mean (95% CI) Steady-State Plasma Amprenavir Pharmacokinetic Parameters by Weight in Pediatric and Adolescent Subjects Aged at Least 4 Weeks to 18 Years Receiving LEXIVA With Ritonavir

Weight	Recommended Dosage Regimen	C_{max}		AUC_{24}		C_{min}	
		n	(mcg/mL)	n	(mcg•hr/mL)	n	(mcg/mL)
<11 kg	LEXIVA 45 mg/kg plus Ritonavir 7 mg/kg b.i.d	12	6.00 (3.88, 9.29)	12	57.3 (34.1, 96.2)	27	1.65 (1.22, 2.24)
11 kg - <15 kg	LEXIVA 30 mg/kg plus Ritonavir 3 mg/kg b.i.d	Not studied[a]					
15 kg - <20 kg	LEXIVA 23 mg/kg plus Ritonavir 3 mg/kg b.i.d.	5	9.54 (4.63, 19.7)	5	121 (54.2, 269)	9	3.56 (2.33, 5.43)
>20 kg - <39 kg	LEXIVA 18 mg/kg plus Ritonavir 3 mg/kg b.i.d.	13	6.24 (5.01, 7.77)	12	97.9 (77.0, 124)	23	2.54 (2.11, 3.06)
≥39 kg	LEXIVA 700 mg plus Ritonavir 100 mg b.i.d.	15	5.03 (4.04, 6.26)	15	72.3 (59.6, 87.6)	42	1.98 (1.72, 2.29)

[a]Recommended dose for pediatric subjects weighing 11 kg to less than 15 kg is based on population pharmacokinetic analysis.

33 grams protein, 58 grams carbohydrate) compared with the fasted state was associated with no significant changes in amprenavir C_{max}, T_{max}, or $AUC_{0-\infty}$ *[see Dosage and Administration (2)]*.

Administration of a single 1,400-mg dose of LEXIVA Oral Suspension in the fed state (standardized high-fat meal: 967 kcal, 67 grams fat, 33 grams protein, 58 grams carbohydrate) compared with the fasted state was associated with a 46% reduction in C_{max}, a 0.72-hour delay in T_{max}, and a 28% reduction in amprenavir $AUC_{0-\infty}$.

Distribution: In vitro, amprenavir is approximately 90% bound to plasma proteins, primarily to alpha$_1$-acid glycoprotein. In vitro, concentration-dependent binding was observed over the concentration range of 1 to 10 mcg per mL, with decreased binding at higher concentrations. The partitioning of amprenavir into erythrocytes is low, but increases as amprenavir concentrations increase, reflecting the higher amount of unbound drug at higher concentrations.

Metabolism: After oral administration, fosamprenavir is rapidly and almost completely hydrolyzed to amprenavir and inorganic phosphate prior to reaching the systemic circulation. This occurs in the gut epithelium during absorption. Amprenavir is metabolized in the liver by the CYP3A4 enzyme system. The 2 major metabolites result from oxidation of the tetrahydrofuran and aniline moieties. Glucuronide conjugates of oxidized metabolites have been identified as minor metabolites in urine and feces.

Amprenavir is both a substrate for and inducer of P-glycoprotein.

Elimination: Excretion of unchanged amprenavir in urine and feces is minimal. Unchanged amprenavir in urine accounts for approximately 1% of the dose; unchanged amprenavir was not detectable in feces. Approximately 14% and 75% of an administered single dose of ^{14}C-amprenavir can be accounted for as metabolites in urine and feces, respectively. Two metabolites accounted for greater than 90% of the radiocarbon in fecal samples. The plasma elimination half-life of amprenavir is approximately 7.7 hours.

Special Populations: Hepatic Impairment: The pharmacokinetics of amprenavir have been studied after the administration of LEXIVA in combination with ritonavir to adult HIV-1–infected subjects with mild, moderate, and severe hepatic impairment. Following 2 weeks of dosing with LEXIVA plus ritonavir, the AUC of amprenavir was increased by approximately 22% in subjects with mild hepatic impairment, by approximately 70% in subjects with moderate hepatic impairment, and by approximately 80% in subjects with severe hepatic impairment compared with HIV-1–infected subjects with normal hepatic function. Protein binding of amprenavir was decreased in subjects with hepatic impairment. The unbound fraction at 2 hours (approximate C_{max}) ranged between a decrease of -7% to an increase of 57% while the unbound fraction at the end of the dosing interval (C_{min}) increased from 50% to 102% *[see Dosage and Administration (2.3)]*.

The pharmacokinetics of amprenavir have been studied after administration of amprenavir given as AGENERASE® Capsules to adult subjects with hepatic impairment. Following administration of a single 600-mg oral dose, the AUC of amprenavir was increased by approximately 2.5-fold in subjects with moderate cirrhosis and by approximately 4.5-fold in subjects with severe cirrhosis compared with healthy volunteers *[see Dosage and Administration (2.3)]*.

Renal Impairment: The impact of renal impairment on amprenavir elimination in adults has not been studied. The renal elimination of unchanged amprenavir represents approximately 1% of the administered dose; therefore, renal impairment is not expected to significantly impact the elimination of amprenavir.

Pediatric Patients: The pharmacokinetics of amprenavir following administration of LEXIVA Oral Suspension and LEXIVA Tablets, with or without ritonavir, have been studied in a total of 212 HIV-1–infected pediatric subjects enrolled in 3 trials. LEXIVA without ritonavir was administered as 30 or 40 mg per kg twice daily to children aged 2 to 5 years. LEXIVA with ritonavir was administered as LEXIVA 30 mg per kg plus ritonavir 6 mg per kg once daily to children aged 2 to 18 years and as LEXIVA 18 to 60 mg per kg plus ritonavir 3 to 10 mg per kg twice daily to children aged at least 4 weeks to 18 years; body weights ranged from 3 to 103 kg.

Amprenavir apparent clearance decreased with increasing weight. Weight-adjusted apparent clearance was higher in children younger than 4 years, suggesting that younger children require higher mg per kg dosing of LEXIVA.

The pharmacokinetics of LEXIVA Oral Suspension in protease inhibitor-naive infants younger than 6 months (n = 9) receiving LEXIVA 45 mg per kg plus ritonavir 10 mg per kg twice daily generally demonstrated lower AUC_{12} and C_{min} than adults receiving twice-daily LEXIVA 700 mg plus ritonavir 100 mg, the dose recommended for protease-experienced adults. The mean steady-state amprenavir AUC_{12}, C_{max}, and C_{min} were 26.6 mcg•hour per mL, 6.25 mcg per mL, and 0.86 mcg per mL, respectively. These data do not support twice-daily dosing of LEXIVA alone or in combination with ritonavir in protease inhibitor-experienced patients younger than 6 months. Because of expected low amprenavir exposure and a requirement for large volume of drug, twice-daily dosing of LEXIVA alone (without ritonavir) in pediatric subjects younger than 2 years was not studied.

Pharmacokinetic parameters for LEXIVA administered with food and with ritonavir in this patient population at the recommended weight-band–based dosage regimens are provided in Table 9.

[See table 9 at top of previous page]

Subjects aged 2 to less than 6 years receiving LEXIVA 30 mg per kg twice daily without ritonavir achieved geometric mean (95% CI) amprenavir C_{max} (n = 9), AUC_{12} (n = 9), and C_{min} (n = 19) of 7.15 (5.05, 10.1), 22.3 (15.3, 32.6), and 0.513 (0.384, 0.686), respectively.

Geriatric Patients: The pharmacokinetics of amprenavir after administration of LEXIVA to patients older than 65 years have not been studied *[see Use in Specific Populations (8.5)]*.

Gender: The pharmacokinetics of amprenavir after administration of LEXIVA do not differ between males and females.

Race: The pharmacokinetics of amprenavir after administration of LEXIVA do not differ between blacks and non-blacks.

Drug Interactions: *[See Contraindications (4), Warnings and Precautions (5.1), Drug Interactions (7).]*

Amprenavir, the active metabolite of fosamprenavir, is metabolized in the liver by the cytochrome P450 enzyme system. Amprenavir inhibits CYP3A4. Data also suggest that amprenavir induces CYP3A4. Caution should be used when coadministering medications that are substrates, inhibitors, or inducers of CYP3A4, or potentially toxic medications that are metabolized by CYP3A4. Amprenavir does not inhibit CYP2D6, CYP1A2, CYP2C9, CYP2C19, CYP2E1, or uridine glucuronosyltransferase (UDPGT).

Drug interaction trials were performed with LEXIVA and other drugs likely to be coadministered or drugs commonly used as probes for pharmacokinetic interactions. The effects of coadministration on AUC, C_{max}, and C_{min} values are summarized in Table 10 (effect of other drugs on amprenavir) and Table 12 (effect of LEXIVA on other drugs). In addition, since LEXIVA delivers comparable amprenavir plasma concentrations as AGENERASE, drug interaction data derived from trials with AGENERASE are provided in Tables 11 and 13. For information regarding clinical recommendations, *[see Drug Interactions (7)]*.

[See table 10 above and on next page]
[See table 11 at top of page 2479]
[See table 12 on pages 2480 and 2481]
[See table 13 on pages 2481 and 2482]

12.4 Microbiology

Mechanism of Action: Fosamprenavir is a prodrug that is rapidly hydrolyzed to amprenavir by cellular phosphatases in the gut epithelium as it is absorbed. Amprenavir is an inhibitor of HIV-1 protease. Amprenavir binds to the active site of HIV-1 protease and thereby prevents the processing of viral Gag and Gag-Pol polyprotein precursors, resulting in the formation of immature non-infectious viral particles.

Antiviral Activity: Fosamprenavir has little or no antiviral activity in cell culture. The antiviral activity of amprenavir was evaluated against HIV-1 IIIB in both acutely and chronically infected lymphoblastic cell lines (MT-4, CEM-CCRF, H9) and in peripheral blood lymphocytes in cell culture. The 50% effective concentration (EC_{50}) of amprenavir ranged from 0.012 to 0.08 microM in acutely infected cells and was 0.41 microM in chronically infected cells (1 microM = 0.50 mcg per mL). The median EC_{50} value of amprenavir against HIV-1 isolates from clades A to G was 0.00095 microM in peripheral blood mononuclear cells (PBMCs). Similarly, the EC_{50} values for amprenavir against monocytes/macrophage tropic HIV-1 isolates (clade B) ranged from 0.003 to 0.075 microM in monocyte/macrophage cultures. The EC_{50} values of amprenavir against HIV-2 isolates grown in PBMCs were higher than those for HIV-1 isolates, and ranged from 0.003 to 0.11 microM. Amprenavir exhibited synergistic anti–HIV–1 activity in combination with the nucleoside reverse transcriptase inhibitors (NRTIs) abacavir, didanosine, lamivudine, stavudine, tenofovir, and zidovudine; the non-nucleoside reverse transcriptase inhibitors (NNRTIs) delavirdine and efavirenz; and the protease inhibitors atazanavir and saquinavir. Amprenavir exhibited additive anti–HIV–1 activity in combination with the NNRTI nevirapine, the protease inhibitors indinavir, lopinavir, nelfinavir, and ritonavir; and the fusion inhibitor enfuvirtide. These drug combinations have not been adequately studied in humans.

Resistance: HIV-1 isolates with decreased susceptibility to amprenavir have been selected in cell culture and obtained

Table 10. Drug Interactions: Pharmacokinetic Parameters for Amprenavir After Administration of LEXIVA in the Presence of the Coadministered Drug(s)

Coadministered Drug(s) and Dose(s)	Dose of **LEXIVA**[a]	n	% Change in **Amprenavir** Pharmacokinetic Parameters (90% CI)		
			C_{max}	AUC	C_{min}
Antacid (MAALOX TC®) 30 mL single dose	1,400 mg single dose	30	↓35 (↓24 to ↓42)	↓18 (↓9 to ↓26)	↑14 (↓7 to ↑39)
Atazanavir 300 mg q.d. for 10 days	700 mg b.i.d. plus ritonavir 100 mg b.i.d. for 10 days	22	↔	↔	↔
Atorvastatin 10 mg q.d. for 4 days	1,400 mg b.i.d. for 2 weeks	16	↓18 (↓34 to ↑1)	↓27 (↓41 to ↓12)	↓12 (↓27 to ↓6)
Atorvastatin 10 mg q.d. for 4 days	700 mg b.i.d. plus ritonavir 100 mg b.i.d. for 2 weeks	16	↔	↔	↔
Efavirenz 600 mg q.d. for 2 weeks	1,400 mg q.d. plus ritonavir 200 mg q.d. for 2 weeks	16	↔	↓13 (↓30 to 7)	↓36 (↓8 to ↓56)
Efavirenz 600 mg q.d. plus additional ritonavir 100 mg q.d. for 2 weeks	1,400 mg q.d. plus ritonavir 200 mg q.d. for 2 weeks	16	↑18 (↑1 to ↑38)	↑11 (0 to ↑24)	↔
Efavirenz 600 mg q.d. for 2 weeks	700 mg b.i.d. plus ritonavir 100 mg b.i.d. for 2 weeks	16	↔	↔	↓17 (↓4 to ↓29)
Esomeprazole 20 mg q.d. for 2 weeks	1,400 mg b.i.d. for 2 weeks	25	↔	↔	↔
Esomeprazole 20 mg q.d. for 2 weeks	700 mg b.i.d. plus ritonavir 100 mg b.i.d. for 2 weeks	23	↔	↔	↔
Ethinyl estradiol/ norethindrone 0.035 mg/0.5 mg q.d. for 21 days	700 mg b.i.d. plus ritonavir[b] 100 mg b.i.d. for 21 days	25	↔[c]	↔[c]	↔[c]
Ketoconazole[d] 200 mg q.d. for 4 days	700 mg b.i.d. plus ritonavir 100 mg b.i.d. for 4 days	15	↔	↔	↔
Lopinavir/ritonavir 533 mg/133 mg b.i.d.	1,400 mg b.i.d. for 2 weeks	18	↓13[e]	↓26[e]	↓42[e]
Lopinavir/ritonavir 400 mg/100 mg b.i.d. for 2 weeks	700 mg b.i.d. plus ritonavir 100 mg b.i.d. for 2 weeks	18	↓58 (↓42 to ↓70)	↓63 (↓51 to ↓72)	↓65 (↓54 to ↓73)
Maraviroc 300 mg b.i.d. for 10 days	700 mg b.i.d. plus ritonavir 100 mg b.i.d. for 20 days	14	↓34 (↓25 to ↓41)	↓35 (↓29 to ↓41)	↓36 (↓27 to ↓43)
Maraviroc 300 mg q.d. for 10 days	1,400 mg q.d. plus ritonavir 100 mg q.d. for 20 days	14	↓29 (↓20 to ↓38)	↓30 (↓23 to ↓36)	↓15 (↓3 to ↓25)
Methadone 70 to 120 mg q.d. for 2 weeks	700 mg b.i.d. plus ritonavir 100 mg b.i.d. for 2 weeks	19	↔[c]	↔[c]	↔[c]
Nevirapine 200 mg b.i.d. for 2 weeks[f]	1,400 mg b.i.d. for 2 weeks	17	↓25 (↓37 to ↓10)	↓33 (↓45 to ↓20)	↓35 (↓50 to ↓15)
Nevirapine 200 mg b.i.d. for 2 weeks[f]	700 mg b.i.d. plus ritonavir 100 mg b.i.d. for 2 weeks	17	↔	↓11 (↓23 to ↑3)	↓19 (↓32 to ↓4)

(Table continued on next page)

from subjects treated with fosamprenavir. Genotypic analysis of isolates from treatment-naive subjects failing amprenavir-containing regimens showed substitutions in the HIV-1 protease gene resulting in amino acid substitutions primarily at positions V32I, M46I/L, I47V, I50V, I54L/M, and I84V, as well as substitutions in the p7/p1 and p1/p6 Gag and Gag-Pol polyprotein precursor cleavage sites. Some of these amprenavir resistance-associated substitu-

Table 10 *(cont.)*. Drug Interactions: Pharmacokinetic Parameters for Amprenavir After Administration of LEXIVA in the Presence of the Coadministered Drug(s)

Coadministered Drug(s) and Dose(s)	Dose of LEXIVA[a]	n	% Change in **Amprenavir** Pharmacokinetic Parameters (90% CI)		
			C_{max}	AUC	C_{min}
Phenytoin 300 mg q.d. for 10 days	700 mg b.i.d. plus ritonavir 100 mg b.i.d. for 10 days	13	↔	↑20 (↑8 to ↑34)	↑19 (↑6 to ↑33)
Raltegravir 400 mg b.i.d. for 14 days	1,400 mg b.i.d. for 14 days (fasted)	14	↓27 (↓46 to ↔)	↓36 (↓53 to ↓13)	↓43[g] (↓59 to ↓21)
	1,400 mg b.i.d. for 14 days[h]	14	↓15 (↓27 to ↓1)	↓17 (↓27 to ↓6)	↓32[g] (↓53 to ↓1)
	700 mg b.i.d. plus ritonavir 100 mg b.i.d. for 14 days (fasted)	14	↓14 (↓39 to ↑20)	↓17 (↓38 to ↑12)	↓20[g] (↓45 to ↑17)
	700 mg b.i.d. plus ritonavir 100 mg b.i.d. for 14 days[h]	12	↓25 (↓42 to ↓2)	↓25 (↓44 to ↔)	↓33[g] (↓52 to ↓7)
Raltegravir 400 mg b.i.d. for 14 days	1,400 mg q.d. plus ritonavir 100 mg q.d. for 14 days (fasted)	13	↓18 (↓34 to ↔)	↓24 (↓41 to ↔)	↓50[g] (↓64 to ↓31)
	1,400 mg q.d. plus ritonavir 100 mg q.d. for 14 days[h]	14	↑27 (↓1 to ↑62)	↑13 (↓7 to ↑38)	17[g] (↓45 to ↑26)
Ranitidine 300 mg single dose (administered 1 hour before fosamprenavir)	1,400 mg single dose	30	51 (↓43 to ↓58)	30 (↓22 to ↓37)	↔ (↓19 to ↑21)
Rifabutin 150 mg q.o.d. for 2 weeks	700 mg b.i.d. plus ritonavir 100 mg b.i.d. for 2 weeks	15	↑36[e] (↑18 to ↑55)	↑35[e] (↑17 to ↑56)	↑17[e] (↓1 to ↑39)
Telaprevir 750 mg q. 8 hr for 10 days	700 mg b.i.d. plus ritonavir 100 mg b.i.d. for 20 days	18	↓35 (↓30 to ↓41)	↓47 (↓42 to ↓51)	↓56 (↓50 to ↓60)
Telaprevir 1,125 mg q. 12 hr for 4 days	700 mg b.i.d. plus ritonavir 100 mg b.i.d. for 24 days	17	↓40[i] (↓33 to ↓45)	↓49[i] (↓45 to ↓53)	↓58[i] (↓53 to ↓63)
Tenofovir 300 mg q.d. for 4 to 48 weeks	700 mg b.i.d. plus ritonavir 100 mg b.i.d. for 4 to 48 weeks	45	NA	NA	↔[j]
Tenofovir 300 mg q.d. for 4 to 48 weeks	1,400 mg q.d. plus ritonavir 200 mg q.d. for 4 to 48 weeks	60	NA	NA	↔[j]

[a]Concomitant medication is also shown in this column where appropriate.
[b]Ritonavir C_{max}, AUC, and C_{min} increased by 63%, 45%, and 13%, respectively, compared with historical control.
[c]Compared with historical control.
[d]Subjects were receiving LEXIVA/ritonavir for 10 days prior to the 4-day treatment period with both ketoconazole and LEXIVA/ritonavir.
[e]Compared with LEXIVA 700 mg/ritonavir 100 mg b.i.d. for 2 weeks.
[f]Subjects were receiving nevirapine for at least 12 weeks prior to trial.
[g]C_{last} ($C_{12\ hr}$ or $C_{24\ hr}$).
[h]Doses of LEXIVA and raltegravir were given with food on pharmacokinetic sampling days and without regard to food all other days.
[i]N = 18 for C_{min}.
[j]Compared with parallel control group.
↑ = Increase; ↓= Decrease; ↔ = No change (↑or ↓ less than or equal to 10%), NA = Not applicable.

tions have also been detected in HIV-1 isolates from antiretroviral-naive subjects treated with LEXIVA. Of the 488 antiretroviral-naive subjects treated with LEXIVA 1,400 mg twice daily or LEXIVA 1,400 mg plus ritonavir 200 mg once daily in Trials APV30001 and APV30002, respectively, 61 subjects (29 receiving LEXIVA and 32 receiving LEXIVA/ritonavir) with virologic failure (plasma HIV-1 RNA greater than 1,000 copies per mL on 2 occasions on or after Week 12) were genotyped. Five of the 29 antiretroviral-naive subjects (17%) receiving LEXIVA without ritonavir in Trial APV30001 had evidence of genotypic resistance to amprenavir: I54L/M (n = 2), I54L + L33F (n = 1), V32I + I47V (n = 1), and M46I + I47V (n = 1). No amprenavir resistance-associated substitutions were detected in antiretroviral-naive subjects treated with LEXIVA/ritonavir for 48 weeks in Trial APV30002. However, the M46I and I50V substitutions were detected in isolates from 1 virologic failure subject receiving LEXIVA/ritonavir once daily at Week 160 (HIV-1 RNA greater than 500 copies per mL). Upon retrospective analysis of stored samples using an ultrasensitive assay, these resistant substitutions were traced back to Week 84 (76 weeks prior to clinical virologic failure).

Cross-Resistance: Varying degrees of cross-resistance among HIV-1 protease inhibitors have been observed. An association between virologic response at 48 weeks (HIV-1 RNA level less than 400 copies per mL) and protease inhibitor-resistance substitutions detected in baseline HIV-1 isolates from protease inhibitor-experienced subjects receiving LEXIVA/ritonavir twice daily (n = 88), or lopinavir/ritonavir twice daily (n = 85) in Trial APV30003 is shown in Table 14. The majority of subjects had previously received either one (47%) or 2 protease inhibitors (36%), most commonly nelfinavir (57%) and indinavir (53%). Out of 102 subjects with baseline phenotypes receiving twice-daily LEXIVA/ritonavir, 54% (n = 55) had resistance to at least one protease inhibitor, with 98% (n = 54) of those having resistance to nelfinavir. Out of 97 subjects with baseline phenotypes in the lopinavir/ritonavir arm, 60% (n = 58) had resistance to at least one protease inhibitor, with 97% (n = 56) of those having resistance to nelfinavir.

[See table 14 at top of page 2482]

The virologic response based upon baseline phenotype was assessed. Baseline isolates from protease inhibitor-experienced subjects responding to LEXIVA/ritonavir twice daily had a median shift in susceptibility to amprenavir relative to a standard wild-type reference strain of 0.7 (range: 0.1 to 5.4, n = 62), and baseline isolates from individuals failing therapy had a median shift in susceptibility of 1.9 (range: 0.2 to 14, n = 29). Because this was a select patient population, these data do not constitute definitive clinical susceptibility break points. Additional data are needed to determine clinically relevant break points for LEXIVA.

Isolates from 15 of the 20 subjects receiving twice-daily LEXIVA/ritonavir up to Week 48 and experiencing virologic failure/ongoing replication were subjected to genotypic analysis. The following amprenavir resistance-associated substitutions were found either alone or in combination: V32I, M46I/L, I47V, I50V, I54L/M, and I84V. Isolates from 4 of the 16 subjects continuing to receive twice-daily LEXIVA/ritonavir up to Week 96 who experienced virologic failure underwent genotypic analysis. Isolates from 2 subjects contained amprenavir resistance-associated substitutions: V32I, M46I, and I47V in 1 isolate and I84V in the other.

13 NONCLINICAL TOXICOLOGY

13.1 Carcinogenesis, Mutagenesis, Impairment of Fertility

In long-term carcinogenicity studies, fosamprenavir was administered orally for up to 104 weeks at doses of 250, 400, or 600 mg per kg per day in mice and at doses of 300, 825, or 2,250 mg per kg per day in rats. Exposures at these doses were 0.3- to 0.7-fold (mice) and 0.7- to 1.4-fold (rats) those in humans given 1,400 mg twice daily of fosamprenavir alone, and 0.2- to 0.3-fold (mice) and 0.3- to 0.7-fold (rats) those in humans given 1,400 mg once daily of fosamprenavir plus 200 mg ritonavir once daily. Exposures in the carcinogenicity studies were 0.1- to 0.3-fold (mice) and 0.3- to 0.6-fold (rats) those in humans given 700 mg of fosamprenavir plus 100 mg ritonavir twice daily. There was an increase in hepatocellular adenomas and hepatocellular carcinomas at all doses in male mice and at 600 mg per kg per day in female mice, and in hepatocellular adenomas and thyroid follicular cell adenomas at all doses in male rats, and at 835 mg per kg per day and 2,250 mg per kg per day in female rats. The relevance of the hepatocellular findings in the rodents for humans is uncertain. Repeat dose studies with fosamprenavir in rats produced effects consistent with enzyme induction, which predisposes rats, but not humans, to thyroid neoplasms. In addition, in rats only there was an increase in interstitial cell hyperplasia at 825 mg per kg per day and 2,250 mg per kg per day, and an increase in uterine endometrial adenocarcinoma at 2,250 mg per kg per day. The incidence of endometrial findings was slightly increased over concurrent controls, but was within background range for female rats. The relevance of the uterine endometrial adenocarcinoma findings in rats for humans is uncertain.

Fosamprenavir was not mutagenic or genotoxic in a battery of in vitro and in vivo assays. These assays included bacterial reverse mutation (Ames), mouse lymphoma, rat micronucleus, and chromosome aberrations in human lymphocytes.

The effects of fosamprenavir on fertility and general reproductive performance were investigated in male (treated for 4 weeks before mating) and female rats (treated for 2 weeks before mating through postpartum day 6). Systemic exposures ($AUC_{0\text{-}24\ hr}$) to amprenavir in these studies were 3 (males) to 4 (females) times higher than exposures in humans following administration of the MRHD of fosamprenavir alone or similar to those seen in humans following administration of fosamprenavir in combination with ritonavir. Fosamprenavir did not impair mating or fertility of male or female rats and did not affect the development and maturation of sperm from treated rats.

14 CLINICAL STUDIES

14.1 Therapy-Naive Adult Trials

APV30001: A randomized, open-label trial evaluated treatment with LEXIVA Tablets (1,400 mg twice daily) versus nelfinavir (1,250 mg twice daily) in 249 antiretroviral treatment-naive subjects. Both groups of subjects also received abacavir (300 mg twice daily) and lamivudine (150 mg twice daily).

The mean age of the subjects in this trial was 37 years (range: 17 to 70 years); 69% of the subjects were male, 20% were CDC Class C (AIDS), 24% were Caucasian, 32% were black, and 44% were Hispanic. At baseline, the median CD4+ cell count was 212 cells per mm^3 (range: 2 to 1,136 cells per mm^3; 18% of subjects had a CD4+ cell count of less than 50 cells per mm^3 and 30% were in the range of 50 to less than 200 cells per mm^3). Baseline median HIV-1 RNA was 4.83 $\log_{10}$ copies per mL (range: 1.69 to 7.41 $\log_{10}$ copies per mL; 45% of subjects had greater than 100,000 copies per mL).

The outcomes of randomized treatment are provided in Table 15.

[See table 15 at top of page 2482]

Treatment response by viral load strata is shown in Table 16.

[See table 16 at top of page 2483]

Through 48 weeks of therapy, the median increases from baseline in CD4+ cell counts were 201 cells per mm^3 in the group receiving LEXIVA and 216 cells per mm^3 in the nelfinavir group.

APV30002: A randomized, open-label trial evaluated treatment with LEXIVA Tablets (1,400 mg once daily) plus ritonavir (200 mg once daily) versus nelfinavir (1,250 mg twice daily) in 649 treatment-naive subjects. Both treatment groups also received abacavir (300 mg twice daily) and lamivudine (150 mg twice daily).

The mean age of the subjects in this trial was 37 years (range: 18 to 69 years); 73% of the subjects were male, 22% were CDC Class C, 53% were Caucasian, 36% were black, and 8% were Hispanic. At baseline, the median CD4+ cell count was 170 cells per mm^3 (range: 1 to 1,055 cells per mm^3; 20% of subjects had a CD4+ cell count of less than 50 cells per mm^3 and 35% were in the range of 50 to less than 200 cells per mm^3). Baseline median HIV-1 RNA was 4.81 $\log_{10}$ copies per mL (range: 2.65 to 7.29 $\log_{10}$ copies per mL; 43% of subjects had greater than 100,000 copies per mL).

The outcomes of randomized treatment are provided in Table 17.

[See table 17 at top of page 2483]

Treatment response by viral load strata is shown in Table 18.

[See table 18 at top of page 2483]

Through 48 weeks of therapy, the median increases from baseline in CD4+ cell counts were 203 cells per mm^3 in the group receiving LEXIVA and 207 cells per mm^3 in the nelfinavir group.

14.2 Protease Inhibitor-Experienced Adult Trials

APV30003: A randomized, open-label, multicenter trial evaluated 2 different regimens of LEXIVA plus ritonavir (LEXIVA Tablets 700 mg twice daily plus ritonavir 100 mg twice daily or LEXIVA Tablets 1,400 mg once daily plus ritonavir 200 mg once daily) versus lopinavir/ritonavir (400 mg/100 mg twice daily) in 315 subjects who had experienced virologic failure to 1 or 2 prior protease inhibitor-containing regimens.

The mean age of the subjects in this trial was 42 years (range: 24 to 72 years); 85% were male, 33% were CDC Class C, 67% were Caucasian, 24% were black, and 9% were Hispanic. The median CD4+ cell count at baseline was 263 cells per mm^3 (range: 2 to 1,171 cells per mm^3). Baseline median plasma HIV-1 RNA level was 4.14 $\log_{10}$ copies per mL (range: 1.69 to 6.41 $\log_{10}$ copies per mL).

The median durations of prior exposure to NRTIs were 257 weeks for subjects receiving LEXIVA/ritonavir twice daily (79% had greater than or equal to 3 prior NRTIs) and 210 weeks for subjects receiving lopinavir/ritonavir (64% had greater than or equal to 3 prior NRTIs). The median durations of prior exposure to protease inhibitors were 149 weeks for subjects receiving LEXIVA/ritonavir twice daily (49% received greater than or equal to 2 prior protease inhibitors) and 130 weeks for subjects receiving lopinavir/ritonavir (40% received greater than or equal to 2 prior protease inhibitors).

The time-averaged changes in plasma HIV-1 RNA from baseline (AAUCMB) at 48 weeks (the endpoint on which the trial was powered) were -1.4 $\log_{10}$ copies per mL for twice-daily LEXIVA/ritonavir and -1.67 $\log_{10}$ copies per mL for the lopinavir/ritonavir group.

Table 11. Drug Interactions: Pharmacokinetic Parameters for Amprenavir After Administration of AGENERASE in the Presence of the Coadministered Drug(s)

Coadministered Drug(s) and Dose(s)	Dose of **AGENERASE**[a]	n	% Change in **Amprenavir** Pharmacokinetic Parameters (90% CI)		
			C_{max}	AUC	C_{min}
Abacavir 300 mg b.i.d. for 2 to 3 weeks	900 mg b.i.d. for 2 to 3 weeks	4	↔[a]	↔[a]	↔[a]
Clarithromycin 500 mg b.i.d. for 4 days	1,200 mg b.i.d. for 4 days	12	↑15 (↑1 to ↑31)	↑18 (↑8 to ↑29)	↑39 (↑31 to ↑47)
Delavirdine 600 mg b.i.d. for 10 days	600 mg b.i.d. for 10 days	9	↑40[b]	↑130[b]	↑125[b]
Ethinyl estradiol/norethindrone 0.035 mg/1 mg for 1 cycle	1,200 mg b.i.d. for 28 days	10	↔	↓22 (↓35 to ↓8)	↓20 (↓41 to ↑8)
Indinavir 800 mg t.i.d. for 2 weeks (fasted)	750 or 800 mg t.i.d. for 2 weeks (fasted)	9	↑18 (↑13 to ↑58)	↑33 (↑2 to ↑73)	↑25 (↓27 to ↑116)
Ketoconazole 400 mg single dose	1,200 mg single dose	12	↓16 (↓25 to ↓6)	↑31 (↑20 to ↑42)	NA
Lamivudine 150 mg single dose	600 mg single dose	11	↔	↔	NA
Methadone 44 to 100 mg q.d. for >30 days	1,200 mg b.i.d. for 10 days	16	↓27[c]	↓30[c]	↓25[c]
Nelfinavir 750 mg t.i.d. for 2 weeks (fed)	750 or 800 mg t.i.d. for 2 weeks (fed)	6	↓14 (↓38 to ↑20)	↔	↑189 (↑52 to ↑448)
Rifabutin 300 mg q.d. for 10 days	1,200 mg b.i.d. for 10 days	5	↔	↓15 (↓28 to 0)	↓15 (↓38 to ↑17)
Rifampin 300 mg q.d. for 4 days	1,200 mg b.i.d. for 4 days	11	↓70 (↓76 to ↓62)	↓82 (↓84 to ↓78)	↓92 (↓95 to ↓89)
Saquinavir 800 mg t.i.d. for 2 weeks (fed)	750 or 800 mg t.i.d. for 2 weeks (fed)	7	↓37 (↓54 to ↓14)	↓32 (↓49 to ↓9)	↓14 (↓52 to ↑54)
Zidovudine 300 mg single dose	600 mg single dose	12	↔	↑13 (↓2 to ↑31)	NA

[a]Compared with parallel control group.
[b]Median percent change; confidence interval not reported.
[c]Compared with historical data.
↑ = Increase; ↓ = Decrease; ↔ = No change (↑or ↓ less than 10%); NA = C_{min} not calculated for single–dose trial.

The proportions of subjects who achieved and maintained confirmed HIV-1 RNA less than 400 copies per mL (secondary efficacy endpoint) were 58% with twice-daily LEXIVA/ritonavir and 61% with lopinavir/ritonavir (95% CI for the difference: -16.6, 10.1). The proportions of subjects with HIV-1 RNA less than 50 copies per mL with twice-daily LEXIVA/ritonavir and with lopinavir/ritonavir were 46% and 50%, respectively (95% CI for the difference: -18.3, 8.9). The proportions of subjects who were virologic failures were 29% with twice-daily LEXIVA/ritonavir and 27% with lopinavir/ritonavir.

The frequency of discontinuations due to adverse events and other reasons, and deaths were similar between treatment arms.

Through 48 weeks of therapy, the median increases from baseline in CD4+ cell counts were 81 cells per mm^3 with twice-daily LEXIVA/ritonavir and 91 cells per mm^3 with lopinavir/ritonavir.

This trial was not large enough to reach a definitive conclusion that LEXIVA/ritonavir and lopinavir/ritonavir are clinically equivalent.

Once-daily administration of LEXIVA plus ritonavir is not recommended for protease inhibitor-experienced patients. Through Week 48, 50% and 37% of subjects receiving LEXIVA 1,400 mg plus ritonavir 200 mg once daily had plasma HIV-1 RNA less than 400 copies per mL and less than 50 copies per mL, respectively.

14.3 Pediatric Trials

Three open-label trials in pediatric subjects aged at least 4 weeks to 18 years were conducted. In one trial (APV29005), twice-daily dosing regimens (LEXIVA with or without ritonavir) were evaluated in combination with other antiretroviral agents in pediatric subjects aged 2 to 18 years. In a second trial (APV20002), twice-daily dosing regimens (LEXIVA with ritonavir) were evaluated in combination with other antiretroviral agents in pediatric subjects aged at least 4 weeks to less than 2 years. A third trial (APV20003) evaluated once-daily dosing of LEXIVA with ritonavir; the pharmacokinetic data from this trial did not support a once-daily dosing regimen in any pediatric patient population.

APV29005: *LEXIVA:* Twenty (18 therapy-naive and 2 therapy-experienced) pediatric subjects received LEXIVA Oral Suspension without ritonavir twice daily. At Week 24, 65% (13/20) achieved HIV-1 RNA less than 400 copies per mL, and the median increase from baseline in CD4+ cell count was 350 cells per mm^3.

LEXIVA plus Ritonavir: Forty-nine protease inhibitor-naive and 40 protease inhibitor-experienced pediatric subjects received LEXIVA Oral Suspension or Tablets with ritonavir twice daily. At Week 24, 71% of protease inhibitor-naive (35/49) and 55% of protease inhibitor-experienced (22/40) subjects achieved HIV-1 RNA less than 400 copies per mL; median increases from baseline in CD4+ cell counts were 184 cells per mm^3 and 150 cells per mm^3 in protease inhibitor-naive and experienced subjects, respectively.

APV20002: Fifty-four pediatric subjects (49 protease inhibitor-naive and 5 protease inhibitor-experienced) received LEXIVA Oral Suspension with ritonavir twice daily. At Week 24, 72% of subjects achieved HIV-1 RNA less than 400 copies per mL. The median increases from baseline in CD4+ cell counts were 400 cells per mm^3 in subjects aged at least 4 weeks to less than 6 months and 278 cells per mm^3 in subjects aged 6 months to 2 years.

16 HOW SUPPLIED/STORAGE AND HANDLING

LEXIVA Tablets, 700 mg, are pink, film-coated, capsule-shaped, biconvex tablets, with "GX LL7" debossed on one face.
Bottle of 60 with child-resistant closure (NDC 49702-207-18).
Store at controlled room temperature of 25°C (77°F); excursions permitted to 15° to 30°C (59° to 86°F) (see USP Controlled Room Temperature). Keep container tightly closed.
LEXIVA Oral Suspension, a white to off-white grape-bubblegum-peppermint–flavored suspension, contains 50 mg of fosamprenavir as fosamprenavir calcium equivalent to approximately 43 mg of amprenavir in each 1 mL.
Bottle of 225 mL with child-resistant closure (NDC 49702-208-53).
This product does not require reconstitution.
Store in refrigerator or at room temperature (5° to 30°C; 41° to 86°F). Shake vigorously before using. Do not freeze.

17 PATIENT COUNSELING INFORMATION

See FDA-approved Patient Labeling (Patient Information)

17.1 Drug Interactions

A statement to patients and healthcare providers is included on the product's bottle label: ALERT: Find out about medicines that should NOT be taken with LEXIVA.
LEXIVA may interact with many drugs; therefore, patients should be advised to report to their healthcare provider the use of any other prescription or nonprescription medication or herbal products, particularly St. John's wort.
Patients receiving PDE5 inhibitors should be advised that they may be at an increased risk of PDE5 inhibitor-associated adverse events, including hypotension, visual changes, and priapism, and should promptly report any symptoms to their healthcare provider.
Patients receiving hormonal contraceptives should be instructed to use alternate contraceptive measures during therapy with LEXIVA because hormonal levels may be altered, and if used in combination with LEXIVA and ritonavir, liver enzyme elevations may occur.

17.2 Sulfa Allergy

Patients should inform their healthcare provider if they have a sulfa allergy. The potential for cross-sensitivity between drugs in the sulfonamide class and fosamprenavir is unknown.

17.3 Redistribution/Accumulation of Body Fat

Patients should be informed that redistribution or accumulation of body fat may occur in patients receiving antiretroviral therapy, including LEXIVA, and that the cause and long-term health effects of these conditions are not known at this time.

17.4 Information About Therapy With LEXIVA

LEXIVA is not a cure for HIV-1 infection and patients may continue to experience illnesses associated with HIV-1 infection, including opportunistic infections. Patients should remain under the care of a physician when using LEXIVA.
Patients should be advised to avoid doing things that can spread HIV-1 infection to others.

- **Do not share needles or other injection equipment.**
- **Do not share personal items that can have blood or body fluids on them, like toothbrushes and razor blades.**
- **Do not have any kind of sex without protection.** Always practice safe sex by using a latex or polyurethane condom to lower the chance of sexual contact with semen, vaginal secretions, or blood.
- **Do not breastfeed.** We do not know if LEXIVA can be passed to your baby in your breast milk and whether it could harm your baby. Also, mothers with HIV-1 should not breastfeed because HIV-1 can be passed to the baby in the breast milk.

Patients should be told that sustained decreases in plasma HIV-1 RNA have been associated with a reduced risk of progression to AIDS and death. Patients should be advised to take LEXIVA every day as prescribed. LEXIVA must always be used in combination with other antiretroviral drugs. Patients should not alter the dose or discontinue therapy without consulting their physician. If a dose is missed, patients should take the dose as soon as possible and then return to their normal schedule. However, if a dose is skipped, the patient should not double the next dose.

17.5 Oral Suspension

Patients should be instructed to shake the bottle vigorously before each use and that refrigeration of the oral suspension may improve the taste for some patients.
LEXIVA and AGENERASE are registered trademarks of ViiV Healthcare.

Table 12. Drug Interactions: Pharmacokinetic Parameters for Coadministered Drug in the Presence of Amprenavir After Administration of LEXIVA

Coadministered Drug(s) and Dose(s)	Dose of LEXIVA[a]	n	% Change in Pharmacokinetic Parameters of Coadministered Drug (90% CI)		
			C_{max}	AUC	C_{min}
Atazanavir 300 mg q.d. for 10 days[b]	700 mg b.i.d. plus ritonavir 100 mg b.i.d. for 10 days	21	↓24 (↓39 to ↓6)	↓22 (↓34 to ↓9)	↔
Atorvastatin 10 mg q.d. for 4 days	1,400 mg b.i.d. for 2 weeks	16	↑304 (↑205 to ↑437)	↑130 (↑100 to ↑164)	↓10 (↓27 to ↑12)
Atorvastatin 10 mg q.d. for 4 days	700 mg b.i.d. plus ritonavir 100 mg b.i.d. for 2 weeks	16	↑184 (↑126 to ↑257)	↑153 (↑115 to ↑199)	↑73 (↑45 to ↑108)
Esomeprazole 20 mg q.d. for 2 weeks	1,400 mg b.i.d. for 2 weeks	25	↔	↑55 (↑39 to ↑73)	ND
Esomeprazole 20 mg q.d. for 2 weeks	700 mg b.i.d. plus ritonavir 100 mg b.i.d. for 2 weeks	23	↔	↔	ND
Ethinyl estradiol[c] 0.035 mg q.d. for 21 days	700 mg b.i.d. plus ritonavir 100 mg b.i.d. for 21 days	25	↓28 (↓21 to ↓35)	↓37 (↓30 to ↓42)	ND
Ketoconazole[d] 200 mg q.d. for 4 days	700 mg b.i.d. plus ritonavir 100 mg b.i.d. for 4 days	15	↑25 (↑0 to ↑56)	↑169 (↑108 to ↑248)	ND
Lopinavir/ritonavir[e] 533 mg/133 mg b.i.d. for 2 weeks	1,400 mg b.i.d. for 2 weeks	18	↔[f]	↔[f]	↔[f]
Lopinavir/ritonavir[e] 400 mg/100 mg b.i.d. for 2 weeks	700 mg b.i.d. plus ritonavir 100 mg b.i.d. for 2 weeks	18	↑30 (↓15 to ↑47)	↑37 (↓20 to ↑55)	↑52 (↓28 to ↑82)
Maraviroc 300 mg b.i.d. for 10 days	700 mg b.i.d. plus ritonavir 100 mg b.i.d. for 20 days	14	↑52 (↑27 to ↑82)	↑149 (↑119 to ↑182)	↑374 (↑303 to ↑457)
Maraviroc 300 mg q.d. for 10 days	1,400 mg q.d. plus ritonavir 100 mg q.d. for 20 days	14	↑45 (↑20 to ↑74)	↑126 (↑99 to ↑158)	↑80 (↑53 to ↑113)
Methadone 70 to 120 mg q.d. for 2 weeks	700 mg b.i.d. plus ritonavir 100 mg b.i.d. for 2 weeks	19	R-Methadone (active)		
			↓21[g] (↓30 to ↓12)	↓18[g] (↓27 to ↓8)	↓11[g] (↓21 to ↑1)
			S-Methadone (inactive)		
			↓43[g] (↓49 to ↓37)	↓43[g] (↓50 to ↓36)	↓41[g] (↓49 to ↓31)
Nevirapine 200 mg b.i.d. for 2 weeks[h]	1,400 mg b.i.d. for 2 weeks	17	↑25 (↑14 to ↑37)	↑29 (↑19 to ↑40)	↑34 (↑20 to ↑49)
Nevirapine 200 mg b.i.d. for 2 weeks[h]	700 mg b.i.d. plus ritonavir 100 mg b.i.d. for 2 weeks	17	↑13 (↑3 to ↑24)	↑14 (↑5 to ↑24)	↑22 (↑9 to ↑35)
Norethindrone[c] 0.5 mg q.d. for 21 days	700 mg b.i.d. plus ritonavir 100 mg b.i.d. for 21 days	25	↓38 (↓32 to ↓44)	↓34 (↓30 to ↓37)	↓26 (↓20 to ↓32)
Phenytoin 300 mg q.d. for 10 days	700 mg b.i.d. plus ritonavir 100 mg b.i.d. for 10 days	14	↓20 (↓12 to ↓27)	↓22 (↓17 to ↓27)	↓29 (↓23 to ↓34)

(Table continued on next page)

The brands listed are trademarks of their respective owners and are not trademarks of ViiV Healthcare. The makers of these brands are not affiliated with and do not endorse ViiV Healthcare or its products.

Manufactured for:

ViiV Healthcare Research Triangle Park, NC 27709	Vertex Pharmaceuticals Incorporated Cambridge, MA 02139

by:
GlaxoSmithKline
Research Triangle Park, NC 27709

LXV:17PI

PHARMACIST-DETACH HERE AND GIVE INSTRUCTIONS TO PATIENT

PATIENT INFORMATION
LEXIVA® (lex-EE-vah)
(fosamprenavir calcium)
Tablets
and
Oral Suspension

Important: LEXIVA can interact with other medicines and cause serious side effects. It is important to know the medicines that should not be taken with LEXIVA. See the section "Who should not take LEXIVA?"

Read this Patient Information before you start taking LEXIVA and each time you get a refill. There may be new information. This information does not take the place of talking with your healthcare provider about your medical condition or treatment.

What is LEXIVA?

LEXIVA is a prescription anti-HIV medicine used with other anti-HIV medicines to treat human immunodeficiency (HIV-1) infections in adults and children 4 weeks of age and older. LEXIVA is a type of anti-HIV medicine called a protease inhibitor. HIV-1 is the virus that causes AIDS (Acquired Immune Deficiency Syndrome).

When used with other anti-HIV medicines, LEXIVA may help:

1. Reduce the amount of HIV-1 in your blood. This is called "viral load".
2. Increase the number of white blood cells called CD4 (T) cells, which help fight off other infections. Reducing the amount of HIV-1 and increasing the CD4 (T) cell count may improve your immune system. This may reduce your risk of death or infections that can happen when your immune system is weak (opportunistic infections).

It is not known if LEXIVA is safe and effective in children less than 4 weeks of age.

LEXIVA does not cure HIV-1 infection or AIDS. People taking LEXIVA may develop infections or other conditions associated with HIV-1 infection, including opportunistic infections (for example, pneumonia and herpes virus infections). You should remain under the care of your healthcare provider when using LEXIVA.

Avoid doing things that can spread HIV-1 infection to others.

- **Do not share needles or other injection equipment.**
- **Do not share personal items that can have blood or body fluids on them, like toothbrushes and razor blades.**
- **Do not have any kind of sex without protection.** Always practice safe sex by using a latex or polyurethane condom to lower the chance of sexual contact with semen, vaginal secretions, or blood.

Ask your healthcare provider if you have any questions on how to prevent passing HIV to other people.

Who should not take LEXIVA?

Do not take LEXIVA if you take any of the following medicines:

- alfuzosin (UROXATRAL®)
- flecainide (TAMBOCOR™)
- propafenone (RYTHMOL SR®)
- rifampin (RIFADIN®, RIFAMATE®, RIFATER®, RIMACTANE®)
- ergot including:
  - dihydroergotamine mesylate (D.H.E. 45®, MIGRANAL®)
  - ergotamine tartrate (CAFERGOT®, MIGERGOT®, ERGOMAR®, MEDIHALER ERGOTAMINE®)
  - methylergonovine (METHERGINE®)
- St. John's wort (*Hypericum perforatum*)
- lovastatin (ADVICOR®, ALTOPREV®, MEVACOR®)
- simvastatin (ZOCOR®, VYTORIN®, SIMCOR®)
- pimozide (ORAP®)
- delavirdine mesylate (RESCRIPTOR®)
- sildenafil (REVATIO®), for treatment of pulmonary arterial hypertension
- triazolam (HALCION®)

Serious problems can happen if you or your child take any of the medicines listed above with LEXIVA.

Do not take LEXIVA if you are allergic to AGENERASE® (amprenavir), fosamprenavir calcium, or any of the ingredients in LEXIVA. See the end of this leaflet for a complete list of ingredients in LEXIVA.

Table 12 *(cont.)*. Drug Interactions: Pharmacokinetic Parameters for Coadministered Drug in the Presence of Amprenavir After Administration of LEXIVA

Coadministered Drug(s) and Dose(s)	Dose of **LEXIVA**[a]	n	% Change in Pharmacokinetic Parameters of **Coadministered Drug** (90% CI)		
			C_{max}	AUC	C_{min}
Rifabutin 150 mg every other day for 2 weeks[i]	700 mg b.i.d. plus ritonavir 100 mg b.i.d. for 2 weeks	15	↓14 (↓28 to ↑4)	↔	↑28 (↑12 to ↑46)
(25-O-desacetylrifabutin metabolite)			↑579 (↑479 to ↑698)	↑1,120 (↑965 to ↑1,300)	↑2,510 (↑1,910 to ↑3,300)
Rifabutin + 25-O-desacetylrifabutin metabolite			NA	↑64 (↑46 to ↑84)	NA
Rosuvastatin 10 mg single dose	700 mg b.i.d. plus ritonavir 100 mg b.i.d. for 7 days		↑45	↑8	NA
Telaprevir 750 mg q. 8 hr for 10 days	700 mg b.i.d. plus ritonavir 100 mg b.i.d. for 20 days	18	↓33 (↓29 to ↓37)	↓32 (↓28 to ↓37)	↓30 (↓23 to ↓36)

[a]Concomitant medication is also shown in this column where appropriate.
[b]Comparison arm of atazanavir 300 mg q.d. plus ritonavir 100 mg q.d. for 10 days.
[c]Administered as a combination oral contraceptive tablet: ethinyl estradiol 0.035 mg/norethindrone 0.5 mg.
[d]Subjects were receiving LEXIVA/ritonavir for 10 days prior to the 4-day treatment period with both ketoconazole and LEXIVA/ritonavir.
[e]Data represent lopinavir concentrations.
[f]Compared with lopinavir 400 mg/ritonavir 100 mg b.i.d. for 2 weeks.
[g]Dose normalized to methadone 100 mg. The unbound concentration of the active moiety, R–methadone, was unchanged.
[h]Subjects were receiving nevirapine for at least 12 weeks prior to trial.
[i]Comparison arm of rifabutin 300 mg q.d. for 2 weeks. AUC is $AUC_{(0-48\ hr)}$.
↑ = Increase; ↓= Decrease; ↔ = No change (↑or ↓less than 10%); ND = Interaction cannot be determined as C_{min} was below the lower limit of quantitation.

Table 13. Drug Interactions: Pharmacokinetic Parameters for Coadministered Drug in the Presence of Amprenavir After Administration of AGENERASE

Coadministered Drug(s) and Dose(s)	Dose of **AGENERASE**	n	% Change in Pharmacokinetic Parameters of **Coadministered Drug** (90% CI)		
			C_{max}	AUC	C_{min}
Abacavir 300 mg b.i.d. for 2 to 3 weeks	900 mg b.i.d for 2 to 3 weeks	4	↔[a]	↔[a]	↔[a]
Clarithromycin 500 mg b.i.d. for 4 days	1,200 mg b.i.d. for 4 days	12	↓10 (↓24 to ↑7)	↔	↔
Delavirdine 600 mg b.i.d. for 10 days	600 mg b.i.d. for 10 days	9	↓47[b]	↓61[b]	↓88[b]
Ethinyl estradiol 0.035 mg for 1 cycle	1,200 mg b.i.d. for 28 days	10	↔	↔	↑32 (↓3 to ↑79)
Indinavir 800 mg t.i.d. for 2 weeks (fasted)	750 mg or 800 mg t.i.d. for 2 weeks (fasted)	9	↓22[a]	↓38[a]	↓27[a]
Ketoconazole 400 mg single dose	1,200 mg single dose	12	↑19 (↑8 to ↑33)	↑44 (↑31 to ↑59)	NA
Lamivudine 150 mg single dose	600 mg single dose	11	↔	↔	NA
Methadone 44 to 100 mg q.d. for >30 days	1,200 mg b.i.d. for 10 days	16	R-Methadone (active)		
			↓25 (↓32 to ↓18)	↓13 (↓21 to ↓5)	↓21 (↓32 to ↓9)
			S-Methadone (inactive)		
			↓48 (↓55 to ↓40)	↓40 (↓46 to ↓32)	↓53 (↓60 to ↓43)
Nelfinavir 750 mg t.i.d. for 2 weeks (fed)	750 mg or 800 mg t.i.d. for 2 weeks (fed)	6	↑12[a]	↑15[a]	↑14[a]

(Table continued on next page)

What should I tell my healthcare provider before taking LEXIVA?

Before taking LEXIVA, tell your healthcare provider if you:

- are allergic to medicines that contain sulfa
- have liver problems, including hepatitis B or C
- have kidney problems
- have high blood sugar (diabetes)
- have hemophilia

Table 13 *(cont.)*. Drug Interactions: Pharmacokinetic Parameters for Coadministered Drug in the Presence of Amprenavir After Administration of AGENERASE

Coadministered Drug(s) and Dose(s)	Dose of AGENERASE	n	% Change in Pharmacokinetic Parameters of Coadministered Drug (90% CI)		
			C_{max}	AUC	C_{min}
Norethindrone 1 mg for 1 cycle	1,200 mg b.i.d. for 28 days	10	↔	↑18 (↑1 to ↑38)	↑45 (↑13 to ↑88)
Rifabutin 300 mg q.d. for 10 days	1,200 mg b.i.d. for 10 days	5	↑119 (↑82 to ↑164)	↑193 (↑156 to ↑235)	↑271 (↑171 to ↑409)
Rifampin 300 mg q.d. for 4 days	1,200 mg b.i.d. for 4 days	11	↔	↔	ND
Saquinavir 800 mg t.i.d. for 2 weeks (fed)	750 mg or 800 mg t.i.d. for 2 weeks (fed)	7	↑21[a]	↓19[a]	↓48[a]
Zidovudine 300 mg single dose	600 mg single dose	12	↑40 (↑14 to ↑71)	↑31 (↑19 to ↑45)	NA

[a]Compared with historical data.
[b]Median percent change; confidence interval not reported.
↑ = Increase; ↓ = Decrease; ↔= No change (↑or ↓ less than 10%); NA = C_{min} not calculated for single-dose trial; ND = Interaction cannot be determined as C_{min} was below the lower limit of quantitation.

Table 14. Responders at Trial Week 48 by Presence of Baseline Protease Inhibitor Resistance-Associated Substitutions[a]

Protease Inhibitor Resistance-Associated Substitutions[b]	LEXIVA/Ritonavir b.i.d. (n = 88)		Lopinavir/Ritonavir b.i.d. (n = 85)	
D30N	21/22	95%	17/19	89%
N88D/S	20/22	91%	12/12	100%
L90M	16/31	52%	17/29	59%
M46I/L	11/22	50%	12/24	50%
V82A/F/T/S	2/9	22%	6/17	35%
I54V	2/11	18%	6/11	55%
I84V	1/6	17%	2/5	40%

[a]Results should be interpreted with caution because the subgroups were small.
[b]Most subjects had greater than 1 protease inhibitor resistance-associated substitution at baseline.

Table 15. Outcomes of Randomized Treatment Through Week 48 (APV30001)

Outcome (Rebound or discontinuation = failure)	LEXIVA 1,400 mg b.i.d. (n = 166)	Nelfinavir 1,250 mg b.i.d. (n = 83)
Responder[a]	66% (57%)	52% (42%)
Virologic failure	19%	32%
Rebound	16%	19%
Never suppressed through Week 48	3%	13%
Clinical progression	1%	1%
Death	0%	1%
Discontinued due to adverse reactions	4%	2%
Discontinued due to other reasons[b]	10%	10%

[a]Subjects achieved and maintained confirmed HIV-1 RNA less than 400 copies per mL (less than 50 copies per mL) through Week 48 (Roche AMPLICOR HIV-1 MONITOR Assay Version 1.5).
[b]Includes consent withdrawn, lost to follow up, protocol violations, those with missing data, and other reasons.

• have any other medical condition
• are pregnant or plan to become pregnant. It is not known if LEXIVA will harm your unborn baby.

Pregnancy Registry. There is a pregnancy registry for women who take antiviral medicines during pregnancy. The purpose of the registry is to collect information about the health of you and your baby. Talk to your healthcare provider about how you can take part in this registry.

• **Do not breastfeed.** We do not know if LEXIVA can be passed to your baby in your breast milk and whether it could harm your baby. Also, mothers with HIV-1 should not breastfeed because HIV-1 can be passed to the baby in the breast milk.

Tell your healthcare provider about all prescription and non-prescription medicines you take. Also tell your healthcare provider about any vitamins , herbal supplements, and dietary supplements you are taking.

Taking LEXIVA with certain other medicines may cause serious side effects. LEXIVA may affect the way other medicines work, and other medicines may affect how LEXIVA works.

Especially tell your healthcare provider if you take estrogen-based contraceptives (birth control pills). LEXIVA may reduce effectiveness of estrogen-based contraceptives. During treatment with LEXIVA, you should use a different contraceptive method.

Know all the medicines that you take. Keep a list of them with you to show healthcare providers and pharmacists when you get a new medicine.

How should I take LEXIVA?

• **Stay under the care of a healthcare provider while taking LEXIVA.**
• Take LEXIVA exactly as prescribed by your healthcare provider.
• Do not change your dose or stop taking LEXIVA without talking with your healthcare provider.
• If your child is taking LEXIVA, your child's healthcare provider will decide the right dose based on your child's weight.
• You can take LEXIVA Tablets with or without food.
• **Adults should take LEXIVA Oral Suspension without food.**
• **Children should take LEXIVA Oral Suspension with food.** If your child vomits within 30 minutes after taking a dose of LEXIVA, the dose should be repeated.
• Shake LEXIVA Oral Suspension well before each use.
• If you miss a dose of LEXIVA, take the next dose as soon as possible and then take your next dose at the regular time. Do not double the next dose. If you take too much LEXIVA, call your healthcare provider or go to the nearest hospital emergency room right away.

What are the possible side effects of LEXIVA?

LEXIVA may cause serious side effects including:

• **Severe skin rash.** LEXIVA may cause severe or life-threatening skin reactions or rash.

If you get a rash with any of the following symptoms, stop taking LEXIVA and call your healthcare provider or get medical help right away:

◦ hives or sores in your mouth, or your skin blisters and peels
◦ trouble swallowing or breathing
◦ swelling of your face, eyes, lips, tongue, or throat

• **Liver problems.** Your healthcare provider should do blood tests before and during your treatment with LEXIVA to check your liver function. Some people with liver problems, including hepatitis B or C, may have an increased risk of developing worsening liver problem during treatment with LEXIVA.
• **Diabetes and high blood sugar (hyperglycemia).** Some people who take protease inhibitors, including LEXIVA, can get high blood sugar, develop diabetes, or your diabetes can get worse. Tell your healthcare provider if you notice an increase in thirst or urinate often while taking LEXIVA.
• **Changes in your immune system (Immune Reconstitution Syndrome)** can happen when you start taking HIV medicines. Your immune system may get stronger and begin to fight infections that have been hidden in your body for a long time. Call your healthcare provider right away if you start having new symptoms after starting your HIV medicine.
• **Changes in body fat.** These changes can happen in people who take antiretroviral therapy. The changes may include an increased amount of fat in the upper back and neck ("buffalo hump"), breast, and around the back, chest, and stomach area. Loss of fat from the legs, arms, and face may also happen. The exact cause and long-term health effects of these conditions are not known.
• **Changes in blood tests** . Some people have changes in blood tests while taking LEXIVA. These include increases seen in liver function tests, blood fat levels, and decreases in white blood cells. Your healthcare provider should do regular blood tests before and during your treatment with LEXIVA.
• **Increased bleeding problems in some people with hemophilia.** Some people with hemophilia have increased bleeding with protease inhibitors, including LEXIVA.
• **Kidney stones.** Some people have developed kidney stones while taking LEXIVA. Tell your healthcare provider right away if you develop signs or symptoms of kidney stones:
◦ pain in your side
◦ blood in your urine
◦ pain when you urinate

The most common side effects of LEXIVA in adults include:

• nausea
• vomiting
• diarrhea
• headache

Vomiting is the most common side effect in children when taking LEXIVA.

Tell your healthcare provider about any side effect that bothers you or that does not go away.

These are not all the possible side effects of LEXIVA. For more information, ask your healthcare provider or pharmacist.

Call your doctor for medical advice about side effects. You may report side effects to FDA at 1-800-FDA-1088.

How should I store LEXIVA?

• Store LEXIVA Tablets at room temperature between 68°F to 77°F (20°C to 25°C).
• Keep the bottle of LEXIVA Tablets tightly closed.
• Store LEXIVA Oral Suspension between 41°F to 86°F (5°C to 30°C). Refrigeration of LEXIVA Oral Suspension may improve taste for some people.
• Do not freeze.

Table 16. Proportions of Responders Through Week 48 by Screening Viral Load (APV30001)

Screening Viral Load HIV-1 RNA (copies/mL)	LEXIVA 1,400 mg b.i.d.		Nelfinavir 1,250 mg b.i.d.	
	<400 copies/mL	n	<400 copies/mL	n
100,000	65%	93	65%	46
>100,000	67%	73	36%	37

Table 17. Outcomes of Randomized Treatment Through Week 48 (APV30002)

Outcome (Rebound or discontinuation = failure)	LEXIVA 1,400 mg q.d./ Ritonavir 200 mg q.d. (n = 322)	Nelfinavir 1,250 mg b.i.d. (n = 327)
Responder[a]	69% (58%)	68% (55%)
Virologic failure	6%	16%
Rebound	5%	8%
Never suppressed through Week 48	1%	8%
Death	1%	0%
Discontinued due to adverse reactions	9%	6%
Discontinued due to other reasons[b]	15%	10%

[a]Subjects achieved and maintained confirmed HIV-1 RNA less than 400 copies per mL (less than 50 copies per mL) through Week 48 (Roche AMPLICOR HIV-1 MONITOR Assay Version 1.5).
[b]Includes consent withdrawn, lost to follow up, protocol violations, those with missing data, and other reasons.

Table 18. Proportions of Responders Through Week 48 by Screening Viral Load (APV30002)

Screening Viral Load HIV-1 RNA	LEXIVA 1,400 mg q.d./ Ritonavir 200 mg q.d.		Nelfinavir 1,250 mg b.i.d.	
(copies/mL)	<400 copies/mL	n	<400 copies/mL	n
100,000	72%	197	73%	194
>100,000	66%	125	64%	133

Keep LEXIVA and all medicines out of the reach of children.

General information about LEXIVA

Medicines are sometimes prescribed for purposes other than those listed in a Patient Information leaflet. Do not use LEXIVA for a condition for which it was not prescribed. Do not give LEXIVA to other people, even if they have the same symptoms you have. It may harm them.

This leaflet summarizes the most important information about LEXIVA. If you would like more information, talk with your healthcare provider. You can ask your pharmacist or healthcare provider for information about LEXIVA that is written for health professionals.

For more information call 877-844-8872 or go to www.LEXIVA.com.

What are the ingredients in LEXIVA?

Tablets:

Active ingredient: fosamprenavir calcium

Inactive ingredients: colloidal silicon dioxide, croscarmellose sodium, magnesium stearate, microcrystalline cellulose, and povidone K30. The tablet film-coating contains the inactive ingredients hypromellose, iron oxide red, titanium dioxide, and triacetin.

Oral Suspension:

Active ingredient: fosamprenavir calcium

Inactive ingredients: artificial grape-bubblegum flavor, calcium chloride dihydrate, hypromellose, methylparaben, natural peppermint flavor, polysorbate 80, propylene glycol, propylparaben, purified water, and sucralose.

This Patient Information has been approved by the U.S. Food and Drug Administration.

LEXIVA and AGENERASE are registered trademarks of ViiV Healthcare.

The brands listed are trademarks of their respective owners and are not trademarks of ViiV Healthcare. The makers of these brands are not affiliated with and do not endorse ViiV Healthcare or its products.

Manufactured for:

ViiV Healthcare Research Triangle Park, NC 27709	Vertex Pharmaceuticals Incorporated Cambridge, MA 02139

by:
GlaxoSmithKline
Research Triangle Park, NC 27709

February 2013
LXV:14PIL

RESCRIPTOR®

℞

[ree-SKRIP-tor]
(delavirdine mesylate)
Tablets

DESCRIPTION

RESCRIPTOR Tablets contain delavirdine mesylate, a synthetic non-nucleoside reverse transcriptase inhibitor (NNRTI) of the human immunodeficiency virus type 1 (HIV-1). The chemical name of delavirdine mesylate is piperazine, 1-[3-[(1-methyl-ethyl)amino]-2- pyridinyl]-4-[[5-[(methylsulfonyl)amino]-1H-indol-2-yl]carbonyl]-, monomethanesulfonate. Its molecular formula is $C_{22}H_{28}N_6O_3S{\bullet}CH_4O_3S$, and its molecular weight is 552.68. The structural formula is:

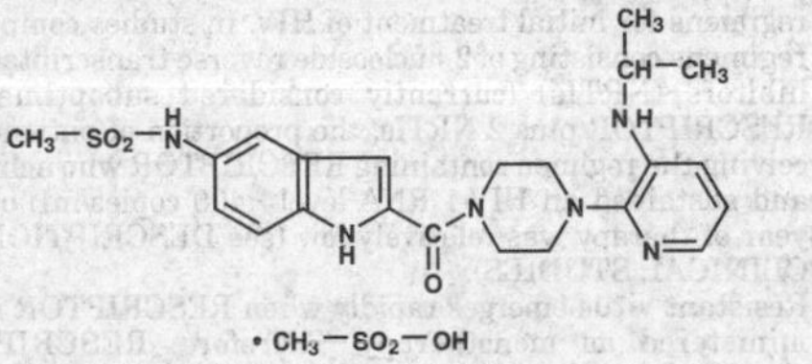

Delavirdine mesylate is an odorless white-to-tan crystalline powder. The aqueous solubility of delavirdine free base at 23°C is 2,942 mcg/mL at pH 1.0, 295 mcg/mL at pH 2.0, and 0.81 mcg/mL at pH 7.4.

Each RESCRIPTOR Tablet, for oral administration, contains 100 or 200 mg of delavirdine mesylate (henceforth referred to as delavirdine). Inactive ingredients consist of carnauba wax, colloidal silicon dioxide, croscarmellose sodium, lactose, magnesium stearate, and microcrystalline cellulose. In addition, the 100 mg tablet contains Opadry White YS-1-7000-E and the 200-mg tablet contains hypromellose and Opadry White YS-1-18202-A.

MICROBIOLOGY

Mechanism of Action

Delavirdine is an NNRTI of HIV-1. Delavirdine binds directly to reverse transcriptase (RT) and blocks RNA-dependent and DNA-dependent DNA polymerase activities. Delavirdine does not compete with template:primer or deoxynucleoside triphosphates. HIV-2 RT and human cellular DNA polymerases α, γ, or δ are not inhibited by delavirdine. In addition, HIV-1 group O, a group of highly divergent strains that are uncommon in North America, may not be inhibited by delavirdine.

In Vitro HIV-1 Susceptibility: In vitro anti-HIV-1 activity of delavirdine was assessed by infecting cell lines of lymphoblastic and monocytic origin and peripheral blood lymphocytes with laboratory and clinical isolates of HIV-1. IC_{50} and IC_{90} values (50% and 90% inhibitory concentrations) for laboratory isolates (n = 5) ranged from 0.005 to 0.030 µM and 0.04 to 0.10 µM, respectively. Mean IC_{50} of clinical isolates (n = 74) was 0.038 µM (range: 0.001 to 0.69 µM); 73 of 74 clinical isolates had an IC_{50} ≤0.18 µM. The IC_{90} of 24 of these clinical isolates ranged from 0.05 to 0.10 µM. In drug combination studies of delavirdine with zidovudine, didanosine, zalcitabine, lamivudine, interferon-α, and protease inhibitors, additive to synergistic anti–HIV-1 activity was observed in cell culture. The relationship between the in vitro susceptibility of HIV-1 RT inhibitors and the inhibition of HIV replication in humans has not been established.

Drug Resistance: Phenotypic analyses of isolates from patients treated with RESCRIPTOR as monotherapy showed a 50- to 500-fold reduced susceptibility in 14 of 15 patients by Week 8 of therapy. Genotypic analysis of HIV-1 isolates from patients receiving RESCRIPTOR plus zidovudine combination therapy (n = 79) showed resistance-conferring mutations in all isolates by Week 24 of therapy. In patients treated with RESCRIPTOR, the mutations in RT occurred predominantly at amino acid positions 103 and less frequently at positions 181 and 236. In a separate study, an average of 86-fold increase in the zidovudine susceptibility of patient isolates (n = 24) was observed after 24 weeks of combination therapy with RESCRIPTOR and zidovudine. The clinical relevance of the phenotypic and the genotypic changes associated with therapy with RESCRIPTOR has not been established.

Cross-Resistance: RESCRIPTOR may confer cross-resistance to other NNRTIs when used alone or in combination. Mutations at positions 103 and/or 181 have been found in resistant virus during treatment with RESCRIPTOR and other NNRTIs. These mutations have been associated with cross-resistance among NNRTIs in vitro.

CLINICAL PHARMACOLOGY

Pharmacokinetics

Absorption and Bioavailability: Delavirdine is rapidly absorbed following oral administration, with peak plasma concentrations occurring at approximately 1 hour. Following administration of delavirdine 400 mg 3 times daily (n = 67, HIV-1–infected patients), the mean ±SD steady-state peak plasma concentration (C_{max}) was 35 ± 20 µM (range: 2 to 100 µM), systemic exposure (AUC) was 180 ± 100 µM•hr (range: 5 to 515 µM•hr), and trough concentration (C_{min}) was 15 ± 10 µM (range: 0.1 to 45 µM). The single-dose bioavailability of delavirdine tablets relative to an oral solution was 85% ± 25% (n = 16, non-HIV–infected subjects). The single-dose bioavailability of delavirdine tablets (100-mg strength) was increased by approximately 20% when a slurry of drug was prepared by allowing delavirdine tablets to disintegrate in water before administration (n = 16, non-HIV–infected subjects). The bioavailability of the 200-mg strength delavirdine tablets has not been evaluated when administered as a slurry because they are not readily dispersed in water (see DOSAGE AND ADMINISTRATION).

Delavirdine may be administered with or without food. In a multiple-dose, crossover study, delavirdine was administered every 8 hours with food or every 8 hours, 1 hour before or 2 hours after a meal (n = 13, HIV-1–infected patients). Patients remained on their typical diet throughout the study; meal content was not standardized. When multiple doses of delavirdine were administered with food, geometric mean C_{max} was reduced by approximately 25%, but AUC and C_{min} were not altered.

Distribution: Delavirdine is extensively bound (approximately 98%) to plasma proteins, primarily albumin. The percentage of delavirdine that is protein-bound is constant over a delavirdine concentration range of 0.5 to 196 µM. In 5 HIV-1–infected patients whose total daily dose of delavirdine ranged from 600 to 1,200 mg, cerebrospinal fluid concentrations of delavirdine averaged 0.4% ± 0.07% of the corresponding plasma delavirdine concentrations; this represents about 20% of the fraction not bound to plasma proteins. Steady-state delavirdine concentrations in saliva (n = 5, HIV-1–infected patients who received delavirdine 400 mg 3 times daily) and semen (n = 5 healthy volunteers who received delavirdine 300 mg 3 times daily) were about 6% and 2%, respectively, of the corresponding plasma delavirdine concentrations collected at the end of a dosing interval.

Metabolism and Elimination: Delavirdine is extensively converted to several inactive metabolites. Delavirdine is primarily metabolized by cytochrome P450 3A (CYP3A), but in vitro data suggest that delavirdine may also be metabolized

Table 1. Pharmacokinetic Parameters for Coadministered Drugs in the Presence of Delavirdine

Coadministered Drug	Dose of Coadministered Drug	Dose of **RESCRIPTOR**	n	% Change in Pharmacokinetic Parameters of **Coadministered Drug** (90% CI)		
				C_{max}	AUC	C_{min}
HIV-Protease Inhibitors						
Indinavir	400 mg t.i.d. for 7 days	400 mg t.i.d. for 7 days	28	↓36[a] (↓52 to ↓14)	↔ [a]	↑118 [a] (↑16 to ↑312)
	600 mg t.i.d. for 7 days	400 mg t.i.d. for 7 days	28	↔	↑53 [a] (↑7 to ↑120)	↑298 [a] (↑104 to ↑678)
Nelfinavir[b]	750 mg t.i.d. for 14 days	400 mg t.i.d. for 7 days	12	↑88 (↑66 to ↑113)	↑107 (↑83 to ↑135)	↑136 (↑103 to ↑175)
Saquinavir	Soft gel capsule 1,000 mg t.i.d. for 28 days	400 mg t.i.d. for 28 days	20	↑98[c] (↑4 to ↑277)	↑121[c] (↑14 to ↑340)	↑199[c] (↑37 to ↑553)
Nucleoside Reverse Transcriptase Inhibitors						
Didanosine (buffered tablets)	125 or 250 mg b.i.d. for 28 days	400 mg t.i.d. for 28 days	9	↓20[d] (↓44 to ↑15)	↓21[d] (↓40 to ↑5)	-
Zidovudine	200 mg t.i.d. for >38 days	100 mg q.i.d. to 400 mg t.i.d. for 8 to 10 days	34	↔	↔	-
Anti-infective Agents						
Clarithromycin	500 mg b.i.d. for 15 days	300 mg t.i.d. for 30 days	6	-	↑100	-
Rifabutin	300 mg q.d. for 15 to 99 days	400 to 1,000 mg t.i.d. for 45 to 129 days	5	↑128 (↑71 to ↑203)	↑230 (↑119 to ↑396)	↑452 (↑246 to ↑781)

↑ Indicates increase.
↓ Indicates decrease.
↔ Indicates no significant change.
- Indicates no data available.
[a] Relative to indinavir 800 mg t.i.d. without RESCRIPTOR.
[b] Plasma concentrations of the nelfinavir active metabolite (nelfinavir hydroxy-t-butylamide) were significantly reduced by delavirdine, which is more than compensated for by increased nelfinavir concentration.
[c] Saquinavir soft gel capsule 1,000 mg t.i.d. plus RESCRIPTOR 400 mg t.i.d. relative to saquinavir soft gel capsule 1,200 mg t.i.d. without RESCRIPTOR.
[d] RESCRIPTOR taken with didanosine (buffered tablets) relative to doses of RESCRIPTOR and didanosine (buffered tablets) separated by at least 1 hour.

by CYP2D6. The major metabolic pathways for delavirdine are N-desalkylation and pyridine hydroxylation. Delavirdine exhibits nonlinear steady-state elimination pharmacokinetics, with apparent oral clearance decreasing by about 22-fold as the total daily dose of delavirdine increases from 60 to 1,200 mg/day. In a study of ^{14}C-delavirdine in 6 healthy volunteers who received multiple doses of delavirdine tablets 300 mg 3 times daily, approximately 44% of the radiolabeled dose was recovered in feces, and approximately 51% of the dose was excreted in urine. Less than 5% of the dose was recovered unchanged in urine. The parent plasma half-life of delavirdine increases with dose; mean half-life following 400 mg 3 times daily is 5.8 hours, with a range of 2 to 11 hours.

In vitro and in vivo studies have shown that delavirdine reduces CYP3A activity and inhibits its own metabolism. In vitro studies have also shown that delavirdine reduces CYP2C9, CYP2D6, and CYP2C19 activity. Inhibition of hepatic CYP3A activity by delavirdine is reversible within 1 week after discontinuation of drug.

Special Populations

Hepatic or Renal Impairment: The pharmacokinetics of delavirdine in patients with hepatic or renal impairment have not been investigated (see PRECAUTIONS).

Age: The pharmacokinetics of delavirdine have not been adequately studied in patients aged <16 years or >65 years.

Gender: Data from population pharmacokinetics suggest that the plasma concentrations of delavirdine tend to be higher in females than in males. However, this difference is not considered to be clinically significant.

Race: No significant differences in the mean trough delavirdine concentrations were observed between different racial or ethnic groups.

Drug Interactions

(See also PRECAUTIONS: Drug Interactions.)

Specific drug interaction studies were performed with delavirdine and a number of drugs. Table 1 summarizes the effects of delavirdine on the geometric mean AUC, C_{max}, and C_{min} of coadministered drugs. Table 2 shows the effects of coadministered drugs on the geometric mean AUC, C_{max}, and C_{min} of delavirdine.

For information regarding clinical recommendations, see CONTRAINDICATIONS, WARNINGS, and PRECAUTIONS: Drug Interactions.

[See table 1 above]
[See table 2 at top of next page]

INDICATIONS AND USAGE

RESCRIPTOR Tablets are indicated for the treatment of HIV-1 infection in combination with at least 2 other active antiretroviral agents when therapy is warranted.

The following should be considered before initiating therapy with RESCRIPTOR in treatment-naive patients. There are insufficient data directly comparing antiretroviral regimens containing RESCRIPTOR with currently preferred 3-drug regimens for initial treatment of HIV. In studies comparing regimens consisting of 2 nucleoside reverse transcriptase inhibitors (NRTIs) (currently considered suboptimal) to RESCRIPTOR plus 2 NRTIs, the proportion of patients receiving the regimen containing RESCRIPTOR who achieved and sustained an HIV-1 RNA level <400 copies/mL over 1 year of therapy was relatively low (see DESCRIPTION OF CLINICAL STUDIES).

Resistant virus emerges rapidly when RESCRIPTOR is administered as monotherapy. Therefore, RESCRIPTOR should always be administered in combination with other antiretroviral agents.

DESCRIPTION OF CLINICAL STUDIES

For clinical Studies 21 Part II and 13C described below, efficacy was evaluated by the percentage of patients with a plasma HIV-1 RNA level <400 copies/mL through Week 52 as measured by the Roche Amplicor® HIV-1 Monitor (standard assay). An intent-to-treat analysis was performed where only subjects who achieved confirmed suppression and sustained it through Week 52 are regarded as responders. All other subjects (including never suppressed, discontinued, and those who rebounded after initial suppression of <400 copies/mL) are considered failures at Week 52. Results of an interim analysis of efficacy conducted for studies 21 Part II and 13C by independent Data and Safety Monitoring Boards (DSMBs) revealed that the triple-therapy arms in both studies produced significantly greater antiviral benefit than the dual-therapy arms, and early termination of the studies was recommended.

Study 21 Part II

Study 21 Part II was a double–blind, randomized, placebo–controlled trial comparing treatment with RESCRIPTOR (400 mg 3 times daily, zidovudine 200 mg 3 times daily, and lamivudine 150 mg twice daily versus RESCRIPTOR 400 mg 3 times daily and zidovudine 200 mg 3 times daily versus zidovudine 200 mg 3 times daily and lamivudine 150 mg twice daily in 373 HIV-1–infected patients (mean age 35 years [range: 17 to 67], 87% male, and 60% Caucasian) who were antiretroviral treatment naive (84%) or had limited nucleoside experience (16%). Mean baseline CD4+ cell count was 359 cells/mm^3 and mean baseline plasma HIV–1 RNA was 4.4 $\log_{10}$ copies/mL.

Results showed that the mean increases from baseline in CD4 cell counts at 52 weeks were 111 cells/mL for RESCRIPTOR + zidovudine + lamivudine, 27 cells/mL for RESCRIPTOR + zidovudine, and 74 cells/mL for zidovudine + lamivudine.

The results of the intent-to-treat analysis of the percentage of patients with a plasma HIV-1 RNA level <400 copies/mL are presented in Figure 1. HIV-1 RNA status and reasons for discontinuation of randomized treatment at 52 weeks are summarized in Table 3. Subjects who were never suppressed before discontinuation were placed in the discontinuation category.

Figure 1. Percentage of Patients With HIV-1 RNA Below 400 copies/mL Standard PCR Assay Protocol 21 Part II: Intent-to-Treat Analysis

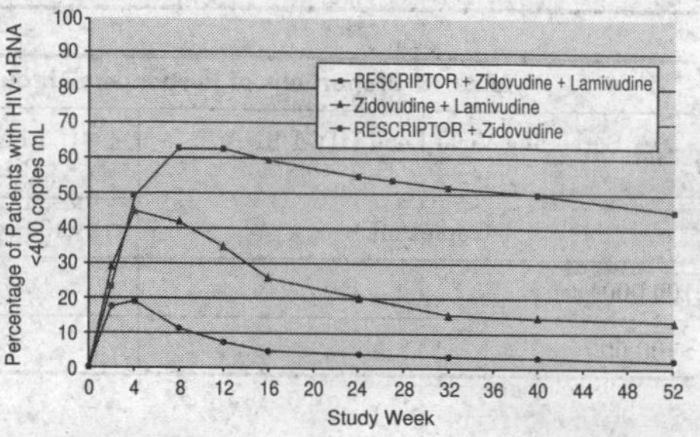

[See table 3 at top of next page]

Study 13C

Study 13C was a double–blind, randomized, placebo–controlled trial comparing treatment with RESCRIPTOR 400 mg 3 times daily, zidovudine 200 mg 3 times daily or 300 mg twice daily, and either didanosine 200 mg twice daily, zalcitabine 0.75 mg 3 times daily, or lamivudine 150 mg twice daily versus zidovudine 200 mg 3 times daily or 300 mg twice daily and either didanosine 200 mg twice daily, zalcitabine 0.75 mg 3 times daily, or lamivudine 150 mg twice daily in 345 HIV-1–infected patients (mean age 35.8 years [range: 18 to 72], 66% male, and 63% Caucasian) who were antiretroviral treatment naive (63%) or had limited antiretroviral experience (37%). Mean baseline CD4+ cell count was 210 cells/mm^3 and mean baseline plasma HIV–1 RNA was 4.9 $\log_{10}$ copies/mL.

Results showed that the mean increases from baseline in CD4+ cell counts at 54 weeks were 102 cells/mL for RESCRIPTOR + zidovudine + didanosine or zalcitabine or lamivudine, and 56 cells/mL for zidovudine + didanosine or zalcitabine or lamivudine.

The results of the intent–to–treat analysis of the percentage of patients with a plasma HIV–1 RNA level 400 copies/mL are presented in Figure 2. HIV–1 RNA status and reasons for discontinuation of randomized treatment at 54 weeks are summarized in Table 4. Subjects who were never suppressed before discontinuation were placed in the discontinuation category.

Figure 2. Percentage of Patients With HIV-1 RNA Below 400 copies/mL Standard PCR Assay Protocol 13C: Intent-to-Treat Analysis

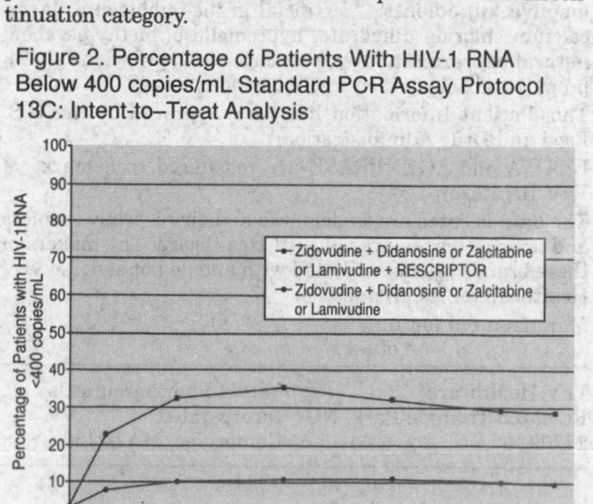

Table 2. Pharmacokinetic Parameters for Delavirdine in the Presence of Coadministered Drugs

Coadministered Drug	Dose of Coadministered Drug	Dose of RESCRIPTOR	n	% Change in **Delavirdine** Pharmacokinetic Parameters (90% CI)		
				C_{max}	AUC	C_{min}
HIV-Protease Inhibitors						
Indinavir	400 or 600 mg t.i.d. for 7 days	400 mg t.i.d. for 7 days	81	No apparent changes based on a comparison to historical data		
Nelfinavir	750 mg t.i.d. for 7 days	400 mg t.i.d. for 14 days	7	↓27 (↓49 to ↑4)	↓31 (↓57 to ↑10)	↓33 (↓70 to ↑49)
Saquinavir	Soft gel capsule 1,000 mg t.i.d. for 28 days	400 mg t.i.d. for 7 to 28 days	23	No apparent changes based on a comparison to historical data		
Nucleoside Reverse Transcriptase Inhibitors						
Didanosine (buffered tablets)	125 or 200 mg b.i.d. for 28 days	400 mg t.i.d. for 28 days	9	↓32[a] (↓48 to↓11)	↓19[a] (↓37 to ↑6)	↔[a]
Zidovudine	200 mg t.i.d. for ≥7 days	400 mg t.i.d. for 7 to 14 days	42	No apparent changes based on a comparison to historical data		
Anti-infective Agents						
Clarithromycin	500 mg b.i.d. for 15 days	300 mg t.i.d. for 30 days	6	↔	↔	↔
Fluconazole	400 mg q.d. for 15 days	300 mg t.i.d. for 30 days	8	↔	↔	↔
Ketoconazole	Various	200 to 400 mg t.i.d.	26	-	-	↑50[b]
Rifabutin	300 mg q.d. for 14 days	400 mg t.i.d. for 28 days	7	↓72 (↓61 to ↓80)	↓82 (↓74 to ↓88)	↓94 (↓90 to ↓96)
Rifampin	600 mg q.d. for 15 days	400 mg t.i.d. for 30 days	7	↓90 (↓94 to ↓83)	↓97 (↓98 to ↓95)	↓100
Sulfamethoxazole or Trimethoprim & Sulfamethoxazole	Various	200 to 400 mg t.i.d.	311	-	-	↔[b]
Other						
Antacid (Maalox® TC)	20 mL	300 mg single dose	12	↓52 (↓68 to ↓29)	↓44 (↓58 to ↓27)	-
Fluoxetine	Various	200 to 400 mg t.i.d.	36	-	-	↑50[b]
Phenytoin, Phenobarbital, Carbamazepine	Various	300 to 400 mg t.i.d.	8	-	-	↓90[b]

↑ Indicates increase.
↓ Indicates decrease.
↔ Indicates no significant change.
- Indicates no data available.
[a] RESCRIPTOR taken with didanosine (buffered tablets) relative to doses of RESCRIPTOR and didanosine (buffered tablets) separated by at least 1 hour.
[b] Population pharmacokinetic data from efficacy studies.

Table 3. Outcomes of Randomized Treatment Through Week 52 for Protocol 21 Part II

Outcome	Zidovudine + Lamivudine (n = 124) %	RESCRIPTOR + Zidovudine (n = 125) %	RESCRIPTOR + Zidovudine + Lamivudine (n = 124) %
HIV-1 RNA <400 copies/mL[a]	14	2	45
HIV-1 RNA ≥400 copies/mL[b,c]	64	52	31
Discontinued due to adverse events[c]	8	13	10
Discontinued due to other reasons[c,d]	14	33	14

[a]Corresponds to rates at Week 52 in proportion curve.
[b]Virologic failures at or before Week 52.
[c]Considered to be treatment failure in the analysis.
[d] Includes discontinuations due to consent withdrawn, loss to follow-up, protocol violations, non-compliance, pregnancy, never treated, and other reasons.

[See table 4 at top of next page]
Results from several smaller supportive studies evaluating the use of RESCRIPTOR in treatment-naive patients suggest that it may have activity when used in combination with protease inhibitors and NRTIs in 3- or 4-drug combinations.

CONTRAINDICATIONS

RESCRIPTOR Tablets are contraindicated in patients with known hypersensitivity to any of its ingredients. Coadministration of RESCRIPTOR is contraindicated with drugs that are highly dependent on CYP3A for clearance and for which elevated plasma concentrations are associated with serious and/or life-threatening events. These drugs are listed in Table 5. **Also, see PRECAUTIONS, Table 6, Drugs That Should Not Be Coadministered With RESCRIPTOR.**

Table 5. Drugs That Are Contraindicated With RESCRIPTOR

Drug Class	Drugs Within Class That Are Contraindicated With RESCRIPTOR
Antihistamines	Astemizole, terfenadine
Ergot derivatives	Dihydroergotamine, ergonovine, ergotamine, methylergonovine
GI motility agent	Cisapride
Neuroleptic	Pimozide
Sedative/hypnotics	Alprazolam, midazolam, triazolam

WARNINGS

ALERT: Find out about medicines that should NOT be taken with RESCRIPTOR. This statement is included on the product's bottle label.

Drug Interactions

Because delavirdine may inhibit the metabolism of many different drugs (e.g., antiarrhythmics, calcium channel blockers, sedative hypnotics, and others), **serious and/or life-threatening drug interactions could result from inappropriate coadministration of some drugs with delavirdine.** In addition, some drugs may markedly reduce delavirdine plasma concentrations, resulting in suboptimal antiviral activity and subsequent emergence of drug resistance. All prescribers should become familiar with the following tables in this package insert: **Table 5, Drugs That Are Contraindicated With RESCRIPTOR, Table 6, Drugs That Should Not Be Coadministered With RESCRIPTOR; and Table 7, Established and Other Potentially Significant Drug Interactions: Alteration in Dose or Regimen May Be Recommended Based on Drug Interaction Studies or Predicted Interaction.** Additional details on drug interactions can be found in Tables 1 and 2 under the CLINICAL PHARMACOLOGY section.

Concomitant use of lovastatin or simvastatin with RESCRIPTOR is not recommended. Caution should be exercised if RESCRIPTOR is used concurrently with other HMG-CoA reductase inhibitors that are also metabolized by the CYP3A4 pathway (e.g., atorvastatin or cerivastatin). The risk of myopathy including rhabdomyolysis may be increased when RESCRIPTOR is used in combination with these drugs.

Particular caution should be used when prescribing sildenafil in patients receiving RESCRIPTOR. Coadministration of sildenafil with RESCRIPTOR is expected to substantially increase sildenafil concentrations and may result in an increase in sildenafil-associated adverse events, including hypotension, visual changes, and priapism (see PRECAUTIONS: Drug Interactions and Information for Patients, and the complete prescribing information for sildenafil).

Concomitant use of St. John's wort (*Hypericum perforatum*) or St. John's wort-containing products and RESCRIPTOR is not recommended. Coadministration of St. John's wort with NNRTIs, including RESCRIPTOR, is expected to substantially decrease NNRTI concentrations and may result in suboptimal levels of RESCRIPTOR and lead to loss of virologic response and possible resistance to RESCRIPTOR or to the class of NNRTIs.

PRECAUTIONS

General

Delavirdine is metabolized primarily by the liver. Therefore, caution should be exercised when administering RESCRIPTOR Tablets to patients with impaired hepatic function.

Immune Reconstitution Syndrome

Immune reconstitution syndrome has been reported in patients treated with combination antiretroviral therapy, including RESCRIPTOR. During the initial phase of the combination antiretroviral treatment, patients whose immune systems respond may develop an inflammatory response to indolent or residual opportunistic infections (such as *Mycobacterium avium* infection, cytomegalovirus, *Pneumocystis jirovecii* pneumonia [PCP], or tuberculosis), which may necessitate further evaluation and treatment.

Autoimmune disorders (such as Graves' disease, polymyositis, and Guillain-Barré syndrome) have also been reported to occur in the setting of immune reconstitution; however, the time to onset is more variable, and can occur many months after initiation of treatment.

Resistance/Cross-Resistance

NNRTIs, when used alone or in combination, may confer cross-resistance to other NNRTIs.

Fat Redistribution

Redistribution/accumulation of body fat including central obesity, dorsocervical fat enlargement (buffalo hump), pe-

Table 4. Outcomes of Randomized Treatment Through Week 54 for Protocol 13C

Outcome	Zidovudine + Didanosine or Zalcitabine or Lamivudine (n = 173) %	Zidovudine + Didanosine or Zalcitabine or Lamivudine + RESCRIPTOR (n = 172) %
HIV–1 RNA 400 copies/mL[a]	10	29
HIV–1 RNA 400 copies/mL[b,c]	69	42
Discontinued due to adverse events[c]	7	12
Discontinued due to other reasons[c,d]	14	17

[a]Corresponds to rates at Week 54 in proportion curve.
[b]Virologic failures at or before Week 54.
[c]Considered to be treatment failure in the analysis.
[d]Includes discontinuations due to consent withdrawn, loss to follow-up, protocol violations, non-compliance, pregnancy, never treated, and other reasons.

Table 6. Drugs That Should Not Be Coadministered With RESCRIPTOR

Drug Class: Drug Name	Clinical Comment
Anticonvulsant agents: Phenytoin, phenobarbital, carbamazepine	May lead to loss of virologic response and possible resistance to RESCRIPTOR or to the class of NNRTIs.
Antihistamines: Astemizole, terfenadine	CONTRAINDICATED due to potential for serious and/or life-threatening reactions such as cardiac arrhythmias.
Antimycobacterials: Rifabutin,[a] rifampin [a]	May lead to loss of virologic response and possible resistance to RESCRIPTOR or to the class of NNRTIs or other coadministered antiviral agents.
Ergot Derivatives: Dihydroergotamine, ergonovine, ergotamine, methylergonovine	CONTRAINDICATED due to potential for serious and/or life-threatening reactions such as acute ergot toxicity characterized by peripheral vasospasm and ischemia of the extremities and other tissues.
GI motility agent: Cisapride	CONTRAINDICATED due to potential for serious and/or life-threatening reactions such as cardiac arrhythmias.
Herbal Products: St. John's wort (*Hypericum perforatum*)	May lead to loss of virologic response and possible resistance to RESCRIPTOR or to the class of NNRTIs.
HMG-CoA reductase inhibitors: Lovastatin, simvastatin	Potential for serious reactions such as risk of myopathy including rhabdomyolysis.
Neuroleptic: Pimozide	CONTRAINDICATED due to potential for serious and/or life-threatening reactions such as cardiac arrhythmias.
Sedative/hypnotics: Alprazolam, midazolam, triazolam	CONTRAINDICATED due to potential for serious and/or life-threatening reactions such as prolonged or increased sedation or respiratory depression.

[a]See CLINICAL PHARMACOLOGY for magnitude of interaction, Tables 1 and 2.

ripheral wasting, facial wasting, breast enlargement, and "cushingoid appearance" have been observed in patients receiving antiretroviral therapy. The mechanism and long-term consequences of these events are currently unknown. A causal relationship has not been established.

Skin Rash

Severe rash, including rare cases of erythema multiforme and Stevens-Johnson syndrome, has been reported in patients receiving RESCRIPTOR. Erythema multiforme and Stevens-Johnson syndrome were rarely seen in clinical trials and resolved after withdrawal of RESCRIPTOR. Any patient experiencing severe rash or rash accompanied by symptoms such as fever, blistering, oral lesions, conjunctivitis, swelling, and muscle or joint aches should discontinue RESCRIPTOR and consult a physician. Two cases of Stevens-Johnson syndrome have been reported through postmarketing surveillance out of a total of 339 surveillance reports.

In Studies 21 Part II and 13C (see DESCRIPTION OF CLINICAL STUDIES), rash (including maculopapular rash) was reported in more patients who were treated with RESCRIPTOR 400 mg 3 times daily (35% and 32%, respectively) than in those who were not treated with RESCRIPTOR (21% and 16%, respectively). The highest intensity of rash reported in these studies was severe (Grade 3), which was observed in approximately 4% of patients treated with RESCRIPTOR in each study and in none of the patients who were not treated with RESCRIPTOR. Also in Studies 21 Part II and 13C, discontinuations due to rash were reported in more patients who received RESCRIPTOR 400 mg 3 times daily (3% and 4%, respectively) than in those who did not receive RESCRIPTOR (0% and 1%, respectively).

In most cases, the duration of the rash was less than 2 weeks and did not require dose reduction or discontinuation of RESCRIPTOR. Most patients were able to resume therapy after rechallenge with RESCRIPTOR following a treatment interruption due to rash. The distribution of the rash was mainly on the upper body and proximal arms, with decreasing intensity of the lesions on the neck and face, and progressively less on the rest of the trunk and limbs.

Occurrence of a delavirdine-associated rash after 1 month is uncommon. Symptomatic relief has been obtained using diphenhydramine hydrochloride, hydroxyzine hydrochloride, and/or topical corticosteroids.

Information for Patients

A statement to patients and healthcare providers is included on the product's bottle label: **ALERT: Find out about medicines that should NOT be taken with RESCRIPTOR**. A patient package insert (PPI) for RESCRIPTOR is available for patient information.

Patients should be informed that RESCRIPTOR is not a cure for HIV–1 infection and that patients may continue to experience illnesses associated with HIV–1 infection, including opportunistic infections. Patients should be advised to remain under the care of a physician while taking RESCRIPTOR.

Patients should be advised to avoid doing things that can spread HIV-1 infection to others.

- **Do not share needles or other injection equipment.**
- **Do not share personal items that can have blood or body fluids on them, like toothbrushes and razor blades.**
- **Do not have any kind of sex without protection.** Always practice safe sex by using a latex or polyurethane condom to lower the chance of sexual contact with semen, vaginal secretions, or blood.
- **Do not breastfeed.** We do not know if RESCRIPTOR can be passed to your baby in your breast milk and whether it could harm your baby. Also, mothers with HIV-1 should not breastfeed because HIV-1 can be passed to the baby in the breast milk.

Patients should be instructed that the major toxicity of RESCRIPTOR is rash and should be advised to promptly notify their physician should rash occur. The majority of rashes associated with RESCRIPTOR occur within 1 to 3 weeks after initiating treatment with RESCRIPTOR. The rash normally resolves in 3 to 14 days and may be treated symptomatically while therapy with RESCRIPTOR is continued. Any patient experiencing severe rash or rash accompanied by symptoms such as fever, blistering, oral lesions, conjunctivitis, swelling, and muscle or joint aches should discontinue medication and consult a physician.

Patients should be informed that redistribution or accumulation of body fat may occur in patients receiving antiretroviral therapy and that the cause and long-term health effects of these conditions are not known at this time.

Patients should be informed to take RESCRIPTOR every day as prescribed. Patients should not alter the dose of RESCRIPTOR without consulting their doctor. If a dose is missed, patients should take the next dose as soon as possible. However, if a dose is skipped, the patient should not double the next dose.

Patients with achlorhydria should take RESCRIPTOR with an acidic beverage (e.g., orange or cranberry juice). However, the effect of an acidic beverage on the absorption of delavirdine in patients with achlorhydria has not been investigated.

Patients taking both RESCRIPTOR and antacids should be advised to take them at least 1 hour apart.

Because RESCRIPTOR may interact with certain drugs, patients should be advised to report to their doctor the use of any prescription, nonprescription medication, or herbal products, particularly St. John's wort.

Patients receiving sildenafil and RESCRIPTOR should be advised that they may be at an increased risk of sildenafil–associated adverse events, including hypotension, visual changes, and prolonged penile erection, and should promptly report any symptoms to their doctor.

Drug Interactions

(See also CONTRAINDICATIONS, WARNINGS, and CLINICAL PHARMACOLOGY: Drug Interactions.)

Delavirdine is an inhibitor of CYP3A isoform and other CYP isoforms to a lesser extent including CYP2C9, CYP2D6, and CYP2C19. Coadministration of RESCRIPTOR and drugs primarily metabolized by CYP3A (e.g., HMG-CoA reductase inhibitors and sildenafil) may result in increased plasma concentrations of the coadministered drug that could increase or prolong both its therapeutic or adverse effects.

Delavirdine is metabolized primarily by CYP3A, but in vitro data suggest that delavirdine may also be metabolized by CYP2D6. Coadministration of RESCRIPTOR and drugs that induce CYP3A, such as rifampin, may decrease delavirdine plasma concentrations and reduce its therapeutic effect. Coadministration of RESCRIPTOR and drugs that inhibit CYP3A may increase delavirdine plasma concentrations. **(See Table 6, Drugs That Should Not Be Coadministered With RESCRIPTOR, and Table 7, Established and Other Potentially Significant Drug Interactions: Alteration in Dose or Regimen May Be Recommended Based on Drug Interaction Studies or Predicted Interaction.)**

[See table 6 above]
[See table 7 on pages 2487 and 2488]

Carcinogenesis, Mutagenesis, Impairment of Fertility

Delavirdine was negative in a battery of genetic toxicology tests which included an Ames assay, an in vitro rat hepatocyte unscheduled DNA synthesis assay, an in vitro chromosome aberration assay in human peripheral lymphocytes, an in vitro mutation assay in Chinese hamster ovary cells, and an in vivo micronucleus test in mice.

Lifetime carcinogenicity studies were conducted in rats at doses of 10, 32, and 100 mg/kg/day and in mice at doses of 62.5, 250, and 500 mg/kg/day for males and 62.5, 125, and 250 mg/kg/day for females. In rats, delavirdine was noncarcinogenic at maximally tolerated doses that produced exposures (AUC) up to 12 (male rats) and 9 (female rats) times human exposure at the recommended clinical dose. In mice, delavirdine produced significant increases in the incidence of hepatocellular adenoma/adenocarcinoma in both males and females, hepatocellular adenoma in females, and mesenchymal urinary bladder tumors in males. The systemic drug exposures (AUC) in female mice were 0.5- to 3-fold and in male mice 0.2- to 4-fold of those in humans at the recommended clinical dose. Given the lack of genotoxic activity of delavirdine, the relevance of urinary bladder and hepatocellular neoplasm in delavirdine-treated mice to humans is not known.

Delavirdine at doses of 20, 100, and 200 mg/kg/day did not cause impairment of fertility in rats when males were treated for 70 days and females were treated for 14 days prior to mating.

Pregnancy

Pregnancy Category C. Delavirdine has been shown to be teratogenic in rats. Delavirdine caused ventricular septal defects in rats at doses of 50, 100, and 200 mg/kg/day when administered during the period of organogenesis. The lowest dose of delavirdine that caused malformations produced systemic exposures in pregnant rats equal to or lower than the expected human exposure to RESCRIPTOR (C_{min} 15 µM) at the recommended dose. Exposure in rats approximately 5-fold higher than the expected human exposure resulted in marked maternal toxicity, embryotoxicity, fetal developmental delay, and reduced pup survival. Additionally, reduced pup survival on postpartum day 0 occurred at an exposure (mean C_{min}) approximately equal to the expected human exposure. Delavirdine was excreted in the milk of lactating rats at a concentration 3 to 5 times that of rat plasma.

Delavirdine at doses of 200 and 400 mg/kg/day administered during the period of organogenesis caused maternal toxicity, embryotoxicity, and abortions in rabbits. The lowest dose of delavirdine that resulted in these toxic effects produced systemic exposures in pregnant rabbits approximately 6-fold higher than the expected human exposure to RESCRIPTOR (C_{min} 15 µM) at the recommended dose. The no-observed-adverse-effect dose in the pregnant rabbit was 100 mg/kg/day. Various malformations were observed at this dose, but the incidence of such malformations was not statistically significantly different from that observed in the control group. Systemic exposures in pregnant rabbits at a dose of 100 mg/kg/day were lower than those expected in humans at the recommended clinical dose. Malformations were not apparent at 200 and 400 mg/kg/day; however, only a limited number of fetuses were available for examination as a result of maternal and embryo death.

No adequate and well-controlled studies in pregnant women have been conducted. RESCRIPTOR should be used during pregnancy only if the potential benefit justifies the potential risk to the fetus. Of 9 pregnancies reported in premarketing clinical studies and postmarketing experience, a total of 10 infants were born (including 1 set of twins). Eight of the infants were born healthy. One infant was born HIV-positive but was otherwise healthy and with no congenital abnormalities detected, and 1 infant was born prematurely (34 to 35 weeks) with a small muscular ventricular septal defect that spontaneously resolved. The patient received approximately 6 weeks of treatment with delavirdine and zidovudine early in the course of the pregnancy.

Antiretroviral Pregnancy Registry: To monitor maternal-fetal outcomes of pregnant women exposed to RESCRIPTOR and other antiretroviral agents, an Antiretroviral Pregnancy Registry has been established. Physicians are encouraged to register patients by calling (800) 258-4263.

Nursing Mothers

The Centers for Disease Control and Prevention recommend that HIV-infected mothers not breastfeed their infants to avoid risking postnatal transmission of HIV. Because of both the potential for HIV transmission and any possible adverse reactions in nursing infants, **mothers should be instructed not to breastfeed if they are receiving RESCRIPTOR.**

Pediatric Use

Safety and effectiveness of delavirdine in combination with other antiretroviral agents have not been established in HIV-1–infected individuals younger than 16 years of age.

Geriatric Use

Clinical studies of RESCRIPTOR did not include sufficient numbers of subjects aged 65 and over to determine whether they respond differently from younger subjects. In general, caution should be taken when dosing RESCRIPTOR in elderly patients due to the greater frequency of decreased hepatic, renal, or cardiac function and of concomitant disease or other drug therapy.

ADVERSE REACTIONS

The safety of RESCRIPTOR Tablets alone and in combination with other therapies has been studied in approximately 6,000 patients receiving RESCRIPTOR. The majority of adverse events were of mild or moderate (i.e., ACTG Grade 1 or 2) intensity. The most frequently reported drug-related adverse event (i.e., events considered by the investigator to be related to the blinded study medication or events with an unknown or missing causal relationship to the blinded medication) among patients receiving RESCRIPTOR was skin rash (see Table 8 and PRECAUTIONS: Skin Rash).

[See table 8 at top of next page]

Adverse events of moderate to severe intensity reported by at least 5% of evaluable patients in any treatment group in the pivotal trials, which includes patients receiving RESCRIPTOR in combination with zidovudine and/or lamivudine in Study 21 Part II for up to 98 weeks and in combination with zidovudine and either lamivudine, didanosine, or zalcitabine in Study 13C for up to 72 weeks are summarized in Table 9.

[See table 9 at top of page 2489]

Other Adverse Events In Phase II/III Studies

Other adverse events that occurred in patients receiving RESCRIPTOR (in combination treatment) in all Phase II and III studies, considered possibly related to treatment, and of at least ACTG Grade 2 in intensity are listed below by body system.

Body as a Whole: Abdominal cramps, abdominal distention, abdominal pain (localized), abscess, allergic reaction, chills, edema (generalized or localized), epidermal cyst, fe-

Table 7. Established and Other Potentially Significant Drug Interactions: Alteration in Dose or Regimen May Be Recommended Based on Drug Interaction Studies or Predicted Interaction

Concomitant Drug Class: Drug Name	Effect on Concentration of Delavirdine or Concomitant Drug	Clinical Comment
HIV-Antiviral Agents: Nucleoside Reverse Transcriptase Inhibitor		
Didanosine[a]	↓Delavirdine ↓Didanosine	Administration of didanosine (buffered tablets) and RESCRIPTOR should be separated by at least 1 hour.
HIV-Antiviral Agents: Non-nucleoside Reverse Transcriptase Inhibitors		
NNRTI	↔Delavirdine ↑NNRTI	Combining NNRTIs has not been shown to be beneficial. RESCRIPTOR should not be coadministered with another NNRTI.
HIV-Antiviral Agents: Protease Inhibitors		
Indinavir[a]	↑Indinavir	A dose reduction of indinavir to 600 mg 3 times daily should be considered when RESCRIPTOR and indinavir are coadministered.
Lopinavir/Ritonavir	↑Lopinavir ↑Ritonavir	Appropriate doses of this combination with respect to safety, efficacy, and pharmacokinetics have not been established.
Nelfinavir[a]	↑Nelfinavir ↓Delavirdine	Appropriate doses of this combination with respect to safety, efficacy, and pharmacokinetics have not been established (see CLINICAL PHARMACOLOGY: Tables 1 and 2).
Ritonavir	↑Ritonavir	Appropriate doses of this combination with respect to safety, efficacy, and pharmacokinetics have not been established.
Saquinavir[a]	↑Saquinavir	A dose reduction of saquinavir (soft gelatin capsules) may be considered when RESCRIPTOR and saquinavir are coadministered (see CLINICAL PHARMACOLOGY: Table 1). Appropriate doses with respect to safety, efficacy, and pharmacokinetics have not been established.
HIV-Antiviral Agents: CCR5 Inhibitor		
Maraviroc	↑Maraviroc	Concomitant use of RESCRIPTOR and maraviroc has not been studied. However, RESCRIPTOR is a potent CYP3A4 inhibitor and the maraviroc dose should be reduced during coadministration. Refer to the full prescribing information for maraviroc (SELZENTRY) for dosing recommendations.
Other Agents		
Acid blockers: Antacids[a]	↓Delavirdine	Doses of an antacid and RESCRIPTOR should be separated by at least 1 hour, because the absorption of delavirdine is reduced when coadministered with antacids.
Histamine H_2-receptor antagonists: Cimetidine, famotidine, nizatidine, ranitidine	↓Delavirdine	These agents increase gastric pH and may reduce the absorption of delavirdine. Although the effect of these drugs on delavirdine absorption has not been evaluated, chronic use of these drugs with RESCRIPTOR is not recommended.
Proton pump inhibitors: Omeprazole, lansoprazole	↓Delavirdine	These agents increase gastric pH and may reduce the absorption of delavirdine. Although the effect of these drugs on delavirdine absorption has not been evaluated, chronic use of these drugs with RESCRIPTOR is not recommended.
Amphetamines	↑Amphetamines	Use with caution.
Antidepressant: Trazodone	↑Trazodone	Concomitant use of trazodone and RESCRIPTOR may increase plasma concentrations of trazodone. Adverse events of nausea, dizziness, hypotension, and syncope have been observed following coadministration of trazodone and ritonavir. If trazodone is used with a CYP3A4 inhibitor such as RESCRIPTOR, the combination should be used with caution and a lower dose of trazodone should be considered.
Antiarrhythmics: Bepridil	↑Antiarrhythmics	Use with caution. Increased bepridil exposure may be associated with life–threatening reactions such as cardiac arrhythmias.
Amiodarone, lidocaine (systemic), quinidine, flecainide, propafenone		Caution is warranted and therapeutic concentration monitoring is recommended, if available, for antiarrhythmics when coadministered with RESCRIPTOR.

(Table continued on next page)

Table 7 *(cont.)*. Established and Other Potentially Significant Drug Interactions: Alteration in Dose or Regimen May Be Recommended Based on Drug Interaction Studies or Predicted Interaction

Concomitant Drug Class: Drug Name	Effect on Concentration of Delavirdine or Concomitant Drug	Clinical Comment
Anticoagulant: Warfarin	↑Warfarin	It is recommended that INR (international normalized ratio) be monitored.
Anti-infective: Clarithromycin[a]	↑Clarithromycin	When coadministered with RESCRIPTOR, clarithromycin should be adjusted in patients with impaired renal function: • For patients with CL_{CR} 30 to 60 mL/min the dose of clarithromycin should be reduced by 50%. • For patients with CL_{CR} <30 mL/min the dose of clarithromycin should be reduced by 75%.
Calcium channel blockers: Amlodipine, diltiazem, felodipine, isradipine, nifedipine, nicardipine, nimodipine, nisoldipine, verapamil	↑Calcium channel blockers	Caution is warranted and clinical monitoring of patients is recommended.
Corticosteroid: Dexamethasone	↓Delavirdine	Use with caution. RESCRIPTOR may be less effective due to decreased delavirdine plasma concentrations in patients taking these agents concomitantly.
Erectile dysfunction agents: Sildenafil	↑Sildenafil	Sildenafil should not exceed a maximum single dose of 25 mg in a 48–hour period.
HMG-CoA reductase inhibitors: Atorvastatin, cerivastatin, fluvastatin	↑Atorvastatin ↑Cerivastatin ↑Fluvastatin	Use lowest possible dose of atorvastatin or cerivastatin, or fluvastatin with careful monitoring, or consider other HMG-CoA reductase inhibitors such as pravastatin in combination with RESCRIPTOR.
Immunosuppressants: Cyclosporine, tacrolimus, rapamycin	↑Immunosuppressants	Therapeutic concentration monitoring is recommended for immunosuppressant agents when coadministered with RESCRIPTOR.
Inhaled/nasal steroid: Fluticasone	↑Fluticasone	Concomitant use of fluticasone and RESCRIPTOR may increase plasma concentrations of fluticasone. Use with caution. Consider alternatives to fluticasone, particularly for long-term use.
Narcotic analgesic: Methadone	↑Methadone	Dosage of methadone may need to be decreased when coadministered with RESCRIPTOR.
Oral contraceptives: Ethinyl estradiol	↑Ethinyl estradiol	Concentrations of ethinyl estradiol may increase. However, the clinical significance is unknown.

↑ Indicates increase.
↓ Indicates decrease.
[a]The interaction between RESCRIPTOR and the drug was evaluated in a clinical study. All other drug interactions shown are predicted.

Table 8. Percent of Patients With Treatment-Emergent Rash in Pivotal Trials (Studies 21 Part II and 13C)[a]

Percent of Patients With:	Description of Rash Grade[b]	RESCRIPTOR 400 mg t.i.d. (n = 412)	Control Group Patients (n = 295)
Grade 1 rash	Erythema, pruritus	69 (16.7%)	35 (11.9%)
Grade 2 rash	Diffuse maculopapular rash, dry desquamation	59 (14.3%)	17 (5.8%)
Grade 3 rash	Vesiculation, moist desquamation, ulceration	18 (4.4%)	0 (0.0%)
Grade 4 rash	Erythema multiforme, Stevens-Johnson syndrome, toxic epidermal necrolysis, necrosis requiring surgery, exfoliative dermatitis	0 (0.0%)	0 (0.0%)
Rash of any grade		146 (35.4%)	52 (17.6%)
Treatment discontinuation as a result of rash		13 (3.2%)	1 (0.3%)

[a]Includes events reported regardless of causality.
[b]ACTG Toxicity Grading System; includes events reported as "rash," "maculopapular rash," and "urticaria."

ver, infection, infection viral, lip edema, malaise, *Mycobacterium* tuberculosis infection, neck rigidity, sebaceous cyst, and redistribution/accumulation of body fat (see PRECAUTIONS: Fat Redistribution).

Cardiovascular System: Abnormal cardiac rate and rhythm, cardiac insufficiency, cardiomyopathy, hypertension, migraine, pallor, peripheral vascular disorder, and postural hypotension.

Digestive System: Anorexia, bloody stool, colitis, constipation, decreased appetite, diarrhea (*Clostridium difficile*), diverticulitis, dry mouth, dyspepsia, dysphagia, enteritis at all levels, eructation, fecal incontinence, flatulence, gagging, gastroenteritis, gastroesophageal reflux, gastrointestinal bleeding, gastrointestinal disorder, gingivitis, gum hemorrhage, hepatomegaly, increased appetite, increased saliva, increased thirst, jaundice, mouth or tongue inflammation or ulcers, nonspecific hepatitis, oral/enteric moniliasis, pancreatitis, rectal disorder, sialadenitis, tooth abscess, and toothache.

Hemic and Lymphatic System: Adenopathy, bruising, eosinophilia, granulocytosis, leukopenia, pancytopenia, purpura, spleen disorder, thrombocytopenia, and prolonged prothrombin time.

Metabolic and Nutritional Disorders: Alcohol intolerance, amylase increased, bilirubinemia, hyperglycemia, hyperkalemia, hypertriglyceridemia, hyperuricemia, hypocalcemia, hyponatremia, hypophosphatemia, increased AST (SGOT), increased gamma glutamyl transpeptidase, increased lipase, increased serum alkaline phosphatase, increased serum creatinine, and weight increase or decrease.

Musculoskeletal System: Arthralgia or arthritis of single and multiple joints, bone disorder, bone pain, myalgia, tendon disorder, tenosynovitis, tetany, and vertigo.

Nervous System: Abnormal coordination, agitation, amnesia, change in dreams, cognitive impairment, confusion, decreased libido, disorientation, dizziness, emotional lability, euphoria, hallucination, hyperesthesia, hyperreflexia, hypertonia, hypesthesia, impaired concentration, manic symptoms, muscle cramp, nervousness, neuropathy, nystagmus, paralysis, paranoid symptoms, restlessness, sleep cycle disorder, somnolence, tingling, tremor, vertigo, and weakness.

Respiratory System: Chest congestion, dyspnea, epistaxis, hiccups, laryngismus, pneumonia, and rhinitis.

Skin and Appendages: Angioedema, dermal leukocytoclastic vasculitis, dermatitis, desquamation, diaphoresis, discolored skin, dry skin, erythema, erythema multiforme, folliculitis, fungal dermatitis, hair loss, herpes zoster or simplex, nail disorder, petechiae, non-application site pruritus, seborrhea, skin hypertrophy, skin disorder, skin nodule, Stevens-Johnson syndrome, urticaria, vesiculobullous rash, and wart.

Special Senses: Blepharitis, blurred vision, conjunctivitis, diplopia, dry eyes, ear pain, parosmia, otitis media, photophobia, taste perversion, and tinnitus.

Urogenital System: Amenorrhea, breast enlargement, calculi of the kidney, chromaturia, epididymitis, hematuria, hemospermia, impaired urination, impotence, kidney pain, metrorrhagia, nocturia, polyuria, proteinuria, testicular pain, urinary tract infection, and vaginal moniliasis.

Postmarketing Experience

Adverse event terms reported from postmarketing surveillance that were not reported in the Phase II and III trials are presented below.

Digestive System: Hepatic failure.

Hemic and Lymphatic System: Hemolytic anemia.

Musculoskeletal System: Rhabdomyolysis.

Urogenital System: Acute kidney failure.

Laboratory Abnormalities

Marked laboratory abnormalities observed in at least 2% of patients during Studies 21 Part II and 13C are summarized in Table 10. Marked laboratory abnormalities are defined as any Grade 3 or 4 abnormality found in patients at any time during study.

[See table 10 at top of page 2490]

OVERDOSAGE

Human experience of acute overdose with RESCRIPTOR is limited.

Management of Overdosage

Treatment of overdosage with RESCRIPTOR should consist of general supportive measures, including monitoring of vital signs and observation of the patient's clinical status. There is no specific antidote for overdosage with RESCRIPTOR. If indicated, elimination of unabsorbed drug should be achieved by emesis or gastric lavage. Since delavirdine is extensively metabolized by the liver and is highly protein-bound, dialysis is unlikely to result in significant removal of the drug.

DOSAGE AND ADMINISTRATION

The recommended dosage for RESCRIPTOR Tablets is 400 mg (four 100-mg or two 200-mg tablets) 3 times daily. RESCRIPTOR should be used in combination with other antiretroviral therapy. The complete prescribing information for other antiretroviral agents should be consulted for information on dosage and administration.

The 100-mg RESCRIPTOR Tablets may be dispersed in water prior to consumption. To prepare a dispersion, add four 100-mg RESCRIPTOR Tablets to at least 3 ounces of water, allow to stand for a few minutes, and then stir until a uniform dispersion occurs (see CLINICAL PHARMACOLOGY: Pharmacokinetics: Absorption and Bioavailability). The dispersion should be consumed promptly. The glass should be rinsed with water and the rinse swallowed to insure the entire dose is consumed. **The 200-mg tablets should be taken as intact tablets, because they are not readily dispersed in water.** Note: The 200-mg tablets are approximately one-third smaller in size than the 100-mg tablets.

RESCRIPTOR Tablets may be administered with or without food (see CLINICAL PHARMACOLOGY: Pharmacokinetics: Absorption and Bioavailability). Patients with achlorhydria should take RESCRIPTOR with an acidic beverage (e.g., orange or cranberry juice). However, the effect of an acidic beverage on the absorption of delavirdine in patients with achlorhydria has not been investigated.
Patients taking both RESCRIPTOR and antacids should be advised to take them at least 1 hour apart.

HOW SUPPLIED

RESCRIPTOR Tablets are available as follows:
100-mg: white, capsule-shaped tablets marked with "U 3761"
Bottles of 360 tablets - NDC 49702-209-24.
200-mg: white, capsule-shaped tablets marked with "RES200"
Bottles of 180 tablets - NDC 49702-225-17.
Store at controlled room temperature 20° to 25°C (68° to 77°F) [see USP]. Keep container tightly closed. Protect from high humidity.

ANIMAL TOXICOLOGY

Toxicities among various organs and organ systems in rats, mice, rabbits, dogs, and monkeys were observed following the administration of delavirdine. Necrotizing vasculitis was the most significant toxicity that occurred in dogs when mean nadir serum concentrations of delavirdine were at least 7-fold higher than the expected human exposure to RESCRIPTOR (C_{min} 15 μM) at the recommended dose. Vasculitis in dogs was not reversible during a 2.5-month recovery period; however, partial resolution of the vascular lesion characterized by reduced inflammation, diminished necrosis, and intimal thickening occurred during this period. Other major target organs included the gastrointestinal tract, endocrine organs, liver, kidneys, bone marrow, lymphoid tissue, lung, and reproductive organs.

Manufactured for
ViiV Healthcare
Research Triangle Park, NC 27709
by
Pfizer Pharmaceuticals LLC
Vega Baja, Puerto Rico 00693

August 2012
RES: 3PI

Patient Information
RESCRIPTOR®
(ree-SKRIP-tor)
(delavirdine mesylate) Tablets
Generic name: delavirdine mesylate (de-LAH-vur-deen MESS-ihl-ate)

ALERT: Find out about medicines that should NOT be taken with RESCRIPTOR. Please also read the section "MEDICINES YOU SHOULD NOT TAKE WITH RESCRIPTOR."

Read this information carefully before taking RESCRIPTOR. Also, read this leaflet each time you renew the prescription, just in case anything has changed. This is a summary and not a replacement for a careful discussion with your healthcare provider (doctor, nurse, pharmacist). You and your healthcare provider should discuss RESCRIPTOR when you start taking this medication and at regular checkups. You should remain under a doctor's care when taking RESCRIPTOR and should not change or stop treatment without first talking with your healthcare provider.

What is RESCRIPTOR and how does it work?

RESCRIPTOR is a medicine used in combination with other anti-HIV medicines to treat people with HIV-1 infection. Infection with HIV-1 leads to the destruction of infection-fighting immune system cells (called CD4+ cells or T cells), which are important to the immune system. After a large number of CD4+ cells have been destroyed, the infected person develops acquired immune deficiency syndrome (AIDS).
RESCRIPTOR helps to block HIV-1 reverse transcriptase, a chemical the virus uses to make more copies of itself. The main goals of anti-HIV medicines like RESCRIPTOR are to decrease the amount of virus in your blood (called viral load) and to increase the number of CD4+ cells as much as possible for as long as possible.
RESCRIPTOR, when taken with other anti-HIV medicines, lowers the HIV-1 viral load in patients. Patients who took RESCRIPTOR as part of combination therapy for HIV-1 also had increases in their CD4+ cell count.

General information about RESCRIPTOR

RESCRIPTOR does not cure HIV-1 or AIDS and you may continue to experience illnesses associated with HIV-1 infection, including opportunistic infections. You should remain under the care of a doctor when using RESCRIPTOR.
Avoid doing things that can spread HIV-1 infection.

- **Do not share needles or other injection equipment.**
- **Do not share personal items that can have blood or body fluids on them, like toothbrushes and razor blades.**

Table 9. Treatment-Emergent Events Regardless of Causality, of Moderate-to-Severe or Life-Threatening Intensity Reported by at Least 5% of Evaluable[a] Patients in Any Treatment Group

	Study 21 Part II			Study 13C	
	Zidovudine + Lamivudine (n = 123)	400 mg t.i.d. RESCRIPTOR + Zidovudine (n = 123)	400 mg t.i.d. RESCRIPTOR + Zidovudine + Lamivudine (n = 119)	Zidovudine + Didanosine, Zalcitabine, or Lamivudine (n = 172)	400 mg t.i.d. RESCRIPTOR + Zidovudine + Didanosine, Zalcitabine, or Lamivudine (n = 170)
Adverse Events	% of pts. (n)	% of pts. (n)	% of pts. (n)	% of pts. (n)	% of pts. (n)
Body as a Whole					
Abdominal pain, generalized	2.4 (3)	3.3 (4)	5.0 (6)	1.7 (3)	2.4 (4)
Asthenia/fatigue	16.3 (20)	15.4 (19)	16.0 (19)	8.1 (14)	5.3 (9)
Fever	2.4 (3)	1.6 (2)	3.4 (4)	6.4 (11)	7.1 (12)
Flu syndrome	4.9 (6)	7.3 (9)	5.0 (6)	5.2 (9)	2.4 (4)
Headache	14.6 (18)	12.2 (15)	16.8 (20)	12.8 (22)	11.2 (19)
Localized pain	4.9 (6)	5.7 (7)	5.0 (6)	2.9 (5)	1.8 (3)
Digestive					
Diarrhea	8.1 (10)	2.4 (3)	4.2 (5)	8.1 (14)	5.9 (10)
Nausea	17.1 (21)	20.3 (25)	16.8 (20)	9.3 (16)	14.7 (25)
Vomiting	8.9 (11)	4.9 (6)	2.5 (3)	4.1 (7)	6.5 (11)
Nervous					
Anxiety	1.6 (2)	2.4 (3)	6.7 (8)	4.1 (7)	3.5 (6)
Depressive symptoms	6.5 (8)	4.9 (6)	12.6 (15)	3.5 (6)	5.9 (10)
Insomnia	4.9 (6)	4.9 (6)	5.0 (6)	2.9 (5)	1.2 (2)
Respiratory					
Bronchitis	4.1 (5)	6.5 (8)	6.7 (8)	3.5 (6)	3.5 (6)
Cough	9.8 (12)	4.1 (5)	5.0 (6)	5.2 (9)	3.5 (6)
Pharyngitis	6.5 (8)	1.6 (2)	5.0 (6)	4.1 (7)	3.5 (6)
Sinusitis	8.9 (11)	7.3 (9)	5.0 (6)	2.3 (4)	1.2 (2)
Upper respiratory infection	11.4 (14)	6.5 (8)	7.6 (9)	8.7 (15)	4.7 (8)
Skin					
Rashes	3.3 (4)	19.5 (24)	13.4 (16)	7.6 (13)	18.8 (32)

[a]Evaluable patients in Study 21 Part II were those who received at least 1 dose of study medication and returned for at least 1 clinic study visit. Evaluable patients in Study 13C were those who received at least 1 dose of study medication.

- **Do not have any kind of sex without protection.** Always practice safe sex by using a latex or polyurethane condom to lower the chance of sexual contact with semen, vaginal secretions, or blood.

How should I take RESCRIPTOR?

- You should stay under a healthcare provider's care when taking RESCRIPTOR. Do not change your treatment or stop treatment without first talking with your healthcare provider.
- You must take RESCRIPTOR every day exactly as your healthcare provider prescribes it. Follow the directions from your healthcare provider, exactly as written on the label.
- **The usual dose of RESCRIPTOR is two 200–mg tablets 3 times a day or four 100–mg tablets 3 times a day, in combination with other anti-HIV-1 medicines. Either way, your total daily dose of RESCRIPTOR remains the same.**
- You can take RESCRIPTOR with or without food.
- If you have trouble swallowing tablets, the 100–mg RESCRIPTOR tablets may be dissolved in water. Place 4 tablets in at least 3 ounces of water and allow the tablets to sit in the water for a few minutes. Then, stir the water until the tablets have dissolved and drink the mixture right away. Add a little more water, swirl, and then drink the rest of the mixture to be sure that you get all the medicine. **The 200–mg tablets must be swallowed whole. They cannot be dissolved in water.**
- Many people find it easier to take their RESCRIPTOR with breakfast, lunch, and dinner, since food does not interfere with RESCRIPTOR. It is a good idea to get into the habit of taking RESCRIPTOR on a regular schedule to make it easier to remember. Figure out things that happen every day at pill-taking time and take your tablets then. By taking your medicine along with activities you do every day, such as getting up in the morning, brushing your teeth, eating lunch, coming home from work in the evening, or watching a favorite TV show, you will find it easier to remember to take every dose.
- When your supply of RESCRIPTOR starts to run low, get more from your healthcare provider or pharmacy. This is very important because the amount of virus in your blood may increase if the medicine is stopped for even a short time. The virus may develop resistance to RESCRIPTOR and become harder to treat.
- Only take medicine that has been prescribed specifically for you. Do not give RESCRIPTOR to others or take medicine prescribed for someone else.

What should I do if I miss a dose of RESCRIPTOR?

If you forget to take a dose of RESCRIPTOR, take it as soon as possible. However, if you skip the dose entirely, do not double the next dose. If you forget a lot of doses, talk to your healthcare provider about how you should continue taking your medicine.

Table 10. Marked Laboratory Abnormalities Reported by ≥2% of Patients

Adverse Events/Toxicity Limits	Study 21 Part II			Study 13C	
	Zidovudine + Lamivudine (n = 123)	400 mg t.i.d. RESCRIPTOR + Zidovudine (n = 123)	400 mg t.i.d. RESCRIPTOR + Zidovudine + Lamivudine (n = 119)	Zidovudine + Didanosine, Zalcitabine, or Lamivudine (n = 172)	400 mg t.i.d. RESCRIPTOR + Zidovudine + Didanosine, Zalcitabine, or Lamivudine (n = 170)
	% pts.	% pts.	% pts.	% pts.	% pts.
Hematology					
Hemoglobin <7 mg/dL	4.1	2.5	0.9	1.7	2.9
Neutrophils <750/mm^3	5.7	4.9	3.4	10.4	7.6
Prothrombin time (PT) >1.5 × ULN	0	0	1.7	2.9	2.4
Activated partial thromboplastin (APTT) >2.33 × ULN	0	0.8	0	5.8	2.4
Chemistry					
Alananine aminotransferase (ALT/SGPT) >5 × ULN	2.5	4.1	5.1	3.5	4.1
Amylase >2 × ULN	0.8	2.5	2.6	3.5	2.9
Aspartate aminotransferase (AST/SGOT) >5 × ULN	1.6	2.5	3.4	3.5	2.3
Bilirubin >2.5 × ULN	0.8	2.5	1.7	1.2	0
Gamma glutamyl transferase (GGT) >5 × ULN	N/A	N/A	N/A	4.1	1.8
Glucose (hypo-/hyperglycemia) <40 mg/dL >250 mg/dL	4.1	0.8	1.7	1.2	0

N/A = not applicable because no predose values were obtained for patients.

Who should not take RESCRIPTOR?

Together with your healthcare provider, you need to decide whether RESCRIPTOR is right for you.

- **Do not take RESCRIPTOR if you are taking certain medicines.** These could cause serious side effects that could cause death. Before you take RESCRIPTOR, you must tell your healthcare provider about all the medicines you are taking or are planning to take. These include other prescription and nonprescription medicines and herbal supplements.
  For more information about medicines you should not take with RESCRIPTOR, please read the section titled **"MEDICINES YOU SHOULD NOT TAKE WITH RESCRIPTOR."**
- **Do not take RESCRIPTOR if you have an allergy to RESCRIPTOR.** Also tell your healthcare provider if you have any known allergies to other medicines, foods, preservatives, or dyes.
- Tell your healthcare provider if you are pregnant or plan to become pregnant. The effects of RESCRIPTOR on pregnant women or their unborn babies are not known.
- If you are breastfeeding, **do not breastfeed.** We do not know if RESCRIPTOR can be passed to your baby in your breast milk and whether it could harm your baby. Also, mothers with HIV-1 should not breastfeed because HIV-1 can be passed to the baby in the breast milk. Talk with your healthcare provider about the best way to feed your baby.
- **Talk with your healthcare provider if you have liver or kidney disease.** RESCRIPTOR has not been studied in people with liver or kidney disease.
- **Certain medical problems may affect the use of RESCRIPTOR.** Be sure to tell your healthcare provider of any other medical problems you may have.

Can I take RESCRIPTOR with other medicines?

RESCRIPTOR may interact with other medicines, including those you take without a prescription. You must tell your healthcare provider about all medicines you are taking or planning to take before you take RESCRIPTOR. It is a good idea to keep a complete list of all the medicines that you take, including nonprescription medicines, herbal remedies and supplements, and street drugs. Update this list when medicines are added or stopped. Give copies of this list to all of your healthcare providers every time you visit or fill a prescription.

MEDICINES YOU SHOULD NOT TAKE WITH RESCRIPTOR

Do not take the following medicines with RESCRIPTOR because they can cause serious problems or death if taken with RESCRIPTOR:

- VERSED® (midazolam) Injection and Syrup (for sedation)
- HALCION® (triazolam) Tablets (for sleep problems)
- XANAX® (alprazolam) Tablets (for anxiety)
- D.H.E. 45® Injection, ERGOMAR®, MIGRANAL®, WIGRAINE®, and CAFERGOT® (for migraine headaches)
- METHERGINE® (for bleeding after childbirth)
- ORAP® (pimozide) Tablets (for seizures)
- PROPULSID® (cisapride) Tablets and Suspension (for heartburn)
- HISMANAL® (astemizole) Tablets (for allergies)
- SELDANE® (terfenadine) Tablets (for allergies)

Do not take the following medicines when you take RESCRIPTOR. They may reduce the levels of RESCRIPTOR in the blood and make it less effective. Talk with your healthcare provider if you are currently taking these medicines because other medicines may have to be given to take their place:

- Rifampin (also known as RIMACTANE®, RIFADIN®, RIFATER®, RIFAMATE®) (to treat tuberculosis)
- Phenobarbital (for seizures)
- DILANTIN® (phenytoin) (for seizures)
- TEGRETOL® (carbamazepine) (for seizures)

Do not take RESCRIPTOR with St. John's wort (*Hypericum perforatum*), an herbal product sold as a dietary supplement, or products containing St. John's wort. Talk with your healthcare provider if you are taking or planning to take St. John's wort. Taking St. John's wort may decrease levels of RESCRIPTOR and lead to increased viral load and possible resistance to RESCRIPTOR or cross-resistance to other anti-HIV medicines.

Do not take RESCRIPTOR with cholesterol-lowering medicines MEVACOR® (lovastatin) or ZOCOR® (simvastatin) because of possible serious reactions. There is also an increased risk of drug interactions between RESCRIPTOR and LIPITOR® (atorvastatin), BAYCOL® (cerivastatin), and LESCOL® (fluvastatin); talk to your healthcare provider before you take any of these cholesterol-reducing medicines with RESCRIPTOR.

Medicines that require dosage adjustments:

It is possible that your healthcare provider may need to increase or decrease the dose of other medicines when you are taking RESCRIPTOR. Remember to tell your healthcare provider all the medicines you are taking or planning to take.

Before you take VIAGRA® (sildenafil) with RESCRIPTOR, talk to your healthcare provider about problems these 2 medicines can cause when taken together. You may get increased side effects of VIAGRA, such as low blood pressure, vision changes, and penis erection lasting more than 4 hours. If an erection lasts longer than 4 hours, get medical help right away to avoid permanent damage to your penis. Your healthcare provider can explain these symptoms to you.

- **If you are taking both VIDEX® (didanosine, ddl) and RESCRIPTOR:** Take VIDEX (buffered tablets) 1 hour before or 1 hour after you take RESCRIPTOR. Taking them together causes lower amounts of RESCRIPTOR in the blood, making both medicines less effective.
- **Protease inhibitors:** A number of healthy volunteers and HIV-1-infected patients were studied while taking RESCRIPTOR with one of these protease inhibitors: CRIXIVAN® (indinavir), INVIRASE® and FORTOVASE® (saquinavir), NORVIR® (ritonavir), or VIRACEPT® (nelfinavir). RESCRIPTOR was shown to increase the amount of these protease inhibitors in the blood. RESCRIPTOR is expected to increase the amount of AGENERASE® (amprenavir) and KALETRA® (lopinavir + ritonavir) in the blood. **As a result, your healthcare provider may choose to lower the dose of one of these medicines or monitor certain lab tests if these protease inhibitors are taken in combination with RESCRIPTOR.**
- **Antacids** should be taken at least 1 hour before or 1 hour after you take RESCRIPTOR because they can slow the absorption of RESCRIPTOR.

Based on your history of taking other anti-HIV medicine, your healthcare provider will direct you on how to take RESCRIPTOR and other anti-HIV medicines. These drugs should be taken in a certain order or at specific times. This will depend on how many times a day each medicine should be taken. It will also depend on whether the medicines should be taken with or without food.

What are the possible side effects of RESCRIPTOR?

- This list of side effects is not complete. If you have questions about side effects, ask your doctor, nurse, or pharmacist. You should report any new or continuing symptoms to your healthcare provider right away. Your healthcare provider may be able to help you manage these side effects.
- The most important common side effect seen in people taking RESCRIPTOR has been a skin rash. The rash occurs mainly on the upper body and upper arms, and sometimes on the neck and face. The rash appears as a red area on the skin with slight bumps, and it can be itchy. The rash tends to occur early, usually within 1 to 3 weeks after you start taking RESCRIPTOR, and it usually lasts less than 2 weeks. Watch your rash carefully and talk to your healthcare provider about how to treat it. If the rash is going to be serious or severe (with fever, blistering, sores in the mouth, redness or swelling of the eyes, or muscle and joint aches), you and your healthcare provider will usually realize it during the first 3 days of the rash. If you have symptoms of a severe rash, you should stop taking RESCRIPTOR and speak with your healthcare provider as soon possible. Be prepared to explain where the rash is, your temperature, and whether or not you have other symptoms.
- Other side effects include headache, nausea, diarrhea, and tiredness. Of these, nausea was the most common.
- Changes in body fat have been seen in some patients taking antiretroviral therapy. These changes may include increased amount of fat in the upper back and neck ("buffalo hump"), breast, and around the trunk. Loss of fat from the legs, arms and face may also happen. The cause and long-term health effects of these conditions are not known at this time.
- Before you start using any medicine, talk with your healthcare provider about what to expect and discuss ways to reduce the side effects you may have.

How do I store RESCRIPTOR?

- Keep RESCRIPTOR and all other medicines out of the reach of children. Keep the bottle closed and store at room temperature (between 68°F and 77°F) away from sources

of moisture such as a sink or other damp place. Heat and moisture may reduce the effectiveness of RESCRIPTOR.
- Do not keep medicine that is out of date or that you no longer need. Be sure that if you throw any medicine away, it is out of the reach of children.

General advice about prescription medicines:
Discuss all questions about your health with your healthcare provider. If you have questions about RESCRIPTOR or any other medicines you are taking, ask your healthcare provider. You can also call 1-877-844-8872 toll free.
AGENERASE and RESCRIPTOR are registered trademarks of ViiV Healthcare.
The brands listed are trademarks of their respective owners and are not trademarks of ViiV Healthcare. The makers of these brands are not affiliated with and do not endorse ViiV Healthcare or its products.
Manufactured for

ViiV Healthcare
Research Triangle Park, NC 27709
by
Pfizer Pharmaceuticals LLC
Vega Baja, Puerto Rico 00693

August 2012
RES: 3PIL

RETROVIR ℞
[re'trō-vir]
(zidovudine)
Tablets, Capsules, and Syrup

HIGHLIGHTS OF PRESCRIBING INFORMATION
These highlights do not include all the information needed to use RETROVIR safely and effectively. See full prescribing information for RETROVIR.
RETROVIR (zidovudine) Tablets, Capsules, and Syrup
Initial U.S. Approval: 1987

WARNING: RISK OF HEMATOLOGICAL TOXICITY, MYOPATHY, LACTIC ACIDOSIS
See full prescribing information for complete boxed warning.
- **Hematologic toxicity including neutropenia and severe anemia have been associated with the use of zidovudine. (5.1)**
- **Symptomatic myopathy associated with prolonged use of zidovudine. (5.2)**
- **Lactic acidosis and severe hepatomegaly with steatosis, including fatal cases, have been reported with the use of nucleoside analogues including RETROVIR. Suspend treatment if clinical or laboratory findings suggestive of lactic acidosis or pronounced hepatotoxicity occur. (5.3)**

—INDICATIONS AND USAGE—
RETROVIR is a nucleoside analogue reverse transcriptase inhibitor indicated for:
- Treatment of Human Immunodeficiency Virus (HIV-1) infection in combination with other antiretroviral agents. (1.1)
- Prevention of maternal-fetal HIV-1 transmission. (1.2)

—DOSAGE AND ADMINISTRATION—
- Treatment of HIV-1 infection:
  Adults: 600 mg/day in divided doses with other antiretroviral agents.
  Pediatric patients (aged 4 weeks to <18 years): Dosage should be calculated based on body weight not to exceed adult dose. (2.1)
- Prevention of maternal-fetal HIV-1 transmission:
  Specific dosage instructions for mother and infant. (2.2)
- Patients with severe anemia and/or neutropenia:
  Dosage interruption may be necessary. (2.3)
- Renal impairment: Recommended dosage in hemodialysis or peritoneal dialysis patients is 100 mg every 6 to 8 hours. (2.4)

—DOSAGE FORMS AND STRENGTHS—
Tablets: 300 mg (3)
Capsules: 100 mg (3)
Syrup: 10 mg/mL (3)

—CONTRAINDICATIONS—
Hypersensitivity to zidovudine (e.g., anaphylaxis, Stevens-Johnson syndrome). (4)

—WARNINGS AND PRECAUTIONS—
- See boxed warning for information about the following: hematologic toxicity, myopathy, and lactic acidosis and severe hepatomegaly (5.1, 5.2, 5.3)
- Exacerbation of anemia has been reported in HIV-1/HCV co-infected patients receiving ribavirin and zidovudine. Coadministration of ribavirin and zidovudine is not advised. (5.4)
- Hepatic decompensation, (some fatal), has occurred in HIV-1/HCV co-infected patients receiving combination antiretroviral therapy and interferon alfa with/without ribavirin. Discontinue zidovudine as medically appropriate and consider dose reduction or discontinuation of interferon alfa, ribavirin, or both. (5.4)
- RETROVIR should not be administered with other zidovudine-containing combination products. (5.5)
- Immune reconstitution syndrome (5.6) and redistribution/accumulation of body fat (5.7) have been reported in patients treated with combination antiretroviral therapy.

—ADVERSE REACTIONS—
- Most commonly reported adverse reactions (incidence ≥15%) in adult HIV-1 clinical trials were headache, malaise, nausea, anorexia, and vomiting. (6.1)
- Most commonly reported adverse reactions (incidence ≥15%) in pediatric HIV-1 clinical trials were fever, cough, and digestive disorders. (6.1)
- Most commonly reported adverse reactions in neonates (incidence ≥15%) in the prevention of maternal-fetal transmission of HIV-1 clinical trial were anemia and neutropenia. (6.1)

To report SUSPECTED ADVERSE REACTIONS, contact ViiV Healthcare at 1-877-844-8872 or FDA at 1-800-FDA-1088 or www.fda.gov/medwatch.

—DRUG INTERACTIONS—
- Stavudine: Concomitant use with zidovudine should be avoided. (7.1)
- Doxorubicin: Use with zidovudine should be avoided. (7.2)
- Bone marrow suppressive/cytotoxic agents: May increase the hematologic toxicity of zidovudine. (7.3)

—USE IN SPECIFIC POPULATIONS—
Pregnancy: Physicians are encouraged to register patients in the Antiretroviral Pregnancy Registry by calling 1-800-258-4263. (8.1)

See 17 for PATIENT COUNSELING INFORMATION
Revised: 05/2013

FULL PRESCRIBING INFORMATION: CONTENTS*

* Sections or subsections omitted from the full prescribing information are not listed

FULL PRESCRIBING INFORMATION

WARNING: RISK OF HEMATOLOGICAL TOXICITY, MYOPATHY, LACTIC ACIDOSIS

Hematologic Toxicity: RETROVIR® (zidovudine) Tablets, Capsules, and Syrup have been associated with hematologic toxicity including neutropenia and severe anemia, particularly in patients with advanced HIV-1 disease *[see Warnings and Precautions (5.1)]*.

Myopathy: Prolonged use of RETROVIR has been associated with symptomatic myopathy *[see Warnings and Precautions (5.2)]*.

Lactic Acidosis and Severe Hepatomegaly: Lactic acidosis and severe hepatomegaly with steatosis, including fatal cases, have been reported with the use of nucleoside analogues alone or in combination, including RETROVIR and other antiretrovirals. Suspend treatment if clinical or laboratory findings suggestive of lactic acidosis or pronounced hepatotoxicity occur *[see Warnings and Precautions (5.3)]*.

1 INDICATIONS AND USAGE
1.1 Treatment of HIV-1
RETROVIR, a nucleoside reverse transcriptase inhibitor, is indicated in combination with other antiretroviral agents for the treatment of HIV-1 infection.

1.2 Prevention of Maternal-Fetal HIV-1 Transmission
RETROVIR is indicated for the prevention of maternal-fetal HIV-1 transmission *[see Dosage and Administration (2.2)]*. The indication is based on a dosing regimen that included 3 components:
1. antepartum therapy of HIV-1 infected mothers
2. intrapartum therapy of HIV-1 infected mothers
3. post-partum therapy of HIV-1 exposed neonate.

Points to consider prior to initiating RETROVIR in pregnant women for the prevention of maternal-fetal HIV-1 transmission include:
- In most cases, RETROVIR for prevention of maternal-fetal HIV-1 transmission should be given in combination with other antiretroviral drugs.
- Prevention of HIV-1 transmission in women who have received RETROVIR for a prolonged period before pregnancy has not been evaluated.
- Because the fetus is most susceptible to the potential teratogenic effects of drugs during the first 10 weeks of gestation and the risks of therapy with RETROVIR during that period are not fully known, women in the first trimester of pregnancy who do not require immediate initiation of antiretroviral therapy for their own health may consider delaying use; this indication is based on use after 14 weeks gestation.

2 DOSAGE AND ADMINISTRATION
2.1 Treatment of HIV-1 Infection
Adults: The recommended oral dose of RETROVIR is 600 mg/day in divided doses in combination with other antiretroviral agents.

Pediatric Patients (Aged 4 Weeks to <18 Years): Healthcare professionals should pay special attention to accurate calculation of the dose of RETROVIR, transcription of the medication order, dispensing information, and dosing instructions to minimize risk for medication dosing errors.

Prescribers should calculate the appropriate dose of RETROVIR for each child based on body weight (kg) and should not exceed the recommended adult dose.

Before prescribing RETROVIR Capsules or Tablets, children should be assessed for the ability to swallow capsules or tablets. If a child is unable to reliably swallow a RETROVIR Capsule or Tablet, the RETROVIR Syrup formulation should be prescribed.

The recommended dosage in pediatric patients aged 4 weeks to <18 years and weighing ≥4 kg is provided in Table 1. RETROVIR Syrup should be used to provide accurate dosage when whole tablets or capsules are not appropriate.

Table 1. Recommended Pediatric Dosage of RETROVIR

Body Weight (kg)	Total Daily Dose	Dosage Regimen and Dose	
		Twice Daily	Three Times Daily
4 to <9	24 mg/kg/day	12 mg/kg	8 mg/kg
≥9 to <30	18 mg/kg/day	9 mg/kg	6 mg/kg
≥30	600 mg/day	300 mg	200 mg

Alternatively, dosing for RETROVIR can be based on body surface area (BSA) for each child. The recommended oral dose of RETROVIR is 480 mg/m^2/day in divided doses (240 mg/m^2 twice daily or 160 mg/m^2 three times daily). In some cases the dose calculated by mg/kg will not be the same as that calculated by BSA.

2.2 Prevention of Maternal-Fetal HIV-1 Transmission

The recommended dosage regimen for administration to pregnant women (>14 weeks of pregnancy) and their neonates is:

Maternal Dosing: 100 mg orally 5 times per day until the start of labor *[see Clinical Studies(14.3)]*. During labor and delivery, intravenous RETROVIR should be administered at 2 mg/kg (total body weight) over 1 hour followed by a continuous intravenous infusion of 1 mg/kg/hour (total body weight) until clamping of the umbilical cord.

Neonatal Dosing: Start neonatal dosing within 12 hours after birth and continue through 6 weeks of age. Neonates unable to receive oral dosing may be administered RETROVIR intravenously. See Table 2.

Table 2. Recommended Neonatal Dosages of RETROVIR

Route	Total Daily Dose	Dose and Dosage Regimen
Oral	8 mg/kg/day	2 mg/kg every 6 hours
IV	6 mg/kg/day	1.5 mg/kg infused over 30 minutes, every 6 hours

2.3 Patients With Severe Anemia and/or Neutropenia

Significant anemia (hemoglobin <7.5 g/dL or reduction >25% of baseline) and/or significant neutropenia (granulocyte count <750 cells/mm^3 or reduction >50% from baseline) may require a dose interruption until evidence of marrow recovery is observed *[see Warnings and Precautions (5.1)]*. In patients who develop significant anemia, dose interruption does not necessarily eliminate the need for transfusion. If marrow recovery occurs following dose interruption, resumption in dose may be appropriate using adjunctive measures such as epoetin alfa at recommended doses, depending on hematologic indices such as serum erythropoetin level and patient tolerance.

2.4 Patients With Renal Impairment

End-Stage Renal Disease: In patients maintained on hemodialysis or peritoneal dialysis, the recommended dosage is 100 mg every 6 to 8 hours *[see Clinical Pharmacology (12.3)]*.

2.5 Patients With Hepatic Impairment

There are insufficient data to recommend dose adjustment of RETROVIR in patients with mild to moderate impaired hepatic function or liver cirrhosis.

3 DOSAGE FORMS AND STRENGTHS

RETROVIR Tablets 300 mg (biconvex, white, round, film-coated) containing 300 mg zidovudine, one side engraved "GX CW3" and "300" on the other side.

RETROVIR Capsules 100 mg (white, opaque cap and body) containing 100 mg zidovudine and printed with "Wellcome" and unicorn logo on cap and "Y9C" and "100" on body.

RETROVIR Syrup (colorless to pale yellow, strawberry-flavored) containing 10 mg zidovudine in each mL.

4 CONTRAINDICATIONS

RETROVIR Tablets, Capsules, and Syrup are contraindicated in patients who have had potentially life-threatening allergic reactions (e.g., anaphylaxis, Stevens-Johnson syndrome) to any of the components of the formulations.

5 WARNINGS AND PRECAUTIONS

5.1 Hematologic Toxicity/Bone Marrow Suppression

RETROVIR should be used with caution in patients who have bone marrow compromise evidenced by granulocyte count <1,000 cells/mm^3 or hemoglobin <9.5 g/dL. Hematologic toxicities appear to be related to pretreatment bone marrow reserve and to dose and duration of therapy. In patients with advanced symptomatic HIV-1 disease, anemia and neutropenia were the most significant adverse events observed. In patients who experience hematologic toxicity, a reduction in hemoglobin may occur as early as 2 to 4 weeks, and neutropenia usually occurs after 6 to 8 weeks. There have been reports of pancytopenia associated with the use of RETROVIR, which was reversible in most instances after discontinuance of the drug. However, significant anemia, in many cases requiring dose adjustment, discontinuation of RETROVIR, and/or blood transfusions, has occurred during treatment with RETROVIR alone or in combination with other antiretrovirals.

Frequent blood counts are strongly recommended to detect severe anemia or neutropenia in patients with poor bone marrow reserve, particularly in patients with advanced HIV-1 disease who are treated with RETROVIR. For HIV-1-infected individuals and patients with asymptomatic or early HIV-1 disease, periodic blood counts are recommended. If anemia or neutropenia develops, dosage interruption may be needed *[see Dosage and Administration (2.3)]*.

5.2 Myopathy

Myopathy and myositis with pathological changes, similar to that produced by HIV-1 disease, have been associated with prolonged use of RETROVIR.

5.3 Lactic Acidosis/Severe Hepatomegaly With Steatosis

Lactic acidosis and severe hepatomegaly with steatosis, including fatal cases, have been reported with the use of nucleoside analogues alone or in combination, including zidovudine and other antiretrovirals. A majority of these cases have been in women. Obesity and prolonged exposure to antiretroviral nucleoside analogues may be risk factors. Particular caution should be exercised when administering RETROVIR to any patient with known risk factors for liver disease; however, cases have also been reported in patients with no known risk factors. Treatment with RETROVIR should be suspended in any patient who develops clinical or laboratory findings suggestive of lactic acidosis or pronounced hepatotoxicity (which may include hepatomegaly and steatosis even in the absence of marked transaminase elevations).

5.4 Use With Interferon- and Ribavirin-Based Regimens in HIV-1/HCV Co-Infected Patients

In vitro studies have shown ribavirin can reduce the phosphorylation of pyrimidine nucleoside analogues such as zidovudine. Although no evidence of a pharmacokinetic or pharmacodynamic interaction (e.g., loss of HIV-1/HCV virologic suppression) was seen when ribavirin was coadministered with zidovudine in HIV-1/HCV co-infected subjects *[see Clinical Pharmacology (12.3)]*, exacerbation of anemia due to ribavirin has been reported when zidovudine is part of the HIV regimen. Coadministration of ribavirin and zidovudine is not advised. Consideration should be given to replacing zidovudine in established combination HIV-1/HCV therapy, especially in patients with a known history of zidovudine-induced anemia.

Hepatic decompensation (some fatal) has occurred in HIV-1/HCV co-infected patients receiving combination antiretroviral therapy for HIV-1 and interferon alfa with or without ribavirin. Patients receiving interferon alfa with or without ribavirin and zidovudine should be closely monitored for treatment-associated toxicities, especially hepatic decompensation, neutropenia, and anemia.

Discontinuation of zidovudine should be considered as medically appropriate. Dose reduction or discontinuation of interferon alfa, ribavirin, or both should also be considered if worsening clinical toxicities are observed, including hepatic decompensation (e.g., Child-Pugh >6) (see the complete prescribing information for interferon and ribavirin).

5.5 Use With Other Zidovudine-Containing Products

RETROVIR should not be administered with combination products that contain zidovudine as one of their components (e.g., COMBIVIR® [lamivudine and zidovudine] Tablets or TRIZIVIR® [abacavir sulfate, lamivudine, and zidovudine] Tablets).

5.6 Immune Reconstitution Syndrome

Immune reconstitution syndrome has been reported in patients treated with combination antiretroviral therapy, including RETROVIR. During the initial phase of combination antiretroviral treatment, patients whose immune systems respond may develop an inflammatory response to indolent or residual opportunistic infections (such as *Mycobacterium avium* infection, cytomegalovirus, *Pneumocystis jirovecii* pneumonia [PCP], or tuberculosis), which may necessitate further evaluation and treatment.

Autoimmune disorders (such as Graves' disease, polymyositis, and Guillain-Barré syndrome) have also been reported to occur in the setting of immune reconstitution; however, the time to onset is more variable, and can occur many months after initiation of treatment.

5.7 Fat Redistribution

Redistribution/accumulation of body fat, including central obesity, dorsocervical fat enlargement (buffalo hump), peripheral wasting, facial wasting, breast enlargement, and "cushingoid appearance," have been observed in patients receiving antiretroviral therapy. The mechanism and long-term consequences of these events are currently unknown. A causal relationship has not been established.

6 ADVERSE REACTIONS

The following adverse reactions are discussed in greater detail in other sections of the labeling:

- Hematologic toxicity, including neutropenia and anemia *[see Boxed Warning, Warnings and Precautions (5.1)]*.
- Symptomatic myopathy *[see Boxed Warning, Warnings and Precautions (5.2)]*.
- Lactic acidosis and severe hepatomegaly with steatosis *[see Boxed Warning, Warnings and Precautions (5.3)]*.
- Hepatic decompensation in patients co-infected with HIV-1 and hepatitis C *[see Warnings and Precautions (5.4)]*.

6.1 Clinical Trials Experience

Because clinical trials are conducted under widely varying conditions, adverse reaction rates observed in the clinical trials of a drug cannot be directly compared with rates in the clinical trials of another drug and may not reflect the rates observed in practice.

Adults: The frequency and severity of adverse reactions associated with the use of RETROVIR are greater in patients with more advanced infection at the time of initiation of therapy.

Table 3 summarizes adverse reactions reported at a statistically significant greater incidence for subjects receiving RETROVIR in a monotherapy trial.

Table 3. Percentage (%) of Subjects With Adverse Reactions[a] in Asymptomatic HIV-1 Infection (ACTG 019)

Adverse Reaction	RETROVIR 500 mg/day (n = 453)	Placebo (n = 428)
Body as a whole		
Asthenia	9%[b]	6%
Headache	63%	53%
Malaise	53%	45%
Gastrointestinal		
Anorexia	20%	11%
Constipation	6%[b]	4%
Nausea	51%	30%
Vomiting	17%	10%

[a] Reported in ≥5% of trial population.

[b] Not statistically significant versus placebo.

In addition to the adverse reactions listed in Table 3, adverse reactions observed at an incidence of ≥5% in any treatment arm in clinical trials (NUCA3001, NUCA3002, NUCB3001, and NUCB3002) were abdominal cramps, abdominal pain, arthralgia, chills, dyspepsia, fatigue, insomnia, musculoskeletal pain, myalgia, and neuropathy. Additionally, in these trials hyperbilirubinemia was reported at an incidence of ≤0.8%.

Selected laboratory abnormalities observed during a clinical trial of monotherapy with RETROVIR are shown in Table 4.

Table 4. Frequencies of Selected (Grade 3/4) Laboratory Abnormalities in Subjects With Asymptomatic HIV-1 Infection (ACTG 019)

Test (Abnormal Level)	RETROVIR 500 mg/day (n = 453)	Placebo (n = 428)
Anemia (Hgb<8 g/dL)	1%	<1%
Granulocytopenia (<750 cells/mm^3)	2%	2%
Thrombocytopenia (platelets<50,000/mm^3)	0%	<1%
ALT (>5 × ULN)	3%	3%
AST (>5 × ULN)	1%	2%

ULN = Upper limit of normal.

Pediatrics: The clinical adverse reactions reported among adult recipients of RETROVIR may also occur in pediatric patients.

Trial ACTG 300: Selected clinical adverse reactions and physical findings with a ≥5% frequency during therapy with EPIVIR® (lamivudine) Oral Suspension 4 mg/kg twice daily plus RETROVIR 160 mg/m^2 3 times daily compared with didanosine in therapy-naive (≤56 days of antiretroviral therapy) pediatric subjects are listed in Table 5.

Table 5. Selected Clinical Adverse Reactions and Physical Findings (≥5% Frequency) in Pediatric Subjects in Trial ACTG 300

Adverse Reaction	EPIVIR plus RETROVIR (n = 236)	Didanosine (n = 235)
Body as a whole		
Fever	25%	32%
Digestive		
Hepatomegaly	11%	11%
Nausea & vomiting	8%	7%
Diarrhea	8%	6%
Stomatitis	6%	12%
Splenomegaly	5%	8%
Respiratory		
Cough	15%	18%
Abnormal breath sounds/wheezing	7%	9%
Ear, Nose, and Throat		
Signs or symptoms of ears[a]	7%	6%
Nasal discharge or congestion	8%	11%
Other		
Skin rashes	12%	14%
Lymphadenopathy	9%	11%

[a] Includes pain, discharge, erythema, or swelling of an ear.

Selected laboratory abnormalities experienced by therapy-naive (≤56 days of antiretroviral therapy) pediatric subjects are listed in Table 6.

Table 6. Frequencies of Selected (Grade 3/4) Laboratory Abnormalities in Pediatric Subjects in Trial ACTG 300

Test (Abnormal Level)	EPIVIR plus RETROVIR	Didanosine
Neutropenia (ANC<400 cells/mm^3)	8%	3%
Anemia (Hgb<7.0 g/dL)	4%	2%
Thrombocytopenia (platelets<50,000/mm^3)	1%	3%
ALT (>10 × ULN)	1%	3%
AST (>10 × ULN)	2%	4%
Lipase (>2.5 × ULN)	3%	3%
Total amylase (>2.5 × ULN)	3%	3%

ULN = Upper limit of normal.
ANC = Absolute neutrophil count.

Macrocytosis was reported in the majority of pediatric subjects receiving RETROVIR 180 mg/m^2 every 6 hours in open-label trials. Additionally, adverse reactions reported at an incidence of <6% in these trials were congestive heart failure, decreased reflexes, ECG abnormality, edema, hematuria, left ventricular dilation, nervousness/irritability, and weight loss.

Use for the Prevention of Maternal-Fetal Transmission of HIV-1: In a randomized, double-blind, placebo-controlled trial in HIV-1-infected women and their neonates conducted to determine the utility of RETROVIR for the prevention of maternal-fetal HIV-1 transmission, RETROVIR Syrup at 2 mg/kg was administered every 6 hours for 6 weeks to neonates beginning within 12 hours following birth. The most commonly reported adverse reactions were anemia (hemoglobin <9.0 g/dL) and neutropenia (<1,000 cells/mm^3). Anemia occurred in 22% of the neonates who received RETROVIR and in 12% of the neonates who received placebo. The mean difference in hemoglobin values was less than 1.0 g/dL for neonates receiving RETROVIR compared with neonates receiving placebo. No neonates with anemia required transfusion and all hemoglobin values spontaneously returned to normal within 6 weeks after completion of therapy with RETROVIR. Neutropenia in neonates was reported with similar frequency in the group that received RETROVIR (21%) and in the group that received placebo (27%). The long-term consequences of in utero and infant exposure to RETROVIR are unknown.

6.2 Postmarketing Experience

In addition to adverse reactions reported from clinical trials, the following reactions have been identified during postmarketing use of RETROVIR. Because they are reported voluntarily from a population of unknown size, estimates of frequency cannot be made. These reactions have been chosen for inclusion due to a combination of their seriousness, frequency of reporting, or potential causal connection to RETROVIR.

Body as a Whole: Back pain, chest pain, flu-like syndrome, generalized pain, redistribution/accumulation of body fat *[see Warnings and Precautions (5.7)]*.

Cardiovascular: Cardiomyopathy, syncope.

Endocrine: Gynecomastia.

Eye: Macular edema.

Gastrointestinal: Dysphagia, flatulence, oral mucosa pigmentation, mouth ulcer.

General: Sensitization reactions including anaphylaxis and angioedema, vasculitis.

Hemic and Lymphatic: Aplastic anemia, hemolytic anemia, leukopenia, lymphadenopathy, pancytopenia with marrow hypoplasia, pure red cell aplasia.

Hepatobiliary Tract and Pancreas: Hepatitis, hepatomegaly with steatosis, jaundice, lactic acidosis, pancreatitis.

Musculoskeletal: Increased CPK, increased LDH, muscle spasm, myopathy and myositis with pathological changes (similar to that produced by HIV-1 disease), rhabdomyolysis, tremor.

Nervous: Anxiety, confusion, depression, dizziness, loss of mental acuity, mania, paresthesia, seizures, somnolence, vertigo.

Respiratory: Dyspnea, rhinitis, sinusitis.

Skin: Changes in skin and nail pigmentation, pruritus, Stevens-Johnson syndrome, toxic epidermal necrolysis, sweat, urticaria.

Special Senses: Amblyopia, hearing loss, photophobia, taste perversion.

Urogenital: Urinary frequency, urinary hesitancy.

7 DRUG INTERACTIONS

7.1 Antiretroviral Agents

Stavudine: Concomitant use of zidovudine with stavudine should be avoided since an antagonistic relationship has been demonstrated in vitro.

Nucleoside Analogues Affecting DNA Replication: Some nucleoside analogues affecting DNA replication, such as ribavirin, antagonize the in vitro antiviral activity of RETROVIR against HIV-1; concomitant use of such drugs should be avoided.

7.2 Doxorubicin

Concomitant use of zidovudine with doxorubicin should be avoided since an antagonistic relationship has been demonstrated in vitro.

7.3 Hematologic/Bone Marrow Suppressive/Cytotoxic Agents

Coadministration of ganciclovir, interferon alfa, ribavirin, and other bone marrow suppressive or cytotoxic agents may increase the hematologic toxicity of zidovudine.

8 USE IN SPECIFIC POPULATIONS

8.1 Pregnancy

Pregnancy Category C.

In humans, treatment with RETROVIR during pregnancy reduced the rate of maternal-fetal HIV-1 transmission from 24.9% for infants born to placebo-treated mothers to 7.8% for infants born to mothers treated with RETROVIR *[see Clinical Studies (14.3)]*. There were no differences in pregnancy-related adverse events between the treatment groups. Animal reproduction studies in rats and rabbits showed evidence of embryotoxicity and increased fetal malformations.

A randomized, double-blind, placebo-controlled trial was conducted in HIV-1-infected pregnant women to determine the utility of RETROVIR for the prevention of maternal-fetal HIV-1-transmission *[see Clinical Studies (14.3)]*. Congenital abnormalities occurred with similar frequency between neonates born to mothers who received RETROVIR and neonates born to mothers who received placebo. The observed abnormalities included problems in embryogenesis (prior to 14 weeks) or were recognized on ultrasound before or immediately after initiation of study drug.

Increased fetal resorptions occurred in pregnant rats and rabbits treated with doses of zidovudine that produced drug plasma concentrations 66 to 226 times (rats) and 12 to 87 times (rabbits) the mean steady-state peak human plasma concentration following a single 100-mg dose of zidovudine. There were no other reported developmental anomalies. In another developmental toxicity study, pregnant rats received zidovudine up to near-lethal doses that produced peak plasma concentrations 350 times peak human plasma concentrations (300 times the daily exposure [AUC] in humans given 600 mg/day zidovudine). This dose was associated with marked maternal toxicity and an increased incidence of fetal malformations. However, there were no signs of teratogenicity at doses up to one-fifth the lethal dose *[see Nonclinical Toxicology (13.2)]*.

Antiretroviral Pregnancy Registry: To monitor maternal-fetal outcomes of pregnant women exposed to RETROVIR, an Antiretroviral Pregnancy Registry has been established. Physicians are encouraged to register patients by calling 1-800-258-4263.

8.3 Nursing Mothers

Zidovudine is excreted in human milk *[see Clinical Pharmacology (12.3)]*.

The Centers for Disease Control and Prevention recommend that HIV-1-infected mothers in the United States not breastfeed their infants to avoid risking postnatal transmission of HIV-1 infection. Because of both the potential for HIV-1 transmission and the potential for serious adverse reactions in nursing infants, mothers should be instructed not to breastfeed if they are receiving RETROVIR.

8.4 Pediatric Use

RETROVIR has been studied in HIV-1-infected pediatric subjects aged ≥6 weeks who had HIV-1-related symptoms or who were asymptomatic with abnormal laboratory values indicating significant HIV-1-related immunosuppression. RETROVIR has also been studied in neonates perinatally exposed to HIV-1 *[see Dosage and Administration (2.1), Adverse Reactions (6.1), Clinical Pharmacology (12.3), Clinical Studies (14.2), (14.3)]*.

8.5 Geriatric Use

Clinical studies of RETROVIR did not include sufficient numbers of subjects aged 65 and over to determine whether they respond differently from younger subjects. Other reported clinical experience has not identified differences in responses between the elderly and younger patients. In general, dose selection for an elderly patient should be cautious, reflecting the greater frequency of decreased hepatic, renal, or cardiac function, and of concomitant disease or other drug therapy.

8.6 Renal Impairment

In patients with severely impaired renal function (CrCl<15 mL/min), dosage reduction is recommended *[see Dosage and Administration (2.4), Clinical Pharmacology (12.3)]*.

8.7 Hepatic Impairment

Zidovudine is eliminated from the body primarily by renal excretion following metabolism in the liver (glucuronidation). Although the data are limited, zidovudine concentrations appear to be increased in patients with severely impaired hepatic function, which may increase the risk of hematologic toxicity *[see Dosage and Administration (2.5), Clinical Pharmacology (12.3)]*.

10 OVERDOSAGE

Acute overdoses of zidovudine have been reported in pediatric patients and adults. These involved exposures up to 50 grams. No specific symptoms or signs have been identified following acute overdosage with zidovudine apart from those listed as adverse events such as fatigue, headache, vomiting, and occasional reports of hematological disturbances. All patients recovered without permanent sequelae. Hemodialysis and peritoneal dialysis appear to have a negligible effect on the removal of zidovudine while elimination of its primary metabolite, 3′-azido-3′-deoxy-5′-*O*-β-*D*-glucopyranuronosylthymidine (GZDV), is enhanced.

11 DESCRIPTION

RETROVIR is the brand name for zidovudine (formerly called azidothymidine [AZT]), a pyrimidine nucleoside analogue active against HIV-1. The chemical name of zidovudine is 3′-azido-3′-deoxythymidine; it has the following structural formula:

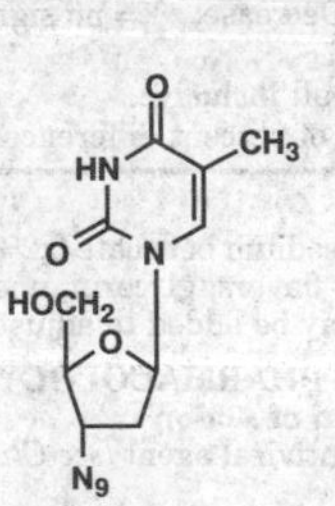

Zidovudine is a white to beige, odorless, crystalline solid with a molecular weight of 267.24 and a solubility of 20.1 mg/mL in water at 25°C. The molecular formula is $C_{10}H_{13}N_5O_4$.

RETROVIR Tablets are for oral administration. Each film-coated tablet contains 300 mg of zidovudine and the inactive ingredients hypromellose, magnesium stearate, microcrystalline cellulose, polyethylene glycol, sodium starch glycolate, and titanium dioxide.

RETROVIR Capsules are for oral administration. Each capsule contains 100 mg of zidovudine and the inactive ingredients corn starch, magnesium stearate, microcrystalline cellulose, and sodium starch glycolate. The 100-mg empty hard gelatin capsule, printed with edible black ink, consists of black iron oxide, dimethylpolysiloxane, gelatin, pharmaceutical shellac, soya lecithin, and titanium dioxide.

RETROVIR Syrup is for oral administration. Each mL of RETROVIR Syrup contains 10 mg of zidovudine and the in-

Table 9. Zidovudine Pharmacokinetic Parameters in Pediatric Subjects[a]

Parameter	Birth to 14 Days	Aged 14 Days to 3 Months	Aged 3 Months to 12 Years
Oral bioavailability (%)	89 ± 19 (n = 15)	61 ± 19 (n = 17)	65 ± 24 (n = 18)
CSF:plasma ratio	no data	no data	0.68 [0.03 to 3.25][b] (n = 38)
CL (L/h/kg)	0.65 ± 0.29 (n = 18)	1.14 ± 0.24 (n = 16)	1.85 ± 0.47 (n = 20)
Elimination half-life (h)	3.1 ± 1.2 (n = 21)	1.9 ± 0.7 (n = 18)	1.5 ± 0.7 (n = 21)

[a] Data presented as mean ± standard deviation except where noted.
[b] Median [range].

Table 10. Effect of Coadministered Drugs on Zidovudine AUC[a]

Note: ROUTINE DOSE MODIFICATION OF ZIDOVUDINE IS NOT WARRANTED WITH COADMINISTRATION OF THE FOLLOWING DRUGS.

Coadministered Drug and Dose	Zidovudine Dose	n	Zidovudine Concentrations		Concentration of Coadministered Drug
			AUC	Variability	
Atovaquone 750 mg q 12 h with food	200 mg q 8 h	14	↑AUC 31%	Range 23% to 78%[b]	↔
Clarithromycin 500 mg twice daily	100 mg q 4 h × 7 days	4	↓AUC 12%	Range ↓34% to ↑14%	Not Reported
Fluconazole 400 mg daily	200 mg q 8 h	12	↑AUC 74%	95% CI: 54% to 98%	Not Reported
Lamivudine 300 mg q 12 h	single 200 mg	12	↑AUC 13%	90% CI: 2% to 27%	↔
Methadone 30 to 90 mg daily	200 mg q 4 h	9	↑AUC 43%	Range 16% to 64%[b]	↔
Nelfinavir 750 mg q 8 h × 7 to 10 days	single 200 mg	11	↓AUC 35%	Range 28% to 41%	↔
Probenecid 500 mg q 6 h × 2 days	2 mg/kg q 8 h × 3 days	3	↑AUC 106%	Range 100% to 170%[b]	Not Assessed
Rifampin 600 mg daily × 14 days	200 mg q 8 h × 14 days	8	↓AUC 47%	90% CI: 41% to 53%	Not Assessed
Ritonavir 300 mg q 6 h × 4 days	200 mg q 8 h × 4 days	9	↓AUC 25%	95% CI: 15% to 34%	↔
Valproic acid 250 mg or 500 mg q 8 h × 4 days	100 mg q 8 h × 4 days	6	↑AUC 80%	Range 64% to 130%[b]	Not Assessed

↑ = Increase; ↓ = Decrease; ↔ = no significant change; AUC = area under the concentration versus time curve; CI = confidence interval.
[a] This table is not all inclusive.
[b] Estimated range of percent difference.

active ingredients sodium benzoate 0.2% (added as a preservative), citric acid, flavors, glycerin, and liquid sucrose. Sodium hydroxide may be added to adjust pH.

12 CLINICAL PHARMACOLOGY

12.1 Mechanism of Action

Zidovudine is an antiviral agent *[see Clinical Pharmacology (12.4)]*.

12.3 Pharmacokinetics

Absorption and Bioavailability: In adults, following oral administration, zidovudine is rapidly absorbed and extensively distributed, with peak serum concentrations occurring within 0.5 to 1.5 hours. The AUC was equivalent when zidovudine was administered as RETROVIR Tablets or Syrup compared with RETROVIR Capsules. The pharmacokinetic properties of zidovudine in fasting adult subjects are summarized in Table 7.

Table 7. Zidovudine Pharmacokinetic Parameters in Fasting Adult Subjects

Parameter	Mean ± SD (except where noted)
Oral bioavailability (%)	64 ± 10 (n = 5)
Apparent volume of distribution (L/kg)	1.6 ± 0.6 (n = 8)
Plasma protein binding (%)	<38
CSF:plasma ratio[a]	0.6 [0.04 to 2.62] (n = 39)
Systemic clearance (L/h/kg)	1.6 ± 0.6 (n = 6)
Renal clearance (L/h/kg)	0.34 ± 0.05 (n = 9)
Elimination half-life (h)[b]	0.5 to 3 (n = 19)

[a] Median [range].
[b] Approximate range.

Distribution: The apparent volume of distribution of zidovudine, following oral administration, is 1.6 ± 0.6 L/kg; and binding to plasma protein is low, <38% (Table 7).

Metabolism and Elimination: Zidovudine is primarily eliminated by hepatic metabolism. The major metabolite of zidovudine is GZDV. GZDV AUC is about 3-fold greater than the zidovudine AUC. Urinary recovery of zidovudine and GZDV accounts for 14% and 74%, respectively, of the dose following oral administration. A second metabolite, 3′-amino-3′-deoxythymidine (AMT), has been identified in the plasma following single-dose intravenous (IV) administration of zidovudine. The AMT AUC was one-fifth of the zidovudine AUC. Pharmacokinetics of zidovudine were dose independent at oral dosing regimens ranging from 2 mg/kg every 8 hours to 10 mg/kg every 4 hours.

Effect of Food on Absorption: RETROVIR may be administered with or without food. The zidovudine AUC was similar when a single dose of zidovudine was administered with food.

Special Populations: *Renal Impairment:* Zidovudine clearance was decreased resulting in increased zidovudine and GZDV half-life and AUC in subjects with impaired renal function (n = 14) following a single 200-mg oral dose (Table 8). Plasma concentrations of AMT were not determined. A dose adjustment should not be necessary for patients with creatinine clearance (CrCl) ≥15 mL/min.

Table 8. Zidovudine Pharmacokinetic Parameters in Subjects With Severe Renal Impairment[a]

Parameter	Control Subjects (Normal Renal Function) (n = 6)	Subjects With Renal Impairment (n = 14)
CrCl (mL/min)	120 ± 8	18 ± 2
Zidovudine AUC (ng•h/mL)	1,400 ± 200	3,100 ± 300
Zidovudine half-life (h)	1.0 ± 0.2	1.4 ± 0.1

[a] Data are expressed as mean ± standard deviation.

Hemodialysis and Peritoneal Dialysis: The pharmacokinetics and tolerance of zidovudine were evaluated in a multiple-dose trial in subjects undergoing hemodialysis (n = 5) or peritoneal dialysis (n = 6) receiving escalating doses up to 200 mg 5 times daily for 8 weeks. Daily doses of 500 mg or less were well tolerated despite significantly elevated GZDV plasma concentrations. Apparent zidovudine oral clearance was approximately 50% of that reported in subjects with normal renal function. Hemodialysis and peritoneal dialysis appeared to have a negligible effect on the removal of zidovudine, whereas GZDV elimination was enhanced. A dosage adjustment is recommended for patients undergoing hemodialysis or peritoneal dialysis *[see Dosage and Administration (2.4)]*.

Hepatic Impairment: Data describing the effect of hepatic impairment on the pharmacokinetics of zidovudine are limited. However, because zidovudine is eliminated primarily by hepatic metabolism, it is expected that zidovudine clearance would be decreased and plasma concentrations would be increased following administration of the recommended adult doses to patients with hepatic impairment *[see Dosage and Administration (2.5)]*.

Pediatric Patients: Zidovudine pharmacokinetics have been evaluated in HIV-1-infected pediatric subjects (Table 9).

Patients Aged 3 Months to 12 Years: Overall, zidovudine pharmacokinetics in pediatric patients older than 3 months are similar to those in adult patients. Proportional increases in plasma zidovudine concentrations were observed following administration of oral solution from 90 to 240 mg/m^2 every 6 hours. Oral bioavailability, terminal half-life, and oral clearance were comparable to adult values. As in adult subjects, the major route of elimination was by metabolism to GZDV. After intravenous dosing, about 29% of the dose was excreted in the urine unchanged, and about 45% of the dose was excreted as GZDV *[see Dosage and Administration (2.1)]*.

Patients Aged Less Than 3 Months: Zidovudine pharmacokinetics have been evaluated in pediatric subjects from birth to 3 months of life. Zidovudine elimination was determined immediately following birth in 8 neonates who were exposed to zidovudine in utero. The half-life was 13.0 ± 5.8 hours. In neonates ≤14 days old, bioavailability was greater, total body clearance was slower, and half-life was longer than in pediatric subjects older than 14 days. For dose recommendations for neonates *[see Dosage and Administration (2.2)]*.

[See table 9 above]

Pregnancy: Zidovudine pharmacokinetics have been studied in a Phase I trial of 8 women during the last trimester of pregnancy. Zidovudine pharmacokinetics were similar to those of nonpregnant adults. Consistent with passive transmission of the drug across the placenta, zidovudine concentrations in neonatal plasma at birth were essentially equal to those in maternal plasma at delivery *[see Use in Specific Populations (8.1)]*.

Although data are limited, methadone maintenance therapy in 5 pregnant women did not appear to alter zidovudine pharmacokinetics.

Nursing Mothers: The Centers for Disease Control and Prevention recommend that HIV-1-infected mothers not breastfeed their infants to avoid risking postnatal transmission of HIV-1. After administration of a single dose of 200 mg zidovudine to 13 HIV-1-infected women, the mean concentration of zidovudine was similar in human milk and serum *[see Use in Specific Populations (8.3)]*.

Geriatric Patients: Zidovudine pharmacokinetics have not been studied in subjects over 65 years of age.

Gender: A pharmacokinetic trial in healthy male (n = 12) and female (n = 12) subjects showed no differences in zidovudine AUC when a single dose of zidovudine was administered as the 300-mg RETROVIR Tablet.

Drug Interactions: *[See Drug Interactions (7)].*

[See table 10 at top of previous page]

Phenytoin: Phenytoin plasma levels have been reported to be low in some patients receiving RETROVIR, while in one case a high level was documented. However, in a pharmacokinetic interaction trial in which 12 HIV-1-positive volunteers received a single 300-mg phenytoin dose alone and during steady-state zidovudine conditions (200 mg every 4 hours), no change in phenytoin kinetics was observed. Although not designed to optimally assess the effect of phenytoin on zidovudine kinetics, a 30% decrease in oral zidovudine clearance was observed with phenytoin.

Ribavirin: In vitro data indicate ribavirin reduces phosphorylation of lamivudine, stavudine, and zidovudine. However, no pharmacokinetic (e.g., plasma concentrations or intracellular triphosphorylated active metabolite concentrations) or pharmacodynamic (e.g., loss of HIV-1/HCV virologic suppression) interaction was observed when ribavirin and lamivudine (n = 18), stavudine (n = 10), or zidovudine (n = 6) were coadministered as part of a multi-drug regimen to HIV-1/HCV co-infected subjects *[see Warnings and Precautions (5.4)]*.

12.4 Microbiology

Mechanism of Action: Zidovudine is a synthetic nucleoside analogue. Intracellularly, zidovudine is phosphorylated to its active 5′-triphosphate metabolite, zidovudine triphosphate (ZDV-TP). The principal mode of action of ZDV-TP is inhibition of reverse transcriptase (RT) via DNA chain termination after incorporation of the nucleotide analogue. ZDV-TP is a weak inhibitor of the cellular DNA polymerases α and γ and has been reported to be incorporated into the DNA of cells in culture.

Antiviral Activity: The antiviral activity of zidovudine against HIV-1 was assessed in a number of cell lines (including monocytes and fresh human peripheral blood lymphocytes). The EC_{50} and EC_{90} values for zidovudine were 0.01 to 0.49 µM (1 µM = 0.27 mcg/mL) and 0.1 to 9 µM, respectively. HIV-1 from therapy-naive subjects with no mutations associated with resistance gave median EC_{50} values of 0.011 µM (range: 0.005 to 0.110 µM) from Virco (n = 92 baseline samples from COL40263) and 0.0017 µM (0.006 to 0.0340 µM) from Monogram Biosciences (n = 135 baseline samples from ESS30009). The EC_{50} values of zidovudine against different HIV-1 clades (A-G) ranged from 0.00018 to 0.02 µM, and against HIV-2 isolates from 0.00049 to 0.004 µM. In cell culture drug combination studies, zidovudine demonstrates synergistic activity with the nucleoside reverse transcriptase inhibitors abacavir, didanosine, and lamivudine; the non-nucleoside reverse transcriptase inhibitors delavirdine and nevirapine; and the protease inhibitors indinavir, nelfinavir, ritonavir, and saquinavir; and additive activity with interferon alfa. Ribavirin has been found to inhibit the phosphorylation of zidovudine in cell culture.

Resistance: Genotypic analyses of the isolates selected in cell culture and recovered from zidovudine-treated subjects showed mutations in the HIV-1 RT gene resulting in 6 amino acid substitutions (M41L, D67N, K70R, L210W, T215Y or F, and K219Q) that confer zidovudine resistance. In general, higher levels of resistance were associated with greater number of amino acid substitutions. In some subjects harboring zidovudine-resistant virus at baseline, phenotypic sensitivity to zidovudine was restored by 12 weeks of treatment with lamivudine and zidovudine. Combination therapy with lamivudine plus zidovudine delayed the emergence of substitutions conferring resistance to zidovudine.

Cross-Resistance: In a study of 167 HIV-1-infected subjects, isolates (n = 2) with multi-drug resistance to didanosine, lamivudine, stavudine, zalcitabine, and zidovudine were recovered from subjects treated for ≥1 year with zidovudine plus didanosine or zidovudine plus zalcitabine. The pattern of resistance-associated amino acid substitutions with such combination therapies was different (A62V, V75I, F77L, F116Y, Q151M) from the pattern with zidovudine monotherapy, with the Q151M substitution being most commonly associated with multi-drug resistance. The substitution at codon 151 in combination with substitutions at 62, 75, 77, and 116 results in a virus with reduced susceptibility to didanosine, lamivudine, stavudine, zalcitabine, and zidovudine. Thymidine analogue mutations (TAMs) are selected by zidovudine and confer cross-resistance to abacavir, didanosine, stavudine, tenofovir, and zalcitabine.

13 NONCLINICAL TOXICOLOGY

13.1 Carcinogenesis, Mutagenesis, Impairment of Fertility

Zidovudine was administered orally at 3 dosage levels to separate groups of mice and rats (60 females and 60 males in each group). Initial single daily doses were 30, 60, and 120 mg/kg/day in mice and 80, 220, and 600 mg/kg/day in rats. The doses in mice were reduced to 20, 30, and 40 mg/kg/day after day 90 because of treatment-related anemia, whereas in rats only the high dose was reduced to 450 mg/kg/day on day 91 and then to 300 mg/kg/day on day 279.

In mice, 7 late-appearing (after 19 months) vaginal neoplasms (5 nonmetastasizing squamous cell carcinomas, 1 squamous cell papilloma, and 1 squamous polyp) occurred in animals given the highest dose. One late-appearing squamous cell papilloma occurred in the vagina of a middle-dose animal. No vaginal tumors were found at the lowest dose.

In rats, 2 late-appearing (after 20 months), nonmetastasizing vaginal squamous cell carcinomas occurred in animals given the highest dose. No vaginal tumors occurred at the low or middle dose in rats. No other drug-related tumors were observed in either sex of either species.

At doses that produced tumors in mice and rats, the estimated drug exposure (as measured by AUC) was approximately 3 times (mouse) and 24 times (rat) the estimated human exposure at the recommended therapeutic dose of 100 mg every 4 hours.

It is not known how predictive the results of rodent carcinogenicity studies may be for humans.

Zidovudine was mutagenic in a 5178Y/TK$^{+/-}$ mouse lymphoma assay, positive in an in vitro cell transformation assay, clastogenic in a cytogenetic assay using cultured human lymphocytes, and positive in mouse and rat micronucleus tests after repeated doses. It was negative in a cytogenetic study in rats given a single dose.

Zidovudine, administered to male and female rats at doses up to 7 times the usual adult dose based on body surface area, had no effect on fertility judged by conception rates.

Two transplacental carcinogenicity studies were conducted in mice. One study administered zidovudine at doses of 20 mg/kg/day or 40 mg/kg/day from gestation day 10 through parturition and lactation with dosing continuing in offspring for 24 months postnatally. The doses of zidovudine administered in this study produced zidovudine exposures approximately 3 times the estimated human exposure at recommended doses. After 24 months, an increase in incidence of vaginal tumors was noted with no increase in tumors in the liver or lung or any other organ in either gender. These findings are consistent with results of the standard oral carcinogenicity study in mice, as described earlier. A second study administered zidovudine at maximum tolerated doses of 12.5 mg/day or 25 mg/day (~1,000 mg/kg nonpregnant body weight or ~450 mg/kg of term body weight) to pregnant mice from days 12 through 18 of gestation. There was an increase in the number of tumors in the lung, liver, and female reproductive tracts in the offspring of mice receiving the higher dose level of zidovudine.

13.2 Reproductive and Developmental Toxicology Studies

Oral teratology studies in the rat and in the rabbit at doses up to 500 mg/kg/day revealed no evidence of teratogenicity with zidovudine. Zidovudine treatment resulted in embryo/fetal toxicity as evidenced by an increase in the incidence of fetal resorptions in rats given 150 or 450 mg/kg/day and rabbits given 500 mg/kg/day. The doses used in the teratology studies resulted in peak zidovudine plasma concentrations (after one-half of the daily dose) in rats 66 to 226 times, and in rabbits 12 to 87 times, mean steady-state peak human plasma concentrations (after one-sixth of the daily dose) achieved with the recommended daily dose (100 mg every 4 hours). In an in vitro experiment with fertilized mouse oocytes, zidovudine exposure resulted in a dose-dependent reduction in blastocyst formation. In an additional teratology study in rats, a dose of 3,000 mg/kg/day (very near the oral median lethal dose in rats of 3,683 mg/kg) caused marked maternal toxicity and an increase in the incidence of fetal malformations. This dose resulted in peak zidovudine plasma concentrations 350 times peak human plasma concentrations. (Estimated AUC in rats at this dose level was 300 times the daily AUC in humans given 600 mg/day.) No evidence of teratogenicity was seen in this experiment at doses of 600 mg/kg/day or less.

14 CLINICAL STUDIES

Therapy with RETROVIR has been shown to prolong survival and decrease the incidence of opportunistic infections in patients with advanced HIV-1 disease and to delay disease progression in asymptomatic HIV-1-infected patients.

14.1 Adults

Combination Therapy: RETROVIR in combination with other antiretroviral agents has been shown to be superior to monotherapy for one or more of the following endpoints: delaying death, delaying development of AIDS, increasing CD4+ cell counts, and decreasing plasma HIV-1 RNA.

The clinical efficacy of a combination regimen that includes RETROVIR was demonstrated in trial ACTG 320. This trial was a multi-center, randomized, double-blind, placebo-controlled trial that compared RETROVIR 600 mg/day plus EPIVIR 300 mg/day to RETROVIR plus EPIVIR plus indinavir 800 mg three times daily. The incidence of AIDS-defining events or death was lower in the triple-drug–containing arm compared with the 2-drug–containing arm (6.1% versus 10.9%, respectively).

Monotherapy: In controlled trials of treatment-naive subjects conducted between 1986 and 1989, monotherapy with RETROVIR, as compared with placebo, reduced the risk of HIV-1 disease progression, as assessed using endpoints that included the occurrence of HIV-1-related illnesses, AIDS-defining events, or death. These trials enrolled subjects with advanced disease (BW 002), and asymptomatic or mildly symptomatic disease in subjects with CD4+ cell counts between 200 and 500 cells/mm^3 (ACTG 016 and ACTG 019). A survival benefit for monotherapy with RETROVIR was not demonstrated in the latter 2 trials. Subsequent trials showed that the clinical benefit of monotherapy with RETROVIR was time limited.

14.2 Pediatric Patients

ACTG 300 was a multi-center, randomized, double-blind trial that provided for comparison of EPIVIR plus RETROVIR to didanosine monotherapy. A total of 471 symptomatic, HIV-1-infected therapy-naive pediatric subjects were enrolled in these 2 treatment arms. The median age was 2.7 years (range: 6 weeks to 14 years), the mean baseline CD4+ cell count was 868 cells/mm^3, and the mean baseline plasma HIV-1 RNA was 5.0 $\log_{10}$ copies/mL. The median duration that subjects remained on trial was approximately 10 months. Results are summarized in Table 11.

Table 11. Number of Subjects (%) Reaching a Primary Clinical Endpoint (Disease Progression or Death)

Endpoint	EPIVIR plus RETROVIR (n = 236)	Didanosine (n = 235)
HIV disease progression or death (total)	15 (6.4%)	37 (15.7%)
Physical growth failure	7 (3.0%)	6 (2.6%)
Central nervous system deterioration	4 (1.7%)	12 (5.1%)
CDC Clinical Category C	2 (0.8%)	8 (3.4%)
Death	2 (0.8%)	11 (4.7%)

14.3 Prevention of Maternal-Fetal HIV-1 Transmission

The utility of RETROVIR for the prevention of maternal-fetal HIV-1 transmission was demonstrated in a randomized, double-blind, placebo-controlled trial (ACTG 076) conducted in HIV-1-infected pregnant women with CD4+ cell counts of 200 to 1,818 cells/mm^3 (median in the treated group: 560 cells/mm^3) who had little or no previous exposure to RETROVIR. Oral RETROVIR was initiated between 14 and 34 weeks of gestation (median 11 weeks of therapy) followed by IV administration of RETROVIR during labor and delivery. Following birth, neonates received oral RETROVIR Syrup for 6 weeks. The trial showed a statistically significant difference in the incidence of HIV-1 infection in the neonates (based on viral culture from peripheral blood) between the group receiving RETROVIR and the group receiving placebo. Of 363 neonates evaluated in the trial, the estimated risk of HIV-1 infection was 7.8% in the group receiving RETROVIR and 24.9% in the placebo group, a relative reduction in transmission risk of 68.7%. RETROVIR was well tolerated by mothers and infants. There was no difference in pregnancy-related adverse events between the treatment groups.

16 HOW SUPPLIED/STORAGE AND HANDLING

RETROVIR Tablets 300 mg (biconvex, white, round, film-coated) containing 300 mg zidovudine, one side engraved "GX CW3" and "300" on the other side.

Bottle of 60 (NDC 49702-214-18).

Store at 15° to 25°C (59° to 77°F).

RETROVIR Capsules 100 mg (white, opaque cap and body) containing 100 mg zidovudine and printed with "Wellcome" and unicorn logo on cap and "Y9C" and "100" on body.

Bottles of 100 (NDC 49702-211-20).

Store at 15° to 25°C (59° to 77°F) and protect from moisture.

RETROVIR Syrup (colorless to pale yellow, strawberry-flavored) containing 10 mg zidovudine in each mL.

Bottle of 240 mL (NDC 49702-212-48) with child-resistant cap.

Store at 15° to 25°C (59° to 77°F).

17 PATIENT COUNSELING INFORMATION

17.1 Advice for the Patient

Neutropenia and Anemia: Patients should be informed that the major toxicities of RETROVIR are neutropenia and/or anemia. The frequency and severity of these toxicities are greater in patients with more advanced disease and in those who initiate therapy later in the course of their infection. Patients should be informed that if toxicity develops, they may require transfusions or drug discontinuation. Patients should be informed of the extreme importance of having their blood counts followed closely while on therapy, especially for patients with advanced symptomatic HIV-1 disease *[see Boxed Warning, Warnings and Precautions (5.1)]*.

Myopathy: Patients should be informed that myopathy and myositis with pathological changes, similar to that produced by HIV-1 disease, have been associated with prolonged use of RETROVIR *[see Boxed Warning, Warnings and Precautions (5.2)]*.

Lactic Acidosis/Hepatomegaly: Patients should be informed that some HIV medicines, including RETROVIR, can cause a rare, but serious condition called lactic acidosis with liver enlargement (hepatomegaly) *[see Boxed Warning, Warnings and Precautions (5.3)]*.

HIV-1/HCV Co-Infection: Patients with HIV-1/HCV co-infection should be informed that hepatic decompensation (some fatal) has occurred in HIV-1/HCV co-infected patients receiving combination antiretroviral therapy for HIV-1 and interferon alfa with or without ribavirin *[see Warnings and Precautions (5.4)]*.

Use With Other Zidovudine-Containing Products: RETROVIR should not be administered with combination products that contain zidovudine as one of their components (e.g., COMBIVIR [lamivudine and zidovudine] Tablets or TRIZIVIR [abacavir sulfate, lamivudine, and zidovudine] Tablets) *[see Warnings and Precautions (5.5)]*.

Redistribution/Accumulation of Body Fat: Patients should be informed that redistribution or accumulation of body fat may occur in patients receiving antiretroviral therapy and that the cause and long-term health effects of these conditions are not known at this time *[see Warnings and Precautions (5.7)]*.

Common Adverse Reactions: Patients should be informed that the most commonly reported adverse reactions in adult patients being treated with RETROVIR were headache, malaise, nausea, anorexia, and vomiting. The most commonly reported adverse reactions in pediatric patients receiving RETROVIR were fever, cough, and digestive disorders. Patients also should be encouraged to contact their physician if they experience muscle weakness, shortness of breath, symptoms of hepatitis or pancreatitis, or any other unexpected adverse events while being treated with RETROVIR *[see Adverse Reactions (6)]*.

Drug Interactions: Patients should be cautioned about the use of other medications, including ganciclovir, interferon alfa, and ribavirin, which may exacerbate the toxicity of RETROVIR *[see Drug Interactions (7)]*.

Pregnancy: Pregnant women considering the use of RETROVIR during pregnancy for prevention of HIV-1 transmission to their infants should be informed that transmission may still occur in some cases despite therapy. The long-term consequences of in utero and infant exposure to RETROVIR are unknown, including the possible risk of cancer *[see Use in Specific Populations (8.1)]*.

HIV-1-infected pregnant women should be informed not to breastfeed to avoid postnatal transmission of HIV to a child who may not yet be infected *[see Use in Specific Populations (8.3)]*.

Information About HIV-1 Infection: RETROVIR is not a cure for HIV-1 infection, and patients may continue to experience illnesses associated with HIV-1 infection, including opportunistic infections. Patients should remain under the care of a physician when using RETROVIR.

Patients should be advised to avoid doing things that can spread HIV-1 infection to others.

- **Do not share needles or other injection equipment.**
- **Do not share personal items that can have blood or body fluids on them, like toothbrushes and razor blades.**
- **Do not have any kind of sex without protection.** Always practice safe sex by using a latex or polyurethane condom or other barrier method to lower the chance of sexual contact with semen, vaginal secretions, or blood.
- **Do not breastfeed.** Zidovudine is excreted in human breast milk. Mothers with HIV-1 should not breastfeed because HIV-1 can be passed to the baby in the breast milk.

Patients should be informed to take all HIV medications exactly as prescribed.

RETROVIR, COMBIVIR, EPIVIR, and TRIZIVIR are registered trademarks of ViiV Healthcare.

Manufactured for:
ViiV Healthcare
Research Triangle Park, NC 27709
by:
GlaxoSmithKline
Research Triangle Park, NC 27709

RTT:8PI

RETROVIR® ℞

[re'trō-vir]
(zidovudine)
IV Infusion
FOR INTRAVENOUS INFUSION ONLY

> **WARNING**
>
> **RETROVIR (ZIDOVUDINE) HAS BEEN ASSOCIATED WITH HEMATOLOGIC TOXICITY, INCLUDING NEUTROPENIA AND SEVERE ANEMIA, PARTICULARLY IN PATIENTS WITH ADVANCED HUMAN IMMUNODEFICIENCY VIRUS (HIV) DISEASE (SEE WARNINGS). PROLONGED USE OF RETROVIR HAS BEEN ASSOCIATED WITH SYMPTOMATIC MYOPATHY.**
>
> **LACTIC ACIDOSIS AND SEVERE HEPATOMEGALY WITH STEATOSIS, INCLUDING FATAL CASES, HAVE BEEN REPORTED WITH THE USE OF NUCLEOSIDE ANALOGUES ALONE OR IN COMBINATION, INCLUDING RETROVIR AND OTHER ANTIRETROVIRALS (SEE WARNINGS).**

DESCRIPTION

RETROVIR is the brand name for zidovudine (formerly called azidothymidine [AZT]), a pyrimidine nucleoside analogue active against HIV. RETROVIR IV Infusion is a sterile solution for intravenous infusion only. Each mL contains 10 mg zidovudine in Water for Injection. Hydrochloric acid and/or sodium hydroxide may have been added to adjust the pH to approximately 5.5. RETROVIR IV Infusion contains no preservatives.

The chemical name of zidovudine is 3′-azido-3′-deoxythymidine; it has the following structural formula:

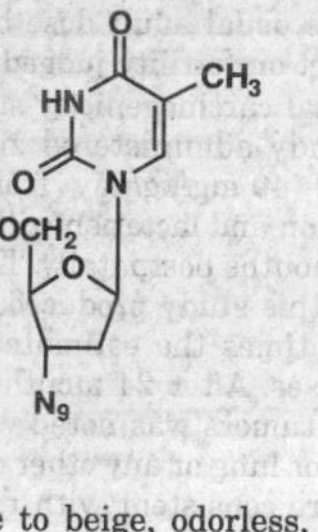

Zidovudine is a white to beige, odorless, crystalline solid with a molecular weight of 267.24 and a solubility of 20.1 mg/mL in water at 25°C. The molecular formula is $C_{10}H_{13}N_5O_4$.

MICROBIOLOGY

Mechanism of Action:

Zidovudine is a synthetic nucleoside analogue. Intracellularly, zidovudine is phosphorylated to its active 5′-triphosphate metabolite, zidovudine triphosphate (ZDV-TP). The principal mode of action of ZDV-TP is inhibition of reverse transcriptase (RT) via DNA chain termination after incorporation of the nucleotide analogue. ZDV-TP is a weak inhibitor of the cellular DNA polymerases α and γ and has been reported to be incorporated into the DNA of cells in culture.

Antiviral Activity:

Activity of zidovudine against HIV-1 was assessed in a number of cell lines (including monocytes and fresh human peripheral blood lymphocytes). The EC_{50} and EC_{90} values for zidovudine were 0.01 to 0.49 μM (1 μM = 0.27 mcg/mL) and 0.1 to 9 μM, respectively. HIV from therapy-naive subjects with no mutations associated with resistance gave median EC_{50} values of 0.011 μM (range: 0.005 to 0.110 μM) from Virco (n = 93 baseline samples from COLA40263) and 0.02 μM (0.01 to 0.03 μM) from Monogram Biosciences (n = 135 baseline samples from ESS30009). The EC_{50} values of zidovudine against different HIV-1 clades (A-G) ranged from 0.00018 to 0.02 μM, and against HIV-2 isolates from 0.00049 to 0.004 μM. In cell culture drug combination studies, zidovudine demonstrates synergistic activity with the nucleoside reverse transcriptase inhibitors (NRTIs) abacavir, didanosine, lamivudine, and zalcitabine; the non-nucleoside reverse transcriptase inhibitors (NNRTIs) delavirdine and nevirapine; and the protease inhibitors (PIs) indinavir, nelfinavir, ritonavir, and saquinavir; and additive activity with interferon alfa. Ribavirin has been found to inhibit the phosphorylation of zidovudine in cell culture.

Resistance:

Genotypic analyses of the isolates selected in cell culture and recovered from zidovudine-treated patients showed mutations in the HIV-1 RT gene resulting in 6 amino acid substitutions (M41L, D67N, K70R, L210W, T215Y or F, and K219Q) that confer zidovudine resistance. In general, higher levels of resistance were associated with greater number of mutations. In some patients harboring zidovudine-resistant virus at baseline, phenotypic sensitivity to zidovudine was restored by 12 weeks of treatment with lamivudine and zidovudine. Combination therapy with lamivudine plus zidovudine delayed the emergence of mutations conferring resistance to zidovudine.

Cross-Resistance:

In a study of 167 HIV-infected patients, isolates (n = 2) with multi-drug resistance to didanosine, lamivudine, stavudine, zalcitabine, and zidovudine were recovered from patients treated for ≥1 year with zidovudine plus didanosine or zidovudine plus zalcitabine. The pattern of resistance-associated mutations with such combination therapies was different (A62V, V75I, F77L, F116Y, Q151M) from the pattern with zidovudine monotherapy, with the Q151M mutation being most commonly associated with multi-drug resistance. The mutation at codon 151 in combination with mutations at 62, 75, 77, and 116 results in a virus with reduced susceptibility to didanosine, lamivudine, stavudine, zalcitabine, and zidovudine. Thymidine analogue mutations (TAMs) are selected by zidovudine and confer cross-resistance to abacavir, didanosine, stavudine, tenofovir, and zalcitabine.

CLINICAL PHARMACOLOGY

Pharmacokinetics:

Adults: The pharmacokinetics of zidovudine have been evaluated in 22 adult HIV-infected patients in a Phase 1 dose-escalation study. Following intravenous (IV) dosing, dose-independent kinetics was observed over the range of 1 to 5 mg/kg. The major metabolite of zidovudine is 3′-azido-3′-deoxy-5′-*O*-β-*D*-glucopyranuronosylthymidine (GZDV). GZDV area under the curve (AUC) is about 3-fold greater than the zidovudine AUC. Urinary recovery of zidovudine and GZDV accounts for 18% and 60%, respectively, following IV dosing. A second metabolite, 3′-amino-3′-deoxythymidine (AMT), has been identified in the plasma following single-dose IV administration of zidovudine. The AMT AUC was one-fifth of the zidovudine AUC.

The mean steady-state peak and trough concentrations of zidovudine at 2.5 mg/kg every 4 hours were 1.06 and 0.12 mcg/mL, respectively.

The zidovudine cerebrospinal fluid (CSF)/plasma concentration ratio was determined in 39 patients receiving chronic therapy with RETROVIR. The median ratio measured in 50 paired samples drawn 1 to 8 hours after the last dose of RETROVIR was 0.6.

Table 1. Zidovudine Pharmacokinetic Parameters Following Intravenous Administration in HIV-Infected Patients

Parameter	Mean ± SD (except where noted)
Apparent volume of distribution (L/kg)	1.6 ± 0.6 (n = 11)
Plasma protein binding (%)	<38
CSF:plasma ratio[a]	0.6 [0.04 to 2.62] (n = 39)
Systemic clearance (L/hr/kg)	1.6 (0.8 to 2.7) (n =18)
Renal clearance (L/hr/kg)	0.34 ± 0.05 (n = 16)
Elimination half-life (hr)[b]	1.1 (0.5 to 2.9) (n = 19)

[a]Median [range].
[b]Approximate range.

Adults With Impaired Renal Function: Zidovudine clearance was decreased resulting in increased zidovudine and GZDV half-life and AUC in patients with impaired renal function (n = 14) following a single 200-mg oral dose (Table 2). Plasma concentrations of AMT were not determined. A dose adjustment should not be necessary for patients with creatinine clearance (CrCl) ≥15 mL/min.

Table 2. Zidovudine Pharmacokinetic Parameters in Patients With Severe Renal Impairment[a]

Parameter	Control Subjects (Normal Renal Function) (n = 6)	Patients With Renal Impairment (n = 14)
CrCl (mL/min)	120 ± 8	18 ± 2
Zidovudine AUC (ng•hr/mL)	1,400 ± 200	3,100 ± 300

Zidovudine half-life (hr)	1.0 ± 0.2	1.4 ± 0.1

[a]Data are expressed as mean ± standard deviation.

The pharmacokinetics and tolerance of oral zidovudine were evaluated in a multiple-dose study in patients undergoing hemodialysis (n = 5) or peritoneal dialysis (n = 6) receiving escalating doses up to 200 mg 5 times daily for 8 weeks. Daily doses of 500 mg or less were well tolerated despite significantly elevated GZDV plasma concentrations. Apparent zidovudine oral clearance was approximately 50% of that reported in patients with normal renal function. Hemodialysis and peritoneal dialysis appeared to have a negligible effect on the removal of zidovudine, whereas GZDV elimination was enhanced. A dosage adjustment is recommended for patients undergoing hemodialysis or peritoneal dialysis (see DOSAGE AND ADMINISTRATION: Dose Adjustment).

Adults With Impaired Hepatic Function: Data describing the effect of hepatic impairment on the pharmacokinetics of zidovudine are limited. However, because zidovudine is eliminated primarily by hepatic metabolism, it is expected that zidovudine clearance would be decreased and plasma concentrations would be increased following administration of the recommended adult doses to patients with hepatic impairment (see DOSAGE AND ADMINISTRATION: Dose Adjustment).

Pediatrics: Zidovudine pharmacokinetics have been evaluated in HIV-infected pediatric patients (Table 3).

Patients Aged 3 Months to 12 Years: Overall, zidovudine pharmacokinetics in pediatric patients >3 months of age are similar to those in adult patients. Proportional increases in plasma zidovudine concentrations were observed following administration of oral solution from 90 to 240 mg/m^2 every 6 hours. Oral bioavailability, terminal half-life, and oral clearance were comparable to adult values. As in adult patients, the major route of elimination was by metabolism to GZDV. After intravenous dosing, about 29% of the dose was excreted in the urine unchanged and about 45% of the dose was excreted as GZDV (see DOSAGE AND ADMINISTRATION: Pediatrics).

Patients Aged Less Than 3 Months: Zidovudine pharmacokinetics have been evaluated in pediatric patients from birth to 3 months of life. Zidovudine elimination was determined immediately following birth in 8 neonates who were exposed to zidovudine in utero. The half-life was 13.0 ± 5.8 hours. In neonates ≤14 days old, bioavailability was greater, total body clearance was slower, and half-life was longer than in pediatric patients >14 days old. For dose recommendations for neonates, see DOSAGE AND ADMINISTRATION: Neonatal Dosing.

[See table 3 above]

Table 3. Zidovudine Pharmacokinetic Parameters in Pediatric Patients[a]

Parameter	Birth to 14 Days	Aged 14 Days to 3 Months	Aged 3 Months to 12 Years
Oral bioavailability (%)	89 ± 19 (n = 15)	61 ± 19 (n = 17)	65 ± 24 (n = 18)
CSF:plasma ratio	no data	no data	0.26 ± 0.17[b] (n = 28)
CL (L/hr/kg)	0.65 ± 0.29 (n = 18)	1.14 ± 0.24 (n = 16)	1.85 ± 0.47 (n = 20)
Elimination half-life (hr)	3.1 ± 1.2 (n = 21)	1.9 ± 0.7 (n = 18)	1.5 ± 0.7 (n = 21)

[a]Data presented as mean ± standard deviation except where noted.
[b]CSF ratio determined at steady-state on constant intravenous infusion.

Pregnancy: Zidovudine pharmacokinetics have been studied in a Phase 1 study of 8 women during the last trimester of pregnancy. As pregnancy progressed, there was no evidence of drug accumulation. Zidovudine pharmacokinetics were similar to those of nonpregnant adults. Consistent with passive transmission of the drug across the placenta, zidovudine concentrations in neonatal plasma at birth were essentially equal to those in maternal plasma at delivery. Although data are limited, methadone maintenance therapy in 5 pregnant women did not appear to alter zidovudine pharmacokinetics. However, in another patient population, a potential for interaction has been identified (see PRECAUTIONS).

Nursing Mothers: **The Centers for Disease Control and Prevention recommend that HIV-infected mothers not breastfeed their infants to avoid risking postnatal transmission of HIV.** After administration of a single dose of 200 mg zidovudine to 13 HIV-infected women, the mean concentration of zidovudine was similar in human milk and serum (see PRECAUTIONS: Nursing Mothers).

Geriatric Patients: Zidovudine pharmacokinetics have not been studied in patients over 65 years of age.

Gender: A pharmacokinetic study in healthy male (n = 12) and female (n = 12) subjects showed no differences in zidovudine exposure (AUC) when a single dose of zidovudine was administered as the 300-mg RETROVIR Tablet.

Drug Interactions:
See Table 4 and PRECAUTIONS: Drug Interactions.

Zidovudine Plus Lamivudine: No clinically significant alterations in lamivudine or zidovudine pharmacokinetics were observed in 12 asymptomatic HIV-infected adult patients given a single oral dose of zidovudine (200 mg) in combination with multiple oral doses of lamivudine (300 mg every 12 hours).

[See table 4 above]

Table 4. Effect of Coadministered Drugs on Zidovudine AUC[a] Note: ROUTINE DOSE MODIFICATION OF ZIDOVUDINE IS NOT WARRANTED WITH COADMINISTRATION OF THE FOLLOWING DRUGS.

Coadministered Drug and Dose	Zidovudine Oral Dose	n	Zidovudine Concentrations		Concentration of Coadministered Drug
			AUC	Variability	
Atovaquone 750 mg q 12 hr with food	200 mg q 8 hr	14	↑AUC 31%	Range 23% to 78%[b]	↔
Fluconazole 400 mg daily	200 mg q 8 hr	12	↑AUC 74%	95% CI: 54% to 98%	Not Reported
Methadone 30 to 90 mg daily	200 mg q 4 hr	9	↑AUC 43%	Range 16% to 64%[b]	↔
Nelfinavir 750 mg q 8 hr × 7 to 10 days	single 200 mg	11	↓AUC 35%	Range 28% to 41%	↔
Probenecid 500 mg q 6 hr × 2 days	2 mg/kg q 8 hr × 3 days	3	↑AUC 106%	Range 100% to 170%[b]	Not Assessed
Rifampin 600 mg daily × 14 days	200 mg q 8 hr × 14 days	8	↓AUC 47%	90% CI: 41% to 53%	Not Assessed
Ritonavir 300 mg q 6 hr × 4 days	200 mg q 8 hr × 4 days	9	↓AUC 25%	95% CI: 15% to 34%	↔
Valproic acid 250 mg or 500 mg q 8 hr × 4 days	100 mg q 8 hr × 4 days	6	↑AUC 80%	Range 64% to 130%[b]	Not Assessed

↑ = Increase; ↓ = Decrease; ↔ = no significant change; AUC = area under the concentration versus time curve; CI = confidence interval.
[a]This table is not all inclusive.
[b]Estimated range of percent difference.

Ribavirin: In vitro data indicate ribavirin reduces phosphorylation of lamivudine, stavudine, and zidovudine. However, no pharmacokinetic (e.g., plasma concentrations or intracellular triphosphorylated active metabolite concentrations) or pharmacodynamic (e.g., loss of HIV/HCV virologic suppression) interaction was observed when ribavirin and lamivudine (n = 18), stavudine (n = 10), or zidovudine (n = 6) were coadministered as part of a multi-drug regimen to HIV/HCV co-infected patients (see WARNINGS).

INDICATIONS AND USAGE

RETROVIR IV Infusion in combination with other antiretroviral agents is indicated for the treatment of HIV infection.

Maternal-Fetal HIV Transmission:
RETROVIR is also indicated for the prevention of maternal-fetal HIV transmission as part of a regimen that includes oral RETROVIR beginning between 14 and 34 weeks of gestation, intravenous RETROVIR during labor, and administration of RETROVIR Syrup to the neonate after birth. The efficacy of this regimen for preventing HIV transmission in women who have received RETROVIR for a prolonged period before pregnancy has not been evaluated. The safety of RETROVIR for the mother or fetus during the first trimester of pregnancy has not been assessed (see Description of Clinical Studies).

Description of Clinical Studies:
Therapy with RETROVIR has been shown to prolong survival and decrease the incidence of opportunistic infections in patients with advanced HIV disease at the initiation of therapy and to delay disease progression in asymptomatic HIV-infected patients.

RETROVIR in combination with other antiretroviral agents has been shown to be superior to monotherapy in one or more of the following endpoints: delaying death, delaying development of AIDS, increasing CD4+ cell counts, and decreasing plasma HIV-1 RNA. The complete prescribing information for each drug should be consulted before combination therapy that includes RETROVIR is initiated.

Pregnant Women and Their Neonates: The utility of RETROVIR for the prevention of maternal-fetal HIV transmission was demonstrated in a randomized, double-blind, placebo-controlled trial (ACTG 076) conducted in HIV-infected pregnant women with CD4+ cell counts of 200 to 1,818 cells/mm^3 (median in the treated group: 560 cells/mm^3) who had little or no previous exposure to RETROVIR. Oral RETROVIR was initiated between 14 and 34 weeks of gestation (median 11 weeks of therapy) followed by intravenous administration of RETROVIR during labor and delivery. Following birth, neonates received oral RETROVIR Syrup for 6 weeks. The study showed a statistically significant difference in the incidence of HIV infection in the neonates (based on viral culture from peripheral blood) between the group receiving RETROVIR and the group receiving placebo. Of 363 neonates evaluated in the study, the estimated risk of HIV infection was 7.8% in the group receiving RETROVIR and 24.9% in the placebo group, a relative reduction in transmission risk of 68.7%. RETROVIR was well tolerated by mothers and infants. There was no difference in pregnancy-related adverse events between the treatment groups.

CONTRAINDICATIONS

RETROVIR IV Infusion is contraindicated for patients who have potentially life-threatening allergic reactions to any of the components of the formulation.

WARNINGS

COMBIVIR® (lamivudine and zidovudine) Tablets and TRIZIVIR® (abacavir sulfate, lamivudine, and zidovudine) Tablets are combination product tablets that contain zidovudine as one of their components. RETROVIR should not be administered concomitantly with COMBIVIR or TRIZIVIR.

The incidence of adverse reactions appears to increase with disease progression; patients should be monitored carefully, especially as disease progression occurs.

Bone Marrow Suppression:
RETROVIR should be used with caution in patients who have bone marrow compromise evidenced by granulocyte count <1,000 cells/mm^3 or hemoglobin <9.5 g/dL. In patients

with advanced symptomatic HIV disease, anemia and neutropenia were the most significant adverse events observed. There have been reports of pancytopenia associated with the use of RETROVIR, which was reversible in most instances, after discontinuance of the drug. However, significant anemia, in many cases requiring dose adjustment, discontinuation of RETROVIR, and/or blood transfusions, has occurred during treatment with RETROVIR alone or in combination with other antiretrovirals.

Frequent blood counts are strongly recommended in patients with advanced HIV disease who are treated with RETROVIR. For HIV-infected individuals and patients with asymptomatic or early HIV disease, periodic blood counts are recommended. If anemia or neutropenia develops, dosage adjustments may be necessary (see DOSAGE AND ADMINISTRATION).

Myopathy:

Myopathy and myositis with pathological changes, similar to that produced by HIV disease, have been associated with prolonged use of RETROVIR.

Lactic Acidosis/Severe Hepatomegaly with Steatosis:

Lactic acidosis and severe hepatomegaly with steatosis, including fatal cases, have been reported with the use of nucleoside analogues alone or in combination, including zidovudine and other antiretrovirals. A majority of these cases have been in women. Obesity and prolonged exposure to antiretroviral nucleoside analogues may be risk factors. Particular caution should be exercised when administering RETROVIR to any patient with known risk factors for liver disease; however, cases have also been reported in patients with no known risk factors. Treatment with RETROVIR should be suspended in any patient who develops clinical or laboratory findings suggestive of lactic acidosis or pronounced hepatotoxicity (which may include hepatomegaly and steatosis even in the absence of marked transaminase elevations).

Use With Interferon- and Ribavirin-Based Regimens:

In vitro studies have shown ribavirin can reduce the phosphorylation of pyrimidine nucleoside analogues such as zidovudine. Although no evidence of a pharmacokinetic or pharmacodynamic interaction (e.g., loss of HIV/HCV virologic suppression) was seen when ribavirin was coadministered with zidovudine in HIV/HCV co-infected patients (see CLINICAL PHARMACOLOGY: Drug Interactions), **hepatic decompensation (some fatal) has occurred in HIV/HCV co-infected patients receiving combination antiretroviral therapy for HIV and interferon alfa with or without ribavirin.** Patients receiving interferon alfa with or without ribavirin and RETROVIR should be closely monitored for treatment-associated toxicities, especially hepatic decompensation, neutropenia, and anemia. Discontinuation of RETROVIR should be considered as medically appropriate. Dose reduction or discontinuation of interferon alfa, ribavirin, or both should also be considered if worsening clinical toxicities are observed, including hepatic decompensation (e.g., Childs Pugh >6) (see the complete prescribing information for interferon and ribavirin).

PRECAUTIONS

General:

Zidovudine is eliminated from the body primarily by renal excretion following metabolism in the liver (glucuronidation). In patients with severely impaired renal function (CrCl<15 mL/min), dosage reduction is recommended. Although the data are limited, zidovudine concentrations appear to be increased in patients with severely impaired hepatic function, which may increase the risk of hematologic toxicity (see CLINICAL PHARMACOLOGY: Pharmacokinetics and DOSAGE AND ADMINISTRATION).

Immune Reconstitution Syndrome:

Immune reconstitution syndrome has been reported in patients treated with combination antiretroviral therapy, including RETROVIR. During the initial phase of combination antiretroviral treatment, patients whose immune system responds may develop an inflammatory response to indolent or residual opportunistic infections (such as *Mycobacterium avium* infection, cytomegalovirus, *Pneumocystis jirovecii* pneumonia [PCP], or tuberculosis), which may necessitate further evaluation and treatment.

Autoimmune disorders (such as Graves' disease, polymyositis, and Guillain-Barré syndrome) have also been reported to occur in the setting of immune reconstitution, however, the time to onset is more variable, and can occur many months after initiation of treatment.

Information for Patients:

RETROVIR is not a cure for HIV-1 infection, and patients may continue to experience illnesses associated with HIV-1 infection, including opportunistic infections. Patients should remain under the care of a physician when using RETROVIR.

Patients should be advised to avoid doing things that can spread HIV-1 infection to others.

- **Do not share needles or other injection equipment.**
- **Do not share personal items that can have blood or body fluids on them, like toothbrushes and razor blades.**
- **Do not have any kind of sex without protection.** Always practice safe sex by using a latex or polyurethane condom or other barrier method to lower the chance of sexual contact with semen, vaginal secretions, or blood.
- **Do not breastfeed.** Zidovudine is excreted in human breast milk. Mothers with HIV-1 should not breastfeed because HIV-1 can be passed to the baby in the breast milk.

The safety and efficacy of RETROVIR in treating women, intravenous drug users, and racial minorities is not significantly different than that observed in white males.

Patients should be informed that the major toxicities of RETROVIR are neutropenia and/or anemia. The frequency and severity of these toxicities are greater in patients with more advanced disease and in those who initiate therapy later in the course of their infection. They should be told that if toxicity develops, they may require transfusions or drug discontinuation. They should be told of the extreme importance of having their blood counts followed closely while on therapy, especially for patients with advanced symptomatic HIV disease. They should be cautioned about the use of other medications, including ganciclovir and interferon alfa, which may exacerbate the toxicity of RETROVIR (see PRECAUTIONS: Drug Interactions). Patients should be informed that other adverse effects of RETROVIR include nausea and vomiting. Patients should also be encouraged to contact their physician if they experience muscle weakness, shortness of breath, symptoms of hepatitis or pancreatitis, or any other unexpected adverse events while being treated with RETROVIR.

Pregnant women considering the use of RETROVIR during pregnancy for prevention of HIV transmission to their infants should be advised that transmission may still occur in some cases despite therapy. The long-term consequences of in utero and neonatal exposure to RETROVIR are unknown, including the possible risk of cancer.

HIV-infected pregnant women should be advised not to breastfeed to avoid postnatal transmission of HIV to a child who may not yet be infected.

Drug Interactions:

See CLINICAL PHARMACOLOGY section (Table 4) for information on zidovudine concentrations when coadministered with other drugs. For patients experiencing pronounced anemia or other severe zidovudine-associated events while receiving chronic administration of zidovudine and some of the drugs (e.g., fluconazole, valproic acid) listed in Table 4, zidovudine dose reduction may be considered.

Antiretroviral Agents: Concomitant use of zidovudine with stavudine should be avoided since an antagonistic relationship has been demonstrated in vitro.

Some nucleoside analogues affecting DNA replication, such as ribavirin, antagonize the in vitro antiviral activity of RETROVIR against HIV; concomitant use of such drugs should be avoided.

Doxorubicin: Concomitant use of zidovudine with doxorubicin should be avoided since an antagonistic relationship has been demonstrated in vitro (see CLINICAL PHARMACOLOGY for additional drug interactions).

Phenytoin: Phenytoin plasma levels have been reported to be low in some patients receiving RETROVIR, while in 1 case a high level was documented. However, in a pharmacokinetic interaction study in which 12 HIV-positive volunteers received a single 300-mg phenytoin dose alone and during steady-state zidovudine conditions (200 mg every 4 hours), no change in phenytoin kinetics was observed. Although not designed to optimally assess the effect of phenytoin on zidovudine kinetics, a 30% decrease in oral zidovudine clearance was observed with phenytoin.

Overlapping Toxicities: Coadministration of ganciclovir, interferon alfa, and other bone marrow suppressive or cytotoxic agents may increase the hematologic toxicity of zidovudine.

Carcinogenesis, Mutagenesis, Impairment of Fertility:

Zidovudine was administered orally at 3 dosage levels to separate groups of mice and rats (60 females and 60 males in each group). Initial single daily doses were 30, 60, and 120 mg/kg/day in mice and 80, 220, and 600 mg/kg/day in rats. The doses in mice were reduced to 20, 30, and 40 mg/kg/day after day 90 because of treatment-related anemia, whereas in rats only the high dose was reduced to 450 mg/kg/day on day 91, and then to 300 mg/kg/day on day 279.

In mice, 7 late-appearing (after 19 months) vaginal neoplasms (5 nonmetastasizing squamous cell carcinomas, 1 squamous cell papilloma, and 1 squamous polyp) occurred in animals given the highest dose. One late-appearing squamous cell papilloma occurred in the vagina of a middle-dose animal. No vaginal tumors were found at the lowest dose.

In rats, 2 late-appearing (after 20 months), nonmetastasizing vaginal squamous cell carcinomas occurred in animals given the highest dose. No vaginal tumors occurred at the low or middle dose in rats. No other drug-related tumors were observed in either sex of either species.

At doses that produced tumors in mice and rats, the estimated drug exposure (as measured by AUC) was approximately 3 times (mouse) and 24 times (rat) the estimated human exposure at the recommended therapeutic dose of 100 mg every 4 hours.

Two transplacental carcinogenicity studies were conducted in mice. One study administered zidovudine at doses of 20 mg/kg/day or 40 mg/kg/day from gestation day 10 through parturition and lactation with dosing continuing in offspring for 24 months postnatally. The doses of zidovudine employed in this study produced zidovudine exposures approximately 3 times the estimated human exposure at recommended doses. After 24 months, an increase in incidence of vaginal tumors was noted with no increase in tumors in the liver or lung or any other organ in either gender. These findings are consistent with results of the standard oral carcinogenicity study in mice, as described earlier. A second study administered zidovudine at maximum tolerated doses of 12.5 mg/day or 25 mg/day (~1,000 mg/kg nonpregnant body weight or ~450 mg/kg of term body weight) to pregnant mice from days 12 through 18 of gestation. There was an increase in the number of tumors in the lung, liver, and female reproductive tracts in the offspring of mice receiving the higher dose level of zidovudine. It is not known how predictive the results of rodent carcinogenicity studies may be for humans.

Zidovudine was mutagenic in a 5178Y/TK$^{+/-}$ mouse lymphoma assay, positive in an in vitro cell transformation assay, clastogenic in a cytogenetic assay using cultured human lymphocytes, and positive in mouse and rat micronucleus tests after repeated doses. It was negative in a cytogenetic study in rats given a single dose.

Zidovudine, administered to male and female rats at doses up to 7 times the usual adult dose based on body surface area considerations, had no effect on fertility judged by conception rates.

Pregnancy:

Pregnancy Category C. Oral teratology studies in the rat and in the rabbit at doses up to 500 mg/kg/day revealed no evidence of teratogenicity with zidovudine. Zidovudine treatment resulted in embryo/fetal toxicity as evidenced by an increase in the incidence of fetal resorptions in rats given 150 or 450 mg/kg/day and rabbits given 500 mg/kg/day. The doses used in the teratology studies resulted in peak zidovudine plasma concentrations (after one half of the daily dose) in rats 66 to 226 times, and in rabbits 12 to 87 times, mean steady-state peak human plasma concentrations (after one sixth of the daily dose) achieved with the recommended daily dose (100 mg every 4 hours). In an in vitro experiment with fertilized mouse oocytes, zidovudine exposure resulted in a dose-dependent reduction in blastocyst formation. In an additional teratology study in rats, a dose of 3,000 mg/kg/day (very near the oral median lethal dose in rats of 3,683 mg/kg) caused marked maternal toxicity and an increase in the incidence of fetal malformations. This dose resulted in peak zidovudine plasma concentrations 350 times peak human plasma concentrations. (Estimated area under the curve [AUC] in rats at this dose level was 300 times the daily AUC in humans given 600 mg per day.) No evidence of teratogenicity was seen in this experiment at doses of 600 mg/kg/day or less.

Two rodent transplacental carcinogenicity studies were conducted (see Carcinogenesis, Mutagenesis, Impairment of Fertility).

A randomized, double-blind, placebo-controlled trial was conducted in HIV-infected pregnant women to determine the utility of RETROVIR for the prevention of maternal-fetal HIV transmission (see INDICATIONS AND USAGE: Description of Clinical Studies). Congenital abnormalities occurred with similar frequency between neonates born to mothers who received RETROVIR and neonates born to mothers who received placebo. Abnormalities were either problems in embryogenesis (prior to 14 weeks) or were recognized on ultrasound before or immediately after initiation of study drug.

Antiretroviral Pregnancy Registry: To monitor maternal-fetal outcomes of pregnant women exposed to RETROVIR, an Antiretroviral Pregnancy Registry has been established. Physicians are encouraged to register patients by calling 1-800-258-4263.

Nursing Mothers:

The Centers for Disease Control and Prevention recommend that HIV-infected mothers not breastfeed their infants to avoid risking postnatal transmission of HIV. Zidovudine is excreted in human milk (see CLINICAL PHARMACOLOGY: Pharmacokinetics: Nursing Mothers). Because of both the potential for HIV transmission and the potential for serious adverse reactions in nursing infants, **mothers should be instructed not to breastfeed if they are receiving RETROVIR** (see Pediatric Use and INDICATIONS AND USAGE: Maternal-Fetal HIV Transmission).

Pediatric Use:

RETROVIR has been studied in HIV-infected pediatric patients over 3 months of age who had HIV-related symptoms or who were asymptomatic with abnormal laboratory values indicating significant HIV-related immunosuppression.

RETROVIR has also been studied in neonates perinatally exposed to HIV (see ADVERSE REACTIONS, DOSAGE AND ADMINISTRATION, INDICATIONS AND USAGE: Description of Clinical Studies, and CLINICAL PHARMACOLOGY: Pharmacokinetics).

Geriatric Use:
Clinical studies of RETROVIR did not include sufficient numbers of subjects aged 65 and over to determine whether they respond differently from younger subjects. Other reported clinical experience has not identified differences in responses between the elderly and younger patients. In general, dose selection for an elderly patient should be cautious, reflecting the greater frequency of decreased hepatic, renal, or cardiac function, and of concomitant disease or other drug therapy.

ADVERSE REACTIONS

The adverse events reported during intravenous administration of RETROVIR IV Infusion are similar to those reported with oral administration; neutropenia and anemia were reported most frequently. Long-term intravenous administration beyond 2 to 4 weeks has not been studied in adults and may enhance hematologic adverse events. Local reaction, pain, and slight irritation during intravenous administration occur infrequently.

Adults:
The frequency and severity of adverse events associated with the use of RETROVIR are greater in patients with more advanced infection at the time of initiation of therapy. Table 5 summarizes events reported at a statistically significantly greater incidence for patients receiving RETROVIR orally in a monotherapy study.

Table 5. Percentage (%) of Patients with Adverse Events[a] in Asymptomatic HIV Infection (ACTG 019)

Adverse Event	RETROVIR 500 mg/day (n = 453)	Placebo (n = 428)
Body as a whole		
Asthenia	8.6%[b]	5.8%
Headache	62.5%	52.6%
Malaise	53.2%	44.9%
Gastrointestinal		
Anorexia	20.1%	10.5%
Constipation	6.4%[b]	3.5%
Nausea	51.4%	29.9%
Vomiting	17.2%	9.8%

[a]Reported in ≥5% of study population.
[b]Not statistically significant versus placebo.

In addition to the adverse events listed in Table 5, other adverse events observed in clinical studies were abdominal cramps, abdominal pain, arthralgia, chills, dyspepsia, fatigue, hyperbilirubinemia, insomnia, musculoskeletal pain, myalgia, and neuropathy.
Selected laboratory abnormalities observed during a clinical study of monotherapy with oral RETROVIR are shown in Table 6.

Table 6. Frequencies of Selected (Grade 3/4) Laboratory Abnormalities in Patients with Asymptomatic HIV Infection (ACTG 019)

Adverse Event	RETROVIR 500 mg/day (n = 453)	Placebo (n = 428)
Anemia (Hgb<8 g/dL)	1.1%	0.2%
Granulocytopenia (<750 cells/mm^3)	1.8%	1.6%
Thrombocytopenia (platelets<50,000/mm^3)	0%	0.5%
ALT (>5 × ULN)	3.1%	2.6%
AST (>5 × ULN)	0.9%	1.6%
Alkaline phosphatase (>5 × ULN)	0%	0%

ULN = Upper limit of normal.

Pediatrics:
Study ACTG300: Selected clinical adverse events and physical findings with a ≥5% frequency during therapy with EPIVIR® (lamivudine) 4 mg/kg twice daily plus RETROVIR 160 mg/m^2 orally 3 times daily compared with didanosine in therapy-naive (≤56 days of antiretroviral therapy) pediatric patients are listed in Table 7.

Table 7. Selected Clinical Adverse Events and Physical Findings (≥5% Frequency) in Pediatric Patients in Study ACTG300

Adverse Event	EPIVIR plus RETROVIR (n = 236)	Didanosine (n = 235)
Body as a Whole		
Fever	25%	32%
Digestive		
Hepatomegaly	11%	11%
Nausea & vomiting	8%	7%
Diarrhea	8%	6%
Stomatitis	6%	12%
Splenomegaly	5%	8%
Respiratory		
Cough	15%	18%
Abnormal breath sounds/ wheezing	7%	9%
Ear, Nose, and Throat		
Signs or symptoms of ears[a]	7%	6%
Nasal discharge or congestion	8%	11%
Other		
Skin rashes	12%	14%
Lymphadenopathy	9%	11%

[a]Includes pain, discharge, erythema, or swelling of an ear.

Selected laboratory abnormalities experienced by therapy-naive (≤56 days of antiretroviral therapy) pediatric patients are listed in Table 8.

Table 8. Frequencies of Selected (Grade 3/4) Laboratory Abnormalities in Pediatric Patients in Study ACTG300

Test (Abnormal Level)	EPIVIR plus RETROVIR	Didanosine
Neutropenia (ANC<400 cells/ mm^3)	8%	3%
Anemia (Hgb<7.0 g/dL)	4%	2%
Thrombocytopenia (platelets<50,000/mm^3)	1%	3%
ALT (>10 × ULN)	1%	3%
AST (>10 × ULN)	2%	4%
Lipase (>2.5 × ULN)	3%	3%
Total amylase (>2.5 × ULN)	3%	3%

ULN = Upper limit of normal.
ANC = Absolute neutrophil count.

Additional adverse events reported in open-label studies in pediatric patients receiving RETROVIR 180 mg/m^2 every 6 hours were congestive heart failure, decreased reflexes, ECG abnormality, edema, hematuria, left ventricular dilation, macrocytosis, nervousness/irritability, and weight loss. The clinical adverse events reported among adult recipients of RETROVIR may also occur in pediatric patients.

Use for the Prevention of Maternal-Fetal Transmission of HIV:
In a randomized, double-blind, placebo-controlled trial in HIV-infected women and their neonates conducted to determine the utility of RETROVIR for the prevention of maternal-fetal HIV transmission, RETROVIR Syrup at 2 mg/kg was administered every 6 hours for 6 weeks to neonates beginning within 12 hours following birth. The most commonly reported adverse experiences were anemia (hemoglobin <9.0 g/dL) and neutropenia (<1,000 cells/mm^3). Anemia occurred in 22% of the neonates who received RETROVIR and in 12% of the neonates who received placebo. The mean difference in hemoglobin values was less than 1.0 g/dL for neonates receiving RETROVIR compared to neonates receiving placebo. No neonates with anemia required transfusion and all hemoglobin values spontaneously returned to normal within 6 weeks after completion of therapy with RETROVIR. Neutropenia was reported with similar frequency in the group that received RETROVIR (21%) and in the group that received placebo (27%). The long-term consequences of in utero and infant exposure to RETROVIR are unknown.

Observed During Clinical Practice:
In addition to adverse events reported from clinical trials, the following events have been identified during use of RETROVIR in clinical practice. Because they are reported voluntarily from a population of unknown size, estimates of frequency cannot be made. These events have been chosen for inclusion due to either their seriousness, frequency of reporting, potential causal connection to RETROVIR, or a combination of these factors.

Body as a Whole: Back pain, chest pain, flu-like syndrome, generalized pain.
Cardiovascular: Cardiomyopathy, syncope.
Endocrine: Gynecomastia.
Eye: Macular edema.
Gastrointestinal: Constipation, dysphagia, flatulence, oral mucosal pigmentation, mouth ulcer.
General: Sensitization reactions including anaphylaxis and angioedema, vasculitis.
Hemic and Lymphatic: Aplastic anemia, hemolytic anemia, leukopenia, lymphadenopathy, pancytopenia with marrow hypoplasia, pure red cell aplasia.
Hepatobiliary Tract and Pancreas: Hepatitis, hepatomegaly with steatosis, jaundice, lactic acidosis, pancreatitis.
Musculoskeletal: Increased CPK, increased LDH, muscle spasm, myopathy and myositis with pathological changes (similar to that produced by HIV disease), rhabdomyolysis, tremor.
Nervous: Anxiety, confusion, depression, dizziness, loss of mental acuity, mania, paresthesia, seizures, somnolence, vertigo.
Respiratory: Cough, dyspnea, rhinitis, sinusitis.
Skin: Changes in skin and nail pigmentation, pruritus, rash, Stevens-Johnson syndrome, toxic epidermal necrolysis, sweat, urticaria.
Special Senses: Amblyopia, hearing loss, photophobia, taste perversion.
Urogenital: Urinary frequency, urinary hesitancy.

OVERDOSAGE

Acute overdoses of zidovudine have been reported in pediatric patients and adults. These involved exposures up to 50 grams. No specific symptoms or signs have been identified following acute overdosage with zidovudine apart from those listed as adverse events such as fatigue, headache, vomiting, and occasional reports of hematological disturbances. All patients recovered without permanent sequelae. Hemodialysis and peritoneal dialysis appear to have a negligible effect on the removal of zidovudine, while elimination of its primary metabolite, GZDV, is enhanced.

DOSAGE AND ADMINISTRATION

Adults:
The recommended intravenous dose is 1 mg/kg infused over 1 hour. This dose should be administered 5 to 6 times daily (5 to 6 mg/kg daily). The effectiveness of this dose compared to higher dosing regimens in improving the neurologic dysfunction associated with HIV disease is unknown. A small randomized study found a greater effect of higher doses of RETROVIR on improvement of neurological symptoms in patients with pre-existing neurological disease.
Patients should receive RETROVIR IV Infusion only until oral therapy can be administered. The intravenous dosing regimen equivalent to the oral administration of 100 mg every 4 hours is approximately 1 mg/kg intravenously every 4 hours.

Maternal-Fetal HIV Transmission:
The recommended dosing regimen for administration to pregnant women (>14 weeks of pregnancy) and their neonates is:
Maternal Dosing: 100 mg orally 5 times per day until the start of labor. During labor and delivery, intravenous RETROVIR should be administered at 2 mg/kg (total body weight) over 1 hour followed by a continuous intravenous infusion of 1 mg/kg/hour (total body weight) until clamping of the umbilical cord.
Neonatal Dosing: Start neonatal dosing within 12 hours after birth and continue through 6 weeks of age. Neonates unable to receive oral dosing may be administered RETROVIR intravenously. See Table 9. (See PRECAUTIONS if hepatic disease or renal insufficiency is present.)

Table 9. Recommended Neonatal Dosages of RETROVIR

Route	Total Daily Dose	Dose and Dosage Regimen
Oral	8 mg/kg/day	2 mg/kg every 6 hours
IV	6 mg/kg/day	1.5 mg/kg infused over 30 minutes, every 6 hours

Monitoring of Patients:
Hematologic toxicities appear to be related to pretreatment bone marrow reserve and to dose and duration of therapy. In patients with poor bone marrow reserve, particularly in patients with advanced symptomatic HIV disease, frequent monitoring of hematologic indices is recommended to detect serious anemia or neutropenia (see WARNINGS). In patients who experience hematologic toxicity, reduction in hemoglobin may occur as early as 2 to 4 weeks, and neutropenia usually occurs after 6 to 8 weeks.

Dose Adjustment:
Anemia: Significant anemia (hemoglobin of <7.5 g/dL or reduction of >25% of baseline) and/or significant neutropenia (granulocyte count of<750 cells/mm^3 or reduction of

>50% from baseline) may require a dose interruption until evidence of marrow recovery is observed (see WARNINGS). In patients who develop significant anemia, dose interruption does not necessarily eliminate the need for transfusion. If marrow recovery occurs following dose interruption, resumption in dose may be appropriate using adjunctive measures such as epoetin alfa at recommended doses, depending on hematologic indices such as serum erythropoetin level and patient tolerance.

For patients experiencing pronounced anemia while receiving chronic coadministration of zidovudine and some of the drugs (e.g., fluconazole, valproic acid) listed in Table 4, zidovudine dose reduction may be considered.

End-Stage Renal Disease: In patients maintained on hemodialysis or peritoneal dialysis (CrCl <15 mL/min), recommended dosing is 1 mg/kg every 6 to 8 hours (see CLINICAL PHARMACOLOGY: Pharmacokinetics).

Hepatic Impairment: There are insufficient data to recommend dose adjustment of RETROVIR in patients with mild to moderate impaired hepatic function or liver cirrhosis. Since RETROVIR is primarily eliminated by hepatic metabolism, a reduction in the daily dose may be necessary in these patients. Frequent monitoring of hematologic toxicities is advised (see CLINICAL PHARMACOLOGY: Pharmacokinetics and PRECAUTIONS: General).

Method of Preparation:

RETROVIR IV Infusion must be diluted prior to administration. The calculated dose should be removed from the 20-mL vial and added to 5% Dextrose Injection solution to achieve a concentration no greater than 4 mg/mL. Admixture in biologic or colloidal fluids (e.g., blood products, protein solutions, etc.) is not recommended.

After dilution, the solution is physically and chemically stable for 24 hours at room temperature and 48 hours if refrigerated at 2° to 8°C (36° to 46°F). Care should be taken during admixture to prevent inadvertent contamination. As an additional precaution, the diluted solution should be administered within 8 hours if stored at 25°C (77°F) or 24 hours if refrigerated at 2° to 8°C to minimize potential administration of a microbially contaminated solution.

Parenteral drug products should be inspected visually for particulate matter and discoloration prior to administration whenever solution and container permit. Should either be observed, the solution should be discarded and fresh solution prepared.

Administration:

RETROVIR IV Infusion is administered intravenously at a constant rate over 1 hour. Rapid infusion or bolus injection should be avoided. RETROVIR IV Infusion should not be given intramuscularly.

HOW SUPPLIED

RETROVIR IV Infusion, 10 mg zidovudine in each mL.
20-mL Single-Use Vial, Tray of 10 (NDC 49702-213-05).

Store vials at 15° to 25°C (59° to 77°F) and protect from light.

Manufactured for:
ViiV Healthcare
Research Triangle Park, NC 27709
by:
GlaxoSmithKline
Research Triangle Park, NC 27709

May 2012
RTV: 3PI

SELZENTRY ℞

[sell-ZEN-tree]
(maraviroc)
Tablets, for oral use

HIGHLIGHTS OF PRESCRIBING INFORMATION

These highlights do not include all the information needed to use SELZENTRY safely and effectively. See full prescribing information for SELZENTRY.
SELZENTRY (maraviroc) Tablets, for oral use
Initial U.S. Approval: 2007

WARNING: HEPATOTOXICITY
See full prescribing information for complete boxed warning.
- **Hepatotoxicity has been reported which may be preceded by severe rash or other features of a systemic allergic reaction (e.g., fever, eosinophilia, or elevated IgE).**
- **Immediately evaluate patients with signs or symptoms of hepatitis or allergic reaction. (5.1)**

RECENT MAJOR CHANGES

Warnings and Precautions, Severe Skin and Hypersensitivity Reactions (5.2) 2/2013
Warnings and Precautions, Immune Reconstitution Syndrome (5.4) 08/2012

INDICATIONS AND USAGE

SELZENTRY is a CCR5 co-receptor antagonist indicated for combination antiretroviral treatment of adults infected with only CCR5-tropic HIV-1.
- In treatment-naive subjects, more subjects treated with SELZENTRY experienced virologic failure and developed lamivudine resistance compared with efavirenz. (12.4,14.3)
- Tropism testing with a highly sensitive tropism assay is required for the appropriate use of SELZENTRY. (1)

DOSAGE AND ADMINISTRATION

When given with potent CYP3A inhibitors (with or without potent CYP3A inducers) including PIs (except tipranavir/ritonavir), delavirdine (2, 7.1)	150 mg twice daily
With NRTIs, tipranavir/ritonavir, nevirapine, raltegravir, and other drugs that are not potent CYP3A inhibitors or CYP3A inducers (2, 7.1)	300 mg twice daily
With potent CYP3A inducers including efavirenz (without a potent CYP3A inhibitor) (2, 7.1)	600 mg twice daily

A more complete list of coadministered drugs is listed in *Dosage and Administration (2)*.
Dose adjustment may be necessary in patients with renal impairment. (2.2)

DOSAGE FORMS AND STRENGTHS

Tablets: 150 mg and 300 mg (3)

CONTRAINDICATIONS

- SELZENTRY should not be used in patients with severe renal impairment or end-stage renal disease (ESRD) (CrCl <30 mL/min) who are taking potent CYP3A inhibitors or inducers. (4)

WARNINGS AND PRECAUTIONS

- Hepatotoxicity accompanied by severe rash or systemic allergic reaction, including potentially life-threatening events, has been reported. Hepatic laboratory parameters including ALT, AST, and bilirubin should be obtained prior to starting SELZENTRY and at other time points during treatment as clinically indicated. If rash or symptoms or signs of hepatitis or allergic reaction develop, hepatic laboratory parameters should be monitored and discontinuation of treatment should be considered. Use caution when administering SELZENTRY to patients with pre-existing liver dysfunction or who are co-infected with viral hepatitis B or C. (5.1)
- Severe and potentially life-threatening skin and hypersensitivity reactions have been reported in patients taking SELZENTRY. This includes cases of Stevens-Johnson syndrome, hypersensitivity reaction, and toxic epidermal necrolysis. Immediately discontinue SELZENTRY and other suspected agents if signs or symptoms of severe skin or hypersensitivity reactions develop and monitor clinical status, including liver aminotransferases, closely. (5.2)
- More cardiovascular events, including myocardial ischemia and/or infarction, were observed in treatment-experienced subjects who received SELZENTRY. Use with caution in patients at increased risk of cardiovascular events. (5.3)
- If patients with severe renal impairment or ESRD receiving SELZENTRY (without concomitant CYP3A inducers or inhibitors) experience postural hypotension, the dose of SELZENTRY should be reduced from 300 mg twice daily to 150 mg twice daily. (5.3)

ADVERSE REACTIONS

The most common adverse events in treatment-experienced subjects (>8% incidence) which occurred at a higher frequency compared with placebo are upper respiratory tract infections, cough, pyrexia, rash, and dizziness. (6)

To report SUSPECTED ADVERSE REACTIONS, contact ViiV Healthcare at 1-877-844-8872 or FDA at 1-800-FDA-1088 or www.fda.gov/medwatch

DRUG INTERACTIONS

- Coadministration with CYP3A inhibitors, including protease inhibitors (except tipranavir/ritonavir) and delavirdine, will increase the concentration of SELZENTRY. (7.1)
- Coadministration with CYP3A inducers, including efavirenz, may decrease the concentration of SELZENTRY. (7.1)

USE IN SPECIFIC POPULATIONS

- SELZENTRY should only be used in pregnant women if the potential benefit justifies the potential risk to the fetus. (8.1)
- There are no data available in pediatric patients; therefore, SELZENTRY should not be used in patients younger than 16 years. (8.4)

See 17 for PATIENT COUNSELING INFORMATION and Medication Guide

Revised: 02/2013

FULL PRESCRIBING INFORMATION: CONTENTS*

*** Sections or subsections omitted from the full prescribing information are not listed**

FULL PRESCRIBING INFORMATION

WARNING: HEPATOTOXICITY
Hepatotoxicity has been reported with use of SELZENTRY®. Severe rash or evidence of a systemic allergic reaction (e.g., fever, eosinophilia, or elevated IgE) prior to the development of hepatotoxicity may occur. Patients with signs or symptoms of hepatitis or allergic reaction following use of SELZENTRY should be evaluated immediately *[see Warnings and Precautions (5.1)]*.

1 INDICATIONS AND USAGE

SELZENTRY, in combination with other antiretroviral agents, is indicated for adult patients infected with only CCR5-tropic HIV-1.

This indication is based on analyses of plasma HIV–1 RNA levels in 2 controlled trials of SELZENTRY in treatment–experienced subjects and one trial in treatment–naive subjects. Both trials in treatment-experienced subjects were conducted in clinically advanced, 3-class antiretroviral–experienced (nucleoside reverse transcriptase inhibitor [NRTI], non-nucleoside reverse transcriptase inhibitor [NNRTI], protease inhibitor [PI], or enfuvirtide) adults with evidence of HIV–1 replication despite ongoing antiretroviral therapy.

The following points should be considered when initiating therapy with SELZENTRY:
- Adult patients infected with only CCR5-tropic HIV-1 should use SELZENTRY.
- Tropism testing must be conducted with a highly sensitive tropism assay that has demonstrated the ability to iden-

tify patients appropriate for use of SELZENTRY. Outgrowth of pre-existing low-level CXCR4- or dual/mixed-tropic HIV-1 not detected by tropism testing at screening has been associated with virologic failure on SELZENTRY *[see Microbiology (12.4), Clinical Studies (14.3)]*.

- Use of SELZENTRY is not recommended in subjects with dual/mixed- or CXCR4-tropic HIV-1 as efficacy was not demonstrated in a Phase 2 trial of this patient group.
- The safety and efficacy of SELZENTRY have not been established in pediatric patients.
- In treatment-naive subjects, more subjects treated with SELZENTRY experienced virologic failure and developed lamivudine resistance compared with efavirenz *[see Microbiology (12.4), Clinical Studies (14.3)]*.

2 DOSAGE AND ADMINISTRATION

2.1 Dose Recommendations for Patients With Normal Renal Function

The recommended dose of SELZENTRY differs based on concomitant medications due to drug interactions (see Table 1). SELZENTRY can be taken with or without food. SELZENTRY must be given in combination with other antiretroviral medications.

Table 1 gives the recommended dose adjustments *[see Drug Interactions (7.1)]*.

Table 1. Recommended Dosing Regimen

Concomitant Medications	Dose of SELZENTRY
Potent CYP3A inhibitors (with or without a potent CYP3A inducer) including: • protease inhibitors (except tipranavir/ritonavir) • delavirdine • ketoconazole, itraconazole, clarithromycin • other potent CYP3A inhibitors (e.g., nefazodone, telithromycin)	150 mg twice daily
Other concomitant medications, including tipranavir/ritonavir, nevirapine, raltegravir, all NRTIs, and enfuvirtide	300 mg twice daily
Potent CYP3A inducers (without a potent CYP3A inhibitor) including: • efavirenz • rifampin • etravirine • carbamazepine, phenobarbital, and phenytoin	600 mg twice daily

2.2 Dose Recommendations for Patients With Renal Impairment

Table 2 provides dosing recommendations for patients based on renal function and concomitant medications.

[See table 2 above]

Table 2. Recommended Dosing Regimens Based on Renal Function

Concomitant Medications[a]	Dose of SELZENTRY Based on Renal Function				
	Normal (CrCl>80 mL/min)	Mild (CrCl >50 and ≤80 mL/min)	Moderate (CrCl ≥30 and ≤50 mL/min)	Severe (CrCl <30 mL/min)	End-Stage Renal Disease On Regular Hemodialysis
Potent CYP3A inhibitors (with or without a CYP3A inducer)[a]	150 mg twice daily	150 mg twice daily	150 mg twice daily	NR	NR
Other concomitant medications[a]	300 mg twice daily	300 mg twice daily	300 mg twice daily	300 mg twice daily[b]	300 mg twice daily[b]
Potent CYP3A Inducers (without a potent CYP3A inhibitor)[a]	600 mg twice daily	600 mg twice daily	600 mg twice daily	NR	NR

NR = Not recommended.

[a]See Table 1 for the list of concomitant medications.

[b]The dose of SELZENTRY should be reduced to 150 mg twice daily if there are any symptoms of postural hypotension *[see Warnings and Precautions (5.3)]*.

3 DOSAGE FORMS AND STRENGTHS

- 150-mg blue, oval, film-coated tablets debossed with "MVC 150" on one side and plain on the other.
- 300-mg blue, oval, film-coated tablets debossed with "MVC 300" on one side and plain on the other.

4 CONTRAINDICATIONS

SELZENTRY should not be used in patients with severe renal impairment or end-stage renal disease (ESRD) (CrCl <30 mL/min) who are taking potent CYP3A inhibitors or inducers.

5 WARNINGS AND PRECAUTIONS

5.1 Hepatotoxicity

Hepatotoxicity with allergic features including life-threatening events has been reported in clinical trials and postmarketing. Severe rash or evidence of systemic allergic reaction including drug-related rash with fever, eosinophilia, elevated IgE, or other systemic symptoms have been reported in conjunction with hepatotoxicity *[see Warnings and Precautions (5.2)]*. These events occurred approximately 1 month after starting treatment. Among reported cases of hepatitis, some were observed in the absence of allergic features or with no pre-existing hepatic disease.

Appropriate laboratory testing including ALT, AST, and bilirubin should be conducted prior to initiating therapy with SELZENTRY and at other timepoints during treatment as clinically indicated. Hepatic laboratory parameters should be obtained in any patient who develops rash, or signs or symptoms of hepatitis, or allergic reaction. Discontinuation of SELZENTRY should be considered in any patient with signs or symptoms of hepatitis, or with increased liver transaminases combined with rash or other systemic symptoms.

Caution should be used when administering SELZENTRY to patients with pre-existing liver dysfunction or who are co-infected with viral hepatitis B or C. The safety and efficacy of SELZENTRY have not been specifically studied in patients with significant underlying liver disorders. In trials of treatment-experienced HIV-1-infected subjects, approximately 6% of subjects were co-infected with hepatitis B and approximately 6% were co-infected with hepatitis C. Due to the small number of co-infected subjects studied, no conclusions can be drawn regarding whether they are at an increased risk for hepatic adverse events with administration of SELZENTRY.

5.2 Severe Skin and Hypersensitivity Reactions

Severe, potentially life-threatening skin and hypersensitivity reactions have been reported in patients taking SELZENTRY, in most cases concomitantly with other drugs associated with these reactions. These include cases of Stevens-Johnson syndrome (SJS), toxic epidermal necrolysis (TEN), and drug rash with eosinophilia and systemic symptoms (DRESS) [see Adverse Reactions (6.2)]. The cases were characterized by features including rash, constitutional findings, and sometimes organ dysfunction, including hepatic failure. Discontinue SELZENTRY and other suspected agents immediately if signs or symptoms of severe skin or hypersensitivity reactions develop (including, but not limited to, severe rash or rash accompanied by fever, malaise, muscle or joint aches, blisters, oral lesions, conjunctivitis, facial edema, lip swelling, eosinophilia). Delay in stopping treatment with SELZENTRY or other suspect drugs after the onset of rash may result in a life-threatening reaction. Clinical status, including liver aminotransferases, should be monitored and appropriate therapy initiated.

5.3 Cardiovascular Events

Use with caution in patients at increased risk for cardiovascular events. Eleven subjects (1.3%) who received SELZENTRY had cardiovascular events, including myocardial ischemia and/or infarction, during the Phase 3 trials in treatment-experienced subjects (total exposure 609 patient-years [300 on SELZENTRY once daily + 309 on SELZENTRY twice daily]), while no subjects who received placebo had such events (total exposure 111 patient-years). These subjects generally had cardiac disease or cardiac risk factors prior to use of SELZENTRY, and the relative contribution of SELZENTRY to these events is not known.

In the Phase 2b/3 trial in treatment-naive subjects, 3 subjects (0.8%) who received SELZENTRY had events related to ischemic heart diseases and 5 subjects (1.4%) who received efavirenz had such events (total exposure 506 and 508 patient-years for SELZENTRY and efavirenz, respectively).

When SELZENTRY was administered to healthy volunteers at doses higher than the recommended dose, symptomatic postural hypotension was seen at a greater frequency than in placebo. However, when SELZENTRY was given at the recommended dose in HIV-1-infected subjects in Phase 3 trials, postural hypotension was seen at a rate similar to placebo (approximately 0.5%). Caution should be used when administering SELZENTRY in patients with a history of postural hypotension or on concomitant medication known to lower blood pressure.

Postural Hypotension in Patients With Renal Impairment: Patients with impaired renal function may have cardiovascular co-morbidities and could be at increased risk of cardiovascular adverse events triggered by postural hypotension. An increased risk of postural hypotension may occur in patients with severe renal insufficiency or in those with ESRD due to increased maraviroc exposure in some patients. SELZENTRY should be used in patients with severe renal impairment or ESRD only if they are not receiving a concomitant potent CYP3A inhibitor or inducer. However, the use of SELZENTRY in these patients should only be considered when no alternative treatment options are available. If patients with severe renal impairment or ESRD experience any symptoms of postural hypotension while taking 300 mg twice daily, the dose should be reduced to 150 mg twice daily *[see Dosage and Administration (2.2)]*.

5.4 Immune Reconstitution Syndrome

Immune reconstitution syndrome has been reported in patients treated with combination antiretroviral therapy, including SELZENTRY. During the initial phase of combination antiretroviral treatment, patients whose immune system responds may develop an inflammatory response to indolent or residual opportunistic infections (such as infection with *Mycobacterium avium* infection, cytomegalovirus, *Pneumocystis* jirovecii pneumonia [PCP], or tuberculosis, or reactivation of *Herpes* simplex and *Herpes* zoster), which may necessitate further evaluation and treatment.

Autoimmune disorders (such as Graves' disease, polymyositis, and Guillain-Barré syndrome) have also been reported to occur in the setting of immune reconstitution; however, the time to onset is more variable, and can occur many months after initiation of treatment.

5.5 Potential Risk of Infection

SELZENTRY antagonizes the CCR5 co-receptor located on some immune cells, and therefore could potentially increase the risk of developing infections. The overall incidence and severity of infection, as well as AIDS-defining category C infections, were comparable in the treatment groups during the Phase 3 treatment-experienced trials of SELZENTRY. While there was a higher rate of certain upper respiratory tract infections reported in the arm receiving SELZENTRY compared with placebo (23% versus 13%), there was a lower rate of pneumonia (2% versus 5%) reported in subjects receiving SELZENTRY. A higher incidence of Herpes virus infections (11 per 100 patient-years) was also reported in the arm receiving SELZENTRY when adjusted for exposure compared with placebo (8 per 100 patient-years).

In the Phase 2b/3 trial in treatment-naive subjects, the incidence of AIDS-defining Category C events when adjusted for exposure was 1.8 for SELZENTRY compared with 2.4 for efavirenz per 100 patient-years of exposure.

Patients should be monitored closely for evidence of infections while receiving SELZENTRY.

5.6 Potential Risk of Malignancy

While no increase in malignancy has been observed with SELZENTRY, due to this drug's mechanism of action it could affect immune surveillance and lead to an increased risk of malignancy.

The exposure-adjusted rate for malignancies per 100 patient-years of exposure in treatment-experienced trials was 4.6 for SELZENTRY compared with 9.3 on placebo. In treatment naive subjects, the rates were 1.0 and 2.4 per 100 patient-years of exposure for SELZENTRY and efavirenz, respectively.

Long-term follow-up is needed to more fully assess this risk.

6 ADVERSE REACTIONS

The following adverse reactions are discussed in other sections of the labeling:

- Hepatotoxicity *[see Boxed Warning, Warnings and Precautions (5.1)]*
- Severe Skin and Hypersensitivity Reactions *[see Warnings and Precautions (5.2)]*
- Cardiovascular events *[see Warnings and Precautions (5.3)]*

6.1 Clinical Trials Experience

Because clinical trials are conducted under widely varying conditions, adverse reaction rates observed in the clinical trials of a drug cannot be directly compared with rates in the clinical trials of another drug and may not reflect the rates observed in practice.

Table 3. Percentage of Subjects With Selected Treatment-Emergent Adverse Events (All Causality)(≥2% on SELZENTRY and at a higher rate compared with placebo) Trials A4001027 and A4001028 (Pooled Analysis, 48 Weeks)

Body System/ Adverse Event	SELZENTRY Twice Daily[a]		Placebo	
	N = 426 (%)	Exposure-adjusted rate (per 100 pt-yrs) PYE = 309[b]	N = 209 (%)	Exposure-adjusted rate (per 100 pt-yrs) PYE = 111[b]
Eye Disorders				
Conjunctivitis	2	3	1	3
Ocular infections, inflammations, and associated manifestations	2	3	1	2
Gastrointestinal Disorders				
Constipation	6	9	3	6
General Disorders and Administration Site Conditions				
Pyrexia	13	20	9	17
Pain and discomfort	4	5	3	5
Infections and Infestations				
Upper respiratory tract infection	23	37	13	27
Herpes infection	8	11	4	8
Sinusitis	7	10	3	6
Bronchitis	7	9	5	9
Folliculitis	4	5	2	4
Pneumonia	2	3	5	10
Anogenital warts	2	3	1	3
Influenza	2	3	0.5	1
Otitis media	2	3	0.5	1
Metabolism and Nutrition Disorders				
Appetite disorders	8	11	7	13
Musculoskeletal and Connective Tissue Disorders				
Joint-related signs and symptoms	7	10	3	5
Muscle pains	3	4	0.5	1
Neoplasms Benign, Malignant, and Unspecified				
Skin neoplasms benign	3	4	1	3
Nervous System Disorders				
Dizziness/postural dizziness	9	13	8	17
Paresthesias and dysesthesias	5	7	3	6
Sensory abnormalities	4	6	1	3
Disturbances in consciousness	4	5	3	6
Peripheral neuropathies	4	5	3	6
Psychiatric Disorders				
Disturbances in initiating and maintaining sleep	8	11	5	10
Depressive disorders	4	6	3	5
Anxiety symptoms	4	5	3	7
Renal and Urinary Disorders				
Bladder and urethral symptoms	5	7	1	3
Urinary tract signs and symptoms	3	4	1	3
Respiratory, Thoracic, and Mediastinal Disorders				
Coughing and associated symptoms	14	21	5	10
Upper respiratory tract signs and symptoms	6	9	3	6
Nasal congestion and inflammations	4	6	3	5
Breathing abnormalities	4	5	2	5
Paranasal sinus disorders	3	4	0.5	1
Skin and Subcutaneous Tissue Disorders				
Rash	11	16	5	11
Apocrine and eccrine gland disorders	5	7	4	7.5
Pruritus	4	5	2	4
Lipodystrophies	3	5	0.5	1
Erythemas	2	3	1	2
Vascular Disorders				
Vascular hypertensive disorders	3	4	2	4

[a]300-mg dose equivalent.
[b]PYE = Patient-years of exposure.

Trials in Treatment-Experienced Subjects: The safety profile of SELZENTRY is primarily based on 840 HIV-1-infected subjects who received at least 1 dose of SELZENTRY during two Phase 3 trials. A total of 426 of these subjects received the indicated twice-daily dosing regimen.

Assessment of treatment-emergent adverse events is based on the pooled data from 2 trials in subjects with CCR5-tropic HIV-1 (A4001027 and A4001028). The median duration of therapy with SELZENTRY for subjects in these trials was 48 weeks, with the total exposure on SELZENTRY twice daily at 309 patient-years versus 111 patient-years on placebo + optimized background therapy (OBT). The population was 89% male and 84% white, with mean age of 46 years (range: 17 to 75 years). Subjects received dose equivalents of 300 mg maraviroc once or twice daily.

The most common adverse events reported with twice-daily therapy with SELZENTRY with frequency rates higher than placebo, regardless of causality, were upper respiratory tract infections, cough, pyrexia, rash, and dizziness. Additional adverse events that occurred with once-daily dosing at a higher rate than both placebo and twice-daily dosing were diarrhea, edema, influenza, esophageal candidiasis, sleep disorders, rhinitis, parasomnias, and urinary abnormalities. In these 2 trials, the rate of discontinuation due to adverse events was 5% for subjects who received SELZENTRY twice daily + OBT as well as those who received placebo + OBT. Most of the adverse events reported were judged to be mild to moderate in severity. The data described below occurred with twice-daily dosing of SELZENTRY.

The total number of subjects reporting infections were 233 (55%) and 84 (40%) in the group receiving SELZENTRY twice daily and the placebo group, respectively. Correcting for the longer duration of exposure on SELZENTRY compared with placebo, the exposure-adjusted frequency (rate per 100 subject-years) of these events was 133 for both SELZENTRY twice daily and placebo.

Dizziness or postural dizziness occurred in 8% of subjects on either SELZENTRY or placebo, with 2 subjects (0.5%) on SELZENTRY permanently discontinuing therapy (1 due to syncope, 1 due to orthostatic hypotension) versus 1 subject on placebo (0.5%) permanently discontinuing therapy due to dizziness.

Treatment-emergent adverse events, regardless of causality, from A4001027 and A4001028 are summarized in Table 3. Selected events occurring at ≥2% of subjects and at a numerically higher rate in subjects treated with SELZENTRY are included; events that occurred at the same or higher rate on placebo are not displayed.

[See table 3 above]

Laboratory Abnormalities: Table 4 shows the treatment-emergent Grade 3-4 laboratory abnormalities that occurred in >2% of subjects receiving SELZENTRY.

[See table 4 at top of next page]

Trial in Treatment–Naive Subjects: *Treatment–Emergent Adverse Events*: Treatment–emergent adverse events, regardless of causality, from Trial A4001026, a double–blind, comparative, controlled trial in which 721 treatment–naive subjects received SELZENTRY 300 mg twice daily (N = 360) or efavirenz (N = 361) in combination with zidovudine/lamivudine for 96 weeks, are summarized in Table 5. Selected events occurring in ≥2% of subjects and at a numerically higher rate in subjects treated with SELZENTRY are included; events that occurred at the same or higher rate on efavirenz are not displayed.

[See table 5 at top of next page]

Laboratory Abnormalities:

[See table 6 at top of page 2504]

Percentages based on total subjects evaluated for each laboratory parameter. If the same subject in a given treatment group had >1 occurrence of the same abnormality, only the most severe is counted.

Less Common Adverse Events in Clinical Trials: The following adverse events occurred in <2% of subjects treated with SELZENTRY. These events have been included because of their seriousness and either increased frequency on SELZENTRY or are potential risks due to the mechanism of action. Events attributed to the patient's underlying HIV infection are not listed.

Blood and Lymphatic System: Marrow depression and hypoplastic anemia.

Cardiac Disorders: Unstable angina, acute cardiac failure, coronary artery disease, coronary artery occlusion, myocardial infarction, myocardial ischemia.

Hepatobiliary Disorders: Hepatic cirrhosis, hepatic failure, cholestatic jaundice, portal vein thrombosis, hypertransaminasemia, jaundice.

Infections and Infestations: Endocarditis, infective myositis, viral meningitis, pneumonia, treponema infections, septic shock, *Clostridium* difficile colitis, meningitis.

Musculoskeletal and Connective Tissue Disorders: Myositis, osteonecrosis, rhabdomyolysis, blood CK increased.

Neoplasms Benign, Malignant, and Unspecified (Including Cysts and Polyps): Abdominal neoplasm, anal cancer, basal cell carcinoma, Bowen's disease, cholangiocarcinoma, diffuse large B-cell lymphoma, lymphoma, metastases to liver, esophageal carcinoma, nasopharyngeal carcinoma, squamous cell carcinoma, squamous cell carcinoma of skin, tongue neoplasm (malignant stage unspecified), anaplastic large cell lymphomas T- and null-cell types, bile duct neoplasms malignant, endocrine neoplasms malignant and unspecified.

Nervous System Disorders: Cerebrovascular accident, convulsions and epilepsy, tremor (excluding congenital), facial palsy, hemianopia, loss of consciousness, visual field defect.

6.2 Postmarketing Experience

The following events have been identified during post-approval use of SELZENTRY and are not listed above. Because these reactions are reported voluntarily from a population of unknown size, it is not possible to estimate their frequency or establish a causal relationship to exposure to SELZENTRY.

Skin and Subcutaneous Tissue Disorders: Stevens–Johnson syndrome (SJS), drug rash with eosinophilia and systemic symptoms (DRESS), toxic epidermal necrolysis (TEN).

7 DRUG INTERACTIONS

7.1 Effect of Concomitant Drugs on the Pharmacokinetics of Maraviroc

Maraviroc is a substrate of CYP3A and P-glycoprotein (P-gp) and hence its pharmacokinetics are likely to be modulated by inhibitors and inducers of these enzymes/transporters. Therefore, a dose adjustment may be required when maraviroc is coadministered with those drugs *[see Dosage and Administration (2)]*.

Concomitant use of maraviroc and St. John's wort (*Hypericum perforatum*) or products containing St. John's wort is not recommended. Coadministration of maraviroc with St. John's wort is expected to substantially decrease maraviroc concentrations and may result in suboptimal levels of maraviroc and lead to loss of virologic response and possible resistance to maraviroc.

For additional drug interaction information, see *Clinical Pharmacology (12.3)*.

8 USE IN SPECIFIC POPULATIONS

8.1 Pregnancy

Pregnancy Category B: The incidence of fetal variations and malformations was not increased in embryofetal toxicity studies performed with maraviroc in rats at exposures (AUC) approximately 20-fold higher and in rabbits at approximately 5-fold higher than human exposures at the recommended daily dose (up to 1,000 mg/kg/day in rats and 75 mg/kg/day in rabbits). During the pre- and postnatal development studies in the offspring, development of the offspring, including fertility and reproductive performance, was not affected by the maternal administration of maraviroc.

However, there are no adequate and well-controlled studies in pregnant women. Because animal reproduction studies are not always predictive of human response, SELZENTRY should be used during pregnancy only if clearly needed.

Antiretroviral Pregnancy Registry: To monitor maternal-fetal outcomes of pregnant women exposed to SELZENTRY and other antiretroviral agents, an Antiretroviral Pregnancy Registry has been established. Physicians are encouraged to register patients by calling 1-800-258-4263.

8.3 Nursing Mothers

The Centers for Disease Control and Prevention recommend that HIV-infected mothers not breastfeed their infants to avoid risking postnatal transmission of HIV infection. Studies in lactating rats indicate that maraviroc is extensively secreted into rat milk. It is not known whether maraviroc is secreted into human milk. Because of the potential for both HIV transmission and serious adverse reactions in nursing infants, mothers should be instructed not to breastfeed if they are receiving SELZENTRY.

8.4 Pediatric Use

The pharmacokinetics, safety and efficacy of maraviroc in patients younger than 16 years have not been established. Therefore, maraviroc should not be used in this patient population.

8.5 Geriatric Use

There were insufficient numbers of subjects aged 65 and over in the clinical trials to determine whether they respond differently from younger subjects. In general, caution should be exercised when administering SELZENTRY in elderly patients, also reflecting the greater frequency of decreased hepatic and renal function, of concomitant disease and other drug therapy.

8.6 Renal Impairment

Recommended doses of SELZENTRY for patients with impaired renal function (CrCl ≤80 mL/min) are based on the results of a pharmacokinetic trial conducted in healthy subjects with various degrees of renal impairment. The pharmacokinetics of maraviroc in subjects with mild and moderate renal impairment was similar to that in subjects with normal renal function *[see Clinical Pharmacology (12.3)]*. A limited number of subjects with mild and moderate renal impairment in the Phase 3 clinical trials (n = 131 and n = 12, respectively) received the same dose of SELZENTRY as that administered to subjects with normal renal function. In these subjects there was no apparent difference in the adverse event profile for maraviroc compared with subjects with normal renal function.

If patients with severe renal impairment or ESRD not receiving a concomitant potent CYP3A inhibitor or inducer experience any symptoms of postural hypotension while taking SELZENTRY 300 mg twice daily, the dose should be reduced to 150 mg twice daily. No trials have been performed in subjects with severe renal impairment or ESRD co-treated with potent CYP3A inhibitors or inducers. Hence, no dose of SELZENTRY can be recommended, and SELZENTRY is contraindicated for these patients *[see Dosage and Administration (2.2), Contraindications (4), Warnings and Precautions (5.2), Clinical Pharmacology (12.3)]*.

8.7 Hepatic Impairment

Maraviroc is principally metabolized by the liver; therefore, caution should be exercised when administering this drug to patients with hepatic impairment, because maraviroc concentrations may be increased. Maraviroc concentrations are higher when SELZENTRY 150 mg is administered with a potent CYP3A inhibitor compared with following administration of 300 mg without a CYP3A inhibitor, so patients with moderate hepatic impairment who receive SELZENTRY 150 mg with a potent CYP3A inhibitor should be monitored closely for maraviroc-associated adverse events. Maraviroc has not been studied in subjects with severe hepatic impairment *[see Warnings and Precautions (5.1), Clinical Pharmacology (12.3)]*.

8.8 Gender

Population pharmacokinetic analysis of pooled Phase 1/2a data indicated gender (female: n = 96, 23.2% of the total population) does not affect maraviroc concentrations. Dosage adjustment based on gender is not necessary.

8.9 Race

Population pharmacokinetic analysis of pooled Phase 1/2a data indicated exposure was 26.5% higher in Asians (N =

Table 4. Maximum Shift in Laboratory Test Values (Without Regard to Baseline)

Incidence ≥2% of Grade 3-4 Abnormalities (ACTG Criteria) Trials A4001027 and A4001028 (Pooled Analysis, 48 Weeks)

Laboratory Parameter Preferred Term	Limit	SELZENTRY Twice Daily + OBT (N = 421)[a] %	Placebo + OBT (N = 207)[a] %
Aspartate aminotransferase	>5.0x ULN	4.8	2.9
Alanine aminotransferase	>5.0x ULN	2.6	3.4
Total bilirubin	>5.0x ULN	5.5	5.3
Amylase	>2.0x ULN	5.7	5.8
Lipase	>2.0x ULN	4.9	6.3
Absolute neutrophil count	<750/mm^3	4.3	2.4

[a]Percentages based on total subjects evaluated for each laboratory parameter.
ULN=upper limit of normal.

Table 5. Percentage of Subjects With Selected Treatment-Emergent Adverse Events (All Causality) (≥2% on SELZENTRY and at a higher rate compared with efavirenz) Trial A4001026 (96 Weeks)

Body System/ Adverse Event	SELZENTRY 300 mg Twice Daily + Zidovudine/Lamivudine (N = 360) %	Efavirenz 600 mg Once Daily + Zidovudine/Lamivudine (N = 361) %
Blood and Lymphatic System Disorders		
Anemias NEC	8	5
Neutropenias	4	3
Ear and Labyrinth Disorders		
Ear disorders NEC	3	2
Gastrointestinal Disorders		
Flatulence, bloating, and distention	10	7
Gastrointestinal atonic and hypomotility disorders NEC	9	5
Gastrointestinal signs and symptoms NEC	3	2
General Disorders and Administration Site Conditions		
Body temperature perception	3	1
Infections and Infestations		
Bronchitis	13	9
Herpes infection	7	6
Upper respiratory tract infection	32	30
Bacterial infections NEC	6	3
Herpes zoster/varicella	5	4
Lower respiratory tract and lung infections	3	2
Neisseria infections	3	0
Tinea infections	4	3
Viral infections NEC	3	2
Musculoskeletal and Connective Tissue Disorders		
Joint-related signs and symptoms	6	5
Nervous System Disorders		
Memory loss (excluding dementia)	3	1
Paresthesias and dysesthesias	4	3
Renal and Urinary Disorders		
Bladder and urethral symptoms	4	3
Reproductive System and Breast Disorders		
Erection and ejaculation conditions and disorders	3	2
Respiratory, Thoracic, and Mediastinal Disorders		
Upper respiratory tract signs and symptoms	9	5
Skin and Subcutaneous Disorders		
Acnes	3	2
Alopecias	2	1
Lipodystrophies	4	3
Nail and nail bed conditions (excluding infections and infestations)	6	2

Table 6. Maximum Shift in Laboratory Test Values (Without Regard to Baseline) Incidence ≥2% of Grade 3-4 Abnormalities (ACTG Criteria) Trial A4001026 (96 Weeks)

Laboratory Parameter Preferred Term	Limit	SELZENTRY 300 mg Twice Daily + Zidovudine/Lamivudine (N = 353)[a] %	Efavirenz 600 mg Once Daily+ Zidovudine/Lamivudine (N = 350)[a] %
Aspartate aminotransferase	>5.0 × ULN	4.0	4.0
Alanine aminotransferase	>5.0 × ULN	3.9	4.0
Creatine kinase		3.9	4.8
Amylase	>2.0 × ULN	4.3	6.0
Absolute neutrophil count	<750/mm³	5.7	4.9
Hemoglobin	<7.0 g/dL	2.9	2.3

[a]N = Total number of subjects evaluable for laboratory abnormalities.
ULN=upper limit of normal.

Table 7. Treatment-Experienced Subjects With Virologic Success by C_{min} Quartile (Q1-Q4)

	150 mg Twice Daily (With CYP3A Inhibitors)			300 mg Twice Daily (Without CYP3A Inhibitors)		
	n	Median C_{min}	% Subjects With Virologic Success	n	Median C_{min}	% Subjects With Virologic Success
Placebo	160	-	30.6	35		28.6
Q1	78	33	52.6	22	13	50.0
Q2	77	87	63.6	22	29	68.2
Q3	78	166	78.2	22	46	63.6
Q4	78	279	74.4	22	97	68.2

Table 9. Mean Maraviroc Pharmacokinetic Parameters

Patient Population	Maraviroc Dose	N	AUC_{12} (ng.hr/mL)	C_{max} (ng/mL)	C_{min} (ng/mL)
Healthy volunteers (Phase 1)	300 mg twice daily	64	2,908	888	43.1
Asymptomatic HIV subjects (Phase 2a)	300 mg twice daily	8	2,550	618	33.6
Treatment-experienced HIV subjects (Phase 3)[a]	300 mg twice daily	94	1,513	266	37.2
	150 mg twice daily (+ CYP3A inhibitor)	375	2,463	332	101
Treatment-naive HIV subjects (Phase 2b/3)[a]	300 mg twice daily	344	1,865	287	60

[a]The estimated exposure is lower compared with other trials possibly due to sparse sampling, food effect, compliance, and concomitant medications.

95) as compared with non-Asians (n = 318). However, a trial designed to evaluate pharmacokinetic differences between Caucasians (n = 12) and Singaporeans (n = 12) showed no difference between these 2 populations. No dose adjustment based on race is needed.

10 OVERDOSAGE

The highest dose administered in clinical trials was 1,200 mg. The dose-limiting adverse event was postural hypotension, which was observed at 600 mg. While the recommended dose for SELZENTRY in patients receiving a CYP3A inducer without a CYP3A inhibitor is 600 mg twice daily, this dose is appropriate due to enhanced metabolism. Prolongation of the QT interval was seen in dogs and monkeys at plasma concentrations 6 and 12 times, respectively, those expected in humans at the intended exposure of 300 mg equivalents twice daily. However, no significant QT prolongation was seen in the trials in treatment-experienced subjects with HIV using the recommended doses of maraviroc or in a specific pharmacokinetic trial to evaluate the potential of maraviroc to prolong the QT interval *[see Clinical Pharmacology (12.3)]*.

There is no specific antidote for overdose with maraviroc. Treatment of overdose should consist of general supportive measures including keeping the patient in a supine position, careful assessment of patient vital signs, blood pressure, and ECG.

If indicated, elimination of unabsorbed active maraviroc should be achieved by emesis. Administration of activated charcoal may also be used to aid in removal of unabsorbed drug. Since maraviroc is moderately protein-bound, dialysis may be beneficial in removal of this medicine.

11 DESCRIPTION

SELZENTRY (maraviroc) is a selective, slowly reversible, small molecule antagonist of the interaction between human CCR5 and HIV-1 gp120. Blocking this interaction prevents CCR5-tropic HIV-1 entry into cells.

SELZENTRY is available as film-coated tablets for oral administration containing either 150 or 300 mg of maraviroc and the following inactive ingredients: dibasic calcium phosphate (anhydrous), magnesium stearate, microcrystalline cellulose, and sodium starch glycolate. The film coat (Opadry® II Blue [85G20583]) contains FD&C blue #2 aluminum lake, soya lecithin, polyethylene glycol (macrogol 3350), polyvinyl alcohol, talc, and titanium dioxide.

Maraviroc is chemically described as 4,4-difluoro-*N*-{(1*S*)-3-[*exo*-3-(3-isopropyl-5-methyl-4*H*-1,2,4-triazol-4-yl)-8-azabicyclo[3.2.1]oct-8-yl]-1-phenylpropyl}cyclohexanecarboxamide.

The molecular formula is $C_{29}H_{41}F_2N_5O$ and the structural formula is:

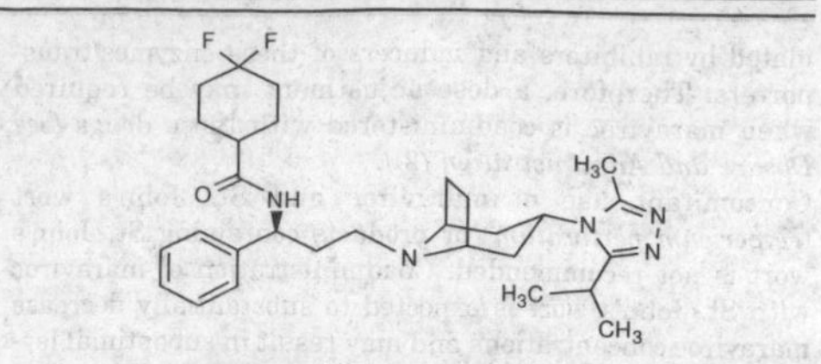

Maraviroc is a white- to pale-colored powder with a molecular weight of 513.67. It is highly soluble across the physiological pH range (pH 1.0 to 7.5).

12 CLINICAL PHARMACOLOGY

12.1 Mechanism of Action

Maraviroc is an antiviral drug *[see Clinical Pharmacology (12.4)]*.

12.2 Pharmacodynamics

Exposure-Response Relationship in Treatment-Experienced Subjects: The relationship between maraviroc, modeled plasma trough concentration (C_{min}) (1 to 9 samples per patient taken on up to 7 visits), and virologic response was evaluated in 973 treatment-experienced HIV-1-infected subjects with varied optimized background antiretroviral regimens in Trials A4001027 and A4001028. The C_{min}, baseline viral load, baseline CD4⁺ cell count, and overall sensitivity score (OSS) were found to be important predictors of virologic success (defined as viral load <400 copies/mL at 24 weeks). Table 7 illustrates the proportions of subjects with virologic success (%) within each C_{min} quartile for 150-mg twice-daily and 300-mg twice-daily groups.

[See table 7 above]

Exposure-Response Relationship in Treatment-Naive Subjects: The relationship between maraviroc, modeled plasma trough concentration (C_{min}) (1 to 12 samples per patient taken on up to 8 visits), and virologic response was evaluated in 294 treatment-naive HIV-1-infected subjects receiving maraviroc 300 mg twice daily in combination with zidovudine/lamivudine in Trial A4001026. Table 8 illustrates the proportion (%) of subjects with virologic success <50 copies/mL at 48 weeks within each C_{min} quartile for the 300-mg twice-daily dose.

Table 8. Treatment-Naive Subjects With Virologic Success by C_{min} Quartile (Q1-Q4)

	300 mg Twice Daily		
	n	Median C_{min}	% Subjects With Virologic Success
Q1	75	23	57.3
Q2	72	39	72.2
Q3	73	56	74.0
Q4	74	81	83.8

Eighteen of 75 (24%) subjects in Q1 had no measurable maraviroc concentration on at least one occasion versus 1 of 73 and 1 of 74 in Q3 and Q4, respectively.

Effects on Electrocardiogram: A placebo-controlled, randomized, crossover trial to evaluate the effect on the QT interval of healthy male and female volunteers was conducted with 3 single oral doses of maraviroc and moxifloxacin. The placebo-adjusted mean maximum (upper 1-sided 95% CI) increases in QTc from baseline after 100, 300, and 900 mg of maraviroc were −2 (0), -1 (1), and 1 (3) msec, respectively, and 13 (15) msec for moxifloxacin 400 mg. No subject in any group had an increase in QTc of ≥60 msec from baseline. No subject experienced an interval exceeding the potentially clinically relevant threshold of 500 msec.

12.3 Pharmacokinetics

[See table 9 above]

Absorption: Peak maraviroc plasma concentrations are attained 0.5 to 4 hours following single oral doses of 1 to 1,200 mg administered to uninfected volunteers. The pharmacokinetics of oral maraviroc are not dose proportional over the dose range.

The absolute bioavailability of a 100–mg dose is 23% and is predicted to be 33% at 300 mg. Maraviroc is a substrate for the efflux transporter P-gp.

Effect of Food on Oral Absorption: Coadministration of a 300–mg tablet with a high–fat breakfast reduced maraviroc C_{max} and AUC by 33% in healthy volunteers. There were no food restrictions in the trials that demonstrated the efficacy and safety of maraviroc *[see Clinical Studies (14)]*. Therefore, maraviroc can be taken with or without food at the recommended dose *[see Dosage and Administration (2)]*.

Distribution: Maraviroc is bound (approximately 76%) to human plasma proteins, and shows moderate affinity for albumin and alpha–1 acid glycoprotein. The volume of distribution of maraviroc is approximately 194 L.

Metabolism: Trials in humans and in vitro studies using human liver microsomes and expressed enzymes have demonstrated that maraviroc is principally metabolized by the cytochrome P450 system to metabolites that are essentially inactive against HIV–1. In vitro studies indicate that CYP3A is the major enzyme responsible for maraviroc metabolism. In vitro studies also indicate that polymorphic enzymes CYP2C9, CYP2D6, and CYP2C19 do not contribute significantly to the metabolism of maraviroc.

Maraviroc is the major circulating component (~42% drug–related radioactivity) following a single oral dose of 300 mg [^{14}C]-maraviroc. The most significant circulating metabolite in humans is a secondary amine (~22% radioactivity) formed by N–dealkylation. This polar metabolite has no significant pharmacological activity. Other metabolites are products of mono–oxidation and are only minor components of plasma drug–related radioactivity.

Excretion: The terminal half–life of maraviroc following oral dosing to steady state in healthy subjects was 14 to 18 hours. A mass balance/excretion trial was conducted using a single 300–mg dose of ^{14}C-labeled maraviroc. Approximately 20% of the radiolabel was recovered in the urine and 76% was recovered in the feces over 168 hours. Maraviroc was the major component present in urine (mean of 8% dose) and feces (mean of 25% dose). The remainder was excreted as metabolites.

Hepatic Impairment: Maraviroc is primarily metabolized and eliminated by the liver. A trial compared the pharmacokinetics of a single 300–mg dose of SELZENTRY in subjects with mild (Child–Pugh Class A, n = 8), and moderate (Child–Pugh Class B, n = 8) hepatic impairment to pharmacokinetics in healthy subjects (n = 8). The mean C_{max} and AUC were 11% and 25% higher, respectively, for subjects with mild hepatic impairment, and 32% and 46% higher, respectively, for subjects with moderate hepatic impairment compared with subjects with normal hepatic function. These changes do not warrant a dose adjustment. Maraviroc concentrations are higher when SELZENTRY 150 mg is administered with a potent CYP3A inhibitor compared with following administration of 300 mg without a CYP3A inhibitor, so patients with moderate hepatic impairment who receive SELZENTRY 150 mg with a potent CYP3A inhibitor should be monitored closely for maraviroc associated adverse events. The pharmacokinetics of maraviroc have not been studied in subjects with severe hepatic impairment *[see Warnings and Precautions (5.1)]*.

Renal Impairment: A trial compared the pharmacokinetics of a single 300–mg dose of SELZENTRY in subjects with severe renal impairment (CLcr <30 mL/min, n = 6) and ESRD (n = 6) to healthy volunteers (n = 6). Geometric mean ratios for maraviroc C_{max} and AUC_{inf} were 2.4–fold and 3.2–fold higher, respectively, for subjects with severe renal impairment, and 1.7–fold and 2.0–fold higher, respectively, for subjects with ESRD as compared with subjects with normal renal function in this trial. Hemodialysis had a minimal effect on maraviroc clearance and exposure in subjects with ESRD. Exposures observed in subjects with severe renal impairment and ESRD were within the range observed in previous 300–mg single–dose trials of SELZENTRY in healthy volunteers with normal renal function. However, maraviroc exposures in the subjects with normal renal function in this trial were 50% lower than that observed in previous trials. Based on the results of this trial, no dose adjustment is recommended for patients with renal impairment receiving SELZENTRY without a potent CYP3A inhibitor or inducer. However, if patients with severe renal impairment or ESRD experience any symptoms of postural hypotension while taking SELZENTRY 300 mg twice daily, their dose should be reduced to 150 mg twice daily *[see Dosage and Administration (2.2); Warnings and Precautions (5.2)]*.

In addition, the trial compared the pharmacokinetics of multiple–dose SELZENTRY in combination with saquinavir/ritonavir 1,000/100 mg twice daily (a potent CYP3A inhibitor combination) for 7 days in subjects with mild renal impairment (CLcr >50 and 80 mL/min, n = 6) and moderate renal impairment (CLcr 30 and 50 mL/min, n = 6) to healthy volunteers with normal renal function (n = 6). Subjects received 150 mg of SELZENTRY at different dose frequencies (healthy volunteers – every 12 hours; mild renal impairment – every 24 hours; moderate renal impairment – every 48 hours). Compared with healthy volunteers (dosed every 12 hours), geometric mean ratios for maraviroc AUC_{tau}, C_{max}, and C_{min} were 50% higher, 20% higher, and 43% lower, respectively, for subjects with mild renal impairment (dosed every 24 hours). Geometric mean ratios for maraviroc AUC_{tau}, C_{max}, and C_{min} were 16% higher, 29% lower, and 85% lower, respectively, for subjects with moderate renal impairment (dosed every 48 hours) compared with healthy volunteers (dosed every 12 hours). Based on the data from this trial, no adjustment in dose is recommended for patients with mild or moderate renal impairment *[see Dosage and Administration (2.2)]*.

Effect of Concomitant Drugs on the Pharmacokinetics of Maraviroc: Maraviroc is a substrate of CYP3A and P-gp and hence its pharmacokinetics are likely to be modulated by inhibitors and inducers of these enzymes/transporters. The CYP3A/P-gp inhibitors ketoconazole, lopinavir/ritonavir, ritonavir, darunavir/ritonavir, saquinavir/ritonavir, and atazanavir ± ritonavir all increased the C_{max} and AUC of maraviroc (see Table 10). The CYP3A inducers rifampin, etravirine, and efavirenz decreased the C_{max} and AUC of maraviroc (see Table 10). Tipranavir/ritonavir (net CYP3A inhibitor/P-gp inducer) did not affect the steady–state pharmacokinetics of maraviroc (see Table 10). Cotrimoxazole and tenofovir did not affect the pharmacokinetics of maraviroc.

[See table 10 above]

Table 10. Effect of Coadministered Agents on the Pharmacokinetics of Maraviroc

Coadministered Drug and Dose	N	Dose of SELZENTRY	Ratio (90% CI) of Maraviroc Pharmacokinetic Parameters With/Without Coadministered Drug (No Effect = 1.00)		
			C_{min}	AUC_{tau}	C_{max}
CYP3A and/or P-gp Inhibitors					
Ketoconazole 400 mg q.d.	12	100 mg b.i.d.	3.75 (3.01, 4.69)	5.00 (3.98, 6.29)	3.38 (2.38, 4.78)
Ritonavir 100 mg b.i.d.	8	100 mg b.i.d.	4.55 (3.37, 6.13)	2.61 (1.92, 3.56)	1.28 (0.79, 2.09)
Saquinavir (soft gel capsules) /ritonavir 1,000 mg/100 mg b.i.d.	11	100 mg b.i.d.	11.3 (8.96, 14.1)	9.77 (7.87, 12.14)	4.78 (3.41, 6.71)
Lopinavir/ritonavir 400 mg/100 mg b.i.d.	11	300 mg b.i.d.	9.24 (7.98, 10.7)	3.95 (3.43, 4.56)	1.97 (1.66, 2.34)
Atazanavir 400 mg q.d.	12	300 mg b.i.d.	4.19 (3.65, 4.80)	3.57 (3.30, 3.87)	2.09 (1.72, 2.55)
Atazanavir/ritonavir 300 mg/100 mg q.d.	12	300 mg b.i.d.	6.67 (5.78, 7.70)	4.88 (4.40, 5.41)	2.67 (2.32, 3.08)
Darunavir/ritonavir 600 mg/100 mg b.i.d.	12	150 mg b.i.d.	8.00 (6.35, 10.1)	4.05 (2.94, 5.59)	2.29 (1.46, 3.59)
CYP3A and/or P-gp Inducers					
Efavirenz 600 mg q.d.	12	100 mg b.i.d.	0.55 (0.43, 0.72)	0.55 (0.49, 0.62)	0.49 (0.38, 0.63)
Efavirenz 600 mg q.d.	12	200 mg b.i.d. (+ efavirenz): 100 mg b.i.d. (alone)	1.09 (0.89, 1.35)	1.15 (0.98, 1.35)	1.16 (0.87, 1.55)
Rifampicin 600 mg q.d.	12	100 mg b.i.d.	0.22 (0.17, 0.28)	0.37 (0.33, 0.41)	0.34 (0.26, 0.43)
Rifampicin 600 mg q.d.	12	200 mg b.i.d. (+ rifampicin): 100 mg b.i.d. (alone)	0.66 (0.54, 0.82)	1.04 (0.89, 1.22)	0.97 (0.72, 1.29)
Etravirine 200 mg b.i.d.	14	300 mg b.i.d.	0.61 (0.53, 0.71)	0.47 (0.38, 0.58)	0.40 (0.28, 0.57)
Nevirapine[a] 200 mg b.i.d. (+ lamivudine 150 mg b.i.d., tenofovir 300 mg q.d.)	8	300 mg single dose	-	1.01 (0.65, 1.55)	1.54 (0.94, 2.51)
CYP3A and/or P-gp Inhibitors and Inducers					
Lopinavir/ritonavir + efavirenz 400 mg/100 mg b.i.d. + 600 mg q.d.	11	300 mg b.i.d.	6.29 (4.72, 8.39)	2.53 (2.24, 2.87)	1.25 (1.01, 1.55)
Saquinavir(soft gel capsules) /ritonavir + efavirenz 1,000 mg/100 mg b.i.d. + 600 mg q.d.	11	100 mg b.i.d.	8.42 (6.46, 10.97)	5.00 (4.26, 5.87)	2.26 (1.64, 3.11)
Darunavir/ritonavir + etravirine 600 mg/100 mg b.i.d. + 200 mg b.i.d.	10	150 mg b.i.d.	5.27 (4.51, 6.15)	3.10 (2.57, 3.74)	1.77 (1.20, 2.60)
Fosamprenavir/ritonavir 700 mg/100 mg b.i.d.	14	300 mg b.i.d.	4.74 (4.03, 5.57)	2.49 (2.19, 2.82)	1.52 (1.27, 1.82)
Fosamprenavir/ritonavir 1,400 mg/100 mg q.d.	14	300 mg q.d.	1.80 (1.53, 2.13)	2.26 (1.99, 2.58)	1.45 (1.20, 1.74)
Tipranavir/ritonavir 500 mg/200 mg b.i.d.	12	150 mg b.i.d.	1.80 (1.55, 2.09)	1.02 (0.85, 1.23)	0.86 (0.61, 1.21)
Other					
Raltegravir 400 mg b.i.d.	17	300 mg b.i.d.	0.90 (0.85, 0.96)	0.86 (0.80, 0.92)	0.79 (0.67, 0.94)

[a]Compared with historical data.

Effect of Maraviroc on the Pharmacokinetics of Concomitant Drugs: Maraviroc is unlikely to inhibit the metabolism of coadministered drugs metabolized by the following cytochrome P enzymes (CYP1A2, CYP2B6, CYP2C8, CYP2C9, CYP2C19, and CYP3A) because maraviroc did not inhibit activity of those enzymes at clinically relevant concentrations in vitro. Maraviroc does not induce CYP1A2 in vitro. In vitro results suggest that maraviroc could inhibit P-gp in the gut. However, maraviroc did not significantly affect the pharmacokinetics of digoxin in vivo, indicating maraviroc may not significantly inhibit or induce P-gp clinically.

Drug interaction trials were performed with maraviroc and other drugs likely to be coadministered or commonly used as probes for pharmacokinetic interactions (see Table 10).

Coadministration of fosamprenavir 700 mg/ritonavir 100 mg twice daily and maraviroc 300 mg twice daily decreased the C_{min} and AUC of amprenavir by 36% and 35%, respectively. Coadministration of fosamprenavir 1,400 mg/ritonavir 100 mg once daily and maraviroc 300 mg once daily decreased the C_{min} and AUC by 15% and 30%, respectively. No dosage adjustment is necessary when SELZENTRY is dosed 150 mg twice daily in combination with fosamprenavir/ritonavir dosed once or twice daily. Fosamprenavir should be given with ritonavir when coadministered with SELZENTRY.

Maraviroc had no effect on the pharmacokinetics of zidovudine or lamivudine. Maraviroc decreased the Cmin and AUC of raltegravir by 27% and 37%, respectively, which is not clinically significant. Maraviroc had no clinically relevant effect on the pharmacokinetics of midazolam, the oral contraceptives ethinylestradiol and levonorgestrel, no effect on the urinary 6β-hydroxycortisol/cortisol ratio, suggesting no induction of CYP3A in vivo. Maraviroc had no effect on the debrisoquine metabolic ratio (MR) at 300 mg twice daily or less in vivo and did not cause inhibition of CYP2D6 in vitro until concentrations >100 µM. However, there was 234% increase in debrisoquine MR on treatment compared with baseline at 600 mg once daily, suggesting potential inhibition of CYP2D6 at higher dose.

12.4 Microbiology

Mechanism of Action: Maraviroc is a member of a therapeutic class called CCR5 co-receptor antagonists. Maraviroc selectively binds to the human chemokine receptor CCR5 present on the cell membrane, preventing the interaction of HIV-1 gp120 and CCR5 necessary for CCR5-tropic HIV-1 to enter cells. CXCR4-tropic and dual-tropic HIV-1 entry is not inhibited by maraviroc.

Antiviral Activity in Cell Culture: Maraviroc inhibits the replication of CCR5-tropic laboratory strains and primary isolates of HIV-1 in models of acute peripheral blood leukocyte infection. The mean EC_{50} value (50% effective concentration) for maraviroc against HIV-1 group M isolates (subtypes A to J and circulating recombinant form AE) and group O isolates ranged from 0.1 to 4.5 nM (0.05 to 2.3 ng/mL) in cell culture.

When used with other antiretroviral agents in cell culture, the combination of maraviroc was not antagonistic with NNRTIs (delavirdine, efavirenz, and nevirapine), NRTIs (abacavir, didanosine, emtricitabine, lamivudine, stavudine, tenofovir, zalcitabine, and zidovudine), or protease inhibitors (amprenavir, atazanavir, darunavir, indinavir, lopinavir, nelfinavir, ritonavir, saquinavir, and tipranavir). Maraviroc was additive/synergistic with the HIV fusion inhibitor enfuvirtide. Maraviroc was not active against CXCR4-tropic and dual-tropic viruses (EC_{50} value >10 µM). The antiviral activity of maraviroc against HIV-2 has not been evaluated.

Resistance in Cell Culture: HIV-1 variants with reduced susceptibility to maraviroc have been selected in cell culture, following serial passage of 2 CCR5-tropic viruses (CC1/85 and RU570). The maraviroc-resistant viruses remained CCR5-tropic with no evidence of a change from a CCR5-tropic virus to a CXCR4-using virus. Two amino acid residue substitutions in the V3-loop region of the HIV-1 envelope glycoprotein (gp160), A316T, and I323V (HXB2 numbering), were shown to be necessary for the maraviroc-resistant phenotype in the HIV-1 isolate CC1/85. In the RU570 isolate a 3-amino acid residue deletion in the V3 loop, ΔQAI (HXB2 positions 315 to 317), was associated with maraviroc resistance. The relevance of the specific gp120 mutations observed in maraviroc-resistant isolates selected in cell culture to clinical maraviroc resistance is not known. Maraviroc-resistant viruses were characterized phenotypically by concentration-response curves that did not reach 100% inhibition in phenotypic drug assays, rather than increases in EC_{50} values.

Cross-Resistance in Cell Culture: Maraviroc had antiviral activity against HIV-1 clinical isolates resistant to NNRTIs, NRTIs, PIs, and the fusion inhibitor enfuvirtide in cell culture (EC_{50} values ranged from 0.7 to 8.9 nM (0.36 to 4.57 ng/mL). Maraviroc-resistant viruses that emerged in cell culture remained susceptible to the enfuvirtide and the protease inhibitor saquinavir.

Clinical Resistance: Virologic failure on maraviroc can result from genotypic and phenotypic resistance to maraviroc, through outgrowth of undetected CXCR4-using virus present before maraviroc treatment (see *Tropism* below), through resistance to background therapy drugs (Table 11), or due to low exposure to maraviroc *[see Clinical Pharmacology (12.2)]*.

Antiretroviral Treatment-Experienced Subjects (Trials A4001027 and A4001028): Week 48 data from treatment-experienced subjects failing maraviroc-containing regimens with CCR5-tropic virus (n = 58) have identified 22 viruses that had decreased susceptibility to maraviroc characterized in phenotypic drug assays by concentration-response curves that did not reach 100% inhibition. Additionally, CCR5-tropic virus from 2 of these treatment-failure subjects had ≥3-fold shifts in EC_{50} values for maraviroc at the time of failure.

Fifteen of these viruses were sequenced in the gp120 encoding region and multiple amino acid substitutions with unique patterns in the heterogeneous V3 loop region were detected. Changes at either amino acid position 308 or 323 (HXB2 numbering) were seen in the V3 loop in 7 of the subjects with decreased maraviroc susceptibility. Substitutions outside the V3 loop of gp120 may also contribute to reduced susceptibility to maraviroc.

Antiretroviral Treatment-Naive Subjects (Trial A4001026): Treatment-naive subjects receiving SELZENTRY had more virologic failures and more treatment-emergent resistance to the background regimen drugs compared with those receiving efavirenz (Table 11).

Table 11. Development of Resistance to Maraviroc or Efavirenz and Background Drugs in Antiretroviral Treatment-Naive Trial A4001026 for Patients with CCR5-Tropic Virus at Screening Using Enhanced Sensitivity TROFILE® Assay

	Maraviroc	Efavirenz
Total N in dataset (as-treated)	273	241
Total virologic failures (as-treated)	85 (31%)	56 (23%)
Evaluable virologic failures with post baseline genotypic and phenotypic data	73	43
• Lamivudine resistance	39 (53%)	13 (30%)
• Zidovudine resistance	2 (3%)	0
• Efavirenz resistance	--	23 (53%)
• Phenotypic resistance to maraviroc[a]	19 (26 %)	

[a]Includes subjects failing with CXCR4- or dual/mixed-tropism because these viruses are not intrinsically susceptible to maraviroc.

In an as-treated analysis of treatment-naive subjects at 96 weeks, 32 subjects failed a maraviroc-containing regimen with CCR5-tropic virus and had a tropism result at failure; 7 of these subjects had evidence of maraviroc phenotypic resistance defined as concentration-response curves that did not reach 95% inhibition. One additional subject had a ≥3-fold shift in the EC_{50} value for maraviroc at the time of failure. A clonal analysis of the V3 loop amino acid envelope sequences was performed from 6 of the 7 subjects. Changes in V3 loop amino acid sequence differed between each of these different subjects, even for those infected with the same virus clade suggesting that that there are multiple diverse pathways to maraviroc resistance. The subjects who failed with CCR5-tropic virus and without a detectable maraviroc shift in susceptibility were not evaluated for genotypic resistance.

Of the 32 maraviroc virologic failures failing with CCR5-tropic virus, 20(63%) also had genotypic and/or phenotypic resistance to background drugs in the regimen (lamivudine, zidovudine).

Tropism: In both treatment-experienced and treatment-naive subjects, detection of CXCR4-using virus prior to initiation of therapy has been associated with a reduced virologic response to maraviroc.

Antiretroviral Treatment-Experienced Subjects: In the majority of cases, treatment failure on maraviroc was associated with detection of CXCR4-using virus (i.e., CXCR4- or dual/mixed-tropic) which was not detected by the tropism assay prior to treatment. CXCR4-using virus was detected at failure in approximately 55% of subjects who failed treatment on maraviroc by Week 48, as compared with 9% of subjects who experienced treatment failure in the placebo arm. To investigate the likely origin of the on-treatment CXCR4-using virus, a detailed clonal analysis was conducted on virus from 20 representative subjects (16 subjects from the maraviroc arms and 4 subjects from the placebo arm) in whom CXCR4-using virus was detected at treatment failure. From analysis of amino acid sequence differences and phylogenetic data, it was determined that CXCR4-using virus in these subjects emerged from a low level of pre-existing CXCR4-using virus not detected by the tropism assay (which is population-based) prior to treatment rather than from a coreceptor switch from CCR5-tropic virus to CXCR4-using virus resulting from mutation in the virus.

Detection of CXCR4-using virus prior to initiation of therapy has been associated with a reduced virological response to maraviroc. Furthermore, subjects failing maraviroc twice daily at Week 48 with CXCR4-using virus had a lower median increase in CD4+ cell counts from baseline (+41 cells/mm^3) than those subjects failing with CCR5-tropic virus (+162 cells/mm^3). The median increase in CD4+ cell count in subjects failing in the placebo arm was +7 cells/mm^3.

Antiretroviral Treatment-Naive Subjects: In a 96-week trial of antiretroviral treatment-naive subjects, 14% (12/85) who had CCR5-tropic virus at screening with an enhanced sensitivity tropism assay (TROFILE) and failed therapy on maraviroc had CXCR4-using virus at the time of treatment failure. A detailed clonal analysis was conducted in 2 previously antiretroviral treatment-naive subjects enrolled in a Phase 2a monotherapy trial who had CXCR4-using virus detected after 10 days treatment with maraviroc. Consistent with the detailed clonal analysis conducted in treatment-experienced subjects, the CXCR4-using variants appear to emerge from outgrowth of a pre-existing undetected CXCR4-using virus. Screening with an enhanced sensitivity tropism assay reduced the number of maraviroc virologic failures with CXCR4- or dual/mixed-tropic virus at failure to 12 compared with 24 when screening with the original tropism assay. All but one (11/12; 92%) of the maraviroc failures failing with CXCR4 or dual/mixed-tropic virus also had genotypic and phenotypic resistance to the background drug lamivudine at failure and 33% (4 /12) developed zidovudine-associated resistance substitutions.

Subjects who had CCR5-tropic virus at baseline and failed maraviroc therapy with CXCR4-using virus had a median increase in CD4+ cell counts from baseline of +113 cells/mm^3 while those subjects failing with CCR5-tropic virus had an increase of +135 cells/mm^3. The median increase in CD4+ cell count in subjects failing in the efavirenz arm was + 95 cells/mm^3.

13 NONCLINICAL TOXICOLOGY

13.1 Carcinogenesis, Mutagenesis, Impairment of Fertility

Carcinogenesis: Long-term oral carcinogenicity studies of maraviroc were carried out in rasH2 transgenic mice (6 months) and in rats for up to 96 weeks (females) and 104 weeks (males). No drug-related increases in tumor incidence were found in mice at 1,500 mg/kg/day and in male and female rats at 900 mg/kg/day. The highest exposures in rats were approximately 11 times those observed in humans at the therapeutic dose of 300 mg twice daily for the treatment of HIV-1 infection.

Mutagenesis: Maraviroc was not genotoxic in the reverse mutation bacterial test (Ames test in *Salmonella* and *E. coli*), a chromosome aberration test in human lymphocytes and rat bone marrow micronucleus test.

Impairment of Fertility: Maraviroc did not impair mating or fertility of male or female rats and did not affect sperm of treated male rats at approximately 20-fold higher exposures (AUC) than in humans given the recommended 300-mg twice daily dose.

14 CLINICAL STUDIES

The clinical efficacy and safety of SELZENTRY are derived from analyses of data from 3 trials in adult subjects infected with CCR5-tropic HIV-1: A4001027 and A4001028 in antiretroviral treatment-experienced adult subjects and A4001026 in treatment-naive subjects. These trials were supported by a 48-week trial in antiretroviral treatment-experienced adult subjects infected with dual/mixed-tropic HIV-1, A4001029.

14.1 Trials in CCR5-Tropic, Treatment-Experienced Subjects

Trials A4001027 and A4001028 were double-blind, randomized, placebo-controlled, multicenter trials in subjects infected with CCR5-tropic HIV-1. Subjects were required to have an HIV-1 RNA of greater than 5,000 copies/mL despite at least 6 months of prior therapy with at least 1 agent from 3 of the 4 antiretroviral drug classes (≥1 NRTI, ≥1 NNRTI, ≥2 PIs, and/or enfuvirtide) or documented resistance to at least 1 member of each class. All subjects received an optimized background regimen consisting of 3 to 6 antiretroviral agents (excluding low-dose ritonavir) selected on the basis of the subject's prior treatment history and baseline genotypic and phenotypic viral resistance measurements. In addition to the optimized background regimen, subjects were then randomized in a 2:2:1 ratio to SELZENTRY 300 mg once daily, SELZENTRY 300 mg twice daily, or placebo. Doses were adjusted based on background therapy as described in *Dosing and Administration*, Table 1.

In the pooled analysis for A4001027 and A4001028, the demographics and baseline characteristics of the treatment groups were comparable (Table 12). Of the 1,043 subjects with a CCR5 tropism result at screening, 7.6% had a dual/mixed-tropism result at the baseline visit 4 to 6 weeks later. This illustrates the background change from CCR5- to dual/mixed-tropism result over time in this treatment-experienced population, prior to a change in antiretroviral regimen or administration of a CCR5 co-receptor antagonist.

[See table 12 above]

The Week 48 results for the pooled Trials A4001027 and A4001028 are shown in Table 13.

[See table 13 at top of next page]

After 48 weeks of therapy, the proportions of subjects with HIV-1 RNA <400 copies/mL receiving SELZENTRY compared with placebo were 56% and 22%, respectively. The mean changes in plasma HIV-1 RNA from baseline to Week 48 were −1.84 $\log_{10}$ copies/mL for subjects receiving SELZENTRY + OBT compared with −0.78 $\log_{10}$ copies/mL for subjects receiving OBT only. The mean increase in CD4+ cell count was higher on SELZENTRY twice daily + OBT (124 cells/mm^3) than on placebo + OBT (60 cells/mm^3).

14.2 Trial in Dual/Mixed-Tropic, Treatment-Experienced Subjects

Trial A4001029 was an exploratory, randomized, double-blind, multicenter trial to determine the safety and efficacy of SELZENTRY in subjects infected with dual/mixed co-receptor tropic HIV-1. The inclusion/exclusion criteria were similar to those for Trials A4001027 and A4001028 above and the subjects were randomized in a 1:1:1 ratio to SELZENTRY once daily, SELZENTRY twice daily, or placebo. No increased risk of infection or HIV disease progression was observed in the subjects who received SELZENTRY. Use of SELZENTRY was not associated with a significant decrease in HIV-1 RNA compared with placebo in these subjects and no adverse effect on CD4+ cell count was noted.

14.3 Trial in Treatment-Naive Subjects

Trial A4001026 is an ongoing, randomized, double-blind, multicenter trial in subjects infected with CCR5-tropic HIV-1 classified by the original TROFILE tropism assay. Subjects were required to have plasma HIV-1 RNA ≥2,000 copies/mL and could not have: 1) previously received any antiretroviral therapy for >14 days, 2) an active or recent opportunistic infection or a suspected primary HIV-1 infection, or 3) phenotypic or genotypic resistance to zidovudine, lamivudine, or efavirenz. Subjects were randomized in a 1:1:1 ratio to SELZENTRY 300 mg once daily, SELZENTRY 300 mg twice daily, or efavirenz 600 mg once daily, each in combination with zidovudine/lamivudine. The efficacy and safety of SELZENTRY are based on the comparison of SELZENTRY twice daily versus efavirenz. In a pre-planned interim analysis at 16 weeks, SELZENTRY 300 mg once daily failed to meet the pre-specified criteria for demonstrating non-inferiority and was discontinued.

The demographic and baseline characteristics of the maraviroc and efavirenz treatment groups were comparable (Table 14). Subjects were stratified by screening HIV-1 RNA levels and by geographic region. The median CD4+ cell counts and mean HIV-1 RNA at baseline were similar for both treatment groups.

[See table 14 at top of next page]

The treatment outcomes at 96 weeks for Trial A4001026 are shown in Table 15. Treatment outcomes are based on re-analysis of the screening samples using a more sensitive tropism assay, Enhanced sensitivity TROFILE HIV tropism assay, which became available after the Week 48 analysis, approximately 15% of the subjects identified as CCR5-tropic in the original analysis had dual/mixed- or CXCR4-tropic virus. Screening with enhanced sensitivity version of the TROFILE tropism assay reduced the number of maraviroc virologic failures with CXCR4- or dual/mixed-tropic virus at failure to 12 compared with 24 when screening with the original TROFILE HIV tropism assay.

[See table 15 at top of next page]

The median increase from baseline in CD4+ cell counts at Week 96 was 184 cells/mm^3 for the arm receiving SELZENTRY compared with 155 cells/mm^3 for the efavirenz arm.

15 REFERENCES

1. IAS-USA Drug Resistance Mutations Figures. http://www.iasusa.org/pub/topics/2006/issue3/125.pdf

16 HOW SUPPLIED/STORAGE AND HANDLING

SELZENTRY film-coated tablets are available as follows: 150- and 300-mg tablets are blue, biconvex, oval, film-coated tablets debossed with "MVC 150" or "MVC 300" on one side and plain on the other.

Table 12. Demographic and Baseline Characteristics of Subjects in Trials A4001027 and A4001028

	SELZENTRY Twice Daily (N = 426)	Placebo (N = 209)
Age (years) Mean (range)	46.3 (21-73)	45.7 (29-72)
Sex		
Male	382 (89.7%)	185 (88.5%)
Female	44 (10.3%)	24 (11.5%)
Race		
White	363 (85.2%)	178 (85.2%)
Black	51 (12.0%)	26 (12.4%)
Other	12 (2.8%)	5 (2.4%)
Region		
U.S.	276 (64.8%)	135 (64.6%)
Non-U.S.	150 (35.2%)	74 (35.4%)
Subjects with previous enfuvirtide use	142 (33.3%)	62 (29.7%)
Subjects with enfuvirtide as part of OBT	182 (42.7%)	91 (43.5%)
Baseline plasma HIV-1 RNA ($\log_{10}$ copies/mL) Mean (range)	4.85 (2.96-6.88)	4.86 (3.46-7.07)
Subjects with screening viral load >100,000 copies/mL	179 (42.0%)	84 (40.2%)
Baseline CD4+ cell count (cells/mm^3) Median (range)	167 (2-820)	171 (1-675)
Subjects with baseline CD4+ cell count ≤200 cells/mm^3)	250 (58.7%)	118 (56.5%)
Subjects with Overall Susceptibility Score (OSS):[a]		
0	57 (13.4%)	35 (16.7%)
1	136 (31.9%)	44 (21.1%)
2	104 (24.4%)	59 (28.2%)
≥3	125 (29.3%)	66 (31.6%)
Subjects with enfuvirtide resistance mutations	90 (21.2%)	45 (21.5%)
Median number of resistance-associated:[b]		
PI mutations	10	10
NNRTI mutations	1	1
NRTI mutations	6	6

[a]OSS - Sum of active drugs in OBT based on combined information from genotypic and phenotypic testing.
[b]Resistance mutations based on IAS guidelines.[1]

Bottle packs 150-mg tablets: 60 tablets (NDC 49702-223-18).

Bottle packs 300-mg tablets: 60 tablets (NDC 49702-224-18).

SELZENTRY film-coated tablets should be stored at 25°C (77°F); excursions permitted between 15°C and 30°C (59°F-86°F) [see USP Controlled Room Temperature].

17 PATIENT COUNSELING INFORMATION

See FDA-approved patient labeling (Medication Guide)

Patients should be informed that liver problems including life-threatening cases have been reported with SELZENTRY. Patients should be informed that if they develop signs or symptoms of hepatitis or allergic reaction following use of SELZENTRY (rash, skin or eyes look yellow, dark urine, vomiting, abdominal pain), they should stop SELZENTRY and seek medical evaluation immediately. Patients should understand that laboratory tests for liver enzymes and bilirubin will be ordered prior to starting SELZENTRY, at other times during treatment, and if they develop severe rash or signs and symptoms of hepatitis or an allergic reaction on treatment *[see Warnings and Precautions (5.1), (5.2)]*.

Patients should be informed that SELZENTRY is not a cure for HIV-1 infection and patients may continue to experience illnesses associated with HIV-1 infection, including opportunistic infections.

Patients should remain under the care of a physician when using SELZENTRY.

Patients should be advised to avoid doing things that can spread HIV-1 infection to others.

- **Do not share needles or other injection equipment.**
- **Do not share personal items that can have blood or body fluids on them, like toothbrushes and razor blades.**
- **Do not have any kind of sex without protection.** Always practice safe sex by using a latex or polyurethane condom to lower the chance of sexual contact with semen, vaginal secretions, or blood.
- **Do not breastfeed.** We do not know if SELZENTRY can be passed to your baby in your breast milk and whether it could harm your baby. Also, mothers with HIV-1 should not breastfeed because HIV-1 can be passed to the baby in the breast milk.

Patients should be advised that it is important to take all their anti–HIV medicines as prescribed and at the same time(s) each day. SELZENTRY must always be used in combination with other antiretroviral drugs. Patients should not alter the dose or discontinue therapy without consulting their physician. If a dose is missed, patients should take the next dose of SELZENTRY as soon as possible and then take their next scheduled dose at its regular time. If it is less than 6 hours before their next scheduled dose, they should not take the missed dose and should instead wait and take the next dose at the regular time.

Patients should be advised that when their supply of SELZENTRY starts to run low, they should ask their doctor or pharmacist for a refill.

Caution should be used when administering SELZENTRY in patients with a history of postural hypotension or on concomitant medication known to lower blood pressure. Patients should be advised that if they experience dizziness while taking SELZENTRY, they should avoid driving or operating machinery.

TROFILE® is a registered trademark of Monogram Biosciences, Inc.

Manufactured for:
ViiV Healthcare
Research Triangle Park, NC 27709
by:
Pfizer Manufacturing Deutschland GmbH
Freiburg, Germany

SEL: 8PI

Table 13. Outcomes of Randomized Treatment at Week 48 Trials A4001027 and A4001028

Outcome	SELZENTRY Twice Daily (N = 426)	Placebo (N = 209)	Mean Difference
Mean change from Baseline to Week 48 in HIV-1 RNA (log_{10} copies/mL)	-1.84	-0.78	-1.05
<400 copies/mL at Week 48	239 (56%)	47 (22%)	34%
<50 copies/mL at Week 48	194 (46%)	35 (17%)	29%
Discontinuations			
Insufficient clinical response	97 (23%)	113 (54%)	
Adverse events	19 (4%)	11 (5%)	
Other	27 (6%)	18 (9%)	
Subjects with treatment-emergent CDC Category C events	22 (5%)	16 (8%)	
Deaths (during trial or within 28 days of last dose)	9 (2%)[a]	1 (0.5%)	

[a]One additional subject died while receiving open-label therapy with SELZENTRY subsequent to discontinuing double-blind placebo due to insufficient response.

Table 14. Demographic and Baseline Characteristics of Subjects in Trial A4001026

	SELZENTRY 300 mg Twice Daily + Zidovudine/Lamivudine (N = 360)	Efavirenz 600 mg Once Daily + Zidovudine/Lamivudine (N = 361)
Age (years)		
Mean	36.7	37.4
Range	20-69	18-77
Female, n%	104 (29)	102 (28)
Race, n%		
White	204 (57)	198 (55)
Black	123 (34)	133 (37)
Asian	6 (2)	5 (1)
Other	27 (8)	25 (7)
Median (range) CD4+ cell count (cells/μL)	241 (5-1,422)	254 (8-1,053)
Median (range) HIV-1 RNA (log_{10} copies/mL)	4.9 (3-7)	4.9 (3-7)

Table 15: Trial Outcome (Snapshot) at Week 96 Using Enhanced Sensitivity Assay[a]

Outcome at Week 96[b]	SELZENTRY 300 mg Twice Daily + Zidovudine/Lamivudine N = 311 n (%)	Efavirenz 600 mg Once Daily + Zidovudine/Lamivudine N = 303 n (%)
Virologic Responders: (HIV-1 RNA <400 copies/mL)	199 (64)	195 (64)
Virologic Failure:		
• Non-sustained HIV-1 RNA suppression	39 (13)	22 (7)
• HIV-1 RNA never suppressed	9 (3)	1 (<1)
Virologic Responders: (HIV-1 RNA <50 copies/mL)	183 (59)	190 (63)
Virologic Failure:		
• Non-sustained HIV-1 RNA suppression	43 (14)	25 (8)
• HIV-1 RNA never suppressed	21 (7)	3 (1)
Discontinuations due to:		
• Adverse events	19 (6)	47 (16)
• Death	2 (1)	2 (1)
• Other[c]	43 (14)	36 (12)

[a]The total number of subjects (Ns) in Table 15 represents the subjects who had a CCR5-tropic virus in the reanalysis of screening samples using the more sensitive tropism assay. This reanalysis reclassified approximately 15% of subjects shown in Table 14 as having dual/mixed- or CXCR4-tropic virus. These numbers are different than those presented in Table 14 because the numbers in Table 14 reflect the subjects with CCR5-tropic virus according to the original tropism assay.
[b]Week 48 results: Virologic responders (<400): 228/311 (73%) in SELZENTRY, 219/303 (72%) in efavirenz; Virologic responders (<50): 213/311 (69 %) in SELZENTRY, 207/303 (68%) in efavirenz
[c]Other reasons for discontinuation include lost to follow-up, withdrawn, protocol violation, and other.

PHARMACIST–DETACH HERE AND GIVE MEDICATION GUIDE TO PATIENT

MEDICATION GUIDE

SELZENTRY® (sell-ZEN-tree) **Tablets**

(maraviroc)

Read the Medication Guide that comes with SELZENTRY before you start taking it and each time you get a refill. There may be new information. This information does not take the place of talking with your healthcare provider about your medical condition or treatment.

What is the most important information I should know about SELZENTRY?

Serious side effects have occurred with SELZENTRY, including liver problems (liver toxicity). An allergic reaction may happen before liver problems occur. Stop taking SELZENTRY and call your healthcare provider right away if you get any of the following symptoms:
- an itchy rash on your body (allergic reaction)
- yellowing of your skin or whites of your eyes (jaundice)
- dark (tea-colored) urine
- vomiting
- upper right stomach area (abdominal) pain

What is SELZENTRY?

SELZENTRY is an anti-HIV medicine called a CCR5 antagonist. HIV-1 (Human Immunodeficiency Virus) is the virus that causes AIDS (Acquired Immune Deficiency Syndrome).

SELZENTRY is used with other anti-HIV medicines in adults with CCR5-tropic HIV-1 infection.

Use of SELZENTRY is not recommended in people with dual/mixed or CXCR4-tropic HIV-1.
- SELZENTRY will not cure HIV-1 infection.
- People taking SELZENTRY may still develop infections, including opportunistic infections or other conditions that happen with HIV-1 infection.
- It is very important that you stay under the care of your healthcare provider during treatment with SELZENTRY.
- The long-term effects of SELZENTRY are not known at this time.

SELZENTRY has not been studied in children less than 16 years of age.

General information about SELZENTRY

SELZENTRY does not cure HIV-1 infection and you may continue to experience illnesses associated with HIV-1 infection, including opportunistic infections. You should remain under the care of a doctor when using SELZENTRY.

Avoid doing things that can spread HIV-1 infection.
- **Do not share needles or other injection equipment.**
- **Do not share personal items that can have blood or body fluids on them, like toothbrushes and razor blades.**
- **Do not have any kind of sex without protection.** Always practice safe sex by using a latex or polyurethane condom to lower the chance of sexual contact with semen, vaginal secretions, or blood.

How does SELZENTRY work?

HIV-1 enters cells in your blood by attaching itself to structures on the surface of the cell called receptors. SELZENTRY blocks a specific receptor called CCR5 that CCR5-tropic HIV-1 uses to enter CD4 or T-cells in your blood. Your healthcare provider will do a blood test to see if you have been infected with CCR5-tropic HIV-1 before prescribing SELZENTRY for you.
- When used with other anti-HIV medicines, SELZENTRY may:
- reduce the amount of HIV-1 in your blood. This is called "viral load".
- increase the number of white blood cells called T (CD4) cells.

SELZENTRY does not work in all people with CCR5-tropic HIV-1 infection.

Who should not take SELZENTRY?

People with severe kidney problems or who are on hemodialysis and are taking certain other medications should not take SELZENTRY. Talk to your healthcare provider before taking this medicine if you have kidney problems.

What should I tell my healthcare provider before taking SELZENTRY?

Before you take SELZENTRY, tell your healthcare provider if you:
- have liver problems including a history of hepatitis B or C.
- have heart problems.
- have kidney problems.
- have low blood pressure or take medicines to lower blood pressure.
- have any other medical condition.
- are pregnant or plan to become pregnant. It is not known if SELZENTRY may harm your unborn baby.
  Antiretroviral Pregnancy Registry. There is a pregnancy registry for women who take antiviral medicines during pregnancy. The purpose of the registry is to collect information about the health of you and your baby. Talk to your healthcare provider about how you can take part in this registry.
- are breastfeeding or plan to breastfeed. **Do not breastfeed.** We do not know if SELZENTRY can be passed to your baby in your breast milk and whether it could harm your baby. Also, mothers with HIV-1 should not breastfeed because HIV-1 can be passed to the baby in the breast milk. Talk with your healthcare provider about the best way to feed your baby.

Tell your healthcare provider about all the medicines you take, including prescription and non-prescription medicines, vitamins, and herbal supplements. Certain other medicines may affect the levels of SELZENTRY in your blood. Your healthcare provider may need to change your dose of SELZENTRY when you take it with certain medicines.

The levels of SELZENTRY in your blood may change and your healthcare provider may need to adjust your dose of SELZENTRY when taking any of the following medications together with SELZENTRY:
- darunavir (PREZISTA®)- delavirdine (RESCRIPTOR®)
- lopinavir/ritonavir (KALETRA®, NORVIR®)- ketoconazole (NIZORAL®)
- atazanavir (REYATAZ®)- itraconazole (SPORANOX®)
- saquinavir (INVIRASE®)- clarithromycin (BIAXIN®)
- nelfinavir (VIRACEPT®)- nefazodone (SERZONE®)
- indinavir (CRIXIVAN®)- telithromycin (KETEK®)
- fosamprenavir (LEXIVA®) - efavirenz (SUSTIVA®, ATRIPLA®)
- etravirine (INTELENCE®)- rifampin (RIFADIN®, RIFATER®)
- carbamezepine (TEGRETOL®)- phenobarbital (LUMINAL®)
- phenytoin (DILANTIN®)
- ritonavir (NORVIR®)

Do not take products that contain St. John's wort (*Hypericum perforatum*). St. John's wort may lower the levels of SELZENTRY in your blood so that it will not work to treat your CCR5-tropic HIV-1 infection.

Know the medicines you take. Keep a list of your medicines. Show the list to your healthcare provider and pharmacist when you get a new medicine.

How should I take SELZENTRY?

Take SELZENTRY exactly as prescribed by your healthcare provider. SELZENTRY comes in 150-mg and 300-mg tablets. Your healthcare provider will prescribe the dose that is right for you.
- Take SELZENTRY 2 times a day.
- Swallow SELZENTRY tablets whole. Do not chew the tablets.
- Take SELZENTRY tablets with or without food.
- Always take SELZENTRY with other anti-HIV drugs as prescribed by your healthcare provider.

Do not change your dose or stop taking SELZENTRY or your other anti-HIV medicines without first talking with your healthcare provider.
- If you take too much SELZENTRY, call your healthcare provider or the poison control center right away.
- If you forget to take SELZENTRY, take the next dose of SELZENTRY as soon as possible and then take your next scheduled dose at its regular time. If it is less than 6 hours before your next dose, do not take the missed dose. Wait and take the next dose at the regular time. Do not take a double dose to make up for a missed dose.
- It is very important to take all your anti-HIV medicines as prescribed. This can help your medicines work better. It also lowers the chance that your medicines will stop working to fight HIV-1 (drug resistance).
- When your SELZENTRY supply starts to run low, ask your healthcare provider or pharmacist for a refill. This is very important because the amount of virus in your blood may increase and SELZENTRY could stop working if it is stopped for even a short period of time.

What are the possible side effects of SELZENTRY?

There have been serious side effects when SELZENTRY has been given with other anti-HIV drugs including:
- **Liver problems.** See "What is the most important information I should know about SELZENTRY?"
- **Serious skin rash and allergic reactions.** Severe and potentially life-threatening skin reactions and allergic reactions have been reported in some patients taking SELZENTRY. If you develop a rash with any of the following symptoms, stop using SELZENTRY and contact your doctor right away:
  - fever
  - generally ill feeling
  - muscle aches
  - blisters or sores in your mouth
  - blisters or peeling of the skin
  - redness or swelling of the eyes
  - swelling of the mouth or face or lips
  - problems breathing
  - yellowing of the skin or whites of your eyes
  - dark or tea colored urine
  - pain, aching, or tenderness on the right side below the ribs
  - loss of appetite
  - nausea/vomiting
- **Heart problems** including heart attack.
- **Low blood pressure when standing up (postural hypotension).** Low blood pressure when standing up can cause dizziness or fainting. Do not drive a car or operate heavy machinery if you have dizziness while taking SELZENTRY.
- **Changes in your immune system.** A condition called Immune Reconstitution Syndrome can happen when you start taking HIV medicines. Your immune system may get stronger and could begin to fight infections that have been hidden in your body such as pneumonia, herpes virus, or tuberculosis. Tell your healthcare provider if you develop new symptoms after starting your HIV medicines.
- **Possible chance of infection or cancer.** SELZENTRY affects other immune system cells and therefore may possibly increase your chance for getting other infections or cancer.

The most common side effects of SELZENTRY include colds, cough, fever, rash, and dizziness.

Tell your healthcare provider about any side effect that bothers you or does not go away.

These are not all of the side effects with SELZENTRY. For more information, ask your healthcare provider or pharmacist.

Call your doctor for medical advice about side effects. You may report side effects to FDA at 1-800-FDA-1088.

How should I store SELZENTRY?
- Store SELZENTRY tablets at room temperature from 59°F to 86°F (15°C to 30°C).
- Safely throw away medicine that is out of date or that you no longer need.

Keep SELZENTRY and all medicines out of the reach of children.

General Information about SELZENTRY

Medicines are sometimes prescribed for conditions that are not mentioned in Medication Guides. Do not use SELZENTRY for a condition for which it was not prescribed. Do not give SELZENTRY to other people, even if they have the same symptoms you have. It may harm them. This Medication Guide summarizes the most important information about SELZENTRY. If you would like more information, talk with your healthcare provider. You can ask your healthcare provider or pharmacist for more information about SELZENTRY that is written for health professionals.

For more information, go to www.selzentry.com.

What are the ingredients in SELZENTRY?

Active ingredient: maraviroc

Inactive ingredients: microcrystalline cellulose, dibasic calcium phosphate (anhydrous), sodium starch glycolate, magnesium stearate

Film-coat: FD&C blue #2 aluminum lake, soya lecithin, polyethylene glycol (macrogol 3350), polyvinyl alcohol, talc, and titanium dioxide

The brands listed are the trademarks or registered marks of their respective owners and are not trademarks of ViiV Healthcare. The makers of these brands are not affiliated with and do not endorse ViiV Healthcare or its products.

This Medication Guide has been approved by the US Food and Drug Administration.

Manufactured for:
ViiV Healthcare
Research Triangle Park, NC 27709
by:
Pfizer Manufacturing Deutschland GmbH
Freiburg, Germany

February 2013
SEL:4MG

TIVICAY ℞
(dolutegravir)
Tablets for Oral Use

HIGHLIGHTS OF PRESCRIBING INFORMATION

These highlights do not include all the information needed to use TIVICAY safely and effectively. See full prescribing information for TIVICAY.

TIVICAY (dolutegravir) Tablets for Oral Use
Initial U.S. Approval: 2013

INDICATIONS AND USAGE

TIVICAY is a human immunodeficiency virus type 1 (HIV-1) integrase strand transfer inhibitor (INSTI) indicated in combination with other antiretroviral agents for the treatment of HIV-1 infection in adults and children aged 12 years and older and weighing at least 40 kg. (1)

The following should be considered prior to initiating TIVICAY:
- Poor virologic response was observed in subjects treated with TIVICAY 50 mg twice daily with an INSTI-resistance Q148 substitution plus 2 or more additional INSTI-resistance substitutions including L74I/M, E138A/D/K/T, G140A/S, Y143H/R, E157Q, G163E/K/Q/R/S, or G193E/R. (12.4)

DOSAGE AND ADMINISTRATION

May be taken without regard to meals. (2)

Adult Population	Recommended Dose
Treatment-naïve or treatment-experienced INSTI-naïve	50 mg once daily
Treatment-naïve or treatment-experienced INSTI-naïve when coadministered with the following potent UGT1A/CYP3A inducers: efavirenz, fosamprenavir/ritonavir, tipranavir/ritonavir, or rifampin	50 mg twice daily
INSTI-experienced with certain INSTI-associated resistance substitutions or clinically suspected INSTI resistance[a] (12.4)	50 mg twice daily

[a] Alternative combinations that do not include metabolic inducers should be considered where possible.

Pediatric Patients: (Treatment-naïve or treatment-experienced, INSTI-naïve, aged 12 years and older, and weighing at least 40 kg). (2.2)
- The recommended dose is TIVICAY 50 mg once daily.
- If efavirenz, fosamprenavir/ritonavir, tipranavir/ritonavir, or rifampin are coadministered, then the dose is TIVICAY 50 mg twice daily.

DOSAGE FORMS AND STRENGTHS

Tablets: 50 mg (3)

CONTRAINDICATIONS

Coadministration with dofetilide is contraindicated. (4)

WARNINGS AND PRECAUTIONS

- Hypersensitivity reactions characterized by rash, constitutional findings, and sometimes organ dysfunction, including liver injury, have been reported. Discontinue TIVICAY and other suspect agents immediately if signs or symptoms of hypersensitivity reactions develop, as a delay in stopping treatment may result in a life-threatening reaction. TIVICAY should not be used in patients who have experienced a previous hypersensitivity reaction to TIVICAY. (5.1)
- Patients with underlying hepatitis B or C may be at increased risk for worsening or development of transaminase elevations with use of TIVICAY. Appropriate laboratory testing prior to initiating therapy and monitoring for hepatotoxicity during therapy with TIVICAY is recommended in patients with underlying hepatic disease such as hepatitis B or C. (5.2)
- Redistribution/accumulation of body fat and immune reconstitution syndrome have been reported in patients treated with combination antiretroviral therapy. (5.3, 5.4)

ADVERSE REACTIONS

The most common adverse reactions of moderate to severe intensity and incidence ≥2% (in those receiving TIVICAY in any one adult trial) are insomnia and headache. (6.1)

To report SUSPECTED ADVERSE REACTIONS, contact ViiV Healthcare at 1-877-844-8872 or FDA at 1-800-FDA-1088 or www.fda.gov/medwatch

DRUG INTERACTIONS

- Drugs that are metabolic inducers may decrease the plasma concentrations of dolutegravir. (7.2, 7.3)
- TIVICAY should be taken 2 hours before or 6 hours after taking cation-containing antacids or laxatives, sucralfate, oral iron supplements, oral calcium supplements, or buffered medications. (7.3)

USE IN SPECIFIC POPULATIONS

- Pregnancy: TIVICAY should be used during pregnancy only if the potential benefit justifies the potential risk. (8.1)
- Nursing mothers: Breastfeeding is not recommended due to the potential for HIV transmission. (8.3)
- Pediatric patients: Safety and efficacy of TIVICAY have not been established in pediatric patients younger than 12 years or weighing less than 40 kg, or in pediatric patients who are INSTI-experienced with documented or clinically suspected resistance to other INSTIs (raltegravir, elvitegravir). (8.4)

See 17 for PATIENT COUNSELING INFORMATION and FDA-approved patient labeling

Revised: 08/2013

FULL PRESCRIBING INFORMATION: CONTENTS*

*** Sections or subsections omitted from the full prescribing information are not listed**

FULL PRESCRIBING INFORMATION

1 INDICATIONS AND USAGE

TIVICAY® is indicated in combination with other antiretroviral agents for the treatment of human immunodeficiency virus type 1 (HIV-1) infection in adults and children aged 12 years and older and weighing at least 40 kg.

The following should be considered prior to initiating treatment with TIVICAY:

- Poor virologic response was observed in subjects treated with TIVICAY 50 mg twice daily with an integrase strand transfer inhibitor (INSTI)-resistance Q148 substitution plus 2 or more additional INSTI-resistance substitutions, including L74I/M, E138A/D/K/T, G140A/S, Y143H/R, E157Q, G163E/K/Q/R/S, or G193E/R *[see Microbiology (12.4)]*.

2 DOSAGE AND ADMINISTRATION

TIVICAY tablets may be taken with or without food.

2.1 Adults

Table 1. Dosing Recommendations for TIVICAY in Adult Patients

Population	Recommended Dose
Treatment-naïve or treatment-experienced INSTI-naïve	50 mg once daily
Treatment-naïve or treatment-experienced INSTI-naïve when coadministered with the following potent UGT1A/CYP3A inducers: efavirenz, fosamprenavir/ritonavir, tipranavir/ritonavir, or rifampin	50 mg twice daily
INSTI-experienced with certain INSTI-associated resistance substitutions or clinically suspected INSTI resistance[a] *[see Microbiology (12.4)]*	50 mg twice daily

[a] Alternative combinations that do not include metabolic inducers should be considered where possible *[see Drug Interactions (7)]*.

The safety and efficacy of doses above 50 mg twice daily have not been evaluated.

2.2 Pediatric Patients

Treatment-Naïve or Treatment-Experienced INSTI-Naïve: The recommended dose of TIVICAY in pediatric patients aged 12 years and older and weighing at least 40 kg is 50 mg administered orally once daily.

If efavirenz, fosamprenavir/ritonavir, tipranavir/ritonavir, or rifampin are coadministered, the recommended dose of TIVICAY is 50 mg twice daily.

Table 2. Treatment-Emergent Adverse Drug Reactions of at Least Moderate Intensity (Grades 2 to 4) and ≥2% Frequency in Treatment-Naïve Subjects in SPRING-2 and SINGLE Trials (Week 48 Analysis)

	SPRING-2		SINGLE	
System Organ Class/ Preferred Term	TIVICAY 50 mg Once Daily + 2 NRTIs (N = 403)	Raltegravir 400 mg Twice Daily + 2 NRTIs (N = 405)	TIVICAY 50 mg + EPZICOM Once Daily (N = 414)	ATRIPLA Once Daily (N = 419)
Psychiatric				
Insomnia	<1%	<1%	3%	2%
Abnormal dreams	<1%	<1%	<1%	2%
Nervous System				
Dizziness	<1%	<1%	<1%	5%
Headache	<1%	<1%	2%	2%
Gastrointestinal				
Nausea	1%	1%	<1%	3%
Diarrhea	<1%	<1%	<1%	2%
Skin and Subcutaneous Tissue				
Rash[a]	0	<1%	<1%	6%
Ear and Labyrinth				
Vertigo	0	<1%	0	2%

[a]Includes pooled terms: rash, rash generalized, rash macular, rash maculo-papular, rash pruritic, and drug eruption.

Safety and efficacy of TIVICAY have not been established in pediatric patients younger than 12 years or weighing less than 40 kg, or in pediatric patients who are INSTI-experienced with documented or clinically suspected resistance to other INSTIs (raltegravir, elvitegravir).

3 DOSAGE FORMS AND STRENGTHS

TIVICAY 50-mg tablets are yellow, round, film-coated, biconvex tablets debossed with SV 572 on one side and 50 on the other side. Each tablet contains 50 mg of dolutegravir (as dolutegravir sodium) *[see Description (11)]*.

4 CONTRAINDICATIONS

Coadministration of TIVICAY with dofetilide is contraindicated due to the potential for increased dofetilide plasma concentrations and the risk for serious and/or life-threatening events *[see Drug Interactions (7)]*.

5 WARNINGS AND PRECAUTIONS

5.1 Hypersensitivity Reactions

Hypersensitivity reactions have been reported and were characterized by rash, constitutional findings, and sometimes organ dysfunction, including liver injury. The events were reported in 1% or fewer subjects receiving TIVICAY in Phase 3 clinical trials. Discontinue TIVICAY and other suspect agents immediately if signs or symptoms of hypersensitivity reactions develop (including, but not limited to, severe rash or rash accompanied by fever, general malaise, fatigue, muscle or joint aches, blisters or peeling of the skin, oral blisters or lesions, conjunctivitis, facial edema, hepatitis, eosinophilia, angioedema, difficulty breathing). Clinical status, including liver aminotransferases, should be monitored and appropriate therapy initiated. Delay in stopping treatment with TIVICAY or other suspect agents after the onset of hypersensitivity may result in a life-threatening reaction. TIVICAY should not be used in patients who have experienced a previous hypersensitivity reaction to TIVICAY.

5.2 Effects on Serum Liver Biochemistries in Patients With Hepatitis B or C Co–infection

Patients with underlying hepatitis B or C may be at increased risk for worsening or development of transaminase elevations with use of TIVICAY *[see Adverse Reactions (6.1)]*. In some cases the elevations in transaminases were consistent with immune reconstitution syndrome or hepatitis B reactivation particularly in the setting where anti-hepatitis therapy was withdrawn. Appropriate laboratory testing prior to initiating therapy and monitoring for hepatotoxicity during therapy with TIVICAY are recommended in patients with underlying hepatic disease such as hepatitis B or C.

5.3 Fat Redistribution

Redistribution/accumulation of body fat, including central obesity, dorsocervical fat enlargement (buffalo hump), peripheral wasting, facial wasting, breast enlargement, and "cushingoid appearance" have been observed in patients receiving antiretroviral therapy. The mechanism and long-term consequences of these events are currently unknown. A causal relationship has not been established.

5.4 Immune Reconstitution Syndrome

Immune reconstitution syndrome has been reported in patients treated with combination antiretroviral therapy, including TIVICAY. During the initial phase of combination antiretroviral treatment, patients whose immune systems respond may develop an inflammatory response to indolent or residual opportunistic infections (such as *Mycobacterium avium* infection, cytomegalovirus, *Pneumocystis jirovecii* pneumonia [PCP], or tuberculosis), which may necessitate further evaluation and treatment.

Autoimmune disorders (such as Graves' disease, polymyositis, and Guillain-Barré syndrome) have also been reported to occur in the setting of immune reconstitution; however, the time to onset is more variable and can occur many months after initiation of treatment.

6 ADVERSE REACTIONS

The following adverse drug reactions (adverse events assessed as causally related by the investigator or ADRs) are discussed in other sections of the labeling:

- Hypersensitivity reactions *[see Warnings and Precautions (5.1)]*.
- Effects on serum liver biochemistries in patients with hepatitis B or C co-infection *[see Warnings and Precautions (5.2)]*.
- Fat Redistribution *[see Warnings and Precautions (5.3)]*.
- Immune Reconstitution Syndrome *[see Warnings and Precautions (5.4)]*.

Because clinical trials are conducted under widely varying conditions, adverse reaction rates observed in the clinical trials of a drug cannot be directly compared with rates in the clinical trials of another drug and may not reflect the rates observed in practice.

6.1 Clinical Trials Experience in Adult Subjects

Treatment–Emergent Adverse Drug Reactions (ADRs): *Treatment-Naïve Subjects*: The safety assessment of TIVICAY in HIV–1–infected treatment-naïve subjects is based on the analyses of 48-week data from 2 ongoing, international, multicenter, double-blind trials, SPRING-2 (ING113086) and SINGLE (ING114467).

In SPRING-2, 822 subjects were randomized and received at least 1 dose of either TIVICAY 50 mg once daily or raltegravir 400 mg twice daily, both in combination with fixed-dose dual nucleoside reverse transcriptase inhibitor (NRTI) treatment (either abacavir sulfate and lamivudine [EPZICOM®] or emtricitabine/tenofovir [TRUVADA®]). There were 808 subjects included in the efficacy and safety analyses. The rate of adverse events leading to discontinuation was 2% in both treatment arms.

In SINGLE, 833 subjects were randomized and received at least 1 dose of either TIVICAY 50 mg with fixed-dose abacavir sulfate and lamivudine (EPZICOM) once daily or fixed-dose efavirenz/emtricitabine/tenofovir (ATRIPLA®) once daily. The rates of adverse events leading to discontinuation were 2% in subjects receiving TIVICAY 50 mg once daily + EPZICOM and 10% in subjects receiving ATRIPLA once daily.

Treatment-emergent ADRs of moderate to severe intensity observed in ≥2% of subjects in either treatment arm are provided in Table 2. Side-by-side tabulation is to simplify presentation; direct comparisons across trials should not be made due to differing trial designs.

[See table 2 above]

In addition, Grade 1 insomnia was reported by 1% and <1% of subjects receiving TIVICAY and raltegravir, respectively, in SPRING-2; whereas in SINGLE the rates were 7% and 3% for TIVICAY and ATRIPLA, respectively. These events were not treatment limiting.

Treatment-Experienced, Integrase Strand Transfer Inhibitor-Naïve Subjects: In an international, multicenter, double-blind trial (ING111762, SAILING), 719 HIV–1–infected, antiretroviral treatment-experienced adults were randomized and received either TIVICAY 50 mg once daily or raltegravir 400 mg twice daily with investigator-selected background regimen consisting of up to 2 agents, including at least one fully active agent. At 24 weeks, the rates of adverse events leading to discontinuation were 2% in subjects receiving TIVICAY 50 mg once daily + background regimen and 4% in subjects receiving raltegravir 400 mg twice daily + background regimen.

The only treatment-emergent ADR of moderate to severe intensity with ≥2% frequency in either treatment group was diarrhea, 1% (5/354) in subjects receiving TIVICAY 50 mg once daily + background regimen and 2% (6/361) in subjects receiving raltegravir 400 mg twice daily + background regimen.

Treatment-Experienced, Integrase Strand Transfer Inhibitor-Experienced Subjects: In a multicenter, open-label, single-arm trial (ING112574, VIKING-3), 183 HIV–1–infected, antiretroviral treatment-experienced adults with virological failure and current or historical evidence of raltegravir and/or elvitegravir resistance received TIVICAY 50 mg twice daily with the current failing background regimen for 7 days and with optimized background therapy from Day 8. The rate of adverse events leading to discontinuation was 3% of subjects at Week 24.

Treatment-emergent ADRs in VIKING-3 were generally similar compared with observations with the 50-mg once-daily dose in adult Phase 3 trials.

Less Common Adverse Reactions Observed in Treatment-Naïve and Treatment-Experienced Trials: The following ADRs occurred in <2% of treatment-naïve or treatment-experienced subjects receiving TIVICAY in a combination regimen in any one trial. These events have been included because of their seriousness and assessment of potential causal relationship.

Gastrointestinal Disorders: Abdominal pain, abdominal discomfort, flatulence, upper abdominal pain, vomiting.

General Disorders: Fatigue.

Hepatobiliary Disorders: Hepatitis.

Musculoskeletal Disorders: Myositis.

Renal and Urinary Disorders: Renal impairment.

Skin and Subcutaneous Tissue Disorders: Pruritus.

Laboratory Abnormalities: *Treatment-Naïve Subjects*: Selected laboratory abnormalities (Grades 2 to 4) with a worsening grade from baseline and representing the worst-grade toxicity in ≥2% of subjects are presented in Table 3. The mean change from baseline observed for selected lipid values is presented in Table 4. Side-by-side tabulation is to simplify presentation; direct comparisons across trials should not be made due to differing trial designs.

[See table 3 above]

[See table 4 above]

Table 3. Selected Laboratory Abnormalities (Grades 2 to 4) in Treatment-Naïve Subjects in SPRING-2 and SINGLE Trials (Week 48 Analysis)

	SPRING-2		SINGLE	
Laboratory Parameter Preferred Term	TIVICAY 50 mg Once Daily + 2 NRTIs (N = 403)	Raltegravir 400 mg Twice Daily + 2 NRTIs (N = 405)	TIVICAY 50 mg + EPZICOM Once Daily (N = 414)	ATRIPLA Once Daily (N = 419)
ALT				
Grade 2 (>2.5-5.0 × ULN)	2%	3%	2%	5%
Grade 3 to 4 (>5.1 × ULN)	2%	1%	<1%	<1%
AST				
Grade 2 (>2.5-5.0 × ULN)	3%	3%	2%	3%
Grade 3 to 4 (>5.1 × ULN)	2%	2%	0	2%
Total Bilirubin				
Grade 2 (1.6-2.5 × ULN)	2%	2%	<1%	0
Grade 3 to 4 (>2.5 × ULN)	<1%	<1%	<1%	0
Creatine kinase				
Grade 2 (6.0-9.9 × ULN)	1%	3%	3%	1%
Grade 3 to 4 (>10.0 × ULN)	4%	3%	3%	4%
Hyperglycemia				
Grade 2 (126-250 mg/dL)	5%	5%	7%	4%
Grade 3 (>251 mg/dL)	<1%	1%	1%	<1%
Lipase				
Grade 2 (>1.5-3.0 × ULN)	5%	6%	8%	7%
Grade 3 to 4 (>3.1 × ULN)	1%	3%	3%	2%
Total neutrophils				
Grade 2 (0.75-0.99 × 109)	3%	3%	2%	4%
Grade 3 to 4 (<0.74 × 109)	2%	1%	2%	3%

ULN = Upper limit of normal.

Table 4. Mean Change From Baseline in Fasted Lipid Values in Treatment-Naïve Subjects in SPRING-2 and SINGLE Trials (Week 48 Analysis)

	SPRING-2		SINGLE	
Laboratory Parameter Preferred Term	TIVICAY 50 mg Once Daily + 2 NRTIs (N = 403)	Raltegravir 400 mg Twice Daily + 2 NRTIs (N = 405)	TIVICAY 50 mg + EPZICOM Once Daily (N = 414)	ATRIPLA Once Daily (N = 419)
Cholesterol (mg/dL)	6.7	8.3	17.1	24.0
HDL cholesterol (mg/dL)	2.8	2.6	5.2	7.9
LDL cholesterol (mg/dL)	2.7	2.8	8.5	13.1
Triglycerides (mg/dL)	7.7	9.8	17.7	18.6

[a] Subjects on lipid-lowering agents at baseline were excluded from these analyses (19 subjects in each arm in SPRING-2, and in SINGLE: TIVICAY n = 27 and ATRIPLA n = 26). Forty-nine subjects initiated a lipid-lowering agent post-baseline; their last fasted on-treatment values (prior to starting the agent) were used regardless if they discontinued the agent (SPRING-2: TIVICAY n = 5, raltegravir n = 8; SINGLE: TIVICAY n = 19 and ATRIPLA: n = 17).

Treatment-Experienced, Integrase Strand Transfer Inhibitor-Naïve Subjects: Laboratory abnormalities observed in SAILING were generally similar compared with observations seen in the treatment-naïve (SPRING-2 and SINGLE) trials.

Treatment-Experienced, Integrase Strand Transfer Inhibitor-Experienced Subjects: The most common treatment-emergent laboratory abnormalities (>5% for Grades 2 to 4 combined) were elevated ALT (8%), AST (6%), cholesterol (8%), hyperglycemia (12%), and lipase (8%). Two percent (3/183) of subjects had a Grade 3 to 4, treatment-emergent hematology laboratory abnormality, with neutropenia (1% [2/183]) being the most frequently reported.

Hepatitis B and/or Hepatitis C Virus Co-infection: In Phase 3 trials, subjects with hepatitis B and/or C virus co-infection were permitted to enroll provided that baseline liver chemistry tests did not exceed 5 times the upper limit of normal. Overall, the safety profile in subjects with hepatitis B and/or C virus co-infection was similar to that observed in subjects without hepatitis B or C co-infection, although the rates of AST and ALT abnormalities were higher in the subgroup with hepatitis B and/or C virus co-infection for all treatment groups. Grades 2 to 4 ALT abnormalities in hepatitis B and/or C co-infected compared with HIV mono-infected subjects receiving TIVICAY were observed in 16% vs. 2% with the 50-mg once-daily dose and 8% vs. 7% with the 50-mg twice-daily dose. Liver chemistry elevations consistent with immune reconstitution syndrome were observed in some subjects with hepatitis B and/or C at the start of therapy with TIVICAY, particularly in the setting where anti-hepatitis therapy was withdrawn *[see Warnings and Precautions (5.2)]*.

Changes in Serum Creatinine: Dolutegravir has been shown to increase serum creatinine due to inhibition of tubular secretion of creatinine without affecting renal glomerular function *[see Clinical Pharmacology (12.2)]*. Increases in serum creatinine occurred within the first 4 weeks of treatment and remained stable through 24 to 48 weeks. In treatment-naïve subjects, a mean change from baseline of 0.11 mg/dL (range: -0.60 mg/dL to 0.62 mg/dL) was observed after 48 weeks of treatment. Creatinine increases were comparable by background NRTIs and were similar in treatment-experienced subjects.

6.2 Clinical Trials Experience in Pediatric Subjects

IMPAACT P1093 is an ongoing multi-center, open-label, non-comparative trial of approximately 160 HIV–1–infected pediatric subjects aged 6 weeks to less than 18 years, of which 23 treatment-experienced, INSTI-naïve subjects aged 12 to less than 18 years were enrolled *[see Use in Specific Populations (8.4), Clinical Studies (14.2)]*.

The adverse reaction profile was similar to that for adults. Grade 2 ADRs reported in at least 1 subject were rash (n = 1), abdominal pain (n = 1), and diarrhea (n = 1). No Grade 3 or 4 ADRs were reported. The Grade 3 laboratory abnormalities were elevated total bilirubin and lipase reported in 1 subject each. No Grade 4 laboratory abnormalities were reported. The changes in mean serum creatinine were similar to those observed in adults.

7 DRUG INTERACTIONS

Refer to Table 5 for established and other potentially significant drug-drug interactions.

7.1 Effect of Dolutegravir on the Pharmacokinetics of Other Agents

In vitro, dolutegravir inhibited the renal organic cation transporter, OCT2 (IC_{50} = 1.93 μM). In vivo, dolutegravir inhibits tubular secretion of creatinine by inhibiting OCT2. Dolutegravir may increase plasma concentrations of drugs eliminated via OCT2 (dofetilide and metformin, Table 5) *[see Contraindications (4), Drug Interactions (7.3)]*.

In vitro, dolutegravir did not inhibit (IC_{50} >50 μM) the following: cytochrome P450 (CYP)1A2, CYP2A6, CYP2B6, CYP2C8, CYP2C9, CYP2C19, CYP2D6, CYP3A, UGT1A1, UGT2B7, P-glycoprotein (P-gp), breast cancer resistance protein (BCRP), organic anion transporter polypeptide (OATP)1B1, OATP1B3, OCT1, or multidrug resistance protein (MRP)2. In vitro, dolutegravir did not induce CYP1A2, CYP2B6, or CYP3A4. Based on these data and the results of drug interaction trials, dolutegravir is not expected to affect the pharmacokinetics of drugs that are substrates of these enzymes or transporters.

In drug interaction trials, dolutegravir did not have a clinically relevant effect on the pharmacokinetics of the following drugs: tenofovir, methadone, midazolam, rilpivirine, and oral contraceptives containing norgestimate and ethinyl estradiol. Using cross-study comparisons to historical pharmacokinetic data for each interacting drug, dolutegravir did not appear to affect the pharmacokinetics of the following drugs: atazanavir, darunavir, efavirenz, etravirine, fosamprenavir, lopinavir, ritonavir, and telaprevir.

7.2 Effect of Other Agents on the Pharmacokinetics of Dolutegravir

Dolutegravir is metabolized by UGT1A1 with some contribution from CYP3A. Dolutegravir is also a substrate of UGT1A3, UGT1A9, BCRP, and P-gp in vitro. Drugs that induce those enzymes and transporters may decrease dolutegravir plasma concentration and reduce the therapeutic effect of dolutegravir.

Table 5. Established and Other Potentially Significant Drug Interactions: Alterations in Dose or Regimen May Be Recommended Based on Drug Interaction Trials or Predicted Interactions [see Dosage and Administration (2)]

Concomitant Drug Class: Drug Name	Effect on Concentration of Dolutegravir and/or Concomitant Drug	Clinical Comment
	HIV-1 Antiviral Agents	
Non-nucleoside reverse transcriptase inhibitor: Etravirine[a]	↓Dolutegravir	TIVICAY should not be used with etravirine without coadministration of atazanavir/ritonavir, darunavir/ ritonavir, or lopinavir/ritonavir.
Non-nucleoside reverse transcriptase inhibitor: Efavirenz[a]	↓Dolutegravir	A dose adjustment of TIVICAY to 50 mg twice daily is recommended in treatment-naïve or treatment-experienced, INSTI-naïve patients. Alternative combinations that do not include metabolic inducers should be considered where possible for INSTI-experienced patients with certain INSTI-associated resistance substitutions or clinically suspected INSTI resistance.[b]
Non-nucleoside reverse transcriptase inhibitor: Nevirapine	↓Dolutegravir	Coadministration with nevirapine should be avoided because there are insufficient data to make dosing recommendations.
Protease Inhibitor: Fosamprenavir/ritonavir[a] Tipranavir/ritonavir[a]	↓Dolutegravir	A dose adjustment of TIVICAY to 50 mg twice daily is recommended in treatment-naïve or treatment-experienced, INSTI-naïve patients. Alternative combinations that do not include metabolic inducers should be considered where possible for INSTI-experienced patients with certain INSTI-associated resistance substitutions or clinically suspected INSTI resistance.[b]
	Other Agents	
Oxcarbazepine Phenytoin Phenobarbital Carbamazepine St. John's wort (*Hypericum perforatum*)	↓Dolutegravir	Coadministration with these metabolic inducers should be avoided because there are insufficient data to make dosing recommendations.
Medications containing polyvalent cations (e.g., Mg, Al, Fe, or Ca) Cation-containing antacids[a] or laxatives Sucralfate Oral iron supplements Oral calcium supplements Buffered medications	↓Dolutegravir	TIVICAY should be administered 2 hours before or 6 hours after taking medications containing polyvalent cations.
Metformin	↑Metformin	Close monitoring is recommended when starting or stopping TIVICAY and metformin together. A dose adjustment of metformin may be necessary.
Rifampin[a]	↓Dolutegravir	A dose adjustment of TIVICAY to 50 mg twice daily is recommended in treatment-naïve or treatment-experienced, INSTI-naïve patients. Alternatives to rifampin should be used where possible for INSTI-experienced patients with certain INSTI-associated resistance substitutions or clinically suspected INSTI resistance.[b]

[a] *See Clinical Pharmacology (12.3)Table 9 for magnitude of interaction.*
[b] The lower dolutegravir exposures observed in INSTI-experienced patients (with certain INSTI-associated resistance substitutions or clinically suspected INSTI resistance *[see Microbiology (12.4)]*) upon coadministration with potent inducers may result in loss of therapeutic effect and development of resistance to TIVICAY or other coadministered antiretroviral agents.

Coadministration of dolutegravir and other drugs that inhibit these enzymes may increase dolutegravir plasma concentration.

Etravirine significantly reduced plasma concentrations of dolutegravir, but the effect of etravirine was mitigated by coadministration of lopinavir/ritonavir or darunavir/ritonavir, and is expected to be mitigated by atazanavir/ritonavir. (Table 5) *[see Drug Interactions (7.3), Clinical Pharmacology (12.3)]*.

Darunavir/ritonavir, lopinavir/ritonavir, rilpivirine, tenofovir, boceprevir, telaprevir, prednisone, rifabutin, and omeprazole had no clinically significant effect on the pharmacokinetics of dolutegravir.

7.3 Established and Other Potentially Significant Drug Interactions

Table 5 provides clinical recommendations as a result of drug interactions with TIVICAY. These recommendations are based on either drug interaction trials or predicted interactions due to the expected magnitude of interaction and potential for serious adverse events or loss of efficacy. *[See Dosage and Administration (2), Clinical Pharmacology (12.3).]*

[See table 5 above]

8 USE IN SPECIFIC POPULATIONS

8.1 Pregnancy

Pregnancy Category B. There are no adequate and well-controlled studies in pregnant women. Because animal reproduction studies are not always predictive of human response, and dolutegravir was shown to cross the placenta in animal studies, this drug should be used during pregnancy only if clearly needed.

Antiretroviral Pregnancy Registry: To monitor maternal-fetal outcomes of pregnant women with HIV exposed to TIVICAY and other antiretroviral agents, an Antiretroviral Pregnancy Registry has been established. Physicians are encouraged to register patients by calling 1-800-258-4263.

Animal Data: Reproduction studies have been performed in rats and rabbits at doses up to 27 times the human dose of 50 mg twice daily and have revealed no evidence of impaired fertility or harm to the fetus due to TIVICAY.

Oral administration of dolutegravir to pregnant rats at doses up to 1,000 mg/kg daily, approximately 27 times the 50-mg twice-daily human clinical exposure based on AUC, from days 6 to 17 of gestation did not elicit maternal toxicity, developmental toxicity, or teratogenicity.

Oral administration of dolutegravir to pregnant rabbits at doses up to 1,000 mg/kg daily, approximately 0.4 times the 50–mg twice-daily human clinical exposure based on AUC, from days 6 to 18 of gestation did not elicit developmental toxicity or teratogenicity. In rabbits, maternal toxicity (decreased food consumption, scant/no feces/urine, suppressed body weight gain) was observed at 1,000 mg/kg.

8.3 Nursing Mothers

The Centers for Disease Control and Prevention recommend that HIV–1–infected mothers in the United States not breastfeed their infants to avoid risking postnatal transmission of HIV-1 infection. Studies in lactating rats and their offspring indicate that dolutegravir was present in rat milk.It is not known whether dolutegravir is excreted in human milk.

Because of both the potential for HIV transmission and the potential for adverse reactions in nursing infants, **mothers should be instructed not to breastfeed if they are receiving TIVICAY.**

8.4 Pediatric Use

TIVICAY is not recommended in pediatric patients younger than 12 years or weighing less than 40 kg. Safety and efficacy of TIVICAY have not been established in pediatric patients who are INSTI-experienced with documented or clinically suspected resistance to other INSTIs (raltegravir, elvitegravir).

The safety, virologic, and immunologic responses in subjects who received TIVICAY were evaluated in 23 treatment-experienced, INSTI-naïve, HIV–1–infected subjects aged 12 to less than 18 years in an open-label, multicenter, dose-finding clinical trial, IMPAACT P1093 *[see Adverse Reactions (6.2), Clinical Pharmacology (12.3), Clinical Studies (14.2)]*. Pharmacokinetic parameters, evaluated in 9 subjects weighing ≥40 kg receiving 50 mg daily and 1 subject (weighing 37 kg) receiving 35 mg once daily, were similar to adults receiving 50 mg once daily. See *Dosage and Administration (2.2)* for dosing recommendations for pediatric patients aged 12 years and older and weighing at least 40 kg. Frequency, type, and severity of adverse drug reactions in pediatric subjects were comparable to those observed in adults *[see Adverse Reactions (6.2)]*.

8.5 Geriatric Use

Clinical trials of TIVICAY did not include sufficient numbers of subjects aged 65 and older to determine whether they respond differently from younger subjects. In general, caution should be exercised in the administration of TIVICAY in elderly patients reflecting the greater frequency of decreased hepatic, renal, or cardiac function, and of concomitant disease or other drug therapy *[see Clinical Pharmacology (12.3)]*.

8.6 Hepatic Impairment

No clinically important pharmacokinetic differences between subjects with moderate hepatic impairment and matching healthy subjects were observed. No dosage adjustment is necessary for patients with mild to moderate hepatic impairment (Child-Pugh Score A or B). The effect of severe hepatic impairment (Child-Pugh Score C) on the pharmacokinetics of dolutegravir has not been studied. Therefore, TIVICAY is not recommended for use in patients with severe hepatic impairment *[see Clinical Pharmacology (12.3)]*.

8.7 Renal Impairment

Dolutegravir plasma concentrations were decreased in subjects with severe renal impairment compared with those in matched healthy controls. However, no dosage adjustment is necessary for treatment-naïve or treatment-experienced and INSTI-naïve patients with mild, moderate, or severe renal impairment or for INSTI-experienced patients (with certain INSTI-associated resistance substitutions or clinically suspected INSTI resistance) with mild or moderate renal impairment. Caution is warranted for INSTI-experienced patients (with certain INSTI-associated resistance substitutions or clinically suspected INSTI resistance *[see Microbiology (12.4)]*) with severe renal impairment, as the decrease in dolutegravir concentrations may result in loss of therapeutic effect and development of resistance to TIVICAY or other coadministered antiretroviral agents *[see Clinical Pharmacology (12.3)]*. Dolutegravir has not been studied in patients on dialysis.

10 OVERDOSAGE

Limited experience with single higher doses (up to 250 mg in healthy subjects) revealed no specific symptoms or signs apart from those listed as adverse reactions. There is no known specific treatment for overdose with TIVICAY. If overdose occurs, the patient should be monitored and standard supportive treatment applied as required. As dolutegravir is highly bound to plasma proteins, it is unlikely that it will be significantly removed by dialysis.

11 DESCRIPTION

TIVICAY contains dolutegravir, as dolutegravir sodium, an HIV INSTI. The chemical name of dolutegravir sodium is sodium (4*R*,12a*S*)-9-{[(2,4-difluorophenyl)methyl]carbamoyl}-4-methyl-6,8-dioxo-3,4,6,8,12,12a-hexahydro-2*H*-pyrido[1′,2′:4,5]pyrazino[2,1-*b*][1,3]oxazin-7-olate. The empirical formula is $C_{20}H_{18}F_2N_3NaO_5$ and the molecular weight is 441.36 g/mol. It has the following structural formula:

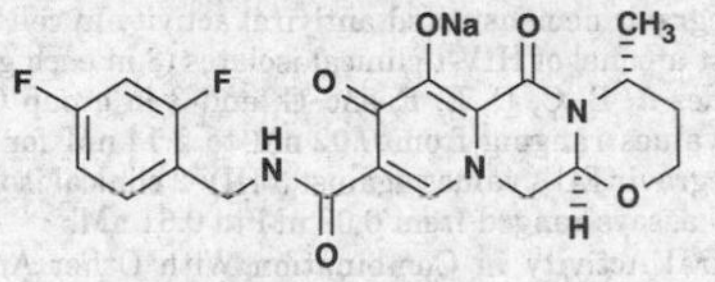

Dolutegravir sodium is a white to light yellow powder and is slightly soluble in water.

Each film-coated tablet of TIVICAY for oral administration contains 52.6 mg of dolutegravir sodium, which is equivalent to 50 mg dolutegravir free acid, and the following inactive ingredients: D-mannitol, microcrystalline cellulose, povidone K29/32, sodium starch glycolate, and sodium stearyl fumarate. The tablet film-coating contains the inactive ingredients iron oxide yellow, macrogol/PEG, polyvinyl alcohol-part hydrolyzed, talc, and titanium dioxide.

12 CLINICAL PHARMACOLOGY

12.1 Mechanism of Action

Dolutegravir is an HIV-1 antiviral agent *[see Microbiology (12.4)]*.

12.2 Pharmacodynamics

In a randomized, dose-ranging trial, HIV-1-infected subjects treated with dolutegravir monotherapy demonstrated rapid and dose-dependent antiviral activity with mean declines from baseline to Day 11 in HIV-1 RNA of 1.5, 2.0, and 2.5 $\log_{10}$ for dolutegravir 2 mg, 10 mg, and 50 mg once daily, respectively. This antiviral response was maintained for 3 to 4 days after the last dose in the 50-mg group.

Effects on Electrocardiogram: In a randomized, placebo-controlled, cross-over trial, 42 healthy subjects received single-dose oral administrations of placebo, dolutegravir 250-mg suspension (exposures approximately 3-fold of the 50-mg once-daily dose at steady state), and moxifloxacin 400 mg (active control) in random sequence. After baseline and placebo adjustment, the maximum mean QTc change based on Fridericia correction method (QTcF) for dolutegravir was 2.4 msec (1-sided 95% upper CI: 4.9 msec). TIVICAY did not prolong the QTc interval over 24 hours postdose.

Effects on Renal Function: The effect of dolutegravir on renal function was evaluated in an open-label, randomized, 3-arm, parallel, placebo-controlled trial in healthy subjects (n = 37) who received dolutegravir 50 mg once daily (n = 12), dolutegravir 50 mg twice daily (n = 13), or placebo once daily (n = 12) for 14 days. A decrease in creatinine clearance, as determined by 24-hour urine collection, was observed with both doses of dolutegravir after 14 days of treatment in subjects who received 50 mg once daily (9% decrease) and 50 mg twice daily (13% decrease). Neither dose of dolutegravir had a significant effect on the actual glomerular filtration rate (determined by the clearance of probe drug, iohexol) or effective renal plasma flow (determined by the clearance of probe drug, para-amino hippurate) compared with the placebo.

12.3 Pharmacokinetics

The pharmacokinetic properties of dolutegravir have been evaluated in healthy adult subjects and HIV-1-infected adult subjects. Exposure to dolutegravir was generally similar between healthy subjects and HIV-1-infected subjects. The non-linear exposure of dolutegravir following 50 mg twice daily compared with 50 mg once daily in HIV-1-infected subjects (Table 6) was attributed to the use of metabolic inducers in the background antiretroviral regimens of subjects receiving dolutegravir 50 mg twice daily in clinical trials. TIVICAY was administered without regard to food in these trials.

Table 6. Dolutegravir Steady-State Pharmacokinetic Parameter Estimates in HIV-1-Infected Adults

Parameter	50 mg Once Daily Geometric Mean[a] (%CV)	50 mg Twice Daily Geometric Mean[b] (%CV)
$AUC_{(0-24)}$ (mcg.h/mL)	53.6 (27)	75.1 (35)
C_{max} (mcg/mL)	3.67 (20)	4.15 (29)
C_{min} (mcg/mL)	1.11 (46)	2.12 (47)

[a]Based on population pharmacokinetic analyses using data from SPRING-1 and SPRING-2.

[b]Based on population pharmacokinetic analyses using data from VIKING (ING112961) and VIKING-3.

Table 7. Dolutegravir Steady-State Pharmacokinetic Parameters in Pediatric Subjects

Age/Weight	Dose of TIVICAY[a]	Dolutegravir Pharmacokinetic Parameter Estimates Geometric Mean (%CV)		
		C_{max} (mcg/mL) (n = 10)	$AUC_{(0-24)}$ (mcg.h/mL) (n = 10)	C_{24} (mcg/mL) (n = 10)
12 to <18 years and ≥40 kg [a]	50 mg once daily	3.49 (38)	46 (43)	0.90 (59)

[a]One subject weighing 37 kg received TIVICAY 35 mg once daily.

Table 8. Summary of Effect of Dolutegravir on the Pharmacokinetics of Coadministered Drugs

Coadministered Drug(s) and Dose(s)	Dose of TIVICAY	n	Geometric Mean Ratio (90% CI) of Pharmacokinetic Parameters of Coadministered Drug With/Without Dolutegravir No Effect = 1.00		
			C_{max}	AUC	C_τ or C_{24}
Ethinyl estradiol 0.035 mg	50 mg twice daily	15	0.99 (0.91 to 1.08)	1.03 (0.96 to 1.11)	1.02 (0.93 to 1.11)
Methadone 16 to 150 mg	50 mg twice daily	11	1.00 (0.94 to 1.06)	0.98 (0.91 to 1.06)	0.99 (0.91 to 1.07)
Midazolam 3 mg	25 mg once daily	10	–	0.95 (0.79 to 1.15)	–
Norgestromin 0.25 mg	50 mg twice daily	15	0.89 (0.82 to 0.97)	0.98 (0.91 to 1.04)	0.93 (0.85 to 1.03)
Rilpivirine 25 mg once daily	50 mg once daily	16	1.10 (0.99 to 1.22)	1.06 (0.98 to 1.16)	1.21 (1.07 to 1.38)
Tenofovir disoproxil fumarate 300 mg once daily	50 mg once daily	15	1.09 (0.97 to 1.23)	1.12 (1.01 to 1.24)	1.19 (1.04 to 1.35)

Absorption: Following oral administration of dolutegravir, peak plasma concentrations were observed 2 to 3 hours postdose. With once-daily dosing, pharmacokinetic steady state is achieved within approximately 5 days with average accumulation ratios for AUC, C_{max}, and $C_{24\ h}$ ranging from 1.2 to 1.5.

Dolutegravir plasma concentrations increased in a less than dose-proportional manner above 50 mg. Dolutegravir is a P-glycoprotein substrate in vitro. The absolute bioavailability of dolutegravir has not been established.

Effects of Food on Oral Absorption: TIVICAY may be taken with or without food. Food increased the extent of absorption and slowed the rate of absorption of dolutegravir. Low-, moderate-, and high-fat meals increased dolutegravir $AUC_{(0-\infty)}$ by 33%, 41%, and 66%; increased C_{max} by 46%, 52%, and 67%; and prolonged T_{max} to 3, 4, and 5 hours from 2 hours under fasted conditions, respectively.

Distribution: Dolutegravir is highly bound (≥98.9%) to human plasma proteins based on in vivo data and binding is independent of plasma concentration of dolutegravir. The apparent volume of distribution (Vd/F) following 50-mg once-daily administration is estimated at 17.4 L based on a population pharmacokinetic analysis.

Cerebrospinal Fluid (CSF): In 11 treatment-naïve subjects on dolutegravir 50 mg daily plus abacavir/lamivudine, the median dolutegravir concentration in CSF was 18 ng/mL (range: 4 ng/mL to 232 ng/mL) 2 to 6 hours postdose after 2 weeks of treatment. The clinical relevance of this finding has not been established.

Metabolism and Elimination: Dolutegravir is primarily metabolized via UGT1A1 with some contribution from CYP3A. After a single oral dose of [^{14}C] dolutegravir, 53% of the total oral dose was excreted unchanged in feces. Thirty-one percent of the total oral dose was excreted in urine, represented by an ether glucuronide of dolutegravir (18.9% of total dose), a metabolite formed by oxidation at the benzylic carbon (3.0% of total dose), and its hydrolytic N-dealkylation product (3.6% of total dose). Renal elimination of unchanged drug was low (<1% of the dose).

Dolutegravir has a terminal half-life of approximately 14 hours and an apparent clearance (CL/F) of 1.0 L/h based on population pharmacokinetic analyses.

Polymorphisms in Drug-Metabolizing Enzymes: In a meta-analysis of healthy subject trials, subjects with UGT1A1 (n = 7) genotypes conferring poor dolutegravir metabolism had a 32% lower clearance of dolutegravir and 46% higher AUC compared with subjects with genotypes associated with normal metabolism via UGT1A1 (n = 41).

Specific Populations: *Hepatic Impairment*: Dolutegravir is primarily metabolized and eliminated by the liver. In a trial comparing 8 subjects with moderate hepatic impairment (Child-Pugh Score B) with 8 matched healthy controls, exposure of dolutegravir from a single 50-mg dose was similar between the 2 groups. No dosage adjustment is necessary for patients with mild to moderate hepatic impairment (Child-Pugh Score A or B). The effect of severe hepatic impairment (Child-Pugh Score C) on the pharmacokinetics of dolutegravir has not been studied. Therefore, TIVICAY is not recommended for use in patients with severe hepatic impairment.

HBV/HCV Co-infection: Population analyses using pooled pharmacokinetic data from adult trials indicated no clinically relevant effect of HCV co-infection on the pharmacokinetics of dolutegravir. There were limited data on HBV co-infection.

Renal Impairment: Renal clearance of unchanged drug is a minor pathway of elimination for dolutegravir. In a trial comparing 8 subjects with severe renal impairment (CrCl <30 mL/min) with 8 matched healthy controls, AUC, C_{max}, and C_{24} of dolutegravir were decreased by 40%, 23%, and 43%, respectively, compared with those in matched healthy subjects. The cause of this decrease is unknown. Population pharmacokinetic analysis using data from SAILING and VIKING-3 trials indicated that mild and moderate renal impairment had no clinically relevant effect on the exposure of dolutegravir. No dosage adjustment is necessary for treatment-naïve or treatment-experienced and INSTI-naïve patients with mild, moderate, or severe renal impairment or for INSTI-experienced patients (with certain INSTI-associated resistance substitutions or clinically suspected INSTI resistance) with mild or moderate renal impairment. Caution is warranted for INSTI-experienced patients (with certain INSTI-associated resistance substitutions or clinically suspected INSTI resistance *[see Microbiology (12.4)]*) with severe renal impairment, as the decrease in dolutegravir concentrations may result in loss of therapeutic effect and development of resistance to TIVICAY or other coadministered antiretroviral agents. Dolutegravir has not been studied in patients requiring dialysis.

Gender: Population analyses using pooled pharmacokinetic data from adult trials indicated gender had no clinically relevant effect on the exposure of dolutegravir.

Race: Population analyses using pooled pharmacokinetic data from adult trials indicated race had no clinically relevant effect on the pharmacokinetics of dolutegravir.

Table 9. Summary of Effect of Coadministered Drugs on the Pharmacokinetics of Dolutegravir

Coadministered Drug(s) and Dose(s)	Dose of **TIVICAY**	n	Geometric Mean Ratio (90% CI) of **Dolutegravir** Pharmacokinetic Parameters With/Without Coadministered Drugs No Effect = 1.00		
			C_{max}	AUC	C_τ or C_{24}
Atazanavir 400 mg once daily	30 mg once daily	12	1.50 (1.40 to 1.59)	1.91 (1.80 to 2.03)	2.80 (2.52 to 3.11)
Atazanavir/ritonavir 300/100 mg once daily	30 mg once daily	12	1.34 (1.25 to 1.42)	1.62 (1.50 to 1.74)	2.21 (1.97 to 2.47)
Tenofovir 300 mg once daily	50 mg once daily	15	0.97 (0.87 to 1.08)	1.01 (0.91 to 1.11)	0.92 (0.82 to 1.04)
Darunavir/ritonavir 600/100 mg twice daily	30 mg once daily	15	0.89 (0.83 to 0.97)	0.78 (0.72 to 0.85)	0.62 (0.56 to 0.69)
Efavirenz 600 mg once daily	50 mg once daily	12	0.61 (0.51 to 0.73)	0.43 (0.35 to 0.54)	0.25 (0.18 to 0.34)
Etravirine 200 mg twice daily	50 mg once daily	16	0.48 (0.43 to 0.54)	0.29 (0.26 to 0.34)	0.12 (0.09 to 0.16)
Etravirine + darunavir/ritonavir 200 mg + 600/100 mg twice daily	50 mg once daily	9	0.88 (0.78 to 1.00)	0.75 (0.69 to 0.81)	0.63 (0.52 to 0.76)
Etravirine + lopinavir/ritonavir 200 mg + 400/100 mg twice daily	50 mg once daily	8	1.07 (1.02 to 1.13)	1.11 (1.02 to 1.20)	1.28 (1.13 to 1.45)
Fosamprenavir/ritonavir 700 mg/100 mg twice daily	50 mg once daily	12	0.76 (0.63 to 0.92)	0.65 (0.54 to 0.78)	0.51 (0.41 to 0.63)
Lopinavir/ritonavir 400/100 mg twice daily	30 mg once daily	15	1.00 (0.94 to 1.07)	0.97 (0.91 to 1.04)	0.94 (0.85 to 1.05)
Antacid (Maalox®) Simultaneous administration	50 mg single dose	16	0.28 (0.23 to 0.33)	0.26 (0.22 to 0.32)	0.26 (0.21 to 0.31)
Antacid (Maalox®) 2 hrs after dolutegravir	50 mg single dose	16	0.82 (0.69 to 0.98)	0.74 (0.62 to 0.90)	0.70 (0.58 to 0.85)
Multivitamin (One-A-Day®) Simultaneous administration	50 mg single dose	16	0.65 (0.54 to 0.77)	0.67 (0.55 to 0.81)	0.68 (0.56 to 0.82)
Omeprazole 40 mg once daily	50 mg single dose	12	0.92 (0.75 to 1.11)	0.97 (0.78 to 1.20)	0.95 (0.75 to 1.21)
Prednisone 60 mg once daily with taper	50 mg once daily	12	1.06 (0.99 to 1.14)	1.11 (1.03 to 1.20)	1.17 (1.06 to 1.28)
Rifampin[a] 600 mg once daily	50 mg twice daily	11	0.57 (0.49 to 0.65)	0.46 (0.38 to 0.55)	0.28 (0.23 to 0.34)
Rifampin[b] 600 mg once daily	50 mg twice daily	11	1.18 (1.03 to 1.37)	1.33 (1.15 to 1.53)	1.22 (1.01 to 1.48)
Rifabutin 300 mg once daily	50 mg once daily	9	1.16 (0.98 to 1.37)	0.95 (0.82 to 1.10)	0.70 (0.57 to 0.87)
Rilpivirine 25 mg once daily	50 mg once daily	16	1.13 (1.06 to 1.21)	1.12 (1.05 to 1.19)	1.22 (1.15 to 1.30)
Tipranavir/ritonavir 500/200 mg twice daily	50 mg once daily	14	0.54 (0.50 to 0.57)	0.41 (0.38 to 0.44)	0.24 (0.21 to 0.27)
Telaprevir 750 mg every 8 hours	50 mg once daily	15	1.18 (1.11 to 1.26)	1.25 (1.19 to 1.31)	1.40 (1.29 to 1.51)
Boceprevir 800 mg every 8 hours	50 mg once daily	13	1.05 (0.96 to 1.15)	1.07 (0.95 to 1.20)	1.08 (0.91 to 1.28)

[a]Comparison is rifampin taken with dolutegravir 50 mg twice daily compared with dolutegravir 50 mg twice daily.
[b]Comparison is rifampin taken with dolutegravir 50 mg twice daily compared with dolutegravir 50 mg once daily.

Geriatric Patients: Population analyses using pooled pharmacokinetic data from adult trials indicated age had no clinically relevant effect on the pharmacokinetics of dolutegravir.

Pediatric Patients: The pharmacokinetics of dolutegravir in HIV–1–infected children (n = 10) aged 12 to less than 18 years were similar to those observed in HIV–1–infected adults who received dolutegravir 50 mg once daily (Table 7) *[see Clinical Studies (14.2)]*.

[See table 7 at top of previous page]

Drug Interactions: Drug interaction trials were performed with TIVICAY and other drugs likely to be coadministered or commonly used as probes for pharmacokinetic interactions. As dolutegravir is not expected to affect the pharmacokinetics of other drugs dependent on hepatic metabolism (Table 8) *[see Drug Interactions (7.1)]*, the primary focus of these drug interaction trials was to evaluate the effect of coadministered drug on dolutegravir (Table 9).

Dosing or regimen recommendations as a result of established and other potentially significant drug-drug interactions with TIVICAY are provided in Table 5 *[see Dosage and Administration (2.1), Drug Interactions (7.3)]*.

[See table 8 at top of previous page]
[See table 9 above]

12.4 Microbiology

Mechanism of Action: Dolutegravir inhibits HIV integrase by binding to the integrase active site and blocking the strand transfer step of retroviral deoxyribonucleic acid (DNA) integration which is essential for the HIV replication cycle. Strand transfer biochemical assays using purified HIV-1 integrase and pre-processed substrate DNA resulted in IC_{50} values of 2.7 nM and 12.6 nM.

Antiviral Activity in Cell Culture: Dolutegravir exhibited antiviral activity against laboratory strains of wild-type HIV-1 with mean EC_{50} values of 0.5 nM (0.21 ng/mL) to 2.1 nM (0.85 ng/mL) in peripheral blood mononuclear cells (PBMCs) and MT-4 cells. Dolutegravir exhibited antiviral activity against 13 clinically diverse clade B isolates with a mean EC_{50} of 0.52 nM in a viral integrase susceptibility assay using the integrase coding region from clinical isolates. Dolutegravir demonstrated antiviral activity in cell culture against a panel of HIV-1 clinical isolates (3 in each group of M clades A, B, C, D, E, F, and G, and 3 in group O) with EC_{50} values ranging from 0.02 nM to 2.14 nM for HIV-1. Dolutegravir EC_{50} values against 3 HIV-2 clinical isolates in PBMC assays ranged from 0.09 nM to 0.61 nM.

Antiviral Activity in Combination With Other Antiviral Agents: The antiviral activity of dolutegravir was not antagonistic when combined with the INSTI, raltegravir; non-nucleoside reverse transcriptase inhibitors (NNRTIs), efavirenz or nevirapine; the nucleoside reverse transcriptase inhibitors (NRTIs), abacavir or stavudine; the protease inhibitors (PIs), amprenavir or lopinavir; the CCR5 co-receptor antagonist, maraviroc; or the fusion inhibitor, enfuvirtide. Dolutegravir antiviral activity was not antagonistic when combined with the HBV reverse transcriptase inhibitor, adefovir, or with the antiviral, ribavirin.

Resistance: *Cell Culture*: Dolutegravir-resistant viruses were selected in cell culture starting from different wild-type HIV-1 strains and clades. Amino acid substitutions E92Q, G118R, S153F or Y, G193E or R263K emerged in different passages and conferred decreased susceptibility to dolutegravir of up to 4-fold. Passage of mutant viruses containing the Q148R or Q148H substitutions selected for additional substitutions in integrase that conferred decreased susceptibility to dolutegravir (fold-change increase of 13 to 46). The additional integrase substitutions included T97A, E138K, G140S, and M154I. Passage of mutant viruses containing both G140S and Q148H selected for L74M, E92Q, and N155H.

Treatment-Naïve Subjects: No subjects in the dolutegravir 50-mg once-daily treatment arms of treatment-naïve trials SPRING-2 and SINGLE had a detectable decrease in susceptibility to dolutegravir or background NRTIs in the resistance analysis subset (n = 6 with HIV-1 RNA >400 copies/mL at failure or last visit through Week 48 and having resistance data). One additional subject in SINGLE with 275 copies/mL HIV-1 RNA had a treatment-emergent INSTI-resistance substitution (E157Q/P) detected at Week 24, but no corresponding decrease in dolutegravir susceptibility. No treatment-emergent genotypic resistance to the background regimen was isolated in the dolutegravir arm in either the SPRING-2 or SINGLE trials.

Treatment-Experienced, Integrase Strand Transfer Inhibitor-Naïve Subjects: In SAILING, viruses from 5 of 15 subjects in the dolutegravir arm with post-baseline resistance data had evidence of treatment-emergent integrase substitutions (1 subject each with L74I/M, Q95Q/L, or V151V/I, and 2 subjects with R263K). However, none of these subjects' isolates had detectable phenotypic decreases in susceptibility to either dolutegravir or raltegravir. In the comparator raltegravir arm, 9 of 32 subjects with post-baseline resistance data had evidence of emergent INSTI-resistance substitutions (L74M, E92E/Q, Q95Q/R, T97A, G140A/S, Y143C/R, Q148H/R, V151I, N155H, E157E/Q, and G163G/R) and raltegravir phenotypic resistance.

Treatment-Experienced, Integrase Strand Transfer Inhibitor-Experienced Subjects: VIKING-3 examined the efficacy of dolutegravir 50 mg twice daily plus optimized background therapy in subjects with prior or current virologic failure on an INSTI- (elvitegravir or raltegravir) containing regimen.

Response by Baseline Genotype: Of the 183 subjects with baseline data, 30% harbored virus with a substitution at Q148, and 33% had no primary INSTI-resistance substitutions (T66A/I/K, E92Q/V, Y143C/H/R, Q148H/K/R and N155H) at baseline, but had historical genotypic evidence of INSTI-resistance substitutions, phenotypic evidence of elvitegravir or raltegravir resistance, or genotypic evidence of INSTI-resistance substitutions at screening.

Response rates by baseline genotype were analyzed using a subset of subjects who had reached Week 24, as well as those who discontinued or rebounded before Week 24 (n = 124) (Table 10). The response rate at Week 24 for subjects with only historic evidence of INSTI-resistance at baseline was 75% (33/44). The response rate at Week 24 to dolutegravir-containing regimens was 36% (13/36) when

Q148 substitutions were present at baseline; Q148 was always present with additional INSTI-resistance substitutions. Diminished virologic responses (25% [7/28]) were observed when ≥3 of the following INSTI-resistance substitutions were present at baseline: L74I/M, E138A/D/K/T, G140A/S, Y143H/R, Q148H/R, E157Q, G163E/K/Q/R/S, or G193E/R.

Table 10. Response by Baseline Integrase Genotype in Subjects with Prior Experience to an Integrase Strand Transfer Inhibitor in VIKING-3

Baseline Genotype	Response at Week 24 (<50 copies/mL) Subset N = 124
Overall Response	64% (79/124)
N155H without a Q148 substitution	80% (16/20)
Y143C/H/R without a Q148 substitution	56% (10/18)
Q148H/R + G140A/S without additional INSTI-resistance substitutions	56% (10/18)
Q148H/R + ≥2 INSTI-resistance substitutions[a,b]	18% (3/17)

[a]INSTI-resistance substitutions include L74I/M, E138A/D/K/T, G140A/S, Y143H/R, E157Q, G163E/K/Q/R/S, or G193E/R.
[b]The most common pathway with Q148H/R + ≥2 INSTI-resistance substitutions had Q148+G140+E138 substitutions (n = 12).

Response by Baseline Phenotype: Response rates by baseline phenotype were analyzed using a subset of subjects who had reached Week 24, as well as those who discontinued or rebounded before Week 24 (n = 120) (See Table 11). These baseline phenotypic groups are based on subjects enrolled in VIKING-3 and are not meant to represent definitive clinical susceptibility cut points for dolutegravir. The data are provided to guide clinicians on the likelihood of virologic success based on pretreatment susceptibility to dolutegravir in INSTI-resistant patients.

Table 11. Response by Baseline Dolutegravir Phenotype (Fold-Change From Reference) in Subjects With Prior Experience to an Integrase Strand Transfer Inhibitor in VIKING-3

Baseline Dolutegravir Phenotype (Fold-Change From Reference)	Response at Week 24 (<50 copies/mL) Subset N = 120
Overall Response	63% (75/120)
<3-fold change	72% (63/87)
3- <10-fold change	42% (10/24)
≥10-fold change	22% (2/9)

Integrase Strand Transfer Inhibitor Treatment-Emergent Resistance: There were 40 subjects on the dolutegravir twice-daily regimen in VIKING-3 with HIV-1 RNA >400 copies/mL at Week 24, the failure timepoint, or the last timepoint on trial who were included in the Week 24 resistance analysis set. In the Week 24 resistance analysis set, 45% (18/40) of the subjects had treatment-emergent INSTI-resistance substitutions in their isolates. The most common treatment-emergent INSTI-resistance substitution was T97A. Other frequently emergent INSTI-resistance substitutions included E138K or A, G140S or A, or Q148H or R or K; substitutions at Q148 were detected in subjects with changes documented at or prior to enrollment in the trial. Substitutions L74M, E92Q, Y143H or C, S147G, V151A, M154I, and N155H each emerged in 1 or 2 subjects' isolates. At failure, the median dolutegravir fold-change from reference was 23-fold (range: 0.92 to 209) for isolates with emergent INSTI-resistance substitutions (n = 18).

Resistance to one or more background drugs in the dolutegravir twice-daily regimen also emerged in 30% (12/40) of the subjects in the Week 24 resistance analysis set.

Cross-Resistance: *Site-Directed Integrase Strand Transfer Inhibitor-Resistant Mutant HIV-1 and HIV-2 Strains*: The susceptibility of dolutegravir was tested against 60 INSTI-resistant site-directed mutant HIV-1 viruses (28 with single substitutions and 32 with 2 or more substitutions) and 6 INSTI-resistant site-directed mutant HIV-2 viruses. The

Table 12. Virologic Outcomes of Randomized Treatment in SPRING-2 and SINGLE at Week 48 (Snapshot Algorithm)

	SPRING-2		SINGLE	
	TIVICAY 50 mg Once Daily + 2 NRTIs (N = 403)	Raltegravir 400 mg Twice Daily + 2 NRTIs (N = 405)	TIVICAY 50 mg + EPZICOM Once Daily (N = 414)	ATRIPLA Once Daily (N = 419)
HIV-1 RNA <50 copies/mL	88%	86%	88%	81%
Treatment difference[a]	2.6% (95% CI: -1.9%, 7.2%)		7.4% (95% CI: 2.5%, 12.3%)	
Virologic nonresponse[b]	5%	7%	5%	6%
No virologic data at Week 48 window	7%	7%	7%	13%
Reasons				
Discontinued study/study drug due to adverse event or death[c]	2%	1%	2%	10%
Discontinued study/study drug for other reasons[d]	5%	6%	5%	3%
Missing data during window but on study	0	0	0	<1%
Proportion (%) of Subjects With HIV-1 RNA <50 copies/mL at Week 48 by Baseline Category				
Plasma viral load (copies/mL)				
≤100,000	91%	90%	90%	83%
>100,000	82%	75%	83%	76%
Gender				
Male	89%	86%	88%	82%
Female	84%	82%	85%	75%
Race				
White	88%	86%	90%	84%
Non white	85%	85%	84%	74%

[a]Adjusted for pre-specified stratification factors.
[b]Includes subjects who changed BR to new class or changed BR not permitted per protocol or due to lack of efficacy prior to Week 48 (for SPRING-2 only), subjects who discontinued prior to Week 48 for lack or loss of efficacy, and subjects who were HIV-1 RNA ≥50 copies/mL in the Week 48 window.
[c]Includes subjects who discontinued due to an adverse event or death at any time point from Day 1 through the Week 48 window if this resulted in no virologic data on treatment during the Week 48 window.
[d]Other includes reasons such as withdrew consent, loss to follow-up, moved, and protocol deviation.
SPRING-2: Virologic outcomes were also comparable across baseline characteristics including CD4+ cell count, age, and use of EPZICOM or TRUVADA as NRTI background regimen. The median change in CD4+ cell counts from baseline for both groups was +230 cells/mm^3 at 48 weeks.
SINGLE: Treatment differences were maintained across baseline characteristics including HIV-1 RNA, CD4+ cell count, age, gender, and race.

single INSTI-resistance substitutions T66K, I151L, and S153Y conferred a >2-fold decrease in dolutegravir susceptibility (range: 2.3-fold to 3.6-fold from reference). Combinations of multiple substitutions T66K/L74M, E92Q/N155H, G140C/Q148R, G140S/Q148H, R or K, Q148R/N155H, T97A/G140S/Q148, and substitutions at E138/G140/Q148 showed a >2-fold decrease in dolutegravir susceptibility (range: 2.5-fold to 21-fold from reference). In HIV-2 mutants, combinations of substitutions A153G/N155H/S163G and E92Q/T97A/N155H/S163D conferred 4-fold decreases in dolutegravir susceptibility, and E92Q/N155H and G140S/Q148R showed 8.5-fold and 17-fold decreases in dolutegravir susceptibility, respectively.

Reverse Transcriptase Inhibitor- and Protease Inhibitor-Resistant Strains: Dolutegravir demonstrated equivalent antiviral activity against 2 NNRTI-resistant, 3 NRTI-resistant, and 2 PI-resistant HIV-1 mutant clones compared with the wild-type strain.

13 NONCLINICAL TOXICOLOGY

13.1 Carcinogenesis, Mutagenesis, Impairment of Fertility

Carcinogenesis: Two-year carcinogenicity studies in mice and rats were conducted with dolutegravir. Mice were administered doses of up to 500 mg/kg, and rats were administered doses of up to 50 mg/kg. In mice, no significant increases in the incidence of drug-related neoplasms were observed at the highest doses tested, resulting in dolutegravir AUC exposures approximately 14-fold higher than those in humans at the recommended dose of 50 mg twice daily. In rats, no increases in the incidence of drug-related neoplasms were observed at the highest dose tested, resulting in dolutegravir AUC exposures 10-fold and 15-fold higher in males and females, respectively, than those in human at the recommended dose of 50 mg twice daily.

Mutagenesis: Dolutegravir was not genotoxic in the bacterial reverse mutation assay, mouse lymphoma assay, or in the in vivo rodent micronucleus assay.

Impairment of Fertility: In a study conducted in rats, there were no effects on mating or fertility with dolutegravir up to 1,000 mg/kg/day. This dose is associated with an exposure that is approximately 24 times higher than the exposure in humans at the recommended dose of 50 mg twice daily.

14 CLINICAL STUDIES

The efficacy of TIVICAY is based on analyses of data from 2 trials, SPRING-2 (ING113086) and SINGLE (ING114467), in treatment-naïve, HIV–1–infected subjects (n = 1,641); one trial, SAILING (ING111762), in treatment-experienced, INSTI-naïve HIV–1–infected subjects (n = 715); and from VIKING-3 (ING112574) trial in INSTI-experienced HIV–1–infected subjects (n = 183). The use of TIVICAY in pediatric patients aged 12 years and older is based on evaluation of safety, pharmacokinetics, and efficacy through 24 weeks in a multi-center, open-label trial in subjects (n = 23) without INSTI resistance.

14.1 Adult Subjects

Treatment-Naïve Subjects: The efficacy of TIVICAY in HIV–1–infected treatment-naïve adults is based on the analyses of 48-week data from 2 randomized, international, multicenter, double-blind, active-controlled trials, SPRING-2 and SINGLE.

In SPRING-2, 822 subjects were randomized and received at least 1 dose of either TIVICAY 50 mg once daily or raltegravir 400 mg twice daily, both in combination with fixed-dose dual NRTI treatment (either abacavir sulfate and lamivudine [EPZICOM] or emtricitabine/tenofovir [TRUVADA]). There were 808 subjects included in the efficacy and safety analyses. At baseline, the median age of subjects was 36 years, 13% female, 15% non-white, 11% had hepatitis B and/or C virus co-infection, 2% were CDC Class C (AIDS), 28% had HIV-1 RNA >100,000 copies/mL, 48% had CD4+ cell count <350 cells/mm^3, and 39% received EPZICOM; these characteristics were similar between treatment groups.

In SINGLE, 833 subjects were randomized and received at least 1 dose of either TIVICAY 50 mg once daily with fixed-dose abacavir sulfate and lamivudine (EPZICOM) or fixed-dose efavirenz/emtricitabine/tenofovir (ATRIPLA). At baseline, the median age of subjects was 35 years, 16% female, 32% non-white, 7% had hepatitis C co-infection (hepatitis B virus co-infection was excluded), 4% were CDC Class C (AIDS), 32% had HIV-1 RNA >100,000 copies/mL, and 53% had CD4+ cell count <350 cells/mm^3; these characteristics were similar between treatment groups.

Week 48 outcomes for SPRING-2 and SINGLE are provided in Table 12. Side-by-side tabulation is to simplify presentation; direct comparisons across trials should not be made due to differing trial designs.

[See table 12 at top of previous page]

The adjusted mean changes in CD4+ cell counts from baseline were 267 cells/mm^3 in the group receiving TIVICAY + EPZICOM and 208 cells/mm^3 for the ATRIPLA group at 48 weeks. The adjusted difference between treatment arms and 95% CI was 58.9 cells/mm^3 (33.4 cells/mm^3, 84.4 cells/mm^3) (adjusted for pre-specified stratification factors: baseline HIV-1 RNA, baseline CD4+ cell count, and multiplicity).

Treatment-Experienced, Integrase Strand Transfer Inhibitor-Naïve Subjects: In the international, multicenter, double-blind trial (SAILING), 719 HIV–1– infected, antiretroviral treatment-experienced adults were randomized and received either TIVICAY 50 mg once daily or raltegravir 400 mg twice daily with investigator selected background regimen consisting of up to 2 agents, including at least 1 fully active agent. There were 715 subjects included in the efficacy and safety analyses. At baseline, the median age was 43 years, 32% were female, 49% non-white, 16% had hepatitis B and/or C virus co-infection, 46% were CDC Class C (AIDS), 20% had HIV-1 RNA >100,000 copies/mL, and 72% had CD4+ cell count <350 cells/mm^3; these characteristics were similar between treatment groups. All subjects had at least 2-class antiretroviral treatment resistance, and 49% of subjects had at least 3-class antiretroviral treatment resistance at baseline. Week 24 outcomes for SAILING are shown in Table 13.

Table 13. Virologic Outcomes of Randomized Treatment in SAILING at 24 Weeks (Snapshot Algorithm)

	TIVICAY 50 mg Once Daily + BR[a] (N = 354)	Raltegravir 400 mg Twice Daily + BR[a] (N = 361)
HIV-1 RNA <50 copies/mL	79%	70%
Adjusted[b] treatment difference	9.7% (95% CI: 3.4%, 15.9%)	
Virologic nonresponse	15%	24%
No virologic data at Week 24 window	6%	6%
Reasons		
Discontinued study/ study drug due to adverse event or death	2%	2%
Discontinued study/ study drug for otherreasons[c]	3%	3%
Missing data during window but on study	<1%	<1%
Proportion (%) With HIV-1 RNA <50 copies/mL at Week 24 by Baseline Category		
Plasma viral load (copies/mL)		
≤50,000 copies/mL	83%	77%
>50,000 copies/mL	70%	53%
Background regimen		
No darunavir use or use of darunavir with primary PI substitutions	79%	67%
Use of darunavir without primary PI substitutions	80%	81%
Gender		
Male	78%	70%
Female	83%	69%
Race		
White	79%	69%
Non-white	80%	71%

[a]BR = Background regimen. Background regimen was restricted to ≤2 antiretroviral treatments with at least 1 fully active agent.

[b]Adjusted for pre-specified stratification factors.

[c]Other includes reasons such as withdrew consent, loss to follow-up, moved, and protocol deviation.

Treatment differences were maintained across the baseline characteristics including CD4+ cell count and age.

The mean changes in CD4+ cell counts from baseline were 114 cells/mm^3 in the group receiving TIVICAY and 106 cells/mm^3 in the raltegravir group.

Treatment-Experienced, Integrase Strand Transfer Inhibitor-Experienced Subjects: VIKING-3 examined the effect of TIVICAY 50 mg twice daily over 7 days of functional monotherapy, followed by optimized background therapy with continued treatment of TIVICAY 50 mg twice daily.

In the multicenter, open-label, single-arm VIKING-3 trial, 183 HIV–1–infected, antiretroviral treatment-experienced adults with virological failure and current or historical evidence of raltegravir and/or elvitegravir resistance received TIVICAY 50 mg twice daily with the current failing background regimen for 7 days, then received TIVICAY with optimized background therapy from Day 8. A total of 183 subjects enrolled: 133 subjects with INSTI resistance at screening and 50 subjects with only historical evidence of resistance (and not at screening). At baseline, median age of subjects was 48 years; 23% were female, 29% non-white, and 20% had hepatitis B and/or C virus co-infection. Median baseline CD4+ cell count was 140 cells/mm^3, median duration of prior antiretroviral treatment was 13 years, and 56% were CDC Class C. Subjects showed multiple-class antiretroviral treatment resistance at baseline: 79% had ≥2 NRTI, 75% ≥1 NNRTI, and 71% ≥2 PI major substitutions; 62% had non-R5 virus.

Mean reduction from baseline in HIV-1 RNA at Day 8 (primary endpoint) was 1.4 $\log_{10}$ (95% CI: 1.3 $\log_{10}$, 1.5 $\log_{10}$). Response at Week 24 was affected by baseline INSTI substitutions *[see Microbiology (12.4)]*.

After the functional monotherapy phase, subjects had the opportunity to re-optimize their background regimen when possible. Week 24 virologic outcomes for VIKING-3 are shown in Table 14.

Table 14. Virologic Outcomes of Treatment of VIKING-3 at 24 Weeks (Snapshot Algorithm)

	TIVICAY 50 mg Twice Daily + Optimized Background Therapy (N = 114)
HIV-1 RNA <50 copies/mL	63%
Virologic nonresponse	32%
No virologic data at Week 24	
Reasons	
Discontinued study/study drug due to adverse event or death	4%
Proportion (%) With HIV-1 RNA <50 copies/mL at Week 24 by Baseline Category	
Gender	
Male	64%
Female	60%
Race	
White	67%
Non-white	52%

Subjects harboring virus with Q148 and with additional Q148-associated secondary substitutions also had a reduced response at Week 24 in a stepwise fashion *[see Microbiology (12.4)]*.

The median change in CD4+ cell count from baseline was 65 cells/mm^3 at Week 24.

14.2 Pediatric Subjects

IMPAACT P1093 is a Phase 1/2, 48-week, multicenter, open-label trial to evaluate the pharmacokinetic parameters, safety, tolerability, and efficacy of TIVICAY in combination treatment regimens in HIV–1–infected infants, children, and adolescents.

The initial dose-finding stage included intensive pharmacokinetic evaluation in 10 INSTI-naïve subjects (aged 12 to 18 years). Dose selection was based upon achieving similar dolutegravir plasma exposure and trough concentration as seen in adults. After dose selection, an additional 13 subjects were enrolled for evaluation of long-term safety, tolerability, and efficacy.

These 23 subjects had a mean age of 14 years (range: 12 to 17), were 78% female and 52% black. At baseline, mean plasma HIV-1 RNA was 4.3 $\log_{10}$ copies/mL, median CD4+ cell count was 466 cells/mm3 (range: 11 to 1,025), and median CD4+% was 22% (range: 1% to 39%). Overall, 17% had baseline plasma HIV-1 RNA >50,000 copies/mL and 39% had a CDC HIV clinical classification of category C. Most subjects had previously used at least 1 NNRTI (52%) or 1 PI (78%).

At 24 weeks, 70% of subjects treated with TIVICAY once daily (35 mg: n = 4, 50 mg: n = 19) plus optimized background therapy achieved a viral load <50 copies/mL. The median CD4+ cell count (percent) increase from baseline to Week 24 was 63 cells/mm3 (5%).

16 HOW SUPPLIED/STORAGE AND HANDLING

TIVICAY Tablets, 50 mg, are yellow, round, film-coated, biconvex tablets debossed with SV 572 on one side and 50 on the other side.

Bottle of 30 tablets with child-resistant closure NDC 49702-228-13.

Store at 25°C (77°F); excursions permitted 15 to 30°C (59° to 86°F) [See USP Controlled Room Temperature].

17 PATIENT COUNSELING INFORMATION

See FDA-approved Patient Labeling (Patient Information).

Drug Interactions: TIVICAY should not be coadministered with dofetilide because interactions between these drugs can result in potentially life-threatening adverse events *[see Contraindications (4)]*.

Hypersensitivity Reactions: Patients should be advised to immediately contact their healthcare provider if they develop rash. Instruct patients to immediately stop taking TIVICAY and other suspect agents, and seek medical attention if they develop a rash associated with any of the following symptoms, as it may be a sign of a more serious reaction such as severe hypersensitivity: fever; generally ill feeling; extreme tiredness; muscle or joint aches; blisters or peeling of the skin; oral blisters or lesions; eye inflammation; facial swelling; swelling of the eyes, lips, tongue, or mouth; breathing difficulty; and/or signs and symptoms of liver problems (e.g., yellowing of the skin or whites of the eyes, dark or tea-colored urine, pale-colored stools or bowel movements, nausea, vomiting, loss of appetite, or pain, aching, or sensitivity on the right side below the ribs). Patients should understand that if hypersensitivity occurs, they will be closely monitored, laboratory tests will be ordered, and appropriate therapy will be initiated. Patients should also be told that it is very important that they remain under a physician's care during treatment with TIVICAY *[see Warnings and Precautions (5.1)]*.

Effects on Serum Liver Biochemistries in Patients With Hepatitis B or C Co-infection: Patients with underlying hepatitis B or C may be at increased risk for worsening or development of transaminase elevations with use of TIVICAY and should be advised that they are recommended to have laboratory testing before and during therapy *[see Warnings and Precautions (5.2)]*.

Fat Redistribution: Patients should be informed that redistribution or accumulation of body fat may occur in patients receiving antiretroviral therapy and that the cause and long–term health effects of these conditions are not known at this time *[see Warnings and Precautions (5.3)]*.

Immune Reconstitution Syndrome: In some patients with advanced HIV infection, signs and symptoms of inflammation from previous infections may occur soon after anti-HIV treatment is started. It is believed that these symptoms are due to an improvement in the body's immune response, enabling the body to fight infections that may have been present with no obvious symptoms. Patients should be advised to inform their healthcare provider immediately of any symptoms of infection *[see Warnings and Precautions (5.4)]*.

Information About HIV–1 Infection: TIVICAY is not a cure for HIV–1 infection and patients may continue to experience illnesses associated with HIV–1 infection, including opportunistic infections. Patients must remain on continuous HIV therapy to control HIV infection and decrease HIV-related illness. Patients should be told that sustained decreases in plasma HIV RNA have been associated with a reduced risk of progression to AIDS and death. Patients should remain under the care of a physician when using TIVICAY.

Patients should be informed to take all HIV medications exactly as prescribed.

Patients should be advised to avoid doing things that can spread HIV-1 infection to others.

- **Do not re-use or share needles or other injection equipment.**
- **Do not share personal items that can have blood or body fluids on them, like toothbrushes and razor blades.**
- Continue to practice safe sex by using a latex or polyurethane condom to lower the chance of sexual contact with semen, vaginal secretions, or blood.
- Female patients should be advised not to breastfeed because it is not known if TIVICAY can be passed to the baby in your breast milk and whether it could harm the baby. Mothers with HIV–1 should not breastfeed because HIV-1 can be passed to the baby in the breast milk.

Physicians should instruct their patients to read the Patient Information before starting TIVICAY and to reread it each time the prescription is renewed. Patients should be instructed to inform their physician or pharmacist if they develop any unusual symptom, or if any known symptom persists or worsens.

Physicians should instruct their patients that if they miss a dose, they should take it as soon as they remember. If they do not remember until it is within 4 hours of the time for the next dose, they should be instructed to skip the missed dose and go back to the regular schedule. Patients should not double their next dose or take more than the prescribed dose.

TIVICAY and EPZICOM are registered trademarks of ViiV Healthcare.

The other brands listed are trademarks of their respective owners and are not trademarks of ViiV Healthcare. The makers of these brands are not affiliated with and do not endorse ViiV Healthcare or its products.

Manufactured for:
ViiV Healthcare
Research Triangle Park, NC 27709
by:
GlaxoSmithKline
Research Triangle Park, NC 27709

TVC:1PI

Patient Information

TIVICAY®(TIV-eh-kay)

(dolutegravir)

Tablets

Read this Patient Information before you start taking TIVICAY and each time you get a refill. There may be new information. This information does not take the place of talking with your healthcare provider about your medical condition or treatment.

What is TIVICAY?

TIVICAY is a prescription HIV medicine that is used with other antiretroviral medicines to treat Human Immunodeficiency Virus-1 (HIV-1) infections in adults and children 12 years of age and older and weighing at least 88 pounds.

HIV-1 is the virus that causes Acquired Immune Deficiency Syndrome (AIDS).

It is not known if TIVICAY is safe and effective in children under 12 years of age or who weigh less than 88 pounds.

When used with other HIV-1 medicines to treat HIV–1 infection, TIVICAY may help:

- Reduce the amount of HIV-1 in your blood. This is called "viral load".
- Increase the number of white blood cells called CD4+ (T) cells in your blood, which help fight off other infections.
- Reduce the amount of HIV-1 and increase the CD4+ (T) cell in your blood which may help improve your immune system. This may reduce your risk of death or getting infections that can happen when your immune system is weak (opportunistic infections).

TIVICAY does not cure HIV-1 infection or AIDS. You must stay on continuous HIV-1 therapy to control HIV-1 infection and decrease HIV-related illnesses.

Avoid doing things that can spread HIV-1 infection to others.

- Do not share or re-use needles or other injection equipment.
- Do not share personal items that can have blood or body fluids on them, like toothbrushes and razor blades.
- Do not have any kind of sex without protection.Always practice safe sex by using a latex or polyurethane condom to lower the chance of sexual contact with any body fluids such as semen, vaginal secretions, or blood.

Ask your healthcare provider if you have any questions about how to prevent passing HIV to other people.

Who should not take TIVICAY?

Do not take TIVICAY if you take dofetilide. Taking TIVICAY and dofetilide can cause side effects that may be life-threatening.

What should I tell my healthcare provider before taking TIVICAY?

Before you take TIVICAY, tell your healthcare provider if you:

- have ever had an allergic reaction to TIVICAY
- have or had liver problems, including hepatitis B or C infection
- have any other medical condition
- are pregnant or plan to become pregnant. It is not known if TIVICAY will harm your unborn baby. Tell your healthcare provider if you become pregnant while taking TIVICAY.
  Pregnancy Registry. There is a pregnancy registry for women who take antiviral medicines during pregnancy. The purpose of the registry is to collect information about the health of you and your baby. Talk to your healthcare provider about how you can take part in this registry.
- are breastfeeding or plan to breastfeed. **Do not breastfeed if you take TIVICAY.**
  - You should not breastfeed if you have HIV-1 because of the risk of passing HIV-1 to your baby.
  - It is not known if TIVICAY passes into your breast milk.
  - Talk to your healthcare provider about the best way to feed your baby.

Tell your healthcare provider about the medicines you take, including prescription and over-the-counter medicines, vitamins, or herbal supplements.

TIVICAY and other medicines may affect each other causing side effects. TIVICAY may affect the way other medicines work, and other medicines may affect how TIVICAY works.

Especially tell your healthcare provider if you take:

- other HIV-1 medicines including: efavirenz (SUSTIVA®), etravirine (INTELENCE®), fosamprenavir (LEXIVA®)/ritonavir (N0RVIR®), nevirapine (VIRAMUNE®), or tipranavir (APTIVUS®)/ritonavir (N0RVIR).
- antacids or laxatives that contain aluminum, magnesium or calcium, sucralfate (CARAFATE®), iron or calcium supplements, or buffered medicines. TIVICAY should be taken at least 2 hours before or 6 hours after you take these medicines.
- anti-seizure medicines:
  - oxcarbazepine (TRILEPTAL®)
  - phenytoin (DILANTIN®, DILANTIN®-125, PHENYTEK®)
  - phenobarbital (LUMINAL®)
  - carbamazepine (CARBATROL®, EQUETRO®, TEGRETOL®, TEGRETOL®-XR, TERIL®, EPITOL®)
- St. John's wort (*Hypericum perforatum*)
- a medicine that contains metformin
- rifampin (RIFATER®, RIFAMATE®, RIMACTANE®, RIFADAN®)

Ask your healthcare provider or pharmacist if you are not sure if your medicine is one that is listed above.

Know the medicines you take. Keep a list of them to show your healthcare provider and pharmacist when you get a new medicine.

How should I take TIVICAY?

- Take TIVICAY exactly as your healthcare provider tells you.
- Do not change your dose or stop taking TIVICAY without talking with your healthcare provider.
- Stay under the care of a healthcare provider while taking TIVICAY.
- You can take TIVICAY with or without food.
- If you miss a dose of TIVICAY, take it as soon as you remember. If it is within 4 hours of your next dose, skip the missed dose and take the next dose at your regular time. Do not take 2 doses at the same time. If you are not sure about your dosing, call your healthcare provider.
- If you take too much TIVICAY, call your healthcare provider or go to the nearest hospital emergency room right away.
- Do not run out of TIVICAY. The virus in your blood may become resistant to other HIV-1 medicines if TIVICAY is stopped for even a short time. When your supply starts to run low, get more from your healthcare provider or pharmacy.

What are the possible side effects of TIVICAY?

TIVICAY may cause serious side effects, including:

- **Allergic reactions.** Call your healthcare provider right away if you develop a rash with TIVICAY. **Stop taking TIVICAY and get medical help right away if you:**
- **develop a rash with any of the following signs or symptoms**
  - fever
  - generally ill feeling
  - extreme tiredness
  - muscle or joint aches
  - blisters or sores in mouth
  - blisters or peeling of the skin
  - redness or swelling of the eyes
  - swelling of the mouth, face, lips, or tongue
  - problems breathing
- **develop any of the following signs or symptoms of liver problems:**
  - yellowing of the skin or whites of the eyes
  - dark or tea-colored urine
  - pale-colored stools or bowel movements
  - nausea or vomiting
  - loss of appetite
  - pain, aching, or tenderness on the right side below the ribs
- **Changes in liver tests.** People with a history of hepatitis B or C virus may have an increased risk of developing new or worsening changes in certain liver tests during treatment with TIVICAY. Your healthcare provider may do tests to check your liver function before and during treatment with TIVICAY.
- **Changes in body fat** can happen in people who take HIV-1 medicines. These changes may include increased amount of fat in the upper back and neck ("buffalo hump"), breast, and around the middle of your body (trunk). Loss of fat from the legs, arms, and face may also happen. The exact cause and long-term health effects of these problems are not known.
- **Changes in your immune system (Immune Reconstitution Syndrome)** can happen when you start taking HIV-1 medicines. Your immune system may get stronger and begin to fight infections that have been hidden in your body for a long time. Tell your healthcare provider right away if you start having new symptoms after starting your HIV-1 medicine.

The most common side effects of TIVICAY include:

- trouble sleeping
- headache

Tell your healthcare provider about any side effect that bothers you or that does not go away.

These are not all the possible side effects of TIVICAY. For more information, ask your healthcare provider or pharmacist.

Call your doctor for medical advice about side effects. You may report side effects to FDA at 1–800–FDA–1088.

How should I store TIVICAY?

- Store TIVICAY at room temperature between 68°F to 77°F (20°C to 25°C).

Keep TIVICAY and all medicines out of the reach of children.

General information about TIVICAY

Medicines are sometimes prescribed for purposes other than those listed in a Patient Information leaflet. Do not use TIVICAY for a condition for which it was not prescribed. Do not give TIVICAY to other people, even if they have the same symptoms you have. It may harm them.

You can ask your pharmacist or healthcare provider for information about TIVICAY that is written for health professionals.

For more information call 1-877-844-8872 or go to www.TIVICAY.com.

What are the ingredients in TIVICAY?

Active ingredient: dolutegravir sodium

Inactive ingredients: d-mannitol, microcrystalline cellulose, povidone K29/32, sodium starch glycolate, and sodium stearyl fumarate. The tablet film-coating contains the inactive ingredients iron oxide yellow, macrogol/PEG, polyvinyl alcohol-part hydrolyzed, talc, and titanium dioxide.

This Patient Information has been approved by the U.S. Food and Drug Administration.

Manufactured for:
ViiV Healthcare
Research Triangle Park, NC 27709
by:
GlaxoSmithKline
Research Triangle Park, NC 27709
August 2013
TVC:1PIL

TIVICAY and LEXIVA are registered trademarks of ViiV Healthcare.

The brands listed are trademarks of their respective owners and are not trademarks of ViiV Healthcare. The makers of these brands are not affiliated with and do not endorse ViiV Healthcare or its products.

TRIZIVIR ℞

[trī' zə-vir]

(abacavir sulfate, lamivudine, and zidovudine)
Tablets, for oral use

HIGHLIGHTS OF PRESCRIBING INFORMATION

These highlights do not include all the information needed to use TRIZIVIR safely and effectively. See full prescribing information for TRIZIVIR.

TRIZIVIR (abacavir sulfate, lamivudine, and zidovudine) Tablets, for oral use
Initial U.S. Approval: 2000

WARNING: RISK OF HYPERSENSITIVITY REACTIONS, HEMATOLOGIC TOXICITY, MYOPATHY, LACTIC ACIDOSIS AND SEVERE HEPATOMEGALY, EXACERBATIONS OF HEPATITIS B

See full prescribing information for complete boxed warning.

- **Serious and sometimes fatal hypersensitivity reactions have been associated with abacavir-containing products. (5.1)**
- **Hypersensitivity to abacavir is a multi-organ clinical syndrome. (5.1)**
- **Patients who carry the HLA-B*5701 allele are at high risk for experiencing a hypersensitivity reaction to abacavir. (5.1)**
- **Discontinue TRIZIVIR as soon as a hypersensitivity reaction is suspected. Regardless of HLA-B*5701 status, permanently discontinue TRIZIVIR if hypersensitivity cannot be ruled out. (5.1)**
- **Following a hypersensitivity reaction to abacavir, NEVER restart TRIZIVIR or any other abacavir-containing product. (5.1)**
- **Hematologic toxicity, including neutropenia and anemia, has been associated with the use of zidovudine, a component of TRIZIVIR. (5.2)**
- **Symptomatic myopathy associated with prolonged use of zidovudine. (5.3)**

- **Lactic acidosis and severe hepatomegaly with steatosis, including fatal cases, have been reported with the use of nucleoside analogues. (5.4)**
- **Severe acute exacerbations of hepatitis B have been reported in patients who are co-infected with hepatitis B virus (HBV) and human immunodeficiency virus (HIV-1) and have discontinued lamivudine, a component of TRIZIVIR. Monitor hepatic function closely in these patients and, if appropriate, initiate anti-hepatitis B treatment. (5.5)**

INDICATIONS AND USAGE

TRIZIVIR, a combination of abacavir, lamivudine, and zidovudine, each nucleoside analogue HIV-1 reverse transcriptase inhibitors, is indicated in combination with other antiretroviral agents for the treatment of HIV-1 infection. (1)

DOSAGE AND ADMINISTRATION

- A medication guide and warning card should be dispensed with each new prescription and refill. (2)
- Adults and Adolescents: 1 tablet twice daily. (2.1)
- Not recommended in adolescents who weigh less than 40 kg. (2.1)
- Do not prescribe for patients requiring dosage adjustment or patients with hepatic impairment. (2.2)

DOSAGE FORMS AND STRENGTHS

Tablets contain 300 mg abacavir, 150 mg of lamivudine, and 300 mg of zidovudine. (3)

CONTRAINDICATIONS

- Previously demonstrated hypersensitivity to abacavir or any other component of the product. (4, 5.1, 6)
- Hepatic impairment. (4)

WARNINGS AND PRECAUTIONS

- See boxed warning for information about the following: hypersensitivity reactions, hematologic toxicity, myopathy, lactic acidosis and severe hepatomegaly, and severe acute exacerbations of hepatitis B. (5.1, 5.2, 5.3, 5.4, 5.5)
- Hepatic decompensation, some fatal, has occurred in HIV-1/HCV co-infected patients receiving combination antiretroviral therapy and interferon alfa with or without ribavirin. Discontinue TRIZIVIR as medically appropriate and consider dose reduction or discontinuation of interferon alfa, ribavirin, or both. (5.6)
- Exacerbation of anemia has been reported in HIV-1/HCV co-infected patients receiving ribavirin and zidovudine. Coadministration of ribavirin and zidovudine is not advised. (5.6)
- Immune reconstitution syndrome (5.7) and redistribution/accumulation of body fat (5.8) have been reported in patients treated with combination antiretroviral therapy.
- TRIZIVIR should not be administered with other products containing abacavir, lamivudine, or zidovudine; or with emtricitabine. (5.11)

ADVERSE REACTIONS

The most commonly reported adverse reactions (incidence ≥10%) in clinical trials were nausea, headache, malaise and fatigue, and nausea and vomiting. (6.1)

To report SUSPECTED ADVERSE REACTIONS, contact ViiV Healthcare at 1-877-844-8872 or FDA at 1-800-FDA-1088 or www.fda.gov/medwatch.

DRUG INTERACTIONS

- Concomitant use with the following drugs should be avoided: stavudine (7.1), doxorubicin (7.2).
- Ethanol: Decreases the elimination of abacavir. (7.3)
- Bone marrow suppressive/cytotoxic agents: May increase the hematologic toxicity of zidovudine. (7.4)
- Methadone: An increased methadone dose may be required in a small number of patients. (7.6)

See 17 for PATIENT COUNSELING INFORMATION and Medication Guide

Revised: 05/2013

FULL PRESCRIBING INFORMATION: CONTENTS*

*** Sections or subsections omitted from the full prescribing information are not listed**

FULL PRESCRIBING INFORMATION

WARNING: RISK OF HYPERSENSITIVITY REACTIONS, HEMATOLOGIC TOXICITY, MYOPATHY, LACTIC ACIDOSIS AND SEVERE HEPATOMEGALY, EXACERBATIONS OF HEPATITIS B

Hypersensitivity Reactions: Serious and sometimes fatal hypersensitivity reactions have been associated with abacavir sulfate, a component of TRIZIVIR. Hypersensitivity to abacavir is a multi-organ clinical syndrome usually characterized by a sign or symptom in 2 or more of the following groups: (1) fever, (2) rash, (3) gastrointestinal (including nausea, vomiting, diarrhea, or abdominal pain), (4) constitutional (including generalized malaise, fatigue, or achiness), and (5) respiratory (including dyspnea, cough, or pharyngitis). Discontinue TRIZIVIR as soon as a hypersensitivity reaction is suspected.

Patients who carry the HLA-B*5701 allele are at high risk for experiencing a hypersensitivity reaction to abacavir. Prior to initiating therapy with abacavir, screening for the HLA-B*5701 allele is recommended; this approach has been found to decrease the risk of hypersensitivity reaction. Screening is also recommended prior to reinitiation of abacavir in patients of unknown HLA-B*5701 status who have previously tolerated abacavir. HLA-B*5701-negative patients may develop a suspected hypersensitivity reaction to abacavir; however, this occurs significantly less frequently than in HLA-B*5701-positive patients.

Regardless of HLA-B*5701 status, permanently discontinue TRIZIVIR if hypersensitivity cannot be ruled out, even when other diagnoses are possible.

Following a hypersensitivity reaction to abacavir, NEVER restart TRIZIVIR or any other abacavir-containing product because more severe symptoms can occur within hours and may include life-threatening hypotension and death.

Reintroduction of TRIZIVIR or any other abacavir-containing product, even in patients who have no identified history or unrecognized symptoms of hypersensitivity to abacavir therapy, can result in serious or fatal hypersensitivity reactions. Such reactions can occur within hours *[see Warnings and Precautions (5.1)]*.

Hematologic Toxicity: Zidovudine, a component of TRIZIVIR, has been associated with hematologic toxicity, including neutropenia and severe anemia, particularly in patients with advanced Human Immunodeficiency Virus (HIV-1) disease *[see Warnings and Precautions (5.2)]*.

Myopathy: Prolonged use of zidovudine has been associated with symptomatic myopathy *[see Warnings and Precautions (5.3)]*.

Lactic Acidosis and Severe Hepatomegaly: Lactic acidosis and severe hepatomegaly with steatosis, including fatal cases, have been reported with the use of nucleoside analogues alone or in combination, including abacavir, lamivudine, zidovudine, and other antiretrovirals *[see Warnings and Precautions (5.4)]*.

Exacerbations of Hepatitis B: Severe acute exacerbations of hepatitis B have been reported in patients who are co-infected with hepatitis B virus (HBV) and HIV-1 and have discontinued lamivudine, which is one component of TRIZIVIR. Hepatic function should be monitored closely with both clinical and laboratory follow-up for at least several months in patients who discontinue TRIZIVIR and are co-infected with HIV-1 and HBV. If appropriate, initiation of anti-hepatitis B therapy may be warranted *[see Warnings and Precautions (5.5)]*.

1 INDICATIONS AND USAGE

TRIZIVIR is indicated in combination with other antiretrovirals or alone for the treatment of HIV-1 infection.

Additional important information on the use of TRIZIVIR for treatment of HIV-1 infection:

- TRIZIVIR is one of multiple products containing abacavir. Before starting TRIZIVIR, review medical history for prior exposure to any abacavir-containing product in order to avoid reintroduction in a patient with a history of hypersensitivity to abacavir *[see Warnings and Precautions (5.1), Adverse Reactions (6)]*.
- TRIZIVIR is a fixed-dose combination of 3 nucleoside analogues: abacavir, lamivudine, and zidovudine and is intended only for patients whose regimen would otherwise include these 3 components.
- Limited data exist on the use of TRIZIVIR alone in patients with higher baseline viral load levels (>100,000 copies/mL) *[see Clinical Studies (14)]*.

2 DOSAGE AND ADMINISTRATION

- A Medication Guide and Warning Card that provide information about recognition of hypersensitivity reactions should be dispensed with each new prescription and refill.
- TRIZIVIR can be taken with or without food.

2.1 Adults and Adolescent Patients

The recommended oral dose of TRIZIVIR is one tablet twice daily.

TRIZIVIR is not recommended in adolescents who weigh less than 40 kg because it is a fixed-dose tablet and cannot be dose adjusted.

2.2 Dosage Adjustment

Because it is a fixed-dose combination, TRIZIVIR should not be prescribed for:

- patients requiring dosage adjustment such as those with creatinine clearance <50 mL/min.
- patients with hepatic impairment.

3 DOSAGE FORMS AND STRENGTHS

TRIZIVIR Tablets contain 300 mg of abacavir as abacavir sulfate, 150 mg of lamivudine, and 300 mg of zidovudine. The tablets are blue-green, capsule-shaped, film-coated, and imprinted with "GX LL1" on one side with no markings on the reverse side.

4 CONTRAINDICATIONS

TRIZIVIR Tablets are contraindicated in patients with:

- previously demonstrated hypersensitivity to abacavir or any other component of the product. NEVER restart TRIZIVIR or any other abacavir-containing product following a hypersensitivity reaction to abacavir, regardless of HLA-B*5701 status *[see Warnings and Precautions (5.1), Adverse Reactions (6)]*.
- hepatic impairment *[see Use in Specific Populations (8.7)]*.

5 WARNINGS AND PRECAUTIONS

5.1 Hypersensitivity Reaction

Serious and sometimes fatal hypersensitivity reactions have been associated with TRIZIVIR and other abacavir-containing products. Patients who carry the HLA-B*5701 allele are at high risk for experiencing a hypersensitivity reaction to abacavir. Prior to initiating therapy with abacavir, screening for the HLA-B*5701 allele is recommended; this approach has been found to decrease the risk of a hypersensitivity reaction. Screening is also recommended prior to reinitiation of abacavir in patients of unknown HLA-B*5701 status who have previously tolerated abacavir. For HLA-B*5701-positive patients, treatment with an abacavir-containing regimen is not recommended and should be considered only with close medical supervision and under exceptional circumstances when the potential benefit outweighs the risk.

HLA-B*5701-negative patients may develop a hypersensitivity reaction to abacavir; however, this occurs significantly less frequently than in HLA-B*5701-positive patients. Regardless of HLA-B*5701 status, permanently discontinue TRIZIVIR if hypersensitivity cannot be ruled out, even when other diagnoses are possible.

Important information on signs and symptoms of hypersensitivity, as well as clinical management, is presented below.

Signs and Symptoms of Hypersensitivity: Hypersensitivity to abacavir is a multi-organ clinical syndrome usually characterized by a sign or symptom in 2 or more of the following groups.

Group 1: Fever
Group 2: Rash
Group 3: Gastrointestinal (including nausea, vomiting, diarrhea, or abdominal pain)
Group 4: Constitutional (including generalized malaise, fatigue, or achiness)
Group 5: Respiratory (including dyspnea, cough, or pharyngitis)

Hypersensitivity to abacavir following the presentation of a single sign or symptom has been reported infrequently.

Hypersensitivity to abacavir was reported in approximately 8% of 2,670 subjects (n = 206) in 9 clinical trials (range: 2% to 9%) with enrollment from November 1999 to February 2002. Data on time to onset and symptoms of suspected hypersensitivity were collected on a detailed data collection module. The frequencies of symptoms are shown in Figure 1. Symptoms usually appeared within the first 6 weeks of treatment with abacavir, although the reaction may occur at any time during therapy. Median time to onset was 9 days; 89% appeared within the first 6 weeks; 95% of subjects reported symptoms from 2 or more of the 5 groups listed above.

A trial with ZIAGEN® (abacavir sulfate) used double-blind ascertainment of suspected hypersensitivity reactions. During the blinded portion of the trial, suspected hypersensitivity to abacavir was reported by investigators in 9% of 324 subjects in the abacavir group and 3% of 325 subjects in the zidovudine group.

Figure 1. Hypersensitivity-Related Symptoms Reported With ≥10% Frequency in Clinical Trials (n = 206 Subjects)

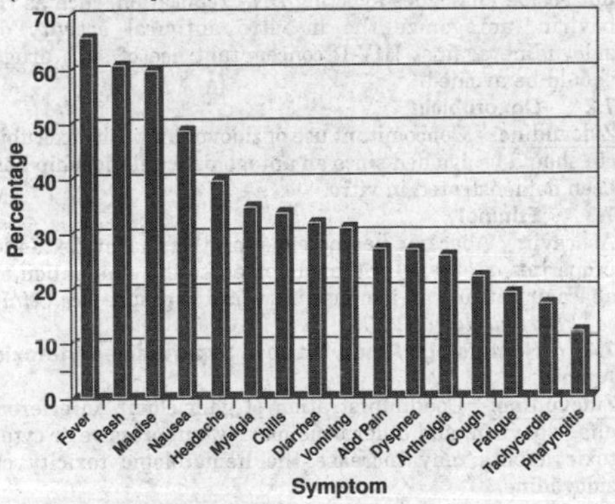

Other less common signs and symptoms of hypersensitivity include lethargy, myolysis, edema, abnormal chest x-ray findings (predominantly infiltrates, which can be localized), and paresthesia. Anaphylaxis, liver failure, renal failure, hypotension, adult respiratory distress syndrome, respiratory failure, and death have occurred in association with hypersensitivity reactions.

Physical findings associated with hypersensitivity to abacavir in some subjects include lymphadenopathy, mucous membrane lesions (conjunctivitis and mouth ulcerations), and rash. The rash usually appears maculopapular or urticarial, but may be variable in appearance. There have been reports of erythema multiforme. Hypersensitivity reactions have occurred without rash.

Laboratory abnormalities associated with hypersensitivity to abacavir in some subjects include elevated liver function tests, elevated creatinine phosphokinase, elevated creatinine, and lymphopenia.

Clinical Management of Hypersensitivity: Discontinue TRIZIVIR as soon as a hypersensitivity reaction is suspected. To minimize the risk of a life-threatening hypersensitivity reaction, permanently discontinue TRIZIVIR if hypersensitivity cannot be ruled out, even when other diagnoses are possible (e.g., acute onset respiratory diseases such as pneumonia, bronchitis, pharyngitis, or influenza; gastroenteritis; or reactions to other medications).

Following a hypersensitivity reaction to abacavir, NEVER restart TRIZIVIR or any other abacavir-containing product because more severe symptoms can occur within hours and may include life-threatening hypotension and death.

When therapy with TRIZIVIR has been discontinued for reasons other than symptoms of a hypersensitivity reaction, and if reinitiation of abacavir is under consideration, carefully evaluate the reason for discontinuation to ensure that the patient did not have symptoms of a hypersensitivity reaction. If the patient is of unknown HLA-B*5701 status, screening for the allele is recommended prior to reinitiation of TRIZIVIR.

If hypersensitivity cannot be ruled out, DO NOT reintroduce TRIZIVIR or any other abacavir-containing product. Even in the absence of the HLA-B*5701 allele, it is important to permanently discontinue abacavir and not rechallenge with abacavir if a hypersensitivity reaction cannot be ruled out on clinical grounds, due to the potential for a severe or even fatal reaction.

If symptoms consistent with hypersensitivity are not identified, reintroduction can be undertaken with continued monitoring for symptoms of a hypersensitivity reaction. Make patients aware that a hypersensitivity reaction can occur with reintroduction of abacavir and that abacavir reintroduction needs to be undertaken only if medical care can be readily accessed by the patient or others.

Risk Factor: *HLA-B*5701 Allele:* Trials have shown that carriage of the HLA-B*5701 allele is associated with a significantly increased risk of a hypersensitivity reaction to abacavir.

CNA106030 (PREDICT-1), a randomized, double-blind trial, evaluated the clinical utility of prospective HLA-B*5701 screening on the incidence of abacavir hypersensitivity reaction in abacavir-naive HIV-1-infected adults (n = 1,650). In this trial, use of pre-therapy screening for the HLA-B*5701 allele and exclusion of subjects with this allele reduced the incidence of clinically suspected abacavir hypersensitivity reactions from 7.8% (66/847) to 3.4% (27/803). Based on this trial, it is estimated that 61% of patients with the HLA-B*5701 allele will develop a clinically suspected hypersensitivity reaction during the course of abacavir treatment compared with 4% of patients who do not have the HLA-B*5701 allele.

Screening for carriage of the HLA-B*5701 allele is recommended prior to initiating treatment with abacavir. Screening is also recommended prior to reinitiation of abacavir in patients of unknown HLA-B*5701 status who have previously tolerated abacavir. For HLA-B*5701-positive patients, initiating or reinitiating treatment with an abacavir-containing regimen is not recommended and should be considered only with close medical supervision and under exceptional circumstances where potential benefit outweighs the risk.

Skin patch testing is used as a research tool and should not be used to aid in the clinical diagnosis of abacavir hypersensitivity.

In any patient treated with abacavir, the clinical diagnosis of hypersensitivity reaction must remain the basis of clinical decision-making. Even in the absence of the HLA-B*5701 allele, it is important to permanently discontinue abacavir and not rechallenge with abacavir if a hypersensitivity reaction cannot be ruled out on clinical grounds, due to the potential for a severe or even fatal reaction.

5.2 Hematologic Toxicity/Bone Marrow Suppression

Zidovudine, a component of TRIZIVIR, has been associated with hematologic toxicity including neutropenia and anemia, particularly in patients with advanced HIV-1 disease. TRIZIVIR should be used with caution in patients who have bone marrow compromise evidenced by granulocyte count less than 1,000 cells/mm^3 or hemoglobin less than 9.5 g/dL.

Frequent blood counts are strongly recommended in patients with advanced HIV-1 disease who are treated with TRIZIVIR. Periodic blood counts are recommended for other HIV-1-infected patients. If anemia or neutropenia develops, dosage interruption may be needed.

5.3 Myopathy

Myopathy and myositis, with pathological changes similar to that produced by HIV-1 disease, have been associated with prolonged use of zidovudine, and therefore may occur with therapy with TRIZIVIR.

5.4 Lactic Acidosis/Hepatomegaly With Steatosis

Lactic acidosis and severe hepatomegaly with steatosis, including fatal cases, have been reported with the use of nucleoside analogues alone or in combination, including abacavir, lamivudine, zidovudine, and other antiretrovirals. A majority of these cases have been in women. Obesity and prolonged nucleoside exposure may be risk factors. Particular caution should be exercised when administering TRIZIVIR to any patient with known risk factors for liver disease; however, cases have also been reported in patients with no known risk factors. Treatment with TRIZIVIR should be suspended in any patient who develops clinical or laboratory findings suggestive of lactic acidosis or pronounced hepatotoxicity (which may include hepatomegaly and steatosis even in the absence of marked transaminase elevations).

5.5 Patients With HIV-1 and Hepatitis B Virus Co-infection

Posttreatment Exacerbations of Hepatitis: In clinical trials in non-HIV-1-infected subjects treated with lamivudine for chronic HBV, clinical and laboratory evidence of exacerbations of hepatitis have occurred after discontinuation of lamivudine. These exacerbations have been detected primarily by serum ALT elevations in addition to re-emergence of hepatitis B viral DNA (HBV DNA). Although most events appear to have been self-limited, fatalities have been reported in some cases. Similar events have been reported from post-marketing experience after changes from lamivudine-containing HIV-1 treatment regimens to non-lamivudine-containing regimens in patients infected with both HIV-1 and HBV. The causal relationship to discontinuation of lamivudine treatment is unknown. Patients should be closely monitored with both clinical and laboratory follow-up for at least several months after stopping treatment. There is insufficient evidence to determine whether reinitiation of lamivudine alters the course of posttreatment exacerbations of hepatitis.

Emergence of Lamivudine-Resistant HBV: Safety and efficacy of lamivudine have not been established for treatment of chronic hepatitis B in subjects dually infected with HIV-1 and HBV. In non-HIV-infected subjects treated with lamivudine for chronic hepatitis B, emergence of lamivudine-resistant HBV has been detected and has been associated with diminished treatment response (see full prescribing information for EPIVIR-HBV® [lamivudine] for additional information). Emergence of hepatitis B virus variants associated with resistance to lamivudine has also been reported in HIV-1-infected subjects who have received lamivudine-containing antiretroviral regimens in the presence of concurrent infection with hepatitis B virus.

5.6 Use With Interferon- and Ribavirin-Based Regimens

In vitro studies have shown ribavirin can reduce the phosphorylation of pyrimidine nucleoside analogues such as lamivudine and zidovudine. Although no evidence of a pharmacokinetic or pharmacodynamic interaction (e.g., loss of HIV-1/HCV virologic suppression) was seen when ribavirin was coadministered with lamivudine or zidovudine in HIV-1/HCV co-infected subjects *[see Clinical Pharmacology (12.3)]*, hepatic decompensation (some fatal) has occurred in HIV-1/HCV co-infected subjects receiving combination antiretroviral therapy for HIV-1 and interferon alfa with or without ribavirin. Patients receiving interferon alfa with or without ribavirin and TRIZIVIR should be closely monitored for treatment-associated toxicities, especially hepatic decompensation, neutropenia, and anemia. Discontinuation of TRIZIVIR should be considered as medically appropriate. Dose reduction or discontinuation of interferon alfa, ribavirin, or both should also be considered if worsening clinical toxicities are observed, including hepatic decompensation (e.g., Child-Pugh greater than 6) (see the complete prescribing information for interferon and ribavirin).

Exacerbation of anemia has been reported in HIV-1/HCV co-infected patients receiving ribavirin and zidovudine. Coadministration of ribavirin and TRIZIVIR is not advised.

5.7 Immune Reconstitution Syndrome

Immune reconstitution syndrome has been reported in patients treated with combination antiretroviral therapy, including TRIZIVIR. During the initial phase of combination antiretroviral treatment, patients whose immune systems respond may develop an inflammatory response to indolent or residual opportunistic infections (such as *Mycobacterium avium* infection, cytomegalovirus, *Pneumocystis jirovecii* pneumonia [PCP], or tuberculosis), which may necessitate further evaluation and treatment.

Autoimmune disorders (such as Graves' disease, polymyositis, and Guillain-Barré syndrome) have also been reported to occur in the setting of immune reconstitution; however, the time to onset is more variable, and can occur many months after initiation of treatment.

5.8 Fat Redistribution

Redistribution/accumulation of body fat including central obesity, dorsocervical fat enlargement (buffalo hump), peripheral wasting, facial wasting, breast enlargement, and "cushingoid appearance" have been observed in patients receiving antiretroviral therapy. The mechanism and long-term consequences of these events are currently unknown. A causal relationship has not been established.

5.9 Myocardial Infarction

In a published prospective, observational, epidemiological trial designed to investigate the rate of myocardial infarction in patients on combination antiretroviral therapy, the use of abacavir within the previous 6 months was correlated with an increased risk of myocardial infarction (MI).[1] In a sponsor-conducted pooled analysis of clinical trials, no excess risk of myocardial infarction was observed in abacavir-treated subjects as compared with control subjects. In totality, the available data from the observational cohort and from clinical trials are inconclusive.

Table 1. Treatment-Emergent (All Causality) Adverse Reactions of at Least Moderate Intensity (Grades 2-4, ≥5% Frequency) in Therapy-Naive Adults (CNA3005) Through 48 Weeks of Treatment

Adverse Reaction	ZIAGEN plus Lamivudine/Zidovudine (n = 262)	Indinavir plus Lamivudine/Zidovudine (n = 264)
Nausea	19%	17%
Headache	13%	9%
Malaise and fatigue	12%	12%
Nausea and vomiting	10%	10%
Hypersensitivity reaction	8%	2%
Diarrhea	7%	5%
Fever and/or chills	6%	3%
Depressive disorders	6%	4%
Musculoskeletal pain	5%	7%
Skin rashes	5%	4%
Ear/nose/throat infections	5%	4%
Viral respiratory infections	5%	5%
Anxiety	5%	3%
Renal signs/symptoms	<1%	5%
Pain (non-site-specific)	<1%	5%

Table 2. Treatment-Emergent Laboratory Abnormalities (Grades 3/4) in CNA3005

Grade 3/4 Laboratory Abnormalities	Number of Subjects by Treatment Group	
	ZIAGEN plus Lamivudine/Zidovudine (n = 262)	Indinavir plus Lamivudine/Zidovudine (n = 264)
Elevated CPK (>4 × ULN)	18 (7%)	18 (7%)
ALT (>5.0 × ULN)	16 (6%)	16 (6%)
Neutropenia (<750/mm^3)	13 (5%)	13 (5%)
Hypertriglyceridemia (>750 mg/dL)	5 (2%)	3 (1%)
Hyperamylasemia (>2.0 × ULN)	5 (2%)	1 (<1%)
Hyperglycemia (>13.9 mmol/L)	2 (<1%)	2 (<1%)
Anemia (Hgb ≤6.9 g/dL)	0 (0%)	3 (1%)

ULN = Upper limit of normal.
n = Number of patients assessed.

As a precaution, the underlying risk of coronary heart disease should be considered when prescribing antiretroviral therapies, including abacavir, and action taken to minimize all modifiable risk factors (e.g., hypertension, hyperlipidemia, diabetes mellitus, smoking).

5.10 Therapy Experienced Patients

In clinical trials, subjects with prolonged prior nucleoside reverse transcriptase inhibitor (NRTI) exposure or who had HIV-1 isolates that contained multiple mutations conferring resistance to NRTIs had limited response to abacavir. The potential for cross-resistance between abacavir and other NRTIs should be considered when choosing new therapeutic regimens in therapy-experienced patients *[see Clinical Pharmacology (12.4)]*.

5.11 Use With Other Abacavir-, Lamivudine-, Zidovudine-, and/or Emtricitabine-Containing Products

TRIZIVIR is a fixed-dose combination of abacavir, lamivudine, and zidovudine and is intended only for patients whose regimen would otherwise include these 3 components. TRIZIVIR should not be administered concomitantly with other abacavir-, lamivudine-, or zidovudine-containing products including ZIAGEN (abacavir sulfate) Tablets and Oral Solution, EPIVIR® (lamivudine) Tablets and Oral Solution, EPIVIR-HBV (lamivudine) Tablets and Oral Solution, RETROVIR® (zidovudine) Tablets, Capsules, Syrup, and IV Infusion, COMBIVIR® (lamivudine and zidovudine) Tablets, EPZICOM® (abacavir sulfate and lamivudine) Tablets; or emtricitabine–containing products, including ATRIPLA® (efavirenz/emtricitabine/tenofovir disoproxil fumarate) Tablets, EMTRIVA® (emtricitabine) Capsules and Oral Solution, TRUVADA® (emtricitabine/tenofovir disoproxil fumarate) Tablets, or COMPLERA® (emtricitabine/rilpirivine/tenofovir disoproxil fumarate) Tablets.

The complete prescribing information for all agents being considered for use with TRIZIVIR should be consulted before combination therapy with TRIZIVIR is initiated.

6 ADVERSE REACTIONS

The following adverse reactions are discussed in greater detail in other sections of the labeling:

- Serious and sometimes fatal hypersensitivity reactions *[see Boxed Warning, Warnings and Precautions (5.1)]*.
- Hematologic toxicity, including neutropenia and anemia *[see Boxed Warning, Warnings and Precautions (5.2)]*.
- Symptomatic myopathy *[see Boxed Warning, Warnings and Precautions (5.3)]*.
- Lactic acidosis and severe hepatomegaly with steatosis *[see Boxed Warning, Warnings and Precautions (5.4)]*.
- Acute exacerbations of hepatitis B *[see Boxed Warning, Warnings and Precautions (5.5)]*.
- Hepatic decompensation in patients co-infected with HIV-1 and hepatitis C *[see Warnings and Precautions (5.6)]*.
- Exacerbation of anemia in HIV-1/HCV co-infected patients receiving ribavirin and zidovudine *[see Warnings and Precautions (5.6)]*.
- Immune reconstitution syndrome *[see Warnings and Precautions (5.7)]*.
- Fat redistribution *[see Warnings and Precautions (5.8)]*.
- Myocardial infarction *[see Warnings and Precautions (5.9)]*.

6.1 Clinical Trials Experience

Because clinical trials are conducted under widely varying conditions, adverse reaction rates observed in the clinical trials of a drug cannot be directly compared with rates in the clinical trials of another drug and may not reflect the rates observed in clinical practice.

Treatment-emergent clinical adverse reactions (rated by the investigator as moderate or severe) with a frequency greater than or equal to 5% during therapy with abacavir 300 mg twice daily, lamivudine 150 mg twice daily, and zidovudine 300 mg twice daily compared with indinavir 800 mg 3 times daily, lamivudine 150 mg twice daily, and zidovudine 300 mg twice daily from CNA3005 are listed in Table 1.

[See table 1 above]

Five subjects receiving abacavir in CNA3005 experienced worsening of pre-existing depression compared to none in the indinavir arm. The background rates of pre-existing depression were similar in the 2 treatment arms.

Laboratory Abnormalities: Laboratory abnormalities in CNA3005 are listed in Table 2.

[See table 2 above]

Other Adverse Events: In addition to adverse reactions in Tables 1 and 2, other adverse events observed in the expanded access program for abacavir were pancreatitis and increased GGT.

6.2 Postmarketing Experience

In addition to adverse reactions reported from clinical trials, the following reactions have been identified during postmarketing use of abacavir, lamivudine, and/or zidovudine. Because they are reported voluntarily from a population of unknown size, estimates of frequency cannot be made. These reactions have been chosen for inclusion due to a combination of their seriousness, frequency of reporting, or potential causal connection to abacavir, lamivudine and/or zidovudine.

Abacavir:
Cardiovascular: Myocardial infarction.
Skin: Suspected Stevens-Johnson syndrome (SJS) and toxic epidermal necrolysis (TEN) have been reported in patients receiving abacavir primarily in combination with medications known to be associated with SJS and TEN, respectively. Because of the overlap of clinical signs and symptoms between hypersensitivity to abacavir and SJS and TEN, and the possibility of multiple drug sensitivities in some patients, abacavir should be discontinued and not restarted in such cases.

There have also been reports of erythema multiforme with abacavir use.

Abacavir, Lamivudine, and/or Zidovudine:
Body as a Whole: Redistribution/accumulation of body fat *[see Warnings and Precautions (5.8)]*.
Cardiovascular: Cardiomyopathy.
Digestive: Stomatitis.
Endocrine and Metabolic: Gynecomastia, hyperglycemia.
Gastrointestinal: Anorexia and/or decreased appetite, abdominal pain, dyspepsia, oral mucosal pigmentation.
General: Vasculitis, weakness.
Hemic and Lymphatic: Aplastic anemia, anemia (including pure red cell aplasia and severe anemias progressing on therapy), lymphadenopathy, splenomegaly, thrombocytopenia.
Hepatic: Lactic acidosis and hepatic steatosis *[see Warnings and Precautions (5.4)]*, elevated bilirubin, elevated transaminases, posttreatment exacerbation of hepatitis B *[see Warnings and Precautions (5.5)]*.
Hypersensitivity: Sensitization reactions (including anaphylaxis), urticaria.
Musculoskeletal: Arthralgia, myalgia, muscle weakness, CPK elevation, rhabdomyolysis.
Nervous: Dizziness, paresthesia, peripheral neuropathy, seizures.
Psychiatric: Insomnia and other sleep disorders.
Respiratory: Abnormal breath sounds/wheezing.
Skin: Alopecia, erythema multiforme, Stevens-Johnson syndrome.

7 DRUG INTERACTIONS

- No drug interaction trials have been conducted using TRIZIVIR Tablets *[see Clinical Pharmacology (12.3)]*.

7.1 Antiretroviral Agents

Zidovudine: *Stavudine:* Concomitant use of zidovudine with stavudine should be avoided since an antagonistic relationship has been demonstrated in vitro.

Nucleoside Analogues Affecting DNA Replication: Some nucleoside analogues affecting DNA replication, such as ribavirin, antagonize the in vitro antiviral activity of zidovudine against HIV-1; concomitant use of such drugs should be avoided.

7.2 Doxorubicin

Zidovudine: Concomitant use of zidovudine with doxorubicin should be avoided since an antagonistic relationship has been demonstrated in vitro.

7.3 Ethanol

Abacavir: Abacavir has no effect on the pharmacokinetic properties of ethanol. Ethanol decreases the elimination of abacavir causing an increase in overall exposure *[see Clinical Pharmacology (12.3)]*.

7.4 Hematologic/Bone Marrow Suppressive/Cytotoxic Agents

Zidovudine: Coadministration of ganciclovir, interferon alfa, ribavirin, and other bone marrow suppressive or cytotoxic agents may increase the hematologic toxicity of zidovudine.

7.5 Interferon- and Ribavirin-Based Regimens

Lamivudine: Although no evidence of a pharmacokinetic or pharmacodynamic interaction (e.g., loss of HIV-1/HCV virologic suppression) was seen when ribavirin was coadministered with lamivudine in HIV-1/HCV co-infected subjects, hepatic decompensation (some fatal) has occurred in HIV-1/HCV co-infected subjects receiving combination antiretroviral therapy for HIV-1 and interferon alfa with or without ribavirin *[see Warnings and Precautions (5.6), Clinical Pharmacology (12.3)]*.

7.6 Methadone

Abacavir: The addition of methadone has no clinically significant effect on the pharmacokinetic properties of abacavir. In a trial of 11 HIV-1-infected subjects receiving methadone-maintenance therapy with 600 mg of ZIAGEN twice daily (twice the currently recommended dose), oral methadone clearance increased *[see Clinical Pharmacology (12.3)]*. This alteration will not result in a methadone dose modification in the majority of patients; however, an increased methadone dose may be required in a small number of patients.

7.7 Trimethoprim/Sulfamethoxazole (TMP/SMX)

Lamivudine: No change in dose of either drug is recommended *[see Clinical Pharmacology (12.3)]*. There is no information regarding the effect on lamivudine pharmacokinetics of higher doses of TMP/SMX such as those used to treat PCP.

8 USE IN SPECIFIC POPULATIONS

8.1 Pregnancy

TRIZIVIR: Pregnancy Category C. There are no adequate and well-controlled studies of TRIZIVIR in pregnant women. Reproduction studies with abacavir, lamivudine, and zidovudine have been performed in animals (see Abacavir, Lamivudine, and Zidovudine sections below). TRIZIVIR should be used during pregnancy only if the potential benefits outweigh the risks.

Abacavir: Studies in pregnant rats showed that abacavir is transferred to the fetus through the placenta. Fetal malformations (increased incidences of fetal anasarca and skeletal malformations) and developmental toxicity (depressed fetal body weight and reduced crown-rump length) were observed in rats at a dose which produced 35 times the human exposure, based on AUC. Embryonic and fetal toxicities (increased resorptions, decreased fetal body weights) and toxicities to the offspring (increased incidence of stillbirth and lower body weights) occurred at half of the above-mentioned dose in separate fertility studies conducted in rats. In the rabbit, no developmental toxicity and no increases in fetal malformations occurred at doses that produced 8.5 times the human exposure at the recommended dose based on AUC.

Lamivudine: Studies in pregnant rats showed that lamivudine is transferred to the fetus through the placenta. Reproduction studies with orally administered lamivudine have been performed in rats and rabbits at doses producing plasma levels up to approximately 35 times that for the recommended adult HIV dose. No evidence of teratogenicity due to lamivudine was observed. Evidence of early embryolethality was seen in the rabbit at exposure levels similar to those observed in humans, but there was no indication of this effect in the rat at exposure levels up to 35 times those in humans.

Zidovudine: Reproduction studies with orally administered zidovudine in the rat and in the rabbit at doses up to 500 mg/kg/day revealed no evidence of teratogenicity with zidovudine. Zidovudine treatment resulted in embryo/fetal toxicity as evidenced by an increase in the incidence of fetal resorptions in rats given 150 or 450 mg/kg/day and rabbits given 500 mg/kg/day. The doses used in the teratology studies resulted in peak zidovudine plasma concentrations (after one half of the daily dose) in rats 66 to 226 times, and in rabbits 12 to 87 times, mean steady-state peak human plasma concentrations (after one sixth of the daily dose) achieved with the recommended daily dose (100 mg every 4 hours). In an additional teratology study in rats, a dose of 3,000 mg/kg/day (very near the oral median lethal dose in rats of approximately 3,700 mg/kg) caused marked maternal toxicity and an increase in the incidence of fetal malformations. This dose resulted in peak zidovudine plasma concentrations 350 times peak human plasma concentrations. No evidence of teratogenicity was seen in this experiment at doses of 600 mg/kg/day or less. Two rodent carcinogenicity studies were conducted *[see Nonclinical Toxicology (13.1)]*.

Antiretroviral Pregnancy Registry: To monitor maternal-fetal outcomes of pregnant women exposed to TRIZIVIR or other antiretroviral agents, an Antiretroviral Pregnancy Registry has been established. Physicians are encouraged to register patients by calling 1-800-258-4263.

8.3 Nursing Mothers

The Centers for Disease Control and Prevention recommend that HIV-1-infected mothers not breastfeed their infants to avoid risking postnatal transmission of HIV infection.

Abacavir, Lamivudine, and Zidovudine: Lamivudine and zidovudine are excreted in human breast milk; abacavir and lamivudine are secreted into the milk of lactating rats.

Because of both the potential for HIV-1 transmission and the potential for serious adverse reactions in nursing infants, mothers should be instructed not to breastfeed if they are receiving TRIZIVIR.

8.4 Pediatric Use

TRIZIVIR is not intended for use in pediatric patients and is not recommended in adolescents who weigh less than 40 kg because it is a fixed-dose tablet that cannot be adjusted for these patient populations.

Therapy-Experienced Pediatric Trial: A randomized, double-blind trial, CNA3006, compared ZIAGEN plus lamivudine and zidovudine versus lamivudine and zidovudine in pediatric subjects, most of whom were extensively pretreated with nucleoside analogue antiretroviral agents. Subjects in this trial had a limited response to abacavir.

8.5 Geriatric Use

Clinical studies of abacavir, lamivudine, and zidovudine did not include sufficient numbers of subjects aged 65 and over to determine whether they respond differently from younger subjects. In general, dose selection for an elderly patient should be cautious, reflecting the greater frequency of decreased hepatic, renal, or cardiac function, and of concomitant disease or other drug therapy *[see Dosage and Administration (2.3), Use in Specific Populations (8.6)]*.

8.6 Patients With Impaired Renal Function

TRIZIVIR is not recommended for patients with impaired renal function (i.e., creatinine clearance <50 mL/min) because TRIZIVIR is a fixed-dose combination and the dosage of the individual components cannot be adjusted.

8.7 Patients With Impaired Hepatic Function

TRIZIVIR is contraindicated for patients with hepatic impairment because TRIZIVIR is a fixed-dose combination and the dosage of the individual components cannot be adjusted.

10 OVERDOSAGE

Abacavir: There is no known antidote for abacavir. It is not known whether abacavir can be removed by peritoneal dialysis or hemodialysis.

Lamivudine: One case of an adult ingesting 6 grams of lamivudine was reported; there were no clinical signs or symptoms noted and hematologic tests remained normal. It is not known whether lamivudine can be removed by peritoneal dialysis or hemodialysis.

Zidovudine: Acute overdoses of zidovudine have been reported in pediatric patients and adults. These involved exposures up to 50 grams. The only consistent findings were nausea and vomiting. Other reported occurrences included headache, dizziness, drowsiness, lethargy, and confusion. Hematologic changes were transient. All patients recovered. Hemodialysis and peritoneal dialysis appear to have a negligible effect on the removal of zidovudine, while elimination of its primary metabolite, 3′-azido-3′-deoxy-5′-*O*-β-*D*-glucopyranuronosylthymidine (GZDV), is enhanced.

11 DESCRIPTION

TRIZIVIR: TRIZIVIR Tablets contain the following 3 synthetic nucleoside analogues: abacavir sulfate (ZIAGEN), lamivudine (also known as EPIVIR or 3TC), and zidovudine (also known as RETROVIR, azidothymidine, or ZDV) with inhibitory activity against HIV-1.

TRIZIVIR Tablets are for oral administration. Each film-coated tablet contains the active ingredients 300 mg of abacavir as abacavir sulfate, 150 mg of lamivudine, and 300 mg of zidovudine, and the inactive ingredients magnesium stearate, microcrystalline cellulose, and sodium starch glycolate. The tablets are coated with a film (OPADRY® green 03B11434) that is made of FD&C Blue No. 2, hypromellose, polyethylene glycol, titanium dioxide, and yellow iron oxide.

Abacavir Sulfate: The chemical name of abacavir sulfate is *(1S,cis)*-4-[2-amino-6-(cyclopropylamino)-9*H*-purin-9-yl]-2-cyclopentene-1-methanol sulfate (salt) (2:1). Abacavir sulfate is the enantiomer with *1S, 4R* absolute configuration on the cyclopentene ring. It has a molecular formula of $(C_{14}H_{18}N_6O)_2 \cdot H_2SO_4$ and a molecular weight of 670.76 daltons. It has the following structural formula:

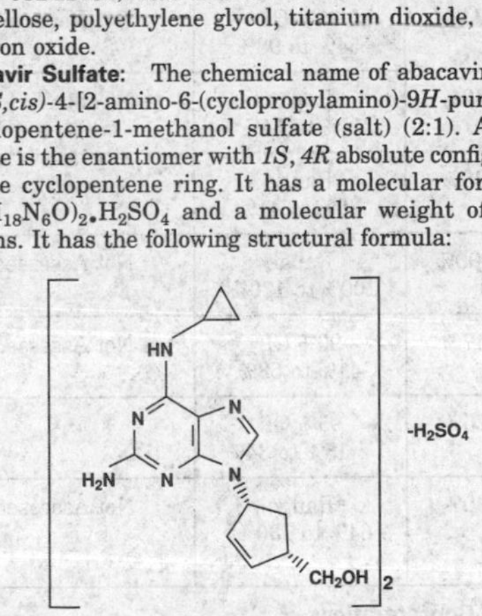

Abacavir sulfate is a white to off-white solid with a solubility of approximately 77 mg/mL in distilled water at 25°C. In vivo, abacavir sulfate dissociates to its free base, abacavir. In this insert, all dosages for ZIAGEN (abacavir sulfate) are expressed in terms of abacavir.

Lamivudine: The chemical name of lamivudine is (2R,cis)-4-amino-1-(2-hydroxymethyl-1,3-oxathiolan-5-yl)-(1H)-pyrimidin-2-one. Lamivudine is the (-)enantiomer of a dideoxy analogue of cytidine. Lamivudine has also been referred to as (-)2′,3′-dideoxy, 3′-thiacytidine. It has a molecular formula of $C_8H_{11}N_3O_3S$ and a molecular weight of 229.3 daltons. It has the following structural formula:

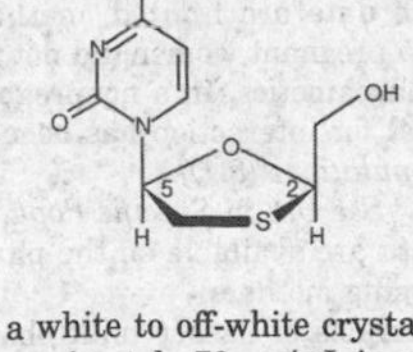

Lamivudine is a white to off-white crystalline solid with a solubility of approximately 70 mg/mL in water at 20°C.

Zidovudine: The chemical name of zidovudine is 3′-azido-3′-deoxythymidine. It has a molecular formula of $C_{10}H_{13}N_5O_4$ and a molecular weight of 267.24 daltons. It has the following structural formula:

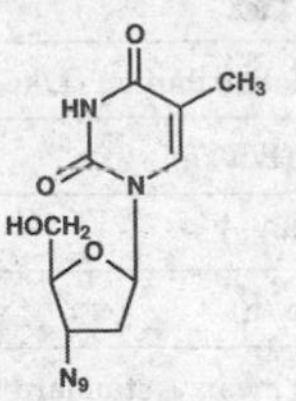

Zidovudine is a white to beige, crystalline solid with a solubility of 20.1 mg/mL in water at 25°C.

12 CLINICAL PHARMACOLOGY

12.1 Mechanism of Action

TRIZIVIR is an antiviral agent *[see Clinical Pharmacology (12.4)]*.

12.3 Pharmacokinetics

Pharmacokinetics in Adults: *TRIZIVIR:* In a single-dose, 3-way crossover bioavailability trial of 1 TRIZIVIR Tablet versus 1 ZIAGEN Tablet (300 mg), 1 EPIVIR Tablet (150 mg), plus 1 RETROVIR Tablet (300 mg) administered simultaneously in healthy subjects (n = 24), there was no difference in the extent of absorption, as measured by the area under the plasma concentration-time curve (AUC) and maximal peak concentration (C_{max}), of all 3 components. One TRIZIVIR Tablet was bioequivalent to 1 ZIAGEN Tablet (300 mg), 1 EPIVIR Tablet (150 mg), plus 1 RETROVIR Tablet (300 mg) following single-dose administration to fasting healthy subjects (n = 24).

Abacavir: Following oral administration, abacavir is rapidly absorbed and extensively distributed. Binding of abacavir to human plasma proteins is approximately 50%. Binding of abacavir to plasma proteins was independent of concentration. Total blood and plasma drug-related radioactivity concentrations are identical, demonstrating that abacavir readily distributes into erythrocytes. The primary routes of elimination of abacavir are metabolism by alcohol dehydrogenase to form the 5′-carboxylic acid and glucuronyl transferase to form the 5′-glucuronide.

Lamivudine: Following oral administration, lamivudine is rapidly absorbed and extensively distributed. Binding to plasma protein is low. Approximately 70% of an intravenous dose of lamivudine is recovered as unchanged drug in the urine. Metabolism of lamivudine is a minor route of elimination. In humans, the only known metabolite is the trans-sulfoxide metabolite (approximately 5% of an oral dose after 12 hours).

Zidovudine: Following oral administration, zidovudine is rapidly absorbed and extensively distributed. Binding to plasma protein is low. Zidovudine is eliminated primarily by hepatic metabolism. The major metabolite of zidovudine is GZDV. GZDV AUC is about 3-fold greater than the zidovudine AUC. Urinary recovery of zidovudine and GZDV accounts for 14% and 74% of the dose following oral administration, respectively. A second metabolite, 3′-amino-3′-deoxythymidine (AMT), has been identified in plasma. The AMT AUC was one-fifth of the zidovudine AUC.

In humans, abacavir, lamivudine, and zidovudine are not significantly metabolized by cytochrome P450 enzymes.

The pharmacokinetic properties of abacavir, lamivudine, and zidovudine in fasting subjects are summarized in Table 3.

[See table 3 at top of next page]

Effect of Food on Absorption of TRIZIVIR: Administration with food in a single-dose bioavailability trial resulted in lower C_{max}, similar to results observed previously for the reference formulations. The average [90% CI] decrease in abacavir, lamivudine, and zidovudine C_{max} was 32% [24% to 38%], 18% [10% to 25%], and 28% [13% to 40%], respectively, when administered with a high-fat meal, compared with administration under fasted conditions. Administration of TRIZIVIR with food did not alter the extent of abacavir, lamivudine, and zidovudine absorption (AUC), as compared with administration under fasted conditions (n = 24) *[see Dosage and Administration (2.1)]*.

Special Populations: *Renal Impairment: TRIZIVIR:* Because lamivudine and zidovudine require dose adjustment in the presence of renal insufficiency, TRIZIVIR is not recommended for use in patients with creatinine clearance <50 mL/min *[see Use in Specific Populations (8.6)]*.

Hepatic Impairment: TRIZIVIR: TRIZIVIR is contraindicated for patients with impaired hepatic function because TRIZIVIR is a fixed-dose combination and the dosage of the individual components cannot be adjusted. Abacavir is contraindicated in patients with moderate to severe hepatic impairment and dose reduction is required in patients with mild hepatic impairment.

Table 3. Pharmacokinetic Parameters[a] for Abacavir, Lamivudine, and Zidovudine in Adults

Parameter	Abacavir		Lamivudine		Zidovudine	
Oral bioavailability (%)	86 ± 25	n = 6	86 ± 16	n = 12	64 ± 10	n = 5
Apparent volume of distribution (L/kg)	0.86 ± 0.15	n = 6	1.3 ± 0.4	n = 20	1.6 ± 0.6	n = 8
Systemic clearance (L/h/kg)	0.80 ± 0.24	n = 6	0.33 ± 0.06	n = 20	1.6 ± 0.6	n = 6
Renal clearance (L/h/kg)	.007 ± .008	n = 6	0.22 ± 0.06	n = 20	0.34 ± 0.05	n = 9
Elimination half-life (h)	1.45 ± 0.32	n = 20	5 to 7[b]		0.5 to 3[b]	

[a] Data presented as mean ± standard deviation except where noted.
[b] Approximate range.

Table 4. Effect of Coadministered Drugs on Abacavir, Lamivudine, and Zidovudine AUC[a] Note: ROUTINE DOSE MODIFICATION OF ABACAVIR, LAMIVUDINE, AND ZIDOVUDINE IS NOT WARRANTED WITH COADMINISTRATION OF THE FOLLOWING DRUGS.

Drugs That May Alter Lamivudine Blood Concentrations

Coadministered Drug and Dose	Lamivudine Dose	n	Lamivudine Concentrations: AUC	Lamivudine Concentrations: Variability	Concentration of Coadministered Drug
Nelfinavir 750 mg q 8 h × 7 to 10 days	single 150 mg	11	↑10%	95% CI: 1% to 20%	↔
Trimethoprim 160 mg/ Sulfamethoxazole 800 mg daily × 5 days	single 300 mg	14	↑43%	90% CI: 32% to 55%	↔

Drugs That May Alter Zidovudine Blood Concentrations

Coadministered Drug and Dose	Zidovudine Dose	n	Zidovudine Concentrations: AUC	Zidovudine Concentrations: Variability	Concentration of Coadministered Drug
Atovaquone 750 mg q 12 h with food	200 mg q 8 h	14	↑31%	Range 23% to 78%[b]	↔
Clarithromycin 500 mg twice daily	100 mg q 4 h × 7 days	4	↓12%	Range ↓34% to ↑14%	Not Reported
Fluconazole 400 mg daily	200 mg q 8 h	12	↑74%	95% CI: 54% to 98%	Not Reported
Methadone 30 to 90 mg daily	200 mg q 4 h	9	↑43%	Range 16% to 64%[b]	↔
Nelfinavir 750 mg q 8 h × 7 to 10 days	single 200 mg	11	↓35%	Range 28% to 41%	↔
Probenecid 500 mg q 6 h × 2 days	2 mg/kg q 8 h × 3 days	3	↑106%	Range 100% to 170%[b]	Not Assessed
Rifampin 600 mg daily × 14 days	200 mg q 8 h × 14 days	8	↓47%	90% CI: 41% to 53%	Not Assessed
Ritonavir 300 mg q 6 h × 4 days	200 mg q 8 h × 4 days	9	↓25%	95% CI: 15% to 34%	↔
Valproic acid 250 mg or 500 mg q 8 h × 4 days	100 mg q 8 h × 4 days	6	↑80%	Range 64% to 130%[b]	Not Assessed

Drugs That May Alter Abacavir Blood Concentrations

Coadministered Drug and Dose	Abacavir Dose	n	Abacavir Concentrations: AUC	Abacavir Concentrations: Variability	Concentration of Coadministered Drug
Ethanol 0.7 g/kg	single 600 mg	24	↑41%	90% CI: 35% to 48%	↔

↑ = Increase; ↓ = Decrease; ↔ = no significant change; AUC = area under the concentration versus time curve; CI = confidence interval.
[a] *See Drug Interactions (7)* for additional information on drug interactions.
[b] Estimated range of percent difference.

Pregnancy: See Use in Specific Populations (8.1).
Abacavir and Lamivudine: No data are available on the pharmacokinetics of abacavir or lamivudine during pregnancy.
Zidovudine: Zidovudine pharmacokinetics have been studied in a Phase 1 trial of 8 women during the last trimester of pregnancy. As pregnancy progressed, there was no evidence of drug accumulation. The pharmacokinetics of zidovudine were similar to that of nonpregnant adults. Consistent with passive transmission of the drug across the placenta, zidovudine concentrations in neonatal plasma at birth were essentially equal to those in maternal plasma at delivery. Although data are limited, methadone maintenance therapy in 5 pregnant women did not appear to alter zidovudine pharmacokinetics. In a nonpregnant adult population, a potential for interaction has been identified *[see Use in Specific Populations (8.1)]*.
Nursing Mothers: See Use in Specific Populations (8.3).
Abacavir: No data are available on the pharmacokinetics of abacavir in nursing mothers.
Lamivudine: Samples of breast milk obtained from 20 mothers receiving lamivudine monotherapy (300 mg twice daily) or combination therapy (150 mg lamivudine twice daily and 300 mg zidovudine twice daily) had measurable concentrations of lamivudine.
Zidovudine: After administration of a single dose of 200 mg zidovudine to 13 HIV–1-infected women, the mean concentration of zidovudine was similar in human milk and serum *[see Use in Specific Populations (8.3)]*.
Pediatric Patients: TRIZIVIR is not intended for use in pediatric patients. TRIZIVIR is not recommended in adolescents who weigh less than 40 kg because it is a fixed-dose tablet that cannot be dose adjusted for this patient population.
Geriatric Patients: The pharmacokinetics of abacavir, lamivudine, and zidovudine have not been studied in subjects over 65 years of age.
Gender:
Abacavir: A population pharmacokinetic analysis in HIV-1-infected male (n = 304) and female (n = 67) subjects showed no gender differences in abacavir AUC normalized for lean body weight.
Lamivudine and Zidovudine: A pharmacokinetic trial in healthy male (n = 12) and female (n = 12) subjects showed no gender differences in zidovudine exposure (AUC_∞) or lamivudine (AUC_∞) normalized for body weight.
Race:
Abacavir: There are no significant differences between blacks and Caucasians in abacavir pharmacokinetics.
Lamivudine: There are no significant racial differences in lamivudine pharmacokinetics.
Zidovudine: The pharmacokinetics of zidovudine with respect to race have not been determined.
Drug Interactions: The drug interactions described below are based on trials conducted with the individual nucleoside analogues.
Cytochrome P450: In humans, abacavir, lamivudine, and zidovudine are not significantly metabolized by cytochrome P450 enzymes; therefore, it is unlikely that clinically significant drug interactions will occur with drugs metabolized through these pathways.
Glucuronyl Transferase: Due to the common metabolic pathways of abacavir and zidovudine via glucuronyl transferase, 15 HIV-1-infected subjects were enrolled in a crossover trial evaluating single doses of abacavir (600 mg), lamivudine (150 mg), and zidovudine (300 mg) alone or in combination. Analysis showed no clinically relevant changes in the pharmacokinetics of abacavir with the addition of lamivudine or zidovudine or the combination of lamivudine and zidovudine. Lamivudine exposure (AUC decreased 15%) and zidovudine exposure (AUC increased 10%) did not show clinically relevant changes with concurrent abacavir.
Lamivudine and Zidovudine: No clinically significant alterations in lamivudine or zidovudine pharmacokinetics were observed in 12 asymptomatic HIV-1-infected adult subjects given a single dose of zidovudine (200 mg) in combination with multiple doses of lamivudine (300 mg q 12 h).
Methadone: In a trial of 11 HIV-1-infected subjects receiving methadone-maintenance therapy (40 mg and 90 mg daily), with 600 mg of ZIAGEN twice daily (twice the currently recommended dose), oral methadone clearance increased 22% (90% CI: 6% to 42%) *[see Drug Interactions (7.6)]*.
Ribavirin: In vitro data indicate ribavirin reduces phosphorylation of lamivudine, stavudine, and zidovudine. However, no pharmacokinetic (e.g., plasma concentrations or intracellular triphosphorylated active metabolite concentrations) or pharmacodynamic (e.g., loss of HIV-1/HCV virologic suppression) interaction was observed when ribavirin and lamivudine (n = 18), stavudine (n = 10), or zidovudine (n = 6) were coadministered as part of a multi-drug regimen to HIV-1/HCV co-infected subjects *[see Warnings and Precautions (5.6)]*.
The effects of other coadministered drugs on abacavir, lamivudine, or zidovudine are provided in Table 4.
[See table 4 above]

12.4 Microbiology

Mechanism of Action: *Abacavir:* Abacavir is a carbocyclic synthetic nucleoside analogue. Abacavir is converted by cellular enzymes to the active metabolite, carbovir triphosphate (CBV-TP), an analogue of deoxyguanosine-5′-triphosphate (dGTP). CBV-TP inhibits the activity of HIV-1 reverse transcriptase (RT) both by competing with the natural substrate dGTP and by its incorporation into viral DNA. The lack of a 3′-OH group in the incorporated nucleotide analogue prevents the formation of the 5′ to 3′ phosphodiester linkage essential for DNA chain elongation, and therefore, the viral DNA growth is terminated. CBV-TP is a weak inhibitor of cellular DNA polymerases α, β, and γ.
Lamivudine: Lamivudine is a synthetic nucleoside analogue. Intracellularly, lamivudine is phosphorylated to its active 5′-triphosphate metabolite, lamivudine triphosphate (3TC-TP). The principal mode of action of 3TC-TP is inhibi-

tion of RT via DNA chain termination after incorporation of the nucleotide analogue. 3TC-TP is a weak inhibitor of cellular DNA polymerases α, β, and γ.

Zidovudine: Zidovudine is a synthetic nucleoside analogue. Intracellularly, zidovudine is phosphorylated to its active 5′-triphosphate metabolite, zidovudine triphosphate (ZDV-TP). The principal mode of action of ZDV-TP is inhibition of RT via DNA chain termination after incorporation of the nucleotide analogue. ZDV-TP is a weak inhibitor of the cellular DNA polymerases α and γ and has been reported to be incorporated into the DNA of cells in culture.

Antiviral Activity: *Abacavir:* The antiviral activity of abacavir against HIV-1 was evaluated against a T-cell tropic laboratory strain HIV-1_{IIIB} in lymphoblastic cell lines, a monocyte/macrophage tropic laboratory strain HIV-1_{BaL} in primary monocytes/macrophages, and clinical isolates in peripheral blood mononuclear cells. The concentration of drug necessary to effect viral replication by 50 percent (EC_{50}) ranged from 3.7 to 5.8 μM (1 μM = 0.28 mcg/mL) and 0.07 to 1.0 μM against HIV-1_{IIIB} and HIV-1_{BaL}, respectively, and was 0.26 ± 0.18 μM against 8 clinical isolates. The EC_{50} values of abacavir against different HIV-1 clades (A-G) ranged from 0.0015 to 1.05 μM, and against HIV-2 isolates, from 0.024 to 0.49 μM. Abacavir had synergistic activity in cell culture in combination with the NRTI zidovudine, the nonnucleoside reverse transcriptase inhibitor (NNRTI) nevirapine, and the protease inhibitor (PI) amprenavir; and additive activity in combination with the NRTIs didanosine, emtricitabine, lamivudine, stavudine, tenofovir, and zalcitabine. Ribavirin (50 μM) had no effect on the anti–HIV-1 activity of abacavir in cell culture.

Lamivudine: The antiviral activity of lamivudine against HIV-1 was assessed in a number of cell lines (including monocytes and fresh human peripheral blood lymphocytes) using standard susceptibility assays. EC_{50} values (50% effective concentrations) were in the range of 0.003 to 15 μM (1 μM = 0.23 mcg/mL). HIV-1 from therapy-naive subjects with no amino acid substitutions associated with resistance gave median EC_{50} values of 0.429 μM (range: 0.200 to 2.007 μM) from Virco (n = 92 baseline samples from COLA40263) and 2.35 μM (1.37 to 3.68 μM) from Monogram Biosciences (n = 135 baseline samples from ESS30009). The EC_{50} values of lamivudine against different HIV-1 clades (A-G) ranged from 0.001 to 0.120 μM, and against HIV-2 isolates from 0.003 to 0.120 μM in peripheral blood mononuclear cells. Ribavirin (50 μM) decreased the anti-HIV-1 activity of lamivudine by 3.5-fold in MT-4 cells.

Zidovudine: The antiviral activity of zidovudine against HIV-1 was assessed in a number of cell lines (including monocytes and fresh human peripheral blood lymphocytes). The EC_{50} and EC_{90} values for zidovudine were 0.01 to 0.49 μM (1 μM = 0.27 mcg/mL) and 0.1 to 9 μM, respectively. HIV-1 from therapy-naive subjects with no amino acid substitutions associated with resistance gave median EC_{50} values of 0.011 μM (range: 0.005 to 0.110 μM) from Virco (n = 92 baseline samples from COLA40263) and 0.0017 μM (0.006 to 0.0340 μM) from Monogram Biosciences (n = 135 baseline samples from ESS30009). The EC_{50} values of zidovudine against different HIV-1 clades (A-G) ranged from 0.00018 to 0.02 μM, and against HIV-2 isolates from 0.00049 to 0.004 μM. In cell culture drug combination studies, zidovudine demonstrates synergistic activity with the NRTIs abacavir, didanosine, lamivudine, and zalcitabine; the NNRTIs delavirdine and nevirapine; and the PIs indinavir, nelfinavir, ritonavir, and saquinavir; and additive activity with interferon alfa. Ribavirin has been found to inhibit the phosphorylation of zidovudine in cell culture.

Resistance: HIV-1 isolates with reduced sensitivity to abacavir, lamivudine, or zidovudine have been selected in cell culture and were also obtained from subjects treated with abacavir, lamivudine, and zidovudine, or the combination of lamivudine and zidovudine.

Abacavir: Genotypic analysis of isolates selected in cell culture and recovered from abacavir-treated subjects demonstrated that amino acid substitutions K65R, L74V, Y115F, and M184V/I in HIV-1 RT contributed to abacavir resistance. In a trial of subjects receiving abacavir once or twice daily in combination with lamivudine and efavirenz once daily, 39% (7/18) of the isolates from subjects who experienced virologic failure in the abacavir once-daily arm had a >2.5-fold decrease in abacavir susceptibility with a median-fold decrease of 1.3 (range: 0.5 to 11) compared with 29% (5/17) of the failure isolates in the twice-daily arm with a median-fold decrease of 0.92 (range: 0.7 to 13).

Lamivudine: Genotypic analysis of isolates selected in cell culture and recovered from lamivudine-treated subjects showed that the resistance was due to a specific amino acid substitution in the HIV-1 RT at codon 184 changing the methionine to either valine or isoleucine (M184V/I).

Zidovudine: Genotypic analyses of the isolates selected in cell culture and recovered from zidovudine-treated subjects showed mutations in the HIV-1 RT gene resulting in 6 amino acid substitutions (M41L, D67N, K70R, L210W, T215Y or F, and K219Q) that confer zidovudine resistance. In general, higher levels of resistance were associated with greater number of mutations. In some subjects harboring zidovudine-resistant virus at baseline, phenotypic sensitivity to zidovudine was restored by 12 weeks of treatment with lamivudine and zidovudine. Combination therapy with lamivudine plus zidovudine delayed the emergence of substitutions conferring resistance to zidovudine.

Cross-Resistance: Cross-resistance has been observed among NRTIs.

Abacavir: Isolates containing abacavir resistance-associated amino acid substitutions, namely, K65R, L74V, Y115F, and M184V, exhibited cross-resistance to didanosine, emtricitabine, lamivudine, tenofovir, and zalcitabine in cell culture and in subjects. The K65R substitution can confer resistance to abacavir, didanosine, emtricitabine, lamivudine, stavudine, tenofovir, and zalcitabine; the L74V substitution can confer resistance to abacavir, didanosine, and zalcitabine; and the M184V substitution can confer resistance to abacavir, didanosine, emtricitabine, lamivudine, and zalcitabine. An increasing number of thymidine analogue mutations (TAMs: M41L, D67N, K70R, L210W, T215Y/F, K219E/R/H/Q/N) is associated with a progressive reduction in abacavir susceptibility.

Lamivudine: Cross-resistance to abacavir, didanosine, tenofovir, and zalcitabine has been observed in some subjects harboring lamivudine-resistant HIV-1 isolates. In some subjects treated with zidovudine plus didanosine or zalcitabine, isolates resistant to multiple drugs, including lamivudine, have emerged (see under Zidovudine below). Cross-resistance between lamivudine and zidovudine has not been reported.

Zidovudine: In a trial of 167 HIV-infected subjects, isolates (n = 2) with multi-drug resistance to didanosine, lamivudine, stavudine, zalcitabine, and zidovudine were recovered from subjects treated for ≥1 year with zidovudine plus didanosine or zidovudine plus zalcitabine. The pattern of resistance-associated amino acid substitutions with such combination therapies was different (A62V, V75I, F77L, F116Y, Q151M) from the pattern with zidovudine monotherapy, with the Q151M substitution being most commonly associated with multi-drug resistance. The substitution at codon 151 in combination with substitutions at 62, 75, 77, and 116 results in a virus with reduced susceptibility to didanosine, lamivudine, stavudine, zalcitabine, and zidovudine. TAMs are selected by zidovudine and confer cross-resistance to abacavir, didanosine, stavudine, tenofovir, and zalcitabine.

13 NONCLINICAL TOXICOLOGY

13.1 Carcinogenesis, Mutagenesis, Impairment of Fertility

Carcinogenicity:

Abacavir: Abacavir was administered orally at 3 dosage levels to separate groups of mice and rats in 2-year carcinogenicity studies. Results showed an increase in the incidence of malignant and non-malignant tumors. Malignant tumors occurred in the preputial gland of males and the clitoral gland of females of both species, and in the liver of female rats. In addition, non-malignant tumors also occurred in the liver and thyroid gland of female rats. These observations were made at systemic exposures in the range of 6 to 32 times the human exposure at the recommended dose. It is not known how predictive the results of rodent carcinogenicity studies may be for humans.

Lamivudine: Long-term carcinogenicity studies with lamivudine in mice and rats showed no evidence of carcinogenic potential at exposures up to 10 times (mice) and 58 times (rats) those observed in humans at the recommended therapeutic dose for HIV-1 infection.

Zidovudine: Zidovudine was administered orally at 3 dosage levels to separate groups of mice and rats (60 females and 60 males in each group). Initial single daily doses were 30, 60, and 120 mg/kg/day in mice and 80, 220, and 600 mg/kg/day in rats. The doses in mice were reduced to 20, 30, and 40 mg/kg/day after day 90 because of treatment-related anemia, whereas in rats only the high dose was reduced to 450 mg/kg per day on day 91 and then to 300 mg/kg/day on day 279.

In mice, 7 late-appearing (after 19 months) vaginal neoplasms (5 nonmetastasizing squamous cell carcinomas, 1 squamous cell papilloma, and 1 squamous polyp) occurred in animals given the highest dose. One late-appearing squamous cell papilloma occurred in the vagina of a middle-dose animal. No vaginal tumors were found at the lowest dose.

In rats, 2 late appearing (after 20 months), nonmetastasizing vaginal squamous cell carcinomas occurred in animals given the highest dose. No vaginal tumors occurred at the low or middle dose in rats. No other drug-related tumors were observed in either sex of either species.

At doses that produced tumors in mice and rats, the estimated drug exposure (as measured by AUC) was approximately 3 times (mouse) and 24 times (rat) the estimated human exposure at the recommended therapeutic dose of 100 mg every 4 hours.

Two transplacental carcinogenicity studies were conducted in mice. One study administered zidovudine at doses of 20 mg/kg/day or 40 mg/kg/day from gestation day 10 through parturition and lactation with dosing continuing in offspring for 24 months postnatally. At these doses, exposures were approximately 3 times the estimated human exposure at the recommended doses. After 24 months at the 40-mg/kg/day dose, an increase in incidence of vaginal tumors was noted with no increase in tumors in the liver or lung or any other organ in either gender. These findings are consistent with results of the standard oral carcinogenicity study in mice, as described earlier. A second study administered zidovudine at maximum tolerated doses of 12.5 mg/day or 25 mg/day (~1,000 mg/kg nonpregnant body weight or ~450 mg/kg of term body weight) to pregnant mice from days 12 through 18 of gestation. There was an increase in the number of tumors in the lung, liver, and female reproductive tracts in the offspring of mice receiving the higher dose level of zidovudine.

It is not known how predictive the results of rodent carcinogenicity studies may be for humans.

Mutagenicity:

Abacavir: Abacavir induced chromosomal aberrations both in the presence and absence of metabolic activation in an in vitro cytogenetic study in human lymphocytes. Abacavir was mutagenic in the absence of metabolic activation, although it was not mutagenic in the presence of metabolic activation in an L5178Y/TK+/- mouse lymphoma assay. Abacavir was clastogenic in males and not clastogenic in females in an in vivo mouse bone marrow micronucleus assay. Abacavir was not mutagenic in bacterial mutagenicity assays in the presence and absence of metabolic activation.

Lamivudine: Lamivudine was mutagenic in an L5178Y/TK+/- mouse lymphoma assay and clastogenic in a cytogenetic assay using cultured human lymphocytes. Lamivudine was negative in a microbial mutagenicity assay, in an in vitro cell transformation assay, in a rat micronucleus test, in a rat bone marrow cytogenetic assay, and in an assay for unscheduled DNA synthesis in rat liver.

Zidovudine: Zidovudine was mutagenic in an L5178Y/TK+/- mouse lymphoma assay, positive in an in vitro cell transformation assay, clastogenic in a cytogenetic assay using cultured human lymphocytes, and positive in mouse and rat micronucleus tests after repeated doses. It was negative in a cytogenetic study in rats given a single dose.

Impairment of Fertility:

Abacavir: Abacavir had no adverse effects on the mating performance or fertility of male and female rats at a dose approximately 8 times the human exposure at the recommended dose based on body surface area comparisons.

Lamivudine: In a study of reproductive performance, lamivudine, administered to male and female rats at doses up to 130 times the usual adult dose based on body surface area considerations, revealed no evidence of impaired fertility judged by conception rates and no effect on the survival, growth, and development to weaning of the offspring.

Zidovudine: Zidovudine, administered to male and female rats at doses up to 7 times the usual adult dose based on body surface area considerations, had no effect on fertility judged by conception rates.

13.2 Animal Toxicology and/or Pharmacology

Myocardial degeneration was found in mice and rats following administration of abacavir for 2 years. The systemic exposures were equivalent to 7 to 24 times the expected systemic exposure in humans. The clinical relevance of this finding has not been determined.

14 CLINICAL STUDIES

The following trial was conducted with the individual components of TRIZIVIR *[see Clinical Pharmacology (12.3)]*.

CNA3005 was a multicenter, double-blind, controlled trial in which 562 HIV-1-infected, therapy-naive adults were randomized to receive either ZIAGEN (300 mg twice daily) plus COMBIVIR (lamivudine 150 mg/zidovudine 300 mg twice daily), or indinavir (800 mg 3 times a day) plus COMBIVIR twice daily. The trial was stratified at randomization by pre-entry plasma HIV-1 RNA 10,000 to 100,000 copies/mL and plasma HIV-1 RNA >100,000 copies/mL. Trial participants were male (87%), Caucasian (73%), black (15%), and Hispanic (9%). At baseline the median age was 36 years, the median pretreatment CD4+ cell count was 360 cells/mm^3, and median plasma HIV-1 RNA was 4.8 log_{10} copies/mL. Proportions of subjects with plasma HIV-1 RNA <400 copies/mL (using Roche AMPLICOR HIV-1 MONITOR® Test) through 48 weeks of treatment are summarized in Table 5.

[See table 5 at top of next page]

Treatment response by plasma HIV-1 RNA strata is shown in Table 6.

[See table 6 at top of next page]

In subjects with baseline viral load >100,000 copies/mL, percentages of subjects with HIV-1 RNA levels <50 copies/mL were 31% in the group receiving abacavir vs. 45% in the group receiving indinavir.

Table 5. Outcomes of Randomized Treatment Through Week 48 (CNA3005)

Outcome	ZIAGEN plus Lamivudine/Zidovudine (n = 262)	Indinavir plus Lamivudine/Zidovudine (n = 265)
Responder[a]	49%	50%
Virologic failure[b]	31%	28%
Discontinued due to adverse reactions	10%	12%
Discontinued due to other reasons[c]	11%	10%

[a] Patients achieved and maintained confirmed HIV-1 RNA <400 copies/mL.
[b] Includes viral rebound and failure to achieve confirmed <400 copies/mL by Week 48.
[c] Includes consent withdrawn, lost to follow-up, protocol violations, those with missing data, clinical progression, and other.

Table 6. Proportions of Responders Through Week 48 By Screening Plasma HIV-1 RNA Levels (CNA3005)

Screening HIV-1 RNA (copies/mL)	ZIAGEN plus Lamivudine/Zidovudine (n = 262)		Indinavir plus Lamivudine/Zidovudine (n = 265)	
	<400 copies/mL	n	<400 copies/mL	N
≥10,000 - ≤100,000	50%	166	48%	165
>100,000	48%	96	52%	100

Through Week 48, an overall mean increase in CD4+ cell count of about 150 cells/mm^3 was observed in both treatment arms. Through Week 48, 9 subjects (3.4%) in the group receiving abacavir sulfate (6 CDC classification C events and 3 deaths) and 3 subjects (1.5%) in the group receiving indinavir (2 CDC classification C events and 1 death) experienced clinical disease progression.

15 REFERENCES

1. Data Collection on Adverse Events of Anti-HIV Drugs (D:A:D) Study Group. *Lancet.* 2008;371 (9622):1417-1426.

16 HOW SUPPLIED/STORAGE AND HANDLING

TRIZIVIR is available as tablets. Each tablet contains 300 mg of abacavir as abacavir sulfate, 150 mg of lamivudine, and 300 mg of zidovudine. The tablets are blue-green capsule-shaped, film-coated, and imprinted with GX LL1 on one side with no markings on the reverse side. They are packaged as follows:

Bottles of 60 Tablets (NDC 49702-217-18).

Store at 25°C (77°F); excursions permitted to 15° to 30°C (59° to 86°F) (see USP Controlled Room Temperature).

17 PATIENT COUNSELING INFORMATION

See FDA-approved patient labeling (Medication Guide)

Hypersensitivity Reaction: Inform patients:

- that a Medication Guide and Warning Card summarizing the symptoms of the abacavir hypersensitivity reaction and other product information will be dispensed by the pharmacist with each new prescription and refill of TRIZIVIR, and encourage the patient to read the Medication Guide and Warning Card every time to obtain any new information that may be present about TRIZIVIR. (The complete text of the Medication Guide is reprinted at the end of this document.)
- to carry the Warning Card with them.
- how to identify a hypersensitivity reaction*[see Warnings and Precautions (5.1), Medication Guide]*.
- that if they develop symptoms consistent with a hypersensitivity reaction they should call their doctor right away to determine if they should stop taking TRIZIVIR.
- that a hypersensitivity reaction can worsen and lead to hospitalization or death if TRIZIVIR is not immediately discontinued.
- to not restart TRIZIVIR or any other abacavir-containing product following a hypersensitivity reaction because more severe symptoms can occur within hours and may include life-threatening hypotension and death.
- that a hypersensitivity reaction is usually reversible if it is detected promptly and TRIZIVIR is stopped right away.
- that if they have interrupted TRIZIVIR for reasons other than symptoms of hypersensitivity (for example, those who have an interruption in drug supply), a serious or fatal hypersensitivity reaction may occur with reintroduction of abacavir.
- to not restart TRIZIVIR or any other abacavir-containing product without medical consultation and that restarting abacavir needs to be undertaken only if medical care can be readily accessed by the patient or others.
- TRIZIVIR should not be coadministered with ATRIPLA, COMBIVIR, COMPLERA, EMTRIVA, EPIVIR, EPIVIR-HBV, EPZICOM, RETROVIR (zidovudine), TRUVADA, or ZIAGEN.

Neutropenia and Anemia: Patients should be informed that the important toxicities associated with zidovudine are neutropenia and/or anemia. They should be told of the extreme importance of having their blood counts followed closely while on therapy, especially for patients with advanced HIV-1 disease *[see Warnings and Precautions (5.2)]*.

Myopathy: Patients should be informed that myopathy and myositis with pathological changes, similar to that produced by HIV-1 disease, have been associated with prolonged use of zidovudine *[see Warnings and Precautions (5.3)]*.

Lactic Acidosis/Hepatomegaly: Inform patients that some HIV medicines, including TRIZIVIR, can cause a rare, but serious condition called lactic acidosis with liver enlargement (hepatomegaly) *[see Warnings and Precautions (5.4)]*.

HIV-1/ HBV Co-Infection: Patients co-infected with HIV-1 and HBV should be informed that deterioration of liver disease has occurred in some cases when treatment with lamivudine was discontinued. Patients should be advised to discuss any changes in regimen with their physician *[see Warnings and Precautions (5.5)]*.

HIV-1/HCV Co-Infection: Patients with HIV-1/HCV co-infection should be informed that hepatic decompensation (some fatal) has occurred in HIV-1/HCV co-infected patients receiving combination antiretroviral therapy for HIV-1 and interferon alfa with or without ribavirin *[see Warnings and Precautions (5.6)]*.

Redistribution/Accumulation of Body Fat: Inform patients that redistribution or accumulation of body fat may occur in patients receiving antiretroviral therapy and that the cause and long-term health effects of these conditions are not known at this time *[see Warnings and Precautions (5.8)]*.

Information About HIV-1 Infection: TRIZIVIR is not a cure for HIV-1 infection and patients may continue to experience illnesses associated with HIV-1 infection, including opportunistic infections. Patients should remain under the care of a physician when using TRIZIVIR.

Patients should be advised to avoid doing things that can spread HIV-1 infection to others.

- **Do not share needles or other injection equipment.**
- **Do not share personal items that can have blood or body fluids on them, like toothbrushes and razor blades.**
- **Do not have any kind of sex without protection.** Always practice safe sex by using a latex or polyurethane condom to lower the chance of sexual contact with semen, vaginal secretions, or blood.
- **Do not breastfeed. Lamivudine and zidovudine are excreted in human breast milk. It is not known if abacavir can be passed to your baby in your breast milk and whether it could harm your baby. Also, mothers with HIV-1 should not breastfeed because HIV-1 can be passed to the baby in the breast milk.**

Patients should be informed to take all HIV medications exactly as prescribed.

COMBIVIR, EPIVIR, EPZICOM, RETROVIR, TRIZIVIR, and ZIAGEN are registered trademarks of ViiV Healthcare. Other brands are trademarks of their respective owners and are not trademarks of ViiV Healthcare. The makers of these brands are not affiliated with and do not endorse ViiV Healthcare or its products.

Manufactured for:
ViiV Healthcare
Research Triangle Park, NC 27709
by:
GlaxoSmithKline
Research Triangle Park, NC 27709
Lamivudine is manufactured under agreement from
Shire Pharmaceuticals Group plc
Basingstoke, UK

TRZ: 7PI

MEDICATION GUIDE

TRIZIVIR® (TRY-zih-veer)

(abacavir sulfate, lamivudine, and zidovudine

Tablets

Read this Medication Guide before you start taking TRIZIVIR and each time you get a refill. There may be new information. This information does not take the place of talking to your healthcare provider about your medical condition or your treatment. Be sure to carry your TRIZIVIR Warning Card with you at all times.

What is the most important information I should know about TRIZIVIR?

1.Serious allergic reaction (hypersensitivity reaction). TRIZIVIR contains abacavir (also contained in ZIAGEN® and EPZICOM®). Patients taking TRIZIVIR may have a serious allergic reaction (hypersensitivity reaction) that can cause death. Your risk of this allergic reaction is much higher if you have a gene variation called HLA-B*5701. Your healthcare provider can determine with a blood test if you have this gene variation.

If you get a symptom from 2 or more of the following groups while taking TRIZIVIR, call your healthcare provider right away to find out if you should stop taking TRIZIVIR.

	Symptom(s)
Group 1	**Fever**
Group 2	**Rash**
Group 3	**Nausea, vomiting, diarrhea, abdominal (stomach area) pain**
Group 4	**Generally ill feeling, extreme tiredness, or achiness**
Group 5	**Shortness of breath, cough, sore throat**

A list of these symptoms is on the Warning Card your pharmacist gives you. **Carry this Warning Card with you at all times.**

If you stop TRIZIVIR because of an allergic reaction, never take TRIZIVIR(abacavir sulfate, lamivudine, and zidovudine)or any other abacavir-containing medicine (ZIAGEN and EPZICOM) again. If you take TRIZIVIR or any other abacavir-containing medicine again after you have had an allergic reaction, **within hours** you may get **life-threatening symptoms** that may include **very low blood pressure or death.** If you stop TRIZIVIR, for any other reason, even for a few days, and you are not allergic to TRIZIVIR, talk with your healthcare provider before taking it again. Taking TRIZIVIR again can cause a serious allergic or life-threatening reaction, even if you never had an allergic reaction to it before.

If your healthcare provider tells you that you can take TRIZIVIR again, start taking it when you are around medical help or people who can call a healthcare provider if you need one.

2. Blood problems. RETROVIR®, one of the medicines in TRIZIVIR, can cause serious blood cell problems. These include reduced numbers of white blood cells (neutropenia) and extremely reduced numbers of red blood cells (anemia). These blood cell problems are especially likely to happen in patients with advanced human immunodeficiency virus (HIV) disease or AIDS. Your doctor should be checking your blood cell counts regularly while you are taking TRIZIVIR. This is especially important if you have advanced HIV or AIDS. This is to make sure that any blood cell problems are found quickly.

3. Lactic Acidosis (buildup of acid in the blood). Some human immunodeficiency virus (HIV) medicines, including TRIZIVIR, can cause a rare but serious condition called lactic acidosis. Lactic acidosis is a serious medical emergency that can cause death and must be treated in the hospital. Call your healthcare provider right away if you get any of the following signs or symptoms of lactic acidosis:

- you feel very weak or tired
- you have unusual (not normal) muscle pain
- you have trouble breathing
- you have stomach pain with nausea and vomiting
- you feel cold, especially in your arms and legs
- you feel dizzy or light-headed
- you have a fast or irregular heartbeat

4. Serious liver problems. Some people who have taken medicines like TRIZIVIR have developed serious liver problems called hepatotoxicity, with liver enlargement (hepatomegaly) and fat in the liver (steatosis). Hepatomegaly with steatosis is a serious medical emergency that can cause death.

Call your healthcare provider right away if you get any of the following signs or symptoms of liver problems:

- your skin or the white part of your eyes turns yellow (jaundice)
- your urine turns dark
- your bowel movements (stools) turn light in color
- you don't feel like eating food for several days or longer
- you feel sick to your stomach (nausea)
- you have lower stomach area (abdominal) pain

You may be more likely to get lactic acidosis or serious liver problems if you are female, very overweight, or have been taking nucleoside analogue medicines for a long time.

5. Use with interferon and ribavirin-based regimens. Worsening of liver disease (sometimes resulting in death) has occurred in patients infected with both HIV and hepatitis C virus who are taking anti-HIV medicines and are also being treated for hepatitis C with interferon with or without ribavirin. If you are taking TRIZIVIR as well as interferon with or without ribavirin and you experience side effects, be sure to tell your healthcare provider.

6. If you have HIV and hepatitis B virus infection, your hepatitis B virus infection may get worse if you stop taking TRIZIVIR.

- Take TRIZIVIR exactly as prescribed.
- Do not run out of TRIZIVIR.
- Do not stop TRIZIVIR without talking to your healthcare provider.

Your healthcare provider should monitor your health and do regular blood tests to check your liver if you stop taking TRIZIVIR.

7. Muscle weakness (myopathy). RETROVIR, one of the medicines in TRIZIVIR, can cause muscle weakness. This can be a serious problem.

What is TRIZIVIR?

TRIZIVIR is a prescription medicine used to treat HIV infection. TRIZIVIR contains 3 medicines: abacavir (ZIAGEN), lamivudine or 3TC (EPIVIR®), and zidovudine, AZT, or ZDV (RETROVIR). All 3 of these medicines are called nucleoside analogue reverse transcriptase inhibitors (NRTIs). When used together, they help lower the amount of HIV in your blood.

- **TRIZIVIR does not cure HIV infection or AIDS.**
- It is not known if TRIZIVIR will help you live longer or have fewer of the medical problems that people get with HIV or AIDS.
- It is very important that you see your healthcare provider regularly while you are taking TRIZIVIR.

Who should not take TRIZIVIR?

Do not take TRIZIVIR if you:

- **are allergic to abacavir or any of the ingredients in TRIZIVIR. See the end of this Medication Guide for a complete list of ingredients in TRIZIVIR.**
- **have certain liver problems.**
- **are an adolescent who weighs less than 90 pounds.**

What should I tell my healthcare provider before taking TRIZIVIR?

Before you take TRIZIVIR, tell your healthcare provider if you:

- **have been tested and know whether or not you have a particular gene variation called HLA-B*5701.**
- **have hepatitis B virus infection or have other liver problems.**
- **have kidney problems.**
- **have low blood cell counts (bone marrow problem).** Ask your doctor if you are not sure.
- **have heart problems, smoke, or have diseases that increase your risk of heart disease such as high blood pressure, high cholesterol, or diabetes.**
- **are pregnant or plan to become pregnant.** It is not known if TRIZIVIR will harm your unborn baby. Talk to your healthcare provider if you are pregnant or plan to become pregnant.

Pregnancy Registry. If you take TRIZIVIR while you are pregnant, talk to your healthcare provider about how you can take part in the Pregnancy Registry for TRIZIVIR. The purpose of the pregnancy registry is to collect information about the health of you and your baby.

- **are breastfeeding or plan to breastfeed. Do not breastfeed.** Lamivudine and zidovudine are excreted in human breast milk. We do not know if abacavir can be passed to your baby in your breast milk and whether it could harm your baby. Also, mothers with HIV-1 should not breastfeed because HIV-1 can be passed to the baby in the breast milk.

Tell your healthcare provider about all the medicines you take, including prescription and nonprescription medicines, vitamins, and herbal supplements.

Especially tell your healthcare provider if you take:

- alcohol
- medicines used to treat hepatitis viruses such as interferon or ribavirin
- methadone
- BACTRIM®, SEPTRA® (trimethoprim [TMP/sulfamethoxazole SMX])
- CYTOVENE®, DHPG (ganciclovir)
- interferon-alfa
- ADRIAMYCIN® (doxorubicin)
- COPEGUS®, REBETOL®, VIRAZOLE® (ribavirin)
- any bone marrow suppressive medicines or cytotoxic medicines. Ask your doctor if you are not sure.
- ATRIPLA® (efavirenz/emtricitabine/tenofovir disoproxil fumarate)
- COMBIVIR® (lamivudine and zidovudine)
- COMPLERA® (emtricitabine/rilpivirine/tenofovir disoproxil fumarate)
- EMTRIVA® (emtricitabine)
- EPIVIR or EPIVIR-HBV® (lamivudine)
- EPZICOM (abacavir sulfate and lamivudine)
- RETROVIR (zidovudine)
- TRUVADA® (emtricitabine/tenofovir disoproxil fumarate)
- ZERIT® (stavudine)
- ZIAGEN (abacavir sulfate)

Ask your healthcare provider if you are not sure if you take one of the medicines listed above.

TRIZIVIR may affect the way other medicines work, and other medicines may affect how TRIZIVIR works.

Know the medicines you take. Keep a list of your medicines with you to show to your healthcare provider and pharmacist when you get a new medicine.

How should I take TRIZIVIR?

- **Take TRIZIVIR exactly as your healthcare provider tells you to take it.**
- TRIZIVIR may be taken with or without food.
- Do not skip doses.
- **Do not let your TRIZIVIR run out.**

If you stop your anti-HIV medicines, even for a short time, the amount of virus in your blood may increase and the virus may become harder to treat.If you take too much TRIZIVIR, call your healthcare provider or poison control center or go to the nearest hospital emergency room right away.

What are the possible side effects of TRIZIVIR?

TRIZIVIR can cause serious side effects including allergic reactions, lactic acidosis, and liver problems. See "What is the most important information I should know about TRIZIVIR?"

- **Blood problems.**
- **Muscle weakness.**
- **Changes in immune system (Immune Reconstitution Syndrome).** Your immune system may get stronger and begin to fight infections that have been hidden in your body for a long time. Tell your healthcare provider if you start having new or worse symptoms of infection after you start taking TRIZIVIR.
- **Changes in body fat (fat redistribution).** Changes in body fat (lipoatrophy or lipodystrophy) can happen in some people taking antiretroviral medicines including TRIZIVIR. These changes may include:
- more fat in or around your trunk, upper back and neck (buffalo hump), breast or chest
- loss of fat in your legs, arms, or face
- **Heart attack (myocardial infarction).** Some HIV medicines including TRIZIVIR may increase your risk of heart attack.

The most common side effects of TRIZIVIR include:

- nausea
- headache
- weakness or tiredness
- vomiting
- diarrhea
- fever and/or chills
- depression
- muscle and joint pain
- skin rashes
- ear, nose, throat infections
- cold symptoms
- nervousness

Tell your healthcare provider if you have any side effect that bothers you or that does not go away.

These are not all the possible side effects of TRIZIVIR. For more information, ask your healthcare provider or pharmacist.

Call your doctor for medical advice about side effects. You may report side effects to FDA at 1-800-FDA-1088.

How should I store TRIZIVIR?

- Store TRIZIVIR at 59°F to 86°F (15°C to 30°C).
- **Keep TRIZIVIR and all medicines out of the reach of children.**

General information for safe and effective use of TRIZIVIR. Avoid doing things that can spread HIV-1 infection to others.

- **Do not share needles or other injection equipment.**
- **Do not share personal items that can have blood or body fluids on them, like toothbrushes and razor blades.**
- **Do not have any kind of sex without protection.** Always practice safe sex by using a latex or polyurethane condom to lower the chance of sexual contact with semen, vaginal secretions, or blood.

Medicines are sometimes prescribed for purposes other than those listed in a Medication Guide. Do not use TRIZIVIR for a condition for which it was not prescribed. Do not give TRIZIVIR to other people, even if they have the same symptoms that you have. It may harm them.

This Medication Guide summarizes the most important information about TRIZIVIR. If you would like more information, talk with your healthcare provider. You can ask your healthcare provider or pharmacist for the information about TRIZIVIR that is written for healthcare professionals.

For more information go to www.TRIZIVIR.com or call 1-877-844-8872.

What are the ingredients in TRIZIVIR?

Active ingredients: abacavir sulfate, lamivudine, and zidovudine

Inactive ingredients: magnesium stearate, microcrystalline cellulose, sodium starch glycolate, and OPADRY® green 03B11434, a film coating made of FD&C Blue No. 2, hypromellose, polyethylene glycol, titanium dioxide, and yellow iron oxide.

This Medication Guide has been approved by the US Food and Drug Administration.

COMBIVIR, EPIVIR, EPZICOM, RETROVIR, TRIZIVIR, and ZIAGEN are registered trademarks of ViiV Healthcare. The brands listed are trademarks of their respective owners and are not trademarks of ViiV Healthcare. The makers of these brands are not affiliated with and do not endorse ViiV Healthcare or its products.

Manufactured for:
ViiV Healthcare
Research Triangle Park, NC 27709
by:
GlaxoSmithKline
Research Triangle Park, NC 27709
Lamivudine is manufactured under agreement from
Shire Pharmaceuticals Group plc
Basingstoke, UK

May 2013
TRZ:7MG

ZIAGEN ℞

[*zī´ ə-jin*]
(abacavir sulfate)
Tablets, for oral use

ZIAGEN

(abacavir sulfate)
Oral Solution

HIGHLIGHTS OF PRESCRIBING INFORMATION

These highlights do not include all the information needed to use ZIAGEN safely and effectively. See full prescribing information for ZIAGEN.

ZIAGEN (abacavir sulfate) Tablets, for oral use
ZIAGEN (abacavir sulfate) Oral Solution
Initial U.S. Approval: 1998

WARNING: HYPERSENSITIVITY REACTIONS, LACTIC ACIDOSIS, AND SEVERE HEPATOMEGALY

See full prescribing information for complete boxed warning.

- **Serious and sometimes fatal hypersensitivity reactions have been associated with ZIAGEN (abacavir sulfate). (5.1)**
- **Hypersensitivity to abacavir is a multi-organ clinical syndrome. (5.1)**
- **Patients who carry the HLA-B*5701 allele are at high risk for experiencing a hypersensitivity reaction to abacavir. (5.1)**
- **Discontinue ZIAGEN as soon as a hypersensitivity reaction is suspected. Regardless of HLA-B*5701 status, permanently discontinue ZIAGEN if hypersensitivity cannot be ruled out, even when other diagnoses are possible. (5.1)**
- **Following a hypersensitivity reaction to abacavir, NEVER restart ZIAGEN or any other abacavir-containing product. (5.1)**
- **Lactic acidosis and severe hepatomegaly with steatosis, including fatal cases, have been reported with the use of nucleoside analogues. (5.2)**

RECENT MAJOR CHANGES

Dosage and Administration (2) 05/2012
Warnings and Precautions, Hypersensitivity Reaction (5.1) 05/2012

Warnings and Precautions, Immune Reconstitution Syndrome (5.3) 11/2011

INDICATIONS AND USAGE

ZIAGEN, a nucleoside analogue, is indicated in combination with other antiretroviral agents for the treatment of HIV-1 infection. (1)

DOSAGE AND ADMINISTRATION

- A medication guide and warning card should be dispensed with each new prescription and refill. (2)
- Adults: 600 mg daily, administered as either 300 mg twice daily or 600 mg once daily. (2.1)
- Pediatric Patients Aged 3 Months and Older: Dose should be calculated on body weight (kg) and should not exceed 300 mg twice daily. (2.2)
- Patients With Hepatic Impairment: Mild hepatic impairment – 200 mg twice daily; moderate/severe hepatic impairment – contraindicated. (2.3)

DOSAGE FORMS AND STRENGTHS

Tablets: 300 mg, scored; Oral Solution: 20 mg/mL (3)

CONTRAINDICATIONS

- Previously demonstrated hypersensitivity to abacavir. (4, 5.1)
- Moderate or severe hepatic impairment. (4)

WARNINGS AND PRECAUTIONS

- Hypersensitivity: Serious and sometimes fatal hypersensitivity reactions have been associated with ZIAGEN and other abacavir-containing products. Read full prescribing information section 5.1 before prescribing ZIAGEN. (5.1)
- Lactic acidosis and severe hepatomegaly with steatosis have been reported with the use of nucleoside analogues. (5.2)
- Immune reconstitution syndrome (5.3) and redistribution/accumulation of body fat have been reported in patients treated with combination antiretroviral therapy. (5.4)

ADVERSE REACTIONS

- **The most commonly reported adverse reactions of at least moderate intensity (incidence ≥10%) in adult HIV-1 clinical trials were nausea, headache, malaise and fatigue, nausea and vomiting, and dreams/sleep disorders. (6.1)**
- **The most commonly reported adverse reactions of at least moderate intensity (incidence ≥5%) in pediatric HIV-1 clinical trials were fever and/or chills, nausea and vomiting, skin rashes, and ear/nose/throat infections. (6.1)**

To report SUSPECTED ADVERSE REACTIONS, contact ViiV Healthcare at 1-877-844-8872 or FDA at 1-800-FDA-1088 or .

DRUG INTERACTIONS

- Ethanol: Decreases elimination of abacavir. (7.1)
- Methadone: An increased methadone dose may be required in a small number of patients. (7.2)

See 17 for PATIENT COUNSELING INFORMATION and Medication Guide

Revised: 06/2013

FULL PRESCRIBING INFORMATION: CONTENTS*

*** Sections or subsections omitted from the full prescribing information are not listed**

FULL PRESCRIBING INFORMATION

WARNING: RISK OF HYPERSENSITIVITY REACTIONS, LACTIC ACIDOSIS, AND SEVERE HEPATOMEGALY

Hypersensitivity Reactions: Serious and sometimes fatal hypersensitivity reactions have been associated with ZIAGEN® (abacavir sulfate).

Hypersensitivity to abacavir is a multi-organ clinical syndrome usually characterized by a sign or symptom in 2 or more of the following groups: (1) fever, (2) rash, (3) gastrointestinal (including nausea, vomiting, diarrhea, or abdominal pain), (4) constitutional (including generalized malaise, fatigue, or achiness), and (5) respiratory (including dyspnea, cough, or pharyngitis). Discontinue ZIAGEN as soon as a hypersensitivity reaction is suspected.

Patients who carry the HLA-B*5701 allele are at high risk for experiencing a hypersensitivity reaction to abacavir. Prior to initiating therapy with abacavir, screening for the HLA-B*5701 allele is recommended; this approach has been found to decrease the risk of hypersensitivity reaction. Screening is also recommended prior to reinitiation of abacavir in patients of unknown HLA-B*5701 status who have previously tolerated abacavir. HLA-B*5701-negative patients may develop a suspected hypersensitivity reaction to abacavir; however, this occurs significantly less frequently than in HLA-B*5701-positive patients.

Regardless of HLA-B*5701 status, permanently discontinue ZIAGEN if hypersensitivity cannot be ruled out, even when other diagnoses are possible.

Following a hypersensitivity reaction to abacavir, NEVER restart ZIAGEN or any other abacavir-containing product because more severe symptoms can occur within hours and may include life-threatening hypotension and death.

Reintroduction of ZIAGEN or any other abacavir-containing product, even in patients who have no identified history or unrecognized symptoms of hypersensitivity to abacavir therapy, can result in serious or fatal hypersensitivity reactions. Such reactions can occur within hours *[see Warnings and Precautions (5.1)]*.

Lactic Acidosis and Severe Hepatomegaly: Lactic acidosis and severe hepatomegaly with steatosis, including fatal cases, have been reported with the use of nucleoside analogues alone or in combination, including ZIAGEN and other antiretrovirals *[see Warnings and Precautions (5.2)]*.

1 INDICATIONS AND USAGE

ZIAGEN Tablets and Oral Solution, in combination with other antiretroviral agents, are indicated for the treatment of human immunodeficiency virus (HIV-1) infection.

Additional important information on the use of ZIAGEN for treatment of HIV-1 infection:

ZIAGEN is one of multiple products containing abacavir. Before starting ZIAGEN, review medical history for prior exposure to any abacavir-containing product in order to avoid reintroduction in a patient with a history of hypersensitivity to abacavir *[see Warnings and Precautions (5.1), Adverse Reactions (6)]*.

2 DOSAGE AND ADMINISTRATION

- A Medication Guide and Warning Card that provide information about recognition of hypersensitivity reactions should be dispensed with each new prescription and refill.
- ZIAGEN may be taken with or without food.

2.1 Adult Patients

The recommended oral dose of ZIAGEN for adults is 600 mg daily, administered as either 300 mg twice daily or 600 mg once daily, in combination with other antiretroviral agents.

2.2 Pediatric Patients

The recommended oral dose of ZIAGEN Oral Solution in HIV-1-infected pediatric patients aged 3 months and older is 8 mg/kg twice daily (up to a maximum of 300 mg twice daily) in combination with other antiretroviral agents.

ZIAGEN is also available as a scored tablet for HIV-1-infected pediatric patients weighing greater than or equal to 14 kg for whom a solid dosage form is appropriate. Before prescribing ZIAGEN Tablets, children should be assessed for the ability to swallow tablets. If a child is unable to reliably swallow ZIAGEN Tablets, the oral solution formulation should be prescribed. The recommended oral dosage of ZIAGEN Tablets for HIV-1-infected pediatric patients is presented in Table 1.

Table 1. Dosing Recommendations for ZIAGEN Tablets in Pediatric Patients

Weight (kg)	Dosage Regimen Using Scored Tablet		Total Daily Dose
	AM Dose	PM Dose	
14 to 21	½ tablet (150 mg)	½ tablet (150 mg)	300 mg
>21 to <30	½ tablet (150 mg)	1 tablet (300 mg)	450 mg
≥30	1 tablet (300 mg)	1 tablet (300 mg)	600 mg

2.3 Patients With Hepatic Impairment

The recommended dose of ZIAGEN in patients with mild hepatic impairment (Child-Pugh score 5 to 6) is 200 mg twice daily. To enable dose reduction, ZIAGEN Oral Solution (10 mL twice daily) should be used for the treatment of these patients. The safety, efficacy, and pharmacokinetic properties of abacavir have not been established in patients with moderate to severe hepatic impairment; therefore, ZIAGEN is contraindicated in these patients.

3 DOSAGE FORMS AND STRENGTHS

ZIAGEN Tablets contain 300 mg of abacavir as abacavir sulfate. The tablets are yellow, biconvex, scored, capsule-shaped, film-coated, and imprinted with "GX 623" on both sides.

ZIAGEN Oral Solution contains 20 mg/mL of abacavir as abacavir sulfate. The solution is a clear to opalescent, yellowish, strawberry-banana-flavored liquid.

4 CONTRAINDICATIONS

ZIAGEN is contraindicated in patients with:

- previously demonstrated hypersensitivity to abacavir or any other component of the products. NEVER restart ZIAGEN or any other abacavir-containing product following a hypersensitivity reaction to abacavir, regardless of HLA-B*5701 status *[see Warnings and Precautions (5.1), Adverse Reactions (6)]*.
- moderate or severe hepatic impairment *[see Dosage and Administration (2.3)]*.

5 WARNINGS AND PRECAUTIONS

5.1 Hypersensitivity Reaction

Serious and sometimes fatal hypersensitivity reactions have been associated with ZIAGEN and other abacavir-containing products. Patients who carry the HLA-B*5701 allele are at high risk for experiencing a hypersensitivity reaction to abacavir. Prior to initiating therapy with abacavir, screening for the HLA-B*5701 allele is recommended; this approach has been found to decrease the risk of a hypersensitivity reaction. Screening is also recommended prior to reinitiation of abacavir in patients of unknown HLA-B*5701 status who have previously tolerated abacavir. For HLA-B*5701-positive patients, treatment with an abacavir-containing regimen is not recommended and should be considered only with close medical supervision and under exceptional circumstances when the potential benefit outweighs the risk.

HLA-B*5701-negative patients may develop a hypersensitivity reaction to abacavir; however, this occurs significantly less frequently than in HLA-B*5701-positive patients. Regardless of HLA-B*5701 status, permanently discontinue ZIAGEN if hypersensitivity cannot be ruled out, even when other diagnoses are possible.

Important information on signs and symptoms of hypersensitivity, as well as clinical management, is presented below.

Signs and Symptoms of Hypersensitivity: Hypersensitivity to abacavir is a multi-organ clinical syndrome usually characterized by a sign or symptom in 2 or more of the following groups.

Group 1: Fever
Group 2: Rash
Group 3: Gastrointestinal (including nausea, vomiting, diarrhea, or abdominal pain)
Group 4: Constitutional (including generalized malaise, fatigue, or achiness)
Group 5: Respiratory (including dyspnea, cough, or pharyngitis).

Hypersensitivity to abacavir following the presentation of a single sign or symptom has been reported infrequently.

Hypersensitivity to abacavir was reported in approximately 8% of 2,670 subjects (n = 206) in 9 clinical trials (range: 2% to 9%) with enrollment from November 1999 to February 2002. Data on time to onset and symptoms of suspected hypersensitivity were collected on a detailed data collection module. The frequencies of symptoms are shown in Figure 1. Symptoms usually appeared within the first 6 weeks of treatment with abacavir, although the reaction may occur at any time during therapy. Median time to onset was 9 days; 89% appeared within the first 6 weeks; 95% of subjects reported symptoms from 2 or more of the 5 groups listed above.

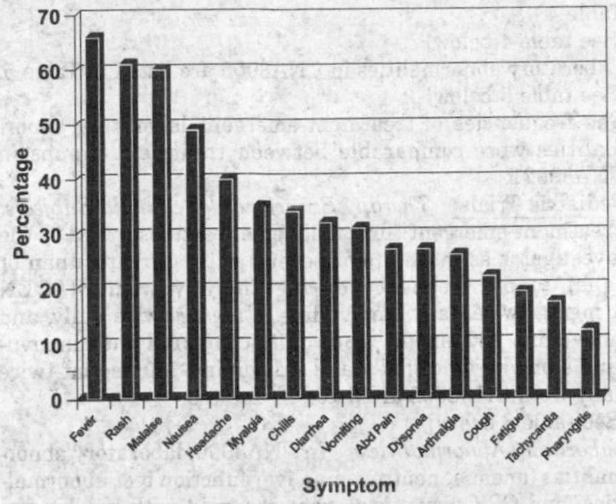

Figure 1. Hypersensitivity-Related Symptoms Reported With ≥10% Frequency in Clinical Trials (n = 206 Subjects)

Other less common signs and symptoms of hypersensitivity include lethargy, myolysis, edema, abnormal chest x-ray findings (predominantly infiltrates, which can be localized), and paresthesia. Anaphylaxis, liver failure, renal failure, hypotension, adult respiratory distress syndrome, respiratory failure, and death have occurred in association with hypersensitivity reactions. In one trial, 4 subjects (11%) receiving ZIAGEN 600 mg once daily experienced hypotension with a hypersensitivity reaction compared with 0 subjects receiving ZIAGEN 300 mg twice daily.

Physical findings associated with hypersensitivity to abacavir in some patients include lymphadenopathy, mucous membrane lesions (conjunctivitis and mouth ulcerations), and rash. The rash usually appears maculopapular or urticarial, but may be variable in appearance. There have been reports of erythema multiforme. Hypersensitivity reactions have occurred without rash.

Laboratory abnormalities associated with hypersensitivity to abacavir in some patients include elevated liver function tests, elevated creatine phosphokinase, elevated creatinine, and lymphopenia.

Clinical Management of Hypersensitivity: Discontinue ZIAGEN as soon as a hypersensitivity reaction is suspected. To minimize the risk of a life-threatening hypersensitivity reaction, permanently discontinue ZIAGEN if hypersensitivity cannot be ruled out, even when other diagnoses are possible (e.g., acute onset respiratory diseases such as pneumonia, bronchitis, pharyngitis, or influenza; gastroenteritis; or reactions to other medications).

Following a hypersensitivity reaction to abacavir, NEVER restart ZIAGEN or any other abacavir-containing product because more severe symptoms can occur within hours and may include life-threatening hypotension and death.

When therapy with ZIAGEN has been discontinued for reasons other than symptoms of a hypersensitivity reaction, and if reinitiation of ZIAGEN or any other abacavir-containing product is under consideration, carefully evaluate the reason for discontinuation of ZIAGEN to ensure that the patient did not have symptoms of a hypersensitivity reaction. If the patient is of unknown HLA-B*5701 status, screening for the allele is recommended prior to reinitiation of ZIAGEN.

If hypersensitivity cannot be ruled out, DO NOT reintroduce ZIAGEN or any other abacavir-containing product. Even in the absence of the HLA-B*5701 allele, it is important to permanently discontinue abacavir and not rechallenge with abacavir if a hypersensitivity reaction cannot be ruled out on clinical grounds, due to the potential for a severe or even fatal reaction.

If symptoms consistent with hypersensitivity are not identified, reintroduction can be undertaken with continued monitoring for symptoms of a hypersensitivity reaction. Make patients aware that a hypersensitivity reaction can occur with reintroduction of ZIAGEN or any other abacavir-containing product and that reintroduction of ZIAGEN or any other abacavir-containing product needs to be undertaken only if medical care can be readily accessed by the patient or others.

Table 2. Treatment-Emergent (All Causality) Adverse Reactions of at Least Moderate Intensity (Grades 2-4, ≥5% Frequency) in Therapy-Naive Adults (CNA30024[a]) Through 48 Weeks of Treatment

Adverse Reaction	ZIAGEN plus Lamivudine plus Efavirenz (n = 324)	Zidovudine plus Lamivudine plus Efavirenz (n = 325)
Dreams/sleep disorders	10%	10%
Drug hypersensitivity	9%	<1%[b]
Headaches/migraine	7%	11%
Nausea	7%	11%
Fatigue/malaise	7%	10%
Diarrhea	7%	6%
Rashes	6%	12%
Abdominal pain/gastritis/gastrointestinal signs and symptoms	6%	8%
Depressive disorders	6%	6%
Dizziness	6%	6%
Musculoskeletal pain	6%	5%
Bronchitis	4%	5%
Vomiting	2%	9%

[a] This trial used double-blind ascertainment of suspected hypersensitivity reactions. During the blinded portion of the trial, suspected hypersensitivity to abacavir was reported by investigators in 9% of 324 subjects in the abacavir group and 3% of 325 subjects in the zidovudine group.

[b] Ten (3%) cases of suspected drug hypersensitivity were reclassified as not being due to abacavir following unblinding.

Risk Factor: *HLA-B*5701 Allele:* Trials have shown that carriage of the HLA-B*5701 allele is associated with a significantly increased risk of a hypersensitivity reaction to abacavir.

CNA106030 (PREDICT-1), a randomized, double-blind trial, evaluated the clinical utility of prospective HLA-B*5701 screening on the incidence of abacavir hypersensitivity reaction in abacavir-naive HIV-1-infected adults (n = 1,650). In this trial, use of pre-therapy screening for the HLA-B*5701 allele and exclusion of subjects with this allele reduced the incidence of clinically suspected abacavir hypersensitivity reactions from 7.8% (66/847) to 3.4% (27/803). Based on this trial, it is estimated that 61% of patients with the HLA-B*5701 allele will develop a clinically suspected hypersensitivity reaction during the course of abacavir treatment compared with 4% of patients who do not have the HLA-B*5701 allele.

Screening for carriage of the HLA -B*5701 allele is recommended prior to initiating treatment with abacavir. Screening is also recommended prior to reinitiation of abacavir in patients of unknown HLA-B*5701 status who have previously tolerated abacavir. For HLA-B*5701-positive patients, initiating or reinitiating treatment with an abacavir-containing regimen is not recommended and should be considered only with close medical supervision and under exceptional circumstances where potential benefit outweighs the risk.

Skin patch testing is used as a research tool and should not be used to aid in the clinical diagnosis of abacavir hypersensitivity.

In any patient treated with abacavir, the clinical diagnosis of hypersensitivity reaction must remain the basis of clinical decision-making. Even in the absence of the HLA B*5701 allele, it is important to permanently discontinue abacavir and not rechallenge with abacavir if a hypersensitivity reaction cannot be ruled out on clinical grounds, due to the potential for a severe or even fatal reaction.

5.2 Lactic Acidosis/Severe Hepatomegaly With Steatosis

Lactic acidosis and severe hepatomegaly with steatosis, including fatal cases, have been reported with the use of nucleoside analogues alone or in combination, including abacavir and other antiretrovirals. A majority of these cases have been in women. Obesity and prolonged nucleoside exposure may be risk factors. Particular caution should be exercised when administering ZIAGEN to any patient with known risk factors for liver disease; however, cases have also been reported in patients with no known risk factors. Treatment with ZIAGEN should be suspended in any patient who develops clinical or laboratory findings suggestive of lactic acidosis or pronounced hepatotoxicity (which may include hepatomegaly and steatosis even in the absence of marked transaminase elevations).

5.3 Immune Reconstitution Syndrome

Immune reconstitution syndrome has been reported in patients treated with combination antiretroviral therapy, including ZIAGEN. During the initial phase of combination antiretroviral treatment, patients whose immune systems respond may develop an inflammatory response to indolent or residual opportunistic infections (such as *Mycobacterium avium* infection, cytomegalovirus, *Pneumocystis jirovecii* pneumonia [PCP], or tuberculosis), which may necessitate further evaluation and treatment.

Autoimmune disorders (such as Graves' disease, polymyositis, and Guillain-Barré syndrome) have also been reported to occur in the setting of immune reconstitution; however, the time to onset is more variable and can occur many months after initiation of treatment.

5.4 Fat Redistribution

Redistribution/accumulation of body fat including central obesity, dorsocervical fat enlargement (buffalo hump), peripheral wasting, facial wasting, breast enlargement, and "cushingoid appearance" have been observed in patients receiving antiretroviral therapy. The mechanism and long-term consequences of these events are currently unknown. A causal relationship has not been established.

5.5 Myocardial Infarction

In a published prospective, observational, epidemiological trial designed to investigate the rate of myocardial infarction in patients on combination antiretroviral therapy, the use of abacavir within the previous 6 months was correlated with an increased risk of myocardial infarction (MI).[1] In a sponsor-conducted pooled analysis of clinical trials, no excess risk of myocardial infarction was observed in abacavir-treated subjects as compared with control subjects. In totality, the available data from the observational cohort and from clinical trials are inconclusive.

As a precaution, the underlying risk of coronary heart disease should be considered when prescribing antiretroviral therapies, including abacavir, and action taken to minimize all modifiable risk factors (e.g., hypertension, hyperlipidemia, diabetes mellitus, smoking).

6 ADVERSE REACTIONS

The following adverse reactions are discussed in greater detail in other sections of the labeling:

- Serious and sometimes fatal hypersensitivity reaction. In one trial, once-daily dosing of abacavir was associated with more severe hypersensitivity reactions *[see Boxed Warning, Warnings and Precautions (5.1)]*.
- Lactic acidosis and severe hepatomegaly *[see Boxed Warning, Warnings and Precautions (5.2)]*.
- Immune reconstitution syndrome *[see Warnings and Precautions (5.3)]*.
- Fat redistribution *[see Warnings and Precautions (5.4)]*.
- Myocardial infarction *[see Warnings and Precautions (5.5)]*.

6.1 Clinical Trials Experience

Because clinical trials are conducted under widely varying conditions, adverse reaction rates observed in the clinical trials of a drug cannot be directly compared with rates in the clinical trials of another drug and may not reflect the rates observed in practice.

Adults: *Therapy-Naive Adults:* Treatment-emergent clinical adverse reactions (rated by the investigator as moderate or severe) with a greater than or equal to 5% frequency during therapy with ZIAGEN 300 mg twice daily, lamivudine 150 mg twice daily, and efavirenz 600 mg daily compared with zidovudine 300 mg twice daily, lamivudine 150 mg twice daily, and efavirenz 600 mg daily from CNA30024 are listed in Table 2.

[See table 2 above]

Treatment-emergent clinical adverse reactions (rated by the investigator as moderate or severe) with a greater than or equal to 5% frequency during therapy with ZIAGEN 300 mg twice daily, lamivudine 150 mg twice daily, and zidovudine 300 mg twice daily compared with indinavir 800 mg 3 times daily, lamivudine 150 mg twice daily, and zidovudine 300 mg twice daily from CNA3005 are listed in Table 3.

Table 3. Treatment-Emergent (All Causality) Adverse Reactions of at Least Moderate Intensity (Grades 2-4, ≥5% Frequency) in Therapy-Naive Adults (CNA3005) Through 48 Weeks of Treatment

Adverse Reaction	ZIAGEN plus Lamivudine/Zidovudine (n = 262)	Indinavir plus Lamivudine/Zidovudine (n = 264)
Nausea	19%	17%
Headache	13%	9%
Malaise and fatigue	12%	12%
Nausea and vomiting	10%	10%
Hypersensitivity reaction	8%	2%
Diarrhea	7%	5%
Fever and/or chills	6%	3%
Depressive disorders	6%	4%
Musculoskeletal pain	5%	7%
Skin rashes	5%	4%
Ear/nose/throat infections	5%	4%
Viral respiratory infections	5%	5%
Anxiety	5%	3%
Renal signs/symptoms	<1%	5%
Pain (non-site-specific)	<1%	5%

Table 4. Laboratory Abnormalities (Grades 3-4) in Therapy-Naive Adults (CNA30024) Through 48 Weeks of Treatment

Grade 3/4 Laboratory Abnormalities	ZIAGEN plus Lamivudine plus Efavirenz (n = 324)	Zidovudine plus Lamivudine plus Efavirenz (n = 325)
Elevated CPK (>4 × ULN)	8%	8%
Elevated ALT (>5 × ULN)	6%	6%
Elevated AST (>5 × ULN)	6%	5%
Hypertriglyceridemia (>750 mg/dL)	6%	5%
Hyperamylasemia (>2 × ULN)	4%	5%
Neutropenia (ANC <750/mm^3)	2%	4%
Anemia (Hgb ≤6.9 gm/dL)	<1%	2%
Thrombocytopenia (Platelets <50,000/mm^3)	1%	<1%
Leukopenia (WBC ≤1,500/mm^3)	<1%	2%

ULN = Upper limit of normal.

n = Number of subjects assessed.

Table 5. Treatment-Emergent Laboratory Abnormalities (Grades 3-4) in CNA3005

Grade 3/4 Laboratory Abnormalities	Number of Subjects by Treatment Group	
	ZIAGEN plus Lamivudine/Zidovudine (n = 262)	Indinavir plus Lamivudine/Zidovudine (n = 264)
Elevated CPK (>4 × ULN)	18 (7%)	18 (7%)
ALT (>5.0 × ULN)	16 (6%)	16 (6%)
Neutropenia (<750/mm^3)	13 (5%)	13 (5%)
Hypertriglyceridemia (>750 mg/dL)	5 (2%)	3 (1%)
Hyperamylasemia (>2.0 × ULN)	5 (2%)	1 (<1%)
Hyperglycemia (>13.9 mmol/L)	2 (<1%)	2 (<1%)
Anemia (Hgb ≤6.9 g/dL)	0 (0%)	3 (1%)

ULN = Upper limit of normal.

n = Number of subjects assessed.

Table 6. Treatment-Emergent (All Causality) Adverse Reactions of at Least Moderate Intensity (Grades 2-4, ≥5% Frequency) in Therapy-Experienced Pediatric Subjects (CNA3006) Through 16 Weeks of Treatment

Adverse Reaction	ZIAGEN plus Lamivudine plus Zidovudine (n = 102)	Lamivudine plus Zidovudine (n = 103)
Fever and/or chills	9%	7%
Nausea and vomiting	9%	2%
Skin rashes	7%	1%
Ear/nose/throat infections	5%	1%
Pneumonia	4%	5%
Headache	1%	5%

[See table 3 above]

Five subjects receiving ZIAGEN in CNA3005 experienced worsening of pre-existing depression compared with none in the indinavir arm. The background rates of pre-existing depression were similar in the 2 treatment arms.

ZIAGEN Once Daily Versus ZIAGEN Twice Daily (CNA30021): Treatment-emergent clinical adverse reactions (rated by the investigator as at least moderate) with a greater than or equal to 5% frequency during therapy with ZIAGEN 600 mg once daily or ZIAGEN 300 mg twice daily, both in combination with lamivudine 300 mg once daily and efavirenz 600 mg once daily from CNA30021, were similar. For hypersensitivity reactions, subjects receiving ZIAGEN once daily showed a rate of 9% in comparison with a rate of 7% for subjects receiving ZIAGEN twice daily. However, subjects receiving ZIAGEN 600 mg once daily, experienced a significantly higher incidence of severe drug hypersensitivity reactions and severe diarrhea compared with subjects who received ZIAGEN 300 mg twice daily. Five percent (5%) of subjects receiving ZIAGEN 600 mg once daily had severe drug hypersensitivity reactions compared with 2% of subjects receiving ZIAGEN 300 mg twice daily. Two percent (2%) of subjects receiving ZIAGEN 600 mg once daily had severe diarrhea while none of the subjects receiving ZIAGEN 300 mg twice daily had this event.

Laboratory Abnormalities: Laboratory abnormalities (Grades 3-4) in therapy-naive adults during therapy with ZIAGEN 300 mg twice daily, lamivudine 150 mg twice daily, and efavirenz 600 mg daily compared with zidovudine 300 mg twice daily, lamivudine 150 mg twice daily, and efavirenz 600 mg daily from CNA30024 are listed in Table 4.

[See table 4 below]

Laboratory abnormalities in CNA3005 are listed in Table 5.

[See table 5 below]

The frequencies of treatment-emergent laboratory abnormalities were comparable between treatment groups in CNA30021.

Pediatric Trials: *Therapy-Experienced Pediatric Subjects:* Treatment-emergent clinical adverse reactions (rated by the investigator as moderate or severe) with a greater than or equal to 5% frequency during therapy with ZIAGEN 8 mg/kg twice daily, lamivudine 4 mg/kg twice daily, and zidovudine 180 mg/m^2 twice daily compared with lamivudine 4 mg/kg twice daily and zidovudine 180 mg/m^2 twice daily from CNA3006 are listed in Table 6.

[See table 6 below]

Laboratory Abnormalities: In CNA3006, laboratory abnormalities (anemia, neutropenia, liver function test abnormalities, and CPK elevations) were observed with similar frequencies as in a trial of therapy-naive adults (CNA30024). Mild elevations of blood glucose were more frequent in pediatric subjects receiving ZIAGEN (CNA3006) as compared with adult subjects (CNA30024).

Other Adverse Events: In addition to adverse reactions and laboratory abnormalities reported in Tables 2, 3, 4, 5, and 6, other adverse reactions observed in the expanded access program were pancreatitis and increased GGT.

6.2 Postmarketing Experience

In addition to adverse reactions reported from clinical trials, the following reactions have been identified during postmarketing use of ZIAGEN. Because they are reported voluntarily from a population of unknown size, estimates of frequency cannot be made. These reactions have been chosen for inclusion due to a combination of their seriousness, frequency of reporting, or potential causal connection to ZIAGEN.

Body as a Whole: Redistribution/accumulation of body fat.

Cardiovascular: Myocardial infarction.

Hepatic: Lactic acidosis and hepatic steatosis.

Skin: Suspected Stevens-Johnson syndrome (SJS) and toxic epidermal necrolysis (TEN) have been reported in patients receiving abacavir primarily in combination with medications known to be associated with SJS and TEN, respectively. Because of the overlap of clinical signs and symptoms between hypersensitivity to abacavir and SJS and TEN, and the possibility of multiple drug sensitivities in some patients, abacavir should be discontinued and not restarted in such cases.

There have also been reports of erythema multiforme with abacavir use.

7 DRUG INTERACTIONS

7.1 Ethanol

Abacavir has no effect on the pharmacokinetic properties of ethanol. Ethanol decreases the elimination of abacavir causing an increase in overall exposure *[see Clinical Pharmacology (12.3)]*.

7.2 Methadone

The addition of methadone has no clinically significant effect on the pharmacokinetic properties of abacavir. In a trial of 11 HIV-1-infected subjects receiving methadone-maintenance therapy with 600 mg of ZIAGEN twice daily (twice the currently recommended dose), oral methadone clearance increased *[see Clinical Pharmacology (12.3)]*. This alteration will not result in a methadone dose modification in the majority of patients; however, an increased methadone dose may be required in a small number of patients.

8 USE IN SPECIFIC POPULATIONS

8.1 Pregnancy

Pregnancy Category C. Studies in pregnant rats showed that abacavir is transferred to the fetus through the placenta. Fetal malformations (increased incidences of fetal anasarca and skeletal malformations) and developmental toxicity (depressed fetal body weight and reduced crown-rump length) were observed in rats at a dose which produced 35 times the human exposure based on AUC. Embryonic and fetal toxicities (increased resorptions, decreased fetal body weights) and toxicities to the offspring (increased incidence of stillbirth and lower body weights) occurred at half of the above-mentioned dose in separate fertility studies conducted in rats. In the rabbit, no developmental toxicity and no increases in fetal malformations occurred at doses that produced 8.5 times the human exposure at the recommended dose based on AUC.

There are no adequate and well-controlled studies in pregnant women. ZIAGEN should be used during pregnancy only if the potential benefits outweigh the risk.

Antiretroviral Pregnancy Registry: To monitor maternal-fetal outcomes of pregnant women exposed to ZIAGEN, an Antiretroviral Pregnancy Registry has been established. Physicians are encouraged to register patients by calling 1-800-258-4263.

8.3 Nursing Mothers

The Centers for Disease Control and Prevention recommend that HIV-1-infected mothers not breastfeed their infants to avoid risking postnatal transmission of HIV-1 infection.

Although it is not known if abacavir is excreted in human milk, abacavir is secreted into the milk of lactating rats. Because of both the potential for HIV-1 transmission and the potential for serious adverse reactions in nursing infants, mothers should be instructed not to breastfeed if they are receiving ZIAGEN.

8.4 Pediatric Use

The safety and effectiveness of ZIAGEN have been established in pediatric patients 3 months to 13 years of age. Use of ZIAGEN in these age-groups is supported by pharmacokinetic trials and evidence from adequate and well-controlled trials of ZIAGEN in adults and pediatric patients *[see Dosage and Administration (2.2), Clinical Pharmacology (12.3), Clinical Studies (14.2)]*.

8.5 Geriatric Use

Clinical studies of ZIAGEN did not include sufficient numbers of patients aged 65 and over to determine whether they respond differently from younger patients. In general, dose selection for an elderly patient should be cautious, reflecting the greater frequency of decreased hepatic, renal, or cardiac function, and of concomitant disease or other drug therapy.

10 OVERDOSAGE

There is no known antidote for ZIAGEN. It is not known whether abacavir can be removed by peritoneal dialysis or hemodialysis.

11 DESCRIPTION

ZIAGEN is the brand name for abacavir sulfate, a synthetic carbocyclic nucleoside analogue with inhibitory activity against HIV-1. The chemical name of abacavir sulfate is (1*S*,*cis*)-4-[2-amino-6-(cyclopropylamino)-9*H*-purin-9-yl]-2-cyclopentene-1-methanol sulfate (salt) (2:1). Abacavir sulfate is the enantiomer with 1*S*, 4*R* absolute configuration on the cyclopentene ring. It has a molecular formula of $(C_{14}H_{18}N_6O)_2 \cdot H_2SO_4$ and a molecular weight of 670.76 daltons. It has the following structural formula:

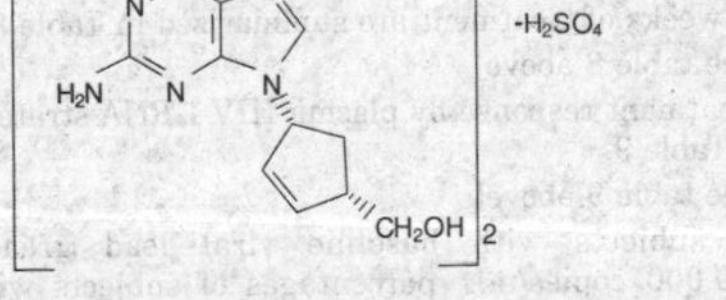

Abacavir sulfate is a white to off-white solid with a solubility of approximately 77 mg/mL in distilled water at 25°C. It has an octanol/water (pH 7.1 to 7.3) partition coefficient (log *P*) of approximately 1.20 at 25°C.

ZIAGEN Tablets are for oral administration. Each tablet contains abacavir sulfate equivalent to 300 mg of abacavir as active ingredient and the following inactive ingredients: colloidal silicon dioxide, magnesium stearate, microcrystalline cellulose, and sodium starch glycolate. The tablets are coated with a film that is made of hypromellose, polysorbate 80, synthetic yellow iron oxide, titanium dioxide, and triacetin.

ZIAGEN Oral Solution is for oral administration. Each milliliter (1 mL) of ZIAGEN Oral Solution contains abacavir sulfate equivalent to 20 mg of abacavir (i.e., 20 mg/mL) as active ingredient and the following inactive ingredients: artificial strawberry and banana flavors, citric acid (anhydrous), methylparaben and propylparaben (added as preservatives), propylene glycol, saccharin sodium, sodium citrate (dihydrate), sorbitol solution, and water.

In vivo, abacavir sulfate dissociates to its free base, abacavir. All dosages for ZIAGEN are expressed in terms of abacavir.

12 CLINICAL PHARMACOLOGY

12.1 Mechanism of Action

Abacavir is an antiviral agent *[See Clinical Pharmacology (12.4)]*.

12.3 Pharmacokinetics

Pharmacokinetics in Adults: The pharmacokinetic properties of abacavir have been studied in asymptomatic, HIV-1-infected adult subjects after administration of a single intravenous (IV) dose of 150 mg and after single and multiple oral doses. The pharmacokinetic properties of abacavir were independent of dose over the range of 300 to 1,200 mg/day.

Absorption and Bioavailability: Abacavir was rapidly and extensively absorbed after oral administration. The geometric mean absolute bioavailability of the tablet was 83%. After oral administration of 300 mg twice daily in 20 subjects, the steady-state peak serum abacavir concentration (C_{max}) was 3.0 ± 0.89 mcg/mL (mean ± SD) and $AUC_{(0\text{-}12\ hr)}$ was 6.02 ± 1.73 mcg•hr/mL. After oral administration of a single dose of 600 mg of abacavir in 20 subjects, C_{max} was 4.26 ± 1.19 mcg/mL (mean ± SD) and AUC_∞ was 11.95 ± 2.51 mcg•hr/mL.

Distribution: The apparent volume of distribution after IV administration of abacavir was 0.86 ± 0.15 L/kg, suggesting that abacavir distributes into extravascular space. In 3 subjects, the CSF $AUC_{(0\text{-}6\ hr)}$ to plasma abacavir $AUC_{(0\text{-}6\ hr)}$ ratio ranged from 27% to 33%.

Binding of abacavir to human plasma proteins is approximately 50%. Binding of abacavir to plasma proteins was independent of concentration. Total blood and plasma drug-related radioactivity concentrations are identical, demonstrating that abacavir readily distributes into erythrocytes.

Metabolism: In humans, abacavir is not significantly metabolized by cytochrome P450 enzymes. The primary routes of elimination of abacavir are metabolism by alcohol dehydrogenase (to form the 5′-carboxylic acid) and glucuronyl transferase (to form the 5′-glucuronide). The metabolites do not have antiviral activity. In vitro experiments reveal that abacavir does not inhibit human CYP3A4, CYP2D6, or CYP2C9 activity at clinically relevant concentrations.

Elimination: Elimination of abacavir was quantified in a mass balance trial following administration of a 600-mg dose of ^{14}C-abacavir: 99% of the radioactivity was recovered, 1.2% was excreted in the urine as abacavir, 30% as the 5′-carboxylic acid metabolite, 36% as the 5′-glucuronide metabolite, and 15% as unidentified minor metabolites in the urine. Fecal elimination accounted for 16% of the dose.

In single-dose trials, the observed elimination half-life ($t_{1/2}$) was 1.54 ± 0.63 hours. After intravenous administration, total clearance was 0.80 ± 0.24 L/hr/kg (mean ± SD).

Effects of Food on Oral Absorption: Bioavailability of abacavir tablets was assessed in the fasting and fed states. There was no significant difference in systemic exposure (AUC_∞) in the fed and fasting states; therefore, ZIAGEN Tablets may be administered with or without food. Systemic exposure to abacavir was comparable after administration of ZIAGEN Oral Solution and ZIAGEN Tablets. Therefore, these products may be used interchangeably.

Special Populations: *Renal Impairment:* The pharmacokinetic properties of ZIAGEN have not been determined in patients with impaired renal function. Renal excretion of unchanged abacavir is a minor route of elimination in humans.

Hepatic Impairment: The pharmacokinetics of abacavir have been studied in subjects with mild hepatic impairment (Child-Pugh score 5 to 6). Results showed that there was a mean increase of 89% in the abacavir AUC and an increase of 58% in the half-life of abacavir after a single dose of 600 mg of abacavir. The AUCs of the metabolites were not modified by mild liver disease; however, the rates of formation and elimination of the metabolites were decreased. A dose of 200 mg (provided by 10 mL of ZIAGEN Oral Solution) administered twice daily is recommended for patients with mild liver disease. The safety, efficacy, and pharmacokinetics of abacavir have not been studied in patients with moderate or severe hepatic impairment; therefore, ZIAGEN is contraindicated in these patients.

Pediatric Patients: The pharmacokinetics of abacavir have been studied after either single or repeat doses of ZIAGEN in 68 pediatric subjects. Following multiple-dose administration of ZIAGEN 8 mg/kg twice daily, steady-state $AUC_{(0\text{-}12\ hr)}$ and C_{max} were 9.8 ± 4.56 mcg•hr/mL and 3.71 ± 1.36 mcg/mL (mean ± SD), respectively *[see Use in Specific Populations (8.4)]*. In addition, to support dosing of ZIAGEN scored tablet (300 mg) for pediatric patients 14 kg to greater than 30 kg, analysis of actual and simulated pharmacokinetic data indicated comparable exposures are expected following administration of 300 mg scored tablet and the 8 mg/kg dosing regimen using oral solution.

Geriatric Patients: The pharmacokinetics of ZIAGEN have not been studied in patients over 65 years of age.

Gender: A population pharmacokinetic analysis in HIV-1-infected male (n = 304) and female (n = 67) subjects showed no gender differences in abacavir AUC normalized for lean body weight.

Race: There are no significant differences between blacks and Caucasians in abacavir pharmacokinetics.

Drug Interactions: In human liver microsomes, abacavir did not inhibit cytochrome P450 isoforms (2C9, 2D6, 3A4). Based on these data, it is unlikely that clinically significant drug interactions will occur between abacavir and drugs metabolized through these pathways.

Lamivudine and/or Zidovudine: Due to the common metabolic pathways of abacavir and zidovudine via glucuronyl transferase, 15 HIV-1-infected subjects were enrolled in a crossover trial evaluating single doses of abacavir (600 mg), lamivudine (150 mg), and zidovudine (300 mg) alone or in combination. Analysis showed no clinically relevant changes in the pharmacokinetics of abacavir with the addition of lamivudine or zidovudine or the combination of lamivudine and zidovudine. Lamivudine exposure (AUC decreased 15%) and zidovudine exposure (AUC increased 10%) did not show clinically relevant changes with concurrent abacavir.

Ethanol: Due to the common metabolic pathways of abacavir and ethanol via alcohol dehydrogenase, the pharmacokinetic interaction between abacavir and ethanol was studied in 24 HIV-1-infected male subjects. Each subject received the following treatments on separate occasions: a single 600-mg dose of abacavir, 0.7 g/kg ethanol (equivalent to 5 alcoholic drinks), and abacavir 600 mg plus 0.7 g/kg ethanol. Coadministration of ethanol and abacavir resulted in a 41% increase in abacavir AUC_∞ and a 26% increase in abacavir $t_{1/2}$. In males, abacavir had no effect on the pharmacokinetic properties of ethanol, so no clinically significant interaction is expected in men. This interaction has not been studied in females.

Methadone: In a trial of 11 HIV-1-infected subjects receiving methadone-maintenance therapy (40 mg and 90 mg daily), with 600 mg of ZIAGEN twice daily (twice the currently recommended dose), oral methadone clearance increased 22% (90% CI: 6% to 42%). This alteration will not result in a methadone dose modification in the majority of patients; however, an increased methadone dose may be required in a small number of patients. The addition of methadone had no clinically significant effect on the pharmacokinetic properties of abacavir.

12.4 Microbiology

Abacavir is a carbocyclic synthetic nucleoside analogue. Abacavir is converted by cellular enzymes to the active metabolite, carbovir triphosphate (CBV-TP), an analogue of deoxyguanosine-5′-triphosphate (dGTP). CBV-TP inhibits the activity of HIV-1 reverse transcriptase (RT) both by competing with the natural substrate dGTP and by its incorporation into viral DNA. The lack of a 3′-OH group in the incorporated nucleotide analogue prevents the formation of the 5′ to 3′ phosphodiester linkage essential for DNA chain elongation, and therefore, the viral DNA growth is terminated. CBV-TP is a weak inhibitor of cellular DNA polymerases α, β, and γ.

Antiviral Activity: The antiviral activity of abacavir against HIV-1 was evaluated against a T-cell tropic laboratory strain HIV-1_{IIIB} in lymphoblastic cell lines, a monocyte/macrophage tropic laboratory strain HIV-1_{BaL} in primary monocytes/macrophages, and clinical isolates in peripheral blood mononuclear cells. The concentration of drug necessary to effect viral replication by 50 percent (EC_{50}) ranged from 3.7 to 5.8 μM (1 μM = 0.28 mcg/mL) and 0.07 to 1.0 μM against HIV-1_{IIIB} and HIV-1_{BaL}, respectively, and was 0.26 ± 0.18 μM against 8 clinical isolates. The EC_{50} values of abacavir against different HIV-1 clades (A-G) ranged from 0.0015 to 1.05 μM, and against HIV-2 isolates, from 0.024 to 0.49 μM. Abacavir had synergistic activity in cell culture in combination with the nucleoside reverse transcriptase inhibitor (NRTI) zidovudine, the non-nucleoside reverse transcriptase inhibitor (NNRTI) nevirapine, and the protease inhibitor (PI) amprenavir; and additive activity in combination with the NRTIs didanosine, emtricitabine, lamivudine, stavudine, tenofovir, and zalcitabine. Ribavirin (50 μM) had no effect on the anti–HIV-1 activity of abacavir in cell culture.

Resistance: HIV-1 isolates with reduced susceptibility to abacavir have been selected in cell culture and were also obtained from subjects treated with abacavir. Genotypic analysis of isolates selected in cell culture and recovered from abacavir-treated subjects demonstrated that amino acid substitutions K65R, L74V, Y115F, and M184V/I in RT contributed to abacavir resistance. In a trial of therapy-naive adults receiving ZIAGEN 600 mg once daily (n = 384) or 300 mg twice daily (n = 386), in a background regimen of lamivudine 300 mg once daily and efavirenz 600 mg once daily (CNA30021), the incidence of virologic failure at 48 weeks was similar between the 2 groups (11% in both arms). Genotypic (n = 38) and phenotypic analyses (n = 35) of virologic failure isolates from this trial showed that the RT substitutions that emerged during abacavir once-daily and twice-daily therapy were K65R, L74V, Y115F, and M184V/I. The substitution M184V/I was the most commonly observed substitution in virologic failure isolates from subjects receiving abacavir once daily (56%, 10/18) and twice daily (40%, 8/20).

Table 7. Outcomes of Randomized Treatment Through Week 48 (CNA30024)

Outcome	ZIAGEN plus Lamivudine plus Efavirenz (n = 324)	Zidovudine plus Lamivudine plus Efavirenz (n = 325)
Responder[a]	69% (73%)	69% (71%)
Virologic failures[b]	6%	4%
Discontinued due to adverse reactions	14%	16%
Discontinued due to other reasons[c]	10%	11%

[a] Subjects achieved and maintained confirmed HIV-1 RNA ≤50 copies/mL (<400 copies/mL) through Week 48 (Roche AMPLICOR Ultrasensitive HIV-1 MONITOR® standard test 1.0 PCR).

[b] Includes viral rebound, insufficient viral response according to the investigator, and failure to achieve confirmed ≤50 copies/mL by Week 48.

[c] Includes consent withdrawn, lost to follow up, protocol violations, those with missing data, clinical progression, and other.

Table 8. Outcomes of Randomized Treatment Through Week 48 (CNA3005)

Outcome	ZIAGEN plus Lamivudine/Zidovudine (n = 262)	Indinavir plus Lamivudine/Zidovudine (n = 265)
Responder[a]	49%	50%
Virologic failure[b]	31%	28%
Discontinued due to adverse reactions	10%	12%
Discontinued due to other reasons[c]	11%	10%

[a] Subjects achieved and maintained confirmed HIV-1 RNA <400 copies/mL.

[b] Includes viral rebound and failure to achieve confirmed <400 copies/mL by Week 48.

[c] Includes consent withdrawn, lost to follow up, protocol violations, those with missing data, clinical progression, and other.

Table 9. Proportions of Responders Through Week 48 By Screening Plasma HIV-1 RNA Levels (CNA3005)

Screening HIV-1 RNA (copies/mL)	ZIAGEN plus Lamivudine/Zidovudine (n = 262)		Indinavir plus Lamivudine/Zidovudine (n = 265)	
	<400 copies/mL	n	<400 copies/mL	n
≥10,000 - ≤100,000	50%	166	48%	165
>100,000	48%	96	52%	100

Table 10. Outcomes of Randomized Treatment Through Week 48 (CNA30021)

Outcome	ZIAGEN 600 mg q.d. plus EPIVIR plus Efavirenz (n = 384)	ZIAGEN 300 mg b.i.d. plus EPIVIR plus Efavirenz (n = 386)
Responder[a]	64% (71%)	65% (72%)
Virologic failure[b]	11% (5%)	11% (5%)
Discontinued due to adverse reactions	13%	11%
Discontinued due to other reasons[c]	11%	13%

[a] Subjects achieved and maintained confirmed HIV-1 RNA <50 copies/mL (<400 copies/mL) through Week 48 (Roche AMPLICOR Ultrasensitive HIV-1 MONITOR standard test version 1.0).

[b] Includes viral rebound, failure to achieve confirmed <50 copies/mL (<400 copies/mL) by Week 48, and insufficient viral load response.

[c] Includes consent withdrawn, lost to follow up, protocol violations, clinical progression, and other.

Thirty-nine percent (7/18) of the isolates from subjects who experienced virologic failure in the abacavir once-daily arm had a greater than 2.5-fold decrease in abacavir susceptibility with a median-fold decrease of 1.3 (range: 0.5 to 11) compared with 29% (5/17) of the failure isolates in the twice-daily arm with a median-fold decrease of 0.92 (range: 0.7 to 13).

Cross-Resistance: Cross-resistance has been observed among NRTIs. Isolates containing abacavir resistance-associated substitutions, namely, K65R, L74V, Y115F, and M184V, exhibited cross-resistance to didanosine, emtricitabine, lamivudine, tenofovir, and zalcitabine in cell culture and in subjects. The K65R substitution can confer resistance to abacavir, didanosine, emtricitabine, lamivudine, stavudine, tenofovir, and zalcitabine; the L74V substitution can confer resistance to abacavir, didanosine, and zalcitabine; and the M184V substitution can confer resistance to abacavir, didanosine, emtricitabine, lamivudine, and zalcitabine. An increasing number of thymidine analogue mutations (TAMs: M41L, D67N, K70R, L210W, T215Y/F, K219E/R/H/Q/N) is associated with a progressive reduction in abacavir susceptibility.

13 NONCLINICAL TOXICOLOGY

13.1 Carcinogenesis, Mutagenesis, Impairment of Fertility

Carcinogenicity: Abacavir was administered orally at 3 dosage levels to separate groups of mice and rats in 2-year carcinogenicity studies. Results showed an increase in the incidence of malignant and non-malignant tumors. Malignant tumors occurred in the preputial gland of males and the clitoral gland of females of both species, and in the liver of female rats. In addition, non-malignant tumors also occurred in the liver and thyroid gland of female rats. These observations were made at systemic exposures in the range of 6 to 32 times the human exposure at the recommended dose. It is not known how predictive the results of rodent carcinogenicity studies may be for humans.

Mutagenicity: Abacavir induced chromosomal aberrations both in the presence and absence of metabolic activation in an in vitro cytogenetic study in human lymphocytes. Abacavir was mutagenic in the absence of metabolic activation, although it was not mutagenic in the presence of metabolic activation in an L5178Y mouse lymphoma assay. Abacavir was clastogenic in males and not clastogenic in females in an in vivo mouse bone marrow micronucleus assay. Abacavir was not mutagenic in bacterial mutagenicity assays in the presence and absence of metabolic activation.

Impairment of Fertility: Abacavir had no adverse effects on the mating performance or fertility of male and female rats at a dose approximately 8 times the human exposure at the recommended dose based on body surface area comparisons.

13.2 Animal Toxicology and/or Pharmacology

Myocardial degeneration was found in mice and rats following administration of abacavir for 2 years. The systemic exposures were equivalent to 7 to 24 times the expected systemic exposure in humans. The clinical relevance of this finding has not been determined.

14 CLINICAL STUDIES

14.1 Adults

Therapy-Naive Adults: CNA30024 was a multicenter, double-blind, controlled trial in which 649 HIV-1-infected, therapy-naive adults were randomized and received either ZIAGEN (300 mg twice daily), lamivudine (150 mg twice daily), and efavirenz (600 mg once daily); or zidovudine (300 mg twice daily), lamivudine (150 mg twice daily), and efavirenz (600 mg once daily). The duration of double-blind treatment was at least 48 weeks. Trial participants were male (81%), Caucasian (51%), black (21%), and Hispanic (26%). The median age was 35 years; the median pretreatment CD4+ cell count was 264 cells/mm^3, and median plasma HIV-1 RNA was 4.79 $\log_{10}$ copies/mL. The outcomes of randomized treatment are provided in Table 7.

[See table 7 above]

After 48 weeks of therapy, the median CD4+ cell count increases from baseline were 209 cells/mm^3 in the group receiving ZIAGEN and 155 cells/mm^3 in the zidovudine group. Through Week 48, 8 subjects (2%) in the group receiving ZIAGEN (5 CDC classification C events and 3 deaths) and 5 subjects (2%) on the zidovudine arm (3 CDC classification C events and 2 deaths) experienced clinical disease progression.

CNA3005 was a multicenter, double-blind, controlled trial in which 562 HIV-1-infected, therapy-naive adults were randomized to receive either ZIAGEN (300 mg twice daily) plus COMBIVIR® (lamivudine 150 mg/zidovudine 300 mg twice daily), or indinavir (800 mg 3 times a day) plus COMBIVIR twice daily. The trial was stratified at randomization by pre-entry plasma HIV-1 RNA 10,000 to 100,000 copies/mL and plasma HIV-1 RNA greater than 100,000 copies/mL. Trial participants were male (87%), Caucasian (73%), black (15%), and Hispanic (9%). At baseline the median age was 36 years; the median baseline CD4+ cell count was 360 cells/mm^3, and median baseline plasma HIV-1 RNA was 4.8 $\log_{10}$ copies/mL. Proportions of subjects with plasma HIV-1 RNA less than 400 copies/mL (using Roche AMPLICOR HIV-1 MONITOR Test) through 48 weeks of treatment are summarized in Table 8.

[See table 8 above]

Treatment response by plasma HIV-1 RNA strata is shown in Table 9.

[See table 9 above]

In subjects with baseline viral load greater than 100,000 copies/mL, percentages of subjects with HIV-1 RNA levels less than 50 copies/mL were 31% in the group receiving abacavir versus 45% in the group receiving indinavir.

Through Week 48, an overall mean increase in CD4+ cell count of about 150 cells/mm^3 was observed in both treatment arms. Through Week 48, 9 subjects (3.4%) in the group receiving abacavir sulfate (6 CDC classification C events and 3 deaths) and 3 subjects (1.5%) in the group receiving indinavir (2 CDC classification C events and 1 death) experienced clinical disease progression.

CNA30021 was an international, multicenter, double-blind, controlled trial in which 770 HIV-1-infected, therapy-naive adults were randomized and received either abacavir 600 mg once daily or abacavir 300 mg twice daily, both in combination with lamivudine 300 mg once daily and efavirenz 600 mg once daily. The double-blind treatment duration was at least 48 weeks. Trial participants had a mean age of 37 years; were male (81%), Caucasian (54%), black (27%), and American Hispanic (15%). The median baseline CD4+ cell count was 262 cells/mm^3 (range 21 to 918 cells/mm^3) and the median baseline plasma HIV-1 RNA was 4.89 $\log_{10}$ copies/mL (range: 2.60 to 6.99 $\log_{10}$ copies/mL).

The outcomes of randomized treatment are provided in Table 10.

[See table 10 above]

After 48 weeks of therapy, the median CD4+ cell count increases from baseline were 188 cells/mm^3 in the group receiving abacavir 600 mg once daily and 200 cells/mm^3 in the group receiving abacavir 300 mg twice daily. Through Week 48, 6 subjects (2%) in the group receiving ZIAGEN 600 mg once daily (4 CDC classification C events and 2 deaths) and 10 subjects (3%) in the group receiving ZIAGEN 300 mg twice daily (7 CDC classification C events and 3 deaths) experienced clinical disease progression. None of the deaths were attributed to trial medications.

14.2 Pediatric Trials

Therapy-Experienced Pediatric Subjects: CNA3006 was a randomized, double-blind trial comparing ZIAGEN 8 mg/kg twice daily plus lamivudine 4 mg/kg twice daily plus zidovudine 180 mg/m^2 twice daily versus lamivudine 4 mg/kg twice daily plus zidovudine 180 mg/m^2 twice daily. Two hundred and five therapy-experienced pediatric subjects were enrolled: female (56%), Caucasian (17%), black (50%), Hispanic (30%), median age of 5.4 years, baseline CD4+ cell percent greater than 15% (median = 27%), and median baseline plasma HIV-1 RNA of 4.6 $\log_{10}$ copies/mL. Eighty percent and 55% of subjects had prior therapy with zidovudine and lamivudine, respectively, most often in combination. The median duration of prior nucleoside analogue therapy was 2 years. At 16 weeks the proportion of subjects responding based on plasma HIV-1 RNA less than or equal to 400 copies/mL was significantly higher in subjects receiving ZIAGEN plus lamivudine plus zidovudine compared with subjects receiving lamivudine plus zidovudine, 13% versus 2%, respectively. Median plasma HIV-1 RNA changes from baseline were -0.53 $\log_{10}$ copies/mL in the group receiving ZIAGEN plus lamivudine plus zidovudine compared with -0.21 $\log_{10}$ copies/mL in the group receiving lamivudine plus zidovudine. Median CD4+ cell count increases from baseline were 69 cells/mm^3 in the group receiving ZIAGEN plus lamivudine plus zidovudine and 9 cells/mm^3 in the group receiving lamivudine plus zidovudine.

15 REFERENCES

1. Data Collection on Adverse Events of Anti-HIV Drugs (D:A:D) Study Group. *Lancet*. 2008;371 (9622):1417-1426.

16 HOW SUPPLIED/STORAGE AND HANDLING

ZIAGEN Tablets, containing abacavir sulfate equivalent to 300 mg abacavir are yellow, biconvex, scored, capsule-shaped, film-coated, and imprinted with "GX 623" on both sides. They are packaged as follows:

Bottles of 60 tablets (NDC 49702-221-18).

Unit dose blister packs of 60 tablets (NDC 49702-221-44). Each pack contains 6 blister cards of 10 tablets each.

Store at controlled room temperature of 20° to 25°C (68° to 77°F) (see USP).

ZIAGEN Oral Solution is a clear to opalescent, yellowish, strawberry-banana-flavored liquid. Each mL of the solution contains abacavir sulfate equivalent to 20 mg of abacavir. It is packaged in plastic bottles as follows:

Bottles of 240 mL (NDC 49702-222-48) with child-resistant closure. This product does not require reconstitution.

Store at controlled room temperature of 20° to 25°C (68° to 77°F) (see USP). DO NOT FREEZE. May be refrigerated.

17 PATIENT COUNSELING INFORMATION

See FDA-approved patient labeling (Medication Guide)

17.1 Information About Therapy With ZIAGEN

Hypersensitivity Reaction: Inform patients:

- that a Medication Guide and Warning Card summarizing the symptoms of the abacavir hypersensitivity reaction and other product information will be dispensed by the pharmacist with each new prescription and refill of ZIAGEN, and encourage the patient to read the Medication Guide and Warning Card every time to obtain any new information that may be present about ZIAGEN. (The complete text of the Medication Guide is reprinted at the end of this document.)
- to carry the Warning Card with them.
- how to identify a hypersensitivity reaction *[see Medication Guide]*.
- that if they develop symptoms consistent with a hypersensitivity reaction they should call their doctor right away to determine if they should stop taking ZIAGEN.
- that a hypersensitivity reaction can worsen and lead to hospitalization or death if ZIAGEN is not immediately discontinued.
- that in one trial, more severe hypersensitivity reactions were seen when ZIAGEN was dosed 600 mg once daily.
- to not restart ZIAGEN or any other abacavir-containing product following a hypersensitivity reaction because more severe symptoms can occur within hours and may include life-threatening hypotension and death.
- that a hypersensitivity reaction is usually reversible if it is detected promptly and ZIAGEN is stopped right away.
- that if they have interrupted ZIAGEN for reasons other than symptoms of hypersensitivity (for example, those who have an interruption in drug supply), a serious or fatal hypersensitivity reaction may occur with reintroduction of abacavir.
- to not restart ZIAGEN or any other abacavir-containing product without medical consultation and that restarting abacavir needs to be undertaken only if medical care can be readily accessed by the patient or others.
- ZIAGEN should not be coadministered with EPZICOM® (abacavir sulfate and lamivudine) Tablets or TRIZIVIR® (abacavir sulfate, lamivudine, and zidovudine) Tablets.

Lactic Acidosis/Hepatomegaly: Inform patients that some HIV medicines, including ZIAGEN, can cause a rare, but serious condition called lactic acidosis with liver enlargement (hepatomegaly) *[see Boxed Warning, Warnings and Precautions (5.2)]*.

Redistribution/Accumulation of Body Fat: Inform patients that redistribution or accumulation of body fat may occur in patients receiving antiretroviral therapy and that the cause and long-term health effects of these conditions are not known at this time *[see Warnings and Precautions (5.4)]*.

Information About HIV-1 Infection: ZIAGEN is not a cure for HIV-1 infection and patients may continue to experience illnesses associated with HIV-1 infection, including opportunistic infections. Patients should remain under the care of a physician when using ZIAGEN.

Patients should be advised to avoid doing things that can spread HIV-1 infection to others.

- **Do not share needles or other injection equipment.**
- **Do not share personal items that can have blood or body fluids on them, like toothbrushes and razor blades.**
- **Do not have any kind of sex without protection.** Always practice safe sex by using a latex or polyurethane condom to lower the chance of sexual contact with semen, vaginal secretions, or blood.
- **Do not breastfeed.** We do not know if ZIAGEN can be passed to your baby in your breast milk and whether it could harm your baby. Also, mothers with HIV-1 should not breastfeed because HIV-1 can be passed to the baby in the breast milk.

Patients should be informed to take all HIV medications exactly as prescribed.

COMBIVIR, EPIVIR, EPZICOM, TRIZIVIR, and ZIAGEN are registered trademarks of ViiV Healthcare.

Manufactured for:
ViiV Healthcare
Research Triangle Park, NC 27709
by:
GlaxoSmithKline
Research Triangle Park, NC 27709

ZGN:6PI

MEDICATION GUIDE
ZIAGEN® (ZY-uh-jen)
(abacavir sulfate)
Tablets and Oral Solution

Read this Medication Guide before you start taking ZIAGEN and each time you get a refill. There may be new information. This information does not take the place of talking to your healthcare provider about your medical condition or your treatment. Be sure to carry your ZIAGEN Warning Card with you at all times.

What is the most important information I should know about ZIAGEN?

1.Serious allergic reaction (hypersensitivity reaction). ZIAGEN contains abacavir (also contained in EPZICOM® and TRIZIVIR®). Patients taking ZIAGEN may have a serious allergic reaction (hypersensitivity reaction) that can cause death. Your risk of this allergic reaction is much higher if you have a gene variation called HLA-B*5701. Your healthcare provider can determine with a blood test if you have this gene variation.

If you get a symptom from 2 or more of the following groups while taking ZIAGEN, call your healthcare provider right away to find out if you should stop taking ZIAGEN.

	Symptom(s)
Group 1	Fever
Group 2	Rash
Group 3	Nausea, vomiting, diarrhea, abdominal (stomach area) pain
Group 4	Generally ill feeling, extreme tiredness, or achiness
Group 5	Shortness of breath, cough, sore throat

A list of these symptoms is on the Warning Card your pharmacist gives you. **Carry this Warning Card with you at all times.**

If you stop ZIAGEN because of an allergic reaction, never take ZIAGEN (abacavir sulfate) or any other abacavir-containing medicine (EPZICOM and TRIZIVIR) again. If you take ZIAGEN or any other abacavir-containing medicine again after you have had an allergic reaction, **within hours** you may get **life-threatening symptoms** that may include **very low blood pressure** or **death**. If you stop ZIAGEN, for any other reason, even for a few days, and you are not allergic to ZIAGEN, talk with your healthcare provider before taking it again. Taking ZIAGEN again can cause a serious allergic or life-threatening reaction, even if you never had an allergic reaction to it before.

If your healthcare provider tells you that you can take ZIAGEN again, start taking it when you are around medical help or people who can call a healthcare provider if you need one.

2. Lactic Acidosis (buildup of acid in the blood). Some human immunodeficiency virus (HIV) medicines, including ZIAGEN, can cause a rare but serious condition called lactic acidosis. Lactic acidosis is a serious medical emergency that can cause death and must be treated in the hospital. Call your healthcare provider right away if you get any of the following signs or symptoms of lactic acidosis:

- you feel very weak or tired
- you have unusual (not normal) muscle pain
- you have trouble breathing
- you have stomach pain with nausea and vomiting
- you feel cold, especially in your arms and legs
- you feel dizzy or light-headed
- you have a fast or irregular heartbeat

3. Serious liver problems. Some people who have taken medicines like ZIAGEN have developed serious liver problems called hepatotoxicity, with liver enlargement (hepatomegaly) and fat in the liver (steatosis). Hepatomegaly with steatosis is a serious medical emergency that can cause death.Call your healthcare provider right away if you get any of the following signs or symptoms of liver problems:

- your skin or the white part of your eyes turns yellow (jaundice)
- your urine turns dark
- your bowel movements (stools) turn light in color
- you don't feel like eating food for several days or longer
- you feel sick to your stomach (nausea)
- you have lower stomach area (abdominal) pain

You may be more likely to get lactic acidosis or serious liver problems if you are female, very overweight, or have been taking nucleoside analogue medicines for a long time.

What is ZIAGEN?

ZIAGEN is a prescription medicine used to treat HIV infection. ZIAGEN is a medicine called a nucleoside analogue reverse transcriptase inhibitor (NRTI). ZIAGEN is always used with other anti-HIV medicines. When used in combination with these other medicines, ZIAGEN helps lower the amount of HIV in your blood.

- **ZIAGEN does not cure HIV infection or AIDS.**
- It is not known if ZIAGEN will help you live longer or have fewer of the medical problems that people get with HIV or AIDS.
- It is very important that you see your doctor regularly while you are taking ZIAGEN.

Who should not take ZIAGEN?

Do not take ZIAGEN if you:

- **are allergic to abacavir or any of the ingredients in ZIAGEN. See the end of this Medication Guide for a complete list of ingredients in ZIAGEN.**
- **have certain liver problems.**

What should I tell my healthcare provider before taking ZIAGEN?

Before you take ZIAGEN, tell your healthcare provider if you:

- **have been tested and know whether or not you have a particular gene variation called HLA-B*5701.**
- **have hepatitis B virus infection or have other liver problems.**
- **have heart problems, smoke, or have diseases that increase your risk of heart disease such as high blood pressure, high cholesterol, or diabetes.**
- **are pregnant or plan to become pregnant.** It is not known if ZIAGEN will harm your unborn baby. Talk to your healthcare provider if you are pregnant or plan to become pregnant.

  Pregnancy Registry. If you take ZIAGEN while you are pregnant, talk to your healthcare provider about how you can take part in the Pregnancy Registry for ZIAGEN. The purpose of the pregnancy registry is to collect information about the health of you and your baby.
- **are breastfeeding or plan to breastfeed. Do not breastfeed.** We do not know if ZIAGEN can be passed to your baby in your breast milk and whether it could harm your baby. Also, mothers with HIV-1 should not breastfeed because HIV-1 can be passed to the baby in the breast milk.

Tell your healthcare provider about all the medicines you take, including prescription and nonprescription medicines, vitamins, and herbal supplements.

Especially tell your healthcare provider if you take:

- alcohol
- methadone
- TRIZIVIR (abacavir sulfate, lamivudine, and zidovudine)
- EPZICOM (abacavir sulfate and lamivudine)

Ask your healthcare provider if you are not sure if you take one of the medicines listed above.

ZIAGEN may affect the way other medicines work, and other medicines may affect how ZIAGEN works.

Know the medicines you take. Keep a list of your medicines with you to show to your healthcare provider and pharmacist when you get a new medicine.

How should I take ZIAGEN?

- **Take ZIAGEN exactly as your healthcare provider tells you to take it.**
- **ZIAGEN is taken by mouth as a tablet or a strawberry- and banana-flavored liquid.**
- ZIAGEN may be taken with or without food.
- Do not skip doses.
- Children aged 3 months and older can also take ZIAGEN. The child's healthcare provider will decide the right dose and whether the child should take the tablet or liquid, based on the child's weight. The dose should not be more than the recommended adult dose.
- **Do not let your ZIAGEN run out.**
  If you stop your anti-HIV medicines, even for a short time, the amount of virus in your blood may increase and the virus may become harder to treat. If you take too much ZIAGEN, call your healthcare provider or poison control center or go to the nearest hospital emergency room right away.

What are the possible side effects of ZIAGEN?

- **ZIAGEN can cause serious side effects including allergic reactions, lactic acidosis, and liver problems. See "What is the most important information I should know about ZIAGEN?"**
- **Changes in immune system (Immune Reconstitution Syndrome).** Your immune system may get stronger and begin to fight infections that have been hidden in your body for a long time. Tell your healthcare provider if you start having new or worse symptoms of infection after you start taking ZIAGEN.
- **Changes in body fat (fat redistribution).** Changes in body fat (lipoatrophy or lipodystrophy) can happen in some people taking antiretroviral medicines including ZIAGEN. These changes may include:
- more fat in or around your trunk, upper back and neck (buffalo hump), breast, or chest
- loss of fat in your legs, arms, or face
- **Heart attack (myocardial infarction).** Some HIV medicines including ZIAGEN may increase your risk of heart attack.

The most common side effects of ZIAGEN in adults include:

- bad dreams or sleep problems
- nausea
- headache
- tiredness
- vomiting

The most common side effects of ZIAGEN in children include:

- fever and chills
- nausea
- vomiting
- rash
- ear, nose, or throat infections

Tell your healthcare provider if you have any side effect that bothers you or that does not go away.

These are not all the possible side effects of ZIAGEN. For more information, ask your healthcare provider or pharmacist.

Call your doctor for medical advice about side effects. You may report side effects to FDA at 1-800-FDA-1088.

How should I store ZIAGEN?

- Store ZIAGEN at room temperature, between 68°F to 77°F (20°C to 25°C).
- Do not freeze ZIAGEN.
- **Keep ZIAGEN and all medicines out of the reach of children.**

General information for safe and effective use of ZIAGEN

Avoid doing things that can spread HIV infection to others.

- **Do not share needles or other injection equipment.**
- **Do not share personal items that can have blood or body fluids on them, like toothbrushes and razor blades.**
- **Do not have any kind of sex without protection.** Always practice safe sex by using a latex or polyurethane condom to lower the chance of sexual contact with semen, vaginal secretions, or blood.

Medicines are sometimes prescribed for purposes other than those listed in a Medication Guide. Do not use ZIAGEN for a condition for which it was not prescribed. Do not give ZIAGEN to other people, even if they have the same symptoms that you have. It may harm them.

This Medication Guide summarizes the most important information about ZIAGEN. If you would like more information, talk with your healthcare provider. You can ask your healthcare provider or pharmacist for the information that is written for healthcare professionals.

For more information go to www.ZIAGEN.com or call 1-877-844-8872.

What are the ingredients in ZIAGEN?

Tablets

Active ingredient: abacavir sulfate

Inactive ingredients: colloidal silicon dioxide, magnesium stearate, microcrystalline cellulose, and sodium starch glycolate, and afilm–coating made of hypromellose, polysorbate 80, synthetic yellow iron oxide, titanium dioxide, and triacetin.

Oral Solution

Active ingredient: abacavir sulfate

Inactive ingredients: artificial strawberry and banana flavors, citric acid (anhydrous), methylparaben and propylparaben (added as preservatives), propylene glycol, saccharin sodium, sodium citrate (dihydrate), sorbitol solution, and water.

This Medication Guide has been approved by the US Food and Drug Administration.

EPZICOM and TRIZIVIR are registered trademarks of ViiV Healthcare.

Manufactured for:
ViiV Healthcare
Research Triangle Park, NC 27709
by:
GlaxoSmithKline
Research Triangle Park, NC 27709

May 2012
ZGN:5MG

WellSpring Pharmaceutical Corporation

5911 N. HONORE AVENUE, STE. 211
SARASOTA, FL 34243

Direct Inquiries to:
phone (941) 312-4727
fax (941) 312-4738

DIBENZYLINE® ℞

[dī-bĕnz-ĭ-lēn]

(phenoxybenzamine hydrochloride, USP)
Capsules 10 mg
adrenergic, alpha-receptor-blocking agent

DESCRIPTION

Each Dibenzyline capsule, with red cap and body, is imprinted WPC 001 and 10 mg, and contains 10 mg of Phenoxybenzamine Hydrochloride USP. Inactive ingredients consist of D&C Red No. 33, FD&C Red No. 3, FD&C Yellow No. 6, Gelatin NF, Lactose NF, Sodium Lauryl Sulfate NF and Silicon Dioxide NF.

Dibenzyline is N-(2-Chloroethyl)-N-(1-methyl-2-phenoxyethyl)benzylamine hydrochloride:

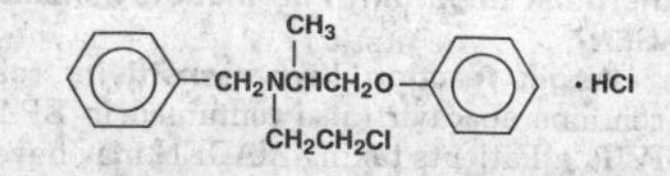

Phenoxybenzamine hydrochloride is a colorless, crystalline powder with a molecular weight of 340.3, which melts between 136°and 141°C. It is soluble in water, alcohol and chloroform; insoluble in ether.

CLINICAL PHARMACOLOGY

Dibenzyline (phenoxybenzamine hydrochloride) is a long-acting, adrenergic, *alpha*-receptor-blocking agent, which can produce and maintain "chemical sympathectomy" by oral administration. It increases blood flow to the skin, mucosa and abdominal viscera, and lowers both supine and erect blood pressures. It has no effect on the parasympathetic system.

Twenty to 30 percent of orally administered phenoxybenzamine appears to be absorbed in the active form.[1]

The half-life of orally administered phenoxybenzamine hydrochloride is not known; however, the half-life of intravenously administered drug is approximately 24 hours. Demonstrable effects with intravenous administration persist for at least 3 to 4 days, and the effects of daily administration are cumulative for nearly a week.[1]

INDICATION AND USAGE

Dibenzyline is indicated in the treatment of pheochromocytoma, to control episodes of hypertension and sweating. If tachycardia is excessive, it may be necessary to use a *beta*-blocking agent concomitantly.

CONTRAINDICATIONS

Conditions where a fall in blood pressure may be undesirable; hypersensitivity to the drug or any of its components.

WARNING

Dibenzyline-induced *alpha*-adrenergic blockade leaves *beta*-adrenergic receptors unopposed. Compounds that stimulate both types of receptors may, therefore, produce an exaggerated hypotensive response and tachycardia.

PRECAUTIONS

General– Administer with caution in patients with marked cerebral or coronary arteriosclerosis or renal damage. Adrenergic blocking effect may aggravate symptoms of respiratory infections.

Drug Interactions [2]

Dibenzyline (phenoxybenzamine hydrochloride) may interact with compounds that stimulate both *alpha*- and *beta*-adrenergic receptors (i.e., epinephrine) to produce an exaggerated hypotensive response and tachycardia.(See WARNING.)

Dibenzyline blocks hyperthermia production by levarterenol, and blocks hypothermia production by reserpine.

Carcinogenesis and Mutagenesis

Case reports of carcinoma in humans after long-term treatment with phenoxybenzamine have been reported. Hence long-term use of phenoxybenzamine is not recommended.[3,4] Carefully weigh the benefits and risks before prescribing this drug.

Phenoxybenzamine hydrochloride showed *in vitro* mutagenic activity in the Ames test and mouse lymphoma assay; it did not show mutagenic activity *in vivo* in the micronucleus test in mice. In rats and mice, repeated intraperitoneal administration of phenoxybenzamine hydrochloride (three times per week for up to 52 weeks) resulted in peritoneal sarcomas. Chronic oral dosing in rats (for up to 2 years) produced malignant tumors of the small intestine and non-glandular stomach, as well as ulcerative and/or erosive gastritis of the glandular stomach. Whereas squamous cell carcinomas of the non-glandular stomach were observed at all tested doses of phenoxybenzamine hydrochloride, there was a no-observed-effect-level of 10 mg/kg for tumors (carcinomas and sarcomas) of the small intestine. This dose is, on a body surface area basis, about twice the maximum recommended human dosage of 20 mg b.i.d.

Pregnancy

Teratogenic Effects - Pregnancy Category C

Adequate reproductive studies in animals have not been performed with Dibenzyline (phenoxybenzamine hydrochloride). It is also not known whether Dibenzyline can cause fetal harm when administered to a pregnant woman. Dibenzyline should be given to a pregnant woman only if clearly needed.

Nursing Mothers

It is not known whether this drug is excreted in human milk. Because many drugs are excreted in human milk, and because of the potential for serious adverse reactions from phenoxybenzamine hydrochloride, a decision should be made whether to discontinue nursing or to discontinue the drug, taking into account the importance of the drug to the mother.

Pediatric Use

Safety and effectiveness in pediatric patients have not been established.

ADVERSE REACTIONS

The following adverse reactions have been observed, but there are insufficient data to support an estimate of their frequency.

Autonomic Nervous System[1]: Postural hypotension, tachycardia, inhibition of ejaculation, nasal congestion, miosis.

Miscellaneous: Gastrointestinal irritation, drowsiness, fatigue.

To report SUSPECTED ADVERSE REACTIONS, contact WellSpring Pharmaceutical Corporation at 1-866-337-4500 or FDA at 1-800-FDA-1088 or www.fda.gov/medwatch.

[1]These so-called "side effects" are actually evidence of adrenergic blockade and vary according to the degree of blockade.

OVERDOSAGE

SYMPTOMS-These are largely the result of blocking of the sympathetic nervous system and of the circulating epinephrine. They may include postural hypotension, resulting in dizziness or fainting; tachycardia, particularly postural; vomiting; lethargy; shock.

TREATMENT

When symptoms and signs of overdosage exist, discontinue the drug. Treatment of circulatory failure, if present, is a prime consideration. In cases of mild overdosage, recumbent position with legs elevated usually restores cerebral circulation. In the more severe cases, the usual measures to combat shock should be instituted. Usual pressor agents are *not* effective. Epinephrine is contraindicated because it stimulates both *alpha*- and *beta*- receptors; since *alpha*- receptors are blocked, the net effect of epinephrine administration is vasodilation and a further drop in blood pressure (epinephrine reversal).

The patient may have to be kept flat for 24 hours or more in the case of overdose, as the effect of the drug is prolonged. Leg bandages and an abdominal binder may shorten the period of disability.

I.V. Infusion of levarterenol bitartrate[2] may be used to combat severe hypotensive reactions, because it stimulates *alpha*-receptors primarily. Although Dibenzyline (phenoxybenzamine hydrochloride) is an *alpha* -adrenergic blocking agent, a sufficient dose of levarterenol bitartrate will overcome this effect.

The oral LD_{50} for phenoxybenzamine hydrochloride is approximately 2000 mg/kg in rats and approximately 500 mg/kg in guinea pigs.

[2] Available as Levophed® Bitartrate (brand of norepinephrine bitartrate) from Abbott Laboratories.

DOSAGE AND ADMINISTRATION

The dosage should be adjusted to fit the needs of each patient. Small initial doses should be *slowly* increased until the desired effect is obtained or the side effects from blockade become troublesome. *After each increase, the patient should be observed on that level before instituting another increase.* The dosage should be carried to a point where symptomatic relief and/or objective improvement are obtained, but not so high that the side effects from blockade become troublesome.

Initially, 10 mg of Dibenzyline (phenoxybenzamine hydrochloride) twice a day. Dosage should be increased every other day, usually to 20 to 40 mg 2 or 3 times a day, until an optimal dosage is obtained, as judged by blood pressure control.

Long-term use of phenoxybenzamine is not recommended (see PRECAUTIONS Carcinogenesis and Mutagenesis)

STORAGE

Store at 25°C (77°F); excursions permitted to 15°- 30°C (59°-86°F) [See USP Controlled Room Temperature].

HOW SUPPLIED

Dibenzyline (phenoxybenzamine hydrochloride) capsules, 10 mg, in bottles of 100 (NDC 65197-001-01).

REFERENCES

1. Weiner, N.: Drugs That Inhibit Adrenergic Nerves and Block Adrenergic Receptors, in Goodman, L., and Gilman, A., *The Pharmacological Basis of Therapeutics*, ed. 6, New York, Macmillan Publishing Co., 1980, p. 179; p. 182.
2. Martin, E.W.: *Drug Interactions Index 1978/1979*, Philadelphia, J.B. Lippincott Co., 1978, pp. 209-210.
3. Nettesheim O, Hoffken G, Gahr M, Breidert M: Haematemesis and dysphagia in a 20-year-old woman with congenital spine malformation and situs inversus partialis [German]. Zeitschrift fur Gastroenterologie. 2003; 41(4):319-24.
4. Vaidyanathan S, Mansour P, Soni BM, Hughes PL, Singh G: Chronic lymphocytic leukaemia, synchronous small cell carcinoma and squamous neoplasia of the urinary bladder in a paraplegic man following long-term phenoxybenzamine therapy. Spinal Cord. 2006;44(3): 188-91.

DATE OF ISSUANCE MARCH 2009

Manufactured for
WellSpring Pharmaceutical Corporation
Sarasota, FL 34243 USA
By WellSpring Pharmaceutical
Canada Corp.
Oakville, Ontario L6H 1M5 Canada
Rev. 03/09

Shown in Product Identification Guide, page 314

DYRENIUM® ℞

(triamterene USP)

Capsules 50 mg and 100 mg potassium-sparing diuretic

Warnings

Abnormal elevation of serum potassium levels (greater than or equal to 5.5 mEq/liter) can occur with all potassium-sparing agents, including Dyrenium. Hyperkalemia is more likely to occur in patients with renal impairment and diabetes (even without evidence of renal impairment), and in the elderly or severely ill. Since uncorrected hyperkalemia may be fatal, serum potassium levels must be monitored at frequent intervals especially in patients receiving Dyrenium, when dosages are changed or with any illness that may influence renal function.

DESCRIPTION

Each capsule for oral use, with opaque red cap and body, contains Triamterene USP, 50 or 100 mg, and is imprinted with the product name, DYRENIUM, strength (50 mg or 100 mg) and WPC 002 (for the 50-mg strength) and WPC 003 (for the 100-mg strength). Inactive ingredients consist of D&C Red No. 33, FD&C Yellow No. 6, Gelatin NF, Lactose NF, Magnesium Stearate NF, Sodium Lauryl Sulfate NF, Titanium Dioxide USP and Silicon Dioxide NF.

Triamterene is 2,4,7-triamino-6-phenyl-pteridine:

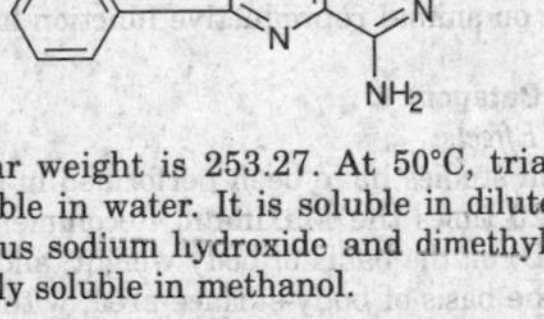

Its molecular weight is 253.27. At 50°C, triamterene is slightly soluble in water. It is soluble in dilute ammonia, dilute aqueous sodium hydroxide and dimethylformamide. It is sparingly soluble in methanol.

CLINICAL PHARMACOLOGY

Triamterene has a unique mode of action; it inhibits the reabsorption of sodium ions in exchange for potassium and hydrogen ions at that segment of the distal tubule under the control of adrenal mineralocorticoids (especially aldosterone). This activity is not directly related to aldosterone secretion or antagonism; it is a result of a direct effect on the renal tubule.

The fraction of filtered sodium reaching this distal tubular exchange site is relatively small, and the amount which is exchanged depends on the level of mineralocorticoid activity. Thus, the degree of natriuresis and diuresis produced by inhibition of the exchange mechanism is necessarily limited. Increasing the amount of available sodium and the level of mineralocorticoid activity by the use of more proximally acting diuretics will increase the degree of diuresis and potassium conservation.

Triamterene occasionally causes increases in serum potassium which can result in hyperkalemia. It does not produce alkalosis, because it does not cause excessive excretion of titratable acid and ammonium.

Triamterene has been shown to cross the placental barrier and appear in the cord blood of animals.

Pharmacokinetics

Onset of action is 2 to 4 hours after ingestion. In normal volunteers the mean peak serum levels were 30 ng/mL at 3 hours. The average percent of drug recovered in the urine (0 to 48 hours) was 21%. Triamterene is primarily metabolized to the sulfate conjugate of hydroxytriamterene. Both the plasma and urine levels of this metabolite greatly exceed triamterene levels. Triamterene is rapidly absorbed, with somewhat less than 50% of the oral dose reaching the urine. Most patients will respond to Dyrenium (triamterene) during the first day of treatment.

Maximum therapeutic effect, however, may not be seen for several days. Duration of diuresis depends on several factors, especially renal function, but it generally tapers off 7 to 9 hours after administration.

INDICATIONS AND USAGE

Dyrenium (triamterene) is indicated in the treatment of edema associated with congestive heart failure, cirrhosis of the liver and the nephrotic syndrome; steroid-induced edema, idiopathic edema and edema due to secondary hyperaldosteronism.

Dyrenium may be used alone or with other diuretics, either for its added diuretic effect or its potassium-sparing potential. It also promotes increased diuresis when patients prove resistant or only partially responsive to thiazides or other diuretics because of secondary hyperaldosteronism.

Usage in Pregnancy. The routine use of diuretics in an otherwise healthy woman is inappropriate and exposes mother and fetus to unnecessary hazard. Diuretics do not prevent development of toxemia of pregnancy, and there is no satisfactory evidence that they are useful in the treatment of developed toxemia.

Edema during pregnancy may arise from pathological causes or from the physiologic and mechanical consequences of pregnancy. Diuretics are indicated in pregnancy (however, see PRECAUTIONS below) when edema is due to pathologic causes, just as they are in the absence of pregnancy. Dependent edema in pregnancy, resulting from restriction of venous return by the expanded uterus, is properly treated through elevation of the lower extremities and use of support hose; use of diuretics to lower intravascular volume in this case is illogical and unnecessary. There is hypervolemia during normal pregnancy which is harmful to neither the fetus nor the mother (in the absence of cardiovascular disease), but which is associated with edema, including generalized edema, in the majority of pregnant women. If this edema produces discomfort, increased recumbency will often provide relief. In rare instances, this edema may cause extreme discomfort which is not relieved by rest. In these cases, a short course of diuretics may provide relief and may be appropriate.

CONTRAINDICATIONS

Anuria. Severe or progressive kidney disease or dysfunction, with the possible exception of nephrosis. Severe hepatic disease. Hypersensitivity to the drug or any of its components.

Dyrenium (triamterene) should not be used in patients with pre-existing elevated serum potassium, as is sometimes seen in patients with impaired renal function or azotemia, or in patients who develop hyperkalemia while on the drug. Patients should not be placed on dietary potassium supplements, potassium salts or potassium-containing salt substitutes in conjunction with Dyrenium.

Dyrenium should not be given to patients receiving other potassium-sparing agents, such as spironolactone, amiloride hydrochloride, or other formulations containing triamterene. Two deaths have been reported in patients receiving concomitant spironolactone and Dyrenium or Dyazide®. Although dosage recommendations were exceeded in one case and in the other serum electrolytes were not properly monitored, these two drugs should not be given concomitantly.

WARNINGS

Abnormal elevation of serum potassium levels (greater than or equal to 5.5 mEq/liter) can occur with all potassium-sparing agents, including Dyrenium. Hyperkalemia is more likely to occur in patients with renal impairment and diabetes (even without evidence of renal impairment), and in the elderly or severely ill. Since uncorrected hyperkalemia may be fatal, serum potassium levels must be monitored at frequent intervals especially in patients receiving Dyrenium, when dosages are changed or with any illness that may influence renal function.

There have been isolated reports of hypersensitivity reactions; therefore, patients should be observed regularly for the possible occurrence of blood dyscrasias, liver damage or other idiosyncratic reactions.

Periodic BUN and serum potassium determinations should be made to check kidney function, especially in patients with suspected or confirmed renal insufficiency. It is particularly important to make serum potassium determinations in elderly or diabetic patients receiving the drug; these patients should be observed carefully for possible serum potassium increases.

If hyperkalemia is present or suspected, an electrocardiogram should be obtained. If the ECG shows no widening of the QRS or arrhythmia in the presence of hyperkalemia, it is usually sufficient to discontinue Dyrenium (triamterene) and any potassium supplementation, and substitute a thiazide alone. Sodium polystyrene sulfonate (Kayexalate®, Sanofi Synthelabo) may be administered to enhance the excretion of excess potassium. **The presence of a widened QRS complex or arrhythmia in association with hyperkalemia requires prompt additional therapy.** For tachyarrhythmia, infuse 44 mEq of sodium bicarbonate or 10 mL of 10% calcium gluconate or calcium chloride over several minutes. For asystole, bradycardia or A-V block transvenous pacing is also recommended.

The effect of calcium and sodium bicarbonate is transient and repeated administration may be required. When indicated by the clinical situation, excess K+ may be removed by dialysis or oral or rectal administration of Kayexalate®. Infusion of glucose and insulin has also been used to treat hyperkalemia.

PRECAUTIONS

General

Dyrenium (triamterene) tends to conserve potassium rather than to promote the excretion as do many diuretics and, occasionally, can cause increases in serum potassium which, in some instances, can result in hyperkalemia. In rare instances, hyperkalemia has been associated with cardiac irregularities.

Electrolyte imbalance often encountered in such diseases as congestive heart failure, renal disease or cirrhosis may be aggravated or caused independently by any effective diuretic agent includingDyrenium. The use of full doses of a diuretic when salt intake is restricted can result in a low-salt syndrome.

Triamterene can cause mild nitrogen retention, which is reversible upon withdrawal of the drug, and is seldom observed with intermittent (every-other-day) therapy.

Triamterene may cause a decreasing alkali reserve, with the possibility of metabolic acidosis.

By the very nature of their illness, cirrhotics with splenomegaly sometimes have marked variations in their blood. Since triamterene is a weak folic acid antagonist, it may contribute to the appearance of megaloblastosis in cases where folic acid stores have been depleted. Therefore, periodic blood studies in these patients are recommended. They should also be observed for exacerbations of underlying liver disease.

Triamterene has elevated uric acid, especially in persons predisposed to gouty arthritis.

Triamterene has been reported in renal stones in association with other calculus components. Dyrenium should be used with caution in patients with histories of renal stones.

Information for Patients

To help avoid stomach upset, it is recommended that the drug be taken after meals.

If a single daily dose is prescribed, it may be preferable to take it in the morning to minimize the effect of increased frequency of urination on nighttime sleep.

If a dose is missed, the patient should not take more than the prescribed dose at the next dosing interval.

Laboratory Tests

Hyperkalemia will rarely occur in patients with adequate urinary output, but it is a possibility if large doses are used for considerable periods of time. If hyperkalemia is observed, Dyrenium (triamterene) should be withdrawn. The normal adult range of serum potassium is 3.5 to 5.0 mEq per liter, with 4.5 mEq often being used for a reference point. Potassium levels persistently above 6 mEq per liter require careful observation and treatment. Normal potassium levels tend to be higher in neonates (7.7 mEq per liter) than in adults. Serum potassium levels do not necessarily indicate true body potassium concentration. A rise in plasma pH may cause a decrease in plasma potassium concentration and an increase in the intracellular potassium concentration. Because Dyrenium conserves potassium, it has been theorized that in patients who have received intensive therapy or been given the drug for prolonged periods, a rebound kaliuresis could occur upon abrupt withdrawal. In such patients, withdrawal of Dyrenium should be gradual.

Drug Interactions

Caution should be used when lithium and diuretics are used concomitantly because diuretic-induced sodium loss may reduce the renal clearance of lithium and increase serum lithium levels with risk of lithium toxicity. Patients receiving such combined therapy should have serum lithium levels monitored closely and the lithium dosage adjusted if necessary.

A possible interaction resulting in acute renal failure has been reported in a few subjects when indomethacin, a nonsteroidal anti-inflammatory agent, was given with triamterene. Caution is advised in administering nonsteroidal anti-inflammatory agents with triamterene.

The effects of the following drugs may be potentiated when given together with triamterene: antihypertensive medication, other diuretics, preanesthetic and anesthetic agents, skeletal muscle relaxants (nondepolarizing).

Potassium-sparing agents should be used with caution in conjunction with angiotensin-converting enzyme (ACE) inhibitors due to an increased risk of hyperkalemia.

The following agents, given together with triamterene, may promote serum potassium accumulation and possibly result in hyperkalemia because of the potassium-sparing nature of triamterene, especially in patients with renal insufficiency: blood from blood bank (may contain up to 30 mEq of potassium per liter of plasma or up to 65 mEq per liter of whole blood when stored for more than 10 days); low-salt milk (may contain up to 60 mEq of potassium per liter); potassium-containing medications (such as parenteral penicillin G potassium); salt substitutes (most contain substantial amounts of potassium).

Dyrenium (triamterene) may raise blood glucose levels; for adult-onset diabetes, dosage adjustments of hypoglycemic agents may be necessary during and/or after therapy; concurrent use with chlorpropamide may increase the risk of severe hyponatremia.

Drug/Laboratory Test Interactions

Triamterene and quinidine have similar fluorescence spectra; thus, triamterene will interfere with the fluorescent measurement of quinidine.

Carcinogenesis, Mutagenesis, Impairment of Fertility

Carcinogenesis: In studies conducted under the auspices of the National Toxicology Program, groups of rats were fed diets containing 0, 150, 300 or 600 ppm of triamterene, and groups of mice were fed diets containing 0, 100, 200 or 400 ppm triamterene. Male and female rats exposed to the highest tested concentration received triamterene at about 25 and 30 mg/kg/day, respectively. Male and female mice exposed to the highest tested concentration received triamterene at about 45 and 60 mg/kg/day, respectively.

There was an increased incidence of hepatocellular neoplasia (primarily adenomas) in male and female mice at the highest dosage level. These doses represent 7.5× and 10× the Maximum Recommended Human Dose (MRHD) of 300 mg/kg/day (or 6 mg/kg/day based on a 50 kg patient) for male and female mice, respectively, when based on body weight and 0.7× and 0.9× the MRHD when based on body-surface area.

Although hepatocellular neoplasia (exclusively adenomas) in the rat study was limited to triamterene-exposed males, incidence was not dose dependent and there was no statistically significant difference from control incidence at any dose level.

Mutagenesis: Triamterene was not mutagenic in bacteria (Salmonella typhimurium strains TA98, TA100, TA1535 or TA1537) with or without metabolic activation. It did not induce chromosomal aberrations in Chinese hamster ovary (CHO) cells *in vitro* with or without metabolic activation, but it did induce sister chromatid exchanges in CHO cells *in vitro* with and without metabolic activation.

Impairment of Fertility: Studies of the effects of triamterene on animal reproductive function have not been conducted.

Pregnancy: Category C

Teratogenic Effects:

Reproduction studies have been performed in rats at doses as high as 20 times the Maximum Recommended Human Dose (MRHD) on the basis of body weight, and 6 times the MRHD on the basis of body-surface area, without evidence of harm to the fetus due to triamterene. Because animal reproduction studies are not always predictive of human response, this drug should be used during pregnancy only if clearly needed.

Nonteratogenic Effects:

Triamterene has been shown to cross the placental barrier and appear in cord blood. The use of triamterene in pregnant women requires that the anticipated benefits be weighed against possible hazards to the fetus. These possible hazards include adverse reactions which have occurred in the adult.

Nursing Mothers:

Triamterene has not been studied in nursing mothers. Triamterene appears in animal milk and is likely present in human milk. If use of the drug product is deemed essential, the patient should stop nursing.

Pediatric Use:

Safety and effectiveness in pediatric patients have not been established.

ADVERSE REACTIONS

Adverse effects are listed in decreasing order of frequency; however, the most serious adverse effects are listed first, regardless of frequency. All adverse effects occur rarely (that is, 1 in 1000, or less).

Hypersensitivity: anaphylaxis, rash, photosensitivity.

Metabolic: hyperkalemia, hypokalemia.

Renal: azotemia, elevated BUN and creatinine, renal stones, acute interstitial nephritis (rare), acute renal failure (one case of irreversible renal failure has been reported).

Gastrointestinal: jaundice and/or liver enzyme abnormalities, nausea and vomiting, diarrhea.

Hematologic: thrombocytopenia, megaloblastic anemia.

Central Nervous System: weakness, fatigue, dizziness, headache, dry mouth.

To report SUSPECTED ADVERSE REACTIONS, contact WellSpring Pharmaceutical Corporation at 1-866-337-4500 or FDA at 1-800-FDA-1088 or www.fda.gov/medwatch.

OVERDOSAGE

In the event of overdosage, it can be theorized that electrolyte imbalance would be the major concern, with particular attention to possible hyperkalemia. Other symptoms that might be seen would be nausea and vomiting, other G.I. disturbances and weakness. It is conceivable that some hypotension could occur. As with an overdose of any drug, immediate evacuation of the stomach should be induced through emesis and gastric lavage. Careful evaluation of the electrolyte pattern and fluid balance should be made. There is no specific antidote.

Reversible acute renal failure following ingestion of 50 tablets of a product containing a combination of 50 mg triamterene and 25 mg hydrochlorothiazide has been reported.

The oral LD50 in mice is 380 mg/kg. The amount of drug in a single dose ordinarily associated with symptoms of overdose or likely to be life-threatening is not known.

Although triamterene is 67% protein bound, there may be some benefit to dialysis in cases of overdosage.

DOSAGE AND ADMINISTRATION

Adult Dosage

Dosage should be titrated to the needs of the individual patient. When used alone, the usual starting dose is 100 mg twice daily after meals. When combined with another diuretic or antihypertensive agent, the total daily dosage of each agent should usually be lowered initially and then adjusted to the patient's needs. The total daily dosage should not exceed 300 mg. Please refer to PRECAUTIONS–General.

When Dyrenium (triamterene) is added to other diuretic therapy or when patients are switched to Dyrenium from other diuretics, all potassium supplementation should be discontinued.

HOW SUPPLIED

Capsules: 50 mg in bottles of 100, and 100 mg in bottles of 100.

STORAGE

Store at 25°C (77°F); excursions permitted to 15° - 30°C (59° - 86°F) [See USP Controlled Room Temperature]. Dispense in a tight, light resistant container.

50 mg 100s: NDC 65197-002-01
100 mg 100s: NDC 65197-003-01
DATE OF ISSUANCE MARCH 2009
©WellSpring, 2009
Manufactured for
WellSpring Pharmaceutical Corporation
Sarasota, FL 34243 USA
By WellSpring Pharmaceutical Canada Corp.
Oakville, Ontario L6H 1M5 Canada
Rev. 03/09

Shown in Product Identification Guide, page 314

Wyeth Pharmaceuticals

A Division of Pfizer
235 EAST 42ND STREET
NEW YORK, NY 10017-5755

For updates to the product information listed below, please check the Pfizer Web site, http://www.pfizerpro.com, or call (800) 438-1985. For complete product listing, please see the Manufacturers' Index.

For Medical Information, Contact:
(800) 438-1985
24 hours a day, 7 days a week

Distribution:
1855 Shelby Oaks Drive North
Memphis, TN 38134
(901) 387-5200

Customer Service:
(800) 533-4535

BENEFIX ℞

[*bĕnĕ-fiks*]

[Coagulation Factor IX (Recombinant)]
For Intravenous Use, Lyophilized Powder for Reconstitution

HIGHLIGHTS OF PRESCRIBING INFORMATION

These highlights do not include all the information needed to use BeneFIX safely and effectively. See full prescribing information for BeneFIX.

BeneFIX [Coagulation Factor IX (Recombinant)] For Intravenous Use, Lyophilized Powder for Reconstitution

Initial U.S. Approval: 1997

INDICATIONS AND USAGE

BeneFIX is an antihemophilic factor (recombinant) indicated for:

- Control and prevention of bleeding episodes in adult and pediatric patients with hemophilia B. (1.1)
- Peri-operative management in adult and pediatric patients with hemophilia B. (1.2)

DOSAGE AND ADMINISTRATION

For Intravenous Use only

The initial estimated dose may be determined using the following formula: (2)

Required units = body weight (kg) × desired factor IX increase (IU/dL or % of normal) × reciprocal of observed recovery (IU/kg per IU/dL)

Average Recovery: Adult and Pediatric (<15 years) Patients

In clinical studies with adult and pediatric (<15 years) patients, one IU of BeneFIX per kilogram of body weight increased the circulating activity of factor IX as follows:

- Adults: 0.8 ± 0.2 IU/dL [range 0.4 to 1.2 IU/dL]. (2.2)
- Pediatric: 0.7 ± 0.3 IU/dL [range 0.2 to 2.1 IU/dL]. (2.2)

Dosing of BeneFIX may differ from that of plasma-derived factor IX products.

Dosage and duration of treatment with BeneFIX depends on the severity of the factor IX deficiency, the location and extent of bleeding, and the patient's clinical condition, age and recovery of factor IX. (2.1)

DOSAGE FORMS AND STRENGTHS

BeneFIX lyophilized powder is available as 250, 500, 1000, 2000, or 3000 IU in single-use vials. (3)

CONTRAINDICATIONS

BeneFIX is contraindicated in patients who have manifested life-threatening, immediate hypersensitivity reactions, including anaphylaxis, to the product or its components, including hamster protein. (4)

WARNINGS AND PRECAUTIONS

- Anaphylaxis and severe hypersensitivity reactions are possible. Should symptoms occur, treatment with the product should be discontinued, and emergency treatment should be sought. Patients may develop hypersensitivity to hamster (CHO) protein as BeneFIX contains trace amounts. (5.2)
- BeneFIX has been associated with the development of thromboembolic complications, including patients receiving continuous infusion through a central venous catheter. (5.3)
- Nephrotic syndrome has been reported following immune tolerance induction with factor IX products in hemophilia B patients with factor IX inhibitors and a history of allergic reactions to factor IX. (5.4)

Development of activity-neutralizing antibodies has been detected in patients receiving factor IX-containing products. If expected plasma factor IX activity levels are not attained, or if patient presents with allergic reaction, or if bleeding is not controlled with an expected dose, an assay that measures factor IX inhibitor concentration should be performed. (5.5)

ADVERSE REACTIONS

The most common adverse reactions (incidence >5%) from clinical trials were nausea, injection site reaction, injection site pain, headache, dizziness and rash. (6.1)

To report SUSPECTED ADVERSE REACTIONS, contact Wyeth Pharmaceuticals Inc. at 1-800-934-5556 or FDA at 1-800-FDA-1088 or www.fda.gov/medwatch

USE IN SPECIFIC POPULATIONS

Pregnancy: No human or animal data. Use only if clearly needed. (8.1)

Pediatric Use: On average, lower recovery has been observed in pediatric patients (<15 years). A dose adjustment may be needed. (12.3, 14)

See 17 for PATIENT COUNSELING INFORMATION and FDA-approved patient labeling

Revised: 03/2012

FULL PRESCRIBING INFORMATION: CONTENTS*

*** Sections or subsections omitted from the full prescribing information are not listed**

FULL PRESCRIBING INFORMATION

1 INDICATIONS AND USAGE

1.1 Control and Prevention of Bleeding Episodes in Hemophilia B

BeneFIX®, Coagulation Factor IX (Recombinant), is indicated for the control and prevention of bleeding episodes in adult and pediatric patients with hemophilia B (congenital factor IX deficiency or Christmas disease).

1.2 Peri-operative Management in Patients with Hemophilia B

BeneFIX, Coagulation Factor IX (Recombinant), is indicated for peri-operative management in adult and pediatric patients with hemophilia B.

BeneFIX, Coagulation Factor IX (Recombinant), is NOT indicated for:

a. treatment of other factor deficiencies (e.g., factors II, VII, VIII, and X),
b. treatment of hemophilia A patients with inhibitors to factor VIII,
c. reversal of coumarin-induced anticoagulation,
d. treatment of bleeding due to low levels of liver-dependent coagulation factors.

2 DOSAGE AND ADMINISTRATION

2.1 General Considerations for Administration

For Intravenous Use after Reconstitution

- **Treatment with BeneFIX, Coagulation Factor IX (Recombinant), should be initiated under the supervision of a physician experienced in the treatment of hemophilia B.**
- **Each vial of BeneFIX has the rFIX potency in the International Units (IU) stated on the vial.**
- **Dosage and duration of treatment for all factor IX products depend on the severity of the factor IX deficiency, the location and extent of bleeding, and the patient's clinical condition, age and recovery of factor IX.**

To ensure that the desired factor IX activity level has been achieved, precise monitoring using the factor IX activity assay is advised. Doses should be titrated using the factor IX activity, pharmacokinetic parameters, such as half-life and recovery, as well as taking the clinical situation into consideration in order to adjust the dose as appropriate.

Dosing of BeneFIX may differ from that of plasma-derived factor IX products [*see Clinical Pharmacology (12)*]. **Subjects at the low end of the observed factor IX recovery may require upward dosage adjustment of BeneFIX to as much as two times (2X) the initial empirically calculated dose in order to achieve the intended rise in circulating factor IX activity.**

The safety and efficacy of BeneFIX administration by continuous infusion have not been established [*see Warnings and Precautions (5.3)*].

Table 4

Type of Hemorrhage	Circulating Factor IX Activity Required [% or (IU/dL)]	Dosing Interval [hours]	Duration of Therapy [days]
Minor			
Uncomplicated hemarthroses, superficial muscle, or soft tissue	20-30	12-24	1-2
Moderate			
Intramuscle or soft tissue with dissection, mucous membranes, dental extractions, or hematuria	25-50	12-24	Treat until bleeding stops and healing begins, about 2 to 7 days
Major			
Pharynx, retropharynx, retroperitoneum, CNS, surgery	50-100	12-24	7-10

Adapted from: Roberts and Eberst[1]

2.2 Method of Calculating Initial Estimated Dose

The method of calculating the factor IX dose is shown in Table 1.

Table 1

number of factor IX IU required (IU)	=	body weight (kg)	×	desired factor IX increase (% or IU/dL)	×	reciprocal of observed recovery (IU/kg per IU/dL)

Average Recovery Adult Patients in Clinical Trial

In adult PTPs, on average, one International Unit (IU) of BeneFIX per kilogram of body weight increased the circulating activity of factor IX by 0.8 ± 0.2 IU/dL (range 0.4 to 1.2 IU/dL). The method of dose estimation is illustrated in Table 2. If you use 0.8 IU/dL average increase of factor IX per IU/kg body weight administered, then:

Table 2

number of factor IX IU required (IU)	=	body weight (kg)	×	desired factor IX increase (% or IU/dL)	×	1.3 (IU/kg per IU/dL)

Average Recovery Pediatric Patients (<15 years) in Clinical Trial

In pediatric patients, on average, one international unit of BeneFIX per kilogram of body weight increased the circulating activity of factor IX by 0.7 ± 0.3 IU/dL (range 0.2 to 2.1 IU/dL; median of 0.6 IU/dL per IU/kg). The method of dose estimation is illustrated in Table 3. If you use 0.7 IU/dL average increase of factor IX per IU/kg body weight administered, then:

Table 3

number of factor IX IU required (IU)	=	body weight (kg)	×	desired factor IX increase (% or IU/dL)	×	1.4 (IU/kg per IU/dL)

Doses administered should be titrated to the patient's clinical response. Patients may vary in their pharmacokinetic (e.g., half-life, *in vivo* recovery) and clinical responses to BeneFIX. Although the dose can be estimated by the calculations above, it is highly recommended that, whenever possible, appropriate laboratory tests, including serial factor IX activity assays, be performed.

2.3 Dosing Guide for Control and Prevention of Bleeding Episodes and Peri-operative Management

[See table 4 above]

2.4 Instructions for Use

BeneFIX is administered by intravenous (IV) infusion after reconstitution of the lyophilized powder with the supplied pre-filled diluent (0.234% sodium chloride solution) syringe. Patients should follow the specific reconstitution and administration procedures provided by their physicians.

For instructions, patients should follow the recommendations in the FDA-Approved Patient Labeling [*see Patient Counseling Information (17)*].

Reconstitution, product administration, and handling of the administration set must be done with caution. Discard all equipment, including any reconstituted BeneFIX product, in an appropriate container. Place needles used for venipuncture in a sharps container after single use. Percutaneous puncture with a needle contaminated with blood from an infected patient can transmit infectious viruses including HIV (AIDS) and hepatitis. Obtain immediate medical attention if injury occurs.

2.5 Preparation and Reconstitution

The procedures below are provided as general guidelines for the reconstitution and administration of BeneFIX.

Preparation

1. Always wash your hands before performing the following procedures.
2. Aseptic technique (meaning clean and germ-free) should be used during the reconstitution procedure.
3. Use all components in the reconstitution and administration of this product as soon as possible after opening their sterile containers to minimize unnecessary exposure to the atmosphere.

   Note: If you use more than one vial of BeneFIX per infusion, each vial should be reconstituted according to the following instructions. The diluent syringe should be removed leaving the vial adapter in place, and a separate large luer lock syringe may be used to draw back the reconstituted contents of each vial. Do not detach the diluent syringes or the large luer lock syringe until you are ready to attach the large luer lock syringe to the next vial adapter.

Reconstitution

1. If refrigerated allow the vial of lyophilized BeneFIX and the pre-filled diluent syringe to reach room temperature.
2. Remove the plastic flip-top cap from the BeneFIX vial to expose the central portions of the rubber stopper.

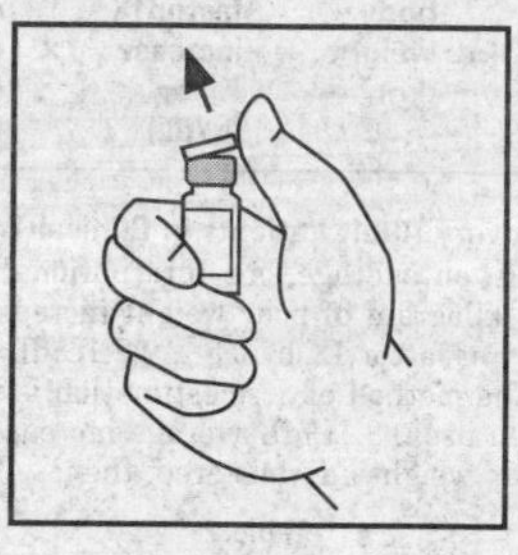

3. Wipe the top of the vial with the alcohol swab provided, or use another antiseptic solution, and allow to dry. After cleaning, do not touch the rubber stopper with your hand or allow it to touch any surface.
4. Peel back the cover from the clear plastic vial adapter package. **Do not remove the adapter from the package.**
5. Place the vial on a flat surface. While holding the adapter in the package, place the vial adapter over the vial and press down firmly on the package until the adapter spike penetrates the vial stopper.

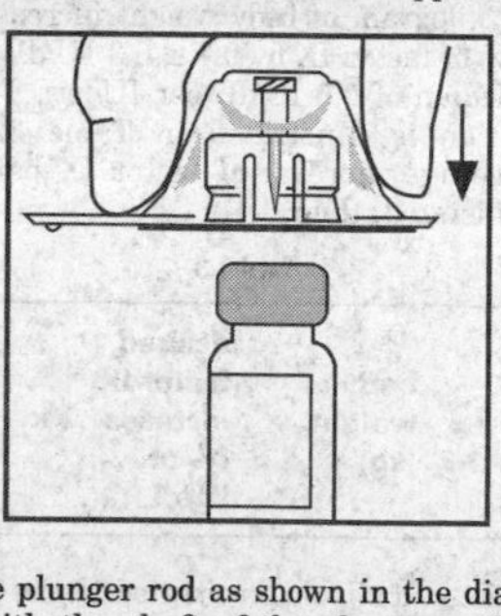

6. Grasp the plunger rod as shown in the diagram. Avoid contact with the shaft of the plunger rod. Attach the threaded end of the plunger rod to the diluent syringe plunger by pushing and turning firmly.

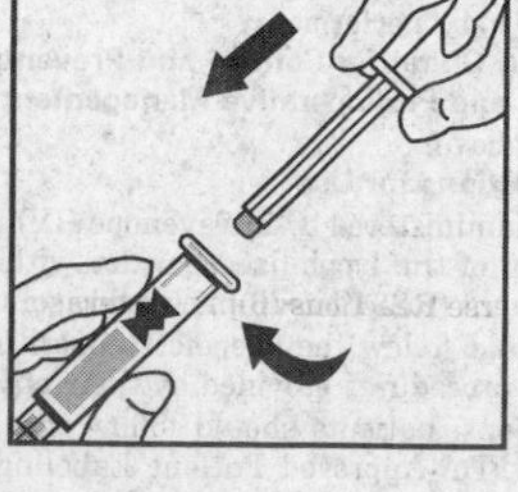

7. Break off the tamper-resistant plastic-tip cap from the diluent syringe by snapping the perforation of the cap. Do not touch the inside of the cap or the syringe tip. The diluent syringe may need to be recapped (if not administering reconstituted BeneFIX immediately), so place the cap on its top on a clean surface in a spot where it would be least likely to become environmentally contaminated.

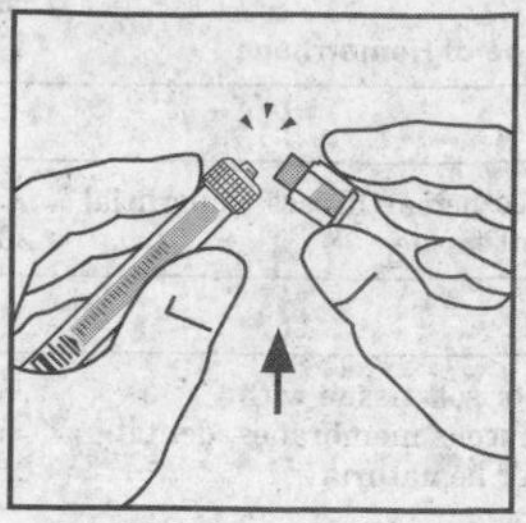

8. Lift the package away from the adapter and discard the package.

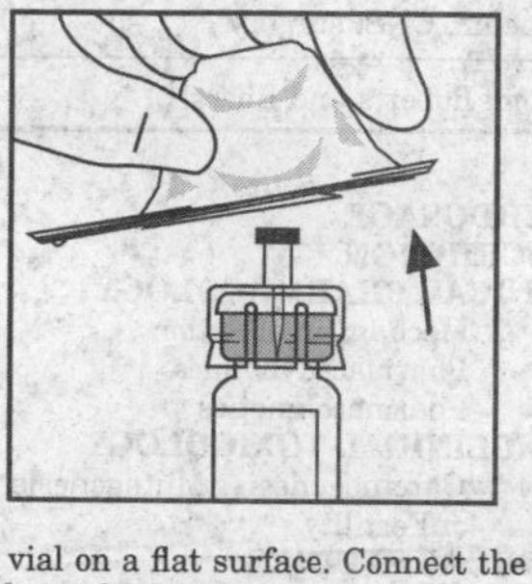

9. Place the vial on a flat surface. Connect the diluent syringe to the vial adapter by inserting the tip into the adapter opening while firmly pushing and turning the syringe clockwise until secured.

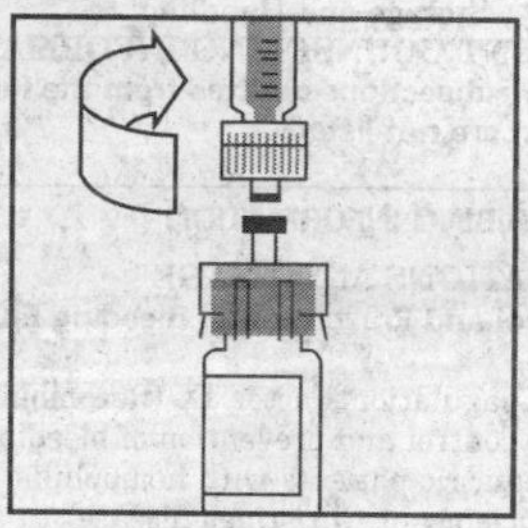

10. Slowly depress the plunger rod to inject all the diluent into the BeneFIX vial.

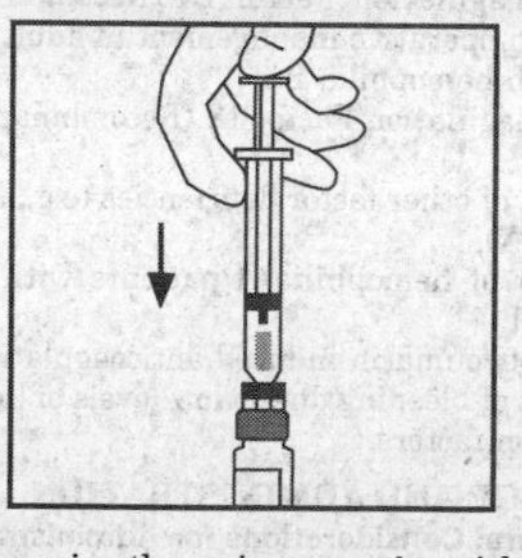

11. Without removing the syringe, **gently** swirl the contents of the vial until the powder is dissolved.

    Note: The final solution should be inspected visually for particulate matter before administration. The solution should appear clear and colorless. If it is not, the solution should be discarded and a new kit should be used.
12. Invert the vial and slowly draw the solution into the syringe.

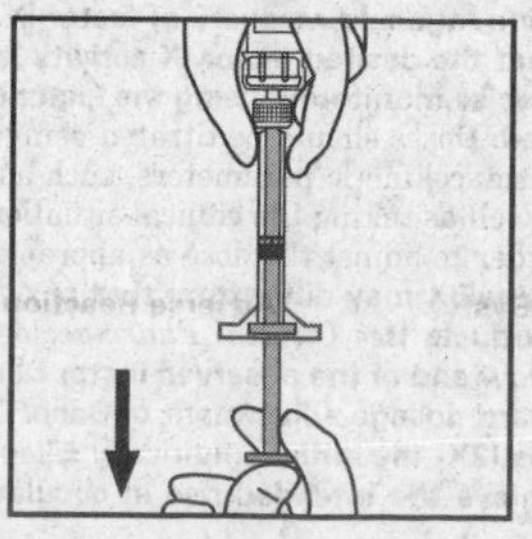

13. Detach the syringe from the vial adapter by gently pulling and turning the syringe counter-clockwise. Discard the vial with the adapter attached.

    Note: If the solution is not to be used immediately, the syringe cap should be carefully replaced. Do not touch the syringe tip or the inside of the cap.

BeneFIX, when reconstituted, contains polysorbate-80, which is known to increase the rate of di-(2-ethylhexyl)phthalate (DEHP) extraction from polyvinyl chloride (PVC). This should be considered during the preparation and administration of BeneFIX, including storage time elapsed in a PVC container following reconstitution. It is important that the recommendations for dosage and administration be followed closely [*see Dosage and Administration (2)*].

Note: The tubing of the infusion set included with this kit does not contain DEHP.

2.6 Administration (Intravenous Injection)

For Intravenous Use only after Reconstitution

BeneFIX is administered by intravenous (IV) infusion after reconstitution with the pre-filled diluent (0.234% sodium chloride solution) syringe.

- BeneFIX should be inspected for particulate matter and discoloration prior to administration, whenever solution and container permit.
- The reconstituted solution may be stored at room temperature prior to administration, but BeneFIX should be administered within 3 hours. BeneFIX should be administered using the tubing provided in this kit, and the pre-filled diluent syringe provided, or a single sterile disposable plastic syringe. In addition, the solution should be withdrawn from the vial using the vial adapter.
- A dose of BeneFIX may be administered over a period of several minutes. The rate of administration, however, should be adapted to the comfort level of each individual patient.

1. Attach the syringe to the luer end of the infusion set tubing provided.
2. Apply a tourniquet and prepare the injections site by wiping the skin well with an alcohol swab provided in the kit.

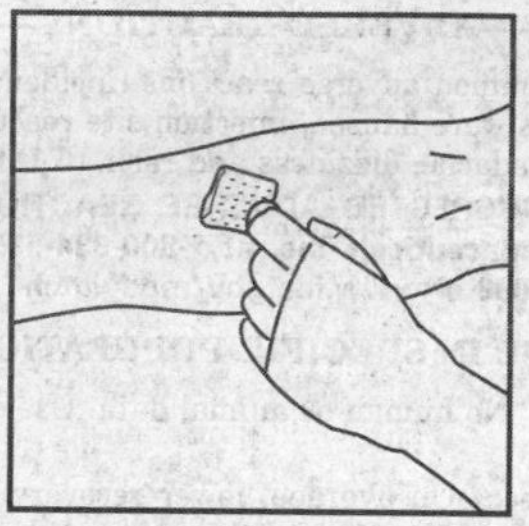

3. Perform venipuncture. Insert the needle on the infusion set tubing into the vein, and remove the tourniquet. The reconstituted BeneFIX product should be injected intravenously over several minutes. The rate of administration should be determined by the patient's comfort level.

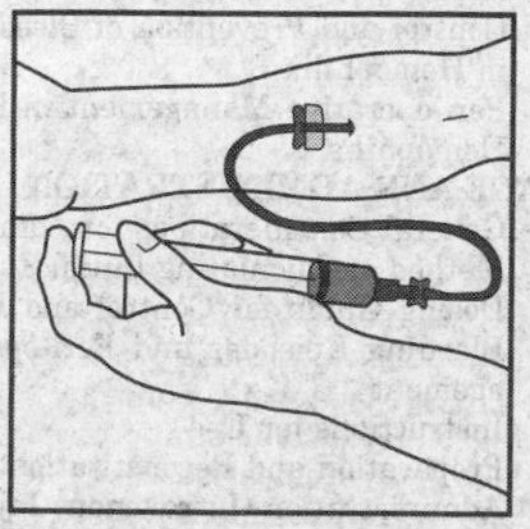

Reconstituted BeneFIX should not be administered in the same tubing or container with other medicinal products. Agglutination of red blood cells in the tubing/syringe has been reported with the administration of BeneFIX. No adverse events have been reported in association with this observation. To minimize the possibility of agglutination, it is important to limit the amount of blood entering the tubing. Blood should not enter the syringe. If red blood cell agglutination is observed in the tubing or syringe, discard all material (tubing, syringe and BeneFIX solution) and resume administration with a new package.

Following completion of BeneFIX treatment, remove the infusion set and discard. Dispose of all unused solution, empty vial(s), and used needles and syringes in an appropriate container for throwing away waste that might hurt others if not handled properly.

The safety and efficacy of administration by continuous infusion have not been established [*see Warnings and Precautions (5.3)*].

3 DOSAGE FORMS AND STRENGTHS

BeneFIX is supplied as a white lyophilized powder in the following dosages:

- 250 IU
- 500 IU
- 1000 IU
- 2000 IU
- 3000 IU

4 CONTRAINDICATIONS

BeneFIX is contraindicated in patients who have manifested life-threatening, immediate hypersensitivity reactions, including anaphylaxis, to the product or its components, including hamster protein.

5 WARNINGS AND PRECAUTIONS

5.1 General

The clinical response to BeneFIX may vary. If bleeding is not controlled with the recommended dose, the plasma level of factor IX should be determined, and a sufficient dose of BeneFIX should be administered to achieve a satisfactory clinical response. If the patient's plasma factor IX level fails to increase as expected or if bleeding is not controlled after the expected dose, the presence of an inhibitor (neutralizing antibodies) should be suspected, and appropriate testing performed [*see Warnings and Precautions (5.6)*].

5.2 Anaphylaxis and Severe Hypersensitivity Reactions

Allergic type hypersensitivity reactions, including anaphylaxis, have been reported with BeneFIX and have manifested as pruritus, rash, urticaria, hives, facial swelling, dizziness, hypotension, nausea, chest discomfort, cough, dyspnea, wheezing, flushing, discomfort (generalized) and fatigue. Frequently, these events have occurred in close temporal association with the development of factor IX inhibitors. Advise patients to discontinue use of the product and contact their physician and/or seek immediate emergency care.

BeneFIX contains trace amounts of hamster (CHO) proteins. Patients treated with this product may develop hypersensitivity to these non-human mammalian proteins.

5.3 Thromboembolic Complications

The safety and efficacy of BeneFIX administration by continuous infusion have not been established [*see Dosage and Administration (2)*]. There have been post-marketing reports of thrombotic events in patients receiving continuous-infusion BeneFIX through a central venous catheter, including life-threatening superior vena cava (SVC) syndrome in critically ill neonates [*see Adverse Reactions (6.2)*].

5.4 Nephrotic Syndrome

Nephrotic syndrome has been reported following immune tolerance induction with factor IX products in hemophilia B patients with factor IX inhibitors and a history of allergic reactions to factor IX. The safety and efficacy of using BeneFIX for immune tolerance induction have not been established.

5.5 Neutralizing Antibodies (Immunogenicity)

Patients using BeneFIX should be monitored for the development of factor IX inhibitors by appropriate clinical observations and laboratory tests. Inhibitors have been reported following administration of BeneFIX [*see Adverse Reactions (6.1)*]. If expected plasma factor IX activity levels are not attained, or if bleeding is not controlled with an expected dose, an assay that measures factor IX inhibitor concentration should be performed.

Patients with factor IX inhibitors may be at an increased risk of anaphylaxis upon subsequent challenge with factor IX.[2] Patients experiencing allergic reactions should be evaluated for the presence of an inhibitor. Patients should be observed closely for signs and symptoms of acute hypersensitivity reactions, particularly during the early phases of initial exposure to product. **Because of the potential for allergic reactions with factor IX concentrates, the initial (approximately 10 - 20) administrations of factor IX should be performed under medical supervision where proper medical care for allergic reactions could be provided.**

5.6 Monitoring Laboratory Tests

- Patients should be monitored for factor IX activity levels by the one-stage clotting assay to confirm that adequate factor IX levels have been achieved and maintained, when clinically indicated [*see Dosage and Administration (2)*].
- Patients should be monitored for the development of inhibitors if expected factor IX activity plasma levels are not attained, or if bleeding is not controlled with the recommended dose of BeneFIX. Assays used to determine if factor IX inhibitor is present should be titered in Bethesda Units (BUs).

6 ADVERSE REACTIONS

The most serious adverse reactions are systemic hypersensitivity reactions, including bronchospastic reactions and/or hypotension and anaphylaxis and the development of high-titer inhibitors necessitating alternative treatments to factor IX replacement therapy.

The most common adverse reactions observed in clinical trials (frequency > 5% of PTPs or PUPs) were headaches, dizziness, nausea, injections site reaction, injection site pain and skin-related hypersensitivity reactions (e.g., rash, hives).

6.1 Clinical Trials Experience

Because clinical trials are conducted under widely varying conditions, adverse reaction rates observed in the clinical trials of a drug cannot be directly compared to rates in the clinical trials of another drug and may not reflect the rates observed in clinical practice.

During uncontrolled open-label clinical studies with BeneFIX, Coagulation Factor IX (Recombinant), conducted in previously treated patients (PTPs), 113 adverse reactions with known or unknown relation to BeneFIX therapy were reported among 38.5% (25 of 65) of subjects (with some subjects reporting more than one event) who received a total of 7,573 infusions. These adverse reactions are summarized in Table 5.

Table 5: Adverse Reactions Reported for PTPs*

Body System	Adverse Reaction	Number of patients (%)
Blood and lymphatic system disorders	Factor IX inhibition[1]	1 (1.5%)
Eye disorders	Blurred vision	1 (1.5%)
Gastrointestinal disorders	Nausea	4 (6.2%)
	Vomiting	1 (1.5%)
General disorders and administration site conditions	Injection site reaction	5 (7.7%)
	Injection site pain	4 (6.2%)
	Fever	2 (3.1%)
Infections and infestations	Cellulitis at IV site	1 (1.5%)
	Phlebitis at IV site	1 (1.5%)
Nervous system disorders	Headache	7 (10.8%)
	Dizziness	5 (7.7%)
	Taste perversion (altered taste)	3 (4.6%)
	Shaking	1 (1.5%)
	Drowsiness	1 (1.5%)
Renal and urinary disorders	Renal infarct[2]	1 (1.5%)
Respiratory, thoracic and mediastinal disorders	Dry cough	1 (1.5%)
	Hypoxia	1 (1.5%)
	Chest tightness	1 (1.5%)
Skin and subcutaneous disorders	Rash	4 (6.2%)
	Hives	2 (3.1%)
Vascular disorders	Flushing	2 (3.1%)

*Adverse reactions reported within 72 hours of an infusion of BeneFIX.

[1]Low-titer transient inhibitor formation.

[2]The renal infarct developed in a hepatitis C antibody-positive patient 12 days after a dose of BeneFIX for a bleeding episode. The relationship of the infarct to the prior administration of BeneFIX is uncertain.

In the 63 previously untreated patients (PUPs), who received a total of 5,538 infusions, 10 adverse reactions were reported among 9.5% of the patients (6 out of 63) having known or unknown relationship to BeneFIX. These events are summarized in Table 6.

Table 6: Adverse Reactions Reported for PUPs*

Body System	Adverse Reaction	Number of Patients (%)
Blood and lymphatic system disorders	Factor IX inhibition[1]	2 (3.2%)
General disorders and administration site conditions	Injection site reaction	1 (1.6%)
	Chills	1 (1.6%)
Respiratory, thoracic and mediastinal disorders	Dyspnea (respiratory distress)	2 (3.2%)
Skin and subcutaneous disorders	Hives	3 (4.8%)
	Rash	1 (1.6%)

*Adverse reactions reported within 72 hours of an infusion of BeneFIX.

[1]Two subjects developed high-titer inhibitor formation during treatment with BeneFIX.

For adverse reactions thought to be related to the administration of BeneFIX, the rate of infusion should be decreased or the infusion stopped.

Immunogenicity

In clinical studies with 65 PTPs (defined as having more than 50 exposure days), a low-titer inhibitor was observed in one patient. The inhibitor was transient, the patient continued on study and had normal factor IX recovery pharmacokinetics at study completion (approximately 15 months after inhibitor detection).

In clinical studies with pediatric PUPs, inhibitor development was observed in 2 out of 63 patients (3.2%), both were high-titer (> 5 BU) inhibitors detected after 7 and 15 exposure days, respectively. Both patients were withdrawn from the study.

6.2 Post-marketing Experience

The following post-marketing adverse reactions have been reported for BeneFIX: inadequate factor IX recovery, inadequate therapeutic response, inhibitor development [*see Clinical Pharmacology (12)*], anaphylaxis [*see Warnings and Precautions (5.2)*], angioedema, dyspnea, hypotension, and thrombosis.

Because these reactions are reported voluntarily from a population of uncertain size, it is not always possible to reliably estimate their frequency or establish a causal relationship to drug exposure.

The safety and efficacy of BeneFIX administration by continuous infusion have not been established [*see Warnings and Precautions (5.3)*]. There have been post-marketing reports of thrombotic events, including life-threatening SVC syndrome in critically ill neonates, while receiving continuous-infusion BeneFIX through a central venous catheter. Cases of peripheral thrombophlebitis and DVT have also been reported. In some, BeneFIX was administered via **continuous infusion, which is not an approved method of administration** [*see Dosage and Administration (2)*].

7 DRUG INTERACTIONS

None known.

8 USE IN SPECIFIC POPULATIONS

8.1 Pregnancy

Pregnancy Category C

Animal reproduction and lactation studies have not been conducted with BeneFIX, Coagulation Factor IX (Recombinant). It is not known whether BeneFIX can affect reproductive capacity or cause fetal harm when given to pregnant women. BeneFIX should be administered to pregnant women only if needed.

8.2 Labor and Delivery

There is no information available on the effect of factor IX replacement therapy on labor and delivery. Use only if needed.

8.3 Nursing Mothers

It is not known whether this drug is excreted into human milk. Because many drugs are excreted into human milk, caution should be exercised if BeneFIX is administered to nursing mothers.

Use only if needed.

8.4 Pediatric Use

Safety, efficacy, and pharmacokinetics of BeneFIX have been evaluated in previously treated (PTP) and previously untreated pediatric patients (PUP) [*see Dosage and Administration (2), Clinical Pharmacology (12.3)*, Clinical Studies (14) and Adverse Reactions (6)]. On average, lower recovery has been observed in pediatric patients (<15 years). A dose adjustment may be needed [*see Dosage and Administration (2) and Clinical Pharmacology (12.3)*].

8.5 Geriatric Use

Clinical studies of BeneFIX did not include sufficient numbers of subjects aged 65 and over to determine whether they respond differently from younger subjects. Dose selection for an elderly patient should be individualized [*see Dosage and Administration (2)*].

Table 10: Efficacy of BeneFIX for on-demand treatment of PTPs and PUPs

	Median dose: IU/kg (range)	Rate of bleeds resolved with 1 infusion	Response to 1st Infusion Rating[c]		
			Excellent/Good	Moderate	No Response
PTPs					
N=55[a]	42.8 (6.5 - 224.6)	81 %	90.9%	7.1%	0.7%
PUPs					
N=54[b]	62.7 (8.2 - 292)	75 %	94.1%	2.9%	1.0%

[a] One subject discontinued the study after one month of treatment due to bleeding episodes that were difficult to control; he did not have a detectable inhibitor.
[b] Three subjects were not successfully treated including one episode in a subject due to delayed time to infusion and insufficient dosing and in 2 subjects due to inhibitor formation.
[c]Response ratings not provided for 1.3% and 2% of 1st infusions for PTPs and PUPs, respectively.

10 OVERDOSAGE

No symptoms of overdose have been reported.

11 DESCRIPTION

BeneFIX, Coagulation Factor IX (Recombinant), is a purified protein produced by recombinant DNA. It has a primary amino acid sequence that is identical to the Ala[148] allelic form of plasma-derived factor IX, and has structural and functional characteristics similar to those of endogenous factor IX. BeneFIX is produced by a genetically engineered Chinese hamster ovary (CHO) cell line that is extensively characterized. No human or animal proteins are added during the purification and formulation processes of BeneFIX.
BeneFIX is not derived from human blood and contains no preservatives, and the manufacture of BeneFIX includes no added animal or human components. The stored cell banks are free of human blood or plasma products. The CHO cell line secretes recombinant factor IX into a defined cell culture medium that does not contain any proteins derived from animal or human sources, and the recombinant factor IX is purified by a chromatography purification process that does not require a monoclonal antibody step. The process also includes a membrane nanofiltration step that has the ability to retain molecules with apparent molecular weights >70,000 Da (such as large proteins and viral particles).
BeneFIX is a single component by SDS-polyacrylamide gel electrophoresis evaluation. The potency (in International Units, IU) is determined using an *in vitro* one-stage clotting assay against the World Health Organization (WHO) International Standard for Factor IX concentrate. One International Unit is the amount of factor IX activity present in 1 mL of pooled, normal human plasma. The specific activity of BeneFIX is greater than or equal to 200 IU per milligram of protein.
BeneFIX is formulated as a sterile, nonpyrogenic, lyophilized powder preparation. BeneFIX is intended for intravenous (IV) injection. It is available in single-use vials containing the labeled amount of factor IX activity, expressed in IU. Each vial contains nominally 250, 500, 1000, 2000, or 3000 IU of Coagulation Factor IX (Recombinant). After reconstitution of the lyophilized drug product, the concentrations of excipients are 0.234% sodium chloride, 8 mM L-histidine, 0.8% sucrose, 208 mM glycine, 0.004% polysorbate 80. All dosage strengths yield a clear, colorless solution upon reconstitution.

12 CLINICAL PHARMACOLOGY

12.1 Mechanism of Action

BeneFIX temporarily replaces the missing clotting factor IX that is needed for effective hemostasis.

12.2 Pharmacodynamics

The activated partial thromboplastin time (aPTT) is prolonged in people with hemophilia B. Treatment with factor IX concentrate may normalize the aPTT by temporarily replacing the factor IX. The administration of BeneFIX, Coagulation Factor IX (Recombinant), increases plasma levels of factor IX, and can temporarily correct the coagulation defect in these patients.

12.3 Pharmacokinetics

After single intravenous (IV) doses of 50 IU/kg of previously marketed BeneFIX, Coagulation Factor IX (Recombinant) [reconstituted with Sterile Water for Injection], in 37 previously treated adult patients (>15 years), each given as a 10-minute infusion, the mean increase from pre-infusion level in circulating factor IX activity was 0.8 ± 0.2 IU/dL per IU/kg infused (range 0.4 to 1.4 IU/dL per IU/kg) and the mean biologic half-life was 18.8 ± 5.4 hours (range 11 to 36 hours). In the original randomized, cross-over pharmacokinetic study in previously treated patients (PTPs), the *in vivo* recovery using previously marketed BeneFIX was statistically significantly less (28% lower, $p<0.05$) than the recovery using a highly purified plasma-derived factor IX product (pdFIX). A summary of pharmacokinetic data for BeneFIX and pdFIX are presented in Table 7.

Table 7: Pharmacokinetic Parameter Estimates for BeneFIX and pdFIX in Previously Treated Patients with Hemophilia B

Parameter	BeneFIX, n = 11	pdFIX, n = 11
	Mean ± SD	Mean ± SD
AUC_∞ (IU•hr/dL)	548 ± 92	928 ± 191
$t_{1/2}$ (hr)	18.1 ± 5.1	17.7 ± 5.3
CL (mL/hr/kg)	8.62 ± 1.7	6.00 ± 1.4
K-value (IU/dL per IU/kg)	0.84 ± 0.30	1.17 ± 0.26
In vivo Recovery (%)	37.8 ± 14.0	52.6 ± 12.4

Abbreviations: AUC_∞ = area under the plasma concentration-time curve from time zero to infinity; K-value = incremental recovery; $t_{1/2}$ = plasma elimination half-life; CL = clearance; SD = standard deviation.

There was no significant difference in biological half-life. Structural differences of the BeneFIX molecule compared with pdFIX were shown to contribute to the lower recovery. In subsequent evaluations for up to 24 months, the pharmacokinetic parameters were similar to the initial results.
In a subsequent randomized, cross-over pharmacokinetic study, BeneFIX reconstituted in 0.234% sodium chloride diluent was shown to be pharmacokinetically equivalent to the previously marketed BeneFIX (reconstituted with Sterile Water for Injection) in 24 previously treated patients (≥12 years) at a dose of 75 IU/kg. In addition, pharmacokinetic parameters were followed up in 23 previously treated patients after repeated administration of BeneFIX for six months and found to be unchanged compared with those obtained at the initial evaluation. A summary of pharmacokinetic data are presented in Table 8:

Table 8: Pharmacokinetic Parameter Estimates for BeneFIX at Baseline (Cross-over phase) and Month 6 (Follow-up phase) in Previously Treated Patients with Hemophilia B

Parameter	Parameters at Initial Visit (Cross-over phase), n = 24 Mean ± SD	Parameters at Month 6 (Follow-up phase), n = 23 Mean ± SD
C_{max} (IU/dL)	54.5 ± 15.0	57.3 ± 13.2
AUC_∞ (IU•hr/dL)	940 ± 237	923 ± 205
$t_{1/2}$ (hr)	22.4 ± 5.3	23.8 ± 6.5
CL (mL/hr/kg)	8.47 ± 2.12	8.54 ± 2.04
K-value (IU/dL per IU/kg)	0.73 ± 0.20	0.76 ± 0.18
In vivo Recovery (%)	34.5 ± 9.3	36.8 ± 8.7

Abbreviations: AUC_∞ = area under the plasma concentration-time curve from time zero to infinity; AUC_t = area under the plasma concentration-time curve from zero to the last measurable concentration; C_{max} = peak concentration; K-value = incremental recovery; $t_{1/2}$ = plasma elimination half-life; CL = clearance; SD = standard deviation.

Pediatric Patients (≤15 years)
Nineteen (19) previously treated pediatric patients (range 4 to ≤15 years) underwent pharmacokinetic evaluations for up to 24 months. Fifty-eight previously untreated patients [PUPs] less than 15 years of age at baseline underwent at least one recovery assessment within 30 minutes post-infusion in the presence or absence of hemorrhage during the study. A total of 202 recovery assessments collected during the 60-month period from these 58 PUPs are combined with 19 recovery assessments from PTPs and were summarized by age group in Table 9. There was one recovery assessment in a neonate, which had a value of 0.46 IU/dL per IU/kg. The overall mean recovery and FIX elimination half-life values were 0.7 ± 0.3 IU/dL per IU/kg and 20.2 ± 4.0 hours, respectively.

Table 9: Summary of BeneFIX Pharmacokinetic Parameters in Pediatric Patients

Age Group	n	K-value (IU/dL per IU/kg)	$t_{1/2}$(h)
Infants (≥1 month to <2 years)	33	0.7 ± 0.4 (0.2, 2.1)	ND
Children (≥2 years to <12 years)	61	0.7 ± 0.2 (0.2, 1.5)	19.8 ± 4.0 (14, 27)[a]
Adolescents (≥12 years to ≤15 years)	9	0.8 ± 0.3 (0.4, 1.4)	21.1 ± 4.5 (15, 28)[b]

[a] n = 13
[b]n = 6
Data presented are mean ± standard deviation (min, max).
Abbreviations: ND = not determined; K-value = incremental recovery; $t_{1/2}$= terminal phase elimination half-life.
Note: The columns are not mutually exclusive; individual patients may be listed under more than 1 age category.

Data from 57 PUP subjects who underwent repeat recovery testing for up to 60 months demonstrated that the average incremental FIX recovery was consistent over time, as shown in Figure 1.

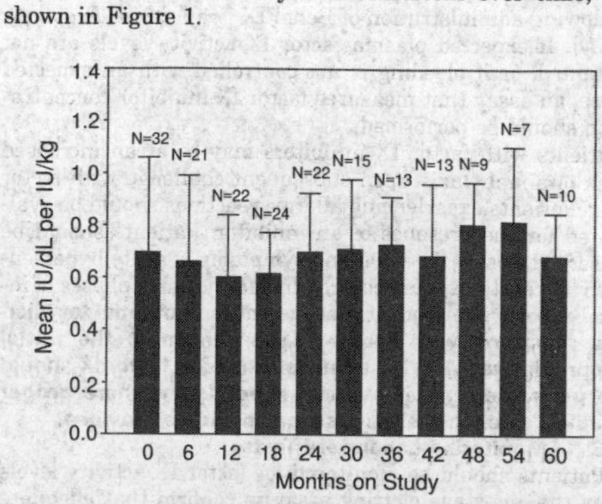

Figure 1. Average Incremental rFIX Recovery over Time

13 NONCLINICAL TOXICOLOGY

13.1 Carcinogenesis, Mutagenesis, Impairment of Fertility

BeneFIX, Coagulation Factor IX (Recombinant), has been shown to be nonmutagenic in the Ames assay and nonclastogenic in a chromosomal aberrations assay. No investigations on carcinogenesis or impairment of fertility have been conducted.

14 CLINICAL STUDIES

Efficacy of BeneFIX has been evaluated in clinical studies in which a total of 128 subjects received BeneFIX either for the treatment of bleeding episodes on an on-demand basis, for the prevention of bleeds (prophylaxis) or for management of hemostasis in the surgical setting (surgical prophylaxis).

Table 11: Efficacy of Prophylaxis of BeneFIX in PTPs and PUPs

	Total exposure (infusions)	Duration of prophylaxis (months) (mean ± SD)	Dose IU/kg (mean ± SD)	Spontaneous bleeds within 48 hrs of infusion	Response rating[a]		
					Excellent	Effective	Inadequate
PTPs							
20	2985	18.2 ± 8.4[b]	40.3 ± 15.2[b]	28	56.0%	37.1%	4.3%
PUPs							
32	3158	14.4 ± 8.1	73.3 ± 33.1	6	91.3%	6.4%	1.7%

[a] Response ratings provided at approximately 3-month intervals. In total, 116 and 172 assessments reported for PTPs and PUPs, respectively. Response ratings not provided for 2.6% and 0.6% of intervals for PTPs and PUPs, respectively.
[b]N = 19

Table 12: Efficacy of BeneFIX for Surgical Procedures in PTPs and PUPs

Surgery Type	Number of Procedures (Number of Subjects)	Response		
		Excellent/Good	Moderate	No Response
Previously Treated Patients				
Ankle surgery	2 (2)	2 (100%)	-	-
Hip prosthesis implant (right)	1 (1)	1 (100%)	-	-
Knee arthroplasty (2 bilateral, 1 right)	3 (3)	3 (100%)	-	-
Knee arthroscopic synovectomy	2 (2)[a]	1 (50%)	-	-
Liver transplantation (orthotopic)	1 (1)	1 (100%)	-	-
Splenectomy	1 (1)	1 (100%)	-	-
External fixation device removal (wrist)	1 (1)	1 (100%)	-	-
Hernia repair	3 (2)	3 (100%)	-	-
Subacromial decompression (left)	1 (1)	1 (100%)	-	-
Calf debridement, dental extraction[b]	1 (1)	1 (100%)	-	-
Lymph node removal, dental extraction[b]	1 (1)	1 (100%)	-	-
Left heel cord lengthening	1 (1)	1 (100%)	-	-
Dental procedures[c]	12 (11)	11 (92%)	1 (8%)	-
Minor procedures	6 (6)	6 (100%)	-	-
Previously Untreated Patients				
Hernia repair	2 (2)	2 (100%)	-	-
Minor procedures	28 (21)[a]	27 (96%)	-	-

[a] Response assessment not provided for 1 procedure.
[b] Includes pulse and continuous-infusion regimens; CI counted as 1 procedure in this summary.
[c]Includes complicated extractions (6), clearance, and fillings.

Fifty-six PTPs and sixty-three PUPs were treated for bleeding episodes on an on-demand basis or for the prevention of bleeds (see Tables 9 and 10). The PTPs were followed over a median interval of 24 months (mean 23.4 ± 5.3 months) and for a median of 83.5. The PUPs were followed over a median interval of 37 months (mean 38.1 ± 16.4 months) and for a median of 89 exposure days.

Fifty-five PTPs and fifty-four PUPs received BeneFIX for the treatment of bleeding episodes (see Table 10). Bleeding episodes that were managed successfully included hemarthrosis and bleeding in soft tissue and muscle. Data concerning the severity of bleeding episodes were not reported. In the PTPs, 88% of total infusions administrated for on-demand treatment were rated as an "excellent" or "good" response.

[See table 10 at top of previous page]

A total of 20 PTPs were treated with BeneFIX for secondary prophylaxis (the regular administration of FIX replacement therapy to prevent bleeding in patients who may have already demonstrated clinical evidence of hemophilic arthropathy or joint disease) at some regular interval during the study with a mean of 2.0 infusions per week (see Table 11). Thirty-two PUPs were administered BeneFIX for routine (primary and secondary) prophylaxis (see Table 11). Twenty-four PUPs were administered BeneFIX at least twice weekly, and eight PUPs were administered BeneFIX once weekly. Seven PTPs experienced a total of 26 spontaneous bleeding episodes within 48 hours after an infusion. Six spontaneous bleeds within 48 hours after an infusion were reported in 5 PUPs. Prophylaxis therapy was rated as "excellent" or "effective" in 93% of PTPs receiving prophylaxis one to two times per week.

[See table 11 above]

Management of hemostasis was evaluated in the surgical setting in both PTPs and PUPs (see Table 12). Thirty-six surgical procedures have been performed in 28 PTPs with 23 major surgical procedures performed (including 6 complicated dental extractions). Thirty surgical procedures have been performed in 23 PUPs. Twenty-eight of these procedures were considered minor. Hemostasis was maintained throughout the surgical period; however, one PTP subject required evacuation of a surgical wound-site hematoma, and another PTP subject who received BeneFIX after a tooth extraction required further surgical intervention due to oozing at the extraction site. There was no clinical evidence of thrombotic complications in any of the subjects.

Among the PTP surgery subjects, the median increase in circulating factor IX activity was 0.7 IU/dL per IU/kg infused (range 0.3 – 1.2 IU/dL; mean 0.8 ± 0.2 IU/dL per IU/kg). The median elimination half-life for the PTP surgery subjects was 19.4 hours (range 10 – 37 hours; mean 21.3 ± 8.1 hours).

[See table 12 below]

Nine of the major surgical procedures were performed in 8 PUPs using a continuous-infusion regimen. Five of the surgical procedures were performed in PUPs using a continuous-infusion regimen over 3 to 5 days. Although circulating factor IX levels targeted to restore and maintain hemostasis were achieved with both pulse replacement and continuous infusion regimens, clinical trial experience with continuous infusion of BeneFIX for surgical prophylaxis in hemophilia B has been too limited to establish the safety and clinical efficacy of administration of the product by continuous infusion.

All subjects participating in the PTP, PUP and surgery studies were monitored for clinical evidence of thrombosis [*see Warnings and Precautions (5.3)*]. No thrombotic complications were reported in PUPs or surgery subjects. One PTP subject experienced a renal infarct 12 days after a dose of BeneFIX for a bleeding episode; the relationship of the infarct to the prior administration of BeneFIX is uncertain. Laboratory studies of thrombogenecity (fibrinopeptide A and prothrombin fragment 1 + 2) were obtained in 41 PTPs and 7 surgery subjects prior to infusion and up to 24 hours following infusion. The results of these studies were inconclusive. Out of 29 PTP subjects noted to have elevated fibrinopeptide A levels post-infusion of BeneFIX, 22 also had elevated levels at baseline. Surgery subjects showed no evidence of significant increase in coagulation activation.

15 REFERENCES

1. Roberts HR, Eberst ME. Current management of hemophilia B. *Hematol Oncol Clin North Am.* 1993;7(6):1269-1280.
2. Shapiro AD, Ragni MV, Lusher JM, et al. Safety and efficacy of monoclonal antibody purified factor IX concentrate in previously untreated patients with hemophilia B. *Thromb Haemost.* 1996;75(1):30-35.

16 HOW SUPPLIED/STORAGE AND HANDLING

16.1 How Supplied

BeneFIX, Coagulation Factor IX (Recombinant), is supplied in kits that include single-use vials which contain nominally 250, 500, 1000, 2000, or 3000 IU per vial with sterile prefilled diluent syringe, vial adapter reconstitution device, sterile infusion set, and two (2) alcohol swabs, one bandage, and one gauze pad. Actual factor IX activity in IU is stated on the label of each vial.

Product labeled "Room Temperature Storage". Store at 2 to 30°C (36 to 86°F).

	NDC number
250 IU	58394-633-03
500 IU	58394-634-03
1000 IU	58394-635-03
2000 IU	58394-636-03
3000 IU	58394-637-03

Product labeled for refrigeration. Store at 2 to 8°C (36 to 46°F).

	NDC number
250 IU	58394-003-06
500 IU	58394-002-06
1000 IU	58394-001-06
2000 IU	58394-008-02

16.2 Storage and Handling

Product kit as packaged for sale: BeneFIX, Coagulation Factor IX (Recombinant), can be stored at room temperature or under refrigeration, at a temperature of 2 to 30°C (36 to 86°F). Do not use BeneFIX after the expiration date on the label.

Different storage conditions are described below:

Product labeled for Room Temperature Storage

Store at 2 to 30°C (36 to 86°F).	If the product kit is labeled for room temperature storage, it can be stored at room temperature (not to exceed 30°C or 86°F) or under refrigeration (2 to 8°C or 36 to 46°F).

Product labeled for Refrigerated Storage

Continuous refrigeration [2 to 8°C (36 to 46°F)]	If the product kit labeled for refrigerated storage has been continuously refrigerated at 2 to 8°C (36 to 46°F), the labeled expiration date on the package is still applicable and the product kit should be stored as labeled on the carton. Prior to the expiration date, the product kit may be stored at room temperature, not to exceed 30°C (86°F), for up to 6 months. If the product kit labeled for refrigerated storage has been removed from refrigeration and stored at room temperature (not to exceed 30°C or 86°F)*, the expiration period should be up to 6 months from the date of removal from refrigeration. Do not use the product once this six month period has elapsed even if the expiration date on the carton has not been exceeded.

*If you have removed the product kit labeled for refrigerated storage from refrigeration as a result of our April 2011 communication on the "Daily Med", and have not recorded the date of removal from refrigeration, the assigned expiration date (printed on the end flap of the product carton) must be reduced by 12 months.

Do not freeze to prevent damage to the diluent syringe.
Product after reconstitution: The product does not contain a preservative and should be used within 3 hours.

17 PATIENT COUNSELING INFORMATION

See FDA-Approved Patient Labeling

Advise patients to report any adverse reactions or problems following BeneFIX administration to their physician or healthcare provider.

- Allergic-type hypersensitivity reactions are possible. Inform patients of the early signs of hypersensitivity reactions [including hives (rash with itching), generalized urticaria, tightness of the chest, wheezing, hypotension] and anaphylaxis. Advise patients to discontinue use of the product and contact their physicians if these symptoms occur.
- Advise patients to contact their physician or treatment facility for further treatment and/or assessment if they experience a lack of a clinical response to factor IX replacement therapy, as in some cases this may be a manifestation of an inhibitor.

FDA-Approved Patient Labeling
BeneFIX® / BEN-uh-fiks/
[Coagulation Factor IX (Recombinant)]

Please read this Patient Leaflet carefully before using BeneFIX and each time you get a refill. There may be new information. This Patient Leaflet does not take the place of talking with your doctor about your medical condition or your treatment.

What is BeneFIX?

BeneFIX is an injectable medicine that is used to help control and prevent bleeding in people with hemophilia B. Hemophilia B is also called congenital factor IX deficiency or Christmas disease.

BeneFIX is **NOT** used to treat hemophilia A.

What should I tell my doctor before using BeneFIX?

Tell your doctor and pharmacist about all of the medicines you take, including all prescription and non-prescription medicines, such as over-the-counter medicines, supplements, or herbal medicines.

Tell your doctor about all of your medical conditions, including if you:

- are pregnant or planning to become pregnant. It is not known if BeneFIX may harm your unborn baby.
- are breastfeeding. It is not known if BeneFIX passes into the milk and if it can harm your baby.

How should I infuse BeneFIX?

The initial administrations of BeneFIX should be administered under proper medical supervision, where proper medical care for severe allergic reactions could be provided.

See the step-by-step instructions for infusing BeneFIX at the end of this leaflet. You should always follow the specific instructions given by your doctor. The steps listed below are general guidelines for using BeneFIX. If you are unsure of the procedures, please call your doctor or pharmacist before using.

Call your doctor right away if bleeding is not controlled after using BeneFIX.

Your doctor will prescribe the dose that you should take.

Your doctor may need to test your blood from time to time.

BeneFIX should not be administered by continuous infusion.

What if I take too much BeneFIX?

Call your doctor if you take too much BeneFIX.

What are the possible side effects of BeneFIX?

Allergic reactions may occur with BeneFIX. Call your doctor or get emergency treatment right away if you have any of the following symptoms:

wheezing
difficulty breathing
chest tightness
turning blue (look at lips and gums)
fast heartbeat
swelling of the face
faintness
rash
hives

Your body can also make antibodies, called "inhibitors," against BeneFIX, which may stop BeneFIX from working properly.

Some common side effects of BeneFIX are nausea, injection site reaction, injection site pain, headache, dizziness and rash.

BeneFIX may increase the risk of thromboembolism (abnormal blood clots) in your body if you have risk factors for developing blood clots, including an indwelling venous catheter through which BeneFIX is given by continuous infusion. There have been reports of severe blood clotting events, including life-threatening blood clots in critically ill neonates, while receiving continuous-infusion BeneFIX through a central venous catheter. The safety and efficacy of BeneFIX administration by continuous infusion have not been established.

These are not all the possible side effects of BeneFIX.

Tell your doctor about any side effect that bothers you or that does not go away.

How should I store BeneFIX?

DO NOT FREEZE BeneFIX kit.

BeneFIX kit can be stored at room temperature (below 86°F) or under refrigeration.

Throw away any unused BeneFIX and diluent after the expiration date indicated on the label.

Different storage conditions are described below.

Product labeled for Room Temperature Storage

Store at 2 to 30°C (36 to 86°F).	If you have the product kit labeled for room temperature storage, it can be stored at room temperature (below 30°C or 86°F) or in the refrigerator (2 to 8°C or 36 to 46°F).

Product labeled for Refrigerated Storage

Continuous refrigeration [2 to 8°C (36 to 46°F)]	If you have the product kit labeled for storage in the refrigerator (2 to 8°C or 36 to 46°F) and you have not taken the kit out of the refrigerator, then the expiration date printed on the package still applies. You can store the product at room temperature (below 30°C or 86°F) for up to 6 months or until it has reached its expiration date, whichever comes first. If you have taken the product kit labeled for storage in the refrigerator out of the refrigerator and stored it at room temperature (below 30°C or 86°F), then use the product within 6 months from the time you took the product out of the refrigerator or until it has reached its expiration date, whichever comes first. If you cannot remember when you took the product out of the refrigerator, then **subtract one year (12 months)** from the date that is printed on the end flap of the carton package. The date you get is your new expiration date. Throw away any product that has gone over the new expiration date.

Freezing should be avoided to prevent damage to the prefilled diluent syringe.

BeneFIX does not contain a preservative. After reconstituting BeneFIX, you can store it at room temperature for up to 3 hours. If you have not used it in 3 hours, throw it away.

Do not use BeneFIX if the reconstituted solution is not clear and colorless.

What else should I know about BeneFIX?

Medicines are sometimes prescribed for purposes other than those listed here. Do not use BeneFIX for a condition for which it was not prescribed. Do not share BeneFIX with other people, even if they have the same symptoms that you have.

This Patient Leaflet summarizes the most important information about BeneFIX. If you would like more information, talk with your doctor. You can ask your doctor or pharmacist for information about BeneFIX that was written for healthcare professionals.

Instructions for Using BeneFIX

BeneFIX is supplied as a powder. Before it can be infused in your vein (intravenous injection), you must reconstitute the powder by mixing it with the liquid diluent supplied. The liquid diluent is 0.234% sodium chloride. BeneFIX should be reconstituted and infused using the infusion set, diluent, syringe, and adapter provided in this kit, and by following the directions below.

RECONSTITUTION

Always wash your hands before performing the following steps. Try to keep everything clean and germ-free while you are reconstituting BeneFIX. Once you open the vials, you should finish reconstituting BeneFIX as soon as possible. This will help keep the infusion set materials germ-free.

Note: If you use more than one vial of BeneFIX per infusion, reconstitute each vial according to steps 1 through 13.

1. If refrigerated, let the vial of BeneFIX and the pre-filled diluent syringe reach room temperature.
2. Remove the plastic flip-top cap from the BeneFIX vial to show the center part of the rubber stopper.

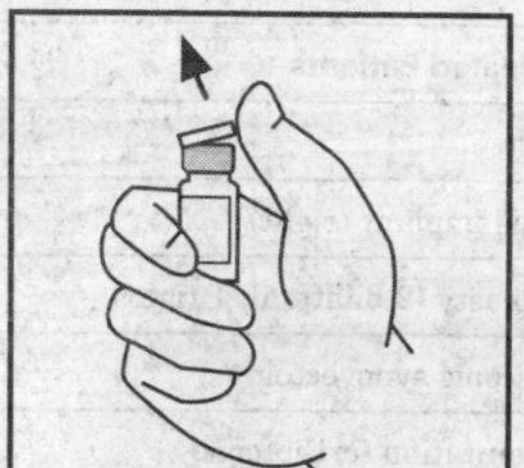

3. Wipe the top of the vial with the alcohol swab provided, or use another antiseptic solution, and allow to dry. After cleaning, do not touch the rubber stopper with your hand or allow it to touch any surface.
4. Peel back the cover from the clear plastic vial adapter package. **Do not remove the adapter from the package.**
5. Place the vial on a flat surface. While holding the adapter in the package, place the vial adapter over the vial. Press down firmly on the package until the adapter snaps into place on top of the vial, with the adapter spike penetrating the vial stopper.

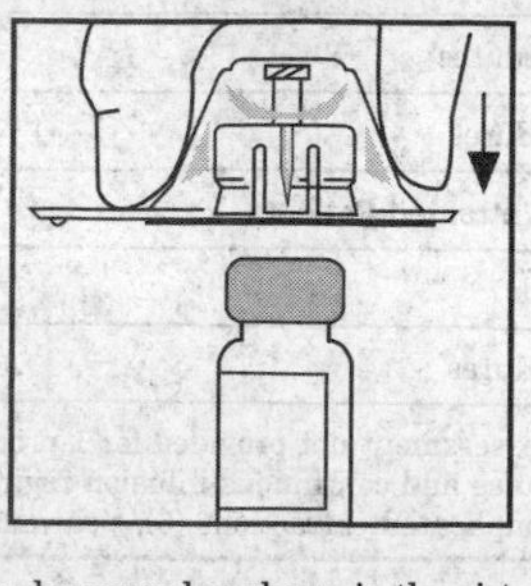

6. Grasp the plunger rod as shown in the picture below. Do not touch the shaft of the plunger rod. Attach the threaded end of the plunger rod to the diluent syringe plunger by pushing and turning firmly.

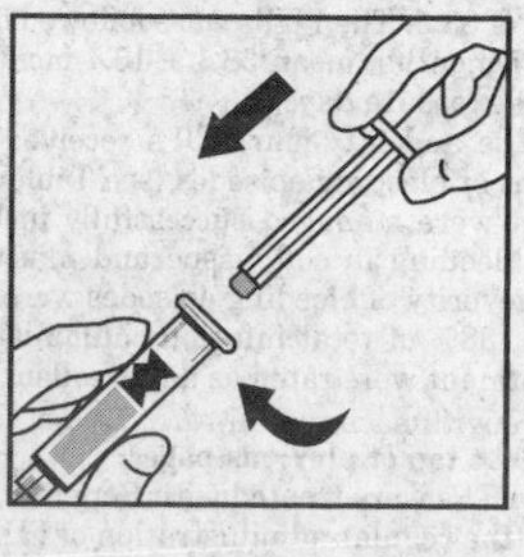

7. Break off the tamper-resistant, plastic-tip cap from the diluent syringe by snapping the perforation of the cap. Do not touch the inside of the cap or the syringe tip. The diluent syringe may need to be recapped (if reconstituted BeneFIX is not used immediately), so place the cap on its tip on a clean surface in a spot where it will stay clean.

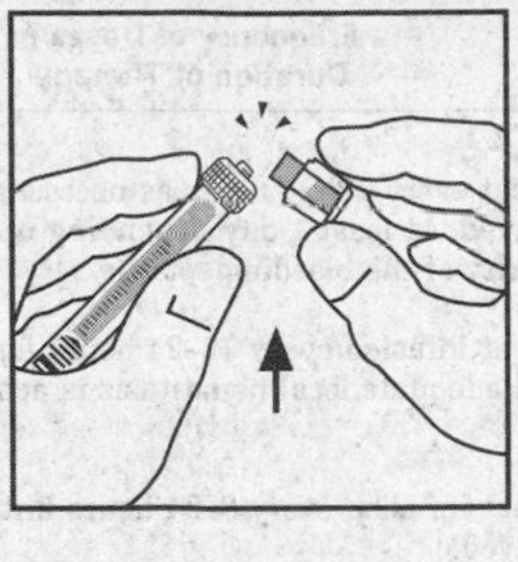

8. Lift the package away from the adapter and discard the package.

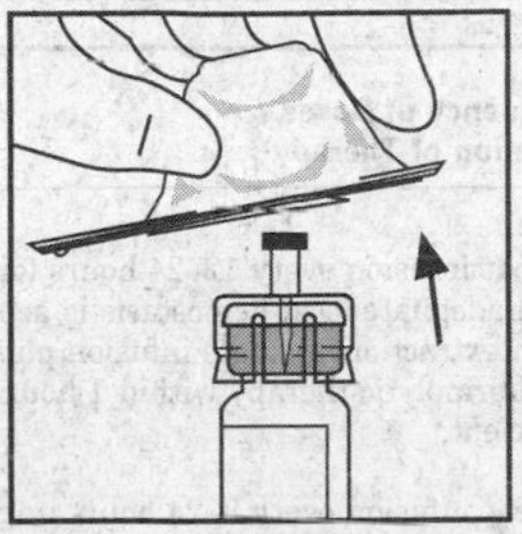

9. Place the vial on a flat surface. Connect the diluent syringe to the vial adapter by inserting the tip of the syringe into the adapter opening while firmly pushing and turning the syringe clockwise until the connection is secured.

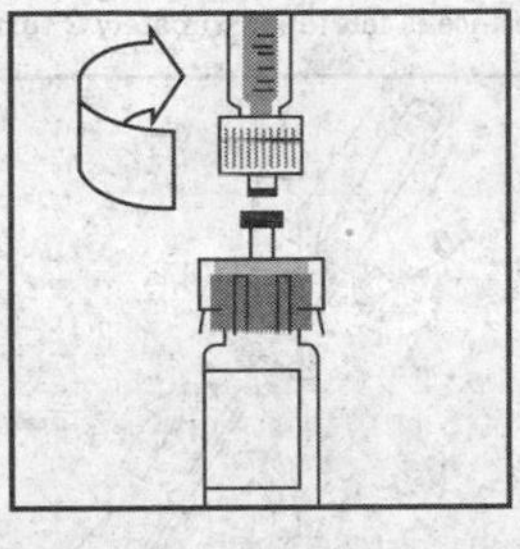

10. Slowly push the plunger rod to inject all the diluent into the BeneFIX vial.

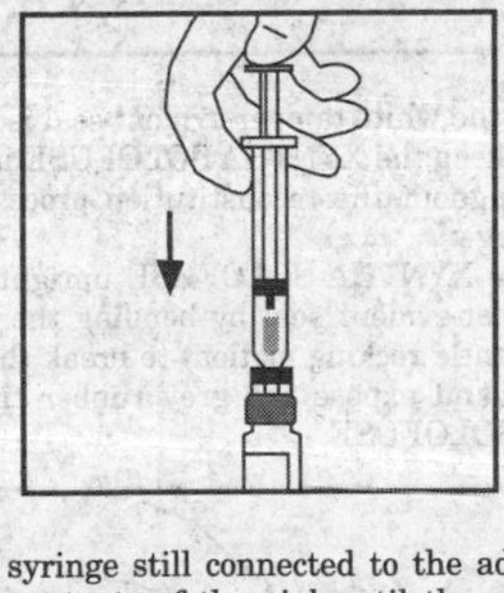

11. With the syringe still connected to the adapter, **gently** swirl the contents of the vial until the powder is dissolved.
    Look at the final solution before infusing it. The solution should be clear to colorless. If it is not, throw away the solution and use a new kit.
12. Make sure the syringe plunger rod is still fully pressed down, then turn over the vial. Slowly pull the solution into the syringe. Turn the syringe upward again and remove any air bubbles by gently tapping the syringe with your finger and slowly pushing air out of the syringe.
    If you reconstituted more than one vial of BeneFIX, remove the diluent syringe from the vial adapter and leave the vial adapter attached to the vial. Quickly attach a separate large luer lock syringe and pull the reconstituted solution as instructed above. Repeat this procedure with each vial in turn. Do not detach the diluent syringes or the large luer lock syringe until you are ready to attach the large luer lock syringe to the next vial adapter.

[See figure at top of next column]

13. Remove the syringe from the vial adapter by gently pulling and turning the syringe counter-clockwise. Throw away the vial with the adapter attached.
    If you are not using the solution right away, you should carefully replace the syringe cap. Do not touch the syringe tip or the inside of the cap.

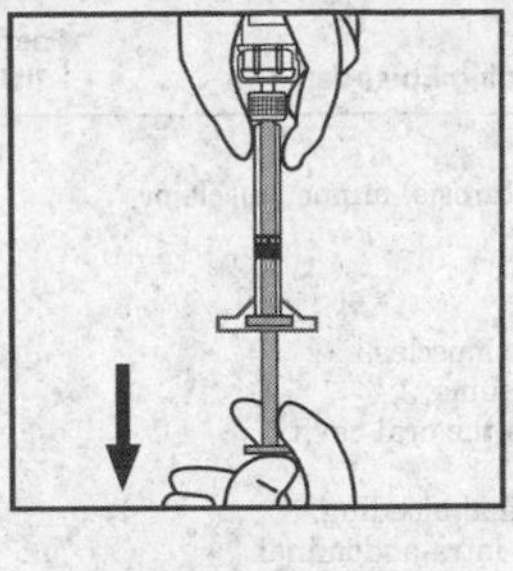

BeneFIX should be infused within 3 hours after reconstitution. The reconstituted solution may be stored at room temperature prior to infusion.

INFUSION (Intravenous Injection)

Continuous infusion is **not** an approved way to administer BeneFIX.

Your doctor or healthcare professional should teach you how to infuse BeneFIX. Once you learn how to self-infuse, you can follow the instructions in this insert.

1. Attach the syringe to the luer end of the provided infusion set tubing.
2. Apply a tourniquet and prepare the injection site by wiping the skin well with an alcohol swab provided in the kit.

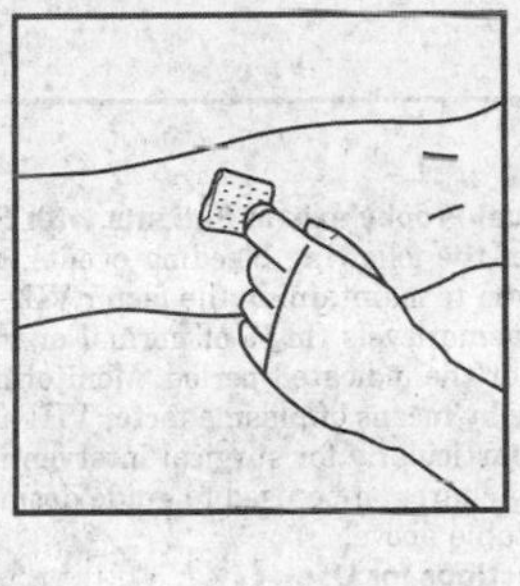

3. Insert the butterfly needle of the infusion set tubing into your vein as instructed by your doctor or healthcare provider. Remove the tourniquet. Infuse the reconstituted BeneFIX product over several minutes. Your comfort level should determine the rate of infusion.

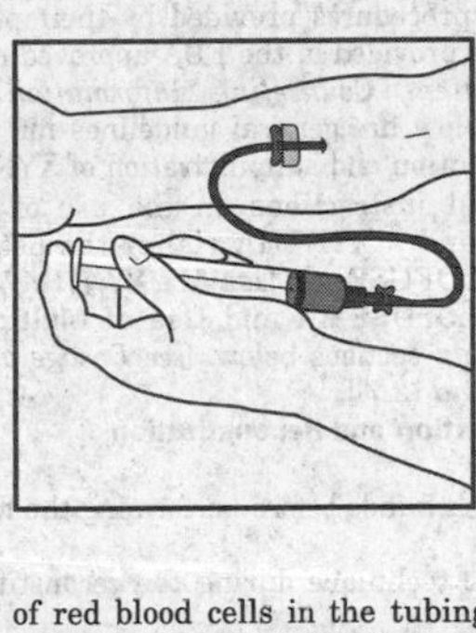

Clumping of red blood cells in the tubing/syringe has been reported with the administration of BeneFIX. No adverse events have been reported in association with this observation. To minimize the possibility of clumping it is important to limit the amount of blood entering the tubing. Blood should not enter the syringe.

Note: If red blood cell clumping is observed in the tubing or syringe, discard all material (tubing, syringe and BeneFIX solution) and continue administration with a new package.

4. After infusing BeneFIX, remove the infusion set and discard. The amount of drug product left in the infusion set will not affect your treatment. Dispose of all unused solution, the empty vial(s), and the used needles and syringes in an appropriate container used for throwing away waste that might hurt others if not handled properly.

It is a good idea to record the lot number from the BeneFIX vial label every time you use BeneFIX. You can use the peel-off label found on the vial to record the lot number.

If you have any questions or concerns about BeneFIX, ask your doctor or healthcare provider.

Distributed by
Wyeth Pharmaceuticals Inc
A subsidiary of Pfizer Inc, Philadelphia, PA 19101
US Govt. License No. 3
LAB-0464-8.0
Revised: 11/2011

XYNTHA® SOLOFUSE™ ℞

[ZIN-tha]

[Antihemophilic Factor (Recombinant), Plasma/Albumin-Free]
For Intravenous Injection - Lyophilized Powder for Solution in Prefilled Dual-Chamber Syringe

HIGHLIGHTS OF PRESCRIBING INFORMATION
These highlights do not include all the information needed to use XYNTHA safely and effectively. See full prescribing information for XYNTHA.
XYNTHA® SOLOFUSE™ [Antihemophilic Factor (Recombinant), Plasma/Albumin-Free]
For Intravenous Injection - Lyophilized Powder for Solution in Prefilled Dual-Chamber Syringe
Initial U.S. Approval: 2008

INDICATIONS AND USAGE

XYNTHA is a recombinant antihemophilic factor indicated for:
- Control and prevention of bleeding episodes in patients with hemophilia A (1.1)
- Surgical prophylaxis in patients with hemophilia A (1.2)

XYNTHA is not indicated in patients with von Willebrand's disease.

DOSAGE AND ADMINISTRATION

For intravenous use after reconstitution only (2)
- The required dosage is determined using the following formula:
  Required units = body weight (kg) × desired factor VIII rise (IU/dL or % of normal) × 0.5 (IU/kg per IU/dL) where IU = International Unit
- Frequency of intravenous injection of the reconstituted product is determined by the type of bleeding episode and the recommendation of the treating physician. (2.1, 2.2)

DOSAGE FORMS AND STRENGTHS

XYNTHA SOLOFUSE is available as lyophilized powder in single-use prefilled dual-chamber syringes of: 250, 500, 1000, 2000 or 3000 IU. (3)

CONTRAINDICATIONS

Do not use in patients who have manifested life-threatening immediate hypersensitivity reactions, including anaphylaxis, to the product or its components, including hamster proteins.

WARNINGS AND PRECAUTIONS

- Anaphylaxis and severe hypersensitivity reactions are possible. Patients may develop hypersensitivity to hamster protein, which is present in trace amounts in XYNTHA. Should such reactions occur, discontinue treatment with the product, and administer appropriate treatment. (5.1)
- Development of activity-neutralizing antibodies has been detected in patients receiving factor VIII-containing products, including XYNTHA. If expected plasma factor VIII activity levels are not attained, or if bleeding is not controlled with an appropriate dose, perform an assay that measures factor VIII inhibitor concentration. (5.2, 5.3, 6.2)

ADVERSE REACTIONS

The most common adverse reactions (≥ 5%) with XYNTHA were headache, pyrexia, nausea, vomiting, diarrhea, and asthenia.

Two patients (n=89), previously treated with factor VIII, developed inhibitors during the safety and efficacy clinical study. (6.2)

In the surgery study (n=30), one low titer persistent inhibitor and one transient false-positive inhibitor were reported. (6.2)

To report SUSPECTED ADVERSE REACTIONS, contact Wyeth Pharmaceuticals Inc. at 1-800-438-1985 or FDA at 1-800-FDA-1088 or www.fda.gov/medwatch

USE IN SPECIFIC POPULATIONS

Pregnancy: No human or animal data. Use only if clearly needed. (8.1)

See 17 for PATIENT COUNSELING INFORMATION, FDA-approved patient labeling, and Medication Guide

Revised: 07/2012

FULL PRESCRIBING INFORMATION: CONTENTS*

FULL PRESCRIBING INFORMATION

1 INDICATIONS AND USAGE

1.1 Control and Prevention of Bleeding Episodes in Hemophilia A

XYNTHA, Antihemophilic Factor (Recombinant), Plasma/Albumin-Free is indicated for the control and prevention of bleeding episodes in patients with hemophilia A (congenital factor VIII deficiency or classic hemophilia).

1.2 Surgical Prophylaxis in Patients with Hemophilia A

XYNTHA, Antihemophilic Factor (Recombinant), Plasma/Albumin-Free is indicated for surgical prophylaxis in patients with hemophilia A.

XYNTHA does not contain von Willebrand factor, and therefore is not indicated in patients with von Willebrand's disease.

2 DOSAGE AND ADMINISTRATION

For intravenous use after reconstitution.

- Initiate treatment with XYNTHA under the supervision of a physician experienced in the treatment of hemophilia A.
- Dosage and duration of treatment depend on the severity of the factor VIII deficiency, the location and extent of bleeding, and the patient's clinical condition. Titrate the administered doses to the patient's clinical response. Careful control of replacement therapy is especially important in cases of major surgery or life-threatening bleeding episodes.
- One International Unit (IU) of factor VIII activity corresponds approximately to the quantity of factor VIII in one milliliter of normal human plasma. The calculation of the required dosage of factor VIII is based upon the empirical finding that, on average, 1 IU of factor VIII per kg body weight raises the plasma factor VIII activity by approximately 2 IU/dL.[2] The required dosage is determined using the following formula:

The expected in vivo peak increase in factor VIII level expressed as IU/dL (or % normal) can be estimated using the following formulas:

Dosage (units) = body weight (kg) × desired factor VIII rise (IU/dL or % of normal) × 0.5 (IU/kg per IU/dL)

or

IU/dL (or % normal) = Total Dose (IU)/body weight (kg) × 2 [IU/dL]/[IU/kg]

The labeled potency of XYNTHA is based on the European Pharmacopoeia chromogenic substrate assay, in which the Wyeth manufacturing standard has been calibrated using a one-stage clotting assay. This method of potency assignment is intended to harmonize XYNTHA with clinical monitoring using a one-stage clotting assay [*see Clinical Pharmacology (12.3)*].

2.1 Control and Prevention of Bleeding Episodes

In the case of the following bleeding events, consideration should be given to maintaining the factor VIII activity at or above the plasma levels (in % of normal or in IU/dL) outlined below for the indicated period.

The following chart can be used to guide dosing in bleeding episodes:

[See first table above]

Type of Bleeding Episode	Factor VIII Level Required (IU/dL or % of normal)	Frequency of Doses / Duration of Therapy
Minor		
Early hemarthrosis, minor muscle or oral bleeds.	20–40	Repeat every 12–24 hours as necessary until resolved. At least 1 day, depending upon the severity of the bleeding episode.
Moderate		
Bleeding into muscles. Mild head trauma. Bleeding into the oral cavity.	30–60	Repeat infusion every 12–24 hours for 3–4 days or until adequate local hemostasis is achieved.
Major		
Gastrointestinal bleeding. Intracranial, intra-abdominal or intrathoracic bleeding. Fractures.	60–100	Repeat infusion every 8–24 hours until bleeding is resolved.

Type of Surgery	Factor VIII Level Required (IU/dL or % of normal)	Frequency of Doses / Duration of Therapy
Minor		
Minor operations, including tooth extraction.	30–60	Repeat infusion every 12–24 hours for 3–4 days or until adequate local hemostasis is achieved. For tooth extraction, a single infusion plus oral antifibrinolytic therapy within 1 hour may be sufficient.
Major		
Major operations.	60–100	Repeat infusion every 8–24 hours until threat is resolved, or in the case of surgery, until adequate local hemostasis and wound healing are achieved.

2.2 Surgical Prophylaxis in Patients with Hemophilia A

In the case of the following bleeding events, consideration should be given to maintaining the factor VIII activity at or above the plasma levels (in % of normal or in IU/dL) outlined below for the indicated period. Monitoring of replacement therapy by means of plasma factor VIII activity is recommended, particularly for surgical intervention.

The following chart can be used to guide dosing in surgery:

[See second table above]

2.3 Instructions for Use

Administer XYNTHA by intravenous infusion after reconstitution of the lyophilized powder with the diluent (0.9% Sodium Chloride). In XYNTHA® SOLOFUSE™, both the XYNTHA powder and the diluent are supplied within the prefilled dual-chamber syringe.

Patients should follow the specific reconstitution and administration procedures provided by their physician. Instructions are provided in the FDA-approved patient labeling [*see Patient Counseling Information (17)*]. The procedures below are general guidelines for the preparation, reconstitution and administration of XYNTHA.

For additional instructions on the use of a XYNTHA SOLOFUSE and a XYNTHA vial or the use of multiple XYNTHA SOLOFUSE, see **Use of a XYNTHA Vial Kit and a XYNTHA SOLOFUSE Kit** and **Use of Multiple XYNTHA SOLOFUSE Kits** sections below. [*see Dosage and Administration (2.6) and (2.7)*]

2.4 Preparation and Reconstitution

Preparation

1. Always wash hands before performing the following procedures.
2. Use aseptic technique during the reconstitution procedures.
3. Use all components for the reconstitution and administration of this product as soon as possible after opening their sterile containers to minimize unnecessary exposure to the atmosphere.

Note:

- If the patient uses one vial of XYNTHA with one XYNTHA SOLOFUSE for the infusion, reconstitute the vial and the syringe according to the instructions for that respective product kit. Use a separate 10 milliliter or larger luer lock syringe (not included in this kit) to draw back the reconstituted contents of the vial and the syringe. [see Dosage and Administration (2.6)]
- If the patient uses multiple XYNTHA SOLOFUSE syringes for the infusion, reconstitute each syringe according to the instructions below. Use a separate 10 milliliter or larger luer lock syringe (not included in this kit) to draw back the reconstituted contents of each syringe. [see Dosage and Administration (2.7)]

Reconstitution

1. Allow the XYNTHA SOLOFUSE Kit to reach room temperature.
2. Remove the contents of the XYNTHA SOLOFUSE Kit and place on a clean surface, making sure you have all the supplies you will need.
3. Grasp the plunger rod as shown in the following diagram. Avoid contact with the shaft of the plunger rod. Screw the plunger rod firmly into the opening in the finger rest of the XYNTHA SOLOFUSE by pushing and turning firmly until resistance is felt (approximately 2 turns).

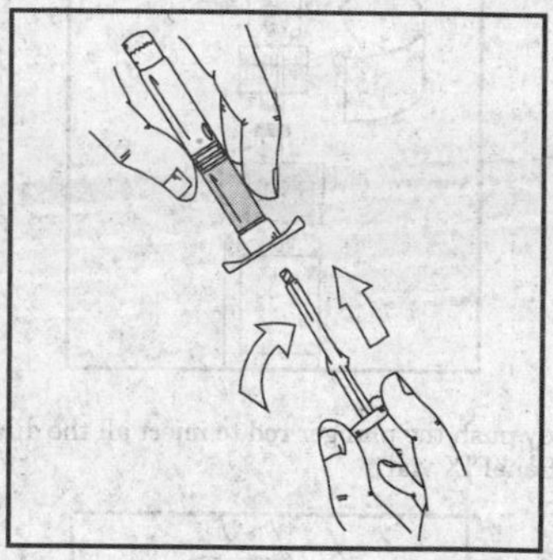

Note: Once the white tamper-evident seal is removed it is important to keep the XYNTHA SOLOFUSE in the upright position throughout the reconstitution process to prevent possible leakage.

4. Holding the XYNTHA SOLOFUSE upright, remove the white tamper-evident seal by bending the seal right to left (or a gentle rocking motion) to break the perforation of the cap and expose the grey rubber tip cap of the XYNTHA SOLOFUSE.

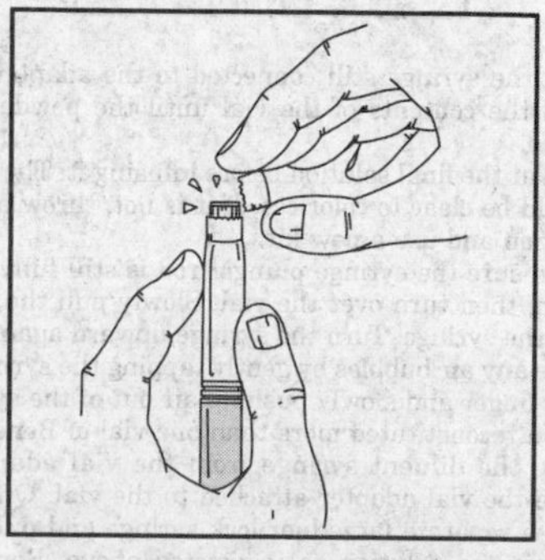

5. Remove the protective blue vented sterile cap from its package. While holding the XYNTHA SOLOFUSE upright, remove the grey rubber tip cap and replace it with the protective blue vented cap (prevents pressure build-up). Avoid touching the open end of both the syringe and the protective blue vented cap.

[See figure at top of next column]

6. **Gently and slowly** advance the plunger rod by pushing until the two stoppers inside the XYNTHA SOLOFUSE meet, and all of the diluent is transferred to the chamber containing the XYNTHA powder.

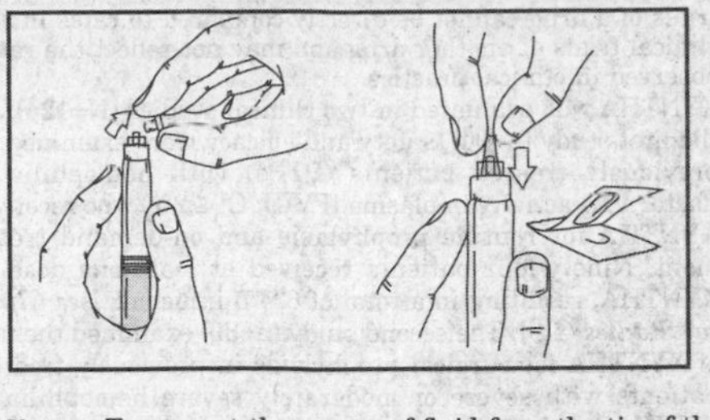

Note: To prevent the escape of fluid from the tip of the syringe, the plunger rod should not be pushed with excessive force.

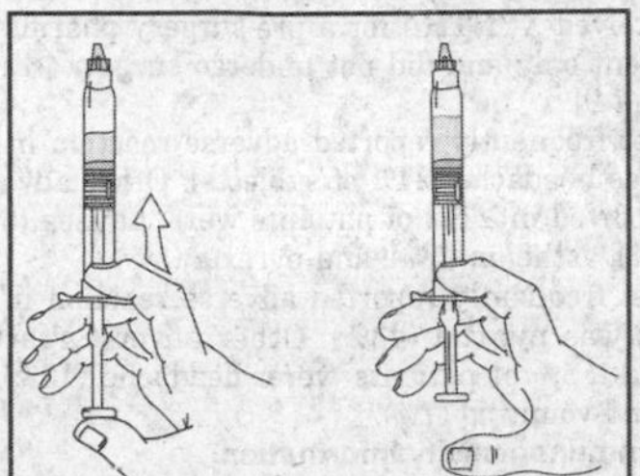

7. With the XYNTHA SOLOFUSE remaining upright, swirl **gently** several times until the powder is dissolved.

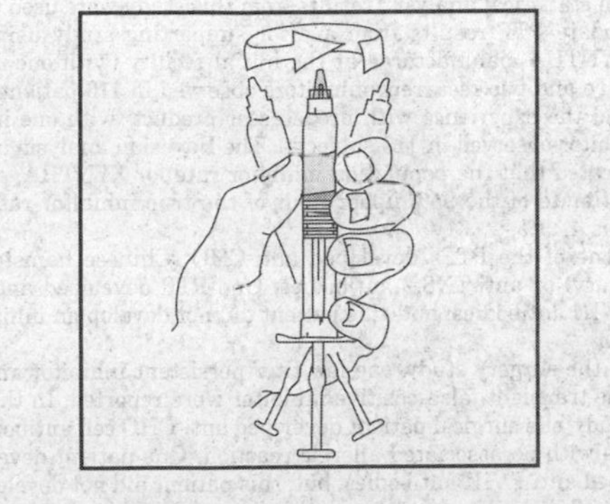

Note: The final solution should be inspected visually for particulate matter before administration. The solution should be clear to slightly opalescent and colorless. If it is not, discard the solution and use a new kit.

8. Holding the XYNTHA SOLOFUSE in an upright position, slowly advance the plunger rod until most, but not all, of the air is removed from the drug product chamber.

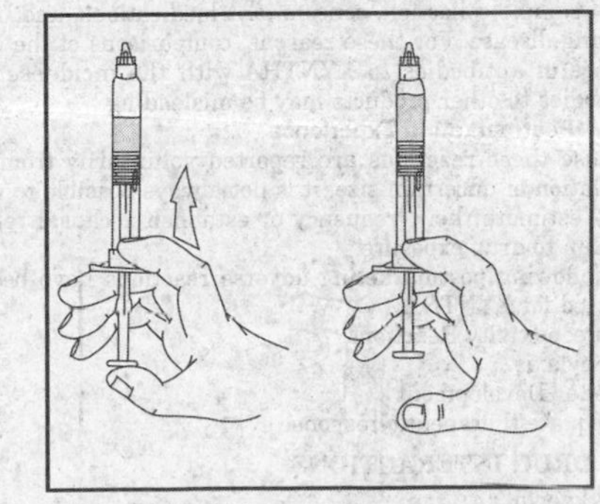

Note:

- If the solution is not to be used immediately, store the syringe upright, leaving the protective blue vent cap on the XYNTHA SOLOFUSE until ready to infuse.
- Store the reconstituted solution at room temperature prior to administration, but use within 3 hours after reconstitution or after removal of the grey rubber tip cap.
- XYNTHA, when reconstituted, contains polysorbate 80, which is known to increase the rate of di-(2-ethylhexyl)phthalate (DEHP) extraction from polyvinyl chloride (PVC). This should be considered during the preparation and administration of XYNTHA, including storage time elapsed in a PVC container following reconstitution. **The tubing of the infusion set included with this kit does not contain DEHP.**

2.5 Administration

Administer XYNTHA by intravenous infusion after reconstitution only.

Inspect the final XYNTHA solution visually for particulate matter and discoloration prior to administration. The solution should be clear to slightly opalescent and colorless. If it is not, discard the solution and use a new kit.

Administer XYNTHA solution using the infusion set included in the kit. Do not administer reconstituted XYNTHA in the same tubing or container with other medicinal products.

1. After removing the protective blue vented cap, firmly attach the intravenous infusion set provided in the kit onto the XYNTHA SOLOFUSE.

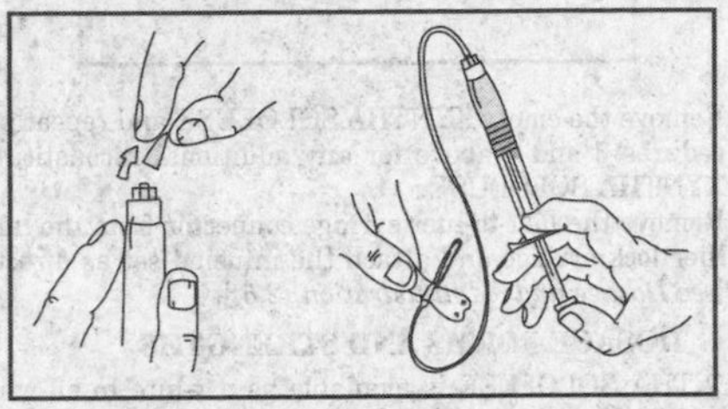

2. Apply a tourniquet and prepare the injection site by wiping the skin well with an alcohol swab provided in the kit.
3. Remove the protective needle cover and perform venipuncture. Insert the needle on the infusion set tubing into the vein, and remove the tourniquet. Verify proper needle placement.
4. Inject the reconstituted XYNTHA intravenously over several minutes. The rate of administration should be determined by the patient's comfort level.

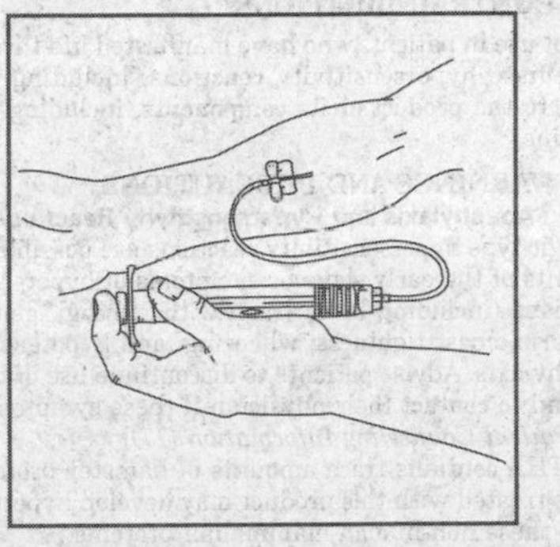

5. After infusing XYNTHA, remove and discard the infusion set. The amount of drug product left in the infusion set will not affect treatment.

Note: Dispose of all unused solution, the empty XYNTHA SOLOFUSE, and other used medical supplies in an appropriate container.

2.6 Use of a XYNTHA Vial Kit with a XYNTHA SOLOFUSE Kit

These instructions are for the use of only one XYNTHA vial kit with one XYNTHA SOLOFUSE Kit. For further information, please contact the Medical Information Department at Wyeth Pharmaceuticals, 1-800-438-1985.

1. Reconstitute the XYNTHA vial using the instructions included with the product kit.
2. Detach the empty diluent syringe from the vial adapter by gently turning and pulling the syringe counterclockwise, leaving the contents in the vial and the vial adapter in place.

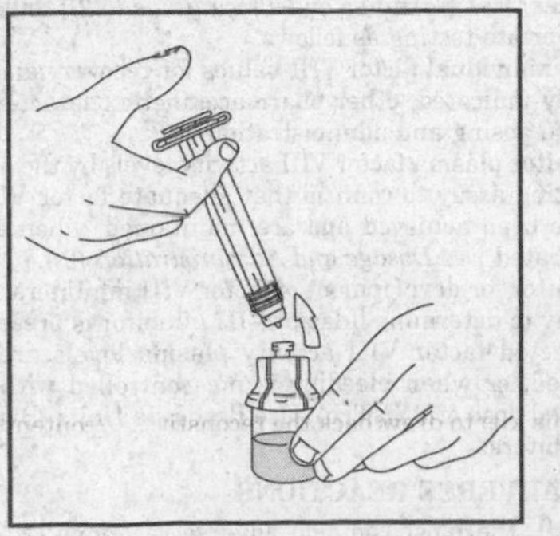

3. Reconstitute the XYNTHA SOLOFUSE using the instructions described in **Preparation and Reconstitution** *[see Dosage and Administration (2.4)]*. Remember to remove most, but not all, of the air from the drug product chamber.

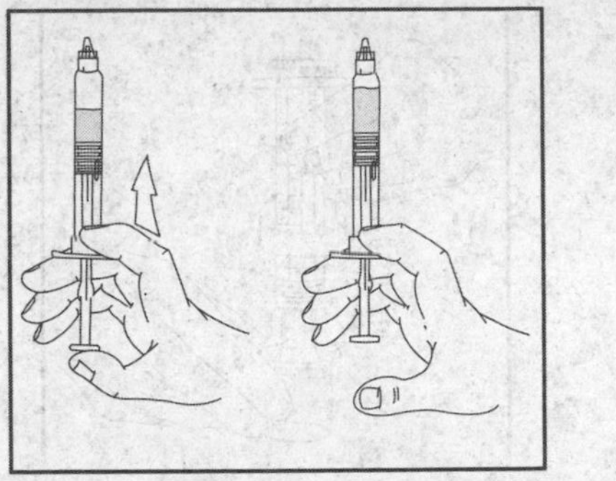

4. After removing the protective blue vented cap, connect the XYNTHA SOLOFUSE to the vial adapter by inserting the tip into the adapter opening while firmly pushing and turning the syringe clockwise until secured.

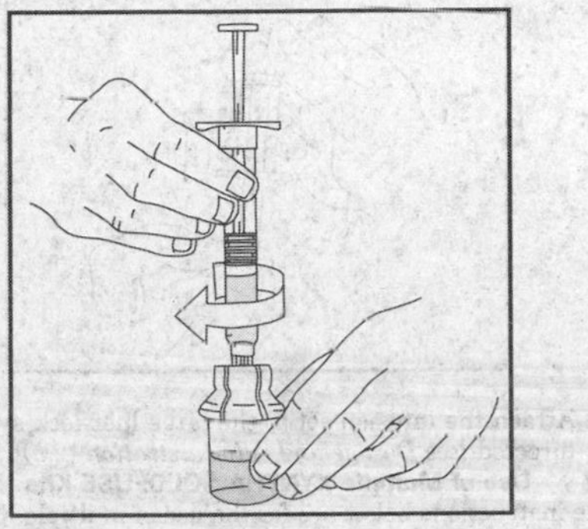

5. Slowly depress the plunger rod of the XYNTHA SOLOFUSE until the contents empty into the XYNTHA vial. The plunger rod may move back slightly after release.

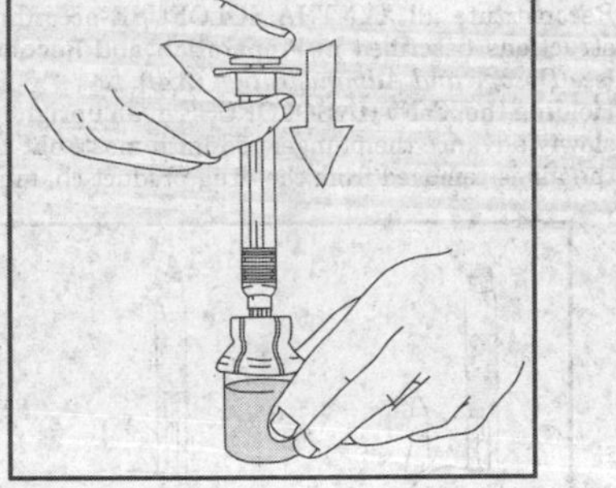

6. Detach and discard the empty XYNTHA SOLOFUSE from the vial adapter.

Note: If the syringe turns without detaching from the vial adapter, grasp the white collar and turn.

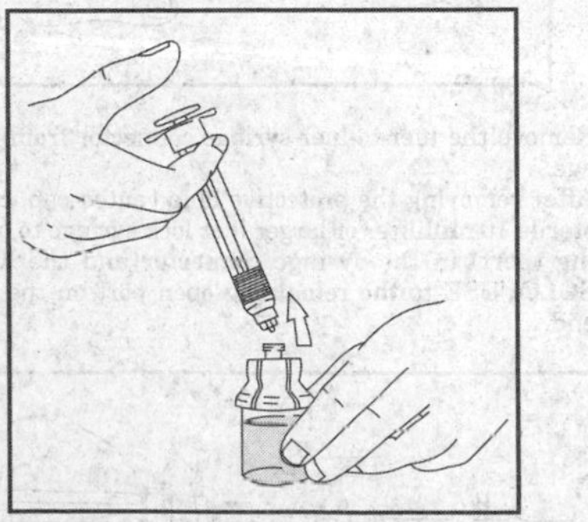

7. Connect a sterile 10 milliliter or larger luer lock syringe to the vial adapter. Inject some air into the vial to make withdrawing the vial contents easier.

[See first figure at top of next column]

8. Invert the vial and slowly draw the solution into the large luer lock syringe.

[See second figure at top of next column]

9. Detach the syringe from the vial adapter by gently turning and pulling the syringe counterclockwise. Discard the empty XYNTHA vial with the adapter attached.

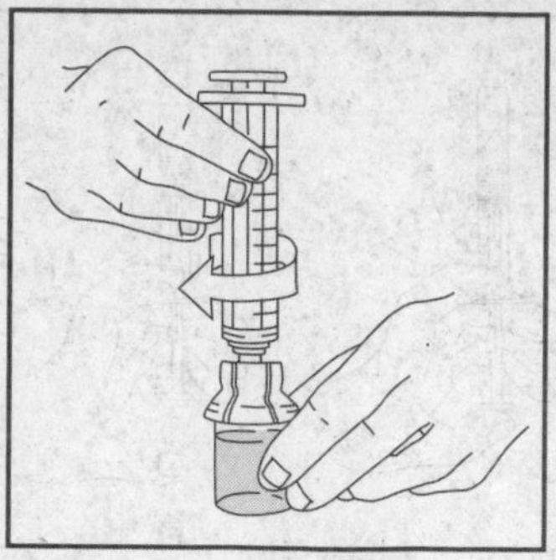

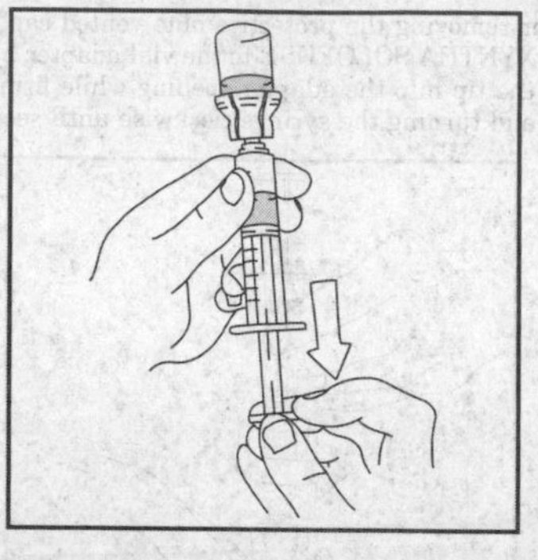

10. Attach the infusion set to the large luer lock syringe as directed [*see Dosage and Administration (2.5)*].

2.7 Use of Multiple XYNTHA SOLOFUSE Kits

The instructions below are for the use of multiple XYNTHA SOLOFUSE kits with a 10 milliliter or larger luer lock syringe. For further information, please contact the Medical Information Department at Wyeth Pharmaceuticals, 1-800-438-1985.

Note: Luer-to-luer syringe connectors are not provided in these kits. Instruct patients to contact their XYNTHA supplier to order.

1. Reconstitute all XYNTHA SOLOFUSE according to instructions described in **Preparation and Reconstitution** [*see Dosage and Administration (2.4)*].
2. Holding the XYNTHA SOLOFUSE in an upright position, slowly advance the plunger rod until most, but not all, of the air is removed from the drug product chamber.

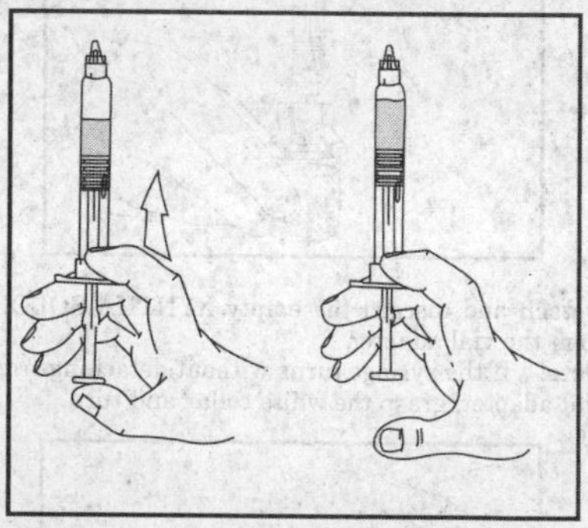

3. Remove the luer-to-luer syringe connector from its package.
4. After removing the protective blue vented cap, connect a sterile 10 milliliter or larger luer lock syringe to one opening (port) in the syringe connector and the XYNTHA SOLOFUSE to the remaining open port on the opposite end.

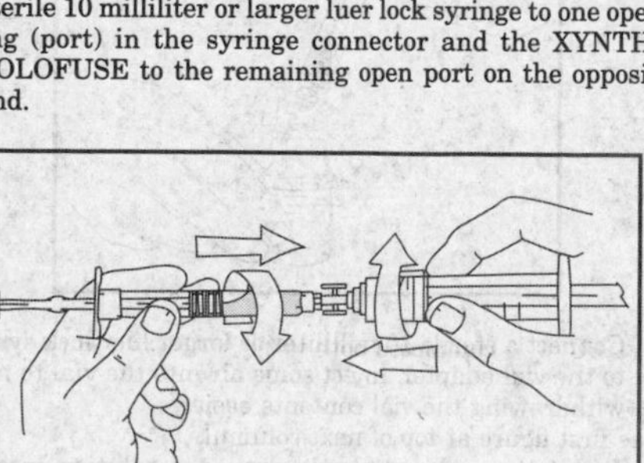

5. With the XYNTHA SOLOFUSE on top, slowly depress the plunger rod until the contents empty into the large luer lock syringe.

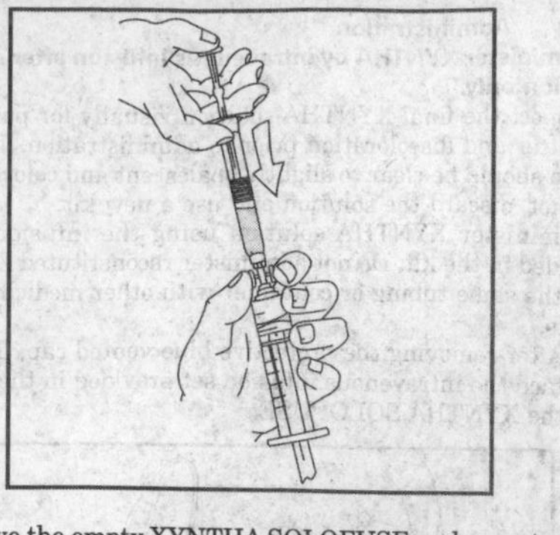

6. Remove the empty XYNTHA SOLOFUSE and repeat procedures 3 and 4 above for any additional reconstituted XYNTHA SOLOFUSE.
7. Remove the luer-to-luer syringe connector from the large luer lock syringe and attach the infusion set as directed [*see Dosage and Administration (2.5)*].

3 DOSAGE FORMS AND STRENGTHS

XYNTHA SOLOFUSE is available as a white to off-white lyophilized powder in the following nominal dosages:

- 250 International Units
- 500 International Units
- 1000 International Units
- 2000 International Units
- 3000 International Units

Each XYNTHA SOLOFUSE has the actual recombinant factor VIII (rFVIII) potency in International Units stated on the label.

4 CONTRAINDICATIONS

Do not use in patients who have manifested life-threatening immediate hypersensitivity reactions, including anaphylaxis, to the product or its components, including hamster proteins.

5 WARNINGS AND PRECAUTIONS

5.1 Anaphylaxis and Hypersensitivity Reactions

Allergic type hypersensitivity reactions are possible. Inform patients of the early signs or symptoms of hypersensitivity reactions (including hives [rash with itching], generalized urticaria, chest tightness, wheezing, and hypotension) and anaphylaxis. Advise patients to discontinue use of the product and to contact their physician if these symptoms occur. [*see Patient Counseling Information (17)*]

XYNTHA contains trace amounts of hamster proteins. Patients treated with this product may develop hypersensitivity to these non-human mammalian proteins.

5.2 Neutralizing Antibodies

Patients using coagulation factor VIII products, including XYNTHA, should be monitored for the development of factor VIII inhibitors by appropriate clinical observations and laboratory tests. Inhibitors have been reported following administration of XYNTHA. If expected factor VIII activity plasma levels are not attained, or if bleeding is not controlled with an appropriate dose, an assay should be performed to determine if a factor VIII inhibitor is present [see Warnings and Precautions (5.3)].[4,5,6,7,8,9,10,11,12]

5.3 Monitoring Laboratory Tests

The clinical response to XYNTHA may vary. If bleeding is not controlled with the recommended dose, determine the plasma level of factor VIII and administer a sufficient dose of XYNTHA to achieve a satisfactory clinical response. If the patient's plasma factor VIII level fails to increase as expected or if bleeding is not controlled after the expected dose, suspect the presence of an inhibitor (neutralizing antibodies) [*see Warnings and Precautions (5.2)*] and perform appropriate testing as follows.

- Use individual factor VIII values for recovery and, if clinically indicated, other pharmacokinetic characteristics to guide dosing and administration.
- Monitor plasma factor VIII activity levels by the one-stage clotting assay to confirm that adequate factor VIII levels have been achieved and are maintained, when clinically indicated [*see Dosage and Administration (2)*].
- Monitor for development of factor VIII inhibitors. Perform assay to determine if factor VIII inhibitor is present when expected factor VIII activity plasma levels are not attained, or when bleeding is not controlled with the expected dose of XYNTHA. Use Bethesda Units (BU) to titer inhibitors.

6 ADVERSE REACTIONS

Overall, the most common adverse reactions (≥ 5%) with XYNTHA were headache, pyrexia, nausea, vomiting, diarrhea, and asthenia.

6.1 Clinical Trials Experience

Because clinical trials are conducted under widely varying conditions, adverse reaction rates observed in the clinical trials of a drug cannot be directly compared to rates in the clinical trials of another drug and may not reflect the rates observed in clinical practice.

XYNTHA was evaluated in two clinical studies (N=124). In the first study (n=94), safety and efficacy were examined in previously treated patients (PTPs) with hemophilia A (factor VIII activity in plasma [FVIII: C] ≤ 2%) who received XYNTHA for routine prophylaxis and on-demand treatment. Ninety-four patients received at least one dose of XYNTHA, resulting in a total of 6,775 infusions [*see Clinical Studies (14)*]. The second study (n=30) examined the use of XYNTHA for surgical prophylaxis in previously treated patients with severe or moderately severe hemophilia A ([FVIII: C] ≤ 2%) who required elective major surgery and were expected to receive XYNTHA replacement therapy for at least 6 days post-surgery. All patients received at least one dose of XYNTHA, resulting in 1161 infusions. One patient received XYNTHA for a pre-surgery pharmacokinetic assessment only and did not undergo surgery [*see Clinical Studies (14)*].

The most frequently reported adverse reaction in PTP patients was headache (24% of subjects). Other adverse reactions reported in ≥ 5% of patients were: nausea (6%), diarrhea (5%), asthenia (5%), and pyrexia (5%).

The most frequently reported adverse reaction in surgical patients was pyrexia (43%). Other adverse reactions reported in ≥ 5% of patients were: headache (13%), nausea (13%), and vomiting (7%).

6.2 Immunogenicity Information

There is a potential for immunogenicity with therapeutic proteins. The clinical studies for XYNTHA examined 94 patients who had previously been treated with factor VIII (PTPs) and 30 surgical patients. In the safety and efficacy study, two subjects with inhibitors were observed in 89 subjects (2.2%) who completed ≥ 50 exposure days. In a Bayesian statistical analysis, results from this study were used to update PTP results from a prior supporting study using XYNTHA manufactured at the initial facility (with one *de novo* and two recurrent inhibitors observed in 110 patients) and the experience with predecessor product (with one inhibitor observed in 113 subjects). The Bayesian analysis indicated that the population inhibitor rate for XYNTHA, an estimate of the 95% upper limit of the true inhibitor rate, was 4.17%.

None of the PTPs developed anti-CHO (Chinese hamster ovary) or anti-TN8.2 antibodies. One PTP developed anti-FVIII antibodies; but, this patient did not develop an inhibitor.

In the surgery study, one low titer persistent inhibitor and one transient false-positive inhibitor were reported. In this study, one surgical patient developed anti-CHO cell antibodies with no associated allergic reaction. One patient developed anti-FVIII antibodies; but, this patient did not develop an inhibitor.

Overall, no allergic manifestation to any immune response was observed during the study.

The detection of antibody formation is highly dependent on the sensitivity and specificity of the assay. Additionally, the observed incidence of antibody, including neutralizing antibody, positivity in an assay may be influenced by several factors, including assay methodology, sample handling, timing of sample collection, concomitant medications, and underlying disease. For these reasons, comparisons of the incidence of antibodies to XYNTHA with the incidence of antibodies to other products may be misleading.

6.3 Postmarketing Experience

Because these reactions are reported voluntarily from a population of uncertain size, it is not always possible to reliably estimate their frequency or establish a causal relationship to drug exposure.

The following postmarketing adverse reactions have been reported for XYNTHA:

Hypersensitivity Reactions
Anaphylaxis
Inhibitor Development
Inadequate therapeutic response

7 DRUG INTERACTIONS

None known.

8 USE IN SPECIFIC POPULATIONS

8.1 Pregnancy

Pregnancy Category C

Animal reproduction studies have not been conducted with XYNTHA. It is not known whether XYNTHA can cause fetal harm when administered to a pregnant woman or can affect reproduction capacity. XYNTHA should be given to a pregnant woman only if clinically indicated.

8.2 Labor and Delivery

There is no information available on the effect of factor VIII replacement therapy on labor and delivery. XYNTHA should be used only if clinically indicated.

8.3 Nursing Mothers

It is not known whether this drug is excreted into human milk. Because many drugs are excreted into human milk, caution should be exercised if XYNTHA is administered to nursing mothers. XYNTHA should be given to nursing mothers only if clinically indicated.

8.4 Pediatric Use

Pharmacokinetics of XYNTHA was studied in 7 previously treated patients 12–16 years of age. Pharmacokinetic parameters in these patients were similar to those obtained for adults after a dose of 50 IU/kg. For these 7 patients, the mean (± SD) C_{max} and AUC_∞ were 1.09 ± 0.21 IU/mL and 11.5 ± 5.2 IU·h/mL, respectively. The mean clearance and plasma half-life values were 5.23 ± 2.36 mL/h/kg and 8.03 ± 2.44 hours (range 3.52 – 10.6 hours), respectively. The mean K-value and *in vivo* recoveries were 2.18 ± 0.41 IU/dL per IU/kg and 112 ± 23%, respectively.

8.5 Geriatric Use

Clinical studies of XYNTHA did not include subjects aged 65 and over. In general, dose selection for an elderly patient should be individualized.

11 DESCRIPTION

The active ingredient in XYNTHA, Antihemophilic Factor (Recombinant), Plasma/Albumin-Free, is a recombinant antihemophilic factor (rAHF), also called coagulation factor VIII, which is produced by recombinant DNA technology. It is secreted by a genetically engineered Chinese hamster ovary (CHO) cell line. The cell line is grown in a chemically defined cell culture medium that contains recombinant insulin, but does not contain any materials derived from human or animal sources.

The rAHF in XYNTHA is a purified glycoprotein, with an approximate molecular mass of 170 kDa consisting of 1,438 amino acids, which does not contain the B-domain.[13] The amino acid sequence of the rAHF is comparable to the 90 + 80 kDa form of human coagulation factor VIII.

The purification process uses a series of chromatography steps, one of which is based on affinity chromatography using a patented synthetic peptide affinity ligand.[14] The process also includes a solvent-detergent viral inactivation step and a virus-retaining nanofiltration step.

The potency expressed in International Units (IU) is determined using the chromogenic assay of the European Pharmacopoeia. The Wyeth manufacturing reference standard for potency has been calibrated against the World Health Organization (WHO) International Standard for factor VIII activity using the one-stage clotting assay. The specific activity of XYNTHA is 5,500 to 9,900 IU per milligram of protein.

XYNTHA is formulated as a sterile, nonpyrogenic, no preservative, lyophilized powder preparation for intravenous injection. Each single-use prefilled dual-chamber syringe (named XYNTHA SOLOFUSE) contains nominally 250, 500, 1000, 2000 or 3000 IU of XYNTHA. Upon reconstitution, the product is a clear to slightly opalescent, colorless solution that contains sodium chloride, sucrose, L-histidine, calcium chloride and polysorbate 80.

12 CLINICAL PHARMACOLOGY

12.1 Mechanism of Action

XYNTHA temporarily replaces the missing clotting factor VIII that is needed for effective hemostasis.

12.2 Pharmacodynamics

The activated partical thromboplastin time (aPTT) is prolonged in patients with hemophilia. Determination of aPTT is a conventional *in vitro* assay for biological activity of factor VIII. Treatment with XYNTHA normalizes the aPTT over the effective dosing period.

12.3 Pharmacokinetics

In a randomized crossover clinical study, 30 previously treated patients (PTP) 12–60 years old received a single infusion of 50 IU/kg of XYNTHA followed by a full-length recombinant FVIII (FLrFVIII) or a single infusion of FLrFVIII followed by XYNTHA. The one-stage clotting assay method was used to determine the concentrations of these two products in blood. XYNTHA was shown to be pharmacokinetically equivalent to FLrFVIII as the 90% confidence intervals for XYNTHA-to-FLrFVIII ratios of the mean values of C_{max} and AUC_∞ were within pre-established limits of 80% to 125%. The pharmacokinetic parameters of XYNTHA in these patients are summarized in Table 1.

In addition, 25 of the same patients later received a single infusion of 50 IU/kg of XYNTHA for a 6-month follow-up pharmacokinetic study. The parameters were comparable between baseline and 6 months, indicating no time-dependent changes in the pharmacokinetic properties of XYNTHA; the 90% confidence intervals for XYNTHA 6 month-to-baseline ratios of the mean values of C_{max} and AUC_∞ were within pre-established limits of 80% to 125%.

In a separate study investigating the efficacy of XYNTHA in patients with hemophilia A undergoing elective major surgery, 8 of 30 patients (≥ 12 years) who received a single 50 IU/kg infusion of XYNTHA as part of their presurgery evaluation participated in a pharmacokinetic evaluation. The pharmacokinetic parameters in these patients also are summarized in Table 1.

Table 1: Mean ± SD XYNTHA Pharmacokinetic Parameters in Previously Treated Patients with Hemophilia A after Single 50 IU/kg Dose

Parameter	Initial Visit (n = 30)	Month 6 (n = 25)	Pre-surgery (n=8)
C_{max} (IU/mL)	1.08 ± 0.22	1.24 ± 0.42	1.08 ± 0.24
AUC_∞ (IU·hr/mL)	13.5 ± 5.6	15.0 ± 7.5	16.0 ± 5.2
$t_{1/2}$ (hr)	11.2 ± 5.0	11.8 ± 6.2*	16.7 ± 5.4
CL (mL/hr/kg)	4.51 ± 2.23	4.04 ± 1.87	3.48 ± 1.25
Vss (mL/kg)	66.1 ± 33.0	67.4 ± 32.6	69.0 ± 20.1
K-value (IU/dL per IU/kg)	2.15 ± 0.44	2.47 ± 0.84	2.17 ± 0.47
In vivo Recovery (%)	103 ± 21	116 ± 40	104 ± 22

Abbreviations: AUC_∞ = area under the plasma concentration-time curve from zero to infinity; C_{max} = peak concentration; K-value = incremental recovery; $t_{1/2}$ = plasma elimination half-life; CL = clearance; n = number of subjects; SD = standard deviation.

* One subject was excluded from the calculation due to lack of a well-defined terminal phase.

Table 2: Time Interval Between Last Prophylaxis Dose of XYNTHA and Start of Bleed

≤ 24 hrs		> 24 ≤ 48 hrs		> 48 ≤ 72 hrs		> 72 hrs		Unknown*		Total Bleeding Episodes
Spon	Traum	Spon	Traum	Spon	Traum	Spon	Traum	Spon	Traum	
13	20	33	44	24	12	18	16	3	4	187

* Bleeds with unknown start time or bleeds in which previous prophylaxis dose was before the start of the safety and efficacy period of the study. Abbreviations: Spon = spontaneous new bleed; Traum = new bleed due to trauma; hrs = hours.

Table 3: Summary of Response to Infusions to Treat New Bleeding Episode by Number of Infusions Needed for Resolution

Response to 1st Infusion	Number of Infusions (%): 1	2	3	4	> 4	Total Number of Bleeds
Excellent	42 (95.5)	2 (4.5)	0 (0.0)	0 (0.0)	0 (0.0)	44
Good	69 (78.4)	16 (18.2)	3 (3.4)	0 (0.0)	0 (0.0)	88
Moderate	24 (53.3)	16 (35.6)	2 (4.4)	0 (0.0)	3 (6.7)	45
No Response	0 (0.0)	0 (0.0)	2 (40.0)	2 (40.0)	1 (20.0)	5
Not Assessed	4 (80.0)	0 (0.0)	0 (0.0)	1 (20.0)	0 (0.0)	5*
Total	139 (74.3)	34 (18.2)	7 (3.7)	3 (1.6)	4 (2.1)	187

* Includes 1 infusion with commercial FVIII that occurred before routine prophylaxis began.

[See table 1 above]

13 NONCLINICAL TOXICOLOGY

13.1 Carcinogenesis, Mutagenesis, Impairment of Fertility

No studies have been conducted with XYNTHA to assess its mutagenic or carcinogenic potential. XYNTHA has been shown to be comparable to the predecessor product with respect to its biochemical and physicochemical properties, as well as its nonclinical *in vivo* pharmacology and toxicology. By inference, predecessor product and XYNTHA would be expected to have equivalent mutagenic and carcinogenic potential. The predecessor product has been shown to be nongenotoxic in the mouse micronucleus assay. No studies have been conducted in animals to assess impairment of fertility or fetal development.

13.2 Animal Toxicology and/or Pharmacology

Preclinical studies evaluating XYNTHA in hemophilia A dogs without inhibitors demonstrated safe and effective restoration of hemostasis. XYNTHA demonstrated a toxicological profile that was similar to the toxicological profile observed with the predecessor product. Toxicity associated with XYNTHA was primarily associated with anti-FVIII neutralizing antibody generation first detectable at 15 days of repeat dosing in high (approximately 735 IU/kg/day) level-dosed, non-human primates.

14 CLINICAL STUDIES

Safety and Efficacy Study

In an open label safety and efficacy study (n=94), subjects received XYNTHA in a routine prophylaxis treatment regimen with on-demand treatment administered as clinically indicated. All 94 subjects were treated with at least one dose and all are included in the intent-to-treat (ITT) population. All subjects had been previously treated (previously treated patients or PTPs) with factor VIII. Eighty-nine (89) subjects accrued ≥ 50 exposure days. Median age for the 94 treated subjects was 24 years (mean 27.7 and range 12–60 years). All subjects had ≥ 150 previous exposure days with baseline FVIII activity level of ≤ 2%.

For routine prophylaxis, XYNTHA was administered at a dose of 30 ± 5 IU/kg 3 times a week with provisions for dose escalation based on pre-specified criteria. Seven dose escalations were prescribed for 6 subjects during the course of the study. Forty-three subjects (43/94 or 45.7%) reported no bleeding while on routine prophylaxis. The median annualized bleeding rate (ABR) for all bleeding episodes was 1.9 (mean 3.9, range 0–42.1).

Fifty-three subjects (53/94) received XYNTHA for on-demand treatment for a total of 187 bleeding episodes (Table 2). Seven of these bleeding episodes occurred in subjects prior to switching to a prophylaxis treatment regimen. One hundred ten of 180 bleeds (110/180 or 61.1%) occurred ≤ 48 hours after the last dose and 38.9% (70/180 bleeds) occurred > 48 hours after the last dose. The majority of bleeds reported to occur ≤ 48 hours after the last prophylaxis dose were traumatic (64/110 bleeds or 58.2%). Forty-two bleeds (42/70 or 60%) reported to occur > 48 hours after the last prophylaxis dose were spontaneous. The on-demand treatment dosing regimen was determined by the investigator. The median dose for on-demand treatment was 30.6 IU/kg (range, 6.4 to 74.4 IU/kg).

[See table 2 above]

The majority of bleeding episodes (173/187 or 92.5%) resolved with 1 or 2 infusions. Subjects rated the outcomes of infusions on a pre-specified four (4) point hemostatic efficacy scale. One hundred thirty-two of 187 bleeding episodes (132/187 or 70.6%) treated with XYNTHA were rated excellent or good in their response to initial treatment, 45 (24.1%) were rated moderate. Five (2.7%) were rated no response, and 5 (2.7%) were not rated.

[See table 3 above]

Of the 94 subjects enrolled in this study, 30 evaluable subjects participated in a randomized crossover pharmacokinetics study. Twenty-five (25/30) of these subjects with FVIII:C ≤ 1% completed both the first (PK1) and the second (PK2) pharmacokinetic assessments [*see Clinical Pharmacology (12.3)*].

Surgical Prophylaxis Study

In an open-label study (n=30) for surgical prophylaxis in subjects with hemophilia A, XYNTHA was administered to 25 efficacy-evaluable PTPs with severe or moderately severe (FVIII:C ≤ 2%) hemophilia A undergoing major surgical procedures (11 total knee replacements, 1 hip replacement, 5 synovectomies, 1 left ulnar nerve transposition release, 1 ventral hernia repair/scar revision, 1 knee arthroscopy, 1 revision and debridement of the knee after a total knee replacement, 1 hip arthroplasty revision, 1 stapes replacement, 1 ankle arthrodesis, and 1 pseudotumor excision).

The results of the hemostatic efficacy ratings for these subjects are presented in Table 4. Investigator's ratings of efficacy at the end of surgery and at the end of the initial postoperative period were "excellent" or "good" for all assessments. Intraoperative blood loss was reported as "normal" or "absent" for all subjects. Thirteen of the subjects (13/25 or 52%) had blood loss in the postoperative period. The postoperative blood loss was rated as "normal" for ten of these cases while three cases were rated "abnormal" (1 due to hemorrhage following surgical trauma to the epigastric artery, 1 due to an 800 mL blood loss after hip replacement surgery, and 1 after an elbow synovectomy where the blood loss could not be measured by the investigator).

Table 4: Summary of Hemostatic Efficacy

Time of Hemostatic Efficacy Assessment	Excellent	Good	Number of subjects
End of surgery	18 (72%)	7 (28%)	25
End of initial postoperative period*	23 (92%)	2 (8%)	25

* Conclusion of initial postoperative period is date of discharge or postoperative Day 6, whichever occurs later.

15 REFERENCES

1. Nilsson IM, Berntorp EE and Freiburghaus C. Treatment of patients with factor VIII and IX inhibitors. *Thromb Haemost*. 1993;70(1):56–59.
2. Hoyer LW. Hemophilia A. *N Engl J Med*. 1994;330:38–47.
3. Juhlin F. Stability and Compatibility of Reconstituted Recombinant Factor VIII SQ, 250 IU/ml, in a System for Continuous Infusion. Pharmacia Document 9610224, 1996.
4. Ehrenforth S, Kreuz W, Scharrer I, et al. Incidence of development of factor VIII and factor IX inhibitors in hemophiliacs. *Lancet*. 1992;339:594–598.
5. Lusher J, Arkin S, Abildgaard CF, Schwartz RS, the Kogenate PUP Study Group. Recombinant factor VIII for the treatment of previously untreated patients with hemophilia A. *N Engl J Med*. 1993;328:453–459.
6. Bray GL, Gomperts ED, Courter S, et al. A multicenter study of recombinant factor VIII (Recombinate): safety, efficacy, and inhibitor risk in previously untreated patients with hemophilia A. *Blood*. 1994;83(9):2428–2435.
7. Kessler C, Sachse K. Factor VIII:C inhibitor associated with monoclonal-antibody purified FVIII concentrate. *Lancet*. 1990;335:1403.
8. Schwartz RS, Abildgaard CF, Aledort LM, et al. Human recombinant DNA-derived antihemophilic factor (factor VIII) in the treatment of hemophilia A. *N Engl J Med*. 1990;323:1800–1805.
9. White GC II, Courter S, Bray GL, et al. A multicenter study of recombinant factor VIII (Recombinate™) in previously treated patients with hemophilia A. *Thromb Haemost*. 1997;77(4):660–667.
10. Gruppo R, Chen H, Schroth P, et al. Safety and immunogenicity of recombinant factor VIII (Recombinate™) in previously untreated patients: A 7.3 year update. *Haemophilia*. 1998;4:228 (Abstract No. 291, XXIII Congress of the WFH, The Hague).
11. Scharrer I, Bray GL, Neutzling O. Incidence of inhibitors in haemophilia A patients - a review of recent studies of recombinant and plasma-derived factor VIII concentrates. *Haemophilia*. 1999;5:145–154.
12. Abshire TC, Brackmann HH, Scharrer I, et al. Sucrose formulated recombinant human antihemophilic Factor VIII is safe and efficacious for treatment of hemophilia A in home therapy: Results of a multicenter, international, clinical investigation. *Thromb Haemost*. 2000;83(6):811–816.
13. Sandberg H, Almstedt A, Brandt J, Castro VM, Gray E, Holmquist L, et al. Structural and Functional Characterization of B-Domain Deleted Recombinant Factor VIII. *Sem Hematol*. 2001;38 (Suppl. 4):4–12.
14. Kelley BD, Tannatt M, Magnusson R, Hagelberg S. Development and Validation of an Affinity Chromatography Step Using a Peptide Ligand for cGMP Production of Factor VIII. *Biotechnol Bioeng*. 2004;87(3):400–412.
15. Mann KG and Ziedens KB. Overview of Hemostasis. In: Lee CA, Berntorp EE and Hoots WK, eds. *Textbook of Hemophilia*. USA, Blackwell Publishing; 2005:1–4.

16 HOW SUPPLIED/STORAGE AND HANDLING

16.1 How Supplied

XYNTHA SOLOFUSE is supplied in a kit that includes the XYNTHA lyophilized powder containing nominally 250, 500, 1000, 2000 or 3000 IU and 4 mL 0.9 % Sodium Chloride solution for reconstitution in a prefilled dual-chamber syringe:

250 International Units Kit: NDC 58394-022-03
500 International Units Kit: NDC 58394-023-03
1000 International Units Kit: NDC 58394-024-03
2000 International Units Kit: NDC 58394-025-03
3000 International Units Kit: NDC 58394-016-03

Each XYNTHA SOLOFUSE Kit contains: one plunger rod for assembly, one sterile infusion set, two alcohol swabs, one bandage, one gauze pad, one vented sterile cap, and one package insert.

Actual factor VIII activity in International Units is stated on the label of each XYNTHA SOLOFUSE.

16.2 Storage and Handling

Product as Packaged for Sale:

- Store XYNTHA SOLOFUSE under refrigeration at a temperature of 2° to 8°C (36° to 46°F) for up to 36 months from the date of manufacture until the expiration date stated on the label. Within the expiration date, XYNTHA SOLOFUSE also may be stored at room temperature not to exceed 25°C (77°F) for up to 3 months.
- Clearly record the starting date at room temperature storage in the space provided on the outer carton. At the end of the 3-month period, immediately use or discard the product. **Do not put the product back into the refrigerator.**
- Do not use XYNTHA SOLOFUSE after the expiration date stated on the label or after 3 months when stored at room temperature, whichever is earlier.
- Do not freeze. (Freezing may damage the XYNTHA SOLOFUSE.)
- During storage, avoid prolonged exposure of XYNTHA SOLOFUSE to light.

Product After Reconstitution:

- Store the reconstituted solution at room temperature prior to administration. Remember to administer XYNTHA SOLOFUSE within 3 hours after reconstitution or after removal of the grey rubber tip cap from the product.

17 PATIENT COUNSELING INFORMATION

See FDA-approved patient labeling (Patient Information and Instructions for Use)

Advise the patients of the following

- Tell their healthcare provider about any adverse reactions or problems that concern them when taking XYNTHA.
- Allergic-type hypersensitivity reactions are possible. Discuss the early signs of hypersensitivity reactions (including hives [rash with itching], generalized urticaria, tightness of the chest, wheezing, hypotension) and anaphylaxis. Advise patients to discontinue use of the product, call their healthcare provider, and go to the emergency department if these symptoms occur.
- Tell their healthcare provider if they experience a lack of a clinical response to factor VIII replacement therapy, as this may be a manifestation of an inhibitor.
- Tell their healthcare provider if they become pregnant or intend to become pregnant during therapy.
- Notify their healthcare provider if they are breastfeeding.
- Local irritation may occur when infusing XYNTHASOLOFUSE.
- Consult their healthcare provider prior to travel and to bring an adequate supply of XYNTHA SOLOFUSE, based on their current regimen, for anticipated treatment when traveling.

FDA-Approved Patient Labeling
Patient Information
XYNTHA® SOLOFUSE™ /ZIN-tha/
[Antihemophilic Factor (Recombinant), Plasma/Albumin-Free]

Please read this patient information carefully before using XYNTHA and each time you get a refill. There may be new information. This leaflet does not take the place of talking with your healthcare provider about your medical problems or your treatment.

What is XYNTHA?

XYNTHA is an injectable medicine that is used to help control and prevent bleeding in people with hemophilia A. Hemophilia A is also called classic hemophilia.

XYNTHA is not used to treat von Willebrand's disease.

What should I tell my healthcare provider before using XYNTHA?

Tell your healthcare provider about all of your medical conditions, including if you:

- are pregnant or planning to become pregnant. It is not known if XYNTHA may harm your unborn baby.
- are breastfeeding. It is not known if XYNTHA passes into your milk and if it can harm your baby.

Tell your healthcare provider about all of the medicines you take, including all prescription and non-prescription medicines, such as over-the-counter medicines, supplements, or herbal remedies.

How should I infuse XYNTHA?

Step-by-step instructions for infusing with XYNTHA SOLOFUSE are provided at the end of this leaflet.

The steps listed below are general guidelines for using XYNTHA SOLOFUSE. Always follow any specific instructions from your healthcare provider. If you are unsure of the procedures, please call your healthcare provider before using.

Call your healthcare provider right away if bleeding is not controlled after using XYNTHA.

Your body can make antibodies against XYNTHA (called "inhibitors") that may stop XYNTHA from working properly. Your healthcare provider may need to take blood tests from time to time to monitor for inhibitors.

Call your healthcare provider right away if you take more than the dose you should take.

Talk to your healthcare provider before traveling. Plan to bring enough XYNTHA SOLOFUSE for your treatment during this time.

What are the possible or reasonably likely side effects of XYNTHA?

Common side effects of XYNTHA are

- headache
- fever
- nausea
- vomiting
- diarrhea
- weakness

Call your healthcare provider or go to the emergency department right away if you have any of the following symptoms because these may be signs of a serious allergic reaction:

- **wheezing**
- **difficulty breathing**
- **chest tightness**
- **turning blue (look at lips and gums)**
- **fast heartbeat**
- **swelling of the face**
- **faintness**
- **rash**
- **hives**

Talk to your healthcare provider about any side effect that bothers you or that does not go away. You may report side effects to FDA at 1-800-FDA-1088.

How should I store XYNTHA SOLOFUSE?

Store in the refrigerator at 36° to 46°F (2° to 8°C).

Do not freeze.

Protect from light.

XYNTHA SOLOFUSE can last at room temperature (below 77°F) for up to 3 months. If you store XYNTHA SOLOFUSE at room temperature, carefully write down the date you put XYNTHA SOLOFUSE at room temperature, so you will know when to throw it away. There is a space on the carton for you to write the date.

Throw away any unused XYNTHA SOLOFUSE after the expiration date.

Infuse within 3 hours after reconstitution or after removal of the grey rubber tip cap from the prefilled dual-chamber syringe. You can keep the reconstituted solution at room temperature before infusion, but if it is not used in 3 hours, throw it away.

Do not use reconstituted XYNTHA if it is not clear to slightly opalescent and colorless.

Dispose of all materials, whether reconstituted or not, in an appropriate medical waste container.

What else should I know about XYNTHA?

Medicines are sometimes prescribed for purposes other than those listed here. Talk to your healthcare provider if you have any concerns. You can ask your healthcare provider for information about XYNTHA SOLOFUSE that was written for healthcare professionals.

Do not share XYNTHA SOLOFUSE with other people, even if they have the same symptoms that you have.

Instructions for Use
XYNTHA® SOLOFUSE™ /ZIN-tha/
[Antihemophilic Factor (Recombinant), Plasma/Albumin-Free]

XYNTHA SOLOFUSE is supplied as a pre-filled dual-chamber syringe with lyophilized XYNTHA powder in one chamber and 0.9% sodium chloride solution in the other chamber. Before you can infuse it (intravenous injection), you must reconstitute the powder by mixing it with the sodium chloride solution.

Reconstitute and infuse XYNTHA SOLOFUSE using the infusion set provided in this kit. Please follow the directions below for the proper use of this product.

PREPARATION AND RECONSTITUTION OF XYNTHA SOLOFUSE

Preparation

1. Always wash your hands before doing the following steps.
2. Keep everything clean and germ-free while you are reconstituting XYNTHA SOLOFUSE.
3. Once the syringes are open, finish reconstituting XYNTHA SOLOFUSE as soon as possible. This will help to keep them germ-free.

4. For additional instructions on the use of a XYNTHA SOLOFUSE and a XYNTHA vial or multiple XYNTHA SOLOFUSE, see the detailed information provided after **INFUSION OF XYNTHA** section.

Reconstitution

1. Allow the XYNTHA SOLOFUSE to reach room temperature.
2. Remove the contents of the XYNTHA SOLOFUSE Kit and place on a clean surface, making sure you have all the supplies you will need.
3. Grasp the plunger rod as shown in the following diagram. Do not touch the shaft of the plunger rod. Screw the plunger rod firmly into the opening in the finger rest of the XYNTHA SOLOFUSE by pushing and turning firmly until resistance is felt (approximately 2 turns).
   Throughout the reconstitution process, it is important to keep the XYNTHA SOLOFUSE upright to prevent possible leakage.

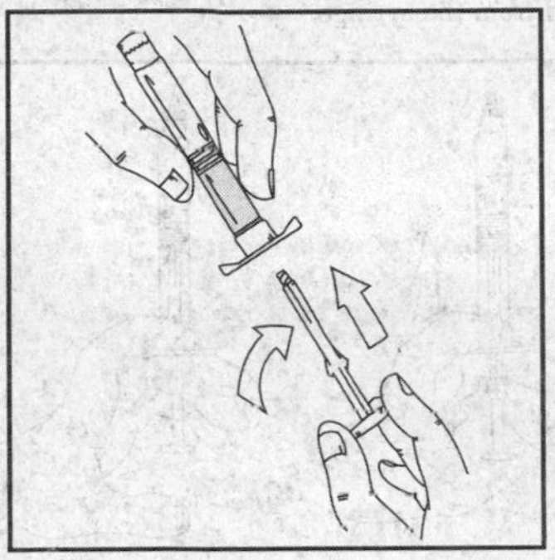

4. Holding the XYNTHA SOLOFUSE upright, remove the white tamper-evident seal by bending the seal right to left (or a gentle rocking motion) to break the perforation of the cap and expose the grey rubber tip cap of the XYNTHA SOLOFUSE.

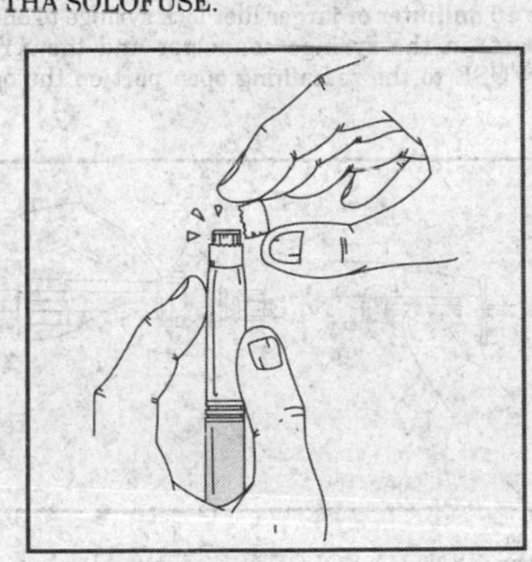

5. Remove the protective blue vented sterile cap from its package. While holding the XYNTHA SOLOFUSE upright, remove the grey rubber tip cap and replace it with the protective blue vented cap (prevents pressure build-up). Avoid touching the open end of both the syringe and the protective blue vented cap.

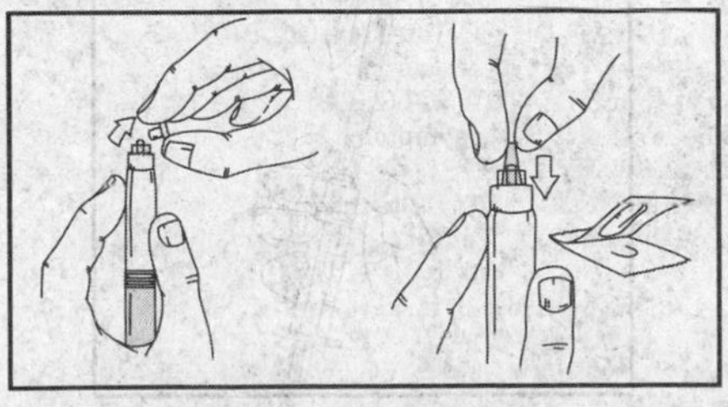

6. **Gently and slowly** push the plunger rod until the two stoppers inside the XYNTHA SOLOFUSE meet, and all of the diluent is transferred to the chamber containing the XYNTHA powder.
   Note: To prevent the escape of fluid from the tip of the syringe, do not push the plunger rod with excessive force.

[See first figure at top of next column]

7. With the XYNTHA SOLOFUSE remaining upright, swirl **gently** several times until the powder is dissolved.

[See second figure at top of next column]

Look carefully at the solution in the XYNTHA SOLOFUSE. The solution should be clear to slightly opalescent and colorless. If it is not, throw away the solution and use a new kit.

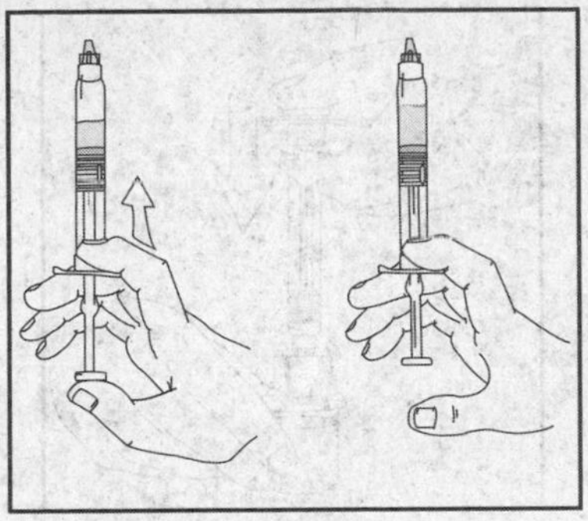

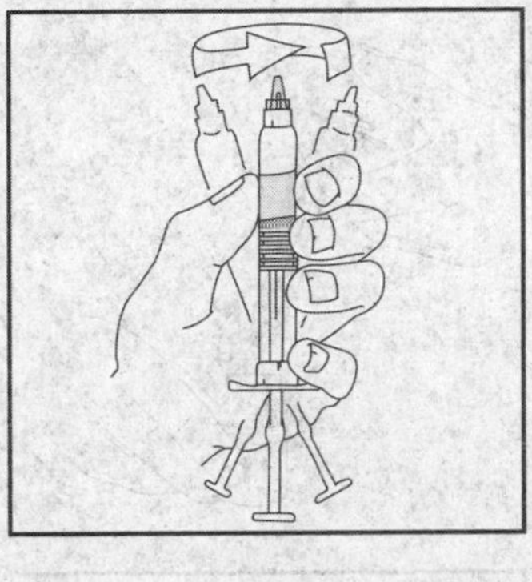

8. Holding the XYNTHA SOLOFUSE in an upright position, slowly advance the plunger rod until most, but not all, of the air is removed from the drug product chamber.

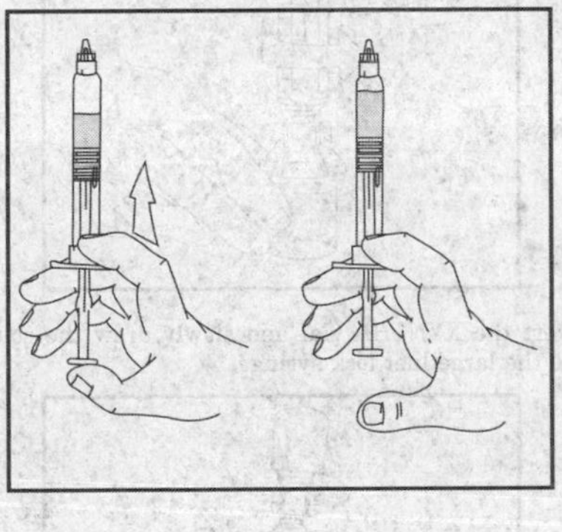

Note:

- If you are not using the solution immediately, store the syringe upright and keep the protective blue vent cap on the XYNTHA SOLOFUSE until ready to infuse.
- Infuse XYNTHA solution within 3 hours after reconstitution or removal of the grey tip cap from the XYNTHA SOLOFUSE. The reconstituted solution may be kept at room temperature for up to 3 hours prior to infusion. If you have not used it in 3 hours, throw it away.
- If more than one XYNTHA SOLOFUSE is needed for each infusion, a luer-to-luer syringe connector can be used (not included in this kit). Please contact your doctor or healthcare provider, or call the Wyeth Medical Information Department at 1-800-438-1985, for additional information.

INFUSION OF XYNTHA

Your healthcare provider will teach you how to infuse XYNTHA yourself. Once you learn how to do this, you can follow the instructions in this insert.

Before XYNTHA can be infused, you must reconstitute it as instructed above in the **PREPARATION AND RECONSTITUTION OF XYNTHA SOLOFUSE** section.

After reconstitution, be sure to look carefully at the XYNTHA solution. The solution should be clear to slightly opalescent and colorless. If it is not, throw away the solution and use a new kit.

Use the infusion set included in the kit to infuse XYNTHA. Do not infuse XYNTHA in the same tubing or container with other medicines.

1. After removing the protective blue vented cap, firmly attach the intravenous infusion set provided in the kit onto the XYNTHA SOLOFUSE.

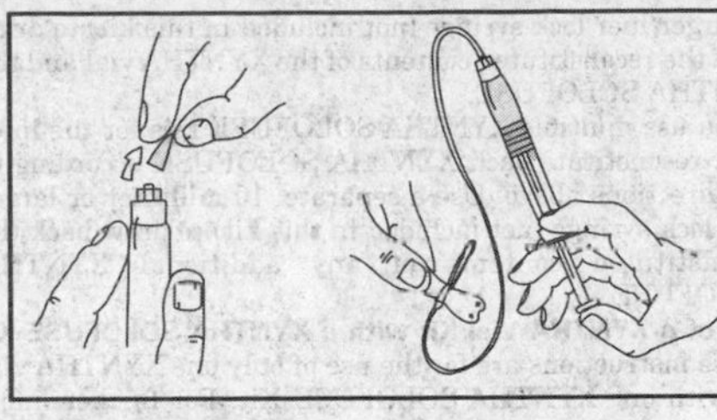

2. Apply a tourniquet and prepare the injection site by wiping the skin well with an alcohol swab provided in the kit.

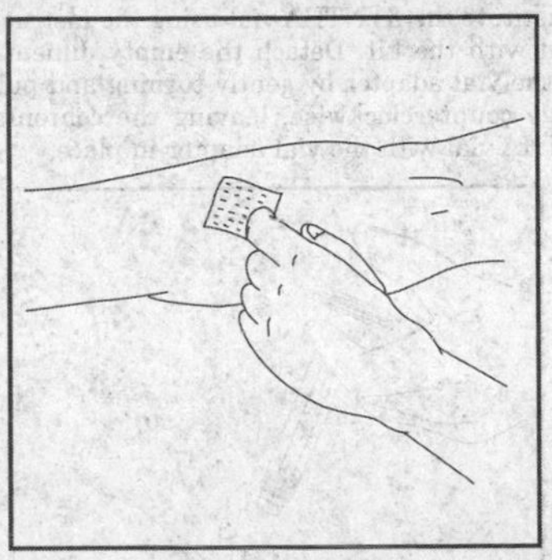

3. Remove the protective needle cover and insert the butterfly needle of the infusion set tubing into your vein as instructed by your healthcare provider. Remove the tourniquet. Verify proper needle placement.
4. Infuse the reconstituted XYNTHA product over several minutes. Your comfort level should determine the rate of infusion.

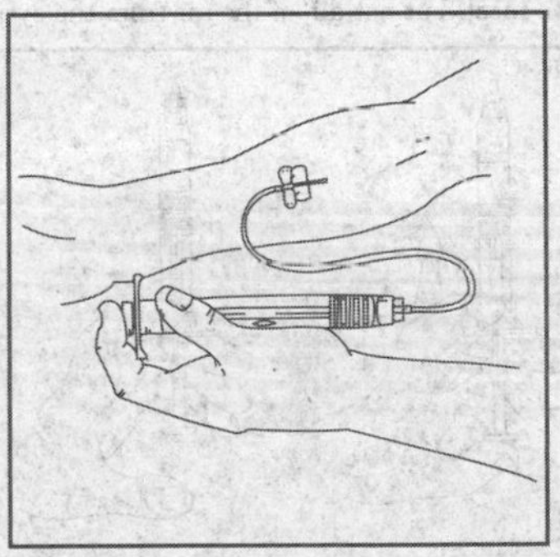

5. After infusing XYNTHA, remove the infusion set and throw it away. The amount of liquid left in the infusion set will not affect your treatment.

Note:

- Throw away all unused solution, the empty XYNTHA SOLOFUSE, and other used medical supplies in an appropriate container.

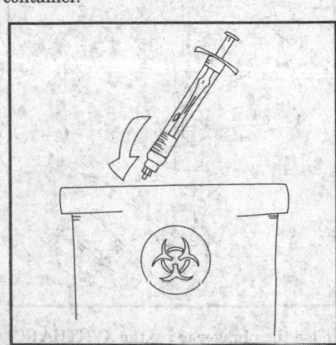

- It is a good idea to record the lot number from the XYNTHA SOLOFUSE label every time you use XYNTHA. You can use the peel-off label found on the XYNTHA SOLOFUSE to record the lot number.

ADDITIONAL INSTRUCTIONS

XYNTHA is also supplied in kits that include single-use vials with lyophilized powder and prefilled diluent syringes. If you use one XYNTHA vial and one XYNTHA SOLOFUSE for the infusion, reconstitute the XYNTHA vial and the XYNTHA SOLOFUSE according to the specific directions for that respective product kit. Use a separate, 10 milliliter or larger luer lock syringe (not included in this kit) to draw back the reconstituted contents of the XYNTHA vial and the XYNTHA SOLOFUSE.

If you use multiple XYNTHA SOLOFUSE kits for the infusion, reconstitute each XYNTHA SOLOFUSE according to the directions above. Use a separate, 10 milliliter or larger luer lock syringe (not included in this kit) to draw back the reconstituted contents of any additional XYNTHA SOLOFUSE.

Use of a XYNTHA Vial Kit with a XYNTHA SOLOFUSE Kit

These instructions are for the use of only one XYNTHA vial kit with one XYNTHA SOLOFUSE Kit. For further information, please contact your healthcare provider or call the Medical Information Department at Wyeth Pharmaceuticals, 1-800-438-1985.

1. Reconstitute the XYNTHA vial using the instructions included with the kit. Detach the empty diluent syringe from the vial adapter by gently turning and pulling the syringe counterclockwise, leaving the contents in the XYNTHA vial with the vial adapter in place.

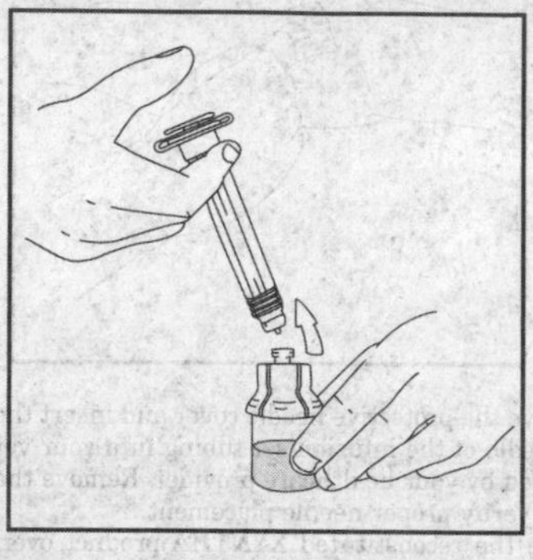

2. Reconstitute the XYNTHA SOLOFUSE using the instructions included with the product kit, remembering to remove most, but not all, of the air from the syringe.

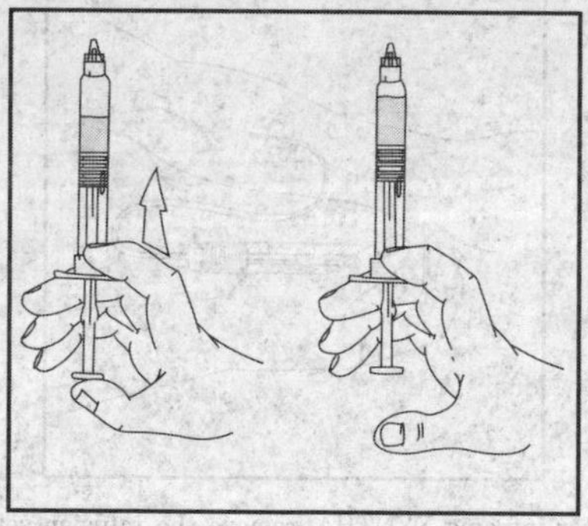

3. After removing the protective blue vented cap, connect the XYNTHA SOLOFUSE to the vial adapter by inserting the tip into the adapter opening while firmly pushing and turning the syringe clockwise until secured.

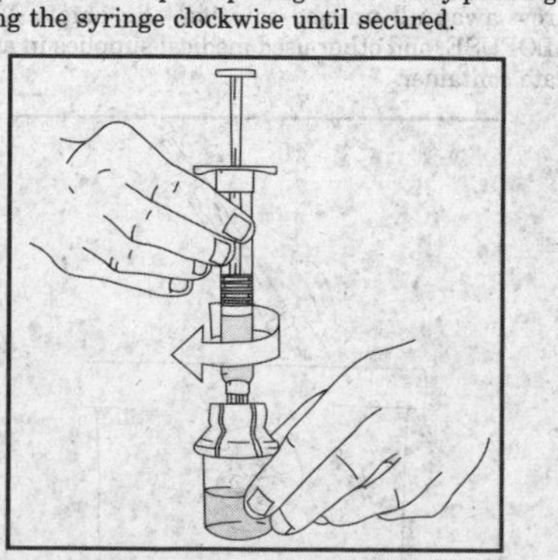

4. Slowly push the plunger rod of the XYNTHA SOLOFUSE to empty the contents into the XYNTHA vial. The plunger rod may move back slightly after release.

[See first figure at top of next column]

5. Detach the empty XYNTHA SOLOFUSE from the vial adapter and throw it away. If the syringe turns without detaching from the vial adapter, grasp the white collar and turn.

[See second figure at top of next column]

6. Connect a sterile 10 milliliter or larger luer lock syringe to the vial adapter. You may want to inject some air into the vial to make withdrawing the vial contents easier.

[See third figure at top of next column]

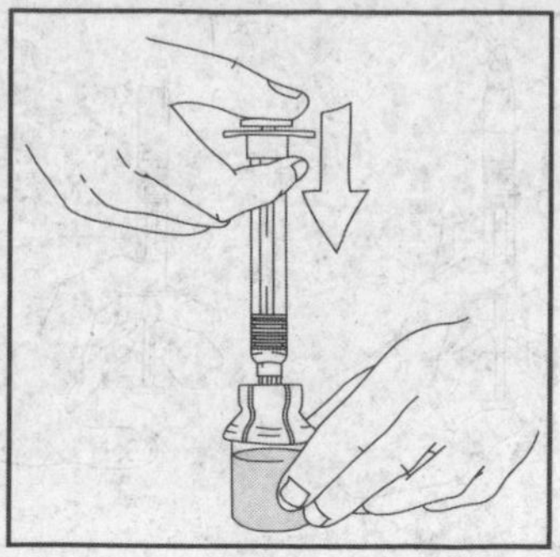

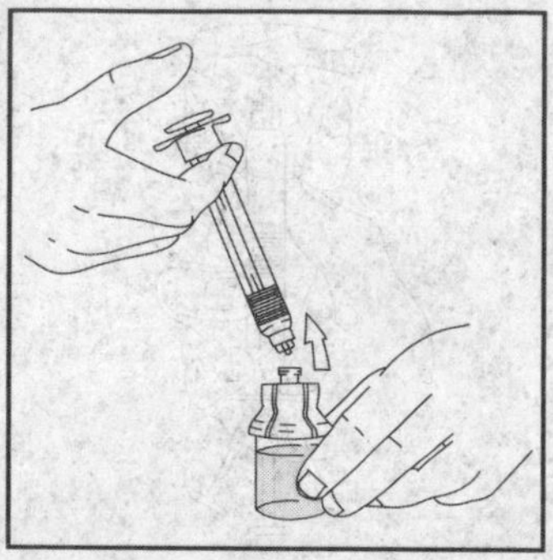

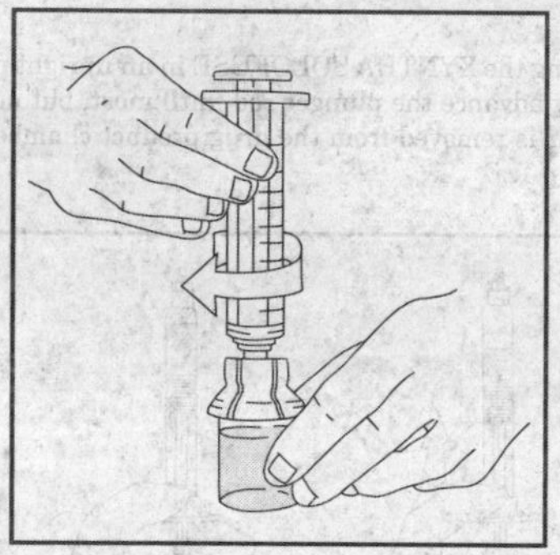

7. Invert the XYNTHA vial and slowly draw the solution into the large luer lock syringe.

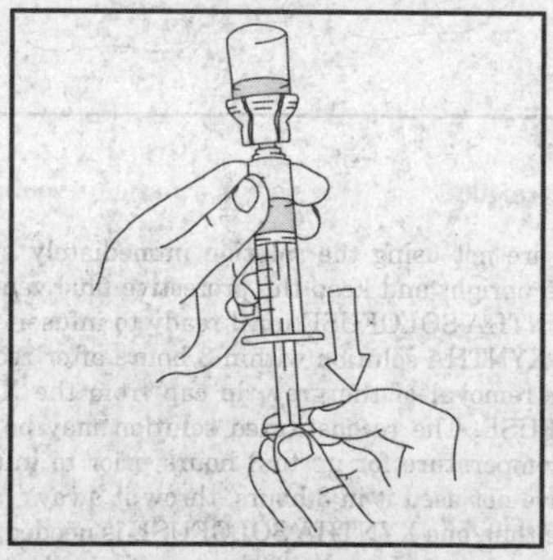

8. Detach the large luer lock syringe from the vial adapter by gently turning and pulling the syringe counterclockwise. Throw away the empty XYNTHA vial with the adapter attached.
9. Attach the infusion set to the large luer lock syringe as directed in the **INFUSION OF XYNTHA** section.

Note: Dispose of all unused solution, the empty XYNTHA SOLOFUSE, and other used medical supplies in an appropriate container.

[See figure at top of next column]

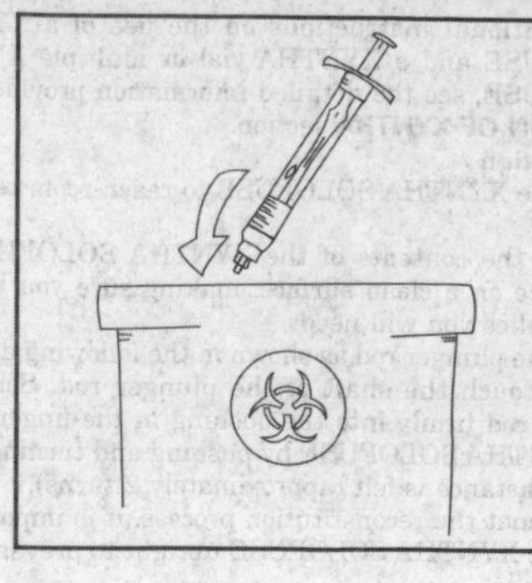

Use of Multiple XYNTHA SOLOFUSE Kits

The instructions below are for the use of multiple XYNTHA SOLOFUSE kits with a 10 milliliter or larger luer lock syringe. For further information, please contact your healthcare provider or call the Medical Information Department at Wyeth Pharmaceuticals, 1-800-438-1985.

Note: Luer-to-luer syringe connectors are not provided in the kits. Contact your XYNTHA supplier to order.

1. Reconstitute all XYNTHA SOLOFUSE according to instructions described in **PREPARATION AND RECONSTITUTION OF XYNTHA SOLOFUSE** section. Holding the XYNTHA SOLOFUSE in an upright position, slowly push the plunger rod until most, but not all, of the air is removed from the syringe.

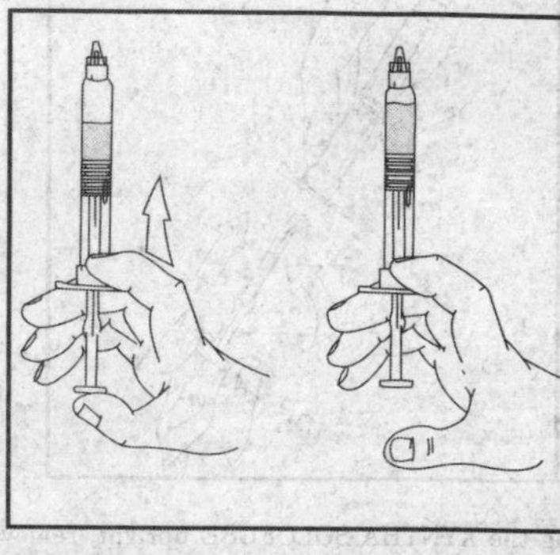

2. Remove the luer-to-luer syringe connector from its package.
3. After removing the protective blue vented cap, connect a sterile 10 milliliter or larger luer lock syringe to one opening (port) in the syringe connector and the XYNTHA SOLOFUSE to the remaining open port on the opposite end.

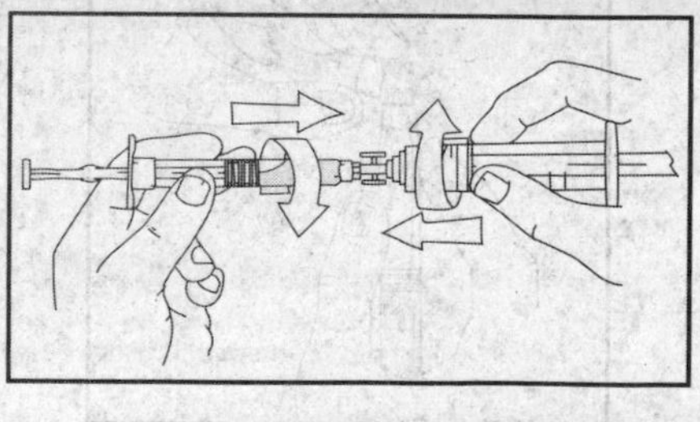

4. With the XYNTHA SOLOFUSE on top, slowly push the plunger rod to empty all the XYNTHA SOLOFUSE content into the large luer lock syringe.

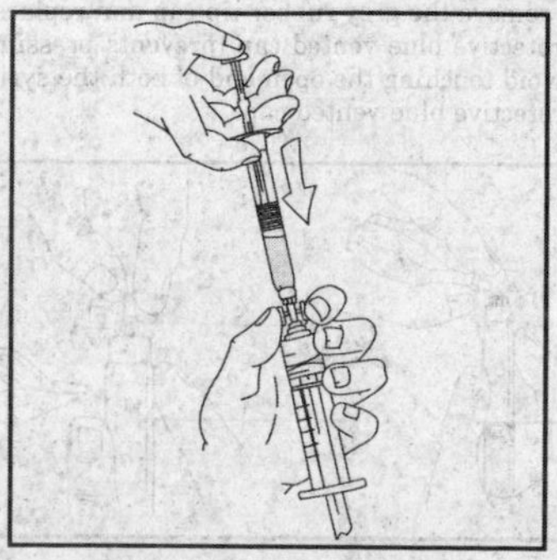

5. Remove the empty XYNTHA SOLOFUSE and repeat procedures 3 and 4 above for any additional XYNTHA SOLOFUSE.
6. Remove the luer-to-luer syringe connector from the large luer lock syringe and attach the infusion set as directed in the **INFUSION OF XYNTHA** section.

Note: Dispose of all unused solution, the empty XYNTHA SOLOFUSE, and other used medical supplies in an appropriate container.

Manufactured by
Wyeth Pharmaceuticals Inc
A subsidiary of Pfizer Inc, Philadelphia, PA 19101
License no: 3
LAB-0500-8.0

Eisai Inc.
100 TICE BLVD.
WOODCLIFF LAKE, NJ 07677

Telephone:
1-888-274-2378

ACIPHEX® ℞
(rabeprazole sodium)
Delayed-Release Tablets, for oral use

ACIPHEX® SPRINKLE™
(rabeprazole sodium)
Delayed-Release Capsules, for oral use

HIGHLIGHTS OF PRESCRIBING INFORMATION
These highlights do not include all the information needed to use ACIPHEX safely and effectively. See full prescribing information for ACIPHEX.
ACIPHEX® (rabeprazole sodium) Delayed-Release Tablets, for oral use
ACIPHEX® Sprinkle™ (rabeprazole sodium) Delayed-Release Capsules, for oral use
Initial U.S. Approval: 1999

RECENT MAJOR CHANGES

Indications and Usage, Pediatric Patients (1.8) 03/2013
Dosage and Administration, Pediatric Patients (2.8) 03/2013
Warnings and Precautions, *Clostridium difficile* associated diarrhea (5.3) 10/2012
Warnings and Precautions, Concomitant use of ACIPHEX with Methotrexate (5.6) 05/2012

INDICATIONS AND USAGE

ACIPHEX is a proton-pump inhibitor (PPI) indicated in adults for:

- Healing of Erosive or Ulcerative Gastroesophageal Reflux Disease (GERD) (1.1)
- Maintenance of Healing of Erosive or Ulcerative GERD (1.2)
- Treatment of Symptomatic GERD (1.3)
- Healing of Duodenal Ulcers (1.4)
- *Helicobacter pylori* Eradication to Reduce the Risk of Duodenal Ulcer Recurrence (1.5)
- Treatment of Pathological Hypersecretory Conditions, Including Zollinger-Ellison Syndrome (1.6)

In adolescent patients 12 years of age and older for:

- Short-term treatment of Symptomatic GERD (1.7)

In pediatric patients 1 to 11 years of age for:

- Treatment of GERD (1.8)

DOSAGE AND ADMINISTRATION

ACIPHEX Delayed-Release Tablets should be swallowed whole. The tablets should not be chewed, crushed or split (2.10).

ACIPHEX Sprinkle Delayed-Release Capsules should be opened and the granule contents sprinkled on a spoonful of soft food or liquid (e.g. apple sauce). Whole dose should be taken within 15 minutes of being sprinkled. The granules should not be chewed or crushed. Dose should be taken 30 minutes before a meal (2.10).

Healing of Erosive or Ulcerative Gastroesophageal Reflux Disease (GERD) (2.1)	20 mg once daily
Maintenance of Healing of Erosive or Ulcerative GERD (2.2)	20 mg once daily
Treatment of Symptomatic GERD in Adults (2.3)	20 mg once daily
Healing of Duodenal Ulcers (2.4)	20 mg once daily after morning meal
***Helicobacter pylori* Eradication to Reduce the Risk of Duodenal Ulcer Recurrence** (2.5) **Three Drug Regimen:** ACIPHEX 20 mg, Amoxicillin 1000 mg, Clarithromycin 500 mg	*All three medications should be taken twice daily with morning and evening meals for 7 days*
Treatment of Pathological Hypersecretory Conditions, Including Zollinger-Ellison Syndrome (2.6)	Starting dose 60 mg once daily then adjust to patient needs
Treatment of Symptomatic GERD in Adolescents 12 Years of Age and Older (2.7)	20 mg once daily
Treatment of GERD in 1 to 11 Years Olds (2.8)	Less than 15 kg: 5 mg once daily *(with the option to increase to 10 mg once daily)*; 15 kg or greater: 10 mg once daily

DOSAGE FORMS AND STRENGTHS

- Delayed-Release Tablets: 20 mg (3)
- Delayed-Release Capsules: 5 mg and 10 mg (3)

CONTRAINDICATIONS

- History of hypersensitivity to rabeprazole (4)

WARNINGS AND PRECAUTIONS

- Symptomatic response to therapy with rabeprazole does not preclude the presence of gastric malignancy (5.1)
- Use with warfarin: monitor for increases in INR and prothombin time (5.2)
- PPI therapy may be associated with increased risk of *Clostridium difficile* associated diarrhea (5.3)
- Bone fracture: Long-term and multiple daily dose PPI therapy may be associated with an increased risk for osteoporosis-related fractures of the hip, wrist, or spine (5.4)
- Hypomagnesemia has been reported rarely with prolonged treatment with PPIs (5.5)

ADVERSE REACTIONS

- In the adult studies (4 to 8 weeks), adverse reactions that occurred at a rate greater than 2% and greater than placebo included pain, pharyngitis, flatulence, infection and constipation (6.1).
- In studies of pediatric and adolescent patients (ages 1 to 16 years, and up to 36 weeks exposure) adverse reactions that occurred at a rate of ≥5% of patients included abdominal pain, diarrhea and headache (6.1).

To report SUSPECTED ADVERSE REACTIONS, contact Eisai Inc. at 1-888-274-2378 or FDA at 1-800-FDA-1088 or *www.fda.gov/medwatch*

DRUG INTERACTIONS

- Increased INR and prothrombin times have been reported with concomitant use with warfarin. Patients need to be monitored (7.2)
- Rabeprazole has been shown to inhibit cyclosporine metabolism *in vitro* (7.3)
- ACIPHEX inhibits gastric acid secretion and may interfere with the absorption of drugs where gastric pH is an important determinant of bioavailability (e.g., ketoconazole, iron salts and digoxin) (7.4)
- ACIPHEX may reduce the plasma levels of atazanavir (7.4)
- Methotrexate: ACIPHEX may increase serum level of methotrexate (7.7)

USE IN SPECIFIC POPULATIONS

- Studies conducted do not support the use of ACIPHEX or the treatment of GERD in pediatric patients younger than 1 year of age (8.4).
- The safety and efficacy of ACIPHEX for the other adult indications have not been established for pediatric patients (8.4).

See 17 for PATIENT COUNSELING INFORMATION and Medication Guide

Revised: 03/2013

FULL PRESCRIBING INFORMATION: CONTENTS*

*** Sections or subsections omitted from the full prescribing information are not listed**

FULL PRESCRIBING INFORMATION

1 INDICATIONS AND USAGE

1.1 Healing of Erosive or Ulcerative GERD in Adults

ACIPHEX is indicated for short-term (4 to 8 weeks) treatment in the healing and symptomatic relief of erosive or ulcerative gastroesophageal reflux disease (GERD). For those patients who have not healed after 8 weeks of treatment, an additional 8-week course of ACIPHEX may be considered.

1.2 Maintenance of Healing of Erosive or Ulcerative GERD in Adults

ACIPHEX is indicated for maintaining healing and reduction in relapse rates of heartburn symptoms in patients with erosive or ulcerative gastroesophageal reflux disease (GERD Maintenance). Controlled studies do not extend beyond 12 months.

1.3 Treatment of Symptomatic GERD in Adults

ACIPHEX is indicated for the treatment of daytime and nighttime heartburn and other symptoms associated with GERD in adults

1.4 Healing of Duodenal Ulcers in Adults

ACIPHEX is indicated for short-term (up to four weeks) treatment in the healing and symptomatic relief of duodenal ulcers. Most patients heal within four weeks.

1.5 *Helicobacter pylori* Eradication to Reduce the Risk of Duodenal Ulcer Recurrence in Adults

ACIPHEX in combination with amoxicillin and clarithromycin as a three drug regimen, is indicated for the treatment of patients with *H. pylori* infection and duodenal ulcer disease (active or history within the past 5 years) to eradicate *H. pylori*. Eradication of *H. pylori* has been shown to reduce the risk of duodenal ulcer recurrence [*see Clinical Studies (14.5)* and *Dosage and Administration (2.5)*].

In patients who fail therapy, susceptibility testing should be done. If resistance to clarithromycin is demonstrated or susceptibility testing is not possible, alternative antimicrobial therapy should be instituted [*see Clinical Pharmacology (12.2)* and the clarithromycin package insert, *Clinical Pharmacology (12.2)*].

1.6 Treatment of Pathological Hypersecretory Conditions, Including Zollinger-Ellison Syndrome in Adults

ACIPHEX is indicated for the long-term treatment of pathological hypersecretory conditions, including Zollinger-Ellison syndrome.

1.7 Short-term Treatment of Symptomatic GERD in Adolescent Patients 12 Years of Age and Older

ACIPHEX is indicated for the treatment of symptomatic GERD in adolescents 12 years of age and above for up to 8 weeks.

1.8 Treatment of GERD in Pediatric Patients 1 to 11 Years of Age

ACIPHEX is indicated for treatment of GERD in children 1 to 11 years of age for up to 12 weeks.

2 DOSAGE AND ADMINISTRATION

2.1 Healing of Erosive or Ulcerative GERD in Adults

The recommended adult oral dose is one ACIPHEX 20 mg Delayed-Release tablet to be taken once daily for four to eight weeks [*see Indications and Usage (1.1)*]. For those patients who have not healed after 8 weeks of treatment, an additional 8-week course of ACIPHEX may be considered.

2.2 Maintenance of Healing of Erosive or Ulcerative GERD in Adults

The recommended adult oral dose is one ACIPHEX 20 mg Delayed-Release tablet to be taken once daily [*see Indications and Usage (1.2)*].

2.3 Treatment of Symptomatic GERD in Adults

The recommended adult oral dose is one ACIPHEX 20 mg Delayed-Release tablet to be taken once daily for 4 weeks [*see Indications and Usage (1.3)*]. If symptoms do not resolve completely after 4 weeks, an additional course of treatment may be considered. The recommended adolescent dosing is one ACIPHEX 20 mg Delayed-Release tablet to be taken once daily for 8 weeks.

2.4 Healing of Duodenal Ulcers in Adults

The recommended adult oral dose is one ACIPHEX 20 mg Delayed-Release tablet to be taken once daily after the morning meal for a period up to four weeks [*see Indications and Usage (1.5)*]. Most patients with duodenal ulcer heal within four weeks. A few patients may require additional therapy to achieve healing.

2.5 *Helicobacter pylori* Eradication to Reduce the Risk of Duodenal Ulcer Recurrence in Adults

TABLE 1 THREE DRUG REGIMEN [a]

ACIPHEX Delayed-Release Tablet	20 mg	Twice Daily for 7 Days
Amoxicillin	1000 mg	Twice Daily for 7 Days
Clarithromycin	500 mg	Twice Daily for 7 Days

All three medications should be taken twice daily with the morning and evening meals.

[a] It is important that patients comply with the full 7-day regimen [*see Clinical Studies (14.5)*].

2.6 Treatment of Pathological Hypersecretory Conditions, Including Zollinger-Ellison Syndrome in Adults

The dosage of ACIPHEX in patients with pathologic hypersecretory conditions varies with the individual patient. The recommended adult oral starting dose is 60 mg once daily. Doses should be adjusted to individual patient needs and should continue for as long as clinically indicated. Some patients may require divided doses. Doses up to 100 mg QD and 60 mg BID have been administered. Some patients with Zollinger-Ellison syndrome have been treated continuously with ACIPHEX for up to one year.

2.7 Short-term Treatment of Symptomatic GERD in Adolescent Patients 12 Years of Age and Older

The recommended oral dose for adolescents 12 years of age and older is one 20 mg Delayed-Release Tablet once daily for up to 8 weeks [*see Use in Specific Populations (8.4)* and *Clinical Studies (14.7)*].

2.8 Treatment of GERD in Pediatric Patients 1 to 11 Years of Age

The recommended dosage of ACIPHEX Sprinkle for pediatric patients 1 to 11 years of age by body weight is:

- Less than 15 kg: 5 mg once daily for up to 12 weeks with the option to increase to 10 mg if inadequate response [*see Clinical Studies (14.7)*].
- 15 kg or more: 10 mg once daily for up to 12 weeks [*see Clinical Studies (14.7)*].

2.9 Elderly, Renal and Hepatic Impaired Patients

No dosage adjustment is necessary in elderly patients, in patients with renal disease or in patients with mild to moderate hepatic impairment. Administration of rabeprazole to patients with mild to moderate liver impairment resulted in increased exposure and decreased elimination. Due to the lack of clinical data on rabeprazole in patients with severe hepatic impairment, caution should be exercised in those patients.

2.10 Administration Recommendations

TABLE 2 Administration Recommendations

Formulation	Population	Instructions
Delayed-Release Tablet	Adults and adolescents 12 years of age and older	Swallow tablets whole. Do not chew, crush or split tablets. Tablets can be taken with or without food.
Delayed-Release Capsule	Pediatric patients 1 to 11 years of age	The dose should be taken 30 minutes before a meal. The granules should not be chewed or crushed. Open capsule and sprinkle entire contents on a small amount of soft food (e.g. applesauce, fruit or vegetable based baby food, or yogurt) or empty contents into a small amount of liquid (e.g. infant formula, apple juice, or pediatric electrolyte solution). The whole dose should be taken within 15 minutes of preparation. Food or liquid should be at or below room temperature. Do not store mixture for future use.

3 DOSAGE FORMS AND STRENGTHS

ACIPHEX Delayed-Release Tablets are provided in strength of 20 mg.

ACIPHEX Sprinkle Delayed-Release Capsules are provided in strengths of 5 and 10 mg. The 5 mg strength is a transparent blue and opaque white No. 2 capsule. The cap of the capsule is imprinted with "↑" and the body is imprinted with "ACX 5mg". The 10 mg strength is a transparent yellow and opaque white No. 2 capsule. The cap of the capsule is imprinted with "↑" and the body is imprinted with "ACX 10mg".

4 CONTRAINDICATIONS

Rabeprazole is contraindicated in patients with known hypersensitivity to rabeprazole, substituted benzimidazoles or to any component of the formulation.

For information about contraindications of antibacterial agents (clarithromycin and amoxicillin) indicated in combination with ACIPHEX, refer to the *Contraindications* section of their package inserts.

5 WARNINGS AND PRECAUTIONS

5.1 Presence of Gastric Malignancy

Symptomatic response to therapy with rabeprazole does not preclude the presence of gastric malignancy.

Patients with healed GERD were treated for up to 40 months with rabeprazole and monitored with serial gastric biopsies. Patients without *H. pylori* infection (221 of 326 patients) had no clinically important pathologic changes in the gastric mucosa. Patients with *H. pylori* infection at baseline (105 of 326 patients) had mild or moderate inflammation in the gastric body or mild inflammation in the gastric antrum. Patients with mild grades of infection or inflammation in the gastric body tended to change to moderate, whereas those graded moderate at baseline tended to remain stable. Patients with mild grades of infection or inflammation in the gastric antrum tended to remain stable. At baseline 8% of patients had atrophy of glands in the gastric body and 15% had atrophy in the gastric antrum. At endpoint, 15% of patients had atrophy of glands in the gastric body and 11% had atrophy in the gastric antrum. Approximately 4% of patients had intestinal metaplasia at some point during follow-up, but no consistent changes were seen.

5.2 Concomitant Use with Warfarin

Steady state interactions of rabeprazole and warfarin have not been adequately evaluated in patients. There have been reports of increased INR and prothrombin time in patients receiving a proton pump inhibitor and warfarin concomitantly. Increases in INR and prothrombin time may lead to abnormal bleeding and even death. Patients treated with a proton pump inhibitor and warfarin concomitantly may need to be monitored for increases in INR and prothrombin time.

5.3 *Clostridium difficile* Associated Diarrhea

Published observational studies suggest that PPI therapy like ACIPHEX may be associated with an increased risk of *Clostridium difficile* associated diarrhea, especially in hospitalized patients. This diagnosis should be considered for diarrhea that does not improve [*see Adverse Reactions (6.2)*].

Patients should use the lowest dose and shortest duration of PPI therapy appropriate to the condition being treated.

Clostridium difficile associated diarrhea (CDAD) has been reported with use of nearly all antibacterial agents. For more information specific to antibacterial agents (clarithromycin and amoxicillin) indicated for use in combination with ACIPHEX, refer to *Warnings* and *Precautions* sections of those package inserts.

5.4 Bone Fracture

Several published observational studies in adults suggest that PPI therapy may be associated with an increased risk for osteoporosis-related fractures of the hip, wrist, or spine. The risk of fracture was increased in patients who received high-dose, defined as multiple daily doses, and long-term PPI therapy (a year or longer). Patients should use the lowest dose and shortest duration of PPI therapy appropriate to the condition being treated. Patients at risk for osteoporosis-related fractures should be managed according to established treatment guidelines [*see Dosage and Administration (2)* and *Adverse Reactions (6.2)*].

5.5 Hypomagnesemia

Hypomagnesemia, symptomatic and asymptomatic, has been reported rarely in patients treated with PPIs for at least three months, in most cases after a year of therapy. Serious adverse events include tetany, arrhythmias, and seizures. In most patients, treatment of hypomagnesemia required magnesium replacement and discontinuation of the PPI.

For patients expected to be on prolonged treatment or who take PPIs with medications such as digoxin or drugs that may cause hypomagnesemia (e.g., diuretics), healthcare professionals may consider monitoring magnesium levels prior to initiation of PPI treatment and periodically [*see Adverse Reactions (6.2)*].

5.6 Concomitant Use of ACIPHEX with Methotrexate

Literature suggests that concomitant use of PPIs with methotrexate (primarily at high dose; see methotrexate prescribing information) may elevate and prolong serum levels of methotrexate and/or its metabolite, possibly leading to methotrexate toxicities. In high-dose methotrexate administration, a temporary withdrawal of the PPI may be considered in some patients [*see Drug Interactions (7.7)*].

6 ADVERSE REACTIONS

Worldwide, over 2900 patients have been treated with rabeprazole in Phase II-III clinical trials involving various dosages and durations of treatment.

Because clinical trials are conducted under varying conditions, adverse reaction rates observed in the clinical trials of a drug cannot be directly compared to rates in the clinical trials of another drug and may not reflect the rates observed in practice.

6.1 Clinical Studies Experience

Adults

The data described below reflect exposure to ACIPHEX in 1064 adult patients exposed for up to 8 weeks. The studies were primarily placebo- and active-controlled trials in adult patients with Erosive or Ulcerative Gastroesophageal Reflux Disease (GERD), Duodenal Ulcers and Gastric Ulcers. The population had a mean age of 53 years (range 18-89 years) and had a ratio of approximately 60% male: 40% female. The racial distribution was 86% Caucasian, 8% African American, 2% Asian and 5% other. Most patients received either 10 mg, 20 mg or 40 mg/day of ACIPHEX.

An analysis of adverse reactions appearing in ≥2% of ACIPHEX patients (n=1064) and with a greater frequency than placebo (n=89) in controlled North American and European acute treatment trials, revealed the following adverse reactions: pain (3% vs. 1%), pharyngitis (3% vs. 2%), flatulence (3% vs. 1%), infection (2% vs. 1%), and constipation (2% vs. 1%).

Three long-term maintenance studies consisted of a total of 740 adult patients; at least 54% of adult patients were exposed to rabeprazole for 6 months while at least 33% were exposed for 12 months. Of the 740 adult patients, 247 (33%) and 241 (33%) patients received 10 mg and 20 mg of ACIPHEX, respectively, while 169 (23%) patients received placebo and 83 (11%) received omeprazole.

The safety profile of rabeprazole in the maintenance studies in adults was consistent with what was observed in the acute studies.

Other adverse reactions seen in controlled clinical trials, which do not meet the above criteria (≥2% of ACIPHEX treated patients and greater than placebo) and for which there is a possibility of a causal relationship to rabeprazole, include the following: headache, abdominal pain, diarrhea, dry mouth, dizziness, peripheral edema, hepatic enzyme increase, hepatitis, hepatic encephalopathy, myalgia, and arthralgia.

Combination Treatment with Amoxicillin and Clarithromycin: In clinical trials using combination therapy with rabeprazole plus amoxicillin and clarithromycin (RAC), no adverse reactions unique to this drug combination were observed. In the U.S. multicenter study, the most frequently reported drug related adverse reactions for patients who received RAC therapy for 7 or 10 days were diarrhea (8% and 7%) and taste perversion (6% and 10%), respectively.

No clinically significant laboratory abnormalities particular to the drug combinations were observed.

For more information on adverse reactions or laboratory changes with amoxicillin or clarithromycin, refer to their respective package prescribing information, *Adverse Reactions* section.

Pediatric

In a multicenter, open-label study of adolescent patients 12 to 16 years of age with a clinical diagnosis of symptomatic GERD or endoscopically proven GERD, the adverse event profile was similar to that of adults. The adverse reactions reported without regard to relationship to ACIPHEX that occurred in ≥2% of 111 patients were headache (9.9%), diarrhea (4.5%), nausea (4.5%), vomiting (3.6%), and abdominal pain (3.6%). The related reported adverse reactions that occurred in ≥2% of patients were headache (5.4%) and nausea (1.8%). There were no adverse reactions reported in this study that were not previously observed in adults.

In a two-part, randomized, multicenter, double-blind, parallel-group study, 127 pediatric patients 1 to 11 years of age with endoscopically proven GERD received either 5 mg or 10 mg (<15 kg body weight) or 10 mg or 20 mg (≥15 kg body weight) rabeprazole. In this study, some patients were exposed to rabeprazole for 36 weeks. Adverse reactions that occurred in ≥5% of patients included abdominal pain (5%), diarrhea (5%), and headache (5%). There were no adverse reactions reported in this study that were not previously observed in trials of adolescents and adults.

6.2 Postmarketing Experience

The following adverse reactions have been identified during post approval use of ACIPHEX. Because these reactions are reported voluntarily from a population of uncertain size, it is not always possible to reliably estimate their frequency or establish a causal relationship to drug exposure: sudden death; coma, hyperammonemia; jaundice; rhabdomyolysis; disorientation and delirium; anaphylaxis; angioedema; bullous and other drug eruptions of the skin; severe dermatologic reactions, including toxic epidermal necrolysis (some fatal), Stevens-Johnson syndrome, and erythema multiforme; interstitial pneumonia; interstitial nephritis; TSH elevations; bone fractures; hypomagnesemia and *Clostridium difficile* associated diarrhea. In addition, agranulocytosis, hemolytic anemia, leukopenia, pancytopenia, and thrombocytopenia have been reported. Increases in prothrombin time/INR in patients treated with concomitant warfarin have been reported.

7 DRUG INTERACTIONS

7.1 Drugs Metabolized by CYP450

Rabeprazole is metabolized by the cytochrome P450 (CYP450) drug metabolizing enzyme system. Studies in healthy subjects have shown that rabeprazole does not have clinically significant interactions with other drugs metabolized by the CYP450 system, such as warfarin and theophylline given as single oral doses, diazepam as a single intravenous dose, and phenytoin given as a single intravenous dose (with supplemental oral dosing). Steady state interactions of rabeprazole and other drugs metabolized by this enzyme system have not been studied in patients.

7.2 Warfarin

There have been reports of increased INR and prothrombin time in patients receiving proton pump inhibitors, including rabeprazole, and warfarin concomitantly. Increases in INR and prothrombin time may lead to abnormal bleeding and even death [*see Warnings and Precautions (5.2)*].

7.3 Cyclosporine

In vitro incubations employing human liver microsomes indicated that rabeprazole inhibited cyclosporine metabolism with an IC_{50} of 62 micromolar, a concentration that is over 50 times higher than the C_{max} in healthy volunteers following 14 days of dosing with 20 mg of rabeprazole. This degree of inhibition is similar to that by omeprazole at equivalent concentrations.

7.4 Compounds Dependent on Gastric pH for Absorption

Rabeprazole produces sustained inhibition of gastric acid secretion. An interaction with compounds which are dependent on gastric pH for absorption may occur due to the magnitude of acid suppression observed with rabeprazole. For example, in normal subjects, co-administration of rabeprazole 20 mg QD resulted in an approximately 30% decrease in the bioavailability of ketoconazole and increases in the AUC and C_{max} for digoxin of 19% and 29%, respectively. Therefore, patients may need to be monitored when such drugs are taken concomitantly with rabeprazole. Co-administration of rabeprazole and antacids produced no clinically relevant changes in plasma rabeprazole concentrations.

Concomitant use of atazanavir and proton pump inhibitors is not recommended. Co-administration of atazanavir with proton pump inhibitors is expected to substantially decrease atazanavir plasma concentrations and thereby reduce its therapeutic effect.

7.5 Drugs Metabolized by CYP2C19

In a clinical study in Japan evaluating rabeprazole in adult patients categorized by CYP2C19 genotype (n=6 per genotype category), gastric acid suppression was higher in poor metabolizers as compared to extensive metabolizers. This could be due to higher rabeprazole plasma levels in poor metabolizers. Whether or not interactions of rabeprazole sodium with other drugs metabolized by CYP2C19 would be different between extensive metabolizers and poor metabolizers has not been studied.

7.6 Combined Administration with Clarithromycin

Combined administration consisting of rabeprazole, amoxicillin, and clarithromycin resulted in increases in plasma concentrations of rabeprazole and 14-hydroxy-clarithromycin [*see Clinical Pharmacology (12.3)*].

Concomitant administration of clarithromycin with other drugs can lead to serious adverse reactions due to drug interactions [*see Warnings and Precautions in prescribing information for clarithromycin*]. Because of these drug interactions, clarithromycin is contraindicated for co-administration with certain drugs [*see Contraindications in prescribing information for clarithromycin*] [*see Drug Interactions in prescribing information for amoxicillin*].

7.7 Methotrexate

Case reports, published population pharmacokinetic studies, and retrospective analyses suggest that concomitant administration of PPIs and methotrexate (primarily at high dose; see methotrexate prescribing information) may elevate and prolong serum levels of methotrexate and/or its metabolite hydroxymethotrexate. However, no formal drug interaction studies of methotrexate with PPIs have been conducted [*see Warnings and Precautions (5.6)*].

7.8 Clopidogrel

Concomitant administration of rabeprazole and clopidogrel in healthy subjects had no clinically meaningful effect on exposure to the active metabolite of clopidogrel [*see Clinical Pharmacology (12.3)*]. No dose adjustment of clopidogrel is necessary when administered with an approved dose of ACIPHEX.

8 USE IN SPECIFIC POPULATIONS

8.1 Pregnancy

Pregnancy Category B

Risk Summary

There are no adequate and well-controlled studies with ACIPHEX in pregnant women. No evidence of teratogenicity was seen in animal reproduction studies with rabeprazole at 13 and 8 times the human exposure at the recommended dose for GERD, in rats and rabbits, respectively. Because animal reproduction studies are not always predictive of human response, this drug should be used during pregnancy only if clearly needed.

Animal Data

Embryo-fetal development studies have been performed in rats at intravenous doses of rabeprazole up to 50 mg/kg/day (plasma AUC of 11.8 µg•hr/mL, about 13 times the human exposure at the recommended oral dose for GERD) and rabbits at intravenous doses up to 30 mg/kg/day (plasma AUC of 7.3 µg•hr/mL, about 8 times the human exposure at the recommended oral dose for GERD) and have revealed no evidence of harm to the fetus due to rabeprazole.

Administration of rabeprazole to rats in late gestation and during lactation at an oral dose of 400 mg/kg/day (about 195-times the human oral dose based on mg/m^2) resulted in decreases in body weight gain of the pups.

8.3 Nursing Mothers

It is not known if ACIPHEX is excreted in human milk; however, rabeprazole is present in rat milk. Because many drugs are excreted in milk, caution should be exercised when ACIPHEX is administered to a nursing woman.

8.4 Pediatric Use

Symptomatic GERD in Adolescent Patients Greater or Equal to 12 Years of Age

In a multicenter, randomized, open-label, parallel-group study, 111 adolescent patients 12 to 16 years of age with a clinical diagnosis of symptomatic GERD, or suspected or endoscopically proven GERD were randomized and treated with either ACIPHEX 10 mg or ACIPHEX 20 mg once daily for up to 8 weeks for the evaluation of safety and efficacy. The adverse event profile in adolescent patients was similar to that of adults. The related reported adverse reactions that occurred in ≥2% of patients were headache (5.4%) and nausea (1.8%). There were no adverse reactions reported in these studies that were not previously observed in adults.

GERD in Pediatric Patients 1 to 11 Years of Age

The use of ACIPHEX for treatment of GERD in pediatric patients 1 to 11 years of age is supported by a randomized, multicenter, double-blind clinical trial which evaluated two dose levels of rabeprazole in 127 pediatric patients with endoscopic and histologic evidence of GERD prior to study treatment. Dosing was determined by body weight: patients weighing 6.0 to 14.9 kg received either 5 or 10 mg and those weighing 15.0 kg or more received 10 or 20 mg of ACIPHEX Sprinkle daily. After 12 weeks of rabeprazole treatment, 81% of patients demonstrated esophageal mucosal healing on endoscopic assessment. In patients who had esophageal mucosal healing at 12 weeks and elected to continue for 24 more weeks of rabeprazole, 90% retained esophageal mucosal healing at 36 weeks. No prespecified formal hypothesis testing for evaluation of efficacy was conducted. The absence of a placebo group does not allow assessment of sustained efficacy through 36 weeks. There were no adverse reactions reported in this study that were not previously observed in adolescents or adults.

Symptomatic GERD in Infants 1 to 11 Months of Age

Studies conducted do not support the use of ACIPHEX Sprinkle for the treatment of GERD in pediatric patients younger than 1 year of age.

In a randomized, multicenter, placebo-controlled withdrawal trial, infants 1 to 11 months of age with a clinical diagnosis of symptomatic GERD, or suspected or endoscopically proven GERD, were treated up to 8 weeks in two treatment periods. In the first treatment period (open-label), 344 infants received 10 mg of ACIPHEX Sprinkle for up to 3 weeks. Infants with clinical response were then eligible to enter the second treatment period, which was double-blind and randomized. Two hundred sixty-eight infants were randomized to receive either placebo or 5 mg or 10 mg ACIPHEX Sprinkle.

This study did not demonstrate efficacy based on assessment of frequency of regurgitation and weight-for-age Z-score. Adverse reactions that occurred in >5% of patients in any treatment group and with a higher rate than placebo included pyrexia (7%) and increased serum gastrin levels (5%). There were no adverse reactions reported in this study that were not previously observed in adolescents and adults.

Neonates <1 Month and Preterm Infants < 44 Weeks Corrected Gestational Age

Use of ACIPHEX Sprinkle in neonates is strongly discouraged at this time for the treatment of GERD, based on the risk of prolonged acid suppression and lack of demonstrated safety and effectiveness in neonates.

Based on population pharmacokinetic analysis, the median (range) for the apparent clearance (CL/F) was 1.05 L/h (0.0543-3.44 L/h) in neonates and 4.46 L/h (0.822-12.4 L/h) in patients 1 to 11 months of age following once daily administration of oral ACIPHEX Sprinkle.

8.5 Geriatric Use

Of the total number of subjects in clinical studies of ACIPHEX, 19% were 65 years and over, while 4% were 75 years and over. No overall differences in safety or effectiveness were observed between these subjects and younger subjects, and other reported clinical experience has not identified differences in responses between the elderly and younger patients, but greater sensitivity of some older individuals cannot be ruled out.

8.6 Gender

Duodenal ulcer and erosive esophagitis healing rates in women are similar to those in men. Adverse reactions and laboratory test abnormalities in women occurred at rates similar to those in men.

10 OVERDOSAGE

Because strategies for the management of overdose are continually evolving, it is advisable to contact a Poison Control Center to determine the latest recommendations for the management of an overdose of any drug. There has been no experience with large overdoses with rabeprazole. Seven reports of accidental overdosage with rabeprazole have been received. The maximum reported overdose was 80 mg. There were no clinical signs or symptoms associated with any reported overdose. Patients with Zollinger-Ellison syndrome have been treated with up to 120 mg rabeprazole QD. No specific antidote for rabeprazole is known. Rabeprazole is extensively protein bound and is not readily dialyzable. In the event of overdosage, treatment should be symptomatic and supportive.

Single oral doses of rabeprazole at 786 mg/kg and 1024 mg/kg were lethal to mice and rats, respectively. The single oral dose of 2000 mg/kg was not lethal to dogs. The major symptoms of acute toxicity were hypoactivity, labored respiration, lateral or prone position and convulsion in mice and rats and watery diarrhea, tremor, convulsion and coma in dogs.

11 DESCRIPTION

The active ingredient in ACIPHEX (rabeprazole sodium) Delayed-Release Tablets and in ACIPHEX Sprinkle (rabeprazole sodium) Delayed-Release Capsules is rabeprazole sodium, which is a proton pump inhibitor. It is a substituted benzimidazole known chemically as 2-[[[4-(3-methoxypropoxy)-3-methyl-2-pyridinyl]-methyl]sulfinyl]-1*H*-benzimidazole sodium salt. It has an empirical formula of $C_{18}H_{20}N_3NaO_3S$ and a molecular weight of 381.42. Rabeprazole sodium is a white to slightly yellowish-white solid. It is very soluble in water and methanol, freely soluble in ethanol, chloroform and ethyl acetate and insoluble in ether and n-hexane. The stability of rabeprazole sodium is a function of pH; it is rapidly degraded in acid media, and is more stable under alkaline conditions. The structural figure is:

FIGURE 1

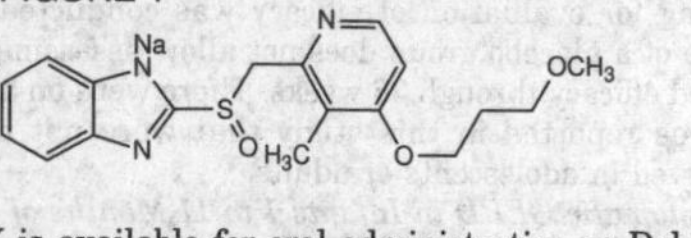

ACIPHEX is available for oral administration as Delayed-Release, enteric-coated tablets containing 20 mg of rabeprazole sodium. ACIPHEX Sprinkle is available for oral administration as 5 mg and 10 mg rabeprazole sodium Delayed-Release Capsules containing enteric coated granules.

Inactive ingredients of the 20 mg tablet are carnauba wax, crospovidone, diacetylated monoglycerides, ethylcellulose, hydroxypropyl cellulose, hypromellose phthalate, magnesium stearate, mannitol, propylene glycol, sodium hydroxide, sodium stearyl fumarate, talc, and titanium dioxide. Iron oxide yellow is the coloring agent for the tablet coating. Iron oxide red is the ink pigment.

ACIPHEX Sprinkle Delayed-Release Capsules contain granules of rabeprazole sodium in a hard hypromellose capsule. Inactive ingredients are colloidal silicon dioxide, diacetylated monoglycerides, ethylcellulose, hydroxypropyl cellulose, hypromellose phthalate, magnesium oxide, magnesium stearate, mannitol, talc, titanium dioxide, carrageenan, potassium chloride, FD&C Blue No. 2 Aluminum Lake (in the 5 mg capsule), FD&C Yellow, No. 6 (in the 10 mg capsule), and gray printing ink.

12 CLINICAL PHARMACOLOGY

12.1 Mechanism of Action

Rabeprazole belongs to a class of antisecretory compounds (substituted benzimidazole proton-pump inhibitors) that do not exhibit anticholinergic or histamine H_2-receptor antagonist properties, but suppress gastric acid secretion by inhibiting the gastric H^+, K^+ATPase at the secretory surface of the gastric parietal cell. Because this enzyme is regarded as the acid (proton) pump within the parietal cell, rabeprazole has been characterized as a gastric proton-pump inhibitor. Rabeprazole blocks the final step of gastric acid secretion.

In gastric parietal cells, rabeprazole is protonated, accumulates, and is transformed to an active sulfenamide. When studied *in vitro*, rabeprazole is chemically activated at pH 1.2 with a half-life of 78 seconds. It inhibits acid transport in porcine gastric vesicles with a half-life of 90 seconds.

12.2 Pharmacodynamics

Antisecretory Activity

The antisecretory effect begins within one hour after oral administration of 20 mg ACIPHEX. The median inhibitory effect of ACIPHEX on 24 hour gastric acidity is 88% of maximal after the first dose. ACIPHEX 20 mg inhibits basal and peptone meal-stimulated acid secretion versus placebo by 86% and 95%, respectively, and increases the percent of a 24-hour period that the gastric pH>3 from 10% to 65% (see table below). This relatively prolonged pharmacodynamic action compared to the short pharmacokinetic half-life (1-2 hours) reflects the sustained inactivation of the H^+, K^+ATPase.

TABLE 3 GASTRIC ACID PARAMETERS ACIPHEX VERSUS PLACEBO AFTER 7 DAYS OF ONCE DAILY DOSING

Parameter	ACIPHEX (20 mg QD)	Placebo
Basal Acid Output (mmol/hr)	0.4*	2.8
Stimulated Acid Output (mmol/hr)	0.6*	13.3
% Time Gastric pH>3	65*	10

*(p<0.01 versus placebo)

TABLE 4 AUC ACIDITY (MMOL·HR/L) ACIPHEX VERSUS PLACEBO ON DAY 7 OF ONCE DAILY DOSING (MEAN±SD)

	Treatment			
AUC interval (hrs)	10 mg RBP (N=24)	20 mg RBP (N=24)	40 mg RBP (N=24)	Placebo (N=24)
08:00 - 13:00	19.6±21.5*	12.9±23*	7.6±14.7*	91.1±39.7
13:00 - 19:00	5.6±9.7*	8.3±29.8*	1.3±5.2*	95.5±48.7
19:00 - 22:00	0.1±0.1*	0.1±0.06*	0.0±0.02*	11.9±12.5
22:00 - 08:00	129.2±84*	109.6±67.2*	76.9±58.4*	479.9±165
AUC 0-24 hours	155.5±90.6*	130.9±81*	85.8±64.3*	678.5±216

*(p<0.001 versus placebo)

TABLE 5 GASTRIC ACID PARAMETERS ACIPHEX ONCE DAILY DOSING VERSUS PLACEBO ON DAY 1 AND DAY 8

	ACIPHEX 20 mg QD		Placebo	
Parameter	Day 1	Day 8	Day 1	Day 8
Mean AUC_{0-24} Acidity	340.8*	176.9*	925.5	862.4
Median trough pH (23-hr)[a]	3.77	3.51	1.27	1.38
% Time Gastric pH>3[b]	54.6*	68.7*	19.1	21.7
% Time Gastric pH>4[b]	44.1*	60.3*	7.6	11.0

[a] No inferential statistics conducted for this parameter.
* (p<0.001 versus placebo)
[b] Gastric pH was measured every hour over a 24-hour period.

Compared to placebo, ACIPHEX, 10 mg, 20 mg, and 40 mg, administered once daily for 7 days significantly decreased intragastric acidity with all doses for each of four meal-related intervals and the 24-hour time period overall. In this study, there were no statistically significant differences between doses; however, there was a significant dose-related decrease in intragastric acidity. The ability of rabeprazole to cause a dose-related decrease in mean intragastric acidity is illustrated below.

[See table 4 above]

After administration of 20 mg ACIPHEX Tablets once daily for eight days, the mean percent of time that gastric pH>3 or gastric pH>4 after a single dose (Day 1) and multiple doses (Day 8) was significantly greater than placebo (see table below). The decrease in gastric acidity and the increase in gastric pH observed with 20 mg ACIPHEX Tablets administered once daily for eight days were compared to the same parameters for placebo, as illustrated below:

[See table 5 above]

Effects on Esophageal Acid Exposure

In patients with gastroesophageal reflux disease (GERD) and moderate to severe esophageal acid exposure, ACIPHEX 20 mg and 40 mg Tablets per day decreased 24-hour esophageal acid exposure. After seven days of treatment, the percentage of time that esophageal pH<4 decreased from baselines of 24.7% for 20 mg and 23.7% for 40 mg, to 5.1% and 2.0%, respectively. Normalization of 24-hour intraesophageal acid exposure was correlated to gastric pH>4 for at least 35% of the 24-hour period; this level was achieved in 90% of subjects receiving ACIPHEX 20 mg and in 100% of subjects receiving ACIPHEX 40 mg. With ACIPHEX 20 mg and 40 mg per day, significant effects on gastric and esophageal pH were noted after one day of treatment, and more pronounced after seven days of treatment.

Effects on Serum Gastrin

In patients given daily doses of ACIPHEX for up to eight weeks to treat ulcerative or erosive esophagitis and in patients treated for up to 52 weeks to prevent recurrence of disease the median fasting gastrin level increased in a dose-related manner. The group median values stayed within the normal range.

In a group of subjects treated daily with ACIPHEX 20 mg tablets for 4 weeks a doubling of mean serum gastrin concentrations were observed. Approximately 35% of these treated subjects developed serum gastrin concentrations above the upper limit of normal. In a study of CYP2C19 genotyped subjects in Japan, poor metabolizers developed statistically significantly higher serum gastrin concentrations than extensive metabolizers.

Effects on Enterochromaffin-like (ECL) Cells

Increased serum gastrin secondary to antisecretory agents stimulates proliferation of gastric ECL cells which, over time, may result in ECL cell hyperplasia in rats and mice and gastric carcinoids in rats, especially in females [*see Nonclinical Toxicology (13.1)*].

In over 400 patients treated with ACIPHEX Tablets (10 or 20 mg/day) for up to one year, the incidence of ECL cell hyperplasia increased with time and dose, which is consistent with the pharmacological action of the proton-pump inhibitor. No patient developed the adenomatoid, dysplastic or neoplastic changes of ECL cells in the gastric mucosa. No patient developed the carcinoid tumors observed in rats.

Endocrine Effects

Studies in humans for up to one year have not revealed clinically significant effects on the endocrine system. In healthy male volunteers treated with ACIPHEX for 13 days, no clinically relevant changes have been detected in the following endocrine parameters examined: 17 β-estradiol, thyroid stimulating hormone, tri-iodothyronine, thyroxine, thyroxine-binding protein, parathyroid hormone, insulin, glucagon, renin, aldosterone, follicle-stimulating hormone, luteotrophic hormone, prolactin, somatotrophic hormone, dehydroepiandrosterone, cortisol-binding globulin, and urinary 6β-hydroxycortisol, serum testosterone and circadian cortisol profile.

Other Effects

In humans treated with ACIPHEX for up to one year, no systemic effects have been observed on the central nervous, lymphoid, hematopoietic, renal, hepatic, cardiovascular, or respiratory systems. No data are available on long-term treatment with ACIPHEX and ocular effects.

Microbiology

The following *in vitro* data are available but the clinical significance is unknown.

Rabeprazole sodium, amoxicillin and clarithromycin as a three drug regimen has been shown to be active against most strains of *Helicobacter pylori in vitro* and in clinical infections as described in the *Clinical Studies* (14) and *Indications and Usage* (1) sections.

Helicobacter pylori

Susceptibility testing of *H. pylori* isolates was performed for amoxicillin and clarithromycin using agar dilution methodology[1], and minimum inhibitory concentrations (MICs) were determined.

Standardized susceptibility test procedures require the use of laboratory control microorganisms to control the technical aspects of the laboratory procedures.

Incidence of Antibiotic-Resistant Organisms Among Clinical Isolates

Pretreatment Resistance: Clarithromycin pretreatment resistance rate (MIC ≥ 1 μg/mL) to *H. pylori* was 9% (51/560) at baseline in all treatment groups combined. A total of > 99% (558/560) of patients had *H. pylori* isolates which were considered to be susceptible (MIC ≤ 0.25 µg/mL) to amoxicillin at baseline. Two patients had baseline *H. pylori* isolates with an amoxicillin MIC of 0.5 µg/mL.

For susceptibility testing information about *Helicobacter pylori, see Microbiology section in prescribing information for clarithromycin and amoxicillin.*

[See table 6 above]

Patients with persistent *H. pylori* infection following rabeprazole, amoxicillin, and clarithromycin therapy will likely have clarithromycin resistant clinical isolates. Therefore, clarithromycin susceptibility testing should be done when possible. If resistance to clarithromycin is demonstrated or susceptibility testing is not possible, alternative antimicrobial therapy should be instituted.

Amoxicillin Susceptibility Test Results and Clinical/Bacteriological Outcomes: In the U.S. multicenter study, a total of >99% (558/560) of patients had *H. pylori* isolates which were considered to be susceptible (MIC ≤ 0.25 µg/mL) to amoxicillin at baseline. The other 2 patients had baseline *H. pylori* isolates with an amoxicillin MIC of 0.5 µg/mL, and both isolates were clarithromycin-resistant at baseline; in one case the *H. pylori* was eradicated. In the 7- and 10-day treatment groups 75% (107/145) and 79% (112/142), respectively, of the patients who had pretreatment amoxicillin susceptible MICs (≤ 0.25 µg/mL) were eradicated of *H. pylori*. No patients developed amoxicillin-resistant *H. pylori* during therapy.

TABLE 6 CLARITHROMYCIN SUSCEPTIBILITY TEST RESULTS AND CLINICAL/BACTERIOLOGIC OUTCOMES[a] FOR A THREE DRUG REGIMEN (RABEPRAZOLE 20 MG TWICE DAILY, AMOXICILLIN 1000 MG TWICE DAILY, AND CLARITHROMYCIN 500 MG TWICE DAILY FOR 7 OR 10 DAYS)

Days of RAC Therapy	Clarithromycin Pretreatment Results	Total Number	*H. pylori* Negative (Eradicated)	*H. pylori* Positive (Persistent) Post-Treatment Susceptibility Results			
				S [b]	I [b]	R [b]	No MIC
7	Susceptible [b]	129	103	2	0	1	23
7	Intermediate [b]	0	0	0	0	0	0
7	Resistant [b]	16	5	2	1	4	4
10	Susceptible [b]	133	111	3	1	2	16
10	Intermediate [b]	0	0	0	0	0	0
10	Resistant [b]	9	1	0	0	5	3

[a] Includes only patients with pretreatment and post-treatment clarithromycin susceptibility test results.

[b] Susceptible (S) MIC ≤ 0.25 µg/mL, Intermediate (I) MIC = 0.5 µg/mL, Resistant (R) MIC ≥ 1 µg/mL

12.3 Pharmacokinetics

ACIPHEX Delayed-Release Tablets and Delayed-Release granules in the capsule formulation are enteric-coated to allow rabeprazole sodium, which is acid labile, to pass through the stomach relatively intact.

After oral administration of 20 mg ACIPHEX tablet, peak plasma concentrations (C_{max}) of rabeprazole occur over a range of 2.0 to 5.0 hours (T_{max}). The rabeprazole C_{max} and AUC are linear over an oral dose range of 10 mg to 40 mg. There is no appreciable accumulation when doses of 10 mg to 40 mg are administered every 24 hours; the pharmacokinetics of rabeprazole is not altered by multiple dosing.

Absorption: Absolute bioavailability for a 20 mg oral tablet of rabeprazole (compared to intravenous administration) is approximately 52%. When ACIPHEX Tablets are administered with a high fat meal, T_{max} is variable; which concomitant food intake may delay the absorption up to 4 hours or longer. However, the C_{max} and the extent of rabeprazole absorption (AUC) are not significantly altered. Thus ACIPHEX Tablets may be taken without regard to timing of meals.

After oral administration to healthy adults of 10 mg ACIPHEX granules sprinkled on applesauce under fasting condition, median time (T_{max}) to peak plasma concentrations (C_{max}) of rabeprazole was 2.5 hours and ranged 1.0 to 6.5 hours. The plasma half-life of rabeprazole ranges from 1 to 2 hours.

In healthy adults, a concomitant high fat meal delayed the absorption of rabeprazole from ACIPHEX granules sprinkled on one Tablespoon of applesauce resulting in the median T_{max} of 4.5 hours and decreased the C_{max} and AUC_{last} on average by 55% and 33%, respectively. ACIPHEX granules should be taken before a meal.

When 10 mg ACIPHEX granules administered under fasting conditions to healthy adults on one Tablespoon (15mL) of applesauce, one Tablespoon (15mL) of yogurt, or when mixed with a small amount (5mL) of liquid infant formula; the type of soft food did not significantly affect T_{max}, C_{max} and AUC of rabeprazole.

Distribution: Rabeprazole is 96.3% bound to human plasma proteins.

Metabolism: Rabeprazole is extensively metabolized. A significant portion of rabeprazole is metabolized via systemic nonenzymatic reduction to a thioether compound. Rabeprazole is also metabolized to sulphone and desmethyl compounds via cytochrome P450 in the liver. The thioether and sulphone are the primary metabolites measured in human plasma. These metabolites were not observed to have significant antisecretory activity. *In vitro* studies have demonstrated that rabeprazole is metabolized in the liver primarily by cytochromes P450 3A (CYP3A) to a sulphone metabolite and cytochrome P450 2C19 (CYP2C19) to desmethyl rabeprazole. CYP2C19 exhibits a known genetic polymorphism due to its deficiency in some sub-populations (e.g. 3 to 5% of Caucasians and 17 to 20% of Asians). Rabeprazole metabolism is slow in these sub-populations, therefore, they are referred to as poor metabolizers of the drug.

Elimination: Following a single 20 mg oral dose of ^{14}C-labeled rabeprazole, approximately 90% of the drug was eliminated in the urine, primarily as thioether carboxylic acid; its glucuronide, and mercapturic acid metabolites. The remainder of the dose was recovered in the feces. Total recovery of radioactivity was 99.8%. No unchanged rabeprazole was recovered in the urine or feces.

Geriatric: In 20 healthy elderly subjects administered 20 mg rabeprazole tablet once daily for seven days, AUC values approximately doubled and the C_{max} increased by 60% compared to values in a parallel younger control group. There was no evidence of drug accumulation after once daily administration [*see Use in Specific Population (8.5)*].

Pediatric: The pharmacokinetics of rabeprazole was studied in pediatric patients with GERD aged up to 16 years in four separate clinical studies.

Patients 12 to 16 Years of Age

The pharmacokinetics of rabeprazole was studied in 12 adolescent patients with GERD 12 to 16 years of age, in a multicenter study. Patients received rabeprazole 20 mg tablets once daily for five or seven days. An approximate 40% increase in exposure was noted following 5 to 7 days of dosing compared with the exposure after 1 day dosing. Pharmacokinetic parameters in adolescent patients with GERD 12 to 16 years of age were within the range observed in healthy adult volunteers.

Patients 1 to 11 Years of Age

In patients with GERD 1 to 11 years of age, following once daily administration of rabeprazole granules at doses from 0.14 to 1 mg/kg, the median time to peak plasma concentration ranged 2-4 hours and the half-life was about 2.5 hour. No appreciable accumulation was noted following 5 days of dosing compared to exposure after a single dose.

Based on population pharmacokinetic analysis, over the body weight range from 7 to 77.3 kg, the apparent rabeprazole clearance increased from 8.0 to 13.5 L/hr, an increase of 68.8%.

The mean estimated total exposure i.e. AUC after a 10 mg dose of ACIPHEX Sprinkle in patients with GERD 1 to 11 years of age is comparable to a 10 mg dose of ACIPHEX Tablets in adolescents and adults.

Patients < 1 Year Old

See section 8.4 Pediatric Use.

Gender and Race: In analyses adjusted for body mass and height, rabeprazole pharmacokinetics showed no clinically significant differences between male and female subjects. In studies that used different formulations of rabeprazole, $AUC_{0-\infty}$ values for healthy Japanese men were approximately 50-60% greater than values derived from pooled data from healthy men in the United States.

Renal Disease: In 10 patients with stable end-stage renal disease requiring maintenance hemodialysis (creatinine clearance ≤5 mL/min/1.73 m^2), no clinically significant differences were observed in the pharmacokinetics of rabeprazole after a single 20 mg oral dose when compared to 10 healthy volunteers [*see Dosage and Administration (2.7)*].

Hepatic Disease: In a single dose study of 10 patients with chronic mild to moderate compensated cirrhosis of the liver who were administered a 20 mg dose of rabeprazole, AUC_{0-24} was approximately doubled, the elimination half-life was 2- to 3-fold higher, and total body clearance was decreased to less than half compared to values in healthy men. In a multiple dose study of 12 patients with mild to moderate hepatic impairment administered 20 mg rabeprazole once daily for eight days, $AUC_{0-\infty}$ and C_{max} values increased approximately 20% compared to values in healthy age- and gender-matched subjects. These increases were not statistically significant.

No information exists on rabeprazole disposition in patients with severe hepatic impairment. Please refer to the *Dosage and Administration (2.7)* for information on dosage adjustment in patients with hepatic impairment.

Combined Administration with Antimicrobials: Sixteen healthy volunteers genotyped as extensive metabolizers with respect to CYP2C19 were given 20 mg rabeprazole sodium, 1000 mg amoxicillin, 500 mg clarithromycin, or all 3 drugs in a four-way crossover study. Each of the four regimens was administered twice daily for 6 days. The AUC and C_{max} for clarithromycin and amoxicillin were not different following combined administration compared to values following single administration. However, the rabeprazole AUC and C_{max} increased by 11% and 34%, respectively, following combined administration. The AUC and C_{max} for 14-hydroxyclarithromycin (active metabolite of clarithromycin) also increased by 42% and 46%, respectively. This increase in exposure to rabeprazole and 14-hydroxyclarithromycin is not expected to produce safety concerns

Concomitant Use with Clopidogrel: Clopidogrel is metabolized to its active metabolite in part by CYP2C19. A study of healthy subjects including CYP2C19 extensive and intermediate metabolizers receiving once daily administration of clopidogrel 75 mg concomitantly with placebo or with ACIPHEX 20 mg (n=36), for 7 days was conducted. The mean AUC of the active metabolite of clopidogrel was reduced by approximately 12% (mean AUC ratio was 88 %, with 90% CI of 81.7 to 95.5%) when ACIPHEX was coadministered compared to administration of clopidogrel with placebo.

13 NONCLINICAL TOXICOLOGY

13.1 Carcinogenesis, Mutagenesis, Impairment of Fertility

In a 88/104-week carcinogenicity study in CD-1 mice, rabeprazole at oral doses up to 100 mg/kg/day did not produce any increased tumor occurrence. The highest tested dose produced a systemic exposure to rabeprazole (AUC) of 1.40 µg•hr/mL which is 1.6 times the human exposure (plasma $AUC_{0-\infty}$ = 0.88 µg•hr/mL) at the recommended dose for GERD (20 mg/day). In a 28-week carcinogenicity study in $p53^{+/-}$ transgenic mice, rabeprazole at oral doses of 20, 60, and 200 mg/kg/day did not cause an increase in the incidence rates of tumors but produced gastric mucosal hyperplasia at all doses. The systemic exposure to rabeprazole at 200 mg/kg/day is about 17-24 times the human exposure at the recommended dose for GERD. In a 104-week carcinogenicity study in Sprague-Dawley rats, males were treated with oral doses of 5, 15, 30 and 60 mg/kg/day and females with 5, 15, 30, 60 and 120 mg/kg/day. Rabeprazole produced gastric enterochromaffin-like (ECL) cell hyperplasia in male and female rats and ECL cell carcinoid tumors in female rats at all doses including the lowest tested dose. The lowest dose (5 mg/kg/day) produced a systemic exposure to rabeprazole (AUC) of about 0.1 µg•hr/mL which is about 0.1 times the human exposure at the recommended dose for GERD. In male rats, no treatment related tumors were observed at doses up to 60 mg/kg/day producing a rabeprazole plasma exposure (AUC) of about 0.2 µg•hr/mL (0.2 times the human exposure at the recommended dose for GERD).

Rabeprazole was positive in the Ames test, the Chinese hamster ovary cell (CHO/HGPRT) forward gene mutation test and the mouse lymphoma cell (L5178Y/TK+/-) forward gene mutation test. Its demethylated-metabolite was also positive in the Ames test. Rabeprazole was negative in the *in vitro* Chinese hamster lung cell chromosome aberration test, the *in vivo* mouse micronucleus test, and the *in vivo* and *ex vivo* rat hepatocyte unscheduled DNA synthesis (UDS) tests.

Rabeprazole at intravenous doses up to 30 mg/kg/day (plasma AUC of 8.8 µg•hr/mL, about 10 times the human exposure at the recommended dose for GERD) was found to have no effect on fertility and reproductive performance of male and female rats.

13.2 Animal Toxicology and/or Pharmacology

Studies in juvenile and young adult rats and dogs were performed. In juvenile animal studies rabeprazole sodium was administered orally to rats for up to 5 weeks and to dogs for

TABLE 7 HEALING OF EROSIVE OR ULCERATIVE GASTROESOPHAGEAL REFLUX DISEASE (GERD) PERCENTAGE OF PATIENTS HEALED

Week	10 mg ACIPHEX QD N=27	20 mg ACIPHEX QD N=25	40 mg ACIPHEX QD N=26	Placebo N=25
4	63%*	56%*	54%*	0%
8	93%*	84%*	85%*	12%

*(p<0.001 versus placebo)

up to 13 weeks, each commencing on Day 7 post-partum and followed by a 13-week recovery period. Rats were dosed at 5, 25 or 150 mg/kg/day and dogs were dosed at 3, 10 or 30 mg/kg/day. The data from these studies were comparable to those reported for young adult animals. Pharmacologically mediated changes, including increased serum gastrin levels and stomach changes, were observed at all dose levels in both rats and dogs. These observations were reversible over the 13-week recovery periods. Although body weights and/or crown-rump lengths were minimally decreased during dosing, no effects on the development parameters were noted in either juvenile rats or dogs.

14 CLINICAL STUDIES

14.1 Healing of Erosive or Ulcerative GERD in Adults

In a U.S., multicenter, randomized, double-blind, placebo-controlled study, 103 patients were treated for up to eight weeks with placebo, 10 mg, 20 mg or 40 mg ACIPHEX QD. For this and all studies of GERD healing, only patients with GERD symptoms and at least grade 2 esophagitis (modified Hetzel-Dent grading scale) were eligible for entry. Endoscopic healing was defined as grade 0 or 1. Each rabeprazole dose was significantly superior to placebo in producing endoscopic healing after four and eight weeks of treatment. The percentage of patients demonstrating endoscopic healing was as follows:

[See table 7 above]

In addition, there was a statistically significant difference in favor of the ACIPHEX 10 mg, 20 mg, and 40 mg doses compared to placebo at Weeks 4 and 8 regarding complete resolution of GERD heartburn frequency (p≤0.026). All ACIPHEX groups reported significantly greater rates of complete resolution of GERD daytime heartburn severity compared to placebo at Weeks 4 and 8 (p≤0.036). Mean reductions from baseline in daily antacid dose were statistically significant for all ACIPHEX groups when compared to placebo at both Weeks 4 and 8 (p≤0.007).

In a North American multicenter, randomized, double-blind, active-controlled study of 336 patients, ACIPHEX was statistically superior to ranitidine with respect to the percentage of patients healed at endoscopy after four and eight weeks of treatment (see table below):

TABLE 8 HEALING OF EROSIVE OR ULCERATIVE GASTROESOPHAGEAL REFLUX DISEASE (GERD) PERCENTAGE OF PATIENTS HEALED

Week	ACIPHEX 20 mg QD N=167	Ranitidine 150 mg QID N=169
4	59%*	36%
8	87%*	66%

*(p<0.001 versus ranitidine)

ACIPHEX 20 mg once daily was significantly more effective than ranitidine 150 mg QID in the percentage of patients with complete resolution of heartburn at Weeks 4 and 8 (p<0.001). ACIPHEX 20 mg once daily was also more effective in complete resolution of daytime heartburn (p≤0.025), and nighttime heartburn (p≤0.012) at both Weeks 4 and 8, with significant differences by the end of the first week of the study.

14.2 Long-term Maintenance of Healing of Erosive or Ulcerative GERD in Adults

The long-term maintenance of healing in patients with erosive or ulcerative GERD previously healed with gastric antisecretory therapy was assessed in two U.S., multicenter, randomized, double-blind, placebo-controlled studies of identical design of 52 weeks duration. The two studies randomized 209 and 285 patients, respectively, to receive either 10 mg or 20 mg of ACIPHEX QD or placebo. As demonstrated in the tables below, ACIPHEX was significantly superior to placebo in both studies with respect to the maintenance of healing of GERD and the proportions of patients remaining free of heartburn symptoms at 52 weeks:

TABLE 9 PERCENT OF PATIENTS IN ENDOSCOPIC REMISSION

	ACIPHEX 10 mg	ACIPHEX 20 mg	Placebo
Study 1	N=66	N=67	N=70
Week 4	83%*	96%*	44%
Week 13	79%*	93%*	39%
Week 26	77%*	93%*	31%
Week 39	76%*	91%*	30%
Week 52	73%*	90%*	29%
Study 2	N=93	N=93	N=99
Week 4	89%*	94%*	40%
Week 13	86%*	91%*	33%
Week 26	85%*	89%*	30%
Week 39	84%*	88%*	29%
Week 52	77%*	86%*	29%
COMBINED STUDIES	N=159	N=160	N=169
Week 4	87%*	94%*	42%
Week 13	83%*	92%*	36%
Week 26	82%*	91%*	31%
Week 39	81%*	89%*	30%
Week 52	75%*	87%*	29%

*(p<0.001 versus placebo)

TABLE 10 PERCENT OF PATIENTS WITHOUT RELAPSE IN HEARTBURN FREQUENCY AND DAYTIME AND NIGHTTIME HEARTBURN SEVERITY AT WEEK 52

	ACIPHEX 10 mg	ACIPHEX 20 mg	Placebo
Heartburn Frequency			
Study 1	46/55 (84%)*	48/52 (92%)*	17/45 (38%)
Study 2	50/72 (69%)*	57/72 (79%)*	22/79 (28%)
Daytime Heartburn Severity			
Study 1	61/64 (95%)*	60/62 (97%)*	42/61 (69%)
Study 2	73/84 (87%)†	82/87 (94%)*	67/90 (74%)
Nighttime Heartburn Severity			
Study 1	57/61 (93%)*	60/61 (98%)*	37/56 (66%)
Study 2	67/80 (84%)	79/87 (91%)†	64/87 (74%)

* p≤0.001 versus placebo
† 0.001<p<0.05 versus placebo

14.3 Treatment of Symptomatic GERD in Adults

Two U.S., multicenter, double-blind, placebo controlled studies were conducted in 316 adult patients with daytime and nighttime heartburn. Patients reported 5 or more periods of moderate to very severe heartburn during the placebo treatment phase the week prior to randomization. Patients were confirmed by endoscopy to have no esophageal erosions.

The percentage of heartburn free daytime and/or nighttime periods was greater with ACIPHEX 20 mg compared to placebo over the 4 weeks of study in Study RAB-USA-2 (47% vs. 23%) and Study RAB-USA-3 (52% vs. 28%). The mean decreases from baseline in average daytime and nighttime heartburn scores were significantly greater for ACIPHEX 20 mg as compared to placebo at week 4. Graphical displays depicting the daily mean daytime and nighttime scores are provided in Figures 2 to 5.

FIGURE 2: MEAN DAYTIME HEARTBURN SCORES RAB-USA-2

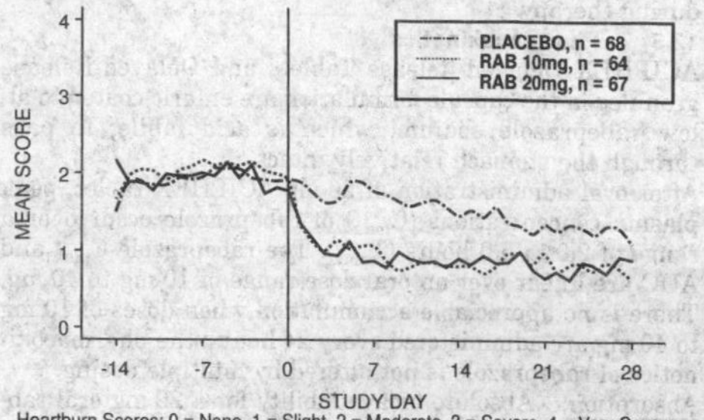

Heartburn Scores: 0 = None, 1 = Slight, 2 = Moderate, 3 = Severe, 4 = Very Severe

FIGURE 3: MEAN NIGHTTIME HEARTBURN SCORES RAB-USA-2

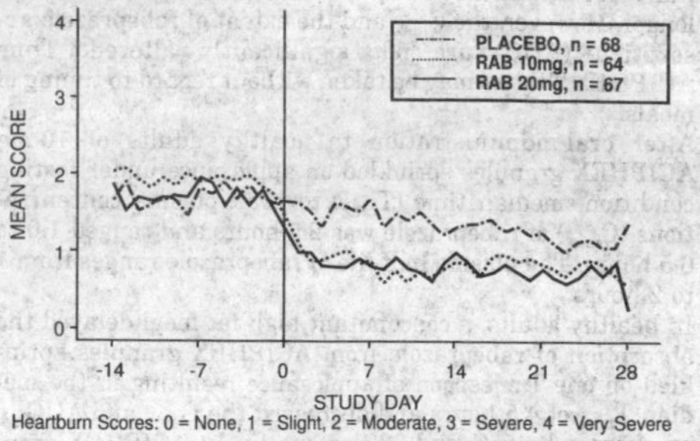

Heartburn Scores: 0 = None, 1 = Slight, 2 = Moderate, 3 = Severe, 4 = Very Severe

FIGURE 4: MEAN DAYTIME HEARTBURN SCORES RAB-USA-3

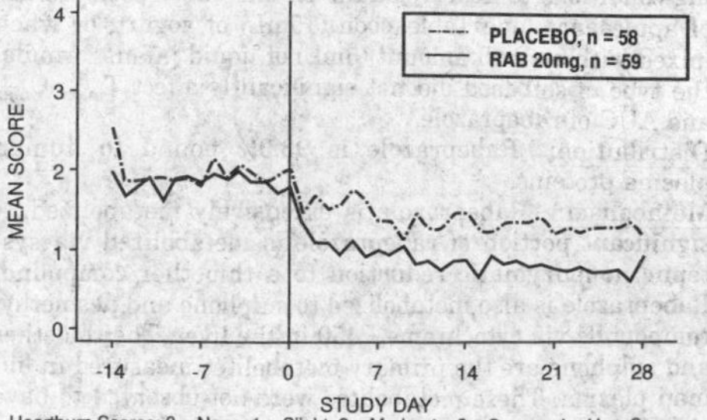

Heartburn Scores: 0 = None, 1 = Slight, 2 = Moderate, 3 = Severe, 4 = Very Severe

FIGURE 5: MEAN NIGHTTIME HEARTBURN SCORES RAB-USA-3

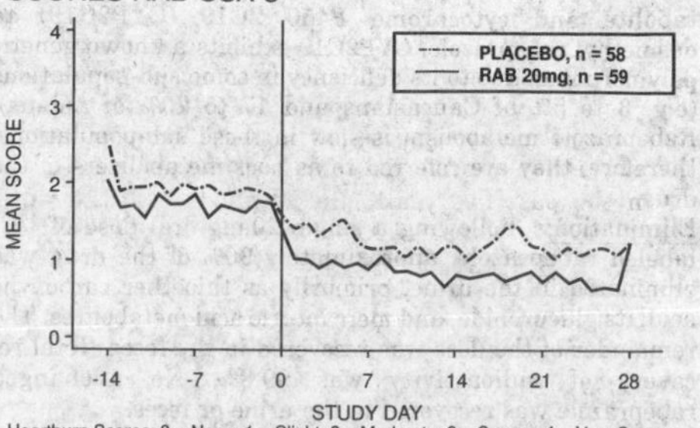

Heartburn Scores: 0 = None, 1 = Slight, 2 = Moderate, 3 = Severe, 4 = Very Severe

In addition, the combined analysis of these two studies showed ACIPHEX 20 mg significantly improved other GERD-associated symptoms (regurgitation, belching and early satiety) by week 4 compared with placebo (all p values < 0.005).

ACIPHEX 20 mg also significantly reduced daily antacid consumption versus placebo over 4 weeks (p<0.001).

14.4 Healing of Duodenal Ulcers in Adults

In a U.S., randomized, double-blind, multicenter study assessing the effectiveness of 20 mg and 40 mg of ACIPHEX QD versus placebo for healing endoscopically defined duodenal ulcers, 100 patients were treated for up to four weeks. ACIPHEX was significantly superior to placebo in producing healing of duodenal ulcers. The percentages of patients with endoscopic healing are presented below:

TABLE 11 HEALING OF DUODENAL ULCERS PERCENTAGE OF PATIENTS HEALED

Week	ACIPHEX 20 mg QD N=34	ACIPHEX 40 mg QD N=33	Placebo N=33
2	44%	42%	21%
4	79%*	91%*	39%

* p≤0.001 versus placebo

At Weeks 2 and 4, significantly more patients in the ACIPHEX 20 and 40 mg groups reported complete resolution of ulcer pain frequency (p≤0.018), daytime pain severity (p≤0.023), and nighttime pain severity (p≤0.035) compared with placebo patients. The only exception was the ACIPHEX 40 mg group versus placebo at Week 2 for duodenal ulcer pain frequency (p=0.094). Significant differences in resolution of daytime and nighttime pain were noted in both ACIPHEX groups relative to placebo by the end of the first week of the study. Significant reductions in daily antacid use were also noted in both ACIPHEX groups compared to placebo at Weeks 2 and 4 (p<0.001).

An international randomized, double-blind, active-controlled trial was conducted in 205 patients comparing 20 mg ACIPHEX QD with 20 mg omeprazole QD. The study was designed to provide at least 80% power to exclude a difference of at least 10% between ACIPHEX and omeprazole, assuming four-week healing response rates of 93% for both groups. In patients with endoscopically defined duodenal ulcers treated for up to four weeks, ACIPHEX was comparable to omeprazole in producing healing of duodenal ulcers. The percentages of patients with endoscopic healing at two and four weeks are presented below:

TABLE 12 HEALING OF DUODENAL ULCERS PERCENTAGE OF PATIENTS HEALED

Week	ACIPHEX 20 mg QD N=102	Omeprazole 20 mg QD N=103	95% Confidence Interval for the Treatment Difference (ACIPHEX - Omeprazole)
2	69%	61%	(-6%, 22%)
4	98%	93%	(-3%, 15%)

ACIPHEX and omeprazole were comparable in providing complete resolution of symptoms.

14.5 *Helicobacter pylori* Eradication in Patients with Peptic Ulcer Disease or Symptomatic Non-Ulcer Disease in Adults

The U.S. multicenter study was a double-blind, parallel-group comparison of rabeprazole, amoxicillin, and clarithromycin for 3, 7, or 10 days vs. omeprazole, amoxicillin and clarithromycin for 10 days. Therapy consisted of rabeprazole 20 mg twice daily, amoxicillin 1000 mg twice daily, and clarithromycin 500 mg twice daily (RAC) or omeprazole 20 mg twice daily, amoxicillin 1000 mg twice daily, and clarithromycin 500 mg twice daily (OAC). Patients with *H. pylori* infection were stratified in a 1:1 ratio for those with peptic ulcer disease (active or a history of ulcer in the past five years) [PUD] and those who were symptomatic but without peptic ulcer disease [NPUD], as determined by upper gastrointestinal endoscopy. The overall *H. pylori* eradication rates, defined as negative ^{13}C-UBT for *H. pylori* ≥ 6 weeks from the end of the treatment are shown in the following table. The eradication rates in the 7 day and 10-day RAC regimens were found to be similar to 10-day OAC regimen using either the Intent-to-Treat (ITT) or Per-Protocol (PP) populations. Eradication rates in the RAC 3-day regimen were inferior to the other regimens.

TABLE 13 HELICOBACTER PYLORI ERADICATION AT ≥ 6 WEEKS AFTER THE END OF TREATMENT

	Treatment Group Percent (%) of Patients Cured (Number of Patients)		Difference (RAC - OAC) [95% Confidence Interval]
	7-day RAC*	**10-day OAC**	
Per Protocol[a]	84.3% (N=166)	81.6% (N=179)	2.8 [- 5.2, 10.7]
Intent-to-Treat[b]	77.3% (N=194)	73.3% (N=206)	4.0 [- 4.4, 12.5]
	10-day RAC*	**10-day OAC**	
Per Protocol[a]	86.0% (N=171)	81.6% (N=179)	4.4 [- 3.3, 12.1]
Intent-to-Treat[b]	78.1% (N=196)	73.3% (N=206)	4.8 [- 3.6, 13.2]
	3-day RAC	**10-day OAC**	
Per Protocol[a]	29.9% (N=167)	81.6% (N=179)	- 51.6 [- 60.6, - 42.6]
Intent-to-Treat[b]	27.3% (N=187)	73.3% (N=206)	- 46.0 [- 54.8, - 37.2]

[a] Patients were included in the analysis if they had *H. pylori* infection documented at baseline, defined as a positive ^{13}C-UBT plus rapid urease test or culture and were not protocol violators. Patients who dropped out of the study due to an adverse event related to the study drug were included in the evaluable analysis as failures of therapy.

[b] Patients were included in the analysis if they had documented *H. pylori* infection at baseline as defined above and took at least one dose of study medication. All dropouts were included as failures of therapy.

* The 95% confidence intervals for the difference in eradication rates for 7-day RAC minus 10-day RAC are (- 9.3, 6.0) in the PP population and (-9.0, 7.5) in the ITT population.

14.6 Pathological Hypersecretory Conditions, Including Zollinger-Ellison Syndrome in Adults

Twelve patients with idiopathic gastric hypersecretion or Zollinger-Ellison syndrome have been treated successfully with ACIPHEX at doses from 20 to 120 mg for up to 12 months. ACIPHEX produced satisfactory inhibition of gastric acid secretion in all patients and complete resolution of signs and symptoms of acid-peptic disease where present. ACIPHEX also prevented recurrence of gastric hypersecretion and manifestations of acid-peptic disease in all patients. The high doses of ACIPHEX used to treat this small cohort of patients with gastric hypersecretion were well tolerated.

14.7 Pediatric GERD

Symptomatic GERD in Adolescents 12 to 16 Years of Age

In a multicenter, randomized, open-label, parallel-group study, 111 adolescent patients 12 to 16 years of age with a clinical diagnosis of symptomatic GERD or suspected or endoscopically proven GERD were randomized and treated with either ACIPHEX 10 mg or ACIPHEX 20 mg once daily for up to 8 weeks for the evaluation of safety and efficacy.

GERD in Pediatric Patients 1 to 11 Years of Age

The use of ACIPHEX Sprinkle in pediatric patients 1 to 11 years of age is supported by a two-part, multicenter, randomized, double-blind, parallel 2 dose arms clinical trial which was conducted in 127 pediatric patients with endoscopic and histologic evidence of GERD prior to study treatment.

Part 1 was 12 weeks in duration. Patients were randomized to one of two rabeprazole dose levels based on body weight. Patients weighing 6.0 to 14.9 kg received either 5 or 10 mg rabeprazole, and those with body weight ≥ 15 kg received either 10 or 20 mg of rabeprazole. Part 2 was a 24-week double-blinded extension of Part 1 (on same dose assigned in Part 1). Endoscopic evaluations were performed at 12 weeks (Part 1) and 36 weeks (Part 2) to assess esophageal healing. No prespecified formal hypothesis testing was conducted.

For Part 1, rates of endoscopic healing were calculated and are shown in Table 14.

TABLE 14 SHORT-TERM (12-WEEK) HEALING RATES IN 1 to 11 YEAR OLD CHILDREN (PART 1)

Endoscopic Classification of GERD At Baseline	Healing Rate at 12 weeks		
	Body Weight <15 kg		Body Weight ≥15 kg
	5 mg dose	10 mg dose	10 mg dose
Erosive[a]	88% (7/8)	83% (5/6)	71% (12/17)
Non-erosive[b]	78% (7/9)	100% (10/10)	81% (17/21)

[a] Hetzel-Dent score ≥2

[b] Hetzel-Dent score = 1

Of the 87 patients with healing in Part 1, 64 patients were enrolled into Part 2. The absence of a placebo group does not allow assessment of sustained efficacy through 36 weeks. Of the 52 patients with available data, healing was observed in 47 (90%) patients at 36 weeks.

15 REFERENCES

1. National Committee for Clinical Laboratory Standards. *Methods for Dilution Antimicrobial Susceptibility Tests for Bacteria That Grow Aerobically*-Fifth Edition. Approved Standard NCCLS Document M7-A5, Vol. 20, No. 2, NCCLS, Wayne, PA, January 2000.

16 HOW SUPPLIED/STORAGE AND HANDLING

ACIPHEX 20 mg is supplied as delayed-release light yellow enteric-coated tablets. The name and strength, in mg, (ACIPHEX 20) is imprinted on one side.

Bottles of 30 (NDC 62856-243-30)

Bottles of 90 (NDC 62856-243-90)

Unit Dose Blisters Package of 100 (10 x 10) (NDC 62856-243-41)

Store at 25°C (77°F); excursions permitted to 15-30°C (59-86°F) [see USP Controlled Room Temperature]. Protect from moisture.

ACIPHEX Sprinkle 5 mg is supplied as transparent blue and opaque white capsules containing enteric coated granules. Identification and strength (ACX 5mg) are imprinted on the body of the capsule. An arrow (↑) imprint on the capsule cap indicates direction for opening a capsule.

Bottles of 30 (NDC 62856-240-30)

ACIPHEX Sprinkle 10 mg is supplied as transparent yellow and opaque white capsules containing enteric coated granules. Identification and strength (ACX 10mg) are imprinted on the body of the capsule. An arrow (↑) imprint on the capsule cap indicates direction for opening a capsule.

Bottles of 30 (NDC 62856-241-30)

Store at 25°C (77°F); excursions permitted to 15-30°C (59-86°F) [see USP Controlled Room Temperature]. Protect from moisture.

17 PATIENT COUNSELING INFORMATION

See FDA-approved patient labeling (Medication Guide)

How to Take ACIPHEX

Patients should be cautioned that ACIPHEX Delayed-Release Tablets should be swallowed whole. The tablets should not be chewed, crushed, or split. ACIPHEX can be taken with or without food.

ACIPHEX Sprinkle Delayed-Release Capsules should be opened and the granule contents sprinkled on a small amount of soft food (e.g. apple sauce, fruit or vegetable based baby food, or yogurt) or empty contents into a small amount of liquid (e.g. infant formula, apple juice, or pediatric electrolyte solution). Food or liquid should be at or below room temperature. The whole dose should be taken within 15 minutes of being sprinkled. The granules should not be chewed or crushed. The dose should be taken 30 minutes before a meal. Do not store mixture for future use.

Advise patient to immediately report and seek care for diarrhea that does not improve. This may be a sign of *Clostridium difficile* associated diarrhea [*see Warnings and Precautions (5.3)*].

MEDICATION GUIDE

ACIPHEX® (a-se-feks)

(rabeprazole sodium)

Delayed-Release Tablets

ACIPHEX(R) Sprinkle™ (a-se-feks spr-en-kle)

(rabeprazole sodium)

Delayed-Release Capsules

Read the Medication Guide that comes with ACIPHEX before you start taking it and each time you get a refill. There may be new information. This Medication Guide does not take the place of talking to your doctor about your medical condition or treatment.

What is the most important information I should know about ACIPHEX?

ACIPHEX may help your acid-related symptoms, but you could still have serious stomach problems. Talk with your doctor.

ACIPHEX can cause serious side effects, including:

- **Diarrhea.** ACIPHEX may increase your risk of getting severe diarrhea. This diarrhea may be caused by an infection (*Clostridium difficile*) in your intestines.
  Call your doctor right away if you have watery stool, stomach pain, and fever that does not go away.
- **Bone fractures.** People who take multiple daily doses of Proton Pump Inhibitor (PPI) medicines for a long period of time (1 year or longer) may have an increased risk of fractures of the hip, wrist, or spine. You should take ACIPHEX exactly as prescribed, at the lowest dose possible for your treatment and for the shortest time needed. Talk to your doctor about your risk of bone fracture if you take ACIPHEX.
  ACIPHEX can have other serious side effects. See **"What are the possible side effects of ACIPHEX?"**

What is ACIPHEX?

ACIPHEX is a prescription medicine called a Proton Pump Inhibitor (PPI). ACIPHEX reduces the amount of acid in your stomach.

ACIPHEX is used in adults:

- for up to 8 weeks to heal acid-related damage to the lining of the esophagus (called erosive esophagitis or EE) and to relieve symptoms, such as heartburn pain. If needed, your doctor may decide to prescribe another 8 weeks of ACIPHEX.
- to maintain the healing of the esophagus and relief of symptoms related to EE. It is not known if ACIPHEX is safe and effective if used longer than 12 months (1 year).
- for 4 weeks to treat daytime and nighttime heartburn and other symptoms that happen with Gastroesophageal Reflux Disease (GERD).
  GERD happens when acid in your stomach backs up into the tube (esophagus) that connects your mouth to your stomach. This may cause a burning feeling in your chest or throat, sour taste, or burping.
- for up to 4 weeks for the healing and relief of duodenal ulcers. The duodenal area is the area where food passes when it leaves the stomach.
- For 7 days with certain antibiotic medicines to treat an infection caused by bacteria called *H. pylori*. Sometimes *H. pylori* bacteria can cause duodenal ulcers. The infection needs to be treated to prevent the ulcers from coming back.
- for the long-term treatment of conditions where your stomach makes too much acid. This includes a rare condition called Zollinger-Ellison syndrome.

ACIPHEX is used in adolescents 12 years of age and older to treat symptoms of Gastroesophageal Reflux Disease (GERD) for up to 8 weeks.

ACIPHEX is used in children 1 to 11 years of age to treat GERD for up to 12 weeks.

ACIPHEX is not effective in treating symptoms of GERD in children 1 month to 11 months of age.

ACIPHEX should not be used to treat GERD in babies younger than 1 month of age.

Who should not take ACIPHEX?

Do not take ACIPHEX if you:

- are allergic to rabeprazole or any of the other ingredients in ACIPHEX. See the end of this Medication Guide for a complete list of ingredients in ACIPHEX.
- are allergic to any other Proton Pump Inhibitor (PPI) medicine.

What should I tell my doctor before taking ACIPHEX?

Before you take ACIPHEX tell your doctor about all of your medical conditions, including if you:

- have been told that you have low magnesium levels in your blood.
- have liver problems.
- have any allergies.
- have any other medical conditions.
- are pregnant or planning to become pregnant. It is not known if ACIPHEX can harm your unborn baby.
- are breastfeeding. It is not known if ACIPHEX passes into your breast milk. Talk to your doctor about the best way to feed your baby if you take ACIPHEX.

Tell your doctor about all the medicines you take, including prescription and non-prescription medicines, vitamins and herbal supplements. ACIPHEX may affect how other medicines work, and other medicines may affect how ACIPHEX works.

Especially tell your doctor if you take:

- atazanavir (Reyataz)
- cyclosporine (Sandimmune, Neoral)
- digoxin (Lanoxin)
- ketoconazole (Nizoral)
- warfarin (Coumadin)
- theophylline (THEO-24 Thelair)
- diazepam (Valium)
- phenytoin (Dilantin)
- an antibiotic that contains amoxicillin or clarithromycin
- a "water pill" (diuretic)
- methotrexate

Ask your doctor or pharmacist for a list of these medicines, if you are not sure.

Know the medicines that you take. Keep a list of them to show your doctor and pharmacist when you get a new medicine.

How should I take ACIPHEX?

- Take ACIPHEX exactly as prescribed. Your doctor will prescribe the dose that is right for you and your medical condition. Do not change your dose or stop taking ACIPHEX unless you talk to your doctor. Take ACIPHEX for as long as it is prescribed even if you feel better.
- ACIPHEX is usually taken one time each day. Your doctor will tell you the time of day to take ACIPHEX, based on your medical condition.
- **ACIPHEX Tablets** can be taken with or without food. Your doctor will tell you whether to take this medicine with or without food based on your medical condition.
- Swallow each **ACIPHEX Tablet** whole with water. **Do not chew, crush, or split ACIPHEX Tablets.** Tell your doctor if you cannot swallow tablets whole.
- **Take a dose of ACIPHEX Sprinkle Delayed-Release Capsules** as follows:
  - Take the dose 30 minutes before a meal.
  - Open the capsule and sprinkle the contents onto a small amount of soft food such as apple sauce, fruit or vegetable based baby food, or yogurt. You may also empty the capsule contents into a small amount of infant formula, apple juice, or a pediatric electrolyte solution such as Pedialyte®. The food or liquid that you use should be at or below room temperature.
  - **Swallow the entire mixture. Do not chew or crush the granules.**
  - Take the entire dose **within 15 minutes**. If you cannot take the dose within 15 minutes of preparing it, throw it away and prepare a new dose. Do not save it for use later.
- If you miss a dose of ACIPHEX, take it as soon as possible. If it is almost time for your next dose, skip the missed dose and go back to your normal schedule. Do not take 2 doses at the same time.
- If you take too much ACIPHEX, call your doctor or Poison Control Center right away, or go to the nearest hospital emergency room.
- Your doctor may prescribe antibiotic medicines with ACIPHEX to help treat a stomach infection and heal stomach (duodenal) ulcers that are caused by bacteria called *H. pylori*. Make sure you read the patient information that comes with an antibiotic before you start taking it.

What are the possible side effects of ACIPHEX?

ACIPHEX can cause serious side effects, including:

- **See "What is the most important information I should know about ACIPHEX?"**
- **Low magnesium levels in your body.** This problem can be serious. Low magnesium can happen in some people who take a Proton Pump inhibitor (PPI) medicine for at least 3 months. If low magnesium levels happen, it is usually after a year of treatment. You may or may not have symptoms of low magnesium.
  Tell your doctor right away if you have any of these symptoms:
  - seizures
  - dizziness
  - abnormal or fast heart beat
  - jitteriness
  - jerking movements or shaking (tremors)
  - muscle weakness
  - spasms of the hands and feet
  - cramps or muscle aches
  - spasm of the voice box

  Your doctor may check the level of magnesium in your body before you start taking ACIPHEX, during treatment, or if you will be taking ACIPHEX for a long period of time.

The most common side effects with ACIPHEX may include:

- headache
- pain
- sore throat
- gas
- infection
- constipation

The most common side effects with ACIPHEX in children include:

- stomach-area (abdomen) pain
- diarrhea
- headache

Other side effects:

Serious allergic reactions. Tell your doctor if you have any of the following symptoms with ACIPHEX:

- rash
- face swelling
- throat tightness
- difficulty breathing

Your doctor may stop ACIPHEX if these symptoms happen.

Tell your doctor if you have any side effect that bothers you or that does not go away. These are not all the side effects of ACIPHEX. For more information, ask your doctor or pharmacist.

Call your doctor for medical advice about side effects. You may report side effects to FDA at 1-800-FDA-1088.

How should I store ACIPHEX?

- Store ACIPHEX Tablets and ACIPHEX Sprinkle Delayed-Release Capsules in a dry place at room temperature between 68(F to 77°F (20°C to 25°C).

Keep ACIPHEX and all medicines out of the reach of children.

General Information about ACIPHEX

Medicines are sometimes prescribed for purposes other than those listed in a Medication Guide. Do not use ACIPHEX for a condition for which it was not prescribed. Do not give ACIPHEX to other people, even if they have the same symptoms that you have. It may harm them.

This Medication Guide summarizes the most important information about ACIPHEX. If you would like more information, talk to your doctor. You can also ask your doctor or pharmacist for information about ACIPHEX that is written for healthcare professionals. For more information, go to http://www.aciphex.com/ or call 1-888-4-ACIPHEX.

What are the ingredients in ACIPHEX?

Active ingredient: rabeprazole sodium

ACIPHEX Delayed-Release Tablets inactive ingredients: carnauba wax, crospovidone, diacetylated monoglycerides, ethylcellulose, hydroxypropyl cellulose, hypromellose phthalate, magnesium stearate, mannitol, propylene glycol, sodium hydroxide, sodium stearyl fumarate, talc, and titanium dioxide. Iron oxide yellow is the coloring agent for the tablet coating. Iron oxide red is the ink pigment.

ACIPHEX Sprinkle Delayed-Release Capsules inactive ingredients: colloidal silicon dioxide, diacetylated monoglycerides, ethylcellulose, hydroxypropyl cellulose, hypromellose phthalate, magnesium oxide, magnesium stearate, mannitol, talc, titanium dioxide, carrageenan, potassium chloride, FD&C Blue No.2 Aluminum Lake (in the 5 mg capsule), FD&C Yellow, No. 6 (in the 10 mg capsule), and gray printing ink.

This Medication Guide has been approved by the U.S. Food and Drug Administration.

Distributed by Eisai Inc., Woodcliff Lake, NJ 07677

Marketed by Janssen Pharmaceuticals Inc., Titusville, NJ 08560

Revised March 2013

Incyte Corporation

Experimental Station
Route 141 & Henry Clay Road
Building E336
Wilmington, DE 19880

Direct Inquiries:
Tel: 1-855-4-INCYTE (1-855-446-2983)
Tel: 302.498.6700
Medical Information Contact
1-855-4-MEDINFO (1-855-463-3463)
medinfo@incyte.com
Normal business hours: 8am to 8pm ET, Mon-Fri

JAKAFI® ℞

(ruxolitinib)
tablets, for oral use

HIGHLIGHTS OF PRESCRIBING INFORMATION

These highlights do not include all the information needed to use JAKAFI safely and effectively. See full prescribing information for JAKAFI.

JAKAFI® (ruxolitinib) tablets, for oral use
Initial U.S. Approval: 2011

RECENT MAJOR CHANGES

Dosage and Administration (2.1 – 2.6)	06/2013
Warnings and Precautions (5.2)	06/2013

INDICATIONS AND USAGE

Jakafi is a kinase inhibitor indicated for treatment of patients with intermediate or high-risk myelofibrosis, including primary myelofibrosis, post-polycythemia vera myelofibrosis and post-essential thrombocythemia myelofibrosis. (1)

DOSAGE AND ADMINISTRATION

- The starting dose of Jakafi is 20 mg given orally twice daily for patients with a platelet count greater than 200 × 10^9/L, and 15 mg twice daily for patients with a platelet count between 100 × 10^9/L and 200 × 10^9/L (2.1)
- The starting dose of Jakafi is 5 mg twice daily for patients with a platelet count between 50 × 10^9/L and less than 100 × 10^9/L. (2.1)
- Monitor complete blood counts every 2 to 4 weeks until doses are stabilized, and then as clinically indicated. Modify or interrupt dosing for thrombocytopenia. (2.1) (2.2)
- Increase dose based on response and as recommended to a maximum of 25 mg twice daily for patients with starting platelet counts 100 × 10^9/L or greater and to a maximum of 10 mg twice daily for patients with starting platelet count between 50 × 10^9/L and less than 100 × 10^9/L. Discontinue after 6 months if no spleen reduction or symptom improvement (2.3) (2.5)

DOSAGE FORMS AND STRENGTHS

Tablets: 5 mg, 10 mg, 15 mg, 20 mg and 25 mg. (3)

CONTRAINDICATIONS

None. (4)

WARNINGS AND PRECAUTIONS

- Thrombocytopenia, Anemia and Neutropenia: Manage by dose reduction, or interruption, or transfusion. (5.1)
- Risk of Infection: Assess patients for signs and symptoms of infection and initiate appropriate treatment promptly. Serious infections should have resolved before starting therapy with Jakafi. (5.2)

ADVERSE REACTIONS

The most common hematologic adverse reactions (incidence > 20%) are thrombocytopenia and anemia. The most common non-hematologic adverse reactions (incidence >10%) are bruising, dizziness and headache. (6.1)

To report SUSPECTED ADVERSE REACTIONS, contact Incyte Corporation at 1-855-463-3463 or FDA at 1-800-FDA-1088 or *www.fda.gov/medwatch*.

DRUG INTERACTIONS

- Strong CYP3A4 Inhibitors: Reduce Jakafi starting dose to 10 mg twice daily for patients with a platelet count greater than or equal to 100 × 10^9/L and concurrent use of strong CYP3A4 inhibitors. Avoid in patients with platelet counts less than 100 × 10^9/L. (2.7) (7.1)

USE IN SPECIFIC POPULATIONS

- Renal Impairment: Reduce Jakafi starting dose to 10 mg twice daily for patients with moderate (CrCl 30-59 mL/min) or severe renal impairment (CrCl 15-29 mL/min) and a platelet count between 100 × 10^9/L and 150 × 10^9/L. Avoid in patients with end stage renal disease (CrCl less than 15 mL/min) not requiring dialysis and in patients with moderate or severe renal impairment and a platelet count less than 100 × 10^9/L. (2.8) (8.6)
- Hepatic Impairment: Reduce Jakafi starting dose to 10 mg twice daily for patients with any degree of hepatic impairment and a platelet count between 100 × 10^9/L and 150 × 10^9/L. Avoid in patients with hepatic impairment with platelet counts less than 100 × 10^9/L. (2.8) (8.7)
- Nursing Mothers: Discontinue nursing or discontinue the drug taking into account the importance of the drug to the mother. (8.3)

See 17 for PATIENT COUNSELING INFORMATION and FDA-approved patient labeling

Revised: 06/2013

FULL PRESCRIBING INFORMATION: CONTENTS*

*** Sections or subsections omitted from the full prescribing information are not listed**

FULL PRESCRIBING INFORMATION

1. INDICATIONS AND USAGE

Jakafi is indicated for treatment of patients with intermediate or high-risk myelofibrosis, including primary myelofibrosis, post-polycythemia vera myelofibrosis and post-essential thrombocythemia myelofibrosis.

2. DOSAGE AND ADMINISTRATION

2.1 Recommended Starting Dose

The recommended starting dose of Jakafi is based on platelet count (*Table 1*). A complete blood count (CBC) and platelet count must be performed before initiating therapy, every 2 to 4 weeks until doses are stabilized, and then as clinically indicated [*see Warnings and Precautions (5.1)*]. Doses may be titrated based on safety and efficacy.

Table 1: Proposed Jakafi Starting Doses

Platelet Count	Starting Dose
Greater than 200 × 10^9/L	20 mg orally twice daily
100 × 10^9/L to 200 × 10^9/L	15 mg orally twice daily
50 × 10^9/L to less than 100 × 10^9/L	5 mg orally twice daily

2.2 Dose Modification Guidelines for Hematologic Toxicity for Patients Starting Treatment with a Platelet Count of 100 × 10^9/L or Greater

Treatment Interruption and Restarting Dosing

Interrupt treatment for platelet counts less than 50 × 10^9/L or absolute neutrophil count (ANC) less than 0.5 × 10^9/L.

After recovery of platelet counts above 50 × 10^9/L and ANC above 0.75 × 10^9/L, dosing may be restarted. Table 2 illustrates the maximum allowable dose that may be used in restarting Jakafi after a previous interruption.

Table 2: Maximum Restarting Doses for Jakafi After Safety Interruption for Thrombocytopenia for Patients Starting Treatment with a Platelet Count of 100 × 10^9/L or Greater

Current Platelet Count	Maximum Dose When Restarting Jakafi Treatment*
Greater than or equal to 125 × 10^9/L	20 mg twice daily
100 to less than 125 × 10^9/L	15 mg twice daily
75 to less than 100 × 10^9/L	10 mg twice daily for at least 2 weeks; if stable, may increase to 15 mg twice daily
50 to less than 75 × 10^9/L	5 mg twice daily for at least 2 weeks; if stable, may increase to 10 mg twice daily
Less than 50 × 10^9/L	Continue hold

*Maximum doses are displayed. When restarting, begin with a dose at least 5 mg twice daily below the dose at interruption.

Following treatment interruption for ANC below 0.5 × 10^9/L, after ANC recovers to 0.75 × 10^9/L or greater, restart dosing at the higher of 5 mg once daily or 5 mg twice daily below the largest dose in the week prior to the treatment interruption.

Dose Reductions

Dose reductions should be considered if the platelet counts decrease as outlined in Table 3 with the goal of avoiding dose interruptions for thrombocytopenia.

[See table 3 above]

Table 3: Dosing Recommendations for Thrombocytopenia for Patients Starting Treatment with a Platelet Count of 100 × 10^9/L or Greater

	Dose at Time of Platelet Decline				
Platelet Count	25 mg twice daily	20 mg twice daily	15 mg twice daily	10 mg twice daily	5 mg twice daily
	New Dose	New Dose	New Dose	New Dose	New Dose
100 to less than 125 × 10^9/L	20 mg twice daily	15 mg twice daily	No Change	No Change	No Change
75 to less than 100 × 10^9/L	10 mg twice daily	10 mg twice daily	10 mg twice daily	No Change	No Change
50 to less than 75 × 10^9/L	5 mg twice daily	5 mg twice daily	5 mg twice daily	5 mg twice daily	No Change
Less than 50 × 10^9/L	Hold	Hold	Hold	Hold	Hold

2.3 Dose Modification Based on Insufficient Response for Patients Starting Treatment with a Platelet Count of 100 × 10^9/L or Greater

If the response is insufficient and platelet and neutrophil counts are adequate, doses may be increased in 5 mg twice daily increments to a maximum of 25 mg twice daily. Doses should not be increased during the first 4 weeks of therapy and not more frequently than every 2 weeks.

Consider dose increases in patients who meet all of the following conditions:

a. Failure to achieve a reduction from pretreatment baseline in either palpable spleen length of 50% or a 35% reduction in spleen volume as measured by CT or MRI;

b. Platelet count greater than 125 × 10^9/L at 4 weeks and platelet count never below 100 × 10^9/L;
c. ANC Levels greater than 0.75 × 10^9/L.

Based on limited clinical data, long-term maintenance at a 5 mg twice daily dose has not shown responses and continued use at this dose should be limited to patients in whom the benefits outweigh the potential risks. Discontinue Jakafi if there is no spleen size reduction or symptom improvement after 6 months of therapy.

2.4 Dose Modifications for Hematologic Toxicity for Patients Starting Treatment with Platelet Counts of 50 × 10^9/L to Less Than 100 × 10^9/L

This section applies only to patients with platelet counts of 50 × 10^9/L to less than 100 × 10^9/L prior to any treatment with ruxolitinib. See Section 2.2 for dose modifications for hematological toxicity in patients whose platelet counts were 100 × 10^9/L or more prior to starting treatment with ruxolitinib.

Treatment Interruption and Restarting Dosing

Interrupt treatment for platelet counts less than 25 × 10^9/L or ANC less than 0.5 × 10^9/L.

After recovery of platelet counts above 35 × 10^9/L and ANC above 0.75 × 10^9/L, dosing may be restarted. Restart dosing at the higher of 5 mg once daily or 5 mg twice daily below the largest dose in the week prior to the decrease in platelet count below 25 × 10^9/L or ANC below 0.5 × 10^9/L that led to dose interruption.

Dose Reductions

Reduce the dose of ruxolitinib for platelet counts less than 35 × 10^9/L as described in Table 4.

Table 4: Dosing Modifications for Thrombocytopenia for Patients with Starting Platelet Count of 50 × 10^9/L to Less Than 100 × 10^9/L

Platelet Count	Dosing Recommendations
Less than 25 × 10^9/L	• Interrupt dosing.
25 × 10^9/L to less than 35 × 10^9/L AND the platelet count decline is less than 20% during the prior four weeks	• Decrease dose by 5 mg once daily. • For patients on 5 mg once daily, maintain dose at 5 mg once daily.
25 × 10^9/L to less than 35 × 10^9/L AND the platelet count decline is 20% or greater during the prior four weeks	• Decrease dose by 5 mg twice daily. • For patients on 5 mg twice daily, decrease the dose to 5 mg once daily. • For patients on 5 mg once daily, maintain dose at 5 mg once daily.

2.5 Dose Modifications Based on Insufficient Response for Patients with Starting Platelet Count of 50 × 10^9/L to Less Than 100 × 10^9/L

Do not increase doses during the first 4 weeks of therapy, and do not increase the dose more frequently than every 2 weeks.

If the response is insufficient as defined in Section 2.3, doses may be increased by increments of 5 mg daily to a maximum of 10 mg twice daily if:
a) the platelet count has remained at least 40 × 10^9/L, and
b) the platelet count has not fallen by more than 20% in the prior 4 weeks, and
c) the ANC is more than 1 × 10^9/L, and
d) the dose has not been reduced or interrupted for an adverse event or hematological toxicity in the prior 4 weeks.

Continuation of treatment for more than 6 months should be limited to patients in whom the benefits outweigh the potential risks. Discontinue Jakafi if there is no spleen size reduction or symptom improvement after 6 months of therapy.

2.6 Dose Modification for Bleeding

Interrupt treatment for bleeding requiring intervention regardless of current platelet count. Once the bleeding event has resolved, consider resuming treatment at the prior dose if the underlying cause of bleeding has been controlled. If the bleeding event has resolved but the underlying cause persists, consider resuming treatment with Jakafi at a lower dose.

2.7 Dose Adjustment with Concomitant Strong CYP3A4 Inhibitors

On the basis of pharmacokinetic studies in healthy volunteers, when administering Jakafi with strong CYP3A4 inhibitors (such as but not limited to boceprevir, clarithromycin, conivaptan, grapefruit juice, indinavir, itraconazole, ketoconazole, lopinavir/ritonavir, mibefradil, nefazodone, nelfinavir, posaconazole, ritonavir, saquinavir, telaprevir, telithromycin, voriconazole), the recommended starting dose is 10 mg twice daily for patients with a platelet count greater than or equal to 100 × 10^9/L. Additional dose modifications should be made with careful monitoring of safety and efficacy.

Concurrent administration of Jakafi with strong CYP3A4 inhibitors should be avoided in patients with platelet counts less than 100 × 10^9/L [*see Drug Interactions (7.1)*].

2.8 Organ Impairment

Renal Impairment

On the basis of pharmacokinetic studies in volunteers with renal impairment, the recommended starting dose is 10 mg twice daily for patients with a platelet count between 100 × 10^9/L and 150 × 10^9/L and moderate (CrCl 30-59 mL/min) or severe renal impairment (CrCl 15-29 mL/min). Additional dose modifications should be made with careful monitoring of safety and efficacy.

The recommended starting dose for patients with end stage renal disease on dialysis is 15 mg for patients with a platelet count between 100 × 10^9/L and 200 × 10^9/L or 20 mg for patients with a platelet count of greater than 200 × 10^9/L. Subsequent doses should be administered on dialysis days following each dialysis session. Additional dose modifications should be made with careful monitoring of safety and efficacy.

Jakafi should be avoided in patients with end stage renal disease (CrCl less than 15 mL/min) not requiring dialysis and in patients with moderate or severe renal impairment with platelet counts less than 100 × 10^9/L [*see Use in Specific Populations (8.6)*].

Hepatic Impairment

On the basis of pharmacokinetic studies in volunteers with hepatic impairment, the recommended starting dose is 10 mg twice daily for patients with a platelet count between 100 × 10^9/L and 150 × 10^9/L. Additional dose modifications should be made with careful monitoring of safety and efficacy.

Jakafi should be avoided in patients with hepatic impairment with platelet counts less than 100 × 10^9/L [*see Use in Specific Populations (8.7)*].

2.9 Method of Administration

Jakafi is dosed orally and can be administered with or without food.

If a dose is missed, the patient should not take an additional dose, but should take the next usual prescribed dose.

When discontinuing Jakafi therapy for reasons other than thrombocytopenia, gradual tapering of the dose of Jakafi may be considered, for example by 5 mg twice daily each week.

For patients unable to ingest tablets, Jakafi can be administered through a nasogastric tube (8 French or greater) as follows:
• Suspend one tablet in approximately 40 mL of water with stirring for approximately 10 minutes.
• Within 6 hours after the tablet has dispersed, the suspension can be administered through a nasogastric tube using an appropriate syringe.

The tube should be rinsed with approximately 75 mL of water. The effect of tube feeding preparations on Jakafi exposure during administration through a nasogastric tube has not been evaluated.

3. DOSAGE FORMS AND STRENGTHS

5 mg tablets - round and white with "INCY" on one side and "5" on the other.
10 mg tablets - round and white with "INCY" on one side and "10" on the other.
15 mg tablets - oval and white with "INCY" on one side and "15" on the other.
20 mg tablets - capsule-shaped and white with "INCY" on one side and "20" on the other.
25 mg tablets - oval and white with "INCY" on one side and "25" on the other.

4. CONTRAINDICATIONS

None.

5. WARNINGS AND PRECAUTIONS

5.1 Thrombocytopenia, Anemia and Neutropenia

Treatment with Jakafi can cause thrombocytopenia, anemia and neutropenia. [*see Dosage and Administration (2.1)*].

Thrombocytopenia was generally reversible and was usually managed by reducing the dose or temporarily interrupting Jakafi. Platelet transfusions may be necessary [*see Dosage and Administration (2.2), and Adverse Reactions (6.1)*].

Patients developing anemia may require blood transfusions and/or dose modifications of Jakafi.

Severe neutropenia (ANC less than 0.5 × 10^9/L) was generally reversible. Withhold Jakafi until recovery [*see Adverse Reactions (6.1)*].

Perform a pre-treatment complete blood count (CBC) and monitor CBCs every 2 to 4 weeks until doses are stabilized, and then as clinically indicated. [*see Dosage and Administration (2.2), and Adverse Reactions (6.1)*].

5.2 Risk of Infection

Serious bacterial, mycobacterial, fungal and viral infections may occur. Active serious infections should have resolved before starting therapy with Jakafi. Observe patients receiving Jakafi for signs and symptoms of infection and initiate appropriate treatment promptly.

PML

Progressive multifocal leukoencephalopathy (PML) has been reported with ruxolitinib treatment for myelofibrosis. If PML is suspected, stop Jakafi and evaluate.

Herpes Zoster

Advise patients about early signs and symptoms of herpes zoster and to seek treatment as early as possible if suspected [*see Adverse Reactions (6.1)*].

6. ADVERSE REACTIONS

The following serious adverse reactions are discussed in greater detail in other sections of the labeling:
• Myelosuppression [*see Warnings and Precautions (5.1)*]
• Risk of Infection [*see Warnings and Precautions (5.2)*]

6.1 Clinical Trials Experience

Because clinical trials are conducted under widely varying conditions, adverse reaction rates observed in the clinical trials of a drug cannot be directly compared to rates in the clinical trials of another drug and may not reflect the rates observed in practice.

The safety of Jakafi was assessed in 617 patients in six clinical studies with a median duration of follow-up of 10.9 months, including 301 patients with myelofibrosis in two Phase 3 studies.

In these two Phase 3 studies, patients had a median duration of exposure to Jakafi of 9.5 months (range 0.5 to 17 months), with 88.7% of patients treated for more than 6 months and 24.6% treated for more than 12 months. One hundred and eleven (111) patients started treatment at 15 mg twice daily and 190 patients started at 20 mg twice daily.

In a double-blind, randomized, placebo-controlled study of Jakafi, 155 patients were treated with Jakafi. The most frequent adverse drug reactions were thrombocytopenia and anemia [*see Table 6*]. Thrombocytopenia, anemia and neutropenia are dose related effects. The three most frequent non-hematologic adverse reactions were bruising, dizziness, and headache [*see Table 5*].

Discontinuation for adverse events, regardless of causality, was observed in 11.0% of patients treated with Jakafi and 10.6% of patients treated with placebo.

Following interruption or discontinuation of Jakafi, symptoms of myelofibrosis generally return to pretreatment levels over a period of approximately 1 week. There have been isolated cases of patients discontinuing Jakafi during acute intercurrent illnesses after which the patient's clinical course continued to worsen; however, it has not been established whether discontinuation of therapy contributed to the clinical course in these patients. When discontinuing therapy for reasons other than thrombocytopenia, gradual tapering of the dose of Jakafi may be considered [*see Dosage and Administration (2.9)*].

Table 5 presents the most common adverse reactions occurring in patients who received Jakafi in the double-blind, placebo-controlled study during randomized treatment.

[See table 5 at top of next page]

Description of Selected Adverse Drug Reactions

Anemia

In the two Phase 3 clinical studies, median time to onset of first CTCAE Grade 2 or higher anemia was approximately 6 weeks. One patient (0.3%) discontinued treatment because of anemia. In patients receiving Jakafi, mean decreases in hemoglobin reached a nadir of approximately 1.5 to 2.0 g/dL below baseline after 8 to 12 weeks of therapy and then gradually recovered to reach a new steady state that was approximately 1.0 g/dL below baseline. This pattern was observed in patients regardless of whether they had received transfusions during therapy.

In the randomized, placebo-controlled study, 60% of patients treated with Jakafi and 38% of patients receiving placebo received red blood cell transfusions during randomized treatment. Among transfused patients, the median number of units transfused per month was 1.2 in patients treated with Jakafi and 1.7 in placebo treated patients.

Thrombocytopenia

In the two Phase 3 clinical studies, in patients who developed Grade 3 or 4 thrombocytopenia, the median time to onset was approximately 8 weeks. Thrombocytopenia was generally reversible with dose reduction or dose interruption. The median time to recovery of platelet counts above 50 × 10^9/L was 14 days. Platelet transfusions were administered to 4.7% of patients receiving Jakafi and to 4.0% of patients receiving control regimens. Discontinuation of treatment because of thrombocytopenia occurred in 0.7% of patients receiving Jakafi and 0.9% of patients receiving control regimens. Patients with a platelet count of 100 × 10^9/L to 200 × 10^9/L before starting Jakafi had a higher frequency of Grade 3 or 4 thrombocytopenia compared to patients with a platelet count greater than 200 × 10^9/L (16.5% versus 7.2%).

Neutropenia

In the two Phase 3 clinical studies, 1.0% of patients reduced or stopped Jakafi because of neutropenia.

Table 6 provides the frequency and severity of clinical hematology abnormalities reported for patients receiving treatment with Jakafi or placebo in the placebo-controlled study. [See table 6 below]

Additional Data from the Placebo-controlled Study

25.2% of patients treated with Jakafi and 7.3% of patients treated with placebo developed newly occurring or worsening Grade 1 abnormalities in alanine transaminase (ALT). The incidence of greater than or equal to Grade 2 elevations was 1.9% for Jakafi with 1.3% Grade 3 and no Grade 4 ALT elevations.

17.4% of patients treated with Jakafi and 6.0% of patients treated with placebo developed newly occurring or worsening Grade 1 abnormalities in aspartate transaminase (AST). The incidence of Grade 2 AST elevations was 0.6% for Jakafi with no Grade 3 or 4 AST elevations.

16.8% of patients treated with Jakafi and 0.7% of patients treated with placebo developed newly occurring or worsening Grade 1 elevations in cholesterol. The incidence of Grade 2 cholesterol elevations was 0.6% for Jakafi with no Grade 3 or 4 cholesterol elevations.

7. DRUG INTERACTIONS

7.1 Drugs That Inhibit or Induce Cytochrome P450 Enzymes

Ruxolitinib is predominantly metabolized by CYP3A4.

Strong CYP3A4 inhibitors: The C_{max} and AUC of ruxolitinib increased 33% and 91%, respectively, with Jakafi administration (10 mg single dose) following ketoconazole 200 mg twice daily for four days, compared to receiving Jakafi alone in healthy subjects. The half-life was also prolonged from 3.7 to 6.0 hours with concurrent use of ketoconazole. The change in the pharmacodynamic marker, pSTAT3 inhibition, was consistent with the corresponding ruxolitinib AUC following concurrent administration with ketoconazole.

When administering Jakafi with strong CYP3A4 inhibitors a dose reduction is recommended [*see Dosage and Administration (2.7)*]. Patients should be closely monitored and the dose titrated based on safety and efficacy.

Mild or moderate CYP3A4 inhibitors: There was an 8% and 27% increase in the C_{max} and AUC of ruxolitinib, respectively, with Jakafi administration (10 mg single dose) following erythromycin, a moderate CYP3A4 inhibitor, at 500 mg twice daily for 4 days, compared to receiving Jakafi alone in healthy subjects. The change in the pharmacodynamic marker, pSTAT3 inhibition was consistent with the corresponding exposure information.

No dose adjustment is recommended when Jakafi is coadministered with mild or moderate CYP3A4 inhibitors (eg, erythromycin).

CYP3A4 inducers: The C_{max} and AUC of ruxolitinib decreased 32% and 61%, respectively, with Jakafi administration (50 mg single dose) following rifampin 600 mg once daily for 10 days, compared to receiving Jakafi alone in healthy subjects. In addition, the relative exposure to ruxolitinib's active metabolites increased approximately 100%. This increase may partially explain the reported disproportionate 10% reduction in the pharmacodynamic marker pSTAT3 inhibition.

No dose adjustment is recommended when Jakafi is coadministered with a CYP3A4 inducer. Patients should be closely monitored and the dose titrated based on safety and efficacy.

8. USE IN SPECIFIC POPULATIONS

8.1 Pregnancy

Pregnancy Category C

There are no adequate and well-controlled studies of Jakafi in pregnant women. In embryofetal toxicity studies, treatment with ruxolitinib resulted in an increase in late resorptions and reduced fetal weights at maternally toxic doses. Jakafi should be used during pregnancy only if the potential benefit justifies the potential risk to the fetus.

Ruxolitinib was administered orally to pregnant rats or rabbits during the period of organogenesis, at doses of 15, 30 or 60 mg/kg/day in rats and 10, 30 or 60 mg/kg/day in rabbits. There was no evidence of teratogenicity. However, decreases of approximately 9% in fetal weights were noted in rats at the highest and maternally toxic dose of 60 mg/kg/day. This dose results in an exposure (AUC) that is approximately 2 times the clinical exposure at the maximum recommended dose of 25 mg twice daily. In rabbits, lower fetal weights of approximately 8% and increased late resorptions were noted at the highest and maternally toxic dose of 60 mg/kg/day. This dose is approximately 7% the clinical exposure at the maximum recommended dose.

In a pre- and post-natal development study in rats, pregnant animals were dosed with ruxolitinib from implantation through lactation at doses up to 30 mg/kg/day. There were no drug-related adverse findings in pups for fertility indices or for maternal or embryofetal survival, growth and development parameters at the highest dose evaluated (34% the clinical exposure at the maximum recommended dose of 25 mg twice daily).

Table 5: Adverse Reactions Occurring in Patients on Jakafi in the Double-blind, Placebo-controlled Study During Randomized Treatment

Adverse Reactions	Jakafi (N=155) All Grades[a] (%)	Jakafi Grade 3 (%)	Jakafi Grade 4 (%)	Placebo (N=151) All Grades (%)	Placebo Grade 3 (%)	Placebo Grade 4 (%)
Bruising[b]	23.2	0.6	0	14.6	0	0
Dizziness[c]	18.1	0.6	0	7.3	0	0
Headache	14.8	0	0	5.3	0	0
Urinary Tract Infections[d]	9.0	0	0	5.3	0.7	0.7
Weight Gain[e]	7.1	0.6	0	1.3	0.7	0
Flatulence	5.2	0	0	0.7	0	0
Herpes Zoster[f]	1.9	0	0	0.7	0	0

[a] National Cancer Institute Common Terminology Criteria for Adverse Events (CTCAE), version 3.0

[b] includes contusion, ecchymosis, hematoma, injection site hematoma, periorbital hematoma, vessel puncture site hematoma, increased tendency to bruise, petechiae, purpura

[c] includes dizziness, postural dizziness, vertigo, balance disorder, Meniere's Disease, labyrinthitis

[d] includes urinary tract infection, cystitis, urosepsis, urinary tract infection bacterial, kidney infection, pyuria, bacteria urine, bacteria urine identified, nitrite urine present

[e] includes weight increased, abnormal weight gain

[f] includes herpes zoster and post-herpetic neuralgia

Table 6: Worst Hematology Laboratory Abnormalities in the Placebo-controlled Study[a]

Laboratory Parameter	Jakafi (N=155) All Grades[b] (%)	Jakafi Grade 3 (%)	Jakafi Grade 4 (%)	Placebo (N=151) All Grades (%)	Placebo Grade 3 (%)	Placebo Grade 4 (%)
Thrombocytopenia	69.7	9.0	3.9	30.5	1.3	0
Anemia	96.1	34.2	11.0	86.8	15.9	3.3
Neutropenia	18.7	5.2	1.9	4.0	0.7	1.3

[a] Presented values are worst Grade values regardless of baseline

[b] National Cancer Institute Common Terminology Criteria for Adverse Events, version 3.0

8.3 Nursing Mothers

It is not known whether ruxolitinib is excreted in human milk. Ruxolitinib and/or its metabolites were excreted in the milk of lactating rats with a concentration that was 13-fold the maternal plasma. Because many drugs are excreted in human milk and because of the potential for serious adverse reactions in nursing infants from Jakafi, a decision should be made to discontinue nursing or to discontinue the drug, taking into account the importance of the drug to the mother.

8.4 Pediatric Use

The safety and effectiveness of Jakafi in pediatric patients have not been established.

8.5 Geriatric Use

Of the total number of myelofibrosis patients in clinical studies with Jakafi, 51.9% were 65 years of age and older. No overall differences in safety or effectiveness of Jakafi were observed between these patients and younger patients.

8.6 Renal Impairment

The safety and pharmacokinetics of single dose Jakafi (25 mg) were evaluated in a study in healthy subjects [CrCl 72-164 mL/min (N=8)] and in subjects with mild [CrCl 53-83 mL/min (N=8)], moderate [CrCl 38-57 mL/min (N=8)], or severe renal impairment [CrCl 15-51 mL/min (N=8)]. Eight (8) additional subjects with end stage renal disease requiring hemodialysis were also enrolled.

The pharmacokinetics of ruxolitinib was similar in subjects with various degrees of renal impairment and in those with normal renal function. However, plasma AUC values of ruxolitinib metabolites increased with increasing severity of renal impairment. This was most marked in the subjects with end stage renal disease requiring hemodialysis. The change in the pharmacodynamic marker, pSTAT3 inhibition, was consistent with the corresponding increase in metabolite exposure. Ruxolitinib is not removed by dialysis; however, the removal of some active metabolites by dialysis cannot be ruled out.

When administering Jakafi to patients with moderate (CrCl 30-59 mL/min) or severe renal impairment (CrCl 15-29 mL/min) with a platelet count between 100×10^9/L and 150×10^9/L and patients with end stage renal disease on dialysis a dose reduction is recommended [*see Dosage and Administration (2.8)*].

8.7 Hepatic Impairment

The safety and pharmacokinetics of single dose Jakafi (25 mg) were evaluated in a study in healthy subjects (N=8) and in subjects with mild [Child-Pugh A (N=8)], moderate [Child-Pugh B (N=8)], or severe hepatic impairment [Child-Pugh C (N=8)]. The mean AUC for ruxolitinib was increased by 87%, 28% and 65%, respectively, in patients with mild, moderate and severe hepatic impairment compared to patients with normal hepatic function. The terminal elimination half-life was prolonged in patients with hepatic impairment compared to healthy controls (4.1-5.0 hours versus 2.8 hours). The change in the pharmacodynamic marker, pSTAT3 inhibition, was consistent with the corresponding increase in ruxolitinib exposure except in the severe (Child-Pugh C) hepatic impairment cohort where the pharmacodynamic activity was more prolonged in some subjects than expected based on plasma concentrations of ruxolitinib.

When administering Jakafi to patients with any degree of hepatic impairment and with a platelet count between 100×10^9/L and 150×10^9/L, a dose reduction is recommended [*see Dosage and Administration (2.8)*].

10. OVERDOSAGE

There is no known antidote for overdoses with Jakafi. Single doses up to 200 mg have been given with acceptable acute tolerability. Higher than recommended repeat doses are associated with increased myelosuppression including leukopenia, anemia and thrombocytopenia. Appropriate supportive treatment should be given.

Hemodialysis is not expected to enhance the elimination of ruxolitinib.

11. DESCRIPTION

Ruxolitinib phosphate is a kinase inhibitor with the chemical name (*R*)-3-(4-(7*H*-pyrrolo[2,3-*d*]pyrimidin-4-yl)-1*H*-

Table 7: Percent of Patients with 35% or Greater Reduction from Baseline in Spleen Volume at Week 24 in Study 1 and at Week 48 in Study 2 (Intent to Treat)

	Study 1		Study 2	
	Jakafi (N=155)	Placebo (N=154)	Jakafi (N=146)	Best Available Therapy (N=73)
Time Points	Week 24		Week 48	
Number (%) of Patients with Spleen Volume Reduction by 35% or More	65 (41.9)	1 (0.7)	41 (28.5)	0
P-value	< 0.0001		< 0.0001	

pyrazol-1-yl)-3-cyclopentylpropanenitrile phosphate and a molecular weight of 404.36. Ruxolitinib phosphate has the following structural formula:

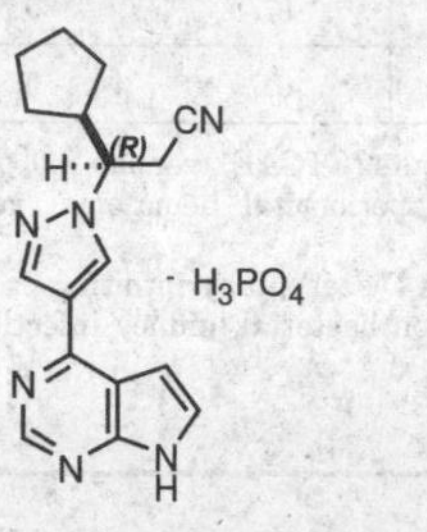

Ruxolitinib phosphate is a white to off-white to light pink powder and is soluble in aqueous buffers across a pH range of 1 to 8.

Jakafi (ruxolitinib) Tablets are for oral administration. Each tablet contains ruxolitinib phosphate equivalent to 5 mg, 10 mg, 15 mg, 20 mg and 25 mg of ruxolitinib free base together with microcrystalline cellulose, lactose monohydrate, magnesium stearate, colloidal silicon dioxide, sodium starch glycolate, povidone and hydroxypropyl cellulose.

12. CLINICAL PHARMACOLOGY

12.1 Mechanism of Action

Ruxolitinib, a kinase inhibitor, inhibits Janus Associated Kinases (JAKs) JAK1 and JAK2 which mediate the signaling of a number of cytokines and growth factors that are important for hematopoiesis and immune function. JAK signaling involves recruitment of STATs (signal transducers and activators of transcription) to cytokine receptors, activation and subsequent localization of STATs to the nucleus leading to modulation of gene expression.

Myelofibrosis (MF) is a myeloproliferative neoplasm (MPN) known to be associated with dysregulated JAK1 and JAK2 signaling. In a mouse model of JAK2V617F-positive MPN, oral administration of ruxolitinib prevented splenomegaly, preferentially decreased JAK2V617F mutant cells in the spleen and decreased circulating inflammatory cytokines (eg, TNF-α, IL-6).

12.2 Pharmacodynamics

Ruxolitinib inhibits cytokine induced STAT3 phosphorylation in whole blood from healthy subjects and MF patients. Jakafi administration resulted in maximal inhibition of STAT3 phosphorylation 2 hours after dosing which returned to near baseline by 10 hours in both healthy subjects and myelofibrosis patients.

12.3 Pharmacokinetics

Absorption

In clinical studies, ruxolitinib is rapidly absorbed after oral Jakafi administration with maximal plasma concentration (C_{max}) achieved within 1 to 2 hours post-dose. Based on a mass balance study in humans, oral absorption of ruxolitinib was estimated to be at least 95%. Mean ruxolitinib C_{max} and total exposure (AUC) increased proportionally over a single dose range of 5 to 200 mg. There were no clinically relevant changes in the pharmacokinetics of ruxolitinib upon administration of Jakafi with a high-fat meal, with the mean C_{max} moderately decreased (24%) and the mean AUC nearly unchanged (4% increase).

Distribution

The apparent volume of distribution of ruxolitinib at steady-state is 53 to 65 L in myelofibrosis patients. Binding to plasma proteins *in vitro* is approximately 97%, mostly to albumin.

Metabolism

In vitro studies suggest that CYP3A4 is the major enzyme responsible for metabolism of ruxolitinib. Ruxolitinib is the predominant entity in humans representing approximately 60% of the drug-related material in circulation. Two major and active metabolites were identified in plasma of healthy subjects representing 25% and 11% of parent AUC. These two metabolites have one-fifth and one-half of ruxolitinib's pharmacological activity, respectively. The sum total of all active metabolites contributes 18% of the overall pharmacodynamics of ruxolitinib.

Elimination

Following a single oral dose of [^{14}C]-labeled ruxolitinib in healthy adult subjects, elimination was predominately through metabolism with 74% of radioactivity excreted in urine and 22% excretion via feces. Unchanged drug accounted for less than 1% of the excreted total radioactivity. The mean elimination half-life of ruxolitinib is approximately 3 hours and the mean half-life of ruxolitinib + metabolites is approximately 5.8 hours.

Effects of Age, Gender, or Race

In healthy subjects, no significant differences in ruxolitinib pharmacokinetics were observed with regard to gender and race. In a population pharmacokinetic evaluation in myelofibrosis patients, no relationship was apparent between oral clearance and patient age or race, and in women, clearance was 17.7 L/h and in men, 22.1 L/h with 39% inter-subject variability.

Drug Interactions

In vitro, ruxolitinib and its M18 metabolite are not inhibitors of CYP1A2, CYP2B6, CYP2C8, CYP2C9, CYP2C19, CYP2D6 or CYP3A4. Ruxolitinib is not an inducer of CYP1A2, CYP2B6 or CYP3A4 at clinically relevant concentrations.

In vitro, ruxolitinib and its M18 metabolite are not inhibitors of the P-gp, BCRP, OATP1B1, OATP1B3, OCT1, OCT2, OAT1 or OAT3 transport systems at clinically relevant concentrations. Ruxolitinib is not a substrate for the P-gp transporter.

12.4 Thorough QT Study

The effect of single dose ruxolitinib 25 mg and 200 mg on QTc interval was evaluated in a randomized, placebo-, and active-controlled (moxifloxacin 400 mg) four-period crossover thorough QT study in 47 healthy subjects. In a study with demonstrated ability to detect small effects, the upper bound of the one-sided 95% confidence interval for the largest placebo adjusted, baseline-corrected QTc based on Fridericia correction method (QTcF) was below 10 ms, the threshold for regulatory concern. The dose of 200 mg is adequate to represent the high exposure clinical scenario.

13. NONCLINICAL TOXICOLOGY

13.1 Carcinogenesis, Mutagenesis, Impairment of Fertility

Ruxolitinib was not carcinogenic in the 6-month Tg.rasH2 transgenic mouse model or in a 2-year carcinogenicity study in the rat.

Ruxolitinib was not mutagenic in a bacterial mutagenicity assay (Ames test) or clastogenic in *in vitro* chromosomal aberration assay (cultured human peripheral blood lymphocytes) or *in vivo* in a rat bone marrow micronucleus assay.

In a fertility study, ruxolitinib was administered to male rats prior to and throughout mating and to female rats prior to mating and up to the implantation day (gestation day 7). Ruxolitinib had no effect on fertility or reproductive function in male or female rats at doses of 10, 30 or 60 mg/kg/day. However, in female rats doses of greater than or equal to 30 mg/kg/day resulted in increased post-implantation loss. The exposure (AUC) at the dose of 30 mg/kg/day is approximately 34% the clinical exposure at the maximum recommended dose of 25 mg twice daily.

14. CLINICAL STUDIES

Two randomized Phase 3 studies (Studies 1 and 2) were conducted in patients with myelofibrosis (either primary myelofibrosis, post-polycythemia vera myelofibrosis or post-essential thrombocythemia-myelofibrosis). In both studies, patients had palpable splenomegaly at least 5 cm below the costal margin and risk category of intermediate 2 (2 prognostic factors) or high risk (3 or more prognostic factors) based on the International Working Group Consensus Criteria (IWG).

The starting dose of Jakafi was based on platelet count. Patients with a platelet count between 100 and 200 × 10^9/L were started on Jakafi 15 mg twice daily and patients with a platelet count greater than 200 × 10^9/L were started on Jakafi 20 mg twice daily. Doses were then individualized based upon tolerability and efficacy with maximum doses of 20 mg twice daily for patients with platelet counts between 100 to less than or equal to 125 × 10^9/L, of 10 mg twice daily for patients with platelet counts between 75 to less than or equal to 100 × 10^9/L, and of 5 mg twice daily for patients with platelet counts between 50 to less than or equal to 75 × 10^9/L.

Study 1

Study 1 was a double-blind, randomized, placebo-controlled study in 309 patients who were refractory to or were not candidates for available therapy. The median age was 68 years (range 40 to 91 years) with 61% of patients older than 65 years and 54% were male. Fifty percent (50%) of patients had primary myelofibrosis, 31% had post-polycythemia vera myelofibrosis and 18% had post-essential thrombocythemia myelofibrosis. Twenty-one percent (21%) of patients had red blood cell transfusions within 8 weeks of enrollment in the study. The median hemoglobin count was 10.5 g/dL and the median platelet count was 251 × 10^9/L. Patients had a median palpable spleen length of 16 cm below the costal margin, with 81% having a spleen length 10 cm or greater below the costal margin. Patients had a median spleen volume as measured by magnetic resonance imaging (MRI) or computed tomography (CT) of 2595 cm^3 (range 478 cm^3 to 8881 cm^3). (The upper limit of normal is approximately 300 cm^3).

Patients were dosed with Jakafi or matching placebo. The primary efficacy endpoint was the proportion of patients achieving greater than or equal to a 35% reduction from baseline in spleen volume at Week 24 as measured by MRI or CT.

Secondary endpoints included duration of a 35% or greater reduction in spleen volume and proportion of patients with a 50% or greater reduction in Total Symptom Score from baseline to Week 24 as measured by the modified Myelofibrosis Symptom Assessment Form (MFSAF) v2.0 diary.

Study 2

Study 2 was an open-label, randomized study in 219 patients. Patients were randomized 2:1 to Jakafi versus best available therapy. Best available therapy was selected by the investigator on a patient-by-patient basis. In the best available therapy arm, the medications received by more than 10% of patients were hydroxyurea (47%) and glucocorticoids (16%). The median age was 66 years (range 35 to 85 years) with 52% of patients older than 65 years and 57% were male. Fifty-three percent (53%) of patients had primary myelofibrosis, 31% had post-polycythemia vera myelofibrosis and 16% had post-essential thrombocythemia myelofibrosis. Twenty-one percent (21%) of patients had red blood cell transfusions within 8 weeks of enrollment in the study. The median hemoglobin count was 10.4 g/dL and the median platelet count was 236 × 10^9/L. Patients had a median palpable spleen length of 15 cm below the costal margin, with 70% having a spleen length 10 cm or greater below the costal margin. Patients had a median spleen volume as measured by MRI or CT of 2381 cm^3 (range 451 cm^3 to 7765 cm^3).

The primary efficacy endpoint was the proportion of patients achieving 35% or greater reduction from baseline in spleen volume at Week 48 as measured by MRI or CT.

A secondary endpoint in Study 2 was the proportion of patients achieving a 35% or greater reduction of spleen volume as measured by MRI or CT from baseline to Week 24.

Study 1 and 2 Efficacy Results

Efficacy analyses of the primary endpoint in Studies 1 and 2 are presented in Table 7 below. A significantly larger proportion of patients in the Jakafi group achieved a 35% or greater reduction in spleen volume from baseline in both studies compared to placebo in Study 1 and best available therapy in Study 2. A similar proportion of patients in the Jakafi group achieved a 50% or greater reduction in palpable spleen length.

[See table 7 above]

Figure 1 shows the percent change from baseline in spleen volume for each patient at Week 24 (Jakafi N=139, placebo N=106) or the last evaluation prior to Week 24 for patients who did not complete 24 weeks of randomized treatment (Jakafi N=16, placebo N=47). One (1) patient (placebo) with a missing baseline spleen volume is not included.

[See figure 1 at top of next page]

In Study 1, myelofibrosis symptoms were a secondary endpoint and were measured using the modified Myelofibrosis Symptom Assessment Form (MFSAF) v2.0 diary. The modified MFSAF is a daily diary capturing the core symptoms of myelofibrosis (abdominal discomfort, pain under left ribs, night sweats, itching, bone/muscle pain and early satiety). Symptom scores ranged from 0 to 10 with 0 representing symptoms "absent" and 10 representing "worst imaginable" symptoms. These scores were added to create the daily total score, which has a maximum of 60.

Table 8 presents assessments of Total Symptom Score from baseline to Week 24 in Study 1 including the proportion of patients with at least a 50% reduction (ie, improvement in symptoms). At baseline, the mean Total Symptom Score was 18.0 in the Jakafi group and 16.5 in the placebo group. A higher proportion of patients in the Jakafi group had a 50% or greater reduction in Total Symptom Score than in the placebo group, with a median time to response of less than 4 weeks.

Table 8: Improvement in Total Symptom Score

	Jakafi (N=148)	Placebo (N=152)
Number (%) of Patients with 50% or Greater Reduction in Total Symptom Score by Week 24	68 (45.9)	8 (5.3)
P-value	< 0.0001	

Figure 2 shows the percent change from baseline in Total Symptom Score for each patient at Week 24 (Jakafi N=129, placebo N=103) or the last evaluation on randomized therapy prior to Week 24 for patients who did not complete 24 weeks of randomized treatment (Jakafi N=16, placebo N=42). Results are excluded for 5 patients with a baseline Total Symptom Score of zero, 8 patients with missing baseline and 6 patients with insufficient post-baseline data.

[See figure 2 below]

Figure 3 displays the proportion of patients with at least a 50% improvement in each of the individual symptoms that comprise the Total Symptom Score indicating that all 6 of the symptoms contributed to the higher Total Symptom Score response rate in the group treated with Jakafi.

Figure 3: Proportion of Patients With 50% or Greater Reduction in Individual Symptom Scores at Week 24

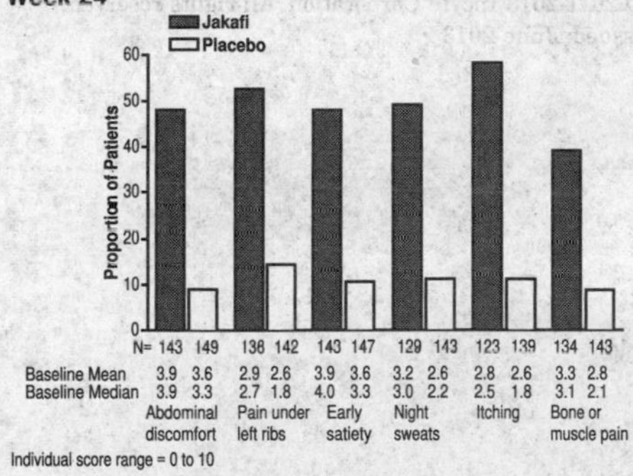

Individual score range = 0 to 10

16. HOW SUPPLIED/STORAGE AND HANDLING

Jakafi (ruxolitinib) Tablets are available as follows:

[See table above]

17. PATIENT COUNSELING INFORMATION

See FDA-approved patient labeling (Patient Information).

Discuss the following with patients prior to treatment with Jakafi:

17.1 Thrombocytopenia, Anemia and Neutropenia

Inform patients that Jakafi is associated with thrombocytopenia, anemia and neutropenia, and of the need to monitor complete blood counts before and during treatment. Advise patients to observe for and report bleeding.

17.2 Infections

Inform patients of the signs and symptoms of infection and to report any such signs and symptoms promptly.

Inform patients regarding the early signs and symptoms of herpes zoster and of progressive multifocal leukoencephalopathy, and advise patients to seek advice of a clinician if such symptoms are observed.

17.3 Drug-drug Interactions

Advise patients to inform their healthcare providers of all medications they are taking, including over-the-counter medications, herbal products and dietary supplements.

17.4 Dialysis

Inform patients on dialysis that their dose should not be taken before dialysis but only following dialysis.

17.5 Compliance

Patients should be advised to continue taking Jakafi every day for as long as their physician tells them and that this is a long-term treatment. Patients should not change dose or stop taking Jakafi without first consulting their physician. Patients should be aware that after discontinuation of treatment, myelofibrosis signs and symptoms are expected to return.

Manufactured by:
DSM Pharmaceuticals, Inc.
Greenville, NC 27834
Manufactured for:
Incyte Corporation
Wilmington, DE 19880

Figure 1: Percent Change from Baseline in Spleen Volume at Week 24 or Last Observation for Each Patient (Study 1)

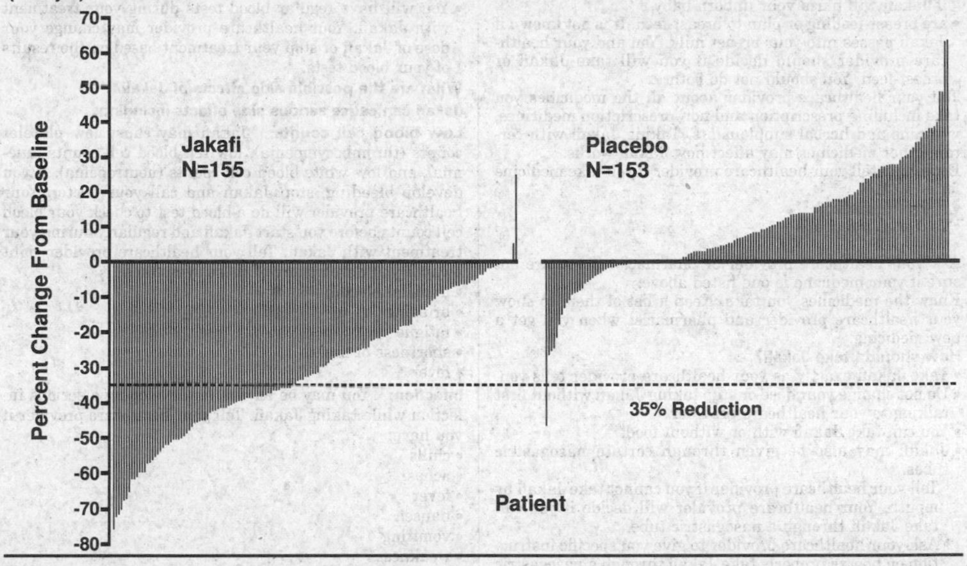

Figure 2: Percent Change from Baseline in Total Symptom Score at Week 24 or Last Observation for Each Patient (Study 1)

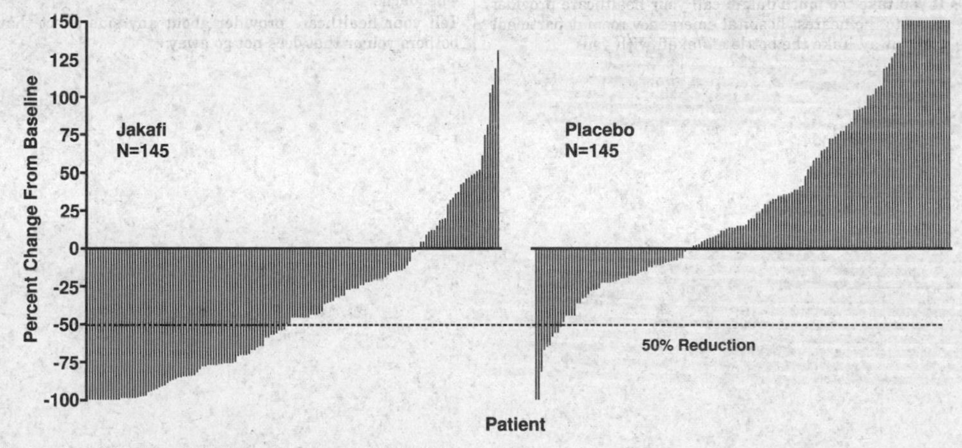

Worsening of Total Sympton Score is truncated at 150%.

Jakafi Trade Presentations

NDC Number	Strength	Description	Tablets per Bottle
50881-005-60	5 mg	Round tablet with "INCY" on one side and "5" on the other	60
50881-010-60	10 mg	Round tablet with "INCY" on one side and "10" on the other	60
50881-015-60	15 mg	Oval tablet with "INCY" on one side and "15" on the other	60
50881-020-60	20 mg	Capsule shaped tablet with "INCY" on one side and "20" on the other	60
50881-025-60	25 mg	Oval tablet with "INCY" on one side and "25" on the other	60

Store at room temperature 20°C to 25°C (68°F to 77°F); excursions permitted between 15°C and 30°C (59°F and 86°F) [see USP Controlled Room Temperature].

Patient Information

Jakafi® (JAK-ah-fye)

(ruxolitinib) Tablets

Read this Patient Information before you start taking Jakafi and each time you get a refill. There may be new information. This information does not take the place of talking to your healthcare provider about your medical condition or treatment.

What is Jakafi?

Jakafi is a prescription medicine used to treat people with intermediate or high-risk myelofibrosis, including primary myelofibrosis, post-polycythemia vera myelofibrosis and post-essential thrombocythemia myelofibrosis.

It is not known if Jakafi is safe or effective in children.

What should I tell my healthcare provider before taking Jakafi?

Before taking Jakafi, tell your healthcare provider if you:

- have an infection.
- have or have had liver or kidney problems.
- are on dialysis. Jakafi should be taken after your dialysis.

- have any other medical conditions.
- are pregnant, or plan to become pregnant. It is not known if Jakafi will harm your unborn baby.
- are breast-feeding or plan to breast-feed. It is not known if Jakafi passes into your breast milk. You and your healthcare provider should decide if you will take Jakafi or breast-feed. You should not do both.

Tell your healthcare provider about all the medicines you take including prescription and non-prescription medicines, vitamins and herbal supplements. Taking Jakafi with certain other medicines may affect how Jakafi works.

Especially tell your healthcare provider if you take medicine for:

- Fungal infections
- Bacterial infections
- HIV-AIDS

Ask your healthcare provider or pharmacist if you are not sure if your medicine is one listed above.

Know the medicines you take. Keep a list of them to show your healthcare provider and pharmacist when you get a new medicine.

How should I take Jakafi?

- Take Jakafi exactly as your healthcare provider tells you.
- Do not change your dose or stop taking Jakafi without first talking to your healthcare provider.
- You can take Jakafi with or without food.
- Jakafi may also be given through certain nasogastric tubes.
  - Tell your healthcare provider if you cannot take Jakafi by mouth. Your healthcare provider will decide if you can take Jakafi through a nasogastric tube.
  - Ask your healthcare provider to give you specific instruction on how to properly take Jakafi through a nasogastric tube.
- Do not drink grapefruit juice while taking Jakafi. Grapefruit juice can affect the amount of Jakafi in your blood.
- If you take too much Jakafi call your healthcare provider or go to the nearest hospital emergency room department right away. Take the bottle of Jakafi with you.
- If you miss a dose of Jakafi, take your next dose at your regular time. Do not take 2 doses at the same time.
- You will have regular blood tests during your treatment with Jakafi. Your healthcare provider may change your dose of Jakafi or stop your treatment based on the results of your blood tests.

What are the possible side effects of Jakafi?

Jakafi can cause serious side effects including:

Low blood cell counts: Jakafi may cause low platelet counts (thrombocytopenia), low red blood cell counts (anemia), and low white blood cell counts (neutropenia). If you develop bleeding, stop Jakafi and call your doctor. Your healthcare provider will do a blood test to check your blood cell counts before you start Jakafi and regularly during your treatment with Jakafi. Tell your healthcare provider right away if you develop any of these symptoms:

- unusual bleeding
- bruising
- fatigue
- shortness of breath
- fever

Infection: You may be at risk for developing a serious infection while taking Jakafi. Tell your healthcare provider if you have:

- chills
- aches
- fever
- nausea
- vomiting
- weakness
- painful skin rash or blisters

The most common side effects of Jakafi include:

- dizziness
- headache

Tell your healthcare provider about any side effect that bothers you or that does not go away.

These are not all the possible side effects of Jakafi. Ask your healthcare provider or pharmacist for more information.

Call your doctor for medical advice about side effects. You may report side effects to FDA at 1-800-FDA-1088.

How should I store Jakafi?

- Store Jakafi at room temperature between 68°F and 77°F (20°C and 25°C).

Keep this and all medicines out of the reach of children.

General information about the safe and effective use of Jakafi:

Medicines are sometimes prescribed for purposes other than those listed in Patient Information. Do not use Jakafi for a condition for which it is not prescribed. Do not give Jakafi to other people, even if they have the same symptoms you have. It may harm them.

This Patient Information leaflet summarizes the most important information about Jakafi. If you would like more information, talk with your healthcare provider. You can ask your healthcare provider or pharmacist for information that is written for healthcare professionals.

For more information call 1-855-463-3463 or go to www.jakafi.com.

What are the ingredients in Jakafi?

Active ingredient: ruxolitinib.

Inactive ingredients: microcrystalline cellulose, lactose monohydrate, magnesium stearate, colloidal silicon dioxide, sodium starch glycolate, povidone and hydroxypropyl cellulose.

This Patient Information has been approved by the U.S. Food and Drug Administration.

U.S. Patent No. 7,598,257; 8,415,362

Issued: June 2013

SECTION 6

DIETARY SUPPLEMENTS

This section presents information on natural remedies and nutritional supplements marketed under the Dietary Supplement Health and Education Act (DSHEA) of 1994. The information on each product described has been provided by the manufacturer and contains the latest information available when *PDR®* went to press. Listings are arranged alphabetically by manufacturer; late submissions appear alphabetically by manufacturer at the end of this section.

The function of PDR Network® is solely the compilation, organization, and distribution of this information on natural remedies and nutritional supplements. PDR Network does not assume, and expressly disclaims, any obligation to obtain and include any information on natural remedies and nutritional supplements other than that provided to it by the manufacturers. It should be understood that by making this material available, PDR Network is not advocating the use of any product described herein; nor is PDR Network responsible for misuse of a product due to typographical error. Additional information on any natural remedy and/or nutritional supplement product may be obtained from the manufacturer.

Products found in this section include herbal preparations, vitamins, minerals, and other substances intended to supplement the diet. The descriptions of these products are designed to provide the information necessary for informed use. Dietary supplements marketed under the DSHEA do not receive formal evaluation or approval from the FDA. The following disclaimer applies to all product information listed in this section, as mandated by the federal government: *These statements have not been evaluated by the Food and Drug Administration. This product is not intended to diagnose, treat, cure, or prevent any disease.*

4Life Research USA, LLC

9850 SOUTH 300 WEST
SANDY, UT 84070

Direct Inquiries to:
(801) 562-3600
Fax: (801) 562-3611
productsupport@4life.com
www.4life.com

4LIFE TRANSFER FACTOR® TRI-FACTOR® FORMULA

PRODUCT DESCRIPTION

4Life Transfer Factor Tri-Factor Formula combines proprietary transfer factors and NanoFactor® molecules extracted from bovine colostrum and chicken egg yolk sources. These molecules contain antigen information which educates, enhances, and helps maintain immune system balance.

TECHNICAL DESCRIPTION

Transfer factors are molecules that communicate antigenic immunological information intercellularly and from a donor to a recipient. They support immune function through cell mediated immunity. Transfer factors, which carry antigen specific information to which all tested immune cells respond, are produced by mononuclear cells and serve to support and improve immune mediated pathways. Mammalian transfer factors, including those of humans are small molecules between 3,500 and 10,000 daltons. (1; 2) Transfer factors are polypeptides that consist of 40 to 44 amino acids (3) and have a conserved region and a variable region. From a molecular biological standpoint, these two properties are analogous to antibodies; however transfer factor's functions of cell mediated immunity (CMI) and non-specific immunological activity differ almost completely from the functions of antibodies. The molecules that have a molecular weight of less than 3,500 daltons modulate immune response but they do not transfer delayed-type hypersensitivity (DTH). (1)

4Life's transfer factors are sourced from the ultra-filtration of colostrum and from egg yolks. (4; 5) The molecules obtained from the spray dried ultra-filtrate of bovine colostrum are of two classes; the transfer factors present in the ultra-filtrate of ≤10,000 daltons and the nanofraction molecules that are present in the nano-filtrate of ≤3,500 daltons.

Transfer factors were first discovered in 1949 by H. Sherwood Lawrence when he demonstrated that CMI could be transferred from one individual to another by way of low molecular weight extracts of white blood cells. Transfer factors could transfer DTH of a specific form from a skin test positive individual to a skin test negative individual who subsequent to the transfer would skin test positive for that antigen. (6) In a subsequent study in 1955 he demonstrated that DTH could be passed serially, first from a skin test positive individual to a test negative individual, who became test positive, then 6 months later from the second individual to another test negative individual who became test positive. (7) At the time antibodies were the focus of immune research and little was known of the importance of DTH and of the involvement of T-cells in immune response. Transfer factors promote wellness via cell mediated immunity. These compounds are components of colostrum, an infant's first meal. They bridge the generational gap by passing cell mediated immunity from mother to infant.

BIOLOGICAL AND PHYSIOLOGICAL ACTION

Transfer factors' preparations contain more than 200 different moieties of polypeptide molecules with a molecular weight of <10,000 daltons; each moiety potentially having a great number of epitotic variations. These antigen specific factors are synthesized in monocytes and stored in the cytoplasm or on the cell membrane. A significant body of evidence indicates that the primary biological function of transfer factors is to recruit and specifically sensitize previously uncommitted lymphocytes. These sensitized T-lymphocytes initiate the events of cell-mediated immunity, thereby, promoting immunity not only at the site of antigen challenge but also throughout the body. (8) The effect of transfer factors on antigen mediated immunity, via B-cells, is not completely understood; however, a clinical test has reported an increase in particular antibodies, such as IgA and IgG, during transfer factor administration.

Clinical studies have demonstrated that transfer factors' unique ability to express DTH and promote cell-mediated immunity can be transferred from a sensitized donor to a non-immune recipient. (1; 9) This antigen specific effect is well documented and is likely produced through activation of the CD3-antigen site of T-cells, increased macrophage activation, and interleukin production—which can also enhance natural killer cell function. (1; 10)

Although the exact mechanism of action is unknown, research has shown that transfer factors will bind to antigens. However, the antigen specificity that is "transferred" to recipients is mediated by T-lymphocytes. (3) Current structure function models propose that transfer factors have a variable region and a conserved amino acid region, which determines the antigenic specificity for an estimated 8^{18} epitopes (1) and serves as a binding target for immune cell receptors respectively. (2; 11) These highly conserved regions presumably allow transfer factors to be administered across a species barrier without any loss of potency. In fact, research has demonstrated that bovine transfer factors are structurally analogous to human-derived transfer factors with equivalent physiological activity. This is further supported by several studies, which used transfer factors extracted from bovine lymph nodes and colostrum to confer cell-mediated immunity to specific antigens in animals and human recipients. (12; 13)

Although most clinical trials with transfer factors have used parental administration; oral administration has also demonstrated successful transfer of DTH and cell mediated immunity I recipients. (14) Dose response studies, which compare in various routes of administration, have been performed in both human and animals. Results of these experiments refute any arguments that the acidic or enzymatic environment of gastrointestinal tract effects oral administration of transfer factors. (14)

CLINICAL AND EXPERIMENTAL STUDIES

Natural Killer Cell Activity

Peripheral blood mononuclear cells were isolated and pooled from several healthy donors. Sixty thousand cells were added to each well of 96-well microtiter plate. Various immune modulating ingredients, including 4Life Transfer Factor Tri-Factor Formula, were added to select wells on the plate and 48 hour incubation started. At the end of the incubation period 30 thousand K562 cells were added to each well. MTT assay techniques were used to determine the cytotoxic index. The various 4Life Transfer Factor products resulted in cytotoxic indices of 80-98%. By comparison, mononuclear cells incubated with IL-2 for the same 48 hour period produced a cytotoxic index of 88%.

CD4 T Helper Cell Research

Multiple studies were performed using the FDA-approved diagnostic CD4 T Helper cell assay kit and/or a T Cell Memory (CD8) assay kit under development by the same company. Similar to the NK cell research described above these *in vitro* studies were preformed on 96-well microtiter plates measuring ATP production via a luciferase-based luminescence reaction.

The CD4 assay utilizes PHA-stimulated cells isolated from whole blood via the use of Dynabeads™. An 18 hour incubation of these isolated, stimulated CD4 cells with the 4Life Transfer Factor products has resulted in a modulation of immune cell activity as exhibited by a decrease in ATP production without a negative impact on cell viability. It is hypothesized that this reduction on ATP production is a result of a redirection in immune cell focus, essentially diminishing the distraction induced by the addition of PHA to the microtiter wells.

Salivary Secretory IgA-Preliminary Investigation

Twenty-four subjects naïve to transfer factor supplementation were enrolled in a small-scale, preliminary test. Twenty-one were included in the final analysis. Salivary samples were collected from each subject weekly at roughly the same time of day and day of the week. Saliva was collected over a 5 minute period via passive drool while subjects chewed on a piece of Parafilm™. The samples were put on ice and then frozen at -70ºC until assay. The commercial Salimetrics™ salivary IgA assay kit was used for analysis. Subjects were given 4Life Transfer Factor Tri-Factor Formula at 2 capsules per day for two weeks and then transitioned to 4Life Transfer Factor RioVida Tri-Factor Formula at 60ml per day for an additional 2 weeks. At the end of the 4 week supplementation period the group showed an average 73% increase in salivary secretory IgA (SIgA) production over their baseline value. Furthermore, none of the 21 subjects showed SIgA production rate less than their baseline value at the end of the test.

Wellness Research

A study conducted with 30 college students found that either 15 or 30 days of transfer factor administered according to label dose helped them maintain their health. Those that took the product for 30 days showed prolonged health maintenance than those who took it for only 15 days. (15)

Longevity Studies

Two studies on the effects of 4Life Transfer Factor products on longevity were conducted. An initial, preliminary study was done on mice. This was followed up with a more intricate study on a small group of older men.

Groups of 20 mice each were compared in terms of organ weights, serum immune parameters, strength (dynamometer and hanging time), and isoproterenol-induced salivary hyperplasia. One group was injected with 4mg/kg of a product containing transfer factors. The treatment group showed improvements in all the aforementioned parameters. Isoproterenol-induced salivary gland hyperplasia declines with age. This diminished response is thought to be a consequence of decreased lymphoid cellular regulation of somatic tissue growth. The increased hyperplasia seen in the treatment animals approximated that seen in the treatment animals approximated that seen in younger, untreated mice. There were no significant changes noted in height, weight, or rectal temperature between the two groups. (16)

Based on the results of this study an additional study was undertaken in 11 older men aged 55-73. Subjects were given 3 capsules per day of a product containing transfer factors 5 days a week for 6 weeks. At the end of the six week study period a determination of biological age using the Kiev method (17; 18) showed a reduction of approximately four years. There were significant improvements in several parameters of cardiovascular function, hearing, balance, vital lung capacity, ability to hold their breath, and some subjective measures. (16)

Safety

In a study of acute toxicity rats were assessed for fourteen days following a single gavage of 4Life Transfer Factor. Five female SD rats were each gavaged with a dose of 2,000mg/kg. No treatment-related mortalities occurred and there were no clinical signs of toxicity. No significant difference in body weight occurred. No gross lesions were found at necropsy in any of the animals. Thus, acute toxicity is considered to be greater than 2,000mg/kg.

Since the discovery of transfer factors in 1949 there have been no reports of allergic reactions (1) or of any side effects resulting from long-term use of 10 years or more. The use of transfer factors is contraindicated in person receiving immunosuppressive therapy, though actual interactions have not been documented.

How Supplied

4Life Transfer Factor® can be found in the following products:

4Life Transfer Factor® Tri-Factor® Formula
4Life® Transfer Factor Plus® Tri-Factor® Formula
4Life Transfer Factor® RioVida® Tri-Factor® Formula
4Life Transfer Factor® Chewable Tri-Factor® Formula
4Life Transfer Factor® Classic
4Life Transfer Factor® Immune Spray
4Life Transfer Factor® KBU®
4Life Transfer Factor® Kids
4Life Transfer Factor® Belle Vie®
4Life Transfer Factor® Cardio
4Life Transfer Factor® GluCoach®
4Life Transfer Factor® MalePro®
4Life Transfer Factor® ReCall®
4Life Transfer Factor Vista®
4Life Transfer Factor Renuvo™
4Life RiteStart® Men
4Life RiteStart® Women

REFERENCES

1. *Progress in Drug Research.* **Fundenberg, H. and G. Pizza.** 1994, Vol. 42. 309-400.
2. **Lawrence, H.S. and W. Borkowsjy.** (1-3), 1996, Biotherapy, Vol. 9, pp. 1-5.
3. **Kirkpatrick, C.H.** 4, 2000, Mol Med, Vol. 6, pp. 332-41.
4. **Hennen, W. and D. Lisonbee.** s.l. : U.P. Office, Editor., 2002, 4Life Research, LC:USA.
5. **Wilson, G. and G. Paddock.** s.l. : U.P. Office, Editor., 1989, Amtron, Inc: USA.
6. **Lawrence, H.S.** 4, 1949, Proc Soc Exp Biol Med, Vol. 71, pp. 516-22.
7. **Lawrence, H.S.** 2, 1955, J Clin Invest, Vol. 34, pp. 219-30.
8. **Levin, A.S., L.E. Spitler, and H.H. Fundenberg.** 1973, Annu Rev Med, Vol. 24, pp. 175-208.
9. **Fudenberg, H. and H. Fudenberg.** 1989, Ann Rev Pharmacol Toxicol, Vol. 29, pp. 475-516.
10. **See, D., S. Mason, and R. Roshan.** 2, 2002, Immunol Invest, Vol. 31, pp. 137-53.
11. *Transfer factor in the age of molecular biology: A review.* **Dwyer, John M.** 1-3, 1996, Biotherapy, Vol. 9, pp. 7-11.
12. **Wilson, G.B., R.T. Newell, and N.M. Burdash.** 1, 1979, Cell Immunol, Vol. 47, pp. 1-18.
13. **Radosevich, J.K., G.H. Scott, and G.B. Olson.** 4, 1985, Am J Vet Res, Vol. 46, pp. 875-8.
14. *Activities and characteristics of transfer factors.* **Kirkpatrick, C.H.** 1-3, 1996, Biotherapy, Vol. 9, pp. 13-6.
15. *in Euromedica Hanover.* **Chizhov, A. et al.** Hanover, Germany : s.n., 2007.
16. *in Euromedica Hannover 2004.* **Klimov, V. and E. Oganova.** Hannover, Germany : s.n., 2004. pp. 15-16.
17. **Agadzhanian, N., et al.** 1996, ATMA.
18. **Chebotarev, D.** 1984, Annals of Gerontology and Geriatrics.

These statements have not been evaluated by the Food and Drug Administration. This product is not intended to diagnose, treat, cure of prevent any disease.

Shown in Product Identification Guide, page 303

A&Z Pharmaceutical Inc.

180 OSER AVENUE, SUITE 300
HAUPPAUGE, NY 11788

Direct Inquiries to:
Telephone: (631) 952-3800
Fax: (631) 952-3900
E-Mail: info@azpharmaceutical.com
Website: www.azpharmaceutical.com

D-CAL OTC

Calcium Supplement / Antacid
Calcium 300 mg
Vitamin D_3 100IU

Supplement Facts

	Adults	Children
■ Serving size	2	1
■ Servings per Container	30	60
■ Amount per Serving		
Calories:	4	2
Calcium (as calcium carbonate)	600 mg (60%DV)	300 mg (37.5%DV)
Vitamin D_3	200 IU (50%DV)	100 IU (25%DV)

Drug Facts

Active ingredient (in each tablet)	***Purpose***
Calcium Carbonate 750 mg	Antacid

Uses

relieves ■ heartburn ■ acid indigestion ■ sour stomach ■ upset stomach due to these symptoms

Warnings

Ask a doctor or pharmacist before use if you are taking a prescription drug. Antacids may interact with certain prescription drugs.

When using this product ■ do not take more than 10 tablets for adults and 5 tablets for chidren in a 24 hour period.

Keep out of reach of children.

Directions

■ **Adults:** chew 2 tablets daily. ■ **Children:** chew 1 tablet daily.
If symptoms persist, ask a doctor.

Other Information

■ store in a dry place
■ do not use if imprinted seal under cap is torn or open

Inactive ingredients cholecalciferol, D&C red #27, flavors, magnesium stearate, maltodextrin, mineral oil, sorbitol

How supplied: bottles of 60 tablets
A&Z Pharmaceutical, Inc
Hauppauge, NY 11788

Shown in Product Identification Guide, page 303

D-CAL® KIDS OTC

Calcium Supplement / Antacid
Granules
Calcium 300mg
Vitamin D_3 100 IU

Supplement Facts

■ Serving size	1g
■ Servings per Container	10
■ Amount per Serving	
Calories: 1	
Calcium (as calcium carbonate)	300 mg (37.5%DV)

Drug Facts

Active Ingredient (in each pouch)	***Purpose***
Calcium Carbonate 750 mg	Antacid

Uses relieves ■ heartburn ■ acid indigestion
■ sour stomach ■ upset stomach due to these symptoms

Warnings

Ask a doctor or pharmacist before use if you are taking a prescription drug. Antacids may interact with certain prescription drugs.

When using this product ■ do not take more than 1 pouch in a 24 hour period

Keep out of reach of children.

Directions

■ find the right dose on chart below based on weight, otherwise use age.
■ pour powder into cup and add 15ml (0.51 oz.) of water, stir and drink.

Dosing Chart

Weight (lbs)	Age	Dose
Under 24	Under 2 yrs	Ask a doctor
24-47	2-5 yrs	1/2 pouch
48-95	6-11 yrs	1 pouch

Other Information

■ store in a dry place ■ do not use if pouch is open or torn

Inactive Ingredients cholecalciferol, dextrose, maltodextrin, sodium citrate

How supplied: 10 1g pouches per carton
A&Z Pharmaceutical, Inc
Hauppauge, NY 11788

Shown in Product Identification Guide, page 303

Alcon Laboratories, Inc.

AND ITS AFFILIATES
CORPORATE HEADQUARTERS
6201 SOUTH FREEWAY
FORT WORTH, TX 76134

Address Inquiries to:
6201 South Freeway
Fort Worth, TX 76134
(800) 757-9195
Outside the U.S. call (817) 568-6725
alcon.medinfo@alcon.com

ICAPS® LUTEIN & OMEGA-3 DS

Eye Vitamin & Mineral Supplement

Directions

Suggested Adult Intake: One softgel daily with a meal or as directed by your physician.

Warnings

DO NOT USE IF THE SAFETY SEAL UNDER THE CAP IS BROKEN OR MISSING.

Caution: Softgels should be consumed whole. Do not consume damaged softgels.

KEEP OUT OF THE REACH OF CHILDREN.

Keep tightly closed in a dry place at controlled room temperature.

Supplement Facts

Serving size: 1 Softgel Servings Per Container: 30		
	Amount Per Serving	% Daily Value
Calories	10	-
Total Fat	0.4 g	0.7%**
Total Carbohydrate	0.03 g	<1%**
Protein	0.32 g	<1%**
Vitamin A (as Retinyl Palmitate)	0.6 mg	20%
Vitamin C (as Niacinamide Ascorbate)	45 mg	75%
Vitamin E (as *d-alpha*-Tocopherol)	10 mg	50%
Thiamin (as Thiamin Mononitrate)	1.2 mg	80%
Riboflavin	1.3 mg	76%
Niacin (as Niacinamide Ascorbate)	16 mg	80%
Vitamin B6 (as Pyridoxine hydrochloride)	1.3 mg	65%
Folic Acid	240 mcg	60%
Vitamin B12 (as Cyanocobalamin)	2.4 mcg	40%
Calcium	1 mg	0.1%
Zinc (as Zinc Oxide)	7 mg	47%
Selenium (as Sodium Selenate)	34 mcg	49%
Copper (as Cupric Gluconate)	0.9 mg	45%
Manganese (as Manganese Sulfate Monohydrate)	2.3 mg	115%
Lutein	10 mg	†
Zeaxanthin	2 mg	†
Omega-3 Fatty Acids	280 mg	†
EPA	148 mg	†
DHA	78 mg	†

** Percent daily values are based on a dict of 2000 calories/day
† Daily Value not established

Other Ingredients: Gelatin, Monounsaturated fatty acids, Beeswax, N-3 fatty acids, Corn oil, Glycerin, Polyunsaturated fatty acids, Sorbitol, Saturated fatty acids, Lecithin (soybean), Silicon dioxide, Sunflower oil, Dicalcium phosphate, Tocopherols, Titanium dioxide, Rosemary, FD&C Red #40, FD&C Yellow #6, Ascorbyl palmitate, FD&C Blue #1, *dl-alpha*-tocopherol, Citric acid, Copper chlorides, Trace metals

Questions or Comments? Call Us. 1-800-757-9195
MedInfo@AlconLabs.com

Distributed by:
ALCON LABORATORIES, INC.
6201 South Freeway
Fort Worth, Texas 76134-2099
Made in The Netherlands

Alto Pharmaceuticals, Inc.

P.O. BOX 271150
TAMPA, FL 33688-1150
3172 LAKE ELLEN DRIVE
TAMPA, FL 33618
www.altopharm.com

Direct Inquiries to:
John J. Cullaro
Customer Service
JOHNC@ALTOPHARM.COM
Tel (800) 330-2891
Fax (813) 968-0527

ZINC-220® DS

DIETARY SUPPLEMENT
(Zinc Sulfate 220 mg. USP)

UNIT DOSE
100 CAPSULES

Supplement Facts
Serving Size 1 Capsule

Amount Per Serving		% Daily Value*
Zinc	50mg	333%
(From Zinc Sulfate Heptahydrate 220mg)		

INGREDIENTS: Each blue and pink capsule contains 50 mg. of elemental zinc. Zinc-220 capsules are gluten free and do not contain dextrose or glucose. Inactive ingredients: rice flour, magnesium stearate, D&C red #22, D&C red #28, FD&C blue #1, titanium dioxide and gelatin (capsule shell).

ACTION AND USES: Zinc-220® Capsules are indicated as a dietary supplement. Normal growth and tissue repair are directly dependent upon an adequate supply of zinc in the diet. Zinc functions as an integral part of a number of enzymes important to protein and carbohydrate metabolism. Zinc-220® Capsules are recommended for deficiencies or the prevention of deficiencies of zinc.

WARNINGS: Zinc-220® if administered in stat dosages of 2 grams (9 capsules) will cause an emetic effect. As with any supplement, if you are pregnant, nursing or taking medication, consult your physician before use.
PRECAUTION: It is recommended that Zinc-220® Capsules be taken with meals to avoid gastric distress.
ADULTS: Take one capsule daily with meals or as directed by a physician.
ALTO®
Pharmaceuticals, Inc.
Tampa, Florida 33688
For Customer Service: 1-800-330-2891
Dist. U.S.A REV 3/11
Shown in Product Identification Guide, page 305

AwarenessLife/PureTrim

25 SOUTH ARIZONA PLACE, SUITE 320
CHANDLER, AZ 85225

Direct Inquiries to:
800-69AWARE
http://www.puretrim.net

LIQUID DAILY COMPLETE — DS

Description
Mediterranean Liquid Supplement. 243 Vitamins, Minerals & Special Nutrients which Provide Energy, Reduce Stress & Supports Healthy Joints*. Contains 100% RDA of key Vitamins and Minerals, and other Nutrients.

Ingredients
A Food-based Blend of Organic Mediterranean Super Seed Blend, Organic Fruit & Vegetable Whole Juice Complex, 100% RDA Of Essential Vitamins & Minerals, With Vitamins D3 & K1, Antioxidants With Resveratrol & Acai Berry, Whole Superfood Green Complex, Proprietary Ocean Blend With Pure Phytoplankton, Ionic Plant Minerals, 34 Mediterranean Herbal Ingredients, Essential Fatty Acid Complex, Vegetarian Wellness Formula

Directions
Take 1 ounce (2 tbsp) only once per day, during or immediately after a meal. Less than 4 calories per ounce, less than 1 gram of sugar.

Warnings
Do not use if Pregnant. Keep out of reach of children.

How Supplied
30 ounces per bottle.
Shown in Product Identification Guide, page 305

LIVERMASTER — DS

Cleanses and supports healthy liver, thyroid, and pancreas.

Mediterranean Ingredients
Vitamin E, Milk Thistle seed, Bless thistle, red beet root, chlorophyll, artichoke leaf extract, pycnogenol, black pepper, rosemary leaf, Eucommia leaf extract, cordyceps, and N-acety-L-Tyrosine with 12 organic vegetables

Directions
1 capsule with water right after your morning meal then take 1 capsule with water right after your evening meal. Take Liver Master for 90 days. You can do up to two 90 days cleanses a year.

Warnings
Do not use if Pregnant. Keep out of reach of children.

How Supplied
60 capsules per box
Shown in Product Identification Guide, page 305

PURETRIM MEDITERRANEAN TRUFFLES — DS

Description
Helps lipid fat binding in the body to promote weight loss. Comes in Sea Salt Caramel or Milk Chocolate flavors. Only 25 calories per Truffle, less than 1 gram of sugar. Helps to control cravings, naturally.

Ingredients
Organic Prickly-pear (Opuntia ficus-indica) [Fruit], Organic Pomegranate (Punica granatum) [Fruit], Organic Thyme (Thymus vulgaris) [Leaf], Organic Cinnamon (Cinnamomum aromaticum) [Bark], Organic Black Seed (Nigella sativa), Organic Milk Thistle (Silybum marianum) [Seed], Organic Olive (Olea europaea) [Leaf], Organic Artichoke (Cynara cardunculus), Organic Lemon Balm (Melissa officinalis) [Herb Top], Organic Sage (Salvia sclarea) [Leaves], Organic Fennel (Foeniculum vulgare) [Leaf], Organic Fenugreek (Trigonella foenum-graecum) [Seed]

Directions
As a dietary supplement, eat 1 Truffle with a FULL glass of water twice daily, any time you feel hungry or start to feel a craving coming on. Do not exceed 4 truffles a day.

Warnings
Do not use if under the age of 18. Do not use if you are pregnant or breastfeeding.

How Supplied
30 Truffles, individually wrapped.
Shown in Product Identification Guide, page 305

PURETRIM MEDITERRANEAN WELLNESS SHAKES — DS

Description
Natural, Vegetarian Weight Loss Shake, High Protein, Low Carbs, Less than 1 gram of Sugar. No Soy, No Whey, No Dairy, and No Aspartame. Less than 200 calories per shake.

Ingredients
21 Gram Protein Blend: NON-GMO Vegetable Pea, Organic Brown Rice, Organic Lentil, and Organic Flaxseed. Blend of Antioxidants, Prebiotics, 500mg of Plant Calcium, 8000mg of Essential Fatty Acids & 1100mg of Super Raw Greens Blend.

Directions
Mix contents of shake in 10-12 oz. of chilled water.
Have 2 shakes a day (one for breakfast & one for your evening meal.) Drink 2 glasses of water after you drink your shake for best results. Once weight loss is achieved, reduce to 1 shake a day for maintenance.

Warnings
Do not use if you are pregnant or nursing. Must be 18 years or older to use. Do not use as a replacement for more than two meals per day.

How Supplied
10 Packets (Net Weight 500g)
Shown in Product Identification Guide, page 305

J.R. Carlson Laboratories, Inc.

600 W. UNIVERSITY DRIVE
ARLINGTON HEIGHTS, IL 60004-1985

Direct Inquiries to:
Customer Service
(888) 234-5656
FAX: (847) 255-1605
www.carlsonlabs.com
For Medical Information Contact:
In Emergencies:
Technical Service
(888) 234-5656
FAX: (847) 255-1605

CARLSON® NORWEGIAN COD LIVER OIL — DS
Dietary Supplement

Carlson Cod Liver Oil comes from the livers of fresh cod fish found in the arctic ocean waters of Norway. The oil is separated from the liver tissues without the use of chemicals. To ensure the freshness of the oil, the air inside the bottle is replaced with nitrogen and natural-source vitamin E is added.

Supplement Facts
Serving Size 1 Teaspoonful (5 ml)

	Amount Per Teaspoonful	% DV
Calories	45	
Calories from Fat	45	
Total Fat	5 g	8% ☆
Saturated Fat	1 g	5% ☆
Cholesterol	20 mg	7%
Vitamin A	850 IU	17%
Vitamin D_3	400 IU	100%
Vitamin E (as d-alpha tocopheryl acetate, d-alpha tocopherol & mixed tocopherols)	10 IU	33%
Omega-3 Fatty Acids*	1,100 mg	†
DHA (Docosahexaenoic Acid)*	500 mg	†
EPA (Eicosapentaenoic Acid)*	400 mg	†
100% Norwegian Cod Liver Oil	4.6 g	†

☆ Percent Daily Values are based on a 2000 calorie diet.
† Daily Value (DV) not established.
* Reported as triglycerides.

Other ingredients: Natural lemon flavor.
Directions: Take one teaspoonful daily AT MEALTIME. After initially opening the bottle, keep refrigerated and preferably use within 100 days.
PURITY GUARANTEED
This product is regularly tested (using AOAC international protocols) for freshness, potency and purity by an independent, FDA-registered laboratory and has been determined to be fresh, fully-potent and free of detrimental levels of mercury, cadmium, lead, PCB's and 28 other contaminants. Manufactured and bottled in Norway for J.R. Carlson Laboratories, Inc.
Arlington Hts., IL 60004-1985 • 847-255-1600 • 888-234-5656 • www.carlsonlabs.com

SUPER DAILY D_3 LIQUID VITAMIN D — OTC
Dietary Supplement

1000 IU per drop
365 drops
0.37 fl. oz. (10.98 ml)

Supplement Facts
Serving Size: 1 drop (0.001 fl.oz./0.027 ml)

	Amount per drop	% Daily Value
Vitamin D_3 (cholecalciferol)	1,000 IU	250%
Vitamin E (d-alpha tocopherol)	1 IU	3%

Other Ingredients: Medium chain triglyceride oil (coconut and palm source).
Directions: Adults take 1 drop daily or as directed by your healthcare professional. May be put on food or mixed in other liquids such as water or juice.
Sugar-free. Corn-free. Wheat-free. Gluten-free. Natural color. Preservative-free.
Store bottle upright. Do not use if security seal is broken or missing. Keep out of reach of children.
Distributed by **Carlson Division of J.R. Carlson Laboratories, Inc.,** Arlington Hts., IL 60004-1985 888-234-5656 • 847-255-1600 • www.carlsonlabs.com
• An F.D.A. Regulated Facility •
1270-1e

CARLSON® SUPER OMEGA-3 GEMS® FISH OIL CONCENTRATE — DS
Dietary Supplement

Medical Scientists Internationally are encouraging people to eat more fish. Fish body oil is the **ONLY MAJOR SOURCE** of the polyunsaturated Omega-3's **EPA** and **DHA**.
For those individuals who do not eat an oily fish diet, Carlson offers Omega-3's in easy-to-swallow soft gelatin capsules. Carlson **SUPER OMEGA-3 GEMS®** soft gels contain 1000 mg (1 gram) of a special concentrate of fish body oils from deep, cold water fish which are especially rich in the important Omega-3's EPA and DHA.
To Promote Cardiovascular, Joint, Brain & Vision Health[1]

Supplement Facts	Serving Size 1 Soft Gel	
	Amount Per Soft Gel	% DV
Calories	10	
Calories from Fat	10	
Total Fat	1 g	2% ☆
Vitamin E Natural (d-Alpha Tocopherol)	10 IU	33%
Norwegian Fish Oil	1000 mg	†
Total Omega-3 Fatty Acids*	600 mg	
EPA (Eicosapentaenoic Acid)*	300 mg	†
DHA (Docosahexaenoic Acid)*	200 mg	†

☆ Percent Daily Values are based on a 2,000 calorie diet.
† Daily Value (DV) not established.
*Reported as ethyl ester.

Other Ingredients: Soft Gel Shell: Beef gelatin, glycerin, water. Contains fish (anchovy and sardine).

[1]**This statement has not been evaluated by the FDA. This product is not intended to diagnose, treat, cure or prevent any disease.**

Directions: Take one soft gel one to five times daily, AT MEALTIME.

PURITY GUARANTEED

This product is regularly tested (using AOAC international protocols) for potency and purity by an independent, FDA registered laboratory and found to be free of detrimental levels of mercury, cadmium, lead, PCB's and 28 other contaminants.

Preservative-free. Cholesterol-free. Gluten-free.

Distributed by Carlson Division of J.R. Carlson Laboratories, Inc., Arlington Heights, IL 60004-1985
888-234-5656 • www.carlsonlabs.com

Shown in Product Identification Guide, page 306

CPH International Corp.

P.O. BOX 11439
OAKLAND, CA 94611

Direct Inquiries:
cphintl@sbcglobal.net
Fax: (510) 352-6009

COROVASIN/CARDIBOSE/VERATROL-CV/RESTROGIN DS

DESCRIPTION

Trans-resveratrol, L-Arginine and Coenzyme Q10 may be recommended for maintaining healthy physiological performance of cardiomyocytes and coronary endothelial cells by increasing normal myocardial energetic efficiency and enhancing cardiac endothelial function.

INGREDIENTS

Trans-Resveratrol, L-Arginine, Coenzyme Q10, Thiamine Mononitrate & Magnesium Oxide.

RECOMMENDED INTAKE

Take one tablet twice daily with water for adults.

WARNINGS

Consult a physician prior to use if pregnant or lactating, or taking a prescription medication.

HOW SUPPLIED

Bottles of 30

*These statements have not been evaluated by the Food and Drug Administration. These products are not intended to diagnose, treat, cure or prevent any disease.

CYTO-SOD/CHELANIL/CARNISOD/PROBIX DS

DESCRIPTION

Natural antioxidant enzymes - SOD and catalase in combination with multiple minerals prepared in chelated forms are regarded as efficient against reactive oxygen species (ROS) for aged men and women to support a healthy metabolic performance.

INGREDIENTS

SOD, Catalase & Minerals.

RECOMMENDED INTAKE

Take one to two tablets daily with water for adults.

WARNINGS

Consult a physician prior to use if pregnant or lactating, or taking a prescription' medication.

HOW SUPPLIED

Bottles of 30

*These statements have not been evaluated by the Food and Drug Administration. These products are not intended to diagnose, treat, cure or prevent any disease.

MACUTEIN MEGA -30MG/OPTIGOLD/CATASOD-OCUXTRA/GLAUCOFIT/NEO-GPX/ERISTINOL DS

DESCRIPTION

Lutein, Zeaxanthin, antioxidant vitamins & trace elements are regarded as beneficial for keeping normal macular function and healthy eyes. The MCT contained in Mega-30mg may enhance the absorption of lutein and zeaxanthin in human intestinal lumen.

INGREDIENTS

Lutein/Zeaxanthin, Vitamins, Minerals & MCT (Mega-30mg tablets).

RECOMMENDED INTAKE

Take one to two tablets daily or one Mega-30mg tablet per day with water for adults.

WARNINGS

Consult a physician prior to use if pregnant or lactating, or taking a prescription medication.

HOW SUPPLIED

Bottles of 30

*These statements have not been evaluated by the Food and Drug Administration. These products are not intended to diagnose, treat, cure or prevent any disease.

NEUROFIT-MEGA/NEUTROPIN/WAXANER/NERVOX-HEXA/TIOWAX DS

DESCRIPTION

Alpha-lipoic acid is regarded as beneficial for maintaining normal nervous function due to its neuroprotective and antioxidant activities. Hexacosanol may be related to the augmentation of secretion of neurotropic factors including NGF, IGF and BDNF on nerve regeneration.

INGREDIENTS

Alpha-lipoic acid, Hexacosanol, Nucleotides & Vitamin B Complex.

RECOMMENDED INTAKE

Take one tablet/capsule twice daily with water for adults.

WARNINGS

Consult a physician prior to use if pregnant or lactating, or taking a prescription medication.

HOW SUPPLIED

Bottles of 30

*These statements have not been evaluated by the Food and Drug Administration. These products are not intended to diagnose, treat, cure or prevent any disease.

TOFIPAN/TOFIPAN-Z/FELAMON/MENOMON DS

DESCRIPTION

Natural dehydroepiandrosterone and vitex agnus-castus may be helpful for menopausal and peri-menopausal women to support healthy endocrinal system.

TOFIPAN-Z is formulated for aged men to maintain healthy and normal androgenic performance.

INGREDIENTS

Natural Dehydroepiandrosterone & Vitex agnus-castus.

RECOMMENDED INTAKE

Take one tablet/capsule twice daily with water for adults.

WARNINGS

Consult a physician prior to use if pregnant or lactating, or taking a prescription medication.

HOW SUPPLIED

Bottles of 30

*These statements have not been evaluated by the Food and Drug Administration. These products are not intended to diagnose, treat, cure or prevent any disease.

Immunotec Inc.

300 JOSEPH CARRIER
VAUDREUIL-DORION, QC
CANADA J7V 5V5

For Direct Inquiries Contact:
450-424-9992 Ext 4453

IMMUNOCAL® DS

Nutraceutical
Glutathione precursor (Bonded cysteine™ supplement)
Powder Sachets

DESCRIPTION and CLINICAL PHARMACOLOGY

IMMUNOCAL® is a U.S. patented natural food protein isolate in the FDA category of GRAS (generally recognized as safe) which assists the body in maintaining optimal concentrations of glutathione (GSH) by supplying the precursors required for intracellular glutathione synthesis. It is clinically proven to raise glutathione values.

Glutathione is a tripeptide made intracellularly from its constituent amino acids L-glutamate, L-cysteine and glycine. The sulfhydryl (thiol) group (SH) of cysteine is responsible for the biological activity of glutathione. Provision of this amino acid is the rate-limiting factor in glutathione synthesis by the cells since bioavailable cysteine is relatively rare in foodstuffs.

Immunocal® is a bovine whey protein isolate specially prepared so as to provide a rich source of bioavailable cysteine. Immunocal® can thus be viewed as a cysteine delivery system.

The disulphide bond in cystine is pepsin and trypsin resistant but may be split by heat, low pH or mechanical stress releasing free cysteine. When subject to heat or shearing forces (inherent in most extraction processes), the fragile disulfide bonds within the peptides are broken and the bioavailablility of cysteine is greatly diminished.

Glutathione is a tightly regulated intracellular constituent and is limited in its production by negative feedback inhibition of its own synthesis through the enzyme gamma-glutamylcysteine synthetase, thus greatly minimizing any possibility of overdosage.

Glutathione has multiple functions:

1. It is the major endogenous antioxidant produced by the cells, participating directly in the neutralization of free radicals and reactive oxygen compounds, as well as maintaining exogenous antioxidants such as vitamins C and E in their reduced (active) forms.
2. Through direct conjugation, it detoxifies many xenobiotics (foreign compounds) and carcinogens, both organic and inorganic.
3. It is essential for the immune system to exert its full potential, e.g. (1) modulating antigen presentation to lymphocytes, thereby influencing cytokine production and type of response (cellular or humoral) that develops, (2) enhancing proliferation of lymphocytes thereby increasing magnitude of response, (3) enhancing killing activity of cytotoxic T cells and NK cells, and (4) regulating apoptosis, thereby maintaining control of the immune response.
4. It plays a fundamental role in numerous metabolic and biochemical reactions such as DNA synthesis and repair, protein synthesis, prostaglandin synthesis, amino acid transport and enzyme activation. Thus, most systems in the body can be affected by the state of the glutathione system, especially the immune system, the nervous system, the gastrointestinal system and the lungs.

INDICATIONS AND USAGE

IMMUNOCAL® is a natural food supplement and as such is limited from stating medical claims per se. Statements have not been evaluated by the FDA. As such, this product is thus not intended to diagnose, cure, prevent or treat any disease.

Glutathione augmentation is a strategy developed to address states of glutathione deficiency, high oxidative stress, immune deficiency, and xenobiotic overload in which glutathione plays a part in the detoxification of the xenobiotic in question. Glutathione deficiency states include, but are not limited to: HIV/AIDS, infectious hepatitis, certain types of cancers, cataracts, Alzheimer's Disease, Parkinsons, chronic obstructive pulmonary disease, asthma, radiation, poisoning by acetominophen and related agents, malnutritive states, arduous physical stress, aging, and has

been associated with sub-optimal immune response. Many clinical pathologies are associated with oxidative stress and are elaborated upon in numerous medical references.
Low glutathione is also strongly implicated in wasting and negative nitrogen balance, notably as seen in cancer, AIDS, sepsis, trauma, burns and even athletic overtraining. Cysteine supplementation can oppose this process and in AIDS, for example, result in improved survival rates.

CONTRAINDICATIONS

IMMUNOCAL® is contraindicated in individuals who develop or have known hypersensitivity to specific milk proteins.

PRECAUTIONS

Each sachet of IMMUNOCAL® contains nine grams of protein. Patients on a protein-restricted diet need to take this into account when calculating their daily protein load. Although a bovine milk derivative, IMMUNOCAL® contains less than 1% lactose and therefore is generally well tolerated by lactose-intolerant individuals.

WARNINGS

Patients undergoing immunosuppressive therapy should discuss the use of this product with their health professional. Individuals with the autosomal-recessive metabolic disorder cystinuria, are at higher risk of developing cysteine nephrolithiasis (1–2% of renal calculi).

ADVERSE REACTIONS

Gastrointestinal bloating and cramps if not sufficiently rehydrated. Transient urticarial-like rash in rare individuals undergoing severe detoxification reaction. Rash abates when product intake stopped or reduced.

OVERDOSAGE

Overdosing on IMMUNOCAL® has not been reported.

DOSAGE AND ADMINISTRATION

For mild to moderate health challenges, 20 grams per day is recommended. Clinical trials in patients with AIDS, COPD, cancer and chronic fatigue syndrome have used 30–40 grams per day without ill effect. IMMUNOCAL® is best administered on an empty stomach or with a light meal. Concomitant intake of another high protein load may adversely affect absorption.

RECONSTITUTION

IMMUNOCAL® is a dehydrated powdered protein isolate. It must be appropriately rehydrated before use. Ideally consumed after mixing. If it is premixed for later consumption, it should be refrigerated and consumed shortly after mixing. DO NOT heat or use a hot liquid to rehydrate the product. DO NOT use a high-speed blender for reconstitution. These methods will decrease the activity of the product.
Proper mixing is imperative. Consult instructions included in packaging.

HOW SUPPLIED

10 grams of bovine milk protein isolate powder per sachet. 30 sachets per box.

STORAGE

Store in a cool dry environment. Refrigeration is not necessary.
Patent no.'s: 5,230,902 - 5,290,571 - 5,456,924 - 5,451,412 - 5,888,552

REFERENCES

1. Baruchel S, Viau G, Olivier R. et al. Nutraceutical modulation of glutathione with a humanized native milk serum protein isolate, Immunocal®: application in AIDS and cancer. *In*: Oxidative Stress in Cancer, AIDS and Neurodegenerative Diseases. Ed.; Montagnier L, Olivier R, Pasquier C. Marcel Dekker Inc. New York, 447–461, 1998
2. Bounous G, Kongshavn P. Influence of protein type in nutritionally adequate diets on the development of immunity. *In* Absorption and Utilization of Amino Acids Vol.II. Ed. M. Friedman. CRC Press, Inc., Fla. 2:219–32, 1989
3. Bounous G, Gold P. The biological activity of undenatured whey proteins: role of glutathione. Clin Invest Med 14:296–309, 1991
4. Bounous G, Baruchel S, Falutz J. Gold P. Whey proteins as a food supplement in HIV-seropositive individuals. Clin Invest Med. 16:3; 204–209, 1992
5. Bounous G. Whey protein concentrate (WPC) and glutathione modulation in cancer treatment. Anticancer Res. 20:4785–4792, 2000
6. Bounous G. Immunoenhancing properties of undenatured milk serum protein isolate in HIV patients. Int. Dairy Fed: Whey: 293–305, 1998
7. Bray T, Taylor C. Enhancement of tissue glutathione for antioxidant and immune functions in malnutrition. Biochem. Pharmacol. 47:2113–2123, 1994.
8. Droge W, Holm E. Role of cysteine and glutathione in HIV infection and other diseases associated with muscle wasting and immunological dysfunction. FASEB J: 11(13):1077–1089, 1997
9. Herzenberg LA, De Rosa SC, Dubs JG et al. Glutathione deficiency is associated with impaired survival in HIV disease. Proc Natl Acad Sci 94:1967–72, 1997
10. Kennedy R, Konok G, Bounous G et al.. The use of a whey protein concentrate in the treatment of patients with metastatic carcinoma: A phase 1-II clinical study. Anticancer Res. 15:2643–50, 1995
11. Lands LC, Grey VL, Smountas AA. Effect of supplementation with a cysteine donor on muscular performance. J. Appl. Physiol. 87:1381–1385, 1999
12. Locigno R, Castronovo V. Reduced glutathione System: Role in cancer development, prevention and treatment. International Journal of Oncology 19:221–236, 2001
13. Lomaestro B, Malone M. Glutathione in health and disease: pharmacotherapeutic issues. Ann Pharmacother 29: 1263–73, 1995
14. Lothian B, Grey V, Kimoff RJ, Lands. Treatment of obstructive airway disease with a cysteine donor protein supplement: a case report. Chest 117:914–916, 2000
15. Meister A. Glutathione. Ann Rev Biochem 52:711–60, 1983
16. Peterson JD, Herzenberg LA, Vasquez KK, Waltenbaugh C. Glutathione levels in antigen-presenting cells modulate Th1 versus Th2 response patterns. Proc. Natl. Acad. Sci. 95:3071–3076, 1998
17. Tozer RG, Tai P, Falconer W, Ducruet T, Karabadjian A, Bounous G, Molson J, Dröge W. Cysteine-rich protein reverses weight loss in lung cancer patients receiving chemotherapy or radiotherapy. Antioxidants & redox signalling. 10: 395–402, 2008.
18. Watanabe A, Higachi K, Yasumura S. et al. Nutritional modulation of glutathione level and cellular immunity in chronic hepatitis B and C. Hepatology. 24:597A, 1996
19. Witschi A, Reddy S, Stofer B, Lauterberg B. The systemic availability of oral glutathione. Eur. J. Clin. Pharmacol. 43:667–669, 1992.

Manufactured by Immunotec Inc.
Tel: 450-424-9992 Ext. 4453
www.immunocal.com

Legacy for Life, LLC

P.O. BOX 14510
OKLAHOMA CITY, OK 73113

Direct Inquiries to:
1-800-557-8477
info@legacyforlife.net
www.LegacyforLife.com

i26® DS

Dietary Supplement
Hyperimmune Egg (HIE) Powder

DESCRIPTION

i26 ("polyvalent hyperimmune" egg) is hyperimmunized whole egg protein("HIE").1 Along with the generation of specific antibodies, increased levels of bioactive molecules are produced.2,3 In vitro, in vivo, and human trials, suggest that the naturally-occurring immune components in hyperimmune egg are utilized by the body to help it achieve immune homeostasis. The biological factors in i26 help the body maintain immune homeostasis by partnering to help it modulate immunological responses, especially those of an autoimmune or inflammatory nature.

BACKGROUND

Upon oral administration of hyperimmune egg, a wide range of immune components, both of a specific and nonspecific nature, are passively transferred to the recipient. Although the intact immunoglobulins are confined to the lumen, other smaller, bioactive immune components may work systemically. This may occur: a) indirectly by activating cells in the GALT which then migrate with the appropriate message, or b) by directly crossing the GI barrier and circulating throughout the body to help it appropriately modulate immunological reactions.
Studies:
Joint Comfort and Flexibilty
An open-label clinical trial conducted at The Hospital for Special Surgery in New York, NYC, demonstrated that the daily consumption of 4.5g of HIE resulted in statistically significant changes in the daily aches and discomfort associated with daily life.4 Combining hyperimmune egg with certain forms of glucosamine-HCl results in a synergistic joint support effect.5
Circulatory and Cardiovascular Health
Hyperimmune egg has been demonstrated to help the body control several key indices of cardiovascular health both in vivo, and in a double-blind, placebo-controlled human trial.6,7
Gastrointestinal Health
In vivo, pre-administration of hyperimmune egg significantly helps the body support healthy digestive function8 and intestinal transit.9 It also appears to help maintain overall health of the gastrointestinal lining.10
Maintaining Healthy Weight in Populations At Risk
Hyperimmune egg helps maintain or increase lean muscle mass in individuals experiencing involuntary weight changes.11,12
Quality of Life
Subjects with poor quality of life, that consumed consuming 6.0g of hyperimmune egg showed marked changes in energy, weight, appetite, sleep quality, gastrointestinal and pulmonary areas as well as blood counts.11-13
Enhanced Athletic Performance, Stamina, Recovery
In a randomized, double-blind, placebo-controlled university trial, subjects utilizing 13.5g daily of hyperimmune egg experienced greater athletic performance as measured by endurance, recovery and strength. Hyperimmune egg appeared to help the body lower intrinsic heart rates, and stimulate muscle growth and repair resulting in better performance. Subjects reported higher levels of both anaerobic and aerobic performance, with less effort when using hyperimmune egg.14,15 Professional athletes report similar findings.

INDICATIONS AND USAGE

i26 is defined under the Dietary Supplements Health and Education Act (DSHEA) as a dietary supplement and as such is not intended to diagnose, prevent, treat, or cure disease. An independent panel of experts has conferred self-affirmed GRAS ("generally recognized as safe") status to hyperimmune egg. The FDA has issued a Food Master File Number for this ingredient.
Statements as to function have not been evaluated by the Food and Drug Administration but the following structure function claims for i26 have been submitted to the Agency:
Balances and supports the immune system
Helps the body maintain:
- digestive tract health
- flexible and healthy joints
- healthy levels of cholesterol
- cardiovascular function and healthy circulatory systems

Helps increase energy levels
Helps enhance a sense of well-being
Note: "Hyperimmune" egg may be used concomitantly with prescription medications.

CONTRAINDICATION

"Hyperimmune" egg is contraindicated in individuals with a history of extreme hypersensitivity, or life-threatening allergy, to orally administered egg.

PRECAUTIONS

Although reactions are rare, it is prudent for individuals with "sensitive" digestive systems to introduce hyperimmune gradually. Start with 0.5g (1/8 of a scoop) of i26/day for 3-4 days successively and double the amount every few days until desired dosage is achieved. Diabetics may wish to monitor their blood glucose levels more frequently while introducing hyperimmune egg into their diets, since some individuals appear to reach glucose homeostasis rapidly as they start to approach immune homeostasis.

ADVERSE REACTIONS

Adverse reactions rarely occur. In two randomized double-blind, placebo-controlled trials (one with the US Military, the other at a University) the hyperimmune egg was well tolerated.
There was 82% compliance in a US Military study and 100% compliance in the University study.

ADMINISTRATION

Recommended servings are 4.5g-9g/daily for maintenance, more as desired. Some of the larger bioactive immune components in hyperimmune egg are heat-labile, but other than high temperature foods or beverages, HIE can be added to almost all foods or beverages (e.g., puddings, yogurts, salads, juices, ice cream, etc.)
The equivalent of one serving (4.5g) of hyperimmune egg is found in: one scoop of i26, 9 capsules, 3 Chewables, 1 scoop of i26 COMPLETE Support, or 2 scoops of i26 FIT.

HOW SUPPLIED

- i26 - pure hyperimmune egg powder (31 servings)
- i26 Capsules – pure hyperimmune egg in capsules (15 servings)
- i26 Chewables- hyperimmune egg in flavored tablets (vanilla, banana) (15 servings)
- i26 COMPLETE Support – hyperimmune egg with vitamins and minerals (chocolate, strawberry, vanilla) (31 servings) [to be reconstituted with liquid]

◦ i26 FIT – hyperimmune egg with protein, fiber, vitamins and minerals (15 servings)
[to be reconstituted with liquid, preferably skim milk]
Stability and Storage
Store in a dry cool location with the lid tightly shut.

REFERENCES

Hens are stimulated multiple times with more than 26 whole inactivated bacteria of human interest including Salmonella, Staphylococcus, Streptococcus, Escherichia coli, Klebsiella pneumoniae, Pseudomonas, Proteus, Propionibacterium acnes, and Hemophilus influenzae.
US Patent # 6,420,337 Highly purified cytokine activating factor and methods of use
US Patent # 7,083,809 Purified cytokine inhibitory factor
Greenblatt HC Adalsteinsson O & L Kagen, Administration to Arthritis Patients of a Dietary Supplement Containing Immune Egg: An Open-Label Pilot Study, 1998 J Med Food 1:171
US Patent # 6,706,267 Glucosamine and egg for reducing inflammation
Wilborn WH Effect of Immune Egg Protein on Serum Cholesterol in Rabbits on Atherogenic Diets 1997 unpublished
Karge WH et al. Pilot Study on the effect of Hyperimmune Egg Protein on Elevated Cholesterol Levels and Cardiovascular Risk Factors 1999 J Med Food 2:51
Jacoby, HI Moore G and G Wnorowski Inhibition of Diarrhea by Immune Egg: A Castor Oil Mouse Model J Nutr Funct 2001 Med Foods 3:47
US Patent # 6,803,035 Anti-diarrheal and method for using the same
US Patent # 5,772,999 Method of Preventing, Countering or Reducing NSAID-Induced Gastrointestinal Damage by Administering Milk or Egg Products from Hyperimmunized Animals
Ambekar R Chungi V Hyperimmune Egg: Its Ability to Maintain Weight and Lean Muscle Mass in Individuals with Cachexia 1998 unpublished
Okullo J An Assessment of Effectiveness and Acceptability of immune26 in the Management of the Sick in Uganda 2002 unpublished
Kizito FB Improvements in Quality of Life for HIV/AIDS Patients Using Hyperimmune Egg (Immune 26™) — The TASO Study 3rd Inter AIDS Soc Conf HIV Pathogenesis and Treatment 2005 Abstract No. MoPe11.2C43
Scheett TM, et al. Hyperimmune Egg Protein Decreases Submaximal Heart Rate and Increases Peak Power 2007 Med Sci Sports Med Exerc 39:S365
Scheett TM, et al. Increased Muscular Strength and Enhanced Muscle Repair with Hyperimmune Egg Protein Supplementation 2007 National Strength Cond Assoc Atlanta, GA

Legacy for Life, LLC
P.O. Box 14510
Oklahoma City, OK 73113
Direct Inquiries to:
1-800-557-8477
info@legacyforlife.net
www.LegacyforLife.com

Shown in Product Identification Guide, page 307

NSE Products, Inc. (Pharmanex)

75 WEST CENTER STREET
PROVO, UT 84601

For Information and Product Support:
Phone: 1-800-487-1000
Website: www.nuskin.com

ageLOC R^2 — DS

Description

ageLOC® R^2 is delivered as alternating Day and Night formulas to help balance two interconnected aspects of youthfulness. ageLOC R^2 Day resets youthful gene expression related to cellular energy production while ageLOC R^2 Night resets youthful gene expression related to cellular purification. Together, ageLOC R^2 targets aging at its source to promote physical vigor, mental acuity, and sexual health, as well as to support the body's ability to neutralize and remove cellular waste and metabolic byproducts.

Benefits

ageLOC R^2 Day and Night were developed to address cellular energy production (primarily mitochondrial functions) and cellular purification mechanisms. The cellular mechanisms of energy production and cellular purification are mutually supporting. ageLOC R^2 Day and Night work synergistically by targeting both mechanisms of cellular energy production and mechanisms of cellular purification.

Ingredients

Each ageLOC R^2 Day capsule provides 378 mg of a proprietary blend of Cordyceps Cs-4 Mushroom Mycelia (*Cordyceps sinensis* [Berk.] Sacc.), Pomegranate (*Punica granatum*) Fruit Extract, and Pharmanex Asian Ginseng Rb1 (*Panax ginseng*) Root Extract. Each ageLOC R^2 Night capsule provides 225 mg of a proprietary blend of Grape (*Vitis vinifera L.*) Seed Extract, Red Orange (*Citrus sinensis*) Fruit Extract, and Broccoli (*Brassica oleracea italica*) Seed Extract.

Recommended Use

Take six (6) ageLOC R^2 Day capsules in the morning, and take two (2) ageLOC R^2 Night capsules in the evening. May be taken with or without meals.

Warnings

Keep this product out of reach of children. Consult a physician prior to use if pregnant or lactating, or taking a prescription medication. Discontinue use of this product 2 weeks prior to and after surgery. Discontinue use and consult a physician if any adverse reactions occur. May contain soy and/or peanuts.

How Supplied

One box of ageLOC R^2 delivers 180 capsules of ageLOC R^2 Day, and 60 capsules of ageLOC R^2 Night, providing a 30 day supply of each.

CORDYMAX® CS-4® — DS

Description

CordyMax® Cs-4® is a dietary supplement used to reduce symptoms of fatigue and to promote vitality and overall well-being.* It is an exclusive fermentation product derived from the renowned *Cordyceps sinensis* mushroom.

Benefits

Numerous scientific studies suggest that CordyMax Cs-4 may promote natural vitality and reduce fatigue.* Cordyceps has been shown in third party research to reduce oxidative stress by scavenging oxygen free radicals in mitochondria, promote efficient utilization of oxygen, elevate energy states (ΔTP) in organs, redistribute blood flow to essential organs, improve liver and kidney functions through metabolizing and excreting toxic substances, and provide a positive benefit for sexual health.*
CordyMax Cs-4, also known as Jin Shui Bao in Chinese, is a cultivated strain of the principle Cordyceps fungal mycelia developed to provide similar benefits delivered by the wild mushroom. It has been profiled extensively by chemical and pharmacological methods. Cs-4 closely mimics the wild mushroom in the temperatures used during fermentation, the similarity of its outward appearance when allowed to grow to maturity, the similarity of its chemical components, and in its beneficial actions as an herbal supplement. Studies have shown that Cs-4® has, in some instances, proven more effective than the wild form.

Ingredients

Each capsule contains 525 mg *Cordyceps sinensis* (Berk.) Sacc. Mycelia (*Paecilomyces hepialid* Chen, Cs-4), standardized 0.14% adenosine and 6% mannitol.

Recommended Use

Take 2 capsules bid or tid with water and food.

Warnings

Keep out of reach of children. Consult a physician prior to use if pregnant or lactating, or using prescription medication. Discontinue use of this product 2 weeks prior to and after surgery. Discontinue use and consult a physician if any adverse reactions occur. May contain soy and/or peanuts.

How Supplied

20-30 day supply, 120 count bottle.

Research using Pharmanex CordyMax Cs-4

CordyMax Cs-4 has been used as the source of Cordyceps in over 11 published studies. Contact Nu Skin for a list of references of studies which have used Pharmanex CordyMax Cs-4.

LIFEPAK® ANTI-AGING FORMULA — DS

Description

LifePak® is a comprehensive nutritional wellness program, delivering the optimum types and amounts of vitamins, minerals, trace elements, antioxidants, and phytonutrients for general health and well-being. LifePak addresses all common nutrient deficiencies, and provides key anti-aging nutrients that promote cellular protection. Additionally, it supports cardiovascular health, bone nutrition, nutrient metabolism, and normal immune function.*

Benefits

Addresses common nutrient deficiencies: LifePak was formulated in consideration of typical dietary intakes, and when consumed with a typical diet ensures meeting the RDAs for all vitamins and minerals.
Provides ingredients that promote cellular protection: LifePak, with its broad spectrum of vitamins and phytonutrients, is optimally formulated to provide comprehensive protection of cellular and mitochondrial DNA as well as the body's lipids and proteins.
Supports cardiovascular health: LifePak addresses many aspects of cardiovascular health by offering the recommended amounts of key cardiovascular nutrients, including vitamin E, vitamin C, carotenoids, flavonoids, B vitamins, magnesium, and calcium.
Supports bone nutrition: LifePak addresses bone health with a comprehensive array of bone nutrients, including nutritionally significant amounts of calcium, magnesium, and vitamin D.
Supports nutrient metabolism: LifePak provides nutritionally meaningful amounts of vitamins and minerals that promote normal glucose metabolism and insulin function, including chromium, zinc, and antioxidants.
Supports normal immune function: LifePak provides nutritionally significant amounts of vitamins A, C, E, and B_6, zinc and selenium. Since the immune system depends on adequate nutritional status of these nutrients, it is expected that LifePak effectively promotes healthy immune function in multiple ways. Deficiency of single nutrients results in altered immune responses, which can be observed even when the deficiency state is relatively mild.
Protects cells with a powerful antioxidant network: LifePak contains more than 40 antioxidants for cell health, including both water- and fat-soluble antioxidants. As part of this antioxidant support, LifePak provides a balanced carotenoid combination in amounts similar to those provided by diets high in fruits and vegetables.
Pharmanex BioPhotonic Scanner:
The BioPhotonic Scanner program may be used in conjunction with LifePak usage. Nu Skin has licensed a scientifically validated method to non-invasively measure the levels of carotenoids present in the skin. These fat-soluble carotenoids have been shown in third party literature to be a reliable indicator of overall antioxidant status. The BioPhotonic Scanner can be used to track overall antioxidant status over time as well as track the effect of LifePak on an individual's skin carotenoid status.

Ingredients

LifePak provides an optimal blend of vitamins, minerals, trace elements, antioxidants, and phytonutrients.
Each LifePak packet contains 1 vitamin capsule, two mineral capsules, and 1 phytonutrient capsule, together providing1250 IU Vitamin A, 6250 IU Beta Carotene, 200 mg Vitamin C, 200 IU Vitamin D, 75 IU Vitamin E, 20 mcg Vitamin K, 3.75 mg Thiamin, 4.25 mg Riboflavin, 17.5 mg Niacin, 5 mg Vitamin B6, 300 mcg Folate, 15 mcg Vitamin B12, 75 mcg Biotin, 15 mg Pantothenic acid, 250 mg Calcium, 50 mcg Iodine, 125 mg Magnesium, 7.5 mg Zinc, 70 mcg Selenium, 0.5 mg Copper, 1 mg Manganese, 100 mcg Chromium, 37.5 mcg Molybdenum, 45 mg Catechins (from green tea), 25 mg Quercetin, 12.5 mg Grape Seed Extract, 12.5 mg Citrus Bioflavonoids, 2.5 mg Resveratrol, 37.5 mg Gamma Tocopherol, 16 mg Beta- and Delta-Tocopherols, 15 mg Alpha-Lipoic Acid, 5 mg Inositol, 2.5 mg Lycopene, 1 mg Alpha Carotene, 1 mg Lutein, 1.5 mg Boron, and 10 mcg Vanadium.

Recommended Use

Take 1 packet bid with water and food.

Warnings

Keep this product out of reach of children. Consult a physician prior to use if pregnant or lactating, or taking a prescription medication. Discontinue use of this product 2 weeks prior to and after surgery. Discontinue use and consult a physician if any adverse reactions occur.

How Supplied

60 individual packets, 30 day supply. Additional LifePak® products include: LifePak® Nano, LifePak Prime, LifePak Women, LifePak Prenatal, LifePak Teen, and Jungamals.

Research using Pharmanex LifePak

LifePak has been used in over 13 published studies. Contact Nu Skin for a list of references of studies which have used Pharmanex LifePak.

MARINEOMEGA DS

Description

MarineOmega is a blend of ultra-pure oils from anchovies and krill; both a source of EPA, DHA and other omega-3 fatty acids. Vitamin E is included to protect important fatty acids against oxidation. Oil derived from wild-caught anchovies delivers omega-3 fatty acids in triglyceride form, and both oils are tested free of harmful levels of toxins PCB's and heavy metals.

Euphasia superba, commonly known as krill, are small shrimp-like crustaceans. Krill oil is rich in EPA and DHA in a unique phospholipid form targeted for use in the brain and in cell membranes throughout the body. Krill oil also contains a unique flavonoid (yet unnamed) and the carotenoid antioxidant astaxanthin.

MarineOmega is delivered in vanilla-infused softgels.

Benefits

Balanced essential fatty acid nutrition is important for normal immune function, cardiovascular health, joint mobility, brain function, and skin health.*

Krill oil provides phospholipids high in EPA and DHA and offers a high ratio of omega-3 to omega-6 fatty acids (15:1) to help compensate for modern diets which significantly favor the omega-6 type.

Phospholipids are an essential component of cell membranes in every cell of the body. They are essential for all vital cell processes and are indispensable nutrients for proper brain function. Krill oil naturally contains 40% phospholipids, while most fish oil sources do not provide any phospholipids.

Ingredients

Each softgel capsule contains 1,100 mg of Marine Lipid Concentrate (150 mg of EPA, 100 mg DHA, and 50 mg of other Omega-3 Fatty Acids), 50 mg of krill oil, and 5 IU of Vitamin E (as Natural Mixed Tocopherols).

Recommended Use

Take 2 softgel capsules bid with water and food.

Warnings

Keep this product out of reach of children. Consult a physician if pregnant or lactating, taking anticoagulants, or taking any other prescription medication. Discontinue use of this product 2 weeks prior to and after surgery. Discontinue use and consult a physician if any adverse reactions occur. Contains shellfish.

How Supplied

30 day supply, 120 count bottle.

REISHIMAX GLp® DS

Description

ReishiMax GLp® is a proprietary, standardized extract of reishi (*Ganoderma lucidum*) mushroom. This standardized product also incorporates cracked spores, a novel technology that releases reishi's active ingredient, providing unique immune activity.*

ReishiMax is produced through solid wood log cultivation. This method is preferred to sawdust and liquid cultivation because it yields both polysaccharides and triterpenes from the fruiting body and is less prone to contamination and quality control issues than other methods.

Reishi spores are minute reproductive cells that are released by the mushroom at maturity. The spores are protected by an extremely hard shell, which prevents the polysaccharides and triterpenes contained in the spore from being absorbed. Pharmanex uses technology which mechanically 'cracks' the spores, making the active ingredients bioavailable.

Benefits

ReishiMax has been demonstrated to support healthy immune system function by stimulating cell-mediated immunity. According to the results of animal and *in vitro* studies, ReishiMax has been demonstrated to stimulate the formation of antibodies, stimulate the proliferation of immune cells, and modulate the functions of T cells. ReishiMax is intended for adults who wish to maintain a healthy immune system.*

In addition to animal and *in vitro* studies conducted with ReishiMax, third party clinical studies have established the ability of reishi mushroom to support immune function in humans.*

Ingredients

Each capsule contains 495 mg of standardized reishi mushroom extract and 5 mg of reishi cracked spores and is standardized to 6% triterpenes and 13.5% polysaccharides.

Warnings

Keep out of reach of children. If you are pregnant or nursing, or taking a prescription medication, including immunosuppressive therapies, consult a physician before using this product. Discontinue use of this product 2 weeks prior to and after surgery. Discontinue use and consult a physician if any adverse reactions occur.

Recommended Use

Take 1-2 capsules bid with water and food.

How Supplied

15-30 day supply, 60 count bottle.

Research using Pharmanex ReishiMax Glp

ReishiMax has been used as the source of reishi mushroom in over 29 published studies. Contact Nu Skin for a list of references of studies which have used Pharmanex ReishiMax Glp.

TEGREEN 97 DS

Description

Tegreen® is a standardized, decaffeinated polyphenol extract of fresh green tea leaves, with proven free radical scavenging and antioxidant properties.*

Benefits

Studies have demonstrated that the polyphenols in green tea, particularly the catechin component, offer potent antioxidant activity through the scavenging of free radicals. More specifically, numerous experiments and studies indicate that green tea polyphenols, especially EGCg, may help block the formation of some potentially toxic compounds such as nitrosamines, suppress the activation of free radicals, detoxify or trap free radicals, inhibit spontaneous and photo-enhanced lipid peroxidation, and increase the activity of natural antioxidants and detoxifying enzymes (e.g., glutathione peroxidase and catalase).*

Antioxidant supplementation may also offer some protective benefits to the skin from free radical damage and the effects of ultraviolet rays. Among the polyphenols that are antioxidants in green tea, EGCg and ECG show the strongest effect in reducing collagenase activity—an enzyme that breaks down collagen.*

Additional third party research shows that green tea supplementation may help improve lipid and glucose metabolism, maintain normal insulin sensitivity, and support a healthy metabolic rate.*

Ingredients

Each capsule contains 250 mg of extract of green tea leaves (*Camellia sinensis*) standardized to a minimum 97% pure polyphenols including 162 mg catechins, of which 95 mg is EGCg.

Recommended Use

Take 1-2 capsules bid with water and food. Maximum recommended dose of 4 capsules daily (1,000 mg). Do not exceed 1,200 mg green tea extract in combination with other green tea-containing supplements.

Warnings

Keep out of reach of children. Consult a physician prior to use if pregnant or lactating, taking anticoagulants, or taking any other prescription medications. Discontinue use of this product 2 weeks prior to and after surgery. Discontinue use and consult a physician if any adverse reactions occur.

How Supplied

30-day supply, 30 and 120 count bottles.

Research using Pharmanex Tegreen 97

Tegreen 97 has been used as the source of green tea in over 13 published studies. Contact Nu Skin for a list of references of studies which have used Pharmanex Tegreen 97.

* These statements have not been evaluated by the Food and Drug Administration. This product is not intended to diagnose, treat, cure or prevent any disease.

Perque Integrative Health

44621 GUILFORD DRIVE, SUITE 150
ASHBURN, VA 20147

Telephone:
1-(800)-525-7372

PERQUE LIFE GUARD™ DS

Tabsules

40 Essential Nutrients Protects Heart, Body, and Brain
Full Disclosure Label
(no hidden or inactive ingredients)

Directions: As a dietary supplement, take two (2) tabsules with meals or as directed by your health professional. ***Best if taken with meals.*** Alternative daily doses as follows:

Low stress, healthy	1-2 tabsules/day
Moderate stress, unwell	3-4 tabsules/day
High stress, training	5-6 tabsules/day

SUPPLEMENT FACTS
Serving size: 2 Tabsules
Servings per container: 90

Energized Nutrients	Amount per serving	% Daily Value
Vitamins:		
Vitamin A (beta-carotene)	5,000 IU	100
Vitamin B-1 (thiamine HCl)	100 mg.	6,666
Vitamin B-2 (riboflavin 40 mg: riboflavin 5'-phosphate, 10 mg)	50 mg.	2,941
Vitamin B-3 (niacin)	25 mg.	125
Vitamin B-3 (niacinamide)	75 mg.	375
Vitamin B-5 (calcium d-pantothenate)	100 mg.	1,000
Vitamin B-6 (pyridoxine HCl, 160 mg. pyridoxol 5'-phosphate, 40 mg	200 mg.	10,000
Vitamin B-12 (hydroxocobalamin)	200 mcg	3,333
Folinate (as calcium folinate)	200 mcg	100
(6S)-5-Methyltetrahydrofolate (as Quatrefolic™)	200 mcg	
PABA (para-aminobenzoic acid)	30 mg.	*
Biotin (pure crystalline)	500 mcg	166
Vitamin C (100% l-ascorbate, fully reduced, corn free)	150 mg.	250
Vitamin D-3 (cholecalciferol)	400 IU	100
Vitamins E (from mixed natural tocopherols)	200 IU	667
Vitamin K-1 (phylloquinone)	500 mcg	625
Elemental Minerals:		
Potassium (as citrate)	99 mg.	3
Calcium (as ascorbate, pantothenate, citrate, fumarate, malate and succinate)	50 mg.	5
Magnesium (as C16 and C18 alkyls†)	100 mg.	25
Zinc (as picolinate)	25 mg.	167
Boron (as ascorbate)	2 mg	*
Chromium (as picolinate 50%, ascorbate 50%)	200 mcg	167
Manganese (as ascorbate)	15 mg.	750
Molybdenum (as ascorbate)	100 mcg	133
Selenium (as I-selenomethionine)	50 mcg	71
Vanadium (as ascorbate)	100 mcg	*
Active Cofactors:		
Quercetin dihydrate (water-soluble bioflavonoid)	100 mg.	*
L-aspartic acid (magnesium aspartate)	50 mg.	*
Trimethylglycine (betaine HCl)	50 mg.	*
Tocotrienols:		
Triacontanol (polycosonol)	774 mcg	*
Hexacosanol (polycosonol)	33 mcg	*
Tetracosanol (polycosonol)	193 mcg	*
Octacosanol (polycosonol)	500 mcg	*
Citrate	59 mg.	*
Fumarate	59 mg.	*
Malate	59 mg.	*
Succinate	59 mg.	*
Vegetable fiber (organic croscarmellose)	170 mg.	*
Natural Vanilla	100 mg.	*

†from whole, untreated palm fruit and leaf

*Daily value not established by FDA

OTHER INGREDIENTS: None

KEEP OUT OF REACH OF CHILDREN. Must be stored with cap on tightly in a cool, dry place . Do not use product if the tamper-resist shrink band around the cap or the inner seal beneath the cap appears to have been tampered with or is missing.

WARNING: Pregnant and nursing mothers need to check with their health professional before taking supplements.
How Supplied: 180 Count
Patents Pending
Researched, uniquely formulated,
& exclusively distributed by:
PERQUE Integrative Health, USA
These statements have not been evaluated by the Food and Drug Administration. This product is not intended to diagnose, treat, cure, or prevent any disease.

PERQUE POTENT C GUARD™ DS
Buffered Ascorbate Powder

Enhances Cell Energy and Helps Reduce Oxidative Stress
Full Disclosure Label
(no hidden or inactive ingredients)
Directions: Take one (1) rounded half-teaspoon mixed with two (2) to four (4) ounces of liquid or as directed by your health professional. Use only dry transfer spoons to remove powder from bottle. Keep tightly capped and moisture free. Please take a few deep, relaxing breaths while the natural effervescence subsides (~1 min.). May be kept on the counter, in refrigerator or freezer to maintain dryness.

SUPPLEMENT FACTS
Serving Size: 1 Rounded Half-Teaspoon
Servings per container: 287

Energized Nutrients	Amount per serving	% Daily Value
Vitamin C (as 100% l-ascorbates, fully reduced and buffered)	1,584 mg.	2,640
Potassium (as ascorbate)	99 mg.	3
Calcium (as ascorbate)	40 mg.	5
Magnesium (as ascorbate)	16 mg.	4
Zinc (as ascorbate)	600 mcg	4

Other Ingredients: None
3/13
KEEP OUT OF REACH OF CHILDREN. Must be stored with cap on tightly in a cool, dry place. Do not use product if the tamper-resist shrink band around the cap or the inner seal beneath the cap appears to have been tampered with or is missing.
WARNING: Pregnant and nursing mothers need to check with their health professional before taking supplements.
How Supplied: 16 oz./454 grams net weight
Patents Pending
Researched, uniquely formulated,
& exclusively distributed by:
PERQUE Integrative Health, USA
These statements have not been evaluated by the Food and Drug Administration. This product is not intended to diagnose, treat, cure, or prevent any disease.

PERQUE REPAIR GUARD™ DS
Tabsules

Eases Oxidative Stress, Pain, and Inflammation
Full Disclosure Label
(no hidden or inactive ingredients)
Directions:
Mild condition: 1 tabsule daily
Moderate condition: 2-4 tabsules daily
Severe condition: 4-12 tabsules daily

SUPPLEMENT FACTS
Serving size:1 Tabsule
Servings per container: 180

Energized Nutrients	Amount per serving	% Daily Value
Quercetin dihydrate (water-soluble bioflavonoid)	1,000 mg.	*
Pomegranate juice powder (high ORAC)	60 mg.	*
OPC (soluble LMW ActiVin®1294™)	10 mg.	*
Magnesium (as c16 and C18 alkyls from whole, untreated palm fruit and leaf)	35 mg.	*
Vegetable fiber (organic croscarmellose)	10 mg.	*
Chlorophyll	100 mcg	*
Turmeric	4 mcg	*

* Daily value not established by FDA

Other Ingredients: None
3/13
KEEP OUT OF REACH OF CHILDREN. Must be stored with cap on tightly in a cool, dry place. Do not use product if the tamper-resist shrink band around the cap or the inner seal beneath the cap appears to have been tampered with or is missing.
WARNING: Pregnant and nursing mothers need to check with their health professional before taking supplements.
How Supplied: 180 Count
U.S Pat. No. 6,620,798
Researched, uniquely formulated,
& exclusively distributed by:
PERQUE Integrative Health, USA
These statements have not been evaluated by the Food and Drug Administration. This product is not intended to diagnose, treat, cure, or prevent any disease.

Synergy WorldWide
1955 WEST GROVE PARKWAY, SUITE 100
PLEASANT GROVE, UT 84062

(801) 769-7800

PROARGI-9+ DS
L-arginine Complexer
Dietary Supplement

ProArgi-9+ is the highest quality l-arginine supplement in the world. This proprietary formulation combines the powerful cardiovascular benefits of l-arginine with a variety of superior heart health ingredients to give your cardiovascular system optimum support.
ProArgi-9+ was formulated in collaboration with leading scientists and cardiovascular specialists who have conducted extensive research on the proper application of l-arginine in promoting heart health. With ProArgi-9+, you're giving your heart the supplementation it needs for a long, healthy life.*
*These statements have not been evaluated by the Food and Drug Administration. This product is not intended to diagnose, treat, cure or prevent any disease.

Supplement Facts
Serving Size: 10.5 g (approx. 1 level scoop)
Servings per container: 30

Amount Per Serving		% Daily Value
Calories 15		
Total Carbohydrate	5 g	2%*
Vitamin C (Ascorbic Acid)	60 mg	100%
Vitamin D3 (Cholecalciferol)	2,500 IU	625%
Vitamin K (Menaquinone)	20 mcg	25%
Vitamin B6 (Pyridoxine HCl)	2 mg	100%
Folate (Folic Acid)	200 mcg	50%
Vitamin B12 (Cyanocobalamin)	6 mcg	100%
Proprietary Blend	6.5 g	**

L-arginine, xylitol, pomegranate fruit concentrate (*Punica granatum*), L-citrulline, d-ribose, grape skin extract (*Vitis vinifera*), red wine extract

*Percent daily values are based on a 2,000 calorie diet.
**Daily value not established.

Other Ingredients: Citric Acid, Malic Acid, Natural Citrus Sweetener, Silicon Dioxide, Natural Citrus and Huckleberry Flavors, Stevia leaf extract (*Slevia rebaudiana*).
DIRECTIONS: Mix 1 serving (1 scoop providing 5 g pure, free form L-arginine) with 4-8 oz. water (depending on individual taste). Stir to dissolve. If water is very cold, mixture will take about one minute to dissolve. One serving (1 scoop) may be taken twice per day.
Store in a cool, dry place. Slight color changes may occur over time due to the natural fruit flavor. There is no change in the efficacy or potency of the product.
Shake Well Before Dispensing
Consult your physician prior to use if you have a preexisting medical condition including: myocardial infarction (heart attack), cardiovascular disease or diabetes, or take medications for any reasons including erectile dysfunction. Not recommended for use in children or pregnant or lactating women.
Manufactured Exclusively for Synergy Worldwide®
Pleasant Grove, UT 84062 • (801) 769-7700
www.synergyworldwide.com
Item Code: Isu74154 ©2012 Made in U.S.A. REV1112
Shown in Product Identification Guide, page 313

TriVita, Inc.
16100 N GREENWAY HAYDEN LOOP
SUITE #950
SCOTTSDALE, AZ 85260

PH: 1.800.991.7116
Fax: 1.480.778.2992

NOPALEA™ SUPERFRUIT FOR WELLNESS DS
Daily Dietary Supplement

SUPPLEMENT FACTS
Serving Size 2 tbsp (1 fl oz)(30 mL)
Servings per Container 32

	Amount per Serving	% Daily Value*
Calories	13	
Calories from Fat	0	
Total Fat	0 g	0%
Saturated Fat	0 g	0%
Cholesterol	0 g	0%
Sodium	2 mg	0%
Total carbohydrate	3.1 g	1%
Dietary Fiber	0 g	0%
Sugars	2.27 g	
Protein	41 mg	0%
Vitamin A	6.8 IU	0%
Vitamin C	1.4 mg	0%
Calcium	3.4 mg	0%
Iron	.04 mg	0%
Proprietary Blend (Nopalea Sonoran Bloom™) Total 907.15 g		†

Water (filtered), Nopal fruit puree (Opuntia ficus indica), Clarified Agave syrup, Beet juice (Beta vulgaris), Cranberry powder (Vaccinium macrocarpon), Papaya powder (Carica papaya fruit with papain), Orange juice crystals (Citrus sinensis), Tomato concentrate (Solanum lycopersicon), Strawberry powder concentrate (Fragaria sp.), Apple powder (Malus domestica), Guava powder (Psidium guajava), Peach fruit powder (Prunus persica), Mango fruit powder (Mangifera indca), Apricot extract (Prunus armeniaca), Acerola powdered extract (Malpighia emarginata), Raspberry powder (Rubus ideaus), Kiwi fruit powder (Actinidia deliciosa), Lemon juice crystals (Citrus limon), Papain from papaya (Carica papaya), Bilberry concentrate (Vaccinium myrtillus), Green Tea extract (Camellia sinensis), Grape Seed extract (Vitis vinifera), Pomegranate extract (Punica granatum with ellagic acid and punicaligans), Bromelain from pineapple (Ananas comosus), Cellulase, Amylase, Protease, Lipase, Maltodextrin, Stevia powder (Stevia rebaudiana), Natural flavors, Guar gum, Silicon dioxide, Cherry Powder, Citric acid, Xanthan gum

* Percent Daily Values are based on a 2,000 calorie diet.
† Daily Value not established.

SUGGESTED USE
When taking Nopalea for the first time, drink 3 to 6 ounces each day, for 30 days. For maintenance, drink 1 to 3 ounces daily depending on your body's inflammation-fighting needs. May be mixed with water or your favorite beverage.

KEEP REFRIGERATED – SHAKE WELL BEFORE USING – PRESERVATIVE FREE
To maintain freshness: Don't drink directly from the container and consume within 30 days of opening. Do not use if safety seal under cap is broken or missing.
To report a serious adverse event or obtain product information, contact: 800.991.7116
Children, women who are pregnant or nursing and all individuals allergic to any food/ingredients should consult their healthcare provider before use.
You should not stop taking any medication without first consulting with a healthcare provider.
What's in Nopalea (Nō-pah lay' uh)
Nopalea is a delicious, nutrient-rich, ready to drink liquid that features the Superfruit of the Nopal cactus. It contains a powerful class of nutrients called Bioflavonoids, which have been scientifically proven to help the body detoxify, reduce inflammation and promote optimal cellular health.

These statements have not been evaluated by the Food and Drug Administration.
This product is not intended to diagnose, treat, cure or prevent any disease.

TRIVITA®
Experience wellness
Manufactured for and distributed by TriVita, Inc.
16100 N Greenway Hayden Loop, Suite 950 Scottsdale, AZ 85260 USA

www.trivita.com
Item 30710 L1204-01
Shown in Product Identification Guide, page 314

Unicity International, Inc.

THE MAKE LIFE BETTER COMPANY
1201 NORTH 800 EAST
OREM, UT 84097

Direct Inquiries to:
(801) 226-2600
www.unicity.com
science.unicity@unicity.com
Products of Unicity International, Inc. are distributed through independent distributors.

BIO-C™ DS
[*bīō sē*]

DESCRIPTION
Bio-C™ is a vitamin C nutritional supplement.
Bio-C™ is a yellow, water-soluble, crystalline powder pressed into a tablet. Each Bio-C™ tablet consists of a proprietary blend of ascorbyl palmitate, calcium ascorbate, ascorbic acid, magnesium ascorbate, and 37.5 mg of citrus bioflavonoids. In addition to the active ingredients, each tablet contains cellulose, stearic acid, silicon dioxide, croscarmellose sodium, and magnesium stearate.
BENEFITS AND RESEARCH
Vitamin C (ascorbic acid) is a water-soluble vitamin that is used in the body to form cartilage, collagen, muscles, and blood vessels. Vitamin C is a potent antioxidant that can protect small molecules such as proteins, carbohydrates, nucleic acids, and lipids from damage caused by free radicals that are generated through the course of normal metabolism or through exposure to external toxins and pollutants (e.g. ultraviolet radiation from the sun or smoking). Vitamin C can also regenerate other antioxidants like vitamin E. Additionally, vitamin C is required for the synthesis of carnitine, a molecule involved in the transport of fats across the mitochondrial membrane, as well as the synthesis of norepinephrine, a neurotransmitter.[1]
USAGE
Take one tablet morning and night with a meal.
SAFETY AND WARNINGS
Bio-C™ is well tolerated. Some gastrointestinal discomfort may be experienced as with any dietary supplement.
HOW SUPPLIED
Available in tablets.
REFERENCES
Carr, AC and Frei B. (1999), American Journal of Clinical Nutrition 96: 1086-1107.
Jacob, RA and Sotoudeh G. (2002), Nutrition in Clinical Care 5: 66-74.
Deruelle F, Baron B. (2008), Journal of Alternative and Complementary Medicine 14:1291-1298.
Levine M, Rumsey SC, Daruwala R, Park JB, Wang Y. (1999), The Journal of the American Medical Association 281: 1415-1423.

[1] THESE STATEMENTS HAVE NOT BEEN EVALUATED BY THE FOOD AND DRUG ADMINISTRATION. THIS PRODUCT IS NOT INTENDED TO DIAGNOSE, TREAT, CURE, OR PREVENT ANY DISEASE.

BIOS LIFE® CARDIO DS
[*bī-ōs līf kärd-ē-ō*]
Advanced Fiber and Nutrient Drink

DESCRIPTION
Bios Life® Cardio is a fiber-based, vitamin rich nutritional supplement. Bios Life® Cardio contains a blend of soluble and insoluble fibers, phytosterols, policosanol, an extract of *Chrysanthemum morifolium*, vitamins, and minerals that when combined with a healthy diet and exercise may lower total serum cholesterol, lower triglyceride levels, and reduce the risk of heart disease.
Bios Life® Cardio is light orange in color. It is a hygroscopic crystalline powder that is generally soluble in water. Each serving of Bios Life® Cardio contains 3 g of fiber, 1 g of phytosterols, 6 mg of policosanol, and 12.5 mg of an extract of *Chrysamthemum morifolium*. In addition to these active ingredients, each serving of Bios Life® Cardio contains maltodextrin, citric acid, orange juice powder, sucralose, and orange flavor.
BENEFITS AND RESEARCH
It's estimated that Americans consume 10-12 g of total fiber per day, less than half the amount of the recommended daily intake. Epidemiological and clinical studies have correlated low daily fiber intake with higher incidences of hyperinsulinemia, hypercholesterolemia, and elevated risks of cardiovascular disease.
Bios Life® Cardio is a nutritional supplement designed to increased daily fiber intake. Each serving of Bios Life® Cardio contains three grams of dietary fiber. When taken three times daily, Bios Life® Cardio contributes to nearly half of the recommended daily value of fiber. Fiber supplementation has been shown to decrease preprandial and postprandial glucose levels and lower LDL cholesterol and apolipoprotein B levels.
In addition to fiber supplementation, Bios Life® Cardio contains a patented blend of phytosterols, policosanol, *Chrysanthemum morifolium*, vitamins, and minerals. This blend of ingredients optimizes cholesterol levels through a combination of four mechanisms. First, the soluble fiber matrix prevents cholesterol reabsorption in the gastrointestinal tract through bile-acid sequestration. Second, the phytosterols reduce dietary absorption of cholesterol. Third, policosanol inhibits hepatic synthesis of cholesterol mediated through HMG-CoA reductase. Fourth, *Chrysanthemum morifolium* provides phytonutrients that enhance conversion of cholesterol to 7-α-hydryoxycholesterol. The four mechanisms provide a synergistic approach to optimizing cholesterol levels. Research has shown that this product may serve as a first line treatment option for mild hypercholesterolemia, as well as adjunct therapy for lipid-lowering pharmaceutical intervention.
SUGGESTED USAGE
Dissolve the contents of one packet or one scoop into 8 to 10 fl. oz. of liquid (water or juice) and stir vigorously. Drink immediately. Use 15-20 minutes prior to meals up to three times daily.
SAFETY AND WARNINGS
Bios Life® Cardio is well tolerated. There may be mild gastrointestinal discomfort, such as increased flatulence or loose stools, during the first month of initial use due to the increased uptake of dietary fiber. This GI disturbance usually disappears within the first thirty days. If the GI discomfort persists, reduce the number of servings of Bios Life® Cardio. If the GI discomfort further persists, stop taking the product and consult your physician. Taking this product without adequate liquid can result in complications. If you are a diabetic, consult a physician for proper use of this product, as the chromium may reduce the need for medication.
HOW SUPPLIED
Bios Life® Cardio is packaged in single-serving foil packets or in bulk canisters.
REFERENCES
Sprecher, DL and Pearce GL (2002), Metabolism 51: 1166–70.
Verdegem, PJE; Freed, S and Joffe D (2005), American Diabetes Assocation 65th Scientific Sessions, San Diego, CA.
Duenas, V; Duenas, J; Burke, E and Verdegem, PJE (2006), 7th International Conference on Arteriosclerosis, Thrombosis, and Vascular Biology, American Heart Association, Denver, CO.
Verdegem, PJE (2007), Current Topics in Nutraceutical Research 5: 1-6
US Patent 6,933,291.
* THESE STATEMENTS HAVE NOT BEEN EVALUATED BY THE FOOD AND DRUG ADMINISTRATION. THIS PRODUCT IS NOT INTENDED TO DIAGNOSE, TREAT, CURE, OR PREVENT ANY DISEASE.
Shown in Product Identification Guide, page 314

BIOS LIFE PROBIONIC® OTC

Description
ProBionic® contains four strands of live, healthy bacteria that enter the digestive system and help balance bacterial populations in the intestinal tract. This supplement is for individuals looking to reduce symptoms of poor digestive health such as constipation, diarrhea, bloating, and inflammatory symptoms associated with Irritable Bowel Syndrome (IBS).
ProBionic® is a water-soluble, light-pink crystalline powder. The proprietary encapsulation used for ProBionic® allows the healthy bacteria to be delivered to the small intestines alive, ensuring the bacteria can confer health benefits for the user. Each packet of ProBionic® contains a 100 mg Probiotic Blend of *Lactobacillus acidophilus LA 02*, *Lactobacillus rhamnosus LR 04*, *Bifidobacterium breve BR 03*, and *Bifidobacterium lactis BS 01*, with a total of 5 billion cells. In addition to these live bacteria, each 2 g packet also contains xylitol, natural berry flavor, citric acid, and silica.
Benefits and Research
The intestinal bacteria of a healthy person will be predominantly good types that help with detoxification, food digestion, waste removal, production of vitamins, and protection from harmful organisms. When the intestinal bacteria is imbalanced and unhealthy bacteria dominate, the body is less able to fight off infection and symptoms of inflammatory conditions such IBS, Chrone's Disease are more severe. The individual strains used in ProBionic® have demonstrated a reduction in symptoms of these conditions.
The proprietary encapsulation used in ProBionic® allows the healthy strains of bacteria to be delivered to the digestive system alive and undisturbed. This also ensures the bacteria will remain alive throughout their shelf life.
Suggested Use
The contents of the packet can be taken dry, or they can be mixed with 8-10 fl. oz. of liquid (water or juice) and drank. Use one packet daily
Safety and Warnings
ProBionic® is generally well tolerated. Some gastrointestinal discomfort may be experienced as with any dietary supplement.
How Supplied
ProBionic® is backaged in single-serving foil packets.
References
Saggioro A. Probiotics in the treatment of Irritable Bowel Syndrome. Journal of Clinical Gastroenterology, 2004; 38(8): S104-106.
Del Piano M, Carmagnola S, Andorno S, Pagliarulo M, Tari R, Mogna L, Strozzi GP, Sforza F, Capurso L. Evaluation of the intestinal colonization by microencapsulated probiotic bacteria in comparison to the same uncoated strains. Under pubblication in supplement of the Journal of Clinical Gastroenterology.
Del Piano M, Carmagnola S, Anderloni A, Andorno S, Ballare M, Balzarini M, Montino F, Orsello M, Pagliarulo M, Stratori M, Tari R, Sforza F, Capurso L. The use of probiotics in healthy volunteers with evacuation disorders and hard stools. A double blind, randomized, placebo-controlled study. Under pubblication in a supplement of the Journal of Clinical Gastroenterology.
Pregliasco F., Anselmi G., Fonte L., Giussani F., Schieppati S., Soletti L. A New Chance of Preventing Winter Diseases by the Administration of Symbiotic Formulations. Journal of Clinical Gastroenterology, 2008; 42(2): 224-233.
* THESE STATEMENTS HAVE NOT BEEN EVALUATED BY THE FOOD AND DRUG ADMINISTRATION. THIS PRODUCT IS NOT INTENDED TO DIAGNOSE, TREAT, CURE, OR PREVENT ANY DISEASE.

BIOS LIFE® VISION ESSENTIALS™ DS

[*bī-ōs līf vizh-uhn ē-sen-shuhls*]

Clinically proven to support healthy eyes and vision.*

DESCRIPTION

Bios Life® Vision Essentials™ is a nutritional supplement for maintaining healthy eyes. Bios Life® Vision Essentials-™contains the following active ingredients: vitamin C, vitamin E, zinc, natural beta carotene, lutein, zeaxanthin, and anthocyanidins from wild bilberry, wild blueberry, strawberry, cranberry, grape seed extract, elderberry, and raspberries.

Bios Life® Vision Essentials™ is a purple crystalline powder that is water-soluble. In addition to the active ingredients, each capsule contains silicon dioxide, microcrystalline cellulose, and is packaged in vegetarian capsules.

BENEFITS AND RESEARCH

Antioxidants from the carotenoid chemical family, such as beta carotene, lutein, and zeaxanthin, play an important role in eye health. Clinical studies have demonstrated that lutein and zeaxanthin are concentrated to the retina and lens of the eye. Low concentrations of these compounds in the retina are associated with age-related macular degeneration (AMD). Supplementation with high levels of lutein can restore the lutein concentration in the retina. Further supplementation of vitamins C, E, and A (in the form of beta-carotene) along with zinc and copper delayed the onset of AMD. Additional support for the eyes comes from a proprietary berry blend included in Bios Life® Vision Essentials™. This proprietary berry blend contains anthocyanidins, antioxidant compounds that support the vasculature within the eye, reducing the risk for diabetic retinopathies.

USAGE

Take two capsules per day with a meal.

SAFETY AND WARNINGS

Bios Life® Vision Essentials™ is well tolerated. Some gastrointestinal discomfort may be experienced as with any dietary supplement.

HOW SUPPLIED

Available in vegetarian capsules.

REFERENCES

Krishnadev N, Meleth AD, Chew EY (2010) "Nutritional supplements for age-related macular degeneration." Current Opinion in Opthamology 21:184-189.

Ma L, Lin XM, Zou ZY, Xu XR, Li Y, Xu R. (2009) "A 12-week lutein supplementation improves visual function in Chinese people with long-term computer display light exposure." British Journal of Nutrition 102: 186-190.

Yagi, A, Fujimoto, K, Michihiro, K, Goh, B, Tsi, D, Nagai, H, (2009) "The effect of lutein supplementation on visual fatigue: A psychophysiological analysis". Applied Ergonomics 40:1047-1054.

Age Related Eye Disease Study Group, (2001) "A randomized, placebo-controlled, clinical trial of high-dose supplementation with vitamins C and E, beta carotene, and zinc for age-related macular degeneration and vision loss: AREDS report no. 8". Archives of Ophthalmology. 10: 1417-36.

* THESE STATEMENTS HAVE NOT BEEN EVALUATED BY THE FOOD AND DRUG ADMINISTRATION. THIS PRODUCT IS NOT INTENDED TO DIAGNOSE, TREAT CURE, OR PREVENT ANY DISEASE.

BONEMATE® PLUS DS

[*bōn-māt plŭs*]

For Strong Bones and Healthy Teeth[1]

DESCRIPTION

BoneMate® Plus is specially formulated to help maintain optimal bone health.[1] It contains three forms of calcium and vitamin D to maximize absorption and aid in the support of healthy bones, teeth, nerves, heart, and muscle tissue.

BoneMate® Plus is a light gray in color and is soluble in water. Each serving of BoneMate® Plus contains the following active ingredients: 600 mg of calcium, 300 mg of magnesium, 30 mg of vitamin C, 2000 IU of vitamin D, 0.5 mg of boron, 5 mg of zinc, 1 mg of manganese, 1 mg of copper, and 20 mcg of vitamin K. In addition, it also contains the inactive ingredients microcrystalline cellulose, croscarmellose sodium, and magnesium stearate, hypromellose, hydroxypropylcellulose, stearic acid.

BENEFITS AND RESEARCH

Calcium is the most common mineral in the body. Almost 99% of the calcium in our body is found in the bones and teeth. Bone is a dynamic tissue that is constantly being remodeled throughout our lives. A chronically low calcium intake in growing individuals may prevent the attainment of optimal peak bone mass. Once peak bone mass has been achieved, inadequate calcium intake may contribute to accelerated bone loss and eventually to osteoporosis.

Vitamin D, a secosteroid that is produced by the body upon exposure to the sun, is required for optimal calcium absorption. To ensure that calcium absorption is not limited by inadequate vitamin D levels, BoneMate® Plus contains 2000 IU of vitamin D per serving. In addition to facilitating calcium absorption, vitamin D has been shown to target over 2000 different genes in the body. Vitamin D deficiency has been associated with increased risks for heart disease, stroke, diabetes, depression, osteoarthritis, chronic pain, and osteoporosis.

USAGE

Take two tablets twice daily with a meal.

SAFETY AND WARNINGS

BoneMate® Plus is well tolerated. Some gastrointestinal discomfort may be experienced as with any dietary supplement. The Food and Nutrition Board of the Institute of Medicine has set the tolerable upper level (UL) of intake for calcium in adults at 2,500 milligrams (mg) of calcium/day.

HOW SUPPLIED

Available as tablets.

REFERENCES

Weaver CM, Heaney RP. Calcium. In: Shils M, Olson JA, Shike M, Ross AC, eds. Modern Nutrition in Health and Disease. 9th ed. Baltimore: Williams & Wilkins; 1999:141-155.

Heaney RP. Calcium, dairy products and osteoporosis. J Am Coll Nutr. 2000;19(2 Suppl):83S-99S.

Food and Nutrition Board, Institute of Medicine. Calcium. Dietary Reference Intakes: Calcium, Phosphorus, Magnesium, Vitamin D, and Fluoride. Washington, D.C.: National Academy Press; 1997:71-145.

Reid IR. Therapy of osteoporosis: calcium, vitamin D, and exercise. Am J Med Sci 1996;312:278-86. Food and Nutrition Board, Institute of Medicine. Calcium. Dietary Reference Intakes: Calcium, Phosphorus, Magnesium, Vitamin D, and Fluoride. Washington, D.C.: National Academy Press; 1997:71-145.

[1] THESE STATEMENTS HAVE NOT BEEN EVALUATED BY THE FOOD AND DRUG ADMINISTRATION. THIS PRODUCT IS NOT INTENDED TO DIAGNOSE, TREAT, CURE, OR PREVENT ANY DISEASE.

CARDIO-BASICS™ DS

Essential Cardiovascular Nutrients*

DESCRIPTION

Cardio-Basics™ is a nutritional supplement that combines multivitamins, minerals, and antioxidants to support the cardiovascular system.

Cardio-Basics™ is a light orange, water-soluble powder pressed into tablets. Each tablet of Cardio-Basics™ contains the following vitamins, minerals, amino acids, and antioxidants: beta-carotene (vitamin A), thiamine (vitamin B1), riboflavin (vitamin B2), niacin (vitamin B3), calcium d-pantothenate (vitamin B5), pyridoxine hydrochloride (vitamin B6), folate (vitamin B9), cyanocobalamin (vitamin B12), ascorbic acid and ascorbyl palmitate (vitamin C), cholecalciferol (vitamin D), d-alpha-tocopherol (vitamin E), biotin, calcium, chromium, copper, magnesium, manganese, molybdenum, phosphorus, potassium, selenium, sodium, zinc, L-arginine, L-carnitine, L-cysteine, L-lysine, L-proline, inositol, coenzyme Q10, and maritime pine extract. In addition to those active ingredients, each tablet also contains cellulose, croscarmellose sodium, stearic acid, silicon dioxide, and magnesium stearate.

BENEFITS AND RESEARCH

According to the Center for Disease Control and Prevention, one American will die every minute as a result of heart disease. Narrowing of the arterial walls can lead to blocked blood flow to the brain. A healthy lifestyle, including being physically active, not smoking, and making good food choices, can lead to a reduction of heart disease. Cardio-Basics™ provides the vitamins, minerals, and antioxidants needed for a healthy heart. In clinical studies, participants using Cardio-Basics™ and Bio-C™ saw a significant reduction in arterial wall thickness, removal of calcification deposits, and a reduced risk for cardiovascular disease when compared to the placebo group. Cardio-Basics™ provides the body with the necessary vitamins and minerals needed to support a healthy vascular system.*

SUGGESTED USE

Take two tablets daily with food.

SAFETY AND WARNINGS

Cardio-Basics™ is well tolerated. Some gastrointestinal discomfort may be experienced as with any dietary supplement.

HOW SUPPLIED

Available in tablets

REFERENCES

Niedzwiekcki, A, Rath, M. (1996) Journal of Applied Nutrition, 48: 67-78.

Jeejeebhoy, F, Keith, M, Freeman, M, Barr, A, McCall, M, Kurian, R, Mazer, D, Errett, L, (2002), American Heart Journal 143: 1092-1100.

Verdgem, PJE, Lonky, S, Curley, S. (2005) 7th Conference on Arteriosclerosis, Thrombosis and Vascular Biology.

Lloyd-Jones D, Adams R, Carnethon M, DeSimone G, Ferguson TB, Flegal K, Ford E, Furie K, Go A, Greenlund K, Haase N, Hailpern S, Ho M, Howard V, Kissela B, Kittner S, Lackland D, Lisabeth L, Marelli A, McDermott M, Meigs J, Mozaffarian D, Nichol G, O'Donnell C, Roger V, Rosamond W, Sacco R, Sorlie P, Stafford R, Steinberger J, Hong Y; (2009) Circulation, 119: 480-486.

* THESE STATEMENTS HAVE NOT BEEN EVALUATED BY THE FOOD AND DRUG ADMINISTRATION. THIS PRODUCT IS NOT INTENDED TO DIAGNOSE, TREAT, CURE, OR PREVENT ANY DISEASE.

CARDIO-ESSENTIALS™ DS

Caring for your heart*

DESCRIPTION

Cardio-Essentials™ is a nutritional supplement for the heart. Cardio-Essentials™ contains Coenzyme Q-10, L-carnitine, L-taurine, and Hawthorn berry.

Cardio-Essentials™ is a light tan, water-soluble powder. Each capsule of Cardio-Essentials™ contains 100 mg of Coenzyme Q-10 and 3.5 g of a blend of L-carnitine, L-taurine, and Hawthorn berry. In addition to these active ingredients, each capsule also contains silicon dioxide, stearic acid, and calcium silicate.

BENEFITS AND RESEARCH

One of the leading causes of congestive heart failure (CHF), left ventricular dysfunction, affects approximately 1.5% of the population in the United States. CHF patients with left ventricular dysfunction have reduced levels of Coenzyme Q-10, L-carnitine, and L-taurine and have an enlarged left ventricle. In a clinical study, the combination of L-carnitine, L-taurine, and Coenzyme Q10 was shown to benefit congestive heart failure patients by reducing left ventricular size. These ingredients are known to be important in providing adequate energy for heart muscle. Cardio-Essentials™ provides adequate amounts of these ingredients, i.e. 100 mg of CoQ10. Hawthorn extract is traditionally used in supporting the heart function.

SUGGESTED USE

Take three capsules twice daily with food.

SAFETY AND WARNINGS

Cardio-Essentials™ is well tolerated. Some gastrointestinal discomfort may be experienced as with any dietary supplement.

HOW SUPPLIED

Available in capsules.

REFERENCES

Lee, JH. et al. (2011) Congestive Heart Failure 4 199-203.

* THESE STATEMENTS HAVE NOT BEEN EVALUATED BY THE FOOD AND DRUG ADMINISTRATION. THIS PRODUCT IS NOT INTENDED TO DIAGNOSE, TREAT, CURE, OR PREVENT ANY DISEASE.

CM PLEX® AND CM PLEX® CREAM DS

[*CM plĕks*]

Supports Joint Health and Mobility*

DESCRIPTION

CM Plex® and CM Plex® Cream are a softgel and topical cream, respectively, that contain a proprietary blend of cetylated fatty acids, soy, and fish oil.

CM Plex® is an opaque lotion that is insoluble in water. One softgel capsule of CM Plex® contains 350 mg of cetylated fatty acids, 160 mg of soy oil, and 25 mg of salmon oil. In addition to these active ingredients, each softgel capsule contains glycerin and St. John's Bread.

CM Plex® Cream is an off-white powder that is insoluble in water. One gram of CM Plex® Cream contains 7.7 mg of cetylated fatty acids and olive oil. In addition to these active ingredients, CM Plex® Cream also contains glyceryl stearate, glycerin, lecithin, tocopheryl acetate, benzyl alcohol, phenoxyethanol, carbomer, PEG-100 stearate, sodium hydroxide, methylparaben, propylparaben, butylparaben, ethylparaben, isobutylparaben, and citrus aurantium bergamia (Bergamot) fruit oil.

BENEFITS AND RESEARCH

Cetyl myristoleate and related fatty acids have been proven to improve joint health through their anti-inflammatory effects. A clinical study indicated that subjects exhibited improvements in knee flexion compared to placebo. A second study indicated the cream is effective for improving knee range of motion, ability to climb stairs, rise from a chair and walk, balance, strength, and endurance.*

SUGGESTED USE

Softgels: Take one to two softgels three times daily with meals.

Cream: Apply generously onto clean skin and gently massage until the cream disappears. Repeat 3 to 4 times daily as necessary. For maximum results, combine both products.

SAFETY AND WARNINGS

CM Plex® Softgels and Cream are well tolerated. Some gastrointestinal discomfort may be experienced with CM Plex® Softgels as with any dietary supplement.

HOW SUPPLIED

CM Plex® is available in softgels and as a topical cream.

REFERENCES

Hesslink, R et al (2002), Journal of Rheumatology 29, 1708–1712.

Kraemer, WJ et al (2004), Journal of Rheumatology 31, 767–774.

* THESE STATEMENTS HAVE NOT BEEN EVALUATED BY THE FOOD AND DRUG ADMINISTRATION. THIS PRODUCT IS NOT INTENDED TO DIAGNOSE, TREAT CURE, OR PREVENT ANY DISEASE.

Shown in Product Identification Guide, page 314

IMMUNIZEN® DS

[*ĭm mōō nĭ zĕn*]

DESCRIPTION

Immunizen® is a nutritional supplement for strengthening and fortifying the immune system.

Immunizen® is a modestly water-soluble, white crystalline powder. Immunizen® consists of a proprietary ingredient blend of colostrum, arabinogalactan, 1,3, 1,6 yeast beta-glucans, and lactoferrin. In addition to the active ingredients, each 835 mg capsule of Immunizen® contains natural gelatin, stearic acid, and silicon dioxide.

BENEFITS AND RESEARCH

Immunizen® combines the positive immune modulating effects of colostrum, arabinogalactans, yeast beta-glucans, and lactoferrin to boost your body's natural defenses to foreign antigens. Colostrum is composed of immunoglobulins that bolster the body's immune system by providing immunity against various pathogens.

Beta-glucans are generally derived from the cell walls of the yeast species *Saccharomyces cerevisiae*. Beta-glucans are potent immuno-modulating agents that prime both the innate and adaptive immune systems.

USAGE

Take six capsules with water one to two hours before a meal for 10 days as needed.

SAFETY AND WARNINGS

Immunizen® is well tolerated. Some gastrointestinal discomfort may be experienced as with any dietary supplement.

HOW SUPPLIED

Available in capsules.

REFERENCES

Lilius EM, Marnila P. (2001), Current Opinion in Infectious Diseases 14:295-300.

Hammarström L, Weiner CK. (2008), Advances in Experimental Medicine and Biology 606: 321-343.

Chan GC, Chan WK, Sze DM. (2009), The Journal of Hematology and Oncology, 2: 25-

* THESE STATEMENTS HAVE NOT BEEN EVALUATED BY THE FOOD AND DRUG ADMINISTRATION. THIS PRODUCT IS NOT INTENDED TO DIAGNOSE, TREAT, CURE, OR PREVENT ANY DISEASE.

OMEGALIFE-3™ DS

[*ōmĕgā-līf 3*]

Omega-3 Fatty Acid Supplementation

DESCRIPTION

OmegaLife-3™ is a blend of omega-3 fatty acids designed to help maintain healthy cardiovascular and cerebral function as well as aid in the prevention of age-related macular degeneration.

OmegaLife-3™ is an amber-colored, semi-viscous, fat-soluble liquid. Each serving of OmegaLife-3™ contains the following active ingredients: 800 mg eicosapentaenoic acid (EPA), 400 mg docosahexaenoic acid (DHA), and vitamin E. In addition, it also contains the inactive ingredients gelatin, glycerin, purified water, and orange oil. OmegaLife-3™ has been molecularly distilled to ensure exceptionally pure oil and includes orange oil to prevent a fishy aftertaste.

BENEFITS AND RESEARCH

Clinical research suggests fish oil can help support proper brain and visual function. In 2002 the FDA approved supplementation of DHA in infant formula. DHA is potentially important in fetal and infant neural development, in that DHA and arachidonic acid have been shown to be incorporated into brain and retinal cell membranes—particularly during the third trimester of pregnancy and early infant life.

DHA is the predominant structural fatty acid in the central nervous system and in the retina of the eyes.

EPA supports the synthesis of important compounds in the body. EPA is the precursor of thromboxane and leukotriene, compounds involved in supporting healthy circulation. They also promote healthy blood vessels.

Evidence is accumulating that increasing intakes of EPA and DHA can decrease the risk of cardiovascular disease by preventing arrhythmias, decreasing the risk of thrombosis, decreasing triglyceride levels, slowing the growth of atherosclerotic plaque, and decreasing inflammation.[1]

The U.S. Food and Drug Administration (FDA) has stated, "Supportive but not conclusive research shows that consumption of EPA and DHA omega-3 fatty acids may reduce the risk of coronary heart disease."

USAGE

Take two softgels twice daily with a meal.

SAFETY AND WARNINGS

OmegaLife-3™ is well tolerated. Some gastrointestinal discomfort may be experienced as with any dietary supplement. Common side effects include a "fishy" taste upon eructation.

HOW SUPPLIED

Available in softgels.

REFERENCES

Barter P, Ginsberg HN. Effectiveness of combined statin plus omega-3 fatty acid therapy for mixed dyslipidemia. Am J Cardiol. 2008 Oct 15:102(8):1040-5

Lee JH, Harris WS, et al. Omega-3 fatty acids for cardioprotection. Mayo Clin Proc. 2008 Mar;83(3):324-32.

SanGiovanni JP, Chew EY, Sperduto RD, et al. The relationship of dietary omega-3 long-chain polyunsaturated fatty acid intake with incident age-related macular degeneration: AREDS report no. 23. Arch Ophthalmol. 2008 Sep;126(9):1274-9.

SanGiovanni JP, Parra-Cabrera S, Colditz GA, Berkey CS, Dwyer JT. Meta-analysis of dietary essential fatty acids and long-chain polyunsaturated fatty acids as they relate to visual resolution acuity in healthy preterm infants. Pediatrics 2000;105:1292-8.

Kris-Etherton PM, Harris WS, Appel LJ. Omega-3 fatty acids and cardiovascular disease: new recommendations from the American Heart Association. Arterioscler Thromb Vasc Biol. 2003;23(2):151-152.

[1] THESE STATEMENTS HAVE NOT BEEN EVALUATED BY THE FOOD AND DRUG ADMINISTRATION. THIS PRODUCT IS NOT INTENDED TO DIAGNOSE, TREAT, CURE, OR PREVENT ANY DISEASE.

UNICITY BALANCE™ DS

(Also known as Bios Life® Slim or Bios Life® S)
Formula for Healthy Cholesterol Support

DESCRIPTION

Unicity Balance (also known as Bios Life® Slim or Bios Life® S) is a fiber-based, vitamin-rich nutritional supplement. Unicity Balance™ contains a blend of soluble and insoluble fibers, Unicity® 7× technology, phytosterols, policosanol, an extract of *Chrysanthemum morifolium*, vitamins, and minerals that when combined with a healthy diet and exercise may lower total serum cholesterol, reduce the risk of heart disease, and help achieve and maintain a healthy body weight.

Unicity Balance™ is light orange in color. It is a hygroscopic crystalline powder that is generally soluble in water. Each serving of Unicity Balance™ contains 4 g of fiber, 1 g of phytosterols, 750 mg of Unicity 7×, 6 mg of policosanol, and 12.5 mg of an extract of *Chrysanthemum morifolium*. In addition to these active ingredients, each serving of Unicity Balance™ contains maltodextrin, citric acid, orange juice powder, sucralose, and orange flavor.

BENEFITS AND RESEARCH

It's estimated that Americans consume 10-12 g of total fiber per day, less than half the amount of the recommended daily intake. Epidemiological and clinical studies have correlated low daily fiber intake with higher incidences of obesity, hyperinsulinemia, hypercholesterolemia, and elevated risks of cardiovascular disease.

Unicity Balance™ is a nutritional supplement designed to increase fiber intake. Each serving of Unicity Balance™ contains four grams of fiber. When taken three times daily, Unicity Balance™ contributes to half of the recommended daily value of fiber. Fiber supplementation has been shown to decrease preprandial and postprandial glucose levels, lower LDL cholesterol and apolipoprotein B levels, increase satiety, and facilitate weight loss.

In addition to fiber supplementation, Unicity Balance™ contains a patented blend of phytosterols, policosanol, *Chrysanthemum morifolium*, vitamins, and minerals. Unicity Balance™ facilitates weight loss through five distinct mechanisms. First, the soluble fiber matrix promotes an increase in satiety. Second, Unicity Balance™ improves cholesterol levels. Reduction in LDL content removes a potent inhibitor of lipolysis. Third, Unicity Balance™ improves blood glucose levels. Maintaining appropriate serum glucose levels reduces hyperinsulinemia and promotes insulin sensitivity. Reducing insulin levels permits fatty acid oxidation to occur. Fourth, Unicity Balance™ restores appropriate leptin signaling. Lastly, Unicity Balance™ reduces triglyceride levels allowing for leptin to cross the blood-brain barrier and affect its mechanism of action. Research has shown that this product may serve as a first line treatment option for mild hypercholesterolemia, as well as adjunct therapy for lipid lowering pharmaceutical intervention.

SUGGESTED USAGE

Dissolve the contents of one packet or one scoop into 8 to 10 fl. oz. of liquid (water or juice) and stir vigorously. Drink immediately. Use 15-20 minutes before meals up to three times daily.

SAFETY AND WARNINGS

Unicity Balance™ is well tolerated. There may be mild gastrointestinal discomfort, such as increased flatulence or loose stools, during the first month of initial use due to the increased uptake of dietary fiber. This GI disturbance usually disappears within the first thirty days. If the GI discomfort persists, reduce the number of servings of Unicity Balance™. If the GI discomfort further persists, stop taking the product and consult your physician. Taking this product without adequate liquid can result in complications. If you are a diabetic, consult a physician for proper use of this product, as the chromium may reduce the need for medication.

HOW SUPPLIED

Unicity Balance™ is packaged in single-serving foil packets or in bulk canisters.

REFERENCES

Sprecher, DL and Pearce GL (2002), Metabolism 51: 1166-70.

Verdegem, PJE; Freed, S and Joffe D (2005), American Diabetes Assocation 65th Scientific Sessions, San Diego, CA.

Slavin, JL, (2005) Nutrition 21: 411-418.

Delzenne NM, Cani PD, (2005) Current Opinion Clincal Nutrition & Metabolic Care 8: 636-640

Duenas, V; Duenas, J; Burke, E and Verdegem, PJE (2006), 7th International Conference on Arteriosclerosis, Thrombosis, and Vascular Biology, American Heart Association, Denver, CO.

Verdegem, PJE (2007), Current Topics in Nutraceutical Research 5: 1-6

US Patent 6,933,291.

* THESE STATEMENTS HAVE NOT BEEN EVALUATED BY THE FOOD AND DRUG ADMINISTRATION. THIS PRODUCT IS NOT INTENDED TO DIAGNOSE, TREAT, CURE, OR PREVENT ANY DISEASE.

Shown in Product Identification Guide, page 314

USANA Health Sciences, Inc.
3838 WEST PARKWAY BOULEVARD
SALT LAKE CITY, UT 84120-6336

Direct Inquiries to:
Ph: (801) 954 7860
Fax: (801) 954 7658

ACTIVE CALCIUM™ DS

COMPOSITION
Each Active Calcium contains the following minerals:

Vitamin D3 (as Cholecalciferol)	100 IU
Vitamin K (as Phylloquinone)	15 mcg
Calcium (as Calcium Citrate and Carbonate)	200 mg
Magnesium (as Magnesium Citrate, Amino Acid Chelate and Oxide)	100 mg
Boron (as Boron Citrate)	0.33 mg
Silicon (as Silicon Amino Acid Complex)	2.25 mg

ADVANTAGES
Each tablet contains a balanced blend of calcium, magnesium, vitamin D, vitamin K, boron and silicon; six nutrients required for bone development, bone remodeling and skeletal health. This non-prescription product meets USP guidelines for potency (as applicable), uniformity and disintegration, and is manufactured according to pharmaceutical cGMP standards.

RECOMMENDED USE
Take 4 tablets by mouth daily, preferably with meals.

SUPPLIED
Capsule-shaped tablet, mottled greenish-white color, with clear film coating, and with USANA imprint. In bottle of 112 tablets.

CHELATED MINERAL DS
[key'-lā-tĕd]
mineral

COMPOSITION
Each Chelated Mineral contains the following minerals:

Calcium (As Calcium Citrate and Carbonate)	67.5 mg
Iodine (As Potassium Iodide)	75 mcg
Magnesium (As Magnesium Citrate and Amino Acid Chelate)	75 mg
Zinc (As Zinc Citrate)	5 mg
Selenium (As L-selenomethionine and Amino Acid Complex)	50 mcg
Copper (As Copper Gluconate)	0.5 mg
Manganese (As Manganese Gluconate)	1.25 mg
Chromium (As Chromium Polynicotinate and Picolinate**)	75 mcg
Molybdenum (As Molybdenum Citrate)	1.25 mcg
Boron (As Boron Citrate)	0.75 mg
Silicon (As Silicon Amino Acid Complex)	1 mg
Vanadium (As Vanadium Citrate)	10 mcg
Ultra trace Minerals	0.75 mg

**Licensed under U.S. Patent 4,315,927.

ADVANTAGES
Each tablet contains a complete and balanced blend of essential minerals in bioavailable forms. The Chelated Mineral is designed to be taken with USANA's Mega Antioxidant to provide a full complement of essential nutrients required for health. This non-prescription product meets USP guidelines for potency (as applicable), uniformity and disintegration, and is manufactured according to pharmaceutical cGMP standards.

RECOMMENDED USE
Take two (2) tablets twice daily, preferably with food.

SUPPLIED
Oblong shaped tablets, off-white color, with clear film coating with USANA imprint. In bottle of 112 tablets

COQUINONE® 30 DS
[cō'-kwi-nōn]

COMPOSITION
Each CoQuinone 30 capsule contains the following:

Coenzyme Q_{10}	30 mg
Alpha Lipoic Acid	12.5 mg

ADVANTAGES
CoQuinone 30 contains a hydrosoluble form of Coenzyme Q_{10} (CoQ_{10}) that is 2.5 times more bioavailable than material supplied in dry tablet/capsule formulas. The higher blood levels of CoQ_{10} supplied enhance mitochondrial production of ATP. CoQ_{10} is a rate-limiting factor in the electron transport chain involved in mitochondrial production of ATP. It is also involved in neutralizing free radicals generated during ATP production. As such, CoQ_{10} helps the body maintain healthy skeletal and cardiac muscle. Alpha lipoic acid is included in the formula as a lipid-soluble antioxidant to recycle CoQ_{10} from the prooxidant form to the antioxidant form. This non-prescription product meets USP guidelines for potency (where applicable), uniformity and disintegration, and is manufactured according to cGMP standards.

RECOMMENDED USE
Take 1 or 2 capsules by mouth daily.

SUPPLIED
Oval shaped, soft gelatin capsule, annatto-colored, opaque, imprinted with USANA in white edible ink. Capsules contain an orange colored liquid. In bottle of 56 soft-gel capsules.

MEGA ANTIOXIDANT DS
[mĕ-gă aenti-ŏx'-si-dĕnt]

COMPOSITION
Each Mega Antioxidant contains the following vitamins and Minerals:

Vitamin A (as Beta Carotene)	3,750 IU
Vitamin C (as Calcium, Potassium, Magnesium, & Zinc Ascorbates)	325 mg
Vitamin D3 (as Cholecalciferol)	450 IU
Vitamin E (as D-alpha Tocopheryl Succinate)	100 IU
Vitamin K (as Phylloquinone)	15 mcg
Thiamin (as Thiamine HCl)	6.75 mg
Riboflavin	6.75 mg
Niacin and Niacinamide	10 mg
Vitamin B6 (as Pyridoxine HCl)	8 mg
Folate (as Folic Acid)	250 mcg
Vitamin B12 (as Cyanocobalamin)	50 mcg
Biotin	75 mcg
Pantothenic Acid (as D-Calcium Pantothenate)	22.5 mg
Olivol ® (Olive Extract)	7.5 mg
Mixed Natural Tocopherols (D-gamma, D-delta, D-beta Tocopherol)	8.5 mg
Bioflavonoid complex (Rutin, Quercetin, Hesperidin, Green Tea Extract-Decaffeinate, Pomegranate Extract, Cinnamon Extract, Bilberry Extract)	49.5 mg
Inositol	37.5 mg
Choline Bitartrate	25 mg
N-Acetyl L-Cysteine	25 mg
Alpha-Lipoic Acid	5 mg
Coenzyme Q10	3 mg
Turmeric Extract	3.75 mg
Lutein	150 mcg
Lycopene	250 mcg

ADVANTAGES
A comprehensive and balanced formula containing the essential vitamins and antioxidants at levels substantially higher than RDA amounts. In addition to the traditionally recognized essential nutrients, the formula contains a unique blend of dietary antioxidants including carotenoids, a bioflavonoid complex, a glutathione complex, and USANA's patented Olivol™ to provide full-spectrum antioxidant protection. This formula is designed to be taken with USANA's Chelated Mineral to provide a full compliment of essential nutrients required for health. This non-prescription product meets USP guidelines for potency (as applicable), uniformity and disintegration, and is manufactured according to pharmaceutical cGMP standards.

RECOMMENDED USE
Take two (2) tablets twice daily, preferably with food.

SUPPLIED
Oblong shaped tablets, mottled orange-brown color, with clear film coating with USANA imprint. In bottle of 112 tablets.

PROCOSA DS

COMPOSITION
Each Procosa tablet contains the following:

Vitamin C (As Calcium Ascorbate)	75 mg
Manganese (As Manganese Gluconate)	1.67 mg
Glucosamine HCL (Vegetarian)	500 mg
Potassium (As Potassium Sulphate)	31.4 mg
Magnesium (As Magnesium Sulphate)	14.5 mg
Meriva Bioavailable Curcumin Complex	82.5 mg

ADVANTAGES
USANA's Procosa is comprehensive joint health formula with a blend of glucosamine, manganese, vitamin C, and silicon — building blocks for healthy cartilage. The combination of glucosamine with Meriva® bioavailable curcumin complex, manganese, vitamin C, and silicon represents a more comprehensive approach to joint health. Over the long term, these ingredients help retain healthy cartilage. Meriva, the new curcumin phytosome used in Procosa, dramatically increases human absorption of curcumin, delivering the same effectiveness at a much lower dose.

RECOMMENDED USE
Take two tablets twice daily, preferably with meals

SUPPLIED
Oblong, orange-colored tablet, scored on one side. In bottle of 120 tablets.

PROFLAVANOL® C 100 DS
[prō-flă' vi-nol]

COMPOSITION
Each Proflavanol C 100 tablet contains the following:

Vitamin C (As Calcium, Potassium, Magnesium, Zinc Ascorbates)	300 mg
Grape Seed Extract (*Vitis Vinifera L.*, Seeds)	100 mg

ADVANTAGES
A potent antioxidant formula combining the proanthocyanidins (bioflavonoids) from standardized grape seed extract with vitamin C in the form of ascorbate salts and ascorbyl palmitate. Proflavanol C 100 is designed to be taken as a stand-alone antioxidant, or preferably in combination with USANA's Mega Antioxidant and Chelated Mineral to provide additional antioxidant protection. This non-prescription product meets USP guidelines for potency (where applicable), uniformity and disintegration, and is manufactured according to pharmaceutical cGMP standards.

RECOMMENDED USE
Take 1–3 tablets by mouth daily.

SUPPLIED
Oblong, bilayer tablet, with clear film coating, with USANA imprint. In bottles of 56 tablets.

USANA BabyCare Prenatal Essentials DS

USANA BabyCare Prenatal Essentials are multivitamin and mineral supplements for women who are pregnant, want to become pregnant, or who have recently given birth. BabyCare Prenatal Essentials are comprised of two products:

- **BabyCare Prenatal Chelated Mineral** is a speckled off-white, water-soluble tablet that contains calcium, iodine, magnesium, zinc, copper, iron. In addition to these active ingredients, each tablet also contains manganese, selenium, molybdenum, and vanadium.
- **BabyCare Prenatal Mega Antioxidant** is an amber color, water-soluble tablet that contains a balanced blend of vitamins A (as beta carotene), C, D, E, B6, B12, folate, thiamin, riboflavin, niacin, biotin, and pantothenic acid. In addition to these active ingredients, each tablet also contains additional natural antioxidant extracts, inositol, choline, and vitamin K.

BabyCare Prenatal Chelated Mineral OTC
Tablets

SUPPLEMENT FACTS

SERVING SIZE: 2 TABLETS

AMOUNT PER SERVING		%DV*
CALCIUM (AS CALCIUM CITRATE AND CALCIUM CARBONATE)	135 mg	10%
IODINE (AS POTASSIUM IODIDE)	150 µg	100%

MAGNESIUM (AS MAGNESIUM CITRATE AND MAGNESIUM AMINO ACID CHELATE)	150 mg	35%
ZINC (AS ZINC CITRATE)	10 mg	70%
COPPER (AS COPPER GLUCONATE)	1 mg	50%
IRON (AS FERROUS FUMERATE USP)	14 mg	80%

*%DV FOR PREGNANT WOMEN

OTHER INGREDIENTS

MICROCRYSTALLINE CELLULOSE, HYDROXYPROPYL CELLULOSE, CROSCARMALLOSE SODIUM, ASCORBYL PALMITATE, MANGANESE GLUCONATE, SELENIUM AMINO ACID COMPLEX, PREGELATINIZED STARCH, SILICON DIOXIDE, DEXTRIN, L-SELENOMETHIONINE, CALCIUM SILICATE, HYDROLIZED RICE PROTEIN, VANADIUM CITRATE, MOLYBDENUM CITRATE, DEXTROSE, SOY LECITHIN, CHROMIUM POLYNICOTINATE, ULTRA TRACE MINERALS, SODIUM CARBOXYMETHYL CELLULOSE, SODIUM CITRATE.

INDICATIONS

USANA PRENATAL CHELATED MINERAL IS A MULTI-MINERAL SUPPLEMENT INDICATED TO IMPROVE THE NUTRITIONAL NEEDS OF WOMEN DURING PREGNANCY. IT ALSO IMPROVES THE NUTRITIONAL BALANCE DURING A MOTHER'S POST NATAL PERIOD FOR LACTATING AND NON-LACTATING WOMEN.

DIRECTIONS

TAKE TWO (2) TABLETS TWICE DAILY WITH FOOD.

WARNINGS

WARNING: ACCIDENTAL OVERDOSE OF IRON CONTAINING PRODUCTS IS A LEADING CAUSE OF FATAL POISONING IN CHILDREN UNDER 6. KEEP THIS PRODUCT OUT OF REACH OF CHILDREN. IN CASE OF ACCIDENTAL OVERDOSE, CALL A DOCTOR OR POISON CONTROL CENTER IMMEDIATELY.
CONSULT YOUR PHYSICIAN IF YOU ARE PREGNANT, NURSING, TAKING A PRESCRIPTION DRUG , OR HAVE A MEDICAL CONDITION.
DO NOT USE IF SAFETY SEAL UNDER CAP IS BROKEN OR MISSING.

STORAGE

STORE BELOW 25° C.

QUESTIONS OR COMMENTS?

FOR INFORMATION, CONTACT 1-800-950-9595

BabyCare Prenatal Mega Antioxidant DS
TABLETS

SUPPLEMENT FACTS

SERVING SIZE: 2 TABLETS

AMOUNT PER SERVING		%DV*
VITAMIN A (AS BETA CAROTENE)	7,500 IU	90%
VITAMIN C (AS CALCIUM, POTASSIUM, MAGNESIUM, & ZINC ASCORBATES)	650 mg	1080%
VITAMIN D3 (AS CHOLECALCIFEROL)	900 IU	225%
VITAMIN E (AS D-ALPHA TOCOPHERYL SUCCINATE)	200 IU	670%
THIAMIN (AS THIAMIN HCl)	13.5 mg	790%
RIBOFLAVIN	13.5 mg	675%
NIACIN (AS NIACIN AND NIACINAMIDE)	20 mg	100%
VITAMIN B6 (AS PYRIDOXINE HCl)	16 mg	640%
FOLATE (AS FOLIC ACID)	500 µg	60%
VITAMIN B12 (AS CYANOCOBALAMIN)	100 µg	1250%
BIOTIN	150 µg	50%
PANTOTHENIC ACID (AS D-CALCIUM PANTOTHENATE)	45 mg	450%

*%DV For Pregnant Women.

OTHER INGREDIENTS

MICROCRYSTALLINE CELLULOSE, INOSITOL, PREGELATINIZED STARCH, RUTIN, MIXED TOCOPHEROLS, CROSCARMALLOSE SODIUM, CHOLINE BITARTRATE, N-ACETYL L-CYSTEINE, HESPERIDIN, OLIVOL®OLEA EUROPAEA (OLIVE FRUIT) EXTRACT[1], ASCORBYL PALMITATE, DEXTRIN, QUERCETIN, ALPHA LIPOIC ACID, SILICON DIOXIDE, CAMELIA SINENSIS (GREEN TEA) EXTRACT, CURCUMA LONGA (TURMERIC) EXTRACT, LUTEIN, COENZYME Q-10, PUNICA GRANATUM (POMEGRANATE) EXTRACT, LYCOPENE, VITAMIN K, DEXTROSE, SOY LECITHIN, CINNAMOMUM CASSIA (CINNAMON) EXTRACT, SODIUM CARBOXYMETHYLCELLULOSE, VACCINIUM MYRTILLUS L. (BILBERRY) EXTRACT, SODIUM CITRATE.

[1]PROTECTED UNDER US PATENTS 6,358,542 OR 6,361,803.

INDICATIONS

USANA PRENATAL MEGA ANTIOXIDANT IS A MULTIVITAMIN SUPPLEMENT INDICATED TO IMPROVE THE NUTRITIONAL NEEDS OF WOMEN DURING PREGNANCY. IT ALSO IMPROVES THE NUTRITIONAL BALANCE DURING A MOTHER'S POST NATAL PERIOD FOR LACTATING AND NON-LACTATING WOMEN.

DIRECTIONS

TAKE TWO (2) TABLETS TWICE DAILY WITH FOOD.

PRECAUTIONS/WARNINGS

FOLIC ACID IS IMPROPER THERAPY IN THE TREATMENT OF PERNICIOUS ANEMIA AND OTHER MEGALOBLASTIC ANEMIAS WHERE VITAMIN B12 IS DEFICIENT. FOLIC ACID ABOVE 1MG DAILY MAY OBSCURE PERNICIOUS ANEMIA IN THAT HEMATOLOGIC REMISSION CAN OCCUR WHILE NEUROLOGICAL MANIFISTATIONS PROGRESS.
KEEP OUT OF REACH OF CHILDREN. CONSULT YOUR PHYSICIAN IF YOU ARE PREGNANT, NURSING, TAKING A PRESCRIPTION DRUG, OR HAVE A MEDICAL CONDITION.
DO NOT USE IF SAFETY SEAL UNDER CAP IS BROKEN OR MISSING.

STORAGE

STORE BELOW 25°C

QUESTIONS OR COMMENTS?

FOR INFORMATION, CONTACT 1-800-950-9595

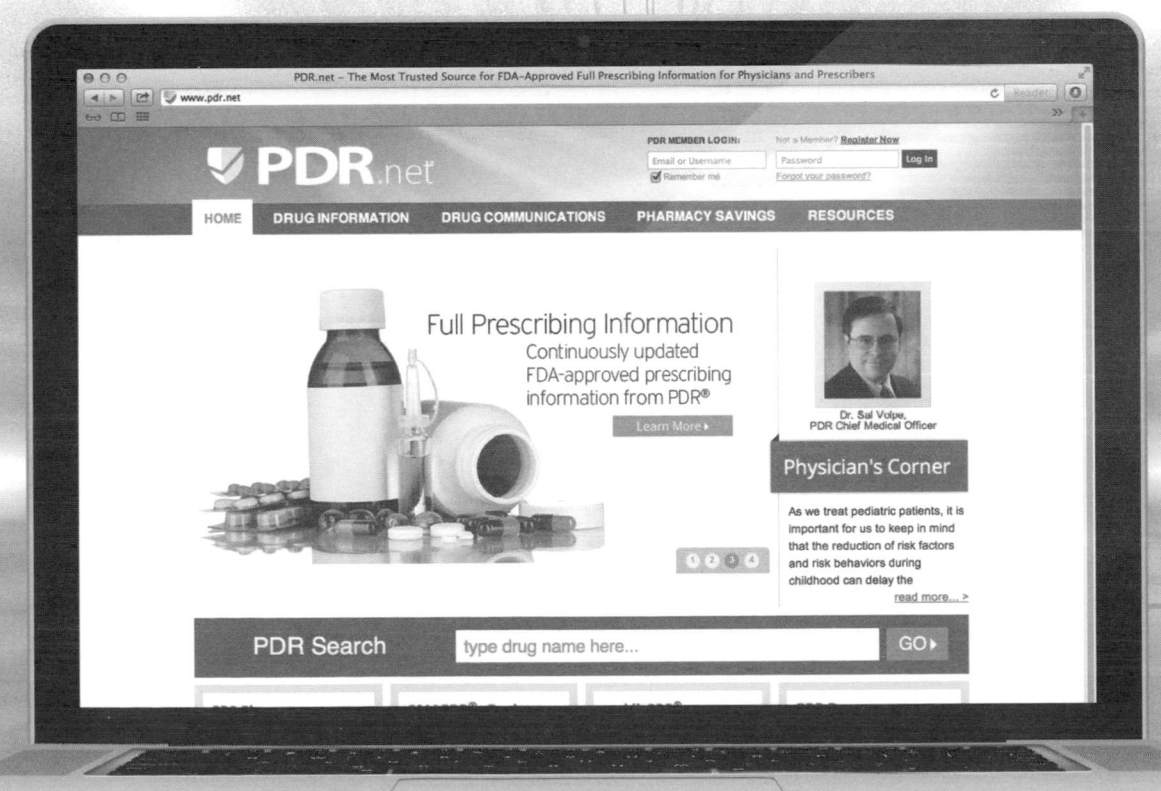

PDR Network®

PDR®: Critical Information When and Where You Need It

With PDR.net® and *mobile*PDR®, we make prescribing information conveniently available to you. Online or on the go, PDR delivers trusted prescribing information to help you provide optimal patient care.

All PDR services are made available to healthcare providers at no charge. Get your PDR today in the format that works for you.

Access PDR anytime online at PDR.net.

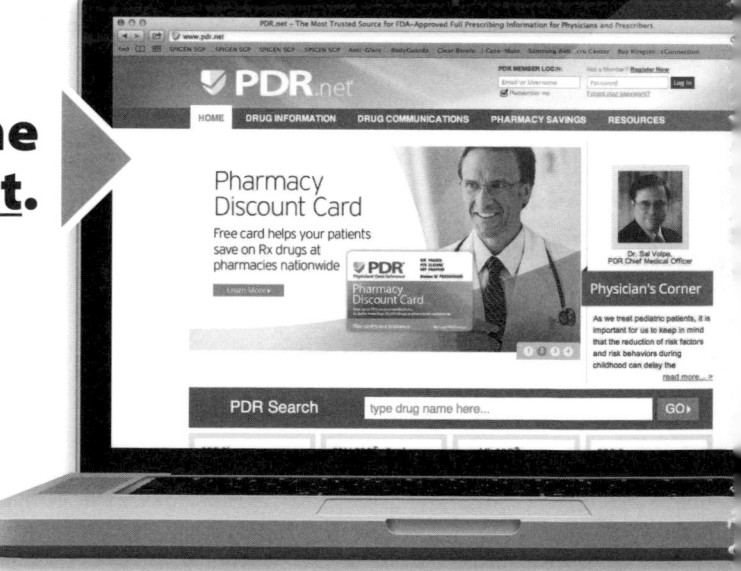

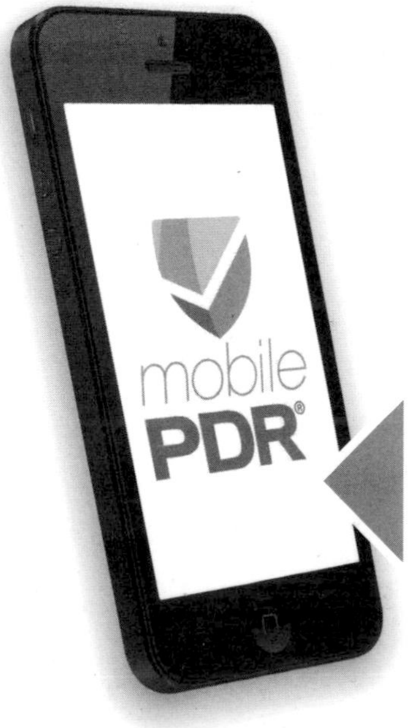

View PDR on the go with *mobile*PDR for your wireless device.